SIXTH EDITION

Principles and Practice of Pediatric Oncology

EDITORS

PHILIP A. PIZZO, M.D.
Dean of the School of Medicine
Carl and Elizabeth Naumann Professor
Professor of Pediatrics and of Microbiology
  and Immunology
Stanford University School of Medicine
Stanford, California

DAVID G. POPLACK, M.D.
Elise C. Young Professor of Pediatric
  Oncology
Head, Hematology–Oncology Section
Department of Pediatrics
Baylor College of Medicine
Director, Texas Children's Cancer Center
Texas Children's Hospital
Houston, Texas

ASSOCIATE EDITORS

PETER C. ADAMSON, M.D.
SUSAN M. BLANEY, M.D.
LEE J. HELMAN, M.D.

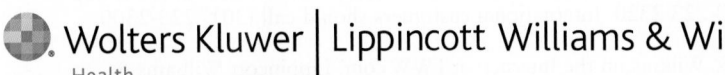

Wolters Kluwer | Lippincott Williams & Wilkins
Health

Philadelphia • Baltimore • New York • London
Buenos Aires • Hong Kong • Sydney • Tokyo

Senior Executive Editor: Jonathan W. Pine, Jr.
Senior Product Manager: Emilie Moyer
Senior Manufacturing Manager: Benjamin Rivera
Senior Marketing Manager: Angela Panetta
Design Coordinator: Teresa Mallon
Production Service: Aptara, Inc.

© 2011 by LIPPINCOTT WILLIAMS & WILKINS, a WOLTERS KLUWER business
Two Commerce Square
2001 Market Street
Philadelphia, PA 19103 USA
LWW.com

Printed in China

Library of Congress Cataloging-in-Publication Data

Principles and practice of pediatric oncology / edited by Philip A. Pizzo and David G. Poplack ; associate editors, Peter Adamson, Susan Blaney, Lee Helman. – 6th ed.
      p. ; cm.
  Includes bibliographical references and index.
  ISBN 978-1-60547-682-7
 1. Cancer in children. I. Pizzo, Philip A. II. Poplack, David G.
  [DNLM: 1. Neoplasms. 2. Child. 3. Infant. QZ 275]
  RC281.C4P65 2011
  618.92′994–dc22

                                                                    2010029712

Care has been taken to confirm the accuracy of the information presented and to describe generally accepted practices. However, the authors, editors, and publisher are not responsible for errors or omissions or for any consequences from application of the information in this book and make no warranty, expressed or implied, with respect to the currency, completeness, or accuracy of the contents of the publication. Application of the information in a particular situation remains the professional responsibility of the practitioner.

The authors, editors, and publisher have exerted every effort to ensure that drug selection and dosage set forth in this text are in accordance with current recommendations and practice at the time of publication. However, in view of ongoing research, changes in government regulations, and the constant flow of information relating to drug therapy and drug reactions, the reader is urged to check the package insert for each drug for any change in indications and dosage and for added warnings and precautions. This is particularly important when the recommended agent is a new or infrequently employed drug.

Some drugs and medical devices presented in the publication have Food and Drug Administration (FDA) clearance for limited use in restricted research settings. It is the responsibility of the health care provider to ascertain the FDA status of each drug or device planned for use in their clinical practice.

To purchase additional copies of this book, call our customer service department at (800) 638-3030 or fax orders to (301) 223-2320. International customers should call (301) 223-2300.

Visit Lippincott Williams & Wilkins on the Internet: at LWW.com. Lippincott Williams & Wilkins customer service representatives are available from 8:30 am to 6:00 pm, EST.

                                10 9 8 7 6 5 4 3 2 1

Contributing Authors

Peter C. Adamson, M.D.
Professor of Pediatrics & Pharmacology
Department of Pediatrics
University of Pennsylvania School of Medicine;
Director, Clinical & Translational Research
Chief, Division of Clinical Pharmacology & Therapeutics
The Children's Hospital of Philadelphia
Philadelphia, Pennsylvania

Bharat Agarwal, M.D., D.N.B., D.C.H.
Professor
Postdoctoral Subspeciality Fellowship Training Programme
National Board of Examinations
New Delhi, India;
Head of Department
Department of Pediatric Hematology & Oncology
B.J. Wadia Hospital for Children
Parel, Mumbai, India

Anurag K. Agrawal, M.D.
Fellow
Pediatric Hematology and Oncology
Children's Hospital and Research Center
Oakland, California

Melissa A. Alderfer
Assistant Professor
Department of Pediatrics
University of Pennsylvania School of Medicine;
Clinical Psychologist
The Cancer Center
The Children's Hospital of Philadelphia
Philadelphia, Pennsylvania

Carl E. Allen, M.D., Ph.D.
Assistant Professor
Hematology–Oncology Section
Department of Pediatrics
Baylor College of Medicine;
Texas Children's Cancer Center
Texas Children's Hospital
Houston, Texas

Arnold J. Altman, M.D.
Hartford Whalers Professor of Childhood Cancer
Department of Pediatrics
University of Connecticut School of Medicine;
Attending Pediatric Hematologist/Oncologist
Connecticut Children's Medical Center
Farmington, Connecticut

Richard J. Andrassy, M.D.
Professor
University of Texas
M.D. Anderson Cancer Center
Houston, Texas

Peter D. Aplan, M.D.
Senior Investigator
Genetics Branch
National Cancer Institute/National Institutes of Health;
Attending Physician
Pediatric Branch
National Institutes of Health Clinical Center
Bethesda, Maryland

Susan D. Apkon, M.D.
Associate Professor
Department of Rehabilitation Medicine
University of Washington;
Director, Rehabilitation Medicine
Seattle Children's Hospital
Seattle, Washington

Daniel A. Arber, M.D.
Professor and Associate Chair for Clinical Services
Department of Pathology
Stanford University
Stanford, California

Saro H. Armenian, D.O., M.P.H.
Assistant Professor
Population Sciences;
Assistant Professor
Department of Pediatrics
City of Hope National Medical Center
Duarte, California

Daniel C. Aronson, M.D., Ph.D.
Professor of Pediatric Surgery
Department of Surgery, Division of Pediatric Surgery
Radboud University Nijmegen;
Chief
Division of Pediatric Surgery
Radboud University Nijmegen Medical Center
Nijmegen, The Netherlands

Rochelle Bagatell, M.D.
Assistant Professor
Department of Pediatrics
University of Pennsylvania School of Medicine;
Division of Oncology
The Children's Hospital of Philadelphia
Philadelphia, Pennsylvania

Frank M. Balis, M.D.
Professor of Pediatrics
Division of Oncology, Department of Pediatrics
University of Pennsylvania;
Director, Cancer Clinical Research
Department of Oncology
The Children's Hospital of Philadelphia
Philadelphia, Pennsylvania

Sonia Arora Ballal, M.D.
Clinical Fellow
Division of Pediatric Gastroenterology and Nutrition
Children's Hospital Boston
Boston, Massachusetts

Ronald Barr, M.B.Ch.B., M.D.
Professor
Pediatrics, Pathology & Medicine
McMaster University;
Member of Staff
Hematology–Oncology
McMaster Children's Hospital
Hamilton, Ontario, Canada

Andrew J. Bauer, M.D.
Associate Professor
Department of Pediatrics
Uniformed Services University
Bethesda, Maryland;
Chief, Pediatric Endocrinology
Department of Pediatrics
Walter Reed Army Medical Center
Washington, District of Columbia

Lori J. Bechard, M.Ed., R.D., L.D.N.
Clinical Nutrition Specialist III
Division of Gastroenterology and Nutrition
Children's Hospital Boston
Boston, Massachusetts

Stacey L. Berg, M.D.
Professor
Hematology–Oncology Section
Department of Pediatrics
Baylor College of Medicine;
Texas Children's Cancer Center
Texas Children's Hospital
Houston, Texas

Smita Bhatia, M.D., M.P.H.
Professor and Chair
Population Sciences
Professor, Department of Pediatrics
City of Hope National Medical Center
Duarte, California

Stefan Bielack, Prof. Dr., M.D.
AO Professor
Pediatric Hematology and Oncology
Universitaetsklinikum Muenster
Muenster, Germany;
Medical Director
Pediatrics (Oncology, Hematology, Immunology)
Klinikum Stuttgart–Olgahospital
Stuttgart, Germany

Amy L. Billett, M.D.
Assistant Professor of Pediatrics
Department of Pediatrics
Harvard Medical School;
Associate in Medicine
Department of Pediatrics
Dana Farber Cancer Institute/Children's Hospital
Boston, Massachusetts

Susan M. Blaney, M.D.
Professor
Hematology–Oncology Section
Department of Pediatrics
Baylor College of Medicine;
Deputy Director, Texas Children's Cancer Center
Texas Children's Hospital
Houston, Texas

W. Archie Bleyer, M.D.
Clinical Research Professor
Department of Radiation Medicine
Oregon Health and Science University
Portland, Oregon;
Medical Director, Clinical Research
Department of Cancer Treatment Center
St. Charles Health System
Bend, Oregon

Catherine M. Bollard, M.D.
Associate Professor
Center for Cell and Gene Therapy
Hematology–Oncology Section
Department of Pediatrics
Baylor College of Medicine;
Texas Children's Cancer Center
Texas Children's Hospital
Houston, Texas

Tobias Bölling, M.D.
Researcher
Department of Radiotherapy
University Hospital of Muenster;
Senior Physician
Department of Radiotherapy
University Hospital of Muenster
Muenster, Germany

Lisa R. Bomgaars, M.D.
Associate Professor
Hematology–Oncology Section
Department of Pediatrics
Baylor College of Medicine
Texas Children's Cancer Center
Texas Children's Hospital
Houston, Texas

Melissa L. Bondy, Ph.D.
Professor
Department of Epidemiology
The University of Texas, MD Anderson Cancer Center
Houston, Texas

Malcolm K. Brenner, M.D., Ph.D.
Professor and Director, Center for Cell and Gene Therapy
Departments of Pediatrics and Medicine
Baylor College of Medicine; The Methodist Hospital
Texas Children's Cancer Center
Texas Children's Hospital,
Houston, Texas

Garrett M. Brodeur, M.D.
Professor
Department of Pediatrics, Division of Oncology
University of Pennsylvania School of Medicine;
Associate Chair for Research
Department of Pediatrics, Division of Oncology
Children's Hospital of Philadelphia
Philadelphia, Pennsylvania

Jacqueline N. Casillas, M.D., M.S.H.S.
Assistant Professor
Department of Pediatrics
University of California, Los Angeles
Los Angeles, California

Patricia Chévez-Barrios, M.D.
Professor
Departments of Pathology and Ophthalmology
Weill College of Medicine of Cornell University;
Director
Ophthalmic Pathology Program
The Methodist Hospital;
Research Co-Director
Retinoblastoma Center of Houston
Houston, Texas

Murali M. Chintagumpala, M.D.
Professor
Hematology–Oncology Section
Department of Pediatrics
Baylor College of Medicine;
Clinical Co-Director
Retinoblastoma Center of Houston
Texas Children's Cancer Center
Texas Children's Hospital
Houston, Texas

Michael L. Cleary, M.D.
Professor
Departments of Pathology and Pediatrics
Stanford University
Stanford, California

Joshua T. Cohen, Ph.D.
Research Associate Professor of Medicine
Department of Medicine
Tufts University School of Medicine;
Institute for Clinical Research and Health Policy Studies
Tufts Medical Center
Boston, Massachusetts

Heather M. Conklin, Ph.D.
Assistant Faculty Member
Department of Behavioral Medicine
St. Jude Children's Research Hospital
Memphis, Tennessee

Todd M. Cooper, D.O.
Assistant Professor
Pediatric Hematology/Oncology;
Assistant Professor
Aflac Cancer Center and Blood Disorders Service
Children's Healthcare of Atlanta/Emory University
Atlanta, Georgia

Christopher Denny, M.D.
Professor
Department of Pediatrics
University of California, Los Angeles, School of Medicine
Los Angeles, California

Jeffrey S. Dome, M.D., Ph.D.
Professor
Department of Pediatrics
George Washington University School of Medicine and
    Health Sciences;
Chief, Division of Oncology
Center for Cancer and Blood Disorders
Children's National Medical Center
Washington, District of Columbia

Zoann Dreyer, M.D.
Associate Professor
Hematology–Oncology Section
Department of Pediatrics
Baylor College of Medicine;
Director, Long-Term Survivor Program
Texas Children's Cancer Center
Texas Children's Hospital
Houston, Texas

Steven DuBois, M.D.
Assistant Professor
Department of Pediatrics
UCSF School of Medicine;
Attending Physician
Division of Pediatric Hematology/Oncology
University of California, San Francisco, Children's Hospital
San Francisco, California

Christopher Duggan, M.D., M.P.H.
Associate Professor of Pediatrics
Harvard Medical School;
Director, Clinical Nutrition Services
Division of Gastroenterology and Nutrition
Children's Hospital Boston
Boston, Massachusetts

Peter F. Ehrlich, M.D.
Associate Professor of Pediatric Surgery
Department of Surgery
University of Michigan;
Staff Surgeon
C.S. Mott Children's Hospital
Ann Arbor, Michigan

Joseph Fay, MBA
Executive Director
Children's Brain Tumor Foundation
New York, New York

Conrad Fernandez, M.D., Hon. B.Sc.
Professor
Department of Pediatrics
Dalhousie University;
Pediatric Oncologist
Department of Pediatrics
IWK Health Centre
Halifax, Nova Scotia, Canada

Michael J. Fisher, M.D.
Assistant Professor
Department of Pediatrics
University of Pennsylvania School of Medicine;
Division of Oncology
Children's Hospital of Philadelphia
Philadelphia, Pennsylvania

James Feusner, M.D., F.A.A.P.
Adjunct Clinical Professor
Department of Pediatrics
University of California, San Francisco
San Francisco, California;
Director of Oncology
Hematology and Oncology
Children's Hospital & Research Center Oakland
Oakland, California

Cecilia Fu, M.D.
Assistant Clinical Professor
Department of Pediatrics, Division of Hematology/Oncology
David Geffen School of Medicine at University of California,
    Los Angeles;
Associate Clinical Professor
Department of Pediatrics, Division of Hematology/Oncology
Mattel Children's Hospital University of California, Los Angeles
Los Angeles, California

Wayne L. Furman, M.D.
Department of Oncology
St. Jude Children's Research Hospital
Memphis, Tennessee

James I. Geller, M.D.
Assistant Professor
Department of Pediatrics
University of Cincinnati;
Assistant Professor
Division of Hematology/Oncology
Cincinnati Children's Hospital Medical Center
Cincinnati, Ohio

Richard Gilbertson, M.D., Ph.D.
Professor
Department of Biology
University of Memphis;
Member
Developmental Neurobiology
St. Jude Children's Research Hospital
Memphis, Tennessee

Dan Gombos, M.D., F.A.C.S.
Associate Professor
Department of Head & Neck Surgery, Section of
    Ophthalmology
MD Anderson Cancer Center;
Clinical Co-Director
Retinoblastoma Center of Houston
Houston, Texas

Julie J. Good, M.D.
Clinical Assistant Professor
Department of Anesthesia
Stanford University
Stanford, California;
Staff Physician
Pediatric Pain Symptom Management and Pediatric Palliative
    Care Team
Lucile Packard Children's Hospital
Palo Alto, California

Richard Gorlick, M.D.
Associate Professor
Department of Molecular Pharmacology and Pediatrics
Albert Einstein College of Medicine of Yeshiva University;
Vice Chairman and Division Chief, Hematology–Oncology
Department of Pediatrics
The Children's Hospital of Montefiore
Bronx, New York

Stephen Gottschalk, M.D.
Assistant Professor
Center for Cell and Gene Therapy
Department of Pediatrics
Baylor College of Medicine
Texas Children's Cancer Center
Texas Children's Hospital
Houston, Texas

Thomas G. Gross, M.D., Ph.D.
Professor
Department of Pediatrics
The Ohio State School of Medicine;
Chief
Hematology/Oncology/BMT
Nationwide Children's Hospital
Columbus, Ohio

Paul E. Grundy
Professor
Department of Pediatrics
University of Alberta;
Director
Pediatrics Oncology
Stollery Children's Hospital
Edmonton, Alberta, Canada

R. Paul Guillerman, M.D.
Associate Professor
Department of Radiology
Baylor College of Medicine;
Staff Radiologist
Department of Diagnostic Imaging
Texas Children's Hospital
Houston, Texas

James G. Gurney, Ph.D.
Associate Professor
Department of Pediatrics
University of Michigan
Ann Arbor, Michigan

Daphne Haas-Kogan, M.D.
Professor, Departments of Radiation Oncology and
    Neurosurgery
Vice-Chair and Program Director, Department of Radiation
    Oncology
Radiation Oncology
University of California
San Francisco, California

Henrik Hasle, M.D., Ph.D.
Associate Professor
Department of Pediatrics
Aarhus University Hospital Skejby;
Senior Consultant
Department of Pediatrics
Aarhus University Hospital Skejby
Aarhus, Denmark

Caroline A. Hastings, M.D.
Associate Clinical Professor
Department of Pediatrics
University of California
San Francisco, California;
Pediatric Hematologist/Oncologist
Hematology and Oncology
Children's Hospital & Research Center Oakland
Oakland, California

Douglas S. Hawkins, M.D.
Associate Professor of Pediatrics
Department of Pediatrics
University of Washington School of Medicine;
Associate Division Chief, Hematology/
    Oncology
Department of Pediatrics
Seattle Children's Hospital
Seattle, Washington

Robert Hayashi, M.D.
Associate Professor of Pediatrics
Division of Pediatric Hematology/Oncology
Washington University School of Medicine
St. Louis, Missouri

Amy Heerema-McKenney, M.D.
Clinical Assistant Professor
Department of Pathology
Stanford University School of Medicine
Stanford, California

Lee J. Helman, M.D.
Scientific Director for Clinical Research
Center for Cancer Research
National Cancer Institute
Bethesda, Maryland

Stephen P. Hersh, M.D., DLFAPA
Clinical Professor
Department of Behavioral Sciences, Psychiatry, and Pediatrics
George Washington University
Washington, District of Columbia;
Director
The Medical Illness Counseling Center
Chevy Chase, Maryland

Helen E. Heslop, M.D., F.R.A.C.P., F.R.C.P.A.
Professor and Dan L. Duncan Chair
Center for Cell and Gene Therapy
Baylor College of Medicine;
Director, Adult Stem Cell Transplant Program
The Methodist Hospital
Texas Children's Cancer Center
Texas Children's Hospital
Houston, Texas

John Hicks, M.D., D.D.S., M.S., Ph.D.
Professor of Pathology
Department of Pathology
Texas Children's Hospital and Baylor College of Medicine;
Attending Pathologist
Department of Pathology
Texas Children's Hospital
Houston, Texas

D. Ashley Hill
Associate Professor
Pathology
George Washington University;
Chief of Pathology
Children's National Medical Center
Washington, District of Columbia

Susan Hilsenbeck, Ph.D.
Professor
Breast Center and Department of Medicine
Baylor College of Medicine
Houston, Texas

Marilyn J. Hockenberry, Ph.D., R.N., P.N.P., F.A.A.N.
Professor
Hematology–Oncology Section
Department of Pediatrics
Baylor College of Medicine;
Nurse Scientist
Texas Children's Cancer Center
Texas Children's Hospital
Houston, Texas

Michael D. Hogarty, M.D.
Associate Professor
Department of Pediatrics
University of Pennsylvania School of Medicine;
Attending Physician
Division of Oncology
The Children's Hospital of Philadelphia
Philadelphia, Pennsylvania

Pancras C.W. Hogendoorn, M.D., Ph.D.
Professor of Pathology
Department of Pathology
Leiden University Medical Center
Leiden, The Netherlands

Melissa M. Hudson, M.D.
Member
Department of Oncology
St. Jude Children's Research Hospital
Memphis, Tennessee

Winston Huh, M.D.
Assistant Professor
Division of Pediatrics;
Clinical Faculty
Division of Pediatrics
University of Texas, MD Anderson Cancer Center
Houston, Texas

Mary Y. Hurwitz, Ph.D.
Associate Professor
Hematology–Oncology Section
Department of Pediatrics
Baylor College of Medicine;
Texas Children's Cancer Center
Texas Children's Hospital
Houston, Texas

Richard L. Hurwitz, M.D.
Associate Professor
Hematology–Oncology Section
Departments of Pediatrics, Ophthalmology,
    and Molecular and Cellular Biology
Baylor College of Medicine;
Co-Director, Retinoblastoma Center of Houston
Texas Children's Cancer Center
Texas Children's Hospital
Houston, Texas

Daniel J. Indelicato, M.D.
Assistant Professor
Department of Radiation Oncology
University of Florida;
Assistant Professor
Department of Radiation Oncology
University of Florida Proton Therapy Institute
Jacksonville, Florida

Tom Jaksic, M.D., Ph.D.
Associate Professor
Department of Surgery
Harvard Medical School;
Senior Surgical Associate
Department of Pediatric Surgery
Children's Hospital Boston
Boston, Massachusetts

Steven Joffe, M.D., M.P.H.
Assistant Professor of Pediatrics
Department of Pediatrics
Harvard Medical School;
Attending in Pediatric Hematology/Oncology
Department of Pediatric Oncology
Dana-Farber Cancer Institute
Boston, Massachusetts

Heribert Jürgens, M.D., Ph.D.
Professor
Department of Pediatric Hematology and Oncology
Westfaelische Wilhelms-Universitaet;
Director
Department of Pediatric Hematology and Oncology
Universitaetsklinikum Muenster
Muenster, Germany

John A. Kalapurakal, M.D.
Professor
Radiation Oncology
Northwestern University;
Professor
Radiation Oncology
Northwestern Memorial Hospital
Chicago, Illinois

Sue C. Kaste, D.O.
Member
Department of Radiological Sciences
St. Jude Children's Research Hospital;
Zull Professor
Department of Radiology
University of Tennessee
Memphis, Tennessee

Kathleen Sakamoto, M.D., Ph.D.
Professor
Department of Pediatrics
University of California, Los Angeles;
Chief
Department of Pediatrics
Mattel Children's Hospital University of California,
    Los Angeles
David Geffen School of Medicine
Los Angeles, California

Jennifer Kesselheim, M.D., M.B.E.
Instructor of Pediatrics
Department of Pediatrics
Harvard Medical School;
Attending in Pediatric Hematology/Oncology
Pediatric Oncology
Dana-Farber Cancer Institute
Boston, Massachusetts

Javed Khan, M.A., M.B.B.Chir., M.R.C.P.
Senior Investigator
Oncogenomics Section;
Attending
Pediatric Oncology Branch
National Cancer Institute
Bethesda, Maryland

Lindsay B. Kilburn, M.D.
Assistant Professor
Hematology–Oncology Section
Department of Pediatrics
Baylor College of Medicine;
Texas Children's Cancer Center
Texas Children's Hospital
Houston, Texas

Nancy E. Kline, Ph.D., R.N., C.P.N.P., F.A.A.N.
Director, Research and Evidence-Based Practice Nursing
Memorial Swan-Kettering Cancer Center
New York, New York

Federico Antillon Klussmann, M.D., M.M.M., Ph.D.
Pediatric Hematology–Oncology Fellowship
Medical School
Universidad Francisco Marroquin;
Medical Director
Unidad Nacional de Oncologia Pediátrica
Guatemala City, Guatemala

Andrew Y. Koh, M.D.
Instructor
Department of Pediatrics
Harvard Medical School;
Department of Medicine, Division of Hematology/Oncology
    and Infectious Diseases
Children's Hospital Boston
Boston, Massachusetts

Robert A. Krance, M.D.
Professor
Center for Cell and Gene Therapy
Department of Pediatrics
Baylor College of Medicine;
Director, Pediatric Stem Cell Transplantation
Texas Children's Cancer Center
Texas Children's Hospital
Houston, Texas

Elliot J. Krane, M.D.
Professor
Departments of Anesthesia and Pediatrics
Stanford University
Stanford, California;
Head of Pediatric Pain Management
Lucile Packard Children's Hospital at Stanford
Palo Alto, California

Matthew J. Krasin, M.D.
Associate Member
Department of Radiological Sciences
St. Jude Children's Research Hospital
Memphis, Tennessee

Larry E. Kun, M.D.
Professor
Department of Radiology & Pediatrics
University of Tennessee
College of Medicine;
Chair
Radiological Sciences
St. Jude Children's Research Hospital
Memphis, Tennessee

Ching C. Lau, M.D., Ph.D.
Associate Professor
Hematology–Oncology Section
Department of Pediatrics
Baylor College of Medicine;
Research Director, Neuro-Oncology Program
Texas Children's Cancer Center
Texas Children's Hospital
Houston, Texas

Laurie D. Leigh, M.A.
Director, School Program
Behavioral Medicine
St Jude Children's Research Hospital
Memphis, Tennessee

Stephen L. Lessnick, M.D., Ph.D.
Associate Professor
Department of Pediatrics, Division of Hematology/Oncology
University of Utah;
Investigator
Center for Children
Huntsman Cancer Institute
Salt Lake City, Utah

Melissa L. Lichte, B.A.
Research Assistant
Institute for Clinical Research and Health Policy Studies
Tufts Medical Center
Boston, Massachusetts

Bertram H. Lubin, M.D.
Adjunct Professor of Pediatrics
Department of Pediatrics
University of California at San Francisco
San Francisco, California;
President, Director of Medical Research
Children's Hospital Oakland Research Institute
Oakland, California

David Malkin, M.D., FRCPC
Professor
Pediatrics & Medical Biophysics
University of Toronto;
Staff Physician & Director, Cancer Genetics Program
Division of Hematology/Oncology
The Hospital for Sick Children
Toronto, Ontario, Canada

Crystal L. Mackall, M.D.
Chief
Pediatric Oncology Branch
National Cancer Institute
Bethesda, Maryland

Marcio H. Malogolowkin, M.D.
Associate Professor of Pediatrics Clinical Schalow
Department of Pediatrics
Keck School of Medicare, University of Southern California;
Director Head, Hematology/Oncology for Clinical Affairs
    Clinical Research
Children's Hospital of Los Angeles
Los Angeles, California

Judith F. Margolin, M.D.
Associate Professor
Hematology–Oncology Section
Department of Pediatrics
Baylor College of Medicine;
Texas Children's Cancer Center
Texas Children's Hospital
Houston, Texas

Neyssa Marina, M.D.
Professor of Pediatrics
Division of Hematology–Oncology
Department of Pediatrics
Stanford University & Lucile Packard Children's Hospital;
Associate Chief of Clinical Affairs
Department of Pediatrics
Lucile Packard Children's Hospital
Palo Alto, California

John M. Maris, M.D.
Associate Professor
Department of Pediatrics
University of Pennsylvania School of Medicine;
Chief, Division of Oncology
Director, Center for Childhood Cancer Research
Department of Pediatrics
Children's Hospital of Philadelphia
Philadelphia, Pennsylvania

Kenneth L. McClain, M.D. Ph.D.
Professor
Hematology–Oncology Section
Department of Pediatrics
Baylor College of Medicine;
Texas Children's Cancer Center
Texas Children's Hospital
Houston, Texas

Thomas W. McLean
Associate Professor
Department of Pediatrics
Wake Forest University;
Brenner Children's Hospital
Winston-Salem, North Carolina

Mary A. McMahon, M.D.
Associate Professor
Departments of Physical Medicine and Rehabilitation and
    Pediatrics
University of Cincinnati College of Medicine;
Attending Pediatric Physiatrist
Division of Pediatric Rehabilitation
Cincinnati Children's Hospital Medical Center
Cincinnati, Ohio

Mary E. (Beth) McCarville, M.D.
Associate Member
Department of Radiological Sciences
St. Jude Children's Research Hospital
Memphis, Tennessee

Anna T. Meadows, M.D.
Professor
Department of Pediatrics
University of Pennsylvania School of Medicine;
Senior Physician
Department of Oncology
The Children's Hospital of Philadelphia
Philadelphia, Pennsylvania

Parth Mehta, M.D.
Assistant Professor
Hematology–Oncology Section
Department of Pediatrics
Baylor College of Medicine
Gaborone, Botswana;
Texas Children's Cancer Center
Texas Children's Hospital
Houston, Texas

Monika Metzger, M.D., M.Sc.
Assistant Professor
Department of Pediatrics
University of Tennessee Health Science Center;
Assistant Member
Department of Oncology
St Jude Children's Research Hospital
Memphis, Tennessee

James Meyer, M.D.
Professor of Radiology
Department of Radiology
University of Pennsylvania School of Medicine;
Associate Radiologist-in-Chief
Department of Radiology
Children's Hospital of Philadelphia
Philadelphia, Pennsylvania

Rebecka L. Meyers, M.D.
Chief, Division of Pediatric Surgery
Professor, Department of Surgery, Division of Pediatric Surgery
University of Utah;
Division of Pediatric Surgery
Primary Children's Medical Center
Salt Lake City, Utah

William H. Meyer, M.D.
CMRI Bon Johnson Professor
Department of Pediatrics
University of Oklahoma Health Sciences Center;
Section Head, Pediatric Hematology/Oncology
Department of Pediatrics
Oklahoma University Medical Center
Oklahoma City, Oklahoma

Linda J. Michaud, M.D., P.T.
Associate Professor
Departments of Physical Medicine and Rehabilitation and
    Pediatrics
University of Cincinnati College of Medicine;
Director
Division of Pediatric Rehabilitation
Cincinnati Children's Hospital Medical Center
Cincinnati, Ohio

Lynn Million, M.D.
Huntsman Cancer Hospital
Radiation Oncology
Salt Lake City, Utah

Grace P. Monaco, J.D.
Director, Medical Care Ombudsman Program
Co-Director, Childhood Cancer Ombudsman Program
Germantown, Maryland

Yael P. Mosse, M.D.
Assistant Professor
Department of Pediatrics
University of Pennsylvania School of Medicine;
Children's Hospital of Philadelphia
Philadelphia, Pennsylvania

Brigitta U. Mueller, M.D., M.H.C.M.
Professor
Hematology–Oncology Section
Department of Pediatrics
Baylor College of Medicine;
Clinical Director
Texas Children's Cancer Center
Texas Children's Hospital
Houston, Texas

M. Fatih Okcu, M.D., M.P.H.
Associate Professor
Hematology–Oncology Section
Department of Pediatrics
Baylor College of Medicine;
Texas Children's Cancer Center
Texas Children's Hospital
Houston, Texas

Thomas A. Olson, M.D.
Associate Professor
Pediatric Hematology/Oncology
Emory University School of Medicine;
Medical Director
Egleston, Aflac Cancer Center and Blood Disorders Service
Children's Healthcare of Atlanta
Atlanta, Georgia

Mihaela Onciu, M.D.
Associate Member
Department of Pathology
St. Jude Children's Research Hospital;
Director, Hematology and Special Hematology Laboratories
Department of Pathology
St. Jude Children's Research Hospital
Memphis, Tennessee

Roger J. Packer, M.D.
Professor
Department of Neurology and Pediatrics
The George Washington University;
Senior Vice President, Neuroscience and Behavioral
    Medicine's Brain Tumor Institute
Children's National Medical Center
Washington, District of Columbia

Alberto S. Pappo, M.D.
Director, Division of Solid Tumor
Department of Oncology
St. Jude Children's Research Hospital
Memphis, Tennessee

Donald "Will" Parsons, M.D., Ph.D.
Assistant Professor
Departments of Pediatrics and Molecular and Human
    Genetics
Baylor College of Medicine;
Texas Children's Cancer Center
Texas Children's Hospital
Houston, Texas

Susan K. Parsons, M.D., M.R.P.
Associate Professor
Department of Medicine and Pediatrics
Tufts University School of Medicine;
Director, The Health Institute for Clinical Research and
    Health Policy Studies
Department of Medicine
Tufts Medical Center
Boston, Massachusetts

Michael Paulussen, M.D., Ph.D.
Professor
Pediatric Hematology/Oncology
University of Basel;
Head
Department of Pediatric Hematology/Oncology
University Children's Hospital
Basel, Switzerland

Sherrie L. Perkins, M.D., Ph.D.
Professor
Department of Pathology
University of Utah;
Chief Medical Officer, Director of Hematopathology
Department of Pathology
ARUP Laboratories
Salt Lake City, Utah

Elizabeth J. Perlman, M.D.
Professor
Department of Pathology
Northwestern University's Feinberg School of Medicine;
Pathologist-in-Chief and Head
Department of Pathology and Laboratory Medicine
Children's Memorial Hospital
Chicago, Illinois

Philip A. Pizzo, M.D.
Dean of the School of Medicine
Carl and Elizabeth Naumann Professor
Professor of Pediatrics and of Microbiology and Immunology
Stanford University School of Medicine
Stanford, California

Sharon E. Plon, M.D., Ph.D.
Professor
Hematology–Oncology Section
Department of Pediatrics
Chief, Baylor Cancer Genetics Clinic
Baylor College of Medicine;
Texas Children's Cancer Center
Texas Children's Hospital
Houston, Texas

Ian Pollack, M.D.
Walter Dandy Professor
Neurological Surgery
University of Pittsburgh School of Medicine;
Professor and Chief
Neurosurgery
Children's Hospital of Pittsburgh
Pittsburgh, Pennsylvania

Brad H. Pollock, M.P.H., Ph.D.
Professor and Chairman
Department of Epidemiology and Biostatistics
University of Texas Health Science Center at San Antonio
San Antonio, Texas

David G. Poplack, M.D.
Elise C. Young Professor of Pediatric Oncology
Head, Hematology–Oncology Section
Department of Pediatrics
Baylor College of Medicine;
Director, Texas Children's Cancer Center
Texas Children's Hospital
Houston, Texas

David W. Pruitt, M.D.
Assistant Professor
Departments of Physical Medicine and Rehabilitation and
    Pediatrics
University of Cincinnati College of Medicine;
Attending Pediatric Physiatrist
Division of Pediatric Rehabilitation
Cincinnati Children's Hospital Medical Center
Cincinnati, Ohio

Karen R. Rabin, M.D.
Assistant Professor
Hematology–Oncology Section
Department of Pediatrics
Baylor College of Medicine;
Texas Children's Cancer Center
Texas Children's Hospital
Houston, Texas

Christina Ullrich, M.D., M.P.H.
Instructor
Department of Pediatrics
Harvard Medical School;
Attending Physician
Pediatric Hematology/Oncology
Psychosocial Oncology and Palliative Care
Dana-Farber Cancer Institute and Children's Hospital
Boston, Massachusetts

Gilbert Vezina, M.D.
Professor
Department of Radiology and Pediatrics
George Washington University Medical Center;
Director
Program in Neuroradiology
Children's National Medical Center
Washington, District of Columbia

Stephan D. Voss, M.D., Ph.D.
Assistant Professor of Radiology
Department of Radiology
Harvard Medical School;
Staff Radiologist
Department of Radiology
Children's Hospital—Boston
Boston, Massachusetts

Steven G. Waguespack, M.D.
Associate Professor
Endocrine Neoplasia & Hormonal Disorders
University of Texas, MD Anderson Cancer Center
Houston, Texas

Susan L. Weiner, Ph.D.
President, Children's Cause for Cancer Advocacy
Silver Spring, Maryland

Christopher B. Weldon, M.D., Ph.D.
Instructor
Department of Surgery
Harvard Medical School;
Assistant in Surgery
Department of Pediatric Surgery
Children's Hospital Boston
Boston, Massachusetts

Leonard H. Wexler, M.D.
Associate Professor
Department of Pediatrics
Weill Medical College of Cornell University;
Associate Attending
Department of Pediatrics
Memorial Sloan-Kettering Cancer Center
New York, New York

Lori S. Wiener, Ph.D., D.C.S.W.
Coordinator
Pediatric Support and Research Program
HIV/AIDS Malignancy Branch
National Cancer Institute
National Institute of Health
Bethesda, Maryland

Robert Wilkinson, M.D.
Professor
Department of Pediatrics
University of Hawaii;
Director
Kapiolani Children's Blood and Cancer Center
Kapiolani Women's and Children's Medicine Center
Honolulu, Hawaii

Joanne Wolfe, M.D., M.P.H.
Assistant Professor
Department of Pediatrics
Harvard Medical School;
Division Chief, Pediatric Palliative Care Service
Department of Psychosocial Oncology and Palliative Care
Dana-Farber Cancer Institute
Boston, Massachusetts

Anita K. Ying, M.D.
Assistant Professor
Endocrine Neoplasia and Hormonal Disorders
The University of Texas, MD Anderson Cancer Center
Houston, Texas

Tina Young-Pouissant, M.D.
Associate Professor
Department of Radiology
Harvard Medical School
Boston, Massachusetts;
Attending Neuroradiologist
Department of Radiology
Children's Hospital Boston
Boston, Massachusetts

Lonnie K. Zeltzer, M.D.
Professor of Pediatrics, Anesthesiology, Psychiatry, and
    Biobehavioral Sciences
Department of Pediatrics
David Geffen School of Medicine at University of California,
    Los Angeles;
Director, Pediatric Pain Program
Department of Pediatrics
Mattel Children's Hospital University of California,
    Los Angeles
Los Angeles, California

Arthur Zimmerman, M.D.
Professor Emeritus
Institute of Pathology
University of Berne
Switzerland
Berne, Switzerland

The five previous editions of the *Principles and Practice of Pediatric Oncology*, now joined by the sixth, have catalogued and chronicled the extraordinary changes that have taken place in the diagnosis, treatment, and long-term care of children with cancer during the past 22 years. When we began our own personal education(s) in science and medicine two decades before the publication of the first edition of *Principles and Practice of Pediatric Oncology,* the treatment of cancer was in its infancy and the prospect for cures a distant aspiration and dream. At that time, there was no consideration of long-term consequences, since survival for most patients was measured in months and years. So much has changed—both in the celebration that the majority of children with cancer can become long-term survivors and in the disappointment that their survival is mired by the consequences of treatments configured in the past. Still, in many ways, pediatric oncology stands as the exemplar in codifying the dramatic changes that have taken place in the discovery and application of new medical knowledge as well as a paradigm for what can be achieved through collaborative clinical and translational research.

From the first pioneering physician–scientists who laid the foundation for the discipline of pediatric oncology, to those now at its leading edge of inquiry, there has been a remarkably integrated relationship between basic sciences, clinical research and patient care in the principles and practice of pediatric oncology. As cancer biology evolved from the study of cellular kinetics to its current molecular and genetic underpinnings, pediatric cancer has served as the equivalent of a model organism. The first edition had a primer of the then still new field of molecular biology. Over the past two decades, modern cancer biology, including genetics and genomics, have become integrated into the diagnosis and treatment of childhood malignancies. Trainees in pediatric oncology today are no longer passive observers of molecular medicine—but more often its leaders and innovators.

The concept of multidisciplinary care had its origins in childhood cancer. This concept of teams of physicians, nurses, social workers, and pharmacists working together to optimize patient care has become the signature of 21st century oncology practice. The locus of care also is shifting from largely in-patient to the more frequent outpatient ambulatory setting—including for the administration of heretofore-intensive therapies including stem cell infusions or even the treatment of complications like fever and neutropenia. Indeed, hospitalization is increasingly reserved for the management of the most intense care situations.

Because of its relative rarity and the need to evaluate patients on a larger scale than that available to regional children's hospitals or treatment centers, pediatric oncologists were pioneers in the development of national cooperative groups and closely linking clinical investigation and clinical trials to the delivery of state-of-the-art patient care. Indeed, the discipline of pediatric oncology stands nearly alone in the close partnership of clinical research and patient care—with the vast majority of children who are diagnosed with cancer receiving treatment on clinical protocols. This stands in stark contrast to adult oncology, and it seems clear that those managing many serious and chronic diseases could learn much from how the care of children with cancer has been organized on a national and international basis. Indeed, in an era when innovation defines state-of-the-art patient care and where quality outcomes, excellence in the patient experience, and attention to cost and efficiency will define the future of medicine, the field of pediatric oncology should be used as a prototype, role model, and testing ground—whose principles for study, evaluation, and organized delivery can be extrapolated to many other diseases, whether in children or adults.

The Sixth Edition of *Principles and Practice of Pediatric Oncology* has been extensively revised and updated to reflect the continued dramatic and significant changes that are occurring in this discipline. Although authors who have contributed to one or more prior editions have prepared the majority of the chapters, new contributors to this edition have written 40% of the chapters. They share in common that each are leaders in their fields and in shaping the future of care for children with cancer. As with prior editions, we have sought to provide the fundamental underpinnings of cancer biology, genetics, and immunology as well as the conceptual context of surgery, chemotherapy, and radiation oncology in discrete chapters. Although each provides an informed introduction for those new to the field, the principles they articulate are suffused in virtually every chapter. Because we also recognize that the diagnosis and management of the child with cancer must be framed in the context of the family, school, and community, we continue to provide informed attention to the broad and interdisciplinary supportive care and psychosocial management of children and their families facing the challenge of childhood cancer.

We have been proud to serve as editors for each of the now six editions of *Principles and Practice of Pediatric Oncology*. In this sixth edition, we are enormously pleased to welcome three associate editors: Peter Adamson, Susan Blaney, and Lee Helman. Each is a national leader in the field and we have had the special privilege of sharing in their education and training at the Pediatric Branch of the National Cancer Institute. We remain indebted to the wonderful support we have received from our staff and assistants, especially Ms. Mira Engel at Stanford University and Ms. Sara Farnum at Texas Children's Hospital. We have also been fortunate in having a continued and outstanding relationship with our publisher, now Wolters Kluwer Health—Lippincott Williams & Wilkins, which has undergone its own evolution over the years. In particular, we want to thank Jonathan Pine, who has worked with us on half of the six editions and also Emilie Moyer who served as our managing editor for the current edition.

The future of books as paper publications is rapidly changing. But in whatever format they appear the power of the knowledge that textbooks contain is transformative. It remains our hope and singular goal that the Sixth Edition of the *Principles and Practice of Pediatric Oncology* will help educate the current and future providers of care to children with cancer and through their accrued knowledge and experience, further transform and improve the lives and futures of their patients.

Contents

SECTION 6 ■ OTHER ISSUES ARISING AT DIAGNOSIS, DURING TREATMENT, AND AFTER CESSATION OF THERAPY

SECTION 1 ■ BIOLOGICAL BASIS OF CHILDHOOD CANCER

CHAPTER 1 ■ EPIDEMIOLOGY OF CHILDHOOD CANCER

MICHAEL E. SCHEURER, MELISSA L. BONDY, AND JAMES G. GURNEY

This chapter provides an update on childhood cancer statistics and an overview of epidemiologic methods, including study designs, potential biases, and statistical measures of effect, with examples from the childhood cancer literature to illustrate these concepts. The information in this chapter is meant to help clinicians better understand the approaches used in epidemiologic research on the causes and consequences of childhood cancer and to interpret and communicate research findings to their patients and colleagues.

CENTRAL CONCEPTS OF EPIDEMIOLOGY

Epidemiology is a key scientific methodology for conducting health-related research. It involves the comparative study of the distribution and determinants of disease and other health-related conditions within defined human populations. Identifying, describing, and interpreting patterns of cancer occurrence (distribution) and studying factors that may cause or contribute to the occurrence, prevention, control, and outcome of cancer (determinants) encompass the activities of epidemiologists.[1,2]

Epidemiology incorporates aspects of research from biologic, clinical, social, and statistical sciences. Two central concepts of epidemiology are as follows:

1. *Disease is not randomly distributed.* Measurable factors influence the patterns and causes of disease within a defined population.
2. *Disease causation is multifactorial.* Few individual agents are necessary or sufficient to cause disease; in fact, disease results from a multitude of endogenous and exogenous factors. Identifying and measuring the relative contribution and interaction of these factors is the principal role of analytic epidemiology.

SURVEILLANCE AND DESCRIPTIVE STUDIES

Public health surveillance involves the systematic collection, analysis, and interpretation of outcome-specific health data and the timely dissemination of the findings to prevent and control disease or injury. Surveillance systems are thus essential to plan, implement, and evaluate public health practice.[3,4] Surveillance systems provide data on disease incidence and mortality on a population basis for policy makers and researchers. In the United States, an exceptionally high-quality cancer surveillance system is funded and coordinated by the National Cancer Institute's (NCI's) Surveillance, Epidemiology, and End Results (SEER) program. The SEER program was established in 1973 and now encompasses nine state and four large metropolitan cancer registries and registries covering the Alaska Native and Arizona American Indian populations (http://www.seer.cancer.gov).

Data from the SEER program enables evaluation, otherwise unachievable, of rare childhood malignancies and of cancer patterns in demographic subgroups. Descriptive analyses from cross-sectional (prevalence) or ecologic (correlational) studies allow investigators to develop hypotheses on the patterns and causes of cancer and then test those hypotheses using analytic approaches.[1,2] The rarity of any specific type of childhood cancer, however, makes it very difficult to recruit enough cases for statistically meaningful studies, even with statewide population-based registries. This problem of conducting good epidemiologic research on rare events has prompted the Children's Oncology Group (COG) to develop a nationwide, volunteer childhood cancer registry, the Childhood Cancer Research Network (CCRN).[5,6] The CCRN allows newly diagnosed childhood cancer patients and their parents to participate in the data registry with or without the option of being recontacted for future research. Initial pilot studies on the feasibility of the registry showed that 96% of participants agreed to fully participate, and only 1% declined participation.[6] About 90% of children with cancer in the United States are treated on the basis of COG protocols; therefore, the CCRN makes it possible to perform essentially population-based research on childhood cancer etiology.

CHILDHOOD CANCER STATISTICS

Childhood cancer is relatively uncommon, with approximately 1 to 2 children in every 10,000 children aged 14 years and younger diagnosed in the United States each year.[7] Despite the rarity of childhood cancer, approximately 15,100 children and adolescents younger than 20 years will be diagnosed with cancer in the United States (~10,700 cases among children 0 to 14 years of age[8] and ~4,400 cases among 15- to 19-year-olds).[9] These numbers correspond to an average annual incidence rate of 18.8 cases per 100,000 person-years for all cancers for children younger than 20 years. The likelihood of a young person reaching adulthood and being diagnosed with cancer during childhood is approximately 1 in 300 for males and 1 in 333 for females.[6] Childhood cancer remains the leading cause of disease-related mortality among children 1 to 14 years of age (Fig. 1.1A), and there were approximately 1,300 cancer-related deaths in 2006 in the United States among children younger than 15 years. The relative contribution of cancer to overall mortality for 15- to 19-year-olds is lower than that for the younger children (Fig. 1.1B), although

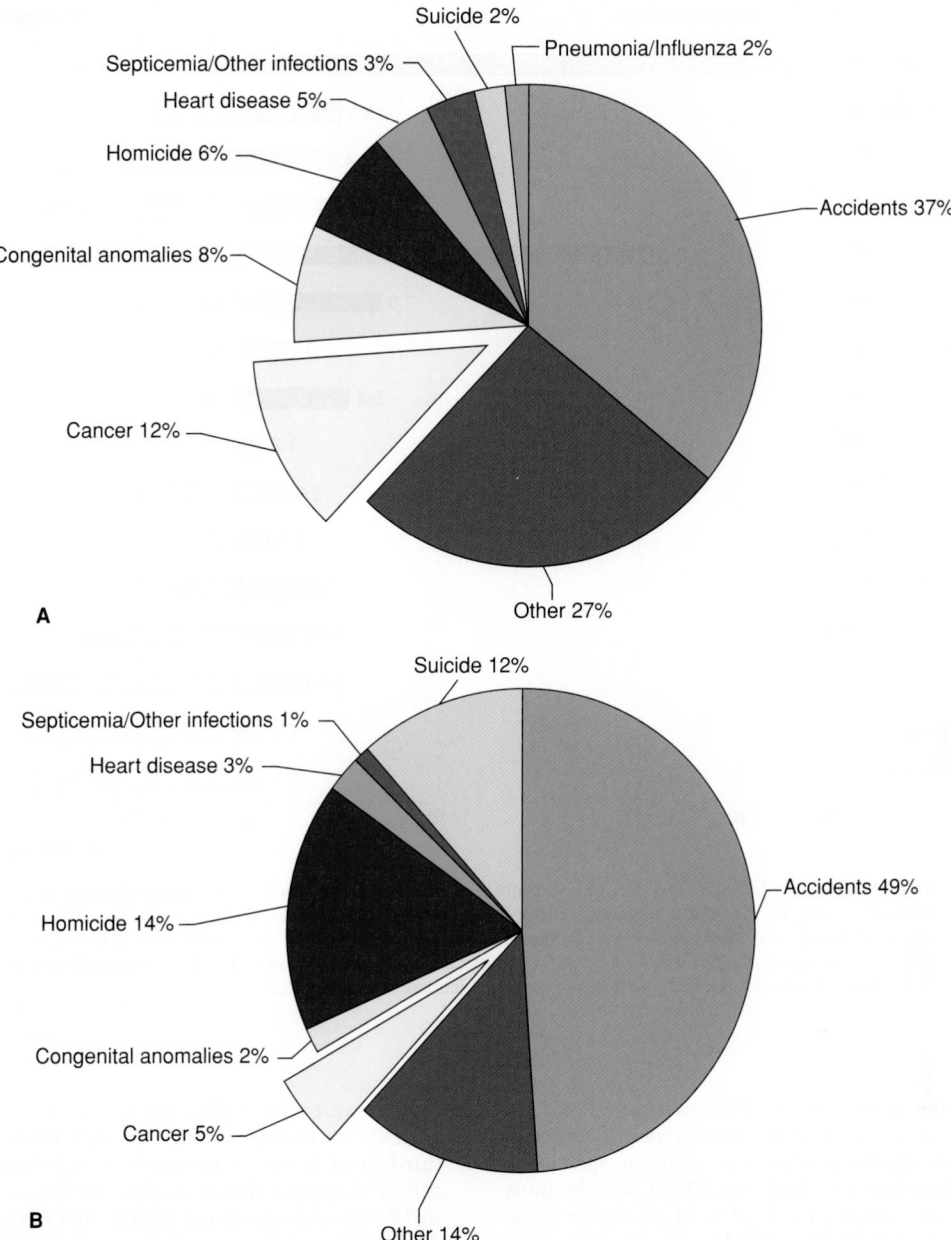

FIGURE 1.1 Leading causes of death in children in the United States, 2006. Causes of death among (**A**) children 1 to 14 years and (**B**) adolescents 15 to 19 years of age. (Death data are from the National Center for Health Statistics public-use file.)

approximately 700 deaths from cancer occurred in 2006 in this age group.

The population-based data for invasive cancer incidence and survival, unless otherwise indicated, are from the SEER program of the NCI. The SEER data for this chapter are based on 58,316 cases of childhood cancer diagnosed among residents of 17 SEER areas that represent approximately 26% of the U.S. population. (More information on the inclusion of these SEER areas and their contribution to case data is available from the SEER Web site.) The mortality data cover all cancer deaths among children in the United States, as provided by the National Center for Health Statistics. The classification scheme used in this chapter is the International Clas-

sification of Childhood Cancer, which allocates tumors into 12 major diagnostic groups that reflect the most prevalent tumors in the pediatric population.[10]

OVERALL CANCER FREQUENCY AND INCIDENCE BY TYPE OF CANCER FOR CHILDREN AND ADOLESCENTS

Figure 1.2 compares the distribution by percentages of the cancers that occurred among 0- to 14-year-olds and 15- to

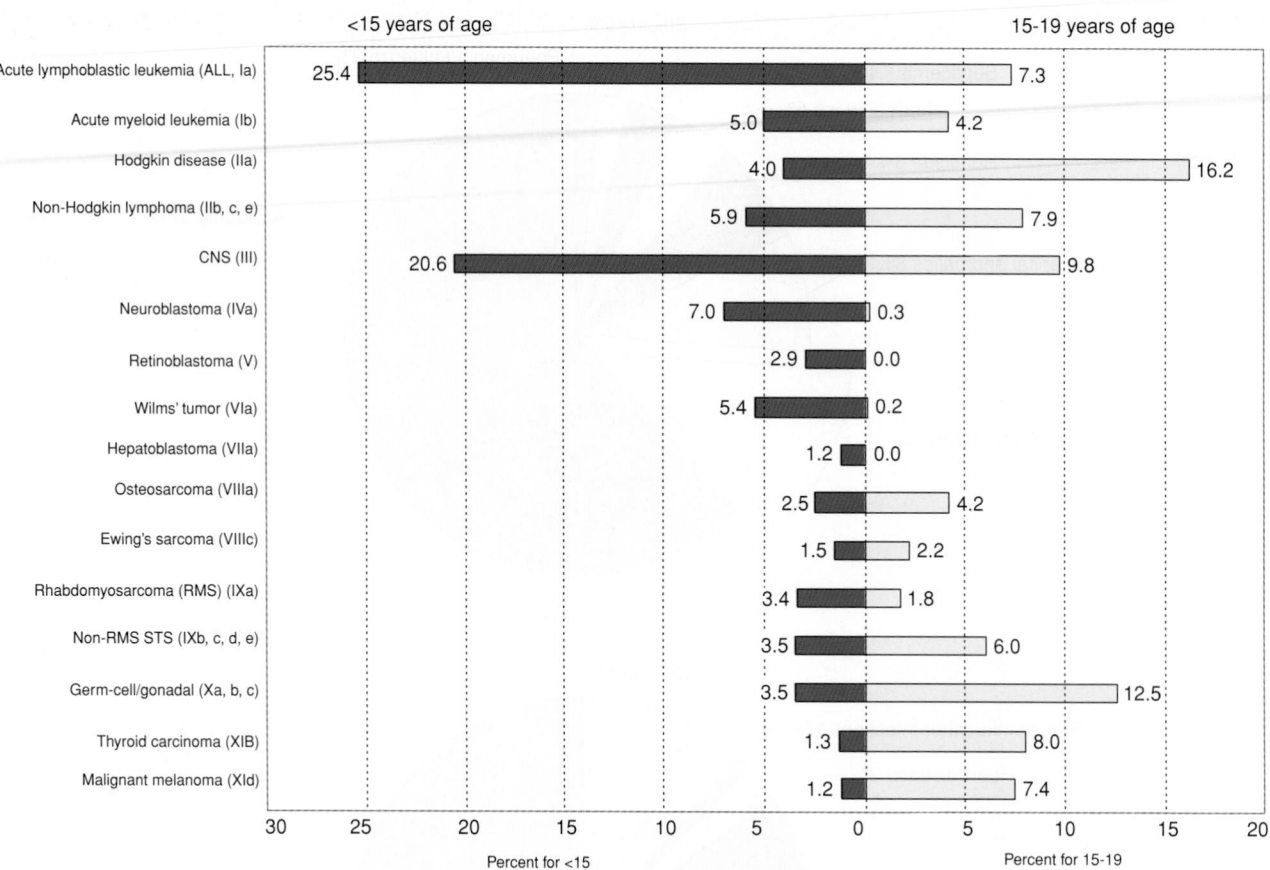

FIGURE 1.2 Distribution of specific cancer diagnoses for children (aged 0 to 14 years) and adolescents (aged 15 to 19 years), 1973 to 2006. Percentage distribution by International Classification of Childhood Cancer diagnostic groups and subgroups for younger than 15 years and 15 to 19 years of age (all races and both sexes). CNS, central nervous system; RMS, rhabdomyosarcoma; STS, soft tissue sarcoma. (Incidence data are from the Surveillance, Epidemiology, and End Results program, National Cancer Institute.)

19-year-olds for the years 1973 to 2006, whereas Table 1.1 provides the annual incidence of the major types of cancer in these two age groups by gender. For children aged 0 to 14 years, acute lymphoblastic leukemia (ALL) was the most common cancer, accounting for 25.4% of all cancer diagnoses. Acute myeloid leukemia (AML) was the next most common type of leukemia in this age group, occurring at a rate one-fifth of that for ALL. Central nervous system (CNS) cancers, primarily occurring in the brain, accounted for 20.6% of cancer diagnoses and together with ALL and AML made up one-half of cancer diagnoses among children younger than 15 years. The most common non-CNS solid tumor in the 0- to 14-year age group was neuroblastoma (7.0%), followed by Wilms' tumor (5.4%) and non-Hodgkin lymphoma (NHL) (5.9%). Other diagnoses that individually represented 2% to 4% of cancer diagnoses in this age group included Hodgkin disease, rhabdomyosarcoma, non-rhabdomyosarcoma soft tissue sarcomas, germ cell tumors, retinoblastoma, and osteosarcoma.

The distribution of cancer diagnoses for 15- to 19-year-olds is significantly different (Fig. 1.2). For example, Hodgkin disease (16.2%) and germ cell tumors (12.5%) were the most frequently diagnosed cancers. The percentages of cases represented by NHL (7.9%), melanoma (7.4%), thyroid cancer (8.0%), non-rhabdomyosarcoma soft tissue sarcoma (6.0%), osteosarcoma (4.2%), and Ewing's sarcoma

(2.2%) were also higher for 15- to 19-year-olds compared with 0- to 14-year-olds. Although CNS tumors were the third most common tumor type, representing 9.8% of all cancer diagnoses (Fig. 1.2), their incidence was lower for 15- to 19-year-olds compared with 0- to 14-year-olds (Table 1.1). ALL accounted for a much lower proportion of cases among 15- to 19-year-olds (7.3%) compared with children 0 to 14 years of age (25.4%) and occurred only slightly more frequently than AML (4.2% of cases) in this age group. The percentages of cases for rhabdomyosarcoma and non-rhabdomyosarcoma soft tissue sarcoma were nearly equal for 0- to 14-year-olds, but the percentage for non-rhabdomyosarcoma soft tissue sarcoma was higher than that for rhabdomyosarcoma for 15- to 19-year-olds (Fig. 1.2). Some cancers that are more common in young children (e.g., CNS cancers, neuroblastoma, retinoblastoma, hepatoblastoma, and Wilms' tumor) occurred at very low rates among 15- to 19-year-olds (Table 1.1).

Variation in Childhood Cancer Incidence by Gender

Table 1.1 shows the incidence of cancer by gender for children (<15 years) and adolescents (15 to 19 years). For both 0- to 14-year-olds and 15- to 19-year-olds, a male predominance

TABLE 1.1

INCIDENCE OF DIFFERENT CANCERS BY GENDER FOR THE 0- TO 14-YEAR-OLD AND 15- TO 19-YEAR-OLD POPULATIONS (1992 TO 2006)

Diagnosis	Age (years)							
	<15 (Both sexes rate)	<15 (Male rate)	<15 (Female rate)	<15 (Male to female ratio)	15–19 (Both sexes rate)	15–19 (Male rate)	15–19 (Female rate)	15–19 (Male to female ratio)
Total	147.7	156.8	138.1	1.1	204.9	215.0	194.3	1.1
Acute lymphoblastic leukemia (Ia)	38.9	42.5	35.1	1.2	15.7	20.6	10.5	2.0
Acute myeloid leukemia (Ib)	7.6	8.1	7.1	1.1	9.3	9.6	8.9	1.1
Hodgkin disease (IIa)	5.4	5.9	4.7	1.3	29.7	27.8	31.7	0.9
Non-Hodgkin lymphoma (IIb,c,e)	8.4	11.2	5.5	2.1	17.2	20.8	13.3	1.6
Central nervous system (III)	30.7	32.8	28.5	1.2	19.6	22.4	16.6	1.3
Neuroblastoma (IVa)	10.3	10.6	9.9	1.1	0.3	0.4	0.2	1.9
Retinoblastoma (V)	4.8	4.9	4.7	1.1	0.1	0.0	0.1	0.9
Wilms' tumor (VIa)	7.6	6.9	8.3	0.8	0.2	0.1	0.3	0.5
Hepatic tumors (VII)	2.4	2.8	2.0	1.4	1.3	1.5	1.1	1.4
Hepatoblastoma (VIIa)	2.0	2.3	1.7	1.4	0.0	0.0	0.0	0.0
Malignant bone tumors (VIII)	5.9	6.1	5.7	1.1	15.5	20.0	10.7	1.9
Osteosarcoma (VIIIa)	3.5	3.2	3.7	0.9	8.8	11.8	5.7	2.1
Ewing's sarcoma (VIIIc)	1.9	2.2	1.6	1.4	4.6	5.7	3.5	1.7
Rhabdomyosarcoma (RMS) (IXa)	4.8	5.4	4.1	1.3	3.7	4.1	3.3	1.2
Non-RMS soft tissue sarcoma (IXb,c,d,e)	5.2	5.4	5.1	1.1	12.4	13.0	11.8	1.1
Germ cell/other gonadal tumors (Xa,b,c)	5.7	5.4	5.9	0.9	27.4	39.3	14.9	2.6
Thyroid carcinoma (XIb)	1.9	1.0	2.9	0.3	16.5	5.3	28.5	0.2
Malignant melanoma (XId)	1.7	1.4	2.0	0.7	15.1	12.2	18.2	0.7

Rates are per 1,000,000 and the <15-year rates are age adjusted to the 2000 U.S. standard. The Roman numerals in parentheses represent the International Classification of Childhood Cancer category for each tumor type.

was most apparent for NHL, with males having incidence rates more than 1.5- to 2.0-fold higher than those for females. For children younger than 15 years, other cancer diagnoses that showed a 1.2-fold or higher male predominance were ALL, CNS tumors, hepatoblastoma, Ewing's sarcoma, and rhabdomyosarcoma. For 15- to 19-year-olds, the patterns of incidence by gender were generally similar to those observed in younger children but with the following exceptions: (a) Hodgkin disease among younger children had a higher incidence rate among males, whereas among adolescents Hodgkin disease had a similar rate between males and females; (b) germ cell tumors had a similar rate between males and females among younger children; however, males had a 2.6-fold higher rate among adolescents; (c) osteosarcoma occurred at similar rates in males and females in the 0- to 14-year-old population, although the rate was 2.1-fold higher in males among 15- to 19-year-olds; and (d) the male

predominance for Ewing's sarcoma was more pronounced in the 15- to 19-year-old group (1.7-fold higher) than in younger children (1.4-fold higher).

Variation in Childhood Cancer Incidence by Race and Ethnicity

For many adult cancers, black Americans have higher incidence rates than do white Americans. However, for children and adolescents, the incidence of cancer among white children was approximately 40% higher than that for black children (Table 1.2; Fig. 1.3). The largest difference in absolute incidence between white children and black children was for ALL (32.5 vs. 15.6 per million). This difference was primarily due to the approximately 2.3-fold higher incidence rate for ALL among 0- to 4-year-old white children compared with 0- to 4-year-old

TABLE 1.2

INCIDENCE OF DIFFERENT CANCERS FOR WHITE, BLACK, AND HISPANIC CHILDREN, 0 TO 19 YEARS OLD (1992 TO 2006)

Cancer type	White	Black	Hispanic	W:B ratio	W:H ratio	B:H ratio
Total	176.9	123.2	153.1	1.4	1.2	0.8
Acute lymphoblastic leukemia (Ia)	32.5	15.6	43.7	2.1	0.7	0.4
Acute myeloid leukemia (Ib)	7.4	7.3	8.8	1.0	0.8	0.8
Hodgkin disease (IIa)	14.0	9.9	9.2	1.4	1.5	1.1
Non-Hodgkin lymphoma (IIb,c,e)	11.6	9.6	8.4	1.2	1.4	1.1
Central nervous system (III)	33.0	22.6	22.7	1.5	1.5	1.0
Neuroblastoma (IVa)	9.2	6.9	6.0	1.3	1.5	1.2
Retinoblastoma (V)	3.2	3.5	4.1	0.9	0.8	0.8
Wilms' tumor (VIa)	6.3	6.9	5.1	0.9	1.2	1.4
Hepatoblastoma (VIIa)	1.5	0.7	1.6	2.1	0.9	0.4
Osteosarcoma (VIIIa)	4.4	5.6	4.8	0.8	0.9	1.2
Ewing's sarcoma (VIIIc)	3.6	0.3	2.1	12.0	1.7	0.1
Rhabdomyosarcoma (RMS) (IXa)	4.8	5.9	3.8	0.8	1.3	1.5
Non-rhabdomyosarcoma STS (IXb,c,d,e)	7.4	7.4	5.8	1.0	1.3	1.3
Germ cell (Xa,b,c)	11.4	5.8	11.7	1.9	1.0	0.5
Thyroid carcinoma (XIb)	6.7	2.0	4.1	3.4	1.6	0.5
Malignant melanoma (XId)	8.4	0.4	1.0	21.0	8.8	0.4

CNS, central nervous system tumors; STS, soft tissue sarcoma.
Rates are per 1,000,000 and are age adjusted to the 2000 U.S. standard. The Roman numerals in parentheses represent the International Classification of Childhood Cancer category for each tumor type.

black children. The higher rates for leukemia were limited to ALL, as white children and black children had identical rates for AML (Table 1.2). The incidence of Ewing's sarcoma in white children was 12 times higher than that for black children. For melanoma, white children had incidence rates 21 times higher than those for black children (Table 1.2).

In contrast to black children, Hispanic children had higher rates of ALL than did white children (43.7 per million vs. 32.5 per million) (Table 1.2). Hispanic children had a higher rate of AML (8.8 per million) compared with both white (7.4 per million) and black (7.3 per million) children. However, overall cancer incidence for Hispanic children

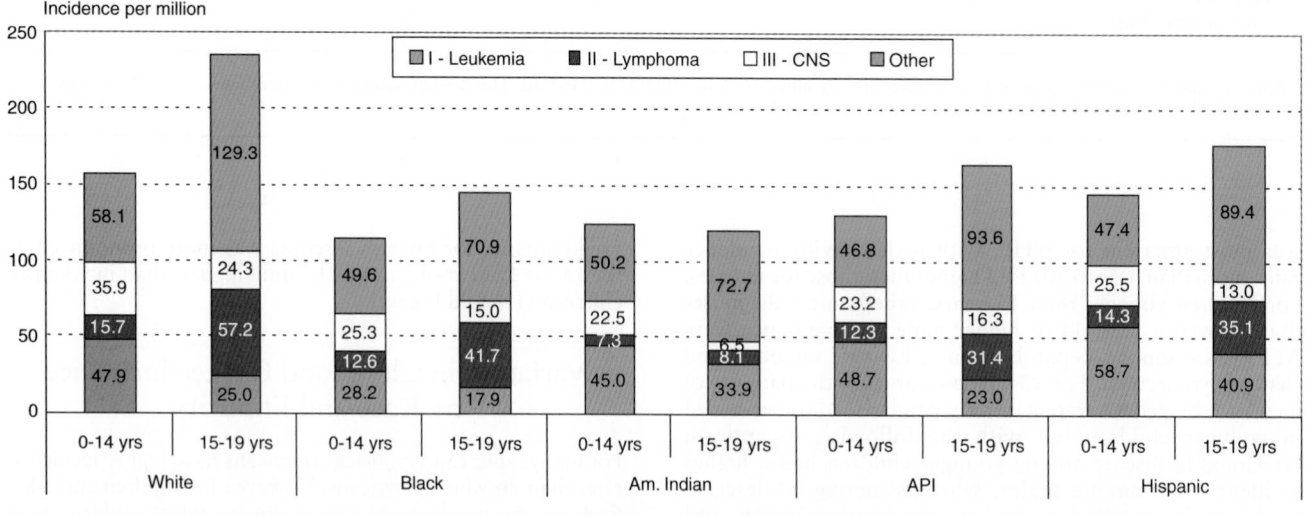

FIGURE 1.3 Age-adjusted incidence rates for childhood cancer by race and ethnicity, 1992 to 2006. Data are for International Classification of Childhood Cancer diagnostic groups (age 0 to 19 years and both sexes). Am. Indian, American Indian or Native American; API, Asian/Pacific Islander; CNS, central nervous system; Hispanic, Hispanic of any race and does not overlap other categories. (Incidence data are from the Surveillance, Epidemiology, and End Results program, National Cancer Institute, and are adjusted to the 2000 U.S. standard population.)

was lower than that for white children because of lower rates for CNS tumors, lymphomas, and other tumors. The incidence of leukemia (Fig. 1.3) was similar for Asian/Pacific Islander children and white children, but Asian/Pacific Islander children had lower rates for CNS tumors and lymphomas.

SURVIVAL AND MORTALITY RATES FOR CHILDREN WITH CANCER

Survival rates for children 0 to 14 years of age have improved dramatically since the 1960s when the overall 5-year survival rate after a cancer diagnosis was estimated as 28%.[9] Improvements in survival rates continued into the early 2000s in the United States (Fig. 1.4), with 3-year survival rates exceeding and 5-year survival rates nearing 80% for children and adolescents diagnosed during this period (Fig. 1.4). In fact, 10-year survival rates have exceeded 75%, looking at those diagnosed in 1996 (the most recent data available for this rate).

The increase in survival rate was most dramatic for ALL, a virtually incurable disease in the early 1960s and for which 5-year survival rates exceeded 80% from 1989 to 1996 (Fig. 1.5A). Survival rates for childhood NHL increased to nearly 80% from 1989 to 1996, up from 20% to 25% in the early 1960s (Fig. 1.5B), and survival rates for Wilms' tumor increased from 33% to 92% during the same period (Fig. 1.5B). Five-year survival rates at or above 90% have also been achieved for Hodgkin disease, thyroid cancer, and melanoma (Fig. 1.6), whereas 5-year survival rates for AML remain approximately 50% (Fig. 1.5A).

Five-year survival rates for 15- to 19-year-olds were similar to those for younger children for most cancer types, including brain tumors, NHL, osteosarcoma, Hodgkin disease, Ewing's sarcoma, AML, and germ cell tumors (Fig. 1.6). Survival rates for 15- to 19-year-olds with ALL were lower than those for younger children, which could be due in part to a higher proportion of cases with unfavorable biology among

15- to 19-year-olds. A similar explanation may explain the lower survival rates for 15- to 19-year-olds with rhabdomyosarcoma. Five-year survival rates near or above 90% were observed for the most common cancers among 15- to 19-year-olds: Hodgkin disease, germ cell tumors, thyroid cancer, and melanoma.

As a result of improved survival, the cancer mortality rates have decreased for children since the 1950s. Mortality rates for all cancers and selected tumors from 1969 to 2004 are shown in Figure 1.7A and B. In the 1950s, childhood cancer mortality rates were stable at approximately 80 per million. The cancer mortality rate for 0- to 19-year-olds began declining in the 1960s and by 1995 had decreased to less than 30 per million. Declines in mortality for leukemias began in the early 1960s, with rates decreasing from 30 to 35 per million to less than 7 per million by 2004 (Fig. 1.7A). For NHL, decline in mortality began in the late 1960s, with rates decreasing from 6 to 7 per million to less than 2 per million by 1994. Mortality due to kidney tumors (primarily Wilms' tumor) decreased by 80% over a similar time period from approximately 4 per million to less than 1 per million by 1989. Mortality rates also declined for Hodgkin disease (data not shown), with rates decreasing from approximately 3 per million in the 1950s and early 1960s to approximately 0.4 per million in the mid-1990s.[7] The brain cancer mortality rate was approximately 10 per million in 1970 and had decreased to approximately 7 per million by 1997 (Fig. 1.7B), remaining fairly constant since then.

Figure 1.8 shows the distribution of causes of cancer death for 0 to 19-year-olds in 2006. Overall, these proportions have remained fairly constant over time. Approximately one-third of cancer-related deaths were caused by leukemias, with ALL accounting for an estimated 50% to 60%, AML for 30% to 40%, and chronic myeloid leukemia for approximately 5% of leukemia-related deaths. CNS tumors were the second leading cause of cancer mortality among children and adolescents, accounting for 24% of cancer-related deaths. The other primary causes of cancer-related mortality were neuroblastoma (classified under endocrine tumors), bone tumors, soft tissue sarcomas, and NHL.

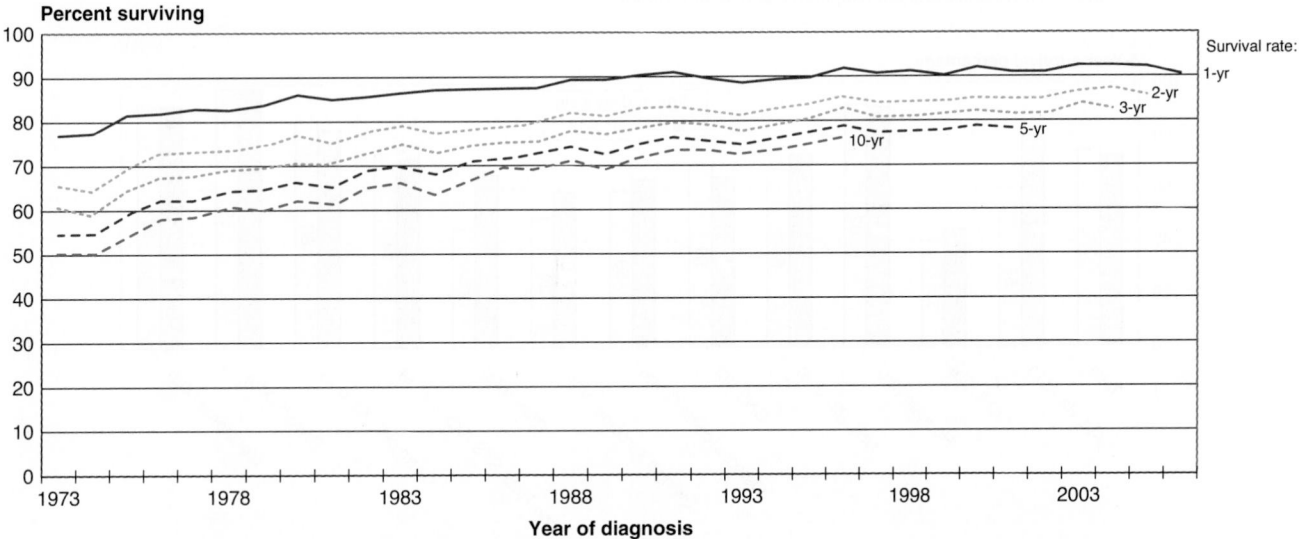

FIGURE 1.4 Trends in relative survival rates for all childhood cancers, age 0 to 19 years (all races and both sexes) for Surveillance, Epidemiology, and End Results (SEER) program regions, 1973 to 2006. (Data are from the SEER program, National Cancer Institute.)

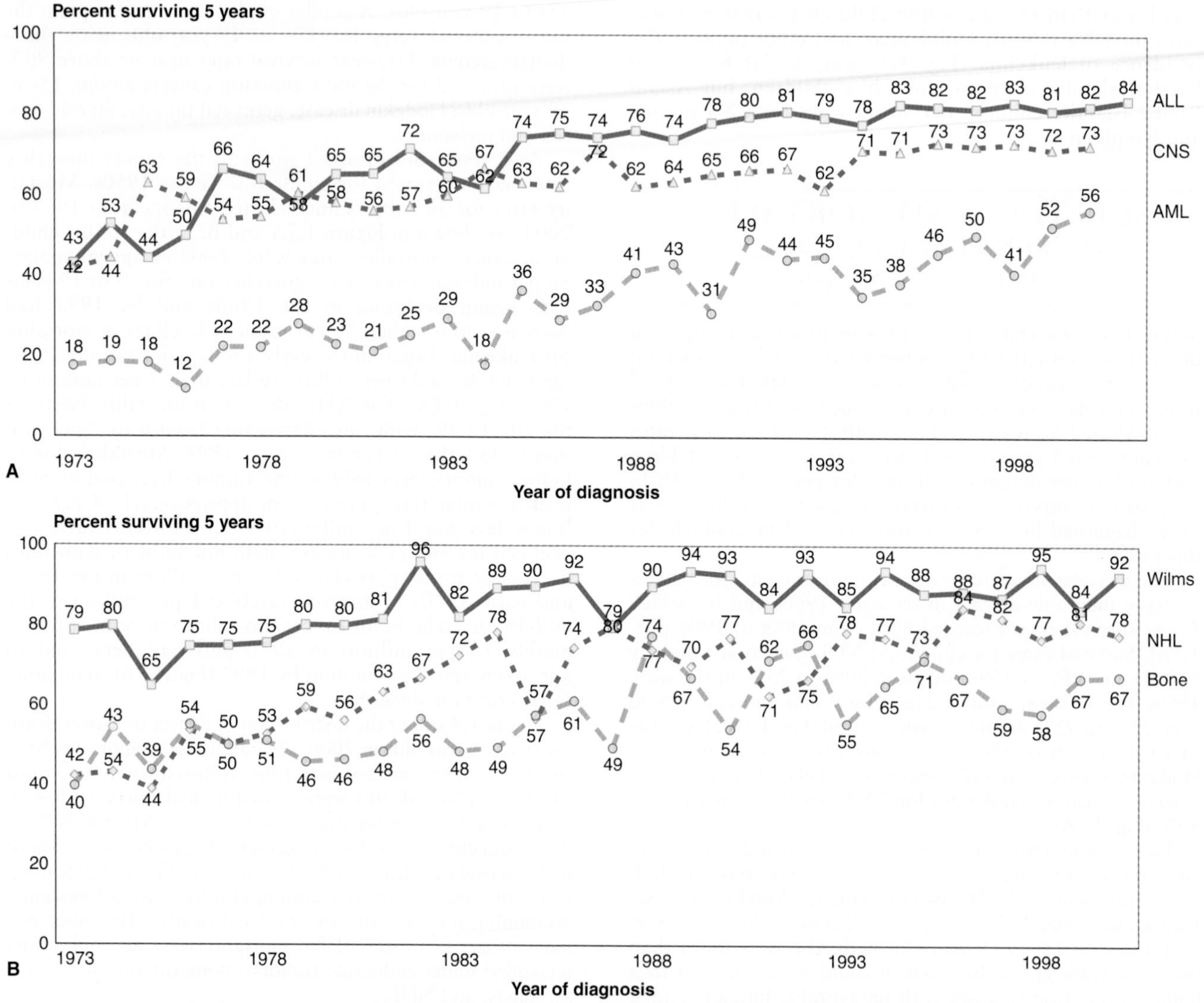

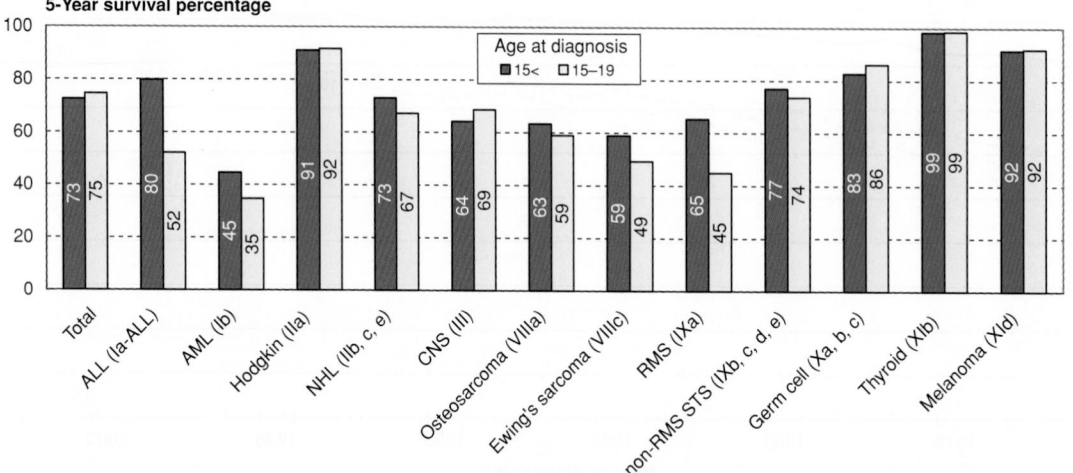

FIGURE 1.5 Five-year relative survival rates for specific cancers of children (aged 0 to 19 years), 1973 to 2006. Data are from the Surveillance, Epidemiology, and End Results (SEER) program regions (nine areas). **A:** ALL, acute lymphoblastic leukemia; AML, acute myeloid leukemia; CNS, central nervous system. **B:** Bone tumors; NHL, non-Hodgkin lymphoma; and Wilms' tumor.

FIGURE 1.6 Five-year survival rates for 0- to 14-year-olds and for 15- to 19-year-olds in Surveillance, Epidemiology, and End Results (SEER) program regions, 1973 to 2006. Rates are for all races and both sexes. ALL, acute lymphoblastic leukemia; AML, acute myeloid leukemia; CNS, central nervous system; NHL, non-Hodgkin lymphoma; non-RMS STS, non-rhabdomyosarcoma soft tissue sarcoma; RMS, rhabdomyosarcoma. (Data are from the SEER program, National Cancer Institute.)

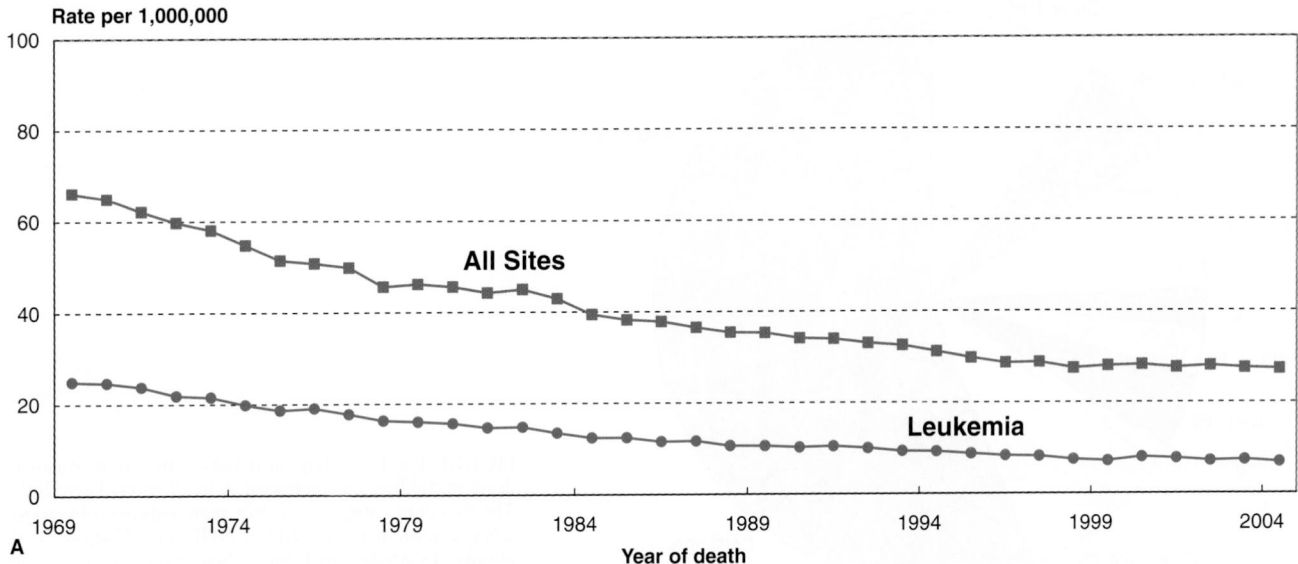

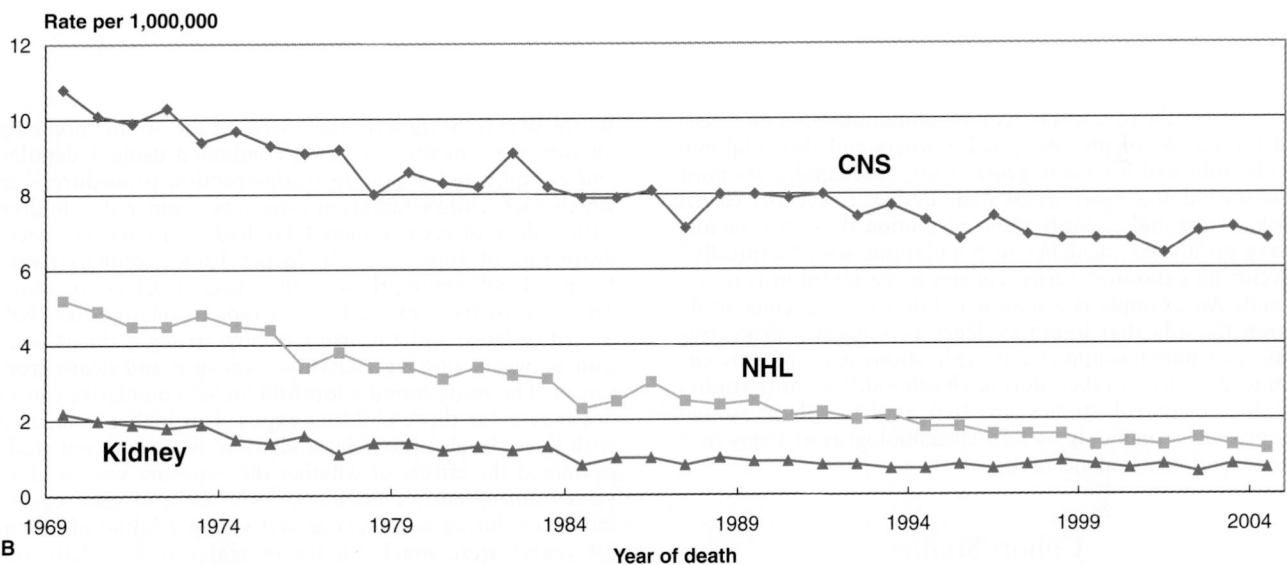

FIGURE 1.7 Mortality rates for children and adolescents (aged 0 to 19 years) in the United States, 1969 to 2004. **A:** Mortality rates for all cancers and for leukemia. **B:** Mortality rates for non-Hodgkin lymphoma (NHL), central nervous system (CNS) tumors, and kidney tumors. (Death data are from the National Center of Health Statistics public-use file.)

ANALYTIC STUDY DESIGNS

Some epidemiologic studies, such as randomized intervention trials and randomized controlled clinical trials, follow the principles of scientific experimentation in which a treatment or intervention of interest and the control condition are randomly assigned.[11] Childhood cancer clinical trials compare one treatment regimen with another, such as the recent study of prophylactic cranial irradiation in children with ALL. This collaborative study from St. Jude Children's Research Hospital and Cook Children's Medical Center showed that prophylactic cranial irradiation could be safely omitted from the standard treatment regimen for children with ALL. Cranial irradiation is beneficial for those ALL patients at high risk for CNS relapse; however, this treatment can lead to a number of

untoward late effects (e.g., second malignancies, cognitive deficits, and endocrinopathy) in this patient population.[12] Well-designed and well-conducted nonexperimental (observational) studies can also provide accurate estimates of treatment effects.[13–15]

Observational analytic studies assess the causal influence of potential risk factors that cannot be evaluated experimentally because the experiment would be unethical or impractical. An obviously unethical experiment would, for example, randomize pregnant mothers to ingesting different kinds and amounts of organophosphate pesticides to measure subsequent incidence rates of NHL in their offspring. As another example, it would be impractical, even if ethical, to randomly allocate newly pregnant mothers to receive high daily doses of vitamins C and E to assess their efficacy in preventing childhood brain cancer. To provide an accurate and reliable

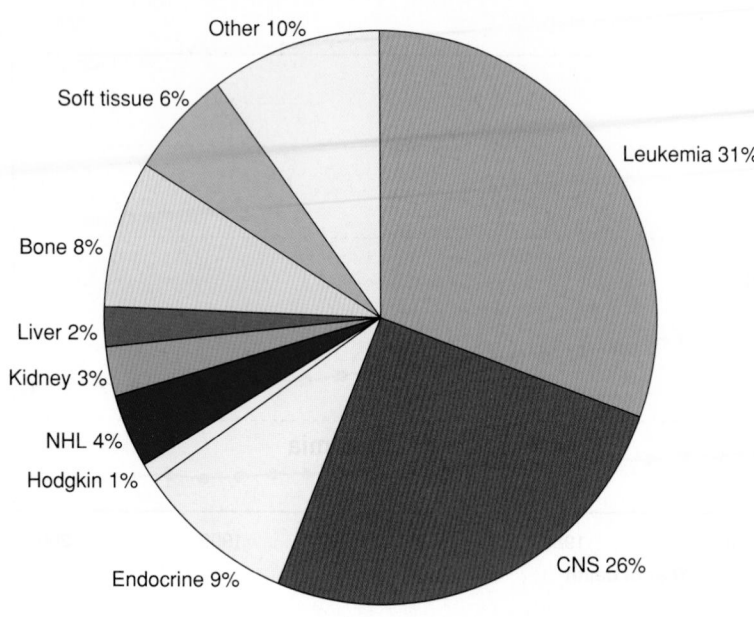

FIGURE 1.8 Percentage distribution by cause of cancer death in children and adolescents 0 to 19 years of age, 2006. The endocrine category primarily represents neuroblastoma. CNS, central nervous system; NHL, non-Hodgkin lymphoma. (Death data are from the National Center for Health Statistics public-use file.)

conclusion, the trial would require thousands, if not hundreds of thousands, of preconceptual mothers and their children to be followed for many years. Thus, epidemiologists must use several nonexperimental study designs to identify causal risk factors and quantify the contribution those risk factors have on disease incidence in populations with "naturally" occurring exposures varied enough to be useful in comparisons. An example is a national childhood leukemia study from Canada that found evidence to suggest a protective effect of immunosuppressant medications (e.g., prednisone, mercaptopurine) taken during childhood.[16] Cohort studies and case-control studies are two analytic observational approaches commonly used by epidemiologists to assess such nonexperimental associations.

Cohort Studies

Cohort studies evaluate subjects initially free of a specific disease of interest and whose exposure status can be classified. Subjects are followed for a defined time period to ascertain differences in rates of end points attributable to exposure, such as new events in or death from a specific disease. The disease rate in the exposed group is then compared statistically with the rate in the unexposed group. A prospective cohort study resembles a clinical trial, but subjects are not randomly allocated to an exposure arm. Rather, as mentioned previously, exposure (or lack of exposure) occurs "naturally" and the investigator uses variations in natural exposure levels to evaluate differences in the risk of subsequent disease occurrence during some follow-up period.

Cohort studies permit efficient study of relatively common diseases with a reasonably short latency period from exposure to disease onset. Cohort studies are usually impractical for rare diseases, such as childhood cancer, as statistically meaningful results could be achieved only by assembling and following for a very long time a huge number of at-risk subjects. One notable exception, however, is a cohort of 3,268 people who were *in utero* and 15,899 who were younger than age 5 and living in Hiroshima or Nagasaki at the time of the atomic bombing during

World War II. Studies on the effects of the atomic bombing on survivors' health are being conducted using a detailed and complicated exposure reconstruction procedure,[17] in which each child's radiation dose was estimated. Children with a dose of greater than 1 Gy had a cumulative cancer death rate of approximately 26 per 1,000, compared with 6.5 per 1,000 among those with a dose of 0.1 Gy or less.[18] The ratio of these rates, 4.0, is a type of relative risk (RR; described later) and a measure of how strong is the association between ionizing radiation exposure and death from cancer. The study found a fourfold higher cumulative cancer death rate for those children exposed to higher compared with lower levels of ionizing radiation. A more recent study examined the effects of whether the exposure was *in utero* versus during early childhood.[19] The rates of solid cancer incidence during adolescence and young adulthood (12 to 29 years) were much higher in males (RR = 5.0) and females (RR = 10.2) who were exposed *in utero* to radiation doses of 0.2 Sv or more. Even though an elevated risk was also seen among males (RR = 2.3) and females (RR = 2.8) who were younger than age 6 at the time of exposure, the association was not as strong. The effect was also not as strong for persons who developed their cancer later in life (ages 30 to 54).

Cohort studies can be prospective or retrospective in nature. Prospective cohort studies involve active follow-up of subjects in real time, as in clinical trials. Retrospective cohort studies use historical records to identify the study population and to reconstruct their exposure and subsequent disease experience. Examples of retrospective cohorts surround the evaluation of excess cancer incidence among those exposed to Salk poliovirus vaccine contaminated with simian virus 40 (SV-40). One birth cohort was inadvertently exposed to the contaminated vaccine during infancy (born 1956 to 1962), one was exposed later in childhood (born 1947 to 1952), and one was unexposed to SV-40 (born 1964 to 1969). Using cancer registry and mortality records, age-specific cancer incidence rates can be calculated for each birth cohort. A study conducted in the United States found no meaningful differences in overall cancer rates or for any specific type of malignancy among the three cohorts.[20] Similar studies have shown no increased incidence of childhood cancers in Denmark[21] or of childhood medulloblastoma in the United States.[22]

The Childhood Cancer Survivors Study (CCSS) was established in 1994 to evaluate medical late effects and psychosocial outcomes as a function of cancer treatment.[23,24] The CCSS includes both retrospective and prospective components and has currently recruited more than 14,000 childhood cancer survivors (or their parents for those deceased) from a consortium of 27 medical centers in the United States and Canada. Eligible subjects survived at least 5 years after diagnosis between 1970 and 1986; efforts are currently underway to extend this cohort to include those diagnosed between 1987 and 1999. This study addresses the important question of the long-term consequences of childhood cancer and its treatment among survivors and serves as a resource for researchers dedicated to identifying modifiable risk factors that could aid in reducing the incidence of these late effects of treatment. To date, the CCSS has produced more than 100 manuscripts on various topics of importance to childhood cancer survivors (i.e., health care utilization, health behaviors, health status, quality of life, etc.) and has contributed invaluably to the development and refinement of epidemiologic methods related to survivorship research.

Case-Control Studies

For rare exposures, such as pesticides or some medications, cohort studies provide the best study design. However, for rare outcomes, such as childhood cancer, case-control studies provide a more efficient strategy to evaluate potential causal associations. A case-control study of childhood cancer identifies and recruits children (or their parents) who are diagnosed within a defined population and time period. A similar group of children without the disease, but from the same defined population (in time, location, and eligibility criteria) that gave rise to the cases, is recruited to serve as controls. The investigator, as completely and accurately as possible, uses self-report, health records, environmental measures, and biologic specimens to reconstruct the cases' prediagnosis exposure experience. Similarly, a "reference" date substituting for a diagnosis date is assigned to each control child, whose exposure experience before that date is reconstructed. The exposure frequency among the case group is then compared statistically with the exposure frequency among the control group. The resultant statistic, known as an *odds ratio* (OR), is analogous to an RR and is a measure of the strength of the association between the exposure and the disease. For example, a population-based case-control study of childhood ALL evaluated household dust in 184 cases and 212 controls of similar birth date, sex, race, and Hispanic ethnicity from northern and central California.[25] Levels of organochlorine pesticides and polychlorinated biphenyls (PCBs) measured in carpet dust from the residences of the cases and controls suggested an increasing risk of childhood ALL with increasing concentrations of PCBs. Relative to homes with the lowest levels of total PCBs in carpet dust, the adjusted OR was 2.8 (95% confidence interval [CI]: 1.4–5.5) for exposure levels of 15.5 ng/g or higher. Thus, in this study, children presumably exposed in their homes to PCB levels of 15.5 ng/g or more were found to have a nearly threefold risk for ALL than were children not so exposed. This study in no way proves a causal relationship between childhood ALL and exposure to PCBs in the home; however, it suggests a possible etiologic agent that should be further explored.

Cluster Investigations

It is common for clinicians to encounter parental concern about multiple cancer occurrences in their child's community. The implication, of course, is that a shared environmental exposure is responsible for the cluster of cancer cases. Cluster investigations use standard epidemiologic study designs, primarily case-control studies, to ascertain whether an unusual number of cancer cases occurred in a specific area (spatial cluster), time (temporal cluster), or both (space-time cluster).[26] The latter, for instance, would be an excess of childhood leukemia in a neighborhood or school over a specific time period. Public health agencies have the responsibility to investigate cancer clusters and communicate findings to the public.[26] Clinicians are well advised to refer cluster inquiries to local health departments or the Centers for Disease Control and Prevention (http://www.cdc.gov or http://www.atsdr.cdc.gov). Such investigations, however, rarely produce evidence that a true childhood cancer cluster exists.[27–30]

MOLECULAR EPIDEMIOLOGY

Classical or traditional epidemiology, as discussed previously, permits epidemiologists to evaluate risks and causal roles of environmental factors in cancer. Molecular epidemiology, a hybrid of epidemiology and molecular biology, enables researchers to assess biologic or genetic characteristics that may influence cancer susceptibility. The concept that risk of cancer from a given exposure differs between subgroups of a population is known in epidemiology as *effect modification*; biostatisticians often refer to this heterogeneity of effect as *interaction*. With the advent of polymerase chain reaction and other advanced laboratory methods, epidemiologists can incorporate molecular markers into their studies to identify specific suspect endogenous or exogenous host factors at the biochemical or molecular level.[31–33] Such studies aim to determine the roles, including interactions, of environmental and genetic factors in the initiation and progression of the carcinogenic process. The approach of incorporating molecular markers in epidemiologic studies of childhood cancer etiology shows promise for reducing cancer risk and providing strategies for prevention.

The addition of molecular parameters to population-based studies aids in the identification of genes and pathways involved in cancer development due to environmental exposures and in the identification of susceptible or resistant subpopulations. In turn, information about molecular mechanisms of carcinogenesis helps improve risk assessment. Past studies of childhood cancer were limited to the examination of only a few candidate genes. However, the exponential growth of scientific technology and the creation of consortia to facilitate the need for larger sample sizes have led to the ability to analyze multiple polymorphisms in the same gene (e.g., haplotypes and diplotypes), multiple genes along the same molecular pathway, and multiple polymorphisms in multiple genes across the entire genome (i.e., genome-wide association studies [GWAS]). In fact, GWAS are quickly becoming the approach of choice for performing association studies of common genetic susceptibility alleles in cancer epidemiology. However, because of the rarity of pediatric cancers, the majority of this work has been conducted for adult tumors. On the other hand, GWAS have proven helpful in identifying genes associated with risk[34] of and treatment outcomes[35] in childhood ALL. It is likely that, as consortia form to investigate other rare childhood cancers, such studies will also contribute to new findings for these other tumors.

In addition to identifying causal factors, studies of childhood cancer etiology aim to determine the critical period of exposure and disease susceptibility. Exposures *in utero* and during the early years of life can disproportionately increase the risk of cancer later in life.[36–38] Laboratory and epidemiologic evidence suggests that differential exposure response or physiologic immaturity raises the risk for infants and children far above that for adults experiencing the same environmental insults. The underlying mechanisms combine to proportionately increase exposure to toxicants and lessen the ability of the child in early stages of development to detoxify or repair damage. The cancer can be initiated *in utero*, with subsequent genetic mutational events and clonal progression occurring later. Adolescence and young adulthood are also sensitive times because of such proliferative surges as hormone outflow and rapid bone growth.

Current studies of molecular epidemiology are based on an understanding of the complex, multistage process of carcinogenesis and heterogeneous responses to carcinogenic exposures. Quantitative methods to measure human exposures to carcinogens improve continuously and have been successfully applied in a number of epidemiologic studies. Genetic predispositions to cancer, both inherited and acquired, have been, and continue to be, identified. The combined approach of correlating genetic polymorphisms with other cancer risk factors is showing considerable promise. For instance, activity of the glutathione *S*-transferase (GST) enzymes is involved in the detoxification of carcinogens such as epoxides and alkylating agents. GST genes are polymorphic, and lack of enzymatic activity potentially increases cancer risk. The *GSTM1* null genotype has been shown to increase the risk of childhood AML and myelodysplasia (AML/MDS),[39] and polymorphisms in *GSTP1* have been associated with ALL/AML/NHL and soft tissue tumors[40] using the case-control study design. These studies illustrate the future of molecular epidemiology as the leader in developing individual risk profiles for patients, including assessment of multiple biomarkers. The field has the near-term potential to have a significant impact on regulatory quantitative risk assessments, which may aid in the determination of allowable exposures and the identification of individuals who will most benefit from cancer prevention strategies.

Molecular epidemiology also holds the key to identifying not only those at risk for the development of a malignancy but also those at risk for adverse events due to the treatment of their primary tumor. Survivorship issues have come to the forefront of cancer epidemiology, as survival for childhood cancers continues to increase and these children move into adulthood. This importance is evidenced by the creation and maintenance of the CCSS (described earlier) as a resource for conducting this type of research. Using the GST enzymes as an example again, researchers have found that ALL patients with the *GSTM1* null genotype will experience less hepatotoxicity from methotrexate[41]; however, they are also at greater risk of severe infection following glucocorticoid administration.[42]

Investigators who conduct molecular epidemiology studies use traditional designs, including case-control and cohort studies, with inclusion of one or more molecular markers to determine exposure associations with disease outcome. Therefore, the methodologic challenges of epidemiologic studies (described later), such as accurate measurement of disease and exposure, appropriate selection of study samples, reduction of potential confounding, and optimization of precision of effect measures, also apply to studies in the rapidly growing and promising field of molecular epidemiology. A serious concern lies with assuring an adequate sample size for study; this is

especially true for studies of childhood tumors. Often, the prevalence of a genetic polymorphism or other biomarker is either quite low or quite high. Hence, the number of cases required to detect an association tends to be very large. Because childhood cancers are rare, it is often necessary to combine data from several studies to obtain adequate statistical power to draw meaningful conclusions. For all of these reasons, it is necessary for investigators to exercise caution when interpreting their study data and the implications of their results.[43]

BIAS AND CAUSAL INFERENCE

All human studies are susceptible to bias of varying degrees (i.e., producing inaccurate measures of the effect of a treatment or exposure on disease). An important goal of any study is to make every effort feasible to minimize the effect of bias.

Three general types of bias can occur:

1. *Selection bias*, when subjects who are sampled, recruited, enrolled, and complete the study are unrepresentative, in that they inaccurately reflect the exposure-disease relationship in the target population
2. *Information (misclassification) bias*, when information collected on exposure, treatment, disease, or other study factors is inaccurate or incomplete
3. *Confounding bias*, when an extraneous factor distorts (increases or decreases) the true magnitude of the exposure-disease association

Selection Bias

Because all human studies include some element of sampling from larger (target) populations and require recruitment from the sample identified, selection bias is a potential source of error. Selection bias may occur when exposure or disease frequency among those in the study is unrepresentative of the target population. Case-control studies are susceptible because it is difficult to identify and recruit controls who provide an accurate accounting of baseline exposure frequency in the population that gave rise to the cases. For instance, selection bias is suspected in the apparent association of some childhood cancer–electromagnetic field (EMF) studies.[44] If lower-income persons are proportionately less likely to participate as controls than higher-income persons, and lower-income persons live in areas with proportionately more high-current power lines, baseline exposure (high EMF) will be underestimated. Unlike controls, if case participation is independent of power line status, the odds of exposure among cases will appear higher than that for controls, resulting in a positive association when none really exists. Cohort studies and randomized trials, on the other hand, are susceptible to selection bias from attrition. If participants lost to the study during the follow-up period represent a different outcome experience than those who remain in the study to completion, the final results may be biased. For this reason, great effort must be expended in prospective studies to assure the most complete follow-up possible of study subjects.

Information Bias

The most important threat to the validity of epidemiologic research of childhood cancer is inaccurate or incomplete information on study participants' exposure relevant to etiology. It is usually impossible, especially in retrospective studies, to directly measure exposure dose and duration during a time thought biologically relevant to cancer initiation or progression. As such, indirect or surrogate measures of exposure are used in lieu of direct measures. Indirect exposure tools include, for instance, self-reported recall of diet, smoking, and alcohol consumption during pregnancy; 24-hour food intake diaries; parental occupational job titles; recall of household pesticide use or inventory of household pesticide products; power line configurations, personal dosimeters or 24-hour measurements of EMF levels in the child's bedroom; pharmacy records among those in self-contained health maintenance organization plans; census tract information; urinary cotinine levels for smoking intake; and medical records.[45]

These proxy measures may usefully approximate real exposure but provide only imprecise information on dose, duration, and exposure time period. When exposure measures are equally inaccurate between study groups (nondifferential error), as is often the case, the cause-effect relationship may be attenuated or completely obscured. Nondifferential misclassification of exposure has no doubt been one reason why few environmental agents are known risks for childhood cancer occurrence.

Differential information bias occurs when accuracy and completeness of exposure information differ between comparison groups. Recall bias in case-control studies, for example, can occur if mothers of children with brain cancer (cases) are more motivated than mothers of healthy children (controls) to recall accurately their history of using household pesticides. This may happen because case mothers want to discover the cause of their children's disease. The control mothers may have hazier memories, and their incomplete or inaccurate recall can lead to underestimates of exposure frequency in the control group, and thus cause exaggeration of the strength of the association between disease and exposure. From a practical standpoint, however, recall bias may be more theoretical than factual. One method sometimes advocated to minimize recall bias is to choose a control group of children with a chronic disease, rather than disease-free. Control mothers might then have equal incentive to recall exposure accurately and completely. Using this approach, one must be sure that the control group's disease is not causally related to the exposure under evaluation, or the resultant risk estimate will be biased as to whether the exposure is causally related to the childhood cancer in question.

Confounding Bias

Randomization in clinical trials, if enough people are in the study, greatly reduces the probability that an extraneous factor will cause bias in the results because such "nuisance" factors should be randomly and evenly distributed among treatment groups. Absent randomization, however, confounding is a threat to validity in observational studies. Confounding requires a variable to be associated with, or a marker for, the disease of interest and for it to occur at a differing frequency between the exposure (or treatment) groups. When these two conditions hold, the extraneous factor may bias the exposure-disease association. Few exogenous risk factors, however, have been identified in the etiology of childhood cancer, and those few represent fairly weak associations. Thus, confounding bias has not been shown empirically to be of major concern in epidemiologic research of childhood cancer, although this possibility cannot be ruled out. Partly because of the implausibility of a biologic connection between nonionizing EMFs and cancer, for instance, some scientists hypothesized that the associations found between power lines and childhood leukemia and brain cancer in early EMF studies were due to confounding by unidentified etiologic agents.[46] A recent methodologic study that carefully examined that possibility found little support for the theory.[47]

Statistical methods to control (adjust for, or correct) confounding, such as stratified analysis or multivariable regression analysis, are at hand, but effective only if data on the potentially confounding variables are collected and accurate. Thus, for statistical analysis, observational studies often collect data on many factors not directly related to the cause-effect relationship being investigated. Design strategies can also minimize or eliminate confounding. A study of asbestos exposure and lung cancer, for example, could minimize confounding from smoking status by recruiting only nonsmokers, although residual confounding may still be present if frequency, duration, or intensity of passive smoke exposure differs between those exposed to asbestos and those not exposed.

Causal Inference

Epidemiologic studies strive to provide the most accurate and precise risk estimate of an exposure-disease association. Concerns about potential bias of effect measures, however, contribute to the critical approach using inference and judgment to evaluate exposure-disease causal relationships. Criteria commonly used to evaluate study results and to help guide judgments on the likelihood that an association indeed is causal and not merely statistical include the following:

1. *Strength of the exposure-disease association.* Large RRs are less likely than small RRs to result from chance or uncontrolled confounding (although this does not preclude other sources of error).
2. *Temporal relationship between exposure and disease onset.* Studies are stronger when they can establish that the exposure appropriately preceded the biologic onset of disease.
3. *Biologic coherence.* When a plausible biologic mechanism or when experimental evidence from animal studies, or both, supports the hypothesized relationship, there is greater confidence in the observed association.
4. *Dose-response gradient.* If exposure intensity or duration is associated with increased disease frequency when it is hypothesized that such a dose gradient should exist, the results appear more coherent and believable.
5. *Consistency of results within and across studies.* If multiple sources of the same exposure type show similar effects, if multiple studies using different target populations and study designs show consistent results, or both, there is greater evidence to favor a true relationship.

These concepts, which are widely applied, were originally derived from two papers by Sir Austin Bradford Hill and reprinted in a monograph on philosophy and epidemiologic reasoning in causal inference.[48]

STATISTICAL MEASURES IN EPIDEMIOLOGY

Epidemiologic analyses generally focus on estimating effect measures, the strength (magnitude) of an exposure-disease association, rather than statistical hypothesis testing using a

p value.[2] The p values provide a measure of probability for observing the study results or results more extreme than those observed, if indeed there is no true association. No direct information from p values is given, however, on the strength, direction, or precision of an effect measure, nor do p values supply information on the extent to which an association (or lack of an association) can be explained by confounding or other bias.

Effect measures for dichotomous outcomes, such as disease occurrence versus no disease, are often estimated using one of several ratio measures of RR.[1,2,49] In a cohort study, in which disease rates can be directly calculated, the ratio of the incidence rate of leukemia among those exposed to an agent can be compared with the rate of leukemia among those not so exposed. The ratio is 1:1 if the rates are the same in the two comparison groups, an RR of 1.0, suggesting no association between exposure and disease. If the exposed group has a higher rate than that of the unexposed group, the ratio will be larger than 1, suggesting an excess risk due to exposure. If the rate is lower in the exposed compared with the unexposed groups, the ratio will be less than 1, suggesting a protective effect from exposure. The further the effect measure is away from the "null" value of 1.0 in either direction, the stronger the association. Notice that an RR of 2.0 (double the risk compared with the reference group) is equivalent in strength to an RR of 0.5 (one-half the risk of the reference group). Rates of disease cannot be calculated directly in case-control studies. Alternatively, exposure frequencies are compared between diseased groups and nondiseased groups. The resultant OR is an effect measure on a ratio scale and, as mentioned previously, functionally equivalent to an RR. Other types of ratio-based RRs are rate ratios, hazard ratios, standardized mortality ratios, standardized incidence ratios, and proportional mortality ratios. CIs are used to measure the precision of an effect measure. Similar to p values, CIs are functions of the variability of the data and the size of the sample. Roughly speaking, a CI provides a likely range in which the true effect measure lies within some level of confidence (often calculated as 95% CI).

RRs are important to help judge whether an association is causal and to estimate the degree to which risk of disease is increased (or decreased) by exposure. RRs, however, do not measure the "absolute" risk from exposure. In other words, an RR does not measure the number of excess cancers that are likely caused by an exposure. Attributable risk measures provide estimates of the actual rate (or number, or percentage) of cases "due to" exposure, assuming there is a causal relationship.[1,2,48] Thus, attributable risks indicate the proportion of the disease preventable if the exposure were removed from the population at risk. Assume for the sake of argument, for example, that living within 50 ft of a high-current power line increases a child's risk of ALL by a factor of 2. The annual rate of ALL in the United States is approximately 34 per million children younger than age 15 years. If 10% of children in the United States lived near high-current power lines, the percentage of childhood ALL cases that could be attributed to the power lines would be 9%. This attributable risk of 9% (sometimes called an *etiologic fraction*) translates to an excess of three ALL cases per million children per year, which is the leukemia rate that hypothetically would be prevented if all children lived away from high-current power lines. Even very large RRs may explain little of the total disease incidence within a population. Children with Down syndrome have an estimated 20-fold excess risk of ALL,[50] but because the prevalence of Down syndrome is only approximately 1.3 per 1,000 live births, the percentage of ALL in

children that can be attributed to Down syndrome is only approximately 2.5%.

RISK FACTORS FOR CHILDHOOD CANCER OCCURRENCE

Environmental risk factors for adult cancer generally involve long latency periods from exposure commencement to clinical onset of disease. Cigarette smoking illustrates this point: Smoking usually starts during adolescence, but associated malignancies do not become apparent until many decades after smoking is initiated. The genetic processes that go awry and lead to childhood cancer are likely different from that of adult malignancies; at the least, the carcinogenic process in children is much shorter in time. Infancy, when embryonal neoplasms such as neuroblastoma predominate, is the age when cancer incidence rates are highest during childhood.[51,52] It is reasonable to surmise, therefore, that many childhood cancers result from aberrations in early developmental processes.

To our dismay from a prevention standpoint, the current evidence to support a major etiologic role for environmental or other exogenous factors in childhood cancer is minimal. A comprehensive review of epidemiologic studies of childhood cancer is available elsewhere[39] and will not be reproduced here. The major types of childhood cancer and the few risk factors that are reasonably well documented are shown in Table 1.3. Many other factors are suspected to increase or decrease risk but are not well established. Even the known risk factors shown in the table explain only a small proportion of childhood cancer cases.

SUMMARY AND FUTURE CONSIDERATIONS

Although knowledge about childhood cancer continues to increase, there is much work to be accomplished before reliable preventative measures can be recommended. In this brief overview, we have discussed the essentials of epidemiologic research approaches in childhood cancer, the role epidemiology plays in understanding the public health impact of childhood cancer, and the ongoing efforts to improve knowledge on the causes of these diseases and the consequences to the children who experience them.

Many of the epidemiologic studies performed to date have provided important clues to the etiology of childhood cancer. The field of molecular epidemiology will continue to expand and take advantage of new "–omic" technologies to elucidate the risk factors for childhood cancer with the goal of preventing these diseases. Current investigations seek to determine the most reliable biomarkers of exposure and disease. Likewise, GWAS have already proven helpful in identifying genes associated with risk of many adult tumors and of childhood ALL. In the near future, these studies will likely contribute to new findings for other childhood cancers. Epigenetic gene expression and the use of copy number variants have been identified as potentially important sources of genetic variation. The possibility of genome-wide sequencing and epigenomics may also become feasible in population-based studies. Such technologies will ultimately offer complete interrogation of genetic variation in the human genome and provide insights into the biology of these tumors, allowing the development of preventive and treatment strategies.

TABLE 1.3

KNOWN RISK FACTORS FOR SELECTED CHILDHOOD CANCERS

Cancer type	Risk factor	Comments
Acute lymphoid leukemia	Ionizing radiation	Although primarily of historical significance, prenatal diagnostic x-ray exposure increases risk. Therapeutic irradiation for cancer treatment also increases risk.
	Race	White children have a twofold higher rate than do black children in the United States.
	Genetic conditions	Down syndrome is associated with an estimated 20-fold increased risk. Neurofibromatosis type 1, Bloom syndrome, ataxia telangiectasia, and Langerhans cell histiocytosis, among others, are associated with an elevated risk.
	Birth weight	>400 g increases risk.
Acute myeloid leukemias	Chemotherapeutic agents	Alkylating agents and epipodophyllotoxins increase risk.
	Genetic conditions	Down syndrome and neurofibromatosis 1 are strongly associated. Familial monosomy 7 and several other genetic syndromes are also associated with increased risk.
Brain cancers	Therapeutic ionizing radiation to the head	With the exception of cancer radiotherapy, higher risk from radiation treatment is essentially of historical importance.
	Genetic conditions	Neurofibromatosis 1 is strongly associated with optic gliomas, and, to a lesser extent with other central nervous system tumors. Tuberous sclerosis and several other genetic syndromes are associated with increased risk.
Hodgkin disease	Family history	Monozygotic twins and siblings of cases are at increased risk.
	Infections	Epstein-Barr virus is associated with increased risk.
Non-Hodgkin lymphoma	Immunodeficiency	Acquired and congenital immunodeficiency disorders and immunosuppressive therapy increase risk.
	Infections	Epstein-Barr virus is associated with Burkitt's lymphoma in African countries.
Osteosarcoma	Ionizing radiation	Cancer radiotherapy and high radium exposure increase risk.
	Chemotherapy	Alkylating agents increase risk.
	Genetic conditions	Increased risk is apparent with Li-Fraumeni syndrome and hereditary retinoblastoma.
Ewing's sarcoma	Race	White children have approximately a ninefold higher incidence rate than do black children in the United States.
Neuroblastoma		No known risk factors.
Retinoblastoma		No known nonhereditary risk factors.
Wilms' tumor	Congenital anomalies	Aniridia and Beckwith-Wiedemann syndrome, as well as other congenital and genetic conditions, increase risk.
	Race	Asian children reportedly have approximately one-half the rates of white and black children.
Rhabdomyosarcoma	Congenital anomalies and genetic conditions	Li-Fraumeni syndrome and neurofibromatosis 1 are believed to be associated with increased risk. There is some concordance with major birth defects.
Hepatoblastoma	Genetic conditions	Beckwith-Wiedemann syndrome, hemihypertrophy, Gardner's syndrome, and family history of adenomatous polyposis increase risk.
Malignant germ cell tumors	Cryptorchidism	Cryptorchidism is a risk factor for testicular germ cell tumors.

Derived from Ries LAG, Smith MA, Gurney JG, eds. Cancer incidence and survival among children and adolescents: United States SEER program 1975–1995. Bethesda, MD: National Cancer Institute, SEER Program, 1999. NIH Pub. No. 99-4649. The publication and additional data are available on the SEER Web site: http://www.seer.cancer.gov.

As research in the field of genomics advances, well-designed studies and new analytic techniques will be critical. With the increasing volume of genomic data comes the need to collect high-quality data on environmental exposures and focus studies onto the evaluation of gene-environment interactions. Such studies require very large sample sizes, which could be accomplished through large consortial studies. In fact, such epidemiologic consortia are now charged with the sole purpose of evaluating risk factors for childhood malignancies.[53,54]

References

1. Koepsell TD, Weiss NS. Epidemiologic methods: studying the occurrence of illness. New York, NY: Oxford University Press, 2003.
2. Rothman K, Greenland S, Lash T, eds. Modern epidemiology. 3rd ed. Philadelphia, PA: Lippincott Williams & Wilkins, 2008.
3. Brookmeyer R, Stroup DF. Monitoring the health of populations: statistical principles and methods for public health surveillance. New York, NY: Oxford University Press, 2004.
4. Thacker SB. Surveillance. In: Gregg MB, ed. Field epidemiology. 3rd ed. New York, NY: Oxford University Press, 2008:38–66.
5. Ross J, Olshan A. Pediatric cancer in the United States: the Children's Oncology Group Epidemiology Research Program. Cancer Epidemiol Biomarkers Prev 2004;13: 1552–1554.
6. Steele JR, Wellemeyer AS, Hansen MJ, et al. Childhood Cancer Research Network: a North American Pediatric Cancer Registry. Cancer Epidemiol Biomarkers Prev 2006;15:1241–1242.
7. Ries LAG, Smith MA, Gurney JG, et al., eds. Cancer incidence and survival among children and adolescents: United States SEER program 1975–1995. Bethesda, MD: National Cancer Institute, SEER Program, 1999. NIH Pub. No. 99-4649.
8. American Cancer Society. Cancer facts and figures, 2009. Atlanta, GA: American Cancer Society, Inc, 2009.
9. Bleyer A, O'Leary M, Barr R, et al. Cancer epidemiology in older adolescents and young adults 15 to 29 years of age, including SEER incidence and survival: 1975–2000. Bethesda, MD: National Cancer Institute, 2006.
10. Steliarova-Foucher E, Stiller C, Lacour B, et al. International classification of childhood cancer, third edition. Cancer 2005;103:1457–1467.
11. Weiss NS. Clinical epidemiology: the study of the outcome of illness. New York, NY: Oxford University Press, 2006.
12. Pui CH, Campana D, Pei D, et al. Treating childhood acute lymphoblastic leukemia without cranial irradiation. N Engl J Med 2009;360:2730–2741.
13. Benson K, Hartz A. A comparison of observational studies and randomized, controlled trials. N Engl J Med 2000;342:1878–1886.
14. Concato J, Shah N, Horwitz R. Randomized, controlled trials, observational studies, and the hierarchy of research designs. N Engl J Med 2000;342:1887–1892.
15. Kunz R. Randomized trials and observational studies: still mostly similar results, still crucial differences. J Clin Epidemiol 2008;61:207–208.
16. MacArthur AC, McBride ML, Spinelli JJ, et al. Risk of childhood leukemia associated with vaccination, infection, and medication use in childhood: the Cross-Canada Childhood Leukemia Study. Am J Epidemiol 2008;167:598–606.
17. Shimizu Y, Schull W, Kato H. Cancer risk among atomic bomb survivors. The RERF Life Span Study. Radiation Effects Research Foundation. JAMA 1990;264:601–604.
18. Shimizu Y, Kato H, Schull W. Studies of the mortality of A-bomb survivors. 9. Mortality, 1950–1985: Part 2. Cancer mortality based on the recently revised doses (DS86). Radiat Res 1990;121:120–141.
19. Preston DL, Cullings H, Suyama A, et al. Solid cancer incidence in atomic bomb survivors exposed in utero or as young children. J Natl Cancer Inst 2008;100:428–436.
20. Strickler H, Rosenberg P, Devesa S, et al. Contamination of poliovirus vaccines with simian virus 40 (1955–1963) and subsequent cancer rates. JAMA 1998;279:292–295.
21. Engels EA, Katki HA, Nielsen NM, et al. Cancer incidence in Denmark following exposure to poliovirus vaccine contaminated with simian virus 40. J Natl Cancer Inst 2003;95:532–539.
22. Strickler HD, Rosenberg PS, Devesa SS, et al. Contamination of poliovirus vaccine with SV40 and the incidence of medulloblastoma. Med Pediatr Oncol 1999;32:77–78.
23. Leisenring WM, Mertens AC, Armstrong GT, et al. Pediatric cancer survivorship research: experience of the Childhood Cancer Survivor Study. J Clin Oncol 2009;27: 2319–2327.
24. Robison LL, Armstrong GT, Boice JD, et al. The Childhood Cancer Survivor Study: a National Cancer Institute-supported resource for outcome and intervention research. J Clin Oncol 2009;27:2308–2318.
25. Ward MH, Colt JS, Metayer C, et al. Residential exposure to polychlorinated biphenyls and organochlorine pesticides and risk of childhood leukemia. Environ Health Perspect 2009;117:1007–1013.
26. Brownson RC. Outbreak and cluster investigations. In: Brownson RC, Petitti DB, eds. Applied epidemiology: theory to practice. New York, NY: Oxford University Press, 1998:71–104.
27. Alexander F. Clusters and clustering of childhood cancer: a review. Eur J Epidemiol 1999;15:847–852.
28. Bithell J. Childhood leukaemia clustering—fact or artefact? Methods Inf Med 2001;40:127–131.
29. Rothman K. A sobering start for the cluster busters' conference. Am J Epidemiol 1990;132:S6–S13.
30. Waller L. A civil action and statistical assessments of the spatial pattern of disease: do we have a cluster? Regul Toxicol Pharmacol 2000;32:174–183.
31. Khoury MJ, Millikan R, Gwinn M. Genetic and molecular epidemiology. In: Rothman K, Greenland S, Lash T, eds. Modern epidemiology. 3rd ed. Philadelphia, PA: Lippincott Williams & Wilkins, 2008:564–579.
32. Rebbeck T, Ambrosone C, Shields P, eds. Molecular epidemiology: applications in cancer and other human diseases. New York, NY: Informa Healthcare, 2008.
33. Schulte P, Perera F, eds. Molecular epidemiology: principles and practices. San Diego, CA: Academic Press, 1993.
34. Trevino LR, Yang W, French D, et al. Germline genomic variants associated with childhood acute lymphoblastic leukemia. Nat Genet 2009;41:1001–1005.
35. Yang JJ, Cheng C, Yang W, et al. Genome-wide interrogation of germline genetic variation associated with treatment response in childhood acute lymphoblastic leukemia. JAMA 2009;301:393–403.
36. Baldwin R, Preston-Martin S. Epidemiology of brain tumors in childhood—a review. Toxicol Appl Pharmacol 2004;199:118–131.
37. Goldman L. Children—unique and vulnerable. Environmental risks facing children and recommendations for response. Environ Health Perspect 1995;103(Suppl 6): 13–18.
38. Perera F, Jedrychowski W, Rauh V, et al. Molecular epidemiologic research on the effects of environmental pollutants on the fetus. Environ Health Perspect 1999;107(Suppl 3):451–460.
39. Davies S, Robison L, Buckley J, et al. Glutathione S-transferase polymorphisms in children with myeloid leukemia: a Children's Cancer Group study. Cancer Epidemiol Biomarkers Prev 2000;9:563–566.
40. Zielinska E, Zubowska M, Bodalski J. Polymorphism within the glutathione S-transferase P1 gene is associated with increased susceptibility to childhood malignant diseases. Pediatr Blood Cancer 2004;43:552–559.
41. Imanishi H, Okamura N, Yagi M, et al. Genetic polymorphisms associated with adverse events and elimination of methotrexate in childhood acute lymphoblastic leukemia and malignant lymphoma. J Hum Genet 2007;52:166–171.
42. Marino S, Verzegnassi F, Tamaro P, et al. Response to glucocorticoids and toxicity in childhood acute lymphoblastic leukemia: role of polymorphisms of genes involved in glucocorticoid response. Pediatr Blood Cancer 2009; 53(6):984–991.
43. Vineis P; International Agency for Research on Cancer. Metabolic polymorphisms and susceptibility to cancer. Lyon, France: International Agency for Research on Cancer; Oxford University Press, 1999.
44. Gurney J, Davis S, Schwartz S, et al. Childhood cancer occurrence in relation to power line configurations: a study of potential selection bias in case-control studies. Epidemiology 1995;6:31–35.
45. Little J; International Agency for Research on Cancer. Epidemiology of childhood cancer. Lyon, France: International Agency for Research on Cancer; Oxford University Press, 1999.
46. Savitz D, Pearce N, Poole C. Methodological issues in the epidemiology of electromagnetic fields and cancer. Epidemiol Rev 1989;11:59–78.
47. Hatch E, Kleinerman R, Linet M, et al. Do confounding or selection factors of residential wiring codes and magnetic fields distort findings of electromagnetic fields studies? Epidemiology 2000;11:189–198.
48. Greenland S. Evolution of epidemiologic ideas: annotated readings on concepts and methods. Chestnut Hill, MA: Epidemiology Resources, 1987.
49. Jewell NP. Statistics for epidemiology. Boca Raton, FL: Chapman & Hall/CRC, 2004.
50. Robison L, Neglia J. Epidemiology of Down syndrome and childhood acute leukemia. Prog Clin Biol Res 1987;246:19–32.
51. Gurney J, Davis S, Severson R, et al. Trends in cancer incidence among children in the U.S. Cancer 1996;78:532–541.
52. Linabery AM, Ross JA. Trends in childhood cancer incidence in the U.S. (1992–2004). Cancer 2008;112:416–432.
53. Bondy ML, Scheurer ME, Malmer B, et al. Brain tumor epidemiology: consensus from the Brain Tumor Epidemiology Consortium. Cancer 2008;113:1953–1968.
54. Brown RC, Dwyer T, Kasten C, et al. Cohort profile: the International Childhood Cancer Cohort Consortium (I4C). Int J Epidemiol 2007;36:724–730.

CHAPTER 2 ■ CHILDHOOD CANCER AND HEREDITY

SHARON E. PLON AND DAVID MALKIN

Questions often arise in the minds of parents when their children are newly diagnosed with cancer: "Did this happen because of something I did or passed on to my child?" and "What are the chances that my other children will develop cancer?" In this chapter, we outline the scientific and clinical evidence that is available to answer these questions with regard to genetic susceptibility. Overall, it is the minority of childhood cancers that are caused by a clearly inherited predisposition. However, the percentage varies significantly with individual tumor types and is a composite of several different genetic factors. Ongoing identification of the genes that are mutated in cancer susceptibility syndromes provides opportunities for genetic testing. After reviewing these syndromes, we discuss the special issues to be considered in genetic testing for cancer susceptibility for the pediatric patient.

INHERITED PREDISPOSITION TO PEDIATRIC CANCERS

Overwhelming evidence demonstrates that cancer is the result of multiple changes in the DNA of the tumor cell, including point mutations, larger-scale copy number changes, and silencing of genes by epigenetic changes. Many of these somatic alterations are discussed in Chapter 3 and in the disease-specific chapters. The proportion of pediatric cancers that have a clear hereditary component is small. *Hereditary* in this case implies a genetic alteration that has been passed on to the child from a parent or that was a new constitutional mutation that occurred in the oocyte or sperm before fertilization. A child therefore can have a hereditary predisposition to cancer despite a negative family history of cancer because of a constitutional chromosome disorder such as trisomy 21 (Down syndrome [DS]) or a *de novo* mutation in a cancer predisposing gene, such as *RB1*.

Estimates of the fraction of hereditary predisposition for an individual cancer were originally based on epidemiologic studies of the number of familial cases and studies of associated syndromes. More recently, these estimates rely on direct molecular testing of a series of cancer patients for mutations as the particular gene involved in a tumor type is discovered. The percentage of cases due to hereditary factors varies widely among tumor types, as illustrated in Table 2.1, with adrenocortical carcinoma, optic glioma, and retinoblastoma having 40% or higher and many other tumor types including leukemia falling in the range of 1% to 10%.[1] Thus, some of the most common pediatric cancers have the lowest hereditary fraction.

Geneticists categorize disorders by the molecular mechanism underlying the cancer susceptibility, including constitutional chromosomal abnormality; mendelian autosomal dominant, recessive, or X-linked patterns; and nonmendelian inheritance, including polygenic, mitochondrial, and imprinting disorders. For any given tumor type, the overall inherited fraction maybe the sum of several different genetic mechanisms. In the following sections, we describe the major types of hereditary disorders that result in genetic susceptibility to childhood cancers.

CONSTITUTIONAL CHROMOSOMAL ABNORMALITIES

Children with constitutional chromosomal abnormalities (abnormal number [i.e., aneuploidy] or structural rearrangements) present with defined clinical phenotypes that can include dysmorphic features, congenital abnormalities, growth failure, and developmental delay. Most chromosome abnormalities result from errors that occurred during male or female meiosis, with both the parents having a normal chromosomal count of 22 pairs of autosomes and the sex chromosome pair. Rarely, these disorders can result when a parent is a carrier for a balanced translocation who has offspring with an unbalanced karyotype. The increased association of specific chromosome disorders with malignancy risk was recognized early.

Down Syndrome

One of the most striking predispositions to cancer caused by a constitutional chromosome abnormality is the increased risk of leukemia in children who have trisomy 21 (reviewed by Rabin and Whitlock[13]). An analysis of the Danish population reveals an estimated cumulative risk for developing leukemia of 2.1% by 5 years and 2.7% by 30 years.[14] This represents at least a 20-fold increase compared with the risk for the general population. Trisomy 21 is also a common finding in the karyotype of leukemia cells from patients without DS. Thus, the presence of an extra chromosome 21 appears to be leukemogenic and may be acquired in the germline or somatically.

In children with DS, the ratio of leukemia subtypes is shifted to 60% lymphoid and 40% myeloid from the ratio in the general population of 80% lymphoid and 20% myeloid.[13] This shift is principally due to the increased incidence of myeloid leukemias in children younger than 2 years. Most striking is the distribution of types of acute myeloid leukemia (AML) among DS children.[15] Approximately 30% of DS children with AML develop acute megakaryocytic leukemia (AMKL or M7). This results in an almost 400-fold excess of AMKL in DS children compared with non-DS (NDS) children. AMKL from children with and without DS show different cytogenetic characteristics, for example, an absence of the characteristic t(1;22)(p13;q13) translocation seen in a proportion of NDS children with AMKL.[16] NDS

TABLE 2.1

HEREDITARY COMPONENT OF SEVERAL PEDIATRIC MALIGNANCIES

Tumor type	Hereditary component (%)[a]
Adrenocortical carcinoma[2,3]	50–80
Optic gliomas[4]	45
Retinoblastoma[5]	40
Pheochromocytoma[6]	40
Rhabdoid/ATRT[7]	25
Wilms' tumor[8,9]	3–5
Central nervous system neoplasms[1,10,11]	<1–3[b]
Leukemia[1,12]	2.5–5

ATRT, atypical teratoid/rhabdoid tumor.
[a]These percentages are approximations from large population studies and may include familial cases and associated syndromes such as Down syndrome.
[b]Studies of pediatric brain tumors vary considerably in detection of a hereditary fraction.

AMKL children tended to present in early infancy and have significant hepatomegaly, but the DS children, on average, presented at 23 months, and a high proportion had myelofibrosis.

In infancy, children with DS can develop transient myeloproliferative disorder (TMD) that can appear similar to leukemia but that is self-limited.[17,18] However, 25% of DS children with this syndrome eventually develop frank AML. Children who are mosaic for trisomy 21 in their blood and bone marrow have also developed TMD and subsequent leukemia.[19] Similarly, children with DS have a higher rate of occurrence of myelodysplasia syndromes (MDS), which are characterized by thrombocytopenia, abnormal megakaryocytopoiesis, and an abnormal karyotype, most commonly trisomy 8.[13]

AMKL samples from DS patients have a distinct pattern of somatic mutation compared with AMKL samples from NDS patients. In particular, somatic mutations in the *GATA1* gene are frequently detected in this group of patients.[20,21] *GATA1* encodes a transcription factor that is essential for maturation of erythroid cells and megakaryocytes.[22,23] *GATA1* mutations are also found in the bone marrow of the majority of TMD patients, suggesting that *GATA1* mutagenesis is an early event in DS myeloid leukemogenesis, probably occurring *in utero*. In contrast *GATA1* mutations are not detected in leukemic cells of NDS patients with AMKL or in DS patients who develop other forms of leukemia.[20,24]

Data from several large Pediatric Oncology Group protocols were compared for the presentation and result of therapy for acute lymphoblastic leukemia (ALL) in children with and without DS.[25] There were no children with DS and t(9;22), t(1;19), or t(4;11) chromosomal translocations, compared with an expected frequency of 10% to 13% in the NDS population. However, the DS children suffered more toxic effects from the chemotherapy, and their overall outcome therefore was not better than that of the NDS patients. Analysis of children with DS and leukemia in the United Kingdom treated between 1980 and 1994 also found a decreased five year disease free survival (57% vs. 75%) for the children with DS.[26] Similar to the *GATA-1/AMKL* story, recently, activating mutations in the *JAK2* kinase have been found in 20% of DS-ALL samples.[27,28]

Despite the well-documented increase in the risk of leukemia in children with DS, a study based on exhaustive analysis of the Danish population found no increased risk of solid tumors in children or adults with DS including significantly fewer cases of breast cancer compared with an age-matched population.[14]

Sex Chromosome Abnormalities

Sex chromosome abnormalities comprise a large group of disorders that result from numerical and structural problems with the X and Y chromosomes. The overall incidence of sex chromosome abnormalities is high, with 47,XXY and Turner syndrome (45,X) each affecting approximately 1 in 2,000 individuals. The diagnosis of these disorders, unlike DS, is often not made until late adolescence or young adulthood, when problems with the transition through puberty and fertility become apparent. However, children with these disorders are at increased risk for certain malignancies during childhood, arguing for earlier diagnosis.

Y Chromosome

Any phenotypic female child with part or all of a Y chromosome is at risk for development of gonadoblastoma. Recent studies suggest that the risk can be as high as 25% for individuals in the late second or third decade and can include gonadoblastoma and dysgerminomas.[29] Children with this problem include girls with androgen resistance syndromes (i.e., testicular feminization) who have a 46,XY karyotype, children with gonadal dysgenesis, and girls with Turner syndrome and a mosaic 45,X, 46,XY karyotype. Mosaicism describes an individual with several different populations of cells, presumably due to a 46,XY zygote losing a Y chromosome in an early mitotic division during development. Approximately 25% of girls with Turner syndrome have some evidence for mosaicism.[30] The *TSPY* gene on the Y chromosome has been implicated as the gene responsible for gonadoblastoma in these conditions (reviewed by Lau[31]).

Phenotypic girls with a Y chromosome component should have prophylactic surgery to remove their gonads (reviewed by Saenger[32]). In most circumstances, these gonads are nonfunctional, and removal does not affect the girls medically. However, the discovery of a sex chromosome karyotype that is not consistent with their phenotypic sex can be devastating for patients and their parents and should be carefully handled by a medical team familiar with these disorders and psychosocial aspects of gender assignment.[33]

47XXY

The clinical phenotype of boys with a 47,XXY karyotype (Klinefelter syndrome) is variable and includes tall stature, infertility, decreased secondary sex characteristics, and gynecomastia. Men with 47,XXY are often not diagnosed until adulthood, making epidemiologic studies of the increased risk of malignancy in childhood difficult. Nonetheless, some studies suggest an increased risk of dysgerminomas[34] and extragonadal germ cell tumors.[35] Men with 47,XXY have an increased risk of breast cancer.[36] There is controversial evidence for an increased risk of leukemia in men with a 47,XXY karyotype, and one large cytogenetic study of men with leukemia demonstrated no increased incidence of 47,XXY.[37]

STRUCTURAL CHROMOSOMAL ABNORMALITIES

Detection and Impact

As cytogenetic techniques were improved in the 1970s, it became clear that many of the complex dysmorphic syndromes were the result of large cytogenetically visible deletions. During the next two decades, detection of deletions by Southern blot analysis and fluorescent *in situ* hybridization (FISH) permitted further progress in identifying the underlying cause of these syndromes. A new method, array comparative genomic hybridization (array CGH), allows detection of small deletions by comparative hybridization of fluorescently labeled DNA from patient and normal control samples onto glass slides containing gridded arrays of human genomic DNA contained in bacterial artificial chromosomes, long oligonucleotides, or cDNAs. Array CGH allows the entire genome to be sampled for deletions or amplification in one experiment.[38] Array CGH is now widely available and has rapidly increased our ability to identify both inherited and somatic interstitial deletions in pediatric cancer.[39]

Interstitial deletions can result in the loss of several contiguous genes, and the varied features of a particular disorder may result from the loss of unrelated neighboring genes, with the size of the deletion impacting how many genes are lost and how many features the child may manifest. Chromosomal deletions may be *de novo* events or inherited from either parent. Deletion syndromes overlap with autosomal dominant disorders that are the result of smaller mutations affecting a single gene within the deleted segment. For example, retinoblastoma can be transmitted as result of an autosomal dominant disorder due to point mutations in the *RB1* gene or can be associated with a cytogenetically visible deletion in a small percentage of cases.[40]

WAGR: Wilms' Tumor, Aniridia, Genital Abnormalities, and Mental Retardation

Patients with Wilms' tumor (WT) commonly exhibit a spectrum of congenital abnormalities and susceptibility to the tumor derives from several different underlying molecular mechanisms.

The WAGR syndrome is named for the components of the disorder: WT; aniridia; genital abnormalities, including hypospadias; and mental retardation associated with cytogenetically detectable deletions at 11p13. Surveys of children with WT in the United Kingdom[41] and France[8] revealed that 3% and 1%, respectively, of children with WT had aniridia.

WT1, the gene responsible for the WT phenotype, lies within the WAGR interval and encodes a zinc finger transcription factor (reviewed by Little[42]). All or part of *WT1* is deleted in children with WAGR and WT.[43] In contrast, point mutations in *WT1* including missense mutations are found in children with the Denys-Drash syndrome, a disorder characterized by severe urogenital abnormalities and WT.[43,44] This is an example where total loss of a gene product results in a less severe disease than does production of a mutant protein due to a missense mutation. It is hypothesized that the mutant protein may have a dominant negative impact on genital development, which may not occur when the gene is deleted. Surprisingly, somatic mutations in the *WT1* gene in sporadic WT are found in only 10% of cases.[42]

PAX6 is the gene responsible for the aniridia phenotype and is deleted in children with WAGR,[45] with point mutations found in isolated aniridia.[46] Array CGH or FISH analysis is performed for infants with aniridia to map out whether the deletion includes the *WT1* gene in order to determine the risk of developing WT and need for surveillance. Screening for the development of WT in children with WAGR or Denys-Drash syndrome is often performed by abdominal ultrasound examinations every 4 months until the age of 5 years, with decreasing frequency of examinations at later ages.[47] The recommendation for serial ultrasound scans is controversial and is based on small numbers of children screened by varying protocols. The National Wilms Tumor Study found more stage 1 tumors in children who had been screened.[47] However, the Childhood Cancer Research Group in Oxford found that eight children who had their WT diagnosed by ultrasound screening did not have more favorable outcomes than those in the group that was not screened, although the screening interval was variable.[9] As discussed later, for Beckwith-Wiedemann syndrome (BWS), there are additional data that show that children who were screened had fewer cases of advanced WT than those unscreened.[48] Parents should be counseled to bring the child in for evaluation if they suspect any change in abdominal girth or feel a mass, regardless of whether ultrasound screening is performed as interval tumors can develop. A long-term analysis of children with WT and either Denys-Drash or WAGR found 62% and 38% rate of renal failure, respectively, 20 years after the diagnosis of WT.[49] Therefore, children with constitutional mutations in the *WT1* gene require long-term follow-up for evidence of declining renal function.

OVERGROWTH DISORDERS AND IMPRINTING ERRORS

Beckwith-Wiedemann Syndrome

The relationship between disorders of increased growth and predisposition to cancer are evident in BWS and hemihyperplasia (HH, previously termed *hemihypertrophy*) linked to a significantly increased risk of developing abdominal tumors, including WT and hepatoblastoma.[50] HH can be a feature of BWS or an isolated finding. HH is defined as asymmetric growth due to overgrowth of one side relative to the other. It can be limited to a limb or the face or can include the whole side. Of 183 children in the BWS Registry, 13 had developed a tumor by age 4.[51] BWS is characterized by excessive intrauterine and postnatal growth, organomegaly, hypoglycemia at birth, macroglossia, and unusual linear ear creases and pitting.[50] For children with isolated HH, the risk of WT is approximately 3%.[47] Children with both BWS and HH had a higher risk of WT than did children with either condition alone.[51,52] Cohort studies have also demonstrated that nephromegaly is associated with an increased risk of WT in children with BWS.[53]

The genetic basis of BWS and HH is complex (reviewed by Weksberg[54]). Rare families have an apparent autosomal dominant pattern that maps to 11p15 with BWS more likely to be inherited from mothers than fathers.[55] Cytogenetically visible rearrangements that result in paternal duplications of 11p15 are also seen. The mechanisms behind these unusual genetics results from *imprinting*, which refers to the fact that certain genes are expressed differently, depending on whether they were inherited from the maternal or paternal chromosome. Disorders of imprinted genes result in unusual pedigrees (e.g., unaffected sisters who can pass on a mutation in an imprinted

TABLE 2.2

BWS GENETIC AND EPIGENETIC SUBGROUPS

Region	DNA	RNA	Karyotype	Frequency (%)	Inheritance
A. Regional	Paternal 11p15 UPD		Normal	10–20	Sporadic
			11p15 Duplication	1	Sporadic
	Disruption of KCNQ1OT1		11p15 Transl/Inver	1	Sporadic
B. Domain 1	H19 Hypermethylation	IGF2 LOI	Normal	2	Sporadic
	Normal H19 methylation	IGF2 LOI	Normal	25–50	Sporadic
C. Domain 2	CDKN1C mutation		Normal	5–10	Sporadic
	CDKN1C mutation		Normal	25	AD
	KvDMR1LOM	KNQ1OT1 LOI	Normal	50	Sporadic
D. Other	Unknown		Normal	5	AD
	Unknown	Unknown	Normal	10–20	Sporadic

BWS, Beckwith-Wiedemann syndrome; UPD, uniparental disomy; LOM, loss of methylation; LOI, loss of imprinting; AD, autosomal dominant.
Adapted from Weksberg R, Smith AC, Squire J, et al. Beckwith-Wiedemann syndrome demonstrates a role for epigenetic control of normal development. Hum Mol Genet 2003;12(spec no 1):R61–R68.

gene to their children, resulting in affected cousins). Apparently, cytogenetically normal children with BWS may inherit two copies of a paternal chromosome 11 and no maternal copy, termed *uniparental disomy* (UPD).[56]

Significant effort has been made to identify which imprinted genes in 11p15 are disrupted in BWS. Imprinted genes implicated in the etiology of BWS include the paternally expressed genes (maternally imprinted) insulin-like growth factor 2 gene (*IGF2*) and RNA transcript, *KCNQ1OT1(LIT1)*,[57,58] and the maternally expressed (paternally imprinted) genes *H19* and *CDKN1C*. Among BWS patients, 25% to 50% have loss of imprinting (biallelic expression) of *IGF2*. Another 50% have an epigenetic mutation that results in loss of imprinting of *KCNQ1OT1*. There are also rare cases of patients with BWS who carry mutations in the *CDKN1C/p57^{KIP2}* gene.[59] These different etiologies may be particularly important in defining the cancer phenotype of different BWS patients. Children with BWS who develop embryonal tumors such as rhabdomyosarcoma (RMS) and hepatoblastoma are more likely to have epigenetic changes in domain 2,[60] whereas WT is more strongly associated with epigenetic alterations in domain 1 or UPD.[61,62] A summary of the molecular defects found in children with BWS is found in Table 2.2.

The risk of having a child with BWS is increased when the pregnancy was initiated by assisted reproductive technologies (ART), including *in vitro* fertilization (IVF). A study of children in the BWS Registry revealed that 4.6% were the result of ART, which appeared increased compared with the general population.[63] A population-based case control study from Australia confirmed a 17-fold relative risk of BWS in pregnancies initiated by IVF.[64] However, the absolute risk of BWS in an ART-associated pregnancy is still very low at 1 in 4,000 pregnancies. BWS in ART pregnancies appears to result from abnormal methylation of *KCNQ1OT1/LIT1*.[65]

Molecular testing for alteration in the genes implicated in BWS is now available in clinically certified laboratories (www.genetests.org). The results of testing improve prediction of cancer risk and the likelihood of the parents having another child with BWS. For example, parents of a child with BWS due to UPD have a very low risk (much less than 1%) of recurrence in another pregnancy.

Overall, given the increased risk of WT and other abdominal malignancy in these conditions, screening by regular serial abdominal ultrasound examinations and serial α-fetoprotein (AFP) levels is recommended for children with BWS, HH, or both (see the preceding section on WAGR for details about screening). Children with BWS who were screened for WT were much less likely to present with advanced disease than those who were not screened (0 of 12 vs. 25 of 59).[48] Screening until age 9 will detect the majority of children with BWS who will develop WT. Although the risk of a second tumor is low (typically WT in the contralateral kidney), it is recommended that children with BWS and WT or hepatoblastoma continue with routine screening by ultrasound and serum AFP levels until age 9.

Other Wilms' Tumor Loci

Using array CGH, a novel gene termed *WTX* was identified on chromosome Xq11.1.[66] *WTX* is inactivated in one-third of WTs, and tumors with *WTX* mutations lack *WT1* mutations. WTX binds WT1 in the nucleus, suggesting a role for WTX in nuclear pathways implicated in the transcriptional regulation of cellular differentiation programs.[67] Whereas autosomal tumor suppressor genes undergo biallelic inactivation, *WTX* is inactivated by a monoallelic "single-hit" event that targets the single X chromosome in WTs in males and the active X chromosome in tumors in females.[68] However, germline mutations of *WTX* do not appear to be associated with WT susceptibility. Rather, this causes a form of X-linked sclerosing bone dysplasia, osteopathia striata congenital with cranial sclerosis.[69] These observations suggest the existence of temporal or spatial constraints on the action of *WTX* during tumorigenesis. Overall, bilateral WT or a family history of WT occurs in 1% to 5% of patients. Although linkage studies have indicated that the gene for familial WT must be distinct from *WT1* and *WTX* and from genes that predispose to BWS, to date, no familial WT gene has been identified.[70]

AUTOSOMAL DOMINANT DISORDERS

Autosomal dominant syndromes comprise the majority of families with single-gene disorders that convey an increased risk of cancer. The features of autosomal dominant inheritance include equal transmission from the father or the mother to a son or daughter, in contrast to an X-linked disorder. Often, there is a multigenerational pattern, and a variable expression of the disorder within a family, with "skipped" generations (at the phenotypic level) because of incomplete penetrance. *Penetrance* is defined as the probability that a person inheriting the mutation will have the disease.

Retinoblastoma

Much of our knowledge of autosomal dominant cancer families was gained from the study of retinoblastoma. In a series of landmark papers in the early 1970s, Knudson and Strong performed statistical analysis of children with retinoblastoma and other pediatric malignancies.[71,72] Knudson hypothesized that bilateral retinoblastoma represented the hereditary form, and those patients had already acquired one "hit" or mutation.[71] The best model consistent with his data indicated that the bilateral form required only one additional hit after birth but that the unilateral form required two hits. Prior to this work, in 1968, Nicholls[73] had proposed that the skin lesions in neurofibromatosis type 1 (NF1) represented two mutational events in the same gene, with the first mutation being inherited and the second mutation occurring somatically.

The most striking features of autosomal dominant cancer predisposition disorders are those initially observed by Knudson: hereditary forms of retinoblastoma present earlier and with a greatly increased percentage of bilateral and multiple primary tumors. Importantly, some patients (about 15%) with unilateral retinoblastoma carry a constitutional mutation. An even milder form, retinoma or retinocytoma, which spontaneously regress, can also be seen in apparently unaffected adults. Approximately 10% of people with a germline mutation in *RB1* do not develop retinoblastoma (i.e., incomplete penetrance).[74] However, the penetrance varies among families, with specific mutations (often missense changes or splice abnormalities) resulting in mutation carriers having a higher likelihood of developing unilateral (as opposed to bilateral) disease. These types of families are said to demonstrate attenuated or low penetrant retinoblastoma.[75,76]

Individuals carrying germline mutations in the *RB1* gene are at increased risk for development of other primary tumors, including osteosarcoma and malignant melanoma in childhood. In a U.K. cohort of long-term survivors, children with bilateral retinoblastoma were found to have 48% risk of developing a second neoplasm by age 50.[77] Further follow-up of this cohort (up to age 84) identified a 68% cumulative incidence of second cancers including many epithelial cancers, for example, lung cancer, at later ages.[78] Few individuals in the U.K. cohort received radiation therapy, confirming that there is a significant risk of second primary cancers in all bilateral retinoblastoma patients. Recent data from a U.S. cohort looking at cumulative cancer mortality (as opposed to incidence) identified 25% and 1% risk for hereditary and nonhereditary retinoblastoma, respectively.[79] For children with hereditary retinoblastoma treated with radiation, there is a substantial increased risk of sarcomas with one estimate of a 13% cumulative risk of developing a sarcoma by age 50.[80]

On the basis of rare cases of patients with cytogenetically visible deletions, the gene mutated in retinoblastoma, *RB1*, was mapped to chromosome 13q14 and eventually isolated.[81] Molecular studies confirmed Knudson's two-hit hypothesis. Retinoblastoma requires loss of both copies (i.e., two hits) of the *RB1* gene for a tumor to develop (Fig. 2.1). Loss of the normal tumor suppressor function of RB1 is consistent with loss of cell cycle control (see Chapter 27 for details). In the familial form, a mutation in one *RB1* gene is inherited; and therefore, all the cells in the body have only one normal allele. If during development that normal copy is mutated or lost, then cell cycle control is disrupted and retinoblastoma can develop. The most common mechanisms by which the second copy is lost are loss of the whole chromosome, large deletions, and gene conversion, normally resulting in loss of heterozygosity (LOH) for markers near the *RB1* locus or silencing of the gene by epigenetic methylation of the *RB1* promoter. In the sporadic form, mutation or loss of both *RB1* genes must

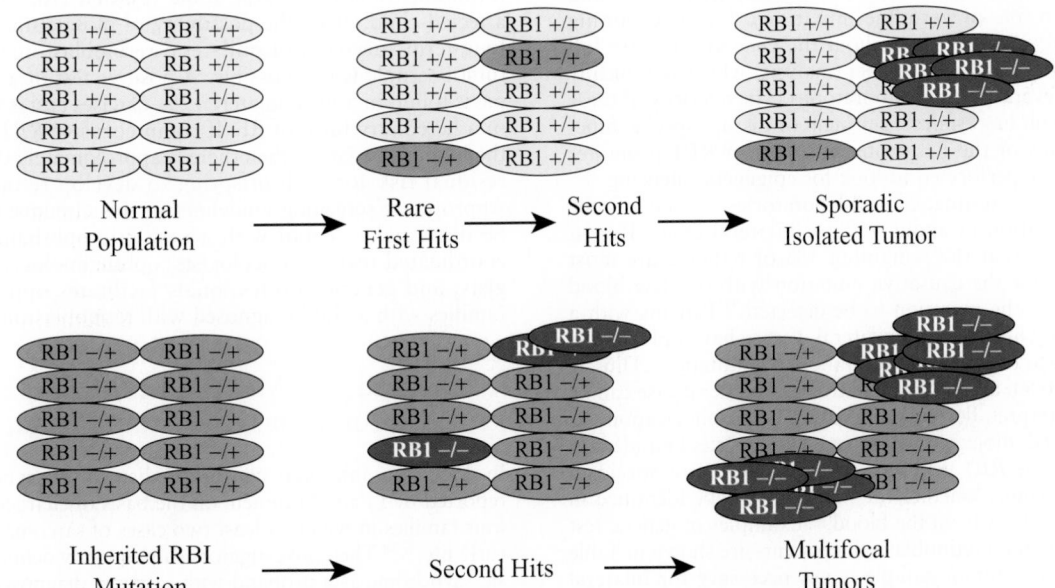

FIGURE 2.1 Knudson's two-hit hypothesis. In all tumors, the same cell must undergo at least two mutations in the *RB1* gene to become malignant. In sporadic, nonhereditary tumors (**top**), the first hit occurs at low frequency, with a rare cell having a second hit in the same gene yield isolated tumors. In hereditary tumors (**bottom**), the first mutation is in a germ cell, such that all body cells have the first mutation. When a second mutation or inactivating event occurs in *RB1*, tumors develop. (Modified from Plon SE. "Cancer Genetics and Molecular Oncology" by Plon, SE in Principles of Molecular Medicine, 2nd Edition, 2006 (Eds. Runge, M.S. and Patterson, C.) The Humana Press, Inc., Totowa, New Jersey. With kind permission of Springer Science+Business Media).

TABLE 2.3

EMPIRICAL RECURRENCE RISKS IN FAMILIES WITH RETINOBLASTOMA IN THE ABSENCE OF GENETIC TESTING

Clinical scenario	Retinoblastoma risk (%)
Offspring of bilateral cases	45
Offspring of unilateral cases	7.5
Sibling of bilateral cases (with unaffected parents)	5–7
Sibling of unilateral cases (with unaffected parents)	1
Sibling of bilateral or unilateral cases (if either parent is affected)	45

TABLE 2.4

EXAMPLES OF *RB1* GENETIC TEST RESULTS FOR TWO PATIENTS WITH UNILATERAL RETINOBLASTOMA

Sample	Allele 1	Allele 2
Patient 1—Hereditary form of RB		
Tumor 1	Q347X	Loss
Blood 1	Q347X	Normal
Patient 2—Sporadic Rb due to somatic mutation		
Tumor 2	Methylation of promoter	567delAG
Blood 2	Normal	Normal

occur in the same somatic retinal cell for retinoblastoma to develop.

Although bilateral retinoblastoma results from constitutional mutations in the *RB1* gene, 80% of patients will have no family history of retinoblastoma. This is due to the majority being the result of a *de novo* mutation in the *RB1* gene. In Table 2.3, the risk is given of having a second child with Rb for parents of a child newly diagnosed with either unilateral or bilateral Rb.[74] Surprisingly, parents of a child with bilateral retinoblastoma who have normal eye examination results retain a 5–7% risk to have a second affected child due to the *de novo* mutation occurring in the father's germline and with a variable percentage of the sperm carrying the mutation (germline mosaicism).[82] More rarely, the mutation occurs during oogenesis. Therefore, if genetic testing is not pursued, all siblings of children with bilateral retinoblastoma should have ophthalmologic surveillance beginning at birth.

The discovery of the *RB1* gene[81] allowed for clinical molecular diagnostics. Several different approaches are used to identify mutations.[83,84] Larger-scale deletions of the entire *RB1* gene (detected by cytogenetics, FISH, or array CGH) are found in fewer than 5% of germline mutations.[40] The remaining mutations are scattered throughout the gene and require full DNA sequence and copy number analysis, which is clinically available in several certified laboratories. The majority of these mutations result in a truncated protein or disrupt specific functional domains of the RB protein. Assays of *RB1* promoter methylation are performed to look for epigenetic silencing.

With extensive testing, clinical laboratories can identify the causative mutation in about 95% of bilateral cases. Recent studies suggest that the remaining 5% of patients are most likely mosaic for the causative mutation with too few blood cells containing the mutation to be detected.[85] Patients with a negative family history and unilateral disease have only a 15% *a priori* chance of having a germline *RB1* mutation. Thus, a negative test from a blood sample from a unilateral case can be difficult to interpret. For unilateral cases, where enucleation has been performed, molecular diagnostic laboratories first identify mutations in the *RB1* gene in a fresh frozen tumor specimen and then determine whether the mutation can be identified in constitutional DNA from the blood.[84] Examples of genetic test results for unilateral retinoblastoma patients are shown in Table 2.4. Testing of a tumor sample is not necessary for bilateral cases where testing is done directly from a blood sample.

Genetic evaluation and testing is recommended for all retinoblastoma patients. Unaffected parents of a child with bilateral disease often are concerned about their risk for having additional children with retinoblastoma. The physician first looks for the mutation in the affected child and then studies both parents and all siblings to ascertain whether they

carry the mutation. If prenatal testing is not pursued, then siblings of the proband should have a careful eye examination at birth and a blood sample sent for analysis of the specific *RB1* mutation found in the affected child. Only those siblings who carry the mutation need subsequent surveillance for retinoblastoma. The adult survivors of childhood retinoblastoma can also use DNA testing for prenatal diagnosis or immediate postnatal diagnosis of their children. Current recommendations for ophthalmic surveillance include examination in the first few days of life and then serial examinations every 3 to 4 months until 3 years of age (see Chapter 27).

In contrast, if genetic testing demonstrates that the child did not inherit the mutation found in the affected relative, the surveillance and anesthesia required for ophthalmic examinations could be avoided, decreasing costs and potential morbidity.[86] Genetic testing of unilateral pediatric patients can be particularly informative for parents. If it can be documented that the child does not carry a constitutional *RB1* mutation then (1) the child is not at substantial risk for secondary malignancies, (2) radiation therapy is associated with less hazard, and (3) the parents have a negligible risk of having another child with retinoblastoma. The child with unilateral retinoblastoma may carry some residual risk of having an affected child, given the possibility of mosaicism.[85] For adult long-term survivors of unilateral retinoblastoma, testing of tumor sample is not possible. A positive test of a blood sample is found in approximately 12% of cases and is informative of a hereditary form of Rb. If comprehensive *RB1* analysis of the blood is negative, then there is approximately 0.5% to 1% residual risk for each offspring to develop retinoblastoma. Appropriate screening guidelines in this circumstance should be discussed in detail with a pediatric ophthalmologist. A coordinated team of oncologists, ophthalmologists, pathologists, and genetics professionals facilitates optimal care of families with a child diagnosed with retinoblastoma.

Inherited p53 Mutations, the Li-Fraumeni Syndrome and Its Variant Phenotypes

In 1969, an inherited cancer predisposition syndrome was reported by Li and Fraumeni on the basis of characterization of four families in which at least two cases of sarcoma occurred in early life.[87,88] These investigators subsequently defined the "classic" syndrome as a proband with sarcoma diagnosed under age 45 years, with a first-degree relative with any cancer under 45 years, plus another first- or second-degree relative with either any cancer under 45 years or a sarcoma at any age.[89,90] An example of a pedigree from a Li-Fraumeni syndrome (LFS) family is shown in Figure 2.2. The list of LFS tumors includes premenopausal breast cancers, brain tumors, leukemias, adrenocortical carcinomas, gastric cancers, lymphomas, and possibly

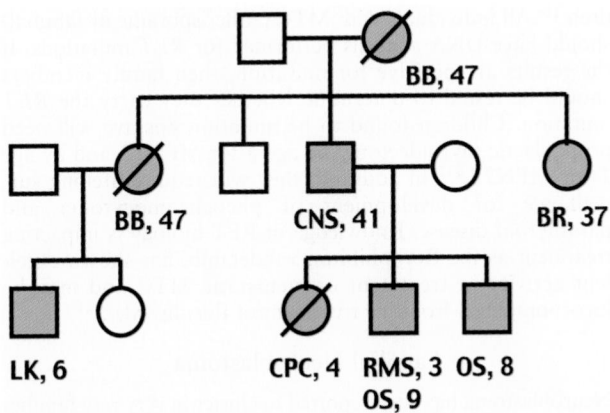

FIGURE 2.2 Pedigree of a family with Li-Fraumeni syndrome. Filled circles/squares represent affected members; circles with slashes represent deceased family members. Numbers represent age at diagnosis. BB, bilateral breast cancer; CNS, brain tumor; BR, unilateral breast cancer; LK, leukemia; CPC, choroid plexus carcinoma; RMS, rhabdomyosarcoma; OS, osteosarcoma.

early-onset lung cancers, choroid plexus carcinomas, and colorectal cancers.[91,92] More recently, the criteria for families that do not quite meet criteria, termed *LFS-like* (LFS-L), are generally accepted to include those outlined by Chompret et al[93] to include all children with adrenocortical carcinomas; a family in which the proband has multiple tumors, two of which are classical LFS tumors and the first occurred before age 36 years; and a family in which the proband has a characteristic LFS tumor diagnosed under age 36 and has at least two first- or second-degree relatives with an LFS component tumor (other than breast cancer if the proband had breast cancer). Hisada and colleagues[94] showed that gene carriers are at significant risk of developing multiple synchronous or metachronous non–therapy-induced neoplasms. In particular, the overall relative risk of occurrence of a second cancer was 5.3 (95% CI = 2.8–7.8), with a cumulative probability of second cancer occurrence of 57%.

Given the high mortality rate for affected members of LFS families, it was not possible to obtain DNA from extended pedigrees to perform linkage analysis. In 1990, Malkin and colleagues[95] took a candidate gene approach based on data from somatic mutation and mouse models of *p53*. These investigators detected heterozygous point mutations in the *P53* gene (also referred to as *TP53*) in constitutional DNA of LFS kindreds.[95] However, numerous subsequent studies have shown that only 60% to 80% of "classic" LFS families harbor detectable germline *p53* mutations,[92,96] while the majority of LFS-L families do not have detectable *p53* mutations (see, e.g., Tinat et al[97]). Mutations occur throughout the *p53* gene, though they are primarily confined to highly conserved regions. More recently, intragenic deletions of the *p53* gene have been reported in a subset of families that had negative sequencing studies.[98] The cancer phenotype in LFS is quite diverse. While specific p53 genotype:phenotype correlations have not been clearly demonstrated, several genetic modifier effects are reported. In particular, the mean age of onset of tumors is significantly less in *p53* mutation carriers who carry an *MDM2* SNP309 G allele compared with those homozygous for the T allele.[98] Similarly, carriers of the *p53* codon 72 arginine allele have an earlier tumor onset than those who harbor a homozygous proline allele.[98] These provide examples of how polymorphisms affecting p53 protein degradation can act as genetic modifiers of mendelian predisposition to cancer. In addition, accelerated telomere shortening as measured in peripheral blood lymphocytes is predictive of earlier tumor onset.[99,100] The cumulative combination of *MDM2* SNP309 and *p53* codon 72 status, telomere length, and possibly specific *p53* mutations may eventually be used as a predictive biomarker for cancer type and the age of onset in LFS.[101] DNA copy number variation (CNV) is strikingly enriched in the constitutional DNA of *p53* mutation carriers, and these CNVs can be inherited and frequently encompass other cancer genes, suggesting that the genomic instability conferred by the *p53* mutation can be transmitted from generation to generation.[102] Regions of DNA showing variability in a number of subjects likely identify other genetic factors that may modulate the cancer phenotype.

Several groups have failed to identify mutations in other tumor suppressor genes, for example, *PTEN*, *p16INK4 a*, and *p19Arf*, or genes in p53-mediated regulatory pathways in LFS, LFS-L families and individuals with the occurrence of multiple tumors who are negative for *P53* mutations. Heterozygous germline mutations in the checkpoint kinase *hCHK2/CHEK2* in one LFS family and one LFS-L family were reported.[103] However, several subsequent studies have failed to identify *CHK2* mutations in a large number of LFS families.[104] Thus, the other genes that result in LFS or LFS-L families are unknown.

Although *p53* behaves as a classic tumor suppressor gene, less than 50% of tumors from *p53*-heterozygous mice and LFS patients have evidence of LOH.[105,106] It remains unclear in these patients how the retained wild-type *p53* allele is functionally inactivated *en route* to malignant transformation of the cell.

A number of studies have analyzed groups of patients with tumors characteristic of LFS, yet lacking characteristic family histories of cancer, for germline *p53* mutations. Such mutations have been identified in approximately 50% to 80% of children with adrenocortical carcinoma,[2,3] 10% of children with osteosarcoma,[107] and 10% of children with RMS.[108,109] The age of onset of tumors in the latter group of patients is strikingly lower (average age approximately 22 months) than in RMS patients with intact constitutional *p53*.[108] One-third of children with sarcomas plus either multiple primary tumors or a significant family history of cancer have germline *p53* mutations. A study of patients with adrenocortical carcinoma in Brazil revealed that 35 or 36 patients carried a specific germline *p53* mutation, R337H, without a family history of cancer, suggesting that it may represent a lower penetrance mutation that imparts a distinct susceptibility to adrenocortical carcinoma.[110]

Presymptomatic molecular testing for *p53* germline mutations in members of Li-Fraumeni kindreds has been met with significant controversy. Because of the variable expressivity, the diverse tumor spectrum, and lack of clear clinical surveillance and preventative or treatment recommendations, it is unclear how to manage the detection of a *p53* mutant carrier. However, women who carry *p53* mutations should begin screening for breast cancer with magnetic resonance imaging (MRI) in their mid-20s, given that the average age of onset is 31 years.[111] Recently, the use of positron emission tomography-computed tomography as a clinical surveillance modality has been reported, identifying presymptomatic lesions in adults,[112] and anecdotal reports of presymptomatic detection of childhood cancers, in particular, adrenocortical carcinoma, have also been noted.[113,114] Furthermore, the concept of predictive genetic testing of a child for a disease that may (or may not) occur in young adulthood poses significant challenges to our perception of the ethics of disclosure of genetic test results, where the potential beneficiary of these results may wish to uphold the right to "not know." Notwithstanding these considerations, presymptomatic and even prenatal genetic testing for *p53* mutation is being performed in carefully selected and counseled situations, taking into account the particular balance of beneficence and harm. These issues are discussed further in the last section of this chapter.

Inheritance of a Mutation in an Oncogene: RET and ALK

A large series of autosomal dominant cancer susceptibility syndromes were identified that resulted from deleterious mutations in tumor suppressor genes. Beginning with multiple endocrine neoplasia (MEN) type 2 in 1993 and continuing with familial neuroblastoma in 2008, it is now clear that some autosomal dominant cancer susceptibility syndromes result from inheritance of a mutation (typically missense mutations) that converts a proto-oncogene to an activated oncogene. These conditions do not require a somatic mutation of the other allele (no "second hit") and do not demonstrate LOH in flanking markers in tumor specimens.

Multiple Endocrine Neoplasia

The MEN disorders represent at least three different diseases, which are all autosomal dominant cancer family syndromes that affect different endocrine organs. MEN type 1 (MEN1) is characterized by parathyroid, pancreatic islet cell, and pituitary gland involvement. Parathyroid involvement is found most frequently, and individuals from MEN1 families can also have their disease complicated by Zollinger-Ellison syndrome. The gene for MEN1 acts as a typical tumor suppressor gene, with inactivating mutations passed down in families.[115] Although most MEN1-associated tumors present in adulthood, by age 15, 28% of mutation carriers have either biochemical or clinical evidence for disease.[116]

Both MEN2A and MEN2B syndromes present in the pediatric period. MEN2A is associated with medullary thyroid carcinoma (MTC), parathyroid adenomas, and pheochromocytomas. MEN2B is a related disorder but with the onset of tumors in infancy, ganglioneuromas of the gastrointestinal (GI) tract, and skeletal abnormalities. Additional families appear to show autosomal dominant MTC without the other features of MEN2A. Because of the life-threatening potential of metastatic MTC, treatment for MEN2 is prophylactic thyroidectomy in childhood.[117]

Analysis of *RET*, at chromosome 10q11.2, in constitutional DNA from multiple MEN2A families revealed a set of highly consistent missense mutations that replace one of a set of conserved cysteines with another amino acid in the extracellular domain of the protein encoded by exons 10 and 11 (reviewed by Raue and Frank-Raue[118]). Families that have isolated MTC or those with the full MEN2A syndrome share the same mutations. However, there is a correlation between disease phenotype and the specific mutation, for example, a mutation in cysteine 634 results in a high risk of pheochromocytomas. Studies of individuals from multiple MEN2B patients demonstrated two specific missense mutations, M918T and A883F, or the association of V804M (with other mutations) in the highly conserved tyrosine kinase domain of the *RET* gene.

These findings are of both scientific and clinical importance. Unlike tumor suppressor genes, predisposition to cancer in MEN2A and MEN2B families is due to inheritance of a mutation that activates the *RET* proto-oncogene as demonstrated by both *in vivo* and *in vitro* assays.[119]

Clinically, the screening, the preventive surgery, and the treatment of MEN2A and MEN2B families have been significantly improved by these genetic discoveries. DNA-based screening results in greatly increased sensitivity and specificity compared with calcitonin assays, particularly for young children.[120] All individuals with MTC (either sporadic or familial) should have DNA analysis performed for *RET* mutations. If the results are positive for mutation, then family members should be tested to determine whether they carry the *RET* mutation. Children found to be mutation positive will need prophylactic thyroidectomy by age 5 for MEN2A and by age 1 for MEN2B.[117] In addition, they will require lifelong surveillance for development of pheochromocytoma and parathyroid disease. Knowledge of RET biology is impacting treatment as the Ret inhibitor, vandetanib, has shown excellent activity in treatment of metastatic MTC and may be incorporated as frontline treatment of this disorder.[121]

Familial Neuroblastoma

Neuroblastoma has been reported to cluster in very rare families and a family history is documented only in 1% to 2% of newly diagnosed cases.[122] Initially, deleterious mutations in one gene, *PHOX2B*, was reported in two families with multiple cases of neuroblastoma.[123] Mutations in *PHOX2B* are also associated with Hirschsprung's disease and congenital central hypoventilation syndrome. Review of larger series of familial neuroblastoma revealed only rare mutations in the *PHOX2B* mutations. By using dense array hybridization techniques that allow genotyping of thousands of single nucleotide polymorphisms, Mosse et al. identified linkage for familial neuroblastoma to chromosome 2p23.[124] Sequence analysis of genes in the interval revealed specific missense mutations in the *ALK* proto-oncogene, resulting in activation of the gene and predisposition to neuroblastoma.[124] These families demonstrate incomplete penetrance (many mutations carriers did not develop tumors) and the grade of tumor varies among family members, from ganglioneuroma to advanced stage IV neuroblastoma. Several groups also identified both constitutional and somatic mutations in *ALK* in approximately 10% of neuroblastoma tumors resulting in the development of clinical trials with inhibitors of Alk kinase.[39,125,126] Clinical testing for *ALK* mutations is now available and is being incorporated into evaluation of familial neuroblastoma.

Atypical Teratoid and Malignant Rhabdoid Tumors and the Rhabdoid Predisposition Syndrome

Malignant rhabdoid tumor (MRT) of the kidney is a rare, aggressive childhood cancer, and it was noted early on that 10% to 15% of presentations in infants are associated with separate primary tumors of the central nervous system (CNS).[127] Although infants' kidney is the most common site for rhabdoid tumors, they occasionally are observed in other sites and in older children and even adults. The tumor is histologically defined by large cells of unknown origin that may resemble benign or malignant skeletal muscle cells. These histologically resemble primitive neuroectodermal tumors (and were previously diagnosed as medulloblastoma or pineoblastoma) or rhabdoid tumors. Because of its potential to differentiate into heterologous elements at the cellular level, this tumor type has been termed *atypical teratoid/rhabdoid tumor* (ATRT).[128]

Cytogenetic analyses of ATRT of the CNS and MRT of the kidney revealed abnormalities of chromosome 22, in particular, loss of one entire copy of the chromosome or deletion or translocation involving 22q11.2.[129,130] In 1998, the *SMARCB1/hSNF5/INI1* gene was isolated from chromosome band 22q11.2 and several rhabdoid tumor cell lines were shown to harbor truncating mutations of this gene.[131] *SMARCB1* encodes a protein that is part of a multiprotein complex involved in chromatin remodeling, an essential process for regulation of gene expression. Biegel and colleagues have reported *hSNF5/INI1* mutations in virtually all

MRTs/ATRTs examined.[7] In this early study, they found that approximately 20% of children with apparently sporadic tumors harbored constitutional mutations of the gene, suggesting a potential hereditary component to the etiology of the disease. Subsequent studies by Severet et al. confirmed this finding and, in sum, approximately 25% of such tumors arise in the context of a constitutional mutation.[132] These studies suggest that *SMARCB1* acts as a classic tumor suppressor gene, namely complete loss of *SMARCB1* function in tumors, resulting either from two somatic events in sporadic cases or an inherited mutation followed by a second somatic silencing event. The dominantly inherited syndrome termed *rhabdoid predisposition syndrome* includes a spectrum of tumors including renal and extrarenal MRT, choroid plexus carcinoma, central PNET, and medulloblastoma.[132] The likelihood of developing a tumor is very high at a very young age and these tumors are often lethal. Thus, in most cases, the constitutional mutation represents a *de novo* dominant mutation in the child diagnosed with the tumor with unaffected siblings or parents. This same paradigm of *de novo* mutation may apply to other rare pediatric tumors with high mortality. A few families have been reported with adult *SMARCB1* mutation carriers without a cancer history, suggesting incomplete penetrance.[133] Unexpected was the recent discovery that a completely different condition, familial schwannomatosis, is also the result of mutations, typically splice site changes, in the *SMARCB1* gene.[134] These families have late childhood and adult onset of multiple schwannomas and occasional meningiomas without evidence for rhabdoid tumors. One family was described with overlap of the two otherwise distinct clinical phenotypes.[135]

Familial Leukemia

Acute leukemias are the most frequent malignancy of childhood. However, knowledge about genetic predisposition to leukemia is very limited compared with many less common malignancies. Some well-described autosomal dominant syndromes, including LFS and NF1, demonstrate an increased risk of leukemia as one of many features as described elsewhere in this chapter. But families that demonstrate a specific predisposition to leukemia are extremely rare (reviewed by Horwitz[136]).

Some progress has been made in mapping loci responsible for these rare families with one leukemia susceptibility gene identified. Familial platelet disorder with predisposition to acute myelogenous leukemia (FPD/AML) is an autosomal dominant syndrome, characterized by both neonatal thrombocytopenia and a very high propensity to develop AML associated with inheritance of deleterious mutations in the *RUNX1/CBFA2/AML1* gene as identified by the laboratory of Gilliland and colleagues.[137]

Many more families and *de novo* cases have been described with *RUNX1* mutations, spanning from point mutations to deletion of the whole gene.[138] Children with large deletions at 21q22 have thrombocytopenia, susceptibility to AML, congenital anomalies and developmental delay.[139] In several cases the AML cells have acquired a trisomy 21 karyotype with the duplicated chromosome 21 carrying the deletion of *RUNX1*. Thus, a gene other than *RUNX1* on chromosome 21 must play a role in tumorigenesis. A recent analysis of multiple leukemia samples from FPD/AML patients reveals second somatic mutations in *RUNX1*, thus following the two-hit hypothesis.[140]

Childhood Cancers Associated With Familial Colon Cancer Syndromes

Although not generally considered a pediatric disease, children of familial colon cancer kindreds can present with GI manifestations in the adolescent period.[141] In addition, there is an increased prevalence of a variety of pediatric malignancies, including hepatoblastoma and brain tumors. The familial colon cancer syndromes are divided into those associated with polyposis (i.e., familial adenomatous polyposis [FAP]) and hereditary nonpolyposis colon cancer (HNPCC).

Familial Adenomatous Polyposis

FAP, also known as *adenomatous polyposis coli* (APC), is associated with carpeting of the colon with thousands of polyps with onset in the second or third decade of extensive polyposis (Fig. 2.3) and a nearly 90% rate of development of malignant colorectal carcinoma (reviewed by Haggitt and Reid[142]). Extracolonic manifestations in some kindreds with polyposis, including desmoid tumors, epidermoid cysts and osteomas of the mandible, was referred to as *Gardner syndrome*. However, with the discovery of the APC gene, these "different" disorders were found in some cases to be caused by identical mutations, and different members of the same family might demonstrate features of Gardner syndrome or isolated colonic polyposis. Thus, the terms Gardner syndrome and FAP are now often used interchangeably.

In addition to the greatly increased risk of colorectal carcinoma, carriers of this disorder have additional cancer risks. Upper GI tract tumors include duodenal and periampullary adenocarcinomas and can result in increased mortality in FAP patients postcolectomy.[143] Approximately 1% of FAP patients develop thyroid cancer, and some authors recommend beginning surveillance at age 15 for thyroid cancer.[144] Of particular importance for pediatric oncologists, approximately 1 child

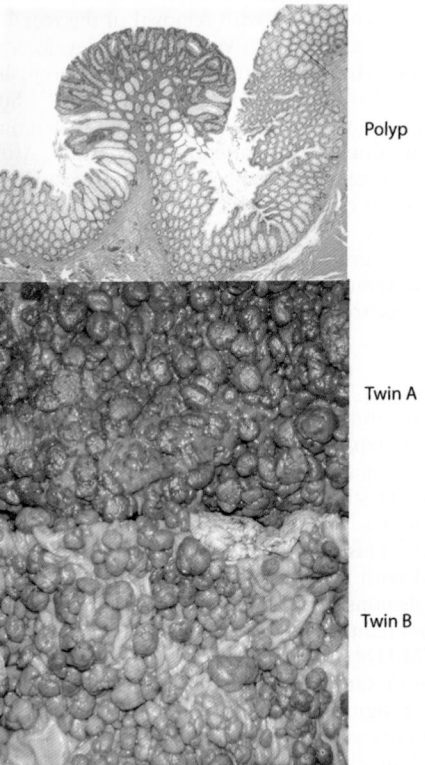

FIGURE 2.3 Carpeting of colonic epithelia with adenomatous polyps. Shown are samples from total colectomy of two twin brothers who were diagnosed with familial adenomatous polyposis due to a *de novo* APC mutation after Twin A presented with abdominal pain and rectal bleeding. (Photographs courtesy of M. Finegold, MD, Baylor College of Medicine/Texas Children's Hospital).

per 250 children with FAP develops hepatoblastoma, compared with 1 per 100,000 in the general population.[145] Familial cases of FAP may not be obvious because the parents of a young child with hepatoblastoma may have unrecognized polyposis even though the parent is at an age when it is essential to perform prophylactic colectomy to prevent invasive colorectal cancer. Thus, a careful family history of colon cancer and polyposis should be taken for any child diagnosed with hepatoblastoma.

Reports from cohorts of patients in Germany and the Children's Oncology Group in the United States suggest that approximately 10% to 15% of hepatoblastoma patients carry mutations in *APC*.[146,147] Thus, some centers now offer *APC* mutation testing (both full sequencing and deletion/rearrangement analysis, described below) for all hepatoblastoma patients, independent of family history. There has not been enough clinical experience to know the mutation yield although one more recent report found mutations in zero of 29 probands with hepatoblastoma.[148]

Deleterious mutations and deletions are found spread throughout the *APC* gene as the causative mutation in 85% to 90% of FAP families.[149] In the workup of a child at risk for polyposis due to an affected parent, it is important to test the affected parent first to identify the specific mutation causing FAP in that family. Subsequently, at-risk family members are tested for that specific mutation. One must also consider a recessive form of colonic polyposis (MYH-associated polyposis) due to inheriting mutations in the *MYH/MUTYH* excision repair gene from both parents.[150] This condition results in somewhat later ages of polyposis and colon cancer compared with classic FAP.

Unlike the situation for LFS, there are clear surveillance and prophylactic surgery guidelines for FAP, and testing of children is considered standard of care.[151,152] Screening by colonoscopy is recommended to begin between the ages of 8 and 10 years for mutation carriers. Prophylactic surgery that includes total colectomy with removal of the rectal mucosa is recommended after extensive polyposis develops or by late adolescence. Modern surgical techniques allow the maintenance of fecal continence in these patients.[153,154] Surgery recommendations are modified if the family is demonstrated to carry a low penetrance or attenuated mutation. After prophylactic surgery, carriers need screening of their upper GI tracts and rectums (if rectal mucosa is left in place) for development of malignancy. Data on the efficacy of nonsteroidal anti-inflammatory drug in reducing colonic polyp risk are controversial and treatment should be conducted in conjunction with a pediatric gastroenterologist.[155]

Familial Juvenile Polyposis

Familial juvenile polyposis (JP) results in multiple hamartomatous polyps in the rectocolon of young children. These lesions often manifest with abdominal pain and rectal bleeding.[156] Recent studies estimate a 39% lifetime risk of colorectal carcinoma with some difference based on the gene involved.[157] This clearly inherited condition stands in contrast to a child with a single, isolated hamartomatous polyp who does not demonstrate cancer risk.[158] JP is inherited as an autosomal dominant trait due to mutations in one of three genes: *SMAD4/MAD4H*, *BMPR1A1*, or rarely *PTEN*.[159,160] Genetic testing for mutations in these three genes is available clinically, although a significant percentage of JP patients still do not have an underlying mutation identified.[159]

Surveillance recommendations for JP include annual complete blood cell count (to detect anemia due to GI blood loss) and semiannual colonoscopy. Prophylactic colectomy is *not* recommended because the risk of colorectal cancer is lower than that seen in FAP. Thus, it is very important to distinguish patients with JP from those with FAP. In addition,

there are a group of *SMAD4* families with JP that also demonstrate clinical features of hereditary hemorrhagic telangiectasias syndrome and require surveillance for visceral and CNS telangiectasias.[161]

Hereditary Nonpolyposis Colon Cancer

The HNPCC or Lynch syndrome describes families with an increased risk of colon cancer and in the absence of polyposis.[162] Extracolonic malignancies include uterine, ovarian, ureteral, biliary tract, and in the upper GI tract cancers. Malignancies can rarely manifest in the second decade of life, and for families with particularly early onset, screening beginning 5 years before the earliest cancer diagnosis or otherwise screening biannually by colonoscopy is recommended to begin around age 25.[163]

Tumors from patients with HNPCC display an unusual DNA pattern, termed *microsatellite instability*, which was identified as changes (both increases and decreases) in the length of repetitive sequences spread throughout the genome.[164] This pattern suggested that the tumor cell is mismatch repair (MMR) deficient and deleterious mutations in one of four different MMR genes, *MSH2*, *MLH1*, *MSH6*, and *PMS2*, were found to be causative for HNPCC (reviewed by Bocker[164]).

Analysis of 25 children younger than 18 years presenting with colorectal carcinoma demonstrated a pattern of colon and uterine cancer in relatives suggestive of HNPCC.[165] A more recent molecular study of patients in a population-based registry found that for those presenting under age 24, more than 75% had microsatellite instability and 50% of those with available germline DNA have documented HNPCC mutations.[166] Thus, mutation in one of the MMR genes (either heterozygous or biallelic) is the predominant cause of childhood and very young adult onset of colon cancer.

Turcot and Mismatch Repair Deficiency Syndrome

Turcot syndrome was first reported as the unusual finding of multiple pediatric brain tumors in families with polyposis and colon cancer.[167] In one study of 14 Turcot syndrome families, there were mutations in *APC* (10 families) or HNPCC loci (4 families).[168] In the families with APC-related mutations, there were more medulloblastomas (92-fold relative risk compared with the general population), and three families with glioblastoma multiforme had microsatellite instability in their tumor specimens, as did the original family studied by Turcot. Two of these families had detectable mutations in the MMR genes *MLH1* and *PMS2*. Thus, the clinical phenotype of these disorders should be enlarged to include pediatric brain tumors. Conversely, careful attention should be paid to a history of colon cancer in relatives of pediatric brain tumor patients.

There is also a third form of Turcot syndrome with autosomal recessive inheritance demonstrating childhood onset of brain tumors (predominantly gliomas), hematopoietic cancers with T cell predominance, and colon cancer. The affected children in these families carry biallelic mutations in one of the MMR genes (reviewed by Wimmer and Etzler[169]). The condition is now referred to as *mismatch repair deficiency syndrome* given that biallelic mutations result in the absence of MMR function and genetic instability in all tissues. These children show a neurofibromatosis-like phenotype (*café au lait* spots and axillary freckling) thought to be due to somatic mutations in the *NF1* gene.[170] Clearly, the identification of this syndrome highlights the need for a careful skin examination in children being diagnosed with gliomas and T cell leukemia/ lymphoma. If molecular testing confirms the diagnosis of MMR deficiency, then surveillance by colonoscopy should begin in early childhood.

TABLE 2.5

DIAGNOSTIC CRITERIA FOR NEUROFIBROMATOSIS TYPE 1 (NF1)

The diagnosis is confirmed if the patient has two or more of the following features:
Six or more café-au-lait spots
  1.5 cm or larger in postpubertal individuals
  0.5 cm or larger in prepubertal individuals
Two or more neurofibromas of any type
One or more plexiform neurofibromas
Freckling of armpits or groin
Optic glioma (tumor of the optic pathway)
Two or more Lisch nodules (benign iris hamartomas)
A distinctive bony lesion
  Dysplasia of the sphenoid bone
  Dysplasia or thinning of long bone cortex
First-degree relative with NF1

From Gutmann DH, Aylsworth A, Carey JC, et al. The diagnostic evaluation and multidisciplinary management of neurofibromatosis 1 and neurofibromatosis 2. JAMA 1997;278:51–57, with permission.

The Phakomatoses

The word *phakomatosis* refers to multiple phacomas (Greek for tumor of the lens) and mato (Greek for spot or spotty) that refers to the patchy nature of these disorders. Although these disorders share many features of the other autosomal dominant disorders, their frequency in the pediatric population and their pleomorphic symptoms deserve additional comment.

Neurofibromatosis Type 1. NF1 is one of the most common genetic disorders in the general population (reviewed by Gutmann and colleagues[171]). Approximately 1 in 2,500 people is affected by this disorder. Table 2.5 lists the diagnostic criteria for *NF1* that were formulated at National Institutes of Health conferences in 1988 and 1997.[171] Many of the criteria, including *café au lait* spots, axillary freckling, and neurofibromas, are detectable by general physical examination. Lisch nodules of the iris, which do not impact vision, are particularly useful in diagnosing NF1 in older children and adults. A careful slit lamp examination reveals Lisch nodules in more than 80% of adults older than 20 years with NF1.[172]

The hallmark of NF1 is the development of benign tumors, including peripheral neurofibromas, plexiform neurofibromas, gliomas of the optic tract, other low-grade gliomas, and pheochromocytomas. The peripheral neurofibromas often do not begin to develop until adolescence and rarely cause significant cosmetic problems until adulthood.[173] In contrast, plexiform neurofibromas are believed to be congenital in nature and can develop within the first few years of life.[174] Plexiform neurofibromas develop most commonly in the craniofacial and paraspinous regions, mediastinum, and retroperitoneum.[173,175] They are deep masses that can be covered by hyperpigmented skin. They can be invasive and can cause significant disability, depending on the structures they invade. Malignant transformation of a plexiform neurofibroma is discussed later. There is no satisfactory treatment for plexiform neurofibromas; partial resection is used if they become too disabling or invade the spinal tract. Clinical studies to determine the efficacy of farnesyl transferase inhibitors in the treatment of plexiform neurofibroma are under way (reviewed by Widemann[176]). Studies of a mouse model of plexiform neurofibromas revealed infiltration of activated mast cells that are sensitive to inhibitors of the c-Kit pathway, such as imatinib.[177,178] Trials of imatinib in patients with NF1 and symptomatic plexiform neurofibromas are under way.

Development of gliomas, especially involving the optic tract, is frequent in young children with NF1. Approximately 15% to 20% of children with NF1 have some optic tract involvement when assayed by MRI or computed tomography scanning.[179] About one-third of these children have lesions that grow large enough to interfere with vision. Conversely, a large percentage (30%–70%) of children with a new finding of optic glioma have NF1.[180] Because of the difficulty in detecting visual changes in young children, MRI of the brain and optic pathway is often performed for a young child with NF1.[181] However, performing scans in asymptomatic children is controversial.[182] If a child does not show any sign of optic pathway involvement by age 6, the prognosis for lack of eye involvement is excellent.[183] Treatment of enlarging optic tract gliomas is described in subsequent chapters. Although treatment guidelines are controversial for patients with NF1, several large series demonstrate that NF1-associated optic gliomas have a more favorable course over long-term follow-up.[184] Children with NF1 are more likely to demonstrate cerebrovascular dysplasia, which should be taken into account when making treatment decisions.[185]

Gliomas can also develop in other parts of the CNS, ranging from very low-grade to high-grade tumors. Indications for imaging include change in headache pattern, seizures, and new neurologic deficits. In several small studies, the presence of an optic glioma in childhood may predispose the person to the later development of other gliomas.[186]

Because NF1 is a common disease, cases of NF1 and malignancy are likely to happen coincidentally. The clearest associations between NF1 and pediatric malignancies are the increased risk of optic gliomas and malignant peripheral nerve sheath tumors (MPNST).[187,188] A large population study of 26,084 children younger than 15 years from Japan revealed a 6- to 8-fold increased incidence of cancer, in particular, gliomas, MPNST, RMSs, and myelogenous leukemia in NF1 patients compared with the non-NF1 patients.[189] In particular, 50% of the patients with MPNST had NF1, a percentage similar to that found in a large Dutch study.[190] In one study, survival among patients with NF1 and MPNST was worse than those with sporadic tumors (33% and 63%, respectively).[191]

The likelihood of a child with NF1 developing MPNST has varied among series with a population-based study from the United Kingdom, demonstrating as high as 8% to 13% lifetime risk.[192] For this reason, physicians, parents, and patients should be particularly concerned and seek prompt evaluation for malignant transformation in a NF1 patient with a plexiform neurofibroma that demonstrates a significant change in growth rate or pain. Although less common than children with MPNST, children with NF1 also have an increased risk of developing GI stromal tumors.[193]

Children with NF1 have an increased risk of several myelogenous disorders, including AML and MDS.[194,195] Moreover, bone marrow from children with NF1 and malignant myeloid disorders shows a loss of the normal *NF1* gene in the malignant cells.[196] Thus, *NF1* appears to be a tumor suppressor gene with regard to malignant myeloid disease.

The gene *NF1*, found at 17q11.2, is a large gene with mutations spread throughout.[197] The *NF1* gene encodes a protein, neurofibronin, which is homologous to the GTPase-activating protein called Gap. This relationship suggests that the NF1 protein normally inhibits the activity of the Ras protein (an oncogene). NF1 follows the two-hit hypothesis in that tumors associated with *NF1*, such as pheochromocytomas,[187,198] show a loss of the remaining normal copy of the *NF1* gene.

Practical molecular testing for *NF1* mutations with detection of more than 95% of NF1 patients is now available clinically.[197] Because of the high *de novo* mutation rate in NF1, most individuals have different mutations, called *private mutations*, scattered throughout a very large gene. Although most patients are diagnosed on the basis of clinical criteria (Table 2.5), molecular testing is useful in some clinical situations. The first is affected adults requesting prenatal diagnosis, which requires knowing their specific mutation. The second is apparently unaffected parents of affected children who are concerned about recurrence risk. Documenting a negative mutation in the parents lowers their risk of having a second child with NF1, although negative skin and eye examinations can already make this likelihood low. A third clinical scenario relevant to pediatricians is a child with a negative family history and multiple *café au lait* spots with or without axillary freckling. The majority of these children will eventually be diagnosed with NF1. However, several groups have recently identified that mutations in *SPRED1* result in Legius syndrome, which demonstrates clinical overlap with NF1, including *café au lait* spots with variable expression of axillary freckling, macrocephaly, and learning disabilities.[199,200] Importantly, these individuals do not demonstrate neurofibromas or CNS tumors. Thus, molecular confirmation of the diagnosis of NF1 versus Legius syndrome by genetic testing is recommended in children with *café au lait* spots and axillary freckling as their only diagnostic criterion. A positive molecular diagnostic study provides the correct diagnosis and the appropriate surveillance.

Neurofibromatosis Type 2

Neurofibromatosis type 2 (NF2) represents a distinct and much rarer disorder than NF1. Because most of the manifestations of NF2 occur in adulthood, they are not discussed in detail here. NF2 is characterized by *café au lait* spots, bilateral vestibular schwannomas, central neurofibromas, and meningiomas (reviewed by Gutmann et al[172]). The disease has a high degree of morbidity and is difficult to treat because of the multiple tumors that develop. Treatment modalities include microsurgery, radiosurgery, and radiation therapy. The gene that is mutated in NF2, also called *NF2*, is found on chromosome 22 and encodes a protein, called *merlin* or *schwannomin*, that is homologous to the band 4.1 protein and appears to play a role in cytoskeletal architecture.[201]

Tuberous Sclerosis Complex

Tuberous sclerosis complex (TSC) is diagnosed clinically on the basis of the characteristic features including benign and neoplastic growths. The classic triad of seizures, mental retardation, and facial angiofibromas (previously called *acne sebaceum*) occur in fewer than 50% of patients with TSC.[202] There is a wide range of phenotypes between and within families, with some adults with TSC having very high degrees of intelligence. Two-thirds of patients are affected due to *de novo* mutations and thus do not have a family history of the disease. Part of the clinical heterogeneity results from the underlying genetic heterogeneity, with causative mutations in two different genes, *TSC1* and *TSC2*, both of which acts as a tumor suppressor gene (reviewed by Kwiatkowski and Manning[203]). *TSC1* is located at chromosome 9q34 and encodes hamartin. *TSC2*, on chromosome 16p13.3, encodes tuberin, which has Rag1-Gap activity. Hamartin and tuberin can physically interact. Thus, the protein products of genes mutated in both NF1 and TSC participate in the regulation of Ras or Ras-related GTPase activity, which may respond to inhibitors of the mTor pathway including rapamycin.[203] A comprehensive analysis of mutations in *TSC1* and *TSC2* in 150 TSC patients revealed 120 mutations, 22 in *TSC1* and 98 in *TSC2*.[204] The majority of *TSC1* mutations are truncating, while for *TSC2*, there are both missense mutations in conserved domains and truncating mutations. Clinically, the degree of mental disability was greater for patients with *TSC2* mutations (67% vs. 31%). It is also not unusual for the first person in the family with TSC to have a milder phenotype due to mosaicism for a TSC mutation. The offspring of this individual may be more severely affected as the child will inherit the mutation in all somatic cells.[205]

TSC is characterized by the growth of normally benign tumors in several different organs. Cardiac rhabdomyomas normally develop *in utero* and are often detected during prenatal ultrasound. The morbidity and mortality associated with these tumors reflect the potential for flow abnormalities in the heart if these tumors grow large enough. They typically regress postnatally and become clinically insignificant.[206] In one study, 50% of children with cardiac rhabdomyomas developed clinical criteria for TSC during childhood.[207]

Later in childhood and early adulthood, individuals with TSC are at risk for the development of giant cell astrocytomas.[202] During adulthood, there is often the slow growth of renal angiomyolipomas. In the British population-based study of childhood cancer,[1] TSC was found to be significantly overrepresented due to an increased risk of brain tumors and RMSs.[208] The TSC consensus conference made specific recommendations for the diagnosis and surveillance of children with TSC including periodic MRI of the brain and renal ultrasounds.[209]

Nevus Basal Cell Carcinoma Syndrome or Gorlin-Goltz Syndrome

Gorlin and Goltz described a number of individuals who had multiple nevoid basal cell epithelioma, odontogenic jaw cysts, and bifid ribs, with the syndrome being inherited in an autosomal dominant fashion.[210] Gorlin-Goltz syndrome or Nevus basal cell carcinoma syndrome (NBCCS) includes the aforementioned features and characteristic palmar and plantar pits, mild facial dysmorphisms including frontal and biparietal bossing, calcification of the falx cerebri, and short fourth metacarpal bones (reviewed by Gorlin[211]). Careful clinical examination and radiographs of ribs, skull, and spine are often sufficient to make the diagnosis. The basal cell carcinomas (BCCs) develop around the time of puberty and can eventually number in the hundreds. There are differences in the number of BCCs in different racial groups, with significantly fewer found in individuals of African American descent.[212] It is estimated that 29% of individuals with a BCC under age 18 have NBCCS syndrome.

Medulloblastoma is a significant feature of NBCCS. Analysis of 105 patients with NBCCS evaluated at National Institutes of Health found four children with the diagnosis of medulloblastoma diagnosed at a mean age of 2.3 years.[212] Conversely, it is estimated that approximately 10% of patients with medulloblastoma diagnosed at age 2 years or under have NBCCS.[213] Because of the high frequency of medulloblastoma, children with NBCCS are recommended to have biannual neurologic examinations and annual MRI examinations up to age 7 for early detection of medulloblastoma.[212] Examination of the parents of medulloblastoma patients may aid in identifying NBCCS in the family.

In children receiving radiation therapy, the skin within the field can become severely affected with hundreds of nevi and BCCs with a latency of approximately 5 years.[212] There have also been reports of secondary meningiomas and ependymomas in the radiation-exposed field of children with NBCCS.[212,214] Thus, use of radiation therapy for treatment of tumors in NBCCS syndrome should be limited when possible.

The gene for NBCCS syndrome, *PTCH*, encodes a homologue of the *Drosophila melanogaster* segment polarity gene.[215,216] Mutations in *PTCH* are found in the majority of NBCCS families and in a large percentage of sporadic BCCs, making it one of the most frequently mutated genes in human cancers.[217] In contrast, analysis of sporadic medulloblastomas has identified *PTCH* mutations in only approximately 10% of cases and rare mutations in other members of the same pathway.[218] Mutations in the *SUFU* gene, another member of the *PTCH* pathway, underlay familial medulloblastomas in the absence or presence of other features of NBCCS.[219,220]

Von Hippel-Lindau Disease

The hallmark of von Hippel-Lindau (VHL) disease is the development of multiple benign and highly malignant tumors in the absence of specific dermatologic or developmental abnormalities. Diagnosis typically occurs during second or third decade, when tumors become clinically apparent. VHL disease is characterized by four common tumor types: cerebellar hemangioblastomas, retinal angiomas, renal cell carcinoma, and pheochromocytomas.[221] Affected individuals also have increased rates of pancreatic carcinoma, epididymal cysts, and endolymphatic sac tumors (ELSTs), which can result in hearing loss.[222] The two leading causes of early mortality are cerebellar lesions and renal cell carcinomas.[221]

The retinal and cerebellar lesions typically develop during the second and third decade of life although they can occur in the first decade and should prompt genetic and clinical evaluation for VHL-associated tumors.[223,224] MRI of both the brain and the spinal cord can reveal the presence of isolated or multiple lesions with signal intensities characteristic of a hemangioblastoma. Multiple cerebellar hemangioblastomas or a first-degree relative with VHL disease and an isolated lesion is sufficient for the diagnosis of VHL disease.

VHL disease is classified into subcategories, depending on the patients' likelihood of developing pheochromocytoma. Type 1 patients have a low risk of developing pheochromocytoma but a high risk of developing RCC. Type 2 patients have a high risk of developing pheochromocytoma, with type 2A patients having an additional lower risk of developing RCC, whereas type 2B patients possess a high risk of developing clear cell RCC. Types 1, 2A, and 2B patients also develop cerebellar and retinal hemangioblastomas. Type 2C patients develop only pheochromocytoma (reviewed by Lonser[221]).

Retinal angiomas can often be asymptomatic and diagnosed on yearly dilated eye examinations. If sufficient in size, they can manifest with new visual defects. Treatment of the retinal lesions at an early stage can yield excellent long-term results.[223] Renal cysts accompanied by renal cell carcinoma are one of the hallmarks of the VHL syndrome. The tumors often develop in the third or fourth decade, but the risk of renal cell carcinoma is lifelong.[225] It is necessary to balance curative intent, tumor removal, maintenance of renal function, potential for transplantation, and the knowledge that the patient is likely to develop other tumors when creating a treatment plan.[221] In particular, the approach to renal cell carcinoma with the avoidance of nephrectomy in VHL patients is designed to preserve as much renal function as possible.[225]

Pheochromocytoma as part of VHL disease can be singular or multiple and may be benign or malignant. They are most likely diagnosed in the second or third decade but can present earlier, and screening for pheochromocytoma is recommended to begin from age 2.

Given the predilection in VHL disease to develop a specific group of tumors, several comprehensive screening protocols have been developed (www.vhl.org).[221,226] The important features are annual surveillance examinations for renal masses, pheochromocytoma, and retinal angiomas, with biannual examination for cerebellar lesions. Screening for pheochromocytoma is improved by use of plasma metanephrines[227] as opposed to urine catecholamines. Any change in hearing or balance or tinnitus should prompt evaluation for an ELST, including computed tomography imaging of the inner auditory canal.[222]

The *VHL* gene, at chromosome 3q25, was cloned in 1994 by using positional methods.[228] The Type 2 VHL families with pheochromocytoma risk tend to have clustering of missense mutations in specific codons.[229] DNA diagnostic assays have been optimized such that more than 98% of patients with VHL disease have a detectable mutation in the *VHL* gene.[230] Testing is used to identify relatives who have not inherited a *VHL* mutation and do not require a surveillance protocol and those who have inherited the mutation and need full screening prior to development of malignancy.

The VHL protein is part of an E3 ubiquitin ligase complex that targets a hypoxia-inducible transcription factor (HIF1α) for ubiquitin-mediated destruction selectively in the presence of oxygen.[231,232] The loss of VHL function results in the overexpression of genes required for angiogenesis under normal oxygen conditions. This has led to clinical trials of thalidomide and antiangiogenesis agents to inhibit tumor growth in patients with VHL.[233,234]

Pheochromocytomas and Paragangliomas

Benign and malignant pheochromocytomas can cause significant morbidity due to the secretion of active catecholamines including norepinephrine, epinephrines, and metanephrines. They typically present in adulthood but can be seen in children, particularly when associated with a genetic predisposition syndrome. As described in this chapter, inherited syndromes associated with a significant risk of pheochromocytoma include VHL, NF1, and MEN2. Extensive mutation analysis of the *RET* and *VHL* genes in case series of patients with pheochromocytoma (both adults and children) suggested that 20% to 30% of patients carry a constitutional mutation in one of these genes.[235] More recent analyses that include *VHL*, *RET*, *SDHD*, and *SDHB* genes (described later) further confirm a high prevalence of 30% to 40% of constitutional mutations.[6,236] Therefore, it is recommended that all patients with pheochromocytoma or paraganglioma should have a genetic evaluation including testing to determine the patient's risk for other tumors (including recurrent pheochromocytoma) and to identify other family members who may be at risk for pheochromocytoma and associated cancers.

Familial Paraganglioma

Paragangliomas arise from chemoreceptor organs distributed throughout the body and are referred to as *glomus tumors*, *chemodectomas*, and *carotid body tumors*. Familial paragangliomas may occur either unilaterally or bilaterally and are transmitted with autosomal dominant inheritance with incomplete penetrance and both intra- and inter-familial variability.[237] Four loci, initially named *PGL1-4*, have been linked to hereditary paraganglioma. Three of the genes, *SDHD (PGL1)*, *SDHC (PGL3)*, and *SDHB (PGL4)* encode subunits of the mitochondrial enzyme II complex (succinate dehydrogenase).[237] This enzyme complex plays a key role in the oxygen-sensing system of paraganglionic tissue.[238] For example, chronic hypoxic stimulation at high altitude has a modifying effect on the development of carotid body paragangliomas due to *SDHD* mutations.[239] Interestingly, even though the SDH genes all function to encode succinate dehydrogenase subunits, only SDHD[237] demonstrates maternal imprinting such that children who inherit a *SDHD* mutation from their father but not from their mother develop paragangliomas. Germline mutations in SDH genes account for 6% and 9% of apparently sporadic paraganglioma and pheochromocytomas, respectively, 29% of pediatric cases, 38% of malignant tumors, and more than 80% of familial aggregations of these tumors.[237] Mutations in one family in the recently identified *SDH5* gene indicate that more genes may yet be implicated in this broad cancer phenotype.[240] Mutations in *SDHD* primarily predispose to mostly benign head and neck paragangliomas[238] and mutations in *SDHB* predispose to abdominal paragangliomas (pheochromocytomas) that may be malignant.[241] The complex inheritance pattern associated with imprinted disorders mandate that genetic evaluation and recurrence risk estimates be performed by a clinician with experience interpreting this pattern of inheritance.

AUTOSOMAL RECESSIVE DISORDERS

This last category of genetic disorders that predispose to cancer has distinct characteristics when compared with the autosomal dominant disorders. Autosomal recessive disorders are much rarer in the general population. Specific ethnic or geographic groups may have an increased risk of autosomal recessive disorders because of a founder effect or increased prevalence of consanguinity. Given the requirement for two mutant alleles, these disorders normally occur in sibships and are not evident in multiple generations. Within a sibship, there is only a one in four chance that a sibling will have the disorder. For this reason, single affected individuals from a small family may appear to be a sporadic case and physicians should not discount the potential for an autosomal recessive condition in a child with a negative family history. Even more complicated, some genetic disorders such as dyskeratosis congenita (associated with bone marrow failure in childhood and adolescent or early adult onset of cancer) can be inherited as autosomal dominant, autosomal recessive, or X-linked disorder, depending on the underlying gene involved.[242]

Generally, the range of expressivity in an autosomal recessive disease may be more limited and the symptoms often more severe than in autosomal dominant disorders. Most of these disorders manifest in childhood, presumably because of the severe nature of the genetic defect. Many of the autosomal recessive

cancer syndromes are caused by mutations in genes that encode DNA repair enzymes or DNA damage checkpoint genes, and they are often referred to as *chromosome breakage syndromes* or *chromosome instability syndromes*. These deficiencies result in increased sensitivity to spontaneous and exogenous DNA damage, which may impact treatment decisions. Significant progress has been made identifying the genes mutated in these disorders. We describe three classes of autosomal recessive disorders later as examples of the severe early-onset presentation and multiple different clinical features of this group of disorders.

Xeroderma Pigmentosum, Cockayne Syndrome, and Trichothiodystrophy

Xeroderma pigmentosum (XP) represents the classic DNA repair defect syndrome. The clinical features of this disorder have been extensively reviewed by Kraemer and colleagues.[243,244] Patients present with cutaneous sensitivity, as revealed by photosensitivity, telangiectasias, and freckling in the first few years of life. Ocular abnormalities are common and are found in ultraviolet light–exposed areas of the cornea, lids, and conjunctivas, including corneal clouding and ocular malignancies. There is a several thousandfold increased risk of basal and squamous cell skin carcinomas in sun-exposed areas, which begin developing around 8 years of age (Fig. 2.4), compared with around the age of 50 for the general U.S. population. There is also a significant increase in melanoma (approximately 5% lifetime risk), and significant but smaller increase in the risk of internal malignancies has also been observed for XP patients.[243]

At the cellular level, the ultraviolet sensitivity in XP patients was found to result from defects in excision repair.[245] This form of repair is essential for repair of the thymine dimers and other structures that results from ultraviolet damage. XP is a group of disorders caused by mutations in at least seven different genes.[246] The determination that multiple genes caused the same clinical disorder was based on complementation assays, in which fibroblasts from different patients are fused together and the heterokaryon cell is then assayed for complementation of the repair defect (reviewed in Bootsma and Hoeijmakers[247]).

Some XP patients have neurologic abnormalities. One group, first reported by DeSanctis and Cacchione,[248] has XP-like dermatologic features and progressive neurologic degeneration beginning around the age of 2 years and accompanied by immature sexual development.[248] These patients tend to cluster in complementation group A. Overall, Kraemer and colleagues[244] found that 18% of reported XP patients had neuro-

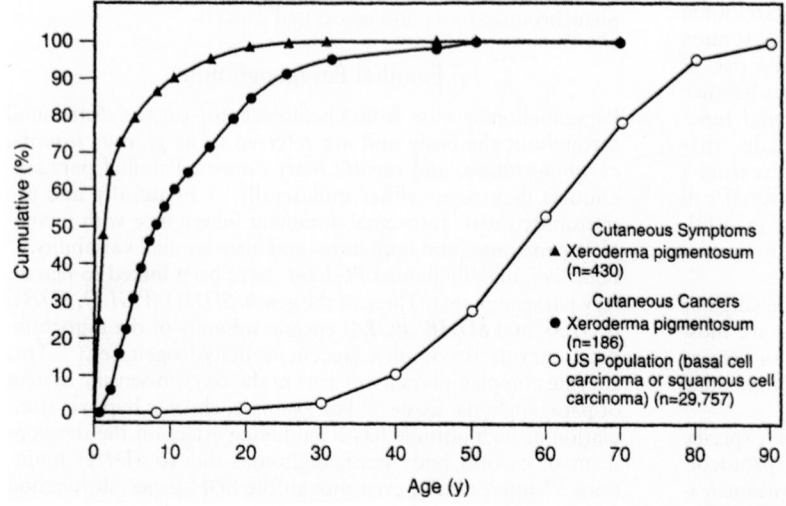

FIGURE 2.4 Age of onset of xeroderma pigmentosum symptoms. The ages at onset of cutaneous symptoms (generally sun sensitivity or pigmentation) was reported for 430 patients. The age at diagnosis of the first skin cancer was reported for 186 patients and is compared with distribution for 29,757 patients with basal cell carcinoma and squamous cell carcinoma in the U.S. general population. (From Kraemer, Myung L, Scotto J. Xeroderma pigmentosum. Arch Dermol 1987;123:241, with permission.)

logic abnormalities, some of which resemble the DeSanctis-Cacchione syndrome and others that have a later onset of neurologic difficulties and that cluster in complementation group D.

Two other disorders can manifest with findings of XP. Trichothiodystrophy (TTD) is a rare disorder that shares an increased risk of skin cancer and repair defects and the findings of brittle hair and ichthyosis. The XP/TTD patients fall in the XP complementation group D.[246] Cockayne syndrome shares some of the ultraviolet hypersensitivity of XP but is also characterized by neurologic deficits, including developmental delay without skin cancer risk. There are at least three complementation groups for Cockayne syndrome.[249]

Utilizing the specific biochemical defects in cells from patients with either XP or Cockayne syndrome, almost all of the genes responsible for this condition have been cloned (reviewed by Cleaver and colleagues[250]). In a normal cell, DNA damage in actively transcribed genes is preferentially repaired before DNA from inactive parts of the genome, a process termed *transcription-coupled repair* (TCR). Cells from patients with Cockayne syndrome are deficient in TCR due to a mutation in the *ERCC2* DNA helicase, which is also a component of active transcription complex TFIIH. The fact that global repair rates are normal in Cockayne cells may explain the lack of cancer predisposition.

A third group of patients who clinically demonstrate ultraviolet sensitivity but have normal nucleotide excision repair *in vitro* are termed *XP^v*. This disorder is due to mutation of a specialized DNA polymerase, polymerase eta, which places two adenine residues opposite a thymine dimer photoproduct, thus restoring the normal base sequence.[251,252]

The Helicase Disorders: Bloom, Werner, and Rothmund-Thomson Syndromes

Three autosomal recessive disorders, although distinct, share some clinical features including a predisposition to malignancy (Table 2.6). Children with Bloom syndrome are very small at birth and remain small[253] and have a photosensitive rash, immunodeficiency, and a very high predisposition to develop a wide variety of malignancies including leukemias/lymphomas and solid tumors.[254] This disorder is more common in children of Ashkenazi descent. Cells from these patients exhibit increased recombination manifested as increased sister chromatid exchange. Werner syndrome is characterized by prema-

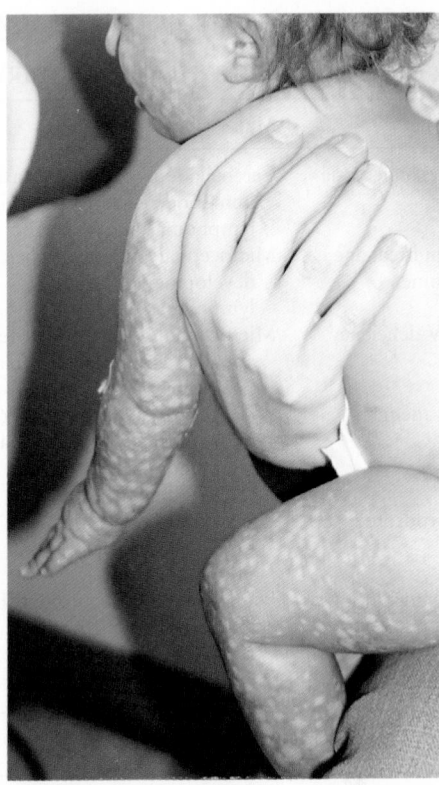

FIGURE 2.5 Poikiloderma rash in Rothmund-Thomson syndrome. Shown is the typical poikilodermatous rash, which begins on the cheeks and spreads to the extremities, sparing the trunk of a child with RTS who carries two deleterious mutations in the *RECQL4* gene. (Photograph courtesy of L.L. Wang, MD, Baylor College of Medicine/Texas Children's Hospital.)

ture aging (including early-onset atherosclerosis, diabetes, and cataracts beginning in the second decade) with increased incidence of soft tissue sarcomas.[255] The premature aging is manifested at a cellular level as early senescence in fibroblasts from these patients. The third disorder in this group, Rothmund-Thomson syndrome (RTS), is characterized by a very distinct rash termed *poikiloderma* (Fig. 2.5), which begins in infancy, and skeletal dysplasias including radial ray abnormalities and

---

TABLE 2.6

FEATURES OF THE CHROMOSOME INSTABILITY SYNDROMES DUE TO MUTATIONS IN GENES ENCODING RECQ HELICASES

Syndrome	Clinical features	Cancer predisposition	Gene/chromosome location
Bloom	Small stature, photosensitive rash, immunodeficiency	Multiple tumor types including leukemia/lymphoma and solid tumors	*BLM* 15q26.1
Werner	Premature ageing, cataracts, diabetes, atherosclerosis	Soft tissue sarcomas and skin cancers	*WRN* 8p11
Rothmund-Thomson	Poikiloderma rash, radial ray defects, cataracts	Osteosarcoma and skin cancers	*RECQL4* 8q24.3[a]

[a]Although *BLM* and *WRN* are the genes mutated in the majority of Bloom and Werner syndrome patients, respectively, approximately 60% of patients with Rothmund-Thomson syndrome carry mutations in the *RECQL4* gene. The risk of osteosarcoma is found in the subset of patients with *RECQL4* mutations.
From Wang LL, Gannavarapu A, Kozinetz CA, et al. Association between osteosarcoma and deleterious mutations in the RECQL4 gene in Rothmund-Thomson syndrome. J Natl Cancer Inst 2003;95:669–674.

CANCER GENETIC DISORDERS THAT REQUIRE MODIFIED TREATMENT REGIMENS

Condition	Major clinical features	Diagnostic test	Treatment requiring adjustment
Ataxia-telangiectasia	Cerebella ataxia, telangiectasias, immunodeficiency, leukemias, lymphomas and solid tumors	Increased α-fetoprotein, sensitivity to ionizing radiation	Radiation therapy, chemotherapeutic agents that produce double strand breaks
Nijmegen breakage syndrome	Microcephaly, immunodeficiency, developmental delay, lymphomas	Sensitivity to ionizing radiation, Polish founder mutation in NBS1	Radiation therapy, chemotherapeutic agents that produce double strand breaks
Ligase IV deficiency	Microcephaly, immunodeficiency, anemia, developmental delay, lymphomas	Sensitivity to ionizing radiation	Radiation therapy, chemotherapeutic agents that produce double strand breaks
Fanconi anemia	Bone marrow failure, radial ray anomalies, microphthalmia, renal anomalies, bronzing of the skin	Chromosome breakage assay after exposure to diepoxybutane	Specialized conditioning regimen prior to bone marrow transplant, sensitivity to cross-linking agents
Bloom syndrome	Short stature, butterfly rash on face, GI intolerance, immunodeficiency	Increased sister chromatid exchange	Some evidence for increased toxicity to chemotherapeutic agents
Gorlin syndrome	Palmar pits, calcification of the falx, odontogenic cysts, basal cell carcinomas, medulloblastoma	Mutation analysis of the *PTCH* gene	Radiation therapy causes development of large numbers of BCC in radiation field

GI, gastrointestinal; BCC, basal cell carcinoma.

cataracts. Children with RTS have a distinct predisposition to the development of osteosarcoma and less frequently skin cancers.[256] Osteosarcoma occurring in individuals with RTS has a similar histologic spectrum and treatment response as that seen in the general population.[257]

All three disorders have been shown to be the result of mutations in RecQ helicase genes which are conserved to bacteria: the *BLM* gene in Bloom syndrome,[258] the *WRN* gene in Werner syndrome,[259] and the *RECQL4* gene in a subset of patients with RTS.[260] Analysis of *RECQL4* mutations in a cohort of RTS patients reveals that there are two types of RTSs. Type 1 RTS (approximately 30% of patients) is not associated with *RECQL4* mutations and does not appear to have an increased risk of osteosarcoma. Type 2 RTS is associated with deleterious mutations in *RECQL4*, with skeletal abnormalities, and with significant osteosarcoma risk.[261,262] Genetic testing for *RECQL4* mutations is now clinically available and will identify those RTS patients at increased risk for developing osteosarcoma.

Ataxia-Telangiectasia

Children with ataxia-telangiectasia (AT) develop ataxia during early years of childhood, with truncal ataxia appearing before appendicular ataxia and eventually requiring a wheelchair for mobility (reviewed by Gatti and colleagues[263]). Choreoathetosis and ocular motor apraxia are also common neurologic findings. Intelligence does not appear to be affected. The oculocutaneous telangiectasias normally begin with the conjunctivas and develop between the ages of 3 and 5 years. Useful biochemical markers for diagnosis include elevated AFP and carcinoembryonic antigen in children with AT.[264]

There is a very high rate of malignancy, particularly the development of leukemias and lymphomas,[265] in AT children. Individuals with AT have immunodeficiency characterized by diminished immunoglobulin G2 and A levels and increased risk of sinopulmonary infections. The major causes of mortality of those with this syndrome are sinopulmonary infection

(especially after significant neurologic degeneration) and malignancy (reviewed by Gatti and colleagues[263]).

In addition to the risk of cancer in the AT homozygous children, heterozygotes carrying one AT mutation appear to have approximately a twofold increased risk of breast cancer.[266] Mothers of children with ATM (a gene mutated in AT) should be advised of this moderate increased risk of breast cancer.

Fibroblasts and lymphocytes from AT patients have multiple cellular defects including increased sensitivity to DNA-damaging agents, particularly ionizing radiation due to defects in DNA repair and cell cycle checkpoints (reviewed by Shiloh[267]). The gene mutated in AT (called *ATM*) was cloned in 1995.[268] After DNA damage, the ATM protein signals through the p53 and BRCA1 tumor suppressor gene products.[269] The finding of ATM in the same molecular pathway as other breast cancer genes further substantiates the epidemiologic data with regard to breast cancer predisposition in heterozygotes.

Children with AT have significantly increased sensitivity to chemotherapy and radiation treatments. Specific treatment regimens have been developed for these children.[270] Specialized clinical centers that are familiar with recommended regimens for these unique children are available through the support of the A-T Children's Project (www.atcp.org). Table 2.7 provides a list of cancer susceptibility syndromes for which alteration in cancer treatment regimen needs to be considered.

ISSUES IN GENETIC TESTING FOR THE PEDIATRIC ONCOLOGY PATIENT

Several studies have suggested that 4% to 10% of childhood cancers result from inherited genetic mutations, making it essential for pediatricians and pediatric oncologists to recognize clinical criteria suggestive of familial cancer syndromes.[1,271] Table 2.8 includes the cancer diagnoses that are frequently the result of genetic susceptibility for which genetics

TABLE 2.8

CANCER DIAGNOSES THAT MERIT A GENETICS EVALUATION INDEPENDENT OF FAMILY HISTORY

Diagnosis	Genetic loci
Retinoblastoma	*RB1*
Adrenocortical carcinoma	*P53*
Pheochromocytoma/paraganglioma	*VHL, NF1, RET, SDHB, SDHD*
Retinal or cerebellar hemangioblastoma	*VHL*
Endolymphatic sac tumors	*VHL*
Hepatoblastoma/desmoid tumors	*APC*
Optic pathway tumor	*NF1*
Medullary thyroid cancer	*RET*
Atypical teratoid and malignant rhabdoid tumor	*SMARCB1/INI1/SNF5*
Acoustic or vestibular schwannomas	*NF2 [F 36] [F 37]*

evaluation should be considered regardless of family history. In addition, as discussed in this chapter, an accurate diagnosis requires an accurate and detailed family history, including all cancers and the age at which they are diagnosed. This is because many cancer predisposition syndromes lack an associated recognized phenotype to identify at-risk individuals. For example, although hemihypertrophy and other features of BWS raise the clinician's alertness to embryonal cancer risk, no known physical features are associated with LFS. It is increasingly important for the pediatric oncologist to recognize that children are part of a network of family members who may be indirectly affected by genetic diagnosis and testing.

In the practice of pediatrics, DNA-based tests for a large number of noncancer conditions, including cystic fibrosis, muscular dystrophy, and hemophilia, have been developed and are currently in use. It has been recommended that as children grow and acquire cognitive and moral skills, they should be permitted to participate in decisions concerning testing.[272] For genetic testing for conditions associated with childhood onset cancers, it is generally accepted that cancer predisposition testing is most helpful for highly penetrant diseases in which individuals at risk for cancer can be identified and followed closely for the development of highly specific tumors,[273] for example, VHL, FAP, and MEN2. For each of these, clear guidelines for clinical surveillance or prophylactic medical interventions in childhood have been established for mutation carriers as discussed in this chapter.

However, for a variety of other cancer-predisposition disorders, the clinical management of carriers is less well defined. Such diseases include LFS. Although predisposition testing may identify asymptomatic carriers, and allow institution of preventive or surveillance programs where available, such testing is associated with the following caveats that must be taken into consideration: (a) the genetic heterogeneity of cancer predisposition, (b) the technical difficulty inherent to gene testing and to test interpretation, and (c) the pyschosocial impact of testing. Both variable degrees of penetrance and expressivity for many conditions, including LFS, suggest that other genetic events play an important role in defining the particular cancer phenotype of individual members of families.

The technical aspects involved in predisposition gene testing and interpretation are complex. Some tests for rare disorders are available only through participation in research studies where results are made less immediately available and confirmation of results is less well controlled than in clinically certified laboratories. Databases are now available to facilitate identification of clinical and research laboratories performing specific genetic tests, for example, www.genetests.org. Fur-

thermore, such testing, particularly of novel genes, tends to be expensive, with different laboratories performing different assays with extra effort by the physician sometimes required to obtain insurance coverage of testing. Given the complexity, genetic testing should be undertaken only by a physician or genetic counselor aware of different testing options and fully capable of interpreting these results. For example, a significant percentage of physicians ordering a genetic test for FAP incorrectly interpreted a negative result in an affected proband.[274]

Genetic testing for any disease, which should now include cancer, has been demonstrated to have profound psychologic and emotional impact on patients and may be further complicated by relationships with parents and other family members.[275] Issues of the "vulnerable child syndrome" in affected carriers and "survivor guilt" in unaffected, noncarrier siblings raise complex psychosocial concerns that may be beyond the general purview of the pediatric oncologist. Furthermore, lessons from studies in adults have demonstrated that although overall patients learning of their increased risk of disease do well, they may experience feelings of shock, depression, grief, altered self-esteem, or even guilt. Limited studies in children, parents and families have yet to clarify the impact of predictive testing for cancer in children or the appropriate timing of testing with regard to cancer diagnosis.

A recent comprehensive study from France explores the perceptions of two groups of genetic services providers for the usage of prenatal diagnosis and preimplantation genetic diagnosis. As parents from cancer susceptibility families are now routinely discussing these options in planning future pregnancies, the need to engage a multidisciplinary team in these discussions is key to providing parents and families the necessary tools with which to make these ethically challenging decisions.[276–278]

In an attempt to address these issues, guidelines for testing have been established by both the American Society of Human Genetics in a statement and the American Society of Clinical Oncology.[151,279,280] These guidelines form a useful foundation on which to build practical testing parameters as better defined genotype:phenotype correlations are generated. While some studies suggest that the benefits to predictive genetic testing for children are still not substantial, further evaluations from different perspectives will continue to evolve in this field.[281]

Based on many of the aforementioned arguments, a number of recommendations established in 1992 for LFS[282] are still applicable to genetic testing in family cancer syndromes that include children. The quality of information provision on cancer genetics is directly related to the knowledge of professionals and their ability to communicate this to a patient and family regardless of their specialty.[283,284] This requirement exists in the face of a relative lack of in-depth education in genetics in medical schools and postgraduate education, which then place pediatricians and pediatric oncologists in a difficult position of integrating rapidly evolving technologies with patient care and unfamiliar and complex genetic testing issues.[285] This unfamiliarity extends to more recent issues with respect to physicians' duty to warn "third parties" (i.e., members of extended families who may be at risk of avoidable harm from a genetically transmissible condition), and its legal ramifications.[286] Therefore, it is incumbent upon pediatric oncologists without additional training to identify appropriate patients and families for referral to a geneticist or genetic counselor with training in cancer genetics. Recently, the multidisciplinary approach taken by several groups[277,287] involving pediatric oncologists, clinical geneticists, genetic counselors, psychologists, and ethicists in establishing cancer genetics clinics and programs whose primary focus is to serve children with cancer and their families provides an intriguing and novel mechanism to optimize care of these families and advance our understanding of the role of genetics in the etiology of childhood cancer.

References

1. Narod SA, Stiller C, Lenoir GM. An estimate of the heritable fraction of childhood cancer. Br J Cancer 1991;63:993–999.
2. Wagner J, Portwine C, Rabin K, et al. High frequency of germline p53 mutations in childhood adrenocortical cancer. J Natl Cancer Inst 1994;86:1707–1710.
3. Varley JM, McGown G, Thorncroft M, et al. Are there low-penetrance TP53 alleles? Evidence from childhood adrenocortical tumors. Am J Hum Genet 1999;65:995–1006.
4. Rush JA, Younge BR, Campbell RJ, et al. Optic glioma: long-term follow-up of 85 histopathologically verified cases. Ophthalmology 1982;89:1213–1219.
5. Lohmann DR, Gallie BL. Retinoblastoma: revisiting the model prototype of inherited cancer. Am J Med Genet C Semin Med Genet 2004;129C:23–28.
6. Neumann HP, Bausch B, McWhinney SR, et al. Germ-line mutations in nonsyndromic pheochromocytoma. N Engl J Med 2002;346:1459–1466.
7. Biegel JA, Zhou JY, Rorke LB, et al. Germ-line and acquired mutations of INI1 in atypical teratoid and rhabdoid tumors. Cancer Res 1999;59:74–79.
8. Bonaiti-Pellie C, Chompret A, Tournade MF, et al. Genetics and epidemiology of Wilms' tumor: the French Wilms' tumor study. Med Pediatr Oncol 1992;20:284–291.
9. Craft AW, Parker L, Stiller C, et al. Screening for Wilms' tumour in patients with aniridia, Beckwith syndrome, or hemihypertrophy. Med Pediatr Oncol 1995;24:231–234.
10. Gold EB, Leviton A, Lopez R, et al. The role of family history in risk of childhood brain tumors. Cancer 1994;73:1302–1311.
11. Farwell J, Flannery JT. Cancer in relatives of children with central-nervous-system neoplasms. N Engl J Med 1984;311:749–753.
12. Gunz FW, Gunz JP, Veale AMO, et al. Familial leukaemia: a study of 909 families. Scand J Haematol 1975;15:117–131.
13. Rabin KR, Whitlock JA. Malignancy in children with trisomy 21. Oncologist 2009;14:164–173.
14. Hasle H, Clemmensen IH, Mikkelsen M. Risks of leukaemia and solid tumours in individuals with Down's syndrome. Lancet 2000;355:165–169.
15. Avet-Loiseau H, Mechinaud F, Harousseau J-L. Clonal hematologic disorders in Down Syndrome: a review. J Pediatr Hematol Oncol 1995;17:19–24.
16. Lu G, Altman AJ, Benn PA. Review of the cytogenetic changes in acute megakaryoblastic leukemia: one disease or several? Cancer Genet Cytogenet 1993;67:81–89.
17. Homans AC, Verissimo AM, Vlacha V. Transient abnormal myelopoiesis of infancy associated with trisomy 21. Am J Pediatr Hematol Oncol 1993;15:392–399.
18. Luna-Fineman S, Shannon KM, Atwater SK, et al. Myelodysplastic and myeloproliferative disorders of childhood: a study of 167 patients. Blood 1999;93:459–466.
19. Brissette MD, Duval-Arnould BJ, Gordon BG, et al. Acute megakaryoblastic leukemia following transient myeloproliferative disorder in a patient without Down Syndrome. Am J Hematol 1994;47:316–319.
20. Wechsler J, Greene M, McDevitt MA, et al. Acquired mutations in GATA1 in the megakaryoblastic leukemia of Down syndrome. Nat Genet 2002;32:148–152.
21. Gurbuxani S, Vyas P, Crispino JD. Recent insights into the mechanisms of myeloid leukemogenesis in Down syndrome. Blood 2004;103:399–406.
22. Izraeli S. Leukaemia—a developmental perspective. Br J Haematol 2004;126:3–10.
23. Cantor AB, Orkin SH. Transcriptional regulation of erythropoiesis: an affair involving multiple partners. Oncogene 2002;21:3368–3376.
24. Hitzler JK, Cheung J, Li Y, et al. GATA1 mutations in transient leukemia and acute megakaryoblastic leukemia of Down syndrome. Blood 2003;101:4301–4304.
25. Pui C-H, Raimondi SC, Borowitz MJ, et al. Immunophenotypes and karyotypes of leukemic cells in children with Down Syndrome and acute lymphoblastic leukemia. J Clin Oncol 1993;11:1361–1367.
26. Stiller CA, Eatock EM. Patterns of care and survival for children with acute lymphoblastic leukaemia diagnosed between 1980 and 1994. Arch Dis Child 1999;81:202–208.
27. Bercovich D, Ganmore I, Scott LM, et al. Mutations of JAK2 in acute lymphoblastic leukaemias associated with Down's syndrome. Lancet 2008;372:1484–1492.
28. Gaikwad A, Rye CL, Devidas M, et al. Prevalence and clinical correlates of JAK2 mutations in Down syndrome acute lymphoblastic leukaemia. Br J Haematol 2009;144:930–932.
29. Canto P, Kofman-Alfaro S, Jimenez AL, et al. Gonadoblastoma in Turner syndrome patients with nonmosaic 45,X karyotype and Y chromosome sequences. Cancer Genet Cytogenet 2004;150:70–72.
30. Hook EB, Warburton D. The distribution of chromosomal genotypes associated with Turner's syndrome: livebirth prevalence rates and evidence for diminished fetal mortality and severity in genotypes associated with structural X abnormalities or mosaicism. Hum Genet 1983;64:24–27.
31. Lau YF. Gonadoblastoma, testicular and prostate cancers, and the TSPY gene. Am J Hum Genet 1999;64:921–927.
32. Saenger P, Wikland KA, Conway GS, et al. Recommendations for the diagnosis and management of Turner syndrome. J Clin Endocrinol Metab 2001;86:3061–3069.
33. Houk CP, Lee PA. Consensus statement on terminology and management: disorders of sex development. Sex Dev 2008;2:172–180.
34. Chaussain JL, Lemerle J, Roger M, et al. Klinefelter syndrome, tumor, and sexual precocity. J Pediatr 1980;97:607–6609.
35. Bussey KJ, Lawce HJ, Olson SB, et al. Chromosome abnormalities of eighty-one pediatric germ cell tumors: sex-, age-, site-, and histopathology-related differences—a Children's Cancer Group study. Genes Chromosomes Cancer 1999;25:134–146.
36. Hultborn R, Hanson C, Kopf I, et al. Prevalence of Klinefelter's syndrome in male breast cancer patients. Anticancer Res 1997;17:4293–4297.
37. Horsman DE, Pantzar JT, Dill FJ, et al. Klinefelter's syndrome and acute leukemia. Cancer Genet Cytogenet 1987;26:375–376.
38. Stankiewicz P, Beaudet AL. Use of array CGH in the evaluation of dysmorphology, malformations, developmental delay, and idiopathic mental retardation. Curr Opin Genet Dev 2007;17:182–192.
39. George RE, Sanda T, Hanna M, et al. Activating mutations in ALK provide a therapeutic target in neuroblastoma. Nature 2008;455:975–978.
40. Turleau C, de Grouchy J, Chavin-Colin F, et al. Cytogenetic forms of retinoblastoma: their incidence in a survey of 66 patients. Cancer Genet Cytogenet 1985;16:321–334.
41. Shannon RS, Mann JR, Harper E, et al. Wilms's tumour and aniridia: clinical and cytogenetic features. Arch Dis Child 1982;57:685–690.
42. Little M, Holmes G, Walsh P. WT1: what has the last decade told us? Bioessays 1999;21:191–202.
43. Huff V. Genotype/phenotype correlations in Wilms' tumor. Med Pediatr Oncol 1996;27:408–414.
44. Pelletier J, Bruening W, Li FP, et al. WT1 mutations contribute to abnormal genital system development and hereditary Wilms' tumour. Nature 1991;353:431–434.
45. Ton CCT, Hirvonen H, Miwa H, et al. Positional cloning and characterization of a paired box- and homeobox-containing gene from the aniridia region. Cell 1991;67:1059–1074.
46. Chao LY, Huff V, Strong LC, et al. Mutation in the PAX6 gene in twenty patients with aniridia. Hum Mutat 2000;15:332–339.
47. Green DM, Breslow NE, Beckwith JB, et al. Screening of children with hemihypertrophy, aniridia, and Beckwith-Wiedemann syndrome in patients with Wilms tumor: a report from the National Wilms Tumor Study. Med Pediatr Oncol 1993;21:188–192.
48. Choyke PL, Siegel MJ, Craft AW, et al. Screening for Wilms tumor in children with Beckwith-Wiedemann syndrome or idiopathic hemihypertrophy. Med Pediatr Oncol 1999;32:196–200.
49. Breslow NE, Takashima JR, Ritchey ML, et al. Renal failure in the Denys-Drash and Wilms' tumor-aniridia syndromes. Cancer Res 2000;60:4030–4032.
50. Elliott M, Bayly R, Cole T, et al. Clinical features and natural history of Beckwith-Wiedemann syndrome: presentation of 74 new cases. Clin Genet 1994;46:168–174.
51. DeBaun MR, Tucker MA. Risk of cancer during the first four years of life in children from The Beckwith-Wiedemann Syndrome Registry. J Pediatr 1998;132:398–400.
52. Wiedemann HR. Tumours and hemihypertrophy associated with Wiedemann-Beckwith syndrome. Eur J Pediatr 1983;141:129.
53. DeBaun MR, Siegel MJ, Choyke PL. Nephromegaly in infancy and early childhood: a risk factor for Wilms tumor in Beckwith-Wiedemann syndrome. J Pediatr 1998;132:401–404.
54. Weksberg R, Smith AC, Squire J, et al. Beckwith-Wiedemann syndrome demonstrates a role for epigenetic control of normal development. Hum Mol Genet 2003;12(spec no 1):R61–R68.
55. Viljoen D, Ramesar R. Evidence for paternal imprinting in familial Beckwith-Wiedemann syndrome. J Med Genet 1992;29:221–225.
56. Slatter RE, Elliott M, Welham K, et al. Mosaic uniparental disomy in Beckwith-Wiedemann syndrome. J Med Genet 1994;31:749–753.
57. Reik W, Constancia M, Dean W, et al. Igf2 imprinting in development and disease. Int J Dev Biol 2000;44:145–150.
58. Lee MP, DeBaun MR, Mitsuya K, et al. Loss of imprinting of a paternally expressed transcript, with antisense orientation to KVLQT1, occurs frequently in Beckwith-Wiedemann syndrome and is independent of insulin-like growth factor II imprinting. Proc Natl Acad Sci U S A 1999;96:5203–5208.
59. Hatada I, Nabetani A, Morisaki H, et al. New p57KIP2 mutations in Beckwith-Wiedemann syndrome. Hum Genet 1997;100:681–683.
60. Weksberg R, Nishikawa J, Caluseriu O, et al. Tumor development in the Beckwith-Wiedemann syndrome is associated with a variety of constitutional molecular 11p15 alterations including imprinting defects of KCNQ1OT1. Hum Mol Genet 2001;10:2989–3000.
61. DeBaun MR, Niemitz EL, McNeil DE, et al. Epigenetic alterations of H19 and LIT1 distinguish patients with Beckwith-Wiedemann syndrome with cancer and birth defects. Am J Hum Genet 2002;70:604–611.
62. Bliek J, Maas SM, Ruijter JM, et al. Increased tumour risk for BWS patients correlates with aberrant H19 and not KCNQ1OT1 methylation: occurrence of KCNQ1OT1 hypomethylation in familial cases of BWS. Hum Mol Genet 2001;10:467–476.
63. DeBaun MR, Niemitz EL, Feinberg AP. Association of in vitro fertilization with Beckwith-Wiedemann syndrome and epigenetic alterations of LIT1 and H19. Am J Hum Genet 2003;72:156–160.
64. Halliday J, Oke K, Breheny S, et al. Beckwith-Wiedemann syndrome and IVF: a case-control study. Am J Hum Genet 2004;75:526–528.
65. Gomes MV, Huber J, Ferriani RA, et al. Abnormal methylation at the KvDMR1 imprinting control region in clinically normal children conceived by assisted reproductive technologies. Mol Hum Reprod 2009;15:471–477.
66. Rivera MN, Kim WJ, Wells J, et al. An X chromosome gene, WTX, is commonly inactivated in Wilms tumor. Science 2007;315:642–645.
67. Rivera MN, Kim WJ, Wells J, et al. The tumor suppressor WTX shuttles to the nucleus and modulates WT1 activity. Proc Natl Acad Sci U S A 2009;106:8338–8343.

68. Huff V. Wilms tumor genetics: a new, UnX-pected twist to the story. Cancer Cell 2007;11:105–107.
69. Jenkins ZA, van KM, Morgan T, et al. Germline mutations in WTX cause a sclerosing skeletal dysplasia but do not predispose to tumorigenesis. Nat Genet 2009;41:95–100.
70. Huff V. Wilms tumor genetics. Am J Med Genet 1998;79:260–267.
71. Knudson AG Jr. Mutation and cancer: statistical study of retinoblastoma. Proc Natl Acad Sci U S A 1971;68:820–823.
72. Knudson AG Jr, Strong LC. Mutation and cancer: neuroblastoma and pheochromocytoma. Am J Hum Genet 1972;24:514–532.
73. Nicholls EM. Somatic variation and multiple neurofibromatosis. Hum Hered 1969;19:473–479.
74. Musarella MA, Gallie BL. A simplified scheme for genetic counseling in retinoblastoma. J Pediatr Ophthalmol Strabismus 1987;24:124–125.
75. Matsunaga E. Hereditary retinoblastoma: penetrance, expressivity and age of onset. Hum Genet 1976;33:1–15.
76. Schubert EL, Strong LC, Hansen MF. A splicing mutation in RB1 in low penetrance retinoblastoma. Hum Genet 1997;100:557–563.
77. MacCarthy A, Bayne AM, Draper GJ, et al. Non-ocular tumours following retinoblastoma in Great Britain 1951 to 2004. Br J Ophthalmol 2009;93:1159–1162.
78. Fletcher O, Easton D, Anderson K, et al. Lifetime risks of common cancers among retinoblastoma survivors. J Natl Cancer Inst 2004;96:357–363.
79. Yu CL, Tucker MA, Abramson DH, et al. Cause-specific mortality in long-term survivors of retinoblastoma. J Natl Cancer Inst 2009;101:581–591.
80. Kleinerman RA, Tucker MA, Abramson DH, et al. Risk of soft tissue sarcomas by individual subtype in survivors of hereditary retinoblastoma. J Natl Cancer Inst 2007;99:24–31.
81. Friend SH, Bernards R, Rogelj S, et al. A human DNA segment with properties of the gene that predisposes to retinoblastoma and osteosarcoma. Nature 1986;323:643–646.
82. Sippel KC, Fraioli RE, Smith GD, et al. Frequency of somatic and germ-line mosaicism in retinoblastoma: implications for genetic counseling. Am J Hum Genet 1998;62: 610–619.
83. Harbour JW. Overview of RB gene mutations in patients with retinoblastoma: implications for clinical genetic screening. Ophthalmology 1998;105:1442–1447.
84. Gallie BL. Predictive testing for retinoblastoma comes of age. Am J Hum Genet 1997;61:279–281.
85. Rushlow D, Piovesan B, Zhang K, et al. Detection of mosaic RB1 mutations in families with retinoblastoma. Hum Mutat 2009;30:842–851.
86. Noorani HZ, Khan HN, Gallie BL, et al. Cost comparison of molecular versus conventional screening of relatives at risk for retinoblastoma. Am J Hum Genet 1996;59: 301–307.
87. Li FP, Fraumeni JF Jr. Soft-tissue sarcomas, breast cancer, and other neoplasms: a familial syndrome? Ann Intern Med 1969;71:747–752.
88. Li FP, Fraumeni JF Jr. Rhabdomyosarcoma in children: epidemiologic study and identification of a familial cancer syndrome. J Natl Cancer Inst 1969;43:1365–1373.
89. Garber JE, Goldstein AM, Kantor AF, et al. Follow-up study of twenty-four families with Li-Fraumeni syndrome. Cancer Res 1991;51:6094–6097.
90. Li FP, Fraumeni JFJ, Mulvihill JJ, et al. A cancer family syndrome in twenty-four kindreds. Cancer Res 1988;48:5358–5362.
91. Garber JE, Burke EM, Lavally BL, et al. Choroid plexus tumors in the breast cancer-sarcoma syndrome. Cancer 1990;66:2658–2660.
92. Kleihues P, Schauble B, zur Hausen A, et al. Tumors associated with p53 germline mutations: a synopsis of 91 families. Am J Pathol 1997;150:1–13.
93. Chompret A, Brugieres L, Ronsin M, et al. P53 germline mutations in childhood cancers and cancer risk for carrier individuals. Br J Cancer 2000;82:1932–1937.
94. Hisada M, Garber JE, Fung CY, et al. Multiple primary cancers in families with Li-Fraumeni syndrome. J Natl Cancer Inst 1998;90:606–611.
95. Malkin D, Li FP, Strong LC, et al. Germ line p53 mutations in a familial syndrome of breast cancer, sarcomas, and other neoplasms. Science 1990;250:1233–1238.
96. Varley JM, McGown G, Thorncroft M, et al. Germ-line mutations of TP53 in Li-Fraumeni families: an extended study of 39 families. Cancer Res 1997;57:3245–3252.
97. Tinat J, Bougeard G, Baert-Desurmont S, et al. 2009 version of the Chompret criteria for Li Fraumeni syndrome. J Clin Oncol 2009;27:e108–e109.
98. Bougeard G, Baert-Desurmont S, Tournier I, et al. Impact of the MDM2 SNP309 and p53 Arg72Pro polymorphism on age of tumour onset in Li-Fraumeni syndrome. J Med Genet 2006;43:531–533.
99. Tabori U, Nanda S, Druker H, Lees J, et al. Younger age of cancer initiation is associated with shorter telomere length in Li-Fraumeni syndrome. Cancer Res 2007;67: 1415–1418.
100. Trkova M, Prochazkova K, Krutilkova V, et al. Telomere length in peripheral blood cells of germline TP53 mutation carriers is shorter than that of normal individuals of corresponding age. Cancer 2007;110:694–702.
101. Tabori U, Malkin D. Risk stratification in cancer predisposition syndromes: lessons learned from novel molecular developments in Li-Fraumeni syndrome. Cancer Res 2008;68:2053–2057.
102. Shlien A, Tabori U, Marshall CR, et al. Excessive genomic DNA copy number variation in the Li-Fraumeni cancer predisposition syndrome. Proc Natl Acad Sci U S A 2008;105:11264–11269.
103. Bell DW, Varley JM, Szydlo TE, et al. Heterozygous germ line hCHK2 mutations in Li-Fraumeni syndrome. Science 1999;286:2528–2531.
104. Sodha N, Houlston RS, Bullock S, et al. Increasing evidence that germline mutations in CHEK2 do not cause Li-Fraumeni syndrome. Hum Mutat 2002;20:460–462.
105. Varley JM, Thorncroft M, McGown G, et al. A novel deletion within exon 6 of TP53 in a family with Li-Fraumeni-like syndrome, and LOH in a benign lesion from a mutation carrier. Cancer Genet Cytogenet 1996;90:14–16.
106. Venkatachalam S, Shi YP, Jones SN, et al. Retention of wild-type p53 in tumors from p53 heterozygous mice: reduction of p53 dosage can promote cancer formation. EMBO J 1998;17:4657–4667.
107. McIntyre JF, Smith-Sorensen B, Friend SH, et al. Germline mutations of the p53 tumor suppressor gene in children with osteosarcoma. J Clin Oncol 1994;12:925–930.
108. Diller L, Sexsmith E, Gottlieb A, Li FP, et al. Germline p53 mutations are frequently detected in young children with rhabdomyosarcoma. J Clin Invest 1995;95:1606–1611.
109. Moutou C, Le Bihan C, Chompret A, et al. Genetic transmission of susceptibility to cancer in families of children with soft tissue sarcomas. Cancer 1996;78:1483–1491.
110. Ribeiro RC, Sandrini F, Figueiredo B, et al. An inherited p53 mutation that contributes in a tissue-specific manner to pediatric adrenal cortical carcinoma. Proc Natl Acad Sci U S A 2001;98:9330–9335.
111. Hwang SJ, Lozano G, Amos CI, et al. Germline p53 mutations in a cohort with childhood sarcoma: sex differences in cancer risk. Am J Hum Genet 2003;72:975–983.
112. Masciari S, Van den Abbeele AD, Diller LR, et al. F18-fluorodeoxyglucose-positron emission tomography/computed tomography screening in Li-Fraumeni syndrome. JAMA 2008;299:1315–1319.
113. Lin MT, Shieh JJ, Chang JH, et al. Early detection of adrenocortical carcinoma in a child with Li-Fraumeni syndrome. Pediatr Blood Cancer 2009;52:541–544.
114. Hwang SM, Lee ES, Shin SH, et al. Genetic counseling can influence the course of a suspected familial cancer syndrome patient: from a case of Li-Fraumeni like syndrome with a germline mutation in the TP53 gene. Korean J Lab Med 2008;28:493–497.
115. Chandrasekharappa SC, Guru SC, Manickam P, et al. Positional cloning of the gene for multiple endocrine neoplasia-type 1. Science 1997;276:404–407.
116. Bassett JH, Forbes SA, Pannett AA, et al. Characterization of mutations in patients with multiple endocrine neoplasia type 1. Am J Hum Genet 1998;62:232–244.
117. Szinnai G, Meier C, Komminoth P, et al. Review of multiple endocrine neoplasia type 2A in children: therapeutic results of early thyroidectomy and prognostic value of codon analysis. Pediatrics 2003;111:E132–E139.
118. Raue F, Frank-Raue K. Multiple endocrine neoplasia type 2: 2007 update. Horm Res 2007;68(suppl 5):101–104.
119. Santoro M, Carlomagno F, Romano A, et al. Activation of RET as a dominant transforming gene by germline mutations of MEN2A and MEN2B. Science 1995;267: 381–383.
120. Decker RA, Peacock ML, Borst MJ, et al. Progress in genetic screening of multiple endocrine neoplasia type 2A: is calcitonin testing obsolete? Surgery 1995;118:257–263.
121. Morabito A, Piccirillo MC, Falasconi F, et al. Vandetanib (ZD6474), a dual inhibitor of vascular endothelial growth factor receptor (VEGFR) and epidermal growth factor receptor (EGFR) tyrosine kinases: current status and future directions. Oncologist 2009;14:378–390.
122. Maris JM, Matthay KK. Molecular biology of neuroblastoma. J Clin Oncol 1999;17: 2264.
123. Trochet D, Bourdeaut F, Janoueix-Lerosey I, et al. Germline mutations of the paired-like homeobox 2B (PHOX2B) gene in neuroblastoma. Am J Hum Genet 2004;74:761–764.
124. Mossé YP, Laudenslager M, Longo L, et al. Identification of ALK as a major familial neuroblastoma predisposition gene. Nature 2008;455:930–935.
125. Janoueix-Lerosey I, Lequin D, Brugieres L, et al. Somatic and germline activating mutations of the ALK kinase receptor in neuroblastoma. Nature 2008;455:967–970.
126. Chen Y, Takita J, Choi YL, et al. Oncogenic mutations of ALK kinase in neuroblastoma. Nature 2008;455:971–974.
127. Bonnin JM, Rubinstein LJ, Palmer NF, et al. The association of embryonal tumors originating in the kidney and in the brain: a report of seven cases. Cancer 1984;54: 2137–2146.
128. Rorke LB, Packer R, Biegel J. Central nervous system atypical teratoid/rhabdoid tumors of infancy and childhood. J Neurooncol 1995;24:21–28.
129. Fort DW, Tonk VS, Tomlinson GE, et al. Rhabdoid tumor of the kidney with primitive neuroectodermal tumor of the central nervous system: associated tumors with different histologic, cytogenetic, and molecular findings. Genes Chromosomes Cancer 1994;11: 146–152.
130. Besnard-Guerin C, Cavenee W, Newsham I. The t(11;22)(p15.5;q11.23) in a retroperitoneal rhabdoid tumor also includes a regional deletion distal to CRYBB2 on 22q. Genes Chromosomes Cancer 1995;13:145–150.
131. Versteege I, Sevenet N, Lange J, et al. Truncating mutations of hSNF5/INI1 in aggressive paediatric cancer. Nature 1998;394:203–206.
132. Sévenet N, Sheridan E, Amram D, et al. Constitutional mutations of the hSNF5/INI1 gene predispose to a variety of cancers. Am J Hum Genet 1999;65:1342–1348.
133. Taylor MD, Gokgoz N, Andrulis IL, et al. Familial posterior fossa brain tumors of infancy secondary to germline mutation of the hSNF5 gene. Am J Hum Genet 2000;66: 1403–1406.
134. Hulsebos TJ, Plomp AS, Wolterman RA, et al. Germline mutation of INI1/SMARCB1 in familial schwannomatosis. Am J Hum Genet 2007;80:805–810.
135. Swensen JJ, Keyser J, Coffin CM, et al. Familial occurrence of schwannomas and malignant rhabdoid tumour associated with a duplication in SMARCB1. J Med Genet 2009;46:68–72.
136. Horwitz M. The genetics of familial leukemia. Leukemia 1997;11:1347–1359.
137. Song WJ, Sullivan MG, Legare RD, et al. Haploinsufficiency of CBFA2 causes familial thrombocytopenia with propensity to develop acute myelogenous leukaemia. Nat Genet 1999;23:166–175.
138. Beri-Dexheimer M, Latger-Cannard V, Philippe C, et al. Clinical phenotype of germline RUNX1 haploinsufficiency: from point mutations to large genomic deletions. Eur J Hum Genet 2008;16:1014–1018.
139. Shinawi M, Erez A, Shardy DL, et al. Syndromic thrombocytopenia and predisposition to acute myelogenous leukemia caused by constitutional microdeletions on chromosome 21q. Blood 2008;112:1042–1047.
140. Preudhomme C, Renneville A, Bourdon V, et al. High frequency of RUNX1 biallelic alteration in acute myeloid leukemia secondary to familial platelet disorder. Blood 2009;113:5583–5587.
141. Vasudevan SA, Patel JC, Wesson DE, et al. Severe dysplasia in children with familial adenomatous polyposis: rare or simply overlooked? J Pediatr Surg 2006;41:658–661.
142. Haggitt RC, Reid BJ. Hereditary gastrointestinal polyposis syndromes. Am J Surg Pathol 1986;10:871–887.
143. Offerhaus GJA, Giardiello FM, Krush AJ, et al. The risk of upper gastrointestinal cancer in familial adenomatous polyposis. Gastroenterology 1992;102:1980–1982.
144. Cetta F, Montalto G, Gori M, et al. Germline mutations of the APC gene in patients with familial adenomatous polyposis-associated thyroid carcinoma: results from a European cooperative study. J Clin Endocrinol Metab 2000;85:286–292.
145. Garber JE, Li FP, Kingston JE, et al. Hepatoblastoma and familial adenomatous polyposis. J Natl Cancer Inst 1988;80:1626–1628.
146. Hirschman BA, Pollock BH, Tomlinson GE. The spectrum of APC mutations in children with hepatoblastoma from familial adenomatous polyposis kindreds. J Pediatr 2005;147:263–266.
147. Aretz S, Koch A, Uhlhaas S, et al. Should children at risk for familial adenomatous polyposis be screened for hepatoblastoma and children with apparently sporadic hepatoblastoma be screened for APC germline mutations? Pediatr Blood Cancer 2006;47: 811–818.
148. Harvey J, Clark S, Hyer W, et al. Germline APC mutations are not commonly seen in children with sporadic hepatoblastoma. J Pediatr Gastroenterol Nutr 2008;47: 675–677.

149. Bertario L, Russo A, Sala P, et al. Multiple approach to the exploration of genotype-phenotype correlations in familial adenomatous polyposis. J Clin Oncol 2003;21:1698–1707.
150. Sampson JR, Dolwani S, Jones S, et al. Autosomal recessive colorectal adenomatous polyposis due to inherited mutations of MYH. Lancet 2003;362:39–41.
151. American Society of Clinical Oncology. American Society of Clinical Oncology policy statement update: genetic testing for cancer susceptibility. J Clin Oncol 2003;21:2397–2406.
152. Heiskanen I, Luostarinen T, Jarvinen HJ. Impact of screening examinations on survival in familial adenomatous polyposis. Scand J Gastroenterol 2000;35:1284–1287.
153. Iwama T, Mishima Y. Factors affecting the risk of rectal cancer following rectum-preserving surgery in patients with familial adenomatous polyposis. Dis Colon Rectum 1994;37:1024–1026.
154. Ziv Y, Church JM, Oakley JR, et al. Surgery for the teenager with familial adenomatous polyposis: ileo-rectal anastomosis or restorative proctocolectomy? Int J Colorectal Dis 1995;10:6–9.
155. Lynch HT, Lynch JF, Lynch PM, et al. Hereditary colorectal cancer syndromes: molecular genetics, genetic counseling, diagnosis and management. Fam Cancer 2008;7:27–39.
156. Desai DC, Murday V, Phillips RK, et al. A survey of phenotypic features in juvenile polyposis. J Med Genet 1998;35:476–481.
157. Brosens LA, van HA, Hylind LM, et al. Risk of colorectal cancer in juvenile polyposis. Gut 2007;56:965–967.
158. Nugent KP, Talbot IC, Hodgson SV, et al. Solitary juvenile polyps: not a marker for subsequent malignancy. Gastroenterology 1993;105:698–700.
159. Howe JR, Sayed MG, Ahmed AF, et al. The prevalence of MADH4 and BMPR1A mutations in juvenile polyposis and absence of BMPR2, BMPR1B, and ACVR1 mutations. J Med Genet 2004;41:484–491.
160. Marsh DJ, Dahia PLM, Zheng Z, et al. Germline mutations in PTEN are present in Bannayan-Zonana syndrome. Nat Genet 1997;16:333–334.
161. Gallione CJ, Richards JA, Letteboer TG, et al. SMAD4 mutations found in unselected HHT patients. J Med Genet 2006;43:793–797.
162. Lynch HT, de la Chapelle A. Genetic susceptibility to non-polyposis colorectal cancer. J Med Genet 1999;36:801–818.
163. Burke W, Petersen G, Lynch P, et al. Recommendations for follow-up care of individuals with an inherited predisposition to cancer, I: hereditary nonpolyposis colon cancer: Cancer Genetics Studies Consortium. JAMA 1997;277:915–919.
164. Bocker T, Ruschoff J, Fishel R. Molecular diagnostics of cancer predisposition: hereditary non-polyposis colorectal carcinoma and mismatch repair defects. Biochim Biophys Acta 1999;1423:1–10.
165. Bhatia S, Pratt CB, Sharp GB, et al. Family history of cancer in children and young adults with colorectal cancer. Med Pediatr Oncol 1999;33:470–475.
166. Durno C, Aronson M, Bapat B, et al. Family history and molecular features of children, adolescents, and young adults with colorectal carcinoma. Gut 2005;54:1146–1150.
167. Turcot J, Depres J, St.Piere E. Malignant tumours of the central nervous system associated with familial polyposis of the colon: report of two cases. Dis Colon Rectum 1959;2:465–468.
168. Hamilton SR, Liu B, Parsons RE, et al. The molecular basis of Turcot's syndrome. N Engl J Med 1995;332:839–847.
169. Wimmer K, Etzler J. Constitutional mismatch repair-deficiency syndrome: have we so far seen only the tip of an iceberg? Hum Genet 2008;124:105–122.
170. Miyaki M, Nishio J, Konishi M, et al. Drastic genetic instability of tumors and normal tissues in Turcot syndrome. Oncogene 1997;15:2877–2881.
171. Gutmann DH, Aylsworth A, Carey JC, et al. The diagnostic evaluation and multidisciplinary management of neurofibromatosis 1 and neurofibromatosis 2. JAMA 1997;278:51–57.
172. Lubs M-LE, Bauer MS, Formas ME, et al. Lisch nodules in neurofibromatosis type 1. N Engl J Med 1991;324:1264–1266.
173. Riccardi V. Neurofibromatosis phenotype, natural history, and pathogenesis. 2nd ed. Baltimore: The Johns Hopkins University Press; 1992.
174. Korf BR. Plexiform neurofibromas. Am J Med Genet 1999;89:31–37.
175. Bass JC, Korobkin M, Francis IR, et al. Retroperitoneal plexiform neurofibromas: CT findings. AJR Am J Roentgenol 1994;163:617–620.
176. Widemann BC. Current status of sporadic and neurofibromatosis type 1-associated malignant peripheral nerve sheath tumors. Curr Oncol Rep 2009;11:322–328.
177. Yang FC, Ingram DA, Chen S, et al. Nf1-dependent tumors require a microenvironment containing Nf1+/– and c-kit-dependent bone marrow. Cell 2008;135:437–448.
178. Lasater EA, Bessler WK, Mead LE, et al. Nf1+/– mice have increased neointima formation via hyperactivation of a Gleevec sensitive molecular pathway. Hum Mol Genet 2008;17:2336–2344.
179. Lewis RA, Gerson LP, Axelson KA, et al. von Recklinghausen neurofibromatosis, II: incidence of optic gliomata. Ophthalmology 1984;91:929–935.
180. Janss AJ, Grundy R, Cnaan A, et al. Optic pathway and hypothalamic/chiasmatic gliomas in children younger than age 5 years with a 6-year follow-up. Cancer 1995;75: 1051–1059.
181. Blazo MA, Lewis RA, Chintagumpala MM, et al. Outcomes of systematic screening for optic pathway tumors in children with Neurofibromatosis Type 1. Am J Med Genet A 2004;127A:224–229.
182. Listernick R, Ferner RE, Liu GT, et al. Optic pathway gliomas in neurofibromatosis-1: controversies and recommendations. Ann Neurol 2007;61:189–198.
183. Listernick R, Charrow J, Greenwald M. Emergence of optic pathway gliomas in children with neurofibromatosis type 1 after normal neuroimaging results. J Pediatr 1992;121:584–587.
184. Guillamo JS, Creange A, Kalifa C, et al. Prognostic factors of CNS tumours in Neurofibromatosis 1 (NF1): a retrospective study of 104 patients. Brain 2003;126: 152–160.
185. Rea D, Brandsema JF, Armstrong D, et al. Cerebral arteriopathy in children with neurofibromatosis type 1 [published online ahead of print August 24, 2009]. Pediatrics DOI: 10.1542/peds.2009-0152.
186. Airewele GE, Sigurdson AJ, Wiley KJ, et al. Neoplasms in neurofibromatosis 1 are related to gender but not to family history of cancer. Genet Epidemiol 2001;20:75–86.
187. Shearer P, Parham D, Kovnar E, et al. Neurofibromatosis type 1 and malignancy: review of 32 pediatric cases treated at a single institution. Med Pediatr Oncol 1994;22:78–83.
188. King AA, DeBaun MR, Riccardi VM, et al. Malignant peripheral nerve sheath tumors in neurofibromatosis 1. Am J Med Genet 2000;93:388–392.
189. Matsui I, Tanimura M, Kobayashi N, et al. Neurofibromatosis type 1 and childhood cancer. Cancer 1993;72:2746–2754.
190. Doorn PF, Molenaar WM, Buter J, et al. Malignant peripheral nerve sheath tumors in patients with and without neurofibromatosis. Eur J Surg Oncol 1995;21:78–82.
191. Porter DE, Prasad V, Foster L, et al. Survival in malignant peripheral nerve sheath tumours: a comparison between sporadic and neurofibromatosis type 1-associated tumours. Sarcoma 2009;2009:756395.
192. Evans DG, Baser ME, McGaughran J, et al. Malignant peripheral nerve sheath tumours in neurofibromatosis 1. J Med Genet 2002;39:311–314.
193. Miettinen M, Fetsch JF, Sobin LH, et al. Gastrointestinal stromal tumors in patients with neurofibromatosis 1: a clinicopathologic and molecular genetic study of 45 cases. Am J Surg Pathol 2006;30:90–96.
194. Brodeur GM. The NF1 gene in myelopoiesis and childhood myelodysplastic syndromes. N Engl J Med 1994;330:637–639.
195. O'Marcaigh AS, Shannon KM. Role of the NF1 gene in leukemogenesis and myeloid growth control. J Pediatr Hematol Oncol 1997;19:551–554.
196. Shannon KM, O'Connell P, Martin GA, et al. Loss of the normal NF1 allele from the bone marrow of children with type 1 neurofibromatosis and malignant myeloid disorders. N Engl J Med 1994;330:597–601.
197. Messiaen LM, Callens T, Mortier G, et al. Exhaustive mutation analysis of the NF1 gene allows identification of 95% of mutations and reveals a high frequency of unusual splicing defects. Hum Mutat 2000;15:541–555.
198. Gutmann DH, Geist RT, Rose K, et al. Loss of neurofibromatosis type I (NF1) gene expression in pheochromocytomas from patients without NF1. Genes Chromosomes Cancer 1995;13:104–109.
199. Spurlock G, Bennett E, Chuzhanova N, et al. SPRED1 mutations (Legius syndrome): another clinically useful genotype for dissecting the neurofibromatosis type 1 phenotype. J Med Genet 2009;46:431–437.
200. Pasmant E, Sabbagh A, Hanna N, et al. SPRED1 germline mutations caused a neurofibromatosis type 1 overlapping phenotype. J Med Genet 2009;46:425–430.
201. Xiao GH, Chernoff J, Testa JR. NF2: the wizardry of merlin. Genes Chromosomes Cancer 2003;38:389–399.
202. Kwiatkowski DJ, Short MP. Tuberous sclerosis. Arch Dermatol 1994;130:348–354.
203. Kwiatkowski DJ, Manning BD. Tuberous sclerosis: a GAP at the crossroads of multiple signaling pathways. Hum Mol Genet 2005;14 (spec no 2):R251–R258.
204. Jones AC, Shyamsundar MM, Thomas MW, et al. Comprehensive mutation analysis of TSC1 and TSC2 and phenotypic correlations in 150 families with tuberous sclerosis. Am J Hum Genet 1999;64:1305–1315.
205. Verhoef S, Bakker L, Tempelaars AM, et al. High rate of mosaicism in tuberous sclerosis complex. Am J Hum Genet 1999;64:1632–1637.
206. Fenoglio JJ Jr, McAllister HA Jr, Ferrans VJ. Cardiac rhabdomyoma: a clinicopathologic and electron microscopic study. Am J Cardiol 1976;38:241–251.
207. Harding CO, Pagon RA. Incidence of tuberous sclerosis in patients with cardiac rhabdomyoma. Am J Med Genet 1990;37:443–446.
208. Armada RC, Longchong RM, Marrero P, et al. Embryonal rhabdomyosarcoma associated with tuberous sclerosis. Med Pediatr Oncol 2002;38:302.
209. Roach ES, DiMario FJ, Kandt RS, et al. Tuberous Sclerosis Consensus Conference: recommendations for diagnostic evaluation: National Tuberous Sclerosis Association. J Child Neurol 1999;14:401–407.
210. Gorlin RJ, Goltz RW. Multiple nevoid basal-cell epithelioma, jaw cysts and bifid rib syndrome. N Engl J Med 1960;262:908–912.
211. Gorlin RJ. Nevoid basal cell carcinoma syndrome. Dermatol Clin 1995;13:113–125.
212. Kimonis VE, Goldstein AM, Pastakia B, et al. Clinical manifestations in 105 persons with nevoid basal cell carcinoma syndrome. Am J Med Genet 1997;69:299–308.
213. Evans DG, Farndon PA, Burnell LD, et al. The incidence of Gorlin syndrome in 173 consecutive cases of medulloblastoma. Br J Cancer 1991;64:959–961.
214. Mack EE, Wilson CB. Meningiomas induced by high-dose cranial irradiation. J Neurosurg 1993;79:28–31.
215. Hahn H, Wicking C, Zaphiropoulous PG, et al. Mutations of the human homolog of Drosophila patched in the nevoid basal cell carcinoma syndrome. Cell 1996;85:841–851.
216. Johnson RL, Rothman AL, Xie J, et al. Human homolog of patched, a candidate gene for the basal cell nevus syndrome. Science 1996;272:1668–1671.
217. Gailani MR, Bale AE. Acquired and inherited basal cell carcinomas and the patched gene. Adv Dermatol 1999;14:261–283.
218. Booth DR. The hedgehog signalling pathway and its role in basal cell carcinoma. Cancer Metastasis Rev 1999;18:261–284.
219. Taylor MD, Liu L, Raffel C, et al. Mutations in SUFU predispose to medulloblastoma. Nat Genet 2002;31:306–310.
220. Pastorino L, Ghiorzo P, Nasti S, et al. Identification of a SUFU germline mutation in a family with Gorlin syndrome. Am J Med Genet A 2009;149A:1539–1543.
221. Lonser RR, Glenn GM, Walther M, et al. von Hippel-Lindau disease. Lancet 2003;361:2059–2067.
222. Lonser RR, Kim HJ, Butman JA, et al. Tumors of the endolymphatic sac in von Hippel-Lindau disease. N Engl J Med 2004;350:2481–2486.
223. Neumann HP, Lips CJ, Hsia YE, et al. Von Hippel-Lindau syndrome. Brain Pathol 1995;5:181–193.
224. Webster AR, Maher ER, Moore AT. Clinical characteristics of ocular angiomatosis in von Hippel-Lindau disease and correlation with germline mutation. Arch Ophthalmol 1999;117:371–378.
225. Bratslavsky G, Liu JJ, Johnson AD, et al. Salvage partial nephrectomy for hereditary renal cancer: feasibility and outcomes. J Urol 2008;179:67–70.
226. Choyke PL, Glenn GM, Walther MM, et al. von Hippel-Lindau disease: genetic, clinical and imaging features. Radiology 1995;194:629–642.
227. Eisenhofer G, Lenders JW, Linehan WM, et al. Plasma normetanephrine and metanephrine for detecting pheochromocytoma in von Hippel-Lindau disease and multiple endocrine neoplasia type 2. N Engl J Med 1999;340:1872–1879.
228. Latif F, Tory K, Gnarra J, et al. Identification of von Hippel-Lindau disease tumor suppressor gene. Science 1993;260:1317–1320.
229. Chen F, Kishida T, Yao M, et al. Germline mutations in the von Hippel-Lindau disease tumor suppressor gene: correlations with phenotype. Hum Mutat 1995;5:66–75.
230. Stolle C, Glenn G, Zbar B, et al. Improved detection of germline mutations in the von Hippel-Lindau disease tumor suppressor gene. Hum Mutat 1998;12:417–423.
231. Ivan M, Kondo K, Yang H, et al. HIFalpha targeted for VHL-mediated destruction by proline hydroxylation: implications for O_2 sensing. Science 2001;292:464–468.
232. Maranchie JK, Vasselli JR, Riss J, et al. The contribution of VHL substrate binding and HIF1-alpha to the phenotype of VHL loss in renal cell carcinoma. Cancer Cell 2002;1:247–255.
233. Sardi I, Sanzo M, Giordano F, et al. Monotherapy with thalidomide for treatment of spinal cord hemangioblastomas in a patient with von Hippel-Lindau disease. Pediatr Blood Cancer 2009;53:464–467.

234. Wong WT, Liang KJ, Hammel K, et al. Intravitreal ranibizumab therapy for retinal capillary hemangioblastoma related to von Hippel-Lindau disease. Ophthalmology 2008;115:1957–1964.

235. Neumann HP, Berger DP, Sigmund G, et al. Pheochromocytomas, multiple endocrine neoplasia type 2, and von Hippel-Lindau disease. N Engl J Med 1993;329:1531–1538.

236. Bryant J, Farmer J, Kessler LJ, et al. Pheochromocytoma: the expanding genetic differential diagnosis. J Natl Cancer Inst 2003;95:1196–1204.

237. Pasini B, Stratakis CA. SDH mutations in tumorigenesis and inherited endocrine tumours: lesson from the phaeochromocytoma-paraganglioma syndromes. J Intern Med 2009;266:19–42.

238. Baysal BE. Hereditary paraganglioma targets diverse paraganglia. J Med Genet 2002;39:617–622.

239. Astrom K, Cohen JE, Willett-Brozick JE, et al. Altitude is a phenotypic modifier in hereditary paraganglioma type 1: evidence for an oxygen-sensing defect. Hum Genet 2003;113:228–237.

240. Hao HX, Khalimonchuk O, Schraders M, et al. SDH5, a gene required for flavination of succinate dehydrogenase, is mutated in paraganglioma. Science 2009;325:1139–1142.

241. Gimenez-Roqueplo AP, Favier J, Rustin P, et al. Mutations in the SDHB gene are associated with extra-adrenal and/or malignant phaeochromocytomas. Cancer Res 2003;63:5615–5621.

242. Alter BP, Giri N, Savage SA, et al. Cancer in dyskeratosis congenita. Blood 2009;113:6549–6557.

243. Kraemer KH, Lee MM, Scotto J. DNA repair protects against cutaneous and internal neoplasia: evidence from xeroderma pigmentosum. Carcinogenesis 1984;5:511–514.

244. Kraemer KH, Lee MM, Scotto J. Xeroderma pigmentosum: cutaneous, ocular, and neurologic abnormalities in 830 published cases. Arch Dermatol 1987;123:241–250.

245. Cleaver JE. Defective repair replication of DNA in xeroderma pigmentosum. Nature 1968;218:652–656.

246. Bootsma D, Hoeijmakers JH. The genetic basis of xeroderma pigmentosum. Ann Genet 1991;34:143–150.

247. Bootsma D, Hoeijmakers JH. DNA repair: engagement with transcription. Nature 1993;363:114–115.

248. DeSanctis C, Cacchione A. Xerodermatic idiocy. Riv Sper Freniatr 1932;56:269–292.

249. Wood RD. DNA repair: seven genes for three diseases. Nature 1991;350:190.

250. Cleaver JE, Thompson LH, Richardson AS, et al. A summary of mutations in the UV-sensitive disorders: xeroderma pigmentosum, Cockayne syndrome, and trichothiodystrophy. Hum Mutat 1999;14:9–22.

251. Johnson RE, Kondratick CM, Prakash S, et al. hRAD30 mutations in the variant form of xeroderma pigmentosum. Science 1999;285:263–265.

252. Johnson RE, Prakash S, Prakash L. Efficient bypass of a thymine-thymine dimer by yeast DNA polymerase, Poleta. Science 1999;283:1001–1004.

253. Keller C, Keller KR, Shew SB, et al. Growth deficiency and malnutrition in Bloom syndrome. J Pediatr 1999;134:472–479.

254. German J. Bloom's syndrome. Dermatol Clin 1995;13:7–18.

255. Shen JC, Loeb LA. The Werner syndrome gene: the molecular basis of RecQ helicase-deficiency diseases. Trends Genet 2000;16:213–220.

256. Wang LL, Levy ML, Lewis RA, et al. Clinical manifestations in a cohort of 41 Rothmund-Thomson syndrome patients. Am J Med Genet 2001;102:11–17.

257. Hicks MJ, Roth JR, Kozinetz CA, et al. Clinicopathologic features of osteosarcoma in patients with Rothmund-Thomson syndrome. J Clin Oncol 2007;25:370–375.

258. Ellis NA, Groden J, Ye TZ, et al. The Bloom's syndrome gene product is homologous to recQ helicases. Cell 1995;83:655–666.

259. Yu CE, Oshima J, Fu YH, et al. Positional cloning of the Werner's syndrome gene. Science 1996;272:258–262.

260. Kitao S, Shimamoto A, Goto M, et al. Mutations in RECQL4 cause a subset of cases of Rothmund-Thomson syndrome. Nat Genet 1999;22:82–84.

261. Wang LL, Gannavarapu A, Kozinetz CA, et al. Association between osteosarcoma and deleterious mutations in the RECQL4 gene in Rothmund-Thomson syndrome. J Natl Cancer Inst 2003;95:669–674.

262. Mehollin-Ray AR, Kozinetz CA, Schlesinger AE, et al. Radiographic abnormalities in Rothmund-Thomson syndrome and genotype-phenotype correlation with RECQL4 mutation status. AJR Am J Roentgenol 2008;191:W62–W66.

263. Gatti RA, Boder E, Vinters HV, et al. Ataxia-telangiectasia: an interdisciplinary approach to pathogenesis. Medicine (Baltimore) 1991;70:99–117.

264. Waldmann R, McIntire K. Serum alpha-fetoprotein levels in patients with ataxia-telangiectasia. Lancet 1972;2:1112–1115.

265. Hecht F, Hecht BK. Cancer in ataxia-telangiectasia patients. Cancer Genet Cytogenet 1990;46:9–19.

266. Walsh T, King MC. Ten genes for inherited breast cancer. Cancer Cell 2007;11:103–105.

267. Shiloh Y. ATM and related protein kinases: safeguarding genome integrity. Nat Rev Cancer 2003;3:155–168.

268. Savitsky K, Bar-Shira A, Gilad S, et al. A single ataxia telangiectasia gene with a product similar to PI-3 kinase. Science 1995;268:1749–1753.

269. Cortez D, Wang Y, Qin J, Elledge SJ. Requirement of ATM-dependent phosphorylation of brca1 in the DNA damage response to double-strand breaks. Science 1999;286:1162–1166.

270. Sandoval C, Swift M. Treatment of lymphoid malignancies in patients with ataxia-telangiectasia. Med Pediatr Oncol 1998;31:491–497.

271. Easton D, Peto J. The contribution of inherited predisposition to cancer incidence. Cancer Surv 1990;9:395–416.

272. Points to consider: ethical, legal, and psychosocial implications of genetic testing in children and adolescents: American Society of Human Genetics Board of Directors, American College of Medical Genetics Board of Directors. Am J Hum Genet 1995;57:1233–1241.

273. Nichols KE, Li FP, Haber DA, et al. Childhood cancer predisposition: applications of molecular testing and future implications. J Pediatr 1998;132:389–397.

274. Giardiello FM, Brensinger JD, Petersen GM, et al. The use and interpretation of commercial APC gene testing for familial adenomatous polyposis. N Engl J Med 1997;336:823–827.

275. Croyle RT, Achilles JS, Lerman C. Psychologic aspects of cancer genetic testing—a research update for clinicians. Cancer 1997;80:569–575.

276. Lammens C, Bleiker E, Aaronson N, et al. Attitude towards pre-implantation genetic diagnosis for hereditary cancer. Fam Cancer 2009;8:457–464.

277. Julian-Reynier C, Chabal F, Frebourg T, et al. Professionals assess the acceptability of preimplantation genetic diagnosis and prenatal diagnosis for managing inherited predisposition to cancer. J Clin Oncol 2009;27:4475–4480.

278. Malkin D. Prenatal diagnosis, preimplantation genetic diagnosis, and cancer: was hamlet wrong? J Clin Oncol 2009;27(27):4446–4447.

279. Statement of the American Society of Clinical Oncology: genetic testing for cancer susceptibility, adopted on February 20, 1996. J Clin Oncol 1996;14:1730–1736.

280. Statement of the American Society of Human Genetics on genetic testing for breast and ovarian cancer predisposition. Am J Hum Genet 1994;55:I–iv.

281. Schwarzbraun T, Obenauf AC, Langmann A, et al. Predictive diagnosis of the cancer prone Li-Fraumeni syndrome by accident: new challenges through whole genome array testing. J Med Genet 2009;46:341–344.

282. Li FP, Garber JE, Friend SH, et al. Recommendations on predictive testing for germ line p53 mutations among cancer-prone individuals. J Natl Cancer Inst 1992;84:1156–1160.

283. Chorley W, MacDermot K. Who should talk to patients with cancer about genetics? BMJ 1997;314:441.

284. Clarke AJ, Gaff C. Challenges in the genetic testing of children for familial cancers. Arch Dis Child 2008;93:911–914.

285. Garber JE, Schrag D. Testing for inherited cancer susceptibility. JAMA 1996;275:1928–1929.

286. McAbee GN, Sherman J, Davidoff-Feldman B. Physician's duty to warn third parties about the risk of genetic diseases. Pediatrics 1998;102:140–142.

287. Malkin D, Smyth K, Shuman C, et al. Establishment of a dedicated cancer genetics program in a tertiary pediatric centre [abstract]. Am J Hum Genet 1999;65(4):A386.

CHAPTER 3 ■ MOLECULAR AND GENETIC BASIS OF CHILDHOOD CANCER

PETER D. APLAN AND JAVED KHAN

INTRODUCTION

The biological behavior of every mammalian cell is determined by the pattern of gene expression within that cell, and the hallmark of cancer is the progressive accumulation of genetic and epigenetic alterations. At the molecular level, cancer is a genetic disease, caused by a combination of inherited (germline) and acquired (somatic) aberrations of the genome. These aberrations lead to alterations of the cell's gene expression profile, which in turn leads to disordered growth, failure of differentiation, or reduced apoptosis. The DNA of cancer cells may acquire point mutations, viral insertions, gene amplifications, deletions, or gene rearrangements, each of which can alter the context and process of normal cellular growth and development. Depending on the genetic locus involved and the mechanism of its disruption, some of these changes may make small or incremental contributions to malignant transformation. Others may be cataclysmic in their unraveling of ordered and regulated growth processes. The identification and characterization of the altered genome, and of the mechanisms by which they are altered, can provide basic insights into the process of oncogenesis and offer the hope of specific therapies if the alteration or its effect can be inhibited or reversed.

This chapter will discuss the principles and, in broad strokes only, the molecular and genetic basis of pediatric cancers. The first sections will focus on the general nature of genetic aberrations associated with cancer. These will be subdivided into inherited (germline) and acquired (somatic) mutations associated with cancer and the mechanisms that generate these aberrations. The following sections will describe the impact of the Human Genome Project (HGP), which has increasingly become a major contributor to the discoveries of the genetic basis of diseases, and tools emanating from the HGP that are available for deciphering the aberrations within the cancer genome. It should be stressed that many of the chromosomal changes and molecular genetic aberrations associated with childhood malignancies overlap with those in adult malignancies, so that the lessons learned from the study of one population are highly relevant to the other. However, childhood cancers often differ from cancers in older patients because of the type of progenitor cells involved and the mechanisms of malignant transformation. Therefore, we have emphasized malignancies that are less common in adults (such as neuroblastoma [NB] and acute lymphoblastic leukemia [ALL]).

GENERAL NATURE OF CANCER-ASSOCIATED GENETIC ABERRATIONS

Cancer is a disease that stems from aberrations within the genome; Figure 3.1 summarizes the broad classification of the alterations that are commonly found with the cancer genome. These alterations can be either germline or somatic. Germline alterations may occur as a result of whole chromosomal changes, usually gains, such as trisomy 21. Most syndromes that result from the loss of whole chromosomes are incompatible with prolonged life. Segmental gains or losses, or copy number variations (CNVs), of germline DNA have been increasingly associated with an increased risk of certain forms of cancer.[1] There are several case reports of cancer arising in patients with constitutional chromosomal rearrangements such as translocations.[2–5] Genome-wide association studies (GWAS) and other genetic linkage studies have identified many genes where single nucleotide variations (SNVs) or single nucleotide polymorphisms (SNPs) are associated with an increased predisposition to cancer. These variations may be in regulatory regions, leading to aberrant gene expression, or may be within the coding regions that alter the function of the protein. These latter mutations may result in loss of function, for example, the Li-Fraumeni syndrome with *TP53* mutations, or gain of function, such as the recently described *ALK* mutations in familial NB.[6,7] Other constitutional alterations that predisposes to cancer include paternal segmental isodisomy found in the Beckwith-Wiedemann syndrome, where the paternal region around the *IGF2* gene is duplicated, leading to overexpression of this growth factor, among other changes (see Table 3.1).

Chromosomal insertion or deletions, breaks, monosomies, trisomies, and translocations occur in nontransformed cells and can be observed as incidental findings during analysis of chromosomes from healthy persons. Their frequency is a function of the age of the individual, the individual's exposure to DNA-interactive agents, the cell type being studied, and whether the cell is being studied directly or after *in vitro* cell culture. The frequency of any incidental abnormality in a routine karyotypic analysis of a normal population of cells hovers around the level of 1%.[72–74] The karyotypically abnormal cells that are observed incidentally do not appear to be clonally proliferative (by definition, they are unique in each metaphase) and therefore are assumed not to confer any selective advantage on the cell in which they occur.

GERMLINE CHROMOSOMAL AND MOLECULAR GENETIC ABERRATIONS

When chromosomal deletions, translocations, amplifications, point mutations, or nondisjunction events occur in a gamete, the abnormality exists in the germline, and the entire organism that develops after conception bears the alteration in each and every cell. A variation on this theme can occur when the alteration or nondisjunction event occurs in a somatic cell early in its lineage development, leading to mosaicism for the

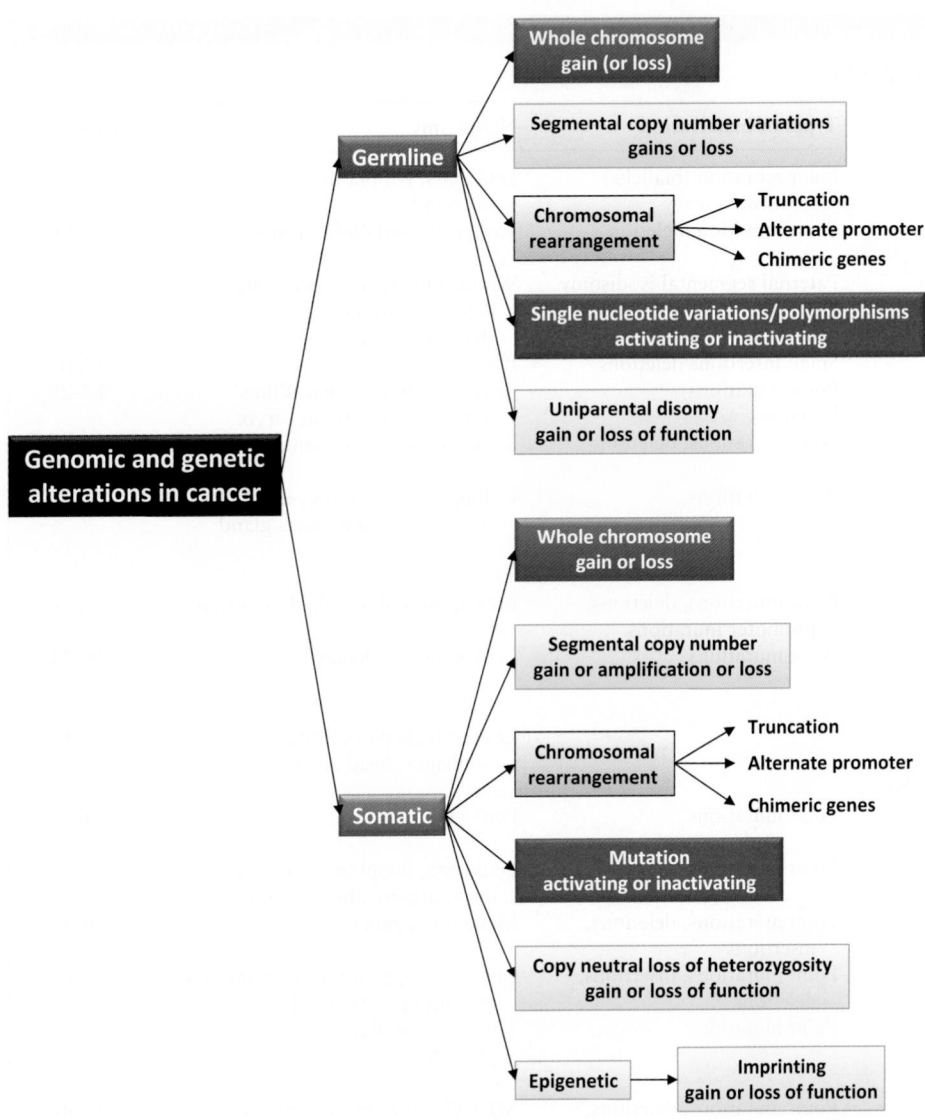

FIGURE 3.1 Summary of the common genomic and genetic alterations found in cancer. These alterations can be either germline (constitutional) or somatic (acquired) and the color scheme reflects similar aberrations that occur in either group. Germline alterations may be a result of copy number alterations, such as whole chromosomal gains (losses usually incompatible with prolonged life), or segmental changes. Constitutional chromosomal rearrangements have been observed in patients with cancer. These rearrangements can result in truncation of a protein, expression of a gene under the control of an alternative promoter, or the production of a chimeric or novel fusion protein not normally found in nature. Single nucleotide variations or single nucleotide polymorphisms are associated with an increased predisposition to cancer. These variations may be in the gene regulatory regions, leading to overexpression or suppression, or may be within the protein-coding regions, leading to expression of mutant proteins. Other constitutional alterations that predisposes to cancer include parental segmental isodisomy. Additional somatic alterations include copy-neutral loss of heterozygosity, where there is no net loss of DNA but uniparental disomy, with only one parental chromosome or region present in two copies. Epigenetic alterations such as silencing of genes by methylation are an increasingly important mechanism of oncogenesis.

entire organism or for particular cell types. A large number of familial cancer syndromes have been identified (see Lindor et al. for a detailed list[75]), and the more common ones impacting childhood cancer are listed in Table 3.1. Although most of these syndromes are rare, it is important to note that they highlight pathways and themes that are common to many types of cancer.

Constitutional deletions can predispose a person to the development of cancer. That such cancers are cell type–specific underscores the fact that one is often dealing with a gene function that makes a contribution to growth or development within only a particular milieu or physiologic context. The classic examples of this phenomenon are the chromosomal abnormalities associated with the hereditary forms of retinoblastoma and Wilms' tumor.

Hereditary and sporadic occurrences of retinoblastoma have been distinguished on the basis of clinical and epidemiologic presentations.[76] The hereditary form (i.e., familial or de novo germline mutation) is estimated to comprise about 40% of affected persons. In this form, the age of onset is earlier, and the frequency of bilateral tumors is increased. There is often a positive family history for this cancer. These observations led Knudson to propose a "two-hit"

mechanism of carcinogenesis, in which the first genetic defect, already present in the germline, must be complemented by an additional spontaneous mutation before a tumor can arise (Fig. 3.2). In the sporadic form, malignant transformation occurs only when two spontaneous mutations take place in the same cell.[77] Support for this concept came from karyotypic analysis of patients with a particular syndrome associated with retinoblastoma. These individuals carried a constitutional deletion of part of the long arm of one allele of chromosome 13.[78,79] This finding not only fit conceptually with the Knudson's model but also pointed directly to the chromosomal region in which the crucial gene was likely to be found.

The involvement, and often the deletion, of one of the two alleles from this region of chromosome 13 in patients with retinoblastoma was proven by molecular analysis. The somatic, unaffected tissue of a particular patient with retinoblastoma showed a heterozygous pattern (with each allele on the two chromosomes 13 contributing its own distinctive pattern). The tumor tissue was likewise analyzed, and one of the two alleles was found to be missing. There had been a "reduction to homozygosity" or loss of heterozygosity (LOH) consistent with an acquired monosomy in the tumor tissue.[80] These kinds

TABLE 3.1

INHERITED PREDISPOSITION TO CANCER

Syndrome	Gene	Types of inactivation	Neoplasms	References
Ataxia–telangiectasia	ATM	Point mutation (biallelic) Haploinsufficiency	Leukemia, lymphoma, breast, ovarian	8,9
Basal cell nevus syndrome (Gorlin syndrome)	PTCH	Point mutation, deletion	Basal cell, medulloblastoma	10,11
Beckwith-Wiedemann syndrome	Multiple	Paternal segmental isodisomy Deletions	Wilms' tumor, neuroblastoma, hepatoblastoma, rhabdomyosarcoma	12–14
Birt-Hogg-Dube syndrome	FLCN	Small insertions/deletions	Renal	15,16
Bloom syndrome	BLM	Point mutations Deletions	Leukemia, lymphoma, Wilms' tumor, colon, breast, cervix	17–20
Hereditary breast/ovarian cancer	BRCA1 BRCA2	Point mutations, deletions	Breast, ovarian, prostate, pancreatic	17,21–23
Hereditary nonpolyposis colon cancer (Lynch syndrome)	MLH1 MSH2 PMS2 MSH6	Point mutations	Colon, uterine, gastric, endometrial, small bowel, sebaceous gland	24–26
Cowden syndrome	PTEN	Point mutations, deletions, promoter mutations	Breast, thyroid, renal, glioblastoma	27,28
Dyskeratosis congenita	DKC1 TERC TERT	Point mutations	Leukemia, esophagus	29–31
Fanconi anemia	Many (FANCA-FANCN)		Leukemia, hepatocellular, esophagus, head and neck, cervix	17,32,33
Familial acute myeloid leukemia	RUNX1 Others	Point mutations	Leukemia	34
Li-Fraumeni syndrome	TP53	Point mutations	Leukemia, lymphoma, breast, osteosarcoma, brain tumors	35–38
Dysplastic nevus syndrome	CDKN2A Others	Point mutations, deletions, insertions	Melanoma, pancreatic	39–41
Multiple endocrine neoplasia type 1	MEN1	Point mutations, insertions, deletions	Parathyroid, pancreas, gastrinomas, insulinoma, carcinoid	42,43
Multiple endocrine neoplasia type 2A and 2B	RET	Point mutations	Thyroid medulla, pheochromocytoma	44,45
Neurofibromatosis type 1	NF1	Point mutations, deletions, translocations	MPNST, pheochromocytoma, astrocytoma, glioma, leukemia	46–48
Neurofibromatosis type 2	NF2	Point mutations	Astrocytoma, melanoma, meningioma	49,50
Nijmegen breakage syndrome	NBS1	Point mutations	Lymphoma, leukemia	51–53
Peutz-Jeghers syndrome	LKB1	Point mutations	Stomach, small intestine, colon, pancreas, uterine, breast	54,55
Familial adenomatous polyposis	APC	Point mutations leading to truncation	Colon, small intestine, thyroid, pancreas, hepatoblastoma, medulloblastoma	56–58
Retinoblastoma	RB	Deletions, point mutations	Retinoblastoma, osteosarcoma, melanoma, pinealoblastoma, lung	59–62
Von Hippel-Lindau	VHL	Point mutations, deletions	Renal cell carcinoma, pancreatic islet cell, pheochromocytoma	63,64
Werner syndrome	WRN	Point mutations	Leukemia, melanoma, osteosarcoma, thyroid	65,66
Xeroderma pigmentosum	Many	Point mutations	Basal cell, melanoma, stomach, leukemia	67,68
WAGR syndrome	WT1	Deletions	Wilms' tumor	69,70
Wiskott-Aldrich syndrome	WASP	Point mutations	Leukemia, lymphoma	71

WAGR, Wilms' tumor characterized by aniridia, genitourinary defects, and mental retardation; MPSNT, malignant peripheral nerve sheath tumors.

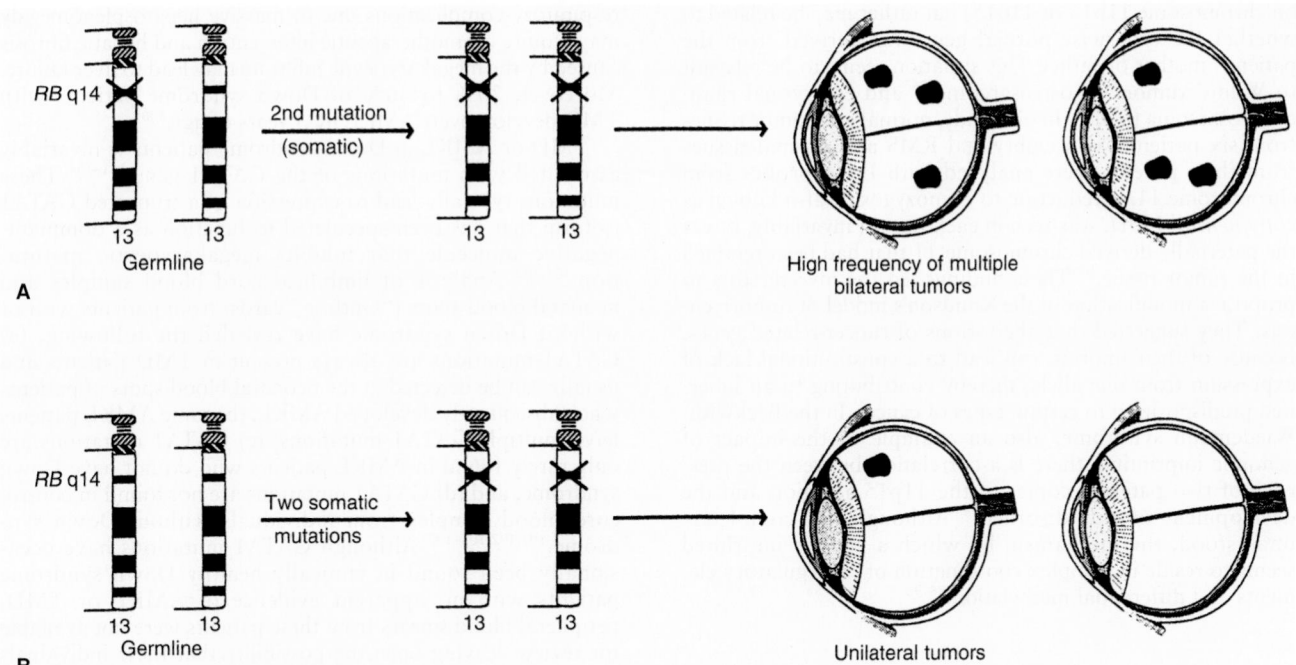

FIGURE 3.2 Knudson's hypothesis illustrated by the development of familial and sporadic retinoblastoma. Children with multiple, bilateral tumors of the eye carry a germ line mutation of the *RB* gene that may be inherited or acquired. A somatic mutation affecting the second *RB* allele leads to tumor formation, usually during the first year of life. By contrast, children with single, unilateral tumors developing after infancy lack germ line mutations of *RB* but have somatic mutations in both *RB* alleles. The "two-hit" model of carcinogenesis, first proposed by Alfred Knudson, has greatly influenced the direction of cancer research during the past three decades.

of analyses led to the successful cloning of the first tumor suppressor gene, *RB*.[60]

Essentially all patients who present with bilateral disease carry a germline mutation of the *RB* gene, which may have been inherited or generated *de novo*. An exception to this scenario has been appreciated with the recognition of families that present with the phenotype of partially penetrant retinoblastoma. In those cases, familial predisposition is clearly evident by pedigree analysis, but tumors may not always be present or may be predominantly unifocal in obligate carriers. In many of these families, the *RB* alteration has been demonstrated to be caused by mutations that lead to an unstable protein that modifies the ability of *RB* to interact with its relevant binding partners.[81]

Another example of a constitutional chromosomal aberration is the rare syndrome of Wilms' tumor characterized by aniridia, genitourinary defects, and mental retardation (WAGR). This variant was found to be correlated with a constitutional deletion of chromosome 11p13,[82] from which a Wilms' tumor susceptibility gene, WT1, has been cloned.[69,70] WT1 encodes a DNA-binding transcription factor whose expression in fetal kidney and embryonic structures suggests its involvement in genitourinary development. Patients with Beckwith-Wiedemann syndrome, which is associated with a chromosomal abnormality distinct from WAGR syndrome, also show an increased susceptibility to the development of Wilms' tumor in the context of macroglossia, somatic gigantism, visceromegaly, hypoglycemia, and abdominal wall defects. They often have constitutional duplications of the 11p15 region, and their Wilms' tumors show LOH in this region.[83] There is evidence that genomic imprinting occurs within this region (see the following section) so that differential loss or

gain of the active allele may contribute to tumorigenesis.[83] Candidate loci for this event include IGF2, H19, and p57^{KIP2}.

Genomic Imprinting

Part of the complexity of neoplasms such as Wilms' tumor may derive from a *de facto* inactivation of one of the two alleles of certain genes, in the absence of a structural deletion or alteration of the locus. The inactivation is imposed because of the origin of the gamete from which it was derived. For example, there can be a cellular "memory" about whether a particular chromosome was derived from the male or the female gamete, and the two chromosomes, or at least certain genes that reside on them, may be activated or suppressed differentially. This mechanism represents a constitutional difference in the expression of the two genes derived from homologous chromosomes in the individual. There may be nothing abnormal about the structure of a gene itself, but it may not be expressed because it resides on the maternally or paternally derived chromosome. For example, a gene not expressed on the paternally derived chromosome but transcribed normally when passed through the female germline has the opportunity to be transferred to the next generation through the female ovum, and because the gene is then maternally derived, it is functional in the offspring.

Genomic imprinting can be invoked to explain a variety of phenomena that appear to violate a simple mendelian model of inheritance. One can appreciate how this effect can complicate cancer genetics, because a particular predisposition to develop a specific kind of cancer (e.g., Wilms' tumor) may not always show linkage with a particular aberrant gene (e.g., one on chromosome 11p13 or 11p15) but rather may be related to whether the otherwise normal gene was derived from the patient's mother or father. This situation seems to be relevant to Wilms' tumor,[84,85] osteosarcoma,[86] and embryonal rhabdomyosarcoma (RMS). In one study, normal and tumor tissues from six patients with embryonal RMS and normal tissues from their parents were analyzed with DNA probes from chromosome 11. A reduction to homozygosity, also known as *copy-neutral LOH*, was seen in each tumor; invariably, it was the paternally derived chromosome 11 that had been retained in the tumor tissue.[87] These findings led the investigators to propose a modification of the Knudson's model of tumorigenesis. They suggested that aberrations of cancer-related genes, because of their imprint, can lead to a constitutional lack of expression from one allele, thereby contributing to an inherited predisposition to certain types of cancer. In the Beckwith-Wiedemann syndrome, also an example of the impact of genomic imprinting, there is a correlation between the presence of two paternal copies of the 11p15.5 region and the development of this disorder.[88] Although not completely understood, the mechanism by which a gene is imprinted seems to reside in complex coordination of *cis*-regulatory elements and differential methylation.[88–90]

Trisomy

Trisomy refers to the presence of an extra copy of a chromosome. Trisomies in the germline result in dramatic deviation from normal growth and development and are, for the most part, incompatible with life.[91] Only trisomies of chromosomes 13, 18, and 21 occur with any frequency in the germline of humans, and each is associated with a defined syndrome.[92]

Although it is possible that an unbalanced number of chromosomes intrinsically leads to aberrant cell division, this seems unlikely, given the vigorous growth of aneuploid cell lines *in vitro*. It would seem more likely that the presence of an extra chromosome poses a basic developmental problem caused by a 50% increase in the dosage of a particular gene or genes. In many instances, there can be a wide tolerance by the organism for twofold variations in the dosage of particular genes, as in the case of many recessive syndromes in which obligate heterozygotes are phenotypically normal. The impact of the trisomies underscores the fine-tuning and dose dependency of certain growth and developmental pathways in higher organisms.

The classic constitutional aneuploidy that demonstrates a predisposition to certain forms of cancer is trisomy 21, or Down syndrome.[93,94] An immediate question is whether the increased risk of leukemia in Down syndrome is directly related to a gene or genes on chromosome 21 or is an indirect effect of some other aspect of the Down phenotype. It would appear that the former might be the case. In trisomy 21 mosaic children, it is the trisomic cell that is at risk for leukemic transformation. In addition, acquired trisomy 21 is a relatively frequent chromosomal abnormality found in the acute leukemias.[95,96] The incidence of both ALL and acute myeloid leukemia (AML), especially acute megakaryoblastic leukemia (AMKL) is increased in patients with Down syndrome.[97]

A related hematopoietic condition, transient myeloproliferative disorder (TMD), is also associated with Down syndrome or trisomy 21 mosaicism.[98,99] TMD classically manifests in newborns or during early infancy as a myeloproliferative disorder that can include hepatosplenomegaly, leukocytosis, and circulating myeloblasts. The morphologic picture is consistent with congenital leukemia except that spontaneous remission occurs. However, this condition is not unequivocally benign, since

respiratory complications due to massive hepatosplenomegaly may require chemotherapeutic intervention and hepatic fibrosis caused by the megakaryocytic infiltrate may lead to liver failure. Moreover, 20% to 30% of Down syndrome patients with TMD develop overt AMKL by 3 years of age.[100]

TMD or AMKL in Down syndrome patients is invariably associated with mutations of the GATA1 gene.[101–104] These mutations typically lead to expression of a truncated GATA1 isoform that has been speculated to function as a dominant-negative molecule that inhibits megakaryocytic maturation.[101,102] Analysis of umbilical cord blood samples and neonatal blood spots ("Guthrie" cards) from patients with or without Down syndrome have revealed the following: (a) GATA1 mutations are always present in TMD patients and usually can be detected in the neonatal blood spots of patients who subsequently developed AMKL, (b) some AMKL patients have multiple GATA1 mutations, (c) GATA1 mutations are only rarely found in AMKL patients who do not have Down syndrome, and (d) GATA1 mutations are not found in control cord blood samples from individuals without Down syndrome.[101,102,105–107] Although GATA1 mutations have occasionally been found in clinically healthy Down syndrome patients with no apparent evidence of AMKL or TMD, peripheral blood smears from these patients were not available for review, leaving open the possibility that these individuals may have had subclinical TMD.[106] In sum, although mutations of GATA1 in the presence of trisomy 21 may be sufficient to cause TMD, additional genetic events are required for TMD to progress to AMKL.

SOMATICALLY ACQUIRED CHROMOSOMAL AND MOLECULAR GENETIC ABERRATIONS

For the past 50 years, cytogeneticists have described an increasing number of specific chromosomal abnormalities associated with malignancy. These abnormalities differ from those discussed previously in that they have been acquired by somatic cells. These acquired aberrations are confined to the malignant clone of a cancer patient, are not found in the normal tissues of that individual, and therefore cannot be transmitted from generation to generation. Moreover, in contrast to constitutional chromosomal abnormalities, cell type–specific or cancer-specific abnormalities often correlate directly with a phenotypic effect. The association of a particular chromosomal abnormality with a specific type of malignancy was first demonstrated in 1960, with the identification of the Philadelphia chromosome (Ph) in the malignant cells of patients with chronic myelogenous leukemia.[108]

Gross chromosomal rearrangements (GCRs) can result in interstitial deletions, amplifications, inversions, and translocations, resulting in the unscheduled expression of proto-oncogenes, generation of oncogenic fusion genes, and deletion of tumor suppressor genes. Given that these GCRs are causal events in malignant transformation, a clearer understanding of their genesis is important in understanding the root causes of childhood cancers. It is not known, for example, whether the regions frequently involved by GCRs represent sites within the genome that are "fragile" and highly susceptible to breakage and religation or simply represent sites near growth-promoting proto-oncogenes, whose deregulation gives cells a growth advantage. The following discussion draws heavily from investigations of the childhood leukemias, which have proved particularly amenable to cytogenetic and molecular analyses.

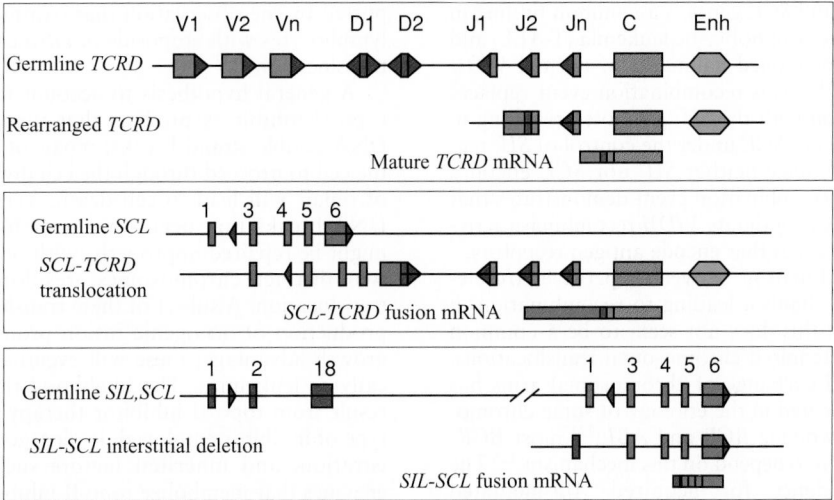

FIGURE 3.3 Chromosomal rearrangements caused by illegitimate V(D)J recombination. The **top panel** depicts normal V(D)J recombination, with one of many V segments (*light blue*) recombining to a D segment (*red*) followed by a J segment (*orange*). Discreet V, D, and J segments are flanked by heptamer/nonamer sequences (*blue triangles*). Splicing of the recombined VDJ segment to the C segment occurs at the RNA level, as depicted. Transcription is regulated by an enhancer region (*green*). The **middle panel** shows a chromosomal translocation mediated by V(D)J recombination. In this case, a cryptic heptamer/nonamer sequence within the *SCL* locus (exons 1–6 depicted, the cryptic heptamer/nonamer is represented by a *triangle* in exon 6) mediates fusion with a *TCRD* D region, resulting in a interchromosomal rearrangement, and subsequent production of a *SCL-TCRD* fusion mRNA. The **bottom panel** shows a V(D)J recombinase-mediated intrachromosomal rearrangement between *SIL* (only exons 1, 2, and 18 are shown for clarity) and *SCL*. Cryptic heptamers within the *SIL* and *SCL* loci are depicted by *blue triangles*. The reconfigured genomic DNA is results in a *SIL-SCL* fusion mRNA, controlled by *SIL* regulatory elements.

Inherited Predisposition to Gross Chromosomal Rearrangements

Several heritable gene defects (see Table 3.1) are known to predispose persons to the development of myeloid and/or lymphoid leukemias; some of these clearly lead to an increased incidence of chromosomal rearrangements. Patients with ataxia-telangiectasia (AT) have mutations of the *ATM* gene and are prone to the acquisition of chromosomal translocations, most commonly involving antigen receptor genes (*IG* or *TCR*).[109] In addition, mice deficient for the ATM protein develop T-cell malignancies, which show chromosomal translocations involving antigen receptor genes.[110] Patients with Nijmegen breakage syndrome, are also predisposed to the development of leukemia and chromosomal translocations affecting antigen receptor genes.[111] It seems likely that the leukemogenic chromosomal translocations associated with these conditions are caused by a specific recombination defect in *V(D)J* recombination (see Fig. 3.3).

Persons with inherited DNA repair defects, such as Bloom syndrome, Fanconi anemia, and Li-Fraumeni syndrome, are predisposed to a spectrum of malignancies, including leukemias, lymphomas, and early-onset adult carcinomas.[34] In contrast to the conditions described earlier, in which the patients develop a malignancy that harbors chromosomal aberrations involving an antigen receptor gene, persons with Bloom, Fanconi, or Li-Fraumeni syndromes have less specific chromosomal aberrations. Although lymphocytes from patients with Bloom syndrome and Fanconi anemia are clearly susceptible to chromosomal breakage *in vitro*, the leukemias developing in patients with Bloom syndrome and Fanconi anemia sometimes, but not always, show clonal chromosomal translocations.[112]

Timing of Leukemogenic Chromosomal Translocations

Several lines of investigation have demonstrated that many of the common chromosomal translocations occur *in utero*, although the leukemia associated with the translocation may not become evident for 10 or more years. Monochorionic twins have been shown to harbor identical *MLL* or *TEL* translocations, indicating that the translocation had arisen in one twin *in utero* and was "metastasized" to the unaffected twin through the shared placenta.[113,114] Moreover, the analysis of neonatal blood spots has demonstrated that clonotypic *TEL-AML1* fusions found in the leukemic cells of children with *TEL-AML1* fusions were present at birth.[115,116]

Molecular Mechanisms Leading to Gross Chromosomal Rearrangements

Some chromosomal translocations seem to be the result of mistakes in normal *V(D)J* recombination (Fig. 3.3).[117] Typically, translocations attributed to illegitimate *V(D)J* recombination juxtapose a proto-oncogene to a locus that codes for an antigen receptor (either an *IG* or a *TCR*) gene. The proto-oncogene present on the translocated chromosome then becomes activated via the regulatory region of the antigen receptor gene. The notion that these translocations are the result of illegitimate *V(D)J* recombinase activity is strengthened by the presence of features associated with normal *V(D)J* recombinase action, such as site-specific DNA cleavage at cryptic heptamer sequences and the addition of nontemplated ("N" region) nucleotides at the translocation breakpoints.[117,118] Interestingly, the site-specific recombination event between the *SIL* and *SCL* genes is a common finding in patients with T-cell acute lymphoblastic leukemia (T-ALL) and shows all of the aforementioned hallmarks of normal *V(D)J* recombinase activity.[119,120] This recombination event replaces the *SCL* promoter region with the *SIL* promoter, resulting in inappropriate expression of *SCL* under the control of *SIL* regulatory elements.[120,121] Since neither *SIL* nor *SCL* encodes antigen receptors, this recombination event demonstrates that translocations caused by illegitimate *V(D)J* recombinase activity are not restricted to genes that encode antigen receptors.

Homologous recombination between repetitive *Alu* elements is a common mechanism leading to recombination in meiotic cells. However, this does not seem to be a common mechanism leading to acquired chromosomal translocations. Although *Alu*-mediated exchange of chromosomal arms has been occasionally implicated in the etiology of some chromosomal translocations involving *BCR* and *ABL*,[122] most *BCR-ABL* fusions do not seem to depend on this mechanism.[123] The most compelling evidence for acquired *Alu*-mediated rearrangement in malignant cells involves the partial tandem duplication of *MLL*; in one series, seven of nine patients with a partial tandem duplication had undergone a rearrangement within *Alu* elements.[124] Additional evidence for *Alu*-mediated rearrangements in malignant cells has recently been reported in the context of *MYB* gene duplication in a subset of leukemia patients.[125]

Numerous chromosomal translocation breakpoints identified in patients with ALL have been mapped within or near extended (200+ consecutive base pair [bp]) tracts of alternating purine and pyrimidine residues (Pu/Py tracts).[126–128] DNA segments consisting of alternating purine and pyrimidine residues are known to form an unusual left-handed helical structure, termed Z-DNA, in solution.[129] Within the genome, Z-DNA segments are preferentially located in internucleosomal regions, presumably because of the higher energy cost of compacting the more rigid Z-DNA into histone-rich nucleosomes.[130] Therefore, it is conceivable that Z-DNA located in internucleosomal regions is more prone to DNA double-strand breaks than is histone-bound nucleosomal DNA. It has been proposed that genomic regions of potential Z-DNA structure may be susceptible to DNA recombination events. This hypothesis is supported by observations that these types of repeat regions are susceptible to "slippage" during DNA replication.[131]

Finally, defective repair of double-strand DNA breaks induced by topoisomerase (topo) II inhibitors has been implicated as a mechanism for chromosomal rearrangement.[132–134] The topo II inhibitors most significantly associated with treatment-related acute myeloid leukemia (t-AML) are the epipodophyllotoxins, such as etoposide (VP-16) and teniposide (VM-26),[135] although the anthracyclines daunorubicin and doxorubicin have also been linked to this disease.[136] t-AML associated with alkylating agent chemotherapy often demonstrates clonal deletions of 7q or 5q, whereas t-AML developing after treatment with topo II inhibitors is characterized by balanced chromosomal translocations involving one of a few genes.[134] The most common chromosomal region involved is 11q23, although recurrent breakpoints involving 21q22, 16p13, 11p15, and 17q21 have also been reported after therapy with topo II inhibitors. The 11q23 translocations result in fusion of the *MLL* gene (also known as *ALL-1* or *HRX*) with a wide spectrum of partner genes; the *MLL* translocation breakpoints generally lie within a 8.3-kb breakpoint cluster region (bcr).[137] The recurrent association of t-AML with *MLL* translocations, short latency periods, and prior exposure to topo II inhibitors has led to the speculation that treatment with topo II inhibitors generates chromosomal translocation involving *MLL*.[135,138] This speculation is supported by the observation that treatment of peripheral blood lymphocytes with etoposide *in vitro* can induce chromosomal translocations.[139]

A general hypothesis to account for t-AML induction by topo II inhibitors predicts that topo II inhibitors generate DNA double-strand breaks; repair of these breaks will allow the cell to proceed through the cell division cycle, while a lack of repair will lead to cell death. Very rarely, double-strand DNA breaks that occur in a hematopoietic progenitor cell might be repaired improperly, with religation of strands from two distinct chromosomes, resulting in a chromosomal translocation. A subset of these translocations will lead to the production of oncogenic fusion proteins that give the cell a growth advantage; these will eventually be recognized clinically as leukemias. The likelihood that a translocation will result from topo II inhibitor therapy has been linked to the type of inhibitor employed, its dosage and schedule of administration, and inherited factors such as subtle defects in enzymes that metabolize topo II inhibitors.[140]

DNA topoisomerase II functions as a homodimer and catalyzes a three-step reaction consisting of double-strand DNA cleavage, strand passage, and DNA religation.[141] During this reaction, a short-lived intermediate consisting of topo II monomers covalently bound to the DNA phosphodiester backbone is stabilized by topo II inhibitors; these short-lived intermediates are recognized as damaged DNA, triggering apoptotic cell death. It has been proposed that a topo II "subunit exchange," in which topo II monomers (subunits) that are covalently bound to DNA exchange partners, might lead to a chromosomal translocation.[142,143] Recently, several chromosomal translocations consistent with this type of subunit exchange, involving the *MLL* or *NUP98* genes, were identified in patients with t-AML or treatment-related myelodysplastic syndrome (t-MDS).[144,145]

An alternative model to account for chromosomal translocations induced by topo II inhibitors suggests that such translocations are initiated by double-strand DNA cleavage, followed by processing of the DNA ends, and created by anomalous joining of these ends to nonhomologous chromosomes (error-prone nonhomologous end joining).[146] In support of this model, nucleotide sequence analysis of translocation breakpoints from patients with t(4;11) translocations shows that DNA sequences flanking the breakpoints have been duplicated, deleted, and inverted during the translocation process,[146] suggesting that the chromosome ends have undergone some type of processing.

In addition, a site within the *MLL* bcr that is uniquely susceptible to DNA double-strand cleavage induced by treatment with topo II poisons has been identified.[138,147] This site-specific *MLL* cleavage can be induced *in vivo* by a wide variety of apoptotic stimuli and *in vitro* by DNAse I.[147,148] Taken together, these observations suggest that this site within the *MLL* bcr represents a region of DNA that is uniquely susceptible to double-strand cleavage, and aberrant repair of the DNA double-strand break leads to a balanced chromosomal translocation.[149]

ONCOGENIC CONSEQUENCES OF GROSS CHROMOSOMAL REARRANGEMENTS— GENERAL THEMES

The cancers of childhood are largely the products of somatically acquired genetic abnormalities that modify protein function. The classes of proteins affected by these changes include growth factors and their receptors, kinase inhibitors, signal transducers, and transcription factors, which may act dominantly as cellular

TABLE 3.2

EXAMPLES OF STRUCTURAL MOTIFS SHARED BY ONCOGENIC TRANSCRIPTION FACTORS AND PROTEINS REGULATING MORPHOGENESIS IN DROSOPHILA EMBRYOS

Human protein	DNA-binding domain	*Drosophila* protein
HLF	bZIP[a]	Giant
PLZF	Zinc finger	Krüppel
AML1	Runt-homology	Runt
PAX3	Paired box	Paired
FKHR	Forkhead	Sloppy-paired
HOXA9	Homeobox	Antennapedia
PBX1	Homeobox	Extradenticle
MLL	A-T hook	Trithorax

[a]Basic region/leucine zipper.
Adapted from Look AT. Oncogenic role of "master" transcription factors in human leukemias and sarcomas: a developmental model. In: Vande Woude G, ed. Advances in cancer research. San Diego, CA: Academic Press, 1995.

oncoproteins or recessively through loss of function, as in the case of tumor suppressors. As described earlier, many of these somatically acquired changes are GCRs. The type of GCR that has been most intensely studied is the nonrandom chromosomal translocations. Through the study of numerous chromosomal translocations, several common themes have emerged.

First, specific translocations are associated with specific forms of leukemia. For instance, the t(15;17)(q22;q12) is exclusively associated with acute promyelocytic leukemia (AML M3), and not other forms of AML.[150,151] Similarly, the t(1;19) is found only in patients with B-cell precursor ALL, and not other forms of leukemia. Although there are numerous exceptions to this generalization (e.g., the t(4;11)(q21;q23) is associated with both AML and B-cell precursor ALL), the recurrent association of specific translocations with specific forms of leukemia strengthens the suspicion that these translocations are causal events for leukemic transformation.

A second theme is that they typically lead to one of two abnormalities (Fig. 3.1). First, the DNA-binding, dimerization, and *trans*-effector regions of discrete proto-oncogenes may be "stitched together" to produce a chimeric protein with altered function. A second mechanism is dysregulated expression of an intact gene, caused by its relocation to sites near promoter/enhancer elements, most commonly those of *TCR* or *IG* genes. The transcription factors involved in leukemia and sarcoma pathogenesis have unique transforming properties that are specific for the different types of progenitors within these distinct developmental pathways.

A third theme is that the genes affected by chromosomal translocations often encode either tyrosine kinases involved in signal transduction or transcription factors. Transcription factors bind to regulatory elements in DNA, such as promoters and enhancers, where they regulate gene transcription. Many of these proteins can be classified on the basis of recurring structural motifs within their DNA- and protein-binding domains, designated as basic region/helix-loop-helix (bHLH), basic region/leucine zipper (bZIP), zinc finger, and homeodomain (helix-turn-helix [HTH]); other motifs with similar functional significance are termed A-T hook, Ets-like, runt homology, and cysteine-rich (LIM).[152,153] The modular organization of transcription factors provides an ideal framework for their multiple functions, particularly binding to DNA in heterodimeric complexes. It also explains why disruption and rearrangement of transcriptional control genes by chromosomal translocations can produce functional hybrid proteins

rather than inert peptides. Tyrosine kinase genes can be aberrantly activated through a variety of mechanisms: truncation of the ligand-binding domain of growth factor receptors, loss or replacement of carboxyl-terminal regulatory tyrosine residues, and point mutations.[154] Such activation can perturb several different signaling pathways that impinge on gene transcription and translation or apoptosis.

In an effort to develop a unifying hypothesis that would account for the tumorigenicity of GCRs, Rabbitts and Boehm emphasized similarities between these oncogenic proteins and the products of so-called master genes, which specify lineage-specific patterns of gene expression during embryologic development.[155] Most intriguing are the similarities between the conserved regions of mammalian transcription factors and those of developmental proteins regulating *Drosophila* embryogenesis (Table 3.2).[156–158] Current observations suggest that aberrant transcription factors may act positively to upregulate critical target genes or negatively to interfere with normal regulatory cascades that coordinate the expression of proteins required to complete cell differentiation.[152,159] A number of the more common recurrent translocations and inversions are discussed in the sections that follow.

CHROMOSOMAL TRANSLOCATIONS AND INVERSIONS LEAD TO ACTIVATION OF PROTO-ONCOGENES AND GENERATION OF ONCOGENIC FUSION GENES

B-Lineage Acute Lymphoblastic Leukemias

TEL-AML1 Fusion Gene in Pro-B Leukemia

Although the most common cytogenetic abnormality found in children with ALL is the t(12;21)(p13;q22) (Table 3.3), this translocation is not easily detected by conventional methods because the rearranged chromosomal fragments closely resemble normal chromosomes. When analyzed by molecular approaches (fluorescent *in situ* hybridization [FISH], Southern blotting, or reverse transcriptase-polymerase chain reaction [RT-PCR]), the t(12;21) is found in about one-fourth of

TABLE 3.3

RECURRENT CHROMOSOMAL TRANSLOCATIONS ASSOCIATED WITH HEMATOLOGIC MALIGNANCIES

Leukemia type	Chromosomal abnormality	Genes involved	Mechanism of activation	Structural motif in chimeric protein[a]	Estimated frequency, %[b]	References
Lymphoid						
B-cell ALL/Burkitt's lymphoma	t(8;14)(q24;q32)	*MYC*	Relocation to IqH locus	bHLHzip	5	160,161
	t(2;8)(p12;q24)	*MYC*	Relocation to IgL locus	bHLHzip	<1	162–166
	t(8;22)(q24;q11)	*MYC*	Relocation to IgL locus	bHLHzip	<1	167,168
B-cell NHL	t(3;11)(q27;q23.1)	*BCL6*	Gene fusion	Zinc finger	1	169
Early-B-cell ALL	t(12;21)(p12;q22)	*TEL-AML1*	Gene fusion	Runt-homology	25	170–172
Pre-B-cell ALL	t(1;19)(q23;p13)	*E2A-PBX1*	Gene fusion	Homeodomain	5	173–175
Pro-B-cell ALL	t(17;19)(q22;p13)	*E2A-HLF*	Gene fusion	bZIP	<1	176,177
	t(4;11)(q21;q23)	*MLL-AF4*	Gene fusion	A-T hook	4	178–180
T-cell ALL	t(8;14)(q24;q11)	*MYC*	Relocation to TCRα/δ locus	bHLHzip	<1	181–183
	t(7;19)(q35;p13)	*LYL1*	Relocation to TCRβ locus	bHLH	<1	184
	t(1;14)(p32;q11)	*SCL(TAL1)*	Relocation to TCRα/δ locus	bHLH	<1	185–187
	t(7;9)(q35;q34)	*TAL2*	Relocation to TCRβ locus	bHLH	<1	187
	t(14;21)(q11;q22)	*BHLHB1*	Relocation to TCRα locus	bHLH	<1	188
	t(11;14)(p15;q11)	*LMO1(RBTN1)*	Relocation to TCRα/δ locus	Cysteine-rich LIM	<1	189,190
	t(11;14)(p13;q11)	*LMO2(RBTN2)*	Relocation to TCRα/δ locus	Cysteine-rich LIM	1	191,192
	t(7;11)(q35;p13)	*LMO2(RBTN2)*	Relocation to TCRβ locus	Cysteine-rich LIM	<1	28
	t(10;14)(q24;q11)	*HOX11*	Relocation to TCRα/δ locus	Homeodomain	<1	193–196
	t(7;10)(q35;q24)	*HOX11*	Relocation to TCRβ locus	Homeodomain	<1	29
	t(5;14)(q35;q32)	*HOX11L2*	Relocation to 14q32	Homeodomain	3	197
	inv(7)(p15;q34)	*HOXA7/9/10*	Relocation to TCRβ locus	Homeodomain	3	198,199
	t(10;11)(p13;q21)	*CALM-AF10*	Gene fusion	Clathrin assembly	2	200,201
	t(4;11)(q21;p15)	*NUP98-RAP1GDS1*	Gene fusion	Nucleoporin	<1	202
	t(9;12)(p24;p13)	*TEL-JAK2*	Gene fusion	Tyrosine kinase	<1	203,204
ALCL	t(2;5)(p23;q35)	*NPM1-ALK*	Gene fusion	Tyrosine kinase	90	205–207
Myeloid						
AML (granulocytic)	t(8;21)(q22;q22)	*AML1-ETO*	Gene fusion	Runt homology	12	208–211
Myelodysplasia	t(3;21)(q26;q22)	*AML1-EAP*	Gene fusion	Runt homology	<1	212
CML, blast crisis	t(3;21)(q26;q22)	*AML1-EV11*	Gene fusion	Runt homology	<1	213
AML (undifferentiated)	t(3;v)(q26;v)	*EV11*	Gene activation	Zinc finger	3	214,215
AML (myelomonocytic)	inv(16)(p13;q22)	*CBFB-MYH11*	Gene fusion	Complex with AML1	12	216
AML (monocytic)	t(9;11)(p21;q23)	*MLL-AF9*	Gene fusion	A-T hook	7	217
AML (promyelocytic)	t(15;17)(q21;q21)	*PML-RARα*	Gene fusion	Zinc finger	7	218–222
	t(11;17)(q23;q21)	*PLZF-RARα*	Gene fusion	Zinc finger	<1	223
AML (undifferentiated)	t(16;21)(p11;q22)	*FUS-ERG*	Gene fusion	Ets-like	<1	224
AML (undifferentiated)	t(6;11)(q21;q23)	*MLL-AF6q21*	Gene fusion	Forkhead	1	225
CMML	t(5;12)(q33;p13)	*TEL-PDGFRB*	Gene fusion	Ets	1	226
AML-M4Eo	t(1;12)(q25;p13)	*ETV6-ARG*	Gene fusion	Ets	1	227
AML, CML	t(7;11)(p15;p15)	*NUP98-HOXA9*	Gene fusion	Homeobox	1.5	228
AML, MDS	t(2;11)(q31;p15)	*NUP98-HOXD13*	Gene fusion	Homeobox	1	229
AML	t(5;14)(q33;q32)	*CEV14-PDGFRB*	Gene fusion	Tyrosine kinase	1	230
AML-M5	t(8;22)(p11;q13)	*P300-MOZ*	Gene fusion	Zinc finger	1	231
AML-M5	t(10;11)(p12;q23)	*MLL-AF10*	Gene fusion	ZIP, A-T hook	1	232,233
AML-M5	t(3;11) complex	*MLL-NRIP3*	Gene fusion			
AML	t(6;9)(p23;q34)	*DEK, NUP214*	Gene fusion	Nucleoporin	<1	234
AML-M7	t(1;22)(p13;q13)	*RBM15, MKL*	Gene fusion	RNA binding	1	235,236
AML	t(11;v)(q23;v)[c]	*MLL*	Gene fusion	AT hook	5	237,238
AML, CMML	t(12;v)(p13;v)[c]	*ETV6*	Gene fusion	Ets	1	171
AML, MDS	t(11;v)(p15;v)[c]	*NUP98*	Gene fusion	Nucleoporin	1	239,240
Ph+ CML, ALL	t(9;22)	*BCR-ABL*	Gene fusion	Tyrosine kinase	100	241

[a]Based on analysis of DNA-binding/protein interaction domain.
[b]Percentage of total cases with childhood lymphoid or myeloid acute leukemia.
[c]"v" represents any of more than 10 chromosomal loci.
ALL, acute lymphoblastic leukemia; NHL, non-Hodgkin lymphoma; ALCL, anaplastic large cell lymphoma; AML, acute myeloid leukemia; CML, chronic myelogenous leukemia; MDS, myelodysplastic syndrome; Ph+, Philadelphia chromosome positive; bHLHzip, basic region/helix-loop-helix/leucine zipper domain; bZIP, basic region/leucine zipper domain; bHLH, basic region/helix-loop-helix.

pediatric B-cell ALL cases[170,242] and about 3% to 4% of adult ALL cases.[243] This rearrangement results in fusion of the oligomerization domain of TEL (ETV6) on chromosome 12 to most of the coding region of AML1 (CBFA2 or RUNX1) on chromosome 21 (Table 3.3).[244] Both AML1 and TEL are also involved in variant translocations associated with both lymphoid and myeloid malignancies. TEL contains a dimerization motif conserved in the ETS family of proteins and has been identified in fusion with many different partners, such as TEL-PDGFRβ in Chronic Myelomonocytic Leukemia (CMML), TEL-MN1 in AML, and TEL-JAK2 in ALL.[171] AML1 (CBF2 A or RUNX1) on chromosome 21 encodes the human homolog of the *Drosophila* runt protein[245] and is involved in the pathogenesis of AML through its fusion with the ETO gene in AML cases with the t(8;21).[246]

Loss of the normal *TEL* allele is frequently observed in ALL patients with a t(12;21), suggesting that TEL loss of function may contribute to leukemic transformation.[247] The vast majority of ALL cases with the *TEL-AML1* (*ETV6-RUNX1*) rearrangement belong to a favorable age group (1–9 years), with 70% to 80% of these cases diagnosed in patients 3 to 6 years of age.[248] Cases of ALL with the t(12;21) have a good prognosis independent of clinical risk factors, such as age and white blood cell (WBC) count at presentation,[172,249] with relapse-free survival rates approaching 90% in studies employing a variety of drug regimens.[250-252] Immunologically, the presence of this translocation is associated with a CD10+ early B-cell progenitor phenotype, an increased frequency of CD13 and CD33 myeloid-associated antigen expression,[253] and a pseudodiploid karyotype.[254]

E2A-PBX1 Fusion Gene in Pre-B Leukemia

The *E2A* (also called *TCF3*) gene, located at 19p13.3, encodes a transcription factor that contains a bHLH DNA-binding and dimerization motif. Its fusion with the *PBX1* homeobox gene as a result of the t(1;19)(q23;p13) occurs in approximately 5% of childhood ALL cases.[173,255,256] E2A-PBX1 hybrids retain the amino-terminal *trans*-activation domain of E2A but not its DNA-binding region, which is replaced by the homeobox DNA-binding and protein-protein interaction domain of PBX1. Thus, the gene targets of E2A-PBX1 are probably those specified by the homeodomain of PBX1; the homeodomain is an approximately 60-amino acid motif first identified in *Drosophila* homeotic selector (Hom) proteins that regulate segment identity during embryogenesis.[257] Evidence suggests that acquisition of the E2A transactivation domain by PBX1 converts the latter into a positive regulator of gene transcription in lymphoid cells, which normally do not express this protein.[258-260]

Reports of *E2A-PBX1* involvement in human disease have been restricted to ALLs with a pre-B-cell phenotype. However, lethally irradiated mice repopulated with bone marrow cells expressing *E2A-PBX1* fusion genes developed AML.[261] Further oncogenic versatility is suggested by the induction of thymic lymphomas in transgenic mice harboring *E2A-PBX1* genes in the germline.[262] In these animals, lymphopenia involving T and B cells preceded malignant transformation, suggesting that E2A-PBX1 proteins can induce apoptosis in murine lymphocyte precursors.

MLL Gene Fusions in Leukemias With 11q23 Rearrangements

An extraordinarily diverse group of chromosomal translocations involve the *MLL* gene (also known as *HRX*, *ALL1*, or *HTRX1*), located at 11q23 (Table 3.3).[178,263-266] *MLL* gene fusions account for as many as 10% of all acute leukemias in children and adults and include B-cell precursor ALL, T-cell ALL, and AML.[267] In addition, as many as 85% of secondary leukemias arising in patients treated with topoisomerase II inhibitors,[132,268] as well as 80% of infant leukemia patients, have rearrangements involving *MLL*.[269-271]

Of the more than 100 different chromosomal loci that have been identified as fusion partners in 11q23 translocations,[267] the most common resides on chromosome 4q21. This site has been implicated in approximately 4% of cases of childhood ALL overall and one-third of such cases in infants.[272] Leukemic blasts carrying the t(4;11)(q21;q23) typically display a pro-B phenotype, with expression of HLA-DR antigens and rearranged *IG* heavy-chain genes.[273,274] Clinical correlates of this rearrangement include an adverse prognosis in patients with WBC counts of more than 100×10^9/L, despite treatment with intensive combination chemotherapy.[269-271]

As mentioned earlier, translocations involving *MLL* can be found in patients with AML as well as those with ALL. A striking example is the t(9;11)(p22;q23), which occurs with high frequency in acute monocytic leukemia,[275] as well as in mixed-lineage leukemias and myeloid leukemias arising after treatment for ALL.[132] Moreover, leukemic lymphoblasts with 11q23 abnormalities can be induced to express monocytic features *in vitro*, strengthening the notion that such lesions arise in uncommitted stem cells or affect genes that control lineage commitment.[276]

The vast majority of *MLL* breakpoints take place within an 8.3 kilobase (kb) bcr[137] and result in a fusion gene that juxtaposes the amino-terminal portion of MLL, containing an A-T hook domain and a DNA methyltransferase (MT) domain, to the carboxyl-terminal portion of the partner gene.[178,263-266,277] The targets of MLL action appear to be the clustered homeodomain *HOX* genes,[237] consistent with the close identity of the MLL protein to that of Trithorax, a *Drosophila* transcription factor known to regulate the actions of a wide spectrum of homeotic genes in the bithorax complex of the fly, which is required throughout embryogenesis for differentiation of the head, thorax, and abdomen.[179,264,266,278] The identity of the fusion partner in 11q23 translocations appears to be of secondary importance to retention of the A-T hook and MT domains of the MLL protein, although it may influence the lineage predilection of the leukemia. The *MLL* gene may participate in leukemogenesis more often than is indicated by studies of 11q23 cytogenetic changes. A tandem duplication of a portion of the *MLL* gene links the intact gene to a duplication of its amino-terminal region.[279]

MYC Activation in B-Cell ALL

ALL often arises from translocations that affect the *IG* genes (Table 3.3). Patients with B-cell ALL or Burkitt's lymphoma commonly display a t(8;14)(q24;q32) translocation that juxtaposes one allele of *MYC*, a bHLH/leucine zipper gene located on chromosome 8, with the *IGH* locus on chromosome 14q32.[160,280,281] This juxtaposition of *MYC* coding sequences to *IGH* enhancer elements results in dysregulated expression of the MYC protein. Although the t(8;14) accounts for most B-cell ALL cases with rearranged *MYC* loci, two variants are also capable of activating MYC. In cells with the t(2;8) or the t(8;22), the *MYC* gene remains on chromosome 8 and portions of the κ or λ light-chain genes on chromosome 2 or 22, respectively, are translocated to a site downstream of *MYC* (reviewed elsewhere),[153] leading to aberrant expression of *MYC*.[161,162,167]

T-Cell Acute Lymphoblastic Leukemia

bHLH, HOX, and Other Developmental Genes

Transcription factor genes are the preferred targets of chromosomal translocations in patients with T-cell ALL (Table 3.3). Notable examples include the bHLH genes *MYC*,[181,182]

SCL(TAL1),[186,282] and *LYL1*,[184] which are essential for the development of other lineages, but, with the exception of *MYC*, are not normally expressed in T-lymphoid cells. When rearranged near enhancers within the *TCRB* locus on chromosome 7q34, or the *TCRA/D* loci on chromosome 14q11, these regulatory genes become active, and their protein products bind inappropriately to the promoter or enhancer elements of downstream target genes.

A useful model of aberrant transcription factor expression in T-cell ALL is provided by *SCL* activation due to the t(1;14)[185,282] or an interstitial deletion upstream of the gene (Fig. 3.3).[120] These chromosomal aberrations characterize 25% of all cases of childhood T-cell ALL and lead to ectopic expression of SCL in the thymus.[283] Because the SCL protein forms a pentameric DNA-binding complex with E2A, LMO2, GATA1, and LDB1,[284] its ectopic expression in T cells might be expected to activate specific sets of target genes that are normally quiescent in T-cell progenitors. Alternatively, SCL might be leukemogenic via a dominant-negative effect, since overexpression of SCL can lead to a functional inactivation of E2A homodimers or E2A-HEB heterodimers, presumably by sequestering E2A in the aforementioned pentameric complex (Fig. 3.4). This model is supported by the observations that E2A-deficient mice develop T-cell ALL[287,288] and that mice expressing the E2A inhibitor Id2 in the thymus develop T-cell ALL.[289] Moreover, mice that express SCL mutant proteins that are unable to bind DNA or activate transcription, but retain the ability to bind E2A, develop a form of T-cell ALL that is indistinguishable from that produced by the full-length SCL protein.[286,290,291]

In addition to genes encoding bHLH proteins, additional classes of regulatory genes are activated by chromosomal translocations in patients with T-cell ALL. These include the t(11;14)(p15;q11) or t(11;14)(p13;q11), which juxtapose the coding sequences of *LMO1* (formerly known as *RBTN1* or *TTG1*) or *LMO2* (formerly known as *RBTN2* or *TTG2*) with regulatory regions of the *TCR* loci.[189,191,192] Although present in high concentrations in the central nervous system (CNS),[189] these proteins are expressed only in the most immature T cells[292] and, as indicated earlier, can bind SCL.[293,294] LMO1 induces thymic lymphomas in transgenic mice[295]; the age of onset and penetrance of the disease is markedly accelerated by coexpression of SCL in the thymus (Fig. 3.4).[286,291]

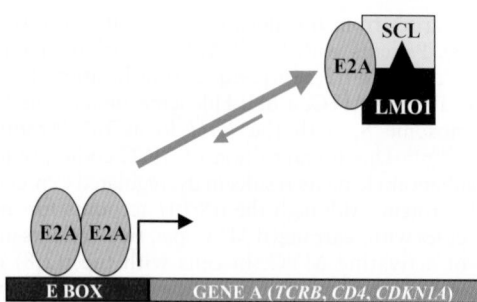

FIGURE 3.4 Dominant negative inhibition leading to disordered gene regulation, impaired differentiation, and leukemia. E2A (*yellow ovals*) normally forms a homodimer in developing thymocytes, binds to an E-box sequence, and activates genes important for the normal differentiation of thymocytes (including *TCRB*, *CD4*, and *CDKN1A*). When SCL (*blue box*) is aberrantly expressed in immature thymocytes, it binds E2A in concert with LMO1 (*black box*) or LMO2. This complex is more stable than the E2A-E2A homodimer.[285] Therefore, E2A molecules are not available to form a homodimer, leading to a functional inactivation of E2A, downregulation of critical developmental genes (such as *TCRB*, *CD4*, and *CDKN1A*), impaired thymocyte differentiation, and ultimately T-cell ALL (see Ref 286 for details).

Tragically, reports from a gene therapy trial of infants with X-linked severe combined immune deficiency demonstrated that four children whose immune system had been successfully reconstituted by a retroviral vector carrying a cDNA for the common γ-chain gene had developed T-cell ALL. Strikingly, the malignant cells from these patients showed that the retroviral particle had integrated near the *LMO2* gene, leading to its overexpression in the malignant lymphoblasts.[296,297] This observation indicates that *LMO2* can be activated iatrogenically by the nearby insertion of a highly active retroviral enhancer.

HOX11 and *HOX11L2* represent two additional developmental control genes that are inappropriately placed under the control of *TCR* loci. Located on 10q24,[193,194] *HOX11* encodes a homeodomain transcription factor that can bind DNA and activate specific target genes.[298] It is most closely related to *Hlx*, a murine homeobox gene expressed in specific hematopoietic cell lineages and during mouse embryogenesis.[299] A specific homeotic role of *HOX11* in mammalian development was demonstrated by ablation of this gene, which blocked the formation of the spleen in otherwise normal mice.[300] Activation of *HOX11* by chromosomal translocations, either the t(10;14)(q24;q11) or the t(7;10)(q35;q24), in developing T cells is thought to interfere with normal regulatory cascades to promote malignant transformation.

More recently, the *HOX11L2* gene, located at 5q35, has been found to be activated by fusion near the *BCL11B* locus as a result of the t(5;14)(q35;q32) or by fusion to the *TCRδ* locus as a result of the t(5;14)(q35;q11). Although neither of these translocations is commonly recognized with use of conventional cytogenetic techniques, almost 20% of childhood T-cell ALL patients demonstrated a *HOX11L2* gene translocation by FISH.[197] Although some studies have suggested that T-cell ALL patients whose lymphoblasts overexpress *HOX11L2* have a poor prognosis, this finding has not been confirmed.[301]

The chromosomal rearrangements inv(7)(p15q34) and t(7;7)(p15;q34) both lead to a fusion of the *HOXA* cluster with *TCRB*.[198,199] The immunophenotypes of T-cell ALL with these translocations were generally negative for cell surface expression of TCR α/β and TCRγ/δ, reflecting differentiation arrest at a relatively immature stage 3.[198] Patients with this fusion overexpressed many *HOXA* cluster genes, particularly *HOXA7*, *HOXA9*, and *HOXA10*.[198,199] Of note, the same *HOXA* cluster genes, (*HOXA7*, *HOXA9*, and *HOXA10*) are frequently overexpressed in patients with AML (see the following sections).

Fusion Genes in T-cell ALL

Although most chromosomal translocations in T-cell ALL patients lead to inappropriate activation of normal cellular proto-oncogenes such as *MYC*, *SCL*, or *LMO2*, some can produce fusion genes (Table 3.3). *MLL-ENL* fusion results from the t(11;19)(q23;p13) translocation and is associated with AML, B-cell precursor ALL, and T-cell ALL. Strikingly, in one series, all 11 T-cell ALL patients with the *MLL-ENL* fusion became long-term survivors, suggesting that this rearrangement is associated with a good prognosis.[302]

The t(10;11)(p13;q21) translocation leads to formation of a *CALM-AF10* fusion gene. This fusion was initially identified in the U937 cell line, which was established from a patient with histiocytic lymphoma and has been shown to differentiate along the macrophage lineage *in vitro*.[303] Subsequently, this fusion was found in patients with a wide spectrum of hematologic malignancies, but most commonly in patients with T-cell ALL.[200,304–306] *CALM-AF10* fusions were identified in 12 (9%) of 131 consecutive patients with T-cell ALL. Of note, all of the patients with *CALM-AF10* fusions had either immature T-cell lymphoblasts that expressed no *TCR* genes or

TCRγ/δ-positive lymphoblasts. None of the patients with *CALM-AF10* fusions expressed *TCRα/β*, suggesting that such fusions are restricted to the *TCRγ/δ* lineage.[201]

An unusual fusion gene resulting in ABL kinase activation has been identified in some patients with T-ALL. A small deletion removes approximately 500 kb of chromosome 9, with breakpoints within an intron of the *NUP214* gene and within the first intron of *ABL*.[307,308] Remarkably, this deleted fragment becomes ligated as a circular episome that encodes a fusion gene between amino-terminal sequences of NUP214 and the ABL kinase. It is maintained and amplified as an episomal structure and is small enough that it does not appear as a double-minute chromatin body and can be visualized cytogenetically only by FISH analysis for the affected genes. The NUP214-ABL fusion typically occurs in the subset of cases with activated HOX11 or HOX11L2 homeobox transcription factors.

Acute Myeloid Leukemia

Core Binding Factor Fusions (AML1-ETO and CBFB-MYH11)

The same general mechanisms responsible for proto-oncogene activation in ALL are active in AML (Table 3.3). A prime example of a chimeric transcription factor in AML patients is the AML1-ETO protein resulting from the t(8;21)(q22;q22).[208,209] In this gene fusion, the sequence-specific DNA-binding and protein-protein interaction properties are encoded by a large domain of the *AML1* (also known as *RUNX1*) gene,[309] which is homologous to the *Drosophila* pair-rule segmentation gene, *runt*. In normal hematopoietic cells, AML1 forms a stable transcription activation complex with the CBFβ protein[310] Intriguingly, CBFβ is also involved in a common chromosomal rearrangement in AML patients, the inv(16)(p13q22), found in association with myelomonocytic AML and increased bone marrow eosinophils (designated M4-Eo in the FAB classification). This rearrangement joins the amino-terminal sequences of the *CBFB* gene to the carboxyl terminus of the smooth muscle myosin heavy-chain gene (*MYH11*), resulting in formation of a CBFB-MYH11 fusion protein.[216] Both *AML1* and *CBFB* are normally expressed in early myeloid cells, suggesting that the oncogenicity of the respective fusion proteins stems from disruption of a transcriptional regulatory complex specific for myeloid developmental processes.[311]

The combinatorial versatility of the *AML1* locus can be seen from its fusion with sequences from the *EVI1* gene in t(3;21)-positive chronic myelogenous leukemia (CML) in blast crisis[213] or the *EAP* gene in patients with myelodysplastic syndrome (MDS).[212] Inclusion of the runt-homologous DNA binding/dimerization domain of AML1 and the zinc-finger DNA-binding domains of EVI1 in the AML1-EVI1 chimeric protein affords numerous opportunities for aberrant regulation of target genes.

PML-RARα Fusions in Promyelocytic Leukemia

Oncologists have long envisioned treatments based on a molecular understanding of oncogenic proteins. Major progress toward this goal has been achieved in patients with acute promyelocytic leukemia (APL; FAB M3) and a t(15;17)(q21;q11-q22) translocation. This translocation leads to a chimeric protein that fuses the ligand- and DNA-binding sequences of the retinoic acid receptor α (*RARA*) gene on chromosome 17 to the *PML* gene on chromosome 15 (Table 3.3).[218-220] In its unaltered form, the RARA protein binds first to the retinoic acid ligand and then to DNA through its zinc-finger region. PML proteins are normally located in novel macromolecular nuclear organelles, called *PML oncogenic domains*

(PODs).[312-314] The PML-RARA fusion proteins disrupt these subnuclear structures, causing normal PML, RXR, and other nuclear proteins to disperse in an abnormal microparticulate pattern,[312-314] and interfere with normal myeloid cell development, leading to arrest of differentiation in the promyelocytic stage. These fundamental observations provide a rationale for use of all-*trans*-retinoic acid to treat patients with APL.[315-318] In pharmacologic doses, the compound binds to the RARA fusion partner, followed by reorganization of PML and its associated proteins into normal-appearing nuclear PODs. Subsequently, the leukemic cells develop into mature myeloid cells with limited life spans. Although retinoic acid treatment of APL does not result in permanent remissions, combination with cytotoxic agents has led to dramatic improvements in long-term remission rates.[210,309,318,319]

NUP98 Fusion Genes in the Myeloid Leukemias

The *NUP98* locus encodes a 98-kDa component of the nuclear pore complex, which mediates nucleocytoplasmic transport of RNA and protein. *NUP98* has been identified in fusion transcripts with more than 20 different partner genes, predominantly in patients with myeloid leukemias and MDS.[202,239,320-326] About half of the *NUP98* partner genes encode homeobox proteins, predominantly of the *abd-b* type (*HOXA7, A9, A11, HOXC11, C13, HOXD11, D13*). The remaining *NUP98* partner genes belong to no recognized gene family, but most are predicted to form coiled-coil structures.[327] *NUP98* gene fusions are associated with a wide spectrum of malignant diseases. Although MDS and AML are the most common diagnoses associated with these fusions, the *NUP98-RAP1GDS1* fusion is seen exclusively in T-cell ALL patients.[202] Many of the *NUP98* fusions, including *NUP98-HOXD13*, *NUP98-TOP1*, and *NUP98-DDX10*, have been identified in patients with t-AML or t-MDS following multiagent chemotherapy.[229,321,328] Several reports have suggested that individuals of East Asian decent are more prone to translocations involving *NUP98*, especially the t(7;11),[329,330] although this observation has not been confirmed in all studies.[228] In addition to acute leukemias, NUP98 translocations have also been recognized in patients with CML, most commonly during evolution to blast crisis.[331] This observation suggests that the products of NUP98 fusion genes might cooperate with receptor tyrosine kinases, such as BCR-ABL, during the course of malignant transformation. This hypothesis is supported by a report showing that NUP98-HOXA9 and BCR-ABL fusion kinase induce acute leukemia in a mouse model.[332]

EVI1 Activation in Myeloid Leukemias With High Platelet Counts

In some cases of AML with high platelet counts, the inv(3)(q21;q26.2) or the t(3;3)(q21;q26.2) moves promoter/enhancer sequences from one site on chromosome 3 into the *EVI1* locus on the same chromosome,[214] leading to increased gene expression. The EVI1 protein binds to promoter/enhancer sequences containing the GATA sequence motif, and its tumorigenicity may come from interference with regulatory signals normally mediated by the GATA family of hematopoietic transcriptional regulators.[333,334] The tissue distribution of EVI1 in oocytes and kidney cells and its dominant interfering effect on normal myelopoiesis suggest an important developmental role in regulatory pathways of proliferation or differentiation.

Chronic Myelogenous Leukemia

The Ph, a product of the t(9;22)(q34;q11) translocation, was originally identified in patients with CML; subsequently, it was found in 3% to 5% of children and 30% to 40% of adults with ALL.[335,336] The t(9;22) produces a *BCR-ABL* fusion gene consisting of 5′ (upstream) sequences from *BCR* and 3′ (downstream) sequences from *ABL*.[337,338] The 8.5-kb fusion transcript found in CML encodes a 210-kDa hybrid protein that is activated as a tyrosine-specific protein kinase, similar to the v-abl protein product.[339,340] In patients with ALL, the *BCR-ABL* rearrangement typically produces a 6.5- to 7.0-kb fusion transcript and a 185- to 190-kDa hybrid protein. [341,342]

The amino-terminal sequences of *ABL* are replaced in oncogenic forms of the gene, by the Moloney virus *gag* gene in the case of the retroviral v-abl[343] and by *BCR* sequences in the *BCR-ABL* fusion gene of CML and ALL.[339,340] Products of both the v-abl and *BCR-ABL* fusion genes can transform pre-B cells, but the latter cannot transform fibroblasts,[344] suggesting that amino-terminal alterations influence the ability of *ABL* to function as a lineage-specific transforming gene.

The poor prognosis of patients with BCR-ABL fusions has been attributed to transformation of a primitive hematopoietic stem cell that is poorly responsive to most forms of chemotherapy.[336,345,346] Responses have been induced in a subset of childhood Ph+ ALL patients with low WBC count by using intensive induction chemotherapy, followed by rotational treatment with pairs of non–cross-resistant drugs.[347] However, treatment of both CML and Ph+ ALL patients has been revolutionized by a tyrosine kinase inhibitor, imatinib mesylate (STI571; Glivec).[348] Remarkably, 98% of patients with chronic phase CML achieved a complete hematologic response with imatinib.[349] The responses seem to be quite durable, with an overall survival of 89% at 5 years.[349] Most relapses seem to be due to emergence of preexisting clones with BCR-ABL mutations.[350] Imatinib has also proven to be a very useful adjunct to conventional cytotoxic chemotherapy in the treatment of Ph+ ALL patients, with complete remission rates of 95% and 3 year survival rates of up to 55%.[351]

Anaplastic Large Cell Lymphoma

The t(2;5)(p23;q35) translocation in anaplastic large cell non-Hodgkin lymphoma (NHL) creates a novel fusion gene in which amino-terminal sequences from the nucleophosmin (*NPM*) nucleolar phosphoprotein gene on chromosome 5q35 are linked to the catalytic domain from a previously unidentified tyrosine kinase gene on chromosome 2p23, called *ALK* for *anaplastic lymphoma kinase* (Table 3.3).[205] Normally expressed in nervous system–derived cells of small intestine, testis, and brain, but not in normal lymphoid cells, ALK shares greatest homology with members of the insulin receptor subfamily of receptor tyrosine kinases. Unscheduled expression of a truncated ALK kinase in activated T lymphocytes probably contributes to the pathogenesis of anaplastic large cell lymphoma.

Soft Tissue Sarcomas

EWS and FUS Fusion Genes

Chimeric transcription factors arising from chromosomal translocations have been identified in a large number of soft tissue sarcomas (see Table 3.4). The first translocation to be characterized at the molecular level in sarcomas was the t(11;22), which is virtually pathognomonic of the Ewing's sarcoma family of tumors (ESFT). The fusion gene created by this rearrangement, *EWS-FLI1*,[358] encodes a chimeric protein containing amino-terminal sequences of EWS linked to the

Ets-like DNA-binding domain of FLI1 (named for Friend leukemia integration site 1).[377] *In vitro* transformation assays[378] suggested that malignant transformation by this protein required the FLI1 DNA-binding domain, suggesting that the chimeric protein acts by disrupting transcriptional regulatory pathways. The fusion gene has been reported to alter the expression of more than 750 genes[358,379,380] and to be involved in transformation, increased proliferation, inhibition of differentiation, and suppression of apoptosis.[381–386] Finally, EWS-FLI1 expression has been shown to be necessary for the oncogenic process in Ewing's sarcoma cells since "knockdown" of EWS-FLI1 decreases proliferation and tumorigenicity of ESFT.[387]

Variant translocations fuse identical *EWS* sequences to the DNA-binding domains of two related Ets family members, *ERG*[360,371,388] and *ETV1* (see Table 3.4).[361] As is the case for EWS-FLI1, the RNA recognition motif of EWS is absent from these variant proteins, replaced by the DNA-binding domains of the fusion partners. The amino-terminal sequences of EWS are rich in glutamine, serine, and tyrosine, making this domain a potent *trans*-activator of gene expression.[378,389] Hence, fusion proteins containing the EWS *trans*-activation domain and an Ets-like DNA-binding domain could act by changing the expression of target genes.

The t(12;22)(q13;q12) results in fusion of the *EWS* gene to the bZIP domain of *ATF1* and leads to an entirely different tumor, the malignant melanoma of the soft parts.[371] In malignant liposarcoma, the t(12;16)(q13;q14) fuses the amino terminus of an *EWS*-related gene called *FUS* (or *TLS*) to the bZIP domain of *CHOP*, initially characterized as a non–DNA-binding, dominant-negative inhibitor of other bZIP proteins of the CAAT-box–binding C/EBP family.[365,366] The abundant EWS and FUS/TLS proteins can form ternary complexes with a variety of RNA-binding proteins, such as A1 and C1/C2.[201] In addition, the amino-terminal sequences of FUS and EWS can be interchanged in chimeric constructs without affecting the results of *trans*-activation and transformation assays.[390]

The ubiquitous involvement of EWS and FUS, combined with the lineage-specific association of the DNA-binding domains of fusion proteins in the malignant solid tumors, in general, suggests that the DNA-binding region specifies the downstream target gene and thus the phenotype of the arrested and transformed malignant mesenchymal progenitor cell. This principle is well illustrated by the Wilms' tumor gene, *WT1*, which gives rise to desmoplastic round cell tumors when it becomes fused to *EWS*.[363]

PAX, SYT, and TFE3 Fusion Genes in Soft Tissue Sarcomas

In patients with alveolar rhabdomyosarcoma (ARMS), translocations affecting chromosome 13q14 fuse either the *PAX3* or the *PAX7* gene with a portion of a forkhead domain gene, *FKHR* (or *FOXO1A*) (Table 3.4).[355–357] The t(2;13) (q35;q14) chromosomal translocation is found in 60% of patients with ARMS [391,392] and results in the fusion of PAX3, a developmental transcription factor required for limb myogenesis,[393] with *FOXO1A*. The paired box and homeodomain regions of the *PAX3* gene are preserved, but the carboxyl-terminal sequences are replaced by a portion of the forkhead DNA-binding sequences from *FOXO1A*. The resultant fusion gene binds to PAX3 targets, is a more potent transactivator than the wild-type PAX3,[394] and causes transformation. In ARMS, the presence of the translocation is critical to the survival of tumors, as downregulation of this gene leads to apoptosis.[395] The PAX3-FOXO1A, but not PAX3, activated a myogenic/myoblastic transcription program, including induction

TABLE 3.4

RECURRENT CHROMOSOMAL TRANSLOCATIONS ASSOCIATED WITH CHILDHOOD SARCOMAS

Sarcoma type	Chromosomal abnormality	Chimeric gene	Structure motif in chimeric protein	Estimated frequency, %	References
Angiomatoid fibrous histiocytoma	t(2;16)(q34;p11)	FUS-CREB1	bZIP	89	352
Angiomatoid fibrous histiocytoma	t(12;16)(q13;p11)	FUS-ATF1	bZIP	11	353
Alveolar soft part sarcoma	t(X;17)(p11;q25)	ASPSCR1-TFE3	Microphthalmia-TFE bHLHzip	100	354
Rhabdomyosarcoma (alveolar)	t(2;2)(q35;p23)	PAX3–NCOA1	Paired box/homeodomain	Rare	
Rhabdomyosarcoma (alveolar)	t(2;13)(q35;q14)	PAX3-FKHR	Paired box/homeodomain	95	355,356
Rhabdomyosarcoma (alveolar)	t(1;13)(p36;q14)	PAX7-FKHR	Paired box/homeodomain	5	357
EWS	t(11;22)(q24;q12)	EWSR1-FLI1	Ets-like	85	358,359
EWS	t(21;22)(q22;q12)	EWSR1-ERG	Ets-like	10	359,360
EWS	t(7;22)(p22;q12)	EWSR1-ETV1	Ets-like	Rare	359,361
EWS	t(17;22)(q12;q12)	EWSR1-ETV4	Ets-like	Rare	359,362
EWS	t(2;22)(q33;q12)	EWSR1-FEV	Ets-like	Rare	359
DSRCT	t(11;22)(p13;q12)	EWSR1-WT1	Zinc finger	95	359,363
Inflammatory myofibroblastic tumor	t(1;2)(q25;p23)	ALK-TPM3	Tyrosine kinase		364
Inflammatory myofibroblastic tumor	t(2;19)(p23;p13)	ALK-TPM4	Tyrosine kinase		364
Inflammatory myofibroblastic tumor	t(2;17)(p23;q23)	ALK-CLTC	Tyrosine kinase		364
Myxoid liposarcoma	t(12;16)(q13;p11)	FUS-DDIT3	bZIP	95	359,365,366
Myxoid liposarcoma Extrasketal	t(12;22)(q13;q12)	EWSR1-ATF1	bZIP	5	359,367
Myxoid chondrosarcoma	t(9;22)(q22;q12)	EWSR1-NR4A3	bZIP	75	359,368
Myxoid chondrosarcoma	t(9;15)(q22;q21)	TFC12-NR4A3	bHLH		369
Myxoid chondrosarcoma	t(9;17)(q22;q11)	TAF15- NR4A3	bZIP		370
Malignant melanoma of soft part	t(12;22)(q13;q12)	EWSR1-ATF1	bZIP	Not known	359,371
Liposarcoma	t(12;16)(q13,p11)	FUS-ATF1	bZIP	Not known	365,366
Synovial sarcoma	t(X;18)(p11;q11)	SYT-SSX1	Kruppel-associated box	65	359,366
Synovial sarcoma	t(X;18)(p11;q11)	SYT-SSX2	Kruppel-associated box	35	359,366
Synovial sarcoma	t(X;18)(p11;q11)	SYT-SSX4	Kruppel-associated box		
Synovial sarcoma	t(X;20)	SS18L1-SSX1	Kruppel-associated box	Rare	
Synovial sarcoma	t(X;20)	SS18L1-SSX2	Kruppel-associated box	Rare	
Dermatofibrosarcoma protuberans	t(17;22)(q22;q13)	COL1A1-PDGFB	Tyrosine kinase	Not known	359,372
Endometrial stromal sarcoma	t(7;17)(p15;q21)	JAZF1-JJAZ1	Polycomb group complexes Zinc finger		373
Congenital fibrosarcoma and mesoblastic nephroma	t(12;15)(p13;q25)	EVT6-NTRK3	HLH, tyrosine kinase	Not known	359,374,375
Small round cell sarcoma	inv 22q	EWSR1-ZSG	Zinc finger	Not known	376

EWS, Ewing's sarcoma; DSRCT, desmoplastic small round cell tumor; bZIP, basic region/leucine zipper domain; bHLHzip, basic region/helix-loop-helix/leucine zipper domain; bHLH, basic region/helix-loop-helix; HLH, helix-loop-helix.

of transcription factors *MyoD*, *Myogenin*, *Slug*, and a battery of other genes involved in muscle function.[396] Notable among this group were the growth factor gene *Igf2* and several other genes (*IGFBP5*, *HSIX1*, and *Slug*) that were also highly expressed in patients with ARMS. The variant translocation, t(1;13)(p36;q14), truncates the *PAX7* gene in a similar fashion,[357] suggesting that a common set of target genes, recognized by both of the PAX proteins, are involved in the pathogenesis of ARMS.

Synovial sarcoma is a highly aggressive soft tissue sarcoma in adolescents and young adults with a mortality rate of more than 50%,[397] which is associated with t(X;18) (p11;q11) translocations (Table 3.4). The translocations result in the fusion of the genes *SYT*, on chromosome 18, and *SSX* (*SSX1*, *SSX2*, or rarely *SSX4*) on the X chromosome. In the SYT-SSX chimeric protein, almost the entire SYT protein is retained except the last eight amino acids, which are replaced by the 78 amino acids from the carboxyl-terminal of SSX. The SSX-derived regions are required for transformation since forced overexpression of wild-type SYT does not induce transformation unlike the SYT-SSX fusion protein.[398]

Alveolar soft part sarcoma (ASPS) is a rare extremity sarcoma presenting in adolescents or young adults. Its clinical course is indolent, but it is chemoresistant and associated with a high risk of metastases to the lung and the CNS.[354] Despite the slow growth, the cancer progresses relentlessly and is usually fatal.[399] ASPS cells have a recurrent chromosomal translocation, der(17)t(X;17)(p11;q25),[400,401] that has been shown to result in the fusion of the *TFE3* transcription factor gene (from Xp11) with a novel gene at 17q25, named *ASPSCR1*.[354] The same translocation has also been described in a small number of renal carcinomas, primarily in children and young adults. *TFE3* has also been reported as a fusion gene partner in other renal carcinomas (*PRCC-TFE3*),[402–404] *PSF-TFE3*, and *NONO-TFE3*.[405] TFE3 is transcription factor and a member of the microphthalmia-TFE bHLH/leucine zipper subfamily; the function of the fusion partner ASPSCR1 remains largely unknown. The *ASPSCR1-TFE3* fusion encodes a chimeric protein that replaces the amino-terminal portion of TFE3 by ASPSCR1 sequences, while retaining the TFE3 DNA-binding region, activation domain, and nuclear localization signal.[354] The function of the *ASPSCR1-TFE3* fusion gene is largely unknown, but, analogous to the PAX3-FOXO1A fusion, the ASPSCR1-TFE3 fusion protein is a more efficient transactivator than the native TFE3.

In summary, many recurrent translocations occur in pediatric soft tissue sarcoma patients, often involving the fusion of transcription factors implicated in the embryonic development of the tissue of origin. The fusion protein is generally more active than the wild-type partner and leads to disordered growth and failure of terminal differentiation. Moreover, although the precise mechanism of oncogenesis is unknown for the majority of these chimeric proteins, they or their target genes remain excellent therapeutic targets since they are uniquely expressed in these cancers and not in normal human cells.

CHROMOSOMAL DELETION LEADS TO INACTIVATION OF TUMOR SUPPRESSOR GENES

In addition to the proto-oncogene–activating lesions described earlier, recurring genetic changes affect a second class of genes, known as *tumor suppressor genes*, whose products normally provide negative controls over cell proliferation or survival. Loss of function of these proteins through deletion or mutational inactivation liberates the cell from growth constraints, contributing to malignant transformation. The cumulative effect of genetic lesions that activate proto-oncogenes or inactivate tumor suppressor genes is a breakdown in the balance between cell proliferation and cell loss due to terminal differentiation or apoptosis, resulting in clonal overgrowth within a specific cell lineage. The available evidence suggests that the progression of tumors to clinically recognizable forms requires both types of changes.[406]

The first indication that negatively acting proteins contribute to cancer came from research with somatic cell hybrids, showing that tumor cells fused to normal cells no longer exhibited malignant growth properties.[407] These observations were supported by epidemiologic studies on the inherited predisposition to develop retinoblastoma, characterized by an early age of onset for bilateral tumors.[77] Knudson's genetic model of carcinogenesis (Fig. 3.2) specifies two rate-limiting mutations, the first of which can be germline (in bilateral tumors) or somatic (in unilateral tumors), with the second invariably being somatic (Table 3.1). Subsequent findings made it clear that both types of inactivating mutations target the alleles of a single susceptibility locus, the *RB* gene, which resides on the long arm of chromosome 13.[80]

Mutations in the "*RB*" pathway

The *RB* gene encodes a ubiquitously expressed 110-kDa nuclear phosphoprotein[60,408,409] that plays a central role in regulating the progression of cells through the first gap (G_1) phase of the cell cycle (reviewed by Weinberg[410]). As discussed in a later section, RB serves as a versatile gatekeeper of the cell cycle, transducing physiologic signals that instruct cells to remain in G_1 or to move past a defined restriction point and prepare for DNA replication. Most commonly, the *RB* locus is disrupted by localized deletions or by point mutations that produce frameshift mutations, which result in truncation of the protein. Other point mutations give rise to stable proteins with single amino acid substitutions in critical domains of the protein.[411–413] Such mutants lose the ability to bind cell cycle regulatory proteins, such as E2F, which then can participate without restraint in cell cycle progression (as reviewed by Nevins[414]). In addition to RB inactivation produced by mutations of genomic DNA, several viral transforming proteins can deplete cells of RB protein by binding to the unphosphorylated form of the protein.[415,416] The net result is analogous to that produced by inactivation of both *RB* alleles in human retinoblastoma.[417]

Mutations resulting in homozygous inactivation of the *RB* gene are invariably found in retinoblastoma[408,418,419] but are not restricted to this tumor. Patients with germline mutations of one *RB* allele characteristically develop bilateral retinoblastoma in the first year of life and are predisposed to develop osteosarcoma and soft tissue sarcomas as well (as reviewed elsewhere[420]) although these tumors occur later in childhood and adolescence. Somatically acquired *RB* mutations figure prominently in the development of many epithelial tumors, such as bladder, prostate, breast, cervical, and small cell lung cancer,[419,421–425] even though germline mutations are not predisposing events. Apparently, the inactivation of *RB* is an early and essential step in the cascade of genetic changes leading to retinoblastoma and possibly to osteosarcoma; in adult carcinomas, *RB* mutations are not rate limiting but contribute to tumor progression.

The *CDKN2A* locus and the closely linked *CDKN2B* locus, both located on chromosome 9p21, are among the genomic regions most commonly deleted in cancer.[426,427] The *CDKN2A* locus encodes two proteins, formed by alternate first exons.[426] The two proteins utilize different reading frames and have no significant amino acid similarity. The CDKN2A protein, known as p16, INK4A, or MTS1, was the first to be discovered and will be referred to here as p16[INK4A]. p16[INK4A] encodes an inhibitor of the cyclin D-CDK4/6 complex, which, in turn, inhibits RB function (Fig. 3.5). Therefore, loss of p16[INK4A] leads to increased CDK4/6 activity, increased phosphorylated RB, and progression through the cell cycle.[428] The second protein encoded at the *CDKN2A* locus is p14[ARF], which encodes a protein that regulates p53 stability, perhaps through an interaction with MDM2.[429] The *CDKN2B* (also know as p15, INK4B, or MTS2) locus encodes a single protein that shares significant amino acid identity with CDKN2A. Because *CDKN2A* and *CDKN2B* are closely linked, genomic deletions often delete both loci. In addition to deletion, *CDKN2A* and *CDKN2B* are frequently inactivated by point mutations or promoter hypermethylation.[430] Thus, inactivation of CDKN2A or CDKN2B leads to the same functional result as inactivation of RB does, namely, loss of cell cycle control. Interestingly, relatively few tumors have mutations in both *RB* and *CDKN2A* or *CDKN2B*, underscoring the fact that *CDKN2A* and *CDKN2B* are in the same pathway as *RB*.[431]

The *TP53* Gene

The *TP53* gene in humans is located on 17p13 and encodes the ubiquitously expressed p53 nuclear protein,[432,433] which is inactivated in a wide variety of human tumors,[434] including carcinomas of the colon,[435] lung,[436] breast,[437] esophagus,[438] stomach,[439] liver,[440,441] anus,[442] ovary,[443] and prostate.[444] In these neoplasms, *TP53* mutations tend to occur as point mutations within four highly conserved domains, producing a protein that lacks normal regulatory functions. Often, the second allele is lost from the malignant clone by deletion, resulting in a reduction to homozygosity for the mutant allele.[434,435] *TP53* is also frequently inactivated in childhood tumors such as osteosarcoma,[445,446] RMS,[446,447] brain tumors,[434] NB,[448,449] CML,[450] Burkitt's lymphoma, and B-cell leukemia and is less frequently inactivated in T-cell or B-cell progenitor ALL.[451,452] Although these tumors can arise from the same types of missense mutations that occur in carcinomas, more often they contain deletions or GCRs of both alleles, resulting in total loss of the p53 protein rather than the production of a faulty protein.

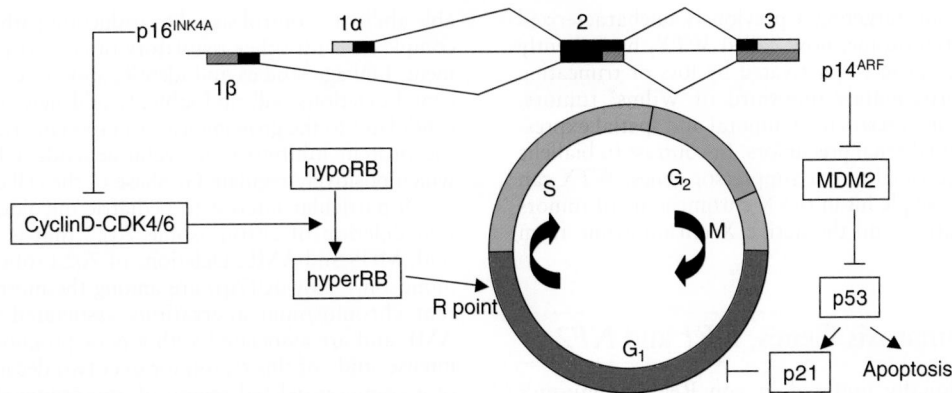

FIGURE 3.5 Cell cycle regulation by *RB*, *TP53*, and *CDKN2A* gene products. The *CDKN2A* locus encodes two proteins (p16[INK4A] and p14[ARF]), via the use of alternate first exons and alternate reading frames, as shown (*black boxes* indicate coding sequences, *blue* and *orange boxes* indicate untranslated regions). The p16INK4A inhibits the cyclin D-CDK interaction, which is required to phosphorylate RB. Phosphorylated RB in turn releases E2Fs and allows passage of the cell cycle through the restriction point ("R") and entry into S phase. Therefore, the net effect of either p16[INK4A] or RB loss is E2F activation, leading to cell cycle progression. p14[ARF] inhibits MDM2, which in turn inhibits p53. p53 activation leads to expression of p21, which inhibits cell cycle progression. Therefore, the net effect of p14[ARF] loss is also cell cycle progression.

Heritable cancer-associated changes of the *TP53* tumor suppressor gene occur in families with Li-Fraumeni syndrome (Table 3.1), an autosomal dominant predisposition for the development of RMS, other soft tissue sarcoma and bone sarcoma, premenopausal breast cancer, brain tumors, adrenocortical cell carcinoma, and acute leukemia.[37,453–455] The Li-Fraumeni syndrome appears to be rare, consistent with its autosomal dominant pattern of inheritance and its high fatality rate.[456] Statistical modeling suggests a 50% probability of invasive cancer by the age of 30 in members of Li-Fraumeni–affected families who carry the mutated *TP53* gene, compared with a 1% risk by the age of 30 in the general population.[456,457] Germline *TP53* mutations could be inherited or could arise as *de novo* mutations early in embryogenesis.

The existence of multiple independent *TP53* mutations in both sporadic and familial tumors[458–460] and the variety of familial tumors that can result from a single point mutation[460,461] suggest that the wild-type p53 gene product is critical for normal cellular DNA damage-response pathways and that alterations in p53 function lead to the transformation of diverse cell types. p53 functions, at least in part, as a transcription factor.[460,462,463] Its conserved domains include an amino-terminal activation domain[464,465] and a central sequence-specific DNA-binding domain.[466,467] Clues to the types of genes targeted by p53 came from the realization that its levels are increased in response to DNA damage.[468] The prevailing view is that p53 functions as a cell cycle checkpoint, blocking cell division in G₁ phase to allow repair of damaged DNA or even triggering apoptosis in cells that have defective genomes not amenable to repair.[469] In this way, the protein is thought to function almost exclusively as a tumor suppressor, preventing the development of malignant clones from cells with damaged genes. Thus, the p53 protein is not essential for normal cell division within any lineage during development; rather it acts as a gatekeeper, stopping the cell cycle and repairing or removing cells with damaged genomes that might otherwise evolve into malignant tumors.

WT1, the Wilms' Tumor Gene

The *WT1* gene, located on chromosome 11p13, encodes a 50-kDa nuclear transcription factor that contains four zinc-finger DNA-binding domains (reviewed elsewhere[470]). Its identification was the logical end of studies demonstrating large constitutional deletions of the 11p13 region in patients who developed the WAGR syndrome, comprising Wilms' tumor, aniridia, genitourinary tract abnormalities, and mental retardation.[82] As predicted by Knudson's hypothesis, tumors from these patients showed mutations of *WT1* in the remaining allele, indicating homozygous loss at this locus.[471] Somatic disruption of both *WT1* alleles has also been demonstrated in patients with unilateral Wilms' tumors.[472] Overall, 5% to 10% of Wilms' tumors have demonstrable homozygous *WT1* mutations,[473] although this number may be underestimated, because approximately 20% of such tumors show an LOH within the region encompassing this gene.[69,70,474]

Unique *WT1* mutations have been demonstrated in individuals with Denys-Drash syndrome, which includes intersex disorders, nephropathy (e.g., mesangial sclerosis), and Wilms' tumor. These constitutional missense mutations affect single amino acid residues that encode the third zinc finger of the protein.[471,475–478] A defective WT1 protein produced from one allele can apparently interfere with the function of normal WT1 produced from the intact allele, producing developmental anomalies and tumor predisposition. An additional form of the protein resulting from a splicing alteration and lacking exon 2 has been identified in tumor cells but not in normal cells and may represent a distinct mechanism for inactivation of *WT1* in Wilms' tumor.[479]

Expression of the *WT1* gene is restricted during development to mesenchymal tissues; specific cells of the collecting system within the kidney; non–germ cell components of the gonads, uterus, and spleen; primitive hematopoietic cells; and the mesothelium.[69,480,481] Targeted disruptions of the *WT1* gene in the mouse result in embryonic lethality secondary to failure of kidney and gonad development.[482] The transcriptional properties of the WT1 protein have been analyzed extensively and the analysis indicates that it is a repressor of several genes encoding proteins important for cell growth control, including insulin-like growth factor II, platelet-derived growth factor, and epidermal growth factor 1.[483–485] The precise mechanism by which WT1 exerts its effects during normal development and prevents tumor formation in the kidney awaits identification of the actual target genes that it regulates *in vivo*.

A somatic deletion targeting a previously uncharacterized gene on the X chromosome, now called *WTX*, has recently been reported. This gene is inactivated by loss or truncating mutations in approximately one-third of Wilms' tumors. *WTX* and *WT1* share a restricted temporal and spatial expression pattern in normal renal precursors. In contrast to biallelic inactivation of autosomal tumor suppressor genes, *WTX* can be inactivated by a single hit in the X chromosome of tumors from male population and the active X chromosome from female population.[486]

Neurofibromatosis Genes, *NF1* and *NF2*

NF1 is constitutionally mutated in von Recklinghausen's (type 1) neurofibromatosis, an inherited condition characterized by abnormal proliferation of cells of neural crest origin (reviewed elsewhere[487]). In addition to benign neurofibromas, patients with type 1 neurofibromatosis are at increased risk for developing malignant tumors such as pheochromocytomas and malignant peripheral nerve sheath tumors (MPNSTs) (see Table 3.1), which involve loss of the normal *NF1* allele, consistent with the interpretation that *NF1* acts as a tumor suppressor gene in cells of neural crest origin.[488–490] Loss of the normal *NF1* allele has been linked to malignant myeloid disorders, such as juvenile myelomonocytic leukemia (JMML), which occur with increased frequency in NF1 patients, suggesting that NF1 may participate in the downregulation of RAS proteins early in myelopoiesis.[491] Reports have also documented loss of expression and somatic deletion of *NF1* in NB and melanoma,[492,493] even though the frequency of these tumors is not increased in neurofibromatosis patients. More recently, gastrointestinal stromal tumors (GISTs) have been identified in NF1 patients.[494] Thus, NF1 mutations can be an early and predisposing event in the progression of some tumor types but a later and non–rate-limiting step in others.

NF1 interacts with GTPase-activating proteins (GAPs), which catalyze the hydrolysis of the activated GTP-bound form of RAS proteins. Loss of NF1 appears to downregulate GTPase activity in MPNSTs, consistent with a mechanism involving constitutive activation of the RAS pathway; however, NBs and melanomas lacking NF1 have normal GTPase activity, suggesting that loss of NF1 function can contribute to tumorigenesis through a separate and unknown mechanism.[492,493]

The spectrum of malignancies associated with neurofibromatosis type 2 include astrocytomas, meningiomas, and melanomas. The gene associated with this condition, *NF2*, is found on the long arm of chromosome 22 and encodes a protein of the "merlin" family, believed to be involved in a linkage of the cellular cytoskeleton to the cellular membrane and with cell-cell and cell-extracellular matrix interactions.[49,495] The mutations in *NF2* result in the formation of a truncated protein. Sporadic meningiomas are associated with mutations of the *NF2* gene, and loss of the chromosome 22 carrying the normal *NF2* gene often accompanies the development of meningiomas.

Other Known Tumor Suppressors

RB, *TP53*, *WT1*, *NF1*, and *NF2* are just five of the earliest tumor suppressor genes to be characterized. Others, such as von Hippel-Lindau (*VHL*),[496] adenomatous polyposis coli (*APC*),[497,498] inhibitor of CDK4 (*p16^INK4A*),[427,499] ARF (p14), AT mutated (*ATM*),[500] and breast cancer 1 (*BRCA1*),[501] were discovered later and less is known about their mechanisms of action. However, some of these proteins have shown a remarkable ability to control signal transduction pathways by forming complexes with other regulators of cell growth and development. Linkage studies and identification of consistent chromosomal deletions will undoubtedly add new tumor suppressor candidates to the growing list. An especially rich source may be the protein inhibitors of cyclin-dependent kinases (CDKs), which positively regulate G_1 phase of the cell cycle.

Of particular interest to pediatric oncologists is the recurrent deletion of chromosome 7q22 that is associated with both MDS and AML. Deletions of 7q22 (often in the form of monosomy 7 or del(7q)) are among the most common recurrent chromosomal aberrations associated with MDS and AML and are associated with a poor prognosis.[502,503] Despite intense study of this region for over two decades and isolation of a common deleted region of approximately 2.5 megabase (mb), no tumor suppressor gene in this region has been identified.[504,505] These observations have led some investigators to suspect that the phenotype caused by this recurrent deletion is due to haploinsufficiency of one or more genes in this region; this hypothesis can be tested by targeted deletions of large chromosomal regions in model organisms.[503]

Gene Amplification

Gene amplification allows a cell to increase the expression of critical genes whose products are ordinarily tightly controlled. The cytogenetic hallmarks of gene amplification are double-minute chromatin bodies and homogeneously staining regions, which contain the amplified DNA sequences, called *amplicons*. Several clinically important examples of proto-oncogene amplification can be found among the solid tumors of children and adults. The *MYCN* gene is amplified 10- to 300-fold in about one-third of childhood NB cases. Overexpression of the MYCN oncoprotein as a result of the DNA amplification has been linked to an advanced stage of disease and a poor prognosis and was the first amplified gene that was used as a marker to stratify patients for therapy.[506,507] Members of the *MYC* gene family, including *MYC*, *MYCN*, and *MYCL*, are also amplified in DNA extracted from small cell lung cancer lines and show higher levels of amplification when the tumor cells have been exposed to chemotherapy.[508,509] Another gene that has been found to be amplified in a subset of NB is *ALK*.[510–512]

More recently, a duplication of the *MYB* gene, leading to overexpression of MYB, has been identified in T-cell ALL samples.[125,513] The duplication seems to be mediated by a recombination between nearby *Alu* elements,[125] similar to the *MLL* partial tandem duplication. In addition to the partial tandem duplication discussed earlier, *MLL* amplification as part of a large amplicon has been noted by a number of investigators, often in the form of segmental "jumping translocations."[514,515]

Point Mutations Leading to Gene Activation or Inactivation

Activating Mutations in RAS and Receptor Tyrosine Kinase (RTK) Genes

Point mutations have received much less attention than chromosomal rearrangements as activators of cellular proto-oncogenes because they are not apparent by cytogenetic methods. However, this is rapidly changing with the advent of high-throughput gene resequencing studies (discussed in a later section). Through the use of experimental systems, it has been possible to predict the types of genes most likely to be activated by point mutations in human tumors. The *RAS* and

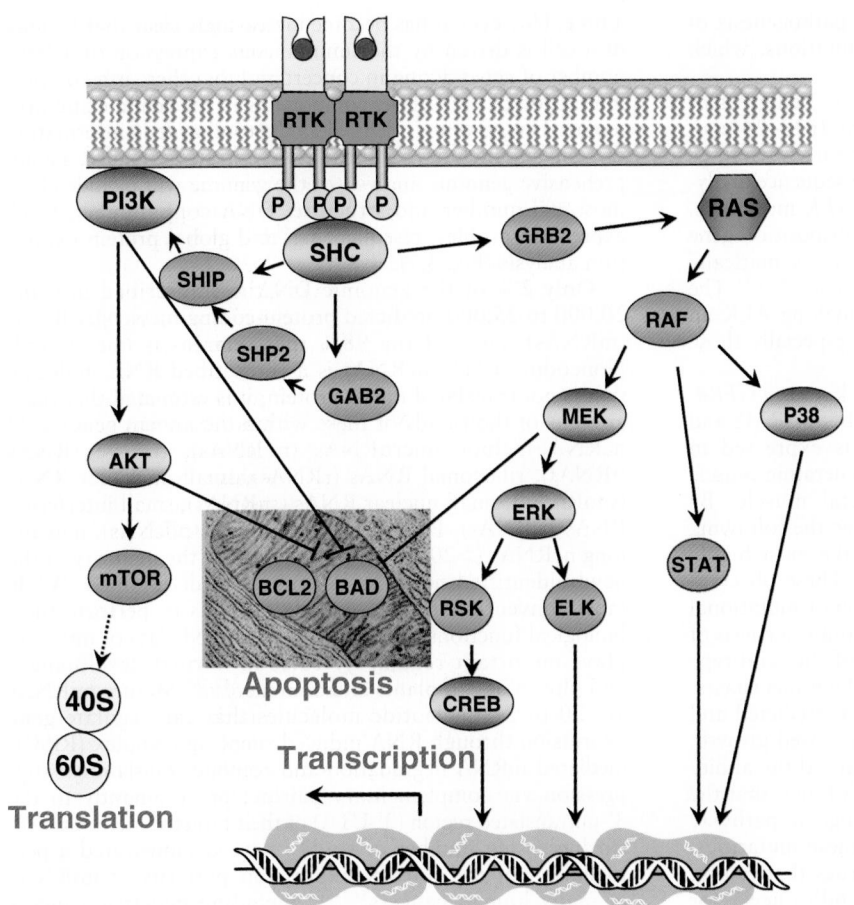

FIGURE 3.6 Signaling pathways initiated by tyrosine kinase receptors. RTK indicates any of numerous represents any of numerous receptor tyrosine kinases, such as EGFR, FLT3, KIT, or PDGFR. Upon activation by ligand (*red circle*) binding, the activated RTK phosphorylates downstream targets, impacting on DNA transcription, translation, and apoptosis, as indicated.

receptor tyrosine kinase gene families, both critical elements in signal transductions pathways, comprise the prototypic genes of this class (Fig. 3.6).

Human tumor DNAs were found to contain activated homologues of *HRAS* or *KRAS*[516,517] after such proto-oncogenes had been identified from comparative studies of viral oncogenes. Gene transfer methods identified an additional *RAS* homologue, called *NRAS*,[518] that had not been previously observed as a component of a transforming retrovirus. These three human genes—*HRAS*, *KRAS*, and *NRAS*—encode 21-kDa proteins localized to the inner surface of the cytoplasmic membrane[519] and function as intermediates in signal transduction pathways that regulate cell proliferation. The somatic mutations that activate *RAS* proto-oncogenes to transforming status usually affect codons 12, 13, or 61.[520] Mutated *RAS* genes also bind guanine nucleotides, but they have diminished capacity to hydrolyze GTP to GDP.[521–523] The transforming properties of activated RAS proteins are likely to result from their constitutive presence in an activated, GTP-bound form, which continuously activates the RAS signal transduction pathway. Human *RAS* genes activated by point mutations are tumorigenic in experimental systems, transforming NIH-3T3 murine fibroblasts *in vitro* and primary cultures of embryo fibroblasts.[524–526] Their role in mammalian tumorigenesis has also been confirmed by studies of oncogene-induced tumors in animal models.[527,528]

Among the childhood cancers, activated *NRAS* genes appear to be preferentially involved in the leukemias, having been detected in myeloid cell lines,[529,530] in fresh leukemic cells from patients with acute and CMLs,[531,532] and in lymphoblastic leukemias with a T-cell immunophenotype.[533] *NRAS* gene mutations involving codon 13 or 61 were found in approxi-

mately 20% of cases of AML, regardless of the morphologic subtype.[531,534] A mutation of codon 12 of the *KRAS* gene was also observed in 2 of 37 AML cases.[535] In a study of lymphoblasts from children with ALL, cells from 2 of 19 patients showed mutated *NRAS* genes; in both cases, the changes involved codon 12.[536]

The importance of RAS pathway activation in pediatric malignancies is highlighted by mutations of additional genes encoding proteins involved in RAS signaling. The association of NF1 deficiency in patients with JMML was discussed earlier, and acquired *PTPN11* mutations have been identified in patients with AML, ALL, and JMML.[537–539] *PTPN11* encodes SHP-2, a protein tyrosine phosphatase with two Src homology 2 (SH2) domains, that transmits signals from growth factor receptors to signaling molecules including KRAS and NRAS.[538] Of note, although most cases of Noonan syndrome are associated with germline mutations of *PTPN11*,[540] some Noonan syndrome patients have germline *KRAS* mutations, underscoring the proposal that *PTPN11* and *KRAS* lie along the same pathway.[541]

Point mutations or internal tandem duplications in receptor tyrosine kinase genes, such as those encoding the gene for *KIT*, and more commonly the *FLT3* receptor tyrosine kinase are associated with myeloid malignancies.[542–544] Similar to *RAS* mutations, mutations of the receptor tyrosine kinase genes are thought to induce constitutive phosphorylation of downstream substrates, resulting in hyperproliferation.[545,546] Analysis of the G-CSF receptor (*CSF4R*) in patients with myeloid leukemia preceded by severe congenital neutropenia, revealed missense mutations, leading to truncation of the carboxyl-terminal cytoplasmic region of the receptor.[547] Presumably, aberrant activation of the cell cycle and survival-signaling functions of this molecule contribute to the pathogenesis of AML in patients with neutrophil elastase mutations, which disrupt normal myeloid cell differentiation.[548,549]

Using a whole-genome linkage approach in pedigrees of patients with NB, a linkage was identified to 2p23–24 containing the *ALK* gene, which had previously been shown to be amplified in a subset of NBs.[510–512] Nucleotide sequence analysis of genes in this region revealed germline *ALK* mutations, suggesting that *ALK* was the familial NB predisposition gene in most of the pedigrees.[7] In addition, *ALK* was somatically mutated in 6% to 12% of sporadic NB tumors.[6,7,550,551] The majority of these mutations are activating, making ALK an ideal target for therapy in patients with NB, especially those harboring these mutations.

Recently, somatic mutations of a receptor kinase, *FGFR4*, have been identified in approximately 7% of both ARMS and embryonal RMS.[552] Interestingly, *FGFR4* is expressed in myoblasts during normal development in regenerating muscle following injury but not in mature skeletal muscle. By microarray-based gene expression analysis (see the following sections), this gene has been reported to be the most highly differentially expressed gene in RMSs.[553–555] These observations led to the hypotheses that overexpression or mutational activation of this gene may be involved in the tumorigenesis of RMS. Investigators found that suppression of the wild-type *FGFR4* in RMS led to reduced growth and lung metastases. Mutations in the tyrosine kinase domain were predicted and confirmed to be activating and resulted in increased growth, resulted in reduced RMS cell death, and enhanced the ability of RMS cells to metastasize. The investigators found that the mutations lead to the activation of the oncogenic pathway involving *STAT3*. When RMS cells harbor these mutations, they are more sensitive to treatment with drugs that inhibit FGFR4 function and thus represent an "Achilles heel" for RMS. This is the first known mutation of a tyrosine receptor kinase in RMS, making FGFR4 or its downstream targets, including STAT3, ideal targets for RMS therapy, in particular those that harbor activating mutations of this gene.[552]

Point Mutations Affecting GATA1, CEBPA, and NOTCH1

Point mutations of *GATA1* (see earlier sections) and *CEBPA*[556] have been identified in patients with myeloid malignancies; *GATA1* and *CEBPA* mutations seem to be confined to myeloid malignancies. In each case, an altered protein is produced, and the altered protein is thought to function as a dominant-negative inhibitor of transcription.[102,556,557] The NOTCH1 transmembrane receptor in human T-cells is a target for activating point mutations that involve the receptor's extracellular heterodimerization domain and/or the carboxyl-terminal PEST domain. Such mutations were found in more than 50% of the clinical samples examined, encompassing all major molecular subtypes of T-ALL. Since activated NOTCH1 appears to play a prominent role in the pathogenesis of this disease, these observations provide a strong rationale for targeted therapies that interfere with NOTCH signaling.[558]

COMPREHENSIVE ANALYSIS OF THE CANCER GENOME

The following section will review the significant impact that the study of the whole genome (genomics) has had on the understanding of the molecular and genetic basis of pediatric cancers. The flow of information within a cell is from DNA to RNA to protein, (Fig. 3.7). The traditional approach used by molecular biologists has been the investigation of one gene at a time. However, it has become increasingly clear that biology of a cell is driven by the simultaneous expression of a large number of genes acting in concert and that there is a complex interaction of each of the components of the genome and proteome. The *genome* is defined as the total genetic information of a cell and includes all of the DNA and RNA. Hence, a comprehensive genomic analysis of the genome will include chromosomal number and structure, DNA copy number, RNA expression profiles, resequencing, and global protein expression analysis (Fig. 3.7).

Only 2% of the genomic DNA is transcribed into the 20,000 to 25,000 predicted protein-coding messenger RNAs (mRNAs), most of the 98% that remains is unexplored. Noncoding RNA (ncRNA) is a transcribed RNA molecule that is not translated into a protein; it is estimated that there are tens of thousands of these within the human genome.[561] ncRNA include microRNAs (miRNAs), transfer RNAs (tRNAs), ribosomal RNAs (rRNAs), small nucleolar RNAs (snoRNAs), small nuclear RNAs (snRNAs), small interfering RNAs (siRNAs), Piwi-interacting RNAs (piRNAs), and the long ncRNAs (>200 bp). The function of the majority of the newly identified ncRNAs has not been determined. While most conventional genes encode proteins to perform their biological functions, the recently discovered class of miRNAs plays important regulatory roles in normal development and physiology of plants and animals.[562,563] Mature miRNAs are 20 to 22 nucleotide molecules that can regulate gene expression through RNA induced silencing complex (RISC)-mediated mRNA degradation and regulate translational suppression via complementary pairing, predominantly to the 3′-untranslated region (3′-UTR) of their targeted mRNAs.[562,564] An increasing number of studies have demonstrated a perturbation of the normal expression patterns of miRNAs in many human cancers[565–568] including pediatric cancers (see later).

The term *proteomics* refers to the study of all proteins within the cell. Although there are estimated to be approximately 20,000 to 25,000 mRNAs in the genome,[569] it is likely that the next generation sequencing of human transcriptomes (see later) will increase this number.[570,571] In addition, it is estimated that perhaps 75% of mRNA transcripts undergo posttranscriptional modification producing multiple splice variant transcripts that make different functional proteins,[570,571] and posttranslational modifications such as phosphorylation alter the function of individual proteins. Thus, it is possible that there may be more than 100,000 individual proteins species within the mammalian proteome. Technologies to measure global protein expression profiles, including protein arrays and mass spectroscopy, have lagged behind genomics in terms of sensitivity, robustness, and reproducibility.[559,560] Nevertheless, it is likely that these methods will improve in the foreseeable future and become a powerful tool for the cancer biologist.

The Human Genome Project and the Discoveries of the Genetic Basis of Disease

The HGP, begun in 1990, was an international effort coordinated by the U.S. Department of Energy and the National Institutes of Health (NIH),[572,573] whose goals included the identification of all the protein-coding genes in human DNA and determination of the sequences of the 3 billion bp that make up the human DNA. The HGP has heralded the way for high-throughput analyses of whole genomes and proteomes and has allowed the identification of fundamental differences between normal and diseased cells, including cancer. Much of these resources, including physical clones, mapping data, and sequence data, produced by both the public[572,573] and the

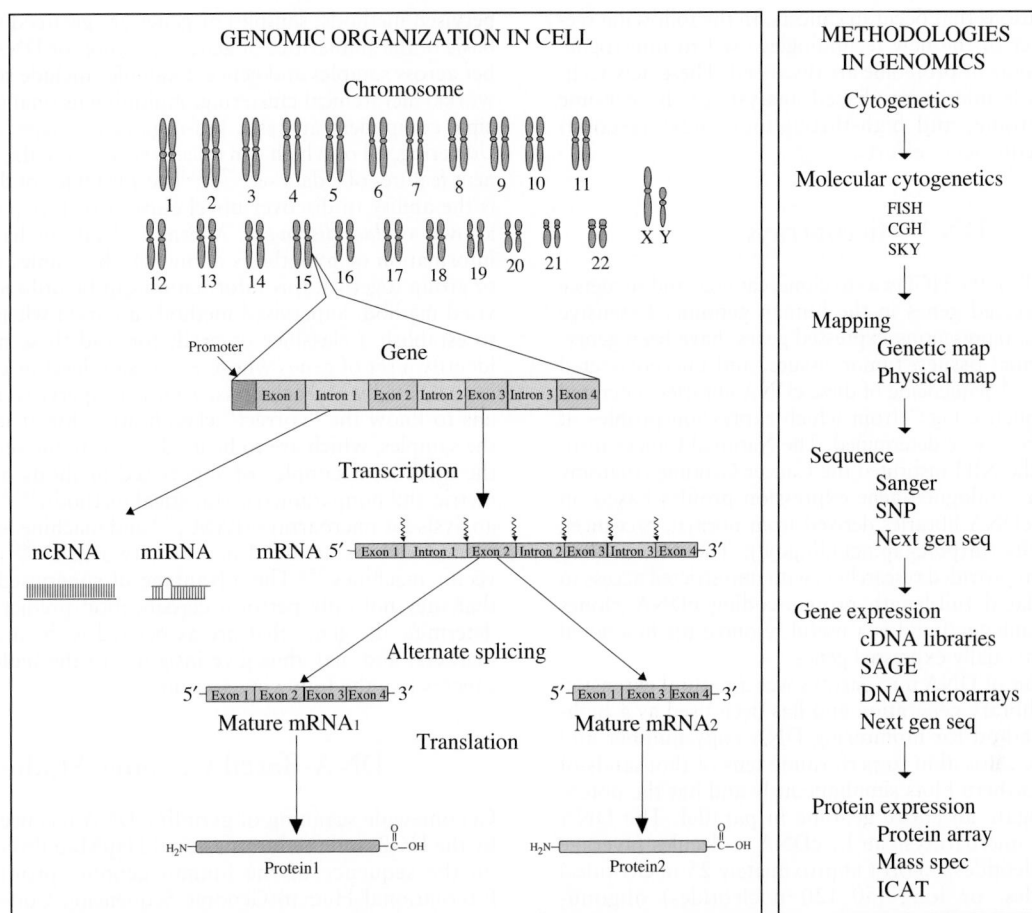

FIGURE 3.7 Whole genome and proteome investigation of cancer. The human genome is contained within 23 chromosomal pairs comprising 3.2 billion pairs of the four nucleotides (adenosine [A], cytidine [C], guanosine [G] and thymidine [T]). Two percent of the genome is transcribed into 20,000 to 25,000 protein-coding messenger RNAs (mRNAs). The genomic sequence contains a promoter region; exons, containing the coding regions; and introns. The introns are spliced out following transcription and alternate splicing can generate several different mRNAs and protein products. Many regions of the genome are also transcribed into noncoding RNA molecules (>10,000), including microRNAs (approximately 700). Shown on the **right** are some of the methodologies in genomics including low-resolution chromosomal structure analysis such as cytogenetics and molecular cytogenetics (fluorescent *in situ* hybridization [FISH], comparative genomic hybridization [CGH], and spectral karyotyping [SKY]). Genetic mapping uses DNA markers to find linkage of a genomic region to an inherited disease to eventually indentify the causal gene. Physical mapping uses clones containing human nucleic acids (e.g., bacterial artificial chromosome) to define physical locations of genes and markers within each chromosome. In parallel to the sequencing of the human genome, many single nucleotide variations or single nucleotide polymorphisms are being detected and catalogued and may contribute to the phenotypic differences found in many patients and their cancers. Increasingly, "next generation" sequencing methods for profiling and discovery of novel genes are replacing traditional genomics methods. Finally, several methods, including protein arrays, mass spectroscopy, and isotope-coded affinity tags (ICAT), are available for detecting which genes are actively being transcribed and translated into proteins.[559,560] (Modified from Whiteford CC, Wei JS, Khan J. Genomics, microarrays and proteomics. In: Raphael E, Pollock RE, Doroshow JH, et al., eds. UICC manual of clinical oncology. 8th ed. 2004:43–62.)

private sectors (http://www.celera.com/), are freely available (http://genome.cse.ucsc.edu/, http://www.ncbi.nlm.nih.gov/, http://www.ensembl.org/). Several key postgenome initiatives focused on increasing our understanding of the molecular or genetic basis of cancer have been launched since the completion of the HGP.

The HGP triggered an explosion of techniques for high-throughput genomewide analysis of the cancer genome, and Figure 3.7 lists some of these methods. Traditional molecular approaches to cancer investigations including cytogenetics;

molecular cytogenetics; Southern, northern, and western blot analyses; immunohistochemistry; and PCR have been successful in identifying alteration in gene expression, losses or gains of large chromosomal regions, and the presence of translocations. However, these methods are limited by either low-resolution, as in the case of cytogenetics, or insufficient throughput, examining a single gene or chromosomal region at a time. In addition, these diagnostic tools are prone to false-negative results due to the technical difficulties on the limited markers examined and also do not provide insight into global, nonrandom, genomic alterations that occur in cancers. In the following sections, a number of the new technologies used to interrogate the cancer genome or proteome are discussed. These new technologies include microarray-based analysis of the genome and transcriptome, and high-throughput "next (second) generation" sequencing efforts.

DNA Microarrays

One of the goals of the HGP was to clone, catalog, and sequence all of the expressed genes in the human genome. Extensive cDNA libraries, representing expressed genes, have been generated from normal tissues, tumor tissues, and microdissected individual cells.[574] Sequencing of these cDNA libraries generated "expressed-sequence tags" from which expression profiles of individual cancers were determined. The National Cancer Institute (NCI) of the NIH instituted the Cancer Genome Anatomy Project, which catalogued gene expression profiles based on sequencing of cDNA libraries derived from normal, precancer, and cancer cells (http://cgap.nci.nih.gov/). The Mammalian Gene Collection provided researchers with unrestricted access to sequence-validated full-length protein-coding cDNA clones (http://mgc.nci.nih.gov/) and is a useful resource for functional studies of differentially expressed genes.

Development of DNA microarrays was a natural extension of the cDNA library generation and has been used as a high-throughput method for monitoring DNA copy number and gene expression. It is akin to performing tens of thousands of Southern or northern blots simultaneously and has the potential to interrogate an entire genome in parallel. The DNA probes on the microarrays can be cDNA molecules (average size 1,500 nucleotides), short (approximately 25 nucleotides) oligonucleotides, or long (50–120 nucleotides) oligonucleotides of known sequences that are immobilized on a solid support such as a glass microscope slide. More than 100,000 of these probes can be placed on a single microarray, giving DNA microarrays the potential to query the entire genome of an organism in a single experiment.

The principle of the microarray technique is demonstrated in Figure 3.8.[575,576] The microarrays are fabricated with DNA from bacterial artificial chromosome (BAC) or cDNA clones, or oligonucleotides. The targets used in DNA microarray experiments are prepared from DNA or RNA that are fluorescently labeled. The fluorescently labeled targets are then hybridized to the microarray slides and imaged. Some microarrays utilize two fluorescent dyes. In these experiments, the test sample (e.g., tumor) is labeled with one dye and the control sample (e.g., normal cell) is labeled with a different colored dye. The two fluorescently labeled samples are then simultaneously hybridized to the microarray slide. Alternatively, Affymetrix and other arrays utilize a single color, in which only the test sample is labeled and hybridized. The targets are then hybridized on microarray slides and imaged. The fluorescence intensity of each spot on the array is quantified and corresponds to the amount of DNA or RNA in the fluorescently labeled test sample. In this manner, a single experiment can easily generate millions of data points. The analysis of this data is greatly aided by computational biology techniques and the accessibility of large, publicly available data sets. The Oncogenomics database (http://pob.abcc.ncifcrf.gov/cgi-bin/JK) houses the largest collection of publically available genomics and proteomic data for pediatric tumor samples, many of which are clinically annotated, and this database is being increasingly used by the scientific community for hypothesis generation and in silico validation of experiments.

Computational analysis of microarray data can be separated into two groups: unsupervised and supervised. In unsupervised methods, samples or genes are grouped solely on the basis of the similarities of gene expression or DNA copy number across samples and genes. Examples include relevance networks, hierarchical clustering, multidimensional scaling, principal component analysis, self-organizing maps, and k-means clustering, all of which can effectively capture the most prominent features of a data set.[577–582] The advantage of these methods is the ability to discover novel clusters or grouping a process known as class discovery. Alternatively, if one has some prior information or hypothesis about which samples are expected to group together, this information can be utilized in a supervised method. Supervised methods are used when one desires to establish a classifier or predictor, and these methods will identify a set of genes whose expression level or copy number is associated with each class. To use a supervised method, one has to know the "correct" classification for at least some of the samples, which are to be used as a training set to calibrate the method. Examples of supervised methods include parametric and nonparametric statistical methods,[581,582] prediction analysis for microarrays (PAM),[583] and machine learning algorithms such as artificial neural networks[553,584] and support vector machines.[585] The advantage of supervised methods is that they not only perform classification prediction but also determine the genes that are associated with each class (biomarkers) and may thus give insight into the biology of these cancers (see the following sections).

DNA-Based Genomic Studies

Genomewide scanning of germline DNA has been facilitated by the HGP, and the International HapMap Project was built on the sequence of the human genome produced by the International Human Genome Sequencing Consortium. The International HapMap Project began with the observation that there are sites within the genome that differ by a single nucleotide across different individuals. If these SNVs occur at a frequency of greater than or equal to 1% in the population, they are referred to as single nucleotide polymorphisms (SNPs). This information could, in theory, be used to discover associations of particular SNPs with disease in order to identify disease loci and genes. However, there are approximately 10 million such SNPs (approximately one site per 300 bases) within the human genome, and mapping all such SNPs would be cost prohibitive. Fortunately, genetic variation among individuals is organized in "DNA neighborhoods," called haplotype blocks. SNP variants that lie close to each other along the DNA molecule form a haplotype block and tend to be inherited together. SNP variants that are far from each other along the DNA molecule tend to be in different haplotype blocks and are less likely to be inherited together. The International HapMap Project has parsed the genome into heritable haplotype units, each of which may contain 10 or more SNPs. Only a few so-called tag SNPs are needed to identify that unique block of genome that represents all of the SNPs associated with that one piece.

The International HapMap Project has enabled investigators to perform genome wide association studies (GWAS) to determine the association of roughly 3 million tag SNPs with human disease and to identify germline alterations associated with cancer and other diseases.[586–589] This approach has identified regions associated with nearly 40 complex diseases or traits.[589] In cancer, this strategy has identified multiple regions associated with prostate,[590–592] breast,[593–595] colorectal,[596–598] and pancreatic cancers.[599] GWAS in pediatric cancers have been hampered by the relative scarcity of childhood cancers and consequent lack of sufficient samples to adequately power these studies. However, a notable exception is the investigation

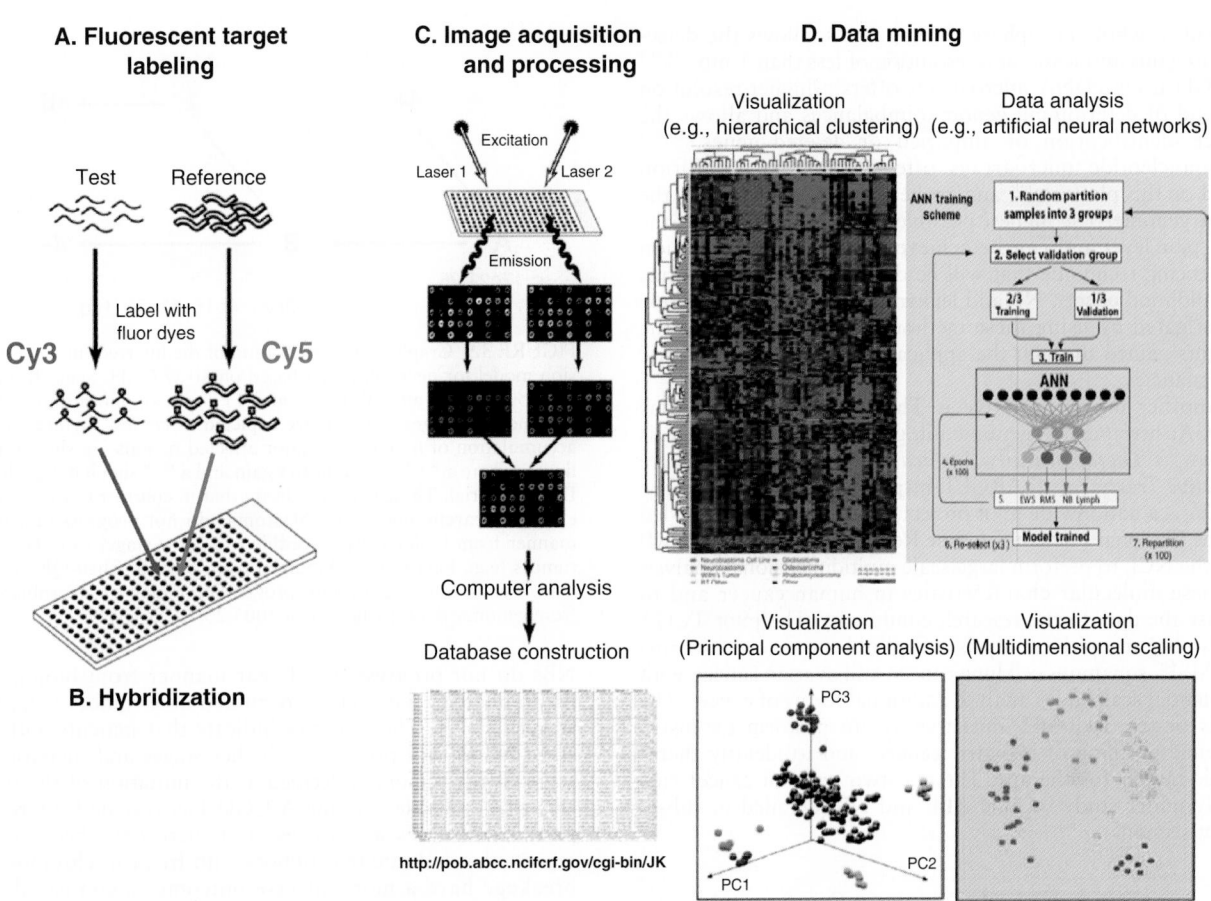

A. Fluorescent target labeling

C. Image acquisition and processing

D. Data mining

FIGURE 3.8 Summary of the DNA microarray technology. **A:** Fluorescent labeling of targets. DNA, mRNA, or microRNA extracted from reference and test samples is fluorescently labeled by utilizing nucleotides tagged for example either Cy3 or Cy5, respectively. Many of the newer oligonucleotide microarrays utilize single-color labeling of test samples. **B:** Hybridization. The probe mixture is hybridized to the microarray on the DNA microarrays. **C:** Image acquisition and processing. Fluorescence intensities at target spots are measured by using laser confocal microscopes with the appropriate excitation lasers and emission filters. Each of the images is arbitrarily assigned a pseudocolor (i.e., Cy5 = red and Cy3 = green). A normalization process is performed to compensate for differential efficiencies of labeling and detection of Cy3 and Cy5, as well as slide-to-slide variation. The fluorescent images thus constitute the raw data from which gene expression values are calculated. All the measurements are stored in a database and can be publically released via the Internet for further processing. **D:** Data mining. Biological information is extracted in this step by using a variety of data-mining tools. The relationships between genes and experiments can be visualized by hierarchical clustering, while principal component analysis and multidimensional scaling allow visualization of the similarity of expression profiles between samples. Algorithms such as artificial neural networks can classify cancers and identify biologically relevant and diagnostic genes. (Modified from Khan J, Wei JS, Ringner M, et al. Classification and diagnostic prediction of cancers using gene expression profiling and artificial neural networks. Nat Med 2001;7:673–679; Whiteford CC, Wei JS, Khan J. Genomics, microarrays and proteomics. In: Raphael E, Pollock RE, Doroshow JH, et al., eds. UICC manual of clinical oncology. 8th ed. 2004:43–62; and Duggan DJ, Bittner M, Chen Y, et al. Expression profiling using cDNA microarrays. Nat Genet 1999;21:10–14.)

of NB, in which researchers have used this strategy to identify common variants in genes or regions associated with increased susceptibility to this cancer.[600,601] Future studies are being planned to apply these types of analyses to other pediatric malignancies in national and international collaborative efforts.

The 1000 Genomes Project builds on the human haplotype map developed by the International HapMap Project to produce a much more comprehensive view of genomic variation. It aims to find all the variants in the genome, including those that contribute to disease risk. It will not only perform whole genome sequencing but also produce a high-resolution map structural variants, including rearrangements, insertions, deletions, or duplications of germline DNA segments. The importance of these structural variants has become increasingly clear from surveys that demonstrate that differences in genome structure may play a role in susceptibility to such conditions as mental retardation and autism.

Genomewide scanning of tumor DNA by using the conventional comparative genomic hybridization (CGH) is an established technique for detecting gain or loss of chromosomal regions.[602] Originally, CGH was performed by hybridizing differentially labeled tumor and normal DNA onto a metaphase preparation of normal human chromosomes. This approach yields a resolution of about 5 to 10 mb. Array-based comparative genomic hybridization (A-CGH), using BAC clones from known genomic regions printed on glass slides instead of whole metaphase chromosomes, allows the detection of gains and losses at a resolution of less than 1 mb.[603,604] A-CGH using cDNA microarrays offers a higher-resolution method of determining genomic imbalances and allows the direct identification of amplified or deleted genes.[510,605] Oligonucleotide microarrays offer the highest-resolution CGH on this platform[606] and probes can be "tiled" across the entire genome. The highest possible CGH resolution is at the base pair level and can be achieved by the next-generation sequencing technique that will be discussed later. Two forms of childhood cancer, NB and leukemia, have been extensively investigated by using these methods and they highlight the insights gained through the application of CGH to pediatric malignancies.

Another major initiative is The Cancer Genome Atlas (TCGA; http://cancergenome.nih.gov/); its pediatric arm is known as *Therapeutically Applicable Research to Generate Effective Treatments* (TARGET; http://target.cancer.gov/). The TCGA is a nationwide pilot project, jointly supported and led by the National Human Genome Research Institute (NHGRI) and the NCI, to perform large-scale multidimensional analysis of these molecular characteristics in human cancer and to release the data to the research community. The pilot TCGA study begun with analysis of glioblastoma multiforme (GBM),[607] squamous cell lung cancer, and ovarian cancer, with a potential scale up to analyze additional forms of cancer. The goals of the TARGET initiative are to perform extensive genomic profiling of pediatric cancers and to identify therapeutic targets for therapy. The first two types of cancer currently under study include ALL and NB (detailed in subsequent sections).

DNA-Based Genomic Studies of Neuroblastoma

NB is a heterogeneous disease whose clinical and biological behavior has been described as enigmatic.[608] For instance, most children presenting under 12 months of age often experience complete regression of their disease with minimal or no therapy, including those patients with metastatic disease. In contrast, older patients more frequently present with metastatic disease and have a cure rate of 30% to 40% despite intensive multimodal therapy. Genomics is a powerful tool that is beginning to unravel the biology of this enigmatic tumor. Genomic alterations in NB have been investigated by cytogenetic and molecular methods, including spectral karyotyping and metaphase comparative genomic hybridization (M-CGH).[609-613] Several genomic alterations have been reported to be associated with different clinical subtypes and prognosis including amplification of the *MYCN* oncogene,[608,614] gains of 17q (>50%), and loss of 1p36 (30%–35%).[608,615-617] Other recurrent changes, including losses of 3p, 4p, 9p, 11q, and 14q, as well as frequent gain of chromosome 7, have also been suggested to have relevance to the development and progression of these tumors.[616,617] Several of these genomic alterations including *MYCN* amplification and loss of 1p36 and 11q23 are already being utilized in risk stratification to guide therapy in patients with NB.[618]

A-CGH using cDNA microarray platforms have been used to systematically identify common genomic alterations in NB of various stages. Initial studies showed that NB tumors have an A-CGH profile specific to stage and *MYCN* amplification status.[510,619] A-CGH profiles of stage 1 and stage 4S tumors have remarkable similarity to each other, identifying a more benign profile.[620] In addition, mathematical progression models based on A-CGH results of NB of different stages have suggested that, in contrast to the common epithelial carcinomas,

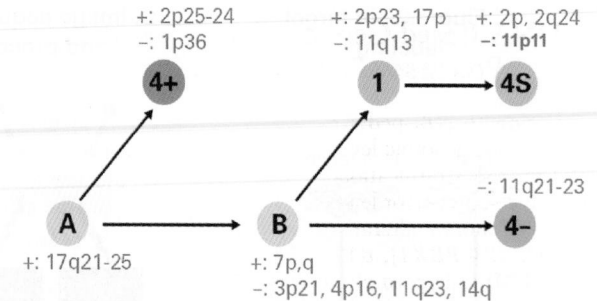

FIGURE 3.9 Graphical representation of the inferred tumor progression model for neuroblastoma based on array-CGH. Stage 1, 4S, 4− (without *MYCN* amplification), and 4+ (with amplification) and two intermediate stages A and B are depicted as *circles*. *Arrows* indicate accumulation of mutations. Major affected regions are shown in the figure, where a "+" sign indicates gain and a "−" sign indicates loss of DNA material. These results indicate that in contrast to the common epithelial carcinomas, neuroblastomas do not progress in a linear manner from biologically favorable (e.g., low stage) to unfavorable tumors (e.g., high stage). (Modified from Bilke S, Chen QR, Westerman F, et al. Inferring a tumor progression model for neuroblastoma from genomic data. J Clin Oncol 2005;23:7322–7331.)

NBs do not progress in a linear manner from biologically favorable (e.g., low stage) to unfavorable tumors (e.g., high stage).[510,619,621] These studies indicate that patients with low stage NB do not progress to higher stages and therefore the stage of the tumors is decided at the initiation of the tumor (Fig. 3.9). Whole-genome A-CGH has revealed interesting patterns of gains and losses, and there have been several reports that indicate that tumors with frequent chromosomal breakage have a more adverse outcome as compared with those that have whole chromosomal gains and losses.[622,623]

Knudson's "two-hit" hypothesis[77] would suggest that if one copy of a gene is lost, the other copy should be silenced by homozygous deletion, methylation, or loss-of-function mutations. However despite whole genome A-CGH scans and extensive sequencing of many genes in regions frequently involved in LOH such as those in 1p36 and 11q23, the identification of "the tumor suppressor" in NB has been elusive with no reports of frequent homozygous deletion or mutations of these regions. Microdeletions in other regions such as *PTPRD* (9p23-p24.3) locus have been reported in a small fraction of tumors. It is plausible that haploinsufficiency or silencing of the remaining allele in these deleted regions may contribute to the process of malignant transformation.[624,625] In addition, it is possible that next-generation sequencing techniques (see the following sections) may identify mutations in as yet unknown genes, for example, an miRNA, or genes not previously sequenced in these frequently lost regions. For many genes, the copy number of genes directly correlates with gene expression levels. For example, investigators have shown that LOH at 1p and 11q was associated with significantly decreased expression of genes mapping to 1p35–36 and all of 11q, respectively.[626] It has also been shown that *WSB1*, which was frequently gained in low-risk stage 4S tumors and unchanged in stage 4 tumors, showed a strong correlation between copy number and expression level, which in turn was associated with outcome.[620]

As discussed earlier, multiple investigators identified amplification of the tyrosine kinase *ALK* gene in a subset of NB by using high-throughput genomic approaches, which led to the exciting discovery that *ALK* was the major familial NB gene. One group found that three separate germline missense mutations in the tyrosine kinase domain of ALK segregated with the disease in eight separate families,[7] and 6% to 12% of sporadic NB tumors had somatic mutations.[6,7,550,551]

DNA-Based Genomic Studies of B-Cell Precursor Pediatric Leukemias

In addition to NB, pediatric leukemia has been extensively studied at the genomic level, and a number of genetic markers useful for risk stratification have been identified. As described earlier, B-cell precursor leukemias can be categorized by several recurrent genomic alterations including t(9;22)[BCR–ABL1], t(1;19)[TCF3–PBX1], t(12;21)[ETV6–RUNX1], rearrangements of MLL, hyperdiploidy, and hypodiploidy. However, in general, single genomic aberrations will not induce leukemia, which are thought to require additional cooperative mutations in order to produce a frank malignancy (see the following section). Investigators have applied high-resolution SNP arrays to investigate pediatric B-cell ALL and found deletions, amplifications, point mutations, and structural rearrangement in genes encoding principal regulators of B-cell lymphocyte development and differentiation in 40% of B-cell precursor ALL cases.[627] They report that the PAX5 gene was the most frequent somatic mutation and also identified deletions of TCF3 (E2A), EBF1, LEF1, IKZF1 (IKAROS), and IKZF3 (AIOLOS). Their findings confirm that mutations in developmental pathways often lead to malignancies within that differentiation lineage.[627] In a follow-up study, as part of the TARGET ALL initiative, the same investigators have shown that patients with high-risk B-cell precursor ALL (excluding known high-risk groups such as BCR-ABL1-positive ALL, hypodiploid ALL, and infant ALL), have recurring copy number abnormalities in genes involved in B-cell development. They report that PAX5 was involved in 31.7% and IKZF1 in 28.6% of patients. The key findings were that genetic alteration of IKZF1 was associated with a very poor outcome in B-cell-precursor ALL, which can be utilized as an additional prognostic marker, and that it contributes to the biological knowledge of this disease.[628]

Gene Expression Profiling for the Investigation of Pediatric Cancers

As described earlier, neoplastic cells have accumulated numerous nonrandom genetic abnormalities. The central hypothesis behind the application of microarrays to investigate cancers is that these genetic alterations result in a perturbation in the gene expression profile that is characteristic to the cancer. The power of the microarray technology is the ability to perform genomewide expression profile analysis of the entire transcriptome including the known and predicted splice variants in a single experiment. The first report on the application of cDNA microarrays for the identification of diagnostic markers in pediatric cancers was in ARMS using cDNA arrays containing 1,238 elements.[577] Up to that point, it had not been clear whether taxonomic classification of cancers based on their gene expression profiles would be possible, because their intrinsic genomic instability would lead to extensive random fluctuations in global gene expression. This study demonstrated that the gene expression profile of ARMS was distinct from other cancers, and it indicated that cancers of a diagnostic type would possess unique gene expression profile specific to that cancer.

A number of statistical techniques have been used to analyze gene expression data to identify genes that distinguish cancers of two different types.[629,630] Investigators used a machine learning algorithm, artificial neural networks (ANNs), to diagnostically classify pediatric cancers belonging to more than two types from gene expression profiles.[553] ANNs are computer-based algorithms, modeled on the structure and behavior of neurons in the human brain,[631] and are trained to recognize and categorize complex patterns through

learning from experience. The input can be any types of data, and any numbers of outputs or categories are possible. ANNs have been applied to clinical problems, such as diagnosing myocardial infarctions and arrhythmias from electrocardiograms,[632] and for interpreting radiographs and magnetic resonance images.[633,634] The investigators hypothesized that ANNs can be trained to diagnose cancers by using gene expression profiles generated by cDNA microarrays as input data and the diagnosis as the output. They used the small round blue cell tumors of childhood (SRBCT), which includes NB, rhabdomyosarcoma (RMS), Burkitt's lymphoma (BL), and EWS (Ewing's sarcoma), as a model, because these cancers can at times present diagnostic difficulties. For example, EWS is diagnosed by immunohistochemical evidence of MIC2 expression[635] and lack of expression of the leukocyte common antigen CD45 (thereby excluding lymphoma), and lack of expression of muscle-specific actin or myogenin (thereby excluding RMS).[636] However, reliance on detection of MIC2 alone can lead to incorrect diagnosis as MIC2 expression does occur occasionally in other tumor types including RMS and NHL.[637] ANN models were trained to recognize cancers in each of the four SRBCT categories based on gene expression data from 6,567 genes. They identified a subset of 93 genes whose expression levels were able to classify these cancers with high sensitivity and specificity (Fig. 3.10). Although the expression of several of these genes had been

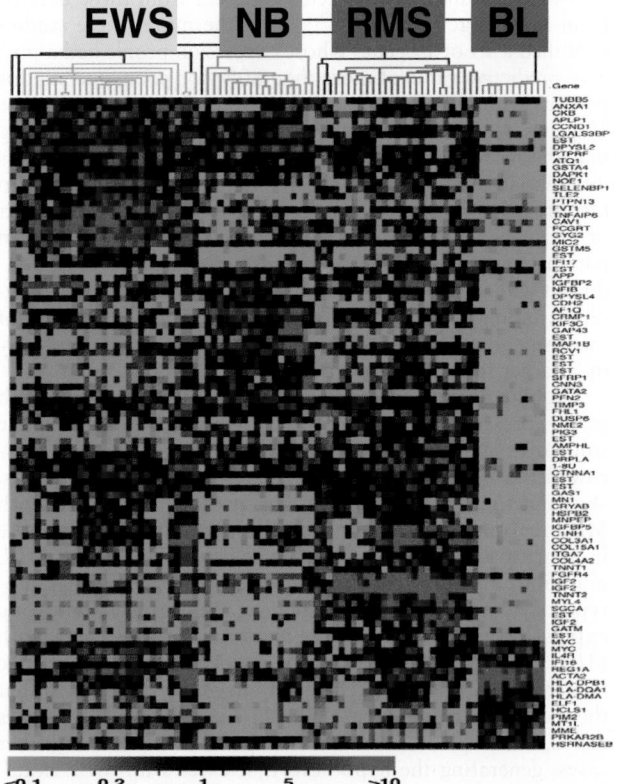

FIGURE 3.10 Identification of mRNA diagnostic signatures in the small round blue cell tumors of childhood. Each row represents one of the 96 cDNA clones (93 unique genes) and each column a separate sample. A pseudocolored representation of the expression level is shown such that a red color indicates high expression and green color low expression, with scale shown below. On the **right** are the gene symbols. Many of these genes had not previously been reported to be expressed in these cancers. (Modified from Khan J, Wei JS, Ringner M, et al. Classification and diagnostic prediction of cancers using gene expression profiling and artificial neural networks. Nat Med 2001;7:673–679).

reported in SRBCT, the majority had not been previously associated with these cancers. These genes are likely to be biologically relevant to these cancers and provide promising targets for therapy. For example, these genes include the FGFR4 receptor tyrosine kinase, which was subsequently found to be mutated in a subset of patients with RMS (see earlier sections). This SRBCT expression signature is being further developed into a clinical assay by using a subset of these genes in a multiplex PCR-based strategy.[638]

Microarray-based gene expression analysis has been applied to identify not only diagnostic biomarkers but also biologically and clinically relevant markers in patients with pediatric malignances; we will now describe in more detail its application for the most commonly studied cancers, including NB and leukemia. Patients with NB in North America are currently stratified by the Children's Oncology Group into high-, intermediate-, and low-risk based on age, tumor staging, histology, MYCN amplification, and DNA ploidy. Although this risk stratification accurately predicts that more than 80% patients with low-risk disease and less than 30% of patients with high-risk disease will survive with modern therapy, it cannot predict the outcome of individual patients with NB. In addition, the current risk stratification gives no insights into the biological reasons as to why more than 60% of patients with high-risk NB will die of disease despite aggressive therapy. Microarray studies demonstrated that NB tumors have a specific gene expression profile compared with normal tissues or other malignancies,[553,639] and that the gene expression profile of low-stage tumors is markedly different from those derived from high-stage tumors.[553,584,640] Furthermore, these studies identified a set of 19 genes whose expression profile had a positive predictive value of more than 80% for poor outcome for patients with NB of all stages.[584] Of note, the majority of these 19 genes are involved in early neural development, suggesting that the more aggressive phenotype is characterized by a less differentiated state. Additional studies have led investigators to identify other prognostic gene sets[641–644] with the recent report of 59 genes whose expression levels can predict outcome in patients with NB.[645] Many of these studies have been conducted with small sample sets. In order to translate these prognostic biomarkers to the clinic and verify the robustness of these signatures, it is necessary to perform a validation study on a larger set of independent samples.

Childhood leukemia has been extensively investigated with gene expression profiling, beginning with a proof of principle study distinguishing ALL from AML.[244] Armstrong et al. narrowed the focus of microarray analysis to infant leukemias, showing that the gene expression profiles associated with MLL-rearranged cases were significantly different from those in nonrearranged cases, providing genetic evidence that MLL mutations are sufficient to generate a distinct molecular subtype of acute leukemia.[646] There was an especially strong expression of myeloid gene expression in ALL cases with MLL rearrangements, suggesting an origin from a primitive hematopoietic stem cell. The most intriguing finding was that the receptor tyrosine kinase gene FLT3, among 12,000 genes tested, best separated MLL-rearranged leukemias from other cases, generating the hypothesis that cases with MLL mutations might depend on FLT3 for survival and therefore could be treated with agents that target this molecule.

Yeoh et al.[647] can be credited with the most comprehensive unsupervised microarray analysis of childhood ALL cases. Their findings confirmed the molecular uniqueness of leukemias with MLL gene fusions and showed, in addition, that each of the recurrent translocations and immunologic subtypes seen in ALL is associated with a unique gene expression pattern, although the biologic significance of this heterogeneity remains unknown. There was also evidence for small subgroups of patients whose gene expression signatures did not correspond to any known molecular abnormalities, suggesting previously unrecognized oncogenic pathways. Alizadeh and colleagues[630] published a landmark study in which they demonstrated the close association of clinical outcome in diffuse large B-cell lymphoma (DLBCL) with distinct gene expression signatures. Using a cDNA microarray with probes for genes expressed in the germinal center, the presumed site of origin of DLBCL, these authors found two subtypes of DLBCL, one sharing many gene profile patterns with normal germinal center B cells and the other showing more similarities to activated B cells in peripheral blood. Importantly, these two previously unrecognized lymphoma subtypes were associated with significantly different overall survival rates.

A novel application of microarray-based gene profiling is illustrated by the work of Ferrando and colleagues[648] who combined this method with RT-PCR analysis to test a provocative hypothesis that aberrant activation of key transcription factor genes is the principal transforming feature of childhood T-cell ALL cases. This combination of gene analysis strategies identified four multistep pathways leading to T-cell ALL induction, each characterized by distinct cytogenetic abnormalities and differentiation arrest at specific stages of normal T-cell development. Importantly, the findings had clinical importance, as HOX11 activation was associated with a significantly better prognosis than the expression of either SCL or LYL1 or, surprisingly, HOX11L2. The hypothesis-driven approach described in this report may be useful in the study of other types of childhood cancers.

Holleman et al.[649] used 14,500 probe sets to identify differentially expressed genes in drug-sensitive and drug-resistant cases of ALL, comparing the results with treatment outcome. Sets of genes sensitive or resistant to vincristine, asparaginase, prednisolone, or daunorubicin were significantly and independently related to clinical outcome in a multivariate analysis. This study illustrates the power of oligonucleotide microarray analysis to detect a relatively small number of previously unrecognized genes associated with drug resistance and treatment outcome in childhood ALL.

Finally, gene expression profiles have been used not only to discover diagnostic and prognostic biomarkers and potential targets for therapy but also to identify targets of transcription factors important for the etiology of pediatric cancers including chimeric fusion genes such as PAX3-FKHR and EWS-FLI1 (see earlier sections) and other proto-oncogenes such as MYCN.[396,640,650,651]

MicroRNA Expression Profiling for the Investigation of Pediatric Cancers

miRNAs are a class of noncoding small RNAs that have important regulatory functions in plants and animals.[562] These highly conserved, approximately 21 to 25 nucleotide RNA molecules regulate the expression of genes through translational inhibition or RNA degradation by preferentially binding to specific target mRNAs.[562] Each miRNA is thought to target as many as 200 genes, and multiple miRNAs can target a single gene. Currently, more than 700 human miRNAs have been identified (release 13.0) (http://microrna.sanger.ac.uk/). miRNAs have diverse functions involved in embryogenesis, metabolism, cell growth, differentiation, and apoptosis.[562] In recent years, there has been an explosion of miRNA studies in the literature, demonstrating the alteration of miRNA expression in various human cancers.[568,651–661] Therefore, it is likely that miRNA expression profiles will be useful in the diagnosis of certain cancers. For instance, Lu et al. demonstrated that miRNA profiles could be used to classify cancers according to their developmental origins and mechanisms of transformation.[568] Furthermore, when comparing the ability of miRNA and mRNA profiles to distinguish poorly differentiated metastatic tumors, miRNA profiles correctly classified 12 out of 17 tumors, but only 1 of 17 tumors was correctly classified by using mRNA profiles.[568] An important practical consideration is that because of the short length of miRNAs, they are more stable and thus more reliably extracted from paraffin sections than are mRNAs.[662] In addition, because of the relatively small number of miRNA species compared with mRNAs, miRNA expression patterns are expected to be less complex. Finally, the majority of pediatric malignancies are thought to arise, at least in part, because of aberrations in normal developmental and differentiation pathways. Given the importance of miRNAs in normal development pathways, it is intriguing to speculate that these molecules may be "drivers" in some cases of pediatric cancer.

miRNAs also have been found to play critical roles in the biology of MYCN amplified NB, which commonly has loss of 1p36.[651] Five miRNAs map to this region and three of these are predicted to target MYCN, by bioinformatic analysis. Investigators found that MYCN has two target sites in the 3'-UTR for miR-34a which is one of the miRNAs that maps to the minimally deleted region of 1p36. They found that MYCN amplified tumors have lower levels of miR-34a, and upon forced overexpression of this miRNA, MYCN protein levels were significantly suppressed. Recently, it has been discovered that p53 directly controls the expression level of members of miR-34 family, and miR-34 family members can mediate some of the functions of p53.[663-665] Intriguingly, despite the fact that 50% of all human cancers harbor mutations inactivating p53, TP53 mutation is rare in NB.[666,667] Therefore, it is possible that the reduction of miR-34a expression from loss of 1p36 has a similar consequence to p53 deficiency, resulting in increased cell growth and suppression of apoptosis, as seen in MYCN-amplified NBs.

Recently, Wei et al. performed microarray-based miRNA profiling on a panel of 57 pediatric cancer xenografts representing 10 cancer types to identify cancer-specific miRNAs as diagnostic and prognostic biomarkers, which may also play critical roles in these diseases.[668] They found that the majority of cancer types clustered together based on unsupervised hierarchical clustering of global miRNA expression profiles. Fourteen miRNAs were significantly differentially expressed between RMS and NB (Fig. 3.11). Currently, the control of miRNA expression is largely unclear, and these researchers found that 36% of the miRNAs map within the coding region of genes, the so-called host genes. For these miRNAs, the study demonstrated that 63% were coregulated with their host gene transcripts and hence under the control of the same promoter. This has led to the speculation that these miRNAs and the host gene are involved in the same biological processes.

Expression of OncomiR-1 was significantly correlated with that of its host gene MIRHG1, and expression levels of MIRHG1 are strongly associated with aggressive NB (higher stages and poor prognosis). The non–protein-coding host gene, MIRHG1 (also known as C13orf25), is of particular interest due to its oncogenic potential in human cancers.[654,658,669] Given that OncomiR-1 has been demonstrated to be directly transactivated by MYC,[670,671] it is possible that OncomiR-1 may mediate at least some of the oncogenic functions of MYC. Several recent studies have indicated that MYCN, another MYC family member, can also upregulate OncomiR-1 expression.[638,669,672] Fontana et al. have demonstrated that MYCN activates OncomiR-1 cluster by directly binding to its promoter and that it promotes cell growth.[669]

Using microRNA to classify cancers

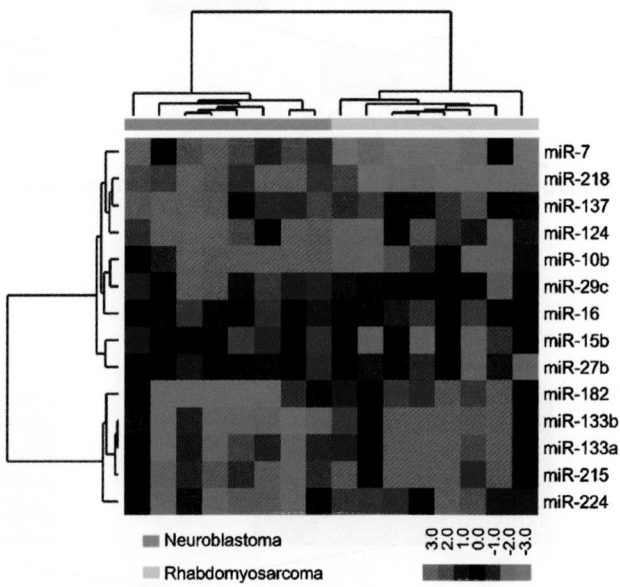

FIGURE 3.11 Differentially expressed cancer-specific microRNAs for neuroblastoma and rhabdomyosarcoma. Comparing the microarray-based microRNA expression profiles of neuroblastoma versus with that of rhabdomyosarcoma identified 14 differentially expressed microRNAs. Samples and microRNAs were hierarchically clustered by using Pearson correlation distance and average linkage. The microRNAs represent diagnostic biomarkers for these two cancer types. (Modified from Wei JS, Johansson P, Chen QR, et al. microRNA profiling identifies cancer-specific and prognostic signatures in pediatric malignancies. Clin Cancer Res 2009;15(17):5560–5568).

This is of particular interest because the MYCN gene is frequently amplified in NB and RMS,[673,674] and this molecular characteristic is used in the clinic to stratify treatment for patients with NB. Of interest, this study showed that the expression level of the MIRHG1 gene predicts the outcome of NB patients independently from MYCN expression. If validated, the expression of host gene MIRHG1 may be used as a molecular maker to further stratify patients with high-risk NB patients who do not have MYCN amplification. It may also be possible to specifically target OncomiR-1 as a potential novel therapy in high-risk NB.

Next-Generation Sequencing Methods

Despite the wide utilization of microarrays in genomic research, this technology has its limitations. First, because of the high background caused by cross-hybridization, it is difficult to detect SNVs or structural alterations such as balanced translocation. Second, prior knowledge of the targeted DNA sequences is required for designing probes on microarrays. Third, it is technically very challenging to detect every mutation in a given tumor sample by using microarray-based strategies or with traditional Sanger sequencing methods. Sanger-based large-scale sequencing projects have identified several genetic alterations that had not previously been associated with neoplasia. In recently published work, Parsons et al. sequenced 20,610 genes from 22 glioblastoma primary tumors or xenografts and identified 44 candidate cancer genes (CANgenes) that may be important for GBM. Of the top 10 alterations predicted in this study, 9 genes already had established

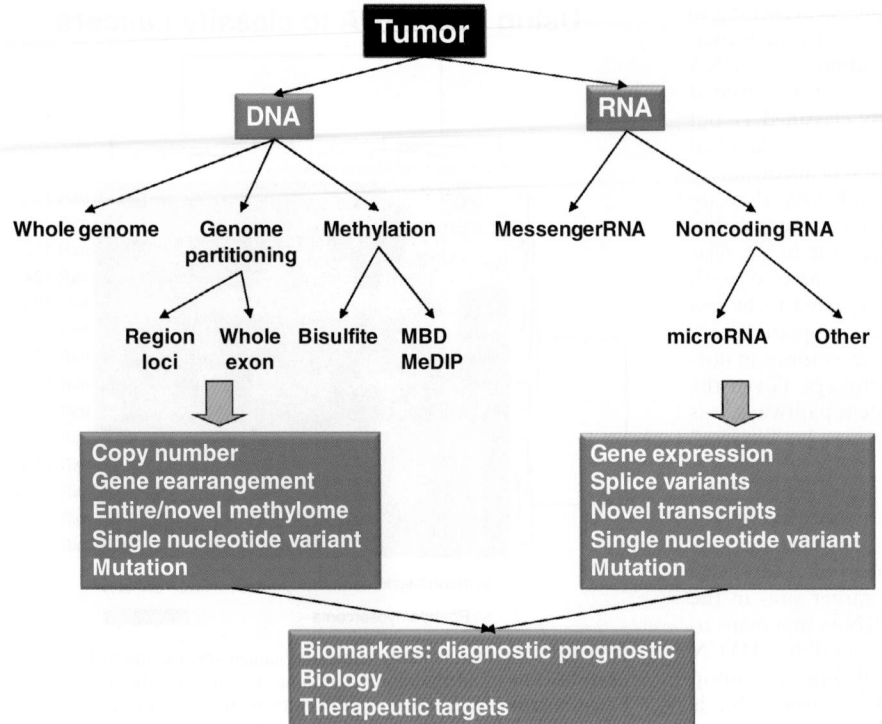

FIGURE 3.12 The application of next-generation sequencing for the comprehensive genomic investigation of cancers. For DNA, it is possible to sequence the entire cancer genome, or the DNA of the whole expressed genome, or a chromosomal region that has been identified by GWAS. These methods can also be used to perform global methylation scans by sequencing either bisulfite-treated DNA or DNA fragments that have been precipitated by an antibody (methylated DNA immunoprecipitation; MeDIP) or protein (methyl-CpG binding protein; MBD) that binds methylated DNA. The power of these techniques is the ability to determine the copy number of every DNA and RNA molecule in the cell, including single nucleotide variants and mutations, and novel transcripts including splice variants. It will also detect all chromosomal rearrangements and novel transcripts produced by these rearrangements including chimeric fusion oncogenes as a result of translocations. With slight modifications, the technique can identify all methylated regions of DNA. In this way, it will be possible to identify diagnostic and prognostic biomarkers, biologically relevant genes, and importantly therapeutic targets, such as kinases activated by mutation.

roles in the pathogenesis of gliomas; however, 1 gene, *IDH1*, has not typically been viewed as an important component of malignant transformation.[675,676] Other more recent Sanger-based sequencing approaches have identified *FGFR4* to be mutated in RMSs.[552]

Next-generation sequencing (also referred to as *massively parallel sequencing* or *deep sequencing*) technology directly identifies millions or even billions of nucleic acid species in parallel in a single experiment. Different from the Sanger method of traditional sequencing, the massively parallel DNA sequencing technology not only generates sequence information for each nucleic acid strand but also determines the abundance of each nucleic acid species due its large capacity, resulting in a digital readout of levels for any sequence, even those at low levels beyond the detection sensitivity of hybridization-based technologies. In addition, next-generation sequencing allows for the detection of mutations in a heterogeneous sample, including those heavily contaminated with normal tissue. With the advent of next-generation sequencing technologies, whole genomes from multiple samples can be readily determined. Thus, this technology has wide-ranging applications for the investigation of both DNA and RNA (Fig. 3.12).[677–681] The method involves firstly fractionating the DNA or RNA to sizes of 200 bp to 3 kb for DNA, 200 bp for mRNA, and less than 200 bp for miRNA. For RNA, the molecules are reverse transcribed into DNA. Adaptors are then ligated onto the DNA, which is then amplified by PCR either in bead-based emulsions or on a solid substrate. The beads are deposited onto glass slides, and by innovative fluorescent or luciferase-based methods, each molecule is sequenced with current lengths 50 to 500 bp in size. By this method, millions of short fragment reads are generated, which are then mapped back to the genome by powerful computer clusters.

With these next-generation sequencing techniques, it is possible to sequence an entire cancer genome in 1 month, a staggeringly short time considering that it took 13 years to sequence a handful of human genomes by the HGP. There are

also hybridization-based methods for purifying the protein-coding exons (the *exome*) or a defined genomic region (termed *genome-partitioning*), using either microarray solid-phase hybridization[682,683] or solution-based methods.[684] These methods are also being modified to perform global methylation scans either by sequencing methylated DNA fragments that have been immunoprecipitated by an antibody or a protein that recognize methylated DNA (methylated DNA immuno-precipitation or methyl-CpG binding protein) or by sequencing bisulfite-modified DNA. Bisulfite genomic sequencing is a widely used technique for analyzing cytosine methylation of DNA. Treatment of genomic DNA with bisulfite deaminates cytosine residues, which become uracil residues. The bisulfite treatment has no effect on 5-methylcytosine residues, and these nucleotide differences can be detected by next-generation sequencing techniques.

In a landmark study, the entire genome of malignant cells from a patient with M1 AML was sequenced, and 10 heterozygous, nonsynonymous SNVs were identified. Among these, 2 were previously implicated in the pathogenesis of AML (*FLT3* and *NPM1*), whereas 8 were alterations in genes not known to be involved in AML pathogenesis, underscoring the limitation of targeted resequencing and validating the importance of unbiased whole-genome sequencing.[677] It seems reasonable to predict that the use of these methods will allow investigators to identify every mutation or SNV in an individual tumor as well as every gene rearrangement with the precise breakpoint. In addition, whole-genome sequencing will allow investigators to determine inherited or acquired copy number variations (CNV), as well as the entire methylome of the malignant cell.

For RNA studies, next-generation sequencing methods make it feasible to determine the gene expression of every gene and identify every splice variants. Novel transcripts and all SNVs or mutations can also be identified via comparison with normal cells from the same individual. Finally, novel gene rearrangements that result in a chimeric fusion gene will be identified by these approaches. The power of this method was demonstrated in a recent report where researchers identified mutations in *FOXL2*, a gene encoding a transcription factor known to be critical for granulosa cell development, in granulosa cell tumors of the ovary.[685]

MECHANISMS OF MALIGNANT CELL TRANSFORMATION, GROWTH, AND CLONAL EXPANSION

Malignant transformation is a complex process in which cells become progressively more abnormal and progressively more independent of normal growth regulation, ultimately culminating in uncontrolled growth and clonal expansion. The exact number of "steps," or mutations, required for malignant transformation of human cells is difficult to determine but is likely to be different for different tissues and has been estimated to involve as few as four or as many as seven discrete events in humans.[686] Genetic analysis of a large series of colon polyps and cancers has identified several specific lesions in common with most colon cancers,[687] suggesting that all or most of these lesions are required for malignant transformation of colonic epithelium. Although primary rodent cells can be transformed by the overexpression of just two genes, *MYC* and a mutant *RAS*,[524] primary human cells are not transformed by overexpression of *MYC* and mutant *RAS* but can be transformed by the simultaneous introduction of four genes: SV40 large T antigen, SV40 small T antigen, *hTERT* (which encodes the catalytic subunit of telomerase), and mutant *RAS*.[688,689] It should again be noted that these human experiments have relied on primary fibroblast and breast epithelial cells and that the results may not be applicable to all cell types.

Weinberg and colleagues[406,690,691] have proposed that six specific pathways need to be disrupted to produce a fully transformed cell. These pathways are loosely defined and include (a) the "RB pathway", including an antiproliferative set of controls regulated in part by RB; (b) the "p53 pathway", an apoptotic pathway regulated in part by p53; (c) a pathway that governs cell proliferation, especially in response to exogenous mitogenic stimuli involving tyrosine kinase receptors; (d) the telomerase pathway, which regulates telomere maintenance; (e) an angiogenesis pathway, which provides a needed blood supply for the growing tumor; and (f) a metastatic pathway, which enables a cancer cell to invade normal tissues. These six pathways are altered by the four previously mentioned genes that can be introduced into primary cells to cause a human cancer.[688,689] The SV40 large T antigen can bind and sequester the RB and TP53 proteins, leading to functional inactivation of both of these pathways. Overexpression of *hTERT* can activate the telomerase pathway. Expression of an activated mutant *RAS* has several effects. It not only leads to independence from mitogenic signals normally required for cellular proliferation[692] but also inhibits apoptosis and is responsible, at least in part,[693] for activation of angiogenesis in tumor cells. However, it is not clear whether any of these four genes (large and small T antigens, *hTERT*, mutant *RAS*) leads to metastasis and invasion.

A simple pathogenic model for AML has been proposed by Gilliland and colleagues, in which AML is caused by two complementary classes of mutations.[694] In this model, one class of mutation affects cellular proliferation and survival and often involves the RAS pathway described earlier. These mutations can involve *RAS* itself or can involve activation of a tyrosine kinase receptor gene that is upstream of *RAS*. The second, complementary class of mutation leads to impaired hematopoietic differentiation and typically involves a known or putative transcription factor. This model is supported by both clinical observations and animal models of leukemia. For instance, patients with acute promyelocytic leukemia usually express a *PML-RARα* fusion gene, which inhibits promyelocytic differentiation, and often express a mutant form of the *FLT3* gene, which leads to increased proliferation and survival of the mutant cells.[695] As another example, patients with CML typically express a *BCR-ABL* fusion gene encoding a tyrosine kinase fusion protein, which confers both a proliferative and a survival advantage to the cells. During blast crisis, as the CML transforms to AML, patients often acquire additional chromosomal abnormalities, including those abnormalities (such as a *NUP98-HOXA9* fusion)[331] able to impair hematopoietic differentiation. This model is further supported by *in vivo* experiments, in which coexpression of a gene leading to increased proliferation and survival (*BCR-ABL*) and a gene that impairs differentiation (*NUP98-HOXA9*) is required to induce acute leukemia.[332] Selected aspects of the multistep nature of childhood cancer induction and progression are discussed in more detail in the sections that follow.

Aberrant Control of the Cell Cycle

Orderly cell division requires a complex set of molecular controls, coordinated in part by the CDKs.[696,697] Many of the signals that drive cells from one phase of the cell cycle to another culminate in the phosphorylation of proteins by CDKs, whose active forms are complexes of a catalytic kinase subunit and a regulatory cyclin subunit. Changes in the components of cyclin-kinase complexes determine the proteins that are activated or inactivated by phosphorylation and hence ensure the integrity of the cell cycle. In mammalian cells, the series of kinase and cyclin subunits that are expressed during progression from the first gap phase (G_1) to mitosis have been designated CDKs 1 through 8 and cyclins A through H.[696-698]

Cells must also depend on other kinases, phosphatases, and inhibitors to regulate the CDKs. Perhaps the most intriguing of these factors are the cyclin-dependent kinase inhibitors (CDKIs)—$p15^{INK4B}$, $p16^{INK4A}$, $p18^{INK4C}$, $p19^{INK4D}$, $p21^{CIP1}$, $p27^{KIP1}$, and $p57^{KIP2}$—which negatively regulate the cell cycle in response to internal and external stimuli.[499] The product of the retinoblastoma tumor suppressor gene, RB, occupies a central position in the interplay among several of the cyclins, CDKs, and CDKIs.[410] In mammalian cells, this protein undergoes phosphorylation at a point approximately two-thirds of the way through G_1 phase, a time coinciding with the cells' advance through a so-called restriction point (R), marked by a transition from mitogen dependence to relative independence from serum factors (see Fig. 3.5).[699]

Considerable evidence indicates that RB phosphorylation by CDKs (i.e., CDK4, CDK6, and possibly CDK2), under regulation of the D cyclins, determines whether a cell can successfully breach the R point and enter the DNA synthetic phase (S). Current models suggest that growth signals originating outside the cell stimulate RB phosphorylation largely through increases in cyclin D levels, leading to activation of CDK4 and CDK6, and then through extended kinase cascades involving cyclin E and CDK2.[499] In its phosphorylated form, RB uncouples from an E2F family partner, enabling the transcription factor to activate a number of genes (e.g., *MYC*) whose products are important components of downstream effector pathways (reviewed elsewhere[414]). Growth inhibitory signals emanating from outside the cell can block RB phosphorylation and hence the passage of cells through G_1.[410]

Because cancer cells show many defects in proliferation, one would predict a carcinogenic role for the proteins affecting

RB function. Evidence to support this notion is quite compelling. Mechanisms causing inactivation of RB include mutations of the *RB* gene that abolish RB function in retinoblastoma, sarcomas, and other tumors.[700] Similar increases in RB phosphorylation may result from amplification of the *CDK4* gene, a common finding in many glioblastomas[701,702] and sarcomas.[703–705] One of the most striking observations is the frequent deletion of the $p16^{INK4A}$ and $p15^{INK4B}$ *CDKI* genes from chromosome 9p21 in cases of childhood ALL with either a T or a B immunophenotype.[427,706] These tandemly linked genes function as specific inhibitors of cyclin D–associated kinases, suggesting that their elimination within cells could remove negative growth regulatory signals emanating from RB, resulting in a proliferative advantage. It should be stressed that the cancer-related molecular changes described previously involve RB inactivation, by which cells are given unrestrained passage into late G_1 phase and subsequently progress unimpeded into S phase.

Escape From Apoptosis

Genetic programs of cell death are crucial to the ordered formation of tissues and organs and to the homeostatic maintenance of rapidly dividing cells. They also play essential roles in the destruction of somatic or germ cells that have suffered DNA damage. Among the myriad intracellular signals that can elicit apoptosis, many are transmitted to the mitochondria, which respond by releasing cytochrome c, a potent catalyst of apoptosis.[707] Whether or not apoptotic signals reach the mitochondria depends on members of the BCL2 family of proteins, which possess either antiapoptotic (BCL2, BCLXL, BCLW) or proapoptotic (BAX, BAK, BID, BIM) function. In response to DNA damage, the p53 tumor suppressor protein induces apoptosis in part by upregulating the expression of proapoptotic BAX and BH3-only protein such as PUMA and NOXA; BAX in turn, collaborates with BAK to elicit the release of cytochrome c from mitochondria. Given the pivotal role of apoptosis in suppressing the growth of potentially harmful cells, it is not surprising that elimination of this mechanism ranks high on the list of acquired attributes of cancer cells. The most frequently inactivated component of the apoptotic machinery in mammalian cells is the *TP53* gene, which is mutated in at least one-half of epithelial tumors and sarcomas. Loss of p53 function increases the chances of the tumor cell survival during the proapoptotic stresses encountered as part of the progression to a full neoplastic phenotype.[708–710] Aberrant activation of the PI3K-AKT/PKB pathway can also block apoptotic responses, through untimely transmission of survival signals activated by IGF1/2 or IL3,[711] RAS signaling,[712] or the loss of the PTEN tumor suppressor, which normally regulates the AKT survival signal.[713]

Overexpression of BCL2 and other antiapoptotic members of this protein family is a hallmark of many types of tumors. In addition, to its direct activation in follicular lymphoma characterized by the t(14;18)(q23;q21),[714] BCL2 has been shown to be upregulated in patients with NHLs, AIDS-related lymphomas, hairy cell leukemia, B-lineage ALL and CLL, and several types of AML, and in general, this overexpression connotes a poor clinical response. Although less compelling than for BCL2, there is also evidence for aberrant upregulation of BCLXL in AML and CML, Hodgkin disease, AIDS-related lymphomas, and multiple myeloma.[715]

Virtually all antineoplastic drugs kill cancer cells by activating apoptotic pathways, yet in clinical practice most human tumors show resistance to chemotherapy. It is now clear that chemoresistance can often be attributed to genetic alterations that disable apoptotic regulators, especially the BCL2 family members, as well as certain components of the death receptor, PI3K-AKT, NF-κB, and ARF-p53 pathways.[406]

Infinite Replication, Telomeres, and Telomerase

There is a particular obstacle to the faithful replication of the ends of chromosomes. DNA polymerases can add nucleotides only onto preexisting nucleotides. There is a requirement for priming, usually provided by short RNA molecules, in the initiation of DNA synthesis. There is also a directionality to DNA synthesis; one of the two strands of the double helix is synthesized in a 5′ to 3′ direction and the other must be synthesized (globally) in a 3′ to 5′ direction. Because DNA polymerases add nucleotides only in a 5′ to 3′ direction, replication of the two strands of a double helix must be accomplished by using distinct mechanisms. The "leading" strand is replicated continuously in a 5′ to 3′ direction, and the opposing strand is replicated by a succession of priming and 5′ to 3′ syntheses of short fragments (Okazaki fragments) that displace the successive primers and are subsequently ligated together (i.e., the lagging strand). However, the 5′ ends of both newly synthesized strands cannot be completely replicated by conventional DNA synthesis. Instead, the 5′ ends of chromosomes are replicated by the action of telomerase, a ribonucleoprotein complex in which the RNA component is used for the recognition and as a template for the extension of telomeric repeats.[716]

The vast majority of nonmalignant cells do not produce telomerase. Therefore, after a certain number of cell divisions, a critical shortening of the chromosome ends is reached, chromosomal instability ensues, and the cells die. Telomere shortening is proposed as a "cellular clock" and a mediator of senescence.[717,718] However, germ cells and other stem cells (e.g., hematopoietic stem cells) maintain the size of their telomeres through the action of telomerase.[719] Given that infinite replication is a hallmark of malignancy, it was not surprising that a survey of more than 100 immortal cell lines demonstrated telomerase activity in most samples.[720–722] Equally striking was the finding of telomerase activity in more than 84% of primary malignancies, comprising more than a dozen distinct tumor types.[719–721] In some cases, levels of telomerase activity may correlate with tumor virulence and prognosis. For example, of 100 NB cases analyzed, 94 had detectable telomerase activity.[723] The higher the activity, the more additional genetic changes were apparent and the poorer the prognosis. Three of the tumors that lacked telomerase activity were classified as stage IVS, a form characterized by spontaneous regression.

OUTLOOK FOR MOLECULARLY TARGETED THERAPIES

The ultimate goal in unraveling the molecular and genetic events that underlie childhood cancer is to develop improved methods for the prevention, diagnosis, monitoring, and treatment of childhood cancer patients. It is hoped that the discovery of critical molecular events in the pathogenesis of childhood cancers will translate into major advances in therapy, based on the paradigm of successful targeting of the PML-RARA fusion protein with retinoic acid. Although few of the subsequently developed agents have proved as effective as retinoic acid, continued progress promises to identify new therapeutic targets within oncogenic pathways whose manipulation should produce significant antitumor effects.

Although it may seem surprising at first glance, a detailed knowledge of cancer pathways is not required in order to use genetic findings in cancer patients to improve therapy. The best example of this principle is the use of risk-directed therapy to select chemotherapy protocols for pediatric leukemia patients. As discussed earlier, genetic characterization of leukemia patients led to the identification of a large number of recurrent genetic aberrations, many of which could be detected by a simple karyotype. Systematic collection of karyotypic data on leukemia patients identified many cytogenetic aberrations, which were important prognostic variables. Armed with the knowledge that specific aberrations predicted a poor outcome with "standard" chemotherapy, investigators were able to select these patients for more intensive therapy. In current treatment schemes for pediatric AML patients, genetic findings have largely supplanted clinical findings; patients with inv(16) and t(8;21) are selected for less intensive therapy, and patients with t(15;17) are treated with differentiation-based therapy.[724–726] Similar findings apply to pediatric ALL patients. The t(12;21) and hyperdiploidy are good prognostic features, and these cytogenetic findings are incorporated into current therapeutic protocols.[727,728]

A number of attractive molecular and genetic targets have been identified. Tyrosine kinases impact signaling pathways that ultimately regulate diverse cellular processes, including cell cycle progression, DNA replication, cell differentiation, and cell death (see Fig. 3.6). Thus, constitutive activation of such enzymes would be expected to confer potent transforming properties. Discovery of the *BCR-ABL* fusion oncogene and demonstration of its transforming potential[108,729] provided formal proof of this concept and suggested that an inhibitor of ABL kinase activity might be an effective therapeutic agent in CML patients, most of whom express this chimeric molecule in their leukemic cells. Imatinib mesylate (Gleevec) inhibits BCR-ABL kinase activity and has proved highly effective in clinical trials, inducing complete hematologic remissions in 97% of CML patients.[730] "Second generation" ABL inhibitors have been identified that are active in patients with imatinib-resistant CML.[731]

Several other cancers, such as GISTs and rare forms of leukemia, express tyrosine kinases that are inhibited by imatinib. More than 90% of GISTs constitutively express *KIT*, which is activated because of somatic mutations, and several lines of evidence indicate that such mutations are an early event in the pathogenesis of these mesenchymal tumors.[732] A subset of patients with CMML positive for *EVT6(TEL)-PDGFRB* fusion oncogenes also respond with complete remissions to imatinib,[733] as do patients with hypereosinophilic syndrome and the FIPL1-PDGFRA fusion protein.[734] Since KIT and PDGFRs are aberrantly expressed in many common tumors, such as gliomas, melanomas, and sarcomas,[730] interest in broader use of imatinib has grown, leading to clinical evaluations that are still under way.

The epidermal growth factor receptor (EGFR) is one of the best-known receptor tyrosine kinase targeted in current efforts to develop more specific cancer therapies. Dysregulation of *EGFR*, by gene overexpression or through somatically acquired activating mutations,[735,736] can disrupt normal activation of downstream kinases such as MAPK and PI3K, leading to aberrant cell signaling that affects cell proliferation and resistance to apoptosis, tumor invasion, and tumor angiogenesis.[737]

Two major strategies have been used to target EGFRs: monoclonal antibodies that compete with the binding of activating ligands to the extracellular domain of the receptor and small-molecule inhibitors of the intracellular tyrosine kinase domain of the receptor.[738] In principle, the inhibition of EGFR signaling should have at least a cytostatic effect on tumor cells, which could prove lethal in combination with therapies directed against other signaling effector molecules, but with the exception of head and neck tumors, complete responses to EGFR-targeted treatment are rarely seen in more than 20% of solid tumor patients.[738,739] Nonetheless, the inhibition of EGFR function may be critical for improving tumor responses to radiation therapy, by virtue of blocking signals that otherwise would inhibit apoptosis. Studies to test brain tumor radiation sensitization with EGFR inhibitors are under way at several institutions.

Experience with tyrosine kinase inhibitors has taught us valuable lessons about the realities of targeted cancer therapy. In both CML and GIST, in which imatinib induces clinical remissions in the majority of patients, the mutant target gene functions as a dominant influence on tumor induction and progression. In other tumor types, where the rationale for use of imatinib is much less compelling, treatment results have been equivocal at best. This has led to a sobering conclusion. While targeted therapies may be highly active in specific subsets of tumors, they clearly will not work in all patients or against all tumors; rather, they are most effective when the tumor is dependent on or driven by the molecule targeted by the drug. Thus, validation of potential molecular targets is a critical step in molecular therapeutics programs. Even with proper screening of candidate molecules, correction of a single genetic aberration may not be sufficient to alter tumor growth. Because many human tumors remain in a preclinical state for years before presentation, they may have acquired multiple cancer-prompting lesions and may not be sensitive to the inhibition of a single oncoprotein. Thus, targeting several different pivotal molecules at once will probably be required in most cases to eradicate all tumor cells and prevent relapse.

Nearly all antineoplastic drugs kill cancer cells by activating apoptotic pathways. Yet, in clinical practice, human tumors can quickly develop resistance to chemotherapy, usually as a result of genetic alterations that disable apoptotic regulators. In the leukemias and lymphomas, BCL2 family members, as well as components of the death receptor—PI3K-AKT, NF-κB, and ARF-p53 pathways[740]—are often altered and are now recognized as the leading contributors to chemoresistance. This realization has stimulated intense interest as a means to selectively disable these prosurvival regulators (BCL2, AFT, or NF-κB) or to reactivate the functions of proapoptotic components (ARF or p53). Genasense, a phosphorothioate antisense oligonucleotide, selectively impairs the expression of *BCL2* mRNA and is being evaluated in clinical trials.[741] Small molecules (so-called BH3 mimetics) that interact with the surface pocket of the BH3 domains of BCL2 family proteins are also under development and perhaps hold the greatest promise for inactivating BCL2 and its related proteins, thus placing the cell on an irreversible course toward destruction when it responds to chemotherapy.[742]

The classes of molecules that have proven to be useful targets for therapy are remarkably limited, consisting primarily of cell surface receptors, transmembrane channels, and tyrosine kinases. Transcription factors and tumor suppressors have generally proven resistant to manipulation. A recent report shows that *NOTCH1*, a gene encoding a transmembrane receptor involved in the regulation of T-cell development, is activated in a large subset of patients with T-ALL.[558] This finding has stimulated trials to test the clinical efficacy of γ-secretase inhibitors in *NOTCH1*-positive cases, since signalling from the membrane-bound activated NOTCH1 receptor is dependent on this enzyme. Sphingosine kinase, which plays a pivotal role in regulating tumor cell growth and apoptosis, also affords an attractive target for therapeutic intervention in the spectrum of solid tumors that overexpress this enzyme.[743]

Despite the difficult challenges posed by the development and testing of targeted therapies, emerging technologies should enable the global analyses of the genetic and epigenetic changes that typify a particular tumor and reveal the lesions that are most critical in maintaining the malignant phenotype and thus are most amenable to therapeutic intervention. In the not-too-distant future, individualized molecular medicine may provide optimal therapy for the cancer patient. Each cancer patient will be treated according to his or her own unique genetic profile, resulting in excellent therapeutic efficacy with minimal toxicity.

SUMMARY

Childhood cancer is ultimately a disorder of genes, whose identity and function have preoccupied cell biologists and geneticists for more than 30 years. The genetic portrait of the diverse group of neoplasms we call pediatric tumors is being rapidly completed. We know that aberrant activation of transcription factor or tyrosine kinase genes by translocation-mediated fusions with normally unrelated partners or by rearrangement to sites near immunoglobulin or T-cell receptor genes can lead to acute leukemia, lymphoma, and sarcoma. It is intriguing that many of these genes have close homologues in the genes controlling *Drosophila* morphogenesis, underscoring their faithful conservation in nature and their relevance to programs of early cell differentiation. The inappropriate expression of specific oncogenes in hematopoietic or mesenchymal progenitor cells could be expected to block normal programs of differentiation.

Rather than inappropriate activation (i.e., gain of function), tumor suppressor genes must be deleted or otherwise inactivated (i.e., loss of function) before their carcinogenic effects become apparent. Although the precise number of steps required to transform normal cells into cancerous ones remains unknown, emerging data indicate that a basic "cancer platform" would consist of disruption or activation of (a) the RB pathway; (b) a cell proliferation pathway involving extracellular signals, including RAS and receptor tyrosine kinases; (c) the telomerase pathway; (d) an apoptotic pathway; (e) an angiogenesis pathway; and (f) a metastatic pathway.

Rapid identification and validation of potential therapeutic targets within pathways controlling tumor growth and survival has led to promising clinical trial results. While none of the antitumor effects have been curative, the responses suggest that detailed genetic profiling of each new childhood cancer patient would not only pay immediate dividends, in terms of improved clinical management, but would soon provide the foundation for a new era of individualized molecular medicine.

ACKNOWLEDGMENTS

The authors thank A. Thomas Look and Ilan R. Kirsch for numerous conversations, advice, and work on prior editions of this chapter and Michael Kuehl, Frederic Kaye, Paul Meltzer, Kevin Shannon, James Downing, Shai Izraeli, R. Keith Humphries, Ying Wei Lin, Chris Slape, Jun Wei, Qingrong Chen, Young Song, Adam Cheuk, members of the Oncogenomics Section of the Pediatric Oncology Branch, and members of the Leukemia Biology Section for their insightful comments and advice. This work was supported by the Intramural Research Program of the National Cancer Institute, National Institutes of Health.

References

1. Diskin SJ, Hou C, Glessner JT, et al. Copy number variation at 1q21.1 associated with neuroblastoma. Nature 2009;459:987–991.
2. Wieland I, Muschke P, Volleth M, et al. High incidence of familial breast cancer segregates with constitutional t(11;22)(q23;q11). Genes Chromosomes Cancer 2006;45:945–949.
3. Laureys G, Versteeg R, Speleman F, et al. Characterisation of the chromosome breakpoints in a patient with a constitutional translocation t(1;17)(p36.31-p36.13;q11.2-q12) and neuroblastoma. Eur J Cancer 1995;31A:523–526.
4. Vandepoele K, Andries V, Van Roy N, et al. A constitutional translocation t(1;17)(p36.2;q11.2) in a neuroblastoma patient disrupts the human NBPF1 and ACCN1 genes. PLoS One 2008;3:e2207.
5. Poland KS, Azim M, Folsom M, et al. A constitutional balanced t(3;8)(p14;q24.1) translocation results in disruption of the TRC8 gene and predisposition to clear cell renal cell carcinoma. Genes Chromosomes Cancer 2007;46:805–812.
6. Janoueix-Lerosey I, Lequin D, Brugieres L, et al. Somatic and germline activating mutations of the ALK kinase receptor in neuroblastoma. Nature 2008;455:967–970.
7. Mosse YP, Laudenslager M, Longo L, et al. Identification of ALK as a major familial neuroblastoma predisposition gene. Nature 2008;455:930–935.
8. Schaffner C, Idler I, Stilgenbauer S, et al. Mantle cell lymphoma is characterized by inactivation of the ATM gene. Proc Natl Acad Sci U S A 2000;97:2773–2778.
9. Bay JO, Uhrhammer N, Pernin D, et al. High incidence of cancer in a family segregating a mutation of the ATM gene: possible role of ATM heterozygosity in cancer. Hum Mutat 1999;14:485–492.
10. Gorlin RJ. Nevoid basal cell carcinoma (Gorlin) syndrome. Genet Med 2004;6:530–539.
11. High A, Zedan W. Basal cell nevus syndrome. Curr Opin Oncol 2005;17:160–166.
12. Weksberg R, Shuman C, Smith AC. Beckwith-Wiedemann syndrome. Am J Med Genet C Semin Med Genet 2005;137C:12–23.
13. Cooper WN, Curley R, Macdonald F, et al. Mitotic recombination and uniparental disomy in Beckwith-Wiedemann syndrome. Genomics 2007;89:613–617.
14. Sparago A, Russo S, Cerrato F, et al. Mechanisms causing imprinting defects in familial Beckwith-Wiedemann syndrome with Wilms' tumour. Hum Mol Genet 2007;16:254–264.
15. Baba M, Hong SB, Sharma N, et al. Folliculin encoded by the BHD gene interacts with a binding protein, FNIP1, and AMPK, and is involved in AMPK and mTOR signaling. Proc Natl Acad Sci U S A 2006;103:15552–15557.
16. Pavlovich CP, Walther MM, Eyler RA, et al. Renal tumors in the Birt-Hogg-Dube syndrome. Am J Surg Pathol 2002;26:1542–1552.
17. Wang W. Emergence of a DNA-damage response network consisting of Fanconi anaemia and BRCA proteins. Nat Rev Genet 2007;8:735–748.
18. Ellis NA, Groden J, Ye TZ, et al. The Bloom's syndrome gene product is homologous to RecQ helicases. Cell 1995;83:655–666.
19. Reliene R, Bishop AJ, Schiestl RH. Involvement of homologous recombination in carcinogenesis. Adv Genet 2007;58:67–87.
20. Hickson ID. RecQ helicases: caretakers of the genome. Nat Rev Cancer 2003;3:169–178.
21. Olopade OI, Grushko TA, Nanda R, et al. Advances in breast cancer: pathways to personalized medicine. Clin Cancer Res 2008;14:7988–7999.
22. De Greve J, Sermijn E, De Brakeleer S, et al. Hereditary breast cancer: from bench to bedside. Curr Opin Oncol 2008;20:605–613.
23. Turnbull C, Rahman N. Genetic predisposition to breast cancer: past, present, and future. Annu Rev Genomics Hum Genet 2008;9:321–345.
24. Hampel H, Frankel WL, Martin E, et al. Screening for the Lynch syndrome (hereditary nonpolyposis colorectal cancer). N Engl J Med 2005;352:1851–1860.
25. Woods MO, Williams P, Careen A, et al. A new variant database for mismatch repair genes associated with Lynch syndrome. Hum Mutat 2007;28:669–673.
26. Wijnen JT, Vasen HF, Khan PM, et al. Clinical findings with implications for genetic testing in families with clustering of colorectal cancer. N Engl J Med 1998;339:511–518.
27. Liaw D, Marsh DJ, Li J, et al. Germline mutations of the PTEN gene in Cowden disease, an inherited breast and thyroid cancer syndrome. Nat Genet 1997;16:64–67.
28. Zhou XP, Waite KA, Pilarski R, et al. Germline PTEN promoter mutations and deletions in Cowden/Bannayan-Riley-Ruvalcaba syndrome result in aberrant PTEN protein and dysregulation of the phosphoinositol-3-kinase/Akt pathway. Am J Hum Genet 2003;73:404–411.
29. Marrone A, Walne A, Tamary H, et al. Telomerase reverse-transcriptase homozygous mutations in autosomal recessive dyskeratosis congenita and Hoyeraal-Hreidarsson syndrome. Blood 2007;110:4198–4205.
30. Vulliamy T, Marrone A, Szydlo R, et al. Disease anticipation is associated with progressive telomere shortening in families with dyskeratosis congenita due to mutations in TERC. Nat Genet 2004;36:447–449.
31. Vulliamy TJ, Dokal I. Dyskeratosis congenita: the diverse clinical presentation of mutations in the telomerase complex. Biochimie 2008;90:122–130.
32. Gurtan AM, D'Andrea AD. Dedicated to the core: understanding the Fanconi anemia complex. DNA Repair (Amst) 2006;5:1119–1125.
33. Alter BP. Cancer in Fanconi anemia, 1927–2001. Cancer 2003;97:425–440.
34. Horwitz M. The genetics of familial leukemia. Leukemia 1997;11:1347–1359.
35. Upton B, Chu Q, Li BD. Li-Fraumeni syndrome: the genetics and treatment considerations for the sarcoma and associated neoplasms. Surg Oncol Clin N Am 2009;18:145–156, ix.
36. Nichols KE, Malkin D, Garber JE, et al. Germ-line p53 mutations predispose to a wide spectrum of early-onset cancers. Cancer Epidemiol Biomarkers Prev 2001;10:83–87.
37. Malkin D, Li FP, Strong LC, et al. Germ line p53 mutations in a familial syndrome of breast cancer, sarcomas, and other neoplasms. Science 1990;250:1233–1238.
38. Olivier M, Goldgar DE, Sodha N, et al. Li-Fraumeni and related syndromes: correlation between tumor type, family structure, and TP53 genotype. Cancer Res 2003;63:6643–6650.
39. Monzon J, Liu L, Brill H, et al. CDKN2A mutations in multiple primary melanomas. N Engl J Med 1998;338:879–887.

40. Greene MH, Clark WH Jr, Tucker MA, et al. Acquired precursors of cutaneous malignant melanoma. The familial dysplastic nevus syndrome. N Engl J Med 1985;312:91–97.
41. Borg A, Sandberg T, Nilsson K, et al. High frequency of multiple melanomas and breast and pancreas carcinomas in CDKN2A mutation-positive melanoma families. J Natl Cancer Inst 2000;92:1260–1266.
42. Brandi ML, Gagel RF, Angeli A, et al. Guidelines for diagnosis and therapy of MEN type 1 and type 2. J Clin Endocrinol Metab 2001;86:5658–5671.
43. Carling T. Multiple endocrine neoplasia syndrome: genetic basis for clinical management. Curr Opin Oncol 2005;17:7–12.
44. Eng C, Clayton D, Schuffenecker I, et al. The relationship between specific RET proto-oncogene mutations and disease phenotype in multiple endocrine neoplasia type 2: international RET mutation consortium analysis. JAMA 1996;276:1575–1579.
45. Neumann HP, Bausch B, McWhinney SR, et al. Germ-line mutations in nonsyndromic pheochromocytoma. N Engl J Med 2002;346:1459–1466.
46. Theos A, Korf BR. Pathophysiology of neurofibromatosis type 1. Ann Intern Med 2006;144:842–849.
47. Ferner RE, Gutmann DH. International consensus statement on malignant peripheral nerve sheath tumors in neurofibromatosis. Cancer Res 2002;62:1573–1577.
48. Widemann BC. Current status of sporadic and neurofibromatosis type 1-associated malignant peripheral nerve sheath tumors. Curr Oncol Rep 2009;11:322–328.
49. Rouleau GA, Merel P, Lutchman M, et al. Alteration in a new gene encoding a putative membrane-organizing protein causes neuro-fibromatosis type 2. Nature 1993;363:515–521.
50. Trofatter JA, MacCollin MM, Rutter JL, et al. A novel moesin-, ezrin-, radixin-like gene is a candidate for the neurofibromatosis 2 tumor suppressor. Cell 1993;72:791–800.
51. Demuth I, Digweed M. The clinical manifestation of a defective response to DNA double-strand breaks as exemplified by Nijmegen breakage syndrome. Oncogene 2007;26:7792–7798.
52. McKinnon PJ, Caldecott KW. DNA strand break repair and human genetic disease. Annu Rev Genomics Hum Genet 2007;8:37–55.
53. Weemaes CM, Hustinx TW, Scheres JM, et al. A new chromosomal instability disorder: the Nijmegen breakage syndrome. Acta Paediatr Scand 1981;70:557–564.
54. Giardiello FM, Welsh SB, Hamilton SR, et al. Increased risk of cancer in the Peutz-Jeghers syndrome. N Engl J Med 1987;316:1511–1514.
55. Hearle N, Schumacher V, Menko FH, et al. Frequency and spectrum of cancers in the Peutz-Jeghers syndrome. Clin Cancer Res 2006;12:3209–3215.
56. Nieuwenhuis MH, Vasen HF. Correlations between mutation site in APC and phenotype of familial adenomatous polyposis (FAP): a review of the literature. Crit Rev Oncol Hematol 2007;61:153–161.
57. Laken SJ, Petersen GM, Gruber SB, et al. Familial colorectal cancer in Ashkenazim due to a hypermutable tract in APC. Nat Genet 1997;17:79–83.
58. Attard TM, Giglio P, Koppula S, et al. Brain tumors in individuals with familial adenomatous polyposis: a cancer registry experience and pooled case report analysis. Cancer 2007;109:761–766.
59. Taylor M, Dehainault C, Desjardins L, et al. Genotype-phenotype correlations in hereditary familial retinoblastoma. Hum Mutat 2007;28:284–293.
60. Friend SH, Bernards R, Rogeli S, et al. A human DNA segment with properties of the gene that predisposes to retinoblastoma and osteosarcoma. Nature 1986;323:643–646.
61. Kleinerman RA, Tucker MA, Abramson DH, et al. Risk of soft tissue sarcomas by individual subtype in survivors of hereditary retinoblastoma. J Natl Cancer Inst 2007;99:24–31.
62. Valverde JR, Alonso J, Palacios I, et al. RB1 gene mutation up-date, a meta-analysis based on 932 reported mutations available in a searchable database. BMC Genet 2005;6:53.
63. Lonser RR, Glenn GM, Walther M, et al. von Hippel-Lindau disease. Lancet 2003;361:2059–2067.
64. Friedrich CA. Genotype-phenotype correlation in von Hippel-Lindau syndrome. Hum Mol Genet 2001;10:763–767.
65. Huang S, Lee L, Hanson NB, et al. The spectrum of WRN mutations in Werner syndrome patients. Hum Mutat 2006;27:558–567.
66. Goto M, Miller RW, Ishikawa Y, et al. Excess of rare cancers in Werner syndrome (adult progeria). Cancer Epidemiol Biomarkers Prev 1996;5:239–246.
67. Kraemer KH, Lee MM, Scotto J. Xeroderma pigmentosum: cutaneous, ocular, and neurologic abnormalities in 830 published cases. Arch Dermatol 1987;123:241–250.
68. Cleaver JE. Cancer in xeroderma pigmentosum and related disorders of DNA repair. Nat Rev Cancer 2005;5:564–573.
69. Call KM, Glaser T, Ito CY, et al. Isolation and characterization of a zinc finger polypeptide gene at the human chromosome 11 Wilms' tumor locus. Cell 1990;60:509–520.
70. Gessler M, Poustka A, Cavenee W, et al. Homozygous deletion in Wilms tumours of a zinc-finger gene identified by chromosome jumping. Nature 1990;343:774–778.
71. Bosticardo M, Marangoni F, Aiuti A, et al. Recent advances in understanding the pathophysiology of Wiskott-Aldrich syndrome. Blood 2009;113:6288–6295.
72. Bochkov NP, Kuleshov NP. Age sensitivity of human chromosomes to alkylating agents. Mutat Res 1972;14:345–353.
73. Therman E. Human chromosomes: structure, behavior, effects. New York: Springer-Verlag, 1986.
74. Sandberg AA. The chromosomes in human cancer and leukemia. 2nd ed. New York: Elsevier, 1990.
75. Lindor NM, McMaster ML, Lindor CJ, et al. Concise handbook of familial cancer susceptibility syndromes—second edition. J Natl Cancer Inst Monogr 2008;(38):1–93.
76. Gallie BL. The misadventures of RB1. In: Kirsch IR, ed. The causes and consequences of chromosomal aberrations. Boca Raton, FL: CRC Press, 1993:429–446.
77. Knudson AG Jr. Mutation and cancer: statistical study of retinoblastoma. Proc Natl Acad Sci U S A 1971;68:820–823.
78. Orye E, Delbeke MJ, Vandaneeble B. Retinoblastoma and long arm deletion of chromosome 13: attempts to define the deleted segment. Clin Genet 1974;5:457–464.
79. Lele KP, Penrose LS, Stallard HB. Chromosome deletion in a case of retinoblastoma. Am J Hum Genet 1963;27:171–174.
80. Cavenee WK, Dryja TP, Phillips RA, et al. Expression of recessive alleles by chromosomal mechanisms in retinoblastoma. Nature 1983;305:779–785.
81. Otterson GA, Modi S, Nguyen K, et al. Temperature-sensitive RB mutations linked to incomplete penetrance of familial retinoblastoma in 12 families. Am J Hum Genet 1999;65:1040–1046.
82. Riccardi VM, Sujanksy E, Smith AC, et al. Chromosomal imbalance in the aniridia-Wilm's tumor association: 11p interstitial deletion. Pediatrics 1978;61:604–610.
83. Reeve AE, Sih AA, Raizis AM, et al. Loss of allelic heterozygosity at a second locus on chromosome 11 in sporadic Wilms' tumor cells. Mol Cell Biol 1989;346:1799–1803.
84. Schroeder WT, Chao LY, Dao DD, et al. Nonrandom loss of maternal chromosome 11 alleles in Wilms tumors. Am J Hum Genet 1987;40:413–420.
85. Mannens M, Slater RM, Heyting C, et al. Regional localization of DNA probes on the short arm of chromosome 11 using aniridia-Wilms' tumor–associated deletions. Hum Genet 1987;75:180–187.
86. Toguchida J, Ishizaki K, Sasaki MS, et al. Preferential mutation of paternally derived RB gene as the initial event in sporadic osteosarcoma. Nature 1989;338:156–158.
87. Scrable H, Witte D, Shimada H, et al. Molecular differential pathology of rhabdomyosarcoma. Genes Chromosomes Cancer 1989;1:23–35.
88. Henry I, Bonaiti-Pellie C, Chehensse V, et al. Uniparental paternal disomy in a genetic cancer-predisposing syndrome. Nature 1991;351:665–667.
89. Tilghman SM. DNA methylation: a phoenix rises. Proc Natl Acad Sci U S A 1993;90:8761–8762.
90. John RM, Surani MA. Genomic imprinting, mammalian evolution, and the mystery of egg-laying mammals. Cell 2000;101:585–588.
91. Niebuhr E. Triploidy in man: cytological and clinical aspects. Hum Genet 1974;21:103–125.
92. Hassold TJ, Jacobs PA. Trisomy in man. Ann Rev Genet 1984;18:69–97.
93. Lejeune J, Turpin R, Gautier M. Le mongolisme, premier example d'aberration autosomique humaine. Ann Genet 1959;1:41–49.
94. Rosner F, Lee SL. Down's syndrome and acute leukemias: myeloblastic or lymphoblastic? Am J Med 1972;53:203–218.
95. Rowley JD. Down syndrome and acute leukemia: increased risk may be due to trisomy 21. Lancet 1981;11:1020–1022.
96. Ferster A, Verhest A, Vamos E, et al. Leukemia in a trisomy 21 mosaic: specific involvement of the trisomic cells. Cancer Genet Cytogenet 1986;20:109–113.
97. Robison LL, Nesbit MEJ, Sather HN, et al. Down syndrome and acute leukemia in children: a 10-year retrospective survey from Children's Cancer Study Group. J Pediatr 1984;105:235–242.
98. Smith AG, Willoughby MLN. Preleukemia in Down's syndrome. Blood 1982;59:870.
99. Seibel NL, Sommer A, Miser J. Transient neonatal leukemoid reactions in mosaic trisomy 21. J Pediatr 1984;104:251–254.
100. Zipursky A, Poon A, Doyle J. Hematologic and oncologic disorders in Down syndrome. In: Lott I, McCoy E, eds. Down syndrome: today's health care issues. New York: John Wiley & Sons, 1991:42–56.
101. Wechsler J, Greene M, McDevitt MA, et al. Acquired mutations in GATA1 in the megakaryoblastic leukemia of Down syndrome. Nat Genet 2002;32:148–152.
102. Rainis L, Bercovich D, Strehl S, et al. Mutations in exon 2 of GATA1 are early events in megakaryocytic malignancies associated with trisomy 21. Blood 2003;102:981–986.
103. Hitzler JK, Cheung J, Li Y, et al. GATA1 mutations in transient leukemia and acute megakaryoblastic leukemia of Down syndrome. Blood 2003;101:4301–4304.
104. Groet J, McElwaine S, Spinelli M, et al. Acquired mutations in GATA1 in neonates with Down's syndrome with transient myeloid disorder. Lancet 2003;361:1617–1620.
105. Greene ME, Mundschau G, Wechsler J, et al. Mutations in GATA1 in both transient myeloproliferative disorder and acute megakaryoblastic leukemia of Down syndrome. Blood Cells Mol Dis 2003;31:351–356.
106. Ahmed M, Sternberg A, Hall G, et al. Natural history of GATA1 mutations in Down syndrome. Blood 2004;103:2480–2489.
107. Harigae H, Xu G, Sugawara T, et al. The GATA1 mutation in an adult patient with acute megakaryoblastic leukemia not accompanying Down syndrome. Blood 2004;103:3242–3243.
108. Nowell PC, Hungerford DA. A minute chromosome in human chronic granulocytic leukemia. Science 1960;132:1497–1499.
109. Rotman G, Shiloh Y. ATM: from gene to function. Hum Mol Genet 1998;7:1555–1563.
110. Liyanage M, Coleman A, du Manoir S, et al. Multicolour spectral karyotyping of mouse chromosomes. Nat Genet 1996;14:312–315.
111. Featherstone C, Jackson SP. DNA repair: the Nijmegen breakage syndrome protein. Curr Biol 1998;8:27.
112. Maarek O, Jonveaux P, Le Coniat M, et al. Fanconi anemia and bone marrow clonal chromosome abnormalities. Leukemia 1996;10:1700–1704.
113. Ford AM, Ridge SA, Cabrera ME, et al. In utero rearrangements in the trithorax-related oncogene in infant leukaemias. Nature 1993;363:358–360.
114. Gill Super HJ, Rothberg PG, Kobayashi H, et al. Clonal, nonconstitutional rearrangements of the MLL gene in infant twins with acute lymphoblastic leukemia: in utero chromosome rearrangement of 11q23. Blood 1994;83:641–644.
115. Gale KB, Ford AM, Repp R, et al. Backtracking leukemia to birth: identification of clonotypic gene fusion sequences in neonatal blood spots. Proc Natl Acad Sci U S A 1997;94:13950–13954.
116. Wiemels JL, Cazzaniga G, Daniotti M, et al. Prenatal origin of acute lymphoblastic leukaemia in children. Lancet 1999;354:1499–1503.
117. Tycko B, Sklar J. Chromosomal translocations in lymphoid neoplasia: a reappraisal of the recombinase model. Cancer Cells 1990;2:1–8.
118. Grawunder U, West RB, Lieber MR. Antigen receptor gene rearrangement. Curr Opin Immunol 1998;10:172–180.
119. Brown L, Cheng JT, Chen Q, et al. Site-specific recombination of the tal-1 gene is a common occurrence in human T cell leukemia. EMBO J 1990;9:3343–3351.
120. Aplan PD, Lombardi DP, Ginsberg AM, et al. Disruption of the human SCL locus by "illegitimate" V-(D)-J recombinase activity. Science 1990;250:1426–1429.
121. Aplan PD, Lombardi DP, Kirsch IR. Structural characterization of SIL, a gene frequently disrupted in T-cell acute lymphoblastic leukemia. Mol Cell Biol 1991;11:5462–5469.
122. Jeffs AR, Benjes SM, Smith TL, et al. The Bcr gene recombines preferentially with Alu elements in complex Bcr-Abl translocations of chronic myeloid leukaemia. Hum Mol Genet 1998;7:767–776.
123. Zhang JG, Goldman JM, Cross CNP. Characterization of genomic BCR-ABL breakpoints in chronic myeloid leukaemia by PCR. Br J Haematol 1995;90:138–146.
124. Strout MP, Marcucci G, Bloomfield CD, et al. The partial tandem duplication of ALL1 (MLL) is consistently generated by Alu-mediated homologous recombination in acute myeloid leukemia. Proc Natl Acad Sci U S A 1998;95:2390–2395.
125. O'Neil J, Tchinda J, Gutierrez A, et al. Alu elements mediate MYB gene tandem duplication in human T-ALL. J Exp Med 2007;204:3059–3066.
126. Aplan PD, Raimondi SC, Kirsch IR. Disruption of the SCL gene by a t(1;3) translocation in a patient with T cell acute lymphoblastic leukemia. J Exp Med 1992;176:1303–1310.
127. Boehm T, Mengle-Gaw L, Kees UR, et al. Alternating purine-pyrimidine tracts may promote chromosomal translocations seen in a variety of human lymphoid tumours. EMBO J 1989;8:2621–2631.

128. Thandla SP, Ploski JE, Raza-Egilmez SZ, et al. ETV6-AML1 translocation breakpoints cluster near a purine/pyrimidine repeat region in the ETV6 gene. Blood 1999;93:293–299.
129. Drew HR, McCall MJ, Calladine CR. Recent studies of DNA in the crystal. Ann Rev Cell Biol 1988;4:1–20.
130. Garner MM, Felsenfeld G. Effect of Z-DNA on nucleosome placement. J Mol Biol 1987;196:581–590.
131. Samadashwily GM, Raca G, Mirkin SM. Trinucleotide repeats affect DNA replication in vivo. Nat Genet 1997;17:298–304.
132. Pui CH, Behm FG, Raimondi SC, et al. Secondary acute myeloid leukemia in children treated for acute lymphoid leukemia. N Engl J Med 1989;321:136–142.
133. Smith MA, McCaffrey RP, Karp JE. The secondary leukemias: challenges and research directions. J Natl Cancer Inst 1996;88:407–418.
134. Pedersen-Bjergaard J, Pedersen M, Roulston D, et al. Different genetic pathways in leukemogenesis for patients presenting with therapy-related myelodysplasia and therapy-related acute myeloid leukemia. Blood 1995;86:3542–3552.
135. Smith MA, Rubinstein L, Ungerleider RS. Therapy-related acute myeloid leukemia following treatment with epipodophyllotoxins: estimating the risks. Med Pediatr Oncol 1994;23:86–98.
136. Felix CA. Secondary leukemias induced by topoisomerase-targeted drugs. Biochim Biophys Acta 1998;1400:233–255.
137. Thirman MJ, Gill HJ, Burnett RC, et al. Rearrangement of the MLL gene in acute lymphoblastic and acute myeloid leukemias with 11q23 chromosomal translocations. N Engl J Med 1993;329:909–914.
138. Aplan PD, Chervinsky DS, Stanulla M, et al. Site-specific DNA cleavage within the MLL breakpoint cluster region induced by topoisomerase II inhibitors. Blood 1996;87:2649–2658.
139. Maraschin J, Dutrillaux B, Aurias A. Chromosome aberrations induced by etoposide (VP-16) are not random. Int J Cancer 1990;46:808–812.
140. Felix CA, Walker AH, Lange BJ, et al. Association of CYP3A4 genotype with treatment-related leukemia. Proc Natl Acad Sci U S A 1998;95:13176–13181.
141. Wang JC. DNA topoisomerases. Ann Rev Biochem 1996;65:635–692.
142. Zhou RH, Wang P, Zou Y, et al. A precise interchromosomal reciprocal exchange between hot spots for cleavable complex formation by topoisomerase II in amsacrine-treated Chinese hamster ovary cells. Cancer Res 1997;57:4699–4702.
143. Baguley BC, Ferguson LR. Mutagenic properties of topoisomerase-targeted drugs. Biochim Biophys Acta 1998;1400:213–222.
144. Lovett BD, Lo Nigro L, Rappaport EF, et al. Near-precise interchromosomal recombination and functional DNA topoisomerase II cleavage sites at MLL and AF-4 genomic breakpoints in treatment-related acute lymphoblastic leukemia with t(4;11) translocation. Proc Natl Acad Sci U S A 2001;98:9802–9807.
145. Ahuja HG, Felix CA, Aplan PD. Potential role for DNA topoisomerase II poisons in the generation of t(11;20)(p15;q11) translocations. Genes Chromosomes Cancer 2000;29: 96–105.
146. Reichel M, Gillert E, Nilson I, et al. Fine structure of translocation breakpoints in leukemic blasts with chromosomal translocation t(4;11): the DNA damage-repair model of translocation. Oncogene 1998;17:3035–3044.
147. Strissel PL, Strick R, Rowley JD, et al. An in vivo topoisomerase II cleavage site and a DNase I hypersensitive site colocalize near exon 9 in the MLL breakpoint cluster region. Blood 1998;92:3793–3803.
148. Stanulla M, Wang J, Chervinsky DS, et al. DNA cleavage within the MLL breakpoint cluster region is a specific event which occurs as part of higher-order chromatin fragmentation during the initial stages of apoptosis. Mol Cell Biol 1997;17:4070–4079.
149. Super HG, Strissel PL, Sobulo OM, et al. Identification of complex genomic breakpoint junctions in the t(9;11) MLL-AF9 fusion gene in acute leukemia. Genes Chromosomes Cancer 1997;20:185–195.
150. Mantadakis E, Samonis G, Kalmanti M. A comprehensive review of acute promyelocytic leukemia in children. Acta Haematol 2008;119:73–82.
151. Wang ZY, Chen Z. Acute promyelocytic leukemia: from highly fatal to highly curable. Blood 2008;111:2505–2515.
152. Look AT. Oncogenic role of "master" transcription factors in human leukemias and sarcomas: a developmental model. In: Vande Woude G, ed. Advances in cancer research. San Diego, CA: Academic Press, 1995:25–57.
153. Rabbitts TH. Translocations, master genes, and differences between the origins of acute and chronic leukemias. Cell 1991;67:641–644.
154. Schlessinger J, Ullrich A. Growth factor signaling by receptor tyrosine kinases. Neuron 1992;9:383–391.
155. Rabbitts TH, Boehm T. Structural and functional chimerism results from chromosomal translocation in lymphoid tumors. Adv Immunol 1991;50:119–146.
156. Nusslein-Volhard C, Wieschaus E. Mutations affecting segment number and polarity in Drosophila. Nature 1980;287:795–801.
157. Nusslein-Volhard C, Frohnhofer HG, Lehmann R. Determination of anteroposterior polarity in Drosophila. Science 1987;238:1675–1681.
158. Levine MS, Harding KW. *Drosophila*: the zygotic contribution. In: Glover DM, Hames BD, eds. Genes and embryos. New York: IRL, 1989:39–94.
159. Rabbitts TH. Chromosomal translocations in human cancer. Nature 1994;372:143–149.
160. Dalla-Favera R, Bregni M, Erikson J, et al. Human c-myc onc gene is located on the region of chromosome 8 that is translocated in Burkitt lymphoma cells. Proc Natl Acad Sci U S A 1982;79:7824–7827.
161. Taub R, Moulding C, Battey J, et al. Activation and somatic mutation of the translocated c-myc gene in Burkitt lymphoma cells. Cell 1984;36:339–348.
162. Emanuel BS, Selden JR, Chaganti RSK, et al. The 2p breakpoint of a 2;8 translocation in Burkitt lymphoma interrupts the V kappa locus. Proc Natl Acad Sci U S A 1984;81: 2444–2446.
163. Erikson J, Nishikura K, ar-Rushdi A, et al. Translocation of an immunoglobulin kappa locus to a region 3′ of an unrearranged *c-myc* oncogene enhances *c-myc* transcription. Proc Natl Acad Sci U S A 1983;80:7581–7585.
164. Rappold GA, Hameister H, Cremer T, et al. *C-myc* and immunoglobulin kappa light chain constant genes are on the 8q+ chromosome of three Burkitt lymphoma lines with t(2;8) translocations. EMBO J 1984;3:2951–2955.
165. Taub R, Kelly K, Battey J, et al. A novel alteration in the structure of an activated c-myc gene in a variant t(2;8) Burkitt lymphoma. Cell 1984;37:511–520.
166. Look AT. Pathobiology of acute lymphoid leukemia cell. In: Hoffman R, Benz EJ Jr, Shattil SJ, Furie B, Cohen HJ, Silberstein LE, eds. Hematology. 2nd ed. New York: Churchill Livingstone, 1995:1047–1066.
167. Hollis GF, Mitchell KF, Battey J, et al. A variant translocation places the lambda immunoglobulin genes 3′ to the *c-myc* oncogene in Burkitt's lymphoma. Nature 1984; 307:752–755.
168. Croce CM, Thierfelder W, Erikson J, et al. Transcriptional activation of an unrearranged and untranslocated c-myc oncogene by translocation of a C lambda locus in Burkitt. Proc Natl Acad Sci U S A 1983;80:6922–6926.
169. Galieque ZS, Quief S, Hildebrand MP, et al. The B cell transcriptional coactivator BOB1/OBF1 gene fuses to the LAZ3/BCL6 gene by t(3;11)(q27;q23.1) chromosomal translocation in a B cell leukemia line (Karpas 231). Leukemia 1996;10:579–587.
170. Faderl S, Kantarjian HM, Manshouri T, et al. The prognostic significance of p16INK4a/p14ARF and p15INK4b deletions in adult acute lymphoblastic leukemia. Clin Cancer Res 1999;5:1855–1861.
171. Golub TR, Barker GF, Stegmaier K, et al. The TEL gene contributes to the pathogenesis of myeloid and lymphoid leukemias by diverse molecular genetic mechanisms. Curr Top Microbiol Immunol 1997;220:67–79.
172. Rubnitz JE, Downing JR, Pui C-H, et al. *TEL* gene rearrangement in acute lymphoblastic leukemia: a new genetic marker with prognostic significance. J Clin Oncol 1997; 15:1150–1157.
173. Kamps MP, Murre C, Sun XH, et al. A new homeobox gene contributes the DNA binding domain of the t(1;19) translocation protein in pre-B ALL. Cell 1990;60:547–555.
174. Nourse J, Mellentin JD, Galili N, et al. Chromosomal translocation t(1;19) results in synthesis of a homeobox fusion mRNA that codes for a potential chimeric transcription factor. Cell 1990;60:535–545.
175. Kamps MP, Look AT, Baltimore D. The human t(1;19) translocation in pre-B ALL produces multiple nuclear E2A-Pbx1 fusion proteins with differing transforming potentials. Genes Dev 1991;5:358–368.
176. Inaba T, Roberts WM, Shapiro LH, Jolly KW, Raimondi SC, Smith SD, Look AT. Fusion of the leucine zipper gene HLF to the E2A gene in human acute B-lineage leukemia. Science. 1992;257:531–534.
177. Hunger SP, Ohyashiki K, Toyama K, et al. Hlf, a novel hepatic bZIP protein, shows altered DNA-binding properties following fusion to E2A in t(17;19) acute lymphoblastic leukemia. Genes Dev 1992;6:1608–1620.
178. Morrissey J, Tkachuk DC, Milatovich A, et al. A serine/proline-rich protein is fused to HRX in t(4;11) acute leukemias. Blood 1993;81:1124–1131.
179. Gu Y, Nakamura T, Alder H, et al. The t(4;11) chromosome translocation of human acute leukemias fuses the ALL-1 gene, related to Drosophila trithorax, to the AF-4 gene. Cell 1992;71:701–708.
180. Domer PH, Fakharzadeh SS, Chen CS, et al. Acute mixed-lineage leukemia t(4;11)(q21;q23) generates an MLL-AF4 fusion product. Proc Natl Acad Sci U S A 1993;90:7884–7888.
181. Finger LR, Harvey RC, Moore RC, et al. A common mechanism of chromosomal translocation in T- and B-cell neoplasia. Science 1986;234:982–985.
182. McKeithan TW, Shima EA, Le Beau MM, et al. Molecular cloning of the breakpoint junction of a human chromosomal 8;14 translocation involving the T-cell receptor alpha-chain gene and sequences on the 3′ side of MYC. Proc Natl Acad Sci U S A 1986;83:6636–6640.
183. Shima EA, Le Beau MM, McKeithan TW, et al. Gene encoding the alpha chain of the T-cell receptor is moved immediately downstream of c-myc in a chromosomal 8;14 translocation in a cell line from a human T-cell leukemia. Proc Natl Acad Sci U S A 1986;83:3439–3443.
184. Mellentin JD, Smith SD, Cleary ML. *Lyl-l*, a novel gene altered by chromosomal translocation in T-cell leukemia, codes for a protein with a helix-loop-helix DNA binding motif. Cell 1989;58:77–83.
185. Begley CG, Aplan PD, Davey MP, et al. Chromosomal translocation in a human leukemic stem-cell line disrupts the T-cell antigen receptor delta-chain diversity region and results in a previously unreported fusion transcript. Proc Natl Acad Sci U S A 1989;86:2031–2035.
186. Chen Q, Cheng JT, Tasi LH, et al. The tal gene undergoes chromosome translocation in T cell leukemia and potentially encodes a helix-loop-helix protein. EMBO J 1990;9:415–424.
187. Xia Y, Brown L, Yang CY, et al. TAL2, a helix-loop-helix gene activated by the (7;9)(q34;q32) translocation in human T-cell leukemia. Proc Natl Acad Sci U S A 1991;88:11416–11420.
188. Wang J, Jani-Sait SN, Escalon EA, et al. The t(14;21)(q11.2;q22) chromosomal translocation associated with T-cell acute lymphoblastic leukemia activates the BHLHB1 gene. Proc Natl Acad Sci U S A 2000;97:3497–3502.
189. Greenberg JM, Boehm T, Sofroniew MV, et al. Segmental and developmental regulation of a presumptive T-cell oncogene in the central nervous system. Nature 1990;344:158–160.
190. McGuire EA, Hockett RD, Pollock KM, et al. The t(11;14)(p15;q11) in a T-cell acute lymphoblastic leukemia cell line activates multiple transcripts, including Ttg-1, a gene encoding a potential zinc finger protein. Mol Cell Biol 1989;9:2124–2132.
191. Boehm T, Foroni L, Kaneko Y, et al. The rhombotin family of cysteine-rich LIM-domain oncogenes: distinct members are involved in T-cell translocations to human chromosomes 11p15 and 11p13. Proc Natl Acad Sci U S A 1991;88:4367–4371.
192. Royer-Pokora B, Loos U, Ludwig WD. TTG-2, a new gene encoding a cysteine-rich protein with the LIM motif, is overexpressed in acute T-cell leukaemia with the t(11;14)(p13;q11). Oncogene 1991;6:1887–1893.
193. Hatano M, Roberts CW, Minden M, et al. Deregulation of a homeobox gene, *HOX11*, by the t(10;14) in T cell leukemia. Science 1991;253:79–82.
194. Dube ID, Kamel-Reid S, Yuan CC, et al. A novel human homeobox gene lies at the chromosome 10 breakpoint in lymphoid neoplasias with chromosomal translocation t(10;14). Blood 1991;78:2996–3003.
195. Kennedy MA, Gonzalez-Sarmiento R, Kees UR, et al. *HOX11*, a homeobox-containing T-cell oncogene on human chromosome 10q24. Proc Natl Acad Sci U S A 1991;88: 8900–8904.
196. Lu M, Gong ZY, Shen WF, et al. The tcl-3 proto-oncogene altered by chromosomal translocation in T-cell leukemia codes for a homeobox protein. EMBO J 1991;10: 2905–2910.
197. Berger R, Dastugue N, Busson M, et al. t(5;14)/HOX11L2-positive T-cell acute lymphoblastic leukemia: a collaborative study of the Groupe Francais de Cytogenetique Hematologique (GFCH). Leukemia 2003;17:1851–1857.
198. Cauwelier B, Cave H, Gervais C, et al. Clinical, cytogenetic and molecular characteristics of 14 T-ALL patients carrying the TCRbeta-HOXA rearrangement: a study of the Groupe Francophone de Cytogenetique Hematologique. Leukemia 2007;21:121–128.
199. Soulier J, Clappier E, Cayuela JM, et al. HOXA genes are included in genetic and biologic networks defining human acute T-cell leukemia (T-ALL). Blood 2005;106:274–286.
200. Carlson KM, Vignon C, Bohlander S, et al. Identification and molecular characterization of CALM/AF10 fusion products in T cell acute lymphoblastic leukemia and acute myeloid leukemia. Leukemia 2000;14:100–104.
201. Asnafi V, Radford-Weiss I, Dastugue N, et al. CALM-AF10 is a common fusion transcript in T-ALL and is specific to the TCRgammadelta lineage. Blood 2003;102:1000–1006.

202. Hussey DJ, Nicola M, Moore S, et al. The (4;11)(q21;p15) translocation fuses the NUP98 and RAP1GDS1 genes and is recurrent in T-cell acute lymphocytic leukemia. Blood 1999;94:2072–2079.
203. Lacronique V, Boureux A, Valle VD, et al. A TEL-JAK2 fusion protein with constitutive kinase activity in human leukemia. Science 1997;278:1309–1312.
204. Carron C, Cormier F, Janin A, et al. TEL-JAK2 transgenic mice develop T-cell leukemia. Blood 2000;95:3891–3899.
205. Morris SW, Kirstein MN, Valentine MB, et al. Fusion of a kinase gene, *ALK*, to a nucleolar protein gene, *NPM*, in non-Hodgkin's lymphoma. Science 1994;263:1281–1284.
206. Benharroch D, Meguerian-Bedoyan Z, Lamant L, et al. ALK-positive lymphoma: A single disease with a broad spectrum of morphology. Blood 1998;91:2076–2084.
207. Damm-Welk C, Klapper W, Oschlies I, et al. Distribution of NPM1-ALK and X-ALK fusion transcripts in paediatric anaplastic large cell lymphoma: a molecular-histological correlation. Br J Haematol 2009;146:306–309.
208. Miyoshi H, Shimizu K, Kozu T, et al. t(8;21) breakpoints on chromosome 21 in acute myeloid leukemia are clustered within a limited region of a single gene, AML1. Proc Natl Acad Sci U S A 1991;88:10431–10434.
209. Gao J, Erickson P, Gardiner K, et al. Isolation of a yeast artificial chromosome spanning the 8;21 translocation breakpoint t(8;21)(q22;q22.3) in acute myelogenous leukemia. Proc Natl Acad Sci U S A 1991;88:4882–4886.
210. Erickson P, Gao J, Chang KS, et al. Identification of breakpoints in t(8;21) acute myelogenous leukemia and isolation of a fusion transcript, AML1/ETO, with similarity to Drosophila segmentation gene, runt. Blood 1992;80:1825–1831.
211. Shimizu K, Miyoshi H, Kozu T, et al. Consistent disruption of the AML1 gene occurs within a single intron in the t(8;21) chromosomal translocation. Cancer Res 1992;52: 6945–6948.
212. Nucifora G, Begy CR, Erickson P, et al. The 3;21 translocation in myelodysplasia results in a fusion transcript between the AML1 gene and the gene for EAP, a highly conserved protein associated with the Epstein-Barr virus small RNA EBER 1. Proc Natl Acad Sci U S A 1993;90:7784–7788.
213. Mitani K, Ogawa S, Tanaka T, et al. Generation of the AML1-EVI-1 fusion gene in the t(3;21)(q26;q22) causes blastic crisis in chronic myelocytic leukemia. EMBO J 1994;13:504–510.
214. Morishita K, Parganas E, Willman CL, et al. Activation of Evi-1 gene expression in human acute myelogenous leukemias by translocations spanning 300–400 kb on chromosome 3q26. Proc Natl Acad Sci U S A 1992;89:3937–3941.
215. Morishita K, Parganas E, Bartholomew C, et al. The human Evi-1 gene is located on chromosome 3q24-q28 but is not rearranged in three cases of acute nonlymphocytic leukemias containing t(3;5)(q25;q34) translocations. Oncogene Res 1990;5:221–231.
216. Liu P, Tarle SA, Hajra A, et al. Fusion between transcription factor CBFβ/PEBP2β and a myosin heavy chain in acute myeloid leukemia. Science 1993;261:1041.
217. Nakamura T, Alder H, Gu Y, et al. Genes on chromosomes 4, 9, and 19 involved in 11q23 abnormalities in acute leukemia share sequence homology and/or common motifs. Proc Natl Acad Sci U S A 1993;90:4631–4635.
218. de Thé H, Chomienne C, Lanotte M, et al. The t(15;17) translocation of acute promyelocytic leukaemia fuses the retinoic acid receptor alpha gene to a novel transcribed locus. Nature 1990;347:558–561.
219. Borrow J, Goddard AD, Sheer D, et al. Molecular analysis of acute promyelocytic leukemia breakpoint cluster region on chromosome 17. Science 1990;249:1577–1580.
220. Longo L, Pandolfi PP, Biondi A, et al. Rearrangements and aberrant expression of the retinoic acid receptor alpha gene in acute promyelocytic leukemias. J Exp Med 1990;172:1571–1575.
221. de Thé H, Lavau C, Marchio A, et al. The PML-RARα fusion mRNA generated by the t(15;17) translocation in acute promyelocytic leukemia encodes a functionally altered RAR. Cell 1991;66:675–684.
222. Kakizuka A, Miller WH Jr, Umesono K, et al. Chromosomal translocation t(15;17) in human acute promyelocytic leukemia fuses RARα with a novel putative transcription factor, PML. Cell 1991;66:663–674.
223. Chen Z, Brand N, Chen A, et al. Fusion between a novel Krüppel-like zinc finger gene and the retinoic acid receptor-α locus due to a variant t(11;17) translocation associated with acute promyelocytic leukaemia. EMBO J 1993;12:1161–1167.
224. Ichikawa H, Shimizu K, Hayashi Y, et al. An RNA-binding protein gene, TLS/FUS, is fused to ERG in human myeloid leukemia with t(16;21) chromosomal translocation. Cancer Res 1994;54:2865–2868.
225. Hillion J, Lecoñiat M, Jonveaux P, et al. AF6q21, a novel partner of the MLL gene in t(6;11)(q21;q23), defines a forkhead transcriptional factor subfamily. Blood 1997;90:3714–3719.
226. Golub TR, Barker GF, Lovett M, et al. Fusion of PDGF receptor beta to a novel ets-like gene, tel, in chronic myelomonocytic leukemia with t(5;12) chromosomal translocation. Cell 1994;77:307–316.
227. Cazzaniga G, Tosi S, Aloisi A, et al. The tyrosine kinase abl-related gene ARG is fused to ETV6 in an AML-M4Eo patient with a t(1;12)(q25;p13): molecular cloning of both reciprocal transcripts. Blood 1999;94:4370–4373.
228. Kwong YL, Pang A. Low frequency of rearrangements of the homeobox gene HOXA9/t(7;11) in adult acute myeloid leukemia. Genes Chromosomes Cancer 1999;25:70–74.
229. Raza-Egilmez SZ, Jani-Sait SN, Grossi M, et al. Nup98-Hoxd13 gene fusion in therapy-related acute myelogenous leukemia. Cancer Res 1998;58:4269–4273.
230. Abe A, Emi N, Mitsune T, et al. Fusion of the platelet-derived growth factor receptor beta to a novel gene CEV14 in acute myelogenous leukemia after clonal evolution. Blood 1997;90:4271–4277.
231. Chaffanet M, Gressin L, Preudhomme C, et al. MOZ is fused to p300 in an acute monocytic leukemia with t(8;22). Genes Chromosomes Cancer 2000;28:138–144.
232. Chaplin T, Bernard O, Beverloo HB, et al. The t(10;11) translocation in acute myeloid leukemia (M5) consistently fuses the leucine zipper motif of AF10 onto the HRX gene. Blood 1995;86:2073–2076.
233. Chaplin T, Ayton P, Bernard OA, et al. A novel class of zinc finger/leucine zipper genes identified from the molecular cloning of the t(10;11) translocation in acute leukemia. Blood 1995;85:1435–1441.
234. Soekarman D, von Lindern M, Daenen S, et al. The translocation (6;9) (p23;q34) shows consistent rearrangement of two genes and defines a myeloproliferative disorder with specific clinical features. Blood 1992;79:2990–2997.
235. Mercher T, Coniat MB, Monni R, et al. Involvement of a human gene related to the Drosophila spen gene in the recurrent t(1;22) translocation of acute megakaryocytic leukemia. Proc Natl Acad Sci U S A 2001;98:5776–5779.
236. Ma Z, Morris SW, Valentine V, et al. Fusion of two novel genes, RBM15 and MKL1, in the t(1;22)(p13;q13) of acute megakaryoblastic leukemia. Nat Genet 2001;28:220–221.
237. Hess JL. MLL: a histone methyltransferase disrupted in leukemia. Trends Mol Med 2004;10:500–507.
238. DiMartino JF, Cleary ML. MLL rearrangements in haematological malignancies: lessons from clinical and biological studies. Br J Haematol 1999;106:614–626.
239. Slape C, Aplan PD. The role of NUP98 gene fusions in hematologic malignancy. Leuk Lymphoma 2004;45:1341–1350.
240. Lam DH, Aplan PD. NUP98 gene fusions in hematologic malignancies. Leukemia 2001;15:1689–1695.
241. Bartram CR, de Klein A, Hagemeijer A, et al. Translocation of c-abl oncogene correlates with the presence of a Philadelphia chromosome in chronic myelocytic leukaemia. Nature 1983;306:277–280.
242. Rubnitz JE, Behm FG, Pui CH, et al. Genetic studies of childhood acute lymphoblastic leukemia with emphasis on p16, MLL, and ETV6 gene abnormalities: results of St Jude Total Therapy Study XII. Leukemia 1997;11:1201–1206.
243. Faderl S, Talpaz M, Estrov Z, et al. Chronic myelogenous leukemia: biology and therapy. Ann Intern Med 1999;131:207–219.
244. Golub TR, Slonim DK, Tamayo P, et al. Molecular classification of cancer: class discovery and class prediction by gene expression monitoring. Science 1999;286:531–537.
245. Lebestky T, Chang T, Hartenstein V, et al. Specification of *Drosophila* hematopoietic lineage by conserved transcription factors. Science 2000;288:146–149.
246. Downing JR. The AML1-ETO chimaeric transcription factor in acute myeloid leukaemia: biology and clinical significance. Br J Haematol 1999;106:296–308.
247. Takeuchi S, Seriu T, Bartram CR, et al. TEL is one of the targets for deletion on 12p in many cases of childhood B-lineage acute lymphoblastic leukemia. Leukemia 1997;11: 1220–1223.
248. Rubnitz JE, Pui CH, Downing JR. The role of TEL fusion genes in pediatric leukemias. Leukemia 1999;13:6–13.
249. Rubnitz JE, Shuster JJ, Land VJ, et al. Case-control study suggests a favorable impact of TEL rearrangement in patients with B-lineage acute lymphoblastic leukemia treated with antimetabolite-based therapy: a Pediatric Oncology Group study. Blood 1997; 89:1143–1146.
250. Borkhardt A, Cazzaniga G, Viehmann S, et al. Incidence and clinical relevance of TEL/AML1 fusion genes in children with acute lymphoblastic leukemia enrolled in the German and Italian multicenter therapy trials. Blood 1997;90:571–577.
251. McLean TW, Ringold S, Neuberg D, et al. TEL/AML-1 dimerizes and is associated with a favorable outcome in childhood acute lymphoblastic leukemia. Blood 1996;88: 4252–4258.
252. Rubnitz JE, Crist WM. Molecular genetics of childhood cancer: implications for pathogenesis, diagnosis, and treatment. Pediatrics 1997;100:101–108.
253. Pui CH, Evans WE. Acute lymphoblastic leukemia. N Engl J Med 1998;33:605–615.
254. Pui CH. Acute lymphoblastic leukemia in children. Curr Opin Oncol 2000;12:3–12.
255. Izraeli S, Kovar H, Gadner H, et al. Unexpected heterogeneity in E2A/PBX1 fusion messenger RNA detected by the polymerase chain reaction in pediatric patients with acute lymphoblastic leukemia. Blood 1992;80:1413–1417.
256. Numata S-I, Kato K, Horibe K. New E2A/PBX1 fusion transcript in a patient with t(1;19)(q23;p13) acute lymphoblastic leukemia. Leukemia 1993;7:1441.
257. McGinnis W, Krumlauf R. Homeobox genes and axial patterning. Cell 1992;68: 283–302.
258. Van Dijk MA, Murre C. Extradenticle raises the DNA binding specificity of homeotic selector gene products. Cell 1994;78:617–624.
259. Lu Q, Wright DD, Kamps MP. Fusion with E2A converts the Pbx1 homeodomain protein into a constitutive transcriptional activator in human leukemias carrying the t(1;19) translocation. Mol Cell Biol 1994;14:3938–3948.
260. LeBrun DL, Cleary ML. Fusion with E2A alters the transcriptional properties of the homeodomain protein PBX1 in t(1;19) leukemias. Oncogene 1994;9:1641–1647.
261. Kamps MP, Baltimore D. E2A-Pbx1, the t(1;19) translocation protein of human pre-B-cell acute lymphocytic leukemia, causes acute myeloid leukemia in mice. Mol Cell Biol 1993;13:351–357.
262. Dedera DA, Waller EK, LeBrun DP, et al. Chimeric homeobox gene E2A-PBX1 induces proliferation, apoptosis, and malignant lymphomas in transgenic mice. Cell 1993;74:833–843.
263. Ziemin-van der Poel S, McCabe NR, Gill HJ, et al. Identification of a gene, MLL, that spans the breakpoint in 11q23 translocations associated with human leukemias. Proc Natl Acad Sci U S A 1991;88:10735–10739.
264. Tkachuk DC, Kohler S, Cleary ML. Involvement of a homolog of Drosophila trithorax by 11q23 chromosomal translocations in acute leukemias. Cell 1992;71:691–700.
265. Adams B, Dorfler P, Aguzzi A, et al. Pax-5 encodes the transcription factor BSAP and is expressed in B lymphocytes, the developing CNS, and adult testis. Genes Dev 1992;6:1589–1607.
266. Djabali M, Selleri L, Parry P, et al. A trithorax-like gene is interrupted by chromosome 11q23 translocations in acute leukemias. Nat Genet 1992;2:113–118.
267. Meyer C, Kowarz E, Hofmann J, et al. New insights to the MLL recombinome of acute leukemias. Leukemia 2009;23(8):1490–1499.
268. DeVore R, Whitlock J, Hainsworth JD, et al. Therapy-related acute nonlymphocytic leukemia with monocytic features and rearrangement of chromosome 11q. Ann Intern Med 1989;110:740–742.
269. Hilden JM, Dinndorf PA, Meerbaum SO, et al. Analysis of prognostic factors of acute lymphoblastic leukemia in infants: report on CCG 1953 from the Children's Oncology Group. Blood 2006;108:441–451.
270. Pieters R, Schrappe M, De Lorenzo P, et al. A treatment protocol for infants younger than 1 year with acute lymphoblastic leukaemia (Interfant-99): an observational study and a multicentre randomised trial. Lancet 2007;370:240–250.
271. Tomizawa D, Koh K, Sato T, et al. Outcome of risk-based therapy for infant acute lymphoblastic leukemia with or without an MLL gene rearrangement, with emphasis on late effects: a final report of two consecutive studies, MLL96 and MLL98, of the Japan Infant Leukemia Study Group. Leukemia 2007;21:2258–2263.
272. Raimondi SC. Current status of cytogenetic research in childhood acute lymphoblastic leukemia. Blood 1993;81:2237–2251.
273. Crist WM, Cleary ML, Grossi CE, et al. Acute leukemias associated with the 4;11 chromosome translocation have rearranged immunoglobulin heavy chain genes. Blood 1985;66:33–38.
274. Mirro J, Kitchingman G, Williams D, et al. Clinical and laboratory characteristics of acute leukemia with the 4;11 translocation. Blood 1986;67:689–697.
275. Diaz MO, Le Beau MM, Pitha P, et al. Interferon and c-ets-1 genes in the translocation (9;11) (p22;q23) in human acute monocytic leukemia. Science 1986;231:265–267.
276. Strong RC, Korsmeyer SJ, Parkin JL, et al. Human acute leukemia cell line with the t(4;11) chromosomal rearrangement exhibits B lineage and monocytic characteristics. Blood 1985;65:21–31.

277. Harper DP, Aplan PD. Chromosomal rearrangements leading to MLL gene fusions: clinical and biological aspects. Cancer Res 2008;68:10024–10027.
278. Chen C-S, Sorensen PHB, Domer PH, et al. Molecular rearrangements on chromosome 11q23 predominate in infant acute lymphoblastic leukemia and are associated with specific biologic variables and poor outcome. Blood 1993;81:2386–2393.
279. Schichman SA, Caligiuri MA, Gu Y, et al. ALL-1 partial duplication in acute leukemia. Proc Natl Acad Sci U S A 1994;91:6236–6239.
280. Taub R, Kirsch I, Morton C, et al. Translocation of the C-*myc* gene into the immunoglobulin heavy chain locus in human Burkitt lymphoma and murine plasmacytoma cells. Proc Natl Acad Sci U S A 1982;79:7837–7841.
281. Adams JM, Gerondakis S, Webb E, et al. Cellular *myc* oncogene is altered by chromosome translocation to an immunoglobulin locus in murine plasmacytomas and is rearranged similarly in Burkitt lymphomas. Proc Natl Acad Sci U S A 1983;80: 1982–1986.
282. Begley CG, Aplan PD, Denning SM, et al. The gene SCL is expressed during early hematopoiesis and encodes a differentiation-related DNA-binding motif. Proc Natl Acad Sci U S A 1989;86:10128–10132.
283. Baer R. TAL1, TAL2, and LYL1: a family of basic helix-loop-helix proteins implicated in T cell acute leukaemia. Semin Cancer Biol 1993;4:341–347.
284. Hsu HL, Cheng JT, Chen Q, et al. Enhancer-binding activity of the tal-1 oncoprotein in association with the E47/E12 helix-loop-helix proteins. Mol Cell Biol 1991;11: 3037–3042.
285. Ryan DP, Duncan JL, Lee C, et al. Assembly of the oncogenic DNA-binding complex LMO2-Ldb1-TAL1-E12. Proteins 2008;70:1461–1474.
286. Chervinsky DS, Zhao XF, Lam DH, et al. Disordered T-cell development and T-cell malignancies in SCL LMO1 double-transgenic mice: parallels with E2A-deficient mice. Mol Cell Biol 1999;19:5025–5035.
287. Yan W, Young AZ, Soares VC, et al. High incidence of T-cell tumors in E2A-null mice and E2A/Id1 double-knockout mice. Mol Cell Biol 1997;17:7317–7327.
288. Bain G, Engel I, Robanus Maandag EC, et al. E2A deficiency leads to abnormalities in alphabeta T-cell development and to rapid development of T-cell lymphomas. Mol Cell Biol 1997;17:4782–4791.
289. Morrow MA, Mayer EW, Perez CA, et al. Overexpression of the helix-loop-helix protein Id2 blocks T cell development at multiple stages. Mol Immunol 1999;36:491–503.
290. O'Neil J, Billa M, Oikemus S, et al. The DNA binding activity of TAL-1 is not required to induce leukemia/lymphoma in mice. Oncogene 2001;20:3897–3905.
291. Aplan PD, Jones CA, Chervinsky DS, et al. An scl gene product lacking the transactivation domain induces bony abnormalities and cooperates with LMO1 to generate T-cell malignancies in transgenic mice. EMBO J 1997;16:2408–2419.
292. Herblot S, Steff A, Hugo P, et al. SCL and LMO1 alter thymocyte differentiation: inhibition of E2A-HEB function and pre-T alpha chain expression. Nat Immunol 2000;1: 138–144.
293. Valge-Archer VE, Osada H, Warren AJ, et al. The LIM protein RBTN2 and the basic helix-loop-helix protein TAL1 are present in a complex in erythroid cells. Proc Natl Acad Sci U S A 1994;91:8617–8621.
294. Wadman I, Li J, Bash RO, et al. Specific in vivo association between the bHLH and LIM proteins implicated in human T cell leukemia. EMBO J 1994;13:4831–4839.
295. McGuire EA, Rintoul CE, Sclar GM, et al. Thymic overexpression of Ttg-1 in transgenic mice results in T-cell acute lymphoblastic leukemia/lymphoma. Mol Cell Biol 1992;12:4186–4196.
296. Hacein-Bey-Abina S, Von Kalle C, Schmidt M, et al. LMO2-associated clonal T cell proliferation in two patients after gene therapy for SCID-X1. Science 2003;302:415–419.
297. McCormack MP, Rabbitts TH. Activation of the T-cell oncogene LMO2 after gene therapy for X-linked severe combined immunodeficiency. N Engl J Med 2004;350:913–922.
298. Dear TN, Sanchez-Garcia I, Rabbitts TH. The HOX11 gene encodes a DNA-binding nuclear transcription factor belonging to a distinct family of homeobox genes. Proc Natl Acad Sci U S A 1993;90:4431–4435.
299. Allen JD, Lints T, Jenkins NA, et al. Novel murine homeobox gene on chromosome 1 expressed in specific hematopoietic lineages and during embryogenesis. Genes Dev 1991;5:509–520.
300. Roberts CWM, Shutter JR, Korsmeyer SJ. *Hox11* controls the genesis of the spleen. Nature 1994;368:747–749.
301. Cave H, Suciu S, Preudhomme C, et al. Clinical significance of HOX11L2 expression linked to t(5;14)(q35;q32), of HOX11 expression, and of SIL-TAL fusion in childhood T-cell malignancies: results of EORTC studies 58881 and 58951. Blood 2004;103: 442–450.
302. Rubnitz JE, Camitta BM, Mahmoud H, et al. Childhood acute lymphoblastic leukemia with the MLL-ENL fusion and t(11;19)(q23;p13.3) translocation. J Clin Oncol 1999;17:191–196.
303. Dreyling MH, Martinez-Climent JA, Zheng M, et al. The t(10;11)(p13;q14) in the U937 cell line results in the fusion of the AF10 gene and CALM, encoding a new member of the AP-3 clathrin assembly protein family. Proc Natl Acad Sci U S A 1996;93: 4804–4809.
304. Kobayashi H, Hosoda F, Maseki N, et al. Hematologic malignancies with the t(10;11)(p13;q21) have the same molecular event and a variety of morphologic or immunologic phenotypes. Genes Chromosomes Cancer 1997;20:253–259.
305. Jones LK, Chaplin T, Shankar A, et al. Identification and molecular characterisation of a CALM-AF10 fusion in acute megakaryoblastic leukaemia. Leukemia 2001;15: 910–914.
306. Caudell D, Aplan PD. The role of CALM-AF10 gene fusion in acute leukemia. Leukemia 2008;22:678–685.
307. Ballerini P, Busson M, Fasola S, et al. NUP214-ABL1 amplification in t(5;14)/HOX11L2-positive ALL present with several forms and may have a prognostic significance. Leukemia 2005;19:468–470.
308. Graux C, Cools J, Melotte C, et al. Fusion of NUP214 to ABL1 on amplified episomes in T-cell acute lymphoblastic leukemia. Nat Genet 2004;36:1084–1089.
309. Meyers S, Downing JR, Hiebert SW. Identification of AML-1 and the (8;21) translocation protein (AML-1/ETO) as sequence specific DNA binding proteins: the runt homology domain is required for DNA binding and protein-protein interactions. Mol Cell Biol 1993;13:6336–6345.
310. Ogawa E, Maruyama M, Kagoshima H, et al. PEBP2/PEA2 represents a family of transcription factors homologous to the products of the Drosophila runt gene and the AML1 gene. Proc Natl Acad Sci U S A 1993;90:6859.
311. Nuchprayoon I, Meyers S, Scott LM, et al. PEBP2/CBF, the murine homolog of the human myeloid AML1 and PEBP2 beta/CBF beta proto-oncoproteins, regulates the murine myeloperoxidase and neutrophil elastase genes in immature myeloid cells. Mol Cell Biol 1994;14:5558–5568.
312. Dyck JA, Maul GG, Miller WH Jr, et al. A novel macromolecular structure is a target of the promyelocyte-retinoic acid receptor oncoprotein. Cell 1994;76:333–343.
313. Weis K, Rambaud S, Lavau C, et al. Retinoic acid regulates aberrant nuclear localization of PML-RAR alpha in acute promyelocytic leukemia cells. Cell 1994;76:345–356.
314. Koken MH, Puvion-Dutilleul F, Guillemin MC, et al. The t(15;17) translocation alters a nuclear body in retinoic acid-reversible fashion. EMBO J 1994;13:1073–1083.
315. Huang ME, Ye YC, Chen SR, et al. Use of all-trans retinoic acid in the treatment of acute promyelocytic leukemia. Blood 1988;72:567–572.
316. Chen ZX, Xue YQ, Zhang R, et al. A clinical and experimental study on all-trans retinoic acid-treated acute promyelocytic leukemia patients. Blood 1991;78: 1413–1419.
317. Warrell RP Jr, Frankel SR, Miller WH Jr, et al. Differentiation therapy of acute promyelocytic leukemia with tretinoin (all-trans-retinoic acid). N Engl J Med 1991;324:1385–1393.
318. Fenaux P, Chastang C, Chomienne C, et al. All transretinoic acid (ATRA) in combination with chemotherapy improves survival in newly diagnosed acute promyelocytic leukemia (APL). Lancet 1994;343:1033.
319. Warrell RP Jr, Maslak P, Eardley A, et al. Treatment of acute promyelocytic leukemia with all-*trans* retinoic acid: an update of the New York experience. Leukemia 1994;8:929–933.
320. Ahuja HG, Hong J, Aplan PD, et al. t(9;11)(p22;p15) in acute myeloid leukemia results in a fusion between NUP98 and the gene encoding transcriptional coactivators p52 and p75-lens epithelium-derived growth factor (LEDGF). Cancer Res 2000;60:6227–6229.
321. Ahuja HG, Felix CA, Aplan PD. The t(11;20)(p15;q11) chromosomal translocation associated with therapy-related myelodysplastic syndrome results in an NUP98-TOP1 fusion. Blood 1999;94:3258–3261.
322. Borrow J, Shearman AM, Stanton VP Jr, et al. The t(7;11)(p15;p15) translocation in acute myeloid leukaemia fuses the genes for nucleoporin NUP98 and class I homeoprotein HOXA9. Nat Genet 1996;12:159–167.
323. Cerveira N, Correia C, Doria S, et al. Frequency of NUP98-NSD1 fusion transcript in childhood acute myeloid leukaemia. Leukemia 2003;17:2244–2247.
324. Hatano Y, Miura I, Kume M, et al. Translocation (1;11)(q23;p15), a novel simple variant of translocation (7;11)(p15;p15), in a patient with AML (M2) accompanied by non-Hodgkin lymphoma and gastric cancer. Cancer Genet Cytogenet 2000;117:19–23.
325. Jaju RJ, Fidler C, Haas OA, et al. A novel gene, NSD1, is fused to NUP98 in the t(5;11)(q35;p15.5) in de novo childhood acute myeloid leukemia. Blood 2001;98: 1264–1267.
326. Romana SP, Radford-Weiss I, Ben Abdelali R, et al. NUP98 rearrangements in hematopoietic malignancies: a study of the Groupe Francophone de Cytogenetique Hematologique. Leukemia 2006;20:696–706.
327. Hussey DJ, Dobrovic A. Recurrent coiled-coil motifs in NUP98 fusion partners provide a clue to leukemogenesis. Blood 2002;99:1097–1098.
328. Arai Y, Hosoda F, Kobayashi H, et al. The inv(11)(p15q22) chromosome translocation of de novo and therapy-related myeloid malignancies results in fusion of the nucleoporin gene, NUP98, with the putative RNA helicase gene, DDX10. Blood 1997;89: 3936–3944.
329. Hatano Y, Miura I, Nakamura T, et al. Molecular heterogeneity of the NUP98/HOXA9 fusion transcript in myelodysplastic syndromes associated with t(7;11)(p15;p15). Br J Haematol 1999;107:600–604.
330. Huang SY, Tang JL, Liang YJ, et al. Clinical, haematological and molecular studies in patients with chromosome translocation t(7;11): a study of four Chinese patients in Taiwan. Br J Haematol 1997;96:682–687.
331. Ahuja HG, Popplewell L, Tcheurekdjian L, et al. NUP98 gene rearrangements and the clonal evolution of chronic myelogenous leukemia. Genes Chromosomes Cancer 2001;30:410–415.
332. Dash AB, Williams IR, Kutok JL, et al. A murine model of CML blast crisis induced by cooperation between BCR/ABL and NUP98/HOXA9. Proc Natl Acad Sci U S A 2002;99:7622–7627.
333. Delwel R, Funabiki T, Kreider BL, et al. Four of the seven zinc fingers of the Evi-1 myeloid-transforming gene are required for sequence-specific binding to GA(C/T)AAGA(T/C)AAGATAA. Mol Cell Biol 1993;13:4291–4300.
334. Perkins AS, Fishel R, Jenkins NA, et al. Evi-1, a murine zinc finger proto-oncogene, encodes a sequence-specific DNA-binding protein. Mol Cell Biol 1991;11:2665–2674.
335. Rowley JD. Biological implications of consistent chromosome rearrangements in leukemia and lymphoma. Cancer Res 1984;44:3159–3168.
336. Ribeiro RC, Abromowitch M, Raimondi SC, et al. Clinical and biologic hallmarks of the Philadelphia chromosome in childhood acute lymphoblastic leukemia. Blood 1987;70:948–953.
337. Gale RP, Canaani E. An 8-kilobase *abl* RNA transcript in chronic myelogenous leukemia. Proc Natl Acad Sci U S A 1984;81:5648–5652.
338. Collins SJ, Kubonishi I, Miyoshi I, et al. Altered transcription of the c-*abl* oncogene in K562 and other chronic myelogenous leukemia cells. Science 1984;225:72–74.
339. Kloetzer W, Kurzrock R, Smith L, et al. The human cellular *abl* gene product in the chronic myelogenous leukemia cell line K562 has an associated tyrosine protein kinase activity. Virology 1985;140:230–238.
340. Konopka JB, Watanabe SM, Witte ON. An alteration of the human c-*abl* protein in K562 leukemia cells unmasks associated tyrosine kinase activity. Cell 1984;37: 1935–1942.
341. Chan LC, Karhi KK, Rayter SI, et al. A novel *abl* protein expressed in Philadelphia chromosome-positive acute lymphoblastic leukaemia. Nature 1987;325:635–637.
342. Kurzrock R, Shtalrid M, Romero P, et al. A novel c-abl protein product in Philadelphia-positive acute lymphoblastic leukemia. Nature 1987;325:631–635.
343. Witte ON, Ponticelli A, Gifford A, et al. Phosphorylation of the Abelson murine leukemia virus transforming protein. J Virol 1981;39:870–878.
344. Daley GQ, McLaughlin J, Witte ON, et al. The CML-specific P210 *bcr/abl* protein, unlike v-*abl*, does not transform NIH/3T3 fibroblasts. Science 1987;237:532–535.
345. Bloomfield CD, Goldman AL, Berger AR, et al. Chromosomal abnormalities identify high-risk and low-risk patients with acute lymphoblastic leukemia. Blood 1986;67: 415–420.
346. Jain K, Arlin Z, Mertelsmann R, et al. Philadelphia chromosome and terminal transferase-positive acute leukemia: similarity of terminal phase of chronic myelogenous leukemia and de novo acute presentation. J Clin Oncol 1983;1:669–676.
347. Roberts WM, Rivera GK, Raimondi SC, et al. Intensive chemotherapy for Philadelphia-chromosome-positive acute lymphoblastic leukaemia. Lancet 1994;343:331–332.
348. Druker BJ. Translation of the Philadelphia chromosome into therapy for CML. Blood 2008;112:4808–4817.
349. Druker BJ, Guilhot F, O'Brien SG, et al. Five-year follow-up of patients receiving imatinib for chronic myeloid leukemia. N Engl J Med 2006;355:2408–2417.

350. O'Hare T, Eide CA, Deininger MW. Bcr-Abl kinase domain mutations, drug resistance, and the road to a cure for chronic myeloid leukemia. Blood 2007;110:2242–2249.

351. Yanada M, Ohno R, Naoe T. Recent advances in the treatment of Philadelphia chromosome-positive acute lymphoblastic leukemia. Int J Hematol 2009;89:3–13.

352. Antonescu CR, Dal Cin P, Nafa K, et al. EWSR1-CREB1 is the predominant gene fusion in angiomatoid fibrous histiocytoma. Genes Chromosomes Cancer 2007;46:1051–1060.

353. Waters BL, Panagopoulos I, Allen EF. Genetic characterization of angiomatoid fibrous histiocytoma identifies fusion of the FUS and ATF-1 genes induced by a chromosomal translocation involving bands 12q13 and 16p11. Cancer Genet Cytogenet 2000;121:109–116.

354. Ladanyi M, Lui MY, Antonescu CR, et al. The der(17)t(X;17)(p11;q25) of human alveolar soft part sarcoma fuses the TFE3 transcription factor gene to ASPL, a novel gene at 17q25. Oncogene 2001;20:48–57.

355. Shapiro DN, Sublett JE, Li B, et al. Fusion of PAX3 to a member of the forkhead family of transcription factors in human alveolar rhabdomyosarcoma. Cancer Res 1993;53:5108–5112.

356. Barr FG, Galili N, Holick J, et al. Rearrangement of the PAX3 paired box gene in the paediatric solid tumour alveolar rhabdomyosarcoma. Nat Genet 1993;3:113–117.

357. Davis RJ, D'Cruz CM, Lovell MA, et al. Fusion of PAX7 to FKHR by the variant t(1;13)(p36;q14) translocation in alveolar rhabdomyosarcoma. Cancer Res 1994;54:2869–2872.

358. Delattre O, Zucman J, Plougastel B, et al. Gene fusion with an ETS DNA-binding domain caused by chromosome translocation in human tumours. Nature 1992;359:162–165.

359. de Alava E, Gerald WL. Molecular biology of the Ewing's sarcoma/primitive neuroectodermal tumor family. J Clin Oncol 2000;18(1):204–213.

360. Sorensen PH, Lessnick SL, Lopez-Terrada D, et al. A second Ewing's sarcoma translocation, t(21;22), fuses the EWS gene to another ETS-family transcription factor, ERG. Nat Genet 1994;6:146–151.

361. Jeon I-S, Davis JN, Braun BS, et al. A variant Ewing's sarcoma translocation (7;22) fuses the EWS gene to the ETS gene ETV1. Oncogene 1995;10:1229–1234.

362. Urano F, Umezawa A, Yabe H, et al. Molecular analysis of Ewing's sarcoma: another fusion gene, EWS-E1AF, available for diagnosis. Jpn J Cancer Res 1998;89:703–711.

363. Ladanyi M, Gerald W. Fusion of the EWS and WT1 genes in the desmoplastic small round cell tumor. Cancer Res 1994;54:2837–2840.

364. Cools J, Wlodarska I, Somers R, et al. Identification of novel fusion partners of ALK, the anaplastic lymphoma kinase, in anaplastic large-cell lymphoma and inflammatory myofibroblastic tumor. Genes Chromosomes Cancer 2002;34:354–362.

365. Crozat A, Aman P, Mandahl N, et al. Fusion of CHOP to a novel RNA-binding protein in human myxoid liposarcoma. Nature 1993;363:640–644.

366. Rabbitts TH, Forster A, Larson R, et al. Fusion of the dominant negative transcription regulator CHOP with a novel gene FUS by translocation t(12;16) in malignant liposarcoma. Nat Genet 1993;4:175–180.

367. Panagopoulos I, Hoglund M, Mertens F, et al. Fusion of the EWS and CHOP genes in myxoid liposarcoma. Oncogene 1996;12:489–494.

368. Clark J, Benjamin H, Gill S, et al. Fusion of the EWS gene to CHN, a member of the steroid/thyroid receptor gene superfamily, in a human myxoid chondrosarcoma. Oncogene 1996;12:229–235.

369. Sjogren H, Wedell B, Meis-Kindblom JM, et al. Fusion of the NH2-terminal domain of the basic helix-loop-helix protein TCF12 to TEC in extraskeletal myxoid chondrosarcoma with translocation t(9;15)(q22;q21). Cancer Res 2000;60:6832–6835.

370. Panagopoulos I, Mencinger M, Dietrich CU, et al. Fusion of the RBP56 and CHN genes in extraskeletal myxoid chondrosarcomas with translocation t(9;17)(q22;q11). Oncogene 1999;18:7594–7598.

371. Zucman J, Delattre O, Desmaze C, et al. EWS and ATF-1 gene fusion induced by t(12;22) translocation in malignant melanoma of soft parts. Nat Genet 1993;4:341–345.

372. Simon MP, Pedeutour F, Sirvent N, et al. Deregulation of the platelet-derived growth factor B-chain gene via fusion with collagen gene COL1A1 in dermatofibrosarcoma protuberans and giant-cell fibroblastoma. Nat Genet 1997;15:95–98.

373. Koontz JI, Soreng AL, Nucci M, et al. Frequent fusion of the JAZF1 and JJAZ1 genes in endometrial stromal tumors. Proc Natl Acad Sci U S A 2001;98:6348–6353.

374. Knezevich SR, McFadden DE, Tao W, et al. A novel ETV6-NTRK3 gene fusion in congenital fibrosarcoma. Nat Genet 1998;18:184–187.

375. Liu Q, Schwaller J, Kutok J, et al. Signal transduction and transforming properties of the TEL-TRKC fusions associated with t(12;15)(p13;q25) in congenital fibrosarcoma and acute myelogenous leukemia. EMBO J 2000;19:1827–1838.

376. Mastrangelo T, Modena P, Tornielli S, et al. A novel zinc finger gene is fused to EWS in small round cell tumor. Oncogene 2000;19:3799–3804.

377. Ben-David Y, Giddens EB, Letwin K, et al. Erythroleukemia induction by Friend murine leukemia virus: insertional activation of a new member of the ets gene family, Fli-1, closely linked to c-ets-1. Genes Dev 1991;5:908–918.

378. May WA, Gishizky ML, Lessnick SL, et al. Ewing sarcoma 11;22 translocation produces a chimeric transcription factor that requires the DNA-binding domain encoded by FLI1 for transformation. Proc Natl Acad Sci U S A 1993;90:5752–5756.

379. Mao X, Miesfeldt S, Yang H, et al. The FLI-1 and chimeric EWS-FLI-1 oncoproteins display similar DNA binding specificities. J Biol Chem 1994;269:18216–18222.

380. Hancock JD, Lessnick SL. A transcriptional profiling meta-analysis reveals a core EWS-FLI gene expression signature. Cell Cycle 2008;7:250–256.

381. Kauer M, Ban J, Kofler R, et al. A molecular function map of Ewing's sarcoma. PLoS One 2009;4:e5415.

382. Owen LA, Kowalewski AA, Lessnick SL. EWS/FLI mediates transcriptional repression via NKX2.2 during oncogenic transformation in Ewing's sarcoma. PLoS One 2008;3:e1965.

383. Dauphinot L, De Oliveira C, Melot T, et al. Analysis of the expression of cell cycle regulators in Ewing cell lines: EWS-FLI-1 modulates p57KIP2 and c-Myc expression. Oncogene 2001;20:3258–3265.

384. Garcia-Aragoncillo E, Carrillo J, Lalli E, et al. DAX1, a direct target of EWS/FLI1 oncoprotein, is a principal regulator of cell-cycle progression in Ewing's tumor cells. Oncogene 2008;27:6034–6043.

385. Ramakrishnan R, Fujimura Y, Zou JP, et al. Role of protein-protein interactions in the antiapoptotic function of EWS-Fli-1. Oncogene 2004;23:7087–7094.

386. Gascoyne DM, Thomas GR, Latchman DS. The effects of Brn-3a on neuronal differentiation and apoptosis are differentially modulated by EWS and its oncogenic derivative EWS/Fli-1. Oncogene 2004;23:3830–3840.

387. Maksimenko A, Malvy C. Oncogene-targeted antisense oligonucleotides for the treatment of Ewing sarcoma. Expert Opin Ther Targets 2005;9:825–830.

388. Delattre O, Zucman J, Melot T, et al. The Ewing family of tumors—a subgroup of small-round-cell tumors defined by specific chimeric transcripts. N Engl J Med 1994;331:294–299.

389. Bailly RA, Bosselut R, Zucman J, et al. DNA-binding and transcriptional activation properties of the EWS-FLI-1 fusion protein resulting from the t(11;22) translocation in Ewing sarcoma. Mol Cell Biol 1994;14:3230–3241.

390. Zinszer H, Albalat R, Ron D. A novel effector domain from the RNA-domain protein TLS or EWS is required for oncogenic transformation by CHOP. Genes Dev 1994;8:2513–2526.

391. Galili N, Davis RJ, Fredericks WJ, et al. Fusion of a fork head domain gene to PAX3 in the solid tumour alveolar rhabdomyosarcoma. Nat Genet 1993;5:230–235.

392. Shapiro DN, Valentine MB, Sublett JE, et al. Chromosomal sublocalization of the 2;13 translocation breakpoint in alveolar rhabdomyosarcoma. Genes Chromosomes Cancer 1992;4:241–249.

393. Bober E, Franz T, Arnold HH, et al. Pax-3 is required for the development of limb muscles: a possible role for the migration of dermomyotomal muscle progenitor cells. Development 1994;120:603–612.

394. Fredericks WJ, Galili N, Mukhopadhyay S, et al. The PAX3-FKHR fusion protein created by the t(2;13) translocation in alveolar rhabdomyosarcomas is a more potent transcriptional activator than PAX3. Mol Cell Biol 1995;15:1522–1535.

395. Bernasconi M, Remppis A, Fredericks WJ, et al. Induction of apoptosis in rhabdomyosarcoma cells through down-regulation of PAX proteins. Proc Natl Acad Sci U S A 1996;93:13164–13169.

396. Khan J, Bittner ML, Saal LH, et al. cDNA microarrays detect activation of a myogenic transcription program by the PAX3-FKHR fusion oncogene. Proc Natl Acad Sci U S A 1999;96:13264–13269.

397. Ferrari A, Gronchi A, Casanova M, et al. Synovial sarcoma: a retrospective analysis of 271 patients of all ages treated at a single institution. Cancer 2004;101:627–634.

398. Nagai M, Tanaka S, Tsuda M, et al. Analysis of transforming activity of human synovial sarcoma-associated chimeric protein SYT-SSX1 bound to chromatin remodeling factor hBRM/hSNF2 alpha. Proc Natl Acad Sci U S A 2001;98:3843–3848.

399. Lazar AJ, Das P, Tuvin D, et al. Angiogenesis-promoting gene patterns in alveolar soft part sarcoma. Clin Cancer Res 2007;13:7314–7321.

400. Heimann P, Devalck C, Debusscher C, et al. Alveolar soft-part sarcoma: further evidence by FISH for the involvement of chromosome band 17q25. Genes Chromosomes Cancer 1998;23:194–197.

401. Joyama S, Ueda T, Shimizu K, et al. Chromosome rearrangement at 17q25 and xp11.2 in alveolar soft-part sarcoma: a case report and review of the literature. Cancer 1999;86:1246–1250.

402. Weterman MA, Wilbrink M, Geurts van Kessel A. Fusion of the transcription factor TFE3 gene to a novel gene, PRCC, in t(X;1)(p11;q21)-positive papillary renal cell carcinomas. Proc Natl Acad Sci U S A 1996;93:15294–15298.

403. Sidhar SK, Clark J, Gill S, et al. The t(X;1)(p11.2;q21.2) translocation in papillary renal cell carcinoma fuses a novel gene PRCC to the TFE3 transcription factor gene. Hum Mol Genet 1996;5:1333–1338.

404. Argani P, Antonescu CR, Couturier J, et al. PRCC-TFE3 renal carcinomas: morphologic, immunohistochemical, ultrastructural, and molecular analysis of an entity associated with the t(X;1)(p11.2;q21). Am J Surg Pathol 2002;26:1553–1566.

405. Clark J, Lu YJ, Sidhar SK, et al. Fusion of splicing factor genes PSF and NonO (p54nrb) to the TFE3 gene in papillary renal cell carcinoma. Oncogene 1997;15:2233–2239.

406. Hanahan D, Weinberg RA. The hallmarks of cancer. Cell 2000;100:57–70.

407. Stanbridge EJ. Suppression of malignancy in human cells. Nature 1976;260:17–20.

408. Lee WH, Shew FY, Hong FD, et al. The retinoblastoma susceptibility gene encodes a nuclear phosphoprotein associated with DNA binding activity. Nature 1987;329:642–645.

409. Lee WH, Bookstein R, Hong F, et al. Human retinoblastoma susceptibility gene: cloning, identification, and sequence. Science 1987;235:1394–1399.

410. Weinberg RA. The retinoblastoma protein and cell cycle control. Cell 1995;81:323–330.

411. Munger K, Scheffner M, Huibregtse JM, et al. Interactions of HPV E6 and E7 oncoproteins with tumour suppressor gene products. Cancer Surv 1992;12:197–217.

412. Livingston DM. Functional analysis of the retinoblastoma gene product and of RB-SV40 T antigen complexes. Cancer Surv 1992;12:153–160.

413. Dyson N, Harlow E. Adenovirus E1A targets key regulators of cell proliferation. Cancer Surv 1992;12:161–195.

414. Nevins JR. E2F: a link between the Rb tumor suppressor protein and viral oncoproteins. Science 1992;258:424–429.

415. Whyte P, Buchkovich KJ, Horowitz JM, et al. Association between an oncogene and an anti-oncogene: the adenovirus E1A proteins bind to the retinoblastoma gene product. Nature 1988;334:124–129.

416. Ludlow JW, DeCaprio JA, Huang CH, et al. SV40 large T antigen binds preferentially to an underphosphorylated member of the retinoblastoma susceptibility gene product family. Cell 1989;56:57–65.

417. Whyte P, Williamson NM, Harlow E. Cellular targets for transformation by the adenovirus E1A protein. Cell 1989;56:67–75.

418. Friend SH, Horowitz JM, Gerber MR, et al. Deletions of a DNA sequence in retinoblastomas and mesenchymal tumors: organization of the sequence and its encoded protein. Proc Natl Acad Sci U S A 1987;84:9059–9063.

419. Lee EY, To H, Shew JY, et al. Inactivation of the retinoblastoma susceptibility gene in human breast cancers. Science 1988;241:218–221.

420. Goodrich DW, Lee WH. Molecular characterization of the retinoblastoma susceptibility gene. Biochim Biophys Acta 1993;1155:43–61.

421. Rygaard K, Sorenson GD, Pettengill OS, et al. Abnormalities in structure and expression of the retinoblastoma gene in small cell lung cancer cell lines and xenografts in nude mice. Cancer Res 1990;50:5312–5317.

422. Cheng J, Scully P, Shew JY, et al. Homozygous deletion of the retinoblastoma gene in an acute lymphoblastic leukemia (T) cell line. Blood 1990;75:730–735.

423. Xu HJ, Hu SX, Hashimoto T, et al. The retinoblastoma susceptibility gene product: a characteristic pattern in normal cells and abnormal expression in malignant cells. Oncogene 1989;4:807–812.

424. Horowitz JM, Park SH, Bogenmann E, et al. Frequent inactivation of the retinoblastoma anti-oncogene is restricted to a subset of human tumor cells. Proc Natl Acad Sci U S A 1990;87:2775–2779.

425. Harbour JW, Lai SL, Whang-Peng J, et al. Abnormalities in structure and expression of the human retinoblastoma gene in SCLC. Science 1988;241:353–357.

426. Rocco JW, Sidransky D. p16(MTS-1/CDKN2/INK4a) in cancer progression. Exp Cell Res 2001;264:42–55.

427. Hirama T, Koeffler HP. Role of the cyclin-dependent kinase inhibitors in the development of cancer. Blood 1995;86:841–854.
428. Benedict WF, Lerner SP, Zhou J, et al. Level of retinoblastoma protein expression correlates with p16 (MTS-1/INK4A/CDKN2) status in bladder cancer. Oncogene 1999;18:1197–1203.
429. Sherr CJ. Divorcing ARF and p53: an unsettled case. Nat Rev Cancer 2006;6:663–673.
430. Herman JG, Civin CI, Issa JP, et al. Distinct patterns of inactivation of p15INK4B and p16INK4A characterize the major types of hematological malignancies. Cancer Res 1997;57:837–841.
431. Otterson GA, Kratzke RA, Coxon A, et al. Absence of p16INK4 protein is restricted to the subset of lung cancer lines that retains wildtype RB. Oncogene 1994;9:3375–3378.
432. Pennica D, Goeddel DV, Hayflick JS, et al. The amino acid sequence of murine p53 determined from a cDNA clone. Virology 1984;134:477–482.
433. Matlashewski G, Lamb P, Pim D, et al. Isolation and characterization of a human p53 cDNA clone: expression of the human p53 gene. EMBO J 1984;3:3257–3262.
434. Nigro JM, Baker SJ, Preisinger AC, et al. Mutations in the p53 gene occur in diverse human tumour types. Nature 1989;342:705–708.
435. Baker SJ, Fearon ER, Nigro JM, et al. Chromosome 17 deletions and p53 gene mutations in colorectal carcinomas. Science 1989;244:217–221.
436. Iggo R, Gatter K, Bartek J, et al. Increased expression of mutant forms of p53 oncogene in primary lung cancer. Lancet 1990;335:675–679.
437. Devilee P, van den BrM, Kuipers-Dijkshoorn N, et al. At least four different chromosomal regions are involved in loss of heterozygosity in human breast carcinoma. Genomics 1989;5:554–560.
438. Hollstein MC, Metcalf RA, Welsh JA, et al. Frequent mutation of the p53 gene in human esophageal cancer. Proc Natl Acad Sci U S A 1990;87:9958–9961.
439. Tamura G, Kihana T, Nomura K, et al. Detection of frequent p53 gene mutations in primary gastric cancer by cell sorting and polymerase chain reaction single-strand conformation polymorphism analysis. Cancer Res 1991;51:3056–3058.
440. Bressac B, Kew M, Wands J, et al. Selective G to T mutations of p53 gene in hepatocellular carcinoma from southern Africa [see comments]. Nature 1991;350:429–431.
441. Hsu IC, Metcalf RA, Sun T, et al. Mutational hotspot in the p53 gene in human hepatocellular carcinomas. Nature 1991;350:427–428.
442. Crook T, Wrede D, Tidy J, et al. Status of c-myc, p53 and retinoblastoma genes in human papillomavirus positive and negative squamous cell carcinomas of the anus. Oncogene 1991;6:1251–1257.
443. Katz JA, Chambers B, Everhart C, et al. Linear growth in children with acute lymphoblastic leukemia treated without cranial irradiation. J Pediatr 1991;118:575–578.
444. Isaacs WB, Carter BS, Ewing CM. Wild-type p53 suppresses growth of human prostate cancer cells containing mutant p53 alleles. Cancer Res 1991;51:4716–4720.
445. Masuda H, Miller C, Koeffler HP, et al. Rearrangement of the p53 gene in human osteogenic sarcomas. Proc Natl Acad Sci U S A 1987;84:7716–7719.
446. Mulligan LM, Matlashewski GJ, Scrable HJ, et al. Mechanisms of p53 loss in human sarcomas. Proc Natl Acad Sci U S A 1990;87:5863–5867.
447. Felix CA, Nau MM, Takahashi T, et al. Hereditary and acquired p53 gene mutations in childhood acute lymphoblastic leukemia. J Clin Invest 1992;89:640–647.
448. Tweddle DA, Pearson AD, Haber M, et al. The p53 pathway and its inactivation in neuroblastoma. Cancer Lett 2003;197:93–98.
449. Keshelava N, Zuo JJ, Chen P, et al. Loss of p53 function confers high-level multidrug resistance in neuroblastoma cell lines. Cancer Res 2001;61:6185–6193.
450. Ahuja H, Bar-Eli M, Advani SH, et al. Alterations in the p53 gene and the clonal evolution of the blast crisis of chronic myelocytic leukemia. Proc Natl Acad Sci U S A 1989;86:6783–6787.
451. Gaidano G, Ballerini P, Gong JZ, et al. p53 mutations in human lymphoid malignancies: association with Burkitt lymphoma and chronic lymphocytic leukemia. Proc Natl Acad Sci U S A 1991;88:5413–5417.
452. Felix CR, Wasserman R, Lange B, et al. Differentiation stages of childhood acute lymphoblastic leukemias with p53 mutations. Leukemia 1994;8:967.
453. Li FP, Fraumeni JF Jr, Mulvihill JJ, et al. A cancer family syndrome in twenty-four kindreds. Cancer Res 1988;48:5358–5362.
454. Srivastava S, Zou Z, Pirollo K, et al. Germ-line transmission of a mutated p53 gene in a cancer-prone family with Li-Fraumeni syndrome. Nature 1990;348:747–749.
455. Frebourg T, Kassel J, Lam KT, et al. Germ-line mutations of the p53 tumor suppressor gene in patients with high risk for cancer inactivate the p53 protein. Proc Natl Acad Sci U S A 1992;89:6413–6417.
456. Strong LC, Williams WR, Tainsky MA. The Li-Fraumeni syndrome: from clinical epidemiology to molecular genetics. Am J Epidemiol 1992;135(2):190–199.
457. Young JL, Perry CL, Asire AJ. National Cancer Institute Monograph 57. Bethesda, MA: U.S. Department of Health and Human Services, 1981.
458. Toguchida J, Yamaguchi T, Dayton SH, et al. Prevalence and spectrum of germline mutations of the p53 gene among patients with sarcoma. N Engl J Med 1992;326:1301–1308.
459. Malkin D, Jolly KW, Barbier N, et al. Germline mutations of the p53 tumor suppressor gene in children and young adults with second malignant neoplasms. N Engl J Med 1992;326:1309–1315.
460. Funk WD, Pak DT, Karas RH, et al. A transcriptionally active DNA-binding site for human p53 protein complexes. Mol Cell Biol 1992;12:2866–2871.
461. Toguchida J, Yamaguchi T, Ritchie B, et al. Mutation spectrum of the p53 gene in bone and soft tissue sarcomas. Cancer Res 1992;52:6194–6199.
462. El-Deiry WS, Kern SE, Pietenpol JA, et al. Definition of a consensus binding site for p53. Nat Genet 1992;1:45–49.
463. Farmer GE, Bargonetti J, Zhu H, et al. Wild-type p53 activates transcription in vitro. Nature 1992;358:83–86.
464. Fields S, Jang SK. Presence of a potent transcription activating sequence in the p53 protein. Science 1990;249:1046–1049.
465. Raycroft L, Schmidt JR, Yoas K, et al. Analysis of p53 mutants for transcriptional activity. Mol Cell Biol 1991;11:6067–6074.
466. Bargonetti J, Friedman PN, Kern SE, et al. Wild-type but not mutant p53 immunopurified proteins bind to sequences adjacent to the SV40 origin of replication. Cell 1991;65:1083–1091.
467. Kern SE, Kinzler KW, Bruskin A, et al. Identification of p53 as a sequence-specific DNA-binding protein. Science 1991;252:1708–1711.
468. Kastan MB, Onyekwere O, Sidransky D, et al. Participation of p53 protein in the cellular response to DNA damage. Cancer Res 1991;51:6304–6311.
469. Hartwell LH, Kastan MB. Cell cycle control and cancer. Science 1994;266:1821–1828.
470. Haber DA, Buckler AJ. WT1: A novel tumor suppressor gene inactivated in Wilms' tumor. New Biol 1992;4:97–106.
471. Baird PN, Santos A, Groves N, et al. Constitutional mutations in the WT1 gene in patients with Denys-Drash syndrome. Hum Mol Genet 1992;1:301–305.
472. Coppes MJ, Campbell CE, Williams BR. The role of WT1 in Wilms tumorigenesis. FASEB J 1993;7:886–895.
473. Little MH, Prosser J, Condie A, et al. Zinc finger point mutations within the WT1 gene in Wilms tumor patients. Proc Natl Acad Sci U S A 1992;89:4791–4795.
474. Coppes MJ, Bonetta L, Huang A, et al. Loss of heterozygosity mapping in Wilms tumor indicates the involvement of three distinct regions and a limited role for nondisjunction or mitotic recombination. Genes Chromosomes Cancer 1992;5:326–334.
475. Huff V, Villalba F, Strong LC, et al. Alteration of the WT1 gene in patients with Wilms' tumor and genitourinary anomalies. Am J Hum Genet 1991;49:44.
476. Pelletier J, Bruening W, Kashtan CE, et al. Germline mutations in the Wilms' tumor suppressor gene are associated with abnormal urogenital development in Denys-Drash syndrome. Cell 1991;67:437–447.
477. Bruening W, Bardeesy N, Silverman BL, et al. Germline intronic and exonic mutations in the Wilms' tumour gene (WT1) affecting urogenital development. Nat Genet 1992;1:144–148.
478. Coppes MJ, Liefers GJ, Higuchi M, et al. Inherited WT1 mutation in Denys-Drash syndrome. Cancer Res 1992;52:6125–6128.
479. Haber DA, Park S, Maheswaran S, et al. WT1-mediated growth suppression of Wilms tumor cells expressing a WT1 splicing variant. Science 1993;262:2057–2059.
480. Pritchard-Jones K, Fleming S, Davidson D, et al. The candidate Wilms' tumour gene is involved in genitourinary development. Nature 1990;346:194–197.
481. Huang A, Campbell CE, Bonetta L, et al. Tissue, developmental, and tumor-specific expression of divergent transcripts in Wilms tumor. Science 1990;250:991–994.
482. Kreidberg JA, Sariola H, Loring JM, et al. WT-1 is required for early kidney development. Cell 1993;74:679–691.
483. Wang ZY, Madden SL, Deuel TF, et al. The Wilms' tumor gene product, WT1, represses transcription of the platelet-derived growth factor A-chain gene. J Biol Chem 1992;267:21999–22002.
484. Madden SL, Cook DM, Morris JF, et al. Transcriptional repression mediated by the WT1 Wilms tumor gene product. Science 1991;253:1550–1553.
485. Drummond IA, Madden SL, Rohwer-Nutter P, et al. Repression of the insulin-like growth factor II gene by the Wilms tumor suppressor WT1. Science 1992;257:674–678.
486. Rivera MN, Kim WJ, Wells J, et al. An X chromosome gene, WTX, is commonly inactivated in Wilms tumor. Science 2007;315:642–645.
487. Riccardi VM. Neurofibromatosis: phenotype, natural history. Baltimore: The Johns Hopkins University Press, 1992.
488. Xu W, Mulligan LM, Ponder MA, et al. Loss of NF1 alleles in phaeochromocytomas from patients with type I neurofibromatosis. Genes Chromosomes Cancer 1992;4:337–342.
489. Skuse GR, Kosciolek BA, Rowley PT. The neurofibroma in von Recklinghausen neurofibromatosis has a unicellular origin. Am J Hum Genet 1990;49:600–607.
490. Glover TW, Stein CK, Legius E, et al. Molecular and cytogenetic analysis of tumors in von Recklinghausen neurofibromatosis. Genes Chromosomes Cancer 1991;3:62–70.
491. Shannon KM, O'Connell P, Martin GA, et al. Loss of the normal NF1 allele from the bone marrow of children with type 1 neurofibromatosis and malignant myeloid disorders. N Engl J Med 1994;330:597–601.
492. Johnson MR, Look AT, DeClue JE, et al. Inactivation of the NF1 gene in human melanoma and neuroblastoma cells lines without impaired regulation of GTP-RAS. Proc Natl Acad Sci U S A 1993;90:5539–5543.
493. The I, Murthy AE, Hannigan GE, et al. Neurofibromatosis type 1 gene mutations in neuroblastoma. Nat Genet 1993;3:62–66.
494. Maertens O, Prenen H, Debiec-Rychter M, et al. Molecular pathogenesis of multiple gastrointestinal stromal tumors in NF1 patients. Hum Mol Genet 2006;15:1015–1023.
495. Pykett MJ, Murphy M, Harnish PR, et al. The neurofibromatosis 2 (NF2) tumor suppressor gene encodes multiple alternatively spliced transcripts. Hum Mol Genet 1994;3:559–564.
496. Latif F, Tory K, Gnarra J, et al. Identification of the von Hippel-Lindau disease tumor suppressor gene. Science 1993;260:1317–1320.
497. Groden J, Thliveris A, Samowitz W, et al. Identification and characterization of the familial adenomatous polyposis coli gene. Cell 1991;66:589–600.
498. Nishisho I, Nakamura Y, Miyoshi Y, et al. Mutations of chromosome 5q21 genes in FAP and colorectal cancer patients. Science 1991;253:665–669.
499. Sherr CJ, Roberts JM. Inhibitors of mammalian G₁ cyclin-dependent kinases. Genes Dev 1995;9:1149–1163.
500. Savitsky K, Bar-Shira A, Gilad S, et al. A single ataxia telangiectasia gene with a product similar to PI-3 kinase [see comments]. Science 1995;268:1749–1753.
501. Miki Y, Swensen J, Shattuck-Eidens D, et al. A strong candidate for the breast and ovarian cancer susceptibility gene BRCA1. Science 1994;266:66–71.
502. Luna-Fineman S, Shannon KM, Lange BJ. Childhood monosomy 7: epidemiology, biology, and mechanistic implications. Blood 1995;85:1985–1999.
503. Wong JC, Le Beau MM, Shannon K. Tumor suppressor gene inactivation in myeloid malignancies. Best Pract Res Clin Haematol 2008;21:601–614.
504. Le Beau MM, Espinosa R III, Davis EM, et al. Cytogenetic and molecular delineation of a region of chromosome 7 commonly deleted in malignant myeloid diseases. Blood 1996;88:1930–1935.
505. Curtiss NP, Bonifas JM, Lauchle JO, et al. Isolation and analysis of candidate myeloid tumor suppressor genes from a commonly deleted segment of 7q22. Genomics 2005;85:600–607.
506. Brodeur GM, Seeger RC, Schwab M, et al. Amplification of N-myc in untreated human neuroblastomas correlates with advanced disease stage. Science 1984;224:1121–1124.
507. Seeger RC, Brodeur GM, Sather H, et al. Association of multiple copies of the N-myc oncogene with rapid progression of neuroblastomas. N Engl J Med 1985;313:1111–1116.
508. Johnson BE, Ihde DC, Makuch RW, et al. Myc family oncogene amplification in tumor cell lines established from small cell lung cancer patients and its relationship to clinical status and course. J Clin Invest 1987;79:1629–1634.
509. Wong AJ, Ruppert JM, Eggleston J, et al. Gene amplification of c-myc and N-myc in small cell carcinoma of the lung. Science 1986;233:461–464.
510. Chen QR, Bilke S, Wei JS, et al. cDNA array-CGH profiling identifies genomic alterations specific to stage and MYCN-amplification in neuroblastoma. BMC Genomics 2004;5:70.
511. Osajima-Hakomori Y, Miyake I, Ohira M, et al. Biological role of anaplastic lymphoma kinase in neuroblastoma. Am J Pathol 2005;167:213–222.
512. George RE, Attiyeh EF, Li S, et al. Genome-wide analysis of neuroblastomas using high-density single nucleotide polymorphism arrays. PLoS One 2007;2:e255.

513. Lahortiga I, De Keersmaecker K, Van Vlierberghe P, et al. Duplication of the MYB oncogene in T cell acute lymphoblastic leukemia. Nat Genet 2007;39:593–595.
514. Felix CA, Megonigal MD, Chervinsky DS, et al. Association of germline p53 mutation with MLL segmental jumping translocation in treatment-related leukemia. Blood 1998;91:4451–4456.
515. Tanaka K, Tanaka T, Kurokawa M, et al. The AML1/ETO(MTG8) and AML1/Evi-1 leukemia-associated chimeric oncoproteins accumulate PEBP2beta(CBFbeta) in the nucleus more efficiently than wild-type AML1. Blood 1998;91:1688–1699.
516. Parada LF, Tabin CJ, Shih C, et al. Human EJ bladder carcinoma oncogene is homologue of Harvey sarcoma virus *ras* gene. Nature 1982;297:474–478.
517. Santos E, Tronick SR, Aaronson SA, et al. T24 human bladder carcinoma oncogene is an activated form of the normal human homologue of BALB- and Harvey-MSV transforming genes. Nature 1982;298:343–347.
518. Shimizu K, Goldfarb M, Perucho M, et al. Isolation and preliminary characterization of the transforming gene of a human neuroblastoma cell line. Proc Natl Acad Sci U S A 1983;80:383–387.
519. Ellis RW, Lowy DR, Scolnick EM. The viral and cellular p21 *ras* gene family. New York: Raven Press, 1982:107–126.
520. Barbacid M. Human oncogenes. In: DeVita VT Jr, Hellman S, Rosenberg SA, eds. Important advances in oncology. Philadelphia: JB Lippincott, 1986:3–22.
521. Gibbs JB, Sigal IS, Poe M, et al. Intrinsic GPTase activity distinguishes normal and oncogenic *ras* p21 molecules. Proc Natl Acad Sci U S A 1984;81:5704–5708.
522. McGrath JP, Capon DJ, Goeddel DV, et al. Comparative biochemical properties of normal and activated human *ras* p21 protein. Nature 1984;310:644–649.
523. Sweet RW, Yokoyama S, Kamata T, et al. The product of *ras* is a GTPase and the T24 oncogenic mutant is deficient in this activity. Nature 1984;311:273–275.
524. Land H, Parada LF, Weinberg RA. Tumorigenic conversion of primary embryo fibroblasts requires at least two cooperation oncogenes. Nature 1983;304:596–602.
525. Land H, Parada LF, Weinberg RA. Cellular oncogenes and multistep carcinogenesis. Science 1983;222:771–778.
526. Parada LF, Land H, Weinberg RA, et al. Cooperation between gene encoding p53 tumour antigen and *ras* in cellular transformation. Nature 1984;312:649–651.
527. Balmain A, Pragnell IB. Mouse skin carcinomas induced *in vivo* by chemical carcinogens have a transforming Harvey-*ras* oncogene. Nature 1983;303:72–74.
528. Sukumar S, Notario V, Martin-Zanca D, et al. Induction of mammary carcinomas in rats by nitroso-methylurea involves malignant activation of H-*ras*-1 locus by single point mutations. Nature 1983;306:658–661.
529. Janssen JWG, Steenvoorden ACM, Collar JG, et al. Oncogene activation in human myeloid leukemia. Cancer Res 1985;45:3262–3267.
530. Murray MJ, Cunningham JM, Parada LF, et al. The HL-60 transforming sequence: a *ras* oncogene coexisting with altered *myc* genes in hematopoietic tumors. Cell 1983;33: 749–757.
531. Bos JL, Toksoz D, Marshall CJ, et al. Amino-acid substitutions at codon 13 of the N-*ras* oncogene in human acute myeloid leukaemia. Nature 1985;315:726–730.
532. Gambke C, Signer E, Moroni C. Activation of N-*ras* gene in bone marrow cells from a patient with acute myeloblastic leukaemia. Nature 1984;307:476–478.
533. Souyri M, Fleissner E. Identification by transfection of transforming sequences in DNA of human T-cell leukemias. Proc Natl Acad Sci U S A 1983;80:6676–6679.
534. Bos JL, Verlaan-de Vries M, van der Eb AJ, et al. Mutations in N-*ras* predominate in acute myeloid leukemia. Blood 1987;69:1237–1241.
535. Bos JL, Fearon ER, Hamilton SR, et al. Prevalence of *ras* gene mutations in human colorectal cancers. Nature 1987;327:293–297.
536. Rodenhuis S, Bos JL, Slater RM, et al. Absence of oncogene amplifications and occasional activation of N-*ras* in lymphoblastic leukemia of childhood. Blood 1986;67:1698–1704.
537. Kratz CP, Niemeyer CM, Castleberry RP, et al. The mutational spectrum of PTPN11 in juvenile myelomonocytic leukemia and Noonan syndrome/myeloproliferative disease. Blood 2005;106:2183–2185.
538. Loh ML, Vattikuti S, Schubbert S, et al. Mutations in PTPN11 implicate the SHP-2 phosphatase in leukemogenesis. Blood 2004;103:2325–2331.
539. Paulsson K, Horvat A, Strombeck B, et al. Mutations of FLT3, NRAS, KRAS, and PTPN11 are frequent and possibly mutually exclusive in high hyperdiploid childhood acute lymphoblastic leukemia. Genes Chromosomes Cancer 2008;47:26–33.
540. Tartaglia M, Mehler EL, Goldberg R, et al. Mutations in PTPN11, encoding the protein tyrosine phosphatase SHP-2, cause Noonan syndrome. Nat Genet 2001;29:465–468.
541. Schubbert S, Zenker M, Rowe SL, et al. Germline KRAS mutations cause Noonan syndrome. Nat Genet 2006;38:331–336.
542. Yokota S, Kiyoi H, Nakao M, et al. Internal tandem duplication of the FLT3 gene is preferentially seen in acute myeloid leukemia and myelodysplastic syndrome among various hematological malignancies: a study on a large series of patients and cell lines. Leukemia 1997;11:1605–1609.
543. Kiyoi H, Naoe T, Nakano Y, et al. Prognostic implication of FLT3 and N-RAS gene mutations in acute myeloid leukemia. Blood 1999;93:3074–3080.
544. Nakao M, Yokota S, Iwai T, et al. Internal tandem duplication of the flt3 gene found in acute myeloid leukemia. Leukemia 1996;10:1911–1918.
545. Stirewalt DL, Radich JP. The role of FLT3 in haematopoietic malignancies. Nat Rev Cancer 2003;3:650–665.
546. John AM, Thomas NS, Mufti GJ, et al. Targeted therapies in myeloid leukemia. Semin Cancer Biol 2004;14:41–62.
547. Dong F, Brynes RK, Tidow N, et al. Mutations in the gene for the granulocyte colony-stimulating-factor receptor in patients with acute myeloid leukemia preceded by severe congenital neutropenia. N Engl J Med 1995;333:487–498.
548. Dale DC, Bos JL, Bolyard AA, et al. Mutations in the gene encoding neutrophil elastase in congenital and cyclic neutropenia. Blood 2000;96:2317–2322.
549. Horwitz M, Benson KF, Person RE, et al. Mutations in ELA2, encoding neutrophil elastase, define a 21-day biological clock in cyclic haematopoiesis. Nat Genet 1999;23:433–436.
550. Chen Y, Takita J, Choi YL, et al. Oncogenic mutations of ALK kinase in neuroblastoma. Nature 2008;455:971–974.
551. George RE, Sanda T, Hanna M, et al. Activating mutations in ALK provide a therapeutic target in neuroblastoma. Nature 2008;455:975–978.
552. Taylor JG, Cheuk AT, Tsang PS, et al. Identification of activating mutations of FGFR4 in human rhabdomyosarcoma which promote metastasis in xenotransplanted models [published online ahead of print October 5, 2009]. J Clin Invest 2009:119;3395–3407. doi:10.1172/JCI39703.
553. Khan J, Wei JS, Ringner M, et al. Classification and diagnostic prediction of cancers using gene expression profiling and artificial neural networks. Nat Med 2001;7: 673–679.
554. Baird K, Davis S, Antonescu CR, et al. Gene expression profiling of human sarcomas: insights into sarcoma biology. Cancer Res 2005;65:9226–9235.
555. Davicioni E, Finckenstein FG, Shahbazian V, et al. Identification of a PAX-FKHR gene expression signature that defines molecular classes and determines the prognosis of alveolar rhabdomyosarcomas. Cancer Res 2006;66:6936–6946.
556. Pabst T, Mueller BU, Zhang P, et al. Dominant-negative mutations of CEBPA, encoding CCAAT/enhancer binding protein-alpha (C/EBPalpha), in acute myeloid leukemia. Nat Genet 2001;27:263–270.
557. Vousden KH, Lu X. Live or let die: the cell's response to p53. Nat Rev Cancer 2002;2:594–604.
558. Weng AP, Ferrando AA, Lee W, et al. Activating mutations of *NOTCH1* in human T cell acute lymphoblastic leukemia. Science 2004;306:269–271.
559. Whiteford CC, Wei JS, Khan J. Genomics, microarrays and proteomics. In: Raphael E, Pollock RE, Doroshow JH, et al., eds. UICC manual of clinical oncology. 8th ed. Hoboken, NJ: John Wiley & Sons Inc. 2004:43–62.
560. Gygi SP, Rist B, Gerber SA, et al. Quantitative analysis of complex protein mixtures using isotope-coded affinity tags. Nat Biotechnol 1999;17:994–999.
561. Wilusz JE, Sunwoo H, Spector DL. Long noncoding RNAs: functional surprises from the RNA world. Genes Dev 2009;23:1494–1504.
562. Bartel DP. MicroRNAs: genomics, biogenesis, mechanism, and function. Cell 2004;116: 281–297.
563. Bartel B, Bartel DP. MicroRNAs: at the root of plant development? Plant Physiol 2003;132:709–717.
564. Ambros V. The functions of animal microRNAs. Nature 2004;431:350–355.
565. Calin GA, Dumitru CD, Shimizu M, et al. Frequent deletions and down-regulation of micro-RNA genes miR15 and miR16 at 13q14 in chronic lymphocytic leukemia. Proc Natl Acad Sci U S A 2002;99:15524–15529.
566. Cimmino A, Calin GA, Fabbri M, et al. miR-15 and miR-16 induce apoptosis by targeting BCL2. Proc Natl Acad Sci U S A 2005;102:13944–13949.
567. Costinean S, Zanesi N, Pekarsky Y, et al. Pre-B cell proliferation and lymphoblastic leukemia/high-grade lymphoma in E(mu)-miR155 transgenic mice. Proc Natl Acad Sci U S A 2006;103:7024–7029.
568. Lu J, Getz G, Miska EA, et al. MicroRNA expression profiles classify human cancers. Nature 2005;435:834–838.
569. Carninci P, Kasukawa T, Katayama S, et al. The transcriptional landscape of the mammalian genome. Science 2005;309:1559–1563.
570. Mortazavi A, Williams BA, McCue K, et al. Mapping and quantifying mammalian transcriptomes by RNA-Seq. Nat Methods 2008;5:621–628.
571. Sultan M, Schulz MH, Richard H, et al. A global view of gene activity and alternative splicing by deep sequencing of the human transcriptome. Science 2008;321:956–960.
572. Lander ES, Linton LM, Birren B, et al. Initial sequencing and analysis of the human genome. Nature 2001;409:860–921.
573. International Human Genome Sequencing Consortium. Finishing the euchromatic sequence of the human genome. Nature 2004;431:931–945.
574. Soares MB, Bonaldo MF, Jelene P, et al. Construction and characterization of a normalized cDNA library. Proc Natl Acad Sci U S A 1994;91:9228–9232.
575. Khan J, Bittner ML, Chen Y, et al. DNA microarray technology: the anticipated impact on the study of human disease. Biochim Biophys Acta 1999;1423:M17–M28.
576. Khan J, Saal LH, Bittner ML, et al. Expression profiling in cancer using cDNA microarrays. Electrophoresis 1999;20:223–229.
577. Khan J, Simon R, Bittner M, et al. Gene expression profiling of alveolar rhabdomyosarcoma with cDNA microarrays. Cancer Res 1998;58:5009–5013.
578. Eisen MB, Spellman PT, Brown PO, et al. Cluster analysis and display of genome-wide expression patterns. Science 1998;95:14863–14868.
579. Tamayo P, Slonim D, Mesirov J, et al. Interpreting patterns of gene expression with self-organizing maps: methods and application to hematopoietic differentiation. Proc Natl Acad Sci U S A 1999;96:2907–2912.
580. Butte AJ, Tamayo P, Slonim D, et al. Discovering functional relationships between RNA expression and chemotherapeutic susceptibility using relevance networks. Proc Natl Acad Sci U S A 2000;97:12182–12186.
581. Quackenbush J. Microarray analysis and tumor classification. N Engl J Med 2006;354:2463–2472.
582. Quackenbush J. Computational analysis of microarray data. Nat Rev Genet 2001;2: 418–427.
583. Tibshirani R, Hastie T, Narasimhan B, et al. Diagnosis of multiple cancer types by shrunken centroids of gene expression. Proc Natl Acad Sci U S A 2002;99:6567–6572.
584. Wei JS, Greer BT, Westermann F, et al. Prediction of clinical outcome using gene expression profiling and artificial neural networks for patients with neuroblastoma. Cancer Res 2004;64:6883–6891.
585. Ringner M, Peterson C, Khan J. Analyzing array data using supervised methods. Pharmacogenomics 2002;3:403–415.
586. International HapMap Consortium. The International HapMap Project. Nature 2003;426:789–796.
587. International HapMap Consortium. A haplotype map of the human genome. Nature 2005;437:1299–1320.
588. Frazer KA, Ballinger DG, Cox DR, et al. A second generation human haplotype map of over 3.1 million SNPs. Nature 2007;449:851–861.
589. Manolio TA, Brooks LD, Collins FS. A HapMap harvest of insights into the genetics of common disease. J Clin Invest 2008;118:1590–1605.
590. Gudmundsson J, Sulem P, Manolescu A, et al. Genome-wide association study identifies a second prostate cancer susceptibility variant at 8q24. Nat Genet 2007;39:631–637.
591. Yeager M, Orr N, Hayes RB, et al. Genome-wide association study of prostate cancer identifies a second risk locus at 8q24. Nat Genet 2007;39:645–649.
592. Gudmundsson J, Sulem P, Steinthorsdottir V, et al. Two variants on chromosome 17 confer prostate cancer risk, and the one in TCF2 protects against type 2 diabetes. Nat Genet 2007;39:977–983.
593. Easton DF, Pooley KA, Dunning AM, et al. Genome-wide association study identifies novel breast cancer susceptibility loci. Nature 2007;447:1087–1093.
594. Stacey SN, Manolescu A, Sulem P, et al. Common variants on chromosomes 2q35 and 16q12 confer susceptibility to estrogen receptor-positive breast cancer. Nat Genet 2007;39:865–869.
595. Hunter DJ, Kraft P, Jacobs KB, et al. A genome-wide association study identifies alleles in FGFR2 associated with risk of sporadic postmenopausal breast cancer. Nat Genet 2007;39:870–874.
596. Zanke BW, Greenwood CM, Rangrej J, et al. Genome-wide association scan identifies a colorectal cancer susceptibility locus on chromosome 8q24. Nat Genet 2007;39: 989–994.

597. Tomlinson I, Webb E, Carvajal-Carmona L, et al. A genome-wide association scan of tag SNPs identifies a susceptibility variant for colorectal cancer at 8q24.21. Nat Genet 2007;39:984–988.
598. Broderick P, Carvajal-Carmona L, Pittman AM, et al. A genome-wide association study shows that common alleles of SMAD7 influence colorectal cancer risk. Nat Genet 2007;39:1315–1317.
599. Amundadottir L, Kraft P, Stolzenberg-Solomon RZ, et al. Genome-wide association study identifies variants in the ABO locus associated with susceptibility to pancreatic cancer. Nat Genet 2009;41:986–990.
600. Capasso M, Devoto M, Hou C, et al. Common variations in BARD1 influence susceptibility to high-risk neuroblastoma. Nat Genet 2009;41:718–723.
601. Maris JM, Mosse YP, Bradfield JP, et al. Chromosome 6p22 locus associated with clinically aggressive neuroblastoma. N Engl J Med 2008;358:2585–2593.
602. Kallioniemi A, Kallioniemi OP, Sudar D, et al. Comparative genomic hybridization for molecular cytogenetic analysis of solid tumors. Science 1992;258:818–821.
603. Pinkel D, Segraves R, Sudar D, et al. High resolution analysis of DNA copy number variation using comparative genomic hybridization to microarrays. Nat Genet 1998;20: 207–211.
604. Bruder CE, Hirvela C, Tapia-Paez I, et al. High resolution deletion analysis of constitutional DNA from neurofibromatosis type 2 (NF2) patients using microarray-CGH. Hum Mol Genet 2001;10:271–282.
605. Pollack JR, Perou CM, Alizadeh AA, et al. Genome-wide analysis of DNA copy-number changes using cDNA microarrays. Nat Genet 1999;23:41–46.
606. Carvalho B, Ouwerkerk E, Meijer GA, et al. High resolution microarray comparative genomic hybridisation analysis using spotted oligonucleotides. J Clin Pathol 2004;57: 644–646.
607. Cancer Genome Atlas Research Network. Comprehensive genomic characterization defines human glioblastoma genes and core pathways. Nature 2008;455:1061–1068.
608. Brodeur GM. Neuroblastoma: biological insights into a clinical enigma. Nat Rev Cancer 2003;3:203–216.
609. Brodeur GM, Azar C, Brother M, et al. Neuroblastoma: effect of genetic factors on prognosis and treatment. Cancer 1992;70:1685–1694.
610. Brinkschmidt C, Christiansen H, Terpe HJ, et al. Comparative genomic hybridization (CGH) analysis of neuroblastomas—an important methodological approach in paediatric tumour pathology. J Pathol 1997;181:394–400.
611. Plantaz D, Vandesompele J, Van Roy N, et al. Comparative genomic hybridization (CGH) analysis of stage 4 neuroblastoma reveals high frequency of 11q deletion in tumors lacking MYCN amplification. Int J Cancer 2001;91:680–686.
612. Cohen N, Betts DR, Trakhtenbrot L, et al. Detection of unidentified chromosome abnormalities in human neuroblastoma by spectral karyotyping (SKY). Genes Chromosomes Cancer 2001;31:201–208.
613. Schleiermacher G, Janoueix-Lerosey I, Combaret V, et al. Combined 24-color karyotyping and comparative genomic hybridization analysis indicates predominant rearrangements of early replicating chromosome regions in neuroblastoma. Cancer Genet Cytogenet 2003;141:32–42.
614. Schwab M, Varmus HE, Bishop JM. Human N-myc gene contributes to neoplastic transformation of mammalian cells in culture. Nature 1985;316:160–162.
615. Maris JM, Matthay KK. Molecular biology of neuroblastoma. J Clin Oncol 1999;17: 2264–1979.
616. Vandesompele J, Speleman F, Van Roy N, et al. Multicentre analysis of patterns of DNA gains and losses in 204 neuroblastoma tumors: how many genetic subgroups are there? Med Pediatr Oncol 2001;36:5–10.
617. Attiyeh EF, London WB, Mosse YP, et al. Chromosome 1p and 11q deletions and outcome in neuroblastoma. N Engl J Med 2005;353:2243–2253.
618. Cohn SL, Pearson AD, London WB, et al. The International Neuroblastoma Risk Group (INRG) classification system: an INRG Task Force report. J Clin Oncol 2009;27:289–297.
619. Chen QR, Bilke S, Khan J. High-resolution cDNA microarray-based comparative genomic hybridization analysis in neuroblastoma. Cancer Lett 2005;228:71–81.
620. Chen QR, Bilke S, Wei JS, et al. Increased WSB1 copy number correlates with its overexpression which associates with increased survival in neuroblastoma. Genes Chromosomes Cancer 2006;45(9):856–862.
621. Bilke S, Chen QR, Westerman F, et al. Inferring a tumor progression model for neuroblastoma from genomic data. J Clin Oncol 2005;23:7322–7331.
622. Bilke S, Chen QR, Wei JS, et al. Whole chromosome alterations predict survival in high-risk neuroblastoma without MYCN amplification. Clin Cancer Res 2008;14:5540–5547.
623. Janoueix-Lerosey I, Schleiermacher G, Michels E, et al. Overall genomic pattern is a predictor of outcome in neuroblastoma. J Clin Oncol 2009;27:1026–1033.
624. Bagchi A, Papazoglu C, Wu Y, et al. CHD5 is a tumor suppressor at human 1p36. Cell 2007;128:459–475.
625. Fujita T, Igarashi J, Okawa ER, et al. CHD5, a tumor suppressor gene deleted from 1p36.31 in neuroblastomas. J Natl Cancer Inst 2008;100:940–949.
626. Wang Q, Diskin S, Rappaport E, et al. Integrative genomics identifies distinct molecular classes of neuroblastoma and shows that multiple genes are targeted by regional alterations in DNA copy number. Cancer Res 2006;66:6050–6062.
627. Mullighan CG, Goorha S, Radtke I, et al. Genome-wide analysis of genetic alterations in acute lymphoblastic leukaemia. Nature 2007;446:758–764.
628. Mullighan CG, Su X, Zhang J, et al. Deletion of IKZF1 and prognosis in acute lymphoblastic leukemia. N Engl J Med 2009;360:470–480.
629. Bittner M, Meltzer P, Chen Y, et al. Molecular classification of cutaneous malignant melanoma by gene expression profiling. Nature 2000;406:536–540.
630. Alizadeh AA, Eisen MB, Davis RE, et al. Distinct types of diffuse large B-cell lymphoma identified by gene expression profiling. Nature 2000;403:503–511.
631. Bishop CM. Neural networks for pattern recognition. Oxford, England: Clarendon Press, 1995.
632. Heden B, Ohlin H, Rittner R, et al. Acute myocardial infarction detected in the 12-lead ECG by artificial neural networks. Circulation 1997;96:1798–1802.
633. Ashizawa K, Ishida T, MacMahon H, et al. Artificial neural networks in chest radiography: application to the differential diagnosis of interstitial lung disease. Acad Radiol 1999;6:2–9.
634. Abdolmaleki P, Buadu LD, Murayama S, et al. Neural network analysis of breast cancer from MRI findings. Radiat Med 1997;15:283–293.
635. Kovar H, Dworzak M, Strehl S, et al. Overexpression of the pseudoautosomal gene MIC2 in Ewing's sarcoma and peripheral primitive neuroectodermal tumor. Oncogene 1990;5:1067–1070.
636. Kumar S, Perlman E, Harris CA, et al. Myogenin is a specific marker for rhabdomyosarcoma: an immunohistochemical study in paraffin-embedded tissues. Mod Pathol 2000;13:988–993.
637. Pizzo PA, Poplack DG. Principles and practice of pediatric oncology. 5th ed. Philadelphia: Lippincott Williams & Wilkins, 2005.
638. Chen QR, Vansant G, Oades K, et al. Diagnosis of the small round blue cell tumors using multiplex polymerase chain reaction. J Mol Diagn 2007;9:80–88.
639. Son CG, Bilke S, Davis S, et al. Database of mRNA gene expression profiles of multiple human organs. Genome Res 2005;15:443–450.
640. Krasnoselsky AL, Whiteford CC, Wei JS, et al. Altered expression of cell cycle genes distinguishes aggressive neuroblastoma. Oncogene 2005;24:1533–1541.
641. Ohira M, Oba S, Nakamura Y, et al. Expression profiling using a tumor-specific cDNA microarray predicts the prognosis of intermediate risk neuroblastomas. Cancer Cell 2005;7:337–350.
642. Schramm A, Schulte JH, Klein-Hitpass L, et al. Prediction of clinical outcome and biological characterization of neuroblastoma by expression profiling. Oncogene 2005;24:7902–7912.
643. Asgharzadeh S, Pique-Regi R, Sposto R, et al. Prognostic significance of gene expression profiles of metastatic neuroblastomas lacking MYCN gene amplification. J Natl Cancer Inst 2006;98:1193–1203.
644. Oberthuer A, Berthold F, Warnat P, et al. Customized oligonucleotide microarray gene expression-based classification of neuroblastoma patients outperforms current clinical risk stratification. J Clin Oncol 2006;24:5070–5078.
645. Vermeulen J, De Preter K, Naranjo A, et al. Predicting outcomes for children with neuroblastoma using a multigene-expression signature: a retrospective SIOPEN/COG/GPOH study. Lancet Oncol 2009;10:663–671.
646. Armstrong SA, Staunton JE, Silverman LB, et al. MLL translocations specify a distinct gene expression profile that distinguishes a unique leukemia. Nat Genet 2002;30: 41–47.
647. Yeoh EJ, Ross ME, Shurtleff SA, et al. Classification, subtype discovery, and prediction of outcome in pediatric acute lymphoblastic leukemia by gene expression profiling. Cancer Cell 2002;1:133–143.
648. Ferrando AA, Look AT. DNA microarrays in the diagnosis and mangement of acute lymphoblastic leukemia. Int J Hematol 2004;80:395–400.
649. Holleman A, Cheok MH, den Boer ML, et al. Gene-expression patterns in drug-resistant acute lymphoblastic leukemia cells and response to treatment. N Engl J Med 2004;351:533–542.
650. Lessnick SL, Dacwag CS, Golub TR. The Ewing's sarcoma oncoprotein EWS/FLI induces a p53-dependent growth arrest in primary human fibroblasts. Cancer Cell 2002;1:393–401.
651. Wei JS, Song YK, Durinck S, et al. The MYCN oncogene is a direct target of miR-34a. Oncogene 2008;27(39):5204–5213.
652. Calin GA, Liu CG, Sevignani C, et al. MicroRNA profiling reveals distinct signatures in B cell chronic lymphocytic leukemias. Proc Natl Acad Sci U S A 2004;101: 11755–11760.
653. Metzler M, Wilda M, Busch K, et al. High expression of precursor microRNA-155/BIC RNA in children with Burkitt lymphoma. Genes Chromosomes Cancer 2004;39: 167–169.
654. Hayashita Y, Osada H, Tatematsu Y, et al. A polycistronic microRNA cluster, miR-17–92, is overexpressed in human lung cancers and enhances cell proliferation. Cancer Res 2005;65:9628–9632.
655. Iorio MV, Ferracin M, Liu CG, et al. MicroRNA gene expression deregulation in human breast cancer. Cancer Res 2005;65:7065–7070.
656. Chan JA, Krichevsky AM, Kosik KS. MicroRNA-21 is an antiapoptotic factor in human glioblastoma cells. Cancer Res 2005;65:6029–6033.
657. He H, Jazdzewski K, Li W, et al. The role of microRNA genes in papillary thyroid carcinoma. Proc Natl Acad Sci U S A 2005;102:19075–19080.
658. He L, Thomson JM, Hemann MT, et al. A microRNA polycistron as a potential human oncogene. Nature 2005;435:828–833.
659. Ota A, Tagawa H, Karnan S, et al. Identification and characterization of a novel gene, C13orf25, as a target for 13q31-q32 amplification in malignant lymphoma. Cancer Res 2004;64:3087–3095.
660. Akao Y, Nakagawa Y, Naoe T. let-7 microRNA functions as a potential growth suppressor in human colon cancer cells. Biol Pharm Bull 2006;29:903–906.
661. Kluiver J, Haralambieva E, de Jong D, et al. Lack of BIC and microRNA miR-155 expression in primary cases of Burkitt lymphoma. Genes Chromosomes Cancer 2006;45:147–153.
662. Li J, Smyth P, Flavin R, et al. Comparison of miRNA expression patterns using total RNA extracted from matched samples of formalin-fixed paraffin-embedded (FFPE) cells and snap frozen cells. BMC Biotechnol 2007;7:36.
663. He L, He X, Lim LP, et al. A microRNA component of the p53 tumour suppressor network. Nature 2007;447:1130–1134.
664. Chang TC, Wentzel EA, Kent OA, et al. Transactivation of miR-34a by p53 broadly influences gene expression and promotes apoptosis. Mol Cell 2007;26:745–752.
665. Raver-Shapira N, Marciano E, Meiri E, et al. Transcriptional activation of miR-34a contributes to p53-mediated apoptosis. Mol Cell 2007;26:731–743.
666. Vogan K, Bernstein M, Leclerc JM, et al. Absence of p53 gene mutations in primary neuroblastomas. Cancer Res 1993;53:5269–5273.
667. Hosoi G, Hara J, Okamura T, et al. Low frequency of the p53 gene mutations in neuroblastoma. Cancer 1994;73:3087–3093.
668. Wei JS, Johansson P, Chen QR, et al. microRNA profiling identifies cancer-specific and prognostic signatures in pediatric malignancies. Clin Cancer Res 2009;15(17):5560–5568.
669. Fontana L, Fiori ME, Albini S, et al. Antagomir-17–5p abolishes the growth of therapy-resistant neuroblastoma through p21 and BIM. PLoS One 2008;3:e2236.
670. O'Donnell KA, Wentzel EA, Zeller KI, et al. c-Myc-regulated microRNAs modulate E2F1 expression. Nature 2005;435:839–843.
671. Nesbit CE, Tersak JM, Prochownik EV. MYC oncogenes and human neoplastic disease. Oncogene 1999;18:3004–3016.
672. Schulte JH, Horn S, Otto T, et al. MYCN regulates oncogenic microRNAs in neuroblastoma. Int J Cancer 2008;122:699–704.
673. Schwab M, Ellison J, Busch M, et al. Enhanced expression of the human gene N-myc consequent to amplification of DNA may contribute to malignant progression of neuroblastoma. Proc Natl Acad Sci U S A 1984;81:4940–4944.
674. Williamson D, Lu YJ, Gordon T, et al. Relationship between MYCN copy number and expression in rhabdomyosarcomas and correlation with adverse prognosis in the alveolar subtype. J Clin Oncol 2005;23:880–888.
675. Parsons DW, Jones S, Zhang X, et al. An integrated genomic analysis of human glioblastoma multiforme. Science 2008;321:1807–1812.
676. Yan H, Parsons DW, Jin G, et al. IDH1 and IDH2 mutations in gliomas. N Engl J Med 2009;360:765–773.

677. Ley TJ, Mardis ER, Ding L, et al. DNA sequencing of a cytogenetically normal acute myeloid leukaemia genome. Nature 2008;456:66–72.

678. Campbell PJ, Stephens PJ, Pleasance ED, et al. Identification of somatically acquired rearrangements in cancer using genome-wide massively parallel paired-end sequencing. Nat Genet 2008;40:722–729.

679. Maher CA, Kumar-Sinha C, Cao X, et al. Transcriptome sequencing to detect gene fusions in cancer. Nature 2009;458(7234):97–101.

680. Visel A, Blow MJ, Li Z, et al. ChIP-seq accurately predicts tissue-specific activity of enhancers. Nature 2009;457:854–858.

681. Brenner S, Johnson M, Bridgham J, et al. Gene expression analysis by massively parallel signature sequencing (MPSS) on microbead arrays. Nat Biotechnol 2000;18:630–634.

682. Hodges E, Xuan Z, Balija V, et al. Genome-wide in situ exon capture for selective resequencing. Nat Genet 2007;39:1522–1527.

683. Okou DT, Steinberg KM, Middle C, et al. Microarray-based genomic selection for high-throughput resequencing. Nat Methods 2007;4:907–909.

684. Gnirke A, Melnikov A, Maguire J, et al. Solution hybrid selection with ultra-long oligonucleotides for massively parallel targeted sequencing. Nat Biotechnol 2009;27: 182–189.

685. Shah SP, Kobel M, Senz J, et al. Mutation of FOXL2 in granulosa-cell tumors of the ovary. N Engl J Med 2009;360:2719–2729.

686. Renan MJ. How many mutations are required for tumorigenesis? Implications from human cancer data. Mol Carcinog 1993;7:139–146.

687. Fearon ER, Vogelstein B. A genetic model for colorectal tumorigenesis. Cell 1990;61:759–767.

688. Hahn WC, Counter CM, Lundberg AS, et al. Creation of human tumour cells with defined genetic elements. Nature 1999;400:464–468.

689. Elenbaas B, Spirio L, Koerner F, et al. Human breast cancer cells generated by oncogenic transformation of primary mammary epithelial cells. Genes Dev 2001;15:50–65.

690. Hahn WC, Weinberg RA. Rules for making human tumor cells. N Engl J Med 2002;347:1593–1603.

691. Rangarajan A, Hong SJ, Gifford A, et al. Species- and cell type-specific requirements for cellular transformation. Cancer Cell 2004;6:171–183.

692. McCormick F. Signalling networks that cause cancer. Trends Cell Biol 1999;9:M53–M66.

693. Wong AK, Chin L. An inducible melanoma model implicates a role for RAS in tumor maintenance and angiogenesis. Cancer Metastasis Rev 2000;19:121–129.

694. Gilliland DG, Tallman MS. Focus on acute leukemias. Cancer Cell 2002;1:417–420.

695. Gilliland DG. Molecular genetics of human leukemias, new insights into therapy. Semin Hematol 2002;39:6–11.

696. Murray AW, Hunt T. The cell cycle: an introduction. New York: Freeman, 1993.

697. Nasmyth K. Control of the yeast cell cycle by the Cdc28 protein kinase. Curr Opin Cell Biol 1993;5:166–179.

698. Sherr CJ. Mammalian G1 cyclins. Cell 1993;73:1059–1065.

699. Pardee AB. G1 events and regulation of cell proliferation. Science 1989;246:603–608.

700. Horowitz JM, Yandell DW, Park SH, et al. Point mutational inactivation of the retinoblastoma antioncogene. Science 1989;243:937–940.

701. He J, Allen JR, Collins VP, et al. CDK4 amplification is an alternative mechanism to p16 gene homozygous deletion in glioma cell lines. Cancer Res 1994;54:5804–5807.

702. Schmidt EE, Ichimura K, Reifenberger G, et al. CDKN2 (p16/MTS1) gene deletion or CDK4 amplification occurs in the majority of glioblastomas. Cancer Res 1994;54: 6321–6324.

703. Roberts WM, Douglass EC, Peiper SC, et al. Amplification of the GLI gene in childhood sarcomas. Cancer Res 1989;49:5407–5413.

704. Ollner JD, Kinzier KW, Meltzer PS, et al. Amplification of a gene encoding a p53-associated protein in human sarcomas. Nature 1992;358:80–83.

705. Khatib ZA, Matsushime H, Valentine M, et al. Coamplification of the CDK4 gene with MDM2 and GLI in human sarcomas. Cancer Res 1993;53:5535–5541.

706. Okuda T, Shurtleff SA, Valentine MB, et al. Frequent deletion of $p16^{INK4a}$/MTS1 and $p15^{INK4b}$/MTS2 in pediatric acute lymphoblastic leukemia. Blood 1995;85:2321–2330.

707. Danial NN, Korsmeyer SJ. Cell death: critical control points. Cell 2004;116:205–219.

708. Sherr CJ. Cancer cell cycles. Science 1996;274:1672–1677.

709. Levine AJ. p53, the cellular gatekeeper for growth and division. Cell 1997;88:323–331.

710. Hollstein M, Sidransky D, Vogelstein B, et al. p53 mutations in human cancers. Science 1991;253:49–53.

711. Evan G, Littlewood T. A matter of life and cell death. Science 1998;281:1317–1322.

712. Downward J. Mechanisms and consequences of activation of protein kinase B/akt. Curr Opin Cell Biol 1998;10:262–267.

713. Cantley LC, Neel BG. New insights into tumor suppression: PTEN suppresses tumor formation by restraining the phosphoinositide 3-kinase/AKT pathway. Proc Natl Acad Sci U S A 1999;96:4240–4245.

714. Korsmeyer SJ. Chromosomal translocations in lymphoid malignancies reveal novel proto-oncogenes. Ann Rev Immunol 1992;10:785–807.

715. Boise LH, Gonzalez-Garcia M, Postena CE, et al. bcl-x, a bcl-2-related gene that functions as a dominant regulator of apoptotic cell death. Cell 1993;74:597–608.

716. Greider CW, Blackburn EH. A telomeric sequence in the RNA of Tetrahymena telomerase required for telomere repeat synthesis. Nature 1989;337:331–337.

717. Olovnikov AM. A theory of marginotomy: the incomplete copying of template margin in enzymic synthesis of polynucleotides and biological significance of the phenomenon. J Theor Biol 1973;41:181–190.

718. Harley CB, Futcher AB, Greider CW. Telomeres shorten during ageing of human fibroblasts. Nature 1990;345:458–460.

719. Rhyu MS. Telomeres, telomerase, and immortality. J Natl Cancer Inst 1995;87: 884–894.

720. Kim NW, Piatyszek MA, Prowse KR, et al. Specific association of human telomerase activity with immortal cells and cancer. Science 1994;266:2011–2015.

721. Shay JW. Telomeres, telomerase, and tumors. Cope 1995;11:46–48.

722. Chadeneau C, Hay K, Hirte HW, et al. Telomerase activity associated with acquisition of malignancy in human colorectal cancer. Cancer Res 1995;55:2533–2536.

723. Hiyama K, Hirai Y, Kyoizumi S, et al. Activation of telomerase in human lymphocytes and hematopoietic progenitor cells. J Immunol 1995;155:3711–3715.

724. Gibson BE, Wheatley K, Hann IM, et al. Treatment strategy and long-term results in paediatric patients treated in consecutive UK AML trials. Leukemia 2005;19: 2130–2138.

725. Grimwade D, Walker H, Oliver F, et al. The importance of diagnostic cytogenetics on outcome in AML: analysis of 1,612 patients entered into the MRC AML 10 trial: the Medical Research Council Adult and Children's Leukaemia Working Parties. Blood 1998;92:2322–2333.

726. Rubnitz JE. Childhood acute myeloid leukemia. Curr Treat Options Oncol 2008;9: 95–105.

727. Pui CH, Sandlund JT, Pei D, et al. Improved outcome for children with acute lymphoblastic leukemia: results of Total Therapy Study XIIIB at St Jude Children's Research Hospital. Blood 2004;104:2690–2696.

728. Pui CH, Schrappe M, Ribeiro RC, et al. Childhood and adolescent lymphoid and myeloid leukemia. Hematol Am Soc Hematol Educ Program 2004:118–145.

729. Heisterkamp N, Jenster G, ten Hoeve J, et al. Acute leukaemia in bcr/abl transgenic mice. Nature 1990;344:251–253.

730. Druker B. Imatinib as a paradigm of targeted therapies. Adv Cancer Res 2004;91:1–30.

731. Shah NP, Tran C, Lee FY, et al. Overriding imatinib resistance with a novel ABL kinase inhibitor. Science 2004;305:399–401.

732. Demetri GD, Titton RL, Ryan DP, et al. Case records of the Massachusetts General Hospital: weekly clinicopathological exercises: case 32-2004: a 68-year-old man with a large retroperitoneal mass. New Engl J Med 2004;351:1779–1787.

733. Apperley JF, Gardembas M, Melo JV, et al. Response to imatinib mesylate in patients with chronic myeloproliferative disease with rearrangements of the platelet-derived growth factor receptor beta. New Engl J Med 2002;347:481–487.

734. Cools J, DeAngelo DJ, Gottib J, et al. A tyrosine kinase careated by fusion of the PDGFRA and FIP1L1 genes as a therapeutic target of imatinib in idiopathic hypereosinophilic syndrome. New Engl J Med 2003;348:1201–1214.

735. Lynch TJ, Bell DW, Sordella R, et al. Activating mutations in the epidermal growth factor receptor underlying responsiveness of non-small-cell lung cancer to gefitinib. N Engl J Med 2004;350:2129–2139.

736. Paez JG, Janne PA, Lee JC, et al. EGFR mutations in lung cancer: correlation with clinical response to gefitinib therapy. Science 2004;304:1497–1500.

737. Yarden Y, Sliwkowski MX. Untangling the ErbB signalling network. Nat Rev Mol Cell Biol 2001;2:127–137.

738. Grunwald V, Hidalgo M. Developing inhibitors of the epidermal growth factor receptor cancer treatment. J Natl Cancer Inst 2003;95:851–867.

739. Wilkinson E. Surprise phase III failure for ZD1839. Lancet Oncol 2002;3:583.

740. Pommier Y, Sordet O, Antony S, et al. Apoptosis defects and chemotherapy resistance: molecular interaction maps and networks. Oncogene 2004;23:2934–2949.

741. Tolcher AW, Kuhn J, Schwartz G, et al. A phase I pharmacokinetic and biological correlative study of oblimersen sodium (genasense, g3139), an antisense oligonucleotide to the bcl-2 mRNA, and of docetaxel in patients with hormone-refractory prostate cancer. Clin Cancer Res 2004;10:5048–5057.

742. Walensky LD, Kung AL, Escher I, et al. Activation of apoptosis in vivo by a hydrocarbon-stapled BH3 helix. Science 2004;305:1411–1413.

743. Nosslinger T, Reisner R, Koller E, et al. Myelodysplastic syndromes, from French-American-British to World Health Organization: comparison of classifications on 431 unselected patients from a single institution. Blood 2001;98:2935–2941.

CHAPTER 4 ■ BIOLOGY OF CHILDHOOD CANCER

CHRISTOPHER DENNY AND KATHLEEN SAKAMOTO

INTRODUCTION

The age-old axiom that pediatric patients are not simply small adults with disease, definitely holds true in oncology. Even when viewed from the broadest perspective, there are fundamental differences between childhood and adult malignancies. First, the incidence of cancer in children is far less than that seen in the adult population. Second, although there is some overlap, children and adults develop different types of cancer. The epithelium-derived tumors that form the majority of adult cancer are rarely seen in normal children. Even when adult and child have the same malignancy by histologic appearance, they may not be equivalent on a biologic level. For example, pediatric patients with pre-B acute lymphoblastic leukemia (ALL) as a group respond very well to current therapy, whereas adults with clinically the same disease fare much worse.

These clinical observations suggest that biologies and perhaps even oncogenic mechanisms of childhood and adult malignancies can be significantly different. Fundamentally, all cancer is thought to arise from cells that have incurred a critical mass of genetic and epigenetic mutations. In adult tumors, a long-held belief has been that these changes may result from cumulative exposures and toxic insults distributed over decades. Given their occurrence at a young age, similar external effects seem less likely to play a major role in the genesis of most childhood cancers.

What sets the pediatric and adult populations apart is that children are in the process of normal growth and development. At a cellular level, an enormously complex program of division and differentiation is being played out. In this developing physiologic milieu, the potential may exist for oncogenic transformation to occur in particular cell populations that are either less vulnerable or not present in a mature adult. This may in part account for the age-related peaks seen with certain pediatric cancers. For example, the highest incidence of osteosarcoma occurs during the skeletal growth spurt in adolescence. Simply put, pediatric cancers may start as errors in normal development.

There is increasing evidence that the study of tumor biology is evolving from a primarily academic exercise to one of immediate therapeutic impact. This is a much anticipated and necessary transition. Current effective treatments for the vast majority of pediatric cancers are triumphs of empiric trial design. Although many viable regimens have been developed, they lack the basic understanding underlying their efficacy such as why L-asparaginase is so effective in ALL and platinum compounds in germ cell neoplasms. From a pragmatic perspective, many pediatric patients continue to benefit from empirically derived regimens. However, when these regimens fall short and the cancer returns, there is usually little insight as to why treatment failed. This leaves few rational options.

Therapies based on the biology of a particular tumor may not only prove to be more effective but just as importantly provide a logical framework in which to work. The expectation is that inhibiting specific molecular pathways that cancer cells need for their continued growth will have greater efficacy with fewer deleterious side effects than is seen with current cytotoxic regimens. Should therapeutic resistance be encountered, follow-up testing could be performed to determine whether the drug is sufficiently inhibiting its molecular target.

In this chapter, we hope to highlight those biologic concepts and molecular pathways that both play dominant roles in oncogenesis and hold the most potential for therapeutic intervention. This chapter was constructed from the bottom-up, starting from the molecular perspective and ending on a more macro level. It is divided into three major sections: (a) cell function—molecular events that occur within individual tumor cells (Signal Transduction, Gene Regulation), (b) cell behavior—responses that normal and cancer cells have to external and internal stimuli (Cell Cycle, Apoptosis), and (c) tumor properties—behaviors that tumor cells display as a group or elicit from their environment (Angiogenesis). There is an arbitrary structure to this schema considering that cross talk among categories is more the rule than the exception. In addition, it must be recognized that no single book chapter could hope to hold all of what is known about pediatric cancer biology. In casting a wide net, we hope to convey salient molecular features and prevalent biologic themes that are common across different pediatric malignancies. It is these elements that will hopefully be the basis of better therapies in the future.

SIGNAL TRANSDUCTION

Overview

In humans, most cells do not exist as independent entities, but as members of populations, that make up normal tissues in the body. To accomplish this, cells have developed finely regulated molecular systems that allow them to respond to environmental cues and to effectively communicate with one another. These systems begin to function at the very earliest stages of embryogenesis and play critical roles in normal growth and development. In adults, signaling modules are cell-based components that are primarily responsible for maintaining physiologic homeostasis within tissues and organ systems. In short, signal transduction systems keep the estimated 10^{13} cells in the human body working in synchrony. Without the ability to send and receive signals among cells, there would be only chaos.

Cell signaling systems have evolved to fulfill a few basic requirements. The ability to respond to specific stimuli is accomplished by the interaction of distinct ligand molecules with their cognate receptors. Signals generated at the cell surface are then propagated through the cytoplasm through a series of interconnected molecular cascades. This allows for multiple different ligand-receptor events to be integrated into a cohesive signal. In most cells, these signals are then passed into the cell nucleus, resulting in alterations in RNA and protein expression and changes in cell behavior.

In such a dynamic system, speed is of the essence. For this reason, most signaling systems rely on enzymatic alterations of component proteins that can be performed in seconds, rather than on modulation of protein levels, which can take minutes to hours. Site-selective phosphorylation of tyrosine, serine, and threonine residues on signaling proteins by protein kinases is a common way that this is accomplished. These posttranslational modifications promote assembly of multiprotein heteromeric complexes with other signaling components like pieces to a jigsaw puzzle. Just as quickly as this system can be activated, it can be turned off through the action of specific protein phosphorylases that return signaling molecules to their dephosphorylated baseline state.

With such exquisite control over cell behavior, it is not surprising that signal transduction systems are frequently subverted in the process of oncogenesis. In fact, the first-described tumor-associated chromosomal abnormality, the Philadelphia chromosome, was later found to encode the BCR/ABL fusion protein, which functions as an aberrant signaling molecule. The fact that so much of signal transduction is governed enzymatically has rendered these systems at least partially accessible to pharmacologic intervention. For this reason, many of the targeted anticancer agents being pioneered today focus on modulating signal transduction pathways.

Receptor Tyrosine Kinases—The Trigger

Receptor tyrosine kinases (RTKs) are a major class of cell surface receptors that initiate signaling cascades (Fig. 4.1). RTKs are constructed in modular fashion and are composed of distinct domains that can be functionally resolved from each other. A typical RTK consists of an extracellular ligand-binding domain followed by a single hydrophobic transmembrane region that is linked to an intracellular protein kinase domain. Binding of the ligand induces RTK dimerization and/or conformational changes that serve to activate intracellular protein kinases, resulting in autophosphorylation at specific tyrosine residues within the RTK. These modifications provide binding surfaces to which intracellular signaling molecules dock and can in turn be phosphorylated by the activated RTK.

Even at this top level, there is inherent complexity built in to this system. Within each RTK family, there can be both multiple RTK members and multiple ligands. For example, in the fibroblast growth factor (FGF) family, there are more than 18 ligands that can bind to four different FGF receptors.[1] If coexpressed in the same cell, different RTKs from the same family may heterodimerize, resulting in activation of signaling pathways that can differ from those activated by their respective homodimers. It is thought that ErbB2, for which no ligand has yet been found, signals primarily by forming heterodimers with other ErbB family members that have been activated by a ligand.[2] Conversely, there are RTK-like molecules that lack functional kinase activity but retain ligand-binding capability. Insulin-like growth factor 2 receptor (IGF-2R) is such an example and appears to serve as a nonsignaling sink that draws insulin-like growth factor 2 (IGF-2) away from signaling through IGF-1R.[3]

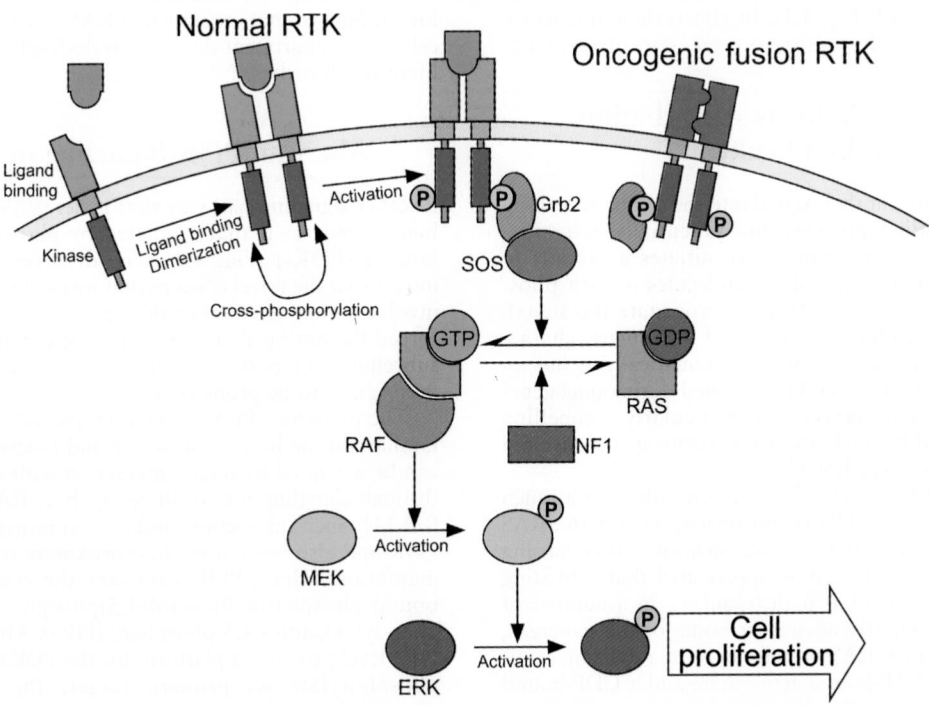

FIGURE 4.1 Normal and abnormal receptor tyrosine kinase (RTK) signaling. Engagement of cell surface RTKs by cognate ligands induces dimerization. RTK cross-phosphorylation activates cytoplasmic kinase domains and also provides docking sites for adapter molecules such as Grb2. Oncogenic fusion RTKs are the chimeric products of tumor-associated chromosomal translocations and promote RTK dimerization and activation in the absence of ligand. The MAPK pathway is frequently activated by RTK stimulation. Recruitment of guanine nucleotide exchange factors (SOS) shifts the equilibrium of the small G protein RAS toward the GTP-bound activated form. This in turn activates a protein kinase cascade (MEK, ERK) that results in gene expression modulation and a cell proliferative stimulus. GTPase-activating proteins (NF1) shift the RAS equilibrium back toward the GDP-bound inactive form, thereby turning off MAPK signaling. Pediatric myeloid malignancies preferentially target the MAPK pathway for inappropriate activation through several mechanisms including (a) activating mutations of FLT3 (an RTK) or RAS, (b) engagement of adapter proteins (Grb2 by BCR/ABL), and (c) loss-of-function mutation of NF1.

Since their discovery, RTKs have been implicated in playing important biologic roles in a wide variety of human malignancies. To a certain extent, this reflects the near-ubiquitous presence of RTKs on normal cells and tissues. Nevertheless, in some instances, data, though primarily correlative, are very suggestive. For example, neuroblastoma patients whose tumors express the neurotrophin receptors TRKA or TRKC have a much better prognosis than the cohort that express TRKB.[4] However, the difficulty comes in trying to gauge to what degree a particular RTK is actively contributing to the biology of a tumor cell on which it is expressed. Numerous tissue culture–based experiments have demonstrated that antagonizing RTK function in model systems may inhibit tumor cell proliferation. However, these results do not necessarily predict clinical response to RTK inhibitors in cancer patients.[5]

Instances where a specific RTK is mutated in a particular human cancer, provide a more compelling argument for direct involvement in oncogenesis. Gene amplifications leading to overexpression of ErbB2 and PDGFR have been described in subpopulations of patients with breast cancer and glioblastoma multiforme (GBM), respectively (for reviews, see Refs 6 and 7). Similarly activating point mutations and internal deletions give rise to mutant forms of c-KIT and EGFR in patients with gastrointestinal stromal tumor (GIST) and non–small cell lung carcinoma.[8,9] Finally, RTK structure can be altered through tumor-associated chromosomal translocations that fuse a portion of the RTK to an unrelated gene, resulting in expression of chimeric proteins.[10-13] In most of these fusions, the extracellular ligand-binding domains of the parent RTKs are replaced by polypeptide sequences that promote receptor dimerization in the absence of a ligand (Fig. 4.1). In effect, these oncogenic fusions behave as RTKs that are in a constant state of activation.

RAS/MAPK Pathway Perturbation in Myeloid Leukemia

Activated RTKs transmit their signal into the cell by recruiting intermediary signaling proteins and potentially activating them through phosphorylation. This initiates a cascade in which these activated intermediate molecules in turn phosphorylate other signaling proteins to propagate the signal. Over the last few decades, the number of molecularly characterized signaling pathways has grown dramatically as has an appreciation for how they can be subverted during oncogenesis through somatic mutation.[14] A particularly compelling example is provided by the RAS/MAPK pathway and myeloid leukemias (for review, see Ref 15).

K-, H-, and NRAS are closely related members of a much larger family of protein GTPases (for review, see Ref 16). RAS proteins were first discovered as active agents in cancer-causing retroviruses in rodents. It is now appreciated that activating RAS mutations are found at high frequency in a number of adult cancers, particularly adenocarcinoma of the pancreas, colon, and biliary tract. RAS proteins exist in a dynamic equilibrium between a GTP-bound active state and a GDP-bound inactive state. The conversion between these two states is catalyzed by specific regulatory molecules. RAS GAPs (GTPase-activating proteins) accelerate hydrolysis of bound GTP to GDP and inactivate RAS. RAS GEFs (guanine nucleotide exchange factors) promote the replacement of RAS GDP with GTP and activate RAS. In normal resting cells, there is approximately 10-fold more inactive RAS than the activated form.

Physiologic activation of many RTKs by ligand binding typically leads to recruitment and activation of numerous signaling molecules, including SOS, a RAS GEF, which shifts the equilibrium toward activated RAS (Fig. 4.1). GTP-binding to RAS induces conformational changes that render it able to bind and activate a number of effector molecules, a major one being RAF, a serine/threonine protein kinase.[17] This initiates a cascade involving sequential activation of protein kinases through phosphorylation: RAF activating MEK, which then activates ERK. ERK then phosphorylates specific transcription factors, which traverse into the nucleus and modulate expression of target genes that can promote cellular proliferation.

In human myeloid leukemias, different somatic mutations occur that result in deregulation of this pathway at numerous levels (for review, see Ref 18). Starting at the cell surface, mutations of the FLT3 or cKIT receptors are found in 30% of acute myelogenous leukemia (AML) patients, which result in unregulated activation of these RTKs. The BCR/ABL fusion, which is present in tumor cells of virtually all chronic myelogenous leukemia (CML) patients, directly recruits SOS resulting in RAS activation. From a reciprocal point of view, loss-of-function mutations in the NF1 gene, which encodes a primary RAS GAP, are found in a subset of juvenile myelomonocytic leukemia (JMML) tumor samples. The loss of this RAS inactivator shifts the equilibrium in favor of the activated RAS. Finally, specific mutations of RAS itself have been found in patients with AML, JMML, and chronic myelomonocytic leukemia (CMML). These mutated RAS proteins are resistant to inactivation by RAS GAPs and thereby promote inappropriate signaling through this pathway.

These tumor-associated mutations together make a compelling albeit correlative argument suggesting that dysregulated activation of RAS/MAPK pathway can promote myeloid leukemia. Recently developed mouse models support this notion. Transgenic mouse strains harboring either germline loss of NF1 or mutant activated RAS restricted to the myeloid cellular compartment develop myelodysplastic and myeloproliferative disorders.[19,20]

Aberrant PI3K Signaling in Gliomas

Another signaling pathway that is deregulated in a variety of human cancers is that regulated by phosphatidylinositol-3-kinases (PI3Ks) (Fig. 4.2). The discovery of this pathway introduced the novel concept that intracellular signaling could involve components other than proteins. In addition, it reinforced the notion that recruitment of complexes to a specific subcellular compartment is necessary, if not sufficient, for certain signals to be propagated.

The numerous PI3Ks have been parsed into three different families on the basis of structure and function. Type 1A PI3K can be activated by direct interaction with activated RTKs or through signaling intermediates such as RAS (for review, see Ref 11). Such interactions induce a conformational change in PI3K and also bring it in close proximity to the inner plasma membrane. Here, PI3K catalyzes the conversion of lipid-bound phosphatidylinositol(4,5)phosphate (PIP2) to phosphatidylinositol(3,4,5)phosphate (PIP3). The local increase in PIP3 level provides a platform for the PDK1 protein kinase to phosphorylate its primary target, the AKT family of serine/threonine kinases.

Once activated, AKT then phosphorylates a number of effector molecules that promote entry into cell cycle and inhibit programmed cell death. Perhaps the most intensively studied AKT effector is mTOR, the catalytic component of the multiprotein complex, mTORC1.[21] MTOR is a highly conserved protein kinase whose normal function is to regulate the cell's response to growth factor and nutrient exposures. Phospho-AKT both directly and through the RAS-like G protein RHEB, derepresses the mTORC1 multiprotein complex. Activation of mTORC1 in turn upregulates metabolic pathways that stimulate ribosomal biogenesis and enhance mRNA

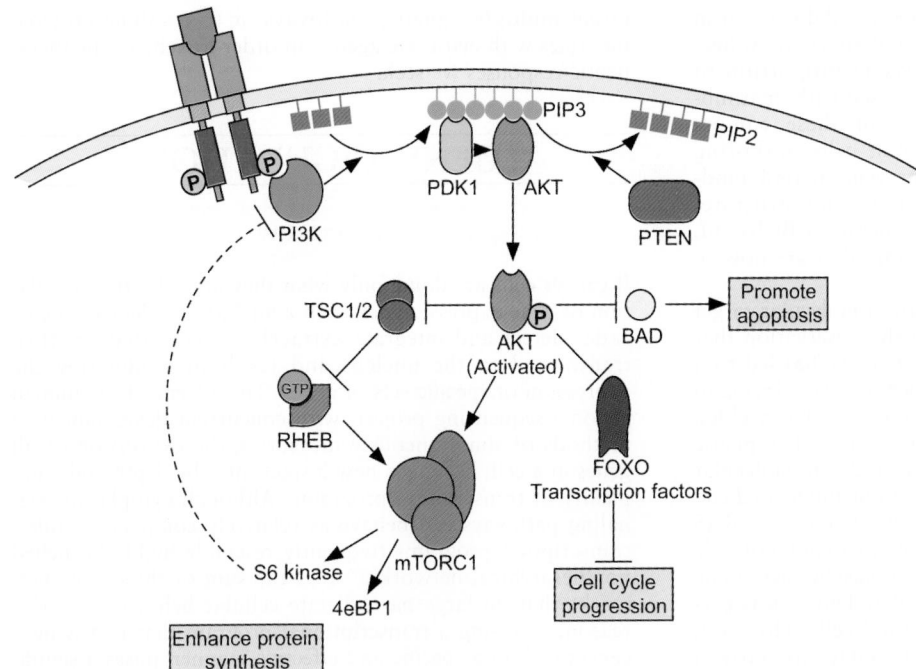

FIGURE 4.2 Regulation of phosphatidylinositol-3-kinase (PI3K) pathway. Activated RTKs recruit PI3K to the inner leaflet of the cytoplasmic membrane, where it converts phosphatidylinositol(4,5)phosphate (PIP2) to phosphatidylinositol(3,4,5)phosphate (PIP3). Lipid-bound PIP3 provides a scaffold to which PDK1 and AKT bind. Having been brought into juxtaposition, PDK1 phosphorylates and activates AKT. Activated AKT then activates the mTORC1 protein complex both directly and through modulation of the RHEB small G protein. MTORC1 then upregulates a number of systems involved in enhancing cell growth. Activated AKT also downregulates FOXO transcription factors, which inhibit cell cycle progression, and BAD, a proapoptotic BH3-only protein. PTEN is a crucial deactivator of the PI3K pathway by hydrolyzing PIP3 to PIP2 and removing the primary means of activating AKT. In some cells, S6 kinase is also a path to negative feedback by inhibiting PI3K.

translation to protein. In essence, mTORC1 activation provides the cell the metabolic wherewithal to grow.

There are negative feedback loops built into the PI3K/AKT system. For example, S6 kinase, which is upregulated by mTORC1, can, in certain cellular contexts, inhibit PI3K recruitment to activated RTKs. However, the primary off switch to the PI3K signaling pathway is the lipid phosphatase PTEN. PTEN catalyzes the dephosphorylation of PIP3, reverting it back to PIP2. Lacking a surface to which they can dock, PDK1 and AKT cease to interact, resulting in the eventual dephosphorylation and inactivation of AKT. It is clear that net AKT activation is a balance of RTK stimulation and PTEN inhibition. Since PTEN is a nonredundant component in this pathway, if it is lost or mutated, there are no other proteins that can fulfill the same regulatory function. In this situation, AKT is inappropriately activated.

Given its unique role, it is not surprising that somatic deletion or loss of function of PTEN is one of the most common mutations found in human cancers.[22] A particularly compelling association is found in brain tumors in which a high proportion of secondary GBMs harbor activating EGFR and/or loss-of-function mutations of PTEN.[23] It now appears that clinical response to EGFR inhibitors may hinge on whether a particular GBM has one or both mutations.[24] Those patients whose tumor had only EGFR mutations, in general, responded well. Those that had both EGFR and PTEN mutated did not. In this context, reducing RTK activation cannot overcome the lack of repression due to loss of PTEN.

Therapeutic Strategies—Biologic Response Is Key

The dominant role that aberrant signaling can have in driving tumor cell growth has stimulated much activity toward developing molecular inhibitors to oncogenic pathway components. Although a wide variety of approaches have been tried, thus far, the greatest successes have come from two generalizable strategies: (a) developing humanized monoclonal antibodies to the extracellular domains of RTKs and (b) creating synthetic small molecules that inhibit the catalytic function of specific protein kinases. In order for these therapies to have the desired anticancer effect, three things must be accomplished. First, the molecular inhibitor must have pharmacologic properties to ensure that it reaches the tumor cell intact and in sufficient concentration. Second, the inhibitor must have a well-defined biochemical specificity and should block only the desired molecular targets. Off-target effects can lead to unacceptable systemic toxicity. Third, once the inhibitor has been delivered on target, it has to be able to elicit the desired cellular response, which for anticancer agents is irreversible growth arrest if not cell death.

Achieving an appropriate biological response has been the main challenge to developing therapeutically effective inhibitors of cell signaling pathways. This probably stems from our early naive notions of how signaling pathways function. Although initially thought to be linear and hierarchical in structure, it is now appreciated that signaling pathways are extensively interconnected and dynamic systems. Under certain circumstances, cell responses depend not only on pathways that are activated but also on the timing of the signaling stimuli. Developing tools that would aid in predicting which signaling molecules should be targeted to achieve an anticancer response for a particular tumor is a challenge that lies immediately ahead.

Many small molecule inhibitors have now been developed for members of the RAS/MAPK and PI3K/AKT signaling pathways.[25] Those targeting the BCR/ABL fusion kinase found in CML are a case study of what to expect when the right inhibitor is matched to the right malignancy. Imatinib, the first BCR/ABL antagonist, was a congener of a small molecule inhibitor of PDGFR.[26,27] Imatinib's clinical potential was demonstrated early on when it was found to inhibit growth of primary bone marrow cultures from CML patients by almost two orders of magnitude greater than normal bone marrow.[28] Clinical trials proved equally promising. Almost 70% of CML patients in chronic phase achieved complete cytogenetic remissions when given imatinib alone. Progression to accelerated phase was also significantly reduced in these patients.[29]

Although imatinib has revolutionized the treatment of CML, with time, its shortcomings have become apparent.

First, response rates in patients with accelerated disease or in blast crisis were generally incomplete and short lived. Second, with longer follow-up, an increasing proportion of patients who had achieved remission relapsed with imatinib-resistant disease. Molecular analyses of these tumors revealed clonal outgrowths of leukemia cells harboring BCR/ABL fusions with mutations that prevent imatinib binding.[30] Knowing these mutations has allowed for structure-based rational design of potent next-generation BCR/ABL inhibitors including dasatinib and nilotinib that are now in clinical trials.[31]

The combination of a well-characterized molecular target in the form of BCR/ABL coupled with the observation that this fusion is necessary for tumor maintenance has led to a paradigm shift in the therapeutic approach to CML. Trying to apply a similar strategy to other malignancies has yielded much more modest success. In many instances, therapeutic failure was not due to the inability of a candidate molecular inhibitor to hit its target but was due to an unanticipated cellular response. For example, to function effectively, most RAS proteins require posttranslational coupling to a lipid molecule to allow them to adhere to the inner cytoplasmic membrane and interact with other signaling molecules. This task is performed by farnesyl transferases in normal cells. However, inhibitors of farnesyl transferase failed to antagonize growth of RAS-transformed cells as hoped because these cells were able to utilize an alternative enzyme system to lipidate RAS.[32,33]

It is now clear that the presence of a particular signaling molecule on or in a tumor cell does not necessarily indicate a vulnerability to inhibitors of the same signaling molecule. For example, imatinib is able to inhibit both PDGFR and cKIT RTKs with approximately the same affinity as BCR/ABL. In fact, dramatic clinical responses in patients with dermatofibrosarcoma that harbor an aberrant ColA1/PDGFR fusion or GISTs that express mutated cKIT have been reported.[34] However, in preclinical studies, imatinib had only modest and transient inhibitory effects on GBMs that express normal PDGFR on their cell surface.[35] Some have suggested that tumor cells that have genetically mutated signaling molecules become "addicted" to them, making these proteins prime targets for pharmacologic targeting. Alternatively, it may be necessary to target multiple signaling pathways or to combine targeted therapies with cytotoxic agents, in order to achieve the therapeutic responses we seek.

GENE REGULATION

Overview

If cancer cells are doing only what they are told, then regulation of gene expression acts as the final arbiter. Signaling cascades detect and integrate extracellular cues that are then transmitted to the nucleus and result in modulating the expression of specific sets of genes. The advent of the human genome sequencing project, with concurrent development of methods of simultaneously measuring the expression of all genes in a cell, has given new insight into the depth and complexity of transcription programs. Although cytoplasmic signaling pathways can behave as relatively compact modules, transcription programs frequently resemble highly branched nonhierarchical networks.[36] It is the sum of these gene networks that, in large part, dictate cellular behavior. For this reason, reversing a transcriptional program that is driving a cancer cell, in a specific and effective manner, poses a significant therapeutic challenge.

Transcription

Many genes are regulated at the level of transcription initiation (Fig. 4.3) (for review, see Ref 37). Two events need to occur in order for transcription of a gene to start. First, the surrounding chromatin needs to be put in a molecular conformation that will allow transcription. This is accomplished by proteins that modify the DNA itself, as well as histones, DNA-binding proteins that are integral in forming the higher-order structure of chromatin in cells. Second, large multiprotein complexes need to be recruited to the core promoter located just upstream of the transcription start site. These complexes include general transcription factors (GTFs) containing the RNA polymerase II holoenzyme (RNAPII) plus coactivator or

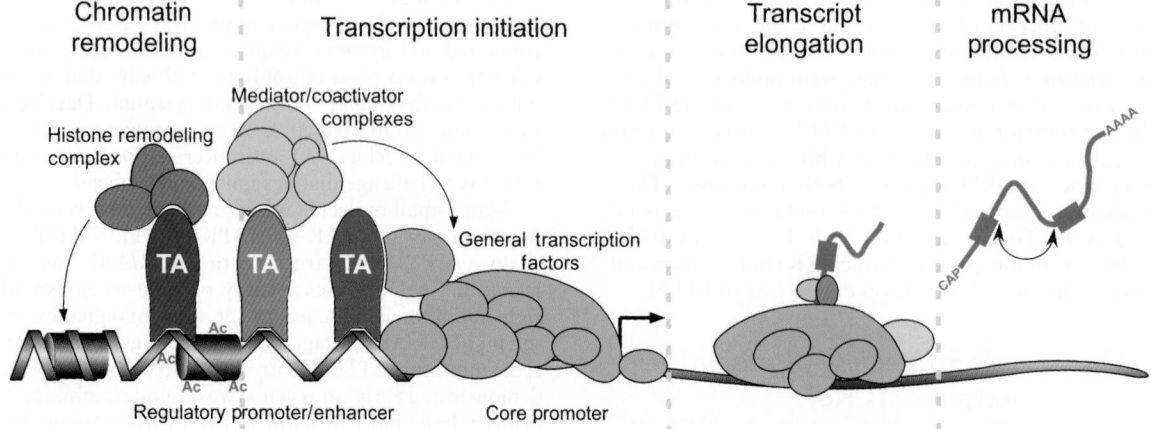

FIGURE 4.3 Mechanisms of gene regulation. Transcription activators bind to specific DNA sequences in regulatory promoters and/or enhancers. Through their transcription activation domains (TA), they interact with other regulatory proteins including (a) members of histone remodeling complex that chemically modify histones (e.g., acetylation, methylation) and promote open chromatin configuration; (b) members of mediator, coactivator, or corepressor complexes; or (c) members of the general transcription factors (GTFs) to enhance transcriptional initiation. Other points of potential regulation include transcript elongation and mRNA processing including alternative splicing.

corepressor complexes. At some genes, these two events occur simultaneously.

Transcriptional activators are key regulators of the transcription process. These proteins are thought to act as links between DNA sequences and basal transcription complex proteins. Transcriptional activators bind to DNA regulatory sequences that are usually located within a gene locus and enhance the recruitment and/or function of transcription complexes. Gene regulatory sequences typically encode binding sites for many different activators. Furthermore, occupancy by multiple activators is usually necessary for upregulating transcription at a particular locus. This combinatorial requirement is an integral feature that allows for specific regulation of a large number of genes by a relatively small number of individual transcriptional activators.

Most transcriptional activators are modular in structure, having well-delineated domains that mediate site-specific binding to particular DNA sequences as well as domains that dictate with which proteins they can interact. Changes in the primary sequences of these domains can have functional consequences due to alteration of protein-DNA or protein-protein specificity. This can result in modulating the expression of a different repertoire of target genes. This is precisely what is thought to happen in certain tumor-associated mutations found in particular pediatric cancers (see later).

Deregulating the Regulators—MYC

Given their integral roles in regulating normal gene expression and therefore cellular behaviors, it is no surprise that transcriptional activators and repressors are potential oncogenic targets. As expected, inappropriate expression of these transcriptional regulators can have profound effects on normal cell growth and differentiation, and many have been implicated in oncogenesis. The difficulty in assessing the significance of potential misexpression of a transcriptional regulator in cancer cells is defining the relevant cellular comparator. Because of their level of aberrant differentiation, cancer cells may express higher levels of certain transcriptional regulators more as a result of the oncogenic process than as a primary cause of it. In these cases, it is important to compare expression levels of candidate deregulated transcription factors to normal progenitor cell populations that are at a similar level of differentiation as the cancer cells.

When misexpression of a transcriptional regulator is a direct result of a tumor-associated chromosomal abnormality, there is usually strong evidence that it is playing a causative role in oncogenesis. The MYC family members of transcription factors are one of the most compelling examples of this (for reviews, see Refs 38 and 39). MYC, a tightly regulated basic region/helix-loop-helix/leucine zipper domain (bHLHzip) protein, binds to DNA targets by forming a heterodimer with MAX, a ubiquitously expressed bHLHzip member (Fig. 4.4). MYC needs MAX in order to bind to DNA at specific genomic sites at MYC target genes. When this happens, MYC is able to interact with GTFs and recruit coactivator complexes that result in modulation of target gene expression. MYC can act as a transcriptional activator or repressor depending on the target gene.

Much effort has been expended in trying to identify and characterize the apparently large number of candidate MYC target genes (for review, see Ref 40). Analyses in several model systems reveal a consistent pattern of upregulation of genes promoting cell cycle (CDK4; cyclins D1, D2, B1), ribosome biosynthesis (rDNA, RNA polymerase III), and metabolism (CAD, ODC). Simultaneously, cell cycle checkpoint regulators (p15^{INK4A}, p21) are downregulated along with genes promoting cell adhesion. In a complementary cell environment, this

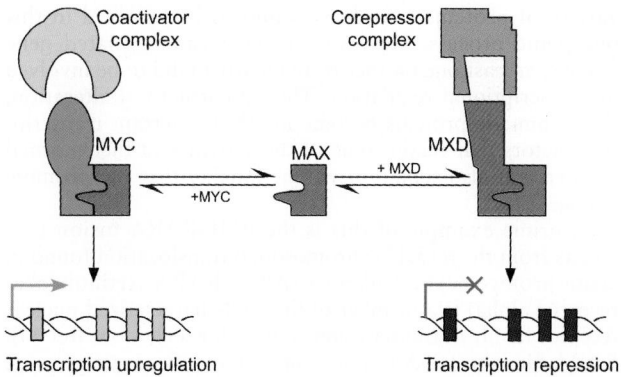

FIGURE 4.4 Mechanism of differential gene regulation by basic region/helix-loop-helix/leucine zipper domain (bHLHzip) proteins. MYC proteins require heterodimerization with MAX to efficiently bind to genomic regulatory sites of target genes. Through its transcriptional activation domain, MYC recruits coactivator complexes that promote upregulation of MYC target genes. The MXD proteins compete with MYC for the limited amount of MAX. MXD/MAX heterodimers recruit corepressor complexes and that transcriptionally downregulate target genes.

repertoire of gene expression changes pushes cells toward growth, mitosis, and enhanced motility, features typically found in aggressive malignancies.

Given these potentially profound effects on cell behavior, it is not surprising that the MYC family is tightly regulated not only at a transcriptional level but also at a functional level. This is accomplished by bHLHzip proteins MNT and MXD1 through MXD4 (formerly MAD1-4). Like MYC, these proteins bind to DNA as MAX heterodimers. However, when bound to genomic response sites, they recruit corepressor complexes that downregulate target gene expression. MNT and MXD not only compete with MYC for the limited amount of MAX but also actively antagonize the biologic effects mediated by MYC. Altering the MYC-MNT/MXD equilibrium could serve as a powerful oncogenic stimulus.

This is in fact what happens in a number of pediatric malignancies.[41] In Burkitt's lymphoma, tumor-associated chromosomal translocations juxtapose immunoglobulin regulatory elements to the cMYC gene (see Chapter 3). As a result, cMYC is inappropriately expressed, which promotes abnormal B-lymphocyte growth. Mouse models harboring immunoglobulin-MYC transgenes develop B-cell malignancies, consistent with cMYC playing a causative role.[42,43] Gene amplification can also serve to deregulate MYC family members. The finding that nMYC amplification confers a very poor prognosis in patients with neuroblastoma is indicative of its importance in the biology of this tumor. The frequent finding of increase in copy number in the region of chromosome 8p, which encodes cMYC, suggests that misexpression of MYC genes may be a common theme in many human cancers.

Transcription Factor Chimerism—"Neither Man nor Beast"

There are now hundreds of chromosomal translocations that have been associated with specific pediatric malignancies (see Chapter 3). Although there are many potential molecular consequences of such genomic rearrangements, the most common outcome is the direct merging of two normally distinct genes. This results in the expression of chimeric transcripts and proteins that correspond to the portions of each partner gene that have been fused into a single molecule. Genes encoding a wide variety of proteins have been found to be involved in this oncogenic process. However, in most cancer-related gene fusions, at least one partner is frequently found to be involved in transcriptional regulation. Through structural alteration, these chimeric proteins become in effect, aberrant transcription factors that retain some of the activities of their normal partners but also acquire new functionality that can promote oncogenesis.

A prime example of this is the PML/RARA fusion that results from the t(15;17) chromosomal translocation found in acute promyelocytic leukemia (APL). RARA (retinoic acid receptor alpha) is a member of the well-characterized nuclear receptor family of transcription factors (for review, see Ref 44). RARA binds to DNA response sites at specific target genes as a heterodimer with RXR, another nuclear receptor member (Fig. 4.5). RAR/RXR heterodimers recruit corepressor complexes, resulting in the transcriptional repression of target genes. Binding to RAR by its cognate ligand all-*trans*-retinoic acid (ATRA) releases these corepressors, resulting in transcriptional upregulation of target genes that promote differentiation of myeloid progenitors.

Fusion of PML to RARA disturbs this regulatory mechanism in several ways. First, PML/RARA more avidly associates with corepressor complexes than with normal RARA. As a result, PML/RARA is relatively resistant to concentrations of ATRA that can derepress RARA under physiologic conditions (for review, see Ref 45). In this way, APL cells are maintained in an undifferentiated state and are able to continue to proliferate. Second, there is evidence that, at least in model systems, PML/RARA may have less restrictive DNA-binding capability than does normal RARA, which could lead to transcriptional modulation of a broader number of target genes.[46,47] Third, PML/RARA may be able to modulate target genes without directly binding to DNA, by interactions mediated through the fused PML domain.[48] Transgenic mouse strains based on expression of the PML/RARA fusion develop acute leukemia with many of the biologic features of APL.[49,50] However, the finding that not all mice developed APL and those that did only did so after a 6- to 14-month latency suggests that though PML/RARA appears necessary for APL oncogenesis, it may not be sufficient.

At about the same time of the initial characterization of PML/RARA, patients with APL were empirically found to respond dramatically when given pharmacologic doses of ATRA. The molecular basis of this response is that these supraphysiologic ATRA levels cause corepressor complexes to dissociate from PML/RARA much the same as seen with normal RARA at lower ATRA levels (Fig. 4.5). The net effect is not cytotoxicity as seen with standard chemotherapy but is one of increasing differentiation of the leukemic blasts. Current multimodal therapy combining ATRA, arsenic trioxide, and cytotoxic chemotherapy have resulted in durable remissions in more than 80% of patients with APL.[51]

RNA Processing—Mix and Match

Gene regulation does not occur only at the level of transcription initiation (Fig. 4.3). A typical mammalian gene is made up of a linear array of exons, which encode peptide sequences, interspersed with relatively long noncoding introns. As genes are transcribed, introns are spliced out of nascent transcripts in the process of forming mature mRNAs. The molecular machinery responsible for recognizing genomic intron-exon boundaries and accurately processing them rivals the transcriptional regulatory system in complexity. Not surprisingly, there is flexibility built in to this system. Variability in intron splicing can result in a single gene giving rise to mRNA isoforms with different exon composition and that correspondingly encode structurally different polypeptides.

It is estimated that alternative exon splicing occurs in more than 75% of human genes.[52] Given the ubiquity of this genetic process, it is tempting to think that mutation of either splicing factors or genomic intron-exon boundaries could play a dominant role in human disease and, in some cases, this appears to be true (for review, see Ref 53). However the jury is still out as to what degree alternative splicing is playing an active role in human cancer. It is clear that transcripts encoding functionally different isoforms of key regulatory proteins are found in certain malignancies (for review, see Ref 54). For example, an alternatively spliced form of HDM2 that cannot interact with p53 is found in a subset of osteosarcomas. However, whether this gene product is actively promoting this tumor's malignant behavior or whether it is simply a consequence of cellular transformation remains to be resolved.

Posttranscriptional Regulation—MicroRNAs Weigh In

Even after a mature mRNA is formed and exported to the cytoplasm, there are additional layers of control. Adaptable cellular systems exist that regulate transcript half-life in the cell and that modulate how efficiently its encoded sequence is translated into protein. Of these regulatory sytems, none are more powerful or pervasive than the heterogeneous group of processes mediated through small noncoding RNAs (for review, see Ref 55). Within this group, it is the microRNAs (miRNAs) that are the most implicated to be playing potentially dominant roles in human oncogenesis.

The miRNA system was discovered through a technological leap rather than in the usual manner where an observation

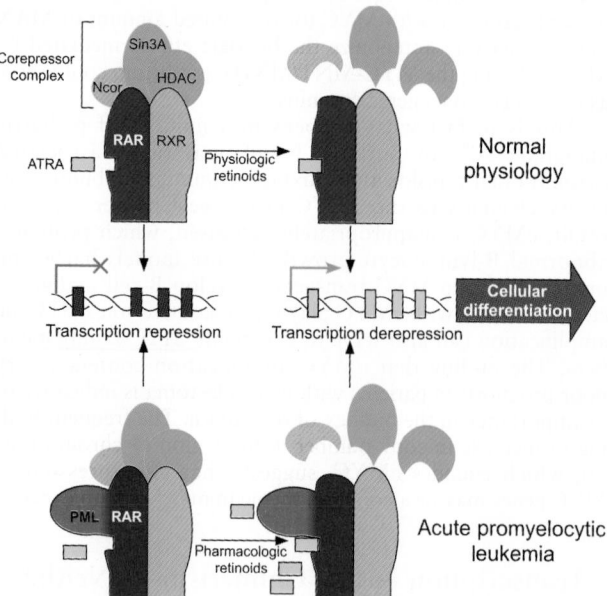

FIGURE 4.5 Gene regulation by normal and aberrant retinoid nuclear receptors. The normal retinoic acid receptor (RAR) binds to genomic regulatory sites as a heterodimer with the structurally related RXR nuclear receptor. Under basal conditions, the RAR/RXR heterodimer recruits corepressor proteins that suppress target gene transcription. Binding of RAR by its cognate ligand, all-*trans*-retinoic acid (ATRA), results in a conformational change that dissociates the corepressor complex and triggers upregulation of target genes that promote cellular differentiation. The PML/RAR fusion can respond in the same manner but much higher levels of ATRA are required to achieve the same effect.

in nature leads to technological development. Just over a decade ago, Fire et al. made the startling discovery of RNA interference (RNAi) in the worm *Caenorhabditis elegans*.[56] They were trying to develop an efficient genetic tool that would allow them to knock down the expression of specific genes in cells. They found that any transcript could be targeted for destruction by simply transducing into cells a double-stranded RNA with the same nucleotide sequence as the target. The remarkable sensitivity and specificity of RNAi could not be accounted for by previously described mechanisms. This suggested to these investigators that RNAi was being mediated by a new physiologic system whose normal purpose was gene silencing. This insight proved to be both prophetic and understated.

Over the subsequent years, there was an explosion of information regarding how miRNAs are formed and the mechanisms through which they regulate mRNA half-life and translation into protein. It is now appreciated that this is an evolutionarily highly conserved system used to regulate gene expression from plants through mammals. In mammals, most miRNAs are encoded within the introns of genes (Fig. 4.6). As these genes are transcribed and their introns spliced out, hairpin-looped miRNAs are excised by the Drosha enzyme complex and exported to the cytoplasm. There, miRNAs are further cleaved by the Dicer endonuclease and incorporated into the multiprotein RNA-induced silencing complex (RISC) as short, approximately 22 base pair (bp) single-stranded RNAs. It is the sequence of this incorporated RNA that both specifies which mRNAs are targeted by the RISC and the molecular consequences of the interaction. Transcripts that have regions of perfect complementarity to the guide sequence are cleaved and rapidly degraded. Transcripts that have only partial homology are not degraded but are inefficiently translated into protein. Most endogenous mammalian miRNAs appear to work primarily through this latter mode of translation inhibition.

Given the way in which miRNAs were discovered, their biochemistry has come well into focus while their biology is still hazy. Estimates of just how many endogenous miRNAs exist in our genome vary from hundreds to thousands.[57] Because miRNAs can target transcripts to which they have only partial nucleotide sequence identity, trying to predict which miRNAs are modulating the expression of which genes has been difficult. Already though there are numerous examples of specific miRNAs being able to modulate the expression of key regulatory genes involved in a wide variety of cellular processes including signal transduction, cell cycle control, differentiation and apoptosis.[58,59]

As with the case with transcription factors, the question of what degree miRNAs actively participate in the process of human oncogenesis is still coming to light. Present evidence is very suggestive but inconclusive.[60–62] High-throughput expression studies have found extensive differences in miRNA expression profiles between normal and cancer cells. In fact, miRNA expression signatures provide an accurate means of classifying human tumors, even cancers of unknown primaries.[63] The finding that certain miRNA genomic clusters are deleted or amplified in particular human malignancies more directly reinforces the notion that misregulation of miRNAs could play an active role in oncogenesis.[64,65]

Treatment Options—Restoring Homeostasis

In spite of the pivotal role that regulation of gene expression plays in human cancer, creation of successful targeted therapies in this venue has been very limited. Although particular transcription factors are clearly valid cancer targets, efforts to develop specific and effective small molecule inhibitors for them have, in general, failed. Nuclear receptor oncogenes such as PML/RARA represent a notable exception probably

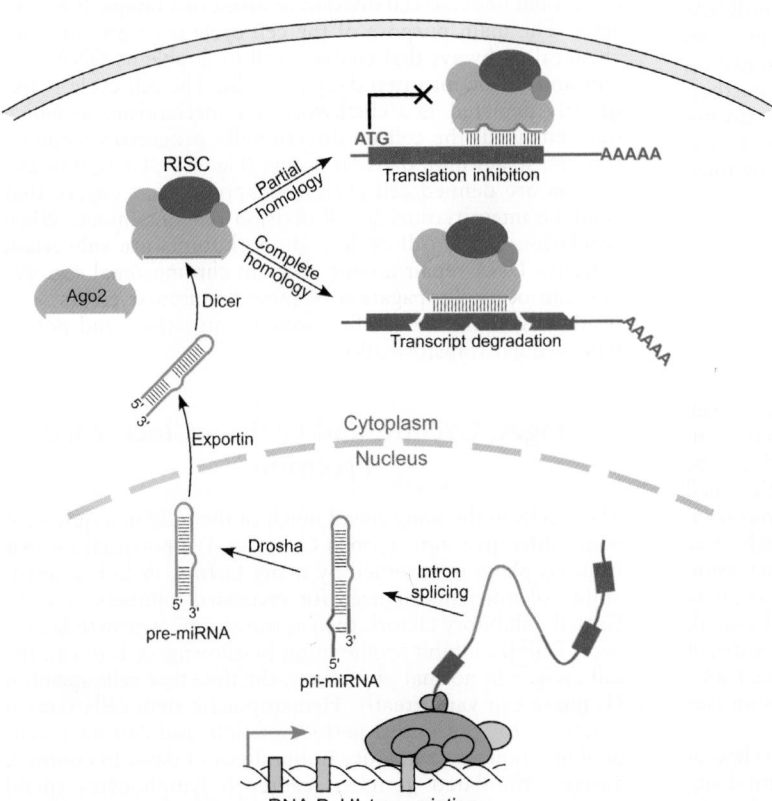

FIGURE 4.6 Metabolism and mechanisms of action of microRNAs (miRNAs). Most mammalian miRNAs originate from intronic genomic sequence that is spliced out in the process of normal RNA polymerase II–mediated transcription. Primary miRNAs are processed by the Drosha complex and then exported into the cytoplasm. There pre-miRNAs are cleaved by Dicer to form a 21 to 22 bp single-stranded RNA molecule (*blue*) that is bound by argonaute 2 (Ago2) and incorporated into the RISC. If this complex encounters a transcript that has a region of complete homology to the RNA guide strand, the transcript is rapidly degraded. On the other hand, if there is only partial homology, the RISC inhibits translation of the target transcript.

because of the preexisting high-affinity relationship between nuclear receptors and their cognate ligands. By contrast, the vast majority of transcription factors function by means of multiple low-affinity interactions in large heterogeneous multiprotein complexes.

Developing molecules that could drive a wedge into select transcription complexes without inhibiting transcription in general and wreaking nonspecific cellular toxicity seems like a daunting proposition. However, the advancing knowledge of transcription biology has led to some preliminary successes in cancer model sytems. For example, investigators have been able to synthesize small molecules that inhibit MYC function by physically blocking MYC-MAX heterodimer formation.[66] These inhibitors are able to antagonize MYC-induced cellular transformation and malignant cell growth in tissue culture models.[67] Taking this strategy a step further, Melnick and coworkers were able to develop short polypeptide inhibitors that block homodimerization of BCL6, a transcription factor that is inappropriately expressed in human B-cell lymphoma.[68] Inhibition of BCL6 by these molecules reduced growth of BCL6-driven lymphoma cell lines both in tissue culture and in murine tumorigenic assays.[69] Although there is a great distance yet to go before such inhibitors are brought into clinical trial, there is hope that by solving transcription factor structures and mapping their interaction surfaces, strategies toward designing specific inhibitors will become more refined.

In contrast to efforts toward functionally antagonizing transcription factors, strategies to harness RNAi to modulate gene expression are galloping forward (for review, see Ref 70). Using an endogenous physiologic system to antagonize malignant cell growth has an appealing feel to it. The already-extensive depth of biochemical knowledge of this system as well as its seemingly programmable nature—that any mRNA can theoretically be targeted by RNAi—weighs in favor of this approach.

However, significant impediments lie ahead. For example, developing RNAi reagents that primarily target only one transcript may prove difficult. It is clear that endogenous miRNAs can downregulate the expression of multiple different genes through translation inhibition. It seems likely that exogenous RNAi constructs will share this similar propensity. Furthermore, because of their negative charge, nucleic acids do not readily enter cells. Therefore, successful *in vivo* RNAi strategies are likely to require an effective means of delivering these constructs intact into cancer cells.

CELL CYCLE

Overview

One of the characteristic behaviors of cancer is abnormal cell growth and proliferation without apparent response to inhibitory signals that arrest normal cells. *Cell growth* can be defined as an increase in cell mass and size rather than cell number. This can be distinguished from *cell proliferation*, which is defined as an increase in cell number. Although these two processes are coordinately regulated during progression of the cell cycle, distinct signal transduction pathways regulate these processes. For example, a major regulator of cell growth is the mTORC1 complex that integrates signals from nutrient sources, growth factors, and energy sources to regulate translation of the mRNAs necessary for cell cycle progression (see the previous section).

Regulation of cell proliferation falls under the purview of the cell cycle. This physiologic system integrates external signals with the internal cellular milieu and decides whether the

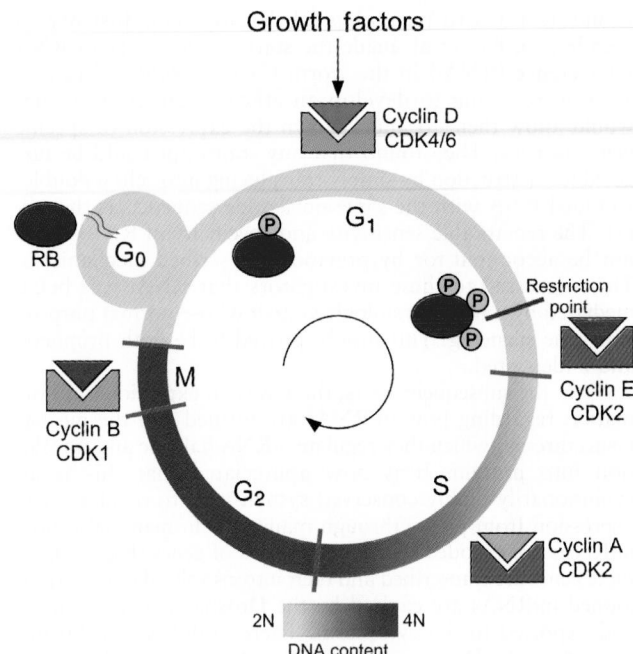

FIGURE 4.7 Normal cell cycle stages and regulation by cyclin-dependent protein kinases (CDKs). Quiescent cells can exist in G_0 phase for extended periods of time. Upon entry into G_1 phase, the retinoblastoma (RB) protein is phosphorylated by the growth factor–responsive cyclin D/CDK4 complex. RB becomes progressively more phosphorylated until the restriction point is met, at which time cyclin E/CDK2 is activated and the cell cycle is no longer responsive to growth factor modulation. The cell's genome is replicated during S phase, and the control shifts to cyclin A/CDK2 complexes. After traversing G_2 phase, the cell undergoes mitosis in M phase under the control of cyclin B/CDK1.

cell should undergo cell division or arrest in a nonproliferative state. The main purpose of the cell cycle is to provide biochemical pathways that enable a cell to double its DNA content and divide into two daughter cells. The cell cycle is frequently depicted as a clockwork-like mechanism, in which once engaged, the cell unidirectionally progresses stepwise through stages until division occurs (Fig. 4.7). Critical to this schema are defined cell cycle checkpoints that ensure that genomic integrity during cell division remains intact. When regulation of the cell cycle and checkpoints are subverted, defective DNA repair and/or aberrant chromosomal segregation can occur. Propagation of these "molecular errors" can result in genomic instability, somatic mutation, and potentially cellular transformation.[71]

Stages, Cyclins, and CDKs—Clockwork Precision

Many cells in the body spend much of their life in a quiescent nonproliferative state, termed G_0 phase. The potential for exit from G_0 phase is governed by many factors, including availability of nutrients or need for increased numbers of cells. Growth inhibitory factors, such as transforming growth factor-beta (TGF-β), inhibit proliferation by allowing cells to exit the cell cycle.[72] In normal physiology, the time that cells spend in G_0 phase can vary greatly. Hematopoietic stem cells remain quiescent for prolonged periods of time and can have cell-doubling times on the order of hundreds of days. In contrast, antigen-stimulated germinal center B lymphocytes spend hardly any time in G_0 phase and double every 6 to 12 hours.

In cells that are not terminally differentiated, the G_0 phase is reversible and cells receiving mitogenic growth factor can reenter the cell cycle to G_1 phase.[71]

Once a cell has decided to divide, it exits G_0 phase and enters the G_1 phase, a period during which the cell cycle prepares for DNA synthesis (Fig. 4.7). This phase, also known as the *first gap* (hence G_1 *phase*), occurs between cell division (M phase) and subsequent DNA synthesis. G_1 phase lasts for approximately 12 to 15 hours and allows cells to produce RNA and proteins and make critical decisions about growth versus quiescence and about whether cell division or differentiation should proceed.[71] For the first two-thirds of the G_1 phase, cells remain responsive to effects of proliferative and antiproliferative stimuli, at which time they pass the restriction (R) point. Traversing the R point, cells no longer need growth factor stimulation, and they make an irreversible commitment to proceeding through cell cycle.[73,74] Before the R point, the cell can still decide whether to remain in G_1 phase or to exit the cell cycle into G_0 phase. The cell cycle can also stop temporarily when genomic, metabolic, or cytoskeletal damages are encountered and resume when the conditions have been remedied. Abnormal regulation of the R point appears to be common in most, if not all, cancer cells.[71]

In cultured mammalian cells, DNA synthesis occurs over a 6- to 8-hour period following G_1 phase, which is known as the S or *synthetic phase*. It is essential that the approximately 6×10^9 bp of DNA in each diploid genome is copied accurately during the S phase. The time of S phase can vary significantly depending on the type of cells. Once cells complete S phase, they enter into the second gap phase or G_2 phase. The G_2 phase lasts for 3 to 5 hours and prepares cells to enter M phase or mitosis followed by cell division. The M phase occurs over 1 hour and consists of four different subphases: prophase, metaphase, anaphase, and telophase. During this time, visible chromosomal condensation occurs, followed by microtubule attachment and centrosome engagement. This leads to chromosomal segregation, followed by cytokinesis or division of cytoplasm from one parent cell into two daughter cells.

Progression through cell cycle is driven through the action of stage-specific cyclin-dependent serine/threonine protein kinases (CDKs).[75] Like protein kinases involved in cell signaling, CDKs function by phosphorylating specific protein substrates that regulate the cell cycle. The unique characteristic of CDKs is their need for noncovalent binding to cyclin partners that boost CDK activity by more than 400,000-fold.[71]

Specific combinations of cyclin/CDK complexes are active at particular stages of the cell cycle (Fig. 4.7). During G_1 phase, cyclins D1, D2, and D3 activate CDK4 and CDK6. The D-type cyclins appear to have additional functions, including programming of differentiation in various cell types.[76] They are also the only cyclins that directly respond to extracellular mitogens, whereas the other cyclins seem to follow a preset program. In late G_1 phase, cyclin E1 and E2 activate CDK2, which then phosphorylates substrates that are necessary to enter S phase.[77] During early S phase, cyclins A1 and A2 partner with CDK2. As the cells traverse G_2 phase, the B-type cyclins (B1 and B2) bind to CDK1 (Cdc2), which initiates the M phase and mitosis.[78]

Early work in frog and sea urchin embryos revealed that the levels of certain cyclins oscillated in a distinctive and reproducible manner during the cell cycle.[79] This regulation is based on the system of rapid protein degradation following posttranslational modification, known as *ubiquitination*. In 2004, the Nobel Prize was awarded to the scientists who discovered this important pathway for protein regulation.[80–82] The ubiquitin-proteasome system consists of a series of enzymatic reactions that result in the attachment of ubiquitin, a small, 76 amino acid polypeptide, onto target proteins.[83] The

E3 ligase is the last step in this process and confers specificity for its particular substrate.[84] Polyubiquitinated cyclins are targeted to the 26S proteasome and are rapidly degraded.

Even at this basic level, the cell cycle is vulnerable to oncogenic perturbations. In particular, abnormal expression of cyclins has been implicated in a number of different cancers. Forced expression of cyclin D has been shown to promote cellular proliferation in tissue culture models. Cyclin D1 amplification or overexpression has been associated with the development of parathyroid adenoma, breast and prostate cancers, lymphoma, and melanoma. High levels of cyclin E is associated with a poor prognosis in patients with breast cancer, whereas lower levels correlate with a good prognosis.

Checkpoints and Cell Cycle Inhibitors— Preserving Genomic Integrity

Cell cycle checkpoints are encountered during G_1 and G_2 phases and provide an internal monitoring system to ensure that the genome is faithfully replicated. In normal cells, if DNA sequence errors are encountered, progression through the cell cycle is halted until these defects are repaired. Genomic errors are detected by the ATM/ATR protein complexes, which signal to p53 and result in cell cycle arrest. Once repaired, the cell continues through the cell cycle. If the genomic errors are too extensive to be repaired, the cell undergoes programmed death or apoptosis (see the following section). Many of these checkpoints are defective in cancer cells, which allows for accumulation of somatic mutations and clonal evolution, leading to increased proliferation.

CKIs

Since CDKs are a primary force driving the cell cycle forward, antagonizing them by means of CDK inhibitors (CKIs) provides an expedient and direct way to apply the brakes to this system. The four INK4 proteins (p16^{INK4A}, p15^{INK4B}, p18^{INK4C}, and p19^{INK4D}) inhibit CDK4 and CDK6 by competitively displacing D cyclins and reverting these CDKs to kinase inactive states (Fig. 4.8). The remaining CKIs (p21$^{Cip1/Waf1}$, p27^{Kip1}, and P57^{Kip2}) work later in cell cycle by noncompetitively inhibiting CDK2 and CDK1 complexes.

Silencing or deletion of CKI genes is seen in a wide variety of pediatric tumors. Virtually all GBMs do not express p16^{INK4A} either through gene deletion or transcriptional silencing of CDKN2A, the gene encoding p16^{INK4A}.[85] Similar evidence of loss of p16 expression is found in about two-thirds of neuroblastoma tumors and approximately one-third of Ewing's sarcomas.[86,87] Finally, deletions of the CDKN2A gene are seen in a subset of pediatric ALL.[88]

RB

Establishment of the G_1 R point is dictated by the tumor suppressor retinoblastoma (RB). The RB gene is one of three family members and encodes a nuclear phosphoprotein. RB is phosphorylated by cyclinD/CDK 4/6 complexes as cells leave the G_0 phase and enter the cell cycle. Moving through G1 phase, RB becomes progressively more phosphorylated until R point is reached. Hyperphosphorylated RB is no longer able to bind and inhibit its primary targets, E2F transcription factors (Fig. 4.8). These derepressed E2Fs are then free to upregulate expression of cell cycle–related genes, including cyclins E, A, and CDK1.[89,90] Beyond the R point, RB remains hyperphosphorylated throughout the rest of the cell cycle until it is dephosphorylated by protein phosphatase type 1 (PP1) at the end of mitosis.

True to its name, homozygous deletions of RB are necessary for the genesis of retinoblastoma.[91] However, loss-of-function

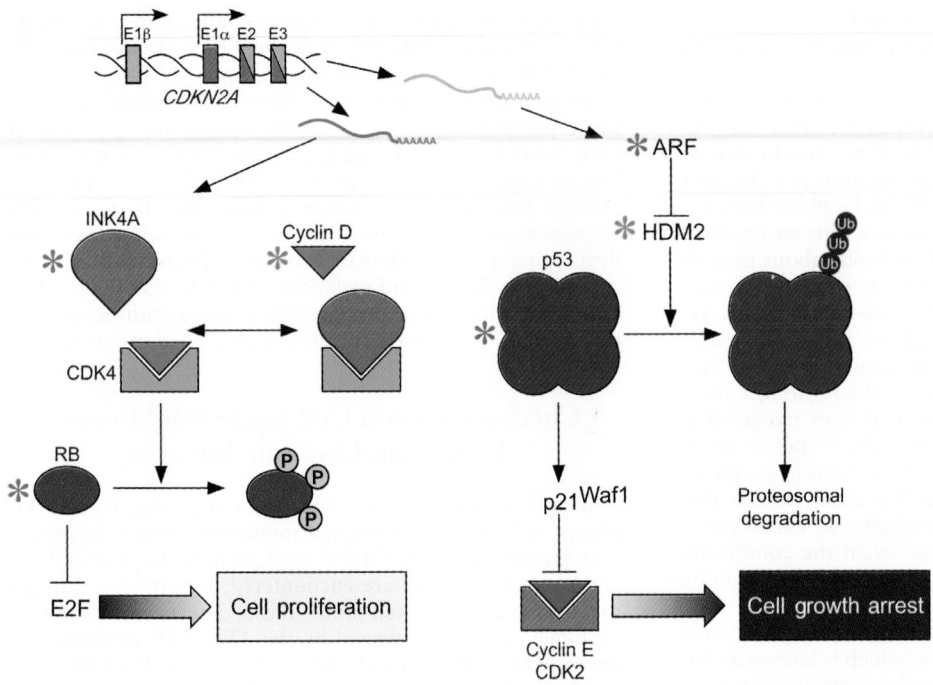

FIGURE 4.8 Two distinct cell cycle regulators are encoded in the CDKN2A gene. Transcription of CDKN2A from the proximal (E1α) promoter results in p16^{ink4A}, a competitive inhibitor of CDK4 that works by displacing for cyclin D. Phosphorylation of RB by cyclin D/CDK4 releases E2F transcription factors, which upregulate genes promoting cell cycle progression. Transcription of CDKN2A from the distal (E1α) promoter results in the formation of p19^{ARF} from an alternative reading frame. P19^{ARF} antagonizes HDM2, an E3 ligase that polyubiquinates p53, a critical cell cycle regulator, and targets it for proteasomal destruction. P53 upregulates p21^{WAF}, which noncompetitively inhibits cyclin E/CDK2 and promotes cell cycle arrest. These cell cycle regulatory components are commonly targeted for either gain-of-function (green asterisks) or loss-of-function (red asterisks) oncogenic mutations.

mutations in RB are also seen in other pediatric cancers, including subsets of osteosarcoma, Burkitt's lymphoma, and GBM. Finally, the oncogenic activity of some DNA virus proteins, including SV40 large T and human papillomavirus E7, is caused, at least in part, through direct inhibition of RB.

P53—The Bridge Between Cell Division and Death

P53 acts as a central hub that cells use to assess the level of external and internal stress and to decide whether to proliferate, quiesce, or die (Fig. 4.8). A variety of external stimuli can induce p53 expression, the best-known being γ irradiation and cytotoxic drugs, such as most chemotherapy, that elicit a genotoxic stress response.[92] The p53 response can come from within cells as well. Depending on cell context, forced expression of oncoproteins such as cMYC result in increased p53 expression and cell cycle arrest if not apoptosis. P53 can even respond to more subtle effects such as "ribosome stress" observed in bone marrow failure syndromes in patients with ribosomal protein subunit mutations, such as Diamond-Blackfan anemia.[93–96] Rising p53 levels transcriptionally modulate specific target genes, such as CDKN1A, which encodes the CKI p21$^{Cip1/Waf1}$, and BH3 proteins, such as BAX, to promote cell cycle arrest and apoptosis.[97]

Like the cyclins, p53 is regulated by controlling the rate of its degradation through the ubiquitin-proteasome system. MDM2 (mouse double minutes) or HDM2 (human ortholog) is the rate-limiting E3 ubiquitin ligase that is upregulated when p53 is phosphorylated or activated in response to stress signals.[98] This results in a negative feedback loop in which MDM2/HDM2 then ubiquitinates p53 and targets the protein for destruction by the 26S proteasome.[99,100] In effect, activated p53 can shut itself off. To add another layer of complexity, CDKN2A not only encodes the CKI p16^{INK4A} but, in an alternative reading frame, also encodes p19^{ARF}, an MDM2/HDM2 inhibitor (Fig. 4.8).[101,102] By binding MDM2/HDM2 and sequestering it in the nucleolus, p19^{ARF} antagonizes p53 destruction by the ubiquitin-proteasome system.

Many cancers cannot live under the strict scrutiny imposed by p53, and for this reason, somatic mutations that inhibit p53 function are some of the most common observations in human malignancies. In many tumors, this is accomplished directly through p53 loss-of-function mutations or deletions. In other cancers such as osteosarcoma, this is accomplished indirectly through amplification and overexpression of MDM2/HDM2 which results in increased destruction of p53.[98] Finally, loss of CDKN2A, as is seen in a subpopulation of Ewing's sarcoma, not only deregulates cell cycle through loss of a CKI but also potentiates the activity of MDM2/HDM2 through loss of p19^{ARF}.[103]

Therapies Targeting Cell Cycle

In many ways, oncologists have been therapeutically targeting the cell cycle for decades through the use of cytotoxic chemotherapy. The *modus operandi* for most of our current systemic anticancer therapies is to damage DNA either by direct chemical disruption or by antagonizing systems involved in its replication or repair. For this reason, it has long been thought that actively proliferating cells are more susceptible to these agents than are quiescent cells. This concept must be applied with caution. The sensitivity that some cancers display to particular chemotherapies that is in apparent excess to their normal cellular counterparts cannot be explained simply on the basis of differing proliferation rates. There must be more to this story.

Considering its central role in cancer biology, therapeutically targeting the cell cycle in tumor cells has great theoretical appeal. Development of small molecules that inhibit the enzymatic function of CDKs is actively being pursued.[104–106] For example, flavopiridol, an inhibitor of CDKs 1, 2, 4, and 7, has been evaluated in both phase 1 and 2 clinical trials. Although no untoward side effects have been seen, the antitumor response in patients with recurrent soft tissue sarcoma was quite limited.[107] Whether this and similar CDK inhibitors will have a greater therapeutic effect when combined with other anticancer agents is a subject of ongoing investigation.

Enhancement of p53 activity is another strategy being pursued. Nutlin-3, a small molecule that inhibits interaction between p53 and the MDM2/HDM2, increases p53 half-life.[108,109] This drug has been shown to induce apoptosis in tumor cells *in vitro* and enhance the effects of chemotherapy.[110–116] Inhibiting the ubiquitin-proteasome machinery directly has also shown promising results. A prime example is bortezomib (PS-341 or Velcade), a small molecule tripeptide that reversibly inhibits the 26S proteasome.[117,118] This drug has been shown to be effective in the treatment of B-cell–type malignancies, including multiple myeloma and non-Hodgkin lymphoma.[119,120] Bortezomib is being studied in clinical trials in pediatric patients with leukemia and a variety of other tumors. While these results are encouraging, it is expected that generalized inhibition of the ubiquitin-proteasome system will alter the levels of many cellular proteins. It may be that the anticancer effects of this drug may, at least in part, be mediated by modulating targets that are not directly involved with cell cycle regulation.

APOPTOSIS

Overview

In multicellular organisms, there is no life without death. Homeostasis requires that cell proliferation be balanced with cell death. Many cells in complex organisms are faced with the decision not only whether to proliferate or quiesce but also to actively cease their existence. This phenomenon, termed *apoptosis*, has been viewed in a social context where the lives of individual cells are sacrificed for the benefit and integrity of the organism as a whole. Apoptosis plays crucial roles in normal development by providing a means for regression and remodeling of tissues. Apoptosis can perform a policing function to ensure that morphogenesis proceeds on track. Errant cells that have mislocalized outside their prescribed environments are induced to die rather than become the nidus for an abnormal morphological event. Apoptosis actively contributes to maintaining the homeostatic balance in mature organisms as well. For example, thymocytes that have rearranged their T-cell receptor loci either in an unproductive manner or in one that recognizes self-antigens undergo apoptosis. This process not only removes nonfunctional T lymphocytes but also prevents development of potentially disease-causing autoimmune T-cell clones.[121]

Not only does apoptosis help maintain structure within cell populations but it also serves as the final solution for irresolvable conflicts within individual cells. Cells faced with irreparable damage to their genome or inappropriate signals to proliferate will frequently opt to engage the apoptosis machinery and die. For example, forced expression of potent proto-oncogenes such as cMYC and activated RAS in normal cell backgrounds frequently does not induce cellular transformation but induces apoptotic death. By actively removing damaged and discordant cells, apoptosis may serve as a primary antioncogenic mechanism in vertebrates.

With this in mind, Green and Evan[122] have put forth a streamlined model of oncogenesis based on the premise that most, if not all, cancers are the product of the same two effects: (a) stimulation of unregulated cell proliferation and (b) inhibition of apoptosis.[122] This is not as easily accomplished as it might seem because both effects need to be achieved in synchrony. Cells in which apoptosis is inhibited but lack a concurrent growth stimulus have no proliferative advantage over normal counterparts. Conversely, cells harboring an oncogenes-driven proliferative stimulus but no inhibition of apoptosis activate the ARF-p53 pathway and undergo programmed cell death.[123] This model prompts the intriguing concept that reestablishing a normal apoptotic response in cancer cells could prove to be a powerful strategy in which to treat human malignancy. Given the complexity of the pathways mediating apoptosis in human cells, this approach, though simple in concept, will probably be more difficult in practice.

Apoptotic Pathways—The Means to the End

Extrinsic

Many normal and cancer cells express surface receptors whose sole purpose is to initiate apoptosis when prompted by extracellular cues.[124] Structurally, these receptors (DR4, DR5, FAS) belong to the TNF (tissue necrosis factor) superfamily and are composed of extracellular ligand-binding domains, a transmembrane region, and an intracellular portion with a characteristic death effector domain (DED). As with most signaling processes, ligand (Apo2L, tumor necrosis factor–related apoptosis-inducing ligand [TRAIL], FASL) binding leads to receptor aggregation, in this case, into trimers, and the formation of multiprotein death-inducing signaling complexes. This in turn initiates a proteolytic cascade involving the caspase family of molecules (Fig. 4.9).

Caspases are cysteine proteases that play integral roles in mediating programmed cell death in virtually all cells.[125] As their name implies, caspases function by cleaving protein substrates at sequence-specific aspartate residues. Caspases are initially synthesized in the cell as enzymatically inactive zymogens consisting of N-terminal prodomains followed by a large subunit and a C-terminal small subunit. The regions between these three domains are punctuated by caspase cleavage sites. Proteolytic cleavage of two procaspase molecules at these sites results in the formation of a tetramer with two active catalytic sites. Since all caspases contain caspase cleavage sites, they, in effect, activate themselves. This, in fact, happens when an active caspase meets an inactive procaspase. This is the common mechanism by which executioner caspases such as caspases 3 and 7 that are located downstream in apoptotic pathways are activated. Once activated, executioner caspases actively promote apoptosis by targeting a wide variety of proteins involved in cell signaling, mitosis, and maintenance of cytoplasmic and nuclear structural integrity.

In contrast, initiator (or apical) caspases that lie at the head of apoptotic signaling pathways rely on aggregation and autoactivation. Aggregation is mediated by specific protein-protein interaction motifs that are encoded into their prodomains. For example, oligomerization of the apoptotic receptor DR4, recruits procaspases 8 and 10 through the interaction of adapter molecules and the DED motifs present in the caspase prodomains. Aggregation induces a conformational change that allows the localized procaspases to activate each other. Once cleaved from their prodomains, activated caspases 8 and 10 are no longer bound to DR4 and can diffuse into the cytoplasm to activate executioner caspases.

Intrinsic

Where the response to a specific external signal to undergo apoptosis is conceptually straight forward, arriving at this fateful decision from intracellular cues is much more complex. There is a wide array of stresses that can push a cell toward apoptosis, ranging from exposure to toxins and hypoxia, to genomic damage, to inappropriate growth signals. Under these circumstances, the cell needs the ability to integrate and weigh these stimuli before committing itself to death. This is accomplished through the interplay of pro- and antiapoptotic members of the BH domain family of proteins and their net effect on producing mitochondrial outer membrane permeabilization (MOMP) (Fig. 4.9).[126–128]

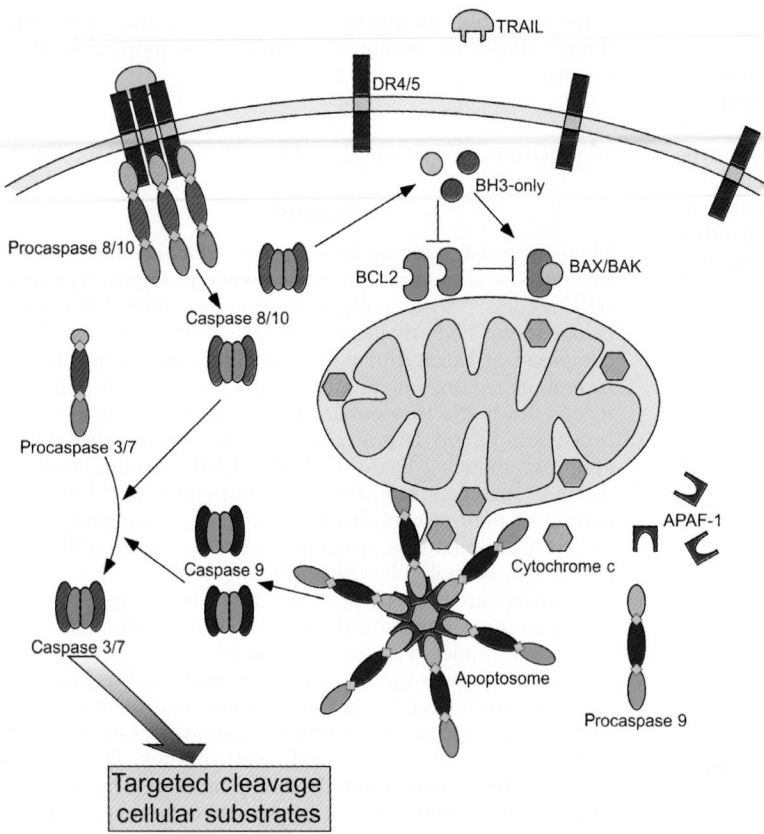

FIGURE 4.9 Extrinsic and intrinsic apoptotic pathways lead to programmed cell death. In the extrinsic pathway, binding of TRAIL at the cell surface induces DR4 or DR5 trimerization. This leads to procaspase 8 and 10 aggregation through interaction with the cytoplasmic domains of DR4/5. Procaspases consist from N- to C-terminus of pro (*gray*), large subunit (*darker color*), and small subunit (*lighter color*) domains. Caspase cleavage sites are between each domain (*yellow diamonds*). Aggregation of initiator procaspases (8, 9, 10) results in autocleavage and formation of activated heterotetramers consisting of two large and two small subunits. In the intrinsic pathway, the balance of antiapoptotic (BCL2) and proapoptotic (BAX, BAK, BH3-only) proteins determine whether mitochondrial outer membrane permeabilization (MOMP) occurs, triggering apoptosis. MOMP releases cytochrome c, which aggregate with APAF-1 and procaspase 9 to form apoptosomes. This activates caspase 9. Both extrinsic and intrinsic pathways result in activation of executioner caspases 3 and 7, which in turn cleave specific cellular substrates, resulting in apoptosis. Activated caspases 8 and 10 can also target the BH3-only protein BID, thereby providing a link between extrinsic and intrinsic apoptotic pathways.

BH proteins can be categorized according to function and the types of BCL2 homology (BH) domains they contain.[129] BAX and BAK are proapoptotic BH1-4 proteins that when activated, homooligomerize on the surface of the mitochondrial outer membrane and directly cause MOMP. BCL2 family proteins (BCL2, BCL-XL, BCLW, A1, MCL) are antiapoptotic BH1-4 proteins that functionally antagonize BAX and BAK. Finally, there is the large class of BH3-only proteins that can promote apoptosis by binding and inhibiting BCL2 proteins. In addition, at least two BH3-only proteins (BID and BIM) can act as direct activators by binding to BAX and BAK and inducing oligomerization.[130,131]

The picture that has emerged from intensive study of these proteins is one of a widely dispersed system that is sensitive to diverse cellular inputs. First, most cells typically express multiple BCL2 family and BH3-only proteins. Second, the regulation of these proteins is incorporated into many signaling pathways and can occur at the transcriptional level or posttranslational level. For example, the BH3-only protein BID is activated by cleavage by caspase 8, thus providing a functional link between the intrinsic and extrinsic apoptotic pathways. A primary mechanism through which activated AKT inhibits apoptosis is through phosphorylation of the BH3-only protein BAD, which targets it for ubiquitination and proteasomal destruction. Finally, each BH3-only protein has a defined repertoire of which BCL2 member proteins it can inhibit. It is through these interactions among BH proteins that pro- and antiapoptotic forces are weighed and the decision to undergo programmed cell death is dictated.

Once BAX or BAK oligomerization and MOMP have occurred, the cell initiates a systematic program of self-destruction. Rupture of the mitochondrial membrane releases a number of proapoptotic proteins, significantly cytochrome c, into the cytoplasm. Cytochrome c, in turn, nucleates a reaction that results in the formation of multi-

protein aggregates, termed *apoptosomes*, consisting of APAF-1 and procaspase 9. Like the other initiator caspases 8 and 10, aggregation of procaspase 9 induces autoproteolytic cleavage resulting in activation. Activated caspase 9 then cleaves and activates executioner caspases 3 and 7. It takes only 10 minutes from MOMP to caspase activation and the irreversible decision to die.[132]

Apoptosis Modulation in Cancer—Life Under Pressure

BCL2 was initially discovered as a gene targeted by the 14;18 chromosomal translocation found in human follicular lymphoma.[133] As a consequence of this rearrangement, the BCL2 genomic locus comes under the transcriptional control of the immunoglobulin heavy chain (IgH) gene. The result is inappropriately high levels of intact BCL2 protein. Transgenic mice harboring an IgH-BCL2 construct develop polyclonal expansions of mature B cells, consistent with a defect in apoptosis.[134] With time, a proportion of these mice incur a secondary mutation, the most frequent being deregulation of cMYC, and progress to overt lymphoma. This model mimics the clinical course of human follicular lymphoma, which generally presents as an indolent disease that can accelerate with time.[135]

Deregulation of BCL2 is a clear example of oncogenic mutation of an apoptotic pathway component. Along similar lines, transcriptional silencing or genomic deletion of caspase 8 is seen in a subpopulation of high risk for neuroblastomas.[136,137] However, these examples may be the exceptions rather than the rule. Loss-of-function mutation of p53 that is seen in many adult tumors clearly has a large impact on a cell's ability to undergo apoptosis. However, as noted previously, there are many pediatric cancers in which p53 mutation is not commonly seen. In the end, directly targeting the apoptotic machinery appears to be an infrequent occurrence in the oncogenesis of pediatric malignancies.

Pediatric tumors may take a more indirect approach to blunting the apoptotic response. Considering that many signaling pathways can modulate the expression of BH3-only and BCL2 family proteins, alteration of these signaling pathways could exert a net antiapoptotic effect. For example, the BCR/ABL fusion protein found in CML, in addition to stimulating growth, also activates AKT which reduces the expression of the proapoptotic BH3-only protein BAD. In similar fashion, growth factor receptors, such as IGFR-1, that are present on a variety of pediatric sarcomas, such as osteosarcoma, rhabdomyosarcoma and Ewing's sarcoma, signal through AKT and exert an antiapoptotic effect.

However, cellular transformation may come at a price (Fig. 4.10). From the perspective of apoptosis signaling, normal cells growing in native environments exist in a relaxed unperturbed state. Both pro- and antiapoptotic factors are present, but BAX and BAK, the primary effectors of MOMP, are inactive for the most part. By contrast, current thinking suggests that cancer cells exist in a state of tension.[138,139] Their inappropriate signals to proliferate engage apoptotic pathways that stimulate activation of BAX and BAK in some cases through upregulation of direct activators BID and BIM. To fend off apoptosis, cancer cells must compensate by increasing expression of antiapoptotic BCL2 family members that bind and counteract BID and BIM. In this scenario, cancer cells are "primed for death." Any perturbation that shifts the antiapoptotic-proapoptotic balance could trigger programmed cell death. While there are many details still to be elucidated, this model may provide a partial explanation of why cytotoxic chemotherapy kills cancer cells primarily through apoptosis. By causing additional genotoxic stress, chemotherapy may, in effect, provide the proapoptotic straw that breaks the cancer's back.

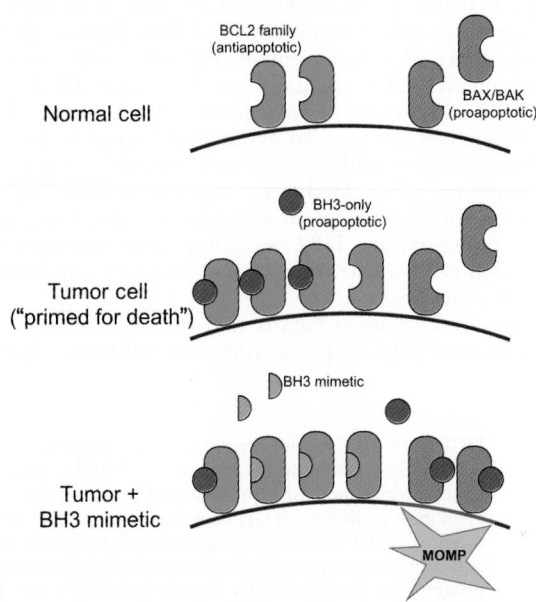

FIGURE 4.10 Model of therapeutic effect of BH3 mimetics on malignant cells. In most normal cells in physiologic conditions, proapoptotic BAX and BAK are not activated. In cancer cells, inappropriate growth signals lead to upregulation of proapoptotic BH3-only proteins. To evade apoptosis, tumor cells upregulate antiapoptotic BCL2 family members. Administration of BH3 mimetics displaces BH3-only proteins from BCL2. Unbound BH3-only proteins then bind to BAX and BAK, activating them, resulting in mitochondrial outer membrane permeabilization (MOMP) and apoptosis.

Anticancer Apoptotic Strategies—Tipping the Balance

The differences in apoptosis engagement between normal and cancer cells has prompted development of targeted therapies aimed at pushing cancer cells toward programmed cell death.[140] Recombinant TRAIL proteins are currently being evaluated for their ability to bind to DR4 and DR5 receptors on cancer cells and stimulate apoptosis through the extrinsic pathway.[141] Using a similar strategy, monoclonal antibodies directed at DR4 or DR5 have been developed that promote receptor aggregation and activation of caspases 8 and 10.

As noted above, many cancers are dependent on BCL2 family proteins to prevent apoptosis, suggesting that these molecules could be potent therapeutic targets. Structural analysis of BCL2 proteins has defined a hydrophobic groove that forms the critical interaction surface to which BH3-only proteins bind. Small molecules have now been synthesized that bind to this groove at high affinity ($Kd < 1$ nM).[142] These BH3 mimetics drive cancer cells toward apoptosis by liberating proapoptotic BH3-only proteins and antagonizing the antiapoptotic activity of BCL2 family members.[127] Of the several BH3 mimetics that have been developed, at present, ABT-737 and its orally available congener ABT-263 show the most promise and have been intensively studied.[143]

Preclinical and early clinical studies using TRAIL agonists and BH3 mimetics have demonstrated common themes. Both classes of drugs are able by themselves to promote apoptosis in a variety of cancer cell lines in tissue culture models.[144] This effect is significantly enhanced when they are combined with cytotoxic chemotherapies, with specific tyrosine kinase inhibitors, or when both TRAIL agonists and BH3 mimetics are used together. Both TRAIL agonists and BH3 mimetics have entered phase 1 to 2 clinical trials. Clinical responses to monotherapy have been modest. However, the general lack of systemic toxicity of these drugs, even with the high-affinity ABT-737 compound, is notable. This is consistent with the idea that most normal cells can tolerate inhibition of BCL2 since unlike cancer cells, they are not primed for death.

At present, modulating apoptosis in cancer cells is a theoretically promising therapeutic approach that has not yet realized its potential. Two hurdles probably need to be cleared in order for this to happen. First, the right apoptosis therapeutics needs to be paired with the right cancer. Considering the combinatorial manner that cells use to regulate apoptosis, cancer cells elude this response through a variety of specific mechanisms. Developing biomarkers that would accurately predict the relative sensitivity of tumors to different apoptosis therapeutics would be a significant step forward. Second, preclinical studies suggest that apoptotic modulators are likely to be most effective when used in combination with other anticancer agents. This reinforces the notion that apoptotic signaling systems integrate anti- and proapoptotic forces within the cell. Combination therapy in effect could provide a greater impetus in driving cancer cells toward their apoptotic threshold, where they would cease by their own hand.

ANGIOGENESIS

Overview

Not all cells in a solid tumor are malignant. Some are simply misguided. To varying degrees, virtually all macroscopic tumor masses are composed of both transformed malignant cells and recruited normal cells that have answered the call.

The vascular epithelial and mesenchymal cells that make up tumor blood vessels are prime examples of the latter. Tumors, like normal tissue structures, require oxygen and nutrients to survive. To grow beyond a 1- to 2-mm size limit imposed by the diffusability of oxygen in tissue, tumors require blood vessels. To address this need, tumors co-opt a normal physiologic response to extended tissue hypoxia which is angiogenesis.

Angiogenesis can be defined as the growth of new blood vessels from preexisting ones and can occur throughout adult life. This contrasts to vasculogenesis, which involves *de novo* formation of blood vessels that occurs during embryogenesis. In normal angiogenesis, tissue hypoxia triggers a series of signaling events that mobilize vascular endothelial cells. This results in the remodeling and growth of vascular structures directed along cytokine gradients and into the area of hypoxia. Although many key components of this complex process have been identified, the interplay between signaling pathways and cell populations is still being clarified.

Long anticipated to be a potential Achilles heel in solid malignancies, tumor-elicited angiogenesis has been the subject of intense scrutiny. Investigations have been spurred by two observations that so far appear to hold true. First, normal angiogenic signaling pathways remain intact in most solid tumors and angiogenic signaling components are not targets for direct oncogenic mutation. Second, many tumors seem to be unable to perform the entire angiogenic program, resulting in a tenuous and incompletely formed vascular system. In this regard, the chaotic nature of a malignant cell tumor mass is frequently reflected in the vascular structures that feed it.

Almost 40 years ago, Folkman[145] first articulated the dynamic interrelationship between tumor growth and angiogenesis and posited that inhibiting angiogenesis could have a significant anticancer impact. Since then, several antiangiogenic compounds have made their way into the clinic and more will undoubtedly soon follow. Initial results indicate that though these agents appear to be hitting their molecular targets, clinical responses have been relatively modest. Recent studies using animal tumorigenesis models have yielded results that were unanticipated if not at odds with certain preconceived notions of how angiogenesis is regulated. Although antiangiogenesis tools are in hand, it appears that more knowledge is needed for them to be used effectively.

Normal Angiogenesis—Engineering Forks in the Road

Angiogenesis starts with a cry for help. Growing cells, having exceeded their oxygen supply, upregulate members of the HIF (hypoxia-inducible factor) family of transcription factors

(Fig. 4.11).[146] Hypoxia leads to polyubiquitination and proteasomal destruction of the von Hippel-Lindau (VHL) protein which actively represses HIF expression under normoxic conditions. As VHL levels fall, HIF levels rise and in turn transcriptionally activate a number of genes involved in angiogenesis including vascular endothelial growth factor (VEGF). This factor is secreted from hypoxic cells and provides a chemotactic gradient, signaling the need for new vascular growth.

VEGF is a lynchpin in initiating angiogenesis (for reviews, see Refs 147–149). There are four related VEGF genes, but it is VEGF-A (frequently abbreviated as "VEGF") that plays the dominant role in angiogenesis. VEGF mediates its effect by binding to cognate VEGF RTKs that are present on the surfaces of a variety of cells including vascular endothelium. VEGF stimulation of VEGFR2 receptors promotes endothelial cell proliferation and viability by activation of MAPK and PI3K signaling pathways, respectively.

With angiogenesis, as with any remodeling project, a certain amount of demolition is needed along with accumulating the necessary building materials. VEGF addresses both needs by simultaneously stimulating vascular endothelial growth and destabilizing vascular structure (Fig. 4.11). Vascular permeability is increased because of loosening of tight junctions between endothelial cells. In addition, VEGF aids in the recruitment of bone marrow–derived endothelial progenitors to an angiogenic locus. In order for normal angiogenesis to occur, VEGF must be precisely regulated with respect to both dose and timing. In animal models, forced overexpression of VEGF can lead to formation of aberrant leaky vascular structures.[150,151] By contrast, haploinsufficient mice that have lost one VEGF allele and therefore express half the normal level of VEGF die in embryogenesis because of vascular abnormalities.[152,153]

The angiopoietin (Ang) family of cytokines work in concert with VEGF. Ang1 and Ang2 work in an antagonistic fashion to maintain and modify blood vessels. Both Ang1 and Ang2 compete as ligands for the TIE2 RTK that is expressed on the surface of vascular endothelial cells. In this context, Ang1 promotes TIE2 signaling while Ang2 turns TIE2 signaling off. In early stages of angiogenesis, Ang2 is upregulated and destabilizes the vascular endothelial barrier by promoting dissociation of endothelium with supporting mesenchymal pericytes. This facilitates vascular remodeling and sprouting. In later stages of angiogenesis, Ang1 predominates, upregulating TIE2 signaling and strengthening endothelial cell-pericyte interactions. This serves to stabilize vascular structures.

There are additional factors that promote angiogenesis, whose explicit roles and regulation are still being clarified.

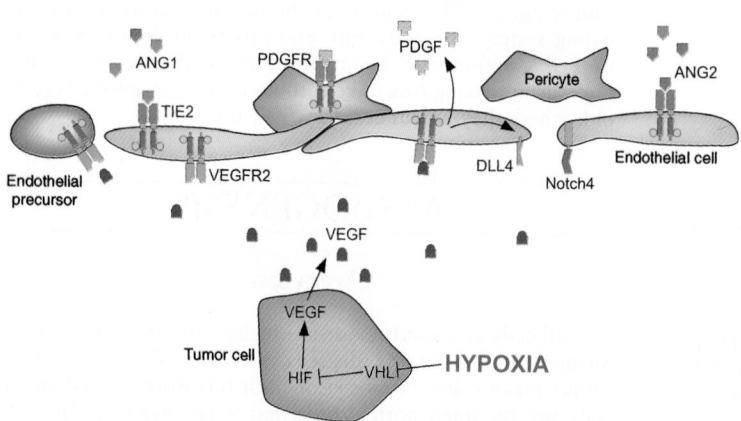

FIGURE 4.11 Cytokine regulation of angiogenesis. Tumor bed hypoxia results in derepression of HIF transcription factors, which increase expression and secretion of vascular cytokines, including VEGF. Signaling through the VEGF2 receptor, VEGF increases vascular endothelial permeability and proliferation as well as recruits circulating endothelial progenitors. Ang2 inhibits signaling through the TIE2 receptor, resulting in reduced endothelial cell-pericyte interaction and destabilized vascular structure. Ang1 competes with Ang2 and has the opposite effect. PDGF secreted by endothelial and other cells enhances pericyte proliferation and survival, which serves to stabilize nascent blood vessels. VEGF stimulation results in upregulation of the Notch ligand delta-like ligand 4 (DLL4) on the surface of endothelial cells. Engagement of DLL4 with Notch4 present on neighboring endothelial cells counteracts the growth stimulatory effects of VEGF and inhibits angiogenesis.

Platelet-derived growth factor-BB (PDGF-BB) secreted by vascular endothelial cells exerts trophic effects on supporting pericytes that express cognate PDGF receptors.[154,155] Enhancing endothelial coverage by pericytes serves to stabilize nascent blood vessels. Members of the FGF family of cytokines can also promote angiogenesis, indicating that there is a certain amount of redundancy in the system.

To balance the angiogenic system, there are molecular components that serve to retard endothelial proliferation and prevent uncontrolled vascular growth. For example, VEGFR activation in endothelial cells leads to upregulation of delta-like ligand 4 (DLL4).[156] Engagement of this cell surface ligand with cognate Notch4 receptors present on neighboring endothelial cells antagonizes vascular growth. Finally, there are a large number of endogenous inhibitors of angiogenesis, many of which are cleavage products of basement membrane and stromal proteins.[157,158] It is thought that these factors are formed as angiogenesis proceeds and they provide a moderating influence against runaway vascular growth. Considering the number and diversity of factors that can impact angiogenesis, it seems clear that this is a process that is sensitive to immediate environment. As a consequence, the set of factors and precise timing that are used to generate new blood vessels are likely to be tissue specific.

Tumor Angiogenesis—The Road to Ruin

It has long been appreciated that tumor vasculature is not normal (for reviews, see Refs 159 and 160). In many tumors, the capillary bed is haphazardly constructed with an assortment of misformed branching structures juxtaposing vessels of random caliber and dimension. There is increased capillary permeability, leading to extravasation of plasma proteins and a proportionate increase in extravascular pressure within many solid tumors. As a result, in spite of an increased number of blood vessels, there is inefficient blood flow through tumor vasculature, leading to poor perfusion and reduced oxygen delivery.

The vasculature of many tumors is not only malformed but also immature. Much of the capillary bed consists of loosely fitted endothelial cells that are sparsely supported by pericytes and smooth muscle cells. The absence of these usual supports renders tumor vasculature unstable and perhaps more susceptible to modulation of angiogenic growth factors. Indeed, this forms the underlying rationale for many of the antiangiogenic therapies currently being pursued.

If, as appears the case, angiogenic pathway components do not seem to be targeted for direct oncogenic mutation, how then has this normal developmental program slipped the track? The answer is certainly multifactorial and, to a certain extent, variable from tumor to tumor. It is clear that oncogenic mutation in some tumor cells can lead to inappropriate expression of angiogenic cytokines. Activated RAS increases the production of VEGF while decreasing the expression of antiangiogenic thrombospondins.[161] Loss of p53 increases levels of the key hypoxic sensor HIF1α by increasing proteasome-mediated destruction of VHL.[162] Increased HIF1α level in turn boosts expression of VEGF. Finally, germline loss of the VHL gene, as found in patients with the von Hipple-Lindau syndrome, leads to uncontrolled VEGF expression, resulting in formation of hemangioblastomas and renal tumors.[163]

Even without directly modulating the regulators of angiogenic cytokines, the ability for many tumors to grow in a relatively hypoxic environment probably leads to abnormal levels of pro- and antiangiogenic factors. At some point, it probably becomes a vicious cycle. The tumor's supranormal hypoxic stimulus leads to an imbalanced angiogenic response, resulting in malformed vasculature. This in turn results in poor nutrient and oxygen delivery, which further exacerbates tumor bed hypoxia.

Targeting Tumor Vasculature—Antagonizing VEGF

Tumor vasculature, given its tenuous structure, has been an attractive target for development of anticancer therapies. Early on, what was sought was a simple scenario of death by asphyxiation. Disruption of tumor vasculature would terminally interrupt oxygen flow to tumor cells, leading irrevocably to their demise. Considering its pivotal role directing angiogenesis, VEGF has been a prime therapeutic target, and a number of inhibitors have been developed (for reviews, see Refs 164 and 165). Bevacizumab (Avastin) is a humanized monoclonal antibody that binds all active isoforms of VEGF-A and prevents subsequent interaction with VEGF receptors.[166] More recently, small molecule inhibitors of the VEGFR2 kinase have been developed, such as sorafenib and sunitinib. These latter compounds are multispecific tyrosine kinase inhibitors and frequently antagonize RTKs in addition to VEGFR. For example, sunitinib, by also inhibiting PDGFR, can target tumor angiogenesis by simultaneously antagonizing two pathways important in this process.[167]

Although VEGF pathway inhibitors performed well in preclinical models, their therapeutic success in the clinic has been much more modest (for review, see Ref 168). These drugs are now approved for use in clear cell renal carcinoma, metastatic colorectal carcinoma, and, more recently, metastatic breast cancer and GBM. Current experience in the pediatric population has been limited to compassionate use and phase 1 trial.[169,170] Although VEGF inhibition has produced some dramatic clinical responses in a variety of different malignancies, as a rule, these are short-lived effects. Resistance to therapy almost invariably develops after weeks to several months of therapy, resulting in tumor regrowth. The causes underlying the quickly developing resistance to anti-VEGF agents are currently being investigated. Compensatory increase in VEGF, alternative angiogenic signaling pathways, and increased recruitment of circulating endothelial progenitors are theories that have all been invoked. Multimodal strategies combining different angiogenesis modulatory agents with or without cytotoxic chemotherapy are being pursued.

However, part of the problem may be that simply trying to turn off the VEGF pathway may have unanticipated biologic effects. Mouse tumorigenesis models have demonstrated that soon after anti-VEGF agents are administered, tumor neovasculature is pruned back and "normalized," resulting in improved perfusion parameters.[171] This suggested that there could be a window of opportunity for delivery of antineoplastic agents after VEGF inhibition.[172] Indeed, increasing tumor perfusion through targeted modulation of perivascular stroma rendered a model of pancreatic carcinoma more susceptible to cytotoxic chemotherapy.[173] Finally, there are recent disconcerting preclinical studies that suggest that use of anti-VEGF agents could promote tumor invasion and metastasis.[174–176] Whether any of these scenarios actually plays out in human patients remains to be seen. However, given how exquisitely VEGF is regulated in normal angiogenesis, a similar level of precision in drug delivery and timing may be necessary if anti-VEGF strategies are to be more successful in treating disease.

References

1. Beenken A, Mohammadi M. The FGF family: biology, pathophysiology and therapy. Nat Rev Drug Discov 2009;8(3):235–253.
2. Hynes NE, Lane HA. ERBB receptors and cancer: the complexity of targeted inhibitors. Nat Rev Cancer 2005;5(5):341–354.
3. Pavelic K, Bukovic D, Pavelic J. The role of insulin-like growth factor 2 and its receptors in human tumors. Mol Med 2002;8(12):771–780.
4. Matsumoto K, Wada RK, Yamashiro JM, et al. Expression of brain-derived neu-rotrophic factor and p145TrkB affects survival, differentiation, and invasiveness of human neuroblastoma cells. Cancer Res 1995;55(8):1798–1806.
5. Gusterson BA, Hunter KD. Should we be surprised at the paucity of response to EGFR inhibitors? Lancet Oncol 2009;10(5):522–527.
6. Baselga J, Swain SM. Novel anticancer targets: revisiting ERBB2 and discovering ERBB3. Nat Rev Cancer 2009;9(7):463–475.
7. Mischel PS, Cloughesy TF. Targeted molecular therapy of GBM. Brain Pathol 2003;13(1):52–61.
8. Tanaka T, Matsuoka M, Sutani A, et al. Frequency of and variables associated with the EGFR mutation and its subtypes. Int J Cancer 2010;126(3):651–655.
9. Miettinen M, Lasota J. Gastrointestinal stromal tumors: review on morphology, molecu-lar pathology, prognosis, and differential diagnosis. Arch Pathol Lab Med 2006;130(10):1466–1478.
10. Tefferi A. Molecular drug targets in myeloproliferative neoplasms: mutant ABL1, JAK2, MPL, KIT, PDGFRA, PDGFRB and FGFR1. J Cell Mol Med 2009;13(2):215–237.
11. Vivanco I, Sawyers CL. The phosphatidylinositol 3-kinase AKT pathway in human can-cer. Nat Rev Cancer 2002;2(7):489–501.
12. Pierotti MA, Greco A. Oncogenic rearrangements of the NTRK1/NGF receptor. Cancer Lett 2006;232(1):90–98.
13. Lannon CL, Sorensen PH. ETV6-NTRK3: a chimeric protein tyrosine kinase with transformation activity in multiple cell lineages. Semin Cancer Biol 2005;15(3):215–223.
14. Steelman LS, Abrams SL, Whelan J, et al. Contributions of the Raf/MEK/ERK, PI3K/PTEN/Akt/mTOR and Jak/STAT pathways to leukemia. Leukemia 2008;22(4):686–707.
15. Schubbert S, Shannon K, Bollag G. Hyperactive Ras in developmental disorders and cancer. Nat Rev Cancer 2007;7(4):295–308.
16. Colicelli J. Human RAS superfamily proteins and related GTPases. Sci STKE 2004;2004(250):RE13.
17. Repasky GA, Chenette EJ, Der CJ. Renewing the conspiracy theory debate: does Raf function alone to mediate Ras oncogenesis? Trends Cell Biol 2004;14(11):639–647.
18. Braun BS, Shannon K. Targeting Ras in myeloid leukemias. Clin Cancer Res 2008;14(8):2249–2252.
19. Sabnis AJ, Cheung LS, Dail M, et al. Oncogenic Kras initiates leukemia in hematopoi-etic stem cells. PLoS Biol 2009;7(3):e59.
20. Le DT, Kong N, Zhu Y, et al. Somatic inactivation of Nf1 in hematopoietic cells results in a progressive myeloproliferative disorder. Blood 2004;103(11):4243–4250.
21. Guertin DA, Sabatini DM. Defining the role of mTOR in cancer. Cancer Cell 2007;12(1):9–22.
22. Endersby R, Baker SJ. PTEN signaling in brain: neuropathology and tumorigenesis. Oncogene 2008;27(41):5416–5430.
23. Ohgaki H, Kleihues P. Genetic pathways to primary and secondary glioblastoma. Am J Pathol 2007;170(5):1445–1453.
24. Mellinghoff IK, Cloughesy TF, Mischel PS. PTEN-mediated resistance to epidermal growth factor receptor kinase inhibitors. Clin Cancer Res 2007;13(2, pt 1):378–381.
25. McCubrey JA, Steelman LS, Abrams SL, et al. Targeting survival cascades induced by activation of Ras/Raf/MEK/ERK, PI3K/PTEN/Akt/mTOR and Jak/STAT pathways for effective leukemia therapy. Leukemia 2008;22(4):708–722.
26. Buchdunger E, Zimmermann J, Mett H, et al. Inhibition of the Abl protein-tyrosine kinase in vitro and in vivo by a 2-phenylaminopyrimidine derivative. Cancer Res 1996;56(1):100–104.
27. Buchdunger E, Zimmermann J, Mett H, et al. Selective inhibition of the platelet-derived growth factor signal transduction pathway by a protein-tyrosine kinase inhibitor of the 2-phenylaminopyrimidine class. Proc Natl Acad Sci U S A 1995;92(7):2558–2562.
28. Druker BJ, Tamura S, Buchdunger E, et al. Effects of a selective inhibitor of the Abl tyrosine kinase on the growth of Bcr-Abl positive cells. Nat Med 1996;2(5):561–566.
29. Druker BJ, Guilhot F, O'Brien SG, et al. Five-year follow-up of patients receiving ima-tinib for chronic myeloid leukemia. N Engl J Med 2006;355(23):2408–2417.
30. Shah NP, Nicoll JM, Nagar B, et al. Multiple BCR-ABL kinase domain mutations confer polyclonal resistance to the tyrosine kinase inhibitor imatinib (STI571) in chronic phase and blast crisis chronic myeloid leukemia. Cancer Cell 2002;2(2):117–125.
31. Shah NP, Tran C, Lee FY, et al. Overriding imatinib resistance with a novel ABL kinase inhibitor. Science 2004;305(5682):399–401.
32. Sousa SF, Fernandes PA, Ramos MJ. Farnesyltransferase inhibitors: a detailed chemical view on an elusive biological problem. Curr Med Chem 2008;15(15):1478–1492.
33. Basso AD, Kirschmeier P, Bishop WR. Lipid posttranslational modifications: farnesyl transferase inhibitors. J Lipid Res 2006;47(1):15–31.
34. Duffaud F, Le Cesne A. Imatinib in the treatment of solid tumours. Target Oncol 2009;4(1):45–56.
35. Kilic T, Alberta JA, Zdunek PR, et al. Intracranial inhibition of platelet-derived growth factor-mediated glioblastoma cell growth by an orally active kinase inhibitor of the 2-phenylaminopyrimidine class. Cancer Res 2000;60(18):5143–5150.
36. Barabasi AL, Oltvai ZN. Network biology: understanding the cell's functional organi-zation. Nat Rev Genet 2004;5(2):101–113.
37. Carey M, Smale ST. Transcriptional regulation in eukaryotes. New York, NY: Cold Spring Harbor Laboratory Press, 1999.
38. Cowling VH, Cole MD. Mechanism of transcriptional activation by the Myc oncopro-teins. Semin Cancer Biol 2006;16(4):242–252.
39. Hurlin PJ, Huang J. The MAX-interacting transcription factor network. Semin Cancer Biol 2006;16(4):265–274.
40. Dang CV, O'Donnell KA, Zeller KI, et al. The c-Myc target gene network. Semin Can-cer Biol 2006;16(4):253.
41. Nesbit CE, Tersak JM, Prochownik EV. MYC oncogenes and human neoplastic disease. Oncogene 1999;18(19):3004–3016.
42. Adams JM, Harris AW, Pinkert CA, et al. The c-myc oncogene driven by immunoglobu-lin enhancers induces lymphoid malignancy in transgenic mice. Nature 1985;318(6046):533–538.
43. Harris AW, Pinkert CA, Crawford M, et al. The E mu-myc transgenic mouse: a model for high-incidence spontaneous lymphoma and leukemia of early B cells. J Exp Med 1988;167(2):353–371.
44. Germain P, Chambon P, Eichele G, et al. International Union of Pharmacology, LX: retinoic acid receptors. Pharmacol Rev 2006;58(4):712–725.
45. Lin RJ, Sternsdorf T, Tini M, et al. Transcriptional regulation in acute promyelocytic leukemia. Oncogene 2001;20(49):7204–7215.
46. Kamashev D, Vitoux D, De The H. PML-RARA-RXR oligomers mediate retinoid and rexinoid/cAMP cross-talk in acute promyelocytic leukemia cell differentiation. J Exp Med 2004;199(8):1163–1174.
47. Zhou J, Peres L, Honore N, et al. Dimerization-induced corepressor binding and relaxed DNA-binding specificity are critical for PML/RARA-induced immortalization. Proc Natl Acad Sci U S A 2006;103(24):9238–9243.
48. van Wageningen S, Breems-de Ridder MC, Nigten J, et al. Gene transactivation without direct DNA binding defines a novel gain-of-function for PML-RARalpha. Blood 2008;111(3):1634–1643.
49. Pollock JL, Westervelt P, Walter MJ, et al. Mouse models of acute promyelocytic leukemia. Curr Opin Hematol 2001;8(4):206–211.
50. Westervelt P, Lane AA, Pollock JL, et al. High-penetrance mouse model of acute promyelocytic leukemia with very low levels of PML-RARalpha expression. Blood 2003;102(5):1857–1865.
51. Sanz MA, Montesinos P, Vellenga E, et al. Risk-adapted treatment of acute promyelo-cytic leukemia with all-trans retinoic acid and anthracycline monochemotherapy: long-term outcome of the LPA 99 multicenter study by the PETHEMA Group. Blood 2008;112(8):3130–3134.
52. Johnson JM, Castle J, Garrett-Engele P, et al. Genome-wide survey of human alternative pre-mRNA splicing with exon junction microarrays. Science 2003;302(5653):2141–2144.
53. Wang GS, Cooper TA. Splicing in disease: disruption of the splicing code and the decod-ing machinery. Nat Rev Genet 2007;8(10):749–761.
54. Venables JP. Aberrant and alternative splicing in cancer. Cancer Res 2004;64(21):7647–7654.
55. Hannon GJ, Rivas FV, Murchison EP, et al. The expanding universe of noncoding RNAs. Cold Spring Harb Symp Quant Biol 2006;71:551–564.
56. Fire A, Xu S, Montgomery MK, et al. Potent and specific genetic interference by double-stranded RNA in Caenorhabditis elegans. Nature 1998;391(6669):806–811.
57. Berezikov E, van Tetering G, Verheul M, et al. Many novel mammalian microRNA can-didates identified by extensive cloning and RAKE analysis. Genome Res 2006;16(10):1289–1298.
58. Felli N, Fontana L, Pelosi E, et al. MicroRNAs 221 and 222 inhibit normal erythro-poiesis and erythroleukemic cell growth via kit receptor down-modulation. Proc Natl Acad Sci U S A 2005;102(50):18081–18086.
59. Georgantas RW III, Hildreth R, Morisot S, et al. CD34+ hematopoietic stem-progenitor cell microRNA expression and function: a circuit diagram of differentiation control. Proc Natl Acad Sci U S A 2007;104(8):2750–2755.
60. Gartel AL, Kandel ES. miRNAs: little known mediators of oncogenesis. Semin Cancer Biol 2008;18(2):103–110.
61. Spizzo R, Nicoloso MS, Croce CM, et al. SnapShot: microRNAs in cancer. Cell 2009;137(3):586–586.e1.
62. Visone R, Croce CM. MiRNAs and cancer. Am J Pathol 2009;174(4):1131–1138.
63. Lu J, Getz G, Miska EA, et al. MicroRNA expression profiles classify human cancers. Nature 2005;435(7043):834.
64. Calin GA, Dumitru CD, Shimizu M, et al. Frequent deletions and down-regulation of micro-RNA genes miR15 and miR16 at 13q14 in chronic lymphocytic leukemia. Proc Natl Acad Sci U S A 2002;99(24):15524–15529.
65. Cimmino A, Calin GA, Fabbri M, et al. miR-15 and miR-16 induce apoptosis by tar-geting BCL2. Proc Natl Acad Sci U S A 2005;102(39):13944–13949.
66. Berg T, Cohen SB, Desharnais J, et al. Small-molecule antagonists of Myc/Max dimer-ization inhibit Myc-induced transformation of chicken embryo fibroblasts. Proc Natl Acad Sci U S A 2002;99(6):3830–3835.
67. Huang MJ, Cheng YC, Liu CR, et al. A small-molecule c-Myc inhibitor, 10058-F4, induces cell-cycle arrest, apoptosis, and myeloid differentiation of human acute myeloid leukemia. Exp Hematol 2006;34(11):1480–1489.
68. Polo JM, Dell'Oso T, Ranuncolo SM, et al. Specific peptide interference reveals BCL6 transcriptional and oncogenic mechanisms in B-cell lymphoma cells. Nat Med 2004;10(12):1329–1335.
69. Cerchietti LC, Yang SN, Shaknovich R, et al. A peptomimetic inhibitor of BCL6 with potent antilymphoma effects in vitro and in vivo. Blood 2009;113(15):3397–3405.
70. Castanotto D, Rossi JJ. The promises and pitfalls of RNA-interference-based therapeu-tics. Nature 2009;457(7228):426–433.
71. Weinberg R. The biology of cancer. New York, NY: Garland Science, 2007.
72. Massague J, Chen YG. Controlling TGF-beta signaling. Genes Dev 2000;14(6):627–644.
73. Planas-Silva MD, Weinberg RA. The restriction point and control of cell proliferation. Curr Opin Cell Biol 1997;9(6):768–772.
74. Hatakeyama M, Weinberg RA. The role of RB in cell cycle control. Prog Cell Cycle Res 1995;1:9–19.
75. Malumbres M, Barbacid M. Cell cycle, CDKs and cancer: a changing paradigm. Nat Rev Cancer 2009;9(3):153–166.
76. Matsushime H, Quelle DE, Shurtleff SA, et al. D-type cyclin-dependent kinase activity in mammalian cells. Mol Cell Biol 1994;14(3):2066–2076.
77. Yamasaki L, Pagano M. Cell cycle, proteolysis and cancer. Curr Opin Cell Biol 2004;16(6):623–628.

78. Guardavaccaro D, Pagano M. Stabilizers and destabilizers controlling cell cycle oscillators. Mol Cell 2006;22(1):1–4.
79. Swenson KI, Farrell KM, Ruderman JV. The clam embryo protein cyclin A induces entry into M phase and the resumption of meiosis in Xenopus oocytes. Cell 1986;47(6):861–870.
80. Behuliak M, Celec P, Gardlik R, et al. Ubiquitin—the kiss of death goes Nobel: will you be quitting? Bratisl Lek Listy 2005;106(3):93–100.
81. Hershko A. The ubiquitin system for protein degradation and some of its roles in the control of the cell division cycle. Cell Death Differ 2005;12(9):1191–1197.
82. Hershko A. Early work on the ubiquitin proteasome system, an interview with Avram Hershko: interview by CDD. Cell Death Differ 2005;12(9):1158–1161.
83. Reinstein E, Ciechanover A. Narrative review: protein degradation and human diseases: the ubiquitin connection. Ann Intern Med 2006;145(9):676–684.
84. Deshaies RJ. SCF and Cullin/Ring H2-based ubiquitin ligases. Annu Rev Cell Dev Biol 1999;15:435–467.
85. Newcomb EW, Alonso M, Sung T, et al. Incidence of p14ARF gene deletion in high-grade adult and pediatric astrocytomas. Hum Pathol 2000;31(1):115–119.
86. Kovar H, Jug G, Aryee DN, et al. Among genes involved in the RB dependent cell cycle regulatory cascade, the p16 tumor suppressor gene is frequently lost in the Ewing family of tumors. Oncogene 1997;15(18):2225–2232.
87. Takita J, Hayashi Y, Kohno T, et al. Deletion map of chromosome 9 and p16 (CDKN2A) gene alterations in neuroblastoma. Cancer Res 1997;57(5):907–912.
88. Okuda T, Shurtleff SA, Valentine MB, et al. Frequent deletion of p16INK4a/MTS1 and p15INK4b/MTS2 in pediatric acute lymphoblastic leukemia. Blood 1995;85(9):2321–2330.
89. Brehm A, Miska EA, McCance DJ, et al. Retinoblastoma protein recruits histone deacetylase to repress transcription. Nature 1998;391(6667):597–601.
90. Kaelin WG Jr. Functions of the retinoblastoma protein. Bioessays 1999;21(11):950–958.
91. Sellers WR, Kaelin WG Jr. Role of the retinoblastoma protein in the pathogenesis of human cancer. J Clin Oncol 1997;15(11):3301–3312.
92. Laptenko O, Prives C. Transcriptional regulation by p53: one protein, many possibilities. Cell Death Differ 2006;13(6):951–961.
93. Danilova N, Sakamoto KM, Lin S. p53 family in development. Mech Dev 2008;125(11/12):919–931.
94. Danilova N, Sakamoto KM, Lin S. Role of p53 family in birth defects: lessons from zebrafish. Birth Defects Res C Embryo Today 2008;84(3):215–227.
95. Danilova N, Sakamoto KM, Lin S. Ribosomal protein S19 deficiency in zebrafish leads to developmental abnormalities and defective erythropoiesis through activation of p53 protein family. Blood 2008;112(13):5228–5237.
96. Gazda HT, Zhong R, Long L, et al. RNA and protein evidence for haplo-insufficiency in Diamond-Blackfan anaemia patients with RPS19 mutations. Br J Haematol 2004;127(1):105–113.
97. Riley T, Sontag E, Chen P, et al. Transcriptional control of human p53-regulated genes. Nat Rev Mol Cell Biol 2008;9(5):402–412.
98. Eischen CM, Lozano G. p53 and MDM2: antagonists or partners in crime? Cancer Cell 2009;15(3):161–162.
99. Vazquez A, Bond EE, Levine AJ, et al. The genetics of the p53 pathway, apoptosis and cancer therapy. Nat Rev Drug Discov 2008;7(12):979–987.
100. Kruse JP, Gu W. Modes of p53 regulation. Cell 2009;137(4):609–622.
101. Sherr CJ. Tumor surveillance via the ARF-p53 pathway. Genes Dev 1998;12(19):2984–2991.
102. Sherr CJ, Weber JD. The ARF/p53 pathway. Curr Opin Genet Dev 2000;10(1):94–99.
103. Brooks CL, Gu W. Dynamics in the p53-Mdm2 ubiquitination pathway. Cell Cycle 2004;3(7):895–899.
104. Alvi AJ, Austen B, Weston VJ, et al. A novel CDK inhibitor, CYC202 (R-roscovitine), overcomes the defect in p53-dependent apoptosis in B-CLL by down-regulation of genes involved in transcription regulation and survival. Blood 2005;105(11):4484–4491.
105. Benson C, White J, De Bono J, et al. A phase I trial of the selective oral cyclin-dependent kinase inhibitor seliciclib (CYC202; R-Roscovitine), administered twice daily for 7 days every 21 days. Br J Cancer 2007;96(1):29–37.
106. Bettayeb K, Oumata N, Echalier A, et al. CR8, a potent and selective, roscovitine-derived inhibitor of cyclin-dependent kinases. Oncogene 2008;27(44):5797–5807.
107. Morris DG, Bramwell VH, Turcotte R, et al. A phase II study of flavopiridol in patients with previously untreated advanced soft tissue sarcoma. Sarcoma 2006;2006:64374.
108. Shangary S, Wang S. Targeting the MDM2-p53 interaction for cancer therapy. Clin Cancer Res 2008;14(17):5318–5324.
109. Shangary S, Wang S. Small-molecule inhibitors of the MDM2-p53 protein-protein interaction to reactivate p53 function: a novel approach for cancer therapy. Annu Rev Pharmacol Toxicol 2009;49:223–241.
110. Ambrosini G, Sambol EB, Carvajal D, et al. Mouse double minute antagonist Nutlin-3a enhances chemotherapy-induced apoptosis in cancer cells with mutant p53 by activating E2F1. Oncogene 2007;26(24):3473–3481.
111. Fry DC, Vassilev LT. Targeting protein-protein interactions for cancer therapy. J Mol Med 2005;83(12):955–963.
112. Klein C, Vassilev LT. Targeting the p53-MDM2 interaction to treat cancer. Br J Cancer 2004;91(8):1415–1419.
113. Kojima K, Konopleva M, Samudio IJ, et al. MDM2 antagonists induce p53-dependent apoptosis in AML: implications for leukemia therapy. Blood 2005;106(9):3150–3159.
114. Stuhmer T, Chatterjee M, Hildebrandt M, et al. Nongenotoxic activation of the p53 pathway as a therapeutic strategy for multiple myeloma. Blood 2005;106(10):3609–3617.
115. Vassilev LT. Small-molecule antagonists of p53-MDM2 binding: research tools and potential therapeutics. Cell Cycle 2004;3(4):419–421.
116. Vassilev LT. MDM2 inhibitors for cancer therapy. Trends Mol Med 2007;13(1):23–31.
117. Adams J. The development of proteasome inhibitors as anticancer drugs. Cancer Cell 2004;5(5):417–421.
118. Adams J. The proteasome: a suitable antineoplastic target. Nat Rev Cancer. 2004;4(5):349–360.
119. Chauhan D, Bianchi G, Anderson KC. Targeting the UPS as therapy in multiple myeloma. BMC Biochem 2008;9(suppl 1):S1.
120. O'Connor OA, Wright J, Moskowitz C, et al. Phase II clinical experience with the novel proteasome inhibitor bortezomib in patients with indolent non-Hodgkin's lymphoma and mantle cell lymphoma. J Clin Oncol 2005;23(4):676–684.
121. Fas SC, Fritzsching B, Suri-Payer E, et al. Death receptor signaling and its function in the immune system. Curr Dir Autoimmun 2006;9:1–17.
122. Green DR, Evan GI. A matter of life and death. Cancer Cell 2002;1(1):19–30.
123. Sherr CJ. Divorcing ARF and p53: an unsettled case. Nat Rev Cancer 2006;6(9):663–673.
124. Zhang L, Fang B. Mechanisms of resistance to TRAIL-induced apoptosis in cancer. Cancer Gene Ther 2005;12(3):228–237.
125. Earnshaw WC, Martins LM, Kaufmann SH. Mammalian caspases: structure, activation, substrates, and functions during apoptosis. Annu Rev Biochem 1999;68:383–424. doi:10.1146/annurev.biochem.68.1.383.
126. Chipuk JE, Green DR. How do BCL-2 proteins induce mitochondrial outer membrane permeabilization? Trends Cell Biol 2008;18(4):157–164.
127. Green DR. Life, death, BH3 profiles, and the salmon mousse. Cancer Cell 2007;12(2):97–99.
128. Green DR, Kroemer G. The pathophysiology of mitochondrial cell death. Science 2004;305(5684):626–629.
129. Youle RJ, Strasser A. The BCL-2 protein family: opposing activities that mediate cell death. Nat Rev Mol Cell Biol 2008;9(1):47–59.
130. Gavathiotis E, Suzuki M, Davis ML, et al. BAX activation is initiated at a novel interaction site. Nature 2008;455(7216):1076–1081.
131. Green DR, Chipuk JE. Apoptosis: stabbed in the BAX. Nature 2008;455(7216):1047–1049.
132. Green DR. Apoptotic pathways: ten minutes to dead. Cell 2005;121(5):671–674.
133. Yang E, Korsmeyer SJ. Molecular thanatopsis: a discourse on the BCL2 family and cell death. Blood 1996;88(2):386–401.
134. McDonnell TJ, Korsmeyer SJ. Progression from lymphoid hyperplasia to high-grade malignant lymphoma in mice transgenic for the t(14; 18). Nature 1991;349(6306):254–256.
135. Tan D, Horning SJ. Follicular lymphoma: clinical features and treatment. Hematol Oncol Clin North Am 2008;22(5):863–882, viii.
136. Iolascon A, Borriello A, Giordani L, et al. Caspase 3 and 8 deficiency in human neuroblastoma. Cancer Genet Cytogenet 2003;146(1):41–47.
137. Teitz T, Wei T, Valentine MB, et al. Caspase 8 is deleted or silenced preferentially in childhood neuroblastomas with amplification of MYCN. Nat Med 2000;6(5):529–535.
138. Certo M, Del Gaizo Moore V, Nishino M, et al. Mitochondria primed by death signals determine cellular addiction to antiapoptotic BCL-2 family members. Cancer Cell 2006;9(5):351–365.
139. Green DR. At the gates of death. Cancer Cell 2006;9(5):328–330.
140. Fesik SW. Promoting apoptosis as a strategy for cancer drug discovery. Nat Rev Cancer 2005;5(11):876–885.
141. Ashkenazi A. Directing cancer cells to self-destruct with pro-apoptotic receptor agonists. Nat Rev Drug Discov 2008;7(12):1001–1012.
142. Lessene G, Czabotar PE, Colman PM. BCL-2 family antagonists for cancer therapy. Nat Rev Drug Discov 2008;7(12):989–1000.
143. Cragg MS, Harris C, Strasser A, et al. Unleashing the power of inhibitors of oncogenic kinases through BH3 mimetics. Nat Rev Cancer 2009;9(5):321–326.
144. Del Gaizo Moore V, Brown JR, Certo M, et al. Chronic lymphocytic leukemia requires BCL2 to sequester prodeath BIM, explaining sensitivity to BCL2 antagonist ABT-737. J Clin Invest 2007;117(1):112–121.
145. Folkman J. Tumor angiogenesis: therapeutic implications. N Engl J Med 1971;285(21):1182–1186.
146. Semenza GL. Targeting HIF-1 for cancer therapy. Nat Rev Cancer 2003;3(10):721–732.
147. Carmeliet P. Mechanisms of angiogenesis and arteriogenesis. Nat Med 2000;6(4):389–395.
148. Yancopoulos GD, Davis S, Gale NW, et al. Vascular-specific growth factors and blood vessel formation. Nature 2000;407(6801):242–248.
149. Breen EC. VEGF in biological control. J Cell Biochem 2007;102(6):1358–1367.
150. Springer ML, Chen AS, Kraft PE, et al. VEGF gene delivery to muscle: potential role for vasculogenesis in adults. Mol Cell 1998;2(5):549–558.
151. Larcher F, Murillas R, Bolontrade M, et al. VEGF/VPF overexpression in skin of transgenic mice induces angiogenesis, vascular hyperpermeability and accelerated tumor development. Oncogene 1998;17(3):303–311.
152. Carmeliet P, Ferreira V, Breier G, et al. Abnormal blood vessel development and lethality in embryos lacking a single VEGF allele. Nature 1996;380(6573):435–439.
153. Ferrara N, Carver-Moore K, Chen H, et al. Heterozygous embryonic lethality induced by targeted inactivation of the VEGF gene. Nature 1996;380(6573):439–442.
154. Reinmuth N, Liu W, Jung YD, et al. Induction of VEGF in perivascular cells defines a potential paracrine mechanism for endothelial cell survival. FASEB J 2001;15(7):1239–1241.
155. Hellstrom M, Kalen M, Lindahl P, et al. Role of PDGF-B and PDGFR-beta in recruitment of vascular smooth muscle cells and pericytes during embryonic blood vessel formation in the mouse. Development 1999;126(14):3047–3055.
156. Noguera-Troise I, Daly C, Papadopoulos NJ, et al. Blockade of Dll4 inhibits tumour growth by promoting non-productive angiogenesis. Nature 2006;444(7122):1032–1037.
157. Ribatti D. Endogenous inhibitors of angiogenesis: a historical review. Leuk Res 2009;33(5):638–644.
158. Grant MA, Kalluri R. Structural basis for the functions of endogenous angiogenesis inhibitors. Cold Spring Harb Symp Quant Biol 2005;70:399–410.
159. Carmeliet P, Jain RK. Angiogenesis in cancer and other diseases. Nature 2000;407(6801):249–257.
160. Kerbel RS. Tumor angiogenesis. N Engl J Med 2008;358(19):2039–2049.
161. Kranenburg O, Gebbink MF, Voest EE. Stimulation of angiogenesis by Ras proteins. Biochim Biophys Acta 2004;1654(1):23–37.
162. Ravi R, Mookerjee B, Bhujwalla ZM, et al. Regulation of tumor angiogenesis by p53-induced degradation of hypoxia-inducible factor 1 alpha. Genes Dev 2000;14(1):34–44.
163. Kaelin WG Jr. The von Hippel-Lindau tumour suppressor protein: O2 sensing and cancer. Nat Rev Cancer 2008;8(11):865–873.
164. Ellis LM, Hicklin DJ. VEGF-targeted therapy: mechanisms of anti-tumour activity. Nat Rev Cancer 2008;8(8):579–591.
165. Heath VL, Bicknell R. Anticancer strategies involving the vasculature. Nat Rev Clin Oncol 2009;6(7):395–404.

166. Ferrara N, Hillan KJ, Gerber HP, et al. Discovery and development of bevacizumab, an anti-VEGF antibody for treating cancer. Nat Rev Drug Discov 2004;3(5): 391–400.

167. Faivre S, Demetri G, Sargent W, et al. Molecular basis for sunitinib efficacy and future clinical development. Nat Rev Drug Discov 2007;6(9):734–745.

168. Ellis LM, Hicklin DJ. Pathways mediating resistance to vascular endothelial growth factor-targeted therapy. Clin Cancer Res 2008;14(20):6371–6375.

169. Benesch M, Windelberg M, Sauseng W, et al. Compassionate use of bevacizumab (Avastin) in children and young adults with refractory or recurrent solid tumors. Ann Oncol 2008;19(4):807–813.

170. Glade Bender JL, Adamson PC, Reid JM, et al. Phase I trial and pharmacokinetic study of bevacizumab in pediatric patients with refractory solid tumors: a Children's Oncology Group Study. J Clin Oncol 2008;26(3):399–405.

171. Tong RT, Boucher Y, Kozin SV, et al. Vascular normalization by vascular endothelial growth factor receptor 2 blockade induces a pressure gradient across the vasculature and improves drug penetration in tumors. Cancer Res 2004;64(11): 3731–3736.

172. Jain RK. Normalizing tumor vasculature with anti-angiogenic therapy: a new paradigm for combination therapy. Nat Med 2001;7(9):987–989.

173. Olive KP, Jacobetz MA, Davidson CJ, et al. Inhibition of Hedgehog signaling enhances delivery of chemotherapy in a mouse model of pancreatic cancer. Science. 2009;324(5933): 1457–1461.

174. Ebos JM, Lee CR, Cruz-Munoz W, et al. Accelerated metastasis after short-term treatment with a potent inhibitor of tumor angiogenesis. Cancer Cell 2009;15(3): 232–239.

175. Loges S, Mazzone M, Hohensinner P, et al. Silencing or fueling metastasis with VEGF inhibitors: antiangiogenesis revisited. Cancer Cell 2009;15(3):167–170.

176. Paez-Ribes M, Allen E, Hudock J, et al. Antiangiogenic therapy elicits malignant progression of tumors to increased local invasion and distant metastasis. Cancer Cell 2009;15(3):220–231.

CHAPTER 5 ■ TUMOR IMMUNOLOGY AND PEDIATRIC CANCER

CRYSTAL L. MACKALL AND PAUL M. SONDEL

The immune system is a complex network of cells and soluble factors that has evolved primarily to respond to infection by foreign, pathogenic organisms. Its hallmarks are its ability to recognize danger, to mobilize a multipronged effector response, and to generate "immunologic memory" that renders future responses to the same organism more efficient. The interface between the immune system and cancer occurs at multiple levels. First, immunodeficient patients have a higher incidence of cancer. Second, cancer itself and many cancer therapies are immunosuppressive and infection is a major comorbidity in cancer patients. Third, a dynamic microenvironment exists at the immune:tumor interface, which sculpts incipient cancers to acquire immune-evasive properties and can positively or negatively affect tumor growth. Fourth, both passive and active immunotherapy can provide substantial antitumor effects. Given the goal of finding less toxic, more effective therapies for childhood cancers, it is essential that the pediatric oncology community learn how to apply current principles of tumor immunology to develop targeted immunotherapies for pediatric cancer. This chapter will review the interface between cancer and the immune system, with emphasis on issues relevant to pediatric cancer.

OVERVIEW OF THE IMMUNE SYSTEM

Immune Tolerance and the Danger Model

Historically, immunologists worked from the premise that the immune system functions primarily by discriminating self from nonself, a model that works well when one considers immune responses to infectious pathogens. The self/nonself model places primary responsibility for preventing autoimmunity at the level of immune cell development, emphasizing that the immune system becomes tolerant to self-antigens during lymphopoiesis through "clonal deletion" of T and B cells that possess antigen-specific receptors recognizing self-antigens. This model holds that the immune repertoire is efficiently cleansed of autoreactive cells during lymphopoiesis, thus eliminating the need for peripheral mechanisms to maintain self-tolerance. However, clinical and experimental data have demonstrated that clonal deletion during lymphopoiesis is not complete, since healthy humans and mice harbor sizable numbers of T cells and B cells expressing receptors that recognize self-antigens. Because many tumor antigens are self-antigens expressed at high levels during development but present at lower levels in adult life, the distinction between a clonal deletion process, which eliminates essentially all "autoreactive" cells, versus a process that leaves room for the induction of immune responses to some self-elements, such as tumor antigens, is directly relevant to tumor immunology.

One poignant demonstration that clonal deletion does not eradicate all self-reactive elements comes from studies of immune responses in patients with melanoma. Most patients with malignant melanoma harbor melanoma-reactive T cells that recognize so-called melanocyte differentiation antigens, molecules highly expressed during melanocyte development and at low levels on normal melanocytes throughout life. The clonal deletion model predicted that cells reactive to such antigens were completely eliminated during lymphopoiesis, but immunotherapy using interleukin-2 (IL-2) or tumor vaccines reproducibly induces immune responses toward these self-antigens that often induce vitiligo, providing direct evidence for autoimmune reactivity directed at normal melanocytes.[1] These insights, and others, raised fundamental questions as to how self-tolerance is maintained in health and how tolerance to tumor antigens could be reversed via immunotherapies.

To explain how immune tolerance is maintained despite the presence of sizable numbers of self-reactive lymphocytes, a newer *danger model* of immune tolerance has been put forth, which can be seen as an extension of the self/nonself model. The "danger model" emphasizes a critical role for innate immune responses in maintaining or breaking self-tolerance. The innate immune system comprises dendritic cells (DCs), neutrophils, monocytes and tissue macrophages, eosinophils, basophils, natural killer (NK) cells, and the complement cascade (Fig. 5.1). Innate immunity serves as the first line of defense against infectious pathogens, and the critical role that neutrophils play in controlling bacterial and fungal infection in cancer patients is well known (Chapter 40). Innate immune cells also play a central role in recognizing danger signals associated with infection and tissue inflammation, and as a result initiate, amplify, and direct adaptive immune responses. Substantial progress has been made in understanding the molecular basis for danger recognition by immune cells, especially in response to infection (Table 5.1). Triggering of pattern recognition receptors, most notably toll-like receptors (TLRs) on the surface of innate immune cells by pathogen-associated molecular proteins (PAMPs) such as bacterial cell wall components, lipopolysaccharide (LPS), viral RNA or DNA, activates innate immune cells and subsequently initiates adaptive immune responses. A more evolving field of study is under way to define the mechanisms whereby tissue damage, in the absence of infection, can initiate inflammation and adaptive immune responses and several damage-associated molecular proteins (DAMPs) released by dead or dying tissues have now been identified. Modulation of DAMPs within neoplastic tissues is an important focus of study in tumor immunology today and will be discussed later in this chapter.

Dendritic Cells

DCs are present in only trace amounts (1%–2% of nucleated cells) in blood, bone marrow, and tissues but are primary sentinels of the immune system. Advances in their characterization

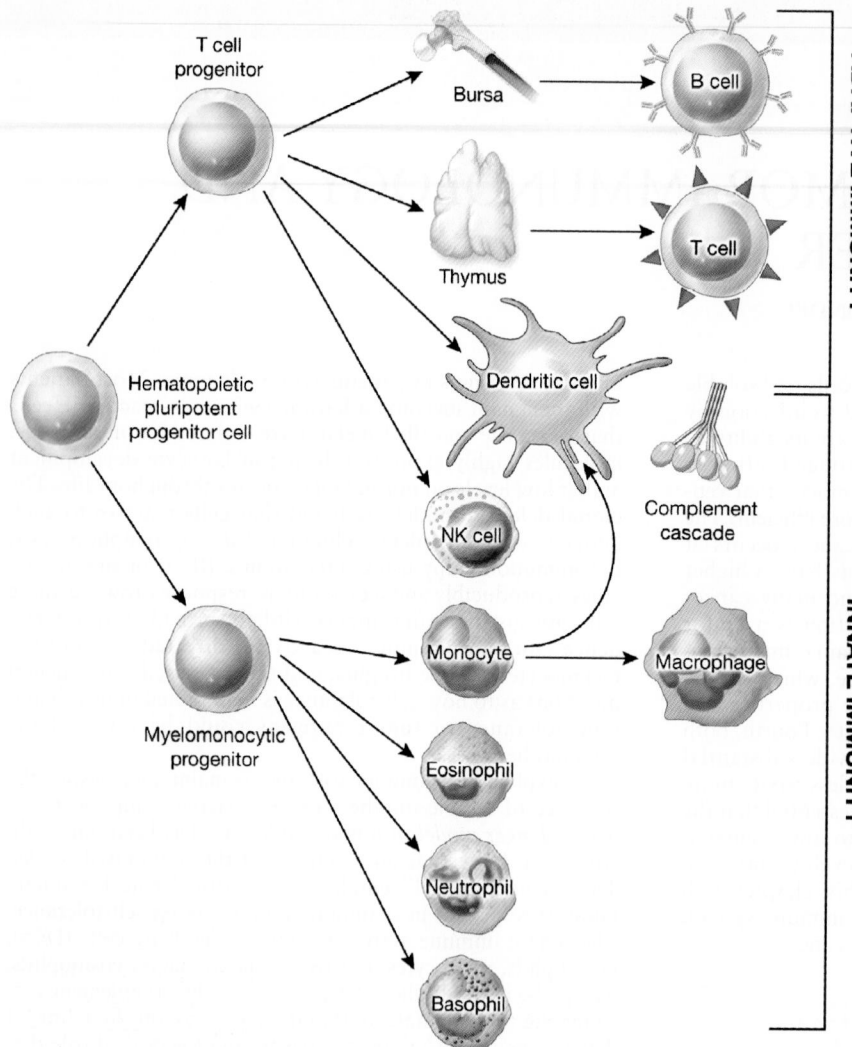

FIGURE 5.1 Innate and adaptive immune systems. All cells of the immune system are derived from pluripotent hematopoietic stem cells that give rise to two distinct progenitors: one for lymphoid cells and the other for myeloid cells. The common lymphoid progenitor has the potential to differentiate into T, B, NK, and lymphoid dendritic cells depending on the microenvironment to which it homes (i.e., the thymus or bone marrow). Immune cells derived from primitive myeloid progenitors include phagocytic effectors (e.g., macrophages, neutrophils, and monocytes) and myeloid dendritic cells. It should be emphasized that the distinction between these systems is somewhat artificial since there is significant cross talk between innate and adaptive immune effectors during the initiation and completion of the immune response.

represent a major advance in immunology over the last three decades. Current models incorporate at least two major lineages of DCs, with differential levels of maturation within each lineage that can be defined by using cell surface markers and functional and morphologic criteria (Fig. 5.2). Both macrophages and myeloid DCs are monocyte progeny residing in tissues, but they are clearly distinct from one another. Macrophages are primarily scavengers, which phagocytize debris but are poor antigen presenters, express low levels of class II major histocompatibility complex (MHC), and do not express sufficient costimulatory molecules to initiate T-cell responses. Myeloid DCs express CD11c and variable levels of MHC class II, depending on their maturational status. Immature myeloid DCs in the skin, termed *Langerhans cells*, are perhaps the most well known and best characterized of the myeloid DCs; however, DCs reside in essentially every tissue of the body where they continually survey the antigenic milieu via macropinocytosis.

Immature myeloid DCs have an exquisite capacity to process exogenous antigen from protein to peptide and to express the peptide on their cell surface in the context of MHC class I (termed *cross-priming*) and MHC class II. In the absence of inflammation, immature DCs do not initiate immune responses and likely contribute to immune tolerance

to self-antigens through as yet poorly understood mechanisms. However, upon contact with danger signals (discussed earlier) immature DCs differentiate into mature DCs, characterized by high-level MHC class I, class II, IL-12 production, and costimulatory molecule expression necessary for T-cell activation, which serves to direct T-cell responses toward a T-helper-1 (Th1) phenotype.[2] T cell and DC cross talk also follows, with DC-expressed costimulatory molecules activating T cells and CD40L on activated CD4[+] cells upregulating B7-1, B7-2, and MHC molecules on DCs.[3] Remarkably, myeloid DCs can be readily generated *in vitro* by incubating monocytes with granulocyte-macrophage colony-stimulating factor (GM-CSF) and IL-4 or by incubating pluripotent hematopoietic progenitor cells with GM-CSF[2,4] and can be matured by using a variety of agents. This ready availability has greatly aided study of these normally rare cells and has also provided opportunity for clinical applications of DC-based immunotherapy for cancer.

Plasmacytoid DCs, DC2, or lymphoid DCs represent a separate lineage, at least some of which are derived from the lymphoid progenitor cells (Fig. 5.1). Plasmacytoid DCs, characterized by expression of IL-3R (CD123) are postulated to play a role in central and peripheral tolerance, but these cells are also a ready source of interferon-α (IFN-α) following activation and

TABLE 5.1

PATHOGEN- AND DAMAGE-ASSOCIATED MOLECULAR PROTEINS THAT PROVIDE DANGER SIGNALS TO ACTIVATE INNATE IMMUNE RESPONSES

Molecule	Source	Receptor
Pathogen-associated molecular proteins (PAMPS)		
Peptidoglycan	Gram-positive bacteria	TLR2
dsRNA	Viruses	TLR3
LPS	Gram-negative bacteria	TLR4
Mannan	Candida	TLR4
Flagellin	Flagellated bacteria	TLR5
ssRNA	RNA viruses	TLR7, 8
CpG	Viruses, bacteria, protozoa	TLR9
Damage-associated molecular proteins (DAMPs, aka alarmins)		
HMGB1	Nuclear protein	RAGE
S100s (aka *calgranulins*)	Calcium-binding proteins	RAGE (S100A12,B); TLRs (S100A8,9)
HSPs	Intracellular chaperones	TLRs
IL-1α	Secreted by activated immune cells	IL-1R
Uric acid	Nucleic acid turnover	?Prion protein [Prp(c)]
Galectins	Surface expression on a variety of cell types	Glycans present on glycoproteins and glycolipids

dsRNA, double-stranded RNA; LPS, lipopolysaccharide; ssRNA, single-stranded RNA; CpG, oligonucleotide with immune-stimulating properties; HMGB1, high-mobility group box 1 protein; HSPs, heat shock proteins; IL-1α, interleukin-1α; TLR, toll-like receptor; RAGE, receptor for advanced glycation endproducts; IL-1R, interleukin-1 receptor.

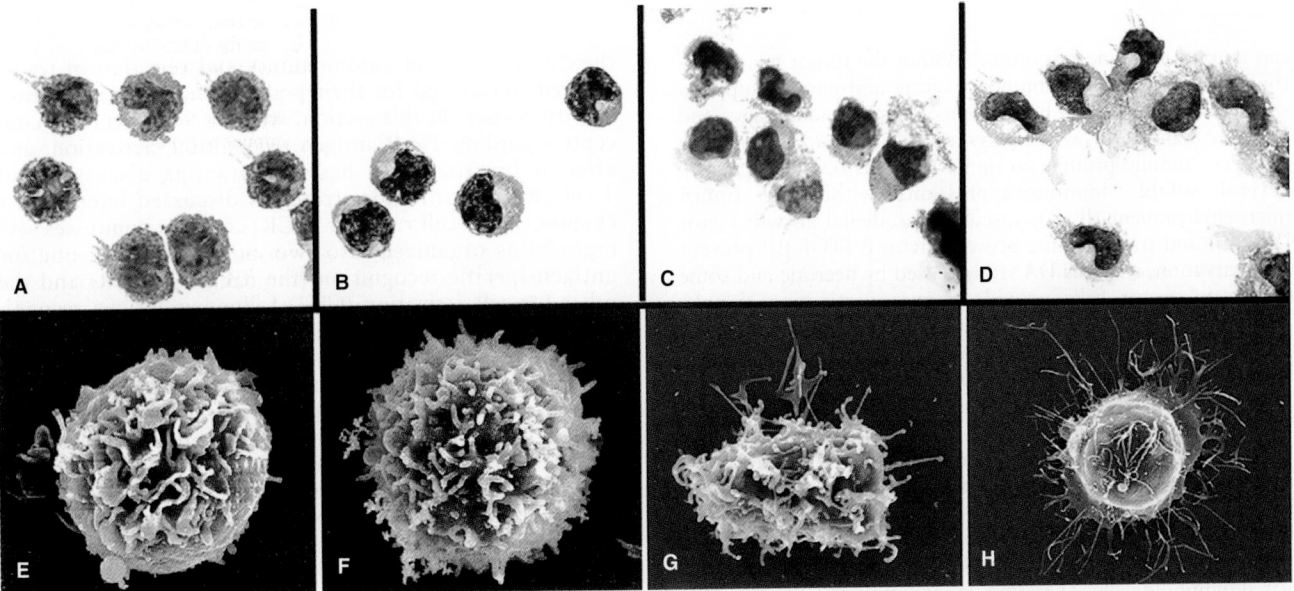

FIGURE 5.2 Morphology of dendritic cell (DC) subsets. Rhesus pre-DC subsets were stained with Giemsa (**A–D**) or examined using scanning electron microscopy (**E–H**) before and after culture with DC maturation-inducing factors GM-CSF and CD40L. **A:** Freshly sorted CD11c+ premyeloid DCs showing a high nucleus-cytoplasm ratio, reniform or multilobulated nuclei, and few prominent dendrites. **B:** Freshly sorted CD123++ prelymphoid DCs with a typical prominent Golgi region and lateralized reniform nucleus. **C:** After culture with rhGM-CSF and rhCD40L for 24 hours, CD11c+ premyeloid DCs showed abundant and well-developed dendrites. **D:** After culture with rhIL-3 and CD40L for 3 days, CD123++ pre-DCs also acquired striking dendritic morphology. **E–H:** SEM images of cells corresponding to populations in panels **A** to **D**. Original magnifications: ×400 (**A–D**), ×7500 (**E**), ×9000 (**F**), ×5000 (**G**), and ×3500 (**H**). (From Coates PT, Barratt-Boyes SM, Zhang L, et al. Dendritic cell subsets in blood and lymphoid tissue of rhesus monkeys and their mobilization with flt3 ligand. Blood 2003;102:2513.)

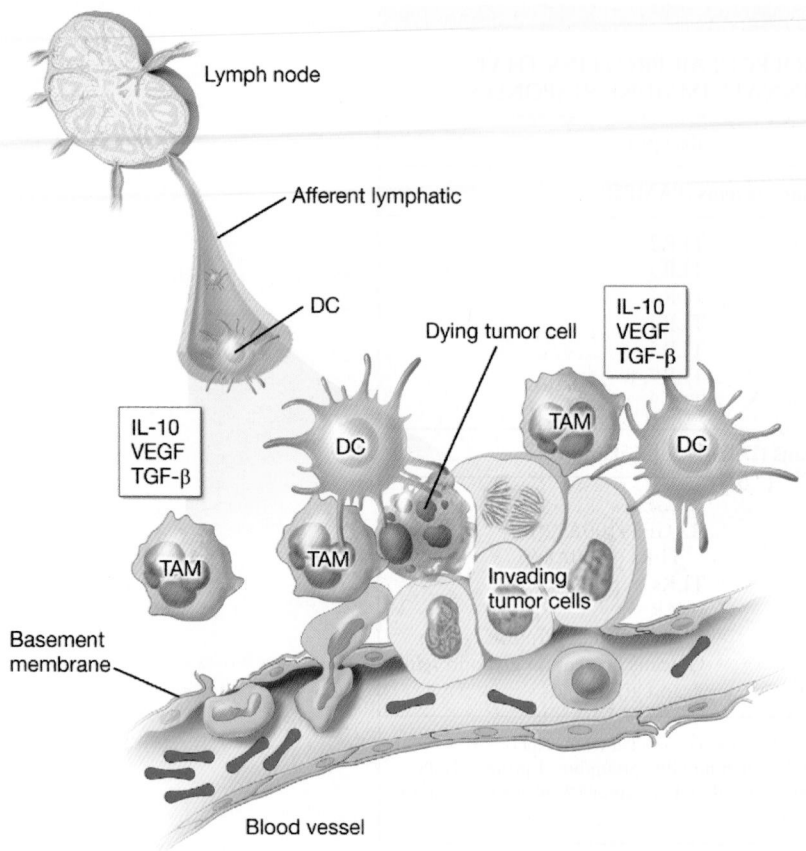

Lymph node

Afferent lymphatic

DC

Dying tumor cell

IL-10
VEGF
TGF-β

TAM

DC

DC

IL-10
VEGF
TGF-β

TAM

TAM

Invading
tumor cells

Basement
membrane

Blood vessel

FIGURE 5.3 The immune: tumor interface. The microenvironment of a growing tumor represents a complex and dynamic interaction between an invading tumor and the inflammatory/immune response. Tumor invasion through the basement membrane is required for metastasis and predicted to induce activation of innate immune effectors that transit from the blood to tissue. If local inflammation is sufficient to activate resident dendritic cells, tumor antigens will be acquired and transported to draining lymph nodes, where T-cell activation can occur. If immunosuppressive mediators predominate, local inflammation is prevented and immune priming does not occur. Immunoactivating elements including HSPs (heat shock proteins; elaborated from dying tumors) and dendritic cell (DC)-activating receptors present on the surface of apoptotic and necrotic tumor cells. Immunosuppressive elements include soluble mediators released by the tumor, including IL-10, VEGF, and TGF-β. TAMs are tumor associated macrophages which contribute to local immunosuppression.

can amplify immune responses.[4] Within the tumor microenvironment, a variety of immunoactivating and immunosuppressive signals are received by tumor-associated macrophages and DCs, the balance of which plays a critical role in determining whether immune priming to tumor antigens occurs (Fig. 5.3). Several soluble immunosuppressants within the tumor microenvironment (IL-10, vascular endothelial growth factor [VEGF], and transforming growth factor-β [TGF-β]) prevent DC activation, whereas DAMPs released by necrotic and some apoptotic tumor cells provide immune activating signals. Tumor-associated macrophages can also be important modulators of immunosuppression within the tumor microenvironment. Tumor-associated macrophages can mediate both protumor (mitogens, growth factors, enzymes, angiogenic stimulants) and antitumor (tumor reactive and immune-activating cytokines, lysozymes, proteases, complement components) effects. Further, in the later stages of the immune response, tumor necrosis factor (TNF)-related apoptosis-inducing ligand (TRAIL) expression by DCs can directly kill TRAIL-sensitive tumors or impair immune surveillance by killing TRAIL-sensitive activated lymphoid cells. Therefore, innate immune responses play a requisite role in initiating adaptive immunity within the tumor microenvironment, and they likely also play important roles in amplifying or suppressing existent antitumor immune responses.

T Lymphocytes

T lymphocytes (designated "T" for their thymic origin) evolved primarily to eradicate viral infections. In modern medicine, however, T-cell responses are also important for their central role in autoimmunity and rejection of transplanted tissues and for their potential for inducing antitumor responses. In this section, we will review current concepts regarding T-cell antigen recognition, activation, and effector function, as a basis for framing discussions of T-cell–based antitumor strategies discussed later in this chapter. The T-cell receptor (TCR) complex comprises several chains organized into two major elements, one for antigen-specific recognition (the αβ or γδ TCR) and the other for cell activation (CD3) following antigen recognition. All T cells express identical CD3 molecules (comprising γ, δ, ε, and ζ chains). CD3 is essential for transmitting T-cell activation signals from the cell surface to the interior, following interaction with antigen. CD3 signaling activates a cascade of tyrosine kinase–based phosphorylation events, which in turn leads to calcium influx and activation of phospholipase C, eventually resulting in cell division and cytokine production. For approximately 95% of T cells, the antigen-specific TCR comprises a unique αβ heterodimer, whereas 5% of T cells recognize antigen through the γδ TCR. Unlike αβ T cells, γδ T cells reside primarily in the gut, show limited TCR diversity, possess potent cytolytic capacity prior to activation, and can recognize virally infected cells in an MHC nonrestricted manner (reviewed in Ref 5). γδ T cells likely serve as a first line of defense against viral and other pathogens.

The αβ TCR heterodimer endows T cells with fine specificity for antigen recognition, since peptides differing in only one amino acid can show widely disparate activation potentials for a given αβ TCR. Genes that are similar in structure to immunoglobulin genes control the expression of the αβ TCR. All nonimmune cells in any individual contain an identical pattern of αβ TCR genes maintained in germline configuration, which is a linear arrangement of segments termed *variable* (V), *diversity* (for β chain only) (D), *junctional* (J), and *constant* (C) regions. Through a process termed *T-cell receptor gene rearrangement*, the VDJ elements of both the α-chain and the β-chain of each unique αβ TCR first rearrange in different combinations, and then "N segment additions" are added to further modify each rearranged chain. TCR rearrangement occurs during the early stages of thymocyte development and results in the TCR diversity that is the hallmark of T-cell immunity. When TCR rearrangement is completed, each individual T cell expresses only one form of the rearranged αβ TCR, and all subsequent progeny of this T cell also express the identical rearranged αβ TCR. From the enormous potential repertoire of TCR specificities that are randomly generated, a carefully controlled series of positive and negative selection events occurs during thymopoiesis, resulting in the survival of a mere fraction of the T cells that begin the process. T cells are selected in the thymus largely on the basis of their TCR-binding affinity for self-MHC. TCR specificities showing intermediate affinity for self-MHC molecules are generally preferred, whereas those with very low or very high affinity do not survive. This maximizes the chance for efficient recognition of antigens from foreign pathogens (presented by self-MHC) while minimizing the chance for autoimmunity. As discussed earlier, the process by which self-reactive cells are clonally deleted is not entirely complete; however, it does delete most T cells with high-affinity receptors for self-antigens, leaving the repertoire of T cells available to recognize most tumor antigens (particularly those that are autologous differentiation antigens) disadvantaged in general, compared with those responding to truly foreign elements.

Molecular analysis of the rearranged TCR-DNA within T-cell populations is useful for a variety of purposes. First, it can distinguish polyclonal reactive processes (i.e., a T-cell response to a viral antigen) from monoclonal malignant expansions (i.e., a T-cell malignancy). Second, molecular monitoring of the unique TCR rearrangements within clonally derived T-cell malignancies by using polymerase chain reaction (PCR) can allow for the sensitive detection of minimal residual neoplastic disease, although this requires that the unique rearrangement for a given individual's leukemia be genetically sequenced (see Chapters 8, 19, and 24). Third, measures of the relative diversity within the TCR repertoire have been used to evaluate the effectiveness of immune reconstitution as immune competence generally correlates with greater TCR diversity. Fourth, during the process of α-chain rearrangement, an element of DNA is frequently excised, which remains as a cytoplasmic remnant of TCR rearrangement, which is termed a *T-cell receptor excision circle* (TREC). Since TRECs do not reproduce as T cells subsequently divide, the existence of TRECs within a given population correlates with the number of recent thymic emigrants, a measure that correlates with thymic function and has been used in the study of immune reconstitution.[6]

T cells recognize peptides derived from cellular proteins, which become accessible on the surface of the target cell via binding to MHC molecules (Fig. 5.4). Crystallographic analysis of human MHC molecules, called *HLA* (human leukocyte antigen), reveals both highly polymorphic and nonpolymorphic regions. The nonpolymorphic region on class I HLA molecules (HLA-A, B, and C) binds to the CD8+ molecule (expressed primarily on cytotoxic T cells) and the nonpolymorphic region on MHC class II molecules (HLA-DR, DP, DQ) bind to the CD4+ molecule (expressed primarily on helper T cells). The polymorphic regions of the HLA molecules form a groove, which binds peptides with varying affinities. In order for a peptide to be visible to a reactive T cell, it must bind avidly within the polymorphic groove of a given

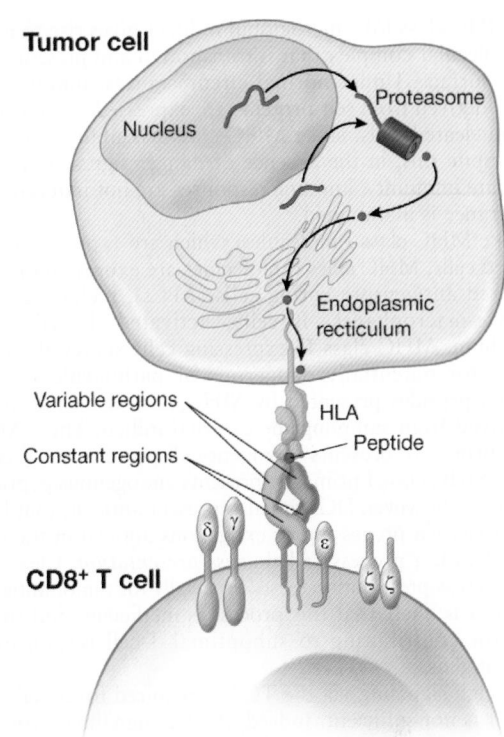

FIGURE 5.4 Peptide recognition by the T-cell receptor (TCR) complex. The α and β polypeptide chains of the TCR is comprised of variable and constant regions (shown in blue), that form a heterodimer anchored in the T-cell membrane. The heterodimer recognizes and binds to peptide associated with an HLA molecule on the surface of a presenting cell *(shown in the figure as a tumor cell)*. The nonpolymorphic CD3 polypeptides (γ, δ, ε, and ζ) are assembled together with the αβ TCR and are involved in signal transduction. Peptides presented by HLA class I molecules are typically derived from the intracellular processing of endogenous proteins that are degraded in the proteasome and subsequently are transported to the endoplasmic reticulum, where they bind nascent MHC molecules prior to transport to the cell surface.

HLA molecule. Peptides bound to MHC class I are typically 9 to 11 amino acid in length, whereas MHC class II binding peptides are typically 13 to 20 amino acid in length. This molecular complex, comprising the polymorphic component of the MHC, with a small peptide within its groove, can then, selectively, be recognized by the polymorphic components of certain αβ TCR. Because the binding of individual peptides varies greatly among the multitudes of MHC alleles that exist across individuals, individual TCRs recognize only specific peptides when presented by a correspondingly specific MHC molecule; they will not recognize the same peptide presented by a genetically distinct MHC molecule. This property has been termed *MHC restriction* and serves as a fundamental dogma of T-cell immunology.[7]

A detailed discussion of the biochemistry and the cell biology of antigen presentation by MHC molecules is beyond the scope of this chapter, but to summarize, endogenous cellular proteins undergo proteolysis and processing in the proteasome. Some peptides derived from this process of normal protein turnover are transported into the endoplasmic reticulum via chaperone molecules, called *transporters of antigen processing* (TAP), that transport peptides into the endoplasmic reticulum via an energy-dependent process. In the endoplasmic reticulum, TAP molecules transfer peptides to unstable MHC class I/β₂-microglobulin dimers. The binding of peptide to the MHC class I/β₂-microglobulin dimer gives rise to a stable trimolecular complex that is transported and presented on the cell surface. Under normal circumstances, innumerable peptides derived from self-proteins are expressed continuously on all nucleated cells, since MHC class I is ubiquitous (Fig. 5.4). Despite this, in the absence of danger signals that activate innate immunity, immune responses are not induced, and self-tolerance is maintained.

Unlike MHC class I molecules, which are expressed on all nucleated cells, MHC class II molecules are expressed only on specialized antigen-presenting cells (APCs), including DCs, monocyte-macrophages, B cells, activated T cells, and endothelium. MHC class II–expressing cells survey the environment for potentially dangerous or pathogenic stimuli; therefore, peptides presented by MHC class II include products derived from sampling the external milieu. Thus, MHC class II primarily presents "exogenous" proteins to T cells, whereas MHC class I primarily presents endogenous peptides. Importantly, however, DCs can also present antigens that have been derived via processing of exogenous antigen in the context of class I, a process called *cross-presentation*. Clear evidence for cross-presentation exists, especially for tumor antigens; however, it is likely that this process is inefficient, and this is one factor contributing to suboptimal T-cell responses to tumor antigens.

Although signaling via the TCR is required for T-cell activation, it is not sufficient. Indeed, if TCR signaling (typically referred to as *signal 1*) is provided in the absence of activating costimulatory signals (signal 2), T cells become anergic and resistant to subsequent activation. Signal 2 can be either stimulatory or inhibitory (Fig. 5.5), with those signals augmenting T-cell activation described as *costimulatory* and those preventing T-cell activation described as *checkpoints*. The most potent costimulatory signals for naive T cells are the B7 family of molecules, which are expressed on the surface of professional APCs. B7-1 (CD80) and B7-2 (CD86) are surface glycoproteins, which interact with CD28 on the surface of T cells. Cross-linking of CD28 during T-cell activation potently enhances proliferation of responding T cells in part, by upregulating IL-2 production. However, CTLA4, a prototypic checkpoint molecule with high affinity for B7-1 and B7-2, competes with CD28 for binding with these molecules. Rather than transmit activation signals to T cells as CD28 does, CTLA4 ligation diminishes T-cell activation. Under normal circumstances, this limits the magnitude of the immune response, thus diminishing the likelihood of autoimmunity and lymphoproliferation. Congenital absence of CTLA4 in mice leads to lethal lymphoproliferation, and inhibition of CTLA4 during the course of an immune response amplifies immunity toward poorly immunogenic tumors in mouse models. Remarkably, blockade of CTLA4 using anti-CTLA4 monoclonal antibodies (mAbs) induces antitumor effects in a variety of malignancies, and these are often associated with autoimmune adverse events such as the development of colitis, iritis, and hypophysitis. These recent clinical results with anti-CTLA4 mAb directly demonstrate that peripheral mechanisms continuously prevent autoimmunity during health, and those therapies that interrupt these immune-inhibitory pathways can directly augment preexisting endogenous antitumor immunity.[8-10] Several ongoing studies are under way to identify the best approach for utilizing CTLA4 blockade in the context of cancer therapy and to identify other checkpoints whereby inhibition can directly augment antitumor immunity.[11] Among these is PD-1, a molecule expressed on exhausted or senescent T cells, which limits their proliferative potential.[12] Mouse models and human studies have shown that tumor-infiltrating lymphocytes are high PD-1 expressers, and preclinical and emerging clinical studies

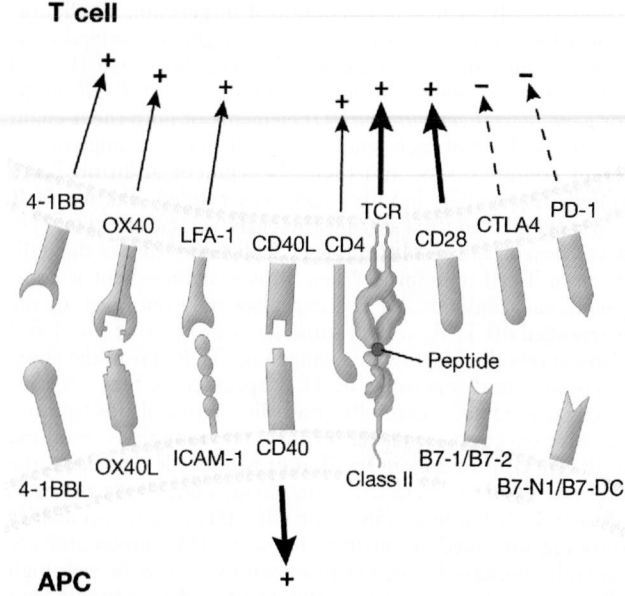

FIGURE 5.5 The T-cell immune synapse. Activation of T lymphocytes by antigen-presenting cell (APC) requires TCR signaling via peptides bound to HLA as well as costimulatory signals delivered by several potential receptor ligand interactions. Many positive costimulators that contribute to T-cell activation have been identified and are shown. A few negative costimulatory molecules (CTLA4, PD-1), also known as checkpoints, have also been described. CTLA4 acts as a negative regulator of T-cell activation and competes with CD28 for binding to CD80 and CD86 on APCs. CD40-CD40L interactions primarily signal the APC, which further upregulates costimulatory molecules. Additional interactions occur between CD4 molecule on the T cell and the nonpolymorphic region of the class II HLA molecule. 4-1BB is primarily a costimulator for CD8⁺ T cells, while OX40 is primarily a costimulator for CD4⁺ T cells.

suggest that blocking PD-1 may enhance T-cell–mediated antitumor effects.

Once activated, T cells participate in immune responses either via secretion of soluble mediators or through cell-to-cell interactions. In general, CD4⁺ cells are described as "helper" T cells (Th) since they primarily amplify and regulate immune responses but are less involved in effector functions. CD4⁺ cells also are rich sources of soluble mediators, including IL-2, a critical cytokine for amplifying CD8⁺ proliferation; IL-10, which dampens immunity by downregulating APC function; IL-4, which provides a critical signal for inducing humoral immunity; and IL-17, which may play an important role in antitumor immunity.[13] A small subset of CD4⁺ cells, which constitutively coexpresses CD25 (the α-chain of the IL-2 receptor [IL-2R]) potently suppress or regulate T-cell immune responses.[14] These are known as *regulatory T cells* (Tregs) and are distinct in function from activated Th, which transiently express CD25. Tregs modulate autoimmunity, graft-vs-host disease (GVHD), and tumor immunity; incorporation of approaches to deplete Tregs can augment antitumor immunity in several animal models. Remarkably IL-2, which has been used as an immune stimulant for many years, selectively expands Tregs, and this immunosuppressive effect of rhIL-2 may serve to limit its effectiveness in the context of antitumor immunity.[15]

CD8⁺ cells serve primarily as effector populations, and in addition to their ability to kill target cells, they are also a rich source of cytokines including IFN-γ. Activated cytolytic CD8⁺ cells, termed *cytolytic T lymphocytes* (CTLs), recognize target

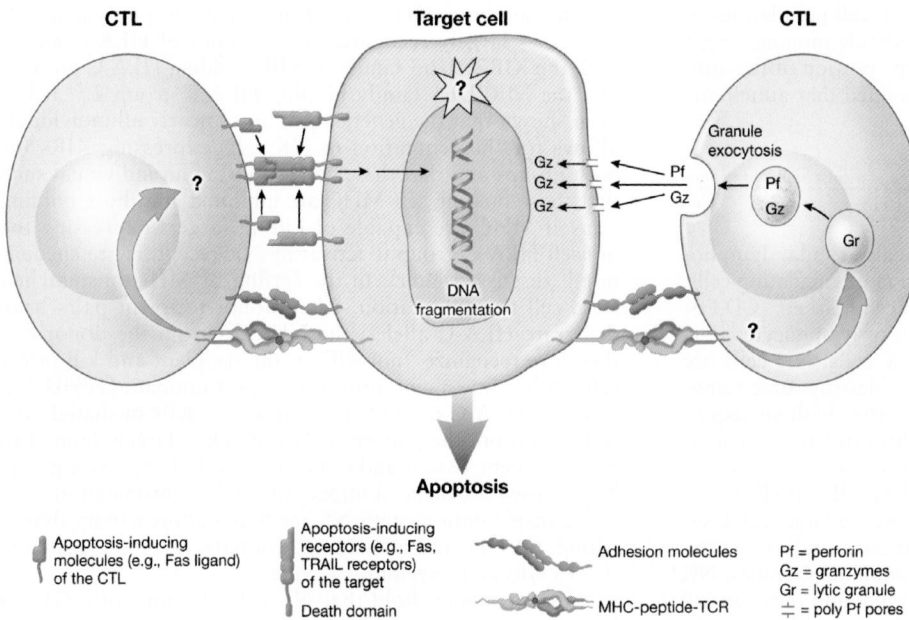

CTL   Target cell   CTL

Granule
exocytosis

Gz
Gz   Pf
Gz   Pf
Gz

Pf
Gz

Gr

DNA
fragmentation

Apoptosis

Apoptosis-inducing molecules (e.g., Fas ligand) of the CTL	Apoptosis-inducing receptors (e.g., Fas, TRAIL receptors) of the target	Adhesion molecules	Pf = perforin
	Death domain	MHC-peptide-TCR	Gz = granzymes
			Gr = lytic granule
			= poly Pf pores

FIGURE 5.6 Mechanisms of lymphocyte-mediated cytolysis. Shown is a schematic diagram of the nonsecretory, receptor (e.g., Fas and TRAIL)-mediated (*left*) and the secretory, perforin/granzyme-mediated (*right*) mechanisms of lymphocytotoxicity. (Adapted from Berke G. Unlocking the secrets of CTL and NK cells. Immunol Today 1995;16:334.)

cells through their T-cell antigen receptor molecules and then cause rapid cellular destruction through one of two pathways. Granule-mediated cytolysis involves perforin (a complement-like molecule) release, which first creates pores in the target membrane, followed by release of granzymes, which then efficiently enter the target cell and induce apoptosis. Alternatively, CD8+ cells can induce apoptosis through TNF receptor family members, including TNF, Fas, or TRAIL receptors (Fig. 5.6).[16,17]

B Lymphocytes

The primary role of B lymphocytes (designated "B" for their bursal origin in fowl) is the production of immunoglobulins, soluble molecules that specifically recognize protein, glycoprotein, and carbohydrate antigens and trigger cellular and molecular responses upon antigen binding. Immunoglobulins bind to whole circulating proteins or molecules expressed on the surface of cells or pathogens. This is to be distinguished from T cells, which do not recognize intact proteins, but rather peptides presented on the cell surface of MHC-bearing cells. Each immunoglobulin molecule consists of light (κ or λ) chains and heavy (M, G, A, D, or E) chains. Intact immunoglobulin molecules have a variable antigen-binding (Fab) end and a constant end (Fc) that can fix and activate complement and bind to Fc receptors expressed by a variety of cells. Memory B cells and plasma cells continue to produce immunoglobulin for years after immunization; therefore, circulating antibody can provide rapid protection against second or subsequent exposure to antigenic pathogens.

Like TCR rearrangement that gives rise to exquisite T-cell diversity, germline and nonimmune cells also contain the same pattern of germline immunoglobulin genes, whereas developing B cells rearrange immunoglobulin genes to generate remarkable B-cell diversity. Immunoglobulin gene rearrangement involves selection from multiple segment possibilities within variable (V), diversity (D), and joining (J) regions. The recombination activating gene proteins, RAG1 and RAG2, are critical in this process. As there are 40 VH regions; 27 D regions, with 3 different reading frames; and 6 JH regions, this could result in 19,440 possible heavy chain combinations. Linking the V and J regions for each of the κ and λ light chains yields 265 different light chain combinations. Random pairing of heavy and light chains would thus yield more than 5 million combinations of distinct immunoglobulin possibilities. These combination estimates may then be expanded by several logs when considering the small substitutions of nucleotides induced by "flexible" insertions at the somatic recombination and splice sites.[18] Thus individuals' immune repertoire might allow 10^{11} different unique antigen-binding combinations within their set of immunoglobulins. While a single B cell and its progeny can secrete many copies of a single specific immunoglobulin molecule, different B cells, having different immunoglobulin gene rearrangement patterns, make distinct immunoglobulin molecules.

Efficient activation of B cells to secrete immunoglobulin molecules usually requires interactions with antigen-specific T cells that have become activated during the course of immune response induction. Some of this T-cell "help" is accomplished via secretion of cytokines such as IL-2, but a substantial component of T-cell help is provided by the cell-associated molecule, CD40L, which is critical for directing B cells to generate antigen-specific immunoglobulin G (IgG). Indeed, humans lacking CD40 have a defect in isotype switch, resulting in an accumulation of IgM molecules, known as the *hyper IgM syndrome*.[19]

Just as molecular characterization of TCR gene patterns can differentiate polyclonal from oligoclonal or monoclonal T-cell populations, the same is possible for immunoglobulin gene rearrangement patterns among B-cell populations. This information has been of use in characterizing a variety of B-cell tumors since monoclonal B-cell tumors consist of a population that all express the identical surface immunoglobulin. The unique structure of a given immunoglobulin's antigen-binding sequence can itself be recognized and is known as its *idiotype*. Identification of a monoclonal population of B cells[20] all with the same idiotype allows malignant cells to be distinguished from normal polyclonal B cells, which do not express the same idiotype. Thus idiotypes can function as tumor-specific markers, and idiotypes have also been the target for individualized immune therapy for some B-cell malignancies, wherein recombinant vaccines are created from the unique idiotype found within the clonal B-cell populations in an individual's lymphoma.[21] Here the peptide immune target for the T cell is derived from the idiotype portion of the antibody itself; T-cell responses can be generated that attack any cell expressing this idiotype.

Natural Killer Cells

Within the population of morphologically similar lymphocytes, there is a relatively small population of circulating cells, which does not express mature T- or B-cell markers (CD3 or immunoglobulin). This third population of lymphocytes (Fig. 5.1) is composed predominantly of NK cells. NK cells are notable for their ability to spontaneously destroy some tumor cells and virally infected populations *in vitro*, without requiring prior immunization or activation. This cytolytic capacity is mediated via the same molecules used by cytolytic T cells (i.e., perforin, granzyme, Fas-Fas ligand, and TRAIL-TRAIL receptor interaction, as shown in Fig. 5.6) to induce target cell lysis. Unlike T cells, which require preactivation to induce expression of their perforin- and granzyme-containing granules, NK cells constitutively express cytolytic granules and thus can kill appropriate targets very rapidly. Indeed, the granules can be observed histologically and have led to the description of NK cells as large granular lymphocytes. The physiologic roles for NK cells are manifold.[22] First, NK cells contribute to a first line of defense against viral pathogens, as hosts lacking NK function show a great susceptibility to infection with herpes viruses.[23,24] Second, NK cells serve a unique position as communicators between innate and adaptive immune responses. To this end, NK cells are highly responsive to IL-12 and respond with the production of high levels of IFN-γ, which plays an important role in directing T helper cell responses toward a Th1 phenotype. The Th1 phenotype has been proposed to be responsible for the induction of cell-mediated immunity and is required for protection against a variety of infections. NK cells can also play a role in preventing the growth of cancer, also described as *immune surveillance*.[25]

The important role that NK cells play in preventing tumor growth and their potential as therapeutic agents in cancer immunotherapy has recently evolved as a result of a better understanding of the components of NK cell recognition. Rather than requiring MHC expression on target cells for induction of cytolysis (as is the case for T cells), NK cell lysis is inhibited by the presence of MHC molecules on the targets they recognize, thereby giving rise to a model for NK cell recognition, termed the *missing self hypothesis*. This model holds that under normal circumstances, NK cells are prevented from granule release by "tonic" engagement of inhibitory receptors on the surface of NK cells, which occurs via their interaction with self MHC. Substantial progress in the identification of these inhibitory receptors has been made in the last several years and include at least three families: (a) the killer inhibitory receptors (KIRs), which are most well characterized in humans and which comprise an immunoglobulin-like molecule; (b) CD94/NKG2 family of lectin-type molecules, which are predominantly characterized in humans; and (c) Ly49 family, which are seen in mice and comprise type II transmembrane protein dimers.

There appears to be great diversity within these systems of NK receptors, with a large diversity of KIRs expressed on individual NK cells and variable specificity for individual KIRs for individual MHC alleles. The recognition pattern of NK KIRs has recently provided an option for exploiting NK-mediated recognition in the context of MHC-mismatched allogeneic stem cell transplantation. Distinct KIR families recognize and, therefore, prevent killing of cells expressing a specific family of MHC class I molecules. In particular, KIR molecules largely recognize two families of HLA-C alleles with the KIR2DL2/3 family of KIRs binding HLA-C group 1 and the KIR2DL1 family binding HLA-C group 2.[26] It has been shown that the genetic makeup of nearly all individuals allows for the generation of NK cells expressing KIRs for both groups and that these coexist within an individual such that those binding self-MHC are inhibited and those binding nonself-MHC are capable of killing targets expressing the nonself HLA-C group if activating NK receptors are encountered (discussed later). In the setting of MHC-mismatched stem cell transplantation, when donor-recipient pairs have disparate HLA-C alleles, the NK cells from the donor can therefore recognize "nonself" in the recipient and kill target cells. While one might intuitively expect rampant GVHD as a result of HLA-C mismatch and resultant KIR-mediated NK-cell activation, the pattern of NK attack is largely limited to hematopoietic tissues and tumor tissues. In fact, investigators have shown a beneficial impact of HLA-C mismatch in stem cell transplantation, with NK-mediated alloreactivity diminishing GVHD and providing dramatic graft-vs-leukemia (GVL) effects in myeloid leukemia.[26]

Current models hold that NK cells do not cause GVHD because activating receptors must also be engaged to generate NK killing and most normal tissues do not express ligands for NK-activating receptors. Among the activating NK receptors is FcγRIII, (CD16), which binds cell-bound IgG molecules recognizing cell surface antigens. Through this interaction, NK cells can recognize, be activated by, and destroy cells that are "opsonized" by antibodies that recognize their cognate antigen on the cell surface, a mechanism designated *antibody-dependent cell-mediated cytotoxicity* (ADCC). Thus, NK cells can mediate destruction of other cells that are coated with antibody via ADCC, a feature of central importance for the efficacy of tumor-directed mAb-based therapy. This property has served as the basis for recent approaches integrating IL-2 infusions into treatment regimens with chimeric mAbs; the goal is to enhance ADCC by increasing the binding of mAbs to NK cells via the IL-2 receptor.[27]

Other activating receptors on NK cells have also recently been characterized. Among these, NKG2D is a C-type lectin receptor found on virtually all human and murine NK cells, which induces potent activation of cytokine release and induction of cell-mediated lysis. NKG2D is activated by tissue-restricted ligands that are overexpressed on cells that have been "stressed" (i.e., virally infected cells, cells exposed to "heat shock," and many types of malignant cells). In humans, the ligands that activate NKG2D are the MHC-like MICA and MICB molecules. Interestingly, while most epithelial cancers overexpress MICA, NK cells from patients with MICA expressing cancers are refractory to MICA-induced stimulation as a result of high levels of soluble MICA found in the serum of these cancer patients. Soluble MICA "strips" functioning NKG2D molecules from the surface of NK cells, leaving them transiently unresponsive to cell-bound MICA on tumor cells.[28] Many other activating NK receptors have been identified, including the NKp44, NKp46 and NKp30 receptors, which are found on distinct clones of human NK cells, and recognize distinct ligands,[29] although a complete delineation of all activating NK receptors and the full understanding of the biology of this system continues to evolve.

The current NK activation model integrates the need for NK recognition of "stressed cells" by activating ligands with the simultaneous requirement for recognition of "missing self". This model explains why NK cells may preferentially attack stressed or neoplastic cells that have downmodulated MHC molecules. In theory, such a model suggests that NK cells provide an "immune surveillance" mechanism selectively targeting tumor cells or virally infected cells that downmodulate MHC molecules. Concurrently, the T-cell arm of the immune system would be poised to lyse MHC-bearing cells that express foreign antigens recognizable by their TCRs. Importantly, however, recent work has shown that certain T-cell subpopulations also express NK-like receptors, suggesting the potential for downmodulation of such NK/T-cell populations via MHC-bearing cells and T-cell costimulation by the "stress" molecules that activate NK cells. With regard to tumor immunology, one could envision a scenario wherein downmodulation of one MHC allele that may be necessary to present a particular tumor-specific peptide may diminish the tumor's capacity to be recognized by classical T cells, while maintenance of another allele, reactive with the KIR receptors, could turn off NK cell–mediated cytolytic responses. In this way, the tumor could subvert both the T-cell and NK-cell immune response.[30]

NK cells also show striking responses to IL-2, a cytokine released by Th cells. *In vitro* and *in vivo*, exposure to IL-2 causes activation and proliferation of NK cells, producing changes readily detectable by molecular and morphologic techniques.[31] Functionally, these IL-2–activated NK cells mediate *in vitro* destruction against an even broader range of tumor cell lines (compared with those killed by fresh NK cells).

Recently, new approaches for expanding NK cells *ex vivo* have been developed, opening the possibility for NK-cell–based adoptive immunotherapy.[32] In addition, IL-15 has been identified as a major growth factor for peripheral NK cell expansion.[33] Preclinical studies with IL-15 have shown effects on NK cells *in vivo*, and it is anticipated that future immunotherapies may incorporate adoptive NK-cell immunotherapy and/or IL-15 as a means for enhancing NK-mediated antitumor immunity. Since the natural evolution of the immune system involved all components working together, one futuristic vision of immunotherapy would integrate an mAb targeting a cell surface receptor, with a therapy designed to augment NK-cell number and function to enhance antibody-mediated ADCC and target tumor cells that have downregulated MHC molecules, with a T-cell–based immunotherapy to target MHC-expressing tumor cells and which could synergize with NK-cell–mediated cytotoxicity. In preclinical studies, such combined immunotherapies have shown promise.[34]

IMMUNE FUNCTION IN CANCER PATIENTS

Immunologic Effects of Cancer and Cancer Therapy

Interactions between cancer and the immune system are complex. It is widely accepted that cancer patients have variable degrees of immunosuppression at the time of clinical presentation, prior to initiation of antineoplastic therapy. The causes of cancer-associated immunosuppression are multifactorial and include anatomic alterations of lymphohematopoietic organs by tumors, immunosuppressive mediators released by tumors (e.g., TGF-β, IL-10, and VEGF), malnutrition, and physiologic stress. Cancer-associated immunosuppression can be clinically significant; combined abnormalities in innate and adaptive immunity, such as those that exist in acute leukemia with pancytopenia, are associated with a high incidence of infectious complications. Patients with solid tumors show subclinical abnormalities in T-cell immunity at the time of diagnosis, prior

to induction of therapy. However, the therapies used to treat malignancy are often the most important factor determining the degree of immunosuppression present. Many commonly administered cancer therapies induce dramatic alterations in both innate and adaptive components of host immunity, which not only predispose patients to infection but also significantly impact the immune:tumor interface.

The most obvious effect of conventional cancer chemotherapy on the immune system is neutrophil depletion, which predisposes patients to bacterial infection (reviewed in Chapter 41). Monocytes are also dramatically depleted following chemotherapy, but they recover rapidly, precede neutrophil recovery, and often "overshoot" to supraphysiologic levels.[35] Less is known about quantitative and qualitative effects of chemotherapy on monocyte-derived macrophages and DCs in tissues.[36–38] In murine models, chemotherapy leads to expansion of "suppressor" macrophages, sometime called *myeloid-derived suppressor cells*, which produce large amounts of inducible nitric oxide synthase, arginase,[39] and TGF-β.[40,41] Similarly, circulating monocytes in humans following cytotoxic chemotherapy suppress T-cell function and can induce apoptosis of a variety of lymphocyte subpopulations.[42–44]

Corticosteroids are commonly administered in the context of cancer chemotherapy, as antineoplastic agents, antiemetics, or prophylaxis against hypersensitivity reactions and they predispose cancer patients to fungal, viral, and other opportunistic infections.[45,46] This is particularly pertinent for patients with brain tumors who are at high risk for opportunistic infections[45,46] largely related to the use of corticosteroids to control cerebral edema. The effects of corticosteroid therapy on host immunity continue to be elucidated, but prevailing evidence demonstrates that the primary immunologic target of corticosteroids are DCs, whereas mature T cells are relatively resistant to corticosteroid-induced lysis. Corticosteroids inhibit the development of immature myeloid DCs from monocytes, inhibit myeloid DC maturation and cytokine secretion,[47–51] and inhibit IFN-α–producing plasmacytoid DCs. Thus, commonly administered antineoplastic therapies substantially alter the innate immune system, predisposing cancer patients to infection, and also potentially modulating antitumor immunity via effects on the immune:tumor interface (Fig. 5.3).

Cytotoxic chemotherapy also depletes lymphocyte populations, but the susceptibility and rate of recovery varies substantially among lymphocyte subsets. NK cells are generally resistant to cytotoxic chemotherapy[35] and even when NK-cell depletion is induced by dose-intensive therapy, it is typically short-lived. Since NK cells are critical for bridging innate and adaptive immunity and are particularly important for antiviral immunity, resistance of NK cells to chemotherapy-induced depletion likely provides a critical secondary role in host defense against viral pathogens following antineoplastic therapy. In contrast to NK cells, B cells are often profoundly depleted following cytotoxic chemotherapy. When cyclic chemotherapy continues for several months, this can result in a complete absence of circulating B cells during the entire period of chemotherapy treatment. B-cell depletion results in diminished circulating IgM and IgA levels, whereas plasma IgG levels typically remain normal since tissue plasma cells are generally resistant to cytotoxic chemotherapy and irradiation.[35] The impact of IgM and IgA deficiency on infectious complications or antitumor immunity has not been well studied. Following cessation of cytotoxic chemotherapy, recovery of B-cell populations and circulating IgM and IgA normally occurs over 3 to 6 months with reconstituting B cells initially resembling those found in cord blood and thereafter developing a mature phenotype over 6 to 12 months.[52,53] Importantly, since optimal B-cell immunity to a complete array of pathogens requires T-cell help, patients with normal B-cell numbers but delayed T-cell immune reconstitution may continue to demonstrate impaired B cell responses to T-dependent antigens.

Cytotoxic chemotherapy can also induce substantial T-cell depletion, and the degree of CD4$^+$ depletion generally correlates with the degree of immunosuppression. Because it is difficult to predict how immunosuppressive a particular regimen will be for an individual patient, quantification of lymphocyte populations by using flow cytometry can be useful to estimate the level of immunosuppression induced by cytotoxic chemotherapy, with increasing risk for opportunistic infections when CD4$^+$ counts are less than 200 cells/µL.[35] Persistent T-cell depletion over time provides more compelling evidence for immunosuppression than isolated, transient decreases in peripheral blood T-cell numbers associated with physiologic stress. In a pediatric oncology population, T-cell immunodeficiency is most severe and most common following allogeneic bone marrow transplantation (BMT),[54–56] in which a variety of factors, including GVHD, contribute to a high incidence of opportunistic complications (reviewed in Ref 57) (discussed in Chapters 16 and 40). Significant T-cell immunosuppression may also be induced by dose-intensive regimens or when particularly immunosuppressive agents are administered in the non-BMT setting. Among individual chemotherapy agents, the purine nucleoside analogs (including clofarabine and fludarabine) are the most potent class of lymphocyte-depleting agents. Similarly, the anti-CD52 mAb (Campath) induces severe T-cell depletion. Cyclophosphamide is also commonly associated with chemotherapy-induced immune suppression, with a substantial dose-response effect, such that severe immunosuppressive effects can be seen when doses greater than 3.0 g/m^2 are administered. Thus, essentially all patients treated with purine nucleoside analogs, Campath, or high-dose cyclophosphamide warrant pneumocystis prophylaxis.[58] More commonly, cyclophosphamide is administered as part of a multiagent regimen where even lower doses can cause significant lymphocyte depletion but wherein monitoring of lymphocyte subsets in individual patients may be necessary to accurately assess the risk of opportunistic complications.

Other classical alkylators can also induce T-cell depletion, although the relative capacity for single agents to do this has not been well studied. For example, ifosfamide is a homologue of cyclophosphamide, with similar antineoplastic effects, but it remains unclear whether ifosfamide is equally T-cell depleting compared with cyclophosphamide. In general, antimetabolites induce less T-cell depletion when compared with alkylators, although definitive studies on the lymphosuppressive effects of individual agents is lacking. Agents that induce minimal immunosuppression are vincristine and actinomycin D as used in the treatment of Wilms' tumor,[59] the topoisomerase I inhibitors topotecan and irinotecan,[60,61] and L-asparaginase. Conflicting reports exist regarding taxane-induced lymphocyte depletion.[60,62]

Unlike regeneration of neutrophils, monocytes, and NK cells, which are predictable and complete in most patients, T-cell regeneration is slow, incomplete, and shows a high level of variability between patients. As a result, T-cell depletion induced by cytotoxic antineoplastic therapy is typically followed by slow and incomplete restoration of peripheral T-cell populations, some of which occurs via thymic-dependent differentiation from hematopoietic stem cells and some of which occurs via thymic-independent expansion of residual mature T cells. Because thymic-dependent progeny have more diverse TCRs and are generally more functional than those generated via thymic-independent pathways, identification of thymic progeny has been of interest to monitor the efficiency of immune reconstitution. While no true definitive marker for recent thymic emigrants has been identified, they are contained within the CD4$^+$CD45RA$^+$CD62hi subset,[63] they have been reported to express CD31,[64] and approximately 20% of recent thymic emigrants are TREC-positive, reflecting "recent" TCR rearrangement.[6] Using these tools to monitor thymic function, it is clear that recovery of CD4$^+$ T-cell populations is highly age-related, especially when comparing children with young adults,[62,65] because children typically show evidence for brisk recovery of thymopoiesis while adults have delayed or absent thymic recovery (Figs. 5.5–5.7). The clinical implication is that children typically experience a shorter period of immunosuppression associated with cytotoxic antineoplastic therapy, than

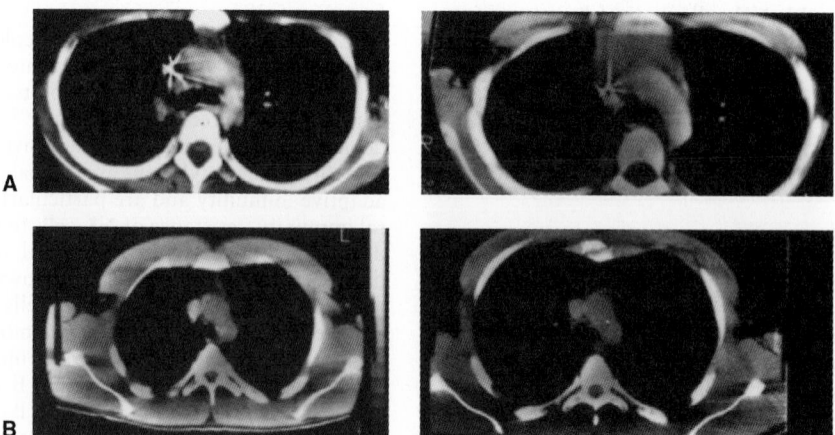

FIGURE 5.7 Thymic rebound following intensive chemotherapy. **Panel A** shows a contrast enhanced CT scan taken pretherapy and 6 months following completion of dose-intensive chemotherapy in an 11-year-old child treated for large cell lymphoma. Enlargement of the thymic shadow compared with baseline is observed. This was associated with a rise in peripheral blood total CD4$^+$ T-cell counts as well as CD45RA$^+$CD4$^+$ T cell counts. Biopsy of the thymus at this time point revealed normal thymic tissue. The hyperplastic organ subsequently returned to baseline size over the ensuing months. In contrast, enlargement of the small amount of thymic tissue present at baseline is not observed in the 19-year-old patient shown in the **bottom panels**. **Left:** Baseline prior to chemotherapy. **Right:** 6 months following completion of chemotherapy. (From Mackall CL, Fleisher TA, Brown MR, et al. Age, thymopoiesis, and CD4+ T-lymphocyte regeneration after intensive chemotherapy. N Engl J Med 1995;332:143–149, with permission.)

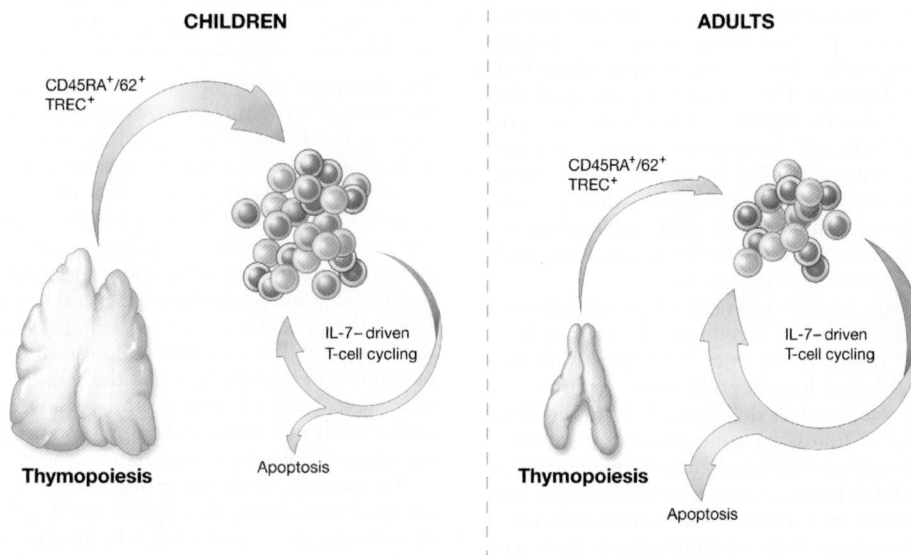

FIGURE 5.8 Pathways of T-cell regeneration following cytotoxic chemotherapy. Shown is a schematic representation of T-cell regeneration, which involves a dynamic interaction of thymic-dependent and thymic-independent pathways. Children primarily regenerate T cells via thymic-dependent pathways, resulting in normalization of peripheral CD4+ T-cell numbers, a diverse T-cell receptor repertoire, and the presence of rising numbers of CD45RA+/CD62L+ cells in the peripheral blood, a substantial proportion of which are TREC+. In contrast, adults primarily regenerate T cells via the peripheral expansion of residual cells via a process of T-cell cycling, which is driven by IL-7 and results in the accumulation of large numbers of activated cells that display a high rate of apoptosis. (Adapted from Mackall CL, Hakim FT, Gress RE: T-cell regeneration: all repertoires are not created equal. Immunology Today 1997;18:245–251, with permission.)

older adolescents and adults. Direct thymic insults, such as GVHD, HIV, or mediastinal irradiation, also substantially diminish thymic reserve, rendering even young patients susceptible to chronic CD4+ depletion.[66,67]

For patients without sufficient thymic reserve to rapidly repopulate T cells via thymic-dependent pathways, the primary pathway of T-cell regeneration is homeostatic peripheral expansion of residual mature T cells (Fig. 5.8). This pathway substantially increases total body T-cell number, but it generally does not completely normalize T-cell numbers. It cannot restore the TCR repertoire diversity, and homeostatically expanding T cells demonstrate limited functional efficacy.[62,68] CD8+ T-cell regeneration occurs more rapidly than CD4+ regeneration, because homeostatic peripheral expansion of CD8+ cells is more efficient than for CD4+ cells.[69] However, the bulk of the CD8+ T cells contained within the recovered populations lack the CD28 coreceptor, are poorly responsive to mitogenic stimuli, and may function primarily as negative regulatory or suppressor populations.[69] Despite these shortcomings, homeostatically expanding cells undergo exaggerated proliferative responses to strong antigens and can uniquely respond to weak, self-antigens, which are typically ignored by "healthier" T cells. Because tumor antigens are weak self-antigens, lymphopenia has been induced in experimental protocols prior to administration of adoptive T-cell immunotherapy for cancer so that the augmented reactivity characteristic of homeostatic peripheral expansion can be exploited for therapeutic benefit.[70,71]

Therapeutic modalities for enhancing immune reconstitution are currently under study and include lymphopoietic growth factors, such as IL-7,[72,73] IL-15, and flt3 ligand,[74] that can increase lymphocyte recovery via thymic-dependent and/or thymic-independent pathways. RhIL7 has completed early trials in humans and shows substantial capacity to augment T-cell recovery, likely through augmenting homeostatic peripheral expansion with preferential expansion of naive T cells. Future studies will likely incorporate such T-cell growth factors to augment immune recovery after lymphocyte-depleting therapies and to direct immune responses in the context of immune-based therapy for cancer.[75] It remains unknown whether the lymphocyte depletion induced by standard cytotoxic chemotherapy increases the risk for tumor recurrence, but several studies have shown improved disease-free survival in patients with higher lymphocyte counts following dose-intensive chemotherapy. Similarly, in a murine model of osteosarcoma, lymphocyte depletion increased the risk for metastatic recurrence and adoptive transfer of T cells to enhance immune reconstitution diminished metastatic recurrence. Together, these data suggest that therapies designed to hasten immune recovery after dose-intensive chemotherapy improve outcomes by diminishing the risk for tumor recurrence.

Modern Concepts of Immune Surveillance

In 1957, F. Macfarlane Burnet proposed the theory of immune surveillance as a first line of defense against cancer,[76] and animal models now provide direct evidence that immune surveillance plays an important role in preventing the development of some primary tumors.[77–81] For instance, mice treated with mutagenic agents and mice genetically engineered to have a predisposition to cancer (via disruption of the p53 gene) develop cancers earlier when there are deficiencies in T cells and/or NK cells compared with immunocompetent mice.[77] These models consistently demonstrate that IFN-γ must be produced within the tumor microenvironment, and tumors must retain sensitivity to IFN-γ signaling in order for immune surveillance to occur. Direct comparison of the growth characteristics of tumors that develop in immunocompetent versus immunodeficient mice reveals important differences. Tumors developing in immunodeficient hosts are "less fit" for subsequent growth in immunocompetent hosts, compared with tumors whose primary growth took place in immunocompetent hosts wherein immune pressure was present. These results suggest that during the early stages of oncogenesis, there is a dynamic interaction between the growing tumor and the immune response, such that the tumor cells which survive have been "imprinted" and "selected" for resistance to host immune responses. Indeed, extensive studies in mouse and human tumors demonstrate a panoply of mechanisms by which tumors evade immune responses, illustrating that acquisition of immune-evasive properties is likely to be a common, and sometimes essential, element of oncogenesis.

In the clinical setting, patients with some immunodeficiencies have an increased incidence of certain neoplasms,[82] including severe combined immunodeficiency (SCID),[82] Wiskott-Aldrich syndrome,[82] X-linked lymphoproliferative syndrome,[83] ataxia-telangiectasia, selective IgA deficiency, HIV and AIDS, and immunosuppression following solid organ transplantation.[84] In immunosuppressed children, lymphoid malignancies (particularly non-Hodgkin lymphomas) are most common, but the incidence of other tumors is also somewhat increased. Current concepts hold that susceptibility to lymphoma in these settings relates to a direct loss of immune surveillance as well as a variety of other factors. For instance, molecular defects that lead to genetic damage in lymphocytes, (e.g., alterations of the ATM gene in ataxia-telangiectasia[85]) may cause DNA damage that predisposes to neoplastic transformation. In addition, patients with lymphocyte depletion have increased serum levels of IL-7, which serve to stimulate residual lymphopoiesis[86,87] and which may increase the incidence of B-cell neoplasms since mice transgenic for IL-7 show a high rate of lymphoma development.[88,89] Finally, immunodeficiency results in impaired immune control of infectious agents that are associated with or stimulate neoplastic differentiation (e.g., Epstein-Barr virus [EBV] as the central factor in inducing posttransplant lymphoproliferative disorder [PTLD] and/or lymphoma).

In summary, modern concepts of immune surveillance emphasize reciprocal interactions between incipient tumor and the immune system whereby immune pressure selects for elements of the primary tumor that are most capable of evading host immune responses.[90] A three-phase model has been put forth wherein initial tumor recognition by the immune system leads to *elimination* of some cancers (and of some cells within cancers), followed by *equilibrium* wherein dynamic interactions between persistent tumor and immune response edit the tumor, followed ultimately by tumor *escape* wherein the immune-edited tumor outstrips immune effector mechanisms and results in clinically evident cancer. Since patients presenting with clinical evidence of cancer are at the last of these three stages, a critical challenge for the field of tumor immunology is to identify specific mechanisms of immune evasion and develop therapies to mitigate, reverse, or circumvent them.

Some studies have hypothesized that true immune tolerance is a mechanism allowing tumors to escape immune recognition and destruction, but sensitive technologies that enable measurement of antigen-specific immune responses more frequently demonstrate that antitumor immune responses coexist with progressively growing tumors. Such ongoing immune responses can potentially impact the clinical course of the tumor, depending upon the relative oncogenic fitness of immune-evading cancer clones[78,90] and the extent of residual immune responses remaining after primary therapy eradicates bulk disease. Delineation of the complex interactions between immune cells and tumor cells at the host:tumor interface represents an area of intense, ongoing research, since development of effective immunotherapy requires approaches that amplify existing antitumor immunity, reverse the mechanisms by which tumors suppress antitumor immunity, or identify alternative pathways to accomplish immune-mediated tumor recognition and destruction that is not abrogated by tumor-induced immune suppression.

IMMUNOTHERAPY OF CANCER

The discipline of tumor immunology seeks to understand how the immune system recognizes neoplastic tissue, identify how tumors evade immune responses, and develop methods to induce, amplify, or circumvent these reactions for preventive or curative therapy. In the last two decades, substantial progress has been made in understanding the basic biology of the immune response, technological advances have identified numerous tumor antigens, and translational medicine has led to clinical grade production of several new molecular and cell-based therapies that are now being tested clinically. In this section, we will review the evolution of our understanding of antitumor immunity, describe the families of tumor antigens that have been identified, and review current approaches under study for immunotherapy of cancer, with an emphasis on issues of relevance to pediatric cancer.

Historically, studies of transplantable syngeneic murine sarcomas demonstrated the capacity for T cells to prevent growth or induce regression of cancer. In the clinical arena, irrefutable evidence that an immune reaction could play an important role in controlling or preventing tumor growth came from at least two separate clinical scenarios. First, following allogeneic BMT, donor-derived T cells play a critical role in mediating a GVL effect, which can prevent or control leukemic relapse (Fig. 5.9). The GVL effect is most potent for chronic myelogenous leukemia (CML), moderately potent for acute myelogenous leukemia (AML), and less potent for acute lymphocytic leukemia (ALL),[91–95] illustrating that susceptibility to immune-based recognition or killing varies by histology, although the factors responsible for these differences remain poorly understood. While T cells play a prominent role in this GVL effect, NK cells have also been shown to be a major component, particularly when transplants involve MHC incompatibility and require T-cell depletion in order to avoid GVHD. In solid tumors, evidence for autologous immune responses are clearly seen in melanoma and renal cell carcinoma, where spontaneous regression has been well described, and regressions can be induced with rhIL-2 therapy, which is a potent immune modulator.

Clear evidence for tumor regressions due to natural acquisition of endogenous immunity are lacking in pediatric tumors, but there is emerging evidence that pediatric tumors are immunogenic and capable of being recognized by the host immune system. One demonstration of tumor immune reactivity comes from patients with opsoclonus-myoclonus syndrome and neuroblastoma.[96–99] Historically, it has been well appreciated that some patients with neuroblastoma present with a clinical syndrome comprising random eye movements, myoclonus, and ataxia. This is associated with the presence of circulating antibodies that bind cerebellar tissues. Patients with this syndrome also tend to have increased lymphocyte infiltrates in their neuroblastoma and an improved oncologic prognosis compared with patients with similar tumors but lacking the syndrome. Together, this has led to a model of opsoclonus-myoclonus as an immune-mediated paraneoplastic syndrome, wherein not only are humoral immune responses associated with improved tumor-free survival but also the immune responses induced toward tumor antigens cross-react with antigens on normal neural tissues to cause neurological disease.

Activation of Innate Immunity

In vitro, macrophages can kill tumor cells by direct cell-cell contact and/or by contact-independent mechanisms through the release of nitric oxide and tumor necrosis factor.[100,101] Activation of monocytes and tissue macrophages occurs following

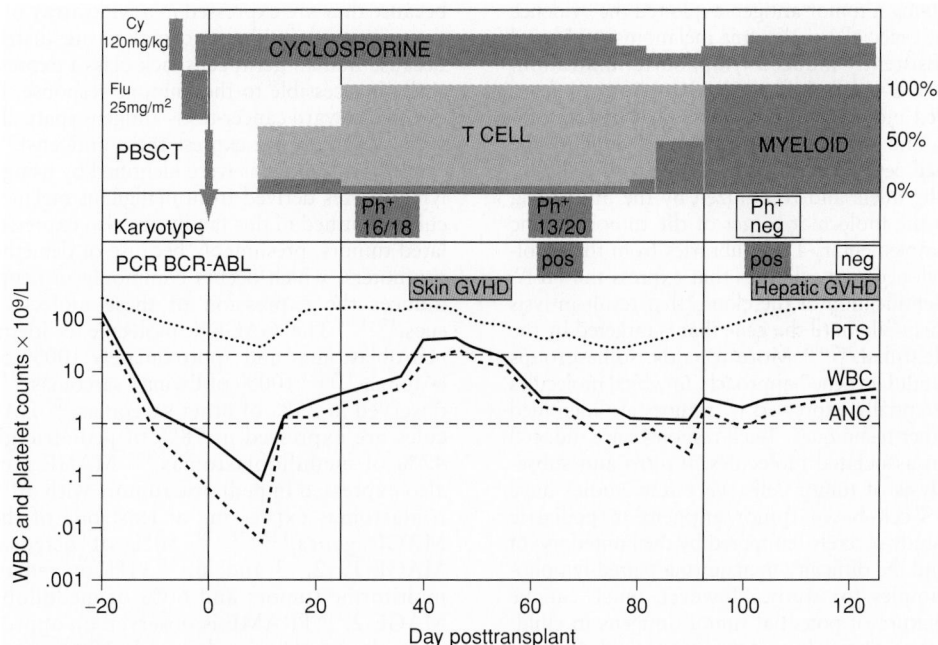

FIGURE 5.9 Graft versus leukemia. This figure shows the clinical course of a 30-year-old patient with Ph[+] chronic myelogenous leukemia (CML) following an HLA sibling-identical peripheral blood stem cell transplant from his sister. He received nonablative conditioning (cyclophosphamide + fludarabine). Following transplant, his white blood cells (WBCs) and platelets counts and absolute neutrophil count (ANC) all dropped and began recovering after 2 weeks. However, by day 30, his WBC count was increasing, with 16 of 18 mitoses showing persistent Ph[+] CML and chimerism studies showing less than 10% donor-derived myeloid cells. He then showed rapid expansion of donor T cells (going from 50%–100% of circulating T cells) with onset of skin graft-vs-host disease (GVHD) on day 35. Oral steroids were started with the cyclosporine, and the GVHD resolved, followed by neutropenia. The WBC count began rising again after day 75, with acquisition of 100% donor chimerism of the myeloid cells, and 20 of 20 mitoses showing normal 46XX, with no Ph[+] cells. Polymerase chain reaction (PCR) for Ph[+] became negative as well. The patients then remained leukemia free. This case demonstrates the onset of GVHD and the onset of a potent antileukemic effect at that same time. Such examples have led to the intentional use of donor-derived lymphocyte infusions following transplant in order to prospectively provide this antileukemic immunotherapy. (From Childs R, Epperson D, Bahceci E, et al. Molecular remission of CML following a non-ablative allogeneic PBSCT: in vivo and in vitro evidence for a graft versus leukemia effect. Br J Haematol 1999;107:396–400.)

administration of the lipophilic agent muramyl tripeptide phosphatidylethanolamine (MTP-PE), an analogue of muramyl dipeptide, which is contained within the cell wall of mycobacteria. When MTP-PE is encapsulated into multilamellar liposomes and administered intravenously, it is efficiently delivered to pulmonary macrophages, circulating monocytes, and monocyte/macrophages within the liver, spleen, nasopharynx, and thyroid.[101] Uptake of MTP-PE by monocytes and macrophages leads to activation with release of IL-1α, IL-1β, IL-7, IL-8, IL-12, and TNF, which can directly or indirectly induce tumor cell death. Because MTP-PE and other monocyte/macrophage-activating agents cannot increase numbers of postmitotic monocytes and macrophages, the number of tumor cells that can be eradicated by MTP-PE is limited by the number of macrophages present within tumor tissue.[101] For this reason, the clinical application of MTP-PE has been focused upon situations where small amounts of residual tumor remain localized to lungs, such as occurs in osteosarcoma. Administration of adjuvant MTP-PE in combination with cisplatin chemotherapy to dogs with spontaneous osteosarcoma resulted in a modest prolongation in median survival time (14.4 months vs. 9.8 months, $p < 0.01$),[102] and improved disease-free survival compared with historical controls was observed following 24 weeks of adjuvant MTP-PE therapy (9 months vs. 4.5 months, $p < 0.03$) in a phase II trial.[101] Peripheral fibrosis, inflammatory cell infiltration, and neovascularization were observed in metastases in MTP-PE recipients but not in control subjects. Further investigation of MTP-PE in osteosar-

coma was therefore undertaken in a phase III clinical trial, where improved 6-year overall survival was noted in patients who received MTP-PE ($p = 0.03$) and there was a trend toward improved event-free survival with MTP-PE as well ($p = 0.08$).[103]

Continuing clinical studies of MTP-PE and similar agents that can activate innate immunity are under way,[104] including systemic administration of CpGs[105] and inhaled GM-CSF for pulmonary metastases from sarcoma, where some evidence for clinical benefit has been reported.[104] Because monocytes recover quickly following cytotoxic chemotherapy, the efficacy of administering agents that augment innate immunity simultaneously with chemotherapy and/or immediately following completion of chemotherapy provide a potential advantage over T-cell–mediated therapies, which may have limited efficacy at this time point due to cytotoxic therapy-induced depletion of T cells.[106] Given that activators of innate immunity are not likely to eradicate bulky tumors but show promise in the adjuvant setting, their use as therapies that can eradicate small numbers of chemoresistant tumor cells, and diminish metastatic recurrence, remain of interest.

T-Cell–Based Immunotherapy

One major advance in T-cell–based immunotherapy for cancer in the last 20 years has been the molecular definition of numerous tumor antigens that can be targeted by T cells. The classical approach for identifying a tumor antigen exploited the evidence that certain tumors, especially malignant melanoma and renal cell carcinoma, consistently induced lymphocyte infiltration. Investigators extracted tumor-infiltrating lymphocytes from these tumors, derived individual T-cell clones that lyse autologous tumor targets, and then used these clones to identify the specific tumor-derived peptide that was presented by the autologous HLA-presenting allele and recognized by the infiltrating T cells. To identify the molecular target of the tumor-specific cytolytic T cells, complementary DNA libraries from the autologous tumor were cloned into cell lines that express the HLA-presenting allele. Identification of the clones that result in lysis was performed sequentially until the gene that is targeted by the T-cell clone was identified.[107,108] More recently, some groups have also used a "candidate gene" approach, in which molecules exclusively or preferentially expressed by tumors are identified by microarray or other techniques. T-cell responses are induced toward these tumor-associated molecules *in vitro* and subsequently tested for lysis of tumor cells. Very few studies have directly identified T-cell–based tumor antigens in pediatric tumors, an area of study severely hampered by the limited use of primary resection and the difficulty in acquiring paired lymphocyte and tumor samples for study. However, much can be learned about the nature of potential tumor antigens in childhood tumors from those defined in adult tumors, and a significant number of the antigens identified in adult cancers are also expressed in pediatric tumors.

Human tumor antigens potentially recognized by autologous T cells can be conveniently divided into different families as shown in Table 5.2. One family of tumor antigens can be described as differentiation antigens, with the most well defined being melanoma-associated differentiation antigens.[109] Seminal reports that identified the melanoma differentiation antigens as T-cell targets provided the important conceptual advance (discussed earlier in this chapter) that some host-reactive immune cells remain present throughout the life of the host and that maintenance of self-tolerance to these antigens occurs via dynamic modulation of their microenvironment.[1,110,111] The corollary of this observation is that autoimmunity is a potential risk of antitumor immunotherapy directed against molecules that are not tumor specific. Beyond the potential for autoimmunity, there is another drawback of targeting differentiation antigens for tumor immunotherapy. The selection against self-reactive T-cell clones of high avidity, which occurs normally during thymopoiesis, results in a T-cell repertoire of low avidity for differentiation antigens; these low-avidity T cells might not be capable of mediating potent antitumor effects *in vivo*.[112,113] Further, immune responses directed toward differentiation antigens that are not critical for tumor cell survival may result in immune escape via selection of antigen-negative clones.[114]

Several antigens have been called *universal* tumor antigens since they are expressed in the majority of tumors, including childhood cancers.[140] Among these, both telomerase and survivin appear widely expressed in pediatric tumors. Telomerase is one of the downstream targets of EWS-Fli1[163] and may be a marker of minimal residual disease in Ewing's sarcoma.[164] Similarly, survivin is expressed in acute leukemia,[165] Ewing's sarcoma family of tumor (ESFT), osteosarcoma, brain tumors, and neuroblastoma,[166,167] and immune responses to survivin have been demonstrated in patients with neuroblastoma.[168] Both of these molecules appear to be involved in critical elements of oncogenesis, suggesting that tumor escape by antigen loss may not readily occur since survivin and/or telomerase deficient tumor cells may be less fit for survival. Like differentiation antigens, such universal antigens are not entirely tumor specific, raising the possibility that targeting them may be limited by tolerance or autoimmunity.

Another family of antigens with widespread expression in pediatric tumors are the cancer-testis antigens, so-named because they are expressed in a wide array of cancer tissues but are restricted in their normal tissue distribution to testes. Because human germ cells lack class I expression and are generally inaccessible to the immune response, immune responses directed toward cancer-testis antigens spare all other normal tissues (which do not express these antigens).[169] Although many cancer-testis antigens were identified by using tumor-infiltrating lymphocytes derived from malignant melanomas, many molecules identified in this family are also expressed in other, nonrelated tumors, presumably because of demethylation of antigen promoters, which occurs commonly in neoplastic tissues and induces the expression of these molecules in normal tissues.[170,171] The GAGE-1 molecule is identified in 82% of neuroblastomas and approximately 100% of stage 4 neuroblastomas,[118,172] 100% of Ewing's sarcomas,[118] and GAGE-1,2 is observed in 25% of other sarcomas.[109] GAGE-3 to -6 molecules are expressed in 78% of pediatric glioblastomas and 47% of medulloblastomas.[116] MAGE family antigens are also expressed in pediatric tumors with 50% to 80% of neuroblastomas expressing at least one of the four identified MAGE genes,[122,172–174] 50% of osteosarcomas express MAGE-1, -2, -3 and -6,[175] 11% of pediatric glioblastoma multiforme tumors and 60% of medulloblastomas express MAGE-2.[116] PRAME is observed on approximately 25% of acute leukemia samples with 100% of those expressing t(8;21) also expressing the PRAME molecule,[176] while XAGE genes are expressed in ESFT and alveolar rhabdomyosarcoma.[177] Although the broad expression of these antigens render them attractive targets for immunotherapy, these molecules do not appear to be required for survival of malignant cells and; therefore, selection of variants within the tumor that lack antigen expression can occur and has been demonstrated in some clinical studies.

The fourth group of tumor antigens includes mutated forms of normal "self" molecules. In pediatric oncology, chromosomal translocations occur in a variety of tumors and provide theoretical targets for T-cell recognition since peptides that span the breakpoint region of the translocation represent novel tumor-specific epitopes that do not exist in normal tissues and hence may be susceptible to immune targeting. Indeed, peptides derived from the breakpoint region of the t(9;22) in CML,[149] t(12;21) in ALL,[150] t(X;18) in synovial cell sarcoma, t(2;13) in rhabdomyosarcoma[178] and t(12;22) in desmoplastic small round cell tumor are immunogenic when presented by some HLA alleles.[148,178] These are attractive candidates as tumor targets because of their absolute tumor specificity and the fact that the translocation directly contributes to the neoplastic state, rendering it less susceptible to immune escape by selection of antigen-negative targets. Potential drawbacks involve the fact that tumor-specific mutations are typically limited to one or a few nucleotides, resulting in a limited number of potential epitopes for immune recognition. As a result, most HLA types will not present immunogenic epitopes, and the breadth of the T-cell response generated to one epitope will be limited. Finally, viral antigens provide strong potential tumor targets for T-cell–based immune responses, since these viral antigens are foreign molecules, for which there should be no central or peripheral tolerance. In pediatric tumors, this is particularly relevant to EBV-associated tumors that include lymphoproliferative disorders, Hodgkin disease, nasopharyngeal carcinoma, and Burkitt's lymphoma.

The multitude of recently identified targets that could serve as T-cell tumor antigens has left many immunologists convinced that the primary limitation of the immune response toward tumors lies not in an absence of targets, but rather the absence of critical costimulation needed to initiate and perpetuate an immune response. Thus, many groups have administered vaccines that seek to present tumor antigens to the

TABLE 5.2

HUMAN TUMOR ANTIGENS RECOGNIZABLE BY AUTOLOGOUS T CELLS

Antigen	Adult tumor expression	Pediatric tumor expression	References
Cancer-testis antigens			
MAGE-1, -2, -3	Melanoma, esophageal, lung, colon, prostate, breast, sarcoma	Gliomas, medulloblastoma, neuroblastoma, osteosarcoma	115–117
GAGE		Gliomas, medulloblastoma, neuroblastoma, ESFT	115–118
BAGE		AML	115, 119
XAGE		ESFT, alveolar rhabdomyosarcoma	120
NY-ESO-1	Lung, bladder, melanoma, cutaneous T-cell lymphoma	Synovial sarcoma, osteosarcoma, neuroblastoma	115, 121, 122
PRAME	Acute myeloid leukemia	AML, Wilms' tumor, neuroblastoma	119, 123–125
MY-BR-1, NW-BR-1	Breast, renal		126
Differentiation/oncofetal antigens: Tissue restricted			
MelanA/MART-1	Melanoma		127
Gp100	Melanoma		127
Tyrosinase	Melanoma		127
ML-IAP (melanoma inhibitor of apoptosis protein)	Melanoma		128
N-Myc		Neuroblastoma	129, 130
Prostate-specific antigen	Prostate cancer		131
Proteinase-3	CML, AML, MDS	CML, AML, MDS	132, 133
CEA	Many epithelial		126
TARP	Breast, prostate		134
WT1	AML, ALL, breast,	AML, ALL, rhabdomyosarcoma	119, 135, 136
Differentiation/oncofetal antigens: Tissue nonrestricted			
OFA/iLRP (oncofetal antigen/immature laminin receptor protein)	"Universal"	"Universal"	137, 138
Survivin	"Universal"	"Universal"	139–141
Telomerase (hTERT)	"Universal"	"Universal"	140, 142, 143
CYP1B1	"Universal"		144, 145
Mutated genes and other "tumor-specific" molecules			
Immunoglobulin idiotype	B cell lymphoma, multiple myeloma		146, 147
Chromosomal translocation breakpoints	Synovial sarcoma t(X;18), ALL t(12;21), CML t(11;22)	Synovial sarcoma t(X;18), CML t(9;22), ALL t(12;21), DSRCT t(11;22)	148–150
MUC-1	Breast and other adenocarcinomas		151
β-catenin	Melanoma		152
Mutant p53	Variable across histologies	Variable across histologies	153, 154
Mutant Ras	Pancreatic, colorectal, melanoma		155, 156
CDK-4	Melanoma		152
TRP-1	Melanoma		152
Viral antigens			
HBV and HCV	Hepatocellular carcinoma	Hepatocellular carcinoma	126
HPV	Cervical carcinoma, squamous cell carcinoma		157, 158
EBV antigens (EBNA, LMP-1, -2)	Hodgkin lymphoma, EBV lymphoproliferative disorder, nasopharyngeal carcinoma	Hodgkin lymphoma, EBV lymphoproliferative disorder, Burkitt's lymphoma	159, 160
HTLV	Adult, HTLV-associated, T-cell leukemia		161
Kaposi's sarcoma	Kaposi's sarcoma–associated herpes virus		162

HBV, hepatitis B virus; HCV, hepatitis C virus; HPV, human papillomavirus; EBV, Epstein-Barr virus; HTLV, human T-lymphotropic virus; CML, chronic myelogenous leukemia; AML, acute myelogenous leukemia; MDS, myelodysplastic syndrome; ALL, acute lymphocytic leukemia; ESFT, Ewing's sarcoma family of tumors; DSRCT, desmoplastic small round cell tumor.

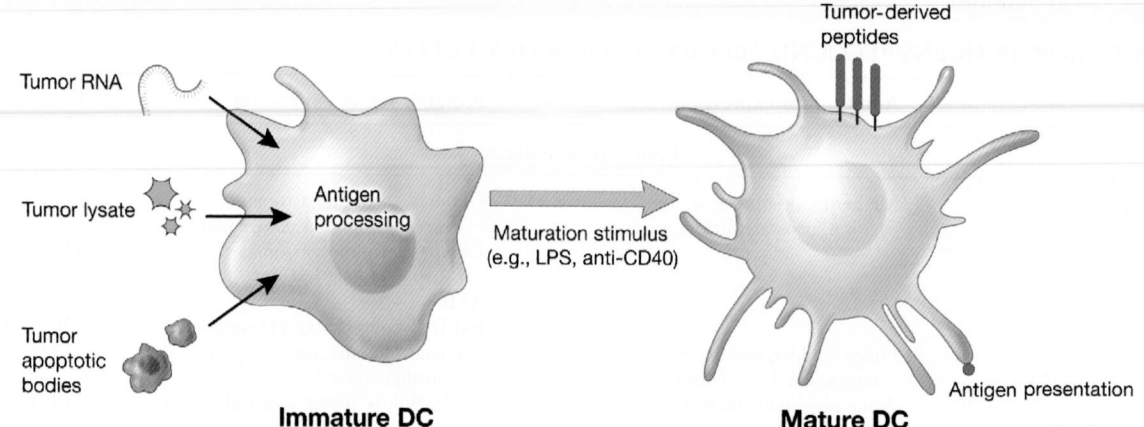

FIGURE 5.10 Approaches currently under study for dendritic cell (DC)-based tumor vaccination. Immature DCs efficiently uptake antigen; and therefore, coincubation of these cells with tumor lysates, tumor RNA, or dead/dying tumor cells leads to their accumulation into the endosomal compartment, followed by antigen processing. Upon maturation of the DC, the processed antigen is presented on the surface of the cell in the context of both MHC class I and MHC class II. Alternatively, mature DCs may be coincubated with peptides that can bind directly to the surface MHC molecules. The antigen-loaded DCs may then be administered intradermally, subcutaneously, or intranodally.

immune system in the context of additional activating or costimulatory signals, which should be recognized as "danger" by the adaptive immune system. Approaches vary from the elemental, such as administration of a peptide that can potentially directly bind to APCs, to genetic modification of tumor cells so that they function as innate immune cells that can deliver requisite costimulatory signals, to the use of cell-based vaccines, which use DCs manipulated to express tumor antigens (Fig. 5.10). The simplest approach to tumor vaccination is to use a tumor-selective peptide as the immunogen. In addition to the initiation of immune response at the tumor site by this peptide, there is evidence that immunization may result in inflammation and subsequent sensitization to other tumor antigens, a phenomenon termed *epitope spreading*, which has been well described.[179] Because peptides alone do not induce the inflammatory response needed for "danger signals" to be generated, peptides are most commonly administered with "adjuvants," irritants which induce local inflammation. Alternatively, GM-CSF may be coadministered subcutaneously with the peptide to recruit DCs to the injection site or the peptides may be loaded onto DCs, which are then administered intradermally, subcutaneously, or intranodally. When large numbers of professional APCs are brought near class I–restricted antigens such as peptides, a process termed *cross-priming* results in pickup of tumor-associated peptides by APCs, presentation by MHC class I, and transfer of the antigen-loaded DC to the draining lymph node, where T-cell sensitization can occur. In the clinical arena, some successful peptide-based vaccines have used peptides that have been altered to enhance their binding to HLA molecules but retain their T-cell specificity. Using this approach, amplification of responses to T-cell antigens can routinely be accomplished, and antitumor immune responses have occurred.[180] However, most tumor vaccine studies have not demonstrated substantial rates of regression in the presence of established tumors. Whether administration of tumor vaccines in the minimal residual disease setting will ultimately affect survival in clinical trials requires randomized trials. Recent results in studies using this antigen-loaded DC vaccine approach in men with advanced prostate cancer has shown benefit over placebo in a large phase III trial (31.7% vs. 23% 3-year survival and 25.8 month vs. 21.7 month median survival), raising the prospect that this

may be the first cancer vaccine approved for general use by the U.S. Food and Drug Administration (FDA).[181]

One of the major limitations of peptide-based vaccines for pediatric oncology lies in the fact that the small size of peptide immunogens (generally 9–20 amino acids in length) limit the HLA-binding capacity for any given peptide. Thus, if individuals with disparate HLA types are to be targeted, vast numbers of individual peptides may need to be developed. Furthermore, peptides are typically developed to generate CD8+-based responses; however, CD4+-based responses may also be important for antitumor immunity. The use of complete proteins (rather than peptides) as immunogens broadens the number of antigens that could potentially be recognized and increases the likelihood that both CD4+ and CD8+ responses may be induced. However, standardization of protein-based vaccination is complex and expensive since it requires clinical-grade protein production. Viral vectors such as vaccinia are well-suited for use in protein vaccination as they allow the insertion of large-sized genes and lead to translation of proteins for a limited period. However, vaccinia-induced inflammation and antivaccinia immunity prevents repetitive use of vaccinia-based vectors. One approach has been initial priming with a vaccinia-based vector, followed by subsequent vaccination with fowlpox, a vector to which most patients have not been previously sensitized.[131]

A third approach for targeting T cells to tumor cells is to utilize whole tumor as the immunogen, or individualized immunotherapy. The complexities of delivering such therapies are greater than delivering off-the-shelf products, but some argue that this may be the most physiologic means for offering the potential for a robust immune response. Approaches have involved transfection of the tumor itself with IL-2, lymphotactin, GM-CSF, or other agents[182] and then injecting the genetically manipulated tumors subcutaneously; clinical responses have been observed with these approaches.[183] Other investigators have used tumor lysates[184,185] or fed apoptotic or necrotic tumor cells to autologous DCs.[186,187] Indeed, a complete tumor response in a pediatric patient with fibrosarcoma was reported by using tumor lysate-pulsed DCs.[185] Alternatively, tumor RNA has been fed to DCs[188,189] or CD40 ligand-activated B cells[168] as a means for whole-cell vaccination. One advantage of the use of whole-cell tumor vaccines is that identification of individual target antigens for individual tumors is not necessary. However, without knowing which tumor antigen is being targeted, it is impossible to monitor whether immune responses against the tumor are being induced. The ability to accurately measure tumor-specific immune responses is a critical surrogate endpoint for evaluating the immunological efficacy of tumor-vaccine trials.

The lack of effectiveness of tumor vaccines as single agents for bulk cancers has led to increasing focus on treatment in the settings of minimal residual disease. In most pediatric patient populations, it is not uncommon for patients with high-risk tumors to be rendered free of visible disease by using standard multimodality therapy. In pediatric oncology, most patient populations are also profoundly lymphopenic upon completion of dose-intensive therapy, which complicates the administration of tumor vaccines in this setting. To circumvent this problem, "consolidative immunotherapy," which combines tumor vaccines with therapies to enhance immune reconstitution, has been piloted in patients with high-risk pediatric sarcomas. In a single-arm study, promising results were seen, although the optimal approaches for vaccination and immune reconstitution require further study. Ultimately, the relative merit of administration of immunotherapy in this setting will require the conduct of controlled randomized studies.

Adoptive Cell Therapy

Tumor vaccines are likely to remain an important component of T-cell–based immunotherapies; however, vaccination alone is limited by the degree to which it can amplify immune responses *in vivo*. Most vaccine studies demonstrate that less than 5% of the $CD8^+$ T-cell repertoire can be induced to be tumor specific, despite repetitive vaccination, and in some studies, even higher levels of antigen-specific T cells were generated without clinical benefit.[190] As a result, many groups have developed adoptive cell therapies, wherein large numbers of *ex vivo* expanded antigen-specific T cells can be propagated and then infused. *Ex vivo* activation allows rapid generation of large numbers of tumor antigen-specific T cells and may overcome tumor-induced immunosuppression. The technology associated with adoptive cell transfer is labor intensive and complex; however; many institutions already have substantial experience in cell processing as a result of the widespread utilization of stem cell transplantation. In pediatric oncology, adoptive cell therapy has been most widely used to target EBV-based malignancies, especially PTLD, which occur following stem cell transplantation.[191–194] Here, the administration of EBV-specific T-cell lines or clones reliably and effectively induces regression of established lymphoma. The approach is even more effective when administered preemptively to prevent the development of PTLD in the setting of a rising EBV load as monitored by PCR. While viral antigens expressed in EBV lymphoproliferative disease tend to be highly immunogenic, presenting a more favorable immunobiologic situation than targeting tumor-associated self-antigens, these results provide important proof-of-principle that adoptive cell therapy can eradicate tumors and prevent tumor growth in humans.[195] Current studies are under way to determine whether other less immunogenic EBV-associated antigens such as those expressed by Hodgkin disease or nonviral tumor antigens may also represent effective targets.[196]

Critical issues that need to be addressed in this field include the optimization of approaches for *ex vivo* expansion and the identification of new approaches to improve *in vivo* expansion, survival and trafficking of the transferred populations. For example, in a murine xenograft model of Ewing's sarcoma, adoptive transfer of anti-CD3/CD28 expanded cells was ineffective, whereas T cells expanded with anti-CD3/4-1BBL effectively controlled tumor growth.[197] These preclinical studies demonstrate that essential cocktails of costimulatory signals, which for $CD8^+$

cells includes 4-1BBL, are needed for efficient *ex vivo* T-cell expansion that can result in meaningful antitumor activity following reinfusion. To provide such signals reproducibly with economical, off-the-shelf reagents, several groups have developed artificial APCs. These vary in their details but comprise either a synthetic matrix or a cell line that has been manipulated to constitutively express essential costimulatory molecules. Depending upon the cell type and target antigen that is undergoing *ex vivo* expansion, one utilizes particular variations of the artificial APC.

Another area of recent focus is the genetic manipulation of T cells to engineer surface expression of either MHC-restricted TCRs or MHC-nonrestricted chimeric antigen receptors[198] (Fig. 5.11). Current approaches are available to reproducibly express either antigen specific TCRs that recognize peptides bound to MHC or MHC-nonrestricted receptors derived from the antigen-binding site of mAbs, which are termed *scFv fragments*. The use of MHC-nonrestricted scFv

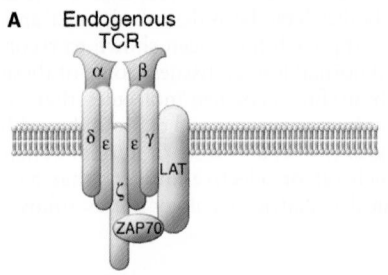

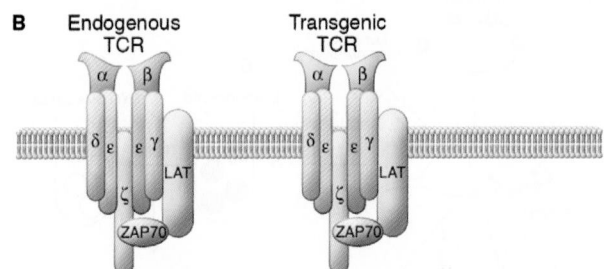

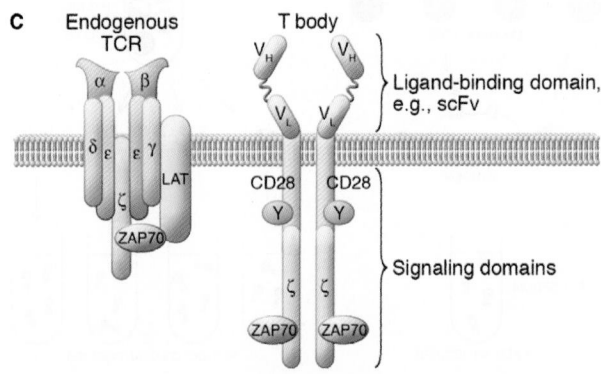

FIGURE 5.11 Genetic engineering of T-cell receptors (TCRs) for adoptive immunotherapy. Panel A shows the normal endogenous TCR. Following cloning of a TCR (**B**), the cloned TCR is expressed in polyclonal T cells and then used for adoptive immunotherapy. All such T cells have two TCRs, one natural and one "transgenic." The antigen-binding region of monoclonal antibodies (mAbs) (Fab region) can also be cloned and attached to the signaling domains of a TCR (**C**), as well as costimulatory molecules, then inserted into T cells or NK cells. The resulting cell has the antigen specificity of the mAb but the killing apparatus and potential for longevity and expansion of the NK and/or T cells. (From June CH. Adoptive T cell therapy for cancer in the clinic. J Clin Invest 2007;117:1466–1476).

fragments eliminates the need to identify epitopes specific for each individual MHC allele. T or NK cells transfected with these engineered antigen receptors can be expanded to the desired cell dose *ex vivo* prior to their infusion. Early studies have demonstrated activity of such genetically engineered T cells in patients with neuroblastoma,[199] and it is anticipated that several other tumors will be targeted with similar approaches during the coming decade.

Antibody Therapy

Of tremendous importance to diagnostic and clinical immunology was the invention of the hybridoma technique that used murine B-cell tumors to make large quantities of mAbs (Fig. 5.12).[200] Since the creation of mAbs in 1975,[201] laboratories worldwide have been immunizing mice with human tumor tissue and screening for antibodies that specifically recognize human cancer cells but not any normal human tissues. While rare tumor-specific antibodies have been described, most antibodies produced by this approach have been shown to recognize both neoplastic and normal human tissues. Some of these, which may be clinically useful, recognize molecules that are overexpressed on certain human tumors and expressed weakly on only a small histologically distinct subset of normal human tissues. Examples of such tumor-selective antigens that have been important in clinical pediatric oncology are as follows:

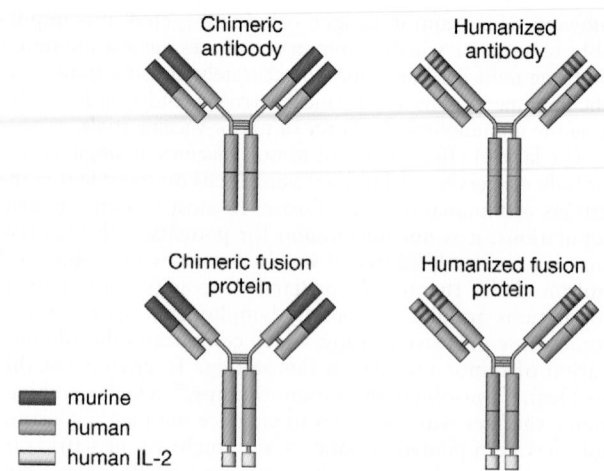

murine
human
human IL-2

FIGURE 5.13 Genetically engineered antibodies and fusion proteins. The chimeric antibody has human constant domains and murine variable domains, which confer antigen specificity. In the humanized antibody, murine framework determinants have replaced the human framework determinants from the three main complementarity-determining regions for both the heavy and light chain variable regions. The remainder of the heavy and light immunoglobulin chains are of human origin. The chimeric fusion protein links a molecule of IL-2 to each of the heavy chains of the chimeric antibody at the carboxyl terminus. In the humanized fusion protein, IL-2 has been linked to each of the heavy chains of the humanized antibody at the carboxyl terminus.

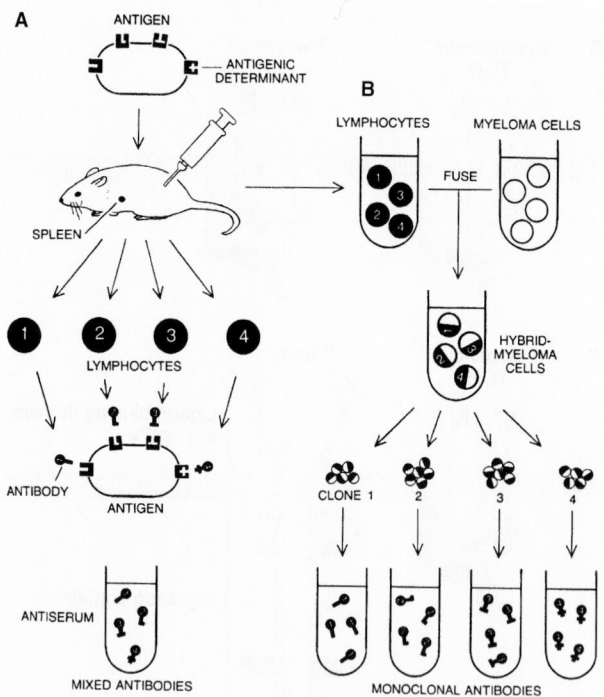

FIGURE 5.12 Generation of monoclonal antibodies. Immune response is initiated (**A**) when an antigen molecule carrying several different antigenic determinants enters the body of an animal. The immune system responds, and lines of B lymphocytes proliferate, each secreting an immunoglobulin molecule that fits a single antigenic determinant or a part of it. A conventional antiserum contains a mixture of these antibodies. **B**: Monoclonal antibodies are derived by fusing lymphocytes from the spleen with malignant myeloma cells. Individual hybrid cells are cloned, and each of the clones secretes a monoclonal antibody that fits a single antigenic determinant on the antibody molecule. (From Milstein C. Monoclonal antibodies. Sci Am 1980;243:66. Reprinted in Paul WE. Immunology: recognition and response. New York, NY: WH Freeman, 1991:125.)

the CD20 molecule expressed on pre-B leukemia and lymphoma, and on certain precursor B cells; the CD33 molecule found on acute myeloid leukemia cells, as well as certain normal myeloid precursors; and the GD2 disialoganglioside, which is overexpressed on neuroblastoma and most osteosarcomas and also expressed weakly on peripheral nerves.[202]

Current genetic engineering techniques allow molecularly modified antibodies to be created with a number of laboratory designer improvements. Chimeric and humanized antibodies are being created that allow mix-and-match combinations of antigen-binding and constant regions, using gene segments from different cells or even different species to provide the desired antigen recognition and biologic function[202] (Fig. 5.13). *In vitro* gene recombination of fully human genes can incorporate steps for cyclical, sequential mutation and recombination to generate immunoglobulins that may not be readily found in immune cells that have superior antigen-binding properties or effector functions.[203] Multiple molecular modifications of these, and other similar tumor-selective mAbs, are being pursued for diagnostic purposes, for *ex vivo* purging of tumor cells from hematopoietic stem cell populations, and several strategies involve direct *in vivo* administration of these tumor-reactive antibodies and their derivatives. Over the past few years, several mAbs have shown antitumor efficacy in patients with cancer, have been FDA-approved, and are generally available (Table 5.3) as effective cancer therapeutics.[204,205]

The molecular mechanism of the antitumor response mediated by the antitumor antibodies in patients is still being characterized, and it clear that mAbs may induce antitumor effects through several pathways (Fig. 5.14): (a) The antibody may bind to the tumor cell surface and activate the complement cascade, resulting in tumor cell lysis; (b) The mAb may bind to the tumor cell via a signaling molecule that causes activation of signals that result, downstream, in apoptosis; (c) The mAb may bind competitively to a critical growth factor receptor that requires continued activation for cell survival; competitive inhibition by the mAb will prevent this requisite

MONOCLONAL ANTIBODIES (mAbs) APPROVED FOR CANCER TREATMENT BY THE FDA

Generic	Brand	Target	Indication	Form
Rituximab	Rituxan	CD20	B-cell NHL	Chimeric mAb
Trastuzumab	Herceptin	Her2/Neu	Breast Cancer	Humanized mAb
Gemtuzumab	Mylotarg	CD33	AML (mAb-toxin)	Humanized mAb linked to calicheamicin
Alemtuzumab	Campath	CD52	B-CLL, CTCL	Humanized mAb
Ibritumomab	Zevalin	CD20	Refractory B NHL (radiolabeled mAb)	Murine mAb linked to ^{90}Y
Tositumomab	Bexxar	CD20	Refractory B NHL (radiolabeled mAb)	Murine mAb linked to ^{131}I
Basiliximab	Simulect	CD25	Anti–graft rejection/GVHD	Chimeric mAb
Daclizumab	Zenapax	CD25	GVHD/anti–graft rejection	Humanized mAb
Bevacizumab	Avastin	VEGF	GI malignancies	Humanized mAb
Edrecolomab	17-1A	EpCam	GI malignancies	Murine mAb
Cetuximab	Erbitux	EGFR	Colorectal and head and neck cancers	Chimeric mAb
Panitumumab	Vectibix	EGFR	Colorectal cancers	Human mAb
Catumaxomab[a] (Europe)	Removab	EpCAM/CD3	Peritoneal ovarian cancer	Bifunctional rat anti-EpCAM linked to murine anti-CD3
Nimotuzumab[a] (Europe)	Theraloc	EGFR	SCCHN and glioma	Human mAb

VEGF, vascular endothelial growth factor; EGFR, epidermal growth factor receptor; NHL, non-Hodgkin lymphoma; AML, acute myelogenous lymphoma; CLL, chronic lymphocytic leukemia; CTCL, cutaneous T-cell lymphoma; GVHD, graft-vs-host disease; GI, gastrointestinal; SCCHN, squamous cell carcinoma of the head and neck; a, approved for clinical use in europe, but not by US-FDA.

growth factor activation, resulting in cell death; (d) The Fab end of the mAb binds to the tumor and its Fc end is recognized by cells of the innate immune system that express FcRs, causing their activation and induction of ADCC; (e) The mAb may be linked to a toxin, drug, or radionuclide that becomes local-ized to the tumor cell via antibody recognition of the antigen on the tumor cell, resulting in its death.

Mechanisms of action critical for antitumor efficacy have been best studied through analyses of the striking anti-tumor activity afforded by the use of the rituximab (Rituxan)

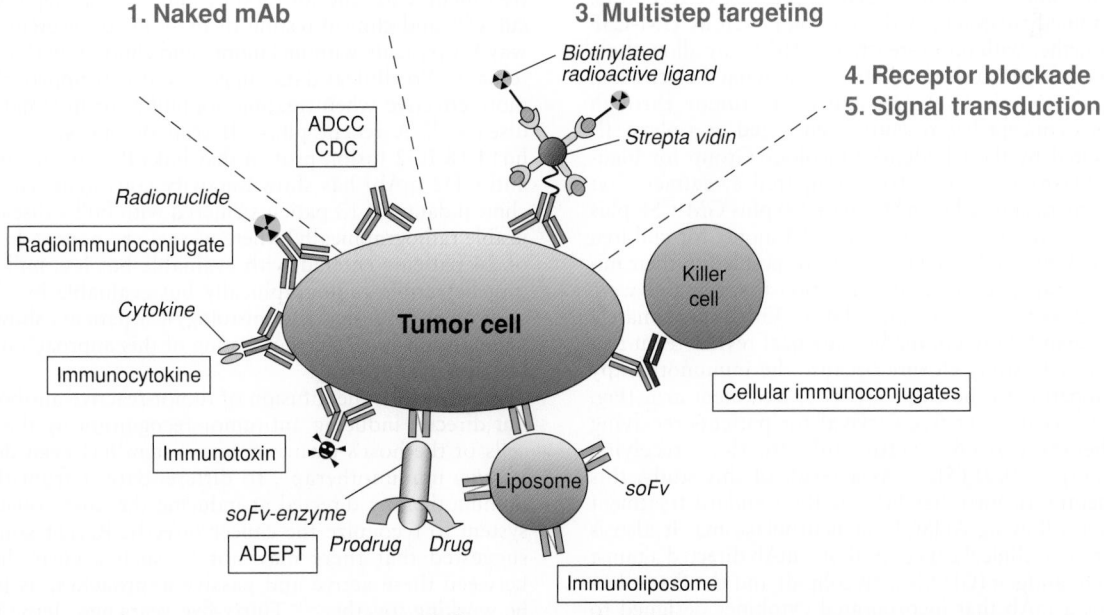

Antitumor applications of mAb

FIGURE 5.14 Effector mechanisms of monoclonal antibodies. ADEPT, antibody-directed enzyme pro-drug therapy; ADCC, antibody-dependent cell-mediated cytotoxicity; CDC, complement-dependent cytotoxicity; mAb, monoclonal antibody; scFv, single-chain Fv fragment. (From Cheung NK, Sondel PM. Neuroblastoma immunology and immunotherapy. In: Cohn S, Cheung NK, eds. Neuroblastoma. New York, NY: Springer, 2005:223–242.)

anti-CD20 mAb. Rituxan can mediate *in vitro* killing against most CD20⁺ B-cell tumors via complement activation. The CD59 cell surface molecule inhibits the formation of the membrane attack complex created by multimers of activated C9, and CD20⁺ B-cell tumors that express CD59 are not destroyed by Rituxan plus complement *in vitro*. However, many patients who have shown beneficial tumor shrinkage following Rituxan treatment have CD20⁺ B-cell tumors that also express CD59, suggesting that complement-mediated destruction is not the main *in vivo* mechanism.[206] Rather, Clynes et al. demonstrated in a mouse model that ADCC was the primary mechanism by which Rituxan exerted its effect *in vivo*.[207] This was because mice genetically engineered to express only activating Fc receptors (FcγRII/III) showed tumor killing with Rituxan, whereas those with inhibitory Fc receptors did not.

Human FcγII on NK cells have two main polymorphisms in the population. Most people have high-affinity binding to the Fc of IgG and have a valine at amino acid position 158, whereas a minority has a receptor with lower affinity for IgG due to a phenylalanine at position 158. Several analyses have shown that patients with the high-affinity FcR have a much greater chance for antitumor efficacy with Rituxan (measured by either tumor shrinkage or time to recurrence/progression).[208,209] A similar analysis has also been conducted for two alleles of the FcγIII expressed on neutrophils and macrophages, and clinical studies indicate better antitumor effects in patients with the more functional FcγIII allele.[210] Further, data consistent with *in vivo* ADCC have come from studies of neuroblastoma and anti-idiotype vaccination.[210,211] Together, the data strongly suggest that ADCC plays an important role in mediating at least some of the beneficial clinical effects of antibody-mediated therapy. Not surprisingly, therefore, many investigators are attempting to enhance the expression of activating Fc receptors on innate immune cells such as NK cells or macrophages in concert with mAb therapy in hopes of improving efficacy. For example, activation of the innate immune system with GM-CSF (neutrophils and macrophages) and IL-2 (NK cells) may have some antitumor activity and is known to activate cells expressing Fc receptors. Thus, combined treatment with cytokines such as GM-CSF and IL-2 together with tumor-reactive mAb[212] may allow these distinct mechanisms to work additively, allowing the activated effector cells to selectively recognize the tumor through ADCC. This concept has recently been tested in a phase III trial sponsored by the Children's Oncology Group for high-risk neuroblastoma.[213] This trial compared a regimen that used the chimeric anti-GD2 mAb (ch14.18) plus GM-CSF plus IL-2 with *cis*-retinoic acid (CRA) to CRA alone, for children with high-risk neuroblastoma that had responded to their initial chemotherapy, surgery, and radiation therapy and were within 100 days of an autologous HSCT. With approximately 2 years' median follow-up, the biostatistical review team recommended early study closure because the immunotherapy arm was superior to the control (CRA) treatment arm (Fig. 5.15). The 2-year event-free survival for patients receiving immunotherapy was 66% versus 46% for those receiving CRA alone (*p* = 0.0115).[214] As a result of this study, this immunotherapy regimen has become the standard treatment for children following AHSCT for neuroblastoma. It also is the first effective clinical cancer trial of a mAb directed against a nonprotein antigen (GD2 is a glycolipid) and the first effective trial of a mAb that incorporated cytokines designed to enhance ADCC. A prior nonrandomized trial of the same ch14.18 mAb in 334 children with high-risk neuroblastoma found this antibody to not provide any clinical benefit.[215] Even though that study was not randomized, and thus did not have

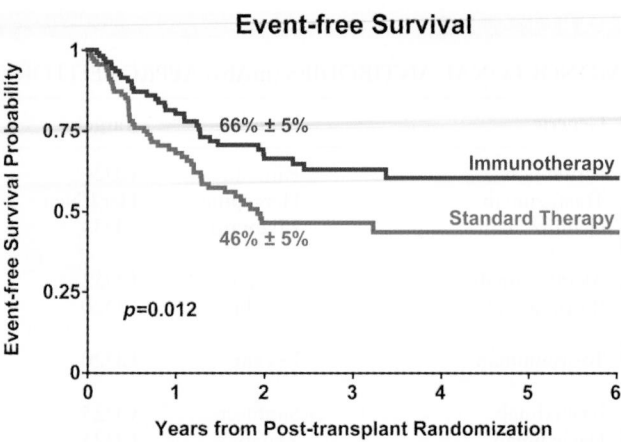

FIGURE 5.15 Activity of immunotherapy in preventing relapse of neuroblastoma. Event free survival for children randomized to cis-retinoic acid (CRA) alone (Standard Therapy) versus Immunotherapy (ch14.18 monoclonal antibody + GM-CSF + IL2 + CRA) for high-risk neuroblastoma.[213] The % values shown indicate data for the 2 year time point. (Data from Children's Oncology Group Operations Office).

the same statistical power as the COG randomized trial, the very different results of these two studies involving the same ch14.18 mAb (in similar doses and schedules) may reflect the use of the GM-CSF and IL-2 in the COG trial, but no cytokines in the Simon et al.[215] trial. Finally, this pediatric study suggests that adding IL-2 plus GM-CSF to treatment with other mAbs that mediate ADCC (such as Herceptin, Rituxan, and Erbitux) may also be appropriate for randomized trial testing in the minimal residual disease setting for high-risk patients.

Novel fusion proteins in which tumor-reactive mAbs are linked to cytokines such as IL-2 (Fig. 5.13) may induce more potent immune reactivity at the sites of tumors *in vivo* than treatment with the antibodies and IL-2 as separate molecules,[216] and clinical testing of these fusion proteins is under way for patients with melanoma and children with neuroblastoma.[217] Preclinical data suggest that this approach will be more effective when treating nonbulky (or minimal residual) disease.[218] A recent phase II trial of one such agent (the hu14.18-IL-2 fusion protein that links IL-2 to the humanized anti-GD2 mAb) has shown activity consistent with the preclinical data. Of 13 patients entered with bulky disease (measurable radiographically), there were no responses. In contrast, of 24 patients entered with evaluable but less bulky disease (not detectable radiographically but evaluable by ¹²⁴I-MIBG scan or by bone marrow histology), 5 patients showed complete responses.[219] Further testing of this approach in neuroblastoma is under way.

Historically, the infusion of tumor-reactive antibody, without directly inducing antitumor recognition by the T and B cells of the host's own immune system has been designated *passive* immunotherapy, to differentiate it from the *active* immunotherapy directed at inducing the host's own immune system to recognize the cancer directly. Recent studies have suggested that there may not be such a clear distinction between these active and passive approaches, as both may be working together.[220] Thirty-five years ago, Jerne proposed an "immune network hypothesis," whereby any immune response turns on a compensatory regulatory response (Fig. 5.16). Within the context of this model, antibody-1 (Ab-1) represents the original antibody induced in response to a

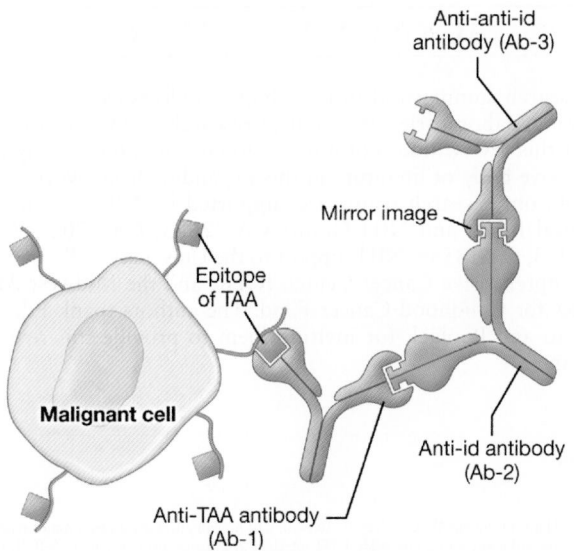

FIGURE 5.16 The immune network: Mimicry of tumor-associated antigens (TAA) by anti-id antibodies. An epitope of a TAA is shown schematically by the *box* attached to a glycoprotein on the membrane of the tumor cell. A monoclonal antibody was made in mice against this TAA. This anti-TAA antibody (Ab-1) has antigen-binding ends (Fab) that allow tight binding of the TAA epitope. When Ab-1 is used as an immunogen, it can induce an antibody directed against it. This anti-idiotypic antibody (Ab-2) has antigen-binding sites that can bind to the antigen binding sites of Ab-1. As such, the antigen binding sites of Ab-2 may interact with the antigen-binding sites of Ab-1 in the same way that the antigen binding sites of Ab-1 interact with the TAA itself. Thus, the antigen-binding sites of both Ab-2 and the TAA are recognized by Ab-1, and the antigen-binding sites of Ab-2 may be immunologically similar in structure to the TAA of the malignant cell. This similarity in structure is referred to as "internal image." If the Ab-2 molecule is recognized as an antigen, the antibody directed against it is an "anti-anti-id antibody" (Ab-3). As the Ab-3 recognizes the internal image of the TAA found on Ab-2, the Ab-3 antibody may directly recognize the TAA itself. This is the rationale behind using an anti-id (Ab-2) to induce an immune response (Ab-3) able to recognize a TAA. (Adapted from Mittleman et al.[213]).

tumor antigen (e.g., GD2). The unique peptide sequence of that Ab-1's antigen-binding component (generated through the somatically derived immunoglobulin gene rearrangement process) can be considered as an antigen itself for the immune system and is designated the *idiotype* of the Ab-1 molecule. Jerne proposed that this could induce the immune system to create an anti-idiotype antibody (Ab-2), which recognizes the idiotype as foreign. Since the antigen-binding portion of the anti-GD2 antibody can specifically interact with the GD2 molecule, and can also specifically interact with the Ab-2 molecule, this implies that the antigen-binding portion of the Ab-2 molecule and the GD2 molecule may have some structural similarity. This concept becomes even more complex when considering the host's immune response against the unique peptide sequence of the antigen-binding portion of the Ab-2 molecule. The anti–Ab-2 molecule (in early descriptions referred to as an *anti-anti-idiotypic* antibody, and now referred to as *Ab-3*) made by the host should recognize the antigen-binding portion of Ab-2 (which has molecular structural similarity to the GD2 itself); thus, the Ab-3 molecule may have direct antitumor recognition capabilities. Sufficient data in a variety of systems have now documented the valid-

ity of this concept. Thus, clinical trials providing passive treatment to patients with antitumor antibody (i.e., Ab-1) suggest that antitumor effects may be influenced by the induction of Ab-3.[221] Furthermore, separate clinical trials are intentionally treating patients with anti-idiotypic antibodies (i.e., Ab-2) in order to induce an Ab-3 response.[220] In such trials the Ab-2 molecule is actually functioning as the antigenic component of a "tumor antigen vaccine." Furthermore, it seems that some patients being "immunized" with Ab-2 molecules are also generating T-cell responses against the initial tumor antigen that had been recognized by the Ab-1 that was the "target" of the Ab-2 molecule.

SUMMARY AND FUTURE DIRECTIONS

The potential importance of the immune system in cancer etiology, pathology, morbidity, and therapy was initially postulated nearly a century ago but remained largely speculative due to inadequate understanding of the basic components of oncogenesis and immune biology. However, advances in the past 25 years have clearly demonstrated that cancer and the immune system interact at multiple levels and that the dynamic interaction between growing tumors and host immunity can both augment and, in some cases, prevent tumor growth. Furthermore, it is now clear that therapies used to treat cancer profoundly alter the ability of the host to initiate or perpetuate immune responses to weak tumor antigens. The challenge for the future is to translate the improved understanding of the reciprocal interactions between tumor and host to better preserve cancer patients' immune defenses to pathogens and to create new immunotherapies that are effective against the malignancies of childhood.

Already, randomized studies have demonstrated benefit to patients by augmentation of innate immunity by using MTP-PE for patients with osteosarcoma and by antibody-mediated antitumor effects in neuroblastoma. It is likely that over the next several years, pediatric oncology will witness many more new clinical initiatives that seek to capitalize on the advances in the understanding of tumor immunology reviewed in this chapter. Among these will be continuing attempts to use tumor vaccines to augment T-cell–mediated responses, which incorporate technological refinements to allow tumor vaccines to be optimized for clinical translation and, thus, be made more widely available. Adjunctive agents that can be used in concert with tumor vaccines, such as cytokines, nonspecific immune stimulants, or approaches that circumvent tumor-induced immune suppression, are likely to be necessary to render tumor vaccine-induced immune responses robust enough to translate into clinical benefit. Finally, adoptive cell therapy remains quite promising and will no doubt benefit from a multitude of technical advances that will make it more readily available and may render it more effective.

With regard to mAb-based therapy, technological advances have created unlimited opportunities for manipulating mAbs and fragments thereof for clinical benefit. As a result, it is anticipated that new molecules targeting already designated tumor antigens will be generated, and new targets for mAb-based therapy will likely be realized. The development of adjunctive approaches to optimize ADCC and other effector mechanisms for mAb-mediated tumor killing have already proven fruitful, and we will likely witness further progress in this arena.

Finally, in virtually all experimental models tested, cancer immunotherapy is most effective when applied in the setting of minimal residual disease. Indeed, both randomized studies demonstrating benefit of immunotherapy in pediatric oncology (MTP-PE in osteosarcoma and ch14.18 plus GM-CSF and IL-2 in neuroblastoma) were effective only in the setting of minimal residual disease. Thus, the most effective application of cancer immunotherapy for the treatment of pediatric malignancies will require that therapies be developed with an eye toward integrating immunotherapy into standard treatment regimens that are already available and that can accomplish significant reductions in disease burden. As such, it is reasonable to envision that immunotherapy for childhood cancers might ultimately find a place as a standard therapy for children with minimal residual disease, known to be at high risk for recurrence, in order to prevent recurrence and prolong disease-free survival.

ACKNOWLEDGMENTS

Research summarized in this chapter reflects experiences of various laboratories and clinical research teams worldwide, but this review does not attempt to cite comprehensively the massive body of literature in this expanding field. Work cited from our research teams are supported by NIH-NCI Intramural funds and NIH Grants CA-32685, CA-87025, CA-81403, CA-13539, NIH support to the University of Wisconsin Comprehensive Cancer Center, ICTR, and the Midwest Athletes for Childhood Cancer Fund. The authors thank Editors Pizzo and Poplack for inviting them to provide this revised chapter.

References

1. Kawakami Y, Rosenberg SA. Immunobiology of human melanoma antigens MART-1 and gp100 and their use for immuno-gene therapy. Int Rev Immunol 1997;14: 173–192.
2. Sallusto F, Lanzavecchia A. Efficient presentation of soluble antigen by culture human dendritic cells in maintained by granulocyte/macrophage colony-stimulating factor plus interleukin-4 and downregulated by tumor necrosis factor alpha. J Exp Med 1994; 179:1109–1118.
3. Ridge JP, Di Rosa F, Matzinger P. A conditioned dendritic cell can be a temporal bridge between a CD4+ T-helper and a T-killer cell [see comments]. Nature 1998;393(6684): 474–478.
4. Banchereau J, Briere F, Caux C, et al. Immunobiology of dendritic cells. Annu Rev Immunol 2000;18:767–811.
5. Lefrançois L. Maturation, selection and specificity of Tcr gamma delta T cells. Immunol Res 1992;11(1):54–65.
6. Douek DC, McFarland RD, Keiser PH, et al. Changes in thymic function with age and during the treatment of HIV infection. Nature 1998;396(6712):690–695.
7. Zinkernagel RM, Doherty PC. MHC-restricted cytotoxic T cells: studies on the biological role of polymorphic major transplantation antigens determining T cell restriction-specificity, function and responsiveness. Adv Immunol 1979;27:51.
8. Kwon ED, Foster BA, Hurwitz AA, et al. Elimination of residual metastatic prostate cancer after surgery and adjunctive cytotoxic T lymphocyte-associated antigen 4 (CTLA-4) blockade immunotherapy. Proc Natl Acad Sci U S A 1999;96(26): 15074–15079.
9. van Elsas A, Hurwitz AA, Allison JP. Combination immunotherapy of B16 melanoma using anti-cytotoxic T lymphocyte-associated antigen 4 (CTLA-4) and granulocyte/macrophage colony-stimulating factor (GM-CSF)-producing vaccines induces rejection of subcutaneous and metastatic tumors accompanied by autoimmune depigmentation. J Exp Med 1999;190(3):355–366.
10. Phan GQ, Yang JC, Sherry RM, et al. Cancer regression and autoimmunity induced by cytotoxic T lymphocyte-associated antigen 4 blockade in patients with metastatic melanoma. Proc Natl Acad Sci U S A 2003;100(14):8372–8377.
11. Fong L, Small EJ. Anti-cytotoxic T-lymphocyte antigen-4 antibody: the first in an emerging class of immunomodulatory antibodies for cancer treatment. J Clin Oncol 2008;26(32):5275–5283.
12. Fourcade J, Kudela P, Sun Z, et al. PD-1 is a regulator of NY-ESO-1-specific CD8+ T cell expansion in melanoma patients. J Immunol 2009;182(9):5240–5249.
13. Bronte V. Th17 and cancer: friends or foes? Blood 2008;112(2):214.
14. Shevach EM. CD4+ CD25+ suppressor T cells: more questions than answers. Nat Rev Immunol 2002;2(6):389–400.
15. Zhang H, Chua KS, Guimond M, et al. Lymphopenia and interleukin-2 therapy alter homeostasis of CD4+CD25+ regulatory T cells. Nat Med 2005;11(11): 1238–1243.
16. Berke G. Unlocking the secrets of CTL and NK cells. Immunol Today 1995;16(7): 343–346.
17. Kontny HU, Hammerle K, Klein R, et al. Sensitivity of Ewing's sarcoma to TRAIL-induced apoptosis. Cell Death Differ 2001;8(5):506–514.
18. Max EE. Immunoglobulins, molecular genetics. In: Paul WE, ed. Fundamental immunology. 5th ed. New York, NY: Lippincott, 2003:107–158.
19. Laman JD, Claassen E, Noelle RJ. Functions of CD40 and its ligand, gp39 (CD40L). Crit Rev Immunol 1996;16(1):59–108.
20. Kwak LW, Taub DD, Duffey PL, et al. Transfer of myeloma idiotype-specific immunity from an actively immunised marrow donor. Lancet 1995;345(8956):1016–1020.
21. Bendandi M, Gocke CD, Kobrin CB, et al. Complete molecular remissions induced by patient-specific vaccination plus granulocyte-monocyte colony-stimulating factor against lymphoma. Nat Med 1999;5(10):1171–1177.
22. Moretta L, Bottino C, Pende D, et al. Human natural killer cells: their origin, receptors and function. Eur J Immunol 2002;32(5):1205–1211.
23. Ashkar AA, Rosenthal KL. Interleukin-15 and natural killer and NKT cells play a critical role in innate protection against genital herpes simplex virus type 2 infection. J Virol 2003;77(18):10168–10171.
24. Pereira RA, Scalzo A, Simmons A. Cutting edge: a NK complex-linked locus governs acute versus latent herpes simplex virus infection of neurons. J Immunol 2001;166(10): 5869–5873.
25. Dunn GP, Old LJ, Schreiber RD. The three Es of cancer immunoediting. Annu Rev Immunol 2004;22:329–360.
26. Ruggeri L, Capanni M, Urbani E, et al. Effectiveness of donor natural killer cell alloreactivity in mismatched hematopoietic transplants. Science 2002;295(5562): 2097–2100.

27. Hank JA, Surfus JE, Gan J, et al. Activation of human effector cells by a tumor reactive recombinant anti-ganglioside GD2 interleukin-2 fusion protein (ch14.18-IL2). Clin Cancer Res 1996;2(12):1951–1959.
28. Doubrovina ES, Doubrovin MM, Vider E, et al. Evasion from NK cell immunity by MHC class I chain-related molecules expressing colon adenocarcinoma. J Immunol 2003;171(12):6891–6899.
29. Moretta A, Bottino C, Vitale M, et al. Activating receptors and coreceptors involved in human natural killer cell-mediated cytolysis. Annu Rev Immunol 2001;19: 197–223.
30. Neal ZC, Imboden M, Rakhmilevich AL, et al. NXS2 murine neuroblastomas express increased levels of MHC class I antigens upon recurrence following NK-dependent immunotherapy. Cancer Immunol Immunother 2004;53(1):41–52.
31. Hank JA, Weil-Hillman G, Surfus JE, et al. Addition of interleukin-2 in vitro augments detection of lymphokine-activated killer activity generated in vivo. Cancer Immunol Immunother 1990;31(1):53–59.
32. Fujisaki H, Kakuda H, Shimasaki N, et al. Expansion of highly cytotoxic human natural killer cells for cancer cell therapy. Cancer Res 2009;69(9):4010–4017.
33. Waldmann TA. The biology of interleukin-2 and interleukin-15: implications for cancer therapy and vaccine design. Nat Rev Immunol 2006;6(8):595–601.
34. Neal ZC, Sondel PM, Bates MK, et al. Flt3-L gene therapy enhances immunocytokine-mediated antitumor effects and induces long-term memory. Cancer Immunol Immunother 2007;56(11):1765–1774.
35. Mackall CL, Fleisher TA, Brown MR, et al. Lymphocyte depletion during treatment with intensive chemotherapy for cancer. Blood 1994;84:2221–2228.
36. Mohty M, Gaugler B, Faucher C, et al. Recovery of lymphocyte and dendritic cell subsets following reduced intensity allogeneic bone marrow transplantation. Hematology 2002;7(3):157–164.
37. Damiani D, Stocchi R, Masolini P, et al. Dendritic cell recovery after autologous stem cell transplantation. Bone Marrow Transplant 2002;30(5):261–266.
38. Santosuosso M, Divangahi M, Zganiacz A, et al. Reduced tissue macrophage population in the lung by anticancer agent cyclophosphamide: restoration by local granulocyte macrophage-colony-stimulating factor gene transfer. Blood 2002;99(4):1246–1252.
39. Rodriguez PC, Ochoa AC. Arginine regulation by myeloid derived suppressor cells and tolerance in cancer: mechanisms and therapeutic perspectives. Immunol Rev 2008;222: 180–191.
40. Angulo I, de las Heras FG, Garcia-Bustos JF, et al. Nitric oxide-producing CD11b(+)Ly-6G(Gr-1)(+)CD31(ER-MP12)(+) cells in the spleen of cyclophosphamide-treated mice: implications for T-cell responses in immunosuppressed mice. Blood 2000;95(1):212–220.
41. Bronte V, Apolloni E, Cabrelle A, et al. Identification of a CD11b(+)/Gr-1(+)/CD31(+) myeloid progenitor capable of activating or suppressing CD8(+) T cells. Blood 2000;96(12):3838–3846.
42. Ino K, Singh RK, Talmadge JE. Monocytes from mobilized stem cells inhibit T cell function. J Leukoc Biol 1997;61(5):583–591.
43. Ageitos AG, Varney ML, Bierman PJ, et al. Comparison of monocyte-dependent T cell inhibitory activity in GM-CSF vs G-CSF mobilized PSC products. Bone Marrow Transplant 1999;23(1):63–69.
44. Varney ML, Ino K, Ageitos AG, et al. Expression of interleukin-10 in isolated CD8+ T cells and monocytes from growth factor-mobilized peripheral blood stem cell products: a mechanism of immune dysfunction. J Interferon Cytokine Res 1999;19(4):351–360.
45. Sepkowitz KA. Pneumocystis carinii pneumonia among patients with neoplastic disease. Semin Respir Infect 1992;7:114–121.
46. Henson JW, Jalaj JK, Walker RW, et al. Pneumocystis carinii pneumonia in patients with primary brain tumors. Arch Neurol 1991;48(4):406–409.
47. Kalthoff FS, Chung J, Musser P, et al. Pimecrolimus does not affect the differentiation, maturation and function of human monocyte-derived dendritic cells, in contrast to corticosteroids. Clin Exp Immunol 2003;133(3):350–359.
48. Piemonti L, Monti P, Allavena P, et al. Glucocorticoids affect human dendritic cell differentiation and maturation. J Immunol 1999;162(11):6473–6481.
49. Woltman AM, de Fijter JW, Kamerling SW, et al. The effect of calcineurin inhibitors and corticosteroids on the differentiation of human dendritic cells. Eur J Immunol 2000;30(7):1807–1812.
50. de Jong EC, Vieira PL, Kalinski P, et al. Corticosteroids inhibit the production of inflammatory mediators in immature monocyte-derived DC and induce the development of tolerogenic DC3. J Leukoc Biol 1999;66(2):201–204.
51. Vieira PL, Kalinski P, Wierenga EA, et al. Glucocorticoids inhibit bioactive IL-12p70 production by in vitro-generated human dendritic cells without affecting their T cell stimulatory potential. J Immunol 1998;161(10):5245–5251.

52. Storek J, Ferrara S, Ku N, et al. B cell reconstitution after human bone marrow transplantation: recapitulation of ontogeny? Bone Marrow Transplant 1993;12: 387–398.

53. Small TN, Keever CA, Weiner-Fedus S, et al. B cell differentiation following autologous, conventional or T cell depleted bone marrow transplantation: a recapitulation of normal B cell ontogeny. Blood 1990;76(8):1647–1656.

54. Mackall CL, Stein D, Fleisher TA, et al. Prolonged CD4 depletion after sequential autologous peripheral blood progenitor cell infusions in children and young adults. Blood 2000;96(2):754–762.

55. Miller RA, Daley J, Ghalie R, et al. Clonal analysis of T cell deficiencies in autotransplant recipients. Blood 1991;77(8):1845–1850.

56. Enright H, Haake R, Weisdorf D, et al. Cytomegalovirus pneumonia after bone marrow transplantation: risk factors and response to therapy. Transplantation 1993;55(6): 1339–1346.

57. Mackall CL, Velardi A, Hakim FT. The immune system in graft-versus-host disease: target and effector organ. In: Ferrara JLM, Cooke KR, Deeg HJ, eds. Graft vs host disease. 3rd ed. New York, NY: Marcel-Dekker, 2004.

58. Schilling PJ, Vadhan-Raj S. Concurrent cytomegalovirus and pneumocystis pneumonia after fludarabine therapy for chronic lymphocytic leukemia. N Engl J Med 1990;323: 833–834.

59. Alanko S, Pelliniemi TT, Salmi TT. Recovery of blood lymphocytes and serum immunoglobulins after treatment of solid tumors in children. Pediatr Hematol Oncol 1994;11:33–45.

60. Kotsakis A, Sarra E, Peraki M, et al. Docetaxel-induced lymphopenia in patients with solid tumors: a prospective phenotypic analysis. Cancer 2000;89(6):1380–1386.

61. Ferrari S, Rovati B, Cucca L, et al. Impact of topotecan-based chemotherapy on the immune system of advanced ovarian cancer patients: an immunophenotypic study. Oncol Rep 2002;9(5):1107–1113.

62. Hakim FT, Cepeda R, Kaimei S, et al. Constraints on CD4 recovery post chemotherapy in adults: thymic insufficiency and apoptotic decline of expanded peripheral CD4 cells. Blood 1997;90:3789–3798.

63. Mackall CL, Granger L, Sheard MA, et al. T cell regeneration after bone marrow transplantation: differential CD45 isoform expression on thymic-derived versus thymic-independent progeny. Blood 1993;82:2585–2594.

64. Kimmig S, Przybylski GK, Schmidt CA, et al. Two subsets of naive T helper cells with distinct T cell receptor excision circle content in human adult peripheral blood. J Exp Med 2002;195(6):789–794.

65. Mackall CL, Fleisher TA, Brown MR, et al. Age, thymopoiesis and CD4+ T lymphocyte regeneration after intensive chemotherapy. N Engl J Med 1995;332:143–149.

66. Weinberg K, Blazar BR, Wagner JE, et al. Factors affecting thymic function after allogeneic hematopoietic stem cell transplantation. Blood 2001;97(5):1458–1466.

67. Watanabe N, De Rosa SC, Cmelak A, et al. Long-term depletion of naive T cells in patients treated for Hodgkin's disease. Blood 1997;90(9):3662–3672.

68. Mackall CL, Hakim FT, Gress RE. T-cell regeneration: all repertoires are not created equal. Immunol Today 1997;18:245–251.

69. Mackall CL, Fleisher TA, Brown MR, et al. Distinctions between CD8+ and CD4+ T cell regenerative pathways result in prolonged T cell subset imbalance after intensive chemotherapy. Blood 1997;89:3700–3707.

70. Gattinoni L, Finkelstein SE, Klebanoff CA, et al. Removal of homeostatic cytokine sinks by lymphodepletion enhances the efficacy of adoptively transferred tumor-specific CD8+ T cells. J Exp Med 2005;202(7):907–912.

71. Dudley ME, Yang JC, Sherry R, et al. Adoptive cell therapy for patients with metastatic melanoma: evaluation of intensive myeloablative chemoradiation preparative regimens. J Clin Oncol 2008;26(32):5233–5239.

72. Mackall CL, Fry TJ, Bare C, et al. IL-7 increases both thymic-dependent and thymic-independent T-cell regeneration after bone marrow transplantation. Blood 2001;97(5): 1491–1497.

73. Fry TJ, Christensen BL, Komschlies KL, et al. Interleukin-7 restores immunity in athymic T-cell-depleted hosts. Blood 2001;97(6):1525–1533.

74. Fry TJ, Sinha M, Milliron M, et al. Flt 3 ligand enhances thymic-dependent and thymic-independent immune reconstitution. Blood 2004;104(9):2794–2800.

75. Sportes C, Hakim FT, Memon SA, et al. Administration of rhIL-7 in humans increases in vivo TCR repertoire diversity by preferential expansion of naive T cell subsets. J Exp Med 2008;205(7):1701–1714.

76. Burnet FM. Cancer—a biological approach. Br Med J 1957;1:841–847.

77. Kaplan DH, Shankaran V, Dighe AS, et al. Demonstration of an interferon gamma-dependent tumor surveillance system in immunocompetent mice. Proc Natl Acad Sci U S A 1998;95(13):7556–7561.

78. Shankaran V, Ikeda H, Bruce AT, et al. IFNgamma and lymphocytes prevent primary tumour development and shape tumour immunogenicity. Nature 2001;410(6832): 1107–1111.

79. Smyth MJ, Crowe NY, Godfrey DI. NK cells and NKT cells collaborate in host protection from methylcholanthrene-induced fibrosarcoma. Int Immunol 2001;13(4): 459–463.

80. Smyth MJ, Cretney E, Takeda K, et al. Tumor necrosis factor-related apoptosis-inducing ligand (TRAIL) contributes to interferon gamma-dependent natural killer cell protection from tumor metastasis. J Exp Med 2001;193(6):661–670.

81. Cretney E, Takeda K, Yagita H, et al. Increased susceptibility to tumor initiation and metastasis in TNF-related apoptosis-inducing ligand-deficient mice. J Immunol 2002;168(3):1356–1361.

82. Filipovich AH, Mathur A, Kamat D, et al. Primary immunodeficiencies: genetic risk factors for lymphoma. Cancer Res 1992;52(19)(suppl):5465s–5467s.

83. Nelson DL, Terhorst C. X-linked lymphoproliferative syndrome. Clin Exp Immunol 2000;122(3):291–295.

84. Penn I. De novo malignancy in pediatric organ transplant recipients. J Pediatr Surg 1994;29(2):221–226, discussion 227–228.

85. Savitsky K, Bar-Shira A, Gilad S, et al. A single ataxia telangiectasia gene with a product similar to PI-3 kinase [see comments]. Science 1995;268(5218):1749–1753.

86. Bolotin E, Annett G, Parkman R, et al. Serum levels of IL-7 in bone marrow transplant recipients: relationship to clinical characteristics and lymphocyte count. Bone Marrow Transplant 1999;23(8):783–788.

87. Fry TJ, Connick E, Falloon J, et al. A potential role for interleukin-7 in T-cell homeostasis. Blood 2001;97(10):2983–2990.

88. Mertsching E, Meyer V, Linares J, et al. Interleukin-7, a non-redundant potent cytokine whose over-expression massively perturbs B-lymphopoiesis. Int Rev Immunol 1998; 16(3/4):285–308.

89. Valenzona HO, Pointer R, Ceredig R, et al. Prelymphomatous B cell hyperplasia in the bone marrow of interleukin-7 transgenic mice: precursor B cell dynamics, microenvironmental organization and osteolysis. Exp Hematol 1996;24(13): 1521–1529.

90. Schreiber H, Wu TH, Nachman J, et al. Immunodominance and tumor escape. Semin Cancer Biol 2002;12(1):25–31.

91. Collins RH, Shpilberg O, Drobyski WR, et al. Donor leukocyte infusions in 140 patients with relapsed malignancy after allogeneic bone marrow transplantation. J Clin Oncol 1997;15(2):433–444.

92. Atra A, Millar B, Shepherd V, et al. Donor lymphocyte infusion for childhood acute lymphoblastic leukaemia relapsing after bone marrow transplantation. Br J Haematol 1997;97(1):165–168.

93. Dazzi F, Szydlo RM, Goldman JM. Donor lymphocyte infusions for relapse of chronic myeloid leukemia after allogeneic stem cell transplant: where we now stand. Exp Hematol 1999;27(10):1477–1486.

94. Porter DL, Collins RH, Hardy C, et al. Treatment of relapsed leukemia after unrelated donor marrow transplantation with unrelated donor leukocyte infusions. Blood 2000; 95(4):1214–1221.

95. Helg C, Starobinski M, Jeannet M, et al. Donor lymphocyte infusion for the treatment of relapse after allogeneic hematopoietic stem cell transplantation. Leuk Lymphoma 1998;29(3/4):301–313.

96. Gambini C, Conte M, Bernini G, et al. Neuroblastic tumors associated with opso-clonus-myoclonus syndrome: histological, immunohistochemical and molecular features of 15 Italian cases. Virchows Arch 2003;442(6):555–562.

97. Cooper R, Khakoo Y, Matthay KK, et al. Opsoclonus-myoclonus-ataxia syndrome in neuroblastoma: histopathologic features—a report from the Children's Cancer Group. Med Pediatr Oncol 2001;36(6):623–629.

98. Rudnick E, Khakoo Y, Antunes NL, et al. Opsoclonus-myoclonus-ataxia syndrome in neuroblastoma: clinical outcome and antineuronal antibodies—a report from the Children's Cancer Group Study. Med Pediatr Oncol 2001;36(6):612–622.

99. Antunes NL, Khakoo Y, Matthay KK, et al. Antineuronal antibodies in patients with neuroblastoma and paraneoplastic opsoclonus-myoclonus. J Pediatr Hematol Oncol 2000;22(4):315–320.

100. Yoshida R, Yoneda Y, Kuriyama M, et al. IFN-gamma- and cell-to-cell contact-dependent cytotoxicity of allograft-induced macrophages against syngeneic tumor cells and cell lines: an application of allografting to cancer treatment. J Immunol 1999;163(1):148–154.

101. Kleinerman ES. Biologic therapy for osteosarcoma using liposome-encapsulated muramyl tripeptide. Hematol Oncol Clin North Am 1995;9(4):927–938.

102. Kurzman ID, MacEwen EG, Rosenthal RC, et al. Adjuvant therapy for osteosarcoma in dogs: results of randomized clinical trials using combined liposome-encapsulated muramyl tripeptide and cisplatin. Clin Cancer Res 1995;1(12):1595–1601.

103. Meyers PA, Schwartz CL, Krailo MD, et al. Osteosarcoma: the addition of muramyl tripeptide to chemotherapy improves overall survival—a report from the Children's Oncology Group. J Clin Oncol 2008;26(4):633–638.

104. Anderson PM, Markovic SN, Sloan JA, et al. Aerosol granulocyte macrophage-colony stimulating factor: a low toxicity, lung-specific biological therapy in patients with lung metastases. Clin Cancer Res 1999;5(9):2316–2323.

105. Vollmer J, Weeratna R, Payette P, et al. Characterization of three CpG oligodeoxynucleotide classes with distinct immunostimulatory activities. Eur J Immunol 2004;34(1): 251–262.

106. Weigel BJ, Rodeberg DA, Krieg AM, et al. CpG oligodeoxynucleotides potentiate the antitumor effects of chemotherapy or tumor resection in an orthotopic murine model of rhabdomyosarcoma. Clin Cancer Res 2003;9(8):3105–3114.

107. van der Bruggen P, Traversari C, Chomez P, et al. A gene encoding an antigen recognized by cytolytic T lymphocytes on a human melanoma. Science 1991;254(5038): 1643–1647.

108. Kawakami Y, Eliyahu S, Delgado CH, et al. Cloning of the gene coding for a shared human melanoma antigen recognized by autologous T cells infiltrating into tumor. Proc Natl Acad Sci U S A 1994;91(9):3515–3519.

109. Van den Eynde BJ, van der Bruggen P. T cell defined tumor antigens. Curr Opin Immunol 1997;9(5):684–693.

110. Rosenberg SA, White DE. Vitiligo in patients with melanoma: normal tissue antigens can be targets for cancer immunotherapy. J Immunother Emphasis Tumor Immunol 1996;19:81–84.

111. Overwijk WW, Lee DS, Surman DR, et al. Vaccination with a recombinant vaccinia virus encoding a "self" antigen induces autoimmune vitiligo and tumor cell destruction in mice: requirement for CD4(+) T lymphocytes. Proc Natl Acad Sci U S A 1999;96(6): 2982–2987.

112. Alexander-Miller MA, Leggatt GR, Berzofsky JA. Selective expansion of high- or low-avidity cytotoxic T lymphocytes and efficacy for adoptive immunotherapy. Proc Natl Acad Sci U S A 1996;93(9):4102–4107.

113. Zeh H Jr, Perry-Lalley D, Dudley ME, et al. High avidity CTLs for two self-antigens demonstrate superior in vitro and in vivo antitumor efficacy. J Immunol 1999;162(2): 989–994.

114. Thurner B, Haendle I, Roder C, et al. Vaccination with mage-3A1 peptide-pulsed mature, monocyte-derived dendritic cells expands specific cytotoxic T cells and induces regression of some metastases in advanced stage IV melanoma. J Exp Med 1999;190(11): 1669–1678.

115. Scanlan MJ, Gure AO, Jungbluth AA, et al. Cancer/testis antigens: an expanding family of targets for cancer immunotherapy. Immunol Rev 2002;188:22–32.

116. Scarcella DL, Chow CW, Gonzales MF, et al. Expression of MAGE and GAGE in high-grade brain tumors: a potential target for specific immunotherapy and diagnostic markers. Clin Cancer Res 1999;5(2):335–341.

117. Sahin U, Koslowski M, Tureci O, et al. Expression of cancer testis genes in human brain tumors. Clin Cancer Res 2000;6(10):3916–3922.

118. Cheung IY, Cheung NK. Molecular detection of GAGE expression in peripheral blood and bone marrow: utility as a tumor marker for neuroblastoma. Clin Cancer Res 1997;3(5):821–826.

119. Greiner J, Ringhoffer M, Taniguchi M, et al. mRNA expression of leukemia-associated antigens in patients with acute myeloid leukemia for the development of specific immunotherapies. Int J Cancer 2004;108(5):704–711.

120. Liu XF, Helman LJ, Yeung C, et al. XAGE-1, a new gene that is frequently expressed in Ewing's sarcoma. Cancer Res 2000;60(17):4752–4755.

121. Rodolfo M, Luksch R, Stockert E, et al. Antigen-specific immunity in neuroblastoma patients: antibody and T-cell recognition of NY-ESO-1 tumor antigen. Cancer Res 2003;63(20):6948–6955.

122. Soling A, Schurr P, Berthold F. Expression and clinical relevance of NY-ESO-1, MAGE-1 and MAGE-3 in neuroblastoma. Anticancer Res 1999;19(3B):2205–2209.
123. Li CM, Guo M, Borczuk A, et al. Gene expression in Wilms' tumor mimics the earliest committed stage in the metanephric mesenchymal-epithelial transition. Am J Pathol 2002;160(6):2181–2190.
124. Oberthuer A, Hero B, Spitz R, et al. The tumor-associated antigen PRAME is universally expressed in high-stage neuroblastoma and associated with poor outcome. Clin Cancer Res 2004;10(13):4307–4313.
125. Steinbach D, Hermann J, Viehmann S, et al. Clinical implications of PRAME gene expression in childhood acute myeloid leukemia. Cancer Genet Cytogenet 2002;133(2): 118–123.
126. Radvanyi L. Discovery and immunologic validation of new antigens for therapeutic cancer vaccines. Int Arch Allergy Immunol 2004;133(2):179–197.
127. Boon T, van der Bruggen P. Human tumor antigens recognized by T lymphocytes. J Exp Med 1996;183(3):725–729.
128. Schmollinger JC, Vonderheide RH, Hoar KM, et al. Melanoma inhibitor of apoptosis protein (ML-IAP) is a target for immune-mediated tumor destruction. Proc Natl Acad Sci U S A 2003;100(6):3398–3403.
129. Sarkar AK, Nuchtern JG. Lysis of MYCN-amplified neuroblastoma cells by MYCN peptide-specific cytotoxic T lymphocytes. Cancer Res 2000;60(7):1908–1913.
130. Sarkar AK, Burlingame SM, Zang YQ, et al. Major histocompatibility complex-restricted lysis of neuroblastoma cells by autologous cytotoxic T lymphocytes. J Immunother 2001;24(4):305–311.
131. Kaufman HL, Wang W, Manola J, et al. Phase II randomized study of vaccine treatment of advanced prostate cancer (E7897): a trial of the Eastern Cooperative Oncology Group. J Clin Oncol 2004;22(11):2122–2132.
132. Molldrem JJ, Lee PP, Wang C, et al. Evidence that specific T lymphocytes may participate in the elimination of chronic myelogenous leukemia. Nat Med 2000;6(9): 1018–1023.
133. Molldrem J. Immune therapy of AML. Cytotherapy 2002;4(5):437–438.
134. Oh S, Terabe M, Pendleton CD, et al. Human CTLs to wild-type and enhanced epitopes of a novel prostate and breast tumor-associated protein, TARP, lyse human breast cancer cells. Cancer Res 2004;64(7):2610–2618.
135. Sugiyama H. Cancer immunotherapy targeting WT1 protein. Int J Hematol 2002;76(2): 127–132.
136. Oka Y, Tsuboi A, Elisseeva OA, et al. WT1 as a novel target antigen for cancer immunotherapy. Curr Cancer Drug Targets 2002;2(1):45–54.
137. Coggin JH Jr, Barsoum AL, Rohrer JW. 37 kiloDalton oncofetal antigen protein and immature laminin receptor protein are identical, universal T-cell inducing immunogens on primary rodent and human cancers. Anticancer Res 1999;19(6C):5535–5542.
138. Siegel S, Wagner A, Kabelitz D, et al. Induction of cytotoxic T-cell responses against the oncofetal antigen-immature laminin receptor for the treatment of hematologic malignancies. Blood 2003;102(13):4416–4423.
139. Andersen MH, thor SP. Survivin—a universal tumor antigen. Histol Histopathol 2002;17(2):669–675.
140. Gordan JD, Vonderheide RH. Universal tumor antigens as targets for immunotherapy. Cytotherapy 2002;4(4):317–327.
141. Altieri DC. Validating survivin as a cancer therapeutic target. Nat Rev Cancer 2003;3(1):46–54.
142. Vonderheide RH, Hahn WC, Schultze JL, et al. The telomerase catalytic subunit is a widely expressed tumor-associated antigen recognized by cytotoxic T lymphocytes. Immunity 1999;10(6):673–679.
143. Vonderheide RH, Domchek SM, Schultze JL, et al. Vaccination of cancer patients against telomerase induces functional antitumor CD8+ T lymphocytes. Clin Cancer Res 2004;10(3):828–839.
144. Maecker B, Sherr DH, Vonderheide RH, et al. The shared tumor-associated antigen cytochrome P450 1B1 is recognized by specific cytotoxic T cells. Blood 2003;102(9): 3287–3294.
145. Murray GI, Taylor MC, McFadyen MC, et al. Tumor-specific expression of cytochrome P450 CYP1B1. Cancer Res 1997;57(14):3026–3031.
146. Kim SB, Kwak LW. The use of idiotype as a target for clinical immunotherapy of B cell malignancies. Cancer Chemother Biol Response Modif 2001;19:289–295.
147. Dar MM, Kwak LW. Vaccination strategies for lymphomas. Curr Oncol Rep 2003;5(5): 380–386.
148. Worley BS, van den Broeke LT, Goletz TJ, et al. Antigenicity of fusion proteins from sarcoma-associated chromosomal translocations. Cancer Res 2001;61(18):6868–6875.
149. Yotnda P, Firat H, Garcia-Pons F, et al. Cytotoxic T cell response against the chimeric p210 BCR-ABL protein in patients with chronic myelogenous leukemia. J Clin Invest 1998;101(10):2290–2296.
150. Yotnda P, Garcia F, Peuchmaur M, et al. Cytotoxic T cell response against the chimeric ETV6-AML1 protein in childhood acute lymphoblastic leukemia. J Clin Invest 1998;102(2):455–462.
151. Finn OJ, Jerome KR, Henderson RA, et al. MUC-1 epithelial tumor mucin-based immunity and cancer vaccines. Immunol Rev 1995;145:61–89.
152. Wang RF, Rosenberg SA. Human tumor antigens recognized by T lymphocytes: implications for cancer therapy. J Leukoc Biol 1996;60(3):296–309.
153. Yanuck M, Carbone DP, Pendleton CD, et al. A mutant p53 tumor suppressor protein is a target for peptide-induced CD8+ cytotoxic T cells. Cancer Res 1993;53: 3257–3261.
154. Maher VE, Worley BS, Contois D, et al. Mutant oncogene and tumor suppressor gene products and fusion proteins created by chromosomal translocations as targets for cancer vaccines. In: Kast WM, ed. Peptide-based cancer vaccines. Georgetown, TX: Landes Biosciences, 2000:17–39.
155. Smith MC, Pendleton CD, Maher VE, et al. Oncogenic mutations in ras create HLA-A2.1 binding peptides but affect their extracellular antigen processing. Int Immunol 1997;9(8):1085–1093.
156. Abrams SI, Hand PH, Tsang KY, et al. Mutant ras epitopes as targets for cancer vaccines. Semin Oncol 1996;23(1):118–134.
157. Koutsky LA, Ault KA, Wheeler CM, et al. A controlled trial of a human papillomavirus type 16 vaccine. N Engl J Med 2002;347(21):1645–1651.
158. Steller MA. Human papillomavirus, it's genes . . . and cancer vaccines. Cancer Cell 2003;3(1):7–8.
159. Roskrow MA, Suzuki N, Gan Y, et al. Epstein-Barr virus (EBV)-specific cytotoxic T lymphocytes for the treatment of patients with EBV-positive relapsed Hodgkin's disease. Blood 1998;91(8):2925–2934.
160. Bollard CM, Straathof KC, Huls MH, et al. The generation and characterization of LMP2-specific CTLs for use as adoptive transfer from patients with relapsed EBV-positive Hodgkin disease. J Immunother 2004;27(4):317–327.
161. Nomura M, Ohashi T, Nishikawa K, et al. Repression of tax expression is associated both with resistance of human T-cell leukemia virus type 1-infected T cells to killing by tax-specific cytotoxic T lymphocytes and with impaired tumorigenicity in a rat model. J Virol 2004;78(8):3827–3836.
162. Kimball LE, Casper C, Koelle DM, et al. Reduced levels of neutralizing antibodies to Kaposi sarcoma-associated herpesvirus in persons with a history of Kaposi sarcoma. J Infect Dis 2004;189(11):2016–2022.
163. Takahashi A, Higashino F, Aoyagi M, et al. EWS/ETS fusions activate telomerase in Ewing's tumors. Cancer Res 2003;63(23):8338–8344.
164. Ohali A, Avigad S, Cohen IJ, et al. Association between telomerase activity and outcome in patients with nonmetastatic Ewing family of tumors. J Clin Oncol 2003;21(20): 3836–3843.
165. Paydas S, Tanriverdi K, Yavuz S, et al. Survivin and aven: two distinct antiapoptotic signals in acute leukemias. Ann Oncol 2003;14(7):1045–1050.
166. Adida C, Berrebi D, Peuchmaur M, et al. Anti-apoptosis gene, survivin, and prognosis of neuroblastoma. Lancet 1998;351(9106):882–883.
167. Islam A, Kageyama H, Hashizume K, et al. Role of survivin, whose gene is mapped to 17q25, in human neuroblastoma and identification of a novel dominant-negative isoform, survivin-beta/2B. Med Pediatr Oncol 2000;35(6):550–553.
168. Coughlin CM, Vance BA, Grupp SA, et al. RNA-transfected CD40-activated B cells induce functional T-cell responses against viral and tumor antigen targets: implications for pediatric immunotherapy. Blood 2004;103(6):2046–2054.
169. Uyttenhove C, Godfraind C, Lethe B, et al. The expression of mouse gene P1A in testis does not prevent safe induction of cytolytic T cells against a P1A-encoded tumor antigen. Int J Cancer 1997;70(3):349–356.
170. De Smet C, De Backer O, Faraoni I, et al. The activation of human gene MAGE-1 in tumor cells is correlated with genome-wide demethylation. Proc Natl Acad Sci U S A 1996;93(14):7149–7153.
171. Weber J, Salgaller M, Samid D, et al. Expression of the MAGE-1 tumor antigen is up-regulated by the demethylating agent 5-aza-2′-deoxycytidine. Cancer Res 1994;54(7): 1766–1771.
172. Cheung IY, Barber D, Cheung NK. Detection of microscopic neuroblastoma in marrow by histology, immunocytology, and reverse transcription-PCR of multiple molecular markers. Clin Cancer Res 1998;4(11):2801–2805.
173. Corrias MV, Scaruffi P, Occhino M, et al. Expression of MAGE-1, MAGE-3 and MART-1 genes in neuroblastoma. Int J Cancer 1996;69(5):403–407.
174. Ishida H, Matsumura T, Salgaller ML, et al. MAGE-1 and MAGE-3 or -6 expression in neuroblastoma-related pediatric solid tumors. Int J Cancer 1996;69(5):375–380.
175. Sudo T, Kuramoto T, Komiya S, et al. Expression of MAGE genes in osteosarcoma. J Orthop Res 1997;15(1):128–132.
176. van Baren N, Chambost H, Ferrant A, et al. PRAME, a gene encoding an antigen recognized on a human melanoma by cytolytic T cells, is expressed in acute leukaemia cells. Br J Haematol 1998;102(5):1376–1379.
177. Brinkmann U, Vasmatzis G, Lee B, et al. Novel genes in the PAGE and GAGE family of tumor antigens found by homology walking in the dbEST database. Cancer Res 1999;59(7):1445–1458.
178. van den Broeke LT, Pendleton CD, et al. Identification and epitope enhancement of a PAX-FKHR fusion protein breakpoint epitope in alveolar rhabdomyosarcoma cells created by a tumorigenic chromosomal translocation inducing CTL capable of lysing human tumors. Cancer Res 2006;66(3):1818–1823.
179. Tatsumi T, Gambotto A, Robbins PD, et al. Interleukin 18 gene transfer expands the repertoire of antitumor Th1-type immunity elicited by dendritic cell-based vaccines in association with enhanced therapeutic efficacy. Cancer Res 2002;62(20): 5853–5858.
180. Rosenberg SA, Yang JC, Schwartzentruber DJ, et al. Immunologic and therapeutic evaluation of a synthetic peptide vaccine for the treatment of patients with metastatic melanoma. Nat Med 1998;4(3):321–327.
181. Finke LH, Wentworth K, Blumenstein B, et al. Lessons from randomized phase III studies with active cancer immunotherapies—outcomes from the 2006 meeting of the Cancer Vaccine Consortium (CVC). Vaccine 2007;25(suppl 2):B97–B109.
182. Bowman L, Grossmann M, Rill D, et al. IL-2 adenovector-transduced autologous tumor cells induce antitumor immune responses in patients with neuroblastoma. Blood 1998;92(6):1941–1949.
183. Brenner MK, Heslop H, Krance R, et al. Phase I study of chemokine and cytokine gene-modified autologous neuroblastoma cells for treatment of relapsed/refractory neuroblastoma using an adenoviral vector. Hum Gene Ther 2000;11(10): 1477–1488.
184. Fields RC, Shimizu K, Mule JJ. Murine dendritic cells pulsed with whole tumor lysates mediate potent antitumor immune responses in vitro and in vivo. Proc Natl Acad Sci U S A 1998;95(16):9482–9487.
185. Geiger JD, Hutchinson RJ, Hohenkirk LF, et al. Vaccination of pediatric solid tumor patients with tumor lysate-pulsed dendritic cells can expand specific T cells and mediate tumor regression. Cancer Res 2001;61(23):8513–8519.
186. Albert ML, Sauter B, Bhardwaj N. Dendritic cells acquire antigen from apoptotic cells and induce class I-restricted CTLs. Nature 1998;392(6671):86–89.
187. Albert ML, Pearce SF, Francisco LM, et al. Immature dendritic cells phagocytose apoptotic cells via alphabeta5 and CD36, and cross-present antigens to cytotoxic T lymphocytes. J Exp Med 1998;188(7):1359–1368.
188. Nair SK, Boczkowski D, Morse M, et al. Induction of primary carcinoembryonic antigen (CEA)-specific cytotoxic T lymphocytes in vitro using human dendritic cells transfected with RNA. Nat Biotechnol 1998;16(4):364–369.
189. Nair SK, Hull S, Coleman D, et al. Induction of carcinoembryonic antigen (CEA)-specific cytotoxic T-lymphocyte responses in vitro using autologous dendritic cells loaded with CEA peptide or CEA RNA in patients with metastatic malignancies expressing CEA. Int J Cancer 1999;82(1):121–124.
190. Rosenberg SA, Yang JC, Restifo NP. Cancer immunotherapy: moving beyond current vaccines. Nat Med 2004;10(9):909–915.
191. Papadopoulos EB, Ladanyi M, Emanuel D, et al. Infusions of donor leukocytes to treat Epstein-Barr virus-associated lymphoproliferative disorders after allogeneic bone marrow transplantation. N Engl J Med 1994;330:1185–1191.
192. Rooney CM, Smith CA, Ng CY, et al. Infusion of cytotoxic T cells for the prevention and treatment of Epstein-Barr virus-induced lymphoma in allogeneic transplant recipients. Blood 1998;92(5):1549–1555.

193. Heslop HE, Ng CY, Li C, et al. Long-term restoration of immunity against Epstein-Barr virus infection by adoptive transfer of gene-modified virus-specific T lymphocytes. Nat Med 1996;2(5):551–555.
194. O'Reilly RJ, Small TN, Papadopoulos E, et al. Biology and adoptive cell therapy of Epstein-Barr virus-associated lymphoproliferative disorders in recipients of marrow allografts. Immunol Rev 1997;157:195–216.
195. Gottschalk S, Edwards OL, Sili U, et al. Generating CTLs against the subdominant Epstein-Barr virus LMP1 antigen for the adoptive immunotherapy of EBV-associated malignancies. Blood 2003;101(5):1905–1912.
196. Bollard CM, Aguilar L, Straathof KC, et al. Cytotoxic T lymphocyte therapy for Epstein-Barr virus+ Hodgkin's disease. J Exp Med 2004;200(12):1623–1633.
197. Zhang H, Merchant MS, Chua KS, et al. Tumor expression of 4-1BB ligand sustains tumor lytic T cells. Cancer Biol Ther 2003;2(5):579–586.
198. June CH. Adoptive T cell therapy for cancer in the clinic. J Clin Invest 2007;117(6):1466–1476.
199. Pule MA, Savoldo B, Myers GD, et al. Virus-specific T cells engineered to coexpress tumor-specific receptors: persistence and antitumor activity in individuals with neuroblastoma. Nat Med 2008;14(11):1264–1270.
200. Milstein C. Monoclonal antibodies. Sci Am 1980;243(4):66–74.
201. Kohler G, Milstein C. Derivation of specific antibody-producing tissue culture and tumor lines by cell fusion. Eur J Immunol 1976;6(7):511–519.
202. Yu AL, Uttenreuther-Fischer MM, Huang CS, et al. Phase I trial of a human-mouse chimeric anti-disialoganglioside monoclonal antibody ch14.18 in patients with refractory neuroblastoma and osteosarcoma. J Clin Oncol 1998;16(6):2169–2180.
203. McCafferty J, Griffiths AD, Winter G, et al. Phage antibodies: filamentous phage displaying antibody variable domains. Nature 1990;348(6301):552–554.
204. Cersosimo RJ. Monoclonal antibodies in the treatment of cancer, part 1. Am J Health Syst Pharm 2003;60(15):1531–1548.
205. Cersosimo RJ. Monoclonal antibodies in the treatment of cancer, part 2. Am J Health Syst Pharm 2003;60(16):1631–1641, quiz 1642–1643.
206. Treon SP, Mitsiades C, Mitsiades N, et al. Tumor cell expression of CD59 is associated with resistance to CD20 serotherapy in patients with B-cell malignancies. J Immunother 2001;24(3):263–271.
207. Clynes RA, Towers TL, Presta LG, et al. Inhibitory Fc receptors modulate in vivo cytotoxicity against tumor targets. Nat Med 2000;6(4):443–446.
208. Cartron G, Dacheux L, Salles G, et al. Therapeutic activity of humanized anti-CD20 monoclonal antibody and polymorphism in IgG Fc receptor FcgammaRIIIa gene. Blood 2002;99(3):754–758.
209. Weng WK, Levy R. Two immunoglobulin G fragment C receptor polymorphisms independently predict response to rituximab in patients with follicular lymphoma. J Clin Oncol 2003;21(21):3940–3947.
210. Weng WK, Czerwinski D, Timmerman J, et al. Clinical outcome of lymphoma patients after idiotype vaccination is correlated with humoral immune response and immunoglobulin G Fc receptor genotype. J Clin Oncol 2004;22(23):4717–4724.
211. Cheung NK, Sowers R, Vickers AJ, et al. FCGR2A polymorphism is correlated with clinical outcome after immunotherapy of neuroblastoma with anti-GD2 antibody and granulocyte macrophage colony-stimulating factor. J Clin Oncol 2006;24(18):2885–2890.
212. Ozkaynak MF, Sondel PM, Krailo MD, et al. Phase I study of chimeric human/murine anti-ganglioside G(D2) monoclonal antibody (ch14.18) with granulocyte-macrophage colony-stimulating factor in children with neuroblastoma immediately after hematopoietic stem-cell transplantation: a Children's Cancer Group Study. J Clin Oncol 2000;18(24):4077–4085.
213. Yu AL, Gilman AL, Ozkaynak MF, et al. A phase III randomized trial of chimeric anti-GD2 antibody + GM-CSF + IL2 immunotherapy of high-risk neuroblastoma (NB) in first response: Children's Oncology Group (COG) study ANBL0032. In: American Society of Clinical Oncology. Orlando, Florida: American Society of Clinical Oncology. 2009. J Clin Oncol. 27(15s), 1322s, abstr 10067z.
214. Yu AL, Gilman MF, Ozkaynak MF, et al. A phase III randomized trial of the chimeric anti-GD2 antibody ch14.18 with GM-CSF and IL2 as immunotherapy following dose intensive chemotherapy for high-risk neuroblastoma: Children's Oncology Group (COG) study ANBL0032. In: American Society of Clinical Oncology. Orlando, Florida: American Society of Clinical Oncology. 2009:15S.
215. Simon T, Hero B, Faldum A, et al. Consolidation treatment with chimeric anti-GD2-antibody ch14.18 in children older than 1 year with metastatic neuroblastoma. J Clin Oncol 2004;22(17):3549–3557.
216. Sondel PM, Gillies SD. Immunocytokines for cancer immunotherapy. In: Morse M, Clay TM, Lyerle HM, eds. Handbook of cancer vaccines. Totowa, NJ: Humana Press, 2003:341–358.
217. King DM, Albertini MR, Schalch H, et al. A phase I clinical trial of the immunocytokine EMD 273063 (hu14.18-IL2) in patients with melanoma. J Clin Oncol 2004;22:4463–4473.
218. Neal ZC, Yang JC, Rakhmilevich AL, et al. Enhanced activity of hu14.18-IL2 immunocytokine against murine NXS2 neuroblastoma when combined with interleukin 2 therapy. Clin Cancer Res 2004;10(14):4839–4847.
219. Shusterman S, London WB, Gillies SD, et al. Anti-neuroblastoma activity of hu14.18-IL2 against minimal residual disease in a Children's Oncology Group study. J Clin Oncol 2008;26(15s);1322s, abstr 3002.
220. Mittelman A, Wang X, Matsumoto K, et al. Antiantiidiotypic response and clinical course of the disease in patients with malignant melanoma immunized with mouse antiidiotypic monoclonal antibody MK2–23. Hybridoma 1995;14(2):175–181.
221. Cheung NK, Guo HF, Heller G, et al. Induction of Ab3 and Ab3′ antibody was associated with long-term survival after anti-G(D2) antibody therapy of stage 4 neuroblastoma. Clin Cancer Res 2000;6(7):2653–2660.

SECTION 2 ■ DIAGNOSIS AND EVALUATION OF THE CHILD WITH CANCER

CHAPTER 6 ■ CLINICAL ASSESSMENT AND DIFFERENTIAL DIAGNOSIS OF THE CHILD WITH SUSPECTED CANCER

LINDSAY B. KILBURN, STUART E. SIEGEL, AND CHARLES P. STEUBER

Cancer, a common disease in adults, is rare in children and adolescents (see Chapter 1). It is often difficult to diagnose childhood cancer in its early stages because many of the presenting signs and symptoms are nonspecific, mimicking more common childhood diseases. However, the incidence of childhood cancer is increasing, with an approximately 1% increase per year overall and for some tumors, such as brain tumors, a 2% increase in incidence per year.[1] Further, cancer remains the leading cause of disease-related mortality in children.

In spite of the inherent difficulties in diagnosis, timely diagnosis of childhood cancer is extremely important. Many pediatric malignancies are highly curable, and with some of them, earlier diagnosis can be associated with a better prognosis, diminished intensity of therapy, and less complications from disease as well as treatment. Patients with solid tumors diagnosed with localized tumors require less aggressive treatment and have better outcomes. Similarly, younger children with B-cell precursor acute lymphoblastic leukemia (ALL) diagnosed prior to the development of high leukocyte counts can be treated with less intense regimens than those with high counts.

Early diagnosis of pediatric cancer requires an astute physician attuned to the subtle or persistent symptoms that may herald the diagnosis of cancer. Furthermore, this increased awareness should extend to the early adult years, as many of the cancers of young adults are more closely related to these rare pediatric tumors (acute leukemia, bone and soft tissue sarcomas, Hodgkin lymphoma, and aggressive non-Hodgkin lymphoma [NHL]) than to the common malignancies of adults (breast cancer, lung cancer, colon cancer, prostate cancer).

The challenge to diagnosing pediatric cancers is that they occur so infrequently and often initially present with symptoms of much more common and less serious illnesses (Table 6.1). The annual incidence of cancer in children is 15 per 100,000. Therefore, the average solo practitioner is likely to encounter only one case every 20 years, and even in practices with multiple providers, one case will be diagnosed every 5 to 7 years.[2] Adding to these early detection difficulties is the fact that once a specific cancer has been diagnosed in a practice not only will there be a long lag time until the next case presents but also that next case is likely to be an entirely different entity with different presenting features.

Consequently, it is important for pediatric oncologists to be involved in educating practitioners who see children and young adults about these diseases, so that in the appropriate context, they will see those warning signs that prompt an evaluation leading to the diagnosis of cancer. This includes educating not only pediatricians but also practitioners in family practice, emergency medicine, internal medicine, and surgery. One study from the emergency department of a large children's hospital revealed that 7.3% of new diagnoses of childhood cancer were made in their emergency department.[3]

As access to routine health care becomes limited for increasing numbers of children, this percentage is only likely to increase.

If a diagnosis of cancer is suspected or confirmed, then referral to a pediatric cancer center is critical. Guidelines for such centers have been published.[4] It is at these centers that the multidisciplinary clinical and investigative resources exist to permit the most accurate diagnosis, to offer the most appropriate therapies, and to provide the best supportive care and long-term follow-up. Diagnosing and treating childhood cancer requires a multidisciplinary team consisting of pediatric oncologists, other pediatric subspecialists, radiation oncologists, surgeons, and pathologists with pediatric expertise. Ideally, the diagnostic procedures, such as biopsy and specialized imaging, should be performed at the pediatric cancer center. As the diagnosis and staging of childhood cancer continues to incorporate more biologic information and techniques, specimens need special handling and processing to permit the whole array of morphologic, histochemical, immunologic, cytogenetic, and molecular testing needed. Furthermore, these centers participate in cooperative group studies that provide for further expert review of the diagnosis as needed. When reviewed by a central panel of pathologists with expertise in childhood cancer, 11% of diagnoses made by pediatric pathologists and 22% of those made by general pathologists were amended.[5] Finally, it is at these centers that tissues are most likely to be collected and stored, after appropriate consent, for biologic studies to elucidate the causes and biologic factors contributing to the clinical outcomes of childhood cancer.

While later chapters will discuss more specific differential diagnoses for individual cancer types, this chapter focuses on some of the more common diagnostic clues to cancer in children, adolescents, and young adults with pediatric malignancies. Cancer can be a great mimic, with its early signs and symptoms often suggesting other disorders. As indicated previously, the occurrence of cancer in children and adolescents is relatively infrequent, and in many cases, for a correct diagnosis to be made, multiple or persistent clues need to be linked together. In other cases, the diagnosis may be more straightforward, provided there is awareness that the sign or symptom points toward a diagnosis of malignancy.

CHILDREN AT RISK

Certain children are at increased risk for developing cancer. They include children with the genetic predispositions to cancer that are discussed in Chapter 2, such as Down syndrome, neurofibromatosis, and Beckwith-Wiedemann syndrome. Very premature infants appear to be at increased risk of developing hepatoblastoma.[6] Certain infectious agents may also predispose

TABLE 6.1

SYMPTOMS AND SIGNS OF CHILDHOOD CANCER
MIMICKING NORMAL CHILDHOOD ILLNESSES

Symptom/sign	Possible malignancy
Generalized malaise, fever, adenopathy	Lymphoma, leukemia, EWS, NBL
Head and neck	
Headache, nausea, vomiting	Brain tumor, leukemia
Febrile seizure	Brain tumor
Earache	STS
Rhinitis	STS
Epistaxis	Leukemia
Pharyngitis	STS
Adenopathy	NBL, thyroid, STS, lymphoma, leukemia
Thorax	
Extrathoracic	
Soft tissue mass	STS, PNET
Bony mass	EWS, NBL
Intrathoracic	
Adenopathy	Lymphoma, leukemia
Abdomen	
External: soft tissue	STS, PNET
Internal: diarrhea, vomiting, hepatomegaly, and/or splenomegaly	NBL, lymphoma, hepatic tumor, leukemia
Genitourinary	
Hematuria	Wilms' tumor, STS
Trouble voiding	Prostatic or bladder STS
Vaginitis	STS
Peritesticular mass	STS
Musculoskeletal	
Soft tissue mass(es)	RMS, other STS, PNET
Bony mass/pain	Osteosarcoma, EWS, NHL, NBL, leukemia

EWS, Ewing's sarcoma; NBL, neuroblastoma; STS, soft tissue sarcoma, including rhabdomyosarcoma; PNET, primitive neuroectodermal tumor; RMS, rhabdomyosarcoma; NHL, non-Hodgkin lymphoma.

to cancer. Epstein-Barr virus (EBV) infection has been associated with B-cell lymphomas, especially Burkitt's lymphoma, as well as less common peripheral T-cell lymphomas, Hodgkin lymphoma, hemophagocytic lymphohistiocytosis, and nasopharyngeal carcinoma.[7–10] Hepatitis B and C infections predispose to hepatocellular carcinoma.[11,12] Human immunodeficiency virus (HIV) infection in pediatric patients has been associated with a number of malignancies, including B-cell lymphomas, leiomyosarcomas, and Kaposi's sarcoma. The latter two malignancies are otherwise not seen in children.[13–15] In addition to HIV, children whose immune systems are otherwise deficient due to inherited immunodeficiency syndromes or are on immunosuppressive therapy, especially solid organ recipients, are at higher risk of malignancy.[16] Posttransplant patients are prone to a posttransplant lymphoproliferative syndrome that can progress to lymphoma.[17] Pediatric solid organ transplant recipients who are on prolonged thiopurine therapy may be predisposed to myelodysplasia and acute myeloid leukemia (AML) in view of the fact that adult recipients treated in this manner are at increased risk for these conditions.[18]

Another group of children at increased risk for developing cancer are those who have survived therapy for another can-

cer.[19,20] For example, children treated for ALL are at increased risk for brain tumors, especially if they received cranial radiation therapy and are thiopurine methyltransferase deficient.[21] Survivors of ALL are also at increased risk for developing AML. Therapy that includes topoisomerase II inhibitors, anthracyclines, and alkylating agents potentiates the risk of AML, as seen in patients with solid tumors treated intensively with these agents.[22,23] Children with Hodgkin lymphoma treated with oncogenic agents such as procarbazine and alkylating agents are also at increased risk for secondary AML and NHL.[24] Patients exposed to radiation therapy as part of their cancer treatment are at increased risk of radiation-related malignancies in the radiation-exposed field.[25] For example, this is the case in patients with Hodgkin lymphoma treated with radiation who are also at increased risk for radiation-related malignancies such as thyroid cancer, bone tumors, and early-onset breast cancer.[26] Similarly, patients who underwent stem cell transplant are at increased risk from high-dose chemotherapy and total-body irradiation for solid tumors such as skin, bone, and thyroid cancers and from their immunosuppression for posttransplant lymphoproliferative disorders.[27] Further, exposure to ionizing radiation outside of cancer therapy, either prenatally or through nuclear accidents such as Chernobyl, also increases the risk for cancer.[28–30]

TIME TO DIAGNOSIS

Various studies have evaluated factors that contribute to the lag time to diagnosis of cancer. A recent review grouped these delays into three categories: disease, patient/parent, and health care related.[31] Cancer type and therefore site of disease and associated symptoms contribute significantly to the timing of diagnosis. For example, Wilms' tumor, which usually presents as an asymptomatic mass often first detected by the parents, tends to be diagnosed quickly, as does childhood acute leukemia. However, for other tumors, such as brain, bone, and Hodgkin lymphoma, diagnosis is often delayed (Table 6.2).[32–36] Some of the differences may relate to clinical presentation and biology, with more aggressive tumors leading to more acute clinical presentation and rapid diagnosis, but they also relate to patient factors such as age. Older children, especially adolescents, are less likely to be supervised when dressing and bathing and to have abnormalities observed by their parents. Signs and symptoms more directly observed by parents in the younger child may not come to attention in older children who are reluctant to discuss their health with parents or practitioners.[37] Other patient/parent-related factors that contribute to delays in diagnosis are ethnicity, parental education, profession, and religion.[34]

As stated previously, the expectation is that earlier diagnosis and treatment will lead to a better outcome with less morbidity. However, studies to date have not substantiated this. There has been a reduction in the incidence of early death (<1 month from diagnosis) in childhood cancer, but this is largely attributed to better supportive care modalities rather than to earlier diagnosis.[38] The only study to address the influence of lag time to disease stage found no significant difference in lag time and the level of the presenting white blood cell (WBC) count in acute leukemia or the level of involvement (stage) in solid tumors.[37] For medulloblastoma, advanced-stage tumors may actually be diagnosed earlier because patients present with more dramatic symptoms of increased intracranial pressure than do patients with less aggressive tumors.[35,39] Patients with head and neck rhabdomyosarcomas often present with vague symptoms or with a swelling or mass initially thought to be due to infection. This may lead to delay in seeking medical care.[40] For patients who experience pain as their initial

TABLE 6.2

DISTRIBUTION OF LAG TIME IN DAYS BY DIAGNOSIS OF COMMON
CHILDHOOD CANCERS

Diagnosis	n	Mean	Median	25th percentile	75th percentile
Brain	194	211	93	38	237
Ewing's sarcoma	82	182	127	79	255
Hodgkin	143	223	136	49	270
Leukemia	908	109	52	20	129
Non-Hodgkin lymphoma	184	117	62	25	141
Neuroblastoma	237	120	58	15	164
Osteosarcoma	67	127	98	40	191
Rhabdomyosarcoma	126	127	55	25	161
Wilms' tumor	223	101	31	9	120

manifestation of cancer, duration of pain was not longer for those presenting with metastatic disease than for those presenting with localized disease.[41] In neuroblastoma, it was hoped that mass screening would result in fewer children being diagnosed with advanced-stage, poorer prognosis tumors and would therefore decrease mortality. However, studies from Japan, United Kingdom, and Canada have demonstrated that screening has had no impact on outcome since it picks up those tumors that are not biologically malignant and have a high probability of regressing.[42]

DIFFERENTIAL DIAGNOSIS

As previously noted, in almost all cases, diseases other than cancer may produce identical nonspecific symptoms at presentation. Although assessment for these findings does not always require an evaluation for cancer, the challenge is to consider cancer in the appropriate context and to connect the dots to establish the diagnosis of malignancy. Table 6.3 lists these signs and symptoms by region of the body, the malignancies they suggest, and the recommended evaluations. Sometimes tumors can present with unusual signs and symptoms that can make early diagnosis even more difficult. The pediatric tumor most commonly associated with unusual signs and symptoms is neuroblastoma (Table 6.4).[43–56] However, unusual presentations have also been reported in association with other pediatric malignancies (Table 6.5).[57–101]

Fever

Fever can be present at diagnosis of many forms of childhood cancer, but it is usually associated with other signs and symptoms that lead to the diagnosis. Occult malignancy, along with infectious and inflammatory disorders, has classically been considered one of the causes of prolonged fever of unknown origin (FUO). However, this is now rarely the case in childhood with at most 10% of patients with prolonged FUO having an underlying malignancy.[102,103] With malignancy, symptoms such as bone pain, mass, weight loss, or pallor often accompany the fever or develop soon thereafter and prompt investigations that lead to the correct diagnosis. Alternatively, investigations performed early in the evaluation of FUO lead to the diagnosis. These investigations commonly are complete blood count (CBC) with differential WBC count, sedimentation rate, and lactic dehydrogenase (LDH) and uric acid levels. If there are no symptoms other than fever and the previously mentioned investigations are not informative, then consultation is sometimes requested to determine whether occult

malignancy is present. Additional tests are rarely diagnostic of malignancy but, when performed, should include chest radiograph, abdominal ultrasound, and bone marrow aspiration.[102–105]

It should also be noted that fever may be associated with the malignancy itself or with associated infection, and appropriate evaluation for infection is warranted for patients with fever in the early evaluation of malignancy. Lymphomas, especially advanced Hodgkin lymphoma and anaplastic large cell lymphoma (ALCL), may have fever as a prominent manifestation of disease. Indeed, ALCL is a great mimic, with its initial features often suggesting an infectious or inflammatory process rather than cancer. Patients with acute leukemia may have fever as a manifestation of the disease itself but are also at high risk of fever from associated infection due to impaired immunity at presentation.

Lymphadenopathy

A diagnosis of lymphoma or another malignancy must always be considered when evaluating the child with an enlarged peripheral lymph node. However, other causes of lymphadenopathy are much more common. One review noted approximately 50% of children older than 5 years seen for well or sick visits had lymphadenopathy.[106] A nodal mass, unlike an abdominal, pelvic, or mediastinal mass, is not always an indication for a detailed workup or for a prompt surgical procedure to establish a diagnosis. The likelihood of malignancy within the node will determine the urgency with which biopsy or other invasive procedures are undertaken. It must be emphasized that not all palpable nodes are pathologically enlarged and that most pathologically enlarged nodes are benign.

Lymph nodes are dynamic structures that can widely fluctuate in size, especially in children, as they are exposed to new viruses and bacteria early in life. When lymph nodes are palpable, a decision must be made as to whether or not they are normal. Factors of importance are age of the child and size and location of the nodes. The nodes of the neck, axilla, and groin are often palpable in normal children. Cervical and axillary nodes greater than 1 cm in diameter are considered enlarged, as are inguinal nodes greater than 1.5 cm in diameter and epitrochlear nodes greater than 0.5 cm in diameter.[107] Palpable supraclavicular nodes should always be considered abnormal, with left-sided (Virchow's) nodes suggesting metastases from an intraabdominal malignancy such as neuroblastoma and right-sided nodes suggesting intrathoracic disease.

In children with head and neck masses, age is an important factor in determining the likely diagnosis. In children younger

TABLE 6.3

UNUSUAL SYMPTOMS AND SIGNS THAT WARRANT IMMEDIATE LABORATORY AND/OR IMAGING STUDIES AND CONSULTATION

Symptoms/signs	Laboratory, imaging studies, and consultations	Major associated tumors
Hypertension	Labs—CXR, abdominal sonogram	Renal or adrenal tumor, neuroblastoma
Weight loss, sudden onset	Labs—abdominal sonogram	Any malignancy
Petechiae	CBC, plt, diff	Leukemia, neuroblastoma
Adenopathy unresponsive to antibiotics	Surgical consultation, CXR, CBC, diff	Leukemia, lymphoma
Endocrine abnormalities		
Growth failure	Hormonal assays	Pituitary tumors
Electrolyte disturbance	CT hypothalamic area	Hypothalamic tumors
Sexual abnormalities	Abdominal CT	Gonadal tumors
Cushing's syndrome	Endocrine consultation	Adrenal tumors
Brain	Neurology or neurosurgery consultation followed by imaging studies	Brain tumor
Headache, vomiting early morning		
Cranial nerve palsy, ataxia		
Dilated pupil, papilledema		
Afebrile seizures		
Hallucinations, aphasia		
Unilateral weakness, paralysis		
Eyes	Ophthalmologist consultation	Retinoblastoma, metastatic rhabdomyosarcoma, neuroblastoma
White spot, proptosis, blindness		
Wandering eye		
Intraorbital hemorrhage		
Ears	CBC, diff, and imaging studies	LCH, rhabdomyosarcoma
Bulging mass external canal		
Mastoid tenderness, swelling		
Puffy face and neck	CBC, diff, and imaging studies	Mediastinal tumors
Pharyngeal mass	CBC, diff, and imaging studies	Rhabdomyosarcoma, lymphoma, nasopharyngeal carcinoma
Periodontal mass, loose teeth	Dental consultation, imaging studies	LCH, Burkitt's lymphoma, neuroblastoma, osteosarcoma
Thorax	CBC, diff, imaging studies	Soft tissue sarcomas, mediastinal tumors, metastatic tumors
Extrathoracic: mass		
Intrathoracic: coughing, SOB without fever or no history of asthma, allergies		
Abdomen/pelvis	CBC, diff	Wilms' tumor, soft tissue sarcoma, neuroblastoma, hepatoblastoma, hepatocarcinoma
Intraabdominal mass	Labs, imaging studies	
Genitourinary	UA, CBC, diff, sonogram of pelvis/abdomen	Germ cell tumor, rhabdomyosarcoma, adrenal tumor
Testes, vagina mass		
Masculinization/feminization		
Musculoskeletal	CBC, diff, imaging studies	Osteosarcoma, Ewing's sarcoma, leukemia, neuroblastoma, soft tissue sarcoma
Soft tissue, bone marrow, and/or pain		

SOB, shortness of breath; labs, laboratory studies, usually hepatic and renal function and electrolytes; CXR, chest x-ray; CBC, complete blood cell count; plt, platelet count; diff, differential count; CT, computed tomography; UA, urinalysis; LCH, Langerhans' cell histiocytosis.

than 6 years, the most common cancers of the head and neck are neuroblastoma, rhabdomyosarcoma, NHL, and leukemia; for those 7 to 13 years old, NHL and Hodgkin lymphoma are equally common followed by thyroid carcinoma and rhabdomyosarcoma; and for those older than 13 years, Hodgkin lymphoma is the most common cancer encountered.[108]

Enlargement of a lymph node may be due to proliferation of its intrinsic cellular components or due to infiltration with cells extrinsic to the node. Benign and malignant adenopathy can be caused by either mechanism. Benign enlargement may result from proliferation of the intrinsic components of the node in response to foreign antigens or from infiltration with granulocytes in response to acute bacterial infection. Neoplastic enlargement may be due to proliferation of intrinsic cellular components as in Hodgkin lymphoma and NHL or due to proliferation of cells that have infiltrated or metastasized to the

TABLE 6.4

UNUSUAL PRESENTATIONS OF CHILDHOOD NEUROBLASTOMA

Unusual signs and symptoms not related directly to tumor growth
Chronic diarrhea[43]
Polymyoclonus-opsoclonus[44]
Cogwheel erythrocytes[45]
Failure to thrive[46]
Cushing's syndrome[47]
Unusual signs and symptoms related directly to tumor growth
Horner's syndrome[48]
Superior vena cava syndrome[49]
Hydrocephalus[50]
Meningeal involvement[51]
Cavernous or lateral sinus involvement[50]
Blindness[52]
Subcutaneous nodules[52]
Leukemoid reaction[53]
Myasthenia gravis[54]
Heterochromia[55]

node, as in leukemia and various solid tumors. Nasopharyngeal carcinoma, thyroid carcinoma, and rhabdomyosarcoma are solid tumors of the head and neck that may metastasize to cervical nodes, and neuroblastoma is the most common intraabdominal tumor to do so.

When evaluating a child with adenopathy, it is important to distinguish between generalized and localized lymph node enlargement. *Generalized adenopathy* is defined as involvement of more than two noncontiguous areas and can be caused by many different disease processes. *Localized adenopathy* is defined as the enlargement of lymph nodes within contiguous anatomic regions and is usually due to one of two processes, infection or malignancy, and the workup is designed to expedite diagnosis of either possibility (Fig. 6.1). Certain characteristics of the node can be helpful in defining the cause of localized adenopathy. Fluctuance, erythema, warmth, and extreme tenderness are signs of suppuration due to a pyogenic bacterial infection, often group A streptococcus or *Staphylococcus aureus*. Patients with such node(s) are usually acutely ill and febrile. Aspiration of these nodes should be considered and once Gram stain and culture are obtained, antibiotic therapy should be promptly instituted. Less acutely ill children, in whom the suppuration is associated with matting of the nodes and their fixation to the skin, may have cat scratch disease or a mycobacterial infection rather than pyogenic adenitis. In these cases, skin tests for mycobacteria, chest radiograph, and serologic testing for antibody to *Bartonella henselae* may be necessary for diagnosis.

In the absence of suppuration, evaluation of localized adenopathy should begin with careful inspection of the regions drained by the node for a focus of infection or for bites or scratches that are portals of entry for microorganisms. The characteristics and location of the nodes should also be considered. Nodes that are more likely to be malignant are those that are large, nontender firm, and rubbery, or are rapidly enlarging, or becoming confluent and fixed, or located in the supraclavicular area.[109,110] If inspection does not clarify the etiology, then CBC and chest radiograph data should be obtained; skin tests for mycobacteria should be placed; and serologic tests should be drawn for infections, especially viral infections such as EBV and cytomegalovirus and, if there are risk factors, for HIV. When CBC and chest radiograph are

TABLE 6.5

UNCOMMON PRESENTATIONS OF CHILDHOOD CANCERS OTHER THAN NEUROBLASTOMA

Cancer	Unusual signs or symptoms
Acute lymphoblastic leukemia	Hypercalcemia[57]
	Cyclic neutropenia[58]
	Eosinophilia[59]
	Pulmonary nodules[60]
	Lupus erythematosus[61]
	Rheumatoid arthritis[62]
	Virus-associated hemophagocytic syndrome[63]
	Bone marrow necrosis[64]
	Skin nodules[65]
	Pericardial effusion[66]
	Aplastic anemia[67]
	Hypoglycemia[68]
	Bilateral renal masses[69]
	Multiple vertebral collapse[70]
	Solid tumors[71]
Acute myelogenous leukemia	Myelofibrosis[72]
	Mediastinal mass[73]
	Clitorism[74]
	Ovarian mass[75,76]
	Pericarditis[76]
	Chloroma[77]
	Bone fractures[78]
Hodgkin or non-Hodgkin lymphoma	Nephrotic syndrome[79]
	Pruritus[80]
	Acute dysautonomia[81]
	Dermatomyositis[82]
	Pontine myelinosis[83]
Germ cell tumor	Parinaud syndrome[84]
Thymoma	Myasthenia gravis[85]
Central nervous system tumor	Diencephalic syndrome[86,87]
Wilms' tumor	Hypoglycemia[88]
	Uterine mass[89]
	Inferior vena cava thrombosis[90]
	Anemia[91,92]
Hepatoma/hepatocellular carcinoma	Erythrocytosis[92]
	Thrombocytosis[93]
Ewing's sarcoma	Superior vena cava syndrome[94]
	Inflammatory syndrome[95]
	Septic arthritis[96]
Rhabdoid tumor	Pericardial effusion[97]
Rhabdomyosarcoma	Pulmonary bronchial cyst[98]
	Cardiac mass[99]
	Leukemia[100]
Chronic myelogenous leukemia	Priapism[101]

normal, invasive procedures can be deferred at least until the skin test and serology results have been evaluated. Significant anemia (hemoglobin levels < 10 g per dL), cytopenias, leukoerythroblastic changes or blasts on smear, or a mass on chest radiograph all point to the need for bone marrow aspiration as the next step in evaluating adenopathy. In patients with only anemia or an abnormal chest radiograph, examination of the marrow may not be diagnostic, but when it is, patients are

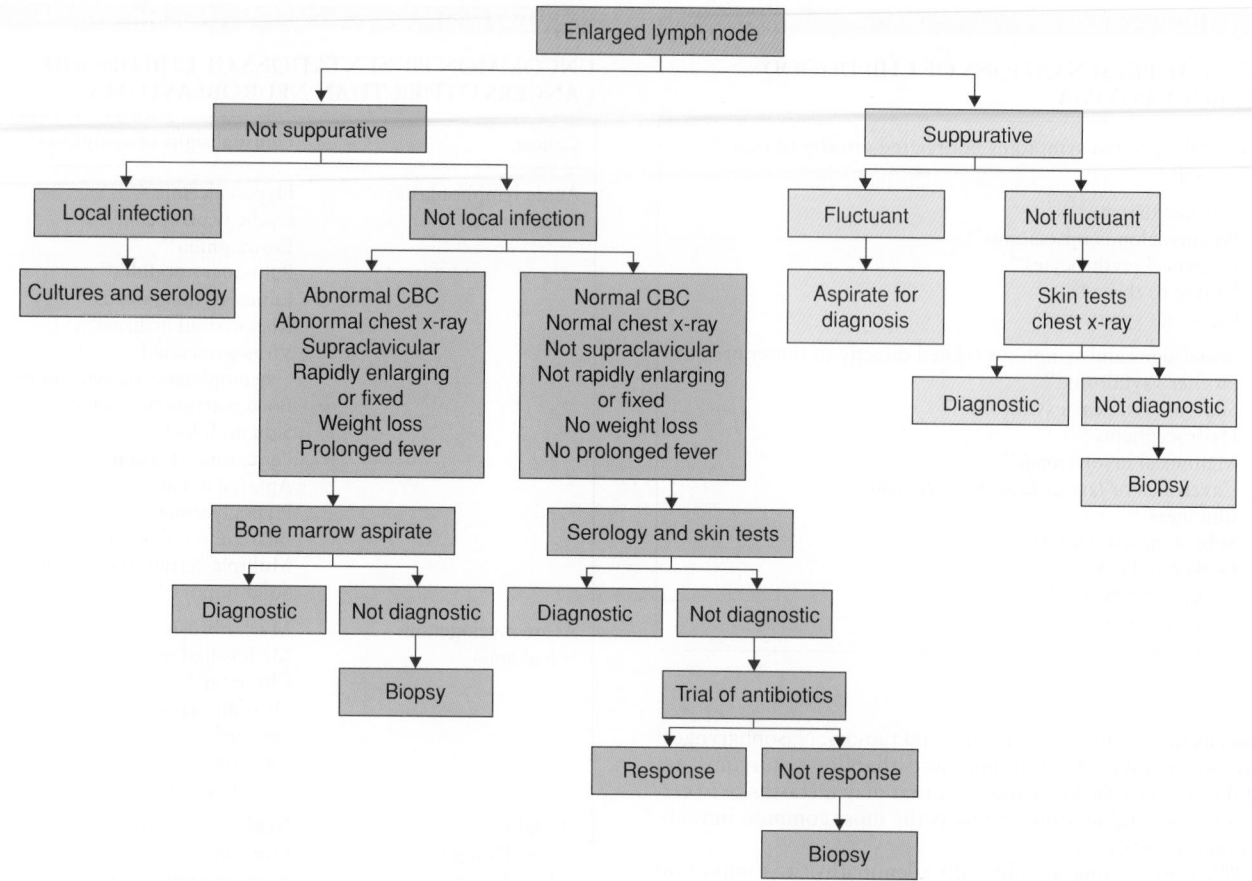

FIGURE 6.1 Evaluation of localized adenopathy in pediatric patients. CBC, complete blood count.

spared the need for biopsy under general anesthesia with its attendant risks. Immediate biopsy of the node is indicated when the marrow does not provide a diagnosis. Patients with normal CBC and chest radiograph findings but who have negative skin tests for mycobacteria and serology findings may be given a 1- to 2-week trial of antibiotic therapy, provided their nodes have not been rapidly enlarging. If the nodes are rapidly enlarging or if their size does not decrease considerably during antibiotic therapy, then biopsy is necessary.[111]

Patients with generalized adenopathy may have systemic infections, disseminated malignancy, autoimmune diseases, drug-induced lymph node hyperplasia, storage diseases, or metabolic diseases. Their evaluation often needs to be more extensive than those for localized adenopathy. In certain situations, such as infectious mononucleosis or drug-induced adenopathy, the clinical picture may be classic enough to permit a specific diagnosis. In many cases, however, the cause of the generalized adenopathy is not readily apparent. In those cases, evaluation should commence, as it did for localized adenopathy, with a CBC and chest radiograph.

Abnormalities on CBC or chest radiograph are indications for prompt bone marrow aspiration. In many cases, the marrow may be sufficiently involved to permit a diagnosis of either leukemia or NHL. Lymph node biopsy should be performed if the marrow is not diagnostic or if involvement is not extensive enough for marrow to be a source of cells for the precise immunologic and histologic diagnosis of the lymphoid malignancy. Patients with normal CBC and chest radiograph may have invasive procedures deferred until the results of other tests for generalized adenopathy are known. In many cases, etiologies are

found that will eliminate the need for marrow aspiration or node biopsy.

Many lymph node biopsies are nondiagnostic. Lake and Oski[112] reported that slightly more than one-half of 75 children with localized or generalized nonsuppurative adenopathy had nondiagnostic biopsies. Thirteen patients (17%) with one or more persistently enlarged nonerythematous and nonfluctuant nodes did have malignancies diagnosed. Only 3 of these patients had NHL, and 9 of the remaining 10 had Hodgkin lymphoma. No single clinical picture consistently predicted the histologic diagnosis. Indeed five children with isolated and asymptomatic cervical adenopathy had malignancy. Knight et al. reviewed biopsies from an even larger group of children and reported remarkably similar results.[113] The majority of the 13% of patients with malignancy had Hodgkin lymphoma; fewer than 2% of patients with peripheral adenopathy had NHL. In both series, certain features were more likely to be associated with malignancy, including weight loss, temperature exceeding 38.5°C for 1 week, arthralgias, supraclavicular adenopathy, generalized adenopathy, and hepatosplenomegaly. Any of these findings was considered an indication for early biopsy. Hemoglobin levels lower than 10 g per dL, an elevated erythrocyte sedimentation rate, or an abnormal chest radiograph were other indications. Torsiglieri et al.[114] reported similar findings in 445 children biopsied for neck masses. The majority of masses were congenital lesions that were not nodal in origin. Of the 45% of children with nodal masses, about one-quarter were malignant, with Hodgkin lymphoma more common than NHL. Less frequently encountered malignancies were thyroid carcinoma, neuroblastoma, rhabdomyosarcoma, Langerhans' cell histiocytosis, and chloroma.[114]

In summary, indications for lymph node biopsy, when other tests have been nondiagnostic, are as follows:

- Chronic, persistent, progressive adenopathy; if an infectious etiology has not been uncovered, a dominant node that persists for 6 weeks should be biopsied[115];
- Any nodes greater than 2.5 cm in diameter in the absence of signs of infection that warrant a trial of antibiotics;
- Supraclavicular adenopathy; and
- Systemic symptoms.

When biopsy is performed, it is important that the tissue be handled properly. It should never be placed directly in formalin. If infection is still considered, then cultures obtained for bacteria, fungi, and acid-fast bacilli. Portions of the nodes should be set aside for routine histology, immunohistochemical stains, immunophenotyping, cytogenetics, and molecular genetic studies. This is best accomplished when a pathologist is present in the operating room to appropriately handle the tissue.

Thoracic Masses

Virtually all primary intrathoracic tumors arise in the mediastinum. Some exceptions include pleuropulmonary blastomas, desmoplastic small round cell tumors, and those rare rhabdomyosarcomas that arise from lung or the intralobar fissures.[116] The mediastinum can be divided into anterior, middle, and posterior compartments, and the location of the mass provides clues to the tumor diagnosis. The anterior mediastinum contains the thymus, heart, anterior pericardium, and anterior mediastinal lymph nodes; the middle mediastinum contains nodes, great vessels, and trachea; and the posterior mediastinum contains descending aorta, esophagus, and sympathetic chain. Mediastinal masses are frequently malignant. A number of series reported 55% to 70% of them to be malignant.[117–119] Patients with mediastinal masses may present with symptoms of compression of respiratory, vascular, or other structures or be asymptomatic with incidental findings on a chest radiograph. Because of the potential for airway and vascular compromise with tumors in this location, careful coordination must be taken in initiating evaluations in order to facilitate a safe and expedient diagnosis.

Anterior masses are common in older patients and, in them, are more likely to be malignant. Common masses include lymphomas, thymic origin masses, teratomas, angiomas, lipomas, and thyroid tumors. One important group of patients are those with T-cell lymphoblastic lymphoma and T-cell ALL. These patients often present with symptoms related to compression of the thoracic contents or related to an associated pleural effusion. In either case, dyspnea is often a prominent manifestation. They may also develop superior vena cava syndrome with edema and plethora of the face and neck due to venous occlusion, wheezing and dyspnea due to airway obstruction, dysphagia due to esophageal compression, and symptoms of increased intracranial pressure produced by diminished cerebral venous return. They may also have cardiac compromise, from a pericardial effusion producing tamponade, or from the mass obstructing outflow from the heart, or from both. These presentations are a medical emergency and require prompt therapeutic measures to relieve the compressive symptoms. Because of the often rapid growth of these types of tumors, rapid evaluation should be sought even in patients without compressive symptoms at initial diagnosis.

For patients with T-cell ALL, the diagnosis can be quickly and safely achieved through examination of the peripheral blood for blasts or by bone marrow aspiration when blasts are not present in the peripheral blood. In cases of lymphoblastic lymphoma with a pleural or pericardial effusion, detection of lymphoblasts in the fluid will often provide a diagnosis.[111] This avoids the need for anesthesia in these patients, which carries considerable risk if they have airway narrowing of 50% or more or have abnormal pulmonary function. Anesthesia or sedation that impairs the respiratory efforts of these critically ill patients can result in fatal obstruction.[109] However, if none of the previous procedures provide a diagnosis, then biopsy of contiguously involved scalene or cervical nodes or, in their absence, biopsy of the mediastinal mass is necessary. If the anesthetic risk is too great, consideration should be given to initiating "gentle" chemotherapy with corticosteroids or radiation therapy and deferring surgery until there is some improvement in the patient's respiratory status. Patients treated in this manner should be adequately hydrated and started on therapy to prevent or treat tumor lysis syndrome. Tumor necrosis may occur with this therapy and may be significant enough to preclude accurate diagnosis. Institution of treatment prior to biopsy will also result in delay in diagnosis of a less common nonlymphoblastic tumor presenting as an anterior mediastinal mass. Germ cell tumor, thymoma, Ewing's sarcoma, and thyroid tumor are all possibilities in this situation, as are those anterior mediastinal lymphomas less responsive to steroids, such as Hodgkin lymphoma and mediastinal large cell lymphoma. In any case, careful coordination with the surgeon, anesthesiologist, and pathologist is critical to allow for safe management and prompt initiation of therapy.

Middle mediastinal masses are often malignant and of nodal origin, although infectious lymphadenopathy including from tuberculosis and histoplasmosis, pericardial cysts, bronchogenic cysts, esophageal lesions, and direct extension of abdominal masses are also encountered. Involvement by Hodgkin lymphoma is common at this site. Other possibilities include nodal metastases from tumors below the diaphragm such as neuroblastoma, rhabdomyosarcoma, or germ cell tumor.

Posterior mediastinal tumors are generally neurogenic in origin and range from neuroblastomas to benign tumors such as ganglioneuroma and neurofibroma. In younger children, tumors of the posterior mediastinum are more likely to be malignant. Many of them are neuroblastomas, some of which are asymptomatic and picked up as incidental findings on chest radiograph, but others can produce symptoms including cord compression, from growth through the intervertebral foramina into the epidural space, or stridor, from airway compression. Posterior mediastinal tumors may also be discovered when a search for an etiology for opsoclonus-myoclonus uncovers an otherwise occult intrathoracic neuroblastoma.

Malignant tumors may also occur outside the thoracic cavity. Extraosseous Ewing's sarcoma and alveolar soft-part sarcoma can present as a chest wall mass, and Ewing's sarcoma and Langerhans' cell histiocytosis can develop in a rib and produce a palpable tumor.

Bone and Joint Pain

Pain is a common symptom of childhood cancer. Miser et al.[41] report that it was one of the initial symptoms of malignancy in more than half of the children and young adults referred to the National Cancer Institute. In one-third of the cases, it was the only symptom. Pain was severe enough to interfere with sleep in the majority of patients. Severe or persistent back pain, often in association with stiffness, is common in adults but rare in children. Its presence demands evaluation, especially if there are any signs of cord compression such as sphincter dysfunction and gait abnormalities.[120] Malignancies causing these symptoms include leukemia, NHL, neuroblastoma, Ewing's sarcoma, Langerhans' cell histiocytosis, and spinal cord tumors.

Patients with primary bone tumors usually present with localized pain at the site of involvement. More than 80% of patients with the two most common primary bone tumors, Ewing's sarcoma and osteosarcoma, complain of pain that may be intermittent initially but over time increases in severity and becomes constant. Pain is often initially attributed to trauma or "growing pains," which may lead to delays in diagnosis.[36] In some cases, there may be an associated soft tissue mass as tumor breaks through the periosteum and infiltrates the surrounding soft tissue, which highlights the importance of a careful clinical examination. Similar presentations are seen with Langerhans' cell histiocytosis and localized NHL of bone.

Diffuse or multifocal bone pain is seen with disseminated malignancy, especially acute leukemia, and also in patients with bony metastases from tumors such as neuroblastoma and Ewing's sarcoma. Bone pain is one of the cardinal manifestations of childhood acute leukemia and is seen more commonly in ALL than in AML.[121] Jonsson et al.[121] report that 40% of newly diagnosed children with ALL had musculoskeletal symptoms at diagnosis, and in almost half of them, they were the only symptoms and were severe. Those patients with severe pain were often diagnosed later than those with less severe or no pain. One of the main reasons for this difference is that patients with severe pain did not present with symptoms of marrow failure and had normal or relatively normal CBCs. Their WBC counts were usually normal, and one-third of them had no blasts detected on peripheral smear.

Some children who present with musculoskeletal pain are referred to rheumatologists or orthopedists because they are thought to have arthritis or bone or joint infections. They may present with a limp, refusal to walk, or arthritis limited to one joint. In children with malignancy, their pain is often disproportionate to the objective signs of inflammation, and morning stiffness is uncommon. In contrast to children with juvenile rheumatoid arthritis, those with leukemia are more likely to have worse pain at night, sometimes waking them from sleep. Although the pain in children with leukemia can be severe, it also tends to shift in location and involve bones as well as joints.[122] Constitutional symptoms such as night sweats and weight loss are also more likely to be present in the child with cancer.[123] Distinguishing musculoskeletal pain due to malignancy from other causes may not always be easy initially and can delay diagnosis. Associated laboratory findings that may suggest malignancy are elevated sedimentation rate, which is unassociated with thrombocytosis due to marrow infiltration, and elevation of serum LDH, as can be frequently seen with leukemia, NHL, Ewing's sarcoma, and neuroblastoma. Finally, careful review of radiographs or other imaging of the involved bones may uncover findings suggestive of leukemia or metastatic tumor.

Intracranial Masses

Because of the anatomic constraints imposed by the rigid skull, the growth of an intracranial mass should cause early signs and symptoms and therefore an early diagnosis. However, previous studies have indicated that patients with brain tumors have significant delays in diagnosis.[35,124] In a study comparing interval from onset of symptoms to the diagnosis, only 38% of brain tumors were diagnosed within the first month after onset of symptoms, in contrast to 84% of Wilms' tumors and 80% of the cases of acute leukemia.[125] Delays were significantly longer for supratentorial tumors (mean time

43.4 weeks) compared with infratentorial tumors (mean time 10.8 weeks).

Signs and symptoms associated with childhood brain tumors are usually nonspecific and can vary from localizing symptoms related to direct effects of tumor on surrounding brain or spinal cord, to obstruction of cerebrospinal fluid flow and resultant hydrocephalus. These symptoms range from more general symptoms such as an enlarging frontal-occipital circumference (FOC) in an infant, chronic or recurrent headaches, vomiting, visual disturbances, and changes in behavior or in school performance to more specific signs such as hemiparesis, cranial nerve palsies, seizures, ataxia, and visual field deficits.

Headache is a common symptom among children and adolescents. Although it is always important to consider a brain tumor when dealing with a pediatric patient with headaches, it is important to recognize that the incidence of brain tumors among children is low. However, the classic triad of headaches, which awaken the child from sleep or are present on arising, vomiting, and papilledema occurs in fewer than a third of the patients.[124,126,127] Therefore, the clinician is frequently faced with the dilemma of ordering expensive imaging studies with some inherent risks (sedation and contrast use) when attempting the early detection of intracranial tumors.

Honig and Charney[126] suggest that the best method of screening for a brain tumor is a careful history and neurologic examination. Their analysis of 76 children with brain tumors indicated the importance of the following symptoms in suggesting a brain tumor: recurrent morning headache; headaches that awaken the child; intense and incapacitating headache; and changes in the quality, frequency, and pattern of the headaches. Further, approximately 95% of children with a headache and a brain tumor had abnormal neurologic findings on clinical examination. This was supported by the findings of Rossi and Vassella[128] who analyzed the signs and symptoms of 67 children with brain tumors and 600 children diagnosed with migraine. In this study, 94% of the children with brain tumors developed progressive neurologic signs and symptoms within 4 months of onset of headache. Again, among the symptoms of headache considered to be alarming, nocturnal headache or headache present on arising, both associated with vomiting, and increasing frequency of headaches showed the greatest sensitivity for the diagnosis of a brain tumor. Wilne et al.[129] also confirmed headache as a common symptom but also highlighted the frequency of visual changes and behavioral and educational symptoms in the context of other neurologic symptoms. Children with these symptoms should undergo neuroradiologic investigation with a computed tomography (CT) or a magnetic resonance imaging (MRI), even in the absence of progressive abnormal neurologic findings.

It should also be noted that in infants, symptoms of an intracranial mass may be quite different and include irritability, increasing FOC or bulging fontanelle, seizures, failure to thrive, and developmental delays or regression.[129,130]

Thus patients with headache and neurologic symptoms, or those children who present with more localizing symptoms such as focal weakness, cranial nerve palsies, ataxia, visual loss, or seizures, should undergo neuroimaging to evaluate for intracranial pathology (Table 6.6).[131] MRI is the best method of assessing for brain tumor; however, CT may be an appropriate initial test in certain settings where MRI is not readily available.

Abdominal Masses

A palpable abdominal mass is one of the most common presenting findings of malignant solid tumors in children. Although there are a variety of benign or pseudotumorous

TABLE 6.6

DIAGNOSTIC STRATEGIES FOR CHILDREN WITH HEADACHE SUSPECTED OF HAVING A BRAIN TUMOR

Risk group[a]	Clinical definition	Probability of brain tumor, %	Diagnostic strategy
Low	HA > 6 months and no neurologic symptoms	0.01	No imaging Clinical follow-up and medical treatment
Intermediate	Migraine[a] HA and no neurologic symptoms	0.4	CT, MRI followed by biopsy or surgery
High	HA < 6 months and one clinical predictor of space occupying lesion[a]	4	MRI followed by biopsy or surgery

HA, headache; CT, computed tomography; MRI, magnetic resonance imaging.
[a]See reference for definitions.

entities that may manifest as abdominal masses, all masses require workup to ensure that an early proper diagnosis is made.

A careful systematic approach to this challenging problem may allow for a rapid and efficient way to establish the diagnosis, dissipate worries, and start appropriate treatment when necessary. The diagnostic considerations and the approach to evaluation are determined by the age of the patient, history, associated symptoms, and physical findings.

Age plays a major role in the diagnostic considerations. A mass found in the neonatal period most often represents a congenital malformation and generally has a good prognosis. In this age period, abnormalities of the genitourinary and gastrointestinal systems should be considered, because malignant tumors are uncommon. Malignant tumors are most often found in older infants and children, with a peak incidence between 1 and 5 years of age. Both Wilms' tumor and neuroblastoma commonly present during these years. Children with Wilms' tumor are more often well appearing at diagnosis than those with neuroblastoma, who may have widespread metastases producing bone pain, fever, and weight loss. NHL can present during these years but is more common in older children and adolescents. Most cases in older children are of Burkitt's lymphoma, which manifests in the abdomen in one of two ways. The first is as a rapidly enlarging abdominal mass producing pain and obstructive symptoms of the gastrointestinal and urinary tracts, often in association with metabolic derangements from tumor lysis.[132] The second is as a much smaller tumor in the ileocecal region that serves as the lead point of an intussusception.[133] Although malignant masses are also found in adolescents, one needs to consider the possibility of inflammatory processes in the differential diagnosis as well as pregnancy in female adolescents.

In obtaining the history, it helps to determine whether symptoms have been referable to the abdominal mass and, if so, their type and duration. Because of the high incidence of renal causes for an abdominal mass, a thorough history that focuses on the urinary tract is particularly important. Associated constitutional symptoms, such as fever, pain, night sweats, and weight loss, are more frequently seen in association with malignant tumors. However, most abdominal masses in children are asymptomatic and found accidentally by the parents or during routine physical examination. Medical or family history may aid in the diagnosis of

hepatoblastoma or hepatocellular carcinoma, as previously noted.

For the child with a mass, a thorough abdominal examination is frequently not easy. Every attempt should be made to have the child relaxed before palpating the abdomen. When examining the abdomen, it is important to remember that a number of structures (i.e., liver edge, spleen, kidneys, aorta, sigmoid colon, feces, and/or spine) are palpable in normal children. A rectal examination is indicated if the child has a normal absolute neutrophil count. Vaginal and pelvic examinations are important in older adolescent females, but bimanual abdominal and rectal examinations are preferred to vaginal examinations in infants and younger girls. Pelvic examinations should be performed by an experienced physician.

Although much has been written about the importance of the size, mobility, and consistency of a mass, such information is unrewarding in determining its nature. However, one should carefully consider the location of the mass and the underlying structures as sites of origin. This approach will help significantly narrow the diagnosis. Table 6.7 describes the most common malignant and benign lesions according to abdominal location. A careful general physical examination should be performed, because many of these abdominal tumors can be associated with important signs and symptoms or syndromes. Aniridia, hemihypertrophy, and genitourinary malformations can occur in association with Wilms' tumor; subcutaneous nodules, periorbital ecchymosis, and opsoclonus-myoclonus may be associated with neuroblastoma; and signs of precocious puberty may be associated with liver, gonadal, and germ cell tumors.

After the physical examination has been completed, appropriate routine laboratory studies should be performed. A CBC should be obtained because it may aid in differentiating an inflammatory condition from a potential malignancy with bone marrow involvement. Urinalysis should be obtained whenever a genitourinary mass is suspected. Tumor markers such as urinary catecholamines, α-fetoprotein, and β-human chorionic gonadotropin should be evaluated when appropriate. All females of childbearing age should have a pregnancy test performed. The workup should then proceed with appropriate imaging studies. Plain abdominal x-ray films and ultrasonography of the abdomen are appropriate initial steps because these are easily obtained, may be diagnostic, and assist in determining the need for further tests such as abdominal CT, with or without contrast, and MRI.

TABLE 6.7

COMMON MALIGNANT AND BENIGN MASSES ACCORDING TO ANATOMIC SITE

Site	Malignant	Benign
Upper abdomen	Wilms' tumor Neuroblastoma Leukemia/lymphoma Hepatoblastoma/HCC Germ cell tumors Sarcomas	Hydronephrosis Multicystic/polycystic kidney Renal vein thrombosis Mesoblastic nephroma Adrenal hemorrhage Pyloric stenosis Splenomegaly Choledochal cyst Storage diseases
Mid abdomen	Non-Hodgkin lymphoma Neuroblastoma/PNET Germ cell tumors Sarcomas	Intestinal duplication Mesenteric cyst Intussusception Lymphoid hyperplasia Appendiceal abscess Fecal material/meconium *Ascaris*
Lower abdomen and pelvis	Ovarian tumors Germ cell tumors Sarcomas	Bladder obstruction Ovarian cyst Hydrometrocolpos Anterior meningomyelocele Pregnancy Pelvic inflammatory disease

HCC, hepatocellular carcinoma; PNET, primitive neuroectodermal tumor.

Other Presentations

Parents and practitioners are often concerned that a lump or swelling may be caused by cancer. Although this is often not the case, there are certain locations where it becomes imperative to consider malignancy. Rhabdomyosarcoma commonly arises on the extremities, especially in older children and adolescents. Another common site for this tumor is head and neck. For some tumors arising inside the head, a mass is not readily apparent because these tumors are located more internally in the nasopharynx or auditory canal. However, for facial or orbital tumors, a mass or swelling may be discernible. Orbital rhabdomyosarcomas may cause proptosis, as can lymphoma, neuroblastoma, retinoblastoma, and Langerhans' cell histiocytosis. Sacrococcygeal teratomas deserve special attention. They often produce a swelling that protrudes between coccyx and rectum, and all are palpable on rectal examination. In neonates, they are usually benign, but they evolve into highly malignant germ cell tumors over the ensuing months. Therefore, their early detection and surgical removal is essential. In general, however, any persistent or enlarging mass regardless of location warrants investigation.

Peripheral Blood Abnormalities

Cytopenias

The cardinal manifestations of acute leukemia are related to bone marrow failure. Few patients have completely normal CBCs at the time of diagnosis. Up to 90% of newly diagnosed children with acute leukemia have anemia or thrombocytopenia or both. Leukocyte counts are quite variable. In approximately one-quarter of children with B-cell precursor ALL, the

WBC count is less than 5,000 per mm^3, and in this leukopenic subset, blasts may not be apparent on peripheral smear.[134] Furthermore, some of these children have leukoerythroblastic changes on peripheral smear that include presence of immature myeloid cells, and they may erroneously be thought to have AML. Similarly, approximately one-third of patients with AML may be leukopenic at diagnosis. This is particularly common with acute promyelocytic leukemia.[135]

Patients with pancytopenia and those with two of three cell lines depressed require bone marrow aspiration and biopsy for diagnosis. The situation is more complex when only a single cell line is depressed. In the absence of renal disease, a readily apparent hemolytic anemia, or features suggestive of transient erythroblastopenia, infants and children with a persistent normocytic and normochromic anemia and a low reticulocyte index should also be considered for bone marrow examination. Patients with isolated and severe thrombocytopenia often have idiopathic thrombocytopenic purpura (ITP). If history is appropriate, organomegaly is not present, and the peripheral blood smear confirms isolated thrombocytopenia as the sole abnormality, then watchful waiting or therapy with intravenous immunoglobulin, corticosteroid, or anti-RhD can be initiated without a bone marrow examination.[136] With a classic presentation of ITP, most investigators no longer consider it necessary to perform a bone marrow aspirate even before commencing corticosteroid therapy.[137] Isolated leukopenia is common with many viral infections and is also a feature of many congenital neutropenias. Unless associated with bone pain or organomegaly, it is very unlikely to be due to leukemia.[138] Neuroblastoma, Ewing's sarcoma, Hodgkin lymphoma, NHL, and rhabdomyosarcoma may all metastasize to the marrow and may present with anemia or thrombocytopenia, and with extensive infiltration, there may be leukoerythroblastic changes. However, pancytopenia due to metastatic disease to the marrow is very uncommon. It has been reported with alveolar rhabdomyosarcoma, especially with t(2;15), and primitive cells have even been found in peripheral blood. Immunologic and cytogenetic studies should easily distinguish this from acute leukemia.[139]

Leukocytosis and Thrombocytosis

Approximately one-half of children with newly diagnosed acute leukemia have WBC counts higher than 20,000 per mm^3. Indeed WBC counts higher than 100,000 per mm^3 are seen in 10% of patients with B-cell precursor ALL, 50% with T-cell ALL, and 30% with AML.[134,135] In all these groups of patients, numerous blasts are present on the differential count, and there should be no confusion with a leukemoid reaction due to infection in which blasts do not predominate, and if there is extreme left shift, they are the least common cells enumerated on differential. In patients with chronic myeloid leukemia (CML), a different blood picture emerges as these patients will have a leukocytosis with few, if any, blasts in the periphery. In those with Philadelphia chromosome–positive CML, the diagnosis is suggested by other abnormalities on smear, such as eosinophilia, basophilia, left shift in myeloid series, and thrombocytosis, and by splenomegaly. In those with juvenile myelomonocytic leukemia, monocytosis, hepatosplenomegaly, and skin lesions point toward the diagnosis. Eosinophilia can be seen as a presenting feature of malignancy as well as of parasitic infections, allergic diatheses, and the hypereosinophilic syndrome. Childhood B-cell precursor ALL can present with eosinophilia as a paraneoplastic phenomenon in association with t(5;14), which results in increased interleukin-3 synthesis.[140] Eosinophilia may also be seen in patients with Hodgkin lymphoma.

The differential diagnosis of thrombocytosis includes infectious (most often), inflammatory, and neoplastic disease. It is commonly observed in patients with CML and in patients with hepatoblastoma and has also been seen in association with neuroblastoma.[141,142] Erythrocytosis has also been reported with Wilms' tumor and brain tumors.

Workup of Cytopenias and Leukocytosis

Bone marrow aspiration and biopsy are indicated in the following situations:

- Significant depression of one or more peripheral blood cell elements without obvious explanation,
- Presence of blasts on peripheral smear,
- Presence of leukoerythroblastic changes on peripheral smear,
- Association with unexplained lymphadenopathy or hepatosplenomegaly, and
- Association with an anterior mediastinal mass.

Bleeding

Bleeding as a presenting symptom of cancer is most frequently due to thrombocytopenia and occurs in children with acute leukemia or less commonly in children with extensive bone marrow infiltration from tumor. For children with leukemia who have bleeding out of proportion to the severity of their thrombocytopenia, evaluation for disseminated intravascular coagulation (DIC) should be obtained. This coagulopathy is present in most patients with acute promyelocytic leukemia and can be severe and life-threatening because of its propensity to cause intracranial hemorrhage.[143] Acute monoblastic leukemia is another form of AML sometimes accompanied by significant DIC and bleeding. DIC is less common in ALL and, when present, is more often seen in patients with T-cell ALL.[144]

DIC can also be seen with solid tumors, such as neuroblastoma, particularly if they are large and necrotic, or in association with infectious complications of cancer. Also, patients with acquired von Willebrand's disease, which has been associated with Wilms' tumor, lymphoma, and Ewing's sarcoma in children, are at risk for bleeding complications.[145–147]

ESTABLISHING THE DIAGNOSIS

With the exception of the rare true emergency, optimal treatment for a malignancy can begin only after the tumor has been accurately diagnosed and the extent of disease precisely defined. Noninvasive imaging techniques, such as CT, diagnostic ultrasound, and MRI, and nuclear medicine scans have dramatically improved the assessment for cancer (see Chapter 9). Increasing use of newer or more specific imaging techniques such as fluorodeoxyglucose positron emission tomography (FDG PET), metaiodobenzylguanidine (MIBG), and newer CT and MRI techniques such as perfusion imaging and spectroscopy are increasingly being used in evaluation of pediatric cancer.[107,115,148,149] However, availability of these imaging techniques is often limited and again highlights the importance of referral to a pediatric cancer center for diagnostic workup of children with suspected cancer. For a few tumors, tumor markers such as plasma or urine catecholamines and α-fetoprotein may potentially provide important clues toward the diagnosis of a cancer. However, the only absolute way to establish the diagnosis of cancer is by pathologic confirmation.

When initiating the evaluation of a child for a suspected cancer, it is important to discuss overall plans and timeline with the parents and the child (if of appropriate age). Most families, and often referring physicians, are frustrated with the length of time that the diagnostic tests, including biopsy and interpretation, may take. For example, routine processing and examining a tissue specimen usually take 2 or 3 days but may take longer if special techniques or preparations are needed to make a definitive diagnosis. The family's frustration and anxiety may be heightened when the signs and symptoms have persisted for months. It helps to prospectively emphasize to the parents that enough time must be taken to ensure the correct diagnosis and to determine the extent of disease accurately. Such care helps ensure proper therapy and prevents later errors and the need to repeat examinations and biopsies after treatment has begun.

Pathologic Diagnosis

When the results of the clinical, laboratory, and imaging studies point to the probability of a neoplasm, the next decision is selection of the quickest and most reliable method to establish the pathologic diagnosis (see Chapter 8). Before obtaining any tissue for pathologic study, the primary physician should confer with a pediatric oncologist, the surgeon, and the pathologist and discuss the optimal site to biopsy, the amount of tissue needed, and the specimens to be obtained. It is important to plan to remove enough tissue initially so that additional biopsies are not necessary.

The basic principles of initial surgery for childhood tumors are outlined in Chapter 12. Excisional and incisional biopsies are the standard techniques for obtaining diagnostic tissue. Most pathologists prefer an excisional biopsy, because it yields a greater amount of tissue with fewer artifactual distortions than does the smaller incisional biopsy. In general, when it appears that the mass is localized to an organ such as the adrenal gland or the kidney, and there is no evidence of metastatic disease, the approach is one of surgical exploration, with the intent of complete resection if possible.

Increasingly, less invasive techniques are being utilized for the diagnosis of pediatric cancer. Fine needle aspiration (FNA) cytology is a cost-efficient and low-morbidity approach to the diagnosis of adults with thyroid, prostate, or breast masses. However, concerns regarding the small sample size obtainable by this approach have limited its acceptance as a primary method for the diagnosis of pediatric tumors. Although FNA can correctly identify a tumor as malignant in almost 100% of the cases, it fails to determine the correct specific diagnosis in 20% of the cases.[150] In a study comparing the use of FNA and needle core biopsy (NCB) in the diagnosis of abdominal and pelvic lesions in children, the correct diagnosis was established in 77% of the FNA and in 95% of the NCB. The complication rates for both procedures were similar, and biopsy-related bleeding was the most severe complication associated with these procedures.[151]

Currently percutaneous imaging-guided (ultrasound or CT) needle biopsy is becoming more commonly used for the diagnosis of malignant tumors in pediatric patients, particularly when complete tumor resection is not possible or indicated for the presumed tumor type. Many studies have shown that this approach is accurate, safe, and cost-effective for the diagnosis of solid tumors in childhood.[152–155] The major advantage of this approach is that a child is spared the morbidity of surgery and therefore possible delay in initiation of therapy.[156]

Minimally invasive surgery (MIS) has become increasingly useful in pediatric surgery for both diagnosis and therapeutic intervention. MIS is another useful method for obtaining diagnostic tissue for diagnosis in children with solid tumors.[157–161] MIS allows for good visualization of the tumor, the pleural surface, and the abdominal cavity without the need for open

TABLE 6.8

PREDOMINANT PEDIATRIC MALIGNANT TUMORS BY AGE AND SITE

Tumors	Newborn (<1 yr)	Infant (1–3 yr)	Child (3–11 yr)	Adolescent and young adult (12–21 yr)
Leukemias	Congenital leukemia AML AMMoL CML-juvenile	ALL AML CML-juvenile	ALL AML	ALL AML
Lymphomas	Very rare	NHL	NHL Hodgkin lymphoma	Hodgkin lymphoma NHL

Central nervous system	Medulloblastoma
	Ependymoma
	Astrocytoma/glioma
	Choroid plexus
	  papilloma
		Medulloblastoma
		Ependymoma
		Astrocytoma/glioma
		Choroid plexus
		  papilloma
			Cerebellar astrocytoma
			Medulloblastoma
			Astrocytoma/glioma
			Ependymoma
			Craniopharyngioma
				Cerebellar astrocytoma
				Astrocytoma
				Craniopharyngioma
				Medulloblastoma

Head and neck	Retinoblastoma Neuroblastoma Rhabdomyosarcoma	Retinoblastoma Neuroblastoma Rhabdomyosarcoma	Rhabdomyosarcoma Lymphoma	Lymphoma Soft tissue sarcoma
Thoracic	Neuroblastoma Teratoma	Neuroblastoma Rhabdomyosarcoma Teratoma	Lymphoma Neuroblastoma	Lymphoma Ewing's sarcoma

Abdominal	Neuroblastoma
	Mesoblastic nephroma
	Hepatoblastoma
	Wilms' tumor (>6 mo)
	Yolk sac tumor of testis
	  (endodermal sinus
	  tumor)
		Neuroblastoma
		Wilms' tumor
		Leukemia
		Hepatoblastoma
		Rhabdomyosarcoma
			Neuroblastoma
			Wilms' tumor
			Lymphoma
			Hepatoma
			Rhabdomyosarcoma
				Lymphoma
				Hepatocellular carcinoma
				Soft tissue sarcoma
				Dysgerminoma

Genitourinary	Teratoma	Rhabdomyosarcoma
		
		Yolk sac tumor of the
		  testis
		Clear cell sarcoma
		  (kidney)
				Teratocarcinoma,
				  teratoma
				Embryonal carcinoma
				  of testis
				Embryonal carcinoma
				  and endodermal sinus
				  tumors of ovary

Extremity	Fibrosarcoma	Fibrosarcoma Rhabdomyosarcoma/ Ewing's sarcoma	Rhabdomyosarcoma	Osteosarcoma Ewing's sarcoma Soft tissue sarcoma

AML, acute myeloid leukemia; AMMoL, acute myelomonocytic leukemia; CML, chronic myeloid leukemia; ALL, acute lymphoblastic leukemia; NHL, non-Hodgkin lymphoma.
Modified from Pizzo PA, Miser JS, Cassidy JR, et al. Solid tumors of childhood. In: De Vita VT Jr, Hellman S, Rosenberg SA, eds. Cancer: Principles and Practice of Oncology. 2nd ed. Philadelphia, PA: JB Lippincott, 1985:1511, with permission.

surgery. MIS is a safe and reliable approach associated with a more prompt recovery, allowing for an earlier initiation of therapy when appropriate.[162]

No matter which technique is utilized, the participation of the pathologist during the surgery of a suspected malignancy allows for frozen-section diagnosis for the establishment of a working differential diagnosis; determination of the need for additional biopsy material, depending on the quality of diagnostic material or need for lymph node or other regional sampling; and review of the surgical margins to determine the adequacy of the excision (e.g., in cases of a partial hepatectomy for hepatoblastoma or resection of a soft tissue sarcoma). In addition, if the lesion is identified as malignant, central venous access and bone marrow aspirate and biopsies, if needed for staging, can be done while the child is still asleep.

Tissue is then appropriately preserved for further testing. This often includes frozen tissue for any pertinent ancillary procedures in addition to the formalin-fixed, paraffin-embedded tissue; the latter is adequate for immunohistochemistry and fluorescence *in situ* hybridization (FISH). The advantage of this approach is that the pathologist can verify that the sample submitted includes material representative of tumor. Cytogenetics, when warranted, requires sterile tissue sample placed in cell culture medium, which can in turn be used for karyotyping and FISH on whole nuclei or on metaphase spreads. Careful coordination of physician performing the biopsy with the pathologist should minimize the potential for inadequate tissue for diagnosis and ensure the appropriate tissue preservation for appropriate diagnostic as well as research studies.

SUMMARY

Throughout this chapter, the emphasis has been on the influence of presenting signs and symptoms in making the early diagnosis of cancer in children. As shown in Table 6.8, the impact of age and site is important and should be considered when evaluating a sick child. The armamentarium of diagnostic tests available to establish the diagnosis of malignant diseases is extensive but their use should be guided by careful consideration of the differential diagnosis. Early diagnosis can improve outcome, but if the physician never considers the possibility of a cancer, delayed diagnosis is the result. Although the incidence of malignant disease in children is low, the impact of cancer makes it imperative that all professionals handling children have a high index of suspicion for cancer.

References

1. Gurney JG, Davis S, Severson RK, et al. Trends in cancer incidence among children in the U.S. Cancer 1996;78(3):532–541.
2. Feltbower RG, Lewis IJ, Picton S, et al. Diagnosing childhood cancer in primary care—a realistic expectation? Br J Cancer 2004;90(10):1882–1884.
3. Jaffe D, Fleisher G, Grosflam J. Detection of cancer in the pediatric emergency department. Pediatr Emerg Care 1985;1(1):11–15.
4. Corrigan JJ, Feig SA. Guidelines for pediatric cancer centers. Pediatrics 2004;113(6):1833–1835.
5. Parkes SE, Muir KR, Cameron AH, et al. The need for specialist review of pathology in paediatric cancer. Br J Cancer 1997;75(8):1156–1159.
6. Tanimura M, Matsui I, Abe J, et al. Increased risk of hepatoblastoma among immature children with a lower birth weight. Cancer Res 1998;58(14):3032–3035.
7. Hjalgrim H, Askling J, Rostgaard K, et al. Characteristics of Hodgkin's lymphoma after infectious mononucleosis. N Engl J Med 2003;349(14):1324–1332.
8. Imashuku S, Hibi S, Morinaga S, et al. Haemophagocytic lymphohistiocytosis in association with granular lymphocyte proliferative disorders in early childhood: characteristic bone marrow morphology. Br J Haematol 1997;96(4):708–714.
9. Pagano JS. The Epstein-Barr virus and nasopharyngeal carcinoma. Cancer 1994;74(9):2397–2398.
10. Thorley-Lawson DA, Gross A. Persistence of the Epstein-Barr virus and the origins of associated lymphomas. N Engl J Med 2004;350(13):1328–1337.
11. Wen WH, Chang MH, Hsu HY, et al. The development of hepatocellular carcinoma among prospectively followed children with chronic hepatitis B virus infection. J Pediatr 2004;144(3):397–399.
12. Wands JR. Prevention of hepatocellular carcinoma. N Engl J Med 2004;351(15):1567–1570.
13. Granovsky MO, Mueller BU, Nicholson HS, et al. Cancer in human immunodeficiency virus-infected children: a case series from the Children's Cancer Group and the National Cancer Institute. J Clin Oncol 1998;16(5):1729–1735.
14. Pollock BH, Jenson HB, Leach CT, et al. Risk factors for pediatric human immunodeficiency virus-related malignancy. JAMA 2003;289(18):2393–2399.
15. Serraino D, Franceschi S. Kaposi's sarcoma and non-Hodgkin's lymphomas in children and adolescents with AIDS. AIDS 1996;10(6):643–647.
16. Paller AS. Immunodeficiency syndromes: X-linked agammaglobulinemia, common variable immunodeficiency, Chediak-Higashi syndrome, Wiskott-Aldrich syndrome, and X-linked lymphoproliferative disorder. Dermatol Clin 1995;13(1):65–71.
17. Penn I. De novo malignancies in pediatric organ transplant recipients. Pediatr Transplant 1998;2(1):56–63.
18. Offman J, Opelz G, Doehler B, et al. Defective DNA mismatch repair in acute myeloid leukemia/myelodysplastic syndrome after organ transplantation. Blood 2004;104(3):822–828.
19. Meadows AT, Friedman DL, Neglia JP, et al. Second neoplasms in survivors of childhood cancer: findings from the Childhood Cancer Survivor Study cohort. J Clin Oncol 2009;27(14):2356–2362.
20. Hijiya N, Ness KK, Ribeiro RC, et al. Acute leukemia as a secondary malignancy in children and adolescents: current findings and issues. Cancer 2009;115(1):23–35.
21. Relling MV, Rubnitz JE, Rivera GK, et al. High incidence of secondary brain tumours after radiotherapy and antimetabolites. Lancet 1999;354(9172):34–39.
22. Kushner BH, Heller G, Cheung NK, et al. High risk of leukemia after short-term dose-intensive chemotherapy in young patients with solid tumors. J Clin Oncol 1998;16(9):3016–3020.
23. Pui CH, Relling MV. Topoisomerase II inhibitor-related acute myeloid leukaemia. Br J Haematol 2000;109(1):13–23.
24. Sankila R, Garwicz S, Olsen JH, et al. Risk of subsequent malignant neoplasms among 1,641 Hodgkin's disease patients diagnosed in childhood and adolescence: a population-based cohort study in the five Nordic countries: Association of the Nordic Cancer Registries and the Nordic Society of Pediatric Hematology and Oncology. J Clin Oncol 1996;14(5):1442–1446.
25. Paulino AC, Fowler BZ. Secondary neoplasms after radiotherapy for a childhood solid tumor. Pediatr Hematol Oncol 2005;22(2):89–101.
26. Bhatia S, Robison LL, Oberlin O, et al. Breast cancer and other second neoplasms after childhood Hodgkin's disease. N Engl J Med 1996;334(12):745–751.
27. Socie G, Curtis RE, Deeg HJ, et al. New malignant diseases after allogeneic marrow transplantation for childhood acute leukemia. J Clin Oncol 2000;18(2):348–357.
28. Boice JD Jr. Cancer following irradiation in childhood and adolescence. Med Pediatr Oncol Suppl 1996;1:29–34.
29. Davis S, Stepanenko V, Rivkind N, et al. Risk of thyroid cancer in the Bryansk Oblast of the Russian Federation after the Chernobyl Power Station accident. Radiat Res 2004;162(3):241–248.
30. Reiners C, Demidchik YE, Drozd VM, et al. Thyroid cancer in infants and adolescents after Chernobyl. Minerva Endocrinol 2008;33(4):381–395.
31. Dang-Tan T, Franco EL. Diagnosis delays in childhood cancer: a review. Cancer 2007;110(4):703–713.
32. Pollock BH, Krischer JP, Vietti TJ. Interval between symptom onset and diagnosis of pediatric solid tumors. J Pediatr 1991;119(5):725–732.
33. Dixon-Woods M, Findlay M, Young B, et al. Parents' accounts of obtaining a diagnosis of childhood cancer. Lancet 2001;357(9257):670–674.
34. Dang-Tan T, Trottier H, Mery LS, et al. Delays in diagnosis and treatment among children and adolescents with cancer in Canada. Pediatr Blood Cancer 2008;51(4):468–474.
35. Dorner L, Fritsch MJ, Stark AM, et al. Posterior fossa tumors in children: how long does it take to establish the diagnosis? Childs Nerv Syst 2007;23(8):887–890.
36. Widhe B, Widhe T. Initial symptoms and clinical features in osteosarcoma and Ewing sarcoma. J Bone Joint Surg Am 2000;82(5):667–674.
37. Saha V, Love S, Eden T, et al. Determinants of symptom interval in childhood cancer. Arch Dis Child 1993;68(6):771–774.
38. Hamre MR, Williams J, Chuba P, et al. Early deaths in childhood cancer. Med Pediatr Oncol 2000;34(5):343–347.
39. Halperin EC, Friedman HS. Is there a correlation between duration of presenting symptoms and stage of medulloblastoma at the time of diagnosis? Cancer 1996;78(4):874–880.
40. Pratt CB, Smith JW, Woerner S, et al. Factors leading to delay in the diagnosis and affecting survival of children with head and neck rhabdomyosarcoma. Pediatrics 1978;61(1):30–34.
41. Miser AW, McCalla J, Dothage JA, et al. Pain as a presenting symptom in children and young adults with newly diagnosed malignancy. Pain 1987;29(1):85–90.
42. Honjo S, Doran HE, Stiller CA, et al. Neuroblastoma trends in Osaka, Japan, and Great Britain 1970–1994, in relation to screening. Int J Cancer 2003;103(4):538–543.
43. Iida Y, Nose O, Kai H, et al. Watery diarrhoea with a vasoactive intestinal peptide-producing ganglioneuroblastoma. Arch Dis Child 1980;55(12):929–936.
44. Altman AJ, Baehner RL. Favorable prognosis for survival in children with coincident opso-myoclonus and neuroblastoma. Cancer 1976;37(2):846–852.
45. Williams TH, House RF Jr, Burgert EO Jr, et al. Unusual manifestations of neuroblastoma: chronic diarrhea, polymyoclonia-opsoclonus, and erythrocyte abnormalities. Cancer 1972;29(2):475–480.
46. Balakrishnan V, Rice MS, Simpson DA. Spinal neuroblastomas: Diagnosis, treatment, and prognosis. J Neurosurg 1974;40(5):631–638.
47. Cummins GE, Cohen D. Cushing's syndrome secondary to ACTH-secreting Wilms' tumor. J Pediatr Surg 1974;9(4):535–539.
48. Beckerman BL, Seaver R. Congenital Horner's syndrome and thoracic neuroblastoma. J Pediatr Ophthalmol Strabismus 1978;15(1):24–25.
49. Familusi JB, Samuel I, Jaiyesimi, et al. Superior vena cava occlusion in a 12-year-old girl with neuroblastoma. Clin Pediatr (Phila) 1977;16(12):1160–1172.

50. Mones RJ. Increased intracranial pressure due to metastatic disease of venous sinuses: a report of six cases. Neurology. 1965;15(11):1000–1007.
51. Farr GH, Hajdu SI. Exfoliative cytology of metastatic neuroblastoma. Acta Cytol 1972;16(3):203–206.
52. Donohue JP, Garrett RA, Baehner RL, et al. The multiple manifestations of neuroblastoma. J Urol 1974;111(2):260–264.
53. D'Angio GJ, Evans AE, Koop CE. Special pattern of widespread neuroblastoma with a favourable prognosis. Lancet 1971;1(7708):1046–1049.
54. Gaffney PC, Hansman CF, Fetterman GH. Experience with smears of aspirates from bone marrow in the diagnosis of neuroblastoma. Am J Clin Pathol 1959;31(3):213–221.
55. Robinson MJ, Howard RM. Neuroblastoma, presenting as myasthenia gravis in a child aged 3 years. Pediatrics 1969;43(1):111–113.
56. Albert DM, Rubenstein RA, Scheie HG. Tumor metastasis to the eye, II: clinical study in infants and children. Am J Ophthalmol 1967;63(4):727–732.
57. Cohn SL, Morgan ER, Mallette LE. The spectrum of metabolic bone disease in lymphoblastic leukemia. Cancer 1987;59(2):346–350.
58. Lensink DB, Barton A, Appelbaum FR, et al. Cyclic neutropenia as a premalignant manifestation of acute lymphoblastic leukemia. Am J Hematol 1986;22(1):9–16.
59. Troxell ML, Mills GM, Allen RC. The hypereosinophilic syndrome in acute lymphocytic leukemia. Cancer 1984;54(6):1058–1061.
60. Corbaton J, Munoz A, Madero L, et al. Pulmonary leukemia in a child presenting with infiltrative and nodular lesions. Pediatr Radiol 1984;14(6):431–432.
61. Saulsbury FT, Sabio H, Conrad D, et al. Acute leukemia with features of systemic lupus erythematosus. J Pediatr 1984;105(1):57–59.
62. Saulsbury FT, Sabio H. Acute leukemia presenting as arthritis in children. Clin Pediatr (Phila) 1985;24(11):625–628.
63. Risdall RJ, McKenna RW, Nesbit ME, et al. Virus-associated hemophagocytic syndrome: a benign histiocytic proliferation distinct from malignant histiocytosis. Cancer 1979;44(3):993–1002.
64. Niebrugge DJ, Benjamin DR. Bone marrow necrosis preceding acute lymphoblastic leukemia in childhood. Cancer 1983;52(11):2162–2164.
65. Dunn NL, McWilliams NB, Mohanakumar T. Clinical and immunological correlates of leukemia cutis in childhood. Cancer 1982;50(10):2049–2051.
66. Mancuso L, Marchi S, Giuliano P, et al. Cardiac tamponade as first manifestation of acute lymphoblastic leukemia in a patient with echographic evidence of mediastinal lymph nodal enlargement. Am Heart J 1985;110(6):1303–1304.
67. de Alarcon PA, Miller ML, Stuart MJ. Erythroid hypoplasia: an unusual presentation of childhood acute lymphocytic leukemia. Am J Dis Child 1978;132(8):763–764.
68. Canivet B, Squara P, Elbaze P, et al. In vitro glucose consumption in severe hyperleukocytosis: a cause of factitious hypoglycemia [in French]. Pathol Biol (Paris) 1982;30(10): 843–846.
69. Ali SH, Yacoub FM, Al-Matar E. Acute lymphoblastic leukemia presenting as bilateral renal enlargement in a child. Med Princ Pract 2008;17(6):504–506.
70. Desmond R, McDerra J, Kelly K, et al. Multiple vertebral collapse as a presentation of childhood acute lymphoblastic leukaemia. Br J Haematol 2009;144(5):627.
71. Urs L, Stevens L, Kahwash SB. Leukemia presenting as solid tumors: report of four pediatric cases and review of the literature. Pediatr Dev Pathol 2008;11(5):370–376.
72. Cairney AE, McKenna R, Arthur DC, et al. Acute megakaryoblastic leukaemia in children. Br J Haematol 1986;63(3):541–554.
73. Banerjee D, Silva E. Mediastinal mass with acute leukemia: myeloblastoma masquerading as lymphoblastic lymphoma. Arch Pathol Lab Med 1981;105(3):126–129.
74. Williams DL, Bell BA, Ragab AH. Clitorism at presentation of acute nonlymphocytic leukemia. J Pediatr 1985;107(5):754–755.
75. Morgan ER, Labotka RJ, Gonzalez-Crussi F, et al. Ovarian granulocytic sarcoma as the primary manifestation of acute infantile myelomonocytic leukemia. Cancer 1981;48(8): 1819–1824.
76. Chu JY, Demello D, O'Connor DM, et al. Pericarditis as presenting manifestation of acute nonlymphocytic leukemia in a young child. Cancer 1983;52(2):322–324.
77. Rajantie J, Tarkkanen A, Rapola J, et al. Orbital granulocytic sarcoma as a presenting sign in acute myelogenous leukemia. Ophthalmologica 1984;189(3):158–161.
78. Alioglu B, Tuncay IC, Ozyurek E, et al. Bone fracture: an unusual presentation of acute megakaryoblastic leukemia. Pediatr Hematol Oncol 2009;26(1):62–69.
79. Powderly WG, Cantwell BM, Fennelly JJ, et al. Renal glomerulopathies associated with Hodgkin's disease. Cancer 1985;56(4):874–875.
80. Gobbi PG, Attardo-Parrinello G, Lattanzio G, et al. Severe pruritus should be a B-symptom in Hodgkin's disease. Cancer 1983;51(10):1934–1936.
81. van Lieshout JJ, Wieling W, van Montfrans GA, et al. Acute dysautonomia associated with Hodgkin's disease. J Neurol Neurosurg Psychiatry 1986;49(7):830–832.
82. Dowsett RJ, Wong RL, Robert NJ, et al. Dermatomyositis and Hodgkin's disease: case report and review of the literature. Am J Med 1986;80(4):719–723.
83. Chintagumpala MM, Mahoney DH Jr, McClain K, et al. Hodgkin's disease associated with central pontine myelinolysis. Med Pediatr Oncol 1993;21(4):311–314.
84. Cho BK, Wang KC, Nam DH, et al. Pineal tumors: experience with 48 cases over 10 years. Childs Nerv Syst 1998;14(1/2):53–58.
85. Furman WL, Buckley PJ, Green AA, et al. Thymoma and myasthenia gravis in a 4-year-old child: case report and review of the literature. Cancer 1985;56(11):2703–2706.
86. Addy DP, Hudson FP. Diencephalic syndrome of infantile emaciation: analysis of literature and report of further 3 cases. Arch Dis Child 1972;47(253):338–343.
87. Fleischman A, Brue C, Poussaint TY, et al. Diencephalic syndrome: a cause of failure to thrive and a model of partial growth hormone resistance. Pediatrics 2005;115(6): e742–e748.
88. Loutfi AH, Mehrez I, Shahbender S, et al. Hypoglycaemia with Wilms' tumour. Arch Dis Child 1964;39:197–203.
89. Bittencourt AL, Britto JF, Fonseca LE Jr. Wilms' tumor of the uterus: the first report of the literature. Cancer 1981;47(10):2496–2499.
90. Slovis TL, Philippart AI, Cushing B, et al. Evaluation of the inferior vena cava by sonography and venography in children with renal and hepatic tumors. Radiology 1981;140(3): 767–772.
91. Ramsay NK, Dehner LP, Coccia PF, et al. Acute hemorrhage into Wilms tumor: a cause of rapidly developing abdominal mass with hypertension, anemia, and fever. J Pediatr 1977;91(5):763–765.
92. Jacobson RJ, Lowenthal MN, Kew MC. Erythrocytosis in hepatocellular cancer. S Afr Med J 1978;53(17):658–660.
93. Nickerson HJ, Silberman TL, McDonald TP. Hepatoblastoma, thrombocytosis, and increased thrombopoietin. Cancer 1980;45(2):315–317.
94. Dvorak PF, Vorlicky LN, Nesbit ME Jr. Ewing's sarcoma of the rib, presenting as the superior mediastinal syndrome. Clin Pediatr (Phila) 1971;10(10):607–610.
95. Wang CC, Schulz MD. Ewing's sarcoma; a study of fifty cases treated at the Massachusetts General Hospital, 1930–1952 inclusive. N Engl J Med 1953;248(14):571–576.
96. Jordanov MI, Block JJ, Gonzalez AL, et al. Transarticular spread of Ewing sarcoma mimicking septic arthritis. Pediatr Radiol 2009;39(4):381–384.
97. Small EJ, Gordon GJ, Dahms BB. Malignant rhabdoid tumor of the heart in an infant. Cancer 1985;55(12):2850–2853.
98. Allan BT, Day DL, Dehner LP. Primary pulmonary rhabdomyosarcoma of the lung in children: report of two cases presenting with spontaneous pneumothorax. Cancer 1987;59(5):1005–1011.
99. Selvaraj T, Kapoor PM, Kiran U. Large rhabdomyosarcoma of the right ventricle obstructing tricuspid valve, pulmonary valve and left ventricular outflow tract. Ann Card Anaesth 2009;12(1):81–82.
100. Shinkoda Y, Nagatoshi Y, Fukano R, et al. Rhabdomyosarcoma masquerading as acute leukemia. Pediatr Blood Cancer 2009;52(2):286–287.
101. Spiers AS. Chronic granulocytic leukemia. Med Clin North Am 1984;68(3):713–727.
102. Chantada G, Casak S, Plata JD, et al. Children with fever of unknown origin in Argentina: an analysis of 113 cases. Pediatr Infect Dis J 1994;13(4):260–263.
103. Pasic S, Minic A, Djuric P, et al. Fever of unknown origin in 185 paediatric patients: a single-centre experience. Acta Paediatr 2006;95(4):463–466.
104. Miller LC, Sisson BA, Tucker LB, et al. Prolonged fevers of unknown origin in children: patterns of presentation and outcome. J Pediatr 1996;129(3):419–423.
105. Steele RW. Fever of unknown origin: a time for patience with your patients. Clin Pediatr (Phila) 2000;39(12):719–720.
106. Herzog LW. Prevalence of lymphadenopathy of the head and neck in infants and children. Clin Pediatr (Phila) 1983;22(7):485–487.
107. Kleis M, Daldrup-Link H, Matthay K, et al. Diagnostic value of PET/CT for the staging and restaging of pediatric tumors. Eur J Nucl Med Mol Imaging 2009;36(1):23–36.
108. Brown RL, Azizkhan RG. Pediatric head and neck lesions. Pediatr Clin North Am 1998;45(4):889–905.
109. Twist CJ, Link MP. Assessment of lymphadenopathy in children. Pediatr Clin North Am 2002;49(5):1009–1025.
110. Oguz A, Karadeniz C, Temel EA, et al. Evaluation of peripheral lymphadenopathy in children. Pediatr Hematol Oncol 2006;23(7):549–561.
111. Quinn JJ. Non-Hodgkin's lymphoma in children. Curr Probl Pediatr 1983;13(4):1–72.
112. Lake AM, Oski FA. Peripheral lymphadenopathy in childhood: ten-year experience with excisional biopsy. Am J Dis Child 1978;132(4):357–359.
113. Knight PJ, Mulne AF, Vassy LE. When is lymph node biopsy indicated in children with enlarged peripheral nodes? Pediatrics 1982;69(4):391–396.
114. Torsiglieri AJ Jr, Tom LW, Ross AJ III, et al. Pediatric neck masses: guidelines for evaluation. Int J Pediatr Otorhinolaryngol 1988;16(3):199–210.
115. Vezina LG. Imaging of central nervous system tumors in children: advances and limitations. J Child Neurol 2008;23(10):1128–1135.
116. Pinot A, Machin G, Trevenen C. Respiratory tract and serosal tumors. In: Pahrham DM, ed. Pediatric neoplasia: morphology and biology. Philadelphia, PA: Lippincott-Raven, 1996:423–447.
117. Grosfeld JL, Skinner MA, Rescorla FJ, et al. Mediastinal tumors in children: experience with 196 cases. Ann Surg Oncol 1994;1(2):121–127.
118. King RM, Telander RL, Smithson WA, et al. Primary mediastinal tumors in children. J Pediatr Surg 1982;17(5):512–520.
119. Massie RJ, Van Asperen PP, Mellis CM. A review of open biopsy for mediastinal masses. J Paediatr Child Health 1997;33(3):230–233.
120. Grattan-Smith PJ, Ryan MM, Procopis PG. Persistent or severe back pain and stiffness are ominous symptoms requiring prompt attention. J Paediatr Child Health 2000;36(3): 208–212.
121. Jonsson OG, Sartain P, Ducore JM, et al. Bone pain as an initial symptom of childhood acute lymphoblastic leukemia: association with nearly normal hematologic indexes. J Pediatr 1990;117(2, pt 1):233–237.
122. Ostrov BE, Goldsmith DP, Athreya BH. Differentiation of systemic juvenile rheumatoid arthritis from acute leukemia near the onset of disease. J Pediatr 1993;122(4): 595–598.
123. Trapani S, Grisolia F, Simonini G, et al. Incidence of occult cancer in children presenting with musculoskeletal symptoms: a 10-year survey in a pediatric rheumatology unit. Semin Arthritis Rheum 2000;29(6):348–359.
124. Edgeworth J, Bullock P, Bailey A, et al. Why are brain tumours still being missed? Arch Dis Child 1996;74(2):148–151.
125. Flores LE, Williams DL, Bell BA, et al. Delay in the diagnosis of pediatric brain tumors. Am J Dis Child 1986;140(7):684–686.
126. Honig PJ, Charney EB. Children with brain tumor headaches: distinguishing features. Am J Dis Child 1982;136(2):121–124.
127. Maytal J, Bienkowski RS, Patel M, et al. The value of brain imaging in children with headaches. Pediatrics 1995;96(3, pt 1):413–416.
128. Rossi LN, Vassella F. Headache in children with brain tumors. Childs Nerv Syst 1989;5(5):307–309.
129. Wilne SH, Ferris RC, Nathwani A, et al. The presenting features of brain tumours: a review of 200 cases. Arch Dis Child 2006;91(6):502–506.
130. Furuta T, Tabuchi A, Adachi Y, et al. Primary brain tumors in children under age 3 years. Brain Tumor Pathol 1998;15(1):7–12.
131. Medina LS, Kuntz KM, Pomeroy S. Children with headache suspected of having a brain tumor: a cost-effectiveness analysis of diagnostic strategies. Pediatrics 2001;108: 255–263.
132. Levine PH, Kamaraju LS, Connelly RR, et al. The American Burkitt's Lymphoma Registry: eight years' experience. Cancer 1982;49(5):1016–1022.
133. Gupta H, Davidoff AM, Pui CH, et al. Clinical implications and surgical management of intussusception in pediatric patients with Burkitt lymphoma. J Pediatr Surg 2007;42(6):998–1001, discussion 1001.
134. Pui CH, Crist W. Acute lymphoblastic leukemia. In: Pui CH, ed. Childhood leukemias. Cambridge, England: Cambridge University Press, 1999:288–312.
135. Weinstein H. Acute myeloid leukemia. In: Pui CH, ed. Childhood leukemias. Cambridge, England: Cambridge University Press 1999:322–335.
136. Calpin C, Dick P, Poon A, et al. Is bone marrow aspiration needed in acute childhood idiopathic thrombocytopenic purpura to rule out leukemia? Arch Pediatr Adolesc Med 1998;152(4):345–347.
137. Klaassen RJ, Doyle JJ, Krahn MD, et al. Initial bone marrow aspiration in childhood idiopathic thrombocytopenia: decision analysis. J Pediatr Hematol Oncol 2001;23(8): 511–518.
138. Kyono W, Coates TD. A practical approach to neutrophil disorders. Pediatr Clin North Am 2002;49(5):929–971, viii.

139. Putti MC, Montaldi A, D'Emilio A, et al. Unusual leukemic presentation of rhab-domyosarcoma: report of two cases with immunological, ultrastructural and cytogenet-ical studies. Haematologica 1991;76(5):368–374.
140. Meeker TC, Hardy D, Willman C, et al. Activation of the interleukin-3 gene by chromo-some translocation in acute lymphocytic leukemia with eosinophilia. Blood 1990;76(2):285–289.
141. Yamaguchi H, Ishii E, Hayashida Y, et al. Mechanism of thrombocytosis in hepatoblas-toma: a case report. Pediatr Hematol Oncol 1996;13(6):539–544.
142. Quinn JJ, Altman AJ. The multiple hematologic manifestations of neuroblastoma. Am J Pediatr Hematol Oncol 1979;1(3):201–205.
143. Barbui T, Finazzi G, Falanga A. The impact of all-trans-retinoic acid on the coagulopathy of acute promyelocytic leukemia. Blood 1998;91(9):3093–3102.
144. Ribeiro RC, Pui CH. The clinical and biological correlates of coagulopathy in children with acute leukemia. J Clin Oncol 1986;4(8):1212–1218.
145. Will A. Paediatric acquired von Willebrand syndrome. Haemophilia 2006;12(3):287–288.
146. Jonge Poerink-Stockschlader AB, Dekker I, Risseeuw-Appel IM, et al. Acquired Von Willebrand disease in children with a Wilms' tumor. Med Pediatr Oncol 1996;26(4):238–243.
147. Baxter PA, Nuchtern JG, Guillerman RP, et al. Acquired von Willebrand syndrome and Wilms tumor: not always benign. Pediatr Blood Cancer 2009;52(3):392–394.
148. Franzius C, Juergens KU. PET/CT in paediatric oncology: indications and pitfalls. Pediatr Radiol 2009;39(suppl 3):446–449.
149. Jadvar H, Connolly LP, Fahey FH, et al. PET and PET/CT in pediatric oncology. Semin Nucl Med 2007;37(5):316–331.
150. Layfield LJ, Glasgow B, Ostrzega N, et al. Fine-needle aspiration cytology and the diagnosis of neoplasms in the pediatric age group. Diagn Cytopathol 1991;7(5):451–461.
151. Hugosson CO, Nyman RS, Cappelen-Smith JM, et al. Ultrasound-guided biopsy of abdominal and pelvic lesions in children: a comparison between fine-needle aspiration and 1.2 mm-needle core biopsy. Pediatr Radiol 1999;29(1):31–36.
152. Shin HJ, Amaral JG, Armstrong D, et al. Image-guided percutaneous biopsy of muscu-loskeletal lesions in children. Pediatr Radiol 2007;37(4):362–369.
153. Sebire NJ, Roebuck DJ. Pathological diagnosis of paediatric tumours from image-guided needle core biopsies: a systematic review. Pediatr Radiol 2006;36(5): 426–431.
154. Sklair-Levy M, Lebensart PD, Applbaum YH, et al. Percutaneous image-guided needle biopsy in children—summary of our experience with 57 children. Pediatr Radiol 2001;31(10):732–736.
155. Skoldenberg EG, Jakobson AA, Elvin A, et al. Diagnosing childhood tumors: a review of 147 cutting needle biopsies in 110 children. J Pediatr Surg 2002;37(1):50–56.
156. Hussain HK, Kingston JE, Domizio P, et al. Imaging-guided core biopsy for the diagno-sis of malignant tumors in pediatric patients. AJR Am J Roentgenol 2001;176(1):43–47.
157. Meehan JJ, Sandler AD. Robotic resection of mediastinal masses in children. J Laparoendosc Adv Surg Tech A 2008;18(1):114–119.
158. Chan KW, Lee KH, Tam YH, et al. Minimal invasive surgery in pediatric solid tumors. J Laparoendosc Adv Surg Tech A 2007;17(6):817–820.
159. Cribbs RK, Wulkan ML, Heiss KF, et al. Minimally invasive surgery and childhood cancer. Surg Oncol 2007;16(3):221–228.
160. Holcomb GW III, Tomita SS, Haase GM, et al. Minimally invasive surgery in children with cancer. Cancer 1995;76(1):121–128.
161. Saenz NC, Conlon KC, Aronson DC, et al. The application of minimal access proce-dures in infants, children, and young adults with pediatric malignancies. J Laparoen-dosc Adv Surg Tech A 1997;7(5):289–294.
162. Waldhausen JH, Tapper D, Sawin RS. Minimally invasive surgery and clinical decision-making for pediatric malignancy. Surg Endosc 2000;14(3):250–253.

CHAPTER 7 ■ PATHOLOGY AND MOLECULAR DIAGNOSIS OF LEUKEMIAS AND LYMPHOMAS

AMY HEEREMA-MCKENNEY, MICHAEL L. CLEARY, AND DANIEL A. ARBER

INTRODUCTION

Hematopoietic neoplasms constitute more than 40% of malignancies in children and represent a wide range of disorders that include acute and chronic leukemias, lymphomas, and histiocytic malignancies. This chapter focuses on the pathologic approach to diagnosis of the more common pediatric hematopoietic neoplasms and their pathologic subclassification by using the most recent World Health Organization's *WHO Classification of Tumours of Haematopoietic and Lymphoid Tissues*[1,2] published in 2008.

It is worth emphasizing that correct pathologic diagnosis and classification requires proper specimen collection and excellent communication between the treating physician and the pathologist or hematologist examining the diagnostic material. Accurate diagnosis also requires correlation with appropriate immunophenotyping and molecular genetic studies, which are now integral components of the classification of these diseases.

SPECIMEN PROCESSING

Bone Marrow and Peripheral Blood

A wide variety of diseases may be diagnosed by the examination of peripheral blood or bone marrow or a combination of the two. While most laboratories are experienced in adequately preparing and staining peripheral blood smears, there is more variability in the quality of bone marrow aspirate smears among laboratories. The latter are preferably prepared at the bedside and may be stained with a variety of Romanowsky stains prior to examination. Smears can also be prepared in the laboratory if the bone marrow aspirate is mixed with EDTA for transport, but such smears are usually of poorer quality when compared with those freshly prepared. Procedures for making bone marrow aspirate smears are published elsewhere,[3–5] but it should be stressed that care must be taken not to crush the marrow cells and that slides are adequately air-dried before staining with quality-controlled reagents, using a well-validated and reproducible procedure. Touch preparations from the biopsy specimen should also be considered in all cases, as they are extremely useful when the aspirate smears contain insufficient particle material for evaluation. Since peripheral blood and bone marrow aspirate materials are ideal for flow cytometry immunophenotyping, an additional sample should be saved in EDTA or heparin when a hematopoietic malignancy is suspected.

Tissue Specimens, Including Lymph Nodes

Fresh tissue specimens, such as lymph node biopsies, also must be handled properly for adequate diagnosis.[6] While lymph node excision provides the best material for diagnosis, smaller biopsies or fine needle aspirations may provide suitable material in some cases. Proper communication between the oncologist, surgeon, and pathologist is essential. If a neoplasm with only rare tumor cells, such as Hodgkin lymphoma, is suspected, then a larger portion of tissue is required. If the initial attempt at diagnosis of a hematopoietic tumor is by fine needle aspiration, a separate sample for flow cytometry is strongly recommended, and it should be confirmed in advance that the laboratory is equipped to handle such specimens. When larger tissue portions are removed, they should be submitted fresh to the pathologist for immediate processing. Depending on the laboratory, samples will be fixed in formalin or other fixatives, and a portion may be submitted fresh for immunophenotyping, cytogenetics studies, or molecular studies or may be frozen and saved for ancillary studies. While many immunophenotypic markers and molecular aberrations can now be assessed on fixed tissues, some of these tests still require fresh or frozen tissue, thus the possible need for such testing should be communicated in advance to the pathologist.

USE OF ANCILLARY STUDIES

Ancillary studies are essential for the proper diagnosis and classification of most hematopoietic tumors and include immunophenotypic, cytogenetic, and molecular genetic studies. While all of these tests are not necessary for each specimen type, an understanding of the utility of the different methods is essential.

Immunophenotyping

Determining the immunophenotype of the neoplastic population is critical for the proper classification of hematopoietic neoplasms. Flow cytometry and immunohistochemistry are the two most common immunophenotypic methods. Some of the more commonly used immunophenotypic markers are listed in Table 7.1. Flow cytometry immunophenotyping is performed on liquid specimens or cell suspensions prepared from solid tissue specimens. It is therefore a preferred method for the immunophenotyping of peripheral blood and bone marrow aspirates and can also be useful in some lymphomas.[7,8] Multicolor flow cytometry is particularly useful for analysis of multiple antigens on a given cell and for rapid evaluation of very large numbers of cells. Since the cells are fresh, a wide range of cell surface and cytoplasmic markers can be readily evaluated by this method.

Immunohistochemical methods are performed on sections of either fixed and paraffin-embedded or frozen tissue, but paraffin-section immunohistochemistry is by far the most commonly used method today.[9] This allows for more definitive correlation between cellular morphology and immunophenotype but usually evaluates only one marker at a time (in contrast to the multiple

TABLE 7.1

SELECTED IMMUNOPHENOTYPING MARKERS IN HEMATOPOIETIC TUMORS

General		B lineage	
	CD45		CD19
Myeloid			CD20
	CD13		CD22
	CD15		CD79a
	CD33		PAX5
	CD117		Kappa/lambda
	Myeloperoxidase	T lineage	
Myelomonocytic			CD2
	CD14		CD3
	CD64		CD5
	CD163		CD7
Megakaryocyte			CD4/CD8
	CD41	Immature lineage	
	CD61		TdT
			CD34

antibodies that can be simultaneously used in flow cytometry). It is ideal for tissue that has already been fixed and unavailable for flow cytometry, tumors in which the cells are fragile and may not survive processing for flow cytometry, and tumors with small numbers of neoplastic cells, such as Hodgkin lymphoma. It is less helpful in acute leukemias[10] because there are fewer antibodies for the acute leukemias that work well in paraffin sections.

Cytogenetic Studies

Cytogenetic studies are of critical importance for many hematopoietic tumors, providing essential prognostic information as well as aiding in their proper classification.[11] These studies are most successful in proliferating tumors, particularly in acute and chronic leukemias, myelodysplastic syndromes (MDSs), and some high-grade lymphomas. Routine karyotype analysis is less commonly performed for lymphomas of small lymphocytes and other tumors with poor cell growth. Molecular-based cytogenetic approaches that incorporate the use of fluorescently labeled DNA probes (fluorescence in situ hybridization, FISH) have significantly enhanced the amount of information that can be gained from cytogenetic studies. Moreover, FISH assays can be applied to resting cells, thus broadening the cellular populations that can be analyzed. Further advances in cytogenetic methodology include spectral karyotyping or SKY analysis, which uses chromosome-specific painting probes that allow for the identification of cryptic chromosomal rearrangements, and the combined use of immunohistochemistry and FISH, which allows the identification of specific genetic lesions within defined cellular populations. These newer approaches are not only advancing our understanding of the genetic alterations within hematopoietic malignancies but are also finding their way into the diagnostic armamentarium.

Molecular Genetic Studies

Molecular genetic studies serve a variety of roles in the evaluation of hematopoietic tumors,[12] including clarification of the precise molecular lesion of a detected karyotypic abnormality, identification of occult cytogenetic aberrations, detection of gene rearrangements that do not cause identifiable karyotype changes, and detection of minimal residual disease. A wide variety of molecular genetic methodologies are now available, including Southern blot hybridization, polymerase chain reaction (PCR) and other amplification methods, FISH analysis, and gene expression array studies. The methodology used for a given aberration or a particular clinical setting can vary between laboratories with, unfortunately, little standardization of methodology achieved to date. This has led to difficulty in comparing results between laboratories and differences in the reported frequencies of specific genetic lesions depending on the methodologies used. Nevertheless, uniform approaches are emerging for the more common genetic abnormalities identified within the pediatric hematopoietic malignancies. The source of patient material required for these molecular assays varies depending on the particular assay used. For example, some FISH and PCR-based tests can be performed on DNA isolated from fixed, paraffin-embedded tissues. By contrast, for the majority of molecular-based assays, fresh or frozen tissue is required.

ACUTE LYMPHOBLASTIC LEUKEMIA/LYMPHOMA (PRECURSOR LYMPHOID NEOPLASMS)

Acute lymphoblastic leukemia (ALL) is the most common hematopoietic tumor of childhood and is defined as a proliferation of immature lymphoid cells or lymphoblasts. A minimal threshold for defining leukemia has not been established for ALL, in contrast to the 20% blasts used for acute myeloid leukemia (AML). Many protocols require that lymphoblasts comprise 25% or more of bone marrow cells.[13] The diagnosis is rarely made in the setting of less than 20% blasts. This disease is biologically similar to lymphoblastic lymphoma, which is usually distinguished from leukemia by evidence of extramedullary disease and less than 25% bone marrow lymphoblasts. In the past, ALL was classified on the basis of the lymphoblast morphology, but more modern classification systems focus on the immunophenotypic and molecular genetic/cytogenetic features of the disease for subclassification. In general, lymphoblasts are cells with a high nuclear to cytoplasmic ratio, with round to convoluted nuclei and lightly basophilic, agranular cytoplasm (Fig. 7.1). The morphology

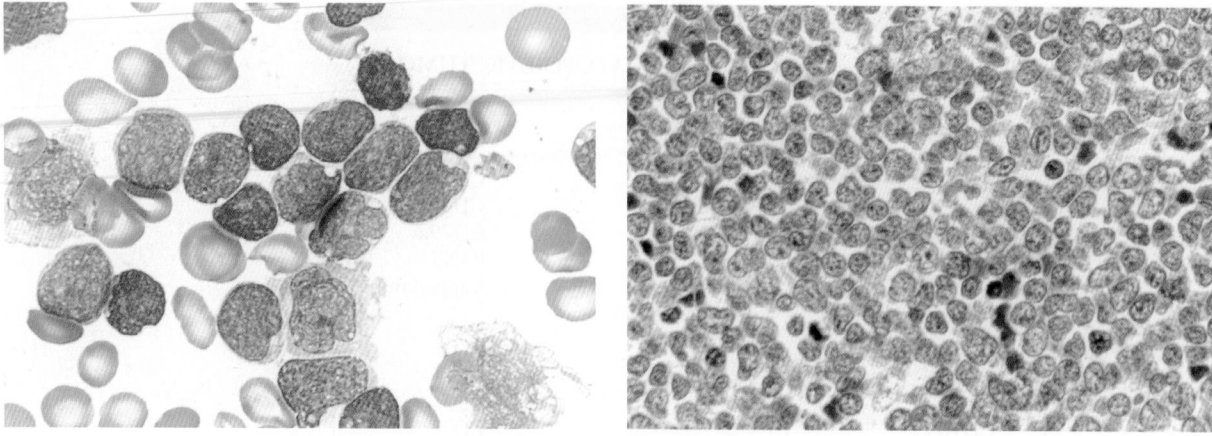

FIGURE 7.1 Acute lymphoblastic leukemia (ALL) and lymphoma. A: ALL shows a monotonous population of bone marrow cells displaying an immature lymphoid appearance with scant cytoplasms, fine nuclear chromatin, and small nucleoli. B: Lymphoblastic lymphoma displays a similar cell composition in tissue sections with monotonous small, irregular cells and a high mitotic rate.

can vary, including the presence of cytoplasmic granules in approximately 5% of cases (Fig. 7.2),[14] and it is not possible to reliably determine lymphoid lineage by morphology or by cytochemistry. For example, some AMLs that are cytochemically negative for myeloperoxidase (MPO) might be misdiagnosed as ALL without additional studies.[15] Therefore, immunophenotypic confirmation of immature lymphoid lineage is necessary for all suspected cases of ALL.

The most clinically and biologically relevant classification schemes for ALL are those that incorporate molecular genetic or cytogenetic features, in conjunction with general immunophenotypic groups.[16–18] The older French-American-British (FAB) classification did not distinguish immunophenotypic disease groups and defined ALL types purely by blast cell morphology with three types, termed *L1, L2,* and *L3* (Fig. 7.3). Lymphoblast morphology is not helpful in subclassifying ALL into clinically important prognostic groups. Burkitt's leukemia/lymphoma, the older FAB L3 type, is classified as a mature B-cell non-Hodgkin lymphoma and should not be termed B-ALL.

The WHO 2008 classification recognizes seven categories of B-ALL with recurrent genetic abnormalities.[1,2] Cases of B-ALL without those genetic aberrancies are classified as B-lymphoblastic leukemia/lymphoma, not otherwise specified (NOS). T-ALL is not further genetically subclassified. Older immunologic classifications of ALL based primarily on the developmental features of normal maturing B and T lymphocytes are not a part of the WHO 2008 classification.[19] Most laboratories no longer perform all of the markers necessary to precisely subdivide these immunophenotypic groups because it is of limited clinical relevance other than to distinguish precursor B versus T lineage. It should be noted that the detection of B-cell or T-cell gene rearrangements is not entirely lineage specific in the precursor lymphoid neoplasms,[20,21] because both types of rearrangements may occur in the same cell type. Thus, gene rearrangement studies are not a reliable means of assigning lineage in ALL. The terminology has changed from the WHO 2001 classification. The terms "precursor B-lymphoblastic leukemia/lymphoblastic lymphoma" and "precursor T-lymphoblastic leukemia/lymphoblastic lymphoma" have been simplified to B-lymphoblastic leukemia/lymphoma and T-lymphoblastic leukemia/lymphoma, respectively.

B-Lymphoblastic Leukemia/Lymphoma

The seven categories of B-ALL with recurrent genetic abnormalities are listed in Table 7.2.[22,23] These tumors characteristically express the B-cell markers CD19 and CD79a, as well as the immature lymphoid marker TdT.[24] Most cases are also CD10 positive, but there is variation in the expression of CD45, CD20, or CD34. Because these are neoplasms of immature B-lineage cells, they do not usually express surface immunoglobulin heavy or light chains; however, the presence of restricted immunoglobulin light or heavy chains in the presence of an otherwise immature cellular immunophenotype (TdT positive) does not preclude a diagnosis of precursor B-cell ALL. The cell lineage (precursor B vs. precursor T) cannot be reliably distinguished by morphologic features alone or distinguished from more immature (minimally differentiated) AMLs. Therefore, immunophenotyping is an essential part of the diagnostic workup. Immunophenotypes show some correlation with genetic disease groups, but they are not reliable predictors of the genetic subclassification.

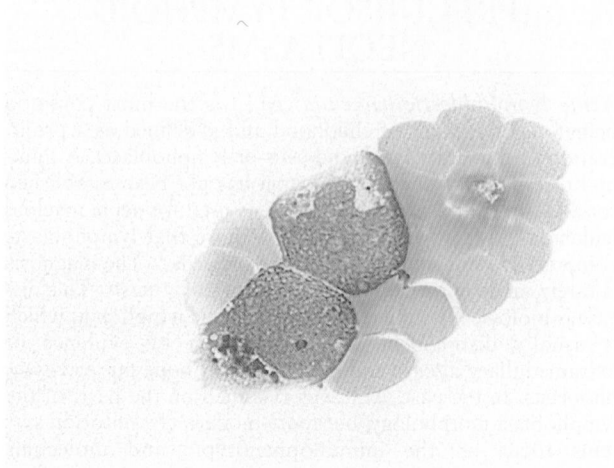

FIGURE 7.2 Acute lymphoblastic leukemia (ALL) with granules. Approximately 5% of pediatric ALLs contain cells with cytoplasmic granules, which may give a false impression of myeloid lineage.

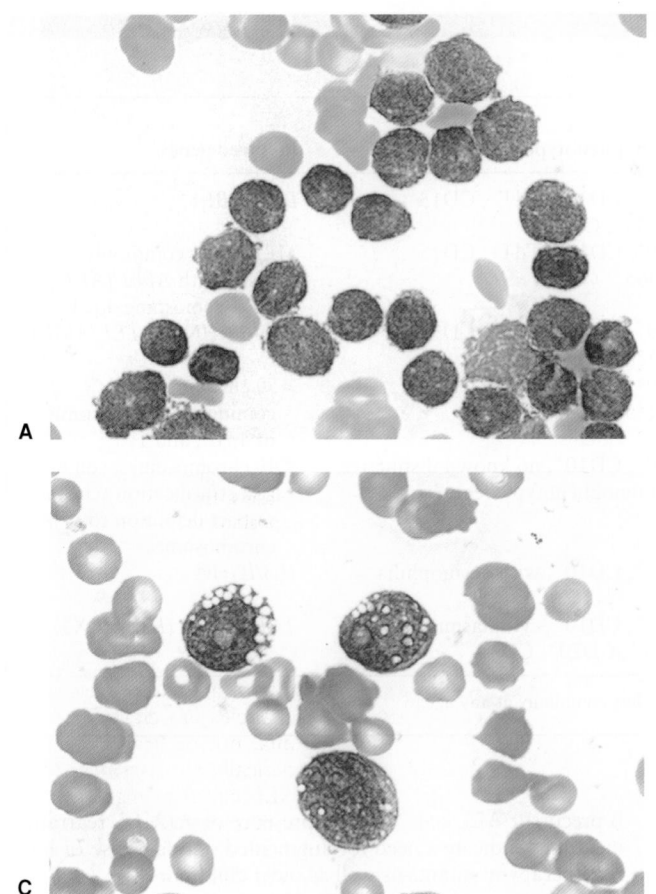

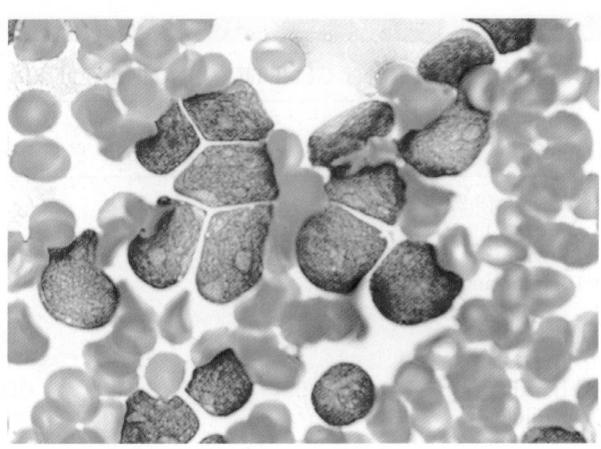

FIGURE 7.3 French-American-British (FAB) Cooperative Group types of acute lymphoblastic leukemia (ALL). **A:** L1 blast cells have fine nuclear chromatin; small, indistinct nucleoli; and generally uniformly sized nuclei with scant cytoplasm. **B:** L2 blasts display more variation in nuclear size, often have more prominent nucleoli and more abundant cytoplasm. **C:** L3 blasts have more mature nuclear chromatin with chromatin clumping, multiple, distinct nucleoli and darkly basophilic and vacuolated cytoplasm. Such cases correlate with Burkitt's lymphoma and are no longer considered as an ALL type.

B-Lymphoblastic Leukemia/Lymphoma With Recurrent Genetic Abnormalities

The frequencies of the seven recurrent genetic aberrations (Table 7.2) vary greatly by age, both compared with adult ALL and among pediatric age groups. These recurrent genetic factors are an important component of risk stratification, together with factors such as patient age, presenting white blood cell (WBC) count, and measures of early treatment response.

B-Lymphoblastic Leukemia/Lymphoma With t(9;22)(q34; q11.2)—BCR/ABL1. The Philadelphia chromosome resulting from the t(9;22)(q34;q11.2) chromosomal translocation is commonly associated with chronic myelogenous leukemia and adult ALL, but it is also a feature of a small proportion (4%) of pediatric B-ALL.[25,26] These children are generally older (>10 years), are African American, and often present with high WBC counts. The Philadelphia chromosome results in a fusion of the *BCR* gene on chromosome 22 and the *ABL1* gene on chromosome 9. At the molecular level, the BCR/ABL1 fusion protein of pediatric ALL (p190) is smaller than the characteristic fusion protein of chronic myelogenous leukemia (p210).[27] Almost 5% to 10% of cases display normal karyotypes with a BCR/ABL1 fusion product detectable by molecular methods. ALLs with t(9;22) are of precursor B-cell lineage (CD10, CD19, and TdT positive) and are often associated with aberrant expression of the myeloid-associated antigens CD13 and CD33, as well as CD38. The dual expression of CD13 and CD33 may cause confusion with acute leukemia of

ambiguous lineage. The 2008 WHO classification proposes strict criteria to distinguish B-ALL with t(9;22) from mixed phenotype acute leukemia (MPAL) with t(9;22), mainly based on evidence of MPO in the blasts of MPAL.[28] Philadelphia chromosome–positive ALL is uniformly considered to have an unfavorable prognosis. Deletions of *IKZF1*, resulting in oncogenic Ikaros isoforms, are common in *BCR-ABL1*–positive B-ALL. They may be important in the development of *BCR-ABL1* ALL and may play a role in resistance to tyrosine kinase inhibitors in these patients.[29–31] Patients with this type of B-ALL may be assigned to "very high-risk" treatment regimens.

B-Lymphoblastic Leukemia/Lymphoma With t(v;11q23)—MLL Rearranged. Precursor B-cell ALL with *MLL* (*HRX/ALL1*) abnormalities, particularly t(4;11)(q21;q23), is the most common ALL type in infants (defined as younger than 1 year) but appears to represent approximately 5% of ALLs in older children or adults (Fig. 7.4).[32–37] It has an unfavorable prognosis and is usually associated with a characteristic pro-B-cell immunophenotype that is CD10 negative with aberrant expression of myeloid-associated antigens CD15 or CD65.[38,39] Other myeloid antigens are not usually expressed (specifically, no more than one marker of monocytic differentiation may be present, such as NSE, CD11c, CD14, CD64, or lysozyme), and the blast cells are routinely MPO negative. These features are necessary to distinguish B-ALL from the diagnosis of MPAL with t(v;11q23)—*MLL* rearranged. Although this ALL phenotype in an infant is characteristic for an underlying *MLL* genetic abnormality, molecular testing is warranted in all infant ALLs

TABLE 7.2

B-ALL WITH RECURRENT GENETIC ABNORMALITIES

Diagnosis	Frequency, %	General age, yr[a]	Immunophenotype	Involved genes
B-ALL with t(9;22) (q34;q11.2)	4	10	CD19+, CD10+, TdT+, CD13+, CD33+, CD38+	*BCR/ABL1*
B-ALL with t(v;11q23), *MLL* rearranged	5	<1	CD19+, CD10−, TdT+, CD15+, CD65+	*MLL*, most commonly fused with *AFF1 (AF4)* on chromosome 4q21
B-ALL with t(12;21) (p13;q22)	25	2–10	CD19+, CD10+, TdT+, CD9−, CD20−, CD13+	*ETV6/RUNX1 (TEL/AML1)*
B-ALL with hyperdiploidy	25	2–10	CD19+, CD10+, TdT+, CD34+, CD45−	>50 chromosomes, commonly with trisomies of 4, 10, and 17
B-ALL with hypodiploidy	1–5	All pediatric	CD19+, CD10+, no known distinctive immunophenotypic features	<46 chromosomes, some risk stratification schema restrict definition to <44 chromosomes
B-ALL with t(5;14) (q31;q32)	<1	All pediatric	CD19+, CD10+, with eosinophilia	*IL3/IGH@*
B-ALL with t(1;19) (q23;p13.3)	5	~5	CD19+, CD10+, cytoplasmic mu+, TdT+, CD20−, CD34−	*TCF3/PBX1 (E2A/PBX1)*

[a]Ages given are for most common age groups, but these disorders may occur less commonly at any age.

to confirm its presence, which is relatively frequent in this age group. The detection of a pro-B immunophenotype with CD15 or CD65 expression and a normal karyotype should prompt additional molecular testing for a potential *MLL* genetic abnormality. High-level expression of the FLT3 receptor tyrosine kinase within the leukemic blasts is a feature of this genetic subtype of ALL. Despite the presence of *FLT3*-activating mutations in only a small subset of cases, small molecule FLT3 inhibitors have been shown to inhibit the growth of the majority of leukemic cell lines and primary leukemic blasts containing *MLL* fusion genes. In cases lacking a *FLT3*-activating mutation, signaling through the receptor appears to be mediated, in part, through the autocrine production of the FLT3 ligand by

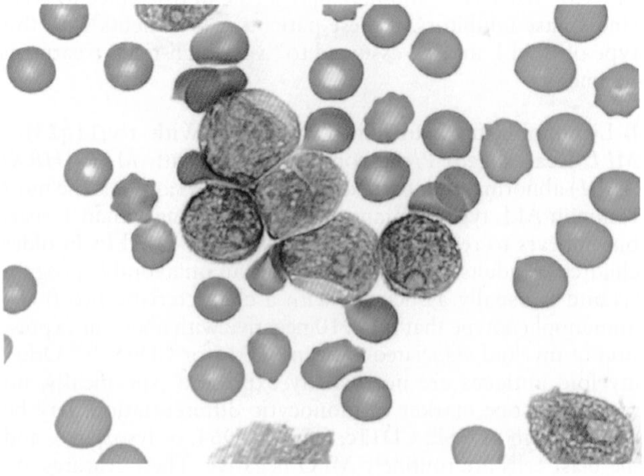

FIGURE 7.4 Infant acute lymphoblastic leukemia with t(4;11). These blasts often have irregular nuclei and nucleoli, which may suggest myeloid lineage. Immunophenotyping is necessary for determination of precursor B-cell lineage.

B-precursor ALL cells.[40,41] The presence of an *MLL* rearrangement may indicate a need for augmented standard-risk or high-risk therapy in infants as well as older children.

B-Lymphoblastic Leukemia/Lymphoma With t(12;21)(p13; q22)—*TEL-AML1 (ETV6-RUNX1)*. B-ALL with t(12;21) (p13;q22) is the most common genetic subtype of ALL in children, particularly in the 2- to 10-year age group, and constitutes at least 20% to 30% of childhood ALL.[42–45] It is extremely uncommon in adult ALL.[46] The disease is associated with relatively low peripheral WBC counts and nonhyperdiploidy. The t(12;21) chromosomal translocation fuses the *ETV6* gene (aka *TEL*) on chromosome 12 with the *RUNX1* (aka *AML1*) gene on chromosome 21.[47] This aberration is not detectable by routine karyotype analysis and requires either RT-PCR or FISH evaluation for detection. The leukemic blasts are of precursor B-cell lineage (CD10, CD19, and TdT positive) and characteristically lack expression of CD9 and CD20, while often showing aberrant expression of the myeloid-associated antigen CD13.[48,49] This genetic subgroup of precursor B-cell leukemia is generally associated with a favorable prognosis, and patients with t(12;21) B-ALL may be eligible for reduced-intensity regimens designed to minimize toxicity while achieving cure.

B-Lymphoblastic Leukemia/Lymphoma With Hyperdiploidy. Blast clones with an abnormal hyperdiploid karyotype of more than 50 chromosomes are seen in 25% of childhood ALL cases. The identification of this subgroup can be made either by routine cytogenetics or by assessing DNA ploidy using flow cytometry. This subgroup has an excellent prognosis attributable to favorable presenting factors such as lower WBC counts and lack of bulky extramedullary disease, as well as a higher sensitivity of the leukemic blasts to methotrexate (MTX) owing to higher intracellular accumulation of MTX-polyglutamates.[50,51] Although hyperdiploid (>50 chromosomes) ALLs have an excellent prognosis, the specific genetic lesions responsible for the aberrant proliferation in these cases remain poorly understood. Interestingly, nearly 100% of hyperdiploid ALLs have trisomy of chromosomes 6, tetrasomy of chromosome 21, and duplication of an X chromosome. Other chromosomes that are frequently trisomic include 4, 10, 14, 17, and 18. Recent studies suggest that an excellent prognosis is best correlated with trisomy of chromosomes 4, 10, and 17.[52] Curiously, studies have revealed a high level of FLT3 expression in hyperdiploid ALLs, similar in level to that seen in ALLs with *MLL* gene rearrangements.[40,41] Moreover, *FLT3*-activating mutations have been identified in 10% to 20% of these cases. As would be expected from these data, hyperdiploid (>50 chromosomes) ALLs show *in vitro* sensitivity to FLT3-specific inhibitors.[53] Whether these agents will yield clinical value remains to be determined.

B-Lymphoblastic Leukemia/Lymphoma With Hypodiploidy. Hypodiploid ALL is defined differently by different authors. The WHO assigns this diagnosis in B-ALL when the chromosome number is less than 46.[22] However, stricter definitions of less than 45 chromosomes or even less than 44 chromosomes may be more clinically significant.[54–56] Leukemias with less than 44 chromosomes are a rare subset comprising less than 1% of B-ALL, with a particularly poor prognosis warranting assignment to very high-risk treatment protocols. Near haploid (23–29 chromosomes) or low hypodiploid B-ALL can be missed by standard karyotyping if the hypodiploid clone has undergone endoreduplication, doubling the number of chromosomes. This discrepancy can be resolved by FISH.

B-Lymphoblastic Leukemia/Lymphoma With t(5;14)(q31; q32)—IL3-IGH@. This very rare subtype of B-ALL occurs both in children and in adults. Too few cases are reported to fully understand any unique prognostic significance. The unusual clinical presentation of reactive eosinophilia in this form of B-ALL warrants its recognition as a diagnostic entity. Patients may present with typical features of ALL or asymptomatic eosinophilia. In the setting of eosinophilia, even small numbers of B lymphoblasts should prompt consideration of this entity and cytogenetic study to confirm the diagnosis. However, the managerial implications of this diagnosis in the setting of less than 20% blasts is unknown.[22] These cases should be distinguished from the rare lymphoblastic leukemias with mutations of *PDGFRA* or *FGFR1* commonly associated with eosinophilia.

Acute Lymphoblastic Leukemia With t(1;19)—E2A/PBX1 (TCF3/PBX1). B-ALL with a balanced or unbalanced t(1;19) (q23;p13.3) chromosomal translocation occurs in approximately 6% of pediatric ALL, with an average age of 5 years, and is more common in cases that express cytoplasmic mu and lack CD34 (often termed *pre-B*).[57–59] This translocation fuses the *TCF3* (aka *E2A*) gene on chromosome 19 to the *PBX1* gene on chromosome 1,[60,61] resulting in the synthesis of a homeobox fusion mRNA that codes for an apparent chimeric transcription factor.[62] A variant chromosomal translocation t(17;19) that fuses the *TCF3* and *HLF* genes may also occur, but it is rare.[63] Up to 25% of cases with underlying *TCF3/PBX1* fusions detected by molecular genetic studies may have normal routine karyotypes. In addition to the presence of cytoplasmic mu and lack of CD34, the blasts are of precursor B-cell lineage (CD10, CD19, and TdT positive), express CD9, and usually lack CD20.[59] This genetic subtype of ALL was originally associated with an unfavorable prognosis; however, treatment with intensive therapeutic approaches has recently yielded excellent long-term results. This genetic subtype is not used to identify high-risk disease in most protocols.[56]

B-Lymphoblastic Leukemia/Lymphoma, Not Otherwise Specified. B-ALL lacking one of the aforementioned recurrent genetic abnormalities is categorized as B-lymphoblastic leukemia/lymphoma, NOS. Additional clinically significant disease subgroups other than those mentioned earlier likely exist and may emerge from future studies. The use of gene expression profiling has confirmed the biologic significance of the ALL subgroups listed previously[64,65] and has identified cases in which the recurring abnormalities mentioned earlier were not detected by other methods. Gene expression profiling studies have identified an additional, novel, subgroup of precursor B-cell ALLs, which represents 4% of pediatric ALLs studied, and further analyses may determine key markers of this new ALL disease subgroup. Somatic missense mutations in the *PTPN11* gene, which encodes a protein tyrosine phosphatase that is frequently altered in juvenile myelomonocytic leukemia (JMML) and acute monoblastic leukemia, were found in a small percentage of children with ALL, characterized by CD10-negative B-lineage immunophenotype.[66] Since these cases have no other recognized genetic aberrations, *PTPN11* mutations might represent a novel primary genetic abnormality. More recently, mutations of *PAX5* and deletions of *IKZF1* have been reported to be common in B-ALL.[29,67] *IKZF1* alterations are associated with a poor prognosis, even when not associated with *BCR-ABL1*, and early studies suggest that these abnormalities are a major prognostic indicator in pediatric B-ALL.

T-Lymphoblastic Leukemia/Lymphoma

T-lymphoblastic tumors constitute approximately 15% of pediatric lymphoblastic leukemia and 85% to 90% of cases that present as lymphoblastic lymphoma.[68] Cases with 25% or more bone marrow involvement are considered to be ALL. Approximately half of T-ALL patients also have a mediastinal mass at the time of presentation, and other organ sites may also be involved. Morphologically, it is not possible to reliably distinguish precursor T-lymphoblasts from precursor B-lymphoblasts, and thus immunophenotyping is required.

T-lymphoblastic neoplasms are TdT positive and usually express CD2, cytoplasmic CD3, CD5, and CD7, although loss of one or more of these T-cell antigens is common.[24] Some cases also express CD1a, CD4, CD8, dual CD4 and CD8, or surface CD3. Surface and/or cytoplasmic CD3 expression is considered the most specific marker for the T lineage. T-lymphoblasts also occasionally express CD79a (a generally specific B-lineage marker) or aberrantly express myeloid antigens such as CD13, CD33, or CD117.[24,69] This aberrant antigen expression is not diagnostic of MPAL (see later).

The 2008 WHO classification does not subclassify T-ALL by recurring cytogenetic abnormalities. A total of 50% to 70% of T-ALL have an abnormal karyotype, most commonly involving the α and δ T-cell receptor loci. Detection of these aberrations at diagnosis may be useful for disease monitoring, but distinct prognostic disease groups defined by recurring cytogenetic abnormalities, as are identified in the precursor B-cell tumors, are not yet part of any major classification scheme for risk group stratification. Improved survival is associated with abnormal karyotype or with t(10;14)(p13;q11).[70] Gene expression profiling studies of T-ALL have identified genetically distinct subgroups that appear to correspond to specific stages of intrathymic maturational arrest but are independent of specific chromosomal translocations.[71] These studies further suggest that expression of *TLX1* (*HOX11*) is associated with a favorable prognosis, whereas expression of *TAL1*, *LYL1* or *TLX3* (*HOX11L2*) is associated with a worse response to therapy. A small subset of T-ALL (5%–6%) contains amplification of the *ABL1* gene on episomal DNA that encodes a *NUP214-ABL1* fusion gene.[72] Recognition of this cryptic rearrangement is important for identifying a T-ALL subgroup that may benefit from imatinib treatment.

ACUTE MYELOID LEUKEMIA

AML is much less common than ALL in childhood. Major changes have occurred in the approach to the classification of AML in recent years.[2,73,74] It is now widely recognized that cytogenetics, and recently gene mutation status, are far more prognostically informative than the older morphologic descriptions of the FAB classification.[15,75–77] The 2008 WHO classification expanded the number of entities with recurrent chromosomal translocations and includes two provisional entities characterized by gene mutations: AML with mutated *NPM1* and AML with mutated *CEBPA*. It retains FAB-like terminology for a morphologic classification of AML, NOS. The diagnosis of AML with multilineage dysplasia has been modified, with specification of a history of prior MDS, MDS-associated cytogenetic abnormalities, or severe multilineage dysplasia. Therapy-related AML (t-AML) remains a category with important biologic and clinical features. Myeloid proliferations of Down syndrome (DS) are now separately classified (Table 7.3).

TABLE 7.3

2008 WORLD HEALTH ORGANIZATION CLASSIFICATION CATEGORIES OF ACUTE MYELOID LEUKEMIA (AML)

AML with recurrent genetic abnormalities
  AML with t(8;21)(q22;q22); (*RUNX1-RUNX1T1*)
  AML with inv(16)(p13.1q22) or t((16;16)(p13.1;q22);
    (*CBFB-MYH11*)
  APL with t(15;17)(q22;q12); (*PML-RARA*)
  AML with t(9;11)(p22;q23); (*MLLT3-MLL*)
  AML with t(6;9)(p23;q34); (*DEK-NUP214*)
  AML with inv(3)(q21q26.2) or t(3;3)(q21;q26.2);
    (*RPN1-EVI1*)
  AML (megakaryoblastic) with t(1;22)(p13;q13);
    (*RBM15-MKL1*)
  Provisional entity: AML with mutated *NPM1*
  Provisional entity: AML with mutated *CEBPA*

AML with myelodysplasia-related changes

Therapy-related myeloid neoplasms

AML, not otherwise specified
  AML with minimal differentiation
  AML without maturation
  AML with maturation
  Acute myelomonocytic leukemia
  Acute monoblastic/monocytic leukemia
  Acute erythroid leukemia
    Pure erythroid leukemia
    Erythroleukemia, erythroid/myeloid
  Acute megakaryoblastic leukemia
  Acute basophilic leukemia
  Acute panmyelosis with myelofibrosis

Myeloid sarcoma

Myeloid proliferations related to Down syndrome
  Transient abnormal myelopoiesis
  AML associated with Down syndrome

APL, acute promyelocytic leukemia.

As in the previous WHO classification, the threshold for AML is 20% (or more) blasts in most AML subtypes, with exception of the two core-binding factor (CBF) AMLs (AML with t(8;21) and AML with inv(16)) and acute promyelocytic leukemia (APL) with t(15;17).

Current models of myeloid leukemogenesis propose two types of requisite genetic events: one to ensure survival and proliferation of the abnormal clone (type I mutations) and another to impair differentiation (type II mutations). Type I mutations are thought to be secondary events, common to many subtypes of AML. They include receptor tyrosine kinase or GTPase alterations such as mutations in *FLT3*, *KIT*, *RAS*, *PTPN11*, and *JAK2*. Type II mutations tend to be more exclusive to one subtype and are thought to be initiating events in myeloid leukemogenesis. Type II mutations include common translocations, such as *PML-RARA*, *RUNX1-RUNX1T1*, *CBFB-MYH11*, *MLL* fusions, and mutations of *CEBPA* and possibly *NPM1*.[78] Many of the type II mutations define categories of AML with recurrent genetic abnormalities in the WHO 2008 classification. The presence of some type I mutations, such as those of *FLT3* and *KIT*, are commonly used to risk stratify patients into those who may or may not benefit from allogeneic stem cell transplantation or to identify patients who may benefit from tyrosine kinase inhibitors.[79–81]

While an initial look at the WHO classification suggests that many leukemia subtypes can be diagnosed only by correlation with cytogenetic results, there are key morphologic and immunophenotypic features in some subtypes of AML that are now well described.[82] Therefore, unlike most subtypes of ALL, many AMLs have morphologic features that are helpful in subclassification. Key features of the more common AML types are summarized in Table 7.4.

Acute Myeloid Leukemia With Recurrent Genetic Abnormalities

Acute Myeloid Leukemia With t(8;21)(q22;q22)—*RUNX1-RUNX1T1*

The t(8;21)(q22;q22) chromosomal translocation is one of the most common recurring cytogenetic abnormalities in AML and is present in 8% to 13% of pediatric AMLs.[83–85] Approximately 10% to 20% of patients may present with extramedullary tumors (myeloid sarcomas), commonly involving the head and neck region in pediatric patients.[86] The t(8;21) results in fusion of the *RUNX1* gene (aka *AML1*) on chromosome 21 with the *RUNX1T1* (aka *ETO*) gene on chromosome 18, and the resulting RUNX1/RUNX1T1 chimeric protein disrupts normal functioning of the CBF transcription factor complex that regulates normal hematopoiesis.[87–89] Despite disruption of CBF by RUNX1/RUNX1T1, this genetic abnormality alone is not sufficient to cause leukemic transformation, underscoring the requirement for additional genetic events consistent with the multistep pathogenesis of acute leukemias.[90]

Blast cells with abundant pink granules and slightly basophilic cytoplasm are characteristic of this disease.[82,91] The blasts usually show perinuclear clearing, or hofs, and a subset have large, irregular pink cytoplasmic granules (Fig. 7.5). Thin Auer rods may also be present. Eosinophils, which are morphologically normal, are often increased in number in the marrow, and maturing granulocytes may show pinker cytoplasm or mild nuclear irregularities than is seen in uninvolved marrows. Despite this granulocytic "dysplasia," there is no evidence of multilineage dysplasia in most cases of AML with t(8;21). The large number of cytoplasmic granules in the neoplastic cells of this leukemia subtype may cause some

TABLE 7.4

COMPARATIVE FEATURES OF COMMON ACUTE MYELOID LEUKEMIA (AML) TYPES WITH RECURRENT GENETIC ABNORMALITIES

Diagnosis	Morphologic features	Immunophenotype	Involved genes
AML with t(8;21)	Perinuclear clearing of blast cytoplasm, large pink granules, dysplastic mature neutrophils	CD13$^+$, CD33$^+$, MPO$^+$, CD34$^+$, CD19$^{+ \text{(weak)}}$	*RUNX1/RUNX1T1*
AML with inv(16)	Eosinophils with large basophilic granules	CD13$^+$, CD33$^+$, CD14$^{+/-}$, CD64$^{+/-}$, CD2$^+$ (subset)	*CBFB/MYH11*
Acute promyelocytic leukemia	Folded blast nuclei, cytoplasmic granules, abundant Auer rods	CD13$^+$, CD33$^+$, MPO^{+++}, CD34$^-$, HLA-DR$^-$, CD2$^+$ (subset)	*PML/RARA*
AML with t(9;11)	Monocytic or myelomonocytic blasts	CD13$^+$, CD33$^+$, MPO$^-$, CD14$^+$, CD64$^+$, CD34$^-$, CD56$^{+/-}$	*MLLT3-MLL*
Acute megakaryoblastic leukemia with t(1;22)	Blasts with cytoplasmic blebs, basophilic cytoplasm, and fine granules	CD13$^+$, CD33$^+$, MPO$^-$, CD41$^+$, CD61$^+$	*RBM15-MKL1*

hesitation in rendering an acute leukemia diagnosis, but the WHO classification considers all cases with this cytogenetic abnormality to represent AML regardless of blast count.

Immunophenotypic studies are often helpful in this specific subtype of AML. The blast cells characteristically express CD13 and CD33, similar to other types of AML, but also usually express CD34 and the B-cell–associated antigen CD19.[92–94] A subset of cases may also express CD56, which is associated with a worse prognosis in some studies.[95] The detection of the distinctive granular blast cell population with perinuclear clearing and large pink cytoplasmic granules in the setting of myeloid antigen expression and CD34 and CD19 expression is highly predictive of the t(8;21),[82] and molecular studies are warranted in this setting if the initial karyotype is normal. AML with t(8;21) and AML with inv(16)/t(16;16) comprise the CBF AMLs and generally have a favorable prognosis in childhood. *FLT3* mutations are uncommon in CBF AML, especially the *FLT3* internal tandem duplication (*FLT3*-ITD) mutations.[96] The presence of a *FLT3*-ITD with a high allelic ratio of abnormal to normal levels of *FLT3* may be used

to assign a patient with CBF leukemia to a high-risk treatment regimen. Mutations in *KIT* are present in 20% to 45% of adult AML with t(8;21) and roughly 20% to 30% of pediatric AML with t(8;21). In adults, exon 8 or 17 mutations are associated with a poor prognosis; in children, the presence of a *KIT* mutation does not seem to significantly affect clinical outcome; however, the number of patients with CBF AML studied is limited.[97]

Acute Myeloid Leukemia With inv(16)(p13.1q22) or t(16;16)(p13.1;q22)—*CBFβ/MYH11*

AML with inv(16)(p13.1q22) or t(16;16)(p13.1;q22) is also a relatively common type of AML (5%–10% of all childhood cases)[83–85] and also tends to occur in children or young adults. Both cytogenetic abnormalities result in a fusion of the *CBFβ* and *MYH11* genes on chromosome 16, which, similar to the t(8;21), disrupts the CBF transcription factor complex.[98]

The bone marrow usually shows a proliferation of myelomonocytic cells with a population of abnormal eosinophils.[99,100] Not all cases, however, will show monocytic differentiation either by morphology or by cytochemistry. The presence of an increase in normal-appearing eosinophils is not sufficient to suggest this diagnosis, as eosinophils may be increased in a variety of AML subtypes. The maturing eosinophils must show abnormal basophilic granules that are large and coarse, which may give the appearance of basophils (Fig. 7.6); however, there are readily identifiable background eosinophilic granules present in the cells as well. Rare cases will have numerous eosinophils and maturing monocytes, making the blast cell count less than 20%. However, the WHO scheme classifies this disease as acute leukemia regardless of the blast cell count. Multilineage dysplasia is usually not present in this AML subtype, but subtle changes have been interpreted as dysplasia in at least one study.[101] The detection of abnormal eosinophils is highly predictive of a chromosome 16 abnormality,[82] which may be subtle on routine karyotype.[102] Therefore, additional studies, such as RT-PCR or FISH should be performed on cases with abnormal eosinophils and an apparently normal karyotype.

AML with inv(16) or t(16;16) shows expression of the expected myeloid antigens (CD13 and CD33), and often monocyte-associated markers, such as CD4, CD14, and CD64. A subset shows aberrant expression of the T-cell–associated marker CD2,[103] but CD2 is not specific for this disease.

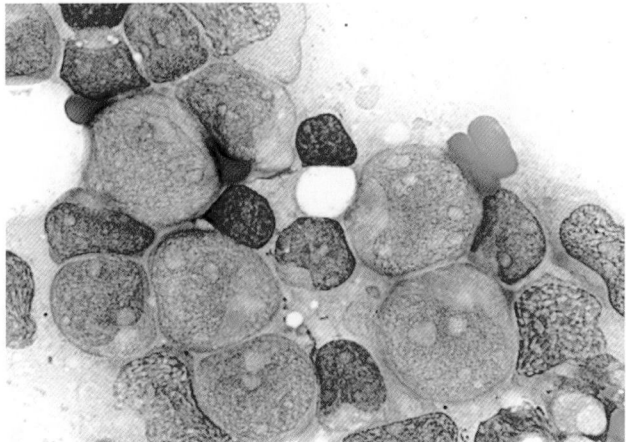

FIGURE 7.5 Acute myeloid leukemia with t(8;21). Large blasts display perinuclear clearing and large pink or salmon-colored cytoplasmic granules.

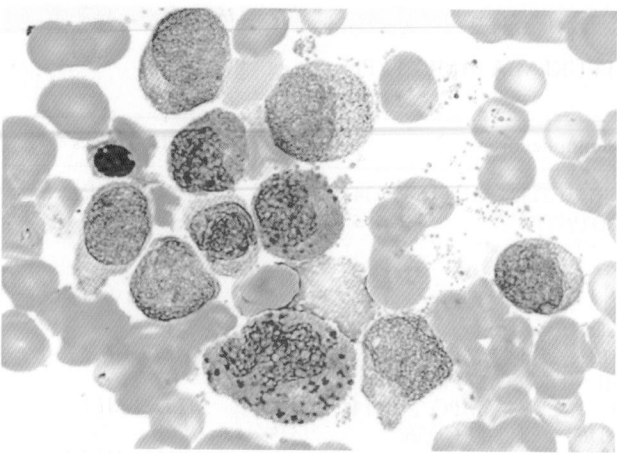

FIGURE 7.6 Acute myeloid leukemia with inv(16). Blast cells contain folded or "monocytoid" nuclear features; abnormal eosinophils contain large, dark-staining granules.

AML with inv(16) or t(16;16) is usually associated with a favorable prognosis with current therapy.[104,105] As in AML with t(8;21), mutations in *KIT* are relatively common but do not have a demonstrated prognostic importance in children. *FLT3-ITD* mutations are uncommon but may adversely affect prognosis and classify the patient as high-risk disease.

Acute Promyelocytic Leukemia/Acute Myeloid Leukemia With t(15;17)(q22;q12)—*PML/RARA*

APL represents 4% to 10% of pediatric AMLs[83,85] and is frequently associated with disseminated intravascular coagulopathy (DIC). These patients are at risk for intracerebral hemorrhage, and recognition of the unique diagnostic features is essential for initiation of rapid therapy. All molecular subtypes contain mutations of the retinoic acid receptor α (*RARA*) gene on chromosome 17.[106] The t(15;17)(q22;q12) is the most common genetic aberration in APL and results in fusion of *RARA* with the *PML* gene on chromosome 15. APL is subdivided into hypergranular and hypogranular (or microgranular) disease (Fig. 7.7). The classic hypergranular APL has "blast" cells that

resemble normal promyelocytes with abundant cytoplasmic granules. In addition, numerous Auer rods are present in individual blasts (so-called faggot cells). In contrast to the blasts of AML with t(8;21) or reactive promyelocyte proliferations, APL cells do not show differing stages of maturation or perinuclear clearing. Hypogranular APL is usually more difficult to recognize[107] and may be mistaken for a myelomonocytic leukemia. The blasts characteristically have folded or bilobed nuclei with very fine to undetectable cytoplasmic granules. Both types of APL show very strong MPO positivity in virtually all blast cells,[82] which is helpful in differentiating hypogranular promyelocytes from myelomonoblasts or monoblasts. *FLT3* mutations are common in APL, present in approximately 40% of patients, with the majority being internal tandem duplication mutations. *FLT3-ITD* in APL is strongly associated with the hypogranular subtype, high WBC counts in peripheral blood, and the bcr-3 breakpoint in *PML*. In one retrospective study, patients with mutant *FLT3* had a higher rate of death during the period of induction chemotherapy but no significant difference in relapse rate or 5-year overall survival.[108]

APL cells express CD33 and CD13, although the latter may be weak and heterogeneous. Unlike most types of AML, APL blasts are typically negative for, or only partially express, HLA-DR. Other AML types, however, may show loss of HLA-DR,[109] thus this immunophenotypic feature alone is nonspecific. A subset of cases, usually of the hypogranular type, aberrantly express CD2,[110,111] which is reportedly associated with a poorer prognosis.[112]

Although *PML/RARA* is the most common fusion gene in APL, chromosomal translocations of *RARA* on chromosome 17 may occur with other genes such as *ZBTB16* (*PLZF*) at 11q23, *NUMA* at 11q13, *NPM1* at 5q35, and *STAT5B* at 17q11.[106] Cases that lack *RARA* translocations or harbor *RARA* translocations involving *ZBTB16* or *STAT5B*, may not respond to all-*trans*-retinoic acid and thus require a different therapeutic approach. With current therapy, APL is considered to have a favorable prognosis.

Acute Myeloid Leukemia With t(9;11)(p22;q23)—*MLLT3-MLL*

The 2008 WHO classification limits the prior category of AML with 11q23 (*MLL*) cytogenetic abnormalities specifically to the t(9;11)(p22;q23) as the only specific subtype of

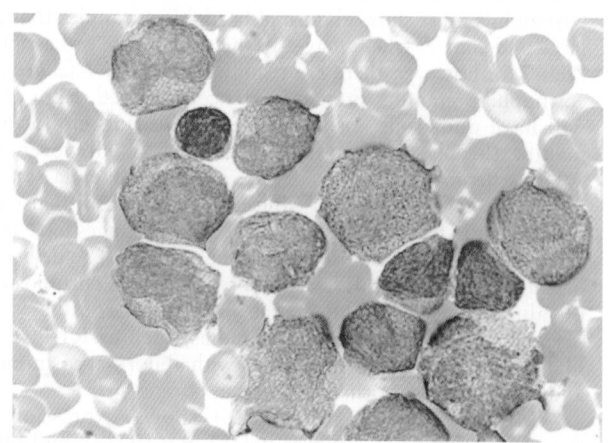

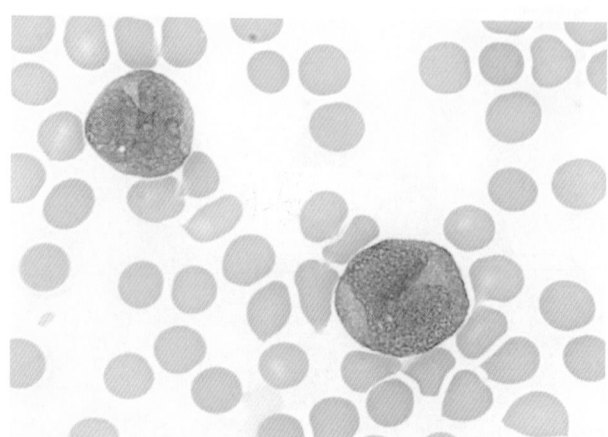

FIGURE 7.7 Acute promyelocytic leukemia. **A:** The hypergranular type shows abundant cytoplasmic granules as well as blasts with numerous Auer rods. **B:** The hypogranular variant shows blasts with basophilic, agranular cytoplasms and characteristic folded nuclei.

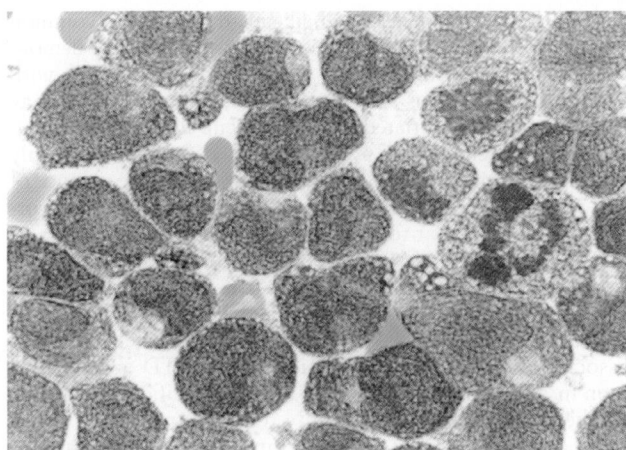

FIGURE 7.8 Acute myeloid leukemia with t(9;11). The blasts are large with folded, monocytoid nuclei, basophilic cytoplasms, and cytoplasmic vacuoles. These features, however, are not specific for the presence of an *MLL* abnormality.

AML with recurrent genetic abnormalities.[113] *MLL* rearrangements are common in pediatric AML, especially in infants, comprising 9% to 22% of pediatric AML cases overall.[83,85] AML with t(9;11) comprises 7% of pediatric AML.[114] Extramedullary disease of the gingiva and skin is described, as well as presentation with DIC. The blasts typically display round to folded, monocytoid nuclei with usually abundant, slightly basophilic, and vacuolated cytoplasm (Fig. 7.8). Promonocytes are frequently present, with more mature-shaped nuclei but retaining immature nuclear chromatin. Occasionally they may lack differentiation or rarely demonstrate megakaryocytic differentiation. Cases morphologically comprising mostly monoblasts and promonocytes are typically MPO negative by cytochemistry. AML with t(9;11) *MLLT3-MLL* most commonly expresses CD33, CD4, CD65, and HLA-DR, with minimal to no CD13, CD14, and CD34 expression, typical of AML with monocytic differentiation. The described morphologic and immunophenotypic features are not specific for this molecular subtype of AML, requiring correlation with cytogenetics or FISH for diagnosis.

While AML with t(9;11)(p22;q23) *MLLT3-MLL* is a consistent clinicopathologic entity with a generally intermediate prognosis, other leukemias with *MLL* rearrangements appear heterogeneous, with more than 80 different translocation partners described. AML with balanced rearrangements of 11q23 other than t(9;11)(p22;q23) are diagnosed as AML, NOS, with the rearrangement stated in the diagnosis line, with exception of those occurring after cytotoxic therapy (which would be considered as t-AML) or the t(11;16)(q23;p13.3) and t(2;11)(p21;q23), which are MDS-associated genetic abnormalities and would be considered AML with myelodysplasia-related changes (AML-MRC). In addition to t(9;11)(p22;q23) *MLL-MLLT3*, the most common *MLL* translocations in AML include t(10;11)(p12;q23) *MLL-MLLT10 (AF10)*, t(11;19)(q23;p13.1) *MLL-ELL*, t(6;11)(q27;q23) *MLL-MLLT4 (AF6)*, and t(11;19)(q23;p13.3) *MLL-MLLT1 (ENL)*. Of these, only the t(11;19)(q23;p13.1) *MLL-ELL* has not been associated with ALL in addition to AML.[115,116] Partial tandem duplication mutations of *MLL* also occur in AML and are more common in patients with normal karyotypes or trisomy of chromosome 11.[117,118] In general, the presence of *MLL* translocations or partial tandem duplications indicates an unfavorable prognosis, but the t(9;11) in childhood AML confers a better prognosis in some

studies.[119] Gene mutations in *KIT* or *FLT3*-ITD are very uncommon in AML with 11q23 translocations. Approximately 20% of AML with t(9;11) will have activating loop domain point mutations in *FLT3*, but these are of uncertain prognostic significance.[96]

Acute Myeloid Leukemia With t(6;9)(p23;q34)—*DEK-NUP214*

AML with t(6;9) is a rare subtype of AML comprising approximately 1% of cases in both children and adults. The blasts of t(6;9) AML may show occasional Auer rods and may exhibit monocytic features. Dyspoiesis of all three lineages may be evident on the peripheral smear and bone marrow aspirate. Basophilia (>2% marrow or blood basophils) is present in roughly half of reported cases, and many cases show an erythroid hyperplasia. By flow cytometry, blasts typically express CD45, CD13, CD33, HLA-DR, and intracytoplasmic MPO, with variable expression of CD34, CD15, CD11c, and TdT. *FLT3*-ITD mutations are common in this type of AML, with a reported frequency of 70%. While the majority of patients with t(6;9) AML may achieve complete remission, survival rates are very poor. Patients may benefit from allogeneic stem cell transplantation. The presence of less than 20% blasts in a patient with the t(6;9)(p23;q34) is not considered diagnostic of AML, and patients should be followed very closely for progression.[120–122]

Acute Myeloid Leukemia With inv(3)(q21q26.2) or t(3;3)(q21;q26.2)—*RPN-EVI1*

AML with inv(3)(q21q26.2) or t(3;3)(q21;q26.2) *RPN1-EVI1* occurs primarily in adults, but rare cases are reported in children in association with monosomy 7.[123] Dysplastic changes of all three lineages are common in the peripheral blood and bone marrow. The bone marrow blasts may show multiple morphologies, including meeting criteria for megakaryoblastic leukemia. MPO activity is often low. Megakaryocytes may be normal or increased in number, frequently with small unilobated and bilobated forms or other dysplastic features. The core biopsy may show decreased cellularity and, occasionally, fibrosis. Blasts may express CD34, CD13, CD33, and HLA-DR, with aberrant CD7 expression reported in some cases. Cases with megakaryocytic differentiation may express CD41 and CD61. Rearrangements of 3q26 lead to abnormal expression of EVI1 (ectopic virus integration-1). Cytogenetics may fail to identify cryptic rearrangements of 3q26 detectable by FISH.[124] Secondary karyotypic abnormalities are present in the majority of cases, including the poor prognosis, MDS-associated abnormalities of −7 and −5q, and complex aberrant karyotypes. *FLT3*-ITD mutations are found in a small subset of patients (13%). Adults with AML with inv(3) or t(3;3) typically have short survival, but too few pediatric cases are reported to know the prognostic significance in children. Patients with inv(3) or t(3;3) may present with less than 20% blasts and should be closely monitored for the development of AML (>20% blasts).

Acute Myeloid (Megakaryoblastic) Leukemia With t(1;22)(p13;q13)—*RBM15-MKL1*

AML with t(1;22) is a disease of infants, with the majority of cases diagnosed in the first 6 months of life.[125–128] Infants typically present with hepatosplenomegaly, and often with extramedullary disease mimicking a solid tumor. Some patients present with bone pain, lytic lesions, and bilaterally symmetric periostitis.[129] The diagnosis can be very difficult, especially in cases without circulating blasts or marrow involvement. The megakaryoblasts show typical morphologies on blood smears and aspirates with a small amount of blue cytoplasm showing

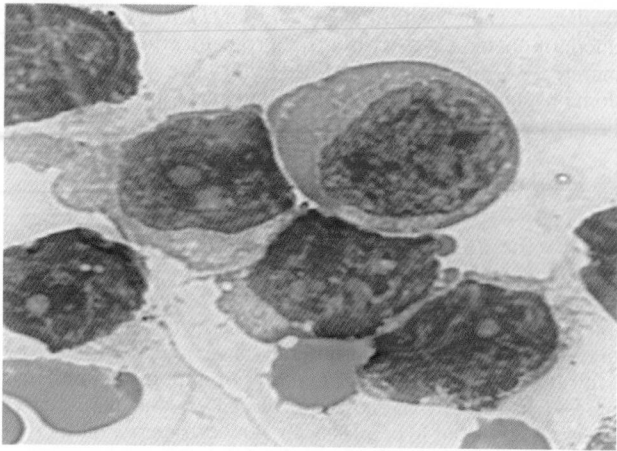

FIGURE 7.9 Infant acute megakaryoblastic leukemia with t(1;22). The blasts have basophilic, finely granular cytoplasms with a suggestion of cytoplasmic blebbing, similar to mature megakaryocytes. These features are not specific for t(1;22), and a diagnosis of acute megakaryoblastic leukemia requires immunophenotypic or electron microscopic confirmation of megakaryocyte lineage.

budding or blebbing (Fig. 7.9). Micromegakaryocytes may be seen in the marrow, but dyserythropoiesis and dysmyelopoiesis are not common. Megakaryoblasts may clump on core biopsies, mimicking metastatic small round blue cell tumor. The marrow may be difficult to aspirate as fibrosis is common. Submission of a core biopsy for flow cytometry and cytogenetics may be necessary. Blasts are commonly CD45 and CD34 negative, and the myeloid antigens CD13 and CD33 are inconsistently expressed. Expression of one or more megakaryocyte antigens (CD41, CD61, Factor VIIIRA, LAT) confirms the blast lineage. Additional chromosomal abnormalities are common in children older than 6 months. Molecular studies or FISH analyses for the translocation are not commonly available for this rare subtype. In patients with less than 20% blasts in the marrow or blood, careful clinical examination for evidence of extramedullary disease is warranted, as the presence of myeloid sarcoma would be diagnostic of AML.

Acute Myeloid Leukemia With Gene Mutations

Two provisional entities in the 2008 WHO classification recognize AML subtypes that typically have a normal karyotype and a favorable prognosis. AML with *NPM1* mutations and AML with *CEBPA* mutations appear to define consistent entities. Unlike mutations in *FLT3* or *KIT*, these mutations are not common to the other subtypes of AML listed earlier. The presence of *FLT3* mutations, particularly internal tandem duplications (*FLT3-ITD*), abrogates the favorable effect of *NPM1* and probably *CEBPA* mutations and must be correlated in the diagnosis.

NPM1 encodes a molecular chaperone for shuttling proteins from the nucleus to the cytoplasm, typically located in the nucleolus.[130] Mutations in exon 12 create a nuclear export motif, resulting in dislocation of the protein to the cytoplasm. The mutation may be detected by PCR or by immunohistochemistry demonstrating abnormal localization of *NPM1* to the cytoplasm. Pediatric AML with *NPM1* mutations comprises

approximately 8% of cases and, like in adults, is most common in cases with a normal karyotype. In adults, cases may demonstrate monocytic morphology and immunophenotype with expression of antigens such as CD4, CD14, or CD64 or may appear as undifferentiated blasts with cup-like nuclear inclusions often lacking CD34 or HLA-DR expression. Roughly 50% of cases may have *FLT3-ITD* mutations. In the absence of *FLT3-ITD*, AML with mutated *NPM1* appears to have a favorable prognosis similar to that of CBF leukemias.[131]

Pediatric AML with mutated *CEBPA* is associated with a normal karyotype in more than 80% of cases and is not associated with CBF mutations or the unfavorable monosomies of chromosome 5 or 7. Unlike the relatively common association with *NPM1* mutations, *FLT3*-ITD is less common in AML with mutated *CEBPA*. No specific morphology has been described in children. N-terminal truncating mutations and basic region leucine zipper (bZip) region mutations are most common and inhibit the normal function of *CEBPA* in promoting myeloblast differentiation. The most common second mutation in cases with one *CEBPA* mutation is a second *CEBPA* mutation. Like *NPM1* mutations, the detection of *CEBPA* mutations in the absence of *FLT3-ITD*, or risk factors such as prior cytotoxic therapy, identifies a subset of AML with a favorable prognosis from a group that would otherwise be classified as having an intermediate risk.[132]

Acute Myeloid Leukemia With Myelodysplasia-Related Changes

AML with multilineage dysplasia (the 2001 WHO category) is traditionally considered rare in pediatric patients. The 2008 WHO classification expands this category with the new name of AML-MRC (see criteria in Table 7.5). The new definition of AML-MRC with cytogenetic abnormalities will encompass more pediatric cases than those recognized by morphologic dysplasia alone in the prior classification. The unbalanced cytogenetic abnormalities of AML-MRC include the subset of pediatric AML with the worst prognosis, that is, monosomy 7 and monosomy 5. Together with the deletions such as in 9q and 11q, an additional 5% to 10% of AML will now be diagnosed as AML-MRC (myelodysplasia-associated cytogenetic abnormality). Cases with complex karyotypes (≥3 unrelated abnormalities, excluding those of AML with recurrent genetic abnormalities mentioned earlier) are also incorporated into this diagnosis, comprising an additional approximately 6% of pediatric AML. The balanced translocations of this category are uncommon in pediatrics. The t(3;5)(q25;q34) tends to occur in young adult men and was found in 5 of 478 pediatric cases, mostly in boys with a median age of 4½ years.[133] The t(3;21)(q26;q22), common to t-AML, was reported in only one patient from the same series. In adults, AML-MRC has a poor prognosis. It is unclear if pediatric AML-MRC, other than the known poor risk −7/7q−, −5/5q− disease types, will have a similar course. Some authors suggest that children with AML arising from MDS and low blast counts (20%–29%) may have more slowly progressive disease, lacking the clinical features of AML and warranting further study for optimal therapy.[134]

Therapy-Related Myeloid Neoplasms

The 2008 WHO classification groups MDS, AML, and myeloproliferative/myelodysplastic overlap syndromes after prior cytotoxic chemotherapy or radiation therapy into one

TABLE 7.5

DIAGNOSIS OF AML WITH MYELODYSPLASIA-RELATED CHANGES

Criteria:
1. ≥20% blood or bone marrow blasts.
2. At least one of the following: history of MDS, MDS-related cytogenetic abnormality, multilineage dysplasia
3. No history of prior cytotoxic therapy for an unrelated disease.
4. No recurrent genetic abnormality as described in AML with recurrent genetic abnormalities

Multilineage dysplasia: Dyplasia present in at least 50% of the components of two bone marrow cell lines.
Dysgranulopoiesis: Hypogranular neutrophils, hyposegmented nuclei (pseudo–Pelger-Huet anomaly)
Dyserythropoiesis: Megaloblastosis, nuclear irregularity, multinucleation, karyorrhexis, ringed sideroblasts, PAS-positive cytoplasmic vacuoles
Dysmegakaryopoiesis: Micromegakaryocytes, hypolobated normally sized forms, multinucleated forms with separated nuclei

MDS-associated cytogenetic abnormalities:
Complex karyotype: (≥3 unrelated abnormalities, none of which are recognized in the AML with recurrent genetic abnormalities subgroup)
Unbalanced abnormalities: −7/del(7q), −5/del(5q), i(17q)/t(17p), −13/del(13q), del(11q), del(12p)/t(12p), del (9q), idic(X)(q13)
Balanced abnormalities:
t(11;16)(q23;p13.3)
t(3;21)(q26.2;q22.1)
t(1;3)(p36.3;q21.1)
t(2;11)(p21;q23)
t(5;12)(q33;p12)
t(5;7)(q33;q11.2)
t(5;17)(q33;p13)
t(5;10)(q33;q21)
t(3;5)(q25;q34)

AML, acute myeloid leukemia; PAS, periodic acid-Schiff; MDS, myelodysplastic syndrome.

biologic category. Alkylating agents and topoisomerase II inhibitors are most commonly implicated in t-AML. Therapy-related disease secondary to alkylating agents tends to occur 5 to 7 years after therapy, with a MDS preceding AML, and is associated with a poor prognosis and MDS-related cytogenetics. In contrast, t-AML after topoisomerase II inhibitors (epipodophyllotoxins, anthracyclines, and mitoxantrone) is associated with a shorter latency of 2 to 3 years, acute onset without prior t-MDS, *MLL* rearrangements, and rearrangements similar to *de novo* AML (e.g., *RUNX1-RUNX1T1*, *CBFB/MYH11*, *PML/RARA*). The prognosis of therapy-related myeloid neoplasms is very poor in general, with overall survival reported at less than 10% for adults. Survival for t-AML in children appears slightly better, though still poor at 24% at 5 years.[135] Median survival is particularly poor for patients with −5 or −7 karyotypes regardless of the blast percentage. Treatment is limited by toxicities of prior treatment as well as drug resistance mechanisms in the neoplastic cells. Some data suggest that secondary APL with t(15;17) and t-AML with inv(16) may have a prognosis more similar to *de novo* AML.[136]

Acute Myeloid Leukemia, Not Otherwise Specified

Cases without the recurrent genetic abnormalities mentioned earlier that do not meet criteria for AML-MRC, lack a history of prior cytotoxic therapy, and do not occur in the setting of DS are classified as AML, NOS and may be subclassified in a manner similar to the older FAB classification. It is not clear whether the subcategories of AML, NOS have prognostic significance. Most of the older literature contained cases with genetic abnormalities now recognized to be of more impor-

tance than the morphology. Minimally differentiated AML has immature blast cells with scant and agranular cytoplasm, which may be mistaken morphologically for lymphoblasts (Fig. 7.10). This disease most commonly occurs in children younger than 3 years.[137] The lack of both MPO (or Sudan black B) and nonspecific esterase in blast cells makes it virtually impossible to reliably distinguish this type of AML from ALL; therefore, all cases of acute leukemia with this cytochemical profile should be immunophenotyped. Interestingly,

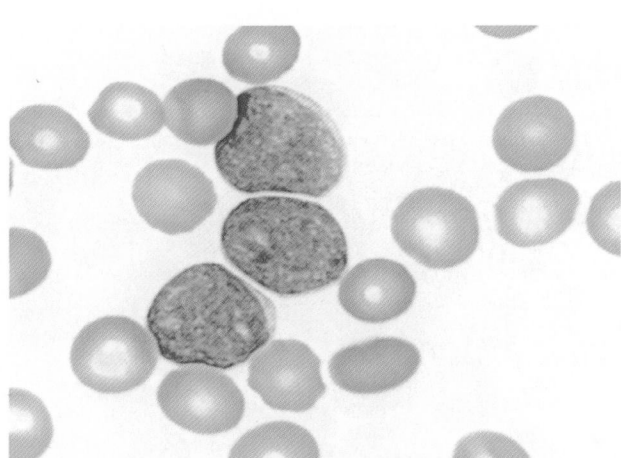

FIGURE 7.10 Acute myeloid leukemia, NOS (minimally differentiated). The blasts have scant, agranular cytoplasms and can be easily mistaken for lymphoblasts. Immunophenotyping studies are required to make this diagnosis.

a subset of minimally differentiated AMLs have point mutations in the *RUNX1* gene that lead either to the production of truncated proteins or to the generation of RUNX1 proteins that lack the ability to bind DNA, CBFB, or both.[138,139] Minimally differentiated AML expresses myeloid-associated antigens, such as CD13 and CD33, similar to other AML types, and approximately half of cases are MPO positive by immunophenotypic methods.[10,137] While older studies cite a worse prognosis for this subtype, many of those cases would now be classified specifically as AML-MRC on the basis of myelodysplasia-associated cytogenetic abnormalities.[140]

Acute monoblastic or monocytic leukemias are also usually MPO negative by cytochemistry but show more than 80% of blast cells positive for nonspecific esterase cytochemistry. Blasts can range from immature cells with round nuclei and abundant slightly basophilic cytoplasm to cells with folded nuclei with immature chromatin and cytoplasmic vacuoles (Fig. 7.11). They express myeloid-associated antigens, such as CD13 and CD33, and usually express monocyte-associated antigens, such as CD14, CD64, and CD4. This category will include cases with 11q23 translocations other than t(9;11). The diagnostic line should list the specific 11q23 translocation in addition to the AML, NOS diagnosis.

Acute erythroid leukemia is relatively uncommon in children compared with adults but warrants mention due to its differing diagnostic criteria when compared with other AML types. In the WHO classification, there are two types of acute erythroid leukemia. One is similar to FAB M6 AML and requires that 50% or more of bone marrow cells are erythroid precursors at any stage of maturation. In addition, 20% or more of the nonerythroid cells must be myeloblasts for this diagnosis. This contrasts with most other AML types, in which the blast cell criterion (20% or more) is applied as a percentage of total cells rather than nonerythroid cells. The second subtype in the WHO system corresponds to what is often called "pure erythroid leukemia." For this diagnosis, more than 80% of marrow cells must be immature erythroid cells. They are usually large with clumped nuclear chromatin, agranular basophilic cytoplasm, and periodic acid-Schiff (PAS)–positive cytoplasmic vacuoles. Cases with similar features but 20% or more total blasts are more appropriately diagnosed as AML-MRC in the presence of sufficient multilineage dysplasia or myelodysplasia-associated cytogenetic abnormalities.[74,141,142]

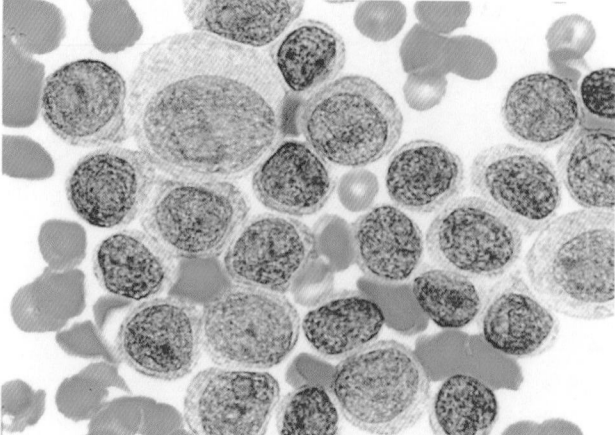

FIGURE 7.11 Acute myeloid leukemia, NOS (monoblastic). The blasts display round uniform nuclei with abundant, vacuolated cytoplasms. Positive nonspecific esterase staining in virtually every blast cell confirmed the diagnosis. The blasts were negative for myeloperoxidase.

Most cases of childhood acute megakaryoblastic leukemia (AMkL) will be recognized as AMkL with t(1;22) or AML-related to DS. Other AMkLs appear to represent a more heterogeneous group that may be similar to the adult disease and characterized by a generally poor prognosis.[143]

Myeloid Sarcoma

Myeloid sarcoma, also known as *extramedullary myeloid tumor* or *granulocytic sarcoma*, is a myeloblast proliferation that occurs outside the bone marrow. It occurs in approximately 10% of pediatric AML, and its presence is generally considered diagnostic of AML, regardless of the marrow blast count. Of note, some presentations in the newborn may warrant a more conservative approach with observation. Myeloid sarcoma occurs in approximately 25% of pediatric AML with t(8;21), particularly head and neck localizations.[86] AML with 11q23 translocations often has myeloid sarcoma in the skin. AMkL with t(1;22) may have bone lesions, in addition to liver and spleen involvement. Congenital leukemia may manifest as skin lesions in the newborn. Some subtypes, in particular, those with t(8;16)(p11;q13) *MYST3/CREBBP*, may demonstrate spontaneous remission.[144,145] In contrast, cases of congenital leukemia with 11q23 translocations tend to have a more consistently aggressive clinical course. Interestingly, both genetic abnormalities are also associated with aggressive AML in adults, commonly t-AML, and appear to share a similar genetic signature.[146]

The diagnosis of myeloid sarcoma can be challenging in the absence of suspicion for hematologic malignancy. Myeloid sarcoma may be confused with other small round blue cell tumors of childhood. The absence of CD45 and the blast marker CD34 on many cases can make recognition of their hematopoietic origin difficult. Myeloid sarcoma is easily confused morphologically with malignant lymphomas, particularly large cell, lymphoblastic, or Burkitt's lymphoma, although they are immunophenotypically distinct from lymphomas by their expression of myeloid or monocytic markers and their lack of expression of specific B- or T-lineage markers.[147] Morphologic clues to the myeloid lineage of the proliferation include a high mitotic rate, large nuclei without the chromatin clearing of large cell lymphomas, and, in a subset of cases, the presence of admixed eosinophilic myelocytes. Despite these morphologic features, immunophenotypic studies are necessary to confirm the diagnosis, and repeat biopsy with flow cytometry may be necessary. Cytogenetic analysis is necessary for optimal classification and risk stratification. Repeat biopsy of the lesion for cytogenetics may be warranted when the blood or bone marrow lacks significant involvement.

MYELOID PROLIFERATIONS RELATED TO DOWN SYNDROME

The presence of an additional chromosome 21 in patients with DS appears to cause hematopoietic instability. *In vitro* studies of trisomy 21 fetal liver hematopoietic stem cells show enhanced proliferation and survival.[148,149] Patients with DS have a 10- to 20-fold increased risk of developing acute leukemia. In the first 4 years of life, DS patients are at risk for developing AML, specifically AMkL. While they remain at risk for acute leukemia throughout their lives, the ratio of AML to ALL becomes similar to that of the general pediatric population after the age of 5 years. While the true incidence is unknown, at least 10% of infants with DS will manifest a transient myeloproliferative disorder often indistinguishable from

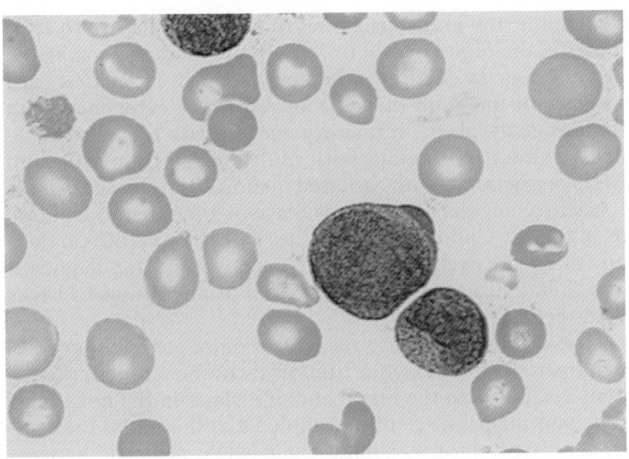

FIGURE 7.12 Transient abnormal myelopoiesis of Down syndrome. The blasts have features similar to acute megakaryoblastic leukemia, and it is not possible to predict the transient nature of this process by morphology.

TABLE 7.6

ASSIGNMENT OF LINEAGE IN MIXED PHENOTYPE ACUTE LEUKEMIA

Lineage	Criteria
Myeloid lineage	• Myeloperoxidase (by flow cytometry, immunohistochemistry or cytochemistry) or • Monocytic differentiation (express at least two of the following: CD11c, CD14, CD64, lysozyme, or NSE)
T lymphoblastic	• Cytoplasmic CD3 by flow cytometry or • Surface CD3 (rare)
B lymphoblastic	• Strong CD19 and strong expression of at least one of the following: CD79a, cytoplasmic CD22, or CD10 or • Weak CD19 and strong expression of at least two of the following: CD79a, cytoplasmic CD22, CD10

AML or MDS, termed *transient abnormal myelopoiesis* (TAM) in the 2008 WHO classification.[150–153] These infants have a marked leukocytosis with numerous peripheral blood and bone marrow blast cells containing basophilic cytoplasm with granules and blebbing suggestive of megakaryoblasts (Fig. 7.12). Some patients will also show peripheral blood basophilia and erythroid dysplasia. The blasts are negative for MPO and express myeloid- and megakaryocyte-associated antigens. TAM may show karyotypic abnormalities in addition to +21, but they do not have the t(1;22) of infant AMkL, and they differ from true AMkL by clinical resolution in 1 to 3 months. Therefore, caution should be taken in diagnosing a proliferation of this type as acute leukemia in a neonate with DS. While TAM may be spontaneously remitting, it is not without risk to the infant, as some cases are complicated by critical illness due to hyperviscosity and organ dysfunction, occasionally with fibrosis of the liver and pancreas. TAM is molecularly characterized by acquired mutations of the *GATA1* gene *in utero*, and some cases have activating mutations in *JAK3*. Almost 10% to 20% of patients with TAM will subsequently develop AML. A gene array study identified three transcriptional differences between the two entities.[154] *CDKN2C* and *PRAME* transcripts were increased in AMkL, whereas expression of the *MYCN* gene was increased in TAM. Confirmation of these transcriptional differences may provide useful molecular markers that distinguish these related but prognostically distinctive diseases. AML associated with DS typically appears in the first 3 years of life, often with a prolonged preleukemic phase resembling MDS with increased blasts. Most cases of DS AML in children younger than 4 years are AMkL. In children younger than 4 years, the prognosis appears good despite the presence of additional karyotypic abnormalities, some of which are myelodysplasia associated.[155]

ACUTE LEUKEMIAS OF AMBIGUOUS LINEAGE

Rare acute leukemias express both myeloid- and lymphoid-associated antigens to a degree that no single lineage can be assigned.[28] Cases that do not express lineage-specific markers are termed *undifferentiated acute leukemia*. Specifically, they lack cytoplasmic CD3 for T lineage, MPO, markers of monocytic, erythroid, megakaryocytic, or blastic plasmacytoid dendritic cell (BPDC) differentiation, and specific markers of B lineage such as cytoplasmic CD22, cytoplasmic CD79a, or strong expression of CD19. Ambiguous lineage may be assigned because one blast population expresses markers definitive for more than one lineage (biphenotypic acute leukemia) or there are two distinct blast populations present: one myeloid and one lymphoid (bilineal acute leukemia). The term MPAL encompasses both types. The 2008 WHO classification clarified criteria for a diagnosis of MPAL, and identified two molecular subtypes: MPAL with t(9;22)(q34;q11.2) *BCR-ABL1* and MPAL with t(v;11q23); *MLL* rearranged. Cases without these cytogenetic abnormalities are described as MPAL, B/myeloid, NOS and MPAL, T/myeloid, NOS, and the very rare category of MPAL, NOS-rare types. The criteria for lineage assignment in the classification of MPAL are detailed in Table 7.6.

BLASTIC PLASMACYTOID DENDRITIC CELL TUMOR

BPDC tumor is a revised entity in the 2008 WHO classification that rarely presents in childhood.[156] Most neoplasms previously called *blastic NK-cell lymphoma* or *CD56⁺ hematodermic neoplasm* are now classified as BPDC tumor. The proliferations typically present in the skin and subsequently rapidly disseminate to the bone marrow. The neoplastic cells of BPDC tumor resemble blasts with immature-appearing chromatin and minimal cytoplasm. Nucleoli can be prominent, and some cases may exhibit cytoplasmic "tail" extensions. Cytoplasmic granules are typically absent. The infiltrates efface normal tissue architecture in the bone marrow or skin. Typically, BPDCs coexpress CD4, CD56, and CD123. Involvement of the skin by AML with monocytic differentiation must be excluded as these antigens are commonly expressed in AML with monocytic or myelomonocytic morphologies. BPDC tumor is MPO and esterase (α-naphthyl butyrate esterase or naphthyl ASD acetate) negative by cytochemistry. BPDCs lack conventional myeloid antigens such as CD13, CD33, CD11b, or MPO, although rare cases are reported to express weak CD33. They lack T-cell markers CD3 and CD5, although some cases may express CD2 or CD7. B-cell markers CD19 and CD20 are not expressed. Some cases may show weak TdT, and exclusion of T- or B-lymphoblastic lineage by other markers is imperative. Cytogenetic studies may show complex karyotypes, with abnormalities of 5q, 12p, 13q, 6q, 15q, and loss of chromosome 9 most frequently observed.[157,158]

MYELODYSPLASTIC SYNDROMES AND MYELOPROLIFERATIVE NEOPLASMS OF CHILDHOOD

Chronic myeloproliferative neoplasms (MPNs) and MDSs in children are uncommon and their classification and nomenclature has often been confusing and inconsistent.[159,160] Clear differences between childhood and adult MDSs are evident, and the myeloproliferative/myelodysplastic condition of chronic myelomonocytic leukemia in adults is not the same as the chronic (juvenile) myelomonocytic leukemia of young children. The 2008 WHO classification of hematopoietic tumors addresses some of these differences by including the uniquely pediatric categories of refractory cytopenia of childhood (RCC) and JMML.[161] Other MPNs such as chronic myelogenous leukemia, polycythemia vera, essential thrombocythemia, primary myelofibrosis, and the newly recognized category of myeloid and lymphoid neoplasms with eosinophilia and abnormalities of *PDGFRA*, *PDGFRB*, and *FGFR1* are rare in childhood and will not be discussed in this chapter. The diagnostic criteria for the rare childhood cases are the same as those used in adults. Algorithms have been proposed to help navigate the complexity of initial diagnosis.[162]

Childhood Myelodysplastic Syndrome

The WHO 2008 classification recognizes that childhood MDSs, while rare, are different from those of adults. In par-ticular, the low-grade categories of MDS lacking 2% to 19% blasts in the blood or 5% to 19% blasts in the bone marrow are different in children. The new category of RCC is used in place of the adult divisions of refractory cytopenias with unilineage dysplasia, refractory anemia with ringed sideroblasts, refractory anemia with multilineage dysplasia, and MDS associated with isolated del(5q). The diagnosis of refractory anemia with excess blasts is the same in children as in adults. Children with a history of prior cytotoxic therapy or DS are excluded from this category and are diagnosed as a therapy-related MDS or myeloid proliferations of DS as described earlier.

The diagnostic criteria for RCC require persistent cytopenia (usually neutropenia and/or thrombocytopenia), less than 2% blasts in the blood and 5% blasts in the bone marrow, and the presence of morphologic dysplasia on the aspirate and core biopsy. Unlike adult MDS, pediatric patients more commonly present with a hypocellular marrow, and the distinction of RCC from inherited bone marrow (BM) failure disorders or acquired aplastic anemia can be challenging. Dysplastic changes must be present in two or more lineages or in more than 10% of the elements of any one lineage. The most reliable diagnostic features of dyserythropoiesis are nuclear abnormalities including nuclear budding, multinuclearity, and internuclear bridges (Fig. 7.13). Nuclear karyorrhexis and megaloblastic changes may also be seen. Dysgranulopoiesis is characterized by abnormal nuclear condensation (pseudo–Pelger-Huet cells) and hypogranularity in the mature forms, sometimes with giant bands. Dysmegakaryopoiesis is evidenced by micromegakaryocytes, forms with separated nuclei, or mature forms with round nuclei. Micromegakaryocytes are considered the strongest indicator of RCC, and immunohistochemistry (CD41, CD61) on core biopsies for their recognition is recommended. Before a diagnosis of RCC can be established, other causes of dyspoiesis must be excluded, including infections, vitamin deficiency, metabolic disorders, inherited bone marrow failure disorders, immune disorders such as autoimmune lymphoproliferative disorder or rheumatic disease, paroxysmal nocturnal hemoglobinuria, and hematologic recovery from acquired aplastic anemia. The most significant prognostic factor is karyotype. Nearly half of the patients with RCC will have monosomy 7, and they have a significantly higher risk of progression.[161]

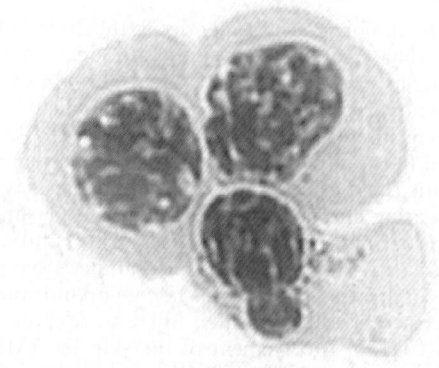
A

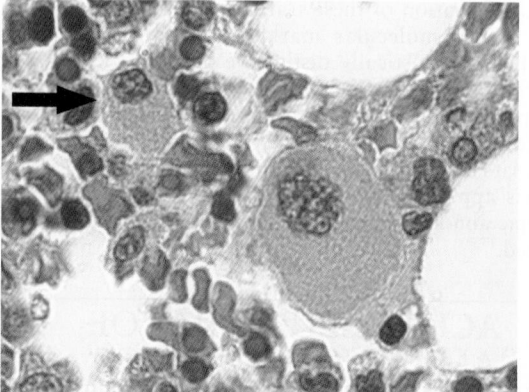
B

FIGURE 7.13 **A:** Nuclear budding and megaloblastic changes evidence dyserythropoiesis in this case of a 15-year-old girl with refractory cytopenia of childhood and monosomy 7. **B:** The marrow of refractory cytopenia of childhood is often hypocellular and shows characteristic micromegakaryocytes (*arrow*).

TABLE 7.7

CRITERIA FOR JUVENILE MYELOMONOCYTIC LEUKEMIA

Required features
  Peripheral blood monocytosis level of $>1 \times 10^9$/L
  Blasts plus promonocytes of >20% in peripheral blood and bone marrow
  No evidence of t(9;22) or *BCR/ABL1*

Plus at least two of the following
  Elevated hemoglobin F level for age
  Immature granulocytes (including promyelocytes and myelocytes) in peripheral blood
  White blood cell count of $>10 \times 10^9$/L
  Clonal chromosomal abnormality
  GM-CSF hypersensitivity of myeloid progenitors *in vitro*

GM-CSF, granulocyte-macrophage colony-stimulating factor.

Juvenile Myelomonocytic Leukemia

JMML is a fatal myelodysplastic/myeloproliferative neoplasm of young children. Allogeneic bone marrow transplantation is currently the only option for cure. Patients are typically diagnosed before age 3, with symptoms related to infiltration of organs by the malignant cells (hepatosplenomegaly, lymphadenopathy), pallor, and skin lesions.[163] Specific laboratory criteria for JMML have been proposed and were adopted by the WHO classification (Table 7.7).[134,164,165] These criteria are useful in excluding other diseases as well as reactive causes of monocytosis in children.

In JMML, the bone marrow (Fig. 7.14) may show fairly nonspecific changes that include hypercellularity with a monocytosis that may be apparent only with nonspecific esterase cytochemical studies. Peripheral blood and marrow monocytes are predominantly mature, with less than 20% having features of either monoblasts or promonocytes. The detection of clonal cytogenetic abnormalities is useful in making this diagnosis, but a single consistent abnormality has not been described. Approximately 25% of patients with JMML

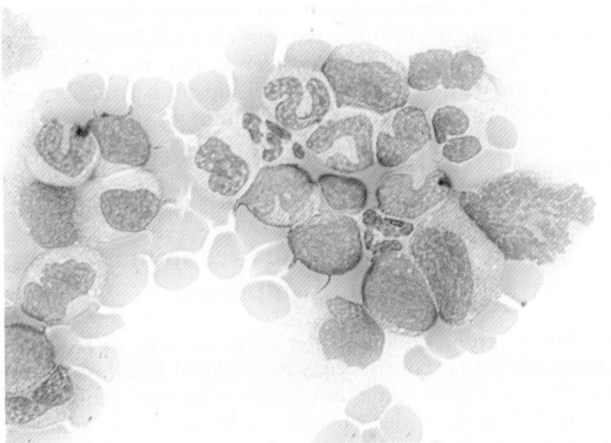

FIGURE 7.14 Juvenile myelomonocytic leukemia. The bone marrow shows an increase in monocytes and blast cells.

have monosomy 7 and such cases were considered as a separate disease (monosomy 7 syndrome) in the past. A recent large study, however, has failed to find significant differences in cases with and without monosomy 7 to warrant a separate designation.[166] Monosomy 7 is also common to RCC, distinguished from JMML by its presentation of bone marrow failure, in contrast to the myeloproliferative features of JMML.[167]

Enhanced colony-forming unit sensitivity to granulocyte-macrophage colony-stimulating factor (GM-CSF) and STAT5 hyperphosphorylation in response to low-dose GM-CSF are distinctive features of JMML, reflecting mutations in the downstream signaling cascade that lead to increased levels of Ras-GTP. These include the mostly mutually exclusive mutations found in *PTPN11* (35% of patients), *KRAS* and *NRAS* (20% of patients), and *NF1* (15%). It is hypothesized that the most recently identified subset with mutations in *CBL* (10%–15%) also affect Ras activation as similar sensitivity to GM-CSF and STAT5 hyperphosphorylation are found in these patients. Although there is an increase of JMML in children with neurofibromatosis type 1,[168] in approximately 15% of patients, mutation of *NF1* occurs in JMML in the absence of a clinical diagnosis of neurofibromatosis.[169–172]

HODGKIN LYMPHOMA

The pathologic classification of Hodgkin lymphoma has also undergone a variety of changes[1,173–175] but is now separated into two main groups: classical Hodgkin lymphoma and nodular lymphocyte predominance Hodgkin lymphoma (NLPHL).[1] Classical Hodgkin lymphoma represents approximately 95% of all cases and frequently occurs in adolescence, while NLPHL is less common in children. Both types of Hodgkin lymphoma are characterized by a proliferation of large neoplastic cells that represent only a minor component of the involved tissue. The two main groups differ by the immunophenotypic features of the neoplastic cell population.

Classical Hodgkin Lymphoma

Classical Hodgkin lymphoma usually presents with enlarged supradiaphragmatic lymph nodes, typically with regional, rather than disseminated, lymph node involvement.[176] Characteristic morphologic and immunophenotypic features of the neoplastic cell population define classical Hodgkin lymphoma. Classic binucleated Reed-Sternberg (RS) cells and their mononuclear variants (often termed *Hodgkin cells*) are large cells with chromatin clearing and large, eosinophilic nuclei (Fig. 7.15). These cells display a characteristic immunophenotype with expression of CD15 and CD30 but lacking CD45 (leukocyte common antigen).[177,178] A majority of cases also express the B-cell transcription factor PAX5, whereas a subset express the B-cell marker CD20. Microdissected Hodgkin and RS cells demonstrate clonal B-cell (immunoglobulin heavy chain) gene rearrangements and molecular changes suggestive that they derive from germinal center B cells.[179–181] A significant subset of cases harbor clonal episomal Epstein-Barr virus (EBV) genomes or express EBV antigens in the neoplastic cells.[182] Surrounding cells in classical Hodgkin lymphoma include small lymphocytes, histiocytes, and eosinophils.

Classical Hodgkin lymphoma is subdivided into several morphologic variants (described later), which have demonstrated prognostic significance in past studies. However, subclassification of classical Hodgkin lymphoma is of less clinical significance with current therapeutic approaches.[183]

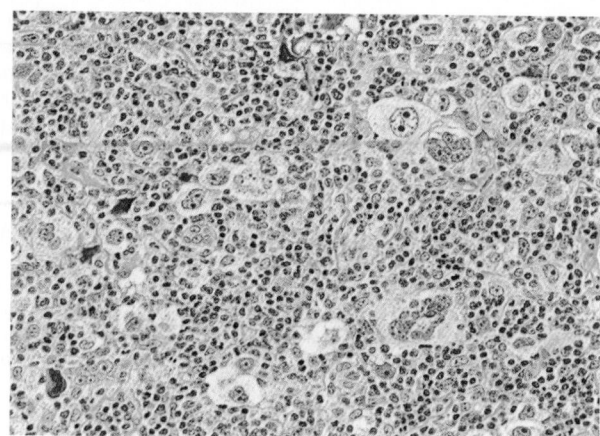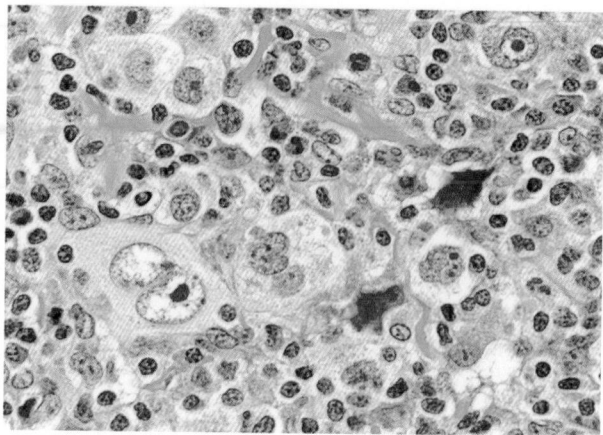

FIGURE 7.15 Classical Hodgkin lymphoma. **A:** Low-power magnification shows scattered large atypical cells, some of which are binucleated, with abundant cytoplasms and prominent eosinophilic nucleoli. **B:** Higher magnification shows characteristic binucleated Reed-Sternberg cells and mononuclear Hodgkin cells.

Nodular Sclerosis Hodgkin Lymphoma

Nodular sclerosis Hodgkin lymphoma (NSHL) is the most common subtype of Hodgkin lymphoma, typically presenting as a mediastinal mass. In addition to the morphologic features described previously for all types of classical Hodgkin lymphoma, NSHL is characterized by a thickened lymph node capsule and broad bands of birefringent collagen. The latter often create a nodular appearance to the lymphoid tissue even in the absence of true lymph node follicles or germinal centers. Zonal areas of necrosis are often present in NSHL, as are lacunar cells, which are Hodgkin cells that show a formalin fixation artifact of cytoplasmic retraction. A syncytial variant of NSHL shows sheets of neoplastic cells that may be confused with metastatic carcinoma.[184]

Because of similarities in the disease site, age distribution, and frequency of admixed fibrosis, the differential diagnosis of NSHL versus mediastinal large B-cell lymphoma, a subtype of non-Hodgkin lymphoma, is often difficult. Different therapies are used to treat these entities. The fibrosis in mediastinal large B-cell lymphoma is often less collagenous than in NSHL. The cells in both may show variable expression of CD20 as well as CD30, but mediastinal large B-cell lymphoma does not typically express CD15 and usually expresses CD45, unlike NSHL. However, some cases are difficult to distinguish, and transcriptional profiling (microarray) studies have also demonstrated many similarities between these two disorders.[185] The 2008 WHO classification recognizes this dilemma with the diagnostic category of B-cell lymphoma, unclassifiable, with features intermediate between diffuse large B-cell lymphoma (DLBCL) and classical Hodgkin lymphoma. In cases morphologically resembling NSHL, strong expression of the B-cell marker CD20 and transcription factors PAX5, with the absence of CD15, place a case into this unclassifiable category of lymphoma.[186]

Mixed Cellularity Hodgkin Lymphoma

Mixed cellularity Hodgkin lymphoma (MCHL) is the second most common type of classical Hodgkin lymphoma and most often involves the cervical lymph nodes but is less frequent than NSHL in children. MCHL often shows fewer Hodgkin cells than does NSHL, without fibrosis or necrosis, and often has a prominent background of histiocytes and eosinophils. MCHL is associated with EBV infection of neoplastic cells in the majority of cases.[187] Infectious mononucleosis, especially in tonsils, may have a cellular composition that mimics MCHL in teenagers and young adults. Because of the rarity of MCHL in this age group and in this location, caution must be exercised to distinguish the two diseases. The tonsil of infectious mononucleosis will often show more pleomorphism of plasmacytoid lymphocytes, admixed with RS-like cells, with abundant cellular or even zonal areas of necrosis.

Other Types of Classical Hodgkin Lymphoma

Lymphocyte-depleted Hodgkin lymphoma consists of a diffuse proliferation of Hodgkin cells with the characteristic immunophenotype of classical Hodgkin lymphoma and a paucity of background small lymphocytes. Although this morphologic subtype may occur with relapse of other types of classical Hodgkin lymphoma, it is extremely uncommon as a primary presentation.

Lymphocyte-rich classical Hodgkin lymphoma is a relatively recently described morphologic subtype of classical Hodgkin lymphoma that was probably classified as lymphocyte predominance or MCHL in the past.[188,189] It is uncommon in children. It is characterized by a nodular or diffuse proliferation of small lymphocytes with admixed cells that are morphologically and immunophenotypically similar to those of the other types of classical Hodgkin lymphoma. These cases differ, however, in that the small lymphocyte population is composed of mostly B lymphocytes, as opposed to the CD4-positive (T lineage) small lymphocytes characteristic of the other types of classical Hodgkin lymphoma.

Nodular Lymphocyte Predominance Hodgkin Lymphoma

NLPHL is rare in children. It is a distinct type of Hodgkin lymphoma[175] that consists of a monoclonal B-cell proliferation[190,191] and most commonly involves cervical, axillary, or inguinal lymph nodes, usually without bone marrow involvement. The proliferation is typically nodular with characteristic large cells that differ in appearance from classic RS cells. They are called *popcorn cells* because of their distinctive nuclear lobulations; nucleoli are smaller than those of RS cells. In contrast to classical Hodgkin lymphoma cells, the neoplastic cells of NLPHL express CD45 and lack CD15 and CD30. They characteristically show uniform expression of CD20 and are accompanied by a background of CD20-positive small B cells. The transcription factors PAX5, OCT-2, and BOB.1 are typically strongly expressed in the neoplastic cells of NLPHL, in contrast to their absence or only weak positivity in classical Hodgkin lymphoma subtypes. The neoplastic cells of NLPHL are typically ringed by CD3+ T-cells expressing CD57 and PD-1.[192] The morphologic appearance of NLPHL is similar to progressive transformation of germinal centers,[193] but the latter entity is associated with reactive germinal centers, while NLPHL usually forms a discrete lymph node mass away from reactive germinal centers.

NON-HODGKIN LYMPHOMA OF CHILDHOOD

Overview of Classifications

The classification of non-Hodgkin lymphoma has evolved dramatically in recent decades to include a very large number of distinct disease entities. While early classification systems, such as the Rappaport classification[194] and the Working Formulation,[195] were based entirely on cell morphology, the more recent classification schemes (REAL and WHO)[1,196] place diseases into categories based on immunophenotypic and, in some cases, cytogenetic or molecular genetic features. Table 7.8 lists

---

TABLE 7.8

WORLD HEALTH ORGANIZATION CLASSIFICATION OF MATURE NON-HODGKIN LYMPHOID NEOPLASMS

Mature B-cell neoplasms	Mature T-cell and natural killer (NK)-cell neoplasms
Chronic lymphocytic leukemia/small lymphocytic lymphoma	T-cell prolymphocytic leukemia
B-cell prolymphocytic leukemia	T-cell large granular lymphocytic leukemia
Splenic marginal zone lymphoma	Chronic lymphoproliferative disorder of NK cells
Hairy cell leukemia	Aggressive NK-cell leukemia
Splenic B-cell lymphoma/leukemia, unclassifiable	EBV-positive T-cell lymphoproliferative diseases of childhood
Splenic diffuse red pulp small B-cell lymphoma	Systemic EBV-positive T-cell lymphoproliferative disease of childhood
Hairy cell leukemia variant	Hydroa vacciniforme–like lymphoma
Lymphoplasmacytic lymphoma	Adult T-cell leukemia/lymphoma
Heavy chain diseases	Extranodal NK/T-cell lymphoma, nasal type
Gamma heavy chain disease	Enteropathy-type T-cell lymphoma
Mu heavy chain disease	Hepatosplenic T-cell lymphoma
Alpha heavy chain disease	Subcutaneous panniculitis-like T-cell lymphoma
Plasma cell neoplasms	Mycosis fungoides
Monoclonal gammopathy of undetermined significance	Sézary syndrome
Plasma cell myeloma	Primary cutaneous CD30-positive T-cell lymphoproliferative disorders
Solitary plasmacytoma of bone	Primary cutaneous peripheral T-cell lymphomas, rare subtypes
Extraosseous plasmacytoma	Primary cutaneous gamma-delta T-cell lymphoma
Monoclonal immunoglobulin deposition diseases	Primary cutaneous CD8-positive aggressive epidermotropic cytotoxic T-cell lymphoma
Extranodal marginal zone lymphoma of mucosa-associated lymphoid tissue	Primary cutaneous CD4-positive small/medium T-cell lymphoma
Nodal marginal zone B-cell lymphoma	Peripheral T-cell lymphoma, not otherwise specified
Follicular lymphoma	Angioimmunoblastic T-cell lymphoma
Mantle cell lymphoma	Anaplastic large cell lymphoma, ALK positive
Diffuse large B-cell lymphoma (DLBCL)	Anaplastic large cell lymphoma, ALK negative
T cell/histiocyte-rich large B-cell lymphoma	
Primary DLBCL of the central nervous system	
Primary cutaneous DLBCL, leg type	
Epstein-Barr virus (EBV)-positive DLBCL of the elderly	
DLBCL associated with chronic inflammation	
Lymphomatoid granulomatosis	
Primary mediastinal (thymic) large B-cell lymphoma	
Intravascular large B-cell lymphoma	
ALK-positive large B-cell lymphoma	
Plasmablastic lymphoma	
Large B-cell lymphoma arising in HHV8-associated multicentric Castleman's disease	
Primary effusion lymphoma	
Burkitt's lymphoma/leukemia	
B-cell lymphoma, unclassifiable, with features intermediate between DLBCL and Burkitt's lymphoma	
B-cell lymphoma, unclassifiable, with features intermediate between DLBCL and classical Hodgkin lymphoma	
Posttransplant lymphoproliferative disorder, polymorphic	

ALK, anaplastic lymphoma receptor protein kinase; HHV-8, human herpes virus-8.

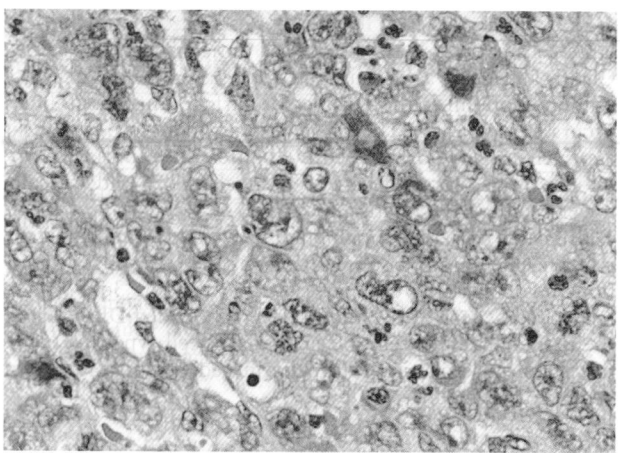

FIGURE 7.18 Anaplastic large cell lymphoma, classic type. Large pleomorphic cells are present, including "hallmark cells" with indented or horseshoe-shaped nuclei and pink cytoplasms. These cells typically express CD3 and CD30.

Most children with ALCL present with lymphadenopathy, but extranodal disease, particularly skin involvement, is also common.[213-218] The most common morphologic type shows a diffuse proliferation of large, pleomorphic cells typically with a sinusoidal pattern of lymph node involvement that might suggest metastatic carcinoma (Fig. 7.18). However, a variety of cellular variants have been described. A small cell variant, which usually has admixed larger cells, may also occur in children and is reportedly more aggressive.[219,220] A lymphohistiocytic variant in which the neoplastic cells may be obscured by numerous histiocytes is also common in children and is often difficult to diagnose as lymphoma on routine histologic sections (Fig. 7.19).[221,222] A monomorphic variant containing uniform, medium-sized cells may mimic DLBCL or a myeloid sarcoma.[223] The neoplastic cells of all types of ALCL usually express at least one T-cell–associated antigen, such as CD2, CD5, or CD3, but some cases may express only the more nonspecific CD43 antigen and are termed *null cell type*. A subset of cases also lacks CD45 (leukocyte common antigen). The

tumor cells in ALCL, however, strongly express CD30 and the majority of pediatric cases express ALK protein. ALK-positive cases have so-called hallmark cells that have eccentric, horseshoe-shaped nuclei with eosinophilic cytoplasm. ALK protein expression correlates with disruption of the *ALK* gene. The most common *ALK* gene abnormality in ALCL is t(2;5)(p23;q35) involving the *NPM1* gene, but *ALK* may also fuse with other genes as well, including *TPM3* at 1p21, *TFG* at 3q21, *ATIC* at 2q35, *CTLC* at 17q23, and *MSN* at Xq11-12.[12,20,224] All of these genetic aberrations result in ALK fusion protein expression. ALK-negative ALCL is more common in adults and does not have the same favorable prognosis as ALK-positive disease. ALK-positive ALCL also differs from primary cutaneous ALCL, which does not express ALK; has a favorable prognosis, and is usually localized to the skin.[225]

ALCL uniformly shows T-cell receptor gene rearrangements, including cases with a null cell immunophenotype. While many cases display evidence of a t(2;5) chromosomal translocation by FISH analysis or *NPM1-ALK* fusion transcripts by RT-PCR, these studies are usually not needed because of the specificity of ALK immunohistochemistry. In fact, ALK immunohistochemistry is superior to these molecular assays because it detects the ALK fusion proteins resulting from all *ALK* chromosomal translocations, some of which evade detection by routine FISH or RT-PCR assays.[226]

The differential diagnosis of ALCL in children includes malignant histiocytosis and classical Hodgkin lymphoma. The lymphohistiocytic variant of ALCL may mimic malignant histiocytosis, although the latter diagnosis is rarely confirmed with modern ancillary methods.[227] The detection of a large cell component that expresses CD30 and ALK confirms the diagnosis of ALCL. Null cell ALCL may mimic classical Hodgkin lymphoma, but ALCL does not express PAX5 or CD15 and is not EBV positive, whereas Hodgkin lymphoma cells do not express ALK.

Hepatosplenic T-Cell Lymphoma

Hepatosplenic T-cell lymphoma, an otherwise rare type of T-cell lymphoma, is relatively common in adolescents with a marked male predominance.[228-230] It is an aggressive T-cell neoplasm that is characterized by a proliferation of medium-sized T cells accompanied by massive enlargement of the liver and spleen and frequent bone marrow involvement. The splenic red pulp and hepatic and marrow sinusoids are expanded by a monotonous proliferation of lymphocytes that may have clear cytoplasm and inconspicuous nucleoli (Fig. 7.20). Admixed histiocytes, sometimes with evidence of hemophagocytosis (Fig. 7.21), may be present.[231,232] The cells express T-cell–associated markers CD2 and CD3 but usually lack CD4 or CD8. Most cases are neoplasms of the less frequent γ/δ T cell that is preferentially localized to the spleen, but α/β T-cell types have also been described with similar clinical and cytogenetic features.[233] The cells also usually express TIA-1, a cytotoxic granule marker. All types show T-cell receptor γ chain gene rearrangements, but the more frequent γ/δ type may not show T-cell receptor β chain rearrangements. This tumor characteristically shows isochromosome 7q, usually in association with trisomy 8.

Immunodeficiency-Associated Lymphoproliferative Disorders

The most common disorders in children from this category are the posttransplant lymphoproliferative disorders (PTLDs), most of which are EBV-associated, and span the spectrum from early, infectious mononucleosis-like lesions to lymphomas indistinguishable from those in nonimmunocompromised

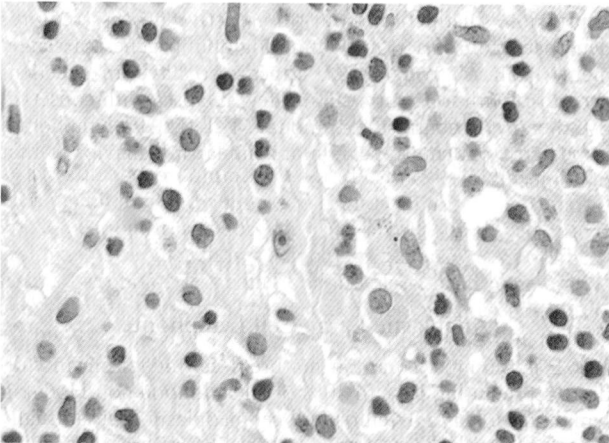

FIGURE 7.19 Anaplastic large cell lymphoma, lymphohistiocytic type. Histiocytes and small lymphocytes predominate with only scattered large cells with prominent nucleoli identified (*center*). These cells invariably express CD30 and ALK-1.

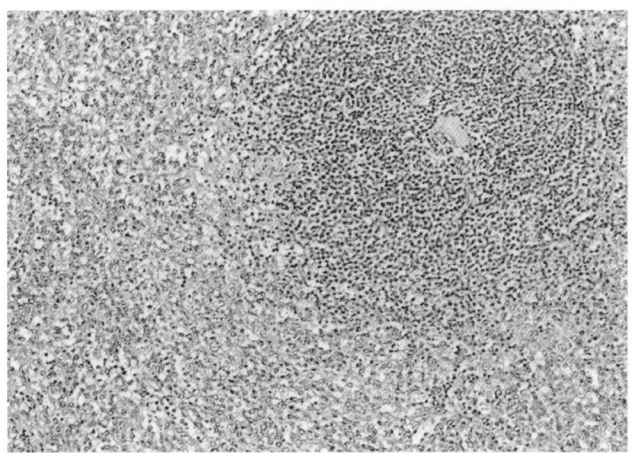

FIGURE 7.20 Hepatosplenic T-cell lymphoma. The splenic red pulp is diffusely infiltrated by medium to large cells, in contrast to the small lymphocytes of the splenic white pulp (*upper right*). The red pulp cells expressed T-cell–associated antigens.

patients. Proliferations composed of a mixture of small and large lymphocytes, immunoblasts, and plasma cells that efface nodal or extranodal tissue architecture are termed *polymorphic PTLD*. This is the most common type of PTLD. The diagnosis is morphologic. Some cases may show light chain monotypia by flow cytometry, and this should be noted as it may reflect possible transformation to monomorphic disease. However, demonstration of clonal B-cell gene rearrangements is common in polymorphic PTLD. Monomorphic PTLD fulfill criteria for one of the B-cell or T/NK-cell neoplasms occurring in an immunocompetent host. Polymorphic and monomorphic diseases are part of a clinical spectrum. Patients may have polymorphic disease at one site and monomorphic disease elsewhere, or a single lesion may show a predominance of atypical large cells suggestive of a polymorphic lesion in transformation.[234]

Children with immunodeficiency disorders are at increased risk for lymphoproliferative disease (LPD). LPDs associated with primary immune disorders include those secondary to ataxia-telangiectasia, Wiskott-Aldrich syndrome, common variable immunodeficiency, severe combined immunodeficiency, X-linked lymphoproliferative disorder, Nijmegen breakage syndrome, hyper-IgM syndrome, and autoimmune lymphoproliferative syndrome. Most cases are EBV-associated, and the lymphoma types resemble those seen in patients without immunodeficiency (e.g., DLBCL, Hodgkin lymphoma, lymphomatoid granulomatosis) and are diagnosed with the same criteria. Certain conditions are characterized with nonneoplastic abnormal lymphoid proliferations, such as CD4-negative/CD8-negative/TCR-α/β–expressing T cells in autoimmune lymphoproliferative syndrome. Children may die from fatal infectious mononucleosis without development of a clonal malignant lymphoma.[235]

OTHER HEMATOPOIETIC TUMORS

Other hematopoietic tumors are rare in children and representative of mostly histiocytic or mast cell tumors. Most cases of histiocytic sarcoma (or malignant histiocytosis) reported in the past have been shown to constitute other tumor types,[236,237] including ALCL and hepatosplenic T-cell lymphoma. Langerhans cell histiocytosis, however, is relatively common in children and represents a clonal proliferation of Langerhans cells, which express CD1a, Langerin, and S100, as well as containing Birbeck granules as demonstrated by electron microscopy.[238–242] These proliferations contain cells with folded nuclei with prominent nuclear grooves and inconspicuous nucleoli. These cells are usually accompanied by eosinophils, histiocytes, and lymphocytes. Cases with malignant cytologic features have also been described as Langerhans cell sarcoma, including cases in children. The clinical and pathologic features of the spectrum of Langerhans histiocytosis are discussed in more detail elsewhere in this volume.

Mastocytosis includes several subtypes of disease (Table 7.10), with cutaneous mast cell disease occurring more commonly in children.[243,244] It may be localized to the skin or may be a systemic disease with or without skin lesions or an associated hematologic malignancy. Cutaneous mast cell disease in children usually occurs in the first 6 months of life. The most common form is urticaria pigmentosa (maculopapular cutaneous mastocytosis) and is characterized by papular lesions. Diffuse cutaneous mastocytosis almost exclusively occurs in children and does not show the defined papules of urticaria pigmentosa. Mastocytoma of the skin typically occurs on the trunk or wrist of infants and is a single lesion and may show extension of mast cells into subcutaneous tissue. Regardless of site of involvement, mastocytosis is characterized by aggregates of mast cells that are round, oval, or even spindled cells

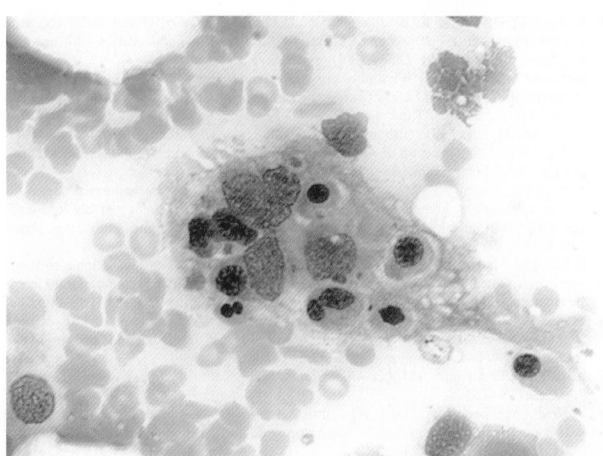

FIGURE 7.21 Hemophagocytosis of bone marrow, secondary to T-cell lymphoma. The bone marrow shows large histiocytes engulfing nucleated red blood cells. The bone marrow was also involved by T-cell lymphoma.

TABLE 7.10

CLASSIFICATION OF MAST CELL DISORDERS

Cutaneous mastocytosis
Indolent systemic mastocytosis
Systemic mastocytosis with associated clonal, hematological non–mast cell lineage disease
Aggressive systemic mastocytosis
Mast cell leukemia
Mast cell sarcoma
Extracutaneous mastocytoma

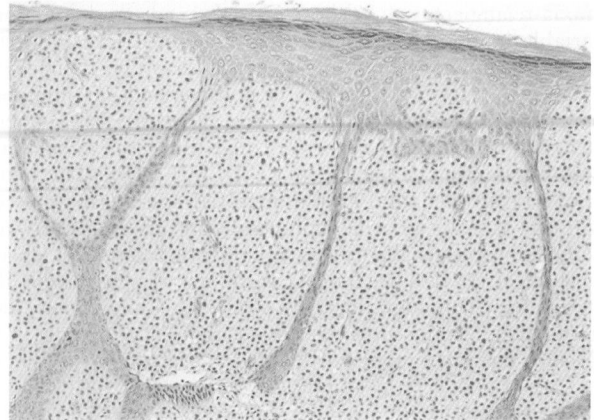

FIGURE 7.22 Cutaneous mastocytoma. The dermis is replaced by monotonous sheets of mast cells with abundant, pink-staining cytoplasms.

with abundant, pink granular cytoplasm and slightly irregular bland nuclei on hematoxylin and eosin stains (Fig. 7.22). On Romanowsky stains, the cells have abundant fine basophilic granules that may obscure the nucleus. Eosinophils and aggregates of small lymphocytes are often admixed with the mast cell proliferation. Outside of the skin, mast cells may be associated with fibrosis, with paratrabecular fibrosis associated with mast cell aggregates common in the bone marrow and patchy fibrotic areas common in the spleen. Because of this, mast cells may be overlooked on tissue sections or confused with granulomas. Mast cells do not mark with most lymphoid markers but show strong expression of CD117 and tryptase.[245] Neoplastic mast cells often express CD2 and CD25.[246] Some cases of systemic mastocytosis are associated with a non–mast cell hematologic malignancy.

FUTURE CONSIDERATIONS

The diagnosis and management of pediatric cancers, which historically have been on the leading edge of efforts to develop risk-adapted therapies, will inevitably evolve in coming years. Advances in the molecular, genetic, and proteomic profiling of pediatric cancers will continue to provide new criteria for diagnostic subclassification. These will need to be validated for their prognostic value in pediatric patients undergoing treatment on appropriately controlled clinical trials. Because multiparameter analysis techniques, such as expression profiling and proteomics, may not be feasible to perform for routine diagnostic workup, a significant challenge will be to identify subsets of genes or gene products that serve as representative surrogate markers and can be readily assessed in the clinical laboratory. Uniform standards will need to be established for their measurement, interpretation, and application. Another ongoing challenge is to correlate new diagnostic criteria with advances in treatment, particularly targeted modalities based on small molecule, immunologic, and cellular therapies employed alone or in combination with conventional chemotherapy. Indeed, it is likely that specific molecular markers will dictate which targeted treatments are employed; thus, advances in diagnosis will continue to evolve hand in hand with advances in therapy. It is also anticipated that molecular diagnosis will serve an increasingly important role in monitoring response to treatment, development of resistance, and early detection of relapse. Finally, genomic and proteomic profiling offers the promise of identifying individuals at increased risk of cancer incidence or relapse months or even years in advance. Appropriate development and utilization of these new technologies and determination of their roles in clinical management decisions will require coordinated efforts among pathologists, clinicians, and laboratory-based investigators.

References

1. Swerdlow SH, Campo E, Harris NL, et al., eds. WHO classification of tumours of haematopoietic and lymphoid tissues. Lyon, France: IARC Press, 2008.
2. Vardiman JW, Thiele J, Arber DA, et al. The 2008 revision of the WHO classification of myeloid neoplasms and acute leukemia: rationale and important changes. Blood 2009;114:937–951.
3. Hyun BH, Gulati GL, Ashton JK. Bone marrow examination: techniques and interpretation. Hematol Oncol Clin North Am 1988;2:513–523.
4. Foucar K. Bone marrow examination: indications and techniques. In: Bone marrow pathology. 2nd ed. Chicago, IL: ASCP Press, 2001:30–49.
5. Brunning RD, McKenna RW. Appendix: bone marrow specimen processing. In: Tumors of the bone marrow. Washington, DC: Armed Forces Institute of Pathology, 1994:475–489.
6. Banks PM. Technical factors in the preparation and evaluation of lymph node biopsies. In: Neoplastic hematopathology. 2nd ed. Philadelphia, PA: Lippincott Williams & Wilkins, 2001:467–482.
7. Schabath R, Ratei R, Ludwig WD. The prognostic significance of antigen expression in leukaemia. Best Pract Res Clin Haematol 2003;16:613–628.
8. Stetler-Stevenson M. Flow cytometry in lymphoma diagnosis and prognosis: useful? Best Pract Res Clin Haematol 2003;16:583–597.
9. Chu PG, Chang KL, Arber DA, et al. Immunophenotyping of hematopoietic neoplasms. Semin Diagn Pathol 2000;17:236–256.
10. Arber DA, Jenkins KA. Paraffin section immunophenotyping of acute leukemias in bone marrow specimens. Am J Clin Pathol 1996;106:462–468.
11. Bain BJ. Overview. Cytogenetic analysis in haematology. Best Pract Res Clin Haematol 2001;14:463–477.
12. Arber DA. Molecular diagnostic approach to non-Hodgkin's lymphoma. J Mol Diagn 2000;2:178–190.
13. Pui CH, Relling MV, Downing JR. Acute lymphoblastic leukemia. N Engl J Med 2004;350:1535–1548.
14. Cerezo L, Shuster JJ, Pullen DJ, et al. Laboratory correlates and prognostic significance of granular acute lymphoblastic leukemia in children: a Pediatric Oncology Group study. Am J Clin Pathol 1991;95:526–531.
15. Bennett JM, Catovsky D, Daniel M-T, et al. Proposal for the recognition of minimally differentiated acute myeloid leukaemia (AML-M0). Br J Haematol 1991;78:325–329.
16. Chessells JM, Swansbury GJ, Reeves B, et al. Cytogenetics and prognosis in childhood lymphoblastic leukaemia: results of MRC UKALL X. Br J Haematol 1997;99:93–100.
17. Forestier E, Johansson B, Gustafsson G, et al. Prognostic impact of karyotypic findings in childhood acute lymphoblastic leukaemia: a Nordic series comparing two treatment periods: for the Nordic Society of Paediatric Haematology and Oncology (NOPHO) Leukaemia Cytogenetic Study Group. Br J Haematol 2000;110:147–153.
18. Pui CH, Campana D, Evans WE. Childhood acute lymphoblastic leukaemia—current status and future perspectives. Lancet Oncol 2001;2:597–607.
19. Bene MC, Castoldi G, Knapp W, et al. Proposal for the immunologic classification of acute leukemias. Leukemia 1995;9:1783–1786.
20. Merker JD, Arber DA. Molecular diagnostics of non-Hodgkin lymphoma. Expert Opin Med Diagn 2007;1:47–63.
21. Brumpt C, Delabesse E, Beldjord K, et al. The incidence of clonal T-cell receptor rearrangements in B-cell precursor acute lymphoblastic leukemia varies with age and genotype. Blood 2000;96:2254–2261.
22. Borowitz MJ, Chan JKC. B lymphoblastic leukaemia/lymphoma with recurrent genetic abnormalities. In: WHO classification of tumours of haematopoietic and lymphoid tissues. Lyon, France: IARC Press, 2008:171–175.
23. Borowitz MJ, Chan JKC. B lymphoblastic leukaemia/lymphoma, not otherwise specified. In: WHO classification of tumours of haematopoietic and lymphoid tissues. Lyon, France: IARC Press, 2008:168–170.
24. Khalidi HS, Chang KL, Medeiros LJ, et al. Acute lymphoblastic leukemia: survey of immunophenotype, French-American-British classification, frequency of myeloid antigen expression, and karyotypic abnormalities in 210 pediatric and adult cases. Am J Clin Pathol 1999;111:467–476.
25. Uckun FM, Nachman JB, Sather HN, et al. Clinical significance of Philadelphia chromosome positive pediatric acute lymphoblastic leukemia in the context of contemporary intensive therapies: a report from the Children's Cancer Group. Cancer 1998;83:2030–2039.
26. Uckun FM, Nachman JB, Sather HN, et al. Poor treatment outcome of Philadelphia chromosome-positive pediatric acute lymphoblastic leukemia despite intensive chemotherapy. Leuk Lymphoma 1999;33:101–106.
27. Advani AS, Pendergast AM. Bcr-Abl variants: biological and clinical aspects. Leuk Res 2002;26:713–720.
28. Borowitz MJ, Bene MC, Harris NL, et al. Acute leukaemias of ambiguous lineage. In: WHO classification of tumours of haematopoietic and lymphoid tissues. Lyon, France: IARC Press, 2008:150–155.
29. Mullighan CG, Su X, Zhang J, et al. Deletion of IKZF1 and prognosis in acute lymphoblastic leukemia. N Engl J Med 2009;360:470–480.
30. Mullighan CG, Miller CB, Radtke I, et al. BCR-ABL1 lymphoblastic leukaemia is characterized by the deletion of Ikaros. Nature 2008;453:110–114.
31. Iacobucci I, Lonetti A, Messa F, et al. Expression of spliced oncogenic Ikaros isoforms in Philadelphia-positive acute lymphoblastic leukemia patients treated with tyrosine

kinase inhibitors: implications for a new mechanism of resistance. Blood 2008;112: 3847–3855.
32. Heerema NA, Arthur DC, Sather H, et al. Cytogenetic features of infants less than 12 months of age at diagnosis of acute lymphoblastic leukemia: impact of the 11q23 breakpoint on outcome: a report of the Childrens Cancer Group. Blood 1994;83:2274–2284.
33. Heerema NA, Sather HN, Ge J, et al. Cytogenetic studies of infant acute lymphoblastic leukemia: poor prognosis of infants with t(4;11)—a report of the Children's Cancer Group. Leukemia 1999;13:679–686.
34. Rubnitz JE, Link MP, Shuster JJ, et al. Frequency and prognostic significance of HRX rearrangements in infant acute lymphoblastic leukemia: a Pediatric Oncology Group study. Blood 1994;84:570–573.
35. Taki T, Ida K, Bessho F, et al. Frequency and clinical significance of the MLL gene rearrangements in infant acute leukemia. Leukemia 1996;10:1303–1307.
36. DiMartino JF, Cleary ML. MLL rearrangements in haematological malignancies: lessons from clinical and biological studies. Br J Haematol 1999;106:614–624.
37. Pui CH, Chessells JM, Camitta B, et al. Clinical heterogeneity in childhood acute lymphoblastic leukemia with 11q23 rearrangements. Leukemia 2003;17:700–706.
38. Pui CH, Rubnitz JE, Hancock ML, et al. Reappraisal of the clinical and biologic significance of myeloid-associated antigen expression in childhood acute lymphoblastic leukemia. J Clin Oncol 1998;16:3768–3773.
39. Lenormand B, Bene MC, Lesesve JF, et al. PreB1 (CD10-) acute lymphoblastic leukemia: immunophenotypic and genomic characteristics, clinical features and outcome in 38 adults and 26 children: the Groupe dEtude Immunologique des Leucemies. Leuk Lymphoma 1998;28:329–342.
40. Armstrong SA, Mabon ME, Silverman LB, et al. FLT3 mutations in childhood acute lymphoblastic leukemia. Blood 2004;103:3544–3546.
41. Taketani T, Taki T, Sugita K, et al. FLT3 mutations in the activation loop of tyrosine kinase domain are frequently found in infant ALL with MLL rearrangements and pediatric ALL with hyperdiploidy. Blood 2004;103:1085–1088.
42. Romana SP, Mauchauffe M, Le Coniat M, et al. The t(12;21) of acute lymphoblastic leukemia results in a tel-AML1 gene fusion. Blood 1995;85:3662–3670.
43. Shurtleff SA, Buijs A, Behm FG, et al. TEL/AML1 fusion resulting from a cryptic t(12;21) is the most common genetic lesion in pediatric ALL and defines a subgroup of patients with an excellent prognosis. Leukemia 1995;9:1985–1989.
44. Golub TR, Barker GF, Bohlander SK, et al. Fusion of the TEL gene on 12p13 to the AML1 gene on 21q22 in acute lymphoblastic leukemia. Proc Natl Acad Sci U S A 1995;92:4917–4921.
45. Borkhardt A, Cazzaniga G, Viehmann S, et al. Incidence and clinical relevance of TEL/AML1 fusion genes in children with acute lymphoblastic leukemia enrolled in the German and Italian multicenter therapy trials: Associazione Italiana Ematologia Oncologia Pediatrica and the Berlin-Frankfurt-Munster Study Group. Blood 1997; 90:571–577.
46. Raynaud S, Mauvieux L, Cayuela JM, et al. TEL/AML1 fusion gene is a rare event in adult acute lymphoblastic leukemia. Leukemia 1996;10:1529–1530.
47. Zelent A, Greaves M, Enver T. Role of the TEL-AML1 fusion gene in the molecular pathogenesis of childhood acute lymphoblastic leukaemia. Oncogene 2004;23: 4275–4283.
48. Borowitz MJ, Rubnitz J, Nash M, et al. Surface antigen phenotype can predict TEL-AML1 rearrangement in childhood B-precursor ALL: a Pediatric Oncology Group study. Leukemia 1998;12:1764–1770.
49. De Zen L, Orfao A, Cazzaniga G, et al. Quantitative multiparametric immunophenotyping in acute lymphoblastic leukemia: correlation with specific genotype, I: ETV6/AML1 ALLs identification. Leukemia 2000;14:1225–1231.
50. Whitehead VM, Vuchich MJ, Lauer SJ, et al. Accumulation of high levels of methotrexate polyglutamates in lymphoblasts from children with hyperdiploid (greater than 50 chromosomes) B-lineage acute lymphoblastic leukemia: a Pediatric Oncology Group study. Blood 1992;80:1316–1323.
51. Whitehead VM, Vuchich MJ, Cooley LD, et al. Accumulation of methotrexate polyglutamates, ploidy and trisomies of both chromosomes 4 and 10 in lymphoblasts from children with B-progenitor cell acute lymphoblastic leukemia: a Pediatric Oncology Group study. Leuk Lymphoma 1998;31:507–519.
52. Sutcliffe MJ, Shuster JJ, Sather HN, et al. High concordance from independent studies by the Children's Cancer Group (CCG) and Pediatric Oncology Group (POG) associating favorable prognosis with combined trisomies 4, 10, and 17 in children with NCI Standard-Risk B-precursor Acute Lymphoblastic Leukemia: a Children's Oncology Group (COG) initiative. Leukemia 2005;19:734–740.
53. Brown P, Levis M, Shurtleff S, et al. FLT3 inhibition selectively kills childhood acute lymphoblastic leukemia cells with high levels of FLT3 expression. Blood 2004;105: 812–820.
54. Trueworthy R, Shuster J, Crist W, et al. Ploidy of lymphoblasts is the strongest predictor of treatment outcome in B-progenitor cell acute lymphoblastic leukemia of childhood: a Pediatric Oncology Group study. J Clin Oncol 1992;10:606–613.
55. Ito C, Kumagai M, Manabe A, et al. Hyperdiploid acute lymphoblastic leukemia with 51 to 65 chromosomes: a distinct biological entity with a marked propensity to undergo apoptosis. Blood 1999;93:315–320.
56. Schultz KR, Pullen DJ, Sather HN, et al. Risk- and response-based classification of childhood B-precursor acute lymphoblastic leukemia: a combined analysis of prognostic markers from the Pediatric Oncology Group (POG) and Children's Cancer Group (CCG). Blood 2007;109:926–935.
57. Crist WM, Carroll AJ, Shuster JJ, et al. Poor prognosis of children with pre-B acute lymphoblastic leukemia is associated with the t(1;19)(q23;p13): a Pediatric Oncology Group study. Blood 1990;76:117–122.
58. Secker-Walker LM, Berger R, Fenaux P, et al. Prognostic significance of the balanced t(1;19) and unbalanced der(19)t(1;19) translocations in acute lymphoblastic leukemia. Leukemia 1992;6:363–369.
59. Borowitz MJ, Hunger SP, Carroll AJ, et al. Predictability of the t(1;19)(q23;p13) from surface antigen phenotype: implications for screening cases of childhood acute lymphoblastic leukemia for molecular analysis: a Pediatric Oncology Group study. Blood 1993;82:1086–1091.
60. Hunger SP, Galili N, Carroll AJ, et al. The t(1;19)(q23;p13) results in consistent fusion of E2A and PBX1 coding sequences in acute lymphoblastic leukemias. Blood 1991;77:687–693.
61. Aspland SE, Bendall HH, Murre C. The role of E2A-PBX1 in leukemogenesis. Oncogene 2001;20:5708–5717.
62. Nourse J, Mellentin JD, Galili N, et al. Chromosomal translocation t(1;19) results in synthesis of a homeobox fusion mRNA that codes for a potential chimeric transcription factor. Cell 1990;60:535–545.
63. Inaba T, Roberts WM, Shapiro LH, et al. Fusion of the leucine zipper gene HLF to the E2A gene in human acute B-lineage leukemia. Science 1992;257:531–534.
64. Yeoh EJ, Ross ME, Shurtleff SA, et al. Classification, subtype discovery, and prediction of outcome in pediatric acute lymphoblastic leukemia by gene expression profiling. Cancer Cell 2002;1:133–143.
65. Ross ME, Zhou X, Song G, et al. Classification of pediatric acute lymphoblastic leukemia by gene expression profiling. Blood 2003;102:2951–2959.
66. Tartaglia M, Martinelli S, Cazzaniga G, et al. Genetic evidence for lineage-related and differentiation stage-related contribution of somatic PTPN11 mutations to leukemogenesis in childhood acute leukemia. Blood 2004;104:307–313.
67. Mullighan CG, Goorha S, Radtke I, et al. Genome-wide analysis of genetic alterations in acute lymphoblastic leukaemia. Nature 2007;446:758–764.
68. Uckun FM, Sensel MG, Sun L, et al. Biology and treatment of childhood T-lineage acute lymphoblastic leukemia. Blood 1998;91:735–746.
69. Pilozzi E, Pulford K, Jones M, et al. Co-expression of CD79a (JCB117) and CD3 by lymphoblastic lymphoma. J Pathol 1998;186:140–143.
70. Schneider NR, Carroll AJ, Shuster JJ, et al. New recurring cytogenetic abnormalities and association of blast cell karyotypes with prognosis in childhood T-cell acute lymphoblastic leukemia: a Pediatric Oncology Group report of 343 cases. Blood 2000;96:2543–2549.
71. Ferrando AA, Neuberg DS, Staunton J, et al. Gene expression signatures define novel oncogenic pathways in T cell acute lymphoblastic leukemia. Cancer Cell 2002;1:75–87.
72. Graux C, Cools J, Melotte C, et al. Fusion of NUP214 to ABL1 on amplified episomes in T-cell acute lymphoblastic leukemia. Nat Genet 2004;36:1084–1089.
73. Head DR. Revised classification of acute myeloid leukemia. Leukemia 1996;10:1826–1831.
74. Arber DA. Realistic pathologic classification of acute myeloid leukemias. Am J Clin Pathol 2001;115:552–560.
75. Bennett JM, Catovsky D, Daniel M-T, et al. Proposals for the classification of the acute leukemias. Br J Haematol 1976;33:451–458.
76. Bennett JM, Catovsky D, Daniel MT, et al. Proposed revised criteria for the classification of acute myeloid leukemia: a report of the French-American-British Cooperative Group. Ann Intern Med 1985;103:626–629.
77. Bennett JM, Catovsky D, Daniel M-T, et al. Criteria for the diagnosis of acute leukemia of megakaryocytic lineage (M7): a report of the French-American-British Cooperative Group. Ann Intern Med 1985;103:460–462.
78. Gilliland DG. Molecular genetics of human leukemias: new insights into therapy. Semin Hematol 2002;39:6–11.
79. Cornelissen JJ, van Putten WL, Verdonck LF, et al. Results of a HOVON/SAKK donor versus no-donor analysis of myeloablative HLA-identical sibling stem cell transplantation in first remission acute myeloid leukemia in young and middle-aged adults: benefits for whom? Blood 2007;109:3658–3666.
80. Lowenberg B. Acute myeloid leukemia: the challenge of capturing disease variety. Hematology Am Soc Hematol Educ Program 2008;1–11.
81. Schlenk RF, Dohner K, Krauter J, et al. Mutations and treatment outcome in cytogenetically normal acute myeloid leukemia. N Engl J Med 2008;358:1909–1918.
82. Arber DA, Carter NH, Ikle D, et al. Value of combined morphologic, cytochemical, and immunophenotypic features in predicting recurrent cytogenetic abnormalities in acute myeloid leukemia. Hum Pathol 2003;34:479–483.
83. Martinez-Climent JA, Lane NJ, et al. Clinical and prognostic significance of chromosomal abnormalities in childhood acute myeloid leukemia de novo. Leukemia 1995; 9:95–101.
84. Wells RJ, Arthur DC, Srivastava A, et al. Prognostic variables in newly diagnosed children and adolescents with acute myeloid leukemia: Children's Cancer Group Study 213. Leukemia 2002;16:601–607.
85. Forestier E, Heim S, Blennow E, et al. Cytogenetic abnormalities in childhood acute myeloid leukaemia: a Nordic series comprising all children enrolled in the NOPHO-93-AML trial between 1993 and 2001. Br J Haematol 2003;121:566–577.
86. Rubnitz JE, Raimondi SC, Halbert AR, et al. Characteristics and outcome of t(8;21)-positive childhood acute myeloid leukemia: a single institution's experience. Leukemia 2002;16:2072–2077.
87. Downing JR, Head DR, Curcio-Brint AM, et al. An AML/ETO fusion transcript is consistently detected by RNA-based polymerase chain reaction in acute myelogenous leukemia containing the (8;21)(q22;q22) translocation. Blood 1993;81:2860–2865.
88. Downing JR. The AML1-ETO chimaeric transcription factor in acute myeloid leukaemia: biology and clinical significance. Br J Haematol 1999;106:296–308.
89. Peterson LF, Zhang DE. The 8;21 translocation in leukemogenesis. Oncogene 2004;23: 4255–4262.
90. Higuchi M, O'Brien D, Kumaravelu P, et al. Expression of a conditional AML1-ETO oncogene bypasses embryonic lethality and establishes a murine model of human t(8;21) acute myeloid leukemia. Cancer Cell 2002;1:63–74.
91. Nakamura H, Kuriyama K, Sadamori N, et al. Morphological subtyping of acute myeloid leukemia with maturation (AML-M2): homogeneous pink-colored cytoplasm of mature neutrophils is most characteristic and AML-M2 with t(8;21). Leukemia 1997;11:651–655.
92. Kita K, Nakase K, Miwa H, et al. Phenotypical characteristics of acute myelocytic leukemia associated with the t(8;21)(q22;q22) chromosomal abnormality: frequent expression of immature B-cell antigen CD19 together with stem cell antigen CD34. Blood 1992;80:470–477.
93. Hurwitz CA, Raimondi SC, Head D, et al. Distinctive immunophenotypic features of t(8;21)(q22;q22) acute myeloblastic leukemia in children. Blood 1992;80:3182–3188.
94. Khoury H, Dalal BI, Nevill TJ, et al. Acute myelogenous leukemia with t(8;21)—identification of a specific immunophenotype. Leuk Lymphoma 2003;44:1713–1718.
95. Baer MR, Stewart CC, Lawrence D, et al. Expression of the neural cell adhesion molecule CD56 is associated with short remission duration and survival in acute myeloid leukemia with t(8;21)(q22;q22). Blood 1997;90:1643–1648.
96. Meshinchi S, Alonzo TA, Stirewalt DL, et al. Clinical implications of FLT3 mutations in pediatric AML. Blood 2006;108:3654–3661.
97. Goemans BF, Zwaan CM, Miller M, et al. Mutations in KIT and RAS are frequent events in pediatric core-binding factor acute myeloid leukemia. Leukemia 2005;19:1536–1542.
98. Shigesada K, van de SB, Liu PP. Mechanism of leukemogenesis by the inv(16) chimeric gene CBFB/PEBP2B-MHY11. Oncogene 2004;23:4297–4307.
99. LeBeau MM, Larson RA, Bitter MA, et al. Association of an inversion of chromosome 16 and abnormal marrow eosinophils in acute myelomonocytic leukemia. N Engl J Med 1983;309:630–636.
100. Larson RA, Williams SF, Le Beau MM, et al. Acute myelomonocytic leukemia with abnormal eosinophils and inv(16) or t(16;16) has a favorable prognosis. Blood 1986;68:1242–1249.
101. Sun X, Medeiros LJ, Lu D, et al. Dysplasia and high proliferation rate are common in acute myeloid leukemia with inv(16)(p13q22). Am J Clin Pathol 2003;120:236–245.

102. Ritter M, Thiede C, Schakel U, et al. Underestimation of inversion (16) in acute myeloid leukaemia using standard cytogenetics as compared with polymerase chain reaction: results of a prospective investigation. Br J Haematol 1997;98:969–972.
103. Adriaansen HJ, te Boekhorst PAW, Hagemeijer AM, et al. Acute myeloid leukemia M4 with bone marrow eosinophilia (M4Eo) and inv(16)(p13q22) exhibits a specific immunophenotype with CD2 expression. Blood 1993;81:3043–3051.
104. Arber DA, Stein AS, Carter NH, et al. Prognostic impact of acute myeloid leukemia classification: importance of detection of recurring cytogenetic abnormalities and multilineage dysplasia on survival. Am J Clin Pathol 2003;119:672–680.
105. Delaunay J, Vey N, Leblanc T, et al. Prognosis of inv(16)/t(16;16) acute myeloid leukemia (AML): a survey of 110 cases from the French AML Intergroup. Blood 2003;102:462–469.
106. Zelent A, Guidez F, Melnick A, et al. Translocations of the RAR alpha gene in acute promyelocytic leukemia. Oncogene 2001;20:7186–7203.
107. Rovelli A, Biondi A, Rajnoldi AC, et al. Microgranular variant of acute promyelocytic leukemia in children. J Clin Oncol 1992;10:1413–1418.
108. Gale RE, Hills R, Pizzey AR, et al. Relationship between FLT3 mutation status, biologic characteristics, and response to targeted therapy in acute promyelocytic leukemia. Blood 2005;106:3768–3776.
109. Wetzler M, McElwain BK, Stewart CC, et al. HLA-DR antigen-negative acute myeloid leukemia. Leukemia 2003;17:707–715.
110. Guglielmi C, Martelli MP, Diverio D, et al. Immunophenotype of adult and childhood acute promyelocytic leukaemia: correlation with morphology, type of PML gene breakpoint and clinical outcome: a cooperative Italian study on 196 cases. Br J Haematol 1998;102:1035–1041.
111. Neame PB, Soamboonsrup P, Leber B, et al. Morphology of acute promyelocytic leukemia with cytogenetic or molecular evidence for the diagnosis: characterization of additional microgranular variants. Am J Hematol 1997;6:131–142.
112. Lin P, Hao S, Medeiros LJ, et al. Expression of CD2 in acute promyelocytic leukemia correlates with short form of PML-RARalpha transcripts and poorer prognosis. Am J Clin Pathol 2004;121:402–407.
113. Arber DA, Brunning RD, Le Beau MM, et al. Acute myeloid leukaemia with recurrent genetic abnormalities. In: WHO classification of tumours of haematopoietic and lymphoid tissues. Lyon, France: IARC Press, 2008:110–123.
114. Ravindranath Y, Chang M, Steuber CP, et al. Pediatric Oncology Group (POG) studies of acute myeloid leukemia (AML): a review of four consecutive childhood AML trials conducted between 1981 and 2000. Leukemia 2005;19:2101–2116.
115. Meyer C, Schneider B, Jakob S, et al. The MLL recombinome of acute leukemias. Leukemia 2006;20:777–784.
116. Shih LY, Liang DC, Fu JF, et al. Characterization of fusion partner genes in 114 patients with de novo acute myeloid leukemia and MLL rearrangement. Leukemia 2006; 20:218–223.
117. Schnittger S, Kinkelin U, Schoch C, et al. Screening for MLL tandem duplication in 387 unselected patients with AML identify a prognostically unfavorable subset of AML. Leukemia 2000;14:796–804.
118. Dohner K, Tobis K, Ulrich R, et al. Prognostic significance of partial tandem duplications of the MLL gene in adult patients 16 to 60 years old with acute myeloid leukemia and normal cytogenetics: a study of the Acute Myeloid Leukemia Study Group Ulm. J Clin Oncol 2002;20:3254–3261.
119. Rubnitz JE, Raimondi SC, Tong X, et al. Favorable impact of the t(9;11) in childhood acute myeloid leukemia. J Clin Oncol 2002;20:2302–2309.
120. Alsabeh R, Brynes RK, Slovak ML, et al. Acute myeloid leukemia with t(6;9)(p23;q34): association with myelodysplasia, basophilia, and initial CD34 negative immunophenotype. Am J Clin Pathol 1997;107:430–437.
121. Slovak ML, Gundacker H, Bloomfield CD, et al. A retrospective study of 69 patients with t(6;9)(p23;q34) AML emphasizes the need for a prospective, multicenter initiative for rare "poor prognosis" myeloid malignancies. Leukemia 2006;20:1295–1297.
122. Oyarzo MP, Lin P, Glassman A, et al. Acute myeloid leukemia with t(6;9)(p23;q34) is associated with dysplasia and a high frequency of flt3 gene mutations. Am J Clin Pathol 2004;122:348–358.
123. Hasle H, Alonzo TA, Auvrignon A, et al. Monosomy 7 and deletion 7q in children and adolescents with acute myeloid leukemia: an international retrospective study. Blood 2007;109:4641–4647.
124. Lugthart S, van Drunen E, van Norden Y, et al. High EVI1 levels predict adverse outcome in acute myeloid leukemia: prevalence of EVI1 overexpression and chromosome 3q26 abnormalities underestimated. Blood 2008;111:4329–4337.
125. Lion T, Haas OA, Harbott J, et al. The translocation t(1;22)(p13;q13) is a nonrandom marker specifically associated with acute megakaryocytic leukemia in young children. Blood 1992;79:3325–3330.
126. Chan WC, Carroll A, Alvarado CS, et al. Acute megakaryoblastic leukemia in infants with t(1;22)(p13;q13) abnormality. Am J Clin Pathol 1992;98:214–221.
127. Bernstein J, Dastugue N, Haas OA, et al. Nineteen cases of the t(1;22)(p13;q13) acute megakaryoblastic leukaemia of infants/children and a review of 39 cases: report from a t(1;22) study group. Leukemia 2000;14:216–218.
128. Duchayne E, Fenneteau O, Pages MP, et al. Acute megakaryoblastic leukaemia: a national clinical and biological study of 53 adult and childhood cases by the Groupe Francais d'Hematologie Cellulaire (GFHC). Leuk Lymphoma 2003;44:49–58.
129. Athale UH, Kaste SC, Razzouk BI, et al. Skeletal manifestations of pediatric acute megakaryoblastic leukemia. J Pediatr Hematol Oncol 2002;24:561–565.
130. Falini B, Nicoletti I, Martelli MF, et al. Acute myeloid leukemia carrying cytoplasmic/mutated nucleophosmin (NPMc+ AML): biologic and clinical features. Blood 2007; 109:874–885.
131. Brown P, McIntyre E, Rau R, et al. The incidence and clinical significance of nucleophosmin mutations in childhood AML. Blood 2007;110:979–985.
132. Ho PA, Alonzo TA, Gerbing RB, et al. Prevalence and prognostic implications of CEBPA mutations in pediatric acute myeloid leukemia (AML): a report from the Children's Oncology Group. Blood 2009;113:6558–6566.
133. Raimondi SC, Chang MN, Ravindranath Y, et al. Chromosomal abnormalities in 478 children with acute myeloid leukemia: clinical characteristics and treatment outcome in a cooperative pediatric oncology group study-POG 8821. Blood 1999;94:3707–3716.
134. Hasle H, Niemeyer CM, Chessells JM, et al. A pediatric approach to the WHO classification of myelodysplastic and myeloproliferative diseases. Leukemia 2003;17:277–282.
135. Hijiya N, Ness KK, Ribeiro RC, et al. Acute leukemia as a secondary malignancy in children and adolescents: current findings and issues. Cancer 2009;115:23–35.
136. Rowley JD, Olney HJ. International workshop on the relationship of prior therapy to balanced chromosome aberrations in therapy-related myelodysplastic syndromes and acute leukemia: overview report. Genes Chromosomes Cancer 2002;33:331–345.
137. Bene MC, Bernier M, Casasnovas RO, et al. Acute myeloid leukaemia M0: haematological, immunophenotypic and cytogenetic characteristics and their prognostic significance: an analysis in 241 patients. Br J Haematol 2001;113:737–745.
138. Preudhomme C, Warot-Loze D, Roumier C, et al. High incidence of biallelic point mutations in the Runt domain of the AML1/PEBP2 alpha B gene in Mo acute myeloid leukemia and in myeloid malignancies with acquired trisomy 21. Blood 2000;96: 2862–2869.
139. Osato M, Yanagida M, Shigesada K, et al. Point mutations of the RUNx1/AML1 gene in sporadic and familial myeloid leukemias. Int J Hematol 2001;74:245–251.
140. Amadori S, Venditti A, Del Poeta G, et al. Minimally differentiated acute myeloid leukemia (AML-M0): a distinct clinico-biologic entity with poor prognosis. Ann Hematol 1996;72:208–215.
141. Park S, Picard F, Azgui Z, et al. Erythroleukemia: a comparison between the previous FAB approach and the WHO classification. Leuk Res 2002;26:423–429.
142. Park S, Picard F, Guesnu M, et al. Erythroleukemia and RAEB-t: a same disease? Leukemia 2004;18:888–890.
143. Athale UH, Razzouk BI, Raimondi SC, et al. Biology and outcome of childhood acute megakaryoblastic leukemia: a single institution's experience. Blood 2001;97: 3727–3732.
144. Wong KF, Yuen HL, Siu LL, et al. t(8;16)(p11;p13) predisposes to a transient but potentially recurring neonatal leukemia. Hum Pathol 2008;39:1702–1707.
145. D'Orazio JA, Pulliam JF, Moscow JA. Spontaneous resolution of a single lesion of myeloid leukemia cutis in an infant: case report and discussion. Pediatr Hematol Oncol 2008;25:457–468.
146. Haferlach T, Kohlmann A, Klein HU, et al. AML with translocation t(8;16)(p11;p13) demonstrates unique cytomorphological, cytogenetic, molecular and prognostic features. Leukemia 2009;23:934–943.
147. Traweek ST, Arber DA, Rappaport H, et al. Extramedullary myeloid cell tumors: an immunohistochemical and morphologic study of 28 cases. Am J Surg Pathol 1993;17: 1011–1019.
148. Chou ST, Opalinska JB, Yao Y, et al. Trisomy 21 enhances human fetal erythro-megakaryocytic development. Blood 2008;112:4503–4506.
149. Tunstall-Pedoe O, Roy A, Karadimitris A, et al. Abnormalities in the myeloid progenitor compartment in Down syndrome fetal liver precede acquisition of GATA1 mutations. Blood 2008;112:4507–4511.
150. Kurahashi H, Hara J, Yumura-Yagi K, et al. Transient abnormal myelopoiesis in Down's syndrome. Leuk Lymphoma 1992;8:465–475.
151. Zipursky A, Brown EJ, Christensen A, et al. Transient myeloproliferative disorder (transient leukemia) and hematologic manifestations of Down syndrome. Clin Lab Med 1999;19:157–167.
152. Isaacs H Jr. Fetal and neonatal leukemia. J Pediatr Hematol Oncol 2003;25:348–361.
153. Baumann I, Niemeyer CM, Brunning RD, et al. Myeloid proliferations related to Down syndrome. In: WHO classification of tumors of haematopoietic and lymphoid tissues. Lyon, France: IARC Press, 2008:142–144.
154. McElwaine S, Mulligan C, Groet J, et al. Microarray transcript profiling distinguishes the transient from the acute type of megakaryoblastic leukaemia (M7) in Down's syndrome, revealing PRAME as a specific discriminating marker. Br J Haematol 2004;125:729–742.
155. Gamis AS, Woods WG, Alonzo TA, et al. Increased age at diagnosis has a significantly negative effect on outcome in children with Down syndrome and acute myeloid leukemia: a report from the Children's Cancer Group Study 2891. J Clin Oncol 2003; 21:3415–3422.
156. Facchetti F, Jones DM, Petrella T. Blastic plasmacytoid dendritic cell neoplasm. In: WHO classification of tumours of heamatopoietic and lymphoid tissues. Lyon, France: IARC Press, 2008:145–147.
157. Feuillard J, Jacob MC, Valensi F, et al. Clinical and biologic features of CD4(+)CD56(+) malignancies. Blood 2002;99:1556–1563.
158. Hu SC, Tsai KB, Chen GS, et al. Infantile CD4+/CD56+ hematodermic neoplasm. Haematologica 2007;92:e91–e93.
159. Emanuel PD. Myelodysplasia and myeloproliferative disorders in childhood: an update. Br J Haematol 1999;105:852–863.
160. Luna-Fineman S, Shannon K, Atwater SK, et al. Myelodysplastic and myeloproliferative disorders of childhood: a study of 167 patients. Blood 1999;93:459–466.
161. Baumann I, Niemeyer CM, Bennett JM, et al. Childhood myelodysplastic syndrome. In: WHO classification of tumours of haematopoietic and lymphoid tissues. Lyon, France: IARC Press, 2008:104–107.
162. Tefferi A, Vardiman JW. Classification and diagnosis of myeloproliferative neoplasms: the 2008 World Health Organization criteria and point-of-care diagnostic algorithms. Leukemia 2008;22:14–22.
163. Aricò M, Biondi A, Pui C-H. Juvenile myelomonocytic leukemia. Blood 1997;90: 479–488.
164. Niemeyer CM, Fenu S, Hasle H, et al. Differentiating juvenile myelomonocytic leukemia from infectious disease. Blood 1998;91:365–367.
165. Baumann I, Bennett JM, Niemeyer CM, et al. Juvenile myelomonocytic leukaemia. In: WHO classification of tumours of haematopoietic and lymphoid tissues. Lyon, France: IARC Press, 2008:82–84.
166. Hasle H, Arico M, Basso G, et al. Myelodysplastic syndrome, juvenile myelomonocytic leukemia, and acute myeloid leukemia associated with complete or partial monosomy 7. Leukemia 1999;13:376–385.
167. Kardos G, Baumann I, Passmore SJ, et al. Refractory anemia in childhood: a retrospective analysis of 67 patients with particular reference to monosomy 7. Blood 2003;102: 1997–2003.
168. Niemeyer CM, Arico M, Basso G, et al. Chronic myelomonocytic leukemia in childhood: a retrospective analysis of 110 cases: European Working Group on Myelodysplastic Syndromes in Childhood (EWOG-MDS). Blood 1997;89:3534–3543.
169. Side L, Emanuel PD, Taylor B, et al. Mutations of the *NF1* gene in children with juvenile myelomonocytic leukemia without clinical evidence of neurofibromatosis, type 1. Blood 1998;92:267–272.
170. Loh ML, Sakai DS, Flotho C, et al. Mutations in CBL occur frequently in juvenile myelomonocytic leukemia. Blood 2009;114:1859–1863.
171. Koike K, Matsuda K. Recent advances in the pathogenesis and management of juvenile myelomonocytic leukaemia. Br J Haematol 2008;141:567–575.
172. Kotecha N, Flores NJ, Irish JM, et al. Single-cell profiling identifies aberrant STAT5 activation in myeloid malignancies with specific clinical and biologic correlates. Cancer Cell 2008;14:335–343.
173. Lukes RJ, Butler JJ. The pathology and nomenclature of Hodgkin's disease. Cancer Res 1966;26:1063–1083.

174. Lukes RJ, Carver LF, Hall TC, et al. Report of the nomenclature committee. Cancer Res 1966;26:1311.
175. Mason DY, Banks PM, Chan J, et al. Nodular lymphocyte predominance Hodgkin's disease: a distinct clinicopathological entity. Am J Surg Pathol 1994;18:526–530.
176. Mauch PM, Kalish LA, Kadin M, et al. Patterns of presentation of Hodgkin's disease: implications for etiology and pathogenesis. Cancer 1993;71:2062–2071.
177. Chittal SM, Caverivière P, Schwarting R, et al. Monoclonal antibodies in the diagnosis of Hodgkin's disease: the search for a rational panel. Am J Surg Pathol 1988;12:9–21.
178. Stein H, Marafioti T, Foss HD, et al. Down-regulation of BOB.1/OBF.1 and Oct2 in classical Hodgkin disease but not in lymphocyte predominant Hodgkin disease correlates with immunoglobulin transcription. Blood 2001;97:496–501.
179. Brauninger A, Hansmann ML, Strickler JG, et al. Identification of common germinal-center B-cell precursors in two patients with both Hodgkin's disease and non-Hodgkin's lymphoma. N Engl J Med 1999;340:1239–1247.
180. Marafioti T, Hummel M, Anagnostopoulos I, et al. Classical Hodgkin's disease and follicular lymphoma originating from the same germinal center B cell. J Clin Oncol 1999;17:3804–3809.
181. Marafioti T, Hummel M, Foss HD, et al. Hodgkin and Reed-Sternberg cells represent an expansion of a single clone originating from a germinal center B-cell with functional immunoglobulin gene rearrangements but defective immunoglobulin transcription. Blood 2000;95:1443–1450.
182. Weiss LM, Chen Y-Y, Liu X-F, et al. Epstein-Barr virus and Hodgkin's disease: a correlative in situ hybridization and polymerase chain reaction study. Am J Pathol 1991;139: 1259–1265.
183. Josting A, Wolf J, Diehl V. Hodgkin disease: prognostic factors and treatment strategies. Curr Opin Oncol 2000;12:403–411.
184. Strickler JG, Michie SA, Warnke RA, et al. The "syncytial variant" of nodular sclerosis Hodgkin's disease. Am J Surg Pathol 1986;10:470–477.
185. Savage KJ, Monti S, Kutok JL, et al. The molecular signature of mediastinal large B-cell lymphoma differs from that of other diffuse large B-cell lymphomas and shares features with classical Hodgkin lymphoma. Blood 2003;102:3871–3879.
186. Jaffe ES, Steinherz P, Swerdlow SH, et al. B-cell lymphoma, unclassifiable, with features intermediate between diffuse large B-cell lymphoma and classical Hodgkin lymphoma. In: WHO classification of tumors of haematopoietic and lymphoid tissues. Lyon, France: IARC Press, 2008:267–268.
187. Chang KL, Chen Y-Y, Shibata D, et al. Description of an in situ hybridization methodology for detection of Epstein-Barr virus RNA in paraffin-embedded tissues, with a survey of normal and neoplastic tissues. Diagn Mol Pathol 1992;1:246–255.
188. Ashton-Key M, Thorpe PA, Allen JP, et al. Follicular Hodgkin's disease. Am J Surg Pathol 1995;19:1294–1299.
189. Anagnostopoulos I, Hansmann ML, Franssila K, et al. European Task Force on Lymphoma project on lymphocyte predominance Hodgkin disease: histologic and immunohistologic analysis of submitted cases reveals 2 types of Hodgkin disease with a nodular growth pattern and abundant lymphocytes. Blood 2000;96:1889–1899.
190. Marafioti T, Hummel M, Anagnostopoulos I, et al. Origin of nodular lymphocyte-predominant Hodgkin's disease from a clonal expansion of highly mutated germinal-center B cells. N Engl J Med 1997;337:453–458.
191. Ohno T, Stribley JA, Wu G, et al. Clonality in nodular lymphocyte-predominant Hodgkin's disease. N Engl J Med 1997;337:459–465.
192. Nam-Cha SH, Roncador G, Sanchez-Verde L, et al. PD-1, a follicular T-cell marker useful for recognizing nodular lymphocyte-predominant Hodgkin lymphoma. Am J Surg Pathol 2008;32:1252–1257.
193. Burns BF, Colby TV, Dorfman RF. Differential diagnostic features of nodular L&H Hodgkin's disease, including progressive transformation of germinal centers. Am J Surg Pathol 1984;8:253–261.
194. Rappaport H. Tumors of the hematopoietic system. Washington, DC: Armed Forces Institute of Pathology, 1966:1–442.
195. National Cancer Institute sponsored study of classifications of non-Hodgkin's lymphomas: summary and description of a working formulation for clinical usage: The Non-Hodgkin's Lymphoma Pathologic Classification Project. Cancer 1982;49: 2112–2135.
196. Harris NL, Jaffe ES, Stein H, et al. A revised European-American classification of lymphoid neoplasms: a proposal from the International Lymphoma Study Group. Blood 1994;84:1361–1392.
197. Wilson JF, Kjeldsberg CR, Sposto R, et al. The pathology of non-Hodgkin's lymphoma of childhood, II: reproducibility and relevance of the histologic classification of "undifferentiated" lymphomas (Burkitt's versus non-Burkitt's). Hum Pathol 1987;18: 1008–1014.
198. Hutchison RE, Murphy SB, Fairclough DL, et al. Diffuse small noncleaved cell lymphoma in children, Burkitt's versus non-Burkitt's types: results from the Pediatric Oncology Group and St. Jude Children's Research Hospital. Cancer 1989;64:23–28.
199. Leoncini L, Rafael M, Stein H, et al. Burkitt lymphoma. In: WHO classification of tumours of haematopoietic and lymphoid tissues. Lyon, France: IARC Press, 2008: 262–264.
200. Gelb AB, van de RM, Warnke RA, et al. Pregnancy-associated lymphomas: a clinicopathologic study. Cancer 1996;78:304–310.
201. Arber DA, Simpson JR, Weiss LM, et al. Non-Hodgkin's lymphoma involving the breast. Am J Surg Pathol 1994;18:288–295.
202. Braziel RM, Arber DA, Slovak ML, et al. The Burkitt-like lymphomas: a Southwest Oncology Group study delineating phenotypic, genotypic, and clinical features. Blood 2001;97:3713–3720.
203. Dalla-Favera R, Bregni M, Erikson J, et al. Human c-*myc onc* gene is located on the region of chromosome 8 that is translocated in Burkitt lymphoma cells. Proc Natl Acad Sci U S A 1982;79:7824–7827.
204. Nakamura N, Nakamine H, Tamaru J, et al. The distinction between Burkitt lymphoma and diffuse large B-cell lymphoma with c-myc rearrangement. Mod Pathol 2002;15:771–776.
205. Stein H, Warnke RA, Chan WC, et al. Diffuse large B-cell lymphoma, not otherwise specified. In: WHO classification of tumors of haematopoietic and lymphoid tissues. Lyon, France: IARC Press, 2008:233–237.
206. Alizadeh AA, Eisen MB, Davis RE, et al. Distinct types of diffuse large B-cell lymphoma identified by gene expression profiling. Nature 2000;403:503–511.
207. Rosenwald A, Wright G, Chan WC, et al. The use of molecular profiling to predict survival after chemotherapy for diffuse large-B-cell lymphoma. N Engl J Med 2002;346: 1937–1947.
208. Lorsbach RB, Shay-Seymore D, Moore J, et al. Clinicopathologic analysis of follicular lymphoma occurring in children. Blood 2002;99:1959–1964.
209. Taddesse-Heath L, Pittaluga S, Sorbara L, et al. Marginal zone B-cell lymphoma in children and young adults. Am J Surg Pathol 2003;27:522–531.
210. Stein H, Foss HD, Durkop H, et al. CD30(+) anaplastic large cell lymphoma: a review of its histopathologic, genetic, and clinical features. Blood 2000;96:3681–3695.
211. Delsol G, Ralfkiaer E, Stein H, et al. Anaplastic large cell lymphoma. In: World Health Organization classification of tumors: pathology and genetics of tumours of haematopoietic and lymphoid tissues. Lyon, France: IARC Press, 2001:230–235.
212. Morris SW, Xue L, Ma Z, et al. Alk+ CD30+ lymphomas: a distinct molecular genetic subtype of non-Hodgkin's lymphoma. Br J Haematol 2001;113:275–295.
213. Kadin ME, Sako D, Berliner N, et al. Childhood Ki-1 lymphoma presenting with skin lesions and peripheral lymphadenopathy. Blood 1986;68:1042–1049.
214. Sandlund JT, Pui CH, Roberts WM, et al. Clinicopathologic features and treatment outcome of children with large-cell lymphoma and the t(2;5)(p23;q35). Blood 1994;84: 2467–2471.
215. Sandlund JT, Pui CH, Santana VM, et al. Clinical features and treatment outcome for children with CD30+ large-cell non-Hodgkin's lymphoma. J Clin Oncol 1994;12: 895–898.
216. Reiter A, Schrappe M, Tiemann M, et al. Successful treatment strategy for Ki-1 anaplastic large-cell lymphoma of childhood: a prospective analysis of 62 patients enrolled in three consecutive Berlin-Frankfurt-Munster group studies. J Clin Oncol 1994;12: 899–908.
217. Brugieres L, Deley MC, Pacquement H, et al. CD30(+) anaplastic large-cell lymphoma in children: analysis of 82 patients enrolled in two consecutive studies of the French Society of Pediatric Oncology. Blood 1998;92:3591–3598.
218. Alessandri AJ, Pritchard SL, Schultz KR, et al. A population-based study of pediatric anaplastic large cell lymphoma. Cancer 2002;94:1830–1835.
219. Hodges KB, Collins RD, Greer JP, et al. Transformation of the small cell variant Ki-1+ lymphoma to anaplastic large cell lymphoma: pathologic and clinical features. Am J Surg Pathol 1999;23:49–58.
220. Kinney MC, Collins RD, Greer JP, et al. A small-cell-predominant variant of primary Ki-1 (CD30)+ T-cell lymphoma. Am J Surg Pathol 1993;17:859–868.
221. Pileri S, Falini B, Delsol G, et al. Lymphohistiocytic T-cell lymphoma (anaplastic large cell lymphoma CD30+/Ki-1+ with a high content of reactive histiocytes). Histopathology 1990;16:383–391.
222. Pileri SA, Pulford K, Mori S, et al. Frequent expression of the NPM-ALK chimeric fusion protein in anaplastic large-cell lymphoma, lympho-histiocytic type. Am J Pathol 1997;150:1207–1211.
223. Chan JK, Ng CS, Hui PK, et al. Anaplastic large cell Ki-1 lymphoma: delineation of two morphological types. Histopathology 1989;15:11–34.
224. Kutok JL, Aster JC. Molecular biology of anaplastic lymphoma kinase-positive anaplastic large-cell lymphoma. J Clin Oncol 2002;20:3691–3702.
225. de Bruin PC, Beljaards RC, van Heerde P, et al. Differences in clinical behaviour and immunophenotype between primary cutaneous and primary nodal anaplastic large cell lymphoma of T-cell or null cell phenotype. Histopathology 1993;23:127–135.
226. Cataldo KA, Jalal SM, Law ME, et al. Detection of t(2;5) in anaplastic large cell lymphoma: comparison of immunohistochemical studies, FISH, and RT-PCR in paraffin-embedded tissue. Am J Surg Pathol 1999;23:1386–1392.
227. Wilson MS, Weiss LM, Gatter KC, et al. Malignant histiocytosis: a reassessment of cases previously reported in 1975 based on paraffin section immunophenotyping studies. Cancer 1990;66:530–536.
228. Cooke CB, Krenacs L, Stetler-Stevenson M, et al. Hepatosplenic T-cell lymphoma: a distinct clinicopathologic entity of cytotoxic γδ T-cell origin. Blood 1996;88:4265–4274.
229. Weidmann E. Hepatosplenic T cell lymphoma: a review on 45 cases since the first report describing the disease as a distinct lymphoma entity in 1990. Leukemia 2000;14:991–997.
230. Gaulard P, Jaffe ES, Krenacs L, et al. Hepatosplenic T-cell lymphoma. In: WHO classification of tumours of haematopoietic and lymphoid tissues. Lyon, France: IARC Press, 2008:292–293.
231. Sun T, Brody J, Susin M, et al. Extranodal T-cell lymphoma mimicking malignant histiocytosis. Am J Hematol 1990;35:269–274.
232. Nosari A, Oreste PL, Biondi A, et al. Hepato-splenic gammadelta T-cell lymphoma: a rare entity mimicking the hemophagocytic syndrome. Am J Hematol 1999;60:61–65.
233. Macon WR, Levy NB, Kurtin PJ, et al. Hepatosplenic alpha beta T-cell lymphomas—a report of 14 cases and comparison with hepatosplenic gamma delta T-cell lymphomas. Am J Surg Pathol 2001;25:285–296.
234. Swerdlow SH, Webber SA, Chadburn A, et al. Post-transplant lymphoproliferative disorders. In: WHO classification of tumours of haematopoietic and lymphoid tissues. Lyon, France: IARC Press, 2008:343–349.
235. van Krieken JH, Onciu M, Elenitoba-Johnson KSJ, et al. Lymphoproliferative diseases associated with primary immune disorders. In: WHO classification of tumours of haematopoietic and lymphoid tissues. Lyon, France: IARC Press, 2009:336–339.
236. Bucsky P, Favara B, Feller AC, et al. Malignant histiocytosis and large cell anaplastic (Ki-1) lymphoma in childhood: guidelines for differential diagnosis—report of the Histiocyte Society. Med Pediatr Oncol 1994;22:200–203.
237. Favara BE, Feller AC. Contemporary classification of histiocytic disorders. Med Pediatr Oncol 1997;29:157–166.
238. Alessi DM, Maceri D. Histiocytosis X of the head and neck in a pediatric population. Arch Otolaryngol Head Neck Surg 1992;118:945–948.
239. Willman CL, Busque L, Griffith BB, et al. Langerhans'-cell histiocytosis (histiocytosis X)—a clonal proliferative disease. N Engl J Med 1994;331:154–160.
240. Angeli SI, Alcalde J, Hoffman HT, et al. Langerhans' cell histiocytosis of the head and neck in children. Ann Otol Rhinol Laryngol 1995;104:173–180.
241. Coppes-Zantinga A, Egeler RM. The Langerhans cell histiocytosis X files revealed. Br J Haematol 2002;116:3–9.
242. Jaffe R, Weiss LM, Facchetti F. Tumours derived from Langerhans cells. In: WHO classification of tumours of haematopoietic and lymphoid tissues. Lyon, France: IARC Press, 2008:358–360.
243. Horny H-P, Metcalfe DD, Bennett JM, et al. Mastocytosis. In: WHO classification of tumours of haematopoietic and lymphoid tissues. Lyon, France: IARC Press, 2008:54–63.
244. Bain BJ. Systemic mastocytosis and other mast cell neoplasms. Br J Haematol 1999; 106:9–17.
245. Yang F, Tran T-A, Carlson JA, et al. Paraffin section immunophenotype of cutaneous and extracutaneous mast cell disease: comparison to other hematopoietic neoplasms. Am J Surg Pathol 2000;24:703–709.
246. Escribano L, Diaz-Agustin B, Lopez A, et al. Immunophenotypic analysis of mast cells in mastocytosis: when and how to do it: Proposals of the Spanish Network on Mastocytosis (REMA). Cytometry B Clin Cytom 2004;58:1–8.

CHAPTER 8 ■ DIAGNOSTIC PATHOLOGY OF PEDIATRIC MALIGNANCIES

TIMOTHY J. TRICHE, JOHN HICKS, AND POUL H.B. SORENSEN

OVERVIEW

Cancer in children and adolescents is distinct from that seen in adults and requires a different approach to diagnosis and treatment. The fact that most pediatric tumors are of either mesenchymal or neuroectodermal origin, whereas the majority of adult cancers are of epithelial origin, sets childhood cancer apart.[1–5] In addition, the primary mode of treatment in adults is surgery, whereas in children, chemotherapy in combination with surgery and radiation therapy is utilized quite successfully. The advent of multimodal therapy protocols brought with it the need to tailor treatment to specific tumor types and subgroups in children. While outcomes have improved dramatically in children, there is an attendant cost with an eightfold increased risk of serious illness related to treatment, and more than 40% will experience significant morbidity or mortality due to sequelae of their therapy.[6] It is of increasing importance to tailor therapy to meet the minimum needs for successful outcome, when adjusted for known risk factors. This is the reason for the widespread use of risk-adjusted therapy in childhood cancer protocols. Outcome in pediatric cancers is directly linked to treatment protocols developed for a specific cancer. Failure to provide an accurate diagnosis for enrollment on a tumor-specific protocol may result in a less than optimal outcome and prognosis. This critical link between a precise diagnosis (including not only diagnosis but also prognostic subgroup, as in neuroblastoma [NB], leukemia, and sarcomas) and optimal outcome places considerable demands on the pediatric pathologist to correctly classify tumors by using a variety of diagnostic tools. During the past decades, there has been a concerted and highly organized approach to childhood cancer treatment. The vast majority of children younger than 16 years in the United Sates (>90%) are enrolled on cooperative group treatment protocols. These protocols have mandated tumor-specific specialized diagnostic methods and biologic marker assessment in conjunction with routine pathologic evaluation.[7] Many pediatric tumors lack morphologic evidence of differentiation that denotes histogenesis or are of ambiguous lineage. These pediatric neoplasms have been referred to as the "small round cell tumors" (SRCTs; although many are not in fact "round," but all are poorly differentiated). Many of these tumors may be classified into appropriate categories when a battery of immunohistochemical, *in situ* hybridization, ultrastructural, and molecular diagnostic procedures are applied.[8] The recent availability of whole-genome techniques has created additional diagnostic tools that provide important insight into histogenesis, pathogenesis, and potential targeted therapy. This may lead to improved survival with reduced treatment-related morbidity and mortality.[9–12] Many of these specialized diagnostic procedures are not familiar to general pathologists who deal primarily with adult cancer patients and may be overlooked in the diagnostic workup of pediatric tumors.

With childhood cancer, a well-defined diagnostic workup and standardized diagnostic modalities are required to accurately classify these tumors. Certain tumor types present particular problems in diagnosis (e.g., the "small round cell" or undifferentiated tumors) or in prognostic classification (leukemia, brain tumors, lymphoma, NB, rhabdomyosarcoma [RMS]). Certain clinical protocols for non-RMS soft tissue sarcomas provide for risk-adjusted therapy based on identification of prognostic subgroups. The intent of this chapter is to provide useful diagnostic and prognostic guidelines for pediatric tumors. In addition, we discuss new diagnostic methods and technologies that improve diagnostic accuracy and enhance our understanding of certain childhood cancers. These are of particular interest, as they are not based on morphology. Rather, they typically depend on the identification of unique genomic defects that are intrinsic to many of these tumors. The quintessential example is the amplified MYCN gene identified in poor prognosis NB more than 20 years ago.[13] Many more examples will be discussed later in this chapter. The final portion of the chapter discusses tumors that can be a diagnostic and oncologic challenge and evolving concepts that are helpful in these difficult to classify tumors.

Unique Challenge of Childhood Cancer Diagnosis: Age, Ethnicity, and Genetic Factors

Epithelial origin cancers (carcinomas) are unusual in children but common in adults. In contrast, retinoblastoma is associated with young children and unknown in adults.[14] It is important to remember that childhood cancer bears little resemblance to adult cancer, as demonstrated by the childhood tumor types illustrated in Figure 8.1. The common carcinomas (breast, lung, colon, prostate) dominate the adult cancer experience but are rarely seen in children. In contrast, mesodermal-derived tumors (leukemia, lymphoma, and sarcoma) and neural tumors (brain and NB) dominate childhood cancer. Pediatric and young adult age groups share certain tumors, such as the Ewing's sarcoma family of tumors (ESFTs), osteosarcoma (OS), synovial sarcoma (SS), and RMS.[5] These tumors possess the same morphology in both the pediatric and adult populations and are treated with similar protocols.

Age Versus Tumor Type

Many pediatric tumors are associated with specific age ranges (Fig. 8.2). Overall cancer incidence is highest just after birth and declines to its lowest point by 10 years of age. This reflects *in utero* oncogenesis and growth for many of these blastemal tumors. These neoplasms represent embryonal tumors that resemble primordial cells from specific organ systems, such as RMS (skeletal muscle), Wilms' tumor (WT) (developing kidney), and NB (sympathetic peripheral nervous system). After

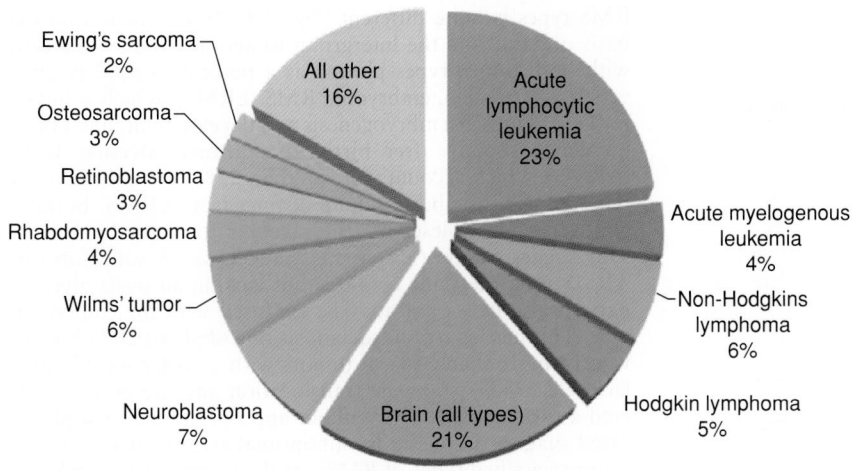

FIGURE 8.1 Distribution of childhood cancer. The first four slices of this pie chart account for approximately one-third of childhood malignancy and are accounted for by acute lymphocytic leukemia (approximately one-fourth) and acute myelogenous leukemia, non-Hodgkin lyphoma, and Hodgkin lymphoma (the remaining three wedges). The next most common category is brain tumors, which account for approximately 20% of all childhood tumors. This is followed by neuroblastoma and Wilms' tumor, which are roughly equal in incidence. Rhabdomyosarcoma, retinoblastoma, osteosarcoma, and Ewing's sarcoma account for the remaining four defined wedges of the pie chart. All other tumors account for less than 20% of all childhood tumors in aggregate. Notably absent from the previous is any significant incidence of carcinoma, the most common form of adult cancer.

the first decade of life, there is a linear increase in nonembryonal cancers that extends into adulthood. These tumors are distinct from childhood embryonal tumors and common adulthood carcinomas. Although environmental and lifestyle factors play major roles in adult carcinomas, these factors are of no known importance in childhood tumor oncogenesis.

Specific childhood tumors have distinct age predilections. Figure 8.3 illustrates this connection with peripheral neuroectodermal tumors, such as NB and the ESFTs. Although these tumors affect persons of different age ranges, they may have similar morphologic features that require nonmorphologic diagnostic methods to determine the precise diagnosis

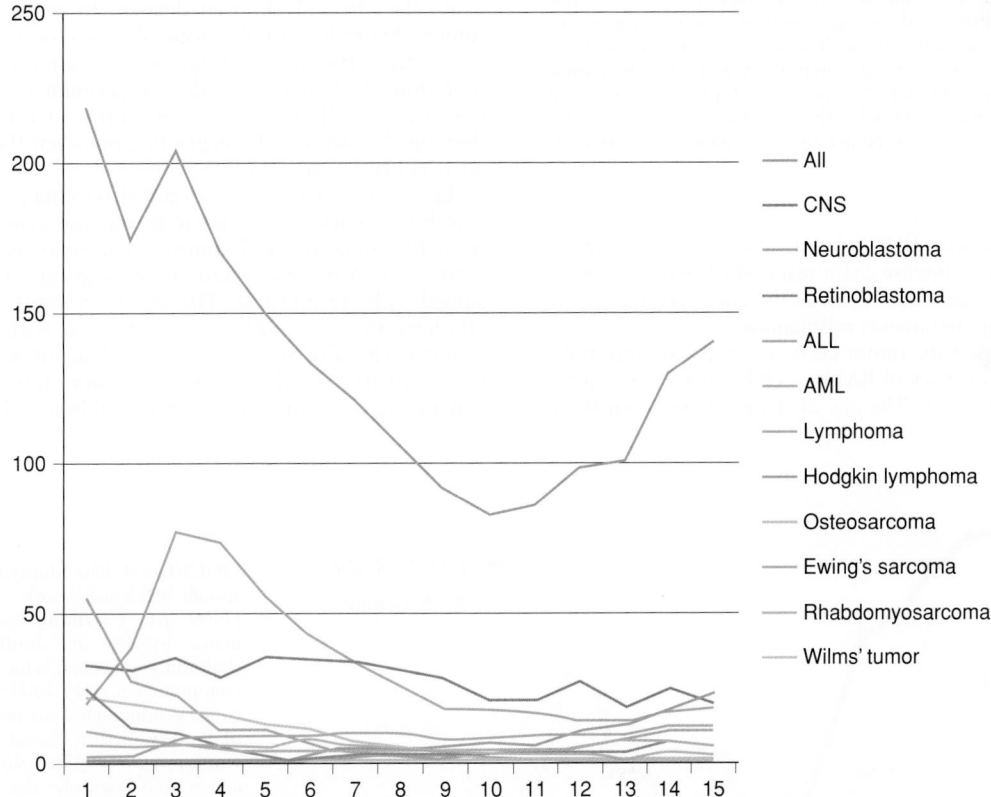

FIGURE 8.2 Childhood cancer: age incidence. That childhood cancer is largely embryonal in character is immediately evident from this chart of age incidence. The **top line,** which represents all forms of childhood cancer, shows a nearly linear increase from birth until approximately 10 years of age at which time the slope of the line reverses and begins to climb steadily toward adult-type incidences found later in life, largely due to the appearance of adult-type malignancies (not detailed here). The overall high incidence at birth is largely attributable to neuroblastoma, which generally presents in the first or second year of life. The large peak seen at approximately 3 years of age is due to the peak incidence of the most common form of childhood cancer, acute lymphocytic leukemia (ALL). Because of the lesser frequency, all the other tumors seem to be relatively constant in incidence (e.g., brain tumors, the next most common malignancy seen here), but in reality, striking differences in ages are found here as well. CNS, central nervous system, AML, acute myeloid leukemia.

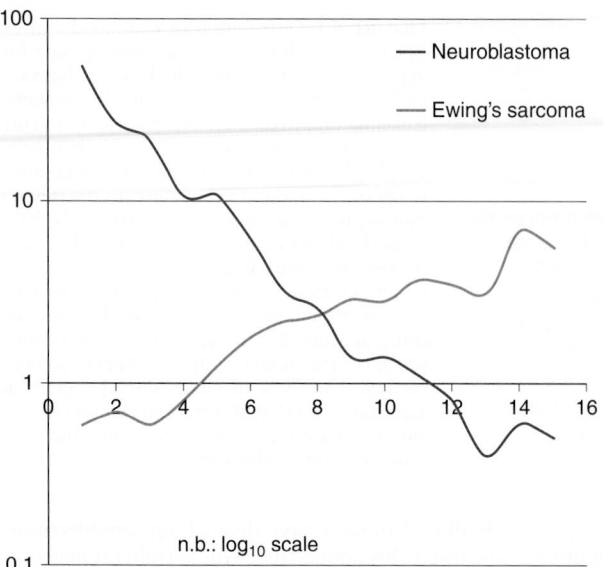

FIGURE 8.3 Neuroblastoma versus Ewing's sarcoma: age-specific incidence. Although the two most common neural tumors in childhood are neuroblastoma and Ewing's sarcoma, respectively, they are strikingly different in their incidence and character (age, incidence rate), despite their common phenotype. This is evident from this graph in which neuroblastoma is clearly a largely congenital tumor most common at birth and declining to extreme rarity by the age of 7 years, versus Ewing's sarcoma with a nearly linear increase from birth when it is exceedingly uncommon to the age of 14 years when it reaches a maximum in the pediatric age group. From this, one would assume that the genetic origins for the two phenotypically similar tumors are distinctly different. Note that the incidence data are plotted on a log₁₀ scale.

(immunohistochemistry [IHC], fluorescence *in situ* hybridization [FISH], and polymerase chain reaction [PCR]; *vide infra*). The patient's age alone may provide the clue that directs the diagnostic workup and avoids misdiagnosis.

Even within a specific tumor class, age plays an important role. The dominant types of RMSs in children are the embryonal and alveolar types. The age at diagnosis between these RMS types is quite different (Fig. 8.4). In this figure, on the basis of data from the Intergroup Rhabdomyosarcoma Study, with both tumor types plotted as a percent of total (y-axis) versus age (x-axis), embryonal RMS (ERMS), which is linked to skeletal muscle embryogenesis and development, has a peak incidence shortly after birth. In contrast, alveolar RMS (ARMS), which accounts for less than 25% of the total, has a bimodal age distribution quite distinct from ERMS. In older children and adolescents, the alveolar form predominates. This suggests a very different pathogenesis. A solid form of ARMS with the same cytology but lacking an overt alveolar pattern also exists and may be confused with the embryonal type. This has led to a misdiagnosis rate of about 20%.[15] Conversely, more than 25% of tumors with alveolar morphology lack a characteristic gene translocation and are best considered a form of ERMS.[16] Without appropriate use of sophisticated diagnostic methods, suboptimal treatment may occur for misclassified types of RMSs, as the prognosis for ERMS is much better than that for ARMS.

Genetic Factors

Genetic factors, such as inherited gene defects, are not uncommon in childhood tumors. The prototypic example is familial versus sporadic retinoblastoma.[17] Children with familial tumors possess a constitutional mutation in one Rb gene allele. With mutation or loss of the remaining normal Rb gene, the affected children develop bilateral and multiple tumors. Sporadic retinoblastoma does not occur bilaterally or as multiple tumors in children with nonfamilial sporadic mutations. Li-Fraumeni syndrome (germline p53 mutation) is another example in which many different tumor types can develop throughout life, depending on when the normal p53 allele is lost or mutated.[18,19]

Ethnicity may be an important determinant of cancer susceptibility. There is no classic mendelian gene defect, as in retinoblastoma and Li-Fraumeni syndrome, ascribed to ethnicity. Yet to be discovered complex genetic traits are presumed to be responsible. The classic example of the role of ethnicity in tumorigenesis is illustrated with ESFTs. This tumor is virtually unknown in individuals of African or (to a lesser extent) Asian descent (Fig. 8.5). In contrast, Ewing's sarcoma is more common than OS in children and young adults

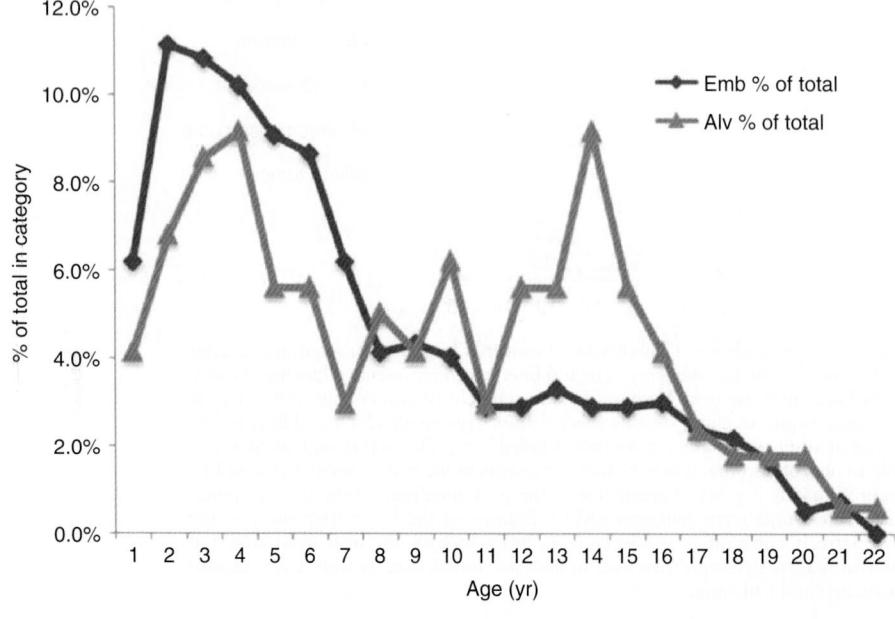

FIGURE 8.4 Rhabdomyosarcoma: age-specific incidence. Another childhood neoplasm with a striking variation in incidence by age is childhood alveolar rhabdomyosarcoma, which although less common than embryonal rhabdomyosarcoma is nonetheless an important source of fatality in this disease because of its worse prognosis. When plotted as percentage of total cases, alveolar rhabdomyosarcoma shows a bimodal age incidence, the first mode roughly corresponding to the peak age incidence of embryonal rhabdomyosarcoma, and the second mode with no parallel increase in embryonal rhabdomyosarcoma seen at approximately 14 years of age. Studies have suggested that the two modes are in fact genetically distinct as well; the first mode includes mostly PAX7-FOXO1A tumors, while the second is largely PAX3 (see text).

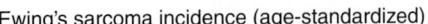

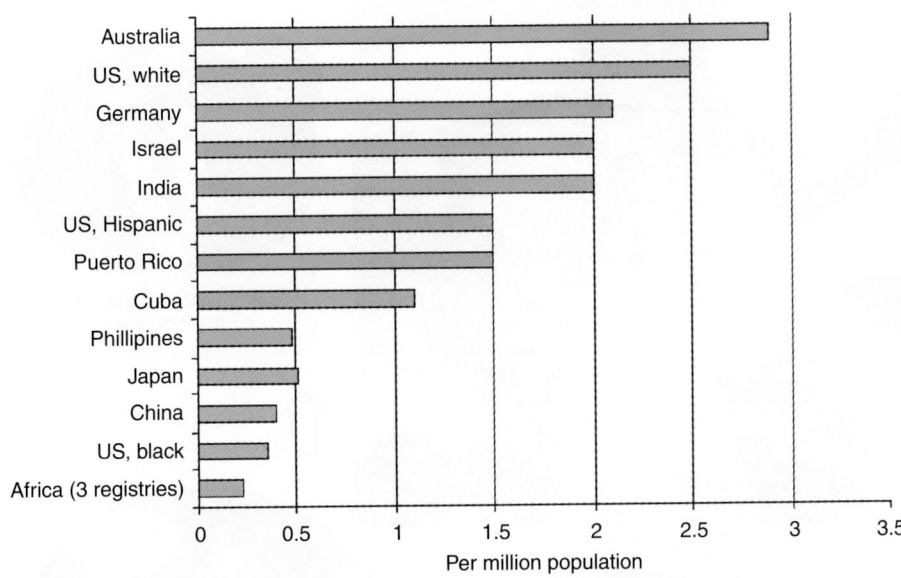

Ewing's sarcoma incidence (age-standardized)

Per million population

FIGURE 8.5 Ewing's sarcoma family of tumors: ethnicity versus incidence. U.S. SEER data from the National Cancer Institute documents striking differences in the incidence of Ewing's sarcoma family tumors among different ethnic groups. Australia reports the highest incidence on a per million population basis, whereas three different African registries report the lowest incidence reported anywhere in the world. U.S. blacks and other Asian populations also have an extremely low incidence of Ewing's sarcoma. These observations have strongly suggested a genetic component to Ewing's susceptibility, but the genetic predisposing factors have not yet been identified. (Data courtesy of Jonathan Buckley, M.D., Ph.D., Preventive Medicine, Keck School of Medicine, USC.)

of northern European descent.[2,20,21] Even more surprising, the tumor is most common in Spanish, Israeli (non-Arabic), and Polynesian (Maori, Hawaiian) populations. Epidemiologic studies have documented other less striking differences in tumor-type incidence among ethnic populations.[5,22] Knowledge of a patient's ethnicity can be a helpful adjunct in diagnosis, particularly with undifferentiated childhood tumors, such as an African American child with a differential diagnosis of NB versus ESFT is far more likely to have NB, based on these criteria.

Current Approach to Childhood Tumor Diagnosis

Pathology has been transformed by new diagnostic technology, instruments, and knowledge gained from advances in immunology, molecular biology, genomics, and proteomics during the past few decades. This has changed the methods used to arrive at a diagnosis. No longer is gross examination and light microscopy, in conjunction with clinical information, the only means to derive the diagnosis. Almost all childhood tumors require some combination of immunochemical, cytogenetic, *in situ* hybridization, ultrastructural, and/or molecular genetic methods to achieve an accurate diagnosis or identification of a prognostic group.[8,23–26] These tools not only have dramatically increased diagnostic precision but also have allowed for improved correlation of diagnosis with clinical behavior, response to therapy, and outcome. Newer genomic methods will further enhance clinically relevant diagnosis and lead to new concepts of tumor classification and targeted "designer" therapy.[23,27,28]

Specific tumor types and their optimal diagnostic evaluation are discussed in detail elsewhere. A brief mention of specific examples will suffice to make the point. No child with suspected leukemia, lymphoma, or NB on a Children's Oncology Group (COG) protocol will fail to have ancillary diagnostic procedures performed to detect gene translocations, antigen expression, or gene amplification, respectively. The availability of advanced diagnostic procedures common to childhood cancer evaluation is unusual in adult cancer centers,

a striking difference often overlooked by adult cancer diagnosticians. This is unfortunate because these advanced diagnostic procedures require special handling (e.g., fresh viable tumor tissue for short-term culture and cytogenetics, fresh frozen tissue for flow cytometry and molecular analysis) that are generally not part of the routine diagnostic workup for adult cancers. In many cases, local institutions lack the facilities to perform these advanced diagnostic studies. In this situation, tissue can still be handled according to prescribed protocols that ensure proper tissue handling and transportation to a central reference laboratory that performs the appropriate studies. The COG, which treats the majority of children with cancer in North America, maintains a central reference facility, the Biopathology Center, in Columbus, Ohio, which receives these specimens from the nearly 250 participating institutions and offers a number of these advanced diagnostic procedures, as well as central pathology review for many of the treatment protocols. If the primary pathologist is not familiar with the proper protocol or diagnostic procedures required, the opportunity to provide additional diagnostic, treatment, and prognostic information derived from specialized tests may be lost. It is useful to have a well-defined protocol and action plan for childhood tumor diagnosis to avoid loss of critically needed diagnostic information.

With routine handling of childhood tumor tissue as prescribed by the COG (Fig. 8.6), optimal evaluation of childhood tumors will be realized.[29] Many pediatric tumors will not be handled by pediatric pathologists familiar with these protocols. It is important for the clinician to discuss the importance of ancillary tests, the availability of reference laboratories, and tumor protocols with the responsible pathologist prior to tumor biopsy or resection. The diagram (Fig. 8.6) illustrates the single most important principle: *Tissue must not be placed into fixative in the operating room!* This single oversight is responsible for most lost diagnostic opportunities. This is also the reason why tissue may not be available for many molecular diagnostics and biomedical research. Fixed tissue has very limited utility for molecular genetic diagnostic procedures and may limit conventional diagnostic techniques, such as immunocytochemistry and electron microscopy (EM). In an attempt to promote nonroutine tissue handling, many childhood cancer protocols specifically request submission of

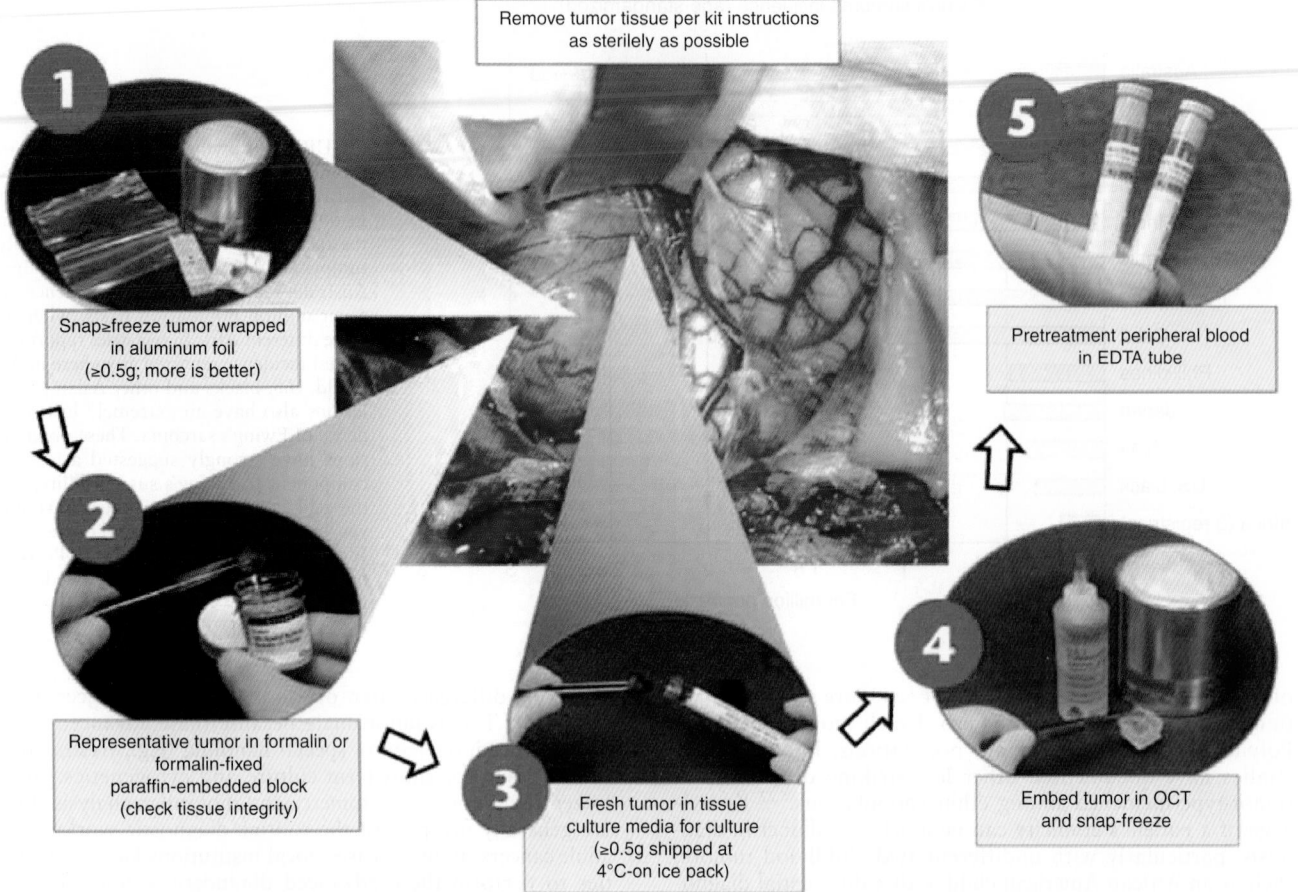

FIGURE 8.6 Tissue handling diagram. Tissue for optimal pathologic and biologic studies requires specialized handling as summarized in this chart. This diagram, which has been used by participating institutions in the Children's Oncology Group for more than 15 years, has been widely adopted and led to significant improvements in diagnostic accuracy in childhood cancer. Note that fresh tissue, not fixed, is required at the outset, for steps 1, 3, and 4. A pretreatment peripheral blood (for DNA from buffy coat and protein from plasma) is required for step 5 and will allow comparison of tumor versus normal DNA, an increasingly important part of the cancer diagnostic workup (see "Molecular Diagnostics" section). Diagram created by Steve Qualman, M.D., for Children's Oncology Group.

fresh frozen or even viable tumor tissue. Despite these efforts, no protocol ever achieves perfect compliance with these protocol requirements. As a result, many of the necessary diagnostic procedures have been (and continue to be) adapted to formalin-fixed, paraffin-embedded (FFPE) tissue. FISH on FFPE tissue for MYCN amplification instead of frozen tissue for DNA extraction and Southern blotting in NB is one example.[30]

The second stage of tissue handling (Fig. 8.6) is simply precautionary: If tissue is divided into multiple forms for specific use as needed in subsequent diagnostic procedures, nothing is lost. If not, the opportunity to perform diagnostic procedures will be lost. Failure to set aside fresh tissue precludes fluorescence-activated cell sorting (FACS-flow cytometry) analysis, which is necessary for the diagnosis of leukemia and lymphoma. Tissue placed in transport or culture medium for cytogenetics and establishment of tumor cell lines is important. Frozen tissue is perhaps even more important, as all manners of molecular diagnostics (particularly for RNA) are now possible. Small tumor portions in cryopreservative matrix (OCT) are invaluable for a "second look" to compare pretreatment and posttreatment tumor for chemosensitivity and new diagnostic methods, such as gene expression profiling. EM, a

mainstay for childhood tumor diagnosis, requires glutaraldehyde fixation for optimal interpretation.

If these procedures are followed, all diagnostic modalities available currently and in the foreseeable future may be employed. Because tissue is not always triaged appropriately, diagnostic techniques that provide similar information from fixed and processed tumor tissue have been developed. Cytogenetic analysis for a chromosomal translocation can now be partially substituted by PCR, FISH, and chromogen *in situ* hybridization (CISH) analyses[31] and single nucleotide polymorphism (SNP) arrays.[32] Gene amplification can be detected by FISH.[30,33,34] Antigen retrieval methods allow monoclonal antibody–mediated detection of scant antigens otherwise detectable only by FACS.[35] These alternative methods sometimes contradict the diagnosis determined by conventional methods and may themselves be open to interpretation: What if the PCR is negative? What if the FISH analysis has a high background due to formalin-induced fluorescence that obscures the signal? What if both are performed but the results disagree with one another? What if the immunocytochemical results are equivocal or contradict the molecular genetic data? It is possible to render an appropriate diagnosis in most cases, but it is clear that adherence to a standardized

TABLE 8.1

TOP TEN DIAGNOSTIC METHODS FOR TUMOR DIAGNOSIS

Method	Comment
1. Light microscopy	Mandatory for all cases
2. Immunohistochemistry	First-choice ancillary diagnostic; widely used
3. Molecular genetic: RT-PCR	Most common molecular Dx; now routine in most pediatric hospitals
4. Molecular genetic: FISH	Rapidly supplanting cytogenetics for many cases with tumors with known genetic abnormalities
5. Molecular genetic: ISH	Specialized use to date (nontumor; EBV typical)
6. Special stains	Still needed in limited number of cases; useful, expensive
7. Electron microscopy	Still widely used to augment light microscopy, especially in undifferentiated pediatric soft tissue tumors
8. Cytogenetics	Needed when no suitable FISH probes available or to identify new translocations and karyotypic prognostic factors
9. Molecular genetic: SKY, CGH	SKY, a useful diagnostic; CGH and SNPs for LOH
10. Molecular genetic: DNA sequencing	Rare case such as Li-Fraumeni (p53 mutation) and other cancer syndromes

RT-PCR, reverse transcriptase polymerase chain reaction; FISH, fluorescence *in situ* hybridization; ISH, *in situ* hybridization; SKY, spectral karyotyping; CGH, comparative genomic hybridization; Dx, diagnosis; EBV, Epstein-Barr virus; SNP, single nucleotide polymorphism; LOH, loss of heterozygosity

tissue handling protocol (Fig. 8.6) can help avoid these pitfalls.

A final comment is also in order. The rapid advances in our understanding of the origins and evolution of cancer are largely dependent on the availability of fresh frozen tumor tissue and increasingly with paired normal tissue. The last few years have witnessed remarkable advances in whole-genome DNA and transcriptome sequencing of cancer (discussed in detail later in this chapter), but all such studies require fresh or frozen tumor tissue. There is an emerging worldwide shortage of suitable tumor specimens to study due to historical methods that require formalin fixation and paraffin embedding. While this remains the foundation of cancer diagnosis, it is no longer sufficient. Clearly, much wider recognition of the need for fresh or frozen tumor tissue will be necessary to meet these emerging needs. At the same time, it is almost certain that there will never be 100% compliance for such requests, which requires the development of molecular testing applicable to FFPE tissue. The general history of molecular biomarkers is to first identify key genomic alterations in optimally handled (fresh or frozen) tissue, then develop testing for these same biomarkers that can circumvent the limitations of FFPE tissue. However, if there is insufficient optimally processed tissue, the reproducibility and utility of such biomarkers will be in doubt. Further, even FFPE tissue must be uniformly processed to obtain consistent results with this universally available diagnostic tissue. Variable time in tissue fixatives, the use of unbuffered fixative, unusual (i.e., heavy metal containing) fixatives, adverse storage conditions, and prolonged exposure to air of unstained sections intended for molecular analysis can each alter the result and introduce uncontrolled variability of the result. This is a problem that has plagued even the rather simple application of prognostic biomarkers for breast cancer.[36–38] It is even more so a problem for childhood cancer.

Interplay of Multiple Diagnostic Techniques in Tumor Diagnosis

The reason for the multiple diagnostic approaches (Fig. 8.6) is that no method alone will suffice for all tumors. Childhood cancer diagnosis is better viewed as a contingency tree. If the initial result suggests a certain diagnosis, then appropriate ancillary diagnostic tests are necessary to confirm the initial diagnostic impression with a high degree of certainty. In most pediatric hospitals, childhood cancers are handled as illustrated in Figure 8.6. After hematoxylin and eosin (H&E) slides prepared from FFPE tissues are examined, the diagnosis either is obvious or requires additional studies. In many cases, tumor protocols mandate special studies, such as MYCN (NMYC) and ploidy studies in NB. Tumor tissue is submitted either at the outset if the diagnosis is equivocal or after the initial studies document an expected or equivocal diagnosis. In the latter instance, failure to follow the tissue handling guidelines (Fig. 8.6) may seriously compromise diagnosis and oncologic management. If diagnostic uncertainty remains, several methods are available that will lead to a specific diagnosis (Table 8.1). Note that these methods are employed judiciously, such that only the rare diagnostic dilemma will require most or all of these methods. The availability of these methods, especially molecular genetics, has led to accurate diagnoses that are linked to therapeutic protocols.

CHILDHOOD TUMOR DIAGNOSIS

Character of Childhood Cancer

The typical SRCT of childhood either lacks definitive morphologic evidence of lineage or histogenesis or has an ambiguous lineage (spindle cell tumors, undifferentiated tumors). This ambiguity, coupled with the need for definitive diagnosis to establish a treatment regimen, invokes the use of a variety of diagnostic methods. For example, the diagnosis of NB is not sufficient alone. It is necessary to indicate the prognostic subgroup class, as defined by the International Neuroblastoma Study Group (Fig. 8.7). NMYC amplification status by FISH (Fig. 8.8), TRKA expression (Fig. 8.9), 1p deletion, and DNA ploidy are important for diagnosis, treatment, and prognosis.[39] More recently, SNP arrays have been employed to detect prognostic DNA copy number variation (CNV) on chromosomes 1, 10, and 17.[40–42] Each of these factors plays an integral part in determining whether a child with NB will be placed on a high-risk, intermediate-risk, or low-risk protocol. Even more recently, ALK gene mutations

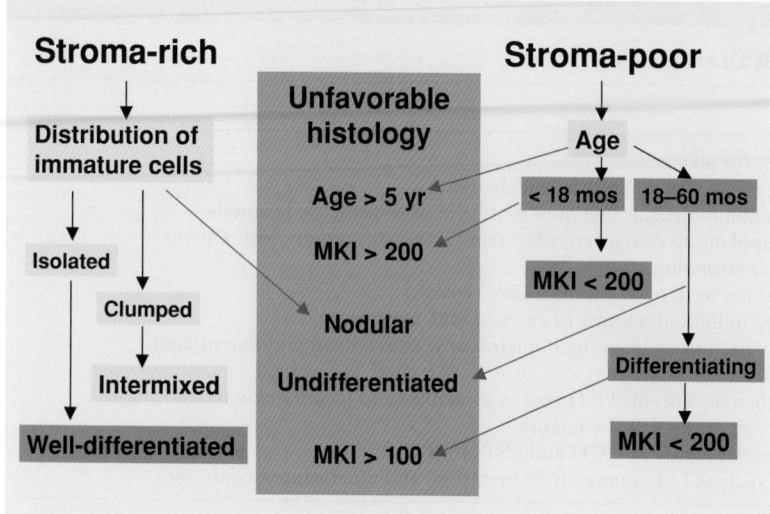

Stroma-rich

Distribution of immature cells

↓

Isolated

↓

Clumped

↓

Intermixed

↓

Well-differentiated

Unfavorable histology

Age > 5 yr

MKI > 200

Nodular

Undifferentiated

MKI > 100

Stroma-poor

↓

Age

< 18 mos   18–60 mos

↓

MKI < 200

Differentiating

↓

MKI < 200

FIGURE 8.7 International Classification System for Neuroblastoma Prognosis and Diagnosis. Although various versions of the standard classification of childhood neuroblastoma based on morphology and associated prognosis have been published by several authors, this version simplifies the classification by describing two basic groups, stroma-rich (**left**) and stroma-poor (**right**). Only one stroma-rich type is associated with a poor prognosis (*nodular*), with clusters or nodules of immature cells set against a well-developed, poorly cellular stoma. In contrast, only two forms of stroma-poor tumors have a favorable prognosis: those in patients younger than 18 months with a mitotic-karyorrhectic nuclei index (MKI) of less than 200 and those in patients aged 18 to 60 months with differentiating tumor cells and an MKI less than 200. All other types in this group are associated with a poor prognosis, as indicated. (Adapted from Shimada H, Ambros IM, Dehner LP, et al. The International Neuroblastoma Pathology Classification (the Shimada system). Cancer 1999; 86(2):364–372.)

may add additional prognostic significance, independent of other factors.[43]

Small Round Cell Tumors of Childhood

SRCTs (Table 8.2) of childhood refer to the "generic" histopathologic appearance of pediatric tumors that do not declare their histogenesis on routine microscopic examination. The histopathology of the most common SRCTs (ESFTs, RMS, NB, lymphoma) is illustrated in Figure 8.10. These tumors are often indistinguishable from each other microscopically. As a group, they have a primitive or embryonal appearance, often present in misleading clinical locations (bone marrow metastases from an occult primary), and lack specific morphologic features that allow for a precise diagnosis without ancillary methods.[44–47]

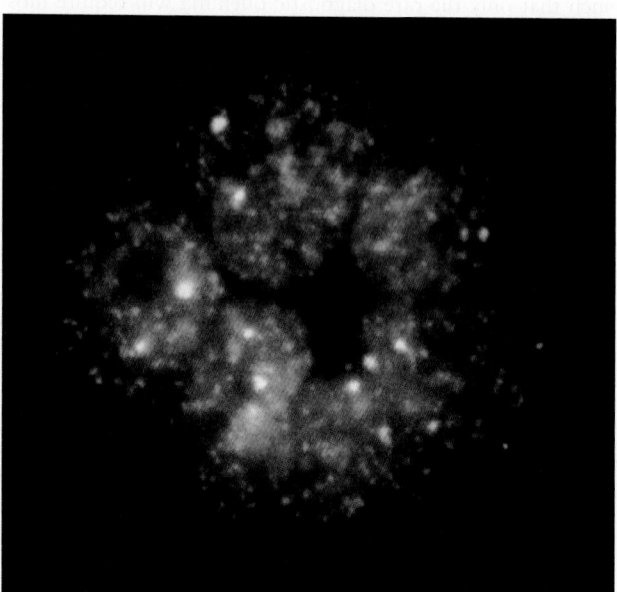

FIGURE 8.8 MYCN amplification in neuroblastoma detected by fluorescence *in situ* hybridization. A touch preparation of a neuroblastoma was incubated with a fluorescent probe for MYCN. Here, one can readily see hundreds of signals in a tumor rosette, each representing at least one copy of MYCN. This clearly documents MYCN amplification in these tumor cells, denoting a poor prognosis group (MYCN amplified).

Because these tumors cannot be distinguished readily from one another, other diagnostic methods must be used to establish a reliable diagnosis. SRCTs serve as a model for demonstrating the benefits of a multimodal approach to tumor diagnosis. At a morphologic level, EM provides unequivocal histogenesis evidence among the most common SRCTs (ESFTs, NB, lymphoma, RMS; Fig. 8.11). Ancillary techniques that are not dependent on morphology are particularly suited for providing a precise diagnosis and for prognostic information with these undifferentiated or poorly differentiated tumors. The most informative methods to emerge in the past few years are based on molecular genetic techniques.[23,40–42,45,48–50] Increasingly, these sophisticated methods offer the potential to confirm the diagnosis while predicting biologic behavior, metastatic potential, tumor recurrence, and sensitivity or resistance to chemotherapy and radiotherapy.[51–54]

A common belief espoused with the advent of "sophisticated" diagnostic methods (EM, immunocytochemistry, molecular genetics) was that "conventional" diagnostic methods (routine H&E studies) would be eliminated in favor of these methods. That has not proved to be the case. No other method besides routine histopathology returns as much information for so little expenditure of time and money. Further, no "sophisticated" test is reliable if the assay is not performed on representative tumor tissue. That cannot be determined without histopathologic examination of the specimen, a fact that has become all too evident in recent genomic studies of cancer that have documented pervasive failure to account for percentage tumor content, or even any tumor at all, in archived specimens that were not quality assured by histopathologic examination.[55] Routine microscopic examination provides information that directs the utilization of appropriate ancillary tests. The discussion that follows is based on the diagnostic workup commencing with routine microscopic evaluation, followed by "more sophisticated" diagnostic methods.

Diagnostic Methodology

The basic approach to tumor diagnosis employs a variety of diverse methods (Table 8.1).[24,56–60] Representative tissue is submitted for formalin fixation, tissue processing, paraffin embedding, and routine H&E staining of the resulting tissue sections. After light microscopic examination of the routinely stained tissue sections, a differential diagnosis is formulated and a series of special studies are selected to provide

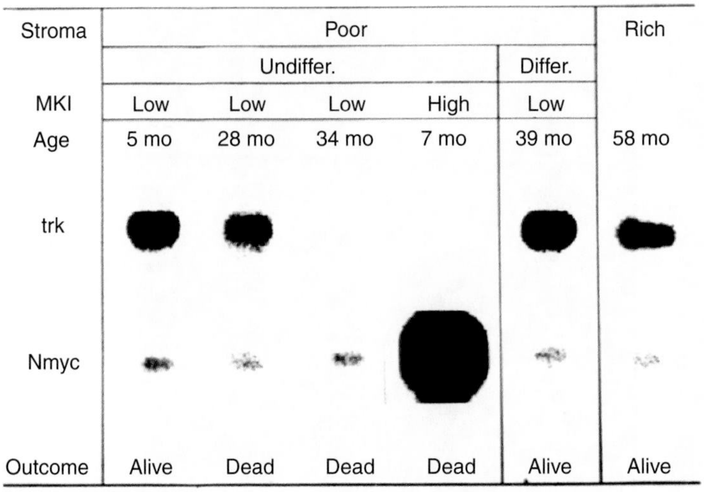

Stroma	Poor					Rich
	Undiffer.				Differ.	
MKI	Low	Low	Low	High	Low	
Age	5 mo	28 mo	34 mo	7 mo	39 mo	58 mo
trk						
Nmyc						
Outcome	Alive	Dead	Dead	Dead	Alive	Alive

FIGURE 8.9 Polymerase chain reaction analysis of *TRKA* and *MYCN*. In this composite blot of *TRKA* (high-affinity nerve growth factor receptor) expression (**upper row**) and *MYCN* copy number determined by Southern blot (**bottom row**), the outcome is compared with Shimada classification. Patients with single-copy *MYCN* that express *TRKA* generally survive. The exception in *lane 2* was associated with a poor-prognosis Shimada category. Sequence analysis of this *TRKA* product revealed an 18 bp deletion that rendered the gene product (a membrane tyrosine kinase receptor) biologically unresponsive to nerve growth factor, the functional equivalent to no *TRKA* expression. Conversely, patients with single-copy *MYCN* who lack *TRKA* expression (*lane 3*) have a poor prognosis, as do those with amplified *MYCN* (*lane 4*). Prognosis therefore correlates more closely with *TRKA* expression of the neuronal isoform than with *MYCN* stats and is best with the Shimada classification system. MKI, mitotic-karyorrhectic index. (Courtesy of H. Shimada, Pathology Department, Children's Hospital, Los Angeles.)

a definitive diagnosis. The most commonly used ancillary diagnostic method is immunocytochemistry. Either concurrent with or subsequent to immunocytochemical study, special histochemical stains (periodic acid-Schiff [PAS], reticulin, trichrome), EM, and molecular studies may be initiated.

Findings from all of these studies are reviewed and interpreted in concert with the clinical history and diagnostic imaging findings. With the vast majority of SRCTs, this multimodal approach will yield a precise and definitive diagnosis that directs further surgical intervention, oncologic

TABLE 8.2

DIFFERENTIAL DIAGNOSIS OF PEDIATRIC BONE AND SOFT TISSUE SOLID TUMORS

A. Small round cell tumors
 1. Peripheral primitive neuroectodermal tumors (Ewing's sarcoma family of tumors)
    - Ewing's tumor (classical, atypical, peripheral primitive neuroectodermal tumor)
    - Askin's tumor (malignant small cell tumor of the thoracopulmonary region)
    - Malignant ectomesenchymoma
    - Biphenotypic sarcoma
 2. Rhabdomyosarcoma (RMS)
    - Alveolar RMS
    - Embryonal RMS
    - Undifferentiated sarcoma (currently in process of reclassification into non-RMS soft tissue tumors)
 3. Neuroblastoma
 4. Desmoplastic small round cell tumor
 5. Lymphoma (B-cell, T-cell, Null)
    - Anaplastic large cell lymphoma
    - Burkitt's lymphoma
 6. Clear cell sarcoma of soft parts (malignant melanoma of soft tissues)
 7. Small cell osteosarcoma
 8. Extrarenal monophasic Wilms' tumor
 9. Extrarenal rhabdoid tumor
 10. Extraskeletal myxoid chondrosarcoma

B. Spindle cell tumors
 1. Congenital infantile fibrosarcoma
 2. Adult-type fibrosarcoma
 3. Fibromatosis
    - Infantile fibromatosis (including aggressive fibromatosis)
    - Other forms of fibromatosis
 4. Myofibromatosis (including hemangiopericytoma-like variant)
 5. Synovial sarcoma
 6. Pleomorphic undifferentiated sarcoma (malignant fibrous histiocytoma)/primitive sarcoma NOS
 7. Spindle cell RMS
 8. Malignant peripheral nerve sheath tumors (including malignant schwannoma, triton tumor)

NOS, not otherwise specified.

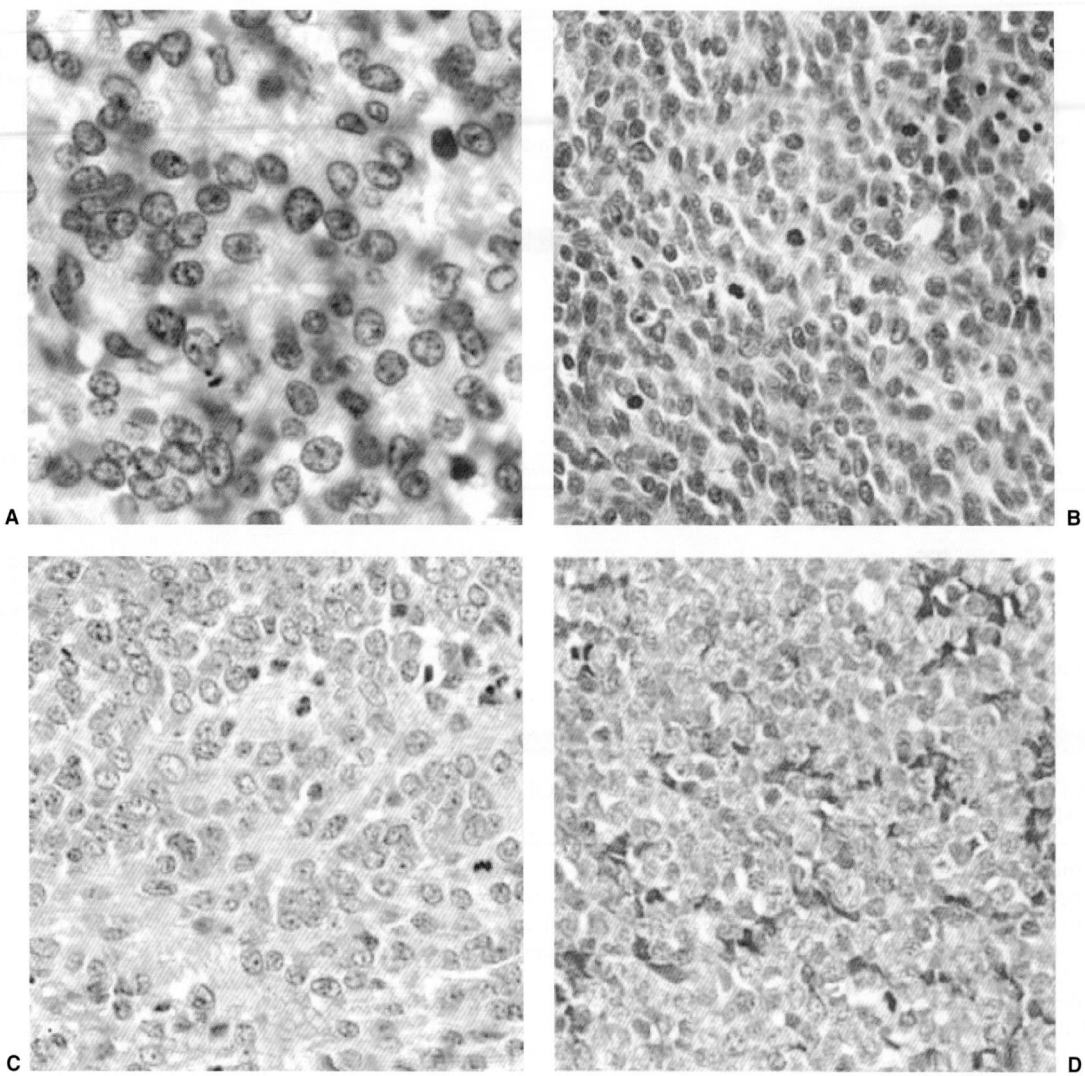

FIGURE 8.10 Histopathology of typical small round cell tumors. Historically, Ewing's sarcoma (**A**), rhabdomyosarcoma (**B**), neuroblastoma (**C**), and lymphoma (**D**) were difficult to distinguish from one another, particularly when undifferentiated rhabdomyosarcoma or neuroblastoma was encountered, as illustrated here. None of the four tumors show light microscopically discernible evidence of differentiation and therefore histogenesis, which is critical to a diagnosis by light microscopy.

management, follow-up, and prognosis. By using these extensive and coordinated methods, it is rare that diagnoses are modified by additional testing, consultative review by pathologists at other institutions, or by expert pathologist reviewers for the COG protocol studies.

Although most tumors require only a few of the procedures listed in Table 8.1, some tumors require all available testing modalities to come to a definitive diagnosis.[24,56,58,60–63] The pathologist plays a critical role in ensuring that adequate tissue is obtained for all diagnostic testing modalities, the COG protocols, and institutional research purposes. Appropriate triaging of tumor tissue (Fig. 8.6) by the pathologist is necessary to make certain that representative viable tumor tissue is available for routine light microscopy, immunocytochemistry, EM, cytogenetics, molecular studies, tumor prognostic markers, and the COG protocol studies. Fresh tumor tissue must be sent from the operating suite to the anatomic pathology grossing station in a sterile container with saline. The tissue must not be exposed to any fixative. A general schema for handling fresh sterile biopsies or resections of pediatric tumors is to (a)

cryopreserve tissue at −70°C with and without cryopreservation matrix for molecular studies; (b) place tumor portions in tissue culture media for cytogenetics, spectral karyotyping (SKY), and comparative genomic hybridization (CGH); (c) perform cytologic imprints (touch preparations) for FISH, CISH, and chimeric translocation detection; (d) fix finely cubed tissue in glutaraldehyde for EM; and (e) submit representative tissue in 10% buffered formalin for routine light microscopic, immunocytochemical, and histochemical analyses. The pathologist is also responsible for determining adequacy of the tumor specimen with respect to the amount of tumor tissue submitted, determining whether viable tumor tissue is submitted, and ensuring that indeed tumorous tissue is submitted and not adjacent reactive tissue. At times, this will require the pathologist to refer to the COG protocols and discuss tissue requirements with the institutional COG clinical research associate and oncologist. For optimal handling of tumor tissue, communication among the surgeon, oncologist, and pathologist is necessary to make certain that tissues are submitted for all required ancillary studies for a particular

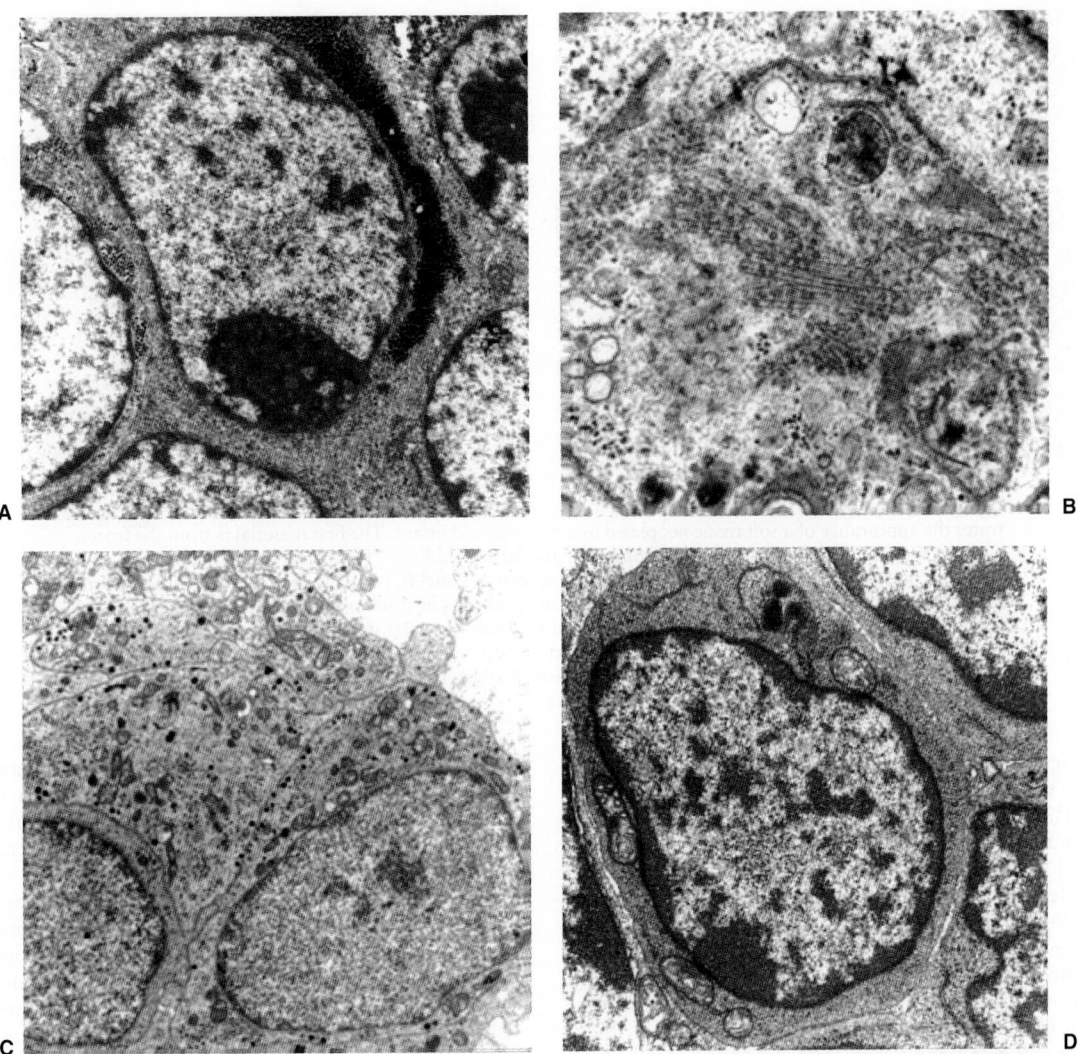

FIGURE 8.11 Electron microscopic features of the same small round cell tumors illustrated in Figure 8.10. **Panel A** illustrates the glycogen-rich cytoplasm that is typical of the usual Ewing's sarcoma in the absence of any other distinctive features, notably neural differentiation. **Panel B** shows the unmistakable actin and myosin bundles of skeletal myogenesis in a childhood rhabdomyosarcoma. **Panel C** shows conspicuous neural differentiation in a neuroblastoma, with innumerable dense core granules (*black dots*). **Panel D** shows a primary lymphoma of bone, with cells devoid of any cell-cell attachments and marginated, dense nuclear heterochromatin, typical of lymphoid cells in general.

tumor type. Finally, the pathologist may perform a frozen section or touch preparations on tumorous tissue to determine a preliminary diagnosis for triaging and immediate surgical management purposes. If the tissue procurement scheme (Fig. 8.6) is performed with pediatric solid tumors, adequate tumor material will be available for diagnosis, oncologic management, prognostic purposes, and oncologic research in the vast majority of cases.

Light Microscopy

FFPE tumor tissue is the most widely studied of all tissues for diagnosis and protocol studies. Attention to optimal fixation, processing, and tissue sectioning are important to allow for optimal light microscopic, immunocytochemical, and histochemical evaluation. This formalin-fixed tissue is also available for DNA extraction to identify tumor-defining translocations by reverse transcriptase PCR (RT-PCR), and tissue can be recovered and subsequently processed for EM if necessary.

When the tissue is properly formalin-fixed and processed, light microscopy will provide overwhelming evidence for the precise diagnosis in the majority of cases via immunocytochemical, histochemical, and ultrastructural methods. The need for optimal fixation, processing, and tissue sectioning is illustrated in Figure 8.12. Initial frozen sections of the tumor tissue were of poor quality and could not be interpreted adequately (Fig. 8.12A). With proper fixation, sectioning, and staining of the same tumor tissue block, diagnostic features defining the tumor became readily apparent (Fig. 8.12B).

Optimal fixation is necessary for routine light microscopy, IHC, and DNA extraction for molecular and FISH studies for identifying tumor-defining translocations and prognostic markers (MYCN). Representative portions of the resected tumor (1 to 3 mm in thickness, approximately 1.5 cm in maximum width and length) should be submitted for formalin-fixation. Tissue portions larger than 3 mm in thickness and larger than 1.5 cm in maximum width and length will not be optimally fixed, resulting in poor tissue preservation with lack

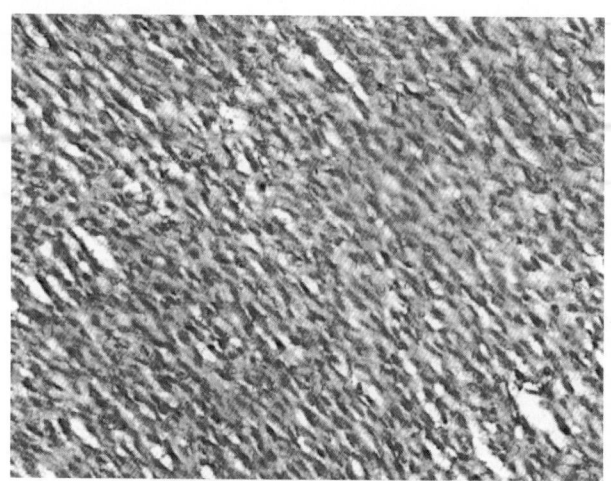
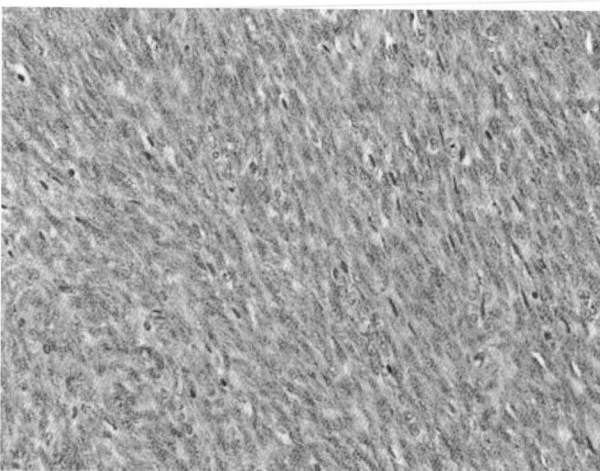

FIGURE 8.12 Poor (**A**) and well-done (**B**) histology of a typical soft tissue tumor. The first panel (**A**) illustrates the appearance of a soft tissue neoplasm in a 9-month-old infant. The first material is from the frozen section, the second, after formalin fixation and paraffin embedding. The correct interpretation became apparent only with proper fixation and embedding as seen in **Panel B**, in which the correct identity as congenital fibrosarcoma became evident. Many diagnostic problems in childhood tumor interpretation benefit from optimal quality histology and can be the useful and necessary first step in the choice of other ancillary diagnostics to confirm the impression gleaned from careful scrutiny of a well-prepared hematoxylin and eosin section. (Photomicrographs courtesy of Dr. Larry Wang, Children's Hospital, Los Angeles).

of tissue antigenicity and degradation of DNA and RNA. Tissue fixation should be conducted with fresh, commercially available 10% buffered formalin for a minimum of 4 hours and a maximum of 24 hours. Following automated tissue processing to allow for tissue dehydration through graded alcohols and xylene and paraffin permeation, the tissue blocks should be made by embedding the tumor tissue portions in low-melting-point paraffin, to protect and preserve the antigenicity of the tissue against excessive heat. The production of tissue sections mounted on coated glass slides requires histotechnologists with the ability to cut wrinkle-free 3-μ thick tissue sections. Placing the tissue sections onto coated glass slides allows for adherence of the tissue sections to the glass infrastructure and allows for immunocytochemistry, in situ hybridization, FISH, in situ PCR, and laser capture microscopic techniques to be performed without loss of tissue sections. The final step in producing high-quality and diagnostically acceptable glass slides of tumor tissue is the staining process. Quality assurance for producing high-quality routine H&E, histochemical, immunochemical, and in situ hybridization staining should be an ongoing process in all anatomic pathology laboratories providing diagnostic services with constant comparison with standardized control tissues.

Immunocytochemistry

Remarkable progress has been made in the development of immunocytochemical antibodies, which are capable of defining undifferentiated neoplasms and allowing for definitive diagnosis.[24,57,62-71] Rapid development and availability of antibodies of recently discovered antigens identified by genomic and proteomic studies of tumors have become a reality in tumor diagnostics. This has resulted in immunocytochemistry being the most frequently employed diagnostic method for SRCTs (Fig. 8.13A–C).[24,64,65,71] In addition, many different antigen retrieval methods have been identified that allow for unmasking and eliminating formalin cross-linking of tumor antigens in FFPE tissue.[24,64,65,68,71,72] The use of enzymatic digestion (protease, pepsin, trypsin), regulation of pH, antigen retrieval solutions (citrate buffer, Tris-HCl, EDTA-NaOH),

and various methods of heat treatment (microwave, pressure cooker, controlled gentle steaming) have been thoroughly explored and refined to optimize antigen retrieval for numerous antibodies. Technical guidelines for individual antibodies are well delineated by the commercial providers of immunocytochemical products, and many of these companies have developed antigen retrieval "kits" to produce optimal results with specific antibodies. Antigen retrieval from formalin-fixed tissue has made it possible to achieve immunoreactivity similar to that previously obtained only with immunocytochemistry performed on frozen tissue. This has occurred while reducing background considerably and decreasing false-negative results. With each antibody lot received, it is necessary to determine the concentration of antibody (titration) necessary to provide diagnostic information, while eliminating background and false-positive results. Monitoring of accurate immunoreactivity requires that known control tissue be run parallel or on the same glass slides as the patient's tissue. This technology is readily available and may be performed either manually or with automated instruments in a reproducible manner, using FFPE tissues.

There are numerous antibodies that are available on a commercial and research basis; however, an exhaustive discussion of the specifics of antibodies and immunoreactivity with tumors is beyond the scope of this chapter. Tables 8.3 to 8.5 provide detailed lists of antibodies that are more commonly employed in pediatric pathology services, along with their common tumor association.[15,24,58,62,63,65-67,69-71,73-88] The immunoreactivity of an antibody with a specific tumor and the pattern of staining are important (Fig. 8.13A–C). Antigen localization in a tissue depends on several factors, most notably the cellular disposition of the antigen. Three basic patterns are observed: nuclear, cytoplasmic, and cell surface (membranous). Certain tumors may be included or eliminated from consideration based on the pattern of staining. For example, cytoplasmic membrane immunoreactivity with CD99 is characteristic for ESFTs and lymphoblastic leukemia/lymphoma (Tables 8.3–8.5). Many different tumors may immunoreact with CD99 in a cytoplasmic or a nuclear pattern but not with a cytoplasmic surface membrane

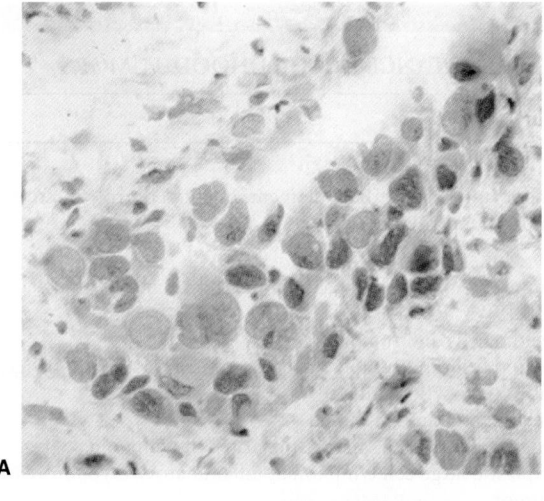

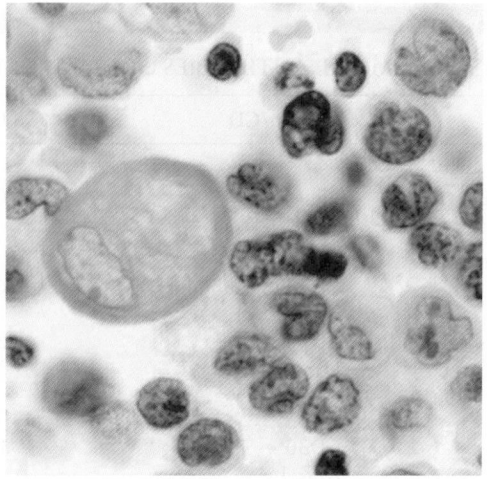

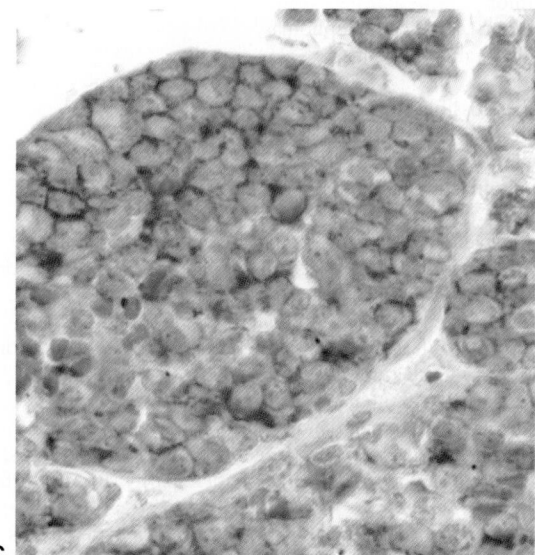

FIGURE 8.13 Immunocytochemistry by cellular localization. Immunocytochemistry is widely utilized on a daily basis in surgical pathology of adult and childhood tissues. In the case of childhood cancer, many specific classes of antigens are detectable. Illustrated here are three categorical examples: (A) an example of nuclear staining for a transcription factor, MyoD, widely used to detect extremely undifferentiated childhood rhabdomyosarcoma; (B) vimentin, ubiquitous intermediate filament found in all mesenchymal tissues and their tumors counterpart. The staining is localized to the cytoplasm. This antigen is most used to verify antigenic preservation sample and is not specific for any given tumor; (C) surface antigen detection, MIC2 (CD99) in Ewing's sarcoma. Here, apparent cytoplasmic as well as cell surface localization is detectable. Such antigens routinely show surface staining that is difficult to photograph but easily detected by focusing up and down through the sample under the light microscope. Many of these antigens are also quite labile and not readily detected in routinely processed tissue.

pattern. Another example is myogenin immunoreactivity.[15,24,57,62,63,75,87] This antibody identifies RMS when a nuclear pattern is present; however, diffuse and intense cytoplasmic myogenin staining is found with mast cells. Within a poorly differentiated tumor, mast cells may be frequently present. Cytoplasmic myogenin immunoreactivity of mast cells in such tumors may result in a mistaken diagnosis of RMS. The pathologist has to be aware of and be up to date with the characteristic immunoreactivity and staining patterns of numerous antibodies with a wide variety of tumors to provide accurate diagnoses.

With any tissue to be preserved for possible immunocytochemistry study, attention must be paid to the length of formalin fixation.[24,56–58,60,62,63] For tumor antigen integrity, formalin fixation (10% buffered formalin) should be for a minimum of 4 hours and a maximum of 24 hours. Exposure to formalin for a shorter or longer period results in significant loss of tumor antigens, making immunocytochemical studies difficult or impossible.

Several antigen retrieval protocols have been developed that allow for unmasking tumor antigens in FFPE tissue.[63,64,68,71,72,89–93] An antigen retrieval solution (10 mM citrate buffer at pH 6.0; 100 mM Tris-HCl at pH 8.0; 1 mM EDTA-NaOH at pH 8.0; 5% urea) and heat treatment (microwave, microwave and pressure cooker, autoclave,

pressure cooker, water bath, steamer, thermal cycler) allow reversing protein cross-linking by formalin fixation. Optimal antigen retrieval intensity from FFPE tissue has been achieved with heat treatment at temperatures of 100°C for 20 minutes, 90°C for 30 minutes, 80°C for 50 minutes, and 70°C for 10 hours. After antigen retrieval, enzyme digestion (trypsin, pronase, proteinase K, pepsin) is usually not necessary prior to reaction of the tissue with the antibody but may be needed for certain antibodies. For most antibodies, heat treatment for 20 to 30 minutes at 100°C with either citrate buffer at pH 6.0 or Tris-HCl buffer at pH 7.0 to pH 8.0 are effective for antigen retrieval. The antibody manufacturer provides general guidelines; however, it is necessary to determine the optimal conditions for the antibody in each institution's immunocytochemistry laboratory. In addition, monitoring for accurate immunoreactivity requires that known control tissue be run parallel, or on the same glass slide as the patient's tissue, and under the same antigen retrieval conditions. Immunoreactivity may be adversely affected if the tissue sections are prepared sometime in advance of staining. Tissue sections should be prepared and should undergo processing for immunostaining without delay to avoid antigen degradation. It is also possible to preserve antigenicity if the tissue sections on glass slides are stored at −70°C until immunocytochemistry is performed.

TABLE 8.3

IMMUNOCYTOCHEMICAL ANTIBODIES OF DIAGNOSTIC IMPORTANCE IN CHILDHOOD TUMORS

Antibody	Antigen/CD	Utility
General		
Antivimentin	Vimentin	Generic anti-intermediate filament, quality control, reactive with most mesenchymal cells
Hematopoietic		
Anti-LCA	CD45 (all subunits)	Common leukocyte antigen; no lineage specificity, unlike CD45RA, RB, and RO
Myeloperoxidase		Myeloid cells and tumors
Muramidase	Lysozyme	Myeloid cells and tumors, histiocytic disorders, macrophages, fibrohistiocytic tumors
LeuM1	CD15	T cells, Hodgkin lymphoma
Ki-1	CD30	Hodgkin lymphoma, anaplastic large cell lymphoma
ALK-1	ALK-1	Anaplastic large cell lymphoma, inflammatory myofibroblastic tumor
NPM	P80NPM/ALK	Anaplastic large cell lymphoma
L26	CD20	B cells, rhabdomyoblasts
UCHL	CD45RO	T cells
T3	CD3	T cells; possibly superior to UCHL1
T6	CD1a	Langerhans' cell histiocytosis and Langerhans' cells
Langerin	CD207	Langerhans' cell histiocytosis, Langerhans' cells
TdT	Terminal deoxynucleotidyl transferase	Lymphoblastic lymphoma, ALL T cell
EBER-1	Epstein-Barr virus (EBV)–encoded RNA-1	EBV-associated B-cell lymphoma, Hodgkin lymphoma, lymphoproliferative disease (including posttransplantation), smooth muscle tumors in HIV/AIDS
EBV-LMP-1	EBV-latent membrane protein-1	EBV-associated B-cell lymphoma, Hodgkin lymphoma, lymphoproliferative disease (including posttransplantation), smooth muscle tumors in HIV/AIDS
Fascin	55K2	Dendritic cell sarcoma, dendritic cells
Factor XIIIa	Factor XIIIa	Dendritic cell sarcoma, dendritic cells
Ham 56, KP-1, PGM1, MAC387	CD68	Histiocytic disorders, macrophages, fibrohistiocytic tumors, sinus histiocytosis with massive lymphadenopathy (Rosai-Dorfman's disease)
Cathepsin B		Histiocytic disorders, macrophages, fibrohistiocytic tumors
Neural		
NSE		Neural antigen, but poorly specific
NB-84		Neuroblastoma
TrkA		Neuroblastoma
PGP 9.5		Neural tumors
TH	Tyrosine hydroxylase	Neuroblastoma
NFTP		Neuronal cells, tumors (e.g., neuroblastoma)
GFAP		Glial cells (gliosis, gliomas)
S-100	S-100A	Nerve sheath tumors, melanoma, neuroblastoma, Langerhans' cells
Chromogranin		Neuroblastoma, neural tumors
Synaptophysin		Neural tumors
Calcitonin		Medullary carcinoma of thyroid
P30/32MIC2	CD99, O13, 12E7, HBA71	Ewing's sarcoma family of tumors, lymphoblastic lymphoma, lymphocytes, endothelial cells
FLI-1		Ewing's sarcoma family of tumors, lymphoblastic lymphoma, lymphocytes
Leu7	CD57	Peripheral nerve sheath tumors, schwann cells, neuroblastomas
P75NTR		Nerve sheath tumors
Neural cell adhesion molecule	NCAM	Neural tumors, neuroendocrine cells, neuroblastic cells, natural killer T cells, sarcomas
Myogenic		
Desmin	Desmin	Myogenic and myofibroblastic tumors
MSA	Muscle-specific actin, HHF5	Myogenic tumors
Myoglobin	Myoglobin	Skeletal muscle tumors
MyoD	MyoD	Skeletal muscle tumors (specific)

(continued)

TABLE 8.3

CONTINUED

Antibody	Antigen/CD	Utility
Myogenin	Myogenin	Skeletal muscle tumors (specific)
Myf-5	Myf-5	Skeletal muscle tumors (specific)
MRF-4-herculin/myf6	MRF-4-herculin/myf6	Skeletal muscle tumors (specific)
Caldesmon		Myogenic tumors
SMA	Smooth muscle actin	Skeletal muscle, smooth muscle, myofibroblasts, pericytes
Smooth muscle myosin heavy chain	SMMHC	Smooth muscle tumors
Calponin		Smooth muscle tumors
Epithelial		
Keratin	Keratins, CAM5.2, AE1/AE3	Carcinoma, synoviosarcoma, germ cell tumors, hepatocellular carcinoma, hepatoblastoma, smooth muscle tumors, epithelioid sarcoma, rhabdoid tumors, atypical teratoid/rhabdoid tumors
EMA	Epithelial membrane antigen	Carcinoma, synoviosarcoma, germ cell tumors, anaplastic large cell lymphoma, rhabdoid tumors, atypical teratoid/rhabdoid tumors
Vascular		
Platelet endothelial cell adhesion molecule 1	CD31 (PECAM-1)	Vascular tumors, endothelium, epithelioid sarcoma
CD34		Vascular tumors, dermatofibrosarcoma protuberans, epithelioid sarcoma, fibroblastic tumors, gastrointestinal stromal tumors, solitary fibrous tumors, endothelium
Factor VIII		Vascular tumors, endothelium
W240		Lymphatic endothelium, lymphatic tumors and malformations
Ulex		Vascular tumors, endothelium
Type IV collagen		Vascular tumors, vessels, nerve sheath tumors, glomus tumors, endothelium
Laminin		Vascular tumors, nerve sheath tumors, synovial sarcoma, endothelium
Thrombomodulin		Vascular tumors, mesothelial tumors, endothelium
Miscellaneous		
α_1-antitrypsin (chymotrypsin)		Phagocytic cells, histiocytic neoplasms
α_1-fetoprotein		Germ cell tumors, hepatic tumors
Human chorionic gonadotropin	β-HCG	Germ cell tumors
Placental alkaline phosphatase (PLAP)	Placental alkaline phosphatase	Germ cell tumors
HMB45	Melanoma antigen	Melanoma, clear cell sarcoma of soft tissues, angiomyolipoma
MelanA	MART-1	Melanoma, clear cell sarcoma of soft tissues, angiomyolipoma
Tyrosinase		Melanoma, clear cell sarcoma of soft tissues, angiomyolipoma
MTF-1	Microphthalmic transcription factor-1	Melanoma, angiomyolipoma, clear cell sarcoma of soft tissue, melanotic schwannoma
HHV-8		Kaposi's sarcoma, B-cell lymphomas (body cavity), Castleman's disease (angiofollicular hyperplasia)
c-KIT	CD117	Gastrointestinal stromal tumors, germ cell tumors, mast cells, hematopoietic cells
Osteocalcin		Osteogenic tumors
Osteonectin		Osteogenic tumors
Osteopontin		Osteogenic tumors
WT-1	Wilms' tumor 1	Wilms' tumor, desmoplastic small round cell tumor, mesothelioma, mesothelial cells
TFE3		Xp11.2 renal tumors, alveolar soft parts sarcoma
INI1/SMARCB1		Rhabdoid tumor, epithelioid sarcoma, atypical teratoid/rhabdoid tumor, small cell (undifferentiated) hepatoblastoma, subset of extramesenchymal myxoid chondrosarcoma
TLE1		Synovial sarcoma
β-catenin		Desmoid, hepatoblastoma, myofibroma, solitary fibrous tumor

(continued)

TABLE 8.3

CONTINUED

Antibody	Antigen/CD	Utility
Proliferation markers, tumor suppressor genes, and others		
Ki-67	MIB-1	Proliferation marker
Bcl-2		Proliferation marker
Minichromosome maintenance protein-7 (MCM-7)		Proliferation marker
Cyclin-dependent kinases 2, 4, 6		Proliferation marker
BAX		Proliferation marker
TRAIL		Proliferation marker
Survivin		Proliferation marker
P21/waf1		Cell cycle regulation
P16 (INK4a)		Cell cycle regulation
P27 (kip1)		Cell cycle regulation
HMDM2		Cell cycle regulation
Cyclin E		Cell cycle regulation
CD44		Prognostic marker
p53		Tumor suppressor gene
PRb		Tumor suppressor gene
ATM		Tumor suppressor gene
PTEN		Tumor suppressor gene

ALL, acute lymphocytic leukemia.

The immunocytochemical results require critical assessment to ensure diagnostic accuracy. These issues have been addressed by many authors in numerous publications but can be summarized here.[15,24,62,63,65–67,69–71,73–88,94] Possible artifacts include the following:

1. Staining at tissue section edges (trapping) or in crevices, while the tissue away from the periphery and tissue section defects have no significant immunoreactivity.
2. Focal staining due to trapping of reagent in an elevated or depressed region of the tissue. It is possible that the tumor is composed of variable cell types with different immunoreactivity to the antibody, resulting in an island of tumor cells with focal staining; however, the staining pattern should follow the cytoplasmic, nuclear, or membranous pattern characteristic for the particular antibody interaction with a specific tumor type. Aberrant expression of a particular antigen(s) by tumor cells may occur (Table 8.5).
3. Diffusion or "leaking" of antigenic proteins from surrounding normal tissue that has been infiltrated by the SRCT. In particular, false-positive immunoreactivity with myogenic antibodies has been reported when an SRCT has invaded skeletal muscle.
4. Poor techniques, such as incomplete paraffin removal, high-melting-point paraffin, prolonged or excessive heat with antigen retrieval, poorly fixed or necrotic tissue, thick section preparation, endogenous biotin with inadequate peroxidase/biotin blocking, incomplete rinsing of slides, desiccation of tissue sections during processing, inadequate incubation time, chromogen staining too intense, and inappropriate concentration of antibody are all factors that may lead to spurious and misleading immunocytochemical findings and interpretations.

If tumor tissue shows immunoreactivity with an antibody but with an inappropriate staining pattern or evidence of artifacts, the immunocytochemical result is suspect and should be used with caution in formulating a diagnosis. Interpretation of immunohistochemical results depends on the knowledge and expertise of the pathologist.

Inmunocytochemical Approach to Small Round Cell Tumors. An immunocytochemical approach to SRCTs, the immunocytochemical profiles of common and relatively infrequent to rare SRCTs, and aberrant immunoreactivity of SRCTs are presented in tabular form (Tables 8.4 and 8.5). On the basis of clinical information, tumor site, cytologic imprints (touch preparations), and frozen section examination, an antibody panel may be ordered immediately following gross examination of the tumor, in order that immunocytochemical studies begin immediately following permanent tissue processing and sectioning. Evaluation of the routinely stained tissue sections the following day may result in additions or deletions to the antibody panel to confirm the diagnostic impression on frozen section evaluation or to eliminate other diagnostic categories from consideration.

Immunocytochemistry plays an important role in allowing the pathologist to place a relatively undifferentiated SRCT into a diagnostic category (Tables 8.3–8.5).[15,24,59,60,63,66,67,69–71,73–88,95–107] When dealing with pediatric tumors, it becomes apparent that there is considerable cross-reactivity among various neoplasms and antibodies (Tables 8.3–8.5). For example, CD99 (MIC2) has been touted as the "Ewing sarcoma marker"; however, it is quite obvious that this antibody is not specific to ESFTs alone (Tables 8.4 and 8.5). In fact, several SRCTs of childhood immunoreact with CD99, but Ewing's sarcoma has a characteristic cytoplasmic membrane staining pattern, whereas other SRCTs more typically have a diffuse cytoplasmic staining pattern. This emphasizes that basing a diagnosis solely on immunocytochemistry, without consideration of clinical information, and histopathologic and ultrastructural features, is fraught with problems.

The initial antibody panel (Table 8.3) for an undifferentiated SRCT would include markers to evaluate myogenic, neural, lymphoid, hematopoietic, germ cell, neural crest, and mesenchymal origins. Pediatric tumors with epithelial differentiation are

TABLE 8.4

IMMUNOCYTOCHEMISTRY APPROACH TO SMALL ROUND CELL TUMORS OF CHILDHOOD

Undifferentiated small round cell tumor immunocytochemistry panel	
Antibody	**Tumor with immunoreactivity to antibody**
Leukocyte common antigen	Leukemia, lymphoma
NB84	Neuroblastoma
Neuron-specific enolase (NSE)	Neuroblastoma, desmoplastic small round cell tumor
S-100 protein	Neuroblastoma, synovial sarcoma, medulloblastoma (primitive neuroectodermal tumor), peripheral nerve sheath tumor, Ewing's sarcoma, liposarcoma, clear cell sarcoma of soft tissues, cutaneous malignant melanoma
Myogenin	Rhabdomyosarcoma
Desmin	Rhabdomyosarcoma, desmoplastic small round cell tumor
Muscle-specific actin	Rhabdomyosarcoma, myofibroma
CD99 (MIC2)	Ewing's sarcoma, lymphoma, leukemia
Pancytokeratin	Rhabdoid tumor, synovial sarcoma, germ cell tumors, hepatoblastoma, carcinoma, desmoplastic small round cell tumor
α-fetoprotein	Hepatoblastoma, endodermal sinus tumor (yolk sac tumor)
CD1a	Langerhans' cell histiocytosis
CD207 (Langerin)	Langerhans' cell histiocytosis
CD30 (Ki-1, Ber-H2)	Anaplastic large cell lymphoma
ALK-1	Anaplastic large cell lymphoma, inflammatory myofibroblastic tumor
INI1/SMARCB1	Rhabdoid, epithelioid sarcoma, atypical teratoid/rhabdoid tumor, small cell (undifferentiated), hepatoblastoma, subset of extraskeletal myxoid chondrosarcoma
TLE1	Synovial sarcoma
Vimentin	Antigen maintenance determination, rhabdoid tumor, fibrosarcoma, spindle cell tumors, mesenchymal tumors, and absent in neuroblastoma,
TFE3	Xp11.2 renal tumors, alveolar soft parts sarcoma

Immunoreactivity of pediatric tumors				
Neuroblastoma neuroblastic			**Stromal cell**	**Cell surface**
NB84	Chromogranin	Protein gene product 9.5	S-100 protein	Leu 7 (CD57)
NSE	Synaptophysin	Microtubule-associated protein (MAP 1/2)	Glial fibrillary protein	TrkA
Dopamine	Peripherin	Vasoactive intestinal protein	Myelin basic protein	NCAM
Neurofilament triple protein	Absence of vimentin			Ganglioside G-D2

Rhabdomyosarcoma		**Ewing's sarcoma/peripheral primitive neuroectodermal tumor**	
Myogenin	Creatine kinase M subunit	CD99	S-100 protein
Desmin	Titin	NSE	Synaptophysin
Muscle-specific actin	Dystrophin	β₂-microglobulin	Neurofilament triple protein
Smooth muscle actin	Calsequestrin	Acetylcholine	Vimentin
Myoglobin	Vimentin		
MyoD1	Myf-3, Myf-4		

Desmoplastic small round cell tumor		**Rhabdoid tumor (renal/extrarenal)**	**Synovial sarcoma**	
Desmin	Vimentin	EMA	EMA	Bcl-2
Cytokeratin	W T-1	Cytokeratin (pancytokeratin)	Cytokeratin	S-100 protein
NSE	Leu-7 (CD57)	Vimentin	Vimentin	TLE1
Epithelial membrane antigen (EMA)		Absence of INI1/SMARCB1		

Wilms' tumor (nephroblastoma)			**Hepatoblastoma**	
Tubular epithelium	**Blastema**	**Stroma**	**Epithelial**	**Mesenchymal**
Cytokeratin	Vimentin	Vimentin	EMA	Desmin
EMA	W T-1	Desmin	Cytokeratin	Muscle-specific actin
W T-1		S-100 protein	α-fetoprotein	S-100 protein
			β-human chorionic gonadotropin (β-HCG)	CEA
			β-catenin	β-catenin
			Absence of INI1/SMARC1 in small cell type	

(continued)

TABLE 8.4

CONTINUED

Medulloblastoma (primitive neuroectodermal tumor)

NSE	S-100 protein	Synaptophysin	NSE
Glial fibrillary acidic protein	Nestin	Tubulin	
Microtubule-associated protein	Neurofilament triple protein	Chromogranin	α_1-antitrypsin

Leukemia/lymphoma	**Myofibroma/myofibromatosis**		**Embryonal sarcoma of liver**
Leukocyte common antigen (LCA), CD99 (MIC2)	Smooth muscle actin	Vimentin	α_1-antitrypsin
CD79a, CD 19/20 (B-Cell)	Muscle-specific actin	S-100	α_1-chymotrypsin
CD3/CD4/CD8/CD45RO (T cell)	Collagen, β-catenin		Vimentin
ALK-NPM, CD30, EMA (anaplastic large cell lymphoma)			

Germ cell tumors

Endodermal sinus tumor	**Embryonal carcinoma**	**Germinoma**	**Choriocarcinoma**
α-fetoprotein	Placental alkaline phosphatase	Placental alkaline phosphatase	β-HCG
Cytokeratin	Cytokeratin		Placental alkaline phosphatase
			Cytokeratin
			Cytokeratin

Intratubular germ cell neoplasia
    PLAP, p53

Pleuropulmonary blastoma	**Mesenchymal chondrosarcoma/chondrosarcoma**
Vimentin	S-100 protein
Desmin	Vimentin
Muscle-specific actin, DICER1	CD99

Langerhans' cell histiocytosis	**Small cell osteosarcoma**	**Malignant peripheral nerve sheath tumor**
CD1a	Vimentin	Leu 7 (CD57)
CD207 (Langerin)	PRb	Glial fibrillary protein
S-100 protein		Collagen type IV
Factor XIIIa		S-100 protein
CD68		

Myxoid liposarcoma/myxoid lipoblastoma	**Dysplastic nevus/cutaneous melanoma/clear cell sarcoma of soft tissues**
S-100 protein	S-100 protein
	HMB-45
	Melan-A
	Tyrosinase
	MTF-1

Proliferation markers

Mib-1 (Ki-67)	p15, p16	Cyclin-dependent kinases
PCNA	Cyclins (A, B, D1, D2)	Bromodeoxyuridine
p53	Bcl-2	WAF/p21/Cip1
PRb	BAX	Caspases
p105		

---

less likely and usually are of a lesser diagnostic challenge. The typical initial panel may include myogenin and desmin (RMS), NB84 (NB), leukocyte common antigen (leukemia, lymphoma), CD99 (ESFTs), vimentin (rhabdoid tumor, antigen preservation confirmation), and α-fetoprotein (germ cell tumors, hepatoblastoma). Expansion of the antibody panel (Tables 8.3–8.5) may be necessary when the immunoreactivity is limited for these markers, or aberrant immunoreactivity (Table 8.5) is present. This panel is for undifferentiated SRCTs and those that display features of a specific tumor type require only a limited panel of antibodies to confirm the suspected diagnosis.[15,24,59,60,63,66,67,69–71,73–88,107]

The most common SRCTs include NB, ESFTs, RMS, and non-Hodgkin lymphoma (NHL)/lymphoid leukemia (Table 8.4).[26,44–47,56,57,63,66,67,70,74,87,102,104,108] Although most of these tumors present with a certain degree of differentiation and

provide diagnostic evidence for their classification on routine histopathologic examination, several tumors will be undifferentiated or poorly differentiated or possess features that overlap with other SRCT categories. With these tumor types, immunocytochemistry is particularly useful in arriving at an accurate diagnosis. NB expresses several antigens that typically immunoreact with several monoclonal or polyclonal antibodies (Table 8.4).[26,44–47,56,57,63,66,67,70,74,87,102,104,108] In particular, NB84, neuron-specific enolase (NSE), PGP9.5, and chromogranin are identified to a high level and support the diagnosis of NB. With differentiation, intermediate filaments associated with neural development become expressed (neurofilament triple proteins, microtubule-associated protein, myelin basic protein). The pathologist should be aware that megakaryocytic leukemia immunoreacts with NB84. NB84-positive megakaryocytic leukemia, particularly involving the

TABLE 8.5

IMMUNOCYTOCHEMICAL WORKUP FOR UNDIFFERENTIATED CHILDHOOD TUMOR

Antibody panel	Tumor type
Myogenin	Rhabdomyosarcoma, DSRCT
Desmin	Rhabdomyosarcoma, DSRCT
NB84	Neuroblastoma
Chromogranin	Neuroblastoma, DSRCT
Leukocyte common antigen	Lymphoma, leukemic infiltrate
CD99 (MIC2)	Ewing's sarcoma family of tumors
α-fetoprotein	Hepatoblastoma, germ cell tumors
Pancytokeratin	Rhabdoid, DSRCT
INI1/SMARCB1	Rhabdoid tumor, epithelioid sarcoma, atypical teratoid/rhabdoid tumor, small cell (undifferentiated) hepatoblastoma, subset of extraskeletal myxoid chondrosarcoma
TLE1	Synovial sarcoma
Vimentin	Antigen preservation, rhabdoid tumor, fibrosarcoma, myofibroma, spindle cell tumors, mesenchymal tumors, but absent in neuroblastoma
TFE3	Xp11.2 renal tumors, alveolar soft parts sarcoma
Antibodies for defining cell of origin	
Myogenic	Desmin, myogenin, MyoD1, muscle-specific actin
Neural	NB84, NSE, S-100 protein
Hematopoietic/lymphoid	LCA, myeloperoxidase
Germ cell	α-fetoprotein, PLAP, β-HCG, keratin
Neural crest	S-100 protein, HMB-45, CD99, NCAM
Mesenchymal	Vimentin, smooth muscle actin
Aberrant immunoreactivity	
Vimentin	Neuroblastoma (absence of vimentin)
Cytokeratin	Ewing's sarcoma family of tumors, rhabdomyosarcoma, lymphoma, lymphoid leukemia
CA-125	Desmoplastic small round cell tumor
Desmin	Ewing's sarcoma family of tumors, malignant peripheral nerve sheath tumor, rhabdoid tumor
Muscle-specific actin	Ewing's sarcoma family of tumors, malignant peripheral nerve sheath tumor, rhabdoid tumor
Smooth muscle actin	Small cell osteosarcoma
Epithelial membrane antigen	Ewing's sarcoma family of tumors, rhabdomyosarcoma, lymphoma, lymphoid leukemia
NB84	Ewing's sarcoma family of tumors, desmoplastic small round cell tumor, megakaryocytic leukemia
S-100 protein	Rhabdomyosarcoma, small cell osteosarcoma
Neuron-specific enolase	Rhabdomyosarcoma, rhabdoid tumor
TrkA	Ewing's sarcoma family of tumors, rhabdomyosarcoma
CD99	Rhabdomyosarcoma, desmoplastic small round cell tumor, synovial sarcoma
CD19/20	Rhabdomyosarcoma
Leu7 (CD57)	Rhabdomyosarcoma, small cell osteosarcoma
CD68	Rhabdomyosarcoma, malignant peripheral nerve sheath tumor
LeuM1 (CD15)	Desmoplastic small round cell tumor
CD 34	Malignant peripheral nerve sheath tumor

DSRCT, desmoplastic small round cell tumor; HCG, human chorionic gonadotropin.

liver, may be mistaken for NB, especially in children thought to have stage IV and stage IV-S NB. Megakaryocytic leukemia may be separated by immunocytochemical study from NB (platelet glycophorin A, CD61, CD43). ESFTs demonstrate a range of neural differentiation (Table 8.4). Classic Ewing's sarcoma lacks neural differentiation and usually expresses only CD99 and vimentin. Atypical Ewing's sarcoma undergoes initial neural differentiation and immunoreacts with CD99 and usually one to two neural markers (NSE, chromogranin, synaptophysin, S-100 protein). Peripheral primitive neuroectodermal tumor possesses pseudorosettes, reacts with CD99, and expresses several neural proteins. As noted previously, lymphoblastic leukemia and lymphoma express membranous CD99 staining identical to that for ESFTs. With leukemic infiltration of soft tissues or extranodal lymphoma, a diagnosis of Ewing's sarcoma may be made incorrectly. Myogenic differentiation is the hallmark of RMS (Tables 8.3–8.5). Many different muscle precursor antibodies are available and may be needed for diagnosis because of the variable degree of differentiation of myoproteins in this tumor (Tables 8.3 and 8.4). Myogenin, polyclonal desmin, myoD1, and muscle-specific actin are expressed in more than 90% of RMSs, whereas myoglobin is expressed in about three-fourths of these tumors. It is interesting to note that high levels of myogenin are expressed preferentially in ARMS when compared with ERMS. This may be particularly useful in discriminating between a solid alveolar pattern and an embryonal pattern. Less than 10% of RMSs immunoreact with smooth muscle actin. In a subtype of RMS named *undifferentiated sarcoma*, vimentin may be the only tumor marker identified. RMS may be particularly troublesome, because CD99 (Ewing's sarcoma marker), CD19 (B-cell lymphocyte), CD20 (B-cell lymphocyte), and NSE (neural marker) may also be expressed. This may lead to erroneous diagnoses of B-cell leukemia, B-cell lymphoma, Ewing's sarcoma, and NB in some cases of RMSs that do not express the expected myogenic markers. Flow cytometry of an undifferentiated or poorly differentiated RMS may lead to a diagnosis of B-cell leukemia or lymphoma due to CD19 and CD20 cell surface antigen detection. NHLs and lymphoid leukemias immunoreact with leukocyte common antigen (CD45) and either a B-cell marker (CD19/CD20) or a T-cell marker (CD3/CD4/CD8/CD45RO). Typically, these lymphoid neoplasms are not a particular diagnostic problem. However, anaplastic large cell lymphoma (ALCL) may resemble a solid tumor and not immunoreact with any lymphoid antibodies but display CD30, cytokeratin, or epithelial membrane antigen (EMA), either alone or in combination. More recently, an antibody to the protein product (ALK-1, ALK-NPM) of the characteristic translocation in ALCL (ALK-NPM) has been cloned and is commercially available to assist with the diagnosis of ALCL.

Less common SRCTs (Table 8.4) include desmoplastic SRCT (DSRCT), small cell (undifferentiated) OS, small cell hepatoblastoma, blastemal predominant WT, malignant peripheral nerve sheath tumor (MPNST), SS, and rhabdoid tumor.[26,44–47,56,57,63,66,67,70,74,87,102,104,108] Although these tend to be infrequent to rare SRCTs, these neoplasms may be confused with the more common SRCTs, such as NB, Ewing's sarcoma, RMS, lymphoma, and leukemia. DSRCT characteristically is polyphenotypic, and this feature is determined by immunocytochemical and ultrastructural investigations (Tables 8.4 and 8.5). Typically, this tumor expresses desmin in a "dot-like," "globoid" or Golgi-like cytoplasmic patterns, NSE, and cytokeratin. Several other neural, myogenic, and epithelial antigens may also be expressed. Of particular interest is the immunoreactivity with tumor suppressor antibody WT-1. The Ewing's sarcoma marker, CD99, may also be expressed in a limited number of cases. In the absence of desmin and cytokeratin staining, the misdiagnosis of extraosseous Ewing's sarcoma could be rendered. Typically, small cell (undifferentiated) OS (Tables 8.4 and 8.5) reacts with only two readily available antibodies, vimentin and retinoblastoma protein, and it may react with p53. Aberrant immunoreaction with smooth muscle actin, Leu7 (CD57), and S-100 protein may confuse this neoplasm with other poorly differentiated peripheral nerve sheath tumors or mesenchymal sarcomas. The small cell variant of hepatoblastoma (Tables 8.4 and 8.5) may be confused with metastatic NB or primary hepatic NB in stage IV-S disease. This tumor has several overlapping features with NB in that both may immunoreact with NSE and chromogranin. In contrast, small cell hepatoblastoma should express cytokeratin and EMA and may also immunoreact with α-fetoprotein, β-human chorionic gonadotropin (β-HCG), carcinoembryonic antigen (CEA), and α₁-antitrypsin. Interestingly, small cell hepatoblastoma has been shown to lack nuclear INI1/SMACRB1 expression, similar to rhabdoid tumor.[109] Blastemal predominant WT (Tables 8.4 and 8.5) may be somewhat difficult to diagnose if the presence of a kidney tumor is not known, and metastatic disease at another site, such as the lung, is considered to be a primary lesion by the clinician. This tumor may have a very undifferentiated appearance and may mimic any of the SRCTs morphologically. Immunocytochemical studies of blastemal WT should demonstrate pancytokeratin and vimentin expression. In addition, more than 40% of WTs will immunoreact with WT-1 antibodies. MPNST (Tables 8.4 and 8.5) may also resemble SRCTs; however, it will typically express markers associated with peripheral nerve derivation, such as S-100 protein and Leu7. It may also immunoreact with HMB-45 and epithelial antibodies. Aberrant immunoreactivity to desmin, muscle-specific actin, and CD68 may confuse this tumor with other SRCTs. It is also well known that rhabdomyoblastic cells may be seen in MPNSTs (triton tumors), and this tumor could be confused with a poorly differentiated spindle cell RMS or malignant ectomesenchymoma (MEM). SS (Tables 8.4 and 8.5) tends to express the epithelial markers, cytokeratin and EMA, and the intermediate filament, vimentin. In addition, bcl-2 and CD99 may also be identified. Confusion with peripheral nerve sheath tumors may occur when SS immunoreacts with S-100 protein. An aberrant expression of CD99 may be seen in this tumor. In poorly differentiated SS, there may be unexpected expression of Leu7 (CD57), nerve growth factor receptor, CD56, type IV collagen, and neurofilament triple protein. There may be a gray zone between poorly differentiated SS and MPNST that can be resolved definitively only by molecular studies for the translocation characteristic for SS (t(X;18), SYT/SSX). Immunocytochemical expression of TLE1 in SS has been proposed as a unique marker of SS, but this has been recently questioned.[110] Extrarenal rhabdoid tumor (Tables 8.4 and 8.5) may mimic RMS; however, this tumor typically expresses cytokeratin and vimentin in a particular pattern and lacks nuclear expression of IN1/SMARCB1.[111] The cytoplasm is engorged with intermediate filaments that displace the nucleus toward the periphery. Rhabdoid tumors may express desmin and muscle-specific actin, whereas RMS may aberrantly immunoreact with pancytokeratin and EMA. The characteristic intermediate filament pattern by immunocytochemistry and EM is useful in differentiating these tumors from one another.

Certain SRCTs express antigens based on their degree of differentiation.[26,44–47,56,57,63,66,67,70,74,87,102,104,108] For example, with RMS, many different muscle precursor antibodies are available and may be needed for diagnosis because of the variable degree of myogenic differentiation in these tumors (Tables 8.3 to 8.5). Myogenic regulator gene proteins (myogenin, myoD1, myf-3, and myf-4) will be expressed as nuclear antigens at an earlier phase of muscle protein differentiation than those associated with later cytoplasmic myogenic maturation (myoglobin). As noted previously, myogenin, myoD1, polyclonal desmin, and muscle-specific actin are expressed in more than 90% of RMSs, whereas myoglobin is expressed variably (29% to 78%). In contrast, less than 10% of RMSs immunoreact with smooth muscle actin.

Cytogenetic, Tumor Suppressor Proteins, and Proliferation Markers. Several antibodies capable of indirectly detecting cytogenetic translocations and tumor suppressor proteins have become available for FFPE tumor tissues (Tables 8.3 and 8.4). Recently, antibodies (Alk-1, p80) to the chimeric protein produced by the translocation (t(2;5), ALK-NPM) associated with ALCL may provide a means for expedited diagnosis via immunocytochemistry.[104,112] The mutated tumor suppressor, WT-1, has been identified in 40% of WTs and in a large proportion of DSRCTs. TP53 protein overexpression in several SRCTs, including RMS and WT, has been associated with unfavorable histology, recurrences, metastatic disease, and decreased survival.[66,80,83] Overexpression of the retinoblastoma gene protein (pRb) may be seen in SRCTs and may have diagnostic value in certain tumors, such as small cell (undifferentiated) OS. FLI-1 and EWS antibodies are also available for immunocytochemical, FISH, and CISH studies and may be helpful in the diagnosis of ESFTs.[66,103]

Many proliferation markers associated with the cell cycle have unfavorable prognostic significance.[24,62,63,78,81,82,113–116] The overexpression of MIB1 (Ki-67), PCNA, bcl-2, p15, p16, and cyclin-dependent kinases are associated with higher grades and stages of tumors, as well as unfavorable outcomes. In the future, semiquantitative and more rigorous quantitative analysis of tumor suppressor gene products and cell cycle proliferation markers may become a standard of care. Prognosis in spindle cell sarcomas is also linked to the expression levels of the cyclin-dependent kinase inhibitor p27 (Kip1) and cyclin E. Decreased metastasis-free survival (odds ratio 21.3) has been determined when there is low expression of p27 and high expression of cyclin E. Survivin, an apoptosis inhibitor, may be helpful in predicting outcome. With nonmalignant tumors, survivin is not expressed. With malignant tumors, detection of survivin and increased expression levels are associated with a more aggressive clinical course and are independent negative predictors of survival in patients with soft tissue sarcomas.

Expression of certain markers may provide a means to predict favorable outcome.[24,59,60,63,74,78,81,82,94,113–116] For example, CD44-positive tumors are associated with improved survival in soft tissue sarcomas (odds ratio of 3.1). This cell surface marker has been shown to be an independent predictor of survival. Also, TrkA overexpression with NBs is known to be associated with improved survival, in contrast to decreased survival noted with MYCN amplification in neuroblastic tumors.

Tissue Microarrays for Immunocytochemical Analysis. During the past decade, technology has been developed that allows for the creation of tissue microarray (TMA) blocks containing several hundred tumor samples and controls in a single paraffin block.[61,117–122] Using a punch biopsy method,

tumor tissue can be removed precisely from a "donor" paraffin tissue block and placed in a "recipient" paraffin tissue block. This allows for rapid analysis of many different tumor types with tissue cores of representative tissues from donor blocks, arrayed into a recipient block. The tissue cores are mapped for specific tumor type identification and data acquisition purposes. Such TMA blocks allow for parallel testing such as (a) routine, immunocytochemical, and *in situ* hybridization staining; (b) DNA and RNA detection for genetic profiling; (c) FISH for genetic markers; and (d) *in situ* PCR for specific genes. Up to 200 markers per block may be analyzed because each block will provide up to 200 consecutive 3-mm tissue sections. An example of a TMA provided by the pediatric Cooperative Human Tissue Network (CHTN) consisting of more than 100 cores of childhood RMS of various types that have been reacted with the alveolar type-specific antibody AP2b is shown in Figure 8.14. Both the low-magnification picture of the glass slide and the individual cores, labeled by type, confirm the type specificity of the antibody. With one slide and one incubation with antibody, it is possible to validate a candidate antibody for potential diagnostic use. The pathologist plays a pivotal role in development of these TMAs. It is necessary to select representative tumor tissue from donor tissue blocks. Because of heterogeneity within the tumor tissue block, the pathologist may select several different areas of the tumor for analysis.

Of interest is the fact that TMAs provide valid and reliable information regarding the lesional tissue as a whole.[61,117–122] It has been shown that 92% of known gene amplifications for a

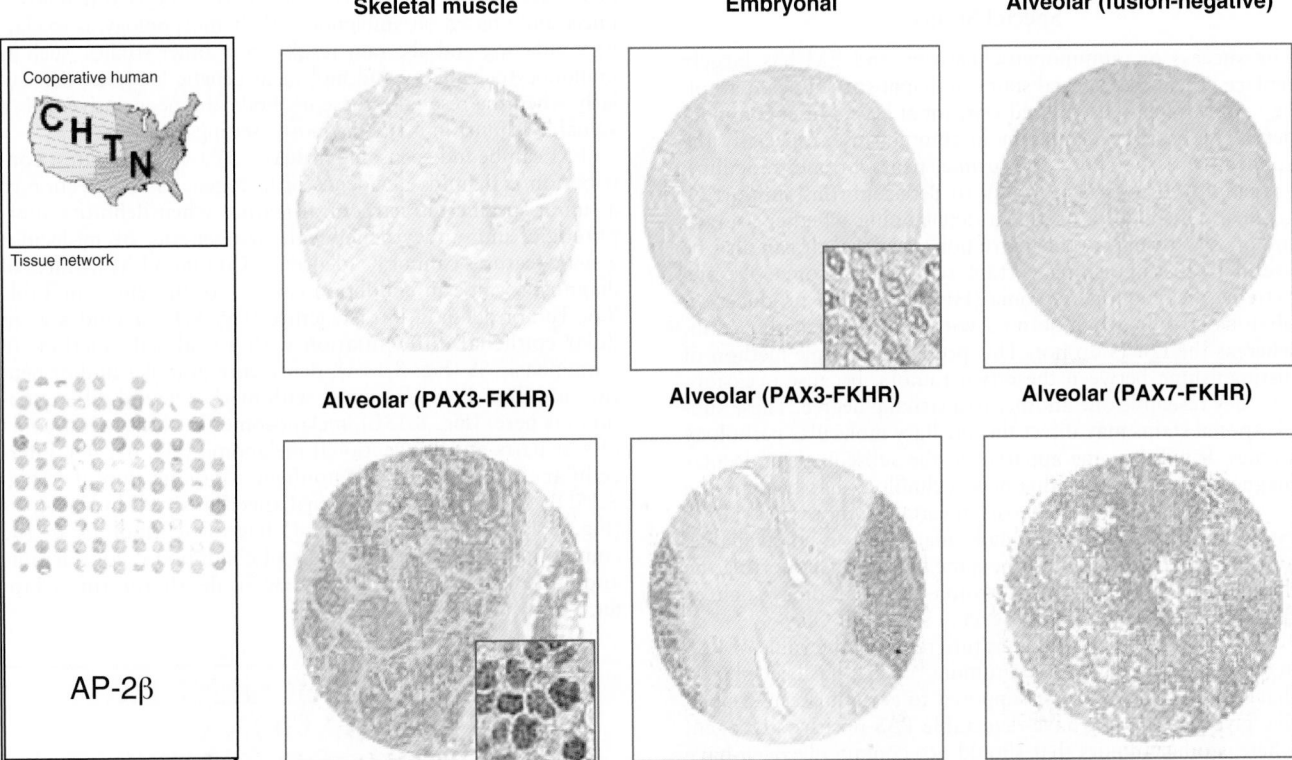

FIGURE 8.14 Tissue microarray (TMA). This TMA with more than 100 cores of childhood rhabdomyosarcoma (RMS) and related control tissues has been reacted with an antibody (TFAP2β) that reacts only with the fusion-positive (e.g., PAX-FOXO1A, PAX 3 or 7) alveolar RMS (ARMS). The ARMS fusion-positive cores are highly reactive; embryonal RMS and fusion-negative ARMS are not, as is also true of other tumors on the array and normal control tissues such as skeletal muscle. Thus, with one slide, an antibody can be evaluated for its specificity and sensitivity, as shown here. (Courtesy of Mike Anderson, Children's Hospital, Los Angeles, Keck School of Medicine, USC.)

specific tumor type are found when at least 25 cases per tumor type are utilized. In addition, only 4% of tissue cores are lost during the sectioning process. Because of this loss, it is recommended that either three cores or two cores from each sample be included in a TMA when using 0.6- or 1.5-mm cores, respectively. It is possible to perform an incredible amount of research in a very short time period. A single marker has been performed on 532 kidney tumor samples over a 3-day period. In a single study, a total of 2,317 tumor specimen cores placed into five recipient TMAs were evaluated by immunocytochemical means for numerous antibodies within a 4-hour time period, and FISH was completed for several tumor markers within a 6-day period. This illustrates well the utility of this technique in defining tumors and obtaining data in a rapid manner.

It is quite obvious that the FFPE tissue blocks from tumors provide a wealth of information that may be "mined" in a relatively short time frame when TMAs are created. The development of tumor-specific TMAs may allow for rapid comparison of the expression of many different antibodies that may be potentially useful in making a diagnosis, directing oncologic management, and predicting metastatic potential, recurrence, and long-term survival. In addition, with TMAs containing a variety of tumors, it is possible to test new antibodies to determine which tumor types react with the antibodies and determine whether these antibodies will be helpful in diagnosis and directing clinical management and predicting prognosis. The added benefit with these TMAs is that FISH, CISH, *in situ* PCR, and molecular studies may also be performed. This opens a large arena for expanding knowledge regarding rare tumors and more conventional tumors, when frozen tissues are not available for in-depth study.

Special Stains

The success of immunocytochemistry and EM has largely replaced the use of special stains in diagnostic surgical pathology. A few remain useful and warrant at least a brief comment here. The basic special stains in common use, especially the connective tissue stains (trichrome, pentachrome, reticulin), are employed most commonly to detect fibrous supporting stroma. This can be useful in determining whether a given tumor is a stroma-producing tumor (sarcoma). It can also be useful in distinguishing certain types of sarcoma. At one extreme, hemangiopericytoma (HPC) generally produces an obvious stroma when stained with a silver reticulin stain, whereas the ESFTs do not. This provides a simple method of distinguishing between these two tumors, because occasionally they resemble one another to a striking degree. These simple special stains may direct the ancillary molecular pathology studies. It will become apparent in the subsequent molecular diagnostic section that this new technology has become the accepted standard for diagnosis in certain tumor types. However, when suitable tissue for molecular studies is not available, a connective tissue stain can be quite helpful in supporting the diagnostic impression of a stroma-poor sarcoma, such as ESFT as opposed to HPC, or even a small cell OS.

The "older" diagnostic literature refers to the value of PAS in the diagnosis of childhood tumors.[123–125] It has been shown that some tumors that are supposed to accumulate PAS-positive glycogen do not have detectable PAS-positive glycogen, whereas other tumors that should not contain glycogen have identifiable glycogen on PAS staining.[126,127] This illustrates that special stains may also give false-negative or false-positive results. It should be noted that formalin fixation and processing extract more than 70% of the glycogen within a cell. If preservation of cytoplasmic glycogen is a goal, it is necessary to use alcohol tissue fixation and tissue processing that contains no formalin. With the current practice of pathology, separate alcohol fixation and dedicated automatic tissue processors for maintaining cytoplasmic glycogen are not currently a standard of practice. The utility of the PAS stain in tumor diagnosis has lost much of its sensitivity and specificity in the face of far more tumor-specific diagnostic methods such as IHC and molecular genetic methods. Still, a strongly positive PAS stain in a suspected Ewing's tumor versus lymphoma versus NB is still strong evidence for a diagnosis of Ewing's tumor. When EM is not available, CD99 results are equivocal, molecular methods yield no conflicting result, and histopathology is equivocal, a strong positive PAS stain can lend credence to a diagnosis of Ewing's sarcoma over the alternatives.

Finally, myeloperoxidase activity demonstrated on tissue sections (von Leder stain) can be an invaluable diagnostic adjunct in the rare case of suspected granulocytic sarcoma (chloroma).[128,129] Often, these tumors present in unusual clinical settings, such as periorbital masses, preceding overt peripheral blood abnormalities suggestive of myeloid leukemia.[130–136] The distinction from more conventional solid tumors of soft tissue such as Langerhans' cell histiocytosis, lymphoma, RMS, and NB (especially periorbital) is generally easily made, because the Leder stain is highly specific for myeloperoxidase activity. Although antibodies against myeloperoxidase have been developed,[129] the Leder stain remains the procedure of choice.

Electron Microscopy

EM no longer plays a major diagnostic role in most adult tumors but is still used in selected cases for childhood tumor diagnosis. Many childhood tumors are studied by EM to improve diagnostic accuracy. The most common reason, beyond diagnostic uncertainty based on ambiguous SRCT morphology, is to clarify conflicting and aberrant results from other studies, such as immunocytochemistry and molecular genetic analyses, particularly when the results of these methods are inconclusive. It is a valuable adjunct in many diagnostic settings.

EM can be indispensable in selected cases. Its greatest contribution is definitive evidence of histogenesis or detection of a tumor-specific ultrastructural feature when definitive morphologic, immunocytochemical, cytogenetic, or molecular genetic features cannot be identified. Common EM features of diagnostic value in childhood cancer are presented in Table 8.6. Tumor-defining ultrastructure (Fig. 8.15) includes glandular epithelial differentiation with apical cell junctions in monophasic SS (Fig. 8.15A), dense core granules and/or neurites in NB or Ewing's tumors with marker neural differentiation (as here) (Fig. 8.15B), melanosomes in clear cell sarcoma of soft parts and conventional melanoma (Fig. 8.15C), intercellular junctions in all nonhematopoietic tumors (Fig. 8.15D), or Birbeck granules in Langerhans' cell histiocytosis (Fig. 8.15E). The spectrum of diagnostic findings in the common and uncommon tumors of childhood is considerable and much too lengthy to review in-depth for this chapter.[24,58,62,63,137–142]

MOLECULAR GENETIC EVALUATION OF CHILDHOOD CANCER

Molecular Genetic Diagnostic Techniques

Molecular genetic diagnostic techniques refer to five major methods currently used to examine the genomic status of cells: (a) PCR, (b) conventional cytogenetics, (c) FISH, (d), SKY, and

TABLE 8.6

ULTRASTRUCTURAL FEATURES FOR SMALL ROUND CELL TUMORS OF CHILDHOOD

Rhabdomyosarcoma
Z-bands
Thick and thin filaments
Myosin-ribosome complexes
Myotubules/myofilaments
Basement membrane
Monoparticulate glycogen
Intercellular junctions, rudimentary

Lymphoma
Polyribosomes
Lack of intercellular junctions
Paucity of organelles

Wilms' tumor, blastemal predominant
Thick, flocculent basement membrane
Cell junctions, well developed
Lumens
Microvilli and cilia
Basilar infolding

Endodermal sinus tumor
Nonmembrane bound
Spheroidal inclusions
Membrane-bound inclusions

Infantile fibrosarcoma
Granular extracellular matrix
Extracellular and intracellular collagen
Intercellular junctions, rudimentary basal lamina
Dilated rough endoplasmic reticulum

Hepatoblastoma
Intercellular junctions
Canaliculi with microvilli
Smooth and rough endoplasmic reticulum

Desmoplastic small round cell tumor
Mesenchymal, rhabdoid, epithelial, and neuroblastic/neural
features
Intermediate filament whirls, neurosecretory dense core
granules
Small glycogen lakes
Focal basal lamina
Rudimentary cell junction

Neuroblastoma
Neurites
Cell processes with fine filaments
Neurosecretory granules
Intercellular junctions, rudimentary
Synaptic-like structures

Ewing's sarcoma/PNET
Focal glycogen aggregates
Neurites, blunted
Pleomorphic neurosecretory granules in PNET
Intercellular junctions, rudimentary

Rhabdoid tumors and atypical teratoid/rhabdoid tumors
Intermediate filament whirls with entrapped organelles
Intercellular junctions, rudimentary

Clear cell sarcoma of soft parts/melanoma
Melanosomes/premelanosomes

Alveolar soft parts sarcoma
Rhomboid crystalline cytoplasmic structures

Myofibroblastic tumors
Spindle cells with peripheral myofilaments
Pinocytotic vesicles
Paucity of collagen
Basal lamina
Dilated rough endoplasmic reticulum
Alveolar soft parts tumor
Rhomboid crystals

PNET, primitive neuroectodermal tumor.

(e) CGH. These methods have certain differences. PCR is applicable largely to extracted DNA or RNA converted into DNA, whereas the other methods detect whole chromosomal genetic status, directly or indirectly.

It is important to note that there are many variations in these methods. In this chapter, the focus is on methods used on a routine basis with childhood tumors. Specific examples of the application of these general methods to childhood tumor diagnosis are discussed.

Karyotypic Analysis (Cytogenetics)

Conventional tumor cytogenetics is in a state of rapid evolution toward integration of molecular techniques. Still, the most common genetic analysis at a whole cell level is the well-established method of G-banding metaphases in karyotypic analysis.[143,144] The vast majority of leukemias and most solid tumors are subjected to karyotypic evaluation.

Standard cytogenetic G-banding readily identifies most tumor-defining gene translocations (Fig. 8.16). In addition, translocations and deletions not previously described in pediatric and adult tumors continue to be discovered. This provides new translocations and genes involved in the oncogenesis of tumors. Unfortunately with tumors, lack of metaphases and failure to grow in short-term culture may lead to uninformative results.[145-147] It must be emphasized that even when metaphases are identified, an occult translocation could be present that is not detectable with standard karyotypic analysis. Further evaluation using PCR to detect occult translocations is definitely justified. Perhaps most importantly, the advent of array CGH and SNP-based molecular cytogenetic methods will increasingly guide decisions as to which method best suits the diagnostic need. For now, our solution is to do all the above, at least until we understand the unique contributions and limitations of each of the techniques.[32,148-150]

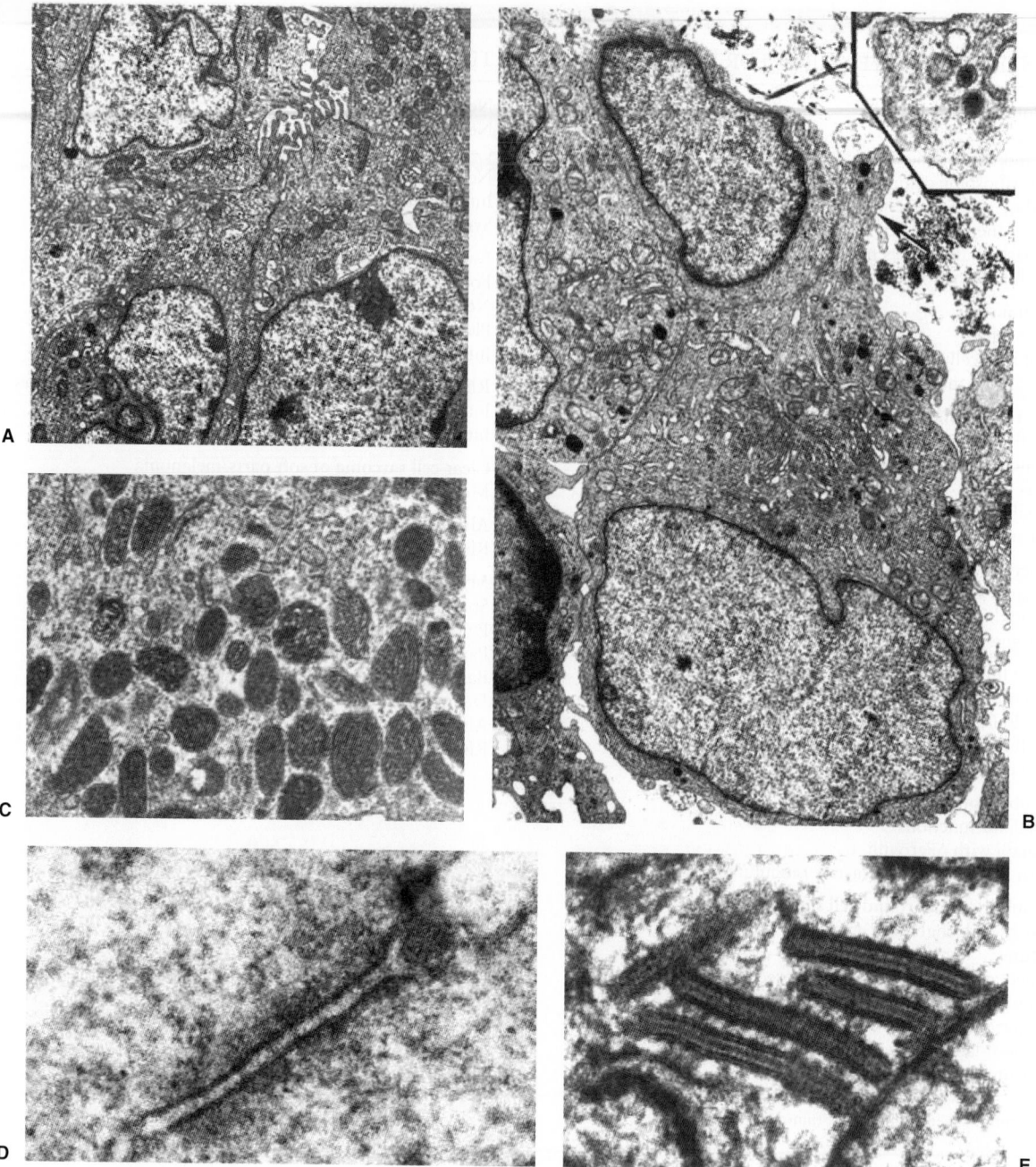

FIGURE 8.15 Tumor ultrastructure. Electron microscopy (EM) remains a valuable adjunctive diagnostic technique, especially when histology is ambiguous and immunocytochemistry is equivocal or contradictory. This composite figure shows five (among many) typical EM findings in childhood tumors that are of diagnostic value: (**A**) glandular differentiation with microvilli (**upper middle**) in a monophasic synovial sarcoma, normally found in the epithelial component; (**B**) marked neural differentiation in a primary bone tumor, establishing the tumor as a Ewing's family tumor with unusually marked neural differentiation; (**C**) typical melanosomes (*arrow*) found in an alveolar soft part sarcoma (melanoma of soft parts) of adolescence; (**D**) a typical cell-cell attachment (*arrow*) in a suspected lymphoma, which is thereby ruled out; and (**E**) Birbeck granules (*arrow*) in an orbital Langerhans' histiocytosis, originally thought to be either metastatic neuroblastoma or orbital rhabdomyosarcoma. In each case, the histopathology and/or immunocytochemistry failed to establish a firm diagnosis, but EM provided the diagnostic information.

Polymerase Chain Reaction

PCR is now commonplace, and this discussion is not intended to review the history of this well-established tool. Modern genomic analysis or most forms of tumor genetics could not be undertaken without it.[151] The purpose here is to discuss how this method has been adapted for detecting genomic alterations and gene expression, even with single tumor cells and FFPE tumor tissue. There are four basic approaches to this technique: (a) conventional PCR, including detection of mRNA, using reverse transcriptase to create complementary DNA (cDNA) from mRNA (RT-PCR); (b) PCR from FFPE

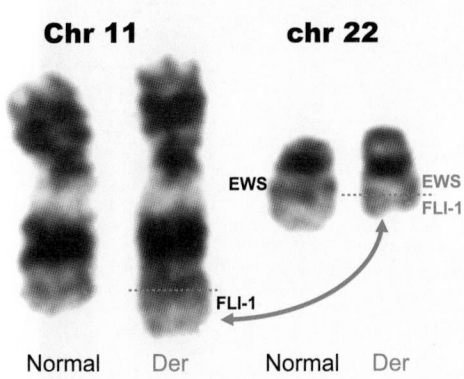

Chr 11   **chr 22**

EWS

EWS
FLI-1

FLI-1

Normal   Der   Normal   Der

FIGURE 8.16 Ewing's sarcoma: cytogenetics. One of the first unequivocal ancillary diagnostics developed in childhood cancer was tumor-specific chromosomal translocations. Ewing's sarcoma routinely shows the chromosomal abnormality illustrated here, a reciprocal translocation of the long arms of chromosome 11 and 22, resulting in the formation of a derivative 11 and 22 paired with a normal 11 and 22. This was the first clue leading to the later identification of a specific chimeric gene in this disease.

tissue by using short primers; (c) quantitative PCR (qPCR); and (d) *in situ* PCR performed on cells or FFPE tissue sections. Creative adaptation of this method includes total mRNA amplification of mRNA extracted from single cells.

PCR is used to detect genomic alterations, gene translocations, amplifications, and deletions, as well as to measure gene (mRNA) expression levels when quantitative methods such as qPCR are employed. Basic PCR is best used to detect alterations in DNA sequences, such as gene fusions, where it is now widely deployed for tumor diagnosis. Although this can be done on genomic DNA, the method of choice is to amplify expressed mRNA sequences. This is quite useful when translocation variants generate huge intronic sequences that may not be reliably amplified, as with the FOXO1A gene involved in ARMS tumorigenesis. This method works reliably and predictably, as documented by the extensive literature on the subject.[152–154] Only a minority of tumors are preserved frozen for analysis by conventional RT-PCR. Therefore, this method has been adapted for FFPE tissues.

A major PCR diagnostic innovation was the introduction of reliable qPCR analysis. This is an important tool because it extends PCR detection of gene expression beyond simply the presence or absence of gene expression. Quantitative levels can be measured and compared, such as MYCN expression (typically associated with MYCN amplification) in NBs or

expression levels of a tumor-specific chimeric gene such as EWS-FLI1 in Ewing's sarcoma (Fig. 8.17).

The emergence of PCR amplification methods allows for generating abundant RNA that stoichiometrically mimics that within the original tumor sample. Several linear amplification methods have been introduced that allow for analysis of the entire expressed gene repertoire from a very small sample or single cells by methods such as microarrays,[155–159] although potentially with bias introduced by nonlinear effects.[160] It is possible to amplify DNA or RNA from minimally invasive procedures, such as fine needle aspiration or laser capture microscopy of single tumor cells or small groups of tumor cells, as a diagnostic procedure in the near future.

Fluorescence *In Situ* Hybridization

The limitations of traditional cytogenetics led to the development of interphase FISH. This technique does not require metaphases and potentially yields diagnostic information from frozen tissue, touch preparations (cytologic imprints), and even FFPE tissue sections (Fig. 8.18).[161–173] Although new translocations and genes cannot be found by this technique, it is an important diagnostic tool because of the rapidity, specificity, and sensitivity in detecting translocations and amplified genes by using commercially available probes. Although FISH has primarily been used to detect genomic alterations, it can also detect gene expression by mRNA hybridization with touch preparations or tissue sections. The mRNA FISH hybridization technique is less sensitive than PCR, requires better RNA preservation, and is not as widely used for diagnostic purposes. It is, however, a very useful diagnostic tool.[174–183]

Spectral Karyotyping

The development of methods to label and detect individual chromosomes, using spectral analysis of emitted fluorescence by assigning computer-generated false colors to individual chromosomes, is a major advance in chromosomal analysis.[184–187] This method also allows metaphase and even interphase chromosome visualization.[188,189] This is particularly important, given the frequent failure of conventional cytogenetics to grow tumor cells. With cell culture failure in conventional cytogenetics, the chance of detecting constitutional chromosomal abnormalities (number, translocation, deletions) is lost. Certain tumors have a high culture failure rate (alveolar soft part sarcoma [ASPS]), and these tumors cannot realistically be analyzed by conventional cytogenetics. Methods such as SKY and FISH are the only practical means of directly visualizing chromosomal abnormalities. Although new, high-resolution methods such as CGH and SNP arrays have become available, these techniques do not allow direct

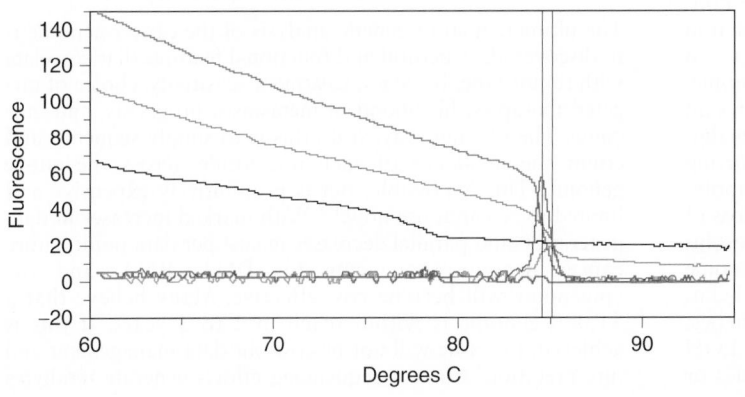

FIGURE 8.17 Quantitative real-time polymerase chain reaction detection of EWS-FLI1 in a presumed Ewing's sarcoma patient. Compared with a positive (**top line**) and negative (**bottom line**) control, two separate assays (**upper:** primary tumor; **lower:** recurrent tumor) for EWS-FLI1 in a patient sample show increased temperature-dependent fluorescence intensity, documenting both the amount and identity of the EWS-FLI1 Ewing's sarcoma–specific chimeric gene and thus confirming the suspected diagnosis. (Courtesy of Betty Schaub, Children's Hospital, Los Angeles)

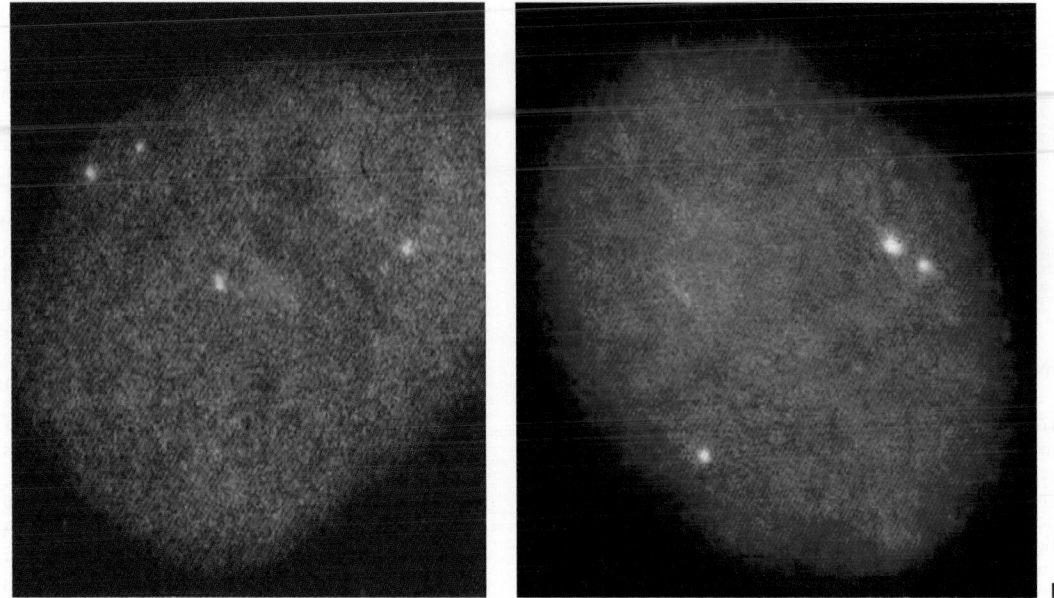

FIGURE 8.18 Ewing's sarcoma: fluorescence *in situ* hybridization (FISH). Once the chimeric gene responsible for Ewing's sarcoma was identified, other forms of molecular cytogenetic analysis, notably FISH, were developed, which routinely and quickly identify the diagnostic translocation, as illustrated here. **Panel A** illustrates the four signals (two from the two copies of EWS, two from the two copies of FLI1) found in nontranslocated cells. **Panel B**, in contrast, illustrates a translocation-positive Ewing's sarcoma family tumor with a typical EWS-FLI1 translocation, which results in three signals: one normal EWS, one FLI1, and one fusion gene, visible as a fused red-green signal.

imaging of chromosomal breaks and fusions such as that allowed by SKY.[190]

SKY has been rapidly deployed to analyze a host of tumors that were previously difficult to analyze by traditional cytogenetic means. Cryptic inversions, translocations, numerical abnormalities, and various chromosomal abnormalities have been readily identified in many childhood tumors, including lymphoma, NB, and RMS.[188,189,191,192] SKY is an important adjunct for chromosomal analysis of tumors, given its enormous scope of application and sensitivity to even minute abnormalities, especially when employed in conjunction with derivative techniques such as SNP arrays for CNV. A drawback is the need for intact fresh tumor cells or tissue for chromosomal analysis.

Single Nucleotide Polymorphism–Based Molecular Cytogenetic Analysis

One of the more exciting developments in genetic analysis of cancer has been the recent emergence of exquisitely sensitive and high-resolution SNP arrays.[32,193,194] It should be noted that the more important content of these arrays is the nonpolymorphic probes. This is because alone or in conjunction with the polymorphic probes, nonpolymorphic probes can interrogate as many as 2 million bases in the human genome. When coupled with suitable analytic software, this allows an unprecedented view of the genome, whether normal or malignant. These arrays are increasingly used to discover recurring and minute CNV patterns (loss or gain, based on nonpolymorphic probe hybridization intensity values) or LOH (loss of heterozygosity in concert with SNPs). The remarkable resolution of 1 to 2 kilobases across the entire nonrepetitive genome of these arrays, coupled with their relative economy has led to their increasing use, often replacing conventional cytogenetics. Often, the results may discover an unknown CNV or LOH abnormality in a tumor that may be of diagnostic values or

prognostic significance when analyzed with clinical information.[194–197] An example of a recurring genomic alteration in Ewing's sarcoma is presented in Figure 8.19. Recurring amplification of chromosome 14q32.33 is seen in all of the 43 tumors demonstrated in Figure 8.19. The variable boundaries and the variable extent of the amplification (pink >1 but <2; red >2) are consistent with a tumor-specific CNV as opposed to a normal CNV, now recognized throughout the genome. The power of this method is evolving, but early data suggest that this approach to cancer "cytogenetics" will become the dominant analysis of the DNA cancer genome. This method may point the way to in-depth DNA sequencing, until DNA sequencing technology becomes cost-effective and reliable. Because of the extraordinary cost (currently approximately $50,000) to sequence a cancer genome, it is likely that SNP-based molecular cytogenetic analysis will be employed in the near future. Additional examples of this potentially diagnostic method for several tumor types will be discussed in the sections that follow.

"Next-Gen" DNA Sequencing

The ultimate goal of genetic analysis of the cancer genome is to discover all structural and functional features that correlate with tumor type, behavior, treatment sensitivity, choice of targeted therapies, likelihood of metastasis, prognosis, and outcome. The obvious way to do this is to simply sequence and count the incidence of each nucleotide across the entire genome. This is possible, but is prohibitively expensive and limited to research use now.[198] With marked increases in data generation and parallel decreases in cost per data point, entire cancer genome sequencing for DNA, RNA, and the epigenome will become cost-effective. Many believe that a $1,000 genome is within reach in 2 to 3 years. If this is achieved, the issue will not be cost but data management and interpretation. Current sequencing efforts generate terabytes

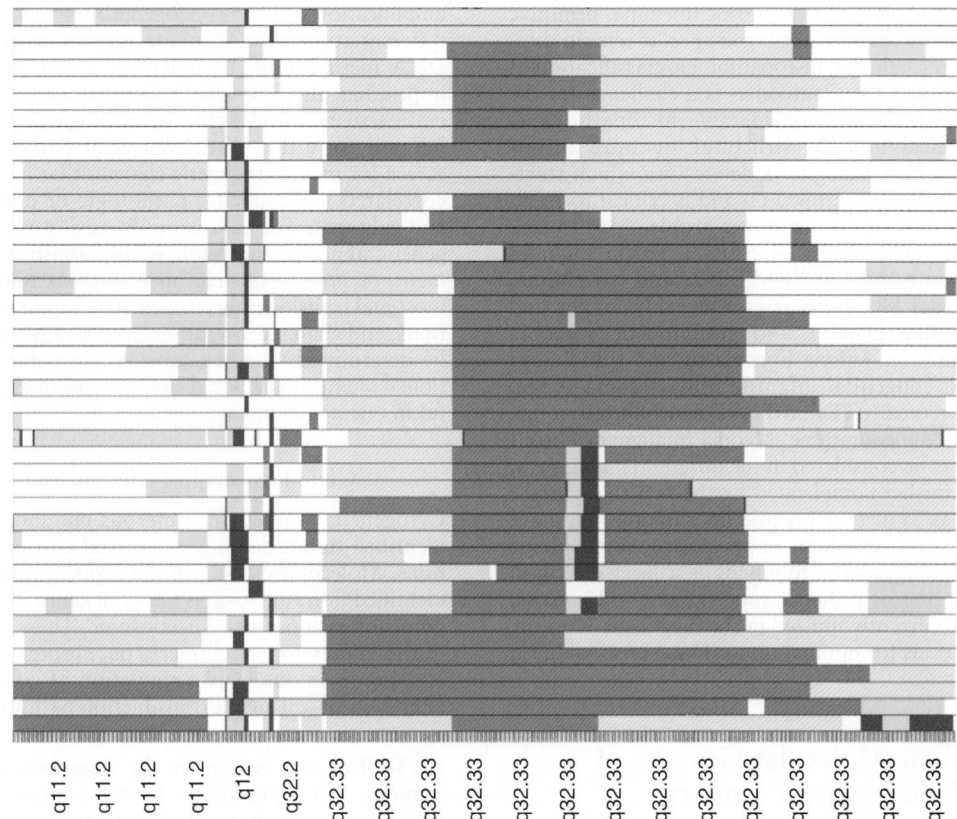

q11.2 q11.2 q11.2 q11.2 q12 q32.2 q32.33 q32.33 q32.33 q32.33 q32.33 q32.33 q32.33 q32.33 q32.33 q32.33 q32.33 q32.33 q32.33

FIGURE 8.19 Copy number variation (CNV) in Ewing's sarcoma detected by single nucleotide polymorphism (SNP) array. Patterns of CNV can be of diagnostic value in tumor diagnosis as well. Here, euploidy (CN = 2) is indicated by white; light and dark blue are areas of genomic loss (CN = 1 and 0, respectively), while pink (CN = 3) and red (CN = 4 and greater) indicate increased copy number. Here, 43 primary Ewing's tumors were compared using Affymetrix SNP 6.0 arrays to detect CNV. Note that all 43 tumors show increased copy number in a region centered around 14q32.33. This appears to be a tumor-specific CNV, as the boundaries are variable and the CNV is not reported in the DGV database of normal genomic variants. If this were a normal CNV, the boundaries would be regular and the degree of copy number increase would be uniform across all tumors, neither of which is true of this CNV. (Image courtesy of Diana Abdueva, Ph.D.; data courtesy of Beth Lawlor, M.D., Ph.D.)

of data within a short time period with a single patient. Data generated will likely rise to petabytes of data within the next few years. At that point, data interpretation will become the dominant theme for cancer diagnosis and management. Already acute lymphocytic leukemia (ALL) has been subjected to an in-depth genetic analysis, with remarkable results.[197,199] NB is in the process of undergoing genetic analysis, and numerous other childhood cancers are close behind. These discoveries were made using current generation technology. When data sets are created using "next generation" DNA and RNA sequencing technology integrated with existing genomic databases, it is all but certain that our understanding of cancer in children and adults will be changed forever. This will lead to unprecedented understanding of "driver" versus "passenger" changes in the genome and allow identification of promising diagnostic, prognostic, and therapeutic targets for future development.[200]

Implications for Tumor Molecular Genetics

The variety of molecular methods currently being applied, or in the development stage, in cancer biology is unprecedented. Given the generally accepted concept that cancer is a disease associated with alteration in a variety of genes, this approach will yield a vast amount of information about the etiology and

mechanisms of cancer. In the future, this may lead to identification of fundamental mechanisms of oncogenesis for specific tumor types and even the child's own tumor. In the meantime, more established methods, such as PCR and correlative FISH with tumor-specific probes, remain the mainstay for molecular genetic diagnosis.

Identification of genetic alterations in human neoplasia has contributed profound insights into the oncogenic process and has been instrumental in the emergence of molecular diagnostics as a distinct field in pathology. Detection of tumor markers in tumor biopsies and resections is rapidly being incorporated into the diagnostic workup. This has led to changes in the way that pathologists handle tumor specimens in the surgical pathology suite to optimize the information derived at the molecular level. As specific tumor markers and genes are discovered for individual tumor types, the pathology community must reevaluate the way in which tumors are classified. This is particularly the case for childhood bone and soft tissue tumors, which tend to possess a primitive appearance and are difficult to differentiate from each other by morphology alone.[201] Tumor-specific chromosomal translocations and gene amplifications characteristic for many pediatric solid tumors play an increasingly important role in the diagnosis, treatment, and prognosis of these tumors. Whereas organ-specific childhood tumors such as WT, hepatoblastoma, and pancreatoblastoma are less of a diagnostic dilemma, primitive pediatric solid tumors that are not organ specific remain difficult to diagnose. In particular, histopathologic classification of pediatric bone and soft tissue sarcomas is a challenge for the surgical pathologist, despite considerable histopathologic, immunohistochemical, and ultrastructural literature on this topic. An accurate initial diagnosis determines which treatment protocol a patient is enrolled on and is critical to prognosis. SRCTs still represent a diagnostic problem due to lack of differentiation. Historically, the SRCT group includes ESFTs, ARMS, some cases of ERMS, NB, and lymphoma. However, the actual SRCT list is considerably longer and includes entities like DSRCT and granulocytic sarcoma (chloroma) (Table 8.2). Among fibroblastic and spindle cell malignancies, SS, congenital infantile fibrosarcoma (CFS), adult-type fibrosarcoma (ATFS), MPNST, neurofibrosarcoma, and undifferentiated pleomorphic sarcoma (malignant fibrous histiocytoma) must be considered in the differential diagnosis. The diagnosis is further complicated by the fact that spindle cell lesions, such as SS or even myxoid liposarcoma, can have a small round cell cytologic appearance and mimic SRCTs.[24,45,46,56,59,63,67,70,141] The following is a brief review of the molecular genetics of pediatric solid tumors, a discussion of molecular tests currently utilized in the diagnostic workup, and recommendations for optimal tumor tissue processing for such studies.

Diagnostic Molecular Genetics of Pediatric Solid Tumors

Molecular studies over the past several decades have expanded the list of genetic abnormalities in pediatric solid tumors, including chromosomal translocations and inversions; amplification of proto-oncogenes involved in cell growth and differentiation; loss of tumor suppressor genes by mutation, DNA methylation, or deletion; abnormalities of genomic imprinting; alterations in DNA repair mechanisms; and telomerase activity. From a clinicopathologic perspective, it is feasible only for a diagnostic molecular pathology laboratory to screen for recurrent genetic changes that have been rigorously correlated with specific pathologic or clinical tumor types and subtypes. The following discussion primarily focuses on genetic abnormalities with well-established diagnostic, treatment, or prognostic relevance, such as tumor-defining chromosomal translocations in pediatric sarcomas, gene amplifications, and genomic alterations in NB (Table 8.7). It remains to be determined whether some of the other previously mentioned alterations will have clinicopathologic correlations useful in oncologic management.

Gene Fusions in Pediatric Solid Tumors

Cytogenetic studies of numerous childhood sarcomas have identified tumor-defining reciprocal chromosomal translocations. Molecular cloning of the translocation breakpoints has identified in-frame fusions between genes located at the breakpoints of each partner chromosome. These gene fusions result in the expression of chimeric oncoproteins that have transforming functions via dysregulation of gene transcription or alteration of cell signal transduction pathways.[50,202,203]

EWS-ETS Gene Fusions in the Diagnosis of Ewing's Family Tumors. The diagnosis of Ewing's tumor and other ESFTs, which occur in bone and soft tissues, has traditionally depended on clinical features along with demonstrable intracellular glycogen accumulation, variable evidence of neural differentiation, and immunocytochemical staining for the

TABLE 8.7

COMMON MOLECULAR TESTS USED IN THE DIAGNOSTIC WORKUP OF PEDIATRIC SOLID TUMORS

Tumor	Cytogenetics	Molecular lesion	Molecular test (reference)
Ewing's family of tumors	t(11;22)(q24;q12)	*EWS-FLI1*	RT-PCR (40,191)
	t(21;22)(q22;q12)	*EWS-ERG*	FISH (184)
	t(7;22)(p22;q12)	*EWS-ETV1*	
	Other 22q12	Other *EWS* fusions	
Alveolar rhabdomyosarcoma	t(2;13)(q35;q14)	*PAX3-FKHR*	RT-PCR (40)
	t(1;13)(p36;q14)	*PAX7-FKHR*	FISH (347)
DSRCT	t(11;22)(p13;q12)	*EWS-WT1*	RT-PCR (40, 491)
CCSSP	t(12;22)(q13;q12)	*EWS-ATF1*	RT-PCR (219)
ALCL	t(2;5)(p23;q35)	*NPM-ALK*	RT-PCR (239)
			IHC (242)
Synovial sarcoma	t(X;18)(p11.2;q11.2)	*SYT-SSX1*	RT-PCR (247, 249)
		SYT-SSX2	FISH (141)
CFS and CMN	t(12;15)(p13;q25)	*ETV6-NTRK3*	RT-PCR (252, 256)
ASPS	t(X;17)(p11;p25)	*ASPL-TFE3*	RT-PCR (274)
IMT	t(1;2)(q22–23;p23)	*TPM3-ALK*	RT-PCR (280)
	t(2;19)(p23;p13.1)	*TPM4-ALK*	
Neuroblastoma	DMs; HSRs	*MYCN* amplif	Differential PCR (119)
			FISH (29, 353, 492)
	1p deletion	?	LOH (285)
	17q amplification	?	CGH and FISH (169)

DSRCT, desmoplastic small round cell tumor; CCSSP, clear cell sarcoma of soft parts; ALCL, anaplastic large cell lymphoma; CFS, congenital fibrosarcoma; CMN, congenital mesoblastic nephroma; ASPS, alveolar soft part sarcoma; IMT, inflammatory myofibroblastic tumor; DMs, double minute chromosomes; HSRs, homogeneously staining regions; RT-PCR, reverse transcriptase polymerase chain reaction; FISH, fluorescence in situ hybridization; IHC, immunohistochemistry; LOH, loss of heterozygosity; CGH, comparative genomic hybridization.

CD99 (MIC2) antigen by using the O13 antibody.[201] Aside from CD99 expression, none of these features are specific. Even MIC2 immunocytochemical staining, although present in more than 95% of ESFTs, has been described in many tumors such as RMS, NB, and lymphoblastic leukemia and lymphoma.[84,204–209] One feature of ESFTs that appears to be consistent is common genetic rearrangements, with approximately 85% of cases showing a t(11;22)(q24;q12) chromosomal translocation (Fig. 8.16).[210] Molecular cloning of the translocation breakpoint has identified an in-frame fusion of the EWS gene from chromosome 22q12 with FLI1 from chromosome 11q24, a member of the ETS family of transcription factors (Fig. 8.20A) that can be detected by a simple EWS-FLI1 PCR reaction and reveals multiple fusion variants (Fig. 8.20B).[211,212] An additional 10% to 15% of ESFTs carry a variant t(21;22)(q22;q12) translocation in which EWS is fused to another ETS gene, ERG from chromosome 21q22.[213] More rarely (<1% of tumors), EWS-FEV, EWS-EVI1, and EWS-ETV1 gene fusions resulting from t(2;22), t(7;22), and t(17;22) translocations, respectively, have been reported.[214–216] Until recently, it was thought that virtually all ESFTs carry some form of EWS-ETS gene fusion and that these rearrangements are pathognomonic of the ESFT.[210] For this reason, the preferred diagnostic PCR reaction utilizes 5′ EWS primers coupled with a generic ETS-domain 3″ primer (Fig. 8.20A). While the overall theme is most likely correct, it is now clear that in a small percentage of ESFTs, different ETS transcription factor genes may be fused to other members of the EWS gene family. For example, gene fusions between the FUS (TLS) gene on chromosome 16p11 with the ERG gene in ESFTs have further highlighted the theme that the transactivation domains of EWS and related proteins are important in ESFT

oncogenesis.[217] More recently, a novel t(2;16) translocation producing an in-frame fusion of FUS and FEV was reported by several groups as another example of this notion.[218] It will be important to assess the incidence of FUS-ERG and FUS-FEV gene fusions in EWS-ETS fusion negative ESFTs to determine the practicality of testing for these fusions to the diagnostic work-up of ESFTs, given the fact that conventional EWS break-apart FISH assays are predicted to be negative in such cases. Also requiring further clarification is the recent description of EWS fusions to the non-ETS gene, NFATc2, in four ESFTs.[219] Such fusions would not be detected by conventional EWS-ETS PCR assays.

Studies of EWS-ETS gene fusions serve as a paradigm for investigating the biology of childhood solid tumor oncogenesis. Expressed EWS-ETS chimeric proteins are oncogenic in NIH3T3 cells[212] and function as aberrant transcription factors binding to ETS consensus sequences of target genes.[212,220–222] Several potentially interesting genes have been implicated as targets of EWS-ETS–mediated transcriptional activation.[223–230] These include those encoding stromelysin 1, cytochrome P450 F1, cytokeratin 15, manic fringe, E2-C, Id2, PIM3, uridine phosphorylase, and p21WAF1/CIP1. How these putative EWS-ETS targets are involved in oncogenesis remains, for the most part, unknown. An interesting possible role for EWS-ETS chimeric oncoproteins is suggested by the recent observation that EWS-FLI1 and other EWS-ETS proteins downregulate expression of the TGFβ type II receptor (TβRII), a putative tumor suppressor gene.[231,232] TGFβ signaling through this receptor induces apoptosis in many cell types; and therefore, repression of TGFβ RII expression may provide ESFT cells with a mechanism to elude a major pathway leading to programmed cell death. Related to this theme is the

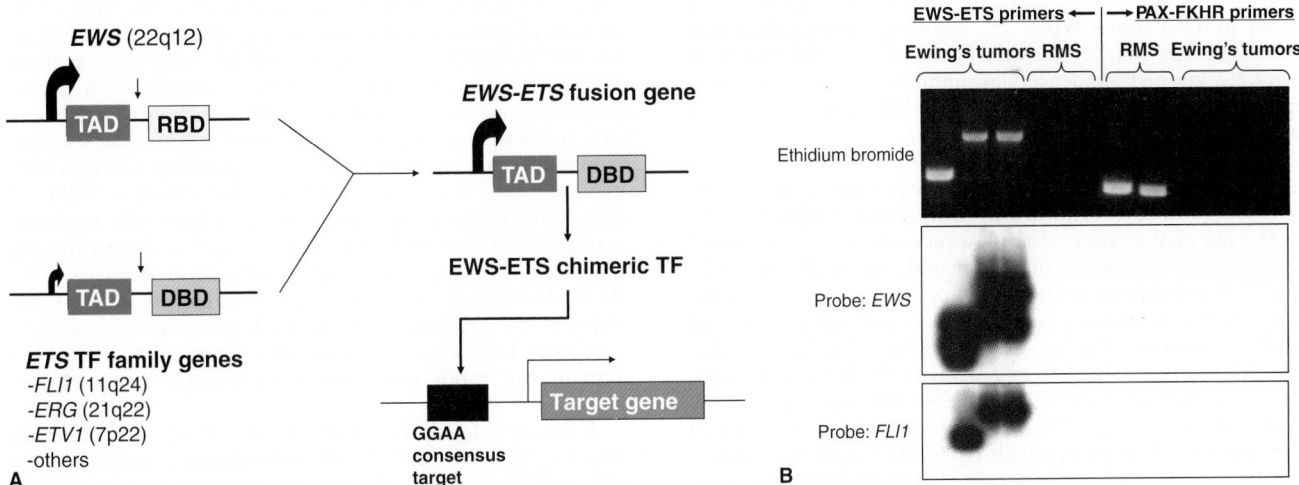

FIGURE 8.20 A: Schematic diagram of EWS-ETS gene fusions in Ewing's family tumors. As a result of chromosomal translocation breakpoints (*small downward arrow*), the EWS gene on chromosome 22q12 becomes fused to one ETS family genes, most often FL11 on 11q24 or ERG on 21q22. This fuses the transcriptional activation domain (TAD) of EWS with the DNA-binding domain (DBD) of the respective ETS gene and places the resulting EWS-ETS fusion gene under the control of the strong EWS promoter. This rearrangement replaces the RNA-binding domain (RBD) of EWS with the ETS DGD, creating a chimeric transcription factor (TF) which binds to ETS concensus GGAA sites on DNA and activates transcription of ET target genes thought to be involved in EWS-ETS induced transformation. B: Reverse transcriptase polymerase chain reaction analysis of Ewing's family tumors. Consensus primers for EWS-ETS fusion transcripts are used in experiments (**left side of figure**) to demonstrate EWS-FL11 transcripts in the three Ewing's tumor samples but not in the two rhabdomyosarcoma (RMS) samples by ethidium bromide staining of agarose gels (**top panel**). This is confirmed by probing the amplification products with oligonucleotide probes for EWS (**middle panel**) and FL11 (**bottom panel**). On the **right** side, primers for the PAX-FOXO1A gene fusions of alveolar RMS are found in the RMS cases but not in the Ewing's tumor samples.

finding that inactivation of the *p16* INK4a locus occurs frequently in ESFTs, suggesting that loss of the pRb pathway may be important in Ewing's sarcoma oncogenesis.[233,234] On the other hand, expression of *EWS-FLI1* in human fibroblasts induces p53-mediated cell death,[235] supporting a role for p53 as a tumor suppressor in ESFTs, although p53 mutations appear to be uncommon in these malignancies.[236] Further studies are necessary to determine the relative roles of the pRb and p53 growth regulatory pathways in ESFT oncogenesis. A recent study discovered that silencing of *EWS-FLI1* fusion gene by using RNA interference (RNAi) results in induction of apoptosis in ESFT cells by a process involving insulin-like growth factor binding protein 3 (IGFBP-3). IGFBP-3 is a repressor of insulin-like growth factor 1 (IGF-1)–mediated proliferation and survival signaling.[237] In fact, ESFTs appear to utilize a number of autocrine growth factor pathways. IGF-1 is expressed by Ewing's sarcomas, and the oncogenicity of EWS-FLI1 requires the presence of an intact IGF-1 receptor (IGF1R) pathway.[238,239] Therefore, an important role of EWS-ETS fusion proteins may be to repress IGFBP-3 or other inhibitors of IGF1R signaling. Moreover, Ewing's sarcoma tumor cells have been found to express neural peptides, such as the bombesin homolog, gastrin-releasing peptide (GRP).[240] The role of GRP in ESFT tumorigenesis remains unclear.

Recent studies of the role that EWS-ETS chimeric proteins play in ESFT oncogenesis have used RNAi to evaluate the effects of knocking down EWS-FLI expression in ESFT cells.[237,241–243] This blocks oncogenic transformation, including xenograft formation in immunodeficient mice, indicating that sustained EWS-FLI expression is required for ESFT oncogenesis. In addition, RNAi studies identified NKX2.2 as an important gene for the transformed phenotype of ESFT cells.[242,243] This homeodomain-containing transcription factor appears to function as a transcriptional repressor in ESFTs through TLE-family corepressor proteins and histone deacetylases.[244] NKX2.2 is expressed in most ESFT cases but only rarely in other tumor types[244,245] and therefore may be a useful diagnostic marker for ESFTs. Moreover, inhibition of NKX2.2 via histone deacetylase inhibitors may represent a tractable approach for the treatment of ESFT patients, but this will require additional investigations.

Other Diagnostic *EWS*-Associated Gene Fusions in Specific Small Round Cell Tumors of Childhood. DSRCT is an aggressive malignancy of adolescence and early adulthood that coexpresses skeletal muscle, neural, and epithelial markers.[246] This tumor most commonly occurs in association with serosal mesothelial-lined surfaces and as such can be confused with extraosseous ESFTs. A characteristic t(11;22)(p13;q12) translocation in DSRCT fuses *EWS* with the *WT1* tumor suppressor gene from 11p13.[48,247] Another *EWS*-associated gene results from the t(12;22)(q13;q12) translocation of clear cell sarcoma of soft parts in which *EWS-ATF1* gene fusion transcripts are expressed in tumor cells.[248] This melanin-producing tumor most commonly occurs in the limbs of young adults and late adolescents.[201] The epithelioid appearance of tumor cells can sometimes cause confusion with other SRCTs and epithelioid sarcoma. Both EWS-W T1 and EWS-ATF1 chimeric products appear to be DNA-binding proteins and function as aberrant transcription factors. *EWS* gene fusions are also observed in the adult sarcoma, extraskeletal myxoid chondrosarcoma, in which *EWS* is fused to the orphan nuclear receptor gene *TEC* (*CHN*).[249,250]

***PAX-FKHR* (FOXO1A) Gene Fusions in the Diagnosis of Alveolar Rhabdomyosarcoma.** Childhood RMS is generally subdivided into ERMS (approximately 65% of cases) and more primitive forms including ARMS (approximately 20%

of cases) and so-called undifferentiated sarcoma (approximately 15% of cases).[251] Currently, undifferentiated sarcoma is in the process of being classified as a separate non-RMS soft tissue sarcoma. The diagnosis of RMS is based on tumor architecture, cellular morphology, and myogenic differentiation in tumor cells.[201] The latter is generally documented by desmin and muscle-specific actin immunostaining and, more recently, expression of myogenin and MyoD family of myogenic transcription factors.[252,253] However, these markers can be expressed in many tumor types.[254,255] Of RMS subtypes, only ARMS is characterized by tumor-defining diagnostic rearrangements. Approximately 60% of ARMS cases demonstrate the t(2;13)(q35;q14) translocation, which fuses the *PAX-3* gene from 2q35 with the *FOXO1A* gene from 13q14. A smaller proportion of ARMS (15%–20%) have the t(1;13)(p36;q14) translocation that fuses *PAX-7* from 1p36 with *FOXO1A*.[256,257] *PAX3* and *PAX7* are members of the PAX family of transcription factors, whereas *FOXO1A* is a member of the forkhead family of developmentally regulated transcription factors.[258] Resulting *PAX3/FOXO1A* and *PAX7/FOXO1A* fusion transcripts can be detected in tumor tissue by RT-PCR.[48] Although several early molecular studies indicate that *PAX3-FOXO1A* and *PAX7-FOXO1A* gene fusions were present in a large majority of ARMS cases,[31,48] others have reported that significantly higher percentages of ARMS cases lack these fusions.[259,260] A total of 171 COG RMS cases were analyzed for the *PAX-FOXO1A* gene fusions. Only *PAX3-FOXO1A* or *PAX7-FOXO1A* gene fusions were expressed in ARMS cases. *PAX3-FOXO1A* and *PAX7-FOXO1A* fusion transcripts were detected in 55% and 22% of ARMS patients, respectively, whereas 23% were fusion negative, indicating that a proportion of ARMS cases either have molecular alterations that are yet to be defined or are not bona fide ARMS, at least as defined by the characteristic PAX:FOXO1A translocation.[260] PAX3-*FOXO1A* and PAX7-*FOXO1A* chimeric oncoproteins, like EWS-ETS chimera, function as aberrant transcription factors.[259] This has lead to translocation-negative ARMS tumors being group with ERMS tumors with respect to treatment, with similar prognosis and survival as ERMS. These fusion proteins activate transcription of genes containing PAX-binding sites but with higher potency than do the corresponding wild-type PAX proteins.[261,262] Expression of *PAX3-FOXO1A* in NIH3T3 cells activates myogenic transcription, including the myogenic transcription factors MyoD and myogenin, demonstrating that this chimeric oncoprotein induces myogenesis.[261,262] PAX3-*FOXO1A* transformation, similar to EWS-FLI1, requires the presence of an intact IGF1R signaling axis.[263] Similar to EWS-FLI1 in human fibroblasts, PAX3-*FOXO1A* activates apoptotic pathways if expressed in non-RMS cell lines.[264]

It was previously reported that in a study of COG RMS patients, those with *PAX7-FOXO1A*–positive tumors had significantly improved outcomes in comparison with patients with PAX3-FOXO1A–positive tumors.[260] *PAX7-FOXO1A* expression was shown to correlate with better patient outcome than *PAX3-FOXO1A* expression in ARMS, but this reached statistical significance only for patients with metastatic disease. However, this notion is not universally accepted. In recent studies, gene expression microarray analysis has been used not only to determine diagnostic subgroups in RMS but also to define a novel prognostic classification scheme.[16,265] Using small metagene subsets for analysis, investigators derived highly reproducible molecular classes of RMS based solely on genomic analysis at diagnosis.[16] Adoption of these molecular criteria may offer a more clinically relevant diagnostic scheme, thus potentially improving patient management and therapeutic outcomes in RMS. Furthermore, these studies were extended to produce a metagene cohort whereby the expression pattern of a small number of genes was highly predictive of outcome.[266] This was independent of individual clinical risk factors, such as patient age, stage, tumor size, and histology, but was correlated with risk classification used by COG as well as biologic subsets of ARMS tumors. This metagene analysis scheme is highly predictive of outcome and appears to provide additional information about outcome for intermediate risk patients.

NPM-ALK **Gene Fusion in Diagnosis of Anaplastic Large Cell Lymphoma.** ALCL (Ki-1 lymphoma, Alkoma) is a distinct clinicopathologic subtype of intermediate grade NHL that may be seen in children[267] (see also Chapter 24). ALCL has a wide range of morphologic appearances, although it is most often described as having large pleomorphic cells expressing CD30 (Ki-1) and ALK1-NPM antigens. A yet to be determined proportion of ALCL cases have a t(2;5)(p23;q35) translocation, which has been cloned.[268] This gene fusion encodes the N-terminal portion of a nonribosomal nucleolar phosphoprotein (nucleophosmin, NPM), fused to the tyrosine kinase domain of a novel transmembrane tyrosine-specific protein kinase (anaplastic lymphoma kinase, ALK).[268] A variant *NPM-ALK* fusion has also been described.[269,270] The incidence of the *NPM-ALK* gene fusion in ALCL is somewhat controversial and remains under investigation.[112,269] The situation is complicated by the fact that ALCL, as originally described, is a heterogeneous disease morphologically, cytogenetically, and clinically. This is reflected in the literature by a wide prevalence range (12%–100%) for this gene fusion in ALCL.[79,269] Current estimates are that approximately 70% of all cases and almost 90% of childhood ALCLs express this gene fusion.[271,272] Neither anaplastic morphology nor CD30 expression accurately predicts the presence of this molecular genetic subtype of lymphoma. Some authors contend that immunostaining for the p80 NPM-ALK (ALK1) chimeric protein is a reliable diagnostic method for identifying cases with the t(2;5)(p23;q35) translocation.[112] Several variant translocations in which ALK is fused to other partners have been reported, both in ALCL and in inflammatory myofibroblastic tumor (IMT).[269,270,273–277] The incidence of these rearrangements in ALCL and IMT remains to be determined.

SYT-SSX **Gene Fusions in Diagnosis of Synovial Sarcoma.** Gene fusions associated with pediatric solid tumors have mainly been identified and characterized in lesions with ambiguous morphology. However, tumor-specific translocations and resulting gene fusions have also been reported in several spindle cell tumors occurring in childhood, namely SS, CFS, and congenital mesoblastic nephroma (CMN). SS is a malignant neoplasm of children and young adults showing variable combinations of spindle cell and epithelial-glandular components. The epithelial-glandular component stains positively for cytokeratin and EMA, causing diagnostic confusion with epithelial tumors if SS is not included in the differential diagnosis.[201] A tumor-defining t(X;18)(p11.2;q11.2) translocation is present in more than 90% of either biphasic or monophasic forms of SS (Fig. 8.21A).[278] Molecular cloning of the translocation breakpoints identified two different rearrangements, namely the fusion of the *SYT* gene from 18q11.2 with either of two closely mapped Xp11.2 genes, *SSX1* or *SSX2* (Fig. 8.21B).[279,280]

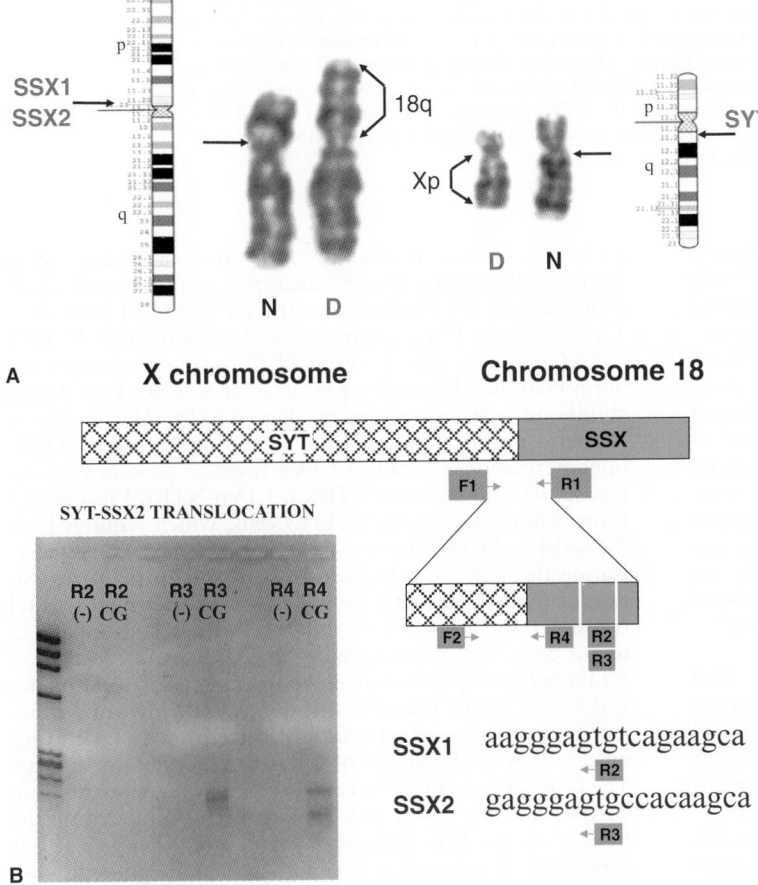

A   **X chromosome**   **Chromosome 18**

FIGURE 8.21 Synovial sarcoma fusion detection. Cytogenetics (**A**) and polymerase chain reaction (PCR) (**B**). An annotated karyotypic analysis of synovial sarcoma is shown. In this disease, the short arm of the X chromosome near the centromere is translocated to the near centromerical long arm of chromosome 18 as illustrated by the *arrows* labeled 18q and Xp, respectively. This results in the formation of derivative chromosomes X and 18 paired with a normal chromosome X and 18 as also labeled here. **B:** This karyotypic abnormality results in the formation of a chimeric gene, illustrated here conventionally labeled SYT-SSX. In reality, two common breakpoints on the X chromosome occur, resulting in the creation of two forms of the chimeric gene, identified as SSX1 and SSX2, respectively. Both can be amplified with universal primary labeled R1 here, which amplifies the sequence distal to the X breakpoint. This can be specifically amplified by using sequence-specific primers as illustrated here (R2 and R3, respectively, for SSX1 and SSX2). In the case of paraffin-embedded material in which mRNA is routinely highly fragmented, the resulting specific amplified signal can be further amplified, resulting in detection that might not otherwise be possible, as illustrated in the three paired lanes of the accompanying PCR gel. (Courtesy of Deborah Schofield, M.D.)

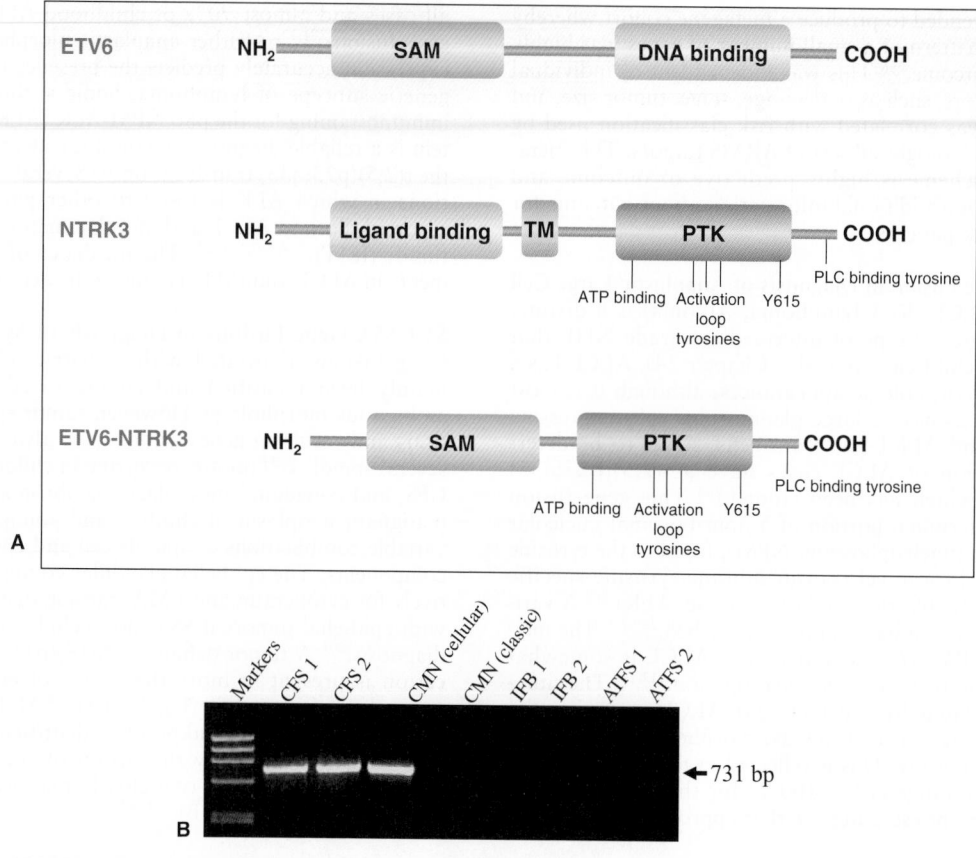

FIGURE 8.22 ETV6-NTRK translocation in congenital infantile fibrosarcoma (CFS). **A:** Schematic diagram of *ETV6-NTRK3* gene fusions in CFS and cellular congenital mesoblastic nephroma (CMN). As a result of t(12;15)(p13;q25) translocations, exons encoding the helix-loop-helix dimerization domain of the 12p13 *ETV6 (TEL)* transcription factor gene are fused to exons encoding the protein tyrosine kinase (PTK) domain of the *NTRK3 (TRKC)* neurotrophin-3 receptor gene on 15q25. This results in expression of a chimeric tyrosine kinase that undergoes ligand-independent dimerization and PTK activation. **B:** Reverse transcriptase polymerase chain reaction (RT-PCR) analysis of the *ETV6-NTRK3* gene fusion in CFS and CMN. With primers from 5′ sequences of the *ETV6* gene and 3′ sequences of the *NTRK3* gene, RT-PCR is used to amplify a 731 bp amplification product in CFS and cellular CMN but not in classic CMN, infantile fibromatosis, or adult-type fibrosarcoma.

Prognostically, analysis of metastasis-free survival showed differences in clinical outcome depending on the *SYT-SSX* fusion type, in that cases with *SYT-SSX2* fusion had superior outcome.[281,282] However, 2 years following diagnosis, the survival curve of patients with tumors containing *SYT-SSX2* began to drop and became almost parallel to that of patients with tumors containing *SYT-SSX1*. These findings indicate that patients with tumors positive for *SYT-SSX2* had a lower risk of early relapse than those with an *SSX1*-specific translocation, but that the cumulative risk of distant metastasis may be similar in both groups.[282–286] It is unclear whether translocation subtype portends better or worse diagnosis. Large tumors, neurovascular invasion, p53 overexpression, high Ki67 expression, and poorly differentiated subtype all portend a poorer outcome and are in aggregate more significant risk factors.[287]

***ETV6-NTRK3* Gene Fusions in Diagnosis of Spindle Cell Tumors of Infancy.** CFS is a cellular spindle cell tumor of the soft tissues, which generally presents before 2 years of age.[288] As the name implies, many cases are congenital. Although CFS shows frankly malignant cytology and a high recurrence rate, it has a very good prognosis with an 80% to 90% overall survival and only a 10% metastatic rate.[288] It must be differentiated from ATFS of older children. ATFS has a poor

prognosis, similar to that for fibrosarcomas occurring in adults.[289] Knezevich et al.[290] identified a t(12;15)(p13;q25) translocation in CFS that fuses the *ETV6 (TEL)* gene from 12p13 with the 15q25 neurotrophin-3 receptor gene, *NTRK3 (TRKC)* (Fig. 8.22A). *ETV6-NTRK3* fusion transcripts are not present in ATFS and appear to be specific for CFS among childhood soft tissue tumors (Fig. 8.22B). The predicted chimeric product contains the sterile alpha motif (SAM) oligomerization domain of ETV6 fused to protein tyrosine kinase (PTK) domain of NTRK3. ETV6-NTRK3 has potent transforming activity in NIH3T3 cells, which requires both the SAM and PTK domains of the fusion protein.[291] Polymerization through the helix-loop-helix domain leads to activation of the NTRK3-PTK domain, which dysregulates signal transduction pathways of the NTRK3 tyrosine kinase in tumor cells.[292,293] Several groups have demonstrated identical *ETV6-NTRK3* gene fusions in another pediatric solid tumor, CMN.[294,295] CMN is an infantile spindle cell tumor of the kidney that is subdivided into classical, mixed, and cellular forms on the basis of the degree of cellularity and mitotic activity. The histogenesis of CMN remains obscure, but a relationship between cellular CMN and CFS has been postulated on the basis of morphologic and ultrastructural similarities.[296] This is supported by similarities in clinical behavior. Although both

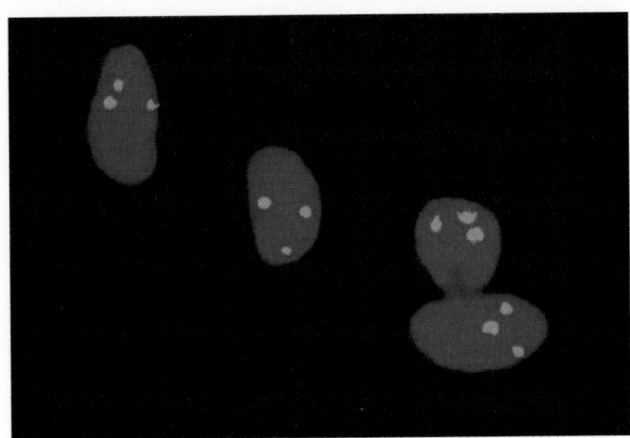

FIGURE 8.23 Trisomy 11 in congenital fibrosarcoma and cellular congenital mesoblastic nephroma (CMN). Four interphase cells from a case of cellular CMN are shown after probing with a centromeric probe for human chromosome 11 (*pink*). Three copies of chromosome 11 are demonstrated for each cell.

classic and cellular forms of CMN occur in very young children and are generally thought to have an excellent prognosis, reports of local recurrences and metastatic spread are almost exclusively associated with the cellular variant.[297–300] These studies indicate that classical and cellular CMN have different genetic features. The finding of *ETV6-NTRK3* fusion transcripts supports the concept that cellular CMN is histogenetically related to CFS. Interestingly, virtually all CFS and cellular CMN cases with the *ETV6-NTRK3* gene fusion carry an extra copy of chromosome 11[295,301] (Fig. 8.23). Trisomy 11 has been previously described for these lesions.[302–305] One intriguing possibility is that the extra copy of chromosome 11 provides cells with an additional copy of the insulin-like growth factor 2 gene (*IGF2*), which is localized to chromosome 11p15.5 and is known to induce antiapoptotic signaling by binding to the IGF-1 receptor.[306] Recent studies indicate that CFS and CMN tumors overexpress IGF2 and that an intact IGF1R signaling axis is required for ETV6-NTRK3 transformation.[307] In fact, ETV6-NTRK3 binds one of the major IGF1R substrates, insulin receptor substrate 1 (IRS-1), an interaction that links the chimeric tyrosine kinase to two pathways essential for its transformation activity, the RAS-MAP kinase mitogenic and the PI3-kinase AKT survival pathway.[307,308] *ETV6-NTRK3* expression has also been reported in a case of acute myeloid leukemia occurring in an adult patient.[309] Moreover, a rare subtype of infiltrating ductal carcinoma of the breast, known as *secretory breast carcinoma* (SBC), is also characterized by *ETV6-NTRK3* gene fusions identical to those of CFS and CMN.[310] This has recently been confirmed in a mouse model.[311] SBC demonstrates a wide age range, including pediatric patients.[312] The gene fusion is, therefore, unique in being expressed in tumors derived from multiple cell lineages, and the resulting chimeric oncoprotein has potent transformation activity in fibroblasts, hematopoietic cells, and breast epithelial cells.

Prognostically, detection of ETV6-NTRK3 fusion transcripts allow CFS and cellular CMN to be differentiated from other childhood spindle cell tumors. These include malignant tumors such as SS, spindle cell RMS, and ATFS of older children. Gene fusion detection also distinguishes CFS and CMN from benign spindle cell lesions such as infantile fibromatosis and myofibromatosis, which lack similar rearrangements.[313] The prognostic significance of the t(12;15) associated ETV6-NTRK3 gene fusion therefore lays in its utility for ensuring a correct diagnosis of CFS/cellular CMN and therefore appropriate management for patients with these diseases.

ASPL-TFE3 **Gene Fusions and Related Gene Fusions in Diagnosis of Alveolar Soft Part Sarcoma and Pediatric Renal Tumors.** Until recently, the molecular genetics of ASPS, a soft tissue malignancy of uncertain histogenesis, was completely unknown. A t(X;17)(p11;p25) translocation, identified by Ladanyi et al.,[314] fuses the TFE3 transcription factor gene from chromosome Xp11 to a previously unknown gene designated *ASPL* from chromosome 17q25. The t(X;17) varies from most other known sarcoma-associated translocations in being nonreciprocal or unbalanced.[143,315] Although the function of the ASPL-TFE3 chimeric protein remains poorly understood, it is believed to act as a transcriptional deregulator.[316] In a fascinating development, identical *ASPL-TFE3* gene fusions were detected in a unique group of primary renal carcinomas occurring predominantly in children and adolescents.[317] Subsequent molecular studies revealed a number of variant translocations involving Xp11 and the TFE3 gene, most commonly the t(1;X)(p11.2;q21).[73] These translocations all fuse *TFE3* to different partner genes, including the *PRCC-TFE3* gene fusion associated with the t(1;X)(p11.2;q21).[318] This has led to the recognition of a new subtype of renal cell carcinoma (RCC) that more frequently affects children and young adults than do other types of RCC, although a few confirmed adult cases have been reported. These tumors show a distinct morphology characterized by papillary architecture composed of clear cells, a combination that is uncommon in adult renal carcinomas.[319] The clinical significance of *TFE3* gene fusion–positive *RCC* remains to be determined. Another distinctive type of renal neoplasm affecting the pediatric population has also recently been identified. These tumors carry a t(6;11)(p21;q12) translocation fusing the *Alpha* gene, an intron-less gene of unknown function at 11q12, to the *TFEB* transcription factor gene at 6p21, such that the entire *TFEB* coding region is preserved.[320] Because TFEB along with TFE3, TFEC, and *Mitf* compose the microphthalmia transcription factor subfamily, it has been hypothesized that t(6;11) renal tumors may be related to *TFE3* gene fusion–positive *RCC*, although it remains unclear whether these lesions are epithelial in their histogenesis.[317]

TPM-ALK **Gene Fusions in Diagnosis of Inflammatory Myofibroblastic Tumors.** IMTs occur occasionally in children. IMTs are benign or low-grade malignant neoplastic mesenchymal proliferations with an inflammatory component consisting primarily of lymphocytes and plasma cells. These tumors can mimic nodular fasciitis, desmoid tumor, and gastrointestinal stromal tumor and lead to misdiagnosis and delay in appropriate oncologic management. Molecular analysis of IMTs demonstrated fusions of tropomyosin 3 or 4 (*TPM3* or *TPM4*) to the *ALK* gene on chromosome 2.[275] Other ALK fusion partners subsequently demonstrated include clathrin heavy chain gene, CLTC,[321] Ran-binding protein 2 (*RANBP2*,[273] and cysteinyl-tRNA synthetase.[274] It is hypothesized that these chimeric proteins function in neoplasia by activating the ALK-PTK signaling pathways.

Other Molecular Genetic Alterations in Pediatric Solid Tumors of Importance to Patient Management

Molecular Genetic Alterations in Neuroblastoma. The diagnosis of NB is generally less problematic than for other SRCTs, given the usual occurrence of a catecholamine-secreting tumor arising in the adrenal gland of a young child and the distinctive neural phenotype in most cases.[322] However, the marked variability in clinical behavior of this tumor, ranging from spontaneous regression to metastatic growth and early death, has prompted an intense search for reliable predictors of prognosis in NB. A number of genetic abnormalities have been identified in NB that correlate to varying degrees with clinical outcome, including *MYCN* amplification, deletion of distal chromosome 1p, deviations from diploid DNA content, expression of neurotrophin receptors (particularly TRKA), amplification of 17q, and detection of telomerase activity.[49,323] Of these, *MYCN* amplification (Figs. 8.8 and 8.9) and 1p deletions, each present in approximately 30% to 50% of NB primary tumors, have in recent years been regarded as the best predictors of poor prognosis. Interestingly, a strong correlation has been found between these two prognostic markers.[324] Brodeur et al.[323] have suggested that NB should be classified into three distinct subsets based on biologic and clinical features. The first includes hyperdiploid tumors that express TRKA (also known as NTRK1), do not overexpress *MYCN*, and are low-stage favorable prognosis tumors occurring in very young children. The second group is near-diploid, non-*MYCN* amplified tumors with 1p deletion, and low TRKA expression. This NB group tends to present as higher-stage lesions in older children and have an intermediate outcome. The third group includes *MYCN*-amplified near-diploid tumors with 1p deletions and low or absent TRKA expression; these tumors present as advanced-stage disease in older children and have a very poor prognosis. This is summarized for TRKA and MYCN in Figure 8.9. Further studies are necessary to confirm the clinical utility of this classification scheme, but it is proposed that the three different subsets represent genetically distinct forms of NB. More recently, it has become apparent that gains of chromosome 17q21-qter may be the most frequent cytogenetic abnormality (>50%) in NB.[325-327] This abnormality has been associated with advanced disease, patients older than 1 year, deletion of chromosome arm 1p, and amplification of the *MYCN* oncogene, all of which have previously been associated with an adverse outcome. In fact, Bown et al.[328] have shown that gain of this region was the most powerful prognostic factor in multivariate analysis of a series of NB patients, strongly indicating that gain of 17q is an important prognostic factor in children with NB. Others have suggested that only a specific region of 17q gain is prognostic.[329] Within the past few years, a large number of whole-genome analyses have been performed and multiple alterations have been identified with apparent prognostic significance, suggesting that a simple 1p-11p-17q CNV analysis is incomplete.[329,330]

Very recently, genetic alterations of the ALK were identified in both familial and sporadic forms of NB.[43,331-334] These alterations include activating mutations in the kinase domain as well as DNA amplification of the *ALK* gene and occur in approximately 15% of sporadic cases. This not only provides further evidence for the genetic etiology of NB (i.e., leading to ALK downstream signaling) but also indicates a heretofore-unrecognized therapeutic opportunity in NB, namely the targeting of the ALK by using blocking antibodies or small molecule kinase inhibitors.

Diagnostic Molecular Genetics of Rhabdoid Tumor. Rhabdoid tumor was first described as an unusual variant of WT in early National Wilms' Tumor Study Group studies.[335] Notable features were an extraordinarily prominent nucleolus and a brightly eosinophilic cytoplasm resembling that of RMS cells (hence the name)[336] (Fig. 8.24A). The cytoplasmic filaments were shown to be nonmyogenic, vimentin intermediate filaments by IHC (Fig. 8.24B). The cytoplasm is filled with whorls of these intermediate filaments with entrapped organelles when examined by EM (Fig. 8.24C). These tumors were first thought to be limited to the kidney, but within a

short time, they were identified in almost every anatomic location.[337-345] These tumor cells often occurred as a component of bona fide tumors of otherwise known lineage, such as SS, with a particularly poor prognosis.[341,343] However, a unique t(11;22) chromosomal translocation was subsequently described that is distinct from that of ESFTs.[341,343,346-352] Numerous attempts to identify a gene fusion analogous to those of ESFTs and ARMS were unsuccessful.[353] Cloning of the chromosome 22q11.2 breakpoint region revealed deletions of the *SNF5* (*INI/SMARCB1*) gene, a member of a family of genes important in chromatin remodeling.[111,354-356] Inactivation of this gene by deletion or mutation was subsequently identified in a large percentage of rhabdoid tumors, including those involving the central nervous system (atypical teratoid/rhabdoid tumor), as well as in some choroid plexus carcinomas and medulloblastomas.[109,337,339,347,354] SNF5/INI1 proteins appear to cause G_0-G_1 arrest through histone deacetylase (HDAC)-dependent transcriptional repression of the cyclin D1 gene and through recruitment to the cyclin D1 promoter.[357] Why most tumors also accumulate unique cytoplasmic whorls of intermediate filaments remains unclear, although recent data suggest a role in actin skeleton organization.[355] *SNF5/INI1* mutations appear to be found in most if not all rhabdoid tumors, suggesting an etiologic role for this defect.[111] Diagnostic testing for *SNF5/INI1* alterations in rhabdoid tumors is offered in specialty laboratories.[354] Absence of SNF5/INI1 protein by immunocytochemistry in tumor cells (Fig. 8.24D, vs. a normal tumor control, E) is supportive of a diagnosis of rhabdoid tumor. Similarly, epithelioid sarcoma also shows the absence of *SNF5/INI1/SMARCB1* protein by immunocytochemistry and deletion of the gene, perhaps providing evidence that this sarcoma is a member of the rhabdoid tumor family.

Molecular Genetic Alterations Characteristic for Wilms' Tumor. WT is the most common renal neoplasm in children, accounting for approximately 90% of pediatric kidney tumors and approximately 5% of all childhood cancers. However, only a few nonrandom cytogenetic alterations have been reported in WT, mainly involving the *WT1* gene on chromosome 11p13 and the *WT2* locus on chromosome 11p15.5.[358-361] These alterations are mostly associated with familial or syndromic forms of WT. Deletions or mutations of *WT1* occur in patients with WAGR syndrome (WT, aniridia, genitourinary malformations, mental retardation), in whom the incidence of WT is 30%, and in Denys-Drash syndrome, in which WTs occur in 90% of cases.[359,362] Alterations of the *WT2* locus are frequently associated with Beckwith-Wiedemann syndrome, an overgrowth syndrome with an increased incidence of WT.[363] Recent studies have identified two familial WT loci, FWT1 (at 17q12–21) and FWT2 (at 19q13). Although these loci appear to be important in familial and syndromic forms of WT, there is currently little evidence that they are commonly mutated in sporadic WT. *WT1* mutations occur only in 5% to 10% of sporadic cases, and *WT2* alterations have yet to be documented in sporadic WT. The finding of activating β-catenin mutations in some WTs has implicated the *Wnt* signaling pathway in this tumor.[364] Moreover, recurrent abnormalities of loci at 16q, 1p, and 7p suggest that other chromosomal regions may harbor WT genes.[358,365,366] Identification and characterization of these and other primary genetic alterations in sporadic WT are paramount to understanding the pathogenesis of this disease. Recent molecular studies led to characterization of an X chromosome gene, *WTX*, which is mutated somatically in approximately 30% of WTs.[367] The WTX gene product appears to negatively regulate the *Wnt* signaling pathway.[368] Another potential WT-related tumor suppressor gene was identified by cloning a balanced nonconstitutional

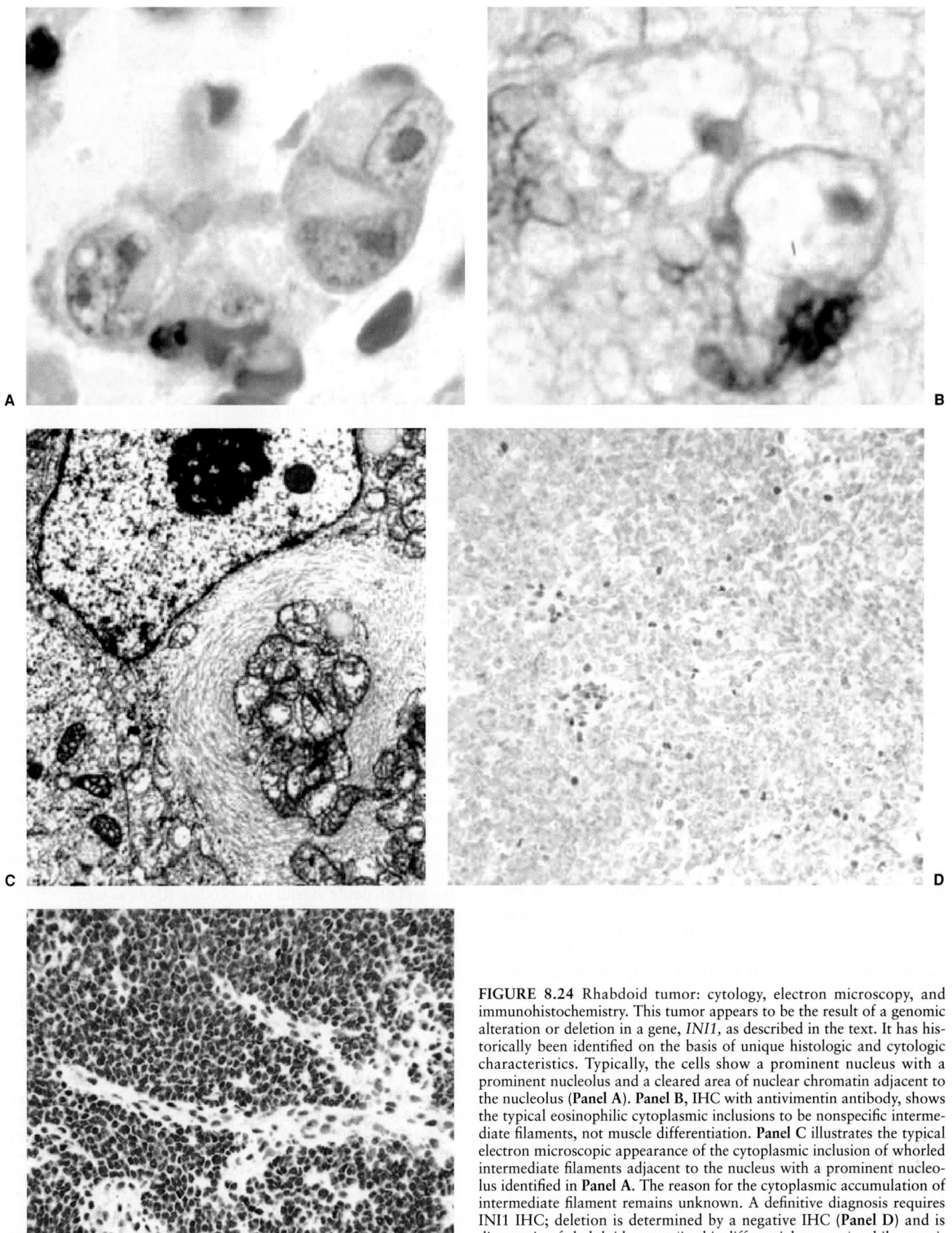

FIGURE 8.24 Rhabdoid tumor: cytology, electron microscopy, and immunohistochemistry. This tumor appears to be the result of a genomic alteration or deletion in a gene, *INI1,* as described in the text. It has historically been identified on the basis of unique histologic and cytologic characteristics. Typically, the cells show a prominent nucleus with a prominent nucleolus and a cleared area of nuclear chromatin adjacent to the nucleolus (**Panel A**). **Panel B**, IHC with antivimentin antibody, shows the typical eosinophilic cytoplasmic inclusions to be nonspecific intermediate filaments, not muscle differentiation. **Panel C** illustrates the typical electron microscopic appearance of the cytoplasmic inclusion of whorled intermediate filaments adjacent to the nucleus with a prominent nucleolus identified in **Panel A**. The reason for the cytoplasmic accumulation of intermediate filament remains unknown. A definitive diagnosis requires INI1 IHC; deletion is determined by a negative IHC (**Panel D**) and is diagnostic of rhabdoid tumor (in this differential context), while a positive result (**Panel E**) effectively rules out the diagnosis.

t(6;15)(q21;q21) translocation in a sporadic WT case, which revealed a 6q21 breakpoint adjacent to a novel gene encoding a HECT domain containing E3 ubiquitin-protein ligase.[369] This gene, designated *HACE1*, is dramatically downregulated at the mRNA and protein levels in more than 75% of 26 sporadic WTs compared with matching normal kidney. Rearrangements of the 6q21 region have been previously reported in WT, including t(5;6)(q21;q21) and t(2;6)(q35;q21) translocations.[365,366,370] Hace1 may not be a specific tumor suppressor for WT, as *HACE1* −/− mice show a broad range of tumor types, particularly in response to environmental stressors.[371] Very recently, another gene mapping to chromosome 6q21 was also shown to be deregulated in WTs with 6q21 rearrangements. The *LIN28B* gene was shown to be overexpressed in two sporadic WTs with t(6;15) translocations in which there was also loss of *HACE1* expression.[372] Further studies are necessary to determine whether *LIN28B* alterations represent a recurrent finding in sporadic WT.

WHOLE-GENOME ANALYSIS

As informative as single gene analyses have been in the study of childhood cancer, recent technologic advances have opened up an entirely new approach to analysis of the functional genome. The power of current technology to elucidate the numerous genomic defects involved in oncogenesis and to identify diagnostic, prognostic, and therapeutic targets is unprecedented. It is important to review the basic technology because these methods will play a major role in the diagnosis of human diseases, both benign and malignant.

The Cancer Genome

The functional human genome is composed of three major categories: DNA, RNA, and protein. Potential diagnostic methods based on each of these categories are illustrated in Figure 8.25 and are discussed later. A brief introduction to issues pertinent to DNA-, RNA-, and protein-based "genomic" diagnostics as applied to childhood cancer is addressed below.

DNA

Among the 3.3 billion nucleotide bases contained within 22 chromosomes and 2 sex chromosomes, there are about 3 million single nucleotide variations or SNPs that occur in 5% or more of the population. There are at least 5 million more that occur with lesser frequency, at the individual patient level, even in the "normal" genome.[194,373] These undoubtedly account for a great deal of human diversity and disease susceptibility, including variations in drug response to cytotoxic chemotherapeutic agents and the likelihood of developing one of the common multigenic diseases, such as cancer.[197,374] These variants may be linked to disease susceptibility. The known racial disparities in susceptibility to specific tumor formation (ESFTs) may be linked to certain SNPs. Evaluation of polymorphic variation (SNPs) within genomes of children with cancer is necessary to determine which specific SNPs may be linked to particular tumors or other diseases. In particular, the task is to distinguish the approximately 5 million "private" or passenger SNPs, perhaps better termed *sequence variants*, from the tumor-related "driver" sequence variants that may number fewer than a hundred in a given tumor.[200]

RNA

The expressed genome is quite compact and composed of approximately 20,000 mRNAs that encode proteins. Some expressed RNAs, such as H19, encode no protein but are known

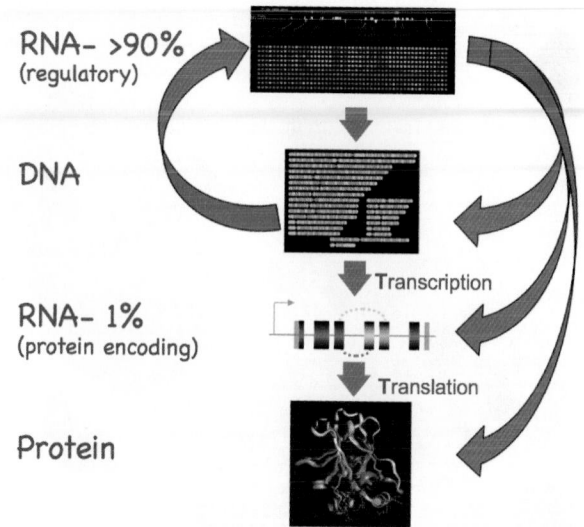

FIGURE 8.25 Functional genome. The traditional static view of the genome as DNA to RNA to protein is now recognized as simplistic. Instead, as shown above, RNA is central to the functional genome, controlling transcriptional, translational, and posttranslational events in the cell. Two major classes of transcripts occur: the coding and noncoding RNAs. The former, transcribed from about only 1% of the DNA genome, are processed into mature messenger RNAs in the nucleus and are exported to the cytoplasm to produce about 20,000 or so annotated genes that are translated into a vast number of different proteins. The latter, or noncoding RNAs, vary enormously in molecular weight, from 21mers (microRNA) to RNA as large as any protein-encoding gene. These RNA transcripts are only now being understood but appear to normally control a wide variety of cellular processes.

to be critical controlling elements in the functional human genome. There are also numerous, largely unidentified noncoding RNAs that are expressed and do not produce protein but are responsible for regulating gene function.[375] One well-known class is micro RNA (miRNA). These miRNAs are increasingly recognized for the role they play in controlling transcription and potentially many other functions in basic cell biology and even cancer.[376,377] For diagnostic purposes, the more than 20,000 protein-encoding mRNAs are the focus of current studies regarding the expressed genome (transcriptome), although in the future, this will no doubt extend to noncoding RNAs as well.[378,379] The methodology to investigate the transcriptome has rapidly become available and has potential clinical utility.

Protein

There is widespread appreciation that DNA (genome) and RNA (transcriptome) are archival genome data and messengers, respectively. Function is generally effected by the protein product (proteome) of expressed mRNAs. Quite intriguing is the fact that 20,000 genes are responsible for the creation of as many as 1.5 million distinct proteins. The incredible diversity of proteins produced is due to translational and post-translational processing (glycosylation, proteolytic cleavage). A large fraction is created by alternative splice variants (exon usage), reading frame shifts, and alternate start sites among the repertoire of expressed genes.[380,381] An example is p16 and p14[mu]/19[hu] (alternate reading frame, ARF) proteins. Both p16 and p14[mu]/19[hu] are transcribed from the same basic encoding exons, but two different exons are transcribed for the second and third encoded exons. A frameshift consequent to an alternate out-of-frame start site encodes an entirely different first exon amino acid sequence for ARF (p14[mu]/19[hu]). This example demonstrates why there are a far greater number of proteins than there are encoding genes. In reality, the scope of alternate splicing is enormous and far outshadows the nominal 20,000 or so protein-encoding genes.[382,383] Alternate splicing may be a major factor in the encoding of multiple proteins from a nominally single gene. The consequence is a major problem for analyzing the proteome (proteins derived from the genome) due to the more than 1.5 million proteins that need to be analyzed. Although nucleotide sequencing technology was used in the human genome project, similar technology is not available for analyzing the entire functional proteome.

Whole-Genome Analytic Methods

Whole-Genome Transcription Profiling

The basic technology for DNA microarrays and gene expression (gene chip) was implemented in the early 1990s.[384–387] The tumor sample is applied to a substrate that contains identified gene sequences of interest, and the sample cDNAs (from the tumor mRNA transcripts) are hybridized to the target sequences. The number of genes analyzed in the older technology has gone from a few hundred genes to thousands of genes and now encompasses the entire human genome (about 20,000 discrete genes) plus vast numbers of unannotated RNA transcripts. Currently available commercial arrays interrogate as many as 1.4 million discrete sequences on a single microarray.

Several types of microarrays have been developed. The first technology was spotted microarrays that employ full-length cDNA clones attached to a glass substrate (typically an ordinary glass slide with a treated surface).[385,387] Current microarrays employ photolithography technology to synthesize short (24- to 60mer) oligonucleotides *in situ*.[386] Alternatively, presynthesized 60mers are attached to the substrate. To adequately represent genes that may be thousands of base pairs in length, multiple short oligonucleotides are chosen throughout the length of the expressed gene sequence and represented as separate "tiles" on the array. In this manner, a single gene may be represented by a number of short 25- to 60mer oligonucleotides from various regions 5′ to 3′ along the length of the gene. To control for nonspecific hybridization, tiles with a single base mismatch are arrayed just below the "perfect match" tile. Hybridization intensity is compared between these two tiles and along the length of the gene. The net values are compiled and a determination of present or absent is calculated and reported, along with a quantitative value. Several rather-sophisticated tools have been developed to account for various hybridization artifacts, with the goal of deriving quantitatively accurate expression values.[388,389]

A variant technology has also been developed, in which spotting technology is used to spot short sequences (often approximately 60mers) on glass slides. In addition, multiple oligonucleotides that represent different regions of the gene, analogous to the photolithography arrays, can be placed in adjacent spots. These oligonucleotides are also chosen from multiple stretches of the entire coding sequence of the gene of interest. This approach combines features from both technologies, specifically the economy of spotted arrays and the predictable performance of short oligonucleotides as synthesized on the photolithography arrays. Both this method and photolithography arrays, unlike cDNA arrays, allow for detection of splice variants, alternate exon usage, message truncation, and chimeric genes formed from the fusion of two normal genes because of chromosomal translocation (assuming features to detect these alterations are inherent in the design of the arrays). This presumes that the chosen oligonucleotides appropriately represent the exon-by-exon sequences

within the gene of interest. An additional challenge is representation of some genes that use the same coding DNA sequence. BCL/BCLX are two genes that are the same except for being out of frame for exon 1, but with the same exons 2 and 3, such as noted previously with p16/INK4a and p14/ARF (human) or p19/ARF (murine).[390–393] The ultimate goal of microarray technology is to detect or monitor genome-wide gene expression as an index of total gene activity. With information gained from pediatric tumors, it is hoped that additional data will be acquired that direct a more accurate diagnosis, predict prognosis, and tailor therapy.

Regardless of the specific method employed, the information returned is similar, resulting in a quasi-quantitative measure of the amount of any given gene being expressed in the tumor sample of interest. When scaled to thousands of genes accessed simultaneously, a snapshot of the activity of the genome in question is obtained. Biologists and physicians have sought such all-encompassing information about disease states, and now it has become a reality. The major question now is how to use this information and integrate it into the clinical practice of pediatric pathology and oncology.[27,394,395]

The great power of this new technology lies in its ability to provide a complex and all-encompassing image of the biologic activity of the cells or tissue in a specific tumor. The major challenge is to analyze the enormous amount of data generated in a meaningful way.[396] The rapid adoption of this technology by life science researchers has fostered a parallel effort to develop suitable data "mining" tools to extract useful information from these arrays. Simple scatter analyses with a list of "outlier" genes that are up- or downregulated in a disease state have limited utility.[397–405] In contrast, clusters of genes statistically associated with a given disease, stage, or clinical behavior can be a powerful analytic tool. An example of the diagnostic utility of gene expression profiling to accurately identify four common pediatric sarcomas is illustrated in Figure 8.26. The power of this tool is noted here by the fact that all 365 cases are clustered by correct tumor type. Tumor cases that do not cluster in a typical fashion proved to be atypical tumors that were difficult to classify. Amazingly, the overall precision of diagnostic microarray profiling (>90%) exceeds that reported in most comparative diagnostic studies with pathologists (60%–70% concordance). As an example (Figs. 8.27 and 8.28), genetic variants of ARMS (PAX3-FOXO1A, PAX7-FOXO1A, translocation negative) are compared with each other and with ERMS and nonmyogenic soft tissue sarcomas with whole-transcriptome expression profiling of 22,000 genes analyzed by similarity matrix (Fig. 8.27) and principal component analysis (Fig. 8.28). The translocation-negative ARMS cases show greater similarity to ERMS than to either PAX3- or PAX7-translocated cases, despite an obvious alveolar architecture. This parallels the observed clinical behavior of these translocation-negative ARMS cases.[260] This suggests that arrays have the potential to identify or "diagnose" specific diseases and identify new diagnostic and prognostic groups within a specific tumor group. This occurs even in the absence of typical "diagnostic" histopathology. Information obtained from analysis of pretreatment biopsy tissue offers the prospect for predicting clinical course and delivering optimal therapy, even in the absence of other diagnostic or prognostic markers prior to therapy or evolution of the disease. Currently, several study cohorts are using this technology to identify prognostic groups based on up- or downregulation of certain genes. Of course, the identification of therapeutic gene targets is especially appealing. It is hoped that targeted therapy can be exploited similar to the imatinib activity against BCR-ABL–positive AML and c-KIT–mutated gastrointestinal stromal tumor.

This is a rapidly evolving field, and several studies have already demonstrated clinically useful applications of this

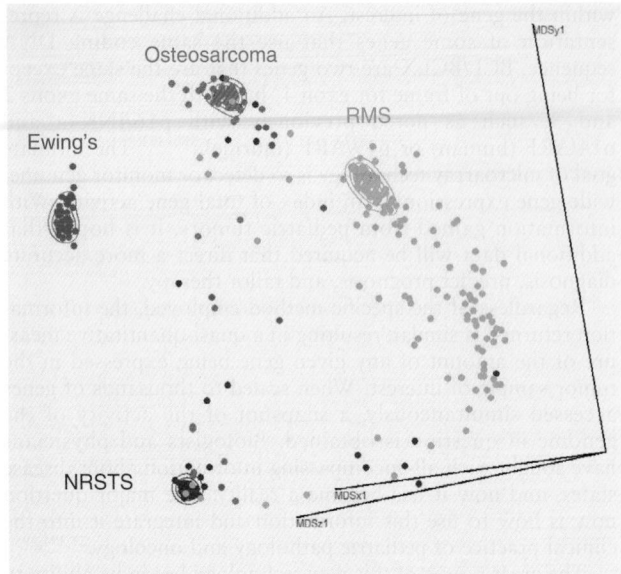

22,000 gene transcripts, 365 cases, multidimensional scaling analysis

FIGURE 8.26 Soft tissue sarcoma diagnostic classification by gene expression profiling. This analysis involved 22,000 gene transcripts, 365 cases, and multidimensional scaling analysis. Comparison of the total gene expression profile of a given tumor with all others in high-dimensional space (the number of genes by the number of samples) followed by dimensionality reduction to two- or three-dimensions allows visual comparison of the overall similarity (diagnostic class) of tumors. Here, four common childhood sarcomas are compared. Generally, most cluster together in this multidimensional scaling three-dimensional comparison. Note, however, that Ewing's sarcoma cluster rather closely; the cases that do not subsequently proved to express little or no *EWS-ETS* fusion gene. Similarly, the tight cluster within rhabdomyosarcoma (RMS) is composed of alveolar subtype that expresses the *PAX-FOXO1A* gene. In other cases, such as osteosarcoma and non-RMS soft tissue sarcoma, there is greater variation and overlap. In general, clustering of typical cases strongly associates with diagnosis, and often aberrant clustering is attributable to incorrect histologic diagnosis. NRSTS, non-myogenic soft tissue sarcoma. (Analysis performed by Daniel Wai, Ph.D., Children's Hospital, Los Angeles, USC.)

technology.[406–417] The current prohibitive cost and technical obstacles that have prevented routine clinical use of microarrays for ancillary diagnostic purposes will likely be ameliorated by rapidly declining costs (approximately $200 for entire coding transcriptome presently), greater availability of central or commercial diagnostic microarrays, the development of validated linear RNA amplification methods, and the development of arrays suitable for FFPE tissues.[418–423]

Whole-Genome DNA Analysis

It is increasingly recognized that individual genomic variations, such as mutations and SNPs, better described as sequence variants, are responsible for profound differences in gene functionality, because of nucleotide changes that result in either amino acid coding changes or changes in promoter regions and overall transcription levels.[386,424,425] SNPs are measured as alterations in overall frequency of a given polymorphism compared with population norms, (Harvey Weinberg equilibria), leading to a measure of deviation from this norm, or linkage disequilibrium.[426–428] These "normal" SNP variants are considered to be associated with complex disease traits, such as early onset of disease, idiosyncratic drug responses, and even disease susceptibility.[193,429] These possible

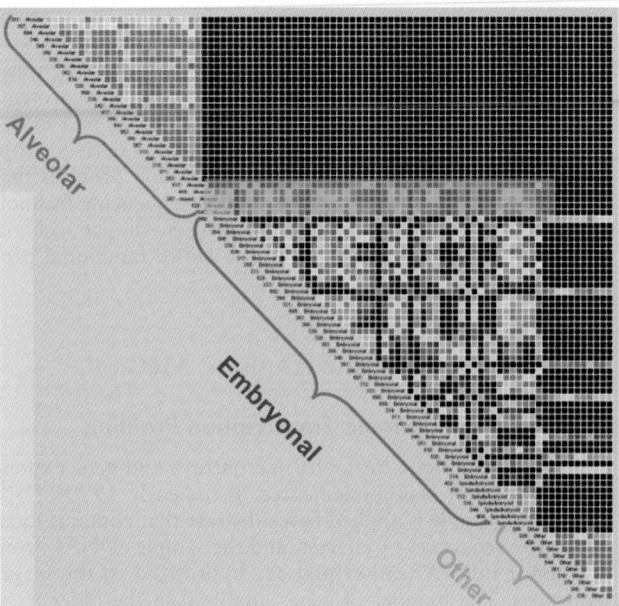

FIGURE 8.27 Similarity matrix. Here, three types of soft tissue sarcomas, alveolar rhabdomyosarcoma, embryonal rhabdomyosarcoma, and nonmyogenic soft tissue sarcomas (other) are compared using all genes differentially expressed by the three groups. Black indicates minimal similarity, while red is marked similarity and yellow is intermediate. Note that most members of each class are quite similar, although there is a group of alveolar cases that better resemble embryonal: these cases have alveolar histology but lack the characteristic PAX-FOXO1A translocation.

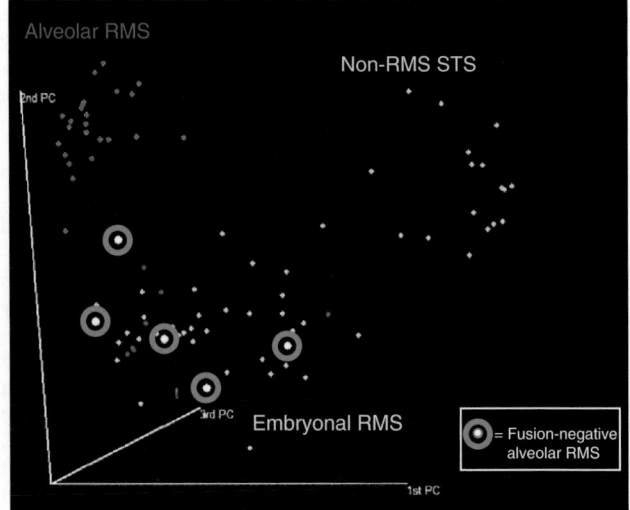

FIGURE 8.28 Rhabdomyosarcoma (RMS) class discovery by gene expression profiling. In this principal component analysis of RMS subtypes, it is apparent that five cases of presumed alveolar RMS (ARMS) cluster with the embryonal subtype. Subsequent investigation confirmed the alveolar histology but documented an absence of PAX-FOXO1A expression. These translocation-negative ARMS appear more similar to embryonal RMS in gene expression profile and prognosis than fusion-positive ARMS, raising the question as to proper diagnostic classification: histology, overall phenotype, or genotype. (Analysis performed by Elai Davicioni, Ph.D. candidate, Children's Hospital, Los Angeles, USC.)

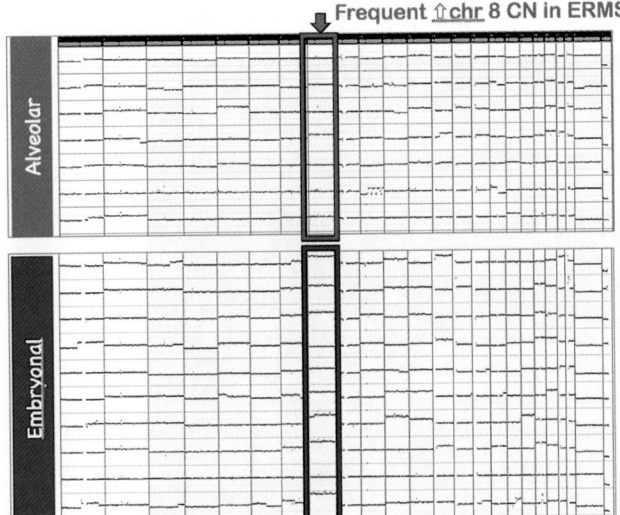

FIGURE 8.29 Genome-wide DNA copy number variation (CNV) in 7 PAX-FOXO1A–positive alveolar rhabdomyosarcoma (RMS) and 10 embryonal RMS cases. Note that only 1 of 7 alveolar RMS cases shows CNV of chromosome 8, but 8 of 10 embryonal RMS cases show marked CNV of that chromosome. This suggests that triploidy of chromosome 8 is widespread in embryonal RMS, as the entire chromosome appears to be involved.

links to disease are of special concern when they occur within coding regions or within regulatory elements of genes associated with disease susceptibility, unique drug responsiveness, or clinical evolution of a disease state.[425,426] Current microarrays and related methods can interrogate millions of SNPs distributed throughout the genome. Although the number of SNPs may exceed 10 million when all human genomic variation is considered (http://www.hapmap.org/abouthapmap. html.en), the task of assessing these sequence variants may be simplified by data suggesting that about a half million well-spaced SNPs will be sufficient to determine the vast majority of a person's haplotype.[430,431] These specific SNPs occur within regulatory and encoding regions of genes or as SNP grouping in large haplotype blocks inherited *in toto* across broad areas of the genome. This would allow assessment of a smaller number of suitably distributed "tag" SNPs to infer the SNP content of virtually the entire genome. It is now possible to

economically assess the haplotype of individuals. The potential of this technology to determine individual haplotypes for disease and risk assessment is staggering; already, studies at densities higher than 500,000 have revealed apparent disease-associated polymorphisms in complex diseases such as age-related macular degeneration.[432–435] There is broad interest in this technology for pharmacogenomics purposes, risk assessment, and disease susceptibility.

Although extremely dense SNP haplotyping is of great interest to biomedical research, the currently available tools are of great value in cancer diagnosis and clinical management. Large-scale genomic loss, gain, and rearrangement are typical of cancer cells and often result in tumor suppressor gene loss or chimeric oncogene creation. It is of great value to assess recurring genomic alterations in tumor cells. In a manner, this is simply a high-resolution variant of karyotyping or CGH, even more so than array CGH.[436,437] The results offer insight into fundamental mechanisms of tumorigenesis that are not possible by alternative means. For example, Figures 8.29 and 8.30 illustrate the use of SNP arrays that interrogate 1.8 million nucleotides across the whole genome. In the first figure, Fig. 8.29, all probes were used in aggregate to assess DNA copy number across all 22 autosomal chromosomes and the X chromosome. The resulting measure of CNV in this group of ERMS versus ARMS cases reveals a consistent increase in signal associated with chromosome 8. This is best interpreted as evidence of trisomy 8. Conversely, if we use only the approximately 1 million polymorphic probes (Fig. 8.30), we can focus on a single chromosome as in case 11 and note the high incidence of LOH observed for this chromosome in ERMS (five of five cases shown here) as opposed to ARMS, where little LOH is noted, save for one case of five and 11pter in a second case. If we examine a larger series of cases and calculate a regional p value for deviation from expected for ERMSs ($n = 512$), compare these with ARMSs ($n = 58$), and plot the resulting p value (in this case, across 5 megabases) as a color code over the karyotype, a striking observation is evident (Fig. 8.31). A recurring allelic loss on the short arm of chromosome 11 (especially in 11pter) is quite apparent with ERMS (A), with red ($p > 0.75$) denoting 11pter, decreasing to negligible (black) toward the centromere. This is compared with a lesser and more uniform loss along all of chromosome 11 in ARMS (B). This is consistent with a known LOH in this region with ERMS and the detailed data noted in the previous two figures.[438,439] With finer-resolution analyses using higher-density SNP arrays, identification of individual genes and their

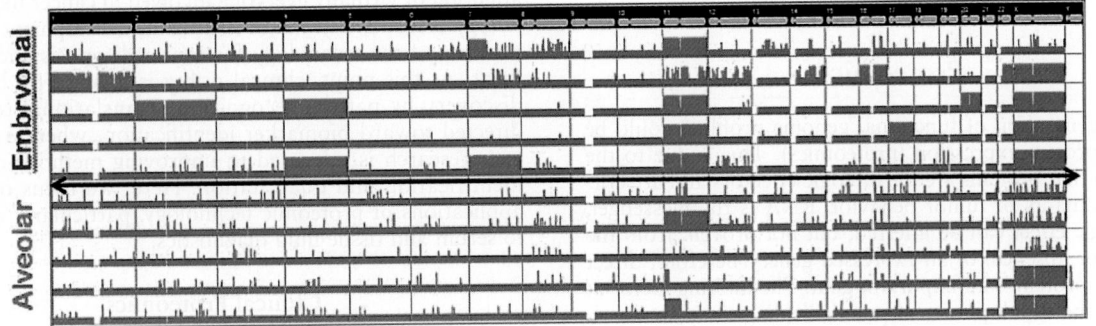

FIGURE 8.30 Loss of heterozygosity (LOH) analysis of five embryonal and five alveolar rhabdomyosarcoma (RMS) cases. Chromosomes are numbered from left (1) to right (X). Note that, unlike the previous figure where chromosome 8 copy number gain was seen in embryonal RMS but not in alveolar RMS, in this analysis of heterozygosity, there is no LOH of chromosome 8 but there is widespread LOH of much of chromosome 11 in embryonal RMS (5/5) and rarely in ARMS (1/5). Apparent LOH of chromosome X is based a result of gender; 6 of the 10 patients are female. SNP 6.0 GeneChip array analysis, with approximately 1 million polymorphic and approximately 1 million nonpolymorphic probes.

A. Embryonal

B. Alveolar

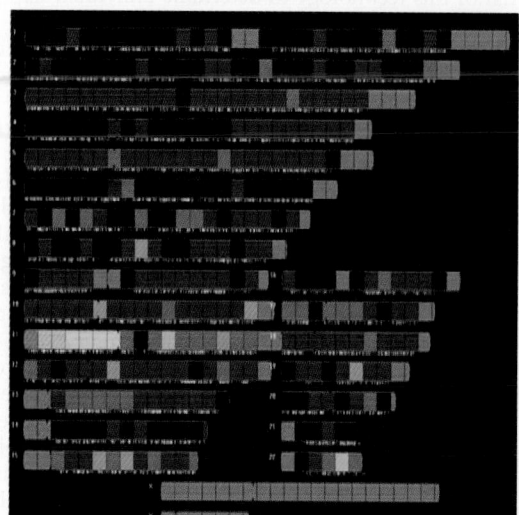
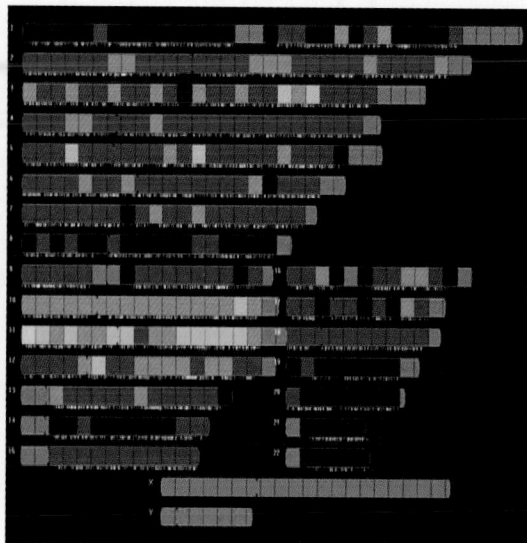

10,000 SNPs, 12 ERMS, 8 ARMS.

LOH proportional to color (e.g., > *p* value):

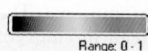

Range: 0 · 1

FIGURE 8.31 Loss of heterozygosity (LOH) in nearly 100 cases of rhabdomyosarcoma (RMS) at low density (10,000 probes). The same two groups of childhood RMSs were compared as in the previous figure. Color-coding shows recurring LOH of terminal chromosome 11p in essentially all embryonal RMS (ERMS) (red) (**A**). In contrast, alveolar RMS (ARMS) (**B**) shows diffuse and less frequent (approximately 505) LOH across chromosome 11, confirming the observations in the previous figure and documenting a fundamental difference in genomic loss and gain between ERMS and ARMS. (Analysis provided by Jonathan Buckley, Ph.D., M.B.B.S., Keck School of Medicine, USC.)

SNPs associated with specific tumors or properties, such as clinical aggressiveness or response to therapy, will be possible. Further, combined analysis with gene expression patterns from the whole-transcriptome profiling will yield insights into gene functionality related to genomic constitution. Such initial analyses where the relative risk for any given genomic feature (gene or RNA expression, miRNA expression, DNA copy number, and methylation status) is considered as a single group and statistically compared with each other are in progress. Similar work has been initiated through the TARGET initiative for ALL and NB, and other pediatric tumors will soon be included.[196,199]

Proteomics

The next generation of functional genome profiling could be based on protein expression (proteomics). This is due to the realization that proteins are the biologic effectors and are critical determinants of tumor behavior. RNA is the messenger, and biologic effect can be inferred, but not proven, from the presence (or absence) of an expressed gene. Therefore, direct analysis of protein is an important goal. The limiting factor at present is the development of practical (diagnostic) technology. In the case of serum proteomics, the confounding effect of abundant, non-diagnostic albumin and globulins, among others, is the limiting factor.[440]

The problem with proteomics is that technology comparable with DNA hybridization currently does not exist. Many competing technologies are being evaluated to accomplish the same result. The pathway from biomarker discovery to iden-

tification and validation is much more difficult with proteomics than the instantaneous discoveries possible with nucleic acids.[336,337,342,343,441] In addition to the presence or absence of a protein, one must also assess posttranslational modifications such as glycosylation and phosphorylation. These are known to dramatically alter the functionality of gene products. These parameters cannot be assessed by a nucleic acid method, as is possible with gene expression and SNP arrays. However, all biomarkers, whether DNA polymorphism, mRNA expression, or protein pattern, have diagnostic value. It is fair to say that proteomics has captured the attention of virtually everyone involved in cancer like no technology before it. The major issue is the development and practical use of the technology for cancer diagnosis and management. At this point, clinical utility is focused on biomarker discovery by pattern recognition. Translational research is directed toward biomarker identification, whereas basic science research is relegated to improving methods of marker identification and quantitation. Here, we focus on clinical applications of proteomic technology, particularly as applied to serum and tissue fluid diagnostics.[442]

Clinical Proteomics

The fundamental issue in clinical proteomics is choice of technology. For diagnostic purposes, simple pattern recognition similar to high-dimensional methods used for gene expression microarrays may suffice. Protein identification may not be necessary or may become a secondary goal once suitable biomarkers are identified. For biomarker discovery, a high-throughput, relatively inexpensive method is desirable.

Traditional methods like one- and two-dimensional protein gel electrophoresis are not suited for protein identification. Fortunately, mass spectrometry (MS) has been adapted to high-throughput protein detection, resulting in practical use of this technology for plasma protein "signatures" to distinguish benign versus malignant bone tumors, for example.[443] MS adaptation has resulted in the emergence of clinical proteomics, which emphasizes biomarker discovery, characterization, and validation of clinical samples (serum, tissue) in a high-throughput system. The ultimate goal of clinical proteomics is to create a multibiomarker diagnostic profile of specific diseases and tumors.[442,444,445] At this point, however, serum-based diagnostic proteomics is still being developed and is not a routine diagnostic technology. Tissue proteomics, a newer approach, is also in development and may yet prove to be a practical diagnostic modality that may be applicable to routine pathology tissues.[446–449]

ISSUES IN THE DIAGNOSIS AND MANAGEMENT OF CHILDHOOD SOFT TISSUE TUMORS

Many tumor-specific issues have been overlooked in the preceding general discussion of childhood tumor diagnosis. A brief consideration of certain specific soft tissue tumors unique to the pediatric age group provides a perspective for childhood cancer in general, where even the diagnosis of benign versus malignant is not always clear cut. This is intended to give the practicing pathologist and interested oncologist a perspective on the integrated use of histopathology, clinical covariates (such as age and site), and molecular pathology testing for the unambiguous diagnosis (and thus prognosis) in this group of tumors or tumor-like lesions. More detailed discussions of specific tumors are found elsewhere in this textbook. Here, the intent is to offer a specific example, using soft tissue tumors, that can be generalized to the diagnosis and management of childhood cancer in general, particularly the issues of morphology, genetic defects, malignancy (or lack thereof), prognosis, and appropriate treatment.

Morphologic Versus Molecular Diagnosis

The increasing use of nonmorphologic assays to assist in the diagnosis of childhood cancer has prompted concerns that routine histopathology might become a secondary diagnostic modality.[27,450] This is a simplistic misunderstanding of the diagnostic process. Pathologists utilize any and all information that might lead to a more precise or clinically relevant diagnosis. The primary challenge arises when information from disparate and seemingly unrelated technologies is difficult to incorporate into the diagnostic process. The origins of this can be traced to EM and IHC, both of which introduced the unavoidable problem of false-positive and false-negative findings. This was only exacerbated with the advent of highly complex assays of protein expression (proteomic analysis), and especially when RNA expression is used as a surrogate for protein expression, with a significant lack of concordance (correlations often < 0.7).[451] While the problem became significant with annotated genes, it will increase only with the incorporation of vast amounts of highly variable data types, such as total RNA, DNA sequence data, methylation data, miRNA data, and histone modifications.

The more important concern is the fundamental nature of a diagnosis. Historically, the intent is to treat the patient with therapy appropriate to risk. The current classifications of childhood cancer are based on the assumption that tumors that appear different under a microscope are different entities, and conversely, those that appear similar are similar. Much of the information reviewed in this chapter conveys the unmistakable message that this is no longer the situation. Tumors with the same histopathologic features are quite different from a molecular standpoint (translocation positive vs. negative ARMSs). Tumors with different histopathologic features may have the same defect (NPM-ALK fusion gene in ALCL and IMT). Even within histopathologically identical tumors, multiple gene defects are observed (Ewing's tumor, with numerous variations in EWS and ETS gene fusions). With the complexity and variation in specific cancer types, the molecular signature may become paramount in determining tumor classification, treatment, and prognosis.

The core purpose of a diagnosis offers both challenges and opportunities for pathologists and oncologists. The ultimate purpose of a diagnosis is to guide therapy, and this requires comprehensive documentation of the morphology, patterns of protein expression (IHC, proteomics), genomic features (RNA expression pattern, DNA abnormalities, other genomic features), and clinical data.[452] While challenging, this integrative approach is the only reasonable approach to improved diagnosis, improved treatment, improved survival with minimal treatment-related morbidity, and mortality. The current challenge is for pathologists to incorporate vast amounts of molecular data with traditional modalities and for oncologists to use that information to design optimal treatment strategies that take advantage of this new knowledge. "Targeted therapy" and "personalized medicine" are catch phrases for this paradigm shift away from the "one size fits all" approach to therapy. This new approach to cancer management is predicated on an intimate knowledge of the unique features of each patient's tumor that allows for better-informed management decisions and improved outcomes.[449,453]

Minimal Diagnostic Criteria for Rhabdomyosarcoma

Two major issues surround the diagnosis of RMS. The first is recognizing poorly or undifferentiated RMS from other SRCTs. The second is determining into which subtype the tumor fits—embryonal, alveolar, or "other," as well as unique subtypes such as spindle cell and botryoid, both of which enjoy exceptional survival rates. These concerns are not trivial, because therapy, recurrence, metastatic disease potential, and survival are intimately linked to an accurate diagnosis. The minimal criteria for diagnosis of RMS plague many pathologists and frustrate oncologists dealing with a controversial case.

Morphologic methods alone for detecting skeletal muscle differentiation in a sarcoma fail with regularity. This became evident when EM and IHC for myogenic proteins became available. The "standard" antibodies for myogenic differentiation (desmin, muscle-specific actin) that are used by many pathologists are not unique to skeletal muscle alone. Desmin occurs in non-RMS cells, including myofibroblasts, whereas muscle-specific actin routinely reacts with smooth muscle. Myogenesis may be assumed, but rhabdomyogenesis cannot be proven. With gene expression profiling, a significant portion of histopathologically defined ERMSs express no skeletal muscle–specific genes, in particular the myogenic transcription factors *MYOD*, *MYF5*, or *MYOGENIN*. However, these tumors are immunoreactive with muscle "specific" markers, such as MSA and desmin. Developmental studies of transcription factors have documented the pivotal role that these genes play in normal skeletal muscle and rhabdomyogenic tumor development. In particular, *MYOD* and *MYOGENIN* are extremely useful markers of "incipient" rhabdomyogenesis. Likewise, *MYF5* serves a similar purpose, but this antibody is less widely employed. Thus, the absence of these myogenic genes (*MYOD, MYOGENIN, MYF5*) among expressed genes argues strongly against rhabdomyogenesis.

The minimal criteria for diagnosis of RMS require expression of at least one of these myogenic markers, transcription factors, or genes. Both gene microarrays and PCR can be useful in detection of these genes in particularly troublesome cases. It must be realized that PCR may be misleading when there is even minute contamination from normal skeletal muscle, leading to a false-positive result in non-RMS tumors. Antibodies have been developed against *MYOD* and *MYOGENIN* protein that are able to detect even minute amounts of transcription factor proteins in the nucleus, with frozen tissue sections or cytologic imprints (Fig. 8.13A). Antigen retrieval methodology has extended this to readily available FFPE tissue sections.[35] A positive result localized to tumor cell nuclei is unequivocal evidence of rhabdomyogenesis, unlike the ambiguous results from desmin and muscle actin antibodies. In summary, demonstrated expression of *MYOD, MYOGENIN,* or *MYF5* is the minimal diagnostic criteria for RMS in poorly differentiated or undifferentiated soft tissue sarcomas. Incorporation of even greater numbers of myogenesis markers can further refine the basic distinction between myogenic and nonmyogenic sarcomas, as recently shown using microarray analysis of a large group of soft tissue sarcomas entered on Intergroup Rhabdomyosarcoma Study IV (IRS IV) treatment protocols.[16]

Molecular Versus Morphologic Classification of Rhabdomyosarcoma

A major challenge that arises when morphologic and molecular data are incorporated into a diagnosis is reconciliation of opposing diagnoses. This is exemplified by ARMS, a morphologic entity with only a 60% to 70% concordance with its unique PAX-FOXO1A gene fusion. The challenge is how to subtype a tumor as either embryonal or alveolar when the histology is alveolar but the fusion gene is absent. This issue is not addressed by the various categories of RMS published by the International Classification of Rhabdomyosarcoma (Table 8.8).

Alveolar Rhabdomyosarcoma With No Alveolar Pattern. This category seems to be a misnomer, because solid ARMS does not need to display an alveolar pattern. The diagnosis of

this type of ARMS is based more on cytologic and molecular genetic features. The difficulty with this diagnosis is apparent by the fact that the older studies of RMS failed to recognize alveolar cytologic features in one-third of ARMS cases with a diagnostic PAX-FOXO1A chimeric gene.[454,455] Recognition and accurate diagnosis of solid ARMS is important, because these tumors have a less favorable prognosis than ERMS and require different treatment protocols. Fortunately, confirmation that these cases are ARMS can be conducted with PCR to identify the characteristic *PAX-FOXO1A* fusion gene. A typical example incorrectly identified as ERMS but confirmed as translocation-positive ARMS lacking an alveolar histologic pattern is shown in Figure 8.32.

Biphenotypic (Rhabdomyogenic and Neural) Sarcomas. This unique tumor possesses *EWS-ETS* gene fusions identical to those found in the ESFTs tumor family and was recognized in a study of myogenic solid tumors arising within soft tissues of children and young adults.[254] These tumors have SRCT morphology with histologic features suggestive of ARMS (Fig. 8.33A). Moreover, biphenotypic sarcomas express myogenic actin and myosin filaments (Fig. 8.33B). In one particular case, the initial presentation was indistinguishable from ESFT; however, after therapy, both Ewing's-like neural differentiation (Fig 8.33C) and frank rhabdomyoblastic elements (Fig. 8.33B) were detected. This case tested positive for EWS-FLI1 fusion transcripts (Fig. 8.34), documenting the ESFT lineage and myogenesis characteristic for a rhabdomyogenic lineage.

It has been suggested that these biphenotypic tumors represent a form of MEMs, a soft tissue tumor with neural sarcomatous and malignant mesenchymal (rhabdomyoblastic) components.[456–458] This is important diagnostically, because at least some apparent RMSs may actually be these pluripotential (i.e., rhabdomyogenic and neurogenic) MEMs. This issue

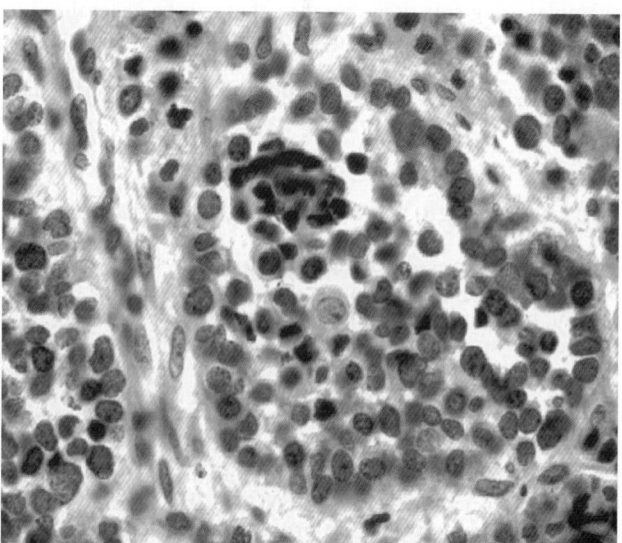

FIGURE 8.32 Solid alveolar rhabdomyosarcoma (ARMS). This tumor was routinely misdiagnosed as a form of embryonal RMS (ERMS). With the International Classification of Rhabdomyosarcoma, more than 15% of all RMS cases have now been reclassified from ERMS to ARMS. Solid ARMS is composed of round poorly differentiated tumor cells, which in some cases (**right side of illustration**) form a vague alveolar pattern. The "true" alveolar character of these tumors is documented with molecular diagnostic means, where a typical PAX3-FOXO1A (50%), PAX7-FOXO1A (25%), or no (25%) translocation is found, similarly to those cases with typical alveolar histology.

TABLE 8.8

INTERNATIONAL CLASSIFICATION OF RHABDOMYOSARCOMA

Diagnosis	Histology	Prognosis
Botryoidal embryonal	Favorable	Superior
Spindle cell embryonal	Favorable	Superior
Embryonal, not otherwise specified	Favorable	Intermediate
Alveolar	Unfavorable	Poor
Solid alveolar	Unfavorable	Poor
Anaplastic/pleomorphic embryonal	Unfavorable	Poor
Undifferentiated sarcoma	Unfavorable	Poor

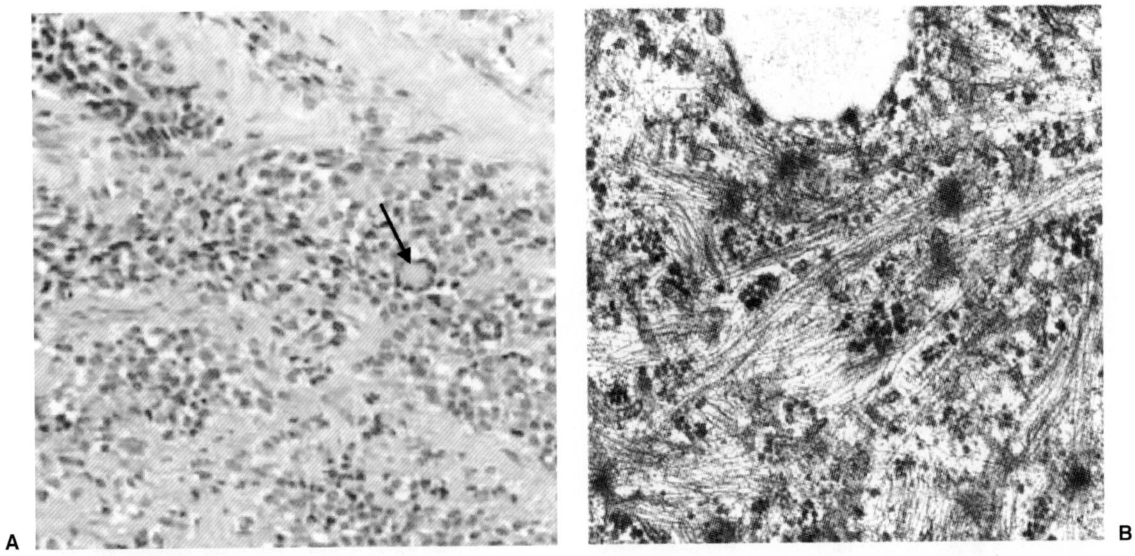

A

B

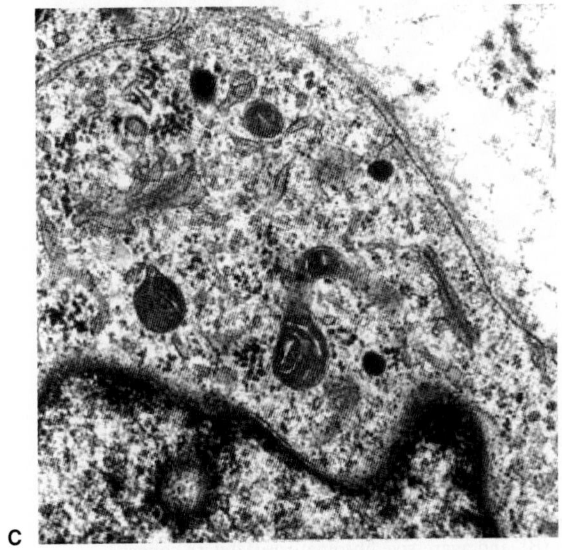

C

FIGURE 8.33 Biphenotypic sarcoma. The three panels show (A) the pretherapy appearance of a tumor, composed entirely of round undifferentiated cells that appeared to be consistent with Ewing's sarcoma. With treatment and subsequent resection, the tumor showed two cell types: (B) cells resembling Ewing's sarcoma and (C) cells with rhabdomyoblastic differentiation. It appears that the tumor at initial biopsy was undifferentiated. With treatment, differentiation was induced and a mixture of Ewing's sarcoma and rhabdomyosarcoma tumor cell types (biphenotypic character) was seen.

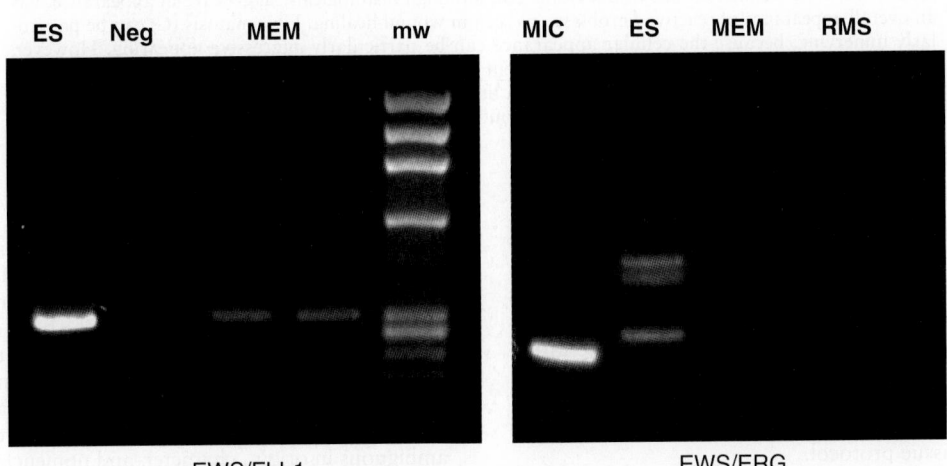

EWS/FLI-1

EWS/ERG

FIGURE 8.34 Polymerase chain reaction (PCR) confirmation of the Ewing's sarcoma translocation. To demonstrate the distinction between undifferentiated rhabdomyosarcoma and biphenotypic sarcoma, PCR analysis of a biphenotypic tumor along with a rhabdomyosarcoma control is illustrated. The results clearly establish that the Ewing's sarcoma—appearing tumor cells at initial biopsy and at posttreatment resection are indeed Ewing's sarcoma—type tumor cells with a portion of the tumor having undergone rhabdomyoblastic differentiation.

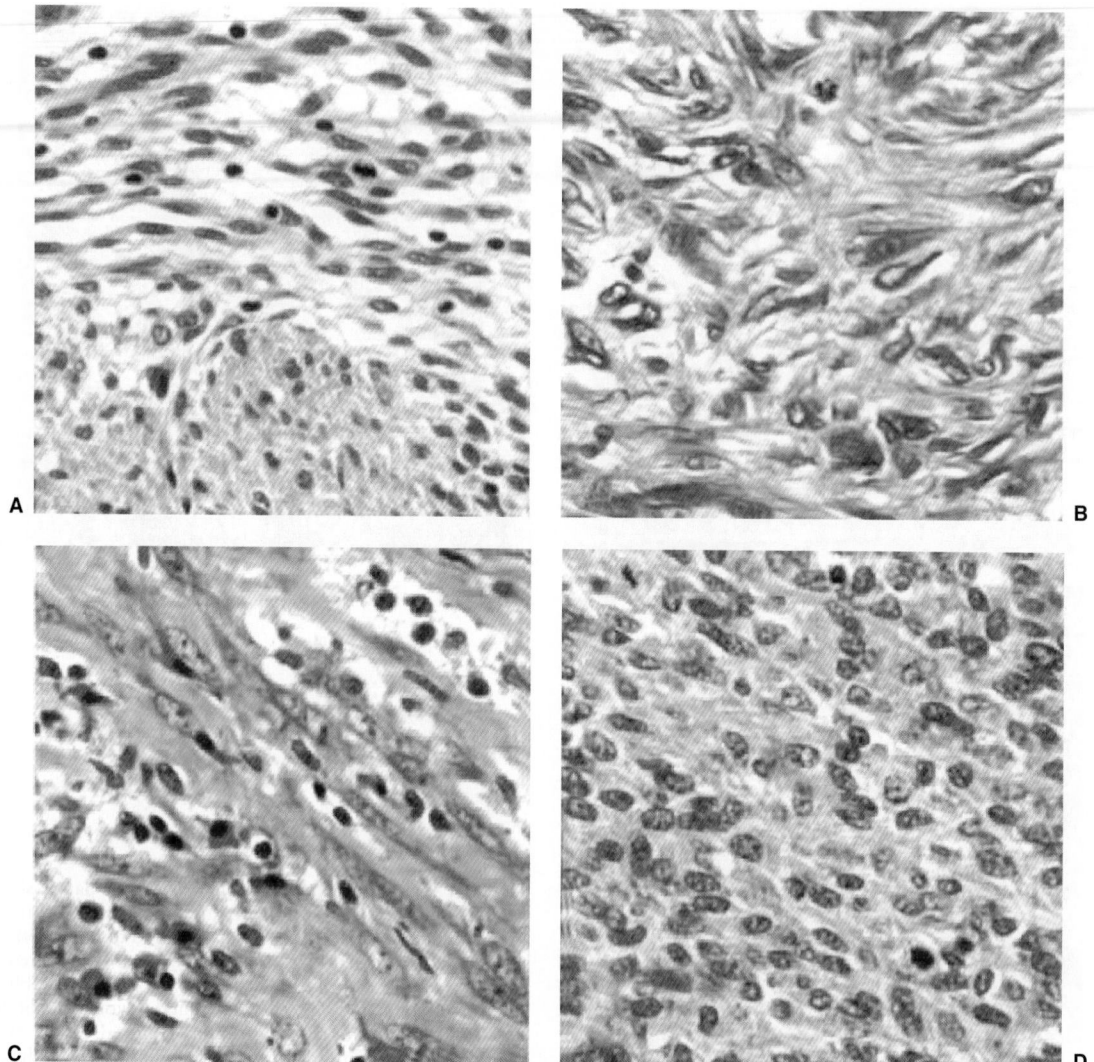

FIGURE 8.35 "Benign" fibrous lesions versus congenital infantile fibrosarcoma. Comparison of the histology of fibrous hamartoma (**A**), fibrous histiocytoma (**B**), and aggressive fibromatosis (**C**) with congenital infantile fibrosarcoma (**D**), which fails to show reliable, objective differences between these four entities. Fibrous hamartoma (**A**) shows areas of smooth muscle differentiation (**bottom center Panel A**) not seen in the other lesions; fibrous histiocytoma (**B**), although histologically aggressive in appearance, has an overall appearance of reactive fibroblasts, as seen in wound healing. Fibromatosis (**C**) can be particularly unnerving, because the cellular appearance can be particularly aggressive appearing. However, coarse bands of normal collagen are inconsistent with a diagnosis of fibrosarcoma. True congenital fibrosarcoma (**D**) is a highly cellular lesion with little or no stroma. Interestingly, the usual criteria for adult sarcoma grading, such as necrosis and mitotic index, are of no value in distinguishing between the four pediatric fibroblastic tumors.

extends to a number of ill-defined soft tissue sarcomas in the pediatric age group, especially those in the first quinquennium, where most of these ambiguous cases occur. The cases described here are unique only in that two clearly defined histogenetic lineages are detectable. In other, less defined entities, two or more lineages are observed. Regardless of the histogenesis, the issue of treatment is of primary importance. Currently, in the COG, such patients may qualify for treatment on a non-RMS soft tissue protocol.

Undifferentiated Soft Tissue Sarcoma. About 15% of cases registered on RMS protocols lack definitive evidence of rhabdomyogenesis on central Intergroup Rhabdomyosarcoma Study Group (IRSG) review. In the past, some of these cases

were not RMS but represented a diverse group of tumors, such as SS, extraosseous Ewing's sarcoma, MPNST, rhabdoid tumors, and CFS or ATFS. With molecular techniques, it is possible to classify these tumors on the basis of the presence of tumor-defining fusion genes. This allows for truly undifferentiated sarcomas to be defined and studied in molecularly homogeneous groups. However, many of these sarcomas lack any diagnostic molecular genetic features and are likely to remain ambiguous in origin, character, and nomenclature.[25]

Fibrous Tumors of Childhood

Unlike adults, children often present with tumoral masses that are neither clearly benign nor malignant. This is particularly true of children in the first few years of life, where benign fibrous lesions (fibromatosis, fibrous histiocytoma, and fibrous hamartoma) are common and coexist with either low-grade malignancies (CFS) or similarly appearing conventional fibrosarcoma (fibrosarcoma), shown in Figure 8.35.[58,459,460] These lesions pose a particularly difficult problem, as the treatment is dependent on diagnosis: the benign lesions are at best surgically removed, with no need for chemotherapy, while congenital fibrosarcoma (with the distinctive ETV6-NTRK gene fusion, described earlier in this chapter), even though "malignant," albeit a very low-grade malignancy is also best treated by surgery alone, while the virtually identical tumor, ATFS (lacking the ETV6-NTRK chimeric gene) is a full-blown malignancy that should be treated with surgical extirpation and chemotherapy, because of its significant potential for metastatic spread. In addition, multiple other fibroblastic neoplasms have been described in this age group,

including low-grade fibromyxoid sarcoma, IMT, and dermatofibrosarcoma protuberans,[461-463] the latter two with characteristic chimeric genes.[273,464-466] While all three are considered neoplasms, they show little malignant potential in most cases and are generally amenable to surgical excision alone, unless extensive disease or (rarely) metastases are present.

Nonmyogenic Spindle Cell Sarcomas in Children

A common diagnostic difficulty in older children is the distinction of CFS, ATFS, monophasic SS, and MPNST from each other (Figs. 8.36 and 8.37). Although these tumors are classified as *nonmyogenic spindle cell sarcomas*, they are quite distinct in their treatment, prognosis, and survival.[467,468] Most

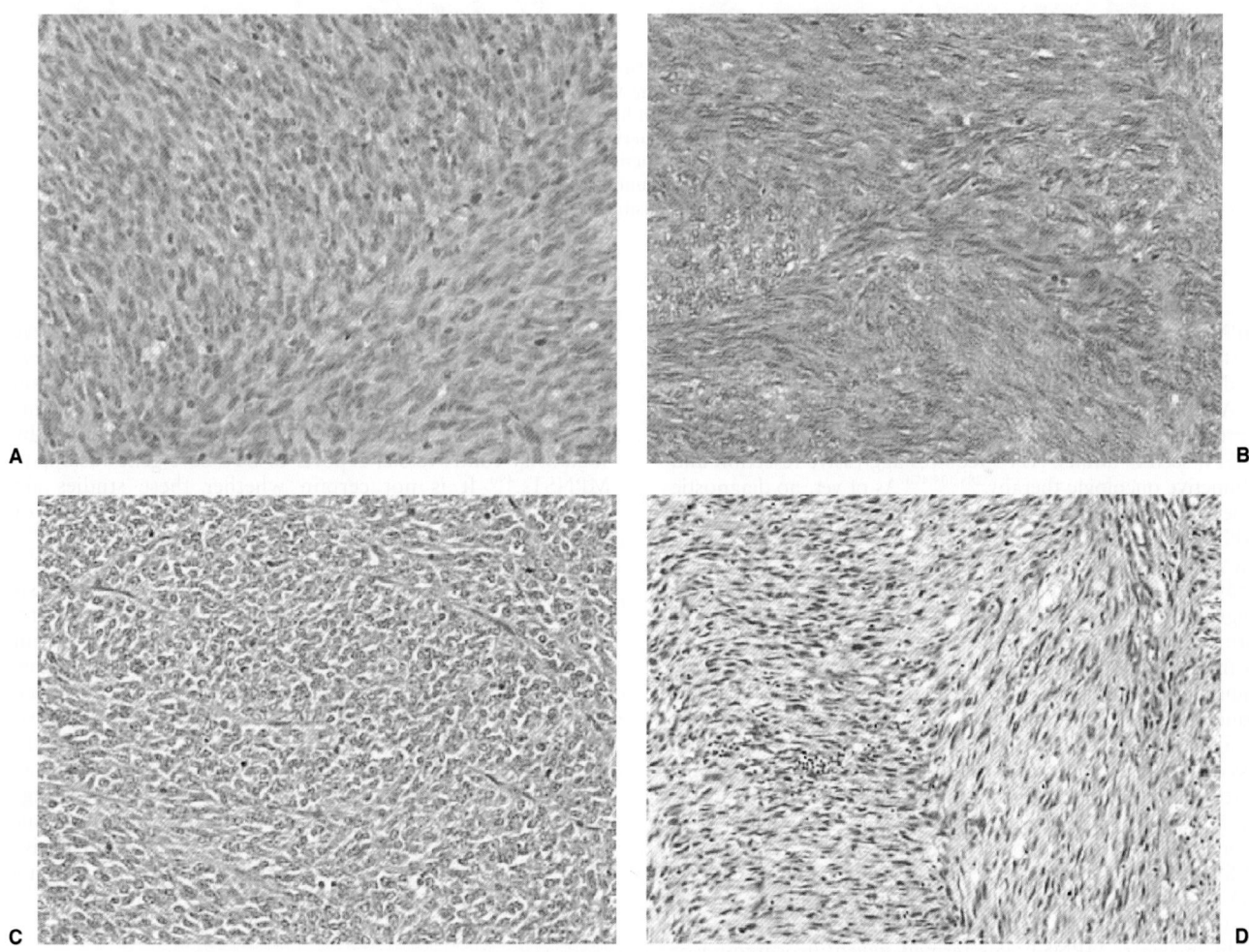

FIGURE 8.36 Common nonmyogenic spindle cell sarcomas in children. Spindle cell tumors, even when clearly malignant, can be difficult to distinguish from one another. Here a typical congenital fibrosarcoma is illustrated in **Panel A,** a typical fibrosarcoma in **Panel B,** a monophasic synovial sarcoma in **Panel C,** and a malignant peripheral nerve sheath tumor (MPNST) in **Panel D.** It can be difficult to distinguish the four in some cases, and monophasic synovial sarcomas have often been identified as fibrosarcoma or malignant peripheral nerve sheath tumor (MPNST) because of their typically fibroblastic appearance, as seen here in **Panel C.** When compared with a conventional fibrosarcoma, striking differences in tumor cytology and tissue organization are evident. Molecular analysis of suspected synoviosarcoma for the diagnostic *SYT-SSX* gene translocation is considered definitive and should be performed on any suspected cases of synoviosarcoma. Unfortunately, there are no unique molecular genetic features so far identified for fibrosarcoma or MPNST. (Photomicrographs courtesy of Dr. Larry Wang, Children's Hospital, Los Angeles).

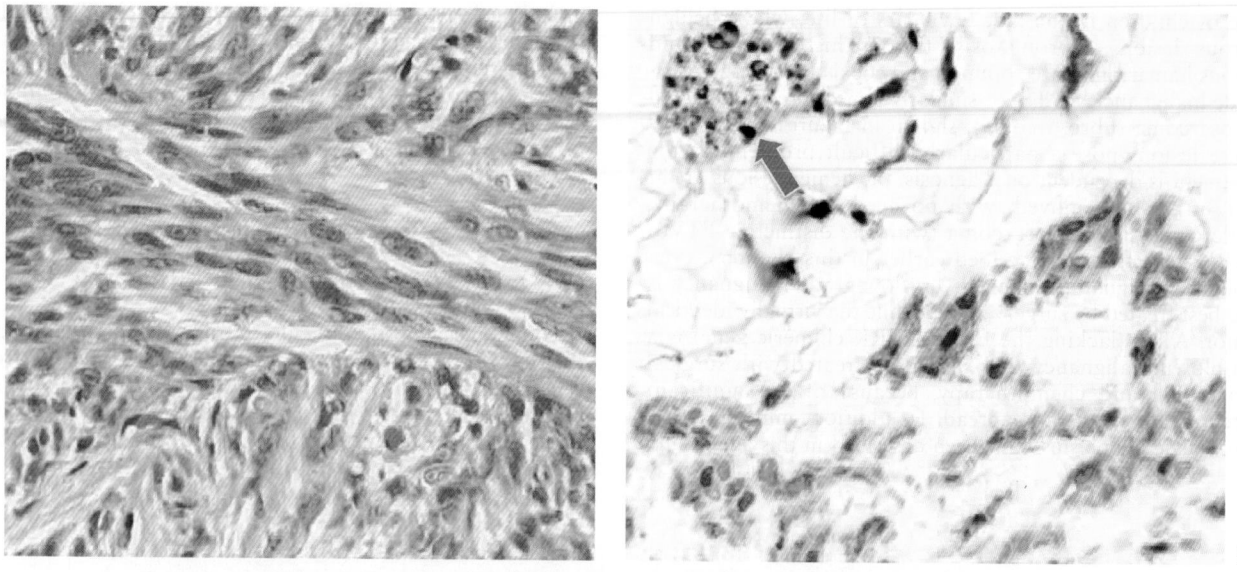

FIGURE 8.37 Malignant peripheral nerve sheath tumor (MPNST). As noted in Figure 8.36 and the accompanying text, it is increasingly recognized that MPNST (hematoxylin and eosin appearance illustrated in **A**) can be difficult to distinguish from both fibrosarcoma and synovial sarcoma (SS). However, an S-100 stain (**B**) will routinely identify malignant nerve sheath tumor in the majority (but not all) cases, is only rarely reactive with SS, and should be nonreactive with all fibrosarcoma. Despite the lack of reactivity in a high percentage of MPNSTs, S-100 immunohistochemistry is routinely performed. However, documented SYT-SSX—positive SS with S-100—positive cells has been reported and a clear distinction between MPNST and SS in all cases is unclear.

MPNSTs are considered to be low-grade malignancies. In contrast, ATFS is a "full blown" malignancy, and SS is a high-grade malignancy with generally poor outcome.[469]

ATFS occurs in adolescents and young adults and does not represent a variant of undifferentiated pleomorphic sarcoma (MFH) seen in adults. ATFS requires aggressive resection and adjunctive oncologic therapy.[288,305,470] As of yet, no diagnostic gene fusion or other distinct biomarkers for ATFS, MPNST, or MFH have been discovered. Consequently, distinction from one another is empirical and most likely often incorrect, especially the diagnosis of MFH, which does not appear to be a single entity.[471] Angiomatoid fibrous histiocytoma, the only form that commonly occurs in children may be the exception to the rule.[472,473] Transcriptional profiling may yet provide some objective diagnostic criteria, but this needs to be confirmed.[245]

SS has for years been recognized in its classic biphasic and less common monophasic form. The monophasic form can be particularly difficult to distinguish from ATFS (Fig. 8.36C vs. A, B, and D).[474] Fortunately, SYT-SSX gene fusions are expressed only in SSs and are detectable in the vast majority of SS cases studied to date.[279,280,475–480] Detection of an SYT-SSX gene fusion is considered to be pathognomonic for SS, distinguishing it from other spindle cell malignancies.

In the past, MPNST was termed *neurofibrosarcoma* or *malignant schwannoma*.[481–486] In contrast to adults affected by MPNST, children with MPNST do not typically have von Recklinghausen's disease or abnormalities of neurofibromatosis type I (NF1) gene. Several features including EM evidence of perineural cell differentiation with basal lamina formation and S-100 immunoreactivity can distinguish this tumor from ATFS and SS, with less than absolute certainty (Fig. 8.37A and B). Other than loss of the neurofibromatosis type I (NF1) gene (17q11.2), no additional recurrent molecular genetic alterations have been defined in MPNST in either pediatric or adult populations.

A diagnostic dilemma may arise when a tumor has nerve sheath features based on immunostaining for neural markers but also has components with divergent differentiation toward skeletal muscle (triton tumors) or glandular elements (glandular/epithelial MPNST).[487–489] This is complicated by somewhat controversial reports of SYT-SSX gene fusions in MPNSTs.[490] It is not certain whether these studies are "flawed," whether there is a link between these tumors, or whether there is expression of neural markers by SS.[77,490–492] This issue has been previously addressed in the literature.[493] Whichever argument is favored, molecular genetic analysis has provoked a reconsideration of how these seemingly unrelated tumors are classified. Given the apparently different behavior of these tumors, it will be important to use both phenotypic and molecular genetic methods to resolve this question.[472,473] We routinely perform SYT-SSX gene fusion analysis on all cases of likely SS, ATFS, and MPNST. Tumor-specific genomic features for MPNST and ATFS would be beneficial, if they exist. If extensive genomic characterization of large numbers of these cases fails to show distinguishing genomic features, it may be necessary to reconsider the noninclusive separation of MPNST, SS, and ATFS, because they occur in a similar age group and at similar anatomic locations.

THE GOLD STANDARD FOR TUMOR CLASSIFICATION

One effect of the rapid incorporation of large-scale biology methods such as gene expression profiling, polymorphism (SNP) analysis, and proteomic analysis has been a reconsideration of the criteria that determine a tumor class or "diagnosis." As discussed previously, what are the minimal criteria necessary for the diagnosis of Ewing's sarcoma or RMS? Does Ewing's sarcoma require a "tumor specific" EWS-ETS chimeric gene for the diagnosis? What if it is not expressed? Likewise, what do we make of a tumor that lacks a diagnostic chimeric gene like Ewing's sarcoma, yet satisfies all other diagnostic criteria from clinical presentation and histopathologic appearance to molecular phenotype as determined by whole-transcriptome profiling? There is currently no consensus, but it is apparent that no single diagnostic modality will "correctly" diagnose all tumors. Rather, the final diagnosis and appropriate treatment must be based on a review of all available information, including clinical history and findings, diagnostic imaging, histopathology, immunocytochemistry, ultrastructure, and various specialized diagnostics (cytogenetics, FISH, CISH, SKY, SNP arrays, RT-PCR, multiplex qPCR, proteomics, gene profiling). Indeed, the advent of highly informative, and sometimes conflicting, diagnostic techniques does not obviate the need for routine diagnostic pathology. New technologies will provide a broader view of the criteria necessary for an accurate diagnosis and better define clinical behavior and treatment response to targeted therapies.[452,453,494] Diagnostic histopathology remains the gold standard for tumor diagnosis, but incorporation of additional specialized diagnostics to allow for further clinically meaningful and predictive categorization has become a necessity.

A FINAL COMMENT

Diagnosis of tumors and tumor-like conditions is especially difficult in children. The rendering of an accurate diagnosis is imperative because therapy, prognosis, and survival are dependent on a precise tumor classification. Many of the most advanced diagnostic modalities were first applied to childhood tumors, owing to the diagnostic challenges associated with pediatric tumors. Molecular genetic analysis of hematopoietic malignancies is considered a standard of care. Likewise, *MYCN* gene amplification and ploidy analysis are mandated for NB protocol enrollment. LOH and gene deletions and gains serve as treatment and prognostic decision points with NB and WT protocols. Gene translocation analysis by several molecular techniques is employed in most cases of RMS, Ewing's sarcomas, SS, DSRCT, and clear cell sarcoma of soft parts. Whole-genome profiling is emerging as a viable diagnostic modality for many cancers, especially pediatric tumors.[16,495,496]

Although ancillary molecular diagnostic techniques were introduced early in childhood cancer diagnosis, this approach is now widespread across all cancers, adult and pediatric alike.[265,449,495,497–499] The high frequency of mesenchymal and blastemal tumors in childhood (leukemia, lymphoma, WT, sarcomas) with recurring genetic abnormalities (translocations, deletions, amplifications, imprinting) contribute to the use of molecular genetic diagnostics in childhood tumors. The prime reason for incorporation of these diagnostic procedures in childhood tumors is the difference that they make in patient management and outcome. Many of the molecular techniques discussed in this chapter have and will continue to contribute to further refinement of risk-based treatment in childhood cancers.

What comes next will be perhaps the most interesting chapter in this ongoing story. The prospect of identifying not just single-gene abnormalities, but wholesale genomic alterations, offer the prospect of identifying diagnostic, prognostic, etiologic, and therapeutic features in a specific tumor. Morphologic diagnosis alone in pediatric tumors is not adequate to guide therapy, provide a meaningful prognosis, and predict event-free and overall survival. Innovative biology-based therapy for Ewing's sarcoma serves as an example. With targeted therapies against IGF1R in Ewing's sarcomas that express IGF1R, it is quite obvious that morphologic diagnosis is only the beginning.[500,501] If treatment response is dictated by IGF1R expression, or other genetic factors, it is imperative to measure IGF1R expression levels in each individual Ewing's sarcoma case.[502,503] Otherwise, response versus nonresponse cannot be related to a tangible, quantitative factor. If IGF1R expression participates in IGF-1 binding, then blocking IGF-1 bind with and IGF1R inhibitor should diminish or halt tumor growth. This personalized medicine approach for tumor therapy is predicated on the relationship between response and receptor display. Correlative molecular and genetic studies will guide decisions in the future as to choice and dose of IGF1R-directed therapy in Ewing's sarcoma. Ultimately, this approach will enhance our understanding of childhood cancer and lead to improved patient management, improved outcome, and reduced morbidity. It is intuitively obvious that rendering a diagnosis needs to move beyond conventional routine histopathologic techniques based on morphology, IHC and EM. Emerging diagnostics that analyze DNA, RNA, and protein for diagnosis, treatment, prognosis, and overall outcome will become the standard of care in the near future.

References

1. Gurney JG, et al. Trends in cancer incidence among children in the U.S. Cancer 1996;78:532–541.
2. Miller RW, Dalager BS. U.S. childhood cancer deaths by cell type, 1960–68. J Pediatr 1974;85(5):664–668.
3. Miller RW. Geographical and ethnic differences in the occurrence of childhood cancer. In: Parkin DM, et al., eds. International incidence of childhood cancer. Lyon, France: Oxford University Press, 1988:3–7.
4. Miller RW. Frequency and environmental epidemiology of childhood cancer. In: Pizzo PA, Poplack DG, eds. Principles and practice of pediatric oncology. Philadelphia, PA: JB Lippincott, 1989:3–18.
5. Parkin DM, et al. eds. International incidence of childhood cancer, vol. II. Lyon, France: International Agency for Research on Cancer, 1998.
6. Oeffinger KC, et al. Chronic health conditions in adult survivors of childhood cancer. N Engl J Med 2006;355(15):1572–1582.
7. Bleyer WA. The U.S. pediatric cancer clinical trials programmes: international implications and the way forward. Eur J Cancer 1997;33:1439–1447.
8. Hill DA, et al. Practical application of molecular genetic testing as an aid to the surgical pathologic diagnosis of sarcomas: a prospective study. Am J Surg Pathol 2002;26(8):965–977.
9. Desper R, Khan J, Schaffer AA. Tumor classification using phylogenetic methods on expression data. J Theor Biol 2004;228(4):477–496.
10. Fu LM, Fu-Liu CS. Multi-class cancer subtype classification based on gene expression signatures with reliability analysis. FEBS Lett 2004;561(1–3):186–190.
11. Khan J, et al. Classification and diagnostic prediction of cancers using gene expression profiling and artificial neural networks. Nat Med 2001;7(6):673–679.
12. Tibshirani R, et al. Diagnosis of multiple cancer types by shrunken centroids of gene expression. Proc Natl Acad Sci U S A 2002;99(10):6567–6572.
13. Seeger RC, et al. Association of multiple copies of the N-myc oncogene with rapid progression of neuroblastomas. N Engl J Med 1985;313(18):1111–1116.
14. Gurney JG, et al. Incidence of cancer in children in the United States: sex-, race-, and 1-year age-specific rates by histologic type. Cancer 1995;75:2186–2195.
15. Qualman SJ, et al. Intergroup Rhabdomyosarcoma Study: update for pathologists. Pediatr Dev Pathol 1998;1(6):550–561.
16. Davicioni E, et al. Molecular classification of rhabdomyosarcoma—genotypic and phenotypic determinants of diagnosis: a report from the Children's Oncology Group. Am J Pathol 2009;174(2):550–564.
17. Hethcote HW, Knudson AG. Model for the incidence of embryonal cancers: application to retinoblastoma. Proc Natl Acad Sci U S A 1978;75(5):2453–2457.
18. Li FP, Fraumeni JF Jr. Rhabdomyosarcoma in children: epidemiologic study and identification of a familial cancer syndrome. J Natl Cancer Inst 1969;43(6):1365–1373.
19. Malkin D, et al. Germ line p53 mutations in a familial syndrome of breast cancer, sarcomas, and other neoplasms. Science 1990;250(4985):1233–1238.
20. Young JL, Miller RW. Incidence of malignant tumors in U.S. children. J Pediatr 1975;86:254–258.
21. Young JJ, et al. Cancer incidence, survival, and mortality for children younger than age 15 years. Cancer 1986;58:598–602.
22. Parkin DM, et al. eds. International incidence of childhood cancer. Lyon, France: Oxford University Press, 1988.
23. Thorner PS, Squire JA. Molecular genetics in the diagnosis and prognosis of solid pediatric tumors. Pediatr Dev Pathol 1998;1(5):337–365.

24. Peydro-Olaya A, et al. Electron microscopy and other ancillary techniques in the diagnosis of small round cell tumors. Semin Diagn Pathol 2003;20(1):25–45.
25. Coffin CM, Dehner LP. Pathologic evaluation of pediatric soft tissue tumors. Am J Clin Pathol 1998;109(4)(suppl 1):S38–S52.
26. Akhtar M, et al. Fine-needle aspiration biopsy diagnosis of small round cell tumors of childhood: a comprehensive approach. Diagn Cytopathol 1999;21(2):81–91.
27. Ladanyi M, et al. Expression profiling of human tumors: the end of surgical pathology? J Mol Diagn 2001;3(3):92–97.
28. Fletcher CD, et al. Diagnostic gold standard for soft tissue tumours: morphology or molecular genetics? Histopathology 2001;39(1):100–103.
29. Grizzle WE, et al. Providing human tissues for research: how to establish a program. Arch Pathol Lab Med 1998;122(12):1065–1076.
30. Misra DN, Dickman PS, Yunis EJ. Fluorescence in situ hybridization (FISH) detection of MYCN oncogene amplification in neuroblastoma using paraffin-embedded tissues. Diagn Mol Pathol 1995;4:128–135.
31. Downing JR, et al. Multiplex RT-PCR assay for the differential diagnosis of alveolar rhabdomyosarcoma and Ewing's sarcoma. Am J Pathol 1995;146:626–634.
32. Rauch A, et al. Molecular karyotyping using an SNP array for genomewide genotyping. J Med Genet 2004;41(12):916–922.
33. Bubendorf L, et al. Survey of gene amplifications during prostate cancer progression by high-throughout fluorescence in situ hybridization on tissue microarrays [published erratum appears in Cancer Res 1999;59(6):1388]. Cancer Res 1999;59(4):803–806.
34. Lee W, et al. Use of FISH to detect chromosomal translocations and deletions: analysis of chromosome rearrangement in synovial sarcoma cells from paraffin-embedded specimens. Am J Pathol 1993;143(1):15–19.
35. Engel ME, Mouton SC, Emms M. Paediatric rhabdomyosarcoma: MyoD1 demonstration in routinely processed tissue sections using wet heat pretreatment (pressure cooking) for antigen retrieval. J Clin Pathol 1997;50(1):37–39.
36. Carlson RW, et al. HER2 testing in breast cancer: NCCN Task Force report and recommendations. J Natl Compr Canc Netw 2006;4(suppl 3):S1–S22, quiz S23–S24.
37. Pusztai L. Current status of prognostic profiling in breast cancer. Oncologist 2008;13(4):350–360.
38. Roukos DH, Murray S, Briasoulis E. Molecular genetic tools shape a roadmap towards a more accurate prognostic prediction and personalized management of cancer. Cancer Biol Ther 2007;6(3):308–312.
39. Katzenstein HM, et al. Prognostic significance of age, MYCN oncogene amplification, tumor cell ploidy, and histology in 110 infants with stage D(S) neuroblastoma: the pediatric oncology group experience—a pediatric oncology group study. J Clin Oncol 1998;16(6):2007–2017.
40. Janoueix-Lerosey I, et al. Overall genomic pattern is a predictor of outcome in neuroblastoma. J Clin Oncol 2009;27(7):1026–1033.
41. Mosse YP, et al. Neuroblastomas have distinct genomic DNA profiles that predict clinical phenotype and regional gene expression. Genes Chromosomes Cancer 2007;46(10):936–949.
42. Spitz R, et al. Oligonucleotide array-based comparative genomic hybridization (aCGH) of 90 neuroblastomas reveals aberration patterns closely associated with relapse pattern and outcome. Genes Chromosomes Cancer 2006;45(12):1130–1142.
43. Mosse YP, et al. Identification of ALK as a major familial neuroblastoma predisposition gene. Nature 2008;455(7215):930–935.
44. Cohn SL. Diagnosis and classification of the small round-cell tumors of childhood [commentary]. Am J Pathol 1999;155:11–15.
45. Lopez-Terrada D. Molecular genetics of small round cell tumors. Semin Diagn Pathol 1996;13:242–249.
46. Meis-Kindblom JM, Stenman G, Kindblom L-G. Differential diagnosis of small round cell tumors. Semin Diagn Pathol 1996;13:213–241.
47. Pohar-Marinsek Z. Difficulties in diagnosing small round cell tumours of childhood from fine needle aspiration cytology samples. Cytopathology 2008;19(2):67–79.
48. Barr FG, et al. Molecular assays for chromosomal translocations in the diagnosis of pediatric soft tissue sarcomas. JAMA 1995;273:553–557.
49. Brodeur GM. Molecular pathology of human neuroblastomas. Semin Diagn Pathol 1994;11:118–125.
50. Ladanyi M. The emerging molecular genetics of sarcoma translocations. Diagn Mol Pathol 1995;4(3):162–173.
51. Coller HA, et al. Expression analysis with oligonucleotide microarrays reveals that MYC regulates genes involved in growth, cell cycle, signaling, and adhesion. Proc Natl Acad Sci U S A 2000;97(7):3260–3265.
52. Golub TR, et al. Molecular classification of cancer: class discovery and class prediction by gene expression monitoring. Science 1999;286(5439):531–537.
53. Perou CM, et al. Molecular portraits of human breast tumours. Nature 2000;406(6797):747–752.
54. Ross DT, et al. Systematic variation in gene expression patterns in human cancer cell lines [see comments]. Nat Genet 2000;24(3):227–235.
55. Heng HH. Cancer genome sequencing: the challenges ahead. Bioessays 2007;29(8):783–794.
56. d'Amore ES, Ninfo V. Soft tissue small round cell tumors: morphological parameters. Semin Diagn Pathol 1996;13(3):184–203.
57. Fisher C. Current aspects of the pathology of soft tissue sarcomas. Semin Radiat Oncol 1999;9(4):315–327.
58. Hicks J, Mierau G. The spectrum of pediatric fibroblastic and myofibroblastic tumors. Ultrastruct Pathol 2004;28(5/6):265–281.
59. Hicks J, Mierau GW. The spectrum of pediatric tumors in infancy, childhood, and adolescence: a comprehensive review with emphasis on special techniques in diagnosis. Ultrastruct Pathol 2005;29(3/4):175–202.
60. Qualman SJ, et al. Protocol for the examination of specimens from patients with Wilms tumor (nephroblastoma) or other renal tumors of childhood. Arch Pathol Lab Med 2003;127(10):1280–1289.
61. Hicks J. Genome, proteome, metabolome: where are we going? Ultrastruct Pathol 2003;27(5):289–294.
62. Hicks J, Mierau G. The spectrum of pediatric tumors in infancy, childhood and adolescence: a comprehensive review with emphasis on special techniques in diagnosis. Ultrastruct Pathol 2005;29(3/4):175–202.
63. Joshi VV, et al. Approach to small round cell tumors of childhood. Pathol Case Rev 2000;5(1):26–41.
64. Chan JK. Advances in immunohistochemistry: impact on surgical pathology practice. Semin Diagn Pathol 2000;17(3):170–177.
65. Coindre JM. Immunohistochemistry in the diagnosis of soft tissue tumours. Histopathology 2003;43(1):1–16.

66. Hibshoosh H, Lattes R. Immunohistochemical and molecular genetic approaches to soft tissue tumor diagnosis: a primer. Semin Oncol 1997;24(5):515–525.
67. Llombart-Bosch A, Contesso G, Peydro-Olaya A. Histology, immunohistochemistry, and electron microscopy of small round cell tumors of bone. Semin Diagn Pathol 1996;13(3):153–170.
68. McNicol AM, Richmond JA. Optimizing immunohistochemistry: antigen retrieval and signal amplification. Histopathology 1998;32(2):97–103.
69. Montesco MC, Alaggio R, Ninfo V. Pediatric-type sarcomas in adult patients. Semin Diagn Pathol 2003;20(4):324–337.
70. Papadimitriou JC, Nikitakis N, Armand R. Immunohistochemical studies in the differential diagnosis of small round cell soft tissue tumors. Arkh Patol 2004;66(2):31–36.
71. Suster S. Recent advances in the application of immunohistochemical markers for the diagnosis of soft tissue tumors. Semin Diagn Pathol 2000;17(3):225–235.
72. Shi SR, Cote RJ, Taylor CR. Antigen retrieval immunohistochemistry: past, present, and future. J Histochem Cytochem 1997;45(3):327–343.
73. Argani P, et al. Aberrant nuclear immunoreactivity for TFE3 in neoplasms with TFE3 gene fusions: a sensitive and specific immunohistochemical assay. Am J Surg Pathol 2003;27(6):750–761.
74. Devoe K, Weidner N. Immunohistochemistry of small round-cell tumors. Semin Diagn Pathol 2000;17(3):216–224.
75. Dias P, et al. Strong immunostaining for myogenin in rhabdomyosarcoma is significantly associated with tumors of the alveolar subclass. Am J Pathol 2000;156(2):399–408.
76. Eusebi V, Bondi A, Rosai J. Immunohistochemical localization of myoglobin in nonmuscular cells. Am J Surg Pathol 1984;8(1):51–55.
77. Folpe AL, et al. Poorly differentiated synovial sarcoma: immunohistochemical distinction from primitive neuroectodermal tumors and high-grade malignant peripheral nerve sheath tumors. Am J Surg Pathol 1998;22(6):673–682.
78. Horowitz ME, et al. Ewing's sarcoma family of tumors: Ewing's sarcoma of bone and soft tissue and the peripheral primitive neuroectodermal tumors. In: Pizzo PA, Poplack DG, eds. Principles and practice of pediatric oncology. Philadelphia, PA: Lippincott, 1997:831–863.
79. Kinney MC, Kadin ME. The pathologic and clinical spectrum of anaplastic large cell lymphoma and correlation with ALK gene dysregulation. Am J Clin Pathol 1999;111(1)(suppl 1):S56–S67.
80. Lee SB, Haber DA. Wilms tumor and the WT1 gene. Exp Cell Res 2001;264(1):74–99.
81. Liapis H, et al. p53 and Ki-67 proliferating cell nuclear antigen in benign and malignant peripheral nerve sheath tumors in children. Pediatr Dev Pathol 1999;2(4):377–384.
82. Linden MD, et al. Clinical application of morphologic and immunocytochemical assessments of cell proliferation. Am J Clin Pathol 1992;97(5)(suppl 1):S4–S13.
83. Ordonez NG. Desmoplastic small round cell tumor, II: an ultrastructural and immunohistochemical study with emphasis on new immunohistochemical markers. Am J Surg Pathol 1998;22(11):1314–1327.
84. Perlman EJ, et al. Ewing's sarcoma—routine diagnostic utilization of MIC2 analysis: a Pediatric Oncology Group/Children's Cancer Group Intergroup Study. Hum Pathol 1994;25:304–307.
85. Pinto A, et al. Undifferentiated rhabdomyosarcoma with lymphoid phenotype expression. Med Pediatr Oncol 1997;28(3):165–170.
86. Riopel M, et al. MIC2 analysis in pediatric lymphomas and leukemias. Hum Pathol 1994;25(4):396–399.
87. Sebire NJ, Malone M, Myogenin and MyoD1 expression in paediatric rhabdomyosarcomas. J Clin Pathol 2003;56(6):412–416.
88. Wang NP, et al. Expression of myogenic regulatory proteins (myogenin and MyoD1) in small blue round cell tumors of childhood. Am J Pathol 1995;147:1799–1810.
89. Agnarsson BA, Kadin ME. The immunophenotype of Reed-Sternberg cells. A study of 50 cases of Hodgkin's disease using fixed frozen tissues. Cancer 1989;63(11):2083–2087.
90. Azumi N, Battifora H. The distribution of vimentin and keratin in epithelial and nonepithelial neoplasms: a comprehensive immunohistochemical study on formalin and alcohol-fixed tumors. Am J Clin Pathol 1987;3:286–296.
91. Norton AJ, Isaacson PG. Monoclonal antibody L26: an antibody that is reactive with normal and neoplastic B lymphocytes in routinely fixed and paraffin wax embedded tissues. J Clin Pathol 1987;40(12):1405–1412.
92. Toth B, et al. Immunophenotyping of acute lymphoblastic leukaemia in routinely processed bone marrow biopsy specimens. J Clin Pathol 1999;52(9):688–692.
93. Trumper L, et al. NPM/ALK fusion mRNA expression in Hodgkin and Reed-Sternberg cells is rare but does occur: results from single-cell cDNA analysis. Ann Oncol 1997;8(Suppl 2):83–87.
94. Qualman SJ, et al. Protocol for the examination of specimens from patients (children and young adults) with rhabdomyosarcoma. Arch Pathol Lab Med 2003;127(10):1290–1297.
95. Fisher C. The comparative roles of electron microscopy and immunohistochemistry in the diagnosis of soft tissue tumours. Histopathology 2006;48(1):32–41.
96. Bakshi NA, et al. ALK-positive anaplastic large cell lymphoma with primary bone involvement in children. Am J Clin Pathol 2006;125(1):57–63.
97. Sigauke E, et al. Absence of expression of SMARCB1/INI1 in malignant rhabdoid tumors of the central nervous system, kidneys and soft tissue: an immunohistochemical study with implications for diagnosis. Mod Pathol 2006;19(5):717–725.
98. Nishio J, et al. Use of a novel FISH assay on paraffin-embedded tissues as an adjunct to diagnosis of alveolar rhabdomyosarcoma. Lab Invest 2006;86(6):547–556.
99. Morotti RA, et al. An immunohistochemical algorithm to facilitate diagnosis and subtyping of rhabdomyosarcoma: the Children's Oncology Group experience. Am J Surg Pathol 2006;30(8):962–968.
100. Mhawech-Fauceglia P, et al. Friend leukaemia integration-1 expression in malignant and benign tumours: a multiple tumour tissue microarray analysis using polyclonal antibody. J Clin Pathol 2007;60(6):694–700.
101. Zhao XF, et al. Pediatric primary bone lymphoma-diffuse large B-cell lymphoma: morphologic and immunohistochemical characteristics of 10 cases. Am J Clin Pathol 2007;127(1):47–54.
102. Wick MR. Immunohistochemical approaches to the diagnosis of undifferentiated malignant tumors. Ann Diagn Pathol 2008;12(1):72–84.
103. Nilsson G, et al. Detection of EWS/FLI-1 by immunostaining: an adjunctive tool in diagnosis of Ewing's sarcoma and primitive neuroectodermal tumour on cytological samples and paraffin-embedded archival material. Sarcoma 1999;3(1):25–32.
104. Willoughby V, et al. A comparative immunohistochemical analysis of small round cell tumors of childhood: utility of peripherin and alpha-internexin as markers for neuroblastomas. Appl Immunohistochem Mol Morphol 2008;16(4):344–348.

105. Houreih MA, et al. Alveolar rhabdomyosarcoma with neuroendocrine/neuronal differentiation: report of 3 cases. Int J Surg Pathol 2009;17(2):135–141.
106. Kreiger PA, et al. Loss of INI1 expression defines a unique subset of pediatric undifferentiated soft tissue sarcomas. Mod Pathol 2009;22(1):142–150.
107. Coindre JM, et al. Immunohistochemical study of rhabdomyosarcoma: unexpected staining with S-100 protein and cytokeratin. J Pathol 1988;155:127–132.
108. Ladanyi M. Diagnosis and classification of small round-cell tumors of childhood [letter; comment]. Am J Pathol 1999;155(6):2181–2182.
109. Russo P, Biegel JA. SMARCB1/INI1 alterations and hepatoblastoma: another extrarenal rhabdoid tumor revealed? Pediatr Blood Cancer 2009;52(3):312–313.
110. Kosemehmetoglu K, Vrana JA, Folpe AL. TLE1 expression is not specific for synovial sarcoma: a whole section study of 163 soft tissue and bone neoplasms. Mod Pathol 2009;22(7):872–878.
111. Roberts CW, Biegel JA. The role of SMARCB1/INI1 in development of rhabdoid tumor. Cancer Biol Ther 2009;8(5):412–416.
112. Huang W, et al. Expression of ALK protein, mRNA and fusion transcripts in anaplastic large cell lymphoma. Exp Mol Pathol 2009;86(2):121–126.
113. Goto Y, et al. The prognosis in spindle-cell sarcoma depends on the expression of cyclin-dependent kinase inhibitor p27(Kip1) and cyclin E. Cancer Sci 2003;94(5):412–417.
114. Kappler M, et al. Elevated expression level of survivin protein in soft-tissue sarcomas is a strong independent predictor of survival. Clin Cancer Res 2003;9(3):1098–1104.
115. Peiper M, et al. CD44s expression is associated with improved survival in soft tissue sarcoma. Anticancer Res 2004;24(2C):1053–1056.
116. Tomek S, et al. Trail-induced apoptosis and interaction with cytotoxic agents in soft tissue sarcoma cell lines. Eur J Cancer 2003;39(9):1318–1329.
117. Hsu FD, et al. Tissue microarrays are an effective quality assurance tool for diagnostic immunohistochemistry. Mod Pathol 2002;15(12):1374–1380.
118. Milanes-Yearsley M, et al. Tissue micro-array: a cost and time-effective method for correlative studies by regional and national cancer study groups. Mod Pathol 2002; 15(12):1366–1373.
119. Nilbert M, Engellau J. Experiences from tissue microarray in soft tissue sarcomas. Acta Orthop Scand Suppl 2004;75(311):29–34.
120. Packeisen J, et al. Demystified ... tissue microarray technology. Mol Pathol 2003; 56(4):198–204.
121. Skacel M, et al. Tissue microarrays: a powerful tool for high-throughput analysis of clinical specimens: a review of the method with validation data. Appl Immunohistochem Mol Morphol 2002;10(1):1–6.
122. Torhorst J, et al. Tissue microarrays for rapid linking of molecular changes to clinical endpoints. Am J Pathol 2001;159(6):2249–2256.
123. Daugaard S, et al. Ewing's sarcoma: a retrospective study of histological and immunohistochemical factors and their relation to prognosis. Virchows Arch A Pathol Anat Histopathol 1989;414(3):243–251.
124. Linnoila RI, et al. Evidence for neural origin and PAS positive variants of the malignant small cell tumor of thoracopulmonary region ("Askin tumor"). Am J Surg Pathol 1986;10:124–133.
125. Schajowicz F. Ewing's sarcoma and reticulum-cell sarcoma of bone. J Bone Joint Surg 1959;41-A(2):349–356.
126. Triche TJ, et al. NSE in neuroblastoma and other round cell tumors of childhood. Prog Clin Biol Res 1985;175:295–317.
127. Carter RL, et al. A comparative study of immunohistochemical staining for neuron-specific enolase, protein gene product 9.5 and S-100 protein in neuroblastoma, Ewing's sarcoma and other round cell tumours in children. Histopathology 1990;16(5):461–467.
128. McCarty KS Jr, et al. Chloroma (granulocytic sarcoma) without evidence of leukemia: facilitated light microscopic diagnosis. Blood 1980;56(1):104–108.
129. Ritter JH, et al. Granulocytic sarcoma: an immunohistologic comparison with peripheral T-cell lymphoma in paraffin sections. J Cutan Pathol 1994;21(3):207–216.
130. Uyesugi WY, Watabe J, Petermann G. Orbital and facial granulocytic sarcoma (chloroma): a case report. Pediatr Radiol 2000;30(4):276–278.
131. Stockl FA, et al. Orbital granulocytic sarcoma. Br J Ophthalmol 1997;81(12): 1084–1088.
132. Rajantie J, et al. Orbital granulocytic sarcoma as a presenting sign in acute myelogenous leukemia. Ophthalmologica 1984;189(3):158–161.
133. Kalmanti M, et al. Ocular granulocytic sarcoma in childhood acute myelogenous leukemia. Acta Paediatr Jpn 1991;33(2):172–176.
134. Ford JG, et al. Granulocytic sarcoma of the eyelid as a presenting sign of leukemia. J Pediatr Ophthalmol Strabismus 1993;30(6):386–387.
135. Davis JL, Parke DW II, Font RL. Granulocytic sarcoma of the orbit: a clinicopathologic study. Ophthalmology 1985;92(12):1758–1762.
136. Bulas RB, Laine FJ, Das Narla L. Bilateral orbital granulocytic sarcoma (chloroma) preceding the blast phase of acute myelogenous leukemia: CT findings. Pediatr Radiol 1995;25(6):488–489.
137. Dickman P. Electron microscopy for diagnosis of tumors in children. In: Rosenberg HS, Bernstein J, eds. Perspectives in pediatric pathology. Basel, Switzerland: S. Karger, 1987:171–213.
138. Erlandson RA. Diagnostic transmission electron microscopy of tumors with clinicopathological, immunohistochemical, and cytogenetic correlations. New York: Raven Press, 1994.
139. Ghadially FN. Diagnostic electron microscopy of tumours. London, England: Butterworths, 1985.
140. Lombardi L, Orazi A. Electron microscopy in an oncologic institution: diagnostic usefulness in surgical pathology. Tumori 1988;74(5):531–535.
141. Mawad JK, et al. Electron microscopy in the diagnosis of small round cell tumors of bone. Ultrastruct Pathol 1994;18:263–268.
142. van Haelst UJ. EM in the study of soft tissue tumors: diagnosis/differential diagnosis and histogenesis. Monogr Ser Eur Org Res Treat Cancer 1986;16(71):71–91.
143. Atkin NB. Solid tumor cytogenetics: progress since 1979. Cancer Genet Cytogenet 1989;40(1):3–12.
144. Sandberg AA, Bridge JA. The cytogenetics of bone and soft tissue tumors. Austin, TX: RG Landes, 1994.
145. Billstrom R, Nilsson PG, Mitelman F. Cytogenetic analysis in 941 consecutive patients with haematologic disorders. Scand J Haematol 1986;37(1):29–40.
146. Neely JE, et al. Characteristics of 85 pediatric tumors heterotransplanted into nude mice. Exp Cell Biol 1983;51(4):217–227.
147. Trent JM, Davis JR, Durie BG. Cytogenetic analysis of leukaemic colonies from acute and chronic myelogenous leukaemia. Br J Cancer 1983;47(1):103–109.
148. Heinrichs S, et al. Accurate detection of uniparental disomy and microdeletions by SNP array analysis in myelodysplastic syndromes with normal cytogenetics. Leukemia 2009.
149. Kawamata N, et al. Identified hidden genomic changes in mantle cell lymphoma using high-resolution single nucleotide polymorphism genomic array. Exp Hematol 2009.
150. Maciejewski JP, Mufti GJ. Whole genome scanning as a cytogenetic tool in hematologic malignancies. Blood 2008;112(4):965–974.
151. McCormick F. The polymerase chain reaction and cancer diagnosis. Cancer Cells 1989;1:56–61.
152. Bustin SA, Mueller R. Real-time reverse transcription PCR (qRT-PCR) and its potential use in clinical diagnosis. Clin Sci (Lond) 2005;109(4):365–379.
153. Murphy J, Bustin SA. Reliability of real-time reverse-transcription PCR in clinical diagnostics: gold standard or substandard? Expert Rev Mol Diagn 2009;9(2):187–197.
154. Yoshida K, et al. Detection of fusion genes in sarcomas using paraffin-embedded tissues. Neuropathology 2005;25(3):263–268.
155. Kralj JG, et al. T7-based linear amplification of low concentration mRNA samples using beads and microfluidics for global gene expression measurements. Lab Chip 2009;9(7):917–924.
156. Morishita S, et al. Real-time reverse transcription loop-mediated isothermal amplification for rapid and simple quantification of WT1 mRNA. Clin Biochem 2009;42(6): 515–520.
157. Klebes A, Kornberg TB. Linear RNA amplification for the production of microarray hybridization probes. Methods Mol Biol 2008;420:303–317.
158. Cikos S, Bukovska A, Koppel J. Relative quantification of mRNA: comparison of methods currently used for real-time PCR data analysis. BMC Mol Biol 2007;8:113.
159. Kurimoto K, et al. Global single-cell cDNA amplification to provide a template for representative high-density oligonucleotide microarray analysis. Nat Protoc 2007;2(3): 739–752.
160. Diboun I, et al. Microarray analysis after RNA amplification can detect pronounced differences in gene expression using limma. BMC Genomics 2006;7:252.
161. Amiel A, et al. Clinical detection of BCR-abl fusion by in situ hybridization in chronic myelogenous leukemia. Cancer Genet Cytogenet 1993;65(1):32–34.
162. Dewald GW, et al. The application of fluorescent in situ hybridization to detect Mbcr/abl fusion in variant Ph chromosomes in CML and ALL. Cancer Genet Cytogenet 1993;71(1):7–14.
163. Caron H, et al. Recurrent 1;17 translocations in human neuroblastoma reveal nonhomologous mitotic recombination during the S/G2 phase as a novel mechanism for loss of heterozygosity. Am J Hum Genet 1994;55(2):341–347.
164. Sacchi N, et al. Interphase cytogenetics of the t(8;21)(q22;q22) associated with acute myelogenous leukemia by two-color fluorescence in situ hybridization. Cancer Genet Cytogenet 1995;79(2):97–103.
165. Janz M, et al. Interphase cytogenetic analysis of distinct X-chromosomal translocation breakpoints in synovial sarcoma. J Pathol 1995;175(4):391–396.
166. McManus AP, et al. Diagnosis of Ewing's sarcoma and related tumours by detection of chromosome 22q12 translocations using fluorescence in situ hybridization on tumour touch imprints. J Pathol 1995;176(2):137–142.
167. Shipley J, et al. Interphase fluorescence in situ hybridization and reverse transcription polymerase chain reaction as a diagnostic aid for synovial sarcoma. Am J Pathol 1996;148(2):559–567.
168. McManus AP, et al. Interphase fluorescence in situ hybridization detection of t(2;13)(q35;q14) in alveolar rhabdomyosarcoma—a diagnostic tool in minimally invasive biopsies. J Pathol 1996;178(4):410–414.
169. Johnson PW, et al. The use of fluorescent in situ hybridization for detection of the t(2;5)(p23;q35) translocation in anaplastic large-cell lymphoma. Ann Oncol 1997;8(suppl 2):65–69.
170. Aoki T, et al. Interphase cytogenetic analysis of myxoid soft tissue tumors by fluorescence in situ hybridization and DNA flow cytometry using paraffin-embedded tissue. Cancer 1997;79(2):284–293.
171. Hagemeijer A, et al. Development of an interphase fluorescent in situ hybridization (FISH) test to detect t(8;21) in AML patients. Leukemia 1998;12(1):96–101.
172. Werner M, et al. Value of fluorescence in situ hybridization for detecting the bcr/abl gene fusion in interphase cells of routine bone marrow specimens. Diagn Mol Pathol 1997;6(5):282–287.
173. Ameye G, et al. The value of interphase fluorescence in situ hybridization for the detection of translocation t(12;21) in childhood acute lymphoblastic leukemia. Ann Hematol 2000;79(5):259–268.
174. Antonescu CR, et al. EWSR1-CREB1 is the predominant gene fusion in angiomatoid fibrous histiocytoma. Genes Chromosomes Cancer 2007;46(12):1051–1060.
175. Attard G, et al. Heterogeneity and clinical significance of ETV1 translocations in human prostate cancer. Br J Cancer 2008;99(2):314–320.
176. Berkova A, et al. A comparison of RT-PCR and FISH techniques in molecular diagnosis of Ewing's sarcoma in paraffin-embedded tissue. Cesk Patol 2008;44(3):67–70.
177. Capodieci P, et al. Gene expression profiling in single cells within tissue. Nat Methods 2005;2(9):663–665.
178. Hallor KH, et al. Fusion of the EWSR1 and ATF1 genes without expression of the MITF-M transcript in angiomatoid fibrous histiocytoma. Genes Chromosomes Cancer 2005;44(1):97–102.
179. Lee YY, et al. Primary pulmonary Ewing's sarcoma/primitive neuroectodermal tumor in a 67-year-old man. J Korean Med Sci 2007;22(suppl):S159–S163.
180. Mazur MA, et al. Intracranial Ewing sarcoma. Pediatr Blood Cancer 2005;45(6): 850–856.
181. Terrier-Lacombe MJ, et al. Superficial primitive Ewing's sarcoma: a clinicopathologic and molecular cytogenetic analysis of 14 cases. Mod Pathol 2009;22(1):87–94.
182. Waugh MS, et al. Desmoplastic small round cell tumor: using FISH as an ancillary technique to support cytologic diagnosis in an unusual case. Diagn Cytopathol 2007;35(8): 516–520.
183. Yang Y, et al. Detection of EWSR1 translocation with nuclear extraction-based fluorescence in situ hybridization for diagnosis of Ewing's sarcoma/primitive neuroectodermal tumor. Anal Quant Cytol Histol 2007;29(4):221–230.
184. Ried T. Images in neuroscience: spectral karyotyping analysis in diagnostic cytogenetics. Am J Psychiatry 1997;154(5):594.
185. Ried T, et al. Tumor cytogenetics revisited: comparative genomic hybridization and spectral karyotyping. J Mol Med 1997;75(11/12):801–814.
186. Schrock E, et al. Multicolor spectral karyotyping of human chromosomes [see comments]. Science 1996;273(5274):494–497.
187. Veldman T, et al. Hidden chromosome abnormalities in haematological malignancies detected by multicolour spectral karyotyping. Nat Genet 1997;15(4):406–410.
188. Tonon G, et al. Spectral karyotyping combined with locus-specific FISH simultaneously defines genes and chromosomes involved in chromosomal translocations. Genes Chromosomes Cancer 2000;27(4):418–423.

189. Zhang FF, et al. Twenty-four-color spectral karyotyping reveals chromosome aberrations in cytogenetically normal acute myeloid leukemia. Genes Chromosomes Cancer 2000;28(3):318–328.
190. Joyama S, et al. Chromosome rearrangement at 17q25 and xp11.2 in alveolar soft-part sarcoma: a case report and review of the literature. Cancer 1999;86(7):1246–1250.
191. Pandita A, et al. Application of comparative genomic hybridization, spectral karyotyping, and microarray analysis in the identification of subtype-specific patterns of genomic changes in rhabdomyosarcoma. Neoplasia 1999;1(3):262–275.
192. Bayani J, et al. Molecular cytogenetic analysis of medulloblastomas and supratentorial primitive neuroectodermal tumors by using conventional banding, comparative genomic hybridization, and spectral karyotyping. J Neurosurg 2000;93(3):437–448.
193. Bacolod MD, et al. Emerging paradigms in cancer genetics: some important findings from high-density single nucleotide polymorphism array studies. Cancer Res 2009;69(3):723–727.
194. Buckley PG, et al. Copy-number polymorphisms: mining the tip of an iceberg. Trends Genet 2005;21(6):315–317.
195. Fix A, et al. Characterization of amplicons in neuroblastoma: high-resolution mapping using DNA microarrays, relationship with outcome, and identification of overexpressed genes. Genes Chromosomes Cancer 2008;47(10):819–834.
196. Maris JM, et al. Chromosome 6p22 locus associated with clinically aggressive neuroblastoma. N Engl J Med 2008;358(24):2585–2593.
197. Yang JJ, et al. Genome-wide interrogation of germline genetic variation associated with treatment response in childhood acute lymphoblastic leukemia. JAMA 2009;301(4):393–403.
198. Tomasson MH, et al. Somatic mutations and germline sequence variants in the expressed tyrosine kinase genes of patients with de novo acute myeloid leukemia. Blood 2008;111(9):4797–4808.
199. Mullighan CG, et al. Deletion of IKZF1 and prognosis in acute lymphoblastic leukemia. N Engl J Med 2009;360(5):470–480.
200. Stratton MR, Campbell PJ, Futreal PA. The cancer genome. Nature 2009;458(7239):719–724.
201. Parham DM, ed. Pediatric neoplasia: morphology and biology. Philadelphia, PA: Lippincott-Raven, 1996.
202. Ladanyi M, Bridge JA. Contribution of molecular genetic data to the classification of sarcomas. Hum Pathol 2000;31(5):532–538.
203. Sorensen PHB, Triche TJ. Gene fusions encoding chimaeric transcription factors in solid tumours. Semin Cancer Biol 1996;7:3–14.
204. Ambros IM, et al. MIC2 is a specific marker for Ewing's sarcoma and peripheral primitive neuroectodermal tumors. Cancer 1991;67:1886–1893.
205. Kovar H, et al. Overexpression of the pseudoautosomal gene MIC2 in Ewing's sarcoma and peripheral primitive neuroectodermal tumor. Oncogene 1990;5(7):1067–1070.
206. Scotlandi K, et al. Immunostaining of the p30/32MIC2 antigen and molecular detection of EWS rearrangements for the diagnosis of Ewing's sarcoma and peripheral neuroectodermal tumor. Hum Pathol 1996;27(4):408–416.
207. Buxton D, et al. Frequent expression of CD99 in anaplastic large cell lymphoma: a clinicopathologic and immunohistochemical study of 160 cases. Am J Clin Pathol 2009; 131(4):574–579.
208. Khoury JD. Ewing sarcoma family of tumors. Adv Anat Pathol 2005;12(4):212–220.
209. Prakash G, et al. MIC-2 positive granulocytic sarcoma of ulna mimicking Ewing sarcoma. Pediatr Blood Cancer 2008;51(6):836–837.
210. Delattre O, et al. The Ewing family of tumors—a subgroup of small-round-cell tumors defined by specific chimeric transcripts. N Engl J Med 1994;331:294–299.
211. Delattre O, et al. Gene fusion with an ETS DNA binding domain caused by chromosome translocation in human cancers. Nature 1992;359:162–165.
212. May WA, et al. Ewing sarcoma 11;22 translocation produces a chimeric transcription factor that requires the DNA-binding domain encoded by FLI1 for transformation. Proc Natl Acad Sci USA 1993;90:5752–5756.
213. Sorensen PHB, et al. A second Ewing's sarcoma translocation, t(21;22), fuses the EWS gene to another ETS-family transcription factor, ERG. Nat Genet 1994;6(2):146–151.
214. Jeon I-S, et al. A variant Ewing's sarcoma translocation (7;22) fuses the EWS gene to the ETS gene ETV1. Oncogene 1995;10:1229–1234.
215. Peter M, et al. A new member of the ETS family fused to EWS in Ewing tumors. Oncogene 1997;14(10):1159–1164.
216. Urano F, et al. A novel chimera gene between EWS and E1A-F, encoding the adenovirus E1A enhancer-binding protein, in extraosseous Ewing's sarcoma. Biochem Biophys Res Commun 1996;219:608–612.
217. Shing DC, et al. FUS/ERG gene fusions in Ewing's tumors. Cancer Res 2003;63(15):4568–4576.
218. Ng TL, et al. Ewing sarcoma with novel translocation t(2;16) producing an in-frame fusion of FUS and FEV. J Mol Diagn 2007;9(4):459–463.
219. Szuhai K, et al. The NFATc2 gene is involved in a novel cloned translocation in a Ewing sarcoma variant that couples its function in immunology to oncology. Clin Cancer Res 2009;15(7):2259–2268.
220. Bailly R-A, et al. DNA-binding and transcriptional activation properties of the EWS-FLI-1 fusion protein resulting from the t(11;22) translocation in Ewing sarcoma. Mol Cell Biol 1994;14:3230–3241.
221. Lessnick SL, et al. Multiple domains mediate transformation by the Ewing's sarcoma EWS/FLI-1 fusion gene. Oncogene 1995;10:423–431.
222. Ohno T, Rao VN, Reddy SP. EWS/Fli-1 chimeric protein is a transcriptional activator. Cancer Res 1993;53:5859–5863.
223. May WA, et al. The Ewing's sarcoma EWS/FLI-1 fusion gene encodes a more potent transcriptional activator and is a more powerful transforming gene than FLI-1. Mol Cell Biol 1993;13:7393–7398.
224. Braun BS, et al. Identification of target genes for the Ewing's sarcoma EWS/FLI fusion protein by representational difference analysis. Mol Cell Biol 1995;15:4623–4630.
225. Thompson AD, et al. EAT-2 is a novel SH2 domain containing protein that is up regulated by Ewing's sarcoma EWS/FLI1 fusion gene. Oncogene 1996;13:2649–2658.
226. May WA, et al. EWS/FLI1-induced manic fringe renders NIH 3T3 cells tumorigenic. Nat Genet 1997;17(4):495–497.
227. Arvand A, et al. EWS/FLI1 up regulates mE2-C, a cyclin-selective ubiquitin conjugating enzyme involved in cyclin B destruction. Oncogene 1998;17(16):2039–2045.
228. Nishimori H, et al. The Id2 gene is a novel target of transcriptional activation by EWS-ETS fusion proteins in Ewing family tumors. Oncogene 2002;21(54):8302–8309.
229. Deneen B, Hamidi H, Denny CT. Functional analysis of the EWS/ETS target gene uridine phosphorylase. Cancer Res 2003;63(14):4268–4274.
230. Nakatani F, et al. Identification of p21WAF1/CIP1 as a direct target of EWS-Fli1 oncogenic fusion protein. J Biol Chem 2003;278(17):15105–15115.
231. Hahm KB, et al. Repression of the gene encoding the TGF-beta type II receptor is a major target of the EWS-FLI1 oncoprotein [published erratum appears in Nat Genet 1999;23(4):481]. Nat Genet 1999;23(2):222–227.
232. Im YH, et al. EWS-FLI1, EWS-ERG, and EWS-ETV1 oncoproteins of Ewing tumor family all suppress transcription of transforming growth factor beta type II receptor gene. Cancer Res 2000;60(6):1536–1540.
233. Kovar H, et al. Among genes involved in the RB dependent cell cycle regulatory cascade, the p16 tumor suppressor gene is frequently lost in the Ewing family of tumors. Oncogene 1997;15(18):2225–2232.
234. Deneen B, Denny CT. Loss of p16 pathways stabilizes EWS/FLI1 expression and complements EWS/FLI1 mediated transformation. Oncogene 2001;20(46):6731–6741.
235. Lessnick SL, Dacwag CS, Golub TR. The Ewing's sarcoma oncoprotein EWS/FLI induces a p53-dependent growth arrest in primary human fibroblasts. Cancer Cell 2002;1(4):393–401.
236. Kovar H, et al. Narrow spectrum of infrequent p53 mutations and absence of MDM2 amplification in Ewing tumours. Oncogene 1993;8(10):2683–2690.
237. Prieur A, et al. EWS/FLI-1 silencing and gene profiling of Ewing cells reveal downstream oncogenic pathways and a crucial role for repression of insulin-like growth factor binding protein 3. Mol Cell Biol 2004;24(16):7275–7283.
238. Yee D, et al. IGF-I expression by tumors of neuroectodermal origin with the t(11;22) chromosomal translocation: a potential autocrine growth factor. J Clin Invest 1990;86:1806–1814.
239. Toretsky JA, et al. The insulin-like growth factor-I receptor is required for EWS/FLI-1 transformation of fibroblasts. J Biol Chem 1997;272(49):30822–30827.
240. Lawlor ER, et al. The Ewing tumor family of peripheral primitive neuroectodermal tumors expresses human gastrin-releasing peptide. Cancer Res 1998;58(11):2469–2476.
241. Kinsey M, Smith R, Lessnick SL. NR0B1 is required for the oncogenic phenotype mediated by EWS/FLI in Ewing's sarcoma. Mol Cancer Res 2006;4(11):851–859.
242. Owen LA, Lessnick SL. Identification of target genes in their native cellular context: an analysis of EWS/FLI in Ewing's sarcoma. Cell Cycle 2006;5(18):2049–2053.
243. Smith R, et al. Expression profiling of EWS/FLI identifies NKX2.2 as a critical target gene in Ewing's sarcoma. Cancer Cell 2006;9(5):405–416.
244. Owen LA, Kowalewski AA, Lessnick SL. EWS/FLI mediates transcriptional repression via NKX2.2 during oncogenic transformation in Ewing's sarcoma. PLoS One 2008;3(4):e1965.
245. Baird K, et al. Gene expression profiling of human sarcomas: insights into sarcoma biology. Cancer Res 2005;65(20):9226–9235.
246. Gerald WL, et al. Clinical, pathologic, and molecular spectrum of tumors associated with t(11;22)(p13;q12): desmoplastic small round-cell tumor and its variants. J Clin Oncol 1998;16(9):3028–3036.
247. Gerald WL, Rosai J, Ladanyi M. Characterization of the genomic breakpoint and chimeric transcripts in the EWS/WT1 gene fusion of desmoplastic small round cell tumor. Proc Natl Acad Sci U S A 1995;92:1028–1032.
248. Zucman J, et al. EWS and ATF-1 gene fusion induced by t(12;22) translocation in malignant melanoma of soft parts. Nat Genet 1993;4(4):341–345.
249. Labelle Y, et al. Oncogenic conversion of a novel orphan nuclear receptor by chromosome translocation. Hum Mol Genet 1995;4(12):2219–2226.
250. Clark J, et al. Fusion of the EWS gene to CHN, a member of the steroid/thyroid receptor gene superfamily, in a human myxoid chondrosarcoma. Oncogene 1996;12:229–235.
251. Newton WA, et al. Classification of rhabdomyosaromas and related sarcomas: pathologic aspects and proposal for a new classification—an Intergroup Rhabdomyosarcoma Study. Cancer 1995;76:1073–1085.
252. Dias P, Dilling M, Houghton P. The molecular basis of skeletal muscle differentiation. Semin Diagn Pathol 1994;11:3–14.
253. Tallini G, et al. Myogenic regulatory protein expression in adult soft tissue sarcomas. Am J Pathol 1994;144:693–701.
254. Sorensen PHB, et al. Biphenotypic sarcomas with myogenic and neural differentiation express the Ewing's sarcoma EWS/FLI1 fusion gene. Cancer Res 1995;55:1385–1392.
255. Wesche WA, et al. Immunohistochemistry of MyoD1 in adult pleomorphic soft tissue sarcomas. Am J Surg Pathol 1995;19:261–269.
256. Davis RJ, et al. Fusion of PAX7 to FKHR by the variant t(1;13)(p36;q14) translocation in alveolar rhabdomyosarcoma. Cancer Res 1994;54:2869–2872.
257. Galili N, et al. Fusion of a fork head domain gene to PAX3 in the solid tumour alveolar rhabdomyosarcoma. Nat Genet 1993;5(3):230–235.
258. Brennan RG. The winged-helix DNA-binding motif: another helix-turn-helix takeoff. Cell 1993;74:773–776.
259. Barr FG. Gene fusions involving PAX and FOX family members in alveolar rhabdomyosarcoma. Oncogene 2001;20(40):5736–5746.
260. Sorensen PH, et al. PAX3-FKHR and PAX7-FKHR gene fusions are prognostic indicators in alveolar rhabdomyosarcoma: a report from the Children's Oncology Group. J Clin Oncol 2002;20(11):2672–2679.
261. Bennicini JL, Edwards RH, Barr FG. Mechanism for transcriptional gain of function resulting from chromosome translocation in alveolar rhabdomyosarcoma. Proc Natl Acad Sci U S A 1996;93(11):5455–5459.
262. Fredericks WJ, et al. The PAX3-FKHR fusion protein created by the t(2;13) translocation in alveolar rhabdomyosarcomas is a more potent transcriptional activator than PAX3. Mol Cell Biol 1995;15:1522–1535.
263. Khan J, et al. cDNA microarrays detect activation of a myogenic transcription program by the PAX3-FKHR fusion oncogene. Proc Natl Acad Sci U S A 1999;96(23):13264–13269.
264. Xia SJ, Barr FG. Analysis of the transforming and growth suppressive activities of the PAX3-FKHR oncoprotein. Oncogene 2004;23(41):6864–6871.
265. Davicioni E, Wai DH, Anderson MJ. Diagnostic and prognostic sarcoma signatures. Mol Diagn Ther 2008;12(6):359–374.
266. Davicioni E, et al. Identification of a PAX-FKHR gene expression signature that defines molecular classes and determines the prognosis of alveolar rhabdomyosarcomas. Cancer Res 2006;66(14):6936–6946.
267. Schnitzer B, et al. Ki-1 lymphomas in children. Cancer 1988;61(6):1213–1221.
268. Morris SW, et al. Fusion of a kinase gene, ALK, to a nucleolar protein gene, NPM, in non-Hodgkin's lymphoma. Science 1994;263(5151):1281–1284.
269. Damm-Welk C, et al. Distribution of NPM1-ALK and X-ALK fusion transcripts in paediatric anaplastic large cell lymphoma: a molecular-histological correlation. Br J Haematol 2009.
270. Ladanyi M, Cavalchire G. Molecular variant of the NPM-ALK rearrangement of Ki-1 lymphoma involving a cryptic ALK splice site. Genes Chromosomes Cancer 1996; 15(3):173–177.

271. Lamant L, et al. High incidence of the t(2;5)(p23;q35) translocation in anaplastic large cell lymphoma and its lack of detection in Hodgkin's disease: comparison of cytogenetic analysis, reverse transcriptase-polymerase chain reaction, and P-80 immunostaining. Blood 1996;87(1):284–291.

272. Sarris AH, et al. Long-range amplification of genomic DNA detects the t(2;5)(p23;q35) in anaplastic large-cell lymphoma, but not in other non-Hodgkin's lymphomas, Hodgkin's disease, or lymphomatoid papulosis. Ann Oncol 1997;8(suppl 2):59–63.

273. Ma Z, et al. Fusion of ALK to the Ran-binding protein 2 (RANBP2) gene in inflammatory myofibroblastic tumor. Genes Chromosomes Cancer 2003;37(1):98–105.

274. Debelenko LV, et al. Identification of CARS-ALK fusion in primary and metastatic lesions of an inflammatory myofibroblastic tumor. Lab Invest 2003;83(9):1255–1265.

275. Lawrence B, et al. TPM3-ALK and TPM4-ALK oncogenes in inflammatory myofibroblastic tumors [see comments]. Am J Pathol 2000;157(2):377–384.

276. Siebert R, et al. Complex variant translocation t(1;2) with TPM3-ALK fusion due to cryptic ALK gene rearrangement in anaplastic large-cell lymphoma [letter]. Blood 1999;94(10):3614–3617.

277. Wlodarska I, et al. The cryptic inv(2)(p23q35) defines a new molecular genetic subtype of ALK-positive anaplastic large-cell lymphoma. Blood 1998;92(8):2688–2695.

278. Turc-Carel C, et al. Translocation x;18 in synovial sarcoma [letter]. Cancer Genet Cytogenet 1986;23(1):93.

279. Clark J, et al. Identification of novel genes, SYT and SSX, involved in the t(X;18)(p11.2;q11.2) translocation found in human synovial sarcoma. Nat Genet 1994;7:502–508.

280. Crew AJ, et al. Fusion of SYT to two genes, SSX1 and SSX2, encoding proteins with homology to the Kruppel-associated box in human synovial sarcoma. EMBO J 1995;14:2333–2340.

281. Kawai A, et al. SYT-SSX gene fusion as a determinant of morphology and prognosis in synovial sarcoma [see comments]. N Engl J Med 1998;338(3):153–160.

282. Ladanyi M, et al. Impact of SYT-SSX fusion type on the clinical behavior of synovial sarcoma: a multi-institutional retrospective study of 243 patients. Cancer Res 2002;62(1):135–140.

283. Guillou L, et al. Histologic grade, but not SYT-SSX fusion type, is an important prognostic factor in patients with synovial sarcoma: a multicenter, retrospective analysis. J Clin Oncol 2004;22(20):4040–4050.

284. Inagaki H, et al. Association of SYT-SSX fusion types with proliferative activity and prognosis in synovial sarcoma. Mod Pathol 2000;13(5):482–488.

285. Mezzelani A, et al. SYT-SSX fusion genes and prognosis in synovial sarcoma. Br J Cancer 2001;85(10):1535–1539.

286. Takenaka S, et al. Prognostic implication of SYT-SSX fusion type in synovial sarcoma: a multi-institutional retrospective analysis in Japan. Oncol Rep 2008;19(2):467–476.

287. Canter RJ, et al. A synovial sarcoma-specific preoperative nomogram supports a survival benefit to ifosfamide-based chemotherapy and improves risk stratification for patients. Clin Cancer Res 2008;14(24):8191–8197.

288. Fisher C. Fibromatosis and fibrosarcoma in infancy and childhood. Eur J Cancer 1996;32A(12):2094–3100.

289. Miser JS, et al. Other soft tissue sarcomas of childhood. In: Pizzo PA, Poplack DG, eds. Principles and practice of pediatric oncology. Philadelphia, PA: Lippincott, 1997:865–888.

290. Knezevich SR, et al. A novel ETV6-NTRK3 gene fusion in congenital fibrosarcoma. Nat Genet 1998;18(2):184–187.

291. Wai DH, et al. The ETV6-NTRK3 gene fusion encodes a chimeric protein tyrosine kinase that transforms NIH3T3 cells. Oncogene 2000;19(7):906–915.

292. Tognon C, et al. The chimeric protein tyrosine kinase ETV6-NTRK3 requires both Ras-Erk1/2 and PI3-kinase-Akt signaling for fibroblast transformation. Cancer Res 2001;61(24):8909–8916.

293. Tognon CE, et al. Mutations in the SAM domain of the ETV6-NTRK3 chimeric tyrosine kinase block polymerization and transformation activity. Mol Cell Biol 2004;24:4636–4650.

294. Argani P, et al. Detection of the ETV6-NTRK3 chimeric RNA of infantile fibrosarcoma/cellular congenital mesoblastic nephroma in paraffin-embedded tissue: application to challenging pediatric renal stromal tumors. Mod Pathol 2000;13(1):29–36.

295. Rubin BP, et al. Congenital mesoblastic nephroma t(12;15) is associated with ETV6-NTRK3 gene fusion: cytogenetic and molecular relationship to congenital (infantile) fibrosarcoma. Am J Pathol 1998;153(5):1451–1458.

296. O'Malley DP, et al. Ultrastructure of cellular congenital mesoblastic nephroma. Ultrastruct Pathol 1996;20(5):417–427.

297. Howell CG, et al. Therapy and outcome in 51 children with mesoblastic nephroma: a report of the National Wilms' Tumor Study. J Pediatr Surg 1982;17(6):826–831.

298. Gonzalez-Crussi F, Sotelo-Avila C, Kidd JM. Malignant mesenchymal nephroma of infancy: report of a case with pulmonary metastases. Am J Surg Pathol 1980;4(2):185–190.

299. Sandstedt B, et al. Mesoblastic nephromas: a study of 29 tumours from the SIOP nephroblastoma file. Histopathology 1985;9(7):741–750.

300. Heidelberger KP, et al. Congenital mesoblastic nephroma metastatic to the brain. Cancer 1993;72(8):2499–2502.

301. Knezevich SR, et al. ETV6-NTRK3 gene fusions and trisomy 11 establish a histogenetic link between mesoblastic nephroma and congenital fibrosarcoma. Cancer Res 1998;58(22):5046–5048.

302. Kaneko Y, et al. Correlation of chromosome abnormalities with histological and clinical features in Wilms' and other childhood renal tumors. Cancer Res 1991;51:5937–5942.

303. Schofield DE, Yunis EJ, Fletcher JA. Chromosome aberrations in mesoblastic nephroma. Am J Pathol 1993;143:714–724.

304. Mascarello JT, et al. Presence or absence of trisomy 11 is correlated with histologic subtype in congenital mesoblastic nephroma. Cancer Genet Cytogenet 1994;77(1):50–54.

305. Schofield DE, et al. Fibrosarcoma in infants and children: application of new techniques. Am J Surg Pathol 1994;18:14–24.

306. Baserga R. The contradictions of the insulin-like growth factor 1 receptor. Oncogene 2000;19(49):5574–5581.

307. Morrison KB, et al. ETV6-NTRK3 transformation requires insulin-like growth factor 1 receptor signaling and is associated with constitutive IRS-1 tyrosine phosphorylation. Oncogene 2002;21:5684–5695.

308. Lannon CL, et al. A highly conserved NTRK3 C-terminal sequence in the ETV6-NTRK3 oncoprotein binds the phosphotyrosine binding domain of insulin receptor substrate-1: an essential interaction for transformation. J Biol Chem 2004;279(8):6225–6234.

309. Eguchi M, et al. Fusion of ETV6 to neurotrophin-3 receptor TRKC in acute myeloid leukemia with t(12;15)(p13;q25). Blood 1999;93(4):1355–1363.

310. Tognon C, et al. Expression of the ETV6-NTRK3 gene fusion as a primary event in human secretory breast carcinoma. Cancer Cell 2002;2(5):367–376.

311. Li Z, et al. ETV6-NTRK3 fusion oncogene initiates breast cancer from committed mammary progenitors via activation of AP1 complex. Cancer Cell 2007;12(6):542–558.

312. Page DL, Anderson TJ, Sakamoto G. Infiltrating carcinoma: major histologic types. In: Page DL, Anderson TJ, eds. Diagnostic histopathology of the breast. Edinburgh, UK: Churchill Livingstone, 1987.

313. Bourgeois JM, et al. Molecular detection of the ETV6-NTRK3 gene fusion differentiates congenital fibrosarcoma from other childhood spindle cell tumors. Am J Surg Pathol 2000;24(7):937–946.

314. Ladanyi M, et al. The der(17)t(X;17)(p11;q25) of human alveolar soft part sarcoma fuses the TFE3 transcription factor gene to ASPL, a novel gene at 17q25. Oncogene 2001;20(1):48–57.

315. Sandberg A, Bridge J. Updates on the cytogenetics and molecular genetics of bone and soft tissue tumors: alveolar soft part sarcoma. Cancer Genet Cytogenet 2002;136(1):1–9.

316. Argani P, Ladanyi M. Recent advances in pediatric renal neoplasia. Adv Anat Pathol 2003;10(5):243–260.

317. Argani P, et al. Primary renal neoplasms with the ASPL-TFE3 gene fusion of alveolar soft part sarcoma: a distinctive tumor entity previously included among renal cell carcinomas of children and adolescents. Am J Pathol 2001;159(1):179–192.

318. Argani P, et al. PRCC-TFE3 renal carcinomas: morphologic, immunohistochemical, ultrastructural, and molecular analysis of an entity associated with the t(X;1)(p11.2;q21). Am J Surg Pathol 2002;26(12):1553–1566.

319. Ruco LP, et al. Letterer-Siwe disease: immunohistochemical evidence for a proliferative disorder involving immature cells of Langerhans lineage. Virchows Arch A Pathol Anat Histopathol 1988;413(3):239–247.

320. Davis IJ, et al. Cloning of an Alpha-TFEB fusion in renal tumors harboring the t(6;11)(p21;q13) chromosome translocation. Proc Natl Acad Sci U S A 2003;100(10):6051–6056.

321. Bridge JA, et al. Fusion of the ALK gene to the clathrin heavy chain gene, CLTC, in inflammatory myofibroblastic tumor. Am J Pathol 2001;159(2):411–415.

322. Triche TJ, Askin FB, Kissane JM. Neuroblastoma, Ewing's sarcoma, and the differential diagnosis of small-, round-, blue-cell tumors. In: Finegold M, ed. Pathology of neoplasia in children and adolescents. Philadelphia, PA: WB Saunders, 1986:145–195.

323. Brodeur GM, et al. Biology and genetics of human neuroblastomas. J Pediatr Hematol Oncol 1997;19(2):93–101.

324. Fong CT, et al. Loss of heterozygosity for the short arm of chromosome 1 in human neuroblastomas: correlation with N-myc amplification. Proc Natl Acad Sci U S A 1989;86(10):3753–3757.

325. Bown N, et al. Gain of chromosome arm 17q and adverse outcome in patients with neuroblastoma [see comments]. N Engl J Med 1999;340(25):1954–1961.

326. Lastowska M, et al. Gain of chromosome arm 17q predicts unfavourable outcome in neuroblastoma patients: U.K. Children's Cancer Study Group and the U.K. Cancer Cytogenetics Group. Eur J Cancer 1997;33(10):1627–1633.

327. Lastowska M, et al. Molecular cytogenetic delineation of 17q translocation breakpoints in neuroblastoma cell lines. Genes Chromosomes Cancer 1998;23(2):116–122.

328. Bown N, et al. 17q gain in neuroblastoma predicts adverse clinical outcome: U.K. Cancer Cytogenetics Group and the U.K. Children's Cancer Study Group. Med Pediatr Oncol 2001;36(1):14–19.

329. Spitz R, et al. Gain of distal chromosome arm 17q is not associated with poor prognosis in neuroblastoma. Clin Cancer Res 2003;9(13):4835–4840.

330. Stallings RL. Origin and functional significance of large-scale chromosomal imbalances in neuroblastoma. Cytogenet Genome Res 2007;118(2/4):110–115.

331. Caren H, et al. High incidence of DNA mutations and gene amplifications of the ALK gene in advanced sporadic neuroblastoma tumours. Biochem J 2008;416(2):153–159.

332. Chen Y, et al. Oncogenic mutations of ALK kinase in neuroblastoma. Nature 2008;455(7215):971–974.

333. George RE, et al. Activating mutations in ALK provide a therapeutic target in neuroblastoma. Nature 2008;455(7215):975–978.

334. Janoueix-Lerosey I, et al. Somatic and germline activating mutations of the ALK kinase receptor in neuroblastoma. Nature 2008;455(7215):967–970.

335. Beckwith JB, Palmer NF. Histopathology and prognosis of Wilm's tumor: results from the First National Wilms Tumor Study. Cancer 1978;41:1937–1948.

336. Rutledge J, et al. Absence of immunoperoxidase staining for myoglobin in the malignant rhabdoid tumor of the kidney. Pediatr Pathol 1983;1(1):93–98.

337. Chang C-H, Ramirez N, Sakr WA. Primitive neuroectodermal tumor of the brain associated with malignant rhabdoid tumor of the liver: a histologic, immunohistochemical, and electron microscopic study. Pediatr Pathol 1989;9:307–319.

338. Chase DR. Rhabdoid versus epithelioid sarcoma. Am J Surg Pathol 1990;14(8):792–794.

339. Gururangan S, et al. Primary extracranial rhabdoid tumors. Cancer 1993;71:2653–2659.

340. Tsokos M, et al. Malignant rhabdoid tumor of the kidney and soft tissues: evidence for a diverse morphological and immunocytochemical phenotype. Arch Pathol Lab Med 1989;113(2):115–120.

341. Tsujimura T, et al. A case of malignant rhabdoid tumor arising from soft parts in the prepubic region. Acta Pathol Jpn 1989;39(10):677–682.

342. Tsuneyoshi M, et al. Malignant soft tissue neoplasms with the histologic features of renal rhabdoid tumors: an ultrastructural and immunohistochemical study. Hum Pathol 1985;16:1235–1242.

343. Tsuneyoshi M, et al. The existence of rhabdoid cells in specified soft tissue sarcomas: histopathological, ultrastructural and immunohistochemical evidence. Virchows Arch A Pathol Anat Histopathol 1987;411(6):509–514.

344. Vogel AM, et al. Rhabdoid tumors of the kidney contain mesenchymal specific and epithelial specific intermediate filament proteins. Lab Invest 1984;50(2):232–238.

345. Weeks DA, Beckwith JB, Mierau GW. Rhabdoid tumor: an entity or a phenotype? [editorial]. Arch Pathol Lab Med 1989;113:113–114.

346. Biegel JA, et al. Narrowing the critical region for a rhabdoid tumor locus in 22q11. Genes Chromosomes Cancer 1996;16:94–105.

347. Biegel JA, et al. Molecular analysis of a partial deletion of 22q in a central nervous system rhabdoid tumor. Genes Chromosomes Cancer 1992;5:104–108.

348. Biegel JA, et al. Monosomy 22 in rhabdoid or atypical tumors of the brain. J Neurosurg 1990;73(5):710–714.

349. Douglass EC, et al. Malignant rhabdoid tumor: a highly malignant childhood tumor with minimal karyotypic changes. Genes Chromosomes Cancer 1990;2(3):210–216.

350. Horie H, Etoh T, Maie M. Cytogenetic characteristics of a malignant rhabdoid tumor arising from the paravertebral region. Acta Pathol Jpn 1992;42:460–465.

351. Sait SNJ, et al. Localization of Beckwith-Wiedemann and rhabdoid tumor chromosome rearrangements to a defined interval in chromosome band 11p15.5. Genes Chromosomes Cancer 1994;11:97–105.

352. Schofield DE, Beckwith JB, Sklar J. Loss of heterozygosity at chromosome regions 22q11-12 and 11p15.5 in renal rhabdoid tumors. Genes Chromosomes Cancer 1996;15:10–17.

353. Newsham I, et al. Molecular sublocalization and characterization of the 11;22 translocation breakpoint in a malignant rhabdoid tumor. Genomics (in press).

354. Biegel JA, et al. Alterations of the hSNF5/INI1 gene in central nervous system atypical teratoid/rhabdoid tumors and renal and extrarenal rhabdoid tumors. Clin Cancer Res 2002;8(11):3461–3467.

355. Medjkane S, et al. The tumor suppressor hSNF5/INI1 modulates cell growth and actin cytoskeleton organization. Cancer Res 2004;64(10):3406–3413.

356. Versteege I, et al. Truncating mutations of hSNF5/INI1 in aggressive paediatric cancer. Nature 1998;394(6689):203–206.

357. Zhang ZK, et al. Cell cycle arrest and repression of cyclin D1 transcription by INI1/hSNF5. Mol Cell Biol 2002;22(16):5975–5988.

358. Coppes MJ, Egeler RM. Genetics of Wilms' tumor. Semin Urol Oncol 1999;17(1):2–10.

359. Hirose M. The role of Wilms' tumor genes. J Med Invest 1999;46(3–4):130–140.

360. Satoh Y, et al. Genetic and epigenetic alterations on the short arm of chromosome 11 are involved in a majority of sporadic Wilms' tumours. Br J Cancer 2006;95(4):541–547.

361. Xin Z, et al. A novel imprinted gene, KCNQ1DN, within the WT2 critical region of human chromosome 11p15.5 and its reduced expression in Wilms' tumors. J Biochem 2000;128(5):847–853.

362. Dome JS, Coppes MJ. Recent advances in Wilms tumor genetics. Curr Opin Pediatr 2002;14(1):5–11.

363. Beckwith JB. Vignettes from the history of overgrowth and related syndromes. Am J Med Genet 1998;79(4):238–248.

364. Koesters R, et al. Mutational activation of the beta-catenin proto-oncogene is a common event in the development of Wilms' tumors. Cancer Res 1999;59(16):3880–3882.

365. Bruce CK, et al. Molecular analysis of region t(5;6)(q21;q21) in Wilms tumor. Cancer Genet Cytogenet 2003;141(2):106–113.

366. Hoban PR, et al. Physical localisation of the breakpoints of a constitutional translocation t(5;6)(q21;q21) in a child with bilateral Wilms' tumour. J Med Genet 1997;34(4):343–345.

367. Rivera MN, et al. An X chromosome gene, WTX, is commonly inactivated in Wilms tumor. Science 2007;315(5812):642–645.

368. Major MB, et al. Wilms tumor suppressor WTX negatively regulates WNT/beta-catenin signaling. Science 2007;316(5827):1043–1046.

369. Anglesio MS, et al. Differential expression of a novel ankyrin containing E3 ubiquitin-protein ligase, Hace1, in sporadic Wilms' tumour versus normal kidney. Hum Mol Genet 2004.

370. Solis V, Pritchard J, Cowell JK. Cytogenetic changes in Wilms' tumors. Cancer Genet Cytogenet 1988;34(2):223–234.

371. Zhang L, et al. The E3 ligase HACE1 is a critical chromosome 6q21 tumor suppressor involved in multiple cancers. Nat Med 2007;13(9):1060–1069.

372. Viswanathan SR, et al. Lin28 promotes transformation and is associated with advanced human malignancies. Nat Genet 2009;41(7):843–848.

373. Takahashi N, et al. Large-scale copy number variants (CNVs) detected in different ethnic human populations. Cytogenet Genome Res 2008;123(1/4):224–233.

374. Rocha JC, et al. Pharmacogenetics of outcome in children with acute lymphoblastic leukemia. Blood 2005;105(12):4752–4758.

375. Guttman M, et al. Chromatin signature reveals over a thousand highly conserved large non-coding RNAs in mammals. Nature 2009;458(7235):223–227.

376. Calin GA, Croce CM. MicroRNA signatures in human cancers. Nat Rev Cancer 2006;6(11):857–866.

377. Garzon R, et al. MicroRNA expression and function in cancer. Trends Mol Med 2006;12(12):580–587.

378. Costa FF. Non-coding RNAs: lost in translation? Gene 2007;386(1/2):1–10.

379. Mercer TR, Dinger ME, Mattick JS. Long non-coding RNAs: insights into functions. Nat Rev Genet 2009;10(3):155–159.

380. de la Grange P, et al. A new advance in alternative splicing databases: from catalogue to detailed analysis of regulation of expression and function of human alternative splicing variants. BMC Bioinformatics 2007;8:180.

381. Bitton DA, et al. Exon level integration of proteomics and microarray data. BMC Bioinformatics 2008;9:118.

382. Birney E, et al. Identification and analysis of functional elements in 1% of the human genome by the ENCODE pilot project. Nature 2007;447(7146):799–816.

383. Willingham AT, et al. Transcriptional landscape of the human and fly genomes: nonlinear and multifunctional modular model of transcriptomes. Cold Spring Harb Symp Quant Biol 2006;71:101–110.

384. DeRisi JL, Iyer VR, Brown PO. Exploring the metabolic and genetic control of gene expression on a genomic scale. Science 1997;278(5338):680–686.

385. Eisen MB, Brown PO. DNA arrays for analysis of gene expression. Methods Enzymol 1999;303:179–205.

386. Lipshutz RJ, et al. Using oligonucleotide probe arrays to access genetic diversity. Biotechniques 1995;19(3):442–447.

387. Schena M, et al. Quantitative monitoring of gene expression patterns with a complementary DNA microarray. Science 1995;270(5235):467–470.

388. Cope LM, et al. A benchmark for Affymetrix GeneChip expression measures. Bioinformatics 2004;20(3):323–331.

389. James AC, et al. Sensitivity and specificity of five abundance estimators for high-density oligonucleotide microarrays. Bioinformatics 2004;20(7):1060–1065.

390. Haber DA. Splicing into senescence: the curious case of p16 and p19ARF. Cell 1999;91:555–558.

391. Kamijo T, et al. Tumor suppression at the mouse INK4e locus mediated by the alternative reading frame product p19ARF. Cell 1999;91:649–659.

392. Quelle DE, et al. Cloning and characterization of murine p16INK4a and p15INK4b genes. Oncogene 1995;11(4):635–645.

393. Quelle DE, et al. Alternative reading frames of the INK4a tumor suppressor gene encode two unrelated proteins capable of inducing cell cycle arrest. Cell 1995;83(6):993–1000.

394. Schofield D, Triche TJ. cDNA microarray analysis of global gene expression in sarcomas. Curr Opin Oncol 2002;14(4):406–411.

395. Triche TJ, Schofield D, Buckley J. DNA microarrays in pediatric cancer. Cancer J 2001;7(1):2–15.

396. Bassett DE Jr, Eisen MB, Boguski MS. Gene expression informatics—it's all in your mine. Nat Genet 1999;21(1)(suppl):51–55.

397. Ermolaeva O, et al. Data management and analysis for gene expression arrays. Nat Genet 1998;20(1):19–23.

398. Tamayo P, et al. Interpreting patterns of gene expression with self-organizing maps: methods and application to hematopoietic differentiation. Proc Natl Acad Sci U S A 1999;96(6):2907–2912.

399. Wittes J, Friedman HP. Searching for evidence of altered gene expression: a comment on statistical analysis of microarray data [editorial; comment]. J Natl Cancer Inst 1999;91(5):400–401.

400. Diehn M, Alizadeh AA, Brown PO. Examining the living genome in health and disease with DNA microarrays. JAMA 2000;283(17):2298–2299.

401. Simon R. Diagnostic and prognostic prediction using gene expression profiles in high-dimensional microarray data. Br J Cancer 2003;89(9):1599–1604.

402. Mjolsness E, Garrett C, Miranker WL. Multiscale optimization in neural nets. Yorktown Heights, NY: IBM TJ Watson Research Center, 1990:20. Research report RC 15910.

403. Lee Y, Lee CK. Classification of multiple cancer types by multicategory support vector machines using gene expression data. Bioinformatics 2003;19(9):1132–1139.

404. Ochs MF, et al. Bayesian decomposition: analyzing microarray data within a biological context. Ann N Y Acad Sci 2004;1020:212–226.

405. Peterson C, Ringner M. Analyzing tumor gene expression profiles. Artif Intell Med 2003;28(1):59–74.

406. Bhattacharjee A, et al. Classification of human lung carcinomas by mRNA expression profiling reveals distinct adenocarcinoma subclasses. Proc Natl Acad Sci U S A 2001;98(24):13790–13795.

407. Iacobuzio-Donahue CA, et al. Exploration of global gene expression patterns in pancreatic adenocarcinoma using cDNA microarrays. Am J Pathol 2003;162(4):1151–1162.

408. Lapointe J, et al. Gene expression profiling identifies clinically relevant subtypes of prostate cancer. Proc Natl Acad Sci U S A 2004;101(3):811–816.

409. Nutt CL, et al. Gene expression-based classification of malignant gliomas correlates better with survival than histological classification. Cancer Res 2003;63(7):1602–1607.

410. Pomeroy SL, et al. Prediction of central nervous system embryonal tumour outcome based on gene expression. Nature 2002;415(6870):436–442.

411. Ramaswamy S, Golub TR. DNA microarrays in clinical oncology. J Clin Oncol 2002;20(7):1932–1941.

412. Ramaswamy S, et al. A molecular signature of metastasis in primary solid tumors. Nat Genet 2003;33(1):49–54.

413. Shipp MA, et al. Diffuse large B-cell lymphoma outcome prediction by gene-expression profiling and supervised machine learning. Nat Med 2002;8(1):68–74.

414. Singh D, et al. Gene expression correlates of clinical prostate cancer behavior. Cancer Cell 2002;1(2):203–209.

415. Sorlie T, et al. Repeated observation of breast tumor subtypes in independent gene expression data sets. Proc Natl Acad Sci U S A 2003;100(14):8418–8423.

416. Yeang CH, et al. Molecular classification of multiple tumor types. Bioinformatics 2001;17(suppl 1):S316–S322.

417. Catchpoole D, et al. Gene expression profiles that segregate patients with childhood acute lymphoblastic leukaemia: an independent validation study identifies that endoglin associates with patient outcome. Leuk Res 2007;31(12):1741–1747.

418. Dumur CI, et al. Evaluation of a linear amplification method for small samples used on high-density oligonucleotide microarray analysis. Anal Biochem 2004;331(2):314–321.

419. Klur S, et al. Evaluation of procedures for amplification of small-size samples for hybridization on microarrays. Genomics 2004;83(3):508–517.

420. Nygaard V, et al. Effects of mRNA amplification on gene expression ratios in cDNA experiments estimated by analysis of variance. BMC Genomics 2003;4(1):11.

421. Schneider J, et al. Systematic analysis of T7 RNA polymerase based in vitro linear RNA amplification for use in microarray experiments. BMC Genomics 2004;5(1):29.

422. Stirewalt DL, et al. Single-stranded linear amplification protocol results in reproducible and reliable microarray data from nanogram amounts of starting RNA. Genomics 2004;83(2):321–331.

423. Zhao H, et al. Optimization and evaluation of T7 based RNA linear amplification protocols for cDNA microarray analysis. BMC Genomics 2002;3(1):31.

424. Fan JB, et al. Parallel genotyping of human SNPs using generic high-density oligonucleotide tag arrays. Genome Res 2000;10(6):853–860.

425. Halushka MK, et al. Patterns of single-nucleotide polymorphisms in candidate genes for blood-pressure homeostasis. Nat Genet 1999;22(3):239–247.

426. Cardon LR, Abecasis GR. Using haplotype blocks to map human complex trait loci. Trends Genet 2003;19(3):135–140.

427. Phillips MS, et al. Chromosome-wide distribution of haplotype blocks and the role of recombination hot spots. Nat Genet 2003;33(3):382–387.

428. Durrant C, et al. Linkage disequilibrium mapping via cladistic analysis of single-nucleotide polymorphism haplotypes. Am J Hum Genet 2004;75(1):35–43.

429. Frazer KA, et al. Human genetic variation and its contribution to complex traits. Nat Rev Genet 2009;10(4):241–251.

430. Hafler DA, De Jager PL. Applying a new generation of genetic maps to understand human inflammatory disease. Nat Rev Immunol 2005;5(1):83–91.

431. Su SC, Kuo CC, Chen T. Inference of missing SNPs and information quantity measurements for haplotype blocks. Bioinformatics 2005;21(9):2001–2007.

432. Dewan A, et al. HTRA1 promoter polymorphism in wet age-related macular degeneration. Science 2006;314(5801):989–992.

433. Haddad S, et al. The genetics of age-related macular degeneration: a review of progress to date. Surv Ophthalmol 2006;51(4):316–363.

434. Klein RJ, et al. Complement factor H polymorphism in age-related macular degeneration. Science 2005;308(5720):385–389.

435. Zareparsi S, et al. Strong association of the Y402H variant in complement factor H at 1q32 with susceptibility to age-related macular degeneration. Am J Hum Genet 2005;77(1):149–153.

436. Bridge J, et al. Novel genomic imbalances in embryonal rhabdomyosarcoma revealed by comparative genomic hybridization and fluorescence in situ hybridization: an Intergroup Rhabdomyosarcoma Study. Genes Chromosomes Cancer 2000;27:337–344.

437. Wong KK, et al. Allelic imbalance analysis by high-density single-nucleotide polymorphic allele (SNP) array with whole genome amplified DNA. Nucleic Acids Res 2004;32(9):e69.

438. Mastrangelo D, et al. Loss of heterozygosity on the long arm of chromosome 11 in orbital embryonal rhabdomyosarcoma (OERMS): a microsatellite study of seven cases. Orbit 1998;17(2):89–95.

439. Visser M, et al. Allelotype of pediatric rhabdomyosarcoma. Oncogene 1997;15(11):1309–1314.

440. Wong SC, et al. Advanced proteomic technologies for cancer biomarker discovery. Expert Rev Proteomics 2009;6(2):123–134.

441. Gaffney EF, Breatnach F. Diverse immunoreactivity and metachronous ultrastructural variability in fatal primitive childhood tumor with rhabdoid features [letter]. Arch Pathol Lab Med 1989;113(12):1322.

442. Rosenblatt KP, et al. Serum proteomics in cancer diagnosis and management. Annu Rev Med 2004;55:97–112.

443. Li Y, et al. Identification of a plasma proteomic signature to distinguish pediatric osteosarcoma from benign osteochondroma. Proteomics 2006;6(11):3426–3435.

444. Petricoin EF, et al. Clinical proteomics: translating benchside promise into bedside reality. Nat Rev Drug Discov 2002;1(9):683–695.

445. Wulfkuhle JD, et al. Proteomic approaches to the diagnosis, treatment, and monitoring of cancer. Adv Exp Med Biol 2003;532:59–68.

446. Craven RA, Banks RE. Laser capture microdissection for proteome analysis. Curr Protoc Protein Sci 2003;Chapter 22:Unit 22.3. doi:10.1002/0471140864.ps2203s31.

447. Ocak S, Chaurand P, Massion PP. Mass spectrometry-based proteomic profiling of lung cancer. Proc Am Thorac Soc 2009;6(2):159–170.

448. Li MX, et al. Proteomic analysis of the stroma-related proteins in nasopharyngeal carcinoma and normal nasopharyngeal epithelial tissues [published online ahead of print February 26, 2009]. Med Oncol 2010;27(1):134–144.

449. Overdevest JB, Theodorescu D, Lee JK. Utilizing the molecular gateway: the path to personalized cancer management. Clin Chem 2009;55(4):684–697.

450. Lakhani SR, Ashworth A. Microarray and histopathological analysis of tumours: the future and the past? Nat Rev Cancer 2001;1(2):151–157.

451. Hack CJ. Integrated transcriptome and proteome data: the challenges ahead. Brief Funct Genomic Proteomic 2004;3(3):212–219.

452. Brown RE. Morphogenomics and morphoproteomics: a role for anatomic pathology in personalized medicine. Arch Pathol Lab Med 2009;133(4):568–579.

453. Phan JH, et al. Convergence of biomarkers, bioinformatics and nanotechnology for individualized cancer treatment. Trends Biotechnol 2009;27(6):350–358.

454. Barr FG, et al. Genetic heterogeneity in the alveolar rhabdomyosarcoma subset without typical gene fusions. Cancer 2002;62(16):4704–4710.

455. Parham DM, et al. Correlation between histology and PAX/FKHR fusion status in alveolar rhabdomyosarcoma: a report from the Children's Oncology Group. Am J Surg Pathol 2007;31(6):895–901.

456. Holimon JL, Rosenblum WI. Gangliorhabdomyosarcoma: a tumor of ectomesenchyme: case report. J Neurosurg 1971;34(3):417–422.

457. Kawamoto EH, et al. Malignant ectomesenchymoma of soft tissue: report of two cases and review of the literature. Cancer 1987;59:1791–1802.

458. Naka A, et al. Ganglioneuroblastoma associated with malignant mesenchymoma. Cancer 1975;35(3):1050–1056.

459. Coffin CM, Dehner LP. Soft tissue tumors in first year of life: a report of 190 cases. Pediatr Pathol 1990;10(4):509–526.

460. Buitendijk S, et al. Pediatric aggressive fibromatosis: a retrospective analysis of 13 patients and review of literature. Cancer 2005;104(5):1090–1099.

461. Billings SD, Giblen G, Fanburg-Smith JC. Superficial low-grade fibromyxoid sarcoma (Evans tumor): a clinicopathologic analysis of 19 cases with a unique observation in the pediatric population. Am J Surg Pathol 2005;29(2):204–210.

462. Weinstein JM, et al. Congenital dermatofibrosarcoma protuberans: variability in presentation. Arch Dermatol 2003;139(2):207–211.

463. Folpe AL, et al. Low-grade fibromyxoid sarcoma and hyalinizing spindle cell tumor with giant rosettes: a clinicopathologic study of 73 cases supporting their identity and assessing the impact of high-grade areas. Am J Surg Pathol 2000;24(10):1353–1360.

464. Li XQ, et al. Expression of anaplastic lymphoma kinase in soft tissue tumors: an immunohistochemical and molecular study of 249 cases. Hum Pathol 2004;35(6):711–721.

465. Sheng WQ, et al. Expression of COL1A1-PDGFB fusion transcripts in superficial adult fibrosarcoma suggests a close relationship to dermatofibrosarcoma protuberans. J Pathol 2001;194(1):88–94.

466. O'Brien KP, et al. Various regions within the alpha-helical domain of the COL1A1 gene are fused to the second exon of the PDGFB gene in dermatofibrosarcomas and giant-cell fibroblastomas. Genes Chromosomes Cancer 1998;23(2):187–193.

467. Spunt SL, Skapek SX, Coffin CM. Pediatric nonrhabdomyosarcoma soft tissue sarcomas. Oncologist 2008;13(6):668–678.

468. Spunt SL, Pappo AS. Childhood nonrhabdomyosarcoma soft tissue sarcomas are not adult-type tumors. J Clin Oncol 2006;24(12):1958–1959, author reply 1959–1960.

469. McCarville MB, et al. Synovial sarcoma in pediatric patients. AJR Am J Roentgenol 2002;179(3):797–801.

470. Enzinger FM, Weiss SW. Fibrosarcoma. In: Soft tissue tumors. St Louis, MO: CV Mosby, 1983:103–124.

471. Nakayama R, et al. Gene expression analysis of soft tissue sarcomas: characterization and reclassification of malignant fibrous histiocytoma. Mod Pathol 2007;20(7):749–759.

472. Fanburg-Smith JC, Miettinen M. Angiomatoid "malignant" fibrous histiocytoma: a clinicopathologic study of 158 cases and further exploration of the myoid phenotype. Hum Pathol 1999;30(11):1336–1343.

473. Hasegawa T, et al. Angiomatoid (malignant) fibrous histiocytoma: a peculiar low-grade tumor showing immunophenotypic heterogeneity and ultrastructural variations. Pathol Int 2000;50(9):731–738.

474. Miettinen M, Lehto V-P, Virtanen I. Monophasic synovial sarcoma of spindle cell type. Virchows Arch B Cell Pathol Incl Mol Pathol 1983;44:187–199.

475. van de Rijn M, et al. Absence of SYT-SSX fusion products in soft tissue tumors other than synovial sarcoma. Am J Clin Pathol 1999;112(1):43–49.

476. Brett D, et al. The SYT protein involved in the t(X;18) synovial sarcoma translocation is a transcriptional activator localised in nuclear bodies. Hum Mol Genet 1997;6:1559–1564.

477. de Leeuw B, et al. Sublocalization of the synovial sarcoma-associated t(X;18) chromosomal breakpoint in Xp11.2 using cosmid cloning and fluorescence in situ hybridization. Oncogene 1993;8(6):1457–1463.

478. Knight JC, et al. Localization of the synovial sarcoma t(X;18)(p11.2;q11.2) breakpoint by fluorescence in situ hybridization. Hum Mol Genet 1992;1(8):633–637.

479. Shipley JM, et al. The t(X;18)(p11.2;q11.2) translocation found in human synovial sarcomas involves two distinct loci on the X chromosome. Oncogene 1994;9:1447–1453.

480. Tureci O, et al. The SSX-2 gene, which is involved in the t(X;18) translocation of synovial sarcomas, codes for the human tumor antigen HOM-MEL-40. Cancer Res 1996;56:4766–4772.

481. deCou JM, et al. Malignant peripheral nerve sheath tumors: the St. Jude Children's Research Hospital experience. Ann Surg Oncol 1995;2(6):524–529.

482. Doorn PF, et al. Malignant peripheral nerve sheath tumors in patients with and without neurofibromatosis. Eur J Surg Oncol 1995;21(1):78–82.

483. Meis JM, et al. Malignant peripheral nerve sheath tumors (malignant schwannomas) in children. Am J Surg Pathol 1992;16:694–707.

484. Meis-Kindblom JM, Enzinger FM. Plexiform malignant peripheral nerve sheath tumor of infancy and childhood [see comments]. Am J Surg Pathol 1994;18(5):479–485.

485. Wanebo JE, et al. Malignant peripheral nerve sheath tumors. Cancer 1993;71:1247–1253.

486. Woodruff JM. Pathology of tumors of the peripheral nerve sheath in type 1 neurofibromatosis. Am J Med Genet 1999;89(1):23–30.

487. Strauss BL, et al. Molecular analysis of malignant triton tumors. Hum Pathol 1999;30(8):984–988.

488. Maeda M, et al. Malignant nerve sheath tumor with rhabdomyoblastic differentiation arising from the acoustic nerve. Acta Pathol Jpn 1993;43:198–203.

489. Robbins P, Papadimitriou J. Glandular peripheral nerve sheath tumours. Pathol Res Pract 1994;190(4):412–415.

490. O'Sullivan MJ, et al. Malignant peripheral nerve sheath tumors with t(X;18): a pathologic and molecular genetic study. Mod Pathol 2000;13(11):1253–1263.

491. Vang R, et al. Malignant peripheral nerve sheath tumor with a t(X;18). Arch Pathol Lab Med 2000;124(6):864–867.

492. O'Connell JX, et al. Intraneural biphasic synovial sarcoma: an alternative "glandular" tumor of peripheral nerve. Mod Pathol 1996;9(7):738–741.

493. O'Sullivan MJ, Kyriakos M, Zhu X, et al. Malignant peripheral nerve sheath tumors with t(X;18): a pathologic and molecular genetic study [comment in Mod Pathol 2001;14(7):733–737]. Mod Pathol 2000;13:1336–1346.

494. Ali-Khan SE, et al. Whole genome scanning: resolving clinical diagnosis and management amidst complex data. Pediatr Res 2009;66(4):357–363.

495. Oesch S, et al. Cannabinoid receptor 1 is a potential drug target for treatment of translocation-positive rhabdomyosarcoma. Mol Cancer Ther 2009;8(7):1838–1845.

496. Ross JS. Multigene classifiers, prognostic factors, and predictors of breast cancer clinical outcome. Adv Anat Pathol 2009;16(4):204–215.

497. Ross JS, et al. Commercialized multigene predictors of clinical outcome for breast cancer. Oncologist 2008;13(5):477–493.

498. Lin J, Li M. Molecular profiling in the age of cancer genomics. Expert Rev Mol Diagn 2008;8(3):263–276.

499. Swanton C, Caldas C. Molecular classification of solid tumours: towards pathway-driven therapeutics. Br J Cancer 2009;100(10):1517–1522.

500. Manara MC, et al. Preclinical in vivo study of new insulin-like growth factor-I receptor–specific inhibitor in Ewing's sarcoma. Clin Cancer Res 2007;13(4):1322–1330.

501. Martins AS, et al. Insulin-like growth factor I receptor pathway inhibition by ADW742, alone or in combination with imatinib, doxorubicin, or vincristine, is a novel therapeutic approach in Ewing tumor. Clin Cancer Res 2006;12(11, pt 1):3532–3540.

502. Huang F, et al. The mechanisms of differential sensitivity to an insulin-like growth factor-1 receptor inhibitor (BMS-536924) and rationale for combining with EGFR/HER2 inhibitors. Cancer Res 2009;69(1):161–170.

503. Yuen JS, Macaulay VM. Targeting the type 1 insulin-like growth factor receptor as a treatment for cancer. Expert Opin Ther Targets 2008;12(5):589–603.

CHAPTER 9 ■ IMAGING STUDIES IN THE DIAGNOSIS AND MANAGEMENT OF PEDIATRIC MALIGNANCIES

R. PAUL GUILLERMAN, MARY E. (BETH) McCARVILLE, SUE C. KASTE,
BARRY L. SHULKIN, AND STEPHAN D. VOSS

INTRODUCTION

Since the publication of previous editions of this chapter, technological advances and refinements of existing imaging methods have expanded the role of radiology in the diagnosis and management of pediatric malignancies. Tumor burden and tumor metabolism can now be better elucidated, but as a result of this progress, radiologists and pediatric oncologists must have increased knowledge and judgment to choose the appropriate sequence of imaging studies for the most prompt, accurate evaluation at the lowest possible cost and risk to the patient. Because critical assessment of diagnostic performance of new imaging technologies lags behind their introduction, clinical decisions often must be made in the absence of evidence-based guidelines. To provide a foundation for such decisions, this chapter discusses the relative merits of currently available imaging modalities and provides general imaging recommendations for tumor diagnosis, staging and risk stratification, therapy response assessment, surveillance for recurrent disease, screening for primary malignancy, and detection of treatment complications. Imaging characteristics and evaluation of particular pediatric malignancies are addressed in detail in the disease-specific chapters.

RELATIVE MERITS OF AVAILABLE IMAGING PROCEDURES

Conventional Radiography and Contrast Fluoroscopy

In an era of sophisticated cross-sectional and functional imaging, conventional radiographs still have value in the evaluation of malignant disease. Conventional radiographs are easy to perform, are rapid, are inexpensive, require no anesthesia or sedation, and deliver a far smaller radiation dose than computed tomography (CT). Conventional chest radiography can identify primary intrathoracic tumors, mediastinal lymphadenopathy, and pulmonary metastases (Fig. 9.1). Chest radiography remains the initial imaging procedure of choice for delineating central vascular catheter placement, detecting a pleural or pericardial effusion or airway compression in association with a mediastinal mass, and identifying pulmonary infections in immunocompromised patients. Coupled with injection of iodinated contrast, chest fluoroscopy is of value in determining whether malfunction of a subclavian central vascular catheter is attributable to fibrin sheath formation, vascular thrombosis, or catheter breakage.

For evaluation of abdominal masses or conditions in pediatric oncology patients, conventional radiographs have been largely superseded by cross-sectional imaging modalities such as CT, ultrasound, and magnetic resonance imaging (MRI). Nevertheless, sufficient information can often be gleaned from abdominal radiographs to warrant their performance before more sophisticated imaging procedures are undertaken. Conventional radiographs of the abdomen are a convenient method for evaluating bowel obstruction or perforation. Conventional radiographs of the abdomen also depict most tumor calcifications and many intra-abdominal masses.

Fluoroscopic studies with barium or water-soluble contrast media are a simple means of evaluating for gastrointestinal (GI) tract lesions (Fig. 9.2). However, with the exception of non-Hodgkin lymphoma (NHL), primary neoplastic involvement of the GI tract is rare in children. In the case of lymphoma, CT is advantageous because it demonstrates not only the bowel wall but also the mesenteric and retroperitoneal lymph nodes and the solid abdominal viscera (Fig. 9.3). Mucosal-based processes (e.g., esophagitis, gastritis, gastro-duodenal ulceration, and colitis) are better seen with barium fluoroscopy studies than advanced cross-sectional imaging. However, contrast enemas are generally contraindicated in neutropenic patients because of the risk of bacteremia. CT and ultrasonography are superior imaging studies for the detection of typhlitis. Oral ingestion or enteric tube infusion of contrast agents is generally safe, even in immunocompromised children, though the presence of oropharyngeal mucositis may hinder the patient's ability to swallow the contrast agent. Barium is an inexpensive and readily available contrast medium for the evaluation of the GI tract. However, when bowel perforation is suspected, the use of barium is contraindicated due to the proclivity of barium to exacerbate peritonitis; water-soluble contrast media should be used in this case.

Conventional radiographs are generally less sensitive than bone scintigraphy or MRI for detecting neoplastic involvement of the skeleton. However, skeletal radiographs should be the first imaging study of a pediatric patient with localized musculoskeletal pain. Bone scintigraphy is generally preferred over conventional radiographic skeletal survey for the detection of bony metastases. An exception is Langerhans' cell histiocytosis, in which the two approaches are complementary. Bone scintigraphy is more sensitive in detecting histiocytic lesions in the ribs, spine, and pelvis, and radiographic skeletal survey is more sensitive in identifying lesions in the skull.[1] Although MRI and bone scintigraphy are highly sensitive, they are less specific than conventional radiography; thus, abnormalities detected by bone scintigraphy or MRI should be correlated with findings on conventional skeletal radiographs.

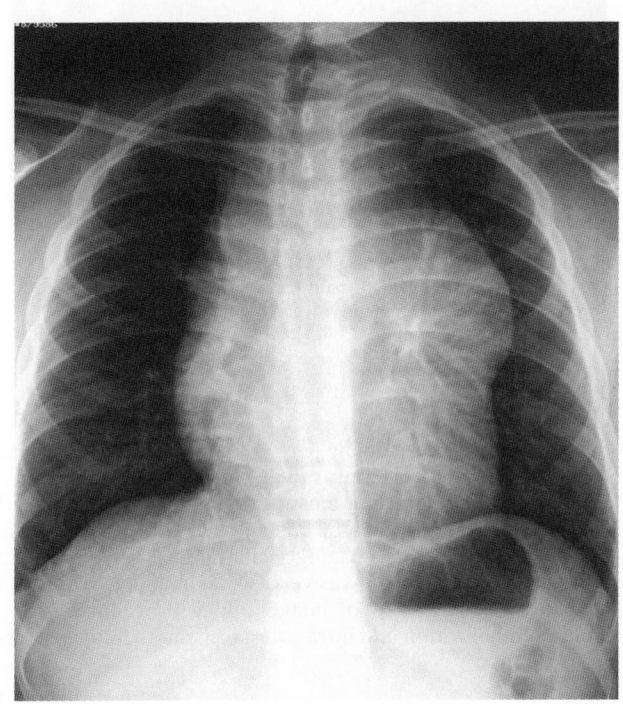

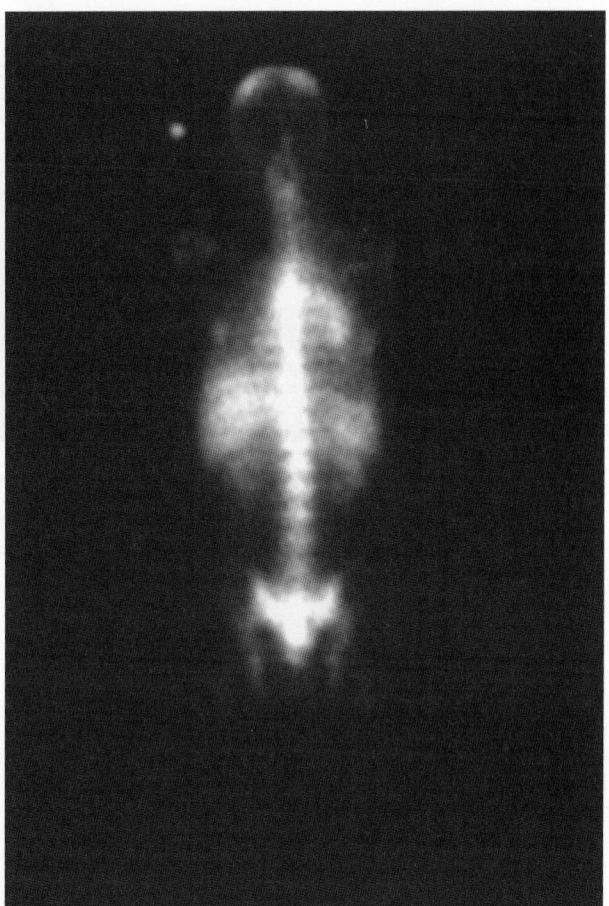

A

B

FIGURE 9.1 Hodgkin lymphoma. Posteroanterior chest radiograph (**A**) shows a large mediastinal mass. Gallium-67 citrate total body imaging (**B**) demonstrates uptake of the radiopharmaceutical by the mediastinal mass, as well as physiologic uptake by the liver, spleen, and bone marrow.

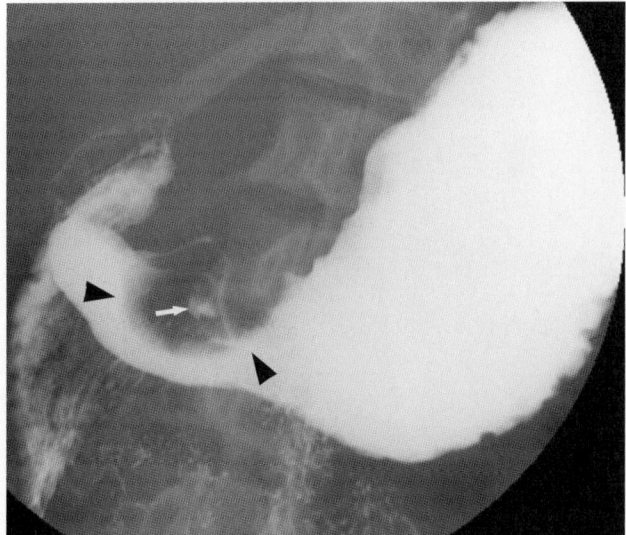

FIGURE 9.2 Gastrointestinal stromal tumor (GIST). Spot view from an upper GI series shows a large filling defect (*arrowheads*) and central barium collection (*arrow*) along the lesser curvature of the stomach, representing a large, ulcerated GIST.

Skull radiographs are not useful for evaluating primary intracranial tumors. Skull radiographs may be included as part of a radiographic survey to detect calvarial metastases, but virtually every lesion of the skull is better depicted by CT or MRI. Even as a mechanism for screening for calvarial metastases, skull radiographs are not as sensitive as CT or bone scintigraphy. In the case of a scalp lump, skull radiographs may be obtained to evaluate for underlying cephalhematoma, fracture, or lytic lesion of the calvarium, but CT or MRI is needed if possible intracranial extension is to be defined.[2]

Spinal radiographs are valuable for identifying vertebral compression fractures secondary to tumor infiltration (Fig. 9.4) or steroid-induced osteoporosis. Spinal radiographs are less sensitive than bone scintigraphy or MRI for the early detection of metastatic disease or osteonecrosis, and CT and MRI better depict bony spinal lesions and associated intraspinal abnormalities.

Spinal CT performed after intrathecal injection of contrast has been nearly completely replaced by spinal MRI. Of particular importance is the high sensitivity of MRI for detecting the extension of paraspinous tumor through the neural foramina into the spinal canal and cord compression by intraspinal tumor (Fig. 9.5). Conventional myelography is occasionally helpful in evaluating patients with metallic orthopedic spinal hardware, because the presence of such hardware degrades the quality of CT and magnetic resonance (MR) images.

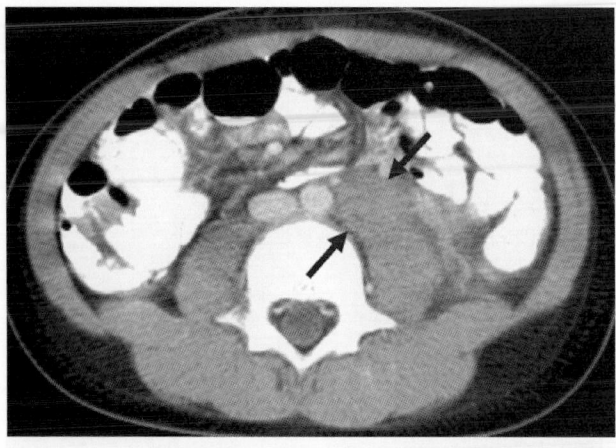
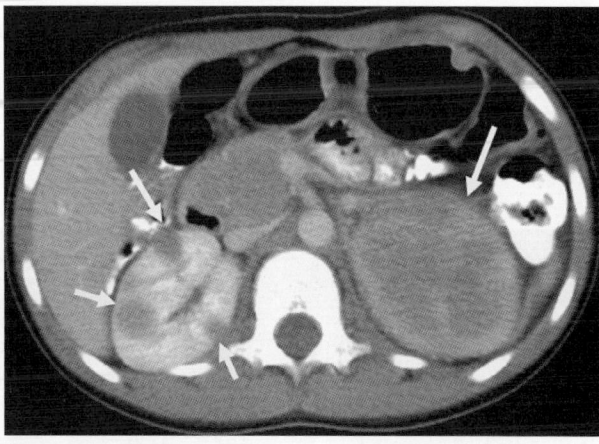

FIGURE 9.3 Burkitt's lymphoma. Axial contrast-enhanced computed tomography (CT) image (**A**) demonstrates retroperitoneal lymphadenopathy (*arrows*) that is easily distinguished from the contrast-enhanced aorta and bowel. Axial contrast-enhanced CT image (**B**) reveals nodular involvement of the right kidney and diffuse involvement of the left kidney (*arrows*).

Angiography

Conventional catheter angiography has been largely superseded by Doppler sonography and CT angiography (CTA) or MR angiography (MRA). Ultrasound, CT, and MRI have replaced inferior vena cavography for the evaluation of intravascular spread of malignancy, as in hepatoblastoma and Wilms' tumor. Although conventional invasive catheter angiography is occasionally performed, particularly when partial hepatectomy or limb-salvage procedures are contemplated, the vasculature of most tumors, including those of the liver and extremities, can be adequately studied by the noninvasive cross-sectional imaging techniques of CTA[3] or MRA[4] (Fig. 9.6). The use of invasive vascular imaging promises to expand in the context of image-guided procedures such as tumor embolization and intra-arterial chemotherapy delivery.[5]

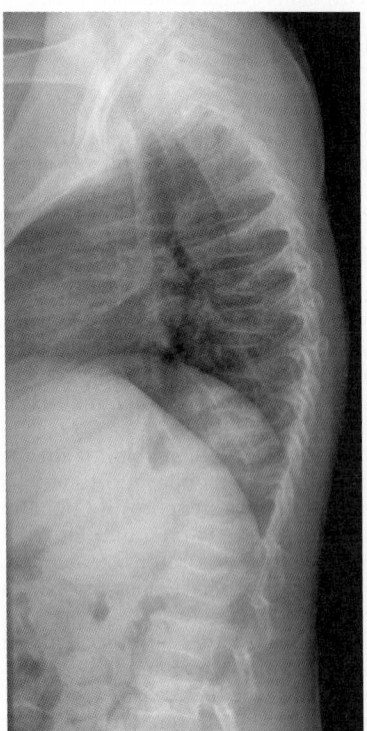
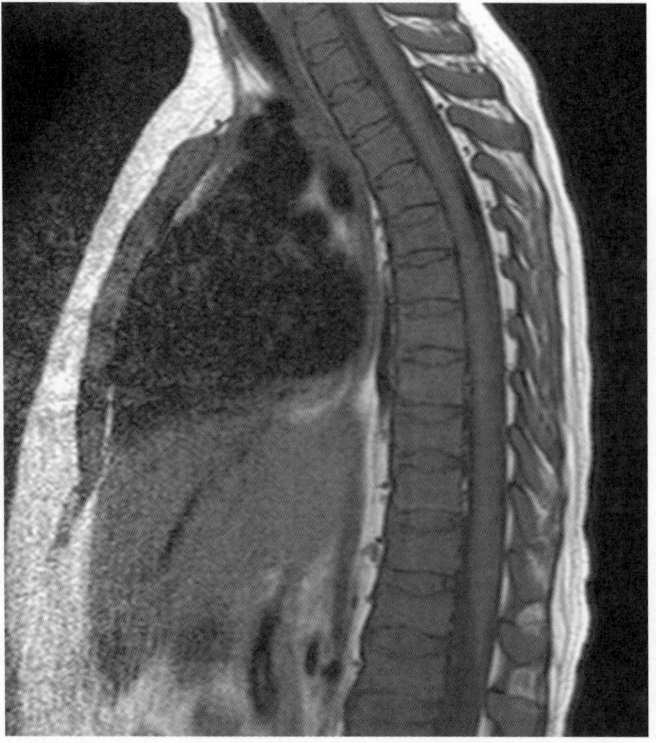

FIGURE 9.4 Acute lymphoblastic leukemia. Lateral radiograph of the thoracic spine (**A**) reveals osteopenia and numerous thoracic vertebral body compression fracture deformities. Sagittal T1-weighted MR image (**B**) shows diffuse abnormal low signal intensity of the bone marrow related to leukemic infiltration.

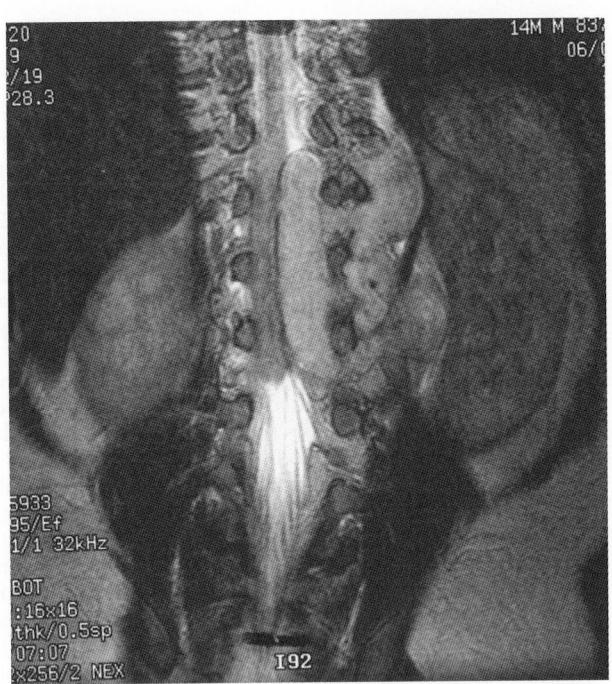
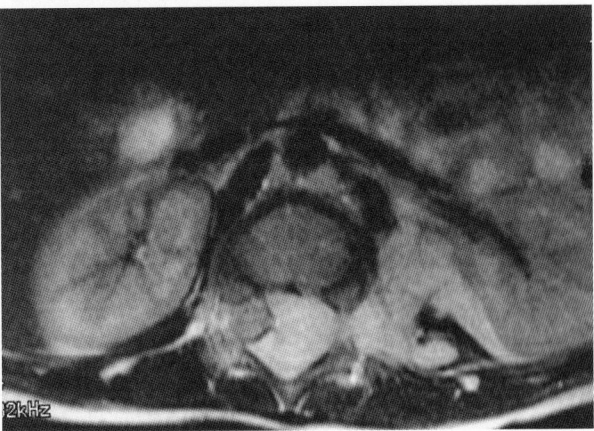

FIGURE 9.5 Neuroblastoma. Left paraspinal neuroblastoma invading several neural foramina and the spinal canal, causing rightward displacement of the thecal sac and spinal cord, as depicted on T2-weighted coronal (**A**) and axial (**B**) magnetic resonance images.

Nuclear Medicine

Although they yield considerably less morphologic information than other imaging modalities, nuclear medicine images provide valuable information about the metabolic and functional status of a spectrum of pediatric tumors. Nuclear medicine examinations are used in the routine evaluation of musculoskeletal tumors, lymphoma, neuroblastoma, and thyroid cancer. A nuclear medicine examination involves administering

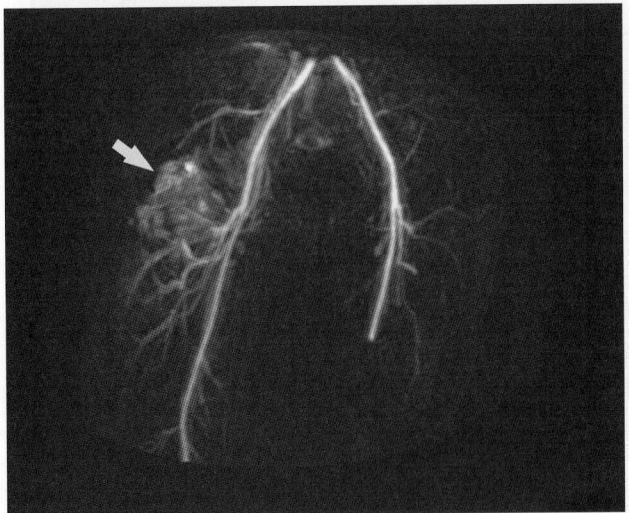

FIGURE 9.6 Osteosarcoma. Gadolinium-enhanced dynamic magnetic resonance angiography image shows a hypervascular proximal right femoral osteosarcoma (*arrow*) supplied by branches of the right profunda femoral artery. Early venous drainage from the mass is also depicted.

a radiopharmaceutical to the patient, allowing an appropriate time interval for the desired selective distribution of the radiopharmaceutical, and using a special camera to detect the radiation emitted from the radiopharmaceutical.

The emission data acquired with conventional gamma cameras are processed to generate planar images of the whole body or selected body regions. Single-photon emission computed tomography (SPECT) applies the mathematical algorithms used in radiographic CT scanning to produce tomographic reconstructions, thereby generating multiplanar and projection images to improve detection and localization of sites of abnormal radiopharmaceutical uptake. Positron emission tomography (PET) incorporates positron-emitting radiopharmaceuticals and coincident detection of the positron-electron annihilation events to achieve superior spatial resolution, higher tumor-to-background uptake ratio, and more readily quantifiable data than conventional gamma camera techniques. The use of image coregistration by combined PET/CT and SPECT/CT scanners allows precise correlation of functional abnormalities with anatomic sites, permitting better differentiation between physiologic and pathologic uptake and more accurate delineation of disease for biopsy and therapy planning.[6]

Although a variety of radiopharmaceuticals can be used, bone scintigraphy is typically performed using a technetium (Tc)-99m-labeled radiopharmaceutical based on a phosphonate, such as methylene diphosphonate (MDP), which accumulates in sites of osteoblastic response. Tc-99m phosphonate–based bone scintigraphy is of less value than MRI in defining the local extent of primary bone tumors. Tc-99m phosphonate–based bone scintigraphy has long been the examination of choice for the detection of bone metastases in children, with the exception of Langerhans' cell histiocytosis, as mentioned earlier.[1] False-negative bone scans can occur in neuroblastoma metastasis to the ends of long bones, where uptake related to tumor can be masked by physiologic physeal uptake. Abnormal uptake can result from nonneoplastic processes potentially leading to false-positive results. For example, increased skeletal uptake of Tc-99m MDP can occur after amputation or limb-salvage procedures or during administration of colony-stimulating factor.[7]

Gallium-67, thallium-201, and Tc-99m sestamibi are nuclear medicine agents that accumulate in viable tumor, less so in inflammatory disease, and not appreciably in necrotic tissue. Uptake of gallium-67 in tumors is thought to be based on its nature as a ferric iron analogue, that of thallium is primarily based on an active ATPase energy-dependent sodium-potassium pump, and that of Tc-99m sestamibi is by diffusion across the cell membrane as a substrate of the MDR (multidrug resistance)-related P-glycoproteins. The efficacy of Tc-99m sestamibi imaging in assessing MDR in tumors before or after chemotherapy is under investigation for hematological malignancies[8] and solid tumors.[9] Tc-99m sestamibi scintigraphy is not useful as an *in vivo* predictor of MDR in neuroblastoma, since P-glycoproteins do not contribute to MDR in neuroblastoma, but instead seem to be a marker of tumor differentiation.[10]

Gallium-67 scintigraphy has been very useful in the assessment of therapy response and residual masses in childhood lymphoma (Fig. 9.1). Normalization of the gallium scan early during therapy is a good predictor of outcome for Hodgkin lymphoma[11] and NHL.[12] Persistent gallium uptake in a residual mass after therapy suggests residual disease; loss of gallium uptake suggests the absence of residual neoplasm.[13] Gallium uptake may be affected by chemotherapy or radiation therapy, and gallium should be injected before initiating therapy to reduce potential false-negative results, but treatment should not be delayed in emergent cases. The addition of SPECT increases the sensitivity of gallium for lymphoma over planar imaging, particularly for small lesions, and aids in the discrimination of pathologic uptake in the mediastinum from adjacent physiologic bone or soft tissue uptake.[14]

Thallium-201 is taken up by virtually all extremity osteosarcomas and Ewing's sarcomas before treatment. Decrease in thallium-201 uptake between the pretreatment and posttreatment scans serves as a noninvasive surrogate marker of histologic response of osteosarcoma to neoadjuvant chemotherapy. In Ewing's sarcoma, thallium-201 scintigraphy more reliably correlates with histologic tumor response than does Tc-99m MDP bone scintigraphy; persistent thallium-201 uptake corresponds to viable tumor, and Tc-99m MDP uptake corresponds to residual or recurrent neoplasm, infection, or pathologic fracture.[15] In some institutions, thallium-201 is also used in the evaluation of patients with brain tumors, lymphoma, rhabdomyosarcoma, and germ cell neoplasms.[16]

Metaiodobenzylguanidine (MIBG) is an analogue of norepinephrine that is concentrated in adrenergic storage vesicles of neural crest–lineage tumors such as neuroblastoma. MIBG labeled with iodine-123 or iodine-131 provides a radiopharmaceutical that is highly sensitive and specific for neuroblastoma (Fig. 9.7).[17] Labeling with iodine-123 is preferable to labeling with iodine-131 in children, due to more favorable radiation dosimetry, more optimal photon energy for gamma camera detection, and the ability to perform SPECT in a shorter acquisition time with the former.[18] Both MIBG and Tc-99m phosphonate–based bone scintigraphy are useful for the detection of skeletal neuroblastoma,[19] but MIBG scintigraphy is better at more fully characterizing the extent of disease because of its superior detection of extraskeletal neuroblastoma.[20] MIBG scintigraphy is favored to identify otherwise occult neuroblastomas in opsoclonus-myoclonus syndrome, which in more than half of cases in children is associated with neuroblastoma, usually small and localized.[21] The use of MIBG scintigraphy to evaluate patients with neuroblastoma is routine, with the International Neuroblastoma Staging System (INSS), the new International Neuroblastoma Risk Group Staging System (INRGSS), and the International Neuroblastoma Response Criteria (INRC) recommending the performance of

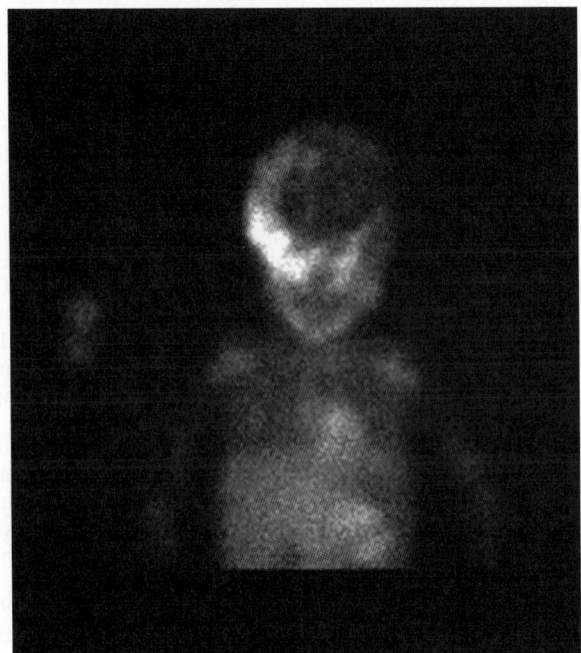
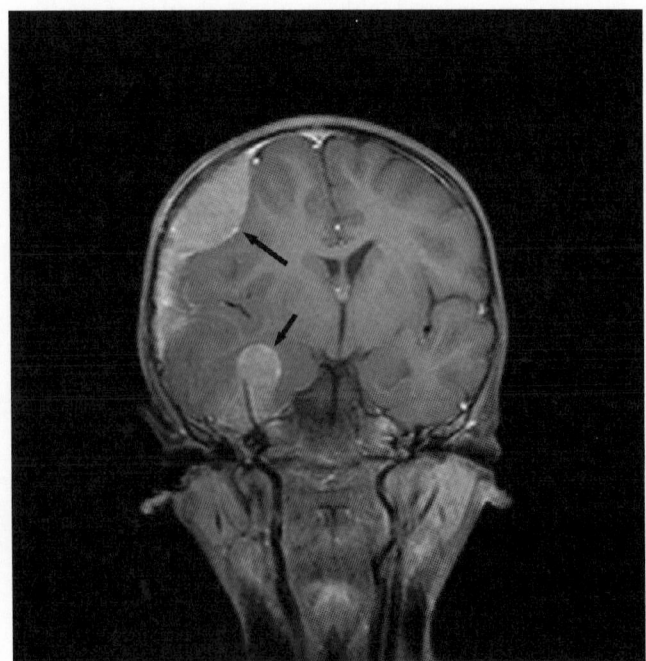

A   **B**

FIGURE 9.7 Neuroblastoma metastatic to the right hemicranium. Abnormal radiopharmaceutical uptake specific for neuroendocrine tumor is depicted on metaiodobenzylguanidine scintigraphy (**A**). Coronal gadolinium-enhanced T1-weighted MR image (**B**) reveals corresponding enhancing intracranial tumor masses (*arrows*).

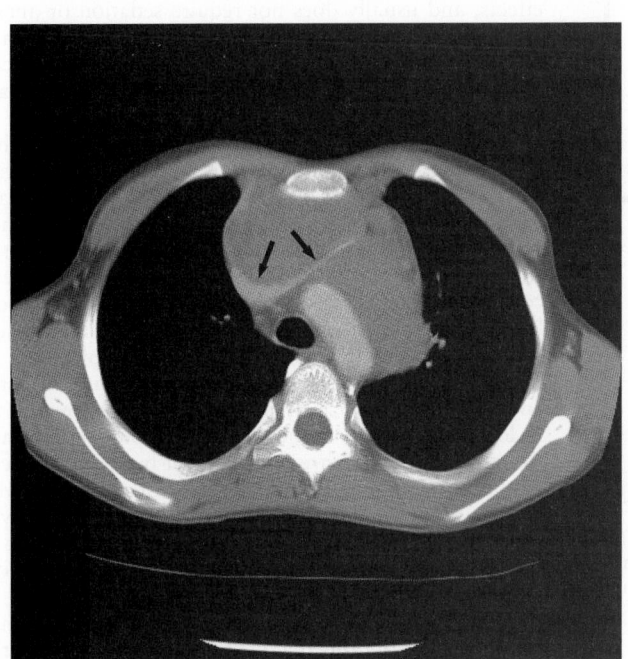
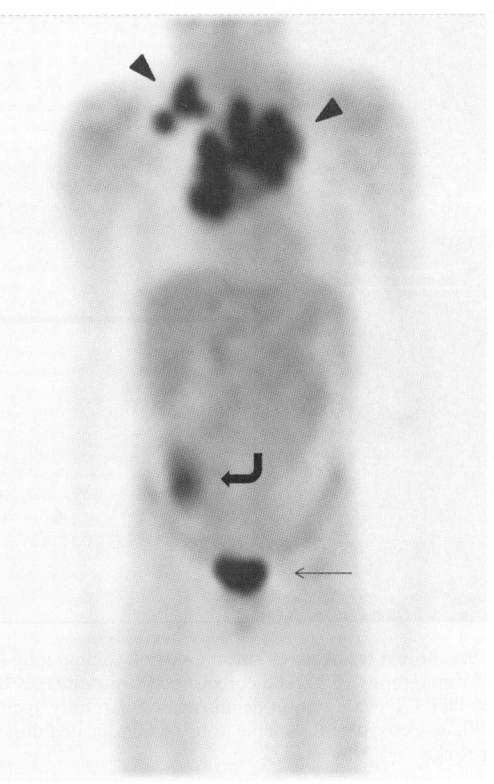

FIGURE 9.8 Hodgkin lymphoma. Contrast-enhanced axial chest computed tomography image (**A**) demonstrates a large anterior mediastinal mass displacing and compressing the left brachiocephalic vein and superior vena cava (*arrows*). Coronal positron emission tomography image (**B**) shows increased fluorodeoxyglucose uptake by the mediastinal mass and by right supraclavicular and infraclavicular lymphadenopathy (*arrowheads*), as well as nonneoplastic uptake by bowel in the right lower abdominal quadrant (*curved arrow*) and excreted activity in the urinary bladder (*straight arrow*).

MIBG scintigraphy in patients with neuroblastoma at the time of initial staging and during therapy. Tc-99m phosphonate–based bone scintigraphy is suggested if the primary tumor is not MIBG-avid or an MIBG examination is unavailable.[22,23]

Flourine-18 fluorodeoxyglucose (FDG) is a glucose analogue, and FDG-PET detects tumor cells that concentrate FDG because of increased glucose transporter activity and glycolysis. The literature supports the use of FDG-PET in the diagnosis and management of adult tumors. Similar success is expected in children, and investigation of the use of FDG-PET is ongoing in the evaluation of childhood lymphoma[24] (Fig. 9.8), neuroblastoma,[25] hepatoblastoma,[26] sarcoma,[27] brain tumors,[28] and Langerhans' cell histiocytosis.[29]

The dissemination of PET imaging was initially limited by the high cost of PET scanners and the lack of financial reimbursement for PET studies by third-party insurers. Insurers now reimburse for PET studies, but the cost of PET and PET/CT scanners remains prohibitive for many children's hospitals. A limitation of PET imaging is the brief half-life (seconds to minutes) of many positron emitters, necessitating that a cyclotron be located in close proximity to the PET scanner to permit administration of the radiopharmaceutical shortly after its creation by the cyclotron. However, F-18, the most widely used positron-emitting isotope at present, has a relatively long half-life of 110 minutes, permitting its production at a central site and distribution to multiple end users, a process commonly used with other medical radionuclides.

Because of the limited availability of PET at most children's hospitals, a large proportion of pediatric PET studies are performed at adult imaging centers. In this setting, there are special considerations in the performance and interpretation of PET imaging of children that must not be neglected. These include fasting, sedation or other motion-suppression techniques, radiopharmaceutical dosing, clearance of excreted radiopharmaceutical from the urinary tract, and awareness of sites of exaggerated physiologic radiopharmaceutical uptake compared with that seen in adults including the thymus, hematopoietic marrow, physes, benign fibro-osseous lesions, and brown fat.[30–32] Uptake of FDG by brown fat is much more prominent in infants and children than in adults, is higher in winter than in warmer seasons, and is higher in those with lower body mass index values. FDG uptake by brown fat is most conspicuous in the lower neck, supraclavicular, and interscapular regions, but it is also seen in the axillary, mediastinal, paravertebral, and perinephric regions. In addition, it can mimic neoplastic uptake and lead to false-positive interpretations.[33,34] FDG-PET/CT fusion images are particularly valuable in distinguishing physiologic uptake in brown fat from pathologic uptake in lymph nodes or other soft tissues[35] (Fig. 9.9). Potentially confounding FDG uptake in brown fat can be reduced by patient warming and premedication with intravenous fentanyl or oral diazepam.[36]

Nuclear medicine plays important roles in the care of pediatric oncology patients, apart from tumor diagnosis, staging, response assessment, and surveillance. Radionuclide ventriculography with Tc-99m–labeled red blood cells is advocated to monitor cardiac function in pediatric patients receiving cardiotoxic anthracycline chemotherapy.[37] Injection of chromium (Cr)-51-EDTA or Tc-99m-DTPA and determination of radioisotope clearance from sequential venous blood samples

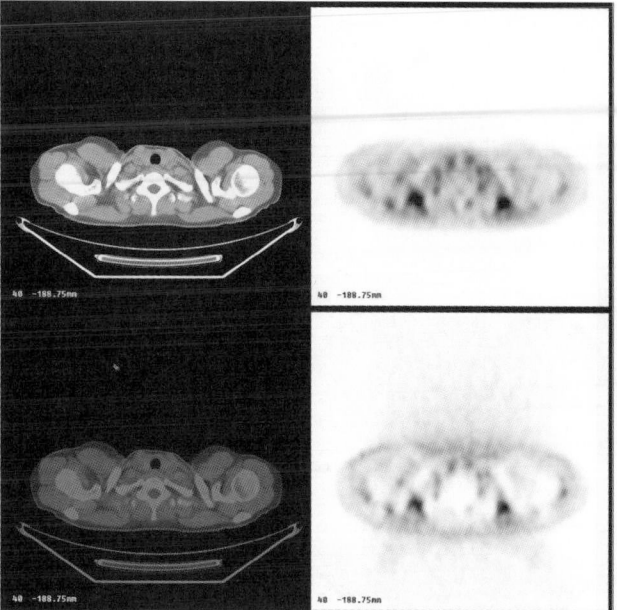

FIGURE 9.9 Brown fat. Axial positron emission tomography (PET), computed tomography (CT), and coregistered fusion images from a combined PET/CT examination demonstrate bilaterally symmetric increased fluorodeoxyglucose uptake in brown fat located dorsally in the lower neck.

is the preferred method of calculating glomerular filtration rate for the purpose of adjusting chemotherapy dosing or evaluating the nephrotoxic effects of chemotherapeutic regimens in pediatric patients.[38] As an aid to the detection of focal infectious processes in the immunocompromised patient, the whole body can be surveyed with nuclear medicine scans using indium-111-oxine– or Tc-99m–hexamethylpropyleneamine oxime–labeled leukocytes or gallium-67 citrate.[39] In such cases, it may be necessary to correlate the nuclear medicine images with ultrasound, CT, or MR images to better localize a lesion. In addition to diagnostic purposes, radiopharmaceuticals can be used in therapy. The targeted treatment of thyroid cancer with iodine-131 is well established, and the treatment of neuroblastoma and pheochromocytoma with iodine-131 MIBG as a relatively nontoxic palliative agent or component of multimodality therapy is under investigation.[40–42]

Ultrasound

Diagnostic ultrasound uses sound waves in the range of 2 to 20 MHz, well above the 20,000 Hz that is the upper limit of normal human aural perception. Higher-frequency sound permits greater imaging resolution but penetrates tissues to a lesser depth than does lower-frequency sound. Thus, high frequencies are used for high-resolution imaging of superficial structures (e.g., testes, thyroid gland, and breasts), and lower frequencies are used for imaging intra-abdominal organs. The fluid in a structure such as the urinary bladder or a simple cyst appears *sonolucent* or *anechoic*. Solid structures, such as the abdominal parenchymal organs or soft tissue tumors, produce echoes of variable number and intensity, resulting in an *echogenic* appearance. Bone, fat, and the interface between air and soft tissue hinder transmission of sound waves and obscure anatomic detail.

Ultrasound is an excellent method for evaluating the abdomen, pelvis, thyroid, breasts, and scrotal contents of chil-

dren. Its utility in other areas of the body depends on the amount of bone or gas present in or near the structure to be imaged. Diagnostic ultrasound is relatively quick and inexpensive, uses no ionizing radiation, has no known adverse effects, and usually does not require sedation or anesthesia. High-quality abdominal ultrasound images are easier to obtain in infants and young children than in older children and adults because of the relative paucity of abdominal fat in younger patients.

Ultrasound is particularly useful in evaluation of the liver, gallbladder, spleen, kidneys, and pelvic organs. Ultrasound can reliably differentiate solid from fluid-filled masses and can usually distinguish the organ of origin of an abdominal or pelvic mass (Fig. 9.10). Imaging of the pancreas, aorta, inferior vena cava, bowel, and retroperitoneal lymph nodes is less consistently successful with ultrasound than with CT or MRI because of intestinal gas. During surgery, high-resolution sonographic imaging can be performed by placing a sterile-dressed ultrasound probe in direct contact with the surface of an organ of interest. Such intraoperative ultrasound is helpful in localizing tumors within the brain, spinal cord, pancreas, liver, or kidneys that are not apparent by visual inspection or palpation. The major disadvantages of conventional ultrasound are inferior resolution compared with CT or MRI for some applications, high dependence on the skill of the sonographer, the limited field of view, and the interference of bone and gas.

Recent advances in ultrasound technology have improved image resolution and diagnostic capability. Broader bandwidth transducers and coded pulse-excitation technologies provide a more favorable compromise between image resolution and penetration depth. Spatial compounding enhances delineation of tumor margins and detection of microcalcifications and low-contrast lesions. Tissue harmonic imaging improves resolution and penetration, particularly in obese patients. Panoramic extended field-of-view imaging allows

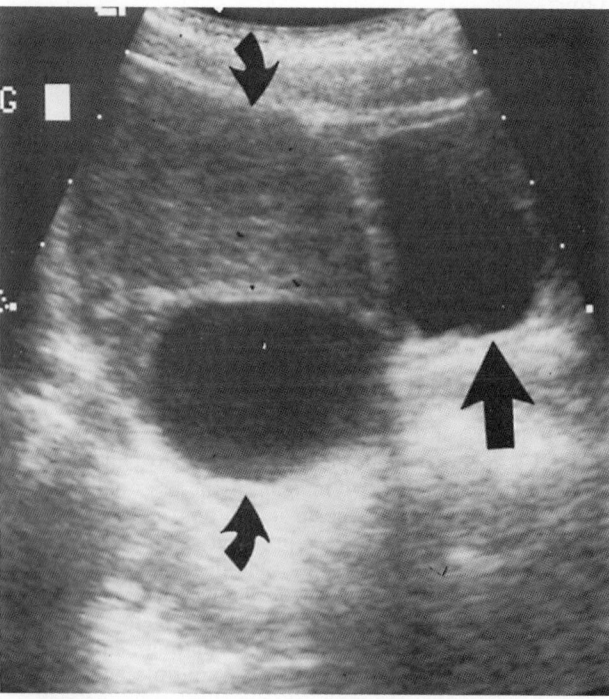

FIGURE 9.10 Ovarian dysgerminoma. Pelvic sonogram discloses a mixed solid and cystic ovarian tumor (*curved arrows*) superior to the urinary bladder (*straight arrow*).

large lesions and major anatomical landmarks to be included on the same image. Three-dimensional (3-D) imaging techniques permit true volumetric analysis. Elastography measures the compressibility or elasticity of tissue and is being clinically evaluated as a means of detecting and differentiating lesions in organs such as the breast, thyroid, and liver.[43]

Blood flow imaging has also progressed with the advent of power Doppler, advanced dynamic flow imaging techniques, and microbubble contrast agents. Although Doppler waveform analysis has limited use in distinguishing malignant from benign disease, the ability of Doppler sonography to detect intravascular thrombus is valuable in assessing thrombotic complications of therapy, guiding placement of central vascular catheters, and therapeutic planning for Wilms' tumor.[44] Microbubble contrast agents confer strong echogenicity to the blood pool that increases the conspicuity of blood vessels and many parenchymal lesions.[45]

Computed Tomography

Since the 1970s, CT has been the preferred imaging modality for the diagnosis and management of many tumors. CT of the head allows rapid identification of tumor masses, intracranial hemorrhage, hydrocephalus, and cerebral and cerebellar complications of anticancer therapy. Although MRI has supplanted CT as the imaging modality of choice for detailed evaluation of the brain and contents of the spinal canal, CT imaging continues to play a major role in the evaluation of intracranial pathology, because it is quicker, less expensive, and more readily available. Although CT remains the primary advanced imaging modality for studying the contents of the thoracic, abdominal, and pelvic cavities, except for the uterus and ovaries, MRI has surpassed CT in the evaluation of most bone and soft tissue masses.

To perform a CT, the body section to be examined is positioned within the CT gantry. Because of geometric considerations in obtaining images at the lowest possible radiation dose, most CT scanning is performed in transaxial cross section, perpendicular to the long axis of the body section being imaged. A fan- or cone-shaped x-ray beam is rotated around the body section of interest. The x-rays strike an array of detectors that convert the energy into electrical signals, and these signals are analyzed to construct images for display. The images can be manipulated to emphasize specific features, for example, images can be windowed to highlight the details of radiodense bones or radiolucent lungs. The images are photographed on film or can be digitally archived on computer storage media and accessed electronically for viewing.

The introduction and dissemination of multidetector (multislice) helical CT scanners and other technologic advances in the field of CT has greatly affected the practice of radiology. During multidetector helical scanning, the x-ray tube and an array of multiple detectors rotate continuously about the patient, collecting data from multiple slices simultaneously while the patient is advanced through the gantry. Because data are acquired in a volumetric fashion, the scan time is reduced, small lesions are not missed because of falling between slices, and the quality of multiplanar and 3-D reconstructions is greatly improved. This provides more accurate assessment of tumor size and relationship to adjacent vital structures and permits "virtual endoscopic" images to be generated[46] (Fig. 9.11). With continued refinement in CT technology, including faster gantry rotation, broader detector arrays (up to 320-slice configuration currently), and dual x-ray tube sources, the scan time has been further reduced so that entire body sections can be imaged in a few seconds or even less than a second; and motion artifact and the need for sedation are decreased. The

individual detectors within the detector arrays have been reduced in size so that slice sections less than 1-mm thick are readily achievable, enhancing the spatial resolution and the quality of image reconstructions.[47] Spectral CT, a technique made feasible by the advent of dual x-ray tube sources and gemstone detectors, exploits the differential attenuation of x-ray beams of differing energy by different tissues and substances, so that solid and cystic masses are better characterized, and CT angiography and perfusion imaging are improved.[48]

High-resolution CT (HRCT) enhances the ability of radiologists to identify subtle interstitial lung disease that is not apparent on chest radiographs or conventional chest CT scans. For HRCT, noncontiguous thin (typically 1.25 mm or less) axial sections are obtained during suspended respiration and images are reconstructed using a high spatial-frequency algorithm that accentuates lung parenchymal detail. In pediatric oncology, HRCT has proven valuable in identifying interstitial lung disease caused by chemotherapeutic agents, thoracic irradiation, and pulmonary Langerhans' cell histiocytosis.[49] Because of the noncontiguous nature of HRCT, the radiation dose is lower than that of a conventional chest CT, but only samples of the lung are surveyed; thus, HRCT is not appropriate for screening the entire lungs for small nodules such as those in metastatic disease or fungal infection.

CT studies performed with iodinated contrast agents are typically more informative than those performed without contrast. After intravenous injection, the contrast agent distributes throughout the vasculature, diffuses into the extravascular interstitial fluid spaces, and is excreted primarily by renal glomerular filtration. The increased radiographic attenuation producing the effect of contrast enhancement is proportional to the iodine concentration achieved. The timing of image acquisition is set by the radiologist in consideration of the clinical indication for the CT examination, because the temporal pattern and intensity of enhancement across tissues vary on the basis of the relative blood volume and flow and the extraction of contrast media by the tissues.

Intravenous contrast agents do not accumulate in normal brain tissue with an intact blood-brain barrier. Thus, the administration of contrast medium increases the conspicuity of brain pathology associated with disruption of the blood-brain barrier. Contrast enhancement is particularly helpful in differentiating neoplastic tissue from surrounding edema. In the body, contrast enhancement is related to the relative differences in vascular delivery and extravascular diffusion of the contrast in normal and pathologic tissues. Intravenous contrast is useful for optimal assessment of the parenchyma of the liver, spleen, and kidneys; evaluation of intratumoral necrosis; and differentiation of blood vessels from other structures such as lymph nodes, particularly in the mediastinum and retroperitoneum.

Acute adverse reactions to intravascular iodinated contrast agents include acute allergic-like anaphylactoid reactions (e.g., urticaria, nasal congestion, bronchospasm, angioedema, cardiopulmonary arrest), chemotoxic reactions (e.g., nephrotoxicity, cardiac depression, arrhythmia), osmotoxic reactions (e.g., changes in plasma volume, vascular permeability, and coagulation), and vasovagal reactions (e.g., bradycardia, hypotension).[50] Other adverse events associated with iodinated contrast administration include extravasation injury and interactions with other drugs and clinical tests. Radiologists and oncologists should be aware of the guidelines for safe use of iodinated contrast that are periodically updated by various organizations.[51] These guidelines address clinical settings in which imaging examination scheduling, patient preparation, and follow-up by the referring clinician may need to be modified from the routine.

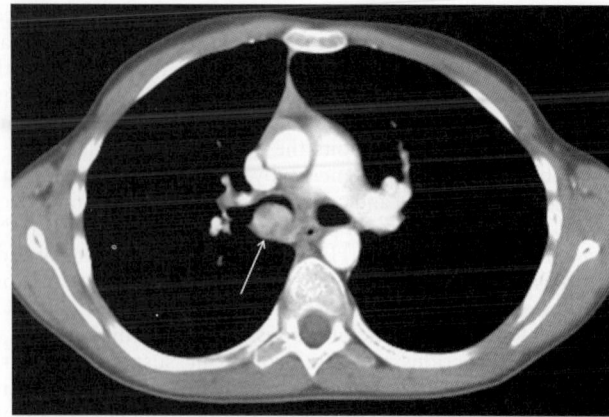

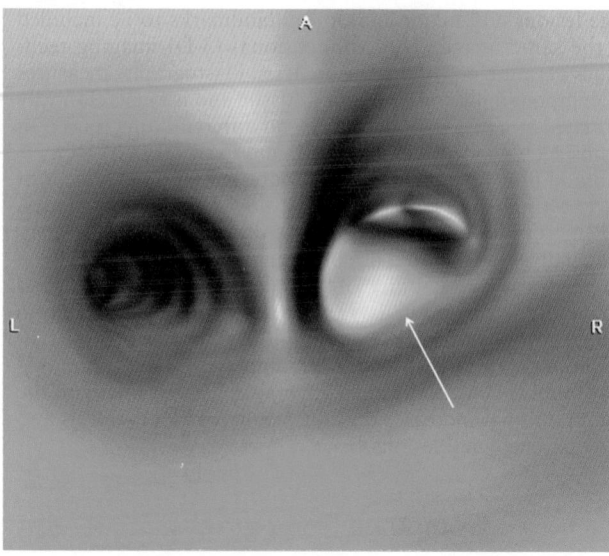

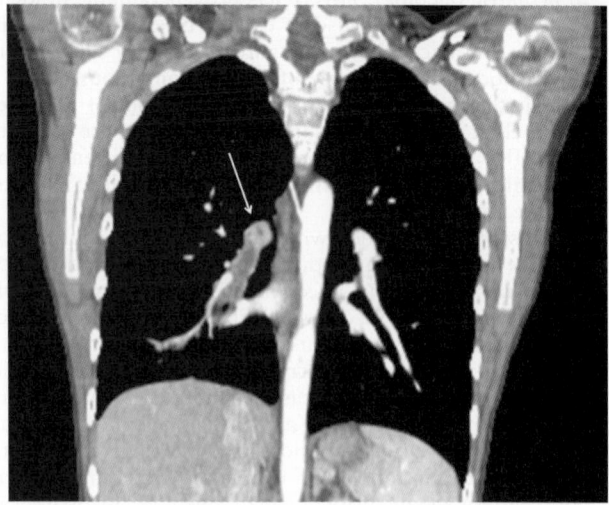

FIGURE 9.11 Bronchial carcinoid. Axial contrast-enhanced computed tomography (CT) image (**A**) and virtual bronchoscopy CT image (**B**) show an enhancing mass (*arrow*) partially occluding the airway lumen near the junction of the right mainstem bronchus and bronchus intermedius. Coronal reformatted CT image (**C**) depicts mucoid impaction of the airway distal to the mass (*arrow*).

Nonionic, low-osmolar iodinated contrast agents are most commonly used in children and have a favorable safety profile; acute allergic-like reactions occur with a frequency of 0.18% per administration and are usually mild.[52] Previous reaction to contrast is the most important risk factor in prediction of an adverse event, and the likelihood of a recurrent reaction is 8% to 25%. A history of other allergies or asthma is associated with a small elevation in the risk of reaction.[53] The overall risk of allergic-like reactions can be reduced by premedication with steroids with or without antihistamines. Premedication should be considered in those with previous allergic-like reaction to iodinated contrast material, multiple (four or more) allergies or a severe allergy to another substance, or asthma with frequent, recent, or severe attacks.[54] Delayed reactions are uncommon and most often cutaneous.[55] Interleukin-2 therapy increases the risk of delayed reactions, and the manifestations (fever, rash, flu-like symptoms, joint pain, flushing, pruritus, emesis, hypotension, dizziness) may resemble a "recall" reaction to interleukin-2.[56]

Contrast-induced nephropathy (CIN) typically manifests as an increasing serum creatinine level within 24 to 48 hours after contrast administration, peaking at 3 to 5 days, and returning to baseline by 10 days. Most cases are nonoliguric; thus, renal insufficiency may be clinically occult. In more severe cases, serum creatinine levels may continue to rise for 5 to 10 days and, in rare cases, dialysis is needed. Risk factors for CIN include preexisting renal insufficiency, diabetes mellitus, dehydration, large volume of injected contrast medium, severe congestive heart failure, concomitant nephrotoxic medications, and a history of contrast-associated acute renal failure.[57] The probability of CIN in patients at risk can be reduced by intravenous volume expansion with isotonic crystalloids for several hours before and after contrast administration, using the minimum contrast dose necessary for a diagnostic examination, and withdrawing nephrotoxic drugs before contrast administration.[58] Theophylline/aminophylline, statins, ascorbic acid, and prostaglandin E_1 are potentially beneficial pharmacologic adjuncts to reduce the likelihood of CIN; N-acetylcysteine has not been shown to be consistently effective; and furosemide and nonsteroidal anti-inflammatory drugs are potentially detrimental.[56,58]

Intravascular iodinated contrast agents transiently inhibit the coagulation cascade. To avoid misleading elevated clotting times, clotting tests should not be performed within 6 hours after intravascular contrast administration. Iodinated contrast agents may also interfere with the determination of blood levels of bilirubin, copper, iron, phosphate, and proteins.[56]

Intravascular iodinated contrast agents are relatively contraindicated or warrant particular caution in patients with renal insufficiency, a history of severe adverse reactions to contrast, severe thyrotoxicosis, suspected or known pheochromocytoma, and those receiving metformin or high-dose methotrexate. In the case of suspected or known pheochromocytoma, the risk of adrenergic hypertensive crisis provoked by intravascular iodinated contrast may be mitigated by pharmacologic adrenergic blockade prior to administration of contrast, although the intravenous administration of nonionic contrast media is most likely safe, even without such blockage.[59] Children and adolescents may be on metformin (dimethylbiguanide) for treatment of non–insulin-dependent (type 2) diabetes mellitus or insulin-resistance syndromes. Renal insufficiency leads to retention of metformin and the development of potentially fatal lactic acidosis. Renal function should be measured in patients on metformin before considering the administration of intravascular contrast, and published guidelines for the safe administration of intravascular contrast agents for elective and emergent radiologic procedures in patients on metformin with normal or impaired renal function should be followed.[51] High-dose methotrexate is used in the treatment of various pediatric malignancies and is associated with mucosal, bone marrow, liver, central nervous system (CNS), and renal toxicity. Both methotrexate and intravenous iodinated contrast are excreted by glomerular filtration, and their combined exposure incurs a higher risk for nephropathy and methotrexate toxicity. To prevent methotrexate toxicity, iodinated contrast should not be administered until the patient's serum methotrexate level is less than 0.1 mmol/L.[60]

Enteric contrast is routinely used for abdominal and pelvic CT scans to help differentiate bowel loops from lymph nodes and soft tissue masses. The use of enteric contrast is especially important in children to increase lesion conspicuity because of the relative lack of retroperitoneal and mesenteric fat surrounding and separating anatomic structures. Orally administered barium suspensions or diluted iodinated agents are typically used for enteric contrast. Significant adverse reactions to enteric contrast are very rare.

The disadvantages of CT include its cost, risk of adverse reaction to contrast media, the need for conscious sedation or general anesthesia in some patients, and the relatively high dose of ionizing radiation. The dose of ionizing radiation can range from less than 1 mSv for a sinus CT to more than 30 mSv for a body CT, particularly if multiple phases are obtained and adult rather than pediatric technique parameters are followed.[61] By comparison, the effective dose for a pediatric chest radiograph is 0.02 to 0.12 mSv.[62] Thus, the effective dose for a pediatric CT is the equivalent of tens to hundreds of chest radiographs. The effective dose of a typical pediatric CT examination is comparable to the average effective dose (3 mSv) of natural background radiation received by a person living in the United States. Equally large or larger effective doses compared with CT are associated with certain nuclear medicine examinations. Assuming the recommended radiopharmaceutical dose, the effective dose range in children is 2.0 to 5.8 mSv for Tc-99m MDP bone scintigraphy, 2.6 to 6.1 mSv for iodine (I)-123 MIBG scintigraphy, 4.9 to 8.6 mSv for fluorine (F)-18 FDG-PET, and 18 to 55 mSv for gallium (Ga)-67 scintigraphy.[63,64] However, the collective effective radiation dose from CT examinations to the population is higher than that from nuclear medicine examinations, because the number of CT examinations performed is much greater than the number of nuclear medicine examinations.

The number of CT examinations performed, including those performed on children, is rapidly increasing.[65,66] Not only is CT the primary method for diagnosis, staging, response evaluation, and surveillance of many pediatric malignancies but it is also a routine method for evaluating complications. This escalating use of CT has prompted public health concerns, because children are at higher risk of radiation-induced malignancy. Unlike conventional radiographs in which overexposure results in poorer image quality, CT images acquired with higher doses of radiation are better in quality. However, in children, CT images of adequate diagnostic quality are often achievable with much lower radiation doses than are used for adults.[3]

Estimates of the risk of radiation-induced malignancy from pediatric CT examinations have received much attention. The lifetime attributable risk of fatal cancer from a pediatric abdominal CT scan is estimated as approximately 0.07% to 0.14%, assuming a linear, no-threshold dose response and applying the cancer mortality data observed in the A-bomb survivor cohort.[65] However, such mathematical modeling has methodological limitations, for example, the radiation doses may differ substantially from those imparted by contemporary CT examinations, the risk of cancer from CT examinations is calculated rather than observed, and no studies have directly linked CT examinations to subsequent increased cancer mortality. Demonstrating an added cancer mortality risk of 0.1% is difficult by epidemiologic methods, because cancer is the cause of death in more than 20% of the overall population, and a very large number of subjects would be required for an adequately powered study.[67] The epidemiologic data are not precise about the risk of cancer from the radiation incurred by one or a few pediatric CT examinations performed with appropriate technique, and the appropriateness of a linear, no-threshold dose-response model for low-dose radiation is subject to dispute. Susceptibility to radiation-induced malignancy is likely inhomogeneously distributed in the population, and a generic statement of the risk of cancer from low doses of ionizing radiation may be an overestimate for some individuals and an underestimate for others, especially those with compromised DNA repair.

Although uncertainty persists about the risk of cancer from ionizing radiation in the dose range associated with diagnostic imaging, the prevailing opinion is to follow the ALARA (as low as reasonably achievable) principle for patient exposure. Although the cancer risk of one or a few CT or nuclear medicine examinations is uncertain, only the least amount of radiation exposure necessary to provide the diagnosis should be used. For CT, this may entail adjusting settings based on the child's size, body region scanned, and clinical indication; minimizing the use of multiphasic examinations; and adopting new dose-reducing technology such as automatic tube current modulation, iterative image reconstruction algorithms, and protective bismuth shields for radiosensitive tissues.[3,68] For nuclear medicine, this may include adjusting the radiopharmaceutical dose based on the patient's weight and compensatorily increasing the duration of imaging to achieve adequate count densities in those who receive a reduced dose.[64]

Clinicians are responsible for judiciously ordering CT and nuclear medicine examinations and considering the use of alternative modalities such as ultrasound and MRI that do not involve ionizing radiation. The most obvious way to reduce radiation exposure is to curtail unnecessary examinations, though this is not an easy task in current clinical practice due to intolerance for uncertainty and medicolegal concerns. Approximately 30% of CT examinations performed in young patients are noncontributory or unjustified.[69] In the context of pediatric oncology, CT examinations are frequently obtained for staging, evaluation of therapy response during treatment, and surveillance after treatment, as well as for evaluation of unexplained fever and complications of therapy. Clinical trial protocols for pediatric cancers often require that multiple radiographs, nuclear medicine examinations, and CT examinations be obtained, resulting in cumulative radiation doses of at least 100 mSv.[70] Further research is needed to determine whether outcomes would be adversely affected by using fewer of these examinations, particularly repetitive low-yield examinations with relatively high-dose radiation. CT revolutionized clinical diagnosis when introduced in the 1970s and remains one of the most valuable diagnostic tests. Given the obvious benefits of diagnostic imaging, the risks of radiation from CT or other radiologic examinations should be kept in proper perspective. The risks of ionizing radiation from radiologic examinations in patients with cancer is generally small compared with the benefits of the information provided by indicated examinations and the much higher risks of complications from the disease and its therapy, particularly in patients with shortened life expectancy from aggressive cancers. Inaccurate or nondiagnostic results due to a poor-quality CT examination or failure to perform a CT examination when indicated carries a high risk of harm to the patient, and overconcern about the long-term effects of radiation could be more harmful than the risk from excess radiation.[66,71]

Magnetic Resonance Imaging

MRI involves interactions between a strong external magnet field, radiofrequency (RF) waves, and the hydrogen nuclei in the body. Once aligned in the strong magnetic field, the body's hydrogen nuclei precess or "wobble" at a frequency proportional to the magnetic field's strength. When the hydrogen nuclei are bombarded with RF waves at the precessional frequency, energy is absorbed by the nuclei. The RF waves are then turned off, and the hydrogen nuclei return to their initial alignment. This results in a release of energy that induces voltage in a wire receiving coil, producing the MR signal. Spatial encoding, the process of localizing the MR signal to generate an image, is accomplished by the use of magnetic field gradients.

As with CT, clinical MR images represent "slices" through the body that are made up of a specified number of volume elements called *voxels*. Unlike CT, in which the slices are almost always obtained in the transaxial plane, MRI slices can be obtained in any desired plane. The imaging volume is restricted to a slice by specific frequencies in the RF pulse and the magnetic field gradient. The same mathematical construct used in CT, the Fourier transformation, processes the signals and assigns each MRI voxel a shade of gray that reflects the amount of hydrogen nuclei and the rate at which equilibrium is reestablished with the magnetic field after RF excitation.

The most common strength of external magnetic fields found on current MRI scanners is 1.5 T, about 30,000 times the strength of the earth's magnetic field. To achieve high-field (1.0–3.0 T) or ultrahigh-field (>3.0 T) strengths, superconducting magnets are used. These require cryogens to maintain the extremely low temperatures necessary for superconducting, contributing to the high costs of higher-field MRI systems. Low-field (≤0.2 T) or mid-field (0.3–1.0 T) strengths are achievable with less costly permanent magnets. High-field systems have higher signal-to-noise ratio, thus better image quality, improved MR spectroscopy, and functional MRI capability. Disadvantages of higher-field systems include the higher magnet cost, the need for greater shielding, which restricts selection of suitable sites for scanner installation, and an increase in some artifacts. Other properties such as longer T1 relaxation times and increased chemical shift and susceptibility can be either an advantage or a disadvantage, depending on the clinical indication.[72] High-field systems typically require that the imaged body part be placed within a long, narrow, tunnel-like bore in the magnet, a setting that can preclude imaging of claustrophobic or very large individuals. Such individuals can be scanned with comparable diagnostic accuracy in most cases, in low- or mid-field systems that employ an "open" geometry in which the imaged body part is placed between two parallel plates that are far less confining.

When placed in the external magnetic field of the MRI scanner, hydrogen nuclei in the body become aligned parallel to the long axis of the external magnetic field, a process known as *longitudinal magnetization*. An RF pulse at a precise frequency, the Larmor frequency, tips the longitudinal magnetization into the transverse plane, a process known as *transverse magnetization*. The longitudinal magnetization recovers partially between RF pulses applied repeatedly at intervals, TR (time to repetition), with time constant T1. Precession of transverse magnetization induces electrical signal in the receive coil, exponentially decaying at time constant T2. The time between the initial pulse and data collection is the TE (time to echo).

To produce a useful diagnostic image, contrast in appearance between normal tissues is needed for anatomic detail, and contrast in appearance between normal and diseased tissue is needed for sensitivity to pathology. The primary sources of tissue contrast in MRI are differences in hydrogen spin densities, T1 relaxation times, and T2 relaxation times. The particular weighting of these sources of tissue contrast is determined by the MRI pulse sequence design. Pulse sequences are continuously being developed and refined for various applications, and a detailed description of the multiple MR sequences available is beyond the scope of this chapter.

In the conventional spin echo pulse sequence, TR and TE are manipulated so that a T1- or T2-weighted image is acquired. An image acquired on a 1.5-T scanner with a short TR (300–600 ms) and short TE (10–20 ms) emphasizes the T1 characteristics of the tissues, and an image acquired with a longer TR (>2,000 ms) and a longer TE (>80 ms) primarily reflects the T2 characteristics of the tissues. On T1-weighted images, substances with short T1 relaxation times (e.g., fat, methemoglobin, melanin, proteinaceous fluid, gadolinium contrast) are depicted with bright signal intensity, and those with longer T1 relaxation times (e.g., edema, tumor, hemosiderin) are depicted with intermediate to low signal intensity. On T2-weighted images, substances with short T2 relaxation times (e.g., white matter, tendon, hemosiderin, fibrosis) are depicted with low to intermediate signal intensity, and substances with longer T2 relaxation times (e.g., edema, tumor, cerebrospinal fluid [CSF]) are depicted with bright signal intensity. Images acquired with TR and TE intermediate to those used for T1- and T2-weighted images are often referred to as *proton-density images*. The signal characteristics on these images reflect a mixture of T1 and T2 relaxation times and the proton density of the imaged tissue.

Pulse sequence development beyond conventional spin echo sequences has been a fertile area for clinical investigation. These efforts have focused primarily on suppressing signal from certain tissues, reducing scanning time, and increasing conspicuity of blood flow. Inversion recovery (IR) sequences permit selective nulling of signal from a specific tissue based on its T1 relaxation time and the chosen inversion time (TI). A variant of the IR sequence, short tau inversion recovery (STIR), selectively suppresses the signal from fat and has proven very valuable in body and musculoskeletal applications, particularly when fat suppression by chemical shift methods is unsuccessful. The fluid-attenuated inversion recovery sequence suppresses signal from the CSF and is highly sensitive for lesions in the brain and spinal cord.

Rapid imaging techniques include low flip angle gradient echo sequences, RF-refocused fast (turbo) spin echo sequences, single shot sequences, echo planar imaging, and parallel imaging simultaneously using multiple receive coils. Rapid imaging techniques allow more body coverage, more sequences performed in less time (improved temporal resolution), or more detailed images obtained in the same time (improved spatial resolution).[73] These are particularly valuable attributes for performing MRI in children, because small structures are commonly imaged, and minimizing patient motion is imperative. Pediatric whole-body MRI scanning with rapid sequences is now feasible in 25 minutes or less of acquisition time and is particularly suited for surveying the bone marrow.[74,75]

Considerable attention has been directed to diffusion-weighted MRI (DWI), a technique that characterizes tissues on the basis of the Brownian molecular motion of constituent water. The initial applications of DWI have primarily been in the field of neuroradiology. DWI is highly sensitive for the detection of acute cerebral ischemia and other processes that are associated with impaired water diffusion. There is an inverse relationship between the apparent diffusion coefficient (ADC) and tumor cellularity due to the restricted diffusion of water molecules among densely packed cells (Fig. 9.12). The ADC is predictive of pediatric brain tumor classification,[76] and assessment of ADC ratios of enhancing regions in the follow-up of treated high-grade gliomas is useful in differentiating radiation effects from tumor recurrence or progression.[77] By exploiting the anisotropic diffusion of water in relation to ordered structures, special applications of DWI termed *diffusion tensor tractography* and *diffusion spectrum imaging* can be used to delineate the course and integrity of important white matter tracts in the brain.[78]

DWI can detect and delineate a wide range of pediatric tumors from adjacent tissues. Solid tumor components tend to show restricted diffusion and correlate with sites of gadolinium contrast enhancement; liquefactive necrotic or cystic components tend to show increased diffusion.[79] The recently introduced technique of diffusion-weighted whole-body imaging with background body signal suppression (DWIBS) allows volumetric diffusion-weighted images of the entire body to be acquired during free breathing, highlights lesions with restricted diffusion, and provides excellent visualization of lymph nodes.[80] However, the use of ADC measurements has not enabled differentiation between malignant and benign extracranial tumors in children.[81]

MRA has become a widely accepted tool for noninvasively depicting blood vessels in children. Depending on the technique, MRA can demonstrate blood flow, with or without the use of intravenous contrast medium, as dark (black blood technique) or light (bright blood technique) signal intensity. The most popular MRA technique currently used in pediatric body imaging is time-resolved gadolinium-enhanced 3-D MRA, a method that relies on the shortening of T1 relaxation time by gadolinium-chelate contrast media within the lumen of the vessel of interest. Timing of injection of contrast and image acquisition allows arteries or veins to be selectively imaged. Time-of-flight, phase contrast, arterial spin labeling, and 3-D steady-state free-precession MRA techniques do not require administration of intravenous contrast and are particularly useful in the setting of renal insufficiency or lack of vascular access, when gadolinium-enhanced MRA may not be feasible. In pediatric oncology, MRA is valuable for depicting vascular anatomy in planning resection or transplantation for liver tumors,[4] detecting intravascular invasion by abdominal tumors,[82] and planning limb salvage procedures in cases of extremity sarcomas.[83] MRA has also proven useful in assessing the venous system for patency before central vascular catheter placement, particularly in children with suspected thrombotic veno-occlusive disease related to prior catheters[84] (Fig. 9.13).

Although the superior soft tissue contrast differentiation of MRI permits identification of most tumors without the administration of contrast agent, intravenously administered gadolinium-chelate contrast agents are used in MRI much like intravenously administered iodinated contrast agents in CT to make tumors more conspicuous, assess tumor vascularity, and evaluate intratumoral necrosis. Gadolinium is a paramagnetic metal that provides enhancement by shortening the T1 and T2 relaxation times. Gadolinium is toxic as a free ion and is usually administered as a chelate to reduce the toxicity and increase elimination, mainly by the kidneys. Intravenous

gadolinium-chelates are by far the most commonly used MRI contrast agents, and seven are currently approved by the U.S. Food and Drug Administration (FDA). Five are classic extracellular contrast agents that act much like iodinated contrast agents for CT and accumulate at sites of increased vascular flow and permeability; one is a hepatocyte agent that is actively transported into hepatocytes and excreted in the bile, facilitating distinction of liver tumors lacking hepatocytes from normal liver parenchyma; and the other binds to serum albumin so that it remains in the intravascular compartment longer to serve as a blood pool imaging agent, thereby improving the quality of MRA. Other available MRI contrast agents include intravenously administered iron-containing compounds for liver, spleen, and bone marrow imaging and a variety of orally administered agents for the GI tract, including perfluorooctylbromide (PFOB) and agents containing barium, iron, manganese, and lipids.[85]

The overall safety profiles of the different gadolinium-chelate MRI contrast agents are comparable.[86] The most common reactions are headache, nausea, urticaria, and taste distortion. Acute allergic-like reactions to gadolinium-chelates are rare in children, occurring with a frequency of 0.04% per administration, and are usually mild.[52] Compared with the other gadolinium-chelate MRI contrast agents, gadodiamide and gadoversetamide have lower stability and higher excess chelate, properties that can interfere with colorimetric assays for serum calcium and result in inappropriate treatment for spurious hypocalcemia.[56] Gadolinium-chelate MRI contrast agents cross the placenta, and their use is not advised during pregnancy, though teratogenesis has not been shown.

Recently, the administration of gadolinium-chelate contrast agents has been associated with the subsequent development of nephrogenic systemic fibrosis (NSF) in patients with acute or chronic renal insufficiency. NSF is characterized by progressive tissue fibrosis, usually starting in the skin of the extremities and advancing over the course of days or weeks to the trunk and extracutaneous structures such as the skeletal muscles, heart, lungs, and esophagus, leading to restricted range of motion, disability, and even death. The risk of NSF is increased by higher gadolinium-chelate doses and greater degrees of renal insufficiency, implying a role of prolonged tissue retention of gadolinium in its pathogenesis, although NSF does not develop in most patients with renal insufficiency, even if they are exposed to high doses of gadolinium-chelates. Because of their lower stability, the nonionic linear gadolinium-chelates release more free gadolinium than the macrocyclic chelates and may pose a greater risk for NSF. Circulating fibrocytes and cytokines are thought to mediate the fibrosing process and other possible associated risk factors include high-dose erythropoietin, systemic inflammation, trauma, metabolic acidosis, lanthanum phosphate binders, hepatorenal syndrome, and the perioperative liver transplantation period. Pediatric cases have been reported, although it is unclear whether the immature kidney function of neonates and infants poses an additional risk factor. Like iodinated contrast agents, gadolinium-chelate MRI contrast agents are removed by dialysis, but dialysis is of unproven efficacy for preventing NSF. To avert NSF, the susceptible population should be defined, and the risk to that population should be minimized. Rather than relying on serum creatinine, one should calculate the glomerular filtration rate or estimate it by using the Schwartz formula. The risk-benefit should be assessed, and alternative imaging techniques that do not entail the use of gadolinium-chelates should be considered for pediatric patients with renal insufficiency.[87,88]

The dynamics of contrast uptake by tumors is under investigation, based on the premise that the rate and intensity of contrast uptake correlates with the density and permeability

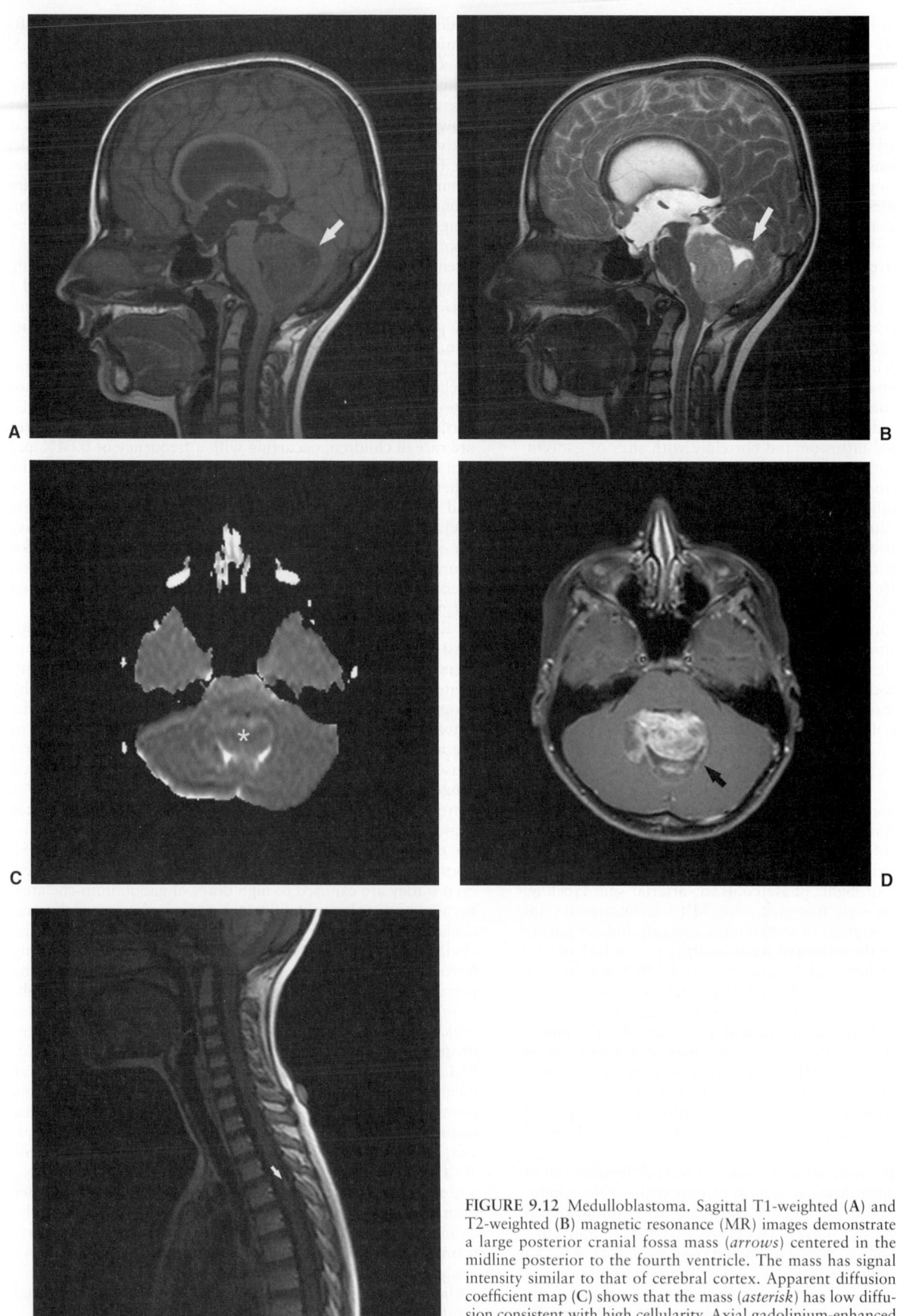

FIGURE 9.12 Medulloblastoma. Sagittal T1-weighted (**A**) and T2-weighted (**B**) magnetic resonance (MR) images demonstrate a large posterior cranial fossa mass (*arrows*) centered in the midline posterior to the fourth ventricle. The mass has signal intensity similar to that of cerebral cortex. Apparent diffusion coefficient map (**C**) shows that the mass (*asterisk*) has low diffusion consistent with high cellularity. Axial gadolinium-enhanced T1-weighted image (**D**) shows considerable though heterogeneous enhancement (*arrow*). Sagittal gadolinium-enhanced T1-weighted MR image (**E**) of the thoracic spine demonstrates a small enhancing focus (*arrow*) at the dorsal margin of the spinal cord at the T4 level that is consistent with a drop metastasis.

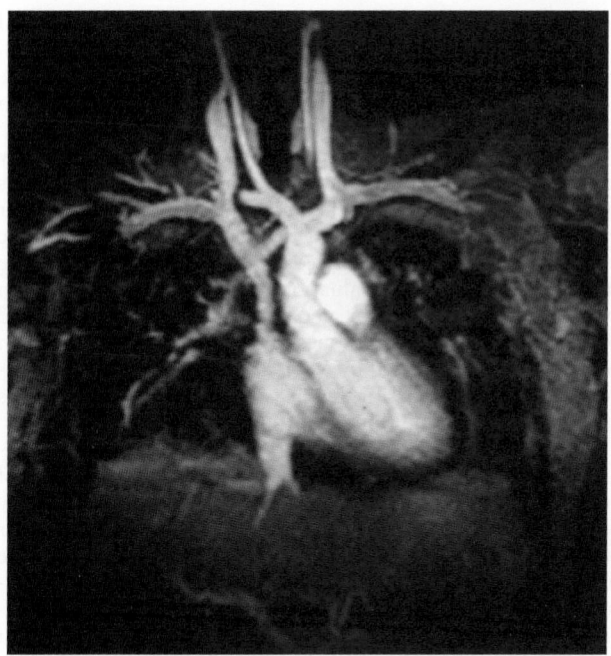

FIGURE 9.13 Patient with a history of bone marrow transplantation for myelodysplastic syndrome after treatment for lymphoma. Magnetic resonance angiogram obtained for planning of central venous catheter placement demonstrates patency of the superior vena cava and brachiocephalic, subclavian, and internal jugular veins.

of the microvasculature of viable tumor. Dynamic contrast-enhanced MRI (DEMRI) consists of rapid sequential MR imaging of a tumor following the bolus administration of intravenous gadolinium-chelate. Selecting a region of interest on all or part of the tumor and plotting a time-intensity curve allows quantitative analysis based on the relative intensity or rate of contrast enhancement (Fig. 9.14). Theoretically, DEMRI can predict accessibility of the tumor to drugs before treatment and viability of residual tumor during or after treatment. Viable tumor tends to exhibit early and intense enhancement, while necrotic and fibrotic areas show slower, less intense, or absent enhancement. In DEMRI of bone

sarcoma, rapid and pronounced contrast uptake into the tumor prior to preoperative chemotherapy, greater decrease in uptake during therapy, and low uptake at the completion of preoperative chemotherapy correspond to a better response and longer disease-free survival.[89] Analysis of contrast uptake by DEMRI can predict clinically important degrees of necrosis in bone sarcomas in response to induction or neoadjuvant preoperative chemotherapy.[90] Response prediction by MRI could facilitate the development of risk-adapted treatment approaches,[91] though static MRI determination of tumor volume at the time of diagnosis is more reliable than DEMRI at predicting clinical outcome in Ewing's sarcoma.[92] The routine application of DEMRI has been hindered by the need for mathematical postprocessing of the imaging data and the lack of a simple standardized approach for use across institutions with varying MRI equipment capabilities.

Magnetic resonance spectroscopy (MRS) allows noninvasive determination of the relative concentrations of various metabolites *in vivo*. MRS is based on the principle that small differences in the resonance frequencies of nuclei are determined by the chemical environment. Each metabolite is identified by the position of its peak (or chemical shift) on a frequency scale, with the area under the peak proportional to the concentration of the metabolite within the voxel. If the metabolite profile at one location is desired, single-voxel methods are used, whereas MRS imaging methods are chosen if the spatial distribution of metabolites is of interest. In single-voxel methods, the spectra are obtained during a short period of time, but the volume of interest is usually large and contains heterogeneous tissue. In multivoxel methods, more time is required to acquire the spectra, but the voxel size is smaller and representative of more homogeneous tissue.[93]

Investigators have focused on proton (^{1}H) and phosphorous (^{31}P) magnetic spectroscopic imaging. The former has received the most attention, particularly in the brain, due to a higher sensitivity resulting in a higher signal-to-noise ratio and allowing a shorter acquisition time and the use of smaller voxels. The ^{1}H-MRS method can be performed on a standard MRI scanner with the appropriate software. In the brain, the principal metabolites measured by ^{1}H-MRS are choline (Cho), N-acetyl aspartate (NAA), lactate (Lac), and creatine (Cr). Cho is a marker for cell membrane turnover; NAA is a neuronal marker; Lac is a marker of anaerobic metabolism; and Cr is involved in energy metabolism and serves as an internal

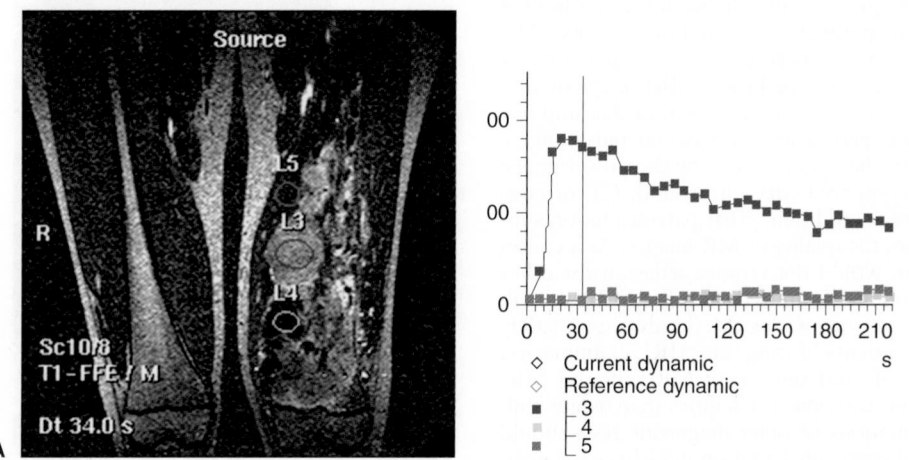

FIGURE 9.14 Osteosarcoma. Coronal T1-weighted fast field echo image (**A**) with regions of interest placed over skeletal muscle and tumor components for dynamic contrast-enhanced magnetic resonance imaging analysis of the rate and intensity of contrast enhancement. **B**: Time-intensity curves showing early and intense enhancement of viable tumor and minimal enhancement of necrotic tumor.

standard because it varies little in normal brain tissue. Pediatric brain tumors generally exhibit elevated Cho levels, decreased or absent NAA levels, and Lac levels that vary with the degree of necrosis.[94] The ^{1}H-MRS method can be used to identify areas in tumors with the highest Cho levels to improve the diagnostic yield of brain biopsies.[95] The maximum tumor Cho:NAA ratio is predictive of outcome in children with recurrent primary brain tumors,[96] and the percentage change in Cho:NAA ratio by ^{1}H-MRS is an important prognostic indicator of tumor progression in children with brain tumors.[97] The ^{31}P-MRS method has been investigated in bone and soft tissue tumors in the extremities and trunk. In comparison with ^{31}P-MRS imaging of benign lesions, that of malignant lesions shows significantly higher mean peak ratios of phosphomonoester to β-nucleoside triphosphate (NTP) and of phosphodiester to NTP, a significantly lower mean peak area ratio of phosphocreatine to NTP, and a higher mean pH.[98]

Despite marked success in the research setting, various technical and physiologic factors have impeded the transfer of MRS to the clinic. MRS is technically far more demanding than MRI and requires an experienced MR spectroscopist for good clinical results. Metabolite profiles vary with age in developing tissues, and the metabolic profiles of differing pathologies often overlap. MRS quality is very susceptible to degradation by patient motion and magnetic field inhomogeneity, such as in the posterior cranial fossa where pediatric brain tumors are common. Although extremely chemically specific, the time necessary to measure the MR signal from a certain volume with a given signal-to-noise ratio increases with the sixth power of the linear dimension of the volume, resulting in the inherently poor sensitivity of MRS. The size of the selected volume has to be relatively large (around 1 cm³ for ^{1}H-MRS and 27 cm³ for ^{31}P-MRS) and care must be taken to minimize partial volume effect and signal contamination from adjacent tissue. Some of these technical limitations of MRS are lessened by the higher signal-to-noise ratio and improved spectral resolution of higher-field MRI systems that are increasingly available.[99]

MRI offers several advantages over CT. MRI delineates normal soft tissues and discriminates abnormal from normal soft tissues better than CT and does so without the use of ionizing radiation. Iodinated contrast agents are not required, beam-hardening artifacts from bone are eliminated, and images can be acquired in any desired plane. The disadvantages of MRI include its relatively high cost, limited availability, insensitivity to the presence of calcifications, and limited ability to assess lung parenchyma and bony cortex. The absence of a widely accepted enteric contrast medium impedes the ability of MRI to evaluate the bowel. MRI image quality is highly susceptible to degradation by normal cardiac and respiratory motion, bowel peristalsis, and vascular pulsations, a disadvantage that is further compounded by the slower image acquisition of MRI compared with ultrasound, CT, or conventional radiography. In addition, gross patient motion substantially compromises the quality of MR images. As a consequence, children who would not require sedation for other imaging modalities often require sedation for MRI, though fast MRI techniques are ameliorating this disadvantage. Safely sedating pediatric patients during an MRI examination requires monitoring of vital signs with MR-safe and MR-compatible monitoring equipment. Facilities that sedate children for MRI examinations or other diagnostic tests should institute standardized protocols based on guidelines for pediatric sedation that have been developed and recommended by professional organizations.[100]

Since its introduction in the 1980s, the role of MRI in the evaluation of pediatric cancers has expanded at a rapid pace.

MRI is now the imaging study of choice for brain and spinal tumors, musculoskeletal tumors, and tumors of the body wall. MRI is complementary to ultrasound in the assessment of the female genital tract and is valuable in the evaluation of certain thoracic, abdominal, and pelvic malignancies.

MRI is superior to CT in detecting CNS tumors, especially in the posterior fossa. Evaluation of multiplanar images allows more precise localization of neoplastic disease as intra-axial or extra-axial. The vertebrae and the contents of the thecal sac can be studied without the need for myelography. MRI is the modality of choice for evaluation of spinal cord compression or intraspinal invasion by neoplastic masses (Figs. 9.5 and 9.15). However, the small bones of the skull and face are often not adequately evaluated by MRI. Therefore, if precise evaluation of the small bones of the face and skull is required, CT is recommended, in addition to or in place of MRI.

Application of MRI to extracranial and extraspinal structures has advanced rapidly. MRI allows direct acquisition of images in the coronal and sagittal planes and has the ability to visualize flowing blood in vessels without the need for intravenous contrast. MRI is equal to or better than CT in the anatomic definition of many abdominal, pelvic, and mediastinal tumors.[101] MRI is generally superior to CT in the evaluation of musculoskeletal tumors, except in the detection of calcification or early cortical bone erosion. MRI is superior to CT, conventional radiographs, or Tc-99m phosphonate–based bone scintigraphy in defining the precise extent of neoplastic infiltration of the bone marrow and extraosseous soft tissues, making MRI the imaging modality of choice for local-regional staging of primary bone tumors[102] (Fig. 9.16). The increased accuracy of MRI in defining the local-regional extent of musculoskeletal tumors is particularly important

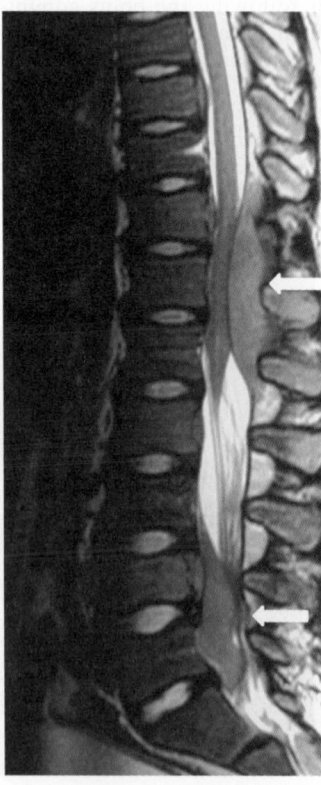

FIGURE 9.15 Burkitt's lymphoma. Sagittal T2-weighted magnetic resonance image shows neoplastic infiltration of vertebral bone marrow and epidural tumor masses (*arrows*) compressing the lower spinal cord and cauda equina.

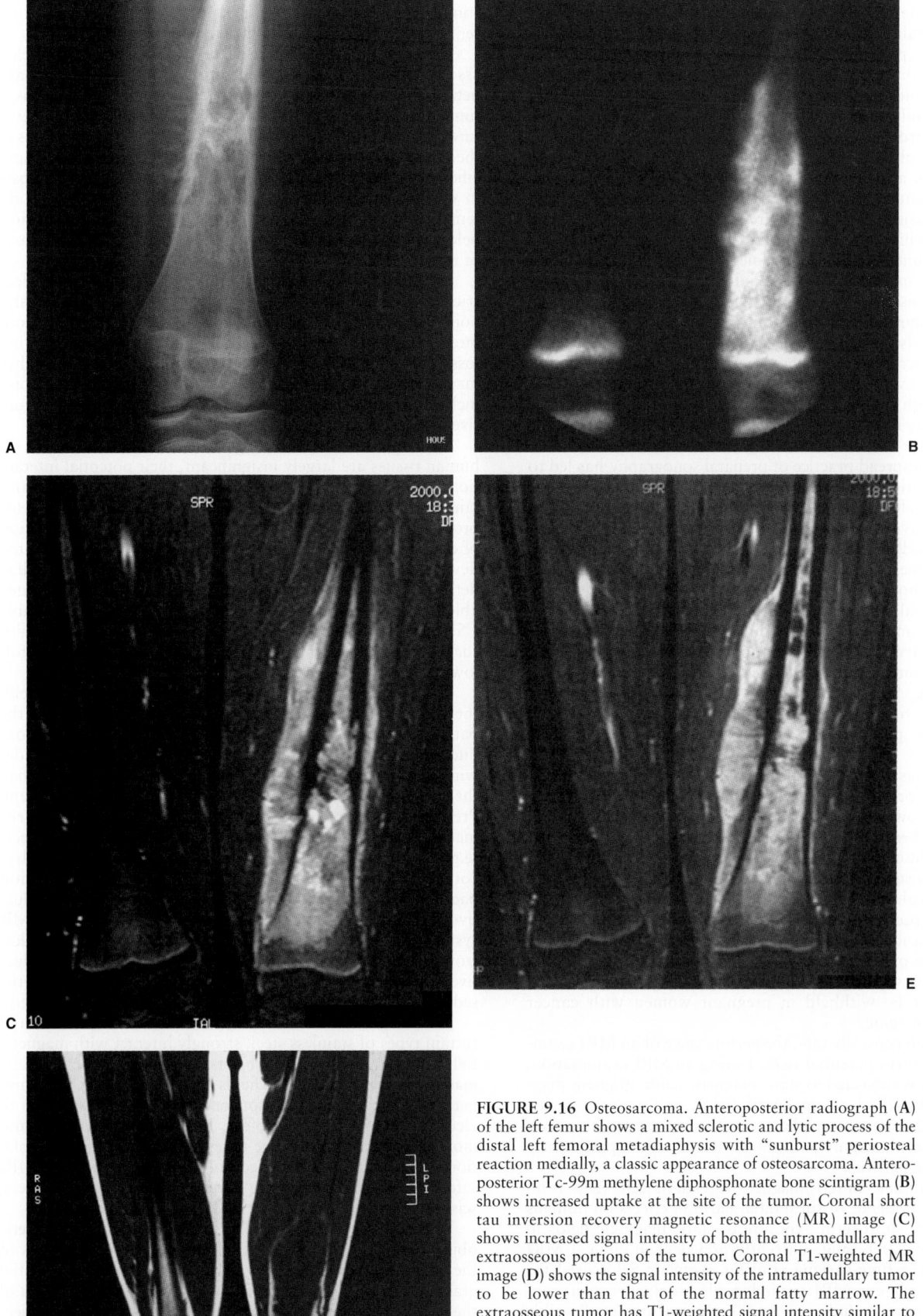

FIGURE 9.16 Osteosarcoma. Anteroposterior radiograph (**A**) of the left femur shows a mixed sclerotic and lytic process of the distal left femoral metadiaphysis with "sunburst" periosteal reaction medially, a classic appearance of osteosarcoma. Anteroposterior Tc-99m methylene diphosphonate bone scintigram (**B**) shows increased uptake at the site of the tumor. Coronal short tau inversion recovery magnetic resonance (MR) image (**C**) shows increased signal intensity of both the intramedullary and extraosseous portions of the tumor. Coronal T1-weighted MR image (**D**) shows the signal intensity of the intramedullary tumor to be lower than that of the normal fatty marrow. The extraosseous tumor has T1-weighted signal intensity similar to that of normal muscle. Coronal gadolinium-enhanced T1-weighted MR image (**E**) shows heterogeneous enhancement of the intramedullary and extraosseous portions of the tumor.

when primary radiation therapy or limb-salvage surgery is being considered.

MRI is valuable for the assessment of bone marrow disease in pediatric patients.[103] The T1 relaxation time in marrow involved with leukemia is longer than that of normal marrow (Fig. 9.4), and marrow from patients with relapsed leukemia shows a similar prolongation of this measure compared with that of marrow from those in remission.[104] The diagnosis of relapsed leukemia can be made by MRI several weeks before it is appreciable by iliac bone marrow aspirate or biopsy, because vertebral marrow, as the primary site of hematopoiesis in children, may reflect the changes of leukemia earlier than iliac crest marrow, and iliac marrow sampling bias could account for initially false-negative results. Although an initial bone marrow biopsy is required for children presenting with new-onset leukemia, MRI may lessen the need for bone marrow aspirates or biopsies during follow-up. MRI of the marrow is also useful in the evaluation and detection of focal areas of macroscopic lymphoma in patients who are symptomatic but have negative bone scans. As many as one-third of patients with lymphoma evaluated by routine bone marrow biopsies may have otherwise occult marrow lymphoma visible by MRI.[105]

The widespread practice of prenatal sonography has led to the recognition of fetal tumors and subsequent pediatric oncology referral. Promoted by the development of fast sequences averting the need for maternal sedation or fetal paralysis and by advances in fetal medicine and surgery, fetal MRI has emerged over the past decade as a useful adjunct to prenatal sonography to better define the extent, composition, and potential complications of fetal tumors. The most common fetal tumors amenable to differentiation by fetal MRI are teratomas, lymphatic malformations, cardiac rhabdomyomas, neuroblastomas, hemangiomas, and mesoblastic nephromas[106] (Fig. 9.17). Fetal MRI is superior to ultrasound in delineating tumor mass effect on the fetal airway and neck vessels for planning of airway management at birth[107] (Fig. 9.18).

There has been no indication that clinical MRI during pregnancy produces deleterious maternal or fetal effects in humans. However, MRI scanning of pregnant women should be undertaken with caution because existing studies of MRI safety in human pregnancy have involved relatively small numbers of subjects and short durations of follow-up, limiting the statistical power for detection of adverse effects. MRI may be used in pregnant women if other forms of diagnostic imaging without ionizing radiation exposure (e.g., ultrasound) are inadequate or if MRI provides important information that would otherwise require exposure to ionizing radiation. MRI should not be withheld in pregnant women with cancer requiring imaging.

Although generally safe, the performance of an MRI examination involves potential risks. During an MRI examination, the patient is subjected to static magnetic fields, gradient magnetic fields, RF electromagnetic fields, and acoustic noise. Intravascular contrast media is often used, and sedation may be necessary to acquire a diagnostic examination, particularly in pediatric patients.

In the absence of ferromagnetic foreign objects, there is no conclusive evidence of substantial harmful effects on humans from acute, short-term exposure to static magnetic fields in the 0.2- to 3.0-T range currently prevalent in clinical MRI systems. The time-varying gradient magnetic fields used for spatial encoding in MRI can induce electrical currents in conductive media, including certain biological tissues. Possible biological effects of induced current include stimulation of nerve or muscles, ventricular fibrillation, magnetophosphenes,

and bone healing. The threshold currents required for cardiac stimulation, though, are much higher than the estimated currents induced during routine MRI.[108]

The main biological effect of the RF electromagnetic fields associated with MRI is the generation of heat related to magnetic induction in tissues. The amount of heat generated is a function of numerous variables, and the rise in body temperature depends on the patient's thermoregulatory system. This is theoretically a concern in 3.0-T scanners capable of high specific absorption rates and in neonates or patients with sepsis in whom thermoregulation is impaired, but changes in body temperature in humans exposed to RF-power deposition below the FDA guidance levels are believed to be minor and of no serious physiologic consequence.[108]

Acoustic noise produced during an MRI arises from electrical current–induced hardware vibrations. The acoustic noise can result in patient annoyance, disruption of sedation, interference with oral communication, and reversible hearing loss. The acoustic noise problem is exacerbated with higher magnetic field strengths. Strategies to mitigate acoustic noise include the use of earplugs, headphones, or antinoise destructive interference techniques.

Although the direct biological effects of MRI fields on human tissues are largely insignificant, their potential interactions with medical devices are an important concern in maintaining the safety of clinical MRI. The electromagnetic fields produced by the MRI system may interfere with the operation of certain electrically, magnetically, or mechanically activated devices, such as cardiac pacemakers, implantable cardiac defibrillators, cochlear implants, neurostimulators, implantable drug-infusion pumps, and programmable or adjustable CSF shunt valves. MRI is contraindicated in patients with such devices, unless highly specific safety guidelines are followed.[108]

When conducting materials are present within the RF field, the induced electrical current may cause a burn injury to the patient. This tends to be problematic primarily when the conductive materials have elongated shapes (e.g., leads, guidewires, and certain catheters), but burns can also occur when the patient is in contact with the RF coils of the MRI system. Precautions against excessive heating and possible burns include ensuring that there are no unnecessary metallic objects (e.g., metallic drug delivery patches, body-piercing jewelry) contacting the patient's skin, using appropriate insulation padding to prevent skin contact, keeping electrically conductive materials that must remain within the RF coil of the MR system (e.g., electrocardiogram leads, pulse oximeter cables) from forming conductive loops, and using MRI-safe conductive devices. These measures are particularly important in the sedated child, where response to thermal stimuli is impaired.

Ferromagnetic materials, such as iron, cobalt, nickel, and certain types of stainless steel, strongly interact with magnetic fields. The interaction of objects containing ferromagnetic materials with the magnetic fields of MRI can result in a number of effects, including distortion of the image, induction of electrical current in the object, heating of the object, and movement of the object. The potential rotational and translational movement of such objects is of primary concern in MRI safety. Projectile injuries have occurred with oxygen canisters, scissors, IV poles, traction weights, and hairpins.

The risk of scanning patients with internal ferromagnetic objects depends on the magnetic and geometric properties of the object, the strength of the static magnetic field and spatial gradient of the MRI system, the retention force of fixation of the object within the body part, and the location of the object relative to vital structures. The presence of a ferromagnetic aneurysm clip is a contraindication to MRI scanning. Most

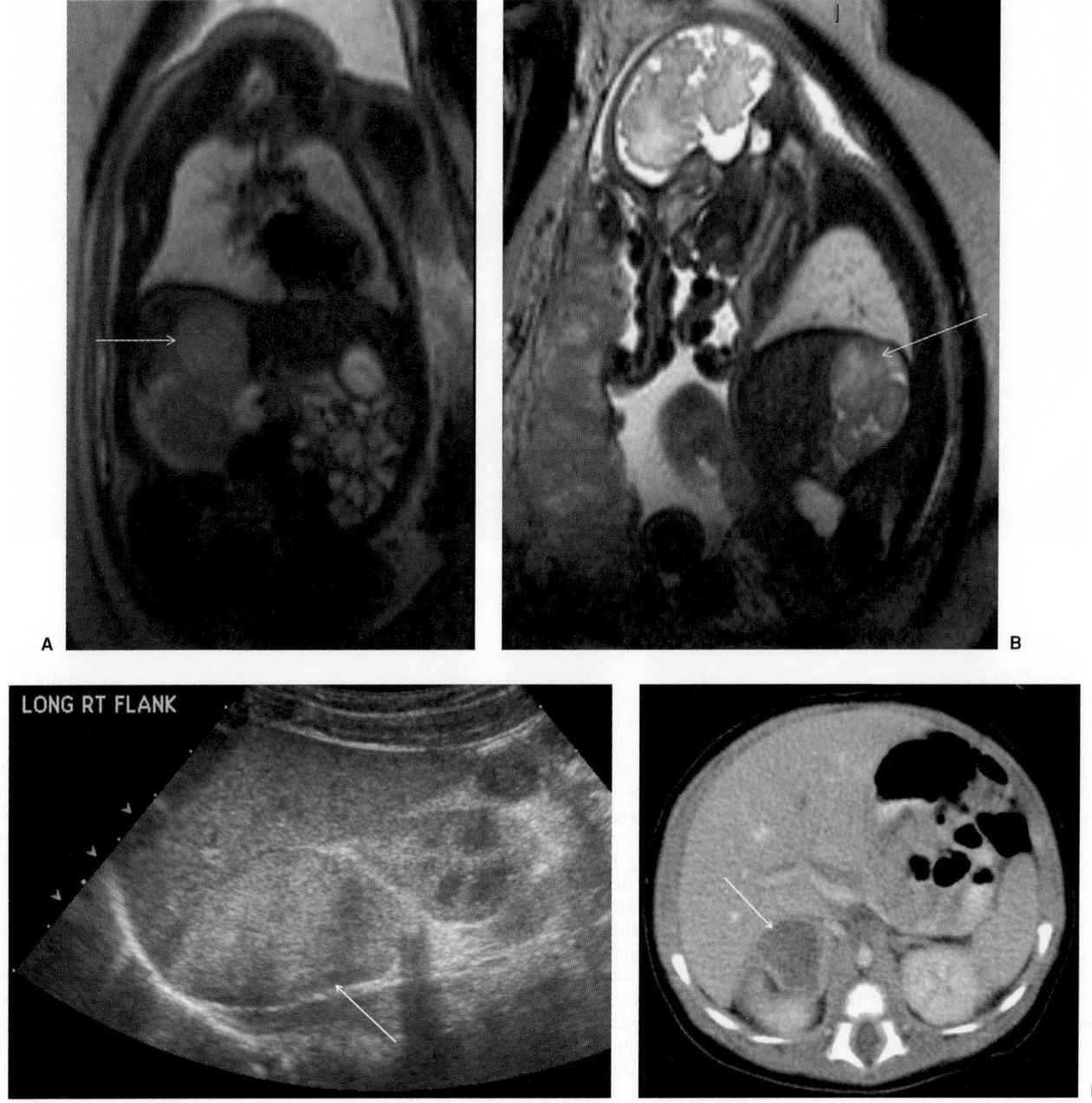

FIGURE 9.17 Prenatally diagnosed neuroblastoma. Fast T2-weighted coronal (**A**) and sagittal (**B**) magnetic resonance images of a 35-week gestational-age fetus reveal a solid right suprarenal mass (*arrow*). Postnatal ultrasound (**C**) and axial contrast-enhanced computed tomography (**D**) images obtained at 1 month of age show no regression of the mass (*arrow*). The mass also exhibited uptake on metaiodobenzylguanidine scintigraphy (not depicted). Subsequent surgical excision and pathologic inspection of the mass confirmed the presence of neuroblastoma.

prosthetic heart valves manufactured after 1964 are not ferromagnetic or experience insignificant deflection forces, but verification of safety is recommended before performing an MRI examination on a child with a prosthetic heart valve. Metal shrapnel near the eye is potentially dangerous and can be detected with radiographs of the orbit as clinically indicated prior to the MRI examination. Hemostatic (ligating) vascular clips were previously thought to not pose a risk for injury from MRI procedures; however, the performance of

MRI is potentially harmful in patients who harbor certain clips used within the GI tract for endoscopic marking, hemostasis, or closure of GI tract luminal perforations.[109]

Many implanted orthopedic devices, including those made of titanium or titanium alloy and used for treatment of scoliosis or internal fixation of fractures, are nonferromagnetic or weakly ferromagnetic and have been demonstrated to be safe for 1.5-T or less MRI systems. For an implanted device that exhibits weakly ferromagnetic qualities (e.g.,

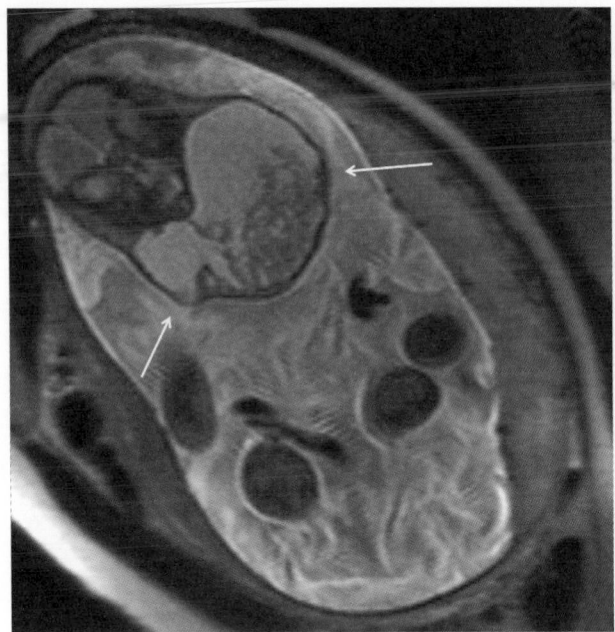
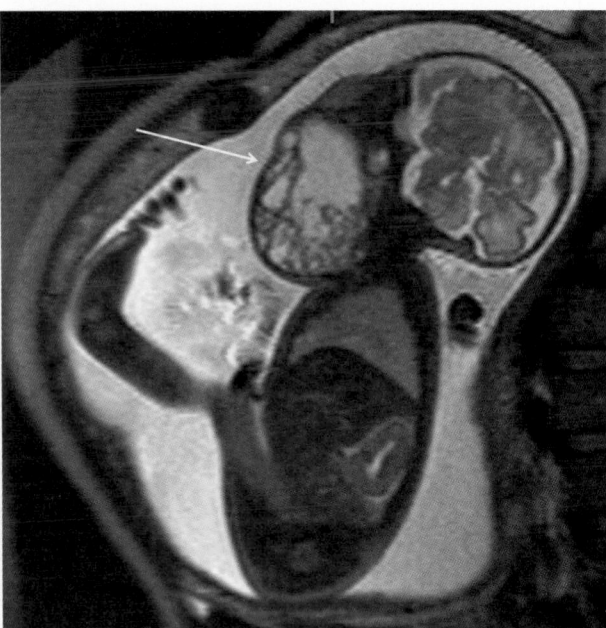

FIGURE 9.18 Prenatally diagnosed teratoma. Fast T2-weighted coronal (**A**) and sagittal (**B**) magnetic resonance images of a 31-week gestational-age fetus demonstrate a large multilocular cystic and solid neck mass (*arrows*) with compression of the airway.

certain intravascular and intracavitary stents, coils, occluders, filters), it is recommended to wait 6 to 8 weeks after implantation before exposure to an MRI operating at 1.5 T or less to provide time for retentive tissue ingrowth to occur. This waiting period may not be necessary in patients with implanted devices that are weakly ferromagnetic but rigidly fixed in the body, such as bone screws.

There are several caveats with regard to conducting MRI examinations in the presence of devices. Although the device may not experience significant motion from magnetic attraction, the device may be subject to heating or malfunction of electrically, magnetically, or mechanically activated components. In 1997, the FDA Center for Devices and Radiological Health proposed definitions for "MR safe" and "MR compatible" devices. *MR-safe* device means that the device presents no additional risk to the patient or other individuals in the MRI environment, and *MR-compatible* device means that operation of the device and quality of the diagnostic information are not significantly affected in the MRI environment. Even if safe, implanted devices can distort images, thereby limiting the diagnostic efficacy of the MRI examination. This is particularly germane in MRI examinations obtained for surveillance of local-regional recurrence of musculoskeletal neoplasms in patients with orthopedic implants. Device labels or product inserts can be misleading, because MR-safe and MR-compatible notations are specific to a particular MRI testing environment. Devices that display only weak magnetic field interactions in a 1.5-T MRI system may display substantially stronger, potentially dangerous interactions in a 3.0-T or higher MRI system. Because of physical differences in the position and magnitude of the highest spatial gradient, movement of a device in newer short-bore MRI systems can be considerably greater and potentially unsafe compared with that in conventional long-bore MRI systems. Therefore, careful consideration must be given to each object relative to the particular MRI system used and the conditions that are present for the individual prior to exposure to the MRI environment.

The MR Task Group of the American Society for Testing and Materials International introduced a new set of terms for devices in 2005.[110] *MR safe* is for items that pose no known hazards in all MRI environments. *MR conditional* is for items that pose no known hazards under specific conditions of use in a specified MRI environment. Any parameter that affects the safety of the item should be listed, and any condition that produces an unsafe condition must be described. *MR unsafe* is for items that pose hazards in all MRI environments. Unfortunately, this new terminology has not been applied retrospectively to devices that previously received FDA-approved labeling using the terms MR safe and MR compatible. Information on the safety of various devices is available at the Institute for Magnetic Resonance Safety, Education, and Research and on the MRIsafety.com Web site.

The risks of MRI fields are incurred not only by the patient being scanned but also by accompanying family members, health care professionals, and others (such as security and housekeeping personnel) who may find themselves in proximity to an MRI scanner. The gauss (G) line specifies the perimeter around an MR scanner within which the static magnetic fields are higher than 5 G. Static magnetic fields not exceeding 5 G are considered safe for the general public; those with cardiac pacemakers, implantable cardiac defibrillators, and other devices susceptible to malfunction in magnetic fields are recommended to stay beyond the 5-G line. Explicit guidelines for safe MRI practice, including screening of patients and personnel, are available from sources such as the American College of Radiology.[109,111]

Interventional Radiology

Like diagnostic radiology, interventional radiology has been the beneficiary of technologic advances that have broadened the contribution of radiologists to the diagnosis and management of pediatric cancers. Refinements in microcatheters, digital fluoroscopy, ultrasound, CT, and MRI have greatly increased the scope of what is feasible for image-guided

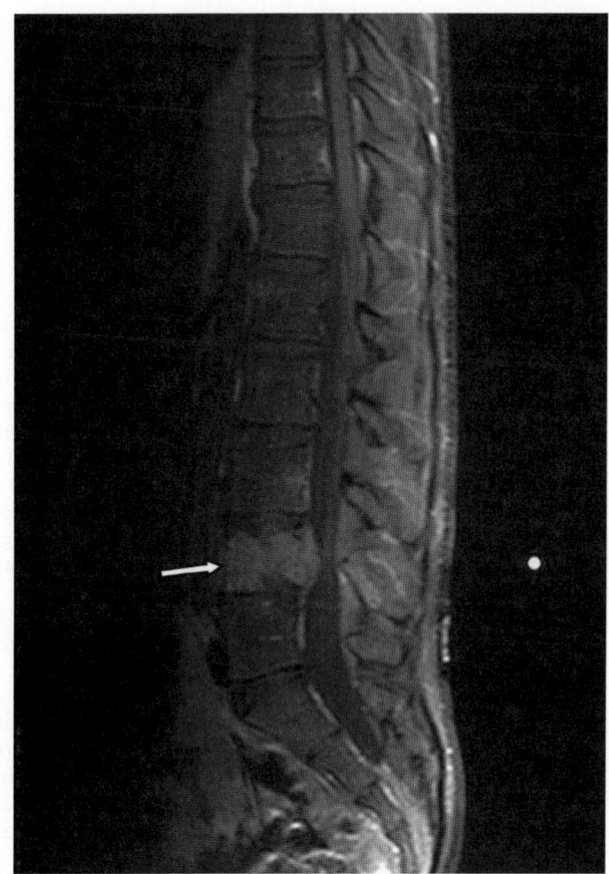

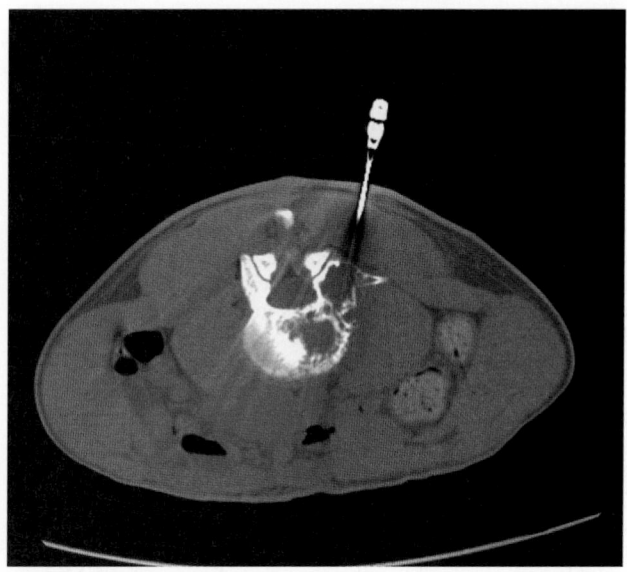

FIGURE 9.19 Alveolar soft parts sarcoma presenting in the spine. A sagittal gadolinium-enhanced T1-weighted image (**A**) demonstrates an enhancing, destructive lesion (*arrow*) of the L4 vertebra. Pathologic specimens adequate for diagnosis obtained via percutaneous computed tomography-guided needle biopsy (**B**) of the involved vertebra.

intervention. Recently developed flat-panel detectors, 3-D rotational angiography, and fast CT and MR fluoroscopy techniques have further facilitated image-guided intervention.

Image-guided percutaneous biopsy or aspiration provides a method of tissue sampling for tumor diagnosis or microorganism culture that is less invasive than surgical methods (Fig. 9.19). Almost any lesion of the neck, trunk, or extremities that is visible by imaging is amenable to sampling by interventional radiology procedures. The choice of imaging modality for guidance and method of tissue sampling depends on the interventional radiologist performing the procedure, the site of the lesion, the condition of the patient, and the type of specimen needed to make the diagnosis. In experienced hands, the procedures are generally safe, although they may require anesthesia in young children. In the case of thin-needle biopsies, cytological examination by an experienced pathologist is necessary to determine whether a lesion is benign or malignant. Often, the precise nature of a malignancy cannot be diagnosed, and for this reason, thin-needle biopsies have been more useful for the determination of recurrent disease than primary diagnosis. If a specific histologic diagnosis is needed from a percutaneous biopsy, larger-bore aspiration needles or cutting needles are used to obtain core biopsy specimens. A recent systematic review of image-guided percutaneous core needle biopsies of pediatric tumors cited a pooled diagnostic accuracy rate of 94% in cases with adequate material.[112] For these procedures, the rate of complications, such as bleeding requiring blood transfusion or pneumothorax requiring chest tube placement, is approximately 1%.[112] These procedures, like all other image-guided interventions, should be performed by an experienced radiologist who is capable of treating potential complications.

The major limitations of percutaneous biopsy are related to sampling problems and specimen inadequacy. Although image-guided percutaneous core needle biopsies of childhood tumors provide an adequate sample for specific diagnosis in 95% of cases,[112] performance of biological studies mandated by some cancer cooperative group clinical trial protocols may require relatively large volumes of tissue. Coordination between the interventional radiologist and pathologist is required for appropriate tissue sampling, handling, and processing to produce adequate specimens for diagnostic pathologic evaluation. Close communication with the oncologist and surgeon is also desirable to plan the path of the biopsy needle through tissue that would be surgically removed if the lesion was malignant, to avoid seeding of the biopsy tract with tumor cells.

Interventional radiology techniques also can be used to localize small lesions for subsequent surgical biopsy or resection. CT or ultrasound can be used to guide needle localization of small soft tissue masses. Preoperative CT localization of pulmonary nodules with methylene blue injection allows small pulmonary nodules or those not located near the pleural surface to be identified and resected thoracoscopically rather than via a more morbid thoracotomy.[113]

There are indications other than tumor diagnosis for image-guided biopsy in pediatric oncology patients. Percutaneous image-guided lung biopsy can help determine the etiology of pulmonary infiltrates or nodules in immunocompromised patients less invasively than open, thoracoscopic, or transbronchial lung biopsy. In pediatric patients who have undergone bone marrow transplantation and in whom graft-versus-host disease (GVHD) or hepatic veno-occlusive disease (HVOD) is a clinical concern, a liver biopsy may be safely performed via a transjugular approach, when percutaneous liver biopsy is contraindicated because of thrombocytopenia, coagulopathy, or ascites.[114]

Interventional radiology plays a role in not only the diagnosis but also the therapy of pediatric oncology patients. Preoperative transcatheter selective arterial chemoembolization can be used to induce surgical resectability of previously unresectable hepatoblastoma, especially in patients without distant metastases.[115] Transcatheter arterial chemoembolization has also been used to successfully treat liver disease in progressive stage 4s neuroblastoma.[116] Transcatheter embolization may be used to occlude arteriovenous shunts in infantile hepatic vascular tumors associated with high-output congestive heart failure refractory to medical therapy.[117] Image-guided tumor ablation with chemical agents (e.g., ethanol, acetic acid), thermal energy (e.g., RF, microwave, laser, cryogen), or radiation (e.g., yttrium-90 microsphere radioembolization) are emerging methods for symptom palliation and local tumor control. Ongoing experience suggests that this technique is a viable therapeutic option in children with primary and metastatic tumors of the liver, lung, kidney, and skeleton that are not amenable to surgery, chemotherapy, or radiotherapy.[114] Multiple lesions may be treated at one session, with the number of lesions treated limited by the patient's overall condition and the potential risk of renal insufficiency induced by tumor lysis, hemoglobinuria, and myoglobinuria. Potential complications and side effects include injury to adjacent structures, such as bile ducts, bowel, and renal collecting systems, and pain or postablation syndrome, which can include low-grade fever and malaise lasting for several days.

Interventional radiologists are active in the treatment of complications of tumors and tumor therapy. Such treatments include, but are not limited to, relief or diversion of biliary and urinary tract obstruction, percutaneous abscess drainage, and angioplasty, stenting, or endovascular fibrinolysis for vascular occlusive disease. In addition, radiologists place chest tubes, enteric feeding tubes, and central vascular catheters. Tunneled central vascular catheter placement in pediatric oncology patients has been associated with a lower rate of infection and mechanical complications when performed by image-guided radiology techniques than by surgery.[118]

Interventional radiology procedures involving fluoroscopy or CT for guidance can be associated with relatively high doses of ionizing radiation. In some instances, high doses can induce skin erythema, desquamation, and epilation. These deterministic effects may not present for up to several weeks after the irradiation. Patients receiving more than 3 Gy skin entrance dose should be identified and asked to return for a follow-up examination in 30 days to monitor for these effects. Pediatric oncology patients undergo repeated diagnostic radiology studies during the course of their disease, and interventional radiology procedures are a potential contributor to large cumulative radiation exposures in these patients. It is important that such procedures be performed by interventional radiologists cognizant of the ALARA principle and methods of radiation dose optimization in these patients.[119]

GENERAL CONCEPTS OF PEDIATRIC TUMOR IMAGING

Imaging plays an important role in guiding clinical management of childhood cancer. This includes detection of conditions requiring emergent or urgent treatment, diagnosis, staging of disease burden and extent for risk stratification, determination of optimal therapy, and assessment of response

to antitumor therapy. Imaging also serves as a method of surveillance for tumor relapse and complications of therapy. Details of the diagnostic imaging of specific tumors are discussed in other chapters of this text. Some basic guidelines for the diagnostic imaging of children with malignancies are offered at this juncture.

Detection of Conditions Requiring Emergent or Urgent Treatment

Although prompt initiation of tumor-specific therapy is an important objective in treating pediatric malignancies, especially tumors that grow rapidly, some patients present with conditions identified by imaging that require urgent or emergent management before definitive diagnostic workup and tumor-specific therapy. For example, spinal MRI obtained for paraplegia or nerve palsy may reveal spinal cord or nerve compression by an intraspinal or perineural tumor (Fig. 9.15). A head CT or MRI performed to evaluate acute neurologic symptoms or signs may demonstrate hydrocephalus or brain herniation related to mass effect from an intracranial tumor or demonstrate cerebral hemorrhage or infarction due to intravascular leukostasis or thrombocytopenia associated with acute leukemia[120] (Fig. 9.20).

Airway obstruction can result from pharyngeal, neck, or thoracic tumors, and substantial narrowing of the airway can occur without signs of respiratory compromise during breathing at rest. Life-threatening upper airway obstruction during general anesthesia or heavy sedation is a potential complication of a large anterior mediastinal mass, most commonly

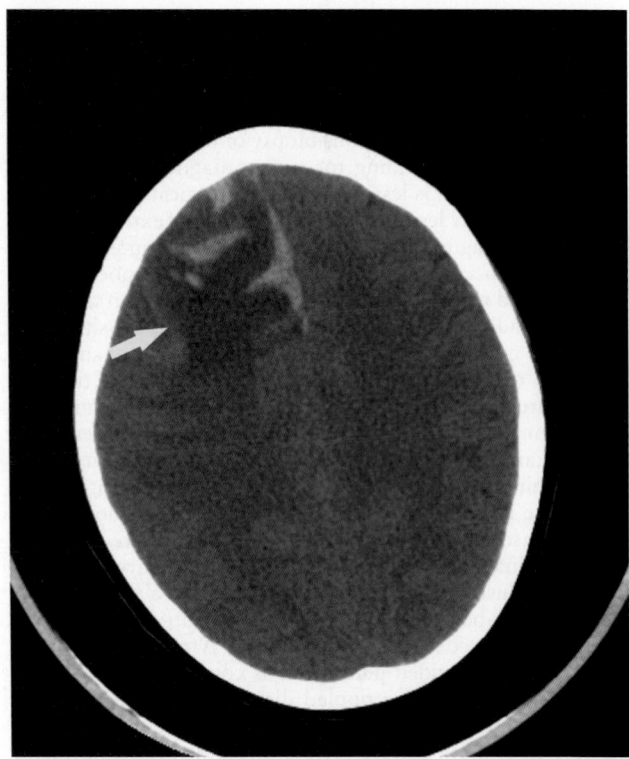

FIGURE 9.20 Acute myelogenous leukemia presenting with cerebral infarction. An axial image from a head computed tomography examination obtained without contrast shows hemorrhagic infarction in the right frontal lobe (*arrow*) consequent to incomplete sagittal sinus and cortical venous thrombosis.

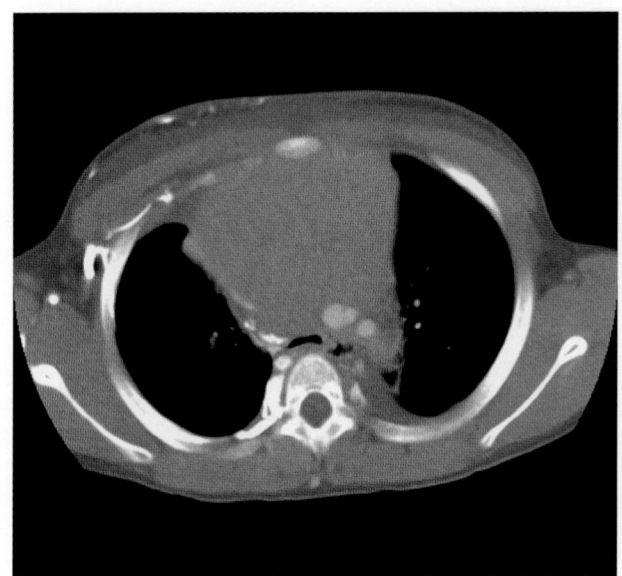 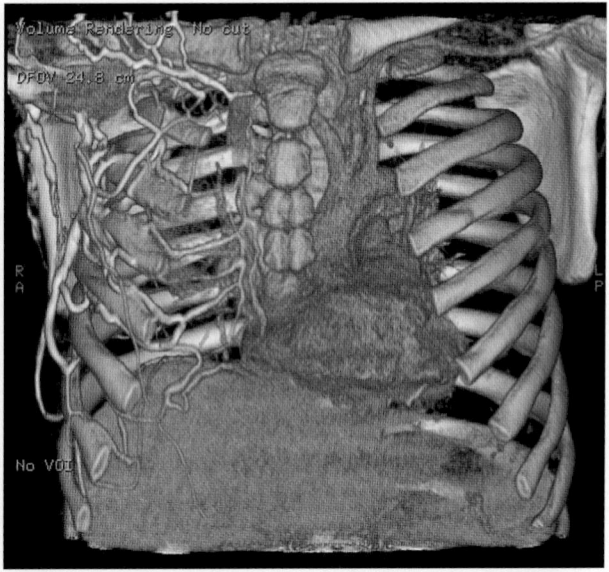

FIGURE 9.21 T-cell acute lymphoblastic leukemia. Axial contrast-enhanced computed tomography (CT) image (**A**) showing a large anterior mediastinal mass effacing the superior vena cava and brachiocephalic veins and displacing and narrowing the airway. Prominent right-sided collateral venous channels are clearly depicted on a three-dimensional volume-rendered CT image (**B**).

lymphoma or acute lymphoblastic leukemia (ALL), and patency of the airway should be assessed before biopsies or other procedures requiring anesthesia or sedation in a patient with a large anterior mediastinal mass[121] (Fig. 9.21). Chest radiographs with a lateral view can provide a gross estimate of the degree of airway compression by a mediastinal mass (Fig. 9.22). Chest CT scan is the most accurate imaging modality for assessing the degree of airway compression and can be used to quantitate the reduction of the cross-sectional area of the trachea and the degree of mainstem bronchi compression to predict the risk of complications with anesthesia or sedation. Those at high risk can be directed toward less invasive interventional radiology procedures requiring only local anesthesia, or steroids can be administered to shrink certain mediastinal masses prior to general anesthesia or deep sedation.[122] Chest imaging can also reveal the presence of a large pericardial or pleural effusion, superior vena cava occlusion, pulmonary mass, or pneumothorax posing risk of cardiorespiratory compromise. Although not necessarily requiring emergent treatment, occlusion or narrowing of the brachiocephalic veins, subclavian veins, or internal jugular veins by an adjacent mass is important to note on imaging, because this may affect the approach to placement of a central vascular catheter, which many pediatric oncology patients require for treatment.

Bowel obstruction, hemorrhage, and perforation are potential complications of GI tract tumors. Intestinal lymphoma may present as an intussusception, particularly in an older child with lymphadenopathy (Fig. 9.23). Such an intussusception may be difficult to treat via fluoroscopy-guided pneumatic or hydrostatic reduction. Also, it may recur after reduction, necessitating surgical intervention. Infants with stage 4s neuroblastoma may present with life-threatening respiratory and cardiovascular compromise related to massive hepatomegaly that is evident on imaging and necessitates remedial measures such as abdominal decompression surgery.[123]

Urinary tract obstruction related to retroperitoneal or pelvic tumors is important to identify, because untreated urinary tract obstruction impairs the diuresis desired to reduce the effects of acute tumor lysis syndrome, especially with a large tumor burden. Detection of urinary tract obstruction by imaging prior to therapy allows remedial measures such as dialysis or urinary diversion to be instituted. Biliary tract obstruction may develop secondary to intraductal, periportal, or pancreatic head masses (Fig. 9.24). Successful biliary drainage can be accomplished by interventional radiology techniques[124] and allow for initial chemotherapy and more conservative surgery, but the presence of malignant biliary tract obstruction does not always mandate an invasive biliary drainage procedure. For tumors such as Burkitt's lymphoma that respond rapidly to chemotherapy, the obstruction also rapidly resolves, and invasive biliary drainage procedures, which are often associated with complications, may be avoided.[125]

Occlusion of the inferior vena cava, hepatic veins, renal veins, pelvic veins, or lower extremity veins in the setting of tumor can arise from thrombosis, extrinsic mass effect, or intravascular tumor extension, as is most frequently encountered in the renal veins and inferior vena cava in children with Wilms' tumor (Fig. 9.25). Although not always possible by imaging, differentiating among the etiologies of vascular occlusion influences the decision about whether anticoagulation should be instituted.

Primary tumor or metastatic disease involving certain skeletal sites can result in morbid complications if not identified by imaging and appropriate remedial measures are not instituted. Tumor involvement of significant weight-bearing sites, such as the proximal femurs, acetabulae, or vertebrae, or sites exposed to significant distractive forces, such as the proximal humeri, portends a risk of pathologic fracture. The telangiectatic form of osteosarcoma is associated with a particularly high rate of pathologic fracture.[126] Restriction of weight-bearing or orthopedic instrumentation can be implemented to prevent a pathologic fracture. Pathologic fracture of a long bone in osteosarcoma or Ewing's sarcoma complicates orthopedic management but does not necessarily mandate amputation instead of a limb-salvage procedure.[127]

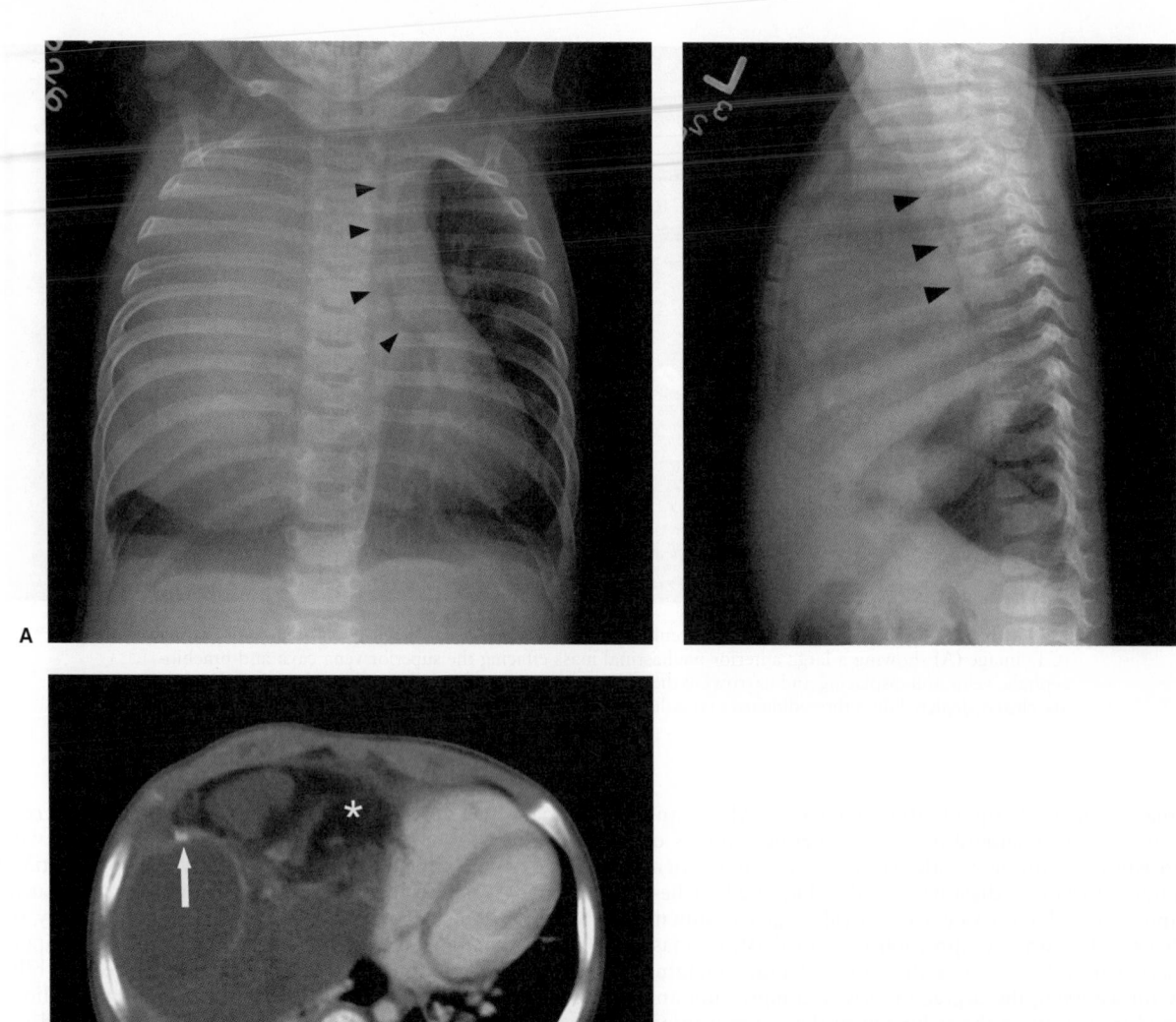

FIGURE 9.22 Teratoma. Anteroposterior (**A**) and lateral (**B**) chest radiographs demonstrate a large anterior mediastinal mass lesion displacing the heart leftward and compressing and displacing the airway (*arrowheads*). An axial contrast-enhanced computed tomography image (**C**) depicts a mixed solid and cystic mass containing fat (*asterisk*) and calcification (*arrow*), characteristic of a teratoma.

Diagnosis

Central Nervous System Tumors

Although cranial CT is a good tool for evaluating the CNS of children with neurologic symptoms and most pediatric CNS tumors can be visualized by CT, MRI is the tool of choice for diagnosis of CNS neoplasms in children. Most CNS tumors in childhood after infancy and prior to the teenage years are located in the posterior cranial fossa, and MRI is superior to CT for evaluation of these lesions, in part because of artifacts related to bone on CT scans. The benefit of MRI over CT in supratentorial tumor diagnosis is not as great, and CT can be used to screen for most of these tumors in the setting of a low clinical likelihood of tumor, but MRI is indicated if there are specific signs or symptoms of a supratentorial mass. Not only is MRI superior to CT for detection of posterior fossa tumors but also it is better for evaluation of tumor extent and presurgical planning. CT remains of some limited value in recognizing intratumoral calcification and in detecting bony involve-

ment of the calvarium, skull base, orbits, or sinonasal apparatus. Ultrasound can be used to screen for a supratentorial mass in young infants.

Although no imaging study can replace the histopathologic diagnosis of CNS tumors, the type of CNS tumor, in many cases, can be predicted prior to surgical intervention by MRI on the basis of the site of origin, signal characteristics, and pattern of spread[78] (Fig. 9.12). PET can help discriminate benign from malignant brain lesions, because higher-grade, aggressive tumors typically have greater FDG uptake than do lower-grade tumors or dysplastic brain tissue, which may appear isometabolic or hypometabolic compared with normal brain tissue.[128]

CNS leukemia can involve the leptomeninges, brain parenchyma, or cerebral vasculature. Abnormal enhancement of the meninges and nerve roots in a child with leukemia suggests leptomeningeal involvement, even if CSF cytologic studies are negative. Small intraparenchymal hemorrhages are occasionally the initial manifestation of acute childhood leukemia.[129]

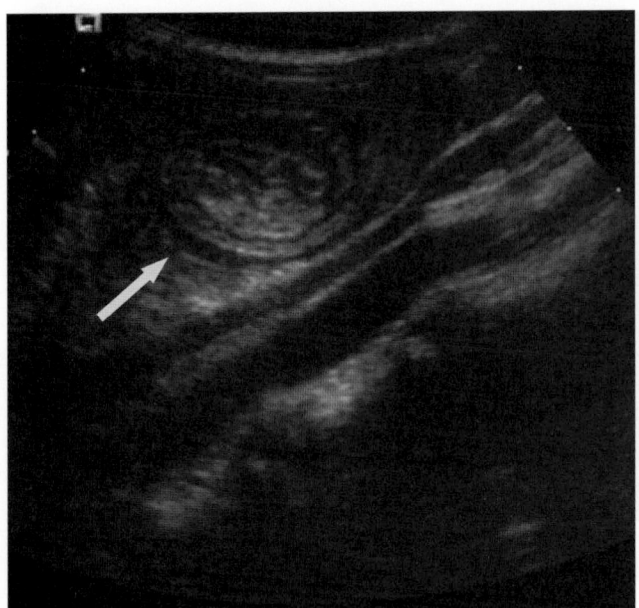 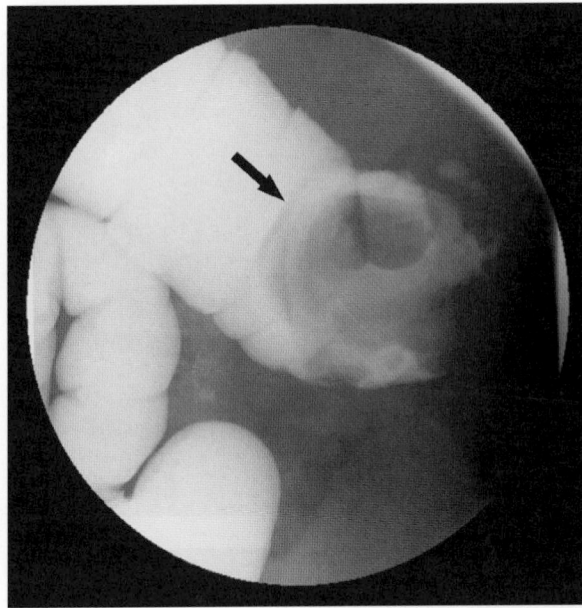

FIGURE 9.23 Burkitt's lymphoma presenting with intussusception in an 8-year-old child. Abdominal ultrasound image (**A**) shows an intussusception (*arrow*). Spot image (**B**) obtained during attempted hydrostatic reduction with water-soluble contrast shows a large filling defect in the colon (*arrow*) representing the intussusceptum in the intussuscipiens. Complete reduction of the intussusception was not possible, and Burkitt's lymphoma was revealed at surgery as the pathologic lead point mass.

Spinal tumors comprise approximately 10% of CNS neoplasms in childhood and are best differentiated by imaging according to their location as intramedullary, extramedullary intradural, or extradural. MRI has also become the modality of choice for diagnosing lesions of the spinal cord and its coverings. Astrocytomas, ependymomas, and gangliogliomas compose the vast majority of intramedullary tumors. Contrast-enhanced MRI helps differentiate intramedullary tumor from adjacent edema or demyelination, and homogeneous gadolinium enhancement on MRI correlates with lower-grade pathology of spinal tumors.[130] MRI sequences sensitive to blood products can detect superficial siderosis of the cord, which suggests ependymoma due to its tendency to hemorrhage. The most common intradural extramedullary tumors are nerve sheath tumors and metastases, most commonly "drop" metastases from primary brain tumors, particularly medulloblastoma, primitive neuroectodermal tumor (PNET), ependymoma, high-grade astrocytoma, and pineoblastoma. Contrast-enhanced MRI is approximately 95% sensitive for the detection of drop metastases. Extradural tumors account for the majority of intraspinal tumors in childhood and are most commonly neuroblastomas, Ewing's sarcomas, rhabdomyosarcomas, lymphomas (Fig. 9.15), histiocytoses, metastases, or primary vertebral bony tumors such as osteoblastomas and aneurysmal bone cysts.[131]

Extracranial Head and Neck Tumors

Most neck masses in children are of a congenital or inflammatory nature rather than neoplastic, and the optimal imaging approach depends on the most likely etiology of the mass, as determined by clinical evaluation. The location of the mass and the nature of the mass as solid or cystic are key factors in formulating an appropriate differential diagnosis. Ultrasound is particularly useful in determining whether a mass is cystic or solid. In the case of a suspected neoplasm in the neck, CT and/or MRI are used to assess for lymphadenopathy, airway compression, vascular encasement, perineural spread, bone involvement, and intracranial or intraspinal extension.[132]

An anterior midline or paramedian cystic mass is typically a thyroglossal duct cyst or dermoid cyst, and the cystic nature can be confirmed with ultrasound. Branchial cleft cysts and thymopharyngeal duct cysts are more laterally located and have characteristic positions in relation to the neck musculature and vasculature. A congenital neck mass with solid and cystic components is most commonly a teratoma.

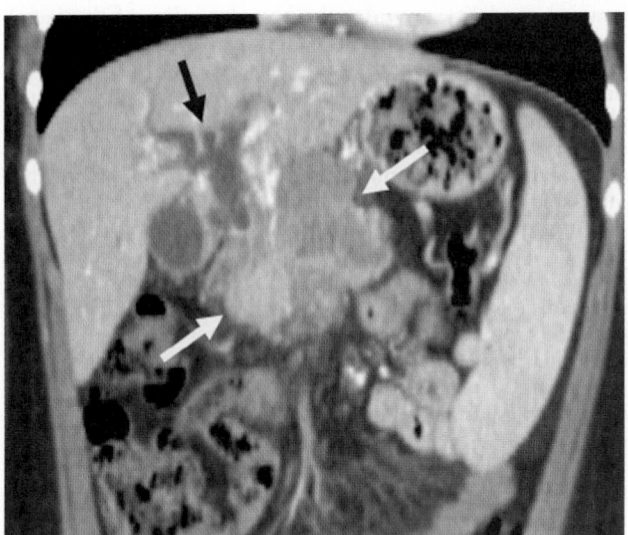

FIGURE 9.24 Pancreatoblastoma in a girl with abdominal pain and jaundice. Coronal contrast-enhanced computed tomography image shows marked biliary ductal dilatation (*black arrow*) due to biliary obstruction by a pancreas head mass (*white arrows*).

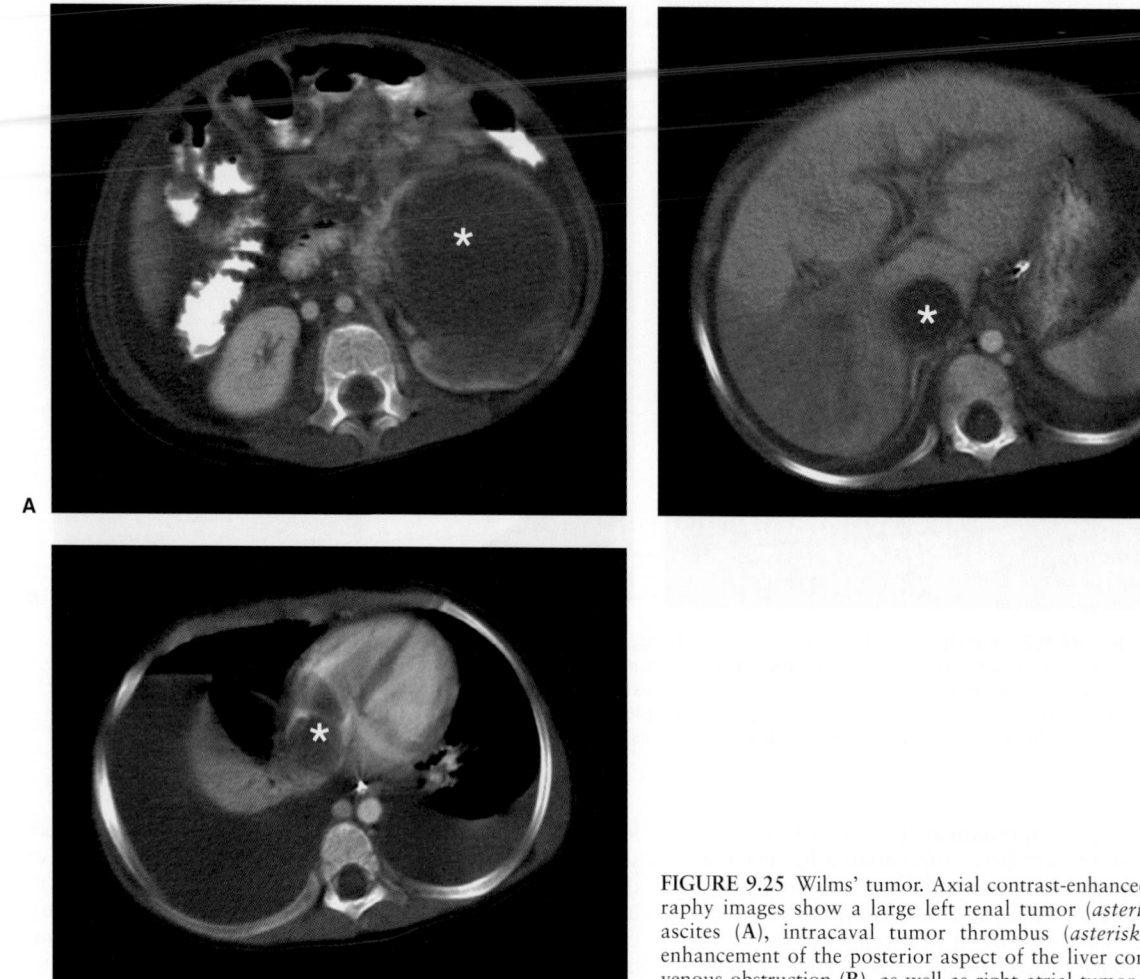

FIGURE 9.25 Wilms' tumor. Axial contrast-enhanced computed tomography images show a large left renal tumor (*asterisk*) with abundant ascites (**A**), intracaval tumor thrombus (*asterisk*), and diminished enhancement of the posterior aspect of the liver consequent to hepatic venous obstruction (**B**), as well as right atrial tumor thrombus (*asterisk*) and large bilateral pleural effusions (**C**).

The two most common solid malignant tumors in the extracranial head and neck in children are lymphoma and rhabdomyosarcoma. CT is used to assess lymphoma, and MRI is preferred to evaluate intracranial extension in solid tumors associated with bony destruction of the skull base or calvarium, including rhabdomyosarcoma, metastatic neuroblastoma, and Langerhans' cell histiocytosis.[133] Parameningeal spread may occur from rhabdomyosarcomas arising in the sinonasal apparatus, middle ear, orbits, or nasopharynx. Nasopharyngeal carcinoma is rare in children and tends to be locally advanced at the time of clinical presentation. The presence of an asymmetric mass with central skull base invasion, parapharyngeal space invasion, or lateral retropharyngeal lymphadenopathy on images distinguishes malignancy from benign adenoidal hypertrophy[134] (Fig. 9.26).

The finding of an intensely enhancing solid mass on CT or MRI in the nasopharyngeal region of an adolescent boy is highly suggestive of juvenile nasal angiofibroma.

A mass in the anterior or inferior periauricular region can represent a parotid gland tumor. The presence of multiple or bilateral parotid masses strongly suggests the diagnosis of Warthin's tumor (papillary cystadenoma lymphomatosum). Warthin's tumor may demonstrate increased uptake on FDG-PET and Tc-99m pertechnetate and Th-201 scintigraphy. Mucoepidermoid carcinoma is the most common malignant salivary gland neoplasm in children and can have a misleadingly benign appearance on ultrasound, CT, and MRI. In the

case of a suspected parotid gland neoplasm, facial nerve involvement should be evaluated with MRI, because this imaging modality provides the best depiction of the facial nerve. To avoid misdiagnosis of infiltrative parotid tumor, it is important to recognize the progressive fatty infiltration that normally occurs as children age. An accessory parotid gland can be confused for a neoplastic mass, but knowledge of its typical location (superficial to the masseter muscle and anterior to the main parotid gland) can help avoid this mistake.[135]

Cervical lymph node enlargement is a common cause of a neck mass in children. Most frequently, this mass represents reactive hyperplasia or lymphadenitis related to head and neck infections. Ultrasound is used to confirm cervical adenitis and evaluate suppurative changes. In the setting of cervical lymph node enlargement in which lymphoma or other neoplasms are a concern, CT or MRI is frequently performed to better define the extent of lymphadenopathy, including possible mediastinal extension.

To avoid unnecessary concern or biopsy, it is important not to confuse fibromatosis colli for a neoplastic mass. Fibromatosis colli classically presents as a mass along the anterior neck during the first few weeks to months after birth, often in association with torticollis. Sonographic demonstration of a heterogeneously echoic mass-like swelling along the sternocleidomastoid muscle and a normal appearance of the adjacent soft tissues help confirm the diagnosis of fibromatosis

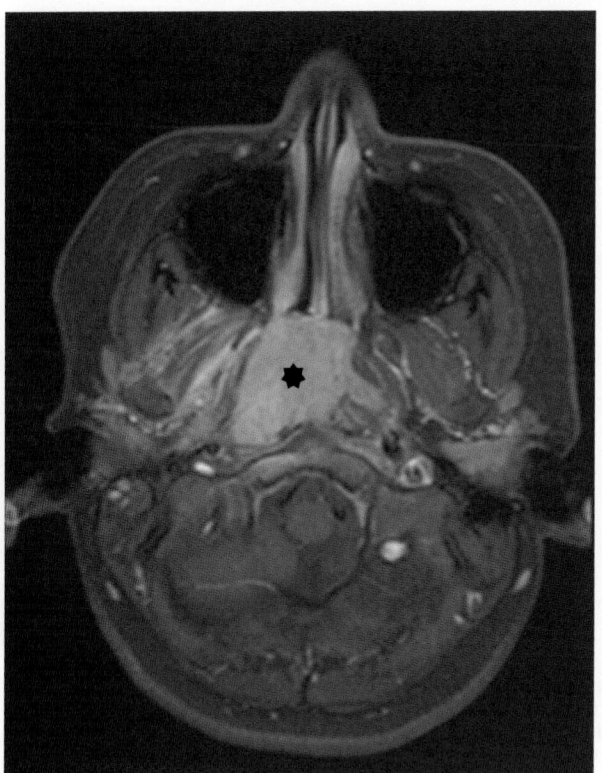

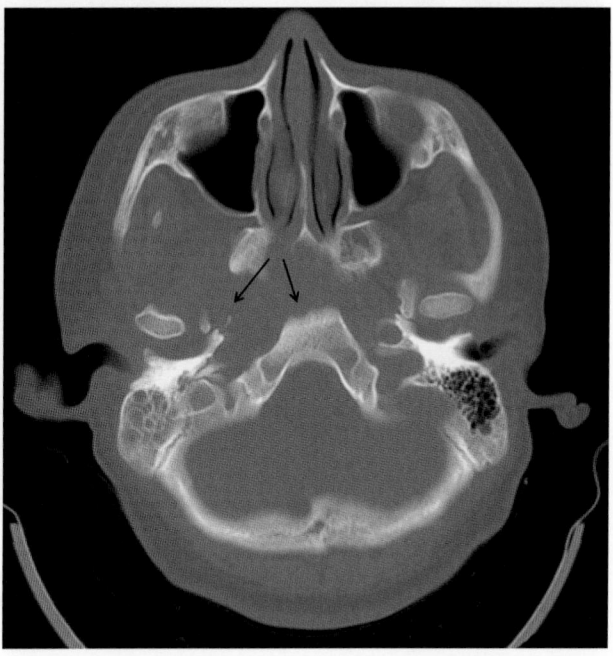

FIGURE 9.26 Nasopharyngeal carcinoma. Axial gadolinium-enhanced T1-weighted magnetic resonance image (**A**) shows a soft tissue mass (*asterisk*) asymmetrically occupying the nasopharynx and invading the skull base. Petroclival sphenoid bone destruction (*arrows*) is better depicted on an axial computed tomography image at bone windows (**B**).

colli.[136] Ectopic cervical thymic rests are usually an incidental finding noted on neck imaging, and misdiagnosis of a neoplasm can be avoided by recognition of their characteristic imaging appearance, although an intrathyroidal location can be difficult to distinguish from other more common causes of a thyroid nodule.[137]

Vascular malformations and vascular tumors are a common cause of an extracranial head or neck mass. Vascular malformations are classified on the basis of their endothelial characteristics as arterial, capillary, venous, lymphatic, or combined.[138] Vascular malformations are present at birth and grow commensurately with the child, in some cases, causing morbid complications due to impingement on vital structures. Vascular malformations are not restricted to the head and neck and are commonly seen in the axillary regions and extremities. MRI is preferred for the imaging of vascular malformations because of its superior ability to depict lesion extent and distinguish venous from lymphatic malformations on the basis of enhancement of the fluid-filled spaces of the former but not of the latter after the administration of the intravenous contrast (Fig. 9.27). The finding of phleboliths within a lesion also helps establish a diagnosis of venous malformation. Hemangiomas of infancy are vascular tumors that appear during early infancy, undergo a proliferative phase, and then involute. Most hemangiomas of infancy occur in the cervicofacial region and have an especially high incidence in premature infants of low birth weight. On MRI or CT, hemangiomas appear as intensely enhancing solid masses with prominent high-flow vessels[139] (Fig. 9.28). Congenital hemangiomas are vascular tumors that arise *in utero* and postnatally can be rapidly involuting or noninvoluting. Kaposiform hemangioendotheliomas are pediatric vascular tumors that

are histologically intermediate between hemangiomas and angiosarcomas and are responsible for most cases of Kasabach-Merritt syndrome with profound thrombocytopenia. MRI is useful for defining their extent.[140]

Thyroid nodules or goiter can present as a neck mass. Neck irradiation for a childhood malignancy is a risk factor for development of thyroid carcinoma.[141] Ultrasound is the preferred modality for evaluating the thyroid gland for nodules (Fig. 9.29). Tiny cysts within the thyroid are frequently seen and usually represent benign colloid cysts. Nearly 70% of solid solitary thyroid nodules represent follicular adenomas. However, thyroid nodules cannot be reliably distinguished as benign or malignant on the basis of sonographic findings. Thyroid scintigraphy is also of limited value in distinguishing benign and malignant thyroid nodules, because not all malignant nodules are "cold," and only 20% of cold nodules in children are malignant.[142,143] An underappreciated cause of a cold thyroid nodule is an intrathyroidal ectopic thymic rest related to aberrant migration of thymic tissue.[144] It is important to avoid CT imaging with iodinated intravenous contrast in patients with suspected or known thyroid cancer when subsequent diagnostic imaging or therapy with radioiodine is to be performed, because contaminant free iodides in the contrast can result in saturation of tissues, decreasing the avidity of thyroid cancer cells for subsequent radioiodine for several weeks.[145] Gadolinium contrast medium does not have the same effect, so gadolinium contrast-enhanced MRI may be performed without reservation in these patients.[146]

Prompt diagnosis and treatment of ocular or orbital tumors is crucial, because these lesions threaten vision. The most common malignant tumor of the globe is retinoblastoma, which usually presents before 2 years of age and is

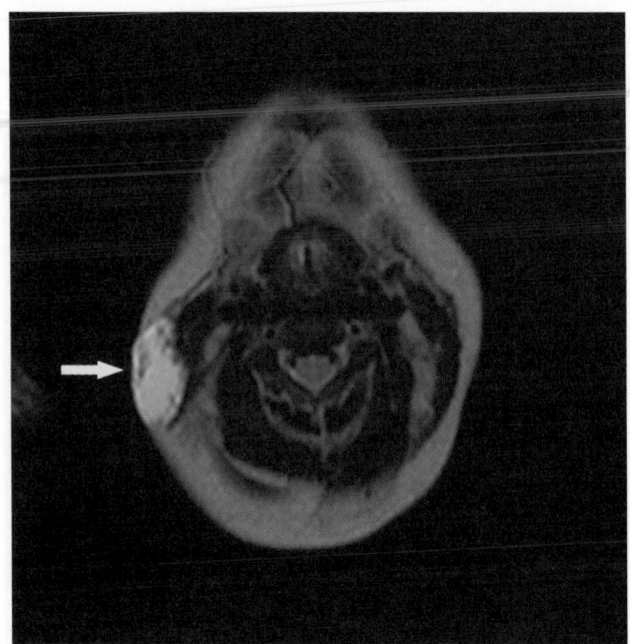
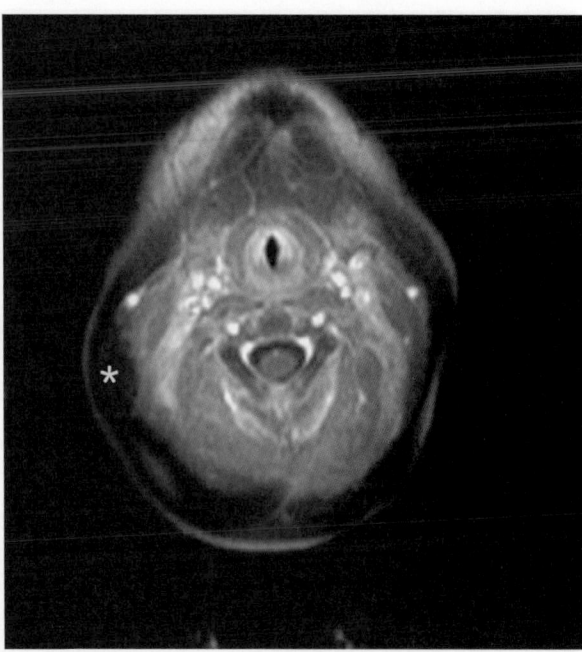

FIGURE 9.27 Lymphatic malformation. Axial T2-weighted magnetic resonance (MR) image (**A**) demonstrates a high-signal intensity lesion (*arrow*) abutting the right sternocleidomastoid muscle. **B:** The lesion (*asterisk*) demonstrates no internal enhancement following gadolinium administration on an axial T1-weighted MR image.

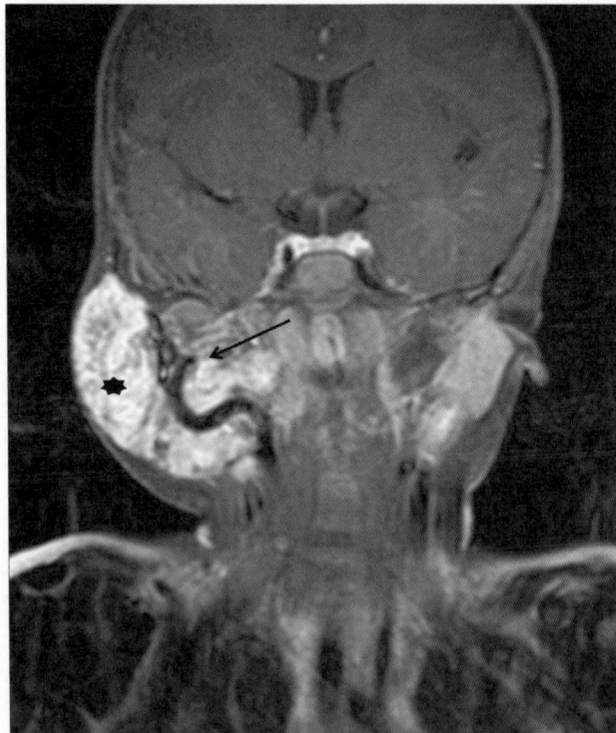

FIGURE 9.28 Hemangioma of infancy in the proliferative phase. A coronal gadolinium-enhanced T1-weighted magnetic resonance image demonstrates an intensely enhancing soft tissue mass (*asterisk*) in the right facial region supplied by branches of an enlarged right external carotid artery (*arrow*).

associated with a mutation in the *RB1* tumor suppressor gene. The germline form is more likely to be multifocal and bilateral and is associated with a high risk of second malignant neoplasms. Those with germline retinoblastoma are at particularly high risk of a midline intracranial tumor, typically in the pineal region and less commonly in the suprasellar cistern or fourth ventricle. Such patients are said to have trilateral retinoblastoma and are at high risk of morbidity and mortality from leptomeningeal tumor dissemination, even in the absence of progression of the midline intracranial tumor.[147]

More than half of patients with retinoblastoma present with leukocoria. This is not a specific finding for retinoblastoma; leukocoria also occurs in nonmalignant processes such as retinal astrocytic hamartomas, Coats' disease, toxocariasis, persistent primary hyperplastic vitreous, and retinopathy of prematurity. Retinoblastomas calcify in approximately 95% of cases, a useful distinction, because other causes of leukocoria

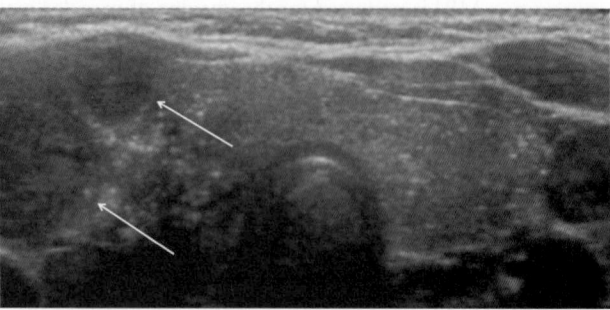

FIGURE 9.29 Multicentric papillary thyroid carcinoma. Thyroid ultrasound examination shows multiple hypoechoic nodules (*arrows*) in the right lobe of the thyroid gland. Sonography is excellent at identifying thyroid nodules but tissue sampling is required to reliably distinguish nodules as benign or malignant in histology.

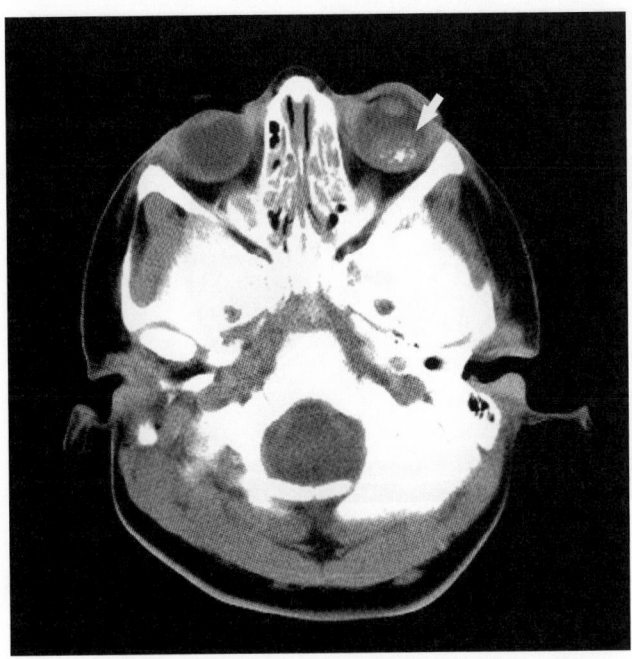

FIGURE 9.30 Retinoblastoma. Axial computed tomography image of the head shows a calcified soft tissue mass (*arrow*) in the left globe, which is characteristic of retinoblastoma.

calcify less frequently and less vigorously. CT is particularly sensitive for detecting these calcifications (Fig. 9.30). However, MRI is the preferred imaging modality for detecting extraocular and intracranial spread and trilateral disease with leptomeningeal dissemination.[148]

As many as half of all cases of acute leukemia involve ocular manifestations, and the most frequent finding is retinal hemorrhage. Retinal hemorrhages related to leukemia are usually bilateral and located in the posterior pole.[129] Orbital chloromas (granulocytic sarcoma, extramedullary leukemia) are seen primarily with acute myelogenous leukemia and can be a presenting sign preceding the blast phase.[149] Extraocular intraorbital malignancies include chloroma, rhabdomyosarcoma, optic nerve glioma, and orbital bony involvement by neuroblastoma metastases and Langerhans' cell histiocytosis.[150] Most extraocular intraorbital masses in childhood are benign; these include hemangiomas, vascular malformations, retro-orbital colobomatous cysts, and dermoid and epidermoid cysts. These lesions often have characteristic imaging features that allow distinction by CT or MRI.

Thoracic Tumors

Most pediatric malignancies involving the pulmonary parenchyma are metastatic in nature and are discussed in the portion of this chapter devoted to tumor staging. Primary malignancies of the lungs and bronchi, such as pleuropulmonary blastomas, bronchial carcinoids (Fig. 9.11), and bronchogenic carcinoma, are very rare in children. They are typically diagnosed by conventional radiography and CT imaging. The cystic form of pleuropulmonary blastoma can be indistinguishable from the large cyst form of congenital cystic adenomatoid or pulmonary airway malformations on imaging and gross pathology (Fig. 9.31), and many previous reports of malignancy developing in a congenital lung cyst most likely represented progression of cystic pleuropulmonary blastoma. A substantial proportion of pleuropulmonary blastomas are associated with a susceptibility syndrome in the patient (or

family) for certain dysplastic or neoplastic conditions, including cystic nephromas, ovarian stromal sex cord tumors, seminomas, and intestinal polyps. Cystic pleuropulmonary blastomas are characterized by multifocality and spontaneous pneumothorax, and excision of congenital lung cysts associated with these conditions during infancy is advocated because of the probability that they represent pleuropulmonary blastoma.[151] Juvenile-onset recurrent respiratory papillomatosis caused by human papilloma virus is associated with airway papillomas and occasional pulmonary involvement manifesting as cavitary lung nodules and an elevated risk of squamous cell bronchogenic carcinoma at an early age[152] (Fig. 9.32). The initial imaging appearance of round pneumonia can be confused with a primary or metastatic pulmonary tumor; however, round pneumonia is usually readily distinguished on clinical grounds, though follow-up imaging is warranted if the clinical presentation or course is not typical.

Primary tumors of the mediastinum are best defined by the compartment in which they arise. Tumors arising in the posterior mediastinum are largely of neurogenic origin, with neuroblastoma being the most common malignant tumor (Fig. 9.33). Rib erosion, widening of spinal neural foramina, and calcification of the mass are conventional radiographic signs that suggest neuroblastoma. Although the differential diagnosis is extensive, common benign lesions have radiographic features that usually differentiate them from neuroblastoma, ganglioneuroma, and ganglioneuroblastoma. Neurenteric cysts, for instance, are associated with congenital anomalies of the thoracic spine, whereas neurofibromas are frequently associated with acute-angle scoliosis and multiple small paraspinous masses at several levels along the spine. Calcifications are also absent in these two benign conditions.

Cross-sectional imaging is essential in the evaluation of a possible posterior mediastinal neuroblastoma. CT is often performed because of logistical issues and is frequently sufficient, although MRI is the best test for detecting nodal or chest wall involvement and intraspinal extension.[153] CT can strongly suggest neuroblastoma by depicting calcification within the mass (90% of neuroblastomas are calcified on CT, but only 50% are calcified on conventional radiographs). MRI is less sensitive than CT for detecting intratumoral calcification.

The middle mediastinum or hilar regions may be involved by lymphadenopathy secondary to leukemia or lymphoma, but this rarely occurs in the absence of anterior mediastinal lymphadenopathy or thymic infiltration. Plexiform neurofibromas and inflammatory myofibroblastic pseudotumors may involve the middle mediastinum or hila as large infiltrating masses. Although nonmalignant, these entities can grow aggressively and cause significant morbidity or mortality due to involvement of the tracheobronchial tree, esophagus, or great vessels.[154] CT and/or MRI are the desired imaging modalities for evaluation of the middle mediastinum and hila.[155] In CT evaluation of the mediastinum, intravenous contrast should be used when feasible to distinguish vascular structures from enlarged nodes or other soft tissue masses. MRI has the advantage of being able to distinguish vascular structures from nodes or other soft tissue masses without the use of intravenous contrast. MRI is particularly useful in depicting and sometimes differentiating benign and malignant cardiac and paracardiac masses, and advances in MRI technology have made MRI superior to echocardiography in the evaluation of many cardiac masses.[156] CT is preferable to MRI when evaluation of the lungs is needed.

The anterior mediastinum is the mediastinal compartment most frequently involved by malignant disease in children. Anterior mediastinal tumor involvement may present as an anterior mediastinal soft tissue mass, lymphadenopathy, or thymic infiltration. Lymphoma and leukemia are by far the

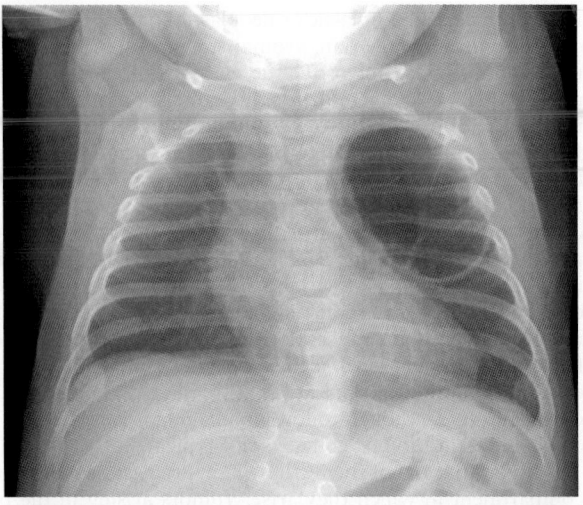

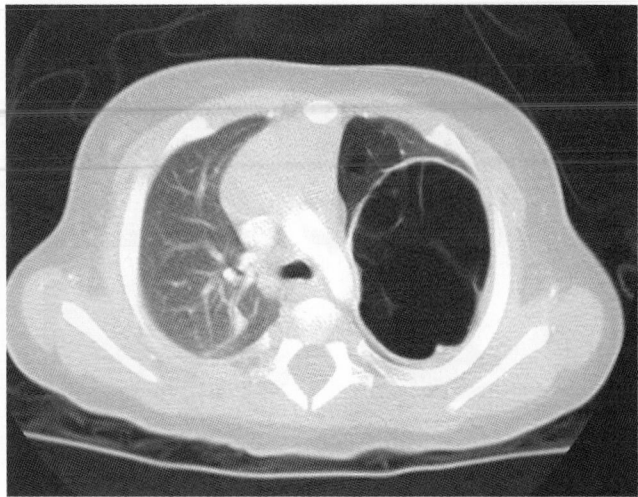

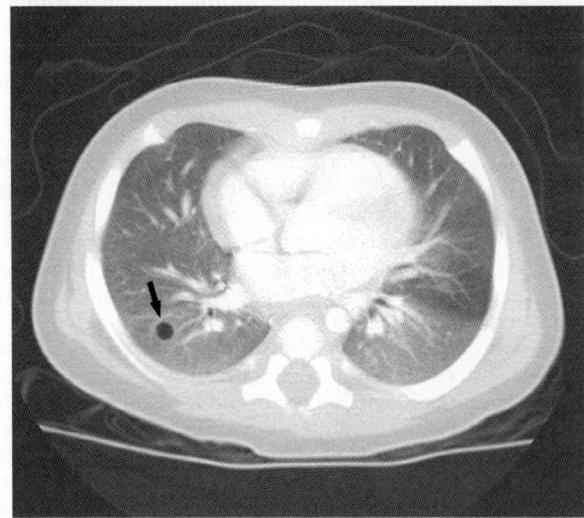

FIGURE 9.31 Bilateral pleuropulmonary blastomas. Frontal chest radiograph (**A**) demonstrates a large cystic lucency in the left mid and upper lung. Contrast-enhanced axial computed tomography images (**B** and **C**) demonstrate the presence of a multilocular cystic lesion of the left lung and a small cystic lesion of the posterior right mid lung (*arrow*) occult to conventional chest radiography. Upon resection and histopathologic inspection, both lesions were found to be pleuropulmonary blastomas.

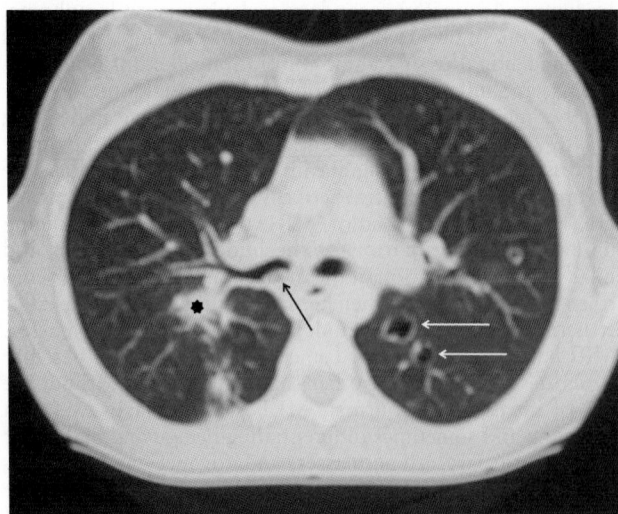

FIGURE 9.32 Bronchogenic carcinoma complicating respiratory papillomatosis. Axial computed tomography image in a teenager with human papilloma virus–associated respiratory papillomatosis shows a right bronchial papilloma (*black arrow*), multiple cavitary lesions (*white arrows*) in the left lung, and a right parahilar mass (*asterisk*) revealed to be squamous cell bronchogenic carcinoma on biopsy.

most common anterior mediastinal neoplasms in children, followed by germ cell tumors, histiocytosis, and thymoma.

Analysis of anterior mediastinal masses in children by conventional chest radiographs is difficult because of the wide range of normal thymic size. The thickness of the thymus decreases with age, and normal pediatric thymus size standards for CT,[157] MRI,[158] and ultrasound[159] have been published. Identifying malignancy within the thymus is complicated, because the normal gland can be quite large, especially in infants and young children. Conversely, the gland can be involved by malignancy without being overtly enlarged. Often, the diagnosis of intrathymic neoplasm is simplified when a prominent thymus is seen in conjunction with lymphadenopathy in other areas of the mediastinum or hila. In the absence of associated lymphadenopathy, the finding of loss of the normal contour or loss of the normal homogeneous parenchymal architecture of the thymus suggests neoplastic infiltration.

In children younger than 5 years, the thymus is quadrilateral in shape with convex lateral margins and undulating borders from costal cartilage impressions. Thereafter, the thymus gradually assumes a triangular shape with straight or concave margins. On CT, the normal attenuation of the thymus approximates that of skeletal muscle. On MRI, the signal intensity of normal thymus is lower than that of fat and slightly greater than that of skeletal muscle on T1-weighted

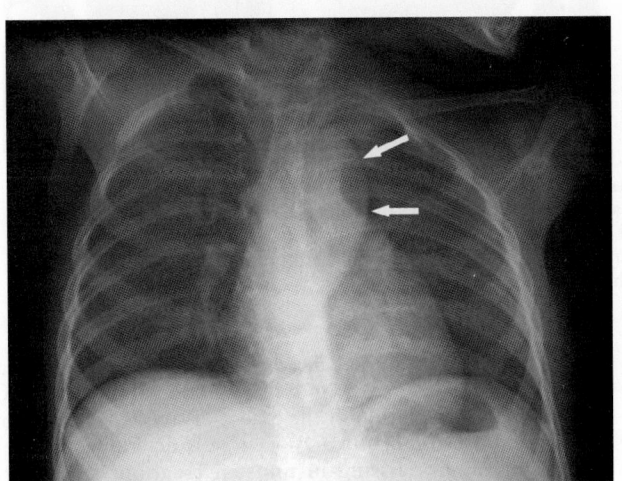

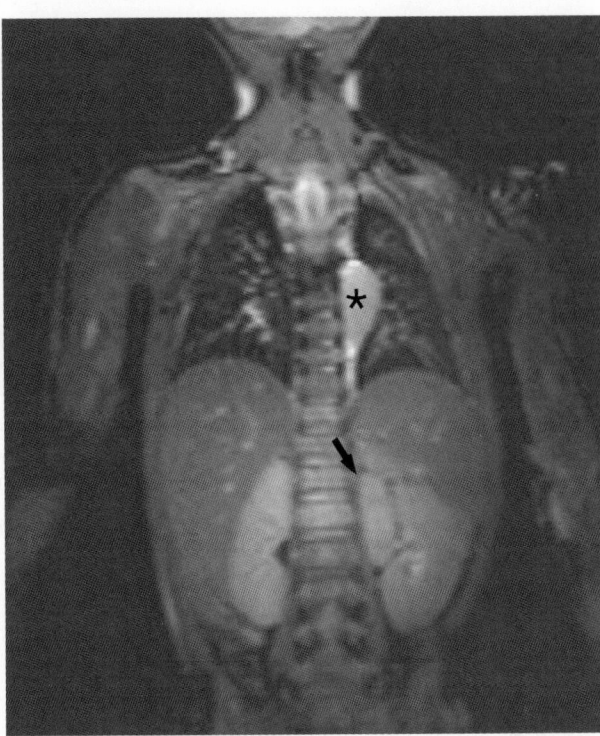

FIGURE 9.33 Neuroblastoma. Frontal chest radiograph (**A**) shows a left mediastinal mass (*arrows*). Coronal T2-weighted magnetic resonance image (**B**) localizes the mass (*asterisk*) to the left paraspinal region and demonstrates a second soft tissue mass adjacent to the left kidney (*arrow*).

images and is greater than that of skeletal muscle and slightly lower than that of fat on T2-weighted images.[158] On ultrasound, the echotexture of the pediatric thymus resembles that of liver parenchyma, and its echogenicity is lower than that of thyroid parenchyma.[159] Before puberty, the thymic parenchyma appears homogeneous. After puberty, fatty infiltration of the thymus occurs.[157] Chemical shift in-phase and opposed-phase gradient-echo MRI can be used to detect the fatty infiltration and possibly distinguish a normal or hyperplastic thymus from neoplastic infiltration.[160] The normal thymus exerts little or no mass effect on adjacent structures and can extend superiorly into the thoracic inlet or posteriorly into the posterior mediastinum. In these cases, normalcy can be established by the findings of homogeneous parenchyma, absence of significant compression of adjacent tracheobronchial structures or mediastinal vessels, and continuity with thymus in the anterior mediastinum.

The high avidity of lymphoma for gallium and FDG suggests a possible role for gallium scintigraphy and FDG-PET in distinguishing lymphoma from other causes of thymic enlargement or an anterior mediastinal mass. However, both methods are of limited use for definitive diagnosis of anterior mediastinal lymphoma due to the nonspecificity of thymic uptake of gallium and FDG. Various infectious and inflammatory conditions of the chest exhibit uptake of FDG.[31,161] Thymic uptake of gallium can occur with lymphoma or nonlymphoid neoplasms, particularly in very young children; this uptake may represent a nonspecific immunologic response.[162] The thymus can demonstrate gallium or FDG uptake as a physiologic phenomenon in children or as a result of rebound thymic hyperplasia after chemotherapy, and this uptake should not be mistaken for recurrent or metastatic thymic malignancy.[163] The pattern of physiologic thymic FDG uptake consists of mild diffuse uptake, most commonly in an inverted V-shape,

whereas lymphomatous involvement of the thymus appears as intense discrete foci of uptake.[164] Rebound thymic hyperplasia most characteristically presents in a child or adolescent as an enlarging thymic mass within 6 to 8 months of completion of chemotherapy for lymphoma and may portend a good prognosis related to bolstered cell-mediated immunity[165] (Fig. 9.34). In rare cases, it may persist for several years.[166] If a child or adolescent has imaging findings compatible with rebound thymic hyperplasia or physiologic thymic radiopharmaceutical uptake, especially if there is no other evidence of recurrence or prior neoplastic involvement of the thymus, observation and imaging follow-up rather than biopsy is advised.[165]

Germ cell tumors are among the most common anterior mediastinal tumors in children. Mature teratomas are the most frequent and typically present as a spherical multilocular cystic mass with thin internal septations and internal fat attenuation (Fig. 9.22). Seminomas are typically homogeneous soft tissue masses indistinguishable from lymphoma. Nonseminomatous malignant germ cell neoplasms are large, locally invasive, heterogeneous masses with central low attenuation and frond-like peripheral soft tissue. In cases of a suspected mediastinal germ cell tumor, a gonadal primary with intervening abdominal lymph node involvement should be excluded.[167]

Langerhans' cell histiocytosis is a proliferative condition that can present with mediastinal and pulmonary abnormalities amenable to detection by chest radiography and CT. The constellation of nodular interstitial lung disease with pneumatocysts and an anterior mediastinal thymic mass with calcifications or cavitation is highly suggestive of Langerhans' cell histiocytosis[168] (Fig. 9.35). Langerhans' cell histiocytosis can also present with low-attenuation thymic cysts,[169] although this is not specific; lymphoma and HIV infection can also be associated with thymic cysts.[170]

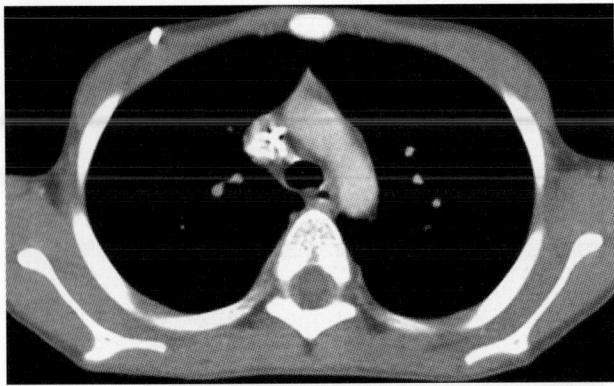
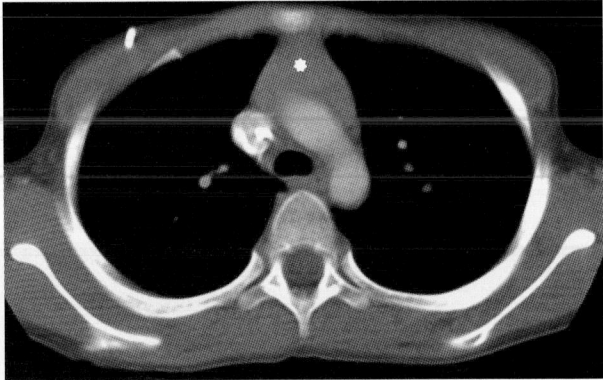

FIGURE 9.34 Rebound thymic hyperplasia in a patient in clinical remission after chemotherapy for Hodgkin lymphoma of the neck. Axial contrast-enhanced computed tomography images of the chest obtained at the time of completion of therapy (**A**) and 3 months after completion of therapy (**B**) demonstrate the development of a homogeneous soft tissue structure with smooth contours in the anterior mediastinum (*asterisk*), which is consistent with rebound thymic hyperplasia.

Pleural involvement by malignant tumors in children is typically from metastatic disease, invasive chest wall neoplasms, lymphoma, or pleuropulmonary blastoma. Pleural masses may be evaluated by CT or MRI. The use of intravenous contrast is important to help distinguish soft tissue masses from pleural effusion (Fig. 9.36).

Chest wall tumors may arise from bone or soft tissues. The most common chest wall malignancies in children are metastatic rib lesions (neuroblastoma, Langerhans' cell histiocytosis, lymphoma, leukemia). The most common pediatric chest wall primary malignancies are rhabdomyosarcoma, extraosseous Ewing's sarcoma, and PNET of the chest (Askin's tumor). Primary bone malignancies, especially Ewing's sarcoma and occasionally osteosarcoma, may arise from the ribs, thoracic vertebrae, or scapulae and manifest as chest wall masses. Nonmalignant chest wall masses include neurofibromas, hemangiomas, vascular malformations, aneurysmal bone cysts, osteochondromas, healing rib fractures, osteomyelitis, and developmental variations of the thoracic cage.[171]

Although conventional chest radiographs may demonstrate a chest wall mass with or without bony destruction, CT allows better evaluation of the extent of tumor, is more sensitive for bony erosion, and may accurately determine the site of origin of tumors arising in unusual locations such as the diaphragm. MRI can also be used to evaluate chest wall tumors. It is superior to CT in assessing the bone marrow of the thoracic skeleton and delineating tumor from soft tissue components of the chest wall, including muscle, fat, lymph nodes, vessels, and nerves.[172] Bone marrow and cortex of the ribs can be evaluated with MRI by using a surface coil, though CT is superior for evaluating cortical bone and tumor matrix calcification. Although the imaging features of malignant chest wall tumors are often nonspecific, differentiation of benign from malignant chest wall masses is usually possible. Imaging findings that suggest a malignant chest wall mass include rib destruction, pleural extension, and large size,[173] though thoracic infectious processes, particularly tuberculosis and actinomyosis, can mimic malignancy. Many benign chest wall masses have features that allow a specific diagnosis. For

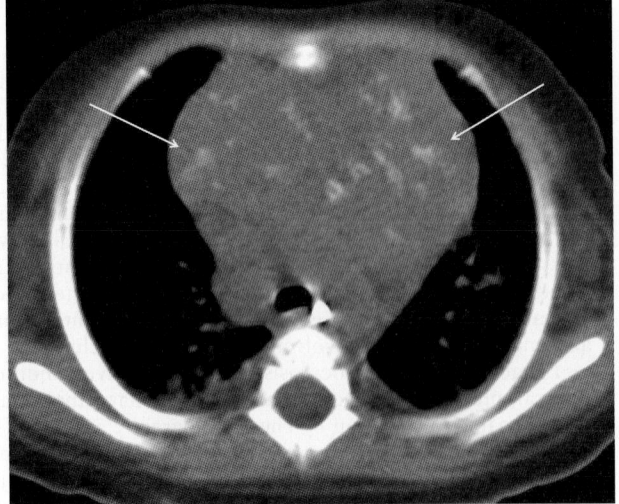
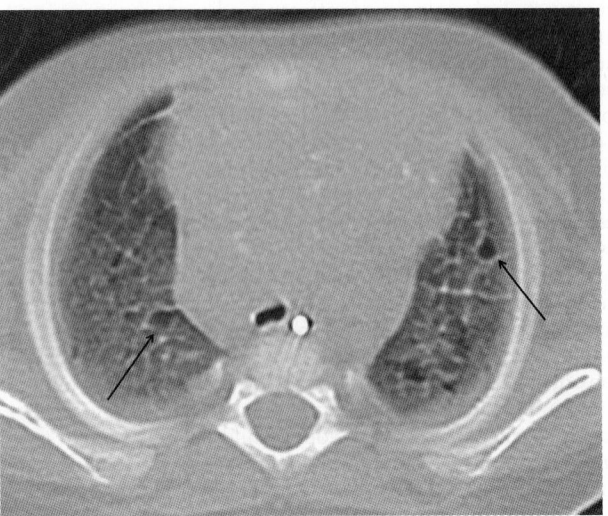

FIGURE 9.35 Langerhans' cell histiocytosis. Axial contrast-enhanced computed tomography (CT) image at soft tissue windows (**A**) demonstrates an enlarged thymus with multiple small calcifications (*arrows*). Axial CT image at lung windows (**B**) demonstrates thickening of the pulmonary interstitium and pneumatocysts (*arrows*).

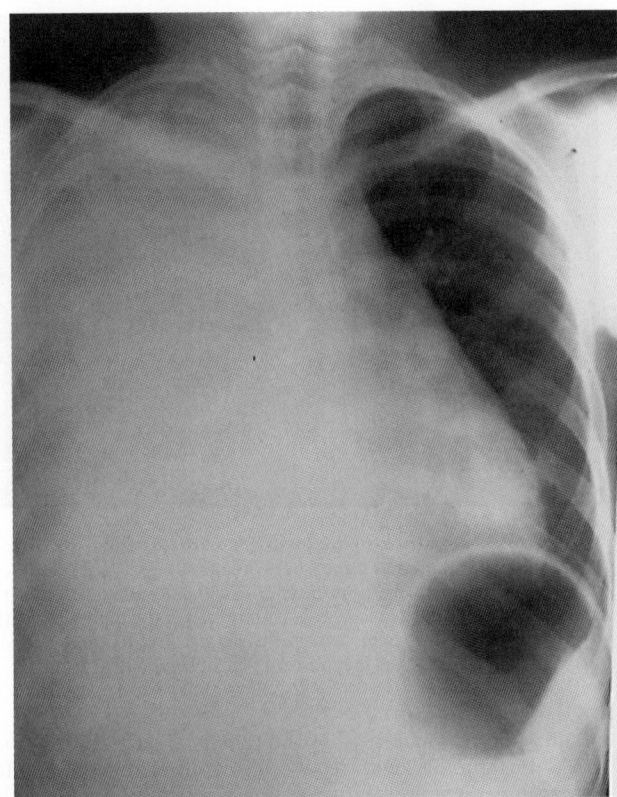

A

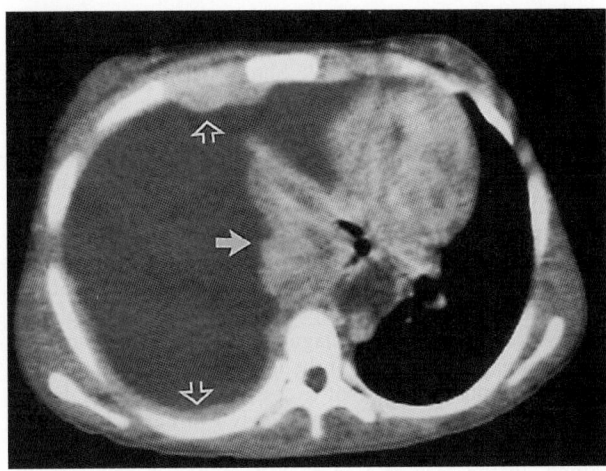

B

FIGURE 9.36 Non-Hodgkin lymphoma. A chest radiograph (**A**) shows complete opacification of the right hemithorax of unclear etiology. Axial computed tomography image (**B**) demonstrates a collapsed right lung (*closed arrow*) and pleural-based soft tissue masses (*open arrows*).

example, the presence of a mass with phleboliths and fluid-filled spaces that enhance with contrast allows a confident diagnosis of a venous vascular malformation. The appearance of signal intensity that is high peripherally and low centrally on T2-weighted MRI images in an intercostal mass strongly suggests neurofibroma.[171]

Palpable breast lumps are rarely malignant in children and adolescents but engender considerable apprehension. Ultrasound is the most appropriate initial imaging modality for the evaluation of a palpable breast lump in a child or adolescent and can reliably determine whether a lump represents normal breast tissue or a discrete solid or fluid-filled mass.[174] Fluid-filled masses include cysts, abscesses, hematomas, and galactoceles. In adolescent males, the vast majority of palpable breast lumps represent gynecomastia. In young females, solid breast masses are most commonly fibroadenomas, with less common etiologies including phyllodes tumors (Fig. 9.37), carcinomas, and metastases. The histology of a solid breast mass cannot be reliably predicted on the basis of the sonographic features alone, and tissue sampling of a solid breast mass is often advised for definitive diagnosis.[175] Assymetric breast enlargement related to asynchronous timing of breast development or premature thelarche can evoke clinical concern. In this setting, an ultrasound examination can confirm the presence of developing breast tissue and exclude the presence of a solid mass, averting unnecessary breast biopsy or surgery and potential damage to the developing breast bud. Occasionally, accessory breast tissue along the course of the primitive milk streak will present as an axillary soft tissue mass in a peripubertal girl and prompt cross-sectional imaging. Appropriate recognition of the characteristic appearance of this breast tissue on imaging will prevent unnecessary biopsy.[176]

Developmental variations in the anterior chest wall are common causes of a palpable chest wall "mass" in a child. These variations occur in as many as one-third of children and include prominent asymmetric convexity of the anterior ribs

or costal cartilages, anterior rib anomalies, sternal tilting, and mild pectus excavatum or carinatum.[177] Multiplanar and 3-D CT reconstructions showing the underlying ribs and costal cartilages are most helpful in diagnosis, as these variations can be difficult to appreciate on axial views alone.[178]

Abdominal Tumors

The multitude of diagnostic imaging studies available for evaluation of abdominal masses in infants and children requires a logical approach to avoid unnecessary expense, radiation, and potential morbidity. Conventional abdominal

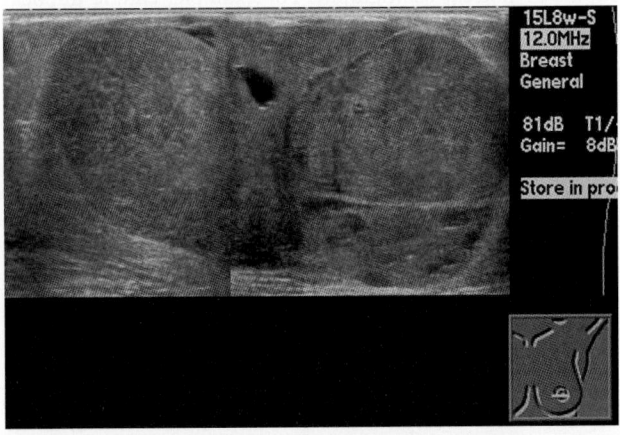

FIGURE 9.37 Phyllodes tumor. Ultrasound image of the left breast of a 10-year-old girl shows a large, predominantly solid breast mass with fluid-filled clefts. Although these findings are suggestive of a phyllodes tumor, similar findings can be seen with giant juvenile fibroadenomas, and tissue sampling is required to characterize the histology as benign or malignant.

radiographs seldom provide a definitive diagnosis but can suggest a mimicking process such as constipation and fecal retention or a distended urinary bladder. The nature of an abdominal mass can sometimes be inferred on abdominal radiographs by the presence or absence of calcifications in the mass and the location of the mass as indicated by the pattern of displacement of bowel loops and other signs of mass effect. More definitive imaging evaluation of a suspected abdominal mass is typically accomplished by ultrasound, CT, or MRI. Ultrasound is most frequently selected on the basis of low comparative cost, absence of ionizing radiation exposure, lack of requirement for intravenous catheter placement or sedation, and high diagnostic efficacy for common pediatric abdominal masses. If the ultrasound examination is technically limited because of excessive bowel gas or body habitus, or if the mass is incompletely evaluated by ultrasound or thought to be neoplastic, CT or MRI is commonly obtained. In the case of a suspected neoplasm, the role of imaging expands to further refine the differential diagnosis, to define the local and regional extent of the mass, and to detect metastases.

In neonates, most abdominal masses are benign. Abdominal ultrasound usually identifies the organ of origin. If the mass is not solid, a benign nature is suggested. Renal abnormalities are the most common palpable abdominal masses that occur during the neonatal period, with hydronephrosis and renal cystic dysplasia accounting for the majority of these. Ultrasound can usually determine a specific diagnosis in these cases. Ultrasound can also be used to diagnosis cephalad extension of an ovarian cyst or hydrometrocolpos, a common cause of an abdominal mass in a female neonate. Ultrasound can differentiate neonatal adrenal hemorrhage that develops central liquefaction and decreases in size over time from an adrenal neuroblastoma that increases in size or has internal blood vessels demonstrable by Doppler.[179] If ultrasound identifies a solid tumor arising from the retroperitoneum or liver, the probability of malignancy increases, and further imaging evaluation by either CT or MRI is usually necessary. Nonmalignant GI tract abnormalities presenting as palpable abdominal masses in neonates, such as large duplication, mesenteric or choledochal cysts, or distended bowel from distal obstruction, may be accompanied by mass effect or bowel dilation evident on conventional abdominal radiographs. Depending on the most likely etiology, diagnosis may be accomplished by the appropriate fluoroscopic GI contrast examination, sonography, or nuclear scintigraphy. For example, enteric duplication cysts exhibit a characteristic echogenic inner mucosal layer and hypoechoic outer muscular layer on sonography.[180]

In older infants and children, the likelihood that an intraabdominal mass represents malignant disease increases. Conventional radiography and ultrasound again are the primary screening imaging modalities, with CT, MRI, and nuclear scintigraphy used for further evaluation. As in neonates, cystic or fluid-filled masses typically are benign, and solid masses are more commonly malignant.

Most solid abdominal tumors in infants and children arise from the kidney or adrenal gland. Mesoblastic nephroma accounts for the majority of solid renal masses in early infancy but is indistinguishable from Wilms' tumor on imaging studies and requires biopsy for definitive diagnosis. Although the classic variant of mesoblastic nephroma is benign, the cellular variant shares biological and clinical features with infantile fibrosarcoma, including aggressive growth and the ability to metastasize.[181] Other renal malignancies of infancy and early childhood that are generally indistinguishable from Wilms' tumor on imaging are malignant rhabdoid tumor and clear cell sarcoma of the kidney, though the latter has a propensity for bone metastases that is unusual for Wilms' tumor. Beyond

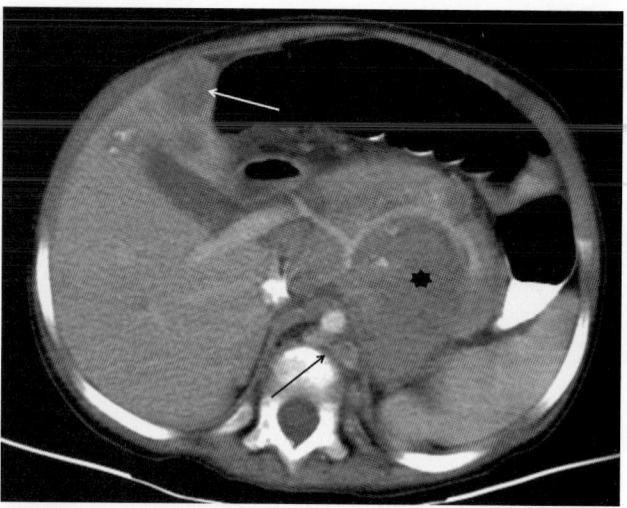

FIGURE 9.38 Neuroblastoma in a 15-month-old child. Axial contrast-enhanced computed tomography image shows a large retroperitoneal mass (*asterisk*) with intratumor calcifications extending to the midline and encasing celiac vessels with retrocrural lymphadenopathy (*black arrow*) and liver metastases (*white arrow*), features that are strongly suggestive of the diagnosis of neuroblastoma.

infancy, the vast majority of solid tumors arising in the kidney are Wilms' tumors, with renal cell carcinomas accounting for a small percentage. Most nonrenal retroperitoneal solid tumors are neuroblastomas arising from the adrenals or sympathetic chain. Wilms' tumors and neuroblastomas may be too large to allow accurate assessment of the organ of origin by ultrasound, but CT or MRI with coronal or sagittal images is usually accurate for this purpose. Vascular encasement, calcification, paravertebral location, intraspinal extension, and liver or bone metastases favor neuroblastoma over Wilms' tumor[182] (Fig. 9.38).

Imaging of Wilms' tumor at diagnosis serves to confirm the presence and location of the mass in the kidney, identify local invasion and vascular extension to determine the potential for surgical resection, discover foci of nephroblastomatosis and contralateral renal tumor, and detect metastatic disease. On CT or MRI, Wilms' tumor appears as a renal mass with internal heterogeneity related to necrosis, hemorrhage, and cyst formation. Striking hypervascularity of Wilms' tumor on imaging is important to note, because it can be associated with acquired von Willebrand syndrome and risk of perioperative bleeding complications.[183] The value of performing any additional imaging beyond ultrasound for abdominal staging of Wilms' tumor is controversial, with arguments for routine MRI or CT[184] or CT only in problematic cases.[185] CT and MRI have similar accuracy for determination of perirenal extension and lymph node involvement[186] but have poor correlation to histologic staging, that is, 75% of stage 1 or 2 tumors are overstaged by these modalities and 40% of stage 3 tumors are understaged.[187] Ultrasound and MRI have been reported to be superior to CT for mapping intravascular extension of Wilms' tumor into the renal vein and inferior vena cava for operative planning,[188,189] but whether this advantage holds true against contemporary multidetector helical CT techniques is unclear (Fig. 9.25). The advantage of MRI over CT to directly image the coronal and sagittal planes has waned with the ability of multidetector helical CT to generate high-quality, thin-section, multiplanar images. At many institutions, CT is the primary imaging modality for evaluation of newly diagnosed Wilms' tumor, because CT is more readily available than MRI, and it allows for concurrent examination of the lungs to evaluate for pulmonary metastases.

Abdominal neuroblastoma typically appears as a heteroge-neous retroperitoneal mass by imaging, and no current imag-ing modality can reliably differentiate neuroblastoma from ganglioneuroblastoma or ganglioneuroma. CT or MRI is used to help define the intra-abdominal extent of neuroblastoma preoperatively, with INSS staging based on the extent of sur-gical resection. Lymph node involvement and midline exten-sion, defined as tumor extending to or beyond the pedicle con-tralateral to the primary tumor, are important factors in INSS staging (Fig. 9.38). Vascular encasement, defined as tumor surrounding at least three quarters of the circumference of a major vessel, and intraspinal extension are also important to note, as vascular encasement may prohibit complete surgical resection, and intraspinal extension may require radiation treatment or a decompressive laminectomy[182] (Fig. 9.5). CT and MRI perform similarly in the evaluation of invasive growth and lymphadenopathy,[190] but the accuracy of CT or MRI in discriminating INSS neuroblastoma stages 1 to 3 is poor.[191] MRI is superior to CT at demonstrating INSS stage 4 disease and could potentially replace the combination of CT and Tc-99m phosphonate–based bone scintigraphy in staging neuroblastoma,[191] but this is of questionable value in the set-ting of routine evaluation of distant disease with MIBG scintigraphy.[192,193] Indium-111 pentetreotide, a somatostatin type 2 receptor agonist, is another radiopharmaceutical with avidity for neuroblastoma, and positive somatostatin receptor scintigraphy predicts better clinical outcome in children with neuroblastoma.[194] The role of FDG-PET in neuroblastoma is evolving. In one study, FDG-PET and bone marrow biopsy alone were deemed sufficient to follow patients with high-risk neuroblastoma in the absence of skull lesions and after resec-tion of the primary tumor.[195] In a more recent study, investi-gators found FDG-PET imaging of value in patients whose tumors failed to accumulate MIBG.[196]

The new INRGSS for neuroblastoma is based on tumor imaging rather than extent of surgical resection and does not use the midline or lymph node status in staging of localized disease. According to the INRGSS, the designation L1 is for localized tumor not involving vital structures and confined to one body compartment, and L2 is for locoregional tumor with one or more image-defined risk factors (IDRFs) on CT or MRI. IDRFs for abdominal neuroblastoma are as follows: ipsilateral tumor extension within two body compartments (e.g., chest-abdomen, abdomen-pelvis), tumor encasing cer-tain vessels (aorta, vena cava, origin of the celiax axis, or superior mesenteric artery, branches of the superior mesenteric artery at the mesenteric root, iliac vessels), tumor invading one or both renal pedicles, tumor infiltrating the porta hepatis and/or the hepatoduodenal ligament, tumor infiltration of adjacent organs/structures (e.g., diaphragm, kidney, liver, duo-denopancreatic block, mesentery), and intraspinal tumor extension, provided that more than one-third of the spinal canal in the axial plane is invaded, and/or the perimedullary leptomeningeal spaces are not visible, and/or the spinal cord signal is abnormal.[23]

The widespread practice of prenatal and perinatal sonog-raphy and growing practice of fetal MRI has lead to increased recognition of suprarenal masses, including neuroblastoma. Perinatal neuroblastomas are predominantly adrenal in origin and frequently cystic, complicating their differentiation from other perinatal suprarenal masses such as adrenal hemor-rhages, extrapulmonary sequestrations, and urinary tract anomalies. Correlation with urinary catecholamines, MIBG scintigraphy, and follow-up imaging are helpful in this regard (Fig. 9.17). The vast majority of perinatal neuroblastomas is associated with favorable disease stage and biologic features and has an excellent prognosis. Although surgery alone is cur-ative for most of these patients, it may be avoided in those

whose tumor shows spontaneous regression over a period of observation.[197] When a small, localized adrenal mass does not regress on follow-up imaging, surgical intervention may be warranted. The management of a perinatal suprarenal mass must strike a balance between surgical intervention and close observation. The Children's Oncology Group is conducting a trial to determine whether expectant observation alone or with surgical resection when warranted of perinatally detected adrenal masses results in a 3-year survival rate of not less than 95%, while sparing at least 75% of patients from resection.

Adrenocortical carcinomas are rare in children and typi-cally present at preschool age or during adolescence with a female predominance. Germline *TP53* mutations are almost always a predisposing factor and virilization with or without hypercortisolism from hormone overproduction is the most common presentation. Cross-sectional imaging usually reveals a large necrotic tumor, and dissemination is most frequently observed to the lymph nodes, liver, and lungs. Vascular inva-sion with intracaval tumor thrombus occurs in 20% of cases and is important to note on imaging for operative planning[198] (Fig. 9.39).

Paragangliomas (pheochromocytomas) in children are more frequently familial, extra-adrenal, and multifocal and are more often associated with hypertension and symptoms of catecholamine excess than they are in adults (Fig. 9.40). Hereditary pheochromocytomas occur in multiple endocrine neoplasia type 2, von Hippel-Lindau syndrome, neurofibro-matosis type 1 (NF1), and familial paraganglioma syndromes with germline mutations of the succinate dehydrogenase (*SDH*) gene. Imaging localization studies should be performed only after a conclusive biochemical diagnosis has been made, unless the clinical suspicion is very high due to a hereditary predisposition for pheochromocytoma. MIBG scintigraphy and abdominal/pelvic MRI or CT are the preferred imaging modalities for diagnosis, with indium-111 octreotide scintig-raphy, FDG-PET, and [^{18}F]-fluorodopamine PET as alterna-tives. Local tumor invasion or metastases, most commonly to bone, lungs, or liver, suggest malignant disease.[199]

Although they are most common in childhood in the sacro-coccygeal region and ovaries, some teratomas develop in the retroperitoneum. Cystic teratomas tend to be benign, and solid teratomas tend to be malignant. Teratomas can be indis-tinguishable from neuroblastomas on imaging studies. The presence of fat within the teratoma is particularly useful, because this suggests a specific diagnosis and CT and MRI are excellent tools for demonstrating fat.[200] Other retroperitoneal malignancies in children, such as fibrosarcoma and rhab-domyosarcoma, can be identified by imaging but have non-specific imaging features.

CT and MRI are excellent methods to evaluate the retroperitoneal lymph nodes. Isolated retroperitoneal lym-phadenopathy is unusual, and associated findings help to clar-ify the etiology. Retroperitoneal lymphadenopathy in children can occur with a variety of malignant processes, including lymphoma or spread from retroperitoneal primary malignan-cies (e.g., Wilms' tumor or neuroblastoma) or from testicular or ovarian malignancies.

Massive intra-abdominal lymphoma in children is nearly always NHL of B-cell origin, most commonly Burkitt's lym-phoma or Burkitt-like lymphoma. The abdomen is the most frequent site of involvement at the time of presentation of spo-radic Burkitt's lymphoma. NHL is the most common pediatric bowel malignancy; it most frequently involves the distal ileum, cecum, and appendix with associated mesenteric and retroperitoneal lymphadenopathy.[201] Intussusception and fis-tula tracts can also occur as complications.[202]

Involvement of the bowel by lymphoma may appear on GI contrast studies as nodular, polypoid, ulcerative, or

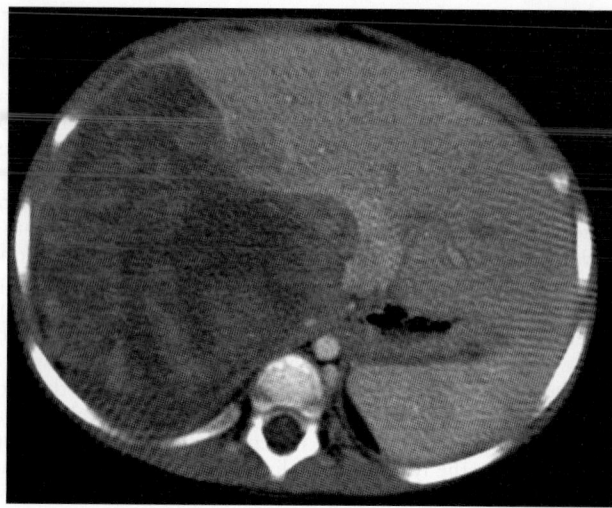

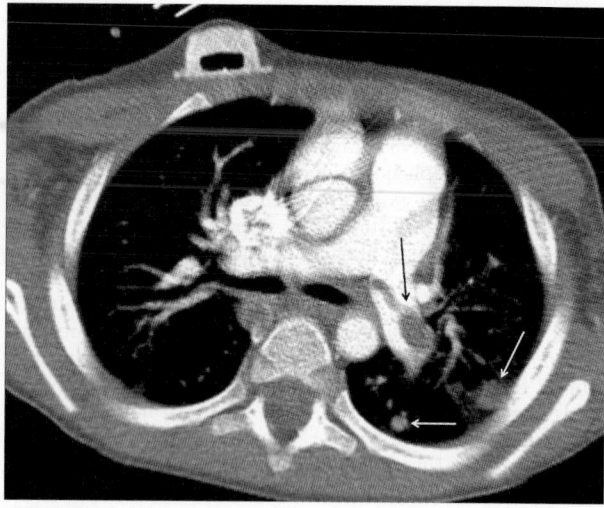

FIGURE 9.39 Adrenocortical carcinoma. Axial contrast-enhanced computed tomography (CT) image of the abdomen (**A**) reveals a large right suprarenal mass invading the liver and inferior vena cava. Axial contrast-enhanced CT image of the chest (**B**) demostrates pulmonary arterial tumor embolus (*black arrow*) and pulmonary metastases (*white arrows*).

infiltrative lesions. Thickening of the bowel wall to more than 1 cm and aneurysmal bowel dilation on CT are particularly suggestive of lymphoma[203] (Fig. 9.41). Conglomerate mesenteric nodal involvement with envelopment of mesenteric vessels and fat produces the "sandwich sign" on ultrasound or CT imaging.[204] Hepatic involvement is more common with NHL than Hodgkin lymphoma and most commonly appears as focal low-attenuation lesions on CT, hypoechoic or anechoic lesions on ultrasound, low-intensity lesions on T1-weighted MRI and high-intensity lesions on T2-weighted MRI. Hepatomegaly often indicates diffuse involvement,[205] although a liver of normal size can be diffusely infiltrated with lymphoma. Splenic size alone is unreliable in determining splenic involvement by lymphoma, because an involved spleen may not be enlarged, and splenomegaly may be present without involvement.[206] FDG-PET and PET-CT are more sensitive than diagnostic CT or gallium scintigraphy for identifying splenic involvement by lymphoma.[24,207] In a

recent study of adults with Hodgkin lymphoma, contrast-enhanced ultrasonography was superior to both diagnostic CT and PET-CT in detecting spleen involvement,[208] and further studies are needed to determine the value of sonography in children with lymphoma. Renal involvement is more common with NHL than Hodgkin lymphoma and is commonly bilateral with concomitant retroperitoneal lymphadenopathy (Fig. 9.3). The most common imaging appearance of pediatric renal lymphoma is multiple soft tissue nodules that are hypoenhancing on CT and hypoechoic on sonography. Less common presentations include direct renal invasion from adjacent nodal masses, a solitary renal mass, or nephromegaly from diffuse infiltration.[209]

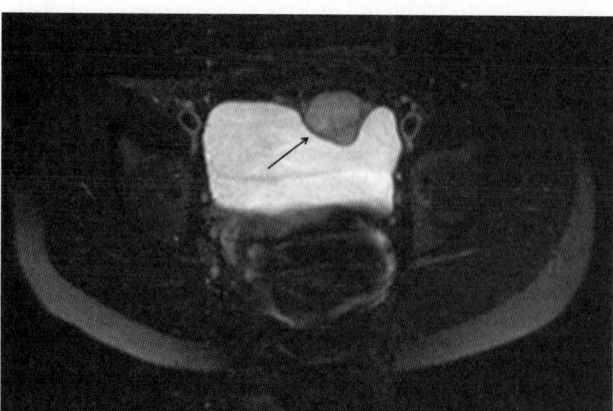

FIGURE 9.40 Extra-adrenal pheochromocytoma (paraganglioma) in a teenager with hypertension and micturitional headache. Axial T2-weighted magnetic resonance image demonstrates a mass (*arrow*) along the left anterior wall of the urinary bladder. An extra-adrenal location and symptoms of catecholamine excess are more common in children than in adults.

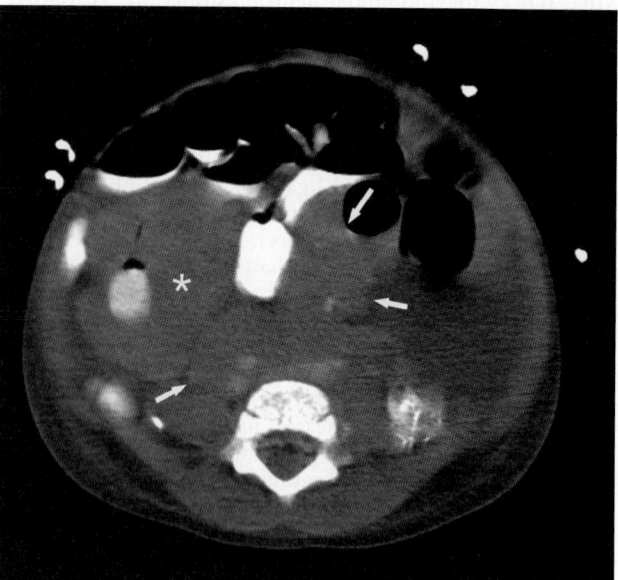

FIGURE 9.41 Burkitt's lymphoma. Axial contrast-enhanced computed tomography image shows pronounced thickening of the bowel wall (*asterisks*) in the right lower abdominal quadrant and retroperitoneal and mesenteric lymphadenopathy (*arrows*).

Primary neoplasms of the bowel are uncommon in children. Pediatric colon cancer is usually poorly differentiated mucinous or signet ring cell carcinoma. Those with familial adenomatous polyposis (FAP), hereditary nonpolyposis colorectal cancer syndrome, or inflammatory bowel disease are at elevated risk. Suspicious findings may be suggested by endoscopy, contrast enema, or CT, but often the diagnosis is made at emergency surgery for bowel obstruction or perforation and at a more advanced stage than diagnosis of adults. Desmoid tumors are associated with FAP and are incited by trauma, particularly abdominal surgery. Although nonmetastasing fibromatoses, these tumors can cause serious morbidity related to compression and invasion of adjacent structures.[210]

Gastrointestinal stromal tumors (GISTs) are rare mesenchymal neoplasms thought to arise from the interstitial cells of Cajal lineage. GISTs can be sporadic or familial and associated with syndromes including NF1, Carney's triad, or paraganglioma-GIST syndrome. Chronic anemia from GI tract bleeding is the most common presentation in children. Unlike adult GISTs, pediatric GISTs are more frequent in female patients, have a higher proportion of gastric and multifocal tumors, and have an indolent course, despite metastases or recurrences.[211,212] GI tract tumors are amenable to diagnosis by contrast fluoroscopy (Fig. 9.2), though CT is preferred to concomitantly evaluate for lymphadenopathy and hepatic and peritoneal metastases. Gastric distention with water as enteric contrast is preferred to maximize the sensitivity of CT for stomach lesions. Pulmonary imaging is also indicated to evaluate for chondromas as part of the Carney's triad.[212]

Malignant liver tumors are the fourth most common pediatric abdominal malignancies. Of pediatric malignant liver tumors, about 90% in patients younger than 5 years are hepatoblastomas, while nearly 90% in patients older than 15 years are hepatocellular carcinoma. Hepatoblastomas are associated with Beckwith-Wiedemann syndrome, FAP, and prematurity, while hepatocellular carcinomas are associated with chronic liver diseases such as hepatitis B and C, tyrosinemia, galactosemia, Wilson's disease, hemochromatosis, and biliary atresia. The age discrepancy and associated conditions are important in formulating a differential diagnosis, because these tumors are difficult to distinguish on the basis of imaging features. Hepatoblastoma and hepatocellular carcinoma generally appear as heterogeneous masses that invade adjacent vessels (Fig. 9.42). The fibrolamellar subtype of hepatocellular carcinoma usually occurs in older adolescents and adults in the absence of chronic liver disease and appears similar to focal nodular hyperplasia on imaging, though the fibrous central scar typically shows calcification and low signal intensity on T2-weighted images in the former and high signal intensity in the latter (Fig. 9.43). Undifferentiated embryonal sarcoma of the liver most commonly presents in children of 6 to 10 years of age and can have a misleadingly cystic appearance on CT and MRI related to myxoid stroma, but its solid nature is revealed by ultrasound. Mesenchymal hamartomas have a variable appearance that ranges from solid to multilocular cystic masses and can spontaneously regress or, in rare cases, undergo malignant transformation.[213] Infantile hepatic hemangiomas (hemangioendotheliomas) exhibit a characteristic enhancement pattern on CT and MRI (Fig. 9.44), can be solitary or multifocal, and can be asymptomatic or complicated by arteriovenous shunting and high-output congestive heart failure.[117] Hepatic adenomas are rare in children but are associated with glycogen storage disease and have a variable appearance on imaging related to hemorrhage. Although CT is superior to MRI for detecting intratumoral calcification, the value of this finding in differentiating pediatric liver tumors is limited, because hepatoblastoma, hepatocellular carcinoma, and hemangioendotheliomas all may exhibit calcifications.

Malignant neoplasms of the spleen are most commonly leukemia, lymphoma, or metastases. Leukemic involvement of the spleen characteristically is diffusely infiltrative and causes splenomegaly rather than a discrete splenic mass. Lymphomatous involvement of the spleen can be nodular or diffusely infiltrative and need not be associated with splenomegaly. Lymphoma isolated to the spleen is unusual. Benign tumors of the spleen are most commonly epithelial or endothelial-lined cysts, and no further imaging is needed if the diagnosis of a cyst is confirmed by ultrasound. Hamartomas are the most common benign solid tumor of the spleen in children and have an echogenic appearance on ultrasound.[214]

Biliary tract neoplasms are rare in children. Porta hepatis lymphadenopathy may cause biliary obstruction, though this is unusual, even with bulky lymphadenopathy. Biliary rhabdomyosarcoma is suspected if a soft tissue mass is detected within a dilated central biliary tract structure on imaging (Fig. 9.45) but may be difficult to distinguish from a hepatocellular tumor if the site of origin is a peripheral bile duct. Disseminated Langerhans' cell histiocytosis is associated with liver abnormalities appreciable on imaging. Hepatomegaly is frequent, but may be attributable to effects of macrophage activation syndrome rather than tumor infiltration.[215] Histiocytic infiltration has a remarkable selectivity for the bile ducts, which manifests on imaging as periportal lesions that are hypoechoic or hyperechoic on ultrasound, low attenuation on CT, and of abnormal signal intensity on T1-weighted, T2-weighted, and contrast-enhanced T1-weighted MRI sequences.[216] Imaging can also reveal sclerosing cholangitis and biliary cirrhosis that occur as complications of hepatic Langerhans' cell histiocytosis.

Neoplastic involvement of the pancreas in childhood most commonly is from lymphoma or local invasion of adjacent retroperitoneal neoplasms such as neuroblastoma. Primary pancreatic neoplasms are very rare in childhood. Islet cell tumors may occur in isolation or as part of a multiple endocrine neoplasia syndrome. Preoperative noninvasive localization of islet cell tumors is desirable for surgical planning but challenging due to the typically small size of the tumors. Thin-section dynamic contrast-enhanced arterial phase CT,[217] MRI,[218] and indium-111-pentetreotide scintigraphy[219] have been touted, though the most effective noninvasive imaging technique has not been established. Combined intraoperative sonography and palpation has a very high sensitivity for pancreatic islet cell tumors.[217] Pancreatoblastoma is typically very large at presentation and has nonspecific features on CT and MRI,[220] although imaging can suggest the diagnosis by demonstrating an origin from the pancreas rather than kidney, adrenal, or liver (Fig. 9.23). The rare solid pseudopapillary tumor of the pancreas (also known as papillary cystic neoplasm of the pancreas, solid and papillary epithelial pancreatic tumor, solid cystic papillary tumor, solid and cystic acinar cell tumor, papillary tumor of the pancreas, or Frantz tumor) should be suspected if a well-marginated, large, encapsulated, solid and cystic mass with areas of hemorrhagic degeneration (best revealed by high signal intensity on T1-weighted MRI images) and progressive peripheral or slightly heterogeneous contrast enhancement is detected in the pancreas of an adolescent girl or a young woman[221] (Fig. 9.46).

Soft tissue peritoneal implants on the mesentery, omentum, and intraperitoneal organ serosal surfaces most typically occur with the spread of ovarian neoplasms. The presence of such peritoneal implants in the absence of an apparent organ-based primary site suggests a diagnosis of desmoplastic small round cell tumor, particularly in adolescents. In cases of desmoplastic small round cell tumor, CT is good for depicting the peritoneal implants, some of which may show

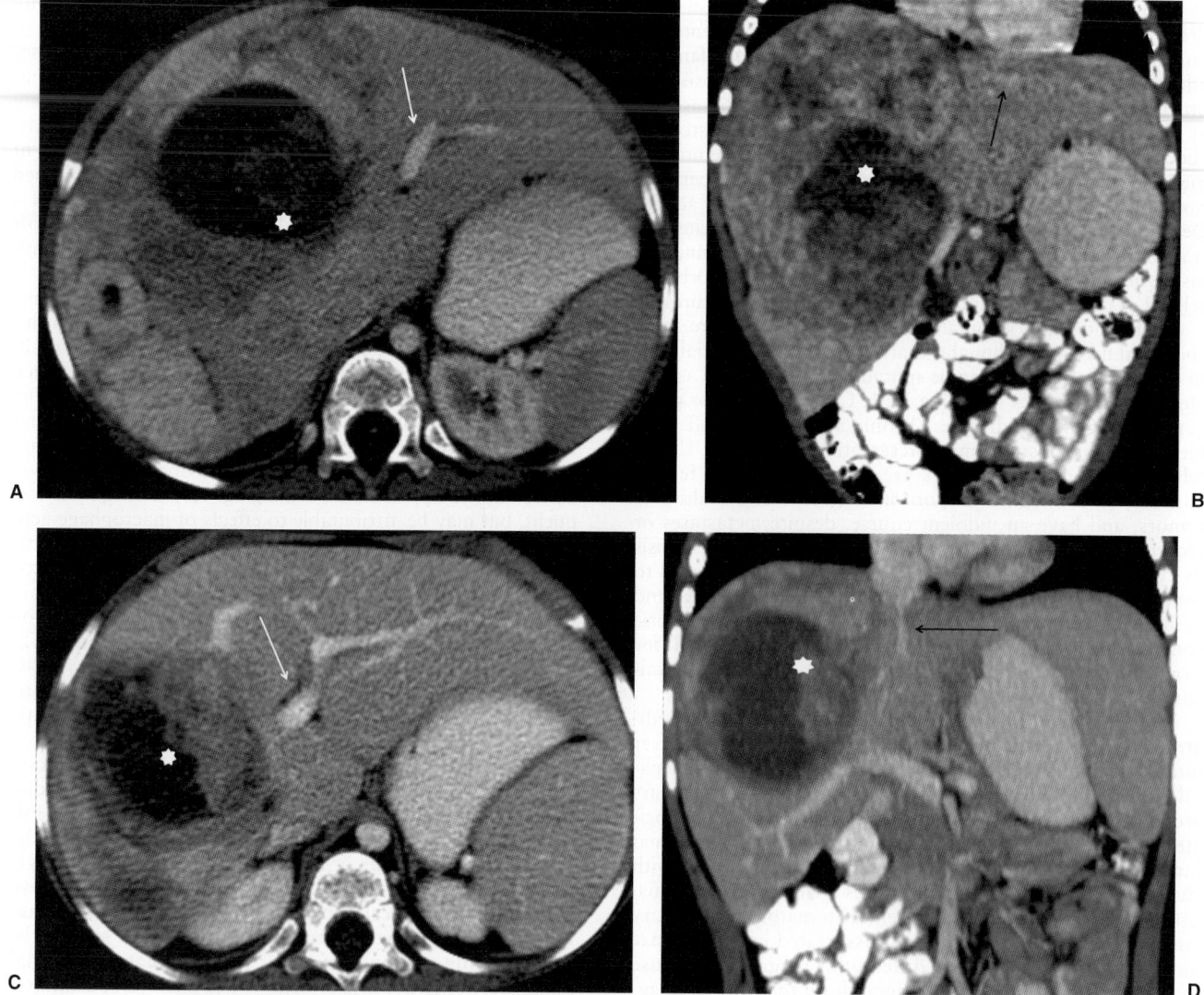

FIGURE 9.42 Hepatoblastoma. Axial (**A**) and coronal (**B**) contrast-enhanced computed tomography (CT) images obtained at diagnosis show a large heterogeneous tumor (*asterisk*) occupying the right hepatic lobe and medial segment left hepatic lobe, with clear planes of separation of the tumor from the left portal vein (*white arrow*) and the left hepatic vein (*black arrow*), corresponding to PRETEXT III classification. Axial (**C**) and coronal (**D**) contrast-enhanced CT images obtained following preoperative chemotherapy show a decrease in size of the tumor (*asterisk*), with visualization of the portal vein bifurcation (*white arrow*) and the middle hepatic vein (*black arrow*). The right hepatic vein is occluded by the tumor. The patient underwent an extended right hepatic lobectomy (right trisegmentectomy) with gross total tumor resection.

calcification, and associated ascites and lymphadenopathy[222] (Fig. 9.47).

Pelvic Tumors

In girls, ultrasound is the initial imaging study of choice for pelvic masses due to its excellent depiction of the ovaries, uterus, and urinary bladder and lack of ionizing radiation or need for intravenous contrast or sedation. With the addition of Doppler to evaluate blood flow, ultrasound is valuable in helping distinguish a vascularized adnexal tumor from a hemorrhagic cyst or enlarged torsed ovary. In boys, ultrasound can be used to screen for bladder masses, but MRI or CT is preferred for the evaluation of extravesical masses. In girls and boys, MRI and CT supply information about the size and extent of the primary tumor, lymphadenopathy, and

intra-pelvic and intra-abdominal metastases. MRI has some advantages over CT in the evaluation of pediatric pelvic tumors, including better soft tissue resolution and the ability to directly image in the sagittal plane. This is a particularly useful attribute for delineating invasion of the posterior aspect of the bladder wall or the anterior aspect of the rectum by rhabdomyosarcoma and for defining the intrapelvic extent of sacrococcygeal teratomas. The ability to evaluate the bladder and assess the upper urinary tracts for obstruction without the use of intravenous contrast is another advantage of MRI.

Most ovarian masses detected by imaging are dominant physiologic follicles or nonneoplastic functional cysts. Ultrasound can readily discriminate dominant follicles or simple functional cysts from complex cysts or solid ovarian masses. The most common etiology of a complex cyst is a hemorrhagic functional cyst, although the differential diagnosis is

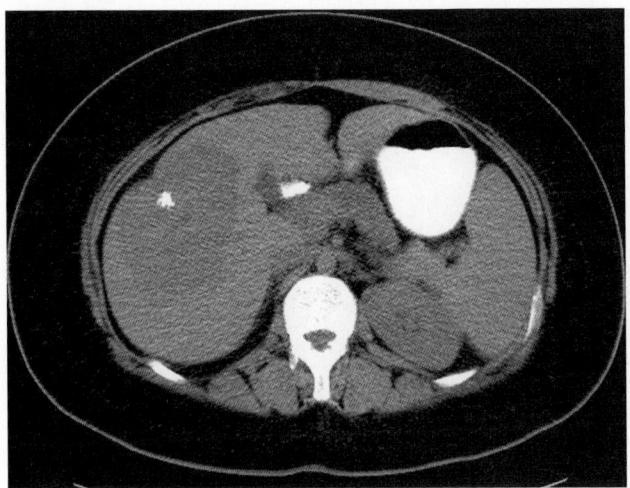

FIGURE 9.43 Fibrolamellar hepatocellular carcinoma in an adolescent girl. Axial nonenhanced computed tomography image of the abdomen shows a low-attenuation hepatic mass with a calcification. The presence of such a calcification can help distinguish fibrolamellar hepatocellular carcinoma from focal nodular hyperplasia.

broad and includes tubo-ovarian abscess, ectopic pregnancy, endometrioma, and cystic neoplasm. If the etiology of a complex cyst is not clarified by clinical correlation, a follow-up pelvic ultrasound in 4 to 6 weeks is typically advised to monitor for involution of the cyst supportive of a diagnosis of a hemorrhagic cyst. Cystic ovarian enlargement can occur with precocious puberty as part of McCune-Albright syndrome with concomitant fibrous dysplasia or van Wyk-Grumbach syndrome with concomitant hypothyroidism.[223] It is important to recognize these conditions to institute appropriate endocrinologic therapy and avoid unnecessary surgery for suspicion of ovarian tumor.

Unlike ovarian neoplasms in adults in whom surface epithelial tumors are most common, those in children are usually germ cell tumors, with teratomas (or dermoid cysts) being the most common form. The imaging appearance of teratomas is highly variable, because it is related to the varied contents, although the appearance often permits a reliable diagnosis. A teratoma is occasionally diagnosed on the basis of teeth-like or bone-like calcifications discovered on an abdominal/pelvic radiograph. Sonographic features most useful in making an accurate diagnosis include an echogenic mural nodule (dermoid plug or Rokitansky nodule containing fat, hair, or calcium), fat-fluid or hair-fluid levels, or shadowing teeth or bone fragments[224] (Fig. 9.48). MRI is particularly valuable in demonstrating fatty components that may not be apparent by other imaging methods.[225] Most ovarian teratomas are benign, and findings on imaging that suggest malignancy include ascites, invasion of neighboring structures, or a solid composition with absence of differentiated hair, fat, or teeth.

Malignant ovarian tumors in childhood typically appear solid or mixed (solid and cystic). In a predominantly cystic mass, the presence of papillary projections or capsular invasion is suggestive of malignancy. Ovarian malignancy can be mimicked on imaging by ovarian torsion and debris-filled hemorrhagic cysts. Differentiation of malignant germ cell, stromal cell, and epithelial cell tumors is usually not possible on the basis of the imaging features of the ovarian mass alone. However, ancillary findings can suggest a specific diagnosis. For example, juvenile granulosa cell tumors frequently produce estrogen, which leads to isosexual pseudoprecocious puberty with breast glandular and endometrial stimulation

evident on imaging studies.[226] Malignant ovarian masses are often very large and can exceed the field of view of standard sonographic images. In this case, abdominal/pelvic CT or MRI can be used to define the full extent of the tumor and detect lymphadenopathy, hematogenous metastases to parenchymal organs such as the liver, and intraperitoneal spread manifesting as ascites and omental or serosal implants (Fig. 9.49).

Rhabdomyosarcoma is the most common intrapelvic malignancy in boys. Defining the site of origin by imaging is important, because rhabdomyosarcomas arising from the bladder/prostate generally have a worse prognosis than those arising from other sites in the pelvis, including the paratesticular region. MRI and/or CT are usually employed to define tumor size and extent for therapeutic planning with the goal of patient survival with an intact, functioning bladder[227] (Fig. 9.50). Rhabdomyosarcoma is by far the most common pediatric bladder malignancy but can be mimicked by inflammatory pseudotumors on imaging, potentially leading to inappropriate choice of therapy.[228] *Paratesticular rhabdomyosarcomas* refer to tumors arising in the spermatic cord, peritesticular appendages, paratesticular tunics, or epididymis. As with other scrotal tumors, ultrasound is the imaging modality of choice for investigation of the primary tumor. Findings of epididymitis can be mimicked by paratesticular rhabdomyosarcoma on sonography; thus, it is important that boys, given a diagnosis of epididymitis on the basis of sonography, receive appropriate clinical follow-up.[229]

The most common primary scrotal neoplasms in boys are testicular germ cell tumors, with endodermal sinus tumor being by far the most common subtype. Testicular tumors are usually heterogeneous in echogenicity on ultrasound, a nonspecific appearance that can be simulated by infarcts or focal orchitis (Fig. 9.51). In boys with premature virilization and a testicular mass, Leydig cell tumor should be suspected. Although ultrasound is the imaging screening examination of choice for testicular tumors, the detection of Leydig cell tumor occult to sonography by MRI has been reported.[230] Leydig cell tumors have a specific appearance of marked and homogeneous contrast enhancement on MRI.[231]

Although primary testicular neoplasms can occasionally be multifocal, this finding on imaging should raise suspicion of other entities such as leukemia, lymphoma, or adrenal rests. Infiltration of the testes is occasionally the presenting manifestation of leukemia, and the testes are a potential sanctuary site for leukemia cells during chemotherapy and an extramedullary relapse site after chemotherapy (Fig. 9.52). Adrenal rests in the testes can enlarge and present as masses in patients with congenital adrenal hyperplasia. The correct diagnosis is prompted by the clinical history and supported by the finding of a spoke-like pattern of vessels radiating from the centers of the rests on sonography.[232]

Skeletal and Extremity Tumors

Acute leukemia is the most common pediatric malignancy; therefore, radiologists who image children encounter this diagnosis frequently. Approximately 40% of children presenting with acute leukemia have at least one radiographic skeletal abnormality. Findings on skeletal radiographs include transverse metaphyseal lucent bands ("leukemic lines"), osteopenia, subperiosteal cortical bone erosion, periostitis, osteosclerosis, and lytic bone lesions.[233] A substantial portion of patients present with so-called aleukemic or subleukemic leukemia with a normal or low white blood cell count and no blasts on peripheral blood smear. Many of these patients have nonspecific bone and joint pain, which clinicians often suspect as osteomyelitis, septic arthritis, or juvenile rheumatoid arthritis, prompting musculoskeletal MRI examinations. MRI suggests the correct

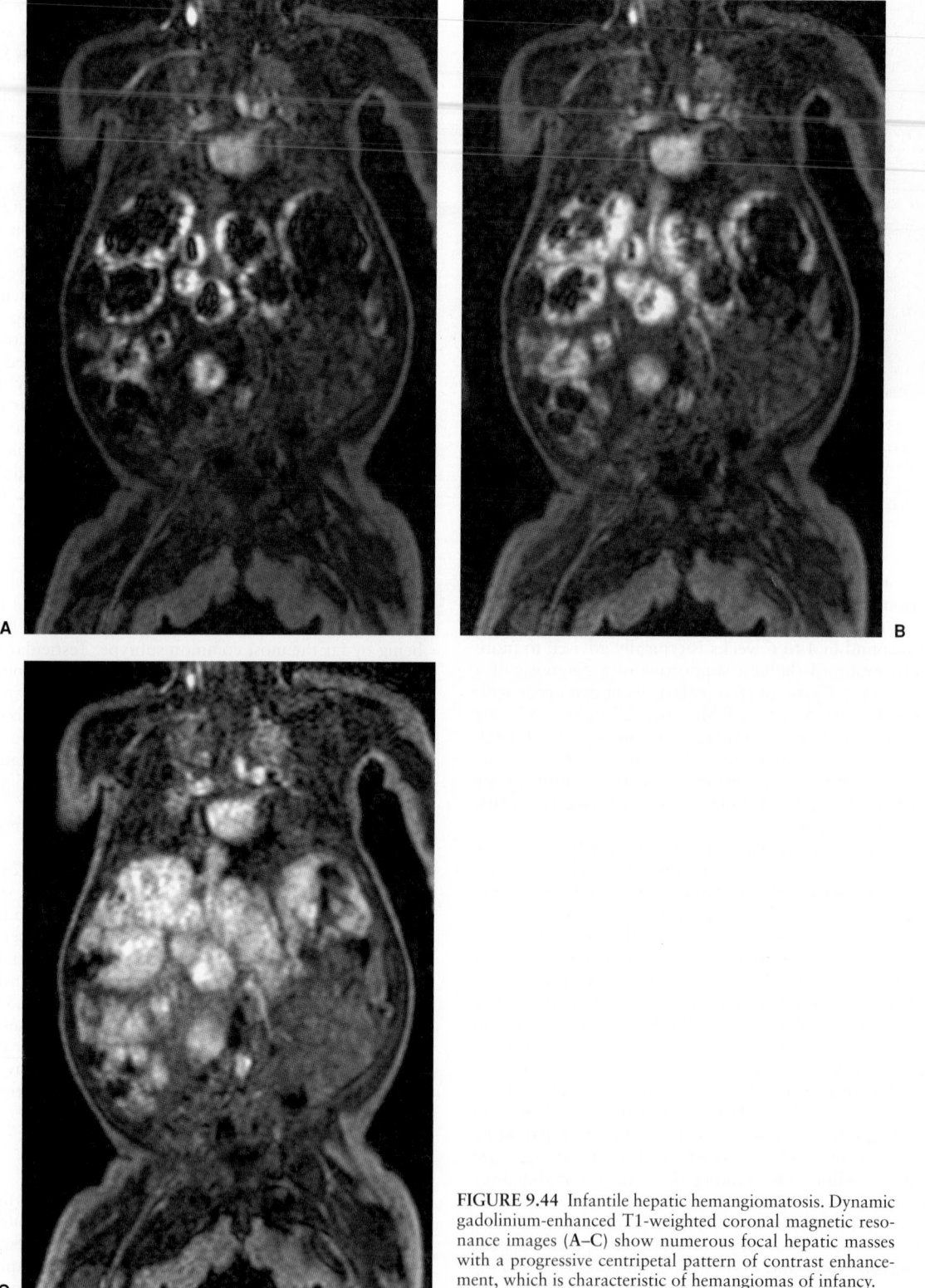

FIGURE 9.44 Infantile hepatic hemangiomatosis. Dynamic gadolinium-enhanced T1-weighted coronal magnetic resonance images (**A–C**) show numerous focal hepatic masses with a progressive centripetal pattern of contrast enhancement, which is characteristic of hemangiomas of infancy.

diagnosis of leukemia by revealing widespread decreased bone marrow signal intensity on T1-weighted sequences and increased signal intensity on fat-suppressed T2-weighted and STIR sequences characteristic of diffuse bone marrow infiltration (Fig. 9.4). The MRI appearance of leukemia can be mimicked by diffuse marrow metastatic disease (neuroblastoma,

rhabdomyosarcoma, or Ewing's sarcoma), myelodysplastic or myeloproliferative syndromes, or conditions associated with red marrow hyperplasia[103] (Fig. 9.53).

Osteosarcoma and Ewing's sarcoma are by far the most common primary bone tumors of childhood, but when destructive bone lesions are encountered, both osteomyelitis

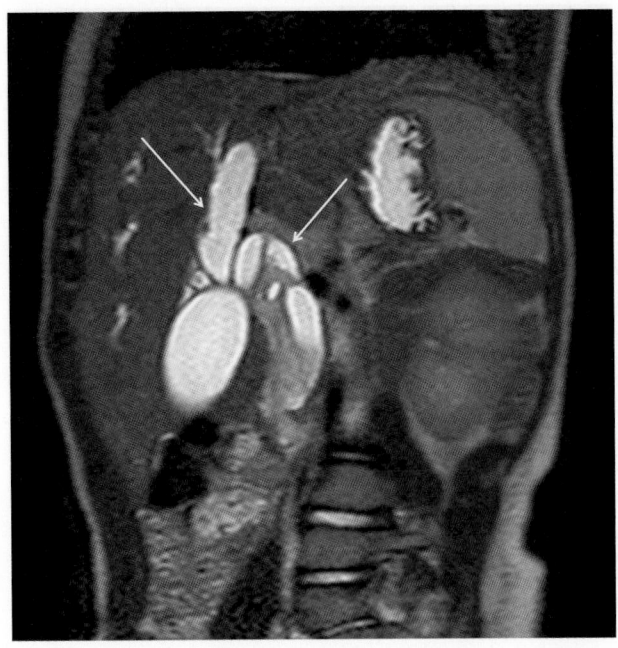
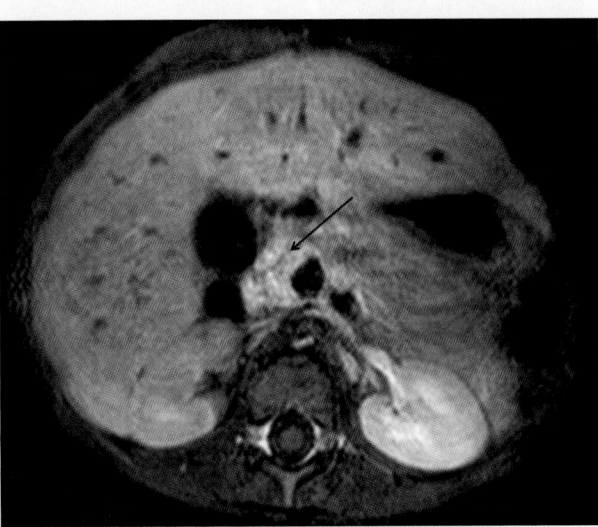

FIGURE 9.45 Biliary rhabdomyosarcoma in a 2-year-old child presenting with jaundice. Coronal oblique heavily T2-weighted magnetic resonance (MR) cholangiopancreatography image (**A**) and an axial gadolinium-enhanced T1-weighted MR image (**B**) show bile duct dilation (*white arrows*) related to an enhancing soft tissue mass (*black arrow*) arising from and obstructing the common duct.

small round cell tumors of childhood must be considered. These tumors include metastatic neuroblastoma, rhabdomyosarcoma, leukemia, lymphoma, and Langerhans' cell histiocytosis. Analysis of the clinical and imaging features may narrow the differential diagnosis, but a specific diagnosis is not always possible. Most osteosarcomas involve the metaphyses of the long bones and produce immature bone appearing as a "cloud-like" matrix with Codman's triangles and spiculated "sunburst" periosteal reaction, allowing diagnosis on conventional radiography (Fig. 9.16). The typical radiographic appearance of Ewing's sarcoma is a permeative lesion of the metadiaphysis of a long bone with lamellar "onion skin" periosteal reaction,

but bone sclerosis can accompany the bone lysis, and involvement of an axial flat bone is more common than with osteosarcoma.[234]

When a combination of clinical information and radiographic appearance makes a primary bone tumor likely, an MRI encompassing the entire bone and adjacent joints should be obtained prior to biopsy to demonstrate the longitudinal extent of intramedullary involvement, assess possible epiphyseal or articular involvement, depict any extraosseous soft tissue mass, and detect skip metastases. This information is crucial for planning the approach to the biopsy and definitive surgical management with limb salvage or amputation.

Although aggressive bone tumors typically have poorly defined margins on radiographs, relatively well-defined areas of abnormal signal intensity are more the norm on MRI. The

FIGURE 9.46 Solid pseudopapillary tumor of the pancreas in an adolescent girl. Axial contrast-enhanced abdominal computed tomography image shows a sharply defined mass of heterogeneous attenuation in the body and tail of the pancreas (*arrows*).

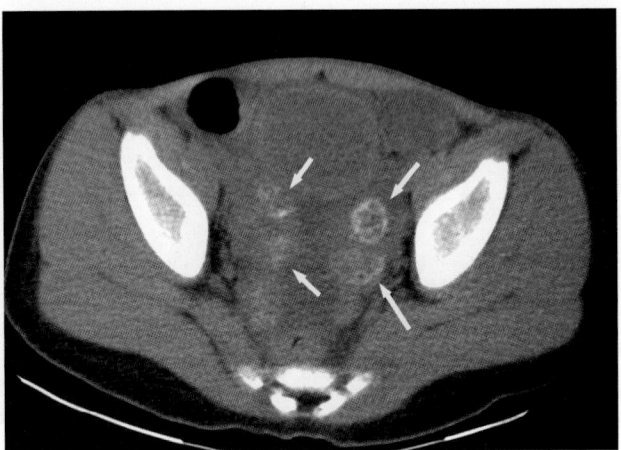

FIGURE 9.47 Desmoplastic small round cell tumor. Axial contrast-enhanced computed tomography image of the pelvis demonstrates multiple, partially calcified peritoneal implants (*arrows*) and ascites.

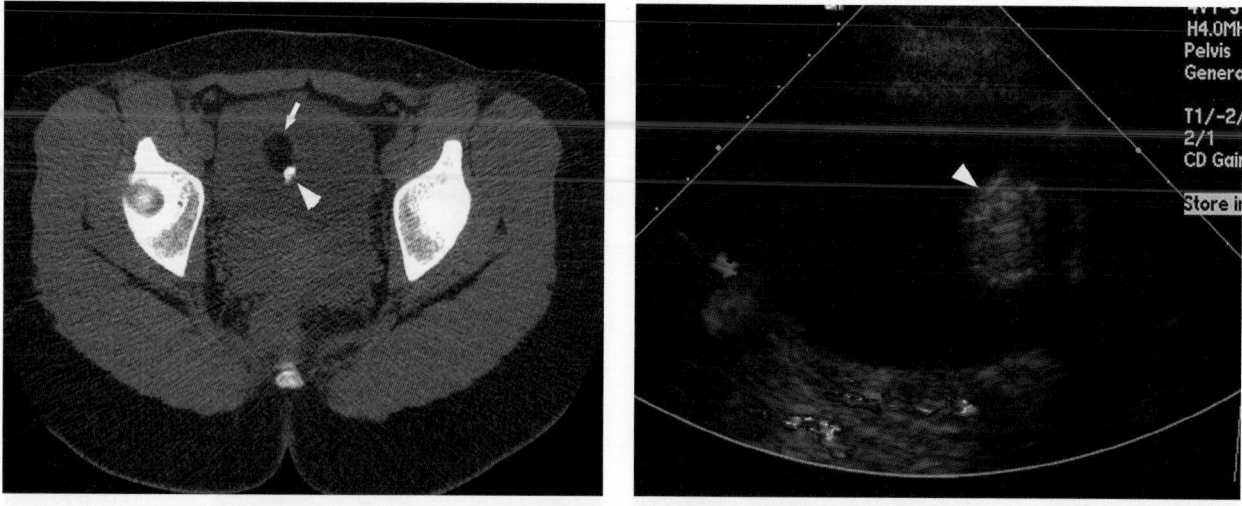

FIGURE 9.48 Mature ovarian teratoma (dermoid tumor). Axial image (**A**) from a noncontrast computed tomography examination performed to assess for possible urolithiasis reveals an intrapelvic structure containing both fat (*arrow*) and calcification (*arrowhead*). Ultrasound image (**B**) depicts a corresponding dermoid cyst containing a characteristic echogenic mural Rokitansky nodule (*arrowhead*).

intramedullary extent of tumor is best defined by unenhanced T1-weighted sequences, and STIR sequences may overestimate tumor extent.[235] Abnormalities of marrow space signal on MRI correlate well enough with tumor to rely on preoperative MRI and pathologic evaluation of the intraoperative specimen to ensure adequate surgical margins in osteosarcoma.[236] Epiphyseal extension is difficult to evaluate by Tc-99m phosphonate–based bone scintigraphy because of physiologic radiopharmaceutical uptake by the physis in children. T1-weighted MRI sequences are more specific but less sensitive than STIR sequences for evaluation of epiphyseal involvement.[237] Contrast-enhanced T1-weighted sequences are useful for depicting the synovium and vasculature. MRI has high sensitivity but only modest specificity for evaluation of intra-articular or neurovascular bundle involvement.[238,239] Although MRI is excellent for delineating normal tissue, it does not adequately discriminate extraosseous soft tissue tumor from peritumoral edema, because both can appear as low or intermediate signal intensity on T1-weighted images and as increased signal intensity on T2-weighted, STIR, or static gadolinium-enhanced T1-weighted images.[240] Skip

metastases are best visualized by MRI, and T1-weighted sequences are more sensitive than Tc-99m phosphonate–based bone scintigraphy.[102] It is important not to confuse physiologic foci of hematopoietic marrow in children for skip metastases.

Although conventional osteosarcoma has characteristic imaging features, less common forms of osteosarcoma can have imaging features that appear similar to benign lesions, and some benign lesions mimic the appearance of malignant lesions. Telangiectatic osteosarcoma can be confused for an aneurysmal bone cyst; both lesions have a pattern of expansile growth with multiple blood-filled cavities, but the presence of thick peripheral, septal, or nodular soft tissue enhancement favors the former.[241] Intracortical osteosarcoma can mimic osteoid osteoma or osteomyelitis, but is exceedingly rare. Parosteal osteosarcoma and myositis ossificans have similar features on MRI, though distinction is usually possible on the basis of a peripheral zone pattern of mineralization in the latter. This pattern is more readily demonstrable by CT than MRI.[242]

A palpable lump in the extremity or trunk of a child is a common reason for referral for diagnostic imaging. For

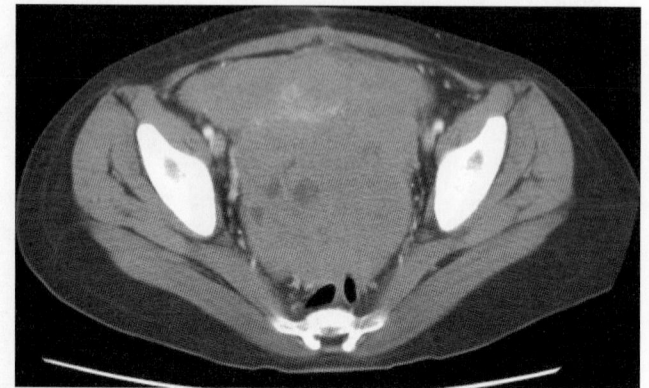
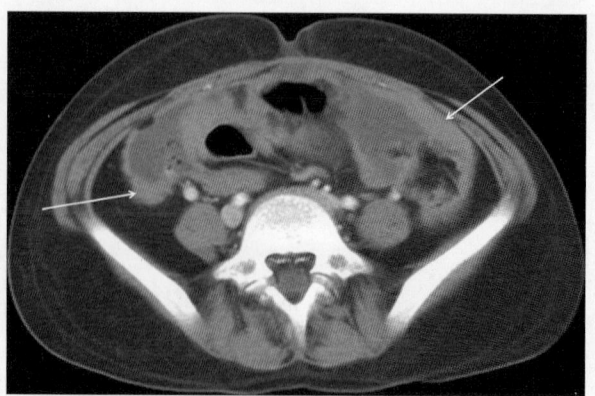

FIGURE 9.49 Immature teratoma. Axial contrast-enhanced computed tomography image of the pelvis (**A**) depicts a predominantly solid mass occupying much of the pelvic cavity. Axial contrast-enhanced image of the abdomen (**B**) demonstrates multiple omental and serosal soft tissue implants (*arrows*) from intraperitoneal tumor spread.

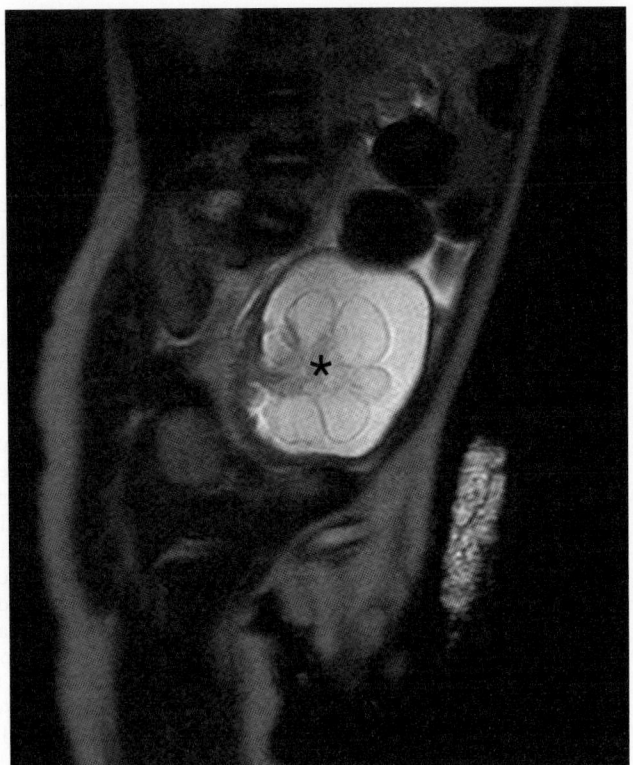

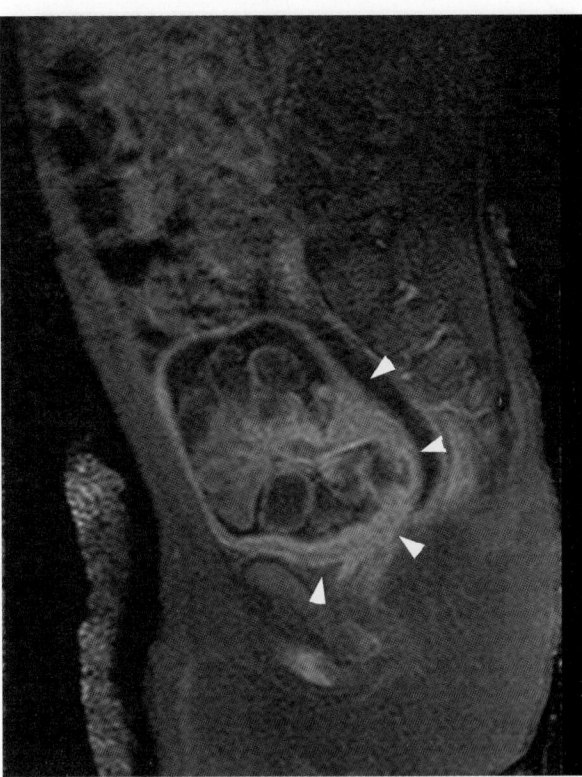

FIGURE 9.50 Embryonal rhabdomyosarcoma of the urinary bladder. An oblique sagittal T2-weighted magnetic resonance (MR) image of the pelvis (**A**) shows a lobulated, pedunculated mass (*asterisk*) arising from the bladder wall and protruding into the bladder lumen. A sagittal gadolinium-enhanced T1-weighted MR image of the pelvis (**B**) demonstrates enhancement of the solid portions of the intraluminal mass and of the invasive intramural component of the mass along the thickened bladder wall (*arrowheads*).

superficial small masses, sonography is often ordered and can confirm the presence of a discrete mass, determine whether the mass is cystic or solid, and if solid, whether the mass is a lymph node or group of nodes. For deep or large nonnodal masses, radiographs are obtained to determine whether there is obvious bony derivation or calcification of the mass, and MRI is performed to define size and extent of the mass and possibly make a specific diagnosis. In some cases, a specific diagnosis is possible on the basis of the MRI features (e.g., hematoma, fat necrosis, vascular malformation, lipoma, muscular herniation, ganglion cyst, pigmented villonodular synovitis), but in many cases, the mass has an indeterminate appearance and a specific diagnosis is not possible. While cer-

tain features on MRI (e.g., size less than 3 cm, homogeneous signal intensity, and absence of neurovascular encasement or osseous invasion) favor a benign versus malignant nature,[243] there is substantial overlap in the appearances of benign and malignant soft tissue masses. For example, infantile fibrosarcoma and rhabdomyosarcoma can be confused for a hemangioma of infancy, and synovial sarcoma and myxoid

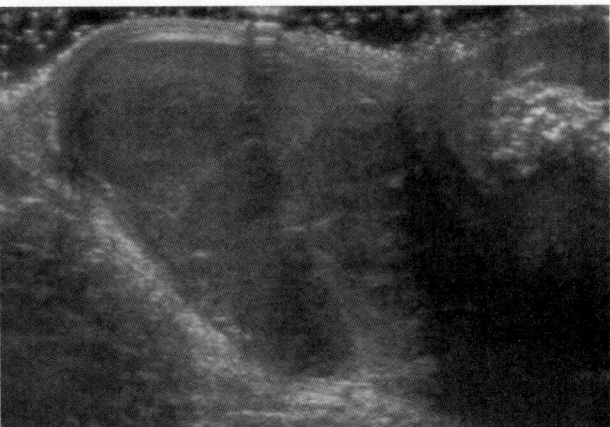

FIGURE 9.51 Malignant testicular germ cell tumor. Ultrasound reveals a well-circumscribed mass of heterogeneous echogenicity (*asterisk*) within the right testicle.

FIGURE 9.52 Testicular relapse of leukemia in a 14-year-old boy with a history of treated acute lymphoblastic leukemia and new painless right testicular enlargement. Sonography shows right testicular enlargement with multiple hypoechoic intratesticular nodules.

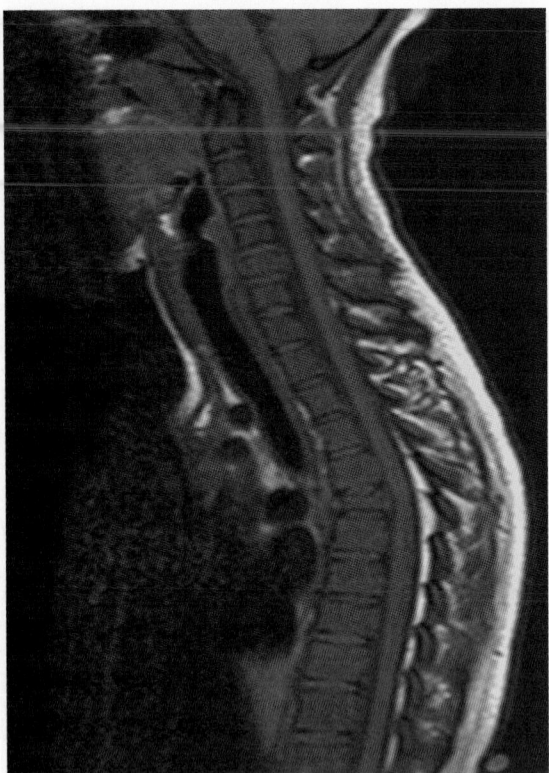

FIGURE 9.53 Diffuse marrow infiltration by metastatic alveolar rhabdomyosarcoma. A sagittal T1-weighted magnetic resonance image of the spine shows diffuse abnormal low signal intensity of the bone marrow and compression deformities of the C6 and T6 vertebral bodies. This diffuse pattern of marrow infiltration mimics leukemia and can also be seen with metastatic disease from other solid tumors such as neuroblastoma and Ewing's sarcoma.

liposarcoma can look like benign cysts. Thus, MRI alone is not always reliable for distinguishing a soft tissue mass as benign or malignant, and biopsy is advised when the imaging appearance is indeterminate.[244]

Tumor Staging and Risk Stratification

Assignment of patients by risk group into stratified prognostic categories is a fundamental feature of the therapeutic protocols of many pediatric malignancies. Treatment intensity can be adapted to minimize toxicity in patients with low-risk disease and maximize the probability of cure in those with high-risk disease. The major determinants of prognosis are tumor biology, tumor volume and extent, and the treatment administered. Imaging studies are invaluable for defining the extent of most solid tumors to establish disease stage at the time of presentation and for assessment of treatment response during and at the completion of therapy. Although imaging studies used in staging depend on tumor type and location, the local extent is usually evaluated by the primary diagnostic modalities discussed previously. This section addresses the evaluation of common sites of metastatic disease.

Lymph Node Involvement

Malignant involvement of a lymph node is suspected on the basis of enlargement of a lymph node in the chain of drainage from the primary tumor and in the absence of an alternative etiology such as infection or granulomatous disease. In children, the threshold of 1 cm at greatest diameter is commonly used to define enlargement,[245] although in healthy children, nodes as large as 2 cm in maximal long axis diameter can be encountered in regions such as the mesentery.[246] The use of nodal size thresholds for determination of malignant involvement is problematic due to variation in normal lymph node size with body site and age, the substantial overlap in size of involved and uninvolved nodes, the paucity of normal lymph node size standards in children, and the inconsistency of measurement methods (e.g., long axis vs. short axis diameter). For borderline enlarged lymph nodes, features such as rounding of the normal ovoid shape and loss of the normal fatty hilum suggest malignant involvement. There is a trade-off of sensitivity and specificity with any selected node size threshold, since nodes may be enlarged because of reactive hyperplasia or neoplasm, and normal-sized nodes may contain tumor deposits. Conventional MRI and CT scans are unable to reliably identify tumor in normal-sized lymph nodes or to distinguish whether lymph nodes are enlarged because of tumor involvement or reactive hyperplasia.[247] A developing technique for characterizing benign and malignant lymph nodes is MRI lymphangiography using ultrasmall superparamagnetic iron oxide (USPIO) nanoparticles.[248] After intravenous administration, USPIO nanoparticles are taken up by macrophages in normally functioning lymph nodes and reduce the signal intensity of these lymph nodes on MRI due to the magnetic properties of the particles. Lymph nodes involved with malignancy take up fewer particles than normal lymph nodes; thus, benign and malignant lymph nodes can be distinguished on the basis of signal intensity.

Sentinel node mapping is an established technique in which Tc-99m–labeled radiocolloids are injected in and around a tumor and transported via draining lymphatic channels to nodes representing the first site of lymphatic metastases. These sentinel nodes can be localized preoperatively by conventional gamma camera scintigraphy or intraoperatively by handheld gamma probes, resulting in more directed lymph node sampling, less morbid surgery, and more accurate staging to direct the patient's treatment. In children and adolescents, sentinel node mapping has been applied most successfully in cases of melanoma, nonrhabdomyosarcoma soft tissue sarcoma, and breast cancer.[249,250]

Combined FDG-PET/CT is a promising technique for evaluating nodal tumor status, since it permits combined metabolic and morphologic imaging for precise localization of viable tumor. FDG-PET coregistered with low-dose unenhanced CT is more sensitive and specific than contrast-enhanced CT alone for evaluation of lymph node involvement in lymphoma,[251] and image fusion enhances the confidence of examination interpretations in pediatric lymphoma.[252] However, these FDG-PET results may not be generalizable to other pediatric malignancies. In a study of pediatric sarcomas, FDG-PET/CT was more accurate for distant metastases but not nodal metastases when compared with FDG-PET alone or conventional imaging with MRI, CT, and Tc-99m phosphonate–based bone scintigraphy.[27] The FDG avidity of malignant nodes in children with rhabdomyosarcoma, osteosarcoma, or Ewing's sarcoma range from mild to intense, and some malignant nodes may not be FDG-avid.[253–255] Furthermore, increased FDG avidity of lymphoid tissues is also seen in nonmalignant processes with increased glycolytic activity, such as mononucleosis, granulomatous disease, and reactive follicular hyperplasia with transforming germinal centers.[31,255,256] When a patient's treatment hinges on detection of nodal involvement, lymph node biopsy may still be needed.

Central Nervous System Metastases

Metastatic disease to the brain, spinal cord, or meninges can be evaluated by CT but is more typically studied by contrast-enhanced MRI. CNS metastases most commonly originate from primary CNS tumors in the form of "drop" metastases. They can also originate from solid tumors outside the CNS, most commonly sarcomas, but the incidence is not high enough to justify routine imaging in patients without clinical signs of neurologic involvement.[257] An exception is clear cell sarcoma of the kidney, which has a relatively high incidence of CNS metastases.[258] Also, in 10% to 15% of young infants with rhabdoid tumors of the kidney, separate primary tumors of the CNS develop, most commonly atypical teratoid/rhabdoid tumors related to a germline *SNF5/INI1* tumor suppressor gene mutation.[259] Imaging should be performed in these patients to evaluate for synchronous or metachronous CNS tumors. Metastases of the bony cranial and vertebral structures most commonly originate from neuroblastoma, lymphoma, or histiocytosis. This can be identified on MRI by changes in the marrow signal. An important caveat in evaluating the CNS for metastatic disease with MRI is recognition of the meningeal enhancement that occurs after craniotomy and lasts for approximately 2 weeks. This enhancement can hide small metastases or be confused for metastatic deposits. To avoid this problem, tumor staging along the craniospinal axis should be performed before resection of a cerebral tumor.[260,261]

Pulmonary Metastases

Pulmonary metastases in children and adolescents are most frequently associated with sarcomas, Wilms' tumor, hepatoblastoma, and gonadal tumors. The incidence of pulmonary metastases detected by CT in pediatric patients at the time of diagnosis of extremity osteosarcoma is 14%.[262] Another study reported that 4% of children with INSS stage 4 neuroblastoma have pulmonary metastasis at diagnosis, and these children have decreased overall survival compared with those without pulmonary metastasis.[263]

Although metastases to the lung can be seen on chest radiographs, CT is a far more sensitive imaging modality for this purpose. CT frequently identifies small pulmonary nodules that are occult on conventional chest radiographs (Fig. 9.54). CT also can identify metastatic lesions at the lung periphery and pleura, a problem for conventional radiographs (Fig. 9.36). The volumetric acquisition of helical CT allows review of images in a "cine" mode, and in sagittal and coronal planes, facilitating discrimination of nodules from vessels sectioned transversely. The use of FDG-PET for the assessment of pulmonary metastases is limited by their often small size and blurring by respiratory motion. CT is superior to FDG-PET in sensitivity for the detection of pulmonary metastases from bone sarcomas.[254]

An exception to the superior sensitivity of CT for lung metastases is the case of differentiated thyroid carcinoma in children, in which CT identifies pulmonary nodules in less than 30% of patients with lung metastases demonstrable by I-131 scanning.[264] Atelectasis can also limit the sensitivity of CT for pulmonary nodules. For this reason, chest CT scan should not be performed for evaluation of pulmonary metastatic disease during the immediate postoperative period. Prone or decubitus positioning or positive-pressure ventilation can be used to reinflate areas of dependent atelectasis. Radiologists' ability to recognize pulmonary nodules is another limiting factor in the sensitivity of chest CT scan for detecting metastases. Computed-aided detection software identifies some pulmonary nodules on CT scan missed by radiologists in pediatric oncology patients and may be useful as a "second reader" to increase the sensitivity of CT for detecting pulmonary metastases.[265]

The major disadvantage of CT in the evaluation of pulmonary metastatic disease is the lack of specificity. Classically, pulmonary metastases are single or multiple, nodular, sharply defined, noncalcified, and predominantly peripherally located. However, nonmetastatic processes can appear indistinguishable from lung metastases on CT (Fig. 9.55). The presence of calcification in a nodule supports a diagnosis of granulomatous disease; however, this inference cannot be made in children with osteosarcoma, the metastases of which also can calcify.[262] The inability of CT to reliably discriminate benign from metastatic disease as a cause of pulmonary nodules in children has been reported by several investigators.[266,267] In children with known solid extrathoracic tumors at initial presentation, the presence of multiple, well-defined pulmonary nodules larger than 5-mm diameter is generally indicative of metastatic disease and 70% of solitary nodules smaller than 5-mm diameter may be benign.[268] In children with sarcomas, having more than three nodules and a bilateral distribution is associated with an increased frequency of recurrent or

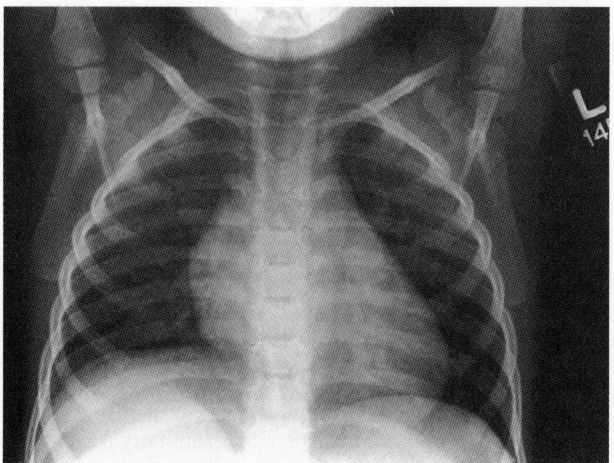 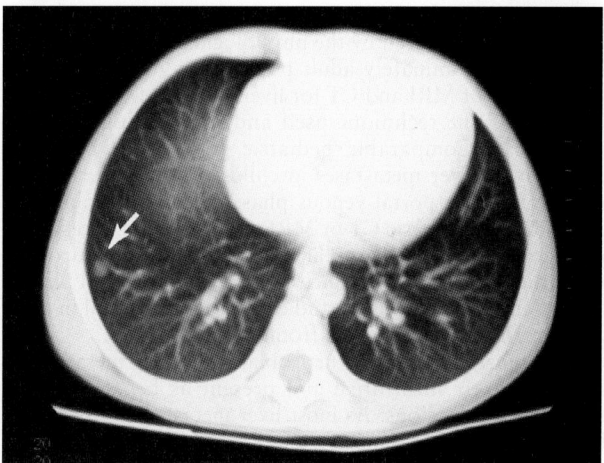

FIGURE 9.54 Wilms' tumor. The lungs appear normal on an anteroposterior chest radiograph (**A**). An axial chest computed tomography image at lung windows (**B**) demonstrates a metastatic right pulmonary nodule (*arrow*) occult to conventional chest radiography.

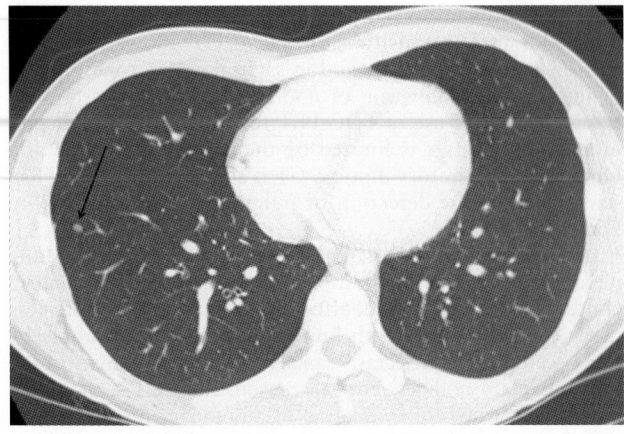

FIGURE 9.55 Intrapulmonary lymph node. An axial chest computed tomography image at lung windows obtained for staging of osteosarcoma shows a well-defined ovoid nodule of the right lower lobe near the pulmonary fissure. Biopsy of the nodule revealed an intrapulmonary lymph node, a potential mimic of pulmonary metastasis.

progressive metastatic disease in the lungs.[269] No increase in the number or a decrease or no change in the size of nodules on follow-up CT examination is reassuring evidence of a benign nature.

The lack of specificity of CT for pulmonary metastases in pediatric oncology patients causes many dilemmas in clinical management, underscored by the ongoing controversy regarding the treatment of children with Wilms' tumor with nodules visible on chest CT but occult on chest radiographs[185,270–272] (Fig. 9.54). Marked interobserver variability in the interpretation of chest CT scans regarding the presence or absence of nodules is another factor limiting the utility of this modality.[273] Despite its shortcomings, CT continues to be used as the primary method for evaluation of pulmonary metastases for most malignancies. When confirmation or refutation of pulmonary metastatic disease is required and the CT findings are nonspecific, CT can localize lesions for subsequent biopsy.

Intra-abdominal Metastases

The liver is the most common abdominal organ involved by metastatic disease, and neuroblastoma, Wilms' tumor, and lymphoma are the most common sources. The liver is best assessed for metastatic disease by CT or MRI. FDG-PET has limited sensitivity for liver metastases, because small FDG-avid lesions are obscured by the physiologic hepatic uptake of FDG.[274] In predominately adult populations, the sensitivity and specificity of MRI and CT for liver metastases has varied, depending on the technique used and the histology of the metastases.[275] Comparable pediatric studies are lacking, although most liver metastases in children are hypovascular and evident in the portal venous phase of contrast enhancement so that multiphasic CT or MRI studies are not necessary. The exceptional hypervascular tumors, such as neuroendocrine tumors, are best depicted in the hepatic arterial phase of enhancement. Multiphasic studies may also be useful in distinguishing liver hemangiomas from liver metastases.

Lymphoma and stage 4s neuroblastoma liver metastases may be diffusely infiltrative and present as hepatomegaly rather than focal lesions. As most liver metastases arise from solid intra-abdominal tumors, the CT and MRI performed to assess the primary tumor usually suffice to evaluate accompanying hepatic metastatic disease (Fig. 9.38). These studies also evaluate lymph nodes and the spleen, adrenal glands, pancreas, and kidneys for possible metastases. Metastases to these other intra-abdominal organs are uncommon in children and are most frequently seen with lymphoma (Fig. 9.3). It is important not to confuse the normal heterogeneous enhancement pattern of the spleen for metastatic disease.[276]

Skeletal Metastases

The skeleton is a frequent site of focal metastases of certain solid tumors in children, especially neuroblastoma, sarcoma, and histiocytosis. On conventional radiographs, skeletal metastatic disease manifests as focal destructive lesions, periosteal reaction, lucent metaphyseal bands, generalized bony demineralization, or pathologic fractures. Tc-99m phosphonate–based bone scintigraphy is generally more sensitive than conventional radiographic surveys for the detection of skeletal metastatic disease and is the customary means of screening for bony metastases. Langerhans' cell histiocytosis is an exception in which Tc-99m phosphonate–based bone scintigraphy is less sensitive than conventional radiographic skeletal series for some disease sites but can serve a complementary role.[1] Tc-99m phosphonate–based bone scintigraphy also does not detect all sites of skeletal involvement by neuroblastoma and is complementary to MIBG-scintigraphy in this regard.[19] Abnormal calcium metabolism often accompanies hepatoblastoma and may cause false-positive uptake on bone scintigraphy.[277]

In the evaluation of bony metastases, CT and MRI are typically used only when the patient presents with symptoms related to the skeleton (e.g., limb pain) but has negative skeletal radiographic and scintigraphic results. MRI is preferable to CT in this setting because of its higher sensitivity to bone marrow disease and superior demonstration of associated extraosseous masses, information that is critical if the lesion is to be irradiated or surgically resected. As a potential alternative imaging modality for the detection of skeletal metastases in children, whole-body MRI has demonstrated superior sensitivity compared with Tc-99m phosphonate–based bone scintigraphy; whole-body MRI can detect tumor deposits in the skeleton before the host osteoblastic response develops.[278-280] The American College of Radiology Imaging Network is currently sponsoring a multi-institutional study to compare the efficacy of fast whole-body MRI with that of CT and Tc-99m phosphonate–based bone scintigraphy for staging and detecting distant metastases in common pediatric small round cell malignancies (rhabdomyosarcoma, Ewing's sarcoma, neuroblastoma, or lymphoma). Growing evidence suggests that FDG-PET is superior to Tc-99m phosphonate–based bone scintigraphy in detecting bone marrow involvement in patients with rhabdomyosarcoma or Ewing's sarcoma[254,280,281] but perhaps not osteosarcoma.[254] In the case of Langerhans' cell histiocytosis, FDG-PET is more sensitive for detecting skeletal involvement than is conventional radiography, Tc-99m phosphonate–based bone scintigraphy, CT, or MRI, with the exception of the spine where MRI is more sensitive.[282] Although the sensitivity of whole-body MRI and FDG-PET for metastatic disease may be high, the specificity is likely to be more modest, and the interpreter of the imaging studies must be cognizant of potential causes of false-positive findings.

Awareness of the effect of therapy with leukocyte colony-stimulating factors such as granulocyte colony-stimulating factor (G-CSF) on the bone marrow is important to avoid false-positive interpretations of marrow metastases. G-CSF causes reconversion of bone marrow from fatty to hematopoietic marrow that coincides temporally with increases in the absolute neutrophil count. This process appears as foci of corresponding bone marrow signal intensity alterations on MRI[283] and increased bone marrow FDG uptake on PET[284]

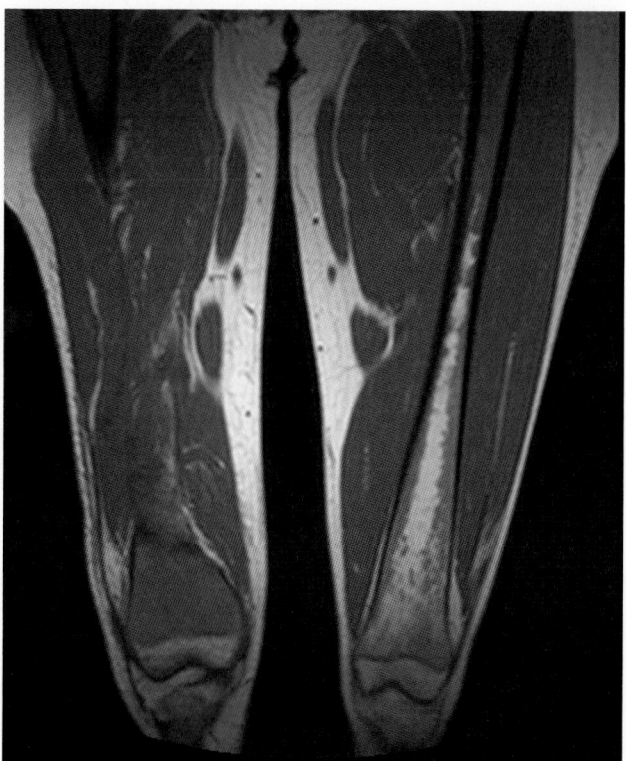

FIGURE 9.56 Granulocyte colony-stimulating factor (G-CSF) effect on the bone marrow. Coronal T1-weighted magnetic resonance image of a patient being treated with G-CSF for myelosuppression related to chemotherapy for Ewing's sarcoma of the distal right femur. Patchy geographic foci of low signal intensity in the bone marrow of the left femur represent granulopoietic marrow hyperplasia. Such marrow hyperplasia can simulate or mask marrow metastases.

that can mimic metastatic infiltration (Fig. 9.56). This can also mask underlying bone marrow metastases. The effect of G-CSF on FDG uptake by the bone marrow varies substantially among individuals and with the intensity of therapy. Patients receiving high-dose chemotherapy followed by bone marrow or stem cell transplantation show less marrow FDG uptake than those receiving low-dose chemotherapy. FDG uptake by the marrow returns to normal within 1 month after the discontinuation of G-CSF treatment in most individuals.[285] Therefore, increased FDG uptake by bone marrow must be correlated with the patient's clinical history to determine whether the uptake is more likely to be related to a benign or malignant process.

Therapeutic Planning

Delineation of the extent of a tumor and its anatomic relationships to vital structures is particularly important when surgery or radiation therapy is planned. Noninvasive imaging studies recommended for tumor diagnosis and staging provide adequate information to guide the pediatric oncology team in selecting the appropriate management course. Invasive diagnostic angiography is rarely needed.

In cases of primary pediatric liver malignancies, high-quality preoperative imaging is crucial to help determine whether partial hepatectomy or liver transplantation should be pursued. Preoperative imaging also identifies anatomic variants of the liver vasculature that may complicate surgery and increase the risk of postoperative complications. To define the extent of tumor and its relationship to the hepatic vasculature, contrast-enhanced multiphasic abdominal CT or MRI is performed, with Doppler sonography as an adjunct if CTA or MRA is not available or is inconclusive for vascular involvement[286] (Fig. 9.42). The PRETEXT (pretreatment extent of disease) staging system[287] predicts operability based on factors such as the liver sections and vasculature involved by tumor and the extrahepatic tumor extent. The PRETEXT system is not highly accurate because it is difficult to distinguish parenchymal compression of a liver section by tumor from parenchymal ingrowth of tumor, but the system has good interobserver reproducibility and prognostic value for children with hepatoblastoma.[288] Intraoperative ultrasound can improve the depiction of tumor extent and assist with the planning of the most appropriate surgical strategy, especially in cases of multifocal hepatoblastoma or hepatocellular carcinoma. Liver transplantation should be strongly considered when complete tumor excision by partial hepatectomy is unlikely, such as in PRETEXT IV tumors (unless a unifocal tumor is clearly downstaged to PRETEXT III after preoperative chemotherapy); multifocal PRETEXT III tumors; and central tumors involving the inferior vena cava, all three hepatic veins, or the main portal vein or its right and left branches. Liver transplantation is a viable option for children with lung metastases that clear with preoperative chemotherapy or surgical resection by the time of transplantation.[286]

Tumor rupture is a major risk factor for abdominal recurrence of Wilms' tumor. The identification of preoperative tumor rupture may indicate the need for immediate surgery to prevent hemorrhagic complications or the need to modify treatment to include flank-only or whole-abdomen radiation therapy, depending on whether rupture is present and whether it is retroperitoneal or intraperitoneal. Clinical signs are insensitive for the detection of preoperative Wilms' tumor rupture, and a reliable diagnostic method is important to ensure that abdominal radiation therapy is administered only when appropriate, to avoid unnecessary toxicity. On CT, an isolated small amount of nonhemorrhagic intraperitoneal fluid is not predictive of rupture, but acute intraperitoneal hemorrhage or peritoneal tumor nodules separate from the primary tumor are accurate indicators of intraperitoneal rupture.[289]

The anatomic and metabolic information gained by MRI and FDG-PET, respectively, improves the diagnostic yield of stereotactic brain biopsy in children with ill-defined, infiltrative brain tumors, reduces tissue sampling in high-risk functional areas,[290] and facilitates tumor resection planning.[291] Use of this information is also being explored for planning of radiation therapy fields in pediatric tumors such as lymphoma.[292]

As part of the preoperative assessment to guide the neurosurgeon and avert injury, blood oxygen level–dependent (BOLD) functional MRI techniques can identify the loci of eloquent cerebral cortical functions,[293] and MR diffusion tensor imaging tractography can localize important white matter tracts relative to the tumor.[78]

Assessment of Therapeutic Response

With any cancer treatment regimen, there is an obvious desire to know whether the treatment is having the intended effect. Tumor response assessment can have different endpoints, depending on the clinical setting. In clinical trials, tumor response assessment serves to determine whether the treatment exhibits encouraging enough results to warrant further testing or serves as a surrogate end point of outcome to estimate pharmacologic effect and treatment benefit. Outside the clinical trial setting, tumor response assessment guides the clinician's decisions about continuation of current therapy.[294]

Cross-sectional imaging techniques are heavily relied upon for determining tumor size and extent. Therapeutic response is typically evaluated with the same imaging modalities used for diagnosis and staging of the tumor. In most instances, CT or MRI is the modality of choice, although ultrasound or scintigraphy may be acceptable (or even desirable) in some settings.

To allow valid comparison of treatment efficacy in clinical trials, tumor response criteria must be uniform and reproducible. The revised WHO criteria[295] assign standardized tumor measurement and treatment response into the categories of complete response, partial response, stable disease, and progressive disease. Following the introduction of these criteria, there was a proliferation of alternative response criteria for solid tumors adopted by the various cancer cooperative groups and other organizations conducting clinical trials. In an effort to more widely standardize tumor response criteria, the Response Evaluation Criteria in Solid Tumors (RECIST) guidelines were developed.[296] A revised version of these guidelines (RECIST 1.1) was recently published[297] and stipulates that only a single dimension is to be used to express lesion size and that the longest diameter of target lesions should be selected only in the axial plane for CT. The guidelines also define measurable disease, with nonmeasurable disease including blastic bone lesions or lytic bone lesions without an identifiable soft tissue component, leptomeningeal spread, ascites, effusions, lymphangitic spread, cystic lesions, and lesions too small to accurately measure (less than 10-mm diameter by CT or MRI). For the purposes of pediatric tumor response assessment, the RECIST 1.1 guidelines have a number of limitations, including the lack of validation in pediatric tumors, disallowance of ultrasound as a measurement technique, limited incorporation of functional tumor assessment (e.g., FDG-PET), preference for CT in body imaging, designation of pathologic measurable lymph nodes as having a short-axis diameter of at least 15 mm and normal nodes as less than 10 mm (normal nodal sizes vary substantially with body region in children), designation of lesions less than 10 mm diameter as too small to accurately measure (current CT and MRI technology can be accurate for smaller sizes) and reliance on a unidimensional measurement approach that results in progressively worse correlation with tumor volume as tumor shape eccentricity increases.[298]

Substantial discordance can occur in response categorization when there is variance in the number of lesions measured[299] or method of measurement.[300] The WHO and RECIST methods of measuring tumor size are crude surrogates for true tumor volume. The imprecision and inaccuracy of these methods is accentuated in tumors with irregular borders or ill-defined margins with adjacent structures. Calculation of true tumor volume is the optimal method of tumor size measurement but has been hindered in routine clinical practice by workflow constraints and the slow implementation of automated image-processing software.

The limitations of using size changes as a measure of tumor response must be recognized. Tumors in rigid confines, such as bone sarcomas, may not grow or shrink like tumors surrounded by soft tissues. Tumor volume provides only a rough estimate of the number of viable neoplastic cells, because tumor masses are composed of variable proportions of viable neoplastic cells, nonneoplastic cellular infiltrate, and extracellular matrix. Also, the number of viable neoplastic cells may not correlate with proclivity for malignant behavior such as invasion and metastasis. Some new therapeutic agents, such as those targeted against tumor angiogenesis, may be more cytostatic than cytotoxic and better assessed either by functional imaging techniques or by measures such as progression-free survival or time to progression than by tumor size reduction.

Metabolic activity and expression of various molecular markers precede changes in tumor size and are evaluable as indicators of response with functional and molecular imaging techniques. For these reasons, tumor response criteria must be adaptable to the specific biological mechanism and goal of therapy. Although the adoption of uniform response criteria facilitates the comparison of trial results, a one-method-fits-all approach is ultimately misguided.

The shortcomings of using size changes as a measure of tumor response is illustrated by the experience with GISTs treated with tyrosine kinase receptor inhibitors. Metabolic response as defined by decreased FDG uptake in GIST lesions predicts a better clinical outcome and precedes a decrease of tumor size on CT by weeks or months, while the lack of metabolic reponse on FDG-PET indicates drug resistance. An apparent increase in GIST size related to fluid accumulation from treatment-related intratumoral hemorrhage or necrosis or an increase in conspicuity of GIST metastases in the liver from diminished tumor enhancement relative to the liver parenchyma can result in misinterpretation of GIST tumor response as progression on CT. Conversely, the development of an enhancing intratumoral nodule within a treated tumor without a change in overall tumor size is indicative of disease progression or recurrence. Revised CT response criteria for GISTs using no growth in tumor size or decreased tumor enhancement show better correlation with FDG-PET results and clinical outcome.[301]

A troublesome clinical dilemma is the detection of a residual mass by imaging after treatment, despite resolution of clinical symptoms and normalization of laboratory tests. Residual masses are especially frequent in mediastinal lymphomas and can be problematic in neuroblastomas, sarcomas, and germ cell tumors[302,303] (Fig. 9.57). The residual mass after treatment may be composed of nonneoplastic scar tissue with or without residual neoplasm, and tumors that are associated with large amounts of fibrosis (e.g., nodular sclerosis Hodgkin lymphoma) are more frequently associated with residual masses than are more cellular tumors. Characterizing a residual mass

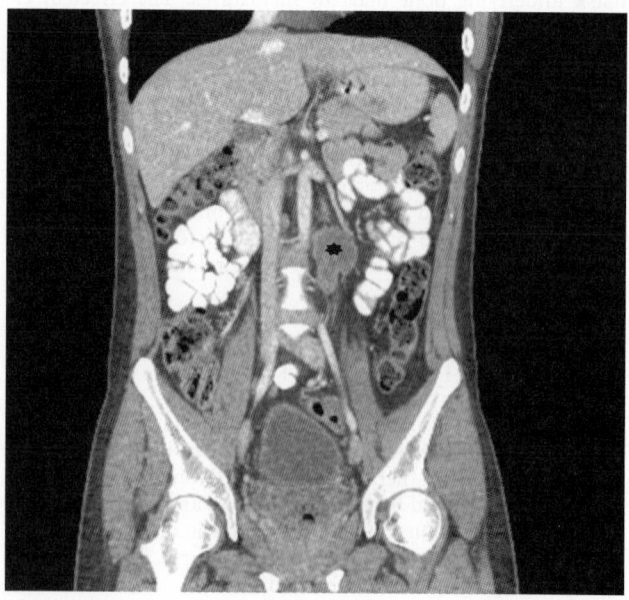

FIGURE 9.57 Residual mass after chemotherapy for metastatic malignant left testicular germ cell tumor. A coronal contrast-enhanced computed tomography image demonstrates a residual nodal soft tissue mass (*asterisk*) in the left para-aortic retroperitoneal region. Biopsy revealed only benign mature teratomatous elements in the mass.

is important, because active residual neoplasm portends a high risk of local relapse if additional therapy is not pursued, while a benign residual mass confers a good prognosis without further treatment. If the residual mass is in the periphery, biopsy can readily be performed, but residual masses are typically in the mediastinum or abdomen, where a noninvasive method of diagnosis is desirable.

Conventional morphologic imaging with CT and MRI is unreliable in assessing whether a residual mass contains viable tumor. FDG-PET more accurately differentiates viable tumor from scar tissue in a residual mass.[304] In a pediatric patient with lymphoma in clinical remission who has a residual mass, FDG-PET has high sensitivity but low specificity. The high-negative predictive value of a negative FDG-PET at the end of therapy for lymphoma may allow for observation and imaging follow-up rather than biopsy,[302] while a positive FDG-PET scan at the end of therapy is not a consistent predictor of relapse in children and adolescents and should not be the sole basis for treatment decisions.[24,305,306] Increased FDG uptake on PET can be observed several weeks or even months after radiation therapy, and the optimal timing for evaluating a residual mass with FDG-PET following completion of radiotherapy in pediatric patients is not clearly defined.[31,307]

FDG-PET is useful for evaluating treatment response in the skeleton, particularly at the primary site. The development of healing sclerosis visible on radiographs may be delayed or absent after the eradication of viable tumor, and residual viable tumor may be indistinguishable from the effects of therapy on MRI or Tc-99m phosphonate–based bone scintigraphy.[255,256] In Langerhans' cell histiocytosis, FDG-PET detects response to therapy more accurately and earlier than other modalities.[282] For restaging of high-risk neuroblastoma before proceeding with bone marrow or stem cell transplantation, residual positivity on MIBG scintigraphy is an important indicator of poor prognosis.[308] Functional imaging studies may eventually serve to predict the risk of relapse in a broad spectrum of pediatric malignancies.[28]

Surveillance for Tumor Recurrence

Recurrent disease is defined as reappearance of tumor in its original location or as metastases in distant sites. The primary objective of tumor surveillance is early detection of recurrence, because salvage therapy is presumably more effective if initiated early. The primary site is usually best followed with the imaging modality used to detect the initial tumor. Selection of the appropriate imaging modality for evaluation of metastatic disease requires knowledge of the natural history of the tumor and may involve a combination of radiography, CT, MRI, and scintigraphy.

A particularly vexing unresolved question is how often and how long follow-up surveillance studies should be obtained. Protocols for imaging surveillance after treatment have been largely based on *ad hoc* assumptions rather than rigorous outcomes research or cost-effectiveness studies. They often entail numerous imaging studies over the course of surveillance, incurring high cumulative costs, radiation exposure, and parental and patient anxiety for questionable benefit in asymptomatic patients. A rational surveillance strategy should be based on knowledge of the frequency, timing, and sites of recurrence; risk factors for recurrence; efficacy of salvage therapy; and efficacy of diagnostic imaging, with diagnostic imaging done more frequently when the risk of recurrence is the highest and less frequently as the risk of recurrence wanes. For example, the same surveillance strategy should not be used for Burkitt's lymphoma, which nearly always reoccurs within the first year after treatment, and Hodgkin lymphoma, which typically reoccurs within the first 3 years and is relatively less common at the sites of initial involvement if radiation therapy was part of the treatment regimen.[309] Certain prognostic indicators should also be considered when planning surveillance strategies, because risk group at presentation and results of laboratory tests or functional imaging studies at the end of therapy can serve as predictors of recurrence. For example, patients with a negative FDG-PET examination at the end of therapy for low-risk Hodgkin lymphoma may not require further imaging unless relapse is clinically suspected.[310]

The efficacy of surveillance by diagnostic imaging depends on the lead time afforded by the imaging study. The lead time is a measure of the ability of an imaging study to detect clinically occult disease and depends on the growth rate of the tumor and the inherent ability of the imaging study to detect it. Unfortunately, the lead time of imaging studies for most pediatric tumors is not well defined. Even if diagnostic imaging is efficacious in detecting relapse earlier than clinical evaluation, the costs of surveillance may be daunting if the risk of recurrence is very small, and a beneficial impact on survival is unlikely, unless there is curative salvage therapy that is more effective if initiated earlier. However, surveillance may still serve to identify disease recurrence in unsuspected sites so that morbid complications can be averted with palliative therapy.[311]

Optimized cancer surveillance strategies can be devised with operations research methodology using data on patterns of recurrence, lead time estimation, and mathematical modeling.[312] Several such analyses have been performed, with strategies offered for surveillance of Ewing's sarcoma[313] and pediatric Hodgkin lymphoma.[314] However, these strategies are based on limited data from a few institutions and may not be generalizable to other practice settings, particularly with differences in relapse rates, efficacy of salvage therapy, and advances made in imaging technology since the time of the analyses. The clinical trial protocols organized by the various cancer cooperative groups should provide a mechanism for collection and analysis of appropriate recurrence data for the various tumor subtypes and risk categories, so that updated optimal surveillance strategies can be derived. The same principles could also be applied to devising optimal strategies for the screening of patients at high risk of developing cancer.

Screening for Primary Malignancy

Screening for certain primary malignancies with imaging is a widely adopted and accepted practice for reducing cancer mortality in adults, as in the case of mammography for breast cancer. In children, screening for primary malignancy with imaging is used on a much more limited basis, mostly because of the much lower incidence of solid tumors in children. However, certain pediatric subpopulations are at relatively high risk for development of solid tumors, and imaging plays a role in their screening.

Children with conditions associated with nephroblastomatosis (multiple or diffuse nephrogenic rests) have an elevated risk for Wilms' tumor. Nephrogenic rests are associated with 99% of bilateral synchronous and 94% of metachronous bilateral Wilms' tumors. Nephrogenic rests are classified histopathologically as dormant/nascent, sclerosing/regressing, hyperplastic, or neoplastic; dormant and sclerosing rests do not have malignant potential. Imaging findings correlate with nephrogenic rest histology. On T2-weighted MRI sequences, sclerosing nephrogenic rests are hypointense compared with normal renal parenchyma, and hyperplastic rests and Wilms' tumor are isointense or hyperintense. On MRI and CT, nephrogenic rests are homogeneous in appearance and tend to

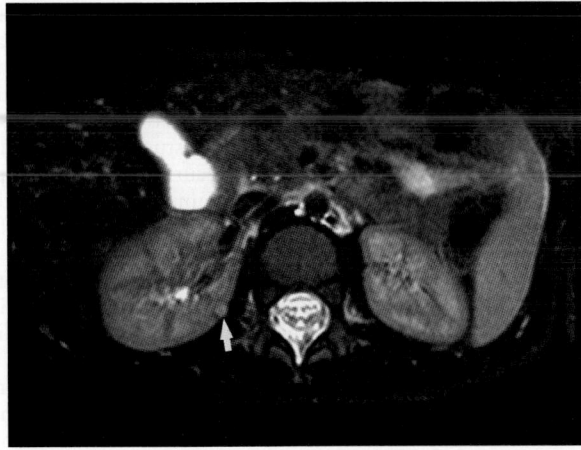
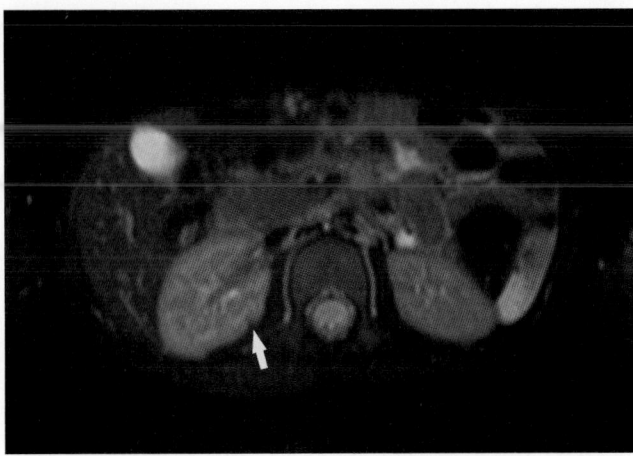

FIGURE 9.58 Nephrogenic rest. Axial T2-weighted magnetic resonance (MR) image (**A**) obtained at the time of presentation of a patient with a right renal lower pole Wilms' tumor (not depicted) shows a small lesion (*arrow*) of nearly isointense signal intensity at the peripheral posteromedial aspect of the mid- to upper-pole region of the right kidney. Fifteen months later, with the patient having undergone partial nephrectomy and chemotherapy, an axial T2-weighted MR image (**B**) demonstrates that the lesion (*arrow*) in the remnant right kidney is smaller and of lower signal intensity, consistent with a sclerosing nephrogenic rest.

be small and lenticular or oval; in contrast, Wilms' tumor is inhomogeneous, particularly on postcontrast images, due to necrosis and hemorrhage (Fig. 9.58). MRI and contrast-enhanced CT are more sensitive than ultrasound for detecting small (less than 2-cm diameter) nephrogenic rests, though the sensitivity of imaging is limited, and nephrogenic rests smaller than 4-mm diameter are generally not detectable by imaging.[315,316] An increase in size or development of inhomogeneity in a nephrogenic rest is suspicious for neoplastic transformation.[317]

The rate of metachronous bilateral Wilms' tumor is similar to the risk (5%) of Wilms' tumor in children with Beckwith-Wiedemann syndrome.[318] In a case series, patients with Beckwith-Wiedemann syndrome or isolated hemihypertrophy screened at 4-month intervals or less when compared with patients not screened had significantly reduced late-stage disease and smaller tumor size.[319] In a cost-effectiveness model analysis, screening children with Beckwith-Wiedemann syndrome for tumors with ultrasound at 4-month intervals up until 4 years of age had an incremental cost per life year saved comparable with the acceptable population-based cancer screening ranges at the time (less than $50,000 per life year saved).[320] Because of the relatively high cure rate for Wilms' tumor, surveillance may not significantly affect overall survival, but detection at earlier stages may avert complications from treatments required for advanced disease such as more extensive surgery or radiation therapy.[321] For surveillance of children with greater than 5% risk of Wilms' tumor, the U.K. Wilms' Tumor Surveillance Working Group recommends that renal ultrasound be obtained at 3- to 4-month intervals until 5 years of age, except in those with Beckwith-Wiedemann syndrome, Simpson-Golabi-Behmel syndrome, or some familial Wilms' tumor pedigrees, in whom the renal ultrasound surveillance should continue until 7 years of age.[322] The brief interval between screening examinations is based on the rapid doubling time of Wilms' tumor cells, which is estimated to be as short as 11 days.[323] Children with Beckwith-Wiedemann syndrome and/or isolated hemihypertrophy are at risk for not only Wilms' tumor but also hepatoblastoma and adrenocortical carcinoma in early childhood, with an overall risk of neoplasia of approximately 6% to 9%. For this reason, some cli-

nicians advocate screening not only the kidneys but also the liver and adrenals with an abdominal ultrasound examination in these children every 3 months until the age of 8 years.[324]

Testicular microlithiasis is an asymptomatic condition in which calcium deposits occur in the seminiferous tubules and appear as punctuate nonshadowing hyperechoic foci by ultrasound (Fig. 9.59). Testicular microlithiasis is associated with testicular neoplasia (particularly germ cell tumors and carcinoma *in situ*), cryptorchidism, varicocele, infertility, Klinefelter syndrome, McCune-Albright syndrome, and pulmonary alveolar microlithiasis. With more frequent use of high-frequency ultrasound transducers, the observation of testicular microlithiasis has increased and has a prevalence of approximately 2% in boys and adolescent males.[325] Testicular microlithiasis is more common in the contralateral testes of patients with testicular germ cell tumors and in their relatives, suggesting that testicular microlithiasis and germ cell tumors have a shared genetic susceptibility and that testicular

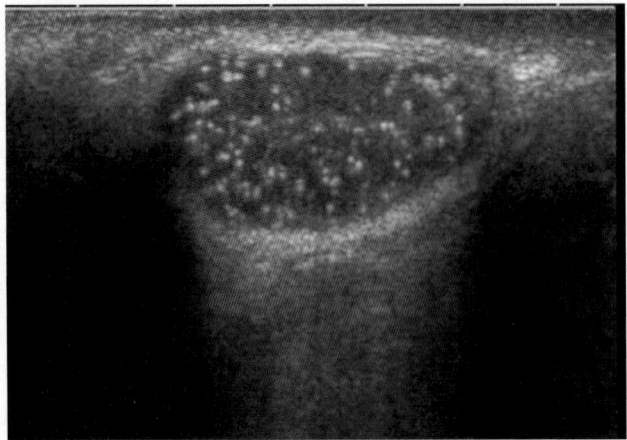

FIGURE 9.59 Testicular microlithiasis. Longitudinal ultrasound image of the left testicle reveals multiple punctate hyperechoic foci within the testicle without an associated soft tissue mass.

microlithiasis is a marker rather than a premalignant lesion. Because of the association of testicular microlithiasis with neoplasia, surveillance with serial scrotal ultrasonography has been recommended, but this has not been demonstrated to be cost-effective or to improve outcomes over surveillance by physical examination alone.[326,327]

Heritable retinoblastoma is a highly penetrant condition that develops in 90% of patients who inherit *RB1* gene mutations, which can be identified by genetic testing;[321] 0.5% to 15% also develop blastomas of the pineal gland or the supra- or parasellar regions (trilateral retinoblastoma). To screen for pineal or sellar region tumors, children harboring a germline *RB1* mutation should undergo brain MRI examinations every 6 months until 5 years of age. Such screening identifies trilateral retinoblastoma at a smaller tumor size and is associated with longer survival.[328]

Patients with NF1 have as much as a 10% lifetime risk of malignant peripheral nerve sheath tumors (MPNST), most of which develop during the second or third decades of life. Most NF1-associated MPNSTs arise within preexisting plexiform neurofibromas, and development in deep cervicothoracic or abdominopelvic locations may not produce symptoms until local growth affects adjacent structures or until distant metastases have occurred, suggesting that individuals with NF1 and plexiform neurofibromas may benefit from imaging surveillance. MRI signs suggestive of malignant transformation of a nerve sheath tumor include rapid growth, irregular margins, and loss of the typical target sign[329] (Fig. 9.60). Benign plexiform neurofibromas can undergo periods of rapid growth that limit the use of MRI in predicting malignant transformation. FDG-PET shows promise as an alternative imaging modality for detecting and discriminating MPNSTs from benign neurofibromas,[330] although guidelines for routine imaging screening await validation. Optic pathway tumors (OPT) occur in 15% to 20% of individuals with NF1, with the greatest risk of development occurring during the first 6 years of life. Although OPTs may be amenable to early detection by MRI surveillance, most are benign and nonprogressive, and routine screening MRI of asymptomatic patients with normal visual examinations may not be warranted. The proposed intervals for follow-up MRI of an NF1-associated OPT range from 3 to 24 months.[331]

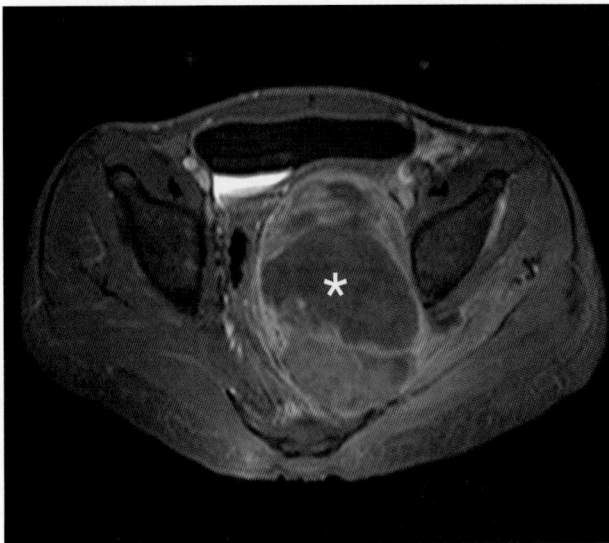

FIGURE 9.60 Malignant peripheral nerve sheath tumor in a patient with NF1. Axial gadolinium-enhanced T1-weighted magnetic resonance image of the pelvis discloses a partially necrotic mass (*asterisk*) arising from the left sacral nerve plexus.

Evaluation of Complications of Therapy and Late Effects

All three primary modalities used in antitumor therapy (surgery, radiation therapy, and chemotherapy), as well as ancillary procedures such as bone marrow or stem cell transplantation, can lead to complications diagnosable by imaging procedures. Most complications of surgery, including infection, bleeding, scarring, organ injury, and bowel obstruction, are not unique to patients with cancer. Complications of radiation therapy and chemotherapy can involve virtually any organ system, and their onset can be acute or delayed. They can be direct effects such as osteonecrosis and pulmonary fibrosis or secondary effects such as infections consequent to immunosuppression. Childhood cancer survivors represent a growing population at risk for late toxic effects of therapy and second malignancies that compromise quality and length of life.[332,333] Guidelines for long-term follow-up of childhood cancer survivors have been developed by the Children's Oncology Group (www.survivorshipguidelines.org), and diagnostic imaging plays a crucial role in diagnosing complications of therapy and monitoring for late effects and second malignancies.

Venous thromboembolic disease is frequently encountered in pediatric oncology patients and is related to multiple risk factors, including malignancy (especially leukemia, lymphoma, and sarcoma), immobilization, infection, genetic prothrombotic disorders, certain chemotherapeutic agents (such as L-asparaginase), and indwelling central vascular catheters. Pulmonary embolus usually originates from migration of bland thrombus in deep or central veins but can also arise from tumor thrombus in malignancies associated with intravascular extension, such as Wilms' tumor, hepatoblastoma, and adrenocortical carcinoma (Fig. 9.39). Although deep venous thrombosis and pulmonary embolism may result in limb swelling or respiratory distress, respectively, many cases of venous thromboembolic disease are initially clinically occult, particularly pericatheter thrombus. If undetected, adverse sequelae such as catheter malfunction, line sepsis, pulmonary embolism, and vascular occlusion with postthrombotic syndrome may ensue.[334] Fibrin sheaths along a catheter can lead to catheter occlusion or drug extravasation and are diagnosable by contrast injection of the catheter under fluoroscopy. Deep venous thrombosis of the extremity and neck vessels is readily amenable to detection by Doppler sonography, and CTA or MRA may be required to detect involvement of intrathoracic or pelvic vessels, particularly in larger patients. Ventilation-perfusion scintigraphy has been largely replaced by CT pulmonary angiography for the diagnosis of pulmonary embolism, although the former incurs a lower radiation dose and is still valuable if there are contraindications to the administration of intravenous iodinated contrast for CT or if chest radiography is clear.[335]

Children receiving chemotherapy or radiation therapy to the CNS are subject to a wide spectrum of complications. White matter disease caused by radiation therapy (or occasionally chemotherapy) manifests on MRI as white matter edema and demyelination within the irradiated region (or diffusely with chemotherapy) and can exhibit mass effect and contrast enhancement. Loss of cerebral white matter fractional anisotropy, as revealed by diffusion tensor MRI, correlates with IQ score deficits in survivors of childhood medulloblastoma or ALL.[336] Parenchymal brain volume loss, which can be associated with steroid therapy, cranial irradiation, or intrathecal chemotherapy, also correlates with neurocognitive deficits.[337] Necrotizing diffuse leukoencephalopathy, seen with combined chemotherapy and radiation therapy, appears as extensive areas of white matter necrosis with marked contrast enhancement and a tendency toward posterior calcification.[338] Mineralizing microangiopathy, most commonly related to combined radiation therapy and chemotherapy with intrathecal methotrexate, appears as dystrophic calcifications on head CT or abnormal signal intensity on MRI in the basal ganglia and subcortical white matter, but the imaging findings do not clearly correlate with clinical symptoms.[339] Radiation-induced vascular malformations, sometimes visible on gradient echo MRI images because of magnetic susceptibility artifact from blood products, appear several years after treatment and have the potential to hemorrhage.[340] Acute encephalopathy related to high-dose or intrathecal methotrexate therapy is associated with waxing and waning stroke-like events and is characterized on MRI by restricted diffusion involving deep cerebral white matter across multiple vascular beds that develop early and resolve as clinical status improves.[341] Head CT readily detects intracranial hemorrhage related to thrombocytopenia or coagulopathy associated with chemotherapy, bone marrow transplantation, or disseminated intravascular coagulation. Head CT and MRI are useful in detecting cerebral hemorrhagic infarction from dural sinus or venous thrombosis, precipitated by leukemic leukostasis, dehydration, or L-asparaginase chemotherapy[342] (Fig. 9.20). Fungal infection, especially invasive aspergillosis in neutropenic patients, can also cause hemorrhagic cerebral infarctions amenable to detection by CT or MRI. Imaging is valuable in screening for fungal paranasal sinusitis that can manifest with only mild symptoms but rapidly invade the CNS in immunosuppressed patients.[343] The characteristic finding of increased diffusion in vasogenic edema at posterior brain regions on DWI helps confirm a diagnosis of reversible posterior leukoencephalopathy in patients with hypertension and predisposing conditions such as cyclosporine therapy.[344] FDG-PET and MRS are useful in distinguishing radiation necrosis from recurrent or residual viable brain tumor, a task that is unable to be reliably accomplished with conventional MRI.[78,345]

Sequelae of neck irradiation include thyroid disorders, carotid artery disease, and esophageal strictures. External irradiation of the thyroid, even at low doses, induces the development of thyroid nodules and carcinomas, and the risk is greater when irradiation occurs at a younger age, in female patients,[346] and when the thyroid is exposed to scatter radiation rather than being in the direct radiation field.[347] Hypothyroidism develops in nearly 40% of childhood cancer survivors who received radiation therapy to the neck; those survivors have decreased thyroid volume compared with those who remain euthyroid.[348] Ultrasonography can screen for nonpalpable thyroid nodules, confirm clinically suspected thyroid nodules, and determine thyroid volume in patients with a history of childhood external neck irradiation.[349] The cumulative incidence of ultrasound-detected abnormalities peaks 10 to 25 years after diagnosis of the primary malignancy.[347]

Acute radiation pneumonitis is well demonstrated by chest radiography, appearing as air space opacities and interstitial thickening within a well-defined anatomic area corresponding to the radiation field. Acute changes usually appear near the end of therapy or within a month of its completion. Acute radiation pneumonitis can progress to chronic interstitial fibrosis with loss of lung volume. Chest CT, particularly with high-resolution technique, is more sensitive than conventional chest radiographs in detecting radiation fibrosis.[350] Pulmonary fibrosis can also arise from exposure to certain chemotherapeutic agents and can simulate metastatic pulmonary nodules.[351] A recently recognized source of pulmonary toxicity is gemcitabine. Gemcitabine-induced severe pulmonary toxicity (GISPT) occurs with an incidence of less than 2% after administration of gemcitabine alone but with a higher frequency

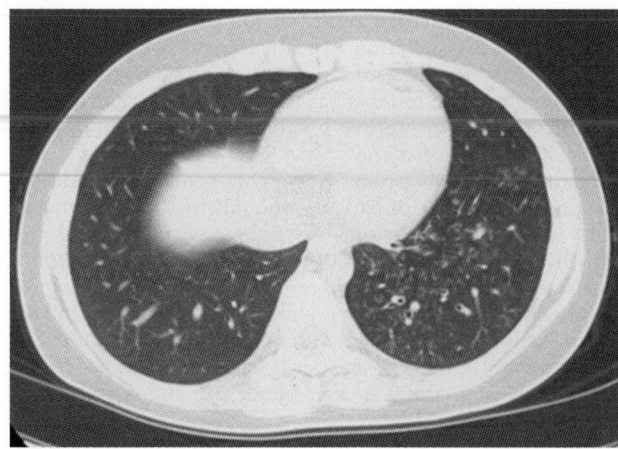

FIGURE 9.61 Atypical mycobacterial infection in an immunocompromised patient with a history of bone marrow transplantation for large cell lymphoma. Axial chest computed tomography image at bone windows shows numerous "tree-in-bud" centrilobular opacities of the left lower lobe. These opacities are produced by the plugging of small airways and are compatible with atypical mycobacterial infection or other infectious/inflammatory processes of the small airways.

when given in combination with other agents such as bleomycin. GISPT is possibly a cytokine-mediated inflammatory reaction of the alveolar capillary wall and manifests as a potentially fatal clinical syndrome of hypoxia with bilateral interstitial or alveolar opacities on chest radiography.[352]

Pulmonary infections are a common cause of morbidity and mortality in immunocompromised patients, and chest imaging is frequently requested to evaluate for these infections. However, the use of routine chest radiography in febrile neutropenic pediatric oncology patients without respiratory symptoms is questionable. Chest CT is more sensitive than conventional chest radiography for detection of pulmonary infections in the immunocompromised host. Nodules with ground-glass halo attenuation suggest aspergillus infection, and tree-in-bud centrilobular opacities suggest atypical mycobacterial infection (Fig. 9.61). However, diagnosis of a specific infectious organism is usually not possible by imaging features alone because they lack specificity.[353,354] Pulmonary cytolytic thrombi (PCT) may be an underrecognized noninfectious etiology of pulmonary nodules in bone marrow or stem cell transplant recipients. The nodules of PCT consist of occlusive vascular lesions associated with hemorrhagic infarcts and may represent a form of acute pulmonary GVHD. The radiologic findings of PCT typically resolve over the course of weeks to months.[355]

Recipients of allogeneic hematopoietic stem cell or bone marrow transplantation are at risk for idiopathic pneumonia syndrome (IPS), bronchiolitis obliterans, and bronchiolitis obliterans with organizing pneumonia (BOOP). IPS is defined as the presence of multilobar opacities on chest radiography or CT, the need for supplemental oxygenation with declining pulse oximetry, and no identifiable pulmonary infection. IPS is associated with hyperacute or acute GVHD and is relatively common, developing in approximately 12% of children 1 to 6 weeks after transplantation.[356] Bronchiolitis obliterans and BOOP are associated with chronic GVHD and develop several months after transplantation. In bronchiolitis obliterans, pulmonary air trapping occurs because of airway occlusion, and chest CT reveals bronchial dilatation, peribronchial thickening, and mosaic lung attenuation. BOOP may be associated with cough and dyspnea and usually demonstrates patchy consolidation or ground-glass attenuation on CT[353] (Fig. 9.62).

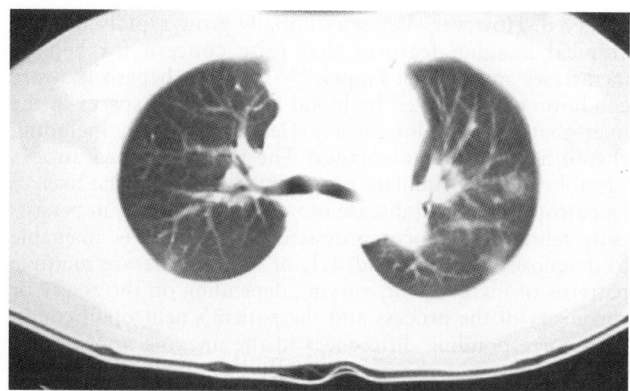

FIGURE 9.62 Bronchiolitis obliterans with organizing pneumonia in a patient with a history of bone marrow transplantation for acute lymphoblastic leukemia. An axial chest computed tomography image at lung windows shows scattered small foci of pulmonary consolidation.

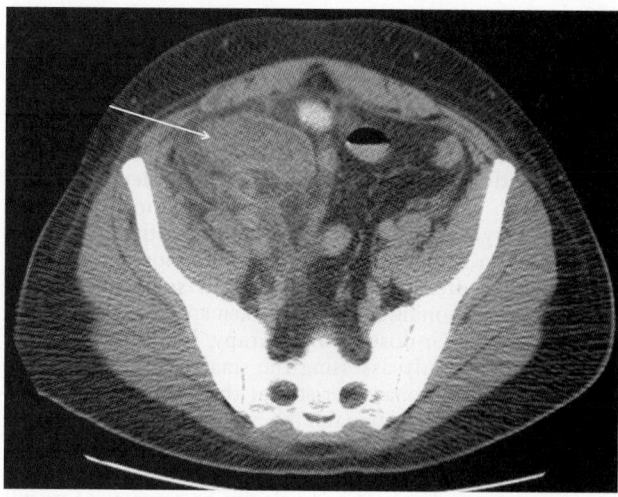

FIGURE 9.63 Typhlitis in a neutropenic patient undergoing chemotherapy for Ewing's sarcoma. An axial computed tomography image of the upper pelvis shows thickening of the wall of the cecum (*arrow*) and marked edema of the pericolonic fat.

Anthracycline chemotherapeutic agents cause a dose-related, irreversible cardiomyopathy; the toxic effect is more pronounced in female patients and those of African descent.[357] Premature coronary artery disease with silent ischemia is a risk of chest irradiation, with a rapid increase over baseline risk for cardiac-related death after about 10 years.[358] Cardiomegaly and pulmonary edema may be seen as relatively late signs of cardiac toxicity on chest radiography, and the early signs of diminished ejection fraction and wall motion abnormalities are evaluable by echocardiography, radionuclide ventriculography, cardiac MRI, or cardiac CT.

Because of the rapid cellular turnover of its mucosa, the GI tract is highly susceptible to toxicity from radiation therapy and chemotherapy. The effects of radiation therapy can be delayed and chronic from compromise of the bowel blood supply, with sequelae of malabsorption and bowel strictures leading to bowel obstruction, evident on abdominal radiographs or contrast fluoroscopy examinations. Other causes of abnormally dilated bowel loops in pediatric oncology patients include severe ileus from vincristine-induced autonomic neuropathy and bowel obstruction from postoperative adhesions or intussusception, most notably after surgery for Wilms' tumor.[359]

Patients undergoing chemotherapy are at particular risk for neutropenic enterocolitis or typhlitis, which involves the cecum but can extend to involve more of the colon, appendix, or ileum. The findings of typhlitis on conventional abdominal radiographs, ultrasound, and CT include bowel wall thickening and pericolonic edema (Fig. 9.63). Bowel wall thickness, as measured by ultrasound, correlates with the duration of typhlitis.[360] The imaging findings of typhlitis overlap with those of other disorders such as *Clostridium difficile* pseudomembranous colitis, cytomegalovirus colitis, ischemic colitis, and GVHD.[361] Correlation of imaging findings with clinical evaluation may be required for differentiation. Although the finding of pneumatosis intestinalis on abdominal radiographs or CT is associated with ischemic or infarcted bowel, "benign pneumatosis" can be seen in a number of settings, including immunosuppressed children, especially if they are on steroids. Benign pneumatosis can be managed conservatively with intravenous antibiotics and bowel rest if the patient otherwise shows no signs of clinical deterioration.[362]

Involvement of the GI tract by GVHD appears as fluid-filled bowel with or without bowel wall thickening, with characteristically increased vascularity by ultrasound and marked bowel wall enhancement by CT or MRI related to mucosal destruction and replacement by highly vascularized granulation tissue.[363,364] Chronic GVHD may manifest in a sclerodermatous form that has a predilection for the extremities, with altered skin pigmentation, indurated plaques, and contractures. This may progress to involve the deeper soft tissues not assessable on physical examination. In these cases, MRI is useful for monitoring the response to immunosuppressive therapy by defining the extent of active disease that appears as increased signal intensity of the involved subcutaneous fat, fascia, or even musculature on STIR and fat-saturated gadolinium-enhanced T1-weighted sequences.[365]

Severe pancreatitis can be induced by L-asparaginase therapy (Fig. 9.64). Sonography and CT are valuable in evaluating complications of pancreatitis that may require treatment by surgery or interventional radiology (i.e., pancreatic necrosis, pseudocyst formation, and arterial pseudoaneurysm).[366]

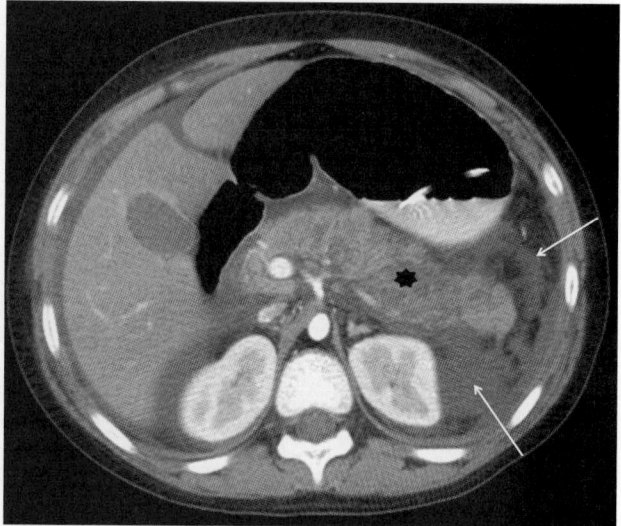

FIGURE 9.64 Pancreatitis induced by L-asparaginase in a patient with acute lymphoblastic leukemia undergoing reinduction chemotherapy. An axial contrast-enhanced abdominal computed tomography image depicts an enlarged, heterogeneously enhancing pancreas (*asterisk*) with extensive peripancreatic fluid (*arrows*) and ascites.

The liver is a common site of complications related to therapy. Hepatic steatosis is frequently observed during chemotherapy and appears as parenchymal hyperechogenicity on sonography, low attenuation on CT, and signal intensity loss on fat-suppressed spin echo and opposed-phase gradient echo MRI. Hepatic steatosis is usually diffuse but can be focal and can simulate focal liver lesions. Hepatic steatosis can also mask liver lesions on CT. Although hepatic steatosis may resolve following cessation of therapy, it can progress to steatohepatitis, fibrosis, and cirrhosis.[367] Doppler ultrasound is often requested to evaluate suspected HVOD following conditioning regimens for hematopoietic cell transplantation or high-dose chemotherapy, but sonography is incapable of directly assessing the small venous and sinusoidal obstruction characteristic of this process. Ancillary findings of HVOD amenable to sonographic assessment include gallbladder wall thickening, ascites, hepatomegaly, elevated hepatic arterial blood flow resistance, patent main hepatic veins, and diminished velocity or reversal of portal venous blood flow (Fig. 9.65). These findings are nonspecific and may not be as useful as clinical parameters in the diagnosis of HVOD.[368] An occasional complication of pediatric cancer therapy is the development of variants of focal nodular hyperplasia or nodular regenerative hyperplasia of the liver, most frequently observed in patients with a history of neuroblastoma treated with cyclophosphamide, busulfan, and melphalan and those with previous HVOD. These lesions may develop in response to localized hepatic vessel injury and can be followed conservatively if asymptomatic and characteristic imaging features of regenerating hepatic nodules are

observed. However, they may initially grow rapidly or have atypical imaging features that raise concern for hepatic metastases and prompt biopsy.[369,370] Peliosis hepatis is a rare condition characterized by blood-filled lacunar spaces in the liver that can develop in a variety of settings, including chemotherapy for malignancy. The imaging appearance is variable and can simulate tumor involvement of the liver.[371] Hepatosplenic fungal disease is a common concern in persistently febrile immunocompromised patients and is amenable to diagnosis by ultrasound, CT, or MRI. There are multiple patterns of involvement, varying depending on the acuity or chronicity of the process and the patient's neutrophil count, with corresponding differences in the imaging appearance. The lesions most characteristically have a "bull's eye" or "wheels-within-wheels" appearance on ultrasound, and a hypoattenuating appearance with or without ring enhancement on CT, with the arterial phase being more sensitive than the portal venous phase.[372] Ultrasound and CT are complementary in sensitivity; MRI or biopsy should be considered if ultrasound and CT are negative, but high clinical concern of hepatosplenic fungal disease persists.[373] The recipient of a liver transplant for treatment of primary hepatic malignancy is subject to a wide array of postoperative complications including hepatic vascular occlusion or pseudoaneurysm, biliary or bowel obstruction or leakage, graft infarction, graft rejection, and infection. Ultrasound is the initial imaging modality for detecting and differentiating these complications, with CT or MRI reserved for cases of an inconclusive or negative ultrasound examination in the setting of a high clinical suspicion.[374]

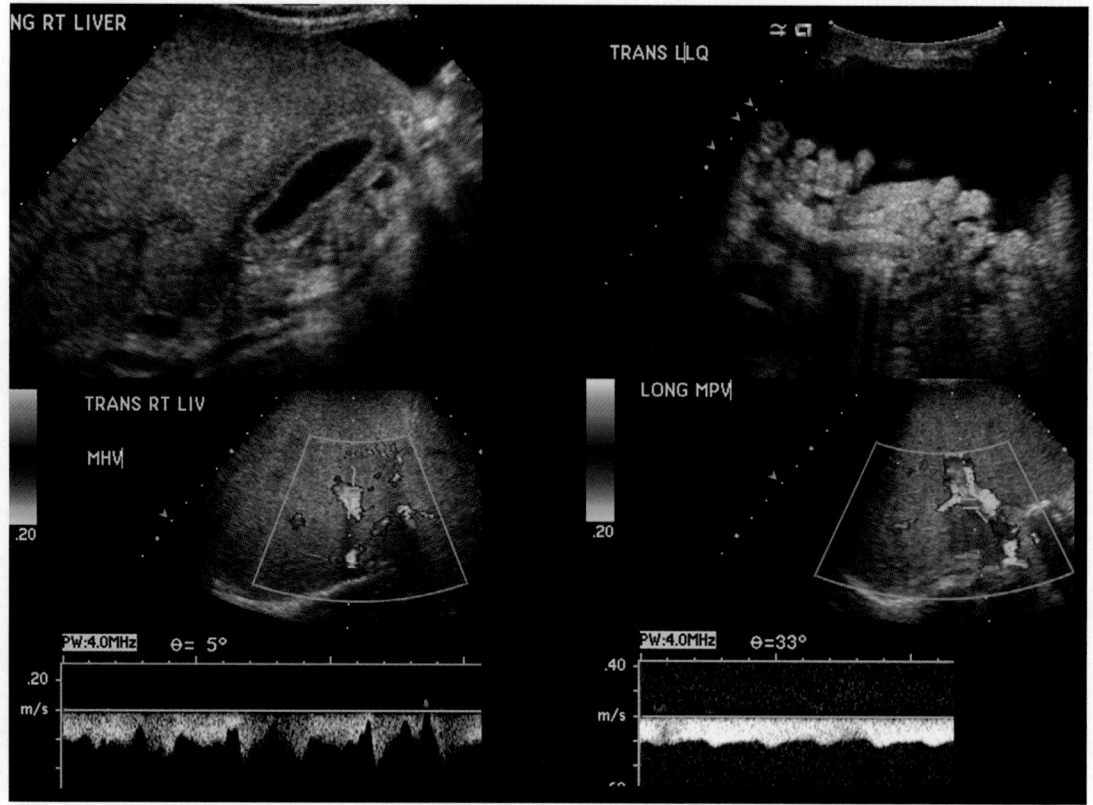

FIGURE 9.65 Hepatic veno-occlusive disease in an infant after bone marrow transplantation. Grayscale and Doppler ultrasound images show hepatomegaly, gall bladder wall thickening, ascites, reversal of portal venous flow, and normal flow in the main hepatic veins. The venous sinusoidal obstruction cannot be directly imaged by sonography, and the diagnosis is inferred from this constellation of findings in the appropriate clinical setting.

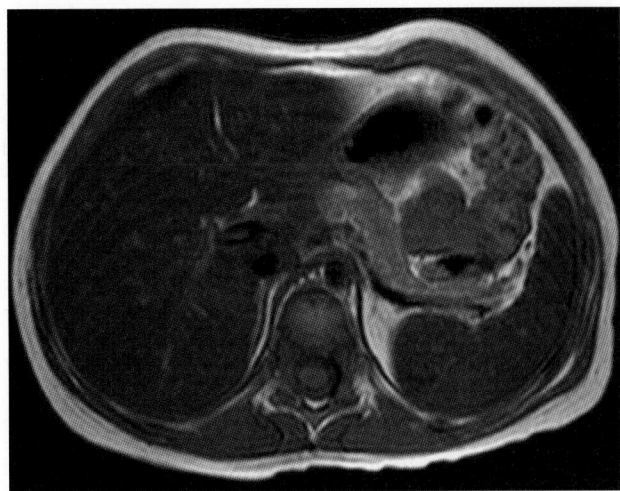

FIGURE 9.66 Hemosiderosis related to numerous blood transfusions in a patient with a history of neuroblastoma and stem cell transplantation. Excess iron deposition in the reticuloendothelial system of the liver and spleen manifests as diffuse, abnormal low signal intensity of these organs on an axial T1-weighted magnetic resonance image.

In hemosiderosis, pathologic levels of iron deposition occur in the reticuloendothelial system of the liver, spleen, and bone marrow, often as a consequence of numerous blood transfusions administered during the course of bone marrow transplantation or chemotherapy-induced marrow depletion in pediatric oncology patients. When iron levels exceed the storage capacity of the reticuloendothelial system, iron accumulates in parenchymal cells of the liver, pancreas, heart, and endocrine glands. By exploiting the superparamagnetic properties of the iron storage complexes of ferritin and hemosiderin, excess iron deposition can be detected on MRI by noting reduced signal intensity of the affected organs, particularly on $T2^*$-weighted gradient echo sequences, but also on T2-weighted spin echo sequences, and, at high iron concentrations, on T1-weighted spin echo sequences (Fig. 9.66). Evidence of iron overload may be seen on MRI within a month after transfusional therapy begins, and the MRI findings of

iron overload regress with iron chelation therapy or cessation of transfusions.[103]

Impaired renal function can occur during therapy secondary to tumor lysis, chemotherapeutic agent nephrotoxicity, or radiation nephritis. Glomerular filtration rate can be calculated by determining the plasma clearance of injected chromium-51-EDTA or Tc-99m-DTPA from multiple blood samples.[38] Serial renal sonography is a simple means to assess renal growth, which may be impaired by radiation nephritis.[375] Hemorrhagic cystitis is a potentially serious complication of chemotherapy (especially after cyclophosphamide or ifosfamide therapy), radiation therapy, or bone marrow transplantation (chiefly from GVHD and BK virus or adenovirus infection). Ultrasound is the imaging modality of choice for the diagnosis and follow-up of hemorrhagic cystitis, but findings may also be appreciable on CT, MRI, or contrast cystography. Typically, there is diffuse thickening and hypervascularity of the bladder wall with or without intraluminal clot, although the entire urothelium is at risk and the renal pelvis and ureters can show urothelial thickening or clot[376] (Fig. 9.67). Dysfunctional voiding can arise from bladder fibrosis or injury to the spinal cord or peripheral nerves from the primary disease or iatrogenic factors, and ultrasound is the initial imaging method of choice to screen for associated bladder wall thickening and urinary tract dilation and assess the bladder capacity and bladder postvoid residual.[377]

Pediatric oncology patients are at risk for a myriad of skeletal complications amenable to diagnosis by imaging. Unless prospectively sought, some of these complications, such as bone mineral density deficits and osteonecrosis, can remain clinically silent until remediation becomes difficult.[378] Children are more prone than adults to skeletal complications of radiation therapy, because growing bone is more sensitive to irradiation than is adult bone. Skeletal irradiation can lead to scoliosis, limb shortening, and overall diminution in height. In the long bones, slipped epiphyses and radiographic changes similar to those seen in patients with rickets can occur, including metaphyseal sclerosis, metaphyseal fraying, and epiphyseal plate widening. The overall incidence of significant orthopedic growth deformities related to radiation therapy for childhood malignancy has decreased over recent decades due to recognition of these effects and modifications in therapy.[379]

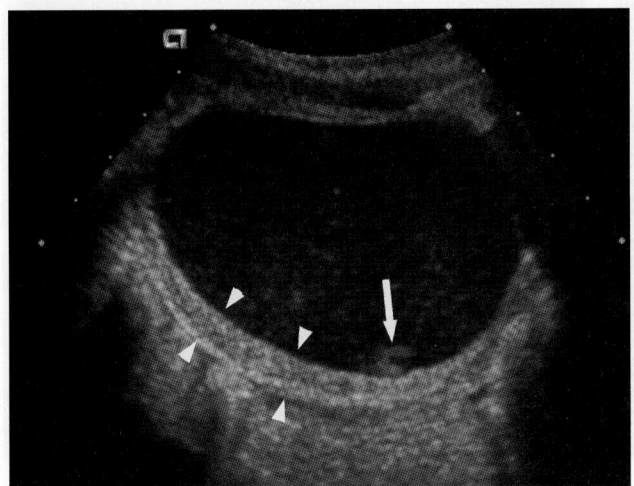
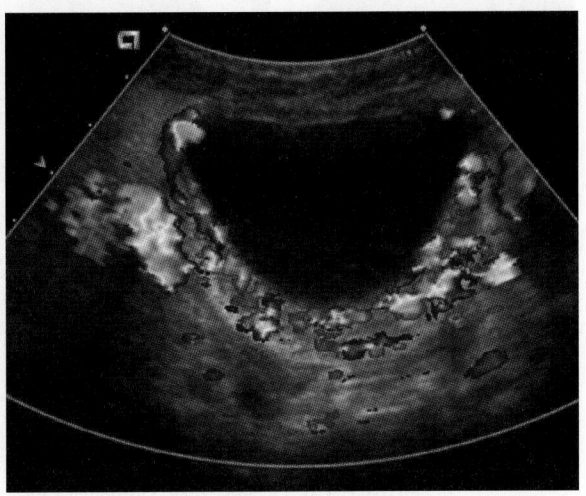

FIGURE 9.67 Hemorrhagic cystitis in a patient after bone marrow transplantation. A: Ultrasound image of the urinary bladder shows bladder wall thickening (arrowheads), echogenic intraluminal debris, and a dependent hyperechoic clot (arrow). B: Doppler sonography reveals marked hyperemia of the bladder wall.

Radiation osteitis is less common in children than adults, and the appearance on radiographs ranges from initial demineralization to subsequent mixed radiolucency and sclerosis or frank radio-osteonecrosis. Because of a similar radiographic appearance, the differentiation between radiation effect and recurrent or metastatic disease can be difficult on conventional radiographs. Radiation osteitis and radio-osteonecrosis generally do not cause cortical bone destruction and tend to be stable over successive examinations, whereas infiltrative tumor shows progression over time with cortical destruction. On MRI, radiation effects manifest as abnormal signal intensity in the bone marrow and periosseous soft tissues corresponding to edema and inflammation in the radiation field without an associated soft tissue mass.[380]

Osteonecrosis is an increasingly recognized toxicity in the growing population of childhood cancer survivors, particularly those with a history of leukemia or lymphoma, allogeneic bone marrow transplantation, or prolonged corticosteroid therapy.[381–384] Bone infarcts occurring within the metaphyses and diaphyses are less clinically significant than those involving the epiphyses, because the latter may progress to collapse of the articular surface and ultimately lead to degenerative arthritis, debilitation, and chronic pain and prompt total joint replacement. The joints most commonly affected by osteonecrosis are the knees, hips, and shoulders, but any joint is at risk.[378] Conventional radiographs are unable to detect osteonecrosis prior to the development of sclerosis, collapse and fragmentation of the articular surface, or subchondral fracture. MRI is the most sensitive imaging method for detecting early osteonecrosis, thereby allowing intervention to minimize joint deterioration[380,385] (Fig. 9.68).

Childhood cancer survivors are at risk of early onset and severe deficits of bone mineral density with attendant complications of insufficiency fractures and thoracic kyphosis with loss of height. Although decreased bone mineral density is a feature of methotrexate osteopathy, it is more frequently associated with prolonged corticosteroid treatment; dexamethasone causes greater bone mineral density deficits than prednisone.[386] Decreased bone mineral density is especially common after treatment for ALL, allogeneic bone marrow transplantation, or brain tumors, but survivors of childhood solid tumors are also at risk.[378,386–388] In these at-risk populations, monitoring of bone mineral density with quantitative CT or dual-energy x-ray absorptiometry is warranted to identify those with bone mineral deficits and institute corrective therapy.[389] Proper performance and interpretation of these techniques differs between the pediatric and adult populations.[387,390–392]

Paradoxic hypertrophy of the sciatic nerve is a peculiar condition that occurs in adolescents after lower extremity amputations for sarcomas. Rather than atrophy of the nerve, which more typically accompanies nerve transection, hypertrophy of the nerve occurs on the side of the amputation and extends from the transected end of the nerve proximally for many centimeters. On MRI, the hypertrophied nerve shares the same signal intensity characteristics as normal nerve, allowing distinction from involvement of the nerve by recurrent tumor and avoiding unnecessary biopsy.[393]

Radiation-induced tumors of bone are most commonly benign, with osteochondroma being the most frequently observed lesion. The development of osteochondromas is particularly common in patients who received total body irradiation at a young age prior to bone marrow transplantation.[394] If the appearance is not convincing on conventional radiographs, MRI can be performed to confirm the diagnosis of an osteochondroma by demonstrating the characteristic cartilaginous cap and bone marrow cavity continuity. Radiation-induced sarcomas arising in bone have a mean latency period for development of just over 10 years and most commonly are osteosarcomas, chondrosarcomas, fibrosarcomas, or malignant fibrous

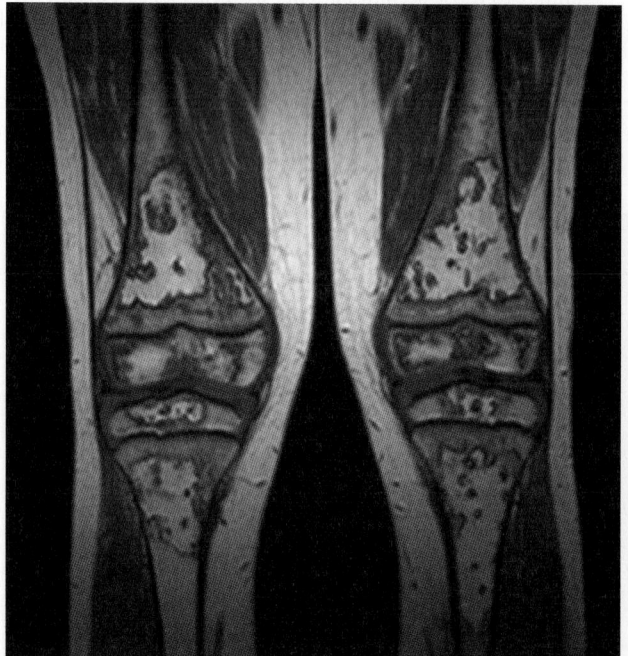
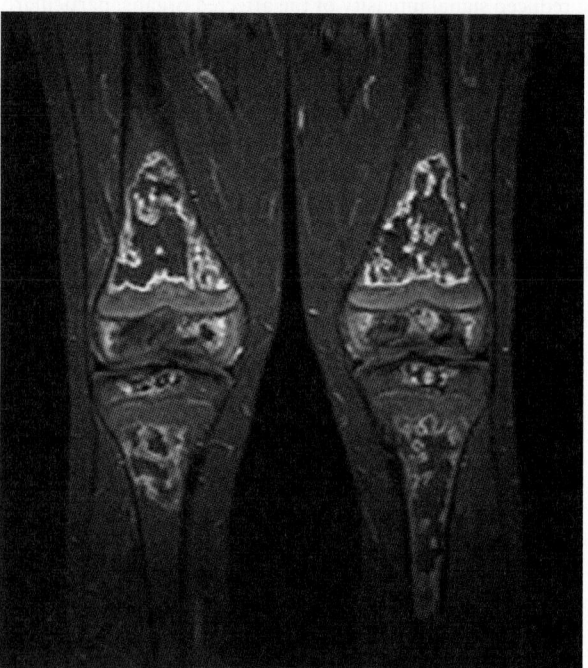

A   **B**

FIGURE 9.68 Osteonecrosis. Coronal T1-weighted (**A**) and short tau inversion recovery (STIR) (**B**) magnetic resonance images of the knees of a patient with acute lymphoblastic leukemia in remission reveal multiple lesions of the femoral and tibial epiphyses and metadiaphyses bilaterally. These lesions show a characteristic geographic shape with an outer low signal intensity rim of sclerosis visible on the T1-weighted image and inner rim of high signal intensity granulation tissue on the STIR image.

histiocytomas. Patients with a history of bilateral or familial retinoblastoma are at especially high risk. Suspicious findings on imaging for radiation-induced bone sarcomas are bone destruction and a soft tissue mass.[380]

The other types of second malignant neoplasms most frequently seen in survivors of childhood cancer include carcinomas (thyroid, skin, breast, GI tract, and renal cell), meningiomas, gliomas, sarcomas, leukemia, and NHL. Risk factors include radiation therapy (the second malignant neoplasms often occur at sites within or contiguous to radiation fields), young age at treatment, certain chemotherapeutic drugs (alkylating agents, epipodophyllotoxins, anthracyclines), bone marrow transplantation, and genetic predisposition (such as NF1, germline retinoblastoma, Li-Fraumeni syndrome).[395,396] One of the most compelling associations is the development of oncocytoid renal cell carcinomas in survivors of childhood neuroblastoma, with a strikingly high standardized incidence ratio of 329.[397]

Imaging surveillance of certain populations at risk for second malignant neoplasm warrants consideration. Women irradiated for Hodgkin lymphoma in childhood and adolescence have a strikingly elevated risk for breast cancer.[398] Screening mammography has been recommended in these women beginning at 25 to 30 years of age or 5 to 8 years after radiation therapy, but the efficacy of mammography is limited in the typically dense breasts of young women and incurs additional ionizing radiation exposure. Breast MRI is a promising method for screening these patients, because it involves no ionizing radiation exposure, is not limited by dense breast tissue, and has been found more sensitive for breast cancer than is mammography, ultrasound, or clinical breast examination in other populations of women at high risk for breast cancer.[399,400]

Children on chronic immunosuppressive therapy after organ, bone marrow, or stem cell transplantation, particularly those with EBV infection, are at risk for posttransplantation lymphoproliferative disorder (PTLD) ranging in spectrum from lymphoid cell hyperplasia to malignant lymphoma. PTLD can involve nearly any organ system, and extranodal and extrasplenic involvement is common. The appearance of PTLD on ultrasound, CT, or MRI can include lymphadenopathy, focal masses, or diffuse infiltration and enlargement of organs[401,402] (Fig. 9.69). Although discovery of these findings in an immunosuppressed patient after transplantation is consistent with a diagnosis of PTLD, the imaging appearance is not specific, and posttransplant spindle cell tumors are capable of producing an identical imaging appearance in immunosuppressed children.[403] At present, the routine use of imaging is not recommended to screen for PTLD. The disease tends to occur in the anatomic region of the transplant in recipients of solid organ transplants, although a complete imaging survey of the head, neck, chest, abdomen, and pelvis is recommended if PTLD is clinically suspected, because the disease can involve various sites. Because the imaging features of PTLD are not reliably predictive of histopathologic subtype, diagnosis depends on tissue biopsy. Imaging can provide guidance for biopsy and is also valuable in treatment follow-up. In a small trial, FDG-PET was deemed superior to CT and MRI for determination of early response of extracerebral PTLD to rituximab therapy.[404]

FUTURE DIRECTIONS

Technologic innovations enhance the role of radiology in the diagnosis and management of childhood cancer by providing better means to define tumor size and extent, evaluate response to therapy, detect recurrent tumor, and diagnose

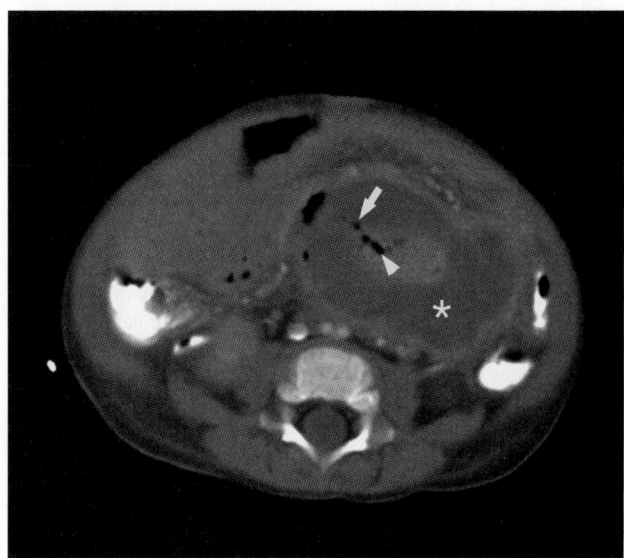

FIGURE 9.69 Posttransplantation lymphoproliferative disorder. An axial contrast-enhanced computed tomography image of the abdomen of a patient with a history of a heart transplant depicts bowel with markedly thickened, hypoattenuating wall (*asterisk*) and both intraluminal (*arrowhead*) and intramural (*arrow*) gas.

complications related to the tumor and its therapy. Fast multidetector CT scanners reduce motion artifact and the need for sedation in children, and novel MRI techniques provide additional tissue characterization without exposure to nontherapeutic ionizing radiation. Imaging software allows volumetric data acquired with MRI and multidetector CT scanners to be reconstructed into exquisite multiplanar and 3-D images for surgical and radiotherapy planning and permits more exacting calculation of true tumor volumes for risk stratification and therapy response assessment. Radiologic images are now nearly uniformly encoded in a digital format for archival, transmission, and display via a PACS (picture archive and communication system), allowing simultaneous access to the images by multiple users at different locations.

While these innovations improve the ability of health care professionals to obtain morphologic information about tumor status, the evolving disciplines of functional and molecular imaging are especially promising, because they offer techniques to evaluate *in vivo* metabolic and biochemical changes that precede morphologic changes. Imaging of glucose metabolism with FDG-PET is currently the most widely adopted of these techniques in oncology, and the use of combined PET/CT scanners and image-fusion software allows precise anatomic localization of sites of abnormal radiopharmaceutical uptake.

In addition to FDG-PET, many functional and molecular imaging techniques are under active investigation for use in oncology. Elasticity, or the tendency of tissue to resist deformation, varies more than x-ray attenuation or magnetic relaxation with physiologic and pathologic processes and can be measured by ultrasound or MR techniques. Ultrasound elastography has shown potential in differentiating benign and malignant lesions of the breast and thyroid,[405] while MR elastography has shown promise in differentiating benign and malignant liver tumors.[406] Apoptosis, a mechanism of tumor cell death, is amenable to imaging with radiolabeled derivatives of annexin, based on the high avidity of annexin for phosphatidylserine expressed on the plasma membrane of apoptotic cells.[407] Cellular proliferation and DNA turnover are amenable to imaging by PET with [^{18}F]-fluorothymidine.[408] The molecular diffusion of water is affected by tumor cellularity and necrosis and is evaluable by DWI. Tumor perfusion and angiogenesis can be assessed by dynamic contrast-enhanced ultrasound, CT, or MRI.[409] Tumor hypoxia can be evaluated by PET with [^{18}F]-fluoromisonidazole-3-fluoro-1-(20-nitro-10-imidazolyl)-2-propanol (F-MISO), 60/64-Cu-diacetyl-bis(N^4-methylthiosemicarbazone [Cu-ATSM]), or by MRI with BOLD techniques.[410] The Warburg effect (aerobic glycolysis), in which there is a shift toward lactate production in cancers even in the presence of adequate oxygen, can by noninvasively quantified by hyperpolarized ^{13}C MRI.[411] These techniques are candidates for determining the response of tumor to therapy prior to morphologic changes such as size reduction, but they must be validated in clinical trials before they can be advocated to replace or complement conventional imaging techniques in routine practice.

Near-infrared fluorescence optical tomographic or endoscopic imaging can be used to visualize microscopic cancer deposits rendered brightly fluorescent by fluorochrome probes activated by enzymes such as cathepsin proteases that are upregulated in tumor or tumor-associated host cells.[412] Antigens and cell surface receptors relatively specific to certain neoplasms potentially can be targeted and selectively imaged by scintigraphy or MRI with radionuclide-, iron particulate-, or gadolinium-conjugated peptides; monoclonal antibodies; polymerized vesicles; or nanoparticles. Examples include the somatostatin receptor expressed on human tumor cells and imaged by 99m-Tc-depreotide or 111-indium-octreotide scintigraphy, and the disialoganglioside GD-2 expressed on neuroblastoma cells and imaged with PET using 64-Cu-anti-GD2 antibody.[413,414] Such imaging techniques provide means of identifying appropriate patients and tumors and assaying pharmacokinetic-pharmacodynamic effects *in vivo* for targeted molecular therapy in early-phase clinical trials.[415]

As cure and long-term survival rates for pediatric cancer improve and an emphasis is placed on reducing adverse late effects of therapy, efforts should be made to reduce the risks and costs of imaging. With concern raised about the potential risk of inducing malignancy in children with ionizing radiation from imaging studies, the radiation dose incurred by imaging should be kept as low as reasonably achievable without compromising diagnostic efficacy.[416] To reduce the number of unnecessary or noncontributory imaging studies, more optimal schedules of imaging studies for surveillance for recurrent tumor need to be devised. Radiologic interpretation has always been a subjective exercise, and radiologists should explore the use of computer-aided detection and diagnostic software to improve diagnostic performance.

Imaging studies are a target of the political focus on controlling the escalating high costs of medical care. In response, rigorous studies of diagnostic efficacy, outcomes, and cost-effectiveness must be conducted to determine the best imaging approaches to the diagnosis and management of the various pediatric malignancies. This is made ever more challenging by the rapid pace of technologic advancements in radiology.

Large cancer cooperative study groups such as the Children's Oncology Group possess the resources to conduct multi-institutional clinical trials on pediatric cancer and provide an opportunity for radiologists to become involved in the development and review of the clinical trial protocols. These protocols considerably influence the selection and timing of imaging studies for staging and risk stratification, therapeutic planning, tumor response assessment, surveillance for recurrence, and detection of early and late complications of therapy.[417] Even if not directly involved with pediatric oncology clinical trials, radiologists participating in the care of children with cancer should have a working knowledge of the most current approaches to the diagnostic imaging and management of pediatric malignancies.

References

1. Dogan AS, Conway JJ, Miller JH, et al. Detection of bone lesions in Langerhans cell histiocytosis: complementary roles of scintigraphy and conventional radiography. J Pediatr Hematol Oncol 1996;18:51–58.
2. Slovis TL. Neoplasms and neoplasm-like lesions of the skull. In: Slovis TL, ed. Caffey's pediatric diagnostic imaging. Philadelphia, PA: Elsevier, 2008:519–533.
3. Frush DP. Pediatric dose reduction in computed tomography. Health Phys 2008;95:518–527.
4. Krishnamurthy R, Guillerman RP. Pediatric abdominal magnetic resonance angiography. Semin Roentgenol 2008;43:60–71.
5. Arcement CM, Towbin RB, Meza MP, et al. Intrahepatic chemoembolization in unresectable pediatric liver malignancies. Pediatr Radiol 2000;30:779–785.
6. Even-Sapir E, Keidar Z, Bar-Shalom R. Hybrid imaging (SPECT/CT and PET/CT)—improving the diagnostic accuracy of functional/metabolic and anatomic imaging. Semin Nucl Med 2009;39:264–275.
7. Stokkel MP, Valdes Olmos RA, Hoefnagel CA, et al. Tumor and therapy associated abnormal changes on bone scintigraphy: old and new phenomena. Clin Nucl Med 1993;18:821–828.
8. Kostakoglu L. Noninvasive detection of multidrug resistance in patients with hematological malignancies: are we there yet? Clin Lymphoma 2002;2:242–248.
9. Burak Z, Moretti JL, Ersoy O, et al. 99mTc-MIBI imaging as a predictor of therapy response in osteosarcoma compared with multidrug resistance-associated protein and P-glycoprotein expression. J Nucl Med 2003;44:1394–1401.
10. De Moerloose B. The prognostic significance of P-glycoprotein in children with acute lymphoblastic leukemia and neuroblastoma [in Dutch]. Verh K Acad Geneeskd Belg 2005;67:45–54.
11. Front D, Bar-Shalom R, Mor M, et al. Hodgkin disease: prediction of outcome with 67Ga scintigraphy after one cycle of chemotherapy. Radiology 1999;210:487–491.
12. Janicek M, Kaplan W, Neuberg D, et al. Early restaging gallium scans predict outcome in poor-prognosis patients with aggressive non-Hodgkin's lymphoma treated with high-dose CHOP chemotherapy. J Clin Oncol 1997;15:1631–1637.
13. Weiner MA, Leventhal BG, Cantor A, et al. Gallium-67 scans as an adjunct to CT scans for the assessment of a residual mediastinal mass in pediatric patients with Hodgkin's disease: a Pediatric Oncology Group study. Cancer 1991;68:2478–2480.
14. Tan TX, Gelfand MJ. Ga-67 scintigraphy in pediatric patients: comparison of extended SPECT of the chest and abdomen with planar imaging. Clin Nucl Med 1996;21:717–719.
15. Goto Y, Ihara K, Kawauchi S, et al. Clinical significance of thallium-201 scintigraphy in bone and soft tissue tumors. J Orthop Sci 2002;7:304–312.
16. Nadel HR. Thallium-201 for oncological imaging in children. Semin Nucl Med 1993;23:243–254.
17. Vik TA, Pfluger T, Kadota R, et al. (123)I-mIBG scintigraphy in patients with known or suspected neuroblastoma: results from a prospective multicenter trial. Pediatr Blood Cancer 2009;52:784–790.
18. Gelfand MJ. Meta-iodobenzylguanidine in children. Semin Nucl Med 1993;23:231–242.
19. Turba E, Fagioli G, Mancini AF, et al. Evaluation of stage 4 neuroblastoma patients by means of MIBG and 99mTc-MDP scintigraphy. J Nucl Biol Med 1993;37:107–114.
20. Shulkin BL, Shapiro B, Hutchinson RJ. Iodine-131-metaiodobenzylguanidine and bone scintigraphy for the detection of neuroblastoma. J Nucl Med 1992;33:1735–1740.
21. Matthay KK, Blaes F, Hero B, et al. Opsoclonus myoclonus syndrome in neuroblastoma: a report from a workshop on the dancing eyes syndrome at the advances in neuroblastoma meeting in Genoa, Italy, 2004. Cancer Lett 2005;228:275–282.
22. Mitjavila M. Meta-iodobenzylguanidine in neuroblastoma: from diagnosis to therapy. Nucl Med Commun 2002;23:3–4.
23. Monclair T, Brodeur GM, Ambros PF, et al. The International Neuroblastoma Risk Group (INRG) staging system: an INRG Task Force report. J Clin Oncol 2009;27:298–303.
24. Hines-Thomas M, Kaste SC, Hudson MM, et al. Comparison of gallium and PET scans at diagnosis and follow-up of pediatric patients with Hodgkin lymphoma. Pediatr Blood Cancer 2008;51:198–203.
25. Shulkin BL, Hutchinson RJ, Castle VP, et al. Neuroblastoma: positron emission tomography with 2-[fluorine-18]-fluoro-2-deoxy-D-glucose compared with metaiodobenzylguanidine scintigraphy. Radiology 1996;199:743–750.
26. Figarola MS, McQuiston SA, Wilson F, et al. Recurrent hepatoblastoma with localization by PET-CT. Pediatr Radiol 2005;35:1254–1258.
27. Tateishi U, Hosono A, Makimoto A, et al. Accuracy of 18F fluorodeoxyglucose positron emission tomography/computed tomography in staging of pediatric sarcomas. J Pediatr Hematol Oncol 2007;29:608–612.
28. Franzius C, Schober O. Assessment of therapy response by FDG PET in pediatric patients. Q J Nucl Med 2003;47:41–45.
29. Kaste SC, Rodriguez-Galindo C, McCarville ME, et al. PET-CT in pediatric Langerhans cell histiocytosis. Pediatr Radiol 2007;37:615–622.
30. Shulkin BL. PET imaging in pediatric oncology. Pediatr Radiol 2004;34:199–204.
31. Kaste SC, Howard SC, McCarville EB, et al. 18F-FDG-avid sites mimicking active disease in pediatric Hodgkin's. Pediatr Radiol 2005;35:141–154.
32. McQuattie S. Pediatric PET/CT imaging: tips and techniques. J Nucl Med Technol 2008;36:171–180.
33. Yeung HW, Grewal RK, Gonen M, et al. Patterns of (18)F-FDG uptake in adipose tissue and muscle: a potential source of false-positives for PET. J Nucl Med 2003;44:1789–1796.

34. Cohade C, Mourtzikos KA, Wahl RL. "USA-Fat": prevalence is related to ambient outdoor temperature-evaluation with 18F-FDG PET/CT. J Nucl Med 2003;44:1267–1270.

35. Truong MT, Erasmus JJ, Munden RF, et al. Focal FDG uptake in mediastinal brown fat mimicking malignancy: a potential pitfall resolved on PET/CT. AJR Am J Roentgenol 2004;183:1127–1132.

36. Gelfand MJ, O'hara SM, Curtwright LA, et al. Pre-medication to block [(18)F]FDG uptake in the brown adipose tissue of pediatric and adolescent patients. Pediatr Radiol 2005;35:984–990.

37. Agarwala S, Kumar R, Bhatnagar V, et al. High incidence of adriamycin cardiotoxicity in children even at low cumulative doses: role of radionuclide cardiac angiography. J Pediatr Surg 2000;35:1786–1789.

38. Gronroos MH, Jahnukainen T, Irjala K, et al. Comparison of glomerular function tests in children with cancer. Pediatr Nephrol 2008;23:797–803.

39. Hughes DK. Nuclear medicine and infection detection: the relative effectiveness of imaging with 111In-oxine-, 99mTc-HMPAO-, and 99mTc-stannous fluoride colloid-labeled leukocytes and with 67 Ga-citrate. J Nucl Med Technol 2003;31:196–201.

40. Kang TI, Brophy P, Hickeson M, et al. Targeted radiotherapy with submyeloablative doses of 131I-MIBG is effective for disease palliation in highly refractory neuroblastoma. J Pediatr Hematol Oncol 2003;25:769–773.

41. Scholz T, Eisenhofer G, Pacak K, et al. Clinical review: current treatment of malignant pheochromocytoma. J Clin Endocrinol Metab 2007;92:1217–1225.

42. Dubois SG, Matthay KK. Radiolabeled metaiodobenzylguanidine for the treatment of neuroblastoma. Nucl Med Biol 2008;35(suppl 1):35S–48S.

43. Gritzmann N, Evans DH. Recent progress in diagnostic ultrasound techniques. Ultraschall Med 2008;29:320–322.

44. Solwa Y, Sanyika C, Hadley GP, et al. Colour Doppler ultrasound assessment of the inferior vena cava in patients with Wilms' tumour. Clin Radiol 1999;54:811–814.

45. Lindner JR. Microbubbles in medical imaging: current applications and future directions. Nat Rev Drug Discov 2004;3:527–532.

46. Donnelly LF, Frush DP. Pediatric multidetector body CT. Radiol Clin North Am 2003;41:637–655.

47. Kalender WA. X-ray computed tomography. Phys Med Biol 2006;51:R29–R43.

48. Johnson TR, Krauss B, Sedlmair M, et al. Material differentiation by dual energy CT: initial experience. Eur Radiol 2007;17:1510–1517.

49. Seely JM, Effmann EL, Muller NL. High-resolution CT of pediatric lung disease: imaging findings. AJR Am J Roentgenol 1997;168:1269–1275.

50. Lasser EC, Lyon SG, Berry CC. Reports on contrast media reactions: analysis of data from reports to the U.S. Food and Drug Administration. Radiology 1997;203:605–610.

51. Thomsen HS. European Society of Urogenital Radiology (ESUR) guidelines on the safe use of iodinated contrast media. Eur J Radiol 2006;60:307–313.

52. Dillman JR, Strouse PJ, Ellis JH, et al. Incidence and severity of acute allergic-like reactions to i.v. nonionic iodinated contrast material in children. AJR Am J Roentgenol 2007;188:1643–1647.

53. Bettmann MA, Heeren T, Greenfield A, et al. Adverse events with radiographic contrast agents: results of the SCVIR Contrast Agent Registry. Radiology 1997;203:611–620.

54. Dillman JR, Ellis JH, Cohan RH, et al. Frequency and severity of acute allergic-like reactions to gadolinium-containing i.v. contrast media in children and adults. AJR Am J Roentgenol 2007;189:1533–1538.

55. Webb JA, Stacul F, Thomsen HS, et al. Late adverse reactions to intravascular iodinated contrast media. Eur Radiol 2003;13:181–184.

56. Morcos SK, Thomsen HS, Exley CM. Contrast media: interactions with other drugs and clinical tests. Eur Radiol 2005;15:1463–1468.

57. Gerlach AT, Pickworth KK. Contrast medium-induced nephrotoxicity: pathophysiology and prevention. Pharmacotherapy 2000;20:540–548.

58. Stacul F, Adam A, Becker CR, et al. Strategies to reduce the risk of contrast-induced nephropathy. Am J Cardiol 2006;98:59K–77K.

59. Bessell-Browne R, O'Malley ME. CT of pheochromocytoma and paraganglioma: risk of adverse events with i.v. administration of nonionic contrast material. AJR Am J Roentgenol 2007;188:970–974.

60. Harned TM, Mascarenhas L. Severe methotrexate toxicity precipitated by intravenous radiographic contrast. J Pediatr Hematol Oncol 2007;29:496–499.

61. Frush DP, Applegate K. Computed tomography and radiation: understanding the issues. J Am Coll Radiol 2004;1:113–119.

62. Hintenlang KM, Williams JL, Hintenlang DE. A survey of radiation dose associated with pediatric plain-film chest X-ray examinations. Pediatr Radiol 2002;32:771–777.

63. Stabin MG, Gelfand MJ. Dosimetry of pediatric nuclear medicine procedures. Q J Nucl Med 1998;42:93–112.

64. Gelfand MJ. Dosimetry of FDG PET/CT and other molecular imaging applications in pediatric patients. Pediatr Radiol 2009;39(suppl 1):46S–56S.

65. Brenner DJ, Hall EJ. Computed tomography—an increasing source of radiation exposure. N Engl J Med 2007;357:2277–2284.

66. Brody AS, Frush DP, Huda W, et al. Radiation risk to children from computed tomography. Pediatr 2007;120:677–682.

67. Linet MS, Kim KP, Rajaraman P. Children's exposure to diagnostic medical radiation and cancer risk: epidemiologic and dosimetric considerations. Pediatr Radiol 2009;39(suppl 1):4S–26S.

68. da Costa e Silva EJ, da Silva GA. Eliminating unenhanced CT when evaluating abdominal neoplasms in children. AJR Am J Roentgenol 2007;189:1211–1214.

69. Oikarinen H, Merilainen S, Paakko E, et al. Unjustified CT examinations in young patients. Eur Radiol 2009;19:1161–1165.

70. Robbins E. Radiation risks from imaging studies in children with cancer. Pediatr Blood Cancer 2008;51:453–457.

71. Brody AS, Guillerman RP. Radiation risk from diagnostic imaging. Pediatr Ann 2002;31:643–647.

72. Dagia C, Ditchfield M. 3T MRI in paediatrics: challenges and clinical applications. Eur J Radiol 2008;68:309–319.

73. MacKenzie JD, Vasanawala SS. Advances in pediatric MR imaging. Magn Reson Imaging Clin N Am 2008;16:385–402, v.

74. Darge K, Jaramillo D, Siegel MJ. Whole-body MRI in children: current status and future applications. Eur J Radiol 2008;68:289–298.

75. Ley S, Ley-Zaporozhan J, Schenk JP. Whole-body MRI in the pediatric patient. Eur J Radiol 2009;70:442–451.

76. Gauvain KM, McKinstry RC, Mukherjee P, et al. Evaluating pediatric brain tumor cellularity with diffusion-tensor imaging. AJR Am J Roentgenol 2001;177:449–454.

77. Hein PA, Eskey CJ, Dunn JF, et al. Diffusion-weighted imaging in the follow-up of treated high-grade gliomas: tumor recurrence versus radiation injury. AJNR Am J Neuroradiol 2004;25:201–209.

78. Vezina LG. Imaging of central nervous system tumors in children: advances and limitations. J Child Neurol 2008;23:1128–1135.

79. Alibek S, Cavallaro A, Aplas A, et al. Diffusion weighted imaging of pediatric and adolescent malignancies with regard to detection and delineation: initial experience. Acad Radiol 2009;16:866–871.

80. Kwee TC, Takahara T, Ochiai R, et al. Diffusion-weighted whole-body imaging with background body signal suppression (DWIBS): features and potential applications in oncology. Eur Radiol 2008;18:1937–1952.

81. Humphries PD, Sebire NJ, Siegel MJ, et al. Tumors in pediatric patients at diffusion-weighted MR imaging: apparent diffusion coefficient and tumor cellularity. Radiology 2007;245:848–854.

82. Pfluger T, Czekalla R, Hundt C, et al. MR angiography versus color Doppler sonography in the evaluation of renal vessels and the inferior vena cava in abdominal masses of pediatric patients. AJR Am J Roentgenol 1999;173:103–108.

83. Lang P, Grampp S, Vahlensieck M, et al. Primary bone tumors: value of MR angiography for preoperative planning and monitoring response to chemotherapy. AJR Am J Roentgenol 1995;165:135–142.

84. Shankar KR, Abernethy LJ, Das KS, et al. Magnetic resonance venography in assessing venous patency after multiple venous catheters. J Pediatr Surg 2002;37:175–179.

85. Geraldes CF, Laurent S. Classification and basic properties of contrast agents for magnetic resonance imaging. Contrast Media Mol Imaging 2009;4:1–23.

86. Kirchin MA, Runge VM. Contrast agents for magnetic resonance imaging: safety update. Top Magn Reson Imaging 2003;14:426–435.

87. Kanal E, Barkovich AJ, Bell C, et al. ACR guidance document for safe MR practices: 2007. AJR Am J Roentgenol 2007;188:1447–1474.

88. Shellock FG, Spinazzi A. MRI safety update 2008, I: MRI contrast agents and nephrogenic systemic fibrosis. AJR Am J Roentgenol 2008;191:1129–1139.

89. Reddick WE, Taylor JS, Fletcher BD. Dynamic MR imaging (DEMRI) of microcirculation in bone sarcoma. J Magn Reson Imaging 1999;10:277–285.

90. Dyke JP, Panicek DM, Healey JH, et al. Osteogenic and Ewing sarcomas: estimation of necrotic fraction during induction chemotherapy with dynamic contrast-enhanced MR imaging. Radiology 2003;228:271–278.

91. Reddick WE, Wang S, Xiong X, et al. Dynamic magnetic resonance imaging of regional contrast access as an additional prognostic factor in pediatric osteosarcoma. Cancer 2001;91:2230–2237.

92. Miller SL, Hoffer FA, Reddick WE, et al. Tumor volume or dynamic contrast-enhanced MRI for prediction of clinical outcome of Ewing sarcoma family of tumors. Pediatr Radiol 2001;31:518–523.

93. Warren KE. NMR spectroscopy and pediatric brain tumors. Oncologist 2004;9:312–318.

94. Tzika AA, Vajapeyam S, Barnes PD. Multivoxel proton MR spectroscopy and hemodynamic MR imaging of childhood brain tumors: preliminary observations. AJNR Am J Neuroradiol 1997;18:203–218.

95. Hall WA, Martin A, Liu H, et al. Improving diagnostic yield in brain biopsy: coupling spectroscopic targeting with real-time needle placement. J Magn Reson Imaging 2001;13:12–15.

96. Warren KE, Frank JA, Black JL, et al. Proton magnetic resonance spectroscopic imaging in children with recurrent primary brain tumors. J Clin Oncol 2000;18:1020–1026.

97. Tzika AA, Astrakas LG, Zarifi MK, et al. Spectroscopic and perfusion magnetic resonance imaging predictors of progression in pediatric brain tumors. Cancer 2004;100:1246–1256.

98. Negendank WG. MR spectroscopy of musculoskeletal soft-tissue tumors. Magn Reson Imaging Clin N Am 1995;3:713–725.

99. Gonen O, Gruber S, Li BS, et al. Multivoxel 3D proton spectroscopy in the brain at 1.5 versus 3.0 T: signal-to-noise ratio and resolution comparison. AJNR Am J Neuroradiol 2001;22:1727–1731.

100. Cote CJ, Wilson S. Guidelines for monitoring and management of pediatric patients during and after sedation for diagnostic and therapeutic procedures: an update. Pediatrics 2006;118:2587–2602.

101. Erasmus JJ, McAdams HP, Donnelly LF, et al. MR imaging of mediastinal masses. Magn Reson Imaging Clin N Am 2000;8:59–89.

102. Bloem JL, Taminiau AH, Eulderink F, et al. Radiologic staging of primary bone sarcoma: MR imaging, scintigraphy, angiography, and CT correlated with pathologic examination. Radiology 1988;169:805–810.

103. Guillerman RP. Normal and abnormal bone marrow. In: Slovis TL, ed. Caffey's pediatric diagnostic imaging. Philadelphia, PA: Elsevier, 2008:2970–2996.

104. Jensen KE, Thomsen C, Henriksen O, et al. Changes in T1 relaxation processes in the bone marrow following treatment in children with acute lymphoblastic leukemia: a magnetic resonance imaging study. Pediatr Radiol 1990;20:464–468.

105. Hoane BR, Shields AF, Porter BA, et al. Detection of lymphomatous bone marrow involvement with magnetic resonance imaging. Blood 1991;78:728–738.

106. Avni FE, Massez A, Cassart M. Tumours of the fetal body: a review. Pediatr Radiol 2009;39(11):1147–57.

107. Coakley FV, Glenn OA, Qayyum A, et al. Fetal MRI: a developing technique for the developing patient. AJR Am J Roentgenol 2004;182:243–252.

108. Shellock FG, Crues JV. MR procedures: biologic effects, safety, and patient care. Radiology 2004;232:635–652.

109. Shellock FG, Spinazzi A. MRI safety update 2008, II: screening patients for MRI. AJR Am J Roentgenol 2008;191:1140–1149.

110. American Society for Testing and Materials International. Standard practice for marking medical devices and other items for safety in the magnetic resonance environment. West Conshohocken, PA: American Society for Testing and Materials International, 2005.

111. Kanal E, Borgstede JP, Barkovich AJ, et al. American College of Radiology White Paper on MR Safety. AJR Am J Roentgenol 2002;178:1335–1347.

112. Sebire NJ, Roebuck DJ. Pathological diagnosis of paediatric tumours from image-guided needle core biopsies: a systematic review. Pediatr Radiol 2006;36:426–431.

113. Partrick DA, Bensard DD, Teitelbaum DH, et al. Successful thoracoscopic lung biopsy in children utilizing preoperative CT-guided localization. J Pediatr Surg 2002;37:970–973.

114. Hoffer FA. Interventional radiology in pediatric oncology. Eur J Radiol 2005;53:3–13.

115. Li JP, Chu JP, Yang JY, et al. Preoperative transcatheter selective arterial chemoembolization in treatment of unresectable hepatoblastoma in infants and children. Cardiovasc Intervent Radiol 2008;31:1117–1123.

116. Weintraub M, Bloom AI, Gross E, et al. Successful treatment of progressive stage 4s hepatic neuroblastoma in a neonate with intra-arterial chemoembolization. Pediatr Blood Cancer 2004;43:148–151.

117. Christison-Lagay ER, Burrow PE, et al. Hepatic hemangiomas: subtype classification and development of a clinical practice algorithm and registry. J Pediatr Surg 2007;42:62–68.
118. Basford TJ, Poenaru D, Silva M. Comparison of delayed complications of central venous catheters placed surgically or radiologically in pediatric oncology patients. J Pediatr Surg 2003;38:788–792.
119. Racadio JM. Controlling radiation exposure during interventional procedures in childhood cancer patients. Pediatr Radiol 2009;39(suppl 1):S71–S73.
120. Vazquez E, Lucaya J, Castellote A, et al. Neuroimaging in pediatric leukemia and lymphoma: differential diagnosis. Radiographics 2002;22:1411–1428.
121. Anghelescu DL, Burgoyne LL, Liu T, et al. Clinical and diagnostic imaging findings predict anesthetic complications in children presenting with malignant mediastinal masses. Paediatr Anaesth 2007;17:1090–1098.
122. Hack HA, Wright NB, Wynn RF. The anaesthetic management of children with anterior mediastinal masses. Anaesthesia 2008;63:837–846.
123. Parisi MT, Fahmy JL, Kaminsky CK, et al. Complications of cancer therapy in children: a radiologist's guide. Radiographics 1999;19:283–297.
124. Roebuck DJ, Stanley P. External and internal-external biliary drainage in children with malignant obstructive jaundice. Pediatr Radiol 2000;30:659–664.
125. Pietsch JB, Shankar S, Ford C, et al. Obstructive jaundice secondary to lymphoma in childhood. J Pediatr Surg 2001;36:1792–1795.
126. Weiss A, Khoury JD, Hoffer FA, et al. Telangiectatic osteosarcoma: the St. Jude Children's Research Hospital's experience. Cancer 2007;109:1627–1637.
127. Bramer JA, Abudu AA, Grimer RJ, et al. Do pathological fractures influence survival and local recurrence rate in bony sarcomas? Eur J Cancer 2007;43:1944–1951.
128. Borgwardt L, Hojgaard L, Carstensen H, et al. Increased fluorine-18 2-fluoro-2-deoxy-D-glucose (FDG) uptake in childhood CNS tumors is correlated with malignancy grade: a study with FDG positron emission tomography/magnetic resonance imaging coregistration and image fusion. J Clin Oncol 2005;23:3030–3037.
129. Ulu EM, Tore HG, Bayrak A, et al. MRI of central nervous system abnormalities in childhood leukemia. Diagn Interv Radiol 2009;15:86–92.
130. Rossi A, Gandolfo C, Morana G, et al. Tumors of the spine in children. Neuroimaging Clin N Am 2007;17:17–35.
131. Hedlund GL, Faerber FN, Piatt J. Spinal cord: tumors and tumor-like conditions. In: Slovis TL, ed. Caffey's pediatric diagnostic imaging. Philadelphia, PA: Elsevier, 2008:998–1018.
132. Cdervantes LF, Medina LS, Effman EL. Neck and upper airway. In: Slovis TL, ed. Caffey's pediatric diagnostic imaging. Philadelphia, PA: Elsevier, 2008:1026–1067.
133. Gujar S, Gandhi D, Mukherji SK. Pediatric head and neck masses. Top Magn Reson Imaging 2004;15:95–101.
134. Stambuk HE, Patel SG, Mosier KM, et al. Nasopharyngeal carcinoma: recognizing the radiographic features in children. AJNR Am J Neuroradiol 2005;26:1575–1579.
135. Lowe LH, Stokes LS, Johnson JE, et al. Swelling at the angle of the mandible: imaging of the pediatric parotid gland and periparotid region. Radiographics 2001;21:1211–1227.
136. Bedi DG, John SD, Swischuk LE. Fibromatosis colli of infancy: variability of sonographic appearance. J Clin Ultrasound 1998;26:345–348.
137. Zielke AM, Swischuk LE, Hernandez JA. Ectopic cervical thymic tissue: can imaging obviate biopsy and surgical removal? Pediatr Radiol 2007;37:1174–1177.
138. Enjolras O, Mulliken JB. Vascular tumors and vascular malformations (new issues). Adv Dermatol 1997;13:375–423.
139. Dubois J, Garel L. Imaging and therapeutic approach of hemangiomas and vascular malformations in the pediatric age group. Pediatr Radiol 1999;29:879–893.
140. Chang MW. Updated classification of hemangiomas and other vascular anomalies. Lymphat Res Biol 2003;1:259–265.
141. Gow KW, Lensing S, Hill DA, et al. Thyroid carcinoma presenting in childhood or after treatment of childhood malignancies: an institutional experience and review of the literature. J Pediatr Surg 2003;38:1574–1580.
142. Hung W. Solitary thyroid nodules in 93 children and adolescents: a 35-years experience. Horm Res 1999;52:15–18.
143. Corrias A, Einaudi S, Chiorboli E, et al. Accuracy of fine needle aspiration biopsy of thyroid nodules in detecting malignancy in childhood: comparison with conventional clinical, laboratory, and imaging approaches. J Clin Endocrinol Metab 2001;86:4644–4648.
144. Megremis S, Stiakaki E, Tritou I, et al. Ectopic intrathyroidal thymus misdiagnosed as a thyroid nodule: sonographic appearance. J Clin Ultrasound 2008;36:443–447.
145. Laurie AJ, Lyon SG, Lasser EC. Contrast material iodides: potential effects on radioactive iodine thyroid uptake. J Nucl Med 1992;33:237–238.
146. Christensen CR, Glowniak JV, Brown PH, et al. The effect of gadolinium contrast media on radioiodine uptake by the thyroid gland. J Nucl Med Technol 2000;28:41–44.
147. Provenzale JM, Gururangan S, Klintworth G. Trilateral retinoblastoma: clinical and radiologic progression. AJR Am J Roentgenol 2004;183:505–511.
148. Kaufman LM, Mafee MF, Song CD. Retinoblastoma and simulating lesions: role of CT, MR imaging and use of Gd-DTPA contrast enhancement. Radiol Clin North Am 1998;36:1101–1117.
149. Bulas RB, Laine FJ, Das NL. Bilateral orbital granulocytic sarcoma (chloroma) preceding the blast phase of acute myelogenous leukemia: CT findings. Pediatr Radiol 1995;25:488–489.
150. Castillo BV Jr, Kaufman L. Pediatric tumors of the eye and orbit. Pediatr Clin North Am 2003;50:149–172.
151. Priest JR, Williams GM, Hill DA, et al. Pulmonary cysts in early childhood and the risk of malignancy. Pediatr Pulmonol 2009;44:14–30.
152. Gelinas JF, Manoukian J, Cote A. Lung involvement in juvenile onset recurrent respiratory papillomatosis: a systematic review of the literature. Int J Pediatr Otorhinolaryngol 2008;72:433–452.
153. Slovis TL, Meza MP, Cushing B, et al. Thoracic neuroblastoma: what is the best imaging modality for evaluating extent of disease? Pediatr Radiol 1997;27:273–275.
154. Hedlund GL, Navoy JF, Galliani CA, et al. Aggressive manifestations of inflammatory pulmonary pseudotumor in children. Pediatr Radiol 1999;29:112–116.
155. Wyttenbach R, Vock P, Tschappeler H. Cross-sectional imaging with CT and/or MRI of pediatric chest tumors. Eur Radiol 1998;8:1040–1046.
156. Hoffmann U, Globits S, Schima W, et al. Usefulness of magnetic resonance imaging of cardiac and paracardiac masses. Am J Cardiol 2003;92:890–895.
157. St Amour TE, Siegel MJ, Glazer HS, et al. CT appearances of the normal and abnormal thymus in childhood. J Comput Assist Tomogr 1987;11:645–650.
158. Siegel MJ, Glazer HS, Wiener JI, et al. Normal and abnormal thymus in childhood: MR imaging. Radiology 1989;172:367–371.
159. Adam EJ, Ignotus PI. Sonography of the thymus in healthy children: frequency of visualization, size, and appearance. AJR Am J Roentgenol 1993;161:153–155.
160. Takahashi K, Inaoka T, Murakami N, et al. Characterization of the normal and hyperplastic thymus on chemical-shift MR imaging. AJR Am J Roentgenol 2003;180:1265–1269.
161. Kavanagh PV, Stevenson AW, Chen MY, et al. Nonneoplastic diseases in the chest showing increased activity on FDG PET. AJR Am J Roentgenol 2004;183:1133–1141.
162. Hibi S, Todo S, Imashuku S. Thymic localization of gallium-67 in pediatric patients with lymphoid and nonlymphoid tumors. J Nucl Med 1987;28:293–297.
163. Jerushalmi J, Frenkel A, Bar-Shalom R, et al. Physiologic thymic uptake of 18F-FDG in children and young adults: a PET/CT evaluation of incidence, patterns, and relationship to treatment. J Nucl Med 2009;50:849–853.
164. Montravers F, McNamara D, Landman-Parker J, et al. [(18)F]FDG in childhood lymphoma: clinical utility and impact on management. Eur J Nucl Med Mol Imaging 2002;29:1155–1165.
165. Guillerman RP, Parker BR. Pediatric lymphoma. In: Guermazi A, ed. Radiological imaging in hematological malignancies. Berlin, Germany: Springer-Verlag, 2004:247–288.
166. Even-Sapir E, Israel O. Gallium-67 scintigraphy: a cornerstone in functional imaging of lymphoma. Eur J Nucl Med Mol Imaging 2003;30(suppl 1):S65–S81.
167. Strollo DC, Rosado-de-Christenson ML. Primary mediastinal malignant germ cell neoplasms: imaging features. Chest Surg Clin N Am 2002;12:645–658.
168. al-Ali F, Gooding CA, Jacques CJ. Calcified mass in anterior part of mediastinum caused by Langerhans' cell histiocytosis. AJR Am J Roentgenol 1994;162:467–468.
169. Donnelly LF, Frush DP. Langerhans' cell histiocytosis showing low-attenuation mediastinal mass and cystic lung disease. AJR Am J Roentgenol 2000;174:877–878.
170. Avila NA, Mueller BU, Carrasquillo JA, et al. Multilocular thymic cysts: imaging features in children with human immunodeficiency virus infection. Radiology 1996;201:130–134.
171. Tateishi U, Gladish GW, Kusumoto M, et al. Chest wall tumors: radiologic findings and pathologic correlation, I: benign tumors. Radiographics 2003;23:1477–1490.
172. Daldrup HE, Link TM, Wortler K, et al. MR imaging of thoracic tumors in pediatric patients. AJR Am J Roentgenol 1998;170:1639–1644.
173. Tateishi U, Gladish GW, Kusumoto M, et al. Chest wall tumors: radiologic findings and pathologic correlation, II: malignant tumors. Radiographics 2003;23:1491–1508.
174. Kronemer KA, Rhee K, Siegel MJ, et al. Gray scale sonography of breast masses in adolescent girls. J Ultrasound Med 2001;20:491–496.
175. Chung EM, Cube R, Hall GJ, et al. From the archives of the AFIP: breast masses in children and adolescents: radiologic-pathologic correlation. Radiographics 2009;29:907–931.
176. Laor T, Collins MH, Emery KH, et al. MRI appearance of accessory breast tissue: a diagnostic consideration for an axillary mass in a peripubertal or pubertal girl. AJR Am J Roentgenol 2004;183:1779–1781.
177. Donnelly LF, Frush DP, Foss JN, et al. Anterior chest wall: frequency of anatomic variations in children. Radiology 1999;212:837–840.
178. Donnelly LF. Use of three-dimensional reconstructed helical CT images in recognition and communication of chest wall anomalies in children. AJR Am J Roentgenol 2001;177:441–445.
179. Deeg KH, Bettendorf U, Hofmann V. Differential diagnosis of neonatal adrenal haemorrhage and congenital neuroblastoma by colour coded Doppler sonography and power Doppler sonography. Eur J Pediatr 1998;157:294–297.
180. Barr LL, Hayden CK Jr, Stansberry SD, et al. Enteric duplication cysts in children: are their ultrasonographic wall characteristics diagnostic? Pediatr Radiol 1990;20:326–328.
181. Bayindir P, Guillerman RP, Hicks MJ, et al. Cellular mesoblastic nephroma (infantile renal fibrosarcoma): institutional review of the clinical, diagnostic imaging, and pathologic features of a distinctive neoplasm of infancy. Pediatr Radiol 2009;39:1066–1074.
182. Meyer JS, Harty MP, Khademian Z. Imaging of neuroblastoma and Wilms' tumor. Magn Reson Imaging Clin N Am 2002;10:275–302.
183. Baxter PA, Nuchtern JG, Guillerman RP, et al. Acquired von Willebrand syndrome and Wilms tumor: not always benign. Pediatr Blood Cancer 2009;52:392–394.
184. Cohen MD. Staging of Wilms' tumour. Clin Radiol 1993;47:77–81.
185. Ditchfield MR, De Campo JF, Waters KD, et al. Wilms' tumor: a rational use of preoperative imaging. Med Pediatr Oncol 1995;24:93–96.
186. Hugosson C, Nyman R, Jacobsson B, et al. Imaging of solid kidney tumours in children. Acta Radiol 1995;36:254–260.
187. Gow KW, Roberts IF, Jamieson DH, et al. Local staging of Wilms' tumor—computerized tomography correlation with histological findings. J Pediatr Surg 2000;35:677–679.
188. Ritchey ML, Kelalis PP, Breslow N, et al. Intracaval and atrial involvement with nephroblastoma: review of National Wilms Tumor Study-3. J Urol 1988;140:1113–1138.
189. Weese DL, Applebaum H, Taber P. Mapping intravascular extension of Wilms' tumor with magnetic resonance imaging. J Pediatr Surg 1991;26:64–67.
190. Hugosson C, Nyman R, Jorulf H, et al. Imaging of abdominal neuroblastoma in children. Acta Radiol 1999;40:534–542.
191. Siegel MJ, Ishwaran H, Fletcher BD, et al. Staging of neuroblastoma at imaging: report of the radiology diagnostic oncology group. Radiology 2002;223:168–175.
192. Cheung NK, Kushner BH. Should we replace bone scintigraphy plus CT with MR imaging for staging of neuroblastoma? Radiology 2003;226:286–287.
193. Hahn K, Charron M, Shulkin BL. Role of MR imaging and iodine 123 MIBG scintigraphy in staging of pediatric neuroblastoma. Radiology 2003;227:908–909.
194. Schilling FH, Bihl H, Jacobsson H, et al. Combined (111)In-pentetreotide scintigraphy and (123)I-mIBG scintigraphy in neuroblastoma provides prognostic information. Med Pediatr Oncol 2000;35:688–691.
195. Kushner BH, Yeung HW, Larson SM, et al. Extending positron emission tomography scan utility to high-risk neuroblastoma: fluorine-18 fluorodeoxyglucose positron emission tomography as sole imaging modality in follow-up of patients. J Clin Oncol 2001;19:3397–3405.
196. Sharp SE, Shulkin BL, Gelfand MJ, et al. 123I-MIBG scintigraphy and 18F-FDG PET in neuroblastoma. J Nucl Med 2009;50:1237–1243.
197. Yamamoto K, Hanada R, Kikuchi A, et al. Spontaneous regression of localized neuroblastoma detected by mass screening. J Clin Oncol 1998;16:1265–1269.
198. Rodriguez-Galindo C, Figueiredo BC, et al. Biology, clinical characteristics, and management of adrenocortical tumors in children. Pediatr Blood Cancer 2005;45:265–273.
199. Havekes B, Romijn JA, Eisenhofer G, et al. Update on pediatric pheochromocytoma. Pediatr Nephrol 2009;24:943–950.

200. Yang DM, Jung DH, Kim H, et al. Retroperitoneal cystic masses: CT, clinical, and pathologic findings and literature review. Radiographics 2004;24:1353–1365.
201. LaQuaglia MP, Stolar CHJ, Krailo M, et al. The role of surgery in abdominal non-Hodgkin's lymphoma: experience from the Children's Cancer Study Group. J Pediatr Surg 1992;27:230–235.
202. Guillerman RP. Primary intestinal non-Hodgkin lymphoma. J Pediatr Hematol Oncol 2000;22:476–478.
203. Siegel MJ, Evans SJ, Balfe DM. Small bowel disease in children: diagnosis with CT. Radiology 1988;169:127–130.
204. Hardy SM. The sandwich sign. Radiology 2003;226:651–652.
205. Halliday T, Baxter G. Lymphoma: pictorial review: II. Eur Radiol 2003;13:1224–1234.
206. Aygun B, Karakas SP, Leonidas J, et al. Reliability of splenic index to assess splenic involvement in pediatric Hodgkin's disease. J Pediatr Hematol Oncol 2004;26:74–76.
207. Miller E, Metser U, Avrahami G, et al. Role of 18F-FDG PET/CT in staging and follow-up of lymphoma in pediatric and young adult patients. J Comput Assist Tomogr 2006;30:689–694.
208. Picardi M, Soricelli A, Pane F, et al. Contrast-enhanced harmonic compound US of the spleen to increase staging accuracy in patients with Hodgkin lymphoma: a prospective study. Radiology 2009;251:574–582.
209. Chepuri NB, Strouse PJ, Yanik GA. CT of renal lymphoma in children. AJR Am J Roentgenol 2003;180:429–431.
210. Durno CA, Gallinger S. Genetic predisposition to colorectal cancer: new pieces in the pediatric puzzle. J Pediatr Gastroenterol Nutr 2006;43:5–15.
211. Kaemmer DA, Otto J, Lassay L, et al. The Gist of literature on pediatric GIST: review of clinical presentation. J Pediatr Hematol Oncol 2009;31:108–112.
212. Pappo AS, Janeway KA. Pediatric gastrointestinal stromal tumors. Hematol Oncol Clin North Am 2009;23:15–34, vii.
213. Moore CW, Lowe LH. Hepatic tumors and tumor-like conditions. In: Slovis TL, ed. Caffey's pediatric diagnostic imaging. Philadelphia, PA: Elsevier, 2008:1929–1948.
214. Spottswood SE, Stein SM, Hill JG. The spleen. In: Slovis TL, ed. Caffey's pediatric diagnostic imaging. Philadelphia, PA: Elsevier, 2008:1970–1982.
215. Jaffe R. Liver involvement in the histiocytic disorders of childhood. Pediatr Dev Pathol 2004;7:214–225.
216. Arakawa A, Matsukawa T, Yamashita Y, et al. Periportal fibrosis in Langerhans' cell histiocytosis mimicking multiple liver tumors: US, CT, and MR findings. J Comput Assist Tomogr 1994;18:157–159.
217. Gouya H, Vignaux O, Augui J, et al. CT, endoscopic sonography, and a combined protocol for preoperative evaluation of pancreatic insulinomas. AJR Am J Roentgenol 2003;181:987–992.
218. Owen NJ, Sohaib SA, Peppercorn PD, et al. MRI of pancreatic neuroendocrine tumours. Br J Radiol 2001;74:968–973.
219. Mirallie E, Pattou F, Malvaux P, et al. Value of endoscopic ultrasonography and somatostatin receptor scintigraphy in the preoperative localization of insulinomas and gastrinomas: experience of 54 cases [in French]. Gastroenterol Clin Biol 2002;26: 360–366.
220. Montemarano H, Lonergan GJ, Bulas DI, et al. Pancreatoblastoma: imaging findings in 10 patients and review of the literature. Radiology 2000;214:476–482.
221. Cantisani V, Mortele KJ, Levy A, et al. MR imaging features of solid pseudopapillary tumor of the pancreas in adult and pediatric patients. AJR Am J Roentgenol 2003;181:395–401.
222. Kim JH, Goo HW, Yoon CH. Intra-abdominal desmoplastic small round-cell tumour: multiphase CT findings in two children. Pediatr Radiol 2003;33:418–421.
223. Browne LP, Boswell HB, Crotty EJ, et al. Van Wyk and Grumbach syndrome revisited: imaging and clinical findings in pre- and postpubertal girls. Pediatr Radiol 2008;38: 538–542.
224. Ekici E, Soysal M, Kara S, et al. The efficiency of ultrasonography in the diagnosis of dermoid cysts. Zentralbl Gynakol 1996;118:136–141.
225. Yamashita Y, Hatanaka Y, Torashima M, et al. Mature cystic teratomas of the ovary without fat in the cystic cavity: MR features in 12 cases. AJR Am J Roentgenol 1994;163:613–616.
226. Outwater EK, Wagner BJ, Mannion C, et al. Sex cord-stromal and steroid cell tumors of the ovary. Radiographics 1998;18:1523–1546.
227. McHugh K, Boothroyd AE. The role of radiology in childhood rhabdomyosarcoma. Clin Radiol 1999;54:2–10.
228. Schneider G, Ahlhelm F, Altmeyer K, et al. Rare pseudotumors of the urinary bladder in childhood. Eur Radiol 2001;11:1024–1029.
229. Mak CW, Chou CK, Su CC, et al. Ultrasound diagnosis of paratesticular rhabdomyosarcoma. Br J Radiol 2004;77:250–252.
230. Kaufman E, Akiya F, Foucar E, et al. Virilization due to Leydig cell tumor diagnosis by magnetic resonance imaging: case management report. Clin Pediatr (Phila) 1990;29: 414–417.
231. Fernandez GC, Tardaguila F, Rivas C, et al. Case report: MRI in the diagnosis of testicular Leydig cell tumour. Br J Radiol 2004;77:521–524.
232. Avila NA, Premkumar A, Shawker TH, et al. Testicular adrenal rest tissue in congenital adrenal hyperplasia: findings at Gray-scale and color Doppler US. Radiology 1996;198:99–104.
233. Sinigaglia R, Gigante C, Bisinella G, et al. Musculoskeletal manifestations in pediatric acute leukemia. J Pediatr Orthop 2008;28:20–28.
234. Kaste SC, Strouse PJ, Fletcher BD, et al. Benign and malignant bone tumors. In: Slovis TL, ed. Caffey's pediatric diagnostic imaging. Philadelphia, PA: Elsevier, 2008:2912–2969.
235. Onikul E, Fletcher BD, Parham DM, et al. Accuracy of MR imaging for estimating intraosseous extent of osteosarcoma. AJR Am J Roentgenol 1996;167:1211–1215.
236. Meyer MS, Spanier SS, Moser M, et al. Evaluating marrow margins for resection of osteosarcoma: a modern approach. Clin Orthop Relat Res 1999;170–175.
237. Hoffer FA, Nikanorov AY, Reddick WE, et al. Accuracy of MR imaging for detecting epiphyseal extension of osteosarcoma. Pediatr Radiol 2000;30:289–298.
238. Schima W, Amann G, Stiglbauer R, et al. Preoperative staging of osteosarcoma: efficacy of MR imaging in detecting joint involvement. AJR Am J Roentgenol 1994;163: 1171–1175.
239. van Trommel MF, Kroon HM, Bloem JL, et al. MR imaging based strategies in limb salvage surgery for osteosarcoma of the distal femur. Skeletal Radiol 1997;26:636–641.
240. Brisse H, Ollivier L, Edeline V, et al. Imaging of malignant tumours of the long bones in children: monitoring response to neoadjuvant chemotherapy and preoperative assessment. Pediatr Radiol 2004;34:595–605.
241. Discepola F, Powell TI, Nahal A. Telangiectatic osteosarcoma: radiologic and pathologic findings. Radiographics 2009;29:380–383.
242. Kransdorf MJ, Meis JM, Jelinek JS. Myositis ossificans: MR appearance with radiologic-pathologic correlation. AJR Am J Roentgenol 1991;157:1243–1248.
243. Berquist TH, Ehman RL, King BF, et al. Value of MR imaging in differentiating benign from malignant soft-tissue masses: study of 95 lesions. AJR Am J Roentgenol 1990;155: 1251–1255.
244. Stein-Wexler R. MR imaging of soft tissue masses in children. Magn Reson Imaging Clin N Am 2009;17:489–507, vi.
245. Grossman M, Shiramizu B. Evaluation of lymphadenopathy in children. Curr Opin Pediatr 1994;6:68–76.
246. Healy MV, Graham PM. Assessment of abdominal lymph nodes in a normal paediatric population: an ultrasound study. Australas Radiol 1993;37:171–172.
247. Wunderbaldinger P. Problems and prospects of modern lymph node imaging. Eur J Radiol 2006;58:325–337.
248. Saksena MA, Saokar A, Harisinghani MG. Lymphotropic nanoparticle enhanced MR imaging (LNMRI) technique for lymph node imaging. Eur J Radiol 2006;58:367–374.
249. Kayton ML, Delgado R, Busam K, et al. Experience with 31 sentinel lymph node biopsies for sarcomas and carcinomas in pediatric patients. Cancer 2008;112:2052–2059.
250. Kayton ML, La Quaglia MP. Sentinel node biopsy for melanocytic tumors in children. Semin Diagn Pathol 2008;25:95–99.
251. Schaefer NG, Hany TF, Taverna C, et al. Non-Hodgkin lymphoma and Hodgkin disease: coregistered FDG PET and CT at staging and restaging—do we need contrast-enhanced CT? Radiology 2004;232:823–829.
252. Furth C, Denecke T, Steffen I, et al. Correlative imaging strategies implementing CT, MRI, and PET for staging of childhood Hodgkin disease. J Pediatr Hematol Oncol 2006;28:501–512.
253. Klem ML, Grewal RK, Wexler LH, et al. PET for staging in rhabdomyosarcoma: an evaluation of PET as an adjunct to current staging tools. J Pediatr Hematol Oncol 2007;29:9–14.
254. Volker T, Denecke T, Steffen I, et al. Positron emission tomography for staging of pediatric sarcoma patients: results of a prospective multicenter trial. J Clin Oncol 2007;25:5435–5441.
255. Ben Arush MW, Bar SR, Postovsky S, et al. Assessing the use of FDG-PET in the detection of regional and metastatic nodes in alveolar rhabdomyosarcoma of extremities. J Pediatr Hematol Oncol 2006;28:440–445.
256. McCarville MB, Christie R, Daw NC, et al. PET/CT in the evaluation of childhood sarcomas. AJR Am J Roentgenol 2005;184:1293–1304.
257. Parasuraman S, Langston J, Rao BN, et al. Brain metastases in pediatric Ewing sarcoma and rhabdomyosarcoma: the St. Jude Children's Research Hospital experience. J Pediatr Hematol Oncol 1999;21:370–377.
258. Green DM, Breslow NE, Beckwith JB, et al. Treatment of children with clear-cell sarcoma of the kidney: a report from the National Wilms' Tumor Study Group. J Clin Oncol 1994;12:2132–2137.
259. Savla J, Chen TT, Schneider NR, et al. Mutations of the hSNF5/INI1 gene in renal rhabdoid tumors with second primary brain tumors. J Natl Cancer Inst 2000;92:648–650.
260. Kaufman BA, Moran CJ, Park TS. Spinal magnetic resonance imaging immediately after craniotomy for detection of metastatic disease. Pediatr Neurosurg 1995;23:171–181.
261. Krampla W, Schatzer R, Urban M, et al. Lumbar meningeal enhancement after surgery in the posterior cranial fossa: a normal finding in children? [in German]. Rofo 2002;174:1511–1515.
262. Kaste SC, Pratt CB, Cain AM, et al. Metastases detected at the time of diagnosis of primary pediatric extremity osteosarcoma at diagnosis: imaging features. Cancer 1999;86: 1602–1608.
263. Dubois SG, London WB, Zhang Y, et al. Lung metastases in neuroblastoma at initial diagnosis: a report from the International Neuroblastoma Risk Group (INRG) project. Pediatr Blood Cancer 2008;51:589–592.
264. Bal CS, Kumar A, Chandra P, et al. Is chest x-ray or high-resolution computed tomography scan of the chest sufficient investigation to detect pulmonary metastasis in pediatric differentiated thyroid cancer? Thyroid 2004;14:217–225.
265. Helm EJ, Silva CT, Roberts HC, et al. Computer-aided detection for the identification of pulmonary nodules in pediatric oncology patients: initial experience. Pediatr Radiol 2009;39:685–693.
266. Rosenfield NS, Keller MS, Markowitz RI, et al. CT differentiation of benign and malignant lung nodules in children. J Pediatr Surg 1992;27:459–461.
267. McCarville MB, Kaste SC, Cain AM, et al. Prognostic factors and imaging patterns of recurrent pulmonary nodules after thoracotomy in children with osteosarcoma. Cancer 2001;91:1170–1176.
268. Grampp S, Bankier AA, Zoubek A, et al. Spiral CT of the lung in children with malignant extra-thoracic tumors: distribution of benign vs malignant pulmonary nodules. Eur Radiol 2000;10:1318–1322.
269. Absalon MJ, McCarville MB, Liu T, et al. Pulmonary nodules discovered during the initial evaluation of pediatric patients with bone and soft-tissue sarcoma. 2008:1147–1153.
270. Cohen MD. Current controversy: is computed tomography scan of the chest needed in patients with Wilms' tumor? Am J Pediatr Hematol Oncol 1994;16:191–193.
271. Owens CM, Veys PA, Pritchard J, et al. Role of chest computed tomography at diagnosis in the management of Wilms' tumor: a study by the United Kingdom Children's Cancer Study Group. J Clin Oncol 2002;20:2768–2773.
272. Green DM. Use of chest computed tomography for staging and treatment of Wilms' tumor in children. J Clin Oncol 2002;20:2763–2764.
273. Wilimas JA, Kaste SC, Kauffman WM, et al. Use of chest computed tomography in the staging of pediatric Wilms' tumor: interobserver variability and prognostic significance. J Clin Oncol 1997;15:2631–2635.
274. Tatsumi M, Miller JH, Wahl RL. 18F-FDG PET/CT in evaluating non-CNS pediatric malignancies. J Nucl Med 2007;48:1923–1931.
275. Choi J. Imaging of hepatic metastases. Cancer Control 2006;13:6–12.
276. Donnelly LF, Foss JN, Frush DP, et al. Heterogeneous splenic enhancement patterns on spiral CT images in children: minimizing misinterpretation. Radiology 1999;210: 493–497.
277. McCarville MB, Kao SC. Imaging recommendations for malignant liver neoplasms in children. Pediatr Blood Cancer 2006;46:2–7.
278. drup-Link HE, Franzius C, Link TM, et al. Whole-body MR imaging for detection of bone metastases in children and young adults: comparison with skeletal scintigraphy and FDG PET. AJR Am J Roentgenol 2001;177:229–236.
279. Goo HW, Choi SH, Ghim T, et al. Whole-body MRI of paediatric malignant tumours: comparison with conventional oncological imaging methods. Pediatr Radiol 2005;35: 766–773.

280. Kumar J, Seith A, Kumar A, et al. Whole-body MR imaging with the use of parallel imaging for detection of skeletal metastases in pediatric patients with small-cell neoplasms: comparison with skeletal scintigraphy and FDG PET/CT. Pediatr Radiol 2008; 38:953–962.
281. Franzius C, Sciuk J, drup-Link HE, et al. FDG-PET for detection of osseous metastases from malignant primary bone tumours: comparison with bone scintigraphy. Eur J Nucl Med 2000;27:1305–1311.
282. Phillips M, Allen C, Gerson P, et al. Comparison of FDG-PET scans to conventional radiography and bone scans in management of Langerhans cell histiocytosis. Pediatr Blood Cancer 2009;52:97–101.
283. Ryan SP, Weinberger E, White KS, et al. MR imaging of bone marrow in children with osteosarcoma: effect of granulocyte colony-stimulating factor. AJR Am J Roentgenol 1995;165:915–920.
284. Hollinger EF, Alibazoglu H, Ali A, et al. Hematopoietic cytokine-mediated FDG uptake simulates the appearance of diffuse metastatic disease on whole-body PET imaging. Clin Nucl Med 1998;23:93–98.
285. Kazama T, Swanston N, Podoloff DA, et al. Effect of colony-stimulating factor and conventional- or high-dose chemotherapy on FDG uptake in bone marrow. Eur J Nucl Med Mol Imaging 2005;32:1406–1411.
286. Finegold MJ, Egler RA, Goss JA, et al. Liver tumors: pediatric population. Liver Transpl 2008;14:1545–1556.
287. Roebuck DJ, Aronson D, Clapuyt P, et al. 2005 PRETEXT: a revised staging system for primary malignant liver tumours of childhood developed by the SIOPEL group. Pediatr Radiol 2007;37:123–132.
288. Aronson DC, Schnater JM, Staalman CR, et al. Predictive value of the pretreatment extent of disease system in hepatoblastoma: results from the International Society of Pediatric Oncology Liver Tumor Study Group SIOPEL-1 study. J Clin Oncol 2005;23: 1245–1252.
289. Brisse HJ, Schleiermacher G, Sarnacki S, et al. Preoperative Wilms tumor rupture: a retrospective study of 57 patients. Cancer 2008;113:202–213.
290. Pirotte B, Goldman S, Salzberg S, et al. Combined positron emission tomography and magnetic resonance imaging for the planning of stereotactic brain biopsies in children: experience in 9 cases. Pediatr Neurosurg 2003;38:146–155.
291. Pirotte B, Goldman S, Dewitte O, et al. Integrated positron emission tomography and magnetic resonance imaging-guided resection of brain tumors: a report of 103 consecutive procedures. J Neurosurg 2006;104:238–253.
292. Krasin MJ, Hudson MM, Kaste SC. Positron emission tomography in pediatric radiation oncology: integration in the treatment-planning process. Pediatr Radiol 2004;34: 214–221.
293. Bogomolny DL, Petrovich NM, Hou BL, et al. Functional MRI in the brain tumor patient. Top Magn Reson Imaging 2004;15:325–335.
294. Therasse P. Measuring the clinical response: what does it mean? Eur J Cancer 2002; 38:1817–1823.
295. Miller AB, Hoogstraten B, Staquet M, et al. Reporting results of cancer treatment. Cancer 1981;47:207–214.
296. Therasse P, Arbuck SG, Eisenhauer EA, et al. New guidelines to evaluate the response to treatment in solid tumors: European Organization for Research and Treatment of Cancer, National Cancer Institute of the United States, National Cancer Institute of Canada. J Natl Cancer Inst 2000;92:205–216.
297. Eisenhauer EA, Therasse P, Bogaerts J, et al. New response evaluation criteria in solid tumours: revised RECIST guideline (version 1.1). Eur J Cancer 2009;45:228–247.
298. McHugh K, Kao S. Can paediatric radiologists resist RECIST (response evaluation criteria in solid tumours)? Pediatr Radiol 2003;33:739–743.
299. Schwartz LH, Mazumdar M, Brown W, et al. Variability in response assessment in solid tumors: effect of number of lesions chosen for measurement. Clin Cancer Res 2003;9: 4318–4323.
300. Mazumdar M, Smith A, Schwartz LH. A statistical simulation study finds discordance between WHO criteria and RECIST guideline. J Clin Epidemiol 2004;57:358–365.
301. Choi H. Response evaluation of gastrointestinal stromal tumors. Oncologist 2008; 13(suppl 2):4–7.
302. Brisse H, Pacquement H, Burdairon E, et al. Outcome of residual mediastinal masses of thoracic lymphomas in children: impact on management and radiological follow-up strategy. Pediatr Radiol 1998;28:444–450.
303. McHugh K, Pritchard J. Problems in the imaging of three common paediatric solid tumours. Eur J Radiol 2001;37:72–78.
304. Mody RJ, Bui C, Hutchinson RJ, et al. Comparison of (18)F Flurodeoxyglucose PET with Ga-67 scintigraphy and conventional imaging modalities in pediatric lymphoma. Leuk Lymphoma 2007;48:699–707.
305. Levine JM, Weiner M, Kelly KM. Routine use of PET scans after completion of therapy in pediatric Hodgkin disease results in a high false positive rate. J Pediatr Hematol Oncol 2006;28:711–714.
306. Meany HJ, Gidvani VK, Minniti CP. Utility of PET scans to predict disease relapse in pediatric patients with Hodgkin lymphoma. Pediatr Blood Cancer 2007;48:399–402.
307. Andre N, Fabre A, Colavolpe C, et al. FDG PET and evaluation of posttherapeutic residual tumors in pediatric oncology: preliminary experience. J Pediatr Hematol Oncol 2008;30:343–346.
308. Matthay KK, Edeline V, Lumbroso J, et al. Correlation of early metastatic response by 123I-metaiodobenzylguanidine scintigraphy with overall response and event-free survival in stage IV neuroblastoma. J Clin Oncol 2003;21:2486–2491.
309. Hudson MM, Onciu M, Donaldson SS. Hodgkin lymphoma. In: Pizzo PA, Poplack DG, eds. Principles and practice of pediatric oncology. Philadelphia, PA: Lippincott Williams & Wilkins, 2006:695–721.
310. Spaepen K, Stroobants S, Verhoef G, et al. Positron emission tomography with [(18)F]FDG for therapy response monitoring in lymphoma patients. Eur J Nucl Med Mol Imaging 2003;30(suppl 1):S97–S105.
311. Weeks JC, Yeap BY, Canellos GP, et al. Value of follow-up procedures in patients with large-cell lymphoma who achieve a complete remission. J Clin Oncol 1991;9: 1196–1203.
312. Dwyer AJ, Prewitt JM, Ecker JG, et al. Use of the hazard rate to schedule follow-up exams efficiently: an optimization approach to patient management. Med Decis Making 1983;3:229–244.
313. Dwyer AJ, Glaubiger DL, Ecker JG, et al. The radiographic follow-up of patients with Ewing sarcoma: a demonstration of a general method. Radiology 1982;145: 327–331.
314. Chang PJ, Parker BR, Donaldson SS, et al. Dynamic probabilistic model for determination of optimal timing of surveillance chest radiography in pediatric Hodgkin disease. Radiology 1989;173:71–75.
315. Gylys-Morin V, Hoffer FA, Kozakewich H, et al. Wilms tumor and nephroblastomatosis: imaging characteristics at gadolinium-enhanced MR imaging. Radiology 1993;188: 517–521.
316. Rohrschneider WK, Weirich A, Rieden K, et al. US, CT and MR imaging characteristics of nephroblastomatosis. Pediatr Radiol 1998;28:435–443.
317. Owens CM, Brisse HJ, Olsen OE, et al. Bilateral disease and new trends in Wilms tumour. Pediatr Radiol 2008;38:30–39.
318. Beckwith JB. Children at increased risk for Wilms tumor: monitoring issues. J Pediatr 1998;132:377–379.
319. Choyke PL, Siegel MJ, Craft AW, et al. Screening for Wilms tumor in children with Beckwith-Wiedemann syndrome or idiopathic hemihypertrophy. Med Pediatr Oncol 1999;32:196–200.
320. McNeil DE, Brown M, Ching A, et al. Screening for Wilms tumor and hepatoblastoma in children with Beckwith-Wiedemann syndromes: a cost-effective model. Med Pediatr Oncol 2001;37:349–356.
321. Rao A, Rothman J, Nichols KE. Genetic testing and tumor surveillance for children with cancer predisposition syndromes. Curr Opin Pediatr 2008;20:1–7.
322. Scott RH, Walker L, Olsen OE, et al. Surveillance for Wilms tumour in at-risk children: pragmatic recommendations for best practice. Arch Dis Child 2006;91:995–999.
323. Craft AW. Growth rate of Wilms' tumour. Lancet 1999;354:1127.
324. Tan TY, Amor DJ. Tumour surveillance in Beckwith-Wiedemann syndrome and hemihyperplasia: a critical review of the evidence and suggested guidelines for local practice. J Paediatr Child Health 2006;42:486–490.
325. Leenen AS, Riebel TW. Testicular microlithiasis in children: sonographic features and clinical implications. Pediatr Radiol 2002;32:575–579.
326. Jaganathan K, Ahmed S, Henderson A, et al. Current management strategies for testicular microlithiasis. Nat Clin Pract Urol 2007;4:492–497.
327. Coffey J, Huddart RA, Elliott F, et al. Testicular microlithiasis as a familial risk factor for testicular germ cell tumour. Br J Cancer 2007;97:1701–1706.
328. Kivela T. Trilateral retinoblastoma: a meta-analysis of hereditary retinoblastoma associated with primary ectopic intracranial retinoblastoma. J Clin Oncol 1999;17: 1829–1837.
329. Bhargava R, Parham DM, Lasater OE, et al. MR imaging differentiation of benign and malignant peripheral nerve sheath tumors: use of the target sign. Pediatr Radiol 1997;27:124–129.
330. Warbey VS, Ferner RE, Dunn JT, et al. [18F]FDG PET/CT in the diagnosis of malignant peripheral nerve sheath tumours in neurofibromatosis type-1. Eur J Nucl Med Mol Imaging 2009;36:751–757.
331. Listernick R, Ferner RE, Liu GT, et al. Optic pathway gliomas in neurofibromatosis-1: controversies and recommendations. Ann Neurol 2007;61:189–198.
332. Landier W, Bhatia S. Cancer survivorship: a pediatric perspective. Oncologist 2008;13: 1181–1192.
333. Robison LL. Treatment-associated subsequent neoplasms among long-term survivors of childhood cancer: the experience of the Childhood Cancer Survivor Study. Pediatr Radiol 2009;39(suppl 1):S32–S37.
334. Monagle P, Chalmers E, Chan A, et al. Antithrombotic therapy in neonates and children: American College of Chest Physicians Evidence-Based Clinical Practice Guidelines (8th edition). Chest 2008;133:887S–968S.
335. Babyn PS, Gahunia HK, Massicotte P. Pulmonary thromboembolism in children. Pediatr Radiol 2005;35:258–274.
336. Leung LH, Ooi GC, Kwong DL, et al. White-matter diffusion anisotropy after chemo-irradiation: a statistical parametric mapping study and histogram analysis. Neuroimage 2004;21:261–268.
337. Reddick WE, White HA, Glass JO, et al. Developmental model relating white matter volume to neurocognitive deficits in pediatric brain tumor survivors. Cancer 2003;97: 2512–2519.
338. Edwards-Brown MK, Jakacki RI. Imaging the central nervous system effects of radiation and chemotherapy of pediatric tumors. Neuroimaging Clin N Am 1999;9: 177–193.
339. Shanley DJ. Mineralizing microangiopathy: CT and MRI. Neuroradiology 1995;37: 331–333.
340. Baumgartner JE, Ater JL, Ha CS, et al. Pathologically proven cavernous angiomas of the brain following radiation therapy for pediatric brain tumors. Pediatr Neurosurg 2003; 39:201–207.
341. Inaba H, Khan RB, Laningham FH, et al. Clinical and radiological characteristics of methotrexate-induced acute encephalopathy in pediatric patients with cancer. Ann Oncol 2008;19:178–184.
342. Fleischhack G, Solymosi L, Reiter A, et al. Imaging methods in diagnosis of cerebrovascular complications with L-asparaginase therapy [in German]. Klin Padiatr 1994;206: 334–341.
343. Kaste SC, Rodriguez-Galindo C, Furman WL, et al. Imaging aspects of neurologic emergencies in children treated for non-CNS malignancies. Pediatr Radiol 2000;30: 558–565.
344. Mukherjee P, McKinstry RC. Reversible posterior leukoencephalopathy syndrome: evaluation with diffusion-tensor MR imaging. Radiology 2001;219:756–765.
345. Chen W. Clinical applications of PET in brain tumors. J Nucl Med 2007;48:1468–1481.
346. DeGroot LJ. Effects of irradiation on the thyroid gland. Endocrinol Metab Clin North Am 1993;22:607–615.
347. Somerville HM, Steinbeck KS, Stevens G, et al. Thyroid neoplasia following irradiation in adolescent and young adult survivors of childhood cancer. Med J Aust 2002;176: 584–587.
348. Bonato C, Severino RF, Elnecave RH. Reduced thyroid volume and hypothyroidism in survivors of childhood cancer treated with radiotherapy. J Pediatr Endocrinol Metab 2008;21:943–949.
349. Brignardello E, Corrias A, Isolato G, et al. Ultrasound screening for thyroid carcinoma in childhood cancer survivors: a case series. J Clin Endocrinol Metab 2008;93: 4840–4843.
350. Park KJ, Chung JY, Chun MS, et al. Radiation-induced lung disease and the impact of radiation methods on imaging features. Radiographics 2000;20:83–98.
351. Ben Arush MW, Roguin A, Zamir E, et al. Bleomycin and cyclophosphamide toxicity simulating metastatic nodules to the lungs in childhood cancer. Pediatr Hematol Oncol 1997;14:381–386.
352. Barlesi F, Villani P, Doddoli C, et al. Gemcitabine-induced severe pulmonary toxicity. Fundam Clin Pharmacol 2004;18:85–91.
353. Worthy SA, Flint JD, Muller NL. Pulmonary complications after bone marrow transplantation: high-resolution CT and pathologic findings. Radiographics 1997;17:1359–1371.

354. Choi YH, Leung AN. Radiologic findings: pulmonary infections after bone marrow transplantation. J Thorac Imaging 1999;14:201–206.

355. Gulbahce HE, Manivel JC, Jessurun J. Pulmonary cytolytic thrombi: a previously unrecognized complication of bone marrow transplantation. Am J Surg Pathol 2000;24:1147–1152.

356. Keates-Baleeiro J, Moore P, Koyama T, et al. Incidence and outcome of idiopathic pneumonia syndrome in pediatric stem cell transplant recipients. Bone Marrow Transplant 2006;38:285–289.

357. Krischer JP, Epstein S, Cuthbertson DD, et al. Clinical cardiotoxicity following anthracycline treatment for childhood cancer: the Pediatric Oncology Group experience. J Clin Oncol 1997;15:1544–1552.

358. Adams MJ, Hardenbergh PH, Constine LS, et al. Radiation-associated cardiovascular disease. Crit Rev Oncol Hematol 2003;45:55–75.

359. Ritchey ML, Kelalis PP, Etzioni R, et al. Small bowel obstruction after nephrectomy for Wilms' tumor: a report of the National Wilms' Tumor Study-3. Ann Surg 1993;218:654–659.

360. McCarville MB, Adelman CS, Li C, et al. Typhlitis in childhood cancer. Cancer 2005;104:380–387.

361. Kirkpatrick ID, Greenberg HM. Gastrointestinal complications in the neutropenic patient: characterization and differentiation with abdominal CT. Radiology 2003;226:668–674.

362. Fenton LZ, Buonomo C. Benign pneumatosis in children. Pediatr Radiol 2000;30:786–793.

363. Donnelly LF, Morris CL. Acute graft-versus-host disease in children: abdominal CT findings. Radiology 1996;199:265–268.

364. Mentzel HJ, Kentouche K, Kosmehl H, et al. US and MRI of gastrointestinal graft-versus-host disease. Pediatr Radiol 2002;32:195–198.

365. Horger M, Bethge W, Boss A, et al. Musculocutaneous chronic graft-versus-host disease: MRI follow-up of patients undergoing immunosuppressive therapy. AJR Am J Roentgenol 2009;192:1401–1406.

366. Sadoff J, Hwang S, Rosenfeld D, et al. Surgical pancreatic complications induced by L-asparaginase. J Pediatr Surg 1997;32:860–863.

367. Robinson PJ. The effects of cancer chemotherapy on liver imaging. Eur Radiol 2009;19:1752–1762.

368. McCarville MB, Hoffer FA, Howard SC, et al. Hepatic veno-occlusive disease in children undergoing bone-marrow transplantation: usefulness of sonographic findings. Pediatr Radiol 2001;31:102–105.

369. Bouyn CI, Leclere J, Raimondo G, et al. Hepatic focal nodular hyperplasia in children previously treated for a solid tumor: incidence, risk factors, and outcome. Cancer 2003;97:3107–3113.

370. Marabelle A, Campagne D, Dechelotte P, et al. Focal nodular hyperplasia of the liver in patients previously treated for pediatric neoplastic diseases. J Pediatr Hematol Oncol 2008;30:546–549.

371. Iannaccone R, Federle MP, Brancatelli G, et al. Peliosis hepatis: spectrum of imaging findings. AJR Am J Roentgenol 2006;187:W43–W52.

372. Metser U, Haider MA, Il-Macky M, et al. Fungal liver infection in immunocompromised patients: depiction with multiphasic contrast-enhanced helical CT. Radiology 2005;235:97–105.

373. Semelka RC, Kelekis NL, Sallah S, et al. Hepatosplenic fungal disease: diagnostic accuracy and spectrum of appearances on MR imaging. AJR Am J Roentgenol 1997;169:1311–1316.

374. Berrocal T, Parron M, varez-Luque A, et al. Pediatric liver transplantation: a pictorial essay of early and late complications. Radiographics 2006;26:1187–1209.

375. MacKenzie JR. Complications of treatment of paediatric malignancies. Eur J Radiol 2001;37:109–119.

376. McCarville MB, Hoffer FA, Gingrich JR, et al. Imaging findings of hemorrhagic cystitis in pediatric oncology patients. Pediatr Radiol 2000;30:131–138.

377. Ritchey M, Ferrer F, Shearer P, et al. Late effects on the urinary bladder in patients treated for cancer in childhood: a report from the Children's Oncology Group. Pediatr Blood Cancer 2009;52:439–446.

378. Kaste SC. Skeletal toxicities of treatment in children with cancer. Pediatr Blood Cancer 2008;50:469–473.

379. Butler MS, Robertson WW Jr, Rate W, et al. Skeletal sequelae of radiation therapy for malignant childhood tumors. Clin Orthop Relat Res 1990;235:240.

380. Roebuck DJ. Skeletal complications in pediatric oncology patients. Radiographics 1999;19:873–885.

381. Mattano LA Jr, Sather HN, Trigg ME, et al. Osteonecrosis as a complication of treating acute lymphoblastic leukemia in children: a report from the Children's Cancer Group. J Clin Oncol 2000;18:3262–3272.

382. Faraci M, Calevo MG, Lanino E, et al. Osteonecrosis after allogeneic stem cell transplantation in childhood: a case-control study in Italy. Haematologica 2006;91:1096–1099.

383. Karimova EJ, Rai SN, Ingle D, et al. MRI of knee osteonecrosis in children with leukemia and lymphoma, II: clinical and imaging patterns. AJR Am J Roentgenol 2006;186:477–482.

384. Kadan-Lottick NS, Dinu I, Wasilewski-Masker K, et al. Osteonecrosis in adult survivors of childhood cancer: a report from the childhood cancer survivor study. J Clin Oncol 2008;26:3038–3045.

385. Karimova EJ, Rai SN, Wu J, et al. Femoral resurfacing in young patients with hematologic cancer and osteonecrosis. Clin Orthop Relat Res 2008;466:3044–3050.

386. Wasilewski-Masker K, Kaste SC, Hudson MM, et al. Bone mineral density deficits in survivors of childhood cancer: long-term follow-up guidelines and review of the literature. Pediatrics 2008;121:e705–e713.

387. Kaste SC. Bone-mineral density deficits from childhood cancer and its therapy: a review of at-risk patient cohorts and available imaging methods. Pediatr Radiol 2004;34:373–378.

388. Muszynska-Roslan K, Konstantynowicz J, Panasiuk A, et al. Is the treatment for childhood solid tumors associated with lower bone mass than that for leukemia and Hodgkin disease? Pediatr Hematol Oncol 2009;26:36–47.

389. Kaste SC, Shidler TJ, Tong X, et al. Bone mineral density and osteonecrosis in survivors of childhood allogeneic bone marrow transplantation. Bone Marrow Transplant 2004;33:435–441.

390. Kaste SC, Tong X, Hendrick JM, et al. QCT versus DXA in 320 survivors of childhood cancer: association of BMD with fracture history. Pediatr Blood Cancer 2006;47:936–943.

391. Lewiecki EM, Gordon CM, Baim S, et al. International Society for Clinical Densitometry 2007 Adult and Pediatric Official Positions. Bone 2008;43:1115–1121.

392. Morris EB, Shelso J, Smeltzer MP, et al. The use of bone age for bone mineral density interpretation in a cohort of pediatric brain tumor patients. Pediatr Radiol 2008;38:1285–1292.

393. Hill SC, Baker AR, Barton NW, et al. Sciatic nerve: paradoxic hypertrophy after amputation in young patients. Radiology 1997;205:559–562.

394. Taitz J, Cohn RJ, White L, et al. Osteochondroma after total body irradiation: an age-related complication. Pediatr Blood Cancer 2004;42:225–229.

395. Vazquez E, Castellote A, Piqueras J, et al. Second malignancies in pediatric patients: imaging findings and differential diagnosis. Radiographics 2003;23:1155–1172.

396. Meadows AT, Friedman DL, Neglia JP, et al. Second neoplasms in survivors of childhood cancer: findings from the Childhood Cancer Survivor Study cohort. J Clin Oncol 2009;27:2356–2362.

397. Bassal M, Mertens AC, Taylor L, et al. Risk of selected subsequent carcinomas in survivors of childhood cancer: a report from the Childhood Cancer Survivor Study. J Clin Oncol 2006;24:476–483.

398. Bhatia S, Robison LL, Oberlin O, et al. Breast cancer and other second neoplasms after childhood Hodgkin's disease. N Engl J Med 1996;334:745–751.

399. Kriege M, Brekelmans CT, Boetes C, et al. Efficacy of MRI and mammography for breast-cancer screening in women with a familial or genetic predisposition. N Engl J Med 2004;351:427–437.

400. Warner E, Plewes DB, Hill KA, et al. Surveillance of BRCA1 and BRCA2 mutation carriers with magnetic resonance imaging, ultrasound, mammography, and clinical breast examination. JAMA 2004;292:1317–1325.

401. Donnelly LF, Frush DP, Marshall KW, et al. Lymphoproliferative disorders: CT findings in immunocompromised children. AJR Am J Roentgenol 1998;171:725–731.

402. Pickhardt PJ, Siegel MJ, Hayashi RJ, et al. Posttransplantation lymphoproliferative disorder in children: clinical, histopathologic, and imaging features. Radiology 2000;217:16–25.

403. Pollock AN, Newman B, Putnam PE, et al. Imaging of post-transplant spindle cell tumors. Pediatr Radiol 1995;25(suppl 1):S118–S121.

404. von FC, Maecker B, Schirg E, et al. Post transplant lymphoproliferative disease in pediatric solid organ transplant patients: a possible role for [18F]-FDG-PET(/CT) in initial staging and therapy monitoring. Eur J Radiol 2007;63:427–435.

405. Rago T, Santini F, Scutari M, et al. Elastography: new developments in ultrasound for predicting malignancy in thyroid nodules. J Clin Endocrinol Metab 2007;92:2917–2922.

406. Venkatesh SK, Yin M, Glockner JF, et al. MR elastography of liver tumors: preliminary results. AJR Am J Roentgenol 2008;190:1534–1540.

407. Blankenberg FG. In vivo detection of apoptosis. J Nucl Med 2008;49(suppl 2):81S–95S.

408. Kenny LM, Aboagye EO, Price PM. Positron emission tomography imaging of cell proliferation in oncology. Clin Oncol (R Coll Radiol) 2004;16:176–185.

409. Padhani AR. Dynamic contrast-enhanced MRI in clinical oncology: current status and future directions. J Magn Reson Imaging 2002;16:407–422.

410. Padhani A. PET imaging of tumour hypoxia. Cancer Imaging 2006;6:S117–S121.

411. Golman K, Zandt RI, Lerche M, et al. Metabolic imaging by hyperpolarized 13C magnetic resonance imaging for in vivo tumor diagnosis. Cancer Res 2006;66:10855–10860.

412. Jaffer FA, Weissleder R. Molecular imaging in the clinical arena. JAMA 2005;293:855–862.

413. Blankenberg FG. Molecular imaging: the latest generation of contrast agents and tissue characterization techniques. J Cell Biochem 2003;90:443–453.

414. Voss SD, Smith SV, DiBartolo N, et al. Positron emission tomography (PET) imaging of neuroblastoma and melanoma with 64Cu-SarAr immunoconjugates. Proc Natl Acad Sci U S A 2007;104:17489–17493.

415. Adamson PC. Imaging in early phase childhood cancer trials. Pediatr Radiol 2009;39(suppl 1):S38–S41.

416. Voss SD, Reaman GH, Kaste SC, et al. The ALARA concept in pediatric oncology. Pediatr Radiol 2009;39:1142–1146.

417. Reaman GH. What, why, and when we image: considerations for diagnostic imaging and clinical research in the Children's Oncology Group. Pediatr Radiol 2009;39(suppl 1):S42–S45.

SECTION 3 ■ PRINCIPLES OF MULTIMODAL THERAPY

CHAPTER 10 ■ GENERAL PRINCIPLES OF CHEMOTHERAPY

PETER C. ADAMSON, ROCHELLE BAGATELL, FRANK M. BALIS, AND SUSAN M. BLANEY

Since the introduction of chemotherapy for the treatment of childhood leukemia more than 50 years ago,[1] the prognosis of childhood cancer has improved dramatically (Fig. 10.1). The 5-year survival rate for this group of diseases, many of which were uniformly fatal in the prechemotherapy era, was 80% for all forms of childhood cancer diagnosed between 1996 and 2004.[2] This striking improvement in survival is a direct result of the incorporation of anticancer drugs into treatment regimens that previously relied only on surgery or radiotherapy for the primary tumor.[3] The multimodality approach, which integrates surgery and radiotherapy to control local disease with chemotherapy to eradicate systemic (metastatic) disease, has become the standard approach to treating most childhood cancers.

PRINCIPLES OF CANCER CHEMOTHERAPY

The ultimate goal of the multimodality treatment approach, in which anticancer drugs play a critical role, is to cure the patient of his or her cancer. The feasibility of achieving cures by the addition of anticancer drugs to surgery or radiation was first demonstrated in chemosensitive childhood cancers, such as Wilms' tumor.[4] However, curing the underlying disease is not the goal of most pharmacological interventions. With the exception of antimicrobial and anticancer chemotherapy, the common classes of drugs (e.g., antihypertensives) are administered with the intent of controlling the disease or the symptoms caused by disease, rather than curing the underlying disease. The model for curing cancer is based on the successful model of curing bacterial infections. This strategy attempts to exploit differences between cancer and normal host cells and eradicate or kill all cancer cells in the body. This "killing paradigm"[5] has had a profound impact on our approach to anticancer drug discovery, drug development, and the design of treatment regimens that incorporate anticancer drugs.

The predominant strategy for anticancer drug discovery has historically been high-throughput *in vitro* screening to evaluate the antiproliferative or cancer cell killing effects of candidate drugs in tumor cell lines.[6] The precise mechanism of action of the candidate drugs was not critical to the selection process, and for many agents (e.g., doxorubicin) the mechanism of action was not defined until after the drugs were in widespread clinical use. This nonmechanistically based screening method identified drugs that are cytotoxic and nonselective. As a result, most conventional anticancer drugs produce substantial toxicity.

In clinical drug development, the initial dose-finding (phase I) clinical trials define the maximum tolerated dose (MTD), which is based on the severity of toxicity, as the optimal dose, rather than using a therapeutic endpoint to establish the optimal dose. This design is based on the premise that the highest tolerable dose will produce the maximum achievable cancer cell kill. In subsequent phase II trials, the MTD is evaluated in small cohorts of patients with different types of cancer to establish whether the drug has activity, which is defined as a 50% or more decrease in the size of measurable tumors in at least 20% to 30% of patients with a specific type of cancer.[7]

Conventional frontline treatment regimens for most types of childhood cancer are composed of multiple anticancer drugs that are administered at their MTD intensity, even though these regimens typically produce substantial toxicity. Methods of rescuing or circumventing anticancer drug toxicity, such as the administration of hematopoietic growth factors and bone marrow or stem cell transplant to alleviate hematological toxicity, have been incorporated into treatment regimens to allow for administration of higher doses of anticancer drugs.

The basic principles that guide our current use of cancer chemotherapy are based on the goal of curing patients by eradicating all cancer cells and on empiric observations made in early clinical trials involving children with drug-sensitive cancers, such as acute lymphoblastic leukemia (ALL), Burkitt's lymphoma, and Wilms' tumor.[8] These principles include the use of multidrug combination regimens (i.e., combination chemotherapy), the administration of chemotherapy before the development of clinically evident metastatic disease (i.e., adjuvant chemotherapy), and the administration of drugs at the maximally tolerated dose rate (i.e., dose intensity).

Combination Chemotherapy

The importance of administering anticancer drugs in combination regimens was first appreciated in the treatment of ALL. Compared with single-agent therapy, the use of drug combinations significantly increased the percentage of patients achieving complete remission and prolonged the duration of their remissions.[9] At best, only 60% of patients treated with a single-agent therapy achieved complete remissions, but standard three- and four-drug combination induction regimens achieve complete remission rates that exceed 95%. Almost all patients on single-agent therapy experienced a relapse within 6 to 9 months, despite continuation of therapy with the same drug. Long-term remissions and cures were only attained after the institution of combination chemotherapy that incorporated the most active single agents.

The primary scientific rationale for the use of combination chemotherapy is to overcome drug resistance to individual agents, the incidence of which can often exceed 50% even in newly diagnosed cancers.[10,11] Because it is not feasible to accurately predict whether a particular patient's tumor will respond to a given drug, administering anticancer drugs in combination ensures a greater chance of achieving a response (i.e., exposing

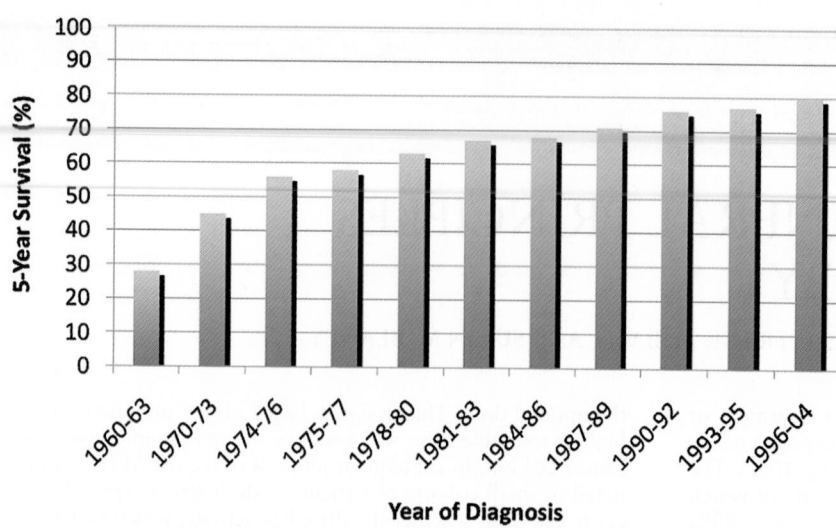

FIGURE 10.1 Five-year survival rate for all childhood cancers diagnosed between 1960 and 2004. (Data from Silverberg E, Boring CC, Squires TS. Cancer statistics, 1990. CA Cancer J Clin 1990;40:9–26; Jemal A, Murray T, Ward E, et al. Cancer statistics, 2005. CA Cancer J Clin 2005;55:10–30; Jemal A, Siegel R, Ward E, et al. Cancer Statistics, 2009. CA Cancer J Clin 2009;59:225–249.

the tumor to at least one active agent). In addition to providing a broader range of coverage against naturally resistant tumor cells, combination chemotherapy also may prevent or delay the development of acquired resistance in initially responsive tumors and provide additive or synergistic cytotoxic effects if agents with different mechanisms of action are selected.

A thorough knowledge of the clinical pharmacology of individual anticancer drugs is required to design effective combination chemotherapy regimens. Traditionally, combination chemotherapy regimens contain drugs with demonstrated single-agent activity against the type of tumor being treated, with a preference for agents that produced complete responses in patients with advanced or recurrent disease; drugs that are non–cross-resistant to overlap against drug-resistant subpopulations of tumor cells; drugs with non-antagonistic (i.e., additive or synergistic) mechanisms of action; and drugs with non-overlapping toxicity profiles, allowing each agent to be administered at its optimal dose and schedule.

Adjuvant Chemotherapy

Anticancer drugs are most effective when administered in the adjuvant setting to patients who are without overt evidence of residual disease after local therapy with surgery or radiation but who are at high risk to relapse at metastatic sites. Before the routine use of adjuvant chemotherapy, relapse at metastatic sites occurred in 60% to 95% of children with localized solid tumors after local therapy. The aim of adjuvant chemotherapy is to prevent metastatic recurrence by eliminating micrometastatic tumor deposits that are present at the time of diagnosis in the lungs, bone, bone marrow, lymph nodes, or other sites.[12] Adjuvant chemotherapy is efficacious for most of the common pediatric cancers, including Wilms' tumor, Ewing's sarcoma, lymphoma, rhabdomyosarcoma, astrocytoma, and osteosarcoma (Table 10.1).[13-19]

TABLE 10.1

BENEFICIAL EFFECTS OF ADJUVANT CHEMOTHERAPY ON SURVIVAL OF PATIENTS WITH COMMON FORMS OF PEDIATRIC CANCER

Tumor	Adjuvant therapy	Survival (%)	
		Without adjuvant chemotherapy	With adjuvant chemotherapy
Wilms' tumor	Vincristine, dactinomycin, ± doxorubicin	40	90
Ewing's sarcoma	Vincristine, dactinomycin, cyclophosphamide	5	50–60
Lymphomas	CHOP, COMP, LSA_2-L_2	<10	50–90
Rhabdomyosarcoma	Vincristine, dactinomycin, cyclophosphamide	10–20	65
Osteosarcoma	HDMTX, doxorubicin, cisplatin, BCD	15	65
Astrocytoma	Prednisone, vincristine, lomustine	20	45

B, bleomycin; C, cyclophosphamide; D, dactinomycin; H, doxorubicin; HDMTX, high-dose methotrexate; LSA_2-L_2, 10-drug regimen; M, methotrexate; O, vincristine; P, prednisone.
From Berg SL, Grissel DL, DeLaney TF, et al. Principles of treatment of pediatric solid tumors. Pediatr Clin North Am 1991;38:249.

Theoretical considerations and experimental evidence support the use of adjuvant chemotherapy.[20–22] Microscopic foci of tumor should be more chemosensitive on a cell-kinetic basis, because a larger fraction of the cells are actively proliferating and potentially susceptible to the cytotoxic effects of the drugs. The smaller burden of tumor cells also implies a lower probability that drug-resistant cells are present. The mathematical modeling experiments of Goldie and Coldman, which assume that a curable tumor is one with no drug-resistant tumor cells and that the development of drug resistance is the result of a random genetic event, predict that the chance for cure is maximized if all available active drugs are given simultaneously in the adjuvant setting, when there is minimal residual disease and the probability that drug-resistant cells are present is low.[10,23]

Clinical experience has demonstrated a correlation between low tumor burden and the efficacy of chemotherapy.[22–24] Children presenting with extensive or disseminated tumors are less likely to be cured than children with the identical type of cancer but with a low tumor burden. For example, the 5-year event-free survival for patients with metastatic Ewing's sarcoma treated on the Children's Cancer Group—Pediatric Oncology Group Ewing's sarcoma trial (INT-0991)—was 22% compared with 69% for children presenting with localized disease.[25]

The selection of appropriate drugs and the optimal timing of drug therapy relative to the definitive local therapy are important considerations in the design of successful adjuvant chemotherapy regimens. Traditionally, drugs have been selected based on their activity in advanced disease. Animal models and clinical experience have shown that regimens producing the most dramatic responses in metastatic or recurrent disease have the greatest likelihood of being curative in the adjuvant setting.[24]

Adjuvant chemotherapy should begin as soon as possible after definitive local therapy. A delay to allow for recovery from surgery or radiation therapy may compromise the chance of curing the patient. One strategy to avoid delays caused by potential adverse interactions between chemotherapy and surgery or irradiation is the administration of the drug therapy before definitive local therapy. This approach, called primary or neoadjuvant chemotherapy, may also improve local control of the primary tumor by shrinking the primary and making it more amenable to surgical resection, in addition to providing earlier therapy for micrometastases.[26,27]

Dose Intensity

Most anticancer drugs have a steep dose-response curve, and a small increment in the dose can significantly enhance the therapeutic effect of a drug in preclinical studies. In animal tumor models, a 2-fold increase in the dose of cyclophosphamide can result in a 10-fold increase in tumor-cell killing.[28,29] Retrospective clinical studies have also demonstrated a relationship between dose intensity of anticancer drugs and disease outcome, but this relationship has not been consistently confirmed in randomized prospective trials.

In a meta-analysis of chemotherapeutic regimens containing cyclophosphamide, methotrexate, and fluorouracil for metastatic breast cancer, Hryniuk and Bush observed a strong correlation between response rate and the relative dose intensity of the various regimens.[30] The relative dose intensity is calculated by normalizing the dose rate (mg/m^2/week) for each agent to the dose rate in an arbitrarily selected standard regimen and then averaging the relative dose intensities for all agents in the regimen to derive the relative dose intensity for the regimen. Over a threefold range in relative dose intensity,

the response rate in metastatic breast cancer ranged from 12% to 84%. Retrospective meta-analyses in stage II breast cancer, ovarian cancer, colorectal cancer, and lymphoma have also demonstrated a correlation between the dose intensity of the drug regimen and disease outcome.[31] However, prospective randomized trials have failed to demonstrate a survival advantage for more dose-intensive regimens, including high-dose chemotherapy with bone marrow or stem cell rescue, compared with standard dose regimens in breast, ovarian, and small-cell lung cancers[32–34] and for more dose-intensive cisplatin in germ cell tumors.[35]

For children with ALL and osteosarcoma, relapse rates are significantly lower in patients receiving more dose-intense chemotherapy.[36–40] In a randomized trial, patients with ALL receiving standard doses of methotrexate and mercaptopurine had a median survival of 15 months compared with 6 months for the group randomized to a half-dose maintenance regimen.[36] In children with high-risk ALL, those who received less than 94% of the protocol-prescribed dose of vincristine, anthracycline, and L-asparaginase during intensification therapy were 5.5 times more likely to experience a subsequent adverse event than patients who received at least 99% of the prescribed dose of these agents.[37] Oral mercaptopurine dose intensity during maintenance therapy is also predictive of event-fee survival in ALL.[38] However, in the latter study, lower mercaptopurine dose intensity was primarily the result of missed doses rather than reductions in the daily dose, leading the authors to conclude that prescribing higher doses of mercaptopurine could be counterproductive if greater hematological toxicity resulted in treatment delays.

Retrospective analyses of osteosarcoma trials demonstrated a twofold higher relapse rate in patients receiving less than 75% of their recommended dose of chemotherapy compared with patients receiving 75% or more in one study[39] and a threefold higher relapse rate in a second study using 80% of the protocol prescribed dose as a cutoff.[40]

Meta-analyses, such as those performed by Hryniuk and Bush, have also been performed for several pediatric tumors.[41,42] Analysis of 44 clinical trials involving 1,592 patients older than 1 year with stage IV neuroblastoma revealed a 5- to 10-fold range in the dose intensity of the individual agents studied.[41] The dose intensity of four drugs (i.e., teniposide, cisplatin, cyclophosphamide, doxorubicin) significantly correlated with response and survival. Similarly, examination of the relation between individual drug dose intensities and disease outcome in osteosarcoma and Ewing's sarcoma suggests that doxorubicin dose intensity is an important determinant of response in osteosarcoma and disease-free survival of patients with Ewing's sarcoma.[42]

Prospective randomized trials to assess the importance of dose intensity in childhood cancers have been performed for a few tumor types. The administered dose intensity of dactinomycin and doxorubicin in pulse-intensive regimens for Wilms' tumor was significantly higher than for the standard treatment regimens, but there was no survival advantage associated with the enhanced dose intensity.[43,44] In a randomized trial of filgrastim in children with high-risk ALL, the treatment interval was shorter with filgrastim, resulting in a slight increase in dose intensity but no impact on event-free survival.[45] A 33% increase in dose intensity was achieved in a five-drug chemotherapy regimen for Ewing's sarcoma by shortening the dosing interval (interval compression) from 21 to 14 days. Compared with the standard every 21-day regimen, event-free survival was higher (76% vs. 65%) on the compressed regimen.[46]

Methods for maximizing dose intensity include greater patient and physician willingness to tolerate drug toxicities; more aggressive supportive care of patients experiencing these side effects; selective rescue of the patient from toxicity, such as with bone marrow or peripheral stem cell transplantation or the administration of filgrastim; the use of regional chemotherapy (e.g., intra-arterial, intrathecal delivery) to achieve high drug concentrations at local tumor sites while minimizing systemic drug exposure; and the development of new treatment schedules, such as long-term continuous infusions, that may allow more drug to be administered over a given period.

CLINICAL PHARMACOLOGY OF ANTICANCER DRUGS

The primary role of the pediatric oncologist is to orchestrate the administration of complex combination chemotherapy regimens to children in the setting of multimodal (i.e., surgery, radiotherapy, and chemotherapy) therapy. Special care must be taken because the anticancer drugs used in these regimens have the lowest therapeutic index of any class of drugs and predictably produce significant, even life-threatening toxicity at therapeutic doses (Fig. 10.2).[47] However, implementing significant dose reductions or delays in therapy to attenuate these toxicities may compromise the therapeutic effect and place the patient at an increased risk for disease recurrence, a uniformly fatal event with most childhood cancers. The cancer chemotherapist must carefully balance the risks of toxicities from therapy against the risk of tumor recurrence from inadequate treatment. Unfortunately, the crucial adjustments in the dose and schedule of chemotherapy needed to achieve this balance often must be made empirically, because therapeutic drug monitoring for most agents is not available.

To ensure that these drugs are used safely and effectively, the pediatric oncologist must have an in-depth knowledge of the clinical pharmacology of these agents, including the mechanisms of drug action, pharmacokinetics, pharmacogenetics, spectrum of toxicities, potential drug interactions, and mechanisms of drug resistance.

Mechanism of Action

Although recent advances in basic research have provided profound insights into the pathogenesis of many forms of childhood cancer and offer hope for the development of specific and selective new cancer treatments, most current conventional anticancer drugs used in the frontline treatment of childhood cancers are cytotoxic agents with nonselective mechanisms of action that target vital macromolecules (e.g., DNA) or metabolic pathways that are critical to both malignant and normal cells, and as a result, they cause many undesirable and potentially severe toxic effects.

Most anticancer drugs produce their cytotoxic effects by interfering at some stage with the synthesis or function of the vital nucleic acids, DNA and RNA (Fig. 10.3). For example, the alkylating agents are chemically reactive compounds that damage DNA by covalently bonding to and cross-linking nucleobases within the DNA,[48] and the antimetabolites block the synthesis of nucleotide precursors or are directly incorporated into DNA as fraudulent bases. The topoisomerases are also an important target of anticancer drugs. These nuclear enzymes maintain the three-dimensional structure of DNA and are critical for DNA replication, transcription, repair, and recombination. The topoisomerases work by cleaving and re-ligating DNA, and agents such as the anthracyclines, epipodophyllotoxins, and camptothecins interfere with re-ligation, resulting in protein-associated DNA strand breaks.[49,50]

Dysregulation of the cell cycle, signal transduction pathways that regulate cell proliferation, and programmed cell death (apoptosis) are common to most forms of cancer.[51–53] These cellular processes are genetically controlled, and mutations to genes involved in these highly complex and interrelated pathways can result in loss of control of DNA replication and cell division and suppression of the apoptotic response to receptor-linked or DNA damage-induced signals. In addition to their role in tumorigenesis, mutations in cell cycle regulatory genes and genes involved in apoptosis may modulate the sensitivity of cancer cells to anticancer drugs.[51,53] The cellular damage produced by most anticancer drugs appears to induce apoptosis in chemosensitive cancer cells. Overexpression of oncogenes that promote apoptosis, such as *MYCC* and *MYCN*, can enhance the chemosensitivity of tumor cells, whereas overexpression of bcl-2, which blocks the apoptotic pathway, can attenuate drug-induced apoptosis and convey pleiotropic resistance to anticancer drugs.[54,55]

The cell cycle is regulated by negative feedback controls or checkpoints that block the cell from proceeding to the next cell cycle event until the prior event is completed and until needed repairs to DNA are performed.[56–59] Normal cells are arrested in G_1 phase in response to DNA damage caused by

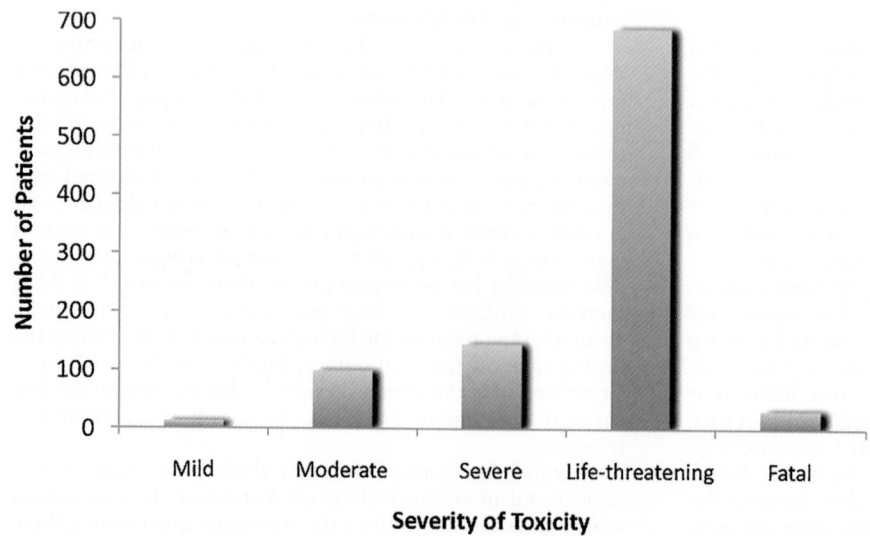

FIGURE 10.2 The worst degree of any toxicity experienced by patients ($n = 1,062$) treated on 1 of the 8 treatment arms of the Intergroup Rhabdomyosarcoma Study III. Seventy-eight percent of patients had at least one severe or life-threatening toxicity, and there were 32 toxicity-related deaths (Adapted from Table 6 in Crist W, Gehan EA, Ragab A, et al. The Third Intergroup Rhabdomyosarcoma Study. J Clin Oncol 1995;13: 610–630.)

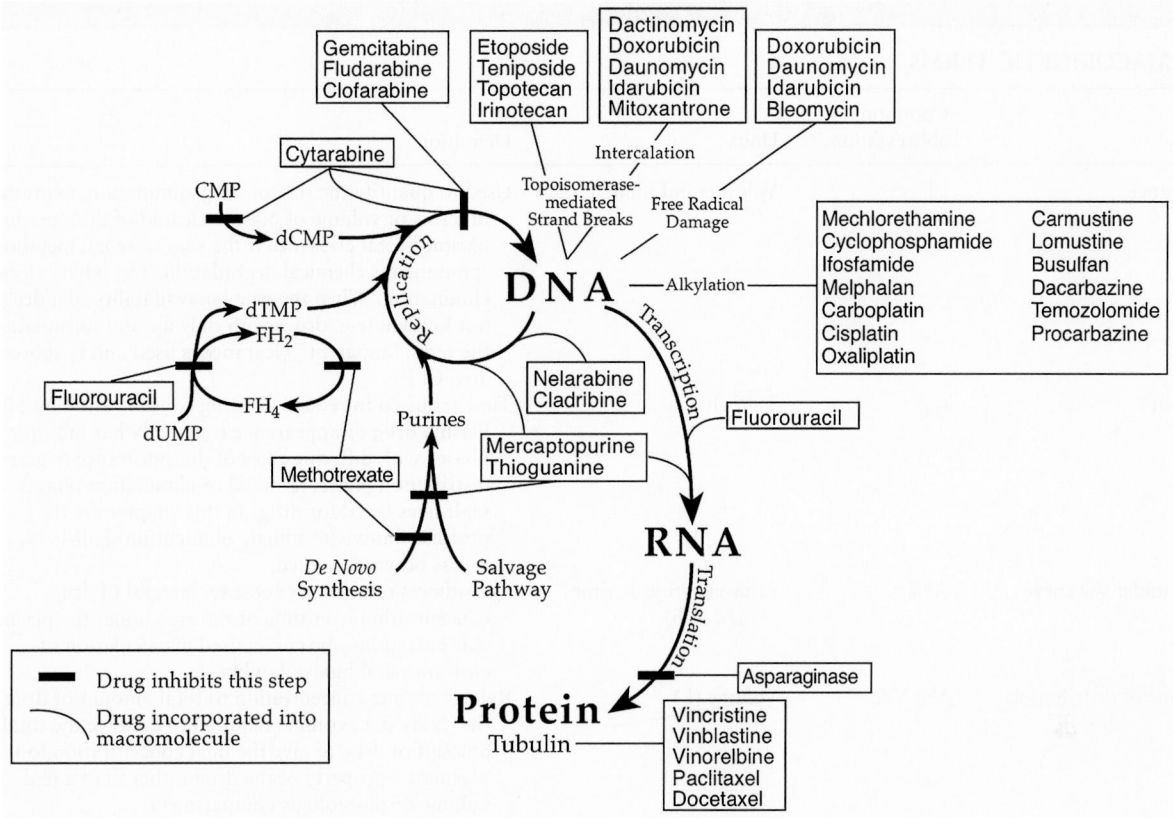

FIGURE 10.3 Site of action of the commonly used cytotoxic anticancer drugs.

cytotoxic drugs, allowing for repair of the DNA damage.[60,61] If this DNA damage is not repaired, the complex process of DNA replication and cell division is disrupted. Mutations in cell cycle regulatory genes that have been implicated in tumorigenesis most frequently involve genes controlling the transition from the G_1 to S phases of the cell cycle,[51] and loss of checkpoint function (e.g., p21) can enhance chemo- and radiosensitivity.[51,62] The same mechanisms that play a role in the pathogenesis of cancer could also sensitize the cancer cell to DNA-damaging anticancer drugs.

TP53 mutations and loss of p53 function, which occur in half of all human cancers, have been associated with enhanced or decreased sensitivity to anticancer drugs in preclinical studies.[63–65] The role of p53 as a dual-effect regulator that induces apoptosis in its activated state and regulates the cell cycle at the G_1/S and G_2/M checkpoints may be responsible for these seemingly contradictory results. Clinical studies correlating p53 mutational status to disease outcomes such as response and survival have also failed to consistently demonstrate a relationship.[65]

A number of new anticancer drugs block the activation of cellular signal transduction pathways by inhibiting protein kinase activity of critical cell membrane receptors and downstream effector proteins.[66,67] Activation of these pathways occurs through sequential phosphorylation of pathway proteins usually on a tyrosine, serine, or threonine moiety. Activating mutations in receptors and effector proteins, such as the BCR-ABL fusion protein created by the t(9;22) translocation in chronic myelogenous leukemia, play a critical role in the pathogenesis of many cancers. New drugs, such as imatinib, that inhibit the protein kinase activity of these constitutively activated signaling proteins block the transduction of the

aberrant signal and, thereby, control cellular proliferation. Examples of cellular receptors that are targeted by this new class of molecularly targeted anticancer drugs include epidermal growth factor receptor (EGFR), vascular endothelial growth factor receptor (VEGFR), insulin-like growth factor receptor (IGFR-1), human epidermal growth factor receptor (HER), KIT, and platelet-derived growth factor receptor (PDGFR).

An understanding of the mechanism of drug action is useful in predicting which tumors may respond to the drug based on their biochemical and cytokinetic profiles and which drug combinations may produce additive or synergistic antitumor effects. Combining agents that together could enhance the inhibition of vital intracellular processes through sequential or concurrent blockade or lead to complementary inhibition of specific metabolic pathways has been a traditional strategy for the design of combination regimens.[68] A drug's schedule of administration may also be influenced by its mechanism of action. For example, the antimetabolites, which are inhibitory only during S phase in the cell cycle, tend to be more cytotoxic if administered by prolonged infusion. This approach ensures that a greater number of tumor cells are exposed to the drug as they pass through S phase.

Pharmacokinetics

The discipline of pharmacokinetics deals with quantitative aspects of drug disposition in the body, including drug absorption, distribution, metabolism, and excretion, referred to as ADME (Table 10.2). Although the pharmacokinetic behavior of most of the commonly used anticancer drugs has been studied in adults, many of these agents have not been extensively

TABLE 10.2

PHARMACOKINETIC TERMS

Term	Common abbreviation	Units	Definition
Clearance	Cl	Vol/time (mL/min)	Used to quantify the rate of drug elimination; expressed in terms of volume of plasma cleared of drug per unit of time. Total clearance is the sum of renal, metabolic, spontaneous chemical degradation, and biliary (fecal) elimination. When the true bioavailability of a drug is not known, (e.g. drugs with only an oral formulation), the term "apparent" clearance is used and is abbreviated Cl/F.
Half-life	$t_{1/2}$	Time (h)	Time required to reduce the drug concentration by 50%. Plasma drug disappearance frequently has multiple phases with differing rates of disappearance (e.g., rapid distribution phase, terminal or elimination phase). Half-lives listed for drugs in this chapter are the postdistributive (terminal, elimination) half-lives, unless otherwise noted.
Area under the curve	AUC	Concentration × time ($\mu M \times h$)	Quantitates total drug exposure; integral of drug concentration over time or the area under the plasma concentration-time curve; used in calculation of clearance and bioavailability.
Volume of distribution	Vd; Vd$_{ss}$	Volume (L)	Relates plasma concentration to total amount of drug in the body (i.e., volume required to dissolve the total amount of drug to give the final concentration found in plasma); a property of the drug rather than a real volume or physiologic compartment.
Bioavailability	F	Fraction (%)	Rate and extent of absorption of a drug, frequently synonymous with the fraction of a dose absorbed when administered by some route other than intravenous.
Biotransformation			Enzymatic metabolism of a drug; may result in the activation of a prodrug, conversion to other biologically active intermediates, or inactivation of a drug.

evaluated in children. As the technology to measure the concentration of these drugs and their metabolites in biologic fluids has improved, a greater emphasis has been placed on studying anticancer drug pharmacokinetics in children with cancer.

Pharmacokinetic studies have revealed substantial interpatient variability in drug disposition and systemic drug exposure with most anticancer drugs.[69,70] Administering a standard dose of etoposide, doxorubicin, or cyclophosphamide to a group of children results in a 2- to 10-fold range in systemic drug exposure, as measured by the area under the plasma drug concentration-time curve (AUC),[71] and substantial variability in systemic drug exposure is also observed with orally administered agents such as methotrexate and mercaptopurine.[72] Assuming that drug effect is more closely related to systemic drug exposure than dose, these differences in drug disposition could account for the variability in toxicities and responses observed with most combination chemotherapy regimens employing standardized doses of individual agents.[73] Variability in anticancer drug disposition in children may result from age-related developmental changes in body composition and excretory organ function, variation in rate of metabolism and excretion of drug by the kidneys or liver, variation in the extent of drug-protein binding, drug interactions, and pharmacogenetics.[74-77]

The most important determinant of variability in anticancer drug pharmacokinetics is the rate of drug metabolism. Drug

metabolizing enzymes are divided into two groups based on the type of reaction that they catalyze. Phase I reactions (e.g., oxidation, hydrolysis, reduction, and demethylation) introduce or expose a functional group (e.g., hydroxyl group) on the drug. Phase I reactions usually diminish the drug's pharmacological activity, but some prodrugs, such as cyclophosphamide, are converted to active metabolites by these enzymes. Phase II conjugation reactions covalently link a highly polar conjugate (e.g., glucuronic acid, sulfate, glutathione, amino acids, or acetate) to the functional group created by the phase I reaction. The conjugated drugs are highly polar, usually devoid of pharmacological activity, and rapidly excreted.

The significant interpatient variation in systemic drug exposure with current dosing methods, the toxic nature of these agents, and the potential importance of dose intensity in cancer chemotherapy point to the need for more precise, individualized dosing methods for anticancer drugs,[70,74,78-80] such as the adaptive dosing techniques that have been successfully applied to individualize carboplatin dose[81] and therapeutic drug monitoring of methotrexate that plays a critical role in determining the duration of leucovorin rescue following high-dose methotrexate therapy.[70,80,82] A prerequisite for these individualized dosing methods is the establishment of the relation between a drug's pharmacokinetics and pharmacodynamics (toxicity or therapeutic effect). Systemic drug exposure (AUC) of anticancer drugs is usually the best correlate of the drug's toxic or therapeutic effects. However, this usually requires plasma sampling at multiple times over a prolonged period, which may not be practical for monitoring large numbers of patients. Through pharmacokinetic modeling, a limited number of sampling times that can reliably estimate the AUC can often be identified, providing a more practical pharmacokinetic monitoring schedule.[70,83–85] Parameters other than AUC, such as peak or trough concentration or average steady-state concentration, can also be evaluated for clinical correlations.

Even though therapeutic drug monitoring has yet to play a significant role in the day-to-day management of the patient with cancer, the pharmacokinetic parameters are important for determining the optimal dose, schedule, and route of administration of the drug. Knowledge of the route of elimination of a drug is also helpful in adjusting the dosage for patients with hepatic or renal dysfunction.[86,87]

Physiologic differences between children and adults can affect drug disposition and must be considered in determining the appropriate dose and schedule of the drug for children. Developmental differences in drug absorption, plasma protein or tissue binding, functional maturation of excretory organs, and distribution of drug in the various tissues of the body (Table 10.3) can result in differences in systemic drug exposure for children compared with adults treated with the same dose.[88,89] The most dramatic changes in excretory organ function and body composition occur during the first few days to months of life, but there are very limited data on the disposition of anticancer drugs in infants.[90]

Pharmacogenetics

In addition to the effects of age, disease, organ function, and drug interactions on the interpatient variability in response to drugs, genetic factors can influence both the efficacy of a drug and the likelihood of toxicity.[91] The field of pharmacogenetics began with the study of drug-metabolizing enzymes, but it now encompasses the study of the influence of genetic variation (polymorphisms) on the entire spectrum of drug action, including drug disposition (absorption, distribution, metabolism, and excretion), drug targets, and treatment modifying genes.[92]

Pharmacogenetically based variability in response to drugs is more apparent for drugs that have a narrow therapeutic index, such as anticancer drugs. The study of mercaptopurine methylation in large measure ushered in the modern era of pharmacogenetics.[93] There are more than 30 families of drug-metabolizing enzymes in humans, and nearly all have genetic variation that, in certain cases, translates into functional changes in the encoded enzyme.[92,94] Phase

TABLE 10.3

PHYSIOLOGIC DIFFERENCES IN CHILDREN THAT MAY INFLUENCE DRUG DISPOSITION

Organ or compartment	Value at birth[a]	Age adult values are reached[b]	Effect on drug disposition[c]
Kidney			
Size	↑		
Renal blood flow	↓	1 yr	↓ Renal excretion
Glomerular filtration	↓	6 mo–1 yr	↓ Renal excretion
Tubular function	↓	1 yr	↓ Tubular secretion
Liver			
Size	↑		
Phase I drug-metabolizing enzymes[d]	↓	Variable (oxidative enzymes increase rapidly after birth)	↓ Metabolic clearance
		↑ Activity in young children	↑ Metabolic clearance
Phase II drug-metabolizing enzymes[e]	↑ Sulfation ↓ other enzymes	Variable (6 mo for glucuronidation)	↓ Metabolic clearance
Biliary excretion	↓	6 mo	↓ Biliary excretion
Gastrointestinal			
Acid secretion	↓	3 mo	Altered drug absorption and stability
Motility	↓	6–8 mo	Delayed absorption
		↑ Transit time in young children	More rapid absorption
Body composition			
Blood volume	↑	Adolescence	
Extracellular fluid	↑	48 mo	↑ Distribution volume
Total body water	↑	4 mo	↑ Distribution volume
Fat	↓	Adolescence	↓ Distribution volume of lipophilic drugs
		↑ From 4 –12 mo of age	↑ Distribution volume of lipophilic drugs
Cerebrospinal fluid volume	↑	3 yr	↑ Distribution volume of intrathecal drugs
Protein binding	↓	1 yr	↑ Free drug levels

[a]↓, decreased; ↑, increased (compared with adult values and relative to body surface area or weight).
[b]Relative to body surface area or weight.
[c]Refer to Table 10.5 to determine which drugs may be affected by alteration of renal, biliary, or metabolic function.
[d]Oxidation, hydrolysis, reduction, and demethylation.
[e]Conjugation, acetylation, and methylation.

I enzymes include the cytochrome P450 (CYP) superfamily of enzymes that catalyze oxidation and demethylation reactions. The CYPs are responsible for 70% to 80% of all phase I drug metabolism (Fig. 10.4) and are categorized into families and subfamilies according to their amino acid sequence similarity. Sequences that are more than 40% identical belong to the same family designated by an initial number (e.g., CYP1); sequences that are more than 55% identical are in the same subfamily designated by a letter suffix (e.g., CYP1A).[95] Subfamilies may contain multiple isoforms (e.g., CYP1A2). Humans have at least 17 families and 39 subfamilies of CYP genes. The CYP1, CYP2, and CYP3 families are primarily responsible for hepatic drug and xenobiotic metabolism in humans, with CYP3A being the most important subfamily, accounting for the metabolism of more than one-third of all drugs (Fig. 10.4).[95,96] A number of CYP genes are known to have functionally relevant polymorphisms.[97,98]

Phase II enzymes also have functionally relevant polymorphisms (Fig. 10.4). Thiopurine methyl transferase (TPMT), which is the enzyme that methylates the thiol group on mercaptopurine and thioguanine, is the classic example for anticancer drugs. Since the original description of enhanced drug toxicity associated with this genetic variation in TPMT, the identification of the gene encoding the enzyme and the DNA sequence variations associated with this inherited trait have been identified[99–104] and studied in diverse populations.[105–107,108] A more recent example is irinotecan, the toxicity of which is a function of the pharmacogenetic variation observed in the phase II enzyme UDP-glucuronosyltransferase.[109–111]

Lastly, genetic differences may also have indirect effects on drug response, as has been observed with methylation of the methylguanine methyltransferase (MGMT) gene promoter. The expression of the DNA repair protein, MGMT, modulates the response of gliomas to carmustine.[112]

Toxicity

In therapeutic doses, actively dividing normal host cells, such as those in the bone marrow or the mucosal epithelium, are sensitive to the cytotoxic effects of anticancer drugs.[113] The nonselective mechanisms of action and resulting low therapeutic indices of these agents mean that a high incidence of potentially severe toxicities must be tolerated to administer effective doses.[114,115] Acute toxicities common to many of the anticancer drugs include myelosuppression, nausea and vomiting, alopecia, orointestinal mucositis, liver function abnormalities, allergic or cutaneous reactions, and local ulceration from subcutaneous drug extravasation. These acute toxicities occur over hours to weeks after a dose and are usually reversible. Many drugs also have unique toxicities affecting specific organs or tissues, such as cardiotoxicity associated with the anthracyclines; hemorrhagic cystitis associated with cyclophosphamide and ifosfamide; peripheral neuropathy from vincristine, cisplatin, and paclitaxel; nephrotoxicity from cisplatin and ifosfamide; and ototoxicity from cisplatin and coagulopathy from L-asparaginase. Many of these latter toxicities are cumulative (i.e., occur after multiple doses), and in some cases they are not completely reversible (e.g., anthracycline cardiotoxicity).

Phase 1

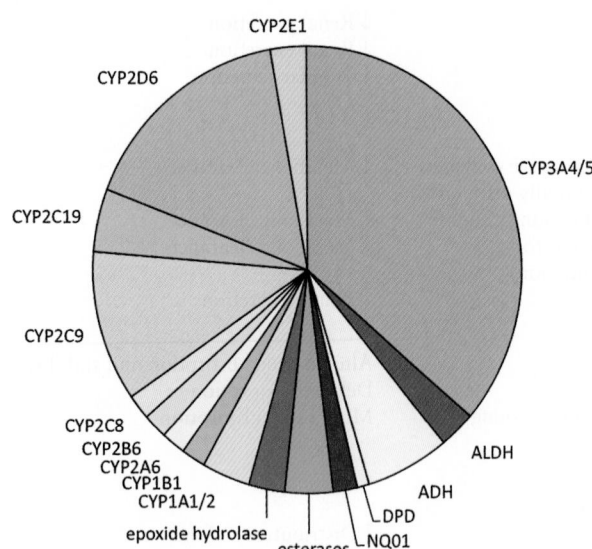

Phase 2

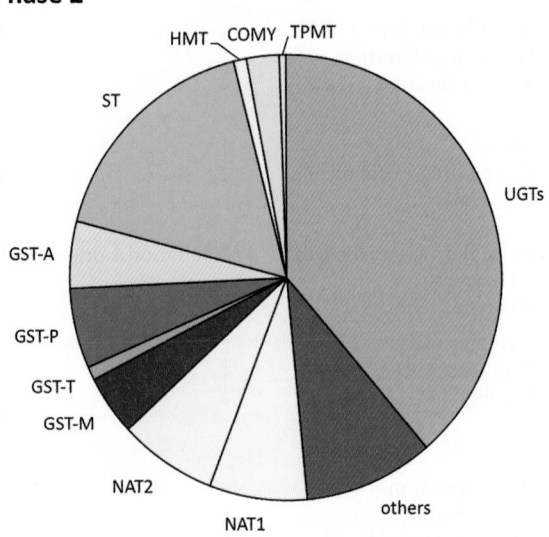

FIGURE 10.4 Phase I and II enzymes involved in drug metabolism. Almost all of the major human enzymes responsible for modification of functional groups or conjugation with endogenous substituents exhibit common polymorphisms at the genomic level. The percentage of phase I and phase II metabolism of drugs that each enzyme contributes is estimated by the relative size of each section of the corresponding chart. ADH, alcohol dehydrogenase; ALDH, aldehyde dehydrogenase; CYP, cytochrome P450; DPD, dihydropyrimidine dehydrogenase; NQO1, NADPH:quinone oxidoreductase or DT diaphorase; COMT, catechol O-methyltransferase; GST, glutathione S-transferase; HMT, histamine methyltransferase; NAT, N-acetyltransferase; STs, sulfotransferases; TPMT, thiopurine methyltransferase; UGTs, uridine 59-triphosphate glucuronosyltransferases. (Adapted from Evans WE, Relling MV. Pharmacogenomics: translating functional genomics into rational therapeutics. Science 1999;286(5439):487–491, with permission. Copyright 1999 AAAS.)

A significant portion of an oncologist's time is spent in providing supportive care for patients experiencing acute and long-term drug toxicities.[116] A number of therapeutic approaches have evolved to attenuate these toxicities, to make the therapy more tolerable, and to safely increase the dose intensity of regimens by circumventing dose-limiting toxicities.[113,117–119] Bone marrow or peripheral stem cell transplantation to rescue patients from myeloablative doses of anticancer drugs is an example of this rescue approach. Other widely used forms of rescue include the administration of leucovorin or glucarpidase[120] to counteract the toxicities of high-dose methotrexate, the use of antiemetics to block nausea and vomiting,[121,122] the use of mesna to prevent the hemorrhagic cystitis caused by the oxazaphosphorines,[123] the use of colony-stimulating factors (e.g., filgrastim) to alleviate myelosuppression,[124–126] and the use of dexrazoxane to prevent anthracycline cardiotoxicity.[127–129]

The toxicity of anticancer drugs has a major impact on the dosing of these agents. The endpoint of the phase I dose-finding studies for most anticancer drugs is the identification of the MTD, which is considered the optimal dose. The dosing interval (every 21 to 28 days) for anticancer drugs is determined by the duration of acute toxicities, and dose modifications are usually based on the severity or duration of toxicities on the prior treatment cycle. The lifetime cumulative dose of the anthracyclines and bleomycin is limited to prevent cardiotoxicity and pulmonary toxicity. This toxicity-based dosing approach for anticancer drugs reflects the lack of data on the relationship between dose and anticancer effect.

The severity, incidence, and time course of toxicities are important factors in designing optimal drug combinations or adjusting doses to avoid overlapping toxicities. For example, nonmyelosuppressive agents such as vincristine, prednisone, L-asparaginase, and high-dose methotrexate with leucovorin rescue often can be administered with traditional myelosuppressive drugs without compromising the dose of other agents. Some regimens administer nonmyelosuppressive agents during the period of marrow suppression from myelotoxic drugs to ensure continuous exposure of the tumor to cytotoxic therapy.[130,131]

The long-term side effects of cancer chemotherapy are also of particular concern to the pediatric oncologist because of the high cure rates and the long life spans of successfully treated patients. The adverse late effects of chemotherapy on growth, development, and reproductive function; possible permanent cardiac, pulmonary, or renal damage; and possible carcinogenic and teratogenic effects are discussed in Chapter 47.

Drug Interactions

In addition to being administered in combination regimens, the anticancer drugs are also administered with antiemetics, antibiotics, analgesics, stool softeners, and other agents used to alleviate the side effects of chemotherapy or the underlying cancer. This degree of polypharmacy introduces a significant risk of drug interactions.[75,132–134] Clinicians must be aware of potential drug interactions, which can alter the disposition of anticancer drugs or alter their effects at the target site in tumor or normal tissues, to avoid unexpected or severe toxicities or antagonism that can diminish a drug's antitumor effect.[75,132] Unfortunately, little information is available about drug interactions involving the anticancer drugs with one another or with other classes of drugs. To some extent, the already high incidence of toxicities and treatment failures and the continued reliance on empirical dosing methods that do not include routine therapeutic drug monitoring obscure the recognition of possible interactions.

Many commonly used anticancer drugs, such as the vinca alkaloids, oxazaphosphorines, epipodophyllotoxins, and taxanes, are metabolized by the CYP3A subfamily of drug-metabolizing enzymes.[135–137] Drugs (e.g., fluconazole) and some foods (e.g., grapefruit juice) can inhibit or induce the activity of CYP3A and other drug-metabolizing enzymes and thereby alter the metabolism and clearance of anticancer drugs. In the case of cyclophosphamide, which is a prodrug that is activated through hydroxylation by CYP3A4, inhibition of this enzyme may reduce the formation of the active metabolite of cyclophosphamide.

Drug Resistance

Although toxic effects of anticancer drugs are usually predictable, the response of any given tumor to individual agents is not. Clinical resistance to anticancer drugs is the primary reason for treatment failure in childhood cancers. Drug resistance can be present at the outset of treatment or can become clinically apparent under the selective pressure of drug exposure.[138] The magnitude of the problem of drug resistance was appreciated early in cancer chemotherapy for childhood cancers. Less than one-half of children with ALL who were treated with single-agent therapy achieved a complete remission, and almost all of the patients who did respond eventually relapsed despite continuation of the drug that produced the remission.[8,139]

The development of most forms of drug resistance has a genetic basis.[10,140] The inherent genetic instability of tumor cells results in the spontaneous generation of drug-resistant clones as a consequence of a mutation, deletion, gene amplification, translocation, or chromosomal rearrangement.[10,140] These genetic alterations are presumed to be random events, which may account for the variability in response observed in most clinical trials. This genetic basis for drug resistance means that resistance can be inherited by subsequent generations of tumor cells, and under the selective pressure of drug exposure, drug-resistant cancer cells become the predominant subpopulation. At a biochemical level, there are a variety of mechanisms by which tumors become drug resistant. In most cases, these alterations in cellular metabolism can be related to an increase, a decrease, or an alteration in some gene product, such as the gene amplification identified in methotrexate-resistant cells that results in overproduction of dihydrofolate reductase (DHFR), the target enzyme of methotrexate.[141]

Genetically based molecular or biochemical alterations in cancer cells can produce anticancer drug resistance that is specific to a single agent or class of agents or provides protection from a broad range of anticancer drugs. In the latter form of resistance, termed multidrug resistance, a single cellular alteration conveys resistance simultaneously to multiple unrelated drugs, including drugs to which the cancer has not been exposed.[142–144] The best-studied multidrug-resistant phenotypes are associated with decreased intracellular drug accumulation and an increase in plasma membrane, adenosine triphosphate (ATP)-dependent drug efflux pumps.[143,145–150]

ATP-dependent drug efflux pumps are part of a family of transporters, the ATP-binding cassette (ABC) transporters.[151] To date, 48 human ABC genes have been identified and classified into seven subfamilies (ABCA to ABCG).[152] The functional protein is usually composed of two nucleotide-binding folds and two transmembrane domains. Most of our knowledge of ABC transporters and their role in drug resistance stems from P-glycoprotein (P-gp), the product of the ABCB1 (MDR1) gene. P-gp is expressed in human tumor specimens, including ALL, neuroblastoma, rhabdomyosarcoma, neuroepithelioma, Ewing's sarcoma, retinoblastoma, and osteosarcoma[153-158] and in a variety of normal human tissues, such as the biliary canaliculi in the liver, the proximal tubules in the kidney, the mucosal lining of the jejunum and colon, the adrenal gland, hematopoietic progenitor cells, and the endothelial cells of blood vessels within the central nervous system (CNS) and testis.[159] P-gp appears to be responsible for excretion of toxic compounds from these normal cells.[153,159,160] Although the presence of P-gp in tumor specimens has been associated with a worse prognosis and a poor response to therapy in some studies, the clinical significance of P-gp expression in childhood cancers remains controversial, in part because of the lack of a universal standard for quantifying expression at an RNA or protein level.[142,143,155,161]

The lack of expression of P-gp in some multidrug resistant cells led to the discovery of ABCC1 (MRP1), initially cloned from a human lung carcinoma cell line.[162] The structural similarity between MRP1 and P-gp underlies the significant overlap in substrate specificity. A notable exception to this are the taxanes, which are poor substrates for MRP1. The second member of the MRP (ABCC) family, MRP2, transports a number of MRP1 substrates as well as cisplatin.[163] MRP4 and MRP5 transport nucleoside analogs.[151,164]

Other mechanisms for multidrug resistance include an enhanced capacity to repair DNA damage produced by alkylating agents[144,165,166]; the detoxification of chemically reactive forms of alkylating agents and anthracyclines by glutathione[167]; decreased levels of topoisomerase II; the target enzyme of the anthracyclines, epipodophyllotoxins, and dactinomycin[168]; and suppression of apoptotic pathways.[52,55] The loss of DNA mismatch repair activity results in multidrug resistance by impairing the cancer cell's ability to detect DNA damage and activate apoptosis.[169]

The mechanism of drug resistance is an important consideration in selecting agents to be included in combination regimens or as second-line therapy in relapsed patients. Ideally, drug combinations should be composed of non–cross-resistant agents, and relapse treatment regimens should avoid the use of drugs that are cross-resistant with drugs used in the frontline regimen. With advances in our understanding of the mechanisms of drug resistance, specific treatment approaches may be devised to prevent the development of or overcome drug resistance in tumor cells.

In the remainder of this chapter, the pharmacological characteristics of the anticancer drugs used to treat pediatric cancers are reviewed. Tables summarize the general pharmacological properties (Table 10.4) and pharmacokinetic parameters (Table 10.5) of the commonly used anticancer drugs.

ALKYLATING AGENTS

The alkylating agents have a broad range of clinical activity in childhood cancers. These drugs are chemically reactive compounds that exert their cytotoxic effect through the covalent bonding of an alkyl group to important cellular macromolecules (Fig. 10.5).[48] Although a number of nucleophilic macromolecules and their precursors are potential targets for alkylation intracellularly, damage to the DNA template and the resulting induction of apoptosis appears to be the major determinant of cytotoxicity.[48,53,170] With the bifunctional alkylating agents that have two alkylating groups, this damage appears to result primarily from interstrand and intrastrand DNA-DNA and DNA-protein cross-links.[170,171]

Alkylating agents have steep dose-response curves in experimental model systems.[172] A log-linear relationship

exists between tumor cell killing and the concentration of the alkylating agent, and this correlation is maintained through 4 to 5 orders of magnitude of cell killing. This steep dose-response relationship for alkylating agents provides a strong rationale for their use in high-dose therapy regimens. Because of the significant myelosuppressive effects of these drugs, high-dose alkylator therapy is generally administered in conjunction with bone marrow or peripheral stem cell transplantation to prevent permanent bone marrow aplasia. The use of melphalan and busulfan in childhood cancers is limited almost exclusively to high-dose transplantation preparative regimens, and other alkylating agents, such as cyclophosphamide and thiotepa, are also frequently incorporated into these regimens.[173-175]

Myelosuppression is the major dose-limiting toxicity for most of the commonly used alkylating agents. Other common acute toxic effects include nausea and vomiting, alopecia, allergic and cutaneous reactions, and gastrointestinal and neurologic toxicity at high doses. Of particular concern to the pediatric oncologist are the potential long-term effects of alkylator therapy. Alkylating agents can produce gonadal atrophy, permanently affecting reproductive function. The nitrogen mustards and the nitrosoureas have been linked to pulmonary fibrosis, and nephrotoxicity of the nitrosoureas, cisplatin, and ifosfamide can permanently impair renal function.[176,177] These agents are also highly carcinogenic, mutagenic, and teratogenic.[178,179]

The pharmacokinetics of the alkylating agents has been difficult to study because the chemical reactivity and inherent chemical instability of the active alkylating species make their measurement in biologic fluids difficult. Spontaneous hydrolysis of alkylating agents or their active metabolites in solution can be a major route of drug elimination. Most alkylating agents also undergo some degree of enzymatic metabolism, which can produce active and inactive metabolites.[180]

Several mechanisms for the development of resistance to alkylating agents have been described, including a decrease in drug uptake or transport by the cell, an increase in intracellular thiol compounds (glutathione) that are capable of detoxifying active alkylating species, enhancement of intracellular enzymatic catabolism to inactive metabolites, and an increase in the capability for repair of DNA damage produced by alkylation.[165,181-183] Loss of DNA mismatch repair capacity induces resistance to the methylating agents procarbazine and temozolomide, busulfan, and the platinum analogs.[169] In vitro studies indicate that resistance to alkylating agents is difficult to induce despite protracted exposure of cells to the drugs and that, after resistance has been induced, it often is not stable without drug in the medium to create continuous selection pressure. Cross-resistance to these drugs is not common in preclinical models.[184-186]

Of the various classes of alkylating agents, the nitrogen mustards and the nitrosoureas are most frequently used in the treatment of the childhood cancers. The chemical structures of these agents and several nonclassical alkylators are shown in Figures 10.6, 10.8, 10.10, and 10.12.

Nitrogen Mustards

The nitrogen mustards were the first class of alkylating agent used to treat cancer and remain the most widely used for childhood cancers. Mechlorethamine (nitrogen mustard), introduced into clinical trials in 1942, was the first drug demonstrated to be effective in the treatment of human cancers. A large number of synthetic nitrogen mustard analogs have since been screened for antitumor activity, and several

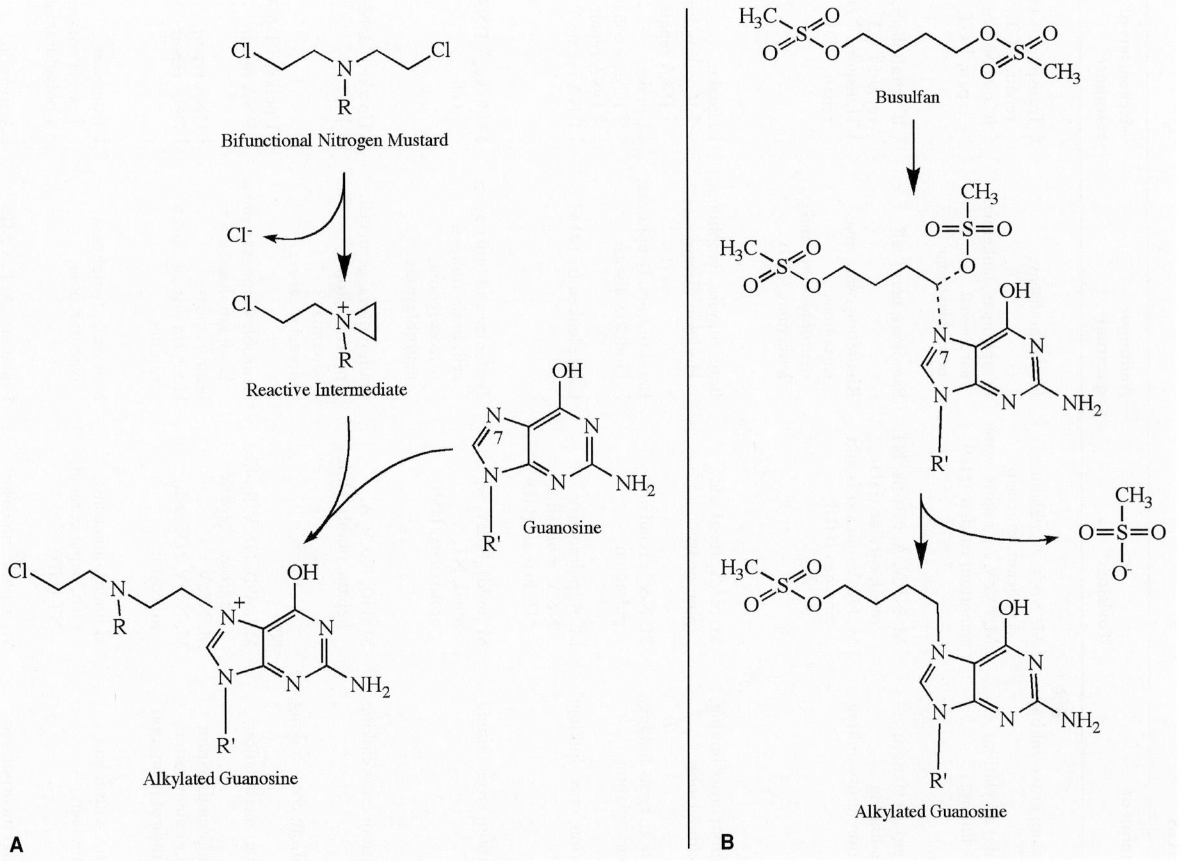

FIGURE 10.5 Mechanisms of alkylation of the nucleophilic N^7 position of guanosine. **A:** The bifunctional nitrogen mustard illustrates the S_N1 type of alkylation reaction, in which a reactive intermediate forms spontaneously and then rapidly reacts with the nucleophilic group. The rate-limiting step for S_N1 alkylation is the formation of the reactive intermediate, and thus the reaction exhibits first-order kinetics (i.e., independent of the target nucleophile concentration). If the second chloroethyl group also reacts with another nucleotide base, a cross-link is formed. **B:** Busulfan exemplifies an S_N2 reaction, characterized by a bimolecular nucleophilic displacement. In this case, the methylsulfonate group on either end of busulfan is displaced by the nucleophilic group on guanosine. The rate of S_N2 alkylation reactions depends on the concentration of the alkylating agent and the target nucleophile, and it therefore follows second-order kinetics.

with greater chemical stability and other pharmacological advantages have largely supplanted mechlorethamine in clinical practice. Cyclophosphamide, its isomer ifosfamide, and melphalan (phenylalanine mustard) are the most widely used in pediatric oncology (Fig. 10.6).

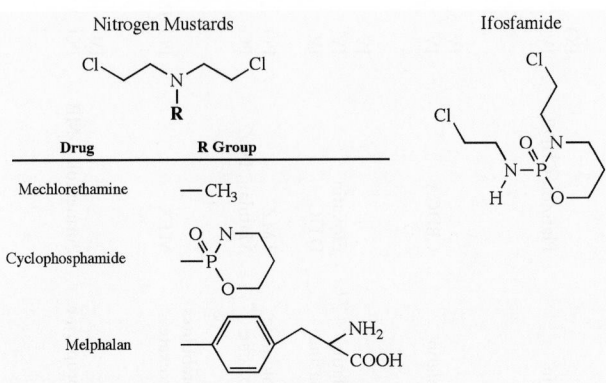

FIGURE 10.6 Chemical structures of the nitrogen mustard alkylating agents and the cyclophosphamide isomer, ifosfamide.

Mechlorethamine

Although the role of mechlorethamine in the treatment of cancer has declined, it is still a model for the chemical reactions of bifunctional alkylators (Fig. 10.5). The spontaneously formed alkylating intermediate is highly chemically reactive, and it rapidly undergoes hydrolysis, leading to inactivation, or it alkylates a wide variety of molecules, with a propensity to react with the N^7 position on guanosine.[170,180,187] Because of this inherent instability, even in aqueous solutions, mechlorethamine must be administered intravenously immediately after preparation to avoid significant loss of activity. Those administering the drug must take precautions, because direct contact with this reactive compound can irritate skin or mucous membranes.

Mechlorethamine has been used primarily in combination with vincristine, prednisone, and procarbazine (MOPP) for the treatment of Hodgkin disease, but the MOPP regimen has been supplanted as standard therapy for this disease.[188] The pharmacokinetics of mechlorethamine in humans has not been well delineated. In animals, the drug disappears from plasma in seconds.[180,189] In addition to its rapid spontaneous hydrolysis, mechlorethamine is rapidly metabolized (N-demethylated) in the liver.[190] As a result of this rapid degradation, renal excretion is not likely to play a role in drug clearance.

TABLE 10.4

PHARMACOLOGIC PROPERTIES OF THE COMMONLY USED ANTICANCER DRUGS

Drug	Synonyms	Route[a]	Dose/m^2	Schedule[b]	Mechanism of action	Toxicities[c]	Antitumor spectrum	Mechanisms of resistance[d]
Alkylating agents								
Mechlorethamine	Mustargen, HN$_2$, nitrogen mustard	IV	6 mg	Weekly × 2, q 28 d	Alkylation; cross-linking	M, N&V, A, phlebitis, vesicant, mucositis	Hodgkin disease	↓ Transport, ↑ DNA repair, ↑ GT
Cyclophosphamide	Cytoxan, CTX	IV PO	250–1,800 mg 100–300 mg	Daily × 1–4 d, q 21–28 d Daily	(Prodrug) alkylation; cross-linking	M, N&V, A, cystitis, water retention; cardiac (HD)	Lymphomas, leukemias, sarcomas, neuroblastoma	↑ IC catabolism, ↑ DNA repair, ↑ GT
Ifosfamide	IFOS, IFEX	IV	1,600–2,400 mg	Daily × 5, q 21–28 d	(Prodrug) alkylation; cross-linking	M, N&V, A, cystitis, NT, renal; cardiac (HD)	Sarcomas, germ cell	↑ IC catabolism, ↑ DNA repair, ↑ GT
Melphalan	Alkeran, L-PAM	IV PO IV	10–35 mg 4–20 mg 140–220 mg	q 21–28 d Daily for 1–21 d Single dose (BMT)	Alkylation; cross-linking	M, N&V; mucositis and diarrhea (HD)	Rhabdomyosarcoma; sarcomas, neuroblastoma and leukemias (HD)	↓ Transport, ↑ DNA repair, ↑ GT
Lomustine	CeeNU, CCNU	PO	100–150 mg	Single dose, q 4–6 wk	Alkylation; cross-linking; carbamoylation	M, N&V, renal and pulmonary	Brain tumors, lymphoma, Hodgkin disease	↓ Uptake, ↑ IC catabolism, ↑ DNA repair
Carmustine	BiCNU, BCNU	IV	200–250 mg	Single dose, q 4–6 wk	Alkylation; cross-linking; carbamoylation	M, N&V, renal and pulmonary	Brain tumors, lymphoma, Hodgkin disease	↓ Uptake, ↑ IC catabolism, ↑ DNA repair
Busulfan	Myleran	PO PO	1.8 mg 37.5 mg	Daily q 6 h for 4 d (BMT)	Alkylation; cross-linking	M, A, pulmonary; N&V, mucositis, NT, hepatic (HD)	CML; leukemias (BMT)	↑ DNA repair, ↑ GT
Cisplatin	Platinol, CDDP	IV IV	50–200 mg 20–40 mg	Over 4–6 h, q 21–28 d Daily × 5, q 21–28 d	Platination; cross-linking	M (mild), N&V, A, renal, NT, ototoxicity, HSR	Testicular and other germ cell, brain tumors, osteosarcoma, neuroblastoma	↓ Uptake, ↑ DNA repair, ↑ GT
Carboplatin	CBDCA	IV IV	400–600 mg 100–175 mg	Single dose or daily × 2, q 28 d Weekly × 4, q 6 wk	Platination; cross-linking	M (Plt), N&V, A, hepatic (mild), HSR	Brain tumors, germ cell, neuroblastoma, sarcomas	↓ Uptake, ↑ DNA repair, ↑ GT
Oxaliplatin	Eloxatin	IV	85–130 mg	Single dose q 21 d	Platination; cross-linking	NT	Colorectal cancer	↓ Uptake, ↑ DNA repair
Dacarbazine	DTIC	IV	250 mg	Daily × 5, q 21–28 d	(Prodrug) methylation	M (mild), N&V, flu-like syndrome, hepatic	Neuroblastoma, sarcomas, Hodgkin disease	↑ DNA repair
Temozolomide	TMZ	PO	200 mg	Daily × 5, q 28 d	(Prodrug) methylation	M, N&V	Brain tumors	↑ DNA repair
Procarbazine	Matulan, PCZ	PO	100 mg	Daily for 10–14 d	(Prodrug) methylation; free radical formation	M, N&V, NT, rash, mucositis	Hodgkin disease, brain tumors	↑ DNA repair
Antimetabolites								
Methotrexate	MTX	PO, IM, SC IV	7.5–30 mg 10–33,000 mg	Weekly or biweekly Bolus or CI (6–42 h)	Interferes with folate metabolism	M (mild), mucositis, rash, hepatic; renal, NT (HD)	Leukemia, lymphoma, osteosarcoma	↓ Transport, ↑ target enzyme, ↓ polyglutamation
Mercaptopurine	Purinethol, 6-MP	PO	75–100 mg	Daily	(Prodrug) incorporated into DNA & RNA; blocks purine synthesis, interconversion	M, hepatic, mucositis	Leukemia (ALL, CML)	↑ Activation, ↑ IC catabolism

(continued)

Drug	Other names	Route	Dose	Schedule	Mechanism	Toxicity	Indication	Resistance
Thioguanine	6-TG	PO	75–100 mg	Daily × 5–7	(Prodrug) incorporated into DNA & RNA; blocks purine synthesis, interconversion,	M, N&V, mucositis, hepatic (VOD)	Leukemia (ALL, AML)	↓ Activation, ↑ IC catabolism
Fludarabine phosphate	F-ara-AMP	PO / IV	40–60 mg / 25 mg	Daily / Daily × 5	(Prodrug) incorporated into DNA; inhibits DNA polymerase, ribonucleotide reductase	M, opportunistic infectious, neurotoxicity (high dose)	Leukemia (AML, CLL), indolent lymphomas	↓ Membrane transport, ↓ IC activation, ↑ IC catabolism
Clofarabine	Clolar	IV	52 mg	Daily × 5	(Prodrug) incorporated into DNA; inhibits DNA polymerase, ribonucleotide reductase	M, hepatic, hypokalemia Systemic inflammatory response syndrome	Leukemia	
Cladribine	2-CdA	IV	8.9 mg	Daily × 5	(Prodrug) incorporated into DNA polymerase, ribonucleotide reductase	M, opportunistic infectious	Leukemia (AML, CLL), indolent lymphomas	↓ Membrane transport, ↓ IC activation, ↑ IC catabolism
Nelarabine	Arranon	IV	400–650 mg	Daily × 5	(Prodrug) incorporated into DNA;	Somnolence, peripheral neuropathy, Guillan-Barre	T-cell leukemia	
Cytarabine	Ara-C, Cytosine arabinoside, Cytosar	IV, SC / IV	100–200 mg / 3,000 mg	q 12 h or CI for 5–7 d / q 12 h for 4 to 8 doses	(Prodrug) incorporated into DNA; inhibits DNA polymerase	M, N&V, mucositis, GI, flu-like syndrome; NT, ocular, skin (HD)	Leukemia, lymphoma	↓ Activation, ↓ transport, ↑ dCTP, ↑ IC catabolism
Gemcitabine	Gemzar, dFdC	IV	1,000 mg	Weekly × 3	(Prodrug) incorporated into DNA; inhibits DNA polymerase, ribonucleotide reductase	M, N&V, hepatic, mucositis, flu-like syndrome, edema, rash	Hodgkin; possibly sarcomas	
Fluorouracil	5-FU	IV / IV	500 mg / 800–1,200 mg	Single or daily × 5 / CI (24–120 h)	(Prodrug) inhibits thymidine synthesis; incorporated into RNA, DNA	M (bolus), mucositis, N&V, diarrhea, skin, NT, ocular, cardiac	Carcinomas, hepatic tumors	↑IC catabolism, ↓ Activation, ↑ target enzyme, altered target enzyme
Antitumor antibiotics								
Doxorubicin	Adriamycin, ADR	IV	45–75 mg	Single, q 21 d	Intercalation; DNA strand breaks (Topo II); free radical formation	M, mucositis, N&V, A, diarrhea, vesicant, cardiac (acute, chronic)	Leukemia (ALL, ANL), lymphomas, most solid tumors	Multidrug resistance, ↓ Topo II
Daunomycin	Daunorubicin, DNR	IV / IV / IV	20–30 mg / 45–90 mg / 30–45 mg	Weekly / CI (24–96 h) / Daily × 3 or weekly	Intercalation; DNA strand breaks (Topo II); free radical formation	M, mucositis, N&V, diarrhea, A, vesicant, cardiac (acute, chronic)	Leukemia (ALL, ANL), lymphomas	Multidrug resistance, ↓ Topo II
Idarubicin	IDA	IV	10–15 mg	Daily or weekly × 3	Intercalation; DNA strand breaks (Topo II); free radical formation	M, mucositis, N&V, diarrhea, A, vesicant, cardiac (acute, chronic)	Leukemia (ALL, ANL), lymphomas	Multidrug resistance, ↓ Topo II
Mitoxantrone	Novantrone, MITO	PO / IV	30–40 mg / 8–12 mg	Daily × 3 / Daily × 3–5 d	Intercalation; DNA strand breaks (Topo II);	M, mucositis, N&V, A, bluish color to urine, veins, sclerae, nails	Leukemia (ALL, ANLL), lymphomas	Multidrug resistance, ↓ Topo II
Bleomycin	Blenoxane, BLEO	IV, IM, SC	10–20 units	Weekly	Free radical-mediated DNA strand breaks	Lung, skin, fever, mucositis, alopecia, hypersensitivity, Raynaud's, N&V	Lymphoma, testicular and other germ cell	↑IC catabolism, ↑DNA repair

291

TABLE 10.4

CONTINUED

Drug	Synonyms	Route[a]	Dose/m²	Schedule[b]	Mechanism of action	Toxicities[c]	Antitumor spectrum	Mechanisms of resistance[d]
Dactinomycin	Cosmegen, ACT-D, actinomycin-D	IV	0.45 mg (15 µg/kg)	Daily × 5, q 3–6 wk	Intercalation; DNA strand breaks (Topo II)	M, N&V, A, mucositis, vesicant, hepatic (VOD)	Wilms' sarcomas	Multidrug resistance, ↓ Topo II
		IV	1.35–1.8 mg (45–60 µg/kg)	Single dose q 3–6 wk				
Plant products								
Vincristine	Oncovin, VCR	IV	1.0–1.5 mg (max, 2.0 mg)	Weekly × 3–6	Mitotic inhibitor; blocks microtubule polymerization	NT, A, SIADH, hypotension, vesicant	Leukemia (ALL), lymphomas, most solid tumors	Multidrug resistance, altered tubulin subunit
Vinblastine	Velban, VLB	IV	3.5–6.0 mg	Weekly × 3–6	Mitotic inhibitor; blocks microtubule polymerization	M, A, mucositis, mild NT, vesicant	Histiocytosis, Hodgkin, testicular	Multidrug resistance, altered tubulin subunit
Vinorelbine	Navelbine	IV	30 mg	Weekly	Mitotic inhibitor; blocks microtubule polymerization	M, mild NT, A, vesicant	?	Multidrug resistance, altered tubulin subunit
Etoposide	VePesid, VP-16	IV	60–120 mg	Daily × 3–5, q 3–6 wk	DNA strand breaks (Topo II)	M, A, N&V, mucositis, mild NT, hypotension, HSR, secondary leukemia; diarrhea (PO)	Leukemias (ALL, ANL), lymphomas, neuroblastoma, sarcomas, brain tumors	Multidrug resistance, ↓ or altered Topo II, ↑ DNA repair
Paclitaxel	Taxol	PO, IV	50 mg, 135–250 mg	Daily × 21 d 4 wk, CI for 3 or 24 h, q 3 wk	Mitotic inhibitor; blocks microtubule depolymerization	M, HSR, A, NT, mucositis, cardiac, EtOH poisoning	?	Multidrug resistance, altered tubulin subunits, ↑ Raf kinase
Docetaxel	Taxotere	IV	100–125 mg	q 3 wk	Mitotic inhibitor; blocks microtubule depolymerization	M, HSR, A, NT, rash, edema, mucositis,	?	Multidrug resistance, altered tubulin subunits
Topotecan	Hycamtin	IV	1.4–4.5 mg	Daily × 5, q 3 wk	DNA strand breaks (Topo I)	M, diarrhea, mucositis, N & V, A, rash, hepatic	Neuroblastoma, rhabdomyosarcoma	↓ or altered Topo I, multidrug resistance
Irinotecan	CPT-11, Camptosar	IV	50 mg	Daily × 5, q 3 wk	(Prodrug) DNA strand breaks (Topo I)	M, diarrhea, N & V, A, hepatic, dehydration, ileus,	Rhabdomyosarcoma	↓ or altered Topo I, multidrug resistance
			125 mg	Weekly × 4, q 6 wk				
Kinase inhibitors								
Imatinib mesylate	Gleevec, STI-571	PO	340 mg	Daily	Inhibits BCR-ABL, VEGF, c-Kit kinases	N & V, Fatigue, M, headache, GI,	Ph + CML	Mutations in bcr-abl
Dasatinib	Sprycel	PO	85	Daily	Inhibits BCR-ABL, c-KIT, PDGF-β receptor, EPHA2, SRC family kinases	Fluid retention events, rash, nausea, bleeding, diarrhea	CML, Ph + ALL	Multidrug resistance
Sorafenib	Nexavar	PO	200	Twice daily	Inhibits VEGFR-2, PDGFR-β, FLT-3, c-KIT, RAF	Rash, hypertension, diarrhea, N&V, bleeding	Renal cell carcinoma, hepatocellular carcinoma	
Sunitinib	Sutent	PO	Adults: 50 mg (flat dosing)	Daily × 4 weeks followed by 2 weeks rest	Inhibits c-KIT, FLT-3, VEGFR2, PDGFR-β	Cardiac, hypertension, diarrhea, N&V, GI, mucositis, bleeding, rash	GIST, renal cell carcinoma	
Bevacizumab	Avastin	IV	5–15 mg/kg	Every 2 weeks	Inhibits VEGF signaling	Infusional reaction, rash, proteinuria, bleeding	Carcinomas, glioblastoma	

Drug	Other names	Route	Dose	Schedule	Mechanism	Toxicity	Uses	Resistance
Erlotinib	Tarceva	PO	85	Daily	Inhibits EGFR signaling	Rash, diarrhea	Carcinomas	
Gefitinib	Iressa	PO	400	Daily	Inhibits EGFR signaling	Rash, diarrhea	Carcinomas	
Cetuximab	Erbitux	IV	Adults: 400 mg/m^2 loading dose, 200 mg/m^2 thereafter	Weekly	Inhibits EGFR signaling	Rash, infusional reaction, diarrhea	Head and neck carcinomas, colorectal carcinoma	
Miscellaneous								
Prednisone	Deltasone, PRED	PO	40 mg	Daily	(Prodrug) receptor-mediated lympholysis	Protean (see text)	Leukemia, lymphomas	Loss or defect in glucocorticoid receptor
Prednisolone		PO, IV	40 mg	Daily	Receptor-mediated lympholysis	Protean	Leukemia, lymphomas	Loss or defect in glucocorticoid receptor
Dexamethasone	Decadron, DEX	PO, IV, IM	6 mg	Daily	Receptor-mediated lympholysis	Protean	Leukemia, lymphomas, brain tumors	Loss or defect in glucocorticoid receptor
Native asparaginase	Elspar, L-ASP	IV, IM	6,000–25,000 IU	3 times per wk	Asparagine depletion; ↓ protein synthesis	HSR, coagulopathy, pancreatitis, hepatic, NT	Leukemia (ALL), lymphoma	↑ IC asparagine synthase
PEG-asparaginase	Oncaspar, PEG-ASP	IV, IM	2,500 IU	Every 1–4 wk	Asparagine depletion; ↓ protein synthesis	HSR, coagulopathy, pancreatitis, hepatic, NT	Leukemia (ALL), lymphoma	↑ IC asparagine synthase
All-*trans*-retinoic acid	ATRA, Tretinoin, Vesanoid	PO	45 mg	Daily for induction; Daily × 7 d q 28 d for maintenance	Differentiation agent	Retinoic acid syndrome, pseudotumor cerebri, cheilitis, conjunctivitis, dry skin, ↑ triglycerides	Acute promyelocytic leukemia	Mutations in *PML-RARα*
13-*cis*-retinoic acid	13cRA, Isotretinoin, Accutane	PO	160 mg	Daily × 14 q 28 d	Differentiation agent	Cheilitis, conjunctivitis, dry mouth, xerosis, pruritus, headache, bone & joint pain, ↑ triglycerides, ↑ Ca++	Minimal residual disease neuroblastoma	
Arsenic	Trisenox, As$_2$O$_3$	IV	0.15 mg/kg	Daily up to 60 doses	Apoptosis; degradation of PML/RAR-alpha	Hepatic, N&V, abdominal pain, musuloskeletal pain, peripheral neuropathy, electrolyte abnormalities, QTc prolongation	Acute promyelocytic leukemia	

[a]IM, intramuscular; IV, intravenous; PO, oral; SC, subcutaneous.
[b]BMT, bone marrow transplant; CI, continuous infusion; d, day; h, hour; wk, week.
[c]A, alopecia; GI, gastrointestinal toxicity; HD, high dose; M, myelosuppression; NT, neurotoxicity; N&V, nausea and vomiting.
[d]↑, increased; ↓, decreased; dCTP, deoxycytidine triphosphate; GT, glutathione-S-transferase; IC, intracellular.

TABLE 10.5

PHARMACOKINETIC PARAMETERS OF THE COMMONLY USED ANTICANCER DRUGS

Drug	Clearance[a] (mL/min/m²)	Half-life[b]	Route of elimination[c]	Volume of distribution (L/m²)[d]	Protein binding (%)	Bioavailability (% absorbed)	CSF: plasma ratio (%)[e]
Alkylating agents							
Mechlorethamine		<1 min	D, m				
Cyclophosphamide							
Parent	35–95	2.5–6.5 h	M, r	15–20	20	90	50
4-OH-cyclophosphamide		4 h	M, R		50		10–20
Ifosfamide							
Parent	50–130	1–5 h	M, r	20		95	30
4-OH-ifosfamide		4 h	M, R				10–20
Melphalan	200–400	0.5–2 h	D, r	20–30	20–30	32–100	10
Lomustine	(Parent drug ND in plasma)		D, M		>90	50–>90	
Carmustine	1,500–2,000	20 min	D, M	90	65–75		>90
Busulfan	70–100	2.5 h	M, d	10–20	30	70	>95
Cisplatin							
Ultrafiltrate	250	40 min	D, r	12	0	<10	<10
Total platinum	3–6	2–5 d	R		>95		<10
Carboplatin							
Ultrafiltrate	70–120	2–3 h	R, d	10	0	10	20–30
Total platinum		2–5 d	R		20–50		
Dacarbazine	450	40 min	M, R	17	20	Variable	15
Temozolomide	90	1.8 h	D	14		100	30
Procarbazine		<10 min	M			Complete	
Antimetabolites							
Methotrexate	100	8–12 h	R, m	11	60	Variable	2–3
Mercaptopurine	800	< 1 h	M, r	22	20	<20 (variable)	25
Thioguanine	1,000–2,000	2 h	M			Low and variable	18
Fludarabine phosphate	70	6–30 h	R	44	20–30	75	
Clofarabine	480	5 h	R, m	170	47		
Cladribine	20–40	7–19 h	R	270–360	20	50	18
Nelarabine	4,300	30 min	M, r	197	<25		
Ara-G metabolite	175	3 h	M, r	50	<25		
Cytarabine	1,000	2–3 h	M	30	10	<20	20
Gemcitabine	2,200	14–62 min	M	16–27	< 10		
Fluorouracil							
Bolus dose	800	10 min	M	15	< 10	0–74 (variable)	48
Infusion	3,600		M				10–20
Antitumor antibiotics							
Doxorubicin	500–1,000	30 h	B, M	800	75	Not absorbed	ND in CSF
Daunomycin	1,000	15–20 h	B, M	1,000		Not absorbed	ND in CSF
Idarubicin	1,000	15–20 h	B, M	1,000		20–30%	ND in CSF[f]
Mitoxantrone	200–600	75 h	B, M	>1,000	78	Not absorbed	Poor
Bleomycin	40	3 h	R, m	10		Not absorbed	
Dactinomycin		36 h	R, B	Large			<10
Plant products							
Vincristine	450	18 h	M, B	350	75	Poor	5
Vinblastine	400	24 h	M, B	800	75	Poor	
Vinorelbine	800	15 h	M, B	550	80–90	25–40 (variable)	
Etoposide	20–25	2–6 h	M, R	5–10	95	50 (variable)	<5
Teniposide	10–15	7–20 h	M, r	7–10	99	40 (variable)	<5
Paclitaxel	150	20 h	M, B	50–100	88–98		ND in CSF
Docetaxel	350	12 h	M, B	100	80		
Topotecan (Lac + HA)[g]	150	3 h	R, m	30	20	30 (variable)	30

(continued)

TABLE 10.5

CONTINUED

Drug	Clearance[a] (mL/min/m²)	Half-life[b]	Route of elimination[c]	Volume of distribution (L/m²)[d]	Protein binding (%)	Bioavailability (% absorbed)	CSF: plasma ratio (%)[e]
Irinotecan (Lac + HA)	250–1,000	4–12 h	M, B, r	90–150	65		15
SN-38 (Lac + HA)		12 h	M, B		96		<10
Kinase inhibitors							
Imatinib	180	9–15 h	M, r	165	95	98	
Dasatanib	3,000	2–3 h	M, r	>1,000[h]	96		
Sorafenib	65[h]	35h[h]	M		99.5	40	
Sunitinib	375[h]	50h[h]	M, r	>1,000[h]	95		
Bevacizumab	0.1	280 h	RES	>1,000			
Erlotinib	50[h]	36 h[h]	M	134[h]	93	60 (100 w/food)	
Gefitinib	243[h]	12 h[h]	M, r	800[h]	90	60	
Cetuximab	0.3[h]	112 h[h]	RES	>1,000[h]			
Miscellaneous							
Prednisolone	250	2.5 h	M	50	70–>95	85	<10
Dexamethasone	200–250	4 h	M	50	70	85	15
Asparaginase							
Escherichia coli	1.4	24 h	M	3		Not absorbed	ND in CSF[i]
Erwinia	3.4	10 h	M	5		Not absorbed	ND in CSF[i]
PEG-asparaginase	0.15	5–7 days	M	2		Not absorbed	ND in CSF[i]
All-*trans*-retinoic acid	300–4,800 (day 1 only)	45 min	M		>99		<10
13-*cis*-retinoic acid	90	10–20 h	M	31	>99	50–75	
Arsenic		12–>24 h	M		75		

[a]For oral drugs, the apparent clearance is reported.
[b]Postdistributive or terminal half-life; min, minutes; h, hours.
[c]B, biliary excretion; D, spontaneous chemical decomposition; M, metabolism (biotransformation); R, renal excretion; RES, reticuloendothelial system; lower case letter (d, m, r, b) indicates that this is a minor route for elimination of the drug.
[d]Volume listed is the steady-state volume of distribution.
[e]ND, not detectable; CSF, cerebrospinal fluid.
[f]The active metabolite idarubicinol is detectable in CSF.
[g]Lac, lactone; HA, hydroxy acid. The combination represents total drug.
[h]Parameter estimate from adult studies.
[i]Asparaginase is ND in CSF, but CSF asparagine is depleted with systemic administration of asparaginase.

In addition to its major clinical toxicities of myelosuppression, nausea, and vomiting, mechlorethamine has an anticholinergic effect, leading to diaphoresis, lacrimation, and diarrhea. It is a potent vesicant, producing a sclerosing thrombophlebitis above the site of administration and severe local tissue damage if extravasated. If extravasation occurs, sodium thiosulfate should be injected into the area as rapidly as possible to neutralize the drug.[191] Neurotoxicity in the form of an acute or delayed encephalopathy has been reported with the use of high doses of mechlorethamine.[192]

Oxazaphosphorines

The oxazaphosphorines, cyclophosphamide and ifosfamide, are inactive prodrugs that require biotransformation by hepatic microsomal oxidative enzymes before expressing alkylating activity.[193,194] Cyclophosphamide is a true nitrogen mustard derivative with a bifunctional bischloroethylamine side chain. Ifosfamide is also bifunctional but has one chloroethyl group shifted to a ring nitrogen (Fig. 10.6). Cyclophosphamide is one of the most widely used anticancer drugs with a broad range of clinical activity that includes the acute

leukemias and a variety of solid tumors (Table 10.5). It is also used in preparative regimens before bone marrow or peripheral stem cell transplantation and as an immunosuppressant in nonmalignant disorders. Ifosfamide has activity as a single agent or in combination with etoposide in sarcomas (e.g., Ewing's sarcoma, rhabdomyosarcoma, osteosarcoma), lymphoma, germ cell tumors, Wilms' tumor, and neuroblastoma.[195–197]

Cyclophosphamide is usually administered as a single-dose bolus or in fractionated doses over 2 to 3 days. Ifosfamide is administered on a fractionated schedule over 5 days, because in the initial trials, the single-dose schedule produced intolerable nephrotoxicity, cystitis, and neurotoxicity. Ifosfamide has also been administered as a continuous 5-day infusion. The maximally tolerated total dose of ifosfamide is approximately three- to fourfold higher than an equitoxic dose of cyclophosphamide.[198]

Biotransformation. The metabolic pathways of cyclophosphamide and ifosfamide are shown in Figure 10.7. The steps in the biotransformation of these two drugs are qualitatively identical. Hydroxylation of the 4-carbon position on the ring

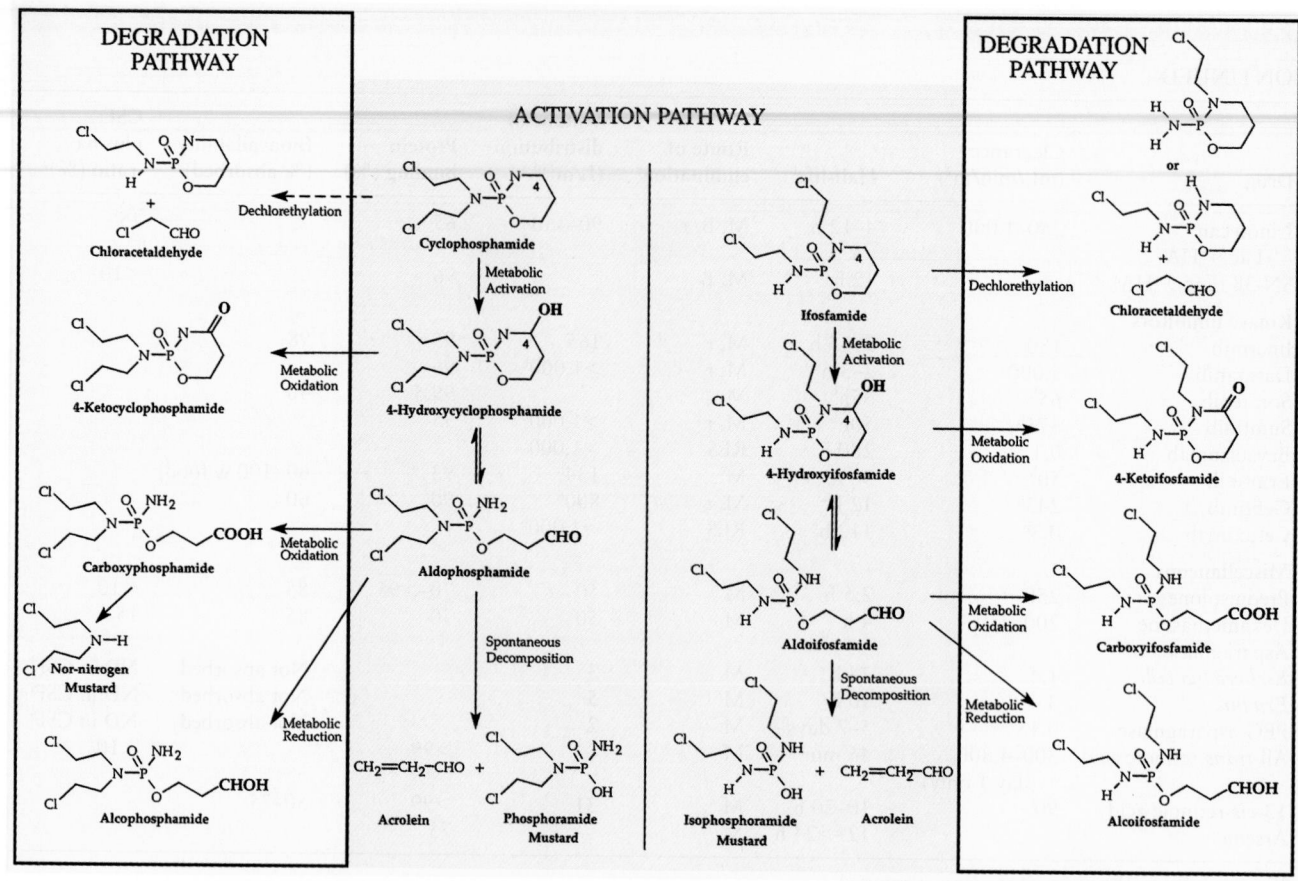

FIGURE 10.7 Metabolic pathways for the oxazaphosphorines, cyclophosphamide and ifosfamide. Both compounds must undergo hydroxylation at position 4 before expressing alkylating activity; this reaction is catalyzed by hepatic microsomal enzymes. The 4-hydroxy metabolites are in spontaneous equilibrium with the open-ring aldehydes (aldophosphamide or aldoifosfamide), which can release acrolein and form the active alkylating mustards (phosphoramide mustard or isophosphoramide mustard). Further oxidation at position 4 of the primary metabolites leads to the formation of inactive metabolites (ketocyclophosphamide and carboxyphosphamide or ketoifosfamide and carboxyifosfamide), which are excreted in the urine. The open-ring aldehyde metabolites can be chemically reduced to an alcohol (alcophosphamide or alcoifosfamide). Inactivation by dechloroethylation leads to formation of the potentially toxic by-product chloroacetaldehyde. This is a minor pathway for cyclophosphamide but more active with ifosfamide.

by hepatic microsomal mixed-function oxidases yields the primary 4-hydroxy metabolites, which are in spontaneous equilibrium with the open-ring aldehydes. Hydroxylation of cyclophosphamide is catalyzed primarily by CYP2B6 with minor contributions from CYP3A4 and CYP2C9, and ifosfamide hydroxylation is catalyzed primarily by CYP3A4 with a minor contribution from CYP2A6.[199] Although not chemically reactive, the 4-hydroxy metabolites are cytotoxic *in vitro* and are thought to be the transport forms of the active alkylating species, phosphoramide mustard and isophosphoramide mustard, which are formed by spontaneous elimination of acrolein from the open-ring aldehydes. Quantitatively, the rate of activation of cyclophosphamide is greater than that of ifosfamide, and this difference in the rate of activation accounts for the difference in clinical pharmacokinetics and MTD of the two isomers.[200–204]

Further oxidation of the hydroxyl group at the 4-carbon position on primary metabolites by aldehyde dehydrogenase leads to inactivation. 4-Ketocyclophosphamide and carboxyphosphamide are the principal urinary metabolites of cyclophosphamide. Aldehyde dehydrogenase is found in

a wide variety of tissues and in cancer cells.[200,204] The chloroethyl side chain can also be enzymatically cleaved by CYP3A4. Less than 10% of the administered dose of cyclophosphamide is metabolized via this pathway, but up to 50% of the ifosfamide is dechloroethylated, resulting in a greater rate of production of the potentially toxic byproduct chloroacetaldehyde compared with cyclophosphamide.[200,201,203]

Pharmacokinetics. The pharmacokinetic behavior of unchanged cyclophosphamide and ifosfamide has been well described. When administrated orally in low doses, 75% to 95% of the cyclophosphamide is absorbed.[205–207] The minimal first-pass metabolism after oral administration indicates that the hepatic extraction ratio for cyclophosphamide is low. Plasma concentrations of the active metabolites, 4-hydroxycyclophosphamide and phosphoramide mustard, after oral administration are equivalent to those achieved with intravenous administration.[207] The oral bioavailability of ifosfamide is greater than 95%.[208–210] Peak concentrations of 4-hydroxy-ifosfamide and chloroacetaldehyde were twofold higher than those achieved with the same dose administered intravenously.[194,211]

Cyclophosphamide and ifosfamide are eliminated primarily by hepatic biotransformation to active and inactive metabolites, which are excreted mainly in the urine. Less than 20% of the dose is excreted as unchanged drug in the urine, and biliary excretion of unchanged drug is minimal.[205,206,212–214] The total body clearance in adults is 30 to 35 mL/min/m^2 and 60 to 80 mL/min/m^2 for cyclophosphamide and ifosfamide, respectively.[205,215,216] Total clearance of cyclophosphamide in children (40 to 50 mL/min/m^2) appears to be higher than in adults.[217–219] The plasma half-life in children (3 to 4 hours) is also reported to be shorter than that in adults (6 to 8 hours).[205,206,216–221] Ifosfamide clearance in children ranges from 50 to 130 mL/min/m^2, similar to that reported in adults, and the half-life of ifosfamide in children is 1 to 5 hours.[222–224] The considerable interpatient variability in the disposition and metabolism of the oxazaphosphorines[217,222,223,225,226] may impact patient outcome. In one study of 36 children with B-cell non-Hodgkin lymphoma, the likelihood of disease recurrence in children with low plasma clearance of the parent prodrug, and thus with decreased capacity to generate active metabolites of cyclophosphamide, was significantly higher than in children with relatively higher clearance.[227]

Cyclophosphamide and ifosfamide can rapidly induce their own metabolism. With infusional or fractionated dosing, there is a decrease in the plasma half-life and an increase in clearance of the parent prodrugs and an increase in metabolite concentrations.[206,208,221,224,228,229] Cyclophosphamide exposure induces the expression of CYP2C9 and CYP3A4 enzyme levels in human hepatocytes.[230] The increase in the rate of metabolism occurs within 12 to 24 hours of the first dose, and a new steady state is achieved by 48 to 72 hours.[231] Over a 5-day course of ifosfamide, the parent drug half-life decreases and the clearance increases by 30% to 50%.[229,232] Although several studies have found that the apparent clearance of ifosfamide and its metabolites is greater when the drug is administered as a continuous infusion,[233–235] an observation that would favor administration of drug on a fractionated schedule, a crossover study in adult patients could not find a significant difference in drug disposition between the two schedules of administration.[236]

The fraction of the cyclophosphamide dose that is converted to active metabolites appears to be constant (60% to 70% of the dose), and there is no evidence of saturation of the activating enzymes over a broad dosage range of 100 to 3,000 mg/m^2.[220,225] However, at doses of 4,000 mg/m^2 used in autologous bone marrow preparative regimens, saturation of drug-activating enzymes becomes apparent.[237,238] Saturation (nonlinearity) of ifosfamide metabolism has also been described at doses exceeding 2,500 mg/m^2. The half-life was prolonged to 15 hours, a higher percentage of the drug is excreted in the urine unchanged, and the AUC of ifosfamide metabolites do not increase in proportion to the dose.[203,213,239]

The activated metabolites of cyclophosphamide and ifosfamide appear in plasma rapidly, reach a peak by 2 hours after the dose, and have a half-life of approximately 4 hours.[180,207,240] At equivalent doses, the plasma concentrations of alkylating metabolites of ifosfamide are approximately one-third that generated from cyclophosphamide, presumably because of a difference in the rate of enzymatic activation.[194,200,201,203] Plasma concentrations of the active metabolites are considerably lower than those of the parent prodrug, because of the chemical instability and reactivity of the active 4-hydroxy metabolites. The plasma concentration of the active 4-hydroxy metabolites is approximately 1% to 3% of that of the parent drug.[203,240–242]

Patients with severe renal function impairment (i.e., creatinine clearance <20 mL/min) have moderately higher parent drug concentrations[243] and significantly higher plasma alkylating activity.[216,220,244] However, in a single anuric patient, Wagner and associates found no change in the disposition of cyclophosphamide and its activated metabolite,[245] and ifosfamide disposition did not appear to be altered in an anuric child.[246] The degree of cyclophosphamide-related hematological toxicity does not correlate with the severity of renal insufficiency.[194,247] There is no strong evidence to support dosage modifications of cyclophosphamide in patients with renal dysfunction; however, ifosfamide dosage adjustment may be indicated because of the increased risk of neurotoxicity in patients with renal dysfunction.[86,246] Cyclophosphamide and ifosfamide can be efficiently removed from blood by dialysis.[246,248] The hemodialysis extraction efficiency for 4-hydroxy-ifosfamide is lower than for the parent drug.[246] Hepatic dysfunction may alter the rate of drug activation and the rate of elimination. With hepatic parenchymal damage, the half-life of cyclophosphamide is prolonged, and peak concentrations of alkylating activity in plasma are lower.[220]

Toxicity. Myelosuppression is the major dose-limiting toxicity of the oxazaphosphorines, but unlike the lipid-soluble alkylating agents, such as the nitrosoureas, they rarely cause cumulative marrow damage. Nausea, vomiting, and alopecia occur in most patients.[48,193]

Hemorrhagic cystitis is a toxicity that is unique to the oxazaphosphorines. It may range from mild dysuria and frequency to severe hemorrhage from bladder epithelial damage. The reported incidence of this complication ranges from 5% to 10% for cyclophosphamide and 20% to 40% for ifosfamide.[48,215] This toxic effect is dose related and appears to be caused by the activated metabolites and by the biologically active by-products, such as acrolein (Fig. 10.7). The incidence and severity of chemical cystitis can be lessened by aggressive hydration and frequent emptying of the bladder, by bladder irrigation, or by the concurrent administration of mesna (2-mercaptoethane sulfonate). After administration, mesna is rapidly oxidized in plasma to a chemically stable and pharmacologically inert disulfide that is then rapidly excreted by the kidneys and converted back to its chemically reduced active form during tubular transport. It is therefore only active in urine and does not interfere with the antitumor effects of cyclophosphamide or ifosfamide.[117,123,249] Although the dose and schedule of mesna varies, it is commonly administered at dose equal to 60% of the total ifosfamide dose, divided into three doses and administered at 0, 4, and 8 hours after ifosfamide.[123] Mesna can be administered orally or intravenously. Mesna also reduces the incidence of oxazaphosphorine-induced bladder cancers in rats, a complication that has been reported in humans.[215,250]

The oxazaphosphorines are also nephrotoxic. Cyclophosphamide can have a direct renal tubular effect that can result in water retention.[251,252] Ifosfamide produces proximal tubular damage resembling Fanconi syndrome, with glucosuria, aminoaciduria, and phosphaturia. Animal studies suggest that it is the ifosfamide metabolite chloroacetaldehyde, acting on mitochondrial NADH:ubiquinone oxidoreductase in the renal tubule, which is the primary mediator of nephrotoxicity.[253] Rickets has been observed in younger children.[254–258] Decreased glomerular filtration rate (GFR) and distal tubular damage manifested by concentrating defects and renal tubular acidosis also have been reported.[259,260] Comprehensive follow-up evaluation of glomerular and tubular function in children previously treated with ifosfamide revealed dysfunction in 78%, including 28% with moderate or severe nephrotoxicity.[261] Cumulative doses of 45 to 80 g/m^2 or greater appear to be the primary risk factor,[261-263] with young children appearing to be at higher risk for proximal renal tubular damage.[264-266]

Other toxic effects of ifosfamide include reversible neurotoxicity characterized by somnolence, disorientation, and lethargy in about 10% to 40% of patients and, more rarely, hallucinations, coma, and seizures.[267-269] The incidence of neurotoxicity was 50% with oral administration, presumably the result of first-pass metabolism of ifosfamide to neurotoxic metabolites.[203] The neurotoxicity has been attributed to the metabolite chloroacetaldehyde (Fig. 10.7), which results from dechloroethylation of ifosfamide.[270] The dechloroethylation pathway accounts for 50% of ifosfamide metabolism but less than 10% for cyclophosphamide. The incidence of neurotoxicity also appears to be greater in children who previously received high cumulative doses of cisplatin. Cisplatin-induced renal damage might have diminished the rate of elimination of neurotoxic metabolites of ifosfamide in these patients.[271] Neurotoxicity may be reversible or preventable with methylene blue,[272,273] but its actual efficacy remains uncertain.[269] Transient hepatic dysfunction has also been reported with ifosfamide.[215] Cardiac toxicity has been observed in patients treated with high doses (≥100 to 200 mg/kg) of cyclophosphamide. Ifosfamide has also been implicated as a cause of cardiomyopathy and arrhythmias at doses of 10 to 18 g/m^2 in a transplant setting.[274]

Although pulmonary toxicity is not commonly associated with the oxazaphosphorines, cases of early- and late-onset interstitial pneumonitis from cyclophosphamide and ifosfamide have been reported.[275-277] Clinical features of drug-induced lung injury typically include fever, cough, dyspnea on exertion, diffuse interstitial infiltrates on chest radiographs, and bilateral pleural thickening usually presenting within weeks to months of drug exposure. Factors that appear to augment oxazaphosphorine lung damage include administration of cyclophosphamide in combination with other cytotoxic drugs and the concurrent use of cyclophosphamide and irradiation. Inspired oxygen has also been shown to enhance lung injury in animals.[278] Oxazaphosphorine-induced lung injury appears to be unresponsive to corticosteroid therapy and the prognosis is poor.

Resistance. Mechanisms of resistance to cyclophosphamide involve intracellular inactivation of the activated metabolites and enhanced repair of DNA adducts.[170,193,279] Elevated concentrations of glutathione, and resulting from increased activity of the enzyme glutathione-S-transferase, can detoxify the biologically active metabolites of the oxazaphosphorines.[280-283] Sensitivity to cyclophosphamide is also inversely correlated with intracellular concentrations of the enzyme aldehyde dehydrogenase, which oxidizes activated cyclophosphamide metabolites to inactive forms.[284] Intracellular levels of this enzyme can be estimated in tissue or tumor specimens by histochemical staining. Enhanced DNA repair by nucleotide excision repair enzymes or O^6-alkylguanine-DNA alkyltransferase may also contribute to resistance.[279]

Drug Interactions. Compounds known to alter the activity of P450 microsomal enzymes can affect the rate of activation and elimination of the oxazaphosphorines. Phenobarbital pretreatment enhances the rate of metabolism of cyclophosphamide and its activated metabolites in animals and in humans[132]; similar induction may also occur with phenytoin.[285] Concurrent allopurinol appears to enhance the myelotoxicity of cyclophosphamide.[286] Busulfan, which is administered with cyclophosphamide in transplant preparatory regimens, can block the conversion of cyclophosphamide to its active metabolite, when cyclophosphamide is administered

less than 24 hours after a dose of busulfan.[287] The neurokinin-1 receptor antagonist aprepitant, a moderate inhibitor of CYP3A4,[288] can inhibit metabolism of cyclophosphamide and thiotepa, but the overall impact is small relative to the overall variability observed.[289] Concurrent fluconazole can block the activation of cyclophosphamide,[217] whereas concurrent itraconazole can increase cyclophosphamide clearance and generation of active metabolites.[290] Dexamethasone and chlorpromazine also appear to induce the metabolism of cyclophosphamide.[217]

Melphalan

Melphalan (L-phenylalanine mustard, Fig. 10.6) is a rationally designed anticancer drug that has the bischloroethylamine moiety attached to the amino acid phenylalanine, with the intention that it would be taken up preferentially by melanin-producing cancers. Although this agent has a broad range of clinical activity in adult cancers (e.g., multiple myeloma, melanoma, breast and ovarian cancers, lymphoma), its use has been limited in the treatment of childhood cancers. At standard doses (35 mg/m^2), melphalan is active against rhabdomyosarcoma.[291] The administration of bone marrow ablative doses (140 to 220 mg/m^2) of melphalan followed by rescue with autologous bone marrow transplant has resulted in high response rates in children with neuroblastoma, Ewing's sarcoma, and acute leukemia.[175,292-294] Melphalan has also been administered intra-arterially by isolated perfusion for cancers localized to an extremity or the liver.[295,296]

Like other chemically reactive compounds, melphalan is rapidly cleared from the body. It is inactivated after spontaneous hydrolysis or alkylation reactions with plasma or tissue proteins. Melphalan does not appear to undergo any appreciable enzymatic degradation.[48,187,297] The absorption of melphalan after oral administration has been reported to be incomplete and highly variable.[297-300] The fraction of a dose absorbed usually ranges from 32% to 100%, but patients with no detectable drug in plasma and urine after an oral dose have been reported.[298-300] Melphalan bioavailability is higher and less variable when the drug is administered in the fasting state.[301] The incidence of myelosuppression is lower with oral than with intravenous melphalan, and poor therapeutic response may be attributable, in part, to poor absorption in some patients receiving oral melphalan.[298,302] The disposition of melphalan after intravenous administration in children and adults is similar.[303] With standard parenteral doses, the terminal half-life ranges from 60 to 120 minutes, with a total clearance exceeding 200 mL/min/m^2.[291,299,300,304,305] Pharmacokinetic parameters in patients receiving high-dose therapy (up to 220 mg/m^2) are similar to those found at standard doses.[303,306-311] Wide interindividual variation in melphalan AUC and clearance has been observed in most studies and has led to the development of pharmacokinetically guided dosing strategies for melphalan.[180]

Renal excretion is a minor route of melphalan elimination, accounting for 20% to 30% of total drug clearance.[86,291,312] However, patients with renal dysfunction have a higher incidence of hematological toxicity.[313] In a group of patients with a wide range of renal function, drug clearance after high-dose melphalan was correlated with creatinine clearance, but the decrease in melphalan clearance in patients with renal dysfunction was insignificant compared with the high degree of interindividual variation in drug disposition.[314] In children previously treated with carboplatin, melphalan clearance was approximately two-third of that observed in other children.[315,316]

At standard doses (5 to 35 mg/m^2), myelosuppression is the primary toxicity, and cumulative marrow damage has been observed with repeated doses.[48,187] Pulmonary fibrosis and secondary leukemia are late effects associated with the chronic administration of melphalan.[187] At high doses with autologous bone marrow or stem cell reinfusion, gastrointestinal toxicity (e.g., mucositis, esophagitis, diarrhea) becomes dose limiting.[175,292,310]

Nitrosoureas

The nitrosoureas are a group of lipid-soluble alkylating agents (Fig. 10.8) that are highly active in experimental tumor models, including intracranially implanted tumors. The 2-chloroethyl derivatives, carmustine (BCNU) and lomustine (CCNU), are the nitrosoureas most widely used in pediatric oncology.[317,318] Rapid spontaneous chemical decomposition of these compounds in solution generates an alkylating intermediate (chloroethyl diazohydroxide) and an isocyanine moiety that can carbamoylate amine groups on proteins. Alkylation, including cross-linking of DNA by the monofunctional lomustine and the bifunctional carmustine, is generally accepted as the primary mechanism of action of the nitrosoureas.[319–321] However, the isocyanates can inhibit DNA repair of alkylator damage and may contribute to the antitumor activity and the toxicity of the nitrosoureas.[317,318] The nitrosoureas alkylate the N^3 position on cytidine and the N^7 and O^6 positions on guanosine,[170] but the primary factor determining tumor cell resistance to the nitrosoureas is the capacity to enzymatically repair O^6-alkyl-guanosine.[322,323] The combination of carmustine and O^6-benzylguanine, an inhibitor of the DNA repair protein O^6-alkylguanine-DNA-alkyltransferase, has been evaluated in phase I and II studies in adults[324–328] and in a phase I study in children.[329] Overall, O^6-benzylguanine increased the myelosuppressive effects of carmustine, resulting in no apparent net improvement in its therapeutic index.

The nitrosoureas have been used primarily to treat patients with brain tumors or lymphomas, and high-dose carmustine has been incorporated into transplant preparative regimens. Delayed and cumulative myelosuppression and other serious long-term cumulative renal and pulmonary toxic effects, which are particularly concerning in children, limit the clinical utility of these agents in combination regimens.[330,331] Carmustine has been incorporated into biodegradable polymer wafers that can be implanted into the tumor cavity after surgical resection for brain tumors. Drug is released slowly from the polymer wafer over 2 weeks, providing prolonged sustained exposure to high concentrations of carmustine locally with a lower risk of systemic toxicity.[332–334]

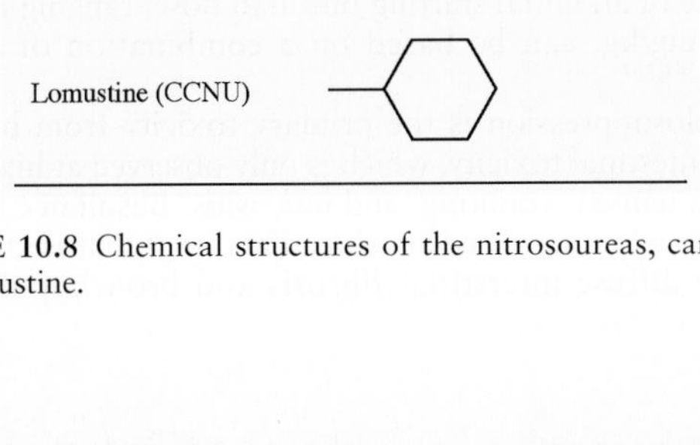

Biotransformation and Pharmacokinetics

In addition to their rapid spontaneous decomposition, nitrosoureas undergo significant hepatic metabolism.[317,335] The cyclohexyl ring of lomustine is hydroxylated at position 4 to yield two isomeric derivatives that are more soluble and have greater alkylating activity than the parent drug.[317,318] Carmustine is inactivated by denitrosation through the action of microsomal enzymes and glutathione conjugation.[317] As a result of this rapid spontaneous and enzymatic degradation, the clearance of nitrosoureas from plasma is extremely rapid. In early studies of carmustine and lomustine, parent drug could not be detected in plasma after intravenous or oral administration.[336,337] With high-dose carmustine administered by intravenous infusion, the half-life was 22 minutes, and clearance exceeded 2,000 mL/min/m².[338] Similar results have been reported with standard doses of the drug (half-life, 22 minutes; clearance, 1,700 mL/min/m²).[339] The half-life of the active 4-hydroxylated metabolites of lomustine is 3 hours.[340] When administered orally, the nitrosoureas are well absorbed, and lomustine is extensively converted to hydroxylated metabolites presystemically during its first pass through the liver.[341] These results confirm that the metabolites of lomustine are primarily responsible for the drug's antitumor activity. Although carmustine is also well absorbed, severe vomiting after oral administration frequently precludes adequate absorption.[342]

The lipid-soluble nitrosoureas are widely distributed and readily penetrate into the CNS. After equilibration, drug concentrations in the cerebrospinal fluid (CSF) approximate those in plasma, which in part accounts for the activity of this group of drugs in treating brain tumors.[337,343] Implantation of carmustine-containing polymer wafers into the tumor bed for brain tumors bypasses the blood-brain barrier and provides local drug concentrations that are higher than those achieved with systemic administration. However, the depth of penetration into the brain parenchyma from the wafer is very limited (5 mm at 30 hours) due to the rapid diffusion of drug into capillaries.[344,345]

Toxicity

Gastrointestinal toxicity (i.e., nausea and vomiting) and cumulative delayed myelosuppression are the most consistent side effects of the nitrosoureas. The nadir of blood counts occurs 4 to 5 weeks after administration, and the platelet count tends to be the most affected. With repeated dosing, chronic marrow hypoplasia develops.[318] With cumulative doses of more than 1,500 mg/m², progressive renal atrophy has been reported.[346,347] Although in children this complication has been primarily associated with semustine (methyl-CCNU), it has also been reported after high cumulative doses of lomustine. Mitchell and Schein recommend that if nitrosourea therapy continues for more than 15 months or if cumulative doses of greater than 1,000 mg/m² are reached, patients should be evaluated for nephrotoxicity and therapy discontinued if renal size or GFR is significantly decreased.[318] Similar cumulative doses (≥1,500 mg/m²) of carmustine are associated with progressive and frequently fatal pulmonary toxicity characterized by cough, dyspnea, tachypnea, and a restrictive-type ventilatory defect.[278,330,348,349] Carmustine-induced pulmonary toxicity can vary substantially in manifestations, outcome, and histopathologic appearance,[330] with the risk of developing significant pulmonary symptoms remaining elevated for many years following completion of therapy.[350] Long-term follow-up of 17 children with brain tumors treated with carmustine revealed that 6 (35%) had died of pulmonary fibrosis and that all of the surviving patients studied had radiographic abnormalities or restrictive defects on spirometry.[331]

FIGURE 10.8 Chemical structures of the nitrosoureas, carmustine and lomustine.

Four of the six patients who died presented with pulmonary symptoms 8 to 13 years after treatment. Females appear to be more susceptible to the complication than males,[330,351] and a history of atopy may increase the risk of pulmonary complications.[352] Pulmonary fibrosis appears less frequent with lomustine, but cases have been reported.[278] CNS toxicity has been reported rarely.[318] High-dose carmustine (300 to 750 mg/m[2]) can produce hypotension, tachycardia, flushing, and confusion.[339]

Drug Interactions

In animals, phenobarbital enhances the microsomal metabolism of the nitrosoureas and significantly reduces the antitumor activity of carmustine and, to a lesser extent, that of lomustine.[353] This potential interaction has not been studied in humans. Carmustine, an inhibitor of glutathione reductase, potentiates the hepatotoxicity of high doses of acetaminophen in animals. Liver damage results from the depletion of intrahepatocyte glutathione by a minor but reactive quinone metabolite of acetaminophen.[354]

Busulfan

The bifunctional alkylating agent busulfan is an alkyl alkane sulfonate (Fig. 10.5). The busulfan alkylation reaction occurs by nucleophilic displacement of the methylsulfonate group on either end of the molecule (Fig. 10.5). Busulfan has a greater propensity to alkylate thiol groups on amino acids and proteins than the nitrogen mustards, but it also can alkylate the N^7 position on guanosine.[48]

Busulfan is not water soluble and is commercially available as an oral formulation (2 and 25 mg tablets) and as an intravenous formulation (Busulfex). Busulfan has been used in conventional doses (1.8 mg/m[2]/day) as palliative therapy for chronic myelogenous leukemia, and high-dose busulfan (16 mg/kg or 600 mg/m[2], in 16 divided doses every 6 hours) is an important component of many bone marrow transplant preparative regimens, usually in combination with cyclophosphamide.[174]

The pharmacokinetics of oral busulfan is highly variable and age dependent.[355,356] Oral busulfan is rapidly absorbed, peaking 1 to 2 hours after the dose, with an average bioavailability of 70% (range, 40 to >90%).[357-359] Pharmacokinetic studies of the intravenous formulation in children suggest that interpatient variability is decreased with this route of administration.[360-362] Children heterozygous or homozygous for the glutathione S-transferase variant GSTA1*B appear to have decreased busulfan clearance,[363] but this finding requires confirmation in larger studies.

Busulfan is a small lipophilic compound that penetrates well across the blood-brain barrier. CSF concentrations at steady state are equivalent to those in plasma.[364,365] The primary route of elimination of busulfan appears to be glutathione conjugation, which is catalyzed by an isoform of glutathione-S-transferase (GSTA1-1).[366,367] Busulfan has a short half-life of 2.5 hours and a clearance in children of 80 mL/min/m[2].[357,368] These pharmacokinetic parameters appear to be linear over the wide dosage range used. Compared with adults, busulfan apparent clearance is more rapid in children, especially children who are 5 years or younger.[357,369,370] The higher apparent clearance in young children is the result of more rapid glutathione conjugation rather than lower bioavailability.[370]

The variability in the disposition of busulfan after oral dosing can result in up to a 20-fold range in systemic drug exposure among patients treated with a fixed dose.[355,371] Factors

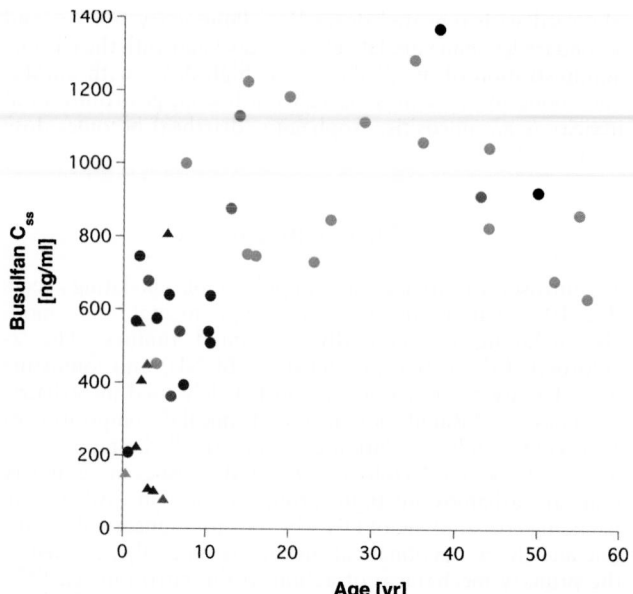

FIGURE 10.9 Plasma busulfan steady state concentrations (C_{ss}) as a function of age. C_{ss} is derived by dividing the AUC by the dosing interval (6 hours). Patients were treated with 16–30 mg/kg of busulfan in combination with cyclophosphamide prior to bone marrow transplant. Triangles represent patients who rejected their graft or had a mixed chimera. Patients who experienced grade 0 treatment-related toxicity are designated in green, grade 1 toxicity in dark blue, grade 2 toxicity in orange, grade 3 toxicity in red, and grade 4 toxicity in black. Young children had substantially lower C_{ss}, less toxicity, and were at greater risk for graft rejection. (From data presented in Tables 1, 2, and 3 in Slattery JT, et al. Graft-rejection and toxicity following bone marrow transplantation in relation to busulfan pharmacokinetics. Bone Marrow Transplant 1995;16:31.)

contributing to this variability include the age-dependent clearance, variable bioavailability, hepatic dysfunction, drug interactions including phenytoin,[372] and circadian rhythmicity.[371] The busulfan AUC in young children treated with 1 mg/kg is less than half the AUC in adults receiving the same dose (Fig. 10.9).[355,365,373] On the every-6-hour oral dosing schedule, busulfan trough plasma concentrations exhibited a marked circadian rhythm with the highest troughs occurring at 6:00 AM.[356,374]

In the transplant setting, busulfan plasma concentrations appear to be predictive of hepatic toxicity and graft rejection.[355] In adults, the risk of developing severe hepatic venoocclusive disease (VOD) is higher when the busulfan AUC exceeds 1,500 μM × min (C_{ss} of 1,000 ng/mL).[369,375,376] In children, targeting a C_{ss} of 600 to 900 ng/mL has been associated with improved engraftment,[377,378] but the upper threshold for increased risk of toxicity has not been well defined. The busulfan AUC or C_{ss} associated with VOD or graft rejection appears dependent on the prior therapy administered,[379] the preparative regimen, and the underlying disease.[355] Therapeutic drug monitoring is now commonly performed following the initial dose of busulfan, as this appears to successfully maintain C_{ss} or AUC in a safe and effective range.[372,378,380] Estimate of an initial starting busulfan dose, ranging from 0.8 to 1.2 mg/kg, can be based on a combination of age and weight.[361,381]

Myelosuppression is the primary toxicity from busulfan. Gastrointestinal toxicity, which is only observed at high doses, includes nausea, vomiting, and mucositis. Busulfan can rarely produce pulmonary toxicity (busulfan lung) that is characterized by diffuse interstitial fibrosis and bronchopulmonary dysplasia. Busulfan lung presents with cough, fever, rales, and dyspnea and usually progresses to respiratory failure.[278,368] Hepatic VOD is observed in up to 40% of patients who are treated with high-dose busulfan without pharmacokinetically guided dosing, and the VOD is severe in 10% of patients.[371,382–384] Seizures have also been reported with high-dose therapy, but they are preventable with prophylactic anticonvulsants.[368,385] Girls who receive high-dose busulfan have a high incidence of severe and persistent ovarian failure.[386]

Nonclassical Alkylating Agents

Platinum Compounds

Cisplatin, carboplatin, and oxaliplatin are heavy metal coordination complexes (Fig. 10.10) that exert their cytotoxic effects by platination of DNA, a mechanism of action that is analagous to alkylation. Reactive equated intermediates are formed in solution in a manner similar to the nitrogen mustards (Fig. 10.5). Chloride is the leaving group that is replaced by a water molecule in cisplatin. Dicarboxycyclobutane is the leaving group in carboplatin, and oxalate is the leaving group in oxaliplatin. These reactive intermediates covalently bind to DNA (N[7]-position of adenine and guanine) and form intrastrand and interstrand DNA cross-links.[387,388] The rate of reaction of these platinum analogs with water to form reactive intermediates is an important determinant of the stability of the compounds in solution and influences the drugs' pharmacokinetics.[387,389–391] Cisplatin is more reactive than carboplatin and is less stable in aqueous solution. The stability of oxaliplatin is intermediate. Chloride-containing solutions such as 0.9% NaCl are required to stabilize cisplatin prior to administration.

Cisplatin is an effective agent for the treatment of testicular tumors and has demonstrated activity against osteosarcoma, neuroblastoma, Wilms' tumor, other germ cell tumors, and brain tumors.[392–395] The drug is administered intravenously on a variety of schedules, including a single dose, infused over 4 to 6 hours; divided doses, usually daily for 5 days; and by continuous infusion for up to 5 days. The divided dose and continuous-infusion schedules may lessen the gastrointestinal and renal toxicities.[392] Other strategies used in an effort to ameliorate the dose-limiting nephrotoxicity of cisplatin include fluid hydration, mannitol diuresis, the use of hypertonic sodium chloride solutions to promote chloruresis, and the coadministration of sodium thiosulfate and amifostine.[396–398] Cisplatin has been administered regionally in a number of trials, including intraperitoneally for ovarian cancer, intravesicularly for bladder cancer, intrapleurally for the malignant pleural effusions, and intra-arterially for brain tumors and for sarcomas of the extremity, including osteosarcoma.[387,390,399]

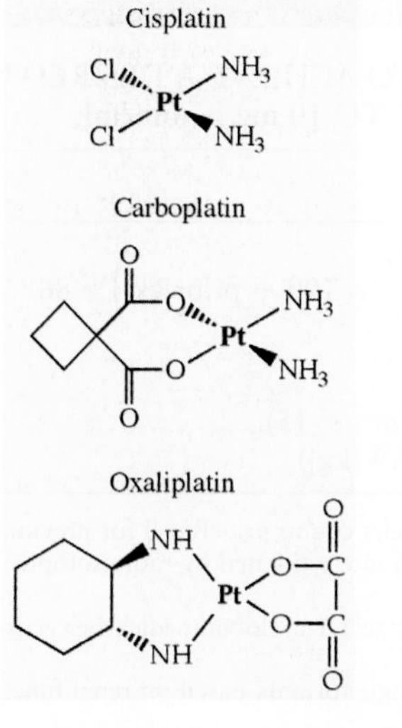

The spectrum of antitumor activity of carboplatin is similar to that of cisplatin in adults, though it may be less efficacious in several solid tumors including testicular cancer.[388,400] Carboplatin is active against brain tumors, neuroblastoma, sarcomas, and germ cell tumors.[401–403] The pharmacokinetic and toxicity profiles of cisplatin and carboplatin are quite different (Tables 10.4 and 10.5).[389,404] In children, carboplatin is administered as a bolus dose of 400 to 600 mg/m^2 or in divided doses of 400 mg/m^2 on 2 consecutive days or 160 mg/m^2 daily for 5 days, every 4 weeks. Adaptive doing formulas that individualize carboplatin dose based on the glomerular filtration rate have also been developed for children and are described below.

Oxaliplatin and 5-fluorouracil are an active combination for the treatment of adults with colorectal carcinoma.[405] As a single agent, oxaliplatin is usually administered at a dose of 130 mg/m^2 every 3 weeks, a dose that is also the recommended phase II dose in children when oxaliplatin is delivered on an every-3-week schedule.[406] Objective responses in children have been seen in rare patients with CNS tumors following treatment with oxaliplatin as a single agent[407] or in combination with etoposide.[408]

Pharmacokinetics. The chemical stability (reactivity) of the platinum analogs is a critical determinant of their pharmacokinetics. The reactive intermediates of cisplatin and carboplatin are rapidly and covalently bound to plasma protein and tissue.[387,390,409] After binding with plasma or tissue proteins, the reactive platinum intermediates are inactivated. Only the free (unbound) platinum species (including the parent drug) are cytotoxic.[410,411] This interaction of platinum compounds with protein is a time-dependent reaction. For cisplatin, more than 90% of total platinum in plasma is protein bound and inactivated within 2 to 4 hours.[390,412] This represents the major route of drug elimination. Oxaliplatin, like cisplatin, is highly protein bound. More than 80% of platinum species were bound to plasma proteins 1 hour after administration of oxaliplatin to pediatric patients enrolled on a phase I trial of this agent.[413] The major route of excretion of oxaliplatin is renal, and there is no evidence of CYP-mediated metabolism.[391] Carboplatin is more chemically stable than cisplatin and oxaliplatin. Only 20% to 40% of total platinum is protein bound at 2 hours following administration of carboplatin, and this slowly increases to 50% over 24 hours.[414–416] Tissue-bound platinum may be retained in the body for a prolonged time and is still measurable in plasma for 10 to 20 years after treatment.[417]

The pharmacokinetic behavior of bound and unbound, active forms of platinum differ appreciably. For cisplatin, after an initial rapid decay, total platinum (≥95% protein bound) persists in plasma and can be detected in urine for many days. The terminal half-life of total platinum ranges from 1 to 5 days.[410,412,418] In contrast, the unbound, active platinum species have a much more rapid decline, with a half-life of less than 1 hour, which is primarily a reflection of the chemical reactivity of cisplatin and the avid binding of the reactive

FIGURE 10.10 The chemical structures of cisplatin, carboplatin, and oxaliplatin, which platinate DNA in a manner analogs to alkylation by the nitrogen mustards. Reactive intermediates are formed after spontaneous elimination of chloride (cisplatin), dicarboxylate cyclobutane (carboplatin), or oxalate (oxaliplatin).

intermediates to tissue and plasma protein.[410,419] In children receiving cisplatin, the half-lives of total and ultrafilterable (unbound) platinum are 44 hours and 40 minutes to 1.5 hours, respectively.[395,420,421]

Approximately 50% of the platinum administered as cisplatin is excreted in the urine over 4 to 5 days, primarily in an inactive form.[412,422,423] Initially, total platinum clearance equals or exceeds creatinine clearance, reflecting excretion of unbound platinum species, but as protein binding becomes extensive, renal clearance of total platinum drops to only a small fraction of creatinine clearance.[410] The renal clearance of the unbound, ultrafilterable species of platinum can actually exceed creatinine clearance, suggesting tubular secretion.[420,424,425] It has been noted that tubular secretion rather than glomerular filtration is increased in obese adults,[426] and the absolute clearance of cisplatin is significantly increased in obese adults compared with lean controls.[427] In children, the clearance of cisplatin was not related to the glomerular filtration rate.[420] Approximately 25% of unbound platinum species is excreted in the urine, and the degree of renal excretion is schedule dependent (greater with short infusions).[428] In patients with impaired renal function, the peak concentration of active, unbound platinum was elevated, but the terminal half-life was not prolonged, presumably because of the rapid reaction of these active species with plasma and tissue protein leading to inactivation.[422,429] However, dosage reductions in patients with renal dysfunction may be indicated because of the drug's nephrotoxic effects, which could further impair renal function.[390,430]

The disposition of carboplatin is characterized by a lower rate and degree of protein binding than for cisplatin. As a result, the terminal half-life of unbound carboplatin is longer (2 to 3 hours), and renal excretion is the primary route of elimination.[389,390,414,416,423,431] By 24 hours, as much as 70% of the total platinum from carboplatin is excreted in the urine, most as parent drug. Carboplatin is dialyzable in patients with severe renal insufficiency.[432,433]

Pharmacokinetic parameters for carboplatin in children are similar to those in adults. The total clearance in children with a normal creatinine clearance is approximately 70 mL/min/m², and the half-life is 2 to 3 hours.[421,434–436] In children younger than 5 years, carboplatin clearance is 120 mL/min/m²,

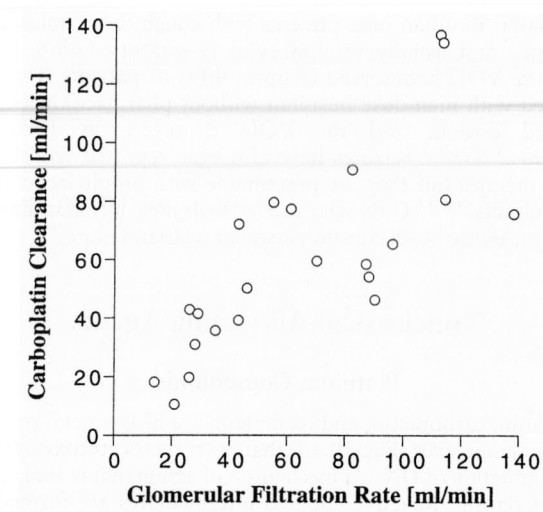

FIGURE 10.11 Relation between carboplatin clearance and glomerular filtration rate as measured by ^{51}Cr-EDTA clearance in 22 children. (Adapted from Newell DR, Pearson ADJ, Balmanno K, et al. Carboplatin pharmacokinetics in children: the development of a pediatric dosing formula. J Clin Oncol 1993;11:2314, with permission.)

but in children younger than 1 year, the clearance is 75 mL/min/m².[437] These age-related differences in carboplatin clearance appear to be related to differences in the glomerular filtration rate. The variability in carboplatin clearance supports the use of the adaptive dosing formulas based on glomerular filtration rate described subsequently.

The total clearance of carboplatin is highly correlated with creatinine clearance (Fig. 10.11),[81,389,414,436,438] and patients with renal dysfunction and higher carboplatin AUCs have a greater probability of experiencing dose-limiting hematological toxicity. These associations allowed the development of adaptive dosing formulas for individualizing carboplatin dose based on creatinine clearance in adults and children (Table 10.6).[81,434,436,438–441] The use of these formulas to calculate an individualized dose decreases the variability in systemic drug

TABLE 10.6

ADAPTIVE DOSING FORMULAS FOR TARGETING CARBOPLATIN DOSE TO ACHIEVE A DESIRED NADIR PLATELET COUNT OR AUC, WITH THE TARGET AUC RANGING FROM 7 TO 10 mg × min/mL

Population	Formula[a]
Adults[b]	$D[\text{mg/m}^2] = 0.091 \times \text{CL}_{CR}[\text{mL/min/m}^2] \times \left(\dfrac{\text{prePlt} - \text{trgtPlt}}{\text{prePlt}} \times 100 - \text{priorRx} \right) + 86$
Adults[c]	$D[\text{mg}] = \text{trgtAUC}[\text{mg} \cdot \text{min/mL}] \times (\text{GFR}[\text{ml/min}] + 25)$
Children[d]	$D[\text{mg/m}^2] = \text{trgtAUC}[\text{mg} \cdot \text{min/mL}] \times (0.93 \times \text{GFR}[\text{mL/min/m}^2] + 15)$
Children[e]	$D[\text{mg}] = \text{trgtAUC}[\text{mg} \cdot \text{min/mL}] \times (\text{GFR}[\text{ml/min}] + 0.36 \times \text{BW}[\text{kg}])$

[a]D, dose; CL$_{CR}$, creatinine clearance; prePlt, pretreatment platelet count; trgtPlt, target nadir platelet count; priorRx, 0 for previously untreated and 17 for previously treated; trgtAUC, target systemic drug exposure (AUC); GFR, glomerular filtration rate estimated by radioisotopic method; BW, body weight. Units for each parameter are listed in the brackets.
[b]Egorin MJ, Van Echo DA, Tipping SJ, et al. Pharmacokinetics and dose reductions of *cis*-diammine(1,1-cyclobutanedicarboxylato)platinum in patients with impaired renal function. Cancer Res 1984;44:5432.
[c]Calvert AH, Newell DR, Gumbrell LA, et al. Carboplatin dosage: prospective evaluation of a single formula based on renal function. J Clin Oncol 1989;7:1748.
[d]Marina NM, Rodman J, Shema SJ, et al. Phase I study of escalated targeted doses of carboplatin combined with ifosfamide and etoposide in children with relapsed solid tumors. J Clin Oncol 1993;11:554.
[e]Newel DR, Pearson ADJ, Balmanno K, et al. Carboplatin pharmacokinetics in children: the development of a pediatric dosing formula. J Clin Oncol 1993;11:2314.

exposure (AUC) and reduces the incidence of severe thrombocytopenia.[414,442,443] Caution must be exercised when using these formulas, however, as the results are expressed either as an absolute dose (mg) or as a dose normalized to body surface area (mg/m²).[444] When administered as a single dose in combination with ifosfamide and etoposide, a targeted carboplatin AUC of up to 10 mg × min/mL was tolerable.[442] In ovarian and testicular cancers in adults, a carboplatin AUC of 5 to 7 mg × min/mL was associated with a higher response rate and a lower risk of disease recurrence.[438,443]

The pharmacokinetic behavior of oxaliplatin in children appears to be similar to that of adults.[406,407,413] Oxaliplatin is rapidly hydrolyzed in a nonenzymatic fashion to a large number of reactive intermediates. The volume of distribution in adults has been shown to exceed 500 L, compared with approximately 20 L for cisplatin and carboplatin. This suggests that the diaminocyclohexane ligand may enhance tissue distribution of oxaliplatin.[391] Adaptive oxaliplatin dosing formulas based on GFR have not been developed, although pediatric pharmacokinetic data identify covariates of such weight and renal function that could potentially be incorporated into a dosing nomogram.[407] Dose reduction does not appear to be necessary in patients with moderate renal or hepatic dysfunction.[445,446]

Toxicity. The toxicity profiles of the platinum analogs are strikingly different. Cisplatin is associated with only mild myelosuppression but produces significant and potentially irreversible nephrotoxicity, ototoxicity, and neurotoxicity. The dose-limiting toxicity of carboplatin is hematological toxicity, primarily thrombocytopenia, and the nonhematological toxicities observed with cisplatin are only seen at doses of carboplatin exceeding 800 mg/m².[387,389,404,447] Dose-limiting toxicities of oxaliplatin include neurotoxicity, thrombocytopenia, and neutropenia.

Nephrotoxicity, manifested as azotemia and electrolyte disturbances (especially hypomagnesemia requiring oral supplementation), was the dose-limiting toxicity in the initial clinical trials with cisplatin.[447-449] The exact mechanism of cisplatin nephrotoxicity is not defined, but patients experience a reduction in renal blood flow and glomerular filtration rate and a loss of tubular function. Pathologic changes are seen primarily in the renal proximal and distal tubule epithelium and collecting ducts.[447,450,451] Renal damage from cisplatin is cumulative.

Although pretreatment hydration, diuresis, chloruresis, and less-toxic dose schedules have reduced the incidence and severity of cisplatin-induced nephrotoxicity, moderate and permanent reductions in the glomerular filtration rate of patients receiving cisplatin have been documented.[452-454] However, in a long-term follow-up study of 40 children who received a median of 500 mg/m² of cisplatin, 22 of the 24 patients with abnormally low end therapy glomerular filtration rates partially recovered, with a median increase in glomerular filtration rate of 13 mL/min/m².[455] The 211 patients participating in the German Late Effects Surveillance System (LESS) had received a somewhat lower cumulative dose of cisplatin (360 mg/m²) but were followed longitudinally (median follow-up time 2 years). None of these patients developed an elevation in creatinine exceeding 1.5 times the upper limit of normal, and the hypomagnesemia detected in 12% of these patients following cisplatin therapy was mild.[456] The long-term nephrotoxic effects of cisplatin in infants are similar to those reported in older children.[457]

In adult patients, pretreatment with the organic thiophosphate amifostine appears to lessen the severity of renal damage by cisplatin without altering the antitumor effect of the drug.[398,458] The proportion of adult patients who suffered a 40% or more reduction in creatinine clearance after at least four courses of cisplatin was 32% when cisplatin was administered

alone and 10% when amifostine was administered prior to cisplatin.[459]

As a result of its nephrotoxic effects, cisplatin can alter its own elimination rate and that of other drugs, such as methotrexate, that rely on renal excretion.[460] In one series, the renal clearance of ultrafilterable platinum fell from almost 500 mL/min with the first course to 150 mL/min by the fourth course in patients receiving repeated doses, probably as a result of decreased renal tubular secretion of the drug.[461] Higher renal cortical concentrations of platinum were found at autopsy in patients who had clinical renal toxicity than in patients without evidence of renal toxicity.[462]

As methods to prevent nephrotoxicity have allowed the administration of higher single and cumulative doses of the drug, ototoxicity and peripheral neuropathy have become more prominent.[447] Cisplatin causes a reversible sensory peripheral neuropathy (i.e., numbness, tingling, and paresthesias) at cumulative doses of 300 to 600 mg/m².[268,447] Lhermitte's sign (an electric shock sensation when the neck is flexed) is common at high cumulative doses of cisplatin.[463] Symptoms may progress after discontinuation of cisplatin and persist for months to years. Seizures and encephalopathy have also been reported in children receiving intensive cisplatin therapy.[464] The irreversible hearing loss is in the high-frequency range and appears to be related to a cumulative dose of cisplatin of greater than 400 mg/m².[403,465-467] Children younger than 5 years also appear more likely to develop cisplatin-related hearing loss compared with older children.[468] Genetic variability also appears to explain some of the variability in platinum-associated neurotoxicity in adults.[469] Amifostine decreases the incidence and severity of platinum-related neurotoxicity and ototoxicity in adults.[458] In a study of children with average risk medulloblastoma, amifostine appeared to have provided some otoprotection,[470] but protective effects have yet to be observed in other pediatric studies.[471-473] Additional toxic effects associated with cisplatin include prominent nausea and vomiting, mild myelosuppression, Raynaud's phenomenon, and hypersensitivity reactions.[392]

Carboplatin's myelosuppressive effects are delayed, affecting the frequency by which the drug can be administered. Platelet nadirs are typically seen up to 3 weeks after the dose and milder granulocyte nadirs are observed 3 to 4 weeks after carboplatin administration. Some patients require 5 to 6 weeks for complete count recovery.[474] Not only are the nephrotoxicity, ototoxicity, and peripheral neuropathy from carboplatin milder than that associated with cisplatin, but the nausea and vomiting, which can be dose limiting with cisplatin, are also less severe.[389,474,475] High cumulative doses of carboplatin are associated with a small drop in glomerular filtration rate and serum magnesium, but these changes are usually not clinically significant.[476] Hypersensitivity reactions to carboplatin are relatively common and the risk increases after multiple cycles of therapy.[477,478]

Myelosuppression due to oxaliplatin is usually mild, and the dose-limiting toxicity in adults is a cumulative peripheral neuropathy. Oxaliplatin is also associated with an unusual acute neurologic toxicity, pharyngolaryngeal dysesthesia, in which patients report difficulty in breathing or swallowing in the absence of laryngeal obstruction, probably related to transient sensory disturbances.[479] The sensory neuropathy associated with oxaliplatin is exacerbated by cold in children as in adults.[406] Although more than one-third of patients enrolled on a phase II study of oxaliplatin in children with CNS tumors developed a sensory neuropathy, it was severe in less than 5% of the patients.[407]

Resistance. Studies in preclinical tumor models have implicated several possible mechanisms of resistance to platinum compounds.[480–482] Decreased drug accumulation may be related to altered drug uptake or the presence of a membrane efflux pump. Increased intracellular levels of thiol-containing compounds, such as glutathione and metallothionein, can react with and inactivate the active equated forms of cisplatin and carboplatin. The enhanced repair of platinum-DNA adducts by the nucleotide excision repair pathway removes the cytotoxic lesion produced by the platinum analogs. Platinum-induced DNA damage activates apoptosis, and expression of cellular proteins that suppress the apoptotic response to this damage or loss of mismatch repair activity may alter sensitivity to the platinum analogs.[169,483]

Dacarbazine

Although dacarbazine (Fig. 10.12) was originally developed as an inhibitor of purine biosynthesis, it does not exert its antitumor effects as an antimetabolite.[484] Dacarbazine is a prodrug that undergoes hepatic microsomal metabolic activation (N-demethylation), which is catalyzed primarily by CYP1A2, to the active metabolite, methyltriazenyl imidazole carboximide (MTIC).[485] MTIC then spontaneously decomposes into a reactive methylating species (methyldiazonium ion) and the primary circulating metabolite aminoimidazole carboxamide (AIC).[484,486] The methyldiazonium ion can methylated nucleophilic sites, including the O^6 and N^7 positions on guanosine, but it cannot form cross-links.

Dacarbazine is generally administered intravenously (150 to 250 mg/m²) on a divided once-daily dosage schedule for 5 days. Absorption after oral administration is slow, incomplete, and variable.[487] After intravenous administration, the drug is rapidly cleared from the plasma, with a terminal half-life of 40 minutes and a total clearance of 450 mL/min/m². One half of the dose is excreted unchanged in the urine, and renal clearance exceeds the GFR, suggesting that the drug is also eliminated by renal tubular secretion.[488] The remainder of the dose presumably undergoes biotransformation. The half-life and renal clearance of the metabolite AIC are similar to that of the parent drug.[488] Methylated DNA adducts in white blood cells of patients treated with dacarbazine (250 to 800 mg/m²) increase rapidly during the first hour after treatment but then decline with a more prolonged half-life (72 hours) than the parent drug.[489]

When dacarbazine was administered as a 1,000 mg/m² infusion over 24 hours, the steady-state plasma concentration was 8.6 µg/mL.[490] Other pharmacokinetic parameters derived from the study of this schedule included a total clearance of 110 mL/min/m², a volume of distribution at steady state of 23 L/m², and a terminal half-life after infusion of 3 hours.

Gastrointestinal toxicity, consisting of moderate-to-severe nausea and vomiting, is the primary toxicity and is frequently dose limiting. Tolerance usually develops over the 5-day course of administration. At standard doses, myelosuppression is mild. Other side effects include a flu-like syndrome with malaise, fever, and myalgias; mild hepatic dysfunction; and local pain at the site of intravenous injection. Rare cases of liver failure and death from VOD and hepatic vein thrombosis (Budd-Chiari syndrome) have been associated with the use of this drug.[491]

Temozolomide

The methylating agent temozolomide is structurally and mechanically related to dacarbazine. Like dacarbazine,

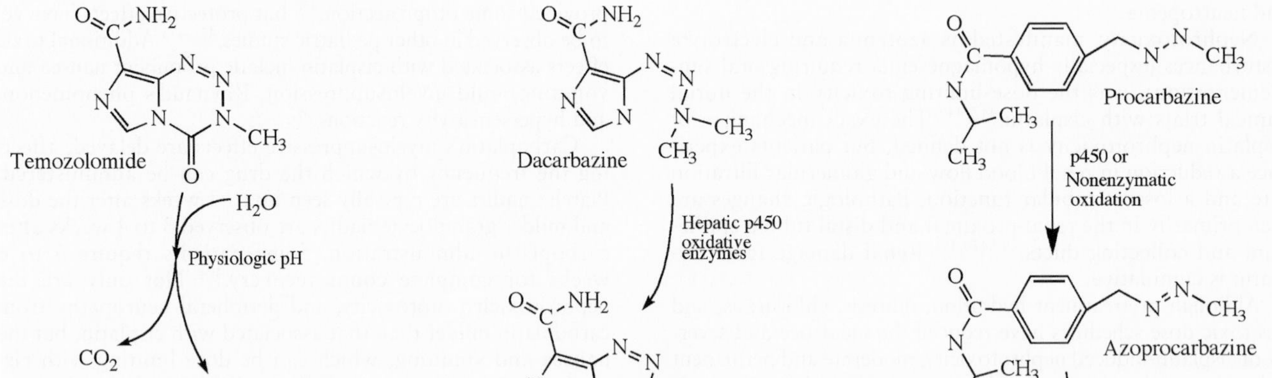

FIGURE 10.12 Chemical structures and activation pathways of the methylating agents, dacarbazine, temozolomide, and procarbazine, which are prodrugs. Dacarbazine requires enzymatically catalyzed activation and temozolomide undergoes spontaneous chemical conversion in solution at physiological pH to the active metabolite, MTIC (MTIC is methyltriazenyl-imidazole carboxamide, HMMTIC is hydroxymethyl-MTIC, and AIC is amino-imidazole carboxamide). The metabolic pathway for procarbazine is highly complex and incompletely shown. In addition to the methyldiazonium ion, free radicals can also be generated from azoprocarbazine.

temozolomide is a prodrug, but temozolomide does not require enzymatic activation in the liver. In solution at physiological pH, temozolomide spontaneously decomposes to MTIC, the same active metabolite that is derived by enzymatic N-demethylation of dacarbazine (Fig. 10.12).[492,493]

Temozolomide is insoluble in aqueous solution and is only available in capsules for oral administration. Based on preclinical studies[492,494] that demonstrated divided dosing schedules had greater antitumor effect than a single bolus dose, and on the initial phase I clinical trial[495] in which responses were only observed on the divided dose schedule, temozolomide is administered as a single daily dose for 5 consecutive days. The recommended dose for children is 200 mg/m²/day (1,000 mg/m²/course) when administered as a single agent, though doses as high as 260 mg/m²/day given daily for 5 days have been well tolerated in children with leukemia.[496–498] A continuous daily dosing schedule is also being investigated, and a dose of 75 mg/m²/day appears to be tolerable for 6 to 7 weeks in adults.[499] Temozolomide is used in children primarily for the treatment of brain tumors but is also undergoing study as part of combination regimens for a number of childhood solid tumors.[500–503]

Absorption of temozolomide from the gastrointestinal tract is rapid and complete.[495,504] The peak concentration of temozolomide is achieved in plasma within 1.5 hours of the dose.[497] When administered with food, the bioavailability is slightly lower but remains 90% or more.[505] Temozolomide is also rapidly eliminated. Its half-life (1.8 hours) is similar to the drug's half-life in a pH 7.4 phosphate buffer solution in vitro,[493] suggesting that decomposition to the active metabolite, MTIC, is the primary route of elimination for temozolomide. A pharmacokinetic study of radiolabeled temozolomide confirmed that AIC, which is the end-product of temozolomide decomposition to MTIC, is primary urinary metabolite.[506] In children, 5% to 15% of the dose of temozolomide was recovered in urine as unchanged drug.[497] The apparent clearance of temozolomide in children is approximately 100 mL/min/m² and the terminal half-life is similar to that observed in adults.[498] The active metabolite, MTIC, is much less stable and has an estimated half-life of 2.5 minutes and clearance exceeding 5,000 mL/min/m².[506,507] There is some evidence that temozolomide clearance is lower in younger children.[508] Temozolomide is widely distributed in tissues and penetrates well across the blood-brain barrier[504] and could therefore be considered the transport form for MTIC.

Myelosuppression is the dose-limiting toxicity of temozolomide. Nadir neutrophil and platelet counts typically occur 21 days after the start of therapy, and recovery of blood counts may take 7 to 10 days.[493,496,497] This delayed myelosuppression necessitates administering temozolomide on a 28-day schedule. The myelosuppression from temozolomide does not appear to be cumulative.[495] Nonhematological toxicities are mild and include nausea and vomiting, which can be controlled by pretreatment with standard antiemetics, headache, fatigue, constipation, and serum transaminase elevations.[504]

The DNA repair protein O⁶-alkylguanine-DNA alkyltransferase (MGMT) removes the methyl adduct from the O⁶-position of guanine. Although this adduct accounts for only 5% of DNA adducts formed by temozolomide,[492] it is thought to be the primary cytotoxic lesion. Tumor cell lines with high levels of this repair protein are resistant to the cytotoxic effect of temozolomide.[492,493,509] Administration of temozolomide itself depletes MGMT.[510] In addition, depletion of MGMT by coadministration of the modulating agent O⁶-benzylguanine markedly enhances the cytotoxic effects of temozolomide.[511] Loss of DNA mismatch repair capacity enhances resistance to temozolomide. Coadministration of O⁶-benzylguanine increases the myelosuppression associated with temozolomide. The combination of O⁶BG (120 mg/m²/day × 5 days) and temozolomide (75 mg/m²/day × 5 days) is well tolerated,

and objective responses in patients with CNS tumors have been observed.[512]

Procarbazine

Procarbazine is a methylhydrazine analog that was originally synthesized as monoamine oxidase inhibitor but was discovered to have antitumor activity in animals. Procarbazine is currently used for the treatment of Hodgkin disease[513] and is also active against brain tumors.[514] Procarbazine is a prodrug that requires metabolic activation in vivo to express its antitumor activity.[484] This activation yields methylating and free radical intermediates, which appear to produce the drug's antitumor effect.

The spontaneous chemical decomposition and biotransformation of procarbazine is complex.[484,486,515] Metabolic activation probably occurs in the liver and is catalyzed by the CYP enzyme complex (Fig. 10.12).[516] In liver perfusion studies, procarbazine is extensively converted to its active ago-metabolite.[517]

The disposition of procarbazine and its active intermediates has not been well characterized in humans. The drug is rapidly and completely absorbed from the gastrointestinal tract,[518] and it undergoes complete first-pass conversion to cytotoxic metabolites, which probably accounts for the activity of the drug when administered orally. After intravenous administration, procarbazine is rapidly metabolized and has a half-life of less than 10 minutes.[519] The metabolites of procarbazine are excreted primarily in the urine. Procarbazine or unidentified metabolites enter the CSF readily.[519] Drugs such as phenobarbital and phenytoin that are capable of inducing hepatic microsomal enzymes can increase the rate of procarbazine activation.[484] Procarbazine can inhibit the biotransformation of the barbiturates, phenothiazines, and other sedatives, resulting in potentiation of their sedative effects. The inhibition of monoamine oxidase by procarbazine can put patients at risk for hypertensive reactions from foods high in tramline (e.g., bananas, wine, cheese). Procarbazine also appears to alter its own metabolism over a 14-day course of therapy. The plasma concentrations of procarbazine metabolites differ markedly between days 1 and 14 of treatment.[520]

The primary toxicities of procarbazine include nausea, vomiting, and myelosuppression. Some patients develop evidence of neurotoxicity consisting of paresthesias, somnolence, depression, or agitation. Neurotoxicity is prominent with high-dose intravenous administration.[521] Patients are also at risk for the long-term toxicities, including azoospermia, ovarian failure, and teratogenic and carcinogenic effects.[484]

ANTIMETABOLITES

The antimetabolites are structural analogs of vital cofactors or intermediates in the biosynthetic pathways of DNA and RNA. By acting as fraudulent substrates for the enzymes in these pathways, antimetabolites inhibit synthesis of the nucleic acids and their building blocks or are incorporated into DNA or RNA, resulting in a defective product. Antimetabolites that are used in the treatment of pediatric cancers include the folate analog methotrexate (Fig. 10.13); the pyrimidine analogs cytarabine, gemcitabine, and fluorouracil (Fig. 10.14); and the purine analogs mercaptopurine, thioguanine, fludarabine, cladribine, clofarabine, and nelarabine (Fig. 10.15).

In general, the clinical pharmacology of these agents is similar to that of the endogenous compounds that they structurally resemble. The absorptive, metabolic, and excretory pathways are frequently shared by the endogenous compound and the antimetabolite. The rate of elimination of the antimetabolites is usually rapid. Most of the antimetabolites are prodrugs that require metabolic activation within the target cell to express

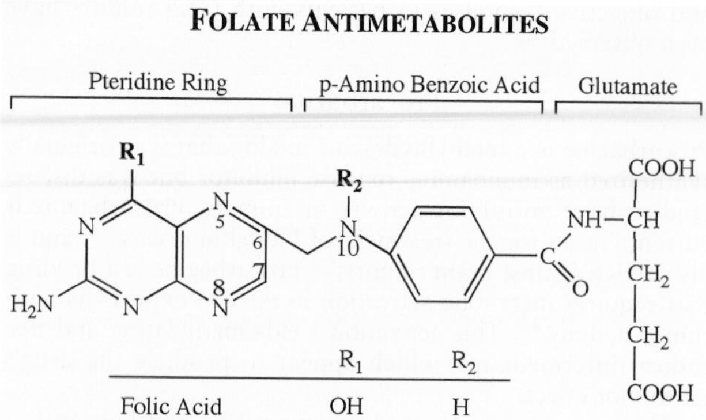

FOLATE ANTIMETABOLITES

FIGURE 10.13 Chemical structures of the antifolate methotrexate compared with the structure of folic acid.

their cytotoxic effects. The purine and pyrimidine analogs, for example, require intracellular conversion to phosphorylated nucleotides, which are the active forms of these drugs. Because most antimetabolites interfere directly with DNA synthesis, they are cell cycle and S phase specific; the maximum cytotoxic effect occurs in cells that are synthesizing DNA. This partially explains the schedule dependence of this class of anticancer drugs. More prolonged drug exposure that results from administering these agents by continuous infusion or by chronic daily dosing increases the chance of exposing a higher proportion of the tumor cell population to the drugs during active DNA replication.

Methotrexate

Methotrexate is the most widely used antimetabolite in childhood cancers. It is effective in the treatment of ALL, non-Hodgkin lymphoma, the histiocytoses, and osteosarcoma.

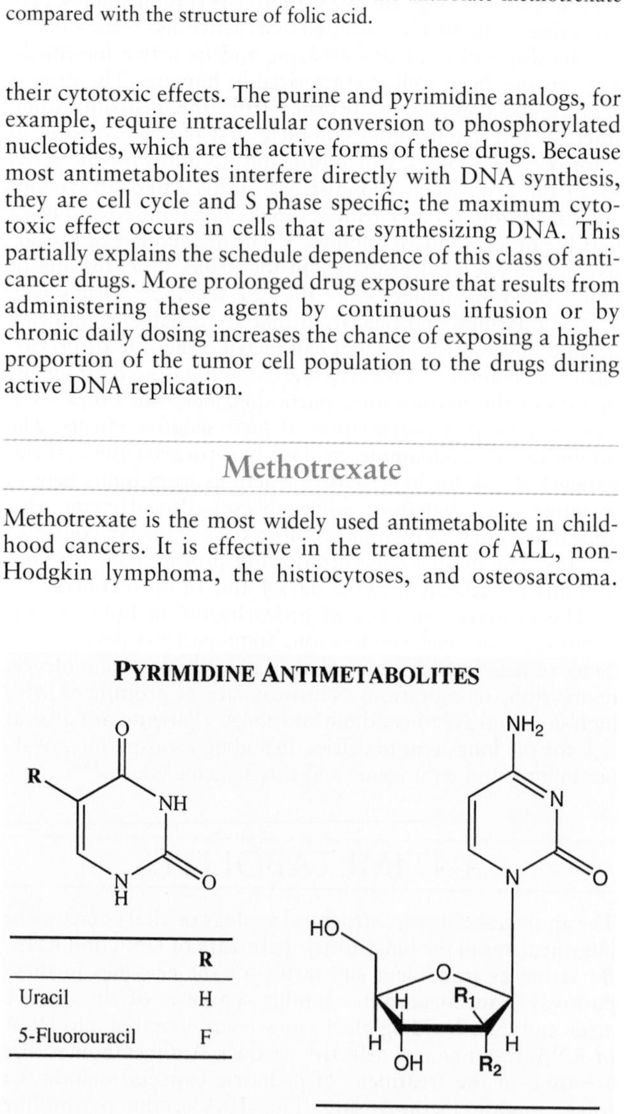

PYRIMIDINE ANTIMETABOLITES

FIGURE 10.14 Chemical structures of commonly used pyrimidine antimetabolites compared with the structures of corresponding endogenous compounds of which they are analogs.

Methotrexate is administered on an intermittent schedule by variety of routes, including oral, intramuscular, subcutaneous, intrathecal, and intravenous. Chronic oral or intramuscular therapy is administered weekly at a dose of 20 mg/m². With intravenous therapy, an extraordinarily wide range of doses has been employed, ranging from a 10 mg bolus to 33,000 mg/m² as a 24-hour infusion. Doses above 300 mg/m², which are usually administered by continuous infusion, must be followed by a course of the rescue agent leucovorin (5-formyl-tetrahydrofolate) to prevent the development of severe toxicities.

The loading and infusion doses required to achieve a desired steady-state plasma concentration ($[MTX]_{plasma}$) can be estimated from the following formulas[522]:

$$\text{Loading dose (mg/m}^2) = 15 \times [MTX]_{plasma} \ (\mu M)$$

$$\text{Infusion dose (mg/m}^2/\text{hr}) = 3 \times [MTX]_{plasma} \ (\mu M)$$

For example, to achieve a steady-state plasma concentration of 10 μM, the loading dose would be 150 mg/m², followed by an infusion of 30 mg/m²/hr. Infusion durations of up to 42 hours are tolerable when followed by leucovorin rescue. In clinical practice, infusion durations range from 4 to 36 hours depending on the type of cancer being treated. Patients who are treated with a high-dose methotrexate infusion must be adequately hydrated and alkalinized to prevent precipitation of methotrexate in acidic urine, and routine monitoring of urinary output, serum creatinine, and plasma methotrexate concentrations is mandatory to determine the duration of leucovorin rescue. For most infusion regimens, 12 to 15 mg/m² of leucovorin should be continued every 6 hours until plasma methotrexate concentration decreases to 0.05 to 0.1 μM.

Mechanism of Action

Methotrexate is a structural analog of folic acid, a required cofactor for the synthesis of purines and thymidine. As a result of the substitution of an amino group for the hydroxyl group at position 4 on the pteridine ring of folic acid (Fig. 10.13), methotrexate is a tight-binding inhibitor of DHFR, the enzyme responsible for converting folates to their active, chemically reduced (tetrahydrofolate) form.[523,524] 10-Formyl-tetrahydrofolate acts as the single carbon donor in the de novo purine synthetic pathway, and 5,10-methylenetetrahydrofolate donates its single-carbon group and is oxidized to dihydrofolate in the conversion of deoxyuridylate (dUMP) to thymidylate (dTMP) by thymidylate synthase. In the presence of methotrexate, intracellular tetrahydrofolate pools are depleted, leading to depletion of purines and thymidylate and inhibition of DNA synthesis. Accumulation of partially oxidized dihydrofolic acid, resulting from the inhibition of DHFR, appears to contribute to the inhibition of de novo purine synthesis.[524-526] A critical determinant of methotrexate cytotoxicity is the rate of thymidylate synthesis, because the synthesis of thymidylate from uridylate is the only reaction that oxidizes the tetrahydrofolate cofactor to the inactive dihydrofolate form. Another determinant is achieving an intracellular methotrexate concentration that is in excess of DHFR binding sites, because intracellular levels of this target enzyme are 20- to 30-fold higher than required to maintain tetrahydrofolate pools.[523,527,528]

Methotrexate shares membrane-transport processes and intracellular metabolic pathways with the naturally occurring folates. It competes with the tetrahydrofolates for an energy-dependent transport system for cell entry. On entry, methotrexate is rapidly and tightly bound to DHFR, and uptake into the target cell is essentially unidirectional until the enzyme binding sites are saturated, allowing for even greater intracellular accumulation of drug.[523]

PURINE ANTIMETABOLITES

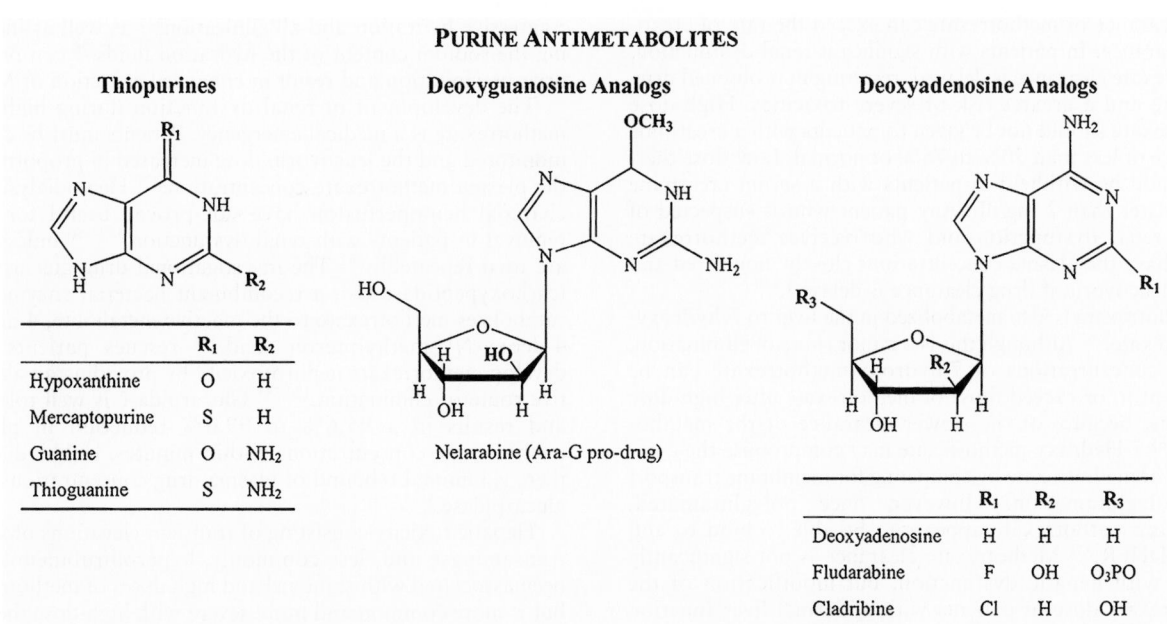

FIGURE 10.15 Chemical structures of commonly used purine antimetabolites compared with the structures of corresponding endogenous compounds of which they are analogs.

With the accumulation of free intracellular drug in excess of DHFR binding sites, methotrexate, like the naturally occurring folates, is metabolized intracellularly to polyglutamated derivatives, which cannot readily efflux from the cell. Methotrexate polyglutamate formation enhances the cytotoxicity of the drug by allowing greater accumulation of free intracellular drug and retention of the drug within the cell, even after extracellular drug is cleared. Methotrexate polyglutamates are also more potent inhibitors of DHFR and are capable of directly inhibiting other enzymes in the synthetic pathways for thymidine (thymidylate synthase) and purines.[524,527,529,530] Methotrexate polyglutamate formation is optimal *in vitro* when cells are exposed to high concentrations for prolonged periods, and children with ALL randomized to receive high-dose methotrexate as initial induction therapy had higher methotrexate polyglutamate levels in their lymphoblasts than patients randomized to low-dose methotrexate.[531,532] The lymphoblasts from children with ALL and good prognostic features, such as B-lineage immunophenotype, hyperdiploidy, young age, low presenting white cell count, and female sex, tend to accumulate methotrexate polyglutamates more efficiently than blasts from higher risk patients, suggesting that ALL in lower risk patients may be more sensitive to methotrexate's antileukemic effect.[532–535]

Pharmacokinetics

At oral doses of 7.5 to 20 mg/m², the rate and extent of absorption of methotrexate is highly variable.[72,536–539] Peak plasma concentrations can occur from 0.5 to 5 hours after oral administration, and the percentage of the dose that is absorbed ranges from 5% to 97%.[536] The AUC of oral methotrexate ranged from 0.63 to 12 μM × hr at a dose of 18 to 22 mg/m², and over a broader dosage range, the AUC correlated poorly with the dose.[72] In patients who are studied after multiple doses, there was also considerable intrapatient variation in the AUC.[72] Absorption of methotrexate is saturable, and as the dose is increased, the fraction of the

dose that is absorbed diminishes.[540–543] Simply increasing the dose in patients who have low plasma concentrations after standard oral doses may not overcome poor bioavailability. The bioavailability of oral methotrexate can also be significantly reduced when administered with food.[544] Despite this variability with oral dosing, there was no relation between the relapse rate and methotrexate pharmacokinetic parameters, such as peak concentration, AUC, and erythrocyte methotrexate concentrations.[38,72,545] When administered intramuscularly or subcutaneously, methotrexate is completely absorbed.[542,543,546,547]

The disposition of methotrexate in children differs from that in adults.[548–551] In one study, children had lower plasma concentrations of methotrexate and excreted the drug in the urine more rapidly after a 6-hour infusion than did adults.[552] The volume of distribution was also greater in children. Within the pediatric age group, the clearance of methotrexate is also age dependent.[553] Children younger than 10 years (n = 94) had a clearance of 160 mL/min/m² compared with 110 mL/min/m² in those older than 10 years (n = 21). Infants (<1 year old) have a slightly lower clearance rate than children,[90] with somewhat more pronounced differences observed in very young (<3 months) infants.[554,555]

The plasma disappearance of methotrexate is multiphasic, with a terminal half-life of 8 to 12 hours.[522,524] Retention of the drug in large extravascular fluid collections, such as ascites or pleural fluid, is associated with prolongation of the half-life as a result of slow release of retained drug into the circulation.[524] This prolonged exposure to the drug can increase the risk for toxicity. Patients who have large extravascular fluid collections and are receiving methotrexate should have their methotrexate concentrations monitored closely.

Methotrexate is eliminated primarily by renal excretion, undergoing glomerular filtration and renal tubular reabsorption and secretion.[556,557] Approximately 70% to 90% of a dose is excreted unchanged in the urine, most within the first 6 hours. Mutations in the drug transporter ABC gene ABCC2 have been associated with impaired methotrexate elimination.[558,559] The renal clearance of methotrexate can exceed the rate of creatinine clearance. In patients with significant renal dysfunction, methotrexate clearance is delayed, resulting in prolonged drug exposure and a greater risk of severe toxicities. High-dose methotrexate should not be given to patients with a creatinine clearance of less than 50% to 75% of normal. Low-dose therapy should be withheld in patients with a serum creatinine level greater than 2 mg/dL. Any patient who is suspected of having renal dysfunction and who receives methotrexate should have the plasma concentrations closely monitored and receive leucovorin if drug clearance is delayed.[560]

Methotrexate is also metabolized in the liver to 7-hydroxy-methotrexate.[561] Although this is a minor route of elimination, plasma concentrations of 7-hydroxy-methotrexate can be equivalent to or exceed those of methotrexate after high-dose infusions, because of the slower clearance of the metabolite.[562–565] 7-Hydroxy-methotrexate may compromise the cytotoxicity of methotrexate by competing for membrane transport and polyglutamation. However, once polyglutamated, 7-hydroxy-methotrexate appears to be able to bind to and inhibit DHFR.[523] Methotrexate clearance is not significantly altered with hepatic dysfunction, but modification of the methotrexate dose in patients with abnormal liver function tests may be indicated to avoid additional hepatic damage.

Total renal and metabolic methotrexate clearance is approximately 100 mL/min/m^2, but it may vary widely among patients.[524,564,566] In patients with normal creatinine clearance, there is not a good correlation between methotrexate clearance and creatinine clearance.[566] Renal tubular dysfunction, which is not measured by creatinine clearance, may account for this disparity. A small test dose of methotrexate can accurately predict the kinetics and steady-state concentration of a high-dose infusion.[567] Optimal management dictates that each course of high-dose methotrexate be closely monitored by following renal function and plasma methotrexate concentration to determine the dose and duration of leucovorin rescue.

Penetration of systemically administered methotrexate into CSF is only 3% in patients without meningeal tumor spread[568,569] but is 20% in patients with leptomeningeal carcinomatosis.[569] At infusion rates exceeding 3,500 mg/m^2 over 24 hours, the CSF methotrexate concentration is typically >1 μM[569]; and high-dose methotrexate infusion regimens are effective for treating and preventing leptomeningeal leukemia.[570]

Toxicity

The primary toxic effects of methotrexate are myelosuppression and orointestinal mucositis, which occur 5 to 14 days after the dose. The development of toxic reactions is related to the concentration of drug and the duration of exposure.[522,524,565] In patients receiving a 6-hour infusion of methotrexate, a 48-hour methotrexate concentration above 1 μM was associated with the development of significant toxicity.[565] These toxicities can be prevented by administration of leucovorin. With the use of therapeutic drug monitoring and continuation of leucovorin rescue until plasma methotrexate concentration has fallen below 0.05 to 0.1 μM, the toxicity of high-dose methotrexate can be avoided in most patients.[522,524] Despite these measures, however, nephrotoxicity still occurs in almost 2% of patients receiving HDMTX infusions.[571]

Nephrotoxicity observed with high-dose methotrexate can delay methotrexate clearance and markedly intensify the drug's other toxic effects.[572,573] An early rise in serum creatinine (1.5 times baseline) within the initial 24 hours can help identify a population of patients at increased risk for delayed MTX elimination.[574] The renal damage may be related to precipitation of methotrexate or 7-hydroxy-methotrexate in acidic urine or to direct toxic effects on the renal tubule.[524,573]

Aggressive hydration and alkalinization[575] as well as increasing the sodium content of the hydration fluids[576] can prevent drug precipitation and result in enhanced excretion of MTX.

The development of renal dysfunction during high-dose methotrexate is a medical emergency. Patients must be closely monitored and the leucovorin dose increased in proportion to the plasma methotrexate concentration.[577] Hemodialysis and charcoal hemoperfusion have not proved useful for drug removal in patients with renal dysfunction,[578–580] unless they are used repeatedly.[581] The investigational drug glucarpidase (carboxypeptidase-G$_2$), a recombinant bacterial enzyme that catabolizes methotrexate to the inactive metabolite, 4-amino-4-deoxy-N^{10}-methylpteroic acid,[582] rescues patients who develop methotrexate nephrotoxicity by providing an alternative route of elimination.[120,583] Glucarpidase is well tolerated and results in a 95.6% to 99.6% reduction in plasma methotrexate concentrations within minutes. Unlike dialysis, there is minimal rebound of plasma drug concentrations after glucarpidase.[584]

Hepatic toxicity consisting of transient elevations of serum transaminase and, less commonly, hyperbilirubinemia, has been associated with standard and high doses of methotrexate but is more common and more severe with high-dose therapy. Hepatic fibrosis has been observed primarily in patients receiving chronic low-dose methotrexate.[549,585] Other side effects include a dermatitis characterized by erythema and desquamation, allergic reactions, and acute pneumonitis.[585–587] Methotrexate osteopathy is a cumulative toxicity that causes bone pain, osteoporosis, and an increased risk for fractures. Neurotoxicity from high-dose methotrexate includes an acute, stroke-like encephalopathy, seizures, and chronic leukoencephalopathy, particularly in association with cranial irradiation.[268,588–591]

Resistance

Mechanisms of resistance to methotrexate identified experimentally include decreased membrane transport, increased levels of the target enzyme DHFR, altered affinity of DHFR for methotrexate, decreased polyglutamation of methotrexate, and decreased thymidylate synthase activity.[524,527,592] Increases in target enzyme levels have been associated with amplification of gene encoding for DHFR, a phenomenon that has also been documented in lymphoblasts from patients whose disease was clinically resistant to methotrexate.[524,593,594] Flow cytometric analysis of lymphoblasts from 29 children with newly diagnosed and relapsed ALL demonstrated heterogeneous expression of elevated DHFR in 11 of 29 specimens and impaired methotrexate transport in 3 of 29 specimens.[595] Newly diagnosed patients whose marrow specimens contained DHFR overproducing subpopulations of lymphoblasts had shorter remission durations than comparable patients whose lymphoblasts only expressed lower DHFR levels. Impaired methotrexate uptake and decreased expression of the reduced folate carrier (the membrane transport protein involved in cellular uptake of methotrexate) appears to occur frequently in osteosarcoma.[596–598] Although inactivating reduced folate carrier mutations do not appear to be a major mechanism of MTX resistance in ALL,[599] a case-control study of gene expression in children with ALL has found an association between higher transcript levels of the human reduced folate carrier gene (heft) and relapse.[600]

Drug Interactions

Several drugs have been associated with increased in toxicity when coadministered with methotrexate.[75,132,133] The most significant interactions involve agents that interfere with methotrexate excretion, primarily by competing for renal tubular secretion. These drugs include probenecid, salicylates, sulfisoxazole, penicillins, ciprofloxacin; the nonsteroidal anti-inflammatory drugs such as indomethacin, ketoprofen, and ibuprofen; and the proton pump inhibitors such as omeprazole, rabeprazole, and pantoprazole.[75,132,601–607] Nephrotoxic drugs, such as the aminoglycosides, vancomycin and cisplatin, may also alter the clearance of methotrexate.[132,608] Pharmacodynamic interactions resulting in synergistic cytotoxic effects have been reported with methotrexate and fluorouracil or cytarabine.[609] The synergistic effects of methotrexate and asparaginase are sequence dependent: asparaginase administration should always follow methotrexate administration. Administering asparaginase prior to or concomitant with methotrexate can directly antagonize methotrexate's effectiveness.[527,610–612]

Thiopurines

Mercaptopurine and thioguanine are thiol-substituted derivatives of the naturally occurring purine bases hypoxanthine and guanine (Fig. 10.15). Mercaptopurine has been used in the treatment of ALL for five decades, primarily for the maintenance of remission. It is also used in the treatment of chronic myelogenous leukemia, histiocytosis, and inflammatory bowel disease. In standard maintenance regimens, mercaptopurine is administered orally at a dose of 60 to 75 mg/m^2/day with upward or downward dose adjustments based on the degree of myelosuppression. Ensuring that patients are receiving their MTD of mercaptopurine appears to be an important factor in the outcome for children with ALL.[38] In a retrospective analysis, when the actual dose of mercaptopurine received increased by 22% as a result of more aggressive prescribing guidelines, the relapse-free survival improved by 18%.[613] Although high-dose intravenous infusions of mercaptopurine (1,000 mg/m^2 over 6 to 24 hours) have been evaluated as an approach to circumvent the pharmacokinetic limitations of oral dosing,[614–617] this route of administration does not offer an advantage over oral dosing in children with ALL.[618] Thioguanine is primarily used in the treatment of acute nonlymphocytic leukemia and is administered orally in doses of 75 to 100 mg/m^2 daily for 5 to 7 days or in doses of 40 to 60 mg/m^2 daily for more prolonged courses.

The thiopurines are prodrugs that must be converted intracellularly to thioguanine nucleotides to exert a cytotoxic effect. The metabolic pathways for activation of mercaptopurine and thioguanine are outlined in Fig. 10.16. The active intracellular metabolites are phosphorylated thioguanine nucleotides, which inhibit *de novo* purine synthesis and purine interconversion and are incorporated into DNA.[619,620] Incorporation of thioguanosine into DNA appears to be the critical determinant of thiopurine cytotoxicity,[621] but there is evidence that for mercaptopurine methylated metabolites also appear to contribute to its overall antiproliferative effects.[622] Thioguanine is 10-fold more potent and less schedule dependent than mercaptopurine against lymphoblastic leukemia cell lines and lymphoblasts from patients with ALL *in vitro*,[623] and can achieve cytotoxic drug concentrations within the CSF with oral dosing.[624] Despite preliminary clinical data suggesting an advantage to thioguanine over mercaptopurine for the treatment of children with ALL,[625] randomized clinical trials failed to demonstrate an overall event-free survival advantage.[626–628]

Biotransformation

The thiopurines are extensively metabolized *in vivo* to active and inactive metabolites (Fig. 10.16).[621,629–632] The activation pathway for thioguanine, which is converted to the nucleotide

thioguanosine monophosphate in a single step, is more direct than that for mercaptopurine, which undergoes a three-step conversion to the thioguanine nucleotide. The primary degradative pathway for mercaptopurine is conversion to the inactive metabolite thiouric acid by the enzyme xanthine oxidase. The oxidation of thioguanine to thiouric acid follows a different metabolic pathway. Thioguanine is initially converted by aldehyde oxidase to 8-hydroxy-thioguanine, which is the primary circulating metabolite of thioguanine.[632,633]

The thiopurines are also subject to S-methylation by the enzyme thiopurine methyltransferase (TPMT).[634] The level of intracellular TPMT activity is an important determinant of the availability of thiopurines for conversion to active thioguanine nucleotides, and as a result, TPMT regulates the cytotoxic effect of these thiopurines.[635] The activity of this enzyme is controlled by a common genetic polymorphism, resulting in a trifocal distribution of intracellular enzyme levels (Fig. 10.17).[621,635] One in 300 patients are deficient of TPMT activity and extremely sensitive to the cytotoxic effects of mercaptopurine, thioguanine, and azathioprine. TMPT activity is also inversely related to the erythrocyte thioguanine nucleotide concentration and the severity of neutropenia, suggesting that TPMT modulates the cytotoxic effect of mercaptopurine.[636]

It is well known that differences in TPMT activity alone cannot account for the wide interpatient variation observed in thiopurine disposition and effect. Of the other enzymes involved in thiopurine metabolism, there is conflicting data as to whether polymorphisms in inosine triphosphate pyrophosphatase (ITPA), which catalyzes conversion of inosine triphosphate (ITP) to inosine monophasophatae (IMP) and hence thiol-ITP to thiol-IMP, can contribute to observed variations in thiopurine pharmacology.[637–642] A recent study in children with ALL has found that children with a polymorphic variation in ITPA accumulate higher concentrations of methylated mercaptopurine metabolites than children with the normal variant.[643]

Pharmacokinetics

The bioavailability of oral mercaptopurine is less than 20% and the resulting plasma drug concentrations are highly variable (Fig. 10.16).[72,644–646] Only one-third of patients achieve plasma concentrations of mercaptopurine above 1 μM.[644] With oral doses ranging from 65 to 85 mg/m^2, the median peak plasma concentration was 0.59 μM (range, 0.13 to 2.3 μM) and the median AUC was 1.8 μM × hr (range, 0.39 to 4.8 μM × hr).[72] Plasma mercaptopurine AUC is not predictive of erythrocyte thioguanine nucleotide concentrations.[72] Significant intrapatient variability has also been observed in patients monitored after multiple doses over the course of maintenance therapy.[72] The bioavailability of mercaptopurine is limited by the extensive first-pass metabolism of the drug by xanthine oxidase in the liver and intestinal mucosa. When mercaptopurine is coadministered with the xanthine oxidase inhibitor allopurinol, the fraction of the dose absorbed increases fivefold.[647]

The bioavailability of oral thioguanine is also poor, and plasma concentrations are variable, with a 30- to 50-fold range in peak plasma concentration and AUC.[624,648,649] The mean (± SD) peak plasma concentration was 0.46 ± 0.68 μM and the AUC ranged from 0.18 to 9.5 μM × hr.[624] The bioavailability was diminished further in nonfasting patients and patients experiencing nausea and vomiting.[649] Plasma thioguanine AUC after an oral dose did not correlate with erythrocyte thioguanine nucleotide concentrations,[624] and although food may incrementally decrease the absorption of the drug, it does not appear to have any impact on the overall accumulation of thioguanine nucleotides.[650]

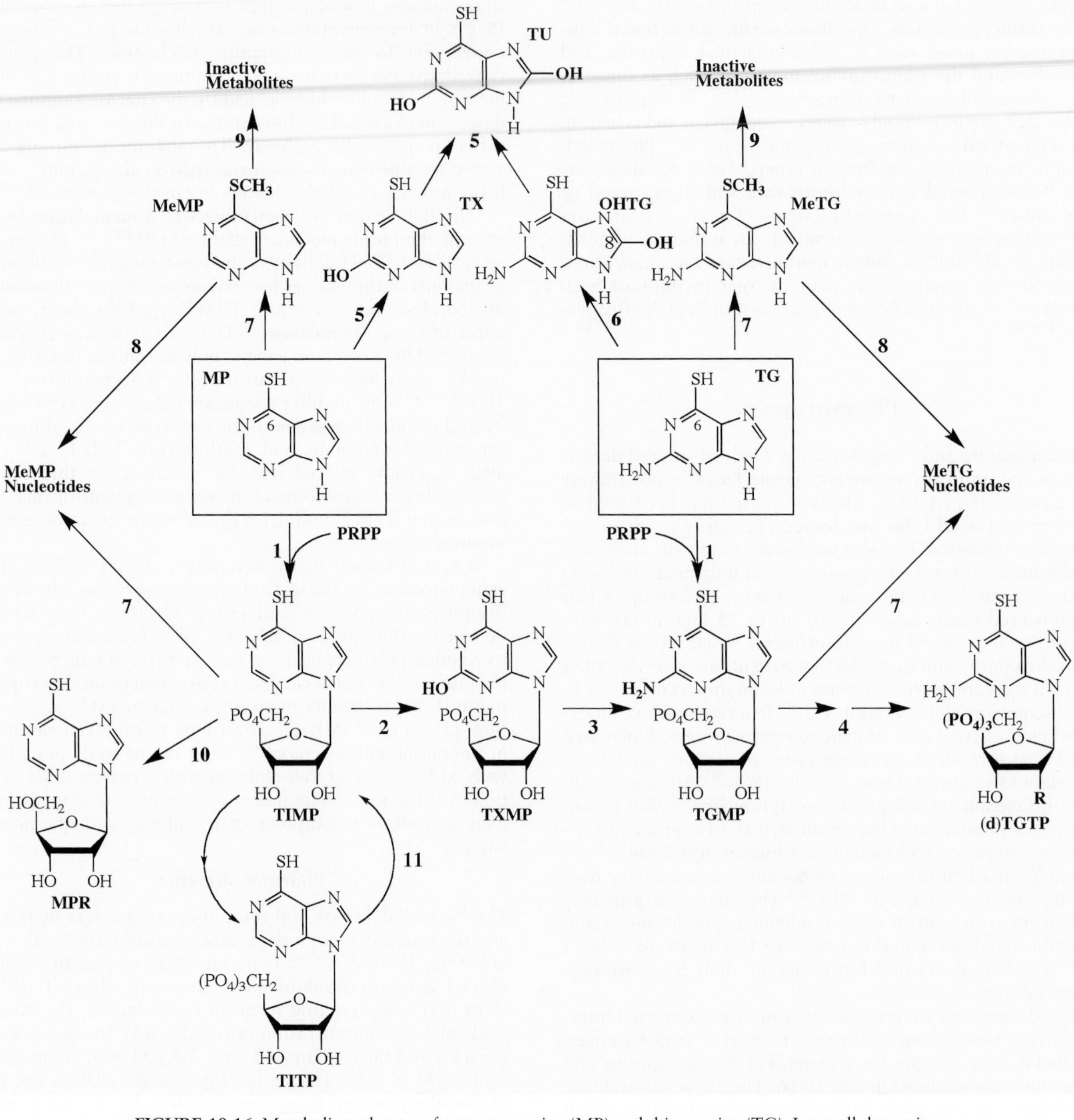

FIGURE 10.16 Metabolic pathways of mercaptopurine (MP) and thioguanine (TG). Intracellular activation of these prodrugs involves conversion to thioguanine nucleotides. For mercaptopurine, this is a three-step process, starting with conversion to thioinosine monophosphate (TIMP), catalyzed by the enzyme hypoxanthine-guanine phosphoribosyl transferase or HGPRT (1). Phosphoribosylpyrophosphate (PRPP) is a required cofactor in this reaction. TIMP is converted to thioxanthosine monophosphate (TXMP) by inosine monophosphate dehydrogenase (2) and then to thioguanine monophosphate (TGMP) by guanosine monophosphate synthetase (3). Thioguanine is converted directly to TGMP by HGPRT. TGMP is phosphorylated by kinases to TGTP (R = OH) and converted to the deoxyribonucleotide dTGTP (R = H) by ribonucleotide reductase (4). dTGTP can then be incorporated into DNA (not shown). There are competing catabolic pathways for the thiopurines, including oxidation to the inactive metabolite, thiouric acid (TU). For MP, this is catalyzed in a two-step reaction by xanthine oxidase (5). The initial oxidation step from TG to 8-hydroxy-thioguanine (OHTG) is catalyzed by aldehyde oxidase (6). The thiopurines also undergo S-methylation, catalyzed by thiopurine methyltransferase or TPMT (7). Methylmercaptopurine (MeMP) and methylthioguanine (MeTG) can be converted to methylated thionucleotides along the same pathways as the parent drug (8). TPMT can also convert TIMP and TGMP to methylated thionucleotides. MeMP and MeTG can also be oxidized or desulfurated to inactivate metabolites (9). Dephosphorylation of TIMP to mercaptopurine riboside is another inactivating step that is catalyzed by several intracellular enzymes (10). Inosine triphosphate pyrophosphatase (ITPA) catalyzes thiol-ITP back to thiol-IMP (11).

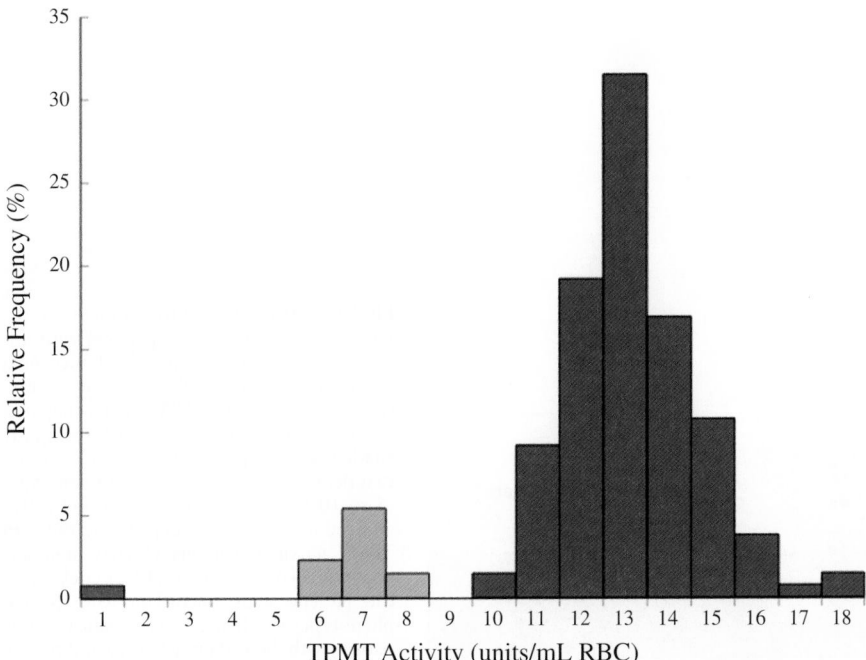

FIGURE 10.17 Frequency distribution histogram of erythrocyte thiopurine methyltransferase (TPMT) activity in 130 unrelated control children, demonstrating a trimodal distribution resulting from a genetic polymorphism (i.e., a low activity allele, TPML, and a high activity allele, TPMTH, at a single genetic locus). One in 300 subjects are TPMT deficient (TPMTL/TPMTL genotype), 11% have intermediate activity (TPMTH/TPMT genotype), and 89% have high activity (TPMTH/TPMTH genotype). Within the predominant high-activity population, there is a wide range of TPMT activity. (Data from Lennard L, Lilleyman JS, Van Loon J, et al. Genetic variation in response to 6-mercaptopurine for childhood acute lymphoblastic leukaemia. Lancet 1990;336:225.)

Erythrocyte levels of thiopurine-derived thioguanine nucleotides have been monitored in children receiving oral therapy. As with plasma concentrations of the parent drug, the erythrocyte metabolite levels are highly variable.[72] Erythrocyte thioguanine nucleotide levels have been correlated with the degree of myelosuppression and the risk of relapse.[651–653] Children with ALL whose erythrocyte thioguanine nucleotide levels were below the median value of 284 pmol/8 $\times$ 10^8 erythrocytes had a twofold higher relapse rate than patients with values above the median.[652,653] However, the differences in erythrocyte thioguanine nucleotide levels in the remission and relapse patients were small, and the range of values overlapped completely (100 to 1,300 pmol/8 $\times$ 10^8 RBC in remission patients and 100 to 800 pmol/8 $\times$ 10^8 RBC in relapsed patients).[652,653] In other studies, no relationship was found between thioguanine nucleotide levels and outcome.[38,72] Erythrocyte thioguanine nucleotide levels in patients receiving daily oral thioguanine are fivefold higher than nucleotide metabolite levels from mercaptopurine therapy,[624,654–656] but differences in leukocyte concentrations of thioguanine nucleotide are less marked.[657]

Toxicity

The common toxic effects of mercaptopurine include myelosuppression, hepatic dysfunction (elevated transaminases, cholestatic jaundice), and mucositis. Myelosuppression is the primary toxic effect of thioguanine. Thioguanine has also been associated with a reversible form of VOD.[625,626,658,659] The long-term outcome for children with leukemia who develop thioguanine-induced VOD has not been determined, but a subset of children appears at risk for developing portal hypertension.[660]

Pharmacogenetics

The molecular basis for polymorphic TPMT activity has been defined,[661] with at least 22 functional variant alleles being described (Fig. 10.18).[662,663] These alleles contain single nucleotide polymorphisms (SNPs) leading to substitution, premature stop codons, or destruction of a splice site. The TPMT*3C, *3A, and *2 account for more than 95% of inher-

ited deficiency.[664] In children who are homozygous TPMT deficient, even a short course of thiopurine administration can result in profound myelosuppression, and erythrocyte thioguanine nucleotide levels in these TPMT-deficient patients are markedly elevated.[665–667] Very low doses of mercaptopurine (5% to 10% of the standard dose) are tolerable in TPMT-deficient patients.[664,666–668] The 11% of patients who are heterozygous at the TPMT locus and have intermediate enzyme activity levels require more frequent mercaptopurine dose reductions for toxicity than homozygous patients with full enzyme activity.[669] In children with ALL, the risk of relapse appears to be related to TPMT, with a lower rate of relapse observed in heterozygotes.[670] Although studies have suggested that children with diminished TPMT activity are at increased risk for developing secondary brain tumors or myeloid leukemias,[670–673] this finding has not been uniformly observed.[674]

Drug Interactions

The classic example of a drug interaction in cancer chemotherapy is the effect of the xanthine oxidase inhibitor allopurinol on the catabolism of mercaptopurine to thiouric acid. When these two agents are administered concurrently, the hematological toxicity of mercaptopurine is significantly enhanced.[675] Allopurinol pretreatment results in a fivefold increase in bioavailability of the oral dose of mercaptopurine,[647] and thus the mercaptopurine dose should be reduced by 75% when coadministered with allopurinol. Because the first step in the oxidation of thioguanine is catalyzed by aldehyde oxidase rather than xanthine oxidase, the coadministration of allopurinol and thioguanine does not require a dose modification. Methotrexate and folates also inhibit xanthine oxidase, and methotrexate can minimally enhance mercaptopurine bioavailability.[676,677]

Deoxyadenosine Analogs

Fludarabine, cladribine, and clofarabine (Fig. 10.15) are analogs of deoxyadenosine and are examples of agents

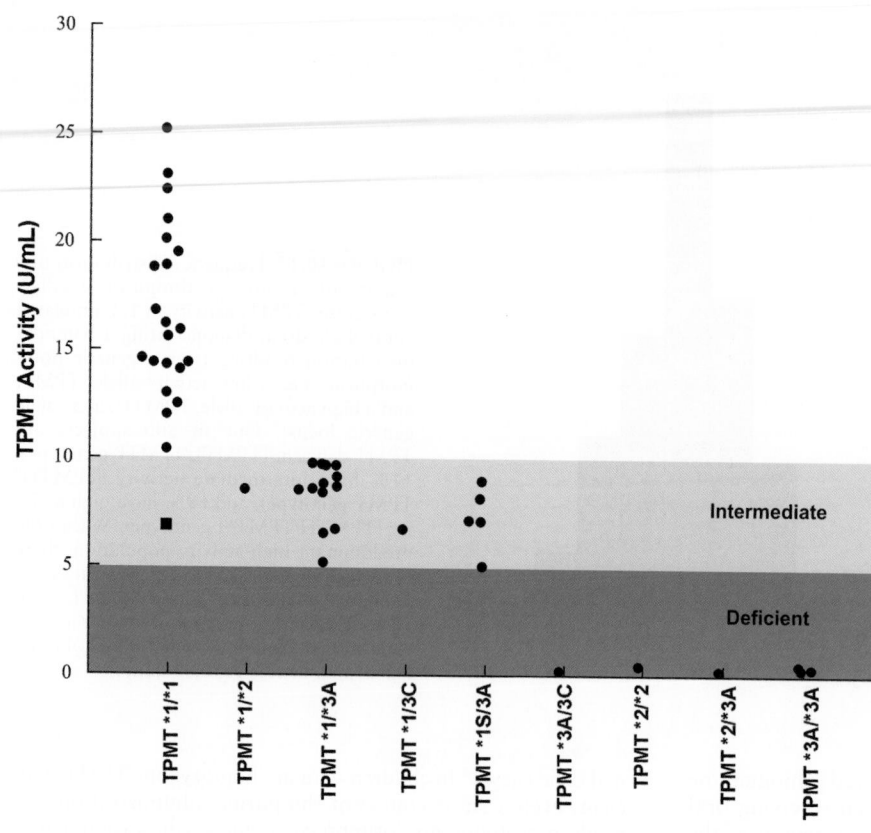

FIGURE 10.18 Thiopurine S-methyltransferase (TPMT) activity in patients with different genotypes. The heavily shaded area depicts the range of TPMT activity in erythrocytes that defines TPMT deficiency (<5 U/mL of packed red blood cells), the lightly shaded area depicts intermediate activity that defines TPMT heterozygous phenotypes (5 to 10 U/mL of packed red blood cells), and the unshaded area depicts the range of TPMT activity in patients who have homozygous wild-type phenotypes. Black circles indicate patients with concordant genotype and phenotype; the black square indicates one patient with discordant genotype and phenotype. (Reprinted from Yates CR, Krynetski EY, Loennechen T, et al. Molecular diagnosis of thiopurine S-methyltransferase deficiency: genetic basis for azathioprine and mercaptopurine intolerance. Ann Intern Med 1997; 126(8):608–614, with permission.)

originally developed through rational drug design based on the observation that patients with adenosine deaminase (ADA) deficiency accumulate deoxyadenosine, which is directly cytotoxic to lymphocytes. The deoxyadenosine analogs have proven particularly useful in adult patients with chronic lymphocytic leukemias; these drugs also have varying degrees of activity in childhood acute leukemias. These drugs are prodrugs that undergo deoxycytidine kinase catalyzed activation to the triphosphate form. The deoxyadenosine analogs inhibit DNA synthesis via inhibition of DNA polymerase and ribonucleotide reductase and via incorporation into DNA.

Fludarabine (Fig. 10.15) was originally developed to circumvent the rapid deamination of the antiviral agent, vidarabine (ara-A), by the ubiquitous enzyme, ADA. Poor solubility of the nucleoside led to synthesis of fludarabine phosphate (9-β-D-arabinofuranosyl-2-fluoroadenine monophosphate, F-ara-AMP). After intravenous administration, fludarabine phosphate is rapidly converted to fludarabine (F-ara-A). F-ara-A has a variable half-life in adults, ranging from 6 to 30 hours, and is primarily excreted unchanged in the urine.[678,679] With conventional fludarabine phosphate doses, myelosuppression and immunosuppression are dose limiting. At high doses, irreversible neurotoxicity can be observed, manifested as cortical blindness, optic neuritis, encephalopathy, and seizures.[680] In children with solid tumors, dose-limiting myelosuppression was observed when fludarabine phosphate was administered as an 8 mg/m² loading dose followed by a continuous infusion of 23.5 mg/m²/day for 5 days,[681,682] similar to the MTD in adult patients treated on a daily × 5 schedule.[683,684] Plasma steady-state concentrations of F-ara-A increase in proportion to the dose. Continuous infusion of 30.5 mg/m²/day achieves a steady-state plasma concentration of 7.2 μM. The terminal half-life of F-ara-A in children averages 12 hours.

Synergy with cytarabine occurs via fludarabine potentiation of intracellular phosphorylation of cytarabine and more rapid accumulation of ara-CTP,[685–687] a finding that has been the basis for a number of regimens that combine these agents in the treatment of leukemias.[688–690] In addition, because of its profound immunosuppressive effects, fludarabine phosphate is used as a component of transplant conditioning regimens, particularly in reduced intensity conditioning regimens.[691]

Another deoxyadenosine analog developed that demonstrated substantial clinical activity was cladribine (Fig. 10.15), which at low doses is particularly active in adult patients with hairy cell leukemia. In children with AML, administration of two courses of high dose (8.9 mg/m²/day for 5 days courses) of cladribine (2-CdA) results in a 40% rate of complete remissions.[692–694] Myelosuppression and immunosuppression are the dose-limiting toxicities, and opportunistic infections occur in 15% to 40% of patients.[695–697] The pharmacokinetics of cladribine have been studied in children treated with 8.9 mg/m²/day administered by continuous infusion for 5 consecutive days.[698] At steady state, 2-CdA has a relatively large volume of distribution (357 L/m²) and an average clearance of 39 L/hr/m². The CSF to plasma drug concentration ratio averages 18%. The terminal half-life in children, 20 hours, appears longer than the 7 hours observed in adult patients,[699] but drug clearances are similar in both populations. Cladribine is resistant to deamination by ADA and renal clearance accounts for 50% of total clearance.

In an effort to further increase the acid stability and improve the solubility of deoxyadenosine analogs, clofarabine (Fig. 10.15) was developed. The drug has been studied on a daily × 5-day schedule with reversible hepatotoxicity being the primary dose-limiting toxicity in adult patients.[700] At a dose of 40 mg/m², median plasma concentration achieved was 1.5 μM; plasma concentrations and intracellular triphosphate concentrations increase in proportion to dose administered.[701]

In children with the leukemia, hepatotoxicity and skin rash were dose limiting resulting in a MTD of 52 mg/m²/day × 5 days. In children treated at the MTD, the median plasma clofarabine concentration at the end of a 1-hour infusion was 1.1 μM (range, 0.4 to 2.3 μM).[702] In a pediatric phase II trial, 12 of 61 children (20%) with refractory ALL achieved a complete response (5 without platelet recovery).[703] The most commonly reported adverse events included hypokalemia, hepatic dysfunction, and infections, with grade 3 or more infections occurring in approximately 70% of children including 20% who developed sepsis or shock. In a pediatric phase II trials of children with AML, only 1 of 42 children achieved a complete remission, although an additional subset was able to proceed to transplant.[704]

Nelarabine

Nelarabine is a water-soluble prodrug of arabinofuranosyl-guanine (ara-G). In the presence of ADA, nelarabine is demethoxylated to ara-G, which is subsequently catabolized intracellularly to a cytotoxic metabolite, ara-GTP.[705] Initial phase I and II trials have focused on patients with T-cell malignancies due to the enhanced accumulation of ara-GTP in T versus B lymphoblasts.[706–708] These studies showed that nelarabine had antitumor activity in patients with recurrent or refractory T-cell malignancies with a response rate of more than 50% for children with T-cell leukemia in first relapse.[709,710]

Nelarabine is generally administered at doses of 400 to 650 mg/m² as a 1-hour infusion daily for 5 consecutive days every 3 weeks. In a phase II trial of 121 children and young adults, the overall response rate at all dose levels was 33%, with a CR + PR rate of 27% of patients in second or subsequent relapse treated at the 650 mg/m²/day dose level.[711] Eighteen percent of patients experience grade 3 or more neurotoxicity, primarily in the form of reversible somnolence and peripheral neuropathy. Severe CNS toxicities associated with nelarabine, although rare, include a Guillan-Barre–like ascending paralysis. The plasma C_{max} and AUC of nelarabine and ara-G increase linearly with dose. The elimination of both agents is monoexponential.[712] The clearance of ara-G is somewhat higher in children versus adults (0.3 L/hr/kg vs. 0.2 L/hr/kg) with a corresponding shorter half-life in children versus adults (2.1 hours vs. 3.0 hours).[712]

Pyrimidine Analogs

Cytarabine

Cytarabine (cytosine arabinoside, ara-C), an arabinose nucleoside analog of deoxycytidine (Fig. 10.14), is active in the treatment of the acute leukemias and lymphoma. After intracellular metabolic activation, cytarabine interferes with DNA replication and repair through inhibition of DNA polymerase and through incorporation into DNA.[713–715] Depending on the dose and schedule of cytarabine used, incorporation into DNA is thought to inhibit chain elongation, result in chain termination or reinitiation at sites of previously replicated segments, or cause DNA strand breaks.[713,714] Inhibition of DNA synthesis or incorporation into DNA by ara-CTP can only occur during the DNA synthesis phase (S phase) of the cell cycle, and more prolonged exposure to cytarabine allows the drug to be incorporated into a larger fraction of the cells as they pass through S phase. Cytarabine incorporation into DNA may also be enhanced by timed re-treatment with cytarabine after recruitment of leukemic cells into an active

phase of DNA synthesis after the first treatment cycle and the simultaneous administration of cytarabine and colony-stimulating factors, which stimulate leukemic cells into S phase.[716–719]

A wide range of doses and schedules for cytarabine has been employed. The standard dose is 100 to 200 mg/m² as a bolus injection every 12 hours or by continuous infusion, and it is usually administered daily for 5 to 7 days. High-dose regimens (3 g/m² every 12 hours for 4 to 12 doses or as a continuous infusion) have also been used with the intention of overcoming resistance mechanisms.[720,721] Low-dose cytarabine regimens (5 to 20 mg/m²/day over several weeks) are used for the treatment of myelodysplastic syndromes.[722]

Biotransformation. After entering cells by the carrier-mediated nucleoside transport system, cytarabine is converted to the active nucleotide, ara-C triphosphate (ara-CTP), by three sequential phosphorylations catalyzed by intracellular kinases.[723,724] Ara-CTP then competes with the natural substrate deoxycytidine triphosphate (dCTP) for DNA replicative and repair enzymes. Cytarabine and ara-CMP can also be catabolized to the inactive by-products uridine arabinoside (ara-U) and ara-UMP by deaminases that are present in high concentrations within cells.[725,726] Cytidine deaminase is a ubiquitous enzyme, and the catabolism of cytarabine to ara-U is the primary route of elimination for the drug. Alterations in these uptake and metabolic pathways within the cancer cell can result in drug resistance, such as a decrease in membrane transport, a decrease in activation by deoxycytidine kinase, an increase in degradation by cytidine deaminase, and an increase in the competing natural substrate, dCTP.[713,720,724]

Pharmacokinetics. The pharmacokinetic behavior of cytarabine is directly related to the activity of the major degradative enzyme, cytidine deaminase. The bioavailability of oral cytarabine is less than 20% because of extensive presystemic metabolism by high levels of this enzyme in gastrointestinal epithelium and liver.[727] The hepatic extraction ratio for cytarabine is estimated to be as high as 80%.[728] Subcutaneously injected cytarabine is completely absorbed.[727]

Drug elimination is rapid with intravenous dosing. Total clearance is 1,000 mL/min/m² or greater, and the postdistributive half-life is 2 to 3 hours.[721,726,727,729,730] Metabolism to ara-U accounts for 80% to 90% of total cytarabine clearance, and renal clearance accounts for less than 10% of total clearance. The ara-U formed is excreted in the urine. Because of the ubiquity of cytidine deaminase (e.g., liver, gastrointestinal tract, plasma, leukocytes), hepatic dysfunction does not significantly alter the rate of elimination of cytarabine. With high-dose prolonged intravenous infusions, the mean steady-state plasma concentration of cytarabine was 5 μM at a dose of 2 g/m²/day, and the steady-state concentration of ara-U was 10-fold higher (60 μM).[721] In these patients, plasma clearance appeared to decrease with increasing dose, suggesting saturation of deaminases at the higher dose levels.[721,731] In children receiving an infusion of 5 g/m²/day, total clearance was 555 mL/min/m²,[731] and at steady state, ara-U plasma concentrations are more than 10-fold higher than steady-state cytarabine concentrations in children.[732]

The pharmacokinetics of cellular ara-CTP, the active intracellular metabolite of cytarabine, has been characterized in the leukemic blasts from patients receiving high-dose cytarabine. After a 3 g/m² dose administered as a short infusion, there was considerable interpatient variability in the amount of ara-CTP accumulated in blasts. However, there was no correlation between the pharmacokinetics of the parent drug in plasma and the cellular concentrations of ara-CTP in leukemic blasts.[733,734] Patients responding to the drug had a significantly slower rate of elimination of ara-CTP. The half-life of ara-CTP was 5.6 hours in responding patients and 3.2 hours in resistant patients. Responding patients also had significantly higher trough concentrations (196 μM vs. 23 μM).[733] This is consistent with earlier studies demonstrating greater *in vitro* ara-CTP formation in the leukemic blasts from patients achieving a complete remission on cytarabine therapy compared with nonresponders.[735] The pharmacokinetics of the active intracellular metabolite appears to be more predictive of outcome than plasma concentrations of the parent drug. The cellular retention of ara-CTP in leukemic blasts was shorter in blasts from patients with T-cell ALL and ANL compared with non–T-cell ALL.[736]

Pharmacogenetics. Population-specific variants may be an important determinant in susceptibility to cytarabine cytotoxicity. Based on results of an unbiased whole-genome approach in lymphoblastoid cell lines, unique pharmacogenetic signatures of 4 SNPs in persons of European ancestry and of 5 SNPs in persons of African ancestry explain more than half of the variability in sensitivity to this agent.[737] Likewise, results of gene sequencing studies have shown that genetic polymorphisms in deoxycytidine kinase, the rate-limiting enzyme in the activation of pyrimidine analogs such as cytarabine, may impact the levels of the active (triphosphate) form of the parent drug.[738] Further functional studies to validate these findings are required.

Toxicity. The primary toxicities of cytarabine are myelosuppression, nausea and vomiting, and gastrointestinal mucosal damage, including life-threatening bowel necrosis.[724,739–741] A syndrome of high fever, malaise, myalgias, joint or bone pain, skin rash, conjunctivitis, and chest pain has also been reported in children receiving cytarabine.[742] Coadministration of corticosteroids appears to relieve these symptoms. Neurotoxicity from cytarabine has been primarily associated with high-dose therapy.[268,743–746] The most common manifestation of neurotoxicity is an acute cerebellar syndrome manifesting 3 to 8 days after initiation of therapy, but seizures and encephalopathy have also been reported.[268,745] Nystagmus, ataxia, dysarthria, dysmetria, and dysdiadochokinesia are the classic cerebellar manifestations. In most cases, these neurologic symptoms resolve within a week, but as many as 30% of patients do not regain full cerebellar function.[268,745] Neuropathological findings include loss of Purkinje cells and a reactive gliosis in the cerebellum. In addition to dose, other risk factors for the development neurotoxicity include advanced age and hepatic or renal dysfunction.[745,747–749] Lowering the dose of cytarabine from 3,000 to 2,000 mg/m² and administering the drug daily instead of every 12 hours is recommended for patients with renal dysfunction.[749] The drug should be immediately withdrawn if nystagmus or ataxia occurs. Skin and ocular toxic effects have also been observed on high-dose regimens.[741]

Gemcitabine

Gemcitabine (dFdC, Gemzar), a difluorinated analog of deoxycytidine (Fig. 10.14), is approved for use as frontline therapy for adult patients with pancreatic cancer and in combination with cisplatin for patients with non–small cell lung cancer.[750] In contrast to cytarabine, gemcitabine has activity against a wide range of solid tumors including breast cancer, bladder carcinoma, ovarian cancer, head and neck cancer, testicular carcinoma, and a variety of sarcomas.[751–756] Although gemcitabine has activity against leukemia and non-Hodgkin lymphoma in adults,[757] it is not active in children with recurrent or refractory leukemias.[758,759] Likewise, gemcitabine as a single agent does not have a clearly defined role in the treatment of childhood solid tumors; at low doses, objective antitumor activity was not observed in tumors of mesenchymal or embryonic origin.[758] In combination with vinorelbine, there is substantial antitumor activity in recurrent Hodgkin lymphoma,[760] and in combination with docetaxel, there is modest antitumor activity in refractory sarcomas of bone.[761]

Similar to cytarabine, gemcitabine is a prodrug that requires intracellular activation by deoxycytidine kinase for its cytotoxic effects. Gemcitabine diphosphate (dFdCDP) inhibits ribonucleotide reductase, and gemcitabine triphosphate (dFdCTP) inhibits DNA polymerase. Intracellular drug concentrations of cells exposed to equimolar concentrations of gemcitabine and cytarabine are up to 20-fold higher for gemcitabine.[762] The intracellular half-life of dFdCTP is 16 hours, which is significantly longer than of ara-CTP (0.7 hours).[762] Gemcitabine is an S phase cell cycle–specific agent that causes cells to accumulate at the G_1-S phase boundary. Gemcitabine is converted by cytidine deaminase to an inactive Uri dine metabolite, dFdU.

The most commonly used dose of gemcitabine is 1,000 mg/m² administered as a 30-minute infusion weekly × 3 weeks every 28 days. However, in one study comparing a standard dosing regimen (2,200 mg/m² over 30 minutes, weekly × 3 every 28 days) with a fixed dose rate infusion regimen (10 mg/m²/min over 150 minutes, weekly × 3 every 28 days), there was a statistically significant increase in median survival for patients who received the fixed dose rate infusion.[763] Furthermore, there was a twofold increase in intracellular gemcitabine triphosphate concentrations for patients receiving the fixed dose rate versus the standard dose.[763] In children with solid tumors, the MTD of gemcitabine administered weekly × 3 weeks was 1,200 mg/m²/dose.[764] In children with relapsed or refractory leukemia, the MTD of gemcitabine was 3,600 mg/m² administered over 6 hours, weekly × 3, every 28 days.[765]

Pharmacokinetic data from one trial suggest that gemcitabine clearance in children may be dose dependent.[764] However, in adults, there is no evidence of dose-dependent clearance over a wide dosage range (53 to 2,500 mg/m²/dose).[750,766] Pharmacokinetic parameters in children and adults are otherwise similar. The half-life and volume of distribution are schedule dependent. In children receiving a 30-minute infusion, the half-life is 14 minutes, whereas in children receiving a 6-hour infusion, the terminal half-life is 62 minutes. Clearance in children is approximately 2.2 L/min/m².[764,765] The volume of distribution is greater with longer infusion durations. The elimination half-life for the inactive deaminated metabolite, dFdU, is approximately 650 minutes. Mild-to-moderate renal insufficiency does not appear to have a significant impact on the pharmacokinetics of gemcitabine.[767]

The primary toxicities associated with gemcitabine administration include myelosuppression, nausea, vomiting, increased serum transaminases, fatigue, fever, diarrhea, mucositis, flu-like symptoms, rash, swelling, and alopecia.[765,766,768] Rarely, gemcitabine may cause somnolence, hypotension, severe pulmonary toxicity, or a thrombotic microangiopathy.[764,765,769,770] Gemcitabine has also been implicated in cases of radiation recall involving the skin and internal organs.[771]

Fluorouracil

The fluorinated pyrimidine fluorouracil (Fig. 10.14) is one of the few rationally designed anticancer drugs. It has been widely used in the treatment of carcinomas of the gastrointestinal tract, breast, ovary, and head and neck, but its use in children, in general, is limited to germ cell and hepatic tumors. Fluorouracil is administered intravenously as a bolus injection

(500 mg/m^2), usually on a daily-for-5-days schedule, or as a continuous infusion (800 to 1,200 mg/m^2 over 24 hours). Protracted low-dose infusional fluorouracil is also effective and well tolerated.[772,773]

Fluorouracil is a prodrug and must be converted intracellularly to nucleotides before expressing cytotoxicity.[774–776] There are several possible pathways for the anabolism of fluorouracil to active intracellular metabolites, and the relative importance of each pathway is tissue and tumor dependent.[777] The deoxyribonucleotides 5-FdUMP is a potent inhibitor of thymidylate synthase, leading to depletion of the DNA precursor, thymidine, and the ribonucleotide FUTP is incorporated into RNA. Inhibition of thymidylate synthase by FdUMP is thought to be the primary mechanism of action in most tumors.[778] Mechanisms of resistance to fluorouracil in preclinical models include an increase in intracellular catabolism by dihydropyrimidine dehydrogenase (DPD), a decrease in the activity of activating enzymes, and an increase in levels of the target enzyme thymidylate synthase.[779–781] A mutant thymidylate synthase with decreased affinity for FdUMP has also been described.[782]

Pharmacokinetics. Bioavailability of oral fluorouracil is highly variable, in part because of a saturable first-pass elimination process.[783,784] Because of this erratic absorption, fluorouracil should not be administered by the oral route, unless it is administered with agents, such as eniluracil,[785] which block the presystemic catabolism of fluorouracil and enhances its bioavailability. Bioavailable fluorouracil prodrugs, such as capecitabine and tegafur-uracil, have also been developed for oral administration. These agents are converted to fluorouracil after absorption and provide more prolonged drug exposure, similar to a prolonged intravenous infusion.[786–789] Subcutaneously administered fluorouracil is well tolerated and has nearly complete bioavailability.[790]

Fluorouracil is eliminated primarily by biotransformation. The degradative pathway is the same as that for the naturally occurring pyrimidines uracil and thymine.[775,785] Less than 10% of the drug is excreted unchanged in the urine. With standard bolus dosing, the elimination of fluorouracil is rapid. The half-life is 6 to 20 minutes, and total clearance is greater than 1,000 mL/min.[776,785,791,792] With a continuous infusion schedule, the pharmacokinetics differ significantly, with clearance values as high as 5,000 mL/min. In children treated with 80 mg/m^2/hr for 12 hours, the mean steady-state concentration of fluorouracil was 6.7 μM and the clearance was 2,500 mL/min/m^2.[793] This schedule-dependent clearance is consistent with a dose-dependent or saturable clearance process.[776,791,794,795] Although the liver is thought to be the principal site of drug catabolism, the high clearance values with infusions exceed the rate of hepatic blood flow, indicating that biotransformation must be taking place in other organs.[791]

Circadian dependency of fluorouracil toxicity appears to be related to rhythmic 3- to 25-fold fluctuations in plasma drug concentrations over the course of the day.[774,796–798] During a continuous intravenous infusion, the plasma fluorouracil concentrations were highest in the late morning and lowest shortly before midnight, and plasma concentrations of fluorouracil were inversely related to the activity of the catabolic enzyme, DPD, in peripheral blood mononuclear cells.[797,798] Adjustments in the dose or rate of fluorouracil infusion may be indicated based on the time of day the drug is being administered.[799,800]

Toxicity. The incidence and severity of clinical toxicities of fluorouracil depend on the dosing schedule. With intravenous bolus dosing, myelosuppression is the primary toxicity, but if the drug is given as a continuous infusion at doses up to 14,000 mg over 24 hours, myelosuppression is less prominent and stomatitis and diarrhea become dose limiting.[801] Protracted low-dose infusions can produce palmar-plantar dysesthesia (hand-foot syndrome). Reversible neurologic toxicity characterized by somnolence, cerebellar ataxia, and headache; ocular toxicity consisting of conjunctivitis and ectropion; dermatitis; and rarely cardiotoxicity, which can include chest pain, arrhythmias, and ischemic changes on ECG, are also reported.[774]

Pharmacogenetics. Inherited partial deficiency of the catabolic enzyme DPD in 1% to 3% of the population is associated with severe fluorouracil toxicity.[781,802–804] The intronic variant, *DPYD*2A*, which is associated with DPD deficiency has been found in approximately half of patients who develop severe neutropenia. In DPD-deficient patients, fluorouracil half-life is markedly prolonged with no evidence of drug catabolism.[803] Genetic polymorphisms in other genes that have been associated with fluorouracil-related treatment outcomes include thymidylate synthase, *TYMS*, and the methylenetetrahydrofolate reductase, *MTHGR* genes.[805–809]

Drug Interactions. Folates are required for the stable binding of 5-FdUMP to its target enzyme, thymidylate synthase, and the combination of leucovorin and fluorouracil is synergistic in experimental systems.[810] This combination has been studied in a large number of clinical trials primarily in adults with gastrointestinal tumors. In randomized clinical trials, the combination results in higher response rates than fluorouracil alone.[810] Pediatric trials of fluorouracil and leucovorin have failed to demonstrate substantial activity against sarcomas.[793,811]

ANTITUMOR ANTIBIOTICS

Most of the current antitumor antibiotics (Fig. 10.19) are natural products that were originally isolated from the microbial broth of a variety of species of the group of soil microorganisms, *Streptomyces*. The agents from this class of anticancer drugs that are used in the treatment of childhood cancers include the anthracyclines, mitoxantrone, dactinomycin, and bleomycin.

The antitumor antibiotics avidly bind to DNA by intercalation, in which a planar, multi-ring portion of the drug inserts between base pairs of the DNA double helix. The anthracyclines, mitoxantrone, and dactinomycin interfere with the topoisomerases, nuclear enzymes that regulate the three-dimensional shape of DNA by cleaving and relegating DNA during replication, transcription, repair, and recombination.

Anthracyclines

The anthracyclines, doxorubicin, daunomycin (daunorubicin), and idarubicin, are highly pigmented compounds composed of a planar tetracyclic anthraquinone nucleus linked to the amino sugar daunosamine (Fig. 10.19). Doxorubicin has a wide range of clinical activity against pediatric cancers, including the acute leukemias, lymphomas, sarcomas of soft tissue and bone, Wilms' tumor, neuroblastoma, and hepatoblastoma. The use of daunomycin and idarubicin is currently limited to the acute leukemias.

Several mechanisms for the antitumor activity of anthracyclines have been proposed.[812–817] These agents intercalate into DNA and induce topoisomerase II–mediated single- and double-strand breaks in DNA. Topoisomerase II–mediated DNA cleavage may also occur by nonintercalative mechanisms.[818]

manifested as the myocarditis-pericarditis syndrome, which in its severest form is characterized by the rapid onset of congestive failure associated with pericarditis.[866] In general, the acute asymptomatic cardiac changes are transient and do not prevent further use of anthracyclines.[818]

Chronic cardiomyopathy can be separated into an early form, which occurs during treatment or within 1 year of completing anthracyclines, and a late form, which occurs more than a year after completing anthracyclines.[863,867] The early form of cardiomyopathy is related to the cumulative dose of anthracyclines. The incidence of clinically apparent congestive heart failure starts increasing after cumulative doses exceed 450 mg/m^2 for doxorubicin and 700 mg/m^2 for daunomycin.[868,869] A maximum lifetime safe cumulative dose has not been defined for idarubicin, but cumulative doses of up to 150 mg/m^2 appear to be well tolerated.[870] Other factors that are reported to increase the risk for the development of a cardiomyopathy include a high dose rate (bolus or short infusion) of doxorubicin administration, prior or concurrent mediastinal irradiation, and preexisting cardiac disease. Children appear to be at higher risk for cardiac toxicity, and those younger than 5 years are at higher risk than older children.[859,871,872] Girls have a significantly higher incidence of abnormal cardiac findings at any given cumulative dose of doxorubicin than boys.[870,872,873] Lowering peak concentrations of anthracycline by administering the drugs on a lower-dose weekly schedule or by 6- to 96-hour continuous infusions appears to reduce the cardiotoxic effects in adults without compromising the antitumor effect.[823,826,874-876] However, prolonged infusions of anthracyclines and divided dosing schedules may not necessarily protect children from late cardiotoxicity.[867,877-879]

Late cardiotoxicity appears to be more common in children[880-883] than in adults and is characterized by a progressive decrease in fractional shortening, left ventricular mass and wall thickness relative to body size, and an increase in left ventricular afterload.[867,880] The probability of abnormal cardiac function is associated with young age at diagnosis, female gender, and cumulative doxorubicin dose.[872] The heart appears unable to grow in proportion to the child leading to a small, poorly compliant left ventricle. Although late anthracycline cardiotoxicity was initially believed to occur primarily in children who received a cumulative doxorubicin dose of 300 mg/m^2 or more,[884] cases following lower cumulative doses have been reported.[872,881-883] A long-term follow-up study in children confirmed that cardiac abnormalities occur at lower total doses and that cardiac abnormalities were both persistent and progressive over time.[885] Maximum lifetime cumulative dose levels designated as safe in adults may not be applicable to children, especially very young children. Long-term monitoring of cardiac function should be performed in children who were previously treated with anthracyclines.

Serial echocardiography and radionuclide cineangiography can detect subclinical decline in left ventricular function at cumulative anthracycline doses below the maximum lifetime limit, and endomyocardial biopsies show a steady increase in damage to myocytes with increasing cumulative dose.[864] The primary pathologic change in the myocardium is the destruction and loss of myofibrils and sarcoplasmic vacillation.[886] Myocardial damage appears to result from the generation of free radicals of the drug (Fig. 10.20) or secondary oxygen-free radicals. These highly reactive species can damage lipid biomembranes and cellular organelles.[818] Myocardium has limited ability to withstand this oxidative stress because of its low levels of catalase, which detoxifies peroxides. In an experimental model, alcohol metabolites were more cardiotoxic than parent anthracyclines, and the former compounds have been shown to accumulate in the heart.[836,837,887,888] Cardiac

doxorubicin and doxorubicinol concentrations in human autopsy hearts were significantly higher than concentrations in skeletal muscle and smooth muscle organs (i.e., bladder and uterus).[888]

Endomyocardial biopsy is the most sensitive and direct method of assessing the degree of anthracycline-induced cardiomyopathy.[886] The results correlate well with cardiac function measured at cardiac catheterization, but the technique is invasive, expensive, and technically demanding. Unfortunately, conventional noninvasive functional studies, such as the electrocardiogram, echocardiogram, and radionuclide cineangiography, may not demonstrate abnormalities until a critical degree of myocardial injury has occurred, and these studies do not appear to be predictive for the late cardiac effects of anthracyclines.[867,888] Cardiac troponin T serum levels may be useful in determining myocardial damage in children receiving anthracyclines, although studies have not been concordant.[889-892]

Children receiving anthracycline therapy should have their cardiac function closely monitored during treatment. Echocardiograms or radionuclide cineangiography are generally recommended before starting therapy and then periodically before courses of anthracyclines. A decline in the shortening fraction to less than 28% by echocardiogram or a 15% point decline in left ventricular ejection fraction (LVEF) or a LVEF less than 45% by cineangiography are indications to discontinue anthracycline therapy. However, the optimal method of screening and the use of screening results to determine anthracycline dose modifications remain controversial.[867,893-895]

Current approaches to the prevention of anthracycline cardiac toxicity include coadministration of agents that protect the myocardium from the cardiotoxic effects of anthracyclines and alterations in the schedule of drug administration to decrease peak drug concentrations. In addition, there is interest in the development of less cardiotoxic anthracycline analogs such as morpholino anthracycline derivatives (idarubicin and epirubicin) as well as liposomal formulations of doxorubicin.[864,896,897] Doxorubicin-containing polyethylene glycol-coated liposomes (Doxil) are currently being used in the treatment of adults with ovarian cancer, multiple myeloma, and Kaposi's sarcoma and a recommended phase II dose for use in children has been identified.[898]

The best studied cardioprotective drug is a chelating agent, dexrazoxane (Zinecard®). This drug undergoes hydrolysis intracellularly to a compound that is similar, in structure, to EDTA and tightly binds iron, a cofactor in anthracycline free radical reactions.[814,818] Preclinical studies demonstrated the ability of dexrazoxane to block the cardiotoxicity of anthracyclines[899] and led to several clinical trials of this drug in patients who were receiving doxorubicin-containing chemotherapy regimens.[899-901] The dexrazoxane dose is determined from the doxorubicin dose as a ratio of 10 mg of dexrazoxane for each 1 mg of doxorubicin. Clinical and subclinical cardiac toxicity, as measured by incidence of congestive heart failure, decline in LVEF on radionuclide cineangiography, and endomyocardial biopsy, was significantly reduced in patients receiving dexrazoxane.[128,902,903] The cardioprotective effect of dexrazoxane has also been demonstrated in children.[129,901,904] In a randomized trial of 206 children with ALL treated with 300 mg/m^2 of doxorubicin,[129] patients treated with doxorubicin alone were more likely than those who received dexrazoxane and doxorubicin to have elevated troponin T levels (50% vs. 21%, $p < 0.001$) and extremely elevated troponin T levels (32% vs. 10%, $p < 0.001$). Importantly, event-free survival at 2.5 years was 83% in both groups, indicating that dexrazoxane does not diminish the antileukemic effect of doxorubicin. Although a greater than anticipated incidence of second malignant neoplasms was observed in children with Hodgkin disease treated with dexrazoxane as a component of multi-agent therapy including administration of other topoisomerase II inhibitors,[905] no increased risk has been observed in adult trials and no such risk was observed in a clinical trial in children with ALL at a median follow-up of 6.2 years.[906]

Drug Interactions

Doxorubicin elimination half-life may be prolonged when coadministered with cyclophosphamide or nitrosoureas, and doxorubicin clearance appears to be enhanced by coadministration with etoposide.[827] The cardioprotectant, dexrazoxane, does not modify doxorubicin pharmacokinetics.[907] Chemosensitizers used to modulate multidrug resistance mediated by P-gp can substantially alter the disposition of the anthracyclines.[908] Doxorubicin-related toxicity is also significantly enhanced when the drug was administered in combination with cyclosporine.[909–911] The mechanism of this interaction is likely to be related, in part, to inhibition of P-gp in the biliary tract and decreased excretion of doxorubicin and doxorubicinol into the bile.

Mitoxantrone

Mitoxantrone is a synthetic anthracenedione that has a planar tricyclic nucleus with two symmetrical para-aminoalkyl side chains but no glycosidic substituent (Fig. 10.19).[818] Mitoxantrone induces topoisomerase II–mediated DNA strand breaks similar to the anthracyclines,[912,913] but it has a diminished capacity to undergo redo reactions compared with the anthracyclines. As a result, it does not appear to induce significant free-radical tissue injury, which is believed to be the mechanism of anthracycline cardiomyopathy.[818] Mitoxantrone is currently used in salvage regimens for the acute leukemias and lymphomas.[914–916] It is usually administered on a daily for 3 to 5 days, weekly, or every 3-week schedule.[917,918]

The plasma concentration-time profile of mitoxantrone resembles that of the anthracyclines, with an initial rapid decline ($t_{1/2}$, 10 minutes) and a prolonged terminal elimination phase ($t_{1/2} > 24$ hours).[913] Mitoxantrone is metabolized by oxidation of the terminal hydroxyl groups on the side chains to the inactive mono- and dicarboxylic acids.[919] Biliary excretion appears to be a major route of elimination for mitoxantrone with renal excretion of parent drug accounting for less than 10% of the administered dose.[913] Mitoxantrone is avidly tissue bound. It has a volume of distribution of 500 to more than 3,000 L/m^2 and can be detected in tissues for weeks after a dose.[913,920] Mitoxantrone clearance is variable and ranges from 100 to 500 $mL/min/m^2$.[913]

The acute toxicities of mitoxantrone include myelosuppression, mucositis, mild nausea and vomiting, diarrhea, and alopecia. Patients may also notice a bluish discoloration of the sclera, fingernails, and urine. Tissue damage from extravasation of mitoxantrone is uncommon. Mitoxantrone appears to be less cardiotoxic than anthracyclines at equivalent myelosuppressive doses in animal models and in some, though not all, clinical trials.[921–924] The long-term cardiac effects in children have not been studied, but there is some evidence of mitoxantrone cardiotoxicity in children.[925]

Bleomycin

Bleomycin is a unique antibiotic that is a mixture of 11 low-molecular-weight (1,500 Da), water-soluble glycopeptides. The major species is bleomycin A_2 (Fig. 10.19), which accounts for 65% of the commercial preparation. Bleomycin

chelates divalent redox-active transition metal ions, such as iron, cobalt, zinc, nickel, or copper, but it is only active in the ferrous form.[926,927] The bleomycin-iron complex binds tightly to DNA with partial intercalation between guanosine-cytosine base pairs. After binding to DNA, the bleomycin-iron complex produces single- and double-strand DNA breaks by a Fe^{2+}-O_2-catalyzed free radical reaction.[928] The bleomycin-Fe coordination complex oxygenates the C4′ hydrogen of deoxyribose and cuts DNA in the minor groove, predominately at the CpT and GpC sequences in actively transcribed chromatin domains.[926,929]

Bleomycin can be administered intravenously, intramuscularly, or subcutaneously at doses of 10 to 20 U/m^2. A unit is a measure of the drug's cytotoxic activity in bacteria and is equivalent to about 1.2 to 1.7 mg of peptide.[930] The drug is active against Hodgkin disease, lymphomas, and testicular cancer and other germ cell tumors. Bleomycin also has been administered regionally into the pleural space for malignant pleural effusions and intravesicularly for bladder tumors.[931,932]

Toxicity

Unlike most other anticancer drugs, bleomycin is not myelosuppressive. The dose-limiting toxicity is an interstitial pneumonitis that can lead to pulmonary fibrosis. Below a total cumulative dose of 450 U, sporadic cases of pulmonary toxicity are reported, with an incidence of 3% to 5%. At cumulative doses above 450 U, the incidence increases with dose.[933,934] Patients with pulmonary toxicity present with a persistent dry cough and exertional dyspnea that can progress to tachypnea, hypoxia, and death.[933,934] The chest x-ray typically shows reticulonodular infiltrates at the base. A decline in the single breath diffusing capacity for carbon monoxide is the most sensitive measure of subclinical damage, but it may not delineate those patients who are at highest risk to develop clinically symptomatic toxicity.[933–935] Pulmonary irradiation and the use of supplemental oxygen may enhance the risk of pulmonary toxicity in patients receiving bleomycin,[927,934,936] but others have found that serum creatinine and age older than 30 years may be more important predictors of pulmonary toxicity than the dose or exposure to supplemental oxygen.[937–939] Concurrent use of G-CSF does not appear to enhance bleomycin pulmonary toxicity.[940] Bleomycin-associated pathologic changes in the lung include edema and cellular infiltration in the perivascular interstitial space, followed by damage to alveolar lining cells and formation of hyaline membranes and fibrosis.[941] These changes may progress even after the drug is stopped. Pulmonary function should be closely monitored in patients receiving bleomycin, and the drug should be discontinued at the first sign of lung damage. High-dose corticosteroids may be of value in decreasing fibroblast activity, although this recommendation is based only on anecdotal experience.[934]

Dermatological toxicity from bleomycin is common. Linear hyperpigmentation of the skin is the most common finding, but other mucocutaneous reactions include erythema, induration, desquamation, and sclerosis of the skin; alopecia; nail hyperpigmentation and deformities; and mucositis.[942] Other side effects include nausea and vomiting, fever, hypersensitivity reactions, and Raynaud's phenomenon.

Pharmacokinetics

Bleomycin is not administered orally, as it would probably be enzymatically degraded in the intestinal tract. Absorption after intramuscular and subcutaneous injection is almost complete, and plasma concentrations with a continuous subcutaneous infusion closely simulate those after an intravenous infusion.[927,930,943,944] With intravenous bolus dosing in children, the drug has a biphasic plasma disappearance curve with a terminal half-life of about 3 hours. Total clearance was 41 mL/min/m^2, and renal clearance accounted for 65% of total drug clearance.[945] Patients with renal failure have prolonged terminal drug half-lives, higher plasma concentrations, and delayed clearance.[927,930,946,947] Bleomycin clearance is diminished in children previously treated with cisplatin, including those in whom the serum creatinine and blood urea nitrogen levels were not increased.[927,945] Concurrent use of other nephrotoxic drugs may also impair bleomycin elimination and augment its toxicity. A 45% to 65% dosage reduction has been recommended for patients with a creatinine clearance of less than 30 mL/min/m^2.[927] In patients undergoing hemodialysis, bleomycin was not detected in the dialysate.[948]

The primary determinants of bleomycin cytotoxicity are cellular uptake, DNA repair activity, concurrent medications that alter DNA conformation (e.g., intercalating agents), and the level of activity of bleomycin hydrolase. The latter is a cysteine proteinase that is found in normal tissues and tumor cells. This proteinase hydrolyzes a terminal carboxamide group within the bleomycin molecule to form an inactive metabolite.[926,929,949] Lung and skin, the tissues with the greatest susceptibility to bleomycin damage, have the lowest levels of this enzyme. In contrast, liver, spleen, intestine, and bone marrow, sites that are less susceptible to bleomycin toxicity, have high levels of this enzyme.[927,930] Bleomycin-resistant cells lines have an increased capacity to hydrolyze bleomycin and an enhanced capacity to repair DNA damage.[950,951]

Pharmacogenetics

Results of a study of men with nonseminomatous testicular cancer who were treated with bleomycin suggest that a polymorphism in the gene coding for bleomycin hydrolase (*BLMH*) may be linked to differential survival in this disease. Although additional studies are needed to confirm this finding, it appears that the homozygous variant G/G of SNP A1450G is associated with an increased risk for disease progression.[952]

Dactinomycin

Dactinomycin (actinomycin D) was one of the first drugs demonstrated to have significant antitumor activity in humans, and it has been in clinical use for more than 40 years. It continues to have a role in the treatment of Wilms' tumor and rhabdomyosarcoma, but it has been supplanted by the anthracyclines in many treatment regimens. Dactinomycin is composed of a planar tricyclic ring chromophore (phenoxazone) to which two identical cyclic polypeptides are attached (Fig. 10.19).[953] The drug intercalates between DNA bases, preferentially binding to the base sequence d(ATGCAT).[954] Dactinomycin binding to DNA causes topoisomerase-mediated single- and double-strand breaks in DNA.[812,955] It also blocks the replication and transcription of the DNA template.[953]

Dactinomycin is administered intravenously, traditionally on a daily-for-5-days schedule at a dose of 15 µg/kg/day. A single bolus dose of 45 to 60 µg/kg is also used for Wilms' tumor. This schedule is more convenient, is equally effective, and is no more toxic than the protracted regimen.[43] A daily-for-3-days schedule on weeks 1, 2, 4, and 5 was more hepatotoxic.[956]

Pharmacokinetics

The recent development of sensitive and precise analytic techniques for quantitation of dactinomycin in blood samples has permitted more detailed studies of the pharmacokinetics of this agent in children.[957,958] After an intravenous bolus injection, plasma dactinomycin concentrations decrease rapidly as a result of its avid tissue binding.[959–961] This distributive phase is followed by a prolonged elimination phase, during which renal and biliary excretion occur, although it is estimated that only 30% of the administered dose is recovered in the urine and stool. Only a small fraction of the dose appears to be metabolized.[959] The median peak plasma concentration in 31 patients determined 15 minutes following a bolus dose was 25.1 ng/mL (range, 3.2 to 99.2 ng/mL). Overall, considerable variability in drug exposure was observed. A large-scale pharmacokinetic study of dactinomycin in children is ongoing.

Toxicity

The primary toxicities of dactinomycin are myelosuppression, orointestinal mucositis, and severe nausea and vomiting. Extravasation of this drug can result in severe local tissue damage and ulceration. Hepatic VOD is a potentially fatal toxicity of dactinomycin in patients with Wilms' tumor. VOD usually occurs during the first 10 weeks of treatment and is characterized by fever, hepatomegaly, ascites, weight gain, jaundice, elevated serum transaminases, and thrombocytopenia.[962] The risk of VOD is similar with 60 µg/kg for 1 day and 15 µg/kg/day for 5 days schedules.[43] The incidence of VOD in Wilms' tumor is approximately 5% and risk factors include low body mass, young age, and concomitant radiation.[956,962,963] Dactinomycin is a radiation sensitizer that can enhance the local toxicity of radiation therapy if administered concurrently. Potentiation of radiation pneumonitis is especially problematic.[964] It can also cause a radiation recall effect if administered up to 2 years after irradiation.[965]

PLANT PRODUCTS

Plant products have been used to treat a variety of diseases for hundreds of years and are still an important source of medically useful drugs.[966] It has been estimated that in recorded history, more than 3,000 species of plants have been used as some form of cancer treatment. However, despite extensive screening in the modern era of cancer treatment, only a few clinically active anticancer drugs have been derived from the higher plants.[967,968] The plant products with indications for the treatment of childhood cancers are the vinca alkaloids derived from leaf extracts of the periwinkle plant, the epipodophyllotoxins, semisynthetic derivatives of podophyllotoxin that was extracted from the roots and rhizomes of the mandrake, and the analogs of camptothecin, derived from the Chinese tree *Camptothecin acuminate*. The taxanes, derived from the yew tree, have clinical activity against a variety of adult cancers but have a very limited role for the treatment of childhood cancers. As with other natural products, these anticancer drugs have novel and complex chemical structures (Fig. 10.21) and potent biological properties.[50,968,969] The biotransformation of these drugs is also complex, and the metabolic pathways have only been partially defined.[970,971]

Vinca Alkaloids

The vinca alkaloids, vincristine, vinblastine, and vinorelbine, are structurally similar alkaloids composed of two multi-ring subunits, vindoline and catharanthine (Fig. 10.21). Despite their structural similarity, these agents, which act as mitotic inhibitors, have differing clinical and toxicological properties. The vinca alkaloids exert their cytotoxic effect by binding to tubulin, a dimeric protein that polymerizes to form microtubules.[970,972] The resulting disruption of the intracellular microtubular system interferes with a number of vital cell

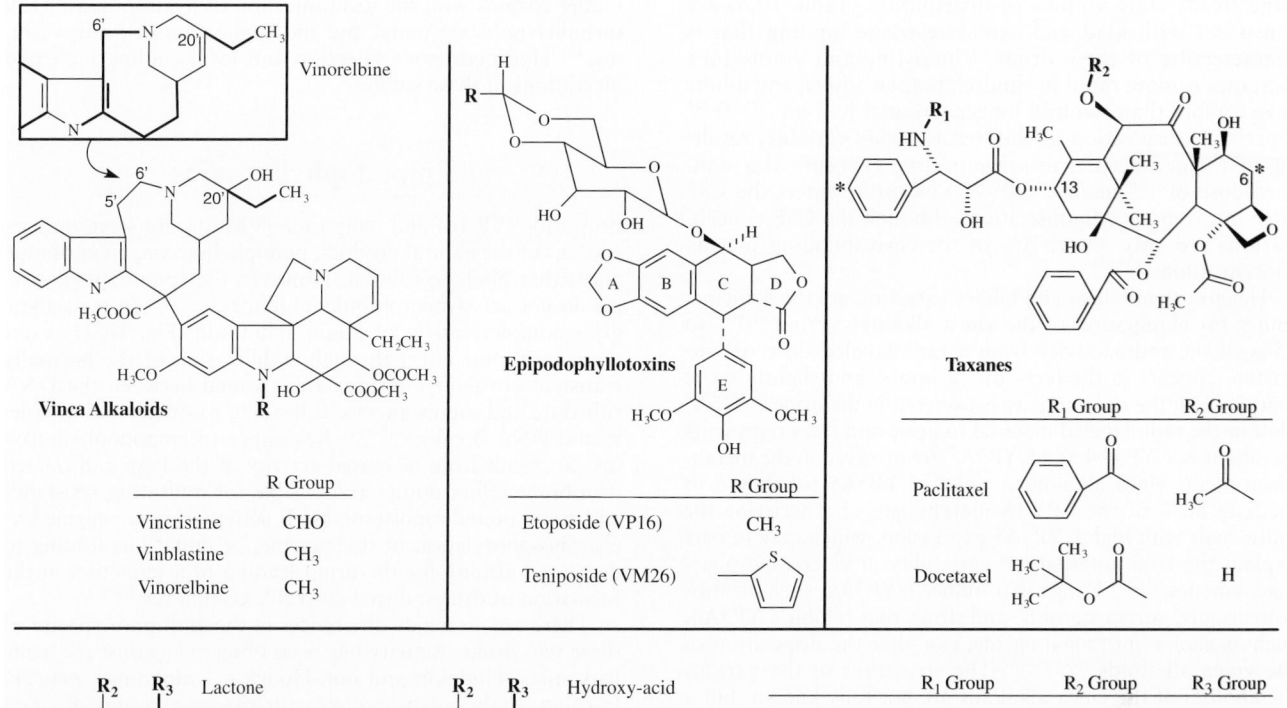

FIGURE 10.21 Chemical structures of the plant alkaloids commonly used in the treatment of childhood cancers: the vinca alkaloids, vincristine and vinblastine, extracted from the periwinkle plant; the epipodophyllotoxins, etoposide and teniposide, synthetic derivatives of the natural product podophyllotoxin which is derived from the mandrake plant (May apple); the taxanes, paclitaxel and docetaxel, derived from the yew tree; and the camptothecins, topotecan and irinotecan, derived from the stem wood of *Camptotheca acuminata*. Vincristine and vinblastine are identical except for the substituent at the R position, whereas the catharanthine ring of vinorelbine is modified. The asterisks on the taxane structure are hydroxylation sites. The hydroxyl group at position 10 of SN-38 is the site of glucuronidation.

functions, including mitosis, maintenance of the cytostructure, movement and transport of solutes such as neurotransmitters in neuronal axons and hormones and proteins in secretory cells, membrane trafficking and transmission of receptor signals, and transport of p53 to the nucleus.[973] The cytotoxic effect of these agents is primarily related to their ability to inhibit mitotic spindle formation, causing metaphase arrest during mitosis. The vinca alkaloids are subject to multidrug resistance, and alterations in the α- and β-tubulin subunits also confer resistance.[974]

Vincristine has a wide spectrum of clinical activity and is currently used in the treatment of ALL, Hodgkin and non-Hodgkin lymphomas, rhabdomyosarcoma, soft tissue sarcomas, Ewing's sarcoma, Wilms' tumor, brain tumors, and neuroblastoma. Vinblastine has been used in the treatment of histiocytosis, testicular cancer, and Hodgkin disease. Vinorelbine has been used in combination with gemcitabine in the treatment of relapsed/refractory Hodgkin disease[760] and is currently being evaluated in the treatment of sarcomas.

Pharmacokinetics

Vincristine and vinblastine are poorly absorbed if administered orally and are therefore administered intravenously as a bolus injection. Oral vinorelbine is bioavailable (29 ± 22%), but the resulting plasma concentrations are variable with the apparent oral clearance and volume of distribution substantially higher in children than in adults receiving similar doses.[975] The standard dose for vincristine is 1.0 to 2.0 mg/m², administered every 1 to 3 weeks. For infants aged 1 year or younger, vincristine dose is scaled to body weight (0.03 to 0.05 mg/kg). Many regimens limit the total single dose of vincristine to 2 mg based on reports of increased neurotoxicity at doses above 2 mg, especially on the weekly schedule. However, this practice of capping the dose may underdose some patients, because there is substantial interpatient variation in the plasma pharmacokinetics of vincristine, with a greater than 10-fold variation in the AUC.[854,976–978] Escalation of the dose beyond the 2 mg maximum may be well tolerated by some patients. Vinblastine doses range from 3.5 to 6.0 mg/m², administered in 1- to 3-week cycles. Vinorelbine is most commonly administered as a 10-minute infusion at a dose of 30 mg/m² weekly for up to 6 weeks.

After bolus administration, the vinca alkaloids manifest a rapid initial decline in plasma concentration (initial half-life of 5 to 10 minutes), followed by a prolonged terminal elimination phase with half-life of approximately 12 to 40 hours.[969,970,979–985] The long terminal half-life and the large steady-state volume of distribution (Table 10.5) are consistent with avid and extensive tissue binding that is characteristic of these drugs. Vincristine and vinorelbine clearance is more rapid in children than in adults, and adults have a more than twofold longer terminal half-life.[975,979,980] Vincristine disposition in children is highly variable, resulting in a wide interpatient range in drug exposure at a standard dose of 1.5 mg/m^2.[979,980,986] Vincristine enters the CSF after intravenous administration, although the CSF concentrations are only 3% to 5% of the corresponding plasma concentrations.[987,988]

Hepatic metabolism and biliary excretion are the principal routes for elimination of the vinca alkaloids. From 70% to 75% of the radioactivity from a radiolabeled dose of vincristine appears in the feces by 72 hours, and slightly more than 10% of the radioactivity is excreted in the urine.[983,989,990] Half of the radiolabeled material in urine and feces represents metabolites. CYP3A4 and CYP3A5 are involved in the metabolism of the vinca alkaloids.[137,991–993] CYP3A5 is believed to mediate 80% of the CPY3A metabolism of vincristine for individuals with high CYP3A5 expression, which may in part explain the large interpatient variability in vincristine pharmacokinetics.[993,994] Drugs that induce CYP3A4, such as anticonvulsants, corticosteroids, and drugs that inhibit CYP3A4, such as azoles antifungal agents, can alter the disposition of the vinca alkaloids.[980,995–997] The structures of the various metabolites of the vinca alkaloids are not fully known, but a desacetyl-metabolite of vincristine, vinblastine, and vinorelbine has been identified.[969]

Dosage modifications of the vinca alkaloids are generally recommended in infants and in patients with delayed biliary excretion as evidenced by an elevated direct bilirubin. Infants appear to manifest increased toxicity with standard doses of vincristine based on body surface area. Infants and younger children have a relatively larger ratio of body surface area to weight, and in a randomized crossover study in infants comparing dosing of vincristine based on body surface area (1.5 mg/m^2) with dosing by body weight (0.05 mg/kg), the dose calculated from body surface area resulted in greater systemic drug exposure (AUC).[998]

Toxicity

Neurotoxicity is the dose-limiting toxicity of vincristine. It is related to the cumulative dose and occurs more commonly on a weekly schedule. Manifestations of the peripheral sensory and motor neuropathy include loss of deep tendon reflexes, neurotic pain (muscular cramping, jaw pain), paresthesias, and wrist and foot drop. Cranial motor nerves may be affected, and autonomic nerve involvement may be responsible for constipation, paralytic ileus, and urinary retention. In most cases, these symptoms are reversible on withdrawal of the drug. Vincristine neurotoxicity can be markedly accentuated in children with Charcot-Marie-Tooth disease.[999] Accidental intrathecal administration of vincristine has been reported and is usually fatal.[1000–1004] Other toxicities associated with vincristine include alopecia, inappropriate antidiuretic hormone syndrome, seizures, and orthostatic hypotension. Nausea and vomiting and myelosuppression are rarely encountered. Vincristine can increase the platelet count.

Myelosuppression is the dose-limiting toxic effect of vinblastine and vinorelbine. Vinblastine also frequently causes mucositis. Neurotoxicity with vinblastine is minimal and is less prominent with vinorelbine than vincristine.[974] Vinorelbine causes constipation in 30% of patients. Vinca alkaloids are vesicants; extreme care must be taken to avoid extravasation during their administration. Ulcerations from vinca alkaloid extravasation were prevented in experimental animal

model systems with the local injection of hyaluronidase (150 turbidity reducing units) and the application of local warming.[191] Hydrocortisone injection and local cooling increased ulcerations in these studies.

Epipodophyllotoxins

Etoposide (VP-16) and teniposide (VM-26) are semisynthetic analogs of the natural product, podophyllotoxin, an antibiotic agent that binds to tubulin. However, the epipodophyllotoxins do not act as microtubule inhibitors.[1005,1006] Instead, these glycosidic derivatives of podophyllotoxin (Fig. 10.21) exert their antitumor effect through stabilization of the normally transient covalent intermediates formed between the DNA substrate and topoisomerase II, leading to single- and double-strand DNA breaks.[1007–1012] Resistance to epipodophyllotoxins can result from increased activity of the P-gp and related membrane efflux pumps responsible for multidrug resistance and from altered topoisomerase II activity (lower enzyme levels, phosphorylation of the enzyme, or mutations leading to decreased affinity for the drug) leading to a reduction in the formation of drug-induced cleavable complexes.[1005]

There are no major differences in the antitumor spectra of these two drugs. Activity has been observed against the acute leukemias, Hodgkin and non-Hodgkin lymphomas, neuroblastoma, rhabdomyosarcoma, soft tissue sarcomas, Ewing's sarcoma, germ cell tumors, and brain tumors.[1013–1015]

Dosage and Toxicity

Because the solubility of the epipodophyllotoxins in water is poor, both are supplied in nonaqueous formulations. Etoposide is formulated in polysorbate 80, polyethylene glycol, and alcohol and teniposide is formulated in Cremophor EL, alcohol, and dimethylacetamide. Before intravenous administration, these agents are diluted in 5% dextrose in water or 0.9% saline to a concentration of less than 0.4 mg/mL and infused over 30 to 60 minutes to avoid the hypotension associated with rapid injections. Etoposide phosphate is a water-soluble prodrug of etoposide that overcomes the formulation difficulties of the parent drug.[1016] Etoposide phosphate is rapidly converted to etoposide *in vivo* by plasma phosphatases and has a toxicity profile, MTD, and pharmacokinetic profile similar to that of etoposide.[1017,1018]

Etoposide is usually administered on a daily schedule for 3 to 5 days at a dose of 60 to 120 mg/m^2/day. Teniposide is administered at a dose of 70 to 180 mg/m^2 daily for 3 days. Both agents have also been administered on a single high-dose schedule (up to 800 mg/m^2 of etoposide and up to 1,000 mg/m^2 of teniposide), and etoposide (2,400 mg/m^2) has been incorporated into bone marrow transplant preparative regimens. A chronic oral low-dose (50 mg/m^2/day) schedule of etoposide has been studied.[1019,1020]

Etoposide antitumor activity is dose and schedule dependent.[1019,1021,1022] In adults with small-cell lung cancers, the response rate in patients treated on a daily-for-5-days schedule is significantly higher than in patients treated with same total dose infused over 24 hours.[1023] The chronic oral dosing schedule is also highly active in a variety of adult cancers.[1024,1025] However, a comparative trial of cisplatin in combination with either 21 days of oral etoposide at 50 mg/m^2/day or 3 days of intravenous etoposide at 130 mg/m^2/day in adults with lung cancer failed to demonstrate a survival advantage for this 21 day oral dosing schedule.[1026]

The primary dose-limiting toxicity of the epipodophyllotoxins is myelosuppression. Other toxicities include alopecia, nausea, vomiting, phlebitis, mild peripheral neuropathy, hepatocellular enzyme elevations, and mucositis. Arrhythmias are relatively rare. Diarrhea was the dose-limiting toxicity in children treated with etoposide on the chronic oral dosing schedule, but myelosuppression and mucositis were also prominent toxicities.[1027] Non–dose-limiting hypersensitivity reactions, characterized by urticaria, flushing, skin rash, angioedema, are common and related to the cumulative dose of etoposide or teniposide.[1028] Severe hypersensitivity reactions, such as bronchospasm and anaphylaxis, are less common and occur less frequently with etoposide than with teniposide.[1029] A severe skin rash has also been reported with high-dose teniposide.[1030]

A distinctive form of secondary acute leukemia, characterized by a short latency period (median time to presentation, 30 months), chromosomal translocations of the MLL gene at chromosome band 11q23, and M4 or M5 FAB morphologic subtype (monocytic or myelomonocytic), occurs in epipodophyllotoxin-treated patients.[1031–1034] The cumulative risk of developing this form of secondary leukemia has been estimated to be 5% to 12% in children with ALL treated with high cumulative doses of epipodophyllotoxins on a weekly or twice-weekly schedule.[1034] In contrast, the incidence of this form of secondary ANLL in survivors of germ cell cancers who were treated with etoposide is less than 1%. The 6-year cumulative incidence of secondary leukemia and myelodysplastic syndrome in patients who were treated on 12 pediatric cooperative group clinical trials was 3.3%, 0.7%, and 2.2% for cumulative etoposide doses of less than 1.5 g/m^2, 1.5 to 2.99 g/m^2, and 3 g/m^2 or more, respectively. Thus, epipodophyllotoxin cumulative dose does not appear to be a significant risk factor for development of secondary leukemia.[1035] However, as discussed later, polymorphisms in CYP isoenzymes may increase the risk of developing a treatment-related leukemia.

Pharmacokinetics and Drug Interactions

The disposition of the epipodophyllotoxins is characterized by a significant degree of intrapatient and interpatient variability.[1036,1037] The bioavailability of oral etoposide is approximately 50% at doses of 200 mg/m^2 or less, but it ranges from 10% to 80%,[1038,1039] and there is considerable dose-to-dose variation within each patient.[1040,1041] Bioavailability is also nonlinear. At higher doses (>200 mg/m^2), the fraction of the dose absorbed decreases.[1042,1043] Because oral absorption is erratic, dose dependent, and associated with increased toxicity, the clinical usefulness of oral administration of standard doses of etoposide has been limited. However, the more efficient absorption of lower doses of etoposide (bioavailability, 70%) suggests that the chronic oral low-dose schedule may circumvent some of these limitations.[1044,1045] The mean bioavailability of etoposide from oral etoposide phosphate is 76% (range, 37% to 144%)[1046]; and the mean bioavailability of teniposide is 40% (range, 20% to 70%).[1047] The absorption of teniposide also appears to decrease as the dose is increased.

The epipodophyllotoxins are extensively metabolized, although specific details of the metabolic pathways have not been fully elucidated. Some of these metabolites retain cytotoxic activity.[1036,1048] Metabolites identified in urine include the hydroxy acid derivatives[1049] and glucuronide and sulfate conjugates.[1036,1050] The epipodophyllotoxins also undergo CYP3A4 and, to a lesser extent, CYP3A5, mediated O-demethylation to the active catechol form, which can be oxidized to a reactive quinone.[994,1051–1053] Patients with the wild-type CYP3A4 genotype appear to produce more potentially DNA-damaging reactive intermediates, which may result in an increased risk of epipodophyllotoxin-related leukemias versus patients with a variant CYP3A4 genotype.[1054]

Renal clearance accounts for 30% to 40% of the total systemic clearance of etoposide but less than 10% of teniposide clearance.[1047,1055–1058] This difference probably reflects the difference in the degree of protein binding of the two drugs (Table 10.5). Biliary excretion is not a major route of elimination for etoposide, accounting for less than 10% of total drug elimination in most studies.[1050] Penetration of the epipodophyllotoxins into the CSF is limited,[1013,1056,1059] but the concentrations achieved may be cytotoxic.[1060]

The clearance of the epipodophyllotoxins is highly variable. For etoposide, the median clearance in children is 26 mL/min/m^2 (range, 14 to 54 mL/min/m^2)[1059]; for teniposide, the median clearance is 13 mL/min/m^2 (range, 4 to 22 mL/min/m^2).[1061] A variety of host- and treatment-related factors such as race, genotype for a variety of drug-metabolizing enzymes, and concomitant medications may impact etoposide clearance.[1062] For example, in children treated for ALL, etoposide clearance is significantly higher after completion of 1 month of prednisone therapy than without prednisone.[1062] Cyclosporine, a modulator of the P-gp, diminishes the renal and nonretail elimination of etoposide and teniposide, resulting in an increase in plasma exposure (AUC) to the drugs and an increase in toxicity.[1063–1065] The concomitant administration of anticonvulsants with etoposide and teniposide in children results in a two- to threefold increase in clearance and a proportional decrease in systemic drug exposure, which could reduce the drugs' efficacy.[1066,1067] The enhanced clearance is presumably the result of induction of hepatic metabolism. Concomitant atovaquone, a hydroxynaphthoquinone with anti-*Pneumocystis carinii* activity, also results in a modest increase in the AUC of etoposide and catechol.[1068]

Etoposide pharmacokinetic parameters including drug clearance are dose independent for doses up to 3,000 mg/m^2.[1056,1059,1069,1070] In infants 3 to 12 months of age, the median clearance was 19 mL/min/m^2, and in children older than 1 year, the median clearance was 18 mL/min/m^2.[1071] Therefore, no special dosing guidelines are required for treating infants, and all patients should receive a dose calculated from body surface area. In children receiving etoposide therapy for 5 consecutive days, the maximum plasma concentration and AUC for total and free etoposide decrease slightly on day 5 versus day 1, the AUC for etoposide catechol is much greater on day 5 than day 1.[1072] Further studies to determine whether the accumulation of this genotoxic metabolite is clinically relevant are warranted.

The pharmacokinetics of etoposide have been evaluated in patients with hepatic and renal dysfunction.[1059,1073–1076] Etoposide clearance was significantly delayed and the terminal half-life prolonged in patients with renal insufficiency, putting them at higher risk for toxic reactions. Overall, there was a good correlation between creatinine and etoposide clearance in these studies, suggesting that etoposide dose modifications could be based on the creatinine clearance. Etoposide clearance was not delayed in patients with abnormal hepatic function. The protein binding of etoposide is highly variable in cancer patients (range, 76% to 97%), and the degree of binding is correlated with the serum albumin level.[1077,1078] Patients with low serum albumin experience more severe hematological toxicity from etoposide, presumably because of higher free-drug concentrations.[1076,1079] A 30% to 40% dosage reduction may be indicated in these patients. The fraction of etoposide bound to protein is higher in pediatric cancer patients than in adults with cancer.[1080]

The wide interpatient variation in plasma concentrations of etoposide and teniposide has prompted investigators to evaluate the relation between plasma drug concentrations and measures of toxicity and response and to develop dosing methods that incorporate dose adjustments based on the plasma drug concentration.[1081–1084] Dose adjustment based on the AUC after the first dose of etoposide are precise in achieving a target AUC for subsequent doses in children.[1084] Attempts to apply therapeutic drug monitoring to low-dose oral etoposide regimens have had limited success because of the marked intrapatient variability in drug absorption and disposition. Because of the variability in the extent of protein binding of etoposide, dosage adjustments based on the nonprotein bound (free) fraction of etoposide may prove more successful than total drug concentration.[1085,1086]

Camptothecins

Topotecan and irinotecan are semisynthetic, water-soluble camptothecin analogs (Fig. 10.21) that produce DNA stand breaks by forming a ternary complex with DNA and topoisomerase I.[50] In aqueous solutions, the camptothecins exist in an equilibrium between the active lactone form and the relatively inactive hydroxy-acid form, which results from reversible hydrolysis of the E-ring. The inactive form predominates at physiologic pH, although the ratio of lactone:hydroxy acid varies for topotecan (10%), irinotecan (25% to 30%) and its active metabolite SN-38 (50% to 65%).[1087,1088] Decreased intracellular levels of topoisomerase I, alterations in the affinity of topoisomerase I for the camptothecin analogs, and expression of MRP are mechanisms of resistance to topotecan and irinotecan,[1089–1095] although the camptothecin analogs are poor substrates for P-gp.[1096]

Topotecan

Topotecan is active against neuroblastoma,[1097,1098] rhabdomyosarcoma,[1099,1100] medulloblastoma,[1101] and Wilms' tumor[1102] but is inactive in osteosarcoma.[1103] Most of the antitumor activity has been observed in phase II window trials[1101,1103] rather than in traditional single-agent phase II studies.[1104–1107]

Topotecan is usually administered intravenously for 5 days at a dose of 1.4 mg/m^2/day every 21 days or 2.0 mg/m^2/day for 5 days followed by filgrastim.[1108] The injectable form of topotecan has also been administered orally once daily for 5 days for 2 consecutive weeks every 28 days at a dose of 1.8 mg/m^2/day[1109] or 0.5 mg/m^2/day twice daily for 21 days.[1097] Continuous infusion schedules of 1 to 21 days duration have also been studied. The dose of topotecan must be substantially reduced when administered in combination with cisplatin, carboplatin, or cyclophosphamide because of enhanced hematological toxicity.[1110,1111] Myelosuppression is the most common topotecan toxicity. Diarrhea becomes dose limiting with more protracted schedules or with oral dosing.[1112] Other toxicities associated with topotecan include nausea and vomiting, alopecia, mucositis, elevated hepatic transaminases, and skin rash.[1108,1113,1114] Typhlitis has also been reported in patients with refractory acute leukemia.[1115]

Pharmacokinetics

The bioavailability of oral topotecan in children is approximately 30%, but there is marked interpatient variability in absorption.[1109,1116] With intravenous administration, the clearance of the lactone form of topotecan is also highly variable.[1113,1117] The terminal half-life of topotecan is 3 to 5 hours, and renal excretion is the primary route of elimination (60% to 70% of total dose).[1113,1118,1119] Impaired renal function decreases topotecan clearance, necessitating a dosage reduction.[1120] N-demethylation is a minor metabolic pathway,[1121] and mild-to-moderate hepatic dysfunction does not appear to impact on drug disposition.[1122] Topotecan penetrates into the CSF better than other topoisomerase I inhibitors.[1123,1124]

Topotecan CSF penetration may be altered with concomitant administration of tyrosine kinase inhibitors such as gefitinib that modulate ABC transporters at the blood-brain and blood-CSF barriers.[1125] Although topotecan penetrates into pleural and ascitic fluid, it is not sequestered in the fluid accumulation and the drug has thus been safely given to patients with large effusions.[1126]

Irinotecan

Irinotecan is a prodrug that is converted by carboxylesterases in the liver and intestinal tract to the active metabolite, 7-ethyl-10-hydroxy camptothecin (SN-38), which is 100- to 1,000-fold more potent than irinotecan. A second active metabolite, 4-piperidinopiperidine (4PP), which is released during the esterolysis of irinotecan to SN-38, has also been identified. The contribution of 4PP to the *in vivo* activity of irinotecan is unlikely to be significant.[1127]

A number of phase I and clinical reports have found that irinotecan has measurable but limited activity in children with neuroblastoma, hepatoblastoma, and some pediatric CNS tumors.[1128–1132] In formal phase II trials, irinotecan was active only in children with rhabdomyosarcoma[1133,1134] and medulloblastoma.[1135]

In adults, irinotecan is administered as a 90-minute intravenous infusion weekly for 4 weeks at a dose of 125 mg/m^2/day. In children, irinotecan has been administered on a number of different schedules[1136–1138] but is most commonly administered as a 60-minute intravenous infusion daily for 5 days at a dose of 50 mg/m^2/day.[1129] The 60-minute intravenous infusion daily for 5 days on 2 consecutive weeks (daily × 5 × 2) every 21 days schedule[1128] is no longer being developed based on results from a randomized trial in children with relapsed rhabdomyosarcoma that found no benefit over the daily × 5 days schedule.[1139]

Myelosuppression and diarrhea are the most common irinotecan-associated toxicities in children and adults. Diarrhea, diaphoresis, and abdominal cramping that are associated with the drug infusion[1129,1140] are responsive to atropine, and delayed diarrhea is responsive to loperamide.[1141] Other toxicities include nausea and vomiting, transient elevations of hepatic transaminases, asthenia, alopecia, malaise, and electrolyte abnormalities.[1128,1138,1142] The combination of irinotecan and oxaliplatin was associated with expected severe diarrhea but unexpected elevations in pancreatic enzymes.[408]

Pharmacokinetics

Oral irinotecan is rapidly absorbed and more efficiently converted to SN-38 due to first-pass metabolism, but plasma drug and metabolite concentrations are highly variable.[1143] The conversion of irinotecan to SN-38 appears to be dose dependent with inefficient (<10% of the dose) conversion after administration of a high intermittent doses[1088,1144] and greater conversion to SN-38 (~50% of the dose) after protracted low-dose administration.[1145] Oxidation of the dipiperidine side chain by CYP3A subfamily enzymes also yields two minor metabolites (APC and NPC).[1146] Induction of these CYP3A catabolic pathways by anticonvulsants can enhance the clearance of irinotecan and reduce the production of SN-38.[1147–1150] Irinotecan and its metabolites are eliminated primarily by biliary excretion.[1146] Renal excretion of the parent drug accounts for 15% to 25% of the dose.[1088]

SN-38 is conjugated to SN-38 glucuronide (SN-38G) by hepatic uridine diphosphate glucuronosyltransferase 1A1 (UGT1A1), the enzyme responsible for bilirubin conjugation.[1151] Newborns, patients who have partial UGT1A1 deficiency (Gilbert or Crigler Najjar syndromes) and patients who are receiving drugs that inhibit UGTA1A, such as valproic acid, are at risk for increased drug-related toxicity.[1152–1154]

SN-38G is secreted into the bile and deconjugated to SN-38 by β-glucuronidase in the gut. This intraluminal formation of SN-38 may be responsible for the delayed diarrhea from irinotecan.[1153] The product of the irinotecan AUC and the ratio of SN-38 and SN-38G AUCs (biliary index) is higher in adults with severe diarrhea after receiving irinotecan on a weekly dosing schedule.[1155] However, there does not appear to be an association between the severity of diarrhea and the biliary index in patients treated on an intermittent dosing schedule.[1146] When administered on protracted dosing schedules, cephalosporins (cefixime, cefpodoxime) allow for greater dose escalation of irinotecan by preventing deglucuronidation by intestinal flora of SN-38G to SN-38.

Pharmacogenetics

Adults with the *UGTA1*28* genotype are at increased risk of neutropenia and an initial dose reduction is recommended.[737,1156] However, in pediatric studies, an association between genotype and toxicity has not been observed, which may be because in children the irinotecan dose and schedule is generally low dose, protracted versus the high dose intermittent schedules in adults.[1135,1157] Other genetic polymorphisms that may contribute to the wide interpatient variability in drug disposition and action are the ABC and solute-linked carrier (SLC) transporter genes.[1158]

Taxanes

The taxanes, paclitaxel and docetaxel, are complex diterpenes (Fig. 10.21) that exert their cytotoxic effect by interfering with microtubule function. However, unlike the vinca alkaloids, the taxanes increase microtubule stability by preventing depolymerization, which results in tubulin bundling.[1159–1161] Taxane-induced cytoskeletal changes lead to cell cycle arrest in the G_2 (premitotic) and M (mitotic) phases and cell death by apoptosis. Because paclitaxel arrests cells in the G_2/M phase, the most radiosensitive phase of the cell cycle, it is also a potent radiosensitizer.[1160,1161] Resistance to taxanes *in vitro* has been ascribed to the development of altered tubulin subunits with impaired ability to polymerize, to the presence of the P-gp, and to elevated levels of Raf-1 kinase, which can suppress paclitaxel-induced apoptosis.[1159,1162,1163]

Paclitaxel is insoluble in water and is formulated in Cremophor EL and ethanol, which has been implicated in the hypersensitivity reactions. As this formulation leaches plasticizers (phthalate) from polyvinylchloride intravenous infusion bags, paclitaxel must be mixed and stored in glass, polypropylene, or polyolefin containers and administered through polyethylene-lined infusion sets. Docetaxel is formulated in polysorbate 80 and ethanol.

Although paclitaxel and docetaxel have a broad spectrum of antitumor activity in adult cancers, they do not appear to be active as single agents against common childhood cancers, with the possible exception of limited docetaxel activity in Ewing's sarcoma.[1164–1167] Modest antitumor activity has also been observed in refractory bone sarcomas when docetaxel is administered in combination with gemcitabine.[761]

Paclitaxel has been administered as a 1-, 3-, 24-, or 96-hour intravenous infusion. The standard adult dose of paclitaxel is 135 or 175 mg/m^2 infused over 3 hours, although doses of up to 250 mg/m^2 are tolerable. Longer infusions appear to be more myelosuppressive.[1168,1169] The recommended dose of paclitaxel administered as a 24-hour infusion every 3 weeks in children is 350 mg/m^2.[1170] The recommended dose of paclitaxel administered as a 3-hour infusion twice weekly × 6 doses, every 28 days, is 50 mg/m^2/dose.[1171] Docetaxel is administered as 1-hour infusion every 3 weeks at a dose of 100 to 125 mg/m^2, but higher doses may be tolerable with filgrastim support.[1172,1173]

Pharmacokinetics

Paclitaxel pharmacokinetics are dose dependent and probably schedule dependent, and complex pharmacokinetic models incorporating capacity-limited elimination and capacity-limited distribution have been devised to describe the disposition of the drug.[1174,1175] Paclitaxel is extensively tissue bound, accounting for its large volume of distribution. Hepatic metabolisms (hydroxylation) by CYP2C8 at the C-6 position on the ring and by CYP3A4 on the C-13 side chain (Fig. 10.21) followed by biliary excretion are the primary routes of paclitaxel elimination (80% of the dose is recovered as parent drug or metabolites in feces).[1176–1179]

Docetaxel also undergoes hepatic metabolism primarily mediated by CY3A4.[1180,1181] At high concentrations, CYP2C8 may play a role in docetaxel elimination.[1182] Drugs or xenobiotics that induce CYP450 enzymes, such as the anticonvulsants, enhance paclitaxel clearance,[1183,1184] and CYP3A4 inhibitors, such as the imidazole antifungal agents, reduce paclitaxel clearance.[1176] Patients with hepatic tumor involvement or biochemical evidence of liver dysfunction (elevated bilirubin or transaminases) are at increased risk for paclitaxel toxicity, presumably because of delayed paclitaxel clearance; dose reductions are recommended for these patients.[1185,1186] Renal excretion accounts for only 5% of total drug clearance.[1176,1187]

Toxicity

Myelosuppression is the primary dose-limiting toxicity of paclitaxel.[1188] Neurotoxicity is also prominent in children and is characterized by a stocking-glove peripheral neuropathy (paresthesias, diffuse myalgias, and loss of fine motor control) and seizures.[1170] Acute encephalopathy and irreversible coma are also associated with paclitaxel.[1189,1190] Ethanol in the formulation can cause toxicity if high doses of paclitaxel are infused over a short period of time.[1191–1193] The incidence of acute hypersensitivity reactions (hypotension, urticaria, and bronchospasm) occurring within minutes of the start of the infusion[1194] has been reduced by administering paclitaxel as a more prolonged infusion and by premedicating patients with corticosteroids and antihistamines (H$_1$ and H$_2$ blockers). Cardiac arrhythmias (bradycardia, atrioventricular conduction disturbances), alopecia, mucositis, radiation-recall dermatitis, pneumonitis, and phlebitis at the injection site are also caused by paclitaxel.[1161,1195]

Docetaxel produces neutropenia without significant thrombocytopenia. Other toxicities include malaise, myalgias, skin rashes (including palmar-plantar erythrodysesthesia), nausea and vomiting, mucositis, diarrhea, alopecia, interstitial pneumonitis, and transient elevations of serum transaminases.[1172,1173,1196] Neurotoxicity is less prominent with docetaxel, but fluid retention, associated with weight gain, edema, and in some cases scleroderma-like skin changes, is a cumulative toxicity that occurs in 20% of patients.[1172,1197,1198] Hypersensitivity reactions, skin rashes, and fluid retention may be ameliorated by premedication with an antihistamine and corticosteroid.

KINASE INHIBITORS

Protein kinases are enzymes that catalyze the transfer of the terminal phosphate of ATP to substrates that usually contain tyrosine, serine, and threonine residues. Phosphorylation of these protein targets leads to activation of signal-transduction pathways that regulate critical processes including growth, differentiation, adhesion, metabolism, and apoptosis. Normal regulation of kinase function may be altered in cancer cells due to mutation, overexpression, or translocation of proto-oncogenes (see Chapter 3). Constitutive activity of these kinases thus has the potential to make cancer cells particularly vulnerable to inhibitors, making kinases attractive targets for anticancer therapeutics.[1199,1200] The most common pharmacologic approaches taken to targeting signal transduction pathways include the development of small molecule inhibitors that target the ATP-binding domain of tyrosine kinases and the development of monoclonal antibodies against the relevant receptors. Kinases of particular interest for the treatment of childhood cancer include BCR-ABL in Ph+ leukemias,[1201,1202] FLT3 in acute myelogenous leukemia,[1203] ALK in neuroblastoma,[1204,1205] the type 1 insulin-like growth factor receptor in sarcomas,[1206,1207] and the VEGFR for a spectrum of pediatric solid tumors.[1208–1210]

BCR-ABL Inhibitors

Imatinib Mesylate

The success of imatinib mesylate (STI-571; Gleevec®) for the treatment of patients with chronic myeloid leukemia (CML) in chronic phase[1202] resulted in a paradigm shift in oncology drug development and ushered in the era of molecularly targeted cancer chemotherapy. Imatinib was identified as an effective inhibitor of ABL kinase activity via high throughput drug screening.[1211] Clinical trials with imatinib began in the late 1990s. Imatinib received accelerated FDA approval for use in adults with Philadelphia chromosome-positive CML in 2001 followed by children in 2003.

Although imatinib targets BCR-ABL, its effects on PDGFR and c-Kit have also been exploited. Imatinib inhibits mutant KIT, which is present in many gastrointestinal stroma tumors (GISTs).[1212] Based on responses observed in adults with KIT positive GIST,[1213] the drug was approved for use in such patients in 2002. Activating mutations of c-Kit are rare in pediatric solid tumors, but expression of the target protein or its ligand is found in Ewing's sarcoma[1214] and medulloblastoma. PDGFR is expressed in rhabdomyosarcoma,[1215] osteosarcoma,[1216] desmoplastic small round cell tumors,[1217] synovial sarcoma,[1218] and medulloblastoma.[1219] Disappointingly, in a pediatric phase II trial of imatinib in children with these types of tumors, only one objective response was observed among 59 evaluable patients with recurrent disease.[1220]

Mechanisms of imatinib resistance have been explored extensively, particularly in the setting of CML. The most common mechanisms include BCR-ABL kinase domain mutations, BCR-ABL amplification and overexpression, impairment of drug transport, and clonal evolution with activation of additional signaling pathways.[1221] Approximately 90 different BCR-ABL mutations that result in alterations in phosphate-binding loop and the activation loop have been identified in adults with imatinib-resistant CML. The majority of these mutations affect six specific amino acid residues, including Gly250, Tyr253, Glu255, Thr315, Met351 and Phe359.[1222]

Imatinib dosing varies with indication. Adults with CML in chronic phase and with GIST are typically treated with a dose of 400 mg/day, whereas adults with CML in blast crisis or accelerated phase are treated with a dose of 600 mg/day administered on a daily basis. Phase I data in children demonstrated that comparable doses of 260 or 340 mg/m²/day are well tolerated and result in drug exposures similar to those observed in adults.[1223] The recommended dose for children with newly diagnosed Philadelphia chromosome-positive

CML is 340 mg/m²/day, while the dose for children with chronic phase CML recurring post–stem cell transplant or postinterferon therapy is 260 mg/m²/day.

Pharmacokinetics. Imatinib (Fig. 10.22) is well absorbed following oral administration and is highly protein bound.[1224] Imatinib exposure (AUC) is dose proportional over a 25- to 1,000-mg dose range. The apparent clearance in adults is 12.5 L/hr and its terminal half-life is approximately 15 hours.[1225] Imatinib is metabolized predominantly by CYP3A4. Peak plasma concentrations of the N-demethylated piperazine derivative of imatinib (CGP74588) are reached within 2 to 4 hours of dosing.[1224] Imatinib and CGP74588 are excreted mainly in feces, with only a small amount of the drug excreted in urine. Wide interpatient variability in the clearance of imatinib is observed in children and adults.[1223,1226] Imatinib penetrates poorly into the CNS[1227–1229] and thus recurrence of disease in this sanctuary site can occur. Drug exposure following imatinib administration in patients with mild and moderate liver dysfunction did not differ significantly from that in patients with normal liver function, but exposures were increased in adults with mild or moderate renal insufficiency.[1230,1231]

Toxicity. The most frequently reported drug-related toxicities in adults are nausea, vomiting, fatigue, diarrhea, musculoskeletal pain, and fluid retention. Although edema is rarely severe, significant fluid retention can occur, manifested as pleural effusion, pericardial effusion, pulmonary edema, ascites, or superficial edema with rapid weight gain. The most common adverse events reported in children were nausea, vomiting, fatigue, diarrhea, and transaminitis.[1223] Hemorrhagic pleural effusions were observed in 7 patients among the 70 children enrolled on a phase II study, with two patients developing hemorrhagic pleural effusions in the absence of disease progression.[1220]

Dasatinib

Point mutations in the kinase domain of the BCR-ABL fusion protein may alter the conformation of the protein, affecting imatinib binding and causing resistance to this agent. Dasatinib, a second-generation kinase inhibitor, binds to the ABL kinase in both its active and inactive conformations.[1232] Dasatinib retains kinase inhibitory activity in cells harboring clinically relevant imatinib resistant BCR-ABL isoforms.[1233] The drug also decreases disease burden in *in vivo* models of CML, including an imatinib "acquired resistance" model.[1233] In addition to binding to the kinase domain of BCR-ABL, dasatinib competes with ATP for binding to additional kinases and kinase families, including the SRC family kinases, c-KIT, EPHA2, and PDGF-β receptor.[1234–1236] Dasatinib is approved for use in adults with Philadelphia chromosome-positive ALL or CML (all phases) who have resistance or intolerance to previous therapy. Recommended doses in adults are 100 mg daily for chronic phase CML and 140 mg daily for accelerated or blast phase CML or for Ph+ ALL. A dose of 85 mg/m² daily has been well tolerated in children.[1237]

Pharmacokinetics. Unlike other small molecule tyrosine kinase inhibitors, dasatinib (Fig. 10.22) has a short half-life (<4 hours) in adults.[1238] In children, the mean terminal half-life is 2.2 hours.[1237] Following oral administration of dasatinib, exposure increases proportionally with dose, though there is considerable interpatient variability in exposure, particularly at higher dose levels. The drug is extensively metabolized prior to elimination, and most metabolites are excreted in feces.[1238] Daily dosing is associated with similar efficacy but

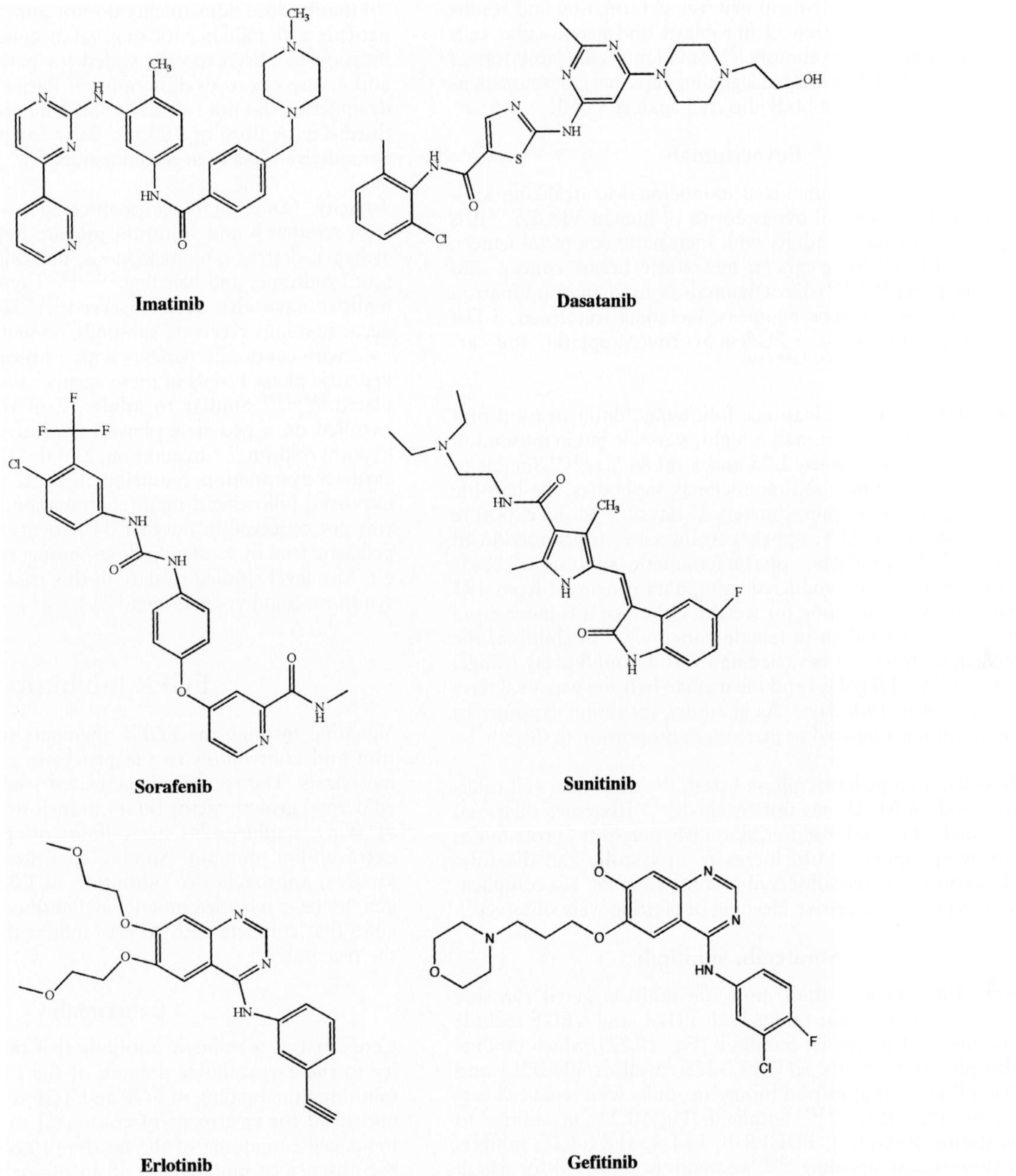

FIGURE 10.22 Chemical structures of small molecule tyrosine kinase inhibitors that have undergone initial clinical evaluation in children with cancer. Imatinib and dasatinib were developed to target BCR-ABL; sorafenib and sunitinib to primarily target VEGF-R; and erlotinib and gefitinib to target EGF-R.

fewer side effects compared with twice daily dosing.[1239] Dosage adjustment does not appear to be necessary in adults with hepatic impairment.[1240] Less than 4% of dasatinib and its metabolites are excreted by the kidney[1238]; however, data are currently unavailable regarding dosing in patients with renal dysfunction.

Toxicity. Notable dasatinib-associated toxicities include thrombocytopenia and pleural effusion.[1239] Other adverse events include pericardial effusion, generalized edema, dyspnea or pulmonary edema, skin rash, flushing, headache, and fatigue.[1241] In children, dose-limiting toxicities were diarrhea, headache, and hypokalemia. Two patients developed pleural

effusions and one patient developed hemangiomatosis with gastrointestinal hemorrhage following repeated courses of dasatinib.[1237]

VEGF Inhibitors

As the role of new blood vessel formation in cancer has become better understood, considerable efforts have been made to develop tyrosine kinase inhibitors that alter the function of angiogenesis-associated kinases such as VEGF and PDGFR. VEGF acts on endothelial cells, promoting their proliferation, survival, migration, and invasion.[1242] PDGF signaling plays a key role in new vessel formation and results in paracrine stimulation of fibroblasts and perivascular cells that support growing tumors.[1243] Small molecule inhibitors of VEGF- and PDGF-mediated signaling have been developed, as has a monoclonal antibody directed against VEGF.

Bevacizumab

Bevacizumab is a humanized monoclonal neutralizing antibody that binds to all five isoforms of human VEGF.[1244] It is approved for use in adults with metastatic colorectal cancer, non–small cell lung cancer, metastatic breast cancer, and glioblastoma.[1245-1247] Bevacizumab is used in combination with various cytotoxic regimens, including irinotecan, 5-FU/leucovorin/irinotecan, 5-FU/leucovorin/oxaliplatin, and carboplatin/paclitaxel.[1245,1246,1248]

Pharmacokinetics. Clearance following administration of a single dose of bevacizumab is highly variable but in most adult patients ranges between 2.75 and 5 mL/kg/day.[1249] Similar to that of other humanized monoclonal antibodies, the half-life of bevacizumab is approximately 21 days.[1249] Serum exposure as measured by AUC appears to increase in proportion to dose.[1249] A population pharmacokinetic analysis of bevacizumab has been conducted using data generated from 491 patients. After adjusting for weight, clearance was more rapid in male patients than in female patients.[1250] In children, the median clearance of bevacizumab was 4.1 mL/kg/day (range, 3.1 to 15.5 mL/kg/day) and the median half-life was 11.8 days (range, 4.4 to 14.6 days). As in adults, the serum exposure to bevacizumab appeared to increase in proportion to dose.[1251]

Toxicity. In a pediatric phase I trial, the drug was well tolerated and an MTD was not reached.[1251] Toxicities observed included infusional reaction, skin rash, mucositis, proteinuria, and lymphopenia. Mild increases in systolic and diastolic blood pressure were observed in most patients. No complications related to excessive bleeding or clotting were observed.

Sorafenib, Sunitinib

Second-generation small molecule multi-targeted tyrosine kinase inhibitors that target both PDGF and VEGF include sunitinib and sorafenib. Sunitinib (Fig. 10.22), which inhibits phosphorylation of c-KIT, FLT-3, as well as VEGFR2 and PDGFR-β,[1252] is approved for use in adults with renal cell carcinoma and GIST.[1253,1254] Sorafenib (Fig. 10.22), in addition to inhibiting VEGFR-2, PDGFR-β, FLT-3, and c-KIT, inhibits RAF-mediated signaling.[1255] Sorafenib is approved for use in adults with renal cell carcinoma and hepatocellular carcinoma.[1256,1257] Preclinical studies and small case series suggest that there may be a role for these agents in the treatment of childhood malignancies.[1258-1260]

Pharmacokinetics. Following administration of sorafenib on a twice-daily schedule, peak plasma concentrations and drug exposure did not appear to increase in proportion to dose.[1261] In adults, the drug has a mean half-life of 24 to 35 hours[1262] and accumulates with multiple doses.[1262,1263] Similar to sorafenib, sunitinib has a long half-life of approximately 40 to 80 hours, with evidence of drug accumulation with multiple doses.[1264] Both sorafenib and sunitinib undergo hepatic metabolism, primarily via CYP3A4, and are excreted in the feces, with a small percentage excreted in urine.[1265,1266] Adjustment of sunitinib dosing is not required for adults with mild hepatic impairment,[1267] but data regarding the pharmacokinetics of sunitinib in patients with severe liver dysfunction or patients with renal impairment have not been published. For sorafenib, dose adjustments do not appear to be required in patients with mild hepatic or renal dysfunction, but dose modification has been recommended for patients with moderate and severe organ dysfunction.[1267] Patients with severe liver dysfunction did not tolerate a sorafenib dose of 200 mg every third day. A dose of 200 mg daily for patients undergoing hemodialysis has been recommended.[1267]

Toxicity. Common toxicities observed in adult patients treated with sorafenib and sunitinib include hypertension, fatigue, asthenia, diarrhea, nausea/emesis, mucositis, skin rash, hand-foot syndrome, and bleeding.[1257,1268] Thyroid function abnormalities have also been observed.[1269] Decreased LVEF can occur in adults receiving sunitinib,[1270] and the drug should be used with caution in patients with a history of cardiac events. Pediatric phase I trials of these agents have recently been completed.[1324,1325] Similar to adults, 2 of the first 12 patients enrolled on a pediatric phase I trial of sunitinib developed hypothyroidism.[1271] In addition, 2 of the 12 patients developed cardiac dysfunction requiring medical therapy. Symptoms improved following drug discontinuation.[1271] Cardiac toxicity was not observed in the first 34 patients treated in a phase I pediatric trial of sorafenib; dose-limiting toxicities at the highest dose level studied to date in this trial included hand-foot syndrome and hyponatremia.[1272]

EGFR Inhibitors

Signaling through the EGFR augments tumor cell proliferation and contributes to the processes of angiogenesis and metastasis. The receptor is activated when ligands including epidermal growth factor (EGF), transforming growth factor α (TGF-α), amphiregulin, betacellulin, or epiregulin bind to the extracellular domain. Similar to other receptor tyrosine kinases, approaches to inhibition of EGFR tyrosine kinase activity have included monoclonal antibodies and small molecules that compete with ATP to inhibit the kinase activity of the receptor.[1273]

Cetuximab

Cetuximab is a chimeric antibody that binds with high affinity to the extracellular domain of the EGFR, competitively inhibiting the binding of EGF and TGF-α to the receptor. It is approved for treatment of colorectal carcinoma and squamous cell carcinoma of the head and neck.[1274,1275] In adults, the absence of mutated KRAS in tumor tissue is associated with an improved response rate and improved progression free survival following treatment with cetuximab.[1276]

Pharmacokinetics. Initial pharmacokinetic studies of cetuximab were designed to identify a dose at which clearance of the antibody became saturated.[1277] As EGFR is widely expressed, saturation of antibody binding sites not only in tumor but also in tissues such as skin and liver is presumably required. Doses of 200 to 400 mg/m² are associated with decreased plasma clearance.[1278] Modeling studies predict that clearance is 90% saturated at a cetuximab dose of 260 mg/m².[1279] The half-life of cetuximab is approximately 7 days, with only limited drug accumulation occurring with weekly administration.[1279] Drug disposition in children and adolescents is similar to that observed in adults.[1280]

Toxicity. In adults, cetuximab is administered as an initial loading dose of 400 mg/m² followed by a weekly maintenance dose of 250 mg/m². An acneiform rash is observed in approximately 80% of adults treated with cetuximab, but grade 3 or greater skin toxicity occurs in less than 10% of patients.[1274] Anaphylactic reactions occur in approximately 1% of patients. In children, cetuximab was well tolerated at a dose of 250 mg/m^2 weekly when delivered in combination with irinotecan.[1281] Mild-to-moderate skin rashes were common.

Erlotinib, Gefitinib

Both gefitinib and erlotinib (Fig. 10.22) compete with ATP for binding to the tyrosine kinase domain of the EGFR. Gefitinib is a low-molecular-weight synthetic anilinoquinazoline that inhibits the *in vitro* growth of cells derived from ovarian, colon, breast, lung, and head and neck carcinomas.[1282] Symptom relief and disease stabilization were observed in substantial numbers of patients with non–small cell lung cancer treated with 250 to 500 mg/day of gefitinib, though objective responses were only observed in a smaller number (12% to 19%) of patients.[1283,1284] The presence of somatic mutations in EGFRs tyrosine kinase domain in these patients has been associated with response.[1285] Erlotinib, a highly specific inhibitor of EGFR-mediated signaling, is approved for use in adults with non–small cell lung cancer and advanced pancreatic cancer. Tumor histology, history of smoking, and expression of EGFR are associated with response.[1286]

Pharmacokinetics. Peak plasma concentrations of gefitinib occur on average 3 hours (range, 1 to 8 hours) following administration of an oral dose.[1287] Although significant interpatient variability is observed,[1287] exposures in general increase in proportion to dose.[1288–1290] Steady-state exposures are two- to eightfold higher than exposures achieved following a single dose.[1287] The mean half-life of gefitinib across dose levels from 50 to 700 mg/day ranged from 37 to 65 hours.[1289] In children, gefitinib is absorbed slowly with peak plasma concentrations occurring between 2 and 8 hours.[1291] The median half-life of gefitinib in pediatric patients is approximately 12 hours.[1291]

Following oral dosing of erlotinib, peak plasma concentrations occur at a median of 3 hours,[1292] with exposures increasing in proportion to dose.[1292] A mean elimination half-life of approximately 24 to 36 hours provides a basis for daily erlotinib dosing.[1292,1293] Interpatient variability in the pharmacokinetics of erlotinib appears to be moderate; total bilirubin, α_1-acid glycoprotein, and smoking status affected clearance in adults.[1293] The clearance of erlotinib in children is similar to that in adults, but the median terminal half-life of approximately 9 hours is shorter than that observed in adult patients with cancer.[501]

Toxicity. In adults, dose-limiting toxicities of gefitinib include diarrhea, skin rash, and somnolence.[1289,1290,1294] Doses up to 600 mg/day were associated with relatively mild, reversible toxicities including nausea, vomiting, asthenia, anorexia, abdominal pain, dry mouth, pharyngitis, cough, and headache. In children, the MTD of gefitinib administered on a daily basis was 400 mg/m^2, and associated toxicities were similar to those observed in adults.[1291] Interstitial lung disease, a toxicity observed in up to 2% of adults treated with this agent, was not observed in patients treated on the phase I pediatric trial.[1295] The toxicity profile of erlotinib is quite similar to that of gefitinib; skin rash and diarrhea were dose limiting in the phase I setting in adults.[1292] The MTD in adults is 150 mg/day on a continuous schedule. In children with solid tumors, the MTD was 85 mg/m^2/day, with dose-limiting rash and hyperbilirubinemia observed following administration of higher doses.[501]

MISCELLANEOUS AGENTS

Corticosteroids

Although they are not generally thought of as anticancer drugs because of the diversity of their other clinical uses, the corticosteroids (prednisone, prednisolone, dexamethasone) play a significant role in the treatment of ALL, lymphoma, and Hodgkin disease and have been incorporated into treatment regimens for the histiocytoses and brain tumors. They are also useful in managing some of the complications of cancer, including hypercalcemia, increased intracranial pressure, anorexia, and chemotherapy-induced nausea and vomiting.

Glucocorticoids induce apoptosis by binding to intracellular glucocorticoid receptors.[1296] The receptor-glucocorticoid complex translocates to the nucleus, dimerizes, and binds to specific DNA response elements. This causes modulation of expression of many genes. Continuous saturation of the receptor by the steroid for many hours to days is needed to induce apoptosis in sensitive cell lines, and in children with ALL, thrice-daily administration is more effective than intermittent schedules.[1296] Glucocorticoid receptor content on leukemic blasts and the duration of receptor occupancy appear to be the critical determinants of response to corticosteroid therapy *in vitro* and *in vivo*. Loss of or defect in the glucocorticoid receptor can lead to drug resistance *in vitro*.[1297–1299] Children with ALL and low levels of glucocorticoid receptor on their lymphoblasts have a poor prognosis when treated on corticosteroid-based regimens.

The chemical structures of the most commonly used synthetic analogs of cortisol, prednisone, prednisolone, and dexamethasone, are shown in Fig. 10.23. The addition of the 1,2-double bond in prednisolone and dexamethasone increases the glucocorticoid and anti-inflammatory potency fourfold and decreases mineralocorticoid activity. Further addition of the fluorine at position 9 in dexamethasone enhances the activity another fivefold. Prednisone is an inactive prodrug analogs to cortisone and requires chemical reduction of the ketone group at position 11 to a hydroxyl group, yielding prednisolone. This activation occurs in the liver.[1300,1301] Prednisolone and dexamethasone are eliminated by the catabolic enzymes that inactivate cortisol by reduction of the 4,5-double bond (hepatic and extrahepatic), hydroxylation at position 6 (hepatic), or reduction of the 3-ketone to a hydroxyl group followed by conjugation with a sulfate or glucuronide (hepatic).[1301]

Pharmacokinetics

The absorption of orally administered prednisone, prednisolone, and dexamethasone is almost complete (>80%).[1300–1302] Prednisone is rapidly converted to prednisolone, which is the predominant form in plasma after an oral dose of prednisone.[1300,1301] In children, variable absorption of prednisone and prednisolone has been reported.[1302,1303] The elimination half-lives are 2.5 hours for prednisolone and 4 hours for dexamethasone, reflecting differences in the rate of catabolism.[1303–1307] Hepatic metabolism is the primary route of elimination; renal clearance accounts for 10% or less of total clearance.[1308,1309] The clearance of prednisolone, due to concentration-dependent plasma protein binding, is dose dependent and increases with increasing dose.[1301,1309,1310] At low concentrations, prednisolone, like cortisol, is more than 95% bound to transcortin, but this specific carrier protein is saturated at higher prednisolone concentrations, so that the relative amount of free drug available for metabolic degradation increases.

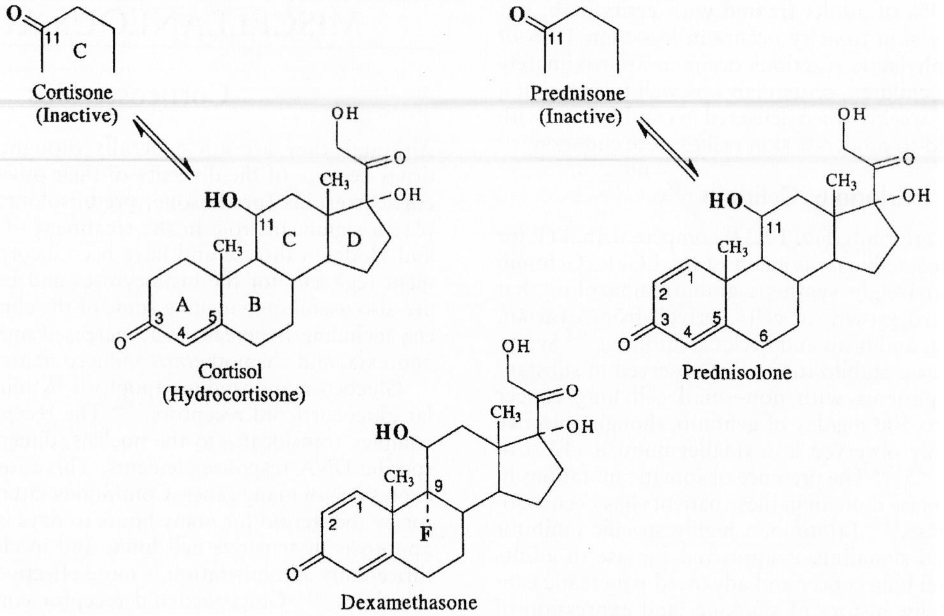

FIGURE 10.23 Chemical structures of the naturally occurring and synthetic corticosteroids commonly used in treating childhood cancers. Reduction of the keto group (cortisone, prednisone) to a hydroxyl group (cortisol, prednisolone) at position 11 is necessary for activity. Addition of the 1,2-double bond (prednisolone, dexamethasone) and the fluorine group at position 9 (dexamethasone) increases glucocorticoid activity.

Dexamethasone is not bound to transcortin, and the degree of protein binding is concentration independent.[1311] Up to a 10-fold range in systemic exposures have been observed following administration of a fixed dexamethasone dose of 8 mg/m²/day, with apparent clearances being greater in younger children.[1312] The lower rate of meningeal relapse in children treated with dexamethasone compared with prednisone may, in part, be explained by this difference in protein binding.[618,1313,1314] The concentration of prednisolone and dexamethasone in the CSF is equivalent to the free drug concentration in plasma, and because prednisolone, unlike dexamethasone, is tightly and extensively bound to transcortin at low concentrations, its free plasma and CSF concentrations are lower at equipotent doses. Diurnal variation in plasma concentrations of prednisolone has also been observed with oral dosing, with higher drug concentrations observed in the morning.[1310]

The capacity to activate prednisone to prednisolone is not impaired in patients with severe hepatic dysfunction, and prednisolone concentrations are elevated in this group, because of delayed catabolism. Unbound prednisolone concentration is also elevated in patients with severe renal dysfunction.[1301]

Toxicity

The corticosteroids have some effect on almost every organ and tissue in the body, and the side effects of these agents are protean. Significant common toxicities include increased appetite, centripedal obesity, immunosuppression, myopathy, osteoporosis, avascular necrosis of bone, peptic ulceration, pancreatitis, psychiatric disorders, cataracts, hypertension, precipitation of diabetes, growth failure, amenorrhea, impaired would healing, and atrophy of subcutaneous tissue.[1297,1311] Although the use of dexamethasone may be associated with fewer thrombotic events than when prednisone is used in intensive leukemia induction regimens,[1315]

its use may increase the rate of serious infections.[1316] Osteonecrosis of weight-bearing joints is a serious complication that occurs in children with leukemia treated with corticosteroids. Risk factors include age older than 10 years, female gender, treatment with two rather than one 21-day course of dexamethasone, and elevated body mass index.[1317–1319] A polymorphism in plasminogen activator inhibitor-1, an inhibitor of fibrinolysis, has recently been associated with an increased risk of developing osteonecrosis, with approximately 27% of heterozygote children developing osteonecrosis versus 12% of children harboring homozygote wild-type variants.[1320]

Drug Interactions

Ketoconazole interferes with the elimination of non–protein-bound prednisolone by inhibiting the catabolic enzyme, 6-β-hydroxylase, leading to a 50% increase in the AUC of unbound prednisolone.[1321] Estrogen-containing oral contraceptives increase transcortin and lower free prednisolone concentrations.[1301] Drugs such as phenytoin, rifampicin, carbamazepine, and barbiturates induce hepatic microsomal enzymes that catabolize prednisolone and result in enhanced prednisolone clearance.[1301] Asparaginase also inhibits dexamethasone clearance, likely through impairing hepatic synthesis of proteins required for drug clearance.[1312]

Asparaginase

Asparaginase is a bacterial enzyme that provides specific nutritional therapy for ALL and lymphoblastic lymphomas. This enzyme rapidly depletes the circulating pool of asparagine by catalyzing the conversion of this amino acid to aspartic acid and ammonia. In most tissues, asparagine is synthesized from aspartic acid and glutamine by the enzyme asparagine

synthase, and normal tissues can respond to asparagine depletion by upregulation of this enzyme. In contrast, sensitive lymphoid cancers do not upregulate asparagine synthase and
therefore depend on exogenous circulating asparagine for protein synthesis.[1322] Asparaginase-resistant lymphoid tumor cells
often have high levels of asparagine synthase rendering them
capable of synthesizing their own asparagine.[1322] Thus,
asparaginase has a selective antileukemic effect.[1322,1323]

The native (unmodified) forms of asparaginase are
derived from *Escherichia coli* or *Erwinia carotovora* and are
administered intravenously or intramuscularly at doses of
6,000 to 25,000 IU/m² on an intermittent schedule (usually
three times each week). Conjugation of poly(ethylene
glycol) to *E. coli* asparaginase (PEG-asparaginase) lowers
the immunogenicity of this foreign protein and prolongs the
drug's half-life, allowing for less frequent administration
(2,500 IU/m² every 2 to 4 weeks).[1324] The k_m of *E. coli*
asparaginase for asparagine is 10 μM, which is approximately 10-fold higher than the minimal concentration of the
amino acid required *in vitro* to support cell growth.[1322] The
continual production and release of asparagine by normal
tissues into the blood stream requires plasma asparaginase
activity exceeding 0.1 IU/mL to suppress the concentration
of asparagine below the critical level of 1 to 3 μM.[1325,1326]
2,500 IU/m² doses of *E. coli* asparaginase appear to be sufficient to deplete serum asparagine,[1327] whereas higher doses
and more frequent administration of *Erwinia* asparaginase
may be required.[1328]

In a randomized trial in standard risk ALL, asparaginase
plasma concentrations were more prolonged with a single
dose of PEG-asparaginase than with 9 to 12 doses of native *E.
coli* asparaginase.[1329] Toxicity of the native and pegylated
enzymes was similar, and the incidence of allergic reactions
and silent antibodies was very low with both preparations.
More prolonged asparaginase treatment regimens improve
disease outcome but are associated with a higher incidence of
allergic reactions.[1330,1331] Children with Philadelphia chromosome-positive leukemia appear to be more resistant to the
effects of PEG-asparaginase.[1332]

Pharmacokinetics

Parenteral administration of asparaginase is required because
of denaturation and peptidase digestion within the intestinal
tract. Peak plasma concentrations of the enzyme are dose
related. Daily administration results in significant accumulation of asparaginase.[1333] Peak concentrations with intramuscular injection are approximately half of those achieved with
intravenous dosing. The time to peak concentration (rate of
absorption) after intramuscular injection is 24 to 48 hours for
E. coli asparaginase, less than 24 hours for *Erwinia* asparaginase, and 72 to 96 hours for PEG-asparaginase.[1334] The volume of distribution for asparaginase approximates plasma
volume, and the rate of elimination is slow. The half-lives for
E. coli asparaginase, *Erwinia* asparaginase, and PEG-asparaginase are 24 to 36 hours, 10 to 15 hours, and 5 to 7 days,
respectively (Fig. 10.24).[1334]

Plasma concentrations of asparagine fall to undetectable
levels within 24 hours of a dose of asparaginase. The duration
of depletion of circulating asparagine is related to the rate of
asparaginase elimination; consequently, it is shorter with
Erwinia asparaginase than with native *E. coli* asparaginase.[1327] PEG-asparaginase depletes serum asparagine for at
least 14 days.[1335,1336] Even though asparaginase distributes primarily within the intravascular space, its effects are more wide
reaching. For example, asparaginase cannot be detected in the
CSF after systemic administration, but CSF levels of
asparagine are depleted for long periods.[1337–1339]

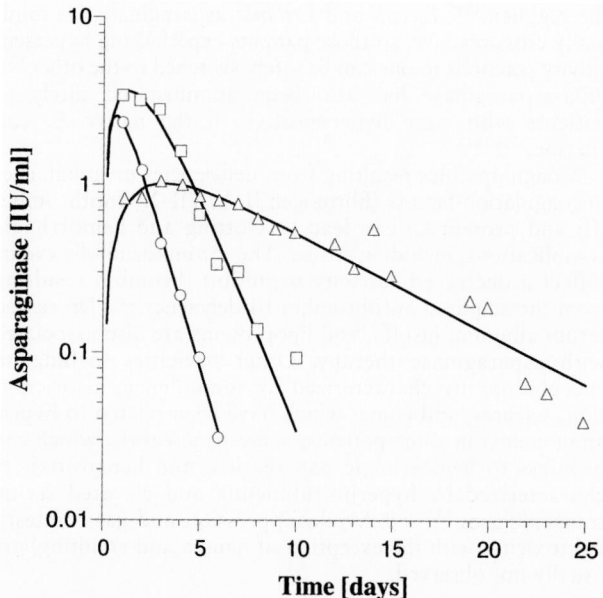

FIGURE 10.24 Disposition of serum asparaginase activity in 10
patients treated intramuscularly with 25,000 IU/m² of native *E. coli*
asparaginase (squares), 10 patients treated intramuscularly with
25,000 IU/m² of native *Erwinia* asparaginase (circles), and 10 patients
treated intramuscularly with 2,500 IU/m² of PEG-asparaginase (triangles). Points represent the mean. (Adapted from Asselin BL, Whitin
JC, Coppola DJ, et al. Comparative pharmacokinetic studies of
three asparaginase preparations. J Clin Oncol 1993;11:1780, with
permission).

Patients who develop antibodies to asparaginase have a
rapid fall in the plasma concentrations of the native enzyme,
indicating that the antibody interferes with the therapeutic
effects of asparaginase.[1323,1340] PEG-asparaginase elimination is
more rapid in one-third of patients who have previously experienced hypersensitivity reactions to native *E. coli* asparaginase.[1334,1341] Many patients who have high antibody titers do
not have a history of clinical hypersensitivity reaction.[1342] Consequently, weekly dosing of PEG-asparaginase is recommended
in children previously treated with native asparaginase.[1334,1343]
In children with relapsed ALL, weekly administration of PEG-
asparaginase resulted in a higher remission induction rate than
biweekly dosing.[1343] Development of antibody to poly(ethylene
glycol) itself may develop in children being treated for ALL,
with anti-PEG antibodies being associated with increased
clearance of PEG-asparaginase.[1344]

Toxicity

The principal side effects of asparaginase are related to sensitization to a bacterial protein or decreased protein synthesis.[1323,1326] Allergic reactions range from local erythema and
swelling at the injection site to urticaria, laryngeal edema,
bronchospasm, or anaphylaxis. Diphenhydramine, epinephrine, and other resuscitative measures must be available when
administering this agent, even for the initial dose. The overall
incidence of hypersensitivity reactions in children is 16% to
33% with native *E. coli* asparaginase.[1323] PEG-asparaginase is
less immunogenic than the native forms, but acute allergic
reactions can occur with repeated administration. The incidence of hypersensitivity reactions is lower (10%) in patients
receiving combination chemotherapy than in those receiving
E. coli asparaginase as a single agent (40%), presumably
because of the immunosuppressive effects of the other drugs in

the regimen.[1345] *E. coli* and *Erwinia* asparaginase are minimally cross-reactive, so those patients experiencing hypersensitivity reactions to one can be safely switched to the other.[1346] PEG-asparaginase has also been administered safely to patients who were hypersensitive to the native *E. coli* enzyme.[1324,1343]

Coagulopathies resulting from deficiencies or imbalances in coagulation factors (fibrinogen II, V, VII–X; antithrombin III; and protein C) can lead to clotting and hemorrhagic complications, including stroke. The thromboembolic events reflect a decreased capacity to inhibit thrombin resulting from the acquired antithrombin III deficiency.[1347] Decreased serum albumin, insulin, and lipoproteins are also associated with asparaginase therapy. Other toxicities include an encephalopathy characterized by somnolence, disorientation, seizures, and coma, which have been related to hyperammonemia in some patients; acute pancreatitis, which can progress to hemorrhagic pancreatitis; and hepatotoxicity characterized by hyperbilirubinemia and elevated serum transaminases.[1323,1326] Myelosuppression and gastrointestinal toxicity (with the exception of nausea and vomiting) are usually not observed.

Drug Interactions

Asparaginase can rescue patients from the toxic effects of methotrexate and cytarabine. The sequential combinations of methotrexate or cytarabine followed by asparaginase have proven effective in consolidation therapy of ALL and in the treatment of children with relapsed leukemia.[1323,1326] Antagonism has been observed if asparaginase is administered before these antimetabolites.[1348] Asparaginase also can decrease the clearance of dexamethasone.[1312]

Retinoids

Retinoids have an established role in the treatment of patients with acute promyelocytic leukemia (APL)[1349,1350] and children with high risk neuroblastoma.[1351] The actions of retinoids are mediated through the nuclear retinoid receptors, which are members of the steroid/thyroid/retinoid hormone receptor family.[1352] Retinoid receptors act as ligand-inducible transcription factors that enhance the transcription of target genes by binding to retinoic acid response elements in the promoter region of retinoid-responsive genes. Two families of retinoid nuclear receptors have been described, the retinoic acid receptors (RARs)[1353,1354] and the retinoid X receptors (RXRs).[1355,1356] The RARs bind the naturally occurring retinoid all-*trans*-retinoic acid (ATRA) with high affinity (Fig. 10.25), whereas the RXRs bind 9-*cis*-retinoic acid (9*c*RA), a naturally occurring, biologically active isomer of ATRA[1357] that is capable of binding and transactivating both the RXRs as well as the RARs. 13-*cis*-retinoic acid (13*c*RA) binds neither class of receptors with high affinity and likely acts as a prodrug for other isomers.

Although 13*c*RA has very limited activity in children with recurrent neuroblastoma,[1358] high-risk patients with treatment induced minimal residual disease benefit from its administration.[1351,1359] As a single agent, daily doses of 45 mg/m^2 of ATRA result in complete response rates of 70% to 92% of patients with newly diagnosed or relapsed APL.[1360–1362] The addition of ATRA to chemotherapeutic regimens for adults[1349,1350,1363] and children[1364] with APL has been responsible for a dramatic improvement in survival, with 5-year disease-free survival ranging from 75% to 85%.[1365,1366]

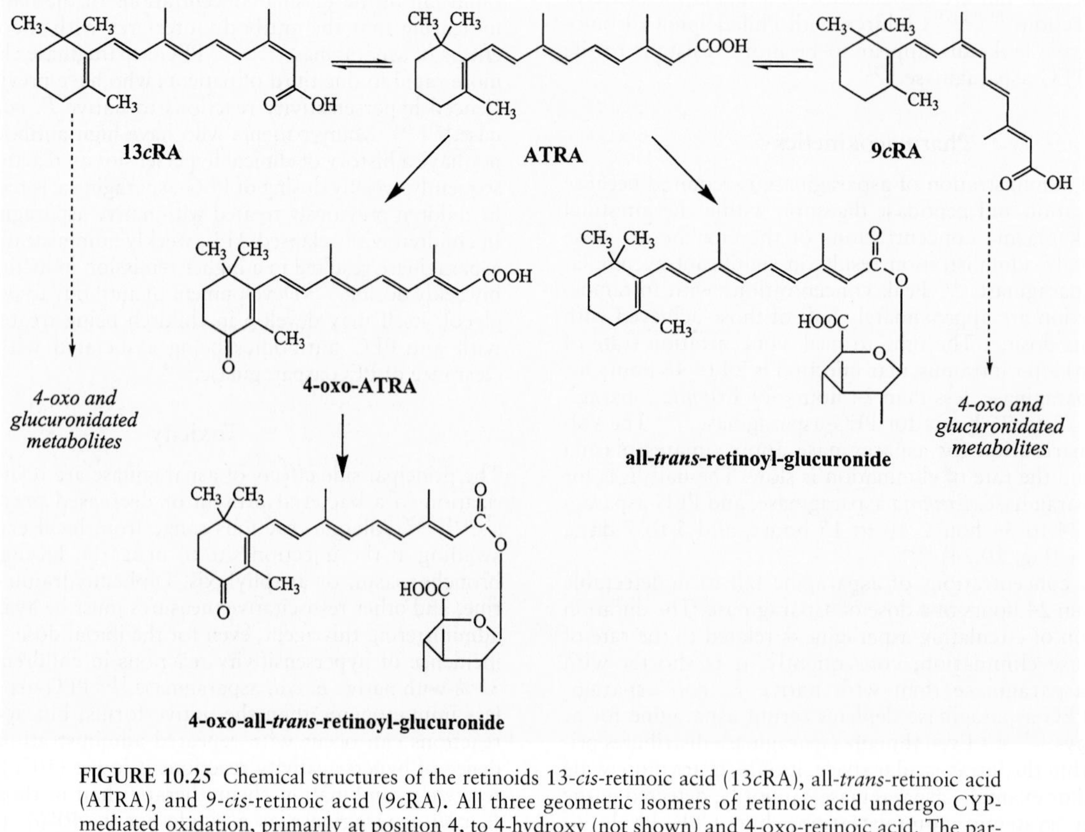

FIGURE 10.25 Chemical structures of the retinoids 13-*cis*-retinoic acid (13*c*RA), all-*trans*-retinoic acid (ATRA), and 9-*cis*-retinoic acid (9*c*RA). All three geometric isomers of retinoic acid undergo CYP-mediated oxidation, primarily at position 4, to 4-hydroxy (not shown) and 4-oxo-retinoic acid. The parent isomers and their oxidized metabolites also undergo glucuronidation.

Pharmacokinetics

The pharmacokinetics of 13cRA following oral administration are highly variable, with peak plasma concentrations occurring within approximately 4 hours and terminal elimination averaging 10 to 20 hours in adult patients with cancer.[1367–1372] The primary 4-oxo-metabolite is formed rapidly and, during chronic administration, its concentration exceeds that of the parent drug by four- to fivefold.[1370,1373] In children, the half-life of elimination appears to be shorter than that observed in adult patients.[1374,1375]

The pharmacokinetics of ATRA, which has been well studied in both adult[1376–1379] and pediatric patients,[1380,1381] differ substantially from 13cRA. Following a 45 mg/m^2 oral dose of ATRA, peak plasma concentrations on the first day of treatment are approximately 1 μM.[1378,1379,1381] The elimination of ATRA, however, is significantly more rapid than that of 13cRA, with a terminal half-life of only approximately 45 minutes.[1378,1381,1382] Furthermore, with daily dosing, there is a significant decrease in plasma ATRA concentrations within days of the start of therapy.[1383] The rapid decrease in plasma drug exposure is related to autoinduction of enzymes CYP2C8, and to lesser extents by CYP3A4, CYP2C9,[1384] and members of the retinoic acid specific CYP26 family[1385–1388] responsible for the 4-hydroxylation of drug (Fig. 10.25). Intermittent schedules of administration can partially overcome the increased clearance of ATRA.[1349,1350,1364,1376,1380]

Toxicity

The embryotoxic and teratogenic effects of retinoids have been well documented and include a characteristic pattern of malformations involving craniofacial, cardiac, thymic, and CNS structures.[1389–1391] A prescriber education program developed to minimize pregnancies among women treated for acne[1392] has been implemented and is required for physicians prescribing 13cRA.[1393]

The most common symptoms associated with retinoid administration include cheilitis, conjunctivitis, dry mouth, xerosis, pruritus, headache, bone and joint pain, epistaxis, and fatigue.[1368] Common laboratory abnormalities include elevated sedimentation rates, elevated triglycerides, and, less commonly, elevations in hepatic transaminases. In children with cancer receiving 13cRA doses of 100 to 200 mg/m^2/day, hypercalcemia was observed in 9 of 39 patients and was dose limiting in 3 children.[1375]

The major adverse effect of ATRA that occurs in 25% of ATRA-treated APL patients in the absence of prophylactic measures is the retinoic acid syndrome.[1394–1397] Retinoic acid syndrome manifests with weight gain, respiratory distress, serous effusions, cardiac, and renal failure and is generally associated with increasing leukocyte counts and subsequent release of several cytokines by maturing blast cells. Prophylaxis, consisting of dexamethasone and, in case of rapidly increasing leukocyte counts, cytotoxic chemotherapy, has reduced drug-related mortality to approximately 1%.[1397]

Children appear more susceptible to the CNS effects of ATRA, manifested by headaches and the development of pseudotumor cerebri.[1364,1380,1381] Doses of 45 mg/m^2/day are generally well tolerated by children, but very young children may remain at increased risk of pseudotumor cerebri even at this dose.

Arsenic

Arsenic is one of the oldest drugs both in the Western as well as in traditional Chinese medicine, with reports of its use dating back more than 2,000 years.[1398] Apart from organic arsenicals in which arsenic atoms are covalently bound to carbon-based molecules, arsenic occurs in three inorganic forms: As_4S_4 (red arsenic, realgar), As_2S_3 (yellow arsenic, orpiment), and As_2O_3 (white arsenic, arsenic trioxide).[1399] In the late 18th and early 19th century, Fowler's solution (potassium bicarbonate–based solution of arsenic) was used to treat a number of diseases including chronic myelogenous leukemia. Its used peaked around 1910 when Ehrlich introduced an organic arsenic–based product for the treatment for tuberculosis and syphilis. The introduction of antibiotics and chemotherapy led to the near abandonment of arsenic-based treatments by the mid 20th century.[1398] It was during the 1970s, in the northeastern region of China, that a crude solution of As_2O_3 was introduced into the treatment of APL,[1398] and in the 1990s results from prospective clinical trials of pure As_2O_3 emerged.[1400,1401]

Numerous investigators have found that arsenic trioxide induces complete, and often durable, remissions in 70% to 90% of adults with newly diagnosed or relapsed APL.[1402–1406] In adults with newly diagnosed APL, the addition of two courses of arsenic trioxide consolidation therapy after remission induction significantly improves the outcome of patients treated with daunorubicin, cytarabine, and oral tretinoin.[1407] The FDA-approved dose for arsenic trioxide in both adults and children with APL for remission induction is 0.15 mg/kg daily, administered intravenously, for up to 60 doses.

Toxicity

In adult patients, adverse events frequently associated with arsenic trioxide administration include elevated hepatic transaminases, abdominal pain, musculoskeletal pain, peripheral neuropathy, hypokalemia, hyperglycemia, and dermatitis. Nearly 40% of adult patients experience cardiac conduction abnormalities, most commonly QTc interval prolongation.[1408] The APL differentiation syndrome, clinically similar to retinoic acid syndrome with fever, dyspnea, pleural effusion, pulmonary infiltrates, and weight gain, occurs in up to 30% of adult patients.[1409,1410]

The toxicity profile of arsenic trioxide in children appears similar to that observed in adults.[1411,1412] In a pediatric phase I trial, frequent non–dose-limiting toxicities observed included elevated serum hepatic transaminases, nausea/vomiting, abdominal pain, constipation, hypomagnesemia, hypocalcemia, hyperglycemia, dermatitis, infection, and headache.[1412] Eight percent of cycles were associated with prolonged QTc interval and 3% with APL differentiation syndrome.

Pharmacokinetics

The metabolism of arsenic trioxide involves reduction of pentavalent arsenic (As^V) to trivalent arsenic (As^{III}) by arsenate reductase, and methylation of trivalent arsenic to monomethylarsonic acid and dimethylarsinic acid by methyltransferases.[1413,1414] Results of current human pharmacokinetic studies are difficult to interpret owing to the differing analytical methodologies employed. In one adult study following administration of 0.15 mg/kg As_2O_3, total peak plasma arsenic concentrations averaged 6.9 μM and the mean terminal half-life averaged 12 hours.[1403] A more recent study found that although the maximum concentration of As^{III} and As^V were similar (0.17 ± 0.11 and 0.13 ± 0.05 μM, respectively), the AUC of As^V was approximately twice that of As^{III}.[1415] With repeated administration, approximately 60% of the dose was excreted in the urine as inorganic arsenic and methylated species. In children, following an intravenous dose of 0.15 mg/kg, the median (range) peak total arsenic concentration was 0.26 (0.11 to 0.37) μM, with a terminal half-life exceeding 24 hours.[1412]

CENTRAL NERVOUS SYSTEM PHARMACOLOGY OF ANTICANCER DRUGS

The penetration of the anticancer drugs into the CNS is relevant to the treatment of childhood cancers, because primary and metastatic tumors of the brain or meninges are common in children and because anticancer drugs are associated with acute and chronic neurotoxicity. The degree of drug penetration across the blood-brain barrier is determined by the physicochemical properties of the drug, such as lipophilicity, molecular size, and degree of ionization, and the free (non-protein bound) drug concentration in plasma.[1416-1418] Most anticancer drugs penetrate poorly into the CSF, which is also used as a surrogate for blood-brain barrier penetration (see Table 10.5). The inability to achieve adequate antileukemic drug concentrations in the CSF probably accounts for the high rate of leptomeningeal relapse in children with ALL after the introduction of effective systemic therapy. Strategies employed to circumvent limited penetration into the CNS are listed in Table 10.7. Regional drug administration, such as intrathecal, intra-arterial, and interstitial implants, is the most commonly used approach.[1416]

Intrathecal Chemotherapy

Poor penetration of systemically administered anticancer drugs into the CSF can be circumvented by direct injection of the agents into the CSF. Intrathecally injected chemotherapy (e.g., methotrexate, cytarabine) is highly effective as primary or preventive therapy for meningeal leukemia and lymphoma. As a form of regional chemotherapy, intrathecal administration has the advantage of delivering very high drug concentrations to the CSF and meninges with low doses and therefore with minimal systemic toxicity.[1416,1419] However, there are disadvantages to intralumbar administration. Repeated lumbar punctures are painful, inconvenient, and technically challenging. In 10% of intralumbar injections, the drug is not delivered into the subarachnoid space but is instead injected or leaks into the subdural or epidural space.[1420] Because of the slow circulation of the CSF, distribution of drugs within the subarachnoid space, specifically to the ventricles, is not uniform. Ventricular methotrexate concentrations after an intralumbar dose are highly variable and are less than 10% of ventricular concentrations after direct intraventricular injection.[1421] The depth of penetration of effective drug concentrations into the brain parenchyma is limited to a few millimeters for the commonly used intrathecal agents. As a result, intrathecal therapy is not likely to be effective for parenchymal brain tumors.[1422] Intrathecal therapy is also associated with unique toxicities, such as chemical arachnoiditis.

The distribution of drug from the lumbar sac to the ventricles can be significantly improved by positioning the patient prone for 60 minutes after intralumbar injection. In animals, ventricular methotrexate concentrations after intralumbar drug administration were more than 20-fold higher when they were placed in the prone position compared with keeping them upright.[1423] Many of the problems associated with intralumbar injection can also be overcome with direct intraventricular administration. This approach entails the surgical placement of a catheter into the lateral ventricle. The catheter is then attached to a subcutaneously implanted reservoir for access.[1424] Administration of drugs directly into the ventricle via this reservoir is more convenient and less painful and allows for more frequent injections. Intraventricular therapy ensures that the drug is delivered to the subarachnoid space and results in better drug distribution throughout the CSF.[1421] Better drug distribution may account for the improved therapeutic results from intraventricular therapy compared with intralumbar administration in the treatment of overt meningeal leukemia.[1425] However, even when methotrexate was infused continuously into the ventricle for prolonged periods in animals, steady-state drug concentrations in the lumbar space were lower than simultaneous ventricular concentrations, presumably because the rate of CSF flow into the lumbar sac is slower than the rate of diffusion or excretion of methotrexate from the CSF.[1426]

Ventricular access devices, which generally are reserved for patients with relapsed leptomeningeal disease, allow for more flexible drug administration schedules, such as the concentration × time (C × T) schedule (daily for 3 consecutive days). C × T methotrexate and cytarabine proved to be effective for inducing and maintaining CSF remission in patients with multiply recurrent leptomeningeal leukemia.[1427]

There are a limited number of agents that are routinely administered intrathecally. The most commonly used agents are the antimetabolites, methotrexate and cytarabine, and the alkylating agent thiotepa. A recently completed phase I clinical trial of intrathecal gemcitabine demonstrated that there was significant neurotoxicity associated precluding intrathecal gemcitabine delivery.[1428] A phase II trial of intrathecal topotecan administered twice weekly in children with leptomeningeal dissemination of CNS or solid tumors was not associated with an adequate progression-free survival,[1429] thus a phase I trial evaluating an alternate dosing schedule is in progress.

Methotrexate

Intrathecal methotrexate has been in clinical use for more than 40 years, primarily for the treatment of the meningeal spread of cancer, especially leukemia and lymphoma. It is also administered adjuvantly to patients with newly diagnosed ALL to prevent meningeal relapse. Acute and delayed neurotoxic reactions to intrathecal methotrexate have been reported. An acute chemical arachnoiditis characterized by headache, nuchal rigidity, vomiting, fever, and CSF pleocytosis can present several hours to days after a dose. A subacute encephalopathy, which may be irreversible in some patients, presents with extremity paresis and cranial nerve palsies, ataxia, visual impairment, seizures, and coma. This syndrome is associated with elevated CSF drug concentrations.[1430] An ascending radiculopathy with loss of primarily motor function

TABLE 10.7

TREATMENT STRATEGIES TO CIRCUMVENT THE BLOOD-BRAIN BARRIER

Strategy	Examples
High-dose systemic chemotherapy	High-dose methotrexate, cytarabine
Identifying drugs that penetrate the blood-brain barrier (cross into CSF)	Thiotepa, topotecan
Disruption of the blood-brain barrier	Osmotic disruption with mannitol
Regional drug administration	
Intrathecal injection	Methotrexate, cytarabine
Intra-arterial injection	Cisplatin
Interstitial therapy	Gliadel

resembling Guillain-Barre syndrome is also associated with intrathecal methotrexate, as well as cytarabine, and occurs days to weeks following a course of therapy.[1431] A chronic, progressive demyelinating encephalopathy (i.e., leukoencephalopathy) that appears months to years after intrathecal methotrexate leads to dementia, spastic paralysis, seizures, and coma in more advanced cases. Severe, often fatal, reactions can result from the inadvertent administration of excessive doses of methotrexate or the administration of the wrong agent (e.g., vincristine) intrathecally. Clinicians administering drugs by this route must take great care.[1432] Intrathecal methotrexate overdose has been treated with CSF drainage and ventriculolumbar perfusion. Intrathecal instillation of the investigational agent glucarpidase (carboxypeptidase-G_2) has also been reported.[1433,1434]

Methotrexate elimination from the CSF after intrathecal injection is biphasic, with a terminal half-life of 14 hours.[1435] Methotrexate is eliminated by passive diffusion out of the CSF, bulk resorption of CSF, and a nonspecific active transport system.[1426] Conditions associated with delayed clearance of methotrexate from the CSF include meningeal leukemia, communicating hydrocephalus, or the lumbar puncture syndrome.[1435]

When methotrexate is administered intrathecally, the volume of the CSF is the initial volume in which the drug is distributed. In young children, CSF volume increases much more rapidly than the body surface area, reaching 80% of the adult volume by the age of 3 years.[1436] An intrathecal dose based on body surface area would underdose young children and overdose adolescents. Bleyer and colleagues recommended an intrathecal dosage schedule for methotrexate based on age instead of body surface area.[1436] This regimen has been less neurotoxic, and because this dosing scheme was incorporated into frontline leukemia protocols, the CNS relapse rate has declined from 12% to 7%.[1437] The greatest decline was observed in the youngest patients, the group in whom the intrathecal methotrexate dosage was increased with the new adaptive dosing regimen.

Cytarabine

Intrathecally administered cytarabine is also of value in the treatment and prevention of meningeal leukemia. The clinical pharmacology of intrathecal cytarabine is quite different from that seen with systemic administration of this agent. With an intraventricular dose of 30 mg, peak concentrations exceed 2 mM and remain above 1 μM for 24 hours.[726,1438] Levels of cytidine deaminase, the enzyme that metabolizes cytarabine to ara-U, are low in brain and CSF, and metabolism to ara-U is therefore only a minor pathway of elimination.[1439] The ratio of ara-U to cytarabine in the CSF is only 0.08. The terminal half-life of cytarabine is 3.5 hours, and the clearance is 0.42 mL/min, similar to the CSF bulk flow rate.[1438] Plasma concentrations of cytarabine after an intrathecal 30-mg dose are less than 1 μM. Leukemic cells in the CSF were found to accumulate significant levels of intracellular ara-CTP after intrathecal cytarabine, and this active metabolite was retained in cells longer (half-life of 8 to 36 hours) than in peripheral lymphoblasts.[1440] Neurotoxicity from intrathecal cytarabine includes arachnoiditis, radiculopathy, seizures, encephalopathy, or myelopathy.[1418,1441]

DepoCyt, which is a liposome-encapsulated formulation of cytarabine, was specifically developed for intrathecal use. Sustained release of cytarabine from the liposomes markedly prolongs the cytarabine half-life (141 hours in adults and 57 hours in children) and the duration of exposure to cytotoxic concentrations (9 days) in CSF.[1442,1443] The recommended dosage in children is 35 mg, which is less than the recommended dose of 50 mg in adults.[1443] When given with concomitant oral dexamethasone, the toxicity profile of DepoCyt is similar to that of unencapsulated cytarabine. Acute drug-related toxicities include fever, headache, back pain, nausea, and encephalopathy.[1442-1444]

Thiotepa

The alkylating agent thiotepa can be safely administered intrathecally at a dose of 10 mg and is sometimes used as a second-line agent for childhood meningeal cancers, although it does not appear to be of substantial benefit.[1445] Thiotepa toxicity is similar to that of intrathecal methotrexate.[1446] However, thiotepa is highly lipophilic and diffuses rapidly out of the CSF leading to limited drug distribution within the subarachnoid space. After intraventricular administration, thiotepa is rapidly cleared from the CSF at a rate 10-fold higher than CSF bulk flow, and exposure in the lumbar CSF is less than 10% of that achieved in the ventricle.[1447]

High-Dose Systemic Therapy for Meningeal and CNS Tumors

Limited CNS penetration of some anticancer agents can be overcome by administering high doses of the drugs systemically. This approach has been successfully applied with methotrexate and cytarabine. The advantages of the systemic approach over intrathecal therapy include sustained CSF drug concentrations with prolonged intravenous infusions and better drug penetration into the deep perivascular spaces and brain parenchyma. However, methotrexate concentrations are not uniform throughout the subarachnoid space at steady state during a continuous intravenous infusion of methotrexate. The lumbar CSF concentrations are higher than ventricular CSF concentrations.[1426] The other disadvantage of this approach is the potential for severe systemic toxicity.[1416]

Very high systemic methotrexate doses can be safely delivered with leucovorin rescue, and therapeutic concentrations of methotrexate can be achieved in the CSF. A dose of 33,600 mg/m^2 administered over 24 hours as a loading dose (6,000 mg/m^2) followed by a continuous infusion (1,200 mg/m^2/hr for 23 hours) results in CSF methotrexate concentrations of 30 to 40 μM.[570] The remission induction rate in patients with overt meningeal leukemia with this regimen is 80%. This regimen has also been successful as preventive therapy for meningeal leukemia in patients with ALL.[1448]

The CSF penetration of cytarabine is more favorable than methotrexate but is dose dependent. The ratio in one study decreased from 33% to 18% with an increase in the dose from 4,000 to 18,000 mg/m^2 administered as a 72-hour infusion.[721] The standard high-dose (3,000 mg/m^2) regimen given every 12 hours results in persistent cytotoxic concentrations of cytarabine in the CSF, in part because the elimination half-life of cytarabine in CSF is eightfold longer than in plasma, because of the low levels of cytidine deaminase in brain and CSF.[1449] High-dose intravenous cytarabine appears to be effective for treating CNS leukemia and lymphoma but is associated with significant systemic toxicity.[1450-1452]

Other agents for which the systemic approach may be applicable include cyclophosphamide and thiotepa. Cyclophosphamide in high doses (80 mg/kg/day for 2 days) appears to be active against brain tumors.[1453] The systemic approach may also be more appropriate for thiotepa. After intravenous administration, plasma and CSF drug concentrations are equivalent, and significant amounts of the active metabolite, TEPA, also penetrate into the CNS.[1447]

PERSPECTIVES

Although a high proportion of children with certain types of cancer are being cured, there are still too many who do not respond or who relapse and eventually succumb to their cancer after a good initial response. Failure of multimodality therapy to cure individual patients may result from *de novo* or acquired resistance to the anticancer drugs that are used in the regimen, or inadequate drug delivery to the cancer. The latter pharmacological limitations of therapy can result from interpatient variability in drug disposition with poor absorption or more rapid drug clearance in a subgroup of patients limiting drug exposure or dose modifications necessitated by acute and chronic toxicity.

Anticancer drug dosing is toxicity based. The optimum dose of most anticancer drugs is the MTD, and after this fixed dose is administered, dose modifications are based on the severity of ensuing toxicity. A more rational approach would be to individualize drug dose and schedule based on specific patient characteristics (adaptive dosing) and on plasma drug concentration (therapeutic drug monitoring). These strategies have been successfully applied to adapting carboplatin dose for renal function and to basing leucovorin rescue on methotrexate plasma concentration after high-dose methotrexate therapy. Although therapeutic and toxic drug concentrations are not known for most anticancer drugs, simply defining the average plasma concentration after a standard drug dose might help to identify outliers and produce rational dose modifications for patients with organ dysfunction.

Those patients who are cured are at risk for significant and often life-threatening acute and long-term toxic effects of the treatment. The severity of the toxicity of the anticancer drugs reflects their nonselective mechanisms of action and the emphasis on dose intensity to maximize tumor cell kill. Methods to circumvent or ameliorate chemotherapy-induced toxicity have improved the tolerability of chemotherapy. Examples of rescuing patients from dose-limiting toxicities include the use of hematopoietic growth factors such as filgrastim to limit the duration of granulocytopenia after myelosuppressive therapy, the administration of mesna to block the urotoxicity of the oxazaphosphorines, leucovorin rescue from high-dose methotrexate, and the prevention of anthracycline cardiotoxicity with dexrazoxane.

The search for more selective and less toxic anticancer drugs and for more effective drug combinations must continue. Imatinib has ushered in the current era of developing agents that target a specific molecular defect. However, the paradigm in chronic myelogenous leukemia, in which the underlying transforming event involves an enzyme (*BCR-ABL* kinase) that can be directly inhibited by a small molecule, may not be readily translated into the majority of other pediatric tumors. Rather, defining the role of an expanding number of agents that target cell signaling pathways that contribute to but are not causative of the malignant process will be the next therapeutic challenge for pediatric cancer drug development. Ongoing advances in our understanding the biology of pediatric cancers may soon identify druggable targets unique to pediatric tumors. Greater resources and efforts will be required to meet these challenges and will require improved integration of advances in the biologic and pharmacologic basic sciences into the design and use of chemotherapeutic regimens.

References

1. Farber S, Diamond LK, Mercer RD, et al. Temporary remissions in acute leukemia in children produced by folic acid antagonist 4-aminopteroylglutamic acid (aminopterin). N Engl J Med 1948;28:787–793.
2. Jemal A, Siegel R, Ward E, et al. Cancer Statistics, 2009. CA Cancer J Clin 2009;59(4):225–249.
3. Hammond GD. Keynote address: the cure of childhood cancers. Cancer 1986;58 (Suppl):407–413.
4. Balis FM. The goal of cancer treatment. Oncologist 1998;3:V.
5. Schipper H, Goh CR, Wang TL. Shifting the cancer paradigm: must we kill to cure? J Clin Oncol 1995;13:801–807.
6. Alley MC, Scudiero DA, Monks A, et al. Feasibility of drug screening with panels of human tumor cell lines using a microculture tetrazolium assay. Cancer Res 1988; 48:589–601.
7. Leventhal BG, Wittes RE. Research methods in clinical oncology. New York, NY: Raven Press, 1988.
8. Bleyer WA. Antineoplastic agents. In: Yaffe SJ, ed. Pediatric pharmacology: therapeutic principles in practice. New York, NY: Grune & Stratton, 1980: 349–377.
9. Henderson EH, Samaha RJ. Evidence that drugs in multiple combinations have materially advanced the treatment of human malignancies. Cancer Res 1969;29: 2272–2280.
10. Goldie JH, Coldman AJ. The genetic origin of drug resistance in neoplasms: implications for systemic therapy. Cancer Res 1984;44:3643–3653.
11. DeVita VT. Principles of chemotherapy. In: DeVita VT, Hellman S, Rosenberg S, eds. Principles and practice of oncology. Philadelphia, PA: JB Lippincott, 1989:276–296.
12. Dawson JW, Taylor I. Principles of adjuvant therapy. Br J Hosp Med 1995;54: 249–254.
13. D'Angio GJ, Evans AE, Breslow N, et al. The treatment of Wilms' tumor: results of the National Wilms' Tumor Study. Cancer 1976;38:633–646.
14. Nesbit ME, Perez CA, Tefft M, et al. Multimodal therapy for the management of primary non-metastatic Ewing's sarcoma of bone: an intergroup study. Natl Cancer Inst Monogr 1981;56:255–262.
15. Link MP. Non-Hodgkin's lymphoma in children. Pediatr Clin North Am 1985; 32:699–720.
16. Ortega JA, Rivard GE, Isaacs H, et al. The influence of chemotherapy on the prognosis of rhabdomyosarcoma. Med Pediatr Oncol 1975;1:227–234.
17. Sposto R, Ertel IJ, Jenkins JD, et al. The effectiveness of chemotherapy for the treatment of high grade astrocytomas in children: results of a randomized trial. A report from the Children's Cancer Study Group. J Neurooncol 1989;7:165–177.
18. Link MP, Goorin AM, Miser AW, et al. The effect of adjuvant chemotherapy on relapse-free survival in patients with osteosarcoma of the extremity. N Engl J Med 1986;314:1600–1606.
19. Eilber F, Giuliano A, Eckardt J, et al. Adjuvant chemotherapy for osteosarcoma: a randomized prospective trial. J Clin Oncol 1987;5:21–26.
20. Berg SL, Grisell DL, DeLaney TF, et al. Principles of treatment of pediatric solid tumors. Pediatr Clin North Am 1991;38:249–267.
21. Martin DS. The scientific basis for adjuvant chemotherapy. Cancer Treat Rev 1981;8:169–189.
22. DeVita VT. The relationship between tumor mass and resistance to chemotherapy. Cancer 1983;51:1209–1220.
23. Goldie JH, Coldman AJ. Theoretical considerations regarding the early use of adjuvant chemotherapy. Recent Results Cancer Res 1986;103:30–35.
24. Wittes RE. Adjuvant chemotherapy—clinical trials and laboratory models. Cancer Treat Rep 1986;70:87–103.
25. Grier HE, Krailo MD, Tarbell NJ, et al. Addition of ifosfamide and etoposide to standard chemotherapy for Ewing's sarcoma and primitive neuroectodermal tumor of bone. N Engl J Med 2003;348:694–701.
26. Rosen G. Neoadjuvant chemotherapy for osteogenic sarcoma: a model for the treatment of other highly malignant neoplasms. Recent Results Cancer Res 1986;103: 148–157.
27. Trimble EL, Ungerleider RS, Abrams JA, et al. Neoadjuvant therapy in cancer treatment. Cancer 1993;72:3515–3524.
28. Frei E, Canellos GP. Dose: a critical factor in cancer chemotherapy. Am J Med 1980;69:585–594.
29. Frei E, Antman K, Teicher B, et al. Bone marrow autotransplantation for solid tumors—prospects. J Clin Oncol 1989;7:515–526.
30. Hryniuk W, Bush H. The importance of dose intensity in chemotherapy of metastatic breast cancer. J Clin Oncol 1984;2:1281–1288.
31. Hryniuk W, Levine MN. Analysis of dose intensity for adjuvant chemotherapy trials in stage II breast cancer. J Clin Oncol 1986;4:1162–1170.
32. MacNeil M, Eisenhauer EA. High-dose chemotherapy: is it standard management for any common solid tumor. Ann Oncol 1999;10:1145–1161.
33. Stadtmauer EA, O'Neill A, Goldstein LJ, et al. Conventional-dose chemotherapy compared with high-dose chemotherapy plus autologous hematopoietic stem-cell transplantation for metastatic breast cancer. N Engl J Med 2000;342:1069–1076.
34. Lippman ME. High-dose chemotherapy plus autologous bone marrow transplantation for metastatic breast cancer. N Engl J Med 2000;342:1119–1120.
35. Nichols CR, Williams SD, Loehrer PJ, et al. Randomized study of cisplatin dose intensity in poor-risk germ cell tumors: a Southeastern Cancer Study Group and Southwest Oncology Group protocol. J Clin Oncol 1991;9:1163–1172.
36. Pinkel D, Hernandez K, Borella L, et al. Drug dosage and remission duration in childhood lymphocytic leukemia. Cancer 1971;27:247–256.
37. Gaynon P, Steinherz P, Bleyer WA, et al. Association of delivered drug dose and outcome for children with acute lymphoblastic leukemia and unfavorable presenting features. Med Pediatr Oncol 1991;19:221–227.
38. Relling MV, Hancock ML, Boyett JM, et al. Prognostic importance of 6-mercaptopurine dose intensity in acute lymphoblastic leukemia. Blood 1999;93:2817–2823.

39. Cortes EP, Holland JF, Glidewell O. Adjuvant treatment of primary osteosarcoma: Cancer and Leukemia Group B experience. Recent Results Cancer Res 1979; 68:16–24.
40. Bacci G, Picci P, Avella M, et al. The importance of dose-intensity in neoadjuvant chemotherapy of osteosarcoma: a retrospective analysis of high-dose methotrexate, cisplatinum and adriamycin used preoperatively. J Chemother 1990;2:127–135.
41. Cheung N-KV, Heller G. Chemotherapy dose intensity correlates strongly with response, median survival, and median progression-free survival in metastatic neuroblastoma. J Clin Oncol 1991;9:1050–1058.
42. Smith MA, Ungerleider RS, Horowitz ME, et al. Influence of doxorubicin dose intensity on response and outcome for patients with osteogenic sarcoma and Ewing's sarcoma. J Natl Cancer Inst 1991;83:1460–1470.
43. Green DM, Breslow NE, Evans I, et al. The effect of chemotherapy dose intensity on the hematological toxicity of the treatment for Wilms' tumor. A report from the National Wilms' Tumor Study. Am J Pediatr Hematol Oncol 1994;16:207–212.
44. Green DM, Breslow NE, Beckwith JB, et al. Comparison between single-dose and divided-dose administration of dactinomycin and doxorubicin for patients with Wilms' tumor: a report from the National Wilms' Tumor Study Group. J Clin Oncol 1998;16:237–245.
45. Michel G, Landman-Parker J, Auclerc MF, et al. Use of recombinant human granulocyte colony-stimulating factor to increase chemotherapy dose-intensity: a randomized trial in very high-risk childhood acute lymphoblastic leukemia. J Clin Oncol 2000;18:1517–1524.
46. Womer RB, West DC, Krailo MD, et al. Randomized comparison of every-two-week v. every-three-week chemotherapy in Ewing sarcoma family tumors (ESFT). J Clin Oncol 2008;26(Suppl):A-10504.
47. Crist W, Gehan EA, Ragab A, et al. The third intergroup rhabdomyosarcoma study. J Clin Oncol 1995;13:610–630.
48. Tew KD, Colvin M, Chabner BA. Alkylating agents. In: Chabner BA, Longo DL, eds. Cancer chemotherapy and biotherapy: principles and practice. Philadelphia, PA: Lippincott-Raven, 1996:297–332.
49. Pommier Y. DNA topoisomerases I and II in cancer chemotherapy: update and perspectives. Cancer Chemother Pharmacol 1993;32:103–108.
50. Takimoto CH, Kieffer LV, Kieffer ME, et al. DNA topoisomerase I poisons. Cancer Chemother Biol Response Modif 1999;18:81–124.
51. Bartek J, Lukas J, Bartkova J. Perspective: defects in cell cycle control and cancer. J Pathol 1999;187:95–99.
52. Reed JC. Dysregulation of apoptosis in cancer. J Clin Oncol 1999;17:2941–2953.
53. Schmitt CA, Lowe SW. Apoptosis and therapy. J Pathol 1999;187:127–137.
54. Lowe SW. Cancer therapy and p53. Curr Opin Oncol 1995;7:547–553.
55. Houghton JA. Apoptosis and drug response. Curr Opin Oncol 1999;11:475–481.
56. Nurse P, Masui Y, Hartwell L. Understanding the cell cycle. Nat Med 1998; 4:1103–1106.
57. Sherr CJ. Cancer cell cycles. Science 1996;274:1672–1677.
58. Hartwell LH, Kastan MB. Cell cycle control and cancer. Science 1994;266: 1821–1828.
59. Hartwell L. 1994 forbeck cancer forum on cell cycle checkpoints. Clin Cancer Res 1995;1:1067.
60. O'Connor PM, Kohn KW. A fundamental role for cell cycle regulation in the chemosensitivity of cancer cells? Semin Cancer Biol 1992;3:409–416.
61. Kohn KW, Jackman J, O'Connor PM. Cell cycle control and cancer chemotherapy. J Cell Biochem 1994;54:440–452.
62. Waldman T, Zhang Y, Dillehay L, et al. Cell-cycle arrest versus cell death in cancer therapy. Nature Med 1997;3:1034–1036.
63. Brown JM, Wouters BG. Apoptosis, p53, and tumor cell sensitivity to anticancer agents. Cancer Res 1999;59:1391–1399.
64. Weller M. Predicting response to cancer chemotherapy: the role of p53. Cell Tissue Res 1998;292:435–445.
65. Ferreira CG, Tolis C, Giaccone G. p53 and chemosensitivity. Ann Oncol 1999;10: 1011–1021.
66. Green MR. Targeting targeted therapy. N Engl J Med 2004;350:2191–2193.
67. Rosa DD, Ismael G, Lago LD, et al. Molecular-targeted therapies: lessons from years of clinical development. Cancer Treat Rev 2008;34:61–80.
68. Wittes RE, Goldin A. Unresolved issues in combination chemotherapy. Cancer Treat Rep 1986;70:105–125.
69. Chabot GG. Factors involved in clinical pharmacology variability in oncology. Anticancer Res 1994;14:2269–2272.
70. Canal P, Chatelut E, Guichard S. Practical treatment guide for dose individualisation in cancer chemotherapy. Drugs 1998;56:1019–1038.
71. Crom W, Glynn-Barnhart A, Rodman J, et al. Pharmacokinetics of anticancer drugs in children. Clin Pharmacokinet 1987;12:168–213.
72. Balis FM, Holcenberg JS, Poplack DG, et al. Pharmacokinetics and pharmacodynamics of oral methotrexate and mercaptopurine in children with lower risk acute lymphoblastic leukemia: a joint Children's Cancer Group and Pediatric Oncology Branch study. Blood 1998;92:3569–3577.
73. Kobayashi K, Ratain M. Individualizing dosing of cancer chemotherapy. Semin Oncol 1993;20:30–42.
74. Gurney H. Dose calculation of anticancer drugs: a review of the current practice and introduction of an alternative. J Clin Oncol 1996;14:2590–2611.
75. McLeod HL. Clinically relevant drug–drug interactions in oncology. Br J Clin Pharmacol 1998;45:539–544.
76. Boddy AV, Ratain MJ. Pharmacogenetics in cancer etiology and chemotherapy. Clin Cancer Res 1997;3:1025–1030.
77. Iyer L, Ratain MJ. Pharmacogenetics and cancer chemotherapy. Eur J Cancer 1998;34:1493–1499.
78. Galpin AJ, Evans WE. Therapeutic drug monitoring in cancer management. Clin Chem 1993;39:2419–2430.
79. Canal P, Gamelin E, Vassal G, et al. Benefits of pharmacological knowledge in the design and monitoring of cancer chemotherapy. Pathol Oncol Res 1998;4: 171–178.
80. Rousseau A, Marquet P, Debord J, et al. Adaptive control methods for the dose individualisation of anticancer agents. Clin Pharmacokinet 2000;38:315–353.
81. Egorin MJ, Van Echo DA, Tipping SJ, et al. Pharmacokinetics and dosage reduction of *cis*-diammine(1,1-cyclobutanedicarboxylate) platinum in patients with impaired renal function. Cancer Res 1984;44:5432–5438.
82. Lennard L. Therapeutic monitoring of antimetabolite cytotoxic drugs. Br J Clin Pharmacol 1999;47:131–143.
83. Panetta JC, Iacono LC, Adamson PC, et al. The importance of pharmacokinetic limited sampling models for childhood cancer drug development. Clin Cancer Res 2003;9:5068–5077.
84. Egorin MJ, Forrest A, Belani CP, et al. A limited sampling strategy for cyclophosphamide pharmacokinetics. Cancer Res 1989;49:3129–3133.
85. Ratain MJ, Vogelzang NJ. Limited sampling model for vinblastine pharmacokinetics. Cancer Treat Rep 1987;71:935–939.
86. Kintzel PE, Dorr RT. Anticancer drug renal toxicity and elimination: dosing guidelines for altered renal function. Cancer Treat Rev 1995;21:33–64.
87. Donelli MG, Zucchetti M, Munzone E, et al. Pharmacokinetics of anticancer agents in patients with impaired liver function. Eur J Cancer 1998;34:33–46.
88. Grochow LB, Baker SD. The relationship of age to the disposition and effects of anticancer drugs. In: Grochow LB, Ames MM, eds. A clinician's guide to chemotherapy pharmacokinetics and pharmacodynamics. Baltimore, MD: Williams & Wilkins, 1998:35–53.
89. Ames MM. Pharmacokinetics of antitumor agents in children. In: Ames MM, Powis G, Kovach JS, eds. Pharmacokinetics of anticancer agents in humans. Amsterdam, The Netherlands: Elsevier, 1983:400–431.
90. McLeod HL, Relling MV, Crom WR, et al. Disposition of antineoplastic agents in the very young child. Br J Cancer Suppl 1992;18:S23–S29.
91. Weinshilboum R. Inheritance and drug response. N Engl J Med 2003;348:529–537.
92. Evans WE, McLeod HL. Pharmacogenomics–drug disposition, drug targets, and side effects. N Engl J Med 2003;348:538–549.
93. Weinshilboum RM, Sladek SL. Mercaptopurine pharmacogenetics: monogenic inheritance of erythrocyte thiopurine methyltransferase activity. Am J Hum Genet 1980;32: 651–662.
94. Evans WE, Relling MV. Pharmacogenomics: translating functional genomics into rational therapeutics. Science 1999;286:487–491.
95. Glue P, Clement RP. Cytochrome P450 enzymes and drug metabolism—basic concepts and methods of assessment. Cell Mol Neurobiol 1999;19:309–323.
96. Omiecinski CJ, Remmel RP, Hosagrahara VP. Concise review of the cytochrome P450s and their roles in toxicology. Toxicol Sci 1999;48:151–156.
97. van der Weide J, Steijns LS. Cytochrome P450 enzyme system: genetic polymorphisms and impact on clinical pharmacology. Ann Clin Biochem 1999;36:722–729.
98. Streetman DS, Bertino JSJ, Nafziger AN. Phenotyping of drug-metabolizing enzymes in adults: a review of in-vivo cytochrome P450 phenotyping probes. Pharmacogenetics 2000;10:187–216.
99. Otterness D, Szumlanski C, Lennard L, et al. Human thiopurine methyltransferase pharmacogenetics: gene sequence polymorphisms. Clin Pharmacol Ther 1997;62: 60–73.
100. Krynetski EY, Tai HL, Yates CR, et al. Genetic polymorphism of thiopurine *S*-methyltransferase: clinical importance and molecular mechanisms. Pharmacogenetics 1996;6:279–290.
101. Tai HL, Krynetski EY, Yates CR, et al. Thiopurine *S*-methyltransferase deficiency: two nucleotide transitions define the most prevalent mutant allele associated with loss of catalytic activity in Caucasians. Am J Hum Genet 1996;58:694–702.
102. Szumlanski C, Otterness D, Her C, et al. Thiopurine methyltransferase pharmacogenetics: human gene cloning and characterization of a common polymorphism. DNA Cell Biol 1996;15:17–30.
103. Lee D, Szumlanski C, Houtman J, et al. Thiopurine methyltransferase pharmacogenetics. Cloning of human liver cDNA and a processed pseudogene on human chromosome 18q21.1. Drug Metab Dispos 1995;23:398–405.
104. Krynetski EY, Schuetz JD, Galpin AJ, et al. A single point mutation leading to loss of catalytic activity in human thiopurine *S*-methyltransferase. Proc Natl Acad Sci U S A 1995;92:949–953.
105. McLeod HL, Lin JS, Scott EP, et al. Thiopurine methyltransferase activity in American white subjects and black subjects. Clin Pharmacol Ther 1994;55:15–20.
106. Collie-Duguid ES, Pritchard SC, Powrie RH, et al. The frequency and distribution of thiopurine methyltransferase alleles in Caucasian and Asian populations. Pharmacogenetics 1999;9:37–42.
107. Chang JG, Lee LS, Chen CM, et al. Molecular analysis of thiopurine *S*-methyltransferase alleles in South-east Asian populations. Pharmacogenetics 2002; 12:191–195.
108. Marinaki AM, Arenas M, Khan ZH, et al. Genetic determinants of the thiopurine methyltransferase intermediate activity phenotype in British Asians and Caucasians. Pharmacogenetics 2003;13:97–105.
109. Iyer L, Das S, Janisch L, et al. UGT1A1*28 polymorphism as a determinant of irinotecan disposition and toxicity. Pharmacogenomics J 2002;2:43–47.
110. Ando Y, Saka H, Ando M, et al. Polymorphisms of UDP-glucuronosyltransferase gene and irinotecan toxicity: a pharmacogenetic analysis. Cancer Res 2000;60: 6921–6926.
111. Iyer L, Hall D, Das S, et al. Phenotype–genotype correlation of in vitro SN-38 (active metabolite of irinotecan) and bilirubin glucuronidation in human liver tissue with UGT1A1 promoter polymorphism. Clin Pharmacol Ther 1999;65:576–582.
112. Esteller M, Garcia-Foncillas J, Andion E, et al. Inactivation of the DNA-repair gene MGMT and the clinical response of gliomas to alkylating agents. N Engl J Med 2000;343:1350–1354.
113. Hoekman K, van der Vijgh WJF, Vermorken JB. Clinical and preclinical modulation of chemotherapy-induced toxicity in patients with cancer. Drugs 1999;57:133–155.
114. Lowenthal RM, Eaton K. Toxicity of chemotherapy. Hematol Oncol Clin North Am 1996;10:967–990.
115. Spiegel RJ. The acute toxicities of chemotherapy. Cancer Treat Rev 1981;8:197–207.
116. Perry MC, Yarbaro JW. Toxicity of chemotherapy. Orlando, FL: Grune & Stratton, 1984.
117. Lewis C. A review of the use of chemoprotectants in cancer chemotherapy. Drug Saf 1994;11:153–162.
118. Zagonel V, Rupolo M, Pinto A. Active protection from chemotherapy toxicity. Crit Rev Oncol Hematol 1998;27:125–127.
119. Links M, Lewis C. Chemoprotectants: a review of their clinical pharmacology and therapeutic efficacy. Drugs 1999;57:293–308.
120. Widemann BC, Balis FM, Murphy RF, et al. Carboxypeptidase-G_2 rescue in patients with high-dose methotrexate-induced renal dysfunction. J Clin Oncol 1997;15: 2125–2134.
121. Roila F, Aapro M, Stewart A. Optimal selection of antiemetics in children receiving cancer chemotherapy. Support Care Cancer 1998;6:215–220.
122. Dicato MA. Medical management of cancer treatment induced emesis. London, England: Martin Dunitz, Ltd., 1998.

123. Siu LL, Moore MJ. Use of mesna to prevent ifosfamide-induced urotoxicity. Support Care Cancer 1998;6:144–154.
124. Steward WP. Granulocyte and granulocyte-macrophage colony stimulating factors. Lancet 1993;342:153–157.
125. Vose JM, Armitage JO. Clinical applications of hematopoietic growth factors. J Clin Oncol 1995;13:1023–1035.
126. Parsons SK. Oncology practice patterns in the use of hematopoietic growth factors. Curr Opin Pediatr 2000;12:10–17.
127. Wiseman LR, Spencer CM. Dexrazoxane. A review of its use as a cardioprotective agent in patients receiving anthracycline-based chemotherapy. Drugs 1998;56: 385–403.
128. Wexler LH. Ameliorating anthracycline cardiotoxicity in children with cancer: clinical trials with dexrazoxane. Semin Oncol 1998;25(4, Suppl 10):86–92.
129. Lipshultz SE, Rifai N, Dalton VM, et al. The effect of dexrazoxane on myocardial injury in doxorubicin-treated children with acute lymphoblastic leukemia. N Engl J Med 2004;351:145–153.
130. Chabner BA. Clinical strategies for cancer treatment: the role of drugs. In: Chabner BA, Collins JM, eds. Cancer chemotherapy principles and practice. Philadelphia, PA: JB Lippincott, 1990:1–15.
131. Magrath IT, Janus C, Edwards BK, et al. An effective therapy for both undifferentiated (including Burkitt's) lymphomas and lymphoblastic lymphomas in children and young adults. Blood 1984;63:1102–1111.
132. Balis FM. Pharmacokinetic drug interactions of commonly used anticancer drugs. Clin Pharmacokinet 1986;11:223–235.
133. Loadman PM, Bibby MC. Pharmacokinetic drug interactions with anticancer drugs. Clin Pharmacokinet 1994;26:486–500.
134. Lokiec F. Drug interactions in cancer chemotherapy. In: Schilsky RL, Milano GA, Ratain MJ, eds. Principles of antineoplastic drug development and pharmacology. Basic and Clinical Oncology. New York, NY: Marcel Dekker, Inc., 1996: 189–202.
135. Dresser GK, Spence JD, Bailey DG. Pharmacokinetic–pharmacodynamic consequences and clinical relevance of cytochrome P450 3A4 inhibition. Clin Pharmacokinet 2000;38:41–57.
136. Fujita K. Cytochrome P450 and anticancer drugs. Curr Drug Metab 2006;7:23–37.
137. Kivisto KT, Kroemer HK, Eichelbaum M. The role of human cytochrome P450 enzymes in the metabolism of anticancer agents: implications for drug interactions. Br J Clin Pharmacol 1995;40:523–530.
138. Anthoney DA, Kaye SB. Drug resistance: the clinical perspective. In: Brown R, Böger-Brown U, eds. Cytotoxic drug resistance mechanisms. Methods in Molecular Medicine. Totowa, NJ: Humana Press, 1999:1–15.
139. Frei E, Freireich EJ, Gehan E, et al. Studies of sequential and combination antimetabolite therapy in acute leukemia: mercaptopurine and methotrexate. Blood 1961;18: 431–454.
140. Goldie JH, Coldman AJ. Drug resistance in cancer mechanisms and models. Cambridge, MA: Cambridge University Press, 1998.
141. Biedler JL, Spengler BA. Metaphase chromosome anomaly: association with drug resistance and cell-specific products. Science 1976;191:185–187.
142. Ling V. Multidrug resistance: molecular mechanisms and clinical relevance. Cancer Chemother Pharmacol 1997;40(Suppl):S3–S8.
143. Bradshaw DM, Arceci RJ. Clinical relevance of transmembrane drug efflux as a mechanism of multidrug resistance. J Clin Oncol 1998;16:3674–3690.
144. Barret JM, Hill BT. DNA repair mechanisms associated with cellular resistance to antitumor drugs: potential novel targets. Anticancer Drugs 1998;9:105–123.
145. Patel NH, Rothenberg ML. Multidrug resistance in cancer chemotherapy. Invest New Drugs 1994;12:1–13.
146. Gottesman MM. How cancer cells evade chemotherapy: sixteenth Richard and Hinda Rosenthal Foundation award lecture. Cancer Res 1993;53:747–754.
147. Schneider E, Paul D, Ivy P, et al. Multidrug resistance. Cancer Chemother Biol Response Modif 1999;18:152–177.
148. List AF. Non-P-glycoprotein drug export mechanisms of multidrug resistance. Semin Hematol 1997;34(Suppl 5):20–24.
149. Hipfner DR, Deeley RG, Cole SPC. Structural, mechanistic and clinical aspects of MRP1. Biochim Biophys Acta 1999;1461:359–376.
150. Borst P, Evers R, Kool M, et al. A family of drug transporters: the multidrug resistance-associated proteins. J Natl Cancer Inst 2000;92:1295–1302.
151. Leonard GD, Fojo T, Bates SE. The role of ABC transporters in clinical practice. Oncologist 2003;8:411–424.
152. Dean M, Rzhetsky A, Allikmets R. The human ATP-binding cassette (ABC) transporter superfamily. Genome Res 2001;11:1156–1166.
153. Fojo AT, Ueda K, Slamon DJ, et al. Expression of a multidrug resistance gene in human tumors and tissues. Proc Natl Acad Sci USA 1987;84:265–269.
154. Rothenberg ML, Mickley LA, Cole DE, et al. Expression of the mdr-1/P-170 gene in patients with acute lymphoblastic leukemia. Blood 1989;74:1388–1395.
155. Chan HS, Grogan TM, Haddad G, et al. P-glycoprotein expression: critical determinant in the response to osteosarcoma chemotherapy. J Natl Cancer Inst 1997;89:1706–1715.
156. Chan HS, Haddad G, Thorner PS, et al. P-glycoprotein expression as a predictor of the outcome of therapy for neuroblastoma. New Engl J Med 1991;325:1608–1614.
157. Chan HS, Thorner PS, Haddad G, et al. Immunohistochemical detection of P-glycoprotein: prognostic correlation in soft tissue sarcoma of childhood. J Clin Oncol 1990;8:689–704.
158. Kuttesch JF. Multidrug resistance in pediatric oncology. Invest New Drugs 1996; 14:55–67.
159. Cordon-Cardo C, O'Brien JP, Boccia J, et al. Expression of the multidrug resistance gene product (P-glycoprotein) in human normal and tumor tissues. J Histochem Cytochem 1990;38:1277–1287.
160. Chaudhary PM, Roninson IB. Expression and activity of P-glycoprotein, a multidrug efflux pump in human hematopoietic stem cell. Cell 1991;66:85–94.
161. Wunder JS, Bull SB, Aneliunas V, et al. MDR1 gene expression and outcome in osteosarcoma: a prospective, multicenter study. J Clin Oncol 2000;18:2685–2994.
162. Cole SP, Chanda ER, Dicke FP, et al. Non-P-glycoprotein-mediated multidrug resistance in a small cell lung cancer cell line: evidence for decreased susceptibility to drug-induced DNA damage and reduced levels of topoisomerase II. Cancer Res 1991;51:3345–3352.
163. Kool M, de Haas M, Scheffer GL, et al. Analysis of expression of cMOAT (MRP2), MRP3, MRP4, and MRP5, homologues of the multidrug resistance-associated protein gene (MRP1), in human cancer cell lines. Cancer Res 1997;57:3537–3547.
164. Kruh GD, Zeng H, Rea PA, et al. MRP subfamily transporters and resistance to anti-cancer agents. J Bioenerg Biomembr 2001;33:493–4501.
165. Chaney SG, Sancar A. DNA repair: enzymatic mechanisms and relevance to drug response. J Natl Cancer Inst 1996;88:1346–1360.
166. Dolan ME. Importance of DNA repair in cancer chemotherapy. In: Schilsky RL, Milano GA, Ratain MJ, eds. Principles of antineoplastic drug development and pharmacology. Basic and Clinical Oncology. New York, NY: Marcel Dekker, Inc., 1996: 523–542.
167. Batist G, Schecter RL, Alaoui-Jamali MA. The glutathione system and drug resistance. In: Schilsky RL, Milano GA, Ratain MJ, eds. Principles of antineoplastic drug development and pharmacology. Basic and Clinical Oncology. New York, NY: Marcel Dekker, Inc., 1996:503–521.
168. Beck WT. DNA topoisomerase and tumor cell resistance to their inhibitors. In: Schilsky RL, Milano GA, Ratain MJ, eds. Principles of antineoplastic drug development and pharmacology. Basic and Clinical Oncology. New York, NY: Marcel Dekker, Inc., 1996:487–501.
169. Fink D, Aebi S, Howell SB. The role of DNA mismatch repair in drug resistance. Clin Cancer Res 1998;4:1–6.
170. Hall AG, Tilby MJ. Mechanisms of action of, and modes of resistance to, alkylating agents used in the treatment of hematological malignancies. Blood Rev 1992;6: 163–173.
171. Kohn KW. Molecular mechanisms of crosslinking by alkylating agents and platinum complexes. In: Sartorelli AC, Lazlo JS, Bertino JR, eds. Molecular actions and targets for cancer chemotherapeutic agents. New York, NY: Academic Press, 1981:3–16.
172. Frei E, Teicher BA, Holden SA, et al. Preclinical studies and clinical correlation of the effect of alkylating dose. Cancer Res 1988;48:6417–6423.
173. Atra A, Pinkerton R. Autologous stem cell transplantation in solid tumours of childhood. Ann Med 1996;28:159–164.
174. Hassan M. The role of busulfan in bone marrow transplantation. Med Oncol 1999;16:166–176.
175. Samuels BL, Bitran JD. High-dose intravenous melphalan: a review. J Clin Oncol 1995;13:1786–1799.
176. Marina N. Long-term survivors of childhood cancer. The medical consequences of cure. Pediatr Clin North Am 1997;44:1021–1042.
177. Schwartz CL. Long-term survivors of childhood cancer: the late effects of therapy. Oncologist 1999;4:45–54.
178. Connors TA. Alkylating drugs, nitrosoureas and dimethyltriazenes. In: Pinedo HM, ed. Cancer chemotherapy, annual 3. New York, NY: Elsevier, 1981:32–74.
179. Mirkes PE. Cyclophosphamide teratogenesis: a review. Teratog Carcinog Mutagen 1985;5:75–88.
180. Lind MJ, Ardiet C. Pharmacokinetics of alkylating agents. Cancer Surv 1993;17: 157–188.
181. Clapper ML, Tew KD. Alkylating agent resistance. Cancer Treat Res 1989;48: 125–150.
182. Wolpert MK, Ruddon RW. A study on the mechanisms of resistance to nitrogen mustard in Ehrlich ascites tumor cells: comparison of uptake of HN2 14C into sensitive and resistant cells. Cancer Res 1969;29:873–879.
183. Redwood WR, Colvin M. Transport of melphalan by sensitive and resistant L1210 cells. Cancer Res 1980;40:1144–1149.
184. Schabel FM, Trader MW, Laster WR, et al. Patterns of resistance and therapeutic synergism among alkylating agents. Antibiot Chemother 1978;23:200–215.
185. Teicher BA, Cucchi CA, Lee JB, et al. Alkylating agents: in vitro studies of cross-resistance patterns in human cell lines. Cancer Res 1986;46:4379–4383.
186. Frei E, Cucchi CA, Rosowsky A, et al. Alkylating agent resistance: in vitro studies with human cell lines. Proc Natl Acad Sci U S A 1985;82:2158–2162.
187. Verweij J, Schellens JHM. Alkylating agents: mitomycin C, nitrogen mustard, chlorambucil, and melphalan. In: Grochow LB, Ames MM, eds. A clinician's guide to chemotherapy pharmacokinetics and pharmacodynamics. Baltimore, MD: Williams & Wilkins, 1998:471–493.
188. Hutchinson RJ, Fryer CJ, Davis PC, et al. MOPP or radiation in addition to ABVD in the treatment of pathologically staged advanced Hodgkin's disease in children: results of the Children's Cancer Group Phase III Trial. J Clin Oncol 1998;16: 897–906.
189. Mellett LB, Woods LA. The fluorometric estimation of mechlorethamine (Mustargen) and its biological disposition in the dog. Cancer Res 1960;20:518–523.
190. Nadkarni MV, Trams EG. Studies on the N-dealkylation of nitrogen mustard and triethylenemelamine by liver homogenates. Cancer Res 1956;16:1069–1075.
191. Dorr RT. Antidotes to vesicant chemotherapy extravasations. Blood Rev 1990; 4:41–60.
192. Shapiro WR, Young DF. Neurological complications of antineoplastic therapy. Acta Neurol Scand 1984;100(Suppl):125–132.
193. Fleming RA. An overview of cyclophosphamide and ifosfamide pharmacology. Pharmacotherapy 1997;17(5, Pt 2):146S–154S.
194. Kaijser GP, Beijnen JH. Oxazaphosphorines: cyclophosphamide and ifosfamide. In: Grochow LB, Ames MM, eds. A clinician's guide to chemotherapy pharmacokinetics and pharmacodynamics. Baltimore, MD: Williams & Wilkins, 1998:229–258.
195. Pratt CB. Ongoing clinical studies of ifosfamide for pediatric cancer in the United States. Semin Oncol 1996;23(3, Suppl 6):84–90.
196. Miser JS, Kinsella TJ, Triche TJ, et al. Ifosfamide with mesna uroprotection and etoposide: an effective regimen in the treatment of recurrent sarcomas and other tumors of children and young adults. J Clin Oncol 1987;5:1191–1198.
197. Jurgens H, Treuner J, Winkler K, et al. Ifosfamide in pediatric malignancies. Semin Oncol 1989;16:46–50.
198. Weiss RB. Ifosfamide vs cyclophosphamide in cancer therapy. Oncology 1990;5: 67–76.
199. Roy P, Yu LJ, Crespi CL, et al. Development of a substrate-activity based approach to identify the major human liver P-450 catalysts of cyclophosphamide and ifosfamide activation based on cDNA-expressed activities and liver microsomal P-450 profiles. Drug Metab Dispos 1999;27:655–666.
200. Colvin OM. An overview of cyclophosphamide development and clinical applications. Curr Pharm Des 1999;5:555–560.
201. Boddy AV, Yule SM. Metabolism and pharmacokinetics of oxazaphosphorines. Clin Pharmacokinet 2000;38:291–304.
202. Ludeman SM. The chemistry of the metabolites of cyclophosphamide. Curr Pharm Des 1999;5:627–643.
203. Wagner T. Ifosfamide clinical pharmacokinetics. Clin Pharmacokinet 1994;26: 439–456.

204. Moore MJ. Clinical pharmacokinetics of cyclophosphamide. Clin Pharmacokinet 1991;20:194–208.
205. Juma FD, Rogers HJ, Trounce JR. Pharmacokinetics of cyclophosphamide and alkylating activity in man after intravenous and oral administration. Br J Clin Pharmacol 1979;8:209–217.
206. D'lncalci M, Bolis G, Facchinetti T, et al. Decreased half-life of cyclophosphamide in patients under continual treatment. Eur J Cancer 1979;15:7–10.
207. Struck RF, Alberts DS, Horne K, et al. Plasma pharmacokinetics of cyclophosphamide and its cytotoxic metabolites after intravenous versus oral administration in a randomized, crossover trial. Cancer Res 1987;47:2723–2726.
208. Aeschlimann C, Küpfer A, Schefer H, et al. Comparative pharmacokinetics of oral and intravenous ifosfamide/mesna/methylene blue therapy. Drug Metab Dispos 1998; 26:883–890.
209. Cerny T, Margison J, Thatcher N, et al. Bioavailability of ifosfamide in patients with bronchial carcinoma. Cancer Chemother Pharmacol 1986;18:261–264.
210. Wagner T, Drings P. Pharmacokinetics and bioavailability of oral ifosfamide. Contrib Oncol 1987;26:53–59.
211. Kurowski V, Cerny T, Kuper A, et al. Metabolism and pharmacokinetics of oral and intravenous ifosfamide. J Cancer Res Clin Oncol 1991;117(Suppl 4):S148–S153.
212. Wagner T, Heydrich D, Jork T, et al. Comparative study on human pharmacokinetics of activated ifosfamide and cyclophosphamide by a modified fluorometric test. J Cancer Res Clin Oncol 1981;100:95–104.
213. Allen LM, Creaven PJ, Nelson RL. Studies on the human pharmacokinetics of ifosfamide (NSC-109724). Cancer Treat Rep 1976;60:451–458.
214. Dooley JS, James CA, Rogers HJ, et al. Biliary elimination of cyclophosphamide in man. Cancer Chemother Pharmacol 1982;9:26–29.
215. Brade WP, Herdrich K, Varini M. Ifosfamide—pharmacology, safety and therapeutic potential. Cancer Treat Rev 1985;12:1–47.
216. Juma FD, Rogers HJ, Trounce JR. Effect of renal insufficiency on the pharmacokinetics of cyclophosphamide and some of its metabolites. Eur J Clin Pharmacol 1981;19: 443–445.
217. Yule SM, Boddy AV, Cole M, et al. Cyclophosphamide pharmacokinetics in children. Br J Clin Pharmacol 1996;41:13–19.
218. Juma FD, Koech DK, Kasili EG, et al. Pharmacokinetics of cyclophosphamide in Kenyan African children with lymphoma. Br J Clin Pharmacol 1984;18:106–107.
219. Tasso MJ, Boddy AV, Price L, et al. Pharmacokinetics and metabolism of cyclophosphamide in paediatric patients. Cancer Chemother Pharmacol 1992;30:207–211.
220. Bagley CM, Bostich FW, DeVita VT. Clinical pharmacology of cyclophosphamide. Cancer Res 1973;33:226–233.
221. Sladek NE, Priest J, Doeden D, et al. Plasma half-life and urinary excretion of cyclophosphamide in children. Cancer Treat Rep 1980;64:1061–1066.
222. Boddy AV, Yule SM, Wyllie R, et al. Intrasubject variation in children of ifosfamide pharmacokinetics and metabolism during repeated administration. Cancer Chemother Pharmacol 1996;38:147–154.
223. Boddy AV, Yule SM, Wyllie R, et al. Pharmacokinetics and metabolism of ifosfamide administered as a continuous infusion in children. Cancer Res 1993;53: 3758–3764.
224. Prasad VK, Corlett SA, Abaasi K, et al. Ifosfamide enantomers: pharmacokinetics in children. Cancer Chemother Pharmacol 1994;34:447–449.
225. Wilkinson PM, O'Neill PA, Thatcher N. Pharmacokinetics of high-dose cyclophosphamide in patients with metastatic bronchogenic carcinoma. Cancer Chemother Pharmacol 1983;11:196–199.
226. Yule SM, Boddy AV, Cole M, et al. Cyclophosphamide metabolism in children. Cancer Res 1995;55:803–809.
227. Yule SM, Price L, McMahon AD, et al. Cyclophosphamide metabolism in children with non-Hodgkin's lymphoma. Clin Cancer Res 2004;10:455–460.
228. Lind MJ, Margson JM, Cerny T, et al. Comparative pharmacokinetics and alkylating activity of fractionated intravenous and oral ifosfamide in patients with bronchogenic carcinoma. Cancer Res 1989;49:753–757.
229. Kurowski V, Wagner T. Comparative pharmacokinetics of ifosfamide, 4-hydroxyifosfamide, chloroacetaldehyde, and 2- and 3-dechloroethylifosfamide in patients on fractionated intravenous ifosfamide therapy. Cancer Chemother Pharmacol 1993;33:36–42.
230. Chang TK, Yu L, Maurel P, et al. Enhanced cyclophosphamide and ifosfamide activation in primary human hepatocyte cultures: response to cytochrome P-450 inducers and autoinduction by oxazaphosphorines. Cancer Res 1997;57:1946–1954.
231. de Jonge ME, Huitema AD, Rodenhuis S, et al. Clinical pharmacokinetics of cyclophosphamide. Clin Pharmacokinet 2005;44:1135–1164.
232. Comandone A, Leone L, Oliva C, et al. Pharmacokinetics of ifosfamide administered according to three different schedules in metastatic soft tissue and bone sarcomas. J Chemother 1998;10:385–393.
233. Boddy AV, Cole M, Pearson ADJ, et al. The kinetics of the auto-induction of ifosfamide metabolism during continuous infusion. Cancer Chemother Pharmacol 1995;36:53–60.
234. Kerbusch T, Mathot RA, Keizer HJ, et al. Influence of dose and infusion duration on pharmacokinetics of ifosfamide and metabolites. Drug Metab Dispos 2001;29: 967–975.
235. Willits I, Price L, Parry A, et al. Pharmacokinetics and metabolism of ifosfamide in relation to DNA damage assessed by the COMET assay in children with cancer. Br J Cancer 2005;92:1626–1635.
236. Brain EG, Rezai K, Weill S, et al. Variations in schedules of ifosfamide administration: a better understanding of its implications on pharmacokinetics through a randomized cross-over study. Cancer Chemother Pharmacol 2007;60:375–381.
237. Chen T-L, Passos-Coelho JL, Noe DA, et al. Nonlinear pharmacokinetics of cyclophosphamide in patients with metastatic breast cancer receiving high-dose chemotherapy followed by autologous bone marrow transplantation. Cancer Res 1995;55(4):810–816.
238. Busse D, Busch FW, Bohnenstengel F, et al. Dose escalation of cyclophosphamide in patients with breast cancer: consequences for pharmacokinetics and metabolism. J Clin Oncol 1997;15:1885–1896.
239. Cerny T, Leyvraz S, von Briel T, et al. Saturable metabolism of continuous high-dose ifosfamide with mesna and GM-CSF: a pharmacokinetic study in advanced sarcoma patients. Swiss Group for Clinical Cancer Research (SAKK). Ann Oncol 1999; 10:1087–1094.
240. Anderson LW, Chen T-L, Colvin OM, et al. Cyclophosphamide and 4-hydroxycyclophosphamide/aldophosphamide kinetics in patients receiving high-dose cyclophosphamide chemotherapy. Clin Cancer Res 1996;2:1481–1487.
241. Ren S, Kalhorn TF, McDonald GB, et al. Pharmacokinetics of cyclophosphamide and its metabolites in bone marrow transplantation patients. Clin Pharmacol Ther 1998;64:289–301.
242. Chan KK, Hong PS, Tutsch K, et al. Clinical pharmacokinetics of cyclophosphamide and metabolites with and without SR-2508. Cancer Res 1994;54:6421–6429.
243. Haubitz M, Bohnenstengel F, Brunkhorst R, et al. Cyclophosphamide pharmacokinetics and dose requirements in patients with renal insufficiency. Kidney Int 2002; 61:1495–1501.
244. Bramwell V, Calvert RT, Edwards G, et al. The disposition of cyclophosphamide in a group of myeloma patients. Cancer Chemother Pharmacol 1979;3:253–259.
245. Wagner T, Heydrich D, Bartels H, et al. Effect of damaged liver parenchyma, renal insufficiency and hemodialysis on the pharmacokinetics of cyclophosphamide and its activated metabolites. Arzneimittelforschung 1980;30:1588–1592.
246. Carlson L, Goren MP, Bush DA, et al. Toxicity, pharmacokinetics, and in vitro hemodialysis clearance of ifosfamide and metabolites in an anephric pediatric patient with Wilms' tumor. Cancer Chemother Pharmacol 1998;41:140–146.
247. Grochow LB, Colvin M. Clinical pharmacokinetics of cyclophosphamide. In: Ames MM, Powis G, Kovach JS, eds. Pharmacokinetics of anticancer agents in humans. Amsterdam, The Netherlands: Elsevier, 1983:135–154.
248. Wang LH, Lee CS, Majeske BL, et al. Clearance and recovery calculations in hemodialysis: application to plasma, red blood cell and dialysate measurements for cyclophosphamide. Clin Pharmacol Ther 1981;29:365–372.
249. Burkert H. Clinical overview of mesna. Cancer Treat Rev 1983;10(Suppl):175–181.
250. Samra Y, Hertz M, Lindner A. Urinary bladder tumors following cyclophosphamide therapy: a report of two cases with a review of the literature. Med Pediatr Oncol 1985;13:86–91.
251. Bode U, Seif SM, Levine AS. Studies on the antidiuretic effect of cyclophosphamide: vasopressin release and sodium excretion. Med Pediatr Oncol 1980;8:295–303.
252. Bressler RB, Huston DP. Water intoxication following moderate-dose intravenous cyclophosphamide. Arch Intern Med 1985;145:548–549.
253. Nissim I, Horyn O, Daikhin Y, et al. Ifosfamide-induced nephrotoxicity: mechanism and prevention. Cancer Res 2006;66:7824–7831.
254. Ho PTC, Zimmerman K, Wexler L, et al. A prospective evaluation of ifosfamide-related nephrotoxicity in children and young adults. Cancer 1995;76:2557–2564.
255. Newbury-Ecob RA, Noble VW, Barbor PRH. Ifosfamide-induced Fanconi syndrome. Lancet 1989;1:1328.
256. Moncrieff M, Foot A. Fanconi syndrome after ifosfamide. Cancer Chemother Pharmacol 1989;23:121–122.
257. Pratt CB, Meyer WH, Jenkins JJ, et al. Ifosfamide, Fanconi's syndrome, and rickets. J Clin Oncol 1991;9:1495–1499.
258. Skinner R, Pearson ADJ, Price L, et al. Nephrotoxicity after ifosfamide. Arch Dis Child 1990;65:732–738.
259. Skinner R, Pearson ADJ, English MW, et al. Risk factors for ifosfamide nephrotoxicity in children. Lancet 1996;348:578–580.
260. Prasad VK, Lewis IJ, Aparicio SR, et al. Progressive glomerular toxicity of ifosfamide in children. Med Pediatr Oncol 1996;27:149–155.
261. Skinner R, Cotterill SJ, Stevens MC. Risk factors for nephrotoxicity after ifosfamide treatment in children: a UKCCSG Late Effects Group study. United Kingdom Children's Cancer Study Group. Br J Cancer 2000;82:1636–1645.
262. Raney B, Ensign LG, Foreman J, et al. Renal toxicity of ifosfamide in pilot regimens of the intergroup rhabdomyosarcoma study for patients with gross residual tumor. Am J Pediatr Hematol Oncol 1994;16:286–295.
263. Lee BS, Lee JH, Kang HG, et al. Ifosfamide nephrotoxicity in pediatric cancer patients. Pediatr Nephrol 2001;16:796–799.
264. Jones DP, Chesney RW. Renal toxicity of cancer chemotherapeutic agents in children: ifosfamide and cisplatin. Curr Opin Pediatr 1995;7:208–213.
265. Loebstein R, Atanackovic G, Bishai R, et al. Risk factors for long-term outcome of ifosfamide-induced nephrotoxicity in children. J Clin Pharmacol 1999;39:454–461.
266. Aleksa K, Woodland C, Koren G. Young age and the risk for ifosfamide-induced nephrotoxicity: a critical review of two opposing studies. Pediatr Nephrol 2001; 16:1153–1158.
267. Pratt CB, Green AA, Horowitz ME, et al. Central nervous system toxicity following the treatment of pediatric patients with ifosfamide/mesna. J Clin Oncol 1986;4: 1253–1261.
268. Tuxen MK, Hansen SW. Neurotoxicity secondary to antineoplastic drugs. Cancer Treat Rev 1994;20:191–214.
269. Sweiss KI, Beri R, Shord SS. Encephalopathy after high-dose ifosfamide: a retrospective cohort study and review of the literature. Drug Saf 2008;31:989–996.
270. Goren M, Wright R, Pratt C, et al. Dechlorethylation of ifosfamide and neurotoxicity [letter]. Lancet 1986;2:1219–1220.
271. Pratt CB, Goren MP, Meyer WH, et al. Ifosfamide neurotoxicity is related to previous cisplatin treatment for pediatric solid tumors. J Clin Oncol 1990;8: 1399–1401.
272. Pelgrims J, De Vos F, Van den Brande J, et al. Methylene blue in the treatment and prevention of ifosfamide-induced encephalopathy: report of 12 cases and a review of the literature. Br J Cancer 2000;82:291–294.
273. Kupfer A, Aeschlimann C, Cerny T. Methylene blue and the neurotoxic mechanisms of ifosfamide encephalopathy. Eur J Clin Pharmacol 1996;50:249–252.
274. Quezado ZMN, Wilson WH, Cunnion RE, et al. High-dose ifosfamide is associated with severe reversible cardiac dysfunction. Ann Intern Med 1993;118:31–36.
275. Malik SW, Myers JL, DeRemee RA, et al. Lung toxicity associated with cyclophosphamide use. Two distinct patterns. Am J Respir Crit Care Med 1996;154(6, Pt 1): 1851–1856.
276. Patel JM. Metabolism and pulmonary toxicity of cyclophosphamide. Pharmacol Ther 1990;47:137–146.
277. Baker WJ, Fistel SJ, Jones RV, et al. Interstitial pneumonitis associated with ifosfamide therapy. Cancer 1990;65:2217–2221.
278. Twohig KJ, Matthay RA. Pulmonary effects of cytotoxic agents other than bleomycin. Clin Chest Med 1990;11:31–54.
279. Gamcsik MP, Dolan ME, Andersson BS, et al. Mechanisms of resistance to the toxicity of cyclophosphamide. Curr Pharm Des 1999;5:587–605.
280. Gurtoo HL, Hipkens JH, Sharma SD. Role of glutathione in the metabolism-dependent toxicity and chemotherapy of cyclophosphamide. Cancer Res 1981;41: 3584–3591.
281. McGown AT, Fox BW. A proposed mechanism of resistance to cyclophosphamide and phosphoramide mustard in a Yoshida cell line in vitro. Cancer Chemother Pharmacol 1986;17:223–226.

282. Crook TR, Souhami RL, Whyman GD, et al. Glutathione depletion as a determinant of sensitivity of human leukemia cells to cyclophosphamide. Cancer Res 1986;46:5035–5038.
283. Tew KD. Glutathione-associated enzymes in anticancer drug resistance. Cancer Res 1994;54:4313–4320.
284. Colvin OM, Hilton J. Cellular resistance to cyclophosphamide. In: Woolley PV, Tew KD, eds. Mechanisms of drug resistance in neoplastic cells. New York, NY: Academic Press, 1988:161–171.
285. de Jonge ME, Huitema AD, van Dam SM, et al. Significant induction of cyclophosphamide and thiotepa metabolism by phenytoin. Cancer Chemother Pharmacol 2005;55:507–510.
286. Boston Collaborative Drug Surveillance Program. Allopurinol and cytotoxic drugs. JAMA 1974;227:1036–1040.
287. Hassan M, Ljungman P, Ringden O, et al. The effect of busulphan on the pharmacokinetics of cyclophosphamide and its 4-hydroxy metabolite: time interval influence on therapeutic efficacy and therapy-related toxicity. Bone Marrow Transplant 2000;25:915–924.
288. Sanchez RI, Wang RW, Newton DJ, et al. Cytochrome P450 3A4 is the major enzyme involved in the metabolism of the substance P receptor antagonist aprepitant. Drug Metab Dispos 2004;32:1287–1292.
289. de Jonge ME, Huitema AD, Holtkamp MJ, et al. Aprepitant inhibits cyclophosphamide bioactivation and thiotepa metabolism. Cancer Chemother Pharmacol 2005;56:370–378.
290. Marr KA, Leisenring W, Crippa F, et al. Cyclophosphamide metabolism is affected by azole antifungals. Blood 2004;103:1557–1559.
291. Horowitz ME, Etcubanas E, Christensen ML, et al. Phase II testing of melphalan in children with newly diagnosed rhabdomyosarcoma: a model for anticancer drug development. J Clin Oncol 1988;6:308–314.
292. Atra A, Whelan JS, Calvagna V, et al. High-dose busulfan/melphalan with autologous stem cell recue in Ewing's sarcoma. Bone Marrow Transplant 1997;20:843–846.
293. McCowage GB, Vowels MR, Shaw PJ, et al. Autologous bone marrow transplantation for advanced neuroblastoma using teniposide, doxorubicin, melphalan, cisplatin, and total-body irradiation. J Clin Oncol 1995;13:2789–2795.
294. Carli M, Colombatti R, Oberlin O, et al. High-dose melphalan with autologous stem-cell rescue in metastatic rhabdomyosarcoma. J Clin Oncol 1999;17:2796–2803.
295. Vahrmeijer AL, Van Der Eb MM, Van Dierendonck JH, et al. Delivery of anticancer drugs via isolated hepatic perfusion: a promising strategy in the treatment of irresectable liver metastases? Semin Surg Oncol 1998;14:262–228.
296. Alexander HRJ, Fraker DL, Bartlett DL. Isolated limb perfusion for malignant melanoma. Semin Surg Oncol 1996;12:416–428.
297. Alberts DS, Chang SV, Chen HS, et al. Comparative pharmacokinetics of chlorambucil and melphalan in man. Recent Results Cancer Res 1980;74:124–131.
298. Alberts DS, Chang SY, Chen HS, et al. Oral melphalan kinetics. Clin Pharmacol Ther 1979;26:737–745.
299. Bosanquet AG, Gilby ED. Pharmacokinetics of oral and intravenous melphalan during routine treatment of multiple myeloma. Eur J Cancer Clin Oncol 1982;18:355–362.
300. Woodhouse KW, Hamilton P, Lennard A, et al. The pharmacokinetics of melphalan in patients with multiple myeloma: an intravenous/oral study using a conventional dose regimen. Eur J Clin Pharmacol 1983;24:283–285.
301. Bosanquet AG, Gilby ED. Comparison of the fed and fasting states on the absorption of melphalan in multiple myeloma. Cancer Chemother Pharmacol 1984;12:183–186.
302. Brox L, Birkett L, Belch A. Pharmacology of intravenous melphalan in patients with multiple myeloma. Cancer Treat Rev 1979;6(Suppl):27–32.
303. Ardiet C, Tranchand B, Biron P, et al. Pharmacokinetics of high dose intravenous melphalan in children and adults with forced diuresis: report in 26 cases. Cancer Chemother Pharmacol 1986;16:300–305.
304. Alberts DS, Chang SY, Chen H-S, et al. Kinetics of intravenous melphalan. Clin Pharmacol Ther 1979;26:73–80.
305. Smith DC, Jodrell DI, Egorin MJ, et al. Phase II trial and pharmacokinetic assessment of intravenous melphalan in patients with advanced prostate cancer. Cancer Chemother Pharmacol 1993;31:363–368.
306. Hersh MR, Ludden TM, Kuhn JG, et al. Pharmacokinetics of high dose melphalan. Invest New Drugs 1983;1:331–334.
307. Taha IAK, Ahmad RA, Rogers DW, et al. Pharmacokinetics of melphalan in children following high-dose intravenous injection. Cancer Chemother Pharmacol 1983;10:212–216.
308. Gouyette A, Hartmann O, Pico JL. Pharmacokinetics of high-dose melphalan in children and adults. Cancer Chemother Pharmacol 1986;16:184–189.
309. Ninane J, Baurain R, de Selys A, et al. High dose melphalan in children with advanced malignant disease. A pharmacokinetic study. Cancer Chemother Pharmacol 1985;15:263–267.
310. Moreau P, Kergueris MF, Milpied N, et al. A pilot study of 220 mg/m^2 melphalan followed by autologous stem cell transplantation in patients with advanced haematological malignancies: pharmacokinetics and toxicity. Br J Haematol 1996;95:527–530.
311. Pinguet F, Martel P, Fabbro M, et al. Pharmacokinetics of high-dose intravenous melphalan in patients undergoing peripheral blood hematopoietic progenitor-cell transplantation. Anticancer Res 1997;17:605–611.
312. Reece PA, Hill HS, Green RM, et al. Renal clearance and protein binding of melphalan in patients with cancer. Cancer Chemother Pharmacol 1988;22:348–352.
313. Cornwell GG, Pajak TF, Mclntyre OR, et al. Influence of renal failure on myelosuppressive effects of melphalan: Cancer and Leukemia Group B experience. Cancer Treat Rep 1982;66:475–481.
314. Kergueris MF, Milpied N, Moreau P, et al. Pharmacokinetics of high-dose melphalan in adults: influence of renal function. Anticancer Res 1994;14:2379–2383.
315. Nath CE, Shaw PJ, Montgomery K, et al. Melphalan pharmacokinetics in children with malignant disease: influence of body weight, renal function, carboplatin therapy and total body irradiation. Br J Clin Pharmacol 2005;59:314–324.
316. Nath CE, Shaw PJ, Montgomery K, et al. Population pharmacokinetics of melphalan in paediatric blood or marrow transplant recipients. Br J Clin Pharmacol 2007;64:151–164.
317. Jones R, Matthes SM, Dufton C, et al. Nitrosoureas. In: Grochow LB, Ames MM, eds. A clinician's guide to chemotherapy pharmacokinetics and pharmacodynamics. Baltimore, MD: Williams & Wilkins, 1998:331–344.
318. Mitchell EP, Schein PS. Contributions of nitrosoureas to cancer treatment. Cancer Treat Rep 1986;70:31–41.
319. Ewig RAG, Kohn KW. DNA damage and repair in mouse leukemia L1210 cells treated with nitrogen mustard, 1,3-*bis*(2-chloroethyl)-1-nitrosourea, and other nitrosoureas. Cancer Res 1977;37:2114–2122.
320. Tew KD, Sudhakar S, Schein PS, et al. Binding of chlorozotocin and 1-(2-chloroethyl)-3-cyclohexyl-1-nitrosourea to chromatin and nucleosomal fractions of HeLa cells. Cancer Res 1978;38:3371–3378.
321. Kann HE. Comparison of biochemical and biological effects of four nitrosoureas with differing carbamoylating activities. Cancer Res 1978;38:2363–2366.
322. Brent TP, Houghton PJ, Houghton JA. O6-Alkylguanine-DNA alkyltransferase activity correlates with the therapeutic response of human rhabdomyosarcoma xenografts to 1-(2-chloroethyl)-3-(*trans*-4-methylcyclohexyl)-1-nitrosourea. Proc Natl Acad Sci U S A 1985;82:2985–2989.
323. Belanich M, Pastor M, Randall T, et al. Retrospective study of the correlation between the DNA repair protein alkyltransferase and survival of brain tumor patients treated with carmustine. Cancer Res 1996;56:783–788.
324. Friedman HS, Pluda J, Quinn JA, et al. Phase I trial of carmustine plus O6-benzylguanine for patients with recurrent or progressive malignant glioma. J Clin Oncol 2000;18:3522–3528.
325. Gajewski TF, Sosman J, Gerson SL, et al. Phase II trial of the O6-alkylguanine DNA alkyltransferase inhibitor O6-benzylguanine and 1,3-*bis*(2-chloroethyl)-1 nitrosourea in advanced melanoma. Clin Cancer Res 2005;11:7861–7865.
326. Quinn JA, Pluda J, Dolan ME, et al. Phase II trial of carmustine plus O(6)-benzylguanine for patients with nitrosourea-resistant recurrent or progressive malignant glioma. J Clin Oncol 2002;20:2277–2283.
327. Ryan CW, Dolan ME, Brockstein BB, et al. A phase II trial of O6-benzylguanine and carmustine in patients with advanced soft tissue sarcoma. Cancer Chemother Pharmacol 2006;58:634–639.
328. Schilsky RL, Dolan ME, Bertucci D, et al. Phase I clinical and pharmacological study of O6-benzylguanine followed by carmustine in patients with advanced cancer. Clin Cancer Res 2000;6:3025–3031.
329. Adams DM, Zhou T, Berg SL, et al. Phase 1 trial of O6-benzylguanine and BCNU in children with CNS tumors: a Children's Oncology Group study. Pediatr Blood Cancer 2008;50:549–553.
330. Schmitz N, Diehl V. Carmustine and the lungs. Lancet 1997;349:1712–1713.
331. O'Driscoll BR, Hasleton PS, Taylor PM, et al. Active lung fibrosis up to 17 years after chemotherapy with carmustine (BCNU) in childhood. N Engl J Med 1990;323:378–382.
332. Engelhard HH. The role of interstitial BCNU chemotherapy in the treatment of malignant glioma. Surg Neurol 2000;53:458–464.
333. Brem H, Piantadosi S, Burger PC, et al. Placebo-controlled trial of safety and efficacy of intraoperative controlled delivery by biodegradable polymers of chemotherapy for recurrent gliomas. Lancet 1995;345:1008–1012.
334. Valtonen S, Timonen U, Toivanen P, et al. Interstitial chemotherapy with carmustine-loaded polymers for high-grade gliomas: a randomized double-blind study. Neurosurgery 1997;41:44–48.
335. Schein PS, Heal J, Green D, et al. Pharmacology of nitrosourea antitumor agents. Antibiot Chemother 1978;23:64–75.
336. DeVita VT, Denham C, Davidson JD, et al. The physiological disposition of the carcinostatic 1,3-*bis*(2-chloroethyl)-1-nitrosourea (BCNU) in man and animals. Clin Pharmacol Ther 1967;8:566–577.
337. Sponzo RW, DeVita VT, Oliverio VT. Physiologic disposition of 1-(2-chloroethyl)-3-cyclohexyl-1-nitrosourea (CCNU) and 1-(2-chloroethyl)-3-(4-methyl cyclohexyl)-1-nitrosourea (MeCCNU) in man. Cancer 1973;31:1154–119.
338. Levin VA, Hoffman W, Weinkam RJ. Pharmacokinetics of BCNU in man: a preliminary study of 20 patients. Cancer Treat Rep 1978;62:1305–1312.
339. Henner WD, Peters WP, Eder JP, et al. Pharmacokinetics and immediate effects of high-dose carmustine in man. Cancer Treat Rep 1986;70:877–880.
340. Kastrissios H, Chao NJ, Blaschke TF. Pharmacokinetics of high-dose oral CCNU in bone marrow transplant patients. Cancer Chemother Pharmacol 1996;38:425–430.
341. Lee FY, Workman P, Roberts JT, et al. Clinical pharmacokinetics of oral CCNU (lomustine). Cancer Chemother Pharmacol 1985;14:125–131.
342. Weiss RB, Issell BF. The nitrosoureas: carmustine (BCNU) and lomustine (CCNU). Cancer Treat Rev 1982;9:313–330.
343. Walker MD, Hilton J. Nitrosourea pharmacodynamics in relation to the central nervous system. Cancer Treat Rep 1976;60:725–728.
344. Fung LK, Ewend MG, Sills A, et al. Pharmacokinetics of interstitial delivery of carmustine, 4-hydroperoxycyclophosphamide, and paclitaxel from a biodegradable polymer implant in the monkey brain. Cancer Res 1998;58:672–684.
345. Wang CC, Li J, Teo CS, et al. The delivery of BCNU to brain tumors. J Control Release 1999;61:21–41.
346. Harmon WE, Cohen HJ, Schneeburger EE. Chronic renal failure in children treated with methyl CCNU. N Engl J Med 1979;300:1200–1203.
347. Ellis ME, Weiss RB, Kuperminc M. Nephrotoxicity of lomustine: a case report and literature review. Cancer Chemother Pharmacol 1985;15:174–175.
348. Aronin PA, Mahaley MS, Rudnick SA, et al. Prediction of BCNU pulmonary toxicity in patients with malignant gliomas: an assessment of risk factors. N Engl J Med 1980;303:183–191.
349. Weinstein AS, Diener-West M, Nelson DF, et al. Pulmonary toxicity of carmustine in patients treated for malignant glioma. Cancer Treat Rep 1986;70:943–946.
350. Mertens AC, Yasui Y, Liu Y, et al. Pulmonary complications in survivors of childhood and adolescent cancer. A report from the Childhood Cancer Survivor Study. Cancer 2002;95:2431–2441.
351. Alessandrino EP, Bernasconi P, Colombo A, et al. Pulmonary toxicity following carmustine-based preparative regimens and autologous peripheral blood progenitor cell transplantation in hematological malignancies. Bone Marrow Transplant 2000;25:309–313.
352. Frankovich J, Donaldson SS, Lee Y, et al. High-dose therapy and autologous hematopoietic cell transplantation in children with primary refractory and relapsed Hodgkin's disease: atopy predicts idiopathic diffuse lung injury syndromes. Biol Blood Marrow Transplant 2001;7:49–57.
353. Levin VA, Sterns J, Byrd A, et al. The effect of phenobarbital pretreatment on the antitumor activity of 1,3-*bis*(2-chloroethyl)-1-nitrosourea (BCNU), 1-(2-chloroethyl)-3-cyclohexyl-1-nitrosourea (CCNU) and 1-(2-chloroethyl)-3-(2,6-dioxo-3-piperidyl)-1-nitrosourea (PCNU), and on the plasma pharmacokinetics and biotransformation of BCNU. J Pharmacol Exp Ther 1979;208:1–6.
354. Kyle ME, Nakae D, Serroni A, et al. 1,3-(2-Chloroethyl)-1-nitrosourea potentiate the toxicity of acetaminophen both in the phenobarbital-induced rat and hepatocyte cultures from such animals. Mol Pharmacol 1988;34:584–589.
355. Slattery JT, Risler LJ. Therapeutic monitoring of busulfan in hematopoietic stem cell transplantation. Ther Drug Monit 1998;20:543–549.

356. Hassan M. Busulfan. In: Grochow LB, Ames MM, eds. A clinician's guide to chemotherapy pharmacokinetics and pharmacodynamics. Baltimore, MD: Williams & Wilkins, 1998:189–208.
357. Hassan M, Ljungman P, Bolme P, et al. Busulfan bioavailability. Blood 1994;84: 2144–2150.
358. Regazzi MB, Locatelli F, Buggia I, et al. Disposition of high-dose busulfan in pediatric patients undergoing bone marrow transplantation. Clin Pharmacol Ther 1993;53: 45–52.
359. Schuler US, Ehrsam M, Schneider A, et al. Pharmacokinetics of intravenous busulfan and evaluation of the bioavailability of the oral formulation in conditioning for haematopoietic stem cell transplantation. Bone Marrow Transplant 1998;22:241–244.
360. Cremers S, Schoemaker R, Bredius R, et al. Pharmacokinetics of intravenous busulfan in children prior to stem cell transplantation. Br J Clin Pharmacol 2002;53:386–389.
361. Booth BP, Rahman A, Dagher R, et al. Population pharmacokinetic-based dosing of intravenous busulfan in pediatric patients. J Clin Pharmacol 2007;47:101–111.
362. Kim AH, Tse JC, Ikeda A, et al. Evaluating pharmacokinetics and pharmacodynamics of intravenous busulfan in pediatric patients receiving bone marrow transplantation [published online ahead of print November 18, 2008]. Pediatr Transplant. DOI: 10.1111/j.1399-3046.2008.01098.x.
363. Johnson L, Orchard PJ, Baker KS, et al. Glutathione *S*-transferase A1 genetic variants reduce busulfan clearance in children undergoing hematopoietic cell transplantation. J Clin Pharmacol 2008;48:1052–1062.
364. Vassal G, Gouyette A, Hartmann O, et al. Pharmacokinetics of high-dose busulfan in children. Cancer Chemother Pharmacol 1989;24:386–390.
365. Vassal G, Deroussent A, Hartmann O, et al. Dose-dependent neurotoxicity of high-dose busulfan in children: a clinical and pharmacological study. Cancer Res 1990;50: 6203–6207.
366. Gibbs JP, Yang JS, Slattery JT. Comparison of human liver and small intestinal glutathione *S*-transferase-catalyzed busulfan conjugation in vitro. Drug Metab Dispos 1998;26:52–55.
367. Czerwinski M, Gibbs JP, Slattery JT. Busulfan conjugation by glutathione *S*-transferases alpha, mu, and pi. Drug Metab Dispos 1996;24:1015–1019.
368. Buggia I, Locatelli F, Regazzi MB, et al. Busulfan. Ann Pharmacother 1994;28: 1055–1062.
369. Slattery JT, Sanders JE, Buckner CD, et al. Graft-rejection and toxicity following bone marrow transplantation in relation to busulfan pharmacokinetics. Bone Marrow Transplant 1995;16:31–42.
370. Gibbs JP, Murray G, Risler L, et al. Age-dependent tetrahydrothiophenium ion formation in young children and adults receiving high-dose busulfan. Cancer Res 1997;57:5509–5516.
371. Vassal G. Pharmacologically-guided dose adjustment of busulfan in high-dose chemotherapy regimens: rationale and pitfalls [review]. Anticancer Res 1994;14: 2363–2370.
372. Sandström M, Karlsson MO, Ljungman P, et al. Population pharmacokinetic analysis resulting in a tool for dose individualization of busulphan in bone marrow transplantation recipients. Bone Marrow Transplant 2001;28:657–664.
373. Grochow LB, Krivit W, Whitley CB, et al. Busulfan disposition in children. Blood 1990;75:1723–1727.
374. Vassal G, Challine D, Koscielny S, et al. Chronopharmacology of high-dose busulfan in children. Cancer Res 1993;53:1534–1537.
375. Grochow LB, Richard JJ, Brundett RB, et al. Pharmacokinetics of busulfan: correlation with veno-occlusive disease in patients undergoing bone marrow transplantation. Cancer Chemother Pharmacol 1989;25:55–61.
376. Dix SP, Wingard JR, Mullins RE, et al. Association of busulfan area under the curve with veno-occlusive disease following BMT. Bone Marrow Transplant 1996;17:225–230.
377. Bolinger AM, Zangwill AB, Slattery JT, et al. An evaluation of engraftment, toxicity and busulfan concentration in children receiving bone marrow transplantation for leukemia or genetic disease. Bone Marrow Transplant 2000;25:925–930.
378. Bolinger AM, Zangwill AB, Slattery JT, et al. Target dose adjustment of busulfan in pediatric patients undergoing bone marrow transplantation. Bone Marrow Transplant 2001;28:1013–1018.
379. Copelan EA, Bechtel TP, Avalos BR, et al. Busulfan levels are influenced by prior treatment and are associated with hepatic veno-occlusive disease and early mortality but not with delayed complications following marrow transplantation. Bone Marrow Transplant 2001;27:1121–1124.
380. Bleyzac N, Souillet G, Magron P, et al. Improved clinical outcome of paediatric bone marrow recipients using a test dose and Bayesian pharmacokinetic individualization of busulfan dosage regimens. Bone Marrow Transplant 2001;28:743–751.
381. Vassal G, Michel G, Esperou H, et al. Prospective validation of a novel IV busulfan fixed dosing for paediatric patients to improve therapeutic AUC targeting without drug monitoring. Cancer Chemother Pharmacol 2008;61:113–123.
382. Bearman SI. The syndrome of hepatic veno-occlusive disease after marrow transplantation. Blood 1995;85:3005–3020.
383. Styler MJ, Crilley P, Biggs J, et al. Hepatic dysfunction following busulfan and cyclophosphamide myeloablation: a retrospective, multicenter analysis. Bone Marrow Transplant 1996;18:171–1716.
384. Vassal G, Koscielny S, Challine D, et al. Busulfan disposition and hepatic veno-occlusive disease in children undergoing bone marrow transplantation. Cancer Chemother Pharmacol 1996;37:247–253.
385. Murphy CP, Harden EA, Thompson JM. Generalized seizures to high-dose busulfan therapy. Ann Pharmacol Ther 1992;26:30–31.
386. Teinturier C, Hartmann O, Valteau-Couanet D, et al. Ovarian function after autologous bone marrow transplantation in childhood: high-dose busulfan is a major cause of ovarian failure. Bone Marrow Transplant 1998;22:989–994.
387. Reed E, Dabholkar M, Chabner BA. Platinum analogues. In: Chabner BA, Longo DL, eds. Cancer chemotherapy and biotherapy principles and practice. Philadelphia, PA: Lippincott-Raven, 1996:357–378.
388. Go RS, Adjei AA. Review of the comparative pharmacology and clinical activity of cisplatin and carboplatin. J Clin Oncol 1999;17:409–422.
389. van der Vijgh WJF. Clinical pharmacokinetics of carboplatin. Clin Pharmacokinet 1991;21:242–261.
390. Canal P. Platinum compounds: pharmacokinetics and pharmacodynamics. In: Grochow LB, Ames MM, eds. A clinician's guide to chemotherapy pharmacokinetics and pharmacodynamics. Baltimore, MD: Williams & Wilkins, 1998:345–373.
391. Graham MA, Lockwood GF, Greenslade D, et al. Clinical pharmacokinetics of oxaliplatin: a critical review. Clin Cancer Res 2000;6:1205–1218.
392. Loehrer PJ, Einhorn LH. Cisplatin. Ann Intern Med 1984;100:704–713.
393. Jaffe N, Knopp J, Chuang VP, et al. Osteosarcoma: intra-arterial treatment in the primary tumor with *cis*-diamminedichloroplatinum (II) (CDP). Angiographic, pathologic, and pharmacologic studies. Cancer 1983;51:402–407.
394. Pratt CB, Hayes A, Green AA, et al. Pharmacokinetic evaluation of cisplatin in children with malignant solid tumors: a phase II study. Cancer Treat Rep 1981;65: 1021–1026.
395. Khan AB, D'Souza B, Wharam M, et al. Cisplatin therapy in recurrent childhood brain tumors. Cancer Treat Rep 1982;66:2013–2020.
396. Pinzani V, Bressolle F, Haug IJ, et al. Cisplatin-induced renal toxicity and toxicity-modulating strategies: a review. Cancer Chemother Pharmacol 1994;35:1–9.
397. Anand AJ, Bashey B. Newer insights into cisplatin nephrotoxicity. Ann Pharmacother 1993;27:1519–1525.
398. Capizzi RL. Amifostine reduces the incidence of cumulative nephrotoxicity from cisplatin: laboratory and clinical aspects. Semin Oncol 1999;26(Suppl 7):72–81.
399. Boyer MW, Moertel CL, Priest JR, et al. Use of intracavitary cisplatin for the treatment of childhood solid tumors in the chest or abdominal cavity. J Clin Oncol 1995; 13:631–636.
400. Lokich J, Anderson N. Carboplatin versus cisplatin in solid tumors: an analysis of the literature. Ann Oncol 1998;9:13–21.
401. Pinkerton CR, Broadbent V, Horwich A, et al. 'JEB'—a carboplatin-based regimen for malignant germ cell tumors in children. Br J Cancer 1990;62:257–262.
402. Doz F, Pinkerton R. What is the place of carboplatin in paediatric oncology? Eur J Cancer 1994;30A:194–201.
403. Gaynon PS. Carboplatin in pediatric malignancies. Semin Oncol 1994;21(Suppl 12):65–76.
404. Wagstaff AJ, Ward A, Benfield P, et al. Carboplatin: a preliminary review of its pharmacodynamic and pharmacokinetic properties and therapeutic efficacy in the treatment of cancer. Drugs 1989;37:162–190.
405. Andre T, Boni C, Mounedji-Boudiaf L, et al. Oxaliplatin, fluorouracil, and leucovorin as adjuvant treatment for colon cancer. N Engl J Med 2004;350:2343–2351.
406. Spunt SL, Freeman BB III, Billups CA, et al. Phase I clinical trial of oxaliplatin in children and adolescents with refractory solid tumors. J Clin Oncol 2007;25:2274–2280.
407. Fouladi M, Blaney SM, Poussaint TY, et al. Phase II study of oxaliplatin in children with recurrent or refractory medulloblastoma, supratentorial primitive neuroectodermal tumors, and atypical teratoid rhabdoid tumors: a pediatric brain tumor consortium study. Cancer 2006;107:2291–2297.
408. McGregor LM, Spunt SL, Furman WL, et al. Phase 1 study of oxaliplatin and irinotecan in pediatric patients with refractory solid tumors: a children's oncology group study. Cancer 2009;115:1765–1775.
409. LeRoy AF, Lutz RJ, Dedrick RL, et al. Pharmacokinetic study of *cis*-diamminedichloroplatinum (II) (DDP) in the beagle dog: thermodynamic and kinetic behavior of DDP in a biologic milieu. Cancer Treat Rep 1979;63:59–71.
410. Gormley PE, Bull JM, LeRoy AF, et al. Kinetics of *cis*-dichlorodiammineplatinum. Clin Pharmacol Ther 1979;25:351–357.
411. Patton TF, Himmelstein KJ, Belt R, et al. Plasma levels and urinary excretion of filterable platinum species following bolus injection and IV infusion of *cis*-dichlorodiammineplatinum (II) in man. Cancer Treat Rep 1978;62:1359–1362.
412. DeConti RC, Toftness BR, Lange RC, et al. Clinical and pharmacologic studies with *cis*-diamminedichloroplatinum (II). Cancer Res 1973;33:1310–1315.
413. Geoerger B, Doz F, Gentet JC, et al. Phase I study of weekly oxaliplatin in relapsed or refractory pediatric solid malignancies. J Clin Oncol 2008;26:4394–4400.
414. Van Echo DA, Egorin MJ, Aisner J. The pharmacology of carboplatin. Semin Oncol 1989;16(Suppl 5):1–6.
415. Van Echo DA, Egorin MJ, Whitacre MY, et al. Phase I and pharmacologic trial of carboplatin daily for 5 days. Cancer Treat Rep 1984;68:1103–1114.
416. Harland SJ, Newell DR, Siddick ZH, et al. Pharmacokinetics of *cis*-diammine-1,1-cyclobutanedicarcoxylate platinum (II) in patients with normal and impaired renal function. Cancer Res 1984;44:1693–1697.
417. Gietema JA, Meinardi MT, Messerschmidt J, et al. Circulating plasma platinum more than 10 years after cisplatin treatment for testicular cancer. Lancet 2000;355: 1075–1076.
418. Vermorken JB, van der Vijgh WJF, Klein I, et al. Pharmacokinetics of free and total platinum species after short-term infusion of cisplatin. Cancer Treat Rep 1984;68: 505–513.
419. Himmelstein KJ, Patton TF, Belt RJ, et al. Clinical kinetics of intact cisplatin and some related species. Clin Pharmacol Ther 1981;29:658–664.
420. Peng B, English MW, Boddy AV, et al. Cisplatin pharmacokinetics in children with cancer. Eur J Cancer 1997;33:1823–1828.
421. Bin P, Boddy AV, English MW, et al. The comparative pharmacokinetics and pharmacodynamics of cisplatin and carboplatin in paediatric patients: a review. Anticancer Res 1994;14:2279–2283.
422. Belt RJ, Himmelstein KJ, Patton TF, et al. Pharmacokinetics of non-protein-bound platinum species following administration of *cis*-dichlorodiamminoplatinum (II). Cancer Treat Rep 1979;63:1515–1521.
423. Oguri S, Sakakibara T, Mase H, et al. Clinical pharmacokinetics of carboplatin. J Clin Pharmacol 1988;28:208–215.
424. Vermorken JB, van der Vijgh WJ, Klein I, et al. Pharmacokinetics of free and total platinum species after rapid and prolonged infusions of cisplatin. Clin Pharmacol Ther 1986;39:136–144.
425. Jacobs C, Kalman SM, Tretton M, et al. Renal handling of *cis*-diamminedichloroplatinum (II). Cancer Treat Rep 1980;64:1223–1226.
426. Blouin RA, Kolpek JH, Mann HJ. Influence of obesity on drug disposition. Clin Pharm 1987;6:706–714.
427. Sparreboom A, Wolff AC, Mathijssen RH, et al. Evaluation of alternate size descriptors for dose calculation of anticancer drugs in the obese. J Clin Oncol 2007;25: 4707–4713.
428. Reece PA, Stafford I, Davy M, et al. Influence of infusion time on unchanged cisplatin disposition in patients with ovarian cancer. Cancer Chemother Pharmacol 1989;24: 256–260.
429. Gorodetsky R, Vexler A, Bar-Khaim Y, et al. Plasma platinum elimination in a hemodialysis patient treated with cisplatin. Ther Drug Monit 1995;17:203–206.
430. Powis G. Effects of disease states on pharmacokinetics of anticancer drugs. In: Ames MM, Powis G, Kovach JS, eds. Pharmacokinetics of anticancer agents in humans. Amsterdam, The Netherlands: Elsevier, 1983:365–397.
431. Calvert AH, Harland SJ, Newell DR, et al. Early clinical studies with *cis*-diammine-1,1-cyclobutane dicarboxylate platinum II. Cancer Chemother Pharmacol 1982;9: 140–147.

432. Motzer RJ, Niedzwiecki D, Isaacs M, et al. Carboplatin-based chemotherapy with pharmacokinetic analysis for patients with hemodialysis-dependent renal insufficiency. Cancer Chemother Pharmacol 1990;27:234–238.
433. Chatelut E, Rostaing L, Gualano V, et al. Pharmacokinetics of carboplatin in a patient suffering from advanced ovarian carcinoma with hemodialysis-dependent renal insufficiency. Nephron 1994;66:157–161.
434. Chatelut E, Boddy AV, Peng B, et al. Population pharmacokinetics of carboplatin in children. Clin Pharmacol Ther 1996;59:436–443.
435. Madden T, Sunderland M, Santana VM, et al. Pharmacokinetics of high-dose carboplatin in pediatric patients with cancer. Clin Pharmacol Ther 1992;51:701–707.
436. Newell DR, Pearson ADJ, Balmanno K, et al. Carboplatin pharmacokinetics in children: the development of a pediatric dosing formula. J Clin Oncol 1993;11(12):2314–2323.
437. Tonda ME, Heideman RL, Petros WP, et al. Carboplatin pharmacokinetics in young children with brain tumors. Cancer Chemother Pharmacol 1996;38:395–400.
438. Duffull SB, Robinson BA. Clinical pharmacokinetics and dose optimisation of carboplatin. Clin Pharmacokinet 1997;33:161–183.
439. Calvert AH, Newell DR, Gumbrell LA, et al. Carboplatin dosage: rospective evaluation of a simple formula based on renal function. J Clin Oncol 1989;7:1748–1756.
440. Marina NM, Rodman J, Shema SJ, et al. Phase I study of escalating targeted doses of carboplatin combined with ifosfamide and etoposide in children with relapsed solid tumors. J Clin Oncol 1993;11:554–560.
441. Chatelut E, Canal P, Brunner V, et al. Prediction of carboplatin clearance from standard morphological and biological patient characteristics. J Natl Cancer Inst 1995;87:573–580.
442. Marina NM, Rodman JH, Murry DJ, et al. Phase I study of escalating targeted doses of carboplatin combined with ifosfamide and etoposide in treatment of newly diagnosed pediatric solid tumors. J Natl Cancer Inst 1994;86:544–548.
443. de Lemos ML. Application of the area under the curve of carboplatin in predicting toxicity and efficacy. Cancer Treat Rev 1998;24:407–414.
444. Liem RI, Higman MA, Chen AR, et al. Misinterpretation of a Calvert-derived formula leading to carboplatin overdose in two children. J Pediatr Hematol Oncol 2003;25:818–821.
445. Takimoto CH, Remick SC, Sharma S, et al. Dose-escalating and pharmacological study of oxaliplatin in adult cancer patients with impaired renal function: a National Cancer Institute Organ Dysfunction Working Group Study. J Clin Oncol 2003;21:2664–2672.
446. Doroshow JH, Synold TW, Gandara D, et al. Pharmacology of oxaliplatin in solid tumor patients with hepatic dysfunction: a preliminary report of the National Cancer Institute Organ Dysfunction Working Group. Semin Oncol 2003;30:14–19.
447. Cvitkovic E. Cumulative toxicities from cisplatin therapy and current cytoprotective measures. Cancer Treat Rev 1998;24:265–281.
448. Meyer KB, Madias NE. Cisplatin nephrotoxicity. Miner Electrolyte Metab 1994;20:201–213.
449. Ariceta G, Rodriguez-Soriano J, Vallo A, et al. Acute and chronic effects of cisplatin therapy on renal magnesium homeostasis. Med Pediatr Oncol 1997;28:35–40.
450. Gonzalez-Vitale JC, Hayes DM, et al. The renal pathology in clinical trials of *cis*-platinum (II) diamminedichloride. Cancer 1977;39:1362–1371.
451. Daugaard G, Abildgaard U. Cisplatin nephrotoxicity. Cancer Chemother Pharmacol 1989;25:1–9.
452. Meijer S, Sleijfer DT, Mulder NH, et al. Some effects of combination chemotherapy with cisplatinum on renal function in patients with nonseminomatous testicular carcinoma. Cancer 1983;51:2035–2040.
453. Womer RB, Pritchard J, Barratt TM. Renal toxicity of cisplatin in children. J Pediatr 1985;106:659–663.
454. Fjeldborg P, Srensen J, Helkjaer PE. The long-term effect of cisplatin on renal function. Cancer 1986;58:2214–2217.
455. Brock PR, Koliouskas DE, Barratt TM, et al. Partial reversibility of cisplatin nephrotoxicity in children. J Pediatr 1991;118:531–534.
456. Stohr W, Paulides M, Bielack S, et al. Nephrotoxicity of cisplatin and carboplatin in sarcoma patients: a report from the late effects surveillance system. Pediatr Blood Cancer 2007;48:140–147.
457. Brock PR, Yeomans EC, Bellman SC, et al. Cisplatin therapy in infants: short and long-term morbidity. Br J Cancer 1992;18:536–540.
458. Markman M. Amifostine in reducing cisplatin toxicity. Semin Oncol 1998;25:522–524.
459. Kemp G, Rose P, Lurain J, et al. Amifostine pretreatment for protection against cyclophosphamide-induced and cisplatin-induced toxicities: results of a randomized control trial in patients with advanced ovarian cancer. J Clin Oncol 1996;14:2101–2112.
460. Crom WR, Pratt CB, Green AA, et al. The effect of prior cisplatin therapy on the pharmacokinetics of high-dose methotrexate. J Clin Oncol 1984;2:655–666.
461. Reece PA, Stafford I, Russell J, et al. Reduced ability to clear ultrafilterable platinum with repeated courses of cisplatin. J Clin Oncol 1986;4:1392–1398.
462. Stewart DJ, Mikhael NZ, Nanji AA, et al. Renal and hepatic concentrations of platinum: relationship to cisplatin time, dose, and nephrotoxicity. J Clin Oncol 1985;3:1251–1256.
463. Mollman JE. Cisplatin neurotoxicity. N Engl J Med 1990;322:126–127.
464. Highley M, Meller ST, Pinkerton CR. Seizures and cortical dysfunction following high-dose cisplatin administration in children. Med Pediatr Oncol1992;20:143–148.
465. McHaney VA, Thibadoux MA, Hayes FA, et al. Hearing loss in children receiving cisplatin chemotherapy. J Pediatr 1983;102:314–317.
466. Cersosimo RJ. Cisplatin neurotoxicity. Cancer Treat Rev 1989;16:195–211.
467. Schaefer SD, Post JD, Close LG, et al. Ototoxicity of low and moderate-dose cisplatin. Cancer 1985;56:1934–1939.
468. Li Y, Womer RB, Silber JH. Predicting cisplatin ototoxicity in children: the influence of age and the cumulative dose. Eur J Cancer 2004;40:2445–2451.
469. McWhinney SR, Goldberg RM, McLeod HL. Platinum neurotoxicity pharmacogenetics. Mol Cancer Ther 2009;8:10–16.
470. Fouladi M, Chintagumpala M, Ashley D, et al. Amifostine protects against cisplatin-induced ototoxicity in children with average-risk medulloblastoma. J Clin Oncol 2008;26:3749–3755.
471. Marina N, Chang KW, Malogolowkin M, et al. Amifostine does not protect against the ototoxicity of high-dose cisplatin combined with etoposide and bleomycin in pediatric germ-cell tumors: a Children's Oncology Group study. Cancer 2005;104:841–847.
472. Katzenstein HM, Chang K, Krailo M, et al. A randomized study of platinum based chemotherapy with or without amifostine for the treatment of children with hepatoblastoma (HB): a report of the Intergroup Hepatoblastoma Study P9645. Proc Am Soc Clin Oncol 2004;23:799.
473. Fisher MJ, Lange BJ, Needle MN, et al. Amifostine for children with medulloblastoma treated with cisplatin-based chemotherapy. Pediatr Blood Cancer 2004;43:780–784.
474. Canetta R, Franks C, Smaldone L, et al. Clinical status of carboplatin. Oncology 1987;1:61–70.
475. Brandt LJ, Broadbent V. Nephrotoxicity following carboplatin use in children: is routine monitoring of renal function necessary. Med Pediatr Oncol 1993;21:31–35.
476. English MW, Skinner R, Pearson AD, et al. Dose-related nephrotoxicity of carboplatin in children. Br J Cancer 1999;81:336–341.
477. Schiavetti A, Varrasso G, Maurizi P, et al. Hypersensitivity to carboplatin in children. Med Pediatr Oncol 1999;32:183–185.
478. Chang SM, Fryberger S, Crouse V, et al. Carboplatin hypersensitivity in children. Cancer 1995;75:1171–1175.
479. Grothey A. Oxaliplatin-safety profile: neurotoxicity. Semin Oncol 2003;30:5–13.
480. Trimmer EE, Essigmann JM. Cisplatin. Essays Biochem 1999;34:191–211.
481. Perez RP. Cellular and molecular determinants of cisplatin resistance. Eur J Oncol 1998;34:1535–1542.
482. Gosland M, Lum B, Schimmelpfennig J, et al. Insights into mechanisms of cisplatin resistance and potential for its clinical reversal. Pharmacotherapy 1996;16:16–39.
483. Branch P, Masson M, Aquilina G, et al. Spontaneous development of drug resistance: mismatch repair and p53 defects in resistance to cisplatin in human tumor cells. Oncogene 2000;19:3138–3145.
484. Friedman HS, Averbuch SD, Kurtzberg J. Nonclassic alkylating agents. In: Chabner BA, Longo DL, eds. Cancer chemotherapy and biotherapy principles and practice. Philadelphia, PA: Lippincott-Raven, 1996:333–356.
485. Reid JM, Kuffel MJ, Miller JK, et al. Metabolic activation of dacarbazine by human cytochromes P450: the role of CYP1A1, CYP1A2, and CYP2E1. Clin Cancer Res 1999;5:2192–2197.
486. Foster BJ. Procarbazine, dacarbazine, and temozolomide. In: Grochow LB, Ames MM, eds. A clinician's guide to chemotherapy pharmacokinetics and pharmacodynamics. Baltimore, MD: Williams & Wilkins, 1998:395–410.
487. Loo TL, Luce JK, Jardine JH, et al. Pharmacologic studies of the antitumor agent 5-(dimethyltriazeno)-imidazole-4-carboxamide. Cancer Res 1968;28:2448–2253.
488. Breithaupt H, Dammann A, Aigner K. Pharmacokinetics of dacarbazine (DTIC) and its metabolite 5-aminoimidazole-4-carboxamide (AIC) following different dose schedules. Cancer Chemother Pharmacol 1982;9:103–109.
489. van Delft JHM, van den Ende AMC, Keizer HJ, et al. Determination of N7-methylguanine in DNA of white blood cells from cancer patients treated with dacarbazine. Carcinogenesis 1992;13:1257–1259.
490. Chabot GG, Flaherty LE, Valdivieso M, et al. Alteration of dacarbazine pharmacokinetics after interleukin-2 administration in melanoma patients. Cancer Chemother Pharmacol 1990;27:157–160.
491. Paschke R, Heine M. Pathophysiological aspects of dacarbazine-induced human liver damage. Hepatogastroenterology 1985;32:273–275.
492. Newlands ES, Stevens MFG, Wedge SR, et al. Temozolomide: a review of its discovery, chemical properties, pre-clinical development and clinical trials. Cancer Treat Rev 1997;23:36–61.
493. Friedman HS, Kerby T, Calvert H. Temozolomide and treatment of malignant glioma. Clin Cancer Res 2000;6:2585–2597.
494. Stevens MF, Hickman JA, Langdon SP, et al. Antitumor activity and pharmacokinetics in mice of 8-carbamoyl-3-methyl-imidazo[5,1-d]-1,2,3,5-tetrazin-4(3H)-one (CCRG 81045; M & B 39831), a novel drug with potential as an alternative to dacarbazine. Cancer Res 1987;47:5846–5852.
495. Newlands ES, Blackledge GR, Slack JA, et al. Phase I trial of temozolomide (CCRG 81045: M&B 39831: NSC 362856). Br J Cancer 1992;65:287–291.
496. Nicholson HS, Krailo M, Ames MM, et al. Phase I study of temozolomide in children and adolescents with recurrent solid tumors: a report from the Children's Cancer Group. J Clin Oncol 1998;16:3037–3043.
497. Estlin EJ, Lashford L, Ablett S, et al. Phase I study of temozolomide in paediatric patients with advanced cancer. United Kingdom Children's Cancer Study Group. Br J Cancer 1998;78:652–661.
498. Horton TM, Thompson PA, Berg SL, et al. Phase I pharmacokinetic and pharmacodynamic study of temozolomide in pediatric patients with refractory or recurrent leukemia: a Children's Oncology Group Study. J Clin Oncol 2007;25:4922–4928.
499. Brock CS, Newlands ES, Wedge SR, et al. Phase I trial of temozolomide using an extended continuous oral schedule. Cancer Res 1998;58:4363–4367.
500. Kushner BH, Kramer K, Modak S, et al. Irinotecan plus temozolomide for relapsed or refractory neuroblastoma. J Clin Oncol 2006;24:5271–5276.
501. Jakacki RI, Hamilton M, Gilbertson RJ, et al. Pediatric phase I and pharmacokinetic study of erlotinib followed by the combination of erlotinib and temozolomide: a Children's Oncology Group Phase I Consortium Study. J Clin Oncol 2008;26:4921–4927.
502. Jakacki RI, Yates A, Blaney SM, et al. A phase I trial of temozolomide and lomustine in newly diagnosed high-grade gliomas of childhood. Neuro Oncol 2008;10:569–576.
503. Wagner LM, Villablanca JG, Stewart CF, et al. Phase I trial of oral irinotecan and temozolomide for children with relapsed high-risk neuroblastoma: a new approach to neuroblastoma therapy consortium study. J Clin Oncol 2009;27:1290–1296.
504. Agarwala SS, Kirkwood JM. Temozolomide, a novel alkylating agent with activity in the central nervous system, may improve the treatment of advanced metastatic melanoma. Oncologist 2000;5:144–151.
505. Brada M, Judson I, Beale P, et al. Phase I dose-escalation and pharmacokinetic study of temozolomide (SCH 52365) for refractory or relapsing malignancies. Br J Cancer 1999;81:1022–1030.
506. Baker SD, Wirth M, Statkevich P, et al. Absorption, metabolism, and excretion of 14C-temozolomide following oral administration to patients with advanced cancer. Clin Cancer Res 1999;5:309–317.
507. Hammond LA, Eckardt JR, Baker SD, et al. Phase I and pharmacokinetic study of temozolomide on a daily-for-5-days schedule in patients with advanced solid malignancies. J Clin Oncol 1999;17:2604–2613.
508. Panetta JC, Kirstein MN, Gajjar A, et al. Population pharmacokinetics of temozolomide and metabolites in infants and children with primary central nervous system tumors. Cancer Chemother Pharmacol 2003;52:435–441.
509. Baer JC, Freeman AA, Newlands ES, et al. Depletion of O6-alkylguanine-DNA alkyltransferase correlates with potentiation of temozolomide and CCNU toxicity in human tumour cells. Br J Cancer 1993;67:1299–1302.

510. Tolcher AW, Gerson SL, Denis L, et al. Marked inactivation of O6-alkylguanine-DNA alkyltransferase activity with protracted temozolomide schedules. Br J Cancer 2003; 88:1004–1011.
511. Wedge SR, Newlands ES. O6-benzylguanine enhances the sensitivity of a glioma xenograft with low O6-alkylguanine-DNA alkyltransferase activity to temozolomide and BCNU. Br J Cancer 1996;73:1049–1052.
512. Warren KE, Aikin AA, Libucha M, et al. Phase I study of O6-benzylguanine and temozolomide administered daily for 5 days to pediatric patients with solid tumors. J Clin Oncol 2005;23:7646–7653.
513. Cramer P, Andrieu JM. Hodgkin's disease in childhood and adolescence: results of chemotherapy-radiotherapy in clinical stages IA-IIB. J Clin Oncol 1985;3:1495–1502.
514. Newton HB, Bromberg J, Junck L, et al. Comparison between BCNU and procarbazine chemotherapy for treatment of gliomas. J Neuro Oncol 1993;15:257–263.
515. Prough RA, Tweedie DJ. Procarbazine. In: Powis G, Prough RA, eds. Metabolism and action of anti-cancer drugs. London: Taylor & Francis, 1987:29–47.
516. Dunn DL, Lubet RA, Prough RA. Oxidative metabolism of *N*-isopropyl-a-(2-methylhydrazino)-*p*-toluamide hydrochloride (procarbazine) by rat liver microsomes. Cancer Res 1979;39:4555–4563.
517. Baggiolini M, Dewald B, Aebi H. Oxidation of *p*-(*N*1-methylhydrazinomethyl)-*N*-isopropylbenzamide to the methylazo derivative and oxidative cleavage of the N2-C bond in the isolated perfused rat liver. Biochem Pharmacol 1969;18: 2187–2196.
518. Oliverio VT, Denham C, DeVita VT, et al. Some pharmacologic properties of a new antitumor agent, *N*-isopropyl-a-(2-methyllydrazino)-*p*-toluamide hydrochloride (NSC-77213). Cancer Chemother Rep 1964;42:1–7.
519. Raaflaub J, Schwartz DE. Uber den metabolismus einer cytostatisch wirksamen methylhydrazin-derivates (Natulan). Experientia 1965;21:44–45.
520. Shiba DA, Weinkam RJ. Quantitative analysis of procarbazine, procarbazine metabolites and chemical degradation products with application to pharmacokinetic studies. J Chromatogr 1982;229:397–407.
521. Chabner BA, Sponzo R, Hubbard S, et al. High-dose intermittent intravenous infusion of procarbazine. Cancer Chemother Rep 1973;57:361–363.
522. Bleyer WA. The clinical pharmacology of methotrexate. Cancer 1978;41:36–51.
523. Goldman ID, Matherly LH. The cellular pharmacology of methotrexate. Pharmacol Ther 1985;28:77–102.
524. Chu E, Allegra CJ. Antifolates. In: Chabner BA, Longo DL, eds. Cancer chemotherapy and biotherapy principles and practice. Philadelphia, PA: Lippincott-Raven, 1996: 109–148.
525. Allegra CJ, Fine RL, Drake JC, et al. Effect of methotrexate on intracellular folate pools in human MCF breast cancer cells. J Biol Chem 1986;261:6478–6485.
526. Baram J, Allegra CJ, Fine RL, et al. Effect of methotrexate on intracellular folate pools in purified myeloid precursor cells from normal human bone marrow. J Clin Invest 1987;79:692–697.
527. Jolivet J, Cowan KH, Curt GA, et al. The pharmacology and clinical use of methotrexate. N Engl J Med 1983;309:1094–1104.
528. White JC. Reversal of methotrexate binding to dihydrofolate reductase by dihydrofolate: studies with purified enzyme and computer modelling using network thermodynamics. J Biol Chem 1979;254:10889–10895.
529. Allegra CJ, Chabner BA, Drake JC, et al. Enhanced inhibition of thymidylate synthetase by methotrexate polyglutamates. J Biol Chem 1985;260:9720–9726.
530. Chabner BA, Allegra CJ, Curt GA, et al. Polyglutamation of methotrexate. Is methotrexate a prodrug? J Clin Invest 1985;76:907–912.
531. Masson E, Relling MV, Synold TW, et al. Accumulation of methotrexate polyglutamates in lymphoblasts is a determinant of antileukemic effects in vivo. A rationale for high-dose methotrexate. J Clin Invest 1996;97:73–80.
532. Synold TW, Relling MV, Boyett JM, et al. Blast cell methotrexate–polyglutamate accumulation in vivo differs by lineage, ploidy, and methotrexate dose in acute lymphoblastic leukemia. J Clin Invest 1994;94:1996–2001.
533. Whitehead VM, Rosenblatt DS, Vuchich M-J, et al. Accumulation of methotrexate polyglutamates in lymphoblasts at diagnosis of childhood acute lymphoblastic leukemia: a pilot prognostic factor analysis. Blood 1990;76:44–49.
534. Whitehead VM, Vuchich MJ, Lauer SJ, et al. Accumulation of high levels of methotrexate polyglutamates in lymphoblasts from children with hyperdiploid (>50 chromosomes) B-lineage acute lymphoblastic leukemia: a Pediatric Oncology Group study. Blood 1992;80:1316–1323.
535. Rots MG, Pieters R, Peters GJ, et al. Role of folylpolyglutamate synthetase and folylpolyglutamate hydrolase in methotrexate accumulation and polyglutamylation in childhood leukemia. Blood 1999;93:1677–1683.
536. Balis FM, Savitch JL, Bleyer WA. Pharmacokinetics of oral methotrexate in children. Cancer Res 1983;43:2342–2345.
537. Kearney PJ, Light PA, Preece A, et al. Unpredictable serum levels after oral methotrexate in children with acute lymphoblastic leukaemia. Cancer Chemother Pharmacol 1979;3:117–120.
538. Pinkerton CR, Welshman SG, Bridges JM. Serum profiles of methotrexate after its administration in children with acute lymphoblastic leukaemia. Br J Cancer 1982; 45:300–303.
539. Pinkerton CR, Welshman SG, Kelly JG, et al. Pharmacokinetics of low-dose methotrexate in children receiving maintenance therapy for acute lymphoblastic leukaemia. Cancer Chemother Pharmacol 1982;10:36–39.
540. Henderson ES, Adamson RH, Oliverio VT. The metabolic fate of tritiated methotrexate II: absorption and excretion in man. Cancer Res 1965;25:1018–1024.
541. Smith DK, Omura GA, Ostroy F. Clinical pharmacology of intermediate-dose oral methotrexate. Cancer Chemother Pharmacol 1980;4:117–120.
542. Balis FM, Mirro J, Reaman GH, et al. Pharmacokinetics of subcutaneous methotrexate. J Clin Oncol 1988;6:1882–1886.
543. Campbell MA, Perrier DG, Dorr RT, et al. Methotrexate: bioavailability and pharmacokinetics. Cancer Treat Rep 1985;69:833–838.
544. Pinkerton CR, Glasgow JFT, Welshman SG, et al. Can food influence the absorption of methotrexate in children with acute lymphoblastic leukaemia? Lancet 1980;2: 944–946.
545. Pearson A, Amineddine H, Yule M, et al. The influence of serum methotrexate concentrations and drug dosage on outcome in childhood acute lymphoblastic leukaemia. Br J Cancer 1991;64:169–173.
546. Edelman J, Biggs DF, Jamali F, et al. Low-dose methotrexate kinetics in arthritis. Clin Pharmacol Ther 1984;35:382–386.
547. Teresi ME, Crom WR, Choi KE, et al. Methotrexate bioavailability after oral and intramuscular administration in children. J Pediatr 1987;110:788–792.
548. Wang YM, Fujimoto T. Clinical pharmacokinetics of methotrexate in children. Clin Pharmacokinet 1984;9:335–348.
549. Bleyer WA. Cancer chemotherapy in infants and children. Pediatr Clin North Am 1985;32:557–574.
550. Pignon T, Lacarelle B, Duffaud F, et al. Pharmacokinetics of high-dose methotrexate in adult osteogenic sarcoma. Cancer Chemother Pharmacol 1994;33:420–424.
551. Najjar TA, al Fawaz IM. Pharmacokinetics of methotrexate in children with acute lymphoblastic leukemia. Chemotherapy 1993;39:242–247.
552. Wang YM, Kim PY, Lantin E, et al. Degradation and clearance of methotrexate in children with osteosarcoma receiving high-dose infusion. Med Pediatr Oncol 1978; 4:221–229.
553. Donelli MG, Zucchetti M, Robatto A, et al. Pharmacokinetics of HD-MTX in infants, children, and adolescents with non-B acute lymphoblastic leukemia. Med Pediatr Oncol 1995;24:154–159.
554. Lonnerholm G, Valsecchi MG, De Lorenzo P, et al. Pharmacokinetics of high-dose methotrexate in infants treated for acute lymphoblastic leukemia. Pediatr Blood Cancer 2009;52:596–601.
555. Thompson PA, Murry DJ, Rosner GL, et al. Methotrexate pharmacokinetics in infants with acute lymphoblastic leukemia. Cancer Chemother Pharmacol 2007;59:847–853.
556. Huffman DH, Wan SH, Azarnoff DL, et al. Pharmacokinetics of methotrexate. Clin Pharmacol Ther 1973;14:572–579.
557. Liegler DG, Henderson ES, Hahn MA, et al. The effect of organic acids on renal clearance of methotrexate in man. Clin Pharmacol Ther 1969;10:849–857.
558. Hulot JS, Villard E, Maguy A, et al. A mutation in the drug transporter gene ABCC2 associated with impaired methotrexate elimination. Pharmacogenet Genomics 2005;15:277–285.
559. Ito K, Oleschuk CJ, Westlake C, et al. Mutation of Trp1254 in the multispecific organic anion transporter, multidrug resistance protein 2 (MRP2) (ABCC2), alters substrate specificity and results in loss of methotrexate transport activity. J Biol Chem 2001;276:38108–114.
560. Balis FM, Holcenberg JS, Bleyer WA. Clinical pharmacokinetics of commonly used anticancer drugs. Clin Pharmacokinet 1983;8:202–232.
561. Jacobs SA, Stoller RG, Chabner BA, et al. 7-Hydroxy-methotrexate as a urinary metabolite in human subjects and Rhesus monkeys receiving high-dose methotrexate. J Clin Invest 1976;57:534–538.
562. Lankelma J, van der Klein E. The role of 7-hydroxy-methotrexate during methotrexate anticancer chemotherapy. Cancer Lett 1980;9:133–142.
563. Erttmann R, Bielack S, Landbeck G. Kinetics of 7-hydroxy-methotrexate after high-dose methotrexate therapy. Cancer Chemother Pharmacol 1985;15:101–104.
564. Wolfrom C, Hepp R, Hartmann R, et al. Pharmacokinetic study of methotrexate, folinic acid and their serum metabolites in children treated with high-dose methotrexate and leucovorin rescue. Eur J Clin Pharmacol 1990;39:377–383.
565. Crom WR. Methotrexate. In: Grochow LB, Ames MM, eds. A clinician's guide to chemotherapy pharmacokinetics and pharmacodynamics. Baltimore, MD: Williams & Wilkins, 1998:311–330.
566. Stoller RG, Hande KR, Jacobs SA, et al. Use of plasma pharmacokinetics to predict and prevent methotrexate toxicity. N Engl J Med 1977;297:630–634.
567. Kerr IG, Jolivet J, Collins JM, et al. Test dose for predicting high-dose methotrexate infusions. Clin Pharmacol Ther 1983;33:44–51.
568. Seidel H, Andersen A, Kvaloy JT, et al. Variability in methotrexate serum and cerebrospinal fluid pharmacokinetics in children with acute lymphocytic leukemia: relation to assay methodology and physiological variables. Leuk Res 2000;24:193–199.
569. Tetef ML, Margolin KA, Doroshow JH, et al. Pharmacokinetics and toxicity of high-dose intravenous methotrexate in the treatment of leptomeningeal carcinomatosis. Cancer Chemother Pharmacol 2000;46:19–26.
570. Balis FM, Savitch JL, Bleyer WA, et al. Remission induction of meningeal leukemia with high-dose intravenous methotrexate. J Clin Oncol 1985;3:485–489.
571. Widemann BC, Balis FM, Kempf-Bielack B, et al. High-dose methotrexate-induced nephrotoxicity in patients with osteosarcoma. Cancer 2004;100:2222–2232.
572. Abelson HT, Fasburg MT, Beardsley GP, et al. Methotrexate-induced renal impairment: clinical studies and rescue from systemic toxicity with high-dose leucovorin and thymidine. J Clin Oncol 1983;1:208–216.
573. Stark AN, Jackson G, Carey PJ, et al. Severe renal toxicity due to intermediate-dose methotrexate. Cancer Chemother Pharmacol 1989;24:243–245.
574. Skärby T, Jönsson P, Hjorth L, et al. High-dose methotrexate: on the relationship of methotrexate elimination time vs renal function and serum methotrexate levels in 1164 courses in 264 Swedish children with acute lymphoblastic leukaemia (ALL). Cancer Chemother Pharmacol 2003;51:311–320.
575. Christensen ML, Rivera GK, Crom WR, et al. Effect of hydration on methotrexate plasma concentrations in children with acute lymphocytic leukemia. J Clin Oncol 1988;6:797–801.
576. Kinoshita A, Kurosawa Y, Kondoh K, et al. Effects of sodium in hydration solution on plasma methotrexate concentrations following high-dose methotrexate in children with acute lymphoblastic leukemia., Cancer Chemother Pharmacol 2003;51(3): 256–260.
577. Bleyer WA. Therapeutic drug monitoring of methotrexate and other antineoplastic drugs. In: Baer DM, Dita WR, eds. Interpretations in therapeutic drug monitoring. Chicago, IL: American Society of Clinical Pathology, 1981:169–181.
578. Langleben A, Hollomby D, Hand R. Case report: management of methotrexate toxicity in an anephric patient. Clin Invest Med 1982;5:129–132.
579. Gibson TP, Reich SD, Krumlovsky FA, et al. Hemoperfusion for methotrexate removal. Clin Pharmacol Ther 1978;23:351–355.
580. Winchester JF, Rahman A, Tilstone WJ, et al. Will hemoperfusion be useful for cancer chemotherapeutic drug removal? Clin Toxicol 1980;17:557–569.
581. Relling MV, Stapleton FB, Ochs J, et al. Removal of methotrexate, leucovorin, and their metabolites by combined hemodialysis and hemoperfusion. Cancer 1988;62: 884–888.
582. Widemann BC, Sung E, Anderson L, et al. Pharmacokinetics and metabolism of the methotrexate metabolite 2,4-diamino-*N*(10)-methylpteroic acid. J Pharmacol Exp Ther 2000;294:894–901.
583. Adamson PC, Balis FM, McCully CL, et al. Methotrexate pharmacokinetics following administration of recombinant carboxypeptidase-G_2 in Rhesus monkeys. J Clin Oncol 1992;10:1359–1364.
584. Widemann BC, Adamson PC. Understanding and managing methotrexate nephrotoxicity. Oncologist 2006;11:694–703.
585. Goodman TA, Polisson RP. Methotrexate: adverse reactions and major toxicities. Rheum Dis Clin North Am 1994;20:513–528.

586. Doyle LA, Berg C, Bottino G, et al. Erythema and desquamation after high-dose methotrexate. Ann Intern Med 1983;98:611–612.
587. Sostman HD, Matthay RA, Putman C, et al. Methotrexate-induced pneumonitis. Medicine (Baltimore) 1976;55(Suppl):371–388.
588. Bleyer WA. Neurologic sequelae of methotrexate and ionizing radiation: a new classification. Cancer Treat Rep 1981;65(Suppl 1):89–98.
589. Packer RJ, Grossman RI, Belasco JB. High dose methotrexate-associated acute neurologic dysfunction. Med Pediatr Oncol 1983;11:159–161.
590. Rubnitz JE, Relling MV, Harrison PL, et al. Transient encephalopathy following high-dose methotrexate treatment in childhood acute lymphoblastic leukemia. Leukemia 1998;12:1176–1181.
591. Mahoney DHJ, Shuster JJ, Nitschke R, et al. Acute neurotoxicity in children with B-precursor acute lymphoid leukemia: an association with intermediate-dose intravenous methotrexate and intrathecal triple therapy—a Pediatric Oncology Group study. J Clin Oncol 1998;16:1712–1722.
592. Bertino JR, Goker E, Gorlick R, et al. Resistance mechanisms to methotrexate in tumors. Stem Cells 1996;14:5–9.
593. Curt GA, Carney DN, Cowan KH, et al. Unstable methotrexate resistance in human small-cell carcinoma associated with double minute chromosomes. N Engl J Med 1983;308:199–202.
594. Horns RC, Dower WJ, Schimke RT. Gene amplification in a leukemic patient treated with methotrexate. J Clin Oncol 1984;2:2–7.
595. Matherly LH, Taub JW, Ravindranath Y, et al. Elevated dihydrofolate reductase and impaired methotrexate transport as elements in methotrexate resistance in childhood acute lymphoblastic leukemia. Blood 1995;85:500–509.
596. Yang R, Sowers R, Mazza B, et al. Sequence alterations in the reduced folate carrier are observed in osteosarcoma tumor samples. Clin Cancer Res 2003;9:837–844.
597. Guo W, Healey JH, Meyers PA, et al. Mechanisms of methotrexate resistance in osteosarcoma. Clin Cancer Res 1999;5:621–627.
598. Ifergan I, Meller I, Issakov J, et al. Reduced folate carrier protein expression in osteosarcoma: implications for the prediction of tumor chemosensitivity. Cancer 2003;98:1958–1966.
599. Kaufman Y, Drori S, Cole PD, et al. Reduced folate carrier mutations are not the mechanism underlying methotrexate resistance in childhood acute lymphoblastic leukemia. Cancer 2004;100:773–782.
600. Ge Y, Haska CL, LaFiura K, et al. Prognostic role of the reduced folate carrier, the major membrane transporter for methotrexate, in childhood acute lymphoblastic leukemia: a report from the Children's Oncology Group. Clin Cancer Res 2007;13:451–457.
601. Basin KS, Escalante A, Beardmore TD. Severe pancytopenia in a patient taking low dose methotrexate and probenecid. J Rheumatol 1991;18:609–610.
602. Cassano WF. Serious methotrexate toxicity caused by interaction with ibuprofen. Am J Pediatr Hematol Oncol 1989;11:481–482.
603. Furst DE, Herman RA, Koehnke R, et al. Effect of aspirin and sulindac on methotrexate clearance. J Pharm Sci 1990;79:782–786.
604. Dalle J-H, Auvrignon A, Vassal G, et al. Interaction between methotrexate and ciprofloxacin. J Pediatr Hematol Oncol 2002;24:321–322.
605. Beorlegui B, Aldaz A, Ortega A, et al. Potential interaction between methotrexate and omeprazole. Ann Pharmacother 2000;34:1024–1027.
606. Troger U, Stotzel B, Martens-Lobenhoffer J, et al. Drug points: severe myalgia from an interaction between treatments with pantoprazole and methotrexate. BMJ 2002; 324:1497.
607. Suzuki K, Doki K, Homma M, et al. Co-administration of proton pump inhibitors delays elimination of plasma methotrexate in high-dose methotrexate therapy. Br J Clin Pharmacol 2009;67:44–49.
608. Blum R, Seymour JF, Toner G. Significant impairment of high-dose methotrexate clearance following vancomycin administration in the absence of overt renal impairment. Ann Oncol 2002;13:327–330.
609. Schornagel JH, McVie JG. The clinical pharmacology of methotrexate. Cancer Treat Rev 1983;10:53–75.
610. Capizzi RL, Summers WP, Bertino JR. L-asparaginase induced alteration of amethopterin (methotrexate) activity in mouse leukemia L5178Y. Ann N Y Acad Sci 1971;186:302–311.
611. Lobel JS, O'Brien RT, McIntosh S, et al. Methotrexate and asparaginase combination chemotherapy in refractory acute lymphoblastic leukemia of childhood. Cancer 1979;43:1089–1094.
612. Capizzi RL. Asparaginase–methotrexate in combination chemotherapy: schedule-dependent differential effects on normal versus neoplastic cells. Cancer Treat Rep 1981;65(Suppl 4):115–121.
613. Hale JP, Lilleyman JS. Importance of 6-mercaptopurine dose in lymphoblastic leukemia. Arch Dis Child 1991;66:462–466.
614. Pinkel D. Intravenous mercaptopurine: life begins at 40. J Clin Oncol 1993;11: 1826–1831.
615. Zimm S, Ettinger LJ, Holcenberg JS, et al. Phase I and clinical pharmacologic study of mercaptopurine administered as a prolonged intravenous infusion. Cancer Res 1985;45:1869–1873.
616. Camitta B, Leventhal B, Lauer S, et al. Intermediate-dose intravenous methotrexate and mercaptopurine therapy for non-T, non-B acute lymphocytic leukemia of childhood: a Pediatric Oncology Group study. J Clin Oncol 1989;7:1539–1544.
617. Mahoney DHJ, Shuster J, Nitschke R, et al. Intermediate-dose intravenous methotrexate with intravenous mercaptopurine is superior to repetitive low-dose oral methotrexate with intravenous mercaptopurine for children with lower-risk B-lineage acute lymphoblastic leukemia: a Pediatric Oncology Group phase III trial. J Clin Oncol 1998; 16:246–254.
618. Bostrom BC, Sensel MR, Sather HN, et al. Dexamethasone versus prednisone and daily oral versus weekly intravenous mercaptopurine for patients with standard-risk acute lymphoblastic leukemia: a report from the Children's Cancer Group. Blood 2003;101:3809–3817.
619. Van Scoik KG, Johnson CA, Porter WR. The pharmacology and metabolism of the thiopurine drugs 6-mercaptopurine and azathioprine. Drug Metab Rev 1985;16:157–174.
620. Bokkerink JP, Stet EH, De Abreu RA, et al. 6-Mercaptopurine: cytotoxicity and biochemical pharmacology in human malignant T-lymphoblasts. Biochem Pharmacol 1993;45:1455–1463.
621. Lennard L. The clinical pharmacology of 6-mercaptopurine. Eur J Clin Pharmacol 1992;43:329–339.
622. Dervieux T, Blanco JG, Krynetski EY, et al. Differing contribution of thiopurine methyltransferase to mercaptopurine versus thioguanine effects in human leukemic cells. Cancer Res 2001;61:5810–5816.
623. Adamson PC, Poplack DG, Balis FM. The cytotoxicity of thioguanine vs mercaptopurine in acute lymphoblastic leukemia. Leukemia Res 1994;11:805–810.
624. Lowe ES, Kitchen BJ, Erdmann G, et al. Plasma pharmacokinetics and cerebrospinal fluid penetration of thioguanine in children with acute lymphoblastic leukemia. Cancer Chemother Pharmacol 2001;47:199–205.
625. Jacobs SS, Stork LC, Bostrom BC, et al. Substitution of oral and intravenous thioguanine for mercaptopurine in a treatment regimen for children with standard risk acute lymphoblastic leukemia: a collaborative Children's Oncology Group/National Cancer Institute pilot trial (CCG-1942). Pediatr Blood Cancer 2007;49:250–255.
626. Vora A, Mitchell CD, Lennard L, et al. Toxicity and efficacy of 6-thioguanine versus 6-mercaptopurine in childhood lymphoblastic leukaemia: a randomised trial. Lancet 2006;368:1339–1348.
627. Harms DO, Gobel U, Spaar HJ, et al. Thioguanine offers no advantage over mercaptopurine in maintenance treatment of childhood ALL: results of the randomized trial COALL-92. Blood 2003;102:2736–2740.
628. Stork LC, Sather H, Hutchinson RJ, et al. Comparison of mercaptopurine (MP) with thioguanine (TG) and IT methotrexate (ITM) with IT "triples" (ITT) in children with SR-ALL: results of CCG-1952. Proc Ann Meet Am Soc Hematol (Blood) 2002;100:36A.
629. Evans WE, Relling MV. Mercaptopurine vs thioguanine for the treatment of acute lymphoblastic leukemia. Leukemia Res 1994;18:811–814.
630. Bostrom B, Erdmann G. Cellular pharmacology of 6-mercaptopurine in acute lymphoblastic leukemia. Am J Pediatr Hematol Oncol 1993;15:80–86.
631. Erdmann GR. 6-Mercaptopurine and 6-thioguanine. In: Grochow LB, Ames MM, eds. A clinician's guide to chemotherapy pharmacokinetics and pharmacodynamics. Baltimore, MD: Williams & Wilkins, 1998:411–425.
632. Kitchen BJ, Moser A, Balis FM, et al. Thioguanine administered as a continuous intravenous infusion to pediatric patients is metabolized to the novel metabolite 8-hydroxy-thioguanine. J Pharmacol Exp Ther 1999;291:870–874.
633. Hande KR, Garrow GC. Purine antimetabolites. In: Chabner BA, Longo DL, eds. Cancer chemotherapy and biotherapy principles and practice. Philadelphia, PA: Lippincott-Raven, 1996:235–252.
634. Weinshilboum RM, Raymond FA, Pazmino P. Human erythrocyte thiopurine methyltransferase: radiochemical microassay and biochemical properties. Clin Chim Acta 1978;85:323–333.
635. Lennard L, Lilleyman JS, Van Loon J, et al. Genetic variation in response to 6-mercaptopurine for childhood acute lymphoblastic leukemia. Lancet 1990;336:225–229.
636. Lennard L, Welch JC, Lilleyman JS. Thiopurine drugs in the treatment of childhood leukaemia: the influence of inherited thiopurine methyltransferase activity on drug metabolism and cytotoxicity. Br J Clin Pharmacol 1997;44:455–461.
637. Gearry RB, Roberts RL, Barclay ML, et al. Lack of association between the ITPA 94C>A polymorphism and adverse effects from azathioprine. Pharmacogenetics 2004;14:779–781.
638. Hindorf U, Lindqvist M, Peterson C, et al. Pharmacogenetics during standardised initiation of thiopurine treatment in inflammatory bowel disease. Gut 2006;55:1423–1431.
639. Marinaki AM, Ansari A, Duley JA, et al. Adverse drug reactions to azathioprine therapy are associated with polymorphism in the gene encoding inosine triphosphate pyrophosphatase (ITPase). Pharmacogenetics 2004;14:181–187.
640. van Dieren JM, van Vuuren AJ, Kusters JG, et al. ITPA genotyping is not predictive for the development of side effects in AZA treated inflammatory bowel disease patients. Gut 2005;54:1664.
641. von Ahsen N, Oellerich M, Armstrong VW. Characterization of the inosine triphosphatase (ITPA) gene: haplotype structure, haplotype-phenotype correlation and promoter function. Ther Drug Monit 2008;30:16–22.
642. Zelinkova Z, Derijks LJ, Stokkers PC, et al. Inosine triphosphate pyrophosphatase and thiopurine *S*-methyltransferase genotypes relationship to azathioprine-induced myelosuppression. Clin Gastroenterol Hepatol 2006;4:44–49.
643. Stocco G, Cheok MH, Crews KR, et al. Genetic polymorphism of inosine triphosphate pyrophosphatase is a determinant of mercaptopurine metabolism and toxicity during treatment for acute lymphoblastic leukemia. Clin Pharmacol Ther 2009;85:164–172.
644. Zimm S, Collins JM, Riccardi R, et al. Variable bioavailability of oral mercaptopurine. Is maintenance chemotherapy in acute lymphoblastic leukemia being optimally delivered? N Engl J Med 1983;308:1005–1009.
645. Lennard L, Keen D, Lilleyman JS. Oral 6-mercaptopurine in childhood leukemia: parent drug pharmacokinetics and active metabolite concentrations. Clin Pharmacol Ther 1986;40:287–292.
646. Sulh H, Koren G, Whalen C, et al. Pharmacokinetic determinants of 6-mercaptopurine myelotoxicity and therapeutic failure in children with acute lymphoblastic leukemia. Clin Pharmacol Ther 1986;40:604–609.
647. Zimm S, Collins J, O'Neill D, et al. Inhibition of first-pass metabolism in cancer chemotherapy: interaction of 6-mercaptopurine and allopurinol. Clin Pharmacol Ther 1983;34:810–817.
648. Lepage GA, Whitecar JP. Pharmacology of thioguanine in man. Cancer Res 1971; 31:1627–16231.
649. Brox LW, Birkett L, Belch A. Clinical pharmacology of oral 6-thioguanine in acute myelogenous leukemia. Cancer Chemother Pharmacol 1981;6:35–38.
650. Lancaster DL, Patel N, Lennard L, et al. 6-Thioguanine in children with acute lymphoblastic leukaemia: influence of food on parent drug pharmacokinetics and 6-thioguanine nucleotide concentrations. Br J Clin Pharmacol 2001;51:531–539.
651. Lennard L, Rees CA, Lilleyman JS, et al. Childhood leukemia: a relationship between intracellular 6-mercaptopurine metabolism and neutropenia. Br J Clin Pharmacol 1983;16:359–363.
652. Lennard L, Lilleyman JS. Variable mercaptopurine metabolism and treatment outcome in childhood lymphoblastic leukemia. J Clin Oncol 1989;7:1816–1823.
653. Lilleyman JS, Lennard L. Mercaptopurine metabolism and risk of relapse in childhood lymphoblastic leukemia. Lancet 1994;343:1188–1190.
654. Lennard L, Davies HA, Lilleyman JS. Is 6-thioguanine more appropriate than 6-mercaptopurine for children with acute lymphoblastic leukemia? Br J Cancer 1993; 68:186–190.
655. Lancaster DL, Lennard L, Rowland K, et al. Thioguanine versus mercaptopurine for therapy of childhood lymphoblastic leukaemia: a comparison of haematological toxicity and drug metabolite concentrations. Br J Haematol 1998;102:439–443.
656. Erb N, Harms DO, Janka-Schaub G. Pharmacokinetics and metabolism of thiopurines in children with acute lymphoblastic leukemia receiving 6-thioguanine versus 6-mercaptopurine. Cancer Chemother Pharmacol 1998;42:266–272.
657. Lancaster DL, Patel N, Lennard L, et al. Leucocyte versus erythrocyte thioguanine nucleotide concentrations in children taking thiopurines for acute lymphoblastic leukaemia. Cancer Chemother Pharmacol 2002;50:33–36.

658. Broxson EH, Dole M, Wong R, et al. Portal hypertension develops in a subset of children with standard risk acute lymphoblastic leukemia treated with oral 6-thioguanine during maintenance therapy. Pediatr Blood Cancer 2005;44:226–231.

659. Stoneham S, Lennard L, Coen P, et al. Veno-occlusive disease in patients receiving thiopurines during maintenance therapy for childhood acute lymphoblastic leukaemia. Br J Haematol 2003;123:100–102.

660. Piel B, Vaidya S, Lancaster D, et al. Chronic hepatotoxicity following 6-thioguanine therapy for childhood acute lymphoblastic leukaemia. Br J Haematol 2004;125:410–411; author reply 412.

661. Evans WE. Pharmacogenetics of thiopurine S-methyltransferase and thiopurine therapy. Ther Drug Monit 2004;26:186–191.

662. Schaeffeler E, Zanger UM, Eichelbaum M, et al. Highly multiplexed genotyping of thiopurine S-methyltransferase variants using MALD-TOF mass spectrometry: reliable genotyping in different ethnic groups. Clin Chem 2008;54:1637–1647.

663. Krynetski E, Evans WE. Drug methylation in cancer therapy: lessons from the TPMT polymorphism. Oncogene 2003;22:7403–7413.

664. McLeod HL, Krynetski EY, Relling MV, et al. Genetic polymorphism of thiopurine methyltransferase and its clinical relevance for childhood acute lymphoblastic leukemia. Leukemia 2000;14:567–572.

665. Lennard L, Van Loon JA, Weinshilboum RM. Pharmacogenetics of acute azathioprine toxicity: relationship to thiopurine methyltransferase genetic polymorphism. Clin Pharmacol Ther 1989;46:149–154.

666. Evans WE, Horner M, Chu YQ, et al. Altered mercaptopurine metabolism, toxic effects, and dosage requirement in a thiopurine methyltransferase-deficient child with acute lymphocytic leukemia. J Pediatr 1991;119:985–989.

667. Lennard L, Gibson BES, Nicole T, et al. Congenital thiopurine methyltransferase deficiency and 6-mercaptopurine toxicity during treatment for acute lymphoblastic leukemia. Arch Dis Child 1993;69:577–579.

668. Lennard L, Lewis IJ, Michelagnoli M, et al. Thiopurine methyltransferase deficiency in childhood lymphoblastic leukaemia: 6-mercaptopurine dosage strategies. Med Pediatr Oncol 1997;29:252–255.

669. Relling MV, Hancock ML, Rivera GK, et al. Mercaptopurine therapy intolerance and heterozygosity at the thiopurine S-methyltransferase gene locus. J Natl Cancer Inst 1999;91:2001–2008.

670. Schmiegelow K, Forestier E, Kristinsson J, et al. Thiopurine methyltransferase activity is related to the risk of relapse of childhood acute lymphoblastic leukemia: results from the NOPHO ALL-92 study. Leukemia 2009;23:557–564.

671. Bo J, Schroder H, Kristinsson J, et al. Possible carcinogenic effect of 6-mercaptopurine on bone marrow stem cells: relation to thiopurine metabolism. Cancer 1999;86:1080–1086.

672. Relling MV, Rubnitz JE, Rivera GK, et al. High incidence of secondary brain tumours after radiotherapy and antimetabolites. Lancet 1999;354:34–39.

673. Relling MV, Yanishevski Y, Nemec J, et al. Etoposide and antimetabolite pharmacology in patients who develop secondary acute myeloid leukemia. Leukemia 1998;12:346–352.

674. Stanulla M, Schaeffeler E, Moricke A, et al. Thiopurine methyltransferase genetics is not a major risk factor for secondary malignant neoplasms after treatment of childhood acute lymphoblastic leukemia on Berlin–Frankfurt–Munster protocols. Blood 2009;114(7):1314–1318.

675. Brooks RJ, Dorr RT, Durie BGM. Interaction of allopurinol with 6-mercaptopurine and allopurinol. Biomedicine 1982;36:217–222.

676. Balis FM, Holcenberg JS, Zimm S, et al. The effect of methotrexate on the bioavailability of oral 6-mercaptopurine. Clin Pharmacol Ther 1987;41:384–387.

677. Innocenti F, Danesi R, Di Paolo A, et al. Clinical and experimental pharmacokinetic interaction between 6-mercaptopurine and methotrexate. Cancer Chemother Pharmacol 1996;37:409–414.

678. Plunkett W, Huang P, Gandhi V. Metabolism and action of fludarabine phosphate. Semin Oncol 1990;17:3–17.

679. Malspeis L, Grever MR, Staubus AE, et al. Pharmacokinetics of 2-F-ara-A (9-beta-D-arabinofuranosyl-2-fluoroadenine) in cancer patients during the phase I clinical investigation of fludarabine phosphate. Semin Oncol 1990;17:18–32.

680. Chun HG, Leyland-Jones BR, Caryk SM, et al. Central nervous system toxicity of fludarabine phosphate. Cancer Treat Rep 1986;70:1225–1228.

681. Dinndorf PA, Avramis VI, Wiersma S, et al. Phase I/II study of idarubicin given with continuous infusion fludarabine followed by continuous infusion cytarabine in children with acute leukemia: a report from the Children's Cancer Group. J Clin Oncol 1997;15:2780–2785.

682. Avramis VI, Champagne J, Sato J, et al. Pharmacology of fludarabine phosphate after a phase I/II trial by a loading bolus and continuous infusion in pediatric patients. Cancer Res 1990;50:7226–7231.

683. Danhauser L, Plunkett W, Keating M, et al. 9-beta-D-arabinofuranosyl-2-fluoroadenine 5′-monophosphate pharmacokinetics in plasma and tumor cells of patients with relapsed leukemia and lymphoma. Cancer Chemother Pharmacol 1986;18:145–152.

684. Hersh MR, Kuhn JG, Phillips JL, et al. Pharmacokinetic study of fludarabine phosphate (NSC 312887). Cancer Chemother Pharmacol 1986;17:277–280.

685. Gandhi V, Plunkett W. Modulation of arabinosylnucleoside metabolism by arabinosylnucleotides in human leukemia cells. Cancer Res 1988;48:329–334.

686. Gandhi V, Kemena A, Keating MJ, et al. Fludarabine infusion potentiates arabinosylcytosine metabolism in lymphocytes of patients with chronic lymphocytic leukemia. Cancer Res 1992;52:897–903.

687. Gandhi V, Nowak B, Keating MJ, et al. Modulation of arabinosylcytosine metabolism by arabinosyl-2-fluoroadenine in lymphocytes from patients with chronic lymphocytic leukemia: implications for combination therapy. Blood 1989;74:2070–2075.

688. Visani G, Tosi P, Zinzani PL, et al. FLAG (fludarabine + high-dose cytarabine + G-CSF): an effective and tolerable protocol for the treatment of 'poor risk' acute myeloid leukemias. Leukemia 1994;8:1842–1846.

689. Huhmann IM, Watzke HH, Geissler K, et al. FLAG (fludarabine, cytosine arabinoside, G-CSF) for refractory and relapsed acute myeloid leukemia. Ann Hematol 1996;73:265–271.

690. McCarthy AJ, Pitcher LA, Hann IM, et al. FLAG (fludarabine, high-dose cytarabine, and G-CSF) for refractory and high-risk relapsed acute leukemia in children. Med Pediatr Oncol 1999;32:411–415.

691. Or R, Shapira MY, Resnick I, et al. Nonmyeloablative allogeneic stem cell transplantation for the treatment of chronic myeloid leukemia in first chronic phase. Blood 2003;101:441–445.

692. Krance RA, Hurwitz CA, Head DR, et al. Experience with 2-chlorodeoxyadenosine in previously untreated children with newly diagnosed acute myeloid leukemia and myelodysplastic diseases. J Clin Oncol 2001;19:2804–2811.

693. Rodriguez-Galindo C, Kelly P, Jeng M, et al. Treatment of children with Langerhans cell histiocytosis with 2-chlorodeoxyadenosine. Am J Hematol 2002;69:179–184.

694. Rubnitz JE, Razzouk BI, Srivastava DK, et al. Phase II trial of cladribine and cytarabine in relapsed or refractory myeloid malignancies. Leuk Res 2004;28:349–352.

695. Van Den Neste E, Delannoy A, Vandercam B, et al. Infectious complications after 2-chlorodeoxyadenosine therapy. Eur J Haematol 1996;56:235–240.

696. Cheson BD. Infectious and immunosuppressive complications of purine analog therapy. J Clin Oncol 1995;13:2431–2448.

697. Betticher DC, Fey MF, von Rohr A, et al. High incidence of infections after 2-chlorodeoxyadenosine (2-CDA) therapy in patients with malignant lymphomas and chronic and acute leukaemias. Ann Oncol 1994;5:57–64.

698. Kearns CM, Blakley RL, Santana VM, et al. Pharmacokinetics of cladribine (2-chlorodeoxyadenosine) in children with acute leukemia. Cancer Res1994;54:1235–1239.

699. Liliemark J, Juliusson G. On the pharmacokinetics of 2-chloro-2′-deoxyadenosine in humans. Cancer Res 1991;51:5570–5572.

700. Kantarjian HM, Gandhi V, Kozuch P, et al. Phase I clinical and pharmacology study of clofarabine in patients with solid and hematologic cancers. J Clin Oncol 2003;21:1167–1173.

701. Gandhi V, Kantarjian H, Faderl S, et al. Pharmacokinetics and pharmacodynamics of plasma clofarabine and cellular clofarabine triphosphate in patients with acute leukemias. Clin Cancer Res 2003;9:6335–6342.

702. Jeha S, Gandhi V, Chan KW, et al. Clofarabine, a novel nucleoside analog, is active in pediatric patients with advanced leukemia. Blood 2004;103:784–789.

703. Jeha S, Gaynon PS, Razzouk BI, et al. Phase II study of clofarabine in pediatric patients with refractory or relapsed acute lymphoblastic leukemia. J Clin Oncol 2006;24:1917–1923.

704. Jeha S, Razzouk B, Gaynon P, et al. Phase II trials of clofarabine in pediatric acute leukemia [ASCO Meeting abstracts]. J Clin Oncol 2005;23:6588.

705. Lambe CU, Averett DR, Paff MT, et al. 2-Amino-6-methoxypurine arabinoside: an agent for T-cell malignancies. Cancer Res 1995;55:3352–3356.

706. Shewach DS, Mitchell BS. Differential metabolism of 9-beta-D-arabinofuranosylguanine in human leukemic cells. Cancer Res 1989;49:6498–6502.

707. Shewach DS, Daddona PE, Ashcraft E, et al. Metabolism and selective cytotoxicity of 9-beta-D-arabinofuranosylguanine in human lymphoblasts. Cancer Res 1985;45:1008–1014.

708. Ullman B, Martin DW Jr. Specific cytotoxicity of arabinosylguanine toward cultured T lymphoblasts. J Clin Invest 1984;74:951–955.

709. Gandhi V, Plunkett W, Rodriguez CO Jr, et al. Compound GW506U78 in refractory hematologic malignancies: relationship between cellular pharmacokinetics and clinical response. J Clin Oncol 1998;16:3607–3615.

710. Kurtzberg J, Ernst TJ, Keating MJ, et al. Phase I study of 506U78 administered on a consecutive 5-day schedule in children and adults with refractory hematologic malignancies. J Clin Oncol 2005;23:3396–3403.

711. Berg SL, Blaney SM, Devidas M, et al. Phase II study of nelarabine (compound 506U78) in children and young adults with refractory T-cell malignancies: a report from the Children's Oncology Group. J Clin Oncol 2005;23:3376–3382.

712. Kisor DF, Plunkett W, Kurtzberg J, et al. Pharmacokinetics of nelarabine and 9-beta-D-arabinofuranosyl guanine in pediatric and adult patients during a phase I study of nelarabine for the treatment of refractory hematologic malignancies. J Clin Oncol 2000;18:995–1003.

713. Grant S. Ara-C: cellular and molecular pharmacology. Adv Cancer Res 1998;72:197–233.

714. Kufe DW, Spriggs DR. Biochemical and cellular pharmacology of cytosine arabinoside. Semin Oncol 1985;12(Suppl 3):34–48.

715. Kufe D, Spriggs D, Egan EM, et al. Relationship among ara-C pools, formation of (ara-C) DNA, and cytotoxicity of human leukemic cells. Blood 1984;64:54–58.

716. Burke PJ, Karp JE, Vaughan WP, et al. Recruitment of quiescent tumor by humoral stimulatory activity: requirement for successful chemotherapy. Blood Cells 1982;8:519–533.

717. Vaughan WP, Karp JE, Burke PJ. Two-cycle-timed sequential chemotherapy for adult acute nonlymphocytic leukemia. Blood 1984;64:975–980.

718. Bettelheim P, Valent P, Andreeff M, et al. Recombinant human granulocyte-macrophage colony-stimulating factor in combination with standard induction chemotherapy in de novo acute myeloid leukemia. Blood 1991;77:700–711.

719. Cannistra SA, DiCarlo J, Groshek P, et al. Simultaneous administration of granulocyte-macrophage colony-stimulating factor and cytosine arabinoside for the treatment of relapsed acute myeloid leukemia. Leukemia 1991;5:230–238.

720. Capizzi RL, Yang J, Rathmell JP, et al. Dose-related pharmacologic effects of high-dose ara-C and its self-potentiation. Semin Oncol 1985;12(2, Suppl 3):65–75.

721. Donehower RC, Karp JE, Burke PJ. Pharmacology and toxicity of high-dose cytarabine by 72-hour continuous infusion. Cancer Treat Rep 1986;70:1059–1065.

722. Cheson BD. Standard and low-dose chemotherapy for the treatment of myelodysplastic syndromes. Leuk Res 1998;22(Suppl 1):S17–S21.

723. Wiley JS, Jones SP, Sawyer WH, et al. Cytosine arabinoside influx and nucleoside transport sites in acute leukemia. J Clin Invest 1982;69:479–489.

724. Chabner BA. Cytidine analogues. In: Chabner BA, Longo DL, eds. Cancer chemotherapy and biotherapy principles and practice. Philadelphia, PA: Lippincott-Raven, 1996:213–233.

725. Chabner BA, Hande KR, Drake JC. Ara-C metabolism: implications for drug resistance and drug interactions. Bull Cancer 1979;66:89–92.

726. Ho DHW, Frei E. Clinical pharmacology of 1-b-D-arabinofuranosylcytosine. Clin Pharmacol Ther 1971;12:944–954.

727. Slevin ML, Piall EM, Aherne GW, et al. The pharmacokinetics of cytosine arabinoside in the plasma and cerebrospinal fluid during conventional and high-dose therapy. Med Pediatr Oncol 1982;10(Suppl 1):157–168.

728. Weiss G, Phillips J, Von Hoff D. A clinical–pharmacological comparison of hepatic arterial and peripheral vein infusion of cytarabine for liver cancer [abstract]. Proc Am Soc Clin Oncol 1986;5:34.

729. Wan SH, Huffman DH, Azarnoff DL, et al. Pharmacokinetics of 1-b-arabinofuranosylcytosine in humans. Cancer Res 1974;34:392–397.

730. Capizzi RL, Yang J-L, Cheng E, et al. Alterations of the pharmacokinetics of high-dose ara-C by its metabolite, high ara-U in patients with acute leukemia. J Clin Oncol 1983;1:763–771.

731. Ochs J, Sinkule JA, Danks MK, et al. Continuous infusion high-dose cytosine arabinoside in refractory childhood leukemia. J Clin Oncol 1984;2:1092–1097.

732. Ozkaynak MF, Avramis VI, Carcich S, et al. Pharmacology of cytarabine given as a continuous infusion followed by mitoxantrone with and without amsacrine/etoposide as reinduction chemotherapy for relapsed or refractory pediatric acute myeloid leukemia. Med Pediatr Oncol 1998;31:475–482.
733. Plunkett W, Iacobani S, Estey E, et al. Pharmacologically directed ara-C therapy for refractory leukemia. Semin Oncol 1985;12(2, Suppl 3):20–30.
734. Liliemark JO, Plunkett W, Dixon DO. Relationship of 1-b-D-arabinofuranosylcytosine in plasma to 1-b-D-arabinofuranosylcytosine 5′-triphosphate levels in leukemic cells during treatment with high-dose 1-b-D-arabinofuranosylcytosine. Cancer Res 1985; 45:5952–5957.
735. Chou T-C, Arlin Z, Clarkson BD, et al. Metabolism of 1-b-D-arabinofuranosylcytosine in human leukemic cells. Cancer Res 1977;37:3561–3570.
736. Boos J, Hohenlochter B, Schulze-Westhoff P, et al. Intracellular retention of cytosine arabinoside triphosphate in blast cells from children with acute myelogenous and lymphoblastic leukemia. Med Pediatr Oncol 1996;26:397–404.
737. Hartford CM, Duan S, Delaney SM, et al. Population-specific genetic variants important in susceptibility to cytarabine arabinoside cytotoxicity. Blood 2009;113: 2145–2153.
738. Lamba JK, Crews K, Pounds S, et al. Pharmacogenetics of deoxycytidine kinase: identification and characterization of novel genetic variants. J Pharmacol Exp Ther 2007;323:935–945.
739. Jones GT, Abramson N. Gastrointestinal necrosis in acute leukemia: a complication of induction therapy. Cancer Invest 1983;1:315–320.
740. Johnson H, Smith TJ, Desforges J. Cytosine arabinoside-induced colitis and peritonitis: nonoperative management. J Clin Oncol 1985;3:607–612.
741. Stentoft J. The toxicity of cytarabine. Drug Saf 1990;5:7–27.
742. Castleberry RP, Crist WM, Holbrook T, et al. The cytosine arabinoside (ara-C) syndrome. Med Pediatr Oncol 1981;9:257–264.
743. Herzig RH, Lazarus HM, Herzig GP, et al. Central nervous system toxicity with high-dose cytosine arabinoside. Semin Oncol 1985;12(2, Suppl 3):233–236.
744. Herzig RH, Wolff SN, Lazarus HM, et al. High-dose cytosine arabinoside therapy for refractory leukemia. Blood 1983;62:361–369.
745. Baker WJ, Royer GL, Weiss RB. Cytarabine and neurologic toxicity. J Clin Oncol 1991;9:679–693.
746. Barnett MJ, Richards MA, Ganesan TS, et al. Central nervous system toxicity of high-dose cytosine arabinoside. Semin Oncol 1985;12(2, Suppl 3):227–232.
747. Rubin EH, Anderson JW, Berg DT, et al. Risk factors for high-dose cytarabine neurotoxicity: an analysis of a Cancer and Leukemia Group B trial with acute myeloid leukemia. J Clin Oncol 1992;10:948–953.
748. Hasle H. Cerebellar toxicity during cytarabine therapy associated with renal insufficiency. Cancer Chemother Pharmacol 1990;27:76–78.
749. Smith GA, Damon LE, Rugo HS, et al. High-dose cytarabine dose modification reduces the incidence of neurotoxicity in patients with renal insufficiency. J Clin Oncol 1997;15:833–839.
750. Storniolo AM, Allerheiligen SR, Pearce HL. Preclinical, pharmacologic, and phase I studies of gemcitabine. Semin Oncol 1997;24:S7-2–S7-7.
751. Catimel G, Vermorken JB, Clavel M, et al. A phase II study of gemcitabine (LY 188011) in patients with advanced squamous cell carcinoma of the head and neck. EORTC Early Clinical Trials Group. Ann Oncol 1994;5:543–547.
752. Fossa A, Santoro A, Hiddemann W, et al. Gemcitabine as a single agent in the treatment of relapsed or refractory aggressive non-Hodgkin's lymphoma. J Clin Oncol 1999;17:3786–3792.
753. Luftner D, Flath B, Akrivakis C, et al. Gemcitabine for palliative treatment in metastatic breast cancer. J Cancer Res Clin Oncol 1998;124:527–531.
754. Ozols RF. The current role of gemcitabine in ovarian cancer. Semin Oncol 2001;28:18–24.
755. Postmus PE, Schramel FM, Smit EF. Evaluation of new drugs in small cell lung cancer: the activity of gemcitabine. Semin Oncol 1998;25:79–82.
756. Leu KM, Ostruszka LJ, Shewach D, et al. Laboratory and clinical evidence of synergistic cytotoxicity of sequential treatment with gemcitabine followed by docetaxel in the treatment of sarcoma. J Clin Oncol 2004;22:1706–1712.
757. Savage DG, Rule SA, Tighe M, et al. Gemcitabine for relapsed or resistant lymphoma. Ann Oncol 2000;11:595–597.
758. Wagner-Bohn A, Henze G, von Stackelberg A, et al. Phase II study of gemcitabine in children with relapsed leukemia. Pediatr Blood Cancer 2006;46:262.
759. Angiolillo AL, Whitlock J, Chen Z, et al. Phase II study of gemcitabine in children with relapsed acute lymphoblastic leukemia or acute myelogenous leukemia (ADVL0022): a Children's Oncology Group Report. Pediatr Blood Cancer 2006;46:193–197.
760. Cole PD, Schwartz CL, Drachtman RA, et al. Phase II study of weekly gemcitabine and vinorelbine for children with recurrent or refractory Hodgkin's disease: a children's oncology group report. J Clin Oncol 2009;27:1456–1461.
761. Navid F, Willert JR, McCarville MB, et al. Combination of gemcitabine and docetaxel in the treatment of children and young adults with refractory bone sarcoma. Cancer 2008;113:419–425.
762. Heinemann V, Hertel LW, Grindey GB, et al. Comparison of the cellular pharmacokinetics and toxicity of 2′,2′-difluorodeoxycytidine and 1-beta-D-arabinofuranosylcytosine. Cancer Res 1988;48:4024–4031.
763. Tempero M, Plunkett W, Ruiz Van Haperen V, et al. Randomized phase II comparison of dose-intense gemcitabine: thirty-minute infusion and fixed dose rate infusion in patients with pancreatic adenocarcinoma. J Clin Oncol 2003;21:3402–3408.
764. Reid JM, Qu W, Safgren SL, et al. Phase I trial and pharmacokinetics of gemcitabine in children with advanced solid tumors. J Clin Oncol 2004;22:2445–2451.
765. Steinherz PG, Seibel NL, Ames MM, et al. Phase I study of gemcitabine (difluorodeoxycytidine) in children with relapsed or refractory leukemia (CCG-0955): a report from the Children's Cancer Group. Leuk Lymphoma 2002;43:1945–1950.
766. Abbruzzese JL, Grunewald R, Weeks EA, et al. A phase I clinical, plasma, and cellular pharmacology study of gemcitabine. J Clin Oncol 1991;9:491–498.
767. Delaloge S, Llombart A, Di Palma M, et al. Gemcitabine in patients with solid tumors and renal impairment: a pharmacokinetic phase I study. Am J Clin Oncol 2004;27:2 89–293.
768. Grunewald R, Abbruzzese JL, Tarassoff P, et al. Saturation of 2′,2′-difluorodeoxycytidine 5′-triphosphate accumulation by mononuclear cells during a phase I trial of gemcitabine. Cancer Chemother Pharmacol 1991;27:258–262.
769. Humphreys BD, Sharman JP, Henderson JM, et al. Gemcitabine-associated thrombotic microangiopathy. Cancer 2004;100:2664–2670.
770. Barlesi F, Villani P, Doddoli C, et al. Gemcitabine-induced severe pulmonary toxicity. Fundam Clin Pharmacol 2004;18:85–91.
771. Friedlander PA, Bansal R, Schwartz L, et al. Gemcitabine-related radiation recall preferentially involves internal tissue and organs. Cancer 2004;100:1793–1799.
772. Lokich JJ, Ahlgren JD, Gullo JJ, et al. A prospective randomized comparison of continuous infusion fluorouracil with a conventional bolus schedule in metastatic colorectal carcinoma: a Mid-Atlantic Oncology Program Study. J Clin Oncol 1989;7:425–432.
773. Leichman CG. Schedule dependency of 5-fluorouracil. Oncology (Huntingt) 1999;13(Suppl 3):26–32.
774. Grem JL. 5-Fluoropyrimidines. In: Chabner BA, Longo DL, eds. Cancer chemotherapy and biotherapy principles and practice. Philadelphia, PA: Lippincott-Raven, 1996:149–211.
775. Myers CE. The pharmacology of the fluoropyrimidines. Pharmacol Rev 1981;33: 1–15.
776. Diasio RB, Harris BE. Clinical pharmacology of 5-fluorouracil. Clin Pharmacokinet 1989;16:215–237.
777. Heidelberger C, Danenberg PV, Moran RG. Fluorinated pyrimidines and their nucleosides. Adv Enzymol 1983;54:58–119.
778. Schilsky RL. Biochemical and clinical pharmacology of 5-fluorouracil. Oncology (Huntingt) 1998;12(Suppl 7):13–18.
779. Mader RM, Muller M, Steger GG. Resistance to 5-fluorouracil. Gen Pharmacol 1998;31:661–666.
780. Houghton JA, Houghton PJ. 5-Halogenated pyrimidines and their nucleosides. Handb Exp Pharmacol 1984;72:515–549.
781. Milano G, Etienne M-C. Dihydropyrimidine dehydrogenase (DPD) and clinical pharmacology of 5-fluorouracil [review]. Anticancer Res 1994;14:2295–2298.
782. Jastreboff MM, Kedzierska B, Rode W. Altered thymidylate synthetase in 5-fluorodeoxyuridine-resistant Ehrlich ascites carcinoma cells. Biochem Pharmacol 1983; 32:2259–2267.
783. Fraile RJ, Baker LH, Buroker TR, et al. Pharmacokinetics of 5-fluorouracil administered orally, by rapid intravenous and by slow infusion. Cancer Res 1980;40: 2223–2228.
784. Christophidis N, Vajda FJE, Lucas I, et al. Fluorouracil therapy in patients with carcinoma of the large bowel: a pharmacokinetic comparison of various rates and routes of administration. Clin Pharmacokinet 1978;3:330–336.
785. Iyer L, Ratain MJ. 5-Fluorouracil pharmacokinetics: causes for variability and strategies for modulation in cancer chemotherapy. Cancer Invest 1999;17:494–506.
786. Diasio RB. Improving fluorouracil chemotherapy with novel orally administered fluoropyrimidines. Drugs 1999;58(Suppl 3):119–126.
787. Hoff PM, Royce M, Medgyesy D, et al. Oral fluoropyrimidines. Semin Oncol 1999; 26:640–646.
788. Pazdur R, Hoff PM, Medgyesy D, et al. The oral fluorouracil prodrugs. Oncology (Huntingt) 1998;12(10, Suppl 7):48–51.
789. Schilsky RL. Pharmacology and clinical status of capecitabine. Oncology 2000;14:1297–1306.
790. Borner MM, Kneer J, Crevoisier C, et al. Bioavailability and feasibility of subcutaneous 5-fluorouracil. Br J Cancer 1993;68:537–539.
791. Collins JM, Dedrick RL, King FG, et al. Nonlinear pharmacokinetic models for 5-fluorouracil in man: intravenous and intraperitoneal routes. Clin Pharmacol Ther 1980;28:235–246.
792. Grem JL, McAtee N, Murphy RF, et al. A pilot study of interferon alfa-2a in combination with 5-fluorouracil plus high-dose leucovorin in metastatic gastrointestinal carcinoma. J Clin Oncol 1991;9:1811–1820.
793. Balis FM, Gillespie A, Belasco J, et al. Phase II trial of sequential methotrexate and 5-fluorouracil with leucovorin in children with sarcomas. Invest New Drugs 1990; 8:181–182.
794. Wagner JG, Gyves JW, Stetson PL, et al. Steady-state nonlinear pharmacokinetics of 5-fluorouracil during hepatic arterial and intravenous infusions in cancer patients. Cancer Res 1986;46:1499–1506.
795. McDermott BJ, van den Berg HW, Murphy RF. Nonlinear pharmacokinetics for the elimination of 5-fluorouracil after intravenous administration in cancer patients. Cancer Chemother Pharmacol 1982;9:173–178.
796. Hrushesky WJM. More evidence for circadian rhythm effects in cancer chemotherapy: the fluoropyrimidine story. Cancer Cells 1990;2:65–68.
797. Harris BE, Song R, Soong S-J, et al. Relationship between dihydropyrimidine dehydrogenase activity and plasma 5-fluorouracil levels with evidence for circadian variation of enzyme activity and plasma drug levels in cancer patients receiving 5-fluorouracil by protracted continuous infusion. Cancer Res 1990;50:197–201.
798. Petit E, Milano G, Levi F, et al. Circadian rhythm varying plasma concentration of 5-fluorouracil during a 5-day continuous venous infusion at a constant rate in cancer patients. Cancer Res 1988;48:1676–1679.
799. Levi F, Brienza S, Metzer G, et al. Implications of chronobiology for 5-fluorouracil (5-FU) efficacy. Adv Exp Med Biol 1993;339:169–183.
800. Bressolle F, Joulia JM, Pinguet F, et al. Circadian rhythm of 5-fluorouracil population pharmacokinetics in patients with metastatic colorectal cancer. Cancer Chemother Pharmacol 1999;44:295–302.
801. MacDonald JS. Toxicity of 5-fluorouracil. Oncology (Huntingt) 1999;13(Suppl 3):33–34.
802. Harris BE, Carpenter JT, Diasio RB. Severe 5-fluorouracil toxicity to dihydropyrimidine dehydrogenase deficiency: a potentially more common pharmacogenetic syndrome. Cancer 1991;68:499–501.
803. Diasio RB, Beavers TL, Carpenter JT. Familial deficiency of dihydropyrimidine dehydrogenase: biochemical basis for familial pyrimidinemia and severe 5-fluorouracil induced toxicity. J Clin Invest 1988;81:47–51.
804. Milano G, Etienne M-C. Fluorinated pyrimidines. In: Grochow LB, Ames MM, eds. A clinician's guide to chemotherapy pharmacokinetics and pharmacodynamics. Baltimore, MD: Williams & Wilkins, 1998:289–300.
805. Huang RS, Ratain MJ. Pharmacogenetics and pharmacogenomics of anticancer agents. CA Cancer J Clin 2009;59:42–55.
806. Marsh S. Thymidylate synthase pharmacogenetics. Invest New Drugs 2005;23:533–537.
807. Etienne-Grimaldi MC, Francoual M, Formento JL, et al. Methylenetetrahydrofolate reductase (MTHFR) variants and fluorouracil-based treatments in colorectal cancer. Pharmacogenomics 2007;8:1561–1566.
808. Lecomte T, Ferraz JM, Zinzindohoue F, et al. Thymidylate synthase gene polymorphism predicts toxicity in colorectal cancer patients receiving 5-fluorouracil-based chemotherapy. Clin Cancer Res 2004;10:5880–5888.
809. Pullarkat ST, Stoehlmacher J, Ghaderi V, et al. Thymidylate synthase gene polymorphism determines response and toxicity of 5-FU chemotherapy. Pharmacogenomics J 2001;1:65–70.

810. Santos GA, Grogan L, Allegra CJ. Preclinical and clinical aspects of biomodulation of 5-fluorouracil. Cancer Treat Rev 1994;20:11–49.
811. Pratt CB, Meyer WH, Howlett N, et al. Phase II study of 5-fluorouracil/leucovorin for pediatric patients with malignant solid tumors. Cancer 1994;74:2593–2598.
812. Pommier Y, Leteurtre F, Fesen MR, et al. Cellular determinants of sensitivity and resistance to DNA topoisomerase inhibitors. Cancer Invest 1994;12:530–542.
813. Cummings J, Anderson L, Willmott N, et al. The molecular pharmacology of doxorubicin in vivo. Eur J Cancer 1991;27:532–535.
814. Keizer HG, Pinedo HM, Schuurhuis GJ, et al. Doxorubicin (adriamycin): a critical review of free radical-dependent mechanisms of cytotoxicity. Pharmacol Ther 1990;47:219–231.
815. Tritton TR. Cell surface actions of adriamycin. Pharmacol Ther 1991;49:292–309.
816. Goormaghtigh E, Ruysschaert JM. Anthracycline glycoside-membrane interactions. Biochim Biophys Acta 1984;779:271–288.
817. Gewirtz DA. A critical evaluation of the mechanism of action proposed for the antitumor effects of the anthracycline antibiotics adriamycin and daunorubicin. Biochem Pharmacol 1999;57:727–741.
818. Doroshow JH. Anthracyclines and anthracenediones. In: Chabner BA, Longo DL, eds. Cancer chemotherapy and biotherapy principles and practice. Philadelphia, PA: Lippincott-Raven, 1996:409–434.
819. Tan B, Piwnica-Worms D, Ratner L. Multidrug resistance transporters and modulation. Curr Opin Oncol 2000;12:450–458.
820. Lampidis TJ, Kolonias D, Podana T, et al. Circumvention of P-GP MDR as a function of anthracycline lipophilicity and charge. Biochemistry 1997;36:2679–2685.
821. Berman E, McBride M. Comparative cellular pharmacology of daunorubicin and idarubicin in human multidrug-resistant leukemia cells. Blood 1992;79:3267–3273.
822. Bielack SS, Erttmann R, Winkler K, et al. Doxorubicin: effect of different schedules on toxicity and antitumor efficacy. Eur J Cancer Clin Oncol 1989;25:873–882.
823. Hortobagyi GN, Frye D, Buzdar AU, et al. Decreased cardiac toxicity of doxorubicin administered by continuous intravenous infusion in combination chemotherapy for metastatic breast cancer. Cancer 1989;63:37–45.
824. Ackland SP, Ratain MJ, Vogelzang NJ, et al. Pharmacokinetics and pharmacodynamics of long-term continuous-infusion doxorubicin. Clin Pharmacol Ther 1989;45:340–347.
825. Legha SS. Infusional schedules for antitumor antibiotics. J Infus Chemother 1991;1:24–27.
826. Shapira J, Gotfried M, Lishner M, et al. Reduced cardiotoxicity of doxorubicin by a 6-hour infusion regimen. A prospective randomized evaluation. Cancer 1990;65:870–873.
827. Robert J. Anthracyclines. In: Grochow LB, Ames MM, eds. A clinician's guide to chemotherapy pharmacokinetics and pharmacodynamics. Baltimore, MD: Williams & Wilkins, 1998:93–173.
828. Kuffel MJ, Reid JM, Ames MM. Anthracyclines and their C13 alcohol metabolites: growth inhibition and DNA damage following incubation with human tumor cells in culture. Cancer Chemother Pharmacol 1992;30:51–57.
829. Stewart DJ, Grewaal D, Green RM, et al. Bioavailability and pharmacology of oral idarubicin. Cancer Chemother Pharmacol 1991;27:308–314.
830. Goebel M. Oral idarubicin—an anthracycline derivative with unique properties. Ann Hematol 1993;66:33–43.
831. Robert J. Clinical pharmacokinetics of idarubicin. Clin Pharmacokinet 1993;24:275–288.
832. Speth PAJ, van Hoesel QGCM, Haanen C. Clinical pharmacokinetics of doxorubicin. Clin Pharmacokinet 1988;15:15–31.
833. Robert J, Rigal-Huguet, Hurteloup P. Comparative pharmacokinetic study of idarubicin and daunomycin in leukemia patients. Hematol Oncol 1992;10:111–116.
834. Greene RF, Collins JM, Jenkins JF, et al. Plasma pharmacokinetics of adriamycin and adriamycinol: implications for the design of in vitro experiments and treatment protocols. Cancer Res 1983;43:3417–3421.
835. Evans WE, Crom WR, Sinkule JA, et al. Pharmacokinetics of anticancer drugs in children. Drug Metab Rev 1983;14:847–886.
836. Timour Q, Nony P, Lang J, et al. Doxorubicin concentrations in plasma and myocardium and their respective roles in cardiotoxicity. Cardiovasc Drugs Ther 1988;1:559–560.
837. Cusack BJ, Young SP, Driskell J, et al. Doxorubicin and doxorubicinol pharmacokinetics and tissue concentrations following bolus injection and continuous infusion doxorubicin in rabbit. Cancer Chemother Pharmacol 1993;32:53–58.
838. Riggs CE. Clinical pharmacology of daunomycin in patients with acute leukemia. Semin Oncol 1984;11(Suppl 3):2–11.
839. Reid JM, Pendergrass TW, Krailo MD, et al. Plasma pharmacokinetics and cerebrospinal fluid concentrations of idarubicin and idarubicinol in pediatric leukemia patients: a Children's Cancer Study Group report. Cancer Res 1990;50:6525–6528.
840. Robert J, Gianni L. Pharmacokinetics and metabolism of anthracyclines. Cancer Surv 1993;17:219–252.
841. Thompson PA, Rosner GL, Matthay KK, et al. Impact of body composition on pharmacokinetics of doxorubicin in children: a Glaser Pediatric Research Network study. Cancer Chemother Pharmacol 2009;64:243–251.
842. Eksborg S, Strandler HYS, Edsmyr F, et al. Pharmacokinetic study of i.v. infusions of adriamycin. Eur J Clin Pharmacol 1985;28:205–212.
843. Ames MM, Spreafico F. Selected pharmacological characteristics of idarubicin and idarubicinol. Leukemia 1992;8:70–75.
844. Crom W, Riley C, Green A, et al. Doxorubicin disposition in children and adolescents with cancer. Drug Intell Clin Pharm 1983;17:448.
845. Mross K, Maessen P, van der Vijgh WJF, et al. Pharmacokinetics and metabolism of epidoxorubicin and doxorubicin in humans. J Clin Oncol 1988;6:517–526.
846. Tamura K. A phase I study of idarubicin hydrochloride in patients with acute leukemia: the Idarubicin Study Group of Japan. Semin Hematol 1996;33(4, Suppl 3):2–11.
847. Yoshida H, Goto M, Honda A, et al. Pharmacokinetics of doxorubicin and its active metabolite in patients with normal renal function and in patients on hemodialysis. Cancer Chemother Pharmacol 1994;33:450–454.
848. Camaggi CM, Strocchi E, Carisi P, et al. Idarubicin metabolism and pharmacokinetics after intravenous and oral administration in cancer patients: a crossover study. Cancer Chemother Pharmacol 1992;30:307–316.
849. Benjamin RS, Wiernik PH, Bachur NR. Adriamycin chemotherapy: efficacy, safety and pharmacologic basis of an intermittent single high-dosage schedule. Cancer 1974;35:19–27.
850. Johnson FL, Balis FM. Hepatopathy following irradiation and chemotherapy for Wilms' tumor. Am J Pediatr Hematol Oncol 1982;4:217–221.
851. Piscitelli SC, Rodvold KA, Rushing DA, et al. Pharmacokinetics and pharmacodynamics of doxorubicin in patients with small cell lung cancer. Clin Pharmacol Ther 1993;53:555–561.
852. Brenner DE, Wiernik PH, Wesley M, et al. Acute doxorubicin toxicity: relationship to pretreatment liver function, response and pharmacokinetics in patients with acute non-lymphocytic leukemia. Cancer 1984;53:1042–1048.
853. Kaye SB, Cummings J, Kerr DJ. How much does liver disease affect the pharmacokinetics of adriamycin? Eur J Cancer Clin Oncol 1985;21:893–895.
854. Sulkes A, Collins JM. Reappraisal of some dosage adjustment guidelines. Cancer Treat Rep 1987;71:229–233.
855. Rodvold KA, Rushing DA, Tewksbury DA. Doxorubicin clearance in the obese. J Clin Oncol 1988;6:1321–1327.
856. Griggs JJ, Sorbero ME, Lyman GH. Undertreatment of obese women receiving breast cancer chemotherapy. Arch Intern Med 2005;165:1267–1273.
857. Rosner GL, Hargis JB, Hollis DR, et al. Relationship between toxicity and obesity in women receiving adjuvant chemotherapy for breast cancer: results from cancer and leukemia group B study 8541. J Clin Oncol 1996;14:3000–3008.
858. Lange BJ, Gerbing RB, Feusner J, et al. Mortality in overweight and underweight children with acute myeloid leukemia. JAMA 2005;293:203–211.
859. Wong KY, Lampkin BC. Anthracycline toxicity. Am J Pediatr Hematol Oncol 1983;5:93–97.
860. Olver IN, Aisner J, Hament A, et al. A prospective study of topical dimethyl sulfoxide for treating anthracycline extravasation. J Clin Oncol 1988;6:1732–1735.
861. Kane RC, McGuinn WD Jr, Dagher R, et al. Dexrazoxane (Totect): FDA review and approval for the treatment of accidental extravasation following intravenous anthracycline chemotherapy. Oncologist 2008;13:445–450.
862. Bowers DG, Lynch JB. Adriamycin extravasation. Plast Reconstr Surg 1978;61:86–92.
863. Giantris A, Abdurrahman L, Hinkle A, et al. Anthracycline-induced cardiotoxicity in children and young adults. Crit Rev Oncol Hematol 1998;27:53–68.
864. Singal PK, Iliskovic N. Doxorubicin-induced cardiomyopathy. N Engl J Med 1998;339:900–905.
865. Singer JW, Narahara KA, Ritchie JL, et al. Time- and dose-dependent changes in ejection fraction determined by radionuclide angiography after anthracycline therapy. Cancer Treat Rep 1978;62:945–948.
866. Bristow MR, Thompson PD, Martin RP, et al. Early anthracycline cardiotoxicity. Am J Med 1978;65:823–832.
867. Grenier MA, Lipshultz SE. Epidemiology of anthracycline cardiotoxicity in children and adults. Semin Oncol 1998;25(4, Suppl 10):72–85.
868. Von Hoff DD, Rozencweig M, Layard MW, et al. Daunomycin-induced cardiotoxicity in children and adults. Am J Med 1977;62:200–205.
869. Von Hoff DD, Layard MW, Basa P, et al. Risk factors for doxorubicin-induced congestive heart failure. Ann Intern Med 1979;91:710–717.
870. Anderlini P, Benjamin RS, Wong FC, et al. Idarubicin cardiotoxicity: a retrospective study in acute myeloid leukemia and myelodysplasia. J Clin Oncol 1995;13:2827–2834.
871. Sallan SE, Clavell LA. Cardiac effects of anthracyclines used in the treatment of childhood acute lymphoblastic leukemia: a 10-year experience. Semin Oncol 1984;11 (Suppl 3):19–21.
872. Lipshultz SE, Lipsitz SR, Mone SM, et al. Female sex and drug dose as risk factors for late cardiotoxic effects of doxorubicin therapy for childhood cancer. N Engl J Med 1995;332:1738–1743.
873. Silber JH, Jakacki RI, Larsen RL, et al. Increased risk of cardiac dysfunction after anthracyclines in girls. Med Pediatr Oncol 1993;21:477–479.
874. Bielack SS, Erttmann R, Kempf-Bielack B, et al. Impact of scheduling on toxicity and clinical efficacy of doxorubicin: what do we know in the mid-nineties? Eur J Cancer 1996;32A:1652–1660.
875. Chlebowski RT, Parloy WS, Pugh RT, et al. Adriamycin given as a weekly schedule without a loading course: clinically effective with reduced incidence of cardiotoxicity. Cancer Treat Rep 1980;64:47–51.
876. Legha SS, Benjamin RS, Mackay B, et al. Reduction of doxorubicin cardiotoxicity by prolonged continuous intravenous infusion. Ann Intern Med 1982;96:133–139.
877. Ewer MS, Jaffe N, Ried H, et al. Doxorubicin cardiotoxicity in children: comparison of a consecutive divided daily dose administration schedule with single dose (rapid) infusion administration. Med Pediatr Oncol 1998;31:512–515.
878. Berrak SG, Ewer MS, Jaffe N, et al. Doxorubicin cardiotoxicity in children: reduced incidence of cardiac dysfunction associated with continuous-infusion schedules. Oncol Rep 2001;8:611–614.
879. Lipshultz SE, Giantris AL, Lipsitz SR, et al. Doxorubicin administration by continuous infusion is not cardioprotective: the Dana-Farber 91-01 Acute Lymphoblastic Leukemia protocol. J Clin Oncol 2002;20:1677–1682.
880. Lipshultz SE, Colan SD, Gelber RD, et al. Late cardiac effects of doxorubicin therapy for acute lymphoblastic leukemia in childhood. N Engl J Med 1991;324:808–815.
881. Steinherz LJ, Steinherz PG, Tan CT. Cardiac failure and dysrhythmias 6–19 years after anthracycline therapy: a series of 15 patients. Med Pediatr Oncol 1995;24:352–361.
882. Goorin AM, Chauvenet AR, Perez-Atayde AR, et al. Initial congestive heart failure, six to ten years after doxorubicin chemotherapy for childhood cancer. J Pediatr 1990;116:144–147.
883. Yeung ST, Yoong C, Spink J, et al. Functional myocardial impairment in children treated with anthracyclines for cancer. Lancet 1991;337:816–818.
884. Nysom K, Holm K, Lipsitz SR, et al. Relationship between cumulative anthracycline dose and late cardiotoxicity in childhood acute lymphoblastic leukemia. J Clin Oncol 1998;16:545–550.
885. Lipshultz SE, Lipsitz SR, Sallan SE, et al. Chronic progressive cardiac dysfunction years after doxorubicin therapy for childhood acute lymphoblastic leukemia. J Clin Oncol 2005;23:2629–2636.
886. Billingham ME, Bristow MR. Evaluation of anthracycline cardiotoxicity: predictive ability and functional correlation of endomyocardial biopsy. Cancer Treat Symp 1984;3:71–76.
887. de Jong J, Schoofs PR, Snabilie AM, et al. The role of biotransformation in anthracycline-induced cardiotoxicity in mice. J Pharmacol Exp Ther 1993;266:1312–1320.
888. Stewart DJ, Grenwaal D, Green RM, et al. Concentrations of doxorubicin and its metabolites in human autopsy heart and other tissues. Anticancer Res 1993;13:1945–1952.
889. Kismet E, Varan A, Ayabakan C, et al. Serum troponin T levels and echocardiographic evaluation in children treated with doxorubicin. Pediatr Blood Cancer 2004;42:220–224.

890. Herman EH, Zhang J, Lipshultz SE, et al. Correlation between serum levels of cardiac troponin-T and the severity of the chronic cardiomyopathy induced by doxorubicin. J Clin Oncol 1999;17:2237–2243.
891. Herman EH, Lipshultz SE, Rifai N, et al. Use of cardiac troponin T levels as an indicator of doxorubicin-induced cardiotoxicity. Cancer Res 1998;58:195–197.
892. Kremer LC, Bastiaansen BA, Offringa M, et al. Troponin T in the first 24 hours after the administration of chemotherapy and the detection of myocardial damage in children. Eur J Cancer 2002;38:686–689.
893. Steinherz LJ, Graham T, Hurwitz R, et al. Guidelines for cardiac monitoring of children during and after anthracycline therapy: report of the cardiology committee of the Children's Cancer Study Group. Pediatrics 1992;89:942–949.
894. Jakacki RI, Larsen RL, Barber G, et al. Comparison of cardiac function tests after anthracycline therapy in childhood. Cancer 1993;72:2739–2745.
895. Lipshultz SE, Sanders SP, Goorin AM, et al. Monitoring for anthracycline cardiotoxicity. Pediatrics 1994;93:433–437.
896. Carlson RW. Reducing the cardiotoxicity of the anthracyclines. Oncology 1992; 6:95–107.
897. Basser RL, Green MD. Strategies for prevention of anthracycline cardiotoxicity. Cancer Treat Rev 1993;19:57–77.
898. Marina NM, Cochrane D, Harney E, et al. Dose escalation and pharmacokinetics of pegylated liposomal doxorubicin (Doxil) in children with solid tumors: a pediatric oncology group study. Clin Cancer Res 2002;8:413–418.
899. Seifert CF, Nesser ME, Thompson DF. Dexrazoxane in the prevention of doxorubicin-induced cardiotoxicity. Ann Pharmacother 1994;28:1063–1072.
900. Speyer JL, Green MD, Kramer E, et al. Protective effect of the bispiperazinedione ICRF-187 against doxorubicin-induced cardiac toxicity in women with advanced breast cancer. N Engl J Med 1988;319:745–752.
901. Wexler LH, Andrich MP, Venzon D, et al. Randomized trial of the cardioprotective agent ICRF-187 in pediatric sarcoma patients treated with doxorubicin. J Clin Oncol 1996;14:362–372.
902. Swain SM, Whaley FS, Gerber MC, et al. Cardioprotection with dexrazoxane for doxorubicin-containing therapy in advanced breast cancer. J Clin Oncol 1997;15: 1318–1332.
903. Speyer JL, Green MD, Zeleniuch-Jacquotte A, et al. ICRF-187 permits longer treatment with doxorubicin in women with breast cancer. J Clin Oncol 1992;10:117–127.
904. Kovacs GT, Erlaky H, Toth K, et al. Subacute cardiotoxicity caused by anthracycline therapy in children: can dexrazoxane prevent this effect? Eur J Pediatr 2007;166: 1187–1188.
905. Tebbi CK, London WB, Friedman D, et al. Dexrazoxane-associated risk for acute myeloid leukemia/myelodysplastic syndrome and other secondary malignancies in pediatric Hodgkin's disease. J Clin Oncol 2007;25:493–500.
906. Barry EV, Vrooman LM, Dahlberg SE, et al. Absence of secondary malignant neoplasms in children with high-risk acute lymphoblastic leukemia treated with dexrazoxane. J Clin Oncol 2008;26:1106–1111.
907. Hochster H, Liebes L, Wadler S, et al. Pharmacokinetics of the cardioprotector ADR-529 (ICRF-187) in escalating doses combined with fixed-dose doxorubicin. J Natl Cancer Inst 1992;84:1725–1730.
908. Lum BL, Fisher GA, Brophy NA, et al. Clinical trials of modulation of multidrug resistance. Pharmacokinetic and pharmacodynamic considerations. Cancer 1993;72:3502–3514.
909. Bartlett NL, Lum BL, Fisher GA, et al. Phase I trial of doxorubicin with cyclosporine as a modulator of multidrug resistance. J Clin Oncol 1994;12:835–842.
910. Rushing DA, Raber SR, Rodvold KA, et al. The effects of cyclosporine on the pharmacokinetics of doxorubicin in patients with small cell lung cancer. Cancer 1994;74:834–841.
911. Sonneveld P, Marie JP, Huisman C, et al. Reversal of multidrug resistance by SDZ PSC 833, combined with VAD (vincristine, doxorubicin, dexamethasone) in refractory multiple myeloma. A phase I study. Leukemia 1996;10:1741–1750.
912. Crespi MD, Ivanier SE, Genovese J, et al. Mitoxantrone affects topoisomerase activities in human breast cancer cells. Biochem Biophys Res Commun 1986;136:521–528.
913. Ehninger G, Schuler U, Proksch B, et al. Pharmacokinetics and metabolism of mitoxantrone. A review. Clin Pharmacokinet 1990;18:365–380.
914. Ungerleider RS, Pratt CB, Vietti TJ, et al. Phase I trial of mitoxantrone in children. Cancer Treat Rep 1985;69:403–407.
915. Starling KA, Mulne AF, Vats TS, et al. Mitoxantrone in refractory acute leukemia in children: a phase I study. Invest New Drugs 1985;3:191–195.
916. Behrendt H, Massar CG, van Leeuwen EF. Mitoxantrone is effective in treating childhood T-cell lymphoma/T-cell acute lymphoblastic leukemia. Cancer 1995;76:339–342.
917. Arlin Z, Case DC, Moore J, et al. Randomized multicenter trial of cytosine arabinoside with mitoxantrone or daunorubicin in previously untreated adult patients with acute nonlymphocytic leukemia. Leukemia 1990;4:177–183.
918. Wells RJ, Gold SH, Krill CE, et al. Cytosine arabinoside and mitoxantrone induction chemotherapy followed by bone marrow transplantation or chemotherapy for relapsed or refractory pediatric acute myeloid leukemia. Leukemia 1994;8: 1626–1630.
919. Chiccarelli FS, Morrison JA, Cosulich DB, et al. Identification of human urinary mitoxantrone metabolites. Cancer Res 1986;46:4858–4861.
920. Alberts DS, Peng YM, Leigh S, et al. Disposition of mitoxantrone in cancer patients. Cancer Res 1985;45:1879–1884.
921. Posner LE, Dukart G, Goldberg T, et al. Mitoxantrone: an overview of safety and toxicity. Invest New Drugs 1985;3:123–132.
922. Herman EH, Zhang J, Hasinoff BB, et al. Comparison of the structural changes induced by doxorubicin and mitoxantrone in the heart, kidney and intestine and characterization of the Fe(III)-mitoxantrone complex. J Mol Cell Cardiol 1997;29:2415–2430.
923. Estorch M, Carrio I, Martinez-Duncker D, et al. Myocyte cell damage after administration of doxorubicin or mitoxantrone in breast cancer patients assessed by indium 111 antimyosin monoclonal antibody studies. J Clin Oncol 1993;11:1264–1268.
924. Aviles A, Neri N, Nambo JM, et al. Late cardiac toxicity secondary to treatment in Hodgkin's disease. A study comparing doxorubicin, epirubicin and mitoxantrone in combined therapy. Leuk Lymphoma 2005;46:1023–1028.
925. Van Dalen EC, Van Der Pal HJ, Bakker PJ, et al. Cumulative incidence and risk factors of mitoxantrone-induced cardiotoxicity in children: a systematic review. Eur J Cancer 2004;40:643–652.
926. Mir LM, Tounekti O, Orlowski S. Bleomycin: revival of an old drug. Gen Pharmacol 1996;27:745–748.
927. Dorr RT. Bleomycin pharmacology: mechanism of action and resistance, and clinical pharmacokinetics. Semin Oncol 1992;19(Suppl 5):3–8.
928. Dedon PC, Goldberg IH. Free-radical mechanisms involved in the formation of sequence-dependent bistranded DNA lesions by the antitumor antibiotics bleomycin, neocarzinostatin, and calicheamicin. Chem Res Toxicol 1992;5:311–332.
929. Bailly C, Henani A, Waring MJ. Altered cleavage of DNA sequences by bleomycin and its deglycosylated derivative in the presence of actinomycin. Nucleic Acid Res 1997; 25:1516–1522.
930. Dorr RT. Bleomycin. In: Grochow LB, Ames MM, eds. A clinician's guide to chemotherapy pharmacokinetics and pharmacodynamics. Baltimore, MD: Williams & Wilkins, 1998:175–187.
931. Patz EF Jr, McAdams HP, Erasmus JJ, et al. Sclerotherapy for malignant pleural effusions: a prospective randomized trial of bleomycin vs doxycycline with small-bore catheter drainage. Chest 1998;113:1305–1311.
932. Bracken RB, Johnson DE, Rodriquez L, et al. Treatment of multiple superficial tumors of bladder with intravesicular bleomycin. Urology 1977;9:161–163.
933. Jules-Elysee K, White DA. Bleomycin-induced pulmonary toxicity. Clin Chest Med 1990;11:1–20.
934. Comis RL. Bleomycin pulmonary toxicity: current status and future directions. Semin Oncol 1992;19(Suppl 5):64–70.
935. Wolkowicz J, Sturgeon J, Rawji M, et al. Bleomycin-induced pulmonary function abnormalities. Chest 1992;101:97–101.
936. Eigen H, Wyszomierski D. Bleomycin lung injury in children. Am J Pediatr Hematol Oncol 1985;7:71–78.
937. Simpson AB, Paul J, Graham J, et al. Fatal bleomycin toxicity in the west of Scotland 1991–1995: a review of patients with germ cell tumors. Brit J Cancer 1998;78: 1061–1066.
938. Kawai K, Hinotsu S, Tombe M, et al. Serum creatinine level during chemotherapy for testicular cancer as a possible predictor of bleomycin-induced pulmonary toxicity. Japanese J Clin Oncol 1998;28:546–550.
939. Donat SM, Levy DA. Bleomycin associated pulmonary toxicity: is perioperative oxygen restriction necessary? J Urol 1998;160:1347–1352.
940. Saxman SB, Nichols CR, Einhorn LH. Pulmonary toxicity in patients with advanced-stage germ cell tumors receiving bleomycin with and without granulocyte colony stimulating factor. Chest 1997;111:657–660.
941. Hay J, Shahzeidi S, Laurent G. Mechanisms of bleomycin-induced lung damage. Arch Toxicol 1991;65:81–94.
942. Mowad CM, Nguyen TV, Elenitsas R, et al. Bleomycin-induced flagellate dermatitis: a clinical and histopathological review. Br J Dermatol 1994;131:700–702.
943. Oken MM, Crooke ST, Elson MK, et al. Pharmacokinetics of bleomycin after im administration in man. Cancer Treat Rep 1981;65:485–489.
944. Harvey VJ, Slevin ML, Aherne GW, et al. Subcutaneous infusions of bleomycin: a practical alternative to intravenous infusion. J Clin Oncol 1987;5:648–650.
945. Yee GC, Crom WR, Lee FH, et al. Bleomycin disposition in children with cancer. Clin Pharmacol Ther 1983;33:668–673.
946. Crooke ST, Comis RL, Einhorn LH, et al. Effects of variation in renal function on the clinical pharmacology of bleomycin administered as an IV bolus. Cancer Treat Rep 1977;61:1631–1636.
947. Alberts DS, Chen H-SG, Liu R, et al. Bleomycin pharmacokinetics in man. I. Intravenous administration. Cancer Chemother Pharmacol 1978;1:177–181.
948. Crooke ST, Luft F, Broughton A, et al. Bleomycin serum pharmacokinetics as determined by a radioimmunoassay and a microbiologic assay in a patient with compromised renal function. Cancer 1977;39:1430–1434.
949. Schwartz DR, Homanics GE, Hoyt DG, et al. The neutral cysteine protease bleomycin hydrolase is essential for epidermal integrity and bleomycin resistance. Proc Natl Acad Sci U S A 1999;96:4680–4685.
950. Zuckerman JE, Raffin TA, Brown JM, et al. In vitro selection and characterization of a bleomycin-resistant subline of B16 melanoma. Cancer Res 1986;46:1748–1753.
951. Sebti SM, Jani JP, Mistry JS, et al. Metabolic inactivation: a mechanism of human tumor resistance to bleomycin. Cancer Res 1991;51:227–232.
952. de Haas EC, Zwart N, Meijer C, et al. Variation in bleomycin hydrolase gene is associated with reduced survival after chemotherapy for testicular germ cell cancer. J Clin Oncol 2008;26:1817–1823.
953. Selman A. Waksman Conference on Actinomycins: their potential for cancer chemotherapy. Cancer Chemother Rep 1974;58:1–123.
954. Myers CE. Anthracyclines and DNA intercalators. In: Holland JF, Frei E, et al., eds. Cancer medicine. Philadelphia, PA: Lea and Febiger, 1993:764–773.
955. Wassermann K, Markovits J, Jaxel C, et al. Effects of morpholinyl doxorubicins, doxorubicin, and actinomycin D on mammalian DNA topoisomerases I and II. Mol Pharmacol 1990;38:38–45.
956. Davidson A, Protchard J. Actinomycin D, hepatic toxicity and Wilms' tumour—a mystery explained? Eur J Cancer 1998;34:1145–1147.
957. Lee JI, Skolnik JM, Barrett JS, et al. A sensitive and selective liquid chromatography–tandem mass spectrometry method for the simultaneous quantification of actinomycin-D and vincristine in children with cancer. J Mass Spectrom 2007;42:761–770.
958. Veal GJ, Errington J, Sludden J, et al. Determination of anti-cancer drug actinomycin D in human plasma by liquid chromatography–mass spectrometry. J Chromatogr B Analyt Technol Biomed Life Sci 2003;795:237–243.
959. Tattersall MHN, Sodergren JE, Sengupta SK, et al. Pharmacokinetics of actinomycin D in patients with malignant melanoma. Clin Pharmacol Ther 1975;17:701–708.
960. Brothman AR, Davis TP, Duffy JJ, et al. Development of an antibody to actinomycin D and its application for the detection of serum levels by radioimmunoassay. Cancer Res 1982;42:1184–1187.
961. Veal GJ, Cole M, Errington J, et al. Pharmacokinetics of dactinomycin in a pediatric patient population: a United Kingdom Children's Cancer Study Group Study. Clin Cancer Res 2005;11:5893–5899.
962. Bisogno G, de Kraker J, Weirich A, et al. Veno-occlusive disease of the liver in children treated for Wilms' tumor. Med Pediatr Oncol 1997;29:245–251.
963. Tornesello A, Piciacchia D, Mastrangelo S, et al. Veno-occlusive disease of the liver in right-sided Wilms' tumours. Eur J Cancer 1998;34:1220–1223.
964. Cohen JJ, Loven D, Schoenfeld T, et al. Dactinomycin potentiation of radiation pneumonitis: a forgotten interaction. Pediatr Hematol Oncol 1991;8:187–192.
965. Verweij J, Schellens JHM, Loo TL, et al. Antitumor antibiotics. In: Chabner BA, Longo DL, eds. Cancer chemotherapy and biotherapy principles and practice. Philadelphia, PA: Lippincott-Raven, 1996:395–407.
966. Cragg GM, Newman DJ. Discovery and development of antineoplastic agents from natural sources. Cancer Invest 1999;17:153–163.
967. Creasy WA. Plant alkaloids. In: Becker FA, ed. Cancer: a comprehensive treatise. Vol 5. New York, NY: Plenum Press, 1977:379–425.

968. Cassady JM, Douros JD. Anticancer agents based on natural product models. New York, NY: Academic Press, 1980.

969. Levêque D, Jehl F, Monteil H. Vinblastine, vincristine and vinorelbine. In: Grochow LB, Ames MM, eds. A clinician's guide to chemotherapy pharmacokinetics and pharmacodynamics. Baltimore, MD: Williams & Wilkins, 1998:459–470.

970. Rahmani R, Zhou X-J. Pharmacokinetics and metabolism of vinca alkaloids. Cancer Surv 1993;17:269–281.

971. Capranico G, Giaccone G, D'Incalci M. DNA topoisomerase II poisons and inhibitors. Cancer Chemother Biol Response Modif 1999;18:125–1243.

972. Owellen RJ, Hartke CA, Dickerson RM, et al. Inhibition of tubulin-microtubule polymerization by drugs of the vinca alkaloid class. Cancer Res 1976;36:1499–1502.

973. Giannakakou P, Sackett DL, Ward Y, et al. p53 is associated with cellular microtubules and is transported to the nucleus by dynein. Nat Cell Biol 2000;2:709–717.

974. Rowinsky EK, Donehower RC. Antimicrotubule agents. In: Chabner BA, Longo DL, eds. Cancer chemotherapy and biotherapy principles and practice. Philadelphia, PA: Lippincott-Raven, 1996:263–296.

975. Johansen M, Kuttesch J, Bleyer WA, et al. Phase I evaluation of oral and intravenous vinorelbine in pediatric cancer patients: a report from the Children's Oncology Group. Clin Cancer Res 2006;12:516–522.

976. Van den Berg HW, Desai ZR, Wilson R, et al. The pharmacokinetics of vincristine in man: reduced drug clearance associated with raised serum alkaline phosphatase and dose-limited elimination. Cancer Chemother Pharmacol 1982;8:215–219.

977. Desai ZR, Van den Berg HW, Bridges JM, et al. Can severe vincristine neurotoxicity be prevented? Cancer Chemother Pharmacol 1982;8:211–214.

978. Frost BM, Lonnerholm G, Koopmans P, et al. Vincristine in childhood leukaemia: no pharmacokinetic rationale for dose reduction in adolescents. Acta Paediatr 2003;92:551–557.

979. de Graaf SSN, Bloemhof H, Vendrig DE, et al. Vincristine disposition in children with acute lymphoblastic leukemia. Med Pediatr Oncol 1995;24:235–240.

980. Crom WR, de Graaf SSN, Synold T, et al. Pharmacokinetics of vincristine in children and adolescents with acute lymphocytic leukemia. J Pediatr 1994;125:642–649.

981. Sethi VS, Kimball JC. Pharmacokinetics of vincristine sulfate in children. Cancer Chemother Pharmacol 1981;6:111–115.

982. Sethi VS, Jackson DV, White DR, et al. Pharmacokinetics of vincristine sulfate in adult cancer patients. Cancer Res 1981;41:3551–3555.

983. Owellen RJ, Root MA, Hains FO. Pharmacokinetics of vindesine and vincristine in humans. Cancer Res 1977;37:2603–2607.

984. Nelson RL, Dyke RW, Root MA. Comparative pharmacokinetics of vindesine, vincristine, and vinblastine in patients with cancer. Cancer Treat Rev 1980;7(Suppl):59–63.

985. Levêque D, Jehl F. Clinical pharmacokinetics of vinorelbine. Clin Pharmacokinet 1996;31:184–197.

986. Gidding CE, Meeuwsen-de Boer GJ, Koopmans P, et al. Vincristine pharmacokinetics after repetitive dosing in children. Cancer Chemother Pharmacol 1999;44:203–209.

987. Jackson DV, Castle MC, Poplack DG, et al. Pharmacokinetics of vincristine in the cerebrospinal fluid of sub-human primates. Cancer Res 1980;40:722–724.

988. Jackson DV, Sethi VS, Spurr CL, et al. Pharmacokinetics of vincristine in the cerebrospinal fluid of humans. Cancer Res 1981;41:1466–1468.

989. Jackson DV, Castle MC, Bender RA. Biliary excretion of vincristine. Clin Pharmacol Ther 1978;24:101–107.

990. Bender RA, Castle MC, Margileth DA, et al. The pharmacokinetics of [3H]-vincristine in man. Clin Pharmacol Ther 1977;22:430–435.

991. Kajita J, Kuwabara T, Kobayashi H, et al. CYP3A4 is mainly responsible for the metabolism of a new vinca alkaloid, vinorelbine, in human liver microsomes. Drug Metab Dispos 2000;28:1121–1127.

992. Zhou XJ, Zhou-Pan XR, Gauthier T, et al. Human liver microsomal cytochrome P450 3A isozymes mediated vindesine biotransformation. Metabolic drug interactions. Biochem Pharmacol 1993;45:853–861.

993. Dennison JB, Mohutsky MA, Barbuch RJ, et al. Apparent high CYP3A5 expression is required for significant metabolism of vincristine by human cryopreserved hepatocytes. J Pharmacol Exp Ther 2008;327:248–257.

994. van Schaik RH. CYP450 pharmacogenetics for personalizing cancer therapy. Drug Resist Updat 2008;11:77–98.

995. Villikka K, Kivisto KT, Maenpaa H, et al. Cytochrome P450-inducing antiepileptics increase the clearance of vincristine in patients with brain tumors. Clin Pharmacol Ther 1999;66:589–593.

996. Gillies J, Hung KA, Fitzsimons E, et al. Severe vincristine toxicity in combination with itraconazole. Clin Lab Haematol 1998;20:123–124.

997. Groninger E, Meeuwsen-de Boar T, Koopmans P, et al. Pharmacokinetics of vincristine monotherapy in childhood acute lymphoblastic leukemia. Pediatr Res 2002;52:113–118.

998. Kohli-Kumar M, McDermott BJ, Gururangan S, et al. Kinetic basis for pediatric dosage of vincristine. Med Pediatr Oncol 18:416, 1990.

999. Neumann Y, Toren A, Rechavi G, et al. Vincristine treatment triggering the expression of asymptomatic Charcot-Marie-Tooth disease. Med Pediatr Oncol 1996;26:280–283.

1000. Shepherd DA, Steuber CP, Starling KA, et al. Accidental intrathecal administration of vincristine. Med Pediatr Oncol 1978;5:85–88.

1001. Slyter H, Liwnicz B, Herrick MK, et al. Fatal myeloencephalopathy caused by intrathecal vincristine. Neurology 1980;30:867–871.

1002. Gaidys WG, Dickerman JD, Walters CL, et al. Intrathecal vincristine. Report of a fatal case despite CNS washout. Cancer 1983;52:799–801.

1003. Bain PG, Lantos PL, Djurovic V, et al. Intrathecal vincristine: a fatal chemotherapeutic error with devastating central nervous system effects. J Neurol 1991;238:230–234.

1004. Fernandez CV, Esau R, Hamilton D, et al. Intrathecal vincristine: an analysis of reasons for recurrent fatal chemotherapeutic error with recommendations for prevention. J Pediatr Hematol Oncol 1998;20:587–590.

1005. Pommier YG, Fesen MR, Goldwasser F. Topoisomerase II inhibitors: the epipodophyllotoxins, m-AMSA, and the ellipticine derivatives. In: Chabner BA, Longo DL, eds. Cancer chemotherapy and biotherapy principles and practice. Philadelphia, PA: Lippincott-Raven, 1996:485–492.

1006. Brewer CF, Loike JD, Horwitz SB, et al. Conformational analysis of podophyllotoxin and its congeners: structure–activity relationship in microtubule assembly. J Med Chem 1979;22:215–221.

1007. Zijlstra JG, de Jong S, de Vries EGE, et al. Topoisomerases, new targets in cancer chemotherapy. Med Oncol Tumor Pharmacother 1990;7:11–18.

1008. Liu LF. DNA topoisomerase poisons as antitumor drugs. Annu Rev Biochem 1989;58:351–375.

1009. Yalowich JC, Goldman ID. Analysis of the inhibitory effects of VP-16-213 (etoposide) and podophyllotoxin on thymidine transport and metabolism in Ehrlich ascites tumor cells in vitro. Cancer Res 1984;44:984–989.

1010. van Maanen JMS, Retel J, de Vries J, et al. Mechanism of action of antitumor drug etoposide: a review. J Natl Cancer Inst 1988;80:1526–1533.

1011. Ross W, Rowe T, Glisson B, et al. Role of topoisomerase II in mediating epipodophyllotoxin-induced DNA cleavage. Cancer Res 1984;44:5857–5860.

1012. Long BH. Mechanisms of action of teniposide (VM-26) and comparison with etoposide (VP-16). Semin Oncol 1992;19(Suppl 6):3–19.

1013. O'Dwyer PJ, Alonso MT, Leyland-Jones B, et al. Teniposide: a review of 12 years of experience. Cancer Treat Rep 1984;68:1455–1466.

1014. O'Dwyer PJ, Leyland-Jones B, Alonso MT, et al. Etoposide (VP-16-213): current status of an active anticancer drug. N Engl J Med 1985;312:692–700.

1015. Schmoll H. Review of etoposide single-agent activity. Cancer Treat Rev 1982;9(Suppl):21–30.

1016. Schacter LP, Igwemezie LN, Seyedsadr M, et al. Clinical and pharmacokinetic overview of parenteral etoposide phosphate. Cancer Chemother Pharmacol 1994;34(Suppl):S58–S63.

1017. Thompson DS, Greco A, Miller AA, et al. A phase I study of etoposide phosphate administered as a daily 30-minute infusion for 5-days. Clin Pharmacol Ther 1995;57:499–507.

1018. Kaul S, Igwemezie LN, Stewart DJ, et al. Pharmacokinetics and bioequivalence of etoposide following intravenous administration of etoposide phosphate and etoposide in patients with solid tumors. J Clin Oncol 1995;13:2835–2841.

1019. Greco FA, Johnson DH, Hainsworth JD. Chronic oral etoposide. Cancer 1991;67:303–309.

1020. Greco FA. Chronic etoposide administration: overview of clinical experience. Cancer Treat Rev 1993;19(Suppl C):35–45.

1021. Cavalli F, Sonntag RW, Jungi F, et al. VP-16-213 monotherapy for remission induction of small cell lung cancer: a randomized trial using three dosage schedules. Cancer Treat Rep 1978;62:473–475.

1022. Henwood JM, Brogden RN. Etoposide: a review of its pharmacodynamic and pharmacokinetic properties, and therapeutic potential in combination chemotherapy of cancer. Drugs 1990;39:438–490.

1023. Slevin ML, Clark PI, Joel SP, et al. A randomized trial to evaluate the effect of schedule on the activity of etoposide in small-cell lung cancer. J Clin Oncol 1989;7:1333–1340.

1024. Johnson DH, Greco FA, Strupp J, et al. Prolonged administration of oral etoposide in patients with relapsed or refractory small-cell lung cancer: a phase II trial. J Clin Oncol 1990;8:1613–1617.

1025. McLeod HL, Evans WE. Clinical pharmacokinetics and pharmacodynamics of epipodophyllotoxins. Cancer Surv 1993;17:253–268.

1026. Miller AA, Herndon JE, Hollis DR, et al. Schedule dependency of 21-day oral versus 3-day intravenous etoposide in combination with intravenous cisplatin in extensive-stage small-cell lung cancer: a randomized phase III study of the Cancer and Leukemia Group B. J Clin Oncol 1995;13:1871–1879.

1027. Mathew P, Ribeiro RC, Sonnichsen D, et al. Phase I study of oral etoposide in children with refractory solid tumors. J Clin Oncol 1994;12:1452–1457.

1028. Kellie SJ, Crist WM, Pui C-H, et al. Hypersensitivity reactions to epipodophyllotoxins in children with acute lymphoblastic leukemia. Cancer 1991;67:1070–1075.

1029. Weiss RB, Bruno S. Hypersensitivity reactions to cancer chemotherapeutic agents. Ann Intern Med 1981;94:66–72.

1030. de Vries EG, Mulder NH, Postmus PE, et al. High-dose teniposide for refractory malignancies: a phase I study. Cancer Treat Rep 1986;70:595–598.

1031. Whitlock JA, Greer JP, Lukens JN. Epipodophyllotoxin-related leukemia. Cancer 1991;68:600–604.

1032. Winick NJ, McKenna RW, Shuster JJ, et al. Secondary acute leukemia in children with acute lymphoblastic leukemia treated with etoposide. J Clin Oncol 1993;11:209–217.

1033. Pui C-H, Behm FG, Raimondi SC, et al. Secondary acute myeloid leukemia in children treated for acute lymphoid leukemia. N Engl J Med 1989;321:136–142.

1034. Smith MA, Rubinstein L, Ungerleider RS. Therapy-related acute myeloid leukemia following treatment with epipodophyllotoxins: estimating the risks. Med Pediatr Oncol 1994;23:86–98.

1035. Smith MA, Rubinstein L, Anderson JR, et al. Secondary leukemia or myelodysplastic syndrome after treatment with epipodophyllotoxins. J Clin Oncol 1999;17:569–577.

1036. Slevin ML. The clinical pharmacology of etoposide. Cancer 1991;67:319–329.

1037. McLeod HL, Evans WE. Epipodophyllotoxins. In: Grochow LB, Ames MM, eds. A clinician's guide to chemotherapy pharmacokinetics and pharmacodynamics. Baltimore, MD: Williams & Wilkins, 1998:259–287.

1038. Cunningham D, McTaggart L, Soupkop M, et al. Etoposide: a pharmacokinetic profile including an assessment of bioavailability. Med Oncol Tumor Pharmacother 1986;3:95–99.

1039. Stewart DJ, Nundy D, Maroun JA, et al. Bioavailability, pharmacokinetics, and clinical effects of an oral preparation of etoposide. Cancer Treat Rep 1985;69:269–273.

1040. Harvey VJ, Slevin ML, Joel SP, et al. Variable bioavailability following repeated oral doses of etoposide. Eur J Cancer Clin Oncol 1985;21:1315–1319.

1041. Smythe RD, Pfeffer M, Scalzo A, et al. Bioavailability and pharmacokinetics of etoposide (VP-16). Semin Oncol 1985;12(Suppl 1):48–51.

1042. Harvey VJ, Slevin ML, Joel SP, et al. The effect of dose on the bioavailability of oral etoposide. Cancer Chemother Pharmacol 1986;16:178–181.

1043. Slevin ML, Joel SP, Whomsley R, et al. The effect of dose on the bioavailability of oral etoposide: confirmation of a clinically relevant observation. Cancer Chemother Pharmacol 1989;24:329–331.

1044. Greco FA. Future directions for etoposide therapy. Cancer 1991;67:315–318.

1045. Hande KR, Krozely MG, Greco FA, et al. Bioavailability of low-dose oral etoposide. J Clin Oncol 1993;11:374–377.

1046. Sessa C, Zucchetti M, Cerny T, et al. Phase I clinical and pharmacokinetic study of oral etoposide phosphate. J Clin Oncol 1995;13:200–209.

1047. Splinter TAW, Holthuis JJM, Kok TC, et al. Absolute bioavailability and pharmacokinetics of oral teniposide. Semin Oncol 1992;19(Suppl 6):28–34.

1048. Evans WE, Sinkule JA, Crom WR, et al. Pharmacokinetics of VM26 and VP16 in children with cancer. In: First International Symposium on the Podophyllotoxins in Cancer Therapy. Southampton, England: Mead Johnson, July 8–9, 1981:51.

1049. Strife RJ, Jarrdine I, Colvin OM. Analysis of the anticancer drugs VP16-213 and VM-26 and their metabolites by high-performance liquid chromatography. J Chromatogr 1980;182:211–220.

1050. Clark PI, Slevin ML. The clinical pharmacology of etoposide and teniposide. Clin Pharmacokinet 1987;12:223–252.

1051. Relling MV, Evans R, Dass C, et al. Human cytochrome P450 metabolism of teniposide and etoposide. J Pharmacol Exp Ther 1992;261:491–496.

1052. Zhuo X, Zheng N, Felix CA, et al. Kinetics and regulation of cytochrome P450-mediated etoposide metabolism. Drug Metab Dispos 2004;32:993–1000.

1053. Relling MV, McLeod HL, Bowman LC, et al. Etoposide pharmacokinetics and pharmacodynamics after acute and chronic exposure to cisplatin. Clin Pharmacol Ther 1994;56:503–511.

1054. Felix CA, Walker AH, Lange BJ, et al. Association of CYP3A4 genotype with treatment-related leukemia. Proc Natl Acad Sci U S A 1998;95:13176–13181.

1055. Allen LM, Creaven PJ. Comparison of the human pharmacokinetics of VM-26 and VP-16, two antineoplastic epipodophyllotoxin glucopyranoside derivatives. Eur J Cancer 1975;11:697–707.

1056. Hande KR, Wedlund PJ, Noone RM, et al. Pharmacokinetics of high-dose etoposide (VP-16-213) administered to cancer patients. Cancer Res 1984;44:379–382.

1057. Holthuis J, Postmus P, Van Oort W, et al. Pharmacokinetics of high-dose etoposide (VP-16-213). Eur J Cancer Clin Oncol 1986;22:1149–1155.

1058. D'Incalci M, Rossi C, Sessa C, et al. Pharmacokinetics of teniposide in patients with ovarian cancer. Cancer Treat Rep 1985;69:73–77.

1059. Lowis SP, Pearson ADJ, Newell DR, et al. Etoposide pharmacokinetics in children: the development and prospective validation of a dosing equation. Cancer Res 1993; 53:4881–4889.

1060. Relling MV, Mahmoud HH, Pui C-H, et al. Etoposide achieves potentially cytotoxic concentrations in CSF of children with acute lymphoblastic leukemia. J Clin Oncol 1996;14:399–404.

1061. Rodman JH, Furman WL, Sunderland M, et al. Escalating teniposide systemic exposure to increase dose intensity for pediatric cancer patients. J Clin Oncol 1993; 11:287–293.

1062. Kishi S, Yang W, Boureau B, et al. Effects of prednisone and genetic polymorphisms on etoposide disposition in children with acute lymphoblastic leukemia. Blood 2004; 103:67–72.

1063. Lum BL, Kaubisch S, Yahanda AM, et al. Alteration of etoposide pharmacokinetics and pharmacodynamics by cyclosporine in a phase I trial to modulate multidrug resistance. J Clin Oncol 1992;10:1635–1642.

1064. Gigante M, Sorio R, Colussi AM, et al. Effect of cyclosporine on teniposide pharmacokinetics and pharmacodynamics in patients with renal cell cancer. Anticancer Drugs 1995;6:479–482.

1065. Bisogno G, Cowie F, Boddy A, et al. High-dose cyclosporin with etoposide—toxicity and pharmacokinetic interaction in children with solid tumours. Br J Cancer 1998;77:2304–2309.

1066. Baker DK, Relling MV, Pui C-H, et al. Increased teniposide clearance with concomitant anticonvulsant therapy. J Clin Oncol 1992;10:311–315.

1067. Rodman JH, Murry DJ, Madden T, et al. Altered etoposide pharmacokinetics and time to engraftment in pediatric patients undergoing autologous bone marrow transplantation. J Clin Oncol 1994;12:2390–2397.

1068. van de Poll ME, Relling MV, Schuetz EG, et al. The effect of atovaquone on etoposide pharmacokinetics in children with acute lymphoblastic leukemia. Cancer Chemother Pharmacol 2001;47:467–472.

1069. Newman EM, Doroshow JH, Forman SJ, et al. Pharmacokinetics of high-dose etoposide. Clin Pharmacol Ther 1988;43:561–564.

1070. Eksborg S, Soderhall S, Frostvik-Stolt M, et al. Plasma pharmacokinetics of etoposide (VP-16) after i.v. administration to children. Anticancer Drugs 2000;11:237–241.

1071. Boos J, Krümpelmann S, Schulze-Westoff P, et al. Steady-state levels and bone marrow toxicity of etoposide in children and infants: does etoposide require age-dependent dose calculations. J Clin Oncol 1995;13:2954–2960.

1072. Zheng N, Felix CA, Pang S, et al. Plasma etoposide catechol increases in pediatric patients undergoing multiple-day chemotherapy with etoposide. Clin Cancer Res 2004;10:2977–2985.

1073. Arbuck SG, Douglass HO, Crom WR, et al. Etoposide pharmacokinetics in patients with normal and abnormal organ function. J Clin Oncol 1986;4:1690–1695.

1074. D'Incalci M, Rossi C, Zucchetti M, et al. Pharmacokinetics of etoposide in patients with abnormal renal and hepatic function. Cancer Res 1986;46:2566–2571.

1075. Hande KR, Wolff SN, Greco FA, et al. Etoposide kinetics in patients with obstructive jaundice. J Clin Oncol 1990;8:1101–1108.

1076. Joel SP, Shah R, Clark PI, et al. Predicting etoposide toxicity: relationship to organ function and protein binding. J Clin Oncol 1996;14:257–267.

1077. Liu B, Earl HM, Poole CJ, et al. Etoposide protein binding. Cancer Chemother Pharmacol 1995;36:506–512.

1078. Nguyen L, Chatelut E, Chevreau C, et al. Population pharmacokinetics of total and unbound etoposide. Cancer Chemother Pharmacol 1998;41:125–132.

1079. Joel SP, Shah R, Slevin ML. Etoposide dosage and pharmacodynamics. Cancer Chemother Pharmacol 1994;34(Suppl):S69–S75.

1080. Liliemark E, Soderhal S, Sirzea F, et al. Higher in vivo protein binding of etoposide in children compared with adult cancer patients. Cancer Lett 1996;106:97–100.

1081. Ratain MJ, Mick R, Schilsky RL, et al. Pharmacologically based dosing of etoposide: a means of safely increasing dose intensity. J Clin Oncol 1991;9:1480–1486.

1082. Rodman JH, Sunderland M, Kavanagh RL, et al. Pharmacokinetics of continuous infusion of methotrexate and teniposide in pediatric cancer patients. Cancer Res 1990;50:4267–4271.

1083. Rodman JH, Abromowitch M, Sinkule JA, et al. Clinical pharmacodynamics of continuous infusion teniposide: systemic exposure as a determinant of response in a phase I trial. J Clin Oncol 1987;5:1007–1014.

1084. Lowis SP, Price L, Pearson AD, et al. A study of the feasibility and accuracy of pharmacokinetically guided etoposide dosing in children. Br J Cancer 1998;77:2318–2323.

1085. Miller AA, Tolley EA, Niell HB. Therapeutic drug monitoring of 21-day oral etoposide in patients with advanced non-small cell lung cancer. Clin Cancer Res 1998; 4:1705–1710.

1086. Perdaems N, Bachaud JM, Rouzaud P, et al. Relation between unbound plasma concentrations and toxicity in a prolonged oral etoposide schedule. Eur J Clin Pharmacol 1998;54:677–683.

1087. Takimoto CH, Arbuck SG. The camptothecins. In: Chabner BA, Longo DL, eds. Cancer chemotherapy and biotherapy principles and practice. Philadelphia, PA: Lippincott-Raven, 1996:463–484.

1088. Chabot GG. Clinical pharmacokinetics of irinotecan. Clin Pharmacokinet 1997;33:245–259.

1089. McLeod HL, Keith WN. Variation in topoisomerase I gene copy number as a mechanism for intrinsic drug sensitivity. Br J Cancer 1996;74:508–512.

1090. Saleem A, Ibrahim N, Patel M, et al. Mechanisms of resistance in a human cell line exposed to sequential topoisomerase poisoning. Cancer Res 1997;57:5100–5106.

1091. Gupta RS, Gupta R, Eng B, et al. Camptothecin-resistant mutants of Chinese hamster ovary cells containing a resistant form of topoisomerase I. Cancer Res 1988; 48:6404–6410.

1092. Benedetti P, Fiorani P, Capuani L, et al. Camptothecin resistance from a single mutation changing glycine 363 of human DNA topoisomerase I to cysteine. Cancer Res 1993;53:4343–4348.

1093. Chen ZS, Furukawa T, Sumizawa T, et al. ATP-dependent efflux of CPT-11 and SN-38 by the multidrug resistance protein (MRP) and its inhibition by PAK-104P. Mol Pharmacol 1999;55:921–928.

1094. Chu XY, Suzuki H, Ueda K, et al. Active efflux of CPT-11 and its metabolites in human KB-derived cell lines. J Pharmacol Exp Ther 1999;288:735–741.

1095. Hendricks CB, Rowinsky EK, Grochow LB, et al. Effect of P-glycoprotein expression on the accumulation and cytotoxicity of topotecan (SK&F 104864), a new camptothecin analogue. Cancer Res 1992;52:2268–2278.

1096. Pommier Y, Gupta M, Valenti M, et al. Cellular resistance to camptothecins. Ann N Y Acad Sci 1996;803:60–73.

1097. Kramer K, Kushner BH, Cheung NK. Oral topotecan for refractory and relapsed neuroblastoma: a retrospective analysis. J Pediatr Hematol Oncol 2003;25:601–605.

1098. Kretschmar CS, Kletzel M, Murray K, et al. Response to paclitaxel, topotecan, and topotecan-cyclophosphamide in children with untreated disseminated neuroblastoma treated in an upfront phase II investigational window: a pediatric oncology group study. J Clin Oncol 2004;22:4119–4126.

1099. Pappo AS, Lyden E, Breneman J, et al. Up-front window trial of topotecan in previously untreated children and adolescents with metastatic rhabdomyosarcoma: an intergroup rhabdomyosarcoma study. J Clin Oncol 2001;19:213–219.

1100. Lager JJ, Lyden ER, Anderson JR, et al. Pooled analysis of phase II window studies in children with contemporary high-risk metastatic rhabdomyosarcoma: a report from the Soft Tissue Sarcoma Committee of the Children's Oncology Group. J Clin Oncol 2006;24:3415–3422.

1101. Stewart CF, Iacono LC, Chintagumpala M, et al. Results of a phase II upfront window of pharmacokinetically guided topotecan in high-risk medulloblastoma and supratentorial primitive neuroectodermal tumor. J Clin Oncol 2004;22:3357–3365.

1102. Metzger ML, Stewart CF, Freeman BB III, et al. Topotecan is active against Wilms' tumor: results of a multi-institutional phase II study. J Clin Oncol 2007;25:3130–316.

1103. Seibel NL, Krailo M, Chen Z, et al. Upfront window trial of topotecan in previously untreated children and adolescents with poor prognosis metastatic osteosarcoma: Children's Cancer Group (CCG) 7943. Cancer 2007;109:1646–1653.

1104. Hawkins DS, Bradfield S, Whitlock JA, et al. Topotecan by 21-day continuous infusion in children with relapsed or refractory solid tumors: a Children's Oncology Group study. Pediatr Blood Cancer 2006;47:790–794.

1105. Blaney SM, Needle MN, Gillespie A, et al. Phase II trial of topotecan administered as 72-hour continuous infusion in children with refractory solid tumors: a collaborative Pediatric Branch, National Cancer Institute, and Children's Cancer Group Study. Clin Cancer Res 1998;4:357–360.

1106. Blaney SM, Phillips PC, Packer RJ, et al. Phase II evaluation of topotecan for pediatric central nervous system tumors. Cancer 1996;78:527–531.

1107. Wagner S, Erdlenbruch B, Langler A, et al. Oral topotecan in children with recurrent or progressive high-grade glioma: a Phase I/II study by the German Society for Pediatric Oncology and Hematology. Cancer 2004;100:1750–1757.

1108. Tubergen DG, Stewart CF, Pratt CB, et al. Phase I trial and pharmacokinetic and pharmacodynamics study of topotecan using a five-day course in children with refractory solid tumors: a Pediatric Oncology Group Study. J Pediatr Hematol Oncol 1996;18:352–361.

1109. Daw NC, Santana VM, Iacono LC, et al. Phase I and pharmacokinetic study of topotecan administered orally once daily for 5 days for 2 consecutive weeks to pediatric patients with refractory solid tumors. J Clin Oncol 2004;22:829–837.

1110. Saylors R, Stewart CF, Zamboni WC, et al. Phase I study of topotecan in combination with cyclophosphamide in pediatric patients with malignant solid tumors: a Pediatric Oncology Group study. J Clin Oncol 1998;16:945–952.

1111. Athale UH, Stewart C, Kuttesch JF, et al. Phase I study of combination topotecan and carboplatin in pediatric solid tumors. J Clin Oncol 2002;20:88–95.

1112. Gerrits CJH, Burris H, Schellens JH, et al. Oral topotecan given once or twice daily for ten days: a phase I pharmacology study in adult patients with solid tumors. Clin Cancer Res 1998;4:1153–1158.

1113. Blaney SM, Balis F, Cole D, et al. Pediatric phase I trial and pharmacokinetic study of topotecan administered as a 24-hour continuous infusion. Cancer Res 1993;43: 1032–1036.

1114. Pratt CB, Stewart C, Santana VM, et al. Phase I study of topotecan for pediatric patients with malignant solid tumors. J Clin Oncol 1994;12:539–543.

1115. Furman WL, Stewart CF, Kirstein M, et al. Protracted intermittent schedule of topotecan in children with refractory acute leukemia: a Pediatric Oncology Group study. J Clin Oncol 2002;20:1617–1624.

1116. Zamboni WC, Bowman LC, Tan M, et al. Interpatient variability in bioavailability of the intravenous formulation of topotecan given orally to children with recurrent solid tumors. Cancer Chemother Pharmacol 1999;43:454–460.

1117. Stewart CF, Zamboni WC, Crom WR, et al. Topoisomerase I interactive drugs in children with cancer. Invest New Drugs 1996;14:37–47.

1118. Stewart CF, Baker SD, Heideman RL, et al. Clinical pharmacodynamics of continuous infusion topotecan in children: systemic exposure predicts hematologic toxicity. J Clin Oncol 1994;12:1946–1954.

1119. Furman WL, Baker SD, Pratt CB, et al. Escalating systemic exposure to topotecan following a 120-hr continuous infusion in children with relapsed acute leukemia. J Clin Oncol 1996;14:1504–1511.

1120. O'Reilly S, Rowinsky EK, Slichenmyer W, et al. Phase I and pharmacologic study of topotecan in patients with impaired renal function. J Clin Oncol 1996;14:3062–3073.

1121. Rosing H, Herben VMM, van Gortel-van Zomeren DM, et al. Isolation and structural confirmation of N-desmethyl topotecan, a metabolite of topotecan. Cancer Chemother Pharmacol 1997;39:498–504.

1122. O'Reilly S, Rowinsky EK, Slichenmyer W, et al. Phase I and pharmacologic studies of topotecan in patients with impaired hepatic function. J Natl Cancer Inst 1996;88: 817–824.

1123. Blaney SM, Cole DE, Balis FM, et al. Plasma and cerebrospinal fluid pharmacokinetic study of topotecan in nonhuman primates. Cancer Res 1993;53:725–727.

1124. Blaney SM, Takimoto C, Murry DJ, et al. Plasma and cerebrospinal fluid pharmacokinetics of 9-aminocamptothecin (9-AC), irinotecan (CPT-11), and SN-38 in nonhuman primates. Cancer Chemother Pharmacol 1998;41:464–468.

1125. Zhuang Y, Fraga CH, Hubbard KE, et al. Topotecan central nervous system penetration is altered by a tyrosine kinase inhibitor. Cancer Res 2006;66:11305–11313.

1126. Gelderblom H, Loos WJ, Verweij J, et al. Topotecan lacks third space sequestration. Clin Cancer Res 2000;6:1288–1292.
1127. Dodds HM, Clarke SJ, Findlay M, et al. Clinical pharmacokinetics of the irinotecan metabolite 4-piperidinopiperidine and its possible clinical importance. Cancer Chemother Pharmacol 2000;45:9–14.
1128. Furman WL, Stewart CF, Poquette CA, et al. Direct translation of a protracted irinotecan schedule from a xenograft model to a phase I trial in children. J Clin Oncol 1999;17:1815–1824.
1129. Blaney S, Berg SL, Pratt C, et al. A phase I study of irinotecan in pediatric patients: a pediatric oncology group study. Clin Cancer Res 2001;7:32–37.
1130. Cosetti M, Wexler LH, Calleja E, et al. Irinotecan for pediatric solid tumors: the Memorial Sloan-Kettering experience. J Pediatr Hematol Oncol 2002;24:101–105.
1131. Katzenstein HM, Rigsby C, Shaw PH, et al. Novel therapeutic approaches in the treatment of children with hepatoblastoma. J Pediatr Hematol Oncol 2002;24:751–755.
1132. Turner CD, Gururangan S, Eastwood J, et al. Phase II study of irinotecan (CPT-11) in children with high-risk malignant brain tumors: the Duke experience. Neuro Oncol 2002;4:102–108.
1133. Vassal G, Couanet D, Stockdale E, et al. Phase II trial of irinotecan in children with relapsed or refractory rhabdomyosarcoma: a joint study of the French Society of Pediatric Oncology and the United Kingdom Children's Cancer Study Group. J Clin Oncol 2007;25:356–361.
1134. Pappo AS, Lyden E, Breitfeld P, et al. Two consecutive phase II window trials of irinotecan alone or in combination with vincristine for the treatment of metastatic rhabdomyosarcoma: the Children's Oncology Group. J Clin Oncol 2007;25: 362–369.
1135. Bomgaars LR, Bernstein M, Krailo M, et al. Phase II trial of irinotecan in children with refractory solid tumors: a Children's Oncology Group Study. J Clin Oncol 2007;25: 4622–4627.
1136. Vassal G, Doz F, Frappaz D, et al. A phase I study of irinotecan as a 3-week schedule in children with refractory or recurrent solid tumors. J Clin Oncol 2003;21:3844–3852.
1137. Mugishima H, Matsunaga T, Yagi K, et al. Phase I study of irinotecan in pediatric patients with malignant solid tumors. J Pediatr Hematol Oncol 2002;24:94–100.
1138. Bomgaars L, Kerr J, Berg S, et al. A phase I study of irinotecan administered on a weekly schedule in pediatric patients. Pediatr Blood Cancer 2006;46:50–55.
1139. Mascarenhas L, Lyden ER, Breitfeld PP, et al. Randomized phase II window study of two schedules of irinotecan (CPT-11) and vincristine (VCR) in rhabdomyosarcoma (RMS) at first relapse/disease progression [Meeting abstracts]. J Clin Oncol 2008; 26:10013.
1140. Rowinsky EK, Grochow LB, Ettinger DS, et al. Phase I and pharmacological study of the novel topoisomerase I inhibitor 7-ethyl-10-[4-(1-piperidino)-1-piperidino]carbonyloxycamptothecin (CPT-11) administered as a ninety-minute infusion every 3 weeks. Cancer Res 1994;54:427–436.
1141. Abigerges D, Armand J-P, Chabot GG, et al. Irinotecan (CPT-11) high-dose escalation using intensive high-dose loperamide to control diarrhea. J Natl Cancer Inst 1994;86:446–449.
1142. Negoro S, Fukuoka M, Masuda N, et al. Phase I study of weekly intravenous infusions of CPT-11, a new derivative of camptothecin, in the treatment of advanced non-small-cell lung cancer. J Natl Cancer Inst 1991;83:1164–1168.
1143. Drengler RL, Kuhn JG, Schaaf LJ, et al. Phase I and pharmacokinetic trial of oral irinotecan administered daily for 5 days every 3 weeks in patients with solid tumors. J Clin Oncol 1999;17:685–696.
1144. Chabot GG, Abigerges D, Catimel G, et al. Population pharmacokinetics and pharmacodynamics of irinotecan (CPT-11) and active metabolite SN-38 during phase I trials. Ann Oncol 1995;6:141–151.
1145. Ma MK, Zamboni WC, Radomski KM, et al. Pharmacokinetics of irinotecan and its metabolites SN-38 and APC in children with recurrent solid tumors after protracted low-dose irinotecan. Clin Cancer Res 2000;6:813–819.
1146. Ratain MJ. Insights into the pharmacokinetics and pharmacodynamics of irinotecan. Clin Cancer Res 2000;6:3393–3394.
1147. Gajjar A, Chintagumpala MM, Bowers DC, et al. Effect of intrapatient dosage escalation of irinotecan on its pharmacokinetics in pediatric patients who have high-grade gliomas and receive enzyme-inducing anticonvulsant therapy. Cancer 2003;97: 2374–2380.
1148. Crews KR, Stewart CF, Jones-Wallace D, et al. Altered irinotecan pharmacokinetics in pediatric high-grade glioma patients receiving enzyme-inducing anticonvulsant therapy. Clin Cancer Res 2002;8:2202–2209.
1149. Murry DJ, Cherrick I, Salama V, et al. Influence of phenytoin on the disposition of irinotecan: a case report. J Pediatr Hematol Oncol 2002;24:130–133.
1150. Prados MD, Yung WK, Jaeckle KA, et al. Phase 1 trial of irinotecan (CPT-11) in patients with recurrent malignant glioma: a North American Brain Tumor Consortium study. Neuro Oncol 2004;6:44–54.
1151. Iyer L, King CD, Roy SK, et al. Genetic predisposition to the metabolism of irinotecan: role of UGT1A1 in the glucuronidation of its active metabolite (SN-38) in human liver microsomes. J Clin Invest 1998;101:847–854.
1152. Wasserman E, Myara A, Lokiec F, et al. Severe CPT-11 toxicity in patients with Gilbert's syndrome: two case reports. Ann Oncol 1997;8:1049–1051.
1153. Kuhn J. Pharmacology of irinotecan. Oncology 1998;6:39–41.
1154. Innocenti F, Undevia SD, Iyer L, et al. Genetic variants in the UDP-glucuronosyltransferase 1A1 gene predict the risk of severe neutropenia of irinotecan. J Clin Oncol 2004;22:1382–1388.
1155. Gupta E, Lestingi TM, Mick R, et al. Metabolic fate of irinotecan in humans: correlation of glucuronidation with diarrhea. Cancer Res 1994;54:3723–3725.
1156. Ratain MJ. From bedside to bench to bedside to clinical practice: an odyssey with irinotecan. Clin Cancer Res 2006;12:1658–1660.
1157. Stewart CF, Panetta JC, O'Shaughnessy MA, et al. UGT1A1 promoter genotype correlates with SN-38 pharmacokinetics, but not severe toxicity in patients receiving low-dose irinotecan. J Clin Oncol 2007;25:2594–2600.
1158. Innocenti F, Kroetz DL, Schuetz E, et al. Comprehensive pharmacogenetic analysis of irinotecan neutropenia and pharmacokinetics. J Clin Oncol 2009;27:2604–2614.
1159. Kumar N. Taxol-induced polymerization of purified tubulin. Mechanism of action. J Biol Chem 1981;256:10435–10441.
1160. Horwitz SB. TAXOL (paclitaxel): mechanism of action. Ann Oncol 1994;5(Suppl 6):S3–S6.
1161. Rowinsky EK, Donehower RC. Paclitaxel (Taxol). New Engl J Med 1995;332: 1004–1014.
1162. Cabral F, Wible L, Brenner S, et al. Taxol-requiring mutant of Chinese hamster ovary cells with impaired mitotic spindle assembly. J Cell Biol 1983;97:30–39.
1163. Horwitz SB, Cohen D, Rao S, et al. Taxol: mechanisms of action and resistance. J Natl Cancer Inst Monogr 1993;15:55–61.
1164. Seibel NL, Reaman GH. New microtubular agents in pediatric oncology. Invest New Drugs 1996;14:49–54.
1165. Hurwitz CA, Strauss LC, Kepner J, et al. Paclitaxel for the treatment of progressive or recurrent childhood brain tumors: a pediatric oncology phase II study. J Pediatr Hematol Oncol 2001;23:277–281.
1166. Franklin JL, Seibel NL, Krailo M, et al. Phase 2 study of docetaxel in the treatment of childhood refractory acute leukemias: a Children's Oncology Group report. Pediatr Blood Cancer 2008;50:533–536.
1167. Zwerdling T, Krailo M, Monteleone P, et al. Phase II investigation of docetaxel in pediatric patients with recurrent solid tumors: a report from the Children's Oncology Group. Cancer 2006;106:1821–1828.
1168. Smith RE, Brown AM, Mamounas EP, et al. Randomized trial of 3-hour versus 24-hour infusion of high-dose paclitaxel in patients with metastatic or locally advanced breast cancer: National Surgical Adjuvant Breast and Bowel Project Protocol B-26. J Clin Oncol 1999;17:3403–3411.
1169. Eisenhauer EA, ten Bokkel Huinink WW, Swenerton KD, et al. European–Canadian randomized trial of paclitaxel in relapsed ovarian cancer: high-dose versus low-dose and long versus short infusion. J Clin Oncol 1994;12:2654–2666.
1170. Hurwitz CA, Relling MV, Weitman SD, et al. Phase I trial of paclitaxel in children with refractory solid tumors: a Pediatric Oncology Group Study. J Clin Oncol 1993; 11:2324–2329.
1171. Hayashi RJ, Blaney S, Sullivan J, et al. Phase 1 study of paclitaxel administered twice weekly to children with refractory solid tumors: a Pediatric Oncology Group study. J Pediatr Hematol Oncol 2003;25:539–542.
1172. Blaney SM, Seibel NL, O'Brien M, et al. Phase I trial of docetaxel administered as a 1-hour infusion in children with refractory solid tumors: a collaborative Pediatric Branch, National Cancer Institute and Children's Cancer Group trial. J Clin Oncol 1997;15:1538–1543.
1173. Seibel NL, Blaney SM, O'Brien M, et al. Phase I trial of docetaxel with filgrastim support in pediatric patients with refractory solid tumors: a collaborative Pediatric Oncology Branch, National Cancer Institute and Children's Cancer Group trial. Clin Cancer Res 1999;5:733–737.
1174. Sonnichsen DS, Hurwitz CA, Pratt CB, et al. Saturable pharmacokinetics and paclitaxel pharmacodynamics in children with solid tumors. J Clin Oncol 1994;12:532–538.
1175. Gianni L, Kearns CM, Giani A, et al. Nonlinear pharmacokinetics and metabolism of paclitaxel and its pharmacokinetic/pharmacodynamic relationships in humans. J Clin Oncol 1995;13:180–190.
1176. Sonnichsen DS, Relling MV. Paclitaxel and docetaxel. In: Grochow LB, Ames MM, eds. A clinician's guide to chemotherapy pharmacokinetics and pharmacodynamics. Baltimore, MD: Williams & Wilkins, 1998:375–394.
1177. Cresteil T, Monsarrat B, Alvinerie P, et al. Taxol metabolism by human liver microsomes: identification of cytochrome P450 isozymes involved in its biotransformation. Cancer Res 1994;54:386–392.
1178. Jamis-Dow CA, Klecker RW, Katki AG, et al. Metabolism of taxol by human and rat liver in vitro: a screen for drug interactions and interspecies differences. Cancer Chemother Pharmacol 1995;36:107–114.
1179. Rowinsky E. The taxanes: dosing and scheduling considerations. Oncology 1997;11(Suppl 2):7–19.
1180. Hirth J, Watkins PB, Strawderman M, et al. The effect of an individual's cytochrome CYP3A4 activity on docetaxel clearance. Clin Cancer Res 2000;6:1255–1258.
1181. Marre F, Sanderink GJ, de Sousa G, et al. Hepatic biotransformation of docetaxel (Taxotere) in vitro: involvement of the CYP3A subfamily in humans. Cancer Res 1996;56:1296–1302.
1182. Komoroski BJ, Parise RA, Egorin MJ, et al. Effect of the St. John's wort constituent hyperforin on docetaxel metabolism by human hepatocyte cultures. Clin Cancer Res 2005;11:6972–6979.
1183. Fetell MR, Grossman SA, Fisher JD, et al. Preirradiation paclitaxel in glioblastoma multiforme: efficacy, pharmacology, and drug interactions. New Approaches to Brain Tumor Therapy Central Nervous System Consortium. J Clin Oncol 1997;3:121–128.
1184. Chang SM, Kuhn JG, Rizzo J, et al. Phase I study of paclitaxel in patients with recurrent malignant glioma: a North American Brain Tumor Consortium report. J Clin Oncol 1998;16:2188–2194.
1185. Venook AP, Egorin MJ, Rosner GL, et al. Phase I and pharmacokinetic trial of paclitaxel in patients with hepatic dysfunction: cancer and leukemia group B 9264. J Clin Oncol 1998;16:1811–1819.
1186. Wilson WH, Berg SL, Bryant G, et al. Paclitaxel in doxorubicin-refractory or mitoxantrone-refractory breast cancer: a phase I/II trial of 96-hour infusion. J Clin Oncol 1994;12:1621–1629.
1187. Rowinsky EK, Wright M, Monsarrat B, et al. Clinical pharmacology and metabolism of TAXOL (paclitaxel): update 1993. Ann Oncol 1994;5(Suppl 6):S7–S16.
1188. Rowinsky EK, Eisenhauer EA, Chaudhry V, et al. Clinical toxicities encountered with paclitaxel (TAXOL®). Semin Oncol 1993;20:1–15.
1189. Perry JR, Warner E. Transient encephalopathy after paclitaxel (Taxol) infusion. Neurology 1996;46:1596–1599.
1190. Nieto Y, Cagnoni P, Bearman S, et al. Acute encephalopathy: a new toxicity associated with high-dose paclitaxel. Clin Cancer Res 1999;5:501–506.
1191. Webster LK, Crinis NA, Morton CG, et al. Plasma alcohol concentrations in patients following paclitaxel infusion. Cancer Chemother Pharmacol 1996;37:499–501.
1192. Wilson DB, Beck TM, Gundlach CA. Paclitaxel formulation as a cause of ethanol intoxication. Ann Pharmacother 1997;31:873–875.
1193. Geller JI, Wall D, Perentesis J, et al. Phase I study of paclitaxel with standard dose ifosfamide in children with refractory solid tumors: a Pediatric Oncology Group study (POG 9376). Pediatr Blood Cancer 2009;52:346–350.
1194. Weiss R, Donehower RC, Wiernik PH, et al. Hypersensitivity reactions from taxol. J Clin Oncol 1990;8:1263–1268.
1195. Woo MH, Relling MV, Sonnichsen DS, et al. Phase I targeted systemic exposure study of paclitaxel in children with refractory acute leukemia. Clin Cancer Res 1999; 5:543–549.
1196. Vukeja S, Baker WJ, Burris HA, et al. Pyridoxine therapy for palmar-plantar erythrodysesthesia associated with taxotere. J Natl Cancer Inst 1993;17:1432–1433.
1197. Semb KA, Aamdal S, Oian P. Capillary protein leak syndrome appears to explain fluid retention in cancer patients who receive docetaxel. J Clin Oncol 1998;16:3426–3432.
1198. Battafarano DF, Zimmerman GC, Older SA, et al. Docetaxel (taxotere) associated scleroderma-like changes of the lower extremities. Cancer 1995;76:110–115.
1199. Weinstein IB. Cancer. Addiction to oncogenes—the Achilles heal of cancer. Science 2002;297:63–64.

1200. Weinstein IB, Joe AK. Mechanisms of disease: oncogene addiction—a rationale for molecular targeting in cancer therapy. Nat Clin Pract Oncol 2006;3:448–457.

1201. Druker BJ, Talpaz M, Resta D, et al. Clinical efficacy and safety of an Abl specific tyrosine kinase inhibitor as targeted therapy for chronic myelogenous leukemia [abstract]. Blood 1999;94(Suppl 1):368a.

1202. Druker BJ, Talpaz M, Resta DJ, et al. Efficacy and safety of a specific inhibitor of the BCR-ABL tyrosine kinase in chronic myeloid leukemia. N Engl J Med 2001;344:1031–1037.

1203. Levis M, Tse KF, Smith BD, et al. A FLT3 tyrosine kinase inhibitor is selectively cytotoxic to acute myeloid leukemia blasts harboring FLT3 internal tandem duplication mutations. Blood 2001;98:885–887.

1204. George RE, Sanda T, Hanna M, et al. Activating mutations in ALK provide a therapeutic target in neuroblastoma. Nature 2008;455:975–978.

1205. Mosse YP, Laudenslager M, Longo L, et al. Identification of ALK as a major familial neuroblastoma predisposition gene. Nature 2008;455:930–935.

1206. Cao L, Yu Y, Darko I, et al. Addiction to elevated insulin-like growth factor I receptor and initial modulation of the AKT pathway define the responsiveness of rhabdomyosarcoma to the targeting antibody. Cancer Res 2008;68:8039–8048.

1207. Toretsky JA, Kalebic T, Blakesley V, et al. The insulin-like growth factor-I receptor is required for EWS/FLI-1 transformation of fibroblasts. J Biol Chem 1997;272:30822–30827.

1208. McCrudden KW, Hopkins B, Frischer J, et al. Anti-VEGF antibody in experimental hepatoblastoma: suppression of tumor growth and altered angiogenesis. J Pediatr Surg 2003;38:308–314; discussion 308–314.

1209. Rowe DH, Huang J, Kayton ML, et al. Anti-VEGF antibody suppresses primary tumor growth and metastasis in an experimental model of Wilms' tumor. J Pediatr Surg 2000;35:30–32; discussion 32–33.

1210. Kim ES, Serur A, Huang J, et al. Potent VEGF blockade causes regression of coopted vessels in a model of neuroblastoma. Proc Natl Acad Sci U S A 2002;99:11399–11404.

1211. Druker BJ. STI571 (Gleevec) as a paradigm for cancer therapy. Trends Mol Med 2002;8:S14–S18.

1212. Tuveson DA, Willis NA, Jacks T, et al. STI571 inactivation of the gastrointestinal stromal tumor c-KIT oncoprotein: biological and clinical implications. Oncogene 2001;20:5054–5058.

1213. Demetri GD, von Mehren M, Blanke CD, et al. Efficacy and safety of imatinib mesylate in advanced gastrointestinal stromal tumors. N Engl J Med 2002;347:472–480.

1214. Bozzi F, Tamborini E, Negri T, et al. Evidence for activation of KIT, PDGFRalpha, and PDGFRbeta receptors in the Ewing sarcoma family of tumors. Cancer 2007;109:1638–1645.

1215. Blandford MC, Barr FG, Lynch JC, et al. Rhabdomyosarcomas utilize developmental, myogenic growth factors for disease advantage: a report from the Children's Oncology Group. Pediatr Blood Cancer 2006;46:329–338.

1216. Kubo T, Piperdi S, Rosenblum J, et al. Platelet-derived growth factor receptor as a prognostic marker and a therapeutic target for imatinib mesylate therapy in osteosarcoma. Cancer 2008;112:2119–2129.

1217. Zhang PJ, Goldblum JR, Pawel BR, et al. PDGF-A, PDGF-Rbeta, TGFbeta3 and bone morphogenic protein-4 in desmoplastic small round cell tumors with EWS-WT1 gene fusion product and their role in stromal desmoplasia: an immunohistochemical study. Mod Pathol 2005;18:382–387.

1218. Tamborini E, Bonadiman L, Greco A, et al. Expression of ligand-activated KIT and platelet-derived growth factor receptor beta tyrosine kinase receptors in synovial sarcoma. Clin Cancer Res 2004;10:938–943.

1219. MacDonald TJ, Brown KM, LaFleur B, et al. Expression profiling of medulloblastoma: PDGFRA and the RAS/MAPK pathway as therapeutic targets for metastatic disease. Nat Genet 2001;29:143–152.

1220. Bond M, Bernstein ML, Pappo A, et al. A phase II study of imatinib mesylate in children with refractory or relapsed solid tumors: a Children's Oncology Group study. Pediatr Blood Cancer 2008;50:254–258.

1221. Volpe G, Panuzzo C, Ulisciani S, et al. Imatinib resistance in CML. Cancer Lett 2009;274:1–9.

1222. Weisberg E, Manley PW, Cowan-Jacob SW, et al. Second generation inhibitors of BCR-ABL for the treatment of imatinib-resistant chronic myeloid leukaemia. Nat Rev Cancer 2007;7:345–356.

1223. Champagne MA, Capdeville R, Krailo M, et al. Imatinib mesylate (STI571) for treatment of children with Philadelphia chromosome-positive leukemia: results from a Children's Oncology Group phase 1 study. Blood 2004;104:2655–2660.

1224. Gleevec® Full Prescribing Information. Novartis oncology 2010. http://www.pharma.us.novartis.com/product/pi/pdf/gleevec-tabs.pdf. Updated 2010. Accessed May 6, 2010.

1225. Peng B, Hayes M, Resta D, et al. Pharmacokinetics and pharmacodynamics of imatinib in a phase I trial with chronic myeloid leukemia patients. J Clin Oncol 2004;22:935–942.

1226. Menon-Andersen D, Mondick JT, Jayaraman B, et al. Population pharmacokinetics of imatinib mesylate and its metabolite in children and young adults. Cancer Chemother Pharmacol 2009;63:229–238.

1227. Dai H, Marbach P, Lemaire M, et al. Distribution of STI-571 to the brain is limited by P-glycoprotein-mediated efflux. J Pharmacol Exp Ther 2003;304:1085–1092.

1228. Neville K, Parise RA, Thompson P, et al. Plasma and cerebrospinal fluid pharmacokinetics of imatinib after administration to nonhuman primates. Clin Cancer Res 2004;10:2525–2529.

1229. Wolff NC, Richardson JA, Egorin M, et al. The CNS is a sanctuary for leukemic cells in mice receiving imatinib mesylate for Bcr/Abl-induced leukemia. Blood 2003;101:5010–5013.

1230. Gibbons J, Egorin MJ, Ramanathan RK, et al. Phase I and pharmacokinetic study of imatinib mesylate in patients with advanced malignancies and varying degrees of renal dysfunction: a study by the National Cancer Institute Organ Dysfunction Working Group. J Clin Oncol 2008;26:570–576.

1231. Ramanathan RK, Egorin MJ, Takimoto CH, et al. Phase I and pharmacokinetic study of imatinib mesylate in patients with advanced malignancies and varying degrees of liver dysfunction: a study by the National Cancer Institute Organ Dysfunction Working Group. J Clin Oncol 2008;26:563–569.

1232. Lombardo LJ, Lee FY, Chen P, et al. Discovery of N-(2-chloro-6-methyl-phenyl)-2-(6-(4-(2-hydroxyethyl)-piperazin-1-yl)-2-methylpyrimidin-4-ylamino)thiazole-5-carboxamide (BMS-354825), a dual Src/Abl kinase inhibitor with potent antitumor activity in preclinical assays. J Med Chem 2004;47:6658–6661.

1233. Shah NP, Tran C, Lee FY, et al. Overriding imatinib resistance with a novel ABL kinase inhibitor. Science 2004;305:399–401.

1234. Schittenhelm MM, Shiraga S, Schroeder A, et al. Dasatinib (BMS-354825), a dual SRC/ABL kinase inhibitor, inhibits the kinase activity of wild-type, juxtamembrane, and activation loop mutant KIT isoforms associated with human malignancies. Cancer Res 2006;66:473–481.

1235. Chang Q, Jorgensen C, Pawson T, et al. Effects of dasatinib on EphA2 receptor tyrosine kinase activity and downstream signalling in pancreatic cancer. Br J Cancer 2008;99:1074–1082.

1236. Chen Z, Lee FY, Bhalla KN, et al. Potent inhibition of platelet-derived growth factor-induced responses in vascular smooth muscle cells by BMS-354825 (dasatinib). Mol Pharmacol 2006;69:1527–1533.

1237. Aplenc R, Strauss LC, Shusterman S, et al. Pediatric phase I trial and pharmacokinetic (PK) study of dasatinib: a report from the Children's Oncology Group Phase I Consortium. J Clin Oncol 2008;26 (suppl 15):3591.

1238. Christopher LJ, Cui D, Wu C, et al. Metabolism and disposition of dasatinib after oral administration to humans. Drug Metab Dispos 2008;36:1357–1364.

1239. Shah NP, Kantarjian HM, Kim DW, et al. Intermittent target inhibition with dasatinib 100 mg once daily preserves efficacy and improves tolerability in imatinib-resistant and -intolerant chronic-phase chronic myeloid leukemia. J Clin Oncol 2008;26:3204–3212.

1240. Sprycel® Full Prescribing Information. Bristol-Myers Squibb Oncology. Available from: http://packageinserts.bms.com/pi/pi_sprycel.pdf. Updated 2010. Accessed May 6, 2010.

1241. Talpaz M, Shah NP, Kantarjian H, et al. Dasatinib in imatinib-resistant Philadelphia chromosome-positive leukemias. N Engl J Med 2006;354:2531–2541.

1242. Ferrara N. Molecular and biological properties of vascular endothelial growth factor. J Mol Med 1999;77:527–543.

1243. Pietras K, Sjoblom T, Rubin K, et al. PDGF receptors as cancer drug targets. Cancer Cell 2003;3:439–443.

1244. Presta LG, Chen H, O'Connor SJ, et al. Humanization of an anti-vascular endothelial growth factor monoclonal antibody for the therapy of solid tumors and other disorders. Cancer Res 1997;57:4593–4599.

1245. Hurwitz H, Fehrenbacher L, Novotny W, et al. Bevacizumab plus irinotecan, fluorouracil, and leucovorin for metastatic colorectal cancer. N Engl J Med 2004;350:2335–2342.

1246. Sandler A, Gray R, Perry MC, et al. Paclitaxel-carboplatin alone or with bevacizumab for non-small-cell lung cancer. N Engl J Med 2006;355:2542–2550.

1247. Miller K, Wang M, Gralow J, et al. Paclitaxel plus bevacizumab versus paclitaxel alone for metastatic breast cancer. N Engl J Med 2007;357:2666–2676.

1248. Saltz LB, Clarke S, Diaz-Rubio E, et al. Bevacizumab in combination with oxaliplatin-based chemotherapy as first-line therapy in metastatic colorectal cancer: a randomized phase III study. J Clin Oncol 2008;26:2013–2019.

1249. Gordon MS, Margolin K, Talpaz M, et al. Phase I safety and pharmacokinetic study of recombinant human anti-vascular endothelial growth factor in patients with advanced cancer. J Clin Oncol 2001;19:843–850.

1250. Lu JF, Bruno R, Eppler S, et al. Clinical pharmacokinetics of bevacizumab in patients with solid tumors. Cancer Chemother Pharmacol 2008;62:779–786.

1251. Glade Bender JL, Adamson PC, Reid JM, et al. Phase I trial and pharmacokinetic study of bevacizumab in pediatric patients with refractory solid tumors: a Children's Oncology Group Study. J Clin Oncol 2008;26:399–405.

1252. Mendel DB, Laird AD, Xin X, et al. In vivo antitumor activity of SU11248, a novel tyrosine kinase inhibitor targeting vascular endothelial growth factor and platelet-derived growth factor receptors: determination of a pharmacokinetic/pharmacodynamic relationship. Clin Cancer Res 2003;9:327–337.

1253. Motzer RJ, Hutson TE, Tomczak P, et al. Sunitinib versus interferon alfa in metastatic renal-cell carcinoma. N Engl J Med 2007;356:115–124.

1254. Demetri GD, van Oosterom AT, Garrett CR, et al. Efficacy and safety of sunitinib in patients with advanced gastrointestinal stromal tumour after failure of imatinib: a randomised controlled trial. Lancet 2006;368:1329–1338.

1255. Wilhelm SM, Adnane L, Newell P, et al. Preclinical overview of sorafenib, a multikinase inhibitor that targets both Raf and VEGF and PDGF receptor tyrosine kinase signaling. Mol Cancer Ther 2008;7:3129–3140.

1256. Escudier B, Eisen T, Stadler WM, et al. Sorafenib in advanced clear-cell renal-cell carcinoma. N Engl J Med 2007;356:125–134.

1257. Llovet JM, Ricci S, Mazzaferro V, et al. Sorafenib in advanced hepatocellular carcinoma. N Engl J Med 2008;359:378–390.

1258. Maris JM, Courtright J, Houghton PJ, et al. Initial testing (stage 1) of sunitinib by the pediatric preclinical testing program. Pediatr Blood Cancer 2008;51:42–48.

1259. Waguespack SG, Sherman SI, Williams MD, et al. The successful use of sorafenib to treat pediatric papillary thyroid carcinoma. Thyroid 2009;19:407–412.

1260. Janeway KA, Albritton KH, Van Den Abbeele AD, et al. Sunitinib treatment in pediatric patients with advanced GIST following failure of imatinib. Pediatr Blood Cancer 2009;52:767–771.

1261. Strumberg D, Richly H, Hilger RA, et al. Phase I clinical and pharmacokinetic study of the Novel Raf kinase and vascular endothelial growth factor receptor inhibitor BAY 43-9006 in patients with advanced refractory solid tumors. J Clin Oncol 2005;23:965–972.

1262. Flaherty KT, Schiller J, Schuchter LM, et al. A phase I trial of the oral, multikinase inhibitor sorafenib in combination with carboplatin and paclitaxel. Clin Cancer Res 2008;14:4836–4842.

1263. Clark JW, Eder JP, Ryan D, et al. Safety and pharmacokinetics of the dual action Raf kinase and vascular endothelial growth factor receptor inhibitor, BAY 43-9006, in patients with advanced, refractory solid tumors. Clin Cancer Res 2005;11:5472–5480.

1264. Faivre S, Delbaldo C, Vera K, et al. Safety, pharmacokinetic, and antitumor activity of SU11248, a novel oral multitarget tyrosine kinase inhibitor, in patients with cancer. J Clin Oncol 2006;24:25–35.

1265. Lathia C, Lettieri J, Cihon F, et al. Lack of effect of ketoconazole-mediated CYP3A inhibition on sorafenib clinical pharmacokinetics. Cancer Chemother Pharmacol 2006;57:685–692.

1266. Deeks ED, Keating GM. Sunitinib. Drugs 2006;66:2255–2266; discussion 2267–2268.

1267. Miller AA, Murry DJ, Owzar K, et al. Phase I and pharmacokinetic study of sorafenib in patients with hepatic or renal dysfunction: CALGB 60301. J Clin Oncol 2009;27:1800–1805.

1268. Escudier B, Lassau N, Angevin E, et al. Phase I trial of sorafenib in combination with IFN alpha-2a in patients with unresectable and/or metastatic renal cell carcinoma or malignant melanoma. Clin Cancer Res 2007;13:1801–1809.

1269. Rini BI, Tamaskar I, Shaheen P, et al. Hypothyroidism in patients with metastatic renal cell carcinoma treated with sunitinib. J Natl Cancer Inst 2007;99:81–83.

1270. Chu TF, Rupnick MA, Kerkela R, et al. Cardiotoxicity associated with tyrosine kinase inhibitor sunitinib. Lancet 2007;370:2011–2019.

1271. DuBois SG, Shusterman S, Ingle AM, et al. A pediatric phase I trial and pharmacokinetic (PK) study of sunitinib: a Children's Oncology Group Phase I Consortium study. J Clin Oncol 2008;26 (suppl 15):3561. ASCO Meeting Abstracts.

1272. Widemann BC, Fox E, Adamson PC, et al. Phase I study of sorafenib in children with refractory solid tumors: a Children's Oncology Group Phase I Consortium trial. J Clin Oncol 2009;27 (suppl 15):10012. ASCO Meeting Abstracts.
1273. Capdevila J, Elez E, Macarulla T, et al. Anti-epidermal growth factor receptor monoclonal antibodies in cancer treatment. Cancer Treat Rev 2009;35:354–363.
1274. Cunningham D, Humblet Y, Siena S, et al. Cetuximab monotherapy and cetuximab plus irinotecan in irinotecan-refractory metastatic colorectal cancer. N Engl J Med 2004;351:337–345.
1275. Bonner JA, Harari PM, Giralt J, et al. Radiotherapy plus cetuximab for squamous-cell carcinoma of the head and neck. N Engl J Med 2006;354:567–578.
1276. Lievre A, Bachet JB, Le Corre D, et al. KRAS mutation status is predictive of response to cetuximab therapy in colorectal cancer. Cancer Res 2006;66:3992–3995.
1277. Mendelsohn J, Baselga J. The EGF receptor family as targets for cancer therapy. Oncogene 2000;19:6550–6565.
1278. Baselga J, Pfister D, Cooper MR, et al. Phase I studies of anti-epidermal growth factor receptor chimeric antibody C225 alone and in combination with cisplatin. J Clin Oncol 2000;18:904–914.
1279. Tan AR, Moore DF, Hidalgo M, et al. Pharmacokinetics of cetuximab after administration of escalating single dosing and weekly fixed dosing in patients with solid tumors. Clin Cancer Res 2006;12:6517–6522.
1280. Trippett TM, Kuttesch J, Herzog C, et al. A phase I study of cetuximab and irinotecan in pediatric patients with refractory solid tumors. J Clin Oncol 2007;25 (suppl 18): 9547. ASCO Meeting Abstracts.
1281. Trippett TM, Herzog C, Whitlock JA, et al. Phase I and pharmacokinetic study of cetuximab and irinotecan in children with refractory solid tumors: a study of the pediatric oncology experimental therapeutic investigators' consortium. J Clin Oncol 2009;27:5102–5108.
1282. Barker AJ, Gibson KH, Grundy W, et al. Studies leading to the identification of ZD1839 (IRESSA): an orally active, selective epidermal growth factor receptor tyrosine kinase inhibitor targeted to the treatment of cancer. Bioorg Med Chem Lett 2001;11:1911–1914.
1283. Kris MG, Natale RB, Herbst RS, et al. Efficacy of gefitinib, an inhibitor of the epidermal growth factor receptor tyrosine kinase, in symptomatic patients with non-small cell lung cancer: a randomized trial. JAMA 2003;290:2149–2158.
1284. Fukuoka M, Yano S, Giaccone G, et al. Multi-institutional randomized phase II trial of gefitinib for previously treated patients with advanced non-small-cell lung cancer (The IDEAL 1 Trial) [corrected]. J Clin Oncol 2003;21:2237–2246.
1285. Lynch TJ, Bell DW, Sordella R, et al. Activating mutations in the epidermal growth factor receptor underlying responsiveness of non-small-cell lung cancer to gefitinib. N Engl J Med 2004;350:2129–2139.
1286. Tsao MS, Sakurada A, Cutz JC, et al. Erlotinib in lung cancer—molecular and clinical predictors of outcome. N Engl J Med 2005;353:133–144.
1287. Swaisland HC, Smith RP, Laight A, et al. Single-dose clinical pharmacokinetic studies of gefitinib. Clin Pharmacokinet 2005;44:1165–1177.
1288. Goss G, Hirte H, Miller WH Jr, et al. A phase I study of oral ZD 1839 given daily in patients with solid tumors: IND.122, a study of the Investigational New Drug Program of the National Cancer Institute of Canada Clinical Trials Group. Invest New Drugs 2005;23:147–155.
1289. Ranson M, Hammond LA, Ferry D, et al. ZD1839, a selective oral epidermal growth factor receptor-tyrosine kinase inhibitor, is well tolerated and active in patients with solid, malignant tumors: results of a phase I trial. J Clin Oncol 2002;20:2240–2250.
1290. Herbst RS, Maddox AM, Rothenberg ML, et al. Selective oral epidermal growth factor receptor tyrosine kinase inhibitor ZD1839 is generally well-tolerated and has activity in non-small-cell lung cancer and other solid tumors: results of a phase I trial. J Clin Oncol 2002;20:3815–3825.
1291. Daw NC, Furman WL, Stewart CF, et al. Phase I and pharmacokinetic study of gefitinib in children with refractory solid tumors: a Children's Oncology Group Study. J Clin Oncol 2005;23:6172–6180.
1292. Hidalgo M, Siu LL, Nemunaitis J, et al. Phase I and pharmacologic study of OSI-774, an epidermal growth factor receptor tyrosine kinase inhibitor, in patients with advanced solid malignancies. J Clin Oncol 2001;19:3267–3279.
1293. Lu JF, Eppler SM, Wolf J, et al. Clinical pharmacokinetics of erlotinib in patients with solid tumors and exposure-safety relationship in patients with non-small cell lung cancer. Clin Pharmacol Ther 2006;80:136–145.
1294. Baselga J, Rischin D, Ranson M, et al. Phase I safety, pharmacokinetic, and pharmacodynamic trial of ZD1839, a selective oral epidermal growth factor receptor tyrosine kinase inhibitor, in patients with five selected solid tumor types. J Clin Oncol 2002;20:4292–4302.
1295. Cohen MH, Williams GA, Sridhara R, et al. United States Food and Drug Administration Drug Approval summary: Gefitinib (ZD1839; Iressa) tablets. Clin Cancer Res 2004;10:1212–1218.
1296. Estlin EJ, Ronghe M, Burke GA, et al. The clinical and cellular pharmacology of vincristine, corticosteroids, L-asparaginase, anthracyclines and cyclophosphamide In relation to childhood acute lymphoblastic leukaemia. Br J Haematol 2000;110:780–790.
1297. Gaynon PS, Carrel AL. Glucocorticosteroid therapy in childhood acute lymphocytic leukemia. Adv Exp Med Biol 1999;457:593–605.
1298. Moalli PA, Rosen ST. Glucocorticoid receptors and resistance to glucocorticoids in hematologic malignancies. Leuk Lymphoma 1994;15:363–374.
1299. Srivastava D, Thompson EB. Two glucocorticoid binding sites on the human glucocorticoid receptor. Endocrinology 1990;127:1770–1778.
1300. Pickup ME. Clinical pharmacokinetics of prednisone and prednisolone. Clin Pharmacokinet 1979;4:111–128.
1301. Frey BM, Frey FJ. Clinical pharmacokinetics of prednisone and prednisolone. Clin Pharmacokinet 1990;19:126–146.
1302. Duggan DE, Yeh KC, Matalia N, et al. Bioavailability of oral dexamethasone. Clin Pharmacol Ther 1975;18:205–209.
1303. Green OC, Winter RJ, Kawahara FS, et al. Pharmacokinetic studies of prednisolone in children. J Pediatr 1978;93:299–303.
1304. Choonara I, Wheeldon J, Rayner P, et al. Pharmacokinetics of prednisolone in children acute lymphoblastic leukemia. Cancer Chemother Pharmacol 1989;23:392–394.
1305. Rose JQ, Nickelsen JA, Ellis EF, et al. Prednisolone disposition in steroid-dependent asthmatic children. J Allergy Immunol 1981;67:188–193.
1306. Richter O, Ern B, Reinhardt D, et al. Pharmacokinetics of dexamethasone in children. Pediatr Pharmacol 1983;3:329–337.
1307. Young MC, Cook N, Read GF, et al. The pharmacokinetics of low-dose dexamethasone in congenital adrenal hyperplasia. Eur J Clin Pharmacol 1989;37:75–77.
1308. Tsuei SE, Moore RG, Ashley JJ, et al. Disposition of synthetic glucocorticoids I: pharmacokinetics of dexamethasone in healthy adults. J Pharmacokinet Biopharm 1979;7: 249–264.
1309. Rose JQ, Yurchak AM, Jusko WJ. Dose-dependent pharmacokinetics of prednisone and prednisolone in man. J Pharmacokinet Biopharm 1981;9:389–405.
1310. Barth J, Damoiseaux M, Mollmann H, et al. Pharmacokinetics and pharmacodynamics of prednisolone after intravenous and oral administration. Int J Clin Pharmacol Ther Toxicol 1992;30:317–324.
1311. Melby JC. Clinical pharmacology of systemic corticosteroids. Annu Rev Pharmacol Toxicol 1977;17:511–527.
1312. Yang L, Panetta JC, Cai X, et al. Asparaginase may influence dexamethasone pharmacokinetics in acute lymphoblastic leukemia. J Clin Oncol 2008;26:1932–1939.
1313. Jones B, Freeman A, Shuster JJ, et al. Lower incidence of meningeal leukemia when prednisone is replaced by dexamethasone in the treatment of acute lymphocytic leukemia. Med Pediatr Oncol 1991;19:269–275.
1314. Balis FM, Lester CM, Chrousos GP, et al. Differences in cerebrospinal fluid penetration of corticosteroids: possible relationship to the prevention of meningeal leukemia. J Clin Oncol 1987;5:202–207.
1315. Nowak-Gottl U, Ahlke E, Fleischhack G, et al. Thromboembolic events in children with acute lymphoblastic leukemia (BFM protocols): prednisone versus dexamethasone administration. Blood 2003;101:2529–2533.
1316. Hurwitz CA, Silverman LB, Schorin MA, et al. Substituting dexamethasone for prednisone complicates remission induction in children with acute lymphoblastic leukemia. Cancer 2000;88:1964–1969.
1317. Mattano LA, Sather HN, Trigg ME, et al. Osteonecrosis as a complication of treating acute lymphoblastic leukemia in children: a report of the Children's Cancer Group. J Clin Oncol 2000;18:3262–3272.
1318. Burger B, Beier R, Zimmermann M, et al. Osteonecrosis: a treatment related toxicity in childhood acute lymphoblastic leukemia (ALL)—experiences from trial ALL-BFM 95. Pediatr Blood Cancer 2005;44:220–225.
1319. Niinimaki RA, Harila-Saari AH, Jartti AE, et al. High body mass index increases the risk for osteonecrosis in children with acute lymphoblastic leukemia. J Clin Oncol 2007;25:1498–1504.
1320. French D, Hamilton LH, Mattano LA Jr, et al. A PAI-1 (SERPINE1) polymorphism predicts osteonecrosis in children with acute lymphoblastic leukemia: a report from the Children's Oncology Group. Blood 2008;111:4496–4499.
1321. Zuurcher RM, Frey BM, Frey FJ. Impact of ketoconazole on the metabolism of prednisolone. Clin Pharmacol Ther 1989;45:366–372.
1322. Broome JD. Studies on the mechanism of tumor inhibition by L-asparaginase. Effects of the enzyme on asparagine levels in the blood, normal tissues and 6C3HED lymphoma of mice: differences in asparagine formation and utilization in asparaginase-sensitive and -resistant lymphoma cells. J Exp Med 1968;127:1055–1072.
1323. Kurtzberg J. L-Asparaginase. In: Holland J, Frei E, et al., eds. Cancer medicine. Baltimore, MD: Williams & Wilkins, 1997:1027–1034.
1324. Ettinger LJ, Kurtzberg J, Voute PA, et al. An open-label, multicenter study of polyethylene glycol-L-asparaginase for the treatment of acute lymphoblastic leukemia. Cancer 1995;75:1176–1181.
1325. Holcenberg J. Therapeutic model for asparaginase and glutaminase treatment. Clin Pharmacol Ther 1975;17:236.
1326. Muller HJ, Boos J. Use of L-asparaginase in childhood ALL. Crit Rev Oncol Hematol 1998;28:97–113.
1327. Ahlke E, Nowak-Gottl U, Schulze-Westhoff P, et al. Dose reduction of asparaginase under pharmacokinetic and pharmacodynamic control during induction therapy in children with acute lymphoblastic leukemia. Br J Haematol 1997;96:675–681.
1328. Vieira Pinheiro JP, Ahkle E, Nowak-Gottl U, et al. Pharmacokinetic dose adjustment of Erwinia asparaginase in protocol II of the paediatric ALL/NHL-BFM treatment protocols. Br J Haematol 1999;104:313–320.
1329. Avramis VI, Sencer S, Periclou AP, et al. A randomized comparison of native *Escherichia coli* asparaginase and polyethylene glycol conjugated asparaginase for treatment of children with newly diagnosed standard-risk acute lymphoblastic leukemia: a Children's Cancer Group study. Blood 2002;99:1986–1994.
1330. Sallan SE, Hitchcock-Bryan S, Gelber R, et al. Influence of intensive asparaginase in the treatment of childhood non-T-cell acute lymphoblastic leukemia. Cancer Res 1983;43:5601–5607.
1331. Amylon MD, Shyuster J, Pullen J, et al. Intensive high-dose asparaginase consolidation improves survival for pediatric patients with T cell acute lymphoblastic leukemia and advanced stage lymphoblastic lymphoma: a Pediatric Oncology Group study. Leukemia 1999;13:335–342.
1332. Appel IM, Kazemier KM, Boos J, et al. Pharmacokinetic, pharmacodynamic and intracellular effects of PEG-asparaginase in newly diagnosed childhood acute lymphoblastic leukemia: results from a single agent window study. Leukemia2008;22:1665–1679.
1333. Ohnuma T, Holland JF, Freeman A, et al. Biochemical and pharmacological studies with asparaginase in man. Cancer Res 1970;30:2297–2305.
1334. Asselin BL, Whitin JC, Coppola DJ, et al. Comparative pharmacokinetic studies of three asparaginase preparations. J Clin Oncol 1993;11:1780–1786.
1335. Douer D, Watkins K, Periclou L, et al. PEG-L-asparaginase: pharmacokinetics and clinical response in newly diagnosed adults with acute lymphoblastic leukemia. Blood 1997;90:334a.
1336. Avramis VI, Periclou P, Majlessipour F, et al. Population pharmacokinetics and pharmacodynamics of PEG-asparaginase in pediatric patients with acute lymphoblastic leukemia: CCG Study 1962. Blood 1999;94:295a.
1337. Berg SL, Balis FM, McCully CL, et al. Pharmacokinetics of PEG-L-asparaginase and plasma and cerebrospinal fluid L-asparagine concentrations in rhesus monkey. Cancer Chemother Pharmacol 1993;32:310–314.
1338. Woo MH, Hak LJ, Storm MC, et al. Cerebrospinal fluid asparagine concentrations after *Escherichia coli* asparaginase in children with acute lymphoblastic leukemia. J Clin Oncol 1999;17:1568–1573.
1339. Riccardi R, Holcenberg JS, Glaubiger DL, et al. L-Asparaginase pharmacokinetics and asparagine levels in cerebrospinal fluid of Rhesus monkeys and humans. Cancer Res 1981;41:4554–4558.
1340. Peterson RG, Handschumacher RE, Mitchell MS. Immunological responses to L-asparaginase. J Clin Invest 1971;50:1080–1089.
1341. Muller HJ, Loning L, Horn A, et al. Pegylated asparaginase (Oncaspar) in children with ALL: drug monitoring in reinduction according to the ALL/NHL-BFM 95 protocols. Br J Haematol 2000;110:379–384.
1342. Asselin BL. The three asparaginases. Comparative pharmacology and optimal use in childhood leukemia. Adv Exp Med Biol 1999;457:621–629.

1343. Abshire TC, Pollock BH, Billett AL, et al. Weekly polyethylene glycol conjugated L-asparaginase compared with biweekly dosing produces superior induction remission rates in childhood relapsed acute lymphoblastic leukemia: a Pediatric Oncology Group Study. Blood 2000;96:1709–1715.
1344. Armstrong JK, Hempel G, Koling S, et al. Antibody against poly(ethylene glycol) adversely affects PEG-asparaginase therapy in acute lymphoblastic leukemia patients. Cancer 2007;110:103–111.
1345. Oettgen HF, Stephenson PA, Schwartz MK, et al. Toxicity of *E. coli* L-asparaginase in man. Cancer 1970;25:253–278.
1346. Billet AL, Carls A, Gelber RD, et al. Allergic reactions to Erwinia asparaginase in children with acute lymphoblastic leukemia who had previous allergic reactions to *Escherichia coli* asparaginase. Cancer 1992;70:201–206.
1347. Andrew M, Brooker L, Mitchell L. Acquired antithrombin III deficiency secondary to asparaginase therapy in childhood acute lymphoblastic leukemia. Blood Coagul Fibrinolysis 1994;5(Suppl 1):S24–S36.
1348. Capizzi RL. Schedule-dependent synergism and antagonism between methotrexate and L-asparaginase. Biochem Pharmacol 1974;23:151–161.
1349. Tallman MS, Andersen JW, Schiffer CA, et al. All-trans-retinoic acid in acute promyelocytic leukemia. N Engl J Med 1997;337:1021–1028.
1350. Fenaux P, Chastang C, Chevret S, et al. A randomized comparison of all transretinoic acid (ATRA) followed by chemotherapy and ATRA plus chemotherapy and the role of maintenance therapy in newly diagnosed acute promyelocytic leukemia. The European APL Group. Blood 1999;94:1192–1200.
1351. Matthay KK, Villablanca JG, Seeger RC, et al. Treatment of high-risk neuroblastoma with intensive chemotherapy, radiotherapy, autologous bone marrow transplantation, and 13-*cis*-retinoic acid. N Engl J Med 1999;341:1165–1173.
1352. Gudas LJ. Retinoids and vertebrate development. J Biol Chem 1994;269: 15399–15402.
1353. Petkovich M, Brand NJ, Krust A, et al. A human retinoic acid receptor which belongs to the family of nuclear receptors. Nature 1987;330:444–450.
1354. Giguere V, Ong ES, Segui P, et al. Identification of a receptor for the morphogen retinoic acid. Nature 1987;330:624–629.
1355. Mangelsdorf DJ, Ong ES, Dyck JA, et al. Nuclear receptor that identifies a novel retinoic acid response pathway. Nature 1990;345:224–229.
1356. Mangelsdorf DJ, Umesono K, Kliewer SA, et al. A direct repeat in the cellular retinol-binding protein type II gene confers differential regulation by RXR and RAR. Cell 1991;66:555–561.
1357. Heyman RA, Mangelsdorf DJ, Dyck JA, et al. 9-*cis* retinoic acid is a high affinity ligand for the retinoid X receptor. Cell 1992;68:397–406.
1358. Finklestein JZ, Krailo MD, Lenarsky C, et al. 13-*cis*-retinoic acid (NSC 122758) in the treatment of children with metastatic neuroblastoma unresponsive to conventional chemotherapy: report from the Children's Cancer Study Group. Med Pediatr Oncol 1992;20:307–311.
1359. Matthay KK, Reynolds CP, Seeger RC, et al. Long-term results for children with high-risk neuroblastoma treated on a randomized trial of myeloablative therapy followed by 13-*cis*-retinoic acid: a Children's Oncology Group study. J Clin Oncol 2009;27:1007–1013.
1360. Huang ME, Ye YC, Chen SR, et al. Use of all-*trans* retinoic acid in the treatment of acute promyelocytic leukemia. Blood 1988;72:567–572.
1361. Huang ME, Huang ME, Ye YC, et al. Use of all-*trans* retinoic acid in the treatment of acute promyelocytic leukemia. Chung Hua I Hsueh Tsa Chih (Taipei) 1988;68: 131–133.
1362. Fenaux P, Chastang C, Chomienne C, et al. Treatment of newly diagnosed acute promyelocytic leukemia (APL) by all transretinoic acid (ATRA) combined with chemotherapy: the European experience. Leuk Lymphoma 1995;16:431–437.
1363. Tallman MS, Andersen JW, Schiffer CA, et al. All-*trans* retinoic acid in acute promyelocytic leukemia: long-term outcome and prognostic factor analysis from the North American Intergroup protocol. Blood 2002;100:4298–4302.
1364. de Botton S, Coiteux V, Chevret S, et al. Outcome of childhood acute promyelocytic leukemia with all-*trans*-retinoic acid and chemotherapy. J Clin Oncol 2004;22: 1404–1412.
1365. Fenaux P, Chevret S, Guerci A, et al. Long-term follow-up confirms the benefit of all-*trans* retinoic acid in acute promyelocytic leukemia. European APL group. Leukemia 2000;14:1371–1377.
1366. Tallmann MS. Curative therapeutic approaches to APL. Ann Hematol 2004;83(Suppl 1):S81–S82.
1367. Kerr IG, Lippman ME, Jenkins J, et al. Pharmacology of 13-*cis*-retinoic acid in humans. Cancer Res 1982;42:2069–2073.
1368. Meyskens FL Jr, Goodman GE, Alberts DS. 13-*Cis*-retinoic acid: pharmacology, toxicology, and clinical applications for the prevention and treatment of human cancer. Crit Rev Oncol Hematol 1985;3:75–101.
1369. Goodman GE, Einspahr JG, Alberts DS, et al. Pharmacokinetics of 13-*cis*-retinoic acid in patients with advanced cancer. Cancer Res 1982;42:2087–2091.
1370. Colburn WA, Vane FM, Shorter HJ. Pharmacokinetics of isotretinoin and its major blood metabolite following a single oral dose to man. Eur J Clin Pharmacol 1983;24: 689–694.
1371. Clamon G, Chabot GG, Valeriote F, et al. Phase I study and pharmacokinetics of weekly high-dose 13-*cis*-retinoic acid. Cancer Res 1985;45:1874–1878.
1372. Brazzell RK, Vane FM, Ehmann CW, et al. Pharmacokinetics of isotretinoin during repetitive dosing to patients. Eur J Clin Pharmacol 1983;24:695–702.
1373. Lucek RW, Colburn WA. Clinical pharmacokinetics of the retinoids. Clin Pharmacokinet 1985;10:38–62.
1374. Khan AA, Villablanca JG, Reynolds CP, et al. Pharmacokinetic studies of 13-*cis*-retinoic acid in pediatric patients with neuroblastoma following bone marrow transplantation. Cancer Chemother Pharmacol 1996;39:34–41.
1375. Villablanca JG, Khan AA, Avramis VI, et al. Phase I trial of 13-*cis*-retinoic acid in children with neuroblastoma following bone marrow transplantation. J Clin Oncol 1995;13:894–901.
1376. Adamson PC, Bailey J, Pluda J, et al. Pharmacokinetics of all-*trans*-retinoic acid administered on an intermittent schedule. J Clin Oncol 1995;13:1238–1241.
1377. Conley BA, Egorin MJ, Sridhara R, et al. Phase I clinical trial of all-*trans*-retinoic acid with correlation of its pharmacokinetics and pharmacodynamics. Cancer Chemother Pharmacol 1997;39:291–299.
1378. Lefebvre P, Thomas G, Gourmel B, et al. Pharmacokinetics of oral all-*trans* retinoic acid in patients with acute promyelocytic leukemia. Leukemia 1991;5:1054–1058.
1379. Muindi J, Frankel SR, Miller WH, Jr, et al. Continuous treatment with all-*trans* retinoic acid causes a progressive reduction in plasma drug concentrations: implications for relapse and retinoid "resistance" in patients with acute promyelocytic leukemia. Blood 1992;79:299–303.
1380. Adamson PC, Reaman G, Finklestein JZ, et al. Phase I trial and pharmacokinetic study of all-*trans*-retinoic acid administered on an intermittent schedule in combination with interferon-alpha2a in pediatric patients with refractory cancer. J Clin Oncol 1997;15:3330–3337.
1381. Smith MA, Adamson PC, Balis FM, et al. Phase I and pharmacokinetic evaluation of all-*trans*-retinoic acid in pediatric patients with cancer. J Clin Oncol 1992;10: 1666–1673.
1382. Muindi J, Frankel SR, Huselton C, et al. Clinical pharmacology of oral all-*trans* retinoic acid in patients with acute promyelocytic leukemia. Cancer Res 1992;52:2138–2142.
1383. Adamson PC. Clinical and pharmacokinetic studies of all-*trans*-retinoic acid in pediatric patients with cancer. Leukemia 1994;8:1813–1816.
1384. McSorley LC, Daly AK. Identification of human cytochrome P450 isoforms that contribute to all-*trans*-retinoic acid 4-hydroxylation. Biochem Pharmacol 2000;60:517–526.
1385. White JA, Beckett-Jones B, Guo YD, et al. cDNA cloning of human retinoic acid-metabolizing enzyme (hP450RAI) identifies a novel family of cytochromes P450. J Biol Chem 1997;272:18538–18541.
1386. Ray WJ, Bain G, Yao M, et al. CYP26, a novel mammalian cytochrome P450, is induced by retinoic acid and defines a new family. J Biol Chem 1997;272:18702–18708.
1387. Haque M, Anreola F. The cloning and characterization of a novel cytochrome P450 family, CYP26, with specificity toward retinoic acid. Nutr Rev 1998;56:84–85.
1388. Ozpolat B, Mehta K, Tari AM, et al. all-*trans*-Retinoic acid-induced expression and regulation of retinoic acid 4-hydroxylase (CYP26) in human promyelocytic leukemia. Am J Hematol 2002;70:39–47.
1389. Lammer EJ, Chen DT, Hoar RM, et al. Retinoic acid embryopathy. N Engl J Med 1985;313:837–841.
1390. Coberly S, Lammer E, Alashari M. Retinoic acid embryopathy: case report and review of literature. Pediatr Pathol Lab Med 1996;16:823–836.
1391. Geelen JA. Hypervitaminosis A induced teratogenesis. CRC Crit Rev Toxicol 1979;6:351–375.
1392. Mitchell AA, Van Bennekom CM, Louik C. A pregnancy-prevention program in women of childbearing age receiving isotretinoin. N Engl J Med 1995;333:101–106.
1393. Accutane risk management program strengthened. FDA Consum 2002;36:8.
1394. Vahdat L, Maslak P, Miller WH Jr, et al. Early mortality and the retinoic acid syndrome in acute promyelocytic leukemia: impact of leukocytosis, low-dose chemotherapy, PMN/RAR-alpha isoform, and CD13 expression in patients treated with all-*trans* retinoic acid. Blood 1994;84:3843–3849.
1395. Frankel SR, Eardley A, Lauwers G, et al. The "retinoic acid syndrome" in acute promyelocytic leukemia. Ann Intern Med 1992;117:292–296.
1396. Fenaux P, De Botton S. Retinoic acid syndrome. Recognition, prevention and management. Drug Saf 1998;18:273–279.
1397. De Botton S, Dombret H, Sanz M, et al. Incidence, clinical features, and outcome of all-*trans*-retinoic acid syndrome in 413 cases of newly diagnosed acute promyelocytic leukemia. The European APL Group. Blood 1998;92:2712–2718.
1398. Zhu J, Chen Z, Lallemand-Breitenbach V, et al. How acute promyelocytic leukaemia revived arsenic. Nat Rev Cancer 2002;2:705–713.
1399. Wang ZY, Chen Z. Acute promyelocytic leukemia: from highly fatal to highly curable. Blood 2008;111:2505–2515.
1400. Chen GQ, Zhu J, Shi XG, et al. In vitro studies on cellular and molecular mechanisms of arsenic trioxide (As2O3) in the treatment of acute promyelocytic leukemia: As2O3 induces NB4 cell apoptosis with downregulation of Bcl-2 expression and modulation of PML-RAR alpha/PML proteins. Blood 1996;88:1052–1061.
1401. Chen GQ, Shi XG, Tang W, et al. Use of arsenic trioxide (As2O3) in the treatment of acute promyelocytic leukemia (APL): I. As2O3 exerts dose-dependent dual effects on APL cells. Blood 1997;89:3345–3353.
1402. Soignet SL, Maslak P, Wang ZG, et al. Complete remission after treatment of acute promyelocytic leukemia with arsenic trioxide [see comments]. N Engl J Med 1998;339:1341–1348.
1403. Shen ZX, Chen GQ, Ni JH, et al. Use of arsenic trioxide (As2O3) in the treatment of acute promyelocytic leukemia (APL): II. Clinical efficacy and pharmacokinetics in relapsed patients. Blood 1997;89:3354–3360.
1404. Soignet S, Frankel SR, Douer D, et al. United States multicenter study of arsenic trioxide in relapsed acute promyelocytic leukemia. J Clin Oncol 2001;19:3852–3860.
1405. Niu C, Yan H, Yu T, et al. Studies on treatment of acute promyelocytic leukemia with arsenic trioxide: remission induction, follow-up, and molecular monitoring in 11 newly diagnosed and 47 relapsed acute promyelocytic leukemia patients. Blood 1999; 94:3315–3324.
1406. Shen Z-X, Zhan-Zhong S, Fang J, et al. All trans retinoic acid/arsenic trioxide combination yields a high quality remission and survival in newly diagnosed acute promyelocytic leukemia. Proc Natl Acad Sci U S A 2004;101:5328–5335.
1407. Powell BL. Effect of consolidation with arsenic trioxide (As2O3) on event-free survival (EFS) and overall survival (OS) among patients with newly diagnosed acute promyelocytic leukemia (APL): North American Intergroup Protocol C9710. ASCO Meeting abstracts 25:2, 2007.
1408. Barbey J, Pessullo JC, Soignet SL. Effect of arsenic trioxide on QT intervalin patients with advanced malignancies. J Clin Oncol 2003;21:3609–3615.
1409. Camacho L, Soignet SL, Chanel S, et al. Leukocytosis and the retinoic acid syndrome in patients with acute promyelocytic leukemia treated with arsenic trioxide. J Clin Oncol 2000;18:2620–2625.
1410. Tallman M, Andersen JW, Schiffer CA, et al. Clinical description of 44 patients with acute promyelocytic leukemia who developed the retinoic acid syndrome. Blood 2000;95:90–95.
1411. George B, Mathews V, Poonkuzhali B, et al. Treatment of children with newly diagnosed acute promyelocytic leukemia with arsenic trioxide: a single center experience. Leukemia 2004;18:1587–1590.
1412. Fox E, Razzouk BI, Widemann BC, et al. Phase 1 trial and pharmacokinetic study of arsenic trioxide in children and adolescents with refractory or relapsed acute leukemia, including acute promyelocytic leukemia or lymphoma. Blood 2008;111:566–573.
1413. Del Razo LM, Styblo M, Cullen WR, et al. Determination of trivalent methylated arsenicals in biological matrices. Toxicol Appl Pharmacol 2001;174:282–293.
1414. Yoshino Y, Yuan B, Miyashita SI, et al. Speciation of arsenic trioxide metabolites in blood cells and plasma of a patient with acute promyelocytic leukemia. Anal Bioanal Chem 2009;393:689–697.
1415. Fujisawa S, Ohno R, Shigeno K, et al. Pharmacokinetics of arsenic species in Japanese patients with relapsed or refractory acute promyelocytic leukemia treated with arsenic trioxide. Cancer Chemother Pharmacol 2007;59:485–493.

1416. Patel M, Blaney SM, Balis FM. Pharmacokinetics of drug delivery to the central nervous system. In: Grochow LB, Ames MM, eds. A clinician's guide to chemotherapy pharmacokinetics and pharmacodynamics. 1st ed. Philadelphia, PA: Williams & Wilkins, 1998:67–90.

1417. Blaney SM, Balis FM, Poplack DG. Current pharmacological treatment approaches to central nervous system leukemia. Drugs 1991;41:702–716.

1418. Berg SL, Poplack DG. Advances in the treatment of meningeal cancers. Crit Rev Oncol Hematol 1995;20:87–98.

1419. Collins JM. Regional therapy: an overview. In: Poplack DG, Massimo L, Cornaglia-Ferraris P, eds. The role of pharmacology in pediatric oncology. Boston, MA: Martinus Nijhoff, 1987:125–135.

1420. Larson SM, Schall GL, DiChiro G. The influence of previous lumbar puncture and pneumoencephalography on the incidence of unsuccessful radioisotope cisternography. J Nucl Med 1971;12:555–557.

1421. Shapiro W, Young D, Metha G. Methotrexate: distribution in cerebrospinal fluid after intravenous, ventricular, and lumbar injections. N Engl J Med 1975;293:161–166.

1422. Blasberg RG, Patlak C, Fenstermacher JD. Intrathecal chemotherapy: brain tissue profiles after ventriculo-cisternal perfusion. J Pharmacol Exp Ther 1975;195:73–83.

1423. Blaney SM, Poplack DG, Godwin K, et al. Effect of body position on ventricular CSF methotrexate concentration following intralumbar administration. J Clin Oncol 1995;13:177–179.

1424. Ommaya AK. Implantable devices for chronic access and drug delivery to the central nervous system. Cancer Drug Deliv 1984;1:169–179.

1425. Bleyer WA, Poplack DG. Intraventricular versus intralumbar methotrexate for central nervous system leukemia: prolonged remission with the Ommaya reservoir. Med Pediatr Oncol 1979;6:207–213.

1426. Balis FM, Blaney SM, McCully C, et al. Methotrexate distribution within the subarachnoid space after intraventricular and intravenous administration. Cancer Chemother Pharmacol 2000;45:259–264.

1427. Moser AM, Adamson PC, Gillespie AJ, et al. Intraventricular concentration times time (CxT) methotrexate and cytarabine for patients with recurrent meningeal leukemia and lymphoma. Cancer 1999;85:511–516.

1428. Bernardi RJ, Bomgaars L, Fox E, et al. Phase I clinical trial of intrathecal gemcitabine in patients with neoplastic meningitis. Cancer Chemother Pharmacol 2008;62:355–361.

1429. Blaney SM, Berg SL, Krailo M, et al. Phase II clinical trial of intrathecal topotecan in children with leptomeningeal dissemination from medulloblastoma or an underlying solid or CNS tumor: a Children's Oncology Group Study. Nara, Japan: Presented at the International Society of Pediatric Neuro-Oncology, 2007.

1430. Bleyer WA, Drake JC, Chabner BA. Neurotoxicity and elevated cerebrospinal-fluid methotrexate concentration in meningeal leukemia. N Engl J Med 1973;289:770–773.

1431. Koh S, Nelson MDJ, Kovanlikaya A, et al. Anterior lumbosacral radiculopathy after intrathecal methotrexate treatment. Pediatr Neurol 1999;21:576–578.

1432. Poplack DG. Massive intrathecal overdose: "check the label twice." N Engl J Med 1984;311:400–402.

1433. O'Marcaigh AS, Johnson CM, Smithson WA, et al. Successful treatment of intrathecal methotrexate overdose by using ventriculolumbar perfusion and intrathecal instillation of carboxypeptidase G₂. Mayo Clin Proc 1996;71:161–165.

1434. Widemann BC, Balis FM, Shalabi A, et al. Treatment of accidental intrathecal methotrexate overdose with intrathecal carboxypeptidase G₂. J Natl Cancer Inst 2004;96:1557–1559.

1435. Bleyer WA, Poplack DG. Clinical studies on the central-nervous-system pharmacology of methotrexate. In: Pinedo HM, ed. Clinical pharmacology of anti-neoplastic drugs. Amsterdam, The Netherlands: Elsevier, 1978:115–131.

1436. Bleyer WA. Clinical pharmacology of intrathecal methotrexate II: an improved dosage regimen derived from age-related pharmacokinetics. Cancer Treat Rep 1977;61:1419–1425.

1437. Bleyer WA, Coccia PF, Sather HN, et al. Reduction in central nervous system leukemia with a pharmacokinetically derived intrathecal methotrexate dosage regimen. J Clin Oncol 1983;1:317–325.

1438. Zimm S, Collins JM, Miser J, et al. Cytosine arabinoside cerebrospinal fluid kinetics. Clin Pharmacol Ther 1984;35:826–830.

1439. Ho DHW. Distribution of kinase and deaminase of 1-b-D-arabinofuranosylcytosine in tissues of man and mouse. Cancer Res 1973;33:2816–2820.

1440. Bekassy AN, Liliemark J, Garwicz S, et al. Pharmacokinetics of cytosine arabinoside in cerebrospinal fluid and of its metabolite in leukemic cells. Med Pediatr Oncol 1990;18:136–142.

1441. Resar LMS, Phillips PC, Kastan MB, et al. Acute neurotoxicity after intrathecal cytosine arabinoside in two adolescents with acute lymphoblastic leukemia of B-cell type. Cancer 1993;71:117–123.

1442. Kim S, Chatelut E, Kim JC, et al. Extended CSF cytarabine exposure following intrathecal administration of DTC 101. J Clin Oncol 1993;11:2186–2193.

1443. Bomgaars L, Geyer JR, Franklin J, et al. Phase I trial of intrathecal liposomal cytarabine in children with neoplastic meningitis. J Clin Oncol 2004;22:3916–3921.

1444. Glantz MJ, Jaeckle KA, Chamberlain MC, et al. A randomized controlled trial comparing intrathecal sustained-release cytarabine (DepoCyt) to intrathecal methotrexate in patients with neoplastic meningitis from solid tumors. Clin Cancer Res 1999;5:3394–3402.

1445. Fisher PG, Kadan-Lottick NS, Korones DN. Intrathecal thiotepa: reappraisal of an established therapy. J Pediatr Hematol Oncol 2002;24:274–278.

1446. Grossman SA, Finkelstein JC, Ruckdeschel JC, et al. Randomized prospective comparison of intraventricular methotrexate and thiotepa in patients with previously untreated neoplastic meningitis. J Clin Oncol 1993;11:561–569.

1447. Strong JM, Collins JM, Lester C, et al. Pharmacokinetics of intraventricular and intravenous N,N',N?-triethylenethiophosphoramide (thiotepa) in Rhesus monkeys and humans. Cancer Res 1986;46:6101–6104.

1448. Nathan PC, Whitcomb T, Wolters PL, et al. Very high-dose methotrexate (33.6 g/m(2)) as central nervous system preventive therapy for childhood acute lymphoblastic leukemia: results of National Cancer Institute/Children's Cancer Group trials CCG-191P, CCG-134P and CCG-144P. Leuk Lymphoma 2006;47:2488–2504.

1449. Lopez JA, Nassif E, Vannicola P, et al. Central nervous system pharmacokinetics of high-dose cytosine arabinoside. J Neurooncol 1985;3:119–124.

1450. Morra E, Lazzarino M, Brusamolino E, et al. The role of systemic high-dose cytarabine in the treatment of central nervous system leukemia. Cancer 1993;72:439–445.

1451. Frick J, Ritch PS, Hansen RM, et al. Successful treatment of meningeal leukemia using systemic high-dose cytosine arabinoside. J Clin Oncol 1984;2:365–368.

1452. Frick JC, Hansen RM, Anderson T, et al. Successful high-dose intravenous cytarabine treatment of parenchymal brain involvement from malignant lymphoma. Ann Intern Med 1986;146:791–792.

1453. Allen JC, Helson L. High-dose cyclophosphamide chemotherapy for recurrent CNS tumors in children. J Neurosurg 1981;55:749–756.

CHAPTER 11 ■ MOLECULARLY TARGETED THERAPIES AND BIOTHERAPEUTICS

MALCOLM A. SMITH

INTRODUCTION

With the approval of the BCR-ABL inhibitor imatinib for the treatment of chronic myeloid leukemia (CML) by the Food and Drug Administration (FDA) on May 10, 2001, the era of molecularly targeted therapy for cancer had undeniably arrived. The remarkable remissions induced by this well-tolerated, orally administered agent in most patients with chronic phase CML raised hopes for a dramatic transformation in the way that cancer is treated. The principle that an agent targeted at the underlying molecular defect(s) of a particular cancer can have potent anticancer activity while producing minimal toxicity has powerful appeal. The activity of all-*trans*-retinoic acid previously demonstrated against acute promyelocytic leukemia supports the validity of this principle. Subsequent to the dramatic successes of imatinib for chronic phase CML, a number of other molecularly targeted agents have shown activity against specific cancers or molecularly defined subsets of patients within a given diagnosis, including epidermal growth factor receptor (EGFR) inhibitors for EGFR-mutated lung cancer, mammalian target of rapamycin (mTOR) inhibitors for mantle cell lymphoma, vascular endothelial growth factor (VEGF) pathway targeted agents against renal cell carcinoma, and HER2-targeted agents for HER2-amplified breast cancer (Table 11.1). These positive examples, however, are counterbalanced by the cautionary observation that many agents advertised as molecularly targeted agents have shown limited activity at tolerable doses and that there remain many cancers (including most pediatric cancers) for which no effective molecularly targeted agents have been identified.

A basic question is how to define "molecularly targeted agent." Identifying the cellular moiety that an agent targets qualifies an agent as "molecularly targeted" only in a tautological sense. By this criterion, most conventional cytotoxic agents can be considered molecularly targeted agents, as illustrated by the high potency with which Vinca alkaloids block tubulin assembly and with which epipodophyllotoxins inhibit topoisomerase II. Rather, the primary distinguishing characteristic of a successful molecularly targeted agent is the dramatic differential dependence of the cancer cell compared with normal cells upon the agent's target for growth and survival. As the degree of differential dependence between cancer cells and normal cells on a specific target or pathway may vary widely, there will be gradations in the extent to which targeted therapies are able to effectively eliminate cancer cells while causing little harm to normal cells.

The prioritization of molecularly targeted agents will differ between adult and pediatric cancers, in part because of the distinctive biology of cancers arising in children compared with those of adults. Another important distinction is that the primary therapeutic goal for childhood cancers is cure, not palliation, whereas for many adult cancers, sustained palliation is an important objective. For adults with cancer, cyto-static agents that slow down tumor growth for a year or two may be considered quite valuable if they can prolong survival while allowing acceptable quality of life. For children, achieving stable disease or delaying disease progression for a year or two is at best a modest success. This fundamental distinction between the relative benefit of cure versus palliation for adults and children with cancer has implications both in terms of cellular pathways targeted for intervention and in terms of the design of clinical trials to evaluate molecularly targeted agents in children. Given the goal of increasing cure rates through the use of molecularly targeted therapies, the identification of critical pathways that promote survival and block apoptosis for specific childhood cancers is a key step in selecting candidate agents for evaluation.

This chapter examines the potential applications of molecularly targeted agents in the treatment of childhood cancers. The chapter addresses general questions relevant to the development of these agents in children with cancer, noting important lessons learned from the development of molecularly targeted agents for adult indications. New technologies that have allowed an extraordinary expansion in the number of cellular targets that can be therapeutically addressed are described, and selected specific molecular targets and pathways with possible relevance to the treatment of childhood cancers are discussed. A key issue that pervades the chapter is the need for effective prioritization methods to determine which new agents should be introduced into the pediatric setting. The large numbers of molecularly targeted agents in development for adult cancers highlights the critical need to make wise decisions about which of these agents should be brought into phase 1 evaluation and then moved forward for phase 2 and 3 evaluations against specific childhood cancers.

BASIC PRINCIPLES FOR THE CLINICAL DEVELOPMENT OF MOLECULARLY TARGETED AGENTS

Identifying Childhood Cancer Therapeutic Targets

Tools for Target Identification

How can the signaling pathways most essential to survival for specific childhood cancers be elucidated? A key strategy for doing this is based on the premise that identification of the recurring genetic changes that occur in a given cancer (or subtype of that cancer) will highlight the gene products and the cellular pathways on which the cancer depends for its growth and survival. Oncogenes that are activated in cancer cells by mutation or by an increase in copy number and tumor

TABLE 11.1

FDA-APPROVED SMALL MOLECULE MOLECULARLY TARGETED AGENTS

Agent	Selected molecular target(s)	Indication
Imatinib	BCR-ABL, PDGFR, KIT	• Multiple indications for patients with Ph⁺ CML and ALL • MDS/MPD associated with PDGFR gene rearrangements • Aggressive systemic mastocytosis without the D816V c-Kit mutation or with c-Kit mutational status unknown • Hypereosinophilic syndrome and/or chronic eosinophilic leukemia with the FIP1L1-PDGFRα fusion kinase • Unresectable, recurrent, and/or metastatic dermatofibrosarcoma protuberans • Kit (CD117) positive GIST
Dasatinib	BCR-ABL, SRC family (SRC, LCK, YES, FYN), KIT, EPHA2, and PDGFR	• CML with resistance or intolerance to prior therapy including imatinib • (Ph + ALL with resistance or intolerance to prior therapy
Nilotinib	BCR-ABL, PDGFR	• Chronic phase and accelerated phase Ph⁺ CML in adult patients resistant to or intolerant to prior therapy that included imatinib
Sorafenib	CRAF, BRAF, KIT, FLT3, RET, VEGFR-1, 2, 3, and PDGFR	• Advanced renal cell carcinoma • Unresectable hepatocellular carcinoma
Sunitinib	PDGFR, VEGFR-1, 2, 3, KIT, FLT3, CSF-1R, and RET	• Advanced renal cell carcinoma • GIST after disease progression on or intolerance to imatinib mesylate
Everolimus	mTOR	• Advanced renal cell carcinoma after failure of treatment with sunitinib or sorafenib
Temsirolimus	mTOR	• Advanced renal cell carcinoma
Vorinostat	HDACs	• CTCL with progressive, persistent, or recurrent disease on or following two systemic therapies
Bortezomib	Proteasome	• Multiple myeloma • Mantle cell lymphoma with at least 1 prior therapy
Erlotinib	EGFR	• Locally advanced or metastatic NSCLC after failure of at least one prior chemotherapy regimen • First-line treatment of patients with locally advanced, unresectable, or metastatic pancreatic cancer, in combination with gemcitabine
Lapatinib	HER2	• Advanced or metastatic breast cancer with HER2 overexpression and with prior therapy including an anthracycline, a taxane, and trastuzumab

Abbreviations: CSF-1R, colony-stimulating factor receptor type 1; CTCL, cutaneous T-cell lymphoma; EGFR, epidermal growth factor receptor; FLT3, FMS-like tyrosine kinase-3; GISTs, gastrointestinal stromal tumors; HDACs, histone deacetylases; HER2, human epidermal receptor type 2; KIT, stem cell factor receptor; mTOR, mammalian target of rapamycin; MDS/MPD, myelodysplastic/myeloproliferative diseases; PDGFR, platelet-derived growth factor receptors; Ph⁺ CML and ALL, Philadelphia chromosome positive chronic myeloid leukemia and acute lymphoblastic leukemia; RET, Rearranged during transfection protooncogene; VEGFR 1, 2, 3, vascular endothelial growth factor receptors 1, 2, and 3.

suppressor genes that are inactivated by mutation or deletion are by definition genes that are important to that cancer. Based upon this premise, a priority for both childhood and adult cancers is comprehensively characterizing the gene expression profiles, the genomic status (in terms of copy number alterations and loss of heterozygosity [LOH]), the epigenetic status (in terms of patterns of promoter methylation), and the gene mutation status of large collections of specimens for a specific cancer diagnosis.

Gene expression profiling is a powerful research tool that can determine the proportion of tumors expressing the mRNA for potential cellular targets and can identify previously unsuspected targets expressed by a particular cancer type. For example, the widespread expression of FMS-like tyrosine

kinase-3 (FLT3) in childhood acute lymphoblastic leukemia (ALL) cases with MLL rearrangement was identified through gene expression profiling, leading to further investigation of FLT3 as a potential therapeutic target for this ALL subtype.[1] Expression profiling can also identify genes that classify subsets of patients with distinct outcomes or clinical characteristics, as exemplified by the identification of a gene expression signature that distinguishes between alveolar and embryonal rhabdomyosarcoma.[2] Particularly important for the identification of new molecular targets is the application of unsupervised clustering methods to identify novel biologically distinctive subsets within a single cancer diagnosis. Relevant examples include gene expression profiling of childhood T-cell ALL, which revealed clinically relevant molecular subtypes of this subset of ALL,[3] and profiling of medulloblastoma which identified distinctive subgroups that have distinctive patterns of gene mutations and chromosomal alterations.[4]

Copy number alterations and LOH can be identified using array-based approaches and are particularly useful in identifying increases in copy number of oncogenes (e.g., MYCN) as well as loss of tumor suppressor genes (e.g., CDKN2A and P53). High density arrays for DNA copy number analysis have provided important insights into the biology of childhood cancers, as exemplified by the identification of BRAF gain in juvenile pilocytic astrocytomas (JPAs).[5] The underlying molecular basis of the BRAF gain was shown to be a gene rearrangement producing tandem duplication of BRAF and resulting in a novel in-frame fusion gene incorporating the kinase domain of the BRAF oncogene.[6] Studies of DNA copy number alterations in pediatric B-precursor ALL identified the prognostic significance of deletions of IKZF1 (IKAROS) as well as the common occurrence of deletions of genes involved in B-cell development.[7,8]

DNA sequencing plays a key role in identifying candidate therapeutic targets, particularly through the identification of activating mutations in genes that drive cancer development. For example, the identification of activating Janus kinase (JAK) family mutations in a subset of B-precursor ALL cases with very high risk of treatment failure has obvious therapeutic implications given the availability of small molecule inhibitors, JAK kinases, that are being studied in the clinic for adult indications.[9,10] In a similar manner, the presence of activating anaplastic lymphoma kinase (ALK) mutations in approximately 10% of patients with high-risk neuroblastoma has driven pediatric clinical development of an ALK inhibitor.[11] Identification of inactivating mutations in tumor suppressor genes can also have important implications for prioritizing molecularly targeted agents for specific populations. For example, approximately 25% of cases of pediatric T-cell ALL have mutations in PTEN,[12] pointing toward the importance of phosphotidylinositol 3-kinase (PI3K)/AKT pathway activation for T-cell ALL.[13] Although the application of DNA sequencing to this point has been focused on a relatively small numbers of candidate genes, advances in sequencing technology will allow future applications to routinely utilize whole genome sequencing.[14] The anticipated sequencing of complete cancer genomes from hundreds of childhood cancer specimens in the coming 5 years will dramatically enhance understanding of the biology of these cancers and should markedly expand the pool of candidate therapeutic targets.

The methods described previously characterize the genome and transcriptome of cancer cells, but additional methods are required to evaluate the proteome, "the protein population of a cell, characterized in terms of localization, posttranslational modifications, interactions, and turnover, at any given time."[15] Of particular importance for targeted therapeutics development is the phosphoproteome, as the phosphorylation status of specific proteins in signaling cascades and networks controls key cellular processes, including metabolism, transcription, cell cycle progression, cytoskeletal rearrangement and cell movement, apoptosis, and differentiation.[16] The human genome codes for more than 500 kinases, which allow cells to rapidly modify the activity and stability of proteins through site-specific phosphorylation.[16] Because of their central role in cellular signal transduction pathways that are aberrantly activated in cancer cells and because of the relative ease with which small molecule inhibitors of their activity can be developed, kinases play a disproportionately large role in cancer drug development.

Monoclonal antibodies that recognize specific phosphorylation sites in proteins are important tools in evaluating the status of signaling pathways. Phosphospecific antibodies can be used to document the activation status of specific proteins using immunoblotting and immunohistochemical methods, as illustrated by the documentation of phospho-ALK in neuroblastoma cell lines containing activating ALK mutations.[11] Application of phosphospecific antibodies to tissue arrays is a particularly efficient way to define phosphorylation profiles of large numbers of clinical specimens, as illustrated by the use of tissue arrays to create a phosphorylation profile of kinases involved in the mTOR and PKC pathways for alveolar and embryonal rhabdomyosarcoma.[17] Phosphospecific muliparameter flow cytometry is an important tool for providing single cell activation state readouts for signaling pathways, both at baseline and following specific stimuli. This method was used to demonstrate a STAT5 signaling signature after exposure to suboptimal concentrations of granulocyte-macrophage colony-stimulating factor (GM-CSF) in samples from patients with juvenile myelomonocytic leukemia (JMML).[18]

The discovery that RNA interference (RNAi), an evolutionarily conserved gene silencing process, occurs in humans has dramatically enhanced the ability of researchers to identify and validate particular molecular targets and signaling pathways.[19] The utility of RNAi lies in its ability to efficiently and selectively silence a target gene through destruction of the gene's mRNA.[20] RNAi is mediated by double-stranded RNA (dsRNA) with sequence homology to the targeted mRNA. dsRNAs can be processed by cellular RNAses into small interfering RNAs (siRNAs) that are approximately 21 to 23 nucleotides long, and these are then incorporated into the RNA-induced silencing complex that recognizes and degrades homologous mRNA. For the purposes of target validation, siRNAs can be introduced into cells either through chemically synthesized short RNA duplexes or as plasmids or viral vectors that produce short hairpin RNAs with sequences complementary to the targeted gene.[19,21] RNAi may be applied for a particular gene of interest to determine the effect of knocking down expression of that gene on a particular biological endpoint.[19] For example, RNAi-mediated knockdown of the EWS/FLI-1 fusion protein correlated with decreased cell proliferation and increased apoptosis.[22,23] Of broader utility is the use of RNAi to perform genome-wide screens to identify previously unsuspected targets for therapeutic exploitation.[24,25]

Genome-wide RNAi screens are uniquely applicable to identifying synthetic lethal interactions, in which the presence of two mutations (neither of which is lethal alone) results in cell death.[26] The cancer drug development equivalent of synthetic lethal interactions is the targeted agent that is not toxic to normal cells but is toxic to cells with an activated oncogene or to cells with tumor suppressor gene deficiency.[27] A genome-wide RNAi screen to identify synthetic lethal interactions with the KRAS oncogene illustrates this point.[28] The screen identified a number of genes involved in the regulation of mitosis, including the mitotic kinase Polo-like kinase 1 (PLK1), as having a synthetic lethal relationship with KRAS, and a small molecule inhibitor of PLK1 (BI-2536) was active against KRAS-mutant colon cancer xenografts.[28]

Oncogene Addiction

The clinical success from pursuing a therapeutic target is dependent on the extent to which cancer cells are differentially dependent upon the activity of the target and its associated signaling pathways for survival and/or proliferation. The term "oncogene addiction" has been used to describe the dependence of cancer cells on specific activated or overexpressed oncogenes for the maintenance of their malignant phenotype,[29] while the term "tumor suppressor hypersensitivity" describes the dependence of the malignant phenotype on the continued silencing of specific tumor suppressor genes.[30]

One of the most direct predictors of whether a cancer cell is "addicted" to a particular protein or pathway for survival and/or proliferation is whether the cancer has activating mutations, increased copy number, or translocations in genes involving the pathway. The clinical efficacy of imatinib (an inhibitor of BCR-ABL, KIT, and platelet-derived growth factor receptor [PDGFR]) against BCR-ABL expressing CML,[31] gastrointestinal stromal tumors (GISTs) with KIT mutations,[32] and hematologic conditions with translocations that create fusion proteins that result in constitutive activation of either PDGFRα[33] or PDGFRβ[34] support the utility of targeting genes with activating mutations. The clinical activity of the hedgehog pathway inhibitor GDC-0449 in patients with advanced basal cell carcinoma,[35] a cancer characterized by activating mutations in the hedgehog pathway, is another example in which the presence of activating mutations predicts for oncogene addiction and clinical activity, as is the activity of the ALK inhibitor PF-02341066 in patients with non-small cell lung cancer (NSCLC) with the EML4-ALK translocation.[36] The modest activity observed to date for FLT3 inhibitors against acute myeloid leukemia (AML) with FLT3 activating mutations illustrates that not all mutations are equal in their ability to predict the clinical benefit that will derive from modulating a specific molecular target.[37]

Target Validation and *In Vitro* and *In Vivo* Testing

Although the presence of mutations, increased copy number, or translocations involving a gene are *a priori* evidence for the importance of the gene for a cancer, functional validation is required before accepting the gene product as a therapeutic target. This requires observing the effect of specifically inhibiting (or activating) the gene product of interest in relevant cancer cell lines and *in vivo* models. Various methods have been used to evaluate the therapeutic potential of modulating the activity of particular proteins or signaling pathways, including blocking antibodies (primarily applicable to protein receptors and their ligands), dominant negative mutants that interfere with function when overexpressed, genetic models in which the pathway's activity is either repressed or overexpressed, nucleic-based methods (e.g., RNAi) to downregulate protein expression, and chemical inhibitors. The example of the insulin-like growth factor I (IGF-I) receptor as a potential therapeutic target for Ewing's sarcoma and rhabdomyosarcoma illustrates how these methods have been applied in the pediatric setting. Data from experiments using blocking antibodies,[38,39] overexpression of a dominant negative IGF-I receptor (IGF-IR),[40,41] and cell lines derived from genetically engineered mice null for IGF-I receptor expression[42] support the validity of targeting IGF-I pathway signaling for these two pediatric cancers.

In vitro testing of candidate targeted agents against panels of molecularly characterized cancer cell lines can provide additional evidence for target specificity and relevance.[43] A hallmark of the *in vitro* sensitivity profile of molecularly targeted agents is that they show highly selective activity against cancer cell lines. As an example, an ALK kinase inhibitor was tested against a panel of 602 cancer cell lines, with most being largely refractory to treatment but with a small subset of lines (approximately 2%) displaying marked sensitivity.[43] The sensitive cell lines were highly enriched for neuroblastoma, anaplastic large cell lymphoma (ALCL), and NSCLC, cancer types now known to contain genomic alterations resulting in ALK activation. Sorafenib is an example of a multitargeted kinase that shows nanomolar range growth inhibition of cell lines that have activation of specific receptor tyrosine kinases, including FLT3, KIT, RET, and PDGFR and that also potently blocks VEGF-R2 signaling.[44] At much higher concentrations

(1 to 10 μM), sorafenib has broad activity against a range of adult cancer cell lines and pediatric cancer cell lines.[45] It is important to cautiously interpret claims of activity based on *in vitro* results using concentrations far in excess of those required to inhibit cell lines with known dependence upon the agent's target(s), as these observations may have limited clinical relevance due to nonspecific toxic effects that preclude achieving such high levels in the clinical setting.

Interpreting the clinical relevance of *in vitro* activity data must also take into consideration the drug concentrations that are achievable in the clinic. When *in vitro* activity requires 72- to 96-hour exposure to concentrations that can only be achieved for brief periods in the clinical setting (or not achieved at all), then skepticism about the presence of a therapeutic window for the agent is warranted. The extent of protein binding must also be considered when relating *in vitro* activity profiles (obtained in low serum conditions) to the clinical setting, as the free drug concentrations upon which activity is dependent will be much lower than measured blood levels for agents with very high levels of protein binding.

A final step in target validation is confirmation of antitumor activity in relevant *in vivo* models.[46] Although genetically engineered models have provided important insights into cancer biology, *in vivo* drug testing has primarily been performed using xenograft models. An exception to this generalization is the central role that genetic models of medulloblastoma heterozygous for Ptch1 have played in the development of hedgehog pathway inhibitors.[47–49] Xenograft models with specific genomic alterations (e.g., ALL xenografts with BCR-ABL, neuroblastoma xenografts with ALK mutations) can be especially useful in confirming the *in vivo* relevance of both therapeutic targets and of agents that block action of the targets. However, the reliability of xenograft models has been questioned,[50] leading to attempts to increase their predictive value, including the following: molecularly characterizing xenografts to confirm that they are biologically similar to the cancers that they are claimed to represent[51]; utilizing panels of xenografts for a given diagnosis to better reflect the clinical heterogeneity within the diagnosis[51–53]; utilizing xenografts established by direct transplantation into immunocompromised mice to reduce the selective pressures forced by the requirement of initial *in vitro* culture[54,55]; and ensuring that the systemic drug exposures at which activity is observed in preclinical models are comparable to those that are achievable in humans.[56] Another important factor in enhancing the predictive value of *in vivo* preclinical models for molecularly targeted agents is the use of clinically relevant criteria for claiming antitumor activity. It is common for reports of *in vivo* testing of new agents to claim activity for tumor growth delay, which in the clinical setting would be defined as progressive disease. Although this level of tumor response may be consistent with an agent's mechanism of action, in the childhood cancer setting in which cure is the primary objective, activity markers based on tumor regression rather than slowing of tumor growth are important to prioritize.

Systematic approaches to testing novel agents against pediatric preclinical models, such as that being employed by the Pediatric Preclinical Testing Program (PPTP), are important for the development of molecularly targeted agents. The PPTP has established a set of molecularly characterized cell lines and xenografts that represent common types of childhood cancers. Standard PPTP testing procedures involve testing novel agents against the 23 cell lines of its *in vitro* panel and against more than 40 solid tumor and ALL xenografts, with most childhood cancers represented by 4 to 8 xenografts. Activity signals have been observed for some targeted agents, including activity of the BCL-2 inhibitor ABT-263 against ALL xenografts and the activity of the Aurora A kinase inhibitor MLN-8237 against neuroblastoma xenografts.[57,58] Conversely, some targeted agents that are effective against adult cancers have limited activity against the PPTP's preclinical models.[59]

Discovering High Priority Combinations Involving Molecularly Targeted Agents

A reasonable assumption is that optimal benefit of molecularly targeted agents will require their use in combination with standard chemotherapy regimens or with other targeted agents. That said, it is important to realize that there are very few examples in which an agent that was ineffective as monotherapy succeeded when used in combination. The concept that a novel agent without activity as a single agent should be tested in combination with known effective agents or with other novel agents should be discouraged except in special situations, as this strategy will be unsuccessful unless the agent produces a change in cancer cells (but not normal cells) that allows other agents to exert their effect in a more potent way.

There are multiple molecular mechanisms by which drug combinations may result in synergistic, additive, or antagonistic effects.[60] An enormous challenge in oncology drug development is how to prioritize among the millions of potential two- or three-drug combinations that could potentially be studied using the hundreds of oncology agents in clinical development. RNAi screens can provide useful information to guide selection of combinations for further evaluation.[61] For example, RNAi chemosensitization screens can identify genes that when suppressed at the translational level sensitize cancer cells to chemotherapy agents, as illustrated by the use of such a screen to demonstrate that suppression of the PDK1 pathway sensitizes breast cancer cells to tamoxifen.[62]

In vitro testing can be used to identify drug combinations that include molecularly targeted agents for possible prioritization for clinical evaluation. As examples, agents that block BCL-2 family signaling potentiate the activity of a range of chemotherapy agents *in vitro*,[63] and mTOR inhibitors potentiate the activity of glucocorticoids against multiple ALL cell lines.[64,65] The cautionary note in assessing the clinical relevance of *in vitro* observations of potentiation or synergy is that these experiments provide no information about whether the potentiation is cancer cell specific. Clinical development of O6-benzylguanine, an agent that robustly potentiated the *in vitro* activity of nitrosoureas against glioblastoma cell lines,[66] illustrates this problem. The agent was unsuccessful in the clinic because it also potentiated the toxic effects of nitrosoureas on normal cells, requiring the use of lower doses of nitrosoureas and resulting in no net benefit.[67]

In vivo combination testing is particularly challenging. "Therapeutic synergy" (also known as "therapeutic enhancement") is a useful concept to apply for *in vivo* combination testing, with a positive claim for therapeutic synergy made when the antitumor effect of the combination is greater than the effect of either of the single agents used at their maximum tolerated doses (MTD).[65,68] Many published combination preclinical studies have failed to compare the combination effect with the effect of the individual agents administered at their MTD, PJ, Morton CL, Gorlick R et al. Stage 2 combination testing of rapamycin with cytotoxic agents by the Pediatric Preclinical Testing Program. Mol.Cancer Ther. 2010;9:101-112[69] which may be one reason for previous incorrect predictions of clinical activity for combinations in which a novel agent is added to a standard agent. In the clinical setting, combinations in which a novel agent is added to a standard agent often require substantial reductions in the dose of the standard agent. Experience with O6-benzylguanine illustrates this, as substantial reductions in nitrosourea dosing were required to safely administer nitrosoureas with O6-benzylguanine. The two-drug combinations using these lower doses of

the nitrosourea were no more effective than the nitrosourea used at its standard single-agent dose.[67,70] The therapeutic synergy concept directly addresses this concern in the preclinical setting by comparing the activity of the combination to the activity of the single agents at their MTD.

Identifying Appropriate Doses and Schedules of Molecularly Targeted Agents

Successful use of a molecularly targeted agent in the clinical setting implies that the activity of the target has been successfully inhibited or blocked by the agent, with the depth of inhibition and the duration of inhibition being sufficient to achieve the desired effect. The depth and duration of inhibition required for antitumor effect can be empirically determined in preclinical *in vivo* models in which pharmacodynamic measures of target inhibition are measured at selected time points following agent administration and correlated to antitumor activity. Pharmacokinetic correlates of antitumor activity can also be determined, so that clinical development of the agent can proceed with both pharmacodynamic and pharmacokinetic benchmarks that need to be met in early phase clinical trials for the agent.[71]

Practical and logistical issues complicate the approach of basing dosing decisions on target effects within tumor tissue.[72] Sequential tumor biopsies are needed to assess target modulation, with pretherapy and posttherapy sampling required. Intratumoral heterogeneity may produce differences between pre- and posttreatment tissues unrelated to agent effects, a factor that is exacerbated by the small size of tissue specimens often obtained with sequential biopsies.[73] Variability may also be introduced by the postexcision processing and storage of biopsy specimens, as changes in the status of signaling pathways in tumor specimens can occur quickly following loss of blood supply.[73] A final source of variability is that associated with the assay procedures themselves. As with any clinical laboratory procedure, obtaining interpretable data requires that issues such as assay sensitivity, specificity, precision, accuracy, and linearity be satisfactorily addressed. It is essential that laboratory methods be adequately studied and validated in preclinical models prior to their application in clinical trials to inform dosing decisions.[73]

Agent effects on surrogate tissues or on blood components may be used to inform dosing decisions. Some on-target effects on surrogate tissues may be clinically evaluable, such as the skin pigmentation changes caused by KIT inhibitors, the characteristic rash associated with EGFR inhibitors, and the rapid decrease in platelets that follows treatment with the BCL-2 inhibitor ABT-263.[74–76] Examples of changes in plasma proteins include the increase in VEGF that occur following treatment with small molecule inhibitors of VEGF-R2 and the compensatory increase in IGF-I and human growth hormone levels that follows administration of antibodies directed against the IGF-IR.[77–79] Both differences between tumor and surrogate tissue in extrinsic factors (e.g., degree of vascularization) and in intrinsic cellular factors (e.g., the activity of drug efflux pumps and other resistance mechanisms) may limit the correlation between surrogate and tumor tissue molecular response to the targeted agent.

The complexities described earlier illustrate the challenges in performing phase 1 studies with dose escalation based on biologic endpoints determined by testing tumor tissue. An argument can be made for developing a targeted agent utilizing the highest dose with acceptable toxicity.[80] Under the assumption that the effect of a targeted agent may plateau (but will not decrease) with increasing dose, this approach ensures that further testing of the agent will be performed at a dose with maximum activity and acceptable toxicity.[80] However, even when dosing decisions are based primarily on toxicity or agent effect on surrogate tissue, it is important to define within one or more adult patient populations the effect of the agent on its target in tumor tissue at the dose and schedule being brought forward for further clinical evaluation. Documenting that the agent consistently achieves its desired target effect in tumor tissue for at least some cancers enhances confidence in the decision to go forward with further clinical development of the agent.

Clinical Trials for Molecularly Targeted Agents in Children

Allowable Risk to Children in Clinical Research

The lessons learned from development of molecularly targeted agents in adults with cancer cannot be simply transferred to the pediatric setting.[81] Unlike adults considering research participation, younger children lack the capacity to decide whether they want to accept risks of harm in return for uncertain benefits or for the common good.[82] In recognition of this lack of capacity, children are afforded special protections from research risk under federal regulation 45 CFR § 46, Subpart D and the related FDA regulation 21 CFR §50, Subpart D. Subpart D defines allowable research based on the risk to subjects associated with the research components of the clinical trial, and it has a direct impact on how molecularly targeted agents can be developed for children with cancer. Children may participate in research that poses greater than minimal risk, but only if "the risk is justified by the anticipated benefit to the subject and the relationship of the risk to benefit is at least as favorable as any available alternative approach" [45 CFR §46.405 and 21 CFR §50.52]. Thus, children with cancer who have exhausted known effective therapy options may participate in phase 1 trials since they offer the potential for direct benefit.[83] However, tissue collection for correlative biological studies is generally performed for research purposes only and is therefore without the prospect of direct benefit. Subpart D stipulates that children with disorders or conditions may participate in research with "no prospect of direct benefit" to individual subjects provided: (a) the risk represents no more than a minor increase over minimal risk, (b) the intervention or procedure presents experiences to subjects that are reasonably commensurate with those inherent in their actual or expected medical setting, and (c) the intervention is likely to yield generalizable knowledge about the subject's disorder that is of vital importance for the understanding or amelioration of the subject's disorder [45 CFR §46.406 and 21 CFR §50.53]. Thus, the risks associated with procedures for collecting tissue for biological studies to evaluate the effects of a molecularly targeted agent in a child receiving the agent must be no greater than a minor increase over minimal risk to be approved under 45 CFR §46.406, effectively ruling out biopsy of solid tumors other than those with superficial locations.

How then should phase 1 studies of molecularly targeted agents be conducted in children? If a molecularly targeted agent studied in adults has a clear dose-limiting toxicity and further development of the agent is using a dose based on tolerability, then it is appropriate for the initial study in children to use the standard pediatric phase 1 design that calls for beginning at approximately 80% of the adult MTD and then escalating dose based on tolerability.[84] Pharmacokinetic data should be obtained to compare with data from adults and to compare with systemic exposures associated with activity in preclinical models (when available). For targeted agents for which an MTD was not defined in adults because of tolerability at doses that met target-effect endpoints or pharmacokinetic

parameter endpoints prior to reaching MTD, then dose escalation in the initial pediatric study can be minimized. The dose tolerated in adults can be studied as the initial dose, with perhaps exploration of one or two higher doses. Comparison of drug levels between children and adults at the tested dose levels can then allow selection of an appropriate dose for further evaluation in children. Another clinical scenario is that of molecularly targeted agents for which clinical development is primarily in combination with standard agents (e.g., the BCL-2 antisense oblimersen). Rather than conduct a phase 1 study of the targeted agent administered alone and then a second phase 1 study in which the targeted agent is used in combination with additional agents, a single phase 1 study of the targeted agent studied in combination with other agents can be performed. For such trials, it is helpful, when possible, to initially administer the agent alone in each patient to evaluate the toxicity and pharmacokinetics of the targeted agent in isolation, followed by administration of the agent in combination with other agents. Correct attribution of adverse events to a new agent that is added to a standard drug regimen can be difficult. This task is made easier when the standard regimen has a well-defined pattern of toxicity and when the new agent and the standard regimen have nonoverlapping toxicity profiles.

How can the effect of molecularly targeted agents on their target be evaluated, either directly or indirectly, in children? As noted earlier, sequential biopsies of tumor tissue will have limited applicability in children because of the research risks associated with biopsy procedures, and hence, alternative methods are required. An indirect estimate of effect can be achieved by targeting drug exposure levels associated with the desired level of tumor target modulation in preclinical models or in adults. This approach is analogous to that taken in the development of the topoisomerase I inhibitor irinotecan, in which systemic exposures of irinotecan associated with anticancer activity against pediatric xenografts were targeted in a phase 1 trial of irinotecan.[85] Achievement of the intended irinotecan serum concentrations in patients was associated with objective responses. Another indirect approach for assessing target modulation is to utilize surrogate tissues (e.g., skin, buccal mucosa, peripheral blood mononuclear cells) for evaluating the biological effects of agents. The caveats described previously for the use of surrogate tissues in adult clinical trials apply equally in the pediatric setting.

The biological effects of targeted agents on cancer cells in children can be directly studied in certain situations. Patients with leukemia provide the greatest opportunities for sequential evaluations of agent effects on cancer cells, given the relative ease with which either peripheral blood or bone marrow can be sampled. An approach taken in recent pediatric phase 1 trials is to add leukemia patients at the conclusion of the trial to receive the dose selected for phase 2 evaluation. The biological effect of the agent under study can then be evaluated by evaluation of pre- and posttreatment blood and/or bone marrow specimens. For patients with solid tumors, circulating cancer cells have been proposed as a potential resource for sequentially evaluating targeted agent effects.[86] Questions about the general applicability of this approach include whether sufficient numbers of circulating cancer cells can be collected to support the necessary laboratory testing and whether cancer cells circulating in the blood respond to treatment in the same way as do cancer cells within tumor masses.

Another approach for studying the effect of targeted agents on tumor tissue for children with solid tumors is to plan administration of the agent around the timing of a clinically indicated surgical procedure. Tumor tissue collected after administration of the agent for a defined period can be analyzed to determine the biological effects of the agent on the tumor. Given the risk to patients that would result from pretreatment tumor biopsies, comparison in most cases will need to be made to tumor tissues collected from patients not receiving the agent, rather than to tumor tissue from the same patient collected prior to treatment. A prerequisite for application of this design is convincing data that administration of the agent is unlikely to complicate either the surgical procedure or the recovery following surgery.

The application of molecular imaging methods, though to date limited, should become increasingly central to the development of molecularly targeted agents in children and may allow childhood cancer researchers to circumvent the inherent limitations resulting from restrictions on performing serial tumor biopsies in children. These imaging methods may allow researchers to sequentially monitor whether an agent had its intended biological effect on its target, and if so, how long this effect was maintained.

Toxicity Concerns for the Use of Molecularly Targeted Agents in Children

There are general issues about toxicities associated with molecularly targeted agents that apply to both adults and children. Although presentations touting the promise of molecularly targeted agents often include reference to their lack of toxicity, this perception does not match reality for many "molecularly targeted" agents. Although these agents often lack the myelosuppression and gastrointestinal toxicities associated with cytotoxic agents that target rapidly cycling cells, many of the agents induce significant mechanism-based adverse events that affect their clinical development. For example, Notch pathway inhibitors cause diarrhea as a result of the goblet cell hyperplasia that occurs when Notch signaling is blocked.[87] Inhibitors of BCL-X$_L$ cause a rapid onset thrombocytopenia as a result of the dependence of platelets on BCL-X$_L$ for survival in the circulation.[88,89] Cardiac toxicity has been associated with trastuzumab and with multitargeted receptor tyrosine kinases.[90] Thus, assumptions of lack of toxicity are misplaced for molecularly targeted agents, and as with conventional cytotoxic agents, the acute and long-term risks from their use will need to be carefully weighed against the evidence for their benefit.

The maxim that children are not simply young adults applies to the clinical development of molecularly targeted agents, just as it does during development of conventional cytotoxic agents. As with any therapeutic agent, children may tolerate molecularly targeted agents differently than adults because of age-related changes in physiology that result in pharmacokinetic differences between children and adults. In addition, molecularly targeted agents may specifically interfere with critical developmental pathways and block the progression from immature to mature adult tissues. For example, the central roles of the Wnt and Hedgehog signaling pathways in bone development will have to be considered as agents blocking these pathways enter clinical evaluation, a point that was emphasized by the permanent defects in bone structure in young mice caused by transient inhibition of the Hedgehog pathway.[91]

The effect of VEGF inhibitors on the growth of immature animals illustrates the distinctive challenges for the pediatric development of molecularly targeted agents.[92] Vascularization of cartilage in long bones is observed during three periods in the life of vertebrates: during late embryonic development, during periods of rapid growth in immature animals as capillary structures invade at the growth plate regions, and during adulthood when angiogenesis is activated for bone remodeling in response to bone injury or other pathologic conditions.[93] Both antibodies that sequester vascular VEGF and small molecule inhibitors of VEGF receptors produce a characteristic

effect on growth plates in immature mice and nonhuman primates.[92,94–98] In these animals, blood vessel invasion of growth plate cartilage is markedly suppressed, concomitant with impaired trabecular bone formation and marked expansion of the hypertrophic chondrocyte zone. Importantly, changes associated with relatively brief intervals of angiogenesis inhibition are reversible.[95,96,98] An infant with cutaneovisceral angiomatosis with thrombocytopenia syndrome receiving bevacizumab developed asymptomatic metaphyseal bone lesions that reversed following cessation of bevacizumab.[99] The limited clinical experience with VEGF pathway inhibitors in children with cancer has shown no evidence for bone effects, but this experience is insufficient, both in terms of the numbers of patients as well as their duration of treatment, to allow conclusions to be made about the impact of this class of agents on bone growth in children.[100,101]

How do the effects of antiangiogenic therapy on growth plates and the potential for detrimental effects on longitudinal bone growth affect development of this class of agents? Most importantly, these observations do not imply that antiangiogenic therapy must be avoided in the pediatric setting. The use of glucocorticoids in children provides a relevant pediatric experience for guiding the development of antiangiogenic agents and for avoiding unacceptable effects on growth. Glucocorticoids exert multiple growth-suppressing effects including interference with endocrine (e.g., endogenous growth hormone secretion) and bone formation processes essential for normal growth.[102,103] Despite the pronounced side effects of glucocorticoids on growth, a tailored approach to the dose, schedule, and duration of glucocorticoid treatment maximizes clinical benefit and minimizes as much as possible deleterious long-term effects. This tailored approach has allowed glucocorticoids to become essential components of the therapeutic armamentarium for a number of serious diseases of childhood. For antiangiogenic agents, it should likewise be possible to evaluate these agents for childhood cancer indications through the use of sequential carefully designed studies in which the potential risks and benefits are appropriately matched for the target study populations.

CLASSES OF MOLECULARLY TARGETED AGENTS

Monoclonal Antibody Approaches to Targeted Therapeutics

The technology for making monoclonal antibodies in mice was first described by Kohler and Milstein in 1975.[104] A 1987 editorial asked the question, "Will monoclonal antibodies find a place in our therapeutic armamentarium?"[105] This question has been answered resoundingly in the affirmative, as monoclonal antibodies are now approved for multiple cancer indications (Table 11.2). Early attempts at therapeutic application utilizing murine monoclonal antibodies were limited by the development of an immune response against the murine antibody.[106] This limitation has been overcome by technologic advances that allow more human-like antibodies (chimeric, humanized, or fully human) to be developed with relative ease against virtually any target antigen. A chimeric monoclonal antibody contains approximately 70% human sequences, with the murine components containing the variable domains responsible for binding to the antigen. Humanized monoclonal antibodies contain more than 90% human sequences, while fully human monoclonal antibodies contain all human sequences. Fully human monoclonal antibodies can be developed using genetically engineered mice with human antibody genes replacing the

TABLE 11.2

MONOCLONAL ANTIBODIES APPROVED BY FDA WITH CANCER-RELATED APPLICATIONS

Antibody generic name (Trade name)	Antigen target	Antibody type	Antibody arming	Disease target(s)	Year approved
Rituximab (Rituxan)	CD20	Chimeric IgG1	None	Non-Hodgkin lymphoma	1997
Trastuzumab (Herceptin)	HER2	Humanized IgG1	None	HER2 overexpressing breast cancer	1998
Gemtuzumab ozogamicin (Mylotarg)	CD33	Humanized IgG4	Calicheamicin	Acute myeloid leukemia	2000
Alemtuzumab (Campath)	CD52	Humanized IgG1	None	Chronic lymphocytic leukemia	2001
^{90}Y-labeled ibritumomab tiuxetan (Zevalin)	CD20	Murine IgG1	^{90}Yttrium	Non-Hodgkin lymphoma	2002
^{131}I-labeled tositumomab (Bexxar)	CD20	Murine IgG2a	^{131}Iodine	Non-Hodgkin lymphoma	2003
Cetuximab (Erbitux)	EGFR	Chimeric IgG1	None	Colorectal cancer SCC of the head and neck	2004 2006
Bevacizumab (Avastin)	VEGF	Humanized IgG1	None	Colorectal cancer NSCLC HER2-negative breast cancer Renal cell carcinoma Glioblastoma	2004 2006 2008 2009 2009
Panitumumab (Vectibix)	EGFR	Human IgG2	None	Colorectal cancer	2006
Ofatumumab (Arzerra)	CD20	Human IgG1	None	Chronic lymphocytic leukemia	2009

Abbreviations: EGFR, epidermal growth factor receptor; HER2, human epidermal receptor type 2; NSCLC, non-small cell lung cancer; SCC, squamous cell carcinoma; VEGF, vascular endothelial growth factor.

murine immunoglobulin genes[107–109] or by using fully human variable domains isolated from phage libraries and converted into complete monoclonal antibodies.[109,110]

After binding to their target antigen, monoclonal antibodies have multiple mechanisms by which they can exert an anticancer effect, including (a) antibody-dependent cell-mediated cytotoxicity (ADCC); (b) complement-dependent cytotoxicity (CDC) through generation of a membrane attack complex or through complement-dependent cellular toxicity; (c) interfering with ligand-receptor interactions, either through binding to the receptor on the cell surface or by binding to the ligand and thereby blocking its ability to interact with the receptor; and (d) modification of signaling pathways to produce apoptosis, as illustrated by agonist antibodies targeted to receptors for the tumor necrosis factor-related apoptosis-inducing ligand (TRAIL) receptors 1 and 2 (also known as DR4 and DR5, respectively) that induce apoptosis in sensitive cells. Monoclonal antibodies can also be conjugated with toxic substances (e.g., radionuclides and highly potent cytotoxic agents) for delivery of these agents to the cancer cell.[111] Some antibodies under clinical evaluation (e.g., rituximab and trastuzumab) are of the IgG1 and IgG3 isotypes and hence have the potential for initiating both ADCC and CDC, whereas other antibodies (e.g., panitumumab, an IgG2 antibody) have limited ability to initiate ADCC and CDC and must work through other mechanisms. The multiple potential mechanisms of action for monoclonal antibodies highlight the potential for differences in therapeutic benefit between small molecule inhibitors of cell surface proteins (e.g., growth factor receptors) and monoclonal antibodies that recognize the same proteins. Examples of specific antibody agents acting through the mechanisms described previously are discussed later.

Rituximab, a chimeric IgG1 monoclonal antibody directed against the B-cell surface antigen CD20, illustrates the multiple mechanisms by which a monoclonal antibody can kill cancer cells.[112] Rituximab was the first monoclonal antibody approved by FDA for a cancer indication, with early studies indicating activity against both indolent lymphomas and aggressive lymphomas in adults.[113] Clinical trials evaluating the addition of rituximab to standard chemotherapy have documented improved outcome for both indolent lymphomas and for aggressive lymphomas.[113] Although experience with rituximab is limited in children with non-Hodgkin lymphoma (NHL), its tolerability and activity appear to be similar to those observed for adults, both when used as a single agent and in combination with chemotherapy.[114,115] The molecular/cellular mechanisms by which rituximab effectively treats many patients with NHL remains controversial despite years of research. A role for complement-mediated lysis is indicated by the inability of rituximab to cure C1q-deficient mice[116] and by the diminished activity of rituximab in a complement-depleted lymphoma xenograft model.[117] Complement activation occurs in patients receiving rituximab and may be associated with the side effects associated with the first infusion,[118] and clinical response to rituximab is correlated with an *ex vivo* measure of CDC susceptibility.[119] ADCC also plays a role in rituximab's antitumor activity, as demonstrated by the reduction of rituximab effect in some murine aggressive lymphoma models when neutrophils or natural killer cells are depleted or when effector cell function is blocked by the absence of effector cell immunoglobulin Fc receptors.[120,121] The association of rituximab clinical response to a polymorphism in FcγRIIIa, an Fc receptor present on NK cells and monocytes, supports a role for ADCC in rituximab clinical activity.[122] Rituximab can additionally modulate signaling pathways that promote the balance between survival and apoptosis, which may explain the ability of rituximab to induce apoptosis and to enhance sensitivity to standard chemotherapy.[123–125]

Bevacizumab, which binds VEGF-A, is another monoclonal antibody that has demonstrated clinical benefit in adults with cancer, having FDA-approved indications for multiple cancer types, including advanced or metastatic colon cancer, NSCLC, breast cancer, renal cell carcinoma, and glioblastoma.[126] Bevacizumab illustrates how ligand binding monoclonal antibodies can potently block receptor protein-tyrosine kinase signaling, in the case of bevacizumab by binding to the ligand (VEGF-A) and preventing VEGF-A from interacting with VEGF-R2 to stimulate signaling required for angiogenesis.[127]

Other monoclonal antibodies that affect receptor protein-tyrosine kinase signaling do so by binding to the receptor protein-tyrosine kinases themselves. For example, the monoclonal antibodies, cetuximab and panitumumab, bind with high affinity to the EGFR, thereby blocking EGF from effectively interacting with the receptor to stimulate downstream signaling.[128,129] Antibody binding to EGFR also leads to rapid internalization of the receptor, further limiting receptor signaling.[129] Of greater relevance in the pediatric setting are the monoclonal antibodies against the insulin-like growth factor receptor 1 (IGF-IR) that have entered clinical evaluation.[130]

The toxicities associated with unmodified monoclonal antibodies can generally be attributed to the action of the antibody on normal cells expressing its target antigen. For example, EGFR-targeted antibodies induce a characteristic skin rash that is also seen with small molecule EGFR inhibitors.[131,132] Similarly, the severe pain that occurs in children with neuroblastoma receiving antibodies targeted at GD2 ganglioside can be attributed to expression of this antigen on nerve cells.[133,134] First dose reactions to antibodies can occur and can be severe, particularly for antibodies targeted at immune cells when large tumor burdens are present.[135,136] In the case of CD52-targeted alemtuzumab, these reactions require utilizing a low starting dose with escalation to the final dose over 1 to 2 weeks.[137]

The antitumor activity of monoclonal antibodies should be increased by interventions that enhance effector cell function, and numerous methods for achieving this have been evaluated in preclinical and clinical studies. One way to achieve increased ADCC is by priming effector cells for greater cytotoxicity through the use of cytokines such as GM-CSF, interleukin 2 (IL-2), and interleukin 12 (IL-12).[138] For example, GM-CSF and IL-2 enhance the *in vitro* antineuroblastoma activity of anti-GD2 monoclonal antibodies (e.g., 14G2a, 3F8, and ch14.18).[139–141] This observation has been used to develop treatment regimens combining anti-GD2 monoclonal antibodies with either GM-CSF[142,143] or IL-2,[144] or both agents.[145] The positive results from the phase 3 evaluation of ch14.18 plus cytokines (GM-CSF and IL-2) for children with high-risk neuroblastoma support the concept that cytokine stimulation of effector cell function can enhance the clinical activity of monoclonal antibodies.[146]

An alternative strategy for enhancing the effectiveness of therapeutic antibodies is through engineering the antibody Fc region to optimize affinity with Fcγ receptors (FcγR) present on immune effector cells.[147] One approach to achieving this is through amino acid engineering in which substitutions are made for specific amino acids in the Fc region that result in increased FcγR binding affinity and increased ADCC.[148] As an example, XmAb5574 is a CD19-targeted monoclonal antibody that has two amino acid substitutions that markedly increase FcγR binding and ADCC and *in vivo* activity compared with a comparable antibody with an unmodified Fc

region.[148,149] Increased ability to activate effector cells can also be achieved through glycoengineering, in which the carbohydrate moieties attached at the primary IgG glycosylation site (Asn297) are altered.[150] IgG normally has a heptasaccharide core attached at ASN297 to which there is variable addition of other sugar residues, including fucose. Although the "core" oligosaccharide is essential for the expression of IgG-Fc effector functions, antibodies bearing oligosaccharides that lack fucose show enhanced FcγR binding, particularly for FcγRIIa, which is the primary FcγR of NK cells.[150] Nonfucosylated monoclonal antibodies have entered clinical evaluation, including MDX-1401 targeting CD30 and RO5072759 (GA101) targeting CD20.[151]

Bispecific antibodies in which one of the component binding sites is directed against a T-cell surface antigen and in which the other component binding site is directed against a chosen target antigen are able to focus T cells to act against cells expressing the target antigen.[152] For example, a class of bispecific antibodies termed BiTEs (bispecific T-cell engagers) recognize both a target antigen as well as CD3.[153] BiTEs show picomolar range potency, strictly target cell-dependent activation of T cells, and support serial lysis by activated T cells allowing activity at low effector to tumor cell ratios.[153] Of particular relevance to the childhood cancer setting is blinatumomab, a CD3/CD19 BiTE that has entered clinical evaluation. Blinatumomab induced objective responses as a single agent at the highest dose tested in seven of seven heavily pretreated patients with follicular and mantle cell lymphoma patients.[154] Blinatumomab was also able to induce molecular remission in a high percentage of adult patients with ALL who were minimal residual disease (MRD)-positive after experiencing molecular failure or molecular relapse after consolidation of frontline therapy.[155]

Enhancement of monoclonal antibody antitumor activity can be accomplished by conjugation with cytotoxic entities such as radionuclides, toxins, chemotherapy agents, and enzymes (for use in pretargeting of prodrugs to tumors via antibody-dependent enzyme-mediated prodrug therapy).[156] Although radionuclide or toxin conjugated antibodies are much more potent than naked antibodies, clinical experience to date has shown enhanced toxic effects toward normal tissues as well.[157] In contrast to naked antibodies that can often be combined with full doses of standard chemotherapy regimens, the normal tissue toxicity associated with conjugated antibodies often requires substantial reductions of either antibody dose or chemotherapy dose when they are studied together. For example, the dose per course of gemtuzumab ozogamicin, a toxin conjugated anti-CD33 antibody, must be reduced by severalfold when combined with standard AML chemotherapy,[158] while rituximab can be given at full dose when combined with NHL chemotherapy regimens.[159]

Conjugation with radionuclides has the theoretical advantage of allowing bystander killing, since the radiation emitted by commonly used radionuclides (e.g., [131]iodine, [90]yttrium) can kill nearby cells that might otherwise not be killed due to low antigen expression, innate resistance to antibody effects, or poor antibody penetration into tumor.[156] Although increasing the antitumor activity of the antibody, radionuclides also increase toxicity to normal tissues, particularly hematopoietic toxicity.[113] Two radioimmunoconjugates are approved by FDA, ^{90}Y-labeled ibritumomab tiuxetan and ^{131}I-labeled tositumomab, with both targeting CD20 and having indications for relapsed or refractory follicular or low-grade lymphoma.[113] The activity of radioconjugated antibodies can exceed that of naked antibodies for radiosensitive tumors, as illustrated by the higher rate of objective responses among patients with recurrent NHL for ^{90}Y-labeled ibritumomab tiuxetan compared with that for rituximab.[160]

Numerous bacterial and plant protein toxins have been evaluated for their ability to enhance the clinical activity of antibodies, including pseudomonas toxin, diphtheria toxin, ricin, gelonin, saporin, and pokeweed antiviral protein.[161] The most favorable clinical results for these immunotoxins have been obtained using BL22, which is composed of the variable domains of the anti-CD22 Mab RFB4 plus a 38 kDa form of Pseudomonas exotoxin called PE38. BL22 demonstrated high levels of activity in patients with recurrent hairy cell leukemia, with an overall complete response rate of approximately 50%.[162] The overall profile of clinical efficacy for immunotoxins is much less promising, however, with renal and hepatic toxicity and vascular leak syndrome limiting the dose of protein toxin immunoconjugates that can be administered to patients and complicating attempts to combine these immunotoxins with standard chemotherapy regimens.[157] A second limitation of protein toxin immunoconjugates is the rapid development of neutralizing antibodies against the toxin component of the immunoconjugate, which can limit the amount of immunoconjugate that can be delivered to the tumor.[163] One strategy for reducing immune responses to immunotoxins is through the engineering of the toxin component to eliminate B-cell epitopes and thereby reduce immunogenicity.[164] Another strategy for avoiding immune reactions is through the development of immunotoxins that utilize cytotoxic human proteins such as granzyme B, a serine protease that is an essential component of the granules released by cytotoxic T cells, proapoptotic BCL-2 family members, and cytotoxic ribonucleases.[165-167]

Immunoconjugates based upon the conjugation of small molecule cytotoxic agents to antibodies are a focus of current research because of their potency, lack of immunogenicity in humans, and clinical convenience.[111] As a consequence of the relatively small amount of antibody that can bind to tumor cells, a requirement for effective ADCs is that the toxic component induce cell death at miniscule concentrations. Calicheamicins and other minor groove binding alkylating agents, maytansinoids (inhibitors of tubulin polymerization with 200- to 1,000-fold greater potency than *Vinca* alkaloids) and auristatins (highly potent inhibitors of tubulin polymerization), are among the small molecule cytotoxic agents under evaluation for conjugation with antibodies.[111] The only ADC approved by FDA for cancer indications is the anti-CD33–targeted antibody gemtuzumab ozogamicin, which has the antitumor antibiotic calicheamicin as its toxin component.[168] Following internalization of the conjugated antibody, calicheamicin can be released from the antibody and travel to the nucleus where it cleaves double-stranded DNA. Gemtuzumab ozogamicin was approved by FDA based on single-agent activity (approximately 30% complete remission) for patients with AML in first relapse who are 60 years of age or older and who are not considered candidates for cytotoxic chemotherapy.[169,170]

The clinical viability of the ADC strategy has been confirmed for agents targeting HER2 and CD30. Trastuzumab-DM1, a HER2-targeted ADC with a maytansinoid cytotoxic component (DM1),[171] has shown greater preclinical activity than nonconjugated trastuzumab and induced objective responses in women with HER2 overexpressing breast cancer previously treated with trastuzumab.[172] Brentuximab vedotin (SGN-35), a CD30-targeted ADC with an auristatin cytotoxic component,[173] is highly active in patients with recurrent Hodgkin lymphoma and has obvious relevance for ALCL.[174] A number of other ADCs are under clinical development that target antigens with relevance in the childhood cancer setting, including SAR3419, composed of the humanized anti-CD19 antibody huB4 conjugated with the potent cytotoxic maytansinoid, DM4[175,176]; inotuzumab ozogamicin (CMC-544),

which is a CD22-specific cytotoxic immunoconjugate of calicheamicin[177]; and IMGN901 (huN901-DM1), which targets CD56 (expressed in neuroblastoma) and contains the maytansinoid DM1 as its toxic component.[178]

The relative lack of toxicity (particularly long-term toxicities) associated with most monoclonal antibody therapies makes them attractive for pediatric evaluation. For unconjugated monoclonal antibodies, the ability to combine antibody therapy with standard chemotherapy using full doses of each modality is an additional favorable feature.

Nucleic Acid–Based Targeted Therapy

Antisense oligonucleotides and their analogs are unmodified or chemically modified single-stranded DNA-like molecules that take advantage of Watson-Crick base pairing to modify expression of specific genes. Because of the flexibility and specificity provided by targeting based on complementary base pairing, antisense agents have the potential for inhibiting expression of virtually any gene, in contrast to monoclonal antibodies that target moieties present at the cell surface or that circulate in the blood. This extraordinary capability, combined with initial promising preclinical results, created high levels of enthusiasm for this technology in the early 1990s. However, only a single antisense agent has been approved by the FDA through 2009. Fomivirsen, a 21-base antisense molecule complementary to mRNA for the major immediate early region (IE2) proteins of cytomegalovirus (CMV), was approved by the FDA in 1998 for use by intravitreal injection for CMV-induced retinitis in patients with AIDS.[179] However, several subsequent pivotal phase 3 trials of first-generation antisense agents failed to demonstrate clinical benefit, including trials of ISIS 2302 targeting intracellular adhesion molecule-1 for Crohn's disease[180]; ISIS 3521 targeting protein kinase C alpha for NSCLC[181]; and oblimersen targeting BCL-2 for melanoma, myeloma, and chronic lymphocytic leukemia (CLL).[182-184] Although these results are discouraging, active clinical programs for nucleic acid–based therapies, including approaches based on RNAi, are seeking to identify strategies by which the exquisite specificity of these strategies can be exploited for clinical benefit.

Antisense molecules can inhibit production of functional protein by their target mRNAs through several distinctive processes. For many antisense agents, the most important process involves RNase H, an ubiquitous endonuclease that recognizes and then cleaves the RNA component of RNA-DNA hybrids. Cleavage of the RNA component of antisense-RNA heteroduplexes by RNase H reduces levels of the target mRNA leading to decreased production of the protein coded by the mRNA.[185] Antisense compounds are divided into classes based on the chemical characteristics of the backbone to which nucleoside bases are attached.[186] Backbone characteristics have major effects on both the sequence specific and the nonsequence-dependent biological activities of antisense molecules.[187] Early generation antisense compounds were *phosphorothioates*, in which a nonbridging oxygen atom in the phosphodiester bond is replaced by a sulfur atom.[188] Phosphorothioate antisense oligonucleotides maintain the ability to stimulate efficient RNA cleavage by RNase H,[189] which is thought to be the key factor explaining their sequence-specific biological activities.[186,190] Phosphorothioate antisense agents produce a characteristic set of sequence-independent side effects related to their polyanionic phosphorothioate backbone,[191] including prolongation of activated partial thromboplastin time,[192,193] complement activation,[192,194] and thrombocytopenia. Phosphorothioate antisense agents can also induce immunostimulatory responses, especially when they contain unmethylated CpG sequences.[195] CpG-dependent immune stimulation is a host mechanism for responding to microbial nucleic acids, and it involves interactions between unmethylated CpG motifs in bacterial DNA and TLR9 receptors in antigen-presenting cells.[196]

Antisense agents with modified sugar phosphate backbones have been developed in efforts to improve upon the efficacy and toxicity profile of phosphorothioate antisense agents.[187] One approach applied in second-generation antisense agents is to include nucleotides on each end of antisense molecules that are modified at the 2′ carbon of their ribose ring with either a methyl group[197,198] or with a methoxyethyl (MOE) group.[199] These modifications increase affinity for target RNA and increase stability due to increased resistance to nuclease activity.[197,198,200] Antisense agents with either the methyl or the MOE modification on all nucleotides do not support RNase H activity.[201] However, hybrid antisense molecules (termed gapmers), which have ends composed of methyl or MOE-modified nucleotides separated by a gap of intervening phosphorothioate-linked nucleotides, maintain the ability to stimulate RNase H cleavage.[198,200] The prolonged tissue stability of these hybrid molecules allow more relaxed dosing schedules (e.g., weekly administration in contrast to the continuous infusion schedules commonly used for phosphorothioate antisense agents).[197,202,203] For example, the 2′MOE gapmer antisense agent OGX-011 targets clusterin, an antiapoptotic protein that is activated after therapeutic stress. Weekly administration of OGX-011 successfully knocked down clusterin expression at both the mRNA and protein level.[204] OGX-011, like many antisense agents, combines well with chemotherapy,[205] and a randomized phase 2 study for patients with prostate cancer provided preliminary evidence for enhanced anticancer activity for docetaxel used with OGX-011 compared with docetaxel alone.[206] Other second-generation antisense agents in clinical development for cancer indications are LY2181308,[207] which targets survivin, and AEG35156, which targets XIAP.[208–210]

Locked nucleic acid (LNA) antisense compounds contain modified nucleotides that have a methylene bridge between the 2′oxygen and the 4′carbon of their ribose sugar.[211] This fixes the LNA base in an orientation that enhances Watson-Click base pairing to mRNA and that has resistance against degradation compared with other oligonucleotides.[211] Because antisense compounds composed entirely of LNAs do not induce RNase H cleavage of their target mRNA, the gapmer strategy is employed in which 3-4 LNA residues bracket a central 7-8 base stretch of DNA residues. EZN-2968 is an LNA antisense agent that targets hypoxia-inducible factor 1α (HIF-1α), a subunit of the transcription factor HIF-1 that plays a critical role in stimulating hypoxia-induced angiogenesis.[212] Proof of principle for specific knockdown of HIF-1α expression has been established *in vitro* and *in vivo*,[212] and the agent is in clinical evaluation.

There is great interest in developing RNAi as an alternative approach for nucleic acid–based targeted therapy.[213] An advantage of using synthetic siRNAs is their potency, as only a few siRNA molecules per cell are required for effective gene silencing.[214] However, there are multiple challenges to converting a powerful laboratory tool into an effective therapeutic modality. The key challenge to address in moving to broadly applicable RNAi-based anticancer agents is the development of technologies to efficiently deliver these agents to cancer cells distributed throughout the body so that clinically meaningful reductions in the targeted gene product can be achieved in the vast majority of cancer cells.[213] Various lipid-based delivery systems are under development,[215] including use of stable nucleic acid-lipid particles (SNALPs) that are designed to facilitate cellular uptake and endosomal release of siRNA.[216] *In vivo* proof of principle for this approach has been demonstrated in nonhuman primates, in which knockdown of apolipoprotein B (ApoB) was induced by intravenously administered ApoB-specific siRNAs encapsulated in SNALPs.[216] *In vivo* anticancer activity against both hepatic and subcutaneous xenografts has been demonstrated using SNALP-incorporated siRNAs targeted to the essential cell-cycle proteins PLK1 and kinesin spindle protein (KSP).[217] This strategy is being translated into the clinic using an agent (ALN-VSP) composed of siRNAs to both KSP and VEGF that are encapsulated in SNALPs. Polymer-mediated delivery systems for siRNA administration are also under development,[215] as illustrated by self-assembling, cyclodextrin polymer-based nanoparticles. Use of this delivery system with an siRNA against EWS-FLI1 produced *in vivo* activity against Ewing's sarcoma xenografts.[218] This delivery strategy has entered clinical evaluation using an agent (CALAA-01) composed of a cyclodextrin-containing polymer containing an siRNA against the M2 subunit of ribonucleotide reductase and using human transferrin (Tf) as a targeting ligand for binding to transferrin receptors (TfR) that are typically upregulated on cancer cells.[219] A third general strategy for siRNA delivery is by conjugation to compounds that enhance cellular delivery and/or uptake.[215]

The same characteristics of specificity and flexibility that make antisense and other nucleic acid–based treatment approaches attractive for adult cancer indications apply equally to childhood cancers. The greatest potential for these approaches may derive from their potential to clinically target pediatric-specific cancer targets. Although development of targeted therapies is inherently resource intensive, the "sameness" of classes of antisense agents because of their common backbone structure can expedite preclinical development and preparation of drug supply for clinical evaluations of new antisense agents.[220] In addition, the sameness within class of nucleic acid–based agents can also facilitate initial clinical evaluations because of their generally predictable pharmacokinetic behavior and toxicity profile. Antisense molecules against childhood cancer targets have been studied in preclinical models. For example, antisense molecules directed against N-Myc have antitumor activity in *in vitro* and *in vivo* models of neuroblastoma.[221–223] Similarly, antisense molecules targeted at the EWS-FLI1 fusion protein have antitumor activity against Ewing's sarcoma cell lines and xenografts.[224–226]

THERAPIES TARGETED TO APOPTOSIS PATHWAYS

A hallmark of cancer is the ability to evade apoptosis (programmed cell death).[227] The acquisition by cancer cells of defects in programmed cell death that provide a survival advantage during tumorigenesis can also provide cancer cells with intrinsic resistance to treatment approaches such as chemotherapy and radiation therapy. An obvious approach to enhancing the effectiveness of cancer therapy is by manipulating the cancer cell's dysregulated apoptosis pathways to favor cell death. Although conceptually simple, achieving clinical benefit through this approach is far from trivial. Apoptotic pathways are complex with multiple steps at which progression toward cell death may be blocked. In addition, for a therapeutic window to exist, the specific apoptosis pathway target of an agent must be one upon which cancer cells are critically dependent and one for which normal cells have much less need. The two primary apoptotic pathways, the extrinsic (death receptor) pathway and intrinsic (mitochondrial) pathway, are described in Figure 11.1.

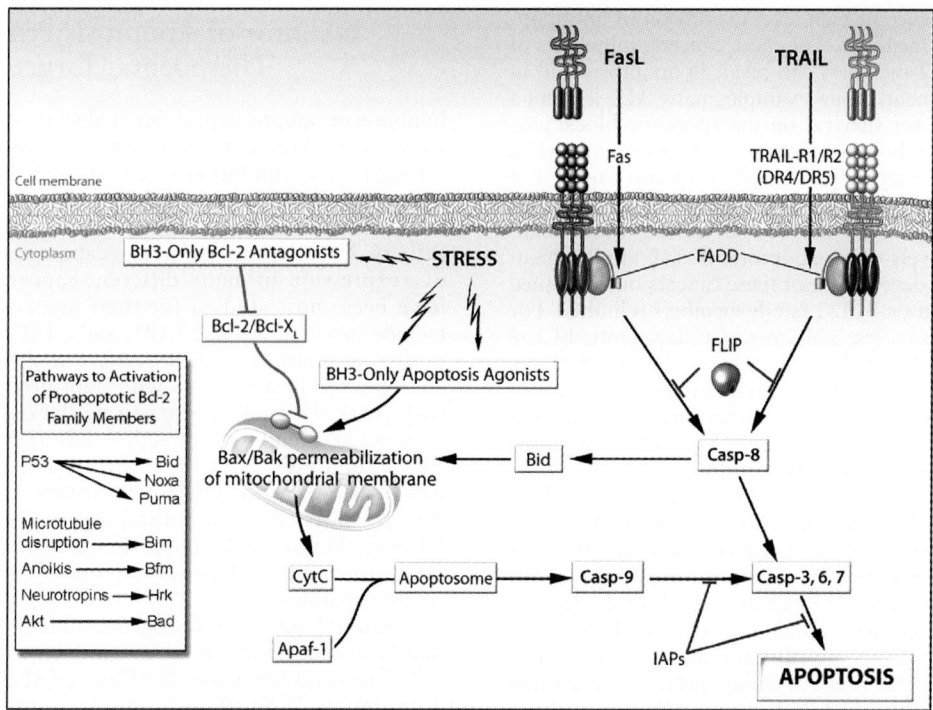

FIGURE 11.1 Simplified schema of extrinsic and intrinsic apoptosis pathways. The extrinsic (death-receptor) pathway is initiated by ligation and clustering of members of the death-receptor superfamily (e.g., tumor necrosis factor [TNF] receptor I, Fas, and the TNF-related apoptosis inducing ligand [TRAIL/Apo-2L] receptors TRAIL-R1 [DR4] and TRAIL-R2 [DR5]). Receptor clustering leads to formation of death-inducing signal complexes (DISC) by recruitment of adapter proteins (e.g., Fas-associated death domain [FADD]), which can then attract procaspase-8. The procaspase-8 that is recruited to the complex is converted by proteolytic cleavage to caspase-8, which can then activate downstream effector caspases leading to apoptosis. The intrinsic (mitochondrial) pathway is responsive to internal toxic stimuli (e.g., DNA damage, disruption of microtubules). These stimuli result in increased levels of proapoptotic BH3-only members of the BCL-2 family (see insert on right side), which inhibit BCL-2 and BCL-X$_L$ function, leading to oligomerization of Bax and Bak in mitochondrial membranes. The interaction of Bax and Bak with the mitochondrial membrane results in the release into the cytoplasm of cytochrome c and other proapoptotic factors, leading to the formation of a cytoplasmic complex (the "apoptosome") that includes cytochrome c, apoptotic protease-activating factor-1 (Apaf-1), and procaspase-9. Formation of the apoptosome results in production of active caspase-9, which then activates downstream effector caspases. Cross-talk between the two apoptosis pathways occurs by caspase-8 cleavage and activation of the BH3-only protein Bid, which can then bind to Bax and Bak, promoting their mitochondrial membrane insertion and oligomerization and leading to activation of the intrinsic pathway. Members of the inhibitor of apoptosis protein (IAP) can suppress apoptosis by binding to and inhibiting caspases.

BCL-2 Family Proteins as Therapeutic Targets

Oligomerization of the proapoptotic BCL-2 family members BAX and BAK in the mitochondrial membrane is a critical step in the mitochondrial apoptosis pathway.[228,229] Whether BAX and BAK oligomerization occurs is dependent upon the overall balance between the expression and activation of the remaining more than 20 BCL-2 family proteins. Each of these proteins contains one or more BCL-2 homology (BH) domains, and they can be divided into those that inhibit apoptosis and those that promote apoptosis. The antiapoptotic group of family members, including BCL-2, BCL-X$_L$, MCL-1, and BFL-1/A1, typically contain BH domains 1–4 and act directly or indirectly to block the apoptosis-inducing activities of BAX and BAK. Among the proapoptotic BCL-2 family members, BAX and BAK contain BH domains 1–3, while the remaining members contain a single BH domain, BH3. These BH3-only proteins include PUMA, NOXA, BIM, BID, BAD,

and others. They are activated in response to a range of cellular stressors to promote apoptosis, as exemplified by the p53-regulated induction of PUMA and NOXA in response to DNA damage. There are two models for BAX and BAK activation, with the direct model positing that activator proteins (e.g., BID and BIM) directly interact with BAX and BAK to promote conformational changes leading to their oligomerization and to apoptosis.[228] The indirect model proposes that the primary role of proapoptotic BH3-only proteins is to displace antiapoptotic members from binding with BAX and BAK, thereby allowing BAX and BAK oligomerization and apoptosis.[230] Regardless of the model, there is the opportunity for therapeutic efficacy if the balance between the activity of pro- and antiapoptotic BCL-2 family members can be selectively shifted in cancer cells to favor apoptosis.

In considering therapeutic applications related to BCL-2 family proteins, an important concept is that some cancers are primed to undergo apoptosis because of their expression of proapoptotic BH-3-only proteins.[231] Because of their high level of expression of BH3-only protein, these cancers are addicted to the concurrent high level expression of antiapoptotic BCL-2 family members. For these cancers, inhibitors of antiapoptotic BCL-2 members can result in apoptosis and in potential clinical benefit. As an example, many ALL leukemia cells are dependent for survival on the apoptotic block provided by BCL-2 family expression.[231] ALL cases with MLL gene rearrangement may be particularly responsive to BCL-2 inhibition.[231,232] CLL is another lymphoid malignancy that appears to be primed for apoptosis.[233] By contrast, other cancers express low levels of proapoptotic BCL-2 family members, and hence the dependence of these cancers on continued activity of antiapoptotic BCL-2 family members is limited. For this latter group of cancers, inhibitors of antiapoptotic BCL-2 family members will have limited activity when used alone. Although BCL-2 inhibitors may potentiate the sensitivity of these cancers to cytotoxic agents, whether this results in clinical benefit will depend upon the relative levels of sensitization in cancer cells versus normal cells.

Agents targeting antiapoptotic BCL-2 family members have entered clinical evaluation. Although the BCL-2 antisense agent, oblimersen (G3139, Genasense), was the first BCL-2 inhibitor to proceed to extensive clinical testing, the results were disappointing,[182–184] likely a result of inadequate levels of target inhibition. Small molecule BCL-2 family inhibitors are now undergoing clinical evaluation, with these inhibitors differing in the range of antiapoptotic members that they effectively inhibit. ABT-263 is an orally bioavailable BH3 mimetic that potently inhibits the prosurvival activity of BCL-2, BCL-X_L, and BCL-W but not that of MCL-1 or BFL-1/BCL2A1.[234] ABT-263 induced regressions as a single agent against small-cell lung cancer and ALL xenograft models.[234,235] The PPTP studied ABT-263 against its childhood cancer preclinical models, and observed limited single-agent activity against solid tumor xenografts, but substantial remission-inducing activity against approximately 50% of the ALL xenografts tested.[57] ABT-263 has entered clinical evaluation, with impressive activity observed in patients with CLL and selected NHLs in the phase 1 setting.[236] ABT-263 has generally been well tolerated, with dose escalation limited by rapid-onset, reversible thrombocytopenia.[74] Thrombocytopenia is an on-target effect of ABT-263, as BCL-X_L blocks the ability of BAK to promote platelet survival.[88] The single-agent activity of ABT-263 against ALL xenografts, its activity in adults with CLL, and its ability to potentiate the cytotoxic effects of standard antileukemia agents,[57,234,237] support testing of ABT-263 for ALL. However, because of the distinctive thrombocytopenia that it induces, it will be challenging to use for remission induction and may have its greatest utility in the postremission setting. ABT-263 generally has lower levels of single-agent activity against nonlymphoid malignancies.[57] For these cancers, an area of research focus is using ABT-263 to potentiate the activity of chemotherapy agents,[63] a strategy whose success in the clinical setting will depend on different levels of potentiation for cancer versus normal cells.

Obatoclax mesylate (GX15–070) is a small molecule pan-BCL-2 family antagonist that is in clinical evaluation. It differs from ABT-263 in that it inhibits MCL-1 activity at concentrations similar to those that inhibit BCL-2 and BCL-X_L.[238] Obatoclax dose escalation in patients is limited by neurotoxicity, and unlike ABT-263, it does not induce thrombocytopenia.[239,240] Obatoclax has shown little clinical activity against CLL,[240] but an ALL patient with MLL gene rearrangement achieved a complete response to obatoclax.[239] AT-101, the negative enantiomer of gossypol, is another BH3-mimetic small molecule BCL-2 family inhibitor that is under clinical evaluation.[241]

Inhibitor of Apoptosis Proteins as Therapeutic Targets

Inhibitor of apoptosis proteins (IAPs) are evolutionarily conserved cytoplasmic proteins that can suppress apoptosis through direct inhibition of caspases.[242] Eight human IAPs have been identified and all share a protein domain, the baculovirus IAP repeat, that is important for their antiapoptotic activity. The relevance of IAPs to cancer is supported by their overexpression in many different cancer types. IAPs that have been most studied for their association with cancer include survivin, XIAP, c-IAP1, and c-IAP2. XIAP is overexpressed in multiple adult cancers,[243] and elevated XIAP levels appear to be associated with poor prognosis for children with AML.[244] XIAP appears to be the only member of the human IAP family that directly binds and inhibits caspases, and it suppresses both the upstream initiator protease caspase-9 as well as the effector proteases caspase-3 and -7.[242] Because of its effect on a distal step in apoptosis pathways, XIAP is able to block apoptosis signaling activated by both the mitochondrial-dependent pathway and by the death-receptor pathway.

Smac/DIABLO is an endogenous inhibitor of IAP proteins that blocks the ability of XIAP to inhibit caspases-3, -7, and -9.[245] Smac also binds to c-IAP1 and c-IAP2 and induces their degradation.[246] Small molecule Smac mimetics have been developed that have these same activities.[245] Smac mimetics induce apoptosis in sensitive cell lines by causing rapid degradation of c-IAP1 and c-IAP2, which induces nuclear factor κB (NF-κB) activation and autocrine tumor necrosis factor α (TNFα) production, which in turn leads to formation of TNFα receptor death-inducing signaling complex with caspase-8 activation and subsequent activation of downstream effector caspases.[245] Concurrent inhibition of XIAP appears to promote the ability of Smac mimetics to induce apoptosis.[247] Smac mimetics show single-agent activity against some cancer cell lines,[248] and they promote apoptosis induced by chemotherapy, TRAIL, and receptor tyrosine kinase inhibition.[249–251] Small molecule Smac mimetics are entering clinical evaluation. An XIAP antisense molecule (AEG35156) is also being studied in the clinical setting.[208,209] Preclinical studies of AEG35156 demonstrated tumor growth inhibition as a single agent and enhancement of the activity of chemotherapy when used in combination in the models tested.[210] In a phase 1/2 trial of AEG35156 in combination with cytarabine and idarubicin in patients with AML, evidence for significant XIAP knockdown was observed, as was preliminary evidence for enhancement of chemotherapy activity by the agent.[209]

Survivin is of particular pediatric interest because of reports of an association between survivin overexpression and poor prognosis in neuroblastoma.[252,253] Survivin maps to chromosome band 17q25, a region that is often represented by chromosome gain in neuroblastoma, a finding that is associated with poor prognosis.[254] Survivin overexpression is common in adult cancers, and survivin expression has been associated with poorer prognosis for some cancers.[255] Although survivin binds to caspases, it appears much less effective than XIAP at potently inhibiting caspase activity.[256] Survivin plays a critical role in chromosome segregation and cytokinesis, and it is a member of the chromosomal passenger complex along with Aurora B kinase, INCENP.[257] Absence of survivin results in abnormal mitoses and cell death.[256] Inhibitors of survivin that are under clinical evaluation include LY2181308,[207] a second-generation antisense agent, and YM155,[258,259] a small molecule survivin inhibitor.

The Death-Receptor Pathway as a Therapeutic Target

Therapeutic strategies based upon activation of TRAIL signaling and activation of the death-receptor pathway have entered clinical evaluation for cancer indications.[260–262] Induction of apoptosis by TRAIL requires binding to one of its receptors, TRAIL-R1 (DR4) or TRAIL-R2 (DR5), with subsequent formation of the TRAIL death-inducing signal complex, followed by recruitment of an adaptor protein Fas-associated death domain (FADD) and the apoptosis initiators, caspase-8 and -10, which then activate the effector caspases-3, -6, and -7.[263] TRAIL-induced apoptosis does not require p53 function, which could allow TRAIL to remain effective against cancer cells that are resistant to chemotherapy and radiation therapy due to loss of p53 function.[260] TRAIL induces apoptosis *in vitro* against a wide range of adult cancer cell lines, and additionally demonstrates *in vivo* activity as a single agent in a variety of xenograft models.[261] However, TRAIL is not universally active in preclinical models, and there is a need for the identification of factors that reliably predict for sensitivity.[260] Impressive antitumor activity has been observed for combinations of TRAIL plus chemotherapy or radiation therapy.[261]

Clinical strategies for activating TRAIL signaling have focused on the use of recombinant human TRAIL (rhApo2L/TRAIL, AMG 951) and on the use of agonist monoclonal antibodies specific for either TRAIL-R1 (mapatumumab/HGS-ETR1) or for TRAIL-R2 (lexatumumab/HGS-ETR2, conatumumab/AMG 655, and apomab).[260–262] These two strategies differ in several important ways. The former activates both TRAIL-R1 and TRAIL-R2 and the latter activates only one or the other TRAIL receptor. Also, rhApo2L/TRAIL has a short half-life, while the agonistic antibodies have prolonged circulation similar to that of other therapeutic monoclonal antibodies.

Mapatumumab (HGS-ETR1) is a fully human IgG1 agonist monoclonal antibody that exclusively targets and activates TRAIL-R1.[262] Mapatumumab induces regressions as a single agent against select TRAIL-R1–expressing adult tumor xenografts of multiple histologies (e.g., colon, non-small cell lung, and renal cancer),[264] and it enhances the antitumor activity of cytotoxic agents against multiple adult cancer cell lines.[264,265] Mapatumumab has been well tolerated in adults with cancer, although signs of single-agent antitumor activity have been limited.[266] Combinations of mapatumumab with cytotoxic agents have been well tolerated,[262,267] with further studies required to determine whether the chemotherapy activity is potentiated by the addition of mapatumumab. The TRAIL-R2 agonist, lexatumumab and conatumumab (AMG 655) and apomab, have also been studied in adults with cancer, and results appear similar to those described for mapatumumab, with good tolerability but limited evidence for single-agent efficacy.[268–271]

TRAIL-induced apoptosis has been noted in preclinical studies employing pediatric cancer cell lines, including those for Ewing's sarcoma,[272–274] rhabdomyosarcoma,[275,276] and high-grade glioma.[277] Neuroblastoma cell lines are generally reported to be resistant to TRAIL-induced apoptosis, which may be the result of lack of caspase-8 expression secondary to promoter methylation as well as due to the absence of both TRAIL-R1 and TRAIL-R2 in some cell lines.[278] The PPTP evaluated the TRAIL-R1 agonist mapatumumab against its *in vitro* cell line panel and against its *in vivo* xenograft panels and observed limited evidence for anticancer activity for this TRAIL-R1–targeted agent. Further study is needed to determine whether TRAIL-R2–targeted agents or approaches that engage both TRAIL-R1 and TRAIL-R2 have greater levels of activity than mapatumumab and also to explore whether a TRAIL pathway targeted agent in combination with cytotoxic chemotherapy is effective against one or more childhood cancers.

TARGETING EXTRACELLULAR SURVIVAL SIGNALING PATHWAYS

The cellular environment provides signals that can promote cell survival and proliferation. Not surprisingly, cancer cells have commandeered these signaling pathways to promote their own survival and growth. In terms of targeted drug development, the signaling pathways initiated by members of the receptor tyrosine kinase family have been most exploited, and the discussion that follows focuses on these pathways. Binding of ligand to receptor tyrosine kinases at the cellular membrane can lead to the activation of multiple-intracellular signaling components as illustrated in Figure 11.2. RAS is activated which in turn activates RAF and subsequently other members of the mitogen-activated protein kinase (MAPK) pathway. PI3K is activated, which leads to activation of AKT which in turn activates multiple downstream proteins that promote survival. Membrane receptors can also activate STAT family proteins. The importance to cancer cells of these signaling pathways is indicated by the variety of activating mutations reported for members of the receptor tyrosine kinase family, including EGFR mutations, translocations resulting in PDGFR activation, KIT mutations in GISTs, ALK mutations in neuroblastoma, ALK fusion proteins NSCLC,[279] and FLT3 mutations in AML. Activating mutations in cancer cells also occur in downstream signaling pathways, as exemplified by mutations of PTEN (which results in AKT activation) in many cancer types and BRAF mutations in melanoma and JPA. Inhibitors of these pathways are discussed briefly later, with a focus on agents being studied in children and on agents of particular pediatric interest that have not yet entered clinical evaluation in children.

Targeting Insulin-Like Growth Factor Receptor 1 Signaling

IGF-IR is a receptor protein tyrosine kinase that has potent effects on both proliferation and survival. IGF-IR is activated by the binding of its ligands, IGF-I and IGF-II. Activation of IGF-IR results in activation of the PI3K-AKT and MAPK signaling pathways. In support of an oncogenic role for IGF-IR, its overexpression can transform immortalized murine fibroblasts, and conversely, targeted disruption of the IGF-IR gene provides resistance to murine fibroblasts against transformation by a number of oncogenes.[280] IGF-IR signaling appears to play an important role in a number of adult cancers, and more than 10 agents (primarily monoclonal antibodies, but also small molecule inhibitors) directly targeting IGF-IR have entered clinical evaluation. IGF-IR has multiple surface epitopes that can be targeted to block IGF-I and/or IGF-II binding and to thereby inhibit IGF-IR signaling.[281] Thus, the anti-IGF-IR antibodies under clinical evaluation may show differences in their relative efficacy in blocking IGF-I versus IGF-II signaling,[282] and these differences could translate into differences in clinical activity. The small molecule inhibitors of IGF-IR have much more prominent effects on the insulin receptor than do anti-IGF-IR monoclonal antibodies, which could result in increased antitumor activity but will also result in greater risk for hyperglycemia.[283]

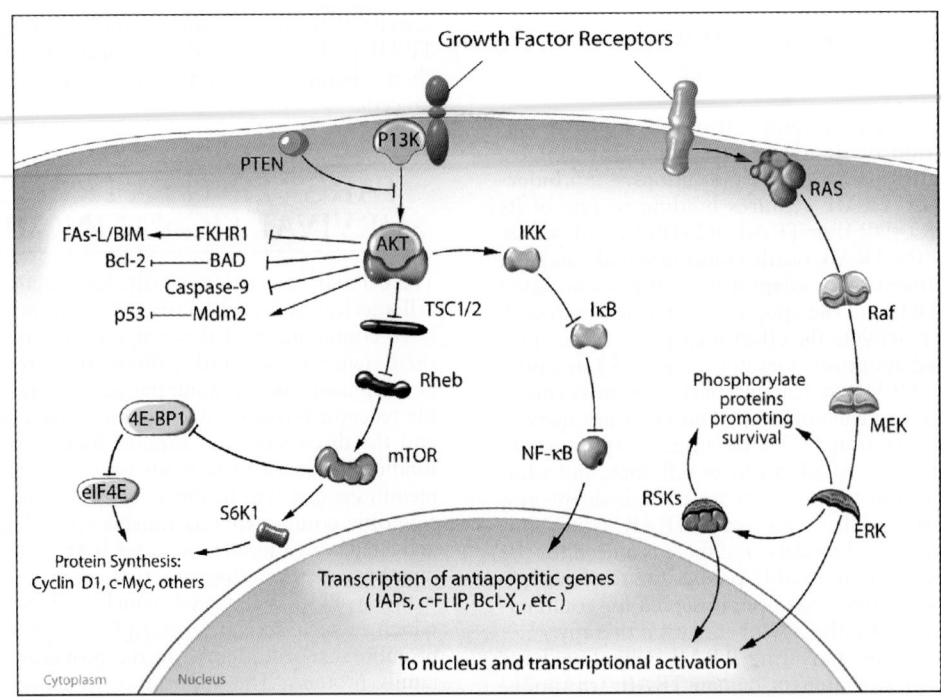

FIGURE 11.2 Simplified schematic of growth factor receptor signaling pathways. Growth factor receptor activation can initiate signaling along multiple intracellular pathways that promote proliferation and survival. The extracellular signal-related kinase (ERK) cascade is initiated when Ras activation leads to Raf membrane recruitment and activation, followed by phosphorylation and activation of MEK1 and MEK2 and then the ERK1 and ERK2. Activated ERK1/2 can translocate to the nucleus and phosphorylate specific transcription factors and can phosphorylate cytoplasmic targets such as cytoskeletal proteins. ERK can also activate members of the 90-kDa ribosomal S6 kinase (RSK) family, which represents an additional amplification step in the mitogen-activated protein kinase (MAPK) catalytic cascades. Growth factor receptor signaling also leads to PI3K and AKT activation. PTEN can reduce the extent of AKT activation, while absence of PTEN can lead to constitutive AKT activation. AKT plays a central role in promoting survival by phosphorylating multiple proteins involved in survival/apoptosis pathways. AKT activates mTOR via the phosphorylation and inhibition of the tuberous sclerosis complex proteins tuberin (Tsc2) and hamartin (Tsc1), which in turn leads to activation of Rheb, a member of the Ras superfamily of GTP-binding proteins, which in turn causes activation of mTOR. Activation of mTOR leads to phosphorylation of eukaryotic initiation factor 4E (eIF4E)-binding protein 1 (4E-BP1) and ribosomal protein S6 kinase 1 (S6K1). Unphosphorylated 4E-BP1 binds to the cap-binding protein eIF4E, thereby reducing translation of mRNAs with complex secondary structures in their 5′untranslated region (e.g., cyclin D1 and c-Myc). Phosphorylation of 4E-BP1 by mTOR frees eIF4E and promotes translation of these mRNAs. Activation of S6K1 leads to increased mRNA translation via downstream effectors that are phosphorylated by S6K1. Growth factor receptor signaling can also lead to nuclear factor κB (NF-κB) pathway activation, in part through AKT phosphorylation and activation of IκB kinase (IKK), which leads to IκB phosphorylation and freeing of NF-κB to translocate to the nucleus. Not pictured is the JAK-STAT pathway, which can also promote proliferation and survival following growth factor receptor activation.

The IGF-IR pathway appears to be important in the survival and growth of a number of childhood cancers. There is particular interest in IGF-IR as a therapeutic target for Ewing's sarcoma, with multiple lines of evidence supporting a central role for IGF-IR signaling for this cancer type. The three most common Ewing's sarcoma fusion proteins (EWS-FLI-1, EWS-ERG, and FUS-ERG) all activate the IGF-I promoter and induce IGF-I expression,[284] and transformation of fibroblasts by the EWS/FLI-1 requires IGF-IR.[42] Growth of Ewing's sarcoma cells *in vitro* and *in vivo* can be inhibited by measures that block signaling through the IGF-IR pathway (e.g., monoclonal antibody or antisense targeted to IGF-IR),[285–287] The objective responses elicited by anti-IGF-IR monoclonal antibodies in patients with Ewing's sarcoma provide clinical validation for IGF-IR as a therapeutic target for this disease.[288,289]

IGF-IR also appears to be important for rhabdomyosarcoma growth and survival. High levels of both IGF-IR and IGF-II expression are common observed for this diagnosis.[290,291] The anti-IGF-IR′ monoclonal antibodies MK-0646 and cixutumumab (IMC-A12) have shown activity against rhabdomyosarcoma xenografts.[291,292] Other pediatric tumors whose growth is affected by IGF-IR targeting include neuroblastoma,[293,294] medulloblastoma,[295] and osteosarcoma.[296] For osteosarcoma, tumor regressions were observed for osteosarcoma xenografts treated with the anti-IGF-IR antibody SCH 717454.[287] In addition, IGF-II is highly expressed in Wilms' tumor[297,298] and hepatoblastoma.[299,300]

Clinical development of IGF-IR–targeted antibodies in the pediatric setting will involve combining these agents with standard chemotherapy regimens. The preclinical rationale for this strategy comes from studies showing that IGF-IR inhibition can potentiate the activity of many cytotoxic agents against cancer cell lines.[301] Also supporting this strategy is the favorable toxicity profiles of anti-IGF-IR monoclonal antibodies, and their documented ability to combine well with some classes of cytotoxic agents in adults with cancer.[302] Given the role of IGF-IR signaling in protecting cardiac myocytes from stress,[303] caution will be needed when developing combinations that include anthracyclines. The combination of an IGF-IR inhibitor with an mTOR inhibitor is also of interest, given promising preclinical activity against selected pediatric sarcomas.[304]

Targeting Anaplastic Lymphoma Kinase

ALK is a receptor tyrosine kinase in the insulin receptor superfamily that is expressed primarily in the developing central and peripheral nervous systems.[305] ALK is an important childhood cancer target because it is activated in several childhood cancers. In ALCL, the t(2;5)(p23;q35) chromosomal rearrangement results in the fusion of NPM at 5q35 with ALK at 2p23, and the resulting fusion protein shows constitutive kinase activity. Multiple other fusion proteins involving ALK have been identified in ALCL, including TPM3-ALK, ATIC-ALK, and CLTC-ALK. ALK fusion proteins are also observed in approximately 50% of cases of inflammatory myofibroblastic tumor, with fusion proteins being more frequent in younger patients.[306] In neuroblastoma, ALK amplification and ALK activating missense mutations are present in 10% to 15% of high-risk cases.[11,307–309] ALK is recognized as a bone fide adult cancer therapeutic target because a small subset of NSCLC cases express an ALK fusion protein (EML 4-ALK).[279]

ALCL, neuroblastoma, and NSLCL cell lines with ALK activation through gene amplification, rearrangement, or mutation often show exquisite sensitivity to small molecule ALK inhibitors.[43,309–311] Cell lines with different ALK activating mutations can show variable patterns of response to specific small molecule inhibitors, as illustrated by the sensitivity of cell lines with the R1275Q mutation (the most common ALK mutation observed in neuroblastoma) to the ALK inhibitor PF-02341066 compared with the relative resistance to this agent observed for cell lines with the F1174L mutation.[312] An in vivo model of ALK + ALCL showed a prompt complete response to treatment with the small molecule ALK inhibitor PF-02341066,[310] and lung tumors arising in a transgenic mouse model of EML4-ALK NSCLC regressed during treatment with an orally administered ALK inhibitor.[313] The response of neuroblastoma xenografts to PF-02341066 mirrored that of the corresponding cell lines, in that xenografts with the R1275Q mutation showed complete tumor regression while xenografts with the F1174L mutation showed progressive disease.[312]

PF-02341066 is the first ALK inhibitor to enter the clinic. The agent was relatively well tolerated in adults with the dose-limiting toxicities being liver enzyme elevations and fatigue.[36] The PF-02341066 adult phase 1 trial included an expansion cohort of 19 patients with NSCLC and the EML4-ALK translocation, and approximately one-half of these patients achieved a partial response.[36] Pediatric clinical testing of PF-02341066 has been initiated and will focus on ALK+ ALCL and ALK-mutant neuroblastoma.

Targeting FMS-Like Tyrosine kinase-3

FLT3 is a receptor tyrosine kinase that is expressed primarily on hematopoietic and neural tissues.[314–316] FLT3, like PDGFR and KIT, is a member of the PDGF receptor subfamily of receptor tyrosine kinases,[317] and it shows lesser degrees of homology with VEGF receptors.[318] These relationships explain the overlapping kinase inhibition profiles observed for small molecule inhibitors of FLT3 such as sorafenib and sunitinib. FLT3 is activated by binding to FLT3 ligand, which induces receptor

dimerization, activation of the receptor's tyrosine kinase activity, and subsequent signaling through multiple downstream pathways (e.g., STAT5, MAPK, and AKT).[319]

Activating mutations of FLT3 have been identified in both pediatric and adult acute leukemias.[319] Internal tandem duplications (ITDs) of the juxtamembrane domain of FLT3 result in constitutive tyrosine kinase activity, as do selected missense activation loop mutations in the FLT3 tyrosine kinase domain.[319] The frequency of FLT3/ITD mutations in AML is age dependent, increasing from 5% to 10% for children younger than 10 years, to approximately 20% in young adults, to more than 35% in AML patients older than 55 years.[319] Presence of a FLT3/ITD mutation is associated with poor prognosis in both adults and children with AML, particularly when there is a high ratio of the mutant allele to the normal allele.[320] FLT3 activation loop mutations (FLT3/ALMs) occur in 6% to 8% of adults and children with AML, but do not appear to be predictive of poor prognosis.[319] FLT3 is commonly overexpressed in infant ALL with MLL rearrangements, and higher levels of expression are associated with poor prognosis.[321,322]

A number of small molecule kinase inhibitors been identified that inhibit FLT3.[37] Clinical evaluation of these agents as FLT3 inhibitors was facilitated because several were already being studied in the clinic for their inhibitory effects against other receptor tyrosine kinases (e.g., lestaurtinib [CEP-701], sunitinib, sorafenib, and midostaurin [PKC412]).[37] These inhibitors cause cell cycle arrest, inhibit proliferation, and induce apoptosis of FLT3-dependent cell lines, including human leukemia-derived cell lines with FLT3/ITD and murine cell lines transfected with FLT3/ITD constructs.[315] Phase 2 studies of these agents in AML patients with FLT3 mutations documented marked reductions in peripheral blood blast count in a substantial percentage of patients, but these reductions were transient and true complete remissions were uncommon.[37] The primary strategy for applying FLT3 inhibitors in the AML setting has been to combine these agents with standard AML chemotherapy agents using either concurrent administration of the inhibitor with chemotherapy,[323] or alternatively using sequential administration with the inhibitor being initiated following completion of chemotherapy.[324,325] The FLT3 inhibitor plus standard agent regimens have been adequately tolerated and have shown promising activity.[323–325] Randomized comparisons in patients with FLT3-mutant AML of standard chemotherapy given with or without a FLT3 inhibitor have been initiated for midostaurin, lestaurtinib, and sorafenib. The pivotal clinical trial of lestaurtinib given in sequence with standard reinduction chemotherapy in patients with relapsed AML expressing FLT3 activating mutations failed to show a benefit for the use of lestaurtinib in terms of remission rate and overall survival (OS).[326] Further research is needed to determine the cause of these disappointing results and to determine how to effectively use FLT3 inhibitors for clinical benefit in patients with FLT3-mutant AML. Clinical trials of lestaurtinib in combination with chemotherapy have also been initiated for infants with ALL that have MLL gene rearrangement, based on preclinical observations of activity for FLT3 inhibitors against this ALL subtype.[327]

Targeting Janus Kinases

The JAK family of protein tyrosine kinases (JAK1–3 and TYK2) are involved in signaling initiated by members of the cytokine receptor superfamily, which themselves lack kinase activity.[328,329] Cytokine receptors bind to JAK family members through their cytoplasmic domains. Ligand binding by the receptors induces their dimerization or oligomerization, bringing the receptor-associated JAKs into close proximity with each other and inducing their cross-phosphorylation and activation. Subsequent signaling events involve JAK phosphorylation of the receptor, recruitment and phosphorylation of STAT proteins, dimerization and nuclear translocation of STAT proteins, and induction of target gene transcription following STAT protein binding to specific regulatory elements.[328,329]

JAK family kinases (JAK1,2,3 and TYK2) have gained increasing recognition in the past 5 years as oncology therapeutic targets following the demonstration that most cases of polycythemia vera and a substantial proportion of essential thrombocytopenia and idiopathic myelofibrosis cases are associated with a specific JAK2 mutation (V617F) that changes an amino acid in the JAK2 pseudokinase domain.[330] JAK-STAT pathway activation is also relevant in the childhood ALL setting. In a ALL cases, activation occurs through fusion proteins in which a JAK family member joins with the oligomerization domain of other proteins such as TEL (ETV6) and PCM1.[331,332] Mutations in JAK1 have been reported in approximately 20% of adults with T-cell ALL[333,334] but appear to be less common in children with T-cell ALL and adults with B-precursor ALL.[333] Activating mutations of JAK2 (primarily at a highly conserved arginine residue, R683) have been reported in 18% to 28% of ALL cases associated with Down syndrome.[335–337] Activating JAK1 and JAK2 mutations occur in a subset of B-precursor ALL cases that have a high rate of treatment failure and that have biological characteristics (e.g., high rate of IFZF1 deletion) similar to those of BCR-ABL ALL, though lacking expression of this fusion protein.[9] JMML, an aggressive myeloproliferative disease associated with GM-CSF hypersensitivity, is another childhood cancer that shows activation of JAK-STAT signaling.[18]

A number of JAK inhibitors have entered clinical evaluation. The inhibitors can be categorized by their relative selectivity (or lack thereof) for JAK family members. INCB018424 is an orally available JAK inhibitor that shows low nanomolar potency against both JAK1 and JAK2.[338] Patients with primary myelofibrosis, postpolycythemia vera, and essential thrombocythemia myelofibrosis (Post-PV/ET MF) enrolled on a phase 1/2 study of INCB018424 showed durable improvements in constitutional symptoms as well as reduced spleen size.[339] The primary adverse effect observed was dose-dependent grade 3 or 4 reversible thrombocytopenia.[339] TG101348 is an orally bioavailable JAK2-selective inhibitor that has also shown evidence of clinical activity in patients with myelofibrosis.[340,341] Other JAK inhibitors under clinical evaluation are CYT387, SB1518, and AZD1480.

Targeting BCR-ABL

Imatinib potently inhibits several receptor tyrosine kinases in addition to ABL (e.g., PDGF receptors and KIT), but in the pediatric setting, the clinical utility of imatinib is related almost exclusively to its ability to inhibit the kinase activity of BCR-ABL in CML and Ph+ ALL. Phase 2 studies of imatinib for children with solid tumors found little or no activity against all histologies evaluated,[342] despite confirmed expression of one or more target receptor tyrosine kinases in many of the cases.[343] The activity of imatinib in pediatric patients with CML is similar to that observed for adults,[344,345] and lessons learned from clinical trials for adults with CML inform treatment of pediatric patients.[346] The strategy of adding imatinib to conventional antileukemia therapy for Ph+ ALL appears to be effective in both the pediatric and adult settings, and substantial improvements in outcome for this patient

population have been observed for multiagent regimens that include imatinib.[347–349]

Dasatinib is both an ABL and an SRC family kinase inhibitor, and it also inhibits other receptor tyrosine kinases including KIT, PDGF receptors, and Ephrin receptors (the EphA and EphB receptor tyrosine kinases).[350] Although dasatinib has not been studied in children with solid tumors, it was evaluated by the PPTP against both ALL and solid tumor xenografts. Very limited activity was observed for datasinib against the PPTP solid tumor panels, while the Ph + ALL xenograft showed a complete remission to dasatinib.[351] Thus, the primary utility for dasatinib in the pediatric setting, similar to that of imatinib, appears to be for patients with BCR-ABL leukemias. Dasatinib does distinguish itself from imatinib in several ways. Dasatinib maintains its activity against several mutant forms of BCR-ABL that induce imatinib resistance, although the T315I BCR-ABL mutation is resistant to both imatinib and dasatinib.[352] Another mechanism of imatinib resistance involves BCR-ABL independent activation of SRC family kinases, and this mechanism of resistance can be overcome by dasatinib.[353,354] Dasatinib is also more potent than imatinib, and unlike imatinib, it is able to induce apoptosis in BCR-ABL leukemia cells after brief exposures.[355,356] This latter characteristic allows dasatinib to be effective with daily dosing, despite its relatively short half-life.[357,358] Dasatinib is being studied in combination with chemotherapy for children with newly diagnosed Ph+ ALL. Other BCR-ABL inhibitors are under clinical evaluation in adults (e.g., nilotinib, bosutinib),[346] but given the small size of the pediatric CML and Ph+ ALL populations, it is unlikely that more than one or two BCR-ABL inhibitors will be extensively studied and used in the pediatric setting.

Targeting the Extracellular Signal-Related Kinase Pathway

The extracellular signal-related kinase (ERK) pathway is one of several MAPK pathways that have been characterized in mammals and that all involve a three-tiered kinase activation sequence.[359] The ERK cascade is initiated when RAS activation leads to RAF recruitment and activation, with downstream phosphorylation of MEK and ERK (see Fig. 11.2). In general, the overall effect of ERK pathway activation is to promote proliferation and survival.[360] The number of cancers associated with abnormalities that result in activation of the ERK cascade (e.g., cancers involving activated growth factors, RAS mutations and RAF mutations) make this cascade a prime target for cancer drug development for both hematological malignancies and for solid tumors, and small molecule inhibitors of RAF and MEK have entered clinical evaluation.[360] Of particular interest for inhibitors of this pathway are cancers with BRAF mutations. These mutations are observed in approximately 60% of melanomas, as well as 40% of thyroid cancers, and 20% of colon cancer and ovarian cancer.[359] Although a large number of missense mutations have been identified in the BRAF gene, a single mutation (V600E) within the activation loop of the kinase domain accounts for the vast majority of cases with BRAF mutations.[361] Mutations of BRAF appear to be uncommon in most childhood cancers,[362,363] with the primary exception being JPA. A high percentage of JPA cases show BRAF activation as a result of a tandem duplication that produces a novel fusion gene (KIAA1549-BRAF) that lacks the BRAF regulatory domain.[6,364] Activating mutations in JPA are less frequent, being identified in approximately 5% of cases. RAS and BRAF mutations are also observed in a subset of childhood ALL cases.[365–367]

RAF inhibitors that have entered clinical evaluation include sorafenib and PLX4032.[359,368] Sorafenib is an orally available ATP-competitive kinase inhibitor, and athough initial reports indicated relative specificity for RAF kinase activity, sorafenib is now recognized to be a potent inhibitor of a number of kinases, including VEGF-R2, PDGFR, KIT, and FLT3.[369] The relative lack of activity of sorafenib against BRAF mutant cell lines is consistent with the limited level of clinical activity observed for sorafenib against BRAF-mutant melanoma,[370] and it is likely that the beneficial clinical effects observed for sorafenib against cancers such as renal cell carcinoma are related to its activity against VEGF-R2 and other non-RAF kinases.[359,360] As a single missense mutation (V600E) accounts for the vast majority of mutant-BRAF cases, an inhibitor selective for this mutation should have broad applicability as well as a wide therapeutic index.[371] PLX4032 is based upon this premise and is a small molecule kinase inhibitor that selectively inhibits mutant (V600E) BRAF compared with wild-type BRAF. The objective response rate for PLX4032 exceeded 50% for patients with BRAF-mutant melanoma in its initial phase 1 clinical trial, providing proof of concept for this drug development strategy.[372]

Two highly selective non–ATP-competitive MEK inhibitors have entered clinical evaluation: PD0325901 and AZD6244.[360,373] Both agents demonstrated impressive in vitro and in vivo activity against preclinical models with mutant BRAF.[374,375] Although PD0325901 demonstrated marked suppression of ERK cascade signaling as well as partial responses in three melanoma patients in its initial phase 1 experience, visual toxicities resulted in cessation of its clinical development.[360] AZD6244 has completed its phase 1 testing, with rash being the most frequent and dose-limiting toxicity and with no serious visual disturbances observed.[376] A randomized phase 2 trial comparing AZD6244 monotherapy against temozolomide for first-line treatment of melanoma showed no difference in progression-free survival (PFS) between the two treatments and fewer than 10% of patients receiving AZD6244 showed objective responses.[377] The PPTP evaluated AZD6244 and found that it was not effective in inducing regressions as a single agent against most of the pediatric preclinical models evaluated. However, complete regressions were induced by AZD6244 against a BRAF-mutant pilocytic astrocytoma xenograft, pointing to the potential utility of MEK inhibition for this disease.[378]

TARGETING MAMMALIAN TARGET OF RAPAMYCIN WITH RAPAMYCIN AND RELATED AGENTS

mTOR (mammalian target of rapamycin) is an important regulator of cell growth and proliferation in response to external factors (e.g., growth factors) and nutritional conditions.[379] mTOR exists in two multiprotein complexes, mTORC1 and mTORC2, with the former including mTOR with raptor, PRAS40, and mLst8 (GβL) and with the latter including mTOR with rictor, Sin1, mLst8, and mAvo3. Rapamycin blocks mTORC1 signaling by first binding to FK506-binding protein 12 (FKBP12), with this drug-protein complex then inhibiting mTORC1 kinase activity. The pathway from growth factor receptor to mTOR proceeds from PI3K through AKT and eventually results in mTORC1-mediated phosphorylation of two proteins that play central roles in promoting the translation of selected mRNA transcripts: eukaryotic initiation factor 4E (eIF4E)-binding protein 1 (4E-BP1) and ribosomal protein S6

kinase 1 (S6K1) (see Fig. 11.2).[380] As mTORC1 promotes the translation of proteins essential to G_1 cell cycle progression, compounds that inhibit mTOR typically cause G_1 arrest in sensitive cells.[381] mTORC1 activity is also responsive to changes in intracellular energy stores. When intracellular energy stores are low, AMP-activated protein kinase activation results in TSC2 phosphorylation and subsequent inhibition of mTORC1 activity.[382]

Rapamycin (sirolimus) was first noted to have significant anticancer activity in preclinical models more than two decades ago.[383,384] Subsequent testing has shown activity of rapamycin against a number of childhood cancer preclinical models, including for rhabdomyosarcoma,[385–387] osteosarcoma,[388] Ewing's sarcoma,[389,390] medulloblastoma,[391] ALL,[392–395] and high-grade glioma.[396] In addition, everolimus inhibits growth of posttransplant lymphoproliferative disorder (PTLD)-like B lymphoblastoid cell lines, both in vitro and in vivo.[397,398] Proof of principle for the ability of rapamycin and its analogs to produce in vivo antitumor activity was provided using preclinical models of tuberous sclerosis complex (TSC), a condition caused by loss of function of TSC1 or TSC2 with resulting mTOR activation.[399,400] An evaluation of rapamycin by the PPTP showed broad in vivo tumor growth inhibition across most of the histologies evaluated, with objective responses (tumor regressions) observed for several diagnoses, including rhabdomyosarcoma, osteosarcoma, and ALL. The activity observed for rapamycin against the ALL PPTP panel is consistent with other reports showing in vivo activity for rapamycin and rapamycin analogs (rapalogs) against ALL xenografts.[395,401] Rapamycin and related mTOR inhibitors also have antiangiogenic activity through inhibition of proliferation of endothelial cells and through impaired VEGF production,[402–404] and hence in vivo activity observed for this class of agents may be related to direct or indirect effects on tumor cells.

Rapalogs that are being studied in the clinic for cancer indications include temsirolimus (CCI-779),[405] everolimus (RAD001),[406] rapamycin,[392] and ridaforolimus (deforolimus, AP23573).[407] The primary diagnoses for which mTOR inhibitors have shown benefit are renal cell carcinoma and various lymphoid malignancies. Temsirolimus at a weekly dose of 25 mg administered intravenously is licensed for treatment of previously untreated, metastatic renal cell carcinoma based on phase 3 trial results showing improved survival for patients receiving temsirolimus compared with that for patients receiving interferon alfa.[408] Everolimus (10 mg daily administered orally) is approved as second-line therapy for renal cell carcinoma following progression on a VEGF-targeted therapy based on results of a phase 3 trial showing improved PFS in a placebo-controlled trial.[409] Although significant improvements in OS and/or PFS were produced by both agents, the overall objective response rates were modest (<10%), supporting primary cytostatic effects and/or antiangiogenesis effects for mTOR inhibitors against renal cell carcinoma.[408,409] Temsirolimus has shown activity against mantle-cell lymphoma and other subtypes of NHL.[410–412] A phase 3 study in refractory mantle-cell lymphoma comparing temsirolimus at a lower and higher dose level to investigator's choice single-agent therapy showed a significant advantage for higher dose, but not lower dose, temsirolimus compared with investigator's choice treatment for both PFS and objective response rate.[411] This study suggests the need to maximize mTOR inhibition for optimal treatment of responsive histologies. Objective responses to rapamycin have been observed in tuberous sclerosis patients with subependymal giant cell astrocytomas, providing evidence for sufficient rapamycin brain penetration for clinical effect.[413] The primary toxicities observed for cancer patients receiving rapalogs include asthenia, mucositis, thrombocytopenia, hypercholesterolemia, and pneumonitis, with higher doses generally being associated with greater levels of toxicity.[379]

Pediatric phase 1 trials of rapalogs have been completed for temsirolimus and everolimus.[414,415] In addition, there is a large body of clinical experience using rapalogs in children undergoing solid organ transplants.[416-419] Pediatric development of rapalogs is now focusing on use of these agents in combination with standard chemotherapy or with other novel agents. The PPTP demonstrated that combinations of rapamycin with cyclophosphamide or vincristine were well tolerated, with the combinations commonly showing significantly greater antitumor activity than the single-agent treatments.[65] The combination of rapalogs with antibodies that block IGF-IR signaling has strong preclinical rationale for selected sarcomas.[304,420] The combination of glucocorticoids with rapalogs is of interest for ALL, given the single-agent activity for rapamycin against a subset of ALL xenografts and given the potentiation by rapamycin of the cytotoxic activity of glucocorticoids against a number of ALL cell lines.[64,65]

TARGETING DEVELOPMENTAL SIGNALING PATHWAYS

Several signaling pathways that play central roles in embryonic development are also involved in tumor development, including the Wnt, Notch, and Hedgehog pathways. In the childhood cancer setting, genomic alterations resulting in activation of these pathways are observed for subsets of selected childhood cancers, including Notch activation in T-cell ALL and ependymoma,[421,422] Hedgehog pathway activation for medulloblastoma,[423] and Wnt pathway activation for Wilms' tumor,[424] hepatoblastoma,[425] and medulloblastoma.[423] Therapeutic development is most advanced for inhibitors of Hedgehog and Notch signaling, as discussed later.

Targeting the Hedgehog Pathway

The Hedgehog signaling pathway is essential to embryonic development, as evidenced by the severe CNS and limb defects associated with pathway mutations or with in utero exposure to pathway inhibitors.[48,49] In adults, the Hedgehog pathway is primarily quiescent. However, there is evidence from studies of immature mice for a continued role for the Hedgehog pathway postnatally, as short-term treatment with pathway inhibitors leads to permanent bone damage.[91] This observation highlights the caution that will be required for appropriate pediatric development of agents targeting important developmental signaling pathways.

Hedgehog pathway signaling is initiated by binding of one of three Hedgehog proteins (Sonic, Indian, or Desert) to the 12-transmembrane receptor patched homologue 1 (PTCH1).[48,49] The normal role of PTCH1 is to tonically repress the activity of Smoothened (SMO). Hedgehog protein binding to PTCH1 leads to SMO de-repression, triggering a cascade of events localized in the cilia that results in nuclear translocation and activation of GLI family zinc-finger transcription factors. Subsequent downstream effects include induction of cyclin expression,[426] upregulation of antiapoptotic proteins such as BCL-2,[427] and induction of transcription of genes such as MYCN that drive cell proliferation.[428] Suppressor of fused (SUFU) is an inhibitor of the Hedgehog pathway that acts downstream of SMO by binding to GLI transcription factors and blocking their ability to stimulate transcription.[429]

A central role of Hedgehog pathway in tumorigenesis is evidenced by the presence of mutations in PTCH1 in basal cell nevus syndrome (Gorlin syndrome), which is characterized by elevated incidence of basal cell carcinoma and medulloblastoma. Genetically engineered mouse models have elegantly demonstrated the ability of genomic alterations in PTCH1, SMO, and SUFU to induce medulloblastoma.[430-432] Medulloblastoma induction in mouse models by upstream activators of Hedgehog signaling (e.g., SMO) requires functional cilia.[433] PTCH1 mutations can be identified in most cases of basal cell carcinoma and are present in approximately 10% of medulloblastoma cases,[423] although a higher proportion of cases show evidence of Hedgehog pathway activation.[434] Hedgehog pathway activation is primarily observed in desmoplastic medulloblastoma cases and appears to be associated with the presence of primary cilia on tumor cells.[423,433]

The Hedgehog pathway inhibitor most advanced in clinical testing is GDC-0449, a potent, orally available, small molecule SMO inhibitor.[435] The agent induced rapid inhibition of Hedgehog pathway signaling and tumor regression in the Ptc1 heterozygous murine model of medulloblastoma.[35] GDC-0449 was well tolerated in adults with locally advanced or metastatic basal-cell carcinoma, and prolonged objective responses were observed in 18 of 33 patients.[35] GDC-0449 treatment also produced rapid (although transient) tumor regression in a young adult with PTCH1-mutant metastatic medulloblastoma.[436] At recurrence, the patient's tumor was shown to have acquired a mutation in SMO that did not effect Hedgehog signaling but that disrupted the ability of GDC-0449 to bind SMO.[437] SMO inhibitors such as GDC-0449 may also have limited activity against medulloblastoma with Hedgehog pathway activation resulting from SUFU mutations.[431] Other Hedgehog pathway inhibitors that have entered clinical evaluation include IPI-926, BMS-833923 (XL139), and PF-04449913. Pediatric evaluations of this class of agents will require careful monitoring for skeletal growth complications, given the bone effects observed for Hedgehog pathway inhibitors in immature mice.[91]

Another potential therapeutic role for Hedgehog pathway inhibitors is targeting cancer stem cells, under the hypothesis that the Hedgehog pathway is required for maintaining this tumor population. Evidence for pathway activation in putative stem cell populations has been described for glioblastoma,[438] multiple myeloma,[439] medulloblastoma,[440] and CML,[441] among others. The concept of combining an agent that depletes the cancer stem cell population with conventional therapy that induces tumor debulking is an attractive, though unproven, application of Hedgehog pathway inhibitors.[49] Because of similarities between cancer stem cells and normal stem cells, implementation of this strategy could lead to reductions in normal self-renewing tissues with resulting long-term consequences, a scenario that is of particular concern in the pediatric setting.

Targeting Notch Pathway Signaling

Notch pathway signaling is implicated in a wide range of developmental and cellular processes, including carcinogenesis. Notch signaling generally requires physical contact between cells and involves a family of four receptors (Notch 1–4) and the ligands, Delta-like (DLL1, DLL3, and DLL4), and Jagged (JAG1 and JAG2).[442] Ligand binding induces proteolytic cleavage of the Notch receptor, extracellularly by an ADAM metalloprotease and intracellularly by γ-secretase. The latter cleavage releases the Notch intracellular domain (NICD) that proceeds to the nuclease where it associates with the DNA binding protein CSL and the transcriptional coactivator

Mastermind to promote transcription of target genes (e.g., HES1, CCND1, and MYC).

The co-optation of Notch signaling for oncogenic purposes is illustrated by T-cell ALL, for which NOTCH1 activating mutations are present in more than 50% of cases.[421] Two types of NOTCH1 mutations are observed in T-cell ALL: mutations in the extracellular heterodimerization domains lead to increased susceptibility to ligand-independent proteolytic cleavage, and mutations in the intracellular domain result in increased NICD stability. Mutations in FBXW7, a ubiquitin ligase implicated in NICD turnover, are also observed in T-cell ALL, and like PEST domain mutations, they lead to increased NICD stability.[421] NOTCH1 mutations have also been reported for a small subset of patients with ependymoma.[422] Notch pathway activation has been described for other childhood cancers, including osteosarcoma, medulloblastoma, and Ewing's sarcoma.[443] By contrast, Notch appears to act as a tumor suppressor gene for selected neuroendocrine tumors and skin cancers.[444,445]

The primary therapeutic strategy being used to block Notch signaling is inhibition of γ-secretase, as Notch proteolytic cleavage by this enzyme is required for Notch signaling.[446] Clinical development of γ-secretase inhibitors was initiated in an effort to identify effective treatments for Alzheimer's disease, as this protease is also involved in production of amyloid-β protein, the protein component of the Alzheimer's cerebral plaques.[447] In vivo studies found that blocking the Notch pathway by inhibition of γ-secretase caused on-target gastrointestinal toxicity as a result of massive goblet cell hyperplasia.[87] The initial clinical experience evaluating a γ-secretase inhibitor (MK-0752) against T-cell ALL was disappointing, as significant gastrointestinal toxicity was observed and none of the patients showed a significant clinical response.[448] These results could be due to inadequate inhibition of Notch signaling because dosing was limited by gastrointestinal toxicity, or they could be related to the limited levels of apoptosis induced in NOTCH1-mutant cell lines by γ-secretase inhibitors.[449,450]

γ-Secretase inhibitors in clinical testing for cancer indications include MK-0752 and RO4929097.[446,451] Successful clinical development of this class of agents will require identifying strategies that can create a therapeutic window by minimizing gastrointestinal toxicity while enhancing anticancer effects.[452] As an example, dexamethasone has been reported to reduce γ-secretase inhibitor induced gastrointestinal toxicity by blocking the induction of KLF4 (a transcription factor responsible for goblet cell differentiation) that occurs when Notch signaling is inhibited.[453] Like Hedgehog pathway inhibitors, Notch pathway inhibitors are being evaluated for their activity against cancer stem cells.[454]

TARGETING MITOTIC KINASES AND KINESINS

The orderly passage of cells through mitosis is driven in large measure by a set of mitotically active kinases and by mitotic kinesins, which are motor proteins that utilize energy from ATP hydrolysis to produce directed mechanical force along microtubules of the emerging mitotic spindle. Both mitotic kinases (e.g., Aurora A and B, and PLK1) and mitotic kinesins (e.g., KSP/HsEg5) have been the focus of successful efforts to develop potent small molecule inhibitors with cytotoxic activity.[455–457] Aurora A is a serine-threonine protein kinase that is involved in centrosome duplication and separation, microtubule-kinetochore attachment, spindle checkpoint, and cytokinesis.[458,459] High level expression of Aurora A kinase is common in cancer cells, and a subset of adult cancers show amplification of the Aurora A gene on chromosome 20.[455] Aurora B is the kinase component of the chromosomal passenger complex, which additionally includes survivin, INCEP, and borealin and Aurora B is required for correct chromosome alignment and segregation as well as for spindle checkpoint function and cytokinesis.[455] PLKs are a group of highly conserved serine-threonine kinases that play key roles at various stages of mitosis, including centrosome maturation, spindle formation, and cytokinesis.[456]

Ispinesib is a small molecule inhibitor of KSP that is not competitive with ATP for binding to KSP, but rather acts as an allosteric inhibitor that binds to the KSP-ADP complex and inhibits ADP release from KSP.[460,461] Potent ATP-competitive inhibitors of Aurora A and B have been developed, differing in their relative specificity for Aurora A versus Aurora B.[455,457] Pan Aurora A and B inhibitors behave like Aurora B inhibitors, as the Aurora B inhibitor phenotype is dominant.[457] Similarly, potent PLK inhibitors (e.g., BI 2536, BI 6727, and GSK 461364) have entered clinical evaluation. Each of these classes of inhibitors has a strong preclinical package, with potent in vitro activity and convincing in vivo activity against a range of xenografts. Given the specificity of these agents for actively dividing cells, they share a similar clinical toxicity profile in which neutropenia and/or thrombocytopenia are common dose-limiting toxicities.[457] A key question for each of these classes of kinase inhibitors is whether a therapeutic window will exist for them against specific cancers, given that normal proliferating tissues are also susceptible to their effects. The high level of in vivo activity of the Aurora A kinase inhibitor MLN8237 observed by the PPTP against neuroblastoma and ALL xenografts at doses producing drug exposures that approximate those tolerable in adults with cancer suggests that clinical benefit against specific cancers may be achievable for Aurora A inhibitors.[58,462] The observation that Aurora A binds MYCN and sequesters it from proteasomal degradation may provide a lead in understanding the in vivo sensitivity of neuroblastoma to Aurora A inhibition.[463,464] MLN8237 has entered pediatric clinical evaluation. Likewise, the observation arising from a genomewide RNAi screen that KRAS mutant cells are hypersensitive to inhibition of PLK1 function supports the potential for a favorable therapeutic index for PLK inhibitors cancers with specific genomic alterations.[28]

TARGETING HISTONE DEACETYLASES

Acetylation of selected lysine residues plays a key role in controlling the function of many proteins, and therapies directed toward modifying protein acetylation patterns can have substantial anticancer activity against specific cancer types.[465,466] The level of protein acetylation is maintained by the counterbalancing actions of histone acetyltransferases and histone deacetylases (HDACs). Histone acetylation alters chromatin structure and induces a local chromatin environment conducive with gene transcription, whereas histone deacetylation is commonly associated with repression of transcription. Although histones were the first proteins identified as targets for HDACs, the activity of a number of nonhistone proteins has subsequently been shown to be modified by acetylation, and these proteins are also substrates for "histone" deacetylases. Additional substrates include nuclear proteins such as p53, myo-D, and E2F1 and cytoplasmic proteins such as a-tubulin and Hsp90.

The HDACs are divided into four families, based on their homology to yeast enzymes.[465,467] Class I enzymes (HDACs 1,

2, 3, and 8) are expressed ubiquitously and are primarily localized to the nucleus. Class II enzymes tend to be expressed in a tissue and/or developmental stage specific manner and are subdivided into two groups: Class IIA enzymes (HDACs 4, 5, 7, and 9) shuttle between the cytoplasm and nucleus in a phosphorylation-dependent manner and Class IIB HDACs (HDACs 6 and 10) are localized to the cytoplasm. HDAC 6 appears to be a major deacetylase for α-tubulin and for Hsp90. HDAC11 is the only member of class IV. Class III HDACs (SIRT 1–7) are structurally related to the yeast sirtuin deacetylase family. Class I, II, and IV enzymes share a common mechanism of action, whereas the sirtuin-related HDACs catalyze a distinctive NAD-dependent reaction.

There are four major groups of HDAC inhibitors that have advanced to clinical evaluation.[468] The short chain fatty acid–related compounds with HDAC inhibitory activity include sodium butyrate and valproic acid. The hydroxamic acid structural class includes vorinostat (suberoylanilide hydroxamic acid, SAHA), belinostat (PXD101), and panobinostat (LBH589). The benzamide structural class includes entinostat (SNDX-275) and MGCD0103, and the cyclic peptides class includes romidepsin (depsipeptide). Most HDAC inhibitors under clinical evaluation inhibit both Class I and II HDACs, although members of the benzamide-based compounds preferentially inhibit Class I HDACs with lesser effect on Class II HDACs.[468] It remains unclear whether there is an advantage to targeting HDAC isotypes versus pan-HDAC inhibition.

There are multiple mechanisms by which HDAC inhibitors may exert anticancer activity in vivo.[465,466] HDAC inhibitors can induce their effects through activation and/or repression of gene transcription following histone hyperacetylation and the resulting effects on chromatin structure. Studies using a variety of HDAC inhibitors have shown that HDAC inhibitors regulate transcription (either upward or downward) for only a small subset of all expressed genes (<10%).[469,470] HDAC inhibitors characteristically induce $p21^{WAF1}$ expression, which can lead to cell cycle arrest in G_1 and reduce expression of genes involved in growth such as cyclin D. Acetylation of nonhistone proteins (e.g., p53, hsp90, HIF-1α, α-tubulin, STAT-3, Ku70) may alter their activity or stability and produce effects on multiple cellular functions, including cell cycle progression, DNA repair, apoptosis, and angiogenesis.[465]

The clinical experience with HDAC inhibitors is notable for the high level of activity observed against cutaneous T-cell lymphoma and peripheral T-cell lymphoma.[471] For example, the objective response rate to vorinostat and to romidepsin in phase 2 studies for CTCL were approximately 30%.[471] The marked efficacy for HDAC inhibitors for these T-cell lymphomas is not understood.[466] By contrast to the activity of HDAC inhibitors in the cutaneous and peripheral T-cell lymphoma setting, objective responses to agents in this class against adult solid tumors have been rare.[466] Preclinical studies have shown a broad range of in vitro activity for HDAC inhibitors, with activity observed against a wide variety of pediatric and adult solid tumor and hematologic malignancy cell lines.[465,472] The broad level of in vitro activity compared with the narrow range of activity observed in the clinical setting for HDAC inhibitors used as single agents may in part be due to differences in the drug concentrations to which cell lines are exposed compared with the drug levels tolerable in the clinical setting.[472]

Pediatric development of HDAC inhibitors has to date focused primarily on vorinostat and depsipeptide.[473,474] Occasional tumor regressions were noted for depsipeptide against a large panel of pediatric xenografts,[475] while for vorinostat, tumor growth delay without regression was the best response.[472] In the pediatric phase 1 experience with vorinostat, toxicities observed were similar to those observed in adults, with thrombocytopenia and neutropenia being dose limiting.[474] Clinical development of vorinostat in the pediatric setting is focusing on combination studies, including combinations of vorinostat with the proteasome inhibitor bortezomib,[476] with isotretinoin,[476,477] and with radiation for children with high grade gliomas.[478]

TARGETING PROTEASOME ACTION

The proteasome is the primary organelle in eukaryotic cells for degradation of intracellular proteins.[479,480] Intracellular proteins are marked for proteasomal degradation by the addition of polyubiquitin chains to specific lysine residues. Polyubiquitinated proteins are recognized by the proteasome and degraded into small polypeptides. Carefully controlled degradation of proteins through the ubiquitin-proteasome pathway is essential for multiple cellular processes, including orderly progression through the cell cycle, p53-mediated responses to cellular stresses, and NF-κB activation.

Compounds have been identified that block the proteolytic activity of proteasomes, with the dipeptidyl boronic acid compound bortezomib (PS-341) being the first to proceed to clinical development.[480] In preclinical studies, bortezomib demonstrated activity against a number of cancer types as evidenced by growth arrest, apoptosis, and restored sensitivity to standard chemotherapy and to radiation therapy.[479] Given the multiple signaling pathways affected by proteasome inhibition, there is probably not a single effect of bortezomib that is responsible for the entirety of its anticancer activity. One effect of bortezomib is to block NF-κB activation by stabilizing IκB and allowing IκB to maintain its inhibitory influence over NF-κB (see Fig. 11.2). However, for myeloma, bortezomib appears to paradoxically induce NF-κB activation in many cases,[481,482] an observation also reported for endometrial carcinoma cell lines.[483] Bortezomib can also stabilize p53, allowing it to function as a proapoptotic transcription factor in cells exposed to bortezomib.[484] Stabilization of the cyclin-dependent kinase inhibitors $p21^{WAF1}$ and $p27^{KIP1}$ may contribute to bortezomib-induced growth inhibition. Proteasome inhibitors also induce formation of aggresomes containing large quantities of ubiquitin-conjugated proteins formation,[485] endoplasmic reticulum stress, and disruption of the unfolded protein response,[486] effects that may be particularly relevant to bortezomib's activity in myeloma cells given their high rates of protein synthesis.[487]

Bortezomib has shown substantial clinical activity against multiple myeloma, and it was approved by FDA in 2003 for the treatment of patients with multiple myeloma who had relapsed following at least two prior lines of therapy,[488] Bortezomib was administered twice weekly for 2 out of every 2 weeks, and it induced objective responses in 28% of patients. A subsequent phase 3 trial demonstrated that bortezomib was significantly more effective than dexamethasone for patients with relapsed multiple myeloma who had received one to three previous therapies.[489,490] Approval in the frontline setting was based on a phase 3 comparison of melphalan and prednisone given with or without bortezomib, with a marked advantage observed for the three-drug combination in terms of PFS and response rate.[491] Bortezomib is also approved for progressive mantle cell lymphoma after at least one prior therapy based on a response rate of approximately 30% in a large single arm study.[492,493] Activity for bortezomib has also been observed for follicular NHL, but it is not active as a single agent against Hodgkin lymphoma or against nonhematologic malignancies.[494] The most common moderate-to-serious adverse events observed in adults receiving bortezomib have been asthenia, peripheral neuropathy, thrombocytopenia, and neutropenia.[479]

A pediatric solid tumor phase 1 study of bortezomib observed thrombocytopenia as its primary dose-limiting toxicity.[495] Given the negative clinical experience for bortezomib in adults with solid tumors and given the lack of significant activity for bortezomib against pediatric solid tumor xenografts,[480,496] there has been little interest in exploring the agent in the pediatric solid tumor setting. There is, however, rationale for pursuing bortezomib for children with ALL. Several reports have documented *in vitro* activity of bortezomib against ALL cell lines,[496,497] although this is a nonspecific observation, as many cancer cell lines are sensitive to bortezomib. Bortezomib showed some activity against the PPTP ALL xenografts, with both of the T-cell ALL xenografts evaluated responding to bortezomib.[496] In a phase 1 study of bortezomib for children with recurrent leukemias, however, there were no responses in nine children with B-precursor ALL, all heavily pretreated.[498] Against ALL cell lines, bortezomib was synergistic with dexamethasone and additive with vincristine, asparaginase, cytarabine, and doxorubicin.[497] Bortezomib can be safely administered with standard reinduction therapy in the recurrent pediatric ALL setting,[499] and this strategy is being pursued further in children with relapsed ALL. Bortezomib is also of interest for AML, based in part on the observation that NF-κB appears to be constitutively activated in primitive AML stem cells and that proteasome inhibitors preferentially induce apoptosis of AML stem cells compared with normal hematopoietic stem cells.[500,501] A phase 1 study adding bortezomib to a standard reinduction regimen using idarubicin and cytarabine demonstrated a good safety profile for the regimen and promising antileukemia activity,[502] and this strategy is being pursued in the pediatric AML setting.

TARGETING ANGIOGENESIS

From 1971 when Folkman proposed targeting angiogenesis as a potential effective strategy for cancer treatment,[503] three decades were required to prove that antiangiogenic therapy could improve survival for patients with cancer. In 2003, results of a phase 3 study were announced demonstrating prolongation of survival when the anti-VEGF monoclonal antibody bevacizumab was added to standard chemotherapy for patients with advanced colon cancer.[504] Subsequently, bevacizumab has been approved for multiple indications involving its use in the metastatic disease setting, and small molecule inhibitors of VEGF-R2 have been approved for use in patients with metastatic renal cell carcinoma.

Although angiogenesis is a complex process involving many factors, VEGF appears to be rate limiting in normal and pathological blood vessel growth.[94,127] VEGF acts primarily by binding to receptors on endothelial cells. VEGF-R2 (also known as Flk-1 or KDR) is a receptor tyrosine kinase and appears to be the VEGF receptor that is the major mediator of endothelial cell mitogenesis, survival, and microvascular permeability.[94,127] Therapeutic approaches to targeting this angiogenic pathway include antibodies directed against VEGF, antibodies targeting VEGF receptors, soluble decoy VEGF receptors (e.g., aflibercept), and small molecule inhibitors of VEGF-R2.[126] Small molecule VEGF-R2 inhibitors under clinical evaluation differ from each other primarily by their relative degree of specificity for VEGF-R2, with multitargeted kinase inhibitors like sunitinib and sorafenib potently inhibit-

ing a wider range of kinases and with more specific agents like cediranib inhibiting a small number of kinases in addition to VEGF-R2.[97,369,505]

The most impressive clinical results for VEGF pathway targeted agents have been for patients with renal cell carcinoma. The most common form of renal cell cancer (the clear cell subtype) is strongly associated with mutations, deletions, and hypermethylation of the von Hippel Lindau (VHL) gene that result in its inactivation.[506] This association may explain the sensitivity of renal cell carcinoma to VEGF pathway inhibition, as loss of VHL function leads to constitutive activation of the transcription factor HIF-1,[507] which in turn leads to overexpression of VEGF.[508] In contrast to many other cancer types for which objective response rates for VEGF pathway targeted agents are in the single digits, for renal cell cancer response rates as high as 30% to 45% have been observed for agents like sunitinib, axitinib, and pazopanib.[509] Both sunitinib and sorafenib improved PFS in phase 3 trials for patients with metastatic renal cell carcinoma, with analyses for overall survival confounded by use of VEGF pathway targeted agents at progression.[510,511] Both agents are approved by FDA for use in patients with metastatic renal cell carcinoma.

Glioblastoma is a tumor characterized by vascular proliferation and high expression of angiogenic factors, and bevacizumab induces objective responses, either as a single agent or in combination with irinotecan, in adults with glioblastoma.[512,513] FDA approval of bevacizumab for adults with progressive glioblastoma following prior therapy was based on objective response rates of 20% to 25% with durations of response of approximately 4 months.[126] Small molecule inhibitors of VEGF-R2 have also shown activity against glioblastoma.[514] Complicating interpretation of clinical results for VEGF pathway targeted agents against glioblastoma is the difficulty in distinguishing between true antitumor response and an antiedema effect, as at least a component of the reduction in enhancement on MRI scans is the result of reduced vascular permeability caused by inhibition of VEGF pathway signaling.[512] Pediatric patients with high-grade gliomas did not show objective responses to bevacizumab.[515]

For adult cancers aside from those with renal cell carcinoma and glioblastoma, bevacizumab has been shown to improve survival and/or progression when used in combination with standard chemotherapy regimens for several cancers when applied in the metastatic disease setting.[126] Of greater relevance in the pediatric setting is the contribution of bevacizumab and other agents targeting the VEGF pathway in the adjuvant setting, as this setting addresses the ability of these agents to cure more patients by working in concert with chemotherapy to eliminate micrometastatic disease. The first study addressing this question was for colorectal cancer, and randomized patients to standard chemotherapy for 6 months with or without 12 months of bevacizumab.[516] The study failed to meet its primary endpoint of improving 3-year disease-free survival, though there was a transient beneficial effect noted for patients receiving bevacizumab. The failure of bevacizumab in the adjuvant setting to aid in controlling micrometastatic disease, if confirmed in other studies, has major implications for the use of this class of agents in the pediatric oncology setting, given the primary focus on curative therapy for children with cancer.

Hypertension and proteinuria are class effects of VEGF pathway targeted agents, and are observed for both large molecule inhibitors and for small molecule inhibitors. For small molecule inhibitors of VEGF-R2 such as sunitinib and sorafenib, other adverse events include hypertension, fatigue, diarrhea, hypothyroidism, and hand-foot syndrome (9%)[369,510,517] As noted previously, growth plate abnormalities are of particular concern in the pediatric population, and ongoing studies in children with agents in this class are monitoring for this adverse effect.

The PPTP has tested several small molecule inhibitors of VEGF-R2, including relatively specific inhibitors (cediranib) and multitargeted kinase inhibitors (sunitinib and sorafenib) that potently block VEGF-R2 signaling.[45,518,519] One conclusion from the *in vitro* testing is that these agents have little direct anticancer effect on pediatric cancer cell lines, with the exception of cell lines with known activating mutations in non-VEGF-R2 receptor tyrosine kinases (e.g., KIT). *In vivo* testing primarily showed tumor growth delay, with very few examples of tumor regression observed. When treatment was stopped, tumors quickly resumed growth, consistent with results from adult cancer models indicating that continuous treatment is necessary for tumor growth inhibition.[519] In a pediatric phase 1 trial of bevacizumab, children with recurrent solid tumors receiving the agent showed few agent-related adverse events and drug disposition appeared to be similar to that observed in adults.[100] Combination studies in which bevacizumab is added to conventional chemotherapy regimens are ongoing in the pediatric population, and pediatric phase 1 trials of small molecule VEGF-R2 inhibitors have also been initiated.

Another approach to blocking angiogenesis is to target the interactions between $\alpha_V\beta_3$ and $\alpha_V\beta_5$ integrin adhesion molecules on sprouting capillary cells and their extracellular matrix ligands.[520] Binding of ligand with endothelial cell $\alpha_V\beta_3$ and $\alpha_V\beta_5$ occurs through specific Arg-Gly-Asp (RGD) motifs and promotes intracellular signaling leading to endothelial cell survival. Cilengitide (EMD 121974), a cyclized pentapeptide that antagonizes $\alpha_V\beta_3$ and $\alpha_V\beta_5$ binding to matrix through the RGD binding site, is in clinical trials.[521] Cilengitide was active against orthotopically implanted medulloblastoma and glioblastoma xenograft lines that express $\alpha_V\beta_3$ and $\alpha_V\beta_5$, but was not active against the same xenografts implanted subcutaneously, suggesting the importance of the extracellular environment for cilengitide effect.[522] Cilengitide is very well tolerated, and it induced objective responses in approximately 10% of adults and children with high-grade gliomas.[523,524] Further testing of cilengitide in the pediatric setting is focusing on the high-grade glioma population.

New targets for antiangiogenic therapy include components of the Notch pathway such as Dll4 and the angiopoietins (Ang-1 and Ang-2) and their receptor (Tie2).[525,526] As with agents targeting the VEGF pathway, the key to novel antiangiogenic agents making important contributions in the pediatric oncology setting will be their ability to promote curative therapy rather than simply slowing tumor growth leading to delayed time to progression.

CONCLUSIONS

Childhood cancer clinical research stands at a crossroads. For decades, there have been consistent improvements in outcome as a result of clinical trials that intensified and refined therapy with standard cytotoxic agents. Advances using this strategy have slowed down for most childhood cancers, and others have stopped altogether.[527] Opportunities for improving outcome through the use of molecularly targeted agents are multiple, but the challenges to success are also substantial. One of the opportunities is the large number of targeted agents in clinical trials that block growth and survival signaling pathways used by cancer cells. This opportunity is the converse of one of the key challenges to successfully employing targeted agents to improve outcome: the selection of truly effective agents to study against specific patient populations from among the scores of agents potentially available for study. There is cause for optimism in addressing this challenge, given the availability of technologies that should allow delineation within the coming decade of all of the recurring genomic and epigenomic alterations present in most childhood cancers. Understanding the genomic alterations that define each childhood cancer will provide invaluable information for prioritizing agents for investigation. Also encouraging is the availability of increasingly sophisticated technologies for target identification and validation, and the presence of molecularly characterized *in vivo* models for developing reliable preclinical assessments of the antitumor activity of novel agents. Another important challenge is the increasing need to study subsets of patients with a particular cancer diagnosis based on the molecular characteristics of their cancer. Meeting this challenge will require pediatric clinical trials infrastructures becoming more proficient in evaluating new therapies in genomically defined subtypes of childhood cancers. Given the relatively limited numbers of children with any given cancer diagnosis and the even smaller number within any given diagnosis that have a specific molecular abnormality, meeting this challenge will increasingly involve international collaborations so that sufficient patient numbers can be enrolled onto clinical trials to define the contribution of novel agents for patient populations whose cancers have specific molecular characteristics. If pediatric oncology researchers can take advantage of the available opportunities related to molecularly targeted agents, then there is cause for optimism that meaningful progress will be made in the coming decade toward having curative therapy available for every child diagnosed with cancer.

References

1. Armstrong SA, Kung AL, Mabon ME, et al. Inhibition of FLT3 in MLL. Validation of a therapeutic target identified by gene expression based classification. Cancer Cell 2003;3:173–183.
2. Davicioni E, Anderson MJ, Finckenstein FG, et al. Molecular classification of rhabdomyosarcoma–genotypic and phenotypic determinants of diagnosis: a report from the Children's Oncology Group. Am J Pathol 2009;174:550–564.
3. Ferrando AA, Neuberg DS, Staunton J, et al. Gene expression signatures define novel oncogenic pathways in T cell acute lymphoblastic leukemia. Cancer Cell 2002;1:75–87.
4. Thompson MC, Fuller C, Hogg TL, et al. Genomics identifies medulloblastoma subgroups that are enriched for specific genetic alterations. J Clin Oncol 2006;24:1924–1931.
5. Pfister S, Janzarik WG, Remke M, et al. BRAF gene duplication constitutes a mechanism of MAPK pathway activation in low-grade astrocytomas. J Clin Invest 2008;118:1739–1749.
6. Jones DT, Kocialkowski S, Liu L, et al. Tandem duplication producing a novel oncogenic BRAF fusion gene defines the majority of pilocytic astrocytomas. Cancer Res 2008;68:8673–8677.
7. Mulligan CG, Su X, Zhang J, et al. Deletion of IKZF1 and prognosis in acute lymphoblastic leukemia. N Engl J Med 2009;360:470–480.
8. Mulligan CG, Goorha S, Radtke I, et al. Genome-wide analysis of genetic alterations in acute lymphoblastic leukaemia. Nature 2007;446:758–764.
9. Mulligan CG, Zhang J, Harvey RC, et al. JAK mutations in high-risk childhood acute lymphoblastic leukemia. Proc Natl Acad Sci U S A 2009;106:9414–9418.
10. Mesa RA, Tefferi A. Emerging drugs for the therapy of primary and post essential thrombocythemia, post polycythemia vera myelofibrosis. Expert Opin Emerg Drugs 2009;14:471–479.
11. Mosse YP, Laudenslager M, Longo L, et al. Identification of ALK as a major familial neuroblastoma predisposition gene. Nature 2008;455: 930–935.
12. Gutierrez A, Sanda T, Grebliunaite R, et al. High frequency of PTEN, PI3K, and AKT abnormalities in T-cell acute lymphoblastic leukemia. Blood 2009;114:647–650.
13. Silva A, Yunes JA, Cardoso BA, et al. PTEN posttranslational inactivation and hyperactivation of the PI3K/Akt pathway sustain primary T cell leukemia viability. J Clin Invest 2008;118:3762–3774.
14. Ley TJ, Mardis ER, Ding L, et al. DNA sequencing of a cytogenetically normal acute myeloid leukaemia genome. Nature 2008;456:66–72.
15. Cristea IM, Gaskell SJ, Whetton AD. Proteomics techniques and their application to hematology. Blood 2004;103:3624–3634.

16. Manning G, Whyte DB, Martinez R, et al. The protein kinase complement of the human genome. Science 2002;298:1912–1934.
17. Cen L, Arnoczky KJ, Hsieh FC, et al. Phosphorylation profiles of protein kinases in alveolar and embryonal rhabdomyosarcoma. Mod Pathol 2007;20:936–946.
18. Kotecha N, Flores NJ, Irish JM, et al. Single-cell profiling identifies aberrant STAT5 activation in myeloid malignancies with specific clinical and biologic correlates. Cancer Cell 2008;14:335–343.
19. Hannon GJ, Rossi JJ. Unlocking the potential of the human genome with RNA interference. Nature 2004;431:371–378.
20. Zamore PD, Haley B. Ribo-gnome: the big world of small RNAs. Science 2005;309:1519–1524.
21. Paddison PJ, Caudy AA, Sachidanandam R, et al. Short hairpin activated gene silencing in mammalian cells. Methods Mol Biol 2004;265: 85–100.
22. Prieur A, Tirode F, Cohen P, et al. EWS/FLI-1 silencing and gene profiling of Ewing cells reveal downstream oncogenic pathways and a crucial role for repression of insulin-like growth factor binding protein 3. Mol Cell Biol 2004;24:7275–7283.
23. Chansky HA, Barahmand-Pour F, Mei Q, et al. Targeting of EWS/FLI-1 by RNA interference attenuates the tumor phenotype of Ewing's sarcoma cells in vitro. J Orthop Res 2004;22:910–917.
24. Paddison PJ, Silva JM, Conklin DS, et al. A resource for large-scale RNA-interference-based screens in mammals. Nature 2004;428:427–431.
25. Berns K, Hijmans EM, Mullenders J, et al. A large-scale RNAi screen in human cells identifies new components of the p53 pathway. Nature 2004;428:431–437.
26. Hartwell LH, Szankasi P, Roberts CJ, et al. Integrating genetic approaches into the discovery of anticancer drugs. Science 1997;278:1064–1068.
27. Canaani D. Methodological approaches in application of synthetic lethality screening towards anticancer therapy. Br J Cancer 2009;100: 1213–1218.
28. Luo J, Emanuele MJ, Li D, et al. A genome-wide RNAi screen identifies multiple synthetic lethal interactions with the Ras oncogene. Cell 2009;137:835–848.
29. Weinstein IB, Joe A. Oncogene addiction. Cancer Res 2008;68:3077–3080.
30. Weinstein IB. Cancer. Addiction to oncogenes—the Achilles heal of cancer. Science 2002;297:63–64.
31. Mauro MJ, O'Dwyer M, Heinrich MC, et al. STI571: a paradigm of new agents for cancer therapeutics. J Clin Oncol 2002;20:325–334.
32. Heinrich MC, Corless CL, Demetri GD, et al. Kinase mutations and imatinib response in patients with metastatic gastrointestinal stromal tumor. J Clin Oncol 2003;21: 4342–4349.
33. Gotlib J, Cools J, Malone JM III, et al. The FIP1L1-PDGFRalpha fusion tyrosine kinase in hypereosinophilic syndrome and chronic eosinophilic leukemia: implications for diagnosis, classification, and management. Blood 2004;103:2879–2891.
34. Apperley JF, Gardembas M, Melo JV, et al. Response to imatinib mesylate in patients with chronic myeloproliferative diseases with rearrangements of the platelet-derived growth factor receptor beta. N Engl J Med 2002;347:481–487.
35. Von Hoff DD, LoRusso PM, Rudin CM, et al. Inhibition of the Hedgehog Pathway in Advanced Basal-Cell Carcinoma. N Engl J Med 2009;361(12): 1164–1172.
36. Kwak EL, Camidge DR, Clark J, et al. Clinical activity observed in a phase I dose escalation trial of an oral c-met and ALK inhibitor, PF-02341066. J Clin Oncol 2009;27:15s (Suppl; abstract 3509).
37. Sanz M, Burnett A, Lo-Coco F, et al. FLT3 inhibition as a targeted therapy for acute myeloid leukemia. Curr Opin Oncol 2009;21(6):594–600.
38. Kalebic T, Tsokos M, Helman LJ. In vivo treatment with antibody against IGF-1 receptor suppresses growth of human rhabdomyosarcoma and down-regulates p34cdc2. Cancer Res 1994;54:5531–5534.
39. Scotlandi K, Benini S, Sarti M, et al. Insulin-like growth factor I receptor-mediated circuit in Ewing's sarcoma/peripheral neuroectodermal tumor: a possible therapeutic target. Cancer Res 1996;56:4570–4574.
40. Scotlandi K, Avnet S, Benini S, et al. Expression of an IGF-I receptor dominant negative mutant induces apoptosis, inhibits tumorigenesis and enhances chemosensitivity in Ewing's sarcoma cells. Int J Cancer 2002;101:11–16.
41. Kalebic T, Blakesley V, Slade C, et al. Expression of a kinase-deficient IGF-I-R suppresses tumorigenicity of rhabdomyosarcoma cells constitutively expressing a wild type IGF-I-R. Int J Cancer 1998;76:223–227.
42. Toretsky JA, Kalebic T, Blakesley V, et al. The insulin-like growth factor-I receptor is required for EWS/FLI-1 transformation of fibroblasts. J Biol Chem 1997;272:30822–30827.
43. McDermott U, Iafrate AJ, Gray NS, et al. Genomic alterations of anaplastic lymphoma kinase may sensitize tumors to anaplastic lymphoma kinase inhibitors. Cancer Res 2008;68:3389–3395.
44. Wilhelm SM, Adnane L, Newell P, et al. Preclinical overview of sorafenib, a multikinase inhibitor that targets both Raf and VEGF and PDGF receptor tyrosine kinase signaling. Mol Cancer Ther 2008;7:3129–3140.
45. Kolb EA, Gorlick R, Houghton PJ, et al. Pediatric Preclinical Testing Program (PPTP) evaluation of the multi-targeted kinase inhibitor sorafenib. In: Proceedings of the 100th Annual Meeting of the American Association for Cancer Research. Philadelphia, PA; 2009. Abstract #3196.
46. Houghton PJ, Adamson PC, Blaney S, et al. Testing of new agents in childhood cancer preclinical models: meeting summary. Clin Cancer Res 2002;8:3646–3657.
47. Romer JT, Kimura H, Magdaleno S, et al. Suppression of the Shh pathway using a small molecule inhibitor eliminates medulloblastoma in Ptc1(+ /−()p53(−/−) mice. Cancer Cell 2004;6:229–240.
48. Gallinari P, Filocamo G, Jones P, et al. Smoothened antagonists: a promising new class of antitumor agents. Expert Opin Drug Discov 2009;4:525–544.
49. Scales SJ, de Sauvage FJ. Mechanisms of Hedgehog pathway activation in cancer and implications for therapy. Trends Pharmacol Sci 2009;30: 303–312.
50. Johnson JI, Decker S, Zaharevitz D, et al. Relationships between drug activity in NCI preclinical in vitro and in vivo models and early clinical trials. Br J Cancer 2001; 84:1424–1431.
51. Neale G, Su X, Morton CL, et al. Molecular characterization of the Pediatric Preclinical Testing Panel. Clin Cancer Res 2008;14:4572–4583.
52. Houghton PJ, Morton CL, Tucker C, et al. The pediatric preclinical testing program: description of models and early testing results. Pediatr Blood Cancer 2007;49:928–940.
53. Yang L, Clarke MJ, Carlson BL, et al. PTEN loss does not predict for response to RAD001 (Everolimus) in a glioblastoma orthotopic xenograft test panel. Clin Cancer Res 2008;14:3993–4001.
54. Garber K. From human to mouse and back: 'tumorgraft' models surge in popularity. J Natl Cancer Inst 2009;101:6–8.
55. Bachmann PS, Lock RB. In vivo models of childhood leukemia for preclinical drug testing. Curr Drug Targets 2007;8:773–783.
56. Santana VM, Furman WL, Billups CA, et al. Improved response in high-risk neuroblastoma with protracted topotecan administration using a pharmacokinetically guided dosing approach. J Clin Oncol 2005;23: 4039–4047.
57. Lock R, Carol H, Houghton PJ, et al. Initial testing (stage 1) of the BH3 mimetic ABT-263 by the pediatric preclinical testing program. Pediatr Blood Cancer 2008;50:1181–1189.
58. Houghton PJ, Morton CL, Maris JM, et al. Pediatric preclinical testing program (PPTP) evaluation of the Aurora A kinase inhibitor MLN8237. In: Proceedings of the 99th Annual Meeting of the American Association for Cancer Research. Philadelphia, PA; 2008. Abstract #2997.
59. Gorlick R, Kolb EA, Houghton PJ, et al. Initial testing (stage 1) of lapatinib by the pediatric preclinical testing program. Pediatr Blood Cancer 2009;53:594–598.
60. Jia J, Zhu F, Ma X, et al. Mechanisms of drug combinations: interaction and network perspectives. Nat Rev Drug Discov 2009;8:111–128.
61. Iorns E, Lord CJ, Turner N, et al. Utilizing RNA interference to enhance cancer drug discovery. Nat Rev Drug Discov 2007;6:556–568.
62. Iorns E, Lord CJ, Ashworth A. Parallel RNAi and compound screens identify the PDK1 pathway as a target for tamoxifen sensitization. Biochem J 2009;417:361–370.
63. Shoemaker AR, Oleksijew A, Bauch J, et al. A small-molecule inhibitor of Bcl-XL potentiates the activity of cytotoxic drugs in vitro and in vivo. Cancer Res 2006;66: 8731–8739.
64. Wei G, Twomey D, Lamb J, et al. Gene expression-based chemical genomics identifies rapamycin as a modulator of MCL1 and glucocorticoid resistance. Cancer Cell 2006; 10:331–342.
65. Houghton PJ, Morton CL, Gorlick R, et al. Stage 2 combination testing of rapamycin with cytotoxic agents by the Pediatric Preclinical Testing Program. Mol Cancer Ther 2010;9:101–112.
66. Dolan ME, Pegg AE. O6-benzylguanine and its role in chemotherapy. Clin Cancer Res 1997;3:837–847.
67. Quinn JA, Pluda J, Dolan ME, et al. Phase II trial of carmustine plus O(6)-benzylguanine for patients with nitrosourea-resistant recurrent or progressive malignant glioma. J Clin Oncol 2002;20:2277–2283.
68. Rose WC, Wild R. Therapeutic synergy of oral taxane BMS-275183 and cetuximab versus human tumor xenografts. Clin Cancer Res 2004;10:7413–7417.
69. Tew KD, Houghton PJ, Houghton JA. Modulation of glutathione. In: Preclinical and clinical modulation of anticancer drugs. Boca Raton, Florida: CRC Press, 1993:13–77.
70. Adams DM, Zhou T, Berg SL, et al. Phase 1 trial of O6-benzylguanine and BCNU in children with CNS tumors: a Children's Oncology Group study. Pediatr Blood Cancer 2008;50:549–553.
71. Yamazaki S, Skaptason J, Romero D, et al. Pharmacokinetic–pharmacodynamic modeling of biomarker response and tumor growth inhibition to an orally available cMet kinase inhibitor in human tumor xenograft mouse models. Drug Metab Dispos 2008;36:1267–1274.
72. Hidalgo M, Messersmith W. Pharmacodynamic studies in drug development. Am Soc Clin Oncol 2004 Ed Book (40th Annual Meeting) 2004;160–163.
73. Kinders RJ, Hollingshead M, Khin S, et al. Preclinical modeling of a phase 0 clinical trial: qualification of a pharmacodynamic assay of poly (ADP-ribose) polymerase in tumor biopsies of mouse xenografts. Clin Cancer Res 2008;14:6877–6885.
74. Roberts A, Gandhi L, O'Connor OA, et al. Reduction in platelet counts as a mechanistic biomarker and guide for adaptive dose-escalation in phase I studies of the Bcl-2 family inhibitor ABT-263. J Clin Oncol 2008;26 (suppl; abstract 3542).
75. Moss KG, Toner GC, Cherrington JM, et al. Hair depigmentation is a biological readout for pharmacological inhibition of KIT in mice and humans. J Pharmacol Exp Ther 2003;307:476–480.
76. Dancey J. Epidermal growth factor receptor inhibitors in clinical development. Int J Radiat Oncol Biol Phys 2004;58:1003–1007.
77. Karp DD, Paz-Ares LG, Novello S, et al. Phase II study of the anti-insulin-like growth factor type 1 receptor antibody CP-751,871 in combination with paclitaxel and carboplatin in previously untreated, locally advanced, or metastatic non-small-cell lung cancer. J Clin Oncol 2009;27: 2516–2522.
78. Lacy MQ, Alsina M, Fonseca R, et al. Phase I, pharmacokinetic and pharmacodynamic study of the anti-insulinlike growth factor type 1 Receptor monoclonal antibody CP-751,871 in patients with multiple myeloma. J Clin Oncol 2008;26:3196–3203.
79. Hurwitz HI, Dowlati A, Saini S, et al. Phase I trial of pazopanib in patients with advanced cancer. Clin Cancer Res 2009;15:4220–4227.
80. Korn EL. Nontoxicity endpoints in phase I trial designs for targeted, non-cytotoxic agents. J Natl Cancer Inst 2004;96:977–978.
81. Anderson BD, Adamson PC, Weiner SL, et al. Tissue collection for correlative studies in childhood cancer clinical trials: ethical considerations and special imperatives. J Clin Oncol 2004;22:4794–4798.
82. Kopelman LM. Children as research subjects: a dilemma. J Med Philos 2000;25: 745–764.
83. Kodish E. Pediatric ethics and early-phase childhood cancer research: conflicted goals and the prospect of benefit. Account Res 2003;10:17–25.
84. Smith M, Bernstein M, Bleyer WA, et al. Conduct of phase I trials in children with cancer. J Clin Oncol 1998;16:966–978.
85. Furman WL, Stewart CF, Poquette CA, et al. Direct translation of a protracted irinotecan schedule from a xenograft model to a phase I trial in children. J Clin Oncol 1999; 17:1815–1824.
86. Seymour L. The design of clinical trials for new molecularly targeted compounds: progress and new initiatives. Curr Pharm Des 2002;8:2279–2284.
87. van Es JH, van Gijn ME, Riccio O, et al. Notch/gamma-secretase inhibition turns proliferative cells in intestinal crypts and adenomas into goblet cells. Nature 2005;435: 959–963.
88. Mason KD, Carpinelli MR, Fletcher JI, et al. Programmed anuclear cell death delimits platelet life span. Cell 2007;128:1173–1186.
89. Zhang H, Nimmer PM, Tahir SK, et al. Bcl-2 family proteins are essential for platelet survival. Cell Death Differ 2007;14:943–951.
90. Chen MH. Cardiac dysfunction induced by novel targeted anticancer therapy: an emerging issue. Curr Cardiol Rep 2009;11:167–174.
91. Kimura H, Ng JM, Curran T. Transient inhibition of the Hedgehog pathway in young mice causes permanent defects in bone structure. Cancer Cell 2008;13:249–260.
92. Hall AP, Westwood FR, Wadsworth PF. Review of the effects of anti-angiogenic compounds on the epiphyseal growth plate. Toxicol Pathol 2006;34:131–147.
93. Gerber HP, Ferrara N. Angiogenesis and bone growth. Trends Cardiovasc Med 2000;10:223–228.
94. Ferrara N, Gerber HP, LeCouter J. The biology of VEGF and its receptors. Nat Med 2003;9:669–676.

95. Gerber HP, Vu TH, Ryan AM, et al. VEGF couples hypertrophic cartilage remodeling, ossification and angiogenesis during endochondral bone formation. Nat Med 1999;5:623–628.

96. Ryan AM, Eppler DB, Hagler KE, et al. Preclinical safety evaluation of rhuMAbVEGF, an antiangiogenic humanized monoclonal antibody. Toxicol Pathol 1999;27:78–86.

97. Wedge SR, Kendrew J, Hennequin LF, et al. AZD2171: a highly potent, orally bioavailable, vascular endothelial growth factor receptor-2 tyrosine kinase inhibitor for the treatment of cancer. Cancer Res 2005;65:4389–4400.

98. Patyna S, Arrigoni C, Terron A, et al. Nonclinical safety evaluation of sunitinib: a potent inhibitor of VEGF, PDGF, KIT, FLT3, and RET receptors. Toxicol Pathol 2008;36:905–916.

99. Smith AR, Hennessy JM, Kurth MA, et al. Reversible skeletal changes after treatment with bevacizumab in a child with cutaneovisceral angiomatosis with thrombocytopenia syndrome. Pediatr Blood Cancer 2008;51:418–420.

100. Glade Bender JL, Adamson PC, Reid JM, et al. Phase I trial and pharmacokinetic study of bevacizumab in pediatric patients with refractory solid tumors: a Children's Oncology Group Study. J Clin Oncol 2008;26:399–405.

101. Modak S, Cheung NK, Abramson SJ, et al. Lack of early bevacizumab-related skeletal radiographic changes in children with neuroblastoma. Pediatr Blood Cancer 2009;52:304–305.

102. Allen DB. Growth suppression by glucocorticoid therapy. Endocrinol Metab Clin North Am 1996;25:699–717.

103. Smink JJ, Buchholz IM, Hamers N, et al. Short-term glucocorticoid treatment of piglets causes changes in growth plate morphology and angiogenesis. Osteoarthritis Cartilage 2003;11:864–871.

104. Kohler G, Milstein C. Continuous cultures of fused cells secreting antibody of predefined specificity. Nature 1975;256:495–497.

105. Levy R. Will monoclonal antibodies find a place in our therapeutic armamentarium? J Clin Oncol 1987;5:527–529.

106. Khazaeli MB, Conry RM, LoBuglio AF. Human immune response to monoclonal antibodies. J Immunother 1994;15:42–52.

107. Green LL, Hardy MC, Maynard-Currie CE, et al. Antigen-specific human monoclonal antibodies from mice engineered with human Ig heavy and light chain YACs. Nat Genet 1994;7:13–21.

108. Wagner SD, Williams GT, Larson T, et al. Antibodies generated from human immunoglobulin miniloci in transgenic mice. Nucleic Acids Res 1994;22:1389–1393.

109. Ezzell C. Magic bullets fly again. Sci Am 2001;285:34–41.

110. Smothers JF, Henikoff S, Carter P. Tech.Sight. Phage display. Affinity selection from biological libraries. Science 2002;298:621–622.

111. Senter PD. Potent antibody drug conjugates for cancer therapy. Curr Opin Chem Biol 2009;13:235–244.

112. Cartron G, Watier H, Golay J, et al. From the bench to the bedside: ways to improve rituximab efficacy. Blood 2004;104:2635–2642.

113. Cheson BD, Leonard JP. Monoclonal antibody therapy for B-cell non-Hodgkin's lymphoma. N Engl J Med 2008;359:613–626.

114. Griffin TC, Weitzman S, Weinstein H, et al. A study of rituximab and ifosfamide, carboplatin, and etoposide chemotherapy in children with recurrent/refractory B-cell (CD20 +) non-Hodgkin lymphoma and mature B-cell acute lymphoblastic leukemia: a report from the Children's Oncology Group. Pediatr Blood Cancer 2009;52:177–181.

115. Attias D, Weitzman S. The efficacy of rituximab in high-grade pediatric B-cell lymphoma/leukemia: a review of available evidence. Curr Opin Pediatr 2008;20:17–22.

116. Di Gaetano N, Cittera E, Nota R, et al. Complement activation determines the therapeutic activity of rituximab in vivo. J Immunol 2003;171: 1581–1587.

117. Cragg MS, Glennie MJ. Antibody specificity controls in vivo effector mechanisms of anti-CD20 reagents. Blood 2004;103:2738–2743.

118. van der Kolk LE, Grillo-Lopez AJ, Baars JW, et al. Complement activation plays a key role in the side-effects of rituximab treatment. Br J Haematol 2001;115:807–811.

119. Mishima Y, Sugimura N, Matsumoto-Mishima Y, et al. An imaging-based rapid evaluation method for complement-dependent cytotoxicity discriminated clinical response to rituximab-containing chemotherapy. Clin Cancer Res 2009;15:3624–3632.

120. Hernandez-Ilizaliturri FJ, Jupudy V, Ostberg J, et al. Neutrophils contribute to the biological antitumor activity of rituximab in a non-Hodgkin's lymphoma severe combined immunodeficiency mouse model. Clin Cancer Res 2003;9:5866–5873.

121. Clynes RA, Towers TL, Presta LG, et al. Inhibitory Fc receptors modulate in vivo cytotoxicity against tumor targets. Nat Med 2000;6:443–446.

122. Cartron G, Dacheux L, Salles G, et al. Therapeutic activity of humanized anti-CD20 monoclonal antibody and polymorphism in IgG Fc receptor FcgammaRIIIa gene. Blood 2002;99:754–758.

123. Shan D, Ledbetter JA, Press OW. Signaling events involved in anti-CD20-induced apoptosis of malignant human B cells. Cancer Immunol Immunother 2000;48:673–683.

124. Chow KU, Sommerlad WD, Boehrer S, et al. Anti-CD20 antibody (IDEC-C2B8, rituximab) enhances efficacy of cytotoxic drugs on neoplastic lymphocytes in vitro: role of cytokines, complement, and caspases. Haematologica 2002;87:33–43.

125. Bonavida B. Rituximab-induced inhibition of antiapoptotic cell survival pathways: implications in chemo/immunoresistance, rituximab unresponsiveness, prognostic and novel therapeutic interventions. Oncogene 2007;26:3629–3636.

126. Grothey A, Galanis E. Targeting angiogenesis: progress with anti-VEGF treatment with large molecules. Nat Rev Clin Oncol 2009;6:507–518.

127. Ferrara N, Hillan KJ, Gerber HP, et al. Discovery and development of bevacizumab, an anti-VEGF antibody for treating cancer. Nat Rev Drug Discov 2004;3:391–400.

128. Goldstein NI, Prewett M, Zuklys K, et al. Biological efficacy of a chimeric antibody to the epidermal growth factor receptor in a human tumor xenograft model. Clin Cancer Res 1995;1:1311–1318.

129. Yang XD, Jia XC, Corvalan JR, et al. Development of ABX-EGF, a fully human anti-EGF receptor monoclonal antibody, for cancer therapy. Crit Rev Oncol Hematol 2001;38:17–23.

130. Burtrum D, Zhu Z, Lu D, et al. A fully human monoclonal antibody to the insulin-like growth factor I receptor blocks ligand-dependent signaling and inhibits human tumor growth in vivo. Cancer Res 2003;63: 8912–8921.

131. Reynolds NA, Wagstaff AJ. Cetuximab: in the treatment of metastatic colorectal cancer. Drugs 2004;64:109–118.

132. Rowinsky EK, Schwartz GH, Gollob JA, et al. Safety, pharmacokinetics, and activity of ABX-EGF, a fully human anti-epidermal growth factor receptor monoclonal antibody in patients with metastatic renal cell cancer. J Clin Oncol 2004;22:3003–3015.

133. Slart R, Yu AL, Yaksh TL, et al. An animal model of pain produced by systemic administration of an immunotherapeutic anti-ganglioside antibody. Pain 1997;69:119–125.

134. Yu AL, Uttenreuther-Fischer MM, Huang CS, et al. Phase I trial of a human-mouse chimeric anti-disialoganglioside monoclonal antibody ch14.18 in patients with refractory neuroblastoma and osteosarcoma. J Clin Oncol 1998;16:2169–2180.

135. Winkler U, Jensen M, Manzke O, et al. Cytokine-release syndrome in patients with B-cell chronic lymphocytic leukemia and high lymphocyte counts after treatment with an anti-CD20 monoclonal antibody (rituximab, IDEC-C2B8). Blood 1999;94:2217–2224.

136. Byrd JC, Waselenko JK, Maneatis TJ, et al. Rituximab therapy in hematologic malignancy patients with circulating blood tumor cells: association with increased infusion-related side effects and rapid blood tumor clearance. J Clin Oncol 1999;17:791–795.

137. Osterborg A, Dyer MJ, Bunjes D, et al. Phase II multicenter study of human CD52 antibody in previously treated chronic lymphocytic leukemia. European Study Group of CAMPATH-1H Treatment in Chronic Lymphocytic Leukemia. J Clin Oncol 1997;15:1567–1574.

138. Sondel PM, Hank JA. Antibody-directed, effector cell-mediated tumor destruction. Hematol Oncol Clin North Am 2001;15:703–721.

139. Kushner BH, Cheung NK. GM-CSF enhances 3F8 monoclonal antibody-dependent cellular cytotoxicity against human melanoma and neuroblastoma. Blood 1989;73:1936–1941.

140. Barker E, Mueller BM, Handgretinger R, et al. Effect of a chimeric anti-ganglioside GD2 antibody on cell-mediated lysis of human neuroblastoma cells. Cancer Res 1991;51:144–149.

141. Hank JA, Surfus J, Gan J, et al. Treatment of neuroblastoma patients with antiganglioside GD2 antibody plus interleukin-2 induces antibody-dependent cellular cytotoxicity against neuroblastoma detected in vitro. J Immunother 1994;15:29–37.

142. Yu AL, Batova A, Alvarado C, et al. Usefulness of a chimeric anti-GD2 (ch14.18) and GM-CSF for refractory neuroblastoma: a POG phase II study. Proc Am Soc Clin Oncol 1997;16:513a.

143. Kushner BH, Kramer K, Cheung NK. Phase II trial of the anti-G(D2) monoclonal antibody 3F8 and granulocyte-macrophage colony-stimulating factor for neuroblastoma. J Clin Oncol 2001;19:4189–4194.

144. Frost JD, Hank JA, Reaman GH, et al. A phase I/IB trial of murine monoclonal anti-GD2 antibody 14.G2a plus interleukin-2 in children with refractory neuroblastoma: a report of the Children's Cancer Group. Cancer 1997;80:317–333.

145. Gilman AL, Ozkaynak MF, Matthay KK, et al. Phase I study of ch14.18 with granulocyte-macrophage colony-stimulating factor and interleukin-2 in children with neuroblastoma after autologous bone marrow transplantation or stem-cell rescue: a report from the Children's Oncology Group. J Clin Oncol 2009;27:85–91.

146. Yu AL, Gilman AL, Ozkaynak MF, et al. A phase III randomized trial of the chimeric anti-GD2 antibody ch14.18 with GM-CSF and IL2 as immunotherapy following dose intensive chemotherapy for high-risk neuroblastoma: Children's Oncology Group (COG) study ANBL0032 . J Clin Oncol 2009;27:15s(Suppl; abstract 10067z).

147. Desjarlais JR, Lazar GA, Zhukovsky EA, Chu SY. Optimizing engagement of the immune system by anti-tumor antibodies: an engineer's perspective. Drug Discov Today 2007;12:898–910.

148. Horton HM, Bernett MJ, Pong E, et al. Potent in vitro and in vivo activity of an Fc-engineered anti-CD19 monoclonal antibody against lymphoma and leukemia. Cancer Res 2008;68:8049–8057.

149. Zalevsky J, Leung IW, Karki S, et al. The impact of Fc engineering on an anti-CD19 antibody: increased Fc(Gamma) receptor affinity enhances B-cell clearing in nonhuman primates. Blood 2009;113:3735–3743.

150. Jefferis R. Glycosylation as a strategy to improve antibody-based therapeutics. Nat Rev Drug Discov 2009;8:226–234.

151. Salles GA, Morschhauser F, Cartron G, et al. A phase I/II study of RO5072759 (GA101) in patients with relapsed/refractory CD20 + malignant disease. Blood (ASH Ann Meet Abstr) 2008;112 [abstract 234].

152. Staerz UD, Kanagawa O, Bevan MJ. Hybrid antibodies can target sites for attack by T cells. Nature 1985;314:628–631.

153. Baeuerle PA, Reinhardt C. Bispecific T-cell engaging antibodies for cancer therapy. Cancer Res 2009;69:4941–4944.

154. Bargou R, Leo E, Zugmaier G, et al. Tumor regression in cancer patients by very low doses of a T cell-engaging antibody. Science 2008;321:974–977.

155. Topp MS, Goekbuget N, Kufer P, et al. Blinatumomab (anti-CD19 BiTE) for targeted therapy of minimal residual disease (MRD) in patients with B-precursor acute lymphoblastic leukemia (ALL): Update of an ongoing phase II study [abstract #482]. Haematologica 2009;94(suppl 2):195.

156. Carter P. Improving the efficacy of antibody-based cancer therapies. Nat Rev Cancer 2001;1:118–129.

157. Frankel AE, Neville DM, Bugge TA, et al. Immunotoxin therapy of hematologic malignancies. Semin Oncol 2003;30:545–557.

158. Kell WJ, Burnett AK, Chopra R, et al. A feasibility study of simultaneous administration of gemtuzumab ozogamicin with intensive chemotherapy in induction and consolidation in younger patients with acute myeloid leukemia. Blood 2003;102:4277–4283.

159. Coiffier B, Lepage E, Briere J, et al. CHOP chemotherapy plus rituximab compared with CHOP alone in elderly patients with diffuse large-B-cell lymphoma. N Engl J Med 2002;346:235–242.

160. Witzig TE, Gordon LI, Cabanillas F, et al. Randomized controlled trial of yttrium-90-labeled ibritumomab tiuxetan radioimmunotherapy versus rituximab immunotherapy for patients with relapsed or refractory low-grade, follicular, or transformed B-cell non-Hodgkin's lymphoma. J Clin Oncol 2002;20:2453–2463.

161. Payne G. Progress in immunoconjugate cancer therapeutics. Cancer Cell 2003;3:207–212.

162. Kreitman RJ, Stetler-Stevenson M, Margulies I, et al. Phase II trial of recombinant immunotoxin RFB4(dsFv)-PE38 (BL22) in patients with hairy cell leukemia. J Clin Oncol 2009;27:2983–2990.

163. Posey JA, Khazaeli MB, Bookman MA, et al. A phase I trial of the single-chain immunotoxin SGN-10 (BR96sFv-PE40) in patients with advanced solid tumors. Clin Cancer Res 2002;8:3092–3099.

164. Onda M, Beers R, Xiang L, et al. An immunotoxin with greatly reduced immunogenicity by identification and removal of B cell epitopes. Proc Natl Acad Sci U S A 2008;105:11311–11316.

165. Mathew M, Verma RS. Humanized immunotoxins: a new generation of immunotoxins for targeted cancer therapy. Cancer Sci 2009;100:1359–1365.

166. Rosenblum MG, Barth S. Development of novel, highly cytotoxic fusion constructs containing granzyme B: unique mechanisms and functions. Curr Pharm Des 2009;15:2676–2692.

167. Stahnke B, Thepen T, Stocker M, et al. Granzyme B-H22(scFv), a human immunotoxin targeting CD64 in acute myeloid leukemia of monocytic subtypes. Mol Cancer Ther 2008;7:2924–2932.

168. Giles F, Estey E, O'Brien S. Gemtuzumab ozogamicin in the treatment of acute myeloid leukemia. Cancer 2003;98:2095–2104.

169. Sievers EL, Larson RA, Stadtmauer EA, et al. Efficacy and safety of gemtuzumab ozogamicin in patients with CD33-positive acute myeloid leukemia in first relapse. J Clin Oncol 2001;19:3244–3254.

170. Bross PF, Beitz J, Chen G, et al. Approval summary: gemtuzumab ozogamicin in relapsed acute myeloid leukemia. Clin Cancer Res 2001;7:1490–1496.

171. Lewis Phillips GD, Li G, Dugger DL, et al. Targeting HER2-positive breast cancer with trastuzumab-DM1, an antibody-cytotoxic drug conjugate. Cancer Res 2008;68:9280–9290.

172. Vogel CL, Burris HA, Limentani S, et al. A phase II study of trastuzumab-DM1 (T-DM1), a HER2 antibody-drug conjugate (ADC), in patients (pts) with HER2 + metastatic breast cancer (MBC): Final results [abstract 1017]. J Clin Oncol 2009;27(suppl):15s.

173. Francisco JA, Cerveny CG, Meyer DL, et al. cAC10-vcMMAE, an anti-CD30-monomethyl auristatin E conjugate with potent and selective antitumor activity. Blood 2003;102:1458–1465.

174. Bartlett N, Forero-Torres A, Rosenblatt J, et al. Complete remissions with weekly dosing of SGN-35, a novel antibody-drug conjugate (ADC) targeting CD30, in a phase I dose-escalation study in patients with relapsed or refractory Hodgkin lymphoma (HL) or systemic anaplastic large cell lymphoma (sALCL). J Clin Oncol 2009;27:15s(Suppl; abstract 1017).

175. Al-Katib AM, Aboukameel A, Mohammad R, et al. Superior antitumor activity of SAR3419 to rituximab in xenograft models for non-Hodgkin's lymphoma. Clin Cancer Res 2009;15:4038–4045.

176. Lock R, Carol H, Houghton P, et al. Pediatric Preclinical Testing Program (PPTP) evaluation of the anti-CD19-DM4 conjugated antibody SAR3419 [abstract #192]. Eur J Cancer Suppl 2008;6:61.

177. DiJoseph JF, Dougher MM, Armellino DC, et al. Therapeutic potential of CD22-specific antibody-targeted chemotherapy using inotuzumab ozogamicin (CMC-544) for the treatment of acute lymphoblastic leukemia. Leukemia 2007;21:2240–2245.

178. Smith SV. Technology evaluation: huN901-DM1, ImmunoGen. Curr Opin Mol Ther 2005;7:394–401.

179. Jabs DA, Griffiths PD. Fomivirsen for the treatment of cytomegalovirus retinitis. Am J Ophthalmol 2002;133:552–556.

180. Yacyshyn BR, Chey WY, Goff J, et al. Double blind, placebo controlled trial of the remission inducing and steroid sparing properties of an ICAM-1 antisense oligodeoxynucleotide, alicaforsen (ISIS 2302), in active steroid dependent Crohn's disease. Gut 2002;51:30–36.

181. Lynch TJ, Raju R, Lind M, et al. Randomized phase III trial of chemotherapy and antisense oligonucleotide LY900003 (ISIS 3521) in patients with advanced NSCLC: initial report [abstract]. Proc Am Soc Clin Oncol 2003;22:623a.

182. Bedikian AY, Millward M, Pehamberger H, et al. Bcl-2 antisense (oblimersen sodium) plus dacarbazine in patients with advanced melanoma: the Oblimersen Melanoma Study Group. J Clin Oncol 2006;24: 4738–4745.

183. Chanan-Khan AA, Niesvizky R, Hohl RJ, et al. Phase III randomised study of dexamethasone with or without oblimersen sodium for patients with advanced multiple myeloma. Leuk Lymphoma 2009;50:559–565.

184. O'Brien S, Moore JO, Boyd TE, et al. Randomized phase III trial of fludarabine plus cyclophosphamide with or without oblimersen sodium (Bcl-2 antisense) in patients with relapsed or refractory chronic lymphocytic leukemia. J Clin Oncol 2007;25:1114–1120.

185. Wu H, Lima WF, Zhang H, et al. Determination of the role of the human RNase H1 in the pharmacology of DNA-like antisense drugs. J Biol Chem 2004;279:17181–17189.

186. Pirollo KF, Rait A, Sleer LS, et al. Antisense therapeutics: from theory to clinical practice. Pharmacol Ther 2003;99:55–77.

187. Kurreck J. Antisense technologies. Improvement through novel chemical modifications. Eur J Biochem 2003;270:1628–1644.

188. Eckstein F. Phosphorothioate oligodeoxynucleotides: what is their origin and what is unique about them? Antisense Nucleic Acid Drug Dev 2000;10:117–121.

189. Cummins L, Graff D, Beaton G, Marshall WS, et al. Biochemical and physicochemical properties of phosphorodithioate DNA. Biochemistry 1996;35:8734–8741.

190. Tamm I, Dorken B, Hartmann G. Antisense therapy in oncology: new hope for an old idea? Lancet 2001;358:489–497.

191. Kandimalla ER, Shaw DR, Agrawal S. Effects of phosphorothioate oligodeoxyribonucleotide and oligoribonucleotides on human complement and coagulation. Bioorg Med Chem Lett 1998;8:2103–2108.

192. Henry SP, Beattie G, Yeh G, et al. Complement activation is responsible for acute toxicities in rhesus monkeys treated with a phosphorothioate oligodeoxynucleotide. Int Immunopharmacol 2002;2:1657–1666.

193. Henry SP, Novotny W, Leeds J, et al. Inhibition of coagulation by a phosphorothioate oligonucleotide. Antisense Nucleic Acid Drug Dev 1997;7:503–510.

194. Henry SP, Giclas PC, Leeds J, et al. Activation of the alternative pathway of complement by a phosphorothioate oligonucleotide: potential mechanism of action. J Pharmacol Exp Ther 1997;281:810–816.

195. Ishii KJ, Gursel I, Gursel M, et al. Immunotherapeutic utility of stimulatory and suppressive oligodeoxynucleotides. Curr Opin Mol Ther 2004;6:166–174.

196. Wagner H. The immunobiology of the TLR9 subfamily. Trends Immunol 2004;25:381–386.

197. Agrawal S, Zhang X, Lu Z, et al. Absorption, tissue distribution and in vivo stability in rats of a hybrid antisense oligonucleotide following oral administration. Biochem Pharmacol 1995;50:571–576.

198. Yu D, Iyer RP, Shaw DR, et al. Hybrid oligonucleotides: synthesis, biophysical properties, stability studies, and biological activity. Bioorg Med Chem 1996;4:1685–1692.

199. Henry SP, Geary RS, Yu R, et al. Drug properties of second-generation antisense oligonucleotides: how do they measure up to their predecessors? Curr Opin Investig Drugs 2001;2:1444–1449.

200. Monia BP, Lesnik EA, Gonzalez C, et al. Evaluation of 2'-modified oligonucleotides containing 2'-deoxy gaps as antisense inhibitors of gene expression. J Biol Chem 1993;268:14514–14522.

201. Inoue H, Hayase Y, Iwai S, Ohtsuka E. Sequence-dependent hydrolysis of RNA using modified oligonucleotide splints and RNase H. FEBS Lett 1987;215:327–330.

202. Zellweger T, Miyake H, Cooper S, et al. Antitumor activity of antisense clusterin oligonucleotides is improved in vitro and in vivo by incorporation of 2'-O-(2-methoxy)ethyl chemistry. J Pharmacol Exp Ther 2001;298:934–940.

203. Geary RS, Yu RZ, Watanabe T, et al. Pharmacokinetics of a tumor necrosis factor-alpha phosphorothioate 2'-O-(2-methoxyethyl) modified antisense oligonucleotide: comparison across species. Drug Metab Dispos 2003;31:1419–1428.

204. Chi KN, Eisenhauer E, Fazli L, et al. A phase I pharmacokinetic and pharmacodynamic study of OGX-011, a 2'-methoxyethyl antisense oligonucleotide to clusterin, in patients with localized prostate cancer. J Natl Cancer Inst 2005;97:1287–1296.

205. Chi KN, Siu LL, Hirte H, et al. A phase I study of OGX-011, a 2'-methoxyethyl phosphorothioate antisense to clusterin, in combination with docetaxel in patients with advanced cancer. Clin Cancer Res 2008;14:833–839.

206. Chi KN, Hotte SJ, Yu E, et al. Mature results of a randomized phase II study of OGX-011 in combination with docetaxel/prednisone versus docetaxel/prednisone in patients with metastatic castration-resistant prostate cancer. J Clin Oncol 2009;27:15s(suppl; abstract 5012).

207. Talbot DC, Davies J, Callies S, et al. First human dose study evaluating safety and pharmacokinetics of LY2181308, an antisense oligonucleotide designed to inhibit survivin. J Clin Oncol 2008;26 (suppl; abstract 3518).

208. Dean E, Jodrell D, Connolly K, et al. Phase I trial of AEG35156 administered as a 7-day and 3-day continuous intravenous infusion in patients with advanced refractory cancer. J Clin Oncol 2009;27:1660–1666.

209. Schimmer AD, Estey EH, Borthakur G, et al. Phase I/II trial of AEG35156 X-linked inhibitor of apoptosis protein antisense oligonucleotide combined with idarubicin and cytarabine in patients with relapsed or primary refractory acute myeloid leukemia. J Clin Oncol 2009;27:4741–4746.

210. LaCasse EC, Cherton-Horvat GG, Hewitt KE, et al. Preclinical characterization of AEG35156/GEM 640, a second-generation antisense oligonucleotide targeting X-linked inhibitor of apoptosis. Clin Cancer Res 2006;12:5231–5241.

211. Vester B, Wengel J. LNA (locked nucleic acid): high-affinity targeting of complementary RNA and DNA. Biochemistry 2004;43:13233–13241.

212. Greenberger LM, Horak ID, Filpula D, et al. A RNA antagonist of hypoxia-inducible factor-1alpha, EZN-2968, inhibits tumor cell growth. Mol Cancer Ther 2008;7:3598–3608.

213. Whitehead KA, Langer R, Anderson DG. Knocking down barriers: advances in siRNA delivery. Nat Rev Drug Discov 2009;8:129–138.

214. Kim DH, Rossi JJ. Strategies for silencing human disease using RNA interference. Nat Rev Genet 2007;8:173–184.

215. Oh YK, Park TG. siRNA delivery systems for cancer treatment. Adv Drug Deliv Rev 2009;61:850–862.

216. Zimmermann TS, Lee AC, Akinc A, et al. RNAi-mediated gene silencing in non-human primates. Nature 2006;441:111–114.

217. Judge AD, Robbins M, Tavakoli I, et al. Confirming the RNAi-mediated mechanism of action of siRNA-based cancer therapeutics in mice. J Clin Invest 2009;119:661–673.

218. Hu-Lieskovan S, Heidel JD, Bartlett DW, et al. Sequence-specific knockdown of EWS-FLI1 by targeted, nonviral delivery of small interfering RNA inhibits tumor growth in a murine model of metastatic Ewing's sarcoma. Cancer Res 2005;65:8984–8992.

219. Davis ME. The first targeted delivery of siRNA in humans via a self-assembling, cyclodextrin polymer-based nanoparticle: from concept to clinic. Mol Pharm 2009;6:659–668.

220. Holmlund JT. Applying antisense technology: Affinitak and other antisense oligonucleotides in clinical development. Ann N Y Acad Sci 2003;1002: 244–251.

221. Burkhart CA, Cheng AJ, Madafiglio J, et al. Effects of MYCN antisense oligonucleotide administration on tumorigenesis in a murine model of neuroblastoma. J Natl Cancer Inst 2003;95:1394–1403.

222. Pession A, Tonelli R, Fronza R, et al. Targeted inhibition of NMYC by peptide nucleic acid in N-myc amplified human neuroblastoma cells: cell-cycle inhibition with induction of neuronal cell differentiation and apoptosis. Int J Oncol 2004;24:265–272.

223. Sun L, Fuselier JA, Murphy WA, et al. Antisense peptide nucleic acids conjugated to somatostatin analogs and targeted at the n-myc oncogene display enhanced cytotoxicity to human neuroblastoma IMR32 cells expressing somatostatin receptors. Peptides 2002;23:1557–1565.

224. Maksimenko A, Lambert G, Bertrand JR, et al. Therapeutic potentialities of EWS-Fli-1 mRNA-targeted vectorized antisense oligonucleotides. Ann N Y Acad Sci 2003;1002: 72–77.

225. Tanaka K, Iwakuma T, Harimaya K, et al. EWS-Fli1 antisense oligodeoxynucleotide inhibits proliferation of human Ewing's sarcoma and primitive neuroectodermal tumor cells. J Clin Invest 1997;99: 239–247.

226. Toretsky JA, Connell Y, Neckers L, et al. Inhibition of EWS-FLI-1 fusion protein with antisense oligodeoxynucleotides. J Neurooncol 1997;31:9–16.

227. Hanahan D, Weinberg RA. The hallmarks of cancer. Cell 2000;100: 57–70.

228. Chonghaile TN, Letai A. Mimicking the BH3 domain to kill cancer cells. Oncogene 2009;27(Suppl 1):S149–S157.

229. Brunelle JK, Letai A. Control of mitochondrial apoptosis by the Bcl-2 family. J Cell Sci 2009;122:437–441.

230. Willis SN, Fletcher JI, Kaufmann T, et al. Apoptosis initiated when BH3 ligands engage multiple Bcl-2 homologs, not Bax or Bak. Science 2007;315:856–859.

231. Del Gaizo Moore V, Schlis KD, et al. BCL-2 dependence and ABT-737 sensitivity in acute lymphoblastic leukemia. Blood 2008;111:2300–2309.

232. Robinson BW, Behling KC, Gupta M, et al. Abundant anti-apoptotic BCL-2 is a molecular target in leukaemias with t(4;11) translocation. Br J Haematol 2008;141:827–839.

233. Del Gaizo Moore V, Brown JR, Certo M, et al. Chronic lymphocytic leukemia requires BCL2 to sequester prodeath BIM, explaining sensitivity to BCL2 antagonist ABT-737. J Clin Invest 2007;117:112–121.

234. Tse C, Shoemaker AR, Adickes J, et al. ABT-263: a potent and orally bioavailable Bcl-2 family inhibitor. Cancer Res 2008;68:3421–3428.

235. Shoemaker AR, Mitten MJ, Adickes J, et al. Activity of the Bcl-2 family inhibitor ABT-263 in a panel of small cell lung cancer xenograft models. Clin Cancer Res 2008; 14:3268–3277.

236. Wilson W, O'Connor O, Roberts AW, et al. ABT-263 activity and safety in patients with relapsed or refractory lymphoid malignancies in particular chronic lymphocytic leukemia (CLL)/small lymphocytic lymphoma (SLL). J Clin Oncol 2009;27:15s(suppl; abstract 8574).

237. Kang MH, Kang YH, Szymanska B, et al. Activity of vincristine, L-ASP, and dexamethasone against acute lymphoblastic leukemia is enhanced by the BH3-mimetic ABT-737 in vitro and in vivo. Blood 2007;110: 2057–2066.

238. Nguyen M, Marcellus RC, Roulston A, et al. Small molecule obatoclax (GX15-070) antagonizes MCL-1 and overcomes MCL-1-mediated resistance to apoptosis. Proc Natl Acad Sci U S A 2007;104:19512–19517.

239. Schimmer AD, O'Brien S, Kantarjian H, et al. A phase I study of the pan bcl-2 family inhibitor obatoclax mesylate in patients with advanced hematologic malignancies. Clin Cancer Res 2008;14:8295–8301.

240. O'Brien SM, Claxton DF, Crump M, et al. Phase I study of obatoclax mesylate (GX15–070), a small molecule pan-Bcl-2 family antagonist, in patients with advanced chronic lymphocytic leukemia. Blood 2009;113:299–305.

241. Liu G, Kelly WK, Wilding G, et al. An open-label, multicenter, phase I/II study of single-agent AT-101 in men with castrate-resistant prostate cancer. Clin Cancer Res 2009;15:3172–3176.

242. Reed JC, Doctor KS, Godzik A. The domains of apoptosis: a genomics perspective. Sci STKE 2004;2004(239):RE9.

243. Nachmias B, Ashhab Y, Ben-Yehuda D. The inhibitor of apoptosis protein family (IAPs): an emerging therapeutic target in cancer. Semin Cancer Biol 2004;14:231–243.

244. Tamm I, Richter S, Oltersdorf D, et al. High expression levels of x-linked inhibitor of apoptosis protein and survivin correlate with poor overall survival in childhood de novo acute myeloid leukemia. Clin Cancer Res 2004;10:3737–3744.

245. Chen DJ, Huerta S. Smac mimetics as new cancer therapeutics. Anticancer Drugs 2009;20:646–658.

246. Yang QH, Du C. Smac/DIABLO selectively reduces the levels of c-IAP1 and c-IAP2 but not that of XIAP and livin in HeLa cells. J Biol Chem 2004;279:16963–16970.

247. Lu J, Bai L, Sun H, et al. SM-164: a novel, bivalent Smac mimetic that induces apoptosis and tumor regression by concurrent removal of the blockade of cIAP-1/2 and XIAP. Cancer Res 2008;68:9384–9393.

248. Gaither A, Porter D, Yao Y, et al. A Smac mimetic rescue screen reveals roles for inhibitor of apoptosis proteins in tumor necrosis factor-alpha signaling. Cancer Res 2007;67:11493–11498.

249. Fulda S. Inhibitor of apoptosis proteins as targets for anticancer therapy. Expert Rev Anticancer Ther 2007;7:1255–1264.

250. Ziegler DS, Wright RD, Kesari S, et al. Resistance of human glioblastoma multiforme cells to growth factor inhibitors is overcome by blockade of inhibitor of apoptosis proteins. J Clin Invest 2008;118:3109–3122.

251. Weisberg E, Kung AL, Wright RD, et al. Potentiation of antileukemic therapies by Smac mimetic, LBW242: effects on mutant FLT3-expressing cells. Mol Cancer Ther 2007;6:1951–1961.

252. Adida C, Berrebi D, Peuchmaur M, et al. Anti-apoptosis gene, survivin, and prognosis of neuroblastoma [letter]. Lancet 1998;351:882–883.

253. Islam A, Kageyama H, Takada N, et al. High expression of Survivin, mapped to 17q25, is significantly associated with poor prognostic factors and promotes cell survival in human neuroblastoma. Oncogene 2000;19:617–623.

254. van Noesel MM, Versteeg R. Pediatric neuroblastomas: genetic and epigenetic 'Danse Macabre'. Gene 2004;325:1–15.

255. Altieri DC. Validating survivin as a cancer therapeutic target. Nat Rev Cancer 2003;3:46–54.

256. Srinivasula SM, Ashwell JD. IAPs: what's in a name? Mol Cell 2008;30:123–135.

257. Lens SM, Vader G, Medema RH. The case for survivin as mitotic regulator. Curr Opin Cell Biol 2006;18:616–622.

258. Giaccone G, Zatloukal P, Roubec J, et al. Multicenter phase II trial of YM155, a small-molecule suppressor of survivin, in patients with advanced, refractory, non-small-cell lung cancer. J Clin Oncol 2009;27:4481–4486.

259. Tolcher AW, Mita A, Lewis LD, et al. Phase I and pharmacokinetic study of YM155, a small-molecule inhibitor of survivin. J Clin Oncol 2008;26: 5198–5203.

260. Ashkenazi A. Directing cancer cells to self-destruct with pro-apoptotic receptor agonists. Nat Rev Drug Discov 2008;7:1001–1012.

261. Ashkenazi A, Holland P, Eckhardt SG. Ligand-based targeting of apoptosis in cancer: the potential of recombinant human apoptosis ligand 2/tumor necrosis factor-related apoptosis-inducing ligand (rhApo2L/TRAIL). J Clin Oncol 2008;26:3621–3630.

262. Mom CH, Verweij J, Oldenhuis CN, et al. Mapatumumab, a fully human agonistic monoclonal antibody that targets TRAIL-R1, in combination with gemcitabine and cisplatin: a phase I study. Clin Cancer Res 2009;15:5584–5590.

263. Wang S. The promise of cancer therapeutics targeting the TNF-related apoptosis-inducing ligand and TRAIL receptor pathway. Oncogene 2008;27:6207–6215.

264. Pukac L, Kanakaraj P, Humphreys R, et al. HGS-ETR1, a fully human TRAIL-receptor 1 monoclonal antibody, induces cell death in multiple tumour types in vitro and in vivo. Br J Cancer 2005;92:1430–1441.

265. Georgakis GV, Li Y, Humphreys R, et al. Activity of selective fully human agonistic antibodies to the TRAIL death receptors TRAIL-R1 and TRAIL-R2 in primary and cultured lymphoma cells: induction of apoptosis and enhancement of doxorubicin- and bortezomib-induced cell death. Br J Haematol 2005;130:501–510.

266. Moretto P, Hotte SJ. Targeting apoptosis: preclinical and early clinical experience with mapatumumab, an agonist monoclonal antibody targeting TRAIL-R1. Expert Opin Investig Drugs 2009;18:311–325.

267. Leong S, Cohen RB, Gustafson DL, et al. Mapatumumab, an antibody targeting TRAIL-R1, in combination with paclitaxel and carboplatin in patients with advanced solid malignancies: results of a phase I and pharmacokinetic study. J Clin Oncol 2009;27:4413–4421.

268. Plummer R, Attard G, Pacey S, et al. Phase 1 and pharmacokinetic study of lexatumumab in patients with advanced cancers. Clin Cancer Res 2007;13:6187–6194.

269. Wakelee HA, Patnaik A, Sikic BI, et al. Phase I and pharmacokinetic study of lexatumumab (HGS-ETR2) given every 2 weeks in patients with advanced solid tumors. Ann Oncol 2010;21:376–1.

270. Camidge DR. Apomab: an agonist monoclonal antibody directed against Death Receptor 5/TRAIL-Receptor 2 for use in the treatment of solid tumors. Expert Opin Biol Ther 2008;8:1167–1176.

271. LoRusso P, Hong D, Heath E, et al. First-in-human study of AMG 655, a pro-apoptotic TRAIL receptor-2 agonist, in adult patients with advanced solid tumors. J Clin Oncol 2007;25:18s(suppl, abstract #3534).

272. Mitsiades N, Poulaki V, Mitsiades C, et al. Ewing's sarcoma family tumors are sensitive to tumor necrosis factor-related apoptosis-inducing ligand and express death receptor 4 and death receptor 5. Cancer Res 2001;61:2704–2712.

273. Kontny HU, Hammerle K, Klein R, et al. Sensitivity of Ewing's sarcoma to TRAIL-induced apoptosis. Cell Death Differ 2001;8:506–514.

274. Kumar A, Jasmin A, Eby MT, et al. Cytotoxicity of tumor necrosis factor related apoptosis-inducing ligand towards Ewing's sarcoma cell lines. Oncogene 2001;20:1010–1014.

275. Petak I, Tillman DM, Vernes R, et al. TRAIL induces apoptosis in pediatric rhabdomyosarcoma (RMS) cell lines. Proc Am Assoc Cancer Res 2000;41:738.

276. Petak I, Vernes R, Szucs KS, et al. A caspase-8-independent component in TRAIL/Apo-2L-induced cell death in human rhabdomyosarcoma cells. Cell Death Differ 2003;10:729–739.

277. Pollack IF, Erff M, Ashkenazi A. Direct stimulation of apoptotic signaling by soluble Apo2l/tumor necrosis factor-related apoptosis-inducing ligand leads to selective killing of glioma cells. Clin Cancer Res 2001;7: 1362–1369.

278. Fulda S. Apoptosis pathways and neuroblastoma therapy. Curr Pharm Des 2009;15:430–435.

279. Soda M, Choi YL, Enomoto M, et al. Identification of the transforming EML4-ALK fusion gene in non-small-cell lung cancer. Nature 2007;448:561–566.

280. Baserga R, Peruzzi F, Reiss K. The IGF-1 receptor in cancer biology. Int J Cancer 2003;107:873–877.

281. Doern A, Cao X, Sereno A, et al. Characterization of inhibitory anti-insulin-like growth factor receptor antibodies with different epitope specificity and ligand-blocking properties: implications for mechanism of action in vivo. J Biol Chem 2009;284:10254–10267.

282. Zhan J, Huang W, Shu L, et al. The IGFI-R targeting antibody SCH717454 differentially blocks IGF-1 and IGF-2 induced signaling. In: Proceedings of the 100th Annual Meeting of the American Association for Cancer Research. Philadelphia, PA; 2009. Abstract #5681.

283. Wittman M, Carboni J, Attar R, et al. Discovery of a (1H-benzoimidazol-2-yl)-1H-pyridin-2-one (BMS-536924) inhibitor of insulin-like growth factor I receptor kinase with in vivo antitumor activity. J Med Chem 2005;48:5639–5643.

284. Cironi L, Riggi N, Provero P, et al. IGF1 is a common target gene of Ewing's sarcoma fusion proteins in mesenchymal progenitor cells. PLoS ONE 2008;3:e2634.

285. Scotlandi K, Benini S, Nanni P, et al. Blockage of insulin-like growth factor-I receptor inhibits the growth of Ewing's sarcoma in athymic mice. Cancer Res 1998;58:4127–4131.

286. Scotlandi K, Maini C, Manara MC, et al. Effectiveness of insulin-like growth factor I receptor antisense strategy against Ewing's sarcoma cells. Cancer Gene Ther 2002;9:296–307.

287. Kolb EA, Gorlick R, Houghton PJ, et al. Initial testing (stage 1) of a monoclonal antibody (SCH 717454) against the IGF-1 receptor by the pediatric preclinical testing program. Pediatr Blood Cancer 2008;50: 1190–1197.

288. Atzori F, Tabernero J, Cervantes A, et al. A phase I, pharmacokinetic (PK) and pharmacodynamic (PD) study of weekly (qW) MK-0646, an insulin-like growth factor-1 receptor (IGF1R) monoclonal antibody (MAb) in patients (pts) with advanced solid tumors. J Clin Oncol 2008;26 (suppl; abstract 3519).

289. Patel S, Pappo A, Crowley J, et al. A SARC global collaborative phase II trial of R1507, a recombinant human monoclonal antibody to the insulin-like growth factor-1 receptor (IGF1R) in patients with recurrent or refractory sarcomas. J Clin Oncol 2009;27: 15s(suppl, abstract 10503).

290. Minniti CP, Tsokos M, Newton WA Jr, et al. Specific expression of insulin-like growth factor-II in rhabdomyosarcoma tumor cells. Am J Clin Pathol 1994;101:198–203.

291. Cao L, Yu Y, Darko I, et al. Addiction to elevated insulin-like growth factor I receptor and initial modulation of the AKT pathway define the responsiveness of rhabdomyosarcoma to the targeting antibody. Cancer Res 2008;68:8039–8048.

292. Kolb EA, Morton C, Houghton PJ, et al. Pediatric Preclinical Testing Program (PPTP) evaluation of the fully human anti-IGF-1R antibody IMC-A12 [abstract #558]. Eur J Cancer Suppl 2008;6:176.

293. Liu X, Turbyville T, Fritz A, et al. Inhibition of insulin-like growth factor I receptor expression in neuroblastoma cells induces the regression of established tumors in mice. Cancer Res 1998;58:5432–5438.

294. Maloney EK, McLaughlin JL, Dagdigian NE, et al. An anti-insulin-like growth factor I receptor antibody that is a potent inhibitor of cancer cell proliferation. Cancer Res 2003;63:5073–5083.

295. Wang JY, Del Valle L, Gordon J, et al. Activation of the IGF-IR system contributes to malignant growth of human and mouse medulloblastomas. Oncogene 2001;20:3857–3868.

296. Kappel CC, Velez-Yanguas MC, Hirschfeld S, et al. Human osteosarcoma cell lines are dependent on insulin-like growth factor I for in vitro growth. Cancer Res 1994;54:2803–2807.

297. Scott J, Cowell J, Robertson ME, et al. Insulin-like growth factor-II gene expression in Wilms' tumour and embryonic tissues. Nature 1985;317: 260–262.

298. Takahashi M, Yang XJ, Lavery TT, et al. Gene expression profiling of favorable histology Wilms tumors and its correlation with clinical features. Cancer Res 2002;62:6598–6605.

299. Gray SG, Eriksson T, Ekstrom C, et al. Altered expression of members of the IGF-axis in hepatoblastomas. Br. J Cancer 2000;82:1561–1567.

300. Nagata T, Takahashi Y, Ishii Y, et al. Transcriptional profiling in hepatoblastomas using high-density oligonucleotide DNA array. Cancer Genet Cytogenet 2003;145:152–160.

301. Martins AS, Mackintosh C, Martin DH, et al. Insulin-like growth factor I receptor pathway inhibition by ADW742, alone or in combination with imatinib, doxorubicin, or vincristine, is a novel therapeutic approach in Ewing tumor. Clin Cancer Res 2006;12:3532–3540.

302. Karp DD, Pollak MN, Cohen RB, et al. Safety, pharmacokinetics, and pharmacodynamics of the insulin-like growth factor type 1 receptor inhibitor figitumumab (CP-751,871) in combination with paclitaxel and carboplatin. J Thorac Oncol 2009;4: 1397–1403.

303. Suleiman MS, Singh RJ, Stewart CE. Apoptosis and the cardiac action of insulin-like growth factor I. Pharmacol Ther 2007;114:278–294.

304. Kurmasheva RT, Dudkin L, Billups C, et al. The insulin-like growth factor-1 receptor-targeting antibody, CP-751,871, suppresses tumor-derived VEGF and synergizes with rapamycin in models of childhood sarcoma. Cancer Res 2009;69:7662–7671.

305. Webb TR, Slavish J, George RE, et al. Anaplastic lymphoma kinase: role in cancer pathogenesis and small-molecule inhibitor development for therapy. Expert Rev Anticancer Ther 2009;9:331–356.

306. Gleason BC, Hornick JL. Inflammatory myofibroblastic tumours: where are we now? J Clin Pathol 2008;61:428–437.

307. Janoueix-Lerosey I, Lequin D, Brugieres L, et al. Somatic and germline activating mutations of the ALK kinase receptor in neuroblastoma. Nature 2008;455:967–970.

308. Chen Y, Takita J, Choi YL, et al. Oncogenic mutations of ALK kinase in neuroblastoma. Nature 2008;455:971–974.

309. George RE, Sanda T, Hanna M, et al. Activating mutations in ALK provide a therapeutic target in neuroblastoma. Nature 2008;455:975–978.

310. Christensen JG, Zou HY, Arango ME, et al. Cytoreductive antitumor activity of PF-2341066, a novel inhibitor of anaplastic lymphoma kinase and c-Met, in experimental models of anaplastic large-cell lymphoma. Mol Cancer Ther 2007;6:3314–3322.

311. Koivunen JP, Mermel C, Zejnullahu K, et al. EML4-ALK fusion gene and efficacy of an ALK kinase inhibitor in lung cancer. Clin Cancer Res 2008;14:4275–4283.

312. Wood AC, Laudenslager M, Haglund EA, et al. Inhibition of ALK mutated neuroblastomas by the selective inhibitor PF-02341066. J Clin Oncol 2009;27:15s(suppl, abstract 10008b).

313. Soda M, Takada S, Takeuchi K, et al. A mouse model for EML4-ALK-positive lung cancer. Proc Natl Acad Sci U S A 2008;105:19893–19897.

314. Gilliland DG, Griffin JD. The roles of FLT3 in hematopoiesis and leukemia. Blood 2002;100:1532–1542.

315. Levis M, Small D. FLT3: ITDoes matter in leukemia. Leukemia 2003;17:1738–1752.
316. Levis M, Small D. Small molecule FLT3 tyrosine kinase inhibitors. Curr Pharm Des 2004;10:1183–1193.
317. Robinson DR, Wu YM, Lin SF. The protein tyrosine kinase family of the human genome. Oncogene 2000;19:5548–5557.
318. van der Geer P, Hunter T, Lindberg RA. Receptor protein-tyrosine kinases and their signal transduction pathways. Annu Rev Cell Biol 1994;10: 251–337.
319. Meshinchi S, Appelbaum FR. Structural and functional alterations of FLT3 in acute myeloid leukemia. Clin Cancer Res 2009;15:4263–4269.
320. Meshinchi S, Alonzo TA, Stirewalt DL, et al. Clinical implications of FLT3 mutations in pediatric AML. Blood 2006;108:3654–3661.
321. Armstrong SA, Staunton JE, Silverman LB, et al. MLL translocations specify a distinct gene expression profile that distinguishes a unique leukemia. Nat Genet 2002;30: 41–47.
322. Ravandi F, Cortes JE, Jones D, et al. Phase I/II study of combination therapy with sorafenib, idarubicin, and cytarabine in younger patients with acute myeloid leukemia. J Clin Oncol 2010;28:1856–1862.
323. Ravandi F, Cortes J, Faderl S, et al. Combination of sorafenib, idarubicin, and cytarabine has a high response rate in patients with newly diagnosed acute myeloid leukemia (AML) younger than 65 years [abstract #768]. Blood 2009;112.
324. Levis M, Smith BD, Beran M, et al. A randomized, open-label study of lestaurtinib (CEP-701), an oral FLT3 inhibitor, administered in sequence with chemotherapy in patients with relapsed AML harboring FLT3 activating mutations: clinical response correlates with successful FLT3 inhibition. Blood (ASH Ann Meet Abstr) 2005;106:(suppl, abstract 403).
325. Stone RM, Fischer T, Paquette R, et al. Phase IB study of PKC412, an oral FLT3 kinase inhibitor, in sequential and simultaneous combinations with daunorubicin and cytarabine (DA) induction and high-dose cytarabine consolidation in newly diagnosed adult patients (pts) with acute myeloid leukemia (AML) under age 61. Blood (ASH Ann Meet Abstr) 2006;108:(suppl, abstract 157).
326. Levis M, Ravandi F, Wang ES et al. Results from a randomized trial of salvage chemotherapy followed by Lestaurtinib for FLT3 Mutant AML Patients in first relapse. Blood (ASH Annu Meet Abstr) 2009;114:(suppl, abstract 788).
327. Brown P, Levis M, McIntyre E, et al. Combinations of the FLT3 inhibitor CEP-701 and chemotherapy synergistically kill infant and childhood MLL-rearranged ALL cells in a sequence-dependent manner. Leukemia 2006;20:1368–1376.
328. Vainchenker W, Dusa A, Constantinescu SN. JAKs in pathology: role of Janus kinases in hematopoietic malignancies and immunodeficiencies. Semin Cell Dev Biol 2008;19:385–393.
329. Benekli M, Baumann H, Wetzler M. Targeting signal transducer and activator of transcription signaling pathway in leukemias. J Clin Oncol 2009;27:4422–4432.
330. Goldman JM. A unifying mutation in chronic myeloproliferative disorders. N Engl J Med 2005;352:1744–1746.
331. Lacronique V, Boureux A, Valle VD, et al. A TEL-JAK2 fusion protein with constitutive kinase activity in human leukemia. Science 1997;278: 1309–1312.
332. Reiter A, Walz C, Watmore A, et al. The t(8;9)(p22;p24) is a recurrent abnormality in chronic and acute leukemia that fuses PCM1 to JAK2. Cancer Res 2005;65:2662–2667.
333. Flex E, Petrangeli V, Stella L, et al. Somatically acquired JAK1 mutations in adult acute lymphoblastic leukemia. J Exp Med 2008;205:751–758.
334. Jeong EG, Kim MS, Nam HK, et al. Somatic mutations of JAK1 and JAK3 in acute leukemias and solid cancers. Clin Cancer Res 2008;14:3716–3721.
335. Bercovich D, Ganmore I, Scott LM, et al. Mutations of JAK2 in acute lymphoblastic leukaemias associated with Down's syndrome. Lancet 2008;372:1484–1492.
336. Gaikwad A, Rye CL, Devidas M, et al. Prevalence and clinical correlates of JAK2 mutations in Down syndrome acute lymphoblastic leukaemia. Br J Haematol 2009;144: 930–932.
337. Kearney L, Gonzalez De CD, Yeung J, et al. Specific JAK2 mutation (JAK2R683) and multiple gene deletions in Down syndrome acute lymphoblastic leukemia. Blood 2009;113:646–648.
338. Quintas-Cardama A, Vaddi K, Liu P, et al. Preclinical characterization of the selective JAK1/2 inhibitor INCB018424: therapeutic implications for the treatment of myeloproliferative neoplasms. Blood 2010;115:3109–3117.
339. Verstovsek S, Kantarjian HM, Pardanani A, et al. A phase I/II study of INCB018424, an oral, selective JAK inhibitor, in patients with primary myelofibrosis (PMF) and post polycythemia vera/essential thrombocythemia myelofibrosis (Post-PV/ET MF). J Clin Oncol 2008;26(suppl, abstract 7004).
340. Wernig G, Kharas MG, Okabe R, et al. Efficacy of TG101348, a selective JAK2 inhibitor, in treatment of a murine model of JAK2V617F-induced polycythemia vera. Cancer Cell 2008;13:311–320.
341. Pardanani AD, Gotlib JR, Jamieson CH, et al. A Phase I Evaluation of TG101348, a Selective JAK2 Inhibitor, in Myelofibrosis: Clinical Response Is Accompanied by Significant Reduction in JAK2V617F Allele Burden. Blood (ASH Annu Meet Abstra) 2009;114:(suppl, abstract 755).
342. Bond M, Bernstein ML, Pappo A, et al. A phase II study of imatinib mesylate in children with refractory or relapsed solid tumors: a Children's Oncology Group study. Pediatr Blood Cancer 2008;50:254–258.
343. Geoerger B, Morland B, Ndiaye A, et al. Target-driven exploratory study of imatinib mesylate in children with solid malignancies by the Innovative Therapies for Children with Cancer (ITCC) European Consortium. Eur J Cancer 2009;45:2342–2351.
344. Champagne MA, Capdeville R, Krailo M, et al. Imatinib mesylate (STI571) for treatment of children with Philadelphia chromosome-positive leukemia: results from a Children's Oncology Group phase 1 study. Blood 2004;104:2655–2660.
345. Champagne MA, Fu C, Chang M, et al. Imatinib in children with newly diagnosed chronic phase chronic myelogenous leukemia (CP CML): AAML0123 COG Study. Blood (ASH Ann Meet Abstr) 2006;108:(suppl, abstract 2140).
346. Quintas-Cardama A, Kantarjian H, Cortes J. Imatinib and beyond—exploring the full potential of targeted therapy for CML. Nat Rev Clin Oncol 2009;6:535–543.
347. Thomas DA, Kantarjian HM, Cortes J, et al. Outcome after Frontline Therapy with the Hyper-CVAD and Imatinib Mesylate Regimen for Adults with De Novo or Minimally Treated Philadelphia Chromosome (Ph) Positive Acute Lymphoblastic Leukemia (ALL). Blood (ASH Annu Meet Abstr) 2008;112:(suppl), abstract 2931).
348. Schultz KR, Bowman WP, Aledo A et al. Improved early event-free survival with imatinib in Philadelphia chromosome-positive acute lymphoblastic leukemia: a Children's Oncology Group study. J Clin Oncol 2009;27:5175–5181.
349. Yanada M, Takeuchi J, Sugiura I, et al. High complete remission rate and promising outcome by combination of imatinib and chemotherapy for newly diagnosed BCR-ABL-positive acute lymphoblastic leukemia: a phase II study by the Japan Adult Leukemia Study Group. J Clin Oncol 2006;24:460–466.
350. Lombardo LJ, Lee FY, Chen P, et al. Discovery of *N*-(2-chloro-6-methyl- phenyl)-2-(6-(4-(2-hydroxyethyl)-piperazin-1-yl)-2-methylpyrimidin-4-ylamino)thiazole-5-carboxamide (BMS-354825), a dual Src/Abl kinase inhibitor with potent antitumor activity in preclinical assays. J Med Chem 2004;47:6658–6661.
351. Kolb EA, Gorlick R, Houghton PJ, et al. Initial testing of dasatinib by the pediatric preclinical testing program. Pediatr Blood Cancer 2007;50:1198–1206.
352. Shah NP, Tran C, Lee FY, et al. Overriding imatinib resistance with a novel ABL kinase inhibitor. Science 2004;305:399–401.
353. Donato NJ, Wu JY, Stapley J, et al. BCR-ABL independence and LYN kinase overexpression in chronic myelogenous leukemia cells selected for resistance to STI571. Blood 2003;101:690–698.
354. Donato NJ, Wu JY, Stapley J, et al. Imatinib mesylate resistance through BCR-ABL independence in chronic myelogenous leukemia. Cancer Res 2004;64:672–677.
355. Shah NP, Kasap C, Weier C, et al. Transient potent BCR-ABL inhibition is sufficient to commit chronic myeloid leukemia cells irreversibly to apoptosis. Cancer Cell 2008; 14:485–493.
356. Snead JL, O'Hare T, Adrian LT, et al. Acute dasatinib exposure commits Bcr-Abl dependent cells to apoptosis. Blood 2009;114:3459–3463.
357. Kantarjian H, Cortes J, Kim DW, et al. Phase 3 study of dasatinib 140 mg once daily versus 70 mg twice daily in patients with chronic myeloid leukemia in accelerated phase resistant or intolerant to imatinib: 15-month median follow-up. Blood 2009;113: 6322–6329.
358. Shah NP, Kantarjian HM, Kim DW, et al. Intermittent target inhibition with dasatinib 100 mg once daily preserves efficacy and improves tolerability in imatinib-resistant and -intolerant chronic-phase chronic myeloid leukemia. J Clin Oncol 2008;26:3204–3212.
359. Montagut C, Settleman J. Targeting the RAF-MEK-ERK pathway in cancer therapy. Cancer Lett 2009;283:125–134.
360. Sebolt-Leopold JS. Advances in the development of cancer therapeutics directed against the RAS-mitogen-activated protein kinase pathway. Clin Cancer Res 2008;14:3651–3656.
361. Garnett MJ, Marais R. Guilty as charged: B-RAF is a human oncogene. Cancer Cell 2004;6:313–319.
362. Miao J, Kusafuka T, Fukuzawa M. Hotspot mutations of BRAF gene are not associated with pediatric solid neoplasms. Oncol Rep 2004;12: 1269–1272.
363. Gilbertson RJ, Langdon JA, Hollander A, et al. Mutational analysis of PDGFR-RAS/MAPK pathway activation in childhood medulloblastoma. Eur J Cancer 2006;42: 646–649.
364. Sievert AJ, Jackson EM, Gai X, et al. Duplication of 7q34 in pediatric low-grade astrocytomas detected by high-density single-nucleotide polymorphism-based genotype arrays results in a novel BRAF fusion gene. Brain Pathol 2009;19:449–458.
365. Gustafsson B, Angelini S, Sander B, et al. Mutations in the BRAF and N-ras genes in childhood acute lymphoblastic leukaemia. Leukemia 2005;19:310–312.
366. Hou P, Liu D, Xing M. The T1790A BRAF mutation (L597Q) in childhood acute lymphoblastic leukemia is a functional oncogene. Leukemia 2007;21:2216–2218.
367. Yamamoto T, Isomura M, Xu Y, et al. PTPN11, RAS and FLT3 mutations in childhood acute lymphoblastic leukemia. Leuk Res 2006;30:1085–1089.
368. Dhomen N, Marais R. BRAF signaling and targeted therapies in melanoma. Hematol Oncol Clin North Am 2009;23:529–545, ix.
369. Wilhelm S, Carter C, Lynch M, et al. Discovery and development of sorafenib: a multikinase inhibitor for treating cancer. Nat Rev Drug Discov 2006;5:835–844.
370. McDermott U, Sharma SV, Dowell L, et al. Identification of genotype-correlated sensitivity to selective kinase inhibitors by using high-throughput tumor cell line profiling. Proc Natl Acad Sci U S A 2007;104: 19936–19941.
371. Tsai J, Lee JT, Wang W, et al. Discovery of a selective inhibitor of oncogenic B-Raf kinase with potent antimelanoma activity. Proc Natl Acad Sci U S A 2008;105:3041–3046.
372. Flaherty K, Puzanov I, Sosman J, et al. Phase I study of PLX4032: proof of concept for V600E BRAF mutation as a therapeutic target in human cancer [abstract 9000]. J Clin Oncol 2009;27(suppl):15s.
373. Yeh TC, Marsh V, Bernat BA, et al. Biological characterization of ARRY-142886 (AZD6244), a potent, highly selective mitogen-activated protein kinase kinase 1/2 inhibitor. Clin Cancer Res 2007;13:1576–1583.
374. Solit DB, Santos E, Pratilas CA, et al. FLT PET as a non-invasive marker of response to MEK inhibition [abstract #2397]. Proc Am Assoc Cancer Res 2006;47.
375. Friday BB, Yu C, Dy GK, et al. BRAF V600E disrupts AZD6244-induced abrogation of negative feedback pathways between extracellular signal-regulated kinase and Raf proteins. Cancer Res 2008;68:6145–6153.
376. Adjei AA, Cohen RB, Franklin W, et al. Phase I pharmacokinetic and pharmacodynamic study of the oral, small-molecule mitogen-activated protein kinase kinase 1/2 inhibitor AZD6244 (ARRY-142886) in patients with advanced cancers. J Clin Oncol 2008;26:2139–2146.
377. Dummer R, Robert C, Chapman PB, et al. AZD6244 (ARRY-142886) vs temozolomide (TMZ) in patients (pts) with advanced melanoma: an open-label, randomized, multicenter, phase II study. J Clin Oncol 2008;26 (suppl; abstract 9033).
378. Kolb EA, Gorlick R, Houghton PJ, et al. Initial Testing (Stage 1) of AZD6244 (ARRY-142886) by the Pediatric Preclinical Testing Program. Pediatr Blood Cancer 2010 (in press).
379. Meric-Bernstam F, Gonzalez-Angulo AM. Targeting the mTOR signaling network for cancer therapy. J Clin Oncol 2009;27:2278–2287.
380. Hay N, Sonenberg N. Upstream and downstream of mTOR. Genes Dev 2004;18: 1926–1945.
381. Bjornsti MA, Houghton PJ. The TOR pathway: a target for cancer therapy. Nat Rev Cancer 2004;4:335–348.
382. Inoki K, Zhu T, Guan KL. TSC2 mediates cellular energy response to control cell growth and survival. Cell 2003;115:577–590.
383. Douros J, Suffness M. New antitumor substances of natural origin. Cancer Treat Rev 1981;8:63–87.
384. Eng CP, Sehgal SN, Vezina C. Activity of rapamycin (AY-22,989) against transplanted tumors. J Antibiot (Tokyo) 1984;37:1231–1237.
385. Hosoi H, Dilling MB, Shikata T, et al. Rapamycin causes poorly reversible inhibition of mTOR and induces p53-independent apoptosis in human rhabdomyosarcoma cells. Cancer Res 1999;59:886–894.
386. Hosoi H, Dilling MB, Liu LN, et al. Studies on the mechanism of resistance to rapamycin in human cancer cells. Mol Pharmacol 1998;54:815–824.
387. Dilling MB, Dias P, Shapiro DN, et al. Rapamycin selectively inhibits the growth of childhood rhabdomyosarcoma cells through inhibition of signaling via the type I insulin-like growth factor receptor. Cancer Res 1994;54:903–907.
388. Albers MW, Williams RT, Brown EJ, et al. FKBP-rapamycin inhibits a cyclin-dependent kinase activity and a cyclin D1-Cdk association in early G_1 of an osteosarcoma cell line. J Biol Chem 1993;268:22825–22829.

389. Mateo-Lozano S, Tirado OM, Notario V. Rapamycin induces the fusion-type independent downregulation of the EWS/FLI-1 proteins and inhibits Ewing's sarcoma cell proliferation. Oncogene 2003;22:9282–9287.

390. Mateo-Lozano S, Gokhale PC, Soldatenkov VA, et al. Combined transcriptional and translational targeting of EWS/FLI-1 in Ewing's sarcoma. Clin Cancer Res 2006;12:6781–6790.

391. Geoerger B, Kerr K, Tang CB, et al. Antitumor activity of the rapamycin analog CCI-779 in human primitive neuroectodermal tumor/medulloblastoma models as single agent and in combination chemotherapy. Cancer Res 2001;61:1527–1532.

392. Brown VI, Fang J, Alcorn K, et al. Rapamycin is active against B-precursor leukemia in vitro and in vivo, an effect that is modulated by IL-7-mediated signaling. Proc Natl Acad Sci U S A 2003;100:15113–15118.

393. Ishizuka T, Sakata N, Johnson GL, et al. Rapamycin potentiates dexamethasone-induced apoptosis and inhibits JNK activity in lymphoblastoid cells. Biochem Biophys Res Commun 1997;230:386–391.

394. Avellino R, Romano S, Parasole R, et al. Rapamycin stimulates apoptosis of childhood acute lymphoblastic leukemia cells. Blood 2005;106:1400–1406.

395. Teachey DT, Obzut DA, Cooperman J, et al. The mTOR inhibitor CCI-779 induces apoptosis and inhibits growth in preclinical models of primary adult human ALL. Blood 2006;107:1149–1155.

396. Houchens DP, Ovejera AA, Riblet SM, et al. Human brain tumor xenografts in nude mice as a chemotherapy model. Eur J Cancer Clin Oncol 1983;19:799–805.

397. Majewski M, Korecka M, Kossev P, et al. The immunosuppressive macrolide RAD inhibits growth of human Epstein-Barr virus-transformed B lymphocytes in vitro and in vivo: a potential approach to prevention and treatment of posttransplant lymphoproliferative disorders. Proc Natl Acad Sci U S A 2000;97:4285–4290.

398. Majewski M, Korecka M, Joergensen J, et al. Immunosuppressive TOR kinase inhibitor everolimus (RAD) suppresses growth of cells derived from posttransplant lymphoproliferative disorder at allograft-protecting doses. Transplantation 2003;75:1710–1717.

399. Kenerson HL, Aicher LD, True LD, et al. Activated mammalian target of rapamycin pathway in the pathogenesis of tuberous sclerosis complex renal tumors. Cancer Res 2002;62:5645–5650.

400. Lee L, Sudentas P, Donohue B, et al. Efficacy of a rapamycin analog (CCI-779) and IFN-gamma in tuberous sclerosis mouse models. Genes Chromosomes Cancer 2005;42:213–227.

401. Teachey DT, Sheen C, Hall J, et al. mTOR inhibitors are synergistic with methotrexate: an effective combination to treat acute lymphoblastic leukemia. Blood 2008;112:2020–2023.

402. Guba M, von Breitenbuch P, Steinbauer M, et al. Rapamycin inhibits primary and metastatic tumor growth by antiangiogenesis: involvement of vascular endothelial growth factor. Nat Med 2002;8:128–135.

403. Kurmasheva RT, Harwood FC, Houghton PJ. Differential regulation of vascular endothelial growth factor by Akt and mammalian target of rapamycin inhibitors in cell lines derived from childhood solid tumors. Mol Cancer Ther 2007;6:1620–1628.

404. Lane HA, Wood JM, McSheehy PM, et al. mTOR inhibitor RAD001 (everolimus) has antiangiogenic/vascular properties distinct from a VEGFR tyrosine kinase inhibitor. Clin Cancer Res 2009;15:1612–1622.

405. Rini BI. Temsirolimus, an inhibitor of mammalian target of rapamycin. Clin Cancer Res 2008;14:1286–1290.

406. Boulay A, Zumstein-Mecker S, Stephan C, et al. Antitumor efficacy of intermittent treatment schedules with the rapamycin derivative RAD001 correlates with prolonged inactivation of ribosomal protein S6 kinase 1 in peripheral blood mononuclear cells. Cancer Res 2004;64:252–261.

407. Mita M, Sankhala K, Abdel-Karim I, Mita A, Giles F. Deforolimus (AP23573) a novel mTOR inhibitor in clinical development. Expert Opin Investig Drugs 2008;17:1947–1954.

408. Hudes G, Carducci M, Tomczak P, et al. Temsirolimus, interferon alfa, or both for advanced renal-cell carcinoma. N Engl J Med 2007;356: 2271–2281.

409. Motzer RJ, Escudier B, Oudard S, et al. Efficacy of everolimus in advanced renal cell carcinoma: a double-blind, randomised, placebo-controlled phase III trial. Lancet 2008;372:449–456.

410. Ansell SM, Inwards DJ, Rowland KM Jr, et al. Low-dose, single-agent temsirolimus for relapsed mantle cell lymphoma: a phase 2 trial in the North Central Cancer Treatment Group. Cancer 2008;113:508–514.

411. Hess G, Herbrecht R, Romaguera J, et al. Phase III study to evaluate temsirolimus compared with investigator's choice therapy for the treatment of relapsed or refractory mantle cell lymphoma. J Clin Oncol 2009;27: 3822–3829.

412. Hess G, Herbrecht R, Romaguera J, et al. Phase III study to evaluate temsirolimus compared with investigator's choice therapy for the treatment of relapsed or refractory mantle cell lymphoma. J Clin Oncol 2009;27:3822–3829.

413. Franz DN, Leonard J, Tudor C, et al. Rapamycin causes regression of astrocytomas in tuberous sclerosis complex. Ann Neurol 2006;59:490–498.

414. Fouladi M, Laningham F, Wu J, et al. Phase I study of everolimus in pediatric patients with refractory solid tumors. J Clin Oncol 2007;25: 4806–4812.

415. Spunt SL, Grupp S, Vik T, et al.: Phase I, safety, pharmacokinetic, exploratory biomarker study of intravenous temsirolimus in children with advanced solid tumors. 2007 PAS Annual Meeting Late-Breaker Abstract Presentations (http://www.pas-meeting.org/2007Toronto/Abstracts/LB%20Sessions%2007.pdf) Abstr #8455.3, 2007.

416. Hoyer PF, Ettenger R, Kovarik JM, et al. Everolimus in pediatric de novo renal transplant patients. Transplantation 2003;75:2082–2085.

417. Kovarik JM, Noe A, Berthier S, et al. Clinical development of an everolimus pediatric formulation: relative bioavailability, food effect, and steady-state pharmacokinetics. J Clin Pharmacol 2003;43:141–147.

418. Sindhi R, Webber S, Venkataramanan R, et al. Sirolimus for rescue and primary immunosuppression in transplanted children receiving tacrolimus. Transplantation 2001;72:851–855.

419. Sindhi R. Sirolimus in pediatric transplant recipients. Transplant Proc 2003;35:113S–114S.

420. Coulter DW, Wilkie MB, Moats-Staats BM. Inhibition of IGF-I receptor signaling in combination with rapamycin or temsirolimus increases MYC-N phosphorylation. Anticancer Res 2009;29:1943–1949.

421. Aster JC, Pear WS, Blacklow SC. Notch signaling in leukemia. Annu Rev Pathol 2008;3:587–613.

422. Puget S, Grill J, Valent A, et al. Candidate genes on chromosome 9q33-34 involved in the progression of childhood ependymomas. J Clin Oncol 2009;27:1884–1892.

423. Gilbertson RJ, Ellison DW. The origins of medulloblastoma subtypes. Annu Rev Pathol 2008;3:341–365.

424. Fukuzawa R, Anaka MR, Weeks RJ, et al. Canonical WNT signalling determines lineage specificity in Wilms tumour. Oncogene 2009;28:1063–1075.

425. Taniguchi K, Roberts LR, Aderca IN, et al. Mutational spectrum of beta-catenin, AXIN1, and AXIN2 in hepatocellular carcinomas and hepatoblastomas. Oncogene 2002;21:4863–4871.

426. Duman-Scheel M, Weng L, Xin S, et al. Hedgehog regulates cell growth and proliferation by inducing Cyclin D and Cyclin E. Nature 2002;417: 299–304.

427. Bar EE, Chaudhry A, Farah MH, et al. Hedgehog signaling promotes medulloblastoma survival via Bcl II. Am J Pathol 2007;170:347–355.

428. Kenney AM, Cole MD, Rowitch DH. Nmyc upregulation by sonic hedgehog signaling promotes proliferation in developing cerebellar granule neuron precursors. Development 2003;130:15–28.

429. Cheng SY, Yue S. Role and regulation of human tumor suppressor SUFU in hedgehog signaling. Adv Cancer Res 2008;101:29–43.

430. Wetmore C, Eberhart DE, Curran T. Loss of p53 but not ARF accelerates medulloblastoma in mice heterozygous for patched. Cancer Res 2001;61:513–516.

431. Lee Y, Kawagoe R, Sasai K, et al. Loss of suppressor-of-fused function promotes tumorigenesis. Oncogene 2007;26:6442–6447.

432. Hatton BA, Villavicencio EH, Tsuchiya KD, et al. The Smo/Smo model: hedgehog-induced medulloblastoma with 90% incidence and leptomeningeal spread. Cancer Res 2008;68:1768–1776.

433. Han YG, Kim HJ, Dlugosz AA, et al. Dual and opposing roles of primary cilia in medulloblastoma development. Nat Med 2009;15:1062–1065.

434. de Bont JM, Packer RJ, Michiels EM, et al. Biological background of pediatric medulloblastoma and ependymoma: a review from a translational research perspective. Neuro Oncol 2008;10:1040–1060.

435. Robarge KD, Brunton SA, Castanedo GM, et al. GDC-0449—a potent inhibitor of the hedgehog pathway. Bioorg Med Chem Lett 2009;19:5576–5581.

436. Rudin CM, Hann CL, Laterra J, et al. Treatment of medulloblastoma with hedgehog pathway inhibitor GDC-0449. N Engl J Med 2009;361:1173–1178.

437. Yauch RL, Dijkgraaf GJ, Alicke B, et al. Smoothened mutation confers resistance to a hedgehog pathway inhibitor in medulloblastoma. Science 2009;326:572–574.

438. Bar EE, Chaudhry A, Lin A, et al. Cyclopamine-mediated hedgehog pathway inhibition depletes stem-like cancer cells in glioblastoma. Stem Cells 2007;25:2524–2533.

439. Peacock CD, Wang Q, Gesell GS, et al. Hedgehog signaling maintains a tumor stem cell compartment in multiple myeloma. Proc Natl Acad Sci U S A 2007;104:4048–4053.

440. Ward RJ, Lee L, Graham K, et al. Multipotent CD15 + cancer stem cells in patched-1-deficient mouse medulloblastoma. Cancer Res 2009;69: 4682–4690.

441. Zhao C, Chen A, Jamieson CH, et al. Hedgehog signalling is essential for maintenance of cancer stem cells in myeloid leukaemia. Nature 2009;458:776–779.

442. Kopan R, Ilagan MX. The canonical Notch signaling pathway: unfolding the activation mechanism. Cell 2009;137:216–233.

443. Zweidler-McKay PA. Notch signaling in pediatric malignancies. Curr Oncol Rep 2008;10:459–468.

444. Dotto GP. Notch tumor suppressor function. Oncogene 2008;27: 5115–5123.

445. Kunnimalaiyaan M, Chen H. Tumor suppressor role of Notch-1 signaling in neuroendocrine tumors. Oncologist 2007;12:535–542.

446. Olson RE, Albright CF. Recent progress in the medicinal chemistry of gamma-secretase inhibitors. Curr Top Med Chem 2008;8:17–33.

447. Wolfe MS. gamma-Secretase in biology and medicine. Semin Cell Dev Biol 2009;20:219–224.

448. DeAngelo DJ, Stone RM, Silverman LB, et al. A phase I clinical trial of the notch inhibitor MK-0752 in patients with T-cell acute lymphoblastic leukemia/lymphoma (T-ALL) and other leukemias [abstract #6585]. J Clin Oncol 2006;24(June 20 suppl).

449. Lewis HD, Leveridge M, Strack PR, et al. Apoptosis in T cell acute lymphoblastic leukemia cells after cell cycle arrest induced by pharmacological inhibition of notch signaling. Chem Biol 2007;14:209–219.

450. Weng AP, Ferrando AA, Lee W, et al. Activating mutations of NOTCH1 in human T cell acute lymphoblastic leukemia. Science 2004;306:269–271.

451. Luistro L, He W, Smith M, et al. Preclinical profile of a potent gamma-secretase inhibitor targeting notch signaling with in vivo efficacy and pharmacodynamic properties. Cancer Res 2009;69:7672–7680.

452. Hyde LA, McHugh NA, Chen J, et al. Studies to investigate the in vivo therapeutic window of the gamma-secretase inhibitor N2-[(2S)-2-(3,5-difluorophenyl)-2-hydroxyethanoyl]-N1-[(7S)-5-methyl-6-oxo-6,7-dihydro-5H-dibenzo[b,d]azepin-7-yl]-L-alaninamide (LY411,575) in the CRND8 mouse. J Pharmacol Exp Ther 2006;319:1133–1143.

453. Real PJ, Tosello V, Palomero T, et al. Gamma-secretase inhibitors reverse glucocorticoid resistance in T cell acute lymphoblastic leukemia. Nat Med 2009;15:50–58.

454. Fan X, Matsui W, Khaki L, et al. Notch pathway inhibition depletes stem-like cells and blocks engraftment in embryonal brain tumors. Cancer Res 2006;66:7445–7452.

455. Gautschi O, Heighway J, Mack PC, et al. Aurora kinases as anticancer drug targets. Clin Cancer Res 2008;14:1639–1648.

456. Schoffski P. Polo-like kinase (PLK) inhibitors in preclinical and early clinical development in oncology. Oncologist 2009;14:559–570.

457. Lapenna S, Giordano A. Cell cycle kinases as therapeutic targets for cancer. Nat Rev Drug Discov 2009;8:547–566.

458. Wysong DR, Chakravarty A, Hoar K, et al. The inhibition of Aurora A abrogates the mitotic delay induced by microtubule perturbing agents. Cell Cycle 2009;8:876–888.

459. Vader G, Lens SM. The Aurora kinase family in cell division and cancer. Biochim Biophys Acta 2008;1786:60–72.

460. Lad L, Luo L, Carson JD, et al. Mechanism of inhibition of human KSP by ispinesib. Biochemistry 2008;47:3576–3585.

461. Johnson RK, McCabe FL, Caulder E, et al. SB-715992, a potent and selective inhibitor of the mitotic kinesin KSP, demonstrates broad-spectrum activity in advanced murine tumors and human tumor xenografts [abstract]. Proc Annu Meet Am Assoc Cancer Res 2002;43:269.

462. Smith MA, Houghton PJ, Morton CL, et al. Pediatric Preclinical Testing Program (PPTP) stage 2 testing of the Aurora A kinase inhibitor MLN8237 [abstract #286]. Eur J Cancer Suppl 2008;6:93.

463. Otto T, Horn S, Brockmann M, et al. Stabilization of N-Myc is a critical function of Aurora A in human neuroblastoma. Cancer Cell 2009;15:67–78.

464. Maris JM. Unholy matrimony: Aurora A and N-Myc as malignant partners in neuroblastoma. Cancer Cell 2009;15:5–6.

465. Schrump DS. Cytotoxicity mediated by histone deacetylase inhibitors in cancer cells: mechanisms and potential clinical implications. Clin Cancer Res 2009;15:3947–3957.

466. Piekarz RL, Bates SE. Epigenetic modifiers: basic understanding and clinical development. Clin Cancer Res 2009;15:3918–3926.

467. Richon VM, Garcia-Vargas J, Hardwick JS. Development of vorinostat: current applications and future perspectives for cancer therapy. Cancer Lett 2009;280:201–210.

468. Batty N, Malouf GG, Issa JP. Histone deacetylase inhibitors as anti-neoplastic agents. Cancer Lett 2009;280:192–200.

469. Van Lint C, Emiliani S, Verdin E. The expression of a small fraction of cellular genes is changed in response to histone hyperacetylation. Gene Expr 1996;5:245–253.

470. Glaser KB, Staver MJ, Waring JF, et al. Gene expression profiling of multiple histone deacetylase (HDAC) inhibitors: defining a common gene set produced by HDAC inhibition in T24 and MDA carcinoma cell lines. Mol Cancer Ther 2003;2:151–163.

471. Prince HM, Bishton MJ, Harrison SJ. Clinical studies of histone deacetylase inhibitors. Clin Cancer Res 2009;15:3958–3969.

472. Keshelava N, Houghton PJ, Morton CL, et al. Initial testing (stage 1) of vorinostat (SAHA) by the Pediatric Preclinical Testing Program. Pediatr Blood Cancer 2009;53:505–508.

473. Fouladi M, Furman WL, Chin T, et al. Phase I study of depsipeptide in pediatric patients with refractory solid tumors: a Children's Oncology Group report. J Clin Oncol 2006;24:3678–3685.

474. Fouladi M, Park JR, Sun J, et al. A phase I trial and pharmacokinetic (PK) study of vorinostat (SAHA) in combination with 13-cis-retinoic acid (13cRA) in children with refractory neuroblastomas, medulloblastomas, primitive neuroectodermal tumors (PNETs), and atypical teratoid rhabdoid tumor [abstract #10012]. J Clin Oncol2008;26.

475. Graham C, Tucker C, Creech J, et al. Evaluation of the antitumor efficacy, pharmacokinetics, and pharmacodynamics of the histone deacetylase inhibitor depsipeptide in childhood cancer models in vivo. Clin Cancer Res 2006;12:223–234.

476. Bots M, Johnstone RW. Rational combinations using HDAC inhibitors. Clin Cancer Res 2009;15:3970–3977.

477. Spiller SE, Ditzler SH, Pullar BJ, et al. Response of preclinical medulloblastoma models to combination therapy with 13-cis-retinoic acid and suberoylanilide hydroxamic acid (SAHA). J Neurooncol 2008;87:133–141.

478. Camphausen K, Tofilon PJ. Inhibition of histone deacetylation: a strategy for tumor radiosensitization. J Clin Oncol 2007;25:4051–4056.

479. Adams J. The proteasome: a suitable antineoplastic target. Nat Rev Cancer 2004;4:349–360.

480. Orlowski RZ, Kuhn DJ. Proteasome inhibitors in cancer therapy: lessons from the first decade. Clin Cancer Res 2008;14:1649–1657.

481. Hideshima T, Ikeda H, Chauhan D, et al. Bortezomib induces canonical nuclear factor-kappaB activation in multiple myeloma cells. Blood 2009;114:1046–1052.

482. Yang DT, Young KH, Kahl BS, et al. Prevalence of bortezomib-resistant constitutive NF-kappaB activity in mantle cell lymphoma. Mol Cancer 2008;7:40.

483. Dolcet X, Llobet D, Encinas M, et al. Proteasome inhibitors induce death but activate NF-kappaB on endometrial carcinoma cell lines and primary culture explants. J Biol Chem 2006;281:22118–22130.

484. Williams SA, McConkey DJ. The proteasome inhibitor bortezomib stabilizes a novel active form of p53 in human LNCaP-Pro5 prostate cancer cells. Cancer Res 2003;63:7338–7344.

485. Nawrocki ST, Carew JS, Pino MS, et al. Aggresome disruption: a novel strategy to enhance bortezomib-induced apoptosis in pancreatic cancer cells. Cancer Res 2006;66:3773–3781.

486. Lee AH, Iwakoshi NN, Anderson KC, et al. Proteasome inhibitors disrupt the unfolded protein response in myeloma cells. Proc Natl Acad Sci U S A 2003;100:9946–9951.

487. Bianchi G, Oliva L, Cascio P, et al. The proteasome load versus capacity balance determines apoptotic sensitivity of multiple myeloma cells to proteasome inhibition. Blood 2009;113:3040–3049.

488. Bross PF, Kane R, Farrell AT, et al. Approval summary for bortezomib for injection in the treatment of multiple myeloma. Clin Cancer Res 2004;10:3954–3964.

489. Richardson PG, Sonneveld P, Schuster MW, et al. Bortezomib or high-dose dexamethasone for relapsed multiple myeloma. N Engl J Med 2005;352:2487–2498.

490. Richardson PG, Sonneveld P, Schuster M, et al. Extended follow-up of a phase 3 trial in relapsed multiple myeloma: final time-to-event results of the APEX trial. Blood 2007;110:3557–3560.

491. San Miguel JF, Schlag R, Khuageva NK, et al. Bortezomib plus melphalan and prednisone for initial treatment of multiple myeloma. N Engl J Med 2008;359:906–917.

492. Kane RC, Dagher R, Farrell A, et al. Bortezomib for the treatment of mantle cell lymphoma. Clin Cancer Res 2007;13:5291–5294.

493. Fisher RI, Bernstein SH, Kahl BS, et al. Multicenter phase II study of bortezomib in patients with relapsed or refractory mantle cell lymphoma. J Clin Oncol 2006;24:4867–4874.

494. Blum KA, Johnson JL, Niedzwiecki D, et al. Single agent bortezomib in the treatment of relapsed and refractory Hodgkin lymphoma: cancer and leukemia Group B protocol 50206. Leuk Lymphoma 2007;48:1313–1319.

495. Blaney SM, Bernstein M, Neville K, et al. Phase I study of the proteasome inhibitor bortezomib in pediatric patients with refractory solid tumors: a Children's Oncology Group study (ADVL0015). J Clin Oncol 2004;22: 4804–4809.

496. Houghton PJ, Morton CL, Kolb EA, et al. Initial testing (stage 1) of the proteasome inhibitor bortezomib by the Pediatric Preclinical Testing Program. Pediatr Blood Cancer 2008;50:37–45.

497. Horton TM, Gannavarapu A, Blaney SM, et al. Bortezomib interactions with chemotherapy agents in acute leukemia in vitro. Cancer Chemother Pharmacol 2006;58:13–23.

498. Horton TM, Pati D, Plon SE, et al. A phase 1 study of the proteasome inhibitor bortezomib in pediatric patients with refractory leukemia: a Children's Oncology Group study. Clin Cancer Res 2007;13: 1516–1522.

499. Messinger YH, Gaynon PS, Raetz E, et al. Remarkable activity of bortezomib combined with chemotherapy in a phase I study of relapsed childhood acute lymphoblastic leukemia (ALL). A report from the Therapeutic Advances in Childhood Leukemia (TACL) Consortium [abstract #1919]. Blood 2008;112.

500. Guzman ML, Neering SJ, Upchurch D, et al. Nuclear factor-kappaB is constitutively activated in primitive human acute myelogenous leukemia cells. Blood 2001;98:2301–2307.

501. Guzman ML, Swiderski CF, Howard DS, et al. Preferential induction of apoptosis for primary human leukemic stem cells. Proc Natl Acad Sci U S A 2002;99:16220–16225.

502. Attar EC, De Angelo DJ, Supko JG, et al. Phase I and pharmacokinetic study of bortezomib in combination with idarubicin and cytarabine in patients with acute myelogenous leukemia. Clin Cancer Res 2008;14: 1446–1454.

503. Folkman J. Tumor angiogenesis: therapeutic implications. N Engl J Med 1971;285:1182–1186.

504. Hurwitz H, Fehrenbacher L, Novotny W, et al. Bevacizumab plus irinotecan, fluorouracil, and leucovorin for metastatic colorectal cancer. N Engl J Med 2004;350:2335–2342.

505. Chow LQ, Eckhardt SG. Sunitinib: from rational design to clinical efficacy. J Clin Oncol 2007;25:884–896.

506. Lonser RR, Glenn GM, Walther M, et al. von Hippel-Lindau disease. Lancet 2003;361:2059–2067.

507. Schofield CJ, Ratcliffe PJ. Oxygen sensing by HIF hydroxylases. Nat Rev Mol Cell Biol 2004;5:343–354.

508. Wiesener MS, Munchenhagen PM, Berger I, et al. Constitutive activation of hypoxia-inducible genes related to overexpression of hypoxia-inducible factor-1alpha in clear cell renal carcinomas. Cancer Res 2001;61: 5215–5222.

509. Rini BI. Vascular endothelial growth factor-targeted therapy in metastatic renal cell carcinoma. Cancer 2009;115:2306–2312.

510. Motzer RJ, Hutson TE, Tomczak P, et al. Overall survival and updated results for sunitinib compared with interferon alfa in patients with metastatic renal cell carcinoma. J Clin Oncol 2009;27:3584–3590.

511. Escudier B, Eisen T, Stadler WM, et al. Sorafenib for treatment of renal cell carcinoma: final efficacy and safety results of the phase III treatment approaches in renal cancer global evaluation trial. J Clin Oncol 2009;27:3312–3318.

512. Kreisl TN, Kim L, Moore K, et al. Phase II trial of single-agent bevacizumab followed by bevacizumab plus irinotecan at tumor progression in recurrent glioblastoma. J Clin Oncol 2009;27:740–745.

513. Friedman HS, Prados MD, Wen PY, et al. Bevacizumab alone and in combination with irinotecan in recurrent glioblastoma. J Clin Oncol 2009;27:4733–4740.

514. Dietrich J, Wang D, Batchelor TT. Cediranib: profile of a novel anti-angiogenic agent in patients with glioblastoma. Expert Opin Investig Drugs 2009;18(10):1549–1557.

515. Gururangan S, Chi S, Onar A, et al. Phase II study of bevacizumab + CPT-11 in children with recurrent malignant glioma and diffuse intrinsic brain stem glioma—a Pediatric Brain Tumor Consortium Study (PBTC -022) [abstract MA-63]. Neuro Oncol 2008;10:833.

516. Wolmark N, Yothers G, O'Connell MJ, et al. A phase III trial comparing mFOLFOX6 to mFOLFOX6 plus bevacizumab in stage II or III carcinoma of the colon: Results of NSABP Protocol C-08 [abstract LBA4]. J Clin Oncol 2009;27(Suppl).

517. Torino F, Corsello SM, Longo R, et al. Hypothyroidism related to tyrosine kinase inhibitors: an emerging toxic effect of targeted therapy. Nat Rev Clin Oncol 2009;6:219–228.

518. Maris JM, Courtright J, Houghton PJ, et al. Initial testing of the VEGFR inhibitor AZD2171 by the pediatric preclinical testing program. Pediatr Blood Cancer 2008;50:581–587.

519. Maris JM, Courtright J, Houghton PJ, et al. Initial testing (stage 1) of sunitinib by the Pediatric Preclinical Testing Program. Pediatr Blood Cancer 2008;51:42–48.

520. Stupack DG, Cheresh DA. Apoptotic cues from the extracellular matrix: regulators of angiogenesis. Oncogene 2003;22:9022–9029.

521. Reardon DA, Nabors LB, Stupp R, et al. Cilengitide: an integrin-targeting arginine-glycine-aspartic acid peptide with promising activity for glioblastoma multiforme. Expert Opin Investig Drugs 2008;17:1225–1235.

522. MacDonald TJ, Taga T, Shimada H, et al. Preferential susceptibility of brain tumors to the antiangiogenic effects of an alpha(v) integrin antagonist. Neurosurgery 2001;48:151–157.

523. Reardon DA, Fink KL, Mikkelsen T, et al. Randomized phase II study of cilengitide, an integrin-targeting arginine-glycine-aspartic acid peptide, in recurrent glioblastoma multiforme. J Clin Oncol 2008;26:5610–5617.

524. MacDonald TJ, Stewart CF, Kocak M, et al. Phase I clinical trial of cilengitide in children with refractory brain tumors: Pediatric Brain Tumor Consortium Study PBTC-012. J Clin Oncol 2008;26:919–924.

525. Noguera-Troise I, Daly C, Papadopoulos NJ, et al. Blockade of Dll4 inhibits tumour growth by promoting non-productive angiogenesis. Nature 2006;444:1032–1037.

526. Herbst RS, Hong D, Chap L, et al. Safety, pharmacokinetics, and antitumor activity of AMG 386, a selective angiopoietin inhibitor, in adult patients with advanced solid tumors. J Clin Oncol 2009;27:3557–3565.

527. Smith MA, Seibel NL, Altekruse SF et al. Outcomes for children and adolescents with cancer: Challenges for the twenty-first century. J Clin Oncol (published online April 19, 2010).

CHAPTER 12 ■ GENERAL PRINCIPLES OF SURGERY

CHRISTOPHER B. WELDON, TOM JAKSIC, AND ROBERT C. SHAMBERGER

Surgery remains a critical component in the multimodal therapy of childhood cancer. Accurate staging and successful resection of tumors is of vital importance, as we strive to minimize the morbidity of treatment as survival rates improve. Decisions regarding biopsy and resection are most accurately made by surgeons who are trained to address these specific issues. This chapter presents an introduction to the significant considerations for surgical patients, including their metabolic response, nutritional support, and vascular access. Critical issues regarding anesthetic management, staging, biopsy, and preoperative adjuvant therapy are also discussed. A brief summary of some of the specific surgical issues for each solid tumor concludes the chapter.

METABOLIC RESPONSE TO MALIGNANCY

Weight loss is frequently seen in children with malignancy. This form of malnutrition, termed *anorexia-cachexia syndrome*, is associated with higher early cancer relapse rates, decreased tolerance to chemotherapy, and a poorer prognosis.[1] Although reduced food intake is an important component of the syndrome, cancer patients, unlike starved individuals, have elevated protein turnover and lose the ability to conserve skeletal muscle mass.[2] The extent of this process may be more pronounced in those patients having malignancies with high cell turnover. Other notable metabolic changes with malignancy include increased rates of gluconeogenesis and lipolysis. There is also a failure to downregulate energy expenditure in reaction to reduced nutrient intake, although actual increases in resting energy expenditure are evident only in patients with large tumor burdens.[3] Surgical stress or infection tends to further exacerbate the net protein catabolism found in these patients.[4]

The pathogenesis of childhood cancer cachexia is complex and is not completely understood. Elaboration of host cytokines in response to the tumor, such as tumor necrosis factor α, interleukin 1, interleukin 6, and interferon gamma, promote catabolism, which in certain instances is further enhanced by specific tumor-generated mediators.[5] The cytokine-independent ubiquitin-proteasome pathway has also been linked to muscle protein loss in cancer patients.[6,7] Compounding this catabolic process is a reduction in enteral intake and, on occasion, malabsorption of nutrients that may be caused by the tumor itself, antineoplastic therapy, or a combination of both. Megestrol and fish oil–supplemented diets have been used to ameliorate anorexia-cachexia syndrome in oncology patients, but the usefulness of these interventions remains uncertain.[8,9]

Nutritional Support

In the absence of efficacious pharmacologic interventions to combat the anorexia-cachexia syndrome, nutritional support remains the primary therapy. Children are particularly susceptible to the deleterious effects of cancer-induced catabolism due to their relatively reduced stores and high baseline requirements. The concern that the provision of nutrition may stimulate tumor growth in children is not supported by clinical data. There is also no evidence that the administration of macronutrients and micronutrients in excess of those recommended for other ill patients is required.

The use of preoperative nutritional support in children with malignancy has not been systematically studied; however, extrapolation from the adult literature would indicate that preoperative nutritional repletion should be considered only in those patients with preexisting malnutrition. Postoperatively, any child who is anticipated to have inadequate nutritional intake for more than 3 days should be considered as a candidate for nutritional support.

Enteral nutritional support is more physiologic, has lower complication rates, and is less costly than parenteral nutrition. Pliable, narrow-bore, nasogastric feeding tubes and percutaneously placed endoscopically guided gastrostomy tubes have facilitated this option in children with cancer. Gastrostomy tubes have been shown to be safe in pediatric cancer patients and should be considered if protracted nutritional support is anticipated.[10] The conversion of gastrostomy tubes to gastrojejunal tubes is occasionally necessary to limit gastroesophageal reflux. Parenteral nutritional support is recommended for those children who are not suitable for enteral nutrition, and adequate amounts of protein, glucose, lipid, trace minerals, and vitamins, commensurate with a metabolic stress state, should be administered.[4]

Vascular Access

Dependable intravascular access in pediatric oncology patients is of vital importance and impacts the child's care daily. Since central venous lines (CVLs) were first described by Dudrick in 1968,[11] they have helped to revolutionize and simplify the delivery and management of pediatric oncologic care. They are utilized for the administration of chemotherapy, intravenous fluids, parenteral nutrition, blood and blood products, antibiotics and other medications, contrast agents for radiographic and imaging studies, and the resuscitation of critically ill oncology patients. Furthermore, they can be used to harvest peripheral stem cells for therapeutic bone marrow transplants or used as an access site for hemodialysis, should it be required. Finally, just as they provide a dependable route of ingress, they are also the primary site of egress for blood sampling for laboratory examination. Phlebotomy can be performed painlessly and repeatedly without undue psychological or physical stress.

Catheters are divided by type and location, but for all, the common objective remains the establishment of dependable and reliable access to the central venous system with the tip of the catheter at the junction of the superior or inferior vena cava and the right atrium as confirmed by radiographic studies both during and after the procedure. The type of catheter can be either temporary or permanent, and catheters can be either external or internal. Regardless of location or catheter type, all CVLs are placed using a percutaneous technique first described by Seldinger[12] or by a cut-down technique depending on operator preference and patient characteristics. Before placing any CVL, coagulation and platelet studies should be assessed to determine the risk of perioperative hemorrhage. The patient's venous anatomy should be confirmed by ultrasound or angiographic studies to ensure patency if there is any question of thrombosis or a history of multiple prior CVLs. The use of antiseptic preparation solutions and sterile technique is mandated for the health care professionals placing and accessing CVLs. Chlorhexidine preparation solutions (2%) are the recommended antiseptic agents for skin preparation.[13] Parenteral antibiotic (single dose of a first-generation cephalosporin 60 minutes before beginning the procedure) administration is a common practice during the placement of a CVL, but there are no data documenting a reduced rate of catheter-related infections in adults or children with antibiotic prophylaxis.[14] Finally, in patients with central lines and a fever, a line infection must always be considered as the source.

Temporary external CVLs can be placed peripherally (called *peripherally inserted central catheter* [PICC]) in an extremity or centrally (femoral, jugular, or subclavian routes), and they can have one to four lumens. PICC lines are generally smaller in caliber than CVLs, and because they are placed peripherally, complications associated with accessing central veins (pneumothorax, hemothorax, etc.) are avoided. However, they have been associated with pericardial tamponade from erosion of a catheter tip through the atrial myocardium into the pericardium.[15] The main advantage of temporary CVLs is that they do not require an anesthetic to remove, and in the case of PICCs, they do not require more than local anesthesia and occasional use of intravenous sedation to place them. However, these catheters do not have a grommet or cuff to prevent bacterial migration down the catheter or to allow fibrous ingrowth to anchor the catheter to the underlying subcutaneous tissues and prevent inadvertent removal. Multiple devices and suturing techniques have been employed to secure these CVLs, but none are infallible.

Permanent external CVLs are catheters that are placed in a similar fashion and location as temporary external CVLs except that the exit skin site of the CVL is distant from its insertion point. These CVLs are tunneled under the skin in the subcutaneous tissue. As an added measure of protection and stability, they have a cuff attached to the catheter wall, which is buried at the skin exit site. This cuff allows for the ingrowth of fibrous tissue (scar) around the catheter, thus securing it to the patient and retarding the migration of microbes along the catheter itself, decreasing the risk of infection.[14,16] These catheters are also made of silicone as opposed to polyurethane or polyethylene. They can have one or multiple lumens. Unfortunately, these CVLs require an anesthetic to both place and remove them in children and adolescents.

Permanent internal CVLs are also known as *implantable venous access devices* or *ports*. Like permanent external CVLs, they sit distant from the introduction site in the subcutaneous tissues. They are commonly secured to the deep fascia on the anterior chest wall with sutures to ensure that they do not migrate. The ports can be single- or double-lumen, and they come in a variety of materials that are not immunogenic. Special ports are now available that allow for high-pressure injections for radiographic imaging. The ports possess silicone membranes that are accessed by special needles that are noncoring. They are self-sealing after the needle is removed. These CVLs have many advantages, including decreased infection rates, increased quality of life for the patients, and minimal pain when they are accessed, requiring only local anesthetic creams.[14,17] However, they do require an anesthetic to place and remove.

Complications of central venous access are mechanical (related to the venous access procedure or the catheter itself), infectious, or infusion related. With percutaneous Seldinger access techniques, the greatest patient risk is pneumothorax, hemorrhage from either arterial puncture or vein laceration, pericardial tamponade secondary to atrial or ventricular penetration, or needle puncture–related neurologic (vagus, phrenic, or sympathetic trunk) or thoracic duct injury. Other mechanical complications include phlebitis, thrombosis, thromboembolism, air embolism, and cardiac arrhythmias. Of concern is the very real risk of a life-endangering event from the vascular access procedure alone, a risk that approximates 1 such event per 1,000 access procedures.[18]

Infectious complications of pediatric central venous access remain most common.[19] Defining such catheter-related bloodstream infections as opposed to local exit-site, tunnel, or pocket infections is important. The local site infections typically account for up to 50% of all central access infections and present with local signs and symptoms, including fever, erythema, tenderness, and drainage. In contrast, bloodstream infections are diagnosed when a presumptive diagnosis of bacteremia or sepsis is made and there is congruence of the cultured organism from a portion of the catheter as well as a remote venous blood culture.[20] However, as transcatheter antibiotics are typically initially administered in an effort to salvage the infected line, the presumption of a catheter-related infection is usually made on clinical suspicion, as it is impossible to culture the catheter without its removal. The pediatric age group has remained a high-risk group for such infections, but these infected CVLs often can be treated effectively with antibiotics alone, although success is dependent on the organism involved.[14,21] The microbiology of such infections are predictable; coagulase-negative staphylococci are the most common offending organisms.[21] In all series, but particularly in immunocompromised oncology patients, the spectrum of causal organisms includes other gram-positive, many gram-negative, and, not infrequently, fungal species. Factors that may protect patients from infection historically included the aseptic techniques of the operating room, the tunnel, and the catheter cuff. To these have been added antibacterial substances bonded to catheters; minocycline and rifampin have decreased the frequency of CVL infections.[22]

Risk factors for the pediatric patient that influence central catheter infections have been carefully analyzed.[19] Early infection occurred in 12% of children (53 of 437), and factors that adversely influenced this rate included moderate (absolute neutrophil count < 1,000/mm^3) or severe (absolute neutrophil count < 500/mm^3) neutropenia and failure to use systemic prophylactic antibiotics. The type of catheter used and the site of placement did not influence the risk of infection. In this series, as in many others, transcatheter antibiotics as an initial therapy in presumed central line infection was effective in treating the infection and preserving the catheter in 70% of the patients.[19] Such transcatheter antibiotic agents worked less well for the child with fungemia. Furthermore, because of the demonstrated relationship between thrombosis and infection, thrombolytic agents, anticoagulants, and antibiotics have all been used to treat the infected catheter.[23]

PRINCIPLES OF PERIOPERATIVE AND ANESTHETIC MANAGEMENT

Although the perioperative and anesthetic management of children with malignancy is generally similar to other ill pediatric patients, the following aspects warrant more detailed consideration: coagulation and transfusion, tumors that result in anterior mediastinal masses, and pheochromocytomas. In patients already treated with chemotherapy, a careful assessment of cardiac, pulmonary, renal, and electrolyte status is particularly warranted. Patients who have received cardiotoxic agents, such as doxorubicin (Adriamycin), require echocardiography to quantitatively document cardiac function before surgery.

Coagulation and Transfusion

Thrombocytopenia is the most commonly encountered clinical coagulation abnormality in children with malignancy requiring surgery. Platelet counts of 150,000 per mm^3 are the lower limit of the normal range in children, whereas normal neonates may have platelet counts as low as 80,000 per mm^3. Patients with platelet counts higher than 10,000 per mm^3 have a low risk of spontaneous bleeding if they are without evidence of other medical complications.[24] If surgery is contemplated, however, a platelet count of 50,000 per mm^3 is usually sought before incision. This guideline is empirically based and has not been formally studied; hence, lower levels may be acceptable to the operating surgeon in specific clinical contexts. In children, the transfusion of 0.1 units of platelet concentrate for each kilogram of body weight may be anticipated to raise the platelet count to 40,000 per mm^3.

No specific hemoglobin concentration or hematocrit level mandates blood transfusion in an oncologic surgical patient. Children with hemoglobin levels of 6 g per dL are often free of adverse physiologic sequelae. The specific clinical scenario governs the need for transfusion, as rapid blood loss, infection, pulmonary dysfunction, cardiomyopathy, and central nervous system compromise may all mandate early transfusion. Immunodeficient patients should receive irradiated blood products to avoid graft-versus-host disease and, if the patients are serologically cytomegalovirus-negative, they should receive cytomegalovirus-negative or leukocyte-poor blood products. Packed red blood cells are the usual blood product used for both acute blood loss and chronic anemia. Although whole blood is a suitable choice with massive hemorrhage, it is rarely available.

Elevations in prothrombin time (PT) and partial thromboplastin time (PTT) are acquired defects in most surgical patients. Vitamin K deficiency manifests with a marked prolongation of the PT and PTT and normal platelet and fibrinogen levels. In older children, this may be due to malabsorption, dietary deficiency, or drug antagonism. The subcutaneous administration of vitamin K results in improvement within several hours and correction within a day. For immediate correction, fresh frozen plasma is required. If the platelet count and fibrinogen level are also low, disseminated intravascular coagulation must be considered, particularly in patients with sepsis or leukemia. Peripheral blood smears, platelet count, thrombin time, fibrin degradation products, fibrin monomers, and D-dimer levels are all useful in confirming the diagnosis. Treatment of disseminated intravascular coagulation consists of correction of the underlying disease and supportive care. If hemorrhagic manifestations are present without major thrombosis, fresh frozen plasma may be indicated. Liver disease with decreased synthetic capacity may also result in an elevated PT and PTT; however, in this instance, correction is refractory to vitamin K.

Evaluation of Anesthetic Risk Produced by an Anterior Mediastinal Mass

Respiratory collapse on induction of general anesthesia is a well-recognized complication of an anterior mediastinal mass (Fig. 12.1). Identification of patients at significant risk remains a major challenge. Orthopnea, respiratory stridor, and wheezing are all ominous signs of significant major airway obstruction (Fig. 12.2). Many patients with no respiratory symptoms, however, have been reported to develop major respiratory complications.[25]

Computed tomography (CT) is useful in defining the cross-sectional area of the trachea, and a reproducible technique for defining the tracheal area has been published.[26-28] The cross-sectional area is measured from the CT slices showing the trachea at its narrowest dimension. The percentage of narrowing is then calculated by comparing the measured area with established standard values.[29]

The use of pulmonary function tests in evaluating children with an anterior mediastinal mass is also important. The predominant distortion of the flow loop for intrathoracic obstruction is a marked reduction in the maximum expiratory flow rate. For extrathoracic obstruction, it is a reduction of the maximum inspiratory flow rate. A fixed lesion usually produces an equal reduction of the inspiratory and expiratory peak flows. The high-flow portion of the forced expiratory loop near total lung capacity, best represented by the peak expiratory flow rate (PEFR), is the first to be distorted.

The PEFR can be easily obtained in patients by using a handheld device and can be obtained in the preoperative area or the emergency department. A prospective evaluation of pulmonary function and tracheal area in 31 children with a mediastinal mass was performed before 34 surgical procedures.[30] The tracheal area (expressed as a percentage of the predicted area) was determined by CT. In this study, criteria for administration of local anesthesia were either a tracheal area of less than 50% of predicted or a PEFR of less than 50% of predicted. All children who were administered anesthetics following these guidelines had an uneventful intraoperative course (Fig. 12.3). The study did not prove that children with a PEFR of less than 50% of predicted would experience respiratory collapse with general anesthesia, because all children who met this criterion were excluded from receiving general anesthesia. It did confirm, however, that general anesthesia could be used safely in children who met the minimum criteria of PEFR and tracheal area of greater than 50% of predicted. As treatment began and the masses shrank, the pulmonary function tests and total lung capacity improved. The patients who had a tracheal area of greater than 50% and yet a PEFR of less than 50%, were found to have either larger masses or compression of the bronchus, which is difficult to quantitate. In a recent review of 55 children at another institution, respiratory complications were found to occur only in those children with a tracheal area of less than 30% or those with associated bronchial compression with tracheal area of less than 70%.[31] Measurement of the PEFR may be the most accurate means of risk assessment.

Among patients with Hodgkin lymphoma and non-Hodgkin lymphoma (NHL) who had their pulmonary status evaluated, those with NHL appeared to be more impaired.[32] Respiratory symptoms were more common in children with NHL than in those with Hodgkin lymphoma. The pulmonary

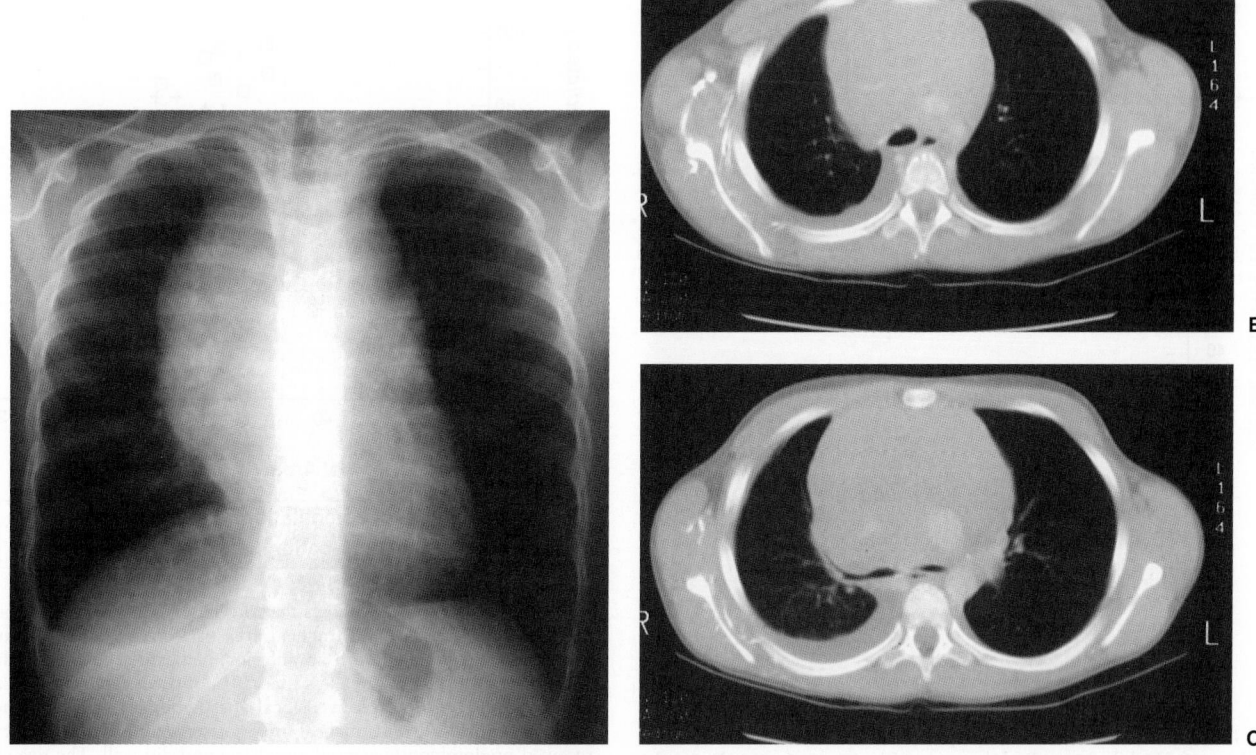

FIGURE 12.1 A: An 11-year-old girl presented with a several-week history of cough and dyspnea on exertion and a 3-day history of puffy eyes and orthopnea. The chest radiograph reveals a large anterior mediastinal mass and a right pleural effusion. **B:** Computed tomogram showed a tracheal area that was 82% of predicted. **C:** However, scans obtained of the lower chest revealed significant narrowing of both bronchi. This finding probably explains the marked reduction in her peak expiratory flow rate, which was 42% of predicted while sitting and only 24% of predicted while in a supine position. The diagnosis of lymphoblastic lymphoma was established by aspiration of her pleural effusion.

function tests were also worse in the NHL cohort, and these tumors were shown to account for a disproportionate number of the larger masses explaining their increased physiologic impact. A correlation between the size of the mass and the impairment in pulmonary function was also noted. Other findings that correlated with acute airway compromise in 8 of 29 pediatric patients in an additional study included anterior location of the mass, histologic diagnosis of lymphoma, signs and symptoms of superior vena cava syndrome, radiographic evidence of vessel compression or displacement, and pericardial and pleural effusion.[33] In a third study of 117 pediatric patients with an anterior mediastinal mass, 11 experienced an anesthesia related complication.[34] Features associated with these complications included orthopnea, upper body edema, great vessel compression or compression of the main-stem bronchus, pleural effusion, tracheal compression, and the diagnosis of lymphoblastic lymphoma.

Inevitably, children will be encountered with significant respiratory compromise who require biopsy but will not tolerate a general anesthetic. The presence of extrathoracic tissue for biopsy, particularly cervical lymphadenopathy, should be sought in all cases, but in some children, it will be entirely lacking. It was demonstrated in the late 1990s that children with lymphoblastic lymphoma have a significantly higher incidence of an associated pleural effusion than do children with Hodgkin lymphoma.[35] This study and others also demonstrated that aspiration of the effusion was diagnostic of

lymphoblastic lymphoma, using cytologic and immunocyto-chemical studies.[36] Cytogenetic evaluation of cells obtained from pleural fluid can be helpful, and diagnostic as well. The t(8;14)(q24;q11) translocation is particularly associated with T-cell lymphoblastic leukemia and the related T-cell lymphoblastic lymphomas, and its identification will facilitate their diagnosis.[37] Immunophenotyping of the cells obtained from pleural fluid can also show a predominance of T-cell versus B-cell markers, supporting the diagnosis of lymphoblastic lymphoma.

Children with significant respiratory compromise and no pleural effusion for aspiration and no extrathoracic disease require either an intrathoracic biopsy under local anesthesia, an image-guided percutaneous needle biopsy, or preliminary treatment with radiotherapy. Shielding of an area of the mass for future biopsy may allow successful diagnosis after the bulk of the mass and airway obstruction have resolved. Needle biopsies are often successful in establishing a diagnosis of NHL but are less helpful in cases of Hodgkin lymphoma. At our institution, biopsies performed under local anesthesia using an extrapleural anterior thoracotomy (Chamberlain procedure) have been performed successfully in four children as young as 10 years of age. This should be conducted with children in a semi-upright position breathing spontaneously. The partially upright position will maximize the compromised respiratory function.[30] The negative intrathoracic pressure exerted by the chest wall during spontaneous ventilation

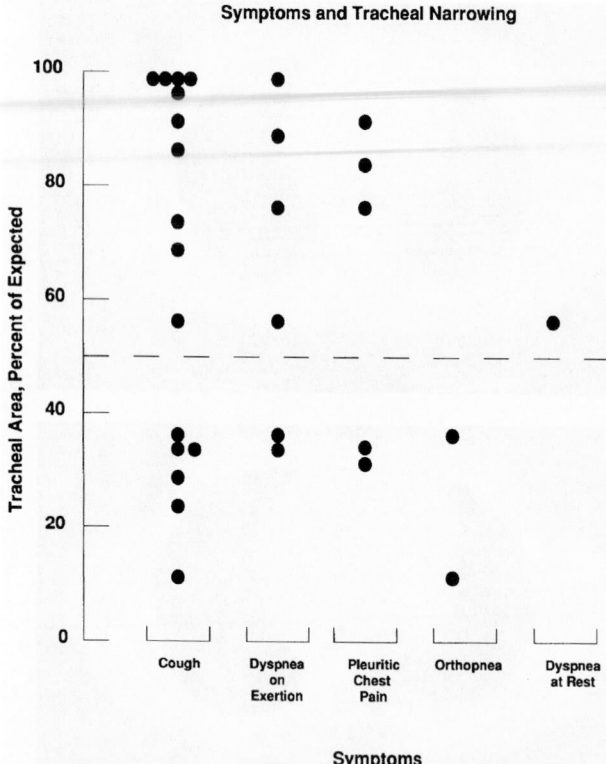

FIGURE 12.2 Correlation of symptoms and tracheal areas from a cohort of 42 children and adolescents with an anterior mediastinal mass. (From Shamberger RC, Holzman RS, Griscom NT, et al. CT quantitation of tracheal cross-sectional area as a guide to the surgical and anesthetic management of children with anterior mediastinal mass. J Pediatr Surg 1991;26:138–142, by permission of the publisher, WB Saunders.)

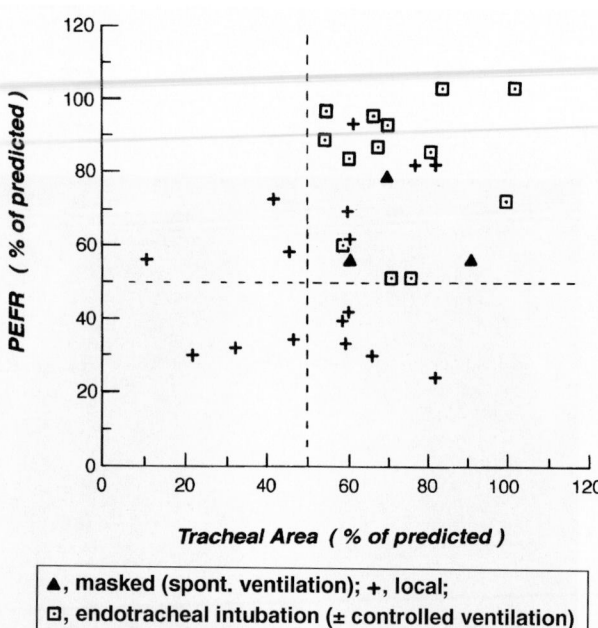

FIGURE 12.3 This graph shows the correlation between peak expiratory flow rate (PEFR) and tracheal area in a cohort of 31 children prospectively evaluated with an anterior mediastinal mass. Children with PEFR and tracheal area less than 50% of predicted (*to left of and below dashed lines*) all received local anesthetic and did well. Those children with PEFR and tracheal area greater than 50% of predicted received predominantly general anesthesia and did well. The five children with tracheal area greater than 50% of predicted (*in lower right box*) might have been considered for general anesthesia if tracheal area was the only parameter considered in assessing risk. Although the study could not demonstrate that these children would have had anesthetic problems, it did confirm that these parameters (>50% of PEFR and tracheal area) were safe for the administration of general anesthesia. (From Shamberger RC, Holzman RS, Griscom NT, et al. Prospective evaluation by computed tomography and pulmonary function tests of children with mediastinal masses. Surgery 1995;118:468–471, by permission of the publisher, Mosby-Year Book.)

minimizes collapse of the trachea. By following these guidelines for the use of general anesthesia, and the biopsy techniques described, a safe biopsy can be obtained in essentially all children and adolescents with an anterior mediastinal mass (Fig. 12.4). An algorithm for the care of children with a "critical airway" was proposed on the basis of a recent review of 40 children.[38] It was found that multiple children had the diagnosis established simultaneously when two procedures were performed, most often a bone marrow biopsy and biopsy of the mediastinal mass. Performing the bone marrow biopsy first would have avoided the risk for the more invasive mediastinal biopsy in these cases. While the use of extracorporeal membrane oxygenation or cardiopulmonary bypass has been described for near total airway collapse, it can be avoided in almost all cases.[39–42]

Management of Pheochromocytomas

Pheochromocytomas in children generally present with hypertension and associated symptoms.[43] Once the diagnosis is confirmed by a 24-hour urine collection for catecholamines or potentially more accurately by measurement of plasma-free metanephrines,[44] localization is then performed. Surgical removal remains the definitive therapy. The principles of preoperative management are blood pressure control and the repletion of intravascular volume. α-Adrenergic blockade should begin at least 1 week before the surgery and is usually accomplished through the use of phenoxybenzamine. This is

an oral long-acting α-adrenergic antagonist that is usually well tolerated by children. The typical starting dose for phenoxybenzamine is 0.20 mg per kg per day divided into a twice-a-day dose. The amine synthesis inhibitor metyrosine may be effective in children with hypertension unresponsive to phenoxybenzamine. More recently doxazosin, a compound related to prazosin, was reported to be as effective as phenoxybenzamine, but with fewer complications.[45] The intravenous administration of phentolamine, with its short half-life, may on occasion also be useful in controlling bouts of hypertension. Patients with pheochromocytoma are intravascular volume constricted because of the α-agonist effect on their vessels. As the α agonists are blocked, adequate intravascular volume expansion is required to correct the fluid and red cell mass deficits and prevent reflex tachycardia. β-Adrenergic blockade should be reserved for the treatment of persistent sinus tachycardia and arrhythmias associated with prior α-blockade and should never precede α-blockade or intravascular volume repletion.

Surgical removal of a pheochromocytoma produces a rapid drop in circulating catecholamines and possible hypotension, which may require further fluid administration. Conversely, the induction of anesthesia or the manipulation of the tumor(s) during resection can result in hypertensive episodes that are best treated with intravenous sodium nitroprusside.

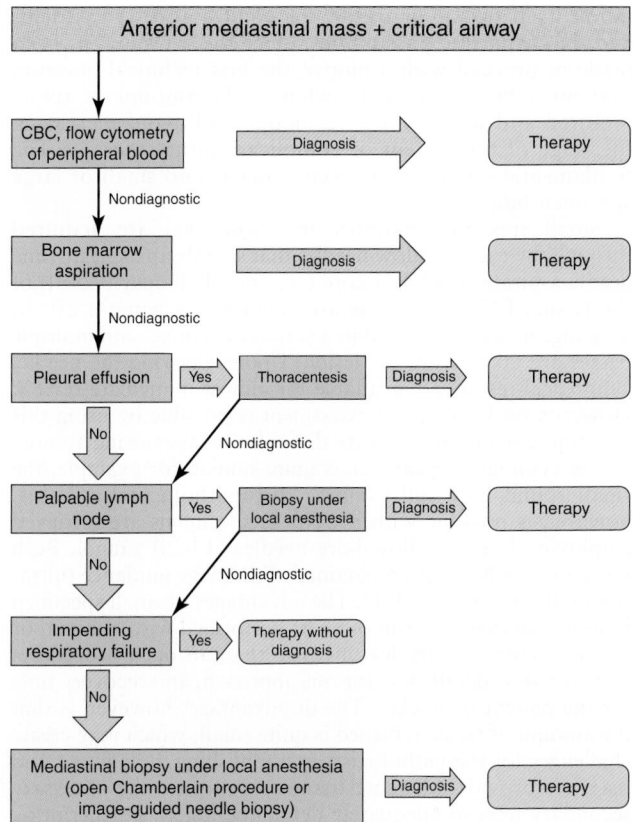

FIGURE 12.4 Algorithm for management of a child or adolescent presenting with an anterior mediastinal mass. CBC, complete blood count.

CANCER SURGERY

Staging

It is critical to establish the correct stage of a tumor for optimal treatment of pediatric solid tumors. All protocols base therapy on the tumor stage, which determines such factors in treatment as use and extent of radiotherapy and intensity of chemotherapy. In an era when cure can be achieved in the majority of patients, efforts to limit therapy and minimize the long-term sequelae of treatment assume a prominent role, particularly in children with low-stage tumors. It has been demonstrated in several tumors that treatment of children based on inadequate or incorrect staging results in an increased incidence of relapse.[46,47] Only in the management of Hodgkin lymphoma has surgical staging decreased in importance as systemic therapy has been used uniformly.

The unique staging system for each of the solid tumors will be presented in the appropriate chapters. These staging systems are not static tools; rather, they have evolved over time as the significance of specific criteria for staging and treatment have been established. Hilar lymph node involvement in Wilms' tumor was initially considered as a criterion for stage II in the first two National Wilms Tumor Study Group (NWTSG) protocols. On the basis of the demonstrated increased incidence of local recurrence in children with hilar lymph node involvement in the NWTS-2, hilar lymph node involvement became a criterion in subsequent studies for stage III.[48,49] A new staging system for neuroblastoma, the International Neuroblastoma Staging System (INSS), was created in the 1990s by a commit-

tee of international experts on neuroblastoma on the basis of the results of prior studies.[50] The treatment for neuroblastoma has progressed even further of late so that not only stage but also the biologic markers of the tumor now determine the intensity of treatment in many protocols.[51]

The surgeon is critical to the proper assignment of stage. A surgical staging system is used for most pediatric solid tumors. In these systems, the extent of residual disease after resection, as well as lymph node involvement, define the stage. In children with Wilms' tumor, lymph nodes must be sampled not only from the perihilar region but also from along the aorta or vena cava to adequately stage the child. It is of note that it has been well established in Wilms' tumor that assessment of lymph node involvement by gross inspection has a very poor correlation with the histology of the node. Othersen et al.[52] demonstrated a false-negative rate of 31.3% and a false-positive rate of 18.1% in a prospective series. In a similar review by Jereb et al.,[53] a false-positive rate of 72% and a false-negative rate of 7% occurred in a series of International Society of Pediatric Oncology (SIOP) patients. An increased incidence of local recurrence occurred in a recent review in children from NWTS-4 in whom lymph node sampling was not performed. The recurrence rate was actually higher than that of children with hilar lymph node involvement who had been appropriately treated.[46] The reason for the increased local recurrence was presumed under treatment of the children; the increased risk of recurrence occurred primarily in children with stage I disease, who receive limited chemotherapy and no radiotherapy.

The new INSS is also a surgically based staging system in which the size of the tumor, extent of residual disease, and involvement of ipsilateral and contralateral nonadherent lymph nodes define the stage.[50] Again, the gross assessment of lymph node involvement in infants and children with neuroblastoma is not adequate for evaluation. Wilson et al.[54] reported a sensitivity of 76% and a specificity of 77% for lymph node involvement by neuroblastoma on the basis of gross inspection of the nodes.

The staging of rhabdomyosarcoma is complex because of the multiple primary sites of involvement and its site-specific response to treatment. Rhabdomyosarcoma is staged on the basis of both tumor, node, metastases (TNM) and clinical group systems by the Intergroup Rhabdomyosarcoma Study (IRS). The TNM system is thought to best define the pretreatment extent of disease and allow comparison between results of various studies.[55] The clinical group system is a surgical staging system in which the extent of resection and the presence of nodal involvement are prime components. An initial incisional biopsy should be performed in most cases of suspected rhabdomyosarcoma. The biopsy site and direction of the incision should always be planned with future resection in mind. Injudicious attempts at initial resection of an extremity lesion that leave residual tumor can greatly complicate future efforts at complete resection.[56]

Children presenting without evidence of distant metastases have an overall 10% incidence of lymphatic spread. The frequency of lymph node involvement is the highest for primary lesions arising in the prostate (41%), paratesticular (26%), and genitourinary sites (24%).[57] Extremity lesions have an intermediate frequency (12%), whereas nonorbital head and neck sites (7%), truncal sites (3%), and the orbit (0%) had the lowest frequency. In extremity and genitourinary sites, it is particularly important to establish the extent of lymph node metastases, as this will guide the use of radiotherapy to treat all involved nodal groups. A representative sample of lymph nodes from the draining nodal group should be biopsied in these lesions. A lymph node resection should not be performed, however, because it may produce lymphedema, which will complicate radiotherapy and subsequent surgical resection of the primary lesion.

Radiologic evaluation of lymph node involvement has been demonstrated to have a low sensitivity. A total of 121 boys with paratesticular rhabdomyosarcoma treated during IRS III had a retroperitoneal lymph node dissection to evaluate nodal status.[58] Lymph nodes were assessed to be negative on the basis of CT in 18% of the boys, 14% of whom had positive nodes when biopsy or retroperitoneal lymph node dissection was performed. Of the clinically positive boys, 94% were confirmed to be positive pathologically. Retroperitoneal relapse occurred in only 2 of the 121 boys, one of whom had pathologically negative lymph nodes and did not receive radiotherapy. Although CT was very accurate, if lymph node abnormalities were identified, it was not extremely sensitive in identifying nodal involvement. In a subsequent study, Wiener et al.[47] from the IRS have reported an increased incidence of retroperitoneal relapse in children treated during IRS IV. In this study, the use of abdominal irradiation was based on thin-cut CT scans in 98% of cases as compared with children treated during IRS III, in which 94% had retroperitoneal biopsy or lymph node dissection. A decreased incidence in stage II disease (positive lymph nodes) from 35% to 17% was found between IRS III and IV, with a corresponding decline in the use of irradiation. This resulted, however, in a fourfold increase in retroperitoneal lymph node recurrence. This is another example of increased local failure resulting from inadequate staging.

Regional lymph node involvement is an extremely important prognostic variable in children with extremity rhabdomyosarcoma. Mandell et al.[59] evaluated children without hematogenous metastasis and found that survival in those without nodal involvement (11 of 12) was significantly better than in those with lymph nodes involved with tumor (1 of 10; $p = 0.001$). Survival has also been shown to be significantly better in patients with distal extremity rhabdomyosarcoma with no evidence of distal metastasis with biopsy-proven negative nodes than in those in whom nodes were not biopsied, just as was seen in Wilms' tumor.[56] These findings highlight the essential nature of proper staging to guide the intensity of therapy and to achieve maximum survival.

Biopsy

A biopsy serves as the basis of diagnosis and treatment of a tumor, and it is the essential starting point of therapeutic interventions. In addition to establishing the histopathological diagnosis, a biopsy can also be utilized to confirm the presence of metastases, to determine therapeutic response, and to document treatment complications.

Before undertaking a biopsy, five objectives must be considered and met. These are as follows: (a) the biopsy procedure, including risks, benefits, limitations, options, and outcomes must be discussed in detail with the patient and family; (b) the oncologist, pathologist, radiologist, and the surgeon must meet to determine the proper technique and quantity of tissue needed from the procedure to provide the maximum information with the least morbidity; (c) the precise biopsy route and site must be selected to facilitate future therapy; (d) a careful and thorough preoperative evaluation must be performed to ensure that the patient has an adequate physiologic reserve for the procedure; and (e) the multidisciplinary team should coordinate multiple procedures under one anesthetic if possible (i.e., a patient who requires a biopsy of a lesion may also need central venous access or a bone marrow biopsy and aspirate).

The type of biopsy a patient requires varies greatly and is dependent on the site of the mass, the characteristics of the lesion itself (cystic or solid), the condition of the patient, and the diagnostic possibilities. Once the decision has been made to proceed with a biopsy, the first technical question that must be answered is: what is the amount of tissue required and what biopsy technique will avoid increasing the stage of the patient or complicate future therapy. The fundamental separation of techniques is into small or large specimen biopsies.

Small specimen biopsies are those that are acquired through the use of hollow needles that sample an aspirate (fine needle aspirate [FNA]) or core (core needle biopsy [CNB]) of the tissue. FNA specimens are acquired by using a 20- to 25-gauge needle connected to a standard syringe, and multiple passes are taken from the lesion. Upon removing the needle, cytological results are available for almost immediate review. However, no histological assessment is possible by using this technique, which may create difficulty in diagnosing tumors whose cytologic appearance is quite similar, for example, the small round blue cell tumors. Histopathological analysis, however, is possible with a CNB as specimens are retrieved employing larger, hollow-bore needles (13–20 gauge). Both FNA and CNB are often obtained with image guidance (ultrasound, fluoroscopy, or CT). The advantages of small specimen biopsies are that they can often be performed with minimal or no anesthesia and are less invasive than an open procedure. Cost is also generally less for this approach, and recovery time for the patient is quicker. The disadvantage, however, is that the amount of tissue returned is quite small, which may create challenges for the pathologists in establishing a diagnosis and may not provide adequate tissue to complete the necessary secondary tests to adequately define the lesion. Furthermore, if imaging modalities are used to assist in this form of biopsy, radiation exposure will occur if CT or fluoroscopy is utilized as opposed to magnetic resonance imaging (MRI) or ultrasound. This issue of radiation exposure is of importance in the pediatric population as there is an increased risk of developing a malignancy from radiation exposure.[60,61] In addition, there is the possibility of tumor spread in needle tracts or of hemorrhage.[62,63] The risk of sampling error, where the specimen harvested may not adequately represent the entirety of the mass, is always a concern with biopsies, and the smaller the sample, the larger the concern. Despite these limitations, small specimen biopsies are an accepted standard of practice in pediatric oncology, and they have recently gained widespread acceptance and usage.[64-67]

In contrast to small specimen sampling techniques, large specimen tissue biopsies involve the removal of all (excisional) or part (incisional) of a lesion. The goal of these procedures is not for local control of the primary site. Large specimen biopsies are preferentially performed over small specimen biopsies in anatomic areas that are difficult to access secondary to proximity to major vessels or nerves or because the lesions cannot be reached without damaging overlying organs. Some disadvantages associated with large specimen biopsy procedures include longer procedure times, anesthetic dosing and recovery periods that can delay the start of adjuvant therapies. They are costlier also. However, the advantages to large specimen biopsies include the ability to obtain large amounts of tissue from multiple areas within the lesion, a detailed anatomic evaluation of the mass and surrounding structures, avoidance of radiation exposure to the patient and the healthcare team, and hemostasis and tumor sampling is controlled and confirmed directly before closing the incision to minimize the complications of tumor spillage and hemorrhage. Regardless of the type of biopsy procedure employed, the goal of this endeavor is the same—to ensure an adequate amount of tissue is available to accurately diagnose and stage a patient with the least amount of morbidity.

PREOPERATIVE ADJUVANT THERAPY

The role of preoperative adjuvant therapy is based on outcomes of completed trials, and its use is very disease specific. Several important questions must be addressed when preoperative therapy is considered. First, will the information regarding stage or histology be lost with the use of preoperative therapy, adversely affecting ultimate therapeutic decisions? Second, will children who do not otherwise require chemotherapy receive it? Third, will adjuvant therapy facilitate surgical resection and decrease the frequency of complications? These issues are considered for several of the solid tumors.

Wilms' Tumor

The two principal multi-institutional groups with therapeutic trials in Wilms' tumor have adopted quite different approaches to the use of adjuvant therapy. Primary nephrectomy has been recommended for patients with Wilms' tumor by the NWTSG. In contrast, initial chemotherapy has been used extensively by members of the SIOP. The potential benefit of preoperative therapy must be balanced against the disadvantages. Treatment without any biopsy has been difficult to support when both NWTSG and SIOP report a 7.6% to 9.9% rate of benign or other malignant diagnosis in children with a prenephrectomy diagnosis of Wilms' tumor.[68-70] Zuppan and colleagues[71] have shown that the histologic diagnosis after preoperative treatment in a group of children followed on NWTSG studies did not appear to have been significantly distorted by pretreatment, but loss of evidence of lymph node involvement has been a significant concern. "Downstaging" of tumors was seen in two consecutive but nonrandomized SIOP studies in which the proportion of low-stage disease increased after preoperative therapy when compared with earlier studies using primary nephrectomy. These findings suggest that the preoperative treatment significantly decreased the apparent stage of disease in children.[72] The proportion of stage I patients at surgery increased from 22% to 48% after chemotherapy. The third SIOP study of Wilms' tumor randomized the use of local radiotherapy (20 Gy) in children treated preoperatively with chemotherapy (vincristine and dactinomycin) who had stage II lymph node–negative disease at resection. All children received vincristine and dactinomycin for 38 weeks. A high rate of stage I tumors (52%) was found in this study, with a low frequency of ruptures (7%). The study randomized the use of abdominal radiotherapy for children with stage II lymph node–negative tumors. The study was closed after randomization of radiotherapy for 123 children. An increased incidence of abdominal recurrence occurred during the first year of follow-up in children not receiving radiation (6 of 59 vs. 0 of 64).[73] This demonstrated that prenephrectomy treatment altered the pathologic findings, which would have led to a diagnosis of lymph node involvement and to the standard administration of abdominal irradiation. The absence of finding lymph node involvement in the posttherapy specimens, however, did not obviate the apparent need for radiotherapy in this cohort to prevent local recurrence.

A major driving force for the use of preoperative therapy by SIOP was the high rate of operative tumor rupture in its early series employing primary resection of the tumor. The rupture rate decreased from 33% (20 of 60) to 4% (3 of 72) with preoperative abdominal irradiation (20 Gy) in the first randomized SIOP study.[74] It must be noted, however, that 33% is an extremely high frequency of rupture. Survival was not affected, and the incidence of local recurrence was not

reported. In NWTS-1 and NWTS-2, operative rupture occurred in 22% and 12% of children, respectively.[68,75] In a subsequent SIOP randomized study, the rate of rupture was essentially the same for children receiving abdominal irradiation (20 Gy) and actinomycin D (9%; 7 of 76) and those receiving vincristine and actinomycin D (6%; 5 of 88).[46]

A second consideration in the use of preoperative chemotherapy in Wilms' tumor has been whether it will allow the safe performance of partial nephrectomy in some cases. This has been evaluated in several centers. McLorie et al.[76] in Toronto obtained percutaneous biopsy in 37 children with Wilms' tumor and then administered multiagent chemotherapy for 4 to 6 weeks. A partial nephrectomy was then performed in nine children (four with unilateral and five with bilateral tumors). Two children experienced intra-abdominal relapse. Only 4 of the 30 unilateral tumors (13.3%) were amenable to a partial nephrectomy. Another analysis of the feasibility of partial nephrectomy was performed at St. Jude Children's Research Hospital.[77] Preoperative CT scans of 43 children with nonmetastatic unilateral Wilms' tumor were reviewed retrospectively. Criteria to allow partial nephrectomy were involvement by the tumor of only one pole and less than one-third of the kidney, a functioning kidney, no involvement of the collecting system or renal vein, and clear margins between the tumor and surrounding structures. Utilizing these criteria, only 2 of 43 scans (4.7%) suggested that partial nephrectomy was feasible.

The primary concern regarding the use of preoperative chemotherapy, as reported in the studies of Cozzi et al.[78] and Moorman-Voestermans et al.,[79] to shrink small tumors to allow partial nephrectomy is that these children may be curable by surgical resection alone, without subjecting them to the toxicity of additional treatments. The issue of inaccurate lymph node staging is also present for all of these patients receiving preoperative chemotherapy.

Preoperative treatment of Wilms' tumor is generally accepted in certain instances. These include the occurrence of Wilms' tumor in a solitary kidney, bilateral renal tumors, a massive tumor that would require resection of other involved organs, and respiratory distress from extensive pulmonary metastasis. Pretreatment biopsy should be obtained. The aim of treatment before surgical resection in the bilateral tumors and when tumor occurs in a solitary kidney is to preserve maximum renal tissue and function. In the NWTSG review of the 55 children who developed renal failure treated on NWTS-1 to NWTS-4, 39 had bilateral tumor involvement. Increasing efforts to preserve renal parenchyma in bilateral cases in the sequence of NWTSG studies resulted in a decline in the incidence of renal failure from 16.4% in NWTS-1 and NWTS-2 to 9.9% in NWTS-3 and 3.8% in NWTS-4, although the frequency may increase in the later studies as the children age.[80] In most cases, preliminary treatment after biopsy and staging produces a significant decrease in the size of the tumor and facilitates resection with preservation of a portion of the kidney. A total of 134 kidneys in 98 children with bilateral Wilms' tumors were managed with renal salvage procedures during NWTS-4.[81] Complete resection of gross disease was accomplished in 118 kidneys (88%). A higher incidence of positive surgical margins (16%; 19 of 134) and local tumor recurrence (8.2%; 11 of 134) occurred in this group of children than in those with complete nephrectomy. This was justified, however, by the desire to preserve renal tissue and thus avoid renal failure. Overall, portions of 72% of the kidneys were preserved, and the 4-year survival rate was 81.7%.

A final indication for preoperative therapy in Wilms' tumor may be in children with intravascular extension of the tumor.

Some studies have demonstrated a decreased incidence or severity of surgical complications in children with atrial extension receiving preoperative chemotherapy compared with children with primary surgical resection.[82]

Neuroblastoma

Therapeutic intervention for patients diagnosed with neuroblastoma is dependent on the risk group to which the patient is assigned at diagnosis by the International Neuroblastoma Classification schema. These determinations are based on the stage of the disease at diagnosis, the patient's age, histopathological classification, quantitative analysis of tumor DNA content, and the presence or absence of MYCN amplification. Patients are categorized into low-, intermediate-, and high-risk cohorts (Table 12.1). Surgery is a mainstay in the treatment of this disease, albeit in conjunction with chemotherapy and radiotherapy. Children classified as low risk receive surgery only in the majority of cases with excellent results.[83,84] For those children who relapse after surgery, results are still excellent with salvage chemotherapy regimens.[83,85] The role of neoadjuvant chemotherapy, therefore, is of limited scope and is employed in cases where tumors cannot be resected without undue morbidity or risk of mortality, or in cases where there is significant neurological, cardiorespiratory, or abdominal visceral compromise at presentation. The success of this approach is highlighted in several studies, including a series by Rubie and colleagues[86] who analyzed 52 patients with localized but unresectable tumors who underwent neoadjuvant chemotherapy. A response rate of greater than 60% was observed, and 51 of 52 children in the study were able to undergo a successful extirpative procedure (Fig. 12.5). Furthermore, whereas surgery was the first modality employed for children presenting with spinal cord compression, neoadjuvant chemotherapy is now the treatment of choice in these children secondary to less morbidity with good response rates (58%) and functional neurological outcome (92%) reported by Rubie and colleagues.[86] Other groups have reported similar outcomes and recommendations.[87,88]

For patients with intermediate-risk disease, neoadjuvant therapy is generally employed prior to attempted operative resection. Surgery is never used as the sole modality of treatment in these children, but it is often undertaken, albeit with some controversy[89,90] in an attempt to acquire a gross total resection and expected better outcomes.[91–93] Exact regimens differ, but common drugs include cyclophosphamide, etoposide, cisplatin, and doxorubicin. Matthay and colleagues[94] reported on the success of this approach of combining neoadjuvant chemotherapy followed by surgery and more adjuvant chemotherapy and radiotherapy in a report documenting 100% event-free survival (EFS) and overall survival (OS) in patients whose tumors had favorable biological characteristics, 90% EFS and 93% OS in infants whose tumors had at least one unfavorable biologic feature and only 54% EFS and 61% OS in older children with tumors that had unfavorable characteristics.[94]

Patients presenting with high-risk disease are treated with neoadjuvant chemotherapy prior to any attempt at surgical extirpation. Current protocols call for 4 to 5 courses of neoadjuvant chemotherapy, followed by surgery and then radiotherapy to treat any residual disease. More adjuvant chemotherapy is then administered followed by autologous hematopoietic stem cell rescue. Finally, biologic therapy employing cis-retinoic acid is used. Despite these modalities, the long-term EFS is only 30%.

Finally, in addition to describing the data documenting where and when neoadjuvant therapy is useful in risk-stratified patients, studies have also described the utility of

---

TABLE 12.1

INSS RISK STRATIFICATION BY AGE, MYCN AMPLIFICATION, PLOIDY, AND SHIMADA CLASSIFICATION[a]

INSS stage	Age, d	MYCN	Ploidy	Histo	Other	Risk
1	Any	Any	Any	Any	Any	Low
2A/2B	Any	NA	Any	Any	>50% rsxn	Low
4S	<365	NA	DI > 1	F	Asympt	Low
2A/2B	Any	NA	Any	Any	<50% rsxn	Inter
2A/2B	Any	NA	Any	Any	Bx only	Inter
3	<547	NA	Any	Any	Any	Inter
3	>547	NA	Any	F	Any	Inter
4	<365	NA	Any	Any	Any	Inter
4	365–547	NA	DI > 1	F	Any	Inter
4S	<365	NA	DI = 1	Any	Any	Inter
4S	<365	?	?	?	Any	Inter
4S	<365	NA	Any	Any	Sympt	Inter
4S	<365	NA	Any	UF	Any	Inter
2A/2B	Any	A	Any	Any	Any	High
3	>547	A	Any	Any	Any	High
3	>547	NA	Any	UF	Any	High
4	<365	A	Any	Any	Any	High
4	365–547	A	Any	Any	Any	High
4	365–547	Any	DI = 1	Any	Any	High
4	365–547	Any	Any	UF	Any	High
4	>547	Any	Any	Any	Any	High
4S	<365	A	Any	Any	Any	High

INSS, International Neuroblastoma Staging System; NA, nonamplified; A, amplified; DI, DNA index; F, favorable; UF, unfavorable; rsxn, resection; asympt, asymptomatic; Bx, biopsy; sympt, symptomatic.
[a]This table depicts the criteria to define a patient with neuroblastoma as being at low, intermediate, or high risk.

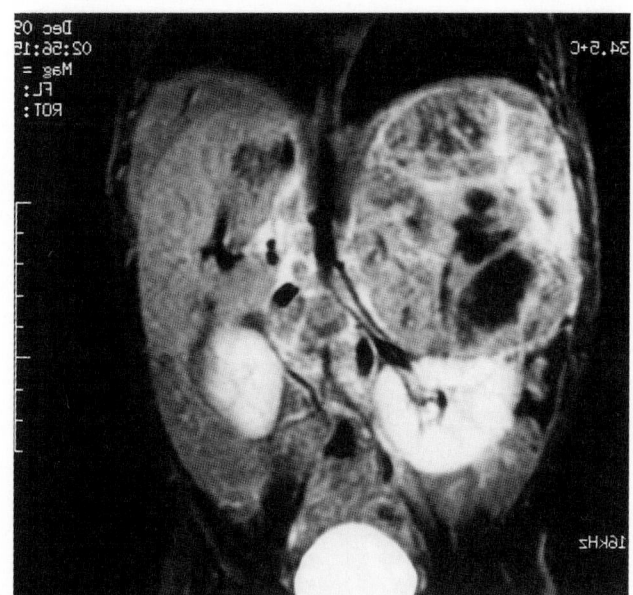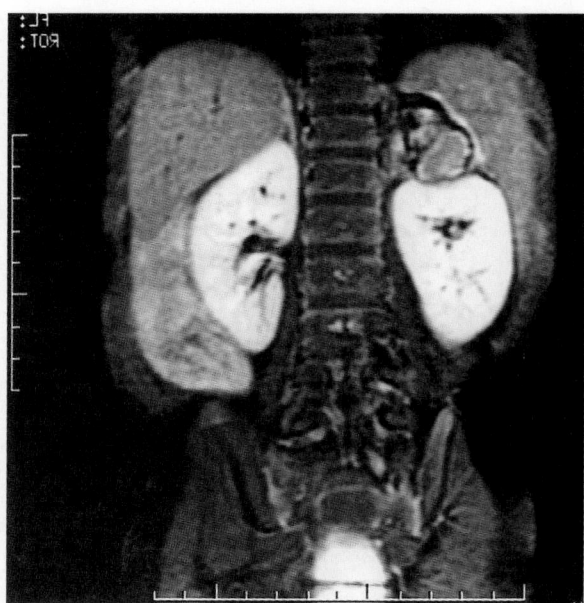

FIGURE 12.5 A: This magnetic resonance imaging scan of a 9-month-old boy with neuroblastoma who presented with a palpable left abdominal mass shows a large left adrenal tumor. The child was not found to have metastatic disease but did have MYCN amplification. **B:** Dramatic response of the tumor to adjuvant chemotherapy is shown in the follow-up scan.

neoadjuvant chemotherapy on surgical outcomes. Neuroblastomas often present as large primary tumors that encircle critical vessels in the abdomen or chest. Although two studies have shown no difference in the surgical complication rate between initial and postinduction resection,[95,96] others have demonstrated a higher incidence of complications, including nephrectomy, in the group undergoing initial resection.[97,98] Preoperative chemotherapy decreases the vascularity and friability of the tumor and facilitates resection, particularly in developing a dissection plane between the tumor and the great vessels (Fig. 12.6). Preoperative therapy may be of particular importance for preservation of renal function. Many current protocols for children with stage IV disease have significant nephrotoxicity, and loss of a kidney from surgery can significantly limit the intensity of therapy. A multi-institutional review of children treated over an 11-year interval demonstrated a 14.9% (52 of 349 children) incidence of nephrectomy or renal infarction as a result of surgery for local control.[99] There was a 25% incidence among those with initial resection (29 children) and a 9.9% incidence in the postchemotherapy resections (23 children). In children undergoing initial resection, the risk of nephrectomy was more than twice of that encountered in children undergoing resection after chemotherapy ($p = 0.012$) strongly supporting the use of neoadjuvant chemotherapy before attempted resection.

Ewing's Sarcoma

Another tumor in which preoperative adjuvant chemotherapy has been found to be of benefit is Ewing's sarcoma/primitive neuroectodermal tumor. Adjuvant therapy is required for all children with this diagnosis because of the very high incidence of local and distant relapse without such therapy. Its use preceding surgery has been of benefit in decreasing the size of the tumor as well as its friability and extremely vascular nature (Fig. 12.7).[100,101] In the North American cooperative group studies, a clear preference of surgeons for resection after

initial therapy was seen, although this was more dominant in sites other than the chest wall (92% vs. 70%).[67] Attempts at resection of the rib primaries was not related to size of the tumor in contrast to tumors at other sites where tumors shorter than 8 cm had primary resection attempted in 18% of cases versus those 8 cm or longer in which only 2% underwent primary resection. More recent multi-institutional studies of children with chest wall primaries have demonstrated a major benefit of preoperative therapy. Complete resection with negative pathologic margins is more frequently achieved in children who have received preoperative chemotherapy.[102] This is of particular importance for children with chest wall primaries because complete resection avoids the use of radiotherapy to the chest with its attendant risks of pulmonary and cardiac injury as well as the risk of second malignant neoplasms seen at all sites. This study showed no added benefit from the addition of radiotherapy in children in whom a complete resection of the tumor was achieved. A randomized controlled trial of the use of preoperative adjuvant therapy in Ewing's sarcoma is difficult to consider at this time, given the clear surgical preference for its use and the established benefit demonstrated in nonrandomized studies for its use in chest wall lesions.

Osteosarcoma

Chemotherapy has been the single greatest therapeutic intervention in the treatment of osteosarcoma in the last four decades. Prior to its use, the mortality of osteosarcoma was nearly 90%. This statistic encompassed those that presented with synchronous metastatic disease (20%) in addition to those that did not and who had adequate local control of the primary lesion. In fact, the 10-year survival of patients treated with surgery alone was only 16% in one series.[103] Most patients developed subsequent metastases to their lungs (95%) and/or bones (15%–30%).[104] For years, it was postulated that these patients had micrometastases that surgery could not

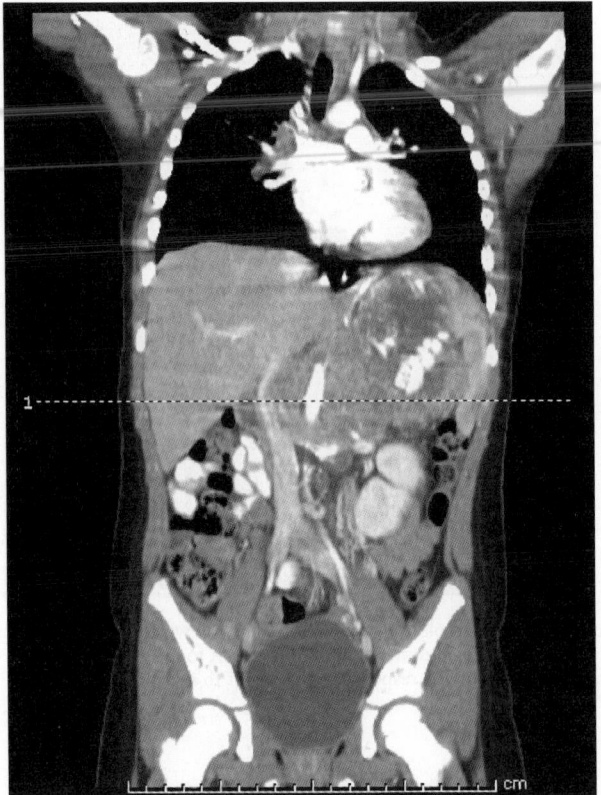

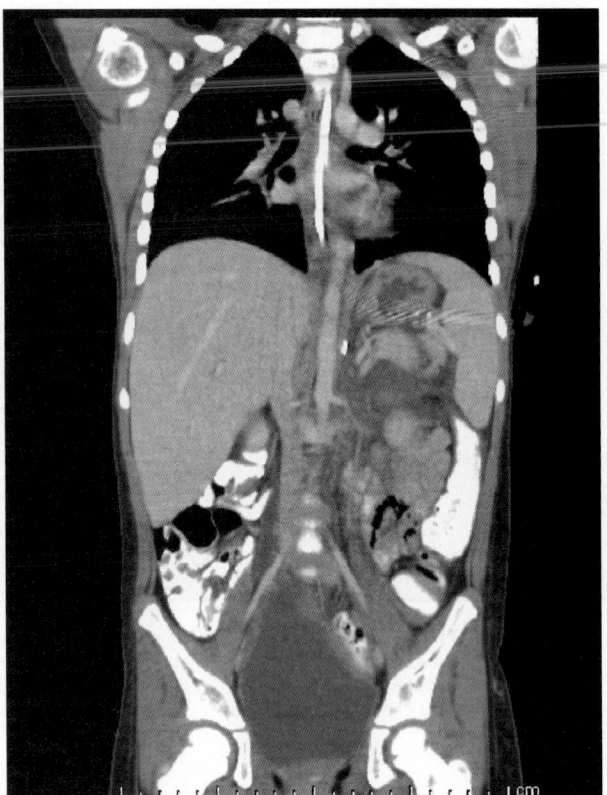

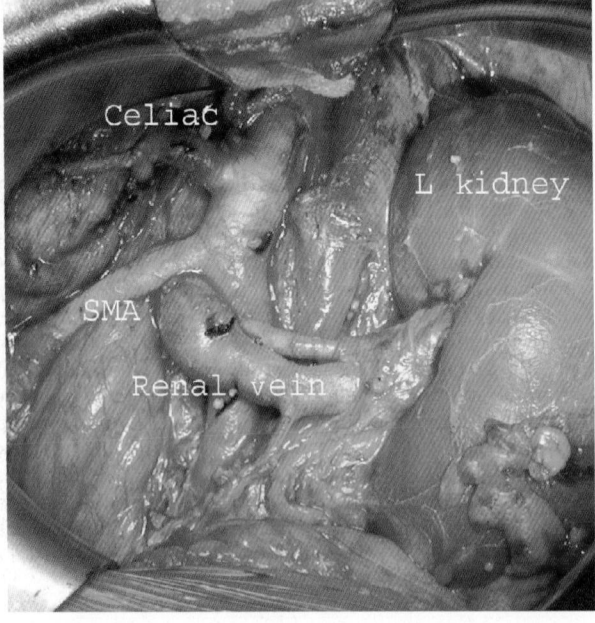

FIGURE 12.6 This abdominal computed tomography (CT) scan (coronal) image demonstrate a large retroperitoneal neuroblastoma involving the aorta and vena cave at presentation (**A**). This intraoperative photograph (**B**) demonstrates the tumor bed after resection of an intra-abdominal neuroblastoma that encircled the aorta, superior mesenteric artery, celiac axis, and renal vessels. Appropriate structures are marked in white. The final image (**C**) is the coronal CT scan postresection. SMA, superior mesenteric artery.

eradicate, and this theory was proven correct in 2005.[105] The utility of chemotherapy was clinically shown to be both relevant and essential to the optimal management of patients who presented with apparent localized disease in several reports from the 1980s.[106,107] These studies were small, randomized trials that demonstrated EFS and OS benefits in the cohort that received chemotherapy over the one that did not. No one specific regimen was employed, and the agents shown to be effective included methotrexate, doxorubicin, bleomycin, cyclophosphamide, dactinomycin, vincristine, and cisplatin.

Building on these trials, the use of neoadjuvant chemotherapy was entertained and explored secondary to the popularity and use of limb-sparing procedures that mandated a specific prosthesis be fabricated for each patient. Construction of this metallic, composite endoprosthesis took many weeks to complete, and hence, chemotherapy was given prior to surgery as a practical matter. Rosen[108] described this approach at his institution, and he also reported a trend in increased survival with neoadjuvant as opposed to adjuvant chemotherapy. The equivalence of neoadjuvant therapy versus adjuvant therapy

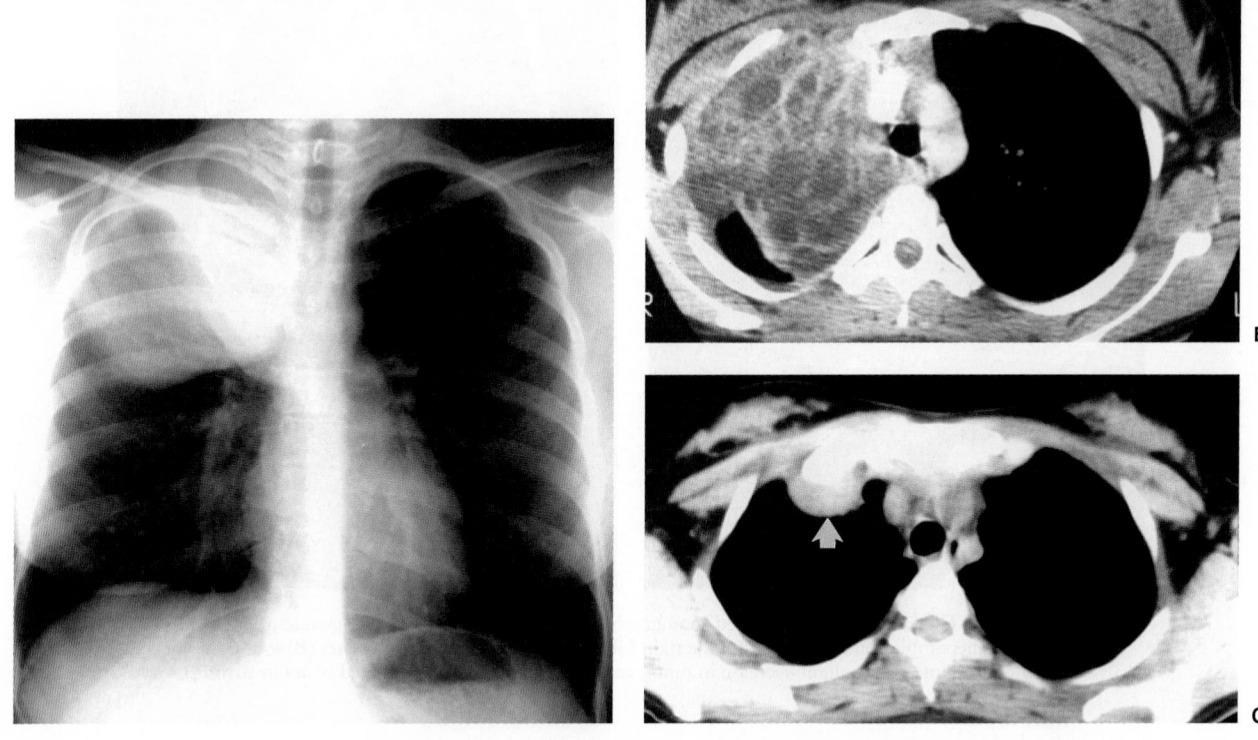

FIGURE 12.7 A: Chest radiograph of a 14-year-old girl with Ewing's sarcoma, who presented with a cough, reveals a mass in the apex of the right chest. B: Computed tomography (CT) scan showed a large mass of varying density without bone erosion. Biopsy was achieved by percutaneous technique. The chest radiograph after 2 months of therapy was normal, and CT scan (C) showed a small residual soft tissue mass (*arrow*). No viable tumor was found in the mass on pathologic examination after resection.

alone was shown in a Pediatric Oncology Group trial,[109] but it was not shown to be superior. The study was criticized for the regimens employed and the types of operations performed for local control, but it set the standard that neoadjuvant therapy worked and was at least equivalent to adjuvant therapy alone.

Even more importantly, a byproduct of these early trials demonstrated that tumor response to neoadjuvant chemotherapy became a significant prognostic and therapeutic factor.[110–112] These studies have documented that patients with a good response to neoadjuvant chemotherapy (>90% necrosis in the specimen as defined by the Memorial Sloan Kettering Group[113]) had a higher survival rate than those that did not (10%–35% difference). Furthermore, these studies implemented different chemotherapy regimens for patients without a good response to the neoadjuvant protocol, and this strategy has been shown to be effective by another group.[114] However, other groups have not had similar success in duplicating these results.[109,115,116] The establishment of the effectiveness of ifosfamide and etoposide in metastatic osteosarcoma patients has led to the development of a multinational, cooperative, prospective, randomized trial of their use in addition to doxorubicin, cisplatin, and methotrexate in patients without a good histological response to neoadjuvant therapy.

Hepatoblastoma

Surgery is the long-standing mainstay in the treatment of hepatoblastoma. However, historical studies document that

resection alone seldom achieved cure despite complete removal of all radiographically identifiable disease. In fact, only 25% of children survived who underwent complete resection of their tumors,[117,118] and this high failure rate was attributed, as in the osteosarcoma patients, to occult metastatic disease not identified radiographically at the time of the initial resection.[119] One of the first studies to document the early success of neoadjuvant chemotherapy was by Weinblatt and colleagues.[120] In fact, more than 75% of the lesions in this series became resectable after neoadjuvant chemotherapy. Subsequent reports documented the efficacy of doxorubicin, cisplatin, vincristine, and 5-fluorouracil alone or in various combinations (Fig. 12.8).[121–124] The ideal timing of surgery was postulated to be between cycle numbers 2 and 4. Resection of the primary tumor at this point was deemed to balance the maximal effect of neoadjuvant therapy to shrink the tumor prior to the development of chemoresistance. Von Schweinitz and colleagues[124] reported that 50% of their patients had evidence of tumor growth after the fourth cycle of neoadjuvant therapy. Ultimately, 5-year survival rates for all patients with hepatoblastoma had increased in just two decades to more than 85% with the addition of neoadjuvant and adjuvant chemotherapy to surgery for hepatoblastoma.

Refinement of this approach has occurred in the last decade, however, as a defined treatment protocol consisting of neoadjuvant chemotherapy and surgical resection or early orthotopic transplant evaluation for those patients with tumors which are too extensive to resect has been developed and reported by the SIOP Liver Tumor Group (SIOPEL)[125,126] This regimen was termed *PLADO*, and it consisted of an

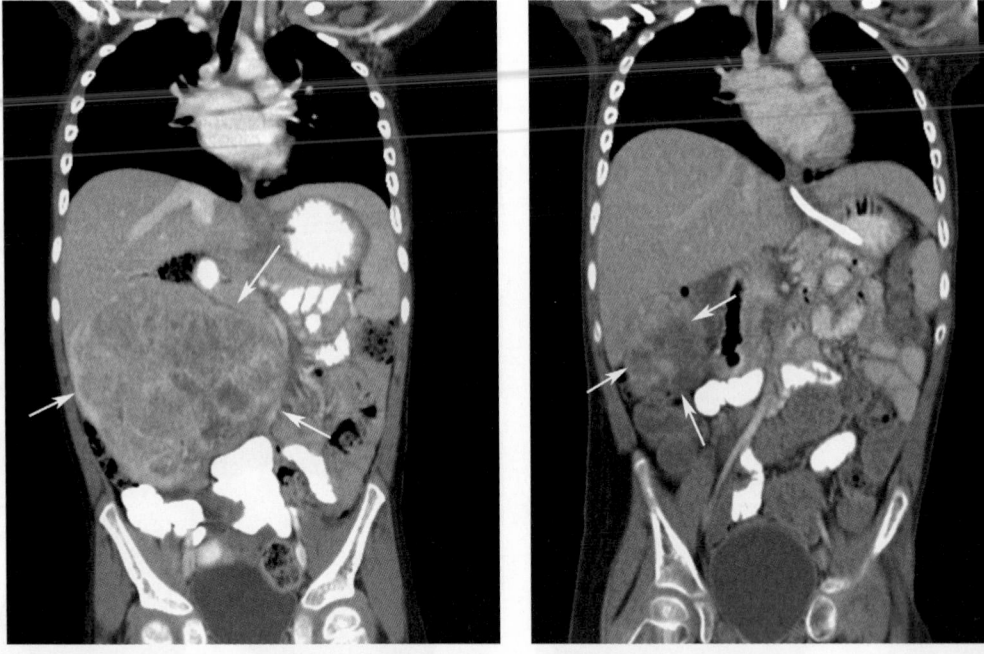

FIGURE 12.8 These abdominal computed tomography scan (coronal) images demonstrate a large, exophytic mass (hepatoblastoma) arising from the right lobe of the liver before (**A**) and after (**B**) four cycles of chemotherapy. Note the resultant decrease in tumor mass by almost 50% (as outlined by *white arrows*).

imaging defined staging protocol (pretreatment extent of disease [PRETEXT]), pretreatment diagnostic biopsy (core needle or incisional biopsy), neoadjuvant chemotherapy of continuous infusion cisplatin (day 1) followed by continuous infusion of doxorubicin (day 2, 3), surgical resection after 4 to 6 cycles (12–20 weeks from diagnosis), and orthotopic liver transplant (OLTX) evaluation and referral for tumors confined to the liver that remained unresectable despite chemotherapy. The only tumors resected primarily were those deemed to be confined to a single section (i.e., right anterior, right posterior, left medial, left lateral) of the liver (PRETEXT I). The overall 5-year survival rate was 75% for the entire cohort, and 85% for those following the complete protocol, including neoadjuvant chemotherapy regardless of PRETEXT stage. PRETEXT stages I to IV had OS rates of 100%, 91%, 58%, and 57%, respectively, which compares favorably to survival reported by North American centers.[127] Finally, ongoing studies attempting to decrease the morbidity of neoadjuvant regimens without sacrificing their cure rates are being undertaken in SIOPEL-3 and SIOPEL-4. In SIOPEL-3, standard risk patients are being prospectively randomized to single agent cisplatin or to cisplatin and doxorubicin. SIOPEL-4 is currently analyzing the addition of carboplatin to a cisplatin and doxorubicin backbone regimen in high-risk patients

MINIMALLY INVASIVE SURGERY

Over the past 15 years, minimally invasive surgical procedures have become common practice. Improved cameras, new trocar systems, and specifically designed instruments now allow a wide spectrum of operations to be performed without the use of large thoracotomy or laparotomy incisions. In the realm of pediatric surgical oncology, these methods have been most broadly applied to biopsies and the excision of selected masses. A CT scan or an MRI scan is often very helpful in

planning the appropriate surgical approach. Oncologic surgical principles, such as adequate exploration, complete excision of a mass with an appropriate margin, and minimizing the risk of a tumor spill, are still paramount. Although rare and possibly technique-related, trocar site tumor implantation has been reported.[128,129]

Thoracoscopic surgery is usually performed under general anesthesia in a full lateral position to allow for visualization of all lobes of the lung. Nodules that are located peripherally in the lung, along the parietal pleura, or on the diaphragm are particularly suitable for removal. In larger patients, a double-lumen endotracheal tube allows for selective lung ventilation and, hence, permits more facile surgery. Thoracoscopic surgery to excise small tumors of the lung is frequently accomplished with the aid of an intracorporeal stapling device. Thoracoscopic lobectomy in children is technically feasible, but experience with such resections for primary malignancies remains limited.[130] Although thoracoscopy is often suitable for the removal of secondary lung tumors, osteogenic sarcoma metastatic to the lung is usually best managed by standard thoracotomy. This is because thoracoscopy and CT scan often miss small intraparenchymal osteogenic sarcoma metastasis that may be easily palpated. The mediastinum is also accessible by minimally invasive techniques for thoracoscopically guided needle biopsies, excisional or incisional biopsies, as well as tumor removal in selected individuals. Laparoscopic surgery is performed under general anesthesia and relies on CO_2 insufflation of the peritoneal cavity to permit visualization. Staging laparoscopy and biopsies of primary and secondary tumors have frequently been performed. If oncologic principles are not compromised, tumor resection may also be considered. Laparoscopic splenectomy, nephrectomy, adrenalectomy, lymph node dissection, and colectomy have all been performed in patients with malignancies. Minimally invasive thyroid excision has also been reported in children with thyroid cancer.[131] In general, no large-scale prospective trials to evaluate the efficacy and complication rate of minimally invasive surgery versus "open" surgery have been completed in pediatric oncology patients.

SPECIFIC TUMOR CONSIDERATIONS

Wilms' Tumor

Resection continues to play a major role in the local control of Wilms' tumor. The importance of complete staging has already been stressed. In most cases, except those previously discussed, including bilateral tumors, the initial management of a renal mass is nephrectomy. Despite the fact that most Wilms' tumors present as a large mass, safe resection is generally feasible. Wilms' tumor, in contrast with neuroblastoma, is less likely to directly invade surrounding organs, complicating resection. It is important that an appropriately sized transverse upper abdominal or thoracoabdominal incision be used. A flank incision does not allow examination of the contralateral kidney or adequate lymph node biopsy, and a small incision in all too many cases results in rupture of the tumor and requires subsequent abdominal irradiation.

The vital importance of lymph node biopsy has already been stressed. There is no role, however, for an extensive lymph node resection, as this has not decreased the incidence of local recurrence or improved long-term EFS.[52,53] One additional consideration during resection of Wilms' tumor is intravascular extension. This has been documented to occur in 4.1% to 6.0% of children treated on NWTS-3 and NWTS-4, respectively, and it should always be suspected.[132] Preoperative imaging should evaluate for intravascular extension, but cannot conclusively exclude its presence. Before ligation of the renal vein, it should be palpated to make certain that there is not intravascular extension of the tumor that might embolize with ligation of the vein. Second, if unexplained hypotension occurs during the course of nephrectomy, the possibility of a pulmonary embolism must always be entertained. Current recommendations from the NWTSG are that children with intravascular extension to the atrium or inferior vena cava extension to the level of the hepatic veins should have a biopsy of the tumor followed by chemotherapy before resection of the tumor.[82]

Neuroblastoma

In operations on patients with neuroblastoma, the goal is to remove all gross disease without compromising organ function or neurovascular structures. During resection, regional lymph nodes should be sampled to adequately assess the stage of the patient. For abdominal lesions, this also consists of contralateral lymph nodes if possible. A key point to remember is that the anatomic midline for determination of laterality of lymph node involvement is the longitudinal axis of the aorta and not the spine. Neuroblastoma is most often located in the abdomen, arising from the adrenal gland or from the sympathetic chain along the spine, but it may also be located in the pelvis along the sacrum or at the bifurcation of the aorta (organ of Zuckerkandl), paraspinous region of the thoracic cavity from the sympathetic chain, in the neck along the cervical spine, and behind the orbit. Neuroblastoma has a propensity to encase vital vascular structures (aorta, vena cava, visceral arteries), nerves (phrenic, vagus, brachial plexus, or recurrent laryngeal) or other organs (kidney), as well as to invade an ipsilateral spinal foramen and grow into the spinal canal. If possible, only the tumor should be removed and not any other structure. As described previously, children who present with symptoms related to spinal cord compression (paralysis, incontinence) should undergo immediate initiation of chemotherapy as opposed to spinal decompression and tumor debulking by surgery or radiation.[87,88] Finally, the extent of the surgical resection in children with stage III and IV disease remains controversial with reports for[91,93,133] and against[89,90] aggressive extirpative procedures. The most telling study in support of these procedures is by LaQuaglia and colleagues[91] who examined a cohort of 141 patients with bulky stage IV disease who had a marked improvement in survival (50% vs. 11%) and decrease in local recurrence (50% vs. 10%) when patients had gross total resections.[91] Whether this was due to a difference in the biology of the tumor facilitating resection or the surgery itself is difficult to establish. In light of the generally poor prognosis for high-risk patients, aggressive extirpative procedures may be warranted.

The timing of surgical intervention is also of critical importance in children with neuroblastoma. Patients with stage I or IIA/B low-risk disease without evidence of organ compromise warrant upfront resections as the only modality of treatment. Outcomes are excellent in this cohort of patients, and if relapse occurs, chemotherapy can then be employed. Patients with advanced disease at presentation (stage III or IV) generally receive neoadjuvant chemotherapy with subsequent operative extirpation followed by adjuvant chemo- and radiotherapy. Patients in the high-risk group, however, still have poor outcomes with most series reporting survival rates of less than 30%.

In addition to knowing when to operate, there are patients with neuroblastoma who may not warrant any operative intervention. The first cohort of patients is in patients with low-risk stage IVs disease. Although stage IV, their prognosis is quite good (85% survival).[134] Treatment is generally supportive if the child is asymptomatic and the disease burden is not great, for these lesions have a tendency to spontaneously regress.[135] In fact, approximately three-fourths of patients, with or without treatment directed at the primary tumor, had spontaneous regression with subsequent cure.[136] If symptoms are present, then chemotherapy may be initiated and surgery to expand the abdominal cavity may be warranted if the child has respiratory dysfunction from abdominal distension due to extensive liver involvement.

The second cohort where observation alone may be warranted is infants with antenatally or perinatally diagnosed adrenal masses. The majority of these lesions are small with favorable biological characteristics with no MYCN amplification. These tumors are generally stage I or II, and surgery alone would be curative in the majority of cases. However, observation of these tumors has also been suggested as a viable alternative secondary to their low risk of progression and likely spontaneous regression. This recommendation is based on a multicenter, nonrandomized study of children younger than 1 year with localized disease.[137] Roughly, 47% (44 of 93) of study subjects had regression of their tumors, with complete regression in 10% (17 subjects). Eleven percent of patients had no change in their tumors (10 of 93), whereas 42% (39 of 93) had progression of their disease. Those who demonstrated progression had salvage chemotherapy and surgery, and the 3-year disease-free survival and OS were not significantly different than those managed with these modalities upfront. On the basis of these data, Children's Oncology Group (COG) is currently performing an observational only study for these lesions by utilizing serial ultrasound, laboratory, and physical examinations to follow these patients. Criteria for intervention are based on radiographic increase in the size of the mass or biologic activity of the lesion as measured by urine catecholamines.

Hepatoblastoma

Despite the progress provided by adjuvant chemotherapy in hepatoblastoma, complete extirpation of the tumor provides the greatest chance for cure. The fundamental goal of surgery is the removal of the tumor with a negative pathologic margin, and results are excellent as described by reports from SIOPEL and COG (CCG/POG).[125-127] Surgical mortality was only 6%, and 92% of patients underwent a complete resection after institution of the PLADO protocol. Overall mortality was 24%, and there were 10 patients who relapsed—5 with local recurrences and 5 with pulmonary metastases. Anatomic hepatic lobectomy is the preferred operation for hepatoblastoma based on the segmental vascular architecture of the liver. These resections correspond to the PRETEXT staging system and may involve right or left lobectomies or, the more technically exacting, extended right or left lobectomy (trisegmentectomy).[138] Nonanatomic resections are appropriate for exophytic tumors that emanate from a superficial portion of the liver. The extent of the resection must leave the child with enough functioning liver parenchyma (20%–25%) for growth and development. Finally, unresectable localized primary or recurrent tumors should be considered for hepatectomy followed by liver transplantation as a therapeutic alternative.

SIOPEL's use of OLTX as primary treatment for local control was recently reviewed.[139] Those patients who were PRETEXT IV or who demonstrated tumor involvement with either the hepatic or portal veins and had no evidence of metastatic disease with a demonstrated response to neoadjuvant chemotherapy were considered for a primary OLTX. Another cohort of patients with intrahepatic recurrence after resection or incomplete resections was eligible for rescue OLTX. Ten-year survival rates for the primary and rescue OLTX groups were 85% and 40%, respectively. The use of primary and rescue OLTX has also been reported by Browne and colleagues,[140] who demonstrated survival rates of 90% and 25%, respectively. These survival rates correlate with the SIOPEL experience. The only deaths reported in the primary group were in the cohort that did not receive post-OLTX chemotherapy; hence, the authors stressed the need for the continuation of adjuvant therapy after transplant. Austin and colleagues[141] reported on the results of OLTX for hepatoblastoma from the United Network of Organ Sharing database. There were 152 orthotopic liver transplants performed in 135 patients, and the actuarial 1-, 5-, and 10-year survival rates were 79%, 69%, and 66%, respectively. More than 54% of patients died of recurrent disease, and the only statistically significant predictors of favorable outcome were the preoperative condition of the patient (intensive care unit [ICU] hospitalization vs. non-ICU hospitalization vs. no hospitalization) and the era when the patient received the transplant (before or after December 31, 1994). These data corroborate SIOPEL's original recommendations for the use of OLTX that include (1) total resection of all gross disease including the retrohepatic vena cava if needed, (2) the use of preoperative chemotherapy to control extrahepatic micrometastases and promote primary tumor regression, (3) the transplantation of patients with synchronous pulmonary metastases if they had responded to neoadjuvant therapy, (4) no transplantation in those patients with evidence of metastatic disease present at surgery, (5) limiting the interval between diagnosis and OLTX to account for the development of chemoresistance and the availability of donors (cadaveric or living), and (5) questioning the need of post-OLTX chemotherapy in the setting of an immunosuppressed patient. This last recommendation, however, has been called into question by several groups who demonstrate improved survival with the addition of chemotherapy after OLTX.[139,142]

Rhabdomyosarcoma

Surgery is a critical component in the management of a patient with rhabdomyosarcoma. General surgical principles have been defined through the IRS Group (IRSG) trials (I–V), and the core premise is to balance the need for total tumor extirpation with a margin of normal, uninvolved tissue while preserving organ function and providing for the least amount of operative morbidity. Certain sites—eye, vagina—are traditionally treated with chemotherapy, followed by radiation for local control to preserve function: results with this approach for these sites have been good. Most lesions will be too large to remove initially, and a pretreatment biopsy will be warranted. Biopsy incisions should be placed so that the entire scar and the traversed tissues can be resected at a later date. Extremity lesions should have a longitudinally oriented incision, and hemorrhage and tissue plane violation should be kept to a minimum so as to avoid unnecessary tumor soilage. Some lesions are inadvertently biopsied by unsuspecting practitioners, often by enucleation of the mass. These patients warrant a pretreatment reexcision to remove the entire lesion (and any associated pseudocapsule with microscopic tumor) and a rim of normal tissue. The exact margin of normal tissue to be excised is not known, but at least 5 mm is warranted,[143] but some studies have documented improved survival in patients with larger, negative margins.[144] The importance of complete tumor excision was also demonstrated by Hays and colleagues[145] when they analyzed the results of IRSG I and II. They demonstrated the success of pretreatment reexcisions. They showed the value of immediately re-resecting tumors (trunk and extremity) that had positive microscopic margins to achieve larger negative tissue margins prior to the initiation of adjuvant therapy by demonstrating a nearly 16% increase in survival (91% vs. 74%) in a cohort of patients undergoing pretreatment reexcision. These measures are reserved for patients who have disease amenable to upfront resections, and radical resections conferring significant organ dysfunction or morbidity should not be attempted primarily.

For lesions too large to remove at presentation, neoadjuvant chemotherapy with "second look operations" to achieve local control with adequate margins are used. The data from IRS III confirmed the utility of this approach by demonstrating that all patients had an improved prognosis save those with pelvic primary and those who did not have complete response to therapy.

Lymph node status and sampling is another critical issue in patients with rhabdomyosarcoma. Regional or distant lymphadenopathy diagnosed clinically or radiographically should be biopsied as the presence of disease will modify therapies and prognosis. Lymphadenectomies of entire compartments are not warranted, however, except for males older than 10 years with paratesticular tumors. IRS IV examined this cohort of patients and demonstrated that relapse and EFS (68% vs. 90%) were greater in older males. They recommended ipsilateral retroperitoneal lymph node sampling to determine the presence of lymph node involvement. If tumor was found, therapy was added in the form of abdominal radiotherapy and intensification of the chemotherapy with cyclophosphamide.[47,58] Finally, for patients with extremity tumors, sentinel lymph node biopsy should be considered to assess lymph node involvement as the incidence was reported to be higher than expected.[59] These procedures involve the administration of a radiolabeled agent (technetium sulfur colloid) and/or an inert dye (lymphozurin blue) to map the lymphatic drainage of the tumor. Once administered, these agents localize to the lymphatics and the draining lymph nodes involved can be determined visually (lymphozurin blue) or via the use of a handheld radiation probe (technetium sulfur colloid).

Ewing's Sarcoma

Local control can be accomplished in Ewing's sarcoma by radiotherapy or surgical resection. No randomized studies have shown the efficacy of one method over another and nonrandomized studies that have suggested a surgical preference have had a regrettable predominance of the smaller, more favorable lesions in the surgical group. Functional evaluations of outcome based on therapy are generally wanting. The ultimate decision between radiotherapy and surgical resection is determined by the relative risks and complications of each modality. As with patients with osteosarcoma, limb preservation using bone allografts or endoprostheses are often feasible and greatly preferable over amputation, although surgical complications are not infrequent.[146-148] These methods are more thoroughly discussed in Chapters 33 and 34.

Osteosarcoma

Surgical considerations in osteosarcoma are many, but they are predicated on accurate staging studies and pretherapy biopsy. The biopsy must be performed with full consideration of the subsequent local control procedure. In osteosarcoma, it is particularly important that the entire biopsy site and tract must be removed and the biopsy must not contaminate vital neurovascular or uninvolved structures complicating subsequent resection and reconstructive procedures.[149] Surgical decisions regarding the treatment of osteosarcoma include both the resection of the primary cancer and reconstruction to provide the best functional outcome with the least morbidity. The success of any operation for osteosarcoma will be dictated by the completeness of the resection—the ability to extirpate the cancer with a rim of normal tissue and bone. These operations are termed *wide excisions*, and they are to encompass the tumor, the reactive zone immediately around the tumor, and a normal tissue margin beyond the reactive zone. There is no defined margin that has been shown to reduce the likelihood of recurrence,[150,151] but a goal of a minimum of 2 to 5 mm in the soft tissues and 1 to 2 cm of uninvolved bone marrow is desirable. Data from several studies have demonstrated that local recurrence is an adverse prognostic factor[152,153] and that tumors with "wide" margins of resection and good response to chemotherapy have a low likelihood of local recurrence,[110,154] thus emphasizing the importance of negative margins.

The goal of all procedures is tumor removal first and functional outcome second. Axial skeleton primaries are challenging tumors in which to obtain a "wide" margin. These tumors—spinal, sacral, and pelvic—have a worse prognosis than extremity tumors due to the challenges of the local control operations.[155,156] "Wide" resection margins are generally easier to achieve in extremity tumors that can be treated with primary amputation or limb-sparing procedures. The preoperative imaging studies, especially MRI, is of vital importance to ensure that there are no bone or marrow skip lesions, that there is no neurovascular involvement, and that enough bone and soft tissue will remain in order to reconstruct the limb. Although limb-sparing procedures have become more common, their limitations are significant. For the active child desiring to compete in athletics, this is not the best option.

TABLE 12.2

GERM CELL TUMOR STAGING CRITERIA

Stage I	Complete resection (negative pathologic margins)
Stage II	Incomplete resection (microscopic positive pathologic margins)
Stage III	Gross disease present or lymph node metastases
Stage IV	Distant metastases

Furthermore, with endoprosthesis or bone allografts, several operations may be needed before and after the achievement of skeletal maturity. Amputations with fixed prosthetics may be a more suitable option for some patients. A special note should be made for the patient with a distal femur tumor that is amenable to a rotationplasty (Van Ness procedure).[157,158] In this procedure, the involved bone and soft tissue is resected *en bloc* with the tumor, and the distal leg, ankle, and foot are spared and rotated 180° with a tibiofemoral osteosynthesis. The nerves are spared, and the femoral/popliteal vessels are either coiled or resected and anastomosed to allow for continued vascular patency. The ankle becomes the "new" knee joint, and it is positioned to match the contralateral knee joint. Results from these operations are excellent, and multiple studies have documented their long-term durability and low functional morbidity.[159-161] Caution must be emphasized regarding the cosmetic outcome of this procedure, however, as it is startling to observe initially. Patients and their families must meet and view the results firsthand before undertaking this operation to fully comprehend the appearance of the extremity after reconstruction.

Germ Cell Tumors

Treatment algorithms traditionally relied on surgery alone for patients with germ cell tumor (GCT), but the mortality with this approach was close to 80%.[162,163] Survival rates drastically improved with the addition of multimodality regimens, and especially with the advent of cisplatin-based treatment espoused by Einhorn and others.[164,165] The COG has added this successful chemotherapy regimen to surgical resection into a stage-stratified, risk-group-defined treatment protocol that focuses on limiting toxicity while producing the greatest survival benefits (Tables 12.2 and 12.3).

TABLE 12.3

GERM CELL TUMOR (GCT) THERAPY BASED ON STAGE AND RISK CLASSIFICATION[a]

Stage	Risk	Treatment
I gonadal	Low	Surgery
Immature teratomas	Low	Surgery
II-IV testes	Inter	Sugery/PEB × 3
II-IV ovary	Inter	Sugery/PEB × 3
I-II nongonadal	Inter	Sugery/PEB × 3
IV ovary	High	Sugery/PEB × 4
III-IV nongonadal	High	Sugery/PEB × 4

[a]Children's Oncology Group risk-stratified GCT treatment protocol.

Sacrococcygeal teratomas can present antenatally or post-natally. The age of the patient at presentation correlates with the incidence of malignancy, low in the newborn and high in children older than 1 year.[166] Lesions can be quite large and exophytic, completely endophytic and small, or a combination of these two presentations. Accurate preoperative axial imaging is critical to determine the extent of the tumor and operative approach. Both abdominal and perineal approaches may be warranted to completely mobilize the tumor, and special attention should be paid to the delineation of the middle sacral artery so that vascular control of this vessel (and the tumor) can be planned. The entire lesion should be removed, including the coccyx. If the coccyx is not removed, recurrence rates of more than 35% have been described.[167] Even with complete extirpation, recurrence rates of up to 20% have been recorded; more than half of the lesions that recur are malignant.[166] Although malignancies are rare, the use of adjuvant therapy has produced dramatic survival benefits.[168-170] Discovery of these lesions *in utero* will necessitate the involvement of a coordinated team of fetal specialists to adequately image and develop therapeutic options for the mother and fetus. Antenatal interventions have been reported in a recent series and fetal survival was greatest in small (10 cm or less), predominantly cystic lesions.

GCT of the trunk includes both the abdominal and the thoracic sites. Abdominal GCT account for only 4% of all GCTs (and they are usually benign (85%).[171] They can be both intraperitoneal and retroperitoneal, and total tumor eradication is the surgical goal. Billmire and colleagues[171] recently reported on the collective experience of the POG/CCG Intergroup results with the malignant variants of these tumors. Their data support the concept of surgical eradication of the tumor before or after the initiation of chemotherapy depending on the size and involvement of other organs at presentation, and this concept of total tumor eradication is also applicable to mediastinal GCTs as well.

Mediastinal GCTs are reported to be more common than abdominal GCTs, but they are also usually benign (86%).[172] The malignant cases of mediastinal GCTs were recently reported by the POG/CCG Intergroup study group.[172] These data documented that the majority of children presented with large tumors (mean diameter of the tumor was greater than 13 cm) and were either stage III or IV at presentation. These data also confirmed the utility of neoadjuvant chemotherapy in facilitating the resection of these lesions, especially in regards to reducing tumor spillage or rupture. However, despite the institution of neoadjuvant chemotherapy, the tumors were still adherent to vital structures that often had to be sacrificed at surgery (e.g., 33% had the phrenic nerve sacrificed).

For testicular GCT, primary therapy—regardless of presentation and stage—involves an inguinal orchiectomy with high-ligation of the spermatic cord at the internal inguinal ring prior to testicular manipulation. Scrotal orchiectomies or transscrotal biopsies are not indicated and will upstage patients (stage I to II) if tumor is otherwise localized to the testis as the risk of local recurrence was greater following this surgical approach.[173] Patients with stage I tumors after adequate surgical resection are treated with observation alone.[173] Recurrences are treated with at least four cycles of PEB chemotherapy, and the outcomes for these patients are excellent. Patients who are stage II to stage IV or greater receive adjuvant chemotherapy (PEB) on current protocols, and any residual disease should be resected to assess for viable tumor and the need for further treatment. Outcomes are reported to be more than 90% for stage II to stage IV patients.

Ovarian GCTs compose a diverse group of histopathological entities, and the majority are benign (80%).[174] They are more common in children with the incidence being reported as more than 60%.[175,176] Tumors may be found incidentally or secondary to the onset of abdominal or pelvic symptoms, and preoperative assessment will be dictated by the patient's presentation. Surgical planning mandates preservation of ovarian tissue if at all possible. Billmire and colleagues[174] recently reviewed the POG/CCG Intergroup experience with malignant ovarian GCTs and documented that almost 60% of all tumors in this series had a cystic component, which is greater than in previously reported studies.[177] From this Intergroup report, the surgical management for these tumors has been defined by COG, and it encompasses six components: (1) collection of ascites or peritoneal washings, (2) examination of the entire peritoneal surface with excision of suspicious lesions, (3) unilateral oophorectomy, (4) examination of the contralateral ovary with biopsy if suspicious, (5) omental examination and biopsy of suspected lesions, and (6) lymph node sampling of suspicious abdominal/pelvic lymph nodes only without a formal pelvic or retroperitoneal lymph node dissection. Tumors that are extremely large or contiguous with other structures should only be biopsied and neoadjuvant therapy utilized to allow for a subsequent resection. Intraoperative tumor spill upstages a patient, and hence intraoperative biopsies are not recommended as localized stage I patients will become stage II and then receive adjuvant chemotherapy unnecessarily. For patients with bilateral tumors, tumor excision and partial oophorectomy (ovarian salvage) should be attempted on at least one side to preserve reproductive function if possible. Furthermore, this study documented the excellent outcome with the use of adjuvant chemotherapy (PEB).

Lymphoma

The role of the surgeon in Hodgkin lymphoma is, in most cases, to establish the diagnosis by biopsy. In the past, staging laparotomy in which the spleen was removed, the liver was biopsied, and multiple abdominal lymph nodes were sampled was frequently used for children with Hodgkin lymphoma to provide the pathologic stage. One series showed that even with current imaging techniques, a change between the clinical and the pathologic stage occurred in 25% of children and adolescents in whom a staging laparotomy was performed.[178] Nonetheless, current Hodgkin lymphoma protocols are based primarily on clinical and not on pathologic staging guidelines. It must be accepted that a significant percentage of children will be understaged using clinical staging, but with improved systemic chemotherapy and the rare use of radiotherapy as a single modality, this seems to be the sole disease in which accurate staging is now considered less important. It does make it exceedingly difficult, however, to compare series in which pathologic staging has been performed with those with clinical staging alone.

In the NHLs, surgery is also important for diagnosis. In the past, it had been claimed that resection of the primary tumor might improve the long-term survival of children with Burkitt's lymphoma.[179] Recent single and multi-institutional studies, however, have refuted this claim.[180,181] Extensive surgery often results in surgical complications that delay the onset of treatment and often allow the regrowth of these rapidly dividing tumors. Anesthetic considerations for biopsy of children with mediastinal involvement of Hodgkin or NHL are discussed earlier in the section on evaluation of anesthetic risk produced by an anterior mediastinal mass.

Metastatic Disease

Although the value of surgery in the treatment of primary malignancies as outlined in this chapter is well established,

TABLE 12.4

SURGICAL THERAPY FOR METASTATIC PULMONARY LESIONS

Lesions to resect	Lesions to biopsy only
Adrenocortical carcinoma	Differentiated thyroid cancer
Hepatoblastoma	Germ cell tumors
Osteosarcoma	Neuroblastoma
	Nephroblastoma

This table depicts the recommended procedures for dealing with pulmonary lesions in the outlined pediatric cancers. The pulmonary lesions encountered in the tumor types listed on the left-hand side of the table should be completely resected. Those lesions found in tumor types listed in the right-hand column should only be biopsied.

the same cannot be said for the treatment of metastatic disease. Several recent works have documented the role of pulmonary metastasectomy in the pediatric population.[182,183] Pulmonary metastasectomy for pediatric cancers has become more prominent in recent years, but evidence-based proof of

its efficacy is limited as there are no tumor-specific, prospective, randomized clinical trials critically evaluating this therapeutic intervention. However, four principles have arisen that must be considered before embarking on this therapeutic endeavor, and they are (a) the primary site must be established and an accurate histopathological diagnosis must be available, (b) the primary tumor site must be controlled before considering pulmonary metastasectomy, (c) the therapeutic benefit of metastasectomy must be analyzed in relation to the availability of effective adjuvant therapies to control microscopic metastases, and (d) the goal of extirpative therapy must be balanced against the patient's underlying pulmonary function and reserve and the extent of pulmonary involvement.

Once these criteria are addressed and the patient deemed an appropriate candidate, pulmonary metastasectomy usually involves "wedge" resections—nonanatomic removal of the cancer with a rim of normal lung tissue around the lesion. Studies have shown that it can be performed with minimal morbidity and mortality.[184] Generalized recommendations regarding the utility of pulmonary metastasectomy in select tumor types are outlined in Table 12.4. Ultimately, when employed properly and for an appropriate primary malignancy, pulmonary metastasectomy is a useful and necessary tool to treat and even cure certain pediatric cancers.

References

1. Murry D, Riva L, Poplack D. Impact of nutrition on pharmacokinetics of anti-neoplastic agents. Int J Cancer Suppl 1998;11:48–51.
2. Picton S. Aspects of altered metabolism in children with cancer. Int J Cancer Suppl 1998;11:62–64.
3. Pencharz P. Aggressive oral, enteral or parenteral nutrition: prescriptive decisions in children with cancer. Int J Cancer Suppl 1998;11:73–75.
4. Shew S, Jaksic T. The metabolic needs of critically ill children and neonates. Semin Pediatr Surg 1999;8:131–139.
5. Tisdale M. Wasting in cancer. J Nutr 1999;129:243S–246S.
6. Lazarus D, Destree A, Mazzola L, et al. A new model of cancer cachexia: contribution of the ubiquitin-proteasome pathway. Am J Physiol 1999;277:E332–E341.
7. Williams A, Sun X, Fischer J, et al. The expression of genes in the ubiquitin-proteasome proteolytic pathway is increased in skeletal muscle from patients with cancer. Surgery 1999;126:744–750.
8. Berenstein E, Ortiz Z. Megestrol acetate for the treatment of anorexia-cachexia syndrome. Cochrane Database Syst Rev 2005;2:CD004310.
9. Dewey A, Baughan C, Dean T, et al. Eicosapentaenoic acid (EPA, an omega-3 fatty acid from fish oils) for the treatment of cancer cachexia. Cochrane Database Syst Rev 2007;1:CD004597.
10. Pedersen A, Kok K, Peterson G, et al. Percutaneous endoscopic gastrostomy in children with cancer. Acta Paediatr 1999;88:849–852.
11. Wilmore D, Dudrick S. Growth and development of an infant receiving all nutrients exclusively by vein. JAMA 1968;203(10):860–864.
12. Seldinger S. Catheter replacement of the needle in percutaneous arteriography: a new technique. Acta Radiol 1053;39(5):368–376.
13. Maki D, Ringer M, Alvarado C. Prospective randomised trial of povidone-iodine, alcohol, and chlorhexidine for prevention of infection associated with central venous and arterial catheters. Lancet 1991;338(8763):339–343.
14. O'Grady N, Alexander M, Dellinger E, et al. Guidelines for the prevention of intravascular catheter-related infections. Centers for Disease Control and Prevention. MMWR Recomm Rep 2002;51(RR-10):1–29 .
15. Nowlen T, Rosenthal G, Johnson G, et al. Pericardial effusion and tamponade in infants with central catheters. Pediatrics 2002;110:137–142.
16. Maki D, Cobb L, Garman J, et al. An attachable silver-impregnated cuff for prevention of infection with central venous catheters: a prospective randomized multicenter trial. Am J Med 1988;85:307–314.
17. Adler A, Yaniv I, Steinberg R, et al. Infectious complications of implantable ports and Hickman catheters in paediatric haematology-oncology patients. J Hosp Infect 2006;62:358–365.
18. Chung D, Ziegler M. Central venous catheter access. Nutrition 1998;14:119–123.
19. Shaul D, Scheer B, Rokhsar S, et al. Risk factors for early infection of central venous catheters in pediatric patients. J Am Coll Surg 1998;186:654–658.
20. Krzywda E, Andris D, Edmiston C. Catheter infections: diagnosis, etiology, treatment, and prevention. Nutr Clin Pract 1999;14:178–190.
21. Mermel L, Farr B, Sheretz R, et al. Guidelines for the management of intravascular catheter-related infections. Clin Infect Dis 2001;32:1249–1272.
22. Darouiche R, Raad I, Heard S, et al. A comparison of two antimicrobial-impregnated central venous catheters. N Engl J Med 1999;340:1–8.
23. Jones G, Konsler G, Dunaway R, et al. Prospective analysis of urokinase in the treatment of catheter sepsis in pediatric hematology-oncology patients. J Pediatr Surg 1993;28:350–357.
24. Rinder H, Arbini A, Snyder E. Optimal dosing and triggers for prophylactic use of platelet transfusions. Curr Opin Hematol 1999;6:437–441.
25. Bray R, Fernandes F. Mediastinal tumour causing airway obstruction in anesthetized children. Anesthesia 1982;37:571–575.

26. Griscom N. Computed tomographic determination of tracheal dimensions in children and adolescents. Radiology 1982;145:361–364.
27. Griscom N. CT measurement of the tracheal lumen in children and adolescents. AJR Am J Roentgenol 1991;156:371–372.
28. Shamberger R, Holzman R, Griscom N, et al. CT quantitation of tracheal cross-sectional area as a guide to the surgical and anesthetic management of children with anterior mediastinal masses. J Pediatr Surg 1991;26:138–142.
29. Griscom N, Wohl M. Dimensions of the growing trachea related to age and gender. AJR Am J Roentgenol 1986;146:233–237.
30. Shamberger R, Holzman R, Griscom N, et al. Prospective evaluation by computed tomography and pulmonary function tests of children with mediastinal masses. Surgery 1995;118:468–471.
31. Hack H, Wright N, Wynn R. The anaesthetic management of children with anterior mediastinal masses. Anaesthesia 2008;63:837–846.
32. King D, Patrick L, Ginn-Pease M, et al. Pulmonary function is compromised in children with mediastinal lymphoma. J Pediatr Surg 1997;32:294–299, discussion 299–300.
33. Lam J, Chui C, Jacobesen A, et al. When is a mediastinal mass critical in a child? An analysis of 29 patients. Pediatr Surg Int 2004;20:180–184.
34. Anghelescu D, Burgoyne L, Liu T, et al. Clinical and diagnostic imaging findings predict anesthetic complications in children presenting with malignant mediastinal masses. Pediatric Anesthesia 2007;17:1090–1098.
35. Chaignaud B, Bonsack T, Kozakewich H, et al. Pleural effusions in lymphoblastic lymphoma: a diagnostic alternative. J Pediatr Surg 1998;33:1355–1357.
36. Petrella T, Mottot C, Cornier F, et al. Diagnosis of two childhood cases of T lymphoblastic lymphoma by immunocytochemical study of pleural fluid. Acta Cytol 1990; 34:580–582.
37. Finger L, Harvey R, Moore R, et al. A common mechanism of chromosomal translocation in T- and B-cell neoplasia. Science 1986;234:982–985.
38. Perger L, Lee E, Shamberger R. Management of children and adolescents with a critical airway due to compression by an anterior mediastinal mass. J Pediatr Surg 2008;43: 1990–1997.
39. Tempe D, Arya R, Dubey S, et al. Mediastinal mass resection: femorofemoral cardiopulmonary bypass before induction of anesthesia in the management of airway obstruction. J Cardiothorac Vasc Anesth 2001;15(2):233–236.
40. Frey T, Chopra A, Lin R, et al. A child with anterior mediastinal mass supported with veno-arterial extracorporeal membrane oxygenation. Pediatr Crit Care Med 2006;7(5): 479–481.
41. Wickiser J, Thompson M, Leavey P, et al. Extracorporeal membrane oxygenation (ECMO) initiation without intubation in two children with mediastinal malignancy. Pediatr Blood Cancer 2007;49(5):751–754.
42. Asai T. Emergency cardiopulmonary bypass in a patient with a mediastinal mass. Anaesthesia 2007;62:850–862.
43. Ein S, Pullerits J, Creighton R, et al. Pediatric pheochromocytoma: a 36-year review. Pediatr Surg Int 1997;12:595–598.
44. Lenders J, Pacak K, Walther M, et al. Biochemical diagnosis of pheochromocytoma: which test is best? JAMA 2002;287(11):1427–1434.
45. Prys-Robert C, Farndon J. Efficacy and safety of doxazosin for perioperative management of patients with pheochromocytoma. World J Surg 2002;26:1037–1042.
46. Shamberger R, Guthrie K, Ritchey M, et al. Surgery-related factors and local recurrence of Wilms' tumor in National Wilms' Tumor Study Group 4. Ann Surg 1999;229: 292–297.
47. Wiener E, Anderson J, Ojimbam J, et al. Controversies in the management of paratesticular rhabdomyosarcoma: is staging retroperitoneal lymph node dissection necessary for adolescents with resected paratesticular rhabdomyosarcoma? Semin Pediatr Surg 2001;10:146–152.

48. Farewell V, D'Angio G, Breslow N, et al. Retrospective validation of a new staging system for Wilms' tumor. Cancer Clin Trials 1981;4:167–171.
49. D'Angio G, Breslow N, Beckwith J, et al. Treatment of Wilms' tumor: results of the Third National Wilms' Tumor Study. Cancer 1989;64:349–360.
50. Brodeur G, Pritchard J, Berthold F, et al. Revisions of the international criteria for neuroblastoma diagnosis, staging, and response to treatment. J Clin Oncol 1993;11: 1466–1477.
51. Matthay K, Perez C, Seeger R, et al. Successful treatment of stage III neuroblastoma based on prospective biologic staging: a Children's Cancer Group Study. J Clin Oncol 1998;16:1256–1264.
52. Othersen HJ, DeLorimer A, Hrabovsky E, et al. Surgical evaluation of lymph node metastases in Wilms' tumor. J Pediatr Surg 1990;25:330–331.
53. Jereb B, Tournade M, Lemerle J, et al. Lymph node invasion and prognosis in nephroblastoma. Cancer 1980;45:1632–1636.
54. Wilson E, Altshuler G, Smith E, et al. Gross observation does not predict regional lymph node metastasis in the surgicopathologic staging of neuroblastoma. Proc Am Soc Clin Oncol 1989;8:304.
55. Rodary C, Flamant F, Donaldson S. An attempt to use a common staging system in rhabdomyosarcoma: a report of an international workshop initiated by the International Society of Pediatric Oncology (SIOP). Med Pediatr Oncol 1989;17:210–215.
56. Andrassy R, Corpron C, Hays D, et al. Extremity sarcomas: an analysis of prognostic factors from the Intergroup Rhabdomyosarcoma Study III. J Pediatr Surg 1996; 31:191–196.
57. Lawrence WJ, Hays D, Heyn R, et al. Lymphatic metastases with childhood rhabdomyosarcoma: a report from the Intergroup Rhabdomyosarcoma Study. Cancer 1987;60:910–915.
58. Wiener E, Lawrence W, Hays D, et al. Retroperitoneal node biopsy in paratesticular rhabdomyosarcoma. J Pediatr Surg 1994;29:171–177, discussion 178.
59. Mandell L, Ghavimi F, LaQuaglia M, et al. Prognostic significance of regional lymph node involvement in childhood extremity rhabdomyosarcoma. Med Pediatr Oncol 1990;18:466–471.
60. Frush D, Donnelly L, Rosen N. Computed tomography and radiation risks: what pediatric health care providers should know. Pediatrics 2003;112:971–972.
61. Brenner D, Elliston C, Hall E, et al. Estimated risks of radiation-induced fatal cancer from pediatric CT. AJR Am J Roentgenol 2001;176(2):289–296.
62. Ayar D, Golla B, Lee J, et al. Needle-track metastasis after transthoracic needle biopsy. J Thorac Imaging 1998;13:2–6.
63. Lundstedt C, Stridbeck H, Andersson R, et al. Tumor seeding occurring after fine-needle biopsy of abdominal malignancies. Acta Radiol 1991;32:518–520.
64. Hoffer F, Chung T, Diller L, et al. Percutaneous biopsy for prognostic testing of neuroblastoma. Radiology 1996;200:213–216.
65. Garrett K, Fuller C, Santana C, et al. Percutaneous biopsy of pediatric solid tumors. Cancer 2005;104:644–652.
66. Hussain H, Kingston J, Domizio P, et al. Imaging-guided core biopsy for the diagnosis of malignant tumors in pediatric patients. AJR Am J Roentgenol 2001;176:43–47.
67. Sklair-Levy M, Lebensart P, Applbaum Y, et al. Percutaneous image-guided needle biopsy in children—summary of our experience with 57 children. Pediatr Radiol 2001;31:732–736.
68. D'Angio G, Evans A, Breslow N, et al. The treatment of Wilms' tumor: results of the National Wilms' Tumor Study. Cancer 1976;38:633–646.
69. Lemerle J, Voute P, Tournade M, et al. Effectiveness of preoperative chemotherapy in Wilms' tumor results of an International Society of Pediatric Oncology (SIOP) clinical trial. J Clin Oncol 1983;1:604–609.
70. Zoeller G, Pekrun A, Lakomek M, et al. Wilms' tumor: the problem of diagnostic accuracy in children undergoing preoperative chemotherapy without histological tumor verification. J Urol 1994;151:169–171.
71. Zuppan C, Beckwith J, Weeks D, et al. The effect of preoperative therapy on the histologic features of Wilms' tumor: an analysis of cases from the Third National Wilms' Tumor Study. Cancer 1991;68:385–394.
72. Voute P, Tournade M, Delemarre J, et al. Preoperative chemotherapy (CT) as first treatment in children with Wilms' tumor: results of the SIOP nephroblastoma trials and studies. Proc Am Soc Clin Oncol 1987;6:223.
73. Tournade M, Com-Nougue C, Voute P, et al. Results of the Sixth International Society of Pediatric Oncology Wilms' Tumor Trial and Study: a risk adapted therapeutic approach in Wilms' tumor. J Clin Oncol 1993;11:1014–1023.
74. Lemerle J, Voute P, Tournade M, et al. Preoperative versus postoperative radiotherapy, single versus multiple course of actinomycin D in the treatment of Wilms' tumor. Cancer 1976;38:647–654.
75. D'Angio G, Evans A, Breslow N, et al. The treatment of Wilms' tumor: results of the Second National Wilms' Tumor Study. Cancer 1981;47:2302–2311.
76. McLorie G, McKenna P, Greenberg M, et al. Reduction in tumor burden allowing partial nephrectomy following preoperative chemotherapy in biopsy proved Wilms' tumor. J Urol 1991;146:509–513.
77. Wilimas J, Magill L, Parham D, et al. Is renal salvage feasible in unilateral Wilms' tumor? Proposed computed tomographic criteria and their relation to surgicopathologic findings. Am J Pediatr Hematol Oncol 1990;12:164–167.
78. Cozzi F, Schiavetti A, Bonanni M, et al. Enucleative surgery for stage I nephroblastoma with a normal contralateral kidney. J Urol 1996;156:1788–1791, discussion 1791–1783.
79. Moorman-Voestermans C, Aronson D, Staalman C, et al. Is partial nephrectomy appropriate treatment for unilateral Wilms' tumor? J Pediatr Surg 1998;33:165–170.
80. Ritchey M, Green D, Thomas P, et al. Renal failure in Wilms' tumor patients: a report from the National Wilms' Tumor Study Group. Med Pediatr Oncol 1996;26:75–80.
81. Horwitz J, Ritchey M, Moksness J, et al. Renal salvage procedures in patients with synchronous bilateral Wilms' tumors: a report from the National Wilms' Tumor Study Group. J Pediatr Surg 1996;31:1020–1025.
82. Shamberger R, Ritchey M, Haase G, et al. Intravascular extension of Wilms' tumor. Ann Surg 2001;234:116–121.
83. Perez C, Matthay K, Atkinson J, et al. Biologic variables in the outcome of stage I and II neuroblastoma treated with surgery as primary therapy: a children's cancer group study. J Clin Oncol 2000;18:18–26.
84. DeBernardi B, Mosseri V, Rubie H, et al. Treatment of localised resectable neuroblastoma: results of the LNESG1 study by the SIOP Europe Neuroblastoma Group. Cancer 2008;99:1027–1033.
85. Alvarado C, London W, Look A, et al. Natural history and biology of stage A neuroblastoma: a Pediatric Oncology Group Study. J Pediatr Hematol Oncol 2000;22: 197–205.
86. Rubie H, Plantaz D, Coze C, et al. Localised and unresectable neuroblastoma in infants: excellent outcome with primary chemotherapy: Neuroblastoma Study Group, Société Française d'Oncologie Pédiatrique. Med Pediatr Oncol 2001;36:247–250.
87. Karzenstein H, Kent P, London W, et al. Treatment and outcome of 83 children with intraspinal neuroblastoma: the Pediatric Oncology Group experience. J Clin Oncol 2001;19:1047–1055.
88. DeBernardi B, Pianca C, Pistamiglio P, et al. Neuroblastoma with symptomatic spinal cord compression at diagnosis: treatment and results with 76 cases. J Clin Oncol 2001;19:183–190.
89. Strother D, van Hoff J, Rao P, et al. Event-free survival of children with biologically favourable neuroblastoma based on the degree of initial tumour resection: results from the Pediatric Oncology Group. Eur J Cancer 1997;33:2121–2125.
90. Kiely E. The surgical challenge of neuroblastoma. J Pediatr Surg 1994;29:128–133.
91. LaQuaglia M, Kushner B, Su W, et al. The impact of gross total resection on local control and survival in high-risk neuroblastoma. J Pediatr Surg 2004;39:412–417.
92. Koh C, Sheu J, Liang D, et al. Complete surgical resection plus chemotherapy prolongs survival in children with stage 4 neuroblastoma. Pediatr Surg Int 2005;21:69–72.
93. Shorter N, Davidoff A, Evans A, et al. The role of surgery in the management of stage IV neuroblastoma: a single institution study. Med Pediatr Oncol 1995;24:287–291.
94. Matthay K, Perez C, Seeger R, et al. Successful treatment of stage III neuroblastoma based on the prospective biologic staging: a Children's Cancer Group Study. J Clin Oncol 1998;16:1256–1264.
95. Kushner B, Cheung N, LaQuaglia M, et al. Survival from locally invasive or widespread neuroblastoma without cytotoxic therapy. J Clin Oncol 1996;14:373–381.
96. Haase G, O'Leary M, Ramsay N, et al. Aggressive surgery combined with intensive chemotherapy improves survival in poor-risk neuroblastoma. J Pediatr Surg 1991;26: 1119–1124.
97. Shamberger R, Smith E, Joshi V, et al. The risk of nephrectomy during local control in abdominal neuroblastoma. J Pediatr Surg 1998;33:161–164.
98. Berthold F, Utsch S, Holschneider A. The impact of preoperative chemotherapy on resectability of primary tumour and complication rate in metastatic neuroblastoma. Z Kinderchir 1989;44:21–24.
99. DeCou J, Bowman L, Rao B, et al. Infants with metastatic neuroblastoma have improved survival with resection of the primary tumor. J Pediatr Surg 1995;30: 937–941.
100. Shamberger R, LaQuaglia M, Krailo M, et al. Ewing's sarcoma of the rib: results of an Intergroup study with analysis of outcome by timing of resection. J Thorac Cardiovasc Surg 2000;119:1154–1156.
101. Shamberger R, Tarbell N, Perez-Atayde A, et al. Malignant small round cell tumor (Ewing's-PNET) of the chest wall in children. J Pediatr Surg 1994;29:179–184, discussion 184–185.
102. Shamberger R, LaQuaglia M, Gebhardt M, et al. Ewing sarcoma/primitive neuroectodermal tumor of the chest wall: impact of initial versus delayed resection on tumor margins, survival, and use of radiation therapy. Ann Surg 2003;238(4):563–567, discussion 567–568.
103. Friedman M, Carter S. The therapy of osteogenic sarcoma: current status and thoughts for the future. J Surg Oncol 1972;4:482–510.
104. Jaffe N, Smith E, Abelson H, et al. Osteogenic sarcoma: alterations in the pattern of pulmonary metastases with adjuvant chemotherapy. J Clin Oncol 1983;1:251–254.
105. Bruland O, Hoifodt H, Saeter G, et al. Hematogenous micrometastases in osteosarcoma patients. Clin Cancer Res 2005;11:4666–4673.
106. Eilber F, Giuliano A, Eckardt J, et al. Adjuvant chemotherapy for osteosarcoma: a randomized prospective trial. J Clin Oncol 1987;5:21–26.
107. Link M, Goorin A, Miser A, et al. The effect of adjuvant chemotherapy on relapse-free survival in patients with osteosarcoma of the extremity. N Engl J Med 1986;314: 1600–1606.
108. Rosen G. Preoperative (neoadjuvant) chemotherapy for osteogenic sarcoma: a ten year experience. Orthopedics 1985;8:659–664.
109. Goorin A, Schwartzentruber D, Devidas M, et al. Presurgical chemotherapy compared with immediate surgery and adjuvant chemotherapy for nonmetastatic osteosarcoma: Pediatric Oncology Group Study POG-8651. J Clin Oncol 2003;21: 1574–1580.
110. Picci P, Sangiorgi L, Rougraff B, et al. Relationship of chemotherapy-induced necrosis and surgical margins to local recurrence in osteosarcoma. J Clin Oncol 1994;12:2699–2705.
111. Bielack S, Kempf-Bielack B, Winkler K. Osteosarcoma: relationship of response to preoperative chemotherapy and type of surgery to local recurrence. J Clin Oncol 1996;12:2699–2705.
112. Bielack S, Kempf-Bielack B, Delling G, et al. Prognostic factors in high-grade osteosarcoma of the extremities or trunk: an analysis of 1,702 patients treated on neoadjuvant cooperative osteosarcoma stud group protocols. J Clin Oncol 2002;20:776–790.
113. Rosen G, Marcove R, Huvos A, et al. Primary osteogenic sarcoma: eight-year experience with adjuvant chemotherapy. J Cancer Res Clin Oncol 1983;106(suppl):55–67.
114. Bacci G, Longhi A, Versari M, et al. Prognostic factors for osteosarcoma of the extremity treated with neoadjuvant chemotherapy: 15-year experience in 789 patients treated at a single institution. Cancer 2006;106:1154–1161.
115. Provisor A, Ettinger L, Nachman J, et al. Treatment of nonmetastatic osteosarcoma of the extremity with preoperative and postoperative chemotherapy: a report from the Children's Cancer Group. J Clin Oncol 1997;15:76–84.
116. Winkler K, Beron G, Delling G, et al. Neoadjuvant chemotherapy of osteosarcoma: results of a randomized cooperative trial (COSS-82) with salvage chemotherapy based on histological tumor response. J Clin Oncol 1988;6:329–337.
117. Exelby P, Filler R, Grosfeld J. Liver tumors in children in the particular reference to hepatoblastoma and hepatocellular carcinoma: American Academy of Pediatrics Surgical Section Study—1974. J Pediatr Surg 1975;10:329–337.
118. Giacomantonio M, Ein S, Mancer K, Stephens C. Thirty years of experience with pediatric primary malignant liver tumors. J Pediatr Surg 1984;19:523–526.
119. Andrassy R, Brennan L, Siegel M, et al. Preoperative chemotherapy for hepatoblastoma in children: report of six cases. J Pediatr Surg 1980;15:517–522.
120. Weinblatt M, Siegel S, Siegel M, et al. Preoperative chemotherapy for unresectable primary hepatic malignancies in children. Cancer 1982;50:1061–1064.
121. Ortega J, Krailo M, Haas J, et al. Effective treatment of unresectable or metastatic hepatoblastoma with cisplatin and continuous infusion doxorubicin chemotherapy: a report from the Children's Cancer Study Group. J Clin Oncol 1991;9:2167–2176.
122. King D, Ortega J, Campbell J, et al. The surgical management of children with incompletely resected hepatic cancer is facilitated by intensive chemotherapy. J Pediatr Surg 1991;26:1074–1080.

123. Reynolds M, Douglass E, Finegold M, et al. Chemotherapy can convert unresectable hepatoblastoma. J Pediatr Surg 1992;27:1083–1084.

124. von Schweinitz D, Hecker H, Harms D, et al. Complete resection before development of drug resistance is essential for survival from advanced hepatoblastoma—a report from the German Cooperative Pediatric Liver Tumor Study HB-89. J Pediatr Surg 1995;30:845–852.

125. Pritchard J, Brown J, Shafford E, et al. Cisplatin, doxorubicin, and delayed surgery for childhood hepatoblastoma: a successful approach—results of the first prospective study of the International Society of Pediatric Oncology. J Clin Oncol 2000;18:3819–3828.

126. Schnater J, Aronson D, Plaschkes J, et al. Surgical view of the treatment of patients with hepatoblastoma: results from the first prospective trial of the International Society of Pediatric Oncology Liver Tumor Study Group. Cancer 2002;94:1111–1120.

127. Ortega J, Douglass E, Feusner J, et al. Randomized comparison of cisplatin-vincristine/fluorouracil and cisplatin/continuous infusion doxorubicin for treatment of pediatric hepatoblastoma: a report from the Children's Cancer Group and the Pediatric Oncology Group. J Clin Oncol 2000;18:2665–2675.

128. Johnstone P, Rohde D, Swartz S, et al. Port site recurrences after laparoscopic and thoracoscopic procedures in malignancy. J Clin Oncol 1996;14:1950–1956.

129. Young-Fadok T. Minimally invasive techniques for colorectal cancer. Surg Oncol 1998;7:165–173.

130. Albanese C, Rothenberg S. Experience with 144 consecutive pediatric thoracoscopic lobectomies. J Laparoendosc Adv Surg Tech A 2007;17:339–241.

131. Spinelli C, Donatini G, Berti P, et al. Minimally invasive thyroidectomy in pediatric patients. J Pediatr Surg 2008;43:1259–1261.

132. Ritchey M, Kelalis P, Breslow N, et al. Intracaval and atrial involvement with nephroblastoma: review of National Wilms' Tumor Study 3. J Urol 1988;140:1113–1117.

133. Castel V, Tovar J, Costa E, et al. The role of surgery in stage IV neuroblastoma. J Pediatr Surg 2002;37:1574–1578.

134. Katzenstein H, Bowman L, Brodeur G, et al. Prognostic significance of age, MYCN oncogene amplification, tumor cell ploidy, and histology in 110 infants with stage D (S) neuroblastoma: the pediatric oncology group experience—a Pediatric Oncology Group Study. J Clin Oncol 1998;16:2007–2017.

135. D'Angio G, Evans A, Koop C. Special pattern of widespread neuroblastoma with a favourable prognosis. Lancet 1971;1:1046–1049.

136. Grosfeld J. Risk-based management: current concepts of treating malignant solid tumors of childhood. J Am Coll Surg 1999;189:407–425.

137. Hero B, Simon T, Spitz R, et al. Localized infant neuroblastomas often show spontaneous regression: results of the prospective trials NB95-S and NB97. J Clin Oncol 2008;26:1504–1510.

138. Iwatsuki S, Starzl T. Personal experience with 411 hepatic resections. Ann Surg 1988;208:421–434.

139. Otte JB, Pritchard J, Aronson DC. Liver transplantation for hepatoblastoma: results from the International Society of Pediatric Oncology (SIOP) study SIOPEL-1 and review of the world experience. Pediatr Blood Cancer 2004;42:74–83.

140. Browne M, Sher D, Grant D, et al. Survival after liver transplantation for hepatoblastoma: a 2-center experience. J Pediatr Surg 2008;43:1973–1981.

141. Austin M, Leys C, Feurer I, et al. Liver transplantation for childhood hepatic malignancy: a review of the United Network for Organ Sharing (UNOS) database. J Pediatr Surg 2006;41:182–186.

142. Srinivasan P, McCall J, Pritchard J, et al. Orthotopic liver transplantation for unresectable hepatoblastoma. Transplantation 2002;74:652–655.

143. Crist W, Gehan E, Ragab A, et al. The Third Intergroup Rhabdomyosarcoma Study. J Clin Oncol 1995;13:610–630.

144. Singer S, Corson J, Gonin R, et al. Prognostic factors predictive of survival and local recurrence for extremity soft tissue sarcoma. Ann Surg 1995;221:165–173.

145. Hays D, Lawrence WJ, Wharam M, et al. Primary reexcision for patients with 'mircoscopic residual' tumor following initial excision of sarcomas of trunk and extremity sites. J Pediatr Surg 1989;24:5–10.

146. Muscolo D, Ayerza M, Aponte-Tinao L, et al. Allograft reconstruction after sarcoma resection in children younger than 10 years old. Clin Orthop Relat Res 2008;466:1856–1862.

147. Baumgart R, Hinterwimmer S, Krammer M, et al. The bioexpandable prosthesis: a new perspective after resection of malignant bone tumors in children. J Pediatr Hematol Oncol 2005;27:452–455.

148. Brigman B, Hornicek F, Gebhardt M, et al. Allografts about the knee in young patients with high-grade sarcoma. Clin Orthop Relat Res 2004;421:232–239.

149. Mankin H, Lange T, Spanier S. The hazards of biopsy in patients with malignant primary bone and soft-tissue tumors. J Bone Joint Surg Am 1982;64:1121–1127.

150. Bacci G, Longhi A, Briccoli A, et al. The role of surgical margins in treatment of Ewing's sarcoma family tumors: experience of a single institution with 512 patients treated with adjuvant and neoadjuvant chemotherapy. Int J Radiation Oncol Biol Phys 2006;65:766–772.

151. Kotz R, Dominkus M, Zettl T, et al. Advances in bone tumour treatment in 30 years with respect to survival and limb salvage: a single institution experience. Int Orthop 2002;26:197–202.

152. Rotdriguez-Galindo C, Shah N, McCarville M, et al. Outcome after local recurrence of osteosarcoma: the St. Jude Children's Research Hospital experience (1970–2000). Cancer 2004;100:1928–1935.

153. Bacci G, Longhi A, Cesari M, et al. Influence of local recurrence on survival in patients with extremity osteosarcoma treated by neoadjuvant chemotherapy: the experience of a single institution with 44 patients. Cancer 2006;106:2701–2706.

154. Picci P, Sangiorgi L, Bahamonde L, et al. Risk factors for local recurrences after limb-salvage surgery for high-grade osteosarcoma of the extremities. Ann Oncol 1997;8:899–903.

155. Bielack S, Wulff B, Delling G, et al. Osteosarcoma of the trunk treated by multimodal therapy: experience of the Cooperative Osteosarcoma Study Group (COSS). Med Pediatr Oncol 1995;24:6–12.

156. Shives T, Dahlin D, Sim F, et al. Osteosarcoma of the spine. J Bone Joint Surg Am 1986;68:660–668.

157. Merkel K, Gebhardt M, Springfield D. Rotationplasty as a reconstructive operation after tumor resection. Clin Orthop Relat Res 1991;270:231–236.

158. Winkelmann W. Rotationplasty. Orthop Clin North Am 1996;27:503–523.

159. Fuchs B, Kotajarvi B, Kaufman K, et al. Functional outcome of patients with rotationplasty about the knee. Clin Orthop Relat Res 2003;415:52–58.

160. Rodl R, Pohlmann U, Gosheger G, et al. Rotationplasty—quality of life after 10 years in 22 patients. Acta Orthop Scand 2002;73:85–88.

161. Veenstra K, Sprangers M, van der Eyken J, et al. Quality of life in survivors with a Van Ness-Borggreve rotationplasty after bone tumour resection. J Surg Oncol 2000;73:192–197.

162. Kurman R, Norris H. Embryonal carcinoma of the ovary: a clinicopathologic entity distinct from endodermal sinus tumor resembling embryonal carcinoma of the adult testis. Cancer 1976;38:2420–2433.

163. Chretien P, Milam J, Foote F, et al. Embryonal adenocarcinomas (a type of malignant teratoma) of the sacrococcygeal region: clinical and pathologic aspects of 21 cases. Cancer 1970;26:522–535.

164. Einhorn L, Donohue J. Cis-diamminedichloroplatinum, vinblastine, and bleomycin combination chemotherapy in disseminated testicular cancer. Ann Intern Med 1977;87:293–298.

165. Roth B, Greist A, Kubilis P, et al. Cisplastin-based combination chemotherapy for disseminated germ cell tumors: long-term follow-up. J Clin Oncol 1988;6:1239–1247.

166. Rescorla F, Sawin R, Coran A, et al. Long-term outcome for infants and children with sacrococcygeal teratoma: a report from the Children's Cancer Group. J Pediatr Surg 1998;33:171–176.

167. Gross R, Clatworth WJ, Meeker IJ. Sacrococcygeal teratomas in infants and children: a report of 40 cases. Surg Gynecol Obstet 1951;92(3):341–354.

168. Rescorla F, Billmire D, Stolar C, et al. The effect of cisplastin dose and surgical resection in children with malignant germ cell tumors at the sacrococcygeal region: a Pediatric Intergroup Trial (POG 9049/CCG 8882). J Pediatr Surg 2001;36:12–17.

169. Gobel U, Schneider D, Calaminus G, et al. Multimodal treatment of malignant sacrococcygeal germ cell tumors: a prospective analysis of 66 patients of the German Cooperative Protocols MAKEI 83/86 and 89. J Clin Oncol 2001;19:1943–1950.

170. Calaminus G, Schneider D, Bokkerink J, et al. Prognostic value of tumor size, metastases, extension into bone, and increased tumor marker in children with malignant sacrococcygeal germ cell tumors: a prospective evaluation of 71 patients treated in the German Cooperative protocols Maligne Keimzelltumoren (MAKEI) 83/86 and MAKEI 89. J Clin Oncol 2003;21:781–786.

171. Billmire D, Vinocur C, Rescorla F, et al. Malignant retroperitoneal and abdominal germ cell tumors: an Intergroup study. J Pediatr Surg 2003;38:315–318.

172. Billmire D, Vinocur C, Rescorla F, et al. Malignant mediastinal germ cell tumors: an Intergroup study. J Pediatr Surg 2001;36:18–24.

173. Schlatter M, Rescorla F, Giller R, et al. Excellent outcome in patients with stage I germ cell tumors of the testes: a study of the Children's Cancer Group/Pediatric Oncology Group. J Pediatr Surg 2003;38:319–324.

174. Billmire D, Vinocur C, Rescorla F, et al. Outcome and staging evaluation in malignant germ cell tumors of the ovary in children and adolescents: an Intergroup study. J Pediatr Surg 2004;39:424–429.

175. Norris H, Jensen R. Relative frequency of ovarian neoplasms in children and adolescents. Cancer 1972;30:713–719.

176. Imai A, Furui T, Tamaya T. Gynecologic tumors and symptoms in childhood and adolescence: 10-years' experience. Int J Gynaecol Obstet 1994;45:227–234.

177. Cohen Z, Shinhar D, Kopernik G, et al. The laparoscopic approach to uterine adnexal torsion in childhood. J Pediatr Surg 1996;31:1557–1559.

178. Breuer C, Tarbell N, Mauch P, et al. The importance of staging laparotomy in pediatric Hodgkin's disease. J Pediatr Surg 1994;29:1085–1089.

179. Ziegler J. Treatment results of 54 American patients with Burkitt's lymphoma are similar to the African experience. N Engl J Med 1977;297:75–80.

180. LaQuaglia M, Stolar C, Krailo M, et al. The role of surgery in abdominal non-Hodgkin's lymphoma: experience from the Children's Cancer Study Group. J Pediatr Surg 1992;27:230–235.

181. Shamberger R, Weinstein H. The role of surgery in abdominal Burkitt's lymphoma. J Pediatr Surg 1992;27:236–240.

182. Kayton M. Pulmonary metastasectomy in pediatric patients. Thorac Surg Clin 2006;16:167–183.

183. Weldon C, Shamberger R. Pediatric pulmonary tumors: primary and metastatic. Semin Pediatr Surg 2008;17:17–29.

184. Pastorino U. History of the surgical management of pulmonary metastases and development of the International Registry. Semin Thorac Cardiovasc Surg 2002;14:18–28.

CHAPTER 13 ■ GENERAL PRINCIPLES OF RADIATION ONCOLOGY

LARRY E. KUN

Radiation oncology is a clinical discipline focused on utilization of radiation therapy as a physical means of producing a biologic effect. The production and targeted delivery of ionizing radiations to a patient relies on the principles and accuracy of *radiation physics*. The goal of radiation physics is to deliver the prescribed radiation dose to a carefully identified target volume, relatively sparing adjacent normal tissues. The *biologic basis of radiation therapy* includes cell- or tissue-specific inherent radiosensitivity but relies primarily on optimally exploiting differences in tumor and normal tissue responses to ionizing radiations based on the time:dose relationship and modifiers of radiation response. Empiric investigations during the past century established the basis for fractionated radiation delivery protracted over several weeks to optimize differences between normal tissues and tumor in both repair of sublethal radiation injury and changes in the tumor microenvironment. The time:dose relationship is defined by the total *dose* (measured in Gray or Gy, the international measure of radiation, defined as that amount of radiation depositing 1 joule of energy in 1 kg, equivalent to 100 rad, the earlier term for absorbed dose where 1 rad is equal to 0.01 Gy or 1 centiGray, cGy), the *number of fractions* (or treatments) required to administer the total dose and the related *dose per fraction*, and the *duration* of treatment (i.e., time in days or weeks to complete the course of therapy). Technological advances in the delivery of radiation therapy and increasing experience with the interactions of radiation therapy and contemporary chemotherapy have led to greater use of irradiation in children and adolescents over the past 10 to 15 years, based on the proven efficacy of local or regional irradiation and the ability to better focus radiation dose with less risk of long-term consequences. Combinations of pharmacologic agents and irradiation aim toward altering the response of the target tumor cell population or the microenvironment to enhance tumor control and/or reduce deleterious effects on normal tissues. Growing, developing tissues in children are more sensitive to late effects of irradiation than are mature, adult tissues—requiring the radiation oncologist to be cognizant of local/regional control data key to recommending radiation therapy and sophisticated in balancing the advantages of technologically advanced radiation therapy and the anticipated late morbidities that limit radiation dose and utilization.

BIOLOGICAL BASIS OF RADIATION THERAPY

Ionizing radiations interact within cells during a picosecond of exposure, producing direct effects on DNA and, more commonly, indirect effects mediated by ionization of water that produces free hydroxyl radicals. Such ionization is relatively "sparsely" distributed along the path of the entrance beam for commonly used radiation beams (therefore termed "low *linear energy transfer* (LET)," as in photons or electrons from linear accelerators and γ rays from radionuclides used in brachytherapy—radiation implants); heavy ions deposit energy more densely and are termed *high linear energy transfer* radiations (e.g., carbon ions from cyclotrons or α particles in brachytherapy). DNA damage is dose dependent and may be lethal (especially double-strand breaks, DSBs) or sublethal (e.g., single-strand breaks, cross-links, or base damage). DNA damage short of DSBs may be repaired via induced genetic mechanisms including strand break repair, mismatch repair, nucleotide excision repair, and base excision repair; repair of sublethal damage is typically complete within 4 to 5 hours and is key as the basis of fractionated irradiation.[1] Cells progressing to mitosis with residual chromosomal aberrations (typically including dicentric and acentric chromosomal fragments) usually undergo cell death due to physical or genetic errors during mitosis or result in abnormal genetic distribution in the surviving progeny that ultimately leads to cell death during subsequent divisions.[2]

Radiation Sensitivity

Relative cellular *radiosensitivity* reflects intrinsic factors, including the cell cycle phase at the time of radiation exposure, activation of apoptotic pathways, accumulation of genetic mutations in oncogenes and tumor suppressor genes, and the proficiency of DNA repair mechanisms (see above). Extrinsic factors determining cellular and tissue radiosensitivity reflect the vasculature and microenvironment determining oxygenation, nutrient availability, and elimination of metabolic waste molecules.[3] *Radiation hypersensitivity* occurs in a few genetic conditions, most notably children with ataxia-telangiectasia (A-T). A mutation of the *ATM* gene removes the usual block before damaged cells enter the cell cycle's S phase, obviating the usual G_1 arrest following radiation exposure and greatly increasing radiosensitivity and genomic instability, the latter associated with later carcinogenesis.[4–6] In the Nijmegen break syndrome (NBS), cells show deficient DSB repair also resulting in enhanced sensitivity to ionizing radiation.[2,7,8] Multigene expression models may correlate with intrinsic radiosensitivity, providing a predictive assay of radiation response in selected tumor types.[9,10]

Classical radiation biology early recognized relationships among tumors of more primitive, rapidly dividing cells and apparent responsiveness to irradiation.[11] The *proliferating stem cell systems* define much of the radiation response for tumors (where the number of clonogenic cells defines the tumor target in achieving tumor sterilization, and the number of surviving clonogenic cells may predict the likelihood of recurrence) and normal tissues (where survival of the repopulating stem cells in skin and intestinal crypts, for example, defines the degree and duration of early radiation response in these tissues).[12–14]

The Four "R's" of Radiation Biology

Fractionated irradiation was experimentally and then clinically found to provide tumor control while reducing the normal tissue effects associated with the single, large fractions used soon after Roentgen's discovery of x-rays in 1895.[15] Forty years later, cell survival assays helped elucidate the four key underlying biologic principles upon which modern radiation parameters are based: *repair* (primarily repair of normal tissue following sublethal radiation damage), *redistribution* (through the cell cycle, where cells in S-G_2 phases are relatively radioresistant), *reoxygenation* (see below), and *repopulation* (where surviving tumor cells often show accelerated repopulation in response to radiation therapy, requiring a relatively brief total duration of therapy to minimize unintended repopulation during the radiation course).[3] In most pediatric tumor settings, *conventionally fractionated* irradiation is the standard, with common total doses of 18 to 65 Gy (determined by the tumor type and presentation) delivered in five daily fractions per week of 150 to 200 cGy (most often 180 cGy in North America) per fraction. For pediatric cancers, a potentially controlling radiation dose can most often be administered using conventional fractionation to dose levels within acceptable tolerance limits of surrounding normal tissues, representing a favorable "therapeutic ratio" as shown in Figure 13.1.

Radiation-Induced Apoptosis

Apoptosis, interphase or programmed cell death, occurs in selected cell lines following irradiation. Radiation-induced apoptosis involves primarily mitochondrial changes with related caspase activation. Accounting for cellular lethality outside reproductive cell death has been uncertain in radiation biology; several investigators have indicated that systems with a high spontaneous apoptotic rate might be more radiosensitive (requiring lower radiation doses to trigger interphase cell death).[2,16] Factors influencing radiation-induced apoptosis include cell type and patient age; hypersensitivity in genetic syndromes (e.g., A-T and NBS) show diminished apoptotic response.[7] The p53 tumor suppressor gene signals apoptosis as a response to irradiation, providing a potential mechanism to exploit in enhancing radiation sensitivity.[3,17]

Oxygen State and Radiation-Induced Lethality

Intratumoral *oxygenation* was noted to affect radiation response early in the 1900's; later *in vitro* studies showed that cells in necrotic tumor foci at the greatest distance from capillaries were yet viable but relatively radiation insensitive due to reduced oxygen concentration.[18] The relative radiosensitivity of euoxic versus hypoxic cells approximates 1.5 to 2.5 (i.e., the dose required for a given reduction in cell survival in a hypoxic environment is 1.5–2.5 times higher than when grown in normally oxygenated conditions). There is a marked difference in the oxygen dependency for radiation effect among low-LET radiations (photons, electrons, protons—all of which show the oxygen effect as mentioned earlier) compared with high-LET radiations (ions, where cell lethality is not related to oxygen content).[12] During a fractionated course of radiation therapy, tumors evidence reoxygenation; this reoxygenation of chronically hypoxic, clonogenic tumor cells

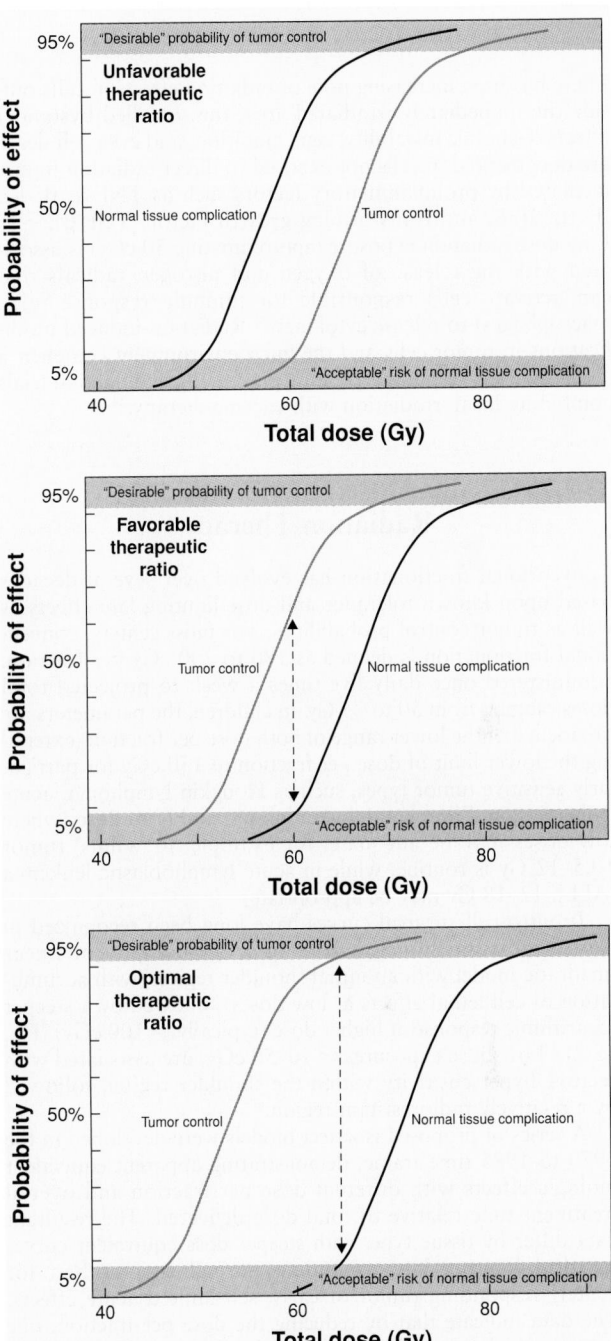

FIGURE 13.1 Dose-response curves representing tumor control and normal tissue complication probabilities, demonstrating tumor- and tissue-specific sigmoid dose responses. Differences in dose-related effects define more or less favorable relationships. (From Gunderson LL, Tepper JE, eds. Clinical radiation oncology. Churchill Livingstone, New York, NY, 2000, with permission.)

is one of the bases underlying fractionation.[19] With preclinical and clinical data substantiating the impact of intralesional hypoxia on tumor control, a number of strategies have been tested to overcome hypoxia, ranging from hyperbaric oxygen to carbogen breathing (an oxygen transporter in blood) to more recent studies of hypoxic cell radiosensitizers. To date, however, only marginal benefit has been apparent with oxygen-enriching methods.[20–23]

Bystander or Abscopal Effects

There has been increasing note of radiation effects in cells outside the immediately irradiated area, the so-called bystander effects. Genomic instability, gene mutation, and even cell death are documented in cells not exposed to direct radiation injury, mediated by proinflammatory factors such as TNF-α, IL-1α, IL-1β, IL-6, and transforming growth factor (TGF-β).[2,24,25] Low-dose radiation exposure (approximating 50 cGy) is associated with the release of oxygen and nitrogen radicals that can activate cells responsible for immune response (e.g., macrophages) to release cytokines.[24] Radiation-induced modifications in tumor cells and the microenvironment can elicit a T-cell immune response, a finding potentially exploited in trials combining local irradiation with vaccine therapy.[24,26]

Time:Dose:Fractionation in Radiation Therapy

Conventional fractionation has evolved over several decades based upon known tolerance and dose-limiting late effects as well as tumor control probabilities. For most centers, conventional fractionation is defined as 180 to 200 cGy per fraction, administered once daily five times a week to projected total doses ranging from 50 to 75 Gy. In children, the parameters are broadened at the lower range of both dose per fraction (extending the lower limit of dose per fraction to 150 cGy for particularly sensitive tumor types, such as Hodgkin lymphoma, acute leukemias, and intracranial germinoma) and total dose (where low doses may be adequate, for example, in Wilms' tumor 10.5–12 Gy is routine, while in acute lymphoblastic leukemia [ALL], 12–18 Gy may be appropriate).

In vitro cell survival curves have long been recognized in classic radiation biology, defining a two-component linear quadratic model with an initial shoulder region (with accumulation of cell lethal effects at low doses) followed by a steeper logarithmic response at higher dose (typically > 100 cGy) (Fig. 13.2).[2] Low-dose exposures (<10–50 cGy) are associated with relative hypersensitivity within the shoulder region, followed by a relatively radioresistant region.[27]

A series of proposed isoeffect models were developed in the 1970 to 1985 time frame, demonstrating apparent equivalent biologic effects with different dose per fraction and overall treatment time relative to total dose delivered. The resultant data differ by tissue type, with steeper dose equivalent curves for dose-limiting late-responding normal tissues than for acutely responding tumor or early, self-limited acute effects. The data indicate that by reducing the dose per fraction, one can go to higher cumulative dose levels with equivalent biologic effect, and that smaller dose per fraction is likely to spare late normal tissue effects while showing little impact upon tumor control. When using smaller dose per fraction, one can accommodate two fractions daily; an interfraction interval of 6 hours or more ensures virtually complete repair of sublethal damage. Relationships are tissue-dependent; for central nervous system (CNS) tissue, where the isoeffect for late reacting phenomena is quite steep compared with the impact of dose per fraction on tumor control, one can roughly equate a conventional fractionation schedule of 54 Gy delivered at 180 cGy once daily, 5 days per week to a *hyperfractionated* schedule of 66 Gy delivered at 110 cGy twice daily, 5 days per week. The result is equivalent normal tissue tolerance and potentially greater antitumor effect.[28–32] Further dose escalation based on observed tolerance led to total doses as high as 75 to 78 Gy in Pediatric Oncology Group (POG) and Children's Cancer Study Group (CCG) trials in brain stem gliomas between 1985 and 1995; unfortunately,

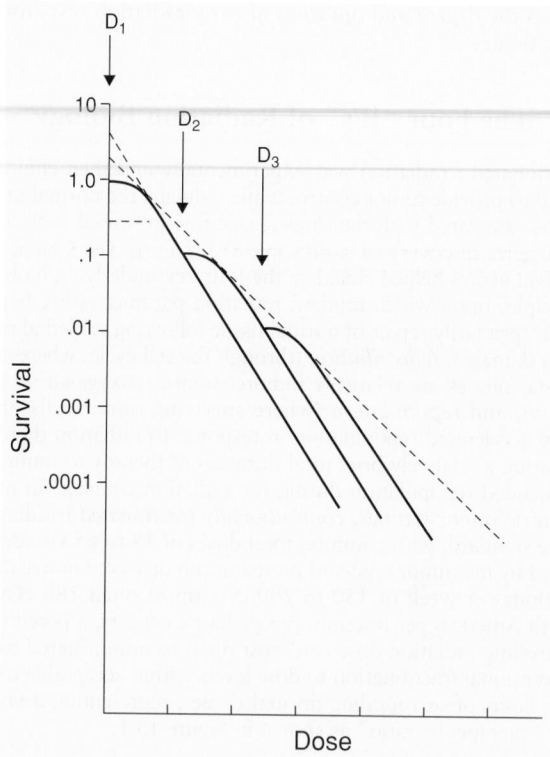

FIGURE 13.2 Cell survival curve from fractionated radiation therapy, demonstrating repeated "less effective" dose in the initial low-dose region ("shoulder") and the combined cell-survival effect (dotted line) reflecting less efficient cell hill and degree of repair in fractionated deliver. (From Cohen ME, Duffner PK. Brain tumors in children: principles of diagnosis and treatment. 2nd ed. Lippincott Williams & Wilkins, Philadelphia, PA, 1994, with permission.)

the population did not include sufficient numbers of long-term survivors to confirm the lack of late effects with numerically higher total dose. Recent investigations of hyperfractionated schedules in children have sought to diminish late toxicity associated with high-dose craniospinal irradiation in advanced (high-risk) medulloblastoma; no unusual toxicities have been reported in that French SIOP trial.[33]

Accelerated fractionation also uses two fractions per day, but each approximates the conventional dose per fraction (150–180 cGy per fraction) to similar or slightly lower total doses than used in conventional fractionation—the goal here to increase tumor control for tumors with rapid repopulation. Although rarely utilized in children, it has had some efficacy in adult head and neck cancers.[34]

There are data indicating the importance of overall treatment duration (time) (or avoiding interruption of a conventionally fractionated schedule), most apparent in pediatrics in medulloblastoma, where prolonged duration of therapy (i.e., interruptions adding days to complete irradiation) negatively impacts disease control.[35] For some of the uniquely sensitive tumors (e.g., Hodgkin lymphoma, germinoma), the duration of therapy does not seem to impact disease control.[36]

PHYSICAL BASIS OF RADIATION THERAPY

Ionizing radiations interact directly with intracellular macromolecules or, more often, indirectly by electron or intranuclear ionization that results in energetic charged particles capable of breaking physical and chemical bonds. The greatest advances in radiation therapy provide sophisticated means of conforming a high-dose radiation volume to the defined tumor target and increasingly sparing critical normal tissues. The convergence of three-dimensional (3-D) imaging identifying the targeted region in anatomic space, 3-D planning for radiation delivery, automated beam direction and shaping, and confirmatory "online" megavoltage imaging allows optimization of radiation planning and delivery in a way that best provides target coverage while limiting "unintended dose" to critical normal tissues. The advances in radiation delivery alone over the past 10 to 20 years have spurred much of the enthusiasm to better utilize radiation therapy in children rather than avoiding a modality that offers considerable efficacy, with increasingly better defined and less pronounced morbidities.

External Beam Irradiation

Photons are electromagnetic radiations without mass and include x-rays (produced electrically) and γ rays (produced by radioactive decay). X-rays are produced at relatively low energy for diagnostic x-rays (typically 50–140 kilovolts [kV]) and at high energies for radiation therapy (approximating 6,000–25,000 kV or 6–25 megavolts [MV]). Photons are produced by *linear accelerators*: electrons are injected into a wave guide that continuously accelerates the electrons by reversing charged plates to ultimately produce an electron beam of up to 6 to 25 M). The electrons then strike a target that stops the beam instantaneously, resulting in bremsstrahlung or x-rays that are then channeled to exit through flattening filters and collimators that define a medical photon beam. The collimators define the field size and, in contemporary multileaf collimators (MLCs), configure the specific beam to the shape planned to encompass the target from a given trajectory aimed at the target from any angle in 3-D space. Photon energy is absorbed exponentially in tissue; the rate of absorption in tissue and the degree of penetration are determined by the beam energy (Table 13.1). The energy of an incident photon beam of 6 MV, for example, is absorbed to 50% of the entry dose by 14 cm; for a 15 MV beam, the dose at 14 cm is 70% of the incident beam.

Electrons are biologically equivalent to photons but are absorbed more superficially, essentially penetrating to a given, limited depth based on the beam energy and then fairly quickly falling toward zero penetrating dose. For a 6 MV electron beam, for example, there is relatively flat deposition of dose between 100% measured just beneath the entry surface and 90% at 2 cm into the tissue; at 4 cm, the dose is only 10% of maximum. For 15 MeV electrons, there is relatively flat deposition of dose to 4 cm, and only 10% remains at 7 cm depth (Table 13.1). Electrons are also produced by linear accelerators, essentially extracting the electron beam directly by removing the target used to create bremsstrahlung; collimation requires beam shaping much closer to the patient to avoid lateral scatter, with current linear accelerators just beginning to introduce technology similar to the autoshaping possible with MLCs for photon beams.

Protons are high-energy, heavy charged particles of particular interest now in radiation oncology, specifically for their potential advantage in pediatric cancer. Protons are essentially equal to photons biologically and are also considered a low LET beam. Measured radiation lethality *in vitro* is used to compare biologic effectiveness of different physical beams, the comparative metric called the *relative biologic effectiveness* or RBE. With megavoltage photons as 1.0, the RBE of protons is estimated at 1.1; thus, a given physical dose of protons (1.8 proton Gy) is essentially equivalent to 2.0 photon Gy.[37]

Interest in protons reflects the relatively favorable physical dose distribution: unlike photons, proton beams enter at 20% to 30% of the maximal dose and reach maximal dose only as they slow down at a depth in tissue related to the incident proton energy. As the protons reach their point of maximal dose, they reach 100% of dose potential in what is called a *Bragg peak* (depositing energy at a given depth in tissue), at which point, all energy is absorbed in matter—there is no further penetration and no exponential exit dose as characterizes photon beams (Table 13.1). Proton beams are produced by high-energy cyclotrons and electronically modulated to produce a "spread out" Bragg peak, the width defined by the width of the tumor at the point of maximal dose. Once modulated to produce a usefully wide Bragg peak, the incident beam is at 70% to 80% of the Bragg peak dose, while the advantage of the abrupt falloff of dose remains (Table 13.1). The lower incident dose and the total lack of exit dose can provide a more sharply conformed dose distribution with potentially greater sparing of normal tissues (see "Radiation Treatment Planning [RTP]" that follows). On the other hand, most currently available proton centers use scatter beam technology, essentially producing a single proton beam of given energy that requires beam compensators (to correct for tissue inhomogeneities within the planned path of the beam) and physical "blocks" to shape the beam to the contour of the target from that trajectory. Both devices generate neutron contamination, a concern regarding secondary carcinogenesis as summarized later. Scanning beam technology is just now being implemented beyond initial use at the Paul Scherrer Institute in Switzerland; the beam is electronically shaped and, ideally, one can alter the energy and intensity across the beam to meet planning parameters for penetration based on the shape of the target along the chosen beam trajectory. There have been several reports of proton-beam radiation therapy (PBRT) in pediatric cancer related to early clinical experience and to dosimetric comparisons of photon irradiation (intensity-modulated radiation therapy or IMRT) and both scatter and scanning beam proton techniques (*v.i.*).

Heavy charged ions include carbon, nitrogen, or other elements in which the electrons have been stripped away during cyclotron acceleration. The mass of the ions exceeds that of protons; such particles show a higher Bragg peak; in addition, the RBE is actually higher in the Bragg peak region as the particles show greater LET as they slow down (Table 13.1). Because the LET is high in the targeted Bragg peak region, there is little oxygen dependency for heavy charged ions.[38] There are currently few centers planning heavy charged ion irradiation, but the potential for yet more conformal physical and biological delivery warrants future interest.

Neutrons are heavy particles without charge. Although offering no physical advantage in dose distribution over photon irradiation, "fast neutrons" (7–14 MV) are of interest because neutron interactions in tissue are not oxygen dependent.[39] Neutrons have an estimated RBE of 2 to 3 compared with photons or protons, with some variation in the RBE based on dose per fraction. Neutron trials just after World War II resulted in unacceptable morbidities, as the variation in RBE was not appreciated. Subsequent trials suggest a benefit when neutrons are used for adult salivary gland tumors.[40] Neutrons are not recommended for children, on the basis of atomic bomb data suggesting that children are particularly sensitive to added carcinogenic risk from neutron irradiation.[39] *Neutron capture therapy* has long had some interest for adult neurosurgeons. Low-energy neutrons (0.1 eV–10 KeV) are absorbed by intratumoral boron to result in unstable radionuclides that immediately undergo disintegration, bathing the local tumor region with energetic, high-LET radiations. There has been little interest in exploiting this in pediatrics.[41–43]

TABLE 13.1

CHARACTERISTICS OF MEDICALLY USEFUL RADIATIONS

Type	Source	Physical properties[a]	Depth-dose curve	Biological characteristics	Use
Photons γ rays	^{60}Co teletherapy	Skin-sparing; slow falloff in dose with depth; absorption independent of tissue density (^{60}Co, 4–10 MeV x-rays); linear accelerator offers superior beam definition		Uniform RBE of 1.0 throughout depth; effectiveness oxygen-dependent	Most common modality for local and wide-field irradiation
Electrons	Linear accelerator (>10 MeV)	Plateau of dose superficially within tissue (1–5 cm); effective range in tissue energy-dependent; increased absorption in bone; relatively poor beam definition		Identical to photons	Often combined with photons for superficial tumors (e.g., parotid bed rhabdomyosarcoma) or to limit dose to a superficial structure (e.g., eye retinoblastoma)

			RBE of 1.1; relative oxygen independence	Favorable dose distribution with *modulated* energies (to broaden the Bragg peak); idealized volume coverage for pediatric CNS tumors (local and potentially for craniospinal irradiation), pediatric sarcomas
			RBE of 1.5–3; Bragg peak RBE for hypoxic cells of 2.5–5; oxygen independence similar to neutrons; late similar to neutrons; late effects in children (CNS, somatic) not yet determined	Focal tumors (e.g., ocular lesions); deep-seated tumors with hypoxic foci and/or potential dosimetric gain re photon therapy (e.g., retroperitoneal, pediatric CNS tumors)
			RBE of 2–3, varies with dose per fraction; dependence on oxygen is one-third to one-half that of photons	Mixed with photons for tumors with known necrotic (hypoxic) fractions (most effective in salivary gland tumors or soft tissue sarcomas in adults; limited enthusiasm for use in children 2° apparent increase in carcinogenicity in the young)
Protons	High-energy cyclotron or synchrotron (>160–250 MeV)	Plateau dose distribution with modulated physical (Bragg) peak; depth of peak and range in tissue distinct and energy-dependent; absorption independent of tissue density; excellent beam definition		
Heavy charged particles ("stripped nuclei" of carbon, neon, argon)	High-energy cyclotron or synchrotron (>5,000 MeV)	Similar to protons		
Neutrons	Cyclotron (>7–14 MeV)	Similar to ⁶⁰Co teletherapy; relatively unfavorable depth-dose characteristics and beam definition	Similar to photons (⁶⁰Co)	

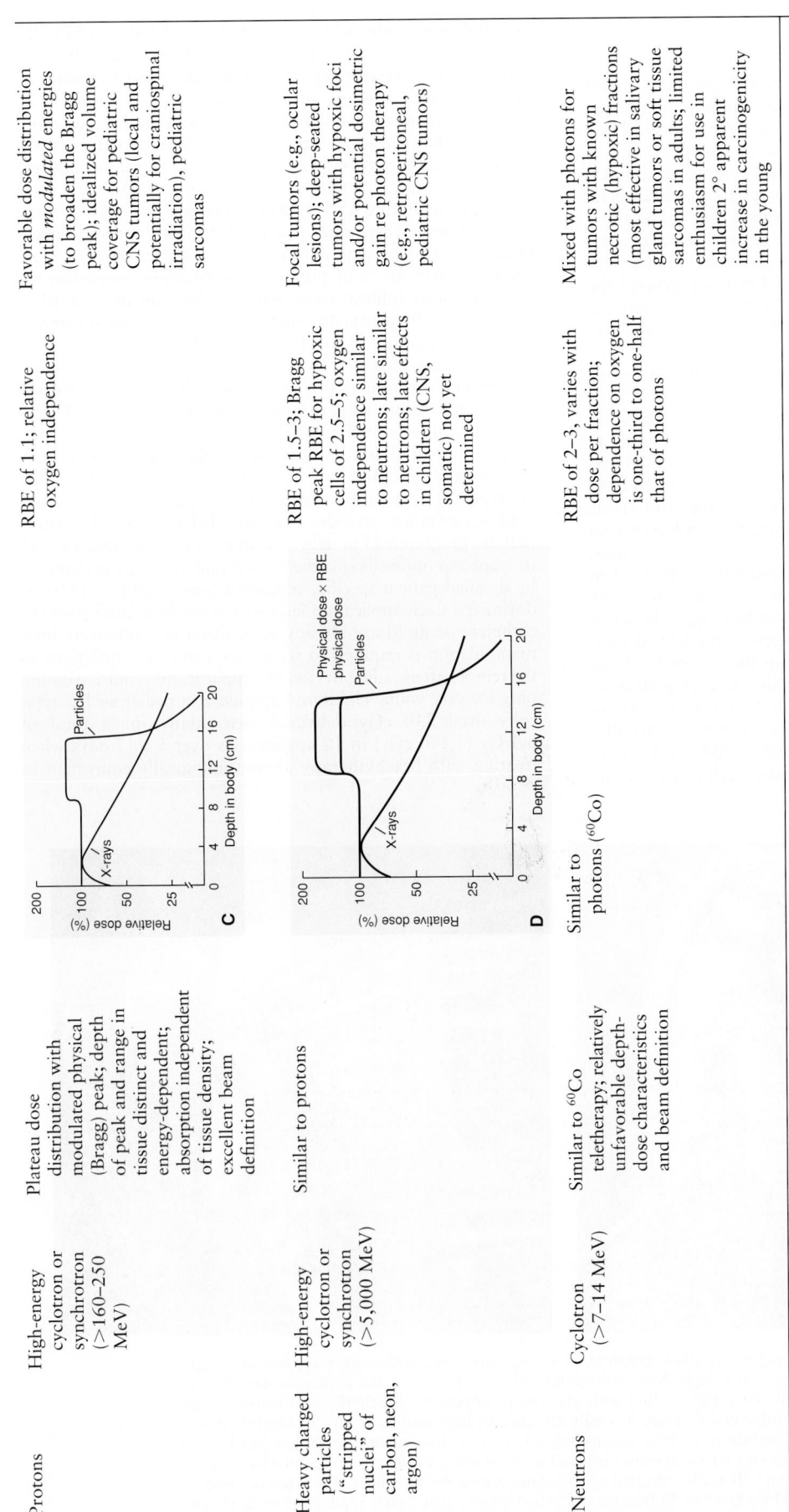

RBE, relative biological effectiveness (RBE = 1 for 250 kV orthovoltage x-rays); CNS, central nervous system.
ᵃBeam definition refers to sharpness of field margins in tissue.

Brachytherapy

The use of radioactive implants or molds provides direct applications of local radiation therapy (or brachytherapy) through *interstitial* (within tissue), *intracavitary* (within body cavities, in pediatrics, primarily vaginal or nasopharyngeal), or *surface mold* (ocular plaques or molds conformed to operative beds) techniques. Radioactive sources are placed directly within or adjacent to the tumor or tumor bed, essentially resulting in "internal" irradiation that delivers a high radiation dose precisely within a confined planning volume with rapid falloff in dose over a very limited distance beyond the application. The dose distribution in brachytherapy applications is governed almost entirely by the inverse square law, explaining the rapid falloff in effective dose (Fig. 13.3). Implants are also completed over a relatively short time frame, typically within 3 to 5 days.

In practice, brachytherapy is limited to tumor beds less than 5 to 10 cm in maximal dimension. The most common uses in pediatrics are for soft tissue sarcomas: rhabdomyosarcomas in specific locations (extremities, vagina, less often head and neck region) and, more commonly, the other soft tissue sarcomas occurring in extremities or along the trunk (synovial cell sarcomas, fibrosarcomas, epithelial cell sarcomas, etc.).[44–46] Afterloading catheters are placed into the tumor bed during surgery for interstitial implants. After a 3- to 5-day immediate postoperative interval to allow healing, radioactive sources are positioned within the catheters at predefined locations to deliver the planned dose within the targeted volume of the implant. Classically, most applications in pediatrics have been manually placed, removable *low-dose rate exposures* using radioisotopes to deliver γ rays (equivalent to photons) at 40 to 90 cGy per hour to a total of 20 to 50 Gy over a continuous exposure time of 2 to 5 days. Such low-dose rate

brachytherapy utilizes iridium 192 (^{192}Ir) or iodine 125 (^{125}I), emitting γ rays of 380 keV or 30 keV, respectively. [192]Ir provides somewhat more homogeneous dose distributions, especially within larger implant volumes, if exposing more peripheral tissues (outside the target volume) to low radiation doses. [125]I has the advantage or more limited penetration and is particularly useful in ocular implants and in young children.

When used as primary postoperative irradiation, a total dose approximating 45 Gy has been typical for most soft tissue sarcomas; when used as a local "boost" within a larger volume treated by external beam radiation therapy (to more broadly cover areas of potential microscopic extension for larger or more infiltrating tumors), an implant dose of 20 to 30 Gy is usually planned.[46] Surface applications, most often as radioactive plaques in focal ocular irradiation for retinoblastoma, use strategically located radioactive seeds imbedded within a gold plaque that is placed directly under the targeted retinal site during surgery and left in place for 3 to 5 days depending upon the planned dose and the dose rate.

For interstitial and intracavitary applications, most centers now utilize *high-dose rate remote afterloading applications* that are repeated on a daily or twice-daily schedule.[47] Remote afterloading equipment provides a self-shielded array of ^{192}Ir sources that are programmed to deliver sources of predetermined length to respective indwelling catheters for time intervals determined by detailed patient-specific, computed tomography (CT)-based dosimetry. Each application lasts only several minutes; since the catheters or mold are already in position and relatively little manipulation is required to secure the catheter connections to the remote afterloading device, the applications require sedation only for very young children. Experience in pediatrics has typically used 340 cGy delivered twice daily for a total of 3.4 Gy (3,400 cGy) in 10 applications over 5 to 7 days when treating with brachytherapy alone (biologically equivalent to

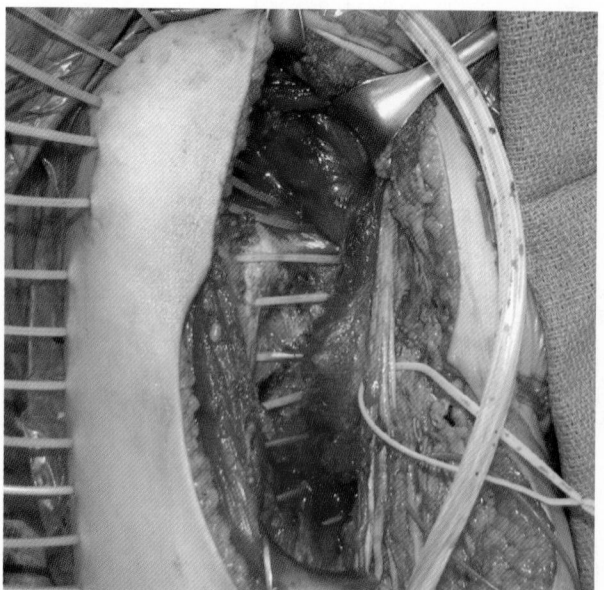
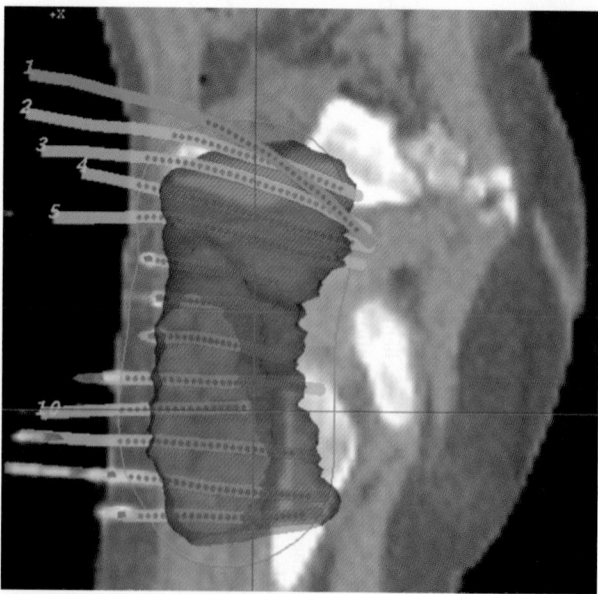

FIGURE 13.3 A: Intraoperative photograph showing operative bed following resection of a high-grade synovial sarcoma of the thigh. Note indwelling catheters inserted in the perpendicular plane to provide coverage for microscopic residual with planned postoperative brachytherapy. Catheters are left in place with accessible end that can be easily attached to high-dose rate unit. **B:** Dosimetry displaying operative bed (red detail in three-dimension), reference isodose volume (green line just beyond red volume) that indicates the region of tumor bed and adjacent microscopic margin covered by intended dose, and catheters (with ^{192}Ir seeds indicated as dark lines within the catheters). The reference isodose volume here received 34 Gy given in 10 fractions of 340 cGy twice daily; each application took 11 minutes. (Courtesy of M. Krasin.)

45 Gy administered via low-dose rate implant) or 300 cGy delivered twice daily for a total of 21 Gy (2100 cGy) in 7 applications over 4 to 6 days when used as a boost (biologically equivalent to 30 Gy low-dose rate brachytherapy).[46] Single applications of high-dose rate brachytherapy have been utilized to provide "boost" irradiation to the tumor bed at the time of surgery, particularly in retroperitoneal, pelvic, or deep-seated extremity sarcomas—a form of *intraoperative radiation therapy*.[48] Such applications allow precise localization and, often, the ability to physically relocate adjacent bowel or kidney away from the radiation implant, further protecting adjacent critical structures.

Radioactive colloids can be instilled directly into cyst cavities, primarily in primary or "salvage" therapy for craniopharyngiomas or, less often, cystic astrocytomas. ^{32}P, ^{90}Y, or ^{186}Re are pure β emitters with extremely limited penetration in tissue (0.5–1.5 mm) providing high doses to the internal cyst wall (200 Gy or 20,000 cGy at the surface). The procedure requires technical experience, wherein the targeted cyst(s) is reduced by aspiration, the volume then calculated based on CT or magnetic resonance imaging (MRI), and physical algorithms employed to determine the amount of colloidal radionuclide that is instilled via stereotactically placed catheter to provide the prescribed dose.[49] Given the short range of β radiations, the key vital structure potentially in range is the visual apparatus (optic nerves, chiasm). In centers adept at this type of intervention, this approach has been safe and effective, with rare reports of late visual loss.[49–51]

Stereotactic Radiosurgery

There are several stereotactic techniques that deliver a precise, relatively small volume of irradiation based on stereotactic coordinates (3-D, image-guided targeting to a defined point in space), precise localization and immobilization, and CT and/or MRI with stereotactic frame or fiducial markers in place. Classical *radiosurgery* is analogous to a surgical procedure, delivering a single high dose of photon irradiation that causes cell death and necrosis within the targeted volume. The procedure relies on the immediate cytolethal effect. With no fractionation, there is no biologic sparing of normal tissues within the targeted volume.[52,53] Initial applications of radiosurgery were limited to intracranial targets, using the Leksell GammaKnife®, a stand-alone radiosurgical device based on triangulating the spherical target defined by collimation and stereotactic positioning to produce a spherical target from 210 ^{60}Co sources strategically placed within a shielded structure, into which the patient is "locked" during the 5- to 12-minute exposure. Specially modified linear accelerators can also deliver radiosurgery, either intracranial or "body" techniques.[53,54] Frameless technology, including CyberKnife®, is based on coordinated orthogonal imaging and both a treatment couch and small, "portable" linear accelerator free to move through all trajectories and locations in 3-D space with fixed anatomic points or surgically placed fiducials to allow real-time image-guided exposure. Both frameless linear accelerator approaches and CyberKnife® permit single- or multiple-fraction radiosurgery, the latter often termed *stereotactic radiotherapy* (implying conventional dose fractionation over several weeks, providing the biologic advantage of fractionation compared with the "ablative" single-dose radiosurgery.[55,56]

Either GammaKnife® or linac radiosurgical programs permit pediatric utilization. Most pediatric experience has been in recurrent tumors, particularly ependymomas and glial neoplasms; as a part of primary therapy, radiosurgical "boost" has been added when standard radiation management and chemotherapy have not achieved early "complete response," particularly in ependymoma, malignant germ cell histiotypes,

and high-grade gliomas.[52,57,58] A few dedicated radiosurgical centers have explored broader use as primary radiation management where anatomic geometry allows high-dose radiosurgery while avoiding excess exposure to critical normal structures; experience with craniopharyngiomas has been of interest, if not broadly adopted.[59] In children with low-grade CNS tumors as a part of neurofibromatosis (NF) (typically type 1 with optic pathway gliomas or tumors located in nonsurgical sites such as the midbrain; also, type 2 with acoustic neuromas), judicious use of radiosurgery has often provided early disease control while preserving broader CNS "radiation tolerance" in anticipation of later requirements for radiation therapy.[52,53,60] With the availability and documentation of precise patient localization and dose deposition, current interest has focused increasingly on spinal body or paravertebral irradiation using rapid fractionation (single exposures or limited number of fractionated treatments) based on what is termed "body radiosurgery."[61] Applications in children have focused primarily on vertebral body irradiation for metastatic disease.

Technical Basis of Radiation Therapy

The ability to better focus radiation dose reflects the introduction of ever more sophisticated technologies. Cross-sectional imaging (CT, MRI) can be imported into RTP systems, enabling 3-D reconstructions or using 3-D MR acquisitions to define overt tumor volumes. Key in this first step of RTP is registering MRI and/or positron emission tomography (PET)/CT imaging to the CT data set that provides the basis for dose calculation. The CT data are obtained at *simulation*—the start of RTP when the patient is positioned ideally for treatment delivery, appropriate molds or casts formed that both allow the patient to be comfortably positioned for therapy and ensure daily reproducibility of the setup and maximal immobilization during treatment. Critical anatomic regions (target volume and/or critical structures) are based on the most informative imaging modality. Diagnostic or radiation therapy–specific MRI or PET/CT studies can be fused to the simulation-obtained reference CT scans. Stereotactic localization based on fiducial markers inserted at the time of surgery or during simulation provides reference points used during simulation and available for "real-time" confirmation or adjustment of patient position during daily irradiation. RTP continues as the physician outlines the *gross target volume* or GTV, typically the initial tumor extent or the postoperative tumor bed as tissues may have reconfigured after surgery; less often, postoperative or postchemotherapy volumes are used to define the GTV, using the residual tumor after chemotherapy or the operative bed and overt residual after surgery.[62] The area(s) of potential microscopic extension (by direct infiltration and/or regional draining lymph nodes) define the expansion of the GTV to form the *clinical target volume* or CTV. In most settings, the CTV is determined by a given 3-D expansion of the GTV (e.g., 0.5–1 cm or more), corrected for anatomic interfaces to identify the final CTV (Fig. 13.4). In practice, the CTV is defined by our best understanding of the degree of tumor infiltration likely in a given direction and then limited by adjacent skull or the midline (falx) or compartmental barrier (e.g., the posterior fossa-defining tentorium in the brain; the mediastinal-pleural surface in targeting thoracic lymph nodes, barriers through which tumor is unlikely to extend). One might expect considerable infiltration of osseous Ewing's sarcoma within the involved medullary cavity, requiring a greater expansion to define the CTV than in a clear cell sarcoma of the kidney, where margins for microscopic extension beyond the renal capsule might be only 1 cm. The CTV can also include the

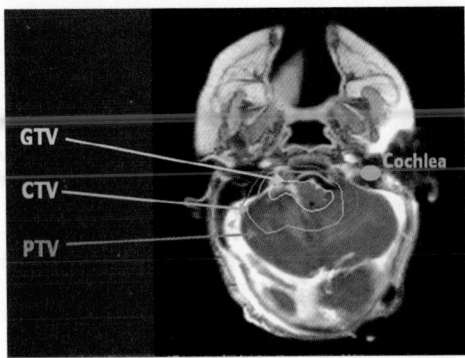

FIGURE 13.4 Defining target volumes for pediatric radiation therapy: the gross tumor volume (GTV) here defines the operative bed and residual tumor for a IVth ventricular ependymoma that surrounded the brain stem and involved the right foramen of Lushka, on the basis of preoperative magnetic resonance imaging and postoperative shift in brain tumor structures; the clinical target volume (CTV) is a 1 cm three-dimensional (3-D) anatomic expansion of the GTV, here corrected for anatomic barriers (the anterior aspect of the tentorium and the prepontine cistern); planning target volume (PTV) is a strict geometric 3-D expansion of the CTV, here using 3 mm for a child treated in an immobilizing mask and sedated (to virtually eliminate movement during therapy) (Courtesy T. Merchant).

immediately adjacent or regional lymph nodes in tumors known to spread via the lymphatic system. Once the CTV is established, a simple geometric expansion of the CTV by 3 to 10 mm provides the *planning target volume* or PTV. The PTV accounts for variation in daily patient setup or any potential movement during therapy (organ movement or degree of patient immobilization) (Fig. 13.4). Dose within the tumor target can be quite homogeneous or show intralesional variations in dose, based on MR spectroscopy or PET to identify regions of greater proliferation or metabolism or focal areas of hypoxia, regions that may require higher radiation doses than otherwise "less active" or "euoxic" areas within the tumor.[63,64]

In addition to target volumes, treatment planning requires identification of critical normal tissues. In developing a treatment plan, one identifies a dose or range of doses sought in the PTV, sometimes recognizing two or more PTVs with different intended dose or doses (e.g., for embryonal brain tumors, a dose of 23.4 or 36 Gy is often prescribed for the entire neuraxis, while the "primary tumor bed" dose is 54 Gy; for nasopharyngeal embryonal rhabdomyosarcoma, a dose of 36–41.4 Gy is typically sought for the nodal region of initial involvement that responded completely to chemotherapy, while the primary tumor dose is 50–55 Gy). Limits are defined for critical structures: in the two prior examples, one would plan to limit the dose to the chiasm to 50 Gy (in both supratentorial embryonal CNS tumors and in nasopharyngeal rhabdomyosarcoma) and the spinal cord to 40 to 45 Gy (in nasopharyngeal tumors where the primary tumor and residual nodal disease require 45–55 Gy and are often contiguous with the spinal cord).

Three-Dimensional Treatment Planning and Delivery: Three-Dimensional Conformal, Intensity-Modulated Radiation Therapy

Standard pediatric radiation therapy requires *3-D conformal* planning/delivery (3D-CRT), anticipating that in certain presentations IMRT may offer advantages.[63,65] Following target volume definition, RTP proceeds to *dosimetry*: determining the array of radiation beams that each provide a proportion of

the dose, including the specific trajectory through which a beam enters the body, encompasses the target (based on the "beam's eye view" of the target's shape and size through the angle at which the beam encompasses the target), and exits beyond the target volume. Sophisticated calculation and display systems enable one to plan and optimize plans that conform the radiation dose to the target along with estimates of the intervening and posttarget exiting dose contributed by each field. As RTP has advanced to more complex field arrays and weighting, the display of target and organ dose uses a format known as *dose-volume histograms*, graphically depicting the radiation dose received by subtended volumes of the identified structure (tumor target or normal tissue) (Fig. 13.5).

In 3-D CRT, a number of trajectories are identified that encompass the PTV and minimize or avoid traversing identified critical normal tissue structures. Each of the beams is shaped to include the size and shape of the target volume in the plane with which the beam intersects the PTV (the so-called beam's eye view). One or more of the beams may

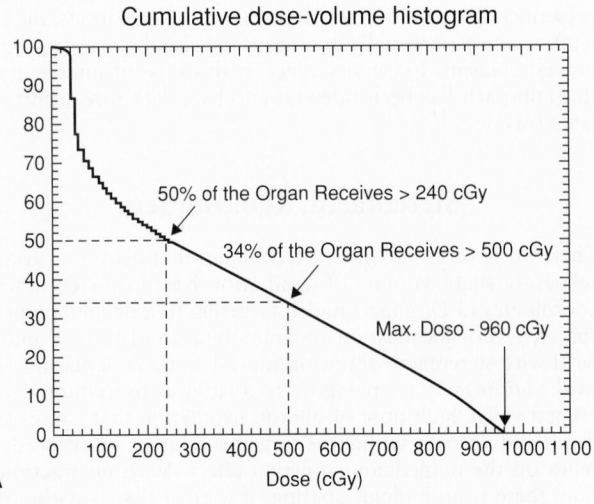

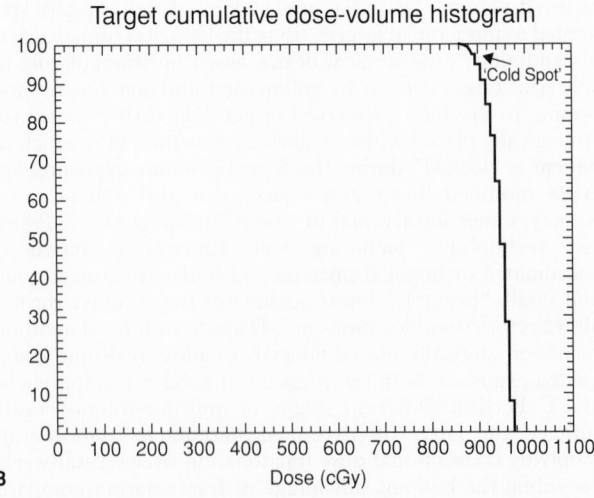

FIGURE 13.5 Dose-volume histograms (DVH). **A:** Nominal DVH indicating dose received in given percentage of indicated structures. The amount of information available in describing three-dimensional dosimetry requires a graphic display to appreciate the relative dose in varying portions of an identified target or normal structure. **B:** For tumor, DVH indicates more than 90% of the projected dose within the identified target; the "cold spot" identifies less than 10% of the target's volume receiving less than 90% of the targeted dose.

include a manual or electronic wedge that modifies the dose across the beam when such will improve the composite dose distribution that accounts for all beams and the body contours through which they traverse. 3-D CRT typically results in highly uniform dose distribution throughout the PTV.

The basis of IMRT is to further optimize radiation therapy to improve the tumor control probability by increasing dose to the target volume while diminishing the likelihood of normal tissue complications by allowing specified dose limits to critical normal structures. While 3D-CRT allows the high-dose region to conform to the target volume to a much greater extent than does the traditional 2-D or planar planning, it is limited in situations where anatomy creates a concave interface between target and normal structure (e.g., around the spine) or where specific structures adjacent to the target volume require relative underdosing (e.g., the cochlea when treating the posterior fossa or a tumor bed within that region, or the spinal cord adjacent to a soft tissue sarcoma). In such circumstances, IMRT offers the advantage of "sculpting" the dose around a given "avoidance" structure.[66] Through multiple beam trajectories, each including multiply shaped, differently weighted "beamlets" that provide "modulation" of dose within the 2-D beam view of each beam angle, one can create a 3-D dose plot that obeys the constraints of minimal and maximal dose within a target volume that has closely conformed dose with (a) greater internal inhomogeneity (specifically, regions of greater dose intensity than one sees with 3D-CRT) but (b) specific areas of "underdosage" as prescribed in adjacent normal tissue structures.[3,51] IMRT delivery requires a MLC aimed through a large number of gantry angles with beam modifications at each trajectory. The result is increased treatment time and complexity, requiring greater attention to immobilization (for children, often sedation/anesthesia) to ensure accurate delivery. Dose delivery through optimized IMRT is quite precise and, when administered in a program that includes *image-guided radiation therapy* (IGRT, see later), can achieve idealized dose conformality to the intended target and meet the demands of limiting normal tissue doses to prescribed dose levels. The longer "beam on" interval and inherent if "minimal" leakage through the MLC result in greater incidental dose to remote normal tissues—resulting in larger normal tissue volumes exposed to very low radiation doses.[67] Specific studies in children show somewhat less unintended dose from IMRT techniques as field volumes are often smaller than in adults, important as survivors of childhood cancer are at risk for late secondary carcinogenesis often related to low-dose radiation exposures (*v.i.*).[68-70]

Proton-Beam Radiation Therapy

IMRT provides excellent dose distribution for most pediatric settings based on widely available linear accelerators. PBRT can often further spare normal tissues, a significant advantage in children with CNS tumors and several other presentations. The physical characteristics of the charged proton beam are discussed earlier; key is the lack of exit dose, sparing underlying normal structures any radiation exposure.[35,67,71,72] In treating medulloblastoma with craniospinal irradiation and boost to the entire posterior fossa, for example, the Harvard group has shown the dose delivered to 90% of the cochlea can be reduced from 100% when using 2-D opposed lateral photon fields to 33% with photon IMRT and 2% with PBRT.[71] Similar comparisons from St. Jude show moderate reductions likely to be important in preserving intellectual function: in treating localized optic charismatic/hypothalamic astrocytomas or craniopharyngiomas, PBRT significantly reduces the volume of normal brain exposed to low- and intermediate-

dose levels in the temporal lobes, dose levels associated with IQ effects in related radiation models.[72,73] Even with posterior fossa ependymomas, where the CTV and PTV expansions require a margin of only 1 to 1.5 cm, substantial sparing of the temporal lobes is seen with PBRT.[72] In craniospinal irradiation, exit exposures from posterior spinal fields can be meaningfully reduced: dose received by 50% of the cardiac volume is reduced from 72% of the PTV dose to 0.5% comparing standard photon irradiation to PBRT.[71] Similar or greater reductions have been reported in paraspinal sarcomas in adults, relevant to common pediatric presentations (e.g., neuroblastoma, vertebral Ewing's sarcoma).[74] In retinoblastoma, more than 500 cGy is delivered to 25% to 70% of the bony orbit with a variety of 2-D and IMRT photon plans compared with 10% with PBRT.[75] In pediatric pelvic sarcomas, the dose to the ovaries and pelvic bones can be substantially reduced depending on the anatomic location and size of the tumor.[75] There are concerns that currently available proton beams, based largely on scatter beam delivery, produce sufficient neutron contamination to potentially increase secondary carcinogenesis, especially in children.[76] PBRT requires enormous capital investment, and there is lively debate both within the field of radiation oncology and within the medical enterprise and government agencies worldwide re cost-benefit issues related to PBRT; often, the only common agreement is in that a potential advantage seems obvious for pediatric cancers.[77-80]

Other charged heavy ions have been preliminarily investigated for radiation delivery. Carbon ions show both physical and biological advantages in dose distributions as noted previously.[77] At higher dose levels, the differential RBE between tumor and normal tissues is further exaggerated, favoring hypofractionated carbon ion regimens (i.e., smaller number of fractions at higher dose/fraction). It will be some time before sufficient data re normal tissue tolerances are available for carbon ion utilization in children.

Image Guidance During Radiation Therapy

Classical radiation delivery requires quality assurance based principally on orthogonal portal films obtained by exposing film to the accelerator's megavoltage beam. Electronic portal imaging devices (EPID) provide digital imaging data that improve the quality assurance process. Kilovoltage x-ray device mounted on the linear accelerator gantry provide greater imaging detail (the lower-energy x-rays produce much greater contrast than does megavoltage imaging). As positioning and RTP are based on cross-sectional imaging, the recent introduction of cone-beam CT (CBCT) enables the radiation therapist (previously, radiation technologist) to obtain an accurate CT image through the center of the volume in the axial plane; the image can be generated by the megavoltage beam or through kilovoltage x-ray as mentioned earlier.[81] CBCTs can be compared (both visually and through computerized registration) with the initial CT image obtained at simulation, allowing accurate repositioning on a daily or regular basis through the course of therapy.

Daily portal imaging data can be used to correct any offsets of the isocenter, balancing added accuracy with the additional exposure. Specific organ-related positioning can be confirmed by CBCT or the use of intralesional radio-opaque fiducial markers or radiofrequency transponders. The former are detectable by CBCT or EPID and the latter by a stereotactic external antenna array integrated with an optical tracking system. Identification of changes in target position (as in prostate cancer, in which significant variability in organ position reflects changes in stool and bladder status) or in pediatric brain tumors with cystic components (e.g., craniopharyngioma, low-grade astrocytoma) in which weekly MRI can reveal changes in cyst volume requiring aspiration or modification of the RTP to accommodate a somewhat larger target volume. Use of individual, essentially "real-time" data with modification of delivery is called *adaptive radiation therapy* and is particularly relevant as one utilizes more limited target volume margins.

Interactions of Radiation Therapy and Chemotherapy

The classic description of interactions between radiation therapy and chemotherapy were published by Steel in 1979.[82] Both spatial cooperation (i.e., radiation therapy for local/regional control, chemotherapy for systemic micrometastases or overt metastatic disease) and toxicity independence (i.e., added effects of radiation therapy and chemotherapy improving tumor control with no "sensitization" or apparent overlapping toxicities) assume no real interaction between the physical and pharmacologic agents. Molecular interactions between the drug(s) and radiation effects define synergistic effects resulting in *radiosensitization* (or local, radiation-induced chemosensitization) or *radiation protection*.

Drug-radiation interactions of particular interest in pediatric oncology include cisplatin and 5-fluorouracil (5-FU). Concurrent use of cisplatin and irradiation shows true radiosensitization at low dose levels (used during the course of irradiation or administered immediately prior to irradiation), based largely on inhibition of repair of sublethal radiation-induced DNA damage.[83] 5-FU is also known to sensitize cells to radiations, presumably through facilitating progression through the S phase in mitosis and abbreviating time to repair radiation damage.[84,85] Capecitabine, a prodrug converted to 5-FU, in part, by thymidine phosphorylase, provides somewhat longer-term exposure, thereby heightening radiosensitization. Capecitabine further increases the ratio of tumor to normal tissue 5-FU concentration as irradiation induces the thymidine phosphorylase activity necessary for interaction.[86]

Attempts to exploit the relative radiosensitivity of well-oxygenated cell systems have been unsuccessful to date. More hypoxic tumors seem to be more resistant to radiocurability, leading to development of hypoxic cytotoxins. Tirapazamine is active against hypoxic cells and potentiates hypoxic cell kill when administered in conjunction with radiation therapy.[87]

Radiation Therapy and Molecular Targeting Agents

Molecular targeting agents, of considerable interest as novel therapeutics, are also of keen interest as potential radiation sensitizers. A significant proportion of cells transformed with the activated *ras* oncogene are noted to be relatively radioresistant. Farnesyl transferase inhibitors (FTIs) cause reversion of ras transformation, inhibiting ras-transformed fibroblasts and human tumor cell lines, respectively. FTIs specifically inhibit *H-ras*-transformed cells *in vitro* with potential radiosensitization; no sensitization was apparent in tumor cells with wild-type ras.[87] Epidermal growth factor receptor (EGFR) is responsible for initiating a cascade of signals from cytoplasm to nucleus, regulating cell division, proliferation, and differentiation; EGFR expression is associated with radioresistance.[87,88] Agents that prevent ligand binding to the receptor appear to result in relative radiosensitization; when administered during irradiation, EGFR inhibitors block cell proliferation.[87] As signaling pathways are targeted (e.g., FTIs—tipifarnib; mTOR inhibitors—rapamycin and temsirolimus; histone deacetylase [HDAC] or HDAC inhibitors—vorinostat and everolimus; P13-K/AKT pathway inhibitors—MN3006), molecular interactions offer potential radiosensitization. Clinical studies of molecular targeting

agents with irradiation in pediatric cancers are advancing from phase I and phase II studies to phase III trials largely in solid tumor and brain tumor trials within Children's Oncology Group, the Pediatric Brain Tumor Consortium, and several large institutional settings.[89–91]

The interaction of radiation therapy and antiangiogenesis agents is a complex one. Both increased expression and inhibition of proangiogenesis factors (e.g., vascular endothelial growth factor [VEGF]) have been related to radiation exposure.[92] Studies have shown that inhibition of receptor tyrosine kinases can sensitize blood vessels to effects of radiations; a component sensitization may be inhibition of pathways that promote endothelial survival and function after radiation exposure.[93] Protein kinase C (PKC) is another pathway linked to tumorigenesis and therapeutic response; PKC inhibitors (e.g., enzastaurin) have been shown to enhance radiation cell kill *in vivo*.[94] Whether angiogenesis inhibition results in relative hypoxia and increased radioresistance has been questioned.[95] Both preclinical and clinical studies seem to show a potential radiosensitizing effect when antiangiogenesis agents are combined with irradiation; the beneficial effect of "trimodal therapy" combining irradiation with both antiangiogenic and cytotoxic chemotherapeutic agents has been noted.[92,96]

Radiation Effects on Normal Tissues

Radiation effects are usually considered in the context of timing relative to therapy: the biologic mechanisms underlying radiation effects on normal tissue differ over time, and the impact in determining radiation indications and parameters differ, especially in children. Radiation effects are divided into *acute* reactions (during the course of radiation therapy; such effects can be ameliorated by modification in radiation intensity), *subacute* reactions (within 3–9 months of treatment), and *late* effects (typically beyond 1 year post-therapy; late effects are dependent on dose per fraction and total dose). Factors associated with radiation-related changes include treatment parameters (total dose, dose per fraction, fractionation schedule), host factors (genetic states predisposing to radiation injury), associated therapies (surgery, chemotherapy—including sequencing and timing of other therapies), and treatment environment (e.g., relative hypoxia, nutritional status). Common radiation-related phenomena, such as progressive fibrosis, are secondary to cytokine production, at least in part mediating acute and late radiation reactions, most notably TGF-β (central to fibroblast recruitment and proliferation).[97] Classical radiobiology has been based on the assumption that tissue-specific differences in radiosensitivity reflect inherent radiosensitivity of targeted visceral replicating cells.[98] Models of radiation effects, from which fractionation schemes have been derived, have utilized the "linear-quadratic formula," based on the ratio of more rapidly proliferating tissues or tissue components (tumors and acutely responding tissues) to slowly or relatively "nonproliferating" components (late-responding tissues).[30] In parallel, classic theory has held that the degree of radiation damage is determined at the time of exposure, with no likelihood of modification by posttherapy intervention.[98] Several pharmacologic interventions, however, have been shown to decrease late normal tissue effects, including corticosteroids, nonsteroidal anti-inflammatory drugs, and angiotensin-converting enzyme (ACE) inhibitors.[99]

Increasingly, the biologic mechanisms determining late effects of irradiation are felt to be secondary to complex interactions in and between parenchymal and endothelial cells with the inflammatory cytokines (particularly TGF-β) mediating much of the late visceral damage.[98–100] Manifestations of late injury reflect radiation-induced reduction in parenchymal cells and TGF-β–induced excessive fibrosis formation.[98] The potential role of TGF-β antagonists (e.g., ACE or ACE inhibitors) in reducing late normal tissue effects is currently under study.[101]

Interpatient variability in normal tissue responses have long been noted. Cellular radiosensitivity assays have been supplanted by patient-specific genetic profiles predicting normal tissue response.[102] The most pronounced examples are inherited syndromes associated with catastrophic response to ionizing radiations: A-T, NBS, and Fanconi's anemia.[103] *ATM* has been the dominant gene associated with hypersensitivity to ionizing radiations, believed related to a key role in detection of DNA DSBs and initiation of genetic signaling leading to cell cycle arrest, DNA repair, or apoptosis.[104] Although markedly heightened radiation effects are associated with homozygotes evidencing the A-T syndrome, reports also suggest that heterozygotes show enhanced reactions, although lesser in degree than those with the full syndrome.[105] Single nucleotide polymorphisms (SNPs) account for a proportion of genetic findings associated with normal tissue radiosensitivity; SNPs are thought to account for nearly 90% of interpatient variability including radiation responsiveness.[103]

Acute Normal Tissue Radiation Effects

Acutely responding tissues demonstrate injury during the course of irradiation, classically based on the rapid proliferation rates of replicating cell systems: epithelial stem cells of skin and the gastrointestinal (GI) tract (e.g., intestinal crypt cells), as well as hematopoietic stem cells. Clinical evidence of radiation injury is apparent only upon completion of the usual survival time of the postmitotic, differentiated cells. The differentiated cells lining the GI mucosa, for example, show a normal life span of 4 to 7 days; the first sign of radiation damage are noted 4 to 7 days after initiating a course of fractionated irradiation. Hematopoietic stem cells replace neutrophils at a median of 12 to 14 days and platelets at 14 to 20 days; one typically notes a fall in the absolute neutrophil count (ANC) at the end of the second week of wide-field irradiation, whereas platelets typically fall between 2 and 3 weeks of therapy.

Acute effects are expected and "normal" during a course of radiation therapy, differing only in degree based on host factors and the microenvironment (*v.s.*). Acute reactions relate to fraction size and dose rate but show little effect from interfraction interval as long as at least 4 to 6 hours are allowed for repair of sublethal damage. Concurrent chemotherapy can accelerate, delay or enhance acute normal issue toxicities, particularly seen with actinomycin D, methotrexate, and cisplatin. There is little correlation between the occurrence or severity of acute effects and the development of dose-limiting late effects.

Acute Epithelial Reactions

Epithelial changes can be seen immediately after radiation exposure. Transient cutaneous erythema and sialadenitis can occur within hours of the initial dose, both more often noted after total body irradiation (TBI) than with focal irradiation. Systemic effects (nausea, vomiting, anorexia, fatigue) occur within a few days of starting therapy; the occurrence and severity are quite variable, in part related to the anatomic region treated, perhaps best correlated with the *integral dose* (dose per fraction multiplied by the volume subtended).

Typical *dry radioepidermitis* presents as hyperpigmentation or erythema about 3 weeks into a course of fractionated irradiation. One sees such reactions along curved surfaces, at exit points, and in cutaneous folds, areas exposed to full photon "buildup" doses (compared with incident skin where direct or *en face* fields enjoy the "surface buildup" effect: surface dose is only 60% to 70% of the full dose level measured 1 to 4 cm into tissue). A variety of lanolin-based ointments are available for management. *Alopecia* also occurs during the third week of cranial irradiation. Only in areas of full buildup, particularly in sensitive individuals or those with certain concurrent pharmacotherapy (e.g., actinomycin D, tipifarnib), does one usually see progression to *moist radioepidermitis* with blotchy or confluent areas of denuded dermis. Moist reactions heal by peripheral cutaneous stem cell "infiltration" and by repopulation from islands of relatively resistant cells within the denuded area. While dry reactions often heal with little or no late sequelae, moist reactions are associated with thin, pale skin and areas of telangiectasia. Hair returns after 2 to 3 months, completely in areas exposed to moderate radiation doses and often incompletely or not at all in areas where surface doses approach 50 Gy.

Mucosal reactions largely mimic cutaneous reactions, appearing earlier (during weeks 2 or 3) in the oral cavity and oropharynx as *radioepithelitis*, initially as patchy areas of enanthema and overlying whitish "pseudomembrane" (exudates) that progresses to confluent areas of enanthema and overlying exudates, sometimes complicated by concurrent candidiasis. Similar changes occur in the hypopharynx and esophagus. Reactions are heightened with concurrent chemotherapy (e.g., methotrexate, actinomycin D, cisplatin) A variety of mouth rinses offer some symptomatic relief; a low threshold for systemic anticandida management is often helpful. Similar changes occur in the esophagus, in which varying degrees of odynophagia are noted during the third week of irradiation. Severe pain should prompt assessment or empiric treatment for superimposed candida overgrowth.

Hematologic Effects

Even local irradiation is associated with prompt, pronounced lymphopenia (related to intermitotic or apoptotic cell death in circulating lymphocyte populations).[106–108] Neutrophils decline 7 to 10 days after initiating irradiation to relatively large volumes (e.g., craniospinal; full thoracic or wide abdominal), reaching a nadir at 2 to 3 weeks into therapy. Neutropenia reflects primary effects on the repopulating uncommitted stem cell population; significant reduction in ANC is typically seen only when substantial proportions of the bone marrow are irradiated (e.g., pelvis, more than 40% of the spinal vertebrae). The ANC usually plateaus at 35% to 45% of initial levels with wide-field irradiation; recovery is apparent within 4 to 6 weeks of therapy. Monocyte levels decrease and recover rapidly during a course of fractionated irradiation.[107] Platelet counts parallel the ANC; it is common to see platelet counts at 35% to 50% of initial levels during wide-field irradiation.

Subacute and Late Visceral Effects

Lung. Post-irradiation pulmonary toxicity can be seen in several pediatric settings, including whole-lung irradiation for metastatic sarcomas or Wilms' tumor, wide-field irradiation for primary thoracic sarcomas or for Hodgkin lymphoma, and in the unique setting of TBI. The pathophysiology is worth detailing, as it is a well-researched model that parallels other visceral effects. Initial radiation injury at the macromolecular and cellular levels results in release of inflammatory cytokines, growth factors, and further reactive oxygen species, with resultant hypoxia, chronic oxidative stress, and fixed tissue damage.[109] Inflammatory and fibrogenic cytokines (including TGF-β, TNF-α, IL-1, and/or IL-6 released from reactive monocytes, pneumocytes, or fibroblasts; KL-6, a lung epithelium–specific protein that correlates with interstitial pneumonitis) may serve as markers of radiation lung injury and be key to potential modulation of post-irradiation inflammatory reactions; such cytokines appear to be active even after radiation exposure.[110,111] Radiation injury is apparent in types I and II alveolar cells, endothelial cells, and stromal fibroblasts. Clinically, the syndrome appears similar to idiopathic interstitial pneumonia: acute pneumonitis is marked by enlarged, atypical type II pneumocytes and edema, with infiltration of inflammatory cells and alveolar macrophages into the alveolar walls and interstitial lung tissues. The timing of the acute pneumonitis phase is within the 1- to 4-month post-irradiation subacute interval. Later, progressive pulmonary fibrosis can be apparent within 6 to 12 months or several years after therapy, marked by accumulation of fibrin and atypical fibroblasts thickening the alveolar interstitial tissues.[110] There is evolving experimental evidence that suppression of the renin-angiotensin system (through captopril, an ACE inhibitor) may ameliorate some of the pulmonary changes.[112]

Radiation parameters associated with lung injury include the volume of lung irradiated above 18 to 20 Gy (unilateral whole lung or substantial pulmonary volume) or 25 to 30 Gy (with volumes limited to <50% of the unilateral lung) (Table 13.2).[113] In combination with chemotherapy (e.g., -bleomycin, actinomycin D), changes typical of postirradiation pneumonitis and fibrosis occur at lower dose levels and with greater frequency.[114] Earlier data confirm significant reduction in total lung capacity and compliance in adults who were exposed to whole-lung irradiation during their childhood.[115–117] Late follow-up among cohorts surviving 5 or more years after initial therapy show a subsequent rate of fatal pulmonary events eight to nine times that of the normal population.[118]

Factors related to pneumonitis in the bone marrow transplant (BMT) setting are complex, noting correlations among the entire conditioning regimen (TBI parameters—total dose, number of fractions, fractions/day, dose rate (cGy/min); also the cytotoxic chemotherapy), the transplant type (syngeneic, allogeneic—matched related donor transplants vs. haploidentical donor vs. matched unrelated donor), and the occurrence and management of graft-versus-host disease.[119,120] Unlike other settings, lung effects in BMT are often apparent within 2 to 3 weeks.

Heart. Cardiac effects following irradiation in children and adolescents are most commonly seen in Hodgkin lymphoma, where there are considerable data re incidence and apparent pathophysiology.[121–124] Such data have been extrapolated to risks in treating thoracic sarcomas and craniospinal irradiation. Postirradiation pericarditis is a subacute effect noted

TABLE 13.2

RADIATION DOSE TOXICITY LEVELS FOR SUBACUTE AND LATE VISCERAL EFFECTS

Organ	Toxicity	Whole organ irradiation			Partial organ irradiation				Chemotherapy effect
		5%–10% incidence dose[a] (Gy)	RT ± CTx	>25%–50% incidence (Gy)	Volume	<5%–10% incidence dose[a] (Gy)	RT ± CTx	>25%–50% incidence (Gy)	
Lung	Subacute pneumonitis or late fibrosis	18–20 15–18	(CTx−) (CTx+)	24–25 21–24	<30% of one lung	25–30 <20	(CTx−) (CTx+)	45–50 >35	++
Heart	Subacute pericarditis	35–40		>50	<50%	40–50		60–70	+/−
	Late cardiomyopathy	45–50	(CTx−)	>60	<25%	<40	(CTx−)	>70	+++
Liver	Subacute hepatopathy	25–30 20–25	(CTx−) (CTx+)	>40 >35	<60%		NA	40	++
Kidney	Subacute or late nephropathy	18–20 16–18	(CTx−) (CTx+)	24–28 22–26	>50%	20–24	NA	>30	+
	Late hypertension	Similar to subacute levels			>50%	20–25	NA	>35	+/−
Small bowel	Subacute enteropathy	15–25	NA	>40	<50%	20–25	NA	>60	+
Brain	Late necrosis	54–60	NA	>65	<50%	Equal to whole brain	NA		+/−
Spinal cord	Subacute or late	40–45	NA	>50	<15%	45–50	NA	>55	−

(CTx−), without prior, concurrent, or subsequent chemotherapy; (CTx+), interaction with one or more chemotherapeutic agents; NA, not applicable.
[a]Dose assumes conventional fractionation (150–200 cGy once daily, 5 days per week); ++, if ≥40% of liver excluded from dose ≥18 Gy, remainder of organ can receive doses up to 40+ Gy; +++, impact of chemotherapy on late necrosis not demonstrated; added subacute toxicities with methotrexate discussed in text.

within 2 months to 1 to 2 years after cardiac irradiation, most often with doses higher than 30 to 35 Gy to most of the heart.[125,126] Signs of pericardial effusion are apparent on imaging with characteristic electrocardiogram findings; symptoms are present in 50% to 75% of cases, typically mild and self-limited. It is uncommon to see evolution toward significant pericardial fibrosis or chronic, constrictive changes.[126,127]

Late cardiac effects include restrictive cardiomyopathy, valvular heart disease, and coronary artery disease; conductive deficits have also been noted. The pathophysiology is classically related to capillary endothelial damage with consequent luminal obstruction, fibrin formation, and platelet thrombi leading to ischemia, myocardial cell death, and fibrosis.[124,126]

As an underlying mechanism, fibrosis affects cardiac function and compliance; following irradiation in very young children, there is relative limitation on growth and development of the heart with diminished left ventricular mass and/or end diastolic dimension.[124,128,129] The frequency of late congestive heart failure and symptomatic angina pectoris with onset beyond 5 to 10 years posttherapy is more common following irradiation in children and adolescents than in young adults 20 to 40 years old.[121] Subclinical cardiovascular disease has been documented in up to 50% to 55% of adults surviving irradiation and/or anthracycline-based chemotherapy in childhood; a similar occurrence of conductive deficits and arrhythmias has been noted.[128,130] Much of the late effects data have been described following radiation doses of 35 to 40 Gy to most of the heart in the context of earlier management of Hodgkin lymphoma; there are yet little data quantifying cardiac changes after current dose levels of 15 to 25 Gy.[128,129]

Late mortality following thoracic irradiation is largely related to an excess risk of myocardial infarction documented as early as 1 to 4 years after irradiation; the peak incidence 15 to 19 years post-therapy has been estimated at 3.5 to 7 times the age-adjusted rate and persists to 25 years after irradiation.[118,122,129]

Kidney. Radiation effects on the kidney are usually subacute and late phenomena; acute changes in renal function are with TBI for BMT (see below). In adults, renal tolerance is typically quoted at 20 to 25 Gy fractionated dose to more than 50% of the functioning renal volume.[131,132] In children, the most common settings where renal tolerance is approached include retroperitoneal tumors (neuroblastoma, sarcomas, Wilms' tumor) or the few instances where full abdominal irradiation is indicated. Renal tolerance defines treatment planning for tumors in this region, requiring limitation of dose to at least 50% of the renal volume to levels typically below 14 to 16 Gy in children whose treatment includes irradiation and chemotherapy, with particular attention to cisplatin. In the TBI setting, protection of even a portion of the kidneys diminishes acute or subacute renal dysfunction.[133]

Late or chronic radiation nephropathy is marked by hypertension, anemia, proteinuria, hematuria, increased serum creatinine, and decreased glomerular filtration rate (GFR). In its more severe clinical presentation, signs mimic the hemolytic-uremic syndrome.[134–136] Chronic, progressive renal dysfunction reflects progressive glomerulosclerosis and tubulointerstitial fibrosis as a result of initial and ongoing chronic inflammatory cytokine responses resulting in aberrant renovascular and renal parenchymal cell function. The kidney has been somewhat unique as animal models have confirmed the systemic hormonal renin-angiotensin-ACE system as central to complex molecular and enzymatic mechanisms responsible for renovascular damage. Even more unique has been documentation in animal models and a recent prospective clinical trial (with TBI) that captopril, an ACE inhibitor, can prevent or ameliorate radiation effects on the kidney; in the clinical

study, the drug was highly effective in preserving GFR at 1 year post-TBI when administered after engraftment and continued for 1 year.[137,138]

Gastrointestinal Tract. Subacute or late enteropathy are relatively uncommon now in children. Earlier reports of frequent radiation-related enteropathy, often requiring surgical management for small bowel obstructive disease, have largely been resolved with more experience in coordinating surgery, abdominal and/or pelvic irradiation, and chemotherapy.[139,140] Children requiring wide abdominal irradiation or pelvic therapy to doses of 45 to 50 Gy or more are yet at risk for late enteropathy or proctitis. Reactions tend to be greater after pre-irradiation surgery (with adhesions often "fixing" bowel into the low abdomen-pelvis). Symptoms often mimic small bowel inflammatory disease, although there is a noted lack of C-reactive protein elevation in radiation-related late bowel injury.[141,142] Animal models have recently shown increased expression of cyclooxygenase 2 (COX-2) in both vascular endothelial cells in the GI tract and in fibroblasts, suggesting a role for COX-2 inhibitors in management.[143]

Endocrine Effects. Endocrine deficits after irradiation have been well documented following cranial and craniospinal irradiation, as well as with cervical nodal irradiation for Hodgkin lymphoma. It is of interest that post-operative, pre-irradiation provocative endocrine testing in children with localized CNS tumors (prior to entry on a St. Jude protocol for local irradiation) showed diminished hormonal secretion in two-thirds of cases, including almost half the children/adolescents with localized posterior fossa tumors.[144] Pre-irradiation deficits were common for growth hormone (GH) and thyroid stimulating hormone (TSH), while reduction in adrenocorticotropic hormone (ACTH) reserve and gonadotropin (corrected for age) was noted in 15% to 20% of cases.[144] From the same program, prospectively studied endocrine status after craniospinal irradiation and chemotherapy for embryonal tumors showed deficits at 4 years post-therapy in growth hormone (93%), TSH (23%), T3-T4 (primary hypothyroidism, 65%), and ACTH (38%).[145] A dose response was not apparent for GH or ACTH or gondotropins (suggesting the median 42–44 Gy to the hypothalamic-pituitary region was higher than the threshold for these hormones), while the frequency of TSH reduction was dose-related, with substantially greater impact following doses approximating 50 Gy.[145]

Primary hypothyroidism after spinal irradiation has been noted to be dose-dependent, approaching 90% following spinal irradiation delivering 30 to 35 Gy to the thyroid in exit.[145,146] Similar data in Hodgkin lymphoma have shown primary hypothyroidism in 75% of children following doses higher than 26 Gy, with a median onset of chemical hypothyroidism 18 to 30 months postirradiation.[147,148] It is of interest that a proportion of cases will show relative recovery of thyroid function 3 to 5 years after documented deficiency.[147,148] There are preliminary clinical data indicating relative protection of thyroid T3-T4 secretion when L-thyroxine is administered to suppress TSH during irradiation.[149]

Gonadal Effects. Precocious puberty is relatively common after low-dose cranial irradiation, attributed to cortical disinhibition of the hypothalamus and imbalance in gonadotropin levels and occurring more frequently in girls.[150–152] Long-term follow-up after 18 to 24 Gy cranial irradiation (preventive therapy in acute leukemia) confirms progression through puberty and menarche, but decreased LH secretion and abbreviated luteal phase, typical of incipient ovarian failure noted even in women in their 20s following irradiation early in childhood.[153,154] Women surviving ALL show lower rates of pregnancy if treatment included low-dose cranial irradiation.[155]

The gonads are particularly radiosensitive; alterations in ovarian endocrine secretions are noted following doses as low as 250 to 400 cGy.[156,157] The maturing ovarian follicles are most radiosensitive, with follicular damage leading to a decrease in the fixed ovarian reserve, ultimately limiting hormone production and resulting in early menopause.[157] The oocytes themselves are similarly sensitive to irradiation; the loss following a total dose of 200 cGy is estimated to approximate 50%.[158] The dose associated with permanent sterility is age-dependent, falling from 18 Gy at 10 years old to 14 Gy at 30 years old.[159] In a large series from the Childhood Cancer Survivor Study (CCSS), it was found that women who had received 30 Gy or more to the hypothalamic-pituitary volume or 5 Gy or more to the pelvis had a pregnancy rate approximating 50% of that seen normally.[160] Women survivors who do get pregnant after pelvic irradiation are at greater risk of spontaneous abortion, preterm delivery, or placental abnormalities secondary to incomplete uterine development or diminished plasticity.[161] Such effects are most apparent following pelvic irradiation in young children with doses in excess of 15 to 30 Gy.

Leydig cell function in boys is decreased after dose levels approximating 24 Gy.[162,163] In adolescents and young adults with Hodgkin lymphoma, pretreatment sperm analyses are normal in only 20% of instances; oligospermia and abnormal morphology or motility are noted in a majority of patients.[164] Following irradiation, azoospermia is noted within 6 to 8 weeks after the start of fractionated doses of 200 cGy.[165] Within 3 to 5 years, some degree of recovery is apparent in young adults whose testicular exposure was less than 200 to 500 cGy; 25% of men at that interval remaining significantly oligospermic.[166] Large-field abdominal irradiation to doses of 35 to 40 Gy result in sufficient intrabody scatter to deliver 200 to 400 cGy to the testes unless specific shielding is provided.

Central Nervous System Effects. The pathophysiology of CNS changes following irradiation is complex. Acute changes are uncommon; radiation "edema" or worsening of tumor-related neurologic signs is a rare event usually associated with high radiation dose (single fraction of 750–1000 cGy).[167] Subacute changes are largely noted in the white matter, classically attributed to both secondary changes (relative ischemia following endothelial cell damage with subsequent changes in small vessel narrowing resulting in focal or more generalized *demyelinization* or *white matter necrosis*) and primary effects (loss of proliferative capacity in the O-2A glial progenitor cells, with failure to replenish the physiologic maturation and replication of oligodendrocytes).[168–170] More recent data show the interdependence of glial, vascular, and neuronal compartments of the nervous system. Direct effects on astrocytes may (a) alter O2-A progenitors' proliferation, differentiation, and migration through secretion of growth factors and (b) similarly impact the terminally differentiated oligodendrocytes, responsible for myelin formation.[171,172] Astrocytes are central to maintaining the blood-brain barrier, and they produce both VEGF and angiotensinogen.[173,174] Microglia respond to radiation damage, inducing local inflammatory effects. Neuronal cells, once considered postmitotic and fixed, are now regarded as the ultimate expression of radiation-induced CNS toxicities.[175] Radiation therapy has been shown to deplete the *subependymal zone* of proliferating neural stem cells in a dose-dependent manner; repopulation is impaired over prolonged intervals post-irradiation.[176]

Clinically, subacute reactions include the so-called somnolence syndrome, notably somnolence, anorexia, and sometimes low-grade fever seen 4 to 8 weeks after large volume brain irradiation either in ALL (where the interaction with methotrexate may increase the apparent frequency of this phenomenon) or primary CNS tumors.[177] In parallel, local irradiation for brain tumors may result in transient exacerbation of neurologic signs associated with the tumor; it is not unusual to see apparent "progression" between 4 to 8 weeks or as long as 8 to 12 months after irradiation, manifest by expansion, increased contrast enhancement, and/or intralesional "necrosis." Although reactive phenomena are usually self-limited and respond to corticosteroids if necessary, on occasion, central necrosis and peripheral reactive gliosis combine to produce a lesion that "balloons out" sufficiently that mass effect results in progressive local neurologic signs requiring surgical intervention[178] (Fig. 13.6). In low-grade tumors, the phenomenon is typically confined and self-limited; in high-grade gliomas or brain stem gliomas, subacute changes mimic the "pseudoprogression" noted in adult malignant gliomas. In areas outside the primary tumor, but typically within the high-dose radiation region, one can see parenchymal areas of focal white matter reactivity or apparent leptomeningeal changes mimicking tumor involvement as a subacute phenomenon; such signs usually abate spontaneously over several months but can progress to frank necrosis.[179] Most important is the recognition of such phenomena and the patience to follow the temporal course, perhaps the most effective test differentiating transitory reactions from tumor progression or extension.[180,181]

Late CNS effects include focal necrosis (a well-defined entity noted within the high-dose volume, typically presenting between 6 and 24 months postirradiation).[169,182] Differentiating focal necrosis from tumor progression remains an important challenge; intralesional necrosis may simply represent the manner in which the tumor is responding to irradiation, while focal necrosis outside the targeted tumor is more likely to be true CNS injury. Current imaging technologies (e.g., diffusion and perfusion studies on MRI, MR spectroscopy, PET) help differentiate active areas of metabolism and/or proliferation (i.e., tumor progression) from areas of limited perfusion, increased lactate on spectroscopy, and lack of PET avidity more likely to represent treatment-related CNS injury/necrosis. Focal necrosis is typically seen only with doses in excess of 60 Gy; the incidence is greatly increased with dose per fraction in excess of 240 to 300 cGy.[169]

Changes in large vessels have been noted following significant radiation dose levels to the circle of Willis in the parasellar region.[183] Focal narrowing of one or more of the six major intracranial vessels is most often seen after irradiation for craniopharyngioma or optic chiasmatic/hypothalamic gliomas, tumors then tend to infiltrate around or adjacent to the major vasculature.[183] Occlusion of the three major vessels emanating from the circle of Willis, sometimes bilaterally, is called *moyamoya syndrome*. The small, convoluted collateral vessels adjacent to the occluded major vessels produce a pattern on angiography termed *puff of smoke* or *moyamoya* in Japanese. The phenomenon is most common in children irradiated before 5 years of age, particularly in the setting of NF-1.[183,184] The median time to the recognition of moyamoya syndrome is 3 to 4 years post-therapy; children and adolescents are at considerable risk for stroke at a relatively young age. Post-irradiation vascular changes can also manifest as cavernomas, most of which are benign, if occasionally associated with intracranial hemorrhage.[185] Preventive antithrombotic therapies or surgical anastamoses to bypass the affected areas or provide new vascular growth into the brain are intended to increase blood flow into the affected cerebral hemisphere.

The spinal cord is often the treatment-limiting organ of interest. Although classically accepted as showing myelopathy at dose levels of 50 Gy or more, recent data have been interpreted to show a 5% risk of myelopathy at 59 Gy, with only a 0.03% risk at 45 Gy and 0.2% at 50 Gy.[186] Radiation myelopathy is an uncommon late event, typically developing toward a complete Brown-Sequard syndrome.

Cranial nerve effects are quite uncommon with conventional doses of irradiation. Noting concerns regarding cisplatin administration and irradiation as ototoxic interventions,

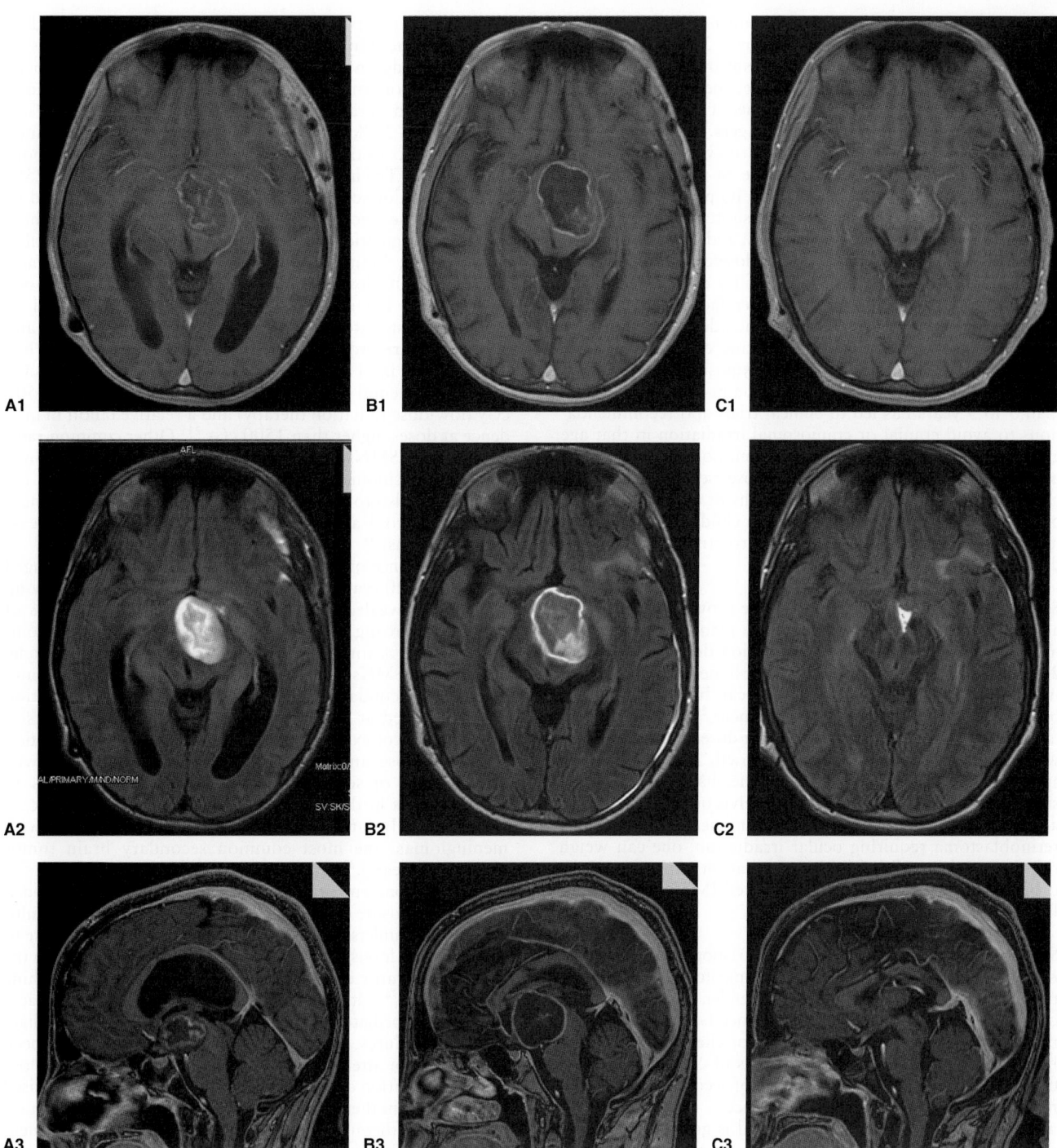

FIGURE 13.6 A: Juvenile pilocytic astrocytoma, left midbrain-anterior thalamic region; presenting magnetic resonance imaging (MRI) prior to radiation therapy. **B:** Imaging 3 months after completion of radiation therapy, at which point, long tract signs increased significantly, requiring corticosteroid management. Note the increased tumor size with enlarging central necrosis. **C:** MRI appearance 3 years after radiation therapy. Intervening peripheral left cerebrovascular accident (CVA, seen on C1, C2) requiring ongoing antiplatelet therapy. The patient has no residual long tract signs and is essentially normal on neurologic examination.

studies have assessed the impact of radiation therapy in *otodoxicity*. Cisplatin-related ototoxicity is early, bilateral, and dose-related, appearing as high-frequency sensorineural loss during a course of cisplatin chemotherapy. Radiation-related ototoxicity is a late, random event occurring as an acute, unilateral, irreversible hearing loss. Radiation oto-toxicity occurs beyond 3–5 years post-therapy following doses of more than 35 to 50 Gy to the cochlea (absent cis-platin).[187,188]

Neurocognitive effects of cranial irradiation have been well documented. Treatment of the whole brain or areas most associated with learning and memory (hippocampus, medial temporal lobes) results in an age-dependent, dose-dependent decline in intelligence quotient (IQ) over 2 to 5 years after radiation therapy.[189,190] The mechanism of intellectual loss has been related to a constant rate of decline beginning immediately after radiation therapy for younger children and noted only after a several year delay in teenagers.[191,192] The pattern of IQ loss seems to be based on difficulties with attention and memory, resulting in gradual decline in assimilating new knowledge and consequent decrease in IQ performance.[193,194] Radiation parameters of dose; volume subtended by relatively low-, intermediate-, or high-dose levels; and specific details of neuroanatomic site-specific radiation dose can be modeled to predict higher or lower likelihood of IQ deficits following cranial or local irradiation.[73,195] Other factors also impact learning and apparent intelligence, including postoperative neurologic deficits, presumably reflecting cerebellar damage in the posterior fossa setting.[196] The exquisite relationship of substantial IQ loss to cranial irradiation in children younger than 3 to 5 years has led to clinical trials and recommendations to avoid cranial or craniospinal irradiation in that age group. Focal posterior fossa irradiation, notably sparing the medial temporal lobes re radiation dose, seems safe even in children younger than 12 to 18 months of age, on the basis of extensive, prospective assessment in children with ependymomas who demonstrated little treatment-related IQ deficit.[197]

Somatic Effects. Late changes in bone growth and integrity as well as soft tissue development are readily apparent primary bone effects noted after radiation doses at or above 20 to 25 Gy to the epiphyseal areas of bone growth.[198–200] In infants, doses as low as 6 to 10 Gy can have an effect on bone growth and soft tissue development.[200,201] It is important to realize that irradiation, even at doses of 36 to 40 Gy, will impede but not ablate bone growth in areas like the spinal column.[202] Growth in long bones has been relatively simple to quantitate; changes in the pelvis or other flat bones are more complex to measure.[203] In unique settings, such as retinoblastoma requiring ocular irradiation, one can weigh the potential benefit of limiting radiation exposure to the orbit (re both growth) by sophisticated IMRT planning or PBRT.[204]

Secondary Malignant Neoplasms. Carcinogenesis following radiation exposure has been well documented for over a century; details regarding host factors (gender, age, genetic susceptibility syndromes), radiation parameters (physical type of radiations, dose), and the influence of chemotherapy have been well documented in large cohorts of children surviving cancer therapies.[205–210] The incidence of secondary malignant neoplasms (SMNs) is of greater concern in children than adults where the likelihood of survival is greater in children and the period of risk extends over decades after cancer therapy.

Radiation-related SMNs are documented at doses as low as 10 cGy. In most pediatric settings, there is a dose response relationship within the therapeutic dose range of 15 to 60 Gy.[208,209] The two disease groups best studied regarding SMN are Hodgkin lymphoma and ALL. Large cohorts of pediatric Hodgkin lymphoma survivors have recently been analyzed to confirm the incidence of secondary solid tumors, largely related to radiation therapy, exceeding 7% to 10% at 20 years and 25% at 30 years posttherapy—a relative incidence of 14 to 18 times that of the normal, age-adjusted population.[211,212] The incidence of breast cancer approaches 25% to 35% in adolescents and young women and is related to radiation dose (increased above 35 Gy) and volume (where supradiaphragmatic irradiation without including the axilla, for example, limits the volume of breast subtended and results in a 20% lower incidence).[213,214] Thyroid cancer is one of the most common SMNs, also more often noted in females; an estimated 85% of thyroid cancers in children and adolescents are radiation-induced.[215] Interestingly, there is a dose-related increase in thyroid cancer between 10 cGy (largely incidental or diagnostic radiation doses) and 1500 cGy (low-dose radiation therapy) and a relative falloff in incidence at doses higher than 1500 cGy.[215] Other common radiation-related SMNs in Hodgkin lymphoma survivors include epithelial carcinomas (GI tract, lung) and sarcomas (soft tissue, bone). Also to be noted is the occurrence of benign neoplasms—thyroid adenomas, osteochondromas, and breast fibroadenomas.[211]

The incidence of SMN after therapy for ALL has averaged 4% at 15 to 20 years post-therapy.[216–218] Long-term follow-up at St. Jude revealed SMN 20 years after therapy in 20% of patients following cranial or craniospinal irradiation compared with 1% for those treated with chemotherapy alone; 20 of the 44 SMNs were benign (basal cell carcinoma, meningioma).[219] Secondary brain tumors after cranial irradiation were estimated at less than 1% to 3% in earlier reports; a unique protocol experience at St. Jude combining irradiation with high-dose antimetabolite therapy ultimately showed an incidence of secondary malignant gliomas of 12% to 20%.[220,221] As in the overall CCSS, secondary gliomas occur relatively early (at a median of 5–9 years) compared with meningiomas, the most common secondary brain tumor (median 17 years).[220–222]

Current concern regarding SMN has focused on the added low-dose exposure inherent in IMRT, where the use of multiple small "beamlets" results in a greater total body exposure to low radiation levels due to minor radiation "leakage" from the linear accelerator collimator during much longer "machine on" intervals.[76,79] It is key to monitor SMNs as IMRT replaces 3-D–CRT in pediatric settings.[76,223,224] Exposure rates for diagnostic procedures, including CT simulation, have also been highlighted for attention to techniques that can minimize "out of field" radiation exposure.[76] Similar concern has been raised re proton beam therapy, where current technology largely uses scatter beam therapy, which is associated with sufficient neutron beam contamination to be of potential concern, especially in children who appear to be more susceptible to neutron-induced carcinogenesis.[76,225] Implementation of scanning beam technologies is now ongoing, a modification that should essentially eliminate concerns re neutron exposure.[71,77]

References

1. Powell S, McMillan TJ. DNA damage and repair following treatment with ionizing radiation. Radiother Oncol 1990;19:95–108.
2. Prise KM, Schettino G, Folkard M, et al. New insights on cell death from radiation exposure. Lancet Oncol 2005;6:520–528.
3. Bernier J, Hall EJ, Giaccia A. Radiation oncology: a century of achievements. Nat Rev Cancer 2004;4:737–747.
4. Painter R, Young B. Radiosensitivity in ataxia-telangiectasia: a new explanation. Proc Natl Acad Sci U S A 1980;77:7315.
5. Taylor AM, Harnden DG, Arlett CF, et al. Ataxia telangiectasia: a human mutation with abnormal radiation sensitivity. Nature 1975;258:427–429.

6. Bakkenist CJ, Kastan MB. DNA damage activates ATM through intermolecular autophosphorylation and dimer dissociation. Nature 2003;421:499–506.
7. Crompton NE, Shi YQ, Emery GC, et al. Sources of variation in patient response to radiation treatment. Int J Radiat Oncol Biol Phys 2001;49:547–554.
8. Demuth I, Digweed M. The clinical manifestation of a defective response to DNA double-strand breaks as exemplified by Nijmegen breakage syndrome. Oncogene 2007;26:7792–7798.
9. Eschrich SA, Pramana J, Zhang H, et al. A gene expression model of intrinsic tumor radiosensitivity: prediction of response and prognosis after chemoradiation. Int J Radiat Oncol Biol Phys 2009;75:489–496.

10. Weller M, Felsberg J, Hartmann C, et al. Molecular predictors of progression-free and overall survival in patients with newly diagnosed glioblastoma: a prospective translational study of the German Glioma Network. J Clin Oncol 2009;27(34):5743–5750.

11. Bergonie J, Tribondeau L. L'interpretation de queiques resultats de la radiotherapie et essai de fixation d'une technique rationnelle. C R Seances Acad Sci 1906;143:983–985.

12. Zeman EM. Radiobiology: biologic basis of radiation oncology. In: Gunderson LL, Tepper JE, eds. Clinical radiation oncology. 2nd ed. Churchill Livingstone, 2007:3–46.

13. Withers HR. The dose-survival relationship for irradiation of epithelial cells of mouse skin. Br J Radiol 1967;40:187–194.

14. Withers HR. Regeneration of intestinal mucosa after irradiation. Cancer 1971; 28:75–81.

15. Coutard H. Principles of x-ray therapy of malignant disease. Lancet 1934;2:1–12.

16. Meyn RE. Apoptosis and response to radiation: implications for radiation therapy. Oncology (Williston Park) 1997;11:349–356.

17. Lowe SW, Ruley HE, Jacks T, et al. p53-dependent apoptosis modulates the cytotoxicity of anticancer agents. Cell 1993;74:957–967.

18. Thomlinson RH, Gray LH. The histological structure of some human lung cancers and the possible implications for radiotherapy. Br J Cancer 1955;9:539–549.

19. Kallman RF. The phenomenon of reoxygenation and its implications for fractionated radiotherapy. Radiology 1972;105:135–142.

20. Gatenby RA, Kessler HB, Rosenblum JS, et al. Oxygen distribution in squamous cell carcinoma metastases and its relationship to outcome of radiation therapy. Int J Radiat Oncol Biol Phys 1988;14:831–838.

21. Dische S. What have we learnt from hyperbaric oxygen? Radiother Oncol 1991;20(suppl 1):71–74.

22. Laurence VM, Ward R, Dennis IF, et al. Carbogen breathing with nicotinamide improves the oxygen status of tumours in patients. Br J Cancer 1995;72:198–205.

23. Overgaard J, Horsman MR. Modification of hypoxia-induced radioresistance in tumors by the use of oxygen and sensitizers. Semin Radiat Oncol 1996;6:10–21.

24. Formenti SC, Demaria S. Systemic effects of local radiotherapy. Lancet Oncol 2009;10:718–726.

25. Barcellos-Hoff MH, Park C, Wright EG. Radiation and the microenvironment—tumorigenesis and therapy. Nat Rev Cancer 2005;5:867–875.

26. Chakraborty M, Abrams SI, Coleman CN, et al. External beam radiation of tumors alters phenotype of tumor cells to render them susceptible to vaccine-mediated T-cell killing. Cancer Res 2004;64:4328–4337.

27. Joiner MC, Marples B, Lambin P, et al. Low-dose hypersensitivity: current status and possible mechanisms. Int J Radiat Oncol Biol Phys 2001;49:379–389.

28. Ellis F. Dose, time and fractionation: a clinical hypothesis. Clin Radiol 1969;20:1–7.

29. Orton CG, Ellis F. A simplification in the use of the NSD concept in practical radiotherapy. Br J Radiol 1973;46:529–537.

30. Thames HD Jr, Withers HR, Peters LJ, et al. Changes in early and late radiation responses with altered dose fractionation: implications for dose-survival relationships. Int J Radiat Oncol Biol Phys 1982;8:219–226.

31. Thames HD, Bentzen SM, Turesson I, et al. Time-dose factors in radiotherapy: a review of the human data. Radiother Oncol 1990;19:219–235.

32. Barendsen GW. Dose fractionation, dose rate and iso-effect relationships for normal tissue responses. Int J Radiat Oncol Biol Phys 1982;8:1981–1997.

33. Carrie C, Muracciole X, Gomez F, et al. Conformal radiotherapy, reduced boost volume, hyperfractionated radiotherapy, and online quality control in standard risk medulloblastoma without chemotherapy: results of the French M-SFOP 98 protocol. Int J Radiat Oncol Biol Phys 2005;63:711–716.

34. Horiot JC, Le FR, N'Guyen T, et al. Hyperfractionation versus conventional fractionation in oropharyngeal carcinoma: final analysis of a randomized trial of the EORTC cooperative group of radiotherapy. Radiother Oncol 1992;25:231–241.

35. Miralbell R, Lomax A, Cella L, et al. Potential reduction of the incidence of radiation-induced second cancers by using proton beams in the treatment of pediatric tumors. Int J Radiat Oncol Biol Phys 2002;54:824–829.

36. Cox JD. Fractionation: a paradigm for clinical research in radiation oncology. Int J Radiat Oncol Biol Phys 1987;13:1271–1281.

37. Paganetti H, Niemierko A, Ancukiewicz M, et al. Relative biological effectiveness (RBE) values for proton beam therapy. Int J Radiat Oncol Biol Phys 2002;53:407–421.

38. Suzuki M, Kase Y, Yamaguchi H, et al. Relative biological effectiveness for cell-killing effect on various human cell lines irradiated with heavy-ion medical accelerator in Chiba (HIMAC) carbon-ion beams. Int J Radiat Oncol Biol Phys 2000;48:241–250.

39. Wambersie A, Richard F, Breteau N. Development of fast neutron therapy worldwide: radiobiological, clinical and technical aspects. Acta Oncol 1994;33:261–274.

40. Laramore GE, Krall JM, Griffin TW, et al. Neutron versus photon irradiation for unresectable salivary gland tumors: final report of an RTOG-MRC randomized clinical trial: Radiation Therapy Oncology Group: Medical Research Council. Int J Radiat Oncol Biol Phys 1993;27:235–240.

41. Barth RF. Boron neutron capture therapy at the crossroads: challenges and opportunities. Appl Radiat Isot 2009;67:S3–S6.

42. Henriksson R, Capala J, Michanek A, et al. Boron neutron capture therapy (BNCT) for glioblastoma multiforme: a phase II study evaluating a prolonged high-dose of boronophenylalanine (BPA). Radiother Oncol 2008;88:183–191.

43. Nakagawa Y, Kageji T, Mizobuchi Y, et al. Clinical results of BNCT for malignant brain tumors in children. Appl Radiat Isot 2009;67:S27–S30.

44. Laskar S, Bahl G, Ann MM, et al. Interstitial brachytherapy for childhood soft tissue sarcoma. Pediatr Blood Cancer 2007;49:649–655.

45. Magne N, Haie-Meder C. Brachytherapy for genital-tract rhabdomyosarcomas in girls: technical aspects, reports, and perspectives. Lancet Oncol 2007;8:725–729.

46. Martinez-Monge R, Cambeiro M, San-Julian M, et al. Use of brachytherapy in children with cancer: the search for an uncomplicated cure. Lancet Oncol 2006;7:157–166.

47. Viani GA, Novaes PE, Jacinto AA, et al. High-dose-rate brachytherapy for soft tissue sarcoma in children: a single institution experience. Radiat Oncol 2008;3:9.

48. Goodman KA, Wolden SL, LaQuaglia MP, et al. Intraoperative high-dose-rate brachytherapy for pediatric solid tumors: a 10-year experience. Brachytherapy 2003;2:139–146.

49. Voges J, Sturm V, Lehrke R, et al. Cystic craniopharyngioma: long-term results after intracavitary irradiation with stereotactically applied colloidal beta-emitting radioactive sources. Neurosurgery 1997;40:263–269.

50. Albright AL, Hadjipanayis CG, Lunsford LD, et al. Individualized treatment of pediatric craniopharyngiomas. Childs Nerv Syst 2005;21:649–654.

51. Derrey S, Blond S, Reyns N, et al. Management of cystic craniopharyngiomas with stereotactic endocavitary irradiation using colloidal 186Re: a retrospective study of 48 consecutive patients. Neurosurgery 2008;63:1045–1052.

52. Hodgson DC, Goumnerova LC, Loeffler JS, et al. Radiosurgery in the management of pediatric brain tumors. Int J Radiat Oncol Biol Phys 2001;50:929–935.

53. Han SR, Yoon SW, Yee GT, et al. Novalis radiosurgery of optic gliomas in children: preliminary report. Pediatr Neurosurg 2007;43:251–257.

54. Keshavarzi S, Meltzer H, Ben-Haim S, et al. Initial clinical experience with frameless optically guided stereotactic radiosurgery/radiotherapy in pediatric patients. Childs Nerv Syst 2009;25:837–844.

55. Calcerrada Diaz-Santos N, Blasco Amaro JA, Cardiel GA, et al. The safety and efficacy of robotic image-guided radiosurgery system treatment for intra- and extracranial lesions: a systematic review of the literature. Radiother Oncol 2008;89:245–253.

56. Adler JR Jr, Murphy MJ, Chang SD, et al. Image-guided robotic radiosurgery. Neurosurgery 1999;44:1299–1306.

57. Flannery T, Kano H, Martin JJ, et al. Boost radiosurgery as a strategy after failure of initial management of pediatric primitive neuroectodermal tumors. J Neurosurg Pediatr 2009;3:205–210.

58. Kano H, Niranjan A, Kondziolka D, et al. Role of stereotactic radiosurgery in the management of pineal parenchymal tumors. Prog Neurol Surg 2009;23:44–58.

59. Kobayashi T. Long-term results of gamma knife radiosurgery for 100 consecutive cases of craniopharyngioma and a treatment strategy. Prog Neurol Surg 2009;22:63–76.

60. Lee M, Kalani MY, Cheshier S, et al. Radiation therapy and CyberKnife radiosurgery in the management of craniopharyngiomas. Neurosurg Focus 2008;24:E4.

61. Dodd RL, Ryu MR, Kamnerdsupaphon P, et al. CyberKnife radiosurgery for benign intradural extramedullary spinal tumors. Neurosurgery 2006;58:674–685.

62. International Committee on Radiation Units. ICRU report 50: prescribing, recording, and reporting photon beam therapy. Bethesda, MD: International Committee on Radiation Units and Measurements, 1993.

63. Moran JM, Elshaikh MA, Lawrence TS. Radiotherapy: what can be achieved by technical improvements in dose delivery? Lancet Oncol 2005;6:51–58.

64. Ling CC, Humm J, Larson S, et al. Towards multidimensional radiotherapy (MD-CRT): biological imaging and biological conformality. Int J Radiat Oncol Biol Phys 2000;47:551–560.

65. Veldeman L, Madani I, Hulstaert F, et al. Evidence behind use of intensity-modulated radiotherapy: a systematic review of comparative clinical studies. Lancet Oncol 2008;9:367–375.

66. Webb S. Advances in three-dimensional conformal radiation therapy physics with intensity modulation. Lancet Oncol 2000;1:30–36.

67. Levin WP, Kooy H, Loeffler JS, et al. Proton beam therapy. Br J Cancer 2005; 93:849–854.

68. Klein EE, Maserang B, Wood R, et al. Peripheral doses from pediatric IMRT. Med Phys 2006;33:2525–2531.

69. Kleinerman RA, Tucker MA, Tarone RE, et al. Risk of new cancers after radiotherapy in long-term survivors of retinoblastoma: an extended follow-up. J Clin Oncol 2005; 23:2272–2279.

70. Kry SF, Salehpour M, Followill DS, et al. The calculated risk of fatal secondary malignancies from intensity-modulated radiation therapy. Int J Radiat Oncol Biol Phys 2005;62:1195–1203.

71. St CW, Adams JA, Bues M, et al. Advantage of protons compared to conventional X-ray or IMRT in the treatment of a pediatric patient with medulloblastoma. Int J Radiat Oncol Biol Phys 2004;58:727–734.

72. Merchant TE, Hua CH, Shukla H, et al. Proton versus photon radiotherapy for common pediatric brain tumors: comparison of models of dose characteristics and their relationship to cognitive function. Pediatr Blood Cancer 2008;51:110–117.

73. Merchant TE, Kiehna EN, Li C, et al. Radiation dosimetry predicts IQ after conformal radiation therapy in pediatric patients with localized ependymoma. Int J Radiat Oncol Biol Phys 2005;63:1546–1554.

74. Weber DC, Trofimov AV, DeLaney TF, et al. A treatment planning comparison of intensity modulated photon and proton therapy for paraspinal sarcomas. Int J Radiat Oncol Biol Phys 2004;58:1596–1606.

75. Lee CT, Bilton SD, Famiglietti RM, et al. Treatment planning with protons for pediatric retinoblastoma, medulloblastoma, and pelvic sarcoma: how do protons compare with other conformal techniques? Int J Radiat Oncol Biol Phys 2005;63:362–372.

76. Hall EJ. Intensity-modulated radiation therapy, protons, and the risk of second cancers. Int J Radiat Oncol Biol Phys 2006;65:1–7.

77. Schulz-Ertner D, Tsujii H. Particle radiation therapy using proton and heavier ion beams. J Clin Oncol 2007;25:953–964.

78. Glatstein E, Glick J, Kaiser L, et al. Should randomized clinical trials be required for proton radiotherapy? An alternative view. J Clin Oncol 2008;26:2438–2439.

79. Suit H, Kooy H, Trofimov A, et al. Should positive phase III clinical trial data be required before proton beam therapy is more widely adopted? No. Radiother Oncol 2008;86:148–153.

80. Lundkvist J, Ekman M, Ericsson SR, et al. Cost-effectiveness of proton radiation in the treatment of childhood medulloblastoma. Cancer 2005;103:793–801.

81. Dawson LA, Jaffray DA. Advances in image-guided radiation therapy. J Clin Oncol 2007;25:938–946.

82. Steel GG. Terminology in the description of drug-radiation interactions. Int J Radiat Oncol Biol Phys 1979;5:1145–1150.

83. Dewit L. Combined treatment of radiation and cisdiamminedichloroplatinum (II): a review of experimental and clinical data. Int J Radiat Oncol Biol Phys 1987;13:403–426.

84. Wilson GD, Bentzen SM, Harari PM. Biologic basis for combining drugs with radiation. Semin Radiat Oncol 2006;16:2–9.

85. Lawrence TS, Davis MA, Loney TL. Fluoropyrimidine-mediated radiosensitization depends on cyclin E-dependent kinase activation. Cancer Res 1996;56:3203–3206.

86. Sawada N, Ishikawa T, Sekiguchi F, et al. X-ray irradiation induces thymidine phosphorylase and enhances the efficacy of capecitabine (Xeloda) in human cancer xenografts. Clin Cancer Res 1999;5:2948–2953.

87. Brown JM. Therapeutic targets in radiotherapy. Int J Radiat Oncol Biol Phys 2001;49:319–326.

88. Chakravarti A, Dicker A, Mehta M. The contribution of epidermal growth factor receptor (EGFR) signaling pathway to radioresistance in human gliomas: a review of preclinical and correlative clinical data. Int J Radiat Oncol Biol Phys 2004;58:927–931.

89. Pollack IF, Jakacki RI, Blaney SM, et al. Phase I trial of imatinib in children with newly diagnosed brainstem and recurrent malignant gliomas: a Pediatric Brain Tumor Consortium report. Neuro Oncol 2007;9:145–160.

90. Haas-Kogan DA, Banerjee A, Kocak M, et al. Phase I trial of tipifarnib in children with newly diagnosed intrinsic diffuse brainstem glioma. Neuro Oncol 2008; 10:341–347.

91. Broniscer A, Baker SJ, Stewart CF, et al. Phase I and pharmacokinetic studies of erlotinib administered concurrently with radiotherapy for children, adolescents, and young adults with high-grade glioma. Clin Cancer Res 2009;15:701–707.
92. O'Reilly MS. Radiation combined with antiangiogenic and antivascular agents. Semin Radiat Oncol 2006;16:45–50.
93. Geng L, Donnelly E, McMahon G, et al. Inhibition of vascular endothelial growth factor receptor signaling leads to reversal of tumor resistance to radiotherapy. Cancer Res 2001;61:2413–2419.
94. Willey CD, Xiao D, Tu T, et al. Enzastaurin (LY317615), a protein kinase C beta selective inhibitor, enhances antiangiogenic effect of radiation. Int J Radiat Oncol Biol Phys, 2009 (Epub ahead of print).
95. Ansiaux R, Dewever J, Gregoire V, et al. Decrease in tumor cell oxygen consumption after treatment with vandetanib (ZACTIMA; ZD6474) and its effect on response to radiotherapy. Radiat Res 2009;172:584–591.
96. Huber PE, Bischof M, Jenne J, et al. Trimodal cancer treatment: beneficial effects of combined antiangiogenesis, radiation, and chemotherapy. Cancer Res 2005;65:3643–3655.
97. Andreassen CN, Alsner J, Overgaard J. Does variability in normal tissue reactions after radiotherapy have a genetic basis—where and how to look for it? Radiother Oncol 2002;64:131–140.
98. Hill RP, Rodemann HP, Hendry JH, et al. Normal tissue radiobiology: from the laboratory to the clinic. Int J Radiat Oncol Biol Phys 2001;49:353–365.
99. Moulder JE, Robbins ME, Cohen EP, et al. Pharmacologic modification of radiation-induced late normal tissue injury. Cancer Treat Res 1998;93:129–151.
100. Yi ES, Bedoya A, Lee H, et al. Radiation-induced lung injury in vivo: expression of transforming growth factor-beta precedes fibrosis. Inflammation 1996;20:339–352.
101. Wang LW, Fu XL, Clough R, et al. Can angiotensin-converting enzyme inhibitors protect against symptomatic radiation pneumonitis? Radiat Res 2000;153:405–410.
102. Baumann M, Holscher T, Begg AC. Towards genetic prediction of radiation responses: ESTRO's GENEPI project. Radiother Oncol 2003;69:121–125.
103. Andreassen CN. Can risk of radiotherapy-induced normal tissue complications be predicted from genetic profiles? Acta Oncol 2005;44:801–815.
104. Angele S, Romestaing P, Moullan N, et al. ATM haplotypes and cellular response to DNA damage: association with breast cancer risk and clinical radiosensitivity. Cancer Res 2003;63:8717–8725.
105. Russell NS, Begg AC. Editorial radiotherapy and oncology 2002: predictive assays for normal tissue damage. Radiother Oncol 2002;64:125–129.
106. Radford IR, Murphy TK. Radiation response of mouse lymphoid and myeloid cell lines, III: different signals can lead to apoptosis and may influence sensitivity to killing by DNA double-strand breakage. Int J Radiat Biol 1994;65:229–239.
107. Plowman PN. The effects of conventionally fractionated, extended portal radiotherapy on the human peripheral blood count. Int J Radiat Oncol Biol Phys 1983;9:829–839.
108. Posner MR, Reinherz E, Lane H, et al. Circulating lymphocyte populations in Hodgkin's disease after mantle and paraaortic irradiation. Blood 1983;61:705–708.
109. Marks LB, Yu X, Vujaskovic Z, et al. Radiation-induced lung injury. Semin Radiat Oncol 2003;13:333–345.
110. Kong FM, Ao X, Wang L, et al. The use of blood biomarkers to predict radiation lung toxicity: a potential strategy to individualize thoracic radiation therapy. Cancer Control 2008;15:140–150.
111. Hara R, Itami J, Komiyama T, et al. Serum levels of KL-6 for predicting the occurrence of radiation pneumonitis after stereotactic radiotherapy for lung tumors. Chest 2004;125:340–344.
112. Ghosh SN, Zhang R, Fish BL, et al. Renin-angiotensin system suppression mitigates experimental radiation pneumonitis. Int J Radiat Oncol Biol Phys 2009;75:1528–1536.
113. Rodrigues G, Lock M, D'Souza D, et al. Prediction of radiation pneumonitis by dose-volume histogram parameters in lung cancer—a systematic review. Radiother Oncol 2004;71:127–138.
114. McDonald S, Rubin P, Phillips TL, et al. Injury to the lung from cancer therapy: clinical syndromes, measurable endpoints, and potential scoring systems. Int J Radiat Oncol Biol Phys 1995;31:1187–1203.
115. Littman P, Meadows AT, Polgar G, et al. Pulmonary function in survivors of Wilm's tumor: patterns of impairment. Cancer 1976;37:2773–2776.
116. Wohl ME, Griscom NT, Traggis DG, et al. Effects of therapeutic irradiation delivered in early childhood upon subsequent lung function. Pediatrics 1975;55:507–516.
117. Jakacki RI, Schramm CM, Donahue BR, et al. Restrictive lung disease following treatment for malignant brain tumors: a potential late effect of craniospinal irradiation. J Clin Oncol 1995;13:1478–1485.
118. Armstrong GT, Liu Q, Yasui Y, et al. Late mortality among 5-year survivors of childhood cancer: a summary from the Childhood Cancer Survivor Study. J Clin Oncol 2009;27:2328–2338.
119. Gopal R, Ha CS, Tucker SL, et al. Comparison of two total body irradiation fractionation regimens with respect to acute and late pulmonary toxicity. Cancer 2001;92:1949–1958.
120. Sampath S, Schultheiss TE, Wong J. Dose response and factors related to interstitial pneumonitis after bone marrow transplant. Int J Radiat Oncol Biol Phys 2005;63: 876–884.
121. Aleman BM, van den Belt-Dusebout AW, De Bruin ML, et al. Late cardiotoxicity after treatment for Hodgkin lymphoma. Blood 2007;109:1878–1886.
122. Swerdlow AJ, Higgins CD, Smith P, et al. Myocardial infarction mortality risk after treatment for Hodgkin disease: a collaborative British cohort study. J Natl Cancer Inst 2007;99:206–214.
123. Adams MJ, Hardenbergh PH, Constine LS, et al. Radiation-associated cardiovascular disease. Crit Rev Oncol Hematol 2003;45:55–75.
124. Adams MJ, Lipshultz SE, Schwartz C, et al. Radiation-associated cardiovascular disease: manifestations and management. Semin Radiat Oncol 2003;13:346–356.
125. Mill WB, Baglan RJ, Kurichety P, et al. Symptomatic radiation-induced pericarditis in Hodgkin's disease. Int J Radiat Oncol Biol Phys 1984;10:2061–2065.
126. Stewart JR, Fajardo LF, Gillette SM, et al. Radiation injury to the heart. Int J Radiat Oncol Biol Phys 1995;31:1205–1211.
127. Green DM, Gingell RL, Pearce J, et al. The effect of mediastinal irradiation on cardiac function of patients treated during childhood and adolescence for Hodgkin's disease. J Clin Oncol 1987;5:239–245.
128. Adams MJ, Lipsitz SR, Colan SD, et al. Cardiovascular status in long-term survivors of Hodgkin's disease treated with chest radiotherapy. J Clin Oncol 2004;22:3139–3148.
129. Hancock SL, Donaldson SS, Hoppe RT. Cardiac disease following treatment of Hodgkin's disease in children and adolescents. J Clin Oncol 1993;11:1208–1215.
130. Heidenreich PA, Hancock SL, Lee BK, et al. Asymptomatic cardiac disease following mediastinal irradiation. J Am Coll Cardiol 2003;42:743–749.
131. Rubin P, Casarett GW. Clinical radiation pathology. Philadelphia, PA: WB Saunders, 1968:1–61.
132. Glatstein E, Fajardo LF, Brown JM. Radiation injury in the mouse kidney, I: sequential light microscopic study. Int J Radiat Oncol Biol Phys 1977;2:933–943.
133. Lawton CA, Cohen EP, Murray KJ, et al. Long-term results of selective renal shielding in patients undergoing total body irradiation in preparation for bone marrow transplantation. Bone Marrow Transplant 1997;20:1069–1074.
134. Cheng JC, Schultheiss TE, Wong JY. Impact of drug therapy, radiation dose, and dose rate on renal toxicity following bone marrow transplantation. Int J Radiat Oncol Biol Phys 2008;71:1436–1443.
135. Kal HB, van Kempen-Harteveld ML. Renal dysfunction after total body irradiation: dose-effect relationship. Int J Radiat Oncol Biol Phys 2006;65:1228–1232.
136. Krochak RJ, Baker DG. Radiation nephritis: clinical manifestations and pathophysiologic mechanisms. Urology 1986;27:389–393.
137. Robbins ME, Diz DI. Pathogenic role of the renin-angiotensin system in modulating radiation-induced late effects. Int J Radiat Oncol Biol Phys 2006;64:6–12.
138. Cohen EP, Irving AA, Drobyski WR, et al. Captopril to mitigate chronic renal failure after hematopoietic stem cell transplantation: a randomized controlled trial. Int J Radiat Oncol Biol Phys 2008;70:1546–1551.
139. Donaldson SS, Jundt S, Ricour C, et al. Radiation enteritis in children: a retrospective review, clinicopathologic correlation, and dietary management. Cancer 1975;35: 1167–1178.
140. Miller AR, Martenson JA, Nelson H, et al. The incidence and clinical consequences of treatment-related bowel injury. Int J Radiat Oncol Biol Phys 1999;43:817–825.
141. Hauer-Jensen M, Wang J, et al. Bowel injury: current and evolving management strategies. Semin Radiat Oncol 2003;13:357–371.
142. Khalid U, Norman AR, Andreyev HJ. Elevated C-reactive protein levels are not a feature of uncomplicated radiation-induced bowel injury. Eur J Cancer Care (Engl) 2007;16:346–350.
143. Keskek M, Gocmen E, Kilic M, et al. Increased expression of cyclooxygenase-2 (COX-2) in radiation-induced small bowel injury in rats. J Surg Res 2006;135:76–84.
144. Merchant TE, Williams T, Smith JM, et al. Preirradiation endocrinopathies in pediatric brain tumor patients determined by dynamic tests of endocrine function. Int J Radiat Oncol Biol Phys 2002;54:45–50.
145. Laughton SJ, Merchant TE, Sklar CA, et al. Endocrine outcomes for children with embryonal brain tumors after risk-adapted craniospinal and conformal primary-site irradiation and high-dose chemotherapy with stem-cell rescue on the SJMB-96 trial. J Clin Oncol 2008;26:1112–1118.
146. Paulino AC. Hypothyroidism in children with medulloblastoma: a comparison of 3600 and 2340 cGy craniospinal radiotherapy. Int J Radiat Oncol Biol Phys 2002;53: 543–547.
147. Constine LS, Donaldson SS, McDougall IR, et al. Thyroid dysfunction after radiotherapy in children with Hodgkin's disease. Cancer 1984;53:878–883.
148. Hancock SL, McDougall IR, Constine LS. Thyroid abnormalities after therapeutic external radiation. Int J Radiat Oncol Biol Phys 1995;31:1165–1170.
149. Massimino M, Gandola L, Collini P, et al. Thyroid-stimulating hormone suppression for protection against hypothyroidism due to craniospinal irradiation for childhood medulloblastoma/primitive neuroectodermal tumor. Int J Radiat Oncol Biol Phys 2007;69:404–410.
150. Leiper AD, Stanhope R, Kitching P, et al. Precocious and premature puberty associated with treatment of acute lymphoblastic leukaemia. Arch Dis Child 1987;62: 1107–1112.
151. Wo JY, Viswanathan AN. Impact of radiotherapy on fertility, pregnancy, and neonatal outcomes in female cancer patients. Int J Radiat Oncol Biol Phys 2009;73:1304–1312.
152. Ogilvy-Stuart AL, Clayton PE, Shalet SM. Cranial irradiation and early puberty. J Clin Endocrinol Metab 1994;78:1282–1286.
153. Bath LE, Anderson RA, Critchley HO, et al. Hypothalamic-pituitary-ovarian dysfunction after prepubertal chemotherapy and cranial irradiation for acute leukaemia. Hum Reprod 2001;16:1838–1844.
154. Bath LE, Wallace WH, Shaw MP, et al. Depletion of ovarian reserve in young women after treatment for cancer in childhood: detection by anti-Mullerian hormone, inhibin B and ovarian ultrasound. Hum Reprod 2003;18:2368–2374.
155. Nygaard R, Clausen N, Siimes MA, et al. Reproduction following treatment for childhood leukemia: a population-based prospective cohort study of fertility and offspring. Med Pediatr Oncol 1991;19:459–466.
156. Horning SJ, Hoppe RT, Kaplan HS, et al. Female reproductive potential after treatment for Hodgkin's disease. N Engl J Med 1981;304:1377–1382.
157. Johnston RJ, Wallace WH. Normal ovarian function and assessment of ovarian reserve in the survivor of childhood cancer. Pediatr Blood Cancer 2009;53:296–302.
158. Wallace WH, Thomson AB, Kelsey TW. The radiosensitivity of the human oocyte. Hum Reprod 2003;18:117–121.
159. Wallace WH, Thomson AB, Saran F, et al. Predicting age of ovarian failure after radiation to a field that includes the ovaries. Int J Radiat Oncol Biol Phys 2005; 62:738–744.
160. Green DM, Kawashima T, Stovall M, et al. Fertility of female survivors of childhood cancer: a report from the childhood cancer survivor study. J Clin Oncol 2009;27: 2677–2685.
161. Larsen EC, Schmiegelow K, Rechnitzer C, et al. Radiotherapy at a young age reduces uterine volume of childhood cancer survivors. Acta Obstet Gynecol Scand 2004; 83:96–102.
162. Delic JI, Hendry JH, Morris ID, et al. Leydig cell function in the pubertal rat following local testicular irradiation. Radiother Oncol 1986;5:29–37.
163. Brauner R, Czernichow P, Cramer P, et al. Leydig-cell function in children after direct testicular irradiation for acute lymphoblastic leukemia. N Engl J Med 1983;309: 25–28.
164. Sieniawski M, Reineke T, Josting A, et al. Assessment of male fertility in patients with Hodgkin's lymphoma treated in the German Hodgkin Study Group (GHSG) clinical trials. Ann Oncol 2008;19:1795–1801.
165. Rowley MJ, Leach DR, Warner GA, et al. Effect of graded doses of ionizing radiation on the human testis. Radiat Res 1974;59:665–678.
166. Pedrick TJ, Hoppe RT. Recovery of spermatogenesis following pelvic irradiation for Hodgkin's disease. Int J Radiat Oncol Biol Phys 1986;12:117–121.

167. Young DF, Posner JB, Chu F, et al. Rapid-course radiation therapy of cerebral metastases: results and complications. Cancer 1974;34:1069–1076.

168. Tofilon PJ, Fike JR. The radioresponse of the central nervous system: a dynamic process. Radiat Res 2000;153:357–370.

169. Sheline GE, Wara WM, Smith V. Therapeutic irradiation and brain injury. Int J Radiat Oncol Biol Phys 1980;6:1215–1228.

170. van der Maazen RW, Verhagen I, Kleiboer BJ, et al. Radiosensitivity of glial progenitor cells of the perinatal and adult rat optic nerve studied by an in vitro clonogenic assay. Radiother Oncol 1991;20:258–264.

171. McMillian MK, Thai L, Hong JS, et al. Brain injury in a dish: a model for reactive gliosis. Trends Neurosci 1994;17:138–142.

172. Barres BA, Schmid R, Sendnter M, et al. Multiple extracellular signals are required for long-term oligodendrocyte survival. Development 1993;118:283–295.

173. Janzer RC, Raff MC. Astrocytes induce blood-brain barrier properties in endothelial cells. Nature 1987;325:253–257.

174. Ijichi A, Sakuma S, Tofilon PJ. Hypoxia-induced vascular endothelial growth factor expression in normal rat astrocyte cultures. Glia 1995;14:87–93.

175. Chiang CS, McBride WH, Withers HR. Radiation-induced astrocytic and microglial responses in mouse brain. Radiother Oncol 1993;29:60–68.

176. Tada E, Yang C, Gobbel GT, et al. Long-term impairment of subependymal repopulation following damage by ionizing irradiation. Exp Neurol 1999;160:66–77.

177. Freeman JE, Johnston PG, Voke JM. Somnolence after prophylactic cranial irradiation in children with acute lymphoblastic leukaemia. Br Med J 1973;4:523–525.

178. Boldrey E, Sheline G. Delayed transitory clinical manifestations after radiation treatment of intracranial tumors. Acta Radiol Ther 1966;5:5.

179. Muscal JA, Jones JY, Paulino AC, et al. Changes mimicking new leptomeningeal disease after intensity-modulated radiotherapy for medulloblastoma. Int J Radiat Oncol Biol Phys 2009;73:214–221.

180. Helton KJ, Edwards M, Steen RG, et al. Neuroimaging-detected late transient treatment-induced lesions in pediatric patients with brain tumors. J Neurosurg 2005;102:179–186.

181. Fouladi M, Chintagumpala M, Laningham FH, et al. White matter lesions detected by magnetic resonance imaging after radiotherapy and high-dose chemotherapy in children with medulloblastoma or primitive neuroectodermal tumor. J Clin Oncol 2004;22:4551–4560.

182. Valk PE, Dillon WP. Radiation injury of the brain. AJNR Am J Neuroradiol 1991;12:45–62.

183. Ullrich NJ, Robertson R, Kinnamon DD, et al. Moyamoya following cranial irradiation for primary brain tumors in children. Neurology 2007;68:932–938.

184. Desai SS, Paulino AC, Mai WY, et al. Radiation-induced moyamoya syndrome. Int J Radiat Oncol Biol Phys 2006;65:1222–1227.

185. Lew SM, Morgan JN, Psaty E, et al. Cumulative incidence of radiation-induced cavernomas in long-term survivors of medulloblastoma. J Neurosurg 2006;104: 103–107.

186. Schultheiss TE. The radiation dose-response of the human spinal cord. Int J Radiat Oncol Biol Phys 2008;71:1455–1459.

187. Hua C, Bass JK, Khan R, et al. Hearing loss after radiotherapy for pediatric brain tumors: effect of cochlear dose. Int J Radiat Oncol Biol Phys 2008;72:892–899.

188. Williams GB, Kun LE, Thompson JW, et al. Hearing loss as a late complication of radiotherapy in children with brain tumors. Ann Otol Rhinol Laryngol 2005;114:328–331.

189. Mulhern RK, Merchant TE, Gajjar A, et al. Late neurocognitive sequelae in survivors of brain tumours in childhood. Lancet Oncol 2004;5:399–408.

190. Nagel BJ, Palmer SL, Reddick WE, et al. Abnormal hippocampal development in children with medulloblastoma treated with risk-adapted irradiation. AJNR Am J Neuroradiol 2004;25:1575–1582.

191. Mulhern RK, Palmer SL, Merchant TE, et al. Neurocognitive consequences of risk-adapted therapy for childhood medulloblastoma. J Clin Oncol 2005;23:5511–5519.

192. Palmer SL, Gajjar A, Reddick WE, et al. Predicting intellectual outcome among children treated with 35–40 Gy craniospinal irradiation for medulloblastoma. Neuropsychology 2003;17:548–555.

193. Palmer SL, Goloubeva O, Reddick WE, et al. Patterns of intellectual development among survivors of pediatric medulloblastoma: a longitudinal analysis. J Clin Oncol 2001;19:2302–2308.

194. Kiehna EN, Mulhern RK, Li C, et al. Changes in attentional performance of children and young adults with localized primary brain tumors after conformal radiation therapy. J Clin Oncol 2006;24:5283–5290.

195. Merchant TE, Kiehna EN, Li C, et al. Modeling radiation dosimetry to predict cognitive outcomes in pediatric patients with CNS embryonal tumors including medulloblastoma. Int J Radiat Oncol Biol Phys 2006;65:210–221.

196. von HK, Kieffer V, Habrand JL, et al. Impairment of intellectual functions after surgery and posterior fossa irradiation in children with ependymoma is related to age and neurologic complications. BMC Cancer 2008;8:15.

197. Merchant TE, Li C, Xiong X, et al. Conformal radiotherapy after surgery for paediatric ependymoma: a prospective study. Lancet Oncol 2009;10:258–266.

198. Eifel PJ, Donaldson SS, Thomas PR. Response of growing bone to irradiation: a proposed late effects scoring system. Int J Radiat Oncol Biol Phys 1995;31: 1301–1307.

199. Gillette EL, Mahler PA, Powers BE, et al. Late radiation injury to muscle and peripheral nerves. Int J Radiat Oncol Biol Phys 1995;31:1309–1318.

200. Probert JC, Parker BR. The effects of radiation therapy on bone growth. Radiology 1975;114:155–162.

201. Gonzalez DG, Breur K. Clinical data from irradiated growing long bones in children. Int J Radiat Oncol Biol Phys 1983;9:841–846.

202. Hartley KA, Li C, Laningham FH, et al. Vertebral body growth after craniospinal irradiation. Int J Radiat Oncol Biol Phys 2008;70:1343–1349.

203. Krasin MJ, Xiong X, Wu S, et al. The effects of external beam irradiation on the growth of flat bones in children: modeling a dose-volume effect. Int J Radiat Oncol Biol Phys 2005;62:1458–1463.

204. Krasin MJ, Crawford BT, Zhu Y, et al. Intensity-modulated radiation therapy for children with intraocular retinoblastoma: potential sparing of the bony orbit. Clin Oncol (R Coll Radiol) 2004;16:215–222.

205. Kohn HI, Fry RJ. Radiation carcinogenesis. N Engl J Med 1984;310:504–511.

206. Li FP, Cassady JR, Jaffe N. Risk of second tumors in survivors of childhood cancer. Cancer 1975;35:1230–1235.

207. Meadows AT, Baum E, Fossati-Bellani F, et al. Second malignant neoplasms in children: an update from the Late Effects Study Group. J Clin Oncol 1985;3:532–538.

208. Hawkins MM. Second primary tumors following radiotherapy for childhood cancer. Int J Radiat Oncol Biol Phys 1990;19:1297–1301.

209. Suit H, Goldberg S, Niemierko A, et al. Secondary carcinogenesis in patients treated with radiation: a review of data on radiation-induced cancers in human, non-human primate, canine and rodent subjects. Radiat Res 2007;167:12–42.

210. Travis LB, Rabkin CS, Brown LM, et al. Cancer survivorship—genetic susceptibility and second primary cancers: research strategies and recommendations. J Natl Cancer Inst 2006;98:15–25.

211. Bhatia S, Yasui Y, Robison LL, et al. High risk of subsequent neoplasms continues with extended follow-up of childhood Hodgkin's disease: report from the Late Effects Study Group. J Clin Oncol 2003;21:4386–4394.

212. Constine LS, Tarbell N, Hudson MM, et al. Subsequent malignancies in children treated for Hodgkin's disease: associations with gender and radiation dose. Int J Radiat Oncol Biol Phys 2008;72:24–33.

213. Crump M, Hodgson D. Secondary breast cancer in Hodgkin's lymphoma survivors. J Clin Oncol 2009;27:4229–4231.

214. De Bruin ML, Sparidans J, van't Veer MB, et al. Breast cancer risk in female survivors of Hodgkin's lymphoma: lower risk after smaller radiation volumes. J Clin Oncol 2009;27:4239–4246.

215. Rubino C, Cailleux AF, de VF, et al. Thyroid cancer after radiation exposure. Eur J Cancer 2002;38:645–647.

216. Neglia JP, Meadows AT, Robison LL, et al. Second neoplasms after acute lymphoblastic leukemia in childhood. N Engl J Med 1991;325:1330–1336.

217. Loning L, Zimmermann M, Reiter A, et al. Secondary neoplasms subsequent to Berlin-Frankfurt-Munster therapy of acute lymphoblastic leukemia in childhood: significantly lower risk without cranial radiotherapy. Blood 2000;95:2770–2775.

218. Kimball Dalton VM, Gelber RD, Li F, et al. Second malignancies in patients treated for childhood acute lymphoblastic leukemia. J Clin Oncol 1998;16:2848–2853.

219. Pui CH, Cheng C, Leung W, et al. Extended follow-up of long-term survivors of childhood acute lymphoblastic leukemia. N Engl J Med 2003;349:640–649.

220. Walter AW, Hancock ML, Pui CH, et al. Secondary brain tumors in children treated for acute lymphoblastic leukemia at St Jude Children's Research Hospital. J Clin Oncol 1998;16:3761–3767.

221. Relling MV, Rubnitz JE, Rivera GK, et al. High incidence of secondary brain tumours after radiotherapy and antimetabolites. Lancet 1999;354:34–39.

222. Neglia JP, Robison LL, Stovall M, et al. New primary neoplasms of the central nervous system in survivors of childhood cancer: a report from the Childhood Cancer Survivor Study. J Natl Cancer Inst 2006;98:1528–1537.

223. Hall EJ, Wuu CS. Radiation-induced second cancers: the impact of 3D-CRT and IMRT. Int J Radiat Oncol Biol Phys 2003;56:83–88.

224. Kun LE, Beltran C. Radiation therapy for children: evolving technologies in the era of ALARA. Pediatr Radiol 2009;39(suppl 1):S65–S70.

225. Brenner DJ, Hall EJ. Secondary neutrons in clinical proton radiotherapy: a charged issue. Radiother Oncol 2008;86:165–170.

CHAPTER 14 ■ CELL AND GENE THERAPIES

STEPHEN GOTTSCHALK, CLIONA M. ROONEY, AND MALCOLM K. BRENNER

INTRODUCTION

A multidisciplinary approach including chemotherapy, radiation, surgery, and/or hematopoietic stem cell transplantation (HSCT) has led to a dramatic improvement in the long-term survival of pediatric malignancies over the last 30 years. However, current treatment modalities kill dividing cells indiscriminately causing considerable short- and long-term side effects. These side effects are of considerable public health concern since currently an estimated 1 in 900 young adults are long-term cancer survivors, increasing to as many as 1 in 250 in the year 2010.[1-3] Cell and gene therapies would be an appealing addition to the treatment armamentarium of pediatric malignancies because both strategies offer the potential of selectively killing malignant cells; thus reducing short- and long-term side effects. In addition, both therapeutic approaches promise to benefit patients, who currently fail multimodal therapy.

Gene therapy refers to a therapeutic approach that aims to treat diseases by replacing, removing, or introducing genetic material into cells. Therapeutic applications of cancer gene therapy include the following: (a) gene repair, (b) prodrug-metabolizing enzyme (PDME) gene therapy, (c) viral oncolysis, (d) modulation of the tumor microenvironment, (e) drug resistance gene therapy, (f) gene marking, and (g) immunotherapy (Table 14.1). Cell therapy involves the administration of autologous or allogeneic cells to produce a desired therapeutic effect. Cell therapies for cancer include HSCT (discussed in Chapter 16) and strategies to manipulate or mobilize the patient's own immune system. Many cell therapy approaches, like the vaccination with genetically modified tumor cells or dendritic cells (DCs) and the adoptive transfer of genetically modified T cells, take advantage of gene transfer technology (Table 14.2). Thus, separating cell and gene therapies that target the immune system is difficult, especially since integration of the two approaches holds the promise of advancing the field of cancer immunotherapy in future. This chapter discusses cell and gene therapy approaches for cancer with special focus on cancer immunotherapy for pediatric malignancies.

The prospect of gene therapy for human diseases was initially welcomed with great enthusiasm fueled by unrealistic expectations from investigators, clinicians, and the general public alike. However, since the first clinical gene therapy trial in 1989, it has become evident that the introduction of gene therapy into clinical practice will be a gradual and progressive process. To a great extent, this is because the current gene transfer technology limits the application of gene therapy. For example, many applications require high-efficiency gene transfer and precise cell targeting. If long-term expression is needed, the transferred gene may have to integrate into a specific site in the genome. Finally, for many applications, the expression of the transferred gene must be regulated. Current methods of gene transfer are a long way from achieving these goals. As a consequence, to date, the practice of human gene therapy is a compromise between the optimal therapeutic and the capability of the available gene transfer technology.

These limitations notwithstanding, more than 1,500 gene therapy trials have been conducted in 28 countries.[4] Of these, 65% have targeted malignancies of which a majority comprises solid tumors occurring in adults, including melanoma, breast cancer, brain tumors, and lung cancer. Although less than 10% of gene therapy clinical trials have been conducted for patients with inherited diseases caused by single gene defects, results from these trials have highlighted the great promise but also the potential pitfalls of current gene therapy approaches. Gene therapy has been used successfully to correct severe combined immunodeficiency (SCID) due to mutations in the common γ chain (γc) or adenosine deaminase (ADA) genes and X-linked chronic granulomatous disease (X-CGD).[5-7] In addition, patients with a rare inherited eye disease, Leber's congenital amaurosis, had significantly improved vision after gene transfer into the retina.[8,9] However, in the γ-SCID and the X-CGD clinical gene transfer trials, a subset of patients developed malignancies.[10,11] Of the γ-SCID patients, 25% developed T-cell leukemias containing a single copy of the retroviral vector inserted in or near the loci of proto-oncogenes (LMO2, BMI1, and CCND2).[10] Analysis of retroviral integration sites near the LMO2 gene in murine leukemias has given credence to a controversial "double hit hypothesis," in which the unregulated expression of the γc transgene by itself acts as an oncogene in conjunction with altered expression of the LMO2 gene in T cells.[12-14] Two treated X-CGD patients developed significant hematological abnormalities due to insertional mutagenesis, which led to activation of growth promoting genes.[11] Although these findings are a concern for the prospect for gene therapy for γc-SCID and X-CGD, it cannot be generalized to the entire field of gene therapy, especially since none of the patients with ADA-SCID developed malignancies after gene transfer after long-term follow up (up to 8 years).[7] Moreover, no malignancies have been reported in 40 gene therapy trials using retroviral vectors involving at least 232 patients.[15] Thus, the prospect for gene therapy remains strong, and the adverse events highlight the urgent need to develop better vectors, which are less toxic, have better targeting capabilities, and allow for transcriptional control of the transgene.[16] In this regard, clinical-grade self-inactivating retroviral and lentiviral vectors are being developed.

CURRENT GENE TRANSFER VECTORS

No single vector will be optimal for all cancer gene therapy applications due to the fundamental differences including the following: (a) vector production, (b) tropism, (c) packaging capacity, (d) integration and duration of transgene expression, and (e) immunogenicity. The demands of each gene therapy application must be matched with the characteristics of the vector; for example, for multidrug resistance gene therapy, genome integration, long-term gene expression, and low immunogenicity of the vector are required, whereas for many

TABLE 14.1

THERAPEUTIC APPLICATIONS OF CANCER GENE THERAPY

Therapeutic application	Comments
Gene repair	Correction of genetic defects associated with the malignant process
Prodrug-metabolizing enzyme gene therapy	Renders the tumor cells sensitive to corresponding cytotoxic agent
Viral oncolysis	Delivery of viruses that selectively replicate in tumor cells
Modulation of the tumor micro-environment	Inhibiting angiogenesis or tumor cell proteinases
Drug resistance gene therapy	Prevention of toxic side effects of chemotherapeutic agents
Gene marking	Assessing efficacy of conventional therapies
Immunotherapy	Generating or boosting immune responses to tumor antigens

cancer immunotherapy approaches, genome integration and long-term gene expression are not required, and a high immunogenicity of the vector is considered advantageous. Advantages and disadvantages of clinically used vectors for cancer gene therapy depend on their application and are listed in Table 14.3.

GENE THERAPY APPLICATION

Gene Repair

There is an attractive elegance to the strategy of introducing genetic material into a pediatric malignancy to correct the specific genetic defects contributing to the neoplastic phenotype. This can be achieved either by introducing the wild-type gene or by silencing the specific genetic defect with zing finger nucleases, ribozymes, antisense RNA, or small interfering RNA.[17,18] A number of mutant oncogenes and fusion tran-

TABLE 14.2

INTEGRATING CELL AND GENE THERAPIES FOR CANCER IMMUNOTHERAPY

Cell therapy	Gene therapy
Dendritic cell vaccine	Expression of antigens, cytokines, chemokines, and costimulatory molecules
Tumor cell vaccine	Expression of cytokines, chemokines, and costimulatory molecules
Cell therapy	Cells as carriers of retroviruses or oncolytic viruses
Adoptive T-cell transfer	Rendering T cells resistant to *in vivo* immunosuppressive environment
	Prodrug-metabolizing enzyme gene transfer as built in "safety switch"
	Expression of chimeric T-cell receptors to target tumor antigens

scripts have been identified in pediatric cancers that are certainly specific to the malignant clone and frequently essential to the malignant process. However, this approach is cumbersome, as most malignancies result from a multiplicity of genetic abnormalities. Unless correction of a single defect is subsequently lethal to the malignant cell, transfer of an individual corrective gene will leave a multiplicity of premalignant cells, with a high risk of later transformation. The biggest obstacle of this approach is that most tumor cells should be transduced, which is not feasible with current vectors for gene transfer. The largest clinical experience with this approach is the correction of the p53 tumor suppressor gene.[19,20] A recombinant adenovirus vector expressing wild-type p53 (Ad-p53) has been evaluated in several clinical trials including adult patients with a variety of malignancies, such as non–small-cell lung cancer (NSCLC), gliomas, ovarian, and bladder cancer. In phase 1 clinical studies, the administration of Ad-p53 was tolerated with minimal toxicity and wild-type p53 expression was observed in tumor cells after injection.[21] In NSCLC patients, combination therapy of Ad-p53 with cisplatin or radiation has demonstrated evidence of tumor regression at the primary injected tumor.[22] To enable the delivery to multiple tumor sites, administration of Ad-p53 by bronchoalveolar lavage has been evaluated with encouraging results.[23]

Prodrug-Metabolizing Enzyme Gene Therapy

Efforts have been made to modify cancer cells with genes that encode enzymes that convert harmless prodrugs into lethal cytotoxins. More than 20 PDME systems have been described; of these, the most widely used has been the herpes simplex virus-derived thymidine kinase (HSV-*tk*), which phosphorylates acyclovir, valacyclovir, or ganciclovir (GCV) to toxic nucleosides.[24] For this approach to be selective for a given malignancy, either the vector or the prodrug must be targeted to the malignant cell. The first clinical studies to test this novel strategy have aimed for both types of selectivity by introducing the HSV-*tk* gene into tumor cells *in vivo* with a retroviral vector. On exposure to GCV, the transduced cells phosphorylate the drug and upon cell division, the phosphorylated GCV is incorporated into DNA with lethal consequences, whereas nondividing cells are unaffected. Initial HSV-*tk* gene transfer trials were preformed in patients with primary and secondary brain tumors. In this case, there is a particularly clear distinction between tumor cells (which divide and are destined to be killed by GCV) and normal neurons, which do not divide.

In the first of two trials performed in pediatric cancer patients, 12 children with progressive supratentorial brain tumors were enrolled.[25] After tumor resection, retroviral producer cells generating retroviral particles encoding the HSV-*tk* gene were injected into the residual tumor. All patients were subsequently treated with GCV. Out of 11 patients, 10 showed disease progression, but 1 patient remained free of progression for 18 months. The second clinical trial targeted pediatric patients with retinoblastoma having vitreous seeds, which are often resistant to nonsurgical therapies requiring enucleation of the eye. Eight patients with vitreous seeds were treated by intravitreous injection of an adenoviral vector encoding the HSV-*tk* transgene.[26] Each injection was followed by GCV treatment for 7 days. One patient treated with 10^8 viral particles had resolution of the tumor seeds around the injection site, and the seven patients treated with doses greater than 10^{10} viral particles had complete resolution of their tumor seeds. Toxicities included transient inflammation, corneal edema, and increased intraocular pressure at 10^{11}

TABLE 14.3

ADVANTAGE AND DISADVANTAGES OF CLINICALLY USED VECTORS FOR CANCER GENE THERAPY

Vector[a]	Advantages	Disadvantages	Cancer gene therapy application
Retrovirus	Stable genome integration[b] Long-term gene expression Low immunogenicity	Integrations only in dividing cells Limited insert size Risk of insertional mutagenesis Inefficient *in vivo* gene delivery	Gene repair, PDME gene therapy, Drug resistance gene therapy, Gene Marking, Immunotherapy
Lentivirus	Stable genome integration[b] Integrates into nondividing cells Long-term gene expression Low immunogenicity	Risk of insertional mutagenesis Inefficient *in vivo* gene delivery	Gene repair, PDME gene therapy, Drug resistance gene therapy, Gene Marking, immunotherapy
Adenovirus	High titer, broad tropism Efficient gene transfer Transduces nondividing cells	Transient gene expression Immunogeneic[c] Strong inflammatory response Liver tropism	Gene repair, viral oncolysis, PDME gene transfer, Modulation of the tumor microenvironment, Immunotherapy
Nonviral DNA delivery	Nonviral Accepts large insert size Low immunogenicity	Transient gene expression Inefficient *in vivo* gene delivery	Gene repair, Modulation of the tumor microenvironment, immunotherapy
Poxviruses and vaccinia virus	High titer, broad tropism Accepts large insert size	Complex viral genome Replicates in target cell Immunogeneic[c]	Viral oncolysis, immunotherapy
Herpesvirus	High titer Accepts large insert size	Complex viral genome May be cytotoxic to cells	Viral oncolysis, PDME gene therapy
Adeno-associated virus	High titer, broad tropism Efficient gene transfer Transduces nondividing cells Limited immunogenicity	Limited insert size	PDME gene therapy, modulation of the tumor microenvironment, immunotherapy

[a]Listed by frequency.
[b]Integration of vector sequences into the genome is a characteristic of retroviruses, lentiviruses and to a limited extent of adeno-associated viruses; depending on the application this may be an advantage or disadvantage.
[c]Immunogenicity is considered advantageous for many cancer immunotherapy applications.
PDME, Prodrug-metabolizing enzyme.

viral particles. Further studies are needed to substantiate these encouraging results. PDME gene therapy has also been successfully used to modulate T-cell therapies and is discussed in detail in the section "Donor Lymphocyte Infusion."

One interesting feature is that transfer of PDME genes may not require all tumor cells to be transduced. An initially puzzling aspect of the original HSV-*tk* retrovirus system was that it worked so well in many preclinical models: even when fewer than 10% of tumor cells were transduced, GCV destroyed nearly 100% of the tumor cell population while sparing normal cells.[27] This phenomenon was termed *bystander effect* and is due to transfer of toxic GCV metabolites from tumor cells expressing HSV-*tk* to neighboring HSV-*tk* negative cells. Gap junctions are intimately involved in the transfer of phosphorylated nucleotides such as GCV metabolites between cells, and several studies have shown that the presence of gap junctions is essential for the "bystander effect."[28]

PDME gene therapy is being actively pursued in combination with other therapeutic approaches, like radiation or the codelivery of genes such as FLT-3 ligand that enhance systemic antitumor immune responses.[29] As discussed in the next section, another promising approach is to use replication-competent viruses to deliver PDME genes into cancer cells.

Viral Oncolysis

Oncolytic viruses selectively replicate in cancer cells, causing cell death while sparing normal cells (Fig. 14.1).[30] Case reports documenting dramatic regression of malignancies after viral infections in the first half of the 20th century gave credence to the concept of using replicating viruses to treat malignancies. However, without detailed knowledge of the molecular biology of viruses and malignancies it proved difficult to develop viruses, whose replication is limited to malignant cells. This has changed over the last two decades, and several oncolytic viruses, which replicate only in tumor cells, have been developed. Genetically engineered adenoviruses are the most widely used oncolytic viruses in clinical trials; other viruses tested in clinical trials include HSV, reovirus, mumps virus, West Nile virus, vaccinia virus, measles virus, and Newcastle disease virus (NDV).[31,32] For other viruses, like vesicular stomatitis virus, only preclinical data are available.[33]

One of the first genetically engineered oncolytic adenoviruses, *dl*1520 (Onyx-015), has a deletion of the viral *E1B* gene, which limits its replication to cells with a defective p53 pathway (i.e., malignant cells).[34] Some controversy remains regarding whether p53 is the sole mechanism that confers specificity; however, in all clinical trials conducted to date,

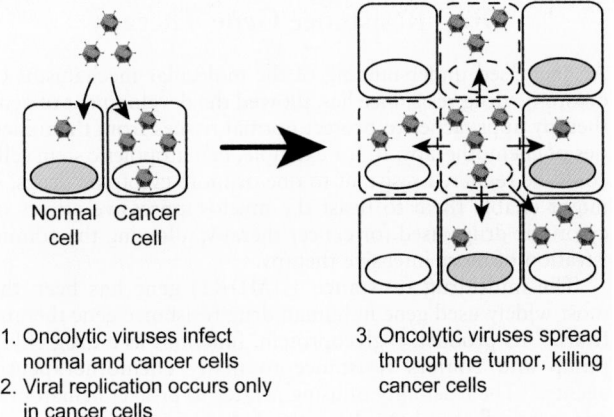

1. Oncolytic viruses infect normal and cancer cells
2. Viral replication occurs only in cancer cells
3. Oncolytic viruses spread through the tumor, killing cancer cells

FIGURE 14.1 Viral oncolysis. Oncolytic viruses selectively replicate in cancer cells, causing cell death while sparing normal cells; for details, see text.

neither nonspecific viral replication nor damage to normal cells was observed. Onyx-015 was tested in multiple phase 1 and 2 clinical trials alone or in combination with chemotherapy. The greatest response rate was observed in patients with head and neck cancer after local injection in combination with systemic cisplatinum and 5-fluorouracil. Out of 37 patients treated, 8 had a complete response (CR) and 11 had partial responses (PRs).[35] H101, another *E1B*-deleted virus was successfully tested in patients with head and neck cancer and in 2005 received marketing approval in China.[36] Two clinical studies have been performed in prostate cancer patients with transcriptionally targeted oncoloytic adenoviruses. No dose limiting toxicities were observed. Out of 43 patients 4 had a PR as judged by a decrease in serum prostate-specific antigen (PSA) levels of greater than 50%.[37,38] One strategy to increase the efficacy of oncolytic adenoviruses is combining this approach with PDME gene therapy (see previous section). An *E1B*-deleted adenoviral vector that encodes a cytosine deaminase/HSV-*tk* fusion (Ad5-CD5/TKrep) has been tested in phase 1 clinical studies.[39,40] In one study, 16 patients were treated with local recurrence of prostate cancer following definitive radiotherapy. No dose limiting toxicity was observed, and patients had a significant increase in progression-free survival using PSA doubling time as a surrogate marker.

HSV type 1 has been genetically engineered to limit replication in malignant cells by deleting one or both copies of the viral ICP34.5 gene. An HSV mutant lacking both copies (HSV1716) has been evaluated in four clinical studies for patients with glioma (3) or melanoma (1).[41–44] Patients with recurrent glioma received direct injections of HSV1716 into the tumor or the resection cavity. No dose limiting toxicies were observed, and tumor resections postinjection in a subset of patients documented viral replication in tumor cells, and neutralizing antibodies did not affect the efficacy of local delivery. Although CRs were not observed, several patients had stable disease (SD) resulting in a prolonged progression-free survival. G207, an ICP34.5 null HSV in which the ICP6 (UL39) gene is also deleted, was tested in two clinical studies in glioma patients with similar results.[45,46] Another attenuated HSV (NV1020) in which one copy of the ICP34.5 gene in addition to ICP0, ICP4, and latency-associated transcripts are deleted was tested in patients with metastatic colorectal carcinoma in the liver.[47] Hepatic arterial injections were well tolerated without significant effects on liver function tests. As for oncolytic adenoviruses, genes have been inserted into oncolytic HSVs to

enhance their antitumor activity. In this regard, the safety of a granulocyte-macrophage colony stimulating factor (GM-CSF) expressing oncolytic HSV (OncoVEX^GM-CSF) has been evaluated with encouraging results in one phase 1 clinical study.[48] In addition, an oncolytic virus derived from HSV type 2 has shown promising results in several preclinical models.[49]

Some viruses serendipitously replicate only in human cancer cells. The best studied examples include NDV and reovirus.[50] NDV is a paramyxovirus that normally replicates only in fowl; however, replication is observed in human cancer cells with defects in the interferon signaling pathway. Several phase 1 clinical trials have been conducted with an attenuated NDV strain, PV701, including trials in which the virus was given systemically. In one study, 79 patients with metastatic solid tumors had SD for 4 to more than 30 months after therapy with one CR and one PR.[51–53] The presence of viral particles was confirmed in biopsies of malignant lesions after therapy. Side effects observed included especially flu-like symptoms. In a follow up study, a "two-step desensitization" with low-dose PV701 prior to high-dose infusion reduced these side effects significantly. In addition, the safety and efficacy of NDV-infected autologous tumor cell vaccines have been evaluated in clinical trials. In one randomized study, colon and rectal cancer patients received adjuvant vaccines or no additional therapy after complete resection of liver metastasis.[54] For colon cancer patients, there was a significant increase in overall survival as well as metastasis-free survival in comparison to controls; no significant differences were observed for rectal cancer patients.

Reoviruses were originally isolated from the intestinal and respiratory tract of healthy individuals and are not considered human pathogens. However, replication of reoviruses with subsequent cell lysis is observed in cancer cells with mutations in the ras oncogene pathway.[55] The safety of reoviruses have been evaluated after local injections as well as after systemic administration.[56,57] Dose limiting toxicities were not observed and viral replication *in vivo* in tumors was confirmed in a subset of patients. Unfortunately, after repeated intravenous administration patients developed neutralizing antibodies. The antitumor activity of local or systemic administration of reoviruses was limited. Although these studies highlight the feasibility of intravenous administration of oncolytic viruses, this approach is at present limited by several factors including the following: (a) the presence or development of neutralizing antibodies in patients' serum, (b) high uptake in noncancerous tissues such as liver and spleen, and (3) the limited ability of viruses to extravasate and penetrate solid tumors. One attractive strategy to overcome these limitations is to use cells as carriers to deliver viruses to tumor sites. In preclinical models, a wide range of cells have been tested with encouraging results, including tumor cells, mesenchymal progenitor cells, and T cells.[58,59]

In summary, oncolytic viruses have been tested in multiple clinical trials for the control of local disease and disseminated disease; some efficacy has been observed and additional clinical trials with improved vectors are in progress. In addition, preclinical studies are being conducted to determine which virus species is best for a particular cancer and how to combine oncolytic viruses with other treatment modalities.

Modulation of the Microenvironment

The tumor microenvironment has become an important therapeutic focus for cancer therapy because of the realization that angiogenesis is a prerequisite for the development of tumors and excessive degradation, and remodeling of the extracellular matrix (ECM) is a hallmark of cancer progression. In addition, inhibitory immune system cells within the tumor microenvironment play an important role in promoting tumor progression. This section focuses on targeting the "non-immune component" of the tumor microenvironment. How to overcome the inhibitory microenvironment is discussed in the section "Immunotherapy" of this chapter. Since the initial proposal by Folkman that tumor growth is dependent on new blood vessel formation, both endogenous and synthetic angiogenesis inhibitors have been described.[60] Many angiogenesis inhibitors have shown efficacy in preclinical murine tumor models, and clinical trials with several inhibitors have been conducted. For example, recombinant human endostatin, the 20 kDa C-terminal fragment of collagen XVIII, has been evaluated in phase 1 clinical trials. Administration was demonstrated to be safe, and minor clinical responses were observed in patients with various solid tumors.[61] Administration of chemotherapy and bevacizumab (Avastin), a humanized monoclonal antibody, designed to inhibit vascular endothelial growth factor, significantly increases survival of patients with metastatic colorectal and was granted Food and Drug Administration (FDA) approval in 2004.[62] Since then, bevacizumab has received FDA approval for other malignancies, including high-grade gliomas.

Gene therapy represents a potentially attractive alternative to the administration of recombinant protein inhibitors of angiogenesis, since it allows for continuous delivery of medication rather than peaks and troughs resulting from intermittent injection. In addition, gene transfer targeting the tumor vasculature can provide high local concentration of angiogenesis inhibitors not achievable by systemic delivery.[63] In animal models, gene transfer vectors containing antiangiogenic genes have been administered systemically or by local injection. For example, persistent high levels of endostatin were achieved after systemic delivery of an adenoviral vector expressing endostatin, which resulted in decreased tumor growth and prevented the development of pulmonary micrometastases in a murine model.[64] In another study, intramuscular injection of adeno-associated viruses (AAV) 2 containing the angiostatin or endostatin gene resulted in decreased tumor growth in a murine model; coinjection of AAV-encoded angiostatin and endostatin genes was superior in comparison with single gene delivery and resulted in complete protection from tumor development.[65] Other antiangiogenic genes are being evaluated alone or in combination with conventional therapies in preclinical models. One phase 1 clinical study with a recombinant adenovirus encoding the human endostatin gene (E10A) has been conducted. Patients with advanced solid tumor received two intratumoral injections of increasing doses of E10A. No dose limiting toxicity was observed, and patients had a decrease in the proangiogenic factors in their serum.[66] Further studies are needed to evaluate the antitumor activity of this approach.

Inhibiting proteinases that remodel the ECM has been an area of intense research.[67] Serine proteinases, matrix metalloproteinases (MMPs), membrane type MMPs, and proteinases belonging to the "a disintegrin and metalloproteinase" family are often overexpressed in many human malignancies and are intimately involved in cell growth, migration, metastasis, and angiogenesis. However, most clinical studies have evaluated synthetic metalloproteinase inhibitors, which have not shown significant benefit in patients with advanced cancer.[68] Several endogenous proteinase inhibitors have been described, including tissue inhibitor of metalloproteinases 1 and 2; however, technical difficulties have prevented their development into useful drugs. Gene transfer has the potential to overcome some of the current limitations of MMP-targeted therapies and may also contribute to a better understanding of the complex interplay between MMPs and their inhibitors in vivo.

Drug Resistance Gene Therapy

An increased understanding of the molecular mechanisms of cytotoxic drug resistance has allowed the development of gene therapy approaches to protect normal tissues from the toxicities of chemotherapy. If, for example, hematopoietic stem cells could be rendered resistant to one or more cytotoxic drugs, it might enable them to resist the myelosuppressive effects of cytotoxic drugs used for cancer therapy, allowing the administration of more intensive therapy.

The multidrug resistance 1 (MDR1) gene has been the most widely used gene in human drug resistance gene therapy trials.[69] Its product, P-glycoprotein, functions as a drug efflux pump and confers resistance to many chemotherapeutic agents.[70] The feasibility of using MDR1 to protect hematopoietic stem cells has been demonstrated in murine experiments. Retroviral transfer of MDR1 to murine hematopoietic progenitors has successfully conferred drug resistance both in vitro and in vivo.[71] Other drug resistance genes tested in animal models include the dihydrofolate reductase gene conferring resistance to methotrexate and the 0^6-methylguanine DNA methyltransferase gene conferring resistance to alkylating agents such as 1,3-bis(2-chloroethyl)-1-nitrosourea.[72,73]

The clinical application of drug resistance gene therapy to date has been unsuccessful. This approach has several pitfalls. The low efficiency of stem cell transduction and poor gene expression observed in the earliest clinical protocols resulted in no selection of gene-modified cells and hence no protection.[74,75] Improved transduction technologies using fibronectin or retronectin and altered combinations of growth factors are potentially promising approaches to enhance in vivo selection.[76] Drug resistance gene therapy also carries the risk of transferring the genes to neoplastic cells that contaminate hematopoietic stem cell grafts, possibly producing drug-resistance relapse. In addition, toxicity to nonprotected organs, including gut, heart, and lungs, may rapidly supervene when marrow resistance allows intensification of cytotoxic drug dosages.

Use of the drug resistance gene therapy approach is likely to be successful in the future only when it becomes possible to target normal tissues in vivo and transduce them with high efficiency.

Gene Marking

Not all gene therapy applications for patients with malignant disease are directly therapeutic in intent. Gene marking of hematopoietic stem cells provides no immediate benefit to patients, but the information from these studies can be used to improve therapies that incorporate high-dose chemotherapy with autologous hematopoietic stem cell rescue.[77]

In the gene marking studies conducted to date, gene transfer has been used to address biologic questions about clinical issues related to HSCT. More specifically, gene transfer has been used after autologous HSCT to determine the source of relapse and to learn more about the biology of normal marrow reconstitution and how to best accelerate this process. One study resolved this issue by gene marking the marrow at the time of harvest with a retroviral vector, and then determining if the marker gene was present in malignant cells at the time of relapse. Among 12 patients with acute myeloid leukemia (AML) who were studied in this manner, four relapsed, two with cells that contained the marker gene.[78] Similar results have been obtained in patients with neuroblastoma and chronic myelogenous leukemia (CML).[79,80] These data show definitively that marrow harvested from patients in apparent clinical remission may contain residual malignant cells and that these cells can contribute to disease recurrence. The implication is that effective purging will be one requirement for improving the outcome of autologous HSCT. These gene marking studies also provided information on normal hematopoietic progenitor cells and showed that marrow autografts contribute to long-term hematopoietic reconstitution after HSCT. Long-term presence of the marker gene, for more than 10 years, has been seen in the mature progeny of transplanted marrow precursor cells, including peripheral blood T and B cells and neutrophils.[81] These results suggest that true stem cells, and not simply lineage-committed progenitors, were transduced by this method. Gene marking has also been used to the track infused Epstein-Barr virus (EBV)-specific T cells *in vivo* (see section "Adoptive Immunotherapy for EBV-LPD Post-HSCT and SOT"). Currently, no human clinical gene marking trials are being conducted because the risks of gene marking studies outweighs their benefit; that is, gene marking studies present no potential benefits to patients, and the use of retroviral vectors is associated with long-term safety concerns.[15] However, the approach of gene marking continues to be used in nonhuman primate models to evaluate whether any increase in progenitor cell numbers and gene transfer efficiency produced by growth factor combinations and cell culture devices *ex vivo* have an effect *in vivo*.

Immunotherapy

Immunotherapy refers to any approach aimed at enhancing the patient's immune system to treat diseases (also see Chapter 5).[82,83] There is now abundant evidence that spontaneously occurring malignancies in humans express antigens that are recognized by the patient's immune system and that the cellular immune response, which is designed to kill virus-infected cells, can also prevent the growth of malignant cells. Nonspecific killer cells such as natural killer (NK) cells and lymphokine-activated killer (LAK) cells recognize cell surface abnormalities, such as low expression of major histocompatibility complex (MHC) class I or carbohydrate abnormalities. T cells recognize "foreign" peptides derived from cytosolic proteins presented on the cell surface by MHC molecules.

Tumor-associated antigens (TAAs) are molecules expressed by tumor cells that can be recognized by the cellular or humoral immune system. They are immunogeneic because they (a) are normally expressed only during fetal development or at immunoprivileged sites, (b) are expressed at higher than normal levels, or (c) contain a novel peptide sequence generated by gene mutation or rearrangement.[84-86] Over the last two decades, numerous TAAs have been identified, and the antigens relevant for pediatric malignancies are listed in Table 14.4.[87-113] Despite expression of immunogeneic TAAs, tumors evade the immune response by a variety of possible mechanisms including the following: (a) releasing inhibitory cytokines, (b) interfering with the antigen-presentation pathway or mutating the antigen, or (c) downregulating cell adhesion or costimulatory molecules resulting in failure to activate specific immune responses either directly or indirectly. Improved understanding of immune escape mechanisms has led to strategies that seek to counteract the immune evasion tactics of tumor cells. This section discusses strategies to generate immune responses to inadequately presented TAAs or to boost the existing responses with the goal of mobilizing the immune system to eradicate the malignancy.

TABLE 14.4

T-CELL DEFINED TUMOR-ASSOCIATED ANTIGENS EXPRESSED IN PEDIATRIC MALIGNANCIES

Antigen	Malignancy	Ref
Mutations/novel epitopes in oncogeneic fusion proteins		
BCR-ABL	Chronic myelogenous leukemia	87, 88
DEK-CAN	Myeloid leukemia	89, 90
PML-RARα	Promyelocytic leukemia	91
ETV6-AML1	Acute lymphoblastic leukemia	92
Cancer testis antigens		
SSX family	Osteosarcoma	93
BAGE family	Rhabdomyosarcoma	94
GAGE family	Brain tumors, rhabdomyosarcoma	94, 95
MAGE family	Brain tumors, neuroblastoma, osteosaroma, rhabdomyosarcoma	94–99
XAGE family	Ewing's sarcoma	100
NY-ESO-1	Osteosarcoma	99
Overexpressed antigens		
HER2	Glioma, medulloblastoma, osteosarcoma	101–103
IL-13Rα2	Glioma, medulloblastoma	103, 105
EphA2	Glioma	106
Papilloma virus binding factor	Osteosarcoma	107
Survivin[a]	Brain tumors, hematopoietic malignancies, neuroblastoma	106, 108–110
Telomerase[a]	Hepatoblatoma	111
WT1	Hematopoietic malignancies, Wilms tumor	112

[a]Universal tumor antigens, most likely overexpressed in other pediatric malignancies.[113]

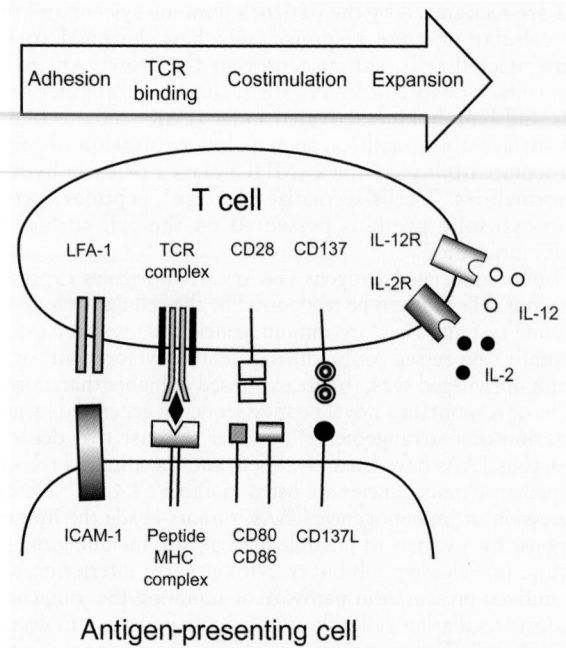

FIGURE 14.2 Requirements for T-cell activation and expansion. *Step 1—Adhesion*: leukocyte function antigen 1 (LFA-1) on T cells and intracellular adhesion molecule 1 (ICAM-1) on target cells/antigen-presenting cells facilitate the interaction between both cells. *Step 2—T-cell receptor (TCR) engagement*: the TCR binds to its cognate peptide presented by the appropriate major histocompatibility complex (MHC) class molecule. *Step 3—Costimulation*: the T-cell receives costimulation, commonly by binding of CD28 to CD80/CD86. In addition, other costimulatory molecules are often required for optimal stimulation including CD134 (OX40) or CD137 (4-1BB). *Step 4—Expansion*: cytokines such as IL-2, produced by T-helper cells, or IL-12, produced by dendritic cells (DCs) are required for optimal expansion.

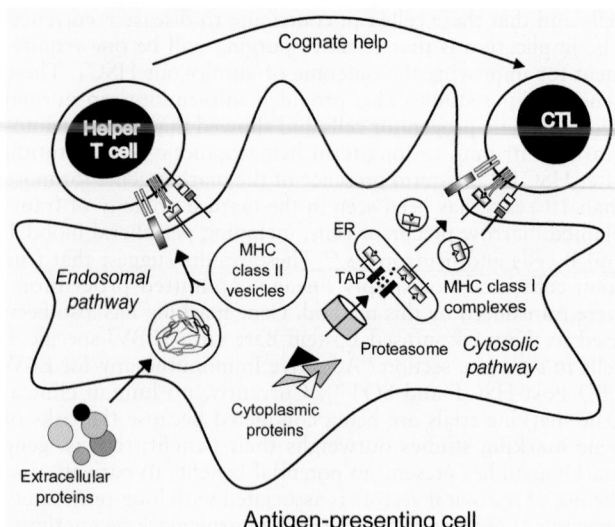

FIGURE 14.3 Major histocompatibility complex (MHC) class I and II processing pathways. *MHC class I processing pathway*: CD8$^+$ cytotoxic T cells (CTLs) recognize peptide presented on MHC class I molecules. For MHC class I molecule loading, intracellular proteins are degraded in the cytosol by the proteasome. The generated peptides are transported into the endoplasmic reticulum (ER) by transporter associated proteins (TAPs) 1 and 2. In the ER the peptides are loaded onto MHC class I molecules and transported to the cell surface. *MHC class II processing pathway*: CD4$^+$ helper T cells recognize peptides on MHC class II molecules. Peptides for MHC class II molecule loading are usually derived from extracellular proteins that are phagocytosed by antigen-presenting cells (APCs). Phagocytosed proteins are degraded in endosomal/lysosomal compartments, where the resulting peptides are loaded onto MHC class II molecules and transported to the cell surface. Helper T cells provide cognate help to CTL for optimal expansion.

Requirements for the Activation and Expansion of Antigen-Specific T Cells

The activation of antigen-specific T lymphocytes is a multistep process requiring antigen-specific triggering of the T-cell receptor (TCR) complex on the T cell and additional signaling via costimulatory molecules.[114] The TCR is triggered by the specific recognition of foreign peptides complexed with MHC class I or class II molecules at the cell surface (Fig. 14.2). CD8$^+$ cytotoxic T cells (CTLs) classically recognize peptides presented on MHC class I molecules, and CD4$^+$ helper T cells recognize peptides in the context of MHC class II molecules. MHC class I peptide loading occurs in the endoplasmic reticulum and requires proteasome-mediated antigen processing in the cytosol. Thus, for class I presentation, antigens must gain access to the cytosol. This is usually a prerogative of endogenously expressed proteins; however, antigen-presenting cells (APCs) have the capacity to phagocytose soluble antigens and present them for MHC class I molecules; a process called "cross-priming." In contrast to MHC class I peptide loading, MHC class II peptides are predominantly derived form phagocytosed soluble antigens (Fig. 14.3). In addition to the described "classical MHC class I and II presentation pathways," recent studies have highlighted the role of autophagy, the degradation of a cell's own components, in antigen presentation.[115] TCR recognition of peptide/MHC complexes results in the formation of a so-called immuno-logical synapse between T cells and the target cells or APC.[116] The immunological synapse consists of a central supramolecular activation cluster (SMAC) containing TCR and peptide MHC complexes and a peripheral SMAC consisting of cell adhesion molecules such as leukocyte function antigen 1 (LFA-1) and its counterpart intracellular adhesion molecule 1. For effective T-cell activation and expansion, other costimulatory signals are necessary. These include receptors belonging to the immunoglobulin superfamily, such as CD28 and ICOS, as well as members of the tumor necrosis factor receptor (TNFR) superfamily such as OX40 (CD134) and 4-1BB (CD137). Inhibition of the CD28 pathway in the presence of antigenic stimulation results in T-cell anergy, and blocking of the TNFR superfamily results in limited expansion of antigen-specific CTL and a reduced frequency of memory T cells.[117] In addition to the discussed costimulatory and adhesion molecules, the CD40/CD154 (CD40L) pathway contributes to the regulation of T-cell activation, both by independently costimulating T cells and at least in part by upregulating ligands for CD28 (CD80/CD86) on APCs.[118] Studies also indicate that the adhesion molecule LFA-1 not only mediates adhesion but also contributes to T-cell activation and differentiation.[119] Finally, CTLs must receive appropriate help before expansion can occur. Antigen-specific T helper cells with Th1 activity must be coactivated by the APCs. Th1 cells release Th1 cytokines, such as IFN-γ, which are also necessary for CTL activation, and IL-2, which is necessary for CTL expansion.

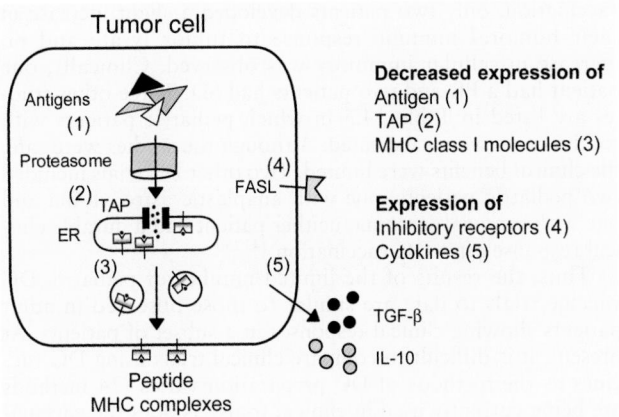

FIGURE 14.4 Immune evasion tactics of tumors. Tumors have developed multiple strategies to evade immune recognition; representative examples are shown, for details see text.

Immune Evasion Strategies of Malignancies and Their Circumvention

Tumor cells use a variety of tactics to avoid immune responses (Fig. 14.4). They can downregulate critical cell surface activation molecules or release inhibitory cytokines and chemokines that inactivate not only T helper cells and CTLs but also local professional APCs that otherwise might compensate for the tumor cell's poor ability to present its own antigens. Tumor cells that present tumor antigen–derived peptides on MHC complexes but do not provide costimulatory signals will anergize antigen-specific T cells. Conversely, a tumor expressing tumor antigens and costimulatory molecules may not present the tumor peptides because of the interference with the antigen-processing pathway. For instance, the expression of peptide transporter molecules TAP-1 and TAP-2 (transporter associated proteins 1 and 2) required for peptide loading of MHC class I complexes is often downregulated in Burkitt's lymphoma and melanoma.[120] Tumors may also inhibit crosspriming by professional APCs by secreting cytokines such as IL-10, which downregulates MHC class II molecule expression on macrophages and DCs and prevents their release of inflammatory cytokines. Even if a CTL receives appropriate activating signals from the tumor cell or APC, the tumor may inhibit or divert the CTL expansion phase. Many tumor cells secrete transforming growth factor β (TGF-β), which inhibits CTL activation in part by inhibiting early signaling events essential to the induction of IFN-γ, GM-CSF, and TNF-α.[121,122] Others secrete chemokines that selectively recruit Th2 cells, regulatory T cells, or myeloid suppressor cells which in turn inhibit Th1 responses, perhaps explaining why some cancer patients, produce tumor-specific antibodies.

Selecting an effective immunotherapy for a particular tumor requires a full understanding of the immune evasion strategies the tumor uses. If a tumor cell does not present a target antigen on its surface because of defective TAP expression, it will not respond to tumor-specific CTLs, regardless of the number of cells infused. If it secretes inhibitory factors, T cells activated by vaccination may fail to expand or will be diverted along the Th2 pathway despite an initial tumor-specific response. For example, although the malignant Reed-Sternberg cells of Hodgkin lymphoma express viral target antigens and have a good antigen-presenting phenotype, they secrete inhibitory cytokines and chemokines.[123] Therefore, a successful immunotherapy approach for Hodgkin lymphoma may require the use of adoptive cell therapy with *ex vivo*–

expanded CTLs to circumvent the *in vivo* immunosuppressive environment (see section "Adoptive immunotherapy with EBV-specific CTL").

Cancer Vaccines

Vaccination has been an effective strategy to protect animals and humans from bacterial and viral infections.[124] Cancer vaccines aim to induce CTL that are able to recognize endogenous antigens. This approach can be especially effective in cases in which the tumor expresses a TAA but fails to activate the immune system, that is, the tumor is antigenic but not immunogenic. To elicit CTL responses *in vivo*, either the TAA must be expressed in professional APCs, or the tumor cell itself must be modified to express APC characteristics and function. The strategy of choice depends on whether (a) the sequence of the TAA is known, (b) CTL epitopes have been identified, and (c) tumor material is available and amenable to genetic modification.

DNA Vaccines. When tumor antigens have been identified and cloned, DNA vaccines injected directly into skin, muscle, or mucosal surfaces have proved capable of inducing both CTL and antibody responses. The type of response depends on the route of immunization, the antigen, and the species immunized. Most of the immune response to DNA vaccines is thought to result from expression of antigen by nonlymphoid tissues and subsequent transfer to and crosspresentation by professional APCs. However, direct antigen presentation by transduced nonlymphoid cells and direct transduction of APCs themselves may also occur. The advantage of DNA vaccines is that they are stable, inexpensive, relatively simple to administer, and do not require adjuvants or viral vectors. Furthermore, the type of immune response elicited may be manipulated by coadministration of (a) cytokines, (b) genes coding for cytokines, costimulatory molecules, or adjuvants, such as the nontoxic region of tetanus toxoid, or (c) DNA sequences such as CpG motifs that activate the immune system.[125,126] Potential disadvantages are the requirement for well-characterized and cloned TAA, which should have no oncogenic potential. Moreover, expression of TAA, which are not exclusively expressed in tumor, might cause autoimmune disease.

Clinical studies with DNA vaccines. So far, clinical trials with DNA vaccines have only been performed in adult patients. DNA vaccines containing TAA genes such as immunoglobulin idiotype (Id) for B-cell lymphomas, tyrosinase epitopes for melanoma, and cancer carcinoembryonic antigen for colorectal cancer have been evaluated.[127–129] All studies were safe, 8% to 43% of patients showed evidence of the induction of a tumor antigen-specific cellular immune response postvaccination; however, no clinical responses were seen. Current efforts focus on how to improve DNA delivery, to induce CD4 helper T-cell responses, and to boost the observed CTL responses.[125,126] In addition, prime/boost vaccine strategies have shown promise in preclinical model as well as one clinical trial in which DNA was used for priming and recombinant vaccinia Ankara (MVA) for boosting antigen-specific immune responses.[130,131]

Dendritic Cell Vaccines. One way to ensure that a TAA is presented in the optimal way is to inject APCs that have been generated and "loaded" with antigen *ex vivo*. Because DCs are the most potent APCs and are capable of inducing primary immune responses and overcoming immune tolerance, they have been used in many preclinical and clinical studies to induce immune responses to tumors.[132] DCs can be generated from precursors in peripheral blood or bone marrow in the presence of cytokines, most commonly IL-4 and GM-CSF.[133] Between 1% and 3% of peripheral blood mononuclear cells

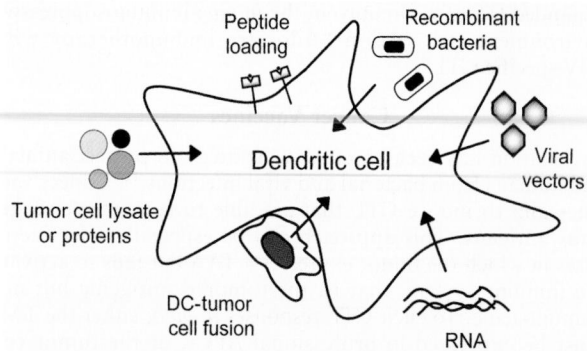

FIGURE 14.5 Antigen loading of dendritic cells (DCs). Different methods to load DCs with antigens have been developed and tested in preclinical models. In clinical DC vaccine trials, loading with peptides or tumor lysates has been the preferred method.

can differentiate into DCs; G-CSF mobilization dramatically increases the DC yield; however, GM-CSF preferentially increased plasmacytoid/CD11$^+$ DC, which stimulate Th2 helper T cells.[134] IL-4/GM-CSF–induced DCs are the so-called immature DCs; they efficiently phagocytose and process dying cells and particulate matter, but for efficient activation of T cells DCs need an additional maturation step. This can be achieved *ex vivo* by the addition of toll-like receptor ligands, cytokine cocktails, or engagement of CD40 or the Fc receptors on the DC surface. Different methods of antigen delivery into DC have been explored, including peptides, tumor lysate, tumor DC cell fusion, RNA, viral vectors, and recombinant bacteria (Fig. 14.5).[135–139] The efficiency of individual delivery systems depends on variables, such as the specific antigen or animal model, and at present the optimal method for antigen delivery into DCs for human clinical trials remains unclear.

Clinical studies with dendritic cell vaccines. More than 170 DC vaccine studies have been published.[140–142] Most human clinical trials using DC vaccines have tested peptide- or tumor lysate–loaded DCs in patients with melanoma, prostate cancer, colorectal cancer, and myeloma. DC-based vaccinations were generally safe, and while CRs are rare, several studies have showed prolonged survival of treated patients. For example, in a phase 3 clinical study (IMmunotherapy for Prostate AdenoCarcinoma Treatment [IMPACT] study), patients with advanced prostate cancer were vaccinated with a DC vaccine targeting prostatic acid phosphatase. Treated patients had a significantly increased 3-year survival in comparison to controls (31.7% vs. 23.0%).[143] FDA approval for the vaccine is expected within the fourth quarter of 2009, making it the first DC vaccine to be approved in the United States for cancer immunotherapy.

DC vaccine trials have been conducted in a small number of pediatric patients (Table 14.5).[144–150] Geiger et al. injected IL-4/GM-CSF–induced DCs loaded with autologous tumor lysate and adjuvant (keyhole limpet hemocyanin; KLH) into 15 pediatric patients with relapsed solid tumors who had failed standard salvage therapies.[144] Six out of 10 evaluable patients had an increase in their cellular immune response to KLH and 3 out of 6 evaluable patients had a greater than 10-fold increase in their cellular immune response to tumor lysate as judged by IFN-γ ELISPOT assays. One of the three patients who had a documented increase in their cellular immune response to tumor lysate had a PR and the two other patients had SD. The overall response rate (SD and PR) was 40%, which is similar to response rates observed in adult DC vaccine trials. Caruso et al. injected DC loaded with tumor RNA into nine patients with recurrent brain tumors.[145] Following

vaccination, only two patients developed a slight increase in their humoral immune response to tumor lysate and no increase in cellular immunity was observed. Clinically, one patient had a PR and two patients had SD. Three other studies are listed in Table 14.5 in which pediatric patients with solid tumors were vaccinated. Although the studies were safe, the clinical benefits were limited. Two other DC trials included two pediatric patients, one with anaplastic astrocytoma and one with synovial sarcoma; neither patient had a durable clinical response after DC vaccination.[149,150]

Thus, the results of the limited number of pediatric DC vaccine trials to date are similar to those observed in adult patients showing clinical responses in a subset of patients. At present, it is difficult to compare clinical trials using DC vaccines as the methods of DC preparation varies (24 methods are being currently used in clinical trials) as does the vaccination routes and schedules of administration. To improve DC vaccination, many variables must be addressed.[155] Strategies that showed promise in preclinical and/or phase 1 clinical studies include the following: (a) the depletion of inhibitory, regulatory T cells with cyclophosphamide or anti-CD25 immunotoxins (Ontak) prior to DC vaccination, (b) combining DC vaccination with the systemic administration of cytokines to enable DC-activated T cells to expand and function *in vivo*, and (c) the genetic modification of DCs to enhance their APC function *in vivo*.[156–159] One caveat concerning the use of DCs with other immunostimulatory molecules to "superactivate" the immune response is that it may break immunologic tolerance to self-antigens and produce autoimmunity. This risk is well illustrated by mice bearing the syngeneic A20 lymphoma that were vaccinated with DCs pulsed with peptides eluted from the tumor in combination with fibroblasts engineered to express CD40 ligand and IL-2. This vaccine protected against lethal doses of the tumor, but the mice developed autoimmune disease.[160,161] A similar although not life-threatening autoimmune response has been observed in melanoma patients who developed vitiligo after vaccination with peptide-pulsed DCs.[162]

Tumor Vaccines. An alternative strategy to DC vaccination is to genetically modify tumor cells to improve their ability to induce an immune response. This strategy, termed *tumor vaccination*, has many variations.[163] Tumors can be modified either *in vivo* or *ex vivo* with a range of gene transfer methods, including viral or nonviral methods. The advantage of *ex vivo* modification is that it permits early evaluation of transgene expression, control of the number of modified tumor cells injected, and escalation of the vaccine dose. *Ex vivo* modification is particularly appropriate for tumors such as neuroblastoma that can be expanded in tissue culture. A potential disadvantage is that the tumor cells growing in culture may not represent the tumor cells that grow *in vivo*. Modification of tumors *in vivo* is more difficult to control because it is impossible to determine the number of tumor cells that have been modified, and there is considerable variation between patients, even when the same dose of viral vector is used. Nevertheless, small numbers of tumor cells modified *in vivo* should be able to induce a specific, systemic immune response that can target unmodified tumors at distant sites.

Tumors can be modified to improve one or multiple phases of CTL activation and expansion (Fig. 14.6). The first phase is the attraction and activation of professional APCs, for which GM-CSF and CD40 ligand are the preferred molecules.[164,165] The second phase is the recruitment of T cells with use of chemokines such as lymphotactin.[166] The third phase, T-cell activation, has been achieved by modifying tumor cells with B7 and CD40 to improve antigen presentation. IL-2 and IL-12 have been used to provide T-cell help to secure the fourth phase, T-cell expansion.[167] In the fifth (or

TABLE 14.5

PEDIATRIC CANCER VACCINE TRIALS

Vaccine	Comments	Ref
Tumor cell lysate–pulsed DC	Fifteen patients with pediatric solid tumors including neuroblastoma (3[a]), fibrosarcoma (1), PNET (2), renal cell cancer (1), osteosarcoma (1), inflammatory myofibroblastic sarcoma (1), hepatic sarcoma (1), desmoplastic round cell sarcoma (1), Ewing's sarcoma (2), clear cell sarcoma (1), Wilm's tumor (1) Outcome: 9 PD, 5 SD, 1 PR	144
Tumor RNA–transfected DC	Seven patients with brain tumors including glioblastoma multiforme (2), astrocytoma (2), and ependymoma (3) Outcome: 1 PR, 2 SD	145
Tumor RNA–transfected DC	Seven patients with stage 4 neuroblastoma; all (4) patients with active disease had PR	146
Tumor cell lysate–pulsed DC	Twenty-two patients with pediatric solid tumors including adrenocortical carcinoma (2), desmoplastic sarcoma (1), Ewing's sarcoma (5), fibrosarcoma (1), hepatocellular carcinoma (3), osteosarcoma (7), renal cell carcinoma (1), Wilm's tumor (2) Outcome for patients with active disease (13): 1 SD, 1 mixed response Outcome for patients with CR (9): 7 remained in CR	147
Peptide-loaded DC/monocytes	Fifteen patients with Ewing's sarcoma (10), PNET (2), and alveolar rhabdomyosarcoma (3); 11 patients had PD after first cycle; 1 patient had mixed response after second cycle	148
Peptide-loaded DC	One patient with synovial sarcoma; transient decrease in growth rate of tumor	149
DC/tumor cell fusion	One patient with anaplastic astrocytoma; progressive disease	150
Autologous neuroblastoma cells expressing IL-2	Ten patients; 1 CR, 1 PR, 3 SD, 5 PD; 4/5 with clinical response had detectable antitumor T-cell response	151
Allogeneic neuroblastoma cells expressing IL-2	Twelve patients; 1 PR, 7 SD, 4 PD; no increase in direct cytotoxic effector function against immunizing cell line	152
Allogeneic neuroblastoma cells expressing IL-2 and Lptn	Twenty-one patients; 2 CR, 1 PR; increased numbers of T and NK cells and eosinophils in peripheral circulation; induction of Th2 helper T cells	153
Leukemia cells/fibroblasts expressing IL-2 and CD40 L	Adjuvant vaccine; 8 patients; T-cell infiltrate at injection site, increased number of circulating Th1-helper cells; 7 out of 8 patients remain in remission	154

[a]Number of patients, PNET, primary neuroectodermal tumor; PD, progressive disease; SD, stable disease; PR, partial response; Lptn, lymphotactin; DC, dendritic cell.

effector) phase, activated CTLs may be anergized or killed by factors released by the tumor or even killed directly by tumor cells. For example, tumor cells expressing FAS ligand can trigger CTL apoptosis by engaging the death receptor, FAS, on CTLs.[168] Influencing this "fifth phase" may not be a real-istic goal of tumor vaccine studies but may be addressed with genetic modification of CTL (see section "Antigen-Specific Cytotoxic T Cells"). Although most tumor vaccine strategies are directed at one or two phases of immune activation, improving one phase usually improves the other phases as well. GM-CSF affords a particularly good example of this principle. Tumors expressing recombinant GM-CSF recruit and activate macrophages and DCs, which in turn secrete inflammatory cytokines that recruit T cells. The activated DCs can then phagocytose dying tumor cells and activate the recruited CD4[+] and CD8[+] T cells. The CD4[+] T cells produce IL-2 and help CTL expansion. So although used primarily to influence the first phase of CTL activation and expansion, GM-CSF also acts on the three subsequent phases. This may explain why GM-CSF has been the most effective cytokine for boosting immune responses to tumors in animal models.[169] The concept of creating immunogeneic tumors to induce long-lasting antitumor immunity has been shown in many preclinical murine tumor models. It is apparent that the success of vaccination with tumor cells depends on a host of interacting factors, including tumor type, type of immune evasion strategy used by the tumor (usually not known), vaccine dose, level of transgene expression, challenge site, and vaccine schedule. Hence, as for DC vaccination, the "best strategy" for translation into human trials has not been identified.

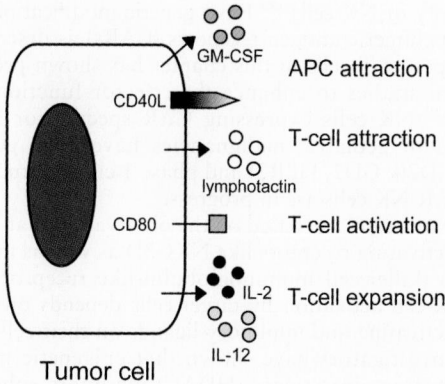

FIGURE 14.6 Genetic modification of tumor cells. Tumor cells can be genetically modified to improve one or multiple phases of cytotoxic T cell (CTL) activation and expansion; representative examples are shown, for details see text.

Clinical studies with tumor vaccines. When used in patients, tumor vaccines have produced little systemic toxicity, with only local inflammation and occasionally patches of vitiligo in melanoma patients.[170] In human clinical trials, tumors have been modified with IL-2, IL-4, IL-7, IFN-γ, GM-CSF, CD40 ligand, and lymphotactin.[137,165,171–174] Infusion of unmodified melanoma cells mixed with IL-2 expressing autologous fibroblasts resulted in infiltration of CD4+ and CD8+ T cells, which produced tumor cell lysis after culture *in vitro*. Some mixed responses and disease stabilization were seen in approximately 10% of patients. One study evaluating the tumor vaccine approach for neuroblastoma injected autologous neuroblastoma cells expanded *ex vivo* and transduced with an adenoviral vector expressing IL-2 into children with advanced disease (Table 14.5).[151–154] Of the 10 children, one had a CR, one had a PR, and three had SD. Four of five responders had an increased frequency of tumor-specific CTLs, compared with only one of five children who did not have a tumor response. Twelve patients for whom no autologous vaccine could be generated, received an allogeneic vaccine consisting of HLA-A2 matched IL-2–transduced neuroblastoma cells. In the allogeneic setting, tumor cells can present antigens through the matched HLA-A2 molecule; in addition, DCs recruited to the vaccination site can phagocytose tumor cells and present shared antigens in association with their own MHC molecules by crosspriming. After vaccination with allogeneic tumor cells expressing IL-2 no patient showed an increase in direct cytotoxic effector function against the immunizing cell line; however, one child had a PR, seven had SD, and four had progressive disease.[152]

A subsequent clinical study with neuroblastoma was developed based upon animal studies showing that the combination of lymphotactin (Lptn), a T-cell chemokine, and IL-2 accelerated and augmented the immune response to neuroblastoma cells.[153] Accordingly, patients received either an autologous or allogeneic vaccine expressing both IL-2 and Lptn. In the allogeneic group, it was possible for the first time to observe specific antitumor immune responses to the immunizing cell line, and 2 out of 21 patients had a CR, which was durable in one. In the autologous group, there was no difference between IL-2 and Lptn versus IL-2 alone. Hence, for the allogeneic setting this study provided preliminary evidence that the combination of two agents acting at different phases of the immune response may be superior to a single agent. If confirmed by other studies, these results indicate that the use of allogeneic tumor cell vaccines, which can be produced in large quantities and do not require custom production such as autologous vaccines, may be feasible.

The concept of combining two molecules, which act at different phases of T-cell activation, has also being evaluated in pediatric and adult patients with high-risk acute lymphoblastic and myelogenous leukemias.[154] Since leukemic blasts are difficult to transduce with current gene transfer technology, blasts were coinjected with autologous fibroblasts secreting IL-2 and CD40 ligand. Seven patients were injected after allogeneic HSCT and one after chemotherapy. Injection site biopsies revealed an increase of CD3+ T cells and in peripheral blood more CD4+ T cells were observed with a TH1 T-cell phenotype. Clinically, seven out of eight patients remain disease free; however, a larger study with long-term follow up is necessary to evaluate if such adjuvant therapy has clinical benefit.

T-Cell Vaccines. Although the supply of autologous DCs and tumor cells for vaccine studies is often limited, autologous T cells can be activated and expanded to great numbers. Depending on the T-cell activation status, T-cells express costimulatory molecules such as CD80 and CD86; in addition, T cells can readily be genetically modified with cytokines or other costimulatory molecules to further enhance their APC

function.[175,176] Although most studies using T cells as APCs have been confined to the preclinical arena, one clinical study using T-cell APCs has been published.[177] Ten melanoma patients received intravenous infusions of genetically modified T cells expressing melanoma-associated antigen 3 (MAGE-A3) or MAGE-A3 and HSV-*tk*. Infusions were well tolerated, and all but one patient who received HSV-*tk*–expressing T cells had an increase in the frequency of tk-specific T cells. In contrast, only three out of nine evaluable patients had an increased frequency of MAGE-A3–specific T cells in their peripheral blood. In two patients, MAGE-A3–specific T cells could be detected at the tumor site. Although this clinical study was not designed to evaluate the antitumor activity of T-cell APCs, the results are encouraging enough to warrant further exploration of this approach.

Adoptive Cell Therapy

Cancer vaccines are widely used to induce antitumor responses; however, as noted above, these may be blocked by *in vivo* immune evasion strategies of malignancies. Generating cells for adoptive immunotherapies *ex vivo* has additional potential advantages over cancer vaccines: (a) the phenotype, activity, and specificity of expanded cells can be analyzed prior to injection, (b) *ex vivo* expanded cells can be gene marked to assess persistence, efficacy, and toxicity, and (c) cells can be genetically modified to change their effector function or modify their antigen specificity.[83,178,179] Adoptive cell transfer strategies have included NK cells, activated T cells, tumor infiltrating lymphocytes (TILs), donor lymphocytes post-HSCT, and tumor-specific T-cell lines and clones (Table 14.6).[180–222]

Natural Killer Cells. NK cells can be activated and expanded *ex vivo* with IL-2 (LAK cells) for adoptive immunotherapy. They have HLA-unrestricted cytotoxicity against a range of human tumor cells *ex vivo*, but their efficacy and persistence *in vivo* remain unclear. In the first clinical applications, published in 1985, LAK cells were infused with IL-2 into patients with advanced malignancies and responses were observed for four types of cancer (renal cell carcinoma, melanoma, adenocarcinoma of the lung, and colorectal carcinoma).[182] These studies demonstrated foremost the feasibility of adoptive cellular therapy for human malignancies. Further studies using IL-2 and LAK cells showed an overall 35% response rate in patients with metastatic renal cell carcinoma. However, LAK cells with IL-2 as therapy for metastatic renal cell carcinoma was subsequently compared with IL-2 alone in randomized clinical trials, which showed that LAK cells with IL-2 was not superior to IL-2 alone.[223,224]

Several strategies are being pursued to enhance the antitumor activity of NK cells.[180] First, genetic modification of NK cells with chimeric antigen receptors (CARs) as described for antigen-specific T cells in this chapter has shown promise in preclinical studies to enhance the effector function of NK cells.[225–228] NK cells expressing CAR specific for antigens expressed in pediatric malignancies have been generated (CD19, CD20, GD2, HER2) and phase 1 clinical studies with CD19-CAR NK cells are in progress.

Other strategies are based on the observation that NK cells express activating receptors like NKG2D as well as inhibitory receptors (killer-cell immunoglobulin-like receptors; KIR). Thus, NK-cell activation by target cells depends on the balance of activating and inhibitory ligands on their cell surface. Several investigators have shown that epigenetic modifiers such as histone deacetylase (HDAC) inhibitors enhance the expression of activating NK-cell ligands on tumor cells resulting in enhanced NK-cell–mediated killing.[229] Since inhibitory ligands are encoded by HLA-C molecules, another strategy

TABLE 14.6

CLINICAL EXPERIENCE WITH ADOPTIVE CELL THERAPIES

Cell therapy	Comments	Ref
NK cells	*LAK cells:* Initial encouraging clinical trials results in melanoma or renal cell cancer patients not confirmed by larger studies	182, 183
	Haplo-identical, KIR-ligand mismatched NK cells: Safe, promising antitumor activity	184, 185
Activated T cells	*Outside HSCT setting:* Safe, limited efficacy	183
	Postautologous HSCT: Safe, rapid immune reconstitution	186–188
	Postallogeneic HSCT: Initial results indicate safety and no increased risk of GVHD in comparison to DLI	189
TIL	Most clinical trials performed with melanoma or renal cell cancer patients; variable responses; use of lymphodepleting chemotherapy and radiation prior to TIL infusion results in increased antitumor effects (response rate up to 72%)	190–193
Donor lymphocyte infusions	Proven efficacy for controlling relapse of CML after HSCT; for other malignancies less efficient; risk of GVHD	194, 195
EBV-specific CTL	*EBV-LPD post-HSCT:* Proven efficacy for prophylaxis and therapy	196–198
	EBV-LPD post-SOT: Safe, antitumor effects, lack of persistence postinfusion	199–202
	EBV-positive Hodgkin disease: CTL persist for up to 1 year postinfusion and home to tumor sites; increase of EBV-specific immunity; variable clinical responses	203–205
	EBV-positive NPC: Increase of EBV-specific immunity; reduction in plasma EBV-DNA levels; clinical responses in patients with small tumor burden	206–209
MART-1- or gp100-specific T cells	T cells home to tumor site, transient clinical responses	210–212
α/β TCR expressing T cells	*Melanoma:* Clinical responses in 19% to 30% of patients; T cells expressing high-affinity α/β TCRs also targeted normal tissues expressing low levels of antigen	213, 214
CAR expressing T cells	*1st Generation CAR in mitogen activated T cells (only zeta signaling domain):* *HIV, ovarian cancer, and renal cancer* Safe, "off-target effects" in renal cancer study, no clinical responses	215–218
	Neuroblastoma Safe, 6 patients with active disease: 1 PR, 5 PD	219
	Non-Hodgkin lymphoma Safe, 5 patients with active disease: 1 PR, 4SD	220
	1st Neuroblastoma Generation CAR in EBV-specific T cells Safe, 8 patients with active disease: 1CR 2 SD, 1 NED, 2 tumor necrosis, 2 PD	221

LAK, lymphocyte activated killer cells; TIL, tumor infiltrating lymphocytes; EBV, Epstein–Barr virus; LPD, lymphoproliferative disease; HSCT, hematopoietic stem cell transplant; SOT, solid organ transplant; TCR, T-cell receptor.

to overcome the presence of inhibitory ligands is the use of haploidentical NK cells, which lack the corresponding KIR.[184,185,230] Indeed, the infusion of haploidentical NK cells is safe and has resulted in promising antitumor effects.[231] Ongoing studies are focused on optimizing KIR-ligand typing for optimal donor selection.

Activated T Cells. Initial studies focused on the adoptive immunotherapy of autologous T cells, which had been activated and expanded with a monoclonal antibody against the TCR (anti-CD3). Most clinical studies have been performed in patients with metastatic renal cell carcinoma but initial encouraging results have not been replicated in larger stud-

ies.[183] A study using autologous, activated T cells as adjuvant therapy after complete resection of hepatocellular carcinoma showed no influence on overall survival; however, infused patients had significantly longer recurrence-free survival.[232] Activation of T cells with anti–CD3- and anti–CD28-coated beads *ex vivo* has the potential to overcome disease-induced anergy and augment CD4$^+$ T-cell responses. Four clinical studies have been conducted with anti–CD3/anti–CD28-activated T cells.[186–189] In three studies, patients received activated T cells postautologous HSCT. T-cell infusions induced a rapid recovery of lymphocyte counts and reversed cytokine activation deficits *in vitro*. In a subset of patients, T-cell infusions were associated with a clinical picture indistinguishable from acute graft-versus-host disease (GVHD).[187] In the fourth study, donor-derived, activated T cells were given to patients after allogeneic HSCT. Infusions were safe and not associated with an increased risk of GVHD. Future studies are necessary to determine if activated T cells have better antitumor activity than donor lymphocyte infusion (DLI) (see section "Donor Lymphocyte Infusion"). In an effort to increase the frequency of antigen-specific T cells in autologous, activated T-cell products, patients have been vaccinated with autologous tumor cells or model antigens prior to leukapheresis and *ex vivo* T-cell activation. Results from two phase 1 clinical studies using this approach are promising.[186,233]

Tumor Infiltrating Lymphocytes. The overall disappointing results of adoptive immunotherapy with LAK cells or anti-CD3 activated autologous T cells resulted in the exploration of TILs as adoptive immunotherapy for malignancies. The success rate of TIL isolation from human solid tumors ranges from 30% to 65% and in most studied malignancies TILs are CD4[+] T cells except in melanoma, in which CD8[+] T cells predominate.[234] Since the number of TILs isolated from tumor biopsies is insufficient for adoptive immunotherapy protocols, they must be expanded *ex vivo* in the presence of IL-2 prior to infusion. Expanded CD8[+] TILs have cytolytic activity against the original tumor and in contrast to LAK cells the killing is MHC class I restricted.[181] The outcome of clinical trials with the adoptive immunotherapy of TIL has been varied most likely reflecting differences in tumor immunogenicity and tumor burden at the time of TIL infusion.[191] In an effort to increase the antitumor efficacy of TILs, patients have been lymphodepleted with fludarabine (Flu) and cyclophosphamide (Cy) with 0, 2, or 12 Gy of total body irradiation (TBI) prior to TIL transfer.[192,193] Lymphodepletion in 93 patients with metastatic, refractory melanoma resulted in increased levels of IL-7 and IL-15, and the objective response rate increased from 49% in patients receiving only Flu/Cy to 72% in patients receiving both Flu/Cy and 12 Gy TBI.

Donor Lymphocyte Infusion. Adoptive immunotherapy with DLIs after HSCT effectively augments the graft-versus-leukemia response and eliminates residual disease, especially CML.[194,195] In 1990, Kolb and coworkers reported three patients with relapsed CML who attained complete cytogenetic remissions after treatment with DLI and IFN-α post-HSCT. In larger series, approximately 70% of all relapsed CML patients treated in chronic phase achieved complete cytogenetic remission, in contrast to only 11% of those in accelerated phase or blast crisis.[235] For patients with other hematologic malignancies relapsing post-HSCT, the rate of response to DLI is much lower, being 29% for AML and 5% for acute lymphoblastic leukemia.[195] This so-called graft-versus-tumor effect may simply be another manifestation of GHVD; however, recent studies indicate that minor histocompatibility antigen-specific T cells present in infused donor lymphocytes can induce durable remissions of malignancies without causing GVHD.[236] Despite the success of DLI, its use is limited by GHVD, a potential life-threatening complication. Infusing CD8-depleted lymphocytes has resulted in a reduction in the incidence of GVHD with preservation of the graft-versus-tumor effect.[237] However, because of varying degrees of alloreactivity with different donor-recipient pairs it may not be possible to define a T-cell dose, which has antitumor activity without causing GVHD in patients. In addition to CD8 depletion, other strategies have been developed to reduce the risk of GVHD after T-cell infusion.

The first strategy employs the transduction of T cells with a PDME gene so that cell death can be induced if GVHD develops (see section "Prodrug-Metabolizing Enzyme Gene Therapy"). Donor-derived T cells transduced with a retroviral vector expressing HSV-*tk*, which renders the cells sensitive to GCV, have been infused into HSCT recipients. Several clinical studies have been conducted using this approach and have shown that the infusion of HSV-*tk* T cells post-HSCT is safe and results in accelerated immune reconstitution. In patient who developed GVHD, the disease was successfully controlled with GCV.[238,239] Drawbacks of this approach are the inherent immunogenicity of HSV-*tk* and the use of nucleoside analogs for inducing T-cell killing, which diminishes their value as antiviral agents. Thus other approaches are being explored for the selective induction of cell killing including the use of inducible FAS or caspase in combination with chemical inducers of dimerization and CD20 with rituximab.[240–243]

The second approach to overcome the problem of alloreactivity is to selectively deplete the T-cell product of alloreactive cells that express activation markers in response to alloantigen. Several studies are evaluating this strategy using an immunotoxin directed against the activation marker CD25. Preclinical studies have shown that this procedure can deplete alloreactive cells while preserving T cells reactive to viruses and TAAs such as the minor histocompatibility antigen HA1 and primary granule enzyme proteinase 3. In two phase 1 clinical studies, patients received alloreactive-depleted T cells and early T-cell expansion was seen with improvements in immune reconstitution against viral pathogens without causing significant GVHD.[244,245] The third approach to prevent GVHD after T-cell infusion is to administer antigen-specific CTLs rather than unmanipulated donor T cells, which is discussed in detail in the following section.

Antigen-Specific T Cells. Currently, antigen-specific T cells for adoptive immunotherapy for malignancies are generated using APCs expressing the antigen of interest or by genetic modification of T cells with viral or nonviral vectors expressing a tumor antigen-specific α/β TCRs or CARs.

Antigen-specific T cells generated by APC stimulation. Developing successful CTL therapies depends on the availability of specific antigens as targets and efficient methods for *ex vivo* T-cell activation and expansion. Riddell et al. pioneered the use of antigen-specific CTLs to prevent CMV reactivation in marrow recipients.[246] Donor-derived CD8[+] T-cell clones activated by coculture with CMV-infected, autologous fibroblasts and specific for the viral tegument proteins pp65 and pp150 proved safe and protected HSCT recipients against the reactivation of CMV. However, the persistence of infused CD8[+] T-cell clones was dependent on the recovery of endogenous CD4[+] CMV-specific T cells.[247] Later studies showed that coinfusion of CD4[+] and CD8[+] CMV-specific T-cell clones was sufficient to ensure persistence of the latter. Since then, studies have been performed with other antigen-specific CTL, including EBV-specific CTL for the adoptive immunotherapy for EBV-associated diseases and MART-1- or gp100-specific CTL for melanoma.[196–201,203–221]

Adoptive immunotherapy with EBV-specific CTL. EBV-associated malignancies provide an excellent model system to test and optimize cellular immunotherapies. EBV is a latent gamma herpes virus and more than 90% of the world's population is EBV positive.[248] During primary infection, EBV establishes lifelong latency in the memory B-cell compartment and the number of latently infected B cells within an individual remains stable over years. Healthy individuals mount a vigorous humoral and cellular immune response to primary infection. Although EBV-specific antibodies neutralize virus infectivity, the cellular immune response, consisting of CD4[+] and CD8[+] T cells, is essential for controlling primary and latent EBV infection.[249] The use of EBV-specific CTL has been evaluated in pediatric patients with EBV-associated lymphoproliferative disease (EBV-LPD) post-HSCT and solid organ transplants (SOTs), as well as in EBV-positive non-Hodgkin and Hodgkin lymphoma and nasopharyngeal carcinoma.

ADOPTIVE IMMUNOTHERAPY FOR EBV-LPD POST-HSCT AND SOT. Donor-derived, polyclonal CTL lines have been developed for prophylaxis and treatment of EBV-LPD in children receiving T cell-depleted HSCT.[196,197] In a subset of patients, these CTL were gene marked with the neomycin resistance gene to allow *in vivo* tracking of the infused cells. The infused CTL expanded several logs *in vivo* after infusion and persisted for up to 7 years, most likely because the CTL lines were infused into a lymphodepleted niche in a regenerating immune system and contained both CD8$^+$ and CD4$^+$ EBV-specific T cells. The infused CTL were safe, reconstituted EBV-specific immunity, and reduced the virus load in patients with elevated EBV-DNA levels at the time of infusion. All patients who received CTL as prophylaxis were protected against EBV-LPD compared with an EBV-LPD incidence of 11.5% in historic controls. The safety and efficacy of EBV-specific CTL, when given as prophylaxis, has been confirmed by other investigators.[198] EBV-specific CTL were also effective in 11 out of 13 patients with bulky disease who received CTL therapy. One patient with extensive disease died 5 days post-CTL transfer and the other nonresponder illustrates one of the recurring problems of immunotherapy: mutation of CTL target epitopes on tumor cells allowing the tumor to escape T-cell recognition.[250] To overcome this limitation, it will be necessary to target multiple epitopes, preferably of essential proteins that cannot be downregulated or mutated.

The success of donor-derived EBV-specific CTL as prophylaxis and treatment of EBV-LPD post-HSCT has fueled the development of adoptive immunotherapy strategies for EBV-LPD post-SOT. Since most EBV-LPD post-SOT are of recipient origin and donors are not HLA matched, the use of donor-derived EBV-specific T cells is of limited value. Therefore, the use of autologous, haploidentical, and partially HLA-matched EBV-specific CTL has been explored. These studies demonstrated that infused EBV-specific CTL (a) can be generated from patients receiving immunosuppressive drugs, even if they had active lymphoma, (b) did not cause graft rejection, (c) increased EBV-specific cellular immune responses *in vivo*, and (d) had antiviral and antitumor effects.[199–202] However, in contrast to HSCT recipients the infused EBV-specific CTL persisted only transiently and did not expand by several orders of magnitude, which may indicate that (a) CTL do not persist because of ongoing immunosuppression and (b) the CTL expansion rate is limited in patients, who have normal lymphocyte counts with a lymphocyte compartment close to or at steady state. Genetically modifying T cells has the potential to render CTLs resistant to immunosuppressive agents such as tacrolimus (FK506), opening the opportunity to improve CTL therapies for patients, who are on chronic immunosuppressive therapy.[251]

ADOPTIVE IMMUNOTHERAPY FOR EBV-POSITIVE LYMPHOMAS. EBV is associated with a subset of non-Hodgkin and Hodgkin lymphomas in immunocompetent individuals.[252] In contrast to EBV-LPD, only a limited number of EBV-derived antigens, EBNA1, LMP1, and LMP2, are present in EBV-positive lymphomas. Nevertheless, the viral antigens provide targets for immunotherapy with CTL and autologous as well as allogeneic EBV-specific CTLs have been evaluated.

Autologous EBV-specific CTLs have been given to patients with EBV-positive Hodgkin lymphoma with multiple relapses or minimal residual disease postautologous HSCT.[203,204] No immediate toxicities were seen. Infused CTL localized to tumor sites and immunological studies showed an increase of LMP2- and EBV-specific cellular immunity after CTL infusion, and

gene-marked CTLs were detected for up to 12 months. Lucas et al. infused six patients with matched or partially matched allogeneic EBV-specific CTL.[205] Three patients received CTL alone and three patients received fludarabine followed by CTL. In the "CTL only" group, all patients had a decrease in measurable disease and two were alive 6 and 22 months after infusion. In the "fludarabine CTL group," two out of three patients had a decrease in tumor size; however, it was impossible to distinguish if the effect was due to fludarabine or CTL infusion.

The clinical experience with autologous and allogeneic EBV-specific CTL indicates that EBV is a legitimate target for the adoptive immunotherapy for EBV-positive lymphomas. One strategy to enhance the antitumor activity of EBV-specific CTL is to increase the frequency of T cells specific for the subdominant EBV antigens LMP1 and LMP2. Twenty-eight patients with EBV-positive non-Hodgkin or Hodgkin lymphoma have been infused with LMP2- or LMP1/LMP2-specific CTL. Fourteen out of 15 patients who were in remission at the time of T-cell infusion remain in remission, and clinical responses were seen in 11 out of 13 patients with active disease including 8 CRs.[253,254]

ADOPTIVE IMMUNOTHERAPY FOR EBV-POSITIVE NASOPHARYNGEAL CARCINOMA. Nasopharyngeal carcinoma (NPC) arises from the epithelial cells of the nasopharynx and almost all nonkeratinizing and undifferentiated NPCs are associated with EBV. However, other environmental or genetic factors must play an important role in oncogenesis, since the incidence of NPC varies 50- to 100-fold from southern China to western countries.[255] As in EBV-positive lymphomas, only a limited number of EBV latent proteins are expressed, being EBNA1, LMP1, and LMP2. The use of autologous EBV-specific CTL for NPC has been evaluated in three clinical trials.[206–208] Three pilot studies using EBV-specific CTL have been published. In one study, four NPC patients with advanced disease were infused and an increase in EBV-specific CTL precursor frequency was observed, as well as a reduction in plasma EBV-DNA levels. Comoli et al. reported 10 patients who received between 2 and 23 CTL infusions. Two patients had a PR for 3 to 4 months and four patients had SD for up to 15 months. We have treated 23 NPC patients with recurrent/refractory disease. Of the 15 patients with active disease, 5 had a CR/Cru, 2 patients had a PR, and 2 patients had SD.

ADOPTIVE IMMUNOTHERAPY WITH TUMOR ANTIGEN-SPECIFIC CTL. In one trial, 10 patients with refractory melanoma received a total of 43 T-cell infusions with either gp100-specific T-cell clones or MART-1–specific T-cell clones.[211] The infused CTL were safe; no *in vivo* expansion of CTL was observed, and the median *in vivo* T-cell survival was 6.7 days without low-dose IL-2 and 16.9 days in the presence of IL-2. Infused CTL localized to tumor sites and had cytotoxic activity as judged by elimination of antigen-positive tumor cells. Minor, mixed, or stable responses were observed in 8 out of 10 patients for up to 21 months. Interestingly, three out of five patients analyzed showed antigen-loss tumor variants at the time of relapse, highlighting the risk of CTL escape mutants with the use of T-cell clones. In a follow up study, patients were lymphodepleted with fludarabine prior to T-cell transfer, which resulted in a 2.9-fold increase in the *in vivo* persistence of adoptively transferred T-cell clones.[210] In clinical studies, localization of infused T-cell clones to tumor sites was demonstrated through biopsies as well as by indium^{111} labeling.[212] Patients have also been infused with T-cell clones specific for HER2 or NY-ESO-1.[222,256] One of these case report highlights the potency of CD4$^+$ T-cell clones; infusion of NY-ESO-1–specific CD4$^+$ T cells resulted in a durable clinical remission in a patient with metastatic melanoma and induced endogenous immune responses against other tumor antigens.[256]

IMPROVING ADOPTIVE IMMUNOTHERAPY WITH ANTIGEN-SPECIFIC CTL. Clinical studies with adoptively transferred CTL have highlighted the need to improve the efficacy of tumor-specific T-cell therapies.[179,257] Expanding CTL *ex vivo* only overcomes the *in vivo* immunosuppressive environment; however, the infused CTL can still be anergized or killed by factors released by the tumor or even killed directly by tumor cells. For example, tumor cells secreting TGF-β are able to anergize infused CTL, and FAS ligand expressing tumor cells trigger CTL apoptosis by engaging the death receptor, FAS, on CTLs. Preclinical studies have shown that CTL can be rendered resistant to the inhibitory effects of TGF-β by expression of a dominant negative TGF-β type II receptor and a phase 1 clinical study is in progress.[258,259] Other preclinical strategies have focused on increasing the effector function of CTLs by expressing the proinflammatory cytokine IL-12 or increasing the homing of CTLs to tumor sites by expressing chemokine receptors.[260–262]

The dramatic expansion of antigen-specific CTL in HSCT recipients was rarely seen in other groups of patients. This may be explained by the homeostatic state of the recipient. After HSCT, the lymphoid compartment is depleted, so that infused, mature, activated T cells expand to fill the void. Most other patients who received CTL have a replete lymphoid compartment, leaving little room for the expansion of infused T cells. As described in the section "Tumor Infiltrating Lymphocytes" studies using chemotherapy and irradiation have confirmed the importance of lymphodepletion to enhance expansion and persistence of adoptively transferred T cells.[192] However, the use of these agents resulted in the extensive and nonspecific destruction of the resident immune system. Monoclonal antibodies that are cytolytic for lymphocytes may be an alternative means of producing lymphodepletion, and we have successfully completed one phase 1 clinical study using CD45 monoclonal antibodies to enhance the expansion of adoptively transferred EBV-specific CTL in NPC patients.[209]

Besides chemotherapy or irradiation, epigenetic modifiers, such as HDAC or DNA methylation inhibitors, have the potential to improve T-cell therapies. Epigenetic modifiers upregulate the expression of TAAs, resulting in better T-cell recognition of tumor cells.[263,264] However, while epigenetic modifiers increase the expression of TAA, they might also inhibit the antigen processing machinery promoting immune escape.[265] Thus, how to best combine epigenetic modifiers with T-cell therapies requires additional studies.

While host conditioning influences the *in vivo* outcome of T-cell infusions, there is increasing evidence that T-cell subsets differ in their *in vivo* fate. For example, Berger et al demonstrated in a nonhuman primate model that T-cell clones derived from central memory T cells are able to reconstitute the memory T-cell pool *in vivo* whereas T-cell clones with the same specificity derived from effector memory T cells did not.[266] In addition, telomere length and the expression of cell surface markers such as CD27 have been correlated with antitumor activity of infused TILs.[267]

Targeting malignancies with genetically modified T cells. Gene transfer allows the rapid generation of antigen-specific T cells for adoptive immunotherapy, and this approach can circumvent tolerance to the self-antigens expressed by tumor cells. Successful gene transfer strategies include the forced expression of α/β TCRs or antigen-specific CARs.

α/β T-CELL RECEPTORS. α/β TCR genes have been cloned for several HLA-restricted epitopes encoded by TAAs.[268–270] Genetic modification of T cells with α/β TCRs requires high expression and correct pairing of two different receptor molecules from a single vector, which has proved problematic for transgenic α/β TCRs. However, in the last 5 years there has been significant progress in overcoming both of these limitations, and three phase 1 clinical studies with α/β TCR T cells for patients with refractory, metastatic melanoma have been completed.[213,214,270,271] Thirty-four patients were infused with T cells expressing a low-affinity MART1-specific α/β TCR T cells and objective clinical responses, including two CRs, were observed.[214] Thirty-six patients then received T cells expressing high-affinity α/β TCR specific for either MART1 or gp100 producing antitumor activity in nine patients including one CR and eight PRs.[213] However, T cells also recognized normal tissues, which expressed low levels of the targeted TAAs, highlighting that as for other targeted therapies, the target selection is critical to prevent "off targets" effects.

CHIMERIC ANTIGEN RECEPTORS. Tumor-specific T cells can also be created by genetically modifying T cells with random specificity to express tumor-specific CARs.[272–274] The concept is based on the observation that engagement of single TCR chains induces cellular activation and proliferation in the presence of growth factors, such as IL-2. T cells with CARs have, conceptually, numerous advantages over immunotherapies based on monoclonal antibodies or T cells alone. They can be directed toward any native TAA or viral-associated antigen, which is expressed on the cell surface, making this strategy potentially applicable to a variety of malignancies and viral diseases. Because CARs provide T-cell activation in a non-MHC restricted manner, there use is not limited by HLA restriction, and they are immune to some of the major mechanisms by which tumors avoid MHC-restricted T-cell recognition, such as downregulation of HLA class I molecules and defects in antigen processing. CAR expressing T cells are more likely to eradicate tumor cells than antibodies alone, since they can migrate through microvascular walls, extravase and penetrate the core of solid tumors to exert their cytolytic activity, sequentially kill a multiplicity of target cells, and recruit additional components of the immune system, thus amplifying the antitumor or antiviral immune response.

CARs can be generated by joining the heavy and light chain variable regions of a monoclonal antibody, expressed as a single-chain Fv (scFv) molecule, to the cytoplasmic TCR ζ or Fc-γ domain and CARs targeting pediatric diseases are listed in Table 14.7.[219–221,275–284] Antigen stimulation of the extracellular component of the chimeric receptor results in phosphorylation of immunoreceptor tyrosine-based activation motifs present in the cytoplasmic domain, initiating TCR signaling. Human T cells genetically engineered to express the recombinant receptor genes were capable of specific lysis and cytokine secretion on exposure to tumor cells expressing the relevant target antigens. In addition, adoptively transferred CAR-transduced cells were protective in murine tumor models.[275,282] Although attempts have been made to translate these encouraging

TABLE 14.7

CHIMERIC ANTIGEN RECEPTORS FOR PEDIATRIC MALIGNANCIES

Specificity of receptor	Tumor	Ref
CD19	Leukemia	275–277
CD20	Lymphoma	220
CD30	Hodgkin disease	278, 279
CD171	Neuroblastoma	219
GD2a	Neuroblastoma	221, 280
HER2	Medulloblastoma, osteosarcoma	281, 282
IL-13 Rα2	Glioblastoma multiforme, Medulloblastoma	105, 283

preclinical experiences into clinical trials, the clinical benefits of adoptively transferred CAR T cells were limited. The most pertinent issue being that CAR T cells failed to expand and rapidly lost their function *in vivo*.[215,216]

Several approaches have been pursued to overcome the limitation of CAR T cells. Incorporation of additional signaling domains from the costimulatory molecules CD28, CD134, and CD137 into CARs as well as the coexpression of cytokines or their receptors have resulted in enhanced effector function of CAR T cells.[285–287] A more pragmatic approach to overcome the signaling defect of CARs with a single ζ signaling domain might be to express the receptors in antigen-specific T cells, which can be activated and expanded through their endogenous TCR. This concept of bispecific T cells was validated in an animal model with alloreactive T cells expressing CARs recognizing folate-binding protein, an ovarian cancer-associated antigen.[288] Clinically relevant examples of this strategy include the expression of CARs in EBV-, Influenza-, or VZV-specific T cells.[276,279,289] In a phase 1 clinical study, EBV-specific T cells expressing a GD2-ζ CAR persisted for significantly longer than autologous GD2-ζ T cells.[221] In addition, the infusion of GD2-specific T cells resulted in tumor necrosis or regression (including a complete remission) in 4/8 patients with refractory/relapsed disease. Currently, several phase 1 clinical trials are in progress testing the safety of T cells expressing CD19-specific CARs.

CONCLUSIONS

Whether cell and gene therapies will prove effective for pediatrics malignancies and improve long-term outcome remain unclear at present, but it is important to remember that most advances in medicine proceed incrementally. The results obtained to date are certainly sufficiently encouraging to justify continued, active exploration of these approaches particularly since the associated toxicities are minor compared with those seen with conventional cancer therapies. Many therapeutic concepts have been tested successfully in preclinical models; however, such models cannot always predict the outcome for human diseases; thus, carefully planned clinical trials are needed to validate these novel therapeutic approaches. Cell and gene therapies will most likely not replace conventional therapies but complement them increasing their potency and hopefully reducing short- and long-term toxicities. The benefits of these new technologies can only increase as current limitations are progressively surmounted.

References

1. Bleyer WA. Cancer in older adolescents and young adults: epidemiology, diagnosis, treatment, survival, and importance of clinical trials. Med Pediatr Oncol 2002;38:1–10.
2. Oeffinger KC, Mertens AC, Hudson MM, et al. Health care of young adult survivors of childhood cancer: a report from the Childhood Cancer Survivor Study. Ann Fam Med 2004;2:61–70.
3. Landier W, Bhatia S. Cancer survivorship: a pediatric perspective. Oncologist 2008;13:1181–1192.
4. Gene Therapy Clinical Trials Worldwide. www.wiley.co.uk/genetherapy/clinical. Accessed August 30, 2009.
5. Hacein-Bey-Abina S, Le Deist F, Carlier F, et al. Sustained correction of X-linked severe combined immunodeficiency by ex vivo gene therapy. N Engl J Med 2002;346:1185–1193.
6. Ott MG, Schmidt M, Schwarzwaelder K, et al. Correction of X-linked chronic granulomatous disease by gene therapy, augmented by insertional activation of MDS1-EVI1, PRDM16 or SETBP1. Nat Med 2006;12: 401–409.
7. Aiuti A, Cattaneo F, Galimberti S, et al. Gene therapy for immunodeficiency due to adenosine deaminase deficiency. N Engl J Med 2009;360:447–458.
8. Bainbridge JW, Smith AJ, Barker SS, et al. Effect of gene therapy on visual function in Leber's congenital amaurosis. N Engl J Med 2008;358: 2231–2239.
9. Maguire AM, Simonelli F, Pierce EA, et al. Safety and efficacy of gene transfer for Leber's congenital amaurosis. N Engl J Med 2008;358: 2240–2248.
10. Hacein-Bey-Abina S, Garrigue A, Wang GP, et al. Insertional oncogenesis in 4 patients after retrovirus-mediated gene therapy of SCID-X1. J Clin Invest 2008;118:3132–3142.
11. Stein S, Ott MG, Schultze-Strasser S, et al. Gene therapy for chronic granulomatous disease: Current status of the German clinical study. Hum Gene Ther 2008;19:1097.
12. Dave UP, Jenkins NA, Copeland NG. Gene therapy insertional mutagenesis insights. Science 2004;303:333.
13. Woods NB, Bottero V, Schmidt M, et al. Gene therapy: therapeutic gene causing lymphoma. Nature 2006;440:1123.
14. Thrasher AJ, Gaspar HB, Baum C, et al. Gene therapy: X-SCID transgene leukaemogenicity. Nature 2006;443:E5–E6.
15. Kohn DB, Sadelain M, Dunbar C, et al. American Society of Gene Therapy (ASGT) ad hoc subcommittee on retroviral-mediated gene transfer to hematopoietic stem cells. Mol Ther 2003;8:180–187.
16. Kohn DB, Candotti F. Gene therapy fulfilling its promise. N Engl J Med 2009;360:518–521.
17. Carroll D. Progress and prospects: zinc-finger nucleases as gene therapy agents. Gene Ther 2008;15:1463–1468.
18. Grimm D, Kay MA. RNAi and gene therapy: a mutual attraction. Hematology Am Soc Hematol Educ Program 2007;1:473–481.
19. McNeish IA, Bell SJ, Lemoine NR. Gene therapy progress and prospects: cancer gene therapy using tumour suppressor genes. Gene Ther 2004;11:497–503.
20. Nemunaitis J, Swisher SG, Timmons T, et al. Adenovirus-mediated p53 gene transfer in sequence with cisplatin to tumors of patients with non-small-cell lung cancer. J Clin Oncol 2000;18:609–622.
21. Clayman GL, El Naggar AK, Lippman SM, et al. Adenovirus-mediated p53 gene transfer in patients with advanced recurrent head and neck squamous cell carcinoma. J Clin Oncol 1998;16:2221–2232.
22. Swisher SG, Roth JA, Komaki R, et al. Induction of p53-regulated genes and tumor regression in lung cancer patients after intratumoral delivery of adenoviral p53 (INGN 201) and radiation therapy. Clin Cancer Res 2003;9:93–101.
23. Keedy V, Wang W, Schiller J, et al. Phase I study of adenovirus p53 administered by bronchoalveolar lavage in patients with bronchioloalveolar cell lung carcinoma: ECOG 6597. J Clin Oncol 2008;26:4166–4171.
24. Niculescu-Duvaz I, Springer CJ. Introduction to the background, principles, and state of the art in suicide gene therapy. Mol Biotechnol 2005;30:71–88.
25. Packer RJ, Raffel C, Villablanca JG, et al. Treatment of progressive or recurrent pediatric malignant supratentorial brain tumors with herpes simplex virus thymidine kinase gene vector-producer cells followed by intravenous ganciclovir administration. J Neurosurg 2000;92:249–254.
26. Chevez-Barrios P, Chintagumpala M, Mieler W, et al. Response of retinoblastoma with vitreous tumor seeding to adenovirus-mediated delivery of thymidine kinase followed by ganciclovir. J Clin Oncol 2005;23:7927–7935.
27. Freeman SM, Abboud CN, Whartenby KA, et al. The "bystander effect": tumor regression when a fraction of the tumor mass is genetically modified. Cancer Res 1993;53:5274–5283.
28. Mesnil M, Yamasaki H. Bystander effect in herpes simplex virus-thymidine kinase/ganciclovir cancer gene therapy: role of gap-junctional intercellular communication. Cancer Res 2000;60:3989–3999.
29. King GD, Muhammad AK, Curtin JF, et al. Flt3L and TK gene therapy eradicate multifocal glioma in a syngeneic glioblastoma model. Neuro Oncol 2008;10:19–31.
30. Chiocca EA. Oncolytic viruses. Nat Rev Cancer 2002;2:938–950.
31. Lin E, Nemunaitis J. Oncolytic viral therapies. Cancer Gene Ther 2004;11:643–664.
32. Liu TC, Galanis E, Kirn D. Clinical trial results with oncolytic virotherapy: a century of promise, a decade of progress. Nat Clin Pract Oncol 2007;4:101–117.
33. Duntsch CD, Zhou Q, Jayakar HR, et al. Recombinant vesicular stomatitis virus vectors as oncolytic agents in the treatment of high-grade gliomas in an organotypic brain tissue slice-glioma coculture model. J Neurosurg 2004;100:1049–1059.
34. Heise C, Sampson-Johannes A, Williams A, et al. ONYX-015, an E1B gene-attenuated adenovirus, causes tumor-specific cytolysis and antitumoral efficacy that can be augmented by standard chemotherapeutic agents [see comments]. Nat Med 1997;3:639–645.
35. Khuri FR, Nemunaitis J, Ganly I, et al. A controlled trial of intratumoral ONYX-015, a selectively-replicating adenovirus, in combination with cisplatin and 5-fluorouracil in patients with recurrent head and neck cancer. Nat Med 2000;6:879–885.
36. Xia ZJ, Chang JH, Zhang L, et al. Phase III randomized clinical trial of intratumoral injection of E1B gene-deleted adenovirus (H101) combined with cisplatin-based chemotherapy in treating squamous cell cancer of head and neck or esophagus [in Chinese]. Ai Zheng 2004;23:1666–1670.
37. Small EJ, Carducci MA, Burke JM, et al. A phase I trial of intravenous CG7870, a replication-selective, prostate-specific antigen-targeted oncolytic adenovirus, for the treatment of hormone-refractory, metastatic prostate cancer. Mol Ther 2006;14:107–117.
38. DeWeese TL, van der PH, Li S, et al. A phase I trial of CV706, a replication-competent, PSA selective oncolytic adenovirus, for the treatment of locally recurrent prostate cancer following radiation therapy. Cancer Res 2001;61:7464–7472.
39. Freytag SO, Stricker H, Pegg J, et al. Phase I study of replication-competent adenovirus-mediated double-suicide gene therapy in combination with conventional-dose three-dimensional conformal radiation therapy for the treatment of newly diagnosed, intermediate- to high-risk prostate cancer. Cancer Res 2003;63:7497–7506.
40. Freytag SO, Stricker H, Peabody J, et al. Five-year follow-up of trial of replication-competent adenovirus-mediated suicide gene therapy for treatment of prostate cancer. Mol Ther 2007;15:636–642.
41. Rampling R, Cruickshank G, Papanastassiou V, et al. Toxicity evaluation of replication-competent herpes simplex virus (ICP 34.5 null mutant 1716) in patients with recurrent malignant glioma. Gene Ther 2000;7:859–866.
42. Papanastassiou V, Rampling R, Fraser M, et al. The potential for efficacy of the modified (ICP 34.5(−)) herpes simplex virus HSV1716 following intratumoural injection into human malignant glioma: a proof of principle study. Gene Ther 2002;9:398–406.

43. Harrow S, Papanastassiou V, Harland J, et al. HSV1716 injection into the brain adjacent to tumour following surgical resection of high-grade glioma: safety data and long-term survival. Gene Ther 2004;11:1648–1658.
44. MacKie RM, Stewart B, Brown SM. Intralesional injection of herpes simplex virus 1716 in metastatic melanoma. Lancet 2001;357:525–526.
45. Markert JM, Medlock MD, Rabkin SD, et al. Conditionally replicating herpes simplex virus mutant, G207 for the treatment of malignant glioma: results of a phase I trial. Gene Ther 2000;7:867–874.
46. Markert JM, Liechty PG, Wang W, et al. Phase Ib trial of mutant herpes simplex virus G207 inoculated pre-and post-tumor resection for recurrent GBM. Mol Ther 2009;17: 199–207.
47. Kemeny N, Brown K, Covey A, et al. Phase I, open-label, dose-escalating study of a genetically engineered herpes simplex virus, NV1020, in subjects with metastatic colorectal carcinoma to the liver. Hum Gene Ther 2006;17:1214–1224.
48. Hu JC, Coffin RS, Davis CJ, et al. A phase I study of OncoVEXGM-CSF, a second-generation oncolytic herpes simplex virus expressing granulocyte macrophage colony-stimulating factor. Clin Cancer Res 2006;12:6737–6747.
49. Li H, Dutuor A, Tao L, et al. Virotherapy with a type 2 herpes simplex virus-derived oncolytic virus induces potent antitumor immunity against neuroblastoma. Clin Cancer Res 2007;13:316–322.
50. Schirrmacher V, Fournier P. Newcastle disease virus: a promising vector for viral therapy, immune therapy, and gene therapy of cancer. Methods Mol Biol 2009;542: 565–605.
51. Pecora AL, Rizvi N, Cohen GI, et al. Phase I trial of intravenous administration of PV701, an oncolytic virus, in patients with advanced solid cancers. J Clin Oncol 2002; 20:2251–2266.
52. Laurie SA, Bell JC, Atkins HL, et al. A phase 1 clinical study of intravenous administration of PV701, an oncolytic virus, using two-step desensitization. Clin Cancer Res 2006;12:2555–2562.
53. Lorence RM, Roberts MS, O'Neil JD, et al. Phase 1 clinical experience using intravenous administration of PV701, an oncolytic Newcastle disease virus. Curr Cancer Drug Targets 2007;7:157–167.
54. Schulze T, Kemmner W, Weitz J, et al. Efficiency of adjuvant active specific immunization with Newcastle disease virus modified tumor cells in colorectal cancer patients following resection of liver metastases: results of a prospective randomized trial. Cancer Immunol Immunother 2009;58:61–69.
55. Kelly K, Nawrocki S, Mita A, et al. Reovirus-based therapy for cancer. Expert Opin Biol Ther 2009;9:817–830.
56. Forsyth P, Roldan G, George D, et al. A phase I trial of intratumoral administration of reovirus in patients with histologically confirmed recurrent malignant gliomas. Mol Ther 2008;16:627–632.
57. Vidal L, Pandha HS, Yap TA, et al. A phase I study of intravenous oncolytic reovirus type 3 Dearing in patients with advanced cancer. Clin Cancer Res 2008;14:7127–7137.
58. Kottke T, Diaz RM, Kaluza K, et al. Use of biological therapy to enhance both virotherapy and adoptive T-cell therapy for cancer. Mol Ther 2008;16:1910–1918.
59. Munguia A, Ota T, Miest T, et al. Cell carriers to deliver oncolytic viruses to sites of myeloma tumor growth. Gene Ther 2008;15:797–806.
60. Folkman J. Tumor angiogenesis: therapeutic implications. N Engl J Med 1971;285: 1182–1186.
61. Eder JP Jr, Supko JG, Clark JW, et al. Phase I clinical trial of recombinant human endostatin administered as a short intravenous infusion repeated daily. J Clin Oncol 2002; 20:3772–3784.
62. Hurwitz H, Fehrenbacher L, Novotny W, et al. Bevacizumab plus irinotecan, fluorouracil, and leucovorin for metastatic colorectal cancer. N Engl J Med 2004;350: 2335–2342.
63. Tandle A, Blazer DG III, Libutti SK. Antiangiogenic gene therapy of cancer: recent developments. J Transl Med 2004;2:22.
64. Sauter BV, Martinet O, Zhang WJ, et al. Adenovirus-mediated gene transfer of endostatin in vivo results in high level of transgene expression and inhibition of tumor growth and metastases. Proc Natl Acad Sci U S A 2000;97:4802–4807.
65. Ponnazhagan S, Mahendra G, Kumar S, et al. Adeno-associated virus 2-mediated antiangiogenic cancer gene therapy: long-term efficacy of a vector encoding angiostatin and endostatin over vectors encoding a single factor. Cancer Res 2004;64:1781–1787.
66. Lin X, Huang H, Li S, et al. A phase I clinical trial of an adenovirus-mediated endostatin gene (E10A) in patients with solid tumors. Cancer Biol Ther 2007;6:648–653.
67. Noel A, Maillard C, Rocks N, et al. Membrane associated proteases and their inhibitors in tumour angiogenesis. J Clin Pathol 2004;57:577–584.
68. Overall CM, Lopez-Otin C. Strategies for MMP inhibition in cancer: innovations for the post-trial era. Nat Rev Cancer 2002;2:657–672.
69. Flasshove M, Moritz T, Bardenheuer W, et al. Hematoprotection by transfer of drug-resistance genes. Acta Haematol 2003;110:93–106.
70. Pastan I, Gottesman MM. Multidrug resistance. Annu Rev Med 1991;42:277–286.
71. Sorrentino BP, McDonagh KT, Woods D, et al. Expression of retroviral vectors containing the human MDR1 cDNA in hematopoietic cells of transplanted mice. Blood 1995;86:491–501.
72. Maze R, Carney JP, Kelley MR, et al. Increasing DNA repair methyltransferase levels via bone marrow stem cell transduction rescues mice from the toxic effects of 1,3-bis(2-chloroethyl)-1-nitrosourea, a chemotherapeutic alkylating agent. Proc Natl Acad Sci U S A 1996;93:206–210.
73. Allay JA, Persons DA, Galipeau J, et al. In vivo selection of retrovirally transduced hematopoietic stem cells. Nat Med 1998;4:1136–1143.
74. Hanania EG, Giles RE, Kavanagh J, et al. Results of MDR-1 vector modification trial indicate that granulocyte/macrophage colony-forming unit cells do not contribute to posttransplant hematopoietic recovery following intensive systemic therapy. Proc Natl Acad Sci U S A 1996;93:15346–15351.
75. Hesdorffer C, Ayello J, Ward M, et al. Phase I trial of retroviral-mediated transfer of the human MDR1 gene as marrow chemoprotection in patients undergoing high-dose chemotherapy and autologous stem-cell transplantation. J Clin Oncol 1998;16: 165–172.
76. Abonour R, Williams DA, Einhorn L, et al. Efficient retrovirus-mediated transfer of the multidrug resistance 1 gene into autologous human long-term repopulating hematopoietic stem cells. Nat Med 2000;6:652–658.
77. Tey SK, Brenner MK. The continuing contribution of gene marking to cell and gene therapy. Mol Ther 2007;15:666–676.
78. Brenner MK, Rill DR, Holladay MS, et al. Gene marking to determine whether autologous marrow infusion restores long-term haemopoiesis in cancer patients. Lancet 1993;342:1134–1137.
79. Rill DR, Santana VM, Roberts WM, et al. Direct demonstration that autologous bone marrow transplantation for solid tumors can return a multiplicity of tumorigenic cells. Blood 1994;84:380–383.
80. Deisseroth AB, Zu Z, Claxton D, et al. Genetic marking shows that Ph+ cells present in autologous transplants of chronic myelogenous leukemia (CML) contribute to relapse after autologous bone marrow in CML. Blood 1994;83:3068–3076.
81. Rill DR, Sycamore DL, Smith SS, et al. Long term in vivo fate of human hemopoietic cells transduced by moloney-based retroviral vectors. Blood 2000;96(11):844a.
82. Finn OJ. Cancer immunology. N Engl J Med 2008;358:2704–2715.
83. Blattman JN, Greenberg PD. Cancer immunotherapy: a treatment for the masses. Science 2004;305:200–205.
84. Renkvist N, Castelli C, Robbins PF, et al. A listing of human tumor antigens recognized by T cells. Cancer Immunol Immunother 2001;50:3–15.
85. van den Eynde BJ, van Der Bruggen P. T cell defined tumor antigens. Curr Opin Immunol 1997;9:684–693.
86. van der Bruggen P, Zhang Y, Chaux P, et al. Tumor-specific shared antigenic peptides recognized by human T cells. Immunol Rev 2002;188: 51–64.
87. Cheever MA, Chen W, Disis M, et al. T-cell immunity to oncogenic proteins including mutated RAS and chimeric BCR-ABL. Ann N Y Acad Sci 1993;690:101–112.
88. Sun JY, Senitzer D, Forman SJ, et al. Identification of new MHC-restriction elements for presentation of the p210(BCR-ABL) fusion region to human cytotoxic T lymphocytes. Cancer Immunol Immunother 2003;52: 761–770.
89. Makita M, Azuma T, Hamaguchi H, et al. Leukemia-associated fusion proteins, dek-can and bcr-abl, represent immunogenic HLA-DR-restricted epitopes recognized by fusion peptide-specific CD4+ T lymphocytes. Leukemia 2002;16:2400–2407.
90. Ohminami H, Yasukawa M, Kaneko S, et al. Fas-independent and nonapoptotic cytotoxicity mediated by a human CD4(+) T-cell clone directed against an acute myelogenous leukemia-associated DEK-CAN fusion peptide. Blood 1999;93:925–935.
91. Gambacorti-Passerini C, Grignani F, Arienti F, et al. Human CD4 lymphocytes specifically recognize a peptide representing the fusion region of the hybrid protein pml/RAR alpha present in acute promyelocytic leukemia cells. Blood 1993;81:1369–1375.
92. Yotnda P, Garcia F, Peuchmaur M, et al. Cytotoxic T cell response against the chimeric ETV6-AML1 protein in childhood acute lymphoblastic leukemia. J Clin Invest 1998; 102:455–462.
93. Naka N, Araki N, Nakanishi H, et al. Expression of SSX genes in human osteosarcomas. Int J Cancer 2002;98:640–642.
94. Dalerba P, Frascella E, Macino B, et al. MAGE, BAGE and GAGE gene expression in human rhabdomyosarcomas. Int J Cancer 2001;93:85–90.
95. Scarcella DL, Chow CW, Gonzales MF, et al. Expression of MAGE and GAGE in high-grade brain tumors: a potential target for specific immunotherapy and diagnostic markers. Clin Cancer Res 1999;5: 335–341.
96. Ishida H, Matsumura T, Salgaller ML, et al. MAGE-1 and MAGE-3 or -6 expression in neuroblastoma-related pediatric solid tumors. Int J Cancer 1996;69:375–380.
97. Sudo T, Kuramoto T, Komiya S, Inoue A, et al. Expression of MAGE genes in osteosarcoma. J Orthop Res 1997;15:128–132.
98. Tanzarella S, Lionello I, Valentinis B, et al. Rhabdomyosarcomas are potential target of MAGE-specific immunotherapies. Cancer Immunol Immunother 2004;53:519–524.
99. Jacobs JF, Brasseur F, Hulsbergen-van de Kaa CA, et al. Cancer-germline gene expression in pediatric solid tumors using quantitative real-time PCR. Int J Cancer 2007; 120:67–74.
100. Liu XF, Helman LJ, Yeung C, et al. XAGE-1, a new gene that is frequently expressed in Ewing's sarcoma. Cancer Res 2000;60:4752–4755.
101. Scotlandi K, Manara MC, Hattinger CM, et al. Prognostic and therapeutic relevance of HER2 expression in osteosarcoma and Ewing's sarcoma. Eur J Cancer 2005;41: 1349–1361.
102. Gajjar A, Hernan R, Kocak M, et al. Clinical, histopathologic, and molecular markers of prognosis: toward a new disease risk stratification system for medulloblastoma. J Clin Oncol 2004;22:984–993.
103. Zhang JG, Eguchi J, Kruse CA, et al. Antigenic profiling of glioma cells to generate allogeneic vaccines or dendritic cell-based therapeutics. Clin Cancer Res 2007;13:566–575.
104. Okano F, Storkus WJ, Chambers WH, et al. Identification of a novel HLA-A*0201-restricted, cytotoxic T lymphocyte epitope in a human glioma-associated antigen, interleukin 13 receptor alpha2 chain. Clin Cancer Res 2002;8:2851–2855.
105. Stastny MJ, Brown CE, Ruel C, et al. Medulloblastomas expressing IL13Ralpha2 are targets for IL13-zetakine+ cytolytic T cells. J Pediatr Hematol Oncol 2007;29:669–677.
106. Okada H, Low KL, Kohanbash G, et al. Expression of glioma-associated antigens in pediatric brain stem and non-brain stem gliomas. J Neurooncol 2008;88:245–250.
107. Tsukahara T, Kawaguchi S, Torigoe T, et al. Prognostic impact and immunogenicity of a novel osteosarcoma antigen, papillomavirus binding factor, in patients with osteosarcoma. Cancer Sci 2008;99:368–375.
108. Islam A, Kageyama H, Takada N, et al. High expression of Survivin, mapped to 17q25, is significantly associated with poor prognostic factors and promotes cell survival in human neuroblastoma. Oncogene 2000;19:617–623.
109. Tamm I, Richter S, Oltersdorf D, et al. High expression levels of x-linked inhibitor of apoptosis protein and survivin correlate with poor overall survival in childhood de novo acute myeloid leukemia. Clin Cancer Res 2004;10:3737–3744.
110. Coughlin CM, Vance BA, Grupp SA, et al. RNA-transfected CD40-activated B cells induce functional T-cell responses against viral and tumor antigen targets: implications for pediatric immunotherapy. Blood 2004;103:2046–2054.
111. Hiyama E, Yamaoka H, Matsunaga T, et al. High expression of telomerase is an independent prognostic indicator of poor outcome in hepatoblastoma. Br J Cancer 2004; 91:972–979.
112. Rosenfeld C, Cheever MA, Gaiger A. WT1 in acute leukemia, chronic myelogenous leukemia and myelodysplastic syndrome: therapeutic potential of WT1 targeted therapies. Leukemia 2003;17:1301–1312.
113. Gordan JD, Vonderheide RH. Universal tumor antigens as targets for immunotherapy. Cytotherapy 2002;4:317–327.
114. Smith-Garvin JE, Koretzky GA, Jordan MS. T cell activation. Annu Rev Immunol 2009;27:591–619.
115. Crotzer VL, Blum JS. Autophagy and its role in MHC-mediated antigen presentation. J Immunol 2009;182:3335–3341.
116. Dustin ML. The cellular context of T cell signaling. Immunity 2009;30:482–492.
117. Croft M. Co-stimulatory members of the TNFR family: keys to effective T-cell immunity? Nat Rev Immunol 2003;3:609–620.

118. Howland KC, Ausubel LJ, London CA, et al. The roles of CD28 and CD40 ligand in T cell activation and tolerance. J Immunol 2000;164:4465–4470.

119. Perez OD, Mitchell D, Jager GC, et al. Leukocyte functional antigen 1 lowers T cell activation thresholds and signaling through cytohesin-1 and Jun-activating binding protein 1. Nat Immunol 2003;4:1083–1092.

120. Khanna R, Burrows SR, Argaet V, et al. Endoplasmic reticulum signal sequence facilitated transport of peptide epitopes restores immunogenicity of an antigen processing defective tumour cell line. Int Immunol 1994;6:639–645.

121. Pentcheva-Hoang T, Corse E, Allison JP. Negative regulators of T-cell activation: potential targets for therapeutic intervention in cancer, autoimmune disease, and persistent infections. Immunol Rev 2009;229:67–87.

122. Liu JQ, Bai XF. Overcoming immune evasion in T cell therapy of cancer: lessons from animal models. Curr Mol Med 2008;8:68–75.

123. Poppema S. Immunobiology and pathophysiology of Hodgkin lymphomas. Hematology Am Soc Hematol Educ Program 2005;231–238.

124. Berzofsky JA, Terabe M, Oh S, et al. Progress on new vaccine strategies for the immunotherapy and prevention of cancer. J Clin Invest 2004;113:1515–1525.

125. Stevenson FK, Ottensmeier CH, Johnson P, et al. DNA vaccines to attack cancer. Proc Natl Acad Sci U S A 2004;101:14646–14652.

126. Stevenson FK. DNA vaccines and adjuvants. Immunol Rev 2004;199:5–8.

127. Timmerman JM, Singh G, Hermanson G, et al. Immunogenicity of a plasmid DNA vaccine encoding chimeric idiotype in patients with B-cell lymphoma. Cancer Res 2002;62:5845–5852.

128. Tagawa ST, Lee P, Snively J, et al. Phase I study of intranodal delivery of a plasmid DNA vaccine for patients with Stage IV melanoma. Cancer 2003;98:144–154.

129. Conry RM, Curiel DT, Strong TV, et al. Safety and immunogenicity of a DNA vaccine encoding carcinoembryonic antigen and hepatitis B surface antigen in colorectal carcinoma patients. Clin Cancer Res 2002;8:2782–2787.

130. McConkey SJ, Reece WH, Moorthy VS, et al. Enhanced T-cell immunogenicity of plasmid DNA vaccines boosted by recombinant modified vaccinia virus Ankara in humans. Nat Med 2003;9:729–735.

131. Woodland DL. Jump-starting the immune system: prime-boosting comes of age. Trends Immunol 2004;25:98–104.

132. Melief CJ. Cancer immunotherapy by dendritic cells. Immunity 2008;29:372–383.

133. Romani N, Reider D, Heuer M, et al. Generation of mature dendritic cells from human blood. An improved method with special regard to clinical applicability. J Immunol Methods 1996;196:137–151.

134. Pulendran B, Banchereau J, Burkeholder S, et al. Flt3-ligand and granulocyte colony-stimulating factor mobilize distinct human dendritic cell subsets in vivo. J Immunol 2000;165:566–572.

135. Boczkowski D, Nair SK, Synder D, et al. Dendritic cells pulsed with RNA are potent antigen-presenting cells in vitro and in vivo. J Exp Med 1996;184:465–472.

136. Radford KJ, Jackson AM, Wang JH, et al. Recombinant E. coli efficiently delivers antigen and maturation signals to human dendritic cells: presentation of MART1 to CD8+ T cells. Int J Cancer 2003;105:811–819.

137. Mackensen A, Herbst B, Chen JL, et al. Phase I study in melanoma patients of a vaccine with peptide-pulsed dendritic cells generated in vitro from CD34(+) hematopoietic progenitor cells. Int J Cancer 2000;86:385–392.

138. Gottschalk S, Edwards OL, Sili U, et al. Generating CTL against the subdominant Epstein-Barr virus LMP1 antigen for the adoptive immunotherapy of EBV-associated malignancies. Blood 2003;101:1905–1912.

139. Wei Y, Sticca RP, Holmes LM, et al. Dendritoma vaccination combined with low dose interleukin-2 in metastatic melanoma patients induced immunological and clinical responses. Int J Oncol 2006;28:585–593.

140. Mater Medical Research Institute. www.mmri.mater.org.au. Accessed August 30, 2009.

141. Ridgway D. The first 1000 dendritic cell vaccinees. Cancer Invest 2003;21:873–886.

142. Nencioni A, Grunebach F, Schmidt SM, et al. The use of dendritic cells in cancer immunotherapy. Crit Rev Oncol Hematol 2008;65:191–199.

143. http://investor.dendreon.com/releasedetail.cfm?ReleaseID=380042. Accessed August 30, 2009.

144. Geiger JD, Hutchinson RJ, Hohenkirk LF, et al. Vaccination of pediatric solid tumor patients with tumor lysate-pulsed dendritic cells can expand specific T cells and mediate tumor regression. Cancer Res 2001;61:8513–8519.

145. Caruso DA, Orme LM, Neale AM, et al. Results of a phase 1 study utilizing monocyte-derived dendritic cells pulsed with tumor RNA in children and young adults with brain cancer. Neuro Oncol 2004;6:236–246.

146. Caruso DA, Orme LM, Amor GM, et al. Results of a phase I study utilizing monocyte-derived dendritic cells pulsed with tumor RNA in children with stage 4 neuroblastoma. Cancer 2005;103:1280–1291.

147. Dohnal AM, Witt V, Hugel H, et al. Phase I study of tumor Ag-loaded IL-12 secreting semi-mature DC for the treatment of pediatric cancer. Cytotherapy 2007;9:755–770.

148. Dagher R, Long LM, Read EJ, et al. Pilot trial of tumor-specific peptide vaccination and continuous infusion interleukin-2 in patients with recurrent Ewing sarcoma and alveolar rhabdomyosarcoma: an inter-institute NIH study. Med Pediatr Oncol 2002;38:158–164.

149. Matsuzaki A, Suminoe A, Hattori H, et al. Immunotherapy with autologous dendritic cells and tumor-specific synthetic peptides for synovial sarcoma. J Pediatr Hematol Oncol 2002;24:220–223.

150. Kikuchi T, Akasaki Y, Irie M, et al. Results of a phase I clinical trial of vaccination of glioma patients with fusions of dendritic and glioma cells. Cancer Immunol Immunother 2001;50:337–344.

151. Bowman L, Grossmann M, Rill D, et al. IL-2 adenovector-transduced autologous tumor cells induce antitumor immune responses in patients with neuroblastoma. Blood 1998;92:1941–1949.

152. Bowman LC, Grossmann M, Rill D, et al. IL-2 gene-modified allogeneic tumor cells for treatment of relapsed neuroblastoma. Hum Gene Ther 1998;9:1303–1311.

153. Rousseau RF, Haight AE, Hirschmann-Jax C, et al. Local and systemic effects of an allogeneic tumor cell vaccine combining transgenic human lymphotactin with interleukin-2 in patients with advanced or refractory neuroblastoma. Blood 2003;101:1718–1726.

154. Rousseau RF, Biagi E, Dutour A, et al. Immunotherapy of high-risk acute leukemia with a recipient (autologous) vaccine expressing transgenic human CD40L and IL-2 after chemotherapy and allogeneic stem cell transplantation. Blood 2006;107:1332–1341.

155. Figdor CG, de Vries IJ, Lesterhuis WJ, et al. Dendritic cell immunotherapy: mapping the way. Nat Med 2004;10:475–480.

156. Terando A, Roessler B, Mule JJ. Chemokine gene modification of human dendritic cell-based tumor vaccines using a recombinant adenoviral vector. Cancer Gene Ther 2004;11:165–173.

157. Steitz J, Bruck J, Lenz J, et al. Depletion of CD25(+) CD4(+) T cells and treatment with tyrosinase-related protein 2-transduced dendritic cells enhance the interferon alpha-induced, CD8(+) T-cell-dependent immune defense of B16 melanoma. Cancer Res 2001;61:8643–8646.

158. Song XT, Evel-Kabler K, Shen L, et al. A20 is an antigen presentation attenuator, and its inhibition overcomes regulatory T cell-mediated suppression. Nat Med 2008;14:258–265.

159. Hanks BA, Jiang J, Singh RA, et al. Re-engineered CD40 receptor enables potent pharmacological activation of dendritic-cell cancer vaccines in vivo. Nat Med 2005;11:130–137.

160. Dilloo D, Brown M, Roskrow M, et al. CD40 ligand induces an anti-leukemia immune response in vivo. Blood 1997;90:1927–1933.

161. Roskrow MA, Dilloo D, Suzuki N, et al. Autoimmune disease induced by dendritic cell immunization against leukemia. Leuk Res 1999;23:549–557.

162. Engelhard VH, Bullock TN, Colella TA, et al. Antigens derived from melanocyte differentiation proteins: self-tolerance, autoimmunity, and use for cancer immunotherapy. Immunol Rev 2002;188:136–146.

163. Ward S, Casey D, Labarthe MC, et al. Immunotherapeutic potential of whole tumour cells. Cancer Immunol Immunother 2002;51:351–357.

164. Loskog A, Dzojic H, Vikman S, et al. Adenovirus CD40 ligand gene therapy counteracts immune escape mechanisms in the tumor Microenvironment. J Immunol 2004;172:7200–7205.

165. Biagi E, Rousseau R, Yvon E, et al. Responses to human CD40 ligand/human interleukin-2 autologous cell vaccine in patients with B-cell chronic lymphocytic leukemia. Clin Cancer Res 2005;11:6916–6923.

166. Dilloo D, Bacon K, Holden W, et al. Combined chemokine and cytokine gene transfer enhances antitumor immunity. Nat Med 1996;2:1090–1095.

167. Liu Y, Ehtesham M, Samoto K, et al. In situ adenoviral interleukin 12 gene transfer confers potent and long-lasting cytotoxic immunity in glioma. Cancer Gene Ther 2002;9:9–15.

168. Abrahams VM, Kamsteeg M, Mor G. The Fas/Fas ligand system and cancer: immune privilege and apoptosis. Mol Biotechnol 2003;25:19–30.

169. Dranoff G, Jaffee E, Lazenby A, et al. Vaccination with irradiated tumor cells engineered to secrete murine granulocyte-macrophage colony-stimulating factor stimulates potent, specific, and long-lasting anti-tumor immunity. Proc Natl Acad Sci U S A 1993;90:3539–3543.

170. Osanto S, Schiphorst PP, Weijl NI, et al. Vaccination of melanoma patients with an allogeneic, genetically modified interleukin 2-producing melanoma cell line. Hum Gene Ther 2000;11:739–750.

171. Moller P, Sun Y, Dorbic T, et al. Vaccination with IL-7 gene-modified autologous melanoma cells can enhance the anti-melanoma lytic activity in peripheral blood of patients with a good clinical performance status: a clinical phase I study. Br J Cancer 1998;77:1907–1916.

172. Kusumoto M, Umeda S, Ikubo A, et al. Phase 1 clinical trial of irradiated autologous melanoma cells adenovirally transduced with human GM-CSF gene. Cancer Immunol Immunother 2001;50:373–381.

173. Kipps TJ. Immune and cell therapy of hematologic malignancies. Int J Hematol 2002;76(Suppl 1):269–273.

174. Wittig B, Marten A, Dorbic T, et al. Therapeutic vaccination against metastatic carcinoma by expression-modulated and immunomodified autologous tumor cells: a first clinical phase I/II trial. Hum Gene Ther 2001;12:267–278.

175. Foster AE, Leen AM, Lee T, et al. Autologous designer antigen-presenting cells by gene modification of T lymphocyte blasts with IL-7 and IL-12. J Immunother 2007;30:506–516.

176. Russo V, Cipponi A, Raccosta L, et al. Lymphocytes genetically modified to express tumor antigens target DCs in vivo and induce antitumor immunity. J Clin Invest 2007;117:3087–3096.

177. Fontana R, Bregni M, Cipponi A, et al. Peripheral blood lymphocytes genetically modified to express the self/tumor antigen MAGE-A3 induce antitumor immune responses in cancer patients. Blood 2009;113:1651–1660.

178. Kapp M, Rasche L, Einsele H, et al. Cellular therapy to control tumor progression. Curr Opin Hematol 2009;16:437–443.

179. Leen AM, Rooney CM, Foster AE. Improving T cell therapy for cancer. Annu Rev Immunol 2007;25:243–265.

180. Ljunggren HG, Malmberg KJ. Prospects for the use of NK cells in immunotherapy of human cancer. Nat Rev Immunol 2007;7:329–339.

181. Rosenberg SA, Restifo NP, Yang JC, et al. Adoptive cell transfer: a clinical path to effective cancer immunotherapy. Nat Rev Cancer 2008;8:299–308.

182. Rosenberg SA, Lotze MT, Muul LM, et al. Observations on the systemic administration of autologous lymphokine-activated killer cells and recombinant interleukin-2 to patients with metastatic cancer. N Engl J Med 1985;313:1485–1492.

183. Bordignon C, Carlo-Stella C, Colombo MP, et al. Cell therapy: achievements and perspectives. Haematologica 1999;84:1110–1149.

184. Ruggeri L, Mancusi A, Burchielli E, et al. NK cell alloreactivity and allogeneic hematopoietic stem cell transplantation. Blood Cells Mol Dis 2008;40:84–90.

185. Ruggeri L, Capanni M, Urbani E, et al. Effectiveness of donor natural killer cell alloreactivity in mismatched hematopoietic transplants. Science 2002;295:2097–2100.

186. Rapoport AP, Stadtmauer EA, Aqui N, et al. Restoration of immunity in lymphopenic individuals with cancer by vaccination and adoptive T-cell transfer. Nat Med 2005;11:1230–1237.

187. Rapoport AP, Stadtmauer EA, Aqui N, et al. Rapid immune recovery and graft-versus-host disease-like engraftment syndrome following adoptive transfer of costimulated autologous T cells. Clin Cancer Res 2009;15:4499–4507.

188. Laport GG, Levine BL, Stadtmauer EA, et al. Adoptive transfer of costimulated T cells induces lymphocytosis in patients with relapsed/refractory non-Hodgkin's lymphoma following CD34+-selected hematopoietic cell transplantation. Blood 2003;102:2004–2013.

189. Porter DL, Levine BL, Bunin N, et al. A phase 1 trial of donor lymphocyte infusions expanded and activated ex vivo via CD3/CD28 costimulation. Blood 2006;107:1325–1331.

190. Rosenberg SA, Packard BS, Aebersold PM, et al. Use of tumor-infiltrating lymphocytes and interleukin-2 in the immunotherapy of patients with metastatic melanoma. A preliminary report. N Engl J Med 1988;319:1676–1680.

191. Ridolfi L, Ridolfi R, Riccobon A, et al. Adjuvant immunotherapy with tumor infiltrating lymphocytes and interleukin-2 in patients with resected stage III and IV melanoma. J Immunother 2003;26:156–162.

192. Dudley ME, Yang JC, Sherry R, et al. Adoptive cell therapy for patients with metastatic melanoma: evaluation of intensive myeloablative chemoradiation preparative regimens. J Clin Oncol 2008;26:5233–5239.

193. Dudley ME, Wunderlich JR, Robbins PF, et al. Cancer regression and autoimmunity in patients after clonal repopulation with antitumor lymphocytes. Science 2002;298: 850–854.

194. Slavin S, Morecki S, Weiss L, et al. Immunotherapy of hematologic malignancies and metastatic solid tumors in experimental animals and man. Crit Rev Oncol Hematol 2003;46:139–163.

195. Kolb HJ. Graft-versus-leukemia effects of transplantation and donor lymphocytes. Blood 2008;112:4371–4383.

196. Rooney CM, Smith CA, Ng CYC, et al. Infusion of cytotoxic T cells for the prevention and treatment of Epstein-Barr virus-induced lymphoma in allogeneic transplant recipients. Blood 1998;92:1549–1555.

197. Heslop HE, Ng CYC, Li C, et al. Long-term restoration of immunity against Epstein-Barr virus infection by adoptive transfer of gene-modified virus-specific T lymphocytes. Nat Med 1996;2:551–555.

198. Gustafsson A, Levitsky V, Zou JZ, et al. Epstein-Barr virus (EBV) load in bone marrow transplant recipients at risk to develop posttransplant lymphoproliferative disease: prophylactic infusion of EBV-specific cytotoxic T cells. Blood 2000;95:807–814.

199. Comoli P, Labirio M, Basso S, et al. Infusion of autologous Epstein-Barr virus (EBV)-specific cytotoxic T cells for prevention of EBV-related lymphoproliferative disorder in solid organ transplant recipients with evidence of active virus replication. Blood 2002;99:2592–2598.

200. Savoldo B, Goss JA, Hammer MM, et al. Treatment of solid organ transplant recipients with autologous Epstein-Barr virus-specific cytotoxic T lymphocytes (CTLs). Blood 2006;108:2942–2949.

201. Haque T, Wilkie GM, Jones MM, et al. Allogeneic cytotoxic T-cell therapy for EBV-positive posttransplantation lymphoproliferative disease: results of a phase 2 multicenter clinical trial. Blood 2007;110:1123–1131.

202. Haque T, Wilkie GM, Taylor C, et al. Treatment of Epstein-Barr-virus-positive post-transplantation lymphoproliferative disease with partly HLA-matched allogeneic cytotoxic T cells. Lancet 2002;360:436–442.

203. Roskrow MA, Suzuki N, Gan Y-J, et al. EBV-specific cytotoxic T lymphocytes for the treatment of patients with EBV positive relapsed Hodgkin's disease. Blood 1998;91: 2925–2934.

204. Bollard CM, Aguilar L, Straathof KC, et al. Cytotoxic T lymphocyte therapy for Epstein-Barr virus+ Hodgkin's disease. J Exp Med 2004;200:1623–1633.

205. Lucas KG, Salzman D, Garcia A, et al. Adoptive immunotherapy with allogeneic Epstein-Barr virus (EBV)-specific cytotoxic T-lymphocytes for recurrent, EBV-positive Hodgkin disease. Cancer 2004;100:1892–1901.

206. Chua D, Huang J, Zheng B, et al. Adoptive transfer of autologous Epstein-Barr virus-specific cytotoxic T cells for nasopharyngeal carcinoma. Int J Cancer 2001;94: 73–80.

207. Comoli P, Pedrazzoli P, Maccario R, et al. Cell therapy of stage IV nasopharyngeal carcinoma with autologous Epstein-Barr virus-targeted cytotoxic T lymphocytes. J Clin Oncol 2005;23:8942–8949.

208. Straathof KC, Bollard CM, Popat U, et al. Treatment of nasopharyngeal carcinoma with Epstein-Barr virus-specific T lymphocytes. Blood 2005;105:1898–1904.

209. Louis CU, Straathof K, Bollard CM, et al. Enhancing the in vivo expansion of adoptively transferred EBV-specific CTL with lymphodepleting CD45 monoclonal antibodies in NPC patients. Blood 2009;113:2442–2450.

210. Wallen H, Thompson JA, Reilly JZ, et al. Fludarabine modulates immune response and extends in vivo survival of adoptively transferred CD8T cells in patients with metastatic melanoma. PLoS One 2009;4:e4749.

211. Yee C, Thompson JA, Byrd D, et al. Adoptive T cell therapy using antigen-specific CD8+ T cell clones for the treatment of patients with metastatic melanoma: in vivo persistence, migration, and antitumor effect of transferred T cells. Proc Natl Acad Sci U S A 2002;99:16168–16173.

212. Meidenbauer N, Marienhagen J, Laumer M, et al. Survival and tumor localization of adoptively transferred melan-A-specific T cells in melanoma patients. J Immunol 2003;170:2161–2169.

213. Johnson LA, Morgan RA, Dudley ME, et al. Gene therapy with human and mouse T-cell receptors mediates cancer regression and targets normal tissues expressing cognate antigen. Blood 2009;114:535–546.

214. Morgan RA, Dudley ME, Wunderlich JR, et al. Cancer regression in patients after transfer of genetically engineered lymphocytes. Science 2006;314:126–129.

215. Mitsuyasu RT, Anton PA, Deeks SG, et al. Prolonged survival and tissue trafficking following adoptive transfer of CD4zeta gene-modified autologous CD4(+) and CD8(+) T cells in human immunodeficiency virus-infected subjects. Blood 2000;96: 785–793.

216. Walker RE, Bechtel CM, Natarajan V, et al. Long-term in vivo survival of receptor-modified syngeneic T cells in patients with human immunodeficiency virus infection. Blood 2000;96:467–474.

217. Kershaw MH, Westwood JA, Parker LL, et al. A phase I study on adoptive immunotherapy using gene-modified T cells for ovarian cancer. Clin Cancer Res 2006; 12:6106–6115.

218. Lamers CH, Sleijfer S, Vulto AG, et al. Treatment of metastatic renal cell carcinoma with autologous T-lymphocytes genetically retargeted against carbonic anhydrase IX: first clinical experience. J Clin Oncol 2006;24:e20–e22.

219. Park JR, Digiusto DL, Slovak M, et al. Adoptive transfer of chimeric antigen receptor re-directed cytolytic T lymphocyte clones in patients with neuroblastoma. Mol Ther 2007;15:825–833.

220. Till BG, Jensen MC, Wang J, et al. Adoptive immunotherapy for indolent non-Hodgkin lymphoma and mantle cell lymphoma using genetically modified autologous CD20-specific T cells. Blood 2008;112:2261–2271.

221. Pule MA, Savoldo B, Myers GD, et al. Virus-specific T cells engineered to coexpress tumor-specific receptors: persistence and antitumor activity in individuals with neuroblastoma. Nat Med 2008;14:1264–1270.

222. Bernhard H, Neudorfer J, Gebhard K, et al. Adoptive transfer of autologous, HER2-specific, cytotoxic T lymphocytes for the treatment of HER2-overexpressing breast cancer. Cancer Immunol Immunother 2008;57:271–280.

223. Rosenberg SA, Lotze MT, Yang JC, et al. Prospective randomized trial of high-dose interleukin-2 alone or in conjunction with lymphokine-activated killer cells for the treatment of patients with advanced cancer. J Natl Cancer Inst 1993;85:622–632.

224. Law TM, Motzer RJ, Mazumdar M, et al. Phase III randomized trial of interleukin-2 with or without lymphokine-activated killer cells in the treatment of patients with advanced renal cell carcinoma. Cancer 1995;76:824–832.

225. Imai C, Iwamoto S, Campana D. Genetic modification of primary natural killer cells overcomes inhibitory signals and induces specific killing of leukemic cells. Blood 2005; 106:376–383.

226. Altvater B, Landmeier S, Pscherer S, et al. 2B4 (CD244) signaling by recombinant antigen-specific chimeric receptors costimulates natural killer cell activation to leukemia and neuroblastoma cells. Clin Cancer Res 2009;15:4857–4866.

227. Tavri S, Jha P, Meier R, et al. Optical imaging of cellular immunotherapy against prostate cancer. Mol Imaging 2009;8:15–26.

228. Muller T, Uherek C, Maki G, et al. Expression of a CD20-specific chimeric antigen receptor enhances cytotoxic activity of NK cells and overcomes NK-resistance of lymphoma and leukemia cells. Cancer Immunol Immunother 2008;57:411–423.

229. Diermayr S, Himmelreich H, Durovic B, et al. NKG2D ligand expression in AML increases in response to HDAC inhibitor valproic acid and contributes to allorecognition by NK-cell lines with single KIR-HLA class I specificities. Blood 2008;111: 1428–1436.

230. Verheyden S, Ferrone S, Mulder A, et al. Role of the inhibitory KIR ligand HLA-Bw4 and HLA-C expression levels in the recognition of leukemic cells by natural killer cells. Cancer Immunol Immunother 2009;58(6):855–865.

231. Miller JS, Soignier Y, Panoskaltsis-Mortari A, et al. Successful adoptive transfer and in vivo expansion of human haploidentical NK cells in patients with cancer. Blood 2005;105:3051–3057.

232. Takayama T, Sekine T, Makuuchi M, et al. Adoptive immunotherapy to lower postsurgical recurrence rates of hepatocellular carcinoma: a randomised trial. Lancet 2000; 356:802–807.

233. Peres E, Wood GW, Poulik J, et al. High-dose chemotherapy and adoptive immunotherapy in the treatment of recurrent pediatric brain tumors. Neuropediatrics 2008;39: 151–156.

234. Balch CM, Riley LB, Bae YJ, et al. Patterns of human tumor-infiltrating lymphocytes in 120 human cancers. Arch Surg 1990;125:200–205.

235. Porter DL, Antin JH. The graft-versus-leukemia effects of allogeneic cell therapy. Annu Rev Med 1999;50:369–386.

236. Marijt WA, Heemskerk MH, Kloosterboer FM, et al. Hematopoiesis-restricted minor histocompatibility antigens HA-1- or HA-2-specific T cells can induce complete remissions of relapsed leukemia. Proc Natl Acad Sci U S A 2003;100:2742–2747.

237. Alyea EP, Canning C, Neuberg D, et al. CD8+ cell depletion of donor lymphocyte infusions using cd8 monoclonal antibody-coated high-density microparticles (CD8-HDM) after allogeneic hematopoietic stem cell transplantation: a pilot study. Bone Marrow Transplant 2004;34:123–128.

238. Ciceri F, Bonini C, Stanghellini MT, et al. Infusion of suicide-gene-engineered donor lymphocytes after family haploidentical haemopoietic stem-cell transplantation for leukaemia (the TK007 trial): a non-randomised phase I-II study. Lancet Oncol 2009;10:489–500.

239. Mercier-Letondal P, Deschamps M, Sauce D, et al. Early immune response against retrovirally transduced herpes simplex virus thymidine kinase-expressing gene-modified T cells coinfused with a T cell-depleted marrow graft: an altered immune response? Hum Gene Ther 2008;19:937–950.

240. Straathof KC, Pule MA, Yotnda P, et al. An inducible caspase 9 safety switch for T-cell therapy. Blood 2005;105:4247–4254.

241. Shariat SF, Desai S, Song W, et al. Adenovirus-mediated transfer of inducible caspases: a novel "death switch" gene therapeutic approach to prostate cancer. Cancer Res 2001; 61:2562–2571.

242. Thomis DC, Marktel S, Bonini C, et al. A Fas-based suicide switch in human T cells for the treatment of graft-versus-host disease. Blood 2001;97:1249–1257.

243. Serafini M, Manganini M, Borleri G, et al. Characterization of CD20-transduced T lymphocytes as an alternative suicide gene therapy approach for the treatment of graft-versus-host disease. Hum Gene Ther 2004;15:63–76.

244. Andre-Schmutz I, Le Deist F, Hacein-Bey-Abina S, et al. Immune reconstitution without graft-versus-host disease after haemopoietic stem-cell transplantation: a phase 1/2 study. Lancet 2002;360:130–137.

245. Amrolia PJ, Muccioli-Casadei G, Huls H, et al. Adoptive immunotherapy with allodepleted donor T-cells improves immune reconstitution after haploidentical stem cell transplantation. Blood 2006;108:1797–1808.

246. Riddell SR, Watanabe KS, Goodrich JM, et al. Restoration of viral immunity in immunodeficient humans by the adoptive transfer of T cell clones. Science 1992;257:238–241.

247. Walter EA, Greenberg PD, Gilbert MJ, et al. Reconstitution of cellular immunity against cytomegalovirus in recipients of allogeneic bone marrow by transfer of T-cell clones from the donor. N Engl J Med 1995;333:1038–1044.

248. Cohen JI. Epstein-Barr virus infection. N Engl J Med 2000;343:481–492.

249. Hislop AD, Taylor GS, Sauce D, et al. Cellular responses to viral infection in humans: lessons from Epstein-Barr virus. Annu Rev Immunol 2007;25:587–617.

250. Gottschalk S, Ng CYC, Smith CA, et al. An Epstein-Barr virus deletion mutant that causes fatal lymphoproliferative disease unresponsive to virus-specific T cell therapy. Blood 2001;97:835–843.

251. De Angelis B, Dotti G, Quintarelli C, et al. Generation of virus-specific cytotoxic T lymphocytes (CTLs) resistant to the immunosuppressive drug Tacrolimus (Fk506). Biol Blood Marrow Transplant 2009;15:377.

252. Heslop HE. Biology and treatment of Epstein-Barr virus-associated non-Hodgkin's lymphomas. Hematology Am Soc Hematol Educ Program 2005;260–266.

253. Bollard CM, Gottschalk S, Leen AM, et al. Complete responses of relapsed lymphoma following genetic modification of tumor-antigen presenting cells and T-lymphocyte transfer. Blood 2007;110:2838–2845.

254. Bollard CM, Stanojevic M, Leen AM, et al. Complete tumor responses in lymphoma patients who receive autologous cytotoxic T lymphocytes targeting EBV latent membrane proteins. Biol Blood Marrow Transplant 2009;15:52.

255. Raab-Traub N. Epstein-Barr virus in the pathogenesis of NPC. Semin Cancer Biol 2002;12:431–441.

256. Hunder NN, Wallen H, Cao J, et al. Treatment of metastatic melanoma with autologous CD4+ T cells against NY-ESO-1. N Engl J Med 2008;358:2698–2703.

257. Berger C, Turtle CJ, Jensen MC, et al. Adoptive transfer of virus-specific and tumor-specific T cell immunity. Curr Opin Immunol 2009;21:224–232.

258. Bollard CM, Rossig C, Calonge MJ, et al. Adapting a transforming growth factor beta-related tumor protection strategy to enhance antitumor immunity. Blood 2002;99: 3179–3187.

259. Foster AE, Dotti G, Lu A, et al. Antitumor activity of EBV-specific T lymphocytes transduced with a dominant negative TGF-β receptor. J Immunother 2008;31:500–505.
260. Wagner HJ, Bollard CM, Vigouroux S, et al. A strategy for treatment of Epstein-Barr virus-positive Hodgkin's disease by targeting interleukin 12 to the tumor environment using tumor antigen-specific T cells. Cancer Gene Ther 2004;11:81–91.
261. Kershaw MH, Wang G, Westwood JA, et al. Redirecting migration of T cells to chemokine secreted from tumors by genetic modification with CXCR2. Hum Gene Ther 2002;13:1971–1980.
262. Di Stasi A, De Angelis B, Rooney CM, et al. T lymphocytes coexpressing CCR4 and a chimeric antigen receptor targeting CD30 have improved homing and antitumor activity in a Hodgkin's tumor model. Blood 2009;113:6392–6402.
263. Schrump DS, Fischette MR, Nguyen DM, et al. Phase I study of decitabine-mediated gene expression in patients with cancers involving the lungs, esophagus, or pleura. Clin Cancer Res 2006;12:5777–5785.
264. Hou M, Wang X, Popov N, et al. The histone deacetylase inhibitor trichostatin A derepresses the telomerase reverse transcriptase (hTERT) gene in human cells. Exp Cell Res 2002;274:25–34.
265. Pellicciotta I, Cortez-Gonzalez X, Sasik R, et al. Presentation of telomerase reverse transcriptase, a self-tumor antigen, is down-regulated by histone deacetylase inhibition. Cancer Res 2008;68:8085–8093.
266. Berger C, Jensen MC, Lansdorp PM, et al. Adoptive transfer of effector CD8+ T cells derived from central memory cells establishes persistent T cell memory in primates. J Clin Invest 2008;118:294–305.
267. Rosenberg SA, Dudley ME. Adoptive cell therapy for the treatment of patients with metastatic melanoma. Curr Opin Immunol 2009;21:233–240.
268. Xue SA, Gao L, Thomas S, et al. Development of a WT1-TCR for clinical trials: engineered patient T cells can eliminate autologous leukemia blasts in NOD/SCID mice. Haematologica 2010;95(1):126–134.
269. Stanislawski T, Voss RH, Lotz C, et al. Circumventing tolerance to a human MDM2-derived tumor antigen by TCR gene transfer. Nat Immunol 2001;2:962–970.
270. Engels B, Uckert W. Redirecting T lymphocyte specificity by T cell receptor gene transfer—a new era for immunotherapy. Mol Aspects Med 2007;28:115–142.
271. Thomas S, Hart DP, Xue SA, et al. T-cell receptor gene therapy for cancer: the progress to date and future objectives. Expert Opin Biol Ther 2007;7:1207–1218.
272. Eshhar Z, Waks T, Gross G, et al. Specific activation and targeting of cytotoxic lymphocytes through chimeric single chains consisting of antibody-binding domains and the gamma or zeta subunits of the immunoglobulin and T-cell receptors. Proc Natl Acad Sci U S A 1993;90:720–724.
273. Pule M, Finney H, Lawson A. Artificial T-cell receptors. Cytotherapy 2003;5:211–226.
274. Sadelain M, Riviere I, Brentjens R. Targeting tumours with genetically enhanced T lymphocytes. Nat Rev Cancer 2003;3:35–45.
275. Brentjens RJ, Latouche JB, Santos E, et al. Eradication of systemic B-cell tumors by genetically targeted human T lymphocytes co-stimulated by CD80 and interleukin-15. Nat Med 2003;9:279–286.
276. Cooper LJ, Al Kadhimi Z, Serrano LM, et al. Enhanced antilymphoma efficacy of CD19-redirected influenza MP1-specific CTLs by cotransfer of T cells modified to present influenza MP1. Blood 2005;105:1622–1631.
277. Imai C, Mihara K, Andreansky M, et al. Chimeric receptors with 4-1BB signaling capacity provoke potent cytotoxicity against acute lymphoblastic leukemia. Leukemia 2004;18:676–684.
278. Hombach A, Heuser C, Sircar R, et al. An anti-CD30 chimeric receptor that mediates CD3-zeta-independent T-cell activation against Hodgkin's lymphoma cells in the presence of soluble CD30. Cancer Res 1998;58:1116–1119.
279. Savoldo B, Rooney CM, Di Stasi A, et al. Epstein Barr virus specific cytotoxic T lymphocytes expressing the anti-CD30zeta artificial chimeric T-cell receptor for immunotherapy of Hodgkin disease. Blood 2007;110:2620–2630.
280. Rossig C, Bollard CM, Nuchtern JG, et al. Targeting of G(D2)-positive tumor cells by human T lymphocytes engineered to express chimeric T-cell receptor genes. Int J Cancer 2001;94:228–236.
281. Ahmed N, Salsman VS, Yvon E, et al. Immunotherapy for osteosarcoma: genetic modification of T cells overcomes low levels of tumor antigen expression. Mol Ther 2009;17:1779–1787.
282. Ahmed N, Ratnayake M, Savoldo B, et al. Regression of experimental medulloblastoma following transfer of HER2-specific T cells. Cancer Res 2007;67:5957–5964.
283. Kahlon KS, Brown C, Cooper LJ, et al. Specific recognition and killing of glioblastoma multiforme by interleukin 13-zetakine redirected cytolytic T cells. Cancer Res 2004;64:9160–9166.
284. Moritz D, Wels W, Mattern J, et al. Cytotoxic T lymphocytes with a grafted recognition specificity for ERBB2-expressing tumor cells. Proc Natl Acad Sci U S A 1994;91:4318–4322.
285. Carpenito C, Milone MC, Hassan R, et al. Control of large, established tumor xenografts with genetically retargeted human T cells containing CD28 and CD137 domains. Proc Natl Acad Sci U S A 2009;106:3360–3365.
286. Maher J, Brentjens RJ, Gunset G, et al. Human T-lymphocyte cytotoxicity and proliferation directed by a single chimeric TCRzeta /CD28 receptor. Nat Biotechnol 2002;20:70–75.
287. Vera JF, Hoyos V, Savoldo B, et al. Genetic manipulation of tumor-specific cytotoxic T lymphocytes to restore responsiveness to IL-7. Mol Ther 2009;17:880–888.
288. Kershaw MH, Westwood JA, Hwu P. Dual-specific T cells combine proliferation and antitumor activity. Nat Biotechnol 2002;20:1221–1227.
289. Landmeier S, Altvater B, Pscherer S, et al. Gene-engineered varicella-zoster virus reactive CD4+ cytotoxic T cells exert tumor-specific effector function. Cancer Res 2007;67:8335–8343.

CHAPTER 15 ■ INFANTS AND ADOLESCENTS WITH CANCER: SPECIAL CONSIDERATIONS

ZOANN DREYER, DANIEL J. INDELICATO, GREGORY H. REAMAN, AND W. ARCHIE BLEYER

The diagnosis and management of cancer in children at the extremes of the pediatric age group pose significant challenges to care providers and clinical investigators. The care of infants with cancer is particularly challenging because of increased vulnerability to the acute complications associated with aggressive, multimodal therapy and the potential long-term sequelae of antineoplastic therapy on growth and development.

Cancer in the first year of life is relatively rare.[1,2] Infants with cancer often have a different clinical presentation from older children with the same disease, and their response to therapy also differs, indicating unique biologic characteristics of cancer in infants that explain the different clinical outcomes.[3–5] Although it is rare, cancer in the newborn and young infant has the potential to provide important insights into early human developmental oncobiology and suggests an intimate relation between oncogenesis and teratogenesis.[6]

Cancer in the population of pediatric patients at the opposite extreme of age (i.e., adolescents and young adults) also presents a unique set of challenges. This group also has a distribution frequency of tumor types that differs from the general pediatric population. They have unique psychosocial, behavioral, and developmental issues, which must be sensitively and adequately addressed during therapy. Furthermore, access of adolescents to clinical trials and, therefore, to acceptable standard of care, is significantly inferior to the experience of younger children.

This chapter reviews the distinct epidemiologic differences between cancer in infants and adolescents and provides guidelines for professionals facing the challenge of treating these patient populations. Some of the unique biologic and clinical features of cancer in infants that have prognostic and therapeutic implications as well as strategies to assure that adolescents and young adults gain access to appropriate multidisciplinary care and to improve their recruitment to clinical trials are also discussed.

CANCER IN INFANTS

Epidemiology

Incidence data from the National Cancer Institute's (NCI's) Surveillance Epidemiology and End Results (SEER 9 www.seer.cancer.gov) program indicate that the overall rate of cancer in U.S. children younger than 1 year is 234 cases per 1 million infants. These data also suggest that the incidence is increasing (Table 15.1).[1,2,7] The most common cancer in infants is neuroblastoma, followed by central nervous system (CNS) tumors, leukemia, retinoblastoma, renal tumors, germ cell tumors (including malignant teratomas), sarcomas, and hepatic tumors.[2] Unlike older children, female infants have a higher incidence of cancer than male infants, although rates for male infants are increasing.[2]

As shown in Table 15.2, there is a difference in the percent distribution of tumor types in newborns and infants compared with all children younger than 15 years.[2,7,8] There have also been changes in the percent distribution over time demonstrating stable rates of leukemia and renal tumors and increased rates of CNS tumors and retinoblastoma.[2]

A report from the International Agency for Research on Cancer that compares population-based registry data from more than 50 nations demonstrates remarkable differences in international rates for cancer in infants.[9] Comparison of incidence data from different nations has limitations, but it does serve to emphasize the contribution of gene-environment interactions to cancer in infants.

Etiology

Although it is a rare event, cancer in infants presents a unique situation to study cancer etiology. In infants, the process of oncogenesis occurs in close temporal relation to embryogenesis. Factors that should be considered as causes of cancer in infants include genetic susceptibility, acquired or constitutional; parental, intrauterine, and immediate postnatal environmental exposures; and transplacental metastasis.[10–14]

Clinical evidence supports an inherited genetic susceptibility to developing cancer in infancy. Familial cases of Wilms' tumor and retinoblastoma occur at an earlier age than sporadic cases. Some genetic syndromes are associated with cancer at an early age, such as Down syndrome with leukemia and familial adenomatous polyposis with infantile hepatoblastoma. Genetic abnormalities have been identified that are frequently found in infants with cancer, such as chromosome band 11q23 breakpoint mutations (location of the MLL gene) in infant acute lymphoblastic leukemia (ALL), low N-myc oncogene copy in good-risk neuroblastoma in infants, and abnormalities in WT1 and the RB1 genes that are more commonly associated with the Wilms' tumors and retinoblastomas that occur in younger children. A report on three pairs of infant twins with concordant leukemia and nonconstitutional gene rearrangements at 11q23 chromosome band breakpoint provides strong evidence for in utero–acquired genetic susceptibility to cancer.[15]

Clinical and molecular evidence suggests that the cause of cancer in infants is related to an acquired or constitutional abnormality of cancer-predisposing genes that are critical during embryogenesis. The activation or suppression of these genes causes dysregulation of the normal developmental process and may lead to a malignant transformation in the infant. The fact that fetal and neonatal malignant tumors clinically manifested in the first few months of life can spontaneously regress or cytodifferentiate supports speculations about the physiologic expression of oncogenes by embryonic cells, and their role in modulation of oncogenesis (see Chapter 2).

TABLE 15.1

INCIDENCE AND SURVIVAL OF INFANTS YOUNGER THAN 1 YEAR, U.S., SEER17, 2000 TO 2006[a]

International Classification of Childhood Cancer (ICCC) category	No. of patients[b]	Incidence per million per year[c]							5-Year survival
	2000–2006	2001	2002	2003	2004	2005	2006		2000–2006 (%)
I Leukemia	357	49	43	40	42	64	48		55.8
I(a) Lymphoid leukemias	160	26	13	15	19	28	24		53.2
I(b) Acute myeloid leukemias	148	17	20	19	16	29	19		51.6
II Lymphoma	61	8	9	9	8	9	4		72.8
II(a) Miscellaneous lymphoreticular neoplasms	51	7	7	9	6	6	4		73.7
III Central nervous system neoplasms	237	34	32	39	35	33	26		46.4
III(a) Ependymomas and choroid plexus tumor	39	4	5	6	7	9	2		49.1
III(b) Astrocytomas	90	12	15	13	14	7	12		67.2
III(c) Intracranial and intraspinal embryonal tumors	78	15	7	16	11	10	9		23.4
III(d) Other gliomas	21	2	5	4	2	4	2		58.0
IV Neuroblastoma and ganglioneuroblastoma	388	51	57	45	53	66	41		88.8
V Retinoblastoma	185	25	29	21	25	19	34		99.1
VI Nephroblastoma, other nonepithelial renal tumors	111	16	28	12	15	12	7		78.3
VII Hepatic tumors	93	13	7	16	14	11	13		74.5
VII(a) Hepatoblastoma	89	12	7	16	13	10	13		76.0
VIII Soft tissue and other extraosseous sarcomas	136	14	21	13	25	18	18		63.9
VIII (a) Rhabdomyosarcomas	44	3	6	3	8	8	5		52.6
VIII (b) Fibrosarcomas, peripheral nerve fibrous	46	5	10	3	8	4	6		95.1
VIII (d) Other specified soft tissue sarcomas	37	5	6	4	6	6	6		46.6
IX Germ cell and trophoblastic neoplasms of gonads	157	25	29	16	17	26	20		83.6
IX(b) Extracranial and extragonadal germ cell tumors	117	17	19	14	11	19	16		83.5
IX(c) Malignant gonadal germ cell tumors	25	5	5	2	5	4	3		100

[a]Surveillance, Epidemiology, and End Results (SEER) Program (www.seer.cancer.gov) SEER*Stat Database: Incidence—SEER 9 Regs Limited-Use, Nov 2008 Sub (1973 to 2006) <Katrina/Rita Population Adjustment> -\ Linked To County Attributes—Total Research Program, Cancer Statistics Branch, released April 2009, based on U.S., 1969 to 2006 Counties, National Cancer Institute, DCCPS, Surveillance the November 2008 submission
[b]All other ICCC categories had <20 patients
[c]Age-adjusted to the 2000 U.S. Std Population (19 age groups—Census P25–1130) standard.

Many studies have shown an association between parental exposure to environmental agents and cancer in very young children (Table 15.3).[16-23] Although these studies are not conclusive, they do suggest that some malignancies occurring in infants can result from preconceptional or *in utero* exposure of the developing fetus to environmental agents. These findings suggest a critical role for the timing of the environmental exposure during gestation and the consequent relation between teratogenesis and carcinogenesis.

Studies that combine current knowledge of the unique genetic determinants of cancers in infants with a focused epidemiologic investigation into specific environmental agents that could disrupt the normal expression or function of cancer-predisposing genes will be important in understanding oncogenesis and the cause of cancer in infants.

Diagnosis

Symptoms and Signs

Recognizing symptoms without having the benefit of subjective patient complaints presents a challenge. In young infants, particularly in newborns, the nonspecific findings of lethargy,

TABLE 15.2

PERCENT DISTRIBUTION OF THE MAJOR TYPES OF CANCER IN CHILDREN, NEWBORNS, AND INFANTS

Histology	Children <15 yr (%)	Newborns <30 d (%)	Infants <1 yr (%)
Leukemia	31	13	14
Central nervous system	18	3	15
Neuroblastoma	8	54	27
Lymphoma	14	0.3	1
Renal	6	13	11
Sarcoma	11	11	5
Hepatic	1.3	0	3
Teratoma	0.4	0	6
Retinoblastoma	4	0	13
Other	6.3	5.7	5

somnolence, irritability, feeding difficulties, vomiting, fever or hypothermia, and failure to thrive could be caused by significant pathology, such as a malignancy. Though extremely rare at this age, it is still important to consider the possibility of this diagnosis.

There are findings on physical examination that should alert the examiner to the diagnosis of cancer in an infant. Table 15.4 summarizes some clinical and laboratory abnormalities commonly associated with cancer and with the more frequent nonmalignant conditions observed in neonates and infants.

Laboratory and Diagnostic Studies

Laboratory techniques that require a minimal amount of blood have facilitated the diagnostic tests necessary for the evaluation of specific organ dysfunction and the existence of

TABLE 15.3

PARENTAL FACTORS ASSOCIATED WITH INCREASED RISK OF CANCER IN INFANTS

Cancer	Risk factor	Reference
ALL	Maternal history of prior fetal loss	17
	Paternal exposure to x-rays	18
	Maternal exposure to naturally-occurring topoisomerase II inhibitors	21–22
AML	Maternal use of marijuana	19
	Maternal exposure to topoisomerase II inhibitors	22–26
CNS (PNET)	Maternal diet deficient in fruits, vegetables, vitamin C, folate, nitrate	20
Hepatic	Maternal occupational exposure to metals, hydrocarbons, paints, and pigments	21
	Paternal occupational exposure to metals	21

ALL, acute lymphoblastic leukemia; AML, acute myelogenous leukemia; CNS, central nervous system; PNET, primitive neuroectodermal tumor.

tumor markers. Radiographic investigations, including ultrasonography, computed tomography, magnetic resonance imaging, and radionuclide scans, are best performed in specialized pediatric centers, which provide technical and interpretive expertise in the diagnosis and management of infants and newborns (see Chapter 9). These radiographic studies provide guidance in determining the nature and extent of the operative procedure (i.e., fine needle aspirate, biopsy, or resection) required to establish a definitive diagnosis.

Pathologic Considerations

The ultimate histopathologic diagnosis of cancer in infants requires the expertise of a pediatric pathologist. Specialized cytochemical, ultrastructural, and immunocytochemical techniques required to establish accurate diagnoses are discussed in Chapter 8. Although the pathologic findings of most tumor types are not unique to this age group, there are potential pitfalls in the pathologic diagnosis. For example, some tumors in infants can appear malignant microscopically but have a benign clinical course (e.g., infantile fibromatoses).[24,25]

Management

Surgery

The surgical management of the infant with cancer encompasses two major facets of care: fastidious attention to metabolic and physiologic details and adaptation of the extent of the surgical procedure to the unique biologic behavior of the specific tumor in this age group. Surgical care during the preoperative, operative, and postoperative periods must focus on temperature regulation; blood volume; fluid and electrolyte control (including calcium and phosphate); gestational development in the case of newborns; and the integrity of cardiac, pulmonary, and renal function.[26] It is critically important that the surgical team work closely with the pediatricians, neonatologists, oncologists, and radiation oncologists.

Maintenance of fluid and caloric intake is imperative. Feeding should be sustained as long as possible without interruption. Strict attention to the integrity of the coagulation system is also required in the young infant. Although vitamin K is routinely given at birth, additional doses may be needed to establish normal levels of vitamin K–dependent clotting factors.

In newborns, particularly those who are premature or small for gestational age, hypoglycemia, hypocalcemia, and environmental temperature must be observed and regulated. The infant's relatively thin skin, with a diminished layer of insulating subcutaneous fat, and the proportionately large surface area to weight ratio create a pronounced vulnerability to large heat losses.[26]

Special attention should be paid to maintaining body temperature while in the operating room including warming intravenous fluids and blood products. Adequate venous access must be ensured and in the critically ill infant, an indwelling temporal, radial, or tibial artery cannula should be placed to monitor arterial blood gases and possible hypotension. During the course of surgery, blood loss must be monitored closely. Prolonged operative procedures require an indwelling urinary catheter to monitor urinary output and to avoid over distention of the bladder.

Radiation Therapy

Radiation therapy plays a major role in the management of many pediatric cancers. Because of the potential for acute and chronic side effects, radiation must be used cautiously in

TABLE 15.4

DIFFERENTIAL DIAGNOSIS OF MALIGNANT AND NONMALIGNANT CONDITIONS IN INFANCY

Feature	Malignancy	Nonmalignant condition
Skin nodules	Neuroblastoma Acute leukemia Reticuloendotheliosis	Congenital viral infections Vasculitis Fibromatosis Neurofibromatosis Xanthoma

Head and neck masses	Rhabdomyosarcoma
	  Orbital
	  Cervical
	Nasopharyngeal
	Neuroblastoma
	Lymphoma
		Brachial cleft cyst
		Thyroglossal duct cyst
		Cystic hygroma
		Fibromatosis
		Hemangioma
		Abscess
		Cellulitis
		Reactive hyperplasia of cervical nodes
		Granulomatous lesions (e.g., atypical tuberculosis)

Abdominal or pelvic masses	Neuroblastoma Wilms' tumor Sarcoma Malignant teratoma Lymphoma Germ cell tumor	Polycystic kidneys Hydronephrosis Benign teratoma Urinary retention Gastrointestinal duplication Intussusception Chordoma Meningomyelocele Horseshoe kidney Splenomegaly Hepatomegaly
Hepatomegaly	Neuroblastoma Acute leukemia Hepatoblastoma	Congenital viral infections Storage diseases Cavernous hemangioma Hemangioendothelioma
Signs/symptoms of increased intracranial pressure	Brain tumors Acute leukemia Retinoblastoma	Intracranial hemorrhage Communicating hydrocephalus Dandy-Walker malformation Vascular malformations
Anemia	Acute leukemia Neuroblastoma (disseminated)	Acute or chronic blood loss Hypoproliferative anemia (nutritional, congenital) Dyserythropoietic anemias Transient erythroblastopenia
Pancytopenia	Acute leukemia Neuroblastoma (disseminated) Retinoblastoma (disseminated)	Congenital viral infections Immune-mediated neutropenia and thrombocytopenia Congenital and acquired aplastic anemias

infants. The severity of the side effects is assumed to be inversely related to the age of the child and directly related to dose though extensive data on infants and newborns are lacking.[27] Acute morbidity is usually reversible. However, pronounced late effects are not readily reversible.

A major late effect of irradiation is growth disturbance. The possibility of bone and soft tissue deformity in children secondary to radiation therapy is recognized, but the normal growth pattern of any organ or structure in the young child can be severely disrupted by therapeutic doses of radiation.[28]

It is generally believed that because of ongoing development, radiation sensitivity of certain structures and organs in infants is increased.[29] Because the brain of the young infant is still immature, the CNS is at high risk. Intellectual functioning is significantly lower in infants with brain tumors who received cranial irradiation as part of their therapy than in infants treated without irradiation.[27,30,31] Other major organ

systems that may be particularly vulnerable to damage include the kidneys, liver, lung, musculoskeletal system, and neuroendocrine system.[29,32]

Decreasing the daily dose of each radiation treatment through hyperfractionation coupled with varied schedules of chemotherapy may be useful in preventing some of the late effects in newborns and infants. Chemotherapy given for systemic benefit probably provides an element of local tumor control as well, which may permit a significant reduction in total dose of radiotherapy required.[33] Image-guidance, intensity-modulated radiation therapy, and, most recently, proton therapy provide technical measures to minimize the risk to surrounding tissues.[34,35] In certain non-CNS cases, brachytherapy may be utilized to isolate the area receiving high-dose radiation.[36] Compared with the other external beam modalities, proton therapy and brachytherapy provide the additional advantage of decreasing the overall integral dose of radiation to normal tissue and thereby reduce the relative risk of second, radiation-induced cancers in survivors.

Chemotherapy

The rationale for the use of cancer chemotherapeutic agents in the newborn and infant is not different from that for older children with cancer though chemotherapy-related toxicities that are of special concern for infants. Infants are known to experience excessive vincristine (VCR)-related neurotoxicity, manifested in extreme cases by hypotonia, poor cry, inability to feed, and fatal flaccid paralysis.[37] Increased myelosuppression in infants with Wilms' tumor given regimens containing VCR, dactinomycin, and doxorubicin (Adriamycin) was seen in the second National Wilms' Tumor Study II (NWTS-II) resulting in the recommendation that dosages of all drugs be reduced by 50% in infants younger than 1 year.[38] Without negative impact on disease control, these infant dose modifications were adopted by several other disease groups including the Intergroup Rhabdomyosarcoma Study (IRS) Committee. In a large group of infants with ALL, however, excessive chemotherapy-related toxicity, other than VCR neurotoxicity, was not observed, and reduction of induction dosages for anticipated toxicity had an unfavorable impact on rates of remission induction and on remission duration.[3] There is a fundamental lack of knowledge regarding optimal dosing of anticancer agents for infants and very young children, often with resultant increased risk of morbidity, mortality, and inferior outcome. Actinomycin-D (AMD) and VCR have been used for the treatment of several childhood cancers for more than 30 years. Despite their longstanding and widespread use in pediatric oncology, there is little pharmacokinetic information from which safe and appropriate age-based pediatric dosing can be derived. The consequences of this lack of fundamental knowledge were evident when the Children's Oncology Group (COG) suspended three active protocols for the treatment of children with rhabdomyosarcoma (RMS) after actinomycin-associated deaths from hepatotoxicity. Age was determined to be the primary risk factor for hepatotoxicity observed.[39]

New strategies must be investigated to improve the therapeutic index of therapy for infants such as identification of genetic polymorphisms, which may impact drug metabolism and risk for toxicity. Ideally, therapeutic drug monitoring will play a role in future studies in children and potentially in infants as well. Because data are lacking on the clinical pharmacology of most chemotherapeutic agents in newborns and infants, the optimal use of chemotherapy in this age group is best accomplished with pharmacokinetic monitoring. Pharmacokinetic analyses in infants are ongoing for widely used agents including VCR, etoposide, and daunorubicin. Analyses of methotrexate pharmacokinetics in infants with leukemia demonstrated that clearance in infants older than 3 months was not different from that in older children aged 1 to 19 years. Analyses are underway in infants younger than 3 months at this time.[40,41] Aspects unique to the pharmacology of the neonate include the rapid change in relative volume of fluid compartments that occurs after birth; different rates of hepatic metabolism; decreased efficiency of renal excretion; decreased protein-binding capacity; increased volume of cerebrospinal fluid, brain, and spinal cord tissue relative to body surface area (BSA); increased permeability of blood-brain barrier; and erratic gastrointestinal absorption.

Rapid changes in the volumes of body water compartments occur during the first 9 months of life. In newborns, total body water constitutes almost 80% of the body weight, and values similar to those in adults (50% to 55%) are seen in the older children. Extracellular water volume is approximately 45% of

body weight at birth but decreases to 20% in older children. Most of the drugs used in cancer chemotherapy are distributed in total body water or extracellular water. The convention of using BSA for drug dosing results in a standardization of the concentration of chemotherapeutic agent originally in the drug's volume of distribution, but it does not account for the changes in the distribution of body water compartments with age. For some drugs, the BSA method therefore may not be optimal for the very small infant (<6.0 kg), for whom calculations of dosage based on body weight may be more physiologic. However, it is also possible that the use of infant dose reductions rather than dosing by BSA may compromise therapeutic intensity and ultimately impact outcome. Thus, it is critical to determine which drugs may be safely dosed based on BSA.

The renal function of very young infants is less than that would be predicted on the basis of body weight or surface area. Renal blood flow is lower in newborns, the ability of the renal tubules to concentrate or acidify the urine is restricted, glomerular filtration rate is low, and the organic ion transport system for active tubular secretion is underdeveloped. The maturation of various renal functions proceeds at different rates; therefore, chemotherapeutic agents that depend on renal excretion for elimination are cleared slowly in the newborn and young infant resulting in prolonged plasma half-lives, with an increased risk of toxic reactions.

Neonates can metabolize drugs, but the ability of the immature liver to metabolize depends on the specific drug.[42] Because of the lower concentration of plasma proteins, the presence of a qualitatively different (fetal) albumin, high serum concentrations of competing substances such as bilirubin and free fatty acids, and lower blood pH, the binding of drugs by plasma proteins is lower in the neonate, resulting in a higher volume of distribution.

Intrathecally administered methotrexate and cytarabine (Ara-C) are widely used for the treatment or prevention of meningeal leukemia. Age-related pharmacokinetic differences exist, and BSA does not accurately reflect the volume of the CNS.[39] The substantially greater ability of drugs to enter the CNS of the newborn compared with the adult has been thought to reflect incomplete myelination. Increased cerebrospinal fluid levels of methotrexate, despite normal renal clearance, have been demonstrated in infants receiving very-high-dose systemic infusions of methotrexate compared with levels in older children.[43]

Low gastric pH and prolonged gastric emptying time in infants may result in relative inefficiency of absorption of orally administered chemotherapeutic agents. Diminished bile acid metabolism due to hepatic immaturity may also result in prolonged clearance of chemotherapeutic agents normally excreted in bile as well as in unanticipated toxicity.[44]

Recommendations for dosage modifications in situations in which excessive myelosuppression should be avoided in newborns and young infants are provided in Table 15.5. These empiric guidelines are based on the very limited data available and must be applied within the context of the specific cancer being treated and the individual clinical situation. Unless otherwise stated, "decreased dose" implies a 50% reduction of the reference dose for older children when calculated on the basis of BSA. For infants weighing less than 6.0 kg, doses calculated on a mg per kg basis, using reference doses in milligrams derived for a 1 m² individual divided by 30 (assuming that a 1 m² individual weighs 30 kg), result in approximately the same 50% reduction.

Pain

The evaluation and management of pain in pediatric oncology patients present a unique challenge. This is especially

TABLE 15.5

DOSAGE MODIFICATIONS OF CHEMOTHERAPEUTIC AGENTS IN INFANTS AND NEWBORNS

Drug	Reason for modification	Dose modification[a]
Vincristine/vinblastine	Decreased biliary excretion	Decrease by 50%; further decrease necessary in presence of jaundice
Actinomycin D	Decreased biliary excretion	—
Adriamycin/daunomycin	Decrease biliary excretion	Consider full dose of daunomycin after 3–6 mo of age in ALL
Cyclophosphamide/ifosfamide	Hepatic activation decreased at birth	—
Prednisone	Protein binding decreased in newborn	Decrease until 1 mo, particularly in presence of hyperbilirubinemia
Methotrexate (i.v. or p.o.)	Renal excretion and renal tubular secretion decreased until 6–8 mo	Decrease proportionately to decrease in GFR (assuming normal of 75–100 mL/min/1.73 m^2); monitor plasma clearance closely for high-dose regimens
Methotrexate (i.t.)	Relative difference in CSF volume	<3 mo, 3 mg; 4–11 mo, 6 mg; 12–23 mo, 8 mg[b]
Ara-C	Clearance dependent on levels of cytidine deaminases; possible increased CSF levels with high-dose regimens	Decrease by 50%, particularly in high-dose regimens
Ara-C (i. t.)	Relative difference in CSF volume	<3 mo, 7.5 mg; 4–11 mo, 15 mg; 12–23 mo, 30 mg[b]
DTIC	Decreased renal excretion	Decrease proportionately to decrease in GFR
Cisplatin	Decreased renal excretion and renal tubular secretion (until 6 mo)	Decrease proportionately to decrease in GFR
VP-16/VM-26	Decreased biliary excretion in neonatal period	Decrease by 50%; decrease further if jaundice is present
6-Mercaptopurine	Clearance dependent on levels of hepatic enzymes; decreased until 3 mo	Decrease by 50% until.3 mo

ALL, acute lymphoblastic leukemia; Ara-C, methotrexate and cytarabine; DTIC, dacarbazine; GFR, glomerularfiltration rates, VM-26, teniposide; VP-16, etoposide.
[a]Many of these modifications have been derived empirically and have not been validated with detailed pharmacokinetic studies.
[b]According to Children's Oncology Group dosing criteria.

true for infants who are nonverbal and have a limited ability to express physical discomfort.[45] Studies have documented that infants have physiologic stress responses to painful procedures and have improved outcomes when pain is treated.[44] Effective pain management in infants depends on a high level of awareness by healthcare providers. Signs of pain in very young infants include cry, grimace, irritable behavior, withdrawal of affected body part, tachycardia, sweating palms or soles, elevated blood pressure. stress hyperglycemia, and decreased oxygen saturation whue older infants may be able to physically resist painful procedures (see Chapter 43).

Supportive Care

Management of the infant with cancer is best accomplished in a specialized pediatric tertiary care setting, where the unique medical, surgical, anesthesia, blood banking, and nutritional requirements of seriously ill newborns and infants can be met. Expertise in critical care medicine is essential.

Because venous access often becomes a problem very early in the management of infants, the elective placement of a tunneled indwelling right atrial catheter (i.e., Hickman and Broviac) or subcutaneous implantable device should be considered to facilitate the administration of parenteral alimentation, blood products, and chemotherapy. Specific guidelines to prevent and treat the infectious and thrombotic occlusive complications of these indwelling catheters are presented in Chapters 12 and 41.

Early empiric institution of nutritional support should be considered before the initiation of intensive therapies. Because there is growing suspicion that a malnourished state impairs ability of the host to tolerate anticancer therapy, possibly decreasing response to treatment, the early use of parenteral alimentation is warranted if less invasive approaches are precluded by gastrointestinal dysfunction.[46] However, chronic parenteral nutrition supplementation can result in hepatotoxicity thus liver enzymes should be closely monitored.

Of great importance in treating infants is the immediate availability of blood products with the lowest possible shelf life and methods to provide maximal transfusion support without the risk of excessive volume overload and unnecessarily increased donor exposures.[47] All blood products administered to infants receiving intensive chemotherapy should be irradiated to prevent graft-versus-host disease. Use of blood products that are cytomegalovirus (CMV) "safe" has also been recommended and may be achieved through leukofiltration or the use of blood products, which have tested negative for CMV (see Chapter 39). Though not clearly proven to reduce the incidence of infections in the infant, many treatment protocols suggest the administration of intravenous immunoglobulin when the plasma IgG level drops below 500 mg/dL.

Potential long-term, treatment-related toxicities in infants warrant the early institution of a coordinated, longitudinal evaluation of growth and specific organ (e.g., lung, liver, and kidney) function to identify subclinical problems that may respond to early therapeutic intervention. Most important, longitudinal assessment of neuropsychological development in infants at risk for neurotoxic sequelae may delineate early signs of learning disabilities that can benefit from remedial intervention.

Specific Neoplasms in Infancy

Neuroblastoma

Neuroblastoma is the most common cancer in infants (see Chapter 31).[1,2] It accounts for more than one third of the malignancies observed in the first year of life and more than one half of those in the neonatal period.[1,2,48] Between 20% and 35% of all neuroblastomas occur in infants younger than 1 year. The incidence of neuroblastoma in infants is probably underestimated because many tumors spontaneously regress before detection. Small neuroblastomas have been found incidentally during routine necropsies of young infants dying of other causes with a frequency 40 times greater than expected for clinically overt neuroblastoma.[49]

More than one half of neuroblastomas in infants present in the abdomen, presumably originating in the adrenal gland. The extent of disease at diagnosis, as demonstrated by the most widely used staging system, is different for infants compared with older children. Most infants present with stage IVS (30%) or local disease (40%), and most older children (55%) present with distant metastases (i.e., stage IV disease).[49,50] Stage IVS patients are a unique group of infants who have small localized primary tumors that do not cross the midline and evidence of distant spread to liver, skin, bone marrow, or combinations of these sites, without radiographic evidence of cortical bone metastases. In general, these patients have particularly good outcomes. However, infants younger than 2 months with stage IVS disease tend to present with very aggressive disease and very large liver masses that quickly result in pulmonary and renal failure. Outcome is usually quite poor in this group.[51]

The patient's age at diagnosis and stage of disease have a dramatic impact on treatment outcome in neuroblastoma. Five-year survival rates for neuroblastoma, derived from SEER data are 83% for children younger than 1 year, 55% for 1 to 4 years and 40% for 5 to 9 years.[52] Historically, survival rates for infants with stage IV disease have been dismal, but regimens using intensive multiagent therapy have improved outcomes.[53,54] However, regardless of stage, the younger the age at diagnosis, the better the survival rate.[55–57]

Although age and stage have important prognostic implications, these two variables alone cannot predict outcome. Other important prognostic variables in infants include serum levels of neuron-specific enolase, serum ferritin, histopathology, cellular DNA content, and metastatic bone marrow disease detected by immunocytology.[58–60] Molecular genetic characteristics of neuroblastoma that are often found in infants and predict a favorable prognosis include tumor cell hyperdiploidy, absence of karyotypic abnormalities (specifically chromosome 1p deletions), no amplification of the MYCN proto-oncogene, and absence of increased TrkA expression.[61–64] Histopathologic classification, biologic variables, and patient age have been combined in the International Neuroblastoma Classification system, established in 1999, to define favorable versus unfavorable tumors. This classification system has now been validated showing the 5-year event-free survival (EFS) was more than three times greater for favorable than for unfavorable disease (90% vs. 27%).[65,66]

The International Neuroblastoma Classification system is used in conjunction with International Neuroblastoma Staging System (INSS) stage, age, ploidy, and MYCN status in the determination of the COG risk category for treatment selection as low-, intermediate-, and high-risk. The primary treatment for low-risk disease (stage I, IIA, or IIB) is surgery alone though chemotherapy and/or radiation therapy may be added if the tumor is unresectable or progresses.[67,68] Some infants

with stage II neuroblastoma have posterior mediastinal primaries not amenable to total surgical resection. Radiation therapy in doses of 900 to 1,800 cGy has been successfully used as an alternative or adjuvant to surgical resection to treat intraspinal disease in these infants but should be reserved for patients failing chemotherapy.[50] Stage III and IV are treated with a combination of surgery, radiation, and intensive multiagent chemotherapy. Infants younger than 1 year with stage IV neuroblastoma have a much improved outcome compared with children older than 1 year. Infants with non–MYCN-amplified tumors have a >90% 4-year EFS, whereas those with MYCN-amplified tumors have a dismal prognosis. Infants with stage III–IV nonamplified disease are considered intermediate risk while those with stage III–IV MYCN-amplified disease are classified as high risk.

Few other clinical situations in pediatric oncology have been as controversial as the management of infants with stage IVS neuroblastoma. The finding of hyperdiploid cells by flow microfluorometric DNA analysis provides convincing evidence that this is a malignant lesion rather than a hyperplastic proliferation resulting from a one-mutation event in germinal cells, as previously proposed.[69] Several studies over the last decade have been unable to prove a significant role for the addition of chemotherapy to observation alone in infants with stage IVS who are older than 2 months and have non–MYCN-amplified disease. In all studies, disease-free survival was greater than 90%. Based on this data, infants aged 2 to 12 months with stage I, IIA, or IIB without MYCN amplification have been observed without further treatment with excellent outcomes.[70,71] However, for those with progression of their disease, surgery and chemotherapy are incorporated.

Because chemotherapy does accelerate tumor regression, an intermediate intensity regimen such as VP-16/carboplatin or VCR/cyclophosphamide is warranted to initiate regression and to prevent life-threatening complications related to mass disease. Radiotherapy in doses of 450 cGy (150-cGy daily fractions using lateral opposing fields) has also been effective.

The biologic and genetic characteristics that have demonstrated prognostic significance in neuroblastoma must be taken into consideration when deciding on treatment options for stage IVS patients. A prospective correlation of clinical and biologic factors with natural history of stage IVS neuroblastoma is being undertaken by the COG to identify stage IVS infants, who may require more intensive therapy. Until these data are available, it is recommended that infants younger than 1 year with clinical stage IVS disease, normal karyotype, nonamplified MYCN, and no complications due to the mass of their disease be closely followed without therapy. Infants with clinical stage IVS, abnormal karyotypes, amplified MYCN, or complications due to the mass of their disease should be aggressively treated.[72]

There has been considerable interest in the early detection of neuroblastoma in infants through mass screening programs using urinary catecholamine measurements at 6 months of age. Despite initial reports of a beneficial impact of such screening on survival,[73] population-based data from controlled studies fail to demonstrate reduced mortality.[74,75] The incidence of the disease in the first year of life has increased considerably in Japan, where a nationwide screening program was instituted in 1985. However, the incidence of neuroblastoma among children older than 1 year has not changed, suggesting that a high proportion of prognostically favorable cases (many of which may have spontaneously regressed) is being detected. Because mass screening has not been shown to reduce mortality, widespread implementation of this practice remains controversial and cannot be recommended.[74–79]

For infants who survive neuroblastoma, potential late effects include endocrinopathies, cardiac dysfunction, renal and ototoxicity postchemotherapy, scoliosis postradiation, ischemic injury to the kidney as a surgical complication, and the risk of development of second malignant neoplasms.

Brain Tumors

Primary tumors of the CNS account for approximately 15% of cancer in infants (see Chapter 27).[2] The most common presenting features of CNS tumors in infants are rapidly expanding head size and bulging fontanelle. Because of the expandability of the cranial vault, symptoms referable to increased intracranial pressure, other than vomiting, are rare in infants. Papilledema is rarely observed. Other clinical signs observed with greater frequency include paresis, seizures, cranial nerve palsies, lethargy, and nuchal rigidity. In contrast to the experience in older children, an increased frequency of supratentorial rather than infratentorial tumors has been observed in infants, partially because of an increased relative frequency of cerebral hemispheric tumors.[80,81] Medulloblastoma and ependymal tumors account for approximately 50% of the histologic subtypes.

Overall, the prognosis for children with brain tumors is poor, and infants represent a subset of patients with particularly high morbidity and mortality.[81] Those with metastatic disease have a particularly dismal prognosis. For patients with medulloblastoma, outcome is strongly influenced by the molecular features of the tumor. High-level expression of neurotrophin-3 receptor TrkC,[82] a low level of myc oncogene transcription,[83] and low-level expression of ErB2 receptor[84] are favorable prognostic indicators. However, analyzing the expression of a panel of genes using gene expression profiling may provide a more accurate prognosis than analyzing the expression of singe gene.[85]

The primary treatment of brain tumors in children has included surgical resection, radiation therapy, and in many cases, chemotherapy. Because of the doses of radiation used, serious sequelae are almost a certainty in infants with primary CNS tumors. Several studies have used various chemotherapy combinations in an attempt to defer radiotherapy in young infants until patients are at least 24 to 36 months of age or even eliminate it completely.[86,87] Early Children's Cancer Group (CCG) and Pediatric Oncology Group (POG) studies in which infants younger than 3 years were treated with intensive chemotherapy in an attempt to delay or defer radiation resulted in extended survival.[87,88] Deferred radiation therapy did not negatively impact progression-free survival, and the extent of surgical resection was an important prognostic factor. Recent studies in infants treated with aggressive chemotherapy who did not receive radiation therapy, unless there was evidence of progressive disease, have been encouraging though the effectiveness of substituting chemotherapy for radiation remains uncertain.[89,90] In one study, infants who did not receive radiation therapy had better neurocognitive outcomes than those who did but still lower than normal age-matched controls. Progression-free survival was approximately 60%.[90] High-dose chemotherapy with stem cell rescue is being evaluated in infants with high-risk CNS tumors.[91–94] Novel approaches using proton therapy and intensity-modulated radiotherapy are being investigated in infants with hopes of improving the long-term outcomes of survivors.[35,95,96] Late effects in infant survivors include a variety of endocrinopathies, neurocognitive deficits, and the risk of second malignant neoplasm. Minimizing radiation exposure (dose and field) may reduce the risk of these late effects.[97,98]

Acute Leukemia

Acute leukemia is the second most common malignancy in the first year of life. According to the SEER 9 program (www.seer.cancer.gov), the 2000 to 2005 respective annual incidences of ALL and acute myelogenous leukemia (AML) were 18 and 17 per million infants. Infant cancer in general and leukemia in particular have unique epidemiologic features. For example, infancy is the only age in which there are more affected girls than boys. In addition, age-specific rates for childhood AML indicate that the highest incidence is in the first year of life. An association of history of maternal fetal loss and acute leukemia at younger ages[99,100] as well as the role of DNA topoisomerase II–interacting compounds in maternal diet, such as soy proteins, with the risk of infant AML, has been observed. There is an association between maternal consumption of DNA topoisomerase II–interacting compounds and increased risk in MLL-rearranged cases of ALL and AML in infants, which suggests distinct etiologic pathways in leukemia in infants.[22,101]

The unique epidemiology of infant leukemia is associated with distinctive clinical and biologic features. ALL in infants has been consistently demonstrated to occur with a constellation of clinical and biologic features, all associated with poor outcome, including hyperleukocytosis, CNS disease at diagnosis, massive hepatomegaly and splenomegaly, CD10 negative immunophenotype, and a poor early response to therapy.[101–104] Virtually, all cases of ALL in this population are of an early pre-B phenotype; infants with this disease have the worst prognosis of pediatric patients with leukemia. Specific adverse prognostic features in this population include age younger than 3 months, white blood cell (WBC) count greater than 200,000 per mL, and MLL gene rearrangement, especially t(4;11). Historically in this group, EFS has been less than 20% with early relapse (<6 months postdiagnosis) the most common event despite the significant morbidity and mortality due to toxicities from treatment.[101–105] However, in the last decade, EFS rates have improved considerably to more than 50% in some trials even in those patients with the MLL gene rearrangement.[106–112] Recent treatment strategies have included more aggressive chemotherapy and in some cases stem cell transplant. In COG, therapy has been shortened and intensified with the incorporation of high doses of cytarabine and methotrexate early in therapy. Dosing most drugs by BSA rather than using traditional infant dose reductions further intensifies therapy delivery likely contributing to improvement in outcome. In the European infant leukemia trial, Interfant 99, addition of late intensification did not improve survival though it did add significant grade 3–4 toxicity.[108]

The most frequent molecular aberration in the pathogenesis of acute leukemia in infants is the MLL translocation. The finding of identical MLL rearrangements in the leukemias from pairs of monozygous twins in which both twins were affected, but not in their constitutional DNA, established that MLL translocations in ALL and AML in infants are nonhereditary, nonconstitutional, *in utero* events.[113] The retrospective finding of leukemia-associated MLL genomic breakpoint junction sequences by polymerase chain reaction analysis of genomic DNAs contained in bloodspots on neonatal Guthrie cards of infants who were diagnosed later with leukemia showed that MLL translocations also occur *in utero* in the nontwin cases, establishing that the time *in utero* is the critical period for the initiating event in acute leukemia in infants.[114]

MLL translocations are present in more than 80% of cases of ALL in infants. The majority of these are the t(4;11) resulting in fusion of the MLL and AF4 genes. The t(11;19) resulting in fusion of MLL with ENL occurs in approximately 13% of cases.[115,116] The MLL-AF4 rearrangement associated with t(4;11) is specifically associated with a poor outcome in ALL in infants when compared with other MLL rearrangements and deletions. In early CCG trials, there were only rare survivors of infant ALL with t(4;11); however, an EFS of ~50%

was found with other MLL translocations or normal karyotypes.[101] The adverse effects of MLL translocations are age dependent, with poorer outcome in infants than in children; however, the general occurrence of MLL gene rearrangements with young age and the constellation of other associated clinical features that portend a poor prognosis make it difficult to fully understand the specific effect of this gene rearrangement on the outcome. The poor clinical response to treatment in infant ALL is mirrored by *in vitro* drug resistance to glucocorticoids and L-asparaginase, drugs used routinely in ALL treatment regimens. In contrast, infant ALL cells exhibit *in vitro* sensitivity to Ara-C.[116] These patterns of sensitivity and resistance have had implications for the design of clinical trials.[101,105]

MLL translocations involve many partner genes that encode diverse types of partner proteins. More than 40 partner genes have been indentified.[113,117,118] Many MLL partner proteins have structural motifs of nuclear transcription factors or other nuclear proteins involved in transcriptional regulation and may play a role in leukemogenesis.[119,120] The function of the MLL gene product, as well as the function of MLL partner proteins and mutant MLL fusion proteins, is critically dependent on protein-protein interactions and may lead to the development of targeted therapies.

The slow onset of clinical disease in mouse models suggests additional genetic changes in leukemia in infants in addition to MLL translocations. FLT3 mutations have emerged as important secondary alterations. The fundamental relationship between the MLL translocation itself and the high level of FLT3 expression observed so often in association with the translocation suggests that FLT3 may be a rational molecular target for the development of new agents. FLT3 inhibition has been shown to selectively kill ALL cells with high levels of expression.[121] In the current COG infant ALL trial, infants with the MLL gene rearrangement are treated on an intensified chemotherapy backbone and randomized to receive or not receive the FTL3 inhibitor, lestaurtinib.

Recently completed parallel clinical trials in infants with ALL (CCG 1953[109] and POG 9407/COG P9407)[110] utilizing similar chemotherapy backbones were directed at evaluating intensive early therapy, including intensive anthracycline exposure, intermediate-dose methotrexate (4 gm/m^2), and cytarabine. Granulocyte-stimulating factor was included to decrease neutropenia for therapy delivery in a dose-intensive fashion. Effective CNS prophylaxis and treatment were obtained without cranial radiation. Infants with MLL rearrangement in their leukemic blasts were eligible for, though not mandated to, bone marrow transplantation from either a five to six or six human leukocyte antigen–matched related or unrelated donor. Fatal induction toxicity associated with the intensive chemotherapy proved to be a major adverse event. While modification of dose and schedule of induction anthracycline had little impact on toxicity, the substitution of prednisone for dexamethasone as the induction steroid significantly reduced induction toxicity to an acceptable level.[122] On CCG 1953, in rank order of significance, CD10 negativity, age less than 6 months, and the MLL rearrangement all had a negative impact on prognosis.[109] On POG 9407 (later renamed COG P9407), age less than 90 days at diagnosis was the prognostic factor of greatest relevance with EFS of less than 20% typical of previous infant trials. However, presenting WBC count (greater or less than 300,000 × 10^9/L) and the presence or absence of the MLL gene rearrangement within blasts had far less impact on EFS than that in previous studies: 64% versus 535(p = 0.61) for WBC count and 52% versus 65% (p = 0.36) for MLL status respectively in infants older than 90 days at diagnosis.[110] There was no advantage for stem cell transplant over intensified chemotherapy alone demonstrated on

this collaborative protocol.[123] However, previous trials have suggested an advantage for stem cell transplant.[124] Multivariate analysis of prognostic factors demonstrates consistency of the significance of t(4;11) over several clinical trials. The EFS in infant ALL remains far inferior to what has been achieved in ALL in children, and novel therapy approaches warrant investigation.

Effective strategies to prevent CNS relapse while eliminating the potential for adverse neurocognitive and neurodevelopmental sequelae are also crucial to current and future clinical trials investigating the optimal management of ALL in infants. Developmental and neuropsychological evaluation of long-term survivors from recent intensive treatment trials has demonstrated mean scores on standardized cognitive and motor tests in the average range, with a normal distribution of scores in comparison with population-based standards.[125,126] These findings suggest a positive early developmental outcome for these children and represent a substantial improvement over the neurocognitive potential of previously treated infants.

The outcome for infants with AML is not significantly different from that for older children (see Chapter 20). However, an excess of myelomonocytic and monoblastic subtypes, which are associated with a less favorable prognosis, has been observed in infants. Infants with AML are more often found to have hyperleukocytosis, CNS leukemia at diagnosis, skin infiltration, and 11q23 abnormalities compared with older children. The same therapeutic strategy is applied to infants and older children with AML. Despite the marked differences in these clinical and laboratory features, no differences in complete remission rate or survival have been observed between infants and children older than 2 years.

Retinoblastoma

The incidence of retinoblastoma is 29 cases per million infants per year in the United States, representing approximately 13% of all cancers in infants (see Chapter 28).[2] Retinoblastoma is usually considered hereditary or nonhereditary (sporadic). Hereditary retinoblastoma represents approximately 40% of all cases, usually presents at a younger age (median, 13 months), and occurs with bilateral disease.[127] Only 10% of hereditary cases have a family history of retinoblastoma. Susceptibility to retinoblastoma is inherited by deletions in the gene on chromosome 13q14, the retinoblastoma gene. Children who have a family history of retinoblastoma or a personal or family history of 13q deletion or 13q deletion mosaicism are at increased risk.[128] Retinoblastoma syndrome has been described in children with microdeletion of 13q14.11 and may also have mental retardation and facial dysmorphia.[129] Sporadic cases are thought to be caused by acquired somatic mutations of this gene.

Infants with retinoblastoma most commonly present with leukocoria. Strabismus, proptosis, blindness, an orbital mass, or other signs and symptoms of distal metastases can also be the initial finding.[130] The International Classification for Intraocular Retinoblastoma is currently used by COG for defining risk and therapy.[131] Depending on the stage of disease, therapeutic options for infants with retinoblastoma include enucleation, irradiation, cryotherapy, and photocoagulation.[130,132,133] Brachytherapy with I-125[134,135] and ruthenium-106 has been used for small tumors and reduces the risk of visual loss by reducing the radiation dose to unaffected tissue.[136] Chemotherapy (systemic and local) currently plays an increasing role in successful attempts to preserve vision. Novel therapies for high-risk disease include pupil thermotherapy,[137] high-dose chemotherapy with stem cell rescue,[138] ophthalmic artery chemoinfusion,[139] and gene therapy.[140] The prognosis for survival and salvation of vision for infants with retinoblastoma depends on the extent of disease at diagnosis. Overall, the survival rate for infants is high (85%).[130,132] In contrast, the mortality rate for retinoblastoma with distant metastasis or extensive local extension at diagnosis is poor. Infants with hereditary retinoblastoma have a worse prognosis for long-term survival because of their increased risk of developing a second malignancy, most often osteosarcoma, later in life.[141–143] The cumulative rate for development of a second malignancy 50 years postdiagnosis is 51% in heritable disease and only 5% in nonhereditary retinoblastoma.[144,145]

Renal Tumors

Renal tumors account for 11% of cancer in infants (see Chapter 30).[2] Although 16% of patients enrolled in the NWTS-II were infants, infantile congeners of Wilms' tumor are the more common renal neoplasms in newborns and infants (Table 15.6).[16] The most common is the congenital mesoblastic nephroma.[146] In the past, this growth was confused with Wilms' tumor, which may account for the more favorable reported prognosis of Wilms' tumor in infants. Mesoblastic nephroma (also known as mesenchymal hamartoma of the kidney) is not encapsulated and infiltrates into normal renal parenchyma. Complete surgical excision, with meticulous nephrectomy, is required. Local recurrences follow inadequate resection, and close follow-up is recommended. Only sparse reports of metastatic spread exist.[147]

The clinical presentation of Wilms' tumor and its management in infants are not different from the experience of older children. The most important prognostic factors include histology (favorable or unfavorable), stage, age, and the presence of biologic markers. Children younger than 24 months generally have lower relapse rates though with improved therapy, the effect of age has been reduced. Tumor-specific loss of heterozygosity (LOH) at chromosome 16q has been associated with a poor prognosis while LOH at 16q and 1p has been independently associated with a higher risk of relapse and death in patients with favorable histology Wilms' tumor.[148,149]

TABLE 15.6

INFANTILE CONGENERS OF WILMS' TUMOR

Renal neoplasm	Histologic and clinical characteristics
Congenital mesoblastic nephroma	Fibromyomatoid tumor; usually benign; often congenital; most common in infants, 6 mo
Well-differentiated epithelial nephroblastoma	Closely packed, well-differentiated tubules; usually benign
Polycystic nephroblastoma or multilocular cystic nephroma	Macrocysts lined by flattened epithelium and fibrous septa; usually benign
Fetal rhabdomyomatous nephroblastoma	Predominantly in skeletal muscle; one-third bilateral; usually benign
Nodular renal blastema/ nephroblastomatosis complex	Nodular or confluent subcortical masses of hamartoid, hyperplastic epithelium; precursor of Wilms' tumor, particularly bilateral, hereditary type

Children younger than 24 months with localized tumors weighing less than 550 g (stage I) and with favorable histology have a reported EFS of 93%.[150] Current management on COG studies is observation alone for this patient population. All other stage I and II patients with favorable histology and without LOH are treated with two chemotherapeutic agents while those with LOH receive three agents. Patients with stage III–IV receive three agents and radiation therapy. Infants receive a 50% dose reduction of all chemotherapeutic agents based on toxic death rates of 6% noted in NWTS-II. The risks and benefits of preoperative chemotherapy versus postoperative chemotherapy continues to be debated between the International Society of Pediatric Oncology (SIOP) and the Wilms' Tumor Study Group (NWTS) though both groups have comparable 5-year overall survival rates of 90%.

Infant survivors of Wilms' tumor are at risk for a variety of late effects including the following: renal impairment especially associated with radiation therapy or bilateral renal involvement[151]; cardiac toxicity associated with anthracycline therapy[152]; hepatotoxicity due to VCR and AMD[153]; muscle atrophy, scoliosis, and short stature related to radiation therapy[154]; and second malignant neoplasms.[155]

Rhabdomyosarcoma

Soft tissue sarcomas are relatively rare in infants; this age group accounts for only 5% of patients in the IRS though overall two thirds of RMSs are diagnosed in children younger than 6 years.[156] No differences in sex ratio or clinical groupings (i.e., stage) were observed. The significant differences in clinical presentation, histopathology, and response are shown in Table 15.7. Most cases are sporadic but RMS has been associated with familial syndromes such as neurofibromatosis, Beckwith-Wiedemann, Li-Fraumeni, and Costello syndromes.[157–161] The association with Li-Fraumeni syndrome is greatest among younger children, which suggests that children who develop RMS under the age of 3 years should be screened for germline p53 mutations.[162]

Unlike neuroblastoma and Wilms' tumor, RMS occurring before 1 year of age is not associated with a more favorable outcome. Aggregate data from Intergroup Rhabdomyosarcoma Study Group (IRSG) studies II to IV demonstrated that, adjusting for known important prognostic variables including stage and histology, infants younger than 1 year had significantly lower failure-free survival rates.[163]

Review of the radiotherapy data for infants with embryonal RMS demonstrated an increased risk of local recurrence in those given total doses below 40 Gy in an attempt to reduce morbidity. In cases of orbital RMS, effective local control was achieved with doses between 30 and 40 Gy; reduction of radiation doses to less than 30 Gy to minimize acute and long-term side effects in infants with soft tissue sarcomas may jeopardize local tumor control.[164] Proton therapy has been used to effectively control orbital and parameningeal RMSs with minimal late effects in young children.[165,166] Unfortunately, this technology is expensive and is limited to a few centers worldwide. The use of high-dose-rate remote brachytherapy as an alternative to external beam radiation therapy was reported to be safe, well tolerated, and effective in the treatment of a small group of very young children with RMS.[36] The efficacy of this treatment option awaits verification.

Conclusion

Improved survival for infants with cancer can be achieved with intensive therapy and the awareness of treatment-related toxicity. The most important challenges that remain include continued investigation of the unique etiologic and biologic

TABLE 15.7

INTERGROUP RHABDOMYOSARCOMA STUDIES III, -IV PILOT AND -IV OUTCOME OF INFANTS AND OLDER CHILDREN

Risk category	<1 yr	1–9 yr	10+ yr
Embryonal failure-free survival (%)			
Stage 1 and stage 2/3; group I/II	78($n = 48$)	84($n = 586$)	74($n = 213$)
Stage 2/3, group III	43($n = 41$)	76($n = 437$)	56($n = 107$)
Group IV	16($n = 13$)	51($n = 145$)	26($n = 62$)
Alveolar or undifferentiated			
Failure-free survival (%)			
Stage 1 and stage 2/3, group I	27($n = 11$)	81($n = 101$)	81($n = 62$)
Stage 2/3, group II	100($n = 3$)	66($n = 40$)	59($n = 36$)
Stage 2/3, group III	55($n = 11$)	61($n = 103$)	42($n = 118$)
Group IV	20($n = 5$)	28($n = 88$)	12($n = 113$)

Revised from Joshi D, Anderson JR, Paidas C, et al. Age is an independent prognostic factor in rhabdomyosarcoma: a report from the Soft Tissue Sarcoma Committee of the Children's Oncology Group. Pediatr Blood Cancer 2004;42:64–73.

characteristics of certain tumor types in infants; the pharmacology of chemotherapeutic agents in the infant population, particularly in newborns; and the design of specific therapeutic strategies, including targeted therapies that provide adequate or increased disease control while lessening potential acute and long-term toxic effects.

CANCER IN ADOLESCENTS AND YOUNG ADULTS

Epidemiology

The most current data from the NCI's SEER program indicate that the overall rate of cancer in 15- to 29-year-olds in the United States is 2.4 times greater than that in younger persons. Among adolescents aged 15 to 19 years, the incidence during the 1980s and early 1990s increased from 172 to 206 new cases per year per million persons, since which it has been stable.[167] The current rate in 15- to 19-year olds is approximately 40% higher than the incidence of cancer in children younger than 15 years, similar to the incidence of cancer among 0- to 4-year-olds, twice that found in 5- to 9-year-olds, and 1.6 times that observed in 10- to 14-year-olds.

The most common cancers in the United States in the 15- to 19-year age group are listed in Table 15.8. Among 15- to 19-year-olds, the seven most common cancer categories account for 91% of the malignancies in this age group (Fig. 15.1). In the order of frequency, they are lymphoma, sarcoma, leukemia, germ cell tumors, brain and spinal cord neoplasms, thyroid carcinoma, and malignant melanoma (Fig. 15.1). The proportion of all cancers that the common malignancies of older adolescents and young adults represent is displayed in Figure 15.2 for each 5-year age group up to the age of 55 years. As emphasized by Smith et al.,[167] this distribution is strikingly different from the patterns in younger and older persons. Many of the common malignancies in children younger than 5 years are virtually absent in 15- to 19-year-olds, including the embryonal malignancies of Wilms' tumor, neuroblastoma, medulloblastoma, ependymoma, hepatoblastoma, and retinoblastoma. Similarly, those cancers that predominate in adults, such as carcinomas of the breast and aerodigestive and genitourinary tracts, are distinctly unusual

among adolescents.[168] Although rare, many of the cancers of younger and older patients have nonetheless been reported to occur in adolescents (see Chapter 38).[169–177]

At least six of the common malignancies in 15- to 19-year-olds increased in incidence between 1975 and 2004 (Table 15.8). Non-Hodgkin lymphoma (NHL), testicular cancer, and thyroid carcinoma in females underwent the greatest increases over this interval. ALL, osteosarcoma, and melanoma also had increments (Table 15.8).

The type of soft tissue sarcoma that occurs in 15- to 19-year-olds is also distinct from that of younger patients. RMS predominates among the sarcomas of childhood, accounting for more than 60% of the soft tissue sarcomas in children younger than 5 years. In 15- to 19-year-olds, RMS accounts for only 25% of the soft tissue sarcomas. Non-RMS soft tissue sarcomas represent 75% of the soft tissue sarcomas. These include synovial sarcoma, liposarcoma, malignant fibrous histiocytoma, and malignant peripheral nerve sheath tumors.

Leukemias and lymphomas are also distributed differently in older adolescents than in young children. ALL declines steadily with age from the 0- to 5-year age bracket upward,

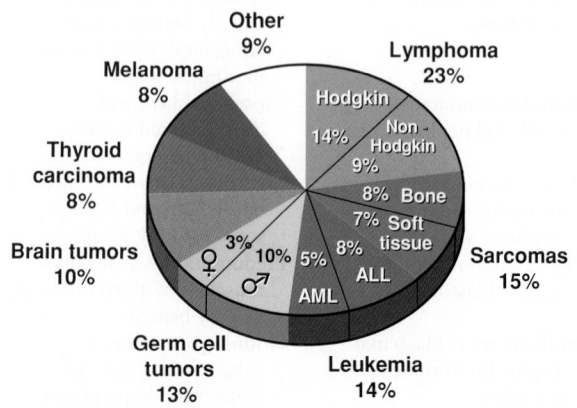

FIGURE 15.1 Types of cancer in 15- to 19-year-olds. Data from U.S. SEER, 2000 to 2006. ALL, acute lymphoblastic leukemia; AML, acute myelogenous leukemia. (SEER17, www.seer.gov. Accessed July 27, 2009.)

TABLE 15.8

AVERAGE ANNUAL AGE-SPECIFIC INCIDENCE RATES PER MILLION ADOLESCENTS 15 TO 19 YEARS OLD FOR SELECTED TUMORS, SEER9, 1975 TO 2004, BY 5-YEAR INTERVALS

	1975–1979	1980–1984	1985–1989	1990–1994	1995–1999	2000–2004
Leukemia	21.7	23.8	21.0	24.7	22.1	29.2
Acute lymphoid leukemia	10.1	12.7	11.6	11.8	11.9	15.7
Acute myeloid leukemia	7.2	6.8	6.6	9.1	8.3	10.1
Lymphomas	48.5	52.3	53.3	52.6	49.9	48.7
Non-Hodgkin lymphoma	11.0	14.3	15.9	16.5	16.1	19.1
Hodgkin lymphoma	37.6	38.0	38.1	36.1	33.8	29.6
CNS tumors	18.8	17.3	21.1	20.8	18.7	21.8
Bone sarcomas	13.3	15.5	15.9	16.7	16.1	16.7
Osteosarcoma	6.5	8.5	9.4	8.3	8.6	8.8
Ewing's sarcoma	4.3	5.8	5.0	6.7	4.9	6.2
Soft tissue sarcomas	14.2	14.3	16.1	11.2	16.2	15.5
Germ cell tumors	19.9	22.9	24.0	27.2	23.9	27.5
Testicular cancer in males	25.6	34.5	31.9	37.1	34.0	41.6
Ovarian cancer in females	14.0	10.9	15.7	16.8	13.2	12.7
Melanoma	12.7	11.4	15.1	16.9	14.9	18.8
Thyroid carcinoma	13.6	14.8	15.4	14.5	18.4	19.1
Thyroid carcinoma in females	23.2	22.4	26.6	26.2	32.2	33.0

such that by age 15 to 19 years, ALL accounts for only 6% of the cancers in contrast to nearly a third of the cancer in children younger than 15 years. In 15- to 29-year-olds, NHL is more common than ALL. NHL increases steadily with age, but the subtype distribution changes from a predominance of lymphoblastic and Burkitt lymphomas during early childhood to a predominance of diffuse large cell lymphoma during adolescence and early adulthood. AML is nearly as common as ALL in 15- to 19-year-olds and more common than ALL in 20- to 29-year-olds. Chronic myelogenous leukemia increases steadily with age from birth on, but it is not as common as either ALL or AML during the 15- to 29-year age range. Juvenile myelomonocytic leukemia is uncommon at all of the four 5-year age groups before age 20 years but especially during the 15- to 19-year interval.

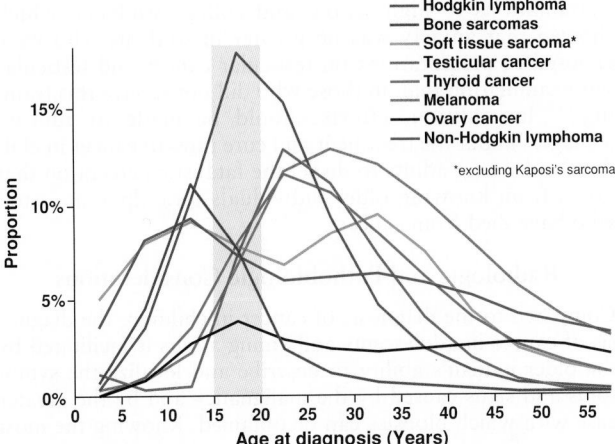

FIGURE 15.2 Proportion of all cancers that predominate in older adolescents and young adults, SEER9, 1975 to 2000. The yellow background designates the 15- to 19-year age range.

Ethnic and racial differences in incidence are particularly apparent among African American and non-Hispanic white adolescents and young adults. Among 15- to 19-year-olds in the United States, the overall incidence of cancer is 50% higher among whites than blacks. Among specific cancers, melanoma and Ewing's sarcoma are strikingly higher in whites, as is the case during any age range. ALL, germ cell tumors, and thyroid cancer are also more common in whites than in blacks, each by at least twofold. Only soft tissue sarcomas, considered as a group, are more common in blacks than in whites among the common cancers in this age group.

Incidence by gender is also different, with an overall incidence equal among males and females aged 15 to 19 years in contrast to a 20% higher rate in boys younger than 15 years. Individual tumor types have unequal sex distributions in the older adolescent populations, however. The most striking difference is in thyroid carcinoma, with females being 10 times more likely to get this disease. The next greatest gender difference is ALL, in which males are more than twice as likely to develop this disease. Females are also 50% more likely to be diagnosed with melanoma and approximately 15% more likely to sustain Hodgkin lymphoma.[167] Males are nearly twice as likely to have NHL or Ewing's sarcoma, 50% more likely to develop osteosarcoma, and 20% to 30% more likely to have brain tumors or NHL.[127]

Etiology

As in younger patients, little is known about the causes of cancer in adolescents and young adults and about the increase in incidence noted prior to the 1990s. Whereas cancers in infants and young children are likely to be strongly influenced by congenital and prenatal factors, and cancers in the elderly are most strongly linked with environmental causes, the cancer in young adults and older adolescents may be a combination of both. Very few cancers in adolescents and young adults have been attributed to environmental or inherited factors. An exception is clear cell adenocarcinoma of the vagina or cervix in adolescent females, with most cases caused by diethylstilbestrol taken prenatally by their mothers in an attempt to prevent spontaneous abortion.[173] Radiation-induced cancer may occur in adolescents and young adults after exposure during early childhood.[145] In fact, many of the adolescent and young adult cancers that have been linked to an identifiable cause are second malignant neoplasms in patients who were treated with chemotherapy and/or radiotherapy for a prior cancer.[178,179]

Skin cancer, lymphoma, sarcoma, and hepatic cancers occur at higher frequency in persons with inherited conditions such as neurofibromatosis, ataxia telangiectasia, Li-Fraumeni syndrome, xeroderma pigmentosa, Fanconi pancytopenia, hereditary dysplastic nevus syndrome, nevoid basal cell carcinoma syndrome, multiple endocrine neoplasia syndromes, and Turner syndrome. Women with BRCA1 and BRCA2 deletions have a higher risk of developing breast cancer at a young age. Collectively, however, these cancers appear to account for only a small proportion of the cancers that occur during adolescence and early adulthood.

Given that the duration of exposure to potential environmental carcinogens is proportional to age, it is not surprising that tobacco-, sunlight-, or diet-related cancers are more likely in older adolescents and young adults than in younger persons. Nonetheless, these environmental agents known to be carcinogens in older adults have not been demonstrated to cause cancer with any significant frequency in adolescents. In most persons, it appears to take considerably longer than one or two decades for these environmentally related cancers to become manifest. The logical hypothesis is that adolescents who get cancer after a carcinogenic exposure must have a predisposing genotype. For example, melanoma is more common among Australian adolescents than among those elsewhere in the world, as described previously. This suggests that solar exposure may be able to induce skin cancer before the end of the second decade of life, at least in that part of the world. That melanomas during adolescence usually occur in nonexposed areas of the body mitigate against this explanation, however.

In the aggregate, both those cancers due to environmental factors and those transmitted vertically via inheritance account for a small proportion of the cancers that occur during adolescence and early adulthood. The vast majority is unexplained, similar to the state of knowledge of cancer during childhood.

Diagnosis

Symptoms and Signs

Because the array of cancer types are clearly different in older adolescents and young adult than that in children, the signs and symptoms of cancer in adolescents are also different from those in younger or older patients.[180] Because of psychological and social factors in adolescents and young adults, adolescents may present with advanced disease that they harbored for months because they are too embarrassed to bring the problem to attention.[181] Similarly, patients in this age range may be at higher risk for a delay in diagnosis, a factor that may impact their cancer survival. In a study of the interval between symptom onset and diagnosis in 2,665 children participating in POG therapeutic protocols between 1982 and 1988, Pollock et al.[182] found by multivariate analysis that for all solid tumors except Hodgkin lymphoma, as age increased, the lag time also increased. The reasons for delay in seeking medical care and obtaining a diagnosis are multiple.[181]

1. Young adults and older adolescents have the lowest rate of primary care use of any age group in the United States.[183] Regardless of health insurance status, adolescents and young adults are more likely than younger children to lack a usual source of care.[184]
   - With a strong self sense of invincibility and immortality, adolescents and young adults ignore symptoms and delay seeking medical attention. When seen, they may be reluctant to provide adequate historical information. Some of the most advanced disease presentations occur in adolescents, with presentation at diagnosis of extraordinarily large masses of the breast, testes, abdomen, pelvis, or extremity.
   - Peer pressure prevents an adolescent from "admitting" symptoms and sharing personal concern.
2. Physicians and other members of the healthcare team do not recognize signs or symptoms of cancer.
   - They are poorly trained to or unwilling to care for adolescents.
   - Adolescents and young adults are not "supposed to" have cancer. Clinical suspicion is low, and symptoms are often attributed to physical exertion, fatigue, and stress.
3. Young adults are the most underinsured nonelderly age group in the United States, falling in the gap between parental coverage and programs designed to provide universal health insurance to children (Medicaid and CHIP) and the coverage supplied by a full-time secure job.[185] During 2002, 30% of all 18- to 24-year-olds had no health insurance for the entire year.[186] Half of all 18- to 24-year-old Americans were uninsured sometime during 2002 to 2003.[187] Uninsured rates among those who seek medical care peak between ages 15 and 17 years (19%) for females and between ages 18 and 21 years (24%) for males. Actual uninsured rates were likely to be higher, because those who do not present for care may not do so because of lack of insurance.[188]

Given the lack of routine care, empowering young adults and older adolescents for self-care and detection is important. However, at this age, it may be most difficult to teach the importance of early detection of cancer, because at no other time in life is the sense of invincibility more pervasive. Adolescents should be taught especially to examine themselves for cancers that increase in incidence during this time period. This is particularly true for testicular self-examination, a subject that is obviously difficult to bring up and teach at this age.[189] Countering this perception, however, is the finding from a preliminary assessment of teaching testicular self-examinations to high school and college students, which showed that anxiety was no greater in students who were exposed to presentations on testicular cancer and testicular self-examination than in those who did not receive this training.[190] In addition, efforts should be made to educate teenagers about the treatment and cure rates of cancer in children and young adults to dispel the fatalistic perception that arises from knowing older individuals (grandparents, etc.) who have died from cancer.

Radiologic and Pathobiologic Considerations

Compared to the diagnosis of cancer in children, the diagnosis of cancer in adolescents and young adults is facilitated by the older patient's ability to describe and localize the symptoms and signs caused by the malignancy and by the greater ease with which biopsies can be obtained. Knowing the most common sites and histology of malignancies in the age group assists in evaluating symptoms and in selecting the most appropriate imaging and biopsy procedures. Noninvasive imaging without the need for sedation, endoscopy, and minimally invasive surgery are all available for patients in this age group. Although these are utilized more often in adolescents and young adults than in children because they are easier to obtain, it is possible that they are underutilized in this group in comparison with older patients owing to lack of insurance and other economic constraints, difficulty taking off from work, transportation limitations, and a lack of understanding on the part of the professional staff as to what diagnostic and staging procedures are appropriate.

From a pathologist's standpoint, the histopathologic findings may seem identical to a cancer known to occur in older (or younger) patients. Nonetheless, the molecular and cellular biology of the tumor may be different, because there is increasing evidence that neoplasms in adolescent and young adult patients have a different molecular profile, mutations, and biochemical pathways, as suggested by novel types of cancer found in adolescent and young adult patients.[191]

Management

As at any age, treatment depends on the type and stage of the tumor. In general, however, the therapeutic management of cancers in adolescents and young adults differs from that in adults because of physiologic, psychological, and social differences.[192–194] Although there is a dearth of publications that address these issues, several provide advice on how to manage individual cancers that occur in this age group.[195–206]

Surgery

In general, surgery is more readily performed in the larger patient, and anesthesia is easier to administer. Another advantage is that young adults are generally healthier than older patients. The main disadvantage in fully grown patients relative to children is that generally the fully grown patient has fewer compensatory mechanisms to overcome deficits and disabilities resulting from surgical resection of large tumors. Decisions to use sedation and anesthesia commonly employed in younger children (e.g., topical anesthetic for venipunctures) should be individualized to the adolescent/young adult patient but should not be dismissed as unnecessary just because of the patient's "maturity."

Radiation Therapy

Compared to children, adolescents and young adults are less vulnerable to the adverse effects of ionizing radiation.[178,179] This is particularly true for the CNS, the cardiovascular system, connective tissue, and the musculoskeletal system, each of which may be irradiated to higher doses and/or larger volumes with less long-term morbidity than in younger patients.[207–210] By analogy, older adolescents who are still maturing may be more vulnerable to radiation toxicities than older persons at those sites and tissues that are still undergoing development, such as the breast and gonads. Breast cancer, for example, is more likely in women who received radiation for Hodgkin lymphoma if the radiation was administered between the onset of puberty and the age of 30 years.[211] Remarkably little is actually known about the differential normal-tissue effects of radiotherapy in patients between 15 and 30 years of age. Such research is complicated by the late-onset nature of many somatic radiation effects combined with the unique challenges of long-term follow-up among adolescent and young adult patients.

Practically speaking, the typical daily course of radiation for cancers in adolescents and young adults extends 4 to 6 weeks. This may interrupt education and career pursuits. Daily transportation to and from treatment may be problematic for adolescent patients and impact compliance. Similar to surgery, radiation may induce functional and cosmetic morbidity during a particularly vulnerable period of social development. The testes and ovaries are exquisitely sensitive to the ionizing effects of radiation so many young patients undergoing pelvic and total body irradiation face the prospect of infertility.

Chemotherapy

The acute and chronic toxicities of chemotherapeutic agents are generally similar in children, adolescents, and young adults. Exceptions are that older patients in this age range may have a greater degree of anticipatory vomiting, have a somewhat less rapid recovery from myeloablative agents, and have fewer stem cells in the peripheral blood available for autologous rescue. The fully grown patient usually requires more stem cells than a smaller patient, such that adolescents and young adults are at a disadvantage for umbilical cord stem cell transplantation. In general, the older patient requires two umbilical cord donors, whereas the child usually fares well with one. In addition, adherence to therapy regimens, particularly oral chemotherapy, is much more problematic in teenagers than in younger or older patients.[212–215]

Adolescents and young adults certainly can tolerate more intensive chemotherapeutic regimens than older adults, because of better organ (especially renal) function. This should encourage those treating patients in this age group to push the limits of dose intensification. Based on this rationale, the University of Texas M.D. Anderson Cancer Center began utilizing the more rigorous pediatric regimen for ALL and AML in the young adult patients many years ago. Others have found the use of pediatric regimens for the treatment of young adults (aged 16 to 48 years) with Ewing's sarcoma "rational and feasible" without excessive dose delays or modifications.[216]

Psychosocial and Supportive Care

The greatest difference in the management of adolescents and young adult patients is in the supportive care, particularly psychosocial care that they require. These patients have special needs that are not only unique to their age group but also broader in scope and more intense than at any other time in life. The challenges include autonomy and independence, peer pressure, education, graduation, social development, sexual maturation, intimacy, marriage, reproduction, fertility, employment, parenting, and insurability.[217]

Young adult and older adolescent patients are on the cusp of autonomy, starting to gain success at independent decision making, when the diagnosis of cancer renders them "out of control" and often throws them back to a dependent role with parents and authority figures (by circumstance and/or by choice). Sometimes the patient has become distanced from his or her nuclear family but has not yet developed a network of adult support relationships. Young adult or adolescent patients usually have many new roles they are just trying to master when the cancer diagnosis hits: high school student, college student, recent graduate, newlywed, new employee, and new parent. Some of the adverse effects of therapy can be devastating to an adolescent's self-image, which is often tenuous under the best of circumstances.[217] Mutilating surgery to the face and extremities, weight gain, alopecia, acne, and stunted growth are examples. Special considerations between the patient, the parents, and the medical staff are necessary to cope with the extra dynamic of psychosocial complexity and to negotiate cancer treatment in adolescents.[218]

Choice of Treatment Setting and Specialist

A central, complex issue is the appropriate specialist to manage the treatment of the young adult and adolescent—a pediatric oncologist or an medical oncologist (medical, radiation, surgical, or gynecologic oncologist). As noted by Leonard et al.[219] in the United Kingdom, medical oncologists are "untutored in arranging ancillary medical, psychological, and educational supports that are so important to people who are facing dangerous diseases and taxing treatment at a vulnerable time in their lives" and "unpracticed in managing rare sarcomas," and pediatric oncologists "have little to no experience in epithelial tumours or some of the other tumours common in late adolescence." The (admittedly biased) American Academy of Pediatrics issued a consensus statement in 1997 in which it indicated that referral to a board-eligible or board-certified pediatric hematologist-oncologist and pediatric subspecialty consultants was the standard of care for all pediatric and adolescent cancer patients.[220] A wider consensus panel that included medical oncologists, the American Federation of Clinical Oncologic Societies, also concluded that "payors must provide ready access to pediatric oncologists, recognizing that childhood cancers are biologically distinct" and that the "likelihood of successful outcome in children is enhanced when treatment is provided by pediatric cancer specialists."[221] However, neither of these statements defines an age cutoff for the recommendation.

At a practical level, the switch from predominantly pediatric specialist management to adult management occurs not at age 21 years or even at age 18 years as might be expected but around age 15 years. A cancer registry review in Utah, a state that has only one pediatric oncology treatment facility, showed that only 36% of oncology patients aged 15 to 19 years were ever seen at the pediatric hospital.[222] A study of the National Cancer Data Base found that for nearly 20,000 cases of cancer in adolescents aged 15 to 19 years, only 34% were treated at centers that had NCI pediatric cooperative group affiliation.[223] Research is only now being done to ascertain the reasons for this practice pattern. The only survey of medical oncologists on the subject had a poor response rate (29%) and concluded that medical oncologists believe that they appropriately treated adolescents as adults.[224]

The answer to which specialist is most appropriate certainly varies according to the type of cancer and from case to case. Patients at any age who have a "pediatric" tumor, such as RMS, Ewing's sarcoma, and osteosarcoma, will probably benefit from the expertise of a pediatric oncologist, at least in the form of consultation. Children younger than 18 years and their parents may benefit from the social and supportive culture of a pediatric hospital regardless of the diagnosis. Individuals between the ages of 16 and 24 years may have varying levels of maturity and independence, and choice of physician and setting for their care should be individually determined. Pediatric oncologists may be less adept at a nonpaternalistic relationship with the patient (and potentially his or her spouse) and less inclined to consider issues such as sexuality, body image, fertility, etc. Medical oncologists are more accustomed to dose delays and adjustments and may be less willing to be aggressive with dosing that can be tolerated by the younger patient.

In the end, the decision should be based in large part on which setting will provide the patient with the best outcome. If these are equivalent, "social" or "supportive" factors should weigh into the decision. Little comparative outcome data are available. Stock et al.[225] compared patients between the ages of 16 and 21 years, who were registered on either a pediatric (CCG) or adult (Cancer and Leukemia Group B, CALGB) treatment protocol between 1988 and 1998. The remarkably significant results were a 6-year EFS of 64% for those treated on the CCG study and 38% for those treated on the CALGB study. For ALL at least, there should be no question that the adolescent with this disease should be treated on

a pediatric regimen by oncologists experienced with this approach.[226] At the University of Texas M.D. Anderson Cancer Center, results of treatment for AML in adults improved substantively after treatment derived from pediatric trials was introduced into the institution's trials.[227] The analysis of data from the National Cancer Data Base revealed that adolescents (aged 15 to 19 years) with NHL, leukemia, liver cancer, and bone tumors have a survival advantage if treated at an NCI pediatric group institution.[223]

The British have pioneered the solution of treating young adult and adolescent patients at a unique "adolescent oncology unit." This provides the adolescent with age-specific nursing care, recreation therapy, and peer companionship. Perhaps it is appropriate to have as a goal centers and oncologists devoted solely to the care of this group of patients.

Lack of Participation in Clinical Trials

In the United States, more than 90% of children with cancer who are younger than 15 years are managed at institutions that participate in NCI-sponsored clinical trials, and 55% to 65% of these young patients are entered into clinical trials. In contrast, only 20% to 35% of 15- to 19-year-olds with cancer are seen at such institutions, and only approximately 10% of the patients are entered into a clinical trial (Fig. 15.3).[181,193,228] Among 20- to 29-year-olds, the participation rate is even lower, with fewer than 10% seen at member institutions of the cooperative groups, either pediatric or adult, and only 1% to 2% entered onto clinical trials of the cooperative groups. Among older patients, the trial participation rate is higher, putatively between 3% and 5%, but still much lower than that in children. The high proportion of older adolescent and young patients, who are not entered into clinical trials, is referred to as the "adolescent and young adult gap." This gap has been observed throughout the United States and spares no geographic region or ethnic group.[228–230]

This dramatic reduction in clinical trials participation in older adolescents may help explain a lower than expected level of progress in older adolescents and young adults, as summarized in the following section. Studies of younger children have shown a survival advantage to children enrolled in clinical trials for ALL,[231] NHL,[232] Wilms' tumor,[233] and medulloblastoma.[234] Although sparse, there is also evidence that older adolescents who participate in clinical trials have a more favorable outcome than those who do not.[181,193,228–230]

In North America, a comparison of 16- to 21-year-olds with ALL or AML showed that the outcome was superior in patients with either cancer treated on cooperative group trials than in those not entered (Fig. 15.4).[235] In France, Holland, and the United Kingdom, older adolescents with ALL treated with pediatric clinical trials have also fared considerably better than those treated on adult leukemia treatment trials (Fig. 15.4).[236–238] In Germany, older adolescents with Ewing's sarcoma, who were treated at pediatric cancer centers, had a better outcome than those treated at other centers.[239] In Italy, young adults with RMS fared better if they were treated according to pediatric standards of therapy than if treated ad hoc or on an adult sarcoma regimen.[240]

On the other hand, a population-based study of 15- to 29-year-olds with acute leukemia in England and Wales showed no difference between patients treated on national clinical trials and those not entered or between those managed at teaching hospitals as opposed to nonteaching hospitals.[241] This observation appears to be exceptional, however, in that subsequent national AML trials in the United Kingdom have shown some of the best results reported to date.[242]

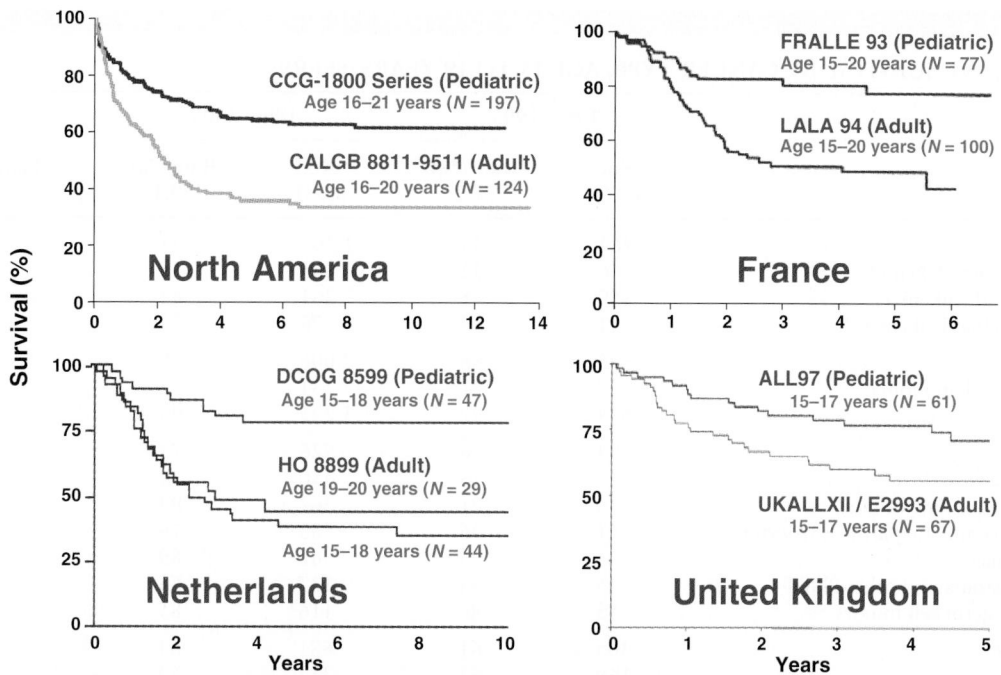

FIGURE 15.3 Pediatric versus adult therapy regimens for 15- to 21-year-olds with acute lymphoblastic leukemia.

Survival

Table 15.9 shows 5-year relative survival rates in the United States for all cancer and for different cancer types in 15- to 19-year-olds diagnosed during the last two decades for which 5-year rates are available in the SEER database: 1986 to 1995 and 1996 to 2005. Overall and in a majority of the cancer, some survival improvement occurred. The gains were modest, however, except for chronic myeloid leukemia, with an overall increase of 1.9% and 13 out of 28 types either demonstrating no change or a decrease.

Moreover, improvement in survival in older adolescents has lagged behind the improvement in younger patients such that the more favorable survival in older adolescents and younger adults than in children has been reversed, with less favorable rates in the adolescent population (Fig. 15.5). In 1980, the 5-year survival rate was 10% higher for 15- to 19-year-olds than in younger patients. By 2000, 15- to 19-year-olds had an overall 5-year survival rate that was 2% lower than younger patients. Thus, the relative improvement in survival was considerably greater in the younger patients than in older adolescents.

Between 1986 to 1995 and 1996 to 2005, the last two decades of survival data available from SEER, 15- to 19-year-olds had the least improvement rate of relative survival improvement of all 5-year age groups up to the age of 85 years (Fig. 15.6). The deficit in 15- to 19-year-olds compared to all other age groups was particularly evident in males (ibid).

The worst outcomes among the common cancers in 15- to 19-year-olds are in AML, ALL, and the sarcomas, particularly RMS, Ewing's sarcoma, and osteosarcoma. Each of these has a considerably lower mean 5-year survival rate than the

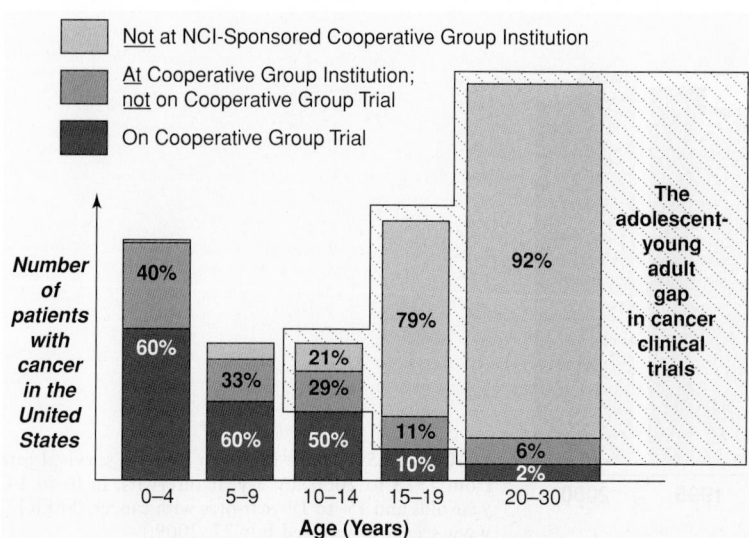

FIGURE 15.4 Adolescent and young adult cancer patients on clinical trials. NCI, National Cancer Institute. (Data from Montello M, Budd T. Cancer Therapy Evaluation Branch, National Cancer Institute, with permission.)

TABLE 15.9

5-YEAR RELATIVE SURVIVAL BY CANCER TYPE, AGE 15 TO 19 YEARS, SEER9[a]

	1986–1995		1996–2005		
	No.	Rate (%)	No.	Rate (%)	Change in rate (%)
All cancer	3,876	77.2	8,661	79.1	1.9
Leukemias	461	45	1,167	55	10
Acute lymphoid leukemia	246	52	685	59	7
Acute myeloid leukemia	150	35	361	44	9
Chronic myeloid leukemia	41	39	76	75	35
Lymphomas	972	86	2,006	88	3
Non-Hodgkin lymphoma	298	71	731	77	6
Hodgkin lymphoma	674	92	1,275	95	2
CNS tumors	394	76	826	73	−3
Astrocytoma	243	76	450	74	−2
Low-grade astrocytic tumors	86	91	262	93	2
Glioblastoma and anaplastic astrocytoma	51	46	103	16	−30
Ependymoma	23	96	62	89	−7
Medulloblastoma and other PNET	45	64	127	63	−1
Intracranial germ cell tumors	55	86	116	85	−1
Bone sarcomas	305	61	681	63	2
Osteosarcoma	169	62	357	63	1
Ewing's sarcoma	105	52	239	55	3
Soft tissue sarcomas	272	67	614	67	0
Fibromatous neoplasms	69	92	150	94	3
Rhabdomyosarcoma	74	48	152	45	−3
Germ cell tumors of gonads	400	92	966	94	3
Melanoma	287	94	700	95	1
Carcinomas	591	85	1,343	86	1
Thyroid carcinoma	288	99	721	99	0
Other carcinoma of head and neck	82	86	164	88	2
Other sites in lip, oral cavity and pharynx	48	96	103	91	−5
Carcinoma of genitourinary tract	105	85	166	84	−1
Carcinoma of colon and rectum	37	56	102	63	7

[a]Cancers with <50 cases excluded; www.seer.gov, accessed July 27, 2009.

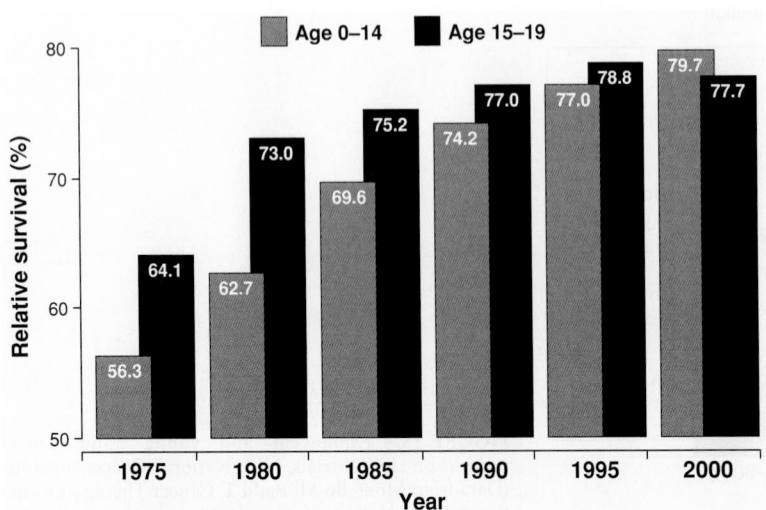

FIGURE 15.5 Change in 5-year relative survival rate from 1975 to 2000, by 5-year intervals, in 0- to 14-year-olds and 15- to 19-year-olds with cancer. (SEER17, www.seer.gov. Accessed July 27, 2009.)

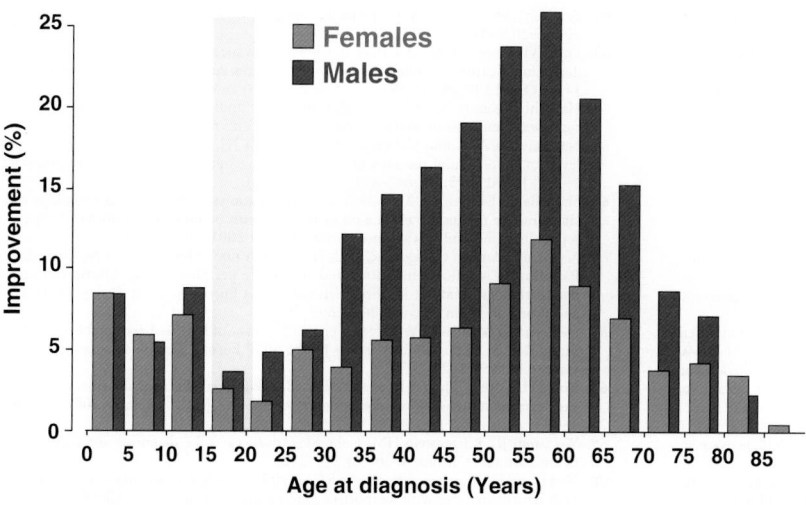

FIGURE 15.6 Percentage change in 5-year relative survival rate from 1986 to 1995 to 1996 to 2005, by age and gender, for all cancer except Kaposi's sarcoma. The yellow background designates the 15- to 19-year age range. (SEER9, www.seer.gov. Accessed April 19, 2009.)

corresponding malignancy in younger patients. With the exceptions of thyroid carcinoma, melanoma, and germ cell tumors, most of the remaining common cancer types in older adolescents have a worse prognosis than the same cancer in younger patients.

The mortality burden is a function of the survival and the incidence rates. More than 80% of the U.S. national cancer mortality burden in 15- to 19-year-olds is due to four malignancy groups: sarcomas, leukemia/lymphomas, CNS tumors, and germ cell tumors. The leukemias are the primary contributor to the cancer mortality burden for cancers developing in 15- to 19-year-olds. Although thyroid carcinoma and melanoma are among the more common cancers in this age group, they contribute little to the overall cancer mortality burden.

Conclusions

Surviving adolescence and young adulthood is difficult enough, even when all is well and health is not limiting.

Adding cancer to this phase of life is extraordinarily more challenging and demanding. There is evidence that progress in diminishing the cancer problem for these patients has lagged behind accomplishments in younger patients. The relative gap in clinical trial participation by older adolescents and young adults with cancer is at least a partial explanation for the relative lack of progress.

Despite the need for adolescent oncology that was recognized two decades ago,[243] a specific discipline for this special target population is evolving.[244,245] This will help bring the problem in focus and begin to address solutions. Meanwhile, resources should be devoted to educating the public, professionals, insurers, and legislators about the special needs of these patients. Meanwhile, a new section on adolescent and young adult cancer statistics has been developed by SEER to include in the annual Cancer Statistics Report.[246] The U.S. NCI, the Lance Armstrong Foundation, and the NCI-sponsored pediatric and adult cooperative groups have launched a national initiative to improve our understanding of the cancers in adolescents and young adults and the accrual of these "orphaned" patients to clinical trials.[247]

References

1. Gurney JG, Severson RK, Davis S, et al. Incidence of cancer in children in the United States. Sex-, race-, and 1-year age-specific rates by histologic type. Cancer 1995;75:2186–2195.
2. Kenney LB, Miller BA, Ries LA, et al. Increased incidence of cancer in infants in the U.S.: 1980–1990. Cancer 1998;82:1396–1400.
3. Reaman G. Biology and treatment of acute leukemia in infants: perspective 2. In: Pui CH, ed. Treatment of acute leukemias: new directions for clinical research. Totowa, NJ: Human Press Inc., 2003:75–86.
4. Campbell AN, Chan HS, O'Brien A, et al. Malignant tumours in the neonate. Arch Dis Child 1987;62:19–23.
5. Iehara T, Hamazaki M, Sawada T. Cytogenetic analysis of infantile neuroblastomas by comparative genomic hybridization. Cancer Lett 2002;178:83–89.
6. Bolande RP. Neoplasia of early life and its relationships to teratogenesis. Perspect Pediatr Pathol 1976;3:145–183.
7. Bader JL, Miller RW. US cancer incidence and mortality in the first year of life. Am J Dis Child 1979;133:157–159.
8. Moore SW, Satge D, Sasco AJ, et al. The epidemiology of neonatal tumours. Report of an international working group. Pediatr Surg Int 2003;19:509–519.
9. Parkin DM, Stiller CA, Draper GJ, et al. The international incidence of childhood cancer. Int J Cancer 1988;42:511–520.
10. Anderson LM. Introduction and overview. Perinatal carcinogenesis: growing a node for epidemiology, risk management, and animal studies. Toxicol Appl Pharmacol 2004; 199:85–90.
11. Rice JM. Causation of nervous system tumors in children: insights from traditional and genetically engineered animal models. Toxicol Appl Pharmacol 2004;199:175–191.
12. Steffen C, Auclerc MF, Auvrignon A, et al. Acute childhood leukaemia and environmental exposure to potential sources of benzene and other hydrocarbons: a case-control study. Occup Environ Med 2004;61:773–778.
13. Perera FP, Tang D, Tu YH, et al. Biomarkers in maternal and newborn blood indicate heightened fetal susceptibility to procarcinogenic DNA damage. Environ Health Perspect 2004;112:1133–1136.
14. Preston RJ. Children as a sensitive subpopulation for the risk assessment process. Toxicol Appl Pharmacol 2004;199:132–141.
15. Gill Super HJ, Rothberg PG, Kobayashi H, et al. Clonal, nonconstitutional rearrangements of the MLL gene in infant twins with acute lymphoblastic leukemia: in utero chromosome rearrangement of 11q23. Blood 1994;83:641–644.
16. Kaye SA, Robison LL, Smithson WA, et al. Maternal reproductive history and birth characteristics in childhood acute lymphoblastic leukemia. Cancer 1991;68:1351–1355.
17. Shu XO, Reaman GH, Lampkin B, et al. Association of paternal diagnostic X-ray exposure with risk of infant leukemia. Investigators of the Childrens Cancer Group. Cancer Epidemiol Biomarkers Prev 1994;3:645–653.
18. Robison LL, Buckley JD, Daigle AE, et al. Maternal drug use and risk of childhood non-lymphoblastic leukemia among offspring. An epidemiologic investigation implicating marijuana (a report from the Childrens Cancer Study Group). Cancer 1989;63:1904–1911.
19. Bunin GR, Kuijten RR, Buckley JD, et al. Relation between maternal diet and subsequent primitive neuroectodermal brain tumors in young children. N Engl J Med 1993;329:536–541.
20. Ross JA, Potter JD, Robison LL. Infant leukemia, topoisomerase II inhibitors, and the MLL gene. J Natl Cancer Inst 1994;86:1678–1680.
21. Greaves MF. Aetiology of acute leukaemia. Lancet 1997;349:344–349.
22. Ross JA, Potter JD, Reaman GH, et al. Maternal exposure to potential inhibitors of DNA topoisomerase II and infant leukemia (United States): a report from the Children's Cancer Group. Cancer Causes Control 1996;7:581–590.

23. Reynolds T. Causes of childhood leukemia beginning to emerge. J Natl Cancer Inst 1998;90:8–10.
24. Ferguson WS. Advances in the adjuvant treatment of infantile fibrosarcoma. Expert Rev Anticancer Ther 2003;3:185–191.
25. Morerio C, Rapella A, Rosanda C, et al. Differential diagnosis of congenital fibrosarcoma. Cancer Genet Cytogenet 2004;152:167–168.
26. De Lorimier AA, Harrison MR. Surgical treatment of tumors in the newborn. Am J Pediatr Hematol Oncol 1981;3:271–277.
27. Moore BD III, Ater JL, Copeland DR. Improved neuropsychological outcome in children with brain tumors diagnosed during infancy and treated without cranial irradiation. J Child Neurol 1992;7:281–290.
28. Xu W, Janss A, Moshang T. Adult height and adult sitting height in childhood medulloblastoma survivors. J Clin Endocrinol Metab 2003;88:4677–4681.
29. Littman PS, D'Angio GJ. Growth considerations in the radiation therapy of children with cancer. Annu Rev Med 1979;30:405–415.
30. Fogelholm R. Ionising radiation in infancy and adult cognitive function: radiation may not solely explain later cognitive function. BMJ 2004;328:581–582.
31. Fouladi M, Gilger E, Kocak M, et al. Intellectual and functional outcome of children 3 years old or younger who have CNS malignancies. J Clin Oncol 2005;23:7152–7160.
32. Merchant TE, Conklin HM, Wu S, et al. Late effects of conformal radiation therapy for pediatric patients with low-grade glioma: prospective evaluation of cognitive, endocrine, and hearing deficits. J Clin Oncol 2009;27:3691–3697.
33. Bradfield SM, Douglas JG, Hawkins DS, et al. Fractionated low-dose radiotherapy after myeloablative stem cell transplantation for local control in patients with high-risk neuroblastoma. Cancer 2004;100:1268–1275.
34. Jain N, Krull KR, Brouwers P, et al. Neuropsychological outcome following intensity-modulated radiation therapy for pediatric medulloblastoma. Pediatr Blood Cancer 2008;51:275–279.
35. Merchant TE, Hua CH, Shukla H, et al. Proton versus photon radiotherapy for common pediatric brain tumors: comparison of models of dose characteristics and their relationship to cognitive function. Pediatr Blood Cancer 2008;51:110–117.
36. Nag S, Tippin DB. Brachytherapy for pediatric tumors. Brachytherapy 2003;2:131–138.
37. Woods WG, O'Leary M, Nesbit ME. Life-threatening neuropathy and hepatotoxicity in infants during induction therapy for acute lymphoblastic leukemia. J Pediatr 1981;98:642–645.
38. Morgan E, Baum E, Breslow N, et al. Chemotherapy-related toxicity in infants treated according to the Second National Wilms' Tumor Study. J Clin Oncol 1988;6:51–55.
39. Bleyer AW. Clinical pharmacology of intrathecal methotrexate. II. An improved dosage regimen derived from age-related pharmacokinetics. Cancer Treat Rep 1977;61:1419–1425.
40. Thompson P, Dreyer Z, Blaney SM, et al. Pharmacokinetics of methotrexate in infants with acute lymphoblastic leukemia. Clin Pharmacol Ther 2004;75:47.
41. Thompson PA, Murry DJ, Rosner GL, et al. Methotrexate pharmacokinetics in infants with acute lymphoblastic leukemia. Cancer Chemother Pharmacol 2007;59:847–853.
42. Neims AH, Warner M, Loughnan PM, et al. Developmental aspects of the hepatic cytochrome P450 monooxygenase system. Annu Rev Pharmacol Toxicol 1976;16:427–445.
43. Bleyer A, Reaman G, Poplack D, et al. Central-nervous system pharmacology of high-dose intravenous methotrexate in infants with acute lymphoblastic leukemia [abstract]. Proc Am Soc Clin Oncol 1984;3:191.
44. Conway A, Moloney-Harmon PA. Ethical issues in the neonatal intensive care unit. Crit Care Nurs Clin North Am 2004;16:271–278.
45. Berman D, Duncan AM, Zeltzer LK. The evaluation and management of pain in the infant and young child with cancer. Br J Cancer Suppl 1992;18:S84–S91.
46. Ramirez I, van Eys J, Carr D, et al. Immunologic evaluation in the nutritional assessment of children with cancer. Am J Clin Nutr 1985;41:1314–1321.
47. Luban NLC. Blood groups and blood component transfusion. In: Baehner RL, Miller DR, McMillan CW, eds. Blood diseases of infancy and childhood. 5th ed. St. Louis, MO: Mosby, 1984:84.
48. Tsuchida Y, Ikeda H, Iehara T, et al. Neonatal neuroblastoma: incidence and clinical outcome. Med Pediatr Oncol 2003;40:391–393.
49. Beckwith JB, Perrin EV. In situ neuroblastomas: a contribution to the natural history of neural crest tumors. Am J Pathol 1963;43:1089–1104.
50. Michalowski MB, Rubie H, Michon J, et al. Neonatal localized neuroblastoma: 52 cases treated from 1990 to 1999. Arch Pediatr 2004;11:782–788.
51. van Noesel MM, Hahlen K, Hakvoort-Cammel FG, et al. Neuroblastoma 4S: a heterogeneous disease with variable risk factors and treatment strategies. Cancer 1997;80:834–843.
52. Goodman MT, Gurney JG, Smith MA, et al. Sympathetic nervous system tumors. In: Ries LA, Smith MA, Gurney JG, et al., eds. Cancer incidence and survival among children and adolescents: United States SEER Program 1975–1995. Bethesta, MD: National Cancer Institute, SEER Program, 1999:65–72.
53. Schmidt ML, Lukens JN, Seeger RC, et al. Biologic factors determine prognosis in infants with stage IV neuroblastoma: A prospective Children's Cancer Group study. J Clin Oncol 2000;18:1260–1268.
54. Paul SR, Tarbell NJ, Korf B, et al. Stage IV neuroblastoma in infants. Long-term survival. Cancer 1991;67:1493–1497.
55. London WB, Castleberry RP, Matthay KK, et al. Evidence for an age cutoff greater than 365 days for neuroblastoma risk group stratification in the Children's Oncology Group. J Clin Oncol 2005;23:6459–6465.
56. Schmidt ML, Lal A, Seeger RC, et al. Favorable prognosis for patients 12 to 18 months of age with stage 4 nonamplified MYCN neuroblastoma: a Children's Cancer Group Study. J Clin Oncol 2005;23:6474–6480.
57. George RE, London WB, Cohn SL, et al. Hyperdiploidy plus nonamplified MYCN confers a favorable prognosis in children 12 to 18 months old with disseminated neuroblastoma: a Pediatric Oncology Group study. J Clin Oncol 2005;23:6466–6473.
58. Look AT, Hayes FA, Nitschke R, et al. Cellular DNA content as a predictor of response to chemotherapy in infants with unresectable neuroblastoma. N Engl J Med 1984;311:231–235.
59. Shimada H, Chatten J, Newton WA Jr, et al. Histopathologic prognostic factors in neuroblastic tumors: definition of subtypes of ganglioneuroblastoma and an age-linked classification of neuroblastomas. J Natl Cancer Inst 1984;73:405–416.
60. Bowman LC, Castleberry RP, Cantor A, et al. Genetic staging of unresectable or metastatic neuroblastoma in infants: a Pediatric Oncology Group study. J Natl Cancer Inst 1997;89:373–380.
61. Brodeur GM. Neuroblastoma: biological insights into a clinical enigma. Nat Rev Cancer 2003;3:203–216.
62. Look AT, Hayes FA, Shuster JJ, et al. Clinical relevance of tumor cell ploidy and N-myc gene amplification in childhood neuroblastoma: a Pediatric Oncology Group study. J Clin Oncol 1991;9:581–591.
63. Hayashi Y, Kanda N, Inaba T, et al. Cytogenetic findings and prognosis in neuroblastoma with emphasis on marker chromosome 1. Cancer 1989;63:126–132.
64. Nakagawara A, Arima-Nakagawara M, Scavarda NJ, et al. Association between high levels of expression of the TRK gene and favorable outcome in human neuroblastoma. N Engl J Med 1993;328:847–854.
65. Shimada H, Umehara S, Monobe Y, et al. International neuroblastoma pathology classification for prognostic evaluation of patients with peripheral neuroblastic tumors: a report from the Children's Cancer Group. Cancer 2001;92:2451–2461.
66. Navarro S, Amann G, Beiske K, et al. Prognostic value of International Neuroblastoma Pathology Classification in localized resectable peripheral neuroblastic tumors: a histopathologic study of localized neuroblastoma European Study Group 94.01 Trial and Protocol. J Clin Oncol 2006;24:695–699.
67. De Bernardi B, Mosseri V, Rubie H, et al. Treatment of localized respectable neuroblastoma. Results of the LNESG1 study by the SIOP Europe Neuroblastoma Group. Br J Cancer 2008;99:1027–1033.
68. Rubie H, Coze C, Plantaz D, et al. Localised and unresectable neuroblastoma in infants: excellent outcome with low-dose primary chemotherapy. Br J Cancer 2003;89:1605–1609.
69. Weinstein JL, Katzenstein HM, Cohn SL. Advances in the diagnosis and treatment of neuroblastoma. Oncologist 2003;8:278–292.
70. Nickerson HJ, Matthay KK, Seeger RC, et al. Favorable biology and outcome of stage IV-S neuroblastoma with supportive care or minimal therapy: a Children's Cancer Group study. J Clin Oncol 2000;18:477–486.
71. Hero B, Simon T, Spitz R, et al. Localized infant neuroblastomas often show spontaneous regression: results of the prospective trials NB95-S and NB97. J Clin Oncol 2008;26:1504–1510.
72. Matthay KK, Yanik G, Messina J, et al. Phase II study on the effect of disease sites, age, and prior therapy on response to iodine-131-metaiodobenzylguanidine therapy in refractory neuroblastoma. J Clin Oncol 2007;25:1054–1060.
73. Noguera R, Canete A, Pellin A, et al. MYCN gain and MYCN amplification in a stage 4S neuroblastoma. Cancer Genet Cytogenet 2003;140:157–161.
74. Naito H, Sasaki M, Yamashiro K, et al. Improvement in prognosis of neuroblastoma through mass population screening. J Pediatr Surg 1990;25:245–248.
75. Woods WG, Gao RN, Shuster JJ, et al. Screening of infants and mortality due to neuroblastoma. N Engl J Med 2002;346:1041–1046.
76. Schilling FH, Spix C, Berthold F, et al. Neuroblastoma screening at one year of age. N Engl J Med 2002;346:1047–1053.
77. Bessho F, Hashizume K, Nakajo T, et al. Mass screening in Japan increased the detection of infants with neuroblastoma without a decrease in cases in older children. J Pediatr 1991;119:237–241.
78. Brodeur GM, Maris JM. Neuroblastoma. In: Pizzo PA, Poplack DG, eds. Principles and practice of pediatric oncology. 5th ed. Philadelphia, PA: Lippincott Williams & Wilkins, 2002:895.
79. Tsubono Y, Hisamichi S. A halt to neuroblastoma screening in Japan. N Engl J Med 2004;350:2010–2011.
80. Farwell JR, Dohrmann GJ, Flannery JT. Intracranial neoplasms in infants. Arch Neurol 1978;35:533–537.
81. Ambrosino MM, Hernanz-Schulman M, Genieser NB, et al. Brain tumors in infants less than a year of age. Pediatr Radiol 1988;19:6–8.
82. Grotzer MA, Janss AJ, Fung K, et al. TrkC expression predicts good clinical outcome in primitive neuroectodermal brain tumors. J Clin Oncol 2000;18:1027–1035.
83. Aldosari N, Bigner SH, Burger PC, et al. MYCC and MYCN oncogene amplification in medulloblastoma. A fluorescence in situ hybridization study on paraffin sections from the Children's Oncology Group. Arch Pathol Lab Med 2002;126:540–544.
84. Gajjar A, Hernan R, Kocak M, et al. Clinical, histopathologic, and molecular markers of prognosis: toward a new disease risk stratification system for medulloblastoma. J Clin Oncol 2004;22:984–993.
85. Liu R, Wang X, Chen GY, et al. The prognostic role of a gene signature from tumorigenic breast-cancer cells. N Engl J Med 2007;356:217–226.
86. Young HK, Johnston H. Intracranial tumors in infants. J Child Neurol 2004;19:424–430.
87. Strauss LC, Killmond TM, Carson BS, et al. Efficacy of postoperative chemotherapy using cisplatin plus etoposide in young children with brain tumors. Med Pediatr Oncol 1991;19:16–21.
88. Geyer JR, Zeltzer PM, Boyett JM, et al. Survival of infants with primitive neuroectodermal tumors or malignant ependymomas of the CNS treated with eight drugs in 1 day: a report from the Childrens Cancer Group. J Clin Oncol 1994;12:1607–1615.
89. Grill J, Sainte-Rose C, Jouvet A, et al. Treatment of medulloblastoma with postoperative chemotherapy alone: an SFOP prospective trial in young children. Lancet Oncol 2005;6:573–580.
90. Rutkowski S, Gerber NU, von Hoff K, et al. Treatment of early childhood medulloblastoma by postoperative chemotherapy and deferred radiotherapy. Neuro Oncol 2009;11:201–210.
91. Duffner PK, Horowitz ME, Krischer JP, et al. Postoperative chemotherapy and delayed radiation in children less than three years of age with malignant brain tumors. N Engl J Med 1993;328:1725–1731.
92. Perez-Martinez A, Quintero V, Vicent MG, et al. High-dose chemotherapy with autologous stem cell rescue as first line of treatment in young children with medulloblastoma and supratentorial primitive neuroectodermal tumors. J Neurooncol 2004;67:101–106.
93. Hilden JM, Meerbaum S, Burger P, et al. Central nervous system atypical teratoid/rhabdoid tumor: results of therapy in children enrolled in a registry. J Clin Oncol 2004;22:2877–2884.
94. Gajjar A, Chintagumpala M, Ashley D, et al. Risk-adapted craniospinal radiotherapy followed by high-dose chemotherapy and stem-cell rescue in children with newly diagnosed medulloblastoma (St Jude Medulloblastoma-96): long-term results from a prospective, multicentre trial. Lancet Oncol 2006;7:813–820.
95. Yuh GE, Loredo LN, Yonemoto LT, et al. Reducing toxicity from craniospinal irradiation: using proton beams to treat medulloblastoma in young children. Cancer J 2004;10:386–390.
96. Miralbell R, Lomax A, Cella L, et al. Potential reduction of the incidence of radiation-induced second cancers by using proton beams in the treatment of pediatric tumors. Int J Radiat Oncol Biol Phys 2002;54:824–829.

97. Xu W, Janss A, Packer RJ, et al. Endocrine outcome in children with medulloblastoma treated with 18 Gy of craniospinal radiation therapy. Neuro Oncol 2004;6: 113–118.
98. Laughton SJ, Merchant TE, Sklar CA, et al. Endocrine outcomes for children with embryonal brain tumors after risk-adapted craniospinal and conformal primary-site irradiation and high-dose chemotherapy with stem-cell rescue on the SJMB-96 trial. J Clin Oncol 2008;26:1112–1118.
99. Bhatia S, Neglia JP. Epidemiology of childhood acute myelogenous leukemia. J Pediatr Hematol Oncol 1995;17:94–100.
100. Yeazel MW, Buckley JD, Woods WG, et al. History of maternal fetal loss and increased risk of childhood acute leukemia at an early age. A report from the Childrens Cancer Group. Cancer 1995;75:1718–1727.
101. Spector LG, Xie Y, Robison LL, et al. Maternal diet and infant leukemia: the DNA topoisomerase II inhibitor hypothesis: a report from the Children's Oncology Group. Cancer Epidemiol Biomarkers Prev 2005;14:651–655.
102. Reaman GH, Sposto R, Sensel MG, et al. Treatment outcome and prognostic factors for infants with acute lymphoblastic leukemia treated on two consecutive trials of the Children's Cancer Group. J Clin Oncol 1999;17:445–455.
103. Reaman G, Zeltzer P, Bleyer WA, et al. Acute lymphoblastic leukemia in infants less than one year of age: a cumulative experience of the Children's Cancer Study Group. J Clin Oncol 1985;3:1513–1521.
104. Reaman GH. Biology and treatment of acute leukemia in infants in treatment of acute leukemias. In: Pui CH, ed. New directions of clinical research. Totowa, NJ: Humana Press, 2003:73–83.
105. Pui CH, Ribeiro RC, Campana D, et al. Prognostic factors in the acute lymphoid and myeloid leukemias of infants. Leukemia 1996;10:952–956.
106. Isoyama K, Eguchi M, Hibi S, et al. Risk-directed treatment of infant acute lymphoblastic leukaemia based on early assessment of MLL gene status: results of the Japan Infant Leukaemia Study (MLL96). Br J Haematol 2002;118:999–1010.
107. Nagayama J, Tomizawa D, Koh K, et al. Infants with acute lymphoblastic leukemia and a germline MLL gene are highly curable with use of chemotherapy alone: results from the Japan Infant Leukemia Study Group. Blood 2006;107:4663–4665.
108. Pieters R, Schrappe M, De Lorenzo P, et al. A treatment protocol for infants younger than 1 year with acute lymphoblastic leukaemia (Interfant-99): an observational study and a multicentre randomised trial. Lancet 2007;370:240–250.
109. Hilden JM, Dinndorf PA, Meerbaum SO, et al. Analysis of prognostic factors of acute lymphoblastic leukemia in infants: report on CCG 1953 from the Children's Oncology Group. Blood 2006;108:441–451.
110. Dreyer Z, Dinndorf PA, Sather W, et al. Shortened intensified therapy in infant ALL: a Pediatric Oncology Group study. In: 20th Annual Meeting of the American Society of Pediatric Hematology-Oncology; May 5, 2007; Toronto, Canada.
111. Kosaka Y, Koh K, Kinukawa N, et al. Infant acute lymphoblastic leukemia with MLL gene rearrangements: outcome following intensive chemotherapy and hematopoietic stem cell transplantation. Blood 2004;104:3527–3534.
112. Campbell M, Cabrera ME, Legues ME, et al. Discordant clinical presentation and outcome in infant twins sharing a common clonal leukaemia. Br J Haematol 1996;93: 166–169.
113. Ford AM, Ridge SA, Cabrera ME, et al. In utero rearrangements in the trithorax-related oncogene in infant leukaemias. Nature 1993;363:358–360.
114. Megonigal MD, Rappaport EF, Jones DH, et al. t(11;22)(q23;q11.2) in acute myeloid leukemia of infant twins fuses MLL with hCDCrel, a cell division cycle gene in the genomic region of deletion in DiGeorge and velocardiofacial syndromes. Proc Natl Acad Sci U S A 1998;95:6413–6418.
115. Gale KB, Ford AM, Repp R, et al. Backtracking leukemia to birth: identification of clonotypic gene fusion sequences in neonatal blood spots. Proc Natl Acad Sci U S A 1997;94:13950–13954.
116. Pui CH, Gaynon PS, Boyett JM, et al. Outcome of treatment in childhood acute lymphoblastic leukaemia with rearrangements of the 11q23 chromosomal region. Lancet 2002;359:1909–1915.
117. LoNigro L, Slater DJ, Mirabile E, et al. Reverse Panhandle PCR identifies RIBOSOMAL PROTEIN S3 (RPS3) as a new partner gene of MLL in a three-way MLL rearrangement in infant acute monoblastic leukemia. Blood 2003;102:184–185b.
118. Pegram LD, Megonigal MD, Lange BJ, et al. t(3;11) translocation in treatment-related acute myeloid leukemia fuses MLL with the GMPS (GUANOSINE 5′ MONOPHOSPHATE SYNTHETASE) gene. Blood 2000;96:4360–4362.
119. Raffini LJ, Slater DJ, Rappaport EF, et al. Panhandle and reverse-panhandle PCR enable cloning of der(11) and der(other) genomic breakpoint junctions of MLL translocations and identify complex translocation of MLL, AF-4, and CDK6. Proc Natl Acad Sci U S A 2002;99:4568–4573.
120. Slater DJ, Hilgenfeld E, Rappaport EF, et al. MLL-SEPTIN6 fusion recurs in novel translocation of chromosomes 3, X, and 11 in infant acute myelomonocytic leukaemia and in t(X;11) in infant acute myeloid leukaemia, and MLL genomic breakpoint in complex MLL-SEPTIN6 rearrangement is a DNA topoisomerase II cleavage site. Oncogene 2002;21:4706–4714.
121. Brown P, Levis M, Shurtleff S, et al. FLT3 inhibition selectively kills childhood acute lymphoblastic leukemia cells with high levels of FLT3 expression. Blood 2005;105: 812–820.
122. Dreyer Z, Dinndorf PA, Hilden JM, et al. Unexpected toxicity with intensified induction in infant acute lymphoid leukemia [abstract]. Blood 2007;110:621a.
123. Dreyer Z, Dinndorf PA, Sather H. Hematopoietic stem cell transplant (HSCT) versus intensive chemotherapy in infant acute lymphoblastic leukemia [abstract]. J Clin Oncol 2007 ASCO Annual Meeting Proceedings 2007;25:9514.
124. Sanders JE, Im HJ, Hoffmeister PA, et al. Allogeneic hematopoietic cell transplantation for infants with acute lymphoblastic leukemia. Blood 2005;105:3749–3756.
125. Kaleita TA, MacLean WE, Reaman GH. Neurodevelopmental outcome of children diagnosed with ALL during infancy: a preliminary report from the Children's Cancer Group [abstract]. Med Pediatr Oncol 1992;20:385–392.
126. Kaleita TA, Reaman GH, MacLean WE, et al. Neurodevelopmental outcome of infants with acute lymphoblastic leukemia: a Children's Cancer Group report. Cancer 1999;85: 1859–1865.
127. Rubenfeld M, Abramson DH, Ellsworth RM, et al. Unilateral vs. bilateral retinoblastoma. Correlations between age at diagnosis and stage of ocular disease. Ophthalmology 1986;93:1016–1019.
128. Kivela T, Tuppurainen K, Riikonen P, et al. Retinoblastoma associated with chromosomal 13q14 deletion mosaicism. Ophthalmology 2003;110:1983–1988.
129. Dryja TP, Morrow JF, Rapaport JM. Quantification of the paternal allele bias for new germline mutations in the retinoblastoma gene. Hum Genet 1997;100:446–449.
130. Jensen RD, Miller RW. Retinoblastoma: epidemiologic characteristics. N Engl J Med 1971;285:307–311.
131. Shields CL, Mashayekhi A, Au AK, et al. The International Classification of Retinoblastoma predicts chemoreduction success. Ophthalmology 2006;113:2276–2280.
132. Friend SH, Dryja TP, Weinberg RA. Oncogenes and tumor-suppressing genes. N Engl J Med 1988;318:618–622.
133. Shields CL, Shields JA. Changing environment of retinoblastoma. Clin Exp Ophthalmol 2004;32:345.
134. Shields CL, Shields JA. Recent developments in the management of retinoblastoma. J Pediatr Ophthalmol Strabismus 1999;36:8–18.
135. Stannard C, Sealy R, Hering E, et al. Postenucleation orbits in retinoblastoma: treatment with 125I brachytherapy. Int J Radiat Oncol Biol Phys 2002;54:1446–1454.
136. Schueler AO, Fluhs D, Anastassiou G, et al. Beta-ray brachytherapy with 106Ru plaques for retinoblastoma. Int J Radiat Oncol Biol Phys 2006;65:1212–1221.
137. Abramson DH, Schefler AC. Transpupillary thermotherapy as initial treatment for small intraocular retinoblastoma: technique and predictors of success. Ophthalmology 2004;111:984–991.
138. Kremens B, Gruhn B, Klingebiel T, et al. High-dose chemotherapy with autologous stem cell rescue in children with nephroblastoma. Bone Marrow Transplant 2002;30: 893–898.
139. Abramson DH, Dunkel IJ, Brodie SE, et al. A phase I/II study of direct intraarterial (ophthalmic artery) chemotherapy with melphalan for intraocular retinoblastoma initial results. Ophthalmology 2008;115:1398–404, 1404.
140. Chevez-Barrios P, Chintagumpala M, Mieler W, et al. Response of retinoblastoma with vitreous tumor seeding to adenovirus-mediated delivery of thymidine kinase followed by ganciclovir. J Clin Oncol 2005;23:7927–7935.
141. Shields CL, Mashayekhi A, Demirci H, et al. Practical approach to management of retinoblastoma. Arch Ophthalmol 2004;122:729–735.
142. Chantada GL, Dunkel IJ, de Davila MT, et al. Retinoblastoma patients with high risk ocular pathological features: who needs adjuvant therapy? Br J Ophthalmol 2004;88: 1069–1073.
143. Abramson DH, Ellsworth RM, Kitchin FD, et al. Second nonocular tumors in retinoblastoma survivors. Are they radiation-induced? Ophthalmology 1984;91:1351–1355.
144. Kleinerman RA, Tucker MA, Abramson DH, et al. Risk of soft tissue sarcomas by individual subtype in survivors of hereditary retinoblastoma. J Natl Cancer Inst 2007;99: 24–31.
145. Kleinerman RA, Tucker MA, Tarone RE, et al. Risk of new cancers after radiotherapy in long-term survivors of retinoblastoma: an extended follow-up. J Clin Oncol 2005;23: 2272–2279.
146. Bolande RP. Congenital mesoblastic nephroma of infancy. Perspect Pediatr Pathol 1973;1:227–250.
147. Heidelberger KP, Ritchey ML, Dauser RC, et al. Congenital mesoblastic nephroma metastatic to the brain. Cancer 1993;72:2499–2502.
148. Grundy PE, Telzerow PE, Breslow N, et al. Loss of heterozygosity for chromosomes 16q and 1p in Wilms' tumors predicts an adverse outcome. Cancer Res 1994;54:2331–2333.
149. Grundy PE, Breslow NE, Li S, et al. Loss of heterozygosity for chromosomes 1p and 16q is an adverse prognostic factor in favorable-histology Wilms tumor: a report from the National Wilms Tumor Study Group. J Clin Oncol 2005;23:7312–7321.
150. Green DM, Breslow NE, Beckwith JB, et al. Treatment outcomes in patients less than 2 years of age with small, stage I, favorable-histology Wilms' tumors: a report from the National Wilms' Tumor Study. J Clin Oncol 1993;11:91–95.
151. Ritchey ML, Coppes MJ. The management of synchronous bilateral Wilms tumor. Hematol Oncol Clin North Am 1995;9:1303–1315.
152. Sorensen K, Levitt G, Sebag-Montefiore D, et al. Cardiac function in Wilms' tumor survivors. J Clin Oncol 1995;13:1546–1556.
153. Green DM, Norkool P, Breslow NE, et al. Severe hepatic toxicity after treatment with vincristine and dactinomycin using single-dose or divided-dose schedules: a report from the National Wilms' Tumor Study. J Clin Oncol 1990;8:1525–1530.
154. Paulino AC, Wen BC, Brown CK, et al. Late effects in children treated with radiation therapy for Wilms' tumor. Int J Radiat Oncol Biol Phys 2000;46:1239–1246.
155. Breslow NE, Takashima JR, Whitton JA, et al. Second malignant neoplasms following treatment for Wilm's tumor: a report from the National Wilms' Tumor Study Group. J Clin Oncol 1995;13:1851–1859.
156. Ragab AH, Heyn R, Tefft M, et al. Infants younger than 1 year of age with rhabdomyosarcoma. Cancer 1986;58:2606–2610.
157. Li FP, Fraumeni JF Jr. Soft-tissue sarcomas, breast cancer, and other neoplasms. A familial syndrome? Ann Intern Med 1969;71:747–752.
158. Hartley AL, Birch JM, Marsden HB, et al. Neurofibromatosis in children with soft tissue sarcoma. Pediatr Hematol Oncol 1988;5:7–16.
159. DeBaun MR, Tucker MA. Risk of cancer during the first four years of life in children from The Beckwith-Wiedemann Syndrome Registry. J Pediatr 1998;132:398–400.
160. Matsui I, Tanimura M, Kobayashi N, et al. Neurofibromatosis type 1 and childhood cancer. Cancer 1993;72:2746–2754.
161. Quezada E, Gripp KW. Costello syndrome and related disorders. Curr Opin Pediatr 2007;19:636–644.
162. Diller L, Sexsmith E, Gottlieb A, et al. Germline p53 mutations are frequently detected in young children with rhabdomyosarcoma. J Clin Invest 1995;95: 1606–1611.
163. Joshi D, Anderson JR, Paidas C, et al. Age is an independent prognostic factor in rhabdomyosarcoma: a report from the Soft Tissue Sarcoma Committee of the Children's Oncology Group. Pediatr Blood Cancer 2004;42:64–73.
164. Tefft M, Wharam M. Radiation therapy and embryonal rhabdomyosarcoma: local control in children less than one year of age and in children with tumors of the orbit. A report from the Intergroup Rhabdomyosarcoma Study (IRS). Proc Am Soc Clin Onc(abs)1986;5:205.
165. Yock T, Schneider R, Friedmann A, et al. Proton radiotherapy for orbital rhabdomyosarcoma: clinical outcome and a dosimetric comparison with photons. Int J Radiat Oncol Biol Phys 2005;63:1161–1168.
166. Kozak KR, Adams J, Krejcarek SJ, et al. A dosimetric comparison of proton and intensity-modulated photon radiotherapy for pediatric parameningeal rhabdomyosarcomas. Int J Radiat Oncol Biol Phys 2009;74:179–186.
167. Smith MA, Gurney JG, Ries LA. Cancer in adolescents 15 to 19 years old. In: Ries LA, Smith MA, Gurney JG, eds. Cancer incidence and survival among children and adolescents: United States Seer Program 1975–1995. Bethesta, MD: National Cancer Institute, SEER Program; 1999:157–164.
168. Ries LAG, Eisner MP, Kosary CL, et al. eds. SEER cancer statistics review, 1975–2001. Bethesda, MD: National Cancer Institute. 2004.

169. Corpron CA, Black CT, Singletary SE, et al. Breast cancer in adolescent females. J Pediatr Surg 1995;30:322–324.
170. Ashikari H, Jun MY, Farrow JH, et al. Breast carcinoma in children and adolescents. Clin Bull 1977;7:55–62.
171. Franks LM, Bollen A, Seeger RC, et al. Neuroblastoma in adults and adolescents: an indolent course with poor survival. Cancer 1997;79:2028–2035.
172. Raney RB Jr, Sinclair L, Uri A, et al. Malignant ovarian tumors in children and adolescents. Cancer 1987;59:1214–1220.
173. Melnick S, Cole P, Anderson D, et al. Rates and risks of diethylstilbestrol-related clear-cell adenocarcinoma of the vagina and cervix. An update. N Engl J Med 1987;316: 514–516.
174. McNall RY, Nowicki PD, Miller B, et al. Adenocarcinoma of the cervix and vagina in pediatric patients. Pediatr Blood Cancer 2004;43:289–294.
175. Indolfi P, Terenziani M, Casale F, et al. Renal cell carcinoma in children: a clinicopathologic study. J Clin Oncol 2003;21:530–535.
176. French CA, Kutok JL, Faquin WC, et al. Midline carcinoma of children and young adults with NUT rearrangement. J Clin Oncol 2004;22:4135–4139.
177. Hamre MR, Chuba P, Bakhshi S, et al. Cutaneous melanoma in childhood and adolescence. Pediatr Hematol Oncol 2002;19:309–317.
178. Meadows AT, Friedman DL, Neglia JP, et al. Second neoplasms in survivors of childhood cancer: findings from the Childhood Cancer Survivor Study cohort. J Clin Oncol 2009;27:2356–2362.
179. Hodgson DC, Gilbert ES, Dores GM, et al. Long-term solid cancer risk among 5-year survivors of Hodgkin's lymphoma. J Clin Oncol 2007;25:1489–1497.
180. Bleyer A. CAUTION! Consider cancer: common symptoms and signs for early detection of cancer in young adults. Semin Oncol 2009;36:207–212.
181. Albritton K, Bleyer WA. The management of cancer in the older adolescent. Eur J Cancer 2003;39:2584–2599.
182. Pollock BH, Krischer JP, Vietti TJ. Interval between symptom onset and diagnosis of pediatric solid tumors. J Pediatr 1991;119:725–732.
183. U.S.Congress, OTA. Adolescent health—Vol. I: summary and policy options, *OTA-H-468*. Washington, DC: U.S. Government Printing Office, 1991.
184. Ziv A, Boulet JR, Slap GB. Utilization of physician offices by adolescents in the United States. Pediatrics 1999;104:35–42.
185. Alliance for Health Reform. Health care coverage in America: understanding the issues & proposed solutions. http://covertheuninsured.org/files/u4/IssuesGuide_0.pdf. Accessed July 18, 2010. Updated March 2008.
186. Mills RJ, Bhandari S. Health insurance coverage in the United States: 2002, Report No. P60–223. Washington, DC: US Department of Commerce, Economics and Statistics Administration, US Census Bureau, 2003:1–21.
187. Stoll K, Jones K. One in three: non-elderly Americans without health insurance, 2002–2003. Washington, DC: Families USA Publication, 2002:1–39.
188. McCormick MC, Kass B, Elixhauser A, et al. Annual review of child health care access and utilization: annual report on access to and utilization of health care for children and youth in the United States—1999 [abstract]. Pediatrics 2000;105:219–230.
189. Friman PC, Finney JW, Glasscock SG, et al. Testicular self-examination: validation of a training strategy for early cancer detection. J Appl Behav Anal 1986;19:87–92.
190. Weist MD, Finney JW. Training in early cancer detection and anxiety in adolescent males: a preliminary report. J Dev Behav Pediatr 1996;17:98–99.
191. Bleyer A, Barr R, Hayes-Lattin B, et al. The distinctive biology of cancer in adolescents and young adults. Nat Rev Cancer 2008;8:288–298.
192. Whyte F, Smith L. A literature review of adolescence and cancer. Eur J Cancer Care (Engl) 1997;6:137–146.
193. Bleyer A. Older adolescents with cancer in North America deficits in outcome and research. Pediatr Clin North Am 2002;49:1027–1042.
194. Freyer DR. Care of the dying adolescent: special considerations. Pediatrics 2004;113: 381–388.
195. Reaman GH, Bonfiglio J, Krailo M, et al. Cancer in adolescents and young adults. Cancer 1993;71:3206–3209.
196. Selby P, Bailey CC, eds. Cancer and the adolescent. London: BMJ Publishing Group, 1996.
197. Yarcheski A, Scoloveno MA, Mahon NE. Social support and well-being in adolescents: the mediating role of hopefulness. Nurs Res 1994;43:288–292.
198. Young MA, Pfefferbaum-Levine B. Perspectives on illness and treatment in adolescence. Cancer Bull 1984;36:275–279.
199. Manne S, Miller D. Social support, social conflict, and adjustment among adolescents with cancer. J Pediatr Psychol 1998;23:121–130.
200. Worchel FF, Copeland DR. Psychological intervention with adolescents. Cancer Bull 1984;36:279–284.
201. Nichols ML. Social support and coping in young adolescents with cancer. Pediatr Nurs 1995;21:235–240.
202. Novakovic B, Fears TR, Wexler LH, et al. Experiences of cancer in children and adolescents. Cancer Nurs 1996;19:54–59.
203. Pelcovitz D, Libov BG, Mandel F, et al. Posttraumatic stress disorder and family functioning in adolescent cancer. J Trauma Stress 1998;11:205–221.
204. Blum RW, Garell D, Hodgman CH, et al. Transition from child-centered to adult health-care systems for adolescents with chronic conditions. A position paper of the Society for Adolescent Medicine. J Adolesc Health 1993;14:570–576.
205. Stoval A, Peacock M. The family of the adolescent with cancer. Cancer Bull 1984;36:285–288.
206. Rait DS, Ostroff JS, Smith K, et al. Lives in a balance: perceived family functioning and the psychosocial adjustment of adolescent cancer survivors. Fam Process 1992;31: 383–397.
207. Mulhern RK, Palmer SL, Merchant TE, et al. Neurocognitive consequences of risk-adapted therapy for childhood medulloblastoma. J Clin Oncol 2005;23: 5511–5519.
208. Hancock SL, Tucker MA, Hoppe RT. Factors affecting late mortality from heart disease after treatment of Hodgkin's disease. JAMA 1993;270:1949–1955.
209. Merchant TE, Nguyen L, Nguyen D, et al. Differential attenuation of clavicle growth after asymmetric mantle radiotherapy. Int J Radiat Oncol Biol Phys 2004;59:556–561.
210. Denys D, Kaste SC, Kun LE, et al. The effects of radiation on craniofacial skeletal growth: a quantitative study. Int J Pediatr Otorhinolaryngol 1998;45:7–13.
211. Clemons M, Loijens L, Goss P. Breast cancer risk following irradiation for Hodgkin's disease. Cancer Treat Rev 2000;26:291–302.
212. Festa RS, Tamaroff MH, Chasalow F, et al. Therapeutic adherence to oral medication regimens by adolescents with cancer. I. Laboratory assessment. J Pediatr 1992;120: 807–811.
213. Tamaroff MH, Festa RS, Adesman AR, et al. Therapeutic adherence to oral medication regimens by adolescents with cancer. II. Clinical and psychologic correlates. J Pediatr 1992;120:812–817.
214. Tebbi CK. Treatment compliance in childhood and adolescence. Cancer 1993;71: 3441–3449.
215. KyngAs HA, Kroll T, Duffy ME. Compliance in adolescents with chronic diseases: a review. J Adolesc Health 2000;26:379–388.
216. Verrill MW, Judson IR, Wiltshaw E, et al. The use of paediatric chemotherapy protocols at full dose is both a rational and feasible treatment strategy in adults with Ewing's family tumours. Ann Oncol 1997;8:1099–1105.
217. Zebrack B, Bleyer A, Albritton K, et al. Assessing the health care needs of adolescent and young adult cancer patients and survivors. Cancer 2006;107:2915–2923.
218. Penson RT, Rauch PK, McAfee SL, et al. Between parent and child: negotiating cancer treatment in adolescents. Oncologist 2002;7:154–162.
219. Leonard RC, Gregor A, Coleman RE, et al. Strategy needed for adolescent patients with cancer. BMJ 1995;311:387.
220. Guidelines for the pediatric cancer center and role of such centers in diagnosis and treatment. American Academy of Pediatrics Section Statement Section on Hematology/Oncology. Pediatrics 1997;99:139–141.
221. Access to quality cancer care. A consensus statement of the American Federation of Clinical Oncologic Societies. J Pediatr Hematol Oncol 1998;20:279–281.
222. Albritton K, Wiggins C. Adolescents with cancer are not referred to Utah's pediatric center [abstract]. Proc Am Soc Clin Oncol 2001;20:248a.
223. Rauck AM, Fremgen AM, Menck HR, et al. Adolescent cancers in the United States: a National Cancer Data Base (NCDB) report [abstract]. Pediatr Hematol Oncol 1999; 21:310.
224. Brady AM, Harvey C. The practice patterns of adult oncologists' care of pediatric oncology patients. Cancer 1993;71:3237–3240.
225. Stock W, Sather H, Dodge RK, et al. Outcome of adolescents and young adults with ALL: a comparison of Children's Cancer Group (CCG) and Cancer and Leukemia Group B (CALGB) regimens [abstract]. Blood 2000;96:476a.
226. Jeha S. Who should be treating adolescents and young adults with acute lymphoblastic leukaemia? Eur J Cancer 2003;39:2579–2583.
227. Kantarjian HM, O'Brien S, Smith TL, et al. Results of treatment with hyper-CVAD, a dose-intensive regimen, in adult acute lymphocytic leukemia. J Clin Oncol 2000;18: 547–561.
228. Bleyer WA, Tejeda H, Murphy SB, et al. National cancer clinical trials: children have equal access; adolescents do not. J Adolesc Health 1997;21:366–373.
229. Bleyer A. Adolescent and young adult (AYA) oncology: the first A. Pediatr Hematol Oncol 2007;24:325–336.
230. Ferrari A, Montello M, Budd T, et al. The challenges of clinical trials for adolescents and young adults with cancer. Pediatr Blood Cancer 2008;50:1101–1104.
231. Meadows AT, Kramer S, Hopson R, et al. Survival in childhood acute lymphocytic leukemia: effect of protocol and place of treatment. Cancer Invest 1983;1:49–55.
232. Wagner HP, Dingeldein-Bettler I, Berchthold W, et al. Childhood NHL in Switzerland: incidence and survival of 120 study and 42 non-study patients. Med Pediatr Oncol 1995;24:281–286.
233. Lennox EL, Stiller CA, Jones PH, et al. Nephroblastoma: treatment during 1970–3 and the effect on survival of inclusion in the first MRC trial. BMJ 1979;2:567–569.
234. Duffner PK, Cohen ME, Flannery JT. Referral patterns of childhood brain tumors in the state of Connecticut. Cancer 1982;50:1636–1640.
235. Nachman J, Sather HN, Buckley JD, et al. Young adults 16–21 years of age at diagnosis entered on Childrens Cancer Group acute lymphoblastic leukemia and acute myeloblastic leukemia protocols. Results of treatment. Cancer 1993;71:3377–3385.
236. Strock W, La M, Sanford B, et al. What determines the outcomes for adolescents and young adults with acute lymphoblastic leukemia treated on cooperative group protocols? A comparison of Children's Cancer Group and Cancer and Leukemia Group B studies. Blood 2008;112:1646–1654.
237. de Bont JM, van der Hold B, Dekker AW, et al. Significant difference in outcome for adolescents with acute lymphoblastic leukemia (ALL) treated on pediatric versus adult ALL protocols [abstract]. Blood 2003;102.
238. Boissel N, Auclerc MF, Lheritier V, et al. Should adolescents with acute lymphoblastic leukemia be treated as old children or young adults? Comparison of the French FRALLE-93 and LALA-94 trials. J Clin Oncol 2003;21:774–780.
239. Paulussen M, Ahrens S, Juergens H. Cure rates in Ewing tumor patients aged over 15 years are better in pediatric oncology units. Results of GPOH CESS/EICESS studies [abstract]. Proc Am Soc Clin Oncol 2003;22.
240. Ferrari A, Dileo P, Casanova M, et al. Rhabdomyosarcoma in adults. A retrospective analysis of 171 patients treated at a single institution. Cancer 2003;98:571–580.
241. Stiller CA, Benjamin S, Cartwright RA, et al. Patterns of care and survival for adolescents and young adults with acute leukaemia—a population-based study. Br J Cancer 1999;79:658–665.
242. Webb DK, Harrison G, Stevens RF, et al. Relationships between age at diagnosis, clinical features, and outcome of therapy in children treated in the Medical Research Council AML 10 and 12 trials for acute myeloid leukemia. Blood 2001;98:1714–1720.
243. Tebbi CK, Stern M. Burgeoning specialty of adolescent oncology. Cancer Bull 1984;36:265–272.
244. Bleyer A, Barr RD, Albritton K, et al. eds. Cancer in Adolescents and Young Adults. Berlin, Heidelberg, New York: Springer, 2007.
245. Bleyer A. Young adult oncology: the patients and their survival challenges. CA Cancer J Clin 2007;57:242–255.
246. Section XXXII: Adolescent and young adult cancer by site incidence, survival and mortality. In: Ries LAG, Melbert D, Krapcho M, et al. eds. SEER Cancer Statistics Review, 1975–2005. Bethesda, MD: National Cancer Institute, 2007.
247. Closing the gap: Research and care imperatives for adolescents and young adults with cancer. Report of the Adolescent and Young Adult Progress Review Group. 2009. www.raibenefit.org/res/Closing_The_Gap_Research_and_Care_Imperatives.pdf. Accessed October 12, 2008.

CHAPTER 16 ■ HEMATOPOIETIC STEM CELL TRANSPLANTATION IN PEDIATRIC ONCOLOGY

CATHERINE M. BOLLARD, ROBERT A. KRANCE, AND HELEN E. HESLOP

Hematopoietic stem cell transplantation (HSCT) is an established treatment approach for many malignant and nonmalignant diseases that affect the hematopoietic and immune systems. The initial human transplants for hematologic malignancy took place in the 1950s[1] and showed transient engraftment only. As increasing information became available in the 1960s about the human leukocyte antigen (HLA) system and typing methods were developed, successful transplants were described for children with immunodeficiency.[2,3] Patients with advanced leukemia also underwent marrow transplantation from matched sibling donors, and a small percentage became long-term survivors.[4] As transplant has become safer, it is now used earlier in the course of malignant diseases with improved outcomes. Over the past decade, indications for HSCT have broadened, and the future suggests even wider applications, especially in correcting genetic disorders and delivering novel treatments for malignancies.

A number of key advances have contributed to making HSCT a more commonly available and successful treatment modality.[5] First, there was improved understanding of the critical role of histocompatibility in allogeneic HSCT and development of molecular methods to more accurately type donors and recipients. These advances along with the increasing numbers of donors in large registries of unrelated donors and cord blood units both expanded access to transplant and allowed recipients to find more closely matched donors.[6–8] Over the last 20 years, there have also been identification of additional sources of stem cells so that bone marrow (BM), peripheral blood (PB), and umbilical cord blood (UCB) are all widely used in clinical practice to provide long-term hematopoietic reconstitution. Finally, there have been improvements in graft-versus-host disease (GVHD) prophylaxis and supportive care during the period of hematopoietic and immune suppression posttransplant.[9–11] HSCT should therefore be considered for patients in whom this procedure is likely to result in superior long-term disease-free survival (DFS) compared with other therapeutic modalities. Potential candidates must also have a suitable source of hematopoietic stem cells (HSCs) available at an appropriate time in the course of the disease. In this chapter, we review the current status of HSCT in pediatric oncology and indications for its use in patients with acute lymphoblastic leukemia (ALL), acute myelogenous leukemia (AML), chronic myelogenous leukemia (CML), myelodysplasia or myeloproliferative syndromes, non-Hodgkin lymphoma (NHL) and Hodgkin disease (HD), and neuroblastoma and other solid tumors. In addition, we provide an overview of HSCT procedures, including conditioning regimens and selection of donor and HSC source, and common early- and late-onset posttransplant complications.

ALLOGENEIC TRANSPLANTATION

In allogeneic transplantation, the recipient receives HSC from a closely matched donor, and alloantigens that differ between donor and recipient are targets for T-cell recognition. The most important criteria for choosing an allogeneic donor is the degree of histocompatibility with the recipient. With increasing genetic differences, there is an increased risk of both graft rejection and of GVHD, although there may also be an increased graft-versus-tumor effect. The most important determinant of alloreactivity is matching at HLA loci, but even when major histocompatibility complex (MHC) antigens are identical, minor histocompatibility antigens, which are naturally processed peptides derived from normal cellular proteins, may evoke a strong MHC-restricted response when different polymorphisms are present in donor and recipient. Natural killer (NK) cells may also contribute to alloreactivity, particularly in the setting of haploidentical transplantation.

Human Leukocyte Antigen Matching

Identification of HLAs and the human MHC was a prerequisite for transplantation of BM between family members. HLAs are cell surface molecules encoded by class I (HLA-A, HLA-B, and HLA-C) and class II (HLA-DR, HLA-DQ, and HLA-DP) genes, a series of closely linked loci known as the MHC on chromosome 6. These antigens present peptides to T lymphocytes and are highly polymorphic. Historically, HLA molecules were typed by alloantisera in complement-dependent cytotoxicity assays. However, serologically identical donors and recipients can have major genotypic differences not detected by this methodology that will be readily detected by alloreactive T cells. Analysis by gene sequencing has revealed multiple alleles for most serologically defined specificities, and more than 3,000 alleles have now been recognized.[12] HLA terminology is designated by the World Health Organization Nomenclature Committee for Factors of the HLA system and is updated at regular intervals.[12] The nomenclature distinguishes the technique used to determine the HLA type and its level of resolution. The broadest designation is based on serologic typing, whereas the highest resolution is based on actual DNA sequence. For example, "HLA A2" designates a specific class I serotype (i.e., determined by reactivity to serologic reagents); antigens (HLA A2) recognized by these reagents can be subdivided into HLA A*02 by additional serologic reagents or by low-resolution molecular techniques. In turn, HLA A*02 can be further classified by intermediate molecular analysis as A*0201/A*0205 or by high-resolution molecular analysis as HLA A*0201. This is incorporated into the nomenclature, resulting in a report confirming the allele as HLA A*0201 on high-resolution typing. The type of assay used and its sensitivity and specificity are important considerations in determining potential histocompatibility, particularly for mismatched family or for any unrelated donor HSCT.

The genetic unit of HLA class I and II regions on one chromosome is referred to as an *HLA haplotype*, and the two HLA haplotypes in one person are called the *HLA genotype*. Class I and class II antigens are codominant and are transmitted as dominantly inherited mendelian traits. Each child expresses one set of paternal and one set of maternal HLAs corresponding to the HLA genes inherited as one paternal and one maternal HLA haplotype. The probability that a child will inherit any one of the four possible HLA genotypes is 0.25. When, by chance, an individual inherits a phenotypically identical HLA allele from each parent, the result is a person homozygous for that locus; a person may be homozygous for one allele at a single HLA locus or for the entire haplotype. Genetic recombination between HLA class I and II regions also occurs infrequently. Thus, although a careful examination of family haplotypes is essential to determining donor suitability, the HLA complex can generally be considered as a single genetic unit that is most often inherited as a block.

The initial BM donors were siblings who shared the patient's HLA genotype. Historically, only approximately 30% of patients have an HLA-matched sibling donor, so that the remaining 70% have to consider alternative donors such as an HLA-mismatched family member, a closely matched unrelated donor (MUD), or a cord blood unit. Development of more precise tissue typing methods using molecular techniques and establishment of large donor registries have facilitated transplants from closely HLA-MUDs.[7,8]

Minor Antigens and Genetic Loci Outside the Major Histocompatibility Complex

The degree of alloreactivity between donor and recipient is also influenced by differences at minor histocompatibility loci. These genes encode polymorphisms of normal cellular genes and have been characterized only in humans over the last 10 to 15 years.[13] Increasing numbers of minor antigens have been identified, and molecular typing for some of these antigens is becoming available. Although less GVHD has been reported in matched sibling transplants when minor antigens are matched,[14] other studies have shown that T cells recognizing minor antigens differentially expressed between donor and recipient mediate antileukemia activity.[15] There is also increasing evidence that genetic loci outside of the MHC may influence the risk of transplant complications such as infection or bronchiolitis obliterans, and several groups are undertaking genome-wide association assays to define genetic variants that might predict these complications.[16,17]

AUTOLOGOUS TRANSPLANTATION

The rationale for autologous transplantation is that dose intensification will increase the response rate of chemosensitive tumors. Hematopoietic toxicity is a limiting factor for dose intensification, which can be overcome by harvesting HSC and then cryopreserving and reinfusing them after doses of chemotherapy and radiotherapy that would otherwise be lethal or require a prolonged period of recovery. For many malignancies occurring in adults, such as NHL, it has been shown in randomized trials or evidence-based reviews that such dose intensification results in improved DFS. Data for some pediatric solid tumors such as neuroblastoma also suggest improved outcome when autologous transplant is used as part of initial therapy in high-risk patients.[18] In other pediatric tumors, autologous transplant remains investigational. One approach that is being investigated is to use reinfusion of autologous HSC to allow courses of high-dose therapy to be given more frequently in so-called tandem transplants.[19]

SOURCE OF HEMATOPOIETIC STEM CELLS

Initial studies used HSCs derived from BM for transplantation. Over the past 10 to 15 years, with the availability of cytokines that can mobilize HSC into the bloodstream, there has been increasing use of mobilized PB.

Autologous Donors

In autologous transplantation in adults, mobilized PB is now the most commonly used product, as it results in faster engraftment. Its use has also increased in pediatrics, although logistic challenges with pheresis in children weighing less than 15 to 20 kg mean that marrow is still more frequently used.[20] Cytokine-mobilized peripheral blood stem cells (PBSCs) can be harvested either after treatment with cytokines alone (most commonly recombinant human granulocyte colony-stimulating factor [G-CSF], 10 to 16 µg/kg/day for 3 to 7 days) or with cytokines given during recovery from chemotherapy. An alternative strategy is to use the chemokine receptor 4 antagonist plerixafor and G-CSF in combination.[21]

Allogeneic Donors

When an allogeneic transplant is indicated, the family is initially typed to determine if there is an HLA-matched sibling. If one of the siblings matches, this is almost always the preferred donor. Rarely, patients will have an identical twin who can serve as the donor. In this setting, there is no alloreactivity and the patients do not require posttransplant immunosuppression, but they have a higher risk of relapse, particularly if they have a myeloid malignancy.[22] In pediatric transplantation, the issue of consenting children by proxy has been debated, but parental consent for the sibling donor is generally considered to be in the donor's best interests.[23] If there is no HLA match in the family, options include the use of a closely MUD, a mismatched family member, or a cord blood unit. All potential allogeneic donors undergo an extensive medical evaluation; in the case of UCB donation, the mother serves as a "surrogate" and the evaluation is adjusted appropriately. Physical examination and screening laboratory tests with complete blood cell count, biochemistry profile, hepatitis screen, and other testing for transmissible infectious agents, including cytomegalovirus (CMV) and human immunodeficiency virus, should be completed. Many donor candidates will have preexisting medical problems that require further evaluation. BM donors are usually admitted to the hospital the morning of the harvest. The aspiration procedure is conducted in an operating room under sterile conditions and with appropriate anesthesia. Marrow is usually harvested only from the posterior iliac crests, but when the recipient is significantly larger than the donor or when large cell volumes are needed, the anterior iliac crests may also be harvested. The total volume of marrow usually collected amounts to 10 to 20 mL/kg of recipient weight to obtain sufficient HSCs for engraftment. BM from children, especially infants, has a higher concentration of nucleated cells and probably a higher proportion of marrow-repopulating cells than marrow from older donors.

As with autologous transplant, cytokine-mobilized allogeneic PBSC harvest has become an alternative to marrow as a source of HSCs. Early phase II studies showed that this source of HSCs resulted in faster engraftment, no increase in acute GVHD (perhaps due to a G-CSF-mediated shift to Th2 helper cells) but an increased incidence of chronic GVHD. In adult patients, both a single-center randomized study and International Bone Marrow Transplant Registry (IBMTR) data have shown that treatment-related mortality rates were lower and leukemia-free survival (LFS) rates were higher with use of blood SC transplants in patients with advanced leukemia, although a difference was not seen for patients with better risk disease.[24,25] However, a retrospective registry review suggested that in pediatric transplants for acute leukemia, the outcome may be worse after PBSC transplant after adjusting for relevant risk factors.[26] Although the results of more studies and specifically studies in children should become available over the next few years, current experience suggests that PB may be the preferred source of SCs for patients with high-risk disease. For patients with low-risk disease, the increased risk of chronic GVHD needs to be balanced against the risk of relapse.

Donor safety is obviously an important issue for pediatric PBSC donors. A review from the Pediatric Bone Marrow Consortium of more than 200 donor collections found that PBSC collection was safe in normal pediatric donors, that target CD34 cell yields were easily achieved, and that children weighing less than 20 kg usually require a single blood product exposure.[27] Although this approach has not shown short-term toxicity, longitudinal studies are needed to establish if there are long-term toxicities that might raise ethical issues for donor safety.[28,29]

Unrelated Donors

Volunteer unrelated donors include healthy persons between 18 and 60 years of age who fulfill health requirements similar to those applied to blood donors. As discussed previously, the outcome after unrelated transplant correlates with the degree of matching and mismatching at HLA class 1, class II, and HLA-C loci are all associated with poorer outcome.[7] With increasing registry size, the chance of finding a donor has increased, so that more than 70% of patients undergo unrelated donor transplantation using an HLA-A, -B, and -C and DRB1 allele MUD.[30] The likelihood of finding a donor matching at these 8 loci (or 10 loci if matching at DQB1 is also included) varies for different ethnic groups and is less for groups with more polymorphism of HLAs.

Historically, the outcome after transplantation from unrelated donors has been inferior to that observed after matched sibling transplantation because of an increased incidence of graft rejection and of GVHD resulting from increased alloreactivity in this setting. Over the past few years, improved results have been reported from several single-center and multicenter studies in defined patient populations, reflecting improvements in donor-recipient matching, GVHD prophylaxis, supportive care, and the timing of transplantation.[31,32] Registry results of unrelated donor transplant in children have also improved over time—for example, children transplanted from 2003 to 2006 have a 2-year survival of 58% compared with 44% for patients transplanted from 1999 to 2002.[33]

Umbilical Cord Blood

Another alternative source of SCs is cord blood. There are several large cord banks where cord blood is collected, cryopreserved, and tested for infectious agents in accordance with standards developed by governmental and specialty oversight organizations.[34] The immediate availability of cryopreserved cord blood units eliminates the usual delay in HSCT when unrelated donor marrow is used. After several studies demonstrated the feasibility of transplants with cord blood from unrelated donors,[35–37] cord blood became an increasing common source of HSCs for pediatric patients requiring transplants. Such transplants have slower engraftment, but they may also induce less GVHD due to the relative naivety of cord T cells. A recent registry study comparing the outcome of cord and marrow transplants in children with acute leukemia found that 5-year LFS was similar for recipients of allele-matched marrow and cord blood mismatched for either one or two antigens.[38] The speed of myeloid engraftment is associated with the mononuclear cell count of the graft, whereas transplantation-related events were associated with the patient's underlying disease and age, the number of leukocytes in the graft, and the degree of HLA disparity.[39] Although the cell count can be limiting for older children, the use of double cord blood transplantation is showing encouraging results in individuals weighing more than 45 kg.[40]

Haploidentical Family Donors

The genetic sharing of one chromosome of the chromosome 6 pair, containing the complete DNA code for the MHC, makes a haploidentical donor in essence a "half-matched donor. There is also a greater likelihood for identity between minor histocompatibility antigens expressed from other chromosomes than could be expected between unrelated individuals. This opens another potential source of donors that increases the access to allogeneic HSCT. In addition, it is more likely that a haploidentical family donor will be readily available compared with the longer task of identifying an unrelated donor. Use of a mismatched family member donor, however, is associated with an increased risk of GVHD due to increased alloreactivity, and this risk increases with the degree of mismatch. Most studies therefore show that transplants from donors mismatched in a single antigen produce results equivalent to those achieved with matched sibling donors. For greater degrees of mismatch, methods have been developed to manipulate or engineer hematopoietic progenitor cells, *ex vivo* or *in vivo*, to eliminate the cells that are thought to mediate alloreactivity. One strategy is to use G-CSF-mobilized, large-volume apheresis and CD34 selection with or without additional T-cell depletion.[41] In a series of studies in children, Lang and Handgretinger have shown that GVHD could be effectively reduced and primary engraftment attained in 83% to 100% of patients after transplantation of high stem cell doses.[42] For patients with ALL in remission, DFS at 3 years ranged between 22% and 48%.[42] A second approach developed by the Dana-Farber group relied on the induction of anergy to inactivate alloreactive T cells in the donor marrow.[43] In a recent update on the outcome of 24 patients who received haploidentical marrow after *ex vivo* induction of alloantigen-specific anergy in donor T cells by allostimulation in the presence of costimulatory blockade, they reported an engraftment rate of 95% and eight long-term survivors.[44] Other groups have administered unmanipulated marrow and relied on *in vivo* agents such as high-dose, cyclophosphamide posttransplant[45] or antithymocyte globulin (ATG)[46] to eliminate alloreactive cells. A recent study using unmanipulated marrow after an ATG containing conditioning regimen in children with hematological malignancies reported a 3-year probability of LFS of 44.7%.[46]

CONDITIONING REGIMENS

In autologous transplant, the aim of the conditioning regimen is to intensify doses of chemotherapy agents that have activity in the particular malignancy. In allogeneic transplant, conditioning regimens must achieve adequate immunosuppression of the recipient to prevent rejection of the donor marrow cells and destroy residual malignant cells while causing minimal toxicity. Historically, patients transplanted for malignancy have received intensive, fully ablative regimens in which hematopoietic reconstitution would not occur without HSC support. Conditioning regimens are discussed in more detail in the following section on indications for transplant, but the most commonly used allogeneic regimens use total body irradiation (TBI) and cyclophosphamide or chemotherapy alone with combinations such as busulfan and cyclophosphamide. Because most fully ablative chemoradiation regimens are at the limits of toxicity, any escalation to attempt reduction of the risk of relapse would likely increase regimen-related toxicity to unacceptable levels, particularly in heavily pretreated patients. Addition of biologic agents, such as monoclonal antibodies reactive with tumor cells or radioconjugates, may provide antileukemic activity without increasing toxicity.[47–49]

As high-dose chemotherapy and allogeneic SC transplantation carry a substantial treatment-related morbidity and mortality in older patients or those who were heavily pretreated prior to HSCT, new approaches for allografting, which have been predominantly conducted in adults, have explored an approach of less intensive conditioning therapy given with the aim of facilitating allogeneic engraftment.[50] This strategy relies on a graft-versus-tumor effect to eradicate malignancy, and a variety of regimens based on low-dose TBI or fludarabine are under investigation. The major problem with submyeloablative regimens is an increased rate of graft failure, ranging from 5% to 30% versus 1% to 5% in patients who underwent full myeloablation prior to HSCT.

TRANSPLANTATION FOR HEMATOPOIETIC MALIGNANCIES

Over the past 5 years, understanding of leukemia biology has continued to progress. One result is that the indications for stem cell transplantation for childhood leukemia have been refined and now are more limited. Improved prognosis for children with leukemia diminishes the value of comparisons between current outcomes and those of previous eras. A sometimes unacknowledged consequence is that the makeup of children still needing transplantation has changed. Therefore, in the current era, compared with the prior, DFS following transplantation may not increase because patients undergoing transplantation may be inherently more resistant to salvage therapy.

For certain leukemias and myelodysplastic diseases, for example, those identified by unfavorable genetic markers, HSCT is the only curative option available and is considered a primary treatment modality. Otherwise, stem cell transplantation (HSCT) for hematopoietic malignancies is widely used as a salvage therapy for patients who fail primary chemotherapy. Because HSCT, particularly from unrelated or mismatched related donors, causes important short-term and long-term morbidity, its role in treating hematopoietic malignancies is under constant scrutiny and reevaluation. Results of clinical trials for leukemias are summarized in Tables 16.1 to 16.3.

Comparison of HSCT to conventional treatments for safety and efficacy is problematic for a number of reasons. First, randomized studies are challenging to conduct because not every patient will have a donor and there may be an inherent selection bias depending on the transplant center. To compensate, statistical constructs have been developed to adjust for potential biases and allow comparisons between nonrandomized cohorts, but such manipulations are never totally satisfactory. An additional consideration is center effect, as the success of HSCT is in part related to the transplant center. Outcomes as reported in registry data are often inferior to that of single centers because the experience and consistency of a single center cannot be duplicated across many institutions. Finally, the measures of treatment outcome are always in flux. As new agents are tried and chemotherapeutic regimens are developed, their effects may alter the survival and outcome following HSCT in unanticipated ways. For example, primary therapy regimens have improved overall survival, but for patients who relapse on these treatments, leukemia may be more resistant to salvage therapy or patients may be more susceptible to the inherent toxicities of HSCT.[86]

ACUTE LYMPHOBLASTIC LEUKEMIA

Acute Lymphoblastic Leukemia First Remission

Cure rates for children with newly diagnosed ALL are projected to reach nearly 90% following current primary chemotherapy treatments.[87] Correspondingly, the role for stem cell transplantation as primary therapy has been reduced. Formerly, children with ALL who had a high initial white count (in excess of 100,000) or the translocation t(4;11) had a high incidence of relapse, but now effective chemotherapy cures many of these patients.[88] More recently, the prognosis for Ph+ ALL, for which less than a quarter of children had achieved long-lasting remission and for which transplantation was recommended if a suitable donor were identified, appears to have markedly improved with the addition of imatinib to traditional chemotherapy regimens.[89] Despite these treatment advances, there are children with ALL for whom transplantation should be considered as primary therapy.

Infants with ALL, particularly those with mutations involving 11q23, the *MLL* gene, initial white blood count >100,000/μL, and younger than 6 months when diagnosed, have a highly unsatisfactory outcome after chemotherapy with event-free survival (EFS) less than 20%.[70,90] Stem cell transplantation may therefore be appropriate for these infants, but reported clinical trials show conflicting results. The Interfant-99 study reported 50% DFS for 37 high-risk infants who achieved complete remission and then underwent allogeneic transplantation.[70] When compared with patients treated with chemotherapy alone (37% DFS) and adjusted for the time to transplant, the difference was not significant. The Japan Infant Leukemia Study Group reported 55% of infants (N = 49) with *MLL* rearrangement remained in complete remission following stem cell transplantation.[67] As in the Interfant-99 study, the interval between remission and transplantation may have biased the outcome in favor of transplantation as almost one-third of infants relapsed at this point. The Children's Cancer Group (CCG) 1953 clinical trial confirmed the worse outcome for infants with *MLL* rearrangement, with 33.6% EFS.[69] Transplantation did not improve the outcome for these infants resulting in 25% EFS, compared with a "time-to-transplant" chemotherapy control group for whom EFS was 58%. Outcome was clearly better in a single-center trial for infants with high-risk disease transplanted in CR1 where 76% DFS was reported.[66]

The one conclusion to draw from these various reports is that the optimal treatment for infant ALL has yet to be devised. For infants older than 6 months at diagnosis and without *MLL* rearrangement, chemotherapy has been effective in treatment for 60% of patients; however, because of the poor results for younger infants with high-risk ALL, in particular those with 11q23 mutations, stem cell transplantation, especially in the context of a clinical trial, is worthy of evaluation. In the studies cited, transplantation from both related and alternative donors did not alter the outcome and thus alternative donor transplantation is reasonable. Because of the risk for early relapse, delay between remission and transplantation must be minimized so that an unrelated cord blood may be the best choice in the absence of a matched related donor. Beyond CR1, stem cell transplantation is problematic. At the Fred Hutchinson Cancer Center, the risk for death was 2.6 times greater for infants transplanted in CR2 or with more advanced disease.[66] Furthermore, infants in relapse will require further intensive chemotherapy, and cumulative toxicity may either prevent transplantation altogether or lead to excessive transplant-related morbidity. If stem cell transplant is appropriate for infants, it will likely be during the initial remission. One major drawback to transplant of infants during initial remission is the concern for impaired growth and neurocognitive development following conditioning therapy with irradiation. Reports have been mixed regarding its impact in these areas, but these concerns must be satisfactorily addressed.[66,91]

High Risk Acute Lymphoblastic Leukemia

In concert with the improved treatment for children with ALL has been the identification of patients most at risk for treatment failure. More than two-thirds of patients with hypodiploid karyotype (<44 chromosomes) are likely to relapse.[92] Likewise, a sizeable portion of children who fail to achieve remission following induction therapy or show leukemic blasts in the blood (>1,000/μL) beyond the first 2 weeks of therapy ultimately fail treatment.[93,94] Fortunately, the numbers of these patients are small probably less than 10% of all newly diagnosed patients.[95] The Berlin-Frankfurt-Munster (BFM) group compared the outcome for children with high-risk T-cell ALL (largely composed of patients who were poor responders to induction therapy) treated with chemotherapy or allogeneic stem cell transplantation (ALL-BFM 90 and 95 trials).[55] The difference in DFS between transplantation and chemotherapy arms was significant at 73% and 51%, respectively; furthermore, DFS was equivalent for patients transplanted from matched related or alternative donors. Similarly, a European pediatric consortium reported a significant difference in DFS, 40% versus 56%, for children with high-risk B- and T-cell ALL in first remission treated with either chemotherapy or matched related donor transplantation.[53] In contrast, in the PETHEMA (Programa de Estudio y Tratamiento de las Hemopatias Malignas) ALL-93 trial for high risk ALL, approximately a third of patients were slow responders or induction failures, and no advantage was found

for allogeneic stem cell transplantation over chemotherapy with 45% DFS for both groups.[54]

Comparisons between these studies and others are made difficult because the definition of high-risk ALL has not been uniform and is continuously being modified as therapy improves or new prognostic findings are used for risk assignment. The recently described mutation of the IKZF1 gene and intrachromosomal amplification of chromosome 21 (iAMP 21) *RUNX1* are associated with relapse in more than half of patients, so these findings are now being incorporated in risk assignment strategies.[96,97] Sensitive measures to detect minimal residual disease (MRD) have become increasingly important, as indicators for patients at heightened risk for relapse for whom transplantation in initial remission may be beneficial. Less than a third of children with B-cell ALL receiving current therapy and showing greater than 1% MRD defined by flow cytometry at the completion of induction treatment remained disease free.[94] Similarly, patients with T-cell ALL and persistent MRD levels at or in excess of one leukemia cell per thousand are unlikely to remain disease free.[98] Studies are underway by cooperative groups in the United States and Europe to evaluate the role of stem transplantation in the setting of persistent MRD.

Treatment design and analysis can also present comparison problems. Outcome can be biased by the time and the logistic process necessary to find a suitable allogeneic donor. Children with high-risk ALL may relapse early before transplantation can be performed. It is unclear whether this is a failure of chemotherapy or transplantation. To adjust for such biases, statisticians utilize "intent-to-treat" analysis, in which all transplant-eligible patients are considered as transplant, regardless whether transplant is performed. "Time-adjusted" analysis excludes from analysis relapse that occurs during the time interval to transplant. These statistical manipulations are never as satisfactory as randomized controlled studies.

Because of its diverse patient constituency and large numbers, registry data provide a measure of transplant outcome. For patients younger than 20 years with ALL in CR1, the CIBMTR (Center for International Blood and Marrow Transplant Research) reports 62% overall probability of survival at 3 years after matched-related donor transplant and 56% after unrelated donor transplant.[99] Although the indications to perform transplantation were not uniform, it is likely that a portion of these patients would fulfill the current understanding of high risk ALL, supporting the contention that stem cell transplantation can be effective for children with high-risk ALL.

A major drawback to transplantation is the unacceptable mortality related to the therapy itself, which may exceed 15%.[26] Improvements in supportive care, especially in the treatment of infections, are notable, but transplant complications from infection, GVHD, and organ toxicity persist. A major goal for transplantation today as it has been for the past 20 years remains reduction in regimen toxicity while preserving antileukemia activity.

Leukemia relapse is the other major obstacle to be overcome. As originally conceived, the conditioning regimen was intended to overcome leukemia cell resistance.[100] Although graft versus leukemia (GVL) may be operative for some patients, much of the curative potential of transplantation for ALL comes from the conditioning therapy.[65,101,102] Unfortunately, there has been no major advance in conditioning therapy for ALL in children. It is reasonably well established that the ablative therapy, which includes TBI, is superior to chemotherapy-only regimens.[56,103] There is little evidence at present that reduced intensity conditioning is a satisfactory alternative. It is also important to recognize the impact of MRD immediately proceeding stem cell transplantation.[104] For patients in first and second remission, there were no

TABLE 16.1

HEMATOPOIETIC STEM CELL TRANSPLANTATION FOR ACUTE LYMPHOBLASTIC LEUKEMIA (ALL)

Ref	Author	Study year	Number of patients	Disease	Status	Donor	Prep	EFS/DFS/LFS	Relapse	TRM	Chemotherapy	Statistical analysis	Comment
51	Satwani	1993–1996	29	Very high risk ALL	CR1	MRD	TBI	EFS 58	35[a]	3[a]			
52	Balduzzi	1995–2000	77	Very high risk ALL	CR1	MRD	TBI-based (busulfan-based <2 y/o)	DFS 56.7	34	9	DFS 40.6	ITT	Transplant superior for very-high risk ALL
53	Ribera	1993–2002	24	Very high risk ALL	CR1	MRD	TBI-based busulfan-based	DFS 45	33[a]	12[a]	DFS 46	ITT	No difference
54	Schrauder	1990–2000	36	High-risk T-cell ALL	CR1	MRD-MUD	TBI-based (busulfan-based <2 y/o)	DFS 67	22[a]	11[a]	DFS 42	TA	Transplant superior for very high risk T cell
55	Gaynon	1995–1998	50	Relapse on therapy or <12 mo off therapy	CR2	MRD	TBI	EFS 29 (EFS 42 actually transplanted)	22[a]	34[a]	EFS 27	ITT	No difference
56	Eapen	1991–1997	186	Pre-B ALL early vs. late relapse (< or > 36 mo)	CR2	MRD	153 TBI-based 33 busulfan-based	Early relapse LFS 41 TBI LFS 8 busulfan; Late relapse LFS 60 TBI LFS 30	Early relapse 44[a] TBI 79[a] busulfan; Late relapse 26[a] TBI 29[a] busulfan		Early relapse LFS 23; Late relapse LFS 59	TA	Transplant superior for early relapse with TBI-based conditioning
57	Roy	1995–2002	43	Relapse on therapy or <24 mo off therapy	CR2	MRD		DFS 69[a] interm DFS 45[a] high risk	15[a] interm 45[a] high risk	15[a] interm 9[a] high risk	DFS 58[a] interm DFS 0[a] high risk		Transplant superior for high risk
58	Smith	1990–2007	87	ALL	CR2	MRD-MUD-cord	TBI-based	LFS 41 MRD LFS 57 MUD LFS 43 cord	50 MRD 17 MUD 33 cord	6 MRD 22 MUD 24 cord			
59	Einsiedel	1987–1990	27	ALL BM relapse (< or >6 mo off therapy)	CR2	MRD	TBI-based	EFS 59		15	EFS 30	TA	Transplant superior for high and intermediate risk analyzed together
60	Borgmann	1983–2001	81	ALL	CR2	MUD	TBI-based	EFS 44 high 39 interm	25	30	0 high 49 inter	TA case control	Transplant superior for high risk

#	Author	Years	Disease	Remission	Donor	Conditioning	Survival			Survival 2		Conclusion
61	Reismuller	1981–1999	62	ALL	CR2	MRD-MUD	TBI-based	EFS 55			EFS 33	TA	Transplant superior
62	Eapen	1990–2000	60	ALL isolated CNS	CR2	MRD	TBI-based	LFS 58	28	22	LFS 66	TA	No difference
63	Harker-Murray	1991–2006	14	ALL isolated CNS	CR2/3	MRD-MUD	TBI-based	LFS 91	7	0			
64	Saarinen-Pihkala	1981–2001	220	ALL	CR2	MRD-MUD	TBI-based busulfan-based	DFS 47[a]	33[a]	20[a]	DFS 31[a]		
65	Kennedy-Nasser	1998–2007	64	ALL	CR2	32 MRD 32 MUD	TBI-based	DFS 67 MRD and MUD	27 MRD 22 MUD				No difference between MRD and MUD
				Infant ALL									
66	Sanders	1982–2003	40	Infant ALL	17 CR1 7 CR2/3 16 relapse	MRD-MUD	TBI-based	DFS 76 CR1 DFS 43 CR2 DFS 8 relapse	12 CR1 43 CR2 69 relapse	17[a] overall			
67	Tomizawa	1995–2001	80	Infant ALL	CR1	MRD-MUD-cord	TBI-based busulfan-based	DFS 47 TBI-based DFS 65 busulfan-based	28[a]	16[a]			No difference by donor type or conditioning
68	Jacobsohn		16	Infant ALL	16 relapse	MRD-MUD-cord	TBI-based	64	19[a]	12			
69	Hilden	1996–2000	37	Infant ALL	CR1 MLL mutation	MRD-MUD	TBI-based	DFS 25			DFS 58	TA case	Chemotherapy superior
70	Pieters	1999–2005	37	Infant ALL	CR1 MLL mutation		TBI-based	DFS 50			DFS 37	TA	No difference

Busulfan-based, busulfan ± cyclophosphamide, ± melphalan; CR1, first remission; CR2, second remission; DFS, probability disease-free survival; EFS, probability event-free survival; ITT, intent to treat; LFS, probability leukemia-free survival; MRD, matched related donor; MUD, matched unrelated donor; TA, time adjusted; TBI-based, total body irradiation ± cyclophosphamide, ± etoposide; TRM, treatment-related mortality; y/o, years old.
[a]Percent incidence.

TABLE 16.2

HEMATOPOIETIC STEM CELL TRANSPLANTATION FOR ACUTE MYELOID LEUKEMIA (AML)

Ref	Author	Study year	Number of patients	Disease	Status	Donor	Conditioning regimen	EFS/DFS/LFS	Relapse	TRM	Chemotherapy	Statistical analysis	Comment
71	Woods	1989–1995	181	AML not risk stratified	CR1	MRD	Busulfan-based	DFS 55	~20	14[a]	DFS 47	ITT	Transplant superior
72	Stevens	1988–1995	85	AML not risk stratified	CR1	MRD	TBI-based	DFS 63[a]	26[a]	9[a]	DFS 54[a]	ITT	No difference in survival
73	Alonzo	1979–1996	373	AML not risk stratified	CR1	MRD	TBI-based busulfan-based	DFS 47	36	17	DFS 34	ITT	Transplant superior except inv(16)
74	Reinhart	1998–2004	63 (36 actually transplanted)	AML high risk	CR1	MRD	Busulfan-based	DFS 43 (as treated DFS 59)	34		DFS 46 (as treated DFS 35)	ITT	No difference
75	Lange	1996–2002	170	AML not risk stratified	CR1	MRD	Busulfan-based	DFS 60			DFS 50	ITT	Transplant superior overall; however, no advantage for t(8;21) or inv(16)
76	Horan		480	AML risk stratified	CR1	MRD	TBI-based busulfan-based	DFS 63 favor DFS 58 inter DFS 33 poor			DFS 61 favor DFS 39 interm DFS 35 poor	ITT	Transplant superior for intermediate risk
77	Bunin	1990–2003	268	AML	>CR1	MUD	TBI-based busulfan-based	LFS 45 CR2 LFS 20 rel LFS 12 PIF	22 CR2 57 rel 51 PIF				Transplant in remission superior to transplant in relapse or with primary refractory disease
78	Fagioli	1989–2004	63	AML	CR2	MRD-MUD-cord	TBI-based busulfan-based	LFS 49	26	25			
79	Abrahamsson	1998–2003	62	AML	CR2	MRD-MUD		Survival 62		20			Survival superior for late relapse (CR1 > 1 yr)
80	Sander	1987–2001	127	AML	CR2	MRD-MUD-AD		os 45					Survival superior for patients in CR2 and late relapse (CR1 > 1 yr)

Busulfan-based, busulfan ± cyclophosphamide, ± melphalan; CR1, first remission; CR2, second remission; DFS, probability disease-free survival; EFS, probability event-free survival; ITT, intent to treat; LFS, probability leukemia-free survival; MRD, matched related donor; MUD, matched unrelated donor; TBI-based, total body irradiation ± cyclophosphamide; ± etoposide; TRM, treatment-related mortality.
[a]Percent incidence.

HEMATOPOIETIC STEM CELL TRANSPLANTATION FOR MYELODYSPLASTIC SYNDROME (MDS) AND SECONDARY MDS-ALL

Ref	Author	Study-year	Number TX	Disease	Status	Donor	Prep	EFS/DFS/LFS	Relapse	TRM
81	Woodard	1991–2004	38	2nd MDS/AML		MRD-MUD	TBI-based	EFS 15	19	60
82	Parikh	1995–2006	23	MDS		Cord	TBI-based	EFS 61	13	27
83	Locatelli		49	Refractory cytopenia		MRD-MUD	Busulfan-based	EFS 77	2	19
84	Strahm	2001–2005	19	Refractory cytopenia		MRD-MUD	RIC	EFS 74		26
85	Yusuf	1976–2001	94	MDS-JMML		MRD-MUD	TBI-based busulfan-based	EFS 41	30	28

AML, acute myelogenous leukemia; busulfan-based, busulfan ± cyclophosphamide, ± melphalan; DFS, probability disease-free survival; EFS, probability event-free survival; ITT, intent to treat; JMML, juvenile myelomonocytic leukemia; LFS, probability leukemia-free survival; MRD, matched related donor; MUD, matched unrelated donor; RIC, reduced intensity conditioning; TBI-based, total body irradiation ± cyclophosphamide, ± etoposide; TRM, treatment-related mortality.

survivors among patients, whose MRD before transplantation ranged from 10^{-2} to 10^{-3} leukemia cells (as measured by PCR for immunoglobulin or T-cell receptor gene rearrangements).[105] For patients without MRD prior to transplant, DFS was reported at 73%. For now, it is unclear how treatment should be tailored for patients with detectable MRD. Additional aggressive therapy may not diminish persistent disease or may cause secondary complications, which ultimately are prohibitive for transplantation.

Acute Lymphoblastic Leukemia Relapse

The principal role for stem cell transplantation in pediatric ALL therapy is as part of therapy after relapse. A recent report from the COG (Children's Oncology Group) examined the outcome for relapse patients treated on COG protocols between 1988 and 2002. For patients with initial remission lasting less than 18 months, the five-year survival was just 21%. In contrast, survival exceeded 78% for patients with isolated CNS relapse provided the initial remission lasted for at least 36 months.[106] Other reports confirm that the interval between diagnosis and relapse is the most important predictor of survival following relapse.[57,61] There is less agreement as to the importance of the site of relapse. For patients with early relapse (i.e. <18 months), in an analysis of patients treated on UKALL (United Kingdom ALL) protocols, the poor overall survival was the same, regardless of whether the site of relapse was marrow or extra medullary.[57] Phenotype may be important, as T-cell leukemia, compared with B-cell leukemia, has been identified as an unfavorable feature at relapse.[59,61] The current practice directs chemotherapy for relapsed patients if relapse is deemed late, usually 6 months after completion of therapy, or relapse is limited to extramedullary sites, such as the CNS or testes. Patients who relapse in the BM while on therapy are unlikely to be cured with chemotherapy alone and are generally directed toward transplantation if a donor is identified.

As reported by the CIBMTR, the 3-year probability of survival following matched related donor transplantation is 54% for children and young adults in second complete remission.[99] For similar patients undergoing transplant from an unrelated donor, the probability of survival at 3 years is 42% and 49%

as reported by the CIBMTR and NMDP (National Marrow Donor Program), respectively.[99,107]

Clinical trials that attempt to compare outcomes for children in CR2 treated with transplantation or chemotherapy suffer from the same limitations as previously identified and also include the availability of a suitable donor, the time required to find a donor, and the distribution of unfavorable features. In the CCG-1941 study, children with a matched related donor were assigned to transplantation.[52] Other patients were randomly allocated between chemotherapy and alternative donor transplantation. Survival analysis was based according to the intent-to-treat analysis. Not unexpectedly, accrual and compliance were problematic. DFS was 29% at 5 years for patients assigned to matched related donor transplantation but was 42% for those actually transplanted. For patients receiving chemotherapy alone, DFS at 5 years was 20%. There was no significant difference in DFS between the various treatments.

Adjusting for the time to transplant, the COG compared chemotherapy alone with matched related donor transplantation. For children with B-cell leukemia whose initial remission was less than 36 months, LFS was significantly superior for patients undergoing transplantation provided conditioning therapy included TBI, 41% versus 23% for chemotherapy.[56] For relapse occurring more than 36 months following initial remission, the LFS was essentially identical for transplantation and chemotherapy, 59% and 60%, respectively.

In the ALL-REZ BFM 87 trial (1987–1990), the EFS for children with BM relapse undergoing matched related donor transplantation was superior (59%) to that achieved with chemotherapy/radiotherapy (30%) adjusted for median time to transplant.[59] Subsequently, the BFM group defined three risk groups for children with relapsed ALL: standard, intermediate, and high. Assignment to risk groups was based upon the duration of CR1, very early relapse (<18 months initial remission), early relapse (initial remission >18 months but <6 months after completion of therapy), late relapse (>6 months after completion of therapy), and also the leukemia phenotype and the site of relapse, BM, isolated extramedullary, or combined. Eighty-one patients transplanted from unrelated donors were matched to 81 patients treated with chemotherapy. The 5-year DFS was superior for high-risk patients undergoing stem cell transplantation (44%) when compared with patients receiving chemotherapy (0%); however, there was no benefit for intermediate risk patients undergoing transplant, who had a DFS of 39% compared with 49% in the chemotherapy cohort.[60] The findings of these and other studies[61] support the practice to recommend transplantation for children whose relapse occurs while on therapy or within 6 months of completing therapy.

Isolated extramedullary relapse, most commonly CNS relapse, has usually been treated with intensive intrathecal and systemic chemotherapy followed by cranial or craniospinal irradiation; however, the duration of initial remission may have prognostic relevance to isolated CNS relapse as well. The UKALL group reported 20% EFS with UKALL R2 protocol therapy for children experiencing an isolated CNS relapse whose initial remission was less than 18 months in duration.[57] It was recommended that children with very early isolated extramedullary disease be placed in the high-risk group. The COG and CIBMTR retrospectively compared the outcome for children with CNS relapse receiving chemotherapy with cranial or craniospinal irradiation or allogeneic transplantation; EFS was similar, 66% and 58% after chemotherapy and transplantation, respectively.[62] Regardless of therapy, initial remission lasting less than 18 months was associated with inferior EFS, as half the patients developed a subsequent occurrence. Transplantation may be effective for these patients. In a single center study reporting on 14 children with very early CNS relapse, the EFS at 5 years was 91% after transplant from both related and unrelated donors.[63]

Transplantation for children beyond second remission can be effective in selected cases. A study by the Nordic Society for Pediatric Hematology and Oncology (NOPHO) considered the outcome for all children with ALL treated on NOPHO studies over a 20-year span. For patients achieving CR3 undergoing transplant, the 10-year survival was 37%; however, the investigators noted that surviving patients manifested "favorable" features, including B-cell phenotype, long-duration CR1 and CR2, or late extramedullary relapse.[64] For patients with high-risk ALL or short duration CR2, transplantation in CR3, if it can be achieved, is unlikely to be successful. As the NOPHO investigators caution patients in CR2 receiving chemotherapy should receive close monitoring for MRD so that they can proceed to immediate transplantation for recurring or persistent disease.

As documented in Table 16.1, transplantation outcomes for childhood ALL have remained relatively steady over the past decade. During this period, improved primary chemotherapy regimens have increased the number of children achieving long-term remission. It may be that current patients who need stem cell transplantation are burdened with leukemia, which is more refractory to treatment. In addition, patients with late relapse (6 to 12 months after cessation of therapy) may be effectively retreated with chemotherapy and are no longer considered for transplantation. Overall, the results following transplantation from both related and unrelated donors, including cord blood, appear to be comparable. For children with BM relapse on therapy or with very early extramedullary relapse, transplantation continues to be beneficial.

ACUTE MYELOID LEUKEMIA

Acute Myeloid Leukemia First Remission

Just as for children with ALL, improvements in the treatment of children with AML have prompted a reconsideration of the indications for stem cell transplantation as part of primary therapy. In part this reconsideration has been prompted by the

recognition that within the disease entity AML, there are morphologic and biologic features, which identify particular patients who are likely to respond to chemotherapy alone. Acute promyelocytic leukemia (APL) with the translocation, t(15;17), was the first AML subtype to manifest an excellent response and prolonged remission with treatments by ATRA-containing regimens. The list of favorable cytogenetic features has expanded and now includes AML with the cytogenetic findings, t(8;21) and inv(16). To achieve a satisfactory outcome, patients must be treated with appropriate agents; for example, high-dose cytosine arabinoside appears a critical component for treating AML with t(8;21) and inv(16).

Current practices for children with *de novo* AML limit allogeneic transplantation in first remission to defined risk groups. COG stratifies patients according to leukemia cell cytogenetics, response to induction therapy, and additional clinical and biologic measures.[77,108] Patients are divided into low-, intermediate- (standard), or high-risk cohorts. The favorable risk group includes patients with the t(8;21) and inv(16) mutations, while patients with monosomy 7, monosomy 5, or 5q deletions are defined as high risk. Leukemia with a normal karyotype or showing other cytogenetic abnormalities is considered as standard or intermediate risk. Patients with APL and Down syndrome children with AML receive alternative chemotherapy.[109] Somewhat similar classification schemes are utilized by the MRC, the BFM, the AIE0P, and other pediatric cooperative groups, and while differences exist, the major risk features are widely agreed upon.[75,110,111] Most investigators support allogeneic transplantation for high-risk patients, with the use of alternative donors if a matched sibling donor is unavailable. Chemotherapy alone is recommended for patients with favorable cytogenetic features. For all other patients, there is no consensus.

The CCG 2891 and 2961 clinical trials, in which all children with a matched related donor were eligible for transplantation, showed a significant advantage for allogeneic transplantation compared with chemotherapy alone: 60% and 61% DFS with transplant versus 48% and 50% DFS with chemotherapy.[112] In MRC AML 10, a similar trial design, DFS at 7 years was 63% versus 54%, transplant versus chemotherapy, but overall survival at 10 years, 68% versus 59%, respectively, was not statistically different.[72,111] In the subsequent MRC AML 12 trial, allogeneic transplant was limited to standard and poor risk patients (*n* = 35) with matched related donors. The 5-year DFS for all patients was 61%.[111] For intermediate- and poor-risk patients, the DFS was 62% and 41%, respectively. Although the risk for relapse was reduced among the transplanted patients, this did not translate into an improved DFS due to the higher numbers of deaths in remission. Investigators from the BFM in the AML 98 trial offered transplant for high-risk AML, which excluded patients with favorable cytogenetics and certain favorable FAB morphotypes. The intent-to-treat analysis showed no significant difference in 5-year DFS between children with and without a donor, 43% versus 47%, respectively; 36/63 eligible patients actually underwent transplantation and compared with patients treated with chemotherapy, only DFS was 59% versus 35%.[74] A risk stratified meta-analysis for 1,373 patients treated on clinical protocols POG 8821, CCG 2891 and 2961, and MRC AML 10 found that for intermediate risk patients, allogeneic transplant in CR1 was superior to chemotherapy, DFS 58% versus 39%.[77] However, DFS was not improved for favorable and poor-risk groups undergoing transplant. Investigators in the UKALL and BFM groups have therefore reserved stem cell transplantation as salvage therapy for relapsed patients, whereas in the United States, patients with intermediate- and high-risk disease and an appropriate donor are recommended for transplantation in CR1.

The clear advantage provided by transplantation in every cooperative group trial is the reduction in relapse rate compared with children who receive chemotherapy only. In the meta-analysis noted above, the incidence of relapse after transplantation was 26% versus 54% with chemotherapy. Unfortunately, treatment related mortality was 16% for transplanted patients, more than twice that for the chemotherapy group (6%). Outcomes achieved by a single center are often superior to that found in cooperative group data as documented in a recent study that reported 74% DFS and only one death from treatment-related mortality in 32 children in CR1 transplanted from matched related donors.[113] The CIBMTR data shows 3-year 65% overall survival for patients younger than 20 years transplanted from matched related donors in CR1; however, these patients were not stratified by risk group.[99]

For children without a matched related donor, alternative donor transplantation may be appropriate for high-risk AML such as that associated with monosomy 7 or a high allelic ratio of FLT3/ITD to wild-type FLT 3. The NMDP data for unrelated donor transplantation indicate 31% overall survival for CR1 patients compared with 51% for CR2 patients.[107] The inferior outcome for CR1 patients reflects the high-risk disease of the recipients. Given these results, it is preferable to enroll patients with high-risk disease without a matched related donor in a clinical trial comparing the benefit from chemotherapy and unrelated donor transplantation. Although autologous stem cell transplantation has been used to treat children with AML in CR1, a number of clinical trials have failed to demonstrate a benefit of autologous transplantation over chemotherapy.[111,112,114] Finally, for patients who fail to achieve remission but who remain well enough to tolerate conditioning therapy, allogeneic transplantation may be effective in up to 20%.[115]

Acute Myeloid Leukemia Relapse

Approximately half the children who relapse during or after chemotherapy only will achieve a second remission. It is generally agreed that after relapse, patients treated with chemotherapy only as primary therapy can be best salvaged with transplantation.[116] Indeed this was the finding of the MRC AML 10 study, which found that for children who relapsed after chemotherapy, salvage therapy with transplantation resulted in equivalent survival compared with patients transplanted in CR1, (59% vs. 68%) at 10 years.[111] This study and others have observed that the likelihood of survival after relapse was better for patients with initial CR1 of more than 1-year duration.[80,117] Leukemia with favorable cytogenetic findings also appeared to respond better to salvage therapy.[118] Among patients treated with chemotherapy only on the CCG 2891 trial, the overall survival for children undergoing transplantation in second remission was 47%, and the BFM group reported 45% overall survival for a similar population.[119,120] According to registry data from the CIBMTR, patients younger than 20 years in second remission transplanted from matched related donors can expect 57% overall survival at 3 years posttransplant.[99] The NMDP reports 45% overall survival at 5 years following unrelated donor transplantation for patients younger than 18 years.[78,107] The results for patients transplanted in relapse as opposed to second remission are inferior as the NMDP report, LFS of just 20%; however, this outcome does not discriminate between relapse patients refractory to reinduction and patients untreated prior to transplantation.

Most children undergoing allogeneic transplantation for acute myeloid leukemia receive ablative conditioning, usually combining busulfan with cyclophosphamide and/or other agents. Alternatively, TBI with cyclophosphamide or other agents has been widely used. There are data from adult AML trials that suggest better LFS and overall survival when TBI-based conditioning is compared with busulfan-based therapy.[121] For children with AML, unlike the data for ALL, no study shows an advantage to the TBI-containing regimen.[114] Because the sequelae and long-term effects following irradiation are usually considered more deleterious when compared with chemotherapy alone, the busulfan-based conditioning regimen has usually been preferred. For children with seriously compromised organ system function reduced intensity conditioning is an option. For patients younger than 20 years transplanted in 2006 and 2007 reported to the CIBMTR, approximately one in six received reduced-intensity conditioning.[99] The Pediatric Blood and Marrow Transplant Consortium (PBMTC) reported data on 47 children with various hematopoietic malignancies treated with reduced intensity conditioning.[122] Sustained engraftment was not statistically different following transplant from related donors (98%) compared with unrelated donors (89%) and unrelated cord blood (90%). Limited data suggest that engraftment and 100 days survival are comparable with that after ablative conditioning when adjusted for patient mix and disease severity, but long-term outcome studies for children are needed.

Secondary Acute Myeloid Leukemia/Myelodysplastic Syndrome

As children with cancer are effectively treated and become survivors, a small but significant number will develop secondary or treatment-related acute myeloid leukemia or myelodysplastic syndrome (MDS). Although the survival for patients with treatment-related leukemia has been dismal, "favorable" cytogenetic findings may justify aggressive therapy for certain patients.[123,124] In CCG 2891, 10/19 of patients with treatment-related AML/MDS achieved remission when assigned to the "intensive-timed" induction.[125] Although no cytogenetic finding predominated, compared with adult treatment-related AML/MDS, disease in children showed underrepresentation of abnormalities of chromosome 5 and 7. At the Fred Hutchinson Cancer Center, the outcome for patients (adults and children) following transplant for treatment-related AML/MDS was similar to that for de novo MDS or AML transforming from MDS when patients were analyzed by cytogenetic risk assignment.[126] For low risk (5q-), relapse-free survival was 40%, but it was less than 20% for high-risk disease (chromosome 7 abnormalities). Overall, the 5-year relapse-free survival for all patients was 29%. In a study of 38 children with therapy-related AML/MDS, the 1-year EFS after transplant was similar for AML and MDS, 28% and 27%, respectively; the 3-year EFS for patients with 11q23 abnormalities (21%) appeared superior to those with monosomy 7 (10%) or other cytogenetic abnormalities (13.3%).[81] Clearly, while the outcome is not optimal, patients with 11q23 abnormalities and cytogenetic findings exclusive of monosomy 7 may benefit from aggressive therapy followed by allogeneic transplantation.

MYELODYSPLASTIC SYNDROME

Refractory Cytopenia and Advanced Myelodysplastic Syndrome

Myelodysplastic syndrome (MDS) accounts for less than 5% of hematopoietic malignancies of childhood.[127] The clinical and biologic features of MDS in children differ in important ways from those seen in adult MDS. Children typically present with cytopenia in more than one hematopoietic lineage, often with marked neutropenia and/or thrombocytopenia, which is identified as refractory cytopenia.[128] It is important to consider the possibility of MDS for children that have been diagnosed with aplastic anemia. Alternatively, adult MDS variants presenting with increased blasts, refractory anemia with excess blasts (RAEB and RAEBt), are uncommon in children and should be distinguished from *de novo* AML. The presence of cytogenetic findings characteristic of AML, for example, t(8;21), support the diagnosis of AML, and patients with *de novo* AML should be treated with chemotherapy; however, monosomy 7 is the most frequent cytogenetic abnormality found in up to 40% of children with MDS. Its presence is associated with poor response to chemotherapy.[129] Children with MDS respond poorly to chemotherapy, and allogeneic stem cell transplantation is the only effective option.

The clinical course for children with refractory cytopenia may be stable without progression for a considerable interval, and transplantation may be delayed until transfusion support is needed or significant neutropenia develops.[130] However, progression to more advanced MDS is associated with reduced survival, and refractory cytopenia with monosomy 7 is associated with early transformation. In this circumstance, transplantation is advisable as soon as practical, using the best available donor. With ablative conditioning, children with refractory cytopenia transplanted before progression have achieved DFS between 59% and 78%; outcomes are similar whether the stem cells are from related, unrelated donors or unrelated cord blood.[82,83,85] After progression, less than 50% survive.[85] Survival is worse for children with advanced MDS, between 20% and 60% depending upon the morphotype.[81,131] In keeping with the adult transplant experience for MDS, reduced intensity conditioning has been used for 19 children with refractory cytopenia transplanted from alternative donors.[84] The 3-year EFS, 74%, compares favorably with that following myeloablative conditioning. Disease control following reduced intensity conditioning has been attributed to donor-derived immunologic mechanisms, and there is evidence that MDS may be sensitive to this approach. For nine children with increasing mixed chimerism posttransplant, the administration of donor lymphocytes resulted in reestablishment of complete chimerism for five patients.[132] Although MDS is uncommon is children, there are treatment options and reason for optimism.

JUVENILE MYELOMONOCYTIC LEUKEMIA

Juvenile myelomonocytic leukemia is a seemingly unique variant of MDS occurring in very young children. It is characterized by, among other things, young age of onset (2 years median age of diagnosis), thrombocytopenia, monocytosis, elevated hemoglobin F, splenomegaly, and marked *in vitro* sensitivity of myeloid progenitors to GM-CSF.[127] In recent years, the understanding of the molecular basis, namely faulty regulation of RAS-dependent signaling, has increased substantively.[133] In spite of this insight into the molecular pathway of disease, no satisfactory alternative therapy to allogeneic stem cell transplantation has been developed. The European Working Group for Myelodysplastic Diseases (EWOG-MDS) has reported 55% and 49% EFS following transplantation from matched related and alternative donors, respectively, using busulfan, cyclophosphamide, and melphalan as conditioning

therapy.[127,134] The overall relapse incidence was 35%, and relapse was the principal reason for failure. Children younger than 2 years achieve significantly superior EFS, 63%, while children 4 years or older at transplant have the highest incidence of relapse (68%). Pretransplant splenectomy does not appear to influence survival or relapse. For patients who relapse, withdrawal of immunosuppression has been reported to be beneficial, but the role for donor lymphocyte infusions has not been adequately established.[127,135]

CHRONIC MYELOID LEUKEMIA

Treatment for the rarest form of leukemia in children, chronic myeloid leukemia, has been transformed by imatinib. The experience for children has paralleled that of adults; more than 80% of patients will achieve a complete cytogenetic response and more than 90% will be alive at 5 years postdiagnosis.[136,137] In spite of this excellent response, patients are not cured and must continue imatinib indefinitely. This presents a dilemma for children, as the long-term effects of the imatinib therapy remain undetermined. The decision to proceed to transplantation is straightforward for patients responding poorly to imatinib treatment. Response is assessed by the steady regression of CML manifestations, beginning with recovery of normal blood counts and ending in a major molecular response (i.e. >3 log reduction in *BCR-ABL*).

Children who have achieved a complete cytogenetic and molecular response to imatinib and who have a matched related donor present a particular dilemma. At this time, there is no established approach. Long-term consequences of imatinib, largely unknown, must be weighed against the risk of transplant regimen-related morbidity and mortality. Data from the European Group for Blood and Marrow Transplantation (EBMT) consortium reported overall and LFS for children following transplantation in first chronic phase from matched related donors of 75% and 63%, respectively, with 20% TRM.[138] Outcome was worse using unrelated donors, survival 65%, DFS 56%, and TRM 35%. For children responding to imatinib, stem cell transplantation should probably be delayed until there is evidence for imatinib resistance. To that end, children in complete cytogenetic and molecular remission will benefit from frequent monitoring every 3 months by quantitative PCR for the *BCR-ABL*. As reported, 10% of patients with a log increase in quantitative PCR developed progressive disease.[136] Patients who never achieve or who lose a major molecular response are probably most at risk. Although patients may respond to increased imatinib dose or alternative tyrosine kinase inhibitors, the concern for sustained response in children is heightened. This would be a reasonable parameter to begin preparation for transplantation.

There has been concern for the possible adverse effect of prior imatinib therapy on transplantation. In a report from the CIBMTR, which compared the outcomes for CML patients undergoing transplantation with or without prior imatinib therapy, there was no statistical difference in survival, LFS or TRM for the two groups.[139] These findings applied to patients undergoing transplant in first chronic phase and with more advanced disease. Finally, because previous experience had shown that delay of transplantation beyond 12 months from diagnosis led to worse outcomes, there is concern that extended imatinib therapy will ultimately diminish the potential curative role for transplantation. Unfortunately, too few patients treated for extended intervals have undergone transplantation to address this point. The answer to this question is most pressing for children with CML.

HODGKIN DISEASE AND NON-HODGKIN LYMPHOMA

With the exception of Hodgkin disease (HD), patients who received minimal previous therapy or patients relapsing years after therapy, pediatric patients with lymphoma who do not enter remission or who subsequently relapse are rarely cured using therapy at conventional doses.[140,141] Autologous HSCT has been used to allow dose escalation of a broad range of active agents. Conditioning regimens are alkylator based, with or without the addition of TBI.[141] Among frequently reported regimens are CBV (cyclophosphamide, carmustine, and etoposide), BEAM (carmustine, etoposide, cytosine arabinoside, and melphalan), BEAC (carmustine, etoposide, cytarabine, and cyclophosphamide), BU/CY (busulphan and cyclophosphamide).[140,142,143] None of these conditioning regimens have been shown to produce a superior outcome in pediatric patients and CBV and BEAM remain the most widely used. The use of TBI as part of the conditioning regimen is becoming less common in the autologous setting due to increased toxicity.[144] However, the role of local radiation therapy either before or after HSCT is still unclear.[144,145]

Many reports of autologous HSCT for both NHL and HD include both adult and pediatric patients. Although an overall DFS of approximately 50% is consistently reported, predictive factors related to disease burden and responsiveness to chemotherapy have been identified.[146] Lymphoma patients with favorable characteristics have a DFS of up to 60% after HSCT, whereas less than 20% of poor-risk patients achieve durable remissions.[140,142] In NHL, progressive disease or lack of response to salvage chemotherapy before HSCT is a negative prognostic factor associated with DFS of less than 10%.[147,148] For patients with relapsed HD, bulky disease at the time of HSCT adversely affects outcome[149–151]; response to prior chemotherapy has also been shown to impact DFS[152] but not all studies.[153]

Virtually all autologous HSCTs for lymphoma now use mobilized PB instead of BM as a hematopoietic SC source. Most reports demonstrate that the time to neutrophil engraftment is shortened and costs reduced, although it has been difficult to show an impact on survival.[154,155] Which SC source is preferable in terms of tumor contamination is a complex issue likely affected by many factors, including the natural history of BM involvement with disease, the degree of BM involvement, and the mechanism by which PBSCs are mobilized.[154,156] Overall, the reported risk of developing secondary leukemia and MDS varies greatly, but it is difficult to ascertain the degree to which autologous HSCT increases this risk beyond that conferred by prior exposure to leukemogenic therapy.[141] Large series of children treated for Hodgkin and non-Hodgkin lymphoma now show an actuarial incidence of secondary malignancy of up to 20% at 10 years post-HSCT with no evidence of a plateau.[157–159] The European BMT Lymphoma registry, reporting on approximately 5,000 patients, found the actuarial risk for MDS/AML at 5 years posttransplant (±95% CI) was 4.6% (3.1 to 6.8) for HD and 3.0% (2.0 to 4.3) for NHL, suggesting that the incidence of MDS/AML may not be greater following an autograft than after conventional chemotherapy.[160] However, there is more recent evidence showing an increased risk of secondary MDS/AML in patients receiving autologous stem cell transplant for NHL or HD. Identified risk factors include age, use of TBI, and/or type of chemotherapy received prior to transplant.[161,162]

The role of allogeneic HSCT has also been investigated, although never in a prospective, randomized manner. Most studies use matched sibling donors although more recently, alternative donor sources including cord blood and haploidentical donor grafts have been used and all suggest a decreased incidence of relapse.[42,163] This is presumably due to graft-versus-lymphoma effect or use of a noncontaminated SC source, or both.[150,164,165] The EBMT retrospectively analyzed 1,185 allogeneic transplants for lymphoma reported to the EBMT registry over a 18-year period and compared these with the results with 14,687 autologous SCT performed over the same period. Actuarial survival at 4 years was approximately 40% for NHL and 25% for HD. After performing a matched analysis, overall survival was better for autologous transplantation.[166] These results were similar to observations in other series where there had been no improvement in overall survival due to an increased toxic death rate (particularly in HD patients) receiving allogeneic transplants.[147] More recently, however, the BFM group reported their results of 20 patients with ALCL who received an allogeneic SCT with TBI/CY/etoposide. They achieved an EFS rate of 75 ± 10% at 3 years after allogeneic transplant.[167]

The use of submyeloablative regimens (generally fludarabine based), however, may reduce transplant-related mortality rates while still achieving a GVL effect in lymphoma patients receiving allografts and warrants further investigation in the pediatric population.[168,169] In one large study from the EBMT, overall survival rates at 1 year for high-grade NHL and HD were 52% and 72%, respectively. However, progression-free survivals were 32% and 55% related to the poor prognosis of patients with chemoresistant disease.[170] In an attempt to enhance the graft-versus-lymphoma effect, Peggs et al. treated 49 patients with relapsed HD with an allogeneic stem cell transplant using a reduced intensity conditioning regimen followed by donor leukocyte infusion (DLI) in 16 patients who had residual disease or disease progression posttransplant. Nine patients showed disease responses including eight complete responses.[171] Further investigations of allogeneic approaches in HD as well as NHL are therefore clearly warranted. However, the further development of approaches to maximize efficacy and minimize the toxicity is critical. Newer strategies such as cellular immunotherapy with antigen specific T cells and NK cells and the use of monoclonal antibodies may enhance the graft-versus-lymphoma effect post-allogeneic transplant while minimizing toxicity.[172–177]

TRANSPLANTATION FOR SOLID TUMORS

HSCT has been used for a variety of solid tumors occurring in children. However, in many cases, the largest reported experience is contained within mixed adult and pediatric series, making the pediatric experience somewhat difficult to assess. Table 16.4 summarizes representative trials of autologous HSCT for solid tumors.

Brain Tumors

CNS tumors comprise the second largest group of pediatric cancers. Because the prognosis is dismal for those children failing surgery, radiation therapy, and/or conventional chemotherapy, several groups have explored the use of autologous SC rescue after high-dose chemotherapy. However, to date, there are no controlled trials published demonstrating that high-dose chemotherapy followed by stem cell rescue improves outcomes in children with CNS tumors. Preparative regimens have used thiotepa and etoposide with or without

TABLE 16.4

OUTCOME OF AUTOLOGOUS STEM CELL TRANSPLANTATION IN PATIENTS WITH SOLID TUMORS

Center/reference	Number of patients	Disease and status	Disease-free survival (%)
MSK[178]	23	Medulloblastoma/recurrent	34
St Jude/Baylor[179]	53 (19 high risk)	Newly diagnosed medulloblastoma or supratentorial PNET	93 (73 high risk)
Rady's Children's Hospital[180]	29	Recurrent/progressive medulloblastoma and germinoma	24
Duke[181]	49	Primary brain/poor prognosis or recurrent	35
MSK[182]	20	Primary brain/recurrent	50
MSK[183]	16	Pontine glioma/resistant	0
Duke[184]	12 (6 children)	Newly diagnosed pineoblastoma	69
UCLA[185,186]	49 (6 brainstem)	PNETs (brainstem and supratentorial)	39 (supratentorial) 0 (brainstem)
UCLA[187]		Ependymoma	0
UCSF[188]	379	Neuroblastoma postinduction without progressive disease	43
CHOP[189]	39	Neuroblastoma postinduction without progressive disease	58
Harvard[190]	52	Neuroblastoma postinduction without progressive disease	63
Northwestern[191]	25	Neuroblastoma postinduction without progressive disease	57
EBMT[192]	63	Ewing's first or second remission	21
MetaEICESS[193]	54	Ewing's first or second remission (single vs. tandem transplants)	22–29
University of Minnesota[194]	36	ES, DSRCT, and other solid tumors (including CNS tumors and rhabdomyosarcoma)	50 (ES) 100 (DSRCT) 6 (other tumors)
Multicenter review[195]	287	Rhabdomyosarcoma CR1 or PR1	24–29
	102	Rhabdomyosarcoma, CR2, PR2, CR3 or with disease	12
German WT group[196]	23	Wilm's tumor poor prognosis/recurrent	48
Northwestern[197]	13	Wilm's tumor after relapse	60

Baylor, Baylor College of Medicine; CHOP, Children's Hospital of Philadelphia; Duke, Duke Comprehensive Cancer Center; DSRCT, desmoplastic small round cell tumor; EBMT, European Group for Blood and Marrow Transplantation; ES, Ewing's sarcoma; German WT group, German Cooperative WT study group; MSK, Memorial Sloan-Kettering Cancer Center; MetaEICESS, Meta European Intergroup Cooperative Ewing' Sarcoma Study; Northwestern, Northwestern University; PNET, primitive neuroectodermal tumor; St Jude, St Jude Children's Research Hospital; UCSF, University of California, San Francisco; WT, Wilm's tumor.

carboplatin, as these agents are known to cross the blood-brain barrier and are dose limited by myelosuppression.

More recently, myeloablative regimens using cyclophosphamide and melphalan have been used.[180] The results for patients with primitive neuroectodermal tumor or medulloblastoma and high-grade gliomas outside of the brainstem are variable, although durable DFS appears achievable for some patients.[180,185,198] Outcome is closely correlated with tumor burden at the time of HSCT, ranging from less than 10% in children with bulky disease to 50% for those with minimal or no disease.[175,198,199]

HSCT has also been used with encouraging preliminary results in infants and young children to avoid or reduce neuroaxis radiation.[182] However, good outcome depended on the ability of surgery or chemotherapy, or both, to produce a state of minimal disease before HSCT.[200] One larger study treated children newly diagnosed with medulloblastoma or supratentorial primitive neuroectodermal tumor (age range: >2 years to <22 years) with four consecutive cycles of high-dose cyclophosphamide, cisplatin, and vincristine, each followed by autologous stem cell rescue after completion of craniospinal irradiation. There were no deaths attributable to the toxicity of high-dose chemotherapy and 2-year progression-free survival

was 93.6% ± 4.7% for average risk patients and 73.7% ± 10.5% for high-risk patients from the start of therapy.[179]

More recently, a report of the Head Start I and II experience for 43 children with newly diagnosed supratentorial primitive neuroectodermal tumors showed that intensified induction chemotherapy followed by autologous stem cell rescue provided an improved EFS of 39% for these poor prognosis patients compared with historical controls. Moreover, 60% of the survivors did not require radiation therapy.[185,201] However, patients with ependymomas and diffuse pontine brain stem tumors show no improvement in either survival or DFS with HSCT, presumably related to the refractory nature of these tumors to pre-HSCT conventional dose chemotherapy.[183,186,187]

Neuroblastoma

Conventional treatment of children with high-risk neuroblastoma has generally resulted in a DFS of less than 20%. Efforts to improve outcome have focused on intensifying induction therapy in addition to using high-dose therapy with autologous SC support for consolidation. Newly diagnosed high-risk patients treated with regimens culminating in HSCT have been reported to have a 3-year DFS of up to 43% after conditioning with myeloablative chemotherapy with or without TBI.[188,202] Purged BM was used as the SC source. Post-HSCT therapy with oral *cis*-retinoic acid, which decreases proliferation and induces differentiation in neuroblastoma cells,[203] further improved survival in this cohort. However, relapse remained a significant problem with 7-year EFS rates reported around 25%.[202] Further intensification of treatment, using PBSC to hasten engraftment, has since been explored in sequential transplants using non–cross-resistant agents and PBSC for rescue. It appears that two to three closely spaced transplants (4 to 6 weeks apart) using both chemotherapy and TBI may increase DFS, but there may be a concern regarding the development of late effects in survivors of these transplants.[189,204,205] The disadvantage of using an autologous product is the risk of tumor cell contamination in the graft, which has been shown to contribute to relapse in children with neuroblastoma.[206,207] For this reason, groups have explored methods to purge the graft of contaminating malignant cells, for example, using CD34 selection.[189,208,209] However, one large study found an increased incidence (5/156 patients or 3.5%) of EBV lymphoproliferative disorder (EBV-LPD) in children undergoing tandem transplants using autologous CD34-selected PB stem cells suggesting that CD34 selection in this setting may not be feasible as the increased immunosuppression unacceptably elevates the risk for EBV-LPD.[210] Although HSCT has thus been effective in newly diagnosed, chemoresponsive patients, those with relapsed or refractory disease have continued to fare poorly. Other strategies have been explored, all of which are considered investigational and should only be performed in the context of a clinical trial. One such approach is allogeneic stem cell transplantation to enhance the graft-versus-tumor effect.[211] Another is the use of cryopreserved SC to circumvent the dose-limiting hematologic toxicity of iodine-131–metaiodobenzylguanidine (131I-MIBG), a targeted radiotherapeutic agent that is able to induce a response in some of these highest risk patients,[212] although data is now surfacing that 131I-MIBG may contribute to the risk of secondary leukemia in this already heavily pretreated patient group.[213]

Another strategy is the use of monoclonal antibodies such as antiganglioside G(D2) as adjuvant therapy postautologous SCT.[214] Recently, the COG conducted a phase III randomized controlled trial for newly diagnosed high-risk NB patients who achieved a clinical response (CR or PR) to induction therapy. The patients received myeloablative conditioning with autologous stem cell rescue and then were randomized to receive six cycles of 13-*cis*-retinoic acid (RA) alone (standard therapy) or six cycles of RA with five cycles of the GD2 antibody ch14.18 combined with alternating doses of GM-CSF and IL-2.[215] A total of 226 patients were enrolled and half (113 patients) were randomized to standard therapy and the other half to immunotherapy. EFS for the immunotherapy group was 66% versus 46% for the standard group which was statistically significant. However, appreciable toxicities were seen in the immunotherapy group with approximately 40% of patients developing grade 3 pain and allergic reactions. Moreover, with a median follow-up of only 2.1 years, further follow-up is required to evaluate whether these differences in EFS are sustained long term.[215] Finally, other immunological approaches such as the use of genetically modified tumor vaccines,[216] the use of autologous tumor-specific T-cell therapy,[217,218] or NK cells[219] posttransplant are additional novel strategies to improve the outcome for this poor prognosis disease while trying to limit treatment-related toxicity.

Sarcomas and Other Solid Tumors

Although most children with Ewing's sarcoma and rhabdomyosarcoma can be cured with conventional therapy, the survival of high-risk patients remains poor. The results of autologous HSCT for such patients, including those with metastatic disease at presentation or those with recurrent disease, have been discouraging.[220] For Ewing's sarcoma, the most common myeloablative agent has been high-dose melphalan, either alone or in combination with TBI. Although most patients demonstrate responsive disease, few have a durable remission.[194]

Like neuroblastoma, this poor response post autografting may be related to contamination of stem cell harvests with tumor cells which appears associated with relapse.[221,222] In 1995, the European BMT Solid Tumor Registry, incorporating data from 21 transplant centers, reported an EFS of 21% at 5 years for new patients with metastatic disease and 32% for those transplanted in CR2.[192] An update from two centers in this cohort (36 patients) reported that the 5-year EFS was 25% and 20% in patients who received autologous SC and allogeneic SC transplants (respectively). Further, twice as many patients died of treatment-related toxicity (40%) after allogeneic versus autologous SCT.[223]

Newer studies have used amifostine with a double alkylator regimen with manageable toxicities but with little change in DFS.[224] Other groups have increased PB stem cell support either using tandem transplants following six cycles of induction chemotherapy followed by conditioning with melphalan/etoposide[193] or using eight cycles of chemotherapy with vincristine, doxorubicin, cyclophosphamide, ifosfamide, and etoposide with stem cell rescue infused after courses 3 and 4 and 6 and 7.[225] Although the toxicity is reduced and the CR rates improved (up to 74%), the 2-year EFS rates were not significantly improved compared with the earlier studies ranging from 29% to 39%.[193,225]

Further, as reported by the United Kingdom Children's Cancer Study Group (UKCCSG), the course of this disease after relapse is usually fatal even using megatherapy with PBSCT; and therefore, more novel strategies for the treatment of Ewing's sarcoma are required.[226,227] The results of HSCT for advanced stage or recurrent rhabdomyosarcoma are even less favorable than for Ewing's sarcoma. HSCT after conditioning regimens based on high-dose alkylator therapy has been well tolerated, but there has been no improvement in DFS.[195,228,229] Smaller cohorts of patients with better results have been reported.[223,230,231] With conventional therapy (surgery and chemotherapy), the prognosis of patients with localized osteosarcoma is approximately 70%[232]; however, the prognosis is poor for patients with metastatic or relapsed disease. Only a few studies have focused on the use of high-dose therapy with stem cell rescue for osteosarcoma, and although complete responses can be induced, the duration of the remissions is short and the overall DFSs poor at around 20%.[233,234]

Although children with metastatic Wilms' tumor have a high likelihood of cure with conventional therapy, as do those who relapse if their histology is favorable, there remains a small group of patients with adverse features who are rarely cured. The European BMT Solid Tumor Registry and, more recently, the German Co-operative Wilms' tumor Study Group reported the outcome of 25 and 23 children, respectively, with Wilms' tumor who were treated with HSCT.[196] Most received melphalan in the conditioning regimen. Morbidity and mortality was decreased in the later study (no toxic deaths) using dosage adjustment based on glomerular filtration rate. The EFSs ranged from 36% to 48.2% with improved outcomes seen in patients who were in CR at the time of HSCT.[196]

Little improvement in outcome was seen for those transplanted with measurable tumor.

In conclusion, curing children with recurrent or refractory solid tumors remains difficult and can result in appreciable toxicity.[235] Therefore, the development of novel strategies are warranted.[189,215,218,219,227]

COMPLICATIONS AFTER STEM CELL TRANSPLANTATION

Posttransplant complications fall into three main categories: those due to alloreactivity (which only occur after allogeneic transplant), the risk of infection during the period of hematopoietic and immune reconstitution, and short- and long-term complications due to toxicities from the conditioning regimen.

GRAFT-VERSUS-HOST DISEASE AND GRAFT FAILURE

Acute Graft-versus-Host Disease

GVHD results from alloreactivity between donor and recipient. The process is initiated by donor T lymphocytes that recognize antigenic disparities between donor and recipient. In the initial phase, chemotherapy and/or radiation given as part of the conditioning regimen results in production of inflammatory cytokines secreted by damaged host cells.[236] After infusion of the HSC product, donor T cells become activated by exposure to host antigens and further activate host dendritic cells and other immune effectors, resulting in a "cytokine storm." Genetic polymorphisms in cytokine genes or promoters may influence the incidence and severity of GVHD.[237]

The classic target organs of acute GVHD are the skin, gastrointestinal (GI) tract, and liver, although the lung may also be affected. GVHD is staged by the degree of organ involvement, and these stages are summed into an overall grade (Table 16.5). The most common organ involved is skin, and patients usually present with a maculopapular rash, often initially localized to palms and soles. It may progress to involve the whole body and in its most severe form produces bullous lesions and extensive epidermal separation. The differential diagnosis includes drug allergy, viral exanthem, or reaction to the conditioning regimen, particularly TBI, and these possibilities are difficult to distinguish both clinically and by skin biopsy in the early posttransplant period. Histologic examination shows changes in the dermal and epidermal layers with dermal perivascular lymphocytic infiltration basal cell vacuolar degeneration with apoptosis (single-cell necrosis) of epidermal cells and, in severe cases, separation of the dermal-epidermal junction.

Liver GVHD presents with abnormal liver function tests, with the most common finding being a rise in the levels of bilirubin and alkaline phosphatase, although this is also a variant where increase in transaminases is the predominant finding. There is a wide differential diagnosis, including veno-occlusive disease, infection, and regimen-related toxicity. Liver biopsy carries a significant risk of bleeding in the early posttransplant period, and a transjugular biopsy may be safer. Histologic examination shows bile duct damage with portal lymphocytic infiltration, which leads to cholestasis. GVHD of the lower GI tract presents as diarrhea, abdominal pain, or cramping, whereas GVHD of the upper GI tract presents with anorexia and nausea. Again, there is a differential diagnosis, including *Clostridium difficile*, CMV, and other infections and histologic study shows crypt cell necrosis.

The two major prophylactic regimens employed to prevent this complication are pharmacologic (administration of immunosuppressive drugs) and immunologic (*in vitro* T-cell depletion of the donor marrow). The most commonly used pharmacologic prophylaxis regimens include the calcineurin inhibitors, cyclosporine and tacrolimus, which block activation of T cells.[236] Both these agents have similar efficacy and

TABLE 16.5

STAGING AND GRADING OF ACUTE GVHD
*(Acute GVHD Grading by the Consensus Conference Criteria[238])

	Staging*				
	Stage 0	Stage 1	Stage 2	Stage 3	Stage 4
Skin	No rash	Rash <25% BSA	25%–50%	>50% generalized erythroderma	Plus bullae and desquamation
Gut	<500 mL diarrhea/day	501–1,000 mL/day	1,001–1,500 mL/day	>1,500 mL/day	Severe abdominal pain and ileus
UGI		Severe nausea/vomiting			
Liver	Bilirubin ≤2 mg/dL	2.1–3 mg/dL	3.1–6 mg/dL	6.1–15 mg/dL	>15 mg/dL

	Grading index of acute GVHD*			
	Skin	Liver	Gut	Upper GI
0	None and	None and	None and	None
I	Stage 1–2 and	None and	None	None
II	Stage 3 and/or	Stage 1 and/or	Stage 1 and/or	Stage 1
III	None—Stage 3 with	Stage 2–3 or	Stage 2–4	N/A
IV	Stage 4 or	Stage 4	N/A	N/A

BSA, body surface area; GVHD, graft-versus-host disease; UGI, upper gastrointestinal.

toxicity profiles including nephrotoxicity, hypertension, and magnesium wasting. More serious adverse effects include transplant-associated thrombotic microangiopathy and posterior reversible encephalopathy syndrome. In most regimens, a calcineurin inhibitor is administered in conjunction with other immunosuppressive agents including mycophenolate mofetil, methotrexate, steroids, or sirolimus.[236] Sirolimus blocks activation of T cells by inhibiting the mammalian target of rapamycin (mTOR) pathway and as it has activity against lymphoid blasts *in vitro* is being evaluated as GVHD prophylaxis in patients with ALL in a current COG study.

Ex vivo T-cell depletion reduces the risk of both acute and chronic GVHD and may allow higher tolerance of mismatching but may also increase the risk of rejection and delay immune reconstitution. A confounding feature for interpreting the value of T-cell depletion is that a variety of methodologies are employed to remove T cells, including physical methods and monoclonal antibodies. Some techniques produce a pan–T-cell depletion, whereas others use antibodies with more restricted T-subset specificities. An IBMTR study shows a better outcome when antibodies with narrow specificities are used.[239] Nevertheless, a large randomized trial comparing pharmacologic immunosuppression with T-cell depletion did not show a significant difference in DFS at 3 years between the two groups, although the range of posttransplant complications differed by mode of prophylaxis.[240]

If the patient develops acute GVHD, the first-line treatment option is steroids, which are usually given in doses up to 2 mg/kg, although some groups use higher dose regimens. If steroids do not control GVHD, second-line treatments are initiated.[241] These include monoclonal antibodies such as daclizumab, Campath, or ATG, which are targeted at the effector cells causing GVHD, or antitumor necrosis factor antibodies such as infliximab targeted at the cytokines that produce tissue damage.[241] Clinical studies are also evaluating the use of immunomodulatory cells such as T regulatory cells or mesenchymal cells to treat GVHD, and mesenchymal cell infusions have shown promise in a phase II study in patients with steroid-resistant, acute GVHD.[242]

Chronic Graft-versus-Host Disease

Chronic GVHD is defined as GVHD occurring after day 100 posttransplant, although this definition is somewhat arbitrary.[243] Chronic GVHD often occurs in a patient who has had preceding acute GVHD, although it may arise *de novo*. Major risk factors for the development of chronic GVHD in pediatric patients are prior acute GVHD, donor-recipient HLA disparity, and increasing patient age. It targets the skin, liver, and GI tract but may also target other organs and shares features with autoimmune diseases such as scleroderma.[244]

In the skin, manifestations range from dry patches or areas of variegated pigmentation to extensive dermal scarring that produces thickened atrophic skin resembling changes seen in scleroderma and joint contractures. The GI tract may also be involved with the oral mucosa showing lichenoid lesions and xerostomia. Esophageal involvement may present with dysphagia, and webs may also occur. Lower GI involvement may result in diarrhea and malabsorption. Chronic GVHD of the liver usually presents as a cholestatic process, which can progress to a syndrome similar to primary biliary cirrhosis. Pulmonary dysfunction can also occur in the setting of chronic GVHD, and there is an association with bronchiolitis obliterans,[16] although it is still debated whether the lung is a primary target. Other manifestations include a sicca syndrome and development of autoantibodies.

The diagnosis of chronic GVHD is usually made clinically with a confirmatory skin biopsy. Chronic GVHD is graded as limited or extensive, with limited disease having localized skin involvement with or without hepatic dysfunction and extensive disease having involvement of any other target organ. A new system based on factors that confer a poor prognosis, including extensive skin involvement, thrombocytopenia, and progressive type of onset, has been proposed but still requires validation.[245]

Treatment of chronic GVHD remains a challenge. Patients with limited chronic GVHD are started on steroids and will often respond well to therapy. For children who fail to respond or who have more extensive disease, the standard treatment is still the combination of prednisone with a calcineurin inhibitor, such as cyclosporine and FK 506.[236] Alternate immunosuppressive agents include mycophenolate, sirolimus, thalidomide, and psoralen ultraviolet irradiation or extracorporeal photopheresis. Although children with limited chronic GVHD have a favorable prognosis, children with extensive chronic GVHD are profoundly immunocompromised, both by the disease and by the agents used as treatment and are at risk of infectious complications, which account for the majority of the mortality associated with chronic GVHD. Children with chronic GVHD require continuing prophylaxis against opportunistic infections and rapid evaluation and treatment of fever, as they may be functionally asplenic.

Graft Failure

Graft failure results from eradication of the incoming donor hematopoietic cells by residual recipient immune system cells, which have survived the conditioning regimen. It is uncommon after fully ablative allogeneic HSCT for hematologic malignancies, occurring in fewer than 1% of recipients of matched sibling grafts and up to 5% of grafts from mismatched donors. Risk factors include T-cell depletion of the donor product, a low nucleated cell dose, and degree of mismatch between donor and recipient. A higher incidence of rejection may be seen when less ablative regimens are used and is also observed after cord blood transplantation.[39] If graft failure occurs, patients may be retransplanted after additional immunosuppressive treatment,[246] although mortality remains significant owing to prolonged neutropenia and consequent infections. Another option is reinfusion of backup autologous marrow if this is available.

Infections

Following transplant, the recipient immune system is reconstituted by donor-derived cells, a process that may take several months and may be delayed by immunosuppressive therapy for GVHD prophylaxis or treatment. The type of infections to which children are susceptible varies depending on time after transplant. During the initial posttransplant period, risk factors include mucositis, neutropenia, and presence of central lines. Patients are at risk of bacterial infection, fungal infection, and infection with respiratory viruses. After engraftment, children may remain at risk of bacterial and fungal infection if they develop GVHD and are also at risk of viral infection, particularly reactivation of herpes viruses such as CMV. Infectious complications occurring later after transplant are mainly seen in allogeneic recipients, and the major risk factor is chronic GVHD. International consensus guidelines on the management of infections posttransplant have recently been published.[247]

Bacterial Infection

In the early posttransplant period, patients are at risk from gram-positive organisms, including coagulase-negative staphylococci, and *Streptococcus viridans* streptococci, and gram-negative bacteria including *Pseudomonas aeruginosa* and Enterobacteriaceae. Most units use prophylactic antibiotics and start empiric intravenous coverage when children develop fevers. Late bacteremia may also occur and is often related to indwelling lines and chronic GVHD. Common pathogens include encapsulated bacteria such as *Streptococcus pneumoniae*, coagulase-negative staphylococci, and *Pseudomonas*.

Fungal Infection

The incidence of invasive *Candida* infection in the period of neutropenia posttransplant has been markedly reduced by antifungal prophylaxis with triazole antimicrobials such as fluconazole and voriconazole. Mold infections with invasive aspergillosis and other molds remain a significant risk in children with GVHD or prolonged neutropenia or in those who have received transplants from alternate donors or cord blood or who are receiving steroid therapy. Amphotericin B, echinocandins such as caspofungin and micafungin, and posaconazole are potential therapies for these pathogens with specific molds exhibiting resistance to particular antifungal agents.[247]

Cytomegalovirus Infection

CMV is a herpes virus, which primarily infects endothelial cells in a range of tissues and, after a lytic cycle, establishes an asymptomatic latent infection. Sixty percent to 70% of high-risk (CMV seropositive) patients will experience CMV reactivation during the first 100 days posttransplant, and historically around half these patients would develop CMV disease, which most commonly targets the lungs, liver, and digestive tract, although children can also present with retinitis or marrow suppression.[248] Over the past 15 to 20 years, the combination of rapid early detection assays for CMV reactivation (including antigenemia assays or polymerase chain reaction) and effective preemptive antiviral therapy with ganciclovir and foscarnet has decreased the incidence of CMV-associated disease in the early posttransplant period.[11] Late or recurrent disease remains a significant problem and has stimulated evaluation of strategies to augment recovery of CMV-specific immunity. Several groups have shown that infusion of CMV-specific cytotoxic T cells can restore CMV immunity and confer protection from CMV disease.[249–252]

Respiratory Viral Infections

Respiratory viral infections are a major cause of morbidity and mortality posttransplant. Respiratory syncytial virus, parainfluenza viruses, and influenza viruses all have a significant incidence of mortality in children who develop lower tract disease in the first month posttransplant.[253] The most important measure in preventing such respiratory infections is to prevent exposure, and recipients should be carefully screened for respiratory tract infections before starting conditioning.[247] The risk of adenovirus infection is higher in recipients who receive T-cell–depleted stem cells from unrelated or HLA-mismatched related donors, and the most common clinical manifestations are hemorrhagic cystitis (HC), gastroenteritis, pneumonitis, and liver failure.[247] Treatment options for adenoviral disease are limited, with some reports of success using cidofovir.[254] Clearance of adenovirus has been shown to be associated with recovery of adenovirus-specific T-cell immunity,[255] and clearance of adenovirus has been reported after infusion of adenovirus specific T cells.[256,257]

Other Infections

Herpes simplex is commonly seen in patients early posttransplant and usually presents as mucositis. Acyclovir is effective as both prophylaxis and therapy. Varicella zoster occurs in up to 50% of children in the first year posttransplant, usually presenting as dermatomal lesions but occasionally with more disseminated disease. It also responds well to acyclovir. Immunocompromised recipients posttransplant who are exposed to individuals with chickenpox or shingles should receive VZIG as soon as possible within 96 hours after contact.[247] Reactivations with other viruses such as HHV6, HHV7, and HHV8 can also occur after transplant.

Pneumocystis pneumonia presents with fever, dyspnea, and cough usually associated with interstitial infiltrates. With effective prophylaxis, the incidence is low, although it can still present late in patients with chronic GVHD. The International Guidelines for Preventing Infectious Complications recommend trimethoprim-sulfamethoxazole as first-line prophylaxis, with dapsone, pentamidine, and atovaquone as options in patients who are allergic or who cannot tolerate trimethoprim-sulfamethoxazole.[247]

Regimen-Related Toxicity

Sinusoidal Obstruction Syndrome (or Veno-Occlusive Disease of the Liver)

Sinusoidal obstruction syndrome also known as hepatic veno-occlusive disease is a syndrome characterized by painful hepatomegaly, weight gain, ascites, and jaundice. The pathogenesis is endothelial cell injury in sinusoidal endothelial cells and hepatocytes with the main histologic features being marked sinusoidal fibrosis, necrosis of pericentral hepatocytes, and narrowing and eventual fibrosis of central veins.[258] Risk factors include preexisting liver disease, the intensity of the conditioning regimen, the amount of previous therapy, the use of radiation, and pretransplant fever. The differential diagnosis is wide, as liver dysfunction posttransplant may also be due to GVHD, infection, or drugs. Ultrasound may show an abnormal portal vein waveform, a hepatic artery resistance index greater than 0.75, or reversal of flow in the portal vein, but this is a late finding. Management is supportive, with careful fluid management. Several studies have evaluated the use of recombinant tissue-type plasminogen activator and heparin, but although responses are reported, these agents carry a risk of hemorrhage.[258] Defibrotide, which is a single-stranded polydeoxyribonucleotide with fibrinolytic, antithrombotic, and antiischemic properties on microvascular endothelium, has shown encouraging results in patients with severe sinusoidal obstruction syndrome with several studies reporting 30% to 60% complete remission rates even among patients with multiorgan failure.[259] Prophylactic strategies including ursodeoxycholic acid and heparin have also been evaluated, but neither agent shows consistent benefit.[258]

Hemorrhagic Cystitis

Hemorrhagic cystitis (HC) is a significant cause of morbidity and, occasionally, mortality in patients undergoing HSCT. In a large pediatric series, the major risk factors were male sex and unrelated donor transplants.[260] The severity of HC can range from mild hematuria to life-threatening bleeding with urinary tract obstruction or renal insufficiency. HC is likely caused by drugs used in conditioning regimens, in particular cyclophosphamide, or in viral infection with adenovirus and BK virus commonly implicated. Most centers use preventative measures including hydration and mesna in patients receiving cyclophosphamide. Mild HC may be treated with hydration, but more severe cases may require continuous bladder irrigation, cystoscopy and clot evacuation, and, more rarely, instillation of astringents or urinary diversion.

Thrombotic Microangiopathy

Transplant-associated microangiopathy (TAM) is a potentially lethal complication seen in patients undergoing HSCT characterized by a clinical syndrome of microangiopathic hemolytic anemia, thrombocytopenia, and renal impairment and histological appearances of renal microvascular injury. Because there are almost always other potential etiologies for these findings posttransplant, there are marked variations in the reported frequency of this complication.[261] In the past, the syndrome was often labeled as transplant-associated thrombotic thrombocytopenic purpura (TTP) or hemolytic uremic syndrome, but the Toxicity Committee of the BMT CTN has recommended that the entity is labeled as TAM, as there are many differences between TAM and classic TTP.[262] In particular, there is no deficiency of ADAMTS13 in TAM and the angiopathic changes are generally confined to the kidney.

The etiology of thrombotic microangiopathy in HSC transplantation is most likely due to a combination of factors that damage microvascular endothelium including calcineurin inhibitors, rapamycin, chemotherapy, and/or total body radiation infections and advanced disease. The acute form is associated with cyclosporine and FK506 therapy, and these agents should be stopped in patients who develop this complication.

Late Complications of Stem Cell Transplantation

Secondary Malignancies

After HSCT, recipients have a two- to sevenfold increased risk of developing a secondary neoplasm, with the most frequently seen malignancies being EBV-related posttransplant lymphoproliferative disease (EBV-PTLD), MDSs, and a variety of solid tumors.[263,264] Children who receive autologous SC transplantation are at risk of developing therapy-related MDS and ALL, a risk likely due to previous exposure to chemotherapy and radiation.[265] Recipients of allogeneic transplant have an increased incidence of PTLD and solid cancers, including malignant melanoma and cancers of the buccal cavity, liver, brain, or other parts of the CNS, thyroid, bone, and connective tissue.[263,264] In a study focusing on children transplanted for ALL, a particularly high incidence was seen with a cumulative risk of solid cancers of 11.0% at 15 years with the highest risk among children younger than 5 years at transplantation.[266]

The most common malignancy after allogeneic transplant is PTLD.[264] Although the overall incidence of PTLD after allogeneic HSCT is approximately 1%, with the majority of cases developing during the first 6 to 12 months after transplantation, the incidence is significantly increased in children with underlying immunodeficiency, in recipients of T-cell–depleted transplants from unrelated donors or HLA-mismatched family members, and in children who receive intensive immunosuppression with T-cell antibodies for the prophylaxis and treatment of GVHD.[267–269] The majority of PTLD is of B-cell origin and is almost always associated with EBV. Over the past decade, progress has been made in better understanding the pathogenesis of PTLD, and early detection strategies, like serial measurement of EBV-DNA load in PB samples, have assisted in the identification of high-risk patients.[270] In addi-

tion, novel immunotherapies have been developed, including the use of monoclonal antibodies and adoptive transfer of EBV-specific T cells.[270]

Endocrine Complications

Children treated with high-dose chemotherapy and/or radiotherapy prior to HSCT are at risk of endocrine dysfunction. The risk will likely be less in recipients who receive subablative regimens, but data are not yet available. The majority of prepubertal boys retain normal Leydig cell function and ability to produce testosterone and will progress normally through puberty posttransplant.[271] However, most will have evidence of germ cell damage, which may be more common in those boys treated during or after puberty, compared with those who were prepubertal at the time of transplant. Sperm banking should be addressed with all eligible male patients before conditioning. Primary gonadal failure has been described in approximately three fourths of postpubertal girls after treatment with fully ablative regimens. Around 50% of prepubertal girls will maintain sufficient ovarian function to enter puberty and menstruate regularly, and the remainder will require ovarian hormone replacement to avoid the side effects of low estrogen production.[271] For women who do conceive after HSCT, there is an increased chance of having an infant with low birth weight and an increased rate of spontaneous abortion for those who have received TBI.[272] There does not appear to be any increased risk of congenital anomalies in children born to survivors of HSCT.[272]

Thyroid dysfunction is well documented after HSCT and is most prevalent after regimens containing TBI but can occur after chemotherapy-only conditioning regimens as well. Thyroid function tests should be checked annually, as it may take many years for thyroid abnormalities to present. In a large recently published series following 791 children transplanted under the age of 18 thyroid abnormalities presented for up to 28 years posttransplant with hypothyroidism being the most common manifestation.[273] Transplant at age younger than 10 years was a significant risk factor.[273] Treatment of thyroid hormone deficiencies allows for optimum growth as well as decreasing the risk of thyroid malignancy.

Growth and Development Complications

Children undergoing HSCT are at risk for growth failure that is preparative regime dependent.[274] Factors predisposing to a decreased growth rate are age at time of transplant, the use of TBI after prior cranial irradiation, busulfan-containing regimens in some studies, and the use of steroids posttransplant.[275] Growth hormone therapy significantly improves final height in children younger than 10 years at HSCT but does not impact the growth of older children.[276]

Children who have received HSCT are also at risk of neurocognitive late effects. In the largest prospective study that followed 102 children longitudinally, there was minimal risk of late neurocognitive sequelae in patients who were 6 years of age or older at the time of transplantation. However, patients who are younger than 6 years and particularly those younger than 3 years at the time of transplant were more likely to show declines in intellectual function with time.[277]

Other Late Complications

A substantial risk of cataract development exists for patients receiving TBI, and annual ophthalmologic evaluation is indicated.[278] The most important bony complication of HSCT is avascular necrosis.

Treatment of Relapse

Relapse remains a major cause of treatment failure following HSCT for pediatric malignancy. Although chemotherapy may induce some responses, it does not result in long-term disease control. With increasing knowledge of the molecular basis of alloreactivity offering the potential to separate graft-versus-tumor responses from GVHD, there has been increasing interest in the use of immunotherapy to treat or prevent relapse. A GVL effect in allogeneic transplant has been documented based on the observations that patients who develop acute or chronic GVHD have a lower risk of relapse.[101]

In addition, the use of donor lymphocyte infusions (DLIs) to treat patients with relapse following an allogeneic transplant has been pivotal in demonstrating the role of GVL reactions in controlling disease.[279] Since the initial reports in the 1980s, a number of studies have documented that reinfusion of unmanipulated leukocytes results in significant clinical responses in relapsed patients, particularly those with CML. Responses have also been noted in other diseases such as AML, but this treatment has been less effective in ALL.[279] DLI is associated with significant morbidity and mortality from GVHD with the incidence depending on cell dose and degree of mismatch. Pancytopenia and BM aplasia are most likely to occur in patients with advanced disease.[279] One means of reducing the risk of GVHD is to administer antigen-specific cytotoxic T-cell lines when a specific antigen is known. Potential targets include minor antigens differentially expressed on hemopoietic cells or lineage-specific antigens, such as WT1, preferentially expressed antigen of melanoma, or proteinase 3.[280,281] In addition to donor lymphocyte infusions, novel post-transplant immunotherapies under investigation include the administration of cytokines, antitumor vaccines, and/or leukemia-specific cytotoxic cells.[282–284] A number of studies are exploring genetic modification of T or NK cells with artificial receptors targeting surface antigens such as CD19 or CD30 in children with relapsed or high-risk hematologic malignancies.[285–287] There is also interest in taking advantage of NK alloreactivity.[287–289]

FUTURE DIRECTIONS

A major challenge will be to redefine indications for transplant, as the outcomes of both HSCT and alternative therapies change and as risk factors continue to be redefined by new information from molecular and proteomics studies. Genome-wide association assays are already starting to yield data about predictive markers after transplant such as an SNP haplotype in TLR4 associated with a two- to fivefold increase in risk of developing invasive aspergillus infection[17] and lipopolysaccharide-binding protein promoter variants that increase the risk for gram-negative sepsis.[290] With increasing use of reduced-intensity transplant as a platform for immunotherapy, it will also be important to define the relative role of fully ablative and reduced-intensity transplant in pediatric malignancies. Several different immunotherapy modalities, such as NK cell infusion, cytotoxic T-cell infusion, and vaccination with dendritic cells or peptides, are being evaluated in clinical trials, and the immunomodulatory effects of mesenchymal cell infusions and regulatory T cells will also be explored. An additional ongoing question concerns the best source of HSC for transplant, and there will be ongoing evaluation of the situations in which PB or marrow is preferred and the relative merits of haploidentical, cord, and unrelated donors for patients who lack a matched sibling. Defining the optimum source for an individual patient will likely depend on a multitude of factors, including the underlying diagnosis and stage of disease, degree of mismatch with potential stem cell sources, and age and size of the patient.

References

1. Thomas ED, Lochte HL, Lu WC, et al. Intravenous infusion of bone marrow in patients receiving radiation and chemotherapy. N Engl J Med 1957;257:491–496.
2. Hong R, Cooper MD, Allan MJ, et al. Immunological restitution in lymphopenic immunological deficiency syndrome. Lancet 1968;1:503–506.
3. Bach FH, Albertini RJ, Joo P, et al. Bone-marrow transplantation in a patient with the Wiskott-Aldrich syndrome. Lancet 1968;2:1364–1366.
4. Thomas ED, Storb R, Clift RA, et al. Bone-marrow transplantation (second of two parts). N Engl J Med 1975;292:895–902.
5. Appelbaum FR. Hematopoietic-cell transplantation at 50. N Engl J Med 2007;357:1472–1475.
6. Dehn J, Arora M, Spellman S, et al. Unrelated donor hematopoietic cell transplantation: factors associated with a better HLA match. Biol Blood Marrow Transplant 2008;14:1334–1340.
7. Lee SJ, Klein J, Haagenson M, et al. High-resolution donor-recipient HLA matching contributes to the success of unrelated donor marrow transplantation. Blood 2007;110:4576–4583.
8. Petersdorf EW, Hansen JA. New advances in hematopoietic cell transplantation. Curr Opin Hematol 2008;15:549–554.
9. Davies SM, Wang D, Wang T, et al. Recent decrease in acute graft-versus-host disease in children receiving unrelated donor bone marrow transplants. Biol Blood Marrow Transplant 2009;15:360–366.
10. Chandrasekar P, Ljungman PT. Antifungal therapy strategies in hematopoietic stem-cell transplant recipients: early treatment options for improving outcomes. Transplantation 2008;86:183–191.
11. Boeckh M, Ljungman P. How we treat cytomegalovirus in hematopoietic cell transplant recipients. Blood 2009;113:5711–5719.
12. Marsh SG. Nomenclature for factors of the HLA system, update June 2009. Tissue Antigens 2009;74(4):364–366.
13. Goulmy E. Minor histocompatibility antigens: from transplantation problems to therapy of cancer. Hum Immunol 2006;67:433–438.
14. Goulmy E, Schipper R, Pool J, et al. Mismatches of minor histocompatibility antigens between HLA-identical donors and recipients and the development of graft-versus-host disease after bone marrow transplantation. N Engl J Med 1996;334:281–285.
15. Marijt WA, Heemskerk MH, Kloosterboer FM, et al. Hematopoiesis-restricted minor histocompatibility antigens HA-1- or HA-2-specific T cells can induce complete remissions of relapsed leukemia. Proc Natl Acad Sci U S A 2003;100:2742–2747.
16. Williams KM, Chien JW, Gladwin MT, et al. Bronchiolitis obliterans after allogeneic hematopoietic stem cell transplantation. JAMA 2009;302:306–314.
17. Bochud PY, Chien JW, Marr KA, et al. Toll-like receptor 4 polymorphisms and aspergillosis in stem-cell transplantation. N Engl J Med 2008;359:1766–1777.
18. Maris JM, Hogarty MD, Bagatell R, et al. Neuroblastoma. Lancet 2007;369:2106–2120.
19. Gajjar A, Chintagumpala M, Ashley D, et al. Risk-adapted craniospinal radiotherapy followed by high-dose chemotherapy and stem-cell rescue in children with newly diagnosed medulloblastoma (St Jude Medulloblastoma-96): long-term results from a prospective, multicentre trial. Lancet Oncol 2006;7:813–820.
20. Lipton JM. Peripheral blood as a stem cell source for hematopoietic cell transplantation in children: is the effort in vein? Pediatr Transplant 2003;7(suppl 3):65–70.
21. Dipersio JF, Uy GL, Yasothan U, et al. Plerixafor. Nat Rev Drug Discov 2009;8:105–106.
22. Gale RP, Horowitz MM, Ash RC, et al. Identical-twin bone marrow transplants for leukemia. Ann Intern Med 1994;120:646–652.
23. Delany L, Month S, Savulescu J, et al. Altruism by proxy: volunteering children for bone marrow donation. BMJ 1996;312:240–243.
24. Bensinger WI, Martin PJ, Storer B, et al. Transplantation of bone marrow as compared with peripheral-blood cells from HLA-identical relatives in patients with hematologic cancers. N Engl J Med 2001;344:175–181.
25. Champlin RE, Schmitz N, Horowitz MM, et al. Blood stem cells compared with bone marrow as a source of hematopoietic cells for allogeneic transplantation. IBMTR Histocompatibility and Stem Cell Sources Working Committee and the European Group for Blood and Marrow Transplantation (EBMT). Blood 2000;95:3702–3709.
26. Eapen M, Horowitz MM, Klein JP, et al. Higher mortality after allogeneic peripheral-blood transplantation compared with bone marrow in children and adolescents: the Histocompatibility and Alternate Stem Cell Source Working Committee of the International Bone Marrow Transplant Registry. J Clin Oncol 2004;22:4872–4880.
27. Pulsipher MA, Levine JE, Hayashi RJ, et al. Safety and efficacy of allogeneic PBSC collection in normal pediatric donors: the pediatric blood and marrow transplant consortium experience (PBMTC) 1996–2003. Bone Marrow Transplant 2005;35:361–367.
28. Pulsipher MA, Chitphakdithai P, Miller JP, et al. Adverse events among 2408 unrelated donors of peripheral blood stem cells: results of a prospective trial from the National Marrow Donor Program. Blood 2009;113:3604–3611.
29. McCullough J, Kahn J, Adamson J, et al. Hematopoietic growth factors—use in normal blood and stem cell donors: clinical and ethical issues. Transfusion 2008;48:2008–2025.
30. Lee SJ, Kamani N, Confer DL. Principles and tools for selection of umbilical cord blood and unrelated adult donor grafts. Biol Blood Marrow Transplant 2008;14:112–119.

31. Eapen M, Rubinstein P, Zhang MJ, et al. Comparable long-term survival after unrelated and HLA-matched sibling donor hematopoietic stem cell transplantations for acute leukemia in children younger than 18 months. J Clin Oncol 2006;24:145–151.
32. Hongeng S, Krance RA, Bowman LC, et al. Outcomes of transplantation with matched-sibling and unrelated-donor bone marrow in children with leukaemia. Lancet 1997; 350:767–771.
33. Macmillan ML, Davies SM, Nelson GO, et al. Twenty years of unrelated donor bone marrow transplantation for pediatric acute leukemia facilitated by the National Marrow Donor Program. Biol Blood Marrow Transplant 2008;14:16–22.
34. Warkentin PI. Voluntary accreditation of cellular therapies: Foundation for the Accreditation of Cellular Therapy (FACT). Cytotherapy 2003;5:299–305.
35. Rubinstein P, Carrier C, Scaradavou A, et al. Outcomes among 562 recipients of placental-blood transplants from unrelated donors. N Engl J Med 1998;339:1565–1577.
36. Kurtzberg J, Laughlin M, Graham ML, et al. Placental blood as a source of hematopoietic stem cells for transplantation into unrelated recipients. N Engl J Med 1996;335: 157–166.
37. Gluckman E, Rocha V, Boyer-Chammard A, et al. Outcome of cord-blood transplantation from related and unrelated donors. Eurocord Transplant Group and the European Blood and Marrow Transplantation Group. N Engl J Med 1997;337:373–381.
38. Eapen M, Rubinstein P, Zhang MJ, et al. Outcomes of transplantation of unrelated donor umbilical cord blood and bone marrow in children with acute leukaemia: a comparison study. Lancet 2007;369:1947–1954.
39. Kurtzberg J. Update on umbilical cord blood transplantation. Curr Opin Pediatr 2009; 21:22–29.
40. Kamani N, Spellman S, Hurley CK, et al. State of the art review: HLA matching and outcome of unrelated donor umbilical cord blood transplants. Biol Blood Marrow Transplant 2008;14:1–6.
41. Aversa F, Tabilio A, Velardi A, et al. Treatment of high-risk acute leukemia with T-cell-depleted stem cells from related donors with one fully mismatched HLA haplotype. N Engl J Med 1998;339:1186–1193.
42. Lang P, Handgretinger R. Haploidentical SCT in children: an update and future perspectives. Bone Marrow Transplant 2008;42(suppl 2):S54–S59.
43. Guinan EC, Boussiotis VA, Neuberg D, et al. Transplantation of anergic histoincompatible bone marrow allografts. N Engl J Med 1999;340:1704–1714.
44. Davies JK, Gribben JG, Brennan LL, et al. Outcome of alloanergized haploidentical bone marrow transplantation after ex vivo costimulatory blockade: results of 2 phase 1 studies. Blood 2008;112:2232–2241.
45. Luznik L, O'Donnell PV, Symons HJ, et al. HLA-haploidentical bone marrow transplantation for hematologic malignancies using nonmyeloablative conditioning and high-dose, posttransplantation cyclophosphamide. Biol Blood Marrow Transplant 2008;14:641–650.
46. Huang X, Liu D, Liu K, et al. Haploidentical hematopoietic stem cell transplantation without in vitro T cell depletion for treatment of hematologic malignancies in children. Biol Blood Marrow Transplant 2008;15:91–94.
47. Krance RA, Kuehnle I, Rill DR, et al. Hematopoietic and immunomodulatory effects of lytic CD45 monoclonal antibodies in patients with hematologic malignancy. Biol Blood Marrow Transplant 2003;9:273–281.
48. Pagel JM, Appelbaum FR, Eary JF, et al. 131I-anti-CD45 antibody plus busulfan and cyclophosphamide before allogeneic hematopoietic cell transplantation for treatment of acute myeloid leukemia in first remission. Blood 2006;107:2184–2191.
49. Straathof KC, Rao K, Eyrich M, et al. Haemopoietic stem cell transplantation with antobody-based minimal-intensity conditioning: a phase 1/2 study. Lancet 2009;324: 912–920.
50. Baron F, Storb R. Allogeneic hematopoietic cell transplantation following nonmyeloablative conditioning as treatment for hematologic malignancies and inherited blood disorders. Mol Ther 2006;13:26–41.
51. Satwani P, Sather H, Ozkaynak F, et al. Allogeneic bone marrow transplantation in first remission for children with ultra-high-risk features of acute lymphoblastic leukemia: a children's oncology group study report. Biol Blood Marrow Transplant 2007;13:218–227.
52. Gaynon PS, Harris RE, Altman AJ, et al. Bone marrow transplantation versus prolonged intensive chemotherapy for children with acute lymphoblastic leukemia and an initial bone marrow relapse within 12 months of the completion of primary therapy: Children's Oncology Group study CCG-1941. J Clin Oncol 2006;24:3150–3156.
53. Balduzzi A, Valsecchi MG, Uderzo C, et al. Chemotherapy versus allogeneic transplantation for very-high-risk childhood acute lymphoblastic leukaemia in first complete remission: comparison by genetic randomisation in an international prospective study. Lancet 2005;366:635–642.
54. Ribera JM, Ortega JJ, Oriol A, et al. Comparison of intensive chemotherapy, allogeneic, or autologous stem-cell transplantation as postremission treatment for children with very high risk acute lymphoblastic leukemia: PETHEMA ALL-93 Trial. J Clin Oncol 2007;25:16–24.
55. Schrauder A, Reiter A, Gadner H, et al. Superiority of allogeneic hematopoietic stem-cell transplantation compared with chemotherapy alone in high-risk childhood T-cell acute lymphoblastic leukemia: results from ALL-BFM 90 and 95. J Clin Oncol 2006;24:5742–5749.
56. Eapen M, Raetz E, Zhang MJ, et al. Outcomes after HLA-matched sibling transplantation or chemotherapy in children with B-precursor acute lymphoblastic leukemia in a second remission: a collaborative study of the Children's Oncology Group and the Center for International Blood and Marrow Transplant Research. Blood 2006;107: 4961–4967.
57. Roy A, Cargill A, Love S, et al. Outcome after first relapse in childhood acute lymphoblastic leukaemia—lessons from the United Kingdom R2 trial. Br J Haematol 2005; 130:67–75.
58. Smith AR, Baker KS, Defor TE, et al. Hematopoietic cell transplantation for children with acute lymphoblastic leukemia in second complete remission: similar outcomes in recipients of unrelated marrow and umbilical cord blood versus marrow from HLA matched sibling donors. Biol Blood Marrow Transplant 2009;15:1086–1093.
59. Einsiedel HG, von Stackelberg A, Hartmann R, et al. Long-term outcome in children with relapsed ALL by risk-stratified salvage therapy: results of trial acute lymphoblastic leukemia-relapse study of the Berlin-Frankfurt-Munster Group 87. J Clin Oncol 2005; 23:7942–7950.
60. Borgmann A, von Stackelberg A, Hartmann R, et al. Unrelated donor stem cell transplantation compared with chemotherapy for children with acute lymphoblastic leukemia in a second remission: a matched-pair analysis. Blood 2003;101:3835–3839.
61. Reismuller B, Attarbaschi A, Peters C, et al. Long-term outcome of initially homogenously treated and relapsed childhood acute lymphoblastic leukaemia in Austria–a population-based report of the Austrian Berlin-Frankfurt-Munster (BFM) Study Group. Br J Haematol 2009;144:559–570.
62. Eapen M, Zhang MJ, Devidas M, et al. Outcomes after HLA-matched sibling transplantation or chemotherapy in children with acute lymphoblastic leukemia in a second remission after an isolated central nervous system relapse: a collaborative study of the Children's Oncology Group and the Center for International Blood and Marrow Transplant Research. Leukemia 2008;22:281–286.
63. Harker-Murray PD, Thomas AJ, Wagner JE, et al. Allogeneic hematopoietic cell transplantation in children with relapsed acute lymphoblastic leukemia isolated to the central nervous system. Biol Blood Marrow Transplant 2008;14:685–692.
64. Saarinen-Pihkala UM, Heilmann C, Winiarski J, et al. Pathways through relapses and deaths of children with acute lymphoblastic leukemia: role of allogeneic stem-cell transplantation in Nordic data. J Clin Oncol 2006;24:5750–5762.
65. Kennedy-Nasser AA, Bollard CM, Myers GD, et al. Comparable outcome of alternative donor and matched sibling donor hematopoietic stem cell transplant for children with acute lymphoblastic leukemia in first or second remission using alemtuzumab in a myeloablative conditioning regimen. Biol Blood Marrow Transplant 2008;14:1245–1252.
66. Sanders JE, Im HJ, Hoffmeister PA, et al. Allogeneic hematopoietic cell transplantation for infants with acute lymphoblastic leukemia. Blood 2005;105:3749–3756.
67. Tomizawa D, Koh K, Sato T, et al. Outcome of risk-based therapy for infant acute lymphoblastic leukemia with or without an MLL gene rearrangement, with emphasis on late effects: a final report of two consecutive studies, MLL96 and MLL98, of the Japan Infant Leukemia Study Group. Leukemia 2007;21:2258–2263.
68. Jacobsohn DA, Hewlett B, Morgan E, et al. Favorable outcome for infant acute lymphoblastic leukemia after hematopoietic stem cell transplantation. Biol Blood Marrow Transplant 2005;11:999–1005.
69. Hilden JM, Dinndorf PA, Meerbaum SO, et al. Analysis of prognostic factors of acute lymphoblastic leukemia in infants: report on CCG 1953 from the Children's Oncology Group. Blood 2006;108:441–451.
70. Pieters R, Schrappe M, De Lorenzo P, et al. A treatment protocol for infants younger than 1 year with acute lymphoblastic leukaemia (Interfant-99): an observational study and a multicentre randomised trial. Lancet 2007;370:240–250.
71. Woods WG, Neudorf S, Gold S, et al. A comparison of allogeneic bone marrow transplantation, autologous bone marrow transplantation, and aggressive chemotherapy in children with acute myeloid leukemia in remission. Blood 2001;97:56–62.
72. Stevens RF, Hann IM, Wheatley K, et al. Marked improvements in outcome with chemotherapy alone in paediatric acute myeloid leukemia: results of the United Kingdom Medical Research Council's 10th AML trial. MRC Childhood Leukaemia Working Party. Br J Haematol 1998;101:130–140.
73. Alonzo TA, Wells RJ, Woods WG, et al. Postremission therapy for children with acute myeloid leukemia: the children's cancer group experience in the transplant era. Leukemia 2005;19:965–970.
74. Reinhardt D. No Improvement of overall-survival in children with high-risk acute myeloid leukemia by stem cell transplantation in 1st complete remission. Blood 2006;108: abstract 320.
75. Pession A, Rondelli R, Basso G, et al. Treatment and long-term results in children with acute myeloid leukaemia treated according to the AIEOP AML protocols. Leukemia 2005;19:2043–2053.
76. Lange BJ, Smith FO, Feusner J, et al. Outcomes in CCG-2961, a children's oncology group phase 3 trial for untreated pediatric acute myeloid leukemia: a report from the children's oncology group. Blood 2008;111:1044–1053.
77. Horan JT, Alonzo TA, Lyman GH, et al. Impact of disease risk on efficacy of matched related bone marrow transplantation for pediatric acute myeloid leukemia: the Children's Oncology Group. J Clin Oncol 2008;26:5797–5801.
78. Bunin NJ, Davies SM, Aplenc R, et al. Unrelated donor bone marrow transplantation for children with acute myeloid leukemia beyond first remission or refractory to chemotherapy. J Clin Oncol 2008;26:4326–4332.
79. Fagioli F, Zecca M, Locatelli F, et al. Allogeneic stem cell transplantation for children with acute myeloid leukemia in second complete remission. J Pediatr Hematol Oncol 2008;30:575–583.
80. Abrahamsson J, Clausen N, Gustafsson G, et al. Improved outcome after relapse in children with acute myeloid leukaemia. Br J Haematol 2007;136:229–236.
81. Woodard P, Barfield R, Hale G, et al. Outcome of hematopoietic stem cell transplantation for pediatric patients with therapy-related acute myeloid leukemia or myelodysplastic syndrome. Pediatr Blood Cancer 2006;47:931–935.
82. Parikh SH, Mendizabal A, Martin PL, et al. Unrelated donor umbilical cord blood transplantation in pediatric myelodysplastic syndrome: a single-center experience. Biol Blood Marrow Transplant 2009;15:948–955.
83. Locatelli F. Hematopoietic stem cell transplantation after a myeloablative conditioning regimen in children with refractory cytopenia: results of a retrospective analysis from the EWOG-MDS group. Leuk Res 2007;31:s39.
84. Strahm B, Locatelli F, Bader P, et al. Reduced intensity conditioning in unrelated donor transplantation for refractory cytopenia in childhood. Bone Marrow Transplant 2007;40:329–333.
85. Yusuf U, Frangoul HA, Gooley TA, et al. Allogeneic bone marrow transplantation in children with myelodysplastic syndrome or juvenile myelomonocytic leukemia: the Seattle experience. Bone Marrow Transplant 2004;33:805–814.
86. Woolfrey AE, Anasetti C, Storer B, et al. Factors associated with outcome after unrelated marrow transplantation for treatment of acute lymphoblastic leukemia in children. Blood 2002;99:2002–2008.
87. Pui CH, Evans WE. Treatment of acute lymphoblastic leukemia. N Engl J Med 2006; 354:166–178.
88. Pui CH, Gaynon PS, Boyett JM, et al. Outcome of treatment in childhood acute lymphoblastic leukaemia with rearrangements of the 11q23 chromosomal region. Lancet 2002;359:1909–1915.
89. Schultz KR, Bowman WP, Slayton W, et al. Improved Early Event Free Survival (EFS) in Children with Philadelphia Chromosome-Positive (Ph+) Acute Lymphoblastic Leukemia (ALL) with Intensive Imatinib in Combination with High Dose Chemotherapy: Children's Oncology Group (COG) Study AALL0031. Blood (ASH Annual Meeting Abstracts) 2007;110:4.
90. van der Linden MH, Valsecchi MG, De Lorenzo P, et al. Outcome of congenital acute lymphoblastic leukemia treated on the Interfant-99 protocol. Blood 2009;114(18): 3764–3768.
91. Leung W, Hudson M, Zhu Y, et al. Late effects in survivors of infant leukemia. Leukemia 2000;14:1185–1190.
92. Nachman JB, Heerema NA, Sather H, et al. Outcome of treatment in children with hypodiploid acute lymphoblastic leukemia. Blood 2007;110:1112–1115.

93. Coustan-Smith E, Ribeiro RC, Stow P, et al. A simplified flow cytometric assay identifies children with acute lymphoblastic leukemia who have a superior clinical outcome. Blood 2006;108:97–102.
94. Borowitz MJ, Devidas M, Hunger SP, et al. Clinical significance of minimal residual disease in childhood acute lymphoblastic leukemia and its relationship to other prognostic factors: a Children's Oncology Group study. Blood 2008;111:5477–5485.
95. Balduzzi A, De Lorenzo P, Schrauder A, et al. Eligibility for allogeneic transplantation in very high risk childhood acute lymphoblastic leukemia: the impact of the waiting time. Haematologica 2008;93:925–929.
96. Moorman AV, Richards SM, Robinson HM, et al. Prognosis of children with acute lymphoblastic leukemia (ALL) and intrachromosomal amplification of chromosome 21 (iAMP21). Blood 2007;109:2327–2330.
97. Mullighan CG, Su X, Zhang J, et al. Deletion of IKZF1 and prognosis in acute lymphoblastic leukemia. N Engl J Med 2009;360:470–480.
98. Willemse MJ, Seriu T, Hettinger K, et al. Detection of minimal residual disease identifies differences in treatment response between T-ALL and precursor B-ALL. Blood 2002; 99:4386–4393.
99. CIBMTR. Current Use and Outcome of Hematopoietic Stem Cell Transplantation 2008. Center for International Blood & Marrow Transplantation Research, 2008.
100. Thomas ED, Sanders JE, Flournoy N, et al. Marrow transplantation for patients with acute lymphoblastic leukemia in remission. Blood 1979;54:468–476.
101. Horowitz MM, Gale RP, Sondel PM, et al. Graft-versus-leukemia reactions after bone marrow transplantation. Blood 1990;75:555–562.
102. Kolb HJ, Holler E. Adoptive immunotherapy with donor lymphocyte transfusions. Curr Opin Oncol 1997;9:139–145.
103. Hahn T, Wall D, Camitta B, et al. The role of cytotoxic therapy with hematopoietic stem cell transplantation in the therapy of acute lymphoblastic leukemia in children: an evidence-based review. Biol Blood Marrow Transplant 2005;11:823–861.
104. Pulsipher MA, Bader P, Klingebiel T, et al. Allogeneic transplantation for pediatric acute lymphoblastic leukemia: the emerging role of peritransplantation minimal residual disease/chimerism monitoring and novel chemotherapeutic, molecular, and immune approaches aimed at preventing relapse. Biol Blood Marrow Transplant 2008;15: 62–71.
105. Knechtli CJ, Goulden NJ, Hancock JP, et al. Minimal residual disease status before allogeneic bone marrow transplantation is an important determinant of successful outcome for children and adolescents with acute lymphoblastic leukemia. Blood 1998;92: 4072–4079.
106. Nguyen K, Devidas M, Cheng SC, et al. Factors influencing survival after relapse from acute lymphoblastic leukemia: a Children's Oncology Group study. Leukemia 2008;22: 2142–2150.
107. NMDP. NMDP Transplantation Outcomes. National Marrow Donor Program, 2007.
108. Franklin J, Alonzo T, Hurwitz CA, et al. COG AAML03P1: Efficacy and Safety in a Pilot Study of Intensive Chemotherapy Including Gemtuzumab in Children Newly Diagnosed with Acute Myeloid Leukemia (AML). Blood (ASH Annual Meeting Abstracts) 2008;112:136.
109. Craze JL, Harrison G, Wheatley K, et al. Improved outcome of acute myeloid leukaemia in Down's syndrome. Arch Dis Child 1999;81:32–37.
110. Creutzig U, Zimmermann M, Ritter J, et al. Treatment strategies and long-term results in paediatric patients treated in four consecutive AML-BFM trials. Leukemia 2005;19:2030–2042.
111. Gibson BE, Wheatley K, Hann IM, et al. Treatment strategy and long-term results in paediatric patients treated in consecutive UK AML trials. Leukemia 2005;19: 2130–2138.
112. Smith FO, Alonzo TA, Gerbing RB, et al. Long-term results of children with acute myeloid leukemia: a report of three consecutive Phase III trials by the Children's Cancer Group: CCG 251, CCG 213 and CCG 2891. Leukemia 2005;19:2054–2062.
113. Gassas A, Afzal S, Ishaqi MK, et al. Pediatric standard-risk AML with fully matched sibling donors: to transplant in first CR or not? Bone Marrow Transplant 2008;42: 393–396.
114. Oliansky DM, Rizzo JD, Aplan PD, et al. The role of cytotoxic therapy with hematopoietic stem cell transplantation in the therapy of acute myeloid leukemia in children: an evidence-based review. Biol Blood Marrow Transplant 2007;13:1–25.
115. Song KW, Lipton J. Is it appropriate to offer allogeneic hematopoietic stem cell transplantation to patients with primary refractory acute myeloid leukemia? Bone Marrow Transplant 2005;36:183–191.
116. Rubnitz JE, Gibson B, Smith FO. Acute myeloid leukemia. Pediatr Clin North Am 2008;55:21–51, ix.
117. Aladjidi N, Auvrignon A, Leblanc T, et al. Outcome in children with relapsed acute myeloid leukemia after initial treatment with the French Leucemie Aique Myeloide Enfant (LAME) 89/91 protocol of the French Society of Pediatric Hematology and Immunology. J Clin Oncol 2003;21:4377–4385.
118. Webb DK, Wheatley K, Harrison G, et al. Outcome for children with relapsed acute myeloid leukaemia following initial therapy in the Medical Research Council (MRC) AML 10 trial. MRC Childhood Leukaemia Working Party. Leukemia 1999;13:25–31.
119. Castellino SM, Alonzo TA, Buxton A, et al. Outcomes in childhood AML in the absence of transplantation in first remission—Children's Cancer Group (CCG) studies 2891 and CCG 213. Pediatr Blood Cancer 2008;50:9–16.
120. Sander A, Zimmermann M, Reinhardt D, et al. Improvement of Survival after Relapse in Pediatric AML Over the Last Two Decades Is Related to a Standardized, Consistent and Intensive Relapse Treatment. Blood (ASH Annual Meeting Abstracts) 2008;112: 963.
121. Ferry C, Socie G. Busulfan-cyclophosphamide versus total body irradiation-cyclophosphamide as preparative regimen before allogeneic hematopoietic stem cell transplantation for acute myeloid leukemia: what have we learned? Exp Hematol 2003;31:1182–1186.
122. Pulsipher MA, Boucher KM, Wall D, et al. Reduced-intensity allogeneic transplantation in pediatric patients ineligible for myeloablative therapy: results of the Pediatric Blood and Marrow Transplant Consortium Study ONC0313. Blood 2009;114:1429–1436.
123. Kern W, Haferlach T, Schnittger S, et al. Prognosis in therapy-related acute myeloid leukemia and impact of karyotype. J Clin Oncol 2004;22:2510–2511.
124. Hijiya N, Ness KK, Ribeiro RC, et al. Acute leukemia as a secondary malignancy in children and adolescents: current findings and issues. Cancer 2009;115:23–35.
125. Barnard DR, Lange B, Alonzo TA, et al. Acute myeloid leukemia and myelodysplastic syndrome in children treated for cancer: comparison with primary presentation. Blood 2002;100:427–434.
126. Chang C, Storer BE, Scott BL, et al. Hematopoietic cell transplantation in patients with myelodysplastic syndrome or acute myeloid leukemia arising from myelodysplastic syndrome: similar outcomes in patients with de novo disease and disease following prior therapy or antecedent hematologic disorders. Blood 2007;110:1379–1387.
127. Niemeyer CM, Kratz CP. Paediatric myelodysplastic syndromes and juvenile myelomonocytic leukaemia: molecular classification and treatment options. Br J Haematol 2008;140:610–624.
128. Niemeyer CM, Baumann I. Myelodysplastic syndrome in children and adolescents. Semin Hematol 2008;45:60–70.
129. Hasle H, Alonzo TA, Auvrignon A, et al. Monosomy 7 and deletion 7q in children and adolescents with acute myeloid leukemia: an international retrospective study. Blood 2007;109:4641–4647.
130. Kardos G, Baumann I, Passmore SJ, et al. Refractory anemia in childhood: a retrospective analysis of 67 patients with particular reference to monosomy 7. Blood 2003;102: 1997–2003.
131. Stary J, Locatelli F, Niemeyer CM. Stem cell transplantation for aplastic anemia and myelodysplastic syndrome. Bone Marrow Transplant 2005;35(suppl 1):S13–S16.
132. Bader P, Niemeyer C, Willasch A, et al. Children with myelodysplastic syndrome (MDS) and increasing mixed chimaerism after allogeneic stem cell transplantation have a poor outcome which can be improved by pre-emptive immunotherapy. Br J Haematol 2005; 128:649–658.
133. Flotho C, Kratz C, Niemeyer CM. Targeting RAS signaling pathways in juvenile myelomonocytic leukemia. Current Drug Targets 2007;8:715–725.
134. Locatelli F, Nollke P, Zecca M, et al. Hematopoietic stem cell transplantation (HSCT) in children with juvenile myelomonocytic leukemia (JMML): results of the EWOG-MDS/EBMT trial. Blood 2005;105:410–419.
135. Yoshimi A, Mohamed M, Bierings M, et al. Second allogeneic hematopoietic stem cell transplantation (HSCT) results in outcome similar to that of first HSCT for patients with juvenile myelomonocytic leukemia. Leukemia 2007;21:556–560.
136. Kantarjian HM, Shan J, Jones D, et al. Significance of increasing levels of minimal residual disease in patients with Philadelphia chromosome-positive chronic myelogenous leukemia in complete cytogenetic response. J Clin Oncol 2009;27:3659–3663.
137. Suttorp M. Innovative approaches of targeted therapy for CML of childhood in combination with paediatric haematopoietic SCT. Bone Marrow Transplant 2008;42 (suppl 2):S40–S46.
138. Cwynarski K, Roberts IA, Iacobelli S, et al. Stem cell transplantation for chronic myeloid leukemia in children. Blood 2003;102:1224–1231.
139. Lee SJ, Kukreja M, Wang T, et al. Impact of prior imatinib mesylate on the outcome of hematopoietic cell transplantation for chronic myeloid leukemia. Blood 2008;112: 3500–3507.
140. Ladenstein R, Pearce R, Hartmann O, et al. High-dose chemotherapy with autologous bone marrow rescue in children with poor-risk Burkitt's lymphoma: a report from the European Lymphoma Bone Marrow Transplantation Registry. Blood 1997;90:2921–2930.
141. Bradley MB, Cairo MS. Stem cell transplantation for pediatric lymphoma: past, present and future. Bone Marrow Transplant 2008;41:149–158.
142. Sandlund JT, Bowman L, Heslop HE, et al. Intensive chemotherapy with hematopoietic stem-cell support for children with recurrent or refractory NHL. Cytotherapy 2002;4: 253–258.
143. Loiseau HA, Hartmann O, Valteau D, et al. High-dose chemotherapy containing busulfan followed by bone marrow transplantation in 24 children with refractory or relapsed non-Hodgkin's lymphoma. Bone Marrow Transplant 1991;8:465–472.
144. Claviez A, Sureda A, Schmitz N. Haematopoietic SCT for children and adolescents with relapsed and refractory Hodgkin's lymphoma. Bone Marrow Transplant 2008;42(suppl 2):S16–S24.
145. Sureda A, Constans M, Iriondo A, et al. Prognostic factors affecting long-term outcome after stem cell transplantation in Hodgkin's lymphoma autografted after a first relapse. Ann Oncol 2005;16:625–633.
146. Majhail NS, Weisdorf DJ, DeFor TE, et al. Long-term results of autologous stem cell transplantation for primary refractory or relapsed Hodgkin's lymphoma. Biol Blood Marrow Transplant 2006;12:1065–1072.
147. Levine JE, Harris RE, Loberiza FR Jr, et al. A comparison of allogeneic and autologous bone marrow transplantation for lymphoblastic lymphoma. Blood 2003;101:2476–2482.
148. Won SC, Han JW, Kwon SY, et al. Autologous peripheral blood stem cell transplantation in children with non-Hodgkin's lymphoma: a report from the Korean society of pediatric hematology-oncology. Ann Hematol 2006;85:787–794.
149. Horning SJ, Chao NJ, Negrin RS, et al. High-dose therapy and autologous hematopoietic progenitor cell transplantation for recurrent or refractory Hodgkin's disease: analysis of the Stanford University results and prognostic indices. Blood 1997;89:801–813.
150. Akpek G, Ambinder RF, Piantadosi S, et al. Long-term results of blood and marrow transplantation for Hodgkin's lymphoma. J Clin Oncol 2001;19:4314–4321.
151. Lieskovsky YE, Donaldson SS, Torres MA, et al. High-dose therapy and autologous hematopoietic stem-cell transplantation for recurrent or refractory pediatric Hodgkin's disease: results and prognostic indices. J Clin Oncol 2004;22:4532–4540.
152. Andre M, Henry-Amar M, Pico JL, et al. Comparison of high-dose therapy and autologous stem-cell transplantation with conventional therapy for Hodgkin's disease induction failure: a case-control study. Societe Francaise de Greffe de Moelle. J Clin Oncol 1999;17:222–229.
153. Stoneham S, Ashley S, Pinkerton CR, et al. Outcome after autologous hemopoietic stem cell transplantation in relapsed or refractory childhood Hodgkin disease. J Pediatr Hematol Oncol 2004;26:740–745.
154. Majolino I, Pearce R, Taghipour G, et al. Peripheral-blood stem-cell transplantation versus autologous bone marrow transplantation in Hodgkin's and non-Hodgkin's lymphomas: a new matched-pair analysis of the European Group for Blood and Marrow Transplantation Registry Data. Lymphoma Working Party of the European Group for Blood and Marrow Transplantation. J Clin Oncol 1997;15:509–517.
155. Hartmann O, Le Corroller AG, Blaise D, et al. Peripheral blood stem cell and bone marrow transplantation for solid tumors and lymphomas: hematologic recovery and costs. A randomized, controlled trial. Ann Intern Med 1997;126:600–607.
156. Leonard BM, Hetu F, Busque L, et al. Lymphoma cell burden in progenitor cell grafts measured by competitive polymerase chain reaction: less than one log difference between bone marrow and peripheral blood sources. Blood 1998;91:331–339.
157. Metayer C, Lynch CF, Clarke EA, et al. Second cancers among long-term survivors of Hodgkin's disease diagnosed in childhood and adolescence. J Clin Oncol 2000;18: 2435–2443.
158. Micallef IN, Lillington DM, Apostolidis J, et al. Therapy-related myelodysplasia and secondary acute myelogenous leukemia after high-dose therapy with autologous

hematopoietic progenitor-cell support for lymphoid malignancies. J Clin Oncol 2000; 18:947–955.
159. Bhatia S, Yasui Y, Robison LL, et al. High risk of subsequent neoplasms continues with extended follow-up of childhood Hodgkin's disease: report from the Late Effects Study Group. J Clin Oncol 2003;21:4386–4394.
160. Milligan DW, Ruiz DEM, Kolb HJ, et al. Secondary leukaemia and myelodysplasia after autografting for lymphoma: results from the EBMT. EBMT Lymphoma and Late Effects Working Parties. European Group for Blood and Marrow Transplantation. Br J Haematol 1999;106:1020–1026.
161. Howe R, Micallef IN, Inwards DJ, et al. Secondary myelodysplastic syndrome and acute myelogenous leukemia are significant complications following autologous stem cell transplantation for lymphoma. Bone Marrow Transplant 2003;32:317–324.
162. Ortega JJ, Olive T, de Heredia CD, et al. Secondary malignancies and quality of life after stem cell transplantation. Bone Marrow Transplant. 2005;35(suppl 1):S83–S87.
163. Majhail NS, Weisdorf DJ, Wagner JE, et al. Comparable results of umbilical cord blood and HLA-matched sibling donor hematopoietic stem cell transplantation after reduced-intensity preparative regimen for advanced Hodgkin lymphoma. Blood 2006;107: 3804–3807.
164. van Besien K, Thall P, Korbling M, et al. Allogeneic transplantation for recurrent or refractory non-Hodgkin's lymphoma with poor prognostic features after conditioning with thiotepa, busulfan, and cyclophosphamide: experience in 44 consecutive patients. Biol Blood Marrow Transplant 1997;3:150–156.
165. Gajewski JL, Phillips GL, Sobocinski KA, et al. Bone marrow transplants from HLA-identical siblings in advanced Hodgkin's disease. J Clin Oncol 1996;14:572–578.
166. Peniket AJ, Ruiz De Elvira MC, Taghipour G, et al. An EBMT registry matched study of allogeneic stem cell transplants for lymphoma: allogeneic transplantation is associated with a lower relapse rate but a higher procedure-related mortality rate than autologous transplantation. Bone Marrow Transplant 2003;31:667–678.
167. Woessmann W, Peters C, Lenhard M, et al. Allogeneic haematopoietic stem cell transplantation in relapsed or refractory anaplastic large cell lymphoma of children and adolescents—a Berlin-Frankfurt-Munster group report. Br J Haematol 2006;133:176–182.
168. Gutman JA, Bearman SI, Nieto Y, et al. Autologous transplantation followed closely by reduced-intensity allogeneic transplantation as consolidative immunotherapy in advanced lymphoma patients: a feasibility study. Bone Marrow Transplant 2005;36: 443–451.
169. Claviez A, Klingebiel T, Beyer J, et al. Allogeneic peripheral blood stem cell transplantation following fludarabine-based conditioning in six children with advanced Hodgkin's disease. Ann Hematol 2004;83:237–241.
170. Robinson SP, Goldstone AH, Mackinnon S, et al. Chemoresistant or aggressive lymphoma predicts for a poor outcome following reduced-intensity allogeneic progenitor cell transplantation: an analysis from the Lymphoma Working Party of the European Group for Blood and Bone Marrow Transplantation. Blood 2002;100:4310–4316.
171. Peggs KS, Hunter A, Chopra R, et al. Clinical evidence of a graft-versus-Hodgkin's-lymphoma effect after reduced-intensity allogeneic transplantation. Lancet 2005;365: 1934–1941.
172. Lucas KG, Salzman D, Garcia A, et al. Adoptive immunotherapy with allogeneic Epstein-Barr virus (EBV)-specific cytotoxic T-lymphocytes for recurrent, EBV-positive Hodgkin disease. Cancer 2004;100:1892–1901.
173. Peggs KS, Thomson K, Hart DP, et al. Dose-escalated donor lymphocyte infusions following reduced intensity transplantation: toxicity, chimerism, and disease responses. Blood 2004;103:1548–1556.
174. Khouri IF, Champlin RE. Nonmyeloablative stem cell transplantation for lymphoma. Semin Oncol 2004;31:22–26.
175. Hale G, Slavin S, Goldman JM, et al. Alemtuzumab (Campath-1H) for treatment of lymphoid malignancies in the age of nonmyeloablative conditioning? Bone Marrow Transplant 2002;30:797–804.
176. Bollard CM, Gottschalk S, Huls MH, et al. In vivo expansion of LMP 1- and 2-specific T-cells in a patient who received donor-derived EBV-specific T-cells after allogeneic stem cell transplantation. Leuk Lymphoma 2006;47:837–842.
177. Miller JS, Soignier Y, Panoskaltsis-Mortari A, et al. Successful adoptive transfer and in vivo expansion of human haploidentical NK cells in patients with cancer. Blood 2005;105:3051–3057.
178. Dunkel IJ, Boyett JM, Yates A, et al. High-dose carboplatin, thiotepa, and etoposide with autologous stem-cell rescue for patients with recurrent medulloblastoma. Children's Cancer Group. J Clin Oncol 1998;16:222–228.
179. Strother D, Ashley D, Kellie SJ, et al. Feasibility of four consecutive high-dose chemotherapy cycles with stem-cell rescue for patients with newly diagnosed medulloblastoma or supratentorial primitive neuroectodermal tumor after craniospinal radiotherapy: results of a collaborative study. J Clin Oncol 2001;19:2696–2704.
180. Kadota RP, Mahoney DH, Doyle J, et al. Dose intensive melphalan and cyclophosphamide with autologous hematopoietic stem cells for recurrent medulloblastoma or germinoma. Pediatr Blood Cancer 2008;51:675–678.
181. Graham ML, Herndon JE, Casey JR, et al. High-dose chemotherapy with autologous stem-cell rescue in patients with recurrent and high-risk pediatric brain tumors. J Clin Oncol 1997;15:1814–1823.
182. Guruangan S, Dunkel IJ, Goldman S, et al. Myeloablative chemotherapy with autologous bone marrow rescue in young children with recurrent malignant brain tumors. J Clin Oncol 1998;16:2486–2493.
183. Dunkel IJ, Garvin JH Jr, Goldman S, et al. High dose chemotherapy with autologous bone marrow rescue for children with diffuse pontine brain stem tumors. Children's Cancer Group. J Neurooncol 1998;37:67–73.
184. Gururangan S, McLaughlin C, Quinn J, et al. High-dose chemotherapy with autologous stem-cell rescue in children and adults with newly diagnosed pineoblastomas. J Clin Oncol 2003;21:2187–2191.
185. Fangusaro J, Finlay J, Sposto R, et al. Intensive chemotherapy followed by consolidative myeloablative chemotherapy with autologous hematopoietic cell rescue (AuHCR) in young children with newly diagnosed supratentorial primitive neuroectodermal tumors (sPNETs): report of the Head Start I and II experience. Pediatr Blood Cancer 2008;50: 312–318.
186. Fangusaro JR, Jubran RF, Allen J, et al. Brainstem primitive neuroectodermal tumors (bstPNET): results of treatment with intensive induction chemotherapy followed by consolidative chemotherapy with autologous hematopoietic cell rescue. Pediatr Blood Cancer 2008;50:715–717.
187. Zacharoulis S, Levy A, Chi SN, et al. Outcome for young children newly diagnosed with ependymoma, treated with intensive induction chemotherapy followed by myeloablative chemotherapy and autologous stem cell rescue. Pediatr Blood Cancer 2007;49: 34–40.
188. Matthay KK, Villablanca JG, Seeger RC, et al. Treatment of high-risk neuroblastoma with intensive chemotherapy, radiotherapy, autologous bone marrow transplantation, and 13-*cis*-retinoic acid. Children's Cancer Group. N Engl J Med 1999;341:1165–1173.
189. Grupp SA, Stern JW, Bunin N, et al. Tandem high-dose therapy in rapid sequence for children with high-risk neuroblastoma. J Clin Oncol 2000;18:2567–2575.
190. Marcus KJ, Shamberger R, Litman H, et al. Primary tumor control in patients with stage 3/4 unfavorable neuroblastoma treated with tandem double autologous stem cell transplants. J Pediatr Hematol Oncol 2003;25:934–940.
191. Kletzel M, Katzenstein HM, Haut PR, et al. Treatment of high-risk neuroblastoma with triple-tandem high-dose therapy and stem-cell rescue: results of the Chicago Pilot II Study. J Clin Oncol 2002;20:2284–2292.
192. Ladenstein R, Lasset C, Pinkerton R, et al. Impact of megatherapy in children with high-risk Ewing's tumours in complete remission: a report from the EBMT Solid Tumour Registry. Bone Marrow Transplant 1995;15:697–705.
193. Burdach S, Meyer-Bahlburg A, Laws HJ, et al. High-dose therapy for patients with primary multifocal and early relapsed Ewing's tumors: results of two consecutive regimens assessing the role of total-body irradiation. J Clin Oncol 2003;21:3072–3078.
194. Fraser CJ, Weigel BJ, Perentesis JP, et al. Autologous stem cell transplantation for high-risk Ewing's sarcoma and other pediatric solid tumors. Bone Marrow Transplant 2006; 37:175–181.
195. Weigel BJ, Breitfeld PP, Hawkins D, et al. Role of high-dose chemotherapy with hematopoietic stem cell rescue in the treatment of metastatic or recurrent rhabdomyosarcoma. J Pediatr Hematol Oncol 2001;23:272–276.
196. Kremens B, Gruhn B, Klingebiel T, et al. High-dose chemotherapy with autologous stem cell rescue in children with nephroblastoma. Bone Marrow Transplant 2002;30: 893–898.
197. Campbell AD, Cohn SL, Reynolds M, et al. Treatment of relapsed Wilms' tumor with high-dose therapy and autologous hematopoietic stem-cell rescue: the experience at Children's Memorial Hospital. J Clin Oncol 2004;22:2885–2890.
198. Papadakis V, Dunkel IJ, Cramer LD, et al. High-dose carmustine, thiotepa and etoposide followed by autologous bone marrow rescue for the treatment of high risk central nervous system tumors. Bone Marrow Transplant 2000;26:153–160.
199. Finlay JL, Goldman S, Wong MC, et al. Pilot study of high-dose thiotepa and etoposide with autologous bone marrow rescue in children and young adults with recurrent CNS tumors. The Children's Cancer Group. J Clin Oncol 1996;14:2495–2503.
200. Mason WP, Grovas A, Halpern S, et al. Intensive chemotherapy and bone marrow rescue for young children with newly diagnosed malignant brain tumors. J Clin Oncol 1998;16:210–221.
201. Cohen KJ. Autologous stem cell rescue in children with brain tumors: the questions mount. Pediatr Blood Cancer 2008;50:191.
202. Zage PE, Kletzel M, Murray K, et al. Outcomes of the POG 9340/9341/9342 trials for children with high-risk neuroblastoma: a report from the Children's Oncology Group. Pediatr Blood Cancer 2008;51:747–753.
203. Villablanca JG, Khan AA, Avramis VI, et al. Phase I trial of 13-*cis*-retinoic acid in children with neuroblastoma following bone marrow transplantation. J Clin Oncol 1995; 13:894–901.
204. Hobbie WL, Moshang T, Carlson CA, et al. Late effects in survivors of tandem peripheral blood stem cell transplant for high-risk neuroblastoma. Pediatr Blood Cancer 2008;51:679–683.
205. George RE, Li S, Medeiros-Nancarrow C, et al. High-risk neuroblastoma treated with tandem autologous peripheral-blood stem cell-supported transplantation: long-term survival update. J Clin Oncol 2006;24:2891–2896.
206. Rill DR, Santana VM, Roberts WM, et al. Direct demonstration that autologous bone marrow transplantation for solid tumors can return a multiplicity of tumorigenic cells. Blood 1994;84:380–383.
207. Handgretinger R, Leung W, Ihm K, et al. Tumour cell contamination of autologous stem cells grafts in high-risk neuroblastoma: the good news? Br J Cancer 2003;88:1874–1877.
208. Kanold J, Halle P, Tchirkov A, et al. Ex vivo expansion of autologous PB CD34+ cells provides a purging effect in children with neuroblastoma. Bone Marrow Transplant 2003;32:485–488.
209. Handgretinger R, Lang P, Ihm K, et al. Isolation and transplantation of highly purified autologous peripheral CD34(+) progenitor cells: purging efficacy, hematopoietic reconstitution and long-term outcome in children with high-risk neuroblastoma. Bone Marrow Transplant 2002;29:731–736.
210. Powell JL, Bunin NJ, Callahan C, et al. An unexpectedly high incidence of Epstein-Barr virus lymphoproliferative disease after CD34+ selected autologous peripheral blood stem cell transplant in neuroblastoma. Bone Marrow Transplant 2004;33:651–657.
211. Inoue M, Nakano T, Yoneda A, et al. Graft-versus-tumor effect in a patient with advanced neuroblastoma who received HLA haplo-identical bone marrow transplantation. Bone Marrow Transplant 2003;32:103–106.
212. Matthay KK, Edeline V, Lumbroso J, et al. Correlation of early metastatic response by 123I-metaiodobenzylguanidine scintigraphy with overall response and event-free survival in stage IV neuroblastoma. J Clin Oncol 2003;21:2486–2491.
213. Weiss B, Vora A, Huberty J, et al. Secondary myelodysplastic syndrome and leukemia following 131I-metaiodobenzylguanidine therapy for relapsed neuroblastoma. J Pediatr Hematol Oncol 2003;25:543–547.
214. Ozkaynak MF, Sondel PM, Krailo MD, et al. Phase I study of chimeric human/murine anti-ganglioside G(D2) monoclonal antibody (ch14.18) with granulocyte-macrophage colony-stimulating factor in children with neuroblastoma immediately after hematopoietic stem-cell transplantation: a Children's Cancer Group Study. J Clin Oncol 2000;18: 4077–4085.
215. Yu AL, Gilman AL, Ozkaynak MF, et al. A phase III randomized trial of the chimeric anti-GD2 antibody ch14.18 with GM-CSF and IL-2 as immunotherapy following dose intensive chemotherapy for high-risk neuroblastoma: Children's Oncology Group (COG) study ANBL0032 [abstract 10067z]. J Clin Oncol 2009;27(suppl).
216. Rousseau RF, Haight AE, Hirschmann-Jax C, et al. Local and systemic effects of an allogeneic tumor cell vaccine combining transgenic human lymphotactin with interleukin-2 in patients with advanced or refractory neuroblastoma. Blood 2003;101: 1718–1726.
217. Gonzales S, Naranjo A, Peng JS, et al. Genetic engineering of T cells for redirected neuroblastoma recognition: preclinical studies supporting the initiation of a FDA-authorized clinical trial [abstract]. Mol Ther 2001;3:S369–S370.
218. Pule MA, Savoldo B, Myers GD, et al. Virus-specific T cells engineered to coexpress tumor-specific receptors: persistence and antitumor activity in individuals with neuroblastoma. Nat Med 2008;14:1264–1270.

219. Lang P, Pfeiffer M, Muller I, et al. Haploidentical stem cell transplantation in patients with pediatric solid tumors: preliminary results of a pilot study and analysis of graft versus tumor effects. Klin Padiatr 2006;218:321–326.
220. Ceschel S, Casotto V, Valsecchi MG, et al. Survival after relapse in children with solid tumors: a follow-up study from the Italian off-therapy registry. Pediatr Blood Cancer 2006;47:560–566.
221. Leung W, Chen AR, Klann RC, et al. Frequent detection of tumor cells in hematopoietic grafts in neuroblastoma and Ewing's sarcoma. Bone Marrow Transplant 1998;22: 971–979.
222. Yaniv I, Cohen IJ, Stein J, et al. Tumor cells are present in stem cell harvests of Ewings sarcoma patients and their persistence following transplantation is associated with relapse. Pediatr Blood Cancer 2004;42:404–409.
223. Burdach S, van Kaick B, Laws HJ, et al. Allogeneic and autologous stem-cell transplantation in advanced Ewing tumors. An update after long-term follow-up from two centers of the European Intergroup study EICESS. Stem-Cell Transplant Programs at Dusseldorf University Medical Center, Germany and St. Anna Kinderspital, Vienna, Austria. Ann Oncol 2000;11:1451–1462.
224. Ozkaynak MF, Sahdev I, Gross TG, et al. A pilot study of addition of amifostine to melphalan, carboplatin, etoposide, and cyclophosphamide with autologous hematopoietic stem cell transplantation in pediatric solid tumors—a pediatric blood and marrow transplant consortium study. J Pediatr Hematol Oncol 2008;30:204–209.
225. Hawkins DS, Felgenhauer J, Park J, et al. Peripheral blood stem cell support reduces the toxicity of intensive chemotherapy for children and adolescents with metastatic sarcomas. Cancer 2002;95:1354–1365.
226. Shankar AG, Ashley S, Craft AW, et al. Outcome after relapse in an unselected cohort of children and adolescents with Ewing sarcoma. Med Pediatr Oncol 2003;40:141–147.
227. Mackall C, Berzofsky J, Helman LJ. Targeting tumor specific translocations in sarcomas in pediatric patients for immunotherapy. Clin Orthop Relat Res 2000;373:25–31.
228. Carli M, Colombatti R, Oberlin O, et al. High-dose melphalan with autologous stem-cell rescue in metastatic rhabdomyosarcoma. J Clin Oncol 1999;17:2796–2803.
229. Koscielniak E, Klingebiel TH, Peters C, et al. Do patients with metastatic and recurrent rhabdomyosarcoma benefit from high-dose therapy with hematopoietic rescue? Report of the German/Austrian Pediatric Bone Marrow Transplantation Group. Bone Marrow Transplant 1997;19:227–231.
230. Boulad F, Kernan NA, LaQuaglia MP, et al. High-dose induction chemoradiotherapy followed by autologous bone marrow transplantation as consolidation therapy in rhabdomyosarcoma, extraosseous Ewing's sarcoma, and undifferentiated sarcoma. J Clin Oncol 1998;16:1697–1706.
231. Matsubara H, Makimoto A, Higa T, et al. Possible benefits of high-dose chemotherapy as intensive consolidation in patients with high-risk rhabdomyosarcoma who achieve complete remission with conventional chemotherapy. Pediatr Hematol Oncol 2003;20: 201–210.
232. Fuchs N, Bielack SS, Epler D, et al. Long-term results of the co-operative German-Austrian-Swiss osteosarcoma study group's protocol COSS-86 of intensive multidrug chemotherapy and surgery for osteosarcoma of the limbs. Ann Oncol 1998;9:893–899.
233. Sauerbrey A, Bielack S, Kempf-Bielack B, et al. High-dose chemotherapy (HDC) and autologous hematopoietic stem cell transplantation (ASCT) as salvage therapy for relapsed osteosarcoma. Bone Marrow Transplant 2001;27:933–937.
234. Fagioli F, Aglietta M, Tienghi A, et al. High-dose chemotherapy in the treatment of relapsed osteosarcoma: an Italian sarcoma group study. J Clin Oncol 2002;20:2150–2156.
235. Ladenstein R, Philip T, Gardner H. Autologous stem cell transplantation for solid tumors in children. Curr Opin Pediatr 1997;9:55–69.
236. Ferrara JL, Levine JE, Reddy P, et al. Graft-versus-host disease. Lancet 2009;373: 1550–1561.
237. Dickinson AM, Middleton PG, Rocha V, et al. Genetic polymorphisms predicting the outcome of bone marrow transplants. Br J Haematol 2004;127:479–490.
238. Przepiorka D, Weisdorf D, Martin P, et al. 1994 Consensus Conference on Acute GVHD Grading. Bone Marrow Transplant 1995;15:825–828.
239. Champlin RE, Passweg JR, Zhang MJ, et al. T-cell depletion of bone marrow transplants for leukemia from donors other than HLA-identical siblings: advantage of T-cell antibodies with narrow specificities. Blood 2000;95:3996–4003.
240. Wagner JE, Thompson JS, Carter SL, et al. Effect of graft-versus-host disease prophylaxis on 3-year disease-free survival in recipients of unrelated donor bone marrow (T-cell Depletion Trial): a multi-centre, randomised phase II–III trial. Lancet 2005;366: 733–741.
241. Deeg HJ. How I treat refractory acute GVHD. Blood 2007;109:4119–4126.
242. Le BK, Frassoni F, Ball L, et al. Mesenchymal stem cells for treatment of steroid-resistant, severe, acute graft-versus-host disease: a phase II study. Lancet 2008;371: 1579–1586.
243. Filipovich AH, Weisdorf D, Pavletic S, et al. National Institutes of Health consensus development project on criteria for clinical trials in chronic graft-versus-host disease: I. Diagnosis and staging working group report. Biol Blood Marrow Transplant 2005;11: 945–956.
244. Pavletic S, Vogelsang GB. Treatment of high-risk chronic GVHD. Biol Blood Marrow Transplant 2008;14:1436–1437.
245. Akpek G, Lee SJ, Flowers ME, et al. Performance of a new clinical grading system for chronic graft-versus-host disease: a multicenter study. Blood 2003;102:802–809.
246. Ahmed N, Leung KS, Rosenblatt H, et al. Successful treatment of stem cell graft failure in pediatric patients using a submyeloablative regimen of campath-1H and fludarabine. Biol Blood Marrow Transplant 2008;14:1298–1304.
247. Tomblyn M, Chiller T, Einsele H, et al. Guidelines for preventing infectious complications among hematopoietic cell transplant recipients: a global perspective. Biol Blood Marrow Transplant 2009;15(10):1143–1238.
248. Boeckh M, Nichols WG, Papanicolaou G, et al. Cytomegalovirus in hematopoietic stem cell transplant recipients: current status, known challenges, and future strategies. Biol Blood Marrow Transplant 2003;9:543–558.
249. Einsele H, Roosnek E, Rufer N, et al. Infusion of cytomegalovirus (CMV)-specific T cells for the treatment of CMV infection not responding to antiviral chemotherapy. Blood 2002;99:3916–3922.
250. Walter EA, Greenberg PD, Gilbert MJ, et al. Reconstitution of cellular immunity against cytomegalovirus in recipients of allogeneic bone marrow by transfer of T-cell clones from the donor. N Engl J Med 1995;333:1038–1044.
251. Peggs KS, Verfuerth S, Pizzey A, et al. Adoptive cellular therapy for early cytomegalovirus infection after allogeneic stem-cell transplantation with virus-specific T-cell lines. Lancet 2003;362:1375–1377.
252. Leen AM, Myers GD, Sili U, et al. Monoculture-derived T lymphocytes specific for multiple viruses expand and produce clinically relevant effects in immunocompromised individuals. Nat Med 2006;12:1160–1166.
253. Boeckh M. The challenge of respiratory virus infections in hematopoietic cell transplant recipients. Br J Haematol 2008;143:455–467.
254. Yusuf U, Hale GA, Carr J, et al. Cidofovir for the treatment of adenoviral infection in pediatric hematopoietic stem cell transplant patients. Transplantation 2006;81:1398–1404.
255. Myers GD, Bollard CM, Wu MF, et al. Reconstitution of adenovirus-specific cell-mediated immunity in pediatric patients after hematopoietic stem cell transplantation. Bone Marrow Transplant 2007;39:677–686.
256. Leen AM, Christin A, Myers GD, et al. Cytotoxic T lymphocyte therapy with donor T cells prevents and treats adenovirus and Epstein-Barr virus infections after haploidentical and matched unrelated stem cell transplant. Blood 2009;114(19)4283–4292.
257. Feuchtinger T, Matthes-Martin S, Richard C, et al. Safe adoptive transfer of virus-specific T-cell immunity for the treatment of systemic adenovirus infection after allogeneic stem cell transplantation. Br J Haematol 2006;134:64–76.
258. McDonald GB. Advances in prevention and treatment of hepatic disorders following hematopoietic cell transplantation. Best Pract Res Clin Haematol 2006;19:341–352.
259. Ho VT, Revta C, Richardson PG. Hepatic veno-occlusive disease after hematopoietic stem cell transplantation: update on defibrotide and other current investigational therapies. Bone Marrow Transplant 2008;41:229–237.
260. Hale GA, Rochester RJ, Heslop HE, et al. Hemorrhagic cystitis after allogeneic bone marrow transplantation in children: clinical characteristics and outcome. Biol Blood Marrow Transplant 2003;9:698–705.
261. Kojouri K, George JN. Thrombotic microangiopathy following allogeneic hematopoietic stem cell transplantation. Curr Opin Oncol 2007;19:148–154.
262. Ho VT, Cutler C, Carter S, et al. Blood and marrow transplant clinical trials network toxicity committee consensus summary: thrombotic microangiopathy after hematopoietic stem cell transplantation. Biol Blood Marrow Transplant 2005;11:571–575.
263. Rizzo JD, Curtis RE, Socie G, et al. Solid cancers after allogeneic hematopoietic cell transplantation. Blood 2009;113:1175–1183.
264. Landgren O, Gilbert ES, Rizzo JD, et al. Risk factors for lymphoproliferative disorders after allogeneic hematopoietic cell transplantation. Blood 2009;113:4992–5001.
265. Gilliland DG, Gribben JG. Evaluation of the risk of therapy-related MDS/AML after autologous stem cell transplantation. Biol Blood Marrow Transplant 2002;8:9–16.
266. Socie G, Curtis RE, Deeg HJ, et al. New malignant diseases after allogeneic marrow transplantation for childhood acute leukemia. J Clin Oncol 2000;18:348–357.
267. Gottschalk S, Rooney CM, Heslop HE. Post-transplant lymphoproliferative disorders. Annu Rev Med 2005;56:29–44.
268. Cohen J, Gandhi M, Naik P, et al. Increased incidence of EBV-related disease following paediatric stem cell transplantation with reduced-intensity conditioning. Br J Haematol 2005;129:229–239.
269. Brunstein CG, Weisdorf DJ, DeFor T, et al. Marked increased risk of Epstein-Barr virus-related complications with the addition of antithymocyte globulin to a nonmyeloablative conditioning prior to unrelated umbilical cord blood transplantation. Blood 2006;108:2874–2880.
270. Heslop HE. How I treat EBV lymphoproliferation. Blood 2009;114(19):4002–4008.
271. Robison LL, Bhatia S. Late-effects among survivors of leukaemia and lymphoma during childhood and adolescence. Br J Haematol 2003;122:345–359.
272. Salooja N, Szydlo RM, Socie G, et al. Pregnancy outcomes after peripheral blood or bone marrow transplantation: a retrospective survey. Lancet 2001;358:271–276.
273. Sanders JE, Hoffmeister PA, Woolfrey AE, et al. Thyroid function following hematopoietic cell transplantation in children: 30 years' experience. Blood 2009;113:306–308.
274. Sanders JE. Growth and development after hematopoietic cell transplant in children. Bone Marrow Transplant 2008;41:223–227.
275. Cohen A, Rovelli A, Bakker B, et al. Final height of patients who underwent bone marrow transplantation for hematological disorders during childhood: a study by the Working Party for Late Effects-EBMT. Blood 1999;93:4109–4115.
276. Sanders JE, Guthrie KA, Hoffmeister PA, et al. Final adult height of patients who received hematopoietic cell transplantation in childhood. Blood 2005;105:1348–1354.
277. Phipps S, Dunavant M, Srivastava DK, et al. Cognitive and academic functioning in survivors of pediatric bone marrow transplantation. J Clin Oncol 2000;18:1004–1011.
278. Dahllof G, Hingorani SR, Sanders JE. Late effects following hematopoietic cell transplantation for children. Biol Blood Marrow Transplant 2008;14:88–93.
279. Kolb HJ. Graft-versus-leukemia effects of transplantation and donor lymphocytes. Blood 2008;112:4371–4383.
280. Falkenburg JH, Heslop HE, Barrett AJ. T cell therapy in allogeneic stem cell transplantation. Biol Blood Marrow Transplant 2008;14:136–141.
281. Quintarelli C, Dotti G, De AB, et al. Cytotoxic T lymphocytes directed to the preferentially expressed antigen of melanoma (PRAME) target chronic myeloid leukemia. Blood 2008;112:1876–1885.
282. Rousseau RF, Biagi E, Dutour A, et al. Immunotherapy of high-risk acute leukemia with a recipient (autologous) vaccine expressing transgenic human CD40L and IL-2 after chemotherapy and allogeneic stem cell transplantation. Blood 2006;107:1332–1341.
283. Singh H, Serrano LM, Pfeiffer T, et al. Combining adoptive cellular and immunocytokine therapies to improve treatment of B-lineage malignancy. Cancer Res 2007;67: 2872–2880.
284. Barrett J, Rezvani K. Immunotherapy: can we include vaccines with stem-cell transplantation? Nat Rev Clin Oncol 2009;6:503–505.
285. Cooper LJ. Adoptive cellular immunotherapy for childhood malignancies. Bone Marrow Transplant 2008;41:183–192.
286. Savoldo B, Rooney CM, Di SA, et al. Epstein Barr virus specific cytotoxic T lymphocytes expressing the anti-CD30zeta artificial chimeric T-cell receptor for immunotherapy of Hodgkin disease. Blood 2007;110:2620–2630.
287. Imai C, Iwamoto S, Campana D. Genetic modification of primary natural killer cells overcomes inhibitory signals and induces specific killing of leukemic cells. Blood 2005;106:376–383.
288. Grzywacz B, Miller JS, Verneris MR. Use of natural killer cells as immunotherapy for leukaemia. Best Pract Res Clin Haematol 2008;21:467–483.
289. Fujisaki H, Kakuda H, Shimasaki N, et al. Expansion of highly cytotoxic human natural killer cells for cancer cell therapy. Cancer Res 2009;69:4010–4017.
290. Chien JW, Boeckh MJ, Hansen JA, et al. Lipopolysaccharide binding protein promoter variants influence the risk for Gram-negative bacteremia and mortality after allogeneic hematopoietic cell transplantation. Blood 2008;111:2462–2469.

CHAPTER 17 ■ CANCER CLINICAL TRIALS: DESIGN, CONDUCT, ANALYSIS, AND REPORTING

SUSAN HILSENBECK, LISA R. BOMGAARS, AND STACEY L. BERG

Outcomes for many forms of childhood cancer have improved greatly over the past 50 years (see Chapter 1). These improvements are largely attributed to the widespread and systematic enrollment of children with cancer onto clinical trials that have elucidated diagnostic and prognostic criteria and identified effective therapy for these diseases. Every pediatric oncologist should understand the essential principles of clinical trial design and conduct to offer the best care to his or her patients and to contribute to further advancements in care for future patients.

A clinical trial is an experiment that attempts to answer a medical question, most often about the effect of a therapeutic intervention on the outcome of a disease. The rationale for conducting clinical trials in pediatric oncology is simple: for a life-threatening illness treated with toxic and expensive therapies, it is critical to evaluate each aspect of therapy and each potential new treatment systematically to make stepwise improvements in the standard of care. Clinical trials produce the data upon which the understanding of current best treatment as well as the choice of most important questions for subsequent trials is based. To generate good data, the clinical trialist must create a study with clearly stated objectives, an experimental design that will permit the objectives to be accomplished, a data analysis plan that will determine the results objectively and definitively, and a reporting plan that will permit dissemination of the results for use by other clinicians.

PLANNING A CLINICAL TRIAL

Objectives

The first step in planning a clinical trial is to define the objectives clearly. In pediatric clinical trials, the choice of primary study objective is especially critical, because the available patient population is not large enough to provide reliable answers to many experimental questions at once, and it may take several years to enroll enough subjects to complete a single clinical trial in a particular disease. The objectives therefore should reflect the most important unanswered question that is feasible to ask about the particular patient population and disease type. A protocol will usually have one major objective and a number of minor ones. For example, the major objective might be "to compare the event-free survival of patients with leukemia receiving best current therapy with or without New Drug X." The secondary objectives might be "to determine the prognostic significance of mutations in the x gene," "to describe the pharmacokinetic behavior of Drug X," etc. It is important to select objectives that can provide useful information regardless of whether the study results are positive or negative; establishing conclusively that a new intervention does not contribute to improved outcomes can be as important as identifying advances in therapy.[1]

The parameters for assessing the effects of interventions on individual patients are generally referred to as *end points*. An end point is a medical event that represents an outcome, either good (e.g., complete remission) or bad (e.g., relapse, death). The results of the clinical trial are based on analyses of the accumulation of end point assessments, the criteria which were predetermined by the investigator. A well-constructed protocol incorporates end points that are objective, practical, and relevant to the clinical situation under study. By defining end points, the researcher indicates precisely which measures of outcome reliably meet the objectives of the protocol. These objectives assist in clarifying what clinical and laboratory data need to be obtained during the trial and provide the basis for statistical analysis.

Trial Design

Cancer clinical trials are conventionally categorized into three types.[2] A *phase 1* trial investigates the adverse events associated with a particular agent or combination of agents and determines the maximum tolerated dose (MTD) or the appropriate dose with a given schedule and route of administration.[3] A *phase 2* trial obtains expanded safety data and estimates the activity of the agent against individual tumor types.[4] A *phase 3* trial assesses the activity of the agent in a comparative fashion, usually with reference to standard therapy or, in some cases, to the natural history of the disease.[5] Some trials, often involving combinations of agents or tests of feasibility of an approach before a large-scale study is launched, are designed to obtain intermediate information before definitive studies are conducted. These trials may be referred to as *pilot studies*.[6] In cancer therapy development in general, and in pediatric trials in specific, the vast majority of clinical trials are early phase.

Phase 1 Trials: Specific Designs

The objective of a phase 1 trial or dose-finding study[7] is to select a dose to carry forward to further evaluation, the so-called recommended phase 2 dose, which is used here synonymously with the "maximum tolerated dose". It is generally assumed that both efficacy and toxicity increase with dose, so the goal is to select the highest tolerable dose with the idea that this will have the highest chance of efficacy.[8] The primary end point of these dose-finding trials is therefore toxicity. The protocol should specify the frequency of monitoring for toxicity and what grading scale is to be used, for example, "toxicity will be assessed after each course and graded using the NCI CTCAE Version 4.0."[9] The grade and types of toxicity that will be deemed dose-limiting toxicities (DLTs) and will determine dose escalation or de-escalation, are also specified ahead of time in the protocol. Common definitions and standards are important to ensure comparability across studies.

491

Phase 1 designs have two parts: specification of the levels of exposure of the agent(s) to be considered (*dose levels*) and rules for moving from one level to the next (*dose escalation*).[10] In adults, the starting dose for "first in human" oncology phase 1 trials is based on animal toxicology studies and generally is one-tenth the dose lethal to 10% of a cohort of mice, expressed in mg/m^2 (0.1 MELD10).[11] Stepwise dose increases are specified in the protocol. Often, a modified Fibonacci scheme is used to determine the levels for successive cohorts.[12] The starting dose is increased by 100% in the second level, and subsequent levels are increased by adding 67%, 50%, 40%, and 33% of the dose established by the preceding cohort. The diminishing proportion increase reflects increasing caution as one becomes farther removed from the starting dose. An alternate version of this scheme is to double the dose until "biologic activity," such as mild myelosuppression, is observed, then to institute the diminishing increases of the Fibonacci series.[13] Phase 1 trials of newer anticancer agents that are intended to modulate or inhibit a specific cellular target associated with the malignant state may not require escalation to DLT. The appropriate phase 1 end point for such agents may be the determination of the dose that best produces the desired response (the "optimal dose") rather than the MTD.[14] For these trials, end points may be related to assessment of the specific modulation or inhibition being sought, although a recent review found that even for newer agents, the most common end point was still MTD.[15]

In children, phase 1 trials usually start after some adult data on the agent of interest are already available. One efficient method is to start children's trials at 80% of the adult phase 2 dose or at 80% of the dose at which biologic activity was observed in adults, bypassing levels that are presumably safe in children but may be too low to be of benefit. Starting doses derived from the adult MTD or recommended phase 2 dose are presumably close to the childhood MTD, and escalation should proceed cautiously, using approximately 30% increases over the preceding dose level. Dose escalation often continues in children beyond the phase 2 dose established for adults, because children often display greater tolerance to chemotherapy.[16]

In practice, it is common to combine two or more agents, or to combine radiation with drugs or biologics. The first time such combinations are used together in people, or in children even if they have been combined in adults, a phase 1 design is often appropriate. It is not always clear what combined doses will be safe and there are a number of proposed strategies for exploring combinations.[10,17]

The second aspect of phase 1 study design is the specification of rules for exploring the different dose levels.[8,10] These have been reviewed by Le Tourneau et al.[10] and fall into two broad categories: algorithmic and model based. The algorithmic designs, which include 3 + 3-like designs and accelerated titration designs, are characterized by prespecified deterministic rules that govern dose escalation or deescalation. Model-based designs, which include the continual reassessment methods (CRMs), fit accumulating data to a likelihood or Bayesian dose-toxicity probability model to estimate the dose level associated with the target rate of DLT and to select the next dose level to be tested. The oldest and still most commonly used phase 1 design is the so-called 3 + 3.[18] In this design, patients are enrolled in cohorts of three, beginning at the lowest dose level, and are then observed for acute toxicity. If any of these patients is inevaluable for toxicity, he or she is replaced. If none of the three evaluable patients experiences DLT, the dose level is escalated. At any dose level, when DLT is observed in one patient, the cohort is expanded to six patients. The MTD is defined as the dose level immediately below that at which two patients (in a cohort of three to six)

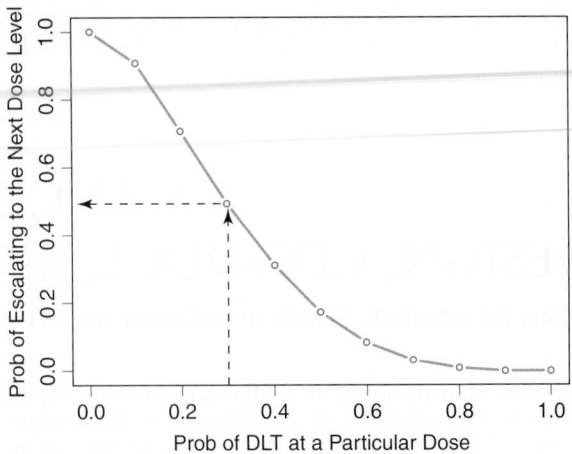

FIGURE 17.1 Graph of probability of escalation to the next dose level in a traditional 3 + 3 phase 1 trial for given probability of DLT at a particular dose level. DLT, dose-limiting toxicity.

experience DLT. If myelosuppression is the DLT, consideration is often given to enrolling patients with limited prior therapy onto the study, because an inappropriately low MTD may be defined if only heavily pretreated patients, who may tolerate therapy less well, are enrolled in the phase 1 trial.[19] Figure 17.1 shows the probability of escalation to the next level for a given probability of DLT at the current dose level. If, for example, the target probability of DLT is 30%, there is a fairly high probability of overshooting or stopping too early. From both past experience and simulations, 3 + 3 designs are widely considered to be safe, but to have a tendency to stop too early when the starting level is far below the true MTD.

The accelerated titration design is actually a family of designs,[13] mostly useful when there is some prior experience, perhaps with related agents, and is designed to move quickly through low, nontoxic levels and then to revert to traditional 3 + 3 escalation once a DLT or multiple lower grade toxicities are observed. In children, a modification of the 3 + 3 called the "rolling 6"[20,21] has been developed to decrease trial duration without increasing the risk of toxicity. In this design, enrollment is not suspended when three subjects have entered a dose cohort. Instead, if toxicity data are available for all three when the fourth subject is entered and there are no DLTs, the fourth participant is enrolled on the subsequent dose level. If data are not yet available for one or more of the first three participants and no DLT has been observed, or if one DLT has been observed, the new subject is entered at the same dose level. Lastly, if two or more DLTs have been observed, the dose level is deescalated. This process is repeated for participants 5 and 6. This design performs especially well in simulations when the accrual rate is relatively slow and when inevaluability rates are not negligible, and is now being tried in several recently opened phase 1 studies of the Children's Oncology Group.

A recognized limitation of the algorithmic designs is the inability to provide formal estimates or confidence/credible intervals for MTDs or to borrow information across dose levels. That is, in the 3 + 3, in essence, only the current dose level information is considered in determining the next dose level; information from other dose levels that have already been studied are ignored. O'Quigley and colleagues[22–24] proposed a new approach to phase 1 studies in cancer aimed at moving to the MTD more quickly and thereby increasing both the efficiency of this early phase of development and the likelihood that patients treated in phase 1 will receive potentially beneficial treatment. This approach, the CRM, targets the dose to an "acceptable" toxicity level selected by the investigators. Either likelihood or Bayesian methods are used to continually update the expected probability of toxicity based on the experience observed up to that point in the study. The original CRM design was criticized on the grounds that it may lead too frequently to treatment at unacceptably toxic levels and may in many cases lead to longer phase 1 trials.[25,26] Modified versions of the CRM (mCRM) often include ad hoc adjustments to the model, cohorts of two or more subjects, starting at the lowest dose level, limiting escalations to a single dose level regardless of the model predicted MTD, and stopping accrual when a certain number of subjects have been treated at the dose level closest to but below the predicted MTD. The Pediatric Brain Tumor Consortium has pioneered the use of a pediatric focused mCRM design, with several ongoing trials, that is expected to be more accurate, reduce excess toxicity, and require fewer patients.[26–29]

Most phase 1 trials are focused on acute toxicity occurring in the first course of therapy, but late or chronic toxicity may also be an important determinant of clinically relevant dose. An enhancement of the CRM called the time-to-event CRM (TiTE-CRM) may prove useful.[30] This design considers toxicity over a longer period of time while still allowing relatively quick escalation decisions. Finally, with biologically targeted agents, higher is not necessarily better, and in theory, it may be desirable to select doses to carry forward that are based on a combined assessment of toxicity and efficacy or biologic response.[31,32] A limitation of this approach is the need for a reliable assay of response and the need to be reasonably certain that the putative biologic response is relevant.

Phase 1 Trials: Sample Size, Subject Population, and Reporting

Sample sizes for phase 1 trials typically range from 15 to 40 subjects and are driven by the number of dose levels studied and the number of subjects at each level. Thus, a study with five dose levels using a 3 + 3 design would enroll at most 30 subjects, although it could conceivably be far fewer. It is common to enroll additional subjects (i.e., 6 to 12) at the MTD level to gain additional insight into the toxicity profile or to obtain additional correlative information such as pharmacokinetic data. Expected sample sizes usually do not vary dramatically among phase 1 designs.

Analysis and reporting of phase 1 trial results are largely descriptive and include detailed summarization of patient characteristics, observed toxicities, MTD, and consequent recommended phase 2 dose. It is common to perform pharmacokinetic studies as part of phase 1 trials, and those results should be summarized. For agents that have already been well studied in adults, pediatric phase 1 pharmacokinetic studies might have limited or sparse sampling. Although frequently omitted, details of the design should be included in reports of phase 1 trials.

Phase 2 Trials: Objectives and End Points

The primary purpose of a "standard" phase 2 trial is to determine whether the new agent(s) is(are) sufficiently promising to warrant further study, usually by comparing the new treatment with a prespecified standard or historical control. More recently, questions addressed by phase 2 studies have become considerably more diverse with objectives ranging from dose refinement and evaluation of early evidence of efficacy to selection of biomarker defined subgroups to definitive comparison. Designs are correspondingly diverse.

Although the gold standard for evaluation of clinical benefit in oncology is improvement in overall survival, this is rarely a feasible outcome in phase 2 trials. It takes too long, and

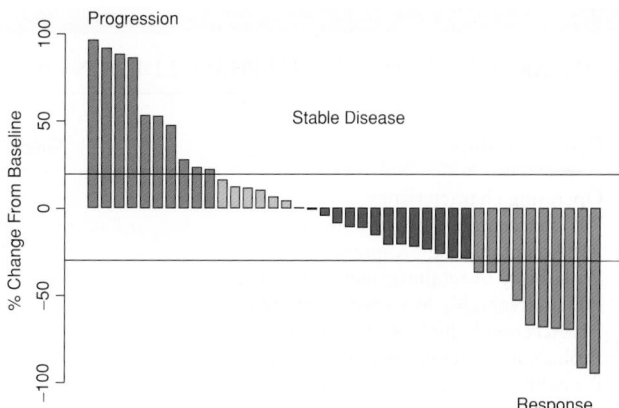

FIGURE 17.2 Example of a waterfall plot showing change in tumor burden (sum of longest diameters) from baseline.

study agent effects are likely to be confounded, with effects of subsequent therapies rendering the survival results uninterpretable. The most common phase 2 end point is objective response, and, in solid tumors, is usually assessed by the Response Evaluation Criteria in Solid Tumors (RECIST) guidelines.[33,34] Objective response, usually defined as confirmed complete or partial response, is a relatively rapidly assessable binary outcome that represents a direct effect of treatment on the cancer and is a surrogate, albeit surprisingly weak, for ultimate clinical benefit. More recently, dissatisfaction with the loss of information due to categorization has resulted in the suggestion to treat response as a continuous variable,[35,36] although this concept is still quite controversial.[37] In this approach, response data are often shown as "waterfall plots," which depict change in tumor size from baseline at a fixed time point (Fig. 17.2), and/or "spider plots," which show individual change trajectories over time.[38] Statistically, continuous outcomes provide more information and thus more power for a fixed sample size than dichotomized versions of the same data, and in theory could allow randomized comparison of two or more treatments. One drawback, however, is that small early differences in tumor size may not reflect clinically meaningful effects, perhaps lowering an already low bar for calling a treatment "active," with the risk that these kinds of phase 2 studies will predict phase 3 success even less well than those using the object response rate to determine drug activity. In addition, accurate measurement of small changes in tumor size is notoriously difficult, and even small errors could seriously bias results. Furthermore, with continuous approaches, it is unclear how to properly consider the appearance of new lesions, which would automatically be deemed progression by RECIST.

Other commonly used end points in phase 2 studies include time to tumor progression (where deaths not due to cancer are censored), progression-free survival (where deaths not due to cancer are events), overall survival, quality of life, change in molecular biomarkers, and change in functional imaging. "Time to" outcomes can be treated as continuous outcomes or, more commonly and conveniently for purposes of design, can be dichotomized by considering status at a fixed time (i.e., 6 months PFS), and can be used in the same kinds of designs that apply to response as an outcome.

Phase 2 Trials: Specific Designs—Single Arm

Most phase 2 trials use a binary or categorical outcome and include only a single arm or disease cohort. In pediatric studies, several different diagnoses may be included, with the agent evaluated separately in each one. The simplest design

TABLE 17.1

COMPARISON OF SINGLE ARM PHASE 2 DESIGNS WITH THE SAME OPERATING CHARACTERISTICS

Design variables	Single stage[39]	Minimax two stage[40]	Admissible two stage[41,42]	Optimal two stage[40]	Toxicity and efficacy[43]
Operating characteristics					
P0. Unacceptably low response rate	10%	10%	10%	10%	10%
P1. Acceptably high response rate	30%	30%	30%	30%	30%
Probability of retaining ineffective drug	5%	5%	5%	5%	5%
P0. Unacceptably low nontoxicity rate	—	—	—	—	60%
P1. Acceptably high nontoxicity rate	—	—	—	—	80%
Probability of retaining a toxic drug	—	—	—	—	10%
Probability of retaining a "good" drug	85%	85%	85%	85%	85%
Sample sizes and decision rules					
N first stage	—	18	13	11	19
Responses required to continue to second stage	—	3	2	2	3
"Nontoxicities" required to continue to second stage	—	—	—	—	13
N	27	27	28	35	43
Responses required to conclude in favor of drug	6	6	6	7	8
"Nontoxicities" required to conclude in favor of drug	—	—	—	—	30
Expected N when drug is bad (or too toxic)	27	20.4	18.7	18.3	26.1

has only one stage, accruing, treating, and evaluating the entire sample before drawing a conclusion. The design can be based on attaining a certain confidence interval or a more formal test of hypothesis, usually selected to have good power but more relaxed one-sided type I error rates. Table 17.1, column 1, illustrates a hypothetical study where the uninteresting response rate is $p_0 = 10\%$, the response rate that would be clinically interesting is $p_1 = 30\%$, the desired probability of spuriously declaring the new treatment to be interesting is $\alpha = 5\%$ (one sided), and the power ($1-\beta$ error) is 85%. The required sample size N, calculated assuming an underlying binomial distribution for the outcome, is 27, and at the end of the trial, we would conclude that the drug is active if six or more responses are observed.

Of particular interest in pediatric oncology, a one-sample log-rank test[44,45] comparing the observed event times with a hypothesized standard can be used when event-free, progression-free, or overall survival is expected to be short relative to accrual, and there is reasonably good historical data on which to base a comparison. Sample sizes are often conservatively estimated using a dichotomization approach (see earlier), and sample size estimation is similar to that used for response. The Children's Oncology Group has several trials that use this estimation and testing methodology, usually in combination with additional group sequential monitoring (see later) for toxicity or efficacy.

Although simple, a disadvantage of one-stage designs is that all the subjects have to be treated before we conclude that the drug is not effective. Multistage or one-sample group sequential designs address this problem by allowing early termination if certain activity criteria are not met in the course of the trial. There are numerous variations with various optimization schemes,[40,46–48] consideration of ordinal response,[49] early disease progression and response,[50] or survival as the primary outcome.[51] The overall goal of these strategies is to use as few patients as possible to obtain the desired information about drug activity. The so-called Simon two-stage design is by far the most common approach.[40] As shown in Table 17.1, column 3, we might accrue 13 patients in the first stage and only if at least two responses are seen would we proceed to stage 2 to accrue the remainder of the sample. Even with only two stages, for given operating characteristics (i.e., p_0, p_1, α, and power), there are many possible choices of stage size and

decision rule, so that some sort of optimization is necessary. Simon defined two approaches: minimizing the maximum sample size (minimax) and minimizing the "expected" sample size when the response rate is poor (optimal). In our example, the optimal design sample is about 25% larger than the minimax, but the first stage is considerably smaller, possibly allowing an early decision with fewer subjects. Bayesian approaches to phase 2 trials have been described that incorporate prior information and continually update the estimated probability of response based on the accumulating observations.[41,52,53] Lee and Liu proposed a predictive probability approach that allows stopping for futility after every subject,[54] and Sargent et al.[55] proposed a design that allows an "inconclusive" result as well as "positive" and "negative" outcomes.

Finally, toxicity information available after phase 1 may be based on very limited sample size. Although toxicity is always monitored in phase 2 studies and early stopping or pausing may considered on an ad hoc basis, it may be prudent to incorporate more formal rules for early stopping in the face of excessive toxicity. Bryant and Day[43] suggested adding a Simon-like decision rule (see Table 17.1) where low rates of "nontoxicity" are considered bad. The approach assumes that toxicity and response are approximately independent and has been shown to have reasonably robust performance.[56]

Phase 2 Trials: Specific Designs—Phase 2 Windows

Both phase 1 and phase 2 studies ideally would be conducted with previously untreated patients to avoid the problems of cumulative toxicity from prior therapy (for phase 1 trials) and acquired tumor drug resistance (for phase 2 trials). Because most childhood cancers are treatable at diagnosis with better-characterized therapies, however, most early phase trials require that there not be known curative therapy available for potential subjects. Thus, most patients in these trials have had prior therapy. One strategy to increase the generalizability of results of phase 2 studies is to perform a brief phase 2 study in patients before standard therapy begins.[57] This design is called a "phase 2 window" or "upfront window"; it usually consists of one or two cycles of the new treatment in a newly diagnosed patient to assess the tumor response rate. The major concern regarding this approach is whether delay in starting standard therapy may compromise patient outcome if the agent used in the upfront window is inactive.[58,59] Limited available data, however, show no difference in outcome between patients who did or did not receive a phase 2 window.[60,61] To avoid compromising the chance for cure, the phase 2 window approach is reserved for patients in high-risk categories where treatment results remain unsatisfactory, such as metastatic osteosarcoma,[62] unresectable rhabdomyosarcoma,[57,63–66] or disseminated neuroblastoma,[60] or poor prognosis brain tumors.[67–69] When this approach is used, it is imperative that patients and their parents be fully informed about the role and optional nature of upfront window research in the patient's overall treatment plan.[70]

Phase 2 Trials: Specific Designs—Multiple Arms

The biggest disadvantage of single arms studies is that they do not permit direct comparison of their results with those of other studies. Formal comparison among interventions is most commonly performed in randomized phase 3 trials, discussed in detail later. Recently, however, the desire to compare outcomes earlier has led to development of randomized phase 2 designs. The concept is controversial, with some arguing that multiple randomized arms should be used sparingly,[15] while others argue that randomization is needed for better, more reliable conclusions.[71] It is clear that randomized phase 2 trials often serve different objectives, that the objectives are unfortunately often unclear in the trial report,[72] and that the advantages and disadvantages of randomization differ depending on the objectives.[73,74] *First*, in some cases, randomization may be used to facilitate the simultaneous conduct of multiple single arm studies without any intent to compare the arms. *Second*, randomization to one or more experimental treatments or a control has been proposed as a way to validate the historical control data used to design the trial.[71,75] This can be reassuring when the control data are as expected, but it is often unclear how to proceed when the controls are not as expected. Single-arm trials may be preferred when available sample size is small,[75] while randomized trials can be beneficial when sample sizes are larger, or there is greater uncertainty about historical controls, for example, when biomarker positive cases are posited to have a different prognosis from the general population. In both the *first* and *second* case, individual arms are usually designed using single arm approaches. A *third* rationale is to select among two or more competitors. Various approaches to "picking the winner" have been proposed,[76] including a proposal by Sargent et al.[77] that allows for a gray area in which outcomes are similar and other considerations might determine whether formal comparative trials should be undertaken. Traditionally, picking the winner or screening designs are only modestly comparative and have no real ability to determine which arm is better. For example, a trial designed to have a high probability (85%) of selecting the treatment that *appears* to be better, when the true response rates are 30% and 10%, would only need nine subjects in each group,[76] even though this is smaller than the sample size required for a single arm trial ($N = 27$) to test whether the response rate of the new treatment is greater than the historical value, and far smaller than the 57 per group that would be needed to compare the response rates of the two treatments definitively (85% power and a one-sided α of 5%). A *fourth* objective of some randomized phase 2 trials is direct, formal comparison. Although the primary end point of such a trial might be progression-free or event-free survival, or change in a biomarker that would not be appropriate for definitive assessment of clinical benefit, and type I error rates might be substantially loosened, in all other respects, formal comparative design concerns apply. Finally, Bayesian adaptive

randomization designs have also been proposed in which the randomization probabilities start out equal among the arms, but after a certain number of enrolled subjects begin to drift in favor of arms with better-observed outcomes.[78,79] Such methods may prove useful for more rapid paired development of targeted therapy and biomarkers.[80] Designs have also been developed to permit seamless transition from a randomized phase 2 study to a definitive phase 3 study, with selection of treatment arms to be studied in phase 3 based on the phase 2 results.[81–83]

Phase 2 Trials: Sample Size, Subject Population, and Reporting

Pediatric phase 2 trials are relatively small, with samples sizes generally in the 15 to 30 subjects per arm range, depending on the response rate of interest. Calculations are design specific but are often based on exact probability calculations using the binomial distribution. These can be computationally intensive. For example, Simon designs require exhaustive examination of possible responses within an approximated target range. Primary end point analyses are also driven by the specifics of the design. In most designs, the parameters for decision making (to accept or reject the new treatment) are determined ahead of time. As in phase 1 reports, patients' characteristics, toxicities, and primary and secondary end points are summarized descriptively.

Phase 3 Trials: Objectives and End Points

The purpose of a phase 3 trial is to definitively compare the efficacy of an experimental therapy with that of a standard or control therapy to determine whether the new therapeutic strategy should be adopted. Because the results of the trial will likely alter clinical practice if positive and because we do not want to miss real improvements, the design must minimize false-positive and false-negative results. Randomized trials are strongly preferred because comparisons based on historical controls trials can be and often are biased due to changes over time in population, therapy, and supportive care. Observed differences in outcome in historically controlled studies are always potentially attributable to causes that are not related to treatment and are always suspect. The most reliable way to generate unbiased comparisons between treatments is to allocate similar patients to different treatment arms by randomization (see later). This helps ensure comparability of the groups, equalizing sources of variability other than treatment. The most common approach is a an active control, two-arm study in which one group of patients receives the current best standard therapy and the other receives the new therapy to be tested. Less commonly, multiple new therapies may be compared or active therapy may be compared with "best supportive care." Improvements in outcome to be detected are generally modest and samples sizes must be large. Large randomized pediatric phase 3 trials are usually feasible only in cooperative group or multicenter settings because of the scarcity of patients. Occasionally, though, even the multicenter approach is inadequate and a carefully done historically controlled trial, however imperfect, may be the only way to evaluate a new therapy.

The ideal end point for evaluation of clinical benefit in oncology is improvement in overall survival, although this may not be practical when deaths tend to occur long after treatment. Consequently, alternative end points are often chosen that are presumed to be early signals of long-term survival, such as the disappearance of detectable tumor or the absence of recurrence or metastases at 3 years. These alternative end points may not always reflect survival, however, as when salvage therapies are effective despite prior treatment failure; or when the influence of an adverse outcome during the first treatment is abrogated by the successful second treatment. As a result, an end point that is widely used in trials of childhood malignancies is "event-free survival." An *event* is defined as "the first occurrence of the major events that represent initial treatment failure: failure to achieve remission (i.e., death in the induction period or nonresponse), relapse at any site after achieving remission, and death in remission without preceding relapse."[84] This end point, also called *failure-free survival* or *time to first event*, is meaningful for studies in any disease population, but it is especially appropriate for trials in which most patients achieve remission and many achieve long-term survival. Increasingly important in studies of children are coprimary or secondary end points regarding adverse and late effects of treatment, such as the occurrence of second malignancies, growth disturbances, neuropsychologic impairment attributed to therapy, and quality of life.

Phase 3 Trials: Sample Size

Sample sizes of phase 3 trials vary widely but can range from as few as several hundred to thousands or even tens of thousands, as in adult prostate or breast cancer prevention trials. The required sample size for a randomized phase 3 study depends on several things: (a) the type of outcome variable (i.e., binary, survival time) and the corresponding statistical method that will be used; (b) the minimum difference in outcome considered important to detect; (c) the expected outcome with standard therapy; (d) the levels of type I and type II errors that are considered acceptable. A type I or α error is the conclusion that the new treatment is better than the standard treatment when in fact it is not. The probability of a type I error is the significance level of the experiment and is denoted by α. A type II or β error is the failure to conclude that the new treatment is different (superior) to the standard when it actually is. The probability of a type II error is denoted by β; its complement $(1-\beta)$ is called the *power* of the experiment. In contrast to phase 2 trials, α in phase 3 trials is usually set to be small (i.e., 5% or even 1%) while β is usually larger than α, although still relatively small (i.e., 20% or 10%). These error rates represent the risk of making two different kinds of mistakes—carrying forward a useless, potentially toxic or expensive therapy or throwing away a potentially useful therapy—and depending on the specific circumstances, the costs associated with these mistakes are different and should help determine the acceptable error rates. Ideally, both error rates should be small, but smaller error rates require larger sample sizes, which may become impractical.

Statistical tests can be one sided or two sided. A one-sided test considers differences in only one direction. For example, if treatments A and B are compared, a one-sided test will permit only two conclusions: A is better than B, or A is not better than B. A two-sided test permits a third conclusion: A is worse than B. Because a two-sided test allows for type I errors in both directions, a larger sample size is required to restrict the overall type I error to the same desired level. Although we are often primarily interested in showing improvement and would not change clinical practice if the new treatment is worse, defining situations in which one-sided tests are appropriate is controversial and most journals require reporting two-sided p values.

The sample size also depends on the type of end point and the statistical methods that will be used. In this regard, phase 3 clinical trials are like many other experiments and a wide range of general statistical references are available.[7,85–87] Sample size considerations for time variables (e.g., event-free survival, overall survival, and remission duration) are especially important in oncology trials and require special consideration.[88] A key feature that distinguishes "time to" variables from other outcomes is the problem of "censored data"—survival times for patients who drop out prior to experiencing an event, or remain alive or event free at the time of study reporting. We thus need to account for the time period over which subjects will be accrued, the expected fraction of dropouts and the amount of follow-up after accrual closes, since these variables will determine the average length of follow-up. Coupled with the hypothesized hazard function (usually for simplicity assumed to be constant), this will determine the expected fraction that will be censored. Somewhat paradoxically, slower accrual will lengthen the average follow-up and reduce censoring, making the total required sample size slightly smaller, although it will take longer to get an answer. In some instances, particularly with pediatric tumors, a substantial cure rate can be anticipated, so the risk of recurrence will decrease over time, and the assumption of constant hazard is untenable. Sposto and Sather developed methods for determining sample sizes in this situation.[89]

The size of the difference we are interested in detecting must be carefully considered, because the required sample size is extremely sensitive to this difference. For example, if we wanted to be 80% certain of observing a statistically significant difference ($\alpha = 5\%$) in 6-month relapse rates when the true event rates were 20% and 40%, 91 patients per arm would be required. For relapse rates of 20% and 30%, however, we would need 313 per arm, and for rates of 20% and 25%, 1,134 per arm. When the difference to be detected is reduced by half, the required sample size more than triples. Reliable detection of small differences, although possibly desirable, is not an achievable goal for most pediatric studies. On the other hand, the specified difference must be small enough so that a study finding "no statistically significant difference" is convincingly negative (see also section "Equivalence Trials," later). If a study is designed only to detect large differences, smaller but clinically meaningful differences may be observed but fail to reach statistical significance. In such a case, the observed difference may be too large to conclude that the two treatments are equivalent but too small to exclude chance as the basis for the difference, and the trial will fail to provide useful information. A properly designed trial should be informative, regardless of the outcome.

Phase 3 Trials: Randomization

The purpose of randomization is to avoid systematic bias in the allocation of patients to treatment in comparative trials. A *bias* is the effect on a study result of some systematic aspect of study design, data collection, or analysis that is unrelated to the actual effect of the treatment under study. For example, a comparison of a medical treatment with a surgical procedure in which treatment assignment depends on a patient's health status (e.g., patients who receive medical treatment are those whose poor condition precludes surgical procedures) is biased. The surgically treated patients are in better shape from the beginning; if their outcomes are better, one has no way to know how much of this superiority is attributable to treatment. Although this is an extreme example, bias can find its way into even the most meticulously randomized trial.

Bias will almost surely be introduced if an investigator knows or can predict which treatment a patient will be assigned. Although we often describe randomization to patients as "flipping a coin," in practice randomization is usually implemented by a computer program that can generate an unpredictable list while still ensuring equal allocation of subjects throughout the study.

When subgroups of patients with identifiably different prognoses are studied in the same trial, a stratified randomization plan may be considered. The purpose of stratification is to ensure that patients with different prognoses are evenly distributed over treatments. The simplest way is to generate separate randomization sequences for each subgroup. However, having too many strata resulting in many small subgroups can cause problems, undoing some of the benefits of randomization. An adaptive allocation method to avoid this, called *minimization*, involves assigning new patients to treatments in a way that tends to minimize the imbalance between treatments on important factors.[90–92]

Registration and randomization are usually accomplished by providing subject information to a central office. Verification of eligibility and the timing of randomization are important. If there is a substantial lag between randomization and initiation of the treatment, some patients may not receive the assigned treatment. Some change their minds; some experience changes in status, making the treatment no longer appropriate; and some die. Including these patients in the analysis dilutes the effect, while leaving them out can introduce bias, especially if the dropouts are not random. Patients should generally be randomized as close in time as possible to the point at which the comparator treatments actually begin.

Phase 3 Trials: Sequential Designs

Historically, the motivation for the use of sequential designs was the desire for efficiency, achieved by terminating an experiment as soon as the answer is "known." In the context of clinical trials, the motivation is primarily ethical. If early results indicate that one treatment is producing substantially improved outcomes, it becomes difficult to justify the continued randomization to the apparently inferior arm. It may also be desirable to stop for futility—that is, when it is clear that the trial will not find a difference or when the new treatment is worse. The problem is how to determine when superiority (or futility) is "known."

Because the type I error increases with more frequent interim monitoring, simple rules, such as stopping the study as soon as the p value reaches 0.05, lead to grossly increased type I (false positive) errors. For example, if the data are reviewed 10 times during the course of a study in which the true efficacies are identical, the probability of declaring a difference is approximately 20%.[93] The fundamental problem here is that of "multiple comparisons." Several different approaches have been developed to deal with the problem of inflating type I errors by frequent evaluation of study results and mainly involve requiring smaller p values at individual looks to compensate for multiple looks. *Group sequential designs* are especially attractive because they are based on analysis of data at a few interim time points, as groups of data are accumulated.[94–97] The simplest approach is to use the same more stringent α level at every look (Fig. 17.3, Pocock). Although the overall α error is, in fact, preserved, this design can seem unnecessarily stringent at the final analysis. An alternative, widely used design was proposed by O'Brien and Fleming.[94] Their method uses a sequence of p values for successive analyses: the first is exceptionally small, with the remainder gradually increasing so the final p value is close to the conventional level (typically 0.05). The O'Brien-Fleming approach could be made more flexible by thinking of the overall study α error rate as something that can be "spent" over the course of the study, allowing the rate of spending, number of looks, and spacing of looks to be flexible.[98]

Originally, these approaches were intended to allow for the possibility of early termination if one treatment appears markedly superior to the other, but it is also desirable to stop in the face of futility if the treatments are not going to be different. Just as multiple looks can inflate the type I error rate, multiple opportunities to stop for futility can inflate the type II error rate (false negative) and reduce study power. Although methods to address this problem are numerous, two widely used approaches involve either setting O'Brien-Fleming–like p value boundaries or calculation of Bayesian-like predictive probabilities. In the first case, the trial is planned to stop if the

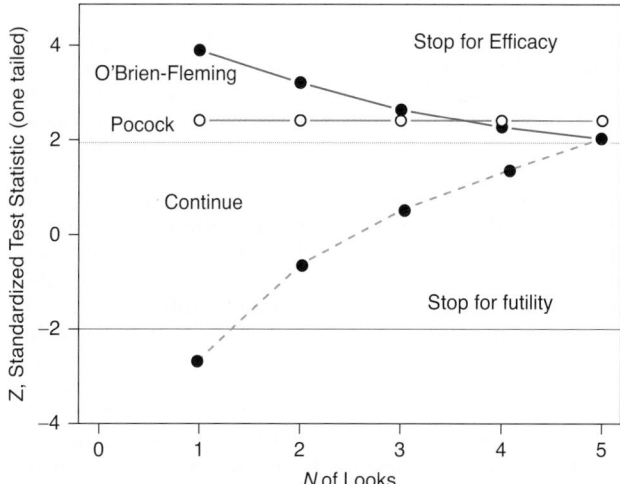

FIGURE 17.3 Example of group sequential monitoring boundaries to protect error rates ($\alpha = 0.025$ one tailed, $\beta = 0.15$, number of looks = 5). Thin dotted lines show the traditional critical value(s) for a single analysis at the end of the trial ($p = 0.025$, one-tailed). Solid lines show efficacy stopping boundaries (critical values) for the Pocock (open) or O'Brien-Fleming strategies. At each look, a test statistic above the critical point will result in a recommendation to stop for efficacy. The dashed line shows stopping boundaries for futility. At each look, a test statistic that is below the critical value (i.e., has a very large p value) will result in a recommendation to stop for futility. Results that fall between the dashed and solid lines (closed circles) will result in study continuation.

observed p value from a one-sided test for superiority exceeds some large (i.e., $p > 0.8$) value, suggesting that a low (significant) p value at the end of the trial will not be achieved. Recently, this method was used to stop a trial of docetaxel in non-small cell lung cancer.[99] Alternatively, one can estimate the probability of declaring a statistically significant result at the end of the trial, given the data accumulated to date (under varying assumptions of how the future data will play out), and stop the trial if the probability is sufficiently small. A trial of biochemotherapy versus interferon-α-2b in melanoma is an example of stopping in this manner.[100]

Phase 3 Trials: Factorial Designs

Phase 3 trials can compare more than two treatments at once. In a factorial design, two or more questions are addressed simultaneously in the same cohort of patients.[101,102] For example, in the National Wilms' Tumor Study III, early stage patients were randomized between postoperative radiotherapy and no postoperative radiotherapy, and also between two different chemotherapy regimens.[103] If the effect of each factor can be assumed to operate independently of the other (i.e., the difference in efficacy of the adjuvant therapy regimens does not depend on whether radiotherapy is used and vice versa), each question can be evaluated by collapsing over the categories of the other question, effectively doubling the sample size/group. This assumption of independent effects is critical and if the data cast doubt on its validity, categories are not collapsible, and the power of the study is drastically reduced.

Phase 3 Trials: Equivalence Trials

An equivalence trial (sometimes called a *noninferiority trial*) is a phase 3 trial whose purpose is to demonstrate that a new treatment is no less efficacious than a standard treatment. This is important if the new treatment is clearly more desirable than the standard in some other way (e.g., less toxic, less invasive, less expensive, or more convenient). In such a case, one would prefer the new treatment as long as efficacy was not reduced. Enough patients must be entered into an equivalence study to demonstrate that a negative result is convincingly negative. A result of "no significant difference" is not sufficient, because one can easily assure such a result by designing a study too small to detect a difference even if it is really there. In general, for these types of studies, the preferred design is one in which the minimal difference of interest (usually denoted as d) is specified as the drug effect under the null hypothesis, and the alternative hypothesis is that there is no difference. Thus, the treatments cannot be accepted as equivalent unless one can rule out with high probability that any decrement in effect is no greater than d. Sample sizes for equivalence trials are usually larger than those in difference-seeking trials because physicians are very reluctant to adopt a new treatment that is less effective than current treatments; the decrement in efficacy that must be ruled out in a noninferiority trial is usually smaller that the targeted increase in efficacy in a superiority study. Sample size considerations and other aspects of equivalence/noninferiority study design are discussed in a number of useful references.[104–108]

Phase 3 Trials: Biomarker Targeted Trials

Molecularly targeted therapies are an increasingly important focus of clinical oncologic research in adults and in pediatrics. The proper design and interpretation of these trials is complex and is an area of active methodologic research. There are several key questions to be asked in considering such a trial. First, how certain are we of the relevance of the putative target or biomarker? If we are very sure, then we might want to limit the trial to subjects exhibiting the target, otherwise we might accrue too many subjects who have no chance of showing the effect of the intervention. Second, how good is the assay for the biomarker? If there is no reliable assay, then it does not matter whether the biomarker is relevant or not, because we cannot measure the effect of intervention on it. Third, how common is the target? If the target is very common, then even if the therapy is of limited or no value in biomarker negative patients, we should see an overall effect. Otherwise, if the biomarker is rare, then any useful effect in the biomarker positive group, no matter how big, will be diluted by lack of benefit in the overall group. Classic examples of this latter issue from adult oncology (breast cancer) include tamoxifen and the estrogen receptor, which is commonly positive, and trastuzumab and Her-2, which is much less commonly positive. The benefit of tamoxifen was observed despite including estrogen receptor negative and positive patients, while trastuzumab was studied only in Her-2–positive subjects and might not have been approved if it had been studied in a broader population less likely to respond.

Phase 0 Trials

Recently, the concept of the "phase 0" trial has been proposed. Phase 0 trials are intended to facilitate more rapid development of molecularly targeted agents by allowing first-in-human studies at extremely low, almost certainly subtherapeutic single doses. The purpose is to allow demonstration of drug-target interactions and to gain pharmacokinetic/pharmacodynamic experience that, in theory, would help better design therapeutic trials; there is no therapeutic intent of the phase 0 trial itself. Very few such trials have been performed, and their use is controversial.[109–112] In particular, the Task Force on Methodology for the Development of Innovative Cancer Therapies reviewed some of the advantages and concerns and urges careful thought before proceeding.[110] In view of the ethical challenges, and the current tendency to develop drugs in adults prior to testing in children, there seems to be little need for phase 0 trials in children at present.

Feasibility Assessment

In addition to the statistical considerations discussed earlier, clinical research in children has unique challenges that must be taken into consideration during study design. Issues that must be considered include developmental differences in physiology and metabolism, which may result in different adverse effects in patients of different ages; wide variability limitations in subjects' physical size, which may limit the amount of blood that can be obtained for research purposes; and the need for palatable drug formulations, especially if young children will be enrolled. In addition, for studies evaluating the adverse effects or toxicities of treatment, prolonged follow-up for years following exposure may be required. Studies requiring subject follow-up beyond the age of 18 years require reconsent when the child reaches the age of majority and may be challenging to perform, given issues with patient relocation during adulthood. Even a statistically well-designed study will fail if these kinds of issues make it impossible to complete.

Protocol Writing

Integral to planning a clinical trial is writing the actual protocol, which can be viewed as an operating manual for the experiment to be conducted. As a procedural guide, the protocol helps to ensure that the investigation is carried out uniformly. This section will discuss common components of a written protocol. Templates containing these elements are available at the NCI's Cancer Trials Web site.[113]

Goals and Objectives

This section of the protocol enumerates the primary and any secondary objectives, as discussed previously.

Background

The background section presents the arguments for conducting the clinical trial and for selecting the specific experimental conditions detailed in subsequent sections and should provide adequate justification for the study. The significance and rationale of the proposed trial should be within the perspective provided by preclinical (*in vitro* and animal) data and previous clinical trials. Phase 2 protocols additionally should include a summary of available data on toxicity in adults and children and a justification of the choice of tumors against which the agent will be assessed. A well-written background section provides collaborating investigators with sufficient information to understand why the trial is being done and what is currently known about the research questions being asked; the goal is not to write a comprehensive review article on all the topics being studied.

Patient Eligibility and Enrollment

The protocol should define the characteristics of the patient population to be studied, including factors such as diagnosis, extent of disease (stage), age restrictions, allowable prior therapy, physiologic and performance status, and any other conditions the investigator wishes to specify, such as the expression of particular biologic markers by malignant cells. In the United States, informed consent must be obtained from patients or parents (depending on patient age) before any research procedures can be performed to establish eligibility (see later).

It is important to note that the population defined by the eligibility criteria is the one to which the study results apply; thus, the criteria should be defined so that what is learned in the trial will be generalizable to a meaningful group of patients. The relatively small number of pediatric patients available for clinical trials must also be considered, because overly restrictive criteria can result in failure to accrue adequate patient numbers.

Strict eligibility criteria, resulting in homogeneity of patients, are more important in phase 1 and phase 2 studies. Phase 1 protocols generally specify patients in whom conventional therapy has failed yet who have sufficiently intact organ function to allow accurate assessment of drug toxicity. Enough time (usually 2 to 4 weeks) should have elapsed since the most recent antitumor therapy to ensure that the short-term effects of that treatment have subsided. The type of DLTs expected, and the mechanisms of drug metabolism and clearance, if known, should be taken into account when determining the criteria for organ function required for a patient to be eligible. For example, if myelosuppression is expected to be dose limiting, subjects with bone marrow involvement by tumor may not be appropriate for dose-finding studies. Regardless of tumor type, performance status sufficient to permit assessment of drug-related effects should be specified.

Phase 2 protocols usually specify histologic diagnoses acceptable for entry, because the end point often depends on the tumor type. Patients are also generally required to have measurable disease, so antitumor response can be assessed accurately.

In phase 3 studies, the issue of generalizability of results obtained in the study population to the affected population as a whole becomes more important. In these trials, it is important to select patients with reasonable potential to show benefit, whether due to decreased toxicity or improved survival, from the experimental therapy. Patients whose prognosis is so good that changes in therapy are unlikely to have an observable positive effect should generally be excluded. It is also appropriate to exclude patients with contraindications to any of the study treatments or those who have other serious conditions that may interfere with administration of therapy.

Treatment Plan

The treatments to be delivered on protocol should be precisely and thoroughly defined to promote uniformity of conditions throughout the experiment. All aspects of therapy should be set forth, including surgical procedures to be used and supportive care guidelines. Provisions for treatment modifications in the event of toxicity should be specified. In complex protocols, a scheme that shows the temporal relationships of chemotherapy and other treatment modalities from study entry through various treatment phases (e.g., induction, consolidation, or maintenance) to discontinuation of therapy is particularly useful. Details about the indications for removal of a patient from therapy may be included here as well.

Drug Information

This section includes details about the mechanism of action, animal and human toxicology data, and pharmaceutical information for each of the drugs used in the clinical trial. This information is included to ensure consistency of preparation and administration of drugs and is an important quality control and safety measure. The protocol is often the only available source of pharmaceutical information for investigational drugs.

Evaluations/Data to Be Collected

The data set required for determination of eligibility and evaluation of treatment effect must be presented in the protocol. This set includes pretreatment, on-treatment, and posttreatment evaluations, indicating specific clinical and laboratory assessments and their timing. These schedules are often presented in tabular form. In comparative trials, the frequency and nature of these assessments must be identical for the regimens being compared with avoid an unbalanced increase in the likelihood of detecting real or chance differences resulting from disparities in medical surveillance. Clinical trials are also used to provide systematic information about the natural history of the disease or to obtain other biologic or correlative samples, independent of therapeutic intervention.[114] Limited resources invariably require careful consideration of the minimum data that can be collected and still support the study objectives.

The design of data collection forms requires the input of a clinician, statistician, data manager, and computer programmer. The designers must ensure that items are unambiguously presented, coding procedures are consistent and straightforward, the form is structured for efficiency in entering and keying the data, and the format of the data allows efficient analysis. Forms should be designed with ease of completion as a primary consideration. Errors are more likely to be made when the form is filled out than at any other point in the data management process. Because delay in completing the data forms increases the potential for errors and for missing data that may become irretrievable, a schedule for collection of data should be established. Proper monitoring of a study cannot be reliably accomplished without a continually current database.

Statistical Considerations

Statistical considerations for each objective of the study are included in the protocol. The targeted effect size and error rates, the estimated number of patients required for assessment of the primary and secondary end points, the anticipated rate of patient accrual, and the expected duration of the trial (including follow-up) are given along with the description of the proposed analysis of outcome data. In describing the study, the availability of patients should be documented whenever possible to show that study objective and sample size plans are realistic.

The definitions of both response (such as complete response, partial response, progressive disease) and toxicity (such as dose limiting toxicity, MTD) end points are presented in this section. These definitions must be clear enough so that treating physicians can apply the criteria consistently to their own patients to determine appropriate clinical actions such as removal of patients from study because of progressive disease as well as to submit their patients' outcomes accurately for further analysis.

Regulatory Affairs

Managing regulatory affairs is a critical part of conducting a clinical trial. In the narrowest sense, this means attention to documentation of compliance with study requirements such as eligibility criteria, drug administration, laboratory and clinical follow-up, and response and toxicity measurement for each individual subject entered onto the trial. In a broader sense, regulatory affairs encompass the sponsors' and investigators' obligations to ensure that the conduct of the study falls within legal and ethical guidelines set forth by the relevant agencies (e.g., in the Good Clinical Practices Guidance document adopted by the US Food and Drug Administration [FDA] as well as regulatory agencies in other countries).[115] Although some regulatory activities, such as obtaining informed consent from subjects, do not take place until the clinical trial is activated, careful consideration of the requirements starting early in the trial design process may circumvent many difficulties and prevent frustrating delays in the initiation of the study.

The sponsor of a clinical trial may be the investigator initiating the trial, a pharmaceutical company, or an entity such as the NCI's Division of Cancer Treatment and Diagnosis. The sponsor is legally responsible for the overall conduct of the trial. Early in the design of the study, the sponsor must consider whether there are special regulatory requirements for the particular type of research in question. For example, if the trial involves an investigational agent, the sponsor must submit to the FDA an Investigational New Drug application. The Investigational New Drug application details the preclinical pharmacology and toxicology experience, the relevant manufacturing information, and details of the proposed clinical trial.

The sponsor of a protocol involving an investigational agent is also responsible for ensuring that individual investigators and participating institutions fulfill their regulatory responsibilities. At each institution, the investigators must obtain appropriate review of the protocol by an Institutional Review Board (IRB). The IRB's duty is to ensure that human subjects participating in clinical trials are protected from research-related risks. The philosophy behind such protection is stated in the Nuremberg Code, the Declaration of Helsinki, and the Belmont Report and codified in the United States in federal law.[116–121] Central to the protection of human subjects is the concept of informed consent, which is discussed in detail in Chapter 46. It is important to note that good scientific design of the clinical trial is an absolute requirement for protection of human subjects, not only because potential benefits will be maximized and risks minimized in a good trial but also because a poorly designed study that is unable to answer the research question cannot offer patients or society any benefit to offset the potential risk of participation.

Once the study is open, the sponsor and investigators are responsible for strict adherence to the principles of good study conduct. The sponsor must ensure that there has been compliance with the protocol requirements, that the data reported are accurate, and that all study procedures have been followed. In particular, adverse event reporting to the appropriate regulatory bodies is an important part of every investigator's obligations, and the procedures for such reporting should be carefully outlined in the study protocol. The accuracy of data submitted on the case report forms for each subject is usually verified using audits of the medical records of some or all participating patients. Finally, compliance with study procedures ensures that appropriate IRB approvals, individual subjects' informed consent, and study drug accountability are all correctly documented.[122]

Informed Consent

All research projects that involve human subjects and are conducted or supported in part or entirely by the US Department of Health and Human Services are subject to regulations regarding the protection of those subjects (see Chapter 46).[119] The Office for Human Research Protection is the government agency charged with ensuring that all research is conducted according to these regulations. International Conference on Harmonization guidelines contain similar recommendations and are often used by sponsors conducting multinational studies.

The documentation for a multicenter clinical trial should include a sample informed consent document, which can be reviewed by the NCI or other appropriate agency for completeness and also can be used by individual sites in a multi-center trial to construct the consent document to be used at that institution. The local version of the consent should not differ substantially from the sample document and must contain all federally required elements.

Federal law prescribes additional protections specifically for children who are subjects of clinical research.[123] Children are defined as persons who have not reached the legal age of consent to treatments or procedures involved in the research; legal age is determined by the applicable law of the jurisdiction in which the research is conducted. Informed consent must be obtained from the parent or guardian before research procedures can begin. The informed consent of one parent is usually adequate if the child is being enrolled onto a study from which he or she may receive direct benefit from the research, such as in a therapeutic trial. In addition to the informed consent of the parent, investigators wishing to enroll children onto clinical trials must obtain assent from the child in a manner appropriate for the child's age and developmental status. Although the process of obtaining informed consent can be difficult and time consuming, it is critical to the ethical conduct of clinical research.

Managing the Clinical Trial

Subject Registration

After consent is obtained, study subjects should be formally registered as study participants before receiving any protocol-directed intervention. Pretreatment registration ensures that all patients who begin treatment can be identified for reporting purposes at the end of the study. In addition, the process of registration can be used to verify that the patient meets the eligibility criteria. Checklists are often used at the time of patient registration or randomization to ensure that the patient actually is eligible and willing to participate before he or she is formally entered on the study. Registration is important, even in studies conducted within a single institution, as a quality control measure to prevent the inadvertent loss of "problem patients," such as those who die or refuse further therapy after only one or two doses of drug, from the reporting process.

Quality Control

All studies should have a clear plan outlining how data quality and study safety will be monitored throughout the clinical trial. *Quality control* refers to all the checks and reviews of data over the course of the study that are designed to make sure that the protocol is appropriately followed and the data submitted are accurate. Much of the responsibility for quality control during the course of the study falls to the central data management personnel.

Data entry procedures should be developed to minimize errors, and a system must be devised to notify physicians or data managers about errors, to request corrected or updated information, and to flag persistent errors. Quality control programs at exemplary clinical research centers also include self-audits, standard operating procedures, recording of study violations and corrective action programs.[124] For cooperative group studies and industry trials, additional quality assurance reviews are routinely performed to ensure the accuracy and integrity of the clinical data.

Complex protocols often require initial training sessions for surgeons, radiotherapists, pathologists, and others who may need more instruction in the experimental procedures than can be reliably transmitted in the written protocol. For such protocols, a study initiation meeting, in which all personnel from treatment providers to data managers discuss the protocol and receive detailed training, can be valuable.

Many aspects of the protocol may require central review. For example, when radiotherapy is an important part of an experimental treatment program, a centralized quality assurance review of the port films is mandatory to ensure that the treatments are administered according to the protocol. Review must be prompt, especially at the beginning of a study, so that problems can be corrected before they affect a large proportion of the study population. Pathology and surgical reports must be reviewed for final determination of patient eligibility. Reports of responses, relapses, or other events of interest may also require review. The responsibility for data reviews is usually shared among the study chairperson, data management staff, and treatment specialists. A position paper on quality assurance in multicenter trials published by a special committee of the Society for Clinical Trials addresses a variety of issues in assuring high-quality clinical trials data and is one of the few published sources of recommendations in this important area.[125]

Subject Follow-Up

For patients entered on phase 1 and phase 2 trials, follow-up is typically limited to the period during which the end points of primary interest (e.g., acute toxicity and tumor response or progression) may be seen. Phase 3 studies, with the goal of defining optimal treatment strategies, require more extensive follow-up. Ideally, all patients enrolled in phase 3 clinical trials of cancer treatment should be followed throughout the remainder of their lives, although this is not always feasible due to limited resources. Extended follow-up has two major purposes. The first is to maintain a check on the treatment comparisons by detecting any late crossing of survival curves and obtaining better estimates of possible cure rates. The second is to detect late adverse effects of the treatment that may not be evident when trial results are initially reported. In pediatric trials, late adverse affects include second malignancies, sterility, and cognitive dysfunction. Follow-up forms should specifically request information about known or suspected adverse effects of the therapies used and the disease studied and information about all other adverse effects noted, regardless of whether an association between the effect and prior treatment appears plausible.

The desirable frequency of follow-up reporting varies with the time since study entry. Patients should be assessed frequently, preferably three or four times a year, as long as the study is in an active stage (i.e., before reporting of results). Without frequent follow-up, one cannot monitor study results reliably. For example, extreme differences observed early in a study might lead to consideration of early termination. Without current follow-up on all patients, one cannot know to what extent the observed difference may be an artifact of delayed reporting. At some point (e.g., 3 to 5 years) after study completion, a large proportion of surviving subjects may be expected to be long-term survivors. It may then be reasonable to request follow-up reporting only on a semiannual or yearly basis.

Data Monitoring Plan

Data from clinical trials must be regularly monitored to check for problems in implementing study procedures, for unexpectedly severe toxicity that may require modification of doses/schedules or even termination of the study, or for early evidence for or against beneficial treatment effects that may also require early termination. Early phase nonrandomized trials are often monitored in real time, as with the modified

CRM, by the investigator or a small team of investigators in conjunction with a data review committee.

Randomized trials usually require a formal data monitoring committee, sometimes called a Data Safety Monitoring Board (DSMB) generally separate from the investigators, to evaluate interim results on a regular basis and to make recommendations to those responsible for the trial (i.e., investigators, IRB, other regulatory agencies, cooperative groups). The voting members of these committees are generally clinicians, statisticians, patient advocates, and other subject matter experts. The committee reviews the accumulating data on a schedule related to the trial design and may recommend modifications to the study design (including early termination) based on the interim results. Although statistical concerns play an important role in aiding committee deliberations, interim monitoring decisions are multifaceted.[126–129] Results of interim analyses, unless they are conclusive, must be kept strictly confidential within the confines of the committee, because disclosure of nondefinitive trends in the accumulating data could lead to changes in subsequent patient selection and enrollment, biasing outcomes.

Data Analysis

The most efficient, most sophisticated statistical analysis cannot compensate for major errors in the design or conduct of a clinical trial. This does not, however, diminish the importance of proper selection and use of analytic procedures even for a well-designed trial.

Hypothesis Testing

At the end of the trial, one has to make a decision, for example, whether the new treatment is better than control. In phase 3 comparative trials, this is most often done based on a statistical test of the null hypothesis (no difference in treatment effect) against an alternative hypothesis (unequal effects). When the data demonstrate a sufficiently large difference in patient outcome, the null hypothesis may be rejected. We compute an appropriate test statistic (Table 17.2) that is essentially a summary of all the data in the study, and compare that to the distribution of possible test statistics that would be expected if the null hypothesis were true. The p value associated with the statistical test of the null hypothesis can be interpreted as follows. If the null hypothesis were true (i.e., if there were truly no difference in treatment effect), the probability of an observed difference as large or larger than this one would be equal to p. Thus, if p is small (i.e., <0.025 one tailed), the observed data may be considered sufficiently inconsistent with the null hypothesis to warrant its rejection. Failure to reject the null hypothesis does not demonstrate that the null hypothesis is true, as discussed in section "Equivalence Trials."

Avoidance of Bias

The most common cause of bias at the analysis stage of clinical trials is the improper exclusion of patients from analysis. This exclusion can affect not only comparisons of treatments but also estimates of the effect of a single regimen. A good rule is that patients who meet the eligibility criteria, who are entered on the study, and who begin treatment should be included in the analysis of study data. This approach is known as *intention to treat*, because analysis includes all patients intended to receive the assigned treatment, whether or not it was ultimately fully administered.[130]

An unbiased estimate of the probability of response to a treatment regimen in a given patient population requires the inclusion of all patients in that population who have been

TABLE 17.2

STATISTICAL TESTS FOR EVALUATING VARIOUS OUTCOME MEASURES

Measurement scale of outcome	Example of an outcome	Examples of relevant tests of hypothesis
Nominal	Response/nonresponse	Chi square, Fisher's exact, logistic regression
Ordinal	Grade of toxicity	Chi square, ordered logistic regression
Interval	Change in T regulatory cells	t Test, Wilcoxon rank sum test, ANOVA, etc.

treated with the regimen. Patients who die or who refuse further therapy after only one or two doses of drug are representative of some fraction of the overall population who may be eligible for this regimen but who will not benefit from it because their disease is too far advanced or because they find the treatment intolerable. When such patients are classified as "inevaluable" and are excluded from study analysis, the resulting response rate will overestimate the proportion of patients in the target population who would actually show tumor regression if treated with the regimen. A response rate has a clear meaning only if the numerator is the number of patients who respond and the denominator is the total number treated. The proportion of responders among patients who receive "adequate" treatment (as defined by each investigator) may have some secondary interest but is not readily interpretable by the medical community at large.

In a randomized study, improper exclusions can clearly bias the treatment comparison. Consider a population of children who have achieved complete response to induction therapy and are then randomized to receive either maintenance therapy or no further treatment. The protocol requires that maintenance therapy begin within 14 days of completion of induction therapy. For some patients, initiation of maintenance therapy is delayed; several other patients become sicker or die in this interval; and a few patients refuse maintenance therapy despite their prior agreement. Some investigators exclude such patients from analysis on the basis that the maintenance therapy may be ineffective if delayed too long (and certainly cannot be effective if not given). It may also be true, however, that patients with poorer prognoses are more likely to present these kinds of problems. Moreover, patients randomized to "no further therapy" are not excluded on the basis of treatment delay or inadequate courses of therapy. Thus, the exclusions may bias the comparison in favor of the maintenance treatment. Additional discussion of this topic is provided by Gail.[131]

Multiple Comparisons and Subsets

The issue of multiple comparisons has already been mentioned in the context of group sequential designs. Similar problems of error inflation arise when examining outcomes in multiple subsets of cases, or when examining multiple outcomes. Depending on the number of tests of hypotheses, the probability of at least one being spuriously significant can be 40% or more. No totally satisfactory way around this dilemma exists. It does not seem realistic to prohibit exploration of data obtained at great expense, nor does it seem reasonable to require that all tests be done at the strict significance levels needed to ensure that the overall significance

level is protected. An intermediate approach may be to consider questions that are not the primary (preplanned) focus of the trial as exploratory, allowing usual significance level but requiring cautious interpretation and subsequent confirmation.[132–134]

An important example of the multiple comparisons problem in clinical trials is the unplanned analysis of data within patient subsets. To speculate that treatment effects may be limited to or more pronounced in some subgroups of patients is reasonable, but confirming this speculation is difficult without extraordinarily large sample sizes. The more subsets considered, the greater the chances of a false positive result. In randomized studies, one can test for the significance of interactions between treatment and covariate (i.e., differential effects in subsets beyond what is expected by chance); however, the power is generally low. "Qualitative interactions" (i.e., beneficial effect in one subset, harmful effect in the other) are of special interest, but even these are difficult to detect reliably. With multiple unplanned subgroup analyses, the increased type 1 error rate and the reduced power due to small subsamples interpretation results in major difficulties.[135–137]

General Analysis

A well-written protocol will include a reasonably detailed "analysis" plan that should be developed in collaboration with an experienced biostatistician and should be used to guide the analysis and reporting of results, just as the treatment plan guides treatment. A few examples linking major types of outcomes to commonly used methods of analysis are shown in Table 17.2. There are many excellent general[138–141] and more specialized[86,135,142] textbooks on the basic principles of statistical analysis of biomedical data. We focus here on a few issues of particular interest in cancer clinical trials and pediatrics in particular.

In reporting the results of a trial, it is desirable to report both point estimates of the effect of therapy (i.e., response rate = 30%) and some measure of the precision of the estimate (i.e., 90% confidence interval of response rate is 40% to 50%), in addition to p values from hypothesis testing. Two similar studies of different sizes that observe the same effect (i.e., hazard ratio = 0.75) will have different p values, and thus smaller p value alone does not imply a larger, more clinical significant effect. Methods for calculation of confidence intervals depend on the type or scale and distribution properties (i.e., normal, binomial) of the data. For example, confidence intervals for response rates are usually based on exact calculations using the binomial distribution. Trials with group sequential monitoring may require special methods to account for the sequential decision making.[143]

Estimation and comparison of survival outcomes is more complex than binary response outcomes but is of special interest in cancer clinical trials where the primary end point is often overall, disease-free, or event-free survival. If all patients have died, so that all survival times are known, one can directly calculate the median survival and the proportion surviving at various times. Complete survival data, as opposed to incomplete or censored survival data, after appropriate transformation can be analyzed using the same parametric (i.e., t tests, analysis of variance [ANOVA]) or nonparametric methods that are appropriate for other interval scaled data. When some data are censored (i.e., some patients are still alive, so their survival times are known only to be longer than the current follow-up time), estimation of survival is more complicated. The Kaplan-Meier method is probably the most commonly used in cancer studies.[144] Estimated survival curves are plotted as a step function, dropping at each point in time, that is, a death, with tick marks to indicate censored observations

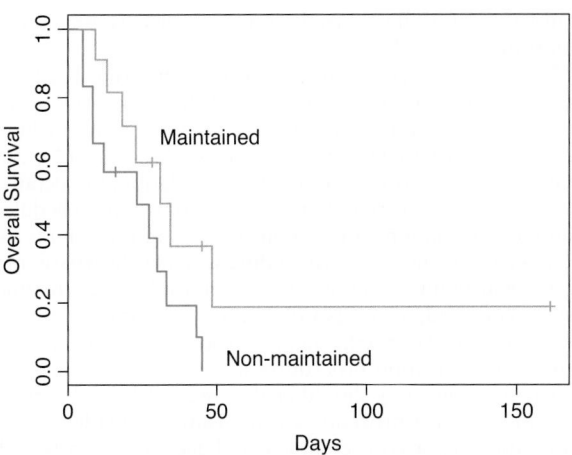

FIGURE 17.4 Kaplan-Meier survival curves for 26 adult patients with AML in complete remission, randomly assigned to maintenance or no maintenance.[145]

(Fig. 17.4). This method can also be used to obtain estimates of median event-free survival, or equivalently, the probability of being alive and event free at particular points in time (e.g., 3 years after diagnosis).

There are several widely used methods for computing confidence intervals and several tests for comparing survival curves including the widely used log-rank test.[86] It might seem tempting in single arm phase 2 studies to try to compare the survival experience of responders with nonresponders, but the fallacious reasoning behind this kind of analysis has been widely discussed.[146–148] One-sample log-rank testing is becoming a more common practice in pediatric oncology. This method allows comparison of the entire experimental group's survival experience with a hypothesized historical control survival distribution.[44] In comparative trials, the log-rank test and a test based on the Cox proportional hazards regression are widely used. Lee and Wang discuss these and other methods for survival analysis in nontechnical terms and provide many excellent examples to illustrate the calculations.[149] The term *proportional hazards* means that the relative superiority of one treatment over another remains constant over time. The assumption of proportional hazards is the basis of the Cox procedure. Although it is not formally required by the log-rank test, marked violation of the assumption compromises interpretability of test results and reduces power. Violations of the assumption to varying degrees are probably common, or even expected, when improvement in long-term survival of pediatric patients may come at the risk of early toxic deaths, but it may still be the appropriate strategy. The additional early deaths may prevent the more toxic regimen from demonstrating a statistically superior survival overall advantage. A number of methods are available to test for non-proportionality.[96,150]

Identification of Prognostic Factors

Recently developed trial designs for codevelopment of biomarkers and targeted therapy have already been discussed. Biomarkers may also be more preliminarily investigated as part of secondary correlative science objectives of the trial. Logistic regression (outcome = response) or Cox regression (outcome = survival) models are widely used. The specific objectives are myriad, including developing predictors of outcome based on known clinical factors and new biomarkers or adjustment for known factors (see later). It should be noted that it is one thing to show that a biomarker is statistically

significantly associated with average outcomes and quite another to show that individual outcomes can be reliably predicted. The former is a common "correlative science" objective in therapeutic clinical trials, the latter more akin to development of a diagnostic test.

The Cox regression model is also useful in dealing with explanatory time-dependent covariates (i.e., covariates that change value over time).[151–153] For example, in a simple bone marrow transplant analysis situation, all patients would start in a chemotherapy "control" group and then certain patients would transition to the BMT group at the times when transplants occur for those patients.[154,155] TDCs can also be used to carry out prognostic factor analysis of serial assessment data such as pharmacologic levels of drug metabolites that are measured at several times during patient follow-up.[156,157]

Evaluating too many factors can lead to serious multiple comparison problems.[158,159] For example, in examining the relationship between a new biomarker and outcome (i.e., disease-free survival), it is common to want to dichotomize the biomarker. If the biomarker has many possible values, it is tempting to try out many possible cutpoints and pick the best one (i.e., most significant), but this can lead to serious overfitting problems. Modern high-dimensional genomic and proteomic technologies vastly increase the number of factors that can be measured on each patients and thus magnify the problem and require even greater care to avoid misleading results.[160–162] Simon and Altman[163] discuss the many pitfalls in the evaluation of prognostic factors and provide detailed guidance for the evaluation of prognostic factors in cancer.

Adjustment for Covariates—Stratified Analysis

Randomization ensures that no systematic bias affects the treatment comparison, but it cannot ensure that the two treatment groups will be identical with regard to prognosis. Even with minimization of stratified randomization as discussed previously, it may happen by chance that more of the patients with a poor prognosis are assigned to one of the treatments. To prevent this type of imbalance from influencing the treatment comparison, one can perform a stratified analysis, essentially analyzing the effects of treatment within and aggregating the results across strata. For example, in a clinical trial of childhood acute lymphoblastic leukemia, one may want to adjust for age by considering outcomes separately for infants (<1 year), children between the ages of 1 and 10 years, and those older than 10 years, because these groups have different prognoses. Even when no imbalances exist, this type of adjusted, or stratified, analysis is more efficient than an unadjusted analysis; by comparing outcomes within homogeneous subgroups, the variability of the overall result is slightly reduced.[164] Both adjusted and unadjusted analyses should be performed and reported whenever important prognostic factors have been identified for the patient population under study.[165,166] For studies intended to provide definitive evaluations, decisions about adjusting for particular covariates should be made before any data analysis to avoid the possibility that the selection of the adjustment strategy may have been influenced by the conclusions that would result.[167]

Meta-Analysis

Meta-analysis is a method for quantitatively summarizing a number of trials by statistically aggregating the results of the several studies. According to Wikipedia, "[t]he first meta-analysis was performed by Karl Pearson in 1904, in an attempt to overcome the problem of reduced statistical power in studies with small sample sizes."[168] Formal meta-analysis has been widely used in the social sciences for many years and is becoming more common in medical research. There are two main approaches, one that seeks to assemble and analyze (stratified by study) individual patient level data from all relevant trials and the other that uses summary statistics for the trials (e.g., hazard ratios) as observations to be summarized in a meta-model. The former requires cooperation of all the individual study investigators and is used relatively infrequently, though the overview analysis regularly conducted by the early breast cancer trialists[169] and a recent analysis of transplant outcomes in pediatric leukemia are notable examples.[170] The meta-model approach, exemplified by a review of neuropsychological sequelae chemotherapy in pediatric acute lymphoblastic leukemia,[171] is more commonly used. A number of methodologic issues in the performance of meta-analyses have been raised. One concern is "publication bias": whether meta-analyses that include only studies that have been published substantially overestimate treatment effects because negative studies are less likely to be published than positive studies.[172] Although publication bias is widely acknowledged to be a real concern, combining peer-reviewed reports with those that have not undergone peer review generates other concerns.[173] Despite the difficulties, some meta-analyses in pediatric cancers have been performed.[174,175] An extensive literature concerning the application of these techniques to clinical trial results is rapidly developing.[176–187]

REPORTING RESULTS OF CLINICAL TRIALS

A useful publication is accurate, medically informative, and convincing to the reader. Accuracy is largely predetermined by the validity of the experimental design, the quality of its execution, and the legitimacy of its statistical analysis. The degree to which a paper is medically informative depends on the importance of the study question and the appropriateness of the experimental conditions. The value of any clinical trials publication is obviously related to the value of the experiment it reports. The ability to convince the reader, however, relates largely to the information the researcher chooses to communicate. Although the general structure of research papers (i.e., background, methods, results, and conclusions) is widely known, the detail presented is often insufficient to persuade a critical readership of the validity or applicability of the conclusions. This deficiency may delay the acceptance of an important advance or, more commonly, as in small studies with limited power, may suggest the acceptance or rejection of a concept based when further investigation is really required.[188] Attempts have been made to standardize the reporting

requirements for clinical trials so that results are presented as uniformly as possible.[189–193]

The methods section is critical to permitting readers to assess the strength and weaknesses of the study. This section should clearly describe the experimental conditions, including the specifics of patient registration procedures, inclusion and exclusion criteria, the target patient population, the details of the treatment regimen and any modifications, the schedule of follow-up evaluations, the definitions of and procedures used to assess major end points (including whether the person making the end point evaluation was "blinded" to the treatment assignment), and, in comparative trials, the nature of the control group and the specific methods used for treatment assignment. Randomization procedures and their timing relative to patient entry on study should be discussed. A brief description of quality control procedures can ensure the reader that the information reported is complete and accurate. Finally, a discussion of the statistical procedures used to analyze the data allows the reader to assess the reliability of the reported results. This description includes identification of analytic procedures used and explanatory material for techniques likely to be unfamiliar to the journal readership. References to articles or books describing all but the simplest and most standard techniques should be provided.

The results section presents the outcome of the experiment; clear and detailed exposition is crucial. A complete description of the patients entered on the study, including age, disease characteristics, nature and amount of prior therapy, and other items considered important in determining eligibility or establishing prognosis, should be provided. Toxicity and compliance information should be included, and outcomes for all patients entered should be reported. Confining information to patients deemed evaluable prevents accurate comparisons across studies whose policies regarding evaluability may differ.[191,194] If feasible, as with small studies, lists of individual end point determinations are useful.

Reports of clinical trials usually conclude with the author's interpretations of the study results. If the data have been analyzed appropriately, the conclusions are usually self-evident. Potential sources of bias, the need for independent confirmation, and any other warnings should be included in the discussion. Claims of patient benefit should be circumspect and based on the demonstrated difference in outcome between experimental and control groups, whose characteristics have been accurately described. Claims of no benefit should be accompanied by a confidence interval around the observed difference; a calculated probability (i.e., power) that a clinically important difference would have been detected with the sample size used may also be of interest.[195] Generalizations to a wider population should be made cautiously.

References

1. Simon R. The design and analysis of clinical trials. In: Levine A, ed. Cancer in the young. New York, NY: Masson, 1982.
2. Muggia FM, Carter SK, Macdonald JS. The cancer therapy evaluation program of the National Cancer Institute. Semin Oncol 1981;8:394–402.
3. Von Hoff DD, Clark JG, Kuhn C III. Design and conduct of phase I trials. In: Buyse M, Staquet M, Sylvester R, eds. Cancer clinical trials: methods and practice. London, England: Oxford University Press, 1983.
4. Carter SK. Clinical aspects in the design and conduct of phase II trials. In: Buyse M, Staquet M, Sylvester R, eds. Cancer clinical trials: methods and practice. London, England: Oxford University Press, 1983.
5. Marsoni S, Wittes R. Clinical development of anticancer agents—a National Cancer Institute perspective. Cancer Treat Rep 1984;68:77–85.
6. Livingstone RB, Carter SK. Experimental design and clinical trials: clinical perspectives. In: Carter SK, Glatstein E, Livingstone RB, eds. Principles of cancer treatment. New York, NY: McGraw-Hill, 1982.
7. Piantadosi S. Clinical trials: a methodologic perspective. Hoboken, NJ: Wiley-Interscience, 2005.
8. Potter DM. Phase I studies of chemotherapeutic agents in cancer patients: a review of the designs. J Biopharm Stat 2006;16:579–604.
9. Institute NC. Common Terminology Criteria for Adverse Events (CTCAE) Version 4.0; 2009.
10. Le Tourneau C, Lee JJ, Siu LL. Dose escalation methods in phase I cancer clinical trials. J Natl Cancer Inst 2009;101:708–720.
11. Grieshaber CK, Marsoni S. Relation of preclinical toxicology to findings in early clinical trials. Cancer Treat Rep 1986;70:65–72.
12. Collins JM, Zaharko DS, Dedrick RL, et al. Potential roles for preclinical pharmacology in phase I clinical trials. Cancer Treat Rep 1986;70:73–80.
13. Simon R, Freidlin B, Rubinstein L, et al. Accelerated titration designs for phase I clinical trials in oncology. J Natl Cancer Inst 1997;89:1138–1147.
14. Herberman RB. Design of clinical trials with biological response modifiers. Cancer Treat Rep 1985;69:1161–1164.
15. Booth CM, Calvert AH, Giaccone G, et al. Endpoints and other considerations in phase I studies of targeted anticancer therapy: recommendations from the task force on Methodology for the Development of Innovative Cancer Therapies (MDICT). Eur J Cancer 2008;44:19–24.
16. Marsoni S, Ungerleider RS, Hurson SB, et al. Tolerance to antineoplastic agents in children and adults. Cancer Treat Rep 1985;69:1263–1269.

17. Thall PF, Millikan RE, Mueller P, et al. Dose-finding with two agents in Phase I oncology trials. Biometrics 2003;59:487–496.
18. Storer BE. Design and analysis of phase I clinical trials. Biometrics 1989;45:925–937.
19. Blaney SM, Seibel NL, O'Brien M, et al. Phase I trial of docetaxel administered as a 1-hour infusion in children with refractory solid tumors: a collaborative pediatric branch, National Cancer Institute and Children's Cancer Group trial. J Clin Oncol 1997;15:1538–1543.
20. Barrett JS, Jayaraman B, Patel D, et al. A SAS-based solution to evaluate study design efficiency of phase I pediatric oncology trials via discrete event simulation. Comput Methods Programs Biomed 2008;90:240–250.
21. Skolnik JM, Barrett JS, Jayaraman B, et al. Shortening the timeline of pediatric phase I trials: the rolling six design. J Clin Oncol 2008;26:190–195.
22. O'Quigley J, Pepe M, Fisher L. Continual reassessment method: a practical design for phase 1 clinical trials in cancer. Biometrics 1990;46:33–48.
23. O'Quigley J, Chevret S. Methods for dose finding studies in cancer clinical trials: a review and results of a Monte Carlo study. Stat Med 1991;10:1647–1664.
24. O'Quigley J. Estimating the probability of toxicity at the recommended dose following a phase I clinical trial in cancer. Biometrics 1992;48:853–862.
25. Korn EL, Midthune D, Chen TT, et al. A comparison of two phase I trial designs. Stat Med 1994;13:1799–1806.
26. Moller S. An extension of the continual reassessment methods using a preliminary up-and-down design in a dose finding study in cancer patients, in order to investigate a greater range of doses. Stat Med 1995;14:911–922; discussion 923.
27. Goodman SN, Zahurak ML, Piantadosi S. Some practical improvements in the continual reassessment method for phase I studies. Stat Med 1995;14:1149–1161.
28. Tighiouart M, Rogatko A, Babb JS. Flexible Bayesian methods for cancer phase I clinical trials. Dose escalation with overdose control. Stat Med 2005;24:2183–2196.
29. Onar A, Kocak M, Boyett JM. Continual reassessment method vs. traditional empirically based design: modifications motivated by Phase I trials in pediatric oncology by the Pediatric Brain Tumor Consortium. J Biopharm Stat 2009;19:437–455.
30. Cheung YK, Chappell R. Sequential designs for phase I clinical trials with late-onset toxicities. Biometrics 2000;56:1177–1182.
31. Zhang W, Sargent DJ, Mandrekar S. An adaptive dose-finding design incorporating both toxicity and efficacy. Stat Med 2006;25:2365–2383.
32. Thall PF, Cook JD. Dose-finding based on efficacy-toxicity trade-offs. Biometrics 2004; 60:684–693.
33. Therasse P, Arbuck SG, Eisenhauer EA, et al. New guidelines to evaluate the response to treatment in solid tumors. European Organization for Research and Treatment of Cancer, National Cancer Institute of the United States, National Cancer Institute of Canada. J Natl Cancer Inst 2000;92:205–216.
34. Eisenhauer EA, Therasse P, Bogaerts J, et al. New response evaluation criteria in solid tumours: revised RECIST guideline (version 1.1). Eur J Cancer 2009;45:228–247.
35. Campbell ME, Grothey A, Sargent DJ, et al. Waterfall plots provide detailed information on magnitude of response to conventional chemotherapy in advanced colorectal cancer (ACRC)—lessons learned from N9741. J Clin Oncol (Meeting Abstracts) 2007; 25:4080.
36. Karrison TG, Maitland ML, Stadler WM, et al. Design of phase II cancer trials using a continuous endpoint of change in tumor size: application to a study of sorafenib and erlotinib in non small-cell lung cancer. J Natl Cancer Inst 2007;99:1455–1461.
37. Rubinstein LV, Dancey JE, Korn EL, et al. Early average change in tumor size in a phase 2 trial: efficient endpoint or false promise? J Natl Cancer Inst 2007;99:1422–1423.
38. Dhani N, Tu D, Sargent DJ, et al. Alternate endpoints for screening phase II studies. Clin Cancer Res 2009;15:1873–1882.
39. A'Hern RP. Sample size tables for exact single-stage phase II designs. Stat Med 2001;20:859–866.
40. Simon R. Optimal two-stage designs for phase II clinical trials. Control Clin Trials 1989;10:1–10.
41. Jung SH, Lee T, Kim K, et al. Admissible two-stage designs for phase II cancer clinical trials. Stat Med 2004;23:561–569.
42. Jung SH, Carey M, Kim KM. Graphical search for two-stage designs for phase II clinical trials. Control Clin Trials 2001;22:367–372.
43. Bryant J, Day R. Incorporating toxicity considerations into the design of two-stage phase II clinical trials. Biometrics 1995;51:1372–1383.
44. Finkelstein DM, Muzikansky A, Schoenfeld DA. Comparing survival of a sample to that of a standard population. J Natl Cancer Inst 2003;95:1434–1439.
45. Woolson RF. Rank tests and the one-sample logrank test for comparing observed survival data to a standard population. Biometrics 1981;37:687–696.
46. Chang MN, Therneau TM, Wieand HS, et al. Designs for group sequential phase II clinical trials. Biometrics 1987;43:865–874.
47. Hanfelt JJ, Slack RS, Gehan EA. A modification of Simon's optimal design for phase II trials when the criterion is median sample size. Control Clin Trials 1999;20:555–566.
48. Ensign LG, Gehan EA, Kamen DS, et al. An optimal three-stage design for phase II clinical trials. Stat Med 1994;13:1727–1736.
49. Panageas KS, Smith A, Gonen M, et al. An optimal two-stage phase II design utilizing complete and partial response information separately. Control Clin Trials 2002;23: 367–379.
50. Zee B, Melnychuk D, Dancey J, et al. Multinomial phase II cancer trials incorporating response and early progression. J Biopharm Stat 1999;9:351–363.
51. Case LD, Morgan TM. Design of Phase II cancer trials evaluating survival probabilities. BMC Med Res Methodol 2003;3:6.
52. Thall PF, Simon R. Practical Bayesian guidelines for phase IIB clinical trials. Biometrics 1994;50:337–349.
53. Tan SB, Machin D. Bayesian two-stage designs for phase II clinical trials. Stat Med 2002;21:1991–2012.
54. Lee JJ, Liu DD. A predictive probability design for phase II cancer clinical trials. Clin Trials 2008;5:93–106.
55. Sargent DJ, Chan V, Goldberg RM. A three-outcome design for phase II clinical trials. Control Clin Trials 2001;22:117–125.
56. Tournoux C, De Rycke Y, Medioni J, et al. Methods of joint evaluation of efficacy and toxicity in phase II clinical trials. Contemp Clin Trials 2007;28:514–524.
57. Horowitz ME, Etcubanas E, Christensen ML, et al. Phase II testing of melphalan in children with newly diagnosed rhabdomyosarcoma: a model for anticancer drug development. J Clin Oncol 1988;6:308–314.
58. Wells RJ. Phase II window therapy. J Clin Oncol 1995;13:302–303.
59. Kadota RP, Kun LE, Langston JW, et al. Cyclophosphamide for the treatment of progressive low-grade astrocytoma: a Pediatric Oncology Group phase II study. J Pediatr Hematol Oncol 1999;21:198–202.
60. Castleberry RP, Cantor AB, Green AA, et al. Phase II investigational window using carboplatin, iproplatin, ifosfamide, and epirubicin in children with untreated disseminated neuroblastoma: a Pediatric Oncology Group study. J Clin Oncol 1994;12:1616–1620.
61. Ettinger DS, Finkelstein DM, Abeloff MD, et al. Justification for evaluating new anticancer drugs in selected untreated patients with extensive-stage small-cell lung cancer: an Eastern Cooperative Oncology Group randomized study. J Natl Cancer Inst 1992; 84:1077–1084.
62. Harris MB, Cantor AB, Goorin AM, et al. Treatment of osteosarcoma with ifosfamide: comparison of response in pediatric patients with recurrent disease versus patients previously untreated: a Pediatric Oncology Group study. Med Pediatr Oncol 1995;24: 87–92.
63. Pappo AS, Etcubanas E, Santana VM, et al. A phase II trial of ifosfamide in previously untreated children and adolescents with unresectable rhabdomyosarcoma. Cancer 1993;71:2119–2125.
64. Pappo AS, Lyden E, Breneman J, et al. Up-front window trial of topotecan in previously untreated children and adolescents with metastatic rhabdomyosarcoma: an intergroup rhabdomyosarcoma study. J Clin Oncol 2001;19:213–219.
65. Walterhouse DO, Lyden ER, Breitfeld PP, et al. Efficacy of topotecan and cyclophosphamide given in a phase II window trial in children with newly diagnosed metastatic rhabdomyosarcoma: a Children's Oncology Group study. J Clin Oncol 2004;22:1398–1403.
66. Pappo AS, Lyden E, Breitfeld P, et al. Two consecutive phase II window trials of irinotecan alone or in combination with vincristine for the treatment of metastatic rhabdomyosarcoma: the Children's Oncology Group. J Clin Oncol 2007;25:362–369.
67. Razzouk BI, Heideman RL, Friedman HS, et al. A phase II evaluation of thiotepa followed by other multiagent chemotherapy regimens in infants and young children with malignant brain tumors. Cancer 1995;75:2762–2767.
68. Stewart CF, Iacono LC, Chintagumpala M, et al. Results of a phase II upfront window of pharmacokinetically guided topotecan in high-risk medulloblastoma and supratentorial primitive neuroectodermal tumor. J Clin Oncol 2004;22:3357–3365.
69. Chintagumpala MM, Friedman HS, Stewart CF, et al. A phase II window trial of procarbazine and topotecan in children with high-grade glioma: a report from the children's oncology group. J Neurooncol 2006;77:193–198.
70. Beauchamp T, Lukens J, Sallan S, et al. Phase II window studies in pediatric oncology: meeting report. Bethesda, MD: National Cancer Institute, 1997.
71. Ratain MJ, Sargent DJ. Optimising the design of phase II oncology trials: the importance of randomisation. Eur J Cancer 2009;45:275–280.
72. Lee JJ, Feng L. Randomized phase II designs in cancer clinical trials: current status and future directions. J Clin Oncol 2005;23:4450–4457.
73. Wieand HS. Randomized phase II trials: what does randomization gain? J Clin Oncol 2005;23:1794–1795.
74. Rubinstein L, Crowley J, Ivy P, et al. Randomized phase II designs. Clin Cancer Res 2009;15:1883–1890.
75. Taylor JM, Braun TM, Li Z. Comparing an experimental agent to a standard agent: relative merits of a one-arm or randomized two-arm Phase II design. Clin Trials 2006;3: 335–348.
76. Simon R, Wittes RE, Ellenberg SS. Randomized phase II clinical trials. Cancer Treat Rep 1985;69:1375–1381.
77. Sargent DJ, Goldberg RM. A flexible design for multiple armed screening trials. Stat Med 2001;20:1051–1060.
78. Huang X, Ning J, Li Y, et al. Using short-term response information to facilitate adaptive randomization for survival clinical trials. Stat Med 2009;28:1680–1689.
79. Giles FJ, Kantarjian HM, Cortes JE, et al. Adaptive randomized study of idarubicin and cytarabine versus troxacitabine and cytarabine versus troxacitabine and idarubicin in untreated patients 50 years or older with adverse karyotype acute myeloid leukemia. J Clin Oncol 2003;21:1722–1727.
80. Barker AD, Sigman CC, Kelloff GJ, et al. I-SPY 2: an adaptive breast cancer trial design in the setting of neoadjuvant chemotherapy. Clin Pharmacol Ther 2009;86:97–100.
81. Inoue LY, Thall PF, Berry DA. Seamlessly expanding a randomized phase II trial to phase III. Biometrics 2002;58:823–831.
82. Thall PF, Simon R, Ellenberg SS. A two-stage design for choosing among several experimental treatments and a control in clinical trials. Biometrics 1989;45:537–547.
83. Schaid DJ, Wieand S, Therneau TM. Optimal two-stage screening designs for survival comparisons. Biometrika 1990;77:507–513.
84. Mastrangelo R, Poplack D, Bleyer A, et al. Report and recommendations of the Rome workshop concerning poor-prognosis acute lymphoblastic leukemia in children: biologic bases for staging, stratification, and treatment. Med Pediatr Oncol 1986;14: 191–194.
85. Fleiss JL, Levin B, Myunghee CP. Statistical methods for rates and proportions. New York, NY: Wiley-Interscience, 2003.
86. Collett D. Modelling survival data in medical research. Bcoa Raton, FL: Chapman & Hall/CRC, 2003.
87. Machin D, Campbell MJ, Say-beng T, et al. Sample size tables for clinical studies. Oxford, UK: BMJ Books, 2008.
88. Wittes J. Sample size calculations for randomized controlled trials. Epidemiol Rev 2002;24:39–53.
89. Sposto R, Sather HN. Determining the duration of comparative clinical trials while allowing for cure. J Chronic Dis 1985;38:683–690.
90. Treasure T, MacRae KD. Minimisation: the platinum standard for trials? BMJ 1998;317:362–363.
91. Pocock SJ, Simon R. Sequential treatment assignment with balancing for prognostic factors in the controlled clinical trial. Biometrics 1975;31:103–115.
92. Taves DR. Minimization: a new method of assigning patients to treatment and control groups. Clin Pharmacol Ther 1974;15:443–453.
93. McPherson K. Statistics: the problem of examining accumulating data more than once. N Engl J Med 1974;290:501–502.
94. O'Brien PC, Fleming TR. A multiple testing procedure for clinical trials. Biometrics 1979;35:549–556.
95. Pocock SJ. Group sequential methods in the design and analysis of clinical trials. Bometrika 1977;64:191–199.
96. Pocock SJ. Interim analyses for randomized clinical trials: the group sequential approach. Biometrics 1982;38:153–162.
97. Fleming TR, Harrington DP, O'Brien PC. Designs for group sequential tests. Control Clin Trials 1984;5:348–361.
98. Reboussin DM, DeMets DL, Kim KM, et al. Computations for group sequential boundaries using the Lan-DeMets spending function method. Control Clin Trials 2000;21: 190–207.

99. Hanna N, Neubauer M, Yiannoutsos C, et al. Phase III study of cisplatin, etoposide, and concurrent chest radiation with or without consolidation docetaxel in patients with inoperable stage III non-small-cell lung cancer: The Hoosier Oncology Group and U.S. Oncology. J Clin Oncol 2008;26:5755–5760.
100. Kim KB, Legha SS, Gonzalez R, et al. A randomized phase III trial of biochemotherapy versus interferon-alpha-2b for adjuvant therapy in patients at high risk for melanoma recurrence. Melanoma Res 2009;19:42–49.
101. Green S, Liu PY, O'Sullivan J. Factorial design considerations. J Clin Oncol 2002;20: 3424–3430.
102. Montgomery AA, Peters TJ, Little P. Design, analysis and presentation of factorial randomised controlled trials. BMC Med Res Methodol 2003;3:26.
103. D'Angio GJ, Breslow N, Beckwith JB, et al. Treatment of Wilms' tumor. Results of the Third National Wilms' Tumor Study. Cancer 1989;64:349–360.
104. Simon R. Bayesian design and analysis of active control clinical trials. Biometrics 1999;55:484–487.
105. Hasselblad V, Kong DF. Statistical methods for comparison to placebo in active-control trials. Drug Inf J 2001;35:435–449.
106. Wang S, Hung H. Assessing treatment efficacy in noninferiority trials. Control Clin Trials 2003;24:147–155.
107. Chan IS. Power and sample size determination for noninferiority trials using an exact method. J Biopharm Stat 2002;12:457–469.
108. DeMets D. Statistical issues in interpreting clinical trials. J Intern Med 2004;255: 529–537.
109. Kummar S, Rubinstein L, Kinders R, et al. Phase 0 clinical trials: conceptions and misconceptions. Cancer J 2008;14:133–137.
110. Kummar S, Doroshow JH, Tomaszewski JE, et al. Phase 0 clinical trials: recommendations from the Task Force on Methodology for the Development of Innovative Cancer Therapies. Eur J Cancer 2009;45:741–746.
111. Abdoler E, Taylor H, Wendler D. The ethics of phase 0 oncology trials. Clin Cancer Res 2008;14:3692–3697.
112. Murgo AJ, Kummar S, Rubinstein L, et al. Designing phase 0 cancer clinical trials. Clin Cancer Res 2008;14:3675–3682.
113. NCI Cancer Therapy Evaluation Program Protocol Templates, Applications and Guidelines. http://ctep.cancer.gov/guidelines/templates.html. Accessed May 7, 2010.
114. Peto R, Pike MC, Armitage P, et al. Design and analysis of randomized clinical trials requiring prolonged observation of each patient. I. Introduction and design. Br J Cancer 1976;34:585–612.
115. International Conference on Harmonisation; Good Clinical Practice: Consolidated Guideline; Notice of Availability," 62 Federal Register 90, May 9, 1997:25691–25709.
116. Shuster E. Fifty years later: the significance of the Nuremberg Code. N Engl J Med 1997;337:1436–1440.
117. National Commission for the Protection of Human Subjects of Biomedical and Behavioral Research. The Belmont report: ethical principles and guidelines for protection of human subjects of research. Washington, DC, 1978.
118. World Medical Association (48th World Medical Assembly). World Medical Association: Declaration of Helsinki IV, as amended by the 48th World Medical Assembly. Somerset West, South Africa: Republic of South Africa, 1996.
119. Title 45, Code of Federal Regulations, Part 46: Health and Welfare, Protection of Human Subjects. October 10, 1999.
120. Title 21, Code of Federal Regulations, Part 50: Food and Drugs, Protection of Human Subjects. April 1, 2000.
121. Title 21, Code of Federal Regulations, Part 56: Food and Drugs, Institutional Review Boards. April 1, 2000.
122. Investigator's Handbook: a manual for participants in clinical trials of investigational agents sponsored by the Division of Cancer Treatment. Bethesda, MD: National Cancer Institute, 1993.
123. Title 45, Code of Federal Regulations, Part 46, Subpart D: Health and welfare, protection of human subjects, additional protections for children involved as subjects in research. October 1, 1999.
124. Zon R, Meropol NJ, Catalano RB, et al. American Society of Clinical Oncology Statement on minimum standards and exemplary attributes of clinical trial sites. J Clin Oncol 2008;26:2562–2567.
125. Knatterud GL, Rockhold FW, George SL, et al. Guidelines for quality assurance in multicenter trials: a position paper. Control Clin Trials 1998;19:477–493.
126. Smith MA, Ungerleider RS, Korn EL, et al. Role of independent data-monitoring committees in randomized clinical trials sponsored by the National Cancer Institute [see comments]. J Clin Oncol 1997;15:2736–2743.
127. Green SJ, Fleming TR, O'Fallon JR. Policies for study monitoring and interim reporting of results. J Clin Oncol 1987;5:1477–1484.
128. US Food and Drug Administration Guidance for Clinical Trial Sponsors: Establishment and Operation of Clinical Trial Data Monitoring Committees, March 2006. Rockville, MD, 2009. PDF–194KB.
129. Ellenberg SS, Fleming TR, DeMets DL. Data monitoring committees in clinical trials: a practical perspective. Chichester: John Wiley, 2002.
130. Lewis JA, Machin D. Intention to treat—who should use ITT? [editorial]. Br J Cancer 1993;68:647–650.
131. Gail MH. Eligibility exclusions, losses to follow-up, removal of randomized patients, and uncounted events in cancer clinical trials. Cancer Treat Rep 1985;69:1107–1113.
132. Simon R. Patient subsets and variation in therapeutic efficacy. Br J Clin Pharmacol 1982;14:473–482.
133. Sather HN. Statistical evaluation of prognostic factors in ALL and treatment results. Med Pediatr Oncol 1986;14:158–165.
134. Armitage P. Importance of prognostic factors in the analysis of data from clinical trials. Control Clin Trials 1981;1:347–353.
135. Green S, Benedetti J, Crowley J. Clinical trials in oncology. Boca Raton, FL: Chapman & Hall, 2003.
136. Yusuf S, Wittes J, Probstfield J, et al. Analysis and interpretation of treatment effects in subgroups of patients in randomized clinical trials. JAMA 1991;266:93–98.
137. Assmann SF, Pocock SJ, Enos LE, et al. Subgroup analysis and other (mis)uses of baseline data in clinical trials [see comments]. Lancet 2000;355:1064–1069.
138. Glantz SA. Primer of biostatistics. New York, NY: McGraw-Hill Medical Pub., 2005.
139. Norman GR, Streiner DL. Biostatistics : the bare essentials. Hamilton, NY: B.C. Decker, 2000.
140. Dawson B, Trapp RG. Basic & clinical biostatistics. New York, NY: Lange Medical Books/McGraw-Hill, Medical Pub. Division, 2004.
141. Rosner B. Fundamentals of biostatistics. Belmont, CA: Thomson-Brooks/Cole, 2006.
142. Crowley J, Ankerst DP. Handbook of statistics in clinical oncology. Boca Raton, FL: Chapman & Hall/CRC, 2006.
143. Myron N. Chang. Improved confidence intervals for a binomial parameter following a group sequential phase II clinical trial. Stat Med 2004;23:2817–2826.
144. Kaplan E, Meier P. Nonparametric estimation from incomplete observations. J Am Stat Assoc 1958;53:457–481.
145. Embury SH, Elias L, Heller PH, et al. Remission maintenance therapy in acute myelogenous leukemia. West J Med 1977;126:267–272.
146. Anderson JR, Cain KC, Gelber RD. Analysis of survival by tumor response. J Clin Oncol 1983;1:710–719.
147. Weiss GB, Bunce H III, Hokanson JA. Comparing survival of responders and nonresponders after treatment: a potential source of confusion in interpreting cancer clinical trials. Control Clin Trials 1983;4:43–52.
148. Mantel N. Responder versus nonresponder comparisons: daunorubicin plus prednisone in treatment of acute nonlymphocytic leukemia [letter]. Cancer Treat Rep 1983;67: 315–316.
149. Lee ET, Wang JW. Statistical methods for survival data analysis. New York, NY: John Wiley, 2003.
150. Therneau TM, Grambsch PM. Modeling survival data : extending the Cox model. New York, NY: Springer, 2000.
151. Crowley J, Hu M. Covariance analysis of heart transplant survival data. J Am Stat Assoc 1972;72:27–36.
152. Gail M. Evaluating serial cancer marker studies in patients at risk of recurrent disease. Biometrics 1984;37:67–78.
153. Altman D, DeStavola B. Practical problems in fitting a proportional hazards model to data with updated measurements of the covariates. Stat Med 1994;13:301–341.
154. Pui C, Gaynon P, Boyett J, et al. Outcome of treatment in childhood acute lymphoblastic leukemia with rearrangements of the 11q23 chromosomal region. Lancet 2002;359: 1909–1915.
155. Arico M, Valsecchi M, Camitta B, et al. Outcome of treatment in children with Philadelphia chromosome-positive acute lymphoblastic leukemia. N Engl J Med 342;998–1006.
156. Schmiegelow K, Bjork O, Glomstein A, et al. Intensification of mercaptopurine/methotrexate chemotherapy may increase the risk of relapse for some children with acute lymphoblastic leukemia. J Clin Oncol 2003;21:1332–1339.
157. Balis F, Holcenberg J, Poplack D, et al. Pharmacokinetics and pharmacodynamics of oral methotrexate in children with lower risk acute lymphoblastic leukemia: a joint Children's Cancer Group and Pediatric Oncology Branch study. Blood 1998;92: 3569–3577.
158. Altman DG, Lausen B, Sauerbrei W, et al. Dangers of using "optimal" cutpoints in the evaluation of prognostic factors [see comments]. J Natl Cancer Inst 1994;86:829–835.
159. Hilsenbeck SG, Clark GM, McGuire WL. Why do so many prognostic factors fail to pan out? Breast Cancer Res Treat 1992;22:197–206.
160. Dobbin KK, Simon RM. Sample size planning for developing classifiers using high-dimensional DNA microarray data. Biostatistics 2007;8:101–117.
161. Simon R, Radmacher MD, Dobbin K, et al. Pitfalls in the use of DNA microarray data for diagnostic and prognostic classification. J Natl Cancer Inst 2003;95:14–18.
162. Simon RM, Dobbin K. Experimental design of DNA microarray experiments. Biotechniques 2003;(suppl):16–21.
163. Simon R, Altman DG. Statistical aspects of prognostic factor studies in oncology [editorial]. Br J Cancer 1994;69:979–985.
164. Green SB, Byar DP. The effect of stratified randomization on size and power of statistical tests in clinical trials. J Chronic Dis 1978;31:445–454.
165. Friedman LM, Furberg CD, DeMets DL. Fundamental of clinical trials. Littleton, MA: John Wright & Sons, 1983.
166. Simon R. Use of statistical regression models. In: Buyse M, Sylvester R, Staquet M, eds. Cancer clinical trials: design, practice, and analysis. London, England: Oxford University Press, 1984.
167. Simon R. Heterogeneity and standardization in clinical trials. In Tagnon HJ, Staquet, MJ, eds. Controversies in cancer. New York, NY: Masson, 1979.
168. http://en.wikipedia.org/wiki/Meta-analysis. Accessed May 7, 2010.
169. Clarke M, Collins R, Darby S, et al. Effects of radiotherapy and of differences in the extent of surgery for early breast cancer on local recurrence and 15-year survival: an overview of the randomised trials. Lancet 2005;366:2087–2106.
170. Horan JT, Alonzo TA, Lyman GH, et al. Impact of disease risk on efficacy of matched related bone marrow transplantation for pediatric acute myeloid leukemia: the Children's Oncology Group. J Clin Oncol 2008;26:5797–5801.
171. Peterson CC, Johnson CE, Ramirez LY, et al. A meta-analysis of the neuropsychological sequelae of chemotherapy-only treatment for pediatric acute lymphoblastic leukemia. Pediatr Blood Cancer 2008;51:99–104.
172. Easterbrook PJ, Berlin JA, Gopalan R, et al. Publication bias in clinical research [see comments]. Lancet 1991;337:867–872.
173. Cook DJ, Guyatt GH, Ryan G, et al. Should unpublished data be included in meta-analyses? Current convictions and controversies. JAMA 1993;269:2749–2753.
174. Clarke M, Gaynon P, Hann I, et al. CNS-directed therapy for childhood acute lymphoblastic leukemia: Childhood ALL Collaborative Group overview of 43 randomized trials. J Clin Oncol 2003;21:1798–1809.
175. Childhood ALL Collaborative Group. Duration and intensity of maintenance chemotherapy in acute lymphoblastic leukemia: overview of 42 trials involving 12,000 randomized children. Lancet 1996;347:1783–1788.
176. Simon R. Overviews of randomized clinical trials. Cancer Treat Rep 1987;71:3–5.
177. Berlin JA, Laird NM, Sacks HS, et al. A comparison of statistical methods for combining event rates from clinical trials. Stat Med 1989;8:141–151.
178. Boissel JP, Blanchard J, Panak E, et al. Considerations for the meta-analysis of randomized clinical trials. Summary of a panel discussion. Control Clin Trials 1989;10: 254–281.
179. Chalmers TC, Berrier J, Sacks HS, et al. Meta-analysis of clinical trials as a scientific discipline. II: Replicate variability and comparison of studies that agree and disagree. Stat Med 1987;6:733–744.
180. Clarke MJ, Stewart LA. Obtaining data from randomised controlled trials: how much do we need for reliable and informative meta-analyses? BMJ 1994;309:1007–1010.
181. DerSimonian R, Laird N. Meta-analysis in clinical trials. Control Clin Trials 1986;7: 177–188.
182. Ellenberg SS. Meta-analysis: the quantitative approach to research review. Semin Oncol 1988;15:472–481.
183. Moher D, Cook DJ, Eastwood S, et al. Improving the quality of reports of meta-analyses of randomised controlled trials: the QUOROM statement. Quality of reporting of meta-analyses [see comments]. Lancet 1999;354:1896–1900.

184. Sacks HS, Berrier J, Reitman D, et al. Meta-analyses of randomized controlled trials. N Engl J Med 1987;316:450–455.
185. Moher D, Pham B, Jones A, et al. Does quality of reports of randomised trials affect estimates of intervention efficacy reported in meta-analyses? [see comments]. Lancet 1998;352:609–613.
186. Thompson SG. Why sources of heterogeneity in meta-analysis should be investigated. BMJ 1994;309:1351–1355.
187. Cook DJ, Sackett DL, Spitzer WO. Methodologic guidelines for systematic reviews of randomized control trials in health care from the Potsdam Consultation on Meta-Analysis. J Clin Epidemiol 1995;48:167–171.
188. DerSimonian R, Charette LJ, McPeek B, et al. Reporting on methods in clinical trials. N Engl J Med 1982;306:1332–1337.
189. Makuch R, Simon R. Sample size requirements for evaluating a conservative therapy. Cancer Treat Rep 1978;62:1037–1040.
190. Altman DG, Gore SM, Gardner MJ, et al. Statistical guidelines for contributors to medical journals. Br Med J (Clin Res Ed) 1983;286:1489–1493.
191. Zelen M. Guidelines for publishing papers on cancer clinical trials: responsibilities of editors and authors. Prog Clin Biol Res 1983;132E:57–68.
192. George SL. Statistics in medical journals: a survey of current policies and proposals for editors. Med Pediatr Oncol 1985;13:109–112.
193. Begg C, Cho M, Eastwood S, et al. Improving the quality of reporting of randomized controlled trials. The CONSORT statement [see comments]. JAMA 1996;276:637–639.
194. Simon R, Wittes RE. Methodologic guidelines for reports of clinical trials. Cancer Treat Rep 1985;69:1–3.
195. Freiman JA, Chalmers TC, Smith H Jr, et al. The importance of beta, the type II error and sample size in the design and interpretation of the randomized control trial. Survey of 71 "negative" trials. N Engl J Med 1978;299:690–694.

CHAPTER 18 ■ REGULATING PATIENT SAFETY IN CANCER TREATMENT

BRIGITTA U. MUELLER AND AMY L. BILLETT

Chemotherapy safety (or the lack thereof) came to the public's attention in 1995, when the case of Betsy Lehman, a *Boston Globe* reporter, who died of an accidental overdose of cyclophosphamide, was prominently featured in the news media.[1]

Betsy Lehman, a 39-year-old woman, was being treated for breast cancer at the Dana Farber Cancer Institute in Boston. She died after receiving a fourfold overdose of cyclophosphamide. This was only discovered several months later during a routine review of her medical records. It was determined that the ordering physician had written "cyclophosphamide 4 g/sq m over four days" with the intention that the patient receive a total of 1 gram per square meter over 4 sequential days. However, the order was interpreted as prescribing 4 grams per square meter for each of 4 sequential days. Betsy Lehman died 3 weeks later from the cardiac complications ensuing from this massive overdose.

In 1980, the American Society of Anesthesiologists was the first professional group to form a patient safety committee after reviewing a television expose of anesthesia incidents. In the 1990s, the literature on medical errors started to become voluminous, and in 2009, PubMed (the search engine of the National Library of Medicine) listed more than 80,000 publications under the search term "medical error."

In 1999, the Institute of Medicine (IOM) published its report *To Err Is Human: Building a Safer Health Care System*, citing an estimated 44,000 to 98,000 deaths in adults per year caused by medical errors.[2] Two out of every 100 hospital admissions result in a preventable adverse drug event (ADE), leading to estimated national costs of $17 billion to $29 billion (lost income, prolonged hospitalizations, disability, excess health care costs).[3–5] Errors are due to many different factors, including lack of teamwork, stress, workload, and clerical mistakes, such as faulty transcriptions.[3,4,6–8] The medical field has only begun to acknowledge this problem, to promote open discussion, and to apply techniques that have been proven effective in other high-risk fields.[9–11]

BACKGROUND

Several studies have demonstrated that errors can occur in every medical setting; however, vulnerable populations and high-risk procedures add additional challenges. Most publications describe interventions in the emergency room or during anesthesia, but few have addressed the special challenges involved in the treatment of children with complex disorders.[12–14] Slonim et al. surveyed hospitalized, non-newborn patients in the United States and found a reported error rate of 1.81 to 2.96 per 100 discharges.[8] An even more disturbing report was published by Kaushal et al., who found 55 medication errors per 100 inpatient admissions at a single, leading pediatric teaching hospital.[15]

Medication errors are made by both junior as well as experienced physicians. In a prospective study over a year, the total and significant error rate, respectively, per 1,000 orders, was 3.30 and 1.76 for attending physicians. A similar rate was found for residents and fellow trainees at any level: the error rate was 2.34 and 1.36 for second-year residents, 1.98 and 0.95 for third-year residents, and 0.81 and 0.54 for fourth-year residents and fellows.[16]

Antineoplastic drugs often have a low therapeutic index and an overdose easily leads to devastating consequences (excessive myelosuppression, renal toxicity, or even death), while underdosing may impact treatment efficacy. Furthermore, certain agents are highly toxic if administered by the wrong route (e.g., vincristine given intrathecally).[17] An analysis of 140 errors reported by nurses in an adult oncology practice revealed multiple sources of mistakes: 39% were due to the wrong dose (body surface area not recalculated, a week's dose given in 1 day, wrong vial used to mix dose); 21% were due to wrong duration of administration or given at wrong time; 18% were due to wrong drug (confused with other drug); and 14% were due to administration of the drug to the wrong patient.[18]

Children who are treated for cancer are of different ages and different body weights and may have specific organ deficiencies. Caregivers, especially nurses and physicians, must adjust their medication orders not only to the underlying disease but also to the age, weight, and height of the child. Although "standard dosing" provides some measure of safety in adults because it brings familiarity with certain doses, the dosing is different for each child and the dosage schedule often changes during the course of the treatment, because the child may lose weight or develop new organ dysfunctions. In a review of oral chemotherapy for children with acute lymphoblastic leukemia, one or more errors were found with 17 of 172 (9.9%) of medications prescribed.[19] Rinke et al. queried a national, voluntary, internet-accessible error reporting system (United States Pharmacopeia MEDMARX database) for all error reports from 1999 through 2004 that involved chemotherapy medications and patients younger than 18 years. Eighty-five percent (264) of the 310 reported pediatric chemotherapy errors reached the patient, and 49 (15.6%) required additional patient monitoring or therapeutic intervention. The most commonly involved chemotherapeutic agents were methotrexate (15.3%), cytarabine (12.1%), and etoposide (8.3%).[20] Pediatric patients were particularly susceptible to the risk of harm in errors involving home medication administration.[13]

Definitions

Understanding the field of patient safety requires an understanding of the terms used (Table 18.1). *Medication errors* are defined as errors that occur at any stage in the medication use

TABLE 18.1

DEFINITIONS OF EVENTS RELATED TO DRUG ADMINISTRATION

Term	Definition	Example(s)
Harm occurred		
Adverse event (AE)	Harm in a patient administered a drug but not necessarily caused by a drug	Traumatic death while receiving Purinethol
Adverse drug event (ADE)	Harm caused by a drug	
Expected ADE (e.g., adverse drug reaction)	A usually predictable or dose-dependent effect of a drug that is not the principal effect for which the drug was chosen (e.g., listed in package insert)	Myelosuppression from chemotherapy Cisplatin-induced emesis in a patient receiving appropriate antiemetics
Unexpected ADE	Not identified in nature, severity, or frequency in the sponsor's brochure or package insert	Common in relatively new drugs
Serious ADE (SAE)	Fatal/life threatening, permanently disabling, leading to or prolonging hospitalization, causing congenital anomaly, any drug overdose	Delayed methotrexate clearance with need for intervention
Sentinel event	Unexpected occurrences involving death or serious physical or psychological injury or risk thereof	Intrathecal administration of vincristine
Preventable ADE	An ADE that could have been prevented by any means	Cisplatin induced emesis in patient not receiving antiemetics
Harm may have occurred		
Medication error	An error that occurs in any stage of the medication process including ordering, transcribing, dispensing, administering, monitoring	30-min delay in mesna administration
Harm did not occur		
Potential ADE (near miss)	A medication error with the potential for harm	A 10-fold overdose of narcotic that is intercepted before administration

process, from ordering to dispensing to administration to monitoring.[21] The vast majority of medication errors are harmless, but 1% to 2% cause injury. However, an additional 5% are "near misses" that fail to cause injury by chance or because they are intercepted before reaching the patient. Medication errors are frequent and cause substantial resource waste due to the need to discard the wrong medication, the additional work in preparing a new dose, and the necessary reporting and cause analysis.

Legal and Financial Implications

Medical malpractice litigation, or personal-injury law (tort), has become not only a large legal and financial enterprise but also a political issue that has been discussed intensively over the last decades.[22,23] Unfortunately, the culture of "finding and punishing the culprits," as practiced by litigators, is in stark contrast to the nonpunitive approach that seeks to find the problems in the system and relies heavily on open reporting.[23]

ADEs are also costly. In a review of 190 ADEs, 60 of them deemed preventable, the additional length of stay associated with the event was 2.2 days, and the increase in cost was $2,595 overall and $4,685 for preventable events.[24] This does not include the costs for malpractice suits or the loss of income suffered by the patients. In an analysis of medication-related malpractice claims, Rothschild et al.[25] found that the mean costs for defending a malpractice claim for preventable and other *outpatient* ADEs was similar (mean $64,700 to $74,200) but was considerably higher for preventable *inpatient* ADEs ($376,500).

RECOGNIZING AND REPORTING OF PROBLEMS

Different techniques have been used to assess error rates in the medical setting. In 2002, a conference entitled "Measuring Medication Safety in Hospitals" was held in Tucson, Arizona, and experts in the field (including physicians, pharmacists, and nurses) discussed the pros and cons of each method.[26] The five main techniques identified were as follows:

1. The *voluntary reporting* method is strongly influenced by the culture of the organization and is most helpful in an environment where reporting is not perceived as being followed by a punitive action. In general, this method does not produce quantitative information, because only a small number of events are being reported, but it can furnish very valuable qualitative information about both errors and "near misses."[27] Another form of voluntary reporting is the Morbidity and Mortality Conference. Although often helpful in better understanding complex cases and the outcome and consequences of different pathologies, these conferences are fraught with hindsight bias, focus on diagnostic errors, and are infrequently and rather randomly used in most academic institutions.[28] Autopsies have been shown to detect potentially fatal misdiagnoses in 20% to 40% of cases but are being used even less often as the frequency of autopsies decreases.[29,30]

2. The *chart review* method is readily available and commonly used but is often inaccurate due to the lack of precise documentation and hindsight bias. It is also very labor intensive and dependent on consensus and confidence of the reviewers.[31]

3. The *observation* method measures actual errors during drug administration and dispensing. This method is more accurate and efficient than chart reviews but does require trained observers (nurses, pharmacists, or pharmacy technicians). Staff members are observed and their activities documented by the observer. The notes are then compared with the written prescription order. In this method, deviations in timing of medication delivery, omission of doses, and the actual dosage administered are determined and can later be reviewed and graded by a medication safety committee in regard to significance.[26,32] Direct observation is extremely labor intensive and rarely practical outside of funded research efforts.

4. The *practitioner intervention* method involves keeping a formal log of interactions that occur daily between pharmacists and nurses or physicians to clarify an order. This method predominantly captures events at the prescribing stage and is also very useful for detecting "near misses."[26] Pharmacists are asked to keep track of any orders that were incorrectly written, that needed clarification, or that violated a safety precaution (e.g., penicillin ordered in a patient with penicillin allergy). Nurses keep track of events where the pharmacy delivered the wrong drug, or at the wrong time, or to the wrong patient. This technique is valuable to measure the amount of "rework" that occurs.

5. *Computerized monitoring* has become more widely available as information technology has matured.[33,34] A data source that has been used for several years is the detecting of adverse events by reviewing the administrative codes used for diagnoses and procedures (ICD-9-CM and CPT codes). However, coding is done weeks to months after discharge, and is generated for reimbursement and legal goals, and is thus not very reliable for detecting adverse events.[35] Laboratory data can be searched more easily, because the data are mostly in numeric form.[36] Examples are the doubling of creatinine levels and high serum drug levels.

Incident Reporting

Internal reporting of adverse events is required by health care institutions, both to meet external regulatory requirements and to provide information to leadership to prevent other such events in the future. Each institution defines what should be reported and how it is carried out based on institutional priorities, relevant state law, and guidelines or requirements from regulatory agencies. Although incident reports themselves are not placed in the patient chart, disclosure to the patient should be documented in a progress note that also describes the event. In some, but not all, states, incident reports are considered peer review material and protected from legal discovery. As an organization focuses on patient safety and a nonpunitive reporting environment, the rate of incident reports tends to increase, a sign of success rather than failure. However, incident reporting vastly underestimates the occurrence of problems.[37]

Root Cause Analysis

Root cause analysis (RCA) is a *retrospective* technique to analyze an error after it occurs. The technique has been widely used in industrial accidents.[38] In 1997, the Joint Commission mandated the use of the RCA technique whenever a sentinel event occurs. The RCA technique can be used to identify what occurred, why it occurred, and to propose changes that would prevent it from happening again. The health care—specific model for an RCA focuses on four major areas: leadership, human factors, information, and the environment. Their Web site (www.jointcommission.org) makes tools available in written format to assist organizations in performing an RCA.

Occurrence Screens

Most, if not all, health care organizations utilize dedicated staff members or automated reports to screen for the occurrence of specific events in the hospital, such as transfer to the intensive care unit, death, readmission within 72 hours, and return to the operating room within 48 hours. These events are reviewed to determine the degree of preventability. Events with a high degree of preventability or events with a fatal outcome can then be further investigated with an RCA.

Adverse Drug Event Reporting

Not all adverse events are due to errors or mistakes. Adverse event collection and reporting is a routine part of every clinical trial. In oncology, the Common Toxicity Criteria (CTC), maintained by the National Cancer Institute, are commonly used to grade the severity of an adverse event. The procedure for the reporting of an ADE or serious adverse event depends on the phase of the clinical trial, the approval status of the drug (investigational vs. noninvestigational), and the seriousness of the event. However, reporting of ADEs does not end with the approval of a drug by the Food and Drug Administration (FDA). A recent study demonstrated that potentially fatal adverse events related to cancer drugs might become apparent only decades after FDA approval of a drug.[39] The Center for Drug Evaluation and Research (CDER) oversees the MedWatch program through which physicians and other health care professionals can report medication errors directly to the FDA. This one-page form, available at http://www.fda.gov/medwatch/, is "intended for use by health professionals and consumers for voluntary reporting of adverse events and product problems related to medications (drugs or biologics, except vaccines), medical devices (including *in vitro* diagnostics), special nutritional products (dietary supplements, infant formulas, medical foods), and other FDA-regulated medical products" (wording from FDA Web site).

Failure Mode and Effects Analysis

In contrast to a retrospective RCA, a failure mode and effects analysis (FMEA) is a *prospective* technique that can be applied to any process without the occurrence of a sentinel event or near miss.[40] This multidisciplinary approach was first developed and applied in the aerospace industry. The analytic approach defines the steps involved in the process of interest and then analyzes each step for potential failures. Three factors are considered:

- Failure modes: what could go wrong?
- Failure causes: why could the failure happen?
- Failure effects: what would be the consequences of each failure?

Consideration of the likelihood of a failure, the severity of the consequences of a failure, and probability of the failure being detected allows each potential failure to be assigned a risk-priority number (RPN = severity × probability × detection). The team can then model or implement changes to those steps with the highest RPN. Repetitive FMEAs can be carried out over time to assess the impact of changes made. This technique has been successfully applied to the chemotherapy administration process in children with cancer and can lead to the more rapid adaptation of safety interventions, such as the use of preprinted order sets.[34] It has also been used during the implementation of computerized order entry systems for pediatric chemotherapy.

Disclosure of Errors

As mentioned earlier, there might be regulatory reporting requirements, especially if an investigational drug or experimental protocol design are involved. Although disclosure to the patient and the family is encouraged and appropriate, this is often the most difficult part for the care providers involved.[41] A recent survey studied the opinions of members of a health plan and found that full disclosure of any errors or mistakes reduced the likelihood of changing physicians and increased patient satisfaction, trust, and positive emotional response.[42] However, the number of people who would seek legal advice was not lowered by full disclosure. The overwhelming majority of responders (98.8%) wanted to be told of an error, and 87% would ask for financial compensation if any harm occurred. Another study confirmed this finding: 76% of surveyed people wanted to be informed immediately of any medical error and to receive full disclosure of the problem's extent.[43] More than 90% of respondents were in favor of reporting errors to government agencies (92%), state medical boards (97%), and hospital committees (99%). The hospital's and/or physician's risk management group thus needs to be notified of any potentially harmful errors to guide any necessary responses in case of media notification or legal action.

PREVENTING ERRORS

National Patient Safety Goals

As of January 1, 2004, all organizations accredited by the Joint Commission are being surveyed for implementation of certain requirements listed in Table 18.2. Compliance with these mandates is required to maintain accreditation.

A "minimum list" of dangerous abbreviations, acronyms, and symbols has been approved by the Joint Commission. As of January 1, 2004, certain items *must* be included on each accredited institution's "do not use" list (Table 18.3).

Promoting a Culture of Safety

An institutional commitment to safety requires multiple components. There must be a governance structure that clearly identifies who is in charge of safety at the institution. In general, that person should be a senior leader who is held accountable by the board of directors to ensure that safety goals are achieved.[44] Executive walk rounds with senior hospital leadership seeking information from staff members through structured questions about safety concerns can be an effective technique to demonstrate commitment of the leadership.[45] Those rounds, however, must be followed by a clear response to the concerns raised. Other components in the governance structure can include a safety committee and/or appointment of a safety officer to lead safety efforts. Such functions work best if well integrated with other standing groups and committees. A robust pharmacy and therapeutics committee can play an invaluable role in promoting safety within the medication process. A multidisciplinary peer review committee that thoroughly reviews critical incidents and near misses can often identify broad issues, such as poor communication, that can impair safety.

Human factors study is the study of humans and their physical and psychological limits in relationship to the tools they use or systems in which they work. All humans have lapses and thus will make errors. Lapses can be promoted by such factors as fatigue, stress, and distractions, and poorly designed medical devices can promote user error.[46,47] These findings were confirmed in a review of 310 pediatric chemotherapy order reports, where the most common error types were due to improper dose or quantity (22.9%), wrong time (22.6%), omission (14.1%), and wrong administration technique, including wrong route (12.2%).[20] A performance deficit was the most common reason (41.3% of 547 cited error causes), followed by problems due to equipment and medication delivery devices (12.4%), lack of communication (8.8%), knowledge deficit (6.8%), and errors in the written order itself (5.5%).[20]

Specific educational components to improve safety in the chemotherapy process have been identified.[48] These components include defined competencies for chemotherapy for all three disciplines involved (physicians/nurse practitioners, nurses, and pharmacists), an ongoing education process for all new protocols, and development and dissemination of multidisciplinary policies for both oncology and non-oncology chemotherapy. Patient (or parent) participation can also help prevent ADEs. Two hundred and nine adult patients on a general medicine unit were enrolled in a study, and 107 of them received drug safety information and their medication list and 102 controls received drug safety information only. A nonsignificant difference was found between intervention patients and controls in the ADE rate (8.4% vs. 2.9%, $p = 0.12$) and close-call rate (7.5% vs. 9.8%, $p = 0.57$), but among nurse respondents, 29% indicated that at least one medication error was prevented when a patient or family member identified a problem.[49]

TABLE 18.2

NATIONAL PATIENT SAFETY GOALS THAT ARE APPLICABLE TO PEDIATRIC ONCOLOGY IN HOSPITALS AND AMBULATORY SETTINGS (COMPLIANCE REQUIRED FOR ACCREDITATION BY JOINT COMMISSION AS OF JANUARY 1, 2009)

Goal 1: Improve the accuracy of patient identification
Goal 2: Improve the effectiveness of communication among caregivers
Goal 3: Improve the safety of using medications
Goal 7: Reduce the risk of health care–associated infections
Goal 8: Accurately and completely reconcile medications across the continuum of care
Goal 9: Reduce the risk of patient harm resulting from falls
Goal 13: Encourage patients' active involvement in their own care as a patient safety strategy
Goal 14: Prevent health care–associated pressure ulcers (decubitus ulcers)
Goal 15: The organization identifies safety risks inherent in its patient population
Goal 16: Improve recognition and response to changes in a patient's condition

TABLE 18.3

REQUIREMENTS AND RECOMMENDATIONS MADE BY THE JOINT COMMISSION

"Do not use" abbreviations	Potential problem	Preferred term
U (for unit)	Mistaken as 0 (zero), 4 (four), or cc	Write "unit"
IU (for international unit)	Mistaken as IV (intravenous) or 10 (ten)	Write "International unit"
Q.D. (once daily) Q.O.D. (every other day)	Mistaken for each other. The period after the Q can be mistaken for an "I" and the "O" can be mistaken for "I"	Write "daily" and "every other day"
Trailing zero (X.0 mg) Lack of leading zero (.X mg)	Decimal point is missed	Never write a zero by itself after a decimal point (X mg), and always use a zero before a decimal point (0.X mg)
MS, MSO_4, $MgSO_4$	Confused for one another. Can mean morphine sulfate or magnesium sulfate	Write "morphine sulfate" or "magnesium sulfate"

Problematic abbreviations	Potential problem	Preferred term
μg (for microgram)	Mistaken for mg (milligrams) resulting in 10-fold dosing overdose	Write "mcg"
H.S. (for half-strength or Latin abbreviation for bedtime)	Mistaken for either half-strength or hour of sleep (at bedtime). q.H.S. mistaken for every hour	Write out "Half-Strength" or "At bedtime"
T.I.W. (for three times a week)	Mistaken for three times a day or twice weekly resulting in an overdose	Write "3 times weekly" or "Three times weekly"
S.C. or S.Q. (for subcutaneous)	Mistaken as SL for sublingual, or "5 every"	Write "Sub-Q," "subQ," or "subcutaneously"
D/C (for discharge)	Interpreted as discontinue whatever medications follow (typically discharge meds)	Write "discharge"
c.c. (for cubic centimeter)	Mistaken for U (units) when poorly written	Write "ml" for milliliters
A.S., A.D., A.U. (Latin abbreviation for left, right, or both ears)	Mistaken for OS, OD, and OU, respectively	Write "Left ear," "Right ear" or "Both ears"

As important as education is the creation of a blame-free environment that is actively and visibly supported and nurtured by leadership. It has become clear that a major shift in culture from a punitive to a nonpunitive environment is necessary to create and maintain positive changes, especially when they emphasize teamwork instead of placing the blame on the end provider.[50,51] This has previously been recognized and implemented in other high-risk and low-error-tolerance industries, such as the aerospace industry and the operation of atomic reactors. A cultural attitude of reporting "near misses" regardless of the individual's organizational position has been fostered. All reports are taken seriously and investigated (and rewarded) whether they come from pilots, mechanics, or maintenance personnel. Over the last few years, reporting of "near-miss" events has become routine in the medical setting as well.[52]

Safeguarding the Medication Process

The medication process is complex and involves multiple steps from the creation of a medication order by a prescriber, transcription by nursing and/or pharmacy, preparation and dispensing by pharmacy, and administration and monitoring by nursing. Each step is error prone in different ways. Accordingly, different safeguards must be implemented to decrease error.

Many institutions rely on vigilance, either by self-checking or checking by others. This strategy tends to be ineffective for many reasons, including fatigue, distractions, and human imperfection.

The medication process generally involves multiple systems with differing potentials to prevent human errors from reaching the patient. An error represents an event that, once set into motion, passes through multiple systems defenses, each with a hole or error in it (Fig. 18.1). The number of layers in the system, and the size of the hole(s) in each one, influences the probability of an error reaching the patient. Thus, the goal is to design systems with as few holes as possible. Several strategies are available to decrease errors. Some of them are addressed in the following sections.

Ordering

A blank piece of paper labeled "order form" provides little support to the prescriber to create a complete, safe order. Instead, the system relies on prescriber vigilance to know, remember, and write down all the necessary components of an order or order set. Even a simple order has multiple elements requiring prescriber vigilance to write correctly. This vigilance is separate from the decision making the prescriber utilizes before writing the order and, in pediatrics, before calculating the final dose to be given.

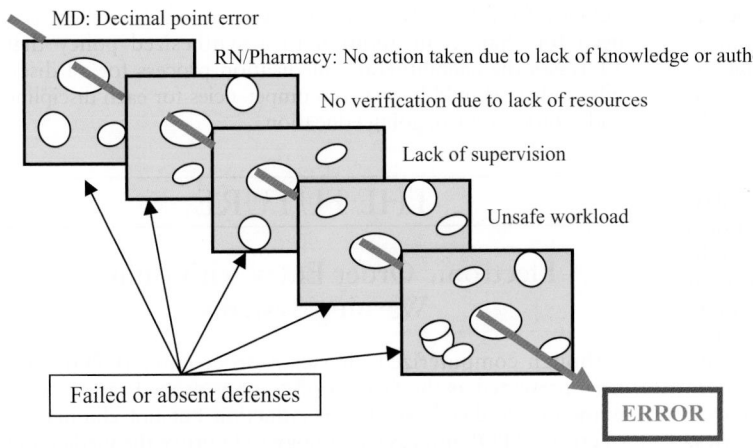

MD: Decimal point error

RN/Pharmacy: No action taken due to lack of knowledge or authority

No verification due to lack of resources

Lack of supervision

Unsafe workload

Failed or absent defenses

ERROR

FIGURE 18.1 An error represents an event that, once set into motion, passes through multiple systems defenses, each with a "hole" or error in it. The number of layers in the system and the size of the hole(s) in each one influence the probability of an error reaching the patient (adapted from Reason's Swiss cheese model).[38]

There are numerous steps that can improve this process, including, but not limited to, prescriber education, ensuring availability of relevant information such as a formulary, ensuring availability and standardization of patient dosing parameters (such as weight in kilograms), ensuring that necessary materials for order writing are available (such as prestamped order sheets, calculators). Clinical pharmacist involvement in work rounds and computerized decision support reduce the number of preventable ADEs at the ordering stage.[53]

Paper order templates, or an order set formatted for a specific aspect of care, can significantly reduce order error by prompting the prescriber to provide necessary information in a standardized format.[54] Templates can target a common process throughout the institution, such as an antibiotic order form, or a repetitive process within a care area such as a postoperative order set that includes a header labeled *"pain"* with suggested dosing options for acetaminophen, codeine, and morphine. Ideally, these order templates are evidence based, an approach that has long been standard practice in oncology.[55,56] Limited decision support can be provided on a paper order template, such as identifying antibiotics that require modification for renal insufficiency. Complex order sets with multiple sections and subheadings can provide more support and standardization. At the Dana Farber Cancer Institute, the intervention rate for complex inpatient chemotherapy orders was immediately reduced by more than 50% for orders written on detailed templates with many sections and detailed orders in each section, compared with a general hospital order form for chemotherapy that included minimal prompts and reminders.[57]

The benefit of the order templates is not just in legibility and prompts for medication orders but in the combined expertise of multiple disciplines to create an order set that meets the needs of all users. Creation of such templates requires leadership support, assigned resources, and a process for approval and regular review and updating by the hospital medication use committee. Templates may be created for such common processes in oncology as initial management of tumor lysis, prehydration for chemotherapy, or admission orders for fever and neutropenia. Templates provide an opportunity to standardize a process, reducing the probability of an error of omission and increasing the likelihood of detection of an error of commission.

Transcription

Improvements in the transcription process for both nursing and pharmacy can utilize both computerized and noncomputerized systems. Direct interfaces between a computerized order entry system and a pharmacy system and/or electronic medication administration record can eliminate the need for transcription entirely, but human assessment and confirmation will still be required. Transcription safety can be promoted by decreasing distractions and by ensuring the appropriate materials are available to staff members. The medication administration record form can be revised, as needed, to support workflow.

Environment

Observation of workflow or interviewing staff members can identify critical environmental factors that increase the probability of error.[58] Medication rooms must be big enough to permit staff members to work without bumping into each other, to allow any necessary paperwork to be laid out on a work surface, and to provide access to reference materials. There should not be multiple medication administration records in one binder, a situation that prevents two nurses from working simultaneously. If this is the case, the storage system should be changed to allow independent access to each patient's record. The area where orders are written should be organized to decrease the probability of an individual making an error. Chemotherapy treatment plans, often research protocols in pediatric oncology, should be easily accessible to staff members so that chemotherapy orders can be created or verified.

Dispensing

Dispensing errors can be decreased by eliminating "look alike, sound alike" medications from the formulary; eliminating or decreasing the availability of multiple concentrations of the same drug; applying unit dosing rules to common medications for larger patients; including both dosage and dose in the order so that intent and calculations are clear to the pharmacist; using visual cues to differentiate similar items that cannot be removed from the area; and utilizing standard concentrations as much as possible. Twenty-four-hour pharmacy coverage decreases medication error.

Chemotherapy-Specific Safeguards

Chemotherapy is a high-risk area for medication errors for multiple reasons. The drugs themselves often have a low therapeutic index and a high probability of expected adverse effects. Treatment plans are complex, may be carried out over a period of months to years, may be modified over time, and may contain conflicting or confusing information.[14,59] The high complexity of the order sets often requires writing orders in advance of a patient visit. Thus, order activation criteria based on patient data may need to be defined.

Chemotherapy orders often require differentiation, specific formatting, and information that are different from general medication orders.[48,60] In addition to standard requirements, such as patient identifiers (name, date of birth, medical record number) and dosing parameter, that is, weight (kg), height (cm), body surface area (m[2]), chemotherapy orders also contain additional elements: a treatment plan (e.g., protocol number), indications about timing within treatment plan (e.g., day, week, cycle, course), and order activation criteria (for orders written before patient visit and test data available). In addition to the usual components of a medication order, any or all of the following may be needed: dosage, calculated dose, any modifications, final dose, specific diluent instructions, and administration guidelines, as well as instructions regarding hydration (prehydration, concurrent or subsequent hydration). Furthermore, the order should include supportive care medications (general or specific), such as antiemetics, hematopoietic growth factors, leucovorin, mesna, and premedications to prevent allergic reactions. Chemotherapy orders will also contain monitoring guidelines for urine output, heme in urine and/or urine pH, monitoring of electrolytes, and possibly drug levels.

Chemotherapy order writing should be limited to staff with specific training or competencies. Each institution should define authorized prescribers for chemotherapy and whether cosignatures are required for some or all prescribers. In one survey, only 7 of 150 centers allowed order writing by house staff.[48] Order writing should require verification of lifetime cumulative dosing of such agents as anthracycline or bleomycin to ensure that safe maximums are not exceeded. Standardization of chemotherapy administration guidelines can make errors more recognizable.[14]

Chemotherapy order writing and verification requires access to the appropriate treatment reference (such as a research protocol, published article, or standardized treatment plan); a work setting without multiple distractions and interruptions; access to patient-specific data (height, weight, and laboratory and other test data); and specific staff competencies such as a dedicated oncology pharmacist.[14,48] Because research protocols undergo frequent modifications, institutions must have a system to ensure that only the current version of the study protocol and the order set are available. Thus, for those patients not being treated on a research protocol, an institutional standard or patient-specific plan must be identified and made available to all staff members who participate in the chemotherapy medication process. Pediatric cancer treatment plans are often complex with multiple treatment arms within a single plan; different phases, each with different medications; or cycles that alternate between two or more chemotherapy combinations. Treatment-specific roadmaps in each patient's chart with dates of treatment already given can be an invaluable tool to avoid errors.

Chemotherapy administration should take place on dedicated oncology inpatient and ambulatory units by nurses with special chemotherapy training. In addition, procedural safeguards specific to certain drugs can be implemented. Such safeguards can include not allowing vincristine into procedure rooms or differentiating chemotherapy for intrathecal administration from other chemotherapy with specific packaging.[61,62]

Policy

Traditionally, many health care institutions have had discipline-specific policies. For example, there could be medical staff, nursing, and pharmacy policies for medication orders. Review and synthesis of these policies, which may be conflicting and/or incomplete, into a single, multidisciplinary policy for medications can provide a starting point for change. In addition, other policies should be reviewed to determine whether there is a need for change. In addition to a synthesized policy that addresses the chemotherapy medication process for all disciplines, there should be specific competencies for each discipline and a process for ongoing education.

THE FUTURE

Electronic Order Entry with Built-in Warning Systems

Although computerized physician order entry (CPOE) has been presented as the "solution" to prevent medication error, numerous studies have shown reduction but not elimination of errors. CPOE utilizes technology to improve the medication order and delivery process and can be developed internally or obtained from a commercial vendor. In general, CPOE systems have the potential to reduce errors in different ways. At the most basic level, the system can prevent errors by forcing entry of generic drug names, ensuring complete orders without missing data such as frequency, ensuring legibility of the order, and providing clear identification of the prescriber through the use of an electronic signature. Such features can significantly reduce medication errors but have a much smaller impact on reducing preventable ADEs.[9,35]

CPOE can enhance workflow by ensuring that relevant data are present when an order is being written, for example, by displaying the most recent creatinine value when a gentamicin order is being written, or by offering predetermined order sets for specific processes. CPOE can also offer alerts and reminders designed to promote safer use of medication such as drug-allergy checking, drug-drug interaction checking, and medication guidelines, requiring deliberate overrides for doses or dosages that exceed predetermined maximums. This decision support may increase or decrease error, depending on its content. CPOE can also enhance reliability of the medication reconciliation process.[63]

By itself, CPOE may not reduce nonorder error unless it is linked to other electronic systems, such as pharmacy system or medication administration record. However, in one study, CPOE alone had a much larger effect on reducing transcription, dispensing, and administration error compared with actual errors in the order. In this study, preventable allergy events occurred because new allergy information was not entered into the system. Of 114 reactions that occurred in hospitalized patients, only 18 were entered into the CPOE system.[9]

CPOE can also serve as a tool to improve physicians' prescribing practice, such as compliance with guidelines for medication use.[64] The incidence of both ADEs and potential adverse events in an inpatient setting was reduced after implementation of a commercial CPOE system.[65]

In high-risk environments, such as pediatric oncology, CPOE can clearly increase the safety of chemotherapy prescriptions. Kim et al. reviewed data from 1,259 pre-CPOE paper and 1,116 post-CPOE pediatric chemotherapy orders. After CPOE deployment, daily chemotherapy orders were less likely to have improper dosing (relative risk [RR], 0.26; 95% confidence interval [CI], 0.11 to 0.61), incorrect dosing calculations (RR, 0.09; 95% CI, 0.03 to 0.34), missing cumulative dose calculations (RR, 0.32; 95% CI, 0.14 to 0.77), and incomplete nursing checklists (RR, 0.51; 95% CI, 0.33 to 0.80).[33]

At present, CPOE is implemented in less than 5% of hospitals.[66] No pediatric-specific data are available. Guidelines to help organizations implement CPOE have been developed.[67] As CPOE and other components of the electronic medical record are implemented in more pediatric institutions, specific pediatric challenges must be addressed, such as unique patient identifier for infants whose name changes; specific pediatric terminology for elements of the history or physical examination; age-based normal ranges; calculation of age in days or months when appropriate; prescribing of medications by weight or body surface area; and immunization support. However, hospital leaders have to remember that implementation of CPOE may, at least temporarily, lead to an increase in error rate, sometimes with fatal consequences. A study by Han et al. found that among 1,942 children, the mortality rate increased significantly from 2.80% (39 of 1,394) before CPOE implementation to 6.57% (36 of 548) after CPOE implementation. Multivariate analysis revealed that CPOE remained independently associated with increased odds of mortality (odds ratio: 3.28; 95% confidence interval: 1.94 to 5.55) after adjustment for other mortality covariables.[68] Chemotherapy ordering in CPOE may raise additional unique challenges that most commercial order entry systems may not be designed to handle. Thus, implementation of CPOE for chemotherapy must be approached with extreme caution. Continued surveillance of error rates is thus mandatory.

Bar Coding

Bar codes, using an automated identification technology that streamlines product identification and data collection, have become prevalent in our daily lives, being used in supermarkets, bookstores, post offices, and many other places. Barcoding technology was first introduced into medical settings about 20 years ago. These early applications were used mainly in clinical laboratories and blood banks.[69] However, widespread application of this technology was slowed down for a variety of reasons, including the lack of industry standards. In addition, there is little systemic research on the benefits, disadvantages, and challenges in implementing barcoding systems.[70] The FDA proposed in 2004 the introduction of rules requiring bar coding on medications, so that bar codes could be cross-matched with a patient's bar-coded wristband in an effort to reduce the number of errors. The FDA estimated that the introduction of this bar-code identification system could result in a 50% increase in the interception of medication errors during the medication dispensing and administration phase. Bar coding reduced the incidence of mislabeled specimens in a large pediatric oncology program.[71]

The use of bar codes to help match patients with their medication orders and administration is thought to be one of the most important mechanisms to decrease adverse medication events.[72] Medication schedules can be computerized and translated into a bar-coded plan. Pharmacy technicians and pharmacists can dispense medications after cross-checking against this schedule, and the nurse can match patient identity and drug order with the medication to be administered. The system not only provides alerts about possible misidentifications but also is integrated with the hospital pharmacy computer system and thus programmed with the patient's specific data (such as weight and age in pediatrics), which prevents overdosing (point-of-care system).

Smart Pumps

Computerized infusion devices (smart pumps) have built-in software that allows the pump to be programmed with institution-established dosage limits, provides warnings to the clinicians when the dosage limits have been exceeded, and allows the downloading of information to a desktop computer. Furthermore, smart pumps can be configured to contain patient-specific data.[73] They can be integrated with a bar-code system, to facilitate the safe recognition of the patient about to receive the infusion, and their computer system can provide data regarding the proper adherence to safety parameters.

Pediatric Labeling Information

A national effort is under way to improve the safety and efficacy of drug therapies for children by providing data that allow specific pediatric labeling of medications. Currently, up to 75% of all drugs used in children have not been studied adequately in this age group,[74] including commonly administered drugs such as heparin, furosemide, and dopamine.

Although more than 100 drugs have been approved for the treatment of malignancies, only 15 have pediatric use information in their labeling, which is less than half of the drugs commonly used in the treatment of childhood cancer.[75] Drugs such as ifosfamide, cisplatin, carboplatin, and etoposide, which are used in many regimens, have never been specifically approved for pediatric use. Having age-appropriate information available when using potent drugs with a narrow therapeutic index would clearly increase the safety of treatment.

Education, Including Simulation Technique: Inclusion in Medical Curriculum

In other high-risk, low—error-tolerant industries, it is standard to use simulation programs not only to train people but also to evaluate and learn from errors that occurred. Several different simulation models have been employed in emergency medicine and anesthesia. Both disciplines lend themselves to the use of mannequins with more or less sophisticated capabilities to simulate real life situations.[76] Other disciplines have been slowed down to adopt such training methods.[77]

Safety education needs to start at the undergraduate level and continue throughout medical practice. Unfortunately, this is not yet the case. Rosebraugh et al.[78] surveyed medical directors of third-year medical students in internal medicine clerkship and residency programs about training provided by their programs in clinical pharmacology and adverse drug reaction. Only 64% of internal medicine residencies had formal lectures covering adverse drug reactions, and only 59% offered lectures on rational drug prescribing. Over half (53%) of medical schools did not have clinical rotations that included clinical pharmacology or adverse drug reaction training. Of those that did, only 8% of the rotations were mandatory.[78]

Massachusetts was the first state to mandate continuing medical education (CME) credits in patient safety to maintain a physician license. Many organizations offer CME credits or provide other helpful tools to address safety issues. Pediatric oncology, due to its high-risk features and complexities, is a field particularly prone to potential errors that can affect the safety of patients (and staff). It is therefore imperative that we take the lead in creating safeguards and an environment that emphasizes recognition and elimination of hazards before an error occurs. The pediatric oncologist, because of the specialty's emphasis on protocol-guided therapy and the use of evidence-based medicine, is in a unique position to take a leadership role in enhancing the safety of the medication process, not only for chemotherapeutic agents but also for the whole field of pediatric medication administration.

References

1. Knox RA. Doctor's orders killed cancer patient. The Boston Globe. March 23, 1995.
2. Kohn LT, Corrigan JM, Donaldson MS. To err is human: building a safer health care system. Washington, DC: National Academic Press, 2000.
3. Brennan TA, Localio AR, Leape LL, et al. Identification of adverse events occurring during hospitalization. A cross-sectional study of litigation, quality assurance, and medical records at two teaching hospitals. Ann Intern Med 1990;112(3):221–226.
4. Leape LL, Brennan TA, Laird N, et al. The nature of adverse events in hospitalized patients. Results of the Harvard Medical Practice Study II. N Engl J Med 1991;324(6):377–384.
5. Thomas EJ, Studdert DM, Newhouse JP, et al. Costs of medical injuries in Utah and Colorado. Inquiry 1999;36(3):255–264.
6. Flores G, Laws MB, Mayo SJ, et al. Errors in medical interpretation and their potential clinical consequences in pediatric encounters. Pediatrics 2003;111(1):6–14.
7. Sexton JB, Thomas EJ, Helmreich RL. Error, stress, and teamwork in medicine and aviation: cross sectional surveys. BMJ 2000;320(7237):745–749.
8. Slonim AD, LaFleur BJ, Ahmed W, et al. Hospital-reported medical errors in children. Pediatrics 2003;111(3):617–621.
9. Bates DW, Leape LL, Cullen DJ, et al. Effect of computerized physician order entry and a team intervention on prevention of serious medication errors. JAMA 1998;280(15): 1311–1316.
10. Bates DW, Teich JM, Lee J, et al. The impact of computerized physician order entry on medication error prevention. J Am Med Inform Assoc 1999;6(4):313–321.
11. Kaushal R, Bates DW. Information technology and medication safety: what is the benefit? Qual Saf Health Care 2002;11(3):261–265.
12. Pichon R, Zelger GL, Wacker P, et al. Analysis and quantification of prescribing and transcription errors in a paediatric oncology service. Pharm World Sci 2002;24(1):12–15.
13. Walsh KE, Dodd KS, Seetharaman K, et al. Medication errors among adults and children with cancer in the outpatient setting. J Clin Oncol 2009;27(6):891–896.
14. Womer RB, Tracy E, Soo-Hoo W, et al. Multidisciplinary systems approach to chemotherapy safety: rebuilding processes and holding the gains. J Clin Oncol 2002;20 (24):4705–4712.
15. Kaushal R, Bates DW, Landrigan C, et al. Medication errors and adverse drug events in pediatric inpatients. JAMA 2001;285(16):2114–2120.
16. Lesar TS, Briceland LL, Delcoure K, et al. Medication prescribing errors in a teaching hospital. JAMA 1990;263(17):2329–2334.
17. Werner RA. Paraplegia and quadriplegia after intrathecal chemotherapy. Arch Phys Med Rehabil 1988;69(12):1054–1056.
18. Schulmeister L. Chemotherapy medication errors: descriptions, severity, and contributing factors. Oncol Nurs Forum 1999;26(6):1033–1042.
19. Taylor JA, Winter L, Geyer LJ, et al. Oral outpatient chemotherapy medication errors in children with acute lymphoblastic leukemia. Cancer 2006;107(6):1400–1406.
20. Rinke ML, Shore AD, Morlock L, et al. Characteristics of pediatric chemotherapy medication errors in a national error reporting database. Cancer 2007;110(1):186–195.
21. Bates DW, Boyle DL, Vander Vliet MB, et al. Relationship between medication errors and adverse drug events. J Gen Intern Med 1995;10(4):199–205.
22. Brennan TA, Mello MM. Patient safety and medical malpractice: a case study. Ann Intern Med 2003;139(4):267–273.
23. Studdert DM, Mello MM, Brennan TA. Medical malpractice. N Engl J Med 2004;350 (3):283–292.
24. Bates DW, Spell N, Cullen DJ, et al. The costs of adverse drug events in hospitalized patients. Adverse Drug Events Prevention Study Group. JAMA 1997;277(4):307–311.
25. Rothschild JM, Federico FA, Gandhi TK, et al. Analysis of medication-related malpractice claims: causes, preventability, and costs. Arch Intern Med 2002;162(21):2414–2420.
26. Schneider PJ. Measuring medication safety in hospitals. Introduction. Am J Health Syst Pharm 2002;59(23):2313–2314.
27. Phillips MA. Voluntary reporting of medication errors. Am J Health Syst Pharm 2002;59(23):2326–2328.
28. Pierluissi E, Fischer MA, Campbell AR, et al. Discussion of medical errors in morbidity and mortality conferences. JAMA 2003;290(21):2838–2842.
29. Cameron HM, McGoogan E. A prospective study of 1152 hospital autopsies: II. Analysis of inaccuracies in clinical diagnoses and their significance. J Pathol 1981;133(4):285–300.
30. Shojania KG, Burton EC, McDonald KM, et al. Changes in rates of autopsy-detected diagnostic errors over time: a systematic review. JAMA 2003;289(21):2849–2856.
31. Kaushal R. Using chart review to screen for medication errors and adverse drug events. Am J Health Syst Pharm 2002;59(23):2323–2325.
32. Flynn EA, Barker KN, Pepper GA, et al. Comparison of methods for detecting medication errors in 36 hospitals and skilled-nursing facilities. Am J Health Syst Pharm 2002;59(5):436–446.
33. Kim GR, Chen AR, Arceci RJ, et al. Error reduction in pediatric chemotherapy: computerized order entry and failure modes and effects analysis. Arch Pediatr Adolesc Med 2006;160(5):495–498.
34. Robinson DL, Heigham M, Clark J. Using failure mode and effects analysis for safe administration of chemotherapy to hospitalized children with cancer. Jt Comm J Qual Patient Saf 2006;32(3):161–166.
35. Bates DW, Evans RS, Murff H, et al. Detecting adverse events using information technology. J Am Med Inform Assoc 2003;10(2):115–128.
36. Bagheri H, Michel F, Lapeyre-Mestre M, et al. Detection and incidence of drug-induced liver injuries in hospital: a prospective analysis from laboratory signals. Br J Clin Pharmacol 2000;50(5):479–484.
37. Cullen DJ, Bates DW, Small SD, et al. The incident reporting system does not detect adverse drug events: a problem for quality improvement. Jt Comm J Qual Improv 1995;21(10): 541–548.
38. Reason J. Human error: models and management. West J Med 2000;172(6):393–396.
39. Ladewski LA, Belknap SM, Nebeker JR, et al. Dissemination of information on potentially fatal adverse drug reactions for cancer drugs from 2000 to 2002: first results from the research on adverse drug events and reports project. J Clin Oncol 2003;21(20):3859–3866.
40. DeRosier J, Stalhandske E, Bagian JP, et al. Using health care failure mode and effect analysis: the VA National Center for Patient Safety's prospective risk analysis system. Jt Comm J Qual Improv 2002;28(5):248–267, 209.
41. Liang BA. A system of medical error disclosure. Qual Saf Health Care 2002;11(1):64–68.
42. Mazor KM, Simon SR, Yood RA, et al. Health plan members' views about disclosure of medical errors. Ann Intern Med 2004;140(6):409–418.
43. Hobgood C, Peck CR, Gilbert B, et al. Medical errors—what and when: what do patients want to know? Acad Emerg Med 2002;9(11):1156–1161.
44. Conway JB. Patient safety: it starts at the top. Trustee 2000;53(5):24.
45. Frankel A, Graydon-Baker E, Neppl C, et al. Patient Safety Leadership WalkRounds. Jt Comm J Qual Saf 2003;29(1):16–26.
46. Weinger MB. Anesthesia equipment and human error. J Clin Monit Comput 1999;15(5): 319–323.
47. Weinger MB, Ancoli-Israel S. Sleep deprivation and clinical performance. JAMA 2002;287(8):955–957.
48. Fischer DS, Alfano S, Knobf MT, et al. Improving the cancer chemotherapy use process. J Clin Oncol 1996;14(12):3148–3155.
49. Weingart SN, Toth M, Eneman J, et al. Lessons from a patient partnership intervention to prevent adverse drug events. Int J Qual Health Care 2004;16(6):499–507.
50. Stump LS. Re-engineering the medication error-reporting process: removing the blame and improving the system. Am J Health Syst Pharm 2000;57(suppl 4):S10–S17.
51. Wilf-Miron R, Lewenhoff I, Benyamini Z, et al. From aviation to medicine: applying concepts of aviation safety to risk management in ambulatory care. Qual Saf Health Care 2003;12(1):35–39.
52. Ardenghi D, Martinengo M, Bocciardo L, et al. Near miss errors in transfusion medicine: the experience of the G. Gaslini Transfusion Medicine Service. Blood transfus 2007;5 (4):210–216.
53. Kucukarslan SN, Peters M, Mlynarek M, et al. Pharmacists on rounding teams reduce preventable adverse drug events in hospital general medicine units. Arch Intern Med 2003;163(17):2014–2018.
54. Wasserfallen JB, Butschi AJ, Muff P, et al. Format of medical order sheet improves security of antibiotics prescription: the experience of an intensive care unit. Crit Care Med 2004;32(3):655–659.
55. Dy SM, Lorenz KA, Naeim A, et al. Evidence-based recommendations for cancer fatigue, anorexia, depression, and dyspnea. J Clin Oncol 2008;26(23):3886–3895.
56. Dy SM, Asch SM, Naeim A, et al. Evidence-based standards for cancer pain management. J Clin Oncol 2008;26(23):3879–3885.
57. Dinning C, Branowicki P, O'Neill JB, et al. Chemotherapy error reduction: a multidisciplinary approach to create templated order sets. J Pediatr Oncol Nurs 2005;22(1):20–30.
58. Rathert C, May DR. Health care work environments, employee satisfaction, and patient safety: care provider perspectives. Health Care Manage Rev 2007;32(1):2–11.
59. Sievers TD, Lagan MA, Bartel SB, et al. Variation in administration of cyclophosphamide and mesna in the treatment of childhood malignancies. J Pediatr Oncol Nurs 2001; 18(1):37–45.
60. Kohler DR, Montello MJ, Green L, et al. Standardizing the expression and nomenclature of cancer treatment regimens. American Society of Health-System Pharmacist (ASHP), American Medical Association (AMA), American Nurses Association (ANA). Am J Health Syst Pharm 1998;55(2):137–144.
61. Anderson RA, Wolff JE, Egeler RM, et al. Infallible measures needed to prevent errors in the administration of chemotherapeutic agents. Med Pediatr Oncol 1999;32(5):401–402.
62. Palmieri C, Barron N, Vigushin DM. The Vincotube System: a design solution to prevent the accidental administration of intrathecal vinca alkaloids. J Clin Oncol 2004; 22(5):965; author reply 965-966.
63. Agrawal A, Wu WY. Reducing medication errors and improving systems reliability using an electronic medication reconciliation system. Jt Comm J Qual Patient Saf 2009; 35(2):106–114.
64. Varkey P, Aponte P, Swanton C, et al. The effect of computerized physician-order entry on outpatient prescription errors. Manag Care Interface 2007;20(3):53–57.
65. Holdsworth MT, Fichtl RE, Raisch DW, et al. Impact of computerized prescriber order entry on the incidence of adverse drug events in pediatric inpatients. Pediatrics 2007;120(5):1058–1066.
66. Pedersen CA, Schneider PJ, Santell JP. ASHP national survey of pharmacy practice in hospital settings: prescribing and transcribing—2001. Am J Health Syst Pharm 2001; 58(23):2251–2266.
67. Gray MD, Felkey BG. Computerized prescriber order-entry systems: evaluation, selection, and implementation. Am J Health Syst Pharm 2004;61(2):190–197.
68. Han YY, Carcillo JA, Venkataraman ST, et al. Unexpected increased mortality after implementation of a commercially sold computerized physician order entry system. Pediatrics 2005;116(6):1506–1512.
69. Murphy MF, Kay JD. Barcode identification for transfusion safety. Curr Opin Hematol 2004;11(5):334–338.
70. Patterson ES, Cook RI, Render ML. Improving patient safety by identifying side effects from introducing bar coding in medication administration. J Am Med Inform Assoc 2002;9(5):540–553.
71. Hayden RT, Patterson DJ, Jay DW, et al. Computer-assisted bar-coding system significantly reduces clinical laboratory specimen identification errors in a pediatric oncology hospital. J Pediatr 2008;152(2):219–224.
72. Bates DW, Cohen M, Leape LL, et al. Reducing the frequency of errors in medicine using information technology. J Am Med Inform Assoc 2001;8(4):299–308.
73. KLAS. Smart pumps: In an area where decimal-point medication errors can be fatal, smart infusion pumps are adding a line of defense. Healthc Inform 2008;25(12):20.
74. Roberts R, Rodriguez W, Murphy D, et al. Pediatric drug labeling: improving the safety and efficacy of pediatric therapies. JAMA 2003;290(7):905–911.
75. Hirschfeld S, Ho PT, Smith M, et al. Regulatory approvals of pediatric oncology drugs: previous experience and new initiatives. J Clin Oncol 2003;21(6):1066–1073.
76. Reznek M, Harter P, Krummel T. Virtual reality and simulation: training the future emergency physician. Acad Emerg Med 2002;9(1):78–87.
77. Wayman KI, Yaeger KA, Sharek PJ, et al. Simulation-based medical error disclosure training for pediatric healthcare professionals. J Healthc Qual 2007;29(4):12–19.
78. Rosebraugh CJ, Honig PK, Yasuda SU, et al. Centers for education and research on therapeutics report: survey of medication errors education during undergraduate and graduate medical education in the United States. Clin Pharmacol Ther 2002;71(1): 4–10.

CHAPTER 19 ■ ACUTE LYMPHOBLASTIC LEUKEMIA

JUDITH F. MARGOLIN, KAREN R. RABIN, C. PHILIP STEUBER, AND DAVID G. POPLACK

INTRODUCTION

Advances in the study and treatment of pediatric acute lymphoblastic leukemia (ALL) are often cited as the paradigm of success in modern, clinical-trial– and translational-research–based medicine.[1] Overall cure rates for pediatric ALL have improved from virtually zero in the 1950s to the current Event Free Survival (EFS) rates of 75% to 85% for this disease (Fig. 19.1). The improved overall cure rate is only part of the story since the cure rates for specific ALL subgroups range from greater than 90% to as low as 40% to 45% (Figs. 19.3, 19.7, 19.8, 19.9, 19.10, 19.12, 19.13, 19.14, 19.15, 19.16, 19.18).[1,2] The advances made have been due to the development of active chemotherapeutic agents, to improvement in our understanding of how to dose and combine these agents more effectively, and to significant advances in supportive care. The triumphs of the past have relied on the identification of therapy- and response-based prognostic factors. Further progress in this field will likely be related to our ability to identify and target specific molecular and genetic abnormalities within the leukemia cells themselves as well as to better understand how to address individual differences in the pharmacogenetics of chemotherapeutic agents.[1,3] Although the improvements in the cure rates have been gratifying to the patients, families, physicians, and researchers, this progress has sometimes come at a significant price in terms of both short- and long-term morbidity. In the future, a goal is to "personalize" ALL therapy such that individualized, targeted treatments can be identified that improve efficacy while minimizing toxicity.

EPIDEMIOLOGY

ALL is the most common malignancy in children. It accounts for one-fourth of all childhood cancers and 72% of all cases of childhood leukemia.[4] Approximately 4,900 children are diagnosed with ALL each year in the United States, with an incidence of 3 to 4 cases per 100,000 white children or 29.2 per million including all U.S. children.[5,6] The peak incidence of ALL occurs between 2 to 5 years of age (Fig. 19.2). This young age peak historically has appeared at different times in different countries. It occurred initially in Great Britain in the 1920s, in the United States in the 1940s, and in Japan in the 1960s. The appearance of these peaks correspond to major periods of industrialization in these countries, suggesting that they may reflect periods of exposure to new environmental leukemogens.[7]

Among children in the United States, ALL is more common among whites than blacks. This disparity appears to be due to the early surge in ALL incidence that occurs in whites, which may reflect differences in susceptibility, environmental exposures, or both.[8] Controversy exists concerning whether outcomes differ among children of different racial and ethnic backgrounds. Early reports indicated that American black children fared significantly worse when compared with white children, but this difference has decreased or even disappeared in more recent studies as outcomes improved for all patients (see section "Prognostic Factors" and Fig. 19.3).[9] Black patients with ALL are more likely to present with unfavorable features (see Prognostic Factors) including higher white blood cell (WBC) counts, higher incidence of disease with T-cell characteristics, and lower incidence of favorable cytogenetics.[10] The incidence of ALL in U.S. Hispanic populations appears to be slightly higher than in Caucasian children, and similar to data which demonstrate slightly worse outcomes in black children, Hispanic children have been reported to have worse outcomes.[8,11] Hispanic children have a relatively lower percentages of cases demonstrating better risk disease features (i.e., a lower incidence of t(12;21) cytogenetics; see Table 19.6) and/or pharmacogenetic differences which may decrease the efficacy of some of the commonly used medications.[8,11] Recent data have shown that the increased incidence of ALL, as well as poorer prognosis, appears to continue into adulthood in Hispanics.[12]

The incidence of ALL is higher among boys than girls, and this difference is greatest among pubertal children.[13] In early studies, male sex was a distinctly poor prognostic factor. At least some of the inferior outcomes in boys have been related to the higher incidence of adverse prognostic features, including a higher percentage of T-cell immunophenotype and fewer cases with a favorable DNA index. Although outcomes have improved with modern therapy, boys continue to have slightly higher incidence and poorer prognosis than girls in most categories of the disease.[13]

There are geographic differences in the frequency and age distribution of ALL. For example, ALL is relatively rare in North Africa and the Middle East where non-Hodgkin lymphoma is the most common childhood malignancy. In India and China, ALL is somewhat more common, but its incidence is still considerably less than in the industrialized West.[14] This geographic variation may reflect, in part, the distribution of different immunologic and cytogenetic ALL subtypes. There appears to be a lower incidence of B-precursor ALL in developing countries and a higher incidence of T-cell ALL in more industrialized countries. Although this may reflect an underdiagnosis of some or all forms of ALL in developing countries, it is also possible that children in industrialized countries have more exposure to leukemogens that cause ALL.[15]

Multiple studies have suggested a link between maternal reproductive history, increasing birth weights and the risk of ALL.[16,17] Recent evidence has implicated increased *in utero* growth rates (more than final birth weight) and Insulin Growth Factor (IGF) pathways in the development of ALL.[18,19] Fetal loss is associated with a higher risk for the development of ALL in subsequent children. It is unclear whether this reflects genetic predisposition, an abnormal intrauterine environment, or a common adverse environmental exposure. Paternal chemical (pesticides and fungicide) exposure, alcohol history, and

Survival Comparison
CCG ALL Study Series

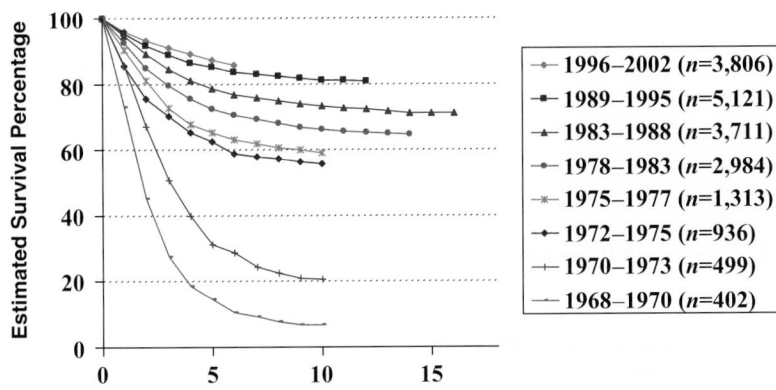

- 1996–2002 (*n*=3,806)
- 1989–1995 (*n*=5,121)
- 1983–1988 (*n*=3,711)
- 1978–1983 (*n*=2,984)
- 1975–1977 (*n*=1,313)
- 1972–1975 (*n*=936)
- 1970–1973 (*n*=499)
- 1968–1970 (*n*=402)

FIGURE 19.1 Improvement in survival of children with acute lymphoblastic leukemia. Curves represent the survival outcomes for patients treated on successive Children's Cancer Group (CCG) clinical trials conducted over the 1968–2002 period. (H. Sather, personal communication, 2004.)

smoking history have been implicated as well.[20] Parental smoking is associated with a higher incidence of ALL, with paternal smoking during the preconception period appearing to carry the highest risk. The mechanism for paternal exposures and ALL risk in offspring is thought to relate directly to DNA damage and carcinogens that can be found in sperm.[21] The susceptibility to DNA mismatch repair after exposure to leukemogens appears to be inherited through a complex set of genotypic variants found in genes involved in the metabolism of specific xenobiotics and repair of the genome.[22] These genotypes have relevance both for the *in utero* development of leukemia as well as in the response and second tumor risk from chemotherapy and radiotherapy delivered later in life.

Numerous reports speak of the occurrence of leukemic *clusters*, observations of a greater than expected number of leukemia cases within a given period for a geographic area (see Chapter 1). Under careful scrutiny, most purported clusters have not been substantiated, but investigators continue to report clusters that point towards environmental and/or infectious contributions to the etiology of at least some cases of ALL.[23]

GENETICS

Genetic factors play a significant role in the etiology of ALL. Evidence for this is based on several observations including: (a) the demonstration of both random and non-random

karyotypic abnormalities in the leukemic cells of the majority children with ALL (Table 19.1), (b) the association between various constitutional chromosomal abnormalities and childhood ALL, (c) the occurrence of familial leukemia, (d) the high incidence of leukemia in identical twins, and (e) the molecular epidemiologic evidence of the importance of various alleles of specific genes (see also Pharmacogenetics).[1]

Constitutional chromosomal abnormalities are associated with an increased incidence of childhood leukemia. Children with trisomy 21 (Down syndrome, DS) are 10 to 20 times more likely to develop leukemia than children without DS.[1,24] Although both ALL and acute myeloid leukemia (AML) occur with increased frequency, ALL predominates in all but the neonatal age group.[25] The age of distribution for ALL in DS is similar to the general population, but the high incidence of AML (megakaryocytic or FAB M7) in children with DS under age 5 causes the overall ratio of AML: ALL in DS to be close to 1:1.[26] The occurrence of leukemia (either ALL or AML) appears to be unrelated to the various other congenital anomalies and medical problems (e.g., congenital heart disease and hypothyroidism) associated with Down syndrome.[27] Controversy exists concerning how the molecular genetic origins of DS-associated leukemias are similar or different from leukemias arising in non-DS children. Some investigators report a high incidence of common ALL cytogenetic changes in leukemic blasts from DS patients, but this is not a consistent finding.[28–30] Several novel somatic genetic alterations have been recently identified which occur markedly more frequently in DS-ALL: Janus kinase 2 (JAK2) activating mutations are found in 20% of DS-ALL, and translocations and interstitial deletions leading to high expression of cytokine receptor-like factor 2 (CRLF2) occur in 50% of DS-ALL.[31,32] Clinical outcomes for DS patients have generally been poorer than for non-DS patients, perhaps due in part to the fact that favorable-prognosis cytogenetic subgroups occur less often in DS children.[33] Outcomes have improved with enhanced supportive care and a better understanding of the characteristic toxicities observed in DS patients, which include more frequent mucositis, hyperglycemia, and infectious complications.[29]

Although other less common preexisting chromosomal abnormalities and specific inherited syndromes have been linked to leukemia, less than 5% of ALL cases (including those in patients with DS) can be linked to any specific genetic cause.[1] Included among these are reports of ALL in children with germline BRCA2 mutations, and in Beckwith-Wiedemann patients.[34,35] Children with neurofibromatosis and those with Shwachman's syndrome are also reported to have an increased risk of leukemia.[36,37]

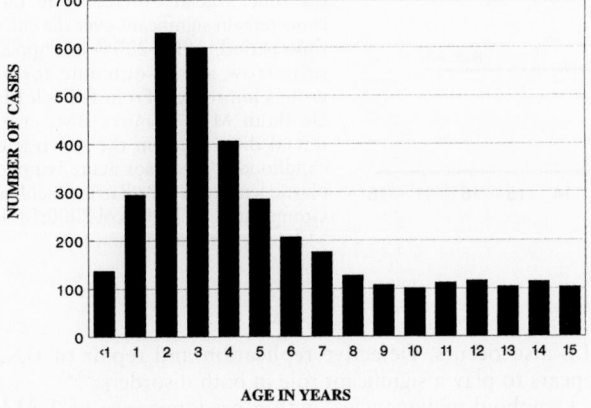

FIGURE 19.2 Age distribution of 3,620 children with acute lymphoblastic leukemia. (Data from the Children's Cancer Group, courtesy of H. Sather.)

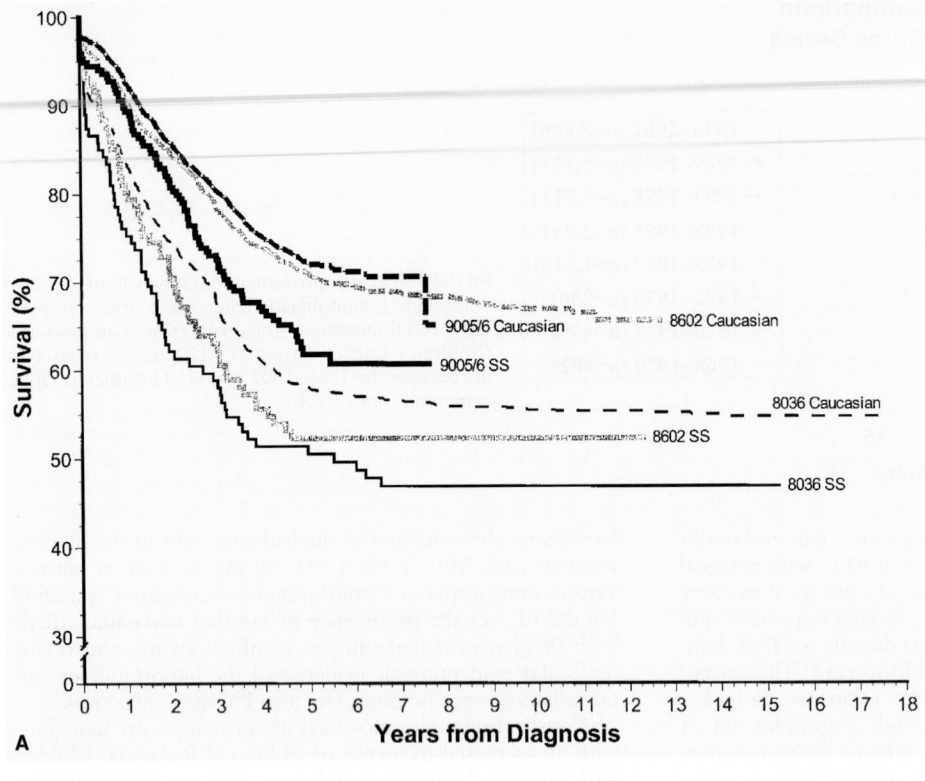

A

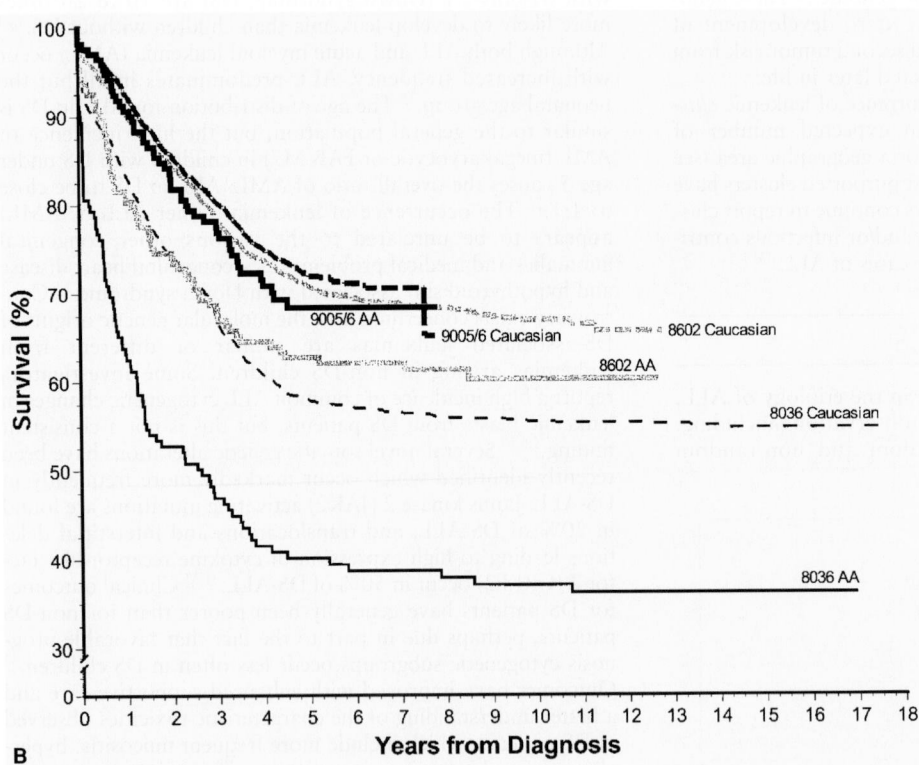

B

FIGURE 19.3 A: Kaplan-Meier analysis of overall survival for Caucasian (4,061 patients) compared with Spanish Surname (SS) (507 patients) on three standard and high-risk Pediatric Oncology Group (POG) protocols, which accrued patients between 1981 and 2005. **B:** Kaplan-Meier estimates of overall survival comparing Caucasian with African-American (AA) children (518 patients) on the same three protocols. POG 8036 was open from 1981 to 1986, POG 8602 was open from 1986 to 1991, and POG 9005/6 spanned 2000 to 2005. Each of these protocols stratified patients according to the valid prognostic indicators of the time. Racial differences in outcome remain significant over the entire time period (1981–2005) but appear to narrow as the outcome for all groups improved. (From Pollock BH, De Baun MR, Camitta BM, et al. Racial differences in the survival of childhood B-precursor acute lymphoblastic leukemia: a Pediatric Oncology Group study. J Clin Oncol 2000;18(4): 813–823, with permission.)

An increased incidence of acute leukemia among those with Bloom's syndrome, Fanconi anemia, and Nijmegen breakage syndrome is well documented.[38,39] These rare, autosomal recessive disorders are characterized by increased chromosomal fragility. Although AML is more common in Bloom's syndrome as well as in patients with Fanconi anemia,

ALL also occurs. Defective replication and repair of DNA appears to play a significant role in both disorders.[40,41]

Lymphoid malignancies, with a predominance of T-ALL, have been reported in patients with ataxia-telangiectasia (AT), an autosomal recessive disorder also characterized by increased chromosomal fragility.[38] However, B- and pre–B-cell

TABLE 19.1

NONRANDOM CHROMOSOMAL TRANSLOCATIONS ASSOCIATED WITH SPECIFIC IMMUNOPHENOTYPES AND FUSION PROTEIN PRODUCTS IN CHILDHOOD ACUTE LYMPHOBLASTIC LEUKEMIA (ALL)

Immunophenotype, disease, and translocation	Affected genes		Protein product transcription factor family	Frequency (%)
Pre–B-cell/early pre–B-cell/ T-cell ALL (myeloid CML)				
			P185$^{BCR-ABL}$	
t(9;22)(q34;q11) Philadelphia chromosome, poor prognosis	*ABL*	*BCR*	Tyrosine kinase (P210$^{BCR-ABL}$ in CML)	3–5
Pre–B-cell/early pre–B-cell ALL				
t(1;19)(q23;p13) associated with high WBC, black race, requires intensive therapy	*PBX1*	*TCF3 (E2A)*	E2A-PBX1 fusion protein (PBX = homeodomain protein)	5–6
t(4;11)(q21;q23), associated with infant ALL as well as infant AML	*AF-4*	*ALL1/MLL/HRX*	ALL1-AF-4 fusion protein	
			A-T hook minor groove binding protein	2
Dic(9;12)(9p11-p12;p12) associated predominantly in boys; good prognosis with antimetabolite therapy	Unknown	Unknown	Unknown	1
T(5;15)(q31;q32)	*IL-3*	*IGH@* (enhancer)	IL-3	<1
T(11;19)(q23:p13)	*ALL1/MLL/ HRX*	*ENL*	ALL1-ENL fusion protein	
			A-T hook minor groove binding protein	<1
t(9;11)(p21-p22;q23)	*AF-9*	*ALL1/MLL/HRX*	ALL1-AF-9 fusion protein	<1
			A-T hook minor groove binding protein	
t(17;19)(q22;p13)	*HLF*	*TCF3 (E2A)*	E2A-HLF fusion protein	<1
			Basic region/leucine zipper DNA binding protein	
			TEL (an ETS transcription factor)	5–10
t(12;v)(p12-p13;V)	*ETV6 (TEL)* or *KIP1*	Unknown	KIP1 (a cyclin-dependent kinase inhibitor) forming fusion proteins with various partners	
t(12;21)(p12;q22)	*ETV6 (TEL)*	*RUNX1 (AML1)*	*ETV6-RUNX1 (TEL-AML1)* fusion protein	16–22 (by molecular techniques; 5 with karyotype)
T-cell ALL				
t(11;14)(p13;q11) associated with males, high WBC count, extramedullary disease	*TTG2/ RHOM2*	*TCRδ*	Cys-rich LIM domain (zinc-finger protein [rhombotin 2])	1
t(11;14)(p15;q11)	*TTG1/ RHOM2*	*TCRδ*	Cys-rich LIM domain (zinc-finger protein [rhombotin 1])	<1
t(10;14)(q24;q11)	*HOX 11/ TCL1*	*TCRδ*	Hox 11 homeodomain protein	<1
t(7;10)(q35;q24)	*HOX 11/ TCL1*	*TCRβ*	Hox 11 homeodomain protein	<1
t(1;14)(p32-p34;q11)	*TAL1/SCL*	*TCR*	TAL1, bHLH protein	<1
t(8;14)(q24;q11)	*MYC*	*TCR*	MYC, bHLH protein	<1
t(7;9)(q34;q32)	*TCRβ*	*TAL2*	bHLH protein	<1
t(7;9)(q34;q34.32)	*TCRβ*	*TAN1*	Unknown	<1
t(7;19)(q35;p13)	*TCRβ*	*LYL1*	bHLH protein	<1
t(1;7)(p34;q34)	*LCK*	*TCRβ*	LY tyrosine kinase	<1
B-cell ALL				
t(8;14)(q24;q32.3) L3 morphology, predominantly boys, favorable prognosis with short-term intensive therapy	*MYC*	*IGH@*	MYC, bHLH protein	1–2
t(8;22)(q24;q11) L3 variant	*MYC*	*IGL@*	MYC, bHLH protein	<1
t(2;8)(p11-p12;q24) L3 variant	*IGK@*	*MYC*	MYC, bHLH protein	<1

AML, acute myeloid leukemia; bHLH, basic helix-loop-helix; CML, chronic myeloid leukemia; Ig, immunoglobulin; IL, interleukin; LIM, transcription factor associated protein-binding domain; TCR, T-cell receptor; WBC, white blood cell.

immunophenotype ALL has been reported occasionally in AT patients.[42] The gene responsible for AT, ataxia-telangiectasia mutated *(ATM)*, is a phosphatidyl kinase that has been cloned, but the mechanism by which it increases the patients' risk for cancer is the subject of active research.[43,44] Care must be taken in examining reports of ALL associated with rare genetic disorders. Klinefelter's syndrome, although linked in the past with both ALL and AML and associated with other tumor types (germ cell tumors), is not currently felt to be etiologically associated with ALL.[45–47]

The importance of *in utero* genetic events has been suspected for many years because of concordance studies on twins with leukemia.[1,48] It has been demonstrated that leukemogenic translocations [e.g., t(4;11) and t(12;21)], hyperdiploidy, and other markers of clonality (e.g., evidence of the same specific immunoglobulin variable, diversity, and joining regions [VDJ] and T-cell receptor [TCR] recombination events) that are found in individual patients' leukemic clones at diagnosis can be detected at birth as minor hematopoietic populations.[1,49] The conditions for rapid growth (i.e., high IGF1 levels as noted above) and expansion in the bone marrow, and in specific lymphoid cell populations, both *in utero* and in the early years of life, may subsequently favor the expansion of these clones.[18,19]

Studies of stored cord blood and neonatal heel-stick (Guthrie) cards have shown that as many as 1 in 100 to 1 in 1,000 newborns have either preleukemic translocations and/or evidence of VDJ recombinant clones present at the level of 10^{-2} to 10^{-4} at the time of birth.[1,49] Clearly, the majority of these children do not eventually develop clinical leukemia, but this is evidence that some of the important initiating events that contribute to leukemogenesis often occur *in utero*. In addition to the research pointing to oncogenic mutations that arise *in utero*, other recent studies have identified inherited, germline single nucleotide polymorphisms (SNPs) that predispose subjects to development of ALL. Genome-wide association studies have recently identified several SNPs associated with a significantly higher risk of developing ALL which occur in genes involved in B-cell transcriptional regulation and differentiation.[50,51] The affected genes include *ARID5B* and *IKZF*, and the *ARID5B* variant SNPs were specifically associated with development of the hyperdiploid subtype of ALL, and with increased accumulation of methotrexate polyglutamates.

Current research in this area utilizes the newest tools of high throughput sequencing, as well as mRNA and microRNA microarrays, DNA copy number alterations, loss of heterozygosity (LOH), and epigenetic changes (e.g., methylation) to uncover cooperating changes that appear to be required for the preleukemic clones identified in the cord blood samples to become frankly leukemic.[52] These studies show promise as tools not only for elucidating the biology of leukemogenesis and potentially identifying children at greatest risk for developing leukemia, but also for the development of new biomarkers and therapeutic targets for the next generation of leukemia treatments.[52]

Multiple cases of leukemia within families have been reported, including aggregates among siblings and groups within the same generation or in several generations. The frequency of leukemia is higher than expected in families of leukemia patients.[53] Siblings of children with leukemia, including ALL, have an approximately two- to four-fold greater risk of developing the disease than do unrelated children in the general population.[53] Although the occurrence of leukemia in identical twins has been used to support the role of *in utero* and genetic factors in the disease, the extent to which this association implicates a genetic susceptibility is ambiguous. The concordance of acute leukemia in monozygotic twins is estimated to be as high as 25%, and although it is often the result of shared *in utero* circulation (since by molecular fingerprinting techniques the leukemic clone can be shown to be identical in the two twins), both patients shared similar exposures to prenatal or postnatal leukemogenic factors.[54] The risk for leukemia concordance among twins (both mono- and dizygotic) is highest in infancy, diminishes with age, and after the age of 7 years, the risk to the unaffected twin is similar to that for persons within the general population.[54]

PATHOGENESIS

In addition to genetic influences, environmental factors, viral infection, and immunodeficiency may predispose children to leukemia.

Environmental Factors

Exposure to ionizing radiation and certain toxic chemicals can facilitate the development of acute leukemia. The high incidence of leukemia in survivors of the atomic bomb explosions in Japan during World War II is well documented.[55,56] The risk of leukemia was dose related and was greatest for those closest to the explosion. For persons who received exposure doses greater than 100 cGy, the dose-response relation for the production of leukemia was linear. The type of leukemia observed was related to the age at exposure. ALL was seen more frequently in children and AML was more common in adults.

Among survivors of the atomic bomb, there was no increase in the incidence of leukemia in children exposed to radiation *in utero*. This experience contrasts with other reports of an increased risk of leukemia in children exposed to diagnostic irradiation *in utero*, particularly during the first trimester.[57] In a study by the National Academy of Sciences, a five-fold increased risk of all childhood cancers was found for children exposed to diagnostic radiation during the first trimester. When exposure occurred during the second and third trimesters, the risk was 1.5 times the baseline. Leukemias comprised approximately half of the cancers in that study; the increased risk for leukemia extends through 12 years of age.[58] A significant leukemogenic effect has been reported in children exposed *in utero* to doses of 0.3 to 0.8 cGy. Prenatal x-ray exposure, however, probably accounts for a very small portion of childhood ALL cases.[59] Changes in obstetrical practices (limiting x-ray exposure because of awareness of potential organ toxicity and carcinogenesis), coupled with improvements in x-ray methodologies and availability of alternate imaging technologies, have significantly removed radiation or lowered radiation doses from routine prenatal procedures. Consequently, the risk of causing childhood ALL from these *in utero* exposures has become so low that it is difficult to measure.[60] Neonatal ultrasound does not seem to pose any leukemogenic risk.[60] The risk of developing leukemia from *ex utero* diagnostic irradiation is also difficult to determine. One study suggested that about 1% of all cases of adult leukemia can be assumed to be a result of exposure to diagnostic radiography.[61] A more recent study utilizing pediatric orthopedic patients who required repeated diagnostic radiographs (e.g., for management of scoliosis) showed a possible 0.8% increased risk over baseline for the development of leukemia.[62]

Therapeutic irradiation has been associated with a higher risk of acute leukemia in patients with ankylosing spondylitis treated with relatively high-dose radiation and neonates administered thymic irradiation (which was once used to treat enlargement of the thymus).[63,64] An increased leukemia incidence rate was also observed in one older study for children who received scalp irradiation for treatment of tinea capitis.[65]

Although the potential of ionizing radiation for causing leukemia is acknowledged, the actual percentage of leukemia cases directly attributable to radiation is usually assumed to be quite small. Some recent data have called this into question, with an estimate of between 8% and 30% of current pediatric ALL cases being related to ionizing radiation from natural, background sources or an occasional diagnostic film.[56,66] Controversy persists about the risks from exposure to ionizing radiation from routine emissions from nuclear power plants or as a result of fallout from atmospheric nuclear testing. Concern regarding the possibility that exposure to electromagnetic fields (EMFs) may be causally related to the development of childhood ALL has not withstood close scientific scrutiny, with the possible exception of rare exposures to very high strength fields.[1,67]

Chronic chemical exposure (e.g., benzene) has been associated with the development of AML in adults.[68] But direct evidence linking specific chemical exposure to the development of childhood ALL has been difficult to establish.[69] However, there does appear to be some association with postnatal exposure to household paint and paint solvents.[69] There is substantial evidence that chemotherapy, particularly with alkylating agents, has leukemogenic potential. In a study of more than 9,000 2-year survivors of childhood cancer, a 14-fold excess of leukemia was observed, primarily attributable to prior therapy with alkylating agents.[70] Most of these cases, however, were secondary AML. Other factors studied for possible association with ALL include exposure to herbicides and pesticides; paternal military experience (particularly with service in Vietnam and/or Cambodia where servicemen were exposed to Agent Orange and other chemicals); maternal use of alcohol, contraceptives, and diethylstilbestrol; household radon exposure; and chemical contamination of groundwater.[69] Whether, and to what degree, any of these exposures contribute to the incidence of childhood ALL is controversial. The evidence that they do contribute is usually in the form of a mild increase in the odds ratio for developing the disease. To date, it appears unlikely that the bulk of ALL is due to any of these individual exposures.

Viral Infection

There has been intense interest in the possible role played by viral infection in the pathogenesis of human leukemia.[71,72] This has been due in large part to the fact that the young age of onset distribution of ALL corresponds to a time when the immune system is developing and is perhaps more vulnerable to the oncogenic effects of particular viruses. Some reports have suggested an increased risk of ALL in children born to mothers recently infected with influenza, varicella, or other viruses, but no definitive link between prenatal viral exposure and leukemic risk has been confirmed. Seasonal variation in ALL incidence rates as well as seasonal variation in the birth dates of specific cohorts of patients have also led to continued interest in the relationship between infectious exposures and the etiology of ALL.[73] No direct association between childhood or maternal viral infections and the subsequent occurrence of ALL has been documented, and those cases that have been investigated have not been shown to be clearly causative.[74] A possible inverse association with hepatitis A virus (as a measure of general hygiene) has been shown. On the basis of this association, it was hypothesized that the increase in ALL rates in the U.S. and Japanese populations, compared to the developing world, may simply be because the children in the developed world are more "immunologically naïve." Thus,

they may be more susceptible to infectious/oncogenic agents acquired either *in utero* or early in life. Both the existence of a rare leukemogenic virus and the possibility that ALL represents a "rare response to a common infection" are the basis for continued studies of a possible viral etiology.[75]

The Epstein-Barr virus (EBV) has been linked to cases of endemic Burkitt's lymphoma, the L3 morphologic subtype of ALL, and to some cases of Hodgkin lymphoma. The EBV association with ALL is discussed further in the subsequent section on molecular genetics and the association of EBV with other cancers is discussed in Chapters 1 and 22–24. The human lymphotropic viruses I and II (HTLV I and II) are retroviruses that are implicated in some cases of adult T-cell and hairy cell leukemia. Cases of childhood malignancies have been linked to human immunodeficiency virus (HIV) infection, but the spectrum of histologies is different from those seen in adult acquired immunodeficiency syndrome (AIDS) patients and does not usually include ALL.[76]

Immunodeficiency

Children with various congenital immunodeficiency diseases, including Wiskott-Aldrich syndrome, congenital hypogammaglobulinemia, and AT (see the Epidemiology and Genetics sections), have an increased risk of developing lymphoid malignancies, as do patients receiving chronic treatment with immunosuppressive drugs. These are usually lymphomas with mature B-cell phenotypes. Although ALL may occur in these circumstances, it is uncommon. Persons with AT and Fanconi anemia have increased chromosomal fragility, frequent abnormalities of chromosomes 14 and 7, which suggests that genetic mechanisms may be related to the increased incidence of cancer associated with these disorders.

Abnormalities of the immune system are frequently observed in newly diagnosed patients with ALL.[77] Abnormally low serum immunoglobulin levels have been observed in as many as 30% of these patients. Whether such abnormalities precede the development of leukemia or are a consequence of the disease is unclear. Similarly, abnormalities of the immune system may persist after therapy, although the effects of therapy versus those of the leukemia may be difficult to discern.[78] In addition to infectious risks or complications, it is conceivable that aberrant immune status may not only be a factor in leukemogenesis, but may also be an important influence on prognosis (see section "Response to Treatment"), susceptibility to relapse, and/or the development of second malignancies after completion of therapy.[79]

Clonal Pathogenesis

ALL, like other lymphoid malignancies, is believed to develop as a consequence of malignant transformation of a single abnormal progenitor cell that has the capability to expand (in a so-called clone of similar progeny cells) by indefinite self-renewal. It is not entirely clear where in the normal course of differentiation the leukemic "clonal event" occurs, and it may actually be highly variable. In pediatric ALL there is evidence that these events occur in committed lymphoid precursors, whereas in AML and Philadelphia chromosome positive (Ph+) ALL (see section "Cytogenetic Classification"), it appears that they may occur in a less differentiated, more primitive hematopoietic cell, because there is evidence of mutation in multiple cell lineages.[80,81] The events that lead to malignant transformation are complex and multifactorial. It has been proposed that ALL results from spontaneous mutation(s), which may occur in lymphoid cells of B- or T-cell lineage or in their precursor stem cells. As noted previously, there is emerging evidence that the causative mutations may occur in a small preleukemic clone years before the presentation of clinical leukemia. During normal lymphoid development, lymphocyte precursors may be at higher risk for spontaneous mutation. The risk of mutation is specifically increased during the process of immunoglobulin and TCR gene rearrangements (when DNA strands are being frequently broken and reannealed in new configurations). The risk is further compounded by the fact that there is often an increased rate of cellular proliferation/immune-based cell expansion in these very same cell populations. Many of the described molecular mutations bear evidence of IgG and TCR recombinase activity.[82]

Other support for the clonal expansion theory comes from classic studies of glucose-6-phosphate dehydrogenase isotypes, cytogenetic profiles, and molecular characterizations.[13] Rearrangement of immunoglobulin and TCR genes also have been studied as a marker of clonality in ALL of pre-B lineage. In most cases, identical patterns of immunoglobulin and TCR gene rearrangement are observed in leukemic cells obtained at diagnosis and relapse. Infrequently, clonal variations occur in serial samples, suggesting polyclonal disease, or clonal progression. In most of these cases, however, the leukemia cells share at least one identical immunoglobulin gene rearrangement, implying a common clonal origin.[13]

The concept of cancer stem cells has been an increasing focus of research over the past decade. Cancer stem cells have been reported in a variety of solid tumors and in AML. The data for cancer stem cells in ALL are less well-developed but constitute an active area of current research.[81] Key features of leukemia stem cells, also termed leukemia initiating cells (LICs), have variously been defined as including the capacity for self-renewal, multipotential differentiation, relatively quiescent cell-cycle status, rarity within the total tumor cell population, a distinctive immunophenotype, and ability to initiate tumors in immunocompromised mice. Some data suggest that the immunophenotype and differentiation stage of LICs differ between different cytogenetically defined ALL subtypes.[81]

Conventional chemotherapy which targets rapidly dividing cells may not eradicate LICs which are, by definition, capable of prolonged quiescence. Thus, leukemia stem cell research holds promise as a novel therapeutic approach; yet it also faces significant challenges: LICs may have changeable and/or patient-specific immunophenotypic markers, and therapeutic responses may be difficult to assess since LICs do not make up the bulk of the leukemic cell burden. It has been suggested that the long-established maintenance backbone of ALL therapy consisting of methotrexate and 6-mercaptopurine may in fact constitute a form of stem cell therapy which already has been in use for decades.[83]

For many years, it has been assumed that cure of ALL necessitated the killing of all leukemic cells. This may not be true, because multiple minimal residual disease (MRD) technologies (see later) occasionally show evidence of persistent viable leukemic cells late in therapy and even in off-therapy patients who do not subsequently clinically relapse. Whether these cells truly represent clonal cells identical to those at leukemic diagnosis, versus a vestige of a preleukemic clone, is controversial. Another hypothesis would accept these cells as being those of the original clone, and the difference (the reason that overt leukemia does not arise) may be related to the fact that the patient's own immune system (or an immune system that has been replaced by a bone marrow or stem cell transplant) has learned to control the proliferation of the remaining leukemic cells.[84]

Molecular Pathogenesis

The molecular underpinnings of leukemogenesis are related to the alteration of key regulatory processes that control hematopoietic proliferation (self-renewal), differentiation, and apoptosis (the molecular signals that lead a cell to death). This can occur through a variety of mechanisms including alterations in cell signaling pathways, with mutations that affect the activity or expression of specific kinases and other proteins, aberrant expression of proto-oncogenes or silencing of suppressor genes, and the expression of chimeric transcription factors encoded by chromosomal translocations.[13]

Chromosomal translocations occur frequently in ALL (Table 19.1 and cytogenetics section) and appear to play a key role in its clonal evolution. Generally, translocations either juxtapose a proto-oncogene with a TCR or immunoglobulin locus, causing its overexpression; or fuse the genes at the translocation breakpoints to form a novel chimeric protein with altered, oncogenic effects.[85]

Genomic studies of global gene expression patterns (see section "Classification by Global Gene Expression") have taken the field of molecular pathogenesis beyond single gene mutations.[86–88] Following on the wave of investigations of gene expression, a new body of work is emerging that utilizes high-resolution, unbiased microarray techniques to investigate alterations of DNA copy number. Genome-wide profiling of DNA copy number and loss of heterozygosity has led to identification of key cryptic deletions and rearrangements too small to have been detected in the past by conventional cytogenetics or candidate gene approaches.[52] Other active areas of investigation include large-scale mutation analysis and characterization of epigenetic modifications such as DNA methylation.[89] Some of these findings are discussed in greater detail in Chapters 3 and 4.

Another potential mechanism in the development of ALL involves mutational events that prevent apoptosis (programmed cell death). Originally cloned from the oncogenic translocation breakpoint t(14;18)(q21;q32) common in adult follicular and diffuse B-cell lymphomas, the Bcl-2 protein is able to prevent apoptosis and immortalize cells in tissue culture and transgenic murine models.[90] Several groups have noticed that increased Bcl-2 levels in leukemic blasts correlate with their ability to grow in tissue culture and with poorer prognosis in both ALL and AML.[91]

CLASSIFICATION OF ALL

Morphologic, immunologic, cytogenetic, biochemical, and molecular genetic characterizations of leukemic lymphoblasts have confirmed that ALL is a biologically heterogeneous disorder (see also Chapter 7). This heterogeneity reflects both the fact that the leukemia may develop at any point during the multiple stages of normal lymphoid differentiation and that individual cases often present a mixture of markers or characteristics of the multiple stages of normal development.[92]

Morphologic Classification

There have been several attempts to classify ALL cells morphologically using criteria such as cell size, nuclear to cytoplasmic ratio, nuclear shape, number and prominence of nucleoli, nature and intensity of cytoplasmic staining, presence of cytoplasmic granules, prominence of cytoplasmic vacuoles, and the character of nuclear chromatin.[92] Most of these efforts were unsuccessful because they were subjective, techni-

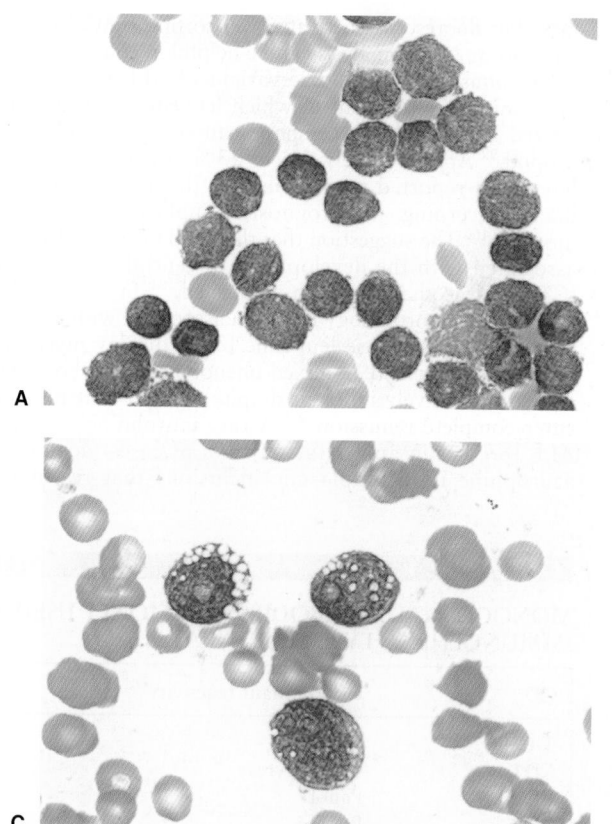
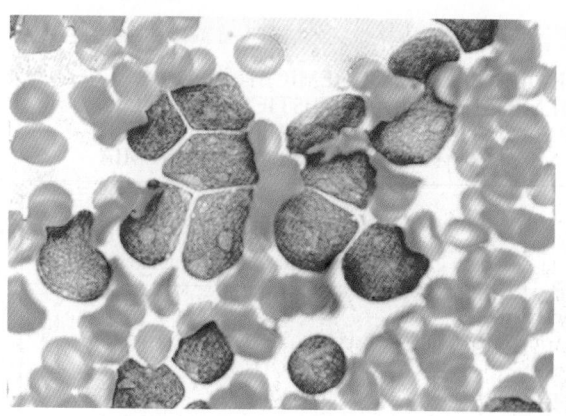

FIGURE 19.4 Morphologic appearance of acute lymphoblastic leukemia cells classified according to the French-American-British system. **A:** L1 morphology. **B:** L2 morphology. **C:** L3 morphology.

cally difficult to reproduce, and often lacked meaningful clinical correlations. One system, however, proposed by the French-American-British (FAB) Cooperative Working Group has become generally accepted. Examination of Romanovsky or Wright-Giemsa stained bone marrow slides and application of the FAB criteria is the first step toward the diagnosis of most patients and provides guidance for the ordering of additional laboratory tests. The FAB system (Fig. 19.4 and Table 19.2) defines three categories of lymphoblasts. L1 lymphoblasts are usually smaller, with scant cytoplasm and inconspicuous nucleoli. Cells of the L2 variety are larger, and they demonstrate considerable heterogeneity in size, prominent nucleoli, and more abundant cytoplasm. Lymphoblasts of the L3 type, notable for their deep cytoplasmic basophilia, are large, frequently display prominent cytoplasmic vacuolation,

and are morphologically identical to Burkitt's lymphoma cells. With the exception of B-cell leukemia (FAB L-3), the FAB classification does not correlate particularly well with immunophenotypic, cytogenetic, and microarray-based classification information (see later).[93]

Approximately 85% of children with ALL have predominant L1 morphology, 14% have L2, and 1% have L3. The L2 subtype is more common in adults.[94] Lymphoblasts of the L3 type possess cell surface immunoglobulin and other characteristic mature B-cell markers. There is, however, no apparent correlation between the FAB L1 and L2 morphologic types and immunologic cell surface markers.[95] Concordance among investigators using the FAB system is relatively high. Since its original description, refinements of the FAB system have been proposed, and several other systems, including the

TABLE 19.2

FRENCH-AMERICAN-BRITISH CLASSIFICATION OF LYMPHOBLASTIC LEUKEMIA

Cytologic features	L1	L2	L3
Cell size	Small cells predominate	Large, heterogeneous in size	Large homogeneous
Nuclear chromatin	Homogeneous in any one case	Variable; heterogeneous in any one case	Finely stippled and homogeneous
Nuclear shape	Not visible or small and inconspicuous; more vesicular	Irregular clefting and indentation common	Regular—oval to round
Nucleoli	Regular; occasional clefting or indenting	One or more present; often large	Prominent; one or more
Amount of cytoplasm	Scanty	Variable; often moderately abundant	Moderately abundant
Basophilia of cytoplasm	Slight or moderate; rarely intense	Variable; deep in some	Very deep
Cytoplasmic vacuolation	Variable	Variable	Often prominent

TABLE 19.3

MORPHOLOGIC, CYTOCHEMICAL, AND BIOCHEMICAL CHARACTERISTICS HELPFUL IN DIFFERENTIATING ACUTE LYMPHOBLASTIC LEUKEMIA FROM ACUTE MYELOID LEUKEMIA

	Acute lymphoblastic leukemia	Acute myeloid leukemia
Characteristic		
Nuclear/cytoplasmic ratio	High	Low
Nuclear chromatin	Clumped	Spongy
Nucleoli	0–2	2–5
Granules	−	+
Auer rods	−	±
Cytoplasm	Blue	Blue-gray
Cytochemical Reaction		
Peroxidase	−	+
Sudan black B	−	+
Periodic acid–Schiff	±	−
Naphthyl ASD chloracetate esterase	−	±
α-Naphthyl acetate esterase	−	±
α-Naphthyl butyrate esterase	−	−
Terminal deoxynucleotidyl transferase	+[a]	−

[a]Terminal deoxynucleotidyl transferase is usually negative in typical French-American-British L3 acute lymphoblastic leukemia.
+, cytochemical stain positive; ±, cytochemical stain equivocal; −, cytochemical stain negative.
Note: Table provides information on characteristics that may be useful in differentiating acute lymphoblastic leukemia from acute myeloid leukemia. Wide variation in morphology is encountered in both disease categories. Diagnostic evaluation should use other studies, including immunophenotyping and cytogenetics.
From Poplack DG. Clinical manifestations of acute lymphoblastic leukemia. In: Hoffman R, Shattil S, Furie B, et al., eds. Hematology: basic principles and practice, 2nd ed. New York: Churchill Livingstone, 1991:1071, with permission.

Morphologic, Immunologic and Cytogenetic Classification of Acute Leukemia (MIC), and World Health Organization (WHO) systems, were proposed that were based on the FAB system but incorporated additional immunologic and cytogenetic criteria.[92] Although the existence of different approaches to FAB classification can confound interstudy comparisons, a variety of individual studies have demonstrated that the FAB classification has prognostic value.[95,96]

L1 morphology has been associated with a higher remission induction rate and better EFS than L2 morphology.[97] In early studies, L2 morphology appeared to be an independent prognostic variable indicative of poor outcome. However, it has subsequently fallen from clinical use because of the stronger predictive values of age, sex, and diagnostic WBC count.[97] Patients with L3 morphology have the worst overall prognosis.[98] Although the FAB classification system appears to have some value as a prognostic indicator, no biologic basis for the morphologic differences delineated by this system has been identified. Generally, the most important morphologic distinctions are those between ALL and AML (Table 19.3). Routine Wright-Giemsa and cytochemical stains are usually adequate for this

task, but fluorescence-activated cell sorting (FACS) (see later) and chromosomal analysis can be helpful in equivocal cases.

An unusual morphologic variant of ALL is the so-called hand mirror cell variant in which leukemic cells are characterized by a hand mirror shape caused by a handle-shaped uropod.[99] Approximately 5% to 23% of pediatric ALL cases have been reported to demonstrate this morphology.[97] The data concerning its prognostic implications have been mixed.[97,100] The suggestion that the hand mirror cell variant is associated with the development of central nervous system (CNS) disease has not been confirmed.[101] In adult ALL, the hand mirror morphology has been associated with a subset of female patients whose leukemic blasts display myeloid and lymphoid antigens (i.e., mixed phenotype) and whose clinical course is relatively indolent despite the fact that they rarely enter complete remission.[102] A rare morphologic variant of ALL (present in approximately 2% of cases) demonstrates azurophilic intracytoplasmic inclusions that resemble the

TABLE 19.4

MONOCLONAL ANTIBODIES COMMONLY USED TO IMMUNOPHENOTYPE LEUKEMIA

CD[a]	Predominant reactivity
T Cell	
CD1	Thymocytes
CD2	Pan-T
CD3	Pan-T
CD4	T helper/inducer
CD5	Pan-T, B-CLL
CD7	Pan-T
CD8	T cytotoxic/suppressor
CDw29	T4+/4B4+ = helper inducer
	T4+/2H4+ = suppressor inducer
B Cell	
CD19	Pan-B
CD20	Pan-B
CD21	C3dR
CD24	Pan-B
	Plasma cells
Myeloid	
CD11c	Monocytes, hairy cell
CD13	Pan-myeloid
CD14	Monocytes
CD15	Monocytes, granulocytes
CD33	Pan-myeloid
Miscellaneous	
CD9	Hematopoietic Progenitor/leukemic blasts
CD10	ALL/Burkitt's/follicular lymphoma
CD34	Hematopoietic genitor cells/human lymphotropic viruses–infected cells
CD41a	Platelets/megakaryocytes
CD45	Pan-leukocyte
	Transferrin receptor/proliferating cells

[a]CD classification number and their predominant reactivity are listed.
ALL, acute lymphoblastic leukemia; B-CLL, B-cell chronic lymphocytic leukemia.
From Poplack DG. Clinical manifestations of acute lymphoblastic leukemia. In: Hoffman R, Shattil S, Furie B, et al., eds. Hematology: basic principles and practice, 2nd ed. New York: Churchill Livingstone, 1991:1072, with permission.

granules of myeloblasts (occasionally appear like Auer rods) in cells that by every other morphologic and immunophenotypic criteria appear to be lymphoid.[103] These granules have recently been shown by electron microscopy to be mitochondria.[103] A standard panel of cytochemical stains (outlined in Table 19.3) coupled with immunophenotype is usually adequate for differentiating ALL from AML.

Cytochemical stains have been studied with respect to their ability to differentiate between various clinical and immunologic subsets of ALL. The periodic acid–Schiff (PAS), acid phosphatase, b-glucuronidase, and acid a-naphthyl acetate esterase reactions have been evaluated.[104] Although some correlations appear strong (i.e., strong focal paranuclear acid phosphatase activity appears to be more common in T-cell disease), the practical use of this type of information is limited and has largely been supplanted by more sophisticated immunologic techniques, such as flow cytometry. In rare cases of acute leukemia that cannot be definitively classified by current immunologic or molecular methods, ultrastructural examination using electron microscopy or detection of platelet peroxidase or myeloperoxidase may be helpful in identifying the megakaryocytic or myeloid nature of the disease.[103,105]

Classification by Immunophenotype

Studies of the immunobiology of ALL have confirmed that leukemic transformation and clonal expansion can occur at different stages of maturation in the process of lymphoid differentiation (Fig. 19.5). In the early 1970s, when the first surface marker methodologies were used to characterize ALL in terms of cell origin and stage of differentiation, three immunologic subsets were delineated: T cells, B cells, and non T/non B cells. Using receptors for sheep erythrocytes, approximately 20% of pediatric patients with ALL were found to T-cell disease.[106] Cell surface immunoglobulin and complement receptors identified ALL of B-cell origin in 1% to 2% of patients.

With these older immunologic methods of characterization, the remaining patients with ALL had no detectable cell surface markers on their blasts, and thus were considered to have non-T, non-B cell or so-called null cell leukemia.[107] The development of heterologous antisera and monoclonal antibodies directed against human leukemia-associated antigens indicated that approximately 80% of patients formerly designated as non-T, non-B cell ALL had a common ALL antigen (CALLA), CD-10, on their cell surface.[108] This leukemic subset is now referred to as *CALLA*+ or *CD 10*+ or *common ALL.*

Most leukemias previously determined to be of the non-T, non-B type are actually of early B-cell lineage. The demonstration of intracytoplasmic immunoglobulin in some of these cells, their reactivity with monoclonal antibodies specific for B-cell associated antigens, and their ability to differentiate *in vitro* into cells with mature B-cell markers confirmed that approximately 80% to 85% of childhood ALL cases develop as a result of the monoclonal proliferation of B-cell precursors.[109] The presence of cytoplasmic immunoglobulin (cIg) has been a useful marker to determine the level of differentiation of leukemic cells of B-cell lineage.[110] cIg is present in approximately 20% to 30% of cases of B-cell precursor ALL.

The use of monoclonal antibodies, improvements in the enzymatic and fluorescent tagging of these antibodies, and the development of multiparameter FACS machines have revolutionized pathologic classifications of many diseases, including ALL. More than 200 different monoclonal antibodies, which can detect antigens associated with the different hematopoietic lineages, are commercially available. Those most helpful in the immunologic classification of ALL are shown in Table 19.4. Using a panel of monoclonal antibodies associated with various stages of B-cell differentiation along with information on the presence or absence of cytoplasmic and surface immunoglobulin, investigators have classified B-lineage ALL into discrete stages according to the degree of differentiation or maturation.[111] However, none of the monoclonal antibodies used in routine clinical immunophenotyping are absolutely

Acute Leukemia
Predominance of blast cells in bone marrow

Assignment of B, T, or Myeloid- Ontogony

B cell	**T cell**	**Myeloid**
Tdt+, PAS+/-, FAB L1,L2	PAS (block positivity)	granules, Auer rods, Sudan Black+ Esterase +/- (See Chapter 20)
Pro-B/early preB CD34+/CD19+ t(4;11)+, t(9;22), hyper-Diploid and others (Table 19.1)	**Pro-T** CD3+/CD7+ Multiple TF /TCR translocations (Table 19.1)	
Common ALL(cALL) CD 34+/-,CD19+/CD10+ FAB L1 (occasionally L2) Hyperdiploid, t(12;21), t(9;22),6q-	**Pre- T** CD2+/CD5+//CD8+ Multiple TF/TCR (Table 19.1)	
Pre-B ALL CD 34-/CD19+/CD20+/CD22+ FAB L1/L2 Cytogenetics frequently similar to cALL but often t(1;19) or t(9;22)	**Common T** CD2+/CD5+/8+ Multiple TF/TCR	
B-ALL CD10+/-CD19+,Tdt- FAB L3 Burkitt translocations: t(8;14) and alternatives t(2;8), t(8;20) between Ig receptors and cmyc (Table 19.1)	**Late T-ALL** TCR α/β +, γ/δ+	

FIGURE 19.5 General guide to the classification of acute lymphoblastic leukemia including morphology with common stains, immunophenotype, and cytogenetic findings. The distinction between lymphoid and myeloid disease, as well as between T- and B-cell lymphoid disease, is usually easily made with standard stains, morphology, and fluorescence-activated cell sorting (FACS). In equivocal cases cytogenetics or electromicroscopy (for ultrastructural detail) can be helpful. (Information drawn from references 105 to 107 and Lilleyman JS et al. Cytomorphology of childhood lymphoblastic leukaemia: a prospective study of 2000 patients. United Kingdom Medical Research Council's Working Party on Childhood Leukaemia, Br J Haematol 1992;81:52–57.)

lineage specific. *Lineage associated* is the preferred terminology. In order to accurately immunophenotype most cases, a panel of multiple antibodies should be used (Table 19.4). The choice of the diagnostic panel may vary among institutions and laboratories but for the characterization of lymphoid leukemias, generally includes antibodies for several T-cell antigens (e.g., CD3, 5, and/or 7) and early-B lineage antigens (e.g., CD10, 19, 20, and 22).

Although improved therapy has overcome many negative factors, there are some prognostic differences between the various precursor B-lineage ALL subgroups, which continue to be true. Mature B-cell ALL has a poorer prognosis compared with the earlier B-lineage subgroups. However, the distinction between patients with pre-B-cell (cIg+) ALL (sometimes referred to as "pro-B cell") and those with early pre-B ALL (cIg−) does not seem to be relevant as long as the patients are stratified and treated according to modern risk criteria (see section "Treatment").[13] Patients with B-cell precursor ALL whose lymphoblasts manifest CALLA (CD10) have a more favorable prognosis than those who are CD10-negative. Expression of the stem cell antigen CD34, present on approximately two thirds of B-cell precursor ALL, also appears to be associated with an improved prognosis.[112]

Identification of immunoglobulin gene rearrangement is helpful in confirming the B-cell precursor lineage of ALL cells otherwise devoid of other B-cell or pre-B-cell markers.[113] There is a hierarchy of immunoglobulin gene rearrangements in B-cell precursor ALL that mirrors different stages of normal B-cell differentiation (Fig. 19.5).[114] Heavy chain rearrangement precedes κ light chain rearrangement, which precedes λ light chain rearrangement. A similar hierarchical pattern of TCR gene rearrangements is present in T-cell development. Study of the δ, γ, β, and α TCR gene rearrangement in T-cell ALL reveals a series of sequential TCR activation events that can be roughly correlated with the sequence of T-cell surface antigen expression in a fashion analogous to the hierarchy of immunoglobulin gene rearrangement found in B-cell precursor ALL.[111] The specificity of immunoglobulin and TCR gene rearrangements are useful markers of clonality that can be used as informative markers for both MRD studies (see later) or in studies to identify preleukemic clones present at the time of birth (see Clonal Pathogenesis section).

Although many cases fit the hypothesis that ALL is a disorder characterized by the clonal expansion of cells representing a specific stage of normal differentiation, it is evident that many B- and T-cell lineage leukemias exhibit a differentiation antigen pattern or immunoglobulin gene rearrangement profile that is not synchronous with any of the normal stages of differentiation.[115] In addition to this asynchrony of antigen expression, leukemic cells from some patients manifest characteristics of more than one lineage. Although once thought to be an unfavorable prognostic sign, the presence of some myeloid antigen marker positivity in cells that predominantly mark as lymphoid has no prognostic meaning.[13]

Heavy chain immunoglobulin gene rearrangement has been observed in approximately 10% to 15% of T-cell ALL cases.[111] This phenomenon of "lineage spillover" indicates that heavy chain rearrangement alone is not a sufficient basis for assigning B-cell lineage.[116] TCR gene rearrangement also occurs with relatively high frequency in B-cell precursor ALL.[116] B-cell precursor ALL devoid of immunoglobulin (or TCR) rearrangement has been described. This germline configuration appears to be a characteristic of some cases of B-cell precursor ALL of infancy.[82]

Although immunophenotyping and cytogenetic analysis have their origin from different scientific disciplines, it has now become apparent that specific combinations of antigen expression correlate with specific molecular genetic changes.[117] As noted previously, not all ALL cases adhere to a specific immunophenotypic lineage. Comparisons between normal and leukemic cells using monoclonal antibodies or molecular genotyping have verified that numerous cases occur in which the leukemic cells express characteristics of more than one hematopoietic lineage.[118] In acute biphenotypic or mixed-lineage leukemia, lymphoid and myeloid characteristics are present on the same leukemia cell. Bilineal or biclonal leukemias are those in which there are two distinct populations of cells, one lymphoid and the other myeloid. "Lineage switch" (or "lineage shift") is the term used to describe a conversion from one phenotype at diagnosis to a different phenotype at relapse.

When initial reports of mixed-lineage leukemias surfaced, it was assumed that dual markers represented an artifact produced by phenotypic markers that lacked specificity. However, numerous well-documented mixed lineage cases exist that meet even the most stringent classification criteria. It is apparent that the simultaneous expression of lymphoid and myeloid markers occurs more commonly than previously believed. In various series of pediatric ALL cases, the incidence of myeloid marker expression has been between 7% and 25%.[119,120]

The biologic basis for the appearance of mixed-lineage leukemias is not understood. It has been suggested that they occur as a result of inappropriate or aberrant gene activation and thus do not represent leukemias derived from a corresponding normal stage of hematopoietic development.[118] Alternatively, it has been proposed that mixed-lineage leukemias represent the clonal expansion of normal, bilineage, or multilineage-potential precursors, which are difficult to detect in normal bone marrow.[118] Mixed-lineage leukemia is sometimes associated with particular cytogenetic and molecular findings. There is a higher incidence of mixed-lineage phenotype seen in the abnormal 11q23 cases, especially in the t(4;11)(q23;q23) cases, and in leukemias containing the Philadelphia chromosome, t(9;22).[121,122] The 11q23 abnormalities and the t(9;22) cytogenetic abnormalities are independently associated with poor prognosis (see section "Cytogenetics").

Although in the past, controversy existed over the preferred treatment of mixed-lineage leukemias, most investigators now agree that with modern chemotherapy regimens, there is no difference in outcomes between myeloid antigen-positive and myeloid antigen-negative ALL. Thus, therapy recommendations should not be altered for this finding, as long as the predominance of the classification evidence (classic morphology, FACS-based immunophenotypic, and cytogenetics) indicates that the patient has ALL.[120]

The optimal treatment of true biclonal disease is less clear. Pre-B/myeloid appears to be slightly more common than T-lymphoid/myeloid, and rare T/B and natural killer (NK) cell combinations have been described.[123]

Historically, therapy for biclonal cases has not shown much success. The general recommendation is that therapy for both types of leukemia (usually pre-B lymphoid and myeloid) be provided in alternating cycles with strong consideration of bone marrow transplantation (BMT) once remission is achieved.[123] The largest published treatment study for biclonal leukemia included 24 patients: 15 were B lymphoid/myeloid, 8 T lymphoid/myeloid, and 1 was a mixed T/B. This study had an unusually high incidence of early deaths (25%) and a 2-year survival rate of 39%. The therapy provided was a mixture of AML and ALL treatments. The authors felt that combining AML/ALL medications in induction had lead to the increase in early deaths, and recommended that AML and ALL therapy be given in separate cycles.[123] The prognosis of biclonal patients is worse in cases where a Philadelphia chromosome is detected or patients are older than 15 years. The development of newer classification schemes based on global gene expression should help to more accurately classify these rare cases, as well as provide information as to which of the available treatment strategies will be most likely to work.

Classification by Global Gene Expression

Microarray technology has made it possible to accurately classify leukemias based on their gene expression profile. This prognostic information is based on complex patterns by globally analyzing the type and amounts of RNA expressed by leukemic cells (Fig. 19.6 and see also Chapter 7).[86,124,125] Although technical problems and controversies exist, microarray technology has improved our understanding of ALL biology and enhanced our ability to define prognostically different patient groups. Using separate test and validation sets, multiple groups have demonstrated that gene expression profiling is useful in defining prognostically significant subsets of pre-B and T-ALL. (Fig. 19.6B). Microarray gene expression profiling also has demonstrated its potential to identify new molecular markers of MRD and potential therapeutic targets as well.[126,127]

When examining similar patient samples on either the same or different microarrays, multiple groups have reported similar and significantly different sets of diagnostically and prognostically important gene expression patterns.[86,125,128,129] Multiple investigators have shown that the six most significant, prognostically important cytogenetically defined subgroups: t(12;21), Ph+ or t(9;22), t(1;19); t(4;11), T-ALL, and hyperdiploidy greater than 50 chromosomes (Fig. 19.6) can be identified by their RNA expression signals.[128–130] In addition to a correlation with known subgroupings, other important relationships are also emerging. For example, the potential value of gene expression profiling in determining outcome on specific therapies was highlighted in a study that identified a set of 124 genes that could differentially predict outcomes on therapy for four of the most common drugs used in ALL induction (prednisolone, vincristine, asparaginase, and daunorubicin).[127] Of interest, 121 of these 124 genes have never been previously identified as being involved in drug resistance (Fig. 19.7A and B).[127] Although these data are intriguing, additional prospective, confirmatory studies will be necessary before this type of information can be used to individualize therapy. Microarray studies identify much of the same information generated at diagnosis by FACS and reverse transcriptase polymerase chain reaction (RT-PCR) for the prognostically significant fusion transcripts from the known chromosomal breakpoints. However, it would be premature to replace these older technologies until it has been truly proven prospectively that this is approach is a valid, as well as economically viable option.[131] It has been predicted that, ultimately, the entire diagnosis and treatment management plan for a patient with ALL may be derived using microarray analysis as a single diagnostic platform at diagnosis. For now, however, the application of global gene expression using microarray technology remains a powerful research tool whose potential role as a diagnostic and treatment assignment tool must be prospectively validated.

CYTOGENETIC CLASSIFICATION

Technical improvements in cytogenetic analysis have increasingly contributed to the understanding of the biology and treatment of ALL. When combining the newer methods of chromosomal banding and standard fluorescent in situ hybridization (FISH), with the molecular genetic techniques of spectral karyotyping (SKY) and comparative genomic hybridization (CGH); abnormalities are detected in the leukemia cells of virtually 100% of cases of pediatric ALL.[132,133] DNA copy number arrays have rapidly emerged as a powerful tool for genome-wide investigation of areas of gain and loss of genetic material. The benefits of these arrays include significantly higher resolution than routine karyotype; genome-wide scope in contrast to the targeting of select lesions by FISH; and lack of requirement for *in vitro* culture prior to analysis. Array comparative genomic hybridization (CGH) detects only DNA copy number alterations, whereas single nucleotide polymorphism (SNP) arrays also detect copy-neutral loss of heterozygosity, also known as uniparental disomy.[134] Array CGH platforms originally utilized large (~200 kb) bacterial artificial chromosome (BAC) derived probes, whereas current CGH and SNP arrays generally utilize small oligonucleotide probes (20–100 nucleotides) which have the capacity to detect much smaller focal copy number abnormalities. The SKY technique (Fig. 19.6D) employs 24-color chromosomal paints (one specific to each chromosome) which allow reliable assignment of chromosomal origin in complex rearrangements that defy standard cytogenetic analysis. Both DNA copy number arrays and SKY are currently used primarily for research rather than clinical applications. These new methods require specific computer and fluorescent microscopy workstations and a licensed clinical cytogeneticist for proper clinical interpretation and correlation with the diagnostic Giemsa-banded karyotype.

The cytogenetic abnormalities reported in ALL involve both chromosomal number (ploidy) and/or structural rearrangements.[13] The following sections discuss the molecular and clinical correlates of specific chromosomal changes in ALL. Their implications for treatment are discussed in the section on treatment.

Ploidy

Ploidy can be determined directly by the classic method of counting the modal number of chromosomes in a metaphase karyotype preparation or by an alternative indirect method of measuring DNA content by flow cytometry. The DNA content by flow cytometry is reported as the DNA index (DI), which is a ratio between the amount of fluorescence seen in a normal diploid cell and the fluorescent content of the bone marrow blasts (in G_0/G_1) at diagnosis. Normal diploid or pseudodiploid cells (cytogenetically abnormal but having a normal DNA content) have a DI of 1.0. Hyperdiploidy represents a chromosome number greater than 46 and DI greater than 1.0, and hypodiploidy represents a chromosome number less than 46 with a DI less than 1.0.

Most cases of ALL exhibit diploidy or hyperdiploidy (Table 19.5). The ploidy of B-lineage ALL karyotypes has long been recognized as a prognostic determinant.[135,136] Although the absolute number of chromosomes chosen as the cut-point for analysis may vary slightly between studies, cases of childhood ALL with higher ploidy have the best prognosis. Cases in the pseudodiploid category (those with a DI = 1.0 or normal chromosome number but other abnormalities) have a relatively poorer prognosis (Fig. 19.8). Those with diploidy and hyperdiploidy with 48 to 53 chromosomes (occasionally referred to as cases with "low hyperdiploidy") have a slightly worse prognosis than the hyperdiploid group with 53 to 58 chromosomes. Prognostically significant hyperdiploidy is commonly determined to be a DI of greater than 1.16 which corresponds to a modal number of

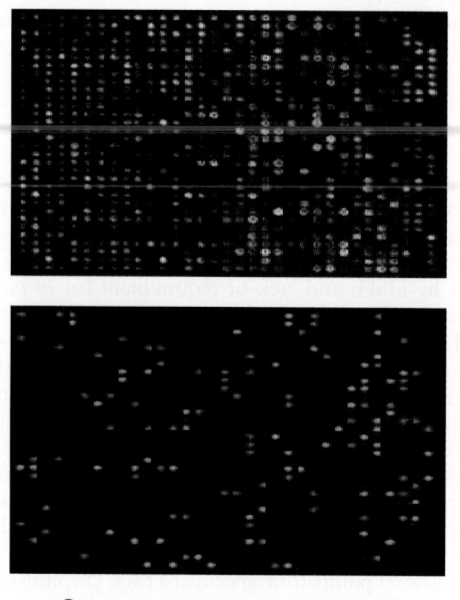

Diagnostic BM Samples (*n*=132)

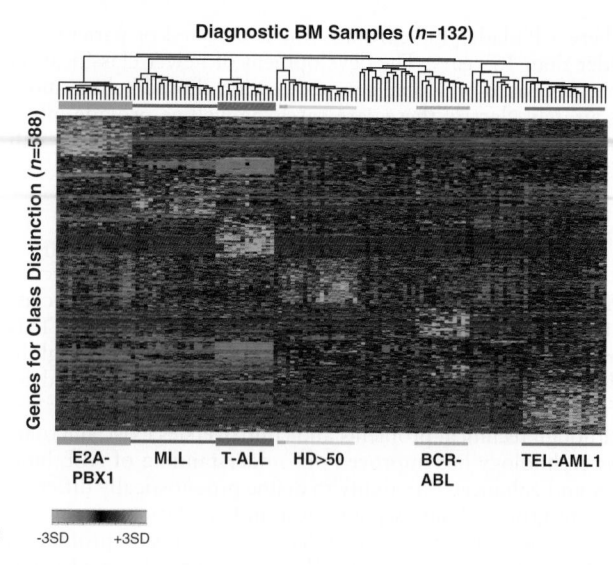

B -3SD +3SD

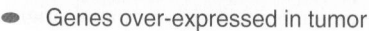

● Genes over-expressed in tumor

● Genes down regulated in tumor

● Genes expressed equally in
A   both normal and tumor cells

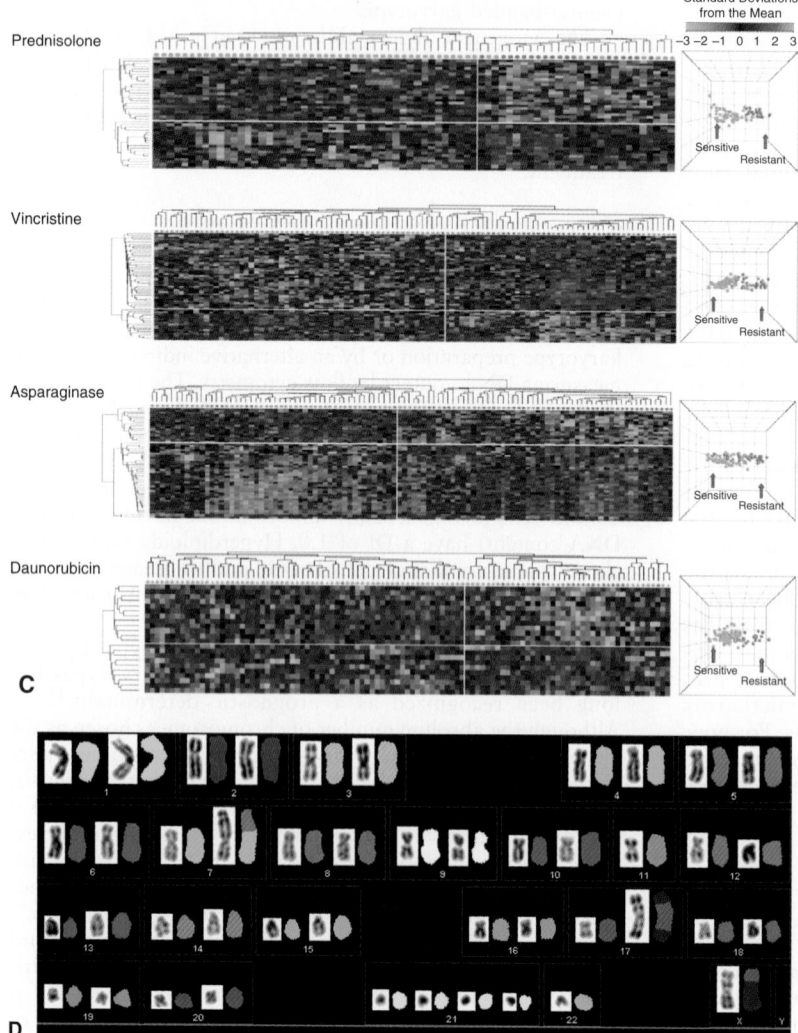

FIGURE 19.6 Application of new techniques for characterizing molecular, cytogenetic, and treatment response potential of acute lymphoblastic leukemia (ALL) blasts. **A:** Complementary DNA/messenger RNA (cDNA/mRNA) microarray. There are several current versions of this technology including spotted cDNA arrays and oligonucleotide arrays. This example is of a cDNA array undergoing competitive hybridization from two sources of fluorescent-labeled RNA. The relative expression of thousands of genes are measured by quantifying the amount of light emitted at the designated wavelengths of each spot on the array. (Array figure courtesy of C.C. Lau, personal communication, 2001.) **B:** Two-dimensional hierarchic cluster analysis (HCA) of 132 pediatric ALL diagnostic bone marrow samples (columns) evaluated using probe sets useful for discriminating six cytogenetically defined subgroups of ALL. The high expression blocks (show as red on actual analysis) readily identify expression patterns common to each of these subgroups. (From Ross ME, Zhou X, Song G, et al. Classification of pediatric acute lymphoblastic leukemia by gene expression profiling. Blood 2003;102:2951–2959, with permission.) **C:** HCA and principal component analysis (PCA) of genes that discriminate between prednisolone and vincristine resistance and drug sensitivity. (From Holleman A, Cheok MH, den Boer ML, et al. Gene-expression patterns in drug-resistant acute lymphoblastic leukemia cells and response to treatment. N Engl J Med 2004;351:533–542, with permission.) **D:** Spectral karyotyping (SKY) on leukemic ALL blast cells. This case is remarkable for aneuploidy (abnormal number) of chromosomes 21 and 22, as well as for several complex marker chromosomes [45,der(X)t(X;17)(p21;q24), -Y,der (7)t (5;7) (a12;p12), and ider(17)(q10)t(X;17)(?q11)]. (SKY results, courtesy of X.Y. Lu, C.P. Harris, C.C. Lau, and R.H. Rao, personal communication, 2004.)

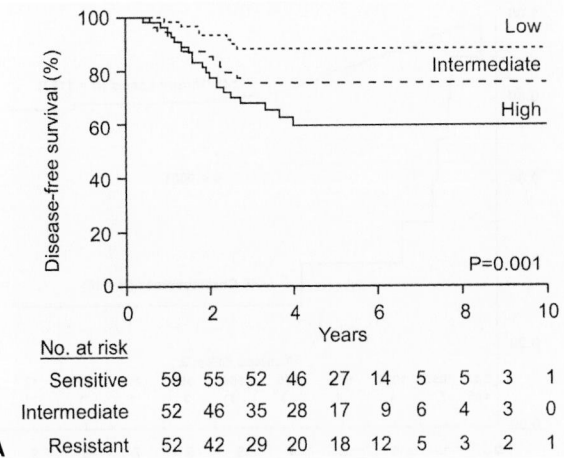

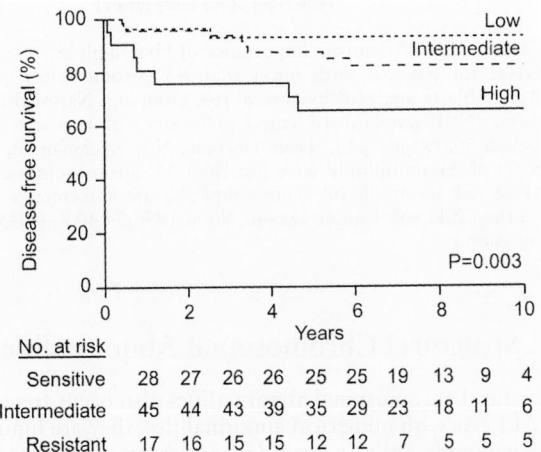

FIGURE 19.7 Kaplan-Meier estimates of disease-free survival among 173 patients in the original study group (**Panel A**) and 98 patients in the validation cohort (**Panel B**), according to whether the pattern of gene expression indicated cellular resistance or sensitivity to the four antileukemic agents. In each panel, patients are grouped according to their combined drug-resistance gene-expression scores for 172 probe sets for prednisolone, vincristine, asparaginase, and daunorubicin. The 33% with the lowest score (indicating sensitivity), the 33% with an intermediate score (indicating an intermediate level of resistance), and the 33% with the highest score (indicating resistance) are shown. (From Holleman A, Cheok MH, den Boer ML, et al. Gene expression patterns in drug-resistant acute lymphoblastic leukemia cells and response to treatment. N Engl J Med 2004; 351:533–542, with permission.)

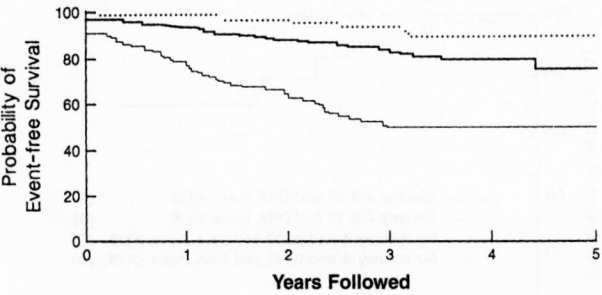

FIGURE 19.8 Ploidy is a prognostic determinant. Results are shown for patients with B-precursor acute lymphoblastic leukemia (infants excluded) treated by the Pediatric Oncology Group. Patients ($n = 114$) with a DNA index greater than 1.16 (i.e., hyperdiploid: [...]) have a better prognosis than those ($n = 353$) with a DNA index less than or equal to 1.16, white blood cell count (WBC) less than 50×10^9 per L, and age younger than 11 years (*bold line*); or a DNA index less than 1.16, WBC less than 50×10^9 per L, and age older than 11 years (*lowest curve*). (From Trueworthy R, Shuster J, Look T, et al. Ploidy of lymphoblasts is the strongest predictor of treatment outcome in B-progenitor cell acute lymphoblastic leukemia of childhood: a Pediatric Oncology Group study. J Clin Oncol 1992;10:606–613, with permission.)

53 chromosomes.[135] The best prognosis occurs for the higher hyperdiploid group with 56 to 67 chromosomes, which is commonly associated with extra copies of specific chromosomes.[137] Patients in the hyperdiploid group usually share a number of the more important favorable prognostic features (see section "Prognostic Factors"), including a favorable age, low initial leukocyte count, and a B-cell precursor phenotype often displaying CALLA (CD10) positivity. An exception to the observation that hyperdiploid ALL cases have a good prognosis may be the relatively rare subset of cases with extreme hyperdiploidy that have near-triploid or near-tetraploid karyotypes (66 to 73 and 82 to 84 chromosomes, respectively).[138] Near-tetraploidy is often associated with a T-cell immunophenotype.[138]

Trisomies of virtually every chromosome have been described in ALL, but the most commonly found include trisomy 4, 6, 10, 14, 17, 18, 21, and X.[137] Combined trisomies of chromosomes 4 and 10 in particular were associated with a very low risk of treatment failure in POG studies (Fig. 19.9).[135,139] The Children's Cancer Group (CCG) found similar correlations with the combination of chromosomes 10 and 17.[137] Trisomy 10 appears to have the larger effect, but in the studies cited, both trisomy 4 and trisomy 17 do appear to have independent positive effects.[137] A combined analysis of POG and CCG data found independent positive prognostic impact of so-called "triple trisomies," the concurrent trisomies of chromosomes 4, 10, and 17, which are used as the basis of stratification on current COG protocols.[140] Trisomy 6 has also been described as a good prognostic finding but does not have as strong a correlation as trisomy 4, 10, and 17.[141] Other trisomies appear to be prognostically neutral in the hyperdiploid context in which they are found. One study suggested that trisomy 5 was related to a slightly worse prognosis in ALL, but this effect vanished when the T-cell cases were removed from the analysis.[137] It is unclear which genes on any of these chromosomes may be responsible for the specific biologic behavior or response to individual therapies in trisomy cases.

Trisomies of chromosomes 8 and 21 are prognostically neutral but warrant some specific comments. Trisomy 8, the most common chromosomal numerical abnormality seen in AML, occurs rarely in ALL and is associated with T-cell

TABLE 19.5

FREQUENCY OF PLOIDY GROUPS IN CHILDHOOD ACUTE LYMPHOBLASTIC LEUKEMIA CASES

Ploidy group	Frequency (%)
Near haploidy	<1.0
Hypodiploidy, 30–40	<1.0
Hypodiploidy, 41–45	6.0
Pseudodiploidy	41.5
Hyperdiploidy, 47–50	15.5
Hyperdiploidy, >50	27.0
Near triploidy	<1.0
Near tetraploidy	1.0
Normal	8.0

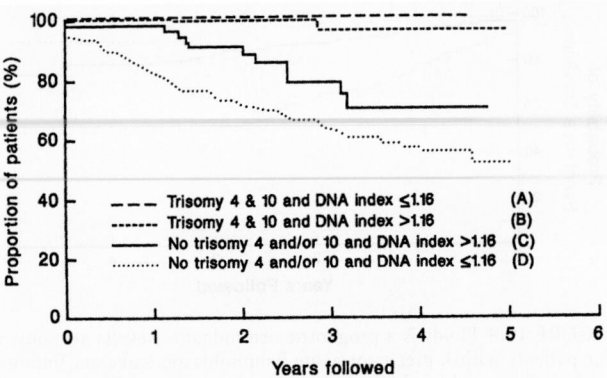

FIGURE 19.9 Prognosis of patients with trisomies of chromosomes 4 and 10. Presence of trisomies of chromosomes 4 and 10 are associated with a low risk of treatment failure. Results are shown for patients with B-precursor acute lymphoblastic leukemia (infants excluded) treated by the Pediatric Oncology Group. Patients with these trisomies have a better prognosis than those of patients in the good-risk (DNA index, greater than 1.16) and poor-risk (DNA index, 1.16 or less) groups. (From Harris MB, Shuster JJ, Carroll A, et al. Trisomy of leukemic cell chromosomes 4 and 10 identifies children with B-progenitor cell acute lymphoblastic leukemia with a very low risk of treatment failure: a Pediatric Oncology Group study. Blood 1992;79:3316–3324, with permission.)

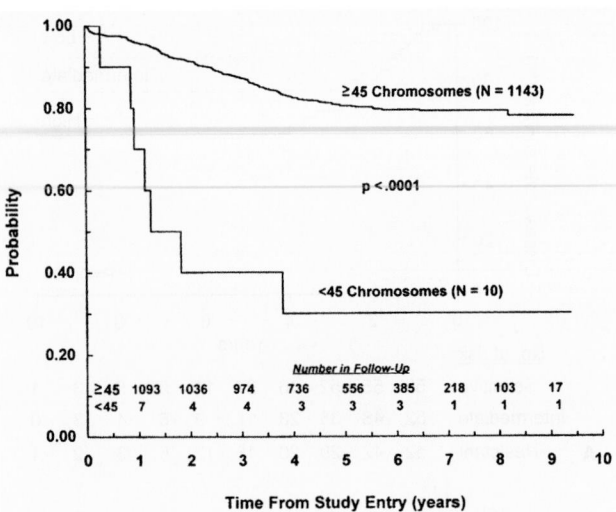

FIGURE 19.10 Prognostic Importance of Hypodiploidy. Event-free survival for patients with fewer than 45 chromosomes in their leukemic blasts analyzed by clinical risk grouping. National Cancer Institute (NCI) standard risk (age 1 to 9 years with leukocyte counts less than 50,000 per μL). (From Heerema NA, Nachman JB, Sather HN, et al. Hypodiploidy with less than 45 chromosomes confers adverse risk in childhood acute lymphoblastic leukemia: a report from the Children's Cancer Group. Blood 1999;94:4036–4045, with permission.)

immunophenotype.[142] When chromosome 8 of leukemic lymphoblasts (i.e., those with trisomies and those without) is examined by FISH, t(8;14)(q24:q32) translocations or duplications of the same 8q24 band may be identified.[143] Chromosome 8q24 is the location of the c-myc gene, which is important for cell growth and the site of many leukemia related translocations (see Table 19.1). The finding of trisomy 8 in leukemic lymphoblasts should prompt a reexamination of the available data to be sure that by morphology, histologic staining, immunophenotype, and karyotype that the patient has pre-B ALL and not L3 ALL, T ALL, or even AML.

Trisomy 21 as an isolated finding in leukemic lymphoblasts (in non-Down syndrome patients) is also a relatively neutral prognostic finding.[137] Chromosome 21 contains a large number of known oncogenic transcription factors and growth factors including *RUNX1* (*AML1*), an oncogene from the *runt* family of *Drosophila* transcription factors. This gene is associated with recurrent translocations such as the t(8;21) which forms the *RUNX1-ETO* fusion in AML (formerly referred to as *AML1-ETO*) and the t(12;21) *ETV6-RUNX1* fusion in ALL (formerly known as *TEL/AML1* based on the older names for the same genes fused by the breakpoint; see further discussion below).[144,145]

The worst prognosis (by ploidy) occurs with hypodiploidy (chromosome number <45 and DI<1.0), with the rare group of patients with near-haploid ALL (24 to 28 chromosomes) demonstrating the worse prognosis. These patients have an EFS of 25%.[146] Independent of other prognostic factors, ploidy greater or less than 45 chromosomes appears to have important prognostic implications that have not been altered by modern therapies (Fig. 19.10).[146] Within the less than 45 chromosome group, other prognostic factors (i.e., National Cancer Institute [NCI] standard vs. poor risk) still appear to have some impact.[146] Hypodiploidy with 45 chromosomes (which occurs frequently with the findings of dicentric chromosomes 9p and/or 12p) has a relatively good prognosis.[147] Hypodiploidy with 44 chromosomes has a prognosis which is poorer, but not as poor as cases with fewer than 44 chromosomes.[148]

Structural Chromosomal Abnormalities

Structural chromosomal abnormalities also occur frequently in ALL. As with numerical abnormalities, they are limited to the leukemic cells, a finding consistent with the clonal nature of the disease. Among the structural abnormalities encountered, translocations are the most common. Translocations that are detectable by standard Giemsa banding techniques occur in about 40% of cases, but that number rises with the use of more sensitive testing methods such as FISH, CGH, and SKY (described above). Multiple recurrent chromosomal translocations linked to altered regulation and function of cellular oncogenes occur in pediatric ALL and are thought to play a pivotal role in leukemogenesis (Table 19.1). Translocations are most frequent in the pseudodiploid and hypodiploid groups, and only rarely occur in other ploidy groups.[149] There appears to be an association between certain translocations and immunophenotype (see Table 19.1 and Classification by Immunophenotype Section). The more common of these, the ones linked to prognosis, and/or to known genes expressed in pediatric ALL are listed in Table 19.1.

The most common ALL translocation, t(12;21), is associated with good prognosis.[150] Twenty-two percent to 25% of pre-B ALL patients in the United States have this abnormality, but the prevalence of this good prognostic finding appears to vary widely between different geographic locations (see Table 19.6).[151] By standard karyotyping, approximately 5% of ALL patients have visible deletions of 12p12-p13 and rearrangements and molecular evidence of loss of heterozygosity involving this same region.[145,150,152] The t(12;21) usually occurs in patients with CALLA-positive B-cell precursor leukemia.[150] The preponderance of reports using more sensitive chromosomal analyses (commonly FISH) now indicate that a much larger percentage of 12p abnormalities occurs in childhood ALL. It results in the fusion of the coding regions of two transcription factors (*TEL* on chromosome 12p13,

FREQUENCY OF *ETV6-RUNX1 (TEL-AML1)* AMONG B LINEAGE ALL PATIENTS BY GEOGRAPHIC LOCATIONS

Author	Year	Country	*n*	B-Lineage ALL (%)
Rubnitz et al.	1997	U.S.	188	26
Eguchi-Ishimae et al.	1998	Japan	74	10
Inamdar et al.	1998	India	46	9
Avigad et al.	1999	Israel	98	24
Garcia-Sanz et al.	1999	Spain	41	3
Spathas et al.	1999	United Kingdom	31	13
Jamil et al.	2000	U.S.	86	17
Magalhaes et al.	2000	Brazil	67	20
Tsang et al.	2001	China	67	18
Liang et al.	2002	Taiwan	165	18
Ozbek et al.	2003	Turkey	219	28
Sazawal et al.	2004	India	35	0
Hill et al.	2005	India	42	7

Note: Incidence of *TEL-AML1* cytogenetic findings differ widely throughout the world. In the US most series show approximately 25% of patients present with this laboratory feature. In India and Spain the incidence is much lower.
Personal communication with P. Buffler and information from Aldrich MC, Luoping Z, Wiemels JL et. al. Cancer Edemiolo Biomarkers Prev 2006;15(3):578–581.

now known as *ETV6*, and *AML1* on chromosome 21q22, now known as *RUNX1*). This t(12;21) fusion appears to be necessary but not sufficient to cause the leukemia, promoting B-progenitor differentiation and self-renewal.[153] The subsequent events that cause progression to true leukemia are not certain. Resistance of t(12;21)+ cells to TGF-β-mediated inhibition of proliferation is one possible mechanism, which may afford a selective proliferative advantage to a t(12;21)+ preleukemic clone in the setting of a dysregulated immune response to infection.[154]

The t(12;21) translocation occurs more often in children 1 to 10 years of age and in CD10 (CALLA)-positive cases. It is generally regarded as a favorable prognostic factor, although some studies have suggested an increased risk of late relapse.[155,156] The presence of a t(12;21) translocation is not a guarantee of successful treatment, however, as 10% of relapsed cases continue to come from this group. Opinion is divided as to whether *ETV6-RUNX1* retains independent prognostic significance or simply tends to occur in cases with other favorable features (e.g., age and response to therapy).[157,158] Relapse in these cases tends to occur late, with excellent chemosensitivity and salvage rates.[159] Relapse may in fact represent an independent "second hit" in the original preleukemic t(12;21)+ clone.[160]

The t(1;19)(q23;p13) is the second most common chromosomal abnormality in childhood ALL.[13] It is found in 6.5% of all children with ALL. It is present in 25% of cytoplasmic IgM heavy chain-positive (cIg+) cases of pre-B-cell ALL and in 1% of cIg-early pre-B-cell ALL cases.[161] This translocation results in the fusion of the transcriptional activation domain of the helix-loop-helix transcription factor *E2A* on chromosome 19p with the DNA binding homeodomain of *PBX1* located on chromosome 1, band q23.[162] The resulting E2A-PBX1 protein is a transcriptional activator that has been associated with a variety of tumors in different animal models, including T-cell ALL and AML.[162,163] The pre-B ALL cases that have the t(1;19)(q23;p13) and express E2A-PBX1 protein had a poor prognosis on the standard therapies of the 1990s but have better outcomes on current therapies. It is no longer used in current prognostic stratification strategies.[1]

Another fusion partner of the *E2A* gene on chromosome 19p13 was originally described as a variant of the t(1;19) (q23;p13).[164] The t(17;19)(q22;p13) occurs in 1% of childhood ALL and appears to define a poor-prognostic group of adolescent patients. These patients have an unusual clinical presentation characterized by hypercalcemia; an increased risk of disseminated intravascular coagulation; and a pre-B (cIgM+), low CD10 positivity immunophenotype.[165,166] The *E2A* fusion partner in this translocation is the hepatic leukemia transcription factor gene (*HLF*) found on chromosome 17q22. The E2A-HLF protein can cause transformation *in vitro*.[167] It is possible to use the known sequence of the *E2A-HLF* fusion in a RT-PCR system for detecting MRD in patients with this type of disease.[165]

The t(8;14)(q24;q32) can be identified in virtually every case of B-cell ALL (FAB L3). In this translocation the myc proto-oncogene, normally located on chromosome 8, is translocated near a transcriptional enhancer of the immunoglobulin heavy chain gene on chromosome 14. The resulting dysregulation of myc expression is believed to be responsible for the uncontrolled proliferation of B cells characteristic of this disorder. In addition to the translocation of myc coding sequences, mutations sometimes occur in the translocated sequences.[168] Two variant translocations, the t(2;8)(p11-p12;q24) and t(8;22) (q24;11) involving the κ and λ light chains, respectively, are observed less commonly. The similarity in the molecular mechanisms associated with these translocations in B-cell ALL and those that occur in Burkitt's lymphoma supports the presumption that B-cell ALL represents a disseminated form of Burkitt's lymphoma. Patients with B-cell ALL respond quite poorly to conventional ALL treatment, but fare better on therapy similar to that used for Burkitt's lymphoma.

Similar translocations [i.e., t(8;14)(q24;q11)] involving TCR loci and the myc gene have been described in some cases of T-cell ALL.[168,169] In these cases, the myc gene is overexpressed, but the resulting leukemic blasts display T-cell immunophenotype.

There are a number of examples of translocations of transcription factor genes to TCR loci in T-cell ALL (Table 19.1

and Chapter 3). These translocations may involve the TCR β at 7q34 or the TCR αδ on 14q11. Rhombotin 1 and 2, *TAL1/SCL*, *TAL2*, *HOX11*, and *LYL1* are the best studied examples of these transcription factor translocations to TCR loci.[168] In most of these translocations, the coding sequences for transcription factor proteins, not normally expressed in T cells, are relocated near the TCR. The translocation breakpoints generally occur at sites of normal VDJ recombination, suggesting that they arise from inappropriate activity of recombinase activating genes (RAGs).[170] These translocations cause inappropriate expression of the translocated transcription factors. The mechanisms that eventually lead from the inappropriate expression of these proteins to frank leukemia vary with the transcription factors involved. Additional cryptic TCR rearrangements, some involving novel putative oncogene partners, continue to be discovered.[171]

TAL1 (also known as *SCL*) is translocated to a TCR in approximately 5% of pediatric T-cell ALL cases. A partial *TAL1* deletion has been described in approximately 25% of pediatric T-cell ALL cases, which causes over-expression of the TAL1 protein.[172] *TAL1* is not expressed in normal T cells, but it appears to be critical to the formation of the entire hematopoietic system.[173] The mechanism by which *TAL1* translocation or partial deletion may cause leukemia is not understood. Translocations involving *TAL1*, *TAL2*, and *LYL1* and the TCRs occur in 30% of T-cell ALL cases (Table 19.1).[13] The genes regulated by these transcription factors are believed to represent a common pathway for the development of T-cell leukemia.

The transcription factor *LMO2* is implicated in T-cell ALL via either fusion with a TCR or partial deletion.[174] Another disturbing instance of *LMO2*-mediated leukemogenesis occurred in a gene therapy trial for X-linked severe combined immunodeficiency (SCID) in which patients underwent retrovirus-mediated gene transfer, and two of 10 patients subsequently developed T-cell ALL. In both cases, the retroviral particle integrated close to the *LMO2* locus and presumably exerted enhancer activity on the *LMO2* promoter.[175,176]

The t(10,14)(q24;q11) and t(7:10)(q35;q24) involve translocations of the transcription factor *HOX11* and TCR loci. *HOX* genes are known to be important regulators of hematopoietic development (see Chapters 3 and 4). Thus, translocations involving different members of this gene family in cases of ALL are not surprising. Despite the heterogeneity of the multiple transcription factor translocations with TCRs in T-cell leukemia, the actual disease associated with these molecular findings is relatively homogenous in clinical and histologic presentation, course, and prognosis.[168,177]

Although T ALL is characterized by multiple transcription factor translocations with TCRs, a partially unifying feature was identified in 2004 with the discovery of somatic activating mutations of the *NOTCH1* gene in over 50% of cases.[178] Since mutated NOTCH1 activity depends on γ-secretase activity, this has led to investigation of γ-secretase inhibitors as a targeted therapy for these cases.[179] Other recent discoveries in molecular genetics of T-cell ALL include identification of episomal amplification of the NUP214-ABL1 fusion protein, a novel mechanism of tyrosine kinase activation; and translocations and duplications involving the *MYB* oncogene.[180–182]

Despite the description of numerous recurrent cytogenetic abnormalities in T-cell ALL, none of these findings appear to identify patients at greater or lesser risk of relapse. Risk stratification strategies for T-cell patients generally rely on clinical features at presentation, and when they are grouped with pre-B ALL patients with similar presentation features, the clinical outcome results appear to be equivalent.

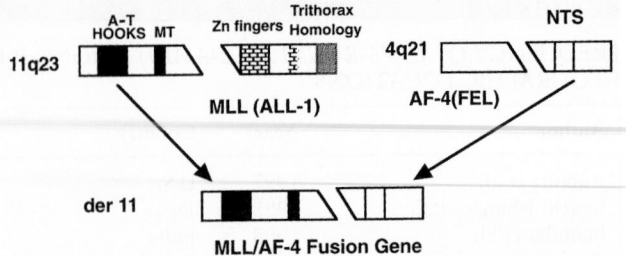

FIGURE 19.11 Schematic representation of the MLL/AF-4 fusion protein created by the t(4:11)(q21;q23) found in up to 70% of infant acute lymphoblastic leukemia (ALL) cases. The translocation involves a reciprocal transfer between the ALL-1 gene (located on band 11q23) and the AF-4 gene (located on band 4q21). The resulting der11 product codes for a protein that is thought to be responsible of the development of the 4:11-positive infant ALL. NTS, nuclear translocation signal; MT, methyl transferase activity; Zn, zinc.

Structural abnormalities (including translocation, deletion, and partial duplication) of chromosome band 11q23 are associated with poor prognosis in both B-lineage ALL and in AML.[1,183] The 11q23 abnormalities are present in 5% to 10% of pediatric and adult cases of ALL, in 60–70% of infant leukemia (i.e., ALL and AML in patients younger than 1 year, see also Chapter 15), and in 85% of secondary leukemias in patients who have received epipodophyllotoxin therapy.[13,184] Virtually all of these 11q23 abnormalities have occurred in the same region of a gene variously named *MLL* (myeloid/lymphoid leukemia gene or mixed lineage leukemia), *Htrx1/HRX*, and *ALL-1*.[185] The MLL1 protein is believed to be an important developmental regulator of pluripotent hematopoietic cells. More than 40 partner genes have been found for *MLL* (see Chapter 3, Table 19.1, and Fig. 19.11), the most common of which are located on chromosomes 4, 6, 9, and 19.[186] ALL patients with rearrangements involving 11q23/*MLL* have significantly poorer treatment outcomes than those of clinically similar patients who do not demonstrate this cytogenetic abnormality (Fig. 19.12).

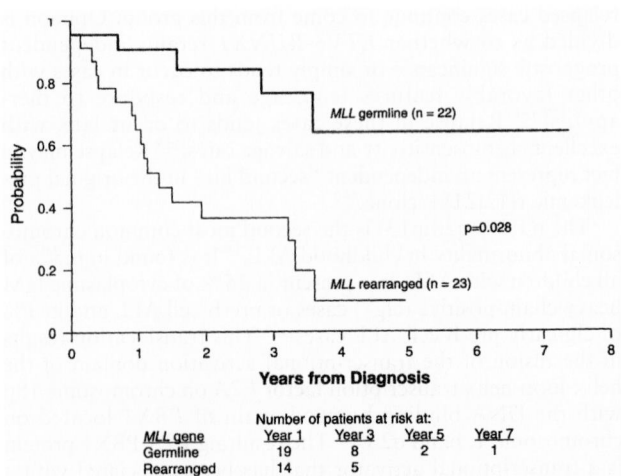

FIGURE 19.12 Event-free survival for patients with acute lymphoblastic leukemia, demonstrating the poorer overall prognosis for those with rearrangements involving 11q23/*MLL*. (From Behm FG, Raimondi SC, Frestedt JL, et al. Rearrangement of the *MLL* gene confers a poor prognosis in childhood acute lymphoblastic leukemia, regardless of presenting age. Blood 1996;87:2870–2877, with permission.)

The t(4;11)(q21;q23) is the most frequent of these translocations (Fig. 19.11 and Table 19.1). It has been reported in up to 5% of pediatric ALL cases, is more common in girls, and as noted occurs in more than 60% of infant leukemias of all types.[13,187] The t(4;11)(q21;q23) generally occurs in B-cell precursor ALL and is somewhat more frequently observed in patients with early pre-B-cell disease (cIg-). A large percentage of these cases manifest a characteristic immunophenotype (i.e., CD10⁻/CD15⁺/CD19⁺). Leukemic cells from patients with t(4;11) may manifest some cytochemical and ultrastructural features of monocytes and thus have biphenotypic characteristics. Because other translocations involving 11q23 have also been associated with characteristics of mixed lineage [e.g., t(11;19)(q23;p12), t(9;11(p21;q23)], it has been suggested by many that leukemias with the 11q23 rearrangement arise from a pluripotent progenitor cell.[13]

The t(9;22)(q34;q11) was one of the first leukemic translocations described and until recently it was the translocation with the worst prognosis in pediatric ALL.[188,189] What has changed this prognosis (at least for some of these patients) is an understanding that a better prognostic subgroups exists within the overall group of pediatric patients with Ph+ ALL, and the successful development and application of ABL tyrosine kinase inhibitors such as imatinib and dasatinib in both adult and pediatric Ph+ ALL (see below).[189–191] The t(9;22) (q34;q11) translocation disrupts the proto-oncogene c-abl on chromosome 9 that encodes the tyrosine kinase ABL, which is part of the RAS signaling pathway (see Chapter 3). The t(9;22) results in the formation of a small marker chromosome, known as the Philadelphia chromosome (Ph), which is found in approximately 5% of childhood ALL and 20% to 30% of adult ALL.[192,193] The typical translocation, t(9;22)(q34;q11), is similar to that observed in chronic myeloid leukemia (CML). In the past, it had been suggested that Ph+ ALL represented CML that lacked a chronic phase and presented in blast crisis. In Ph+ ALL, unlike in CML, the translocation usually cannot be detected in multiple cell lineages.[80]

Cytogenetic and molecular differences distinguish Ph+ ALL from CML. In CML, the c-abl gene on chromosome 9 is translocated to a 5.8-kb span of chromosome 22 known as the major breakpoint cluster region (M-bcr).[194] In Ph+ ALL, however, the breakpoints on chromosome 22 usually occur upstream from the M-bcr at a site referred to as the minor breakpoint cluster region (m-bcr or bcr-2).[195,196] The translocation places the c-abl coding sequences under the transcriptional control of bcr (break point cluster region) on chromosome 22. There are differences between the BCR-ABL gene products expressed in the two diseases. In most cases of Ph+ ALL, a unique p185 BCR-ABL protein with tyrosine kinase activity has been observed that is distinct from the p210 BCR-ABL protein typically found in CML.[197] However, the p210 BCR-ABL protein also has been detected in some cases of Ph+ ALL.[198] Both fusion products have been shown to encode active tyrosine kinases, immortalize cell lines transfected with fusion protein cDNA constructs, and cause leukemias in transgenic mice.[197] In mice, the p185 fusion protein appears to produce more aggressive disease with shorter latencies than the p210. This is consistent with differences in the natural history of ALL and CML.

The Ph chromosome has been observed both in B-cell precursor ALL and in T-cell ALL. Children with Ph+ ALL tend to be older, have higher initial leukocyte counts, and are more likely to display FAB L2 morphology. Occasionally, leukemic blasts may have the BCR-ABL translocation, but either they have had inadequate cytogenetics studies or they do not demonstrate the Ph chromosome on karyotype. PCR techniques have proven useful in diagnosing BCR-ABL positive,

Ph chromosome negative ALL and CML.[199] The BCR-ABL fusion protein confers the poor prognosis. Quantitative PCR and colony assays have been useful in measuring MRD during therapy and after BMT for BCR-ABL positive disease.[199,200]

Clinically, Ph+ ALL patients respond poorly to conventional (non-tyrosine kinase inhibitor inclusive) therapy. On standard therapies these patients have a distinctly lower remission induction rate, a higher frequency of CNS leukemia, and early recurrence of their disease.[201] A subgroup of children with Ph+ ALL who also have partial or complete monosomy 7 may have an even poorer prognosis.[202] Patients with both Ph+ and monosomy 7 had a 31% induction failure rate in an early study.[202] Although the induction response rate using more intensive chemotherapy has improved, these patients continue to fail later in therapy even on modern, intensive regimens.[203] Some cases of Ph+ ALL exhibit mixed-lineage characteristics. It has been suggested that, because of its poor prognosis, children with Ph+ ALL require an alternative to conventional ALL treatment. Early BMT with an HLA-identical sibling (and in some cases with an alternative donor) has been the recommendation of many groups, and the results appear to have improved somewhat over time (see BMT section and Fig. 19.13).[1,204] As noted above, there appears to be a subgroup of Ph+ ALL pediatric patients who present with NCI low-risk features (see section "Prognostic Factors"), who appear to do well with intensive conventional therapies.[189] Recent data has demonstrated that the addition of abl tyrosine kinase inhibitors and close monitoring of MRD status appears to benefit this group, and may also improve outcomes in Ph+ patients with higher risk presenting features.[205] In the context of a very aggressive conventional chemotherapy regimen with the addition of increasing amounts of the tyrosine kinase inhibitor Imatinib researchers were able to achieve a 3 year EFS in PH+ ALL of 80% (Fig. 19.14A). Furthermore, increased duration of therapy (cohort 5 in this study, and Figure 19.14B) with Imatinib seemed able to overcome high levels of end induction MRD.[205] The question of which patients with Ph+ ALL should be treated with BMT continues to be studied, but it now appears that many will be cured with out transplant.

Although monosomy 7 and deletions of 7q are primarily associated with myeloid disorders, they are also found in approximately 4% of pediatric ALL cases.[203] These abnormalities are more likely to be observed in poor risk patients (see section "Prognostic Factors") with hypodiploidy (loss of other chromosomal material as well as material from chromosome 7). Monosomy 7 and del7q in ALL confer a worse prognosis, although it is not clear whether this adds anything further to the negative impact in Ph+ cases treated with TK inhibitor containing regimens.[206] Secondary cytogenetic aberrations of many different types are found in 61% of childhood Ph+ ALL cases, but none have been definitively shown to confer additional positive or negative prognostic significance.[206]

Deletions of chromosomal band 9p21–22 are common in pediatric ALL, occurring in approximately 20% of B-lineage and 50% of T-ALL.[207,208] The reported incidence of deletions in the 9p21–22 region has increased with the increasing use of PCR, and newer interphase FISH techniques capable of detecting lesions not visible using classic cytogenetic techniques. Two separate regions are the targets of these deletions at 9p22. At one locus, the interferon cluster and interferon-β1 gene are fully or partially deleted. The second locus at 9p21 is the site of two cyclin D kinase inhibitors (CDKIs): p16 and p15. p16 is a potent tumor suppressor, which has been shown to be important in a variety of adult solid tumors.[209] It is thought that deletion of p16, p15, or both

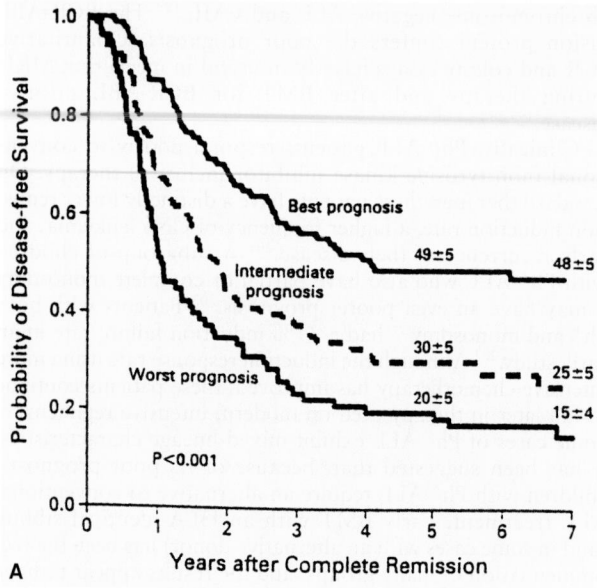

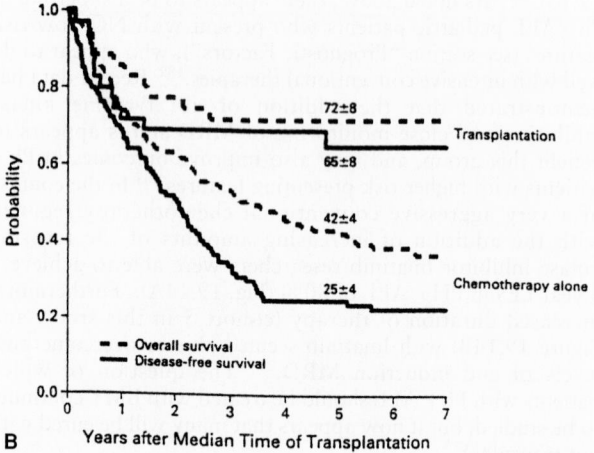

FIGURE 19.13 A: Outcomes for subgroups of pediatric patients with Philadelphia chromosome–positive ALL treated with either chemotherapy alone or bone marrow transplant. A: $N = 326$ patients classified by modified Rome–National Cancer Institute criteria as follows: best prognosis (age 10 years or younger with a leukocyte count less than 50,000/mm^3), intermediate prognosis (intermediate-risk features), and worst prognosis (any age with a leucocyte count greater than 100,000/mm^3). Outcomes analyzed regardless of therapy. B: Disease-free survival and overall survival for $n = 267$ patients treated with either HLA-matched related transplants or chemotherapy alone. (From Arico M, Valsecchi MG, Camitta B, et al. Outcome of treatment in children with Philadelphia chromosome–positive acute lymphoblastic leukemia. N Engl J Med 2000;342:998–1006, with permission.)

allows cells to progress through the G1 cell cycle checkpoint in an uncontrolled way, ultimately resulting in leukemia. Deletions of large portions of 9p (including the 9p21–22 region) are associated with T-cell ALL but do not (with current therapies) seem to be linked with prognosis.[1,207] As already noted, trisomy 8 and del 9p are frequently seen in T-ALL.[210]

Other frequently described structural abnormalities in T-ALL include del 6q and breakpoints at the known immunoglobulin and TCR genes (Table 19.1). The ploidy findings in T-ALL are very different than the ones described

previously for common pre-B ALL. The majority (86% in one study) of T-ALL cases are pseudodiploid or diploid.[210]

The reciprocal translocation of the long arms of chromosomes 5 and 14, t(5;14)(q31;q32), has been characterized by a B-lineage phenotype and hypereosinophilia.[211] The immunoglobulin heavy chain gene and the promotor region of the interleukin-3 (IL-3) gene are joined by this translocation.[149] Overexpression of the IL-3 gene may be involved in the pathogenesis of the hypereosinophilia and leukemia observed in these patients.[212]

Unique translocations, observed in single cases, make up approximately one half of the chromosomal translocations seen in ALL.[195] Whether all translocations are intimately involved in the leukemogenic process is unknown. It appears likely that some translocations, through induction of altered gene expression, confer a growth advantage on cells of a particular phenotype.

Chromosomal studies of bone marrow obtained during remission in ALL are karyotypically normal. The persistence or reappearance of aneuploidy during clinical and morphologic remission heralds relapse.[213] In the majority of patients at relapse, the leukemic clone is cytogenetically related to that observed at diagnosis, although evidence of clonal evolution is common.[213]

Mutation and Loss-of-Heterozygosity (LOH) for Specific Oncogenes

DNA mutations or alterations in protein expression have been described in primary ALL and cell lines for *p53, MDM2, p15, p16;* in the interferon genes located on 9p; *WT1* (i.e., the Wilms tumor gene located at 11p13); in the *ETV6 (TEL)* and *KIP1* loci on 12p12-p13; *PTPN11;* and others.[152,214–216] Although the abnormalities detected in most of these genes may not be as definitively leukemogenic as the *BCR-ABL* and other fusion gene mutations described above (Table 19.1), they are commonly observed in pediatric ALL and appear to contribute both to the development of leukemia and (in some cases) to the response to specific chemotherapeutic agents.[1] FLT-3 is another signaling kinase that appears to have increasing importance not only in AML (in which internal tandem duplication [ITD] has been discovered to have prognostic relevance) but also in ALL.[86,217,218] Increased levels and activity of FLT-3 have been found in both *MLL* rearranged and hyperdiploid cases of ALL. Small molecule inhibitors of FLT-3 are being developed and clinically assessed as possible therapeutic agents for treatment of leukemias of all types.[219]

Mutations and loss-of-heterozygosity (LOH) of the wild-type allele in oncogenes known to be important in other cancers (i.e., p53 and the *RAS* family members N-, K-, and H-RAS) have been demonstrated in small but varying percentages (0.2% to 15%) of pediatric ALL cases.[214,220] The mutation rates of these genes tend to be higher in relapsed cases. Thus far, the mutational status in these genes has not shown particular correlation with outcome. There is evidence that the *p53* and *RB* (retinoblastoma) pathways (through mutation and/or transcriptional silencing of the *p53* target *p21CIP1*) and the cyclin kinase inhibitors *p16INK4a, p15INK4b* and related *INK4* family members collaborate in leukemogenesis.[13]

The Homeobox-containing transcription factors (*Hox*) genes represent an oncogene family of known importance in leukemogenesis. Multiple *Hox* family members and their DNA binding cofactor known as *MEIS1* have been found in microarray and other global gene expression studies to

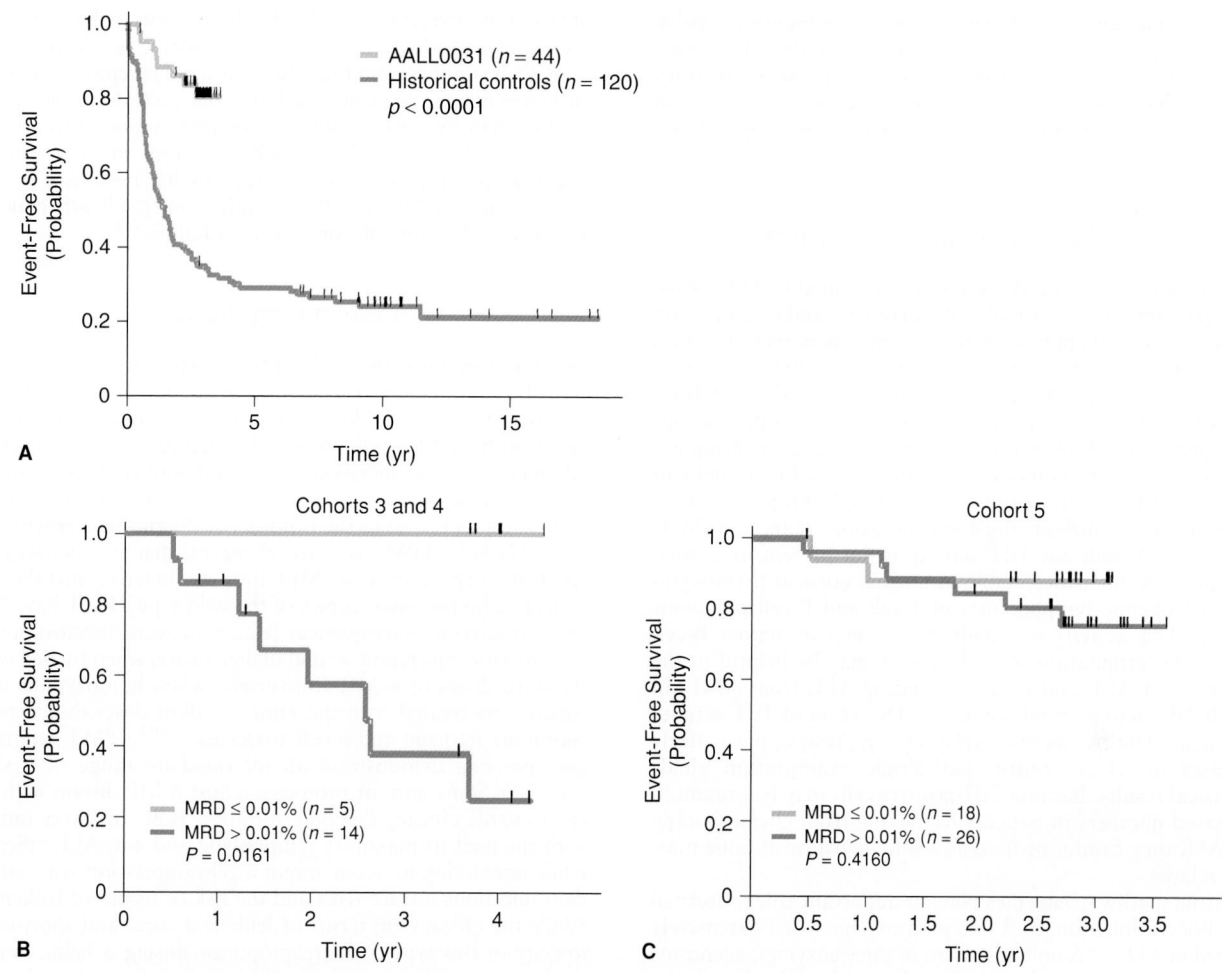

FIGURE 19.14 A: Early event-free survival in Philadelphia chromosome-positive ALL patients treated with Imatinib. Treated patients in cohort 5 (highest dose Imatinib, $N = 44$) were compared with patients previously treated on Pediatric Oncology Group (POG) protocols AlinC 14, 15, and 18 from January 1986 through November 1999 ($N = 120$). **B:** Impact of end of Induction MRD on outcomes with lower (cohort 3 and 4) versus **C:** higher amounts of Imatinib therapy (cohort 5).

be overexpressed in patterns than can be correlated with specific ALL subtypes.[13,218,221] Other Hox family members (i.e., PBX1) are involved in specific oncogenic translocations.

Recent Molecular Findings at Diagnosis and Relapse

Recently, genome-wide investigations of ALL have identified abnormalities of genes involved in regulation of B-cell development in 40% of cases, the most common being deletions and mutations of the lymphoid transcription factor *PAX5*.[222] Deletions and inactivating mutations of the Ikaros Zinc Finger protein I *(IKZF1)*, another lymphoid transcription factor, have been identified in 84% of BCR-ABL+ ALL.[223] IZKF1 alterations have also been associated with very poor outcome in as many as 39% of BCR-ABL-negative ALL cases lacking other cytogenetic abnormalities.[224] Activating mutations in Janus kinase (JAK) family members, predominantly *JAK2*, are also common in BCR-ABL-negative ALL cases with poor outcomes, as well as occurring in 20% of Down syndrome associated ALL.[31,225]

Another recently identified poor prognostic lesion is intrachromosomal amplification of chromosome 21, in which three or more copies of a region including *RUNX1* (also known as *AML1*) are duplicated in tandem along the long arm of chromosome 21.[226,227] Although this lesion has only been identified in 2% of ALL, it is notable because clinical outcomes appear particularly poor.[228] While the immunoglobulin heavy chain *(IGH@)* is well-known for its involvement in the t(8;14) translocation juxtaposing it to the *MYC* oncogene in Burkitt's leukemia and lymphoma, additional translocations have recently been identified involving several members of the CCAAT/Enhancer Binding Protein *(CEBP)* family of transcription factors as well as additional partner genes, all associated with relatively older age, low initial leukocyte count, and a relatively good prognosis.[229]

In the majority of patients at relapse, the leukemic clone is cytogenetically related to that observed at diagnosis, although evidence of clonal evolution is common. Genomic studies of matched diagnosis and relapse pairs demonstrate that the relapse clone demonstrates both acquisition and loss of copy number abnormalities compared to the diagnostic clone.[230,231] Interestingly, the relapse clone may often be detectable at a low level at diagnosis, and in many cases appears not to evolve from the diagnostic clone, but rather to be indirectly related via a shared ancestral clone.[230] Gene expression profiles between diagnosis and relapse tend to be more divergent in late (>18 months off therapy) compared to early relapse cases.[88]

Biochemical Characterization

Various biochemical markers have been studied in ALL. Some have been found to be useful in the diagnosis and classification of the disease; others have been evaluated as potential targets for selective therapy. Terminal deoxynucleotidyl transferase (TdT) is an unusual DNA-polymerizing enzyme that catalyzes the polymerization of deoxynucleoside monophosphates into a single-strand DNA primer without the need for template instruction.[232] TdT is found in the nucleus and is thought to play a role in immunoglobulin and T-cell antigen receptor rearrangement, influencing the generation of immunologic diversity.[233] Significant TdT activity is not present in normal lymphocytes but is detectable in normal cortical thymocytes and in leukemic lymphoblasts of T-cell and B-cell precursor lineage. TdT activity is usually not present in mature B-cell ALL.[234] Determination of TdT activity may be helpful in the diagnosis of ALL and in differentiating ALL from AML, in which TdT activity rarely occurs.[235] Detection of TdT activity may help identify sanctuary relapses (e.g., testes), particularly in cases in which routine pathologic examination yields equivocal results. Because TdT-positive cells may be present in increased numbers in patients recovering from chemotherapy or BMT, they cannot be used as a sole indicator of bone marrow relapse.

Purine pathway enzymes play an important role in normal lymphocyte function, and this pathway has been extensively studied in ALL.[236] A unique pattern of three enzymes, adenosine deaminase, 5'-nucleotidase, and purine nucleoside phosphorylase, has been observed in ALL.[237] Abnormal lymphocyte function and the absence or reduction in activity of each of these enzymes is also a characteristic of certain immunodeficiency disorders. Among the acute leukemias, the activity of adenosine deaminase, which catalyzes the conversion of adenosine to inosine, is highest in ALL. This is particularly true in T-cell ALL, in which decreased 5'-nucleotidase and purine nucleoside phosphorylase activity is noted.[232,238] Investigators have attempted to take advantage of the unique biochemical profile of T-cell ALL. A potent inhibitor of adenosine deaminase, 2'-deoxycoformycin, as well as several other purine analogs singly and in combination, have demonstrated activity against a broad spectrum of lymphoid malignancies.[239] Nelarabine and Clofarabine are purine analogs that have shown promise in phase trials with relapsed ALL patients (T cell and pre-B ALL respectively), and are incorporated in several ongoing front-line trials for high risk T cell ALL and/or relapsed pre-B ALL.[240-242]

Elevated serum levels of lactate dehydrogenase (LDH) have been observed in ALL at diagnosis.[243] LDH levels reportedly normalize during remission and increase again at relapse. Abnormalities in lysosomal enzymes also have been observed in ALL.[244] Glucocorticoid receptors have been identified on leukemic lymphoblasts, and the distribution of glucocorticoid receptor number appears to differ significantly among the major immunologic subtypes of ALL. The greatest numbers of receptor sites per cell are seen in early B lineage ALL. T-cell ALL has significantly lower receptor numbers, and B-cell ALL has the lowest.[245] Glucocorticoid receptor content correlates with sensitivity to steroid treatment *in vitro*, and attempts have been made to correlate receptor number with response to therapy

in vivo. Lower receptor number has been associated with poorer responses to induction therapy and shorter remission durations.[246] It is not certain that glucocorticoid receptor number is an independent prognostic variable that provides more information than the technically less complex, more conventional prognostic factors.[247] Nevertheless, a poor *in vivo* clinical response to initial corticosteroid therapy has been used by the Berlin-Frankfurt-Munster (BFM) study group to identify patients at particularly high risk for treatment failure.[248]

Pharmacogenetics

Pharmacogenomics, the study of the genetic basis for the differences between individual responses to specific drugs, is a growing area of research.[249] In addition to unique biochemical/enzymatic profiles, ALL cells from individual patients demonstrate differences in drug metabolism and response that have important effects on disease outcome and toxicity. Perhaps one of the best examples relates to the isoforms of thiopurine methyltransferase *(TPMT)*. TPMT is a crucial enzyme that metabolizes parent 6-mercaptopurine (6-MP) into an inactive metabolite. Patients who have two copies of the wild-type TPMT have low rates of adverse consequences (e.g., mucositis, myelosuppression, hepatic injury, and second malignancies) when treated with standard doses of 6-MP. Conversely, when homozygous null patients are treated with the same standard doses they experience more frequent and severe toxicities.[250-252] TPMT heterozygote patients demonstrate an intermediate range of toxicities.[250-252] Some current protocols adjust 6-MP dosing with an eye towards efficacy (keeping the total WBC in lower ranges with the goal to maximize lympholytic and anti-ALL efficacy, while attempting to avoid severe myelosuppression with attendant infectious disease risks and the risk of recurrent leukemia. While the efficacy (in terms of leukemia cure) and short-term toxicity of this type of Mercaptopurine dosing is being tested, the longer term consequences of these strategies will need to be monitored. Newer data demonstrate that there may be risks of increased second malignant neoplasms (SMN) from higher and more prolonged Mercaptopurine levels, and additional pharmacogenetic factors (e.g., genetic polymorphisms in inosine triphosphate pyrophosphatase [ITPA], which also regulates 6-MP efficacy and toxicity).[253,254]

Polymorphisms in folate pathway enzymes such as the reduced folate carrier (RFC) and methyltetrahydrofolate reductase (MTHFR) have also been associated with toxicities and survival outcomes.[255] Efforts to control for some of these factors using more individualized pharmacokinetically based dosing schedules have shown promise.[256]

It appears that some of the biochemical pathways implicated in the etiology of the disease (see the discussion of environmental factors and genotype in section "Epidemiology") may also influence both treatment response and toxicities. The glutathione S-transferase (GST) genes encode at least four different subfamilies of cytosolic proteins, some of which display known genetic polymorphisms. GST genotypes that confer lower enzyme activities may enhance the efficacy and toxicity of chemotherapy. The enzymatic null genotypes of GST have been associated with a decreased risk of toxicity and lower overall survival for patients treated for AML.[257] These same GST null mutations have been linked in small series to the development of several adult solid tumors and pediatric ALL.[257,258]

Other germline genetic polymorphisms have also been associated with differential sensitivity of leukemic blasts to chemotherapeutic agents; risk of particular toxicities in the host; and overall survival. For example, specific genetic polymorphisms have been associated with risk of CNS relapse; risk of persistent MRD; osteonecrosis; and susceptibility to obesity in female ALL survivors.[259–262] In addition to these studies which utilized the candidate-gene approach, genome-wide association studies are yielding unbiased, genome-wide analyses of single nucleotide polymorphisms that correlate with drug metabolism and response to therapy.[3,127]

CLINICAL PRESENTATION

The presenting signs and symptoms of a child with ALL reflect the impact of bone marrow infiltration with leukemic cells and the extent of extramedullary disease spread. The typical symptoms and clinical findings (Table 19.7) are manifestations of the underlying anemia, thrombocytopenia, and neutropenia, which in turn reflect the failure of normal hematopoiesis. Pallor, fatigue, bone pain, petechiae, purpura, bleeding, and fever are commonly present. Lymphadenopathy, hepatomegaly, and splenomegaly are frequent manifestations of extramedullary leukemic spread. Hepatosplenomegaly occurs in approximately two thirds of the patients and is usually asymptomatic. Lymphadenopathy, usually painless, may be localized or generalized.

The duration of symptoms in children presenting with ALL may vary from days to months. Anorexia is common, but significant weight loss is infrequent. Bone pain, particularly affecting the long bones, is common and reflects leukemic involvement of the periosteum and bone. Young children may present with a limp or refusal to walk. Bone tenderness is frequently observed. These symptoms and the presence of arthralgias, resulting from leukemic infiltration of a joint, may make the delineation between ALL and nonmalignant disorders (e.g., juvenile rheumatoid arthritis [JRA] or osteomyelitis) difficult.[1,2,262]

TABLE 19.7

CLINICAL AND LABORATORY FEATURES AT DIAGNOSIS IN CHILDREN WITH ACUTE LYMPHOBLASTIC LEUKEMIA

Clinical and laboratory features	Percentage of patients
Symptoms and Physical Findings	
Fever	61
Bleeding (e.g., petechiae or purpura)	48
Bone pain	23
Lymphadenopathy	50
Splenomegaly	63
Hepatosplenomegaly	68
Laboratory Features	
Leukocyte count (mm³)	
<10,000	53
10,000–49,000	30
>50,000	17
Hemoglobin (g/dL)	
<7.0	43
7.0–11.0	45
>11.0	12
Platelet count (mm³)	
<20,000	28
20,000–99,000	47
>100,000	25
Lymphoblast morphology	
L1	84
L2	15
L3	1

TABLE 19.8

DIFFERENTIAL DIAGNOSIS IN CHILDHOOD ACUTE LYMPHOBLASTIC LEUKEMIA

Nonmalignant conditions
  Juvenile rheumatoid arthritis
  Infectious mononucleosis
  Idiopathic thrombocytopenic purpura
  Pertussis; parapertussis
  Aplastic anemia
  Acute infectious lymphocytosis
Malignancies
  Neuroblastoma
  Retinoblastoma
  Rhabdomyosarcoma
Unusual presentations
  Hypereosinophilic syndrome

T-cell ALL represents approximately 15% of ALL cases and is noted for its distinctive clinical features. It frequently occurs in older boys, who present with high initial leukocyte counts and commonly have a mediastinal mass. Approximately one half of children with T-cell ALL have mediastinal masses, and one third to one half have initial leukocyte counts greater than 100,000/mm³.[264,265] Patients with T-cell leukemia also have a higher incidence of CNS leukemia at diagnosis (10% to 15%).[265,266]

Even when there is involvement, signs or symptoms of CNS involvement are rarely observed at the time of the initial diagnosis. A number of presenting clinical features and laboratory findings have prognostic importance. These are elaborated in the sections on prognostic factors and treatment.

The child with ALL typically presents with nonspecific symptoms. Thus, ALL may mimic a variety of other nonmalignant (Table 19.8), as well as malignant conditions. These include infectious mononucleosis, idiopathic thrombocytopenic purpura, acute infectious lymphocytosis, JRA, pertussis and parapertussis, and certain viral illnesses (i.e., cytomegalovirus and EBV infections), all of which may have similar clinical features. Childhood ALL must be differentiated from other pediatric malignancies that may present with bone marrow involvement, including particularly neuroblastoma, and non-Hodgkin lymphoma. Under light microscopy, neuroblastoma may be difficult to differentiate morphologically from ALL, especially if typical neuroblastoma pseudorosettes are not present. Additional laboratory and clinical evaluation can differentiate these two disorders.

Rarely, ALL patients present with signs and symptoms of unusual extramedullary site involvement (i.e., ocular, urinary bladder, pancreas) or uncommon endocrinologic manifestations.[267,268] The involvement of such unusual extramedullary sites usually occurs in relapsed or refractory patients, but the presence of such involvement at diagnosis is possible. Symptomatic signs of hypercalcemia—lethargy, anorexia, muscle weakness, nausea, vomiting, and constipation—have been described in scattered cases.[269,270] Hypercalcemic presentations with and without bone pain have been described, and many of the ALL patients presenting with hypercalcemia will have normal or near-normal peripheral blood counts.[269]

Bone pain can be severe and is often associated with close to normal peripheral blood counts.[271] This finding may contribute to delay in the diagnosis of these patients (18% to 23% of patients). Bone pain with or without hypercalcemia is one of the factors that can mislead a physician into treating the patient with steroids (usually for suspected JRA). A careful physical examination can help distinguish joint from bone pain, and plain x-ray films or magnetic resonance imaging (MRI) can be helpful. The observation of "leukemic lines" on plain radiographs or evidence of T2-weighted changes in the bone marrow on MRI warrants a diagnostic bone marrow aspirate.[270]

Clinicians must also consider ALL among the differential diagnosis of the rare patients who present with hypereosinophilia. Cases of ALL occurring in association with symptomatic hypereosinophilia have been reported, and in rare instances, eosinophilia has preceded the diagnosis of ALL by many months.[272] In symptomatic patients with eosinophilia, the classic findings of the hypereosinophilic syndrome (i.e., Loeffler's syndrome of hypereosinophilia, pulmonary infiltrates, cardiomegaly, and congestive failure) have been observed. The pathogenesis of ALL occurring with hypereosinophilia is not fully defined, but a characteristic translocation, t(5;14), is associated with this syndrome.[210] ALL presenting with hypereosinophilia must be differentiated from eosinophilic myeloid leukemia (FAB M4Eo, see Chapter 20), which has a characteristic chromsomal abnormality involving inversion of chromosome 16.[273]

Leukemia or Lymphoma?

ALL and childhood non-Hodgkin lymphoma are closely related disorders, and distinguishing between the two may be difficult. Many patients who present with features characteristic of a lymphoma, such as an anterior mediastinal mass, massive lymphadenopathy, or both, may have bone marrow involvement. The malignant T cells of lymphoblastic lymphoma are indistinguishable from those of T-cell ALL, and the malignant B cells of Burkitt's lymphoma are similar to those from children with B-cell ALL. As previously discussed, B-cell ALL shares immunologic and molecular genetic features of Burkitt's lymphoma and is considered to be a disseminated form of that disease. Most institutions treat patients with advanced B-cell disorders with similar chemotherapy regimens.

The distinction between T-cell ALL and T-cell lymphoblastic lymphoma is also ill-defined. There is some evidence that these disorders arise from different stages of T-cell differentiation and consequently have immunophenotypes reflecting different stages of T-cell maturation.[107] Because this distinction does not occur in every case, it does not provide a reliable basis for delineating between the two diseases. In the absence of more refined biologic criteria, the percentage of blasts in the bone marrow is conventionally used to differentiate between T-cell ALL and T-cell non-Hodgkin lymphoma. This arbitrary method is confounded by the fact that different institutions and study groups use different criteria. For some, more than 25% blast cells in a bone marrow establishes the diagnosis of leukemia; for others, any evidence of abnormal bone marrow infiltration, regardless of percentage, is used to define leukemia. Because of these differences, meaningful comparisons of treatment results obtained by different groups can be difficult.

Hematologic Abnormalities at Presentation

An elevated leukocyte count (>10,000/mm³) occurs in approximately one half of patients with ALL. In approximately 20% of patients, the initial leukocyte count is greater than 50,000/mm³ (Table 19.7). The degree of leukocyte count elevation at diagnosis remains one of the most important predictors of prognosis in ALL.[11] Neutropenia (<500 granulo-

cytes per mm³) is a common phenomenon and is associated with an increased risk of serious infection.[274] Anemia (hemoglobin <10 g/dL) exists in approximately 80% of patients at diagnosis. Even if the anemia is severe, the erythrocytes usually manifest a normocytic, normochromic pattern and the reticulocyte count is low. Thrombocytopenia occurs in most patients; approximately 75% have fewer than 100,000 platelets per mm³. Isolated thrombocytopenia, however, is a rare event. The severity and the degree of bleeding correlate with the degree of thrombocytopenia.[275] Severe hemorrhage is rare even with platelet counts less than 20,000/mm³, unless fever and infection (both of which can affect platelet survival and function) are present.[275]

Rarely, ALL may initially manifest with pancytopenia and must be differentiated from aplastic anemia.[276,277] An aplastic presentation may represent a true preleukemic state.[277] Another explanation is that there is inhibition of normal hematopoietic progenitors by leukemic cells, causing a period of aplasia, which is followed by a definitive diagnosis of ALL.[278]

To definitively establish the diagnosis of leukemia, a bone marrow aspirate is generally necessary. Although leukemia cells may be present in the peripheral blood at diagnosis, attempts to establish the diagnosis on the basis of morphologic assessment of these cells alone may be misleading. Under most circumstances, a bone marrow aspirate provides sufficient material to establish the diagnosis. Occasionally, bone marrow biopsy may be required. A small subset of patients with leukocytosis may not be candidates for bone marrow aspiration, and the diagnosis may be established using peripheral blood. Although more than 5% lymphoblasts in the bone marrow is highly suggestive of leukemia, a minimum of 25% blast cells is required by the standard hematopathology criteria before the diagnosis is confirmed.[92,93,279] Usually, most cells in the marrow aspirate are leukemic lymphoblasts. In some situations (e.g., in preleukemic states or to differentiate an aplastic presentation of ALL from aplastic anemia) multiple bone marrow aspirates and biopsy specimens may be required.

Definitive diagnosis of the specific leukemic cell type has classically been made by morphologic assessment of bone marrow aspirate slides stained with Romanovsky dye and by the use of special histochemical stains (e.g., PAS, myeloperoxidase, Sudan black), which are helpful in differentiating ALL from AML (Table 19.3). TdT analysis may also contribute important diagnostic information. However at present, few if any centers rely solely on morphologic or cytochemical information to make the diagnosis of ALL. Most routinely employ immunophenotyping, using a panel of monoclonal antibodies (Table 19.4), and cytogenetic studies. Both traditional karyotyping and the use of molecular cytogenetic technologies (i.e., RT-PCR, FISH, and increasingly microarray-based methods) are used for identification of chromosomal features. In a few cases, ultrastructural evaluation (i.e., by electron microscopy) may be helpful.[92,279]

Related Abnormal Laboratory Findings

A variety of other abnormal laboratory study results are frequently seen in newly diagnosed patients with ALL. Many of these findings and their degree of abnormality reflect the leukemic cell burden, the extent of extramedullary spread, or the excessive proliferation and destruction of the leukemic cells. Increased serum uric acid levels, most common in patients with a large leukemic cell burden, reflect increased anabolism and catabolism of purines. A major complication of hyperuricemia is uric acid nephropathy and subsequent renal failure. The risk of this complication is greatest immediately after initiation of treatment, when leukemic cell lysis releases large quantities of uric acid. Adequate hydration, alkalinization, and the use of the xanthine oxidase inhibitor allopurinol have traditionally been required to prevent this potentially serious complication. Alternatively, the high uric acid level can be ameliorated with simple hydration and the therapeutic use of recombinant urate oxidase.[280] Use of this highly effective agent has become much more common, particularly during induction in patients with large tumor burdens. The only significant side effect of urate oxidase is an approximately 5% incidence of acute hypersensitivity reactions.[280]

Various metabolic abnormalities may be encountered, including decreased and increased serum levels of calcium and increased levels of potassium and phosphorus. Renal stones (both of the $CaPO_4$ and precipitated uric acid types) may occur and are principally treated with hydration. These abnormalities are more frequent in patients with bulky extramedullary disease (i.e., extensive lymphadenopathy, hepatosplenomegaly) and high initial leukocyte counts.[281] Kidneys may be infiltrated with leukemic cells and are often enlarged at diagnosis.[282] Although kidney infiltration and dysfunction can complicate the initial therapy, it does not usually affect outcome.[283] Hypercalcemia may result from leukemic infiltration of bone. Although the mechanism(s) of this phenomenon are not entirely clear, the release of a parathormone-like substance from lymphoblasts has been reported.[284] Elevated serum phosphorus levels can occur as a result of leukemic cell lysis and may induce hypocalcemia.

Hepatic dysfunction resulting from leukemic infiltration of the liver is usually mild regardless of the degree of hepatomegaly. Leukemic cell lysis, ineffective hematopoiesis, and liver involvement are associated with elevation of serum LDH. Approximately 5% to 10% of newly diagnosed patients, usually those with T-cell ALL, have an anterior mediastinal mass detected on chest radiographs.

Skeletal changes, particularly in the long bones, are common and include transverse radiolucent metaphyseal growth arrest lines, periosteal elevation with reactive subperiosteal cortical thickening, osteolytic lesions, and diffuse osteoporosis.[285] Such radiologically documented bone changes may be seen in asymptomatic patients. When present, bone pain usually resolves quickly after initiation of antileukemic therapy. Rarely, ALL may masquerade as osteomyelitis.[286]

Coagulation abnormalities may occur but are usually not a feature of the disease, and at presentation, disseminated intravascular coagulation is encountered infrequently.[287] When coagulopathies occur at diagnosis or early in therapy, they are usually associated with concomitant infection, or with therapy (e.g., L-asparaginase) rather than with the leukemia itself.[288] Both *Escherichia coli* and *Erwinia* L-asparaginase may produce thromboses and/or hemorrhagic infarction.[289]

Patterns of Spread

Extramedullary involvement may be readily detectable clinically or demonstrable solely by diagnostic tests and procedures. Extramedullary disease is significant because it may cause morbidity at a localized site, and it often represents a significant percentage of the total body leukemia burden. Many patients have some evidence of extramedullary involvement at diagnosis (Table 19.7). The most common sites of extramedullary spread are the CNS, testes, liver, kidneys, lymph nodes, and spleen. However, virtually any site in the body can become involved either at initial presentation or relapse (e.g., skin, the ocular anterior chamber, pleural and pericardial spaces, and ovarian involvement have all been described).[290] From a clinical point of view, the two most important sites of extramedullary involvement are the CNS and the testes.

Central Nervous System Leukemia

CNS leukemia is found at diagnosis of fewer than 5% of children with ALL.[291] With the institution of CNS preventive therapy, routine lumbar punctures (LPs) with intrathecal therapy have become an integral part of ALL treatment protocols. As a consequence, symptomatic CNS relapse is observed less frequently, and the diagnosis is most often made in the presymptomatic patient. Diagnosis of CNS leukemia requires cytologic confirmation of leukemic cells in the cerebrospinal fluid (CSF). CSF obtained by LP must be examined after cytocentrifugation, a procedure that concentrates the leukemic cells and increases diagnostic sensitivity. Leukemic cells found in the CSF are usually cytogenetically identical to those found in the bone marrow. In symptomatic patients, CSF pressure is usually increased, and elevated CSF protein and hypoglycorrhachia are common. With CNS leukemia now more frequently diagnosed in the asymptomatic patient, CSF pressure may be normal, CSF leukemic cell counts relatively low, and abnormalities in CSF chemistry determinations absent.

In the absence of significant pleocytosis, the diagnosis of meningeal leukemia is problematic.[292] Controversy exists about the meaning of blast cells in situations in which the total CSF WBC count is low, such as fewer than 5 WBCs per mm^3 with blast cells. This clinical finding is identified in as many as 19% of patients at initial presentation, and has been associated with a significantly higher likelihood of CNS relapse when compared with patients without detectable CSF lymphoblasts.[293] However, other investigators have been unable to confirm this finding.[294,295] In an effort to evaluate the importance of low WBC count, lymphoblast-positive, initial CSF samples, NCI-sponsored studies are prospectively gathering data on these patients.[296] The consensus criteria for grading CNS involvement at diagnosis are outlined in Table 19.9.[296] CNS-1 status is defined as no evidence of leukemic lymphoblasts in the CSF. CNS-2 and CNS-3 are respectively defined as less than 5 WBC per mm^3 and $\geq$5 WBC per mm^3 (or with cranial nerve palsy) and blasts on CSF cytospin preparations. In suspicious but equivocal cases, TdT determination is an additional means of confirming the diagnosis of CNS leukemia.[297] The results of cranial computed tomographic (CT) scans, electroencephalography, plain skull radiographs, and MRI may be abnormal for those with CNS leukemia but are frequently normal. None of these imaging methods has sufficient diagnostic sensitivity to be indicated for routine use, but should be employed as symptoms clinically indicate.

The NCI-derived criteria for grading CNS involvement at diagnosis originally assumed cell counts that were not affected by the LP procedure. In recent years, it has become apparent that "bloody" taps or contamination of CSF with peripheral

TABLE 19.9

DEFINITIONS OF CENTRAL NERVOUS SYSTEM (CNS) DISEASE STATUS AT DIAGNOSIS BASED ON CEREBROSPINAL FLUID FINDINGS

Status	Cerebrospinal fluid findings
CNS-1	No lymphoblasts
CNS-2	<5 WBCs/μL with definable blasts on cytocentrifuge examination
CNS-3	≥5 WBCs/μL with blast cells (or cranial nerve palsy)

WBC, white blood cell.

blood elements (which do include leukemic blasts in newly diagnosed patients) may pose a serious risk of later CNS disease and relapse.[298,299] This problem can be partially ameliorated by reducing the numbers of LPs early in therapy and by having them performed by experienced practitioners.[298,299] Effective sedation/anesthesia, adequate platelet counts, and normal coagulation panels help reduce the chance of a traumatic/bloody LP.

CNS leukemia may result from hematogenous spread of circulating leukemia cells or by direct extension from involved cranial bone marrow.[300] Hematogenous spread may occur by means of migration of circulating leukemia cells through venous endothelium or as a consequence of petechial hemorrhages in cases of severe thrombocytopenia. The choroid plexus, with its abundant capillaries, is often a site of leukemic infiltration. Direct extension of leukemia cells may occur from involved cranial bone marrow through bridging veins to the superficial arachnoid. Eventually, infiltration of the deep arachnoid, the pia glial membrane, and the brain parenchyma itself may occur. Direct spread from involved cranial bone marrow may also occur along the perineurium.

The signs and symptoms of clinically overt CNS leukemia include headache, nausea and vomiting, lethargy, irritability, nuchal rigidity, papilledema, and other manifestations of increased intracranial pressure. Cranial nerve involvement, most frequently involving the seventh, third, fourth, and sixth cranial nerves, may occur with other symptoms or as an isolated event. Infiltration of the optic nerve can result in visual disturbances. Eighth cranial nerve involvement, manifested by hyperacusis, tinnitus, vertigo, and even deafness, has been observed. A more unusual manifestation of CNS leukemia is the hypothalamic-obesity syndrome, in which destruction of the ventromedial nucleus of the hypothalamus, the satiety center, results in hyperphagia, pathologic weight gain, and diabetes insipidus. Leukemic subdural involvement and spinal epidural leukemia with spinal cord compression also have been observed. Intracranial leukemic cell masses occur relatively rarely. The numerous neurologic manifestations of overt CNS leukemia make it obligatory for clinicians to exhaustively investigate any neurologic signs or symptoms in the child with ALL to exclude the possibility of CNS leukemia.

The potential clinical impact of CNS leukemia did not become fully apparent until the late 1950s and early 1960s. With improved systemic therapy and longer survival, the CNS became the most common site of initial relapse.[301] Initial bone marrow remissions of short duration could be obtained in most patients, but CNS recurrence was common.[302] The significance of this increasing rate of CNS relapse was two-fold. First, CNS leukemia itself was difficult to eradicate. Second, CNS relapse was usually followed by the rapid development of bone marrow disease.[303] Most patients who experienced a CNS relapse during the era before CNS preventive therapy died as a consequence of marrow relapse rather than of CNS disease. The recognition of this phenomenon led to the development of effective CNS preventive therapy, an applied strategy that contributed significantly to improving the prognosis of children with ALL. Unfortunately, the successful prevention of CNS relapse has come at the price of neurologic toxicities, acute and chronic, which have become more apparent with time as larger numbers of these children have survived.

Testicular Leukemia

Clinically demonstrable testicular disease is rarely present at initial diagnosis, but occult testicular disease can be diagnosed by biopsy in 25% of newly diagnosed boys.[304] The possibility of occult testicular disease, together with the fact that testicular recurrence is frequently followed by systemic relapse, prompted several centers to advocate routine bilateral testicular biopsy at some time during maintenance chemotherapy or immediately before its cessation. This practice has been questioned because of studies indicating that testicular biopsies at diagnosis, after induction, during maintenance, or before cessation of chemotherapy are associated with a significant false-negative rate and do not accurately predict for eventual testicular relapse.[305-307] Routine testicular biopsies at the end of therapy for detection of occult disease are no longer recommended. Noninvasive screening for occult testicular disease using trans-scrotal ultrasound and MRI has been evaluated; neither technique is sufficiently sensitive.[308]

Clinically, overt testicular involvement usually appears as painless testicular enlargement, most often unilateral. The diagnosis must be established by testicular biopsy. When testicular leukemia is suspected clinically, bilateral biopsies are indicated because disease frequently affects the contralateral testis.[309] Wedge biopsies are the preferred diagnostic technique, because this procedure is less likely to result in sampling error. Histologic interpretation is frequently difficult. The incidence of false-negative results from testicular biopsies obtained during maintenance therapy or before stopping all treatment approaches 10%.[306,310] Although it has been suggested that TdT determination may help discriminate between leukemic lymphoblasts and reactive lymphocytes in equivocal biopsy specimens, the value of TdT determination appears to be limited.[311] Immunophenotyping of testicular biopsy specimens may help confirm leukemia cells, but it has not been demonstrated to improve the overall detection rate.[312]

Before the introduction of effective chemotherapy for ALL, clinically evident testicular relapse was a rare event. Paradoxically, with improved therapy and prolonged survival, the incidence of testicular involvement increased. In the 1970s and 1980s, the incidence of overt testicular relapse at some time during the disease course was reported to be as high as 16%, although the actual figure was probably less than 10%.[313] In boys who had successfully completed a full course of chemotherapy for their disease, overt testicular recurrence was a principal cause of relapse during the later phases of therapy and the first 2 years off therapy.[309] The reported incidence in this setting varied but was approximately 10%.[314] With the introduction of more intensive therapies, the incidence of testicular relapse has declined toward 5%.[315] The incidence of testicular relapse after BMT performed after a chemotherapy preparative regimen with or without total body irradiation (TBI) with a testicular "boost" dose is similarly lower than 4%.[316]

The occurrence of isolated testicular relapse led many investigators to consider the testes to be a sanctuary site for extramedullary disease. It has been suggested that leukemic testes are protected from therapeutic concentrations of systemically administered chemotherapy by the blood–testes barrier.[317] Animal studies, however, have questioned the role of the blood-testes barrier in the development of testicular leukemia.[318] The leukemia often can be demonstrated in the liver, spleen, and abdominal lymph nodes in patients studied by exploratory laparotomy at the time of a presumed isolated testicular relapse.[319] This raises the possibility that the term "isolated" testicular relapse may be a misnomer.

In testicular relapse, the disease is usually located within the interstitial spaces; in advanced cases, leukemic infiltration of the tubules may occur.[320] Several factors have been associated with an increased likelihood of developing testicular relapse, including a high initial leukocyte count (>20,000/mm³), T-cell disease, prominent lymphadenopathy, splenomegaly, and significant

TABLE 19.10

FACTORS ASSOCIATED WITH PROGNOSIS FOR PATIENTS WITH ACUTE LYMPHOBLASTIC LEUKEMIA

Initial white blood cell count
Sex
Rapidity of leukemic cytoreduction
Cytogenetics/ploidy
Immunologic subtype
French-American-British morphology
Mediastinal mass
Organomegaly and lymphadenopathy
Hemoglobin level
Race
Platelet count
Serum immunoglobulins
Myeloid antigen expression on leukemic cells
Nutritional status

thrombocytopenia (<30,000/mm³).[320] The time to development of overt testicular relapse ranges from 2 months to several years but has become less of a problem with the modern intensification of therapy. In fact, these data on testicular relapse were all collected during a time when systemic therapy was significantly less effective than what is now available, rendering the prediction of testicular relapse in the current context difficult. However, from the historical data it can be seen that testicular relapse, when it does occur, should be taken as a sign that the systemic control of the disease has also failed.

PROGNOSTIC FACTORS

Certain clinical and laboratory features exhibited at diagnosis as well as rate of early response to induction therapy have prognostic value. The identification of such factors has become essential in the design and analysis of modern therapeutic trials. It is common practice to assign patients on the basis of prognostic factors into different risk groups and to tailor treatment accordingly. Prognostic characteristics of childhood ALL have included (Table 19.10): the initial leukocyte count, age at diagnosis, sex, race, degree of organomegaly and lymphadenopathy, presence of a mediastinal mass, initial hemoglobin level, initial platelet count, FAB morphologic classification, cytogenetics, immunophenotype, expression of myeloid antigens on leukemic cells, serum immunoglobulin levels, CNS disease at diagnosis, the length of time to attainment of remission, rapid versus slow response to induction therapy, glucocorticoid receptor levels, and HLA type and nutritional status.[13,97,321]

Because they are readily available and relatively independent predictors of prognosis, the parameters of initial leukocyte count and age at diagnosis have traditionally provided the most reliable basis for patient stratification. The relative value of other clinical and laboratory features as prognostic indicators varies. To a certain extent, intensity of therapy has become an important prognostic factor. As modern therapy for ALL has become more intensive as well as more successful, many clinical and laboratory features that were once important prognostic features have lost statistical significance after appropriate multivariate analysis. Differences in treatment approaches between large cooperative groups have resulted in differences in published, statistically significant, prognostic factors and emphasizes the importance of the treatment regimen itself as an important variable influencing outcome. To facilitate comparisons among the results from different groups, an NCI workshop developed a set of consensus prognostic factors for age and WBC count outlined in Table 19.11.[296] Although all of the groups remain free to stratify their patients into different risk-group directed therapy, there is now a strong commitment to record and report the common data so that the results of studies done on differing groups of patients can be more easily compared.

Leukocyte Count and Age

The initial WBC count and age are the two characteristics universally accepted as prognostic factors. In most cases, initial leukocyte count retains its importance after adjustment for other criteria. There is a linear relation between the initial leukocyte count and outcome in children with ALL; children with the highest leukocyte counts tend to have a poor prognosis.[13,322] These relationships have continued to be true despite the response improvements (see later) seen in specific subgroups and the general increase in treatment intensity over

TABLE 19.11

UNIFORM AGE AND WHITE BLOOD CELL COUNT CRITERIA FOR B-PRECURSOR ACUTE LYMPHOCYTIC LEUKEMIA STANDARD AND HIGH-RISK COHORTS AT THE CANCER TREATMENT AND EVALUATION PROGRAM/NATIONAL CANCER INSTITUTE WORKSHOP

Risk	Definition	4-year event-free survival (%)	Percentage of B-precursor patients
Standard	WBC count, <50,000/mL and age 1.00–9.99 yr	80.3	68
High	WBC count, ≥50,000/mL or age ≥10.00 yr	63.9	32

WBC, white blood cell.
Note: Table describes the event-free survival and percentages of patients with pediatric B-precursor acute lymphoblastic leukemia treated by the Pediatric Oncology Group (ALINC-14) and Children's Cancer Group (-100 and 1800 series) Protocols by the Uniform Age and WBC Count Criteria.
From Smith M, Arthur D, Camitta B, et al. Uniform approach to risk classification and treatment assignment for children with acute lymphoblastic leukemia. J Clin Oncol 1996;14:18, with permission.

the past several decades. Although there is no sharp dividing line, and the data are influenced by the specific therapy given, patients with an initial leukocyte count greater than 50,000 cells per mm³ (approximately 20% of children with ALL) are recognized as having poorer prognosis.[296] The biologic basis for higher initial leukocyte counts is unclear, although there are definite associations between certain biologic features and this pattern of presentation. Patients with T-cell ALL and infants with t(4;11) often have a high initial leukocyte count and increased lymphoblast proliferative activity.

There is also a relation between age at diagnosis and outcome. Similar to the WBC data, the difference is on a continuum. Patients who are younger at diagnosis (<1 to 2 years) and older patients (>9 to 10 years) have an inferior prognosis compared with children in the intermediate age group. The worst prognosis has traditionally been for infants with ALL who are younger than 1 year at diagnosis (see later and Chapter 15).[323,324] Adolescents with ALL also fare poorly, having a lower remission induction rate and EFS than younger children, excluding infants.[325] Adolescents tend to have a greater constellation of other poor-risk features including T-cell immunophenotype.[326] In the Dana Farber Cancer Institute (DFCI) 91–01 study, age was the only statistically significant prognostic factor.[327]

Historically, infants (i.e., younger than 12 months) with ALL have had a very poor prognosis (EFS <10% to 20%), worse than virtually any other subset of leukemia patients. They have an increased incidence of poor prognostic features, including high initial leukocyte count, massive organomegaly, thrombocytopenia, CNS leukemia involvement at diagnosis, and failure to clear peripheral blasts by Day 14 of induction therapy.[323] Although their complete remission rate appears to be no different than for older children, the EFS and disease-free survival for patients in this age group has been extremely poor due to early bone marrow and extramedullary relapse. The CNS relapse rate in infants is particularly high.

ALL of infancy appears to be biologically unique. The leukemic cells appear to arise from a very early stage of commitment to B-cell differentiation. They usually express the HLA-DR antigen, are CALLA (CD10) negative, and do not express mature B-cell antigens.[328] There is often a high level of myeloperoxidase gene expression. Although there are data regarding the immunoglobulin and TCR gene configuration in these patients suggesting that the ALL in infancy represents an earlier stage of B-cell development than found in the B-cell precursor ALL of older children, this finding has not been universal.[329,330] Infants with ALL also have an increased incidence of chromosomal abnormalities that are associated with a poor prognosis (Figs. 19.11 and 19.12, and the section "cytogenetics"). Structural abnormalities of chromosome 11, particularly rearrangement of band 11q23 within the MLL/ALL-1 gene, are frequently observed. The t(4;11) abnormality is particularly common. In addition to myeloperoxidase, the leukemic cells from infants with ALL frequently express other myeloid markers (e.g., CD15 positive), suggesting that in many infants the leukemia arises in a multipotent precursor cell.[331,332] Leukemic blasts from t(4;11)⁺ infants have been shown to have a unique gene expression profile when analyzed by microarray.[130,221] Infants with rearrangement of 11q23/MLL have a particularly poor prognosis (Fig. 19.15). Because of their poor prognosis, infants are stratified separately from other early pre-B ALL patients for treatment. Modest increases in EFS for infants (which still average EFS 17% to 40% in most studies) have been achieved by significantly increasing the dose intensity of the regimens used to treat them.[324,333,334] It has been suggested that there may be chemoresponsive subgroups of infants (similar to BFM approaches with older children) with ALL that can be determined on the basis of initial prednisone responsiveness.[335]

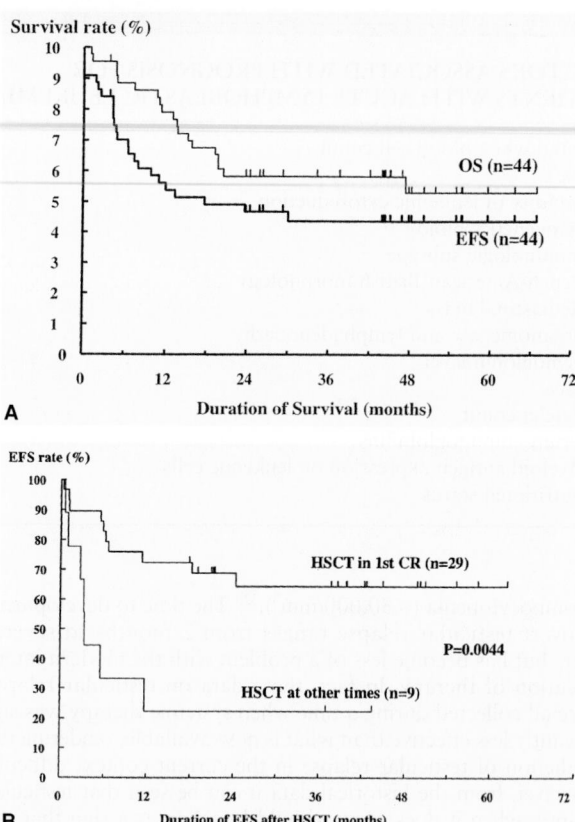

FIGURE 19.15 A: Overall survival (OS) and B: event-free survival (EFS) rates for 44 infants with MLL-positive ALL. The tick marks represent patients still at risk of death or other adverse events. (From Kosaka Y, Koh K, Kinukawa N, et al. Infant acute lymphoblastic leukemia with MLL gene rearrangements: outcome following intensive chemotherapy and hematopoietic stem cell transplantation. Blood 2004;104:3527–3534, with permission.)

Results of a recent study using intensive induction/consolidation followed by hematopoietic stem cell transplant (HSCT) has shown promising results for the treatment of t(4;11) infant ALL (Fig. 19.15).[324] High FLT3 expression is associated with MLL rearrangement, and has provided an opportunity for the introduction of FLT3 inhibitors for treatment of infant MLL-rearranged ALL, a novel targeted therapeutic approach which is sorely needed in this group.[219]

Cytogenetic Factors

As discussed in Cytogenetic Classification above, cytogenetic abnormalities in chromosomal number and structure are common in pediatric ALL (see section on Molecular Pathogenesis) and some have prognostic significance. One interesting association between cytogenetic status and treatment response involves the metabolism of methotrexate (MTX). Hyperdiploid lymphoblasts accumulate increased amounts of MTX and MTX polyglutamates, and they have higher basal apoptotic rates compared with leukemic cells with lower ploidy and normal cells.[336,337] These characteristics may contribute to the better outcomes observed for patients with hyperdiploid lymphoblasts. The prognostic significance of both ploidy and structural cytogenetic changes are presented with the specific associated cytogenetic findings discussed previously and in Figures 19.8, 19.9, 19.10, 19.12, and 19.14.

Sex

The prognostic importance of gender has been well documented (see also section "Epidemiology") and persists on modern chemotherapy protocols.[338,339] In most studies, girls have a better prognosis than boys. Although, this may be partially due to the risk of testicular relapse, the higher incidence of T-cell disease in boys, and the lower incidence of favorable DNA index in boys versus girls (17.8% vs. 25.1%), there are likely to be other genetic, metabolic, and endocrine effects that contribute to this difference.[339]

Immunophenotype

The prognostic implications of the common B- and T-cell immunophenotypes are discussed in the pathobiology section. In the analyses of current therapies immunophenotype is frequently not an independent prognostic variable.[202] Immunophenotype determined directly by FACS analysis or indirectly by RNA/cDNA expression arrays is strongly correlated with the cytogenetic and emerging gene expression groupings that appear to be the most important for determining response on current therapies.[125,128,130,340] CD10 negativity, however, retains prognostic value. Immunophenotype remains important in current classification schemes; however, it may assert increasing importance in the future as more immunospecific therapies are developed.[341,342]

Race

The effect of race on prognosis has been a controversial topic. Although older studies reported significantly poorer outcomes in black versus white patients, several studies in the late 1980s and early 1990s, reported equivalent results when patients had been carefully stratified for risk group at diagnosis.[8–10] Originally, the differences seen between black and white racial groups was attributed to socioeconomic factors. However, newer studies that account for some of these variables have recently demonstrated, small but statistically significant, poorer outcomes for black and other minority children in specific subgroups when compared to white children.[11] These differences vary between studies, and, like many prognostic factors, change with the actual treatment protocols applied.

A study using SEER epidemiologic data on 4,952 ALL patients suggested that black, Hispanic, and American Indian/Alaskan Native children have a worse outcome than whites or Asian/Pacific Islanders.[11] An analysis of the differences between black and white patients revealed that, at least for these two groups, the main differences in outcomes was in the 1- to 9-year-old age group. Essentially equivalent results were observed in the higher risk younger-than-1-year and older-than-10-year categories in which the overall prognosis is poorer.[11] These children were treated on a variety of different protocols. Large CCG and POG studies examining this issue provide data on 8,447 and 5,086 patients diagnosed and treated from the early 1980s to mid-1990s and show continued inferior outcomes for black versus white patients, but these differences have greatly diminished as outcomes have improved for all groups (Fig. 19.3).[8,9]

Data for other ethnic groups have been limited. One report showed a surprisingly good outcome (90.9% EFS) for high-risk Asian children treated in several Children's Cancer Study Group (CCSG) trials.[9] Further study is required both to confirm this finding and to explore its biologic basis. With the newer information concerning pharmacogenomics (see later), it is not surprising that race and ethnicity may have specific impact on both the incidence and the outcomes of therapy.

Leukemic Cell Burden

Leukemic cell burden can be assessed indirectly by evaluation of the extent of extramedullary disease. The degree of hepatosplenomegaly and lymphadenopathy at patient presentation, have emerged in many univariate analyses as important prognostic variables. Although, in some studies, multivariate analyses reveal that some of these features, such as presence of a mediastinal mass, may tend to be dependent variables, other features such as the initial leukocyte count retain significance even after adjustment for other independent variables. The BFM study group has used a measurement of hepatosplenomegaly combined with the initial leukocyte count to compute a "risk factor index," which forms (along with response to initial glucocorticoids therapy) part of the basis for subsequent treatment stratification.[343]

Response to Treatment

Rapidity of response to treatment is a very important indicator of prognosis. It is established that patients who do not achieve a complete remission within the usual 4- to 6-week induction period have a high rate of relapse and shortened survival.[344] Multiple groups have shown the prognostic importance of the rapidity of clearance of blasts (in peripheral blood and bone marrow) during induction therapy.[1] Residual leukemia demonstrable in bone marrow on day 14 of induction is an independent predictor of inferior outcome.[345,346] Patients with residual disease in their bone marrow on day 14 have a lower rate of complete remission and a greater likelihood of early (within the first 24 months of therapy) and late relapse.[347] Day 7 marrow status has also been correlated with treatment outcome.[348] Patients who have an intermediate marrow response to initial chemotherapy (i.e., M1, <5% blasts by day 14) do less well than but have a superior EFS compared with slow responders (i.e., M1 status by day 28).[349] Rapid early responders (i.e., those with an M1 marrow on day 7) have the best EFS (Fig. 19.16). Similar early responses in infants may not have the same prognostic implication.[350] Others have reported that the failure to clear peripheral leukemic blasts by day 8 of therapy correlates significantly with a poorer 5-year EFS.[351]

In recent years, using a variety of technologies it has become possible to quantify and track the presence of small amounts of residual leukemia (see section "Minimal Residual Disease") in bone marrow, peripheral blood, and CSF.[352] The availability of sensitive molecular methods is prompting a redefinition of remission status. In this context, the definition of rapid early and late responses are also being reexamined in a variety of ongoing and planned clinical trials.[84] Generally, the faster a patient is rendered MRD negative, the better the prognosis. MRD levels that are undetectable or at least less than 10^{-4} at the end of a standard induction (or preferably earlier) are associated with the best prognosis.[353,354]

Interestingly, some recent data suggest that in addition to quantification of leukemia cell response to therapy, the measure of host absolute lymphocyte count (ALC) during induction may also have prognostic impact. Lower ALC during induction has been shown to have independent prognostic impact, predicting poorer relapse-free and overall survival.[355] This association suggests that host immune status may play an important role in disease control and ultimate outcome.

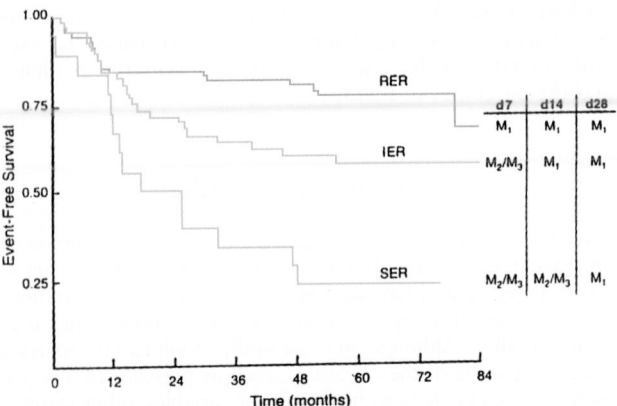

FIGURE 19.16 Event-free survival (EFS) and rapidity of cytoreduction during induction treatment. Rapid early responders (RER), those whose bone marrow aspirate was rated M1 by day 7, have the best EFS. Patients who are M2 or M3 on day 7 can be separated by their day 14 marrow results into an intermediate response group (IER) (M1 on day 14) and a slow early response (SER) group. (From Steinherz PG, Gaynon PS, Breneman JC, et al. Cytoreduction and prognosis in acute lymphoblastic leukemia—the importance of early marrow response: report from the Children's Cancer Group. J Clin Oncol 1996;14:389–398, with permission.)

Nutritional Status

Some studies have suggested that nutritional status is a significant prognostic factor.[356–358] Undernutrition, defined as both height and weight for age below two standard deviations, has been described as a significant predictor of treatment failure.[359,360] In one study, in which weight for age was used to define under-nutrition, more than a three-fold higher 5-year disease-free survival was observed in well-nourished children.[360] The difficulty of using nutritional status as a prognostic factor is that it is rarely independent from other issues related to socioeconomic and even racial status.[361,362] To avoid known problems with assessing nutritional status with variation in weight for age or weight for age tables, it has been suggested that arm circumferences and tricep skin fold thickness may be the best way to assess nutritional status at diagnosis.[361] This may be may be more relevant for the developing world setting since undernutrition (not frank malnutrition) is a more common problem in the developed world.[356,357] It has also been reported that children who were undernourished have less tolerance for chemotherapy and received suboptimal doses.[363] One report from the developing world observed that patients with normal nutritional status at diagnosis who can be maintained above the third percentile for weight will do as well as their better nourished counterparts on similarly intensive treatment.[364] Additional studies to define the prognostic role of nutritional status and effective nutritional interventions during therapy are needed.

TREATMENT

The recognition that ALL is a heterogeneous disease and that children can be stratified into various risk groups has profoundly influenced therapy. Although combination chemotherapy remains the primary therapeutic modality, it is no longer considered appropriate, in the context of current biologic knowledge, for all patients with ALL to be treated on a single treatment regimen. The initial evaluation of the patient with ALL requires sophisticated laboratory techniques to derive appropriate cytogenetic, immunologic, or molecular information. As our understanding of the disease has improved,

the approach to its treatment has become more complex. This circumstance, coupled with the increased intensity of many current treatment regimens, emphasizes the need for children with ALL to be evaluated and managed at established pediatric cancer centers where state-of-the-art treatment protocols are available.[365] Although the specific approaches to patients in various risk groups and the terminology describing the phases of therapy may vary between clinical trials, modern ALL treatment regimens divide therapy into four to five main treatment elements: remission induction, CNS preventive therapy/consolidation, delayed intensification (sometimes divided into reinduction and reconsolidation phases), and maintenance (sometimes labeled as continuation) therapy.

Induction Therapy

The aim of initial ALL treatment is induction of remission. By the standard definition, patients in remission have no evidence of leukemia when evaluated by physical examination and hematologic assessment (light microscopy) of bone marrow and peripheral blood. Peripheral blood values must be within the defined range of normality, and the bone marrow must be of normal cellularity, with fewer than 5% lymphoblasts.[84] Complete remission status also assumes the absence of detectable CNS or extramedullary disease by traditional light microscopy on CSF and physical examination findings. Achievement of a traditionally defined remission is a basic premise of antileukemic treatment and a known prerequisite for prolonged survival.[366] Contemporary treatment regimens include some assessment of MRD often during the Induction period (usually on Day 8 or 15), and at the end of Induction (Day 29–36). In clinically overt ALL, the leukemic cell burden is estimated to be approximately 10^{12} leukemic cells (Fig. 19.17).[367] To induce a complete remission, chemotherapy must reduce the total number of leukemic cells by 99%, leaving fewer than 10^{10} blasts.[368] In actual fact, most patients who undergo a successful remission induction have their total body leukemia burden reduced even further.[84] As noted previously, the rapidity of this response (i.e., by day 7 to 14 vs. day 28) as well as the total reduction in leukemic cell burden are also important factors in determining eventual treatment success (see sections "Prognostic Factors" and "Minimal Residual Disease").[369] Results with slow-responding, high-risk patients, suggest that intervention with intensification of chemotherapy (both in induction and later consolidation phases) may be able to rescue slow responders so that their EFS is comparable to similarly grouped patients who had more rapid initial responses to therapy.[347]

Although the basic two-drug combination of vincristine and a glucocorticoid induces remissions in approximately 85% of children with ALL, the addition of L-asparaginase, an anthracycline, or both improved the remission induction rate to approximately 95%.[370] Prednisone and prednisolone have been the most common glucocorticoids used for this purpose. In the mid- to late 1990s several cooperative groups switched to dexamethasone, because of both laboratory data implying it is a more potent cytotoxic agent and studies indicating it has the pharmacologic advantage of better CNS penetration and exposure.[371,372] It now appears that dexamethasone is also more effective in inducing marrow remission, treating the CNS, and maintaining remissions.[327,371,372] There are data, however, that suggest that dexamethasone may increase both acute (life-threatening infection), as well as non-life threatening problems like avascular necrosis, sleep disturbance/fatigue, as well as longer-term complications (i.e., detrimental neurocognitive sequelae) complication rates.[373–376]

The addition of L-asparaginase to vincristine and a glucocorticoid not only improved induction response rates but also significantly prolonged remission duration.[377] Whether the added leukemic cytoreduction theoretically achieved by including a fourth induction (i.e., an anthracycline) agent leads to an additional improvement in remission duration is controversial. The results of one randomized study indicated that adding daunorubicin (daunomycin) to the three-drug combination of vincristine, prednisone, and L-asparaginase did not improve remission duration for high-risk/slow-responding patients.[378] However, protocols using this four-drug induction combination with intensive consolidation and maintenance therapy uniformly demonstrate improved overall remission duration, even for high-risk patients.[343,379] Because the use of a fourth drug or additional drugs during induction may increase the incidence of complications, many centers reserve the use of induction drug combinations employing four or more agents for patients in the higher risk or relapse populations. A recent meta-analysis indicated that anthracyclines did not produce an improvement in EFS in childhood ALL despite their improved control of bone marrow relapse, due to the concomitant increase in treatment related mortality.[380]

Failure of induction therapy is an uncommon event, occurring in fewer than 5% of children with ALL treated with current regimens.[381] Induction failure is defined as the presence of overt leukemia (certainly >25% but in many current protocols >1% to 5%) in the marrow at the end of the induction phase. The overall EFS for these patients is only 16%.[381] A rare patient may demonstrate severe marrow aplasia at the end of an induction period and hence does not meet the established cellularity criteria for achieving M1 status. The few patients with prolonged postinduction aplasia have a better prognosis than those who fail induction and demonstrate an EFS comparable to that of the patients who were clearly in a standard remission with cellular marrows at the end of induction.[381] A patient with marrow aplasia at the end of induction should simply be supported (e.g., with blood products and antibiotics as needed) until the marrow either recovers in remission (M1) or demonstrates enough blasts that refractory disease is diagnosed. Improved supportive care has decreased the mortality rate during induction therapy to approximately 3% or less.[381,382]

There are occasional patients who demonstrate an M2 marrow (>5% but <25% leukemic blasts) at the end of a standard induction. Although many of these patients will eventually go into remission (either with an extension of the standard induction or with institution of more intensive treatments), this slow response to initial therapy is indicative of poor prognosis (see section "Minimal Residual Disease"), and should be considered in subsequent therapy recommendations.[84,349]

Central Nervous System Preventive Therapy

The recognition that the development of CNS leukemia recurrence constituted a major obstacle to overall treatment success stimulated efforts to prevent CNS disease. The concept of CNS preventive therapy is based on the premise that the CNS acts as a sanctuary site in which leukemic cells, undetected at diagnosis, reside protected by the blood-brain barrier from therapeutic concentrations of systemically administered antileukemic drugs. According to this view, prevention of CNS relapse is more appropriately called presymptomatic CNS therapy than CNS prophylaxis, a term that is widely used. CNS prophylaxis can be accomplished utilizing a variety of modalities. Radiation (either cranial or cranial spinal), intrathecal (IT) chemotherapy, or high-dose systemic chemotherapy and often a combination

of these are used to ensure that the CNS remains free of disease. Although there are experts who feel radiation can be completely removed from the CNS prophylaxis schema of current front line therapies, most cooperative group trials currently advocate the use of prophylactic radiation in specific "high risk for CNS relapse" situations (i.e., for patients who present with CNS 3 status).[383]

The introduction of CNS irradiation as preventive therapy was based on murine studies that demonstrated cures of murine L1210 leukemia when cranial radiation was added to systemic treatment with cyclophosphamide.[384] The first documentation of the value of CNS preventive therapy evolved from a series of studies performed at St. Jude Children's Research Hospital. Although relatively low doses of craniospinal radiation (500 or 1,200 cGy) demonstrated no preventive effect (studies I to III), the administration of 2,400 cGy cranial irradiation plus five concurrent doses of IT MTX or 2,400 cGy of craniospinal irradiation alone (studies V to VII) reduced the incidence of CNS relapse from greater than 50% to approximately 10%.[385] Because the spinal component of craniospinal irradiation is associated with excessive myelosuppression and retardation of spinal growth, cranial irradiation (2,400 cGy) plus IT MTX became the standard form of CNS preventive therapy in the 1970s.

As combined cranial radiation and IT MTX became widely employed, concerns subsequently developed about the adverse effects of this CNS preventive therapy regimen (see section "Late Effects of Treatment"). The identification of brain abnormalities on CT scans, altered intellectual and psychomotor function, and neuroendocrine dysfunction in patients treated with 2,400 cGy of cranial irradiation and IT chemotherapy prompted a reappraisal of CNS preventive therapy strategies and further stimulated investigation into alternative methods of CNS preventive therapy.[386–389] The use of a lower dose of cranial irradiation (1,800 cGy) with IT MTX was shown to be as effective as 2,400 cGy and it is currently used in most CNS preventive therapy regimens that continue to administer cranial irradiation.[390]

It is unclear, however, that the use of 1,800 cGy plus IT MTX significantly reduces the incidence of adverse CNS sequelae. There is evidence that 1,800 cGy may also have significant negative effects on neurocognitive function.[391] There is evidence that children with ALL treated with 1,800 cGy of cranial irradiation and IT MTX demonstrated greater adverse neuropsychological effects than those treated with IT MTX alone.[392] In an attempt to decrease neurotoxicity of the radiation, some have advocated "hyperfractionation" (the delivery of the same total dose of radiation therapy (XRT) split into smaller fractions over the same period of time). Although there is a theoretical advantage to hyperfractionation, no advantage for ALL patients in the setting of CNS prophylaxis has been demonstrated.[393] Various schema for successfully and safely reducing the amount of cranial radiation to 1,200 cGY in combination with specific systemic an IT therapies have been devised.[383,394] However, the need to do this may have been eliminated with the successful introduction of current highly effective CNS prophylaxis that is provided when patients are stratified to more intensive intrathecal and systemic therapy regimens based, in part, on their risk of CNS relapse.[383,395]

A variety of patient characteristics are associated with an increased risk of CNS leukemia, including a high initial leukocyte count, T-cell disease, very young age, thrombocytopenia, lymphadenopathy, hepatomegaly, splenomegaly, black race, and presence of the t(1;19) translocation in the leukemic lymphoblasts.[383,390] The highest rates of CNS relapse occur in infants and patients with extremely high leukocyte counts or lymphomatous presentations.[390] Although no single factor or group of factors can predict with absolute certainty whether an individual patient will relapse in the CNS, the recognition that patients differ in their risk for developing CNS leukemia has permitted investigators to successfully modify recommendations for CNS preventive therapy. Cranial irradiation is clearly unnecessary for patients with a variety of good prognostic indicators. IT MTX alone, given periodically throughout the treatment, provides adequate CNS preventive therapy for these patients.[383,390] Maintenance IT triple chemotherapy (including age based dosing of AraC, Methotrexate, and Hydrocortisone), the combination of IT and moderate-dose intravenous (IV) MTX, and high-dose IV MTX alone all appear to provide equivalent protection to that offered by cranial irradiation and IT MTX for patients at an intermediate risk of CNS relapse.[394]

With current CNS preventive therapy regimens, the incidence of CNS relapse is less than 10% overall and below 5% for good-risk patients.[383] The intensity of systemic chemotherapy appears to influence the efficacy of CNS preventive therapy regimens. The Associazione Italiana di Ematologia ed Oncologia Pediatrica (AIEOP) and COG groups have respectively demonstrated that, when intensive systemic therapy is used, IT MTX alone, administered from the start of treatment throughout maintenance therapy, is equivalent to 1,800 cGy of cranial irradiation in intermediate and even high-risk patients who were rapid early responders (RER) during induction.[347,396] Maintenance IT MTX was significantly less effective than 1,800 cGy of cranial irradiation when less intensive systemic chemotherapy is used.[394]

IT MTX or cranial irradiation alone can produce a wide spectrum of acute or subacute neurotoxic sequelae.[388,397] IT MTX may be associated with an acute arachnoiditis, characterized by headaches, nausea and vomiting, meningismus, and other signs of increased intracranial pressure occurring 12 to 24 hours after administration.[398] These reactions usually are not severe, are self-limited, and have been reduced in frequency by the use of an IT MTX dosing schedule based on the relation of age to CNS volume.[399] A subacute form of MTX neurotoxicity characterized by varying degrees of encephalopathy, myelopathy, and even paraplegia has been observed more rarely.[400] Studies employing frequent pulses of intermediate-dose MTX together with triple IT therapy reportedly are associated with an increased incidence of neurotoxicity including seizures and CT scan abnormalities.[401] Between 5 and 7 weeks after cranial irradiation, some patients develop a subacute neurotoxic reaction characterized by somnolence, lethargy, anorexia, fever, and irritability. These somnolence symptoms, can be reduced by the simultaneous administration of dexamethasone.[402] Somnolence symptoms may be accompanied by electroencephalographic abnormalities and CSF pleocytosis, usually reverse within 1 to 3 weeks, and are not directly predictive of subsequent adverse neurologic events.[403]

The desirability of avoiding cranial irradiation in CNS preventive therapy regimens results from concerns that radiotherapy is primarily responsible for many of the long-term adverse CNS sequelae observed in patients treated with cranial irradiation and IT chemotherapy. Although patients at low and intermediate risks of CNS relapse may receive equally effective therapy with the alternatives to irradiation previously discussed, many centers continue to administer cranial irradiation plus IT MTX to patients at particularly high risk for CNS relapse. Some centers have completely eliminated cranial irradiation for all but CNS relapsed patients.[383] At the present time, only 10% to 15% of ALL patients (in the highest risk categories) receive either prophylactic or therapeutic cranial irradiation. This is a marked improvement over the 100% use of this modality in the late 1960s and early 1970s.

Postinduction Therapy

After complete remission has been achieved, subsequent therapy is required. Early studies demonstrated that without additional therapy, most patients relapse within a median of 1 to 2 months. The actual duration of an unmaintained remission varies with the biology of the individual case, as well as with the intensity and duration of the induction therapy. As shown in Figure 19.17, patients in complete remission theoretically have a leukemic cell burden in the range of 10^{10}. Although successful induction will produce a two log (99%) to four log or greater decrease in the total body burden of leukemia cells, a significant amount of additional therapy is necessary before the leukemia is totally eradicated.

Using a variety of methods, including cytomorphology, biochemistry, in vitro cell culture, cytogenetic analysis, flow cytometry, and molecular biologic approaches (such as Southern blot and PCR analysis of immunoglobulin and TCR gene rearrangements), investigators have documented that occult leukemic disease is often present in patients during otherwise apparent remission (see also section "Minimal Residual Disease").[84] At relapse, lymphoblasts usually demonstrate chromosomal and immunoglobulin gene rearrangement patterns identical to those obtained at the time of original diagnosis.[404] Several mechanisms have been proposed to explain this persistence of leukemic cells during remission. These include the development of biochemical drug resistance, the residence of leukemic cells in physiologic or pharmacologic sanctuary sites (e.g., CNS, testes), and the maintenance of a population of leukemia cells in a metabolically quiescent state (i.e., G_0 of cell cycle) in which they are less vulnerable to chemotherapy.

To be effective in preventing relapse, postinduction therapy must suppress leukemic growth and provide continuing leukemic cytoreduction, without permitting the emergence of drug-resistant clones.[385,405] Postinduction therapy usually consists of consolidative (therapy used to "consolidate' or reinforce remission in both the CNS and marrow compartments), other intensified phases (frequently termed "interim maintenance" which are often more intensive than standard maintenance, reinduction/reconsolidation schema), and maintenance (sometimes called "continuation") phase.

Consolidation therapy is a period of intensified treatment administered immediately after remission induction, and it is a common component of many therapy protocols, particularly

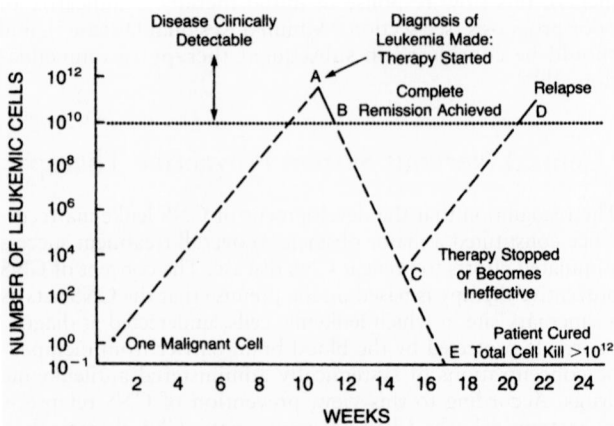

FIGURE 19.17 Schematic representation of the results of therapy in a patient with leukemia. (Adapted from Valeriote F, Vietti TJ, Fernback DJ, eds. Clinical pediatric oncology. St. Louis: CV Mosby, 1977:1182.)

for higher-risk patients.[406,407] Consolidative regimens frequently employ weekly IT and/or high dose chemotherapy infusions to improve leukemic cytoreduction both in the CNS and other sanctuary sites, as well as continue to strengthen the remission (lower the amount of any remaining MRD) in the bone marrow. Several regimens use one or multiple periods where therapy is "intensified" with additional agents. These schedules are designed to minimize the development of drug cross-resistance. The evidence that intensification has improved treatment success, even in patients with a poor prognosis, is substantial. The dual strategies of graded intensity (less intensive for those patients at lowest risk of relapse and higher intensity treatments for those at greater risk) as well as allowing the marrow to recover between higher intensity cycles with periods of less drug intensity combined with important improvements in supportive care (see below) are all responsible for bringing the overall cure rate to it's current 80% to 85%.[1] Treatment protocols and the definitions of high risk vs. low risk often differ between cooperative groups. Most ALL protocols limit the intensive phase treatments to the first 6 to 8 months, but occasionally the intensive phases may last as long as 1 year. After the completion of 6 to 12 months of more intensive treatment lower doses of active agents (maintenance or continuation phases) are used to prevent relapse.

Drugs and dosages particularly effective as induction and consolidation phases are not always useful for maintenance therapy. For example, continued intensive treatments with vincristine and prednisone did not prolong remission duration in early trials. In contrast, maintenance treatment with MTX and 6-mercaptopurine (6-MP) substantially prolongs remission.[408] The combination of MTX and 6-MP, administered continuously in a variety of schedules, has been used most widely and constitutes the principal element in most maintenance therapy regimens. The optimal schedule of administration of these two drugs is different. MTX is more effective administered intermittently, but daily administration of 6-MP appears optimal. Various combinations have been studied in which other agents are added to standard 6-MP and MTX regimens. Addition of intermittent pulses of vincristine and prednisone to 6-MP and MTX maintenance chemotherapy appears to have prolonged remission duration for some patients, although the value of this approach after intensive induction therapy is unclear.[2,409] Changing the pulse medications from monthly vincristine and prednisone to vincristine and dexamethasone (for projected better CNS coverage) did not make a difference at least in the context of a modern regimen for intermediate risk patients.[410] The choice of appropriate maintenance chemotherapy appears to differ according to risk group. 6-MP and MTX may provide adequate maintenance therapy for certain good-risk patients, but more intensive maintenance therapy appears to be more effective for poor-risk patients.

Drug dosage is an important factor in maintenance chemotherapy. Its influence during maintenance was demonstrated in a randomized study in which patients receiving chemotherapy with 6-MP, MTX, and cyclophosphamide at full dose had significantly longer remission duration than patients receiving therapy at one-half dose.[411] Subsequent clinical studies have confirmed this finding, and demonstrated a correlation between cumulative 6-MP dose and prognosis in children with average-risk ALL.[412,413] A Danish study reported a lower relapse rate among patients who had lower leukocyte counts while receiving maintenance therapy with 6-MP and MTX, suggesting that more intensive therapy with these two agents is beneficial.[414] In another study, patients who tolerated only low doses of 6-MP because of neutropenia and those who received higher doses of MTX had a lower rate of

relapse, indicating that the use of these agents in maximally tolerated doses during maintenance may be associated with improved treatment outcome.[415] The results from several cooperative group trials testing this question (i.e., standard vs. dose intensive 6-MP/6-thioguanine (6TG)/MTX) are not yet available.

The frequency of drug administration also appears to influence the length of remission. Patients who receive maintenance therapy on a continuous rather than an interrupted schedule have longer remission durations. There is some evidence that some interrupted schedules may be useful in maintenance therapy, but they tend to utilized higher doses of 6MP and MTX (often iv) at regular (i.e., every 2 to 4 weeks) intervals.[416] Although this might be of some utility in settings where it might be desirable to administer more of the therapy in a controlled setting, for most settings it would be more costly. Studies of the clinical pharmacology of orally administered 6-MP and MTX have documented that their bioavailability after oral administration may be limited and highly variable, suggesting a possible explanation for treatment failures that occur during oral maintenance therapy with these agents.[417] Compliance problems also may diminish the efficacy of maintenance therapy. The possible problems associated with oral administration of 6-MP and MTX theoretically could be circumvented by parenteral administration. However, data on the relative effectiveness of parenteral or oral maintenance therapy are conflicting. Results of a Medical Research Council leukemia trial (UKALL-VII study) indicated a significantly longer actuarial relapse-free survival rate for patients who received MTX intramuscularly compared with those given the drug orally.[418] In another study, which randomized children with non–T-cell ALL to receive MTX during maintenance as a single oral dose or as an intramuscular injection, the route of administration appeared to have no real influence on relapse rate.[419]

There is evidence that intracellular metabolism of 6-MP and MTX may influence the levels of cytotoxic metabolites of 6-MP, and higher levels of these have been associated with a lower relapse rate.[420] Studies have demonstrated that the lymphoblasts from children with low-risk ALL more efficiently accumulate MTX intracellular metabolites indicating that these patients may be more sensitive to MTX therapy.[337] An association has also been found between high levels of lymphoblast dihydrofolate reductase and shorter remission duration.[421]

Duration of Treatment

The optimal length of maintenance chemotherapy has not been established. Most centers treat patients with early B-lineage and T-cell ALL for a total of approximately 2 to 3 years. Data from several studies support this approach.[412,422] The British Medical Research Council (MRC) examined the effect of variation in length of treatment on duration of remission and demonstrated that 19 months of therapy was less effective in preventing relapse than 3 years of treatment.[423] One trial tested shortening maintenance to 6 months and found that this was not enough therapy (due to increased relapse rates) in both low and intermediate risk patients.[424] However in very high-risk patients who had received significantly more intensive treatment early in therapy 6 months of maintenance after intensive induction, consolidative and reintensified (i.e., a Delayed Intensification phase which frequently includes a reinduction and re consolidative subphases) may be adequate.[425]

Although poorly understood, there appears to be gender related impact on outcomes.[426] The tendency for a greater percentage of males to relapse after cessation of chemotherapy was observed in a long-term follow-up study of patients treated on the CCSG 141 protocol. In that study, patients in complete continuous remission for 3 years were randomized to discontinue therapy, to receive a 4-week course of reinduction chemotherapy and then discontinue therapy or to continue therapy for a total of 5 years. No significant difference was found in disease-free survival for the different treatment regimens. However, a higher incidence of late relapse occurred among males, even after excluding patients with occult testicular disease. This is consistent with other studies that have demonstrated that sex is a significant predictor of relapse, even when isolated testicular relapse is excluded.[338,339] On modern protocols the difference in outcomes between boys in girls has lessened. Although, a large proportion of the sex-based differences can be accounted for by the slight increase in higher risk disease presentation features in boys versus girls, small differences in outcomes continue to persist.[338,339]

It is likely that the intensity of therapy has a bearing on the optimal duration of therapy. The current practice of treating patients with early B-lineage ALL for 2.5 to 3 years of maintenance chemotherapy is derived from studies in which patients were treated with a variety of older chemotherapeutic regimens, many of which incorporated fewer agents and were less intensive than those currently in use. For this reason, conclusions about the duration of maintenance based on those studies may not be directly applicable to current treatment programs. It is logical to question whether patients receiving more intensive therapy earlier in their course of treatment may ultimately require a shorter overall duration of therapy. In an attempt to address this question, the BFM study group, which uses an intensive chemotherapy regimen, randomized patients to receive 18 or 24 months of total duration of therapy. A therapeutic advantage was observed in all risk categories for patients who received longer treatment.[426] On the other hand, the MRC UKALL-VIII trial, using less intensive therapy, observed no outcome advantage between patients randomized to receive 3 years and those receiving 2 years of maintenance treatment.[412]

Supportive Care

Optimal management of the child with ALL requires appropriate attention to several areas of supportive care, including the rational use of blood component therapy; an aggressive approach to detection and treatment of infectious complications; careful attention to the metabolic and nutritional needs of the patient; and comprehensive, continuous psychosocial support for patient and family. Advances in supportive care modalities have permitted the safe use of more intensive and more effective therapies on current protocols, and hence have played important role(s) in the improvement in outcomes. Because these topics are thoroughly addressed in Chapters 38 to 49, they are discussed only briefly here.

The importance of adequate hematologic supportive care cannot be overemphasized, because despite huge improvements in the purity and safety of multiple blood products and the implementation of very effective guidelines for their use, hemorrhage remains the leading cause of early deaths (death before remission) in pediatric leukemia (both myeloid and lymphoid).[427] Before the systematic use of platelet transfusions, hemorrhage was the leading cause of death in patients with this disease. The use of prophylactic platelet transfusions and aggressive platelet transfusion support has markedly reduced the incidence of significant bleeding. The use of a platelet count of 20,000/mm^3 as a threshold for transfusion in adult leukemia patients (primarily with AML) has been questionable. Others have found that the use of 10,000/mm^3 in the absence of fever,

trauma, or reason for clotting factor consumption resulted in 20% to 30% less transfusion exposure and cost without a significant increase in serious hemorrhage.[428-430]

However, all of these studies were done on relatively small numbers of patients that included very few children. Erythrocyte transfusions are also frequently required to treat anemia and, as with all blood products, they must be appropriately screeded to exclude the possiblility of viral contamination particularly with hepatitis virus or HIV. Modern blood banking and transfusion techniques including the irradiation of all cellular blood products, white cell depletion, and more comprehensive viral and donor screening have improved the safety and efficacy of transfusion of these children.

The granulocytopenia that occurs as a consequence of therapy-induced marrow hypoplasia, or with disease progression, places patients at risk for potentially life-threatening infections, but the value of granulocyte transfusions is limited and not well defined. An aggressive approach to diagnosis and rapid empiric therapeutic intervention are important principles for the successful management of the severely neutropenic (<500 granulocytes per mm^3) patient with fever (see Chapter 40). The early empiric use of broad-spectrum antibiotics has dramatically reduced overall mortality. Granulocytopenia, chemotherapy-induced immunosuppression, disruption of normal anatomic barriers by invasive procedures, or therapy-induced complications (e.g., mucositis) increase susceptibility to bacterial, fungal, viral, and parasitic infections.[431]

Hematopoietic growth factors, including granulocyte colony stimulating factor (G-CSF), play a significant role in reducing the complications of granulocytopenia after cancer chemotherapy. G-CSF has already been shown to ameliorate the leukopenia incurred by chemotherapy for ALL.[432] The long-term benefits of using growth factors during intensive phases of ALL therapy remains controversial.[433,434] Receptors for G-CSF and other known factors (e.g., granulocyte-macrophage colony-stimulating factor, IL-3) have been identified in leukemic lymphoblasts, raising concern that their use might stimulate leukemic cell growth.[435] For these reasons (as well as the significant financial cost) G-CSF and other growth factors are not routinely used in most standard risk ALL regimens, but they are used often in the BMT, relapse, and occasionally in front-line high risk protocols that use more intensive chemotherapy.[436,437]

To date, there has not been a large amount of research or consensus guidelines published in pediatric oncology both for the type of blood products, hematopoietic growth factors, and threshold values that should be applied in commonly encountered clinical situations (see Chapter 39). Consequently, there is a large degree of heterogeneity in this area of Pediatric Oncology practice.[438]

Although the risk of infections may be greater for patients undergoing intensive induction or reinduction therapy, the child with leukemia is susceptible to various forms of infections while undergoing maintenance chemotherapy as well.[439] *Pneumocystis carinii* pneumonia is an extremely serious, potentially life-threatening complication that commonly affects children undergoing maintenance chemotherapy. The prophylactic use of trimethoprim-sulfamethoxazole, instituted early in therapy, dramatically reduces the incidence of this type of infection and is used routinely in most centers.[440] When trimethoprim-sulfamethoxazole cannot be tolerated because of count suppression or allergy, dapsone or pentamidine (IV or aerosolized) can be substituted.[441]

The leukemic child undergoing treatment is also at risk for disseminated varicella if exposure to an infected person occurs. Administration of zoster immune globulin to such patients within 96 hours after exposure appears to have a protective effect.[442] Immunization of children with ALL with a live, attenuated varicella vaccine has been advocated by some but may not work because of the immune suppression by the disease and/or chemotherapy, and is not currently recommended.[443] The immunization of varicella-susceptible, household contacts of patients with ALL who have not had varicella is currently a recommended practice.[444] Other viral infections also place the leukemic child at risk. Measles tends to run a more complicated, atypical course in the leukemic host.[445] Nonimmunized children exposed to the measles virus should be treated with gamma globulin. Because of the risk of dissemination, immunization against measles or the use of any vaccines containing a live virus, except possibly in the case of varicella vaccine, is contraindicated in patients receiving chemotherapy.

Nutrition

Adequate nutrition is a concern for the patient with leukemia. Multiple studies have suggested that malnutrition is an adverse prognostic factor (see previously and Chapter 41).[358,359] Severe malnutrition was shown in one study to increase the risk of death during induction 2.5-fold.[358] It has been reported that improving nutrition in undernourished patients during chemotherapy improves prognosis.[446] It may be that this effect is due to the relationship between nutritional status and the ability to tolerate standard maintenance chemotherapy. Under-nutrition is common at diagnosis, and it frequently becomes worse during the intensive phases of chemotherapy.[357] In most centers, if normal enteral alimentation is prevented by complications of disease or therapy, IV hyperalimentation is considered. It is clear that the problems with obesity and poor cardiovascular fitness in ALL survivors are likely to be related both to the effects of the chemotherapy (especially steroids) as well as habits developed during the treatment period. Efforts to intervene with nutritional and exercise programs both on therapy and off treatment periods are beginning to show promise, and are the topics of future research.[447]

TREATMENT OF RELAPSE

Most relapsed leukemias at any site retain their original immunophenotypes and karyotypes, but changes in these and other laboratory parameters have been observed.[448–450] Prior to treating relapse, it is helpful to ascertain whether the cells are indeed from the original leukemia. The presence of a different cell lineage at the time of relapse, a so-called lineage switch (e.g., lymphoid to myeloid), is a relatively rare event. Lineage switch may result from chemotherapeutic eradication of one clone and subsequent expansion of a second clone of an originally biclonal leukemia. Alternatively, chemotherapy may induce modulation of antigen expression in a leukemic clone that retains the potential for lymphoid and myeloid differentiation. Lineage switch must be differentiated from the development of a secondary leukemia. Molecular and cytogenetic studies are helpful in documenting similarity with the original clone. In relapse situations, in approximately 30% of the cases, the karyotype will have undergone changes visible with standard Giemsa banding (e.g., clonal evolution).[448] However, there is usually evidence of the original clone within the predominant clone at relapse. Lineage switch usually occurs within months of the initial diagnosis. Secondary acute leukemias tend to occur years later.[451] Lineage shift from lymphoid to nonlymphoid disease is more common than the reverse, although both have been described.[452] In general, both secondary leukemias and relapse of the original leukemia

represent disease which is less responsive, and relapse protocols (often including at least the consideration of BMT) are much more intensive than those used on most de novo cases. Relapse may occur in the bone marrow, in isolated extramedullary sites, or both.

Bone Marrow Relapse

Bone marrow relapse is the principal form of treatment failure in patients with ALL. The two approaches to the treatment of bone marrow relapse are chemotherapy and BMT. Depending on initial chemotherapy regimen employed, second complete remissions can usually be induced in most patients who experience a marrow relapse. The chemotherapeutic approach to the relapsed patient should include aggressive multidrug reinduction therapy followed by intensive systemic consolidation and maintenance chemotherapy. The combination of vincristine, prednisone, and L-asparaginase produces complete remissions in approximately 70% to 75% of patients treated for an initial bone marrow relapse, but is much lower with subsequent relapses and/or when the patient has prior exposure to multiple chemotherapeutic agents at high dose (i.e., if the patient has relapsed after having received the intensive phases of a higher risk modern protocol).

The addition of daunorubicin increases the reinduction rate to 80% to 90% in patients who have received less intensive, lower risk therapy in the past. By using regimens that incorporate agents that were not used during the patient's initial treatment as well as by increasing the dose intensity of all agents to maximally tolerated levels, reinduction rates greater than 90% have been reported.[453,454] Administration of an intensive course of cytarabine and teniposide or high-dose ifosfamide with etoposide can induce complete remission in approximately one third of patients not achieving complete responses with the four-drug reinduction regimen of L-asparaginase, vincristine, daunorubicin, and prednisone.[455] Wherever possible, new agents (drugs not used in the initial therapy) and new combinations of agents should be introduced to try to overcome any drug resistance the leukemic clone may have acquired during the first treatment course.

Although most patients with ALL who suffer a bone marrow relapse will be able to obtain a second Complete Remission (CR2), after modern therapy the cure rates with or without Bone Marrow Transplant (BMT) tend to be in the 30% to 40% range, with patients who relapse early (variously defined as <6 months, <18 months on, or 2 to 3 months after completing their initial treatment protocol) obtaining EFS results as low as 10% in contrast to patients who relapse years after completing their original course who have demonstrated cure rates as high as 50%.[456,457] As initial treatment protocols have become more intensive (and more successful) the outcome results for relapse protocols have remained the same or actually worsened.[315,458]

At the time of a marrow relapse, the CNS must also be checked (with an LP) and consideration given to how, if the CNS is not involved, a second course of CNS preventive therapy should be administered. The need for a second course of CNS preventive therapy for patients in second remission is well established. Without it, almost 50% of patients in second bone marrow remission experience a CNS relapse.[459] For patients who received cranial irradiation as part of their initial CNS preventive therapy, IT chemotherapy is usually used as a second form of CNS preventive therapy.[459] The relative value of single, double, or triple agent IT therapy in this circumstance has not been established. Although it is common for triple intrathecal medications (Hydrocortisone, Methotrexate, and Ara C) to be used in these situations, the data that this is a safe and effective method of CNS prophylaxis have been developed only in the primary, not the relapse context.[460] In the primary treatment setting, the combination of triple IT therapy with extensive use of intermediate dose iv Methotrexate has demonstrated to have increased rate (approximately 11.2% of patients demonstrated some form of acute neurotoxicity) of complications.[401] If the CNS is involved at the time of relapse, a plan for active CNS treatment must be developed, and will often involve radiotherapy if this modality was not used during previous treatment.[461,462]

The use of BMT as a therapeutic approach for ALL patients who have suffered a bone marrow relapse or are assessed to be at an extremely high risk of relapse (i.e., severe hypodiploidy at diagnosis) has increased in recent years. This approach, discussed in Chapter 16, involves the administration of intensive cytoreductive therapy, usually employing Total Body Irradiation (TBI) combined with high-dose chemotherapy in doses lethal to normal bone marrow, and subsequent hematopoietic "rescue" with IV-infused bone marrow or purified peripheral blood stem cells obtained from a compatible donor. To some degree, the initial interest in BMT was generated by the unfavorable treatment results obtained in relapsed patients treated with conventional chemotherapy. The earliest experiences with BMT involved multiply relapsed patients refractory to conventional chemotherapy, who were usually transplanted in relapse. Results in this group of patients were disappointing; approximately 10% of those receiving marrow from an HLA-matched sibling in that setting, achieved prolonged disease-free survival.[463]

Although, these earlier results were discouraging, continual innovation and technologic refinements have given BMT a significant role in the treatment of childhood ALL. Currently, allogeneic marrow transplantation is routinely advocated for patients in second remission who relapsed during or shortly after (with in 6 months) of completing their initial therapy.[464] In this group of patients, overall disease-free survivals range from approximately 40% to more than 60%.[465,466] Currently, most groups are reporting results equivalent to these using matched unrelated donors (MUDs).[467,468] The difficulty of obtaining matched unrelated grafts in a timely fashion has stimulated promising research using either matched unrelated cord blood or haplo-identical donors (a parent or occasionally from a sibling).[469–471]

Other factors that should prompt consideration of BMT (even in first complete remission) include the presence of unfavorable cytogenetics (i.e., t(9;22), t(4;11) or unfavorable ploidy (severe hypodiploidy or triploidy) of the leukemic blasts. Transplantation should be considered in patients who do not respond rapidly to their initial treatment.[472] The value of BMT for infants with or without the t(4;11) translocation has been controversial because of the high morbidity and mortality rates of BMT in these very young patients (see discussion on infant leukemia).[324] Although non-TBI containing regimens are often chosen for young children, they do not seem to be as effective as those that contain TBI.[465]

Better results are obtained for patients transplanted in remission than in those transplanted in relapse or partial remission. In most studies, patients transplanted in earlier remissions fare significantly better than patients transplanted after multiple relapses. The length of first remission and high-risk features at diagnosis are predictive factors.[473] Most studies that have compared the efficacy of allogeneic marrow transplantation with chemotherapy for patients who had experienced a previous relapse indicate that transplantation is associated with a superior outcome.[474] The outlook for patients who relapse after BMT is poor. Although complete remission can be obtained in as many as 50% to 70% of patients, the duration is usually short.[404,475]

Minimal Residual Disease

Multiple studies have demonstrated a strong association between persistent levels of MRD at the end of induction, persistent or rising MRD levels at later time points in therapy, and the risk of relapse in both pre-B and T-cell ALL[352,476] This is true not only for newly diagnosed ALL cases but also for relapsed patients treated with salvage chemotherapy or BMT[352,477] Numerous techniques have been developed to detect MRD and to predict clinical outcome. These include various types of quantitative PCR or RT-PCR, cell culture/soft agar cloning techniques, FACS analysis for abnormal immunophenotypes, or combinations of these.[352] PCR technology has greatly enhanced the ability to detect residual leukemic cells and is currently the most sensitive method. Targets for PCR detection include leukemia-specific translocations and clonal antigen receptor or immunoglobulin gene rearrangements that are specific to a particular leukemic clone. The leukemia cell specific changes can be targeted at the DNA level with PCR or at the level of gene expression with RT-PCR and quantitative real time RT-PCR. Using *in vitro* artificial dilution experiments, the genomic (DNA) PCR approach can detect as few as one leukemic cell in 10^5 (10^{-5}) to 10^6 (10^{-6}) normal bone marrow cells.[352,478] The 10^{-4} and 10^{-5} sensitivity is also within the range of current FACS equipment which can detect the complex (multiple antigens on the same cell) immunophenotype patterns that allow the leukemic cells to be clearly distinguished from normal cells.[352,354] FACS has the added advantage of detecting intact cells, in contrast to PCR and RT-PCR, in which contaminating nucleic acid material from dead cells can complicate interpretation.

RT-PCR is generally applied to cases that have translocations [i.e., t(12;21)] from which a fusion transcript is expressed. However, only approximately 40% of pre-B ALL patients (and a lower percentage of T-cell cases) have these types of translocations. The majority of patients who do not have a detectable chromosomal translocation that can be used for RT-PCR MRD studies (approximately 60% of ALL patients), can be followed by DNA-based PCR of unique Ig or TCR receptor rearrangements. Unfortunately, however, the latter is a costly and laborious approach that has been associated with a higher false positive rate than other methodologies.[478]

Detection of MRD by flow cytometry is in many ways the most accessible of the technologies; however, to perform the needed assays accurately requires multicolor (several laser) equipment/reagents and an operator with considerable skill and experience in MRD assays.

Early studies suggested that PCR may be useful in identifying patients likely to relapse when the amount of detectable leukemic cells in their marrow seemed to be rising.[479,480] In Ph+ ALL, the detection of PCR-positive bcr-abl transcripts after BMT or intensive therapy was the first situation in which increasing amounts of PCR+ cells were found to be associated with a decreased disease-free survival.[481]

More recently, measurement of MRD is being applied to assessment of rate of response to induction therapy (see sections "Prognostic Factors" and "Treatment"). It is becoming clearer that the rapid (i.e., within the first 2 to 4 weeks) lowering of MRD levels to below 10^{-4} correlates well with relapse-free survival.[84,352] Conversely, patients in whom MRD does not clear below this point by the end of induction, have a higher risk of relapse. Clinicians should be aware that a negative MRD analysis does not guarantee the absence of relapse, nor does a positive level of MRD or serially rising MRD levels convey (at this point) anything other than increased risk of relapse. Because there is wide variability in the accuracy and sensitivity of current MRD assessment techniques, use of MRD results to guide clinical decisions is best applied in the context of formal clinical trials.

Extramedullary Relapse

Central Nervous System Relapse

Despite the success of CNS preventive therapy in dramatically reducing the incidence of CNS recurrence, CNS relapse remains a significant cause of treatment failure in ALL. CNS recurrence is observed in fewer than 10% of patients. In the past, the outcome for these patients was generally poor, with most patients suffering subsequent CNS relapses or recurrences at other sites, such as bone marrow and/or testes.[390] CNS relapse may occur as an isolated event, with a bone marrow relapse, or with recurrence at another extramedullary site (e.g., testes). Because periodic LP surveillance for CNS leukemia is performed in most ALL treatment protocols, it is relatively infrequent for patients to present with overt CNS symptoms. More commonly, the diagnosis of meningeal recurrence is based on a routine examination of CSF. The criteria for diagnosing a CSF relapse have been modified over the years.[482] The generally accepted criteria has included more than five leukocytes per microliter, with unequivocal blasts demonstrable in a cytocentrifuge preparation. Although this has been a useful working definition, the significance of blast cells in a cytocentrifuge sample when the CSF leukocyte count is less than or equal to five leukocytes per microliter is not clear. A study by Odom et al. suggested that positive low-cell-count CSF samples obtained on surveillance LPs performed during remission indicated a high likelihood of impending CNS relapse.[483] A CCG study, however, did not confirm these findings.[295] Although this may be true for small amounts of leukemic blasts seen on surveillance LPs, it is becoming clear that small amounts of leukemic cells seen on the initial diagnostic LP (even if they are thought to be the result of even minor "red cell contamination" at the time of the procedure) portend a worse prognosis.[298,383]

During the 1990s intensive treatment plans improved the results for patients with an isolated CNS relapse as high as 70% EFS.[462,484] Despite general decrease in general salvage rates on modern intensive therapies, it is possible (utilizing intensive combinations of chemo and radio-therapy) to maintain these CNS salvage rates.[461] There is evidence that if both cranial/spinal XRT and IT chemotherapy are used as CNS prophylaxis in the context of moderately intensive systemic therapy during the initial treatment regimen, the rate of CNS relapse can be reduced as low as 1% to 2%.[485] Since the majority of children are able to avoid CNS relapse and are cured with current regimens that do not employ radiation, combinations of CNS and XRT prophylaxis which have worse intellectual and growth long-term effects should be avoided in the primary treatment setting. Nevertheless, there remain specific high-risk situations and relapse situations where combined modality treatment may still be required for cure.[383]

Many successful treatment regimens for CNS relapse have used IT chemotherapy while repeating a systemic induction chemotherapy regimen, followed by consolidation chemo and radiotherapy with craniospinal irradiation and maintenance IT chemotherapy.[46] IT MTX alone induces CNS remissions in more than 90% of CNS relapsed patients; however, unless followed by maintenance IT therapy or craniospinal irradiation, relapse occurs within 3 to 4 months.[486] Therapy for CNS relapse must contain vigorous systemic therapy to prevent further relapses of all types. Cranial irradiation alone has little value in the treatment of overt CNS disease, because it does not adequately treat sites of disease along the spinal axis. Furthermore, when cranial irradiation is combined with IT MTX alone, it increases toxicity and does not prolong remission duration.[486] Craniospinal irradiation alone, administered in adequate doses (2,400 cGy to both sites), can induce complete remissions and prolong disease-free survival. Most centers, however, do not use craniospinal irradiation alone. The higher spinal irradiation dose required to achieve equivalent disease control if IT therapy is omitted is associated with prolonged bone marrow suppression, which compromises the ability to deliver adequate systemic chemotherapy. A common approach is first to induce a CSF remission with IT chemotherapy, reinstitute systemic therapy, and then later administer craniospinal irradiation, at doses of 2,400 to 3,000 cGy to the cranial vault and 1,200 to 1,800 cGy to the spinal axis.[487] Factors influencing outcome for patients with CNS relapse include whether the relapse occurred more than or less than 18 months (83% and 46% EFS, respectively; Fig. 19.18) from the initial diagnosis and whether the patient received CNS directed irradiation during the initial treatment regimen.[462,484]

The role of craniospinal irradiation to treat CNS recurrence in a patient who originally received cranial irradiation as part of CNS preventive therapy is less certain. Results from at least one trial demonstrated a continuous complete remission rate of less than 10% for these patients.[488] Other investigators have demonstrated substantially better results with this approach. However, craniospinal irradiation administered in this setting is known to pose a significantly greater risk of delayed neurotoxicity, which must be weighted against the risk of progressive disease.[487]

Several attempts have been made to improve on the use of single-agent IT MTX for CNS relapse. Trials of triple IT therapy consisting of simultaneously administered IT cytarabine, hydrocortisone, and MTX have been advocated produce remission

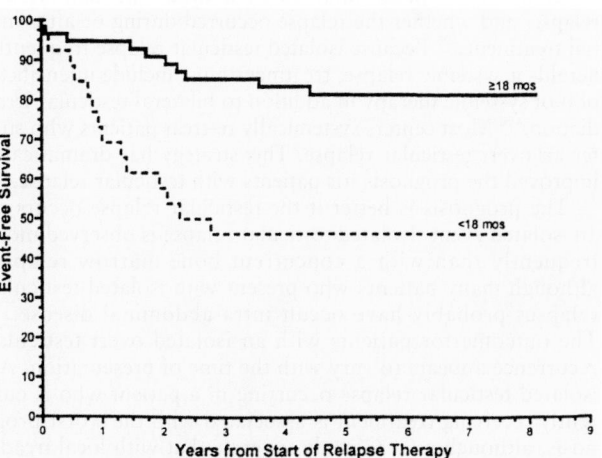

FIGURE 19.18 Event-free survival (EFS) for patients who have isolated central nervous system (CNS) relapses greater than or equal to or less than 18 months from initial diagnosis. The 4-year cumulative EFS rate for patients with first remission at greater than or equal to 18 months was 83.3% ± 5.3%, and, for patients with a first remission at less than 18 months, it was 46.2% ± 10.2%. For all patients (*n* = 83) the EFS after a first isolated CNS relapse was 71.1% ± 5.3%. (From Ritchey AK, Pollock BH, Lauer SJ, et al. Improved survival of children with isolated CNS relapse of acute lymphoblastic leukemia: a pediatric oncology group study. J Clin Oncol 1999;17: 3745–3752, with permission.)

durations similar to those achieved with MTX alone.[390] The use of intraventricular chemotherapy, administered by means of an intraventricular subcutaneous reservoir (i.e., an Omaya reservoir), more completely distributes drug within the CNS, minimizes patient discomfort, and avoids the problems of inadequate delivery of drug into the CSF that may occur with unsuccessful LPs.[489] Early studies demonstrated longer remission durations and fewer additional CNS relapses with intraventricular than with intralumbar therapy in CNS-relapsed patients.[490]

Testicular Relapse

With the increase in intensity of many protocols, the incidence of testicular relapse appears to be decreasing from the 10% to 15% seen in the 1970s and 1980s to 2% to 5% on more recent trials.[491,492] Optimal therapy for testicular relapse includes the use of systemic chemotherapy and the administration of local radiotherapy. Radiation dose appears to be a crucial factor in local control. Doses less than 1,200 cGy are generally suboptimal; doses of 2,400 cGy to both testes have been considered adequate.[493] Reports of local recurrence in patients treated with 2,400 cGy, however, suggest that higher doses may be better.[494] Bilateral testicular radiotherapy is indicated for all patients; unilateral treatment may be followed by relapse in the contralateral testis.[313]

Radiation therapy adversely affects normal testicular function. Sterility is an expected consequence at the radiation doses used.[495] Studies also indicate that testicular endocrine function is impaired at doses of 2,400 cGy. Elevated follicle-stimulating hormone and luteinizing hormone levels, decreased testosterone levels, and delayed sexual maturation have been observed after gonadal irradiation. For this reason, such patients must be carefully followed for signs of delayed sexual maturation and may require androgen replacement therapy.[496]

The impact of a testicular relapse on prognosis depends whether it was overt (clinically detectable) or occult (detected on routine testicular biopsy), whether the recurrence was an isolated event or accompanied by a simultaneous marrow relapse, and whether the relapse occurred during or after initial treatment.[497] Because isolated testicular relapse frequently heralds a systemic relapse, treatment must include intensification of systemic therapy in addition to bilateral testicular irradiation.[498] Most centers systemically re-treat patients who suffer an overt testicular relapse. This strategy has dramatically improved the prognosis for patients with testicular relapse.[498]

The prognosis is better if the testicular relapse occurs as an isolated event. Isolated testicular relapse is observed more frequently than with a concurrent bone marrow relapse, although many patients who present with isolated testicular relapses probably have occult intra-abdominal disease.[319] The outcome for patients with an isolated overt testicular recurrence appears to vary with the time of presentation. An isolated testicular relapse occurring in a patient who is currently receiving treatment is associated with the worst prognosis, although a CCG study suggests that with local irradiation and intensive systemic re-treatment prolonged EFS can be obtained in nearly one half of such patients.[498] In contrast, a late, isolated, overt testicular relapse that occurs off therapy has an even better prognosis. Prolonged disease-free survival can be obtained for more than two thirds of such patients.[309]

The practice of elective testicular biopsy during apparent remission can detect microscopic testicular leukemia in approximately 10% to 15% of boys with ALL. The disease-free survival for patients with occult testicular leukemia treated with testicular irradiation and systemic and CNS chemotherapy is approximately 60% to 70%. The treatment results for occult testicular leukemia and an isolated overt testicular relapse that occurs off therapy are similar.[305] For this reason, documentation of occult disease by performing testicular biopsies in patients on therapy or at the end of therapy is no longer advocated.[305] Most of these data were generated on older protocols which had higher rates of testicular relapse. It is not clear what the current salvage rate for testicular relapse is (now a far less common event) in the context of current therapies. Presumably, patients who originally received the low dose, antimetabolite dependent therapies will continue to have high testicular relapse salvage rates, but the prognosis for a patient who has any relapse after receiving the more intensive higher risk protocols is more guarded.

Other Sites of Relapse

Leukemia may occasionally recur at other sites (e.g., ovary, skin, and various ocular anatomic locations).[499–501] If feasible, the appropriate treatment may include local measures for disease control (e.g., local applications of chemotherapy and/or radiation therapy) and intensification of systemic chemotherapy.

Late Effects of Treatment

A large spectrum of long-term sequelae are observed in survivors of ALL. The dramatic improvements in the survival of children with ALL has focused increasing attention on these late effects of antileukemic therapy. A number of adverse sequelae have been identified. These are discussed in more detail in Chapter 47. The greatest risk for second neoplasms as well as other adverse long-term sequelae occur in patients who received cranial or craniospinal irradiation (Fig. 19.19). The risk in these individuals may not level off, even after 25 years of EFS.[502]

Despite early reports suggesting that CNS preventive therapy with lower dose cranial irradiation and IT chemotherapy was devoid of significant long-term side effects, a large body of evidence indicates that this treatment can produce abnormal brain scans (Fig. 19.20), impaired intellectual and psychomotor functions, and neuroendocrine abnormalities.[503,504] Four neuropathologically distinct forms of delayed CNS toxicity have been identified in patients with ALL: cortical atrophy, necrotizing leukoencephalopathy, subacute leukoencephalopathy, and mineralizing microangiopathy.[505]

Cortical atrophy, the most common histopathologic manifestation of CNS treatment, is a well-recognized delayed toxicity of whole brain irradiation. Radiation produces multiple microscopic areas of focal necrosis that eventually cause the loss of cortical tissue and generalized cortical atrophy.[506] Necrotizing leukoencephalopathy, a particularly severe form of delayed neurotoxicity, is relatively uncommon. It occurs most frequently in patients who have received large cumulative doses of cranial irradiation and IT and systemic MTX (e.g., for treatment of recurrent meningeal leukemia), but it also has been observed in patients who have not received cranial irradiation (Fig. 19.20).[507] Subacute leukoencephalopathy is characterized pathologically by multifocal demyelination. Patients with this syndrome may present with a variety of clinical findings, ranging from poor school performance and mild confusion to lethargy, dysarthria, dysphasia, ataxia, spasticity, or progressive dementia.[508]

Mineralizing microangiopathy, a degenerative mineralizing disorder of the small vessels, is accompanied by dystrophic calcification of brain tissue, primarily gray matter. It also occurs more frequently in patients who have received greater cumulative doses of cranial irradiation and IV MTX, particularly in younger children (<6 years). The intracerebral calcifications

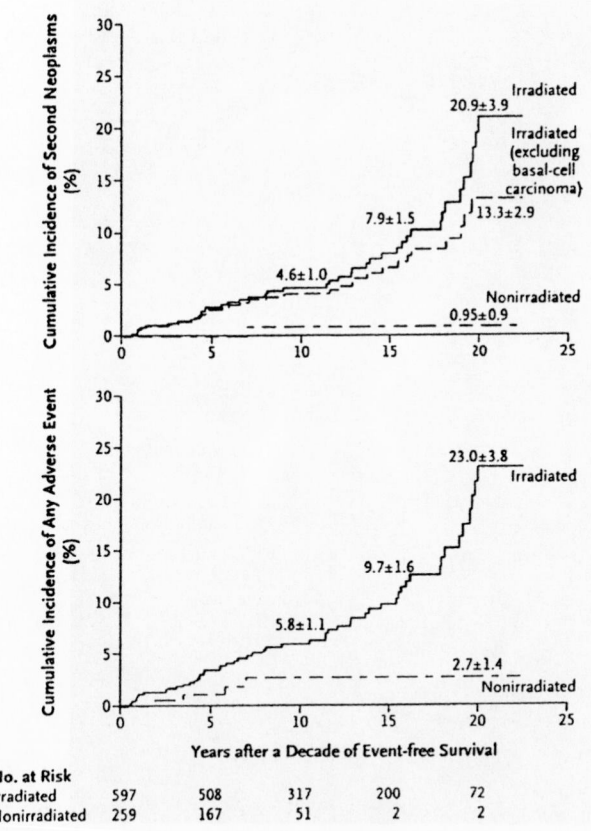

FIGURE 19.19 Mean (±SE) cumulative incidence of second neoplasms or any adverse event among patients attaining 10 or more years of event-free survival, according to whether or not they received cranial or craniospinal radiation. (From Pui C-H, Cheng C, Leung W, et al. Extended follow-up of long-term survivors of childhood acute lymphoblastic leukemia. N Engl J Med 2003;349;640–649, with permission.)

of mineralizing microangiopathy can be demonstrated on CT and MRI scans.

The mechanism(s) underlying this damage are unknown but may relate to chronic effects on the cerebral vasculature of CNS irradiation and/or chemotherapy.[509] MTX and the rises in homocysteine induced by MTX have been linked to both acute (seizures) and chronic neurologic toxicity. Homocysteine is further metabolized to the excitatory amino acid neurotransmitters homocysteic acid and cysteine sulfinic acid, which may also cause seizures and excitotoxic neuronal death.[509]

Numerous studies have demonstrated abnormal CT brain scans in asymptomatic ALL patients who have received CNS preventive therapy, particularly with cranial irradiation and IT chemotherapy. Abnormal CT scan findings identified include ventricular dilatation and widening of the subarachnoid spaces (i.e., cerebral cortical atrophy), decreased attenuation coefficient (i.e., hypodensity of white matter indicating localized edema, demyelination, or both), and intracerebral calcifications (i.e., mineralizing microangiography).[506] The incidence of these abnormalities appears to correlate with the intensity of CNS preventive therapy. Studies have documented a significant association between these abnormalities and neuropsychologic dysfunction.[510] The observation that CT scan lesions may first appear as late as 7 to 9 years after initiation of CNS preventive therapy is of concern and emphasizes the importance of long-term follow-up examination.

Furthermore, a variety of studies have identified the existence of functional CNS impairment in some survivors of childhood ALL. In addition to significantly impaired academic achievement, problems with poor body image and depression, decreased IQ scores, increased distractibility, and abnormalities in memory and frontal lobe functions have all been variously documented.[503,511] Studies of interventions for the important psychological and psychosocial consequences of the disease and its treatment are still in the early phases and must adjust to the differences generated by the vast changes in upfront modalities of treatment, while still caring for the survivors from earlier periods.[512,513] Careful follow-up with comprehensive neuropsychometric testing may permit early identification of developing deficits and possibly allow therapeutic intervention.

Although new approaches to CNS preventive therapy may offer the possibility of reducing or preventing adverse CNS sequelae, a large number of patients currently being followed by pediatric oncologists remain at risk for developing late CNS toxicity. Diagnostic MRI or CT scans of the brain every 2 to 3 years have been recommended for patients who have received cranial irradiation.[514] Patients who were very young at the time of diagnosis or cranial radiation therapy appear to be at the greatest risk. The finding of an apparent increased incidence of CT and MRI abnormalities in nonirradiated patients treated with intermediate-dose MTX and 6-MP indicates the importance of carefully following all patients who have received any form of CNS preventive therapy.[515]

Neuroendocrine abnormalities, primarily involving the hypothalamic pituitary axis, also have been documented in children who have received cranial radiotherapy with CNS preventive therapy. The principal finding is decreased growth hormone output measured by response to provocative stimuli or by analysis of basal pulsatile growth hormone (GH) secretion.[516,517] The incidence of impaired GH responses to provocative stimuli may be 50% or greater. Blunted spontaneous basal pulsatile secretion of GH is a consistent finding in children with ALL who have received 2,400 cGy of cranial irradiation and IT MTX. The effect of 1,800 cGy cranial irradiation on pulsatile GH secretion seems to be less severe. The use of therapeutic GH appears to be safe and does not contribute to relapse or formation of second cancers but has only moderate efficacy in impacting final adult height.[518]

Short stature occurs in some children with ALL, although there is disagreement about its frequency.[519] In many children, "catch-up growth" occurs after discontinuation of therapy; others have persistent short stature. A study of children with ALL treated without cranial irradiation reported that, although an initial decline in height and growth velocity was observed after diagnosis, compensatory increases occur during further treatment. The negative impact of cranial irradiation on growth is well known. Several studies have documented significant reduction in linear growth during and after therapy in patients who have received 2,400 cGy or more of cranial irradiation.[519,520] The data from these studies demonstrate that the final height of adults who received 2,400 cGy cranial irradiation as children is significantly reduced. Decreases have been reported for patients treated with 1,800 cGy, although this has not been a universal finding. The impact of 1,800 cGy on final adult height is reported to be modest, although girls treated with this approach at a young age maybe at risk for significant growth failure. The development of short stature after cranial irradiation requires ongoing comprehensive endocrine evaluation. If GH deficiency is documented, GH replacement may be appropriate.

Although abnormal GH output resulting from cranial irradiation may explain the short stature in some children, others have normal hypothalamic-pituitary function, suggesting that growth delay in children with ALL may be multifactorial.[521]

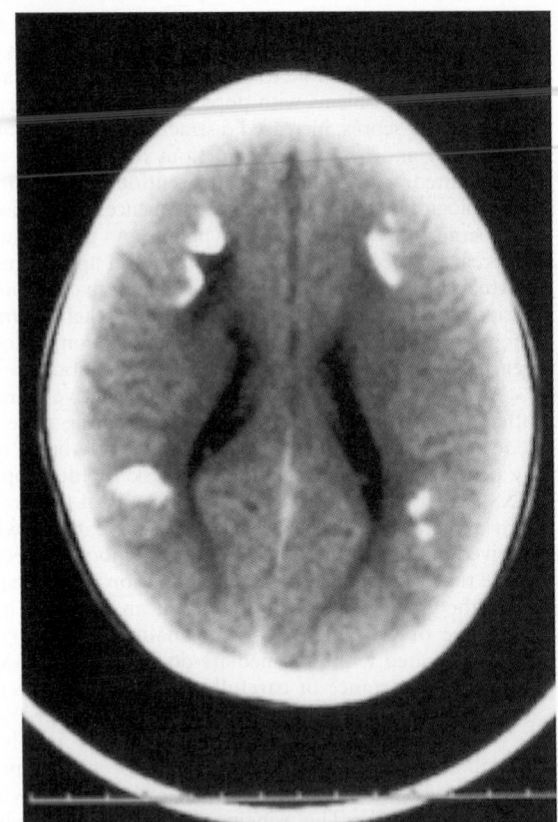 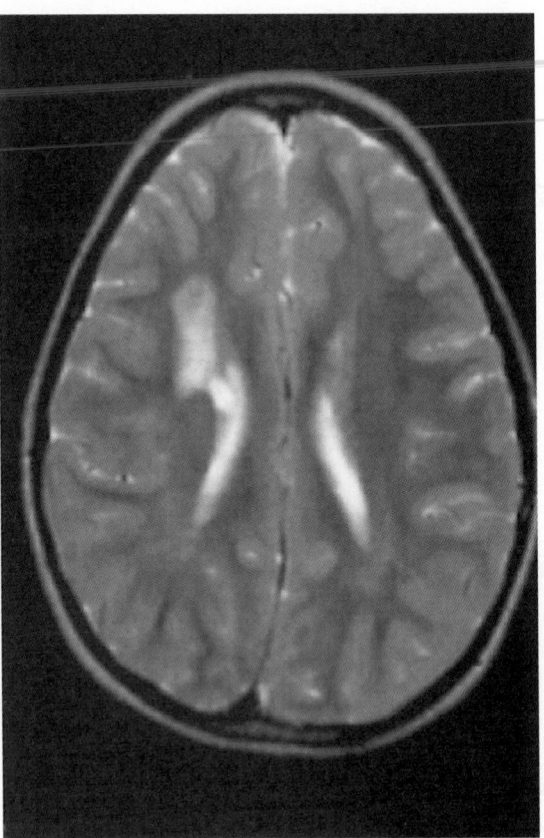

FIGURE 19.20 Radiographic measurement of the late effects of chemotherapy and radiotherapy on the central nervous system (CNS). **A:** Computed tomographic image of a patient with acute lymphoblastic leukemia (ALL) and CNS sequelae. Notice the intracerebral calcifications (discrete bright white areas). **B:** Magnetic resonance image of the same patient showing leukoencephalopathy (hypolucent, demyelinated tracts). This patient was originally diagnosed with standard-risk ALL and did not have CNS disease at any time. The patient received standard-risk therapy, which included intrathecal therapy with cytarabine, methotrexate, and hydrocortisone. No radiation therapy was administered. The patient has mild learning and motor disabilities approximately 5 years from diagnosis. Images were obtained several months after completion of therapy.

Effects of therapy on multiple organ systems cardiac, liver, as well as lung, dental and bone growth itself undoubtedly contribute to the growth problems of some children, both during and after ALL therapy.[522,523] Bone growth and mineralization can be significantly impaired, which predisposes these patients to an increased risk of fractures.[524] However, it does appear that these problems may be improving with modern therapies that do not include cranial radiation or result in long hospitalizations that promote demineralization.[525]

There appears to be a prevalence of obesity among children who have successfully completed therapy for ALL, although the effects of treatment can be difficult to separate from familial genetics and psychosocial issues that can lead to obesity.[526–528] Obesity at diagnosis has been found to be a mild poor prognostic factor on modern therapies.[529] Cranial irradiation is associated with the later development of obesity, but it seems likely that corticosteroids and other drugs are contributing factors.

Chemotherapy may produce long-term side effects in other organs. Patients receiving maintenance treatment frequently have elevated liver function tests, primarily a reflection of MTX hepatotoxicity. After chemotherapy stops, the test results of most patients usually return to normal, and persistent liver function abnormalities are rare.[530]

Many current ALL treatment regimens use anthracyclines. Treatment with these agents carries the potential risk of cardiomyopathy, but because the total cumulative doses of these agents in most protocols is considerably lower than 550 mg/m^2, clinically significant cardiomyopathy in patients undergoing active treatment is a relatively rare occurrence. However, studies suggest that patients exposed to anthracyclines for treatment of ALL may be at a greater risk for late-onset congestive heart failure than previously appreciated.[531,532] Exercise or pregnancy may provoke the occurrence of late-onset cardiomyopathy, or it may be spontaneous. In a study from the DFCI, more than one half of the group of long-term ALL patients who had received significant cumulative anthracycline dosages demonstrated evidence of abnormal left ventricular function.[533] Children younger at the time of treatment and with a greater cumulative anthracycline dose had a greater incidence of subclinical cardiac damage. This and similar reports have heightened concern about late anthracycline cardiotoxicity and emphasized the importance of careful monitoring and follow-up of children at risk.[534] There may be, in fact, no safe anthracycline dose that will avoid some possibility of cardiotoxicity, and the routine use of any amount of such agents in the initial treatment of lower or standard risk ALL patients is the subject of increasing debate.[535]

Other chemotherapeutic agents and modalities (i.e., radiation fields that include the cardiac region) may exacerbate anthracycline cardiac toxicity. Studies aimed at reducing and possibly circumventing anthracycline cardiotoxicity by administering these agents by continuous infusion or together with the cardioprotective agent dexrazoxane (Zinecard), have demonstrated only modest improvements in short-term, subclinical measurements of cardiac toxicity (see Chapters 10 and 47).[536] The contribution towards cure of the anthracyclines is unclear (even in high risk ALL where they are routinely used), and treatments without any anthracycline component have been successful in both high and low risk patients.[380]

Multiple other toxicities are associated with antileukemic agents. Hemorrhagic cystitis and bladder fibrosis from cyclophosphamide treatment, avascular necrosis secondary to steroid treatment, and significant sequelae of L-asparaginase-induced thrombosis and hemorrhagic infarction are encountered in ALL, but the frequency of these problems has been reduced either by avoidance of the agents, or by modification of the frequency and dosages that have been shown to cause these problems.

The reproductive capacity and sexual function of patients with ALL treated with prolonged chemotherapy has been studied.[537–539] Primary gonadal damage has been documented in patients of both sexes treated on a cyclophosphamide-containing intensive ALL treatment regimens. Cyclophosphamide, ifosfamide, and other alkylating agents continue to be used in many intensification schema and BMT preparative regimens. Although alkylating agent therapy can impair reproductive function, little information exists about the reproductive status of patients treated with other commonly used chemotherapies. In most cases, girls with leukemia retain intact reproductive function. However, the timing of chemotherapy in relation to puberty may be important.[540] A study of prepubertal boys who received chemotherapy for ALL, not including cyclophosphamide, also revealed no evidence of subsequent significant gonadal dysfunction.[541] Although this evidence is encouraging, additional information on a larger number of patients treated in the periods before, during, and after puberty is required before definitive conclusions about the reproductive capacity of these patients can be drawn.

More information is needed on the outcome of pregnancy after treatment for leukemia. Although our knowledge of the teratogenicity and mutagenicity of antileukemic therapy is incomplete, some data indicate that normal births occur in most cases in which women receive chemotherapy before gestation or after the first trimester.[542] Chemotherapy administered to men close to or before the time of insemination does not appear to result in fetal damage. Although available information suggests reason for cautious optimism, additional long-term follow-up of the offspring of survivors of childhood leukemia is needed.

The risk of second malignant neoplasm (SMN) in children with ALL has been estimated to be between 3% to 12% in the 5 to 24 years after their primary diagnosis.[543,544] This represents a 6- to 10-fold increase in risk (compared to the general population) for the development of future tumors. The non-hematopoietic SMNs tend to occur 5 to 10 years after the original ALL and, in many cases, occur within or in close proximity to the radiation fields used in the original therapy. Although a causal relation between the development of secondary brain tumors and cranial irradiation is likely, CNS tumors have also been reported for a small number of patients who have not received cranial irradiation.[545]

Investigators at St. Jude Children's Research Hospital reported an unexpected high incidence of secondary AML

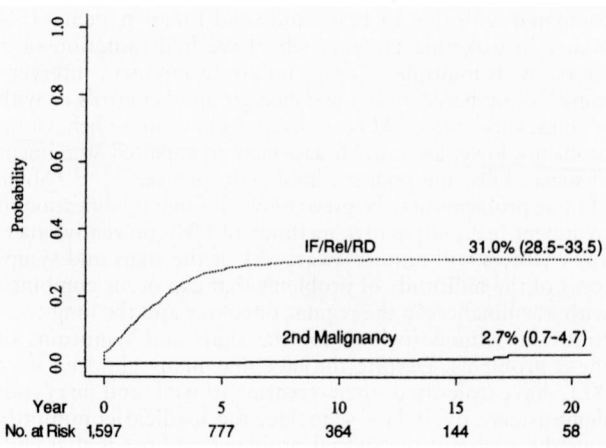

FIGURE 19.21 Risk of induction failure (IF), relapse (Rel), and remission death (RD) far exceeds the risk of second malignancies in patients treated for acute lymphoblastic leukemia. (From Kimball Dalton VM, Gelber RD, Li F, et al. Second malignancies in patients treated for childhood acute lymphoblastic leukemia. J Clin Oncol 1998;16:2848–2853, with permission.)

among a large group of patients treated with intensive chemotherapy, particularly those with T-cell ALL.[546] These leukemias developed a median of 3 years after the diagnosis of ALL and were predominantly characterized by an 11q23 chromosomal abnormality. The risk of developing secondary AML within 6 years of achieving initial remission in this study was estimated to be 5%. There appears to be a strong relation between prior exposure to epipodophyllotoxins and other topoisomerase II inhibitors, anthracyclines, and actinomycin D, and the development of these secondary AML with 11q23 abnormalities.[546] Similar secondary leukemias have been observed in other cancer patients treated with these drugs. Concern over these secondary myeloid leukemias has led to a reappraisal of the role of the epipodophyllotoxins in the treatment of ALL.[547]

Despite the degree of increase in risk of SMNs, the risk of other first events (i.e., induction failure, relapse, or death from another cause) remains 10-fold higher than the risk of developing a SMN (Fig. 19.21).[543] Most reported SMNs are brain tumors (gliomas of varying histologic grades) occurring in patients who received cranial radiation and hematopoietic tumors (primarily AML or myelodysplastic syndrome [MDS]) in all other patients.[543] Other reported tumors include thyroid tumors, melanoma, dysgerminoma, ganglioneuroblastoma, leiomyosarcoma, mucoepidermoid carcinoma of the parotid, osteosarcoma, adenocarcinoma of the colon, and testicular carcinoma.[543,548,549]

Physicians should be aware of the effects of previous chemotherapy on the immune system of children treated for ALL. Earlier studies suggested that recovery of the immune system occurs within the first year after completion of chemotherapy. More recent studies show that a significant percentage of patients have persistence of abnormally low immunoglobulins and other evidence of immune suppression as late as 2 years after completion of treatment.[550] As many as one third of patients have low antibody titers to clinically significant viruses to which they had been previously immunized.[562]

The psychosocial status of long-term survivors of ALL is an area of considerable concern. Posttraumatic stress disorder (PTSD) has been described in as many as 20% of young adult survivors of childhood cancer.[551,552] The rate and severity of PTSD is lower in the survivors of pediatric leukemia when compared with that of brain and solid tumor patients. It is higher in leukemia patients who have had radiation or a course with multiple relapses requiring intensive interventions.[552] Compared with a matched group of controls or with siblings, survivors of ALL are likely to have more behavioral problems, lower levels of life satisfaction, impaired attainment of social skills, and poorer school performance.[371,470,553] Some of these problems may be preventable through modification of treatment (e.g., alternative methods of CNS preventive therapy). Others will require awareness of the signs and symptoms of the multitude of problems that can occur combined with a willingness in the regular oncology and the long-term follow-up clinics to look for the signs and symptoms of these problems. Despite the fact that many children with ALL have tolerated their treatment well and may not demonstrate overt late sequelae, the medical community must be aware of the special problems and needs that children with ALL may incur as they are reincorporated into mainstream society.

FUTURE CHALLENGES

Although there has been dramatic progress in the treatment of ALL in the past half century, overall approximately 10% to 15% of patients with ALL who have access to the most advanced therapies still die of their disease. In addition, a number of those who are cured have suffered significant acute toxicities and/or long-term adverse sequelae. Hope for future progress lies in the improved understanding of the biology of ALL that is likely to come from the application of new molecular and genomic technologies to the study of this disease, which will allow for more individualized therapy. As new therapies emerge, international cooperative trials will likely be required to confirm their effectiveness with statistical certainty. This is particularly true in rare subgroups of patients in which the only way to develop a statistically significant sample would require an international effort.[554] In the near term, the therapeutic strategies developed over the past 60 years are likely to remain the mainstays of therapy. However, there continues to be significant progress in the development of new drugs and treatment strategies for this disease (see Chapters 11 and 14). It is conceivable that better understanding of the mechanism(s) of leukemogenesis may allow for preventive, intervention strategies.

A major challenge for the immediate future is to ensure that effective treatment of ALL be made more available to affected children worldwide. This point was emphasized in the Ponte di Legno Working Group publication that declared the "right of children with leukemia to have full access *to essential treatment for acute lymphoblastic leukemia.*"[554] Despite the impressive successes to date, ultimate control of this disease will not occur until every form of ALL becomes curable and every child with ALL has access to curative therapy.

References

1. Pui CH, Robison LL, Look AT. Acute lymphoblastic leukaemia. Lancet 2008;371:1030–1043.
2. Stanulla M, Schrappe M. Treatment of childhood acute lymphoblastic leukemia. Semin Hematol 2009;46:52–63.
3. Yang JJ, Cheng C, Yang W, et al. Genome-wide interrogation of germline genetic variation associated with treatment response in childhood acute lymphoblastic leukemia. JAMA 2009;301:393–403.
4. Stat bite: estimated new leukemia cases in 2008. J Natl Cancer Inst 2008;100:531.
5. Jemal A, Tiwari RC, Murray T, et al. Cancer statistics, 2004. CA Cancer J Clin 2004;54:8–29.
6. Jemal A, Siegel R, Ward E, Hao Y, et al. Cancer statistics, 2009. CA Cancer J Clin 2009;59:225–249.
7. Hrusak O, Trka J, Zuna J, Polouckova A, et al. Acute lymphoblastic leukemia incidence during socioeconomic transition: selective increase in children from 1 to 4 years. Leukemia 2002;16:720–725.
8. Pollock BH, DeBaun MR, Camitta BM, et al. Racial differences in the survival of childhood B-precursor acute lymphoblastic leukemia: a Pediatric Oncology Group Study. J Clin Oncol 2000;18:813–823.
9. Bhatia S, Sather HN, Heerema NA, et al. Racial and ethnic differences in survival of children with acute lymphoblastic leukemia. Blood 2002;100:1957–1964.
10. Carroll WL. Race and outcome in childhood acute lymphoblastic leukemia. JAMA 2003;290:2061–2063.
11. Kadan-Lottick NS, Ness KK, Bhatia S, et al. Survival variability by race and ethnicity in childhood acute lymphoblastic leukemia. JAMA 2003;290:2008–2014.
12. Pullarkat ST, Danley K, Bernstein L, et al. High lifetime incidence of adult acute lymphoblastic leukemia among Hispanics in California. Cancer Epidemiol Biomarkers Prev 2009;18:611–615.
13. Pui CH, Relling MV, Downing JR. Acute lymphoblastic leukemia. N Engl J Med 2004;350:1535–1548.
14. Greaves MF, Colman SM, Beard ME, et al. Geographical distribution of acute lymphoblastic leukaemia subtypes: second report of the collaborative group study. Leukemia 1993;7:27–34.
15. Ramot B, Magrath I. Hypothesis: the environment is a major determinant of the immunological sub-type of lymphoma and acute lymphoblastic leukaemia in children. Br J Haematol 1982;50:183–189.
16. Ross JA, Potter JD, Shu XO, et al. Evaluating the relationships among maternal reproductive history, birth characteristics, and infant leukemia: a report from the Children's Cancer Group. Ann Epidemiol 1997;7:172–179.
17. Caughey RW, Michels KB. Birth weight and childhood leukemia: a meta-analysis and review of the current evidence. Int J Cancer 2009;124:2658–2670.
18. Callan AC, Milne E. Involvement of the IGF system in fetal growth and childhood cancer: an overview of potential mechanisms. Cancer Causes Control 2009;20(10):1783–1798.
19. Milne E, Laurvick CL, Blair E, et al. Fetal growth and the risk of childhood CNS tumors and lymphomas in Western Australia. Int J Cancer 2008;123:436–443.
20. Lee KM, Ward MH, Han S, et al. Paternal smoking, genetic polymorphisms in CYP1A1 and childhood leukemia risk. Leuk Res 2009;33:250–258.
21. Zenzes MT, Puy LA, Bielecki R, et al. Detection of benzo[a]pyrene diol epoxide-DNA adducts in embryos from smoking couples: evidence for transmission by spermatozoa. Mol Hum Reprod 1999;5:125–131.
22. Mathonnet G, Krajinovic M, Labuda D, et al. Role of DNA mismatch repair genetic polymorphisms in the risk of childhood acute lymphoblastic leukaemia. Br J Haematol 2003;123:45–48.

23. McNally RJ, Alexander FE, Vincent TJ, et al. Spatial clustering of childhood cancer in Great Britain during the period 1969–1993. Int J Cancer 2009;124:932–936.
24. Zwaan MC, Reinhardt D, Hitzler J, et al. Acute leukemias in children with Down syndrome. Pediatr Clin North Am 2008;55:53–70, x.
25. Avet-Loiseau H, Mechinaud F, Harousseau JL. Clonal hematologic disorders in Down syndrome. A review. J Pediatr Hematol Oncol 1995;17:19–24.
26. Hasle H. Pattern of malignant disorders in individuals with Down's syndrome. Lancet Oncol 2001;2:429–436.
27. Linabery AM, Blair CK, Gamis AS, et al. Congenital abnormalities and acute leukemia among children with Down syndrome: a Children's Oncology Group study. Cancer Epidemiol Biomarkers Prev 2008;17:2572–2577.
28. Rabin KR, Whitlock JA. Malignancy in children with trisomy 21. Oncologist 2009;14:164–173.
29. Arico M, Ziino O, Valsecchi MG, et al. Acute lymphoblastic leukemia and Down syndrome: presenting features and treatment outcome in the experience of the Italian Association of Pediatric Hematology and Oncology (AIEOP). Cancer 2008;113:515–521.
30. Forestier E, Izraeli S, Beverloo B, et al. Cytogenetic features of acute lymphoblastic and myeloid leukemias in pediatric patients with Down syndrome: an iBFM-SG study. Blood 2008;111:1575–1583.
31. Bercovich D, Ganmore I, Scott LM, et al. Mutations of JAK2 in acute lymphoblastic leukaemias associated with Down's syndrome. Lancet 2008;372:1484–1492.
32. Russell LJ, Capasso M, Vater I, et al. Deregulated expression of cytokine receptor gene, CRLF2, is involved in lymphoid transformation in B cell precursor acute lymphoblastic leukemia. Blood 2009;114(13):2688–2698.
33. Whitlock JA, Sather HN, Gaynon P, et al. Clinical characteristics and outcome of children with Down syndrome and acute lymphoblastic leukemia: a Children's Cancer Group study. Blood 2005;106:4043–4049.
34. Wagner JE, Tolar J, Levran O, et al. Germline mutations in BRCA2: shared genetic susceptibility to breast cancer, early onset leukemia, and Fanconi anemia. Blood 2004;103:3226–3229.
35. Khatib Z, Levi A, Pefkarou A, et al. Acute lymphocytic leukemia in a child with Beckwith-Wiedemann syndrome. J Pediatr Hematol Oncol 2004;26:45–47.
36. Shearer P, Parham D, Kovnar E, et al. Neurofibromatosis type I and malignancy: review of 32 pediatric cases treated at a single institution. Med Pediatr Oncol 1994;22:78–83.
37. Woods WG, Roloff JS, Lukens JN, et al. The occurrence of leukemia in patients with the Shwachman syndrome. J Pediatr 1981;99:425–428.
38. Duker NJ. Chromosome breakage syndromes and cancer. Am J Med Genet 2002;115:125–129.
39. Tischkowitz M, Dokal I. Fanconi anaemia and leukaemia – clinical and molecular aspects. Br J Haematol 2004;126:176–191.
40. Killen MW, Stults DM, Adachi N, et al. Loss of Bloom syndrome protein destabilizes human gene cluster architecture. Hum Mol Genet 2009;18(18):3417–3428.
41. Guo R, Xu D, Wang W. Identification and analysis of new proteins involved in the DNA damage response network of Fanconi anemia and Bloom syndrome. Methods 2009;48:72–79.
42. Yamada Y, Inoue R, Fukao T, et al. Ataxia telangiectasia associated with B-cell lymphoma: the effect of a half-dose of the drugs administered according to the acute lymphoblastic leukemia standard risk protocol. Pediatr Hematol Oncol 1998;15:425–429.
43. Savitsky K, Bar-Shira A, Gilad S, et al. A single ataxia telangiectasia gene with a product similar to PI-3 kinase. Science 1995;268:1749–1753.

44. Gumy Pause F, Wacker P, Maillet P, et al. ATM gene alterations in childhood acute lymphoblastic leukemias. Hum Mutat 2003;21:554.
45. Hasle H, Mellemgaard A, Nielsen J, et al. Cancer incidence in men with Klinefelter syndrome. Br J Cancer 1995;71:416–420.
46. Keung YK, Buss D, Chauvenet A, et al. Hematologic malignancies and Klinefelter syndrome. a chance association? Cancer Genet Cytogenet 2002;139:9–13.
47. Machatschek JN, Schrauder A, Helm F, et al. Acute lymphoblastic leukemia and Klinefelter syndrome in children: two cases and review of the literature. Pediatr Hematol Oncol 2004;21:621–626.
48. Greaves MF, Wiemels J. Origins of chromosome translocations in childhood leukaemia. Nat Rev Cancer 2003;3:639–649.
49. Wiemels J, Kang M, Greaves M. Backtracking of leukemic clones to birth. Methods Mol Biol 2009;538:7–27.
50. Papaemmanuil E, Hosking FJ, Vijayakrishnan J, et al. Loci on 7p12.2, 10q21.2 and 14q11.2 are associated with risk of childhood acute lymphoblastic leukemia. Nat Genet 2009;41:1006–1010.
51. Trevino LR, Yang W, French D, et al. Germline genomic variants associated with childhood acute lymphoblastic leukemia. Nat Genet 2009;41:1001–1005.
52. Mullighan CG, Downing JR. Global genomic characterization of acute lymphoblastic leukemia. Semin Hematol 2009;46:3–15.
53. Infante-Rivard C, Guiguet M. Family history of hematopoietic and other cancers in children with acute lymphoblastic leukemia. Cancer Detect Prev 2004;28:83–87.
54. Greaves MF, Maia AT, Wiemels JL, et al. Leukemia in twins: lessons in natural history. Blood 2003;102:2321–2333.
55. Moloney WC. Leukemia in survivors of atomic bombing. N Engl J Med 1955;253:88–90.
56. Wakeford R, Kendall GM, Little MP. The proportion of childhood leukaemia incidence in Great Britain that may be caused by natural background ionizing radiation. Leukemia 2009;23:770–776.
57. Brill AB, Tomonaga M, Heyssel RM. Leukemia in man following exposure to ionizing radiation. A summary of the findings in Hiroshima and Nagasaki, and a comparison with other human experience. Ann Intern Med 1962;56:590–609.
58. National Research Council. Health Effects of Low Dose Irradiation. National Academic Press 1990:352–354.
59. Neglia JP, Robison LL. Epidemiology of the childhood acute leukemias. Pediatr Clin North Am 1988;35:675–692.
60. Shu XO, Potter JD, Linet MS, et al. Diagnostic X-rays and ultrasound exposure and risk of childhood acute lymphoblastic leukemia by immunophenotype. Cancer Epidemiol Biomarkers Prev 2002;11:177–185.
61. Evans JS, Wennberg JE, McNeil BJ. The influence of diagnostic radiography on the incidence of breast cancer and leukemia. N Engl J Med 1986;315:810–815.
62. Bone CM, Hsieh GH. The risk of carcinogenesis from radiographs to pediatric orthopaedic patients. J Pediatr Orthop 2000;20:251–254.
63. Brown WM, Doll R. Mortality from cancer and other causes after radiotherapy for ankylosing spondylitis. Br Med J 1965;5474:1327–1332.
64. Murray R, Heckel P, Hempelmann LH. Leukemia in children exposed to ionizing radiation. N Engl J Med 1959;261:585–589.
65. Davies AM, Modan B, Djaldetti M, et al. Epidemiological observations on leukemia in Israel. Arch Intern Med 1961;108:86–90.
66. Little MP, Wakeford R, Tawn EJ, et al. Risks associated with low doses and low dose rates of ionizing radiation: why linearity may be (almost) the best we can do. Radiology 2009;251:6–12.
67. Ahlbom A, Day N, Feychting M, et al. A pooled analysis of magnetic fields and childhood leukaemia. Br J Cancer 2000;83:692–698.
68. Akyol Erikci A, Ozyurt M, Terekeci H, et al. Oesophageal aspergillosis in a case of acute lymphoblastic leukaemia successfully treated with caspofungin alone due to liposomal amphotericin B induced severe hepatotoxicity. Mycoses 2009;52:84–86.
69. Buffler PA, Kwan ML, Reynolds P, et al. Environmental and genetic risk factors for childhood leukemia: appraising the evidence. Cancer Invest 2005;23:60–75.
70. Tucker MA, Meadows AT, Boice JD Jr, et al. Leukemia after therapy with alkylating agents for childhood cancer. J Natl Cancer Inst 1987;78:459–464.
71. Greaves M, Buffler PA. Infections in early life and risk of childhood ALL. Br J Cancer 2009;100:863.
72. Greaves MF. Biological models for leukaemia and lymphoma. IARC Sci Publ 2004: 351–372.
73. Nyari TA, Kajtar P, Bartyik K, et al. Seasonal variation of childhood acute lymphoblastic leukaemia is different between girls and boys. Pathol Oncol Res 2008;14:423–428.
74. Smith MA, Strickler HD, Granovsky M, et al. Investigation of leukemia cells from children with common acute lymphoblastic leukemia for genomic sequences of the primate polyomaviruses JC virus, BK virus, and simian virus 40. Med Pediatr Oncol 1999;33: 441–443.
75. Greaves MF, Alexander FE. An infectious etiology for common acute lymphoblastic leukemia in childhood? Leukemia 1993;7:349–360.
76. McClain KL, Leach CT, Jenson HB, et al. Association of Epstein-Barr virus with leiomyosarcomas in children with AIDS. N Engl J Med 1995;332:12–18.
77. Konior GS, Leventhal BG. Immunocompetence and prognosis in acute leukemia. Semin Oncol 1976;3:283–288.
78. Mustafa MM, Buchanan GR, Winick NJ, et al. Immune recovery in children with malignancy after cessation of chemotherapy. J Pediatr Hematol Oncol 1998;20: 451–457.
79. Leung W. Immunotherapy in acute leukemia. Semin Hematol 2009;46:89–99.
80. Kasprzyk A, Harrison CJ, Secker-Walker LM. Investigation of clonal involvement of myeloid cells in Philadelphia-positive and high hyperdiploid acute lymphoblastic leukemia. Leukemia 1999;13:2000–2006.
81. Bernt KM, Armstrong SA. Leukemia stem cells and human acute lymphoblastic leukemia. Semin Hematol 2009;46:33–38.
82. Felix CA, Reaman GH, Korsmeyer SJ, et al. Immunoglobulin and T cell receptor gene configuration in acute lymphoblastic leukemia of infancy. Blood 1987;70:536–541.
83. Kamen BA. Serendipity-methotrexate and 6-mercaptopurine for continuation therapy for patients with acute lymphoblastic leukemia: the leukemic stem cell and beyond? J Pediatr Hematol Oncol 2009;31:383–384.
84. Pui CH, Campana D. New definition of remission in childhood acute lymphoblastic leukemia. Leukemia 2000;14:783–785.
85. Rabbitts TH. Chromosomal translocations in human cancer. Nature 1994;372: 143–149.
86. Yeoh EJ, Ross ME, Shurtleff SA, et al. Classification, subtype discovery, and prediction of outcome in pediatric acute lymphoblastic leukemia by gene expression profiling. Cancer Cell 2002;1:133–143.
87. Lugthart S, Cheok MH, den Boer ML, et al. Identification of genes associated with chemotherapy crossresistance and treatment response in childhood acute lymphoblastic leukemia. Cancer Cell 2005;7:375–386.
88. Bhojwani D, Kang H, Menezes RX, et al. Gene expression signatures predictive of early response and outcome in high-risk childhood acute lymphoblastic leukemia: A Children's Oncology Group Study [corrected]. J Clin Oncol 2008;26:4376–4384.
89. Neff T, Armstrong SA. Chromatin maps, histone modifications and leukemia. Leukemia 2009;23:1243–1251.
90. Vaux DL, Cory S, Adams JM. Bcl-2 gene promotes haemopoietic cell survival and cooperates with c-myc to immortalize pre-B cells. Nature 1988;335:440–442.
91. Campana D, Coustan-Smith E, Manabe A, et al. Prolonged survival of B-lineage acute lymphoblastic leukemia cells is accompanied by overexpression of bcl-2 protein. Blood 1993;81:1025–1031.
92. Behm F. Classification of acute leukemias: perspective 2. In: Treatment of acute leukemias: new directions for clinical research. Totowa, NJ: Humana Press, 2003:43.
93. Bennett JM, Catovsky D, Daniel MT, et al. The morphological classification of acute lymphoblastic leukaemia: concordance among observers and clinical correlations. Br J Haematol 1981;47:553–561.
94. Brearley RL, Johnson SA, Lister TA. Acute lymphoblastic leukaemia in adults: clinicopathological correlations with the French-American-British (FAB) co-operative group classification. Eur J Cancer 1979;15:909–914.
95. Pullen DJ, Falletta JM, Crist WM, et al. Southwest Oncology Group experience with immunological phenotyping in acute lymphocytic leukemia of childhood. Cancer Res 1981;41:4802–4809.
96. Miller DR, Krailo M, Bleyer WA, et al. Prognostic implications of blast cell morphology in childhood acute lymphoblastic leukemia: a report from the Childrens Cancer Study Group. Cancer Treat Rep 1985;69:1211–1221.
97. Lilleyman JS, Hann IM, Stevens RF, et al. Cytomorphology of childhood lymphoblastic leukaemia: a prospective study of 2000 patients. United Kingdom Medical Research Council's Working Party on Childhood Leukaemia. Br J Haematol 1992;81:52–57.
98. Magrath IT, Ziegler JL. Bone marrow involvement in Burkitt's lymphoma and its relationship to acute B-cell leukemia. Leuk Res 1980;4:33–59.
99. Schumacher HR, Champion JE, Thomas WJ, et al. Acute lymphoblastic leukemia–hand mirror variant. An analysis of a large group of patients. Am J Hematol 1979;7:11–17.
100. Sjogren U, Garwicz S. Prognostic significance of amoeboid movement configuration in lymphoid cells from children with acute lymphoblastic leukaemia. Scand J Haematol 1980;24:335–339.
101. Hogeman PH, Veerman AJ, Huismans DR, et al. Handmirror cells and central nervous system relapse in childhood acute lymphoblastic leukaemia. Acta Haematol 1984;72: 181–189.
102. Wibowo A, Pankowsky D, Mikhael A, et al. Adult acute leukemia: hand mirror cell variant. Hematopathol Mol Hematol 1996;10:85–98.
103. Hodson D, Gatward G, Erber W. Azurophilic granules in acute lymphoblastic leukaemia resulting from abundant mitochondria. Br J Haematol 2004;125:265.
104. McKenna RW, Brynes RK, Nesbit ME, et al. Cycochemical profiles in acute lymphoblastic leukemia. Am J Pediatr Hematol Oncol 1979;1:263–275.
105. Heil G, Gunsilius E, Raghavachar A, et al. Ultrastructural demonstration of peroxidase expression in acute unclassified leukemias: correlation to immunophenotype and treatment outcome. Blood 1991;77:1305–1312.
106. Mirro J Jr, Kitchingman G, Behm FG, et al. T cell differentiation stages identified by molecular and immunologic analysis of the T cell receptor complex in childhood lymphoblastic leukemia. Blood 1987;69:908–912.
107. Roper M, Crist WM, Metzgar R, et al. Monoclonal antibody characterization of surface antigens in childhood T-cell lymphoid malignancies. Blood 1983;61:830–837.
108. Melnick SJ. Acute lymphoblastic leukemia. Clin Lab Med 1999;19:169–186, vii.
109. Williams DL, Raimondi S, Rivera G, et al. Presence of clonal chromosome abnormalities in virtually all cases of acute lymphoblastic leukemia. N Engl J Med 1985;313: 640–641.
110. Vogler LB, Crist WM, Bockman DE, et al. Pre-B-cell leukemia. A new phenotype of childhood lymphoblastic leukemia. N Engl J Med 1978;298:872–878.
111. Felix CA, Poplack DG. Characterization of acute lymphoblastic leukemia of childhood by immunoglobulin and T-cell receptor gene patterns. Leukemia 1991;5:1015–1025.
112. Uckun FM, Gaynon P, Sather H, et al. Clinical features and treatment outcome of children with biphenotypic CD2+ CD19+ acute lymphoblastic leukemia: a Children's Cancer Group study. Blood 1997;89:2488–2493.
113. Greaves MF, Janossy G, Peto J, et al. Immunologically defined subclasses of acute lymphoblastic leukaemia in children: their relationship to presentation features and prognosis. Br J Haematol 1981;48:179–197.
114. Korsmeyer SJ, Hieter PA, Ravetch JV, et al. Developmental hierarchy of immunoglobulin gene rearrangements in human leukemic pre-B-cells. Proc Natl Acad Sci U S A 1981;78:7096–7100.
115. Borowitz MJ. Immunologic markers in childhood acute lymphoblastic leukemia. Hematol Oncol Clin North Am 1990;4:743–765.
116. Felix CA, Poplack DG, Reaman GH, et al. Characterization of immunoglobulin and T-cell receptor gene patterns in B-cell precursor acute lymphoblastic leukemia of childhood. J Clin Oncol 1990;8:431–442.
117. Borowitz MJ, Rubnitz J, Nash M, et al. Surface antigen phenotype can predict TEL-AML1 rearrangement in childhood B-precursor ALL: a Pediatric Oncology Group study. Leukemia 1998;12:1764–1770.
118. Altman AJ. Clinical features and biological implications of acute mixed lineage (hybrid) leukemias. Am J Pediatr Hematol Oncol 1990;12:123–133.
119. Wiersma SR, Ortega J, Sobel E, et al. Clinical importance of myeloid-antigen expression in acute lymphoblastic leukemia of childhood. N Engl J Med 1991;324:800–808.
120. Pui CH, Behm FG, Singh B, et al. Myeloid-associated antigen expression lacks prognostic value in childhood acute lymphoblastic leukemia treated with intensive multiagent chemotherapy. Blood 1990;75:198–202.
121. Parkin JL, Arthur DC, Abramson CS, et al. Acute leukemia associated with the t(4;11) chromosome rearrangement: ultrastructural and immunologic characteristics. Blood 1982;60:1321–1331.
122. Hirsch-Ginsberg C, Childs C, Chang KS, et al. Phenotypic and molecular heterogeneity in Philadelphia chromosome-positive acute leukemia. Blood 1988;71:186–195.
123. Killick S, Matutes E, Powles RL, et al. Outcome of biphenotypic acute leukemia. Haematologica 1999;84:699–706.
124. Golub TR, Slonim DK, Tamayo P, et al. Molecular classification of cancer: class discovery and class prediction by gene expression monitoring. Science 1999;286:531–537.
125. Moos PJ, Raetz EA, Carlson MA, et al. Identification of gene expression profiles that segregate patients with childhood leukemia. Clin Cancer Res 2002;8:3118–3130.

126. Chen JS, Coustan-Smith E, Suzuki T, et al. Identification of novel markers for monitoring minimal residual disease in acute lymphoblastic leukemia. Blood 2001;97:2115–2120.
127. Holleman A, Cheok MH, den Boer ML, et al. Gene-expression patterns in drug-resistant acute lymphoblastic leukemia cells and response to treatment. N Engl J Med 2004;351:533–542.
128. Fine BM, Stanulla M, Schrappe M, et al. Gene expression patterns associated with recurrent chromosomal translocations in acute lymphoblastic leukemia. Blood 2004;103:1043–1049.
129. Armstrong SA, Golub TR, Korsmeyer SJ. MLL-rearranged leukemias: insights from gene expression profiling. Semin Hematol 2003;40:268–273.
130. Ross ME, Zhou X, Song G, et al. Classification of pediatric acute lymphoblastic leukemia by gene expression profiling. Blood 2003;102:2951–2959.
131. Willenbrock H, Juncker AS, Schmiegelow K, et al. Prediction of immunophenotype, treatment response, and relapse in childhood acute lymphoblastic leukemia using DNA microarrays. Leukemia 2004;18:1270–1277.
132. Lu XY, Harris CP, Cooley L, et al. The utility of spectral karyotyping in the cytogenetic analysis of newly diagnosed pediatric acute lymphoblastic leukemia. Leukemia 2002;16:2222–2227.
133. Rabin KR, Man TK, Yu A, et al. Clinical utility of array comparative genomic hybridization for detection of chromosomal abnormalities in pediatric acute lymphoblastic leukemia. Pediatr Blood Cancer 2008;51:171–177.
134. Mullighan CG, Downing JR. Genome-wide profiling of genetic alterations in acute lymphoblastic leukemia: recent insights and future directions. Leukemia 2009;23:1209–1218.
135. Trueworthy R, Shuster J, Look T, et al. Ploidy of lymphoblasts is the strongest predictor of treatment outcome in B-progenitor cell acute lymphoblastic leukemia of childhood: a Pediatric Oncology Group study. J Clin Oncol 1992;10:606–613.
136. Look AT, Roberson PK, Williams DL, et al. Prognostic importance of blast cell DNA content in childhood acute lymphoblastic leukemia. Blood 1985;65:1079–1086.
137. Heerema NA, Sather HN, Sensel MG, et al. Prognostic impact of trisomies of chromosomes 10, 17, and 5 among children with acute lymphoblastic leukemia and high hyperdiploidy (>50 chromosomes). J Clin Oncol 2000;18:1876–1887.
138. Pui CH, Carroll AJ, Head D, et al. Near-triploid and near-tetraploid acute lymphoblastic leukemia of childhood. Blood 1990;76:590–596.
139. Harris MB, Shuster JJ, Carroll A, et al. Trisomy of leukemic cell chromosomes 4 and 10 identifies children with B-progenitor cell acute lymphoblastic leukemia with a very low risk of treatment failure: a Pediatric Oncology Group study. Blood 1992;79:3316–3324.
140. Sutcliffe MJ, Shuster JJ, Sather HN, et al. High concordance from independent studies by the Children's Cancer Group (CCG) and Pediatric Oncology Group (POG) associating favorable prognosis with combined trisomies 4, 10, and 17 in children with NCI Standard-Risk B-precursor Acute Lymphoblastic Leukemia: a Children's Oncology Group (COG) initiative. Leukemia 2005;19:734–740.
141. Jackson JF, Boyett J, Pullen J, et al. Favorable prognosis associated with hyperdiploidy in children with acute lymphocytic leukemia correlates with extra chromosome 6. A Pediatric Oncology Group study. Cancer 1990;66:1183–1189.
142. Pettenati MJ, Rao N, Wofford M, et al. Presenting characteristics of trisomy 8 as the primary cytogenetic abnormality associated with childhood acute lymphoblastic leukemia. A Pediatric Oncology Group (POG) Study (8600/8493). Cancer Genet Cytogenet 1994;75:6–10.
143. Nishida K, Ritterbach J, Repp R, et al. Characterization of chromosome 8 abnormalities by fluorescence in situ hybridization in childhood B-acute lymphoblastic leukemia/non-Hodgkin lymphoma. Cancer Genet Cytogenet 1995;79:8–14.
144. Guerrasio A, Rosso C, Martinelli G, et al. Polyclonal haemopoieses associated with long-term persistence of the AML1-ETO transcript in patients with FAB M2 acute myeloid leukaemia in continuous clinical remission. Br J Haematol 1995;90:364–368.
145. Raimondi SC, Shurtleff SA, Downing JR, et al. 12p abnormalities and the TEL gene (ETV6) in childhood acute lymphoblastic leukemia. Blood 1997;90:4559–4566.
146. Heerema NA, Nachman JB, Sather HN, et al. Hypodiploidy with less than 45 chromosomes confers adverse risk in childhood acute lymphoblastic leukemia: a report from the children's cancer group. Blood 1999;94:4036–4045.
147. Raimondi SC, Zhou Y, Mathew S, et al. Reassessment of the prognostic significance of hypodiploidy in pediatric patients with acute lymphoblastic leukemia. Cancer 2003;98:2715–2722.
148. Nachman JB, Heerema NA, Sather H, et al. Outcome of treatment in children with hypodiploid acute lymphoblastic leukemia. Blood 2007;110:1112–1115.
149. Pui CH, Crist WM, Look AT. Biology and clinical significance of cytogenetic abnormalities in childhood acute lymphoblastic leukemia. Blood 1990;76:1449–1463.
150. Shurtleff SA, Buijs A, Behm FG, et al. TEL/AML1 fusion resulting from a cryptic t(12;21) is the most common genetic lesion in pediatric ALL and defines a subgroup of patients with an excellent prognosis. Leukemia 1995;9:1985–1989.
151. Aldrich MC, Zhang L, Wiemels JL, et al. Cytogenetics of Hispanic and White children with acute lymphoblastic leukemia in California. Cancer Epidemiol Biomarkers Prev 2006;15:578–581.
152. Stegmaier K, Pendse S, Barker GF, et al. Frequent loss of heterozygosity at the TEL gene locus in acute lymphoblastic leukemia of childhood. Blood 1995;86:38–44.
153. Morrow M, Horton S, Kioussis D, et al. TEL-AML1 promotes development of specific hematopoietic lineages consistent with preleukemic activity. Blood 2004;103:3890–3896.
154. Ford AM, Palmi C, Bueno C, et al. The TEL-AML1 leukemia fusion gene dysregulates the TGF-beta pathway in early B lineage progenitor cells. J Clin Invest 2009;119:826–836.
155. Loh ML, Rubnitz JE. TEL/AML1-positive pediatric leukemia: prognostic significance and therapeutic approaches. Curr Opin Hematol 2002;9:345–352.
156. Rubnitz JE, Behm FG, Wichlan D, et al. Low frequency of TEL-AML1 in relapsed acute lymphoblastic leukemia supports a favorable prognosis for this genetic subgroup. Leukemia 1999;13:19–21.
157. Loh ML, Goldwasser MA, Silverman LB, et al. Prospective analysis of TEL/AML1-positive patients treated on Dana-Farber Cancer Institute Consortium Protocol 95-01. Blood 2006;107:4508–4513.
158. Rubnitz JE, Wichlan D, Devidas M, et al. Prospective analysis of TEL gene rearrangements in childhood acute lymphoblastic leukemia: a Children's Oncology Group study. J Clin Oncol 2008;26:2186–2191.
159. Seeger K, Adams HP, Buchwald D, et al. TEL-AML1 fusion transcript in relapsed childhood acute lymphoblastic leukemia. The Berlin-Frankfurt-Munster Study Group. Blood 1998;91:1716–1722.
160. Zuna J, Ford AM, Peham M, et al. TEL deletion analysis supports a novel view of relapse in childhood acute lymphoblastic leukemia. Clin Cancer Res 2004;10:5355–5360.
161. Pui CH, Raimondi SC, Hancock ML, et al. Immunologic, cytogenetic, and clinical characterization of childhood acute lymphoblastic leukemia with the t(1;19) (q23; p13) or its derivative. J Clin Oncol 1994;12:2601–2606.
162. Kamps MP, Baltimore D. E2A-Pbx1, the t(1;19) translocation protein of human pre-B-cell acute lymphocytic leukemia, causes acute myeloid leukemia in mice. Mol Cell Biol 1993;13:351–357.
163. Dedera DA, Waller EK, LeBrun DP, et al. Chimeric homeobox gene E2A-PBX1 induces proliferation, apoptosis, and malignant lymphomas in transgenic mice. Cell 1993;74:833–843.
164. Lai JL, Fenaux P, Estienne MH, et al. Translocation t(1;19)(q23;p13) in acute lymphoblastic leukemia. A report on six new cases and an unusual t(17;19)(q11;q13), with special reference to prognostic factors. Cancer Genet Cytogenet 1989;37:9–17.
165. Devaraj PE, Foroni L, Sekhar M, et al. E2A/HLF fusion cDNAs and the use of RT-PCR for the detection of minimal residual disease in t(17;19)(q22;p13) acute lymphoblastic leukemia. Leukemia 1994;8:1131–1138.
166. Raimondi SC, Privitera E, Williams DL, et al. New recurring chromosomal translocations in childhood acute lymphoblastic leukemia. Blood 1991;77:2016–2022.
167. Yoshihara T, Inaba T, Shapiro LH, et al. E2A-HLF-mediated cell transformation requires both the trans-activation domains of E2A and the leucine zipper dimerization domain of HLF. Mol Cell Biol 1995;15:3247–3255.
168. Cline MJ. The molecular basis of leukemia. N Engl J Med 1994;330:328–336.
169. Harrison CJ. Cytogenetics of paediatric and adolescent acute lymphoblastic leukaemia. Br J Haematol 2009;144:147–156.
170. Rabbitts TH. Chromosomal translocation master genes, mouse models and experimental therapeutics. Oncogene 2001;20:5763–5777.
171. Cauwelier B, Dastugue N, Cools J, et al. Molecular cytogenetic study of 126 unselected T-ALL cases reveals high incidence of TCRbeta locus rearrangements and putative new T-cell oncogenes. Leukemia 2006;20:1238–1244.
172. Xia Y, Brown L, Tsan JT, et al. The translocation (1;14)(p34;q11) in human T-cell leukemia: chromosome breakage 25 kilobase pairs downstream of the TAL1 protooncogene. Genes Chromosomes Cancer 1992;4:211–216.
173. Aplan PD, Nakahara K, Orkin SH, et al. The SCL gene product: a positive regulator of erythroid differentiation. EMBO J 1992;11:4073–4081.
174. Van Vlierberghe P, van Grotel M, Beverloo HB, et al. The cryptic chromosomal deletion del(11)(p12p13) as a new activation mechanism of LMO2 in pediatric T-cell acute lymphoblastic leukemia. Blood 2006;108:3520–3529.
175. Hacein-Bey-Abina S, Von Kalle C, Schmidt M, et al. LMO2-associated clonal T cell proliferation in two patients after gene therapy for SCID-X1. Science 2003;302:415–419.
176. Hacein-Bey-Abina S, von Kalle C, Schmidt M, et al. A serious adverse event after successful gene therapy for X-linked severe combined immunodeficiency. N Engl J Med 2003;348:255–256.
177. Rabbitts TH, Boehm T. Structural and functional chimerism results from chromosomal translocation in lymphoid tumors. Adv Immunol 1991;50:119–146.
178. Weng AP, Ferrando AA, Lee W, et al. Activating mutations of NOTCH1 in human T cell acute lymphoblastic leukemia. Science 2004;306:269–271.
179. Real PJ, Tosello V, Palomero T, et al. Gamma-secretase inhibitors reverse glucocorticoid resistance in T cell acute lymphoblastic leukemia. Nat Med 2009;15:50–58.
180. Graux C, Cools J, Melotte C, et al. Fusion of NUP214 to ABL1 on amplified episomes in T-cell acute lymphoblastic leukemia. Nat Genet 2004;36:1084–1089.
181. Lahortiga I, De Keersmaecker K, Van Vlierberghe P, et al. Duplication of the MYB oncogene in T cell acute lymphoblastic leukemia. Nat Genet 2007;39:593–595.
182. Clappier E, Cuccuini W, Kalota A, et al. The C-MYB locus is involved in chromosomal translocation and genomic duplications in human T-cell acute leukemia (T-ALL), the translocation defining a new T-ALL subtype in very young children. Blood 2007;110:1251–1261.
183. Chen CS, Sorensen PH, Domer PH, et al. Molecular rearrangements on chromosome 11q23 predominate in infant acute lymphoblastic leukemia and are associated with specific biologic variables and poor outcome. Blood 1993;81:2386–2393.
184. Ford AM, Ridge SA, Cabrera ME, et al. In utero rearrangements in the trithorax-related oncogene in infant leukaemias. Nature 1993;363:358–360.
185. Thirman MJ, Gill HJ, Burnett RC, et al. Rearrangement of the MLL gene in acute lymphoblastic and acute myeloid leukemias with 11q23 chromosomal translocations. N Engl J Med 1993;329:909–914.
186. Behm FG, Raimondi SC, Frestedt JL, et al. Rearrangement of the MLL gene confers a poor prognosis in childhood acute lymphoblastic leukemia, regardless of presenting age. Blood 1996;87:2870–2877.
187. Raimondi SC, Peiper SC, Kitchingman GR, et al. Childhood acute lymphoblastic leukemia with chromosomal breakpoints at 11q23. Blood 1989;73:1627–1634.
188. Nowell PC. Molecular monitoring of pre-B acute lymphocytic leukemia. J Clin Oncol 1987;5:692–693.
189. Arico M, Valsecchi MG, Camitta B, et al. Outcome of treatment in children with Philadelphia chromosome-positive acute lymphoblastic leukemia. N Engl J Med 2000;342:998–1006.
190. Gandemer V, Auclerc MF, Perel Y, et al. Impact of age, leukocyte count and day 21-bone marrow response to chemotherapy on the long-term outcome of children with Philadelphia chromosome-positive acute lymphoblastic leukemia in the pre-imatinib era: results of the FRALLE 93 study. BMC Cancer 2009;9:14.
191. Ohno R. Treatment of adult patients with Philadelphia chromosome-positive acute lymphoblastic leukemia. Curr Oncol Rep 2008;10:379–387.
192. Burmeister T, Schwartz S, Bartram CR, et al. Patients' age and BCR-ABL frequency in adult B-precursor ALL: a retrospective analysis from the GMALL study group. Blood 2008;112:918–919.
193. Kohlmann A, Schoch C, Schnittger S, et al. Pediatric acute lymphoblastic leukemia (ALL) gene expression signatures classify an independent cohort of adult ALL patients. Leukemia 2004;18:63–71.
194. Groffen J, Stephenson JR, Heisterkamp N, et al. Philadelphia chromosomal breakpoints are clustered within a limited region, bcr, on chromosome 22. Cell 1984;36:93–99.
195. Look AT. The emerging genetics of acute lymphoblastic leukemia: clinical and biologic implications. Semin Oncol 1985;12:92–104.
196. Cannizzaro LA, Nowell PC, Belasco JB, et al. The breakpoint in 22q11 in a case of Ph-positive acute lymphocytic leukemia interrupts the immunoglobulin light chain gene cluster. Cancer Genet Cytogenet 1985;18:173–177.
197. Lugo TG, Pendergast AM, Muller AJ, et al. Tyrosine kinase activity and transformation potency of bcr-abl oncogene products. Science 1990;247:1079–1082.

198. Suryanarayan K, Hunger SP, Kohler S, et al. Consistent involvement of the bcr gene by 9;22 breakpoints in pediatric acute leukemias. Blood 1991;77:324–330.
199. Lin F, Chase A, Bungey J, et al. Correlation between the proportion of Philadelphia chromosome-positive metaphase cells and levels of BCR-ABL mRNA in chronic myeloid leukaemia. Genes Chromosomes Cancer 1995;13:110–114.
200. Talpaz M, Kantarjian H, Liang J, et al. Percentage of Philadelphia chromosome (Ph)-negative and Ph-positive cells found after autologous transplantation for chronic myelogenous leukemia depends on percentage of diploid cells induced by conventional-dose chemotherapy before collection of autologous cells. Blood 1995;85:3257–3263.
201. Pui CH, Howard SC. Current management and challenges of malignant disease in the CNS in paediatric leukaemia. Lancet Oncol 2008;9:257–268.
202. Russo C, Carroll A, Kohler S, et al. Philadelphia chromosome and monosomy 7 in childhood acute lymphoblastic leukemia: a Pediatric Oncology Group study. Blood 1991;77:1050–1056.
203. Heerema NA, Nachman JB, Sather HN, et al. Deletion of 7p or monosomy 7 in pediatric acute lymphoblastic leukemia is an adverse prognostic factor: a report from the Children's Cancer Group. Leukemia 2004;18:939–947.
204. Roberts WM, Rivera GK, Raimondi SC, et al. Intensive chemotherapy for Philadelphia-chromosome-positive acute lymphoblastic leukaemia. Lancet 1994;343:331–332.
205. Schultz KR, Bowman WP, Aledo A, et al. Improved early event-free survival with Imatinib in Philadelphia chromsome-positive ALL: A children's oncology group study. J Clin Oncol 2009;27:5275–5181.
206. Heerema NA, Harbott J, Galimberti S, et al. Secondary cytogenetic aberrations in childhood Philadelphia chromosome positive acute lymphoblastic leukemia are nonrandom and may be associated with outcome. Leukemia 2004;18:693–702.
207. Sulong S, Moorman AV, Irving JA, et al. A comprehensive analysis of the CDKN2A gene in childhood acute lymphoblastic leukemia reveals genomic deletion, copy number neutral loss of heterozygosity, and association with specific cytogenetic subgroups. Blood 2009;113:100–107.
208. Okuda T, Shurtleff SA, Valentine MB, et al. Frequent deletion of p16INK4a/MTS1 and p15INK4b/MTS2 in pediatric acute lymphoblastic leukemia. Blood 1995;85:2321–2330.
209. Hirama T, Koeffler HP. Role of the cyclin-dependent kinase inhibitors in the development of cancer. Blood 1995;86:841–854.
210. Heerema NA, Sather HN, Sensel MG, et al. Frequency and clinical significance of cytogenetic abnormalities in pediatric T-lineage acute lymphoblastic leukemia: a report from the Children's Cancer Group. J Clin Oncol 1998;16:1270–1278.
211. Hogan TF, Koss W, Murgo AJ, et al. Acute lymphoblastic leukemia with chromosomal 5;14 translocation and hypereosinophilia: case report and literature review. J Clin Oncol 1987;5:382–390.
212. Meeker TC, Hardy D, Willman C, et al. Activation of the interleukin-3 gene by chromosome translocation in acute lymphocytic leukemia with eosinophilia. Blood 1990; 76:285–289.
213. Secker-Walker LM, Alimena G, Bloomfield CD, et al. Cytogenetic studies of 21 patients with acute lymphoblastic leukemia in relapse. Cancer Genet Cytogenet 1989;40:163–169.
214. Felix CA, Nau MM, Takahashi T, et al. Hereditary and acquired p53 gene mutations in childhood acute lymphoblastic leukemia. J Clin Invest 1992;89:640–647.
215. Mekki Y, Catallo R, Bertrand Y, et al. Enhanced expression of p16ink4a is associated with a poor prognosis in childhood acute lymphoblastic leukemia. Leukemia 1999;13: 181–189.
216. Patmasiriwat P, Fraizer G, Kantarjian H, et al. WT1 and GATA1 expression in myelodysplastic syndrome and acute leukemia. Leukemia 1999;13:891–900.
217. Levis M, Small D. FLT3: ITDoes matter in leukemia. Leukemia 2003;17:1738–1752.
218. Qiu J, Gunaratne P, Peterson LE, et al. Novel potential ALL low-risk markers revealed by gene expression profiling with new high-throughput SSH-CCS-PCR. Leukemia 2003;17:1891–1900.
219. Brown P, Small D. FLT3 inhibitors: a paradigm for the development of targeted therapeutics for paediatric cancer. Eur J Cancer 2004;40:707–721, discussion 722–724.
220. Perentesis JP, Bhatia S, Boyle E, et al. RAS oncogene mutations and outcome of therapy for childhood acute lymphoblastic leukemia. Leukemia 2004;18:685–692.
221. Armstrong SA, Staunton JE, Silverman LB, et al. MLL translocations specify a distinct gene expression profile that distinguishes a unique leukemia. Nat Genet 2002;30:41–47.
222. Mullighan CG, Goorha S, Radtke I, et al. Genome-wide analysis of genetic alterations in acute lymphoblastic leukaemia. Nature 2007;446:758–764.
223. Mullighan CG, Miller CB, Radtke I, et al. BCR-ABL1 lymphoblastic leukaemia is characterized by the deletion of Ikaros. Nature 2008;453:110–114.
224. Mullighan CG, Su X, Zhang J, et al. Deletion of IKZF1 and prognosis in acute lymphoblastic leukemia. N Engl J Med 2009;360:470–480.
225. Mullighan CG, Zhang J, Harvey RC, et al. JAK mutations in high-risk childhood acute lymphoblastic leukemia. Proc Natl Acad Sci U S A 2009;106:9414–9418.
226. Harewood L, Robinson H, Harris R, et al. Amplification of AML1 on a duplicated chromosome 21 in acute lymphoblastic leukemia: a study of 20 cases. Leukemia 2003;17:547–553.
227. Soulier J, Trakhtenbrot L, Najfeld V, et al. Amplification of band q22 of chromosome 21, including AML1, in older children with acute lymphoblastic leukemia: an emerging molecular cytogenetic subgroup. Leukemia 2003;17:1679–1682.
228. Moorman AV, Richards SM, Robinson HM, et al. Prognosis of children with acute lymphoblastic leukemia (ALL) and intrachromosomal amplification of chromosome 21 (iAMP21). Blood 2007;109:2327–2330.
229. Akasaka T, Balasas T, Russell LJ, et al. Five members of the CEBP transcription factor family are targeted by recurrent IGH translocations in B-cell precursor acute lymphoblastic leukemia (BCP-ALL). Blood 2007;109:3451–3461.
230. Mullighan CG, Phillips LA, Su X, et al. Genomic analysis of the clonal origins of relapsed acute lymphoblastic leukemia. Science 2008;322:1377–1380.
231. Yang JJ, Bhojwani D, Yang W, et al. Genome-wide copy number profiling reveals molecular evolution from diagnosis to relapse in childhood acute lymphoblastic leukemia. Blood 2008;112:4178–4183.
232. Hoffbrand AV, Drexler HG, Ganeshaguru K, et al. Biochemical aspects of acute leukaemia. Clin Haematol 1986;15:669–694.
233. Desiderio SV, Yancopoulos GD, Paskind M, et al. Insertion of N regions into heavy-chain genes is correlated with expression of terminal deoxytransferase in B cells. Nature 1984;311:752–755.
234. Drexler HG, Menon M, Minowada J. Incidence of TdT positivity in cases of leukemia and lymphoma. Acta Haematol 1986;75:12–17.
235. Hutton JJ, Coleman MS, Moffitt S, et al. Prognostic significance of terminal transferase activity in childhood acute lymphoblastic leukemia: a prospective analysis of 164 patients. Blood 1982;60:1267–1276.
236. Poplack DG, Blatt J, Reaman G. Purine pathway enzyme abnormalities in acute lymphoblastic leukemia. Cancer Res 1981;41:4821–4823.
237. Babusikova O, Cap J, Hrivnakova A, et al. Purine metabolism enzyme pattern, cytochemical characteristics and clinicopathologic features of CD10-positive childhood T-cell leukemia. Neoplasma 1991;38:595–602.
238. Reaman GH, Levin N, Muchmore A, et al. Diminished lymphoblast 5′-nucleotidase activity in acute lymphoblastic leukemia with T-cell characteristics. N Engl J Med 1979;300:1374–1377.
239. Johnson SA, Thomas W. Therapeutic potential of purine analogue combinations in the treatment of lymphoid malignancies. Hematol Oncol 2000;18:141–153.
240. Sanford M, Lyseng-Williamson KA. Nelarabine. Drugs 2008;68:439–447.
241. Jeha S, Gaynon PS, Razzouk BI, et al. Phase II study of clofarabine in pediatric patients with refractory or relapsed acute lymphoblastic leukemia. J Clin Oncol 2006;24:1917–1923.
242. McGregor BA, Brown AW, Osswald MB, et al. The use of higher dose clofarabine in adults with relapsed acute lymphoblastic leukemia. Am J Hematol 2009;84:228–230.
243. Kornberg A, Polliack A. Serum lactic dehydrogenase (LDH) levels in acute leukemia: marked elevations in lymphoblastic leukemia. Blood 1980;56:351–355.
244. Radzun HJ, Parwaresch MR, Kulenkampff C, et al. Lysosomal acid esterase: activity and isoenzymes in separated normal human blood cells. Blood 1980;55:891–897.
245. Quddus FF, Leventhal BG, Boyett JM, et al. Glucocorticoid receptors in immunological subtypes of childhood acute lymphocytic leukemia cells: a Pediatric Oncology Group Study. Cancer Res 1985;45:6482–6486.
246. Mastrangelo R, Malandrino R, Riccardi R, et al. Clinical implications of glucocorticoid receptor studies in childhood acute lymphoblastic leukemia. Blood 1980;56:1036–1040.
247. Pui CH, Ochs J, Kalwinsky DK, et al. Impact of treatment efficacy on the prognostic value of glucocorticoid receptor levels in childhood acute lymphoblastic leukemia. Leuk Res 1984;8:345–350.
248. Schrappe M. Risk-adapted stratification and treatment of childhood acute lymphoblastic leukaemia. Radiat Prot Dosimetry 2008;132:130–133.
249. Evans WE, Relling MV. Pharmacogenomics: translating functional genomics into rational therapeutics. Science 1999;286:487–491.
250. McLeod HL, Krynetski EY, Relling MV, et al. Genetic polymorphism of thiopurine methyltransferase and its clinical relevance for childhood acute lymphoblastic leukemia. Leukemia 2000;14:567–572.
251. Karas-Kuzelicki N, Jazbec J, Milek M, et al. Heterozygosity at the TPMT gene locus, augmented by mutated MTHFR gene, predisposes to 6-MP related toxicities in childhood ALL patients. Leukemia 2009;23:971–974.
252. Relling MV, Hancock ML, Rivera GK, et al. Mercaptopurine therapy intolerance and heterozygosity at the thiopurine S-methyltransferase gene locus. J Natl Cancer Inst 1999;91:2001–2008.
253. Schmiegelow K, Al-Modhwahi I, Andersen MK, et al. Methotrexate/6-mercaptopurine maintenance therapy influences the risk of a second malignant neoplasm after childhood acute lymphoblastic leukemia: results from the NOPHO ALL-92 study. Blood 2009;113:6077–6084.
254. Stocco G, Cheok MH, Crews KR, et al. Genetic polymorphism of inosine triphosphate pyrophosphatase is a determinant of mercaptopurine metabolism and toxicity during treatment for acute lymphoblastic leukemia. Clin Pharmacol Ther 2009;85:164–172.
255. de Jonge R, Tissing WJ, Hooijberg JH, et al. Polymorphisms in folate-related genes and risk of pediatric acute lymphoblastic leukemia. Blood 2009;113:2284–2289.
256. Evans WE, Relling MV, Rodman JH, et al. Conventional compared with individualized chemotherapy for childhood acute lymphoblastic leukemia. N Engl J Med 1998;338: 499–505.
257. Davies SM, Robison LL, Buckley JD, et al. Glutathione S-transferase polymorphisms and outcome of chemotherapy in childhood acute myeloid leukemia. J Clin Oncol 2001;19:1279–1287.
258. Hall AG, Autzen P, Cattan AR, et al. Expression of mu class glutathione S-transferase correlates with event-free survival in childhood acute lymphoblastic leukemia. Cancer Res 1994;54:5251–5254.
259. Rocha JC, Cheng C, Liu W, et al. Pharmacogenetics of outcome in children with acute lymphoblastic leukemia. Blood 2005;105:4752–4758.
260. Davies SM, Borowitz MJ, Rosner GL, et al. Pharmacogenetics of minimal residual disease response in children with B-precursor acute lymphoblastic leukemia: a report from the Children's Oncology Group. Blood 2008;111:2984–2990.
261. French D, Hamilton LH, Mattano LA Jr, et al. A PAI-1 (SERPINE1) polymorphism predicts osteonecrosis in children with acute lymphoblastic leukemia: a report from the Children's Oncology Group. Blood 2008;111:4496–4499.
262. Ross JA, Oeffinger KC, Davies SM, et al. Genetic variation in the leptin receptor gene and obesity in survivors of childhood acute lymphoblastic leukemia: a report from the Childhood Cancer Survivor Study. J Clin Oncol 2004;22:3558–3562.
263. Jones OY, Spencer CH, Bowyer SL, et al. A multicenter case-control study on predictive factors distinguishing childhood leukemia from juvenile rheumatoid arthritis. Pediatrics 2006;117:e840–e844.
264. Crist WM, Shuster JJ, Falletta J, et al. Clinical features and outcome in childhood T-cell leukemia-lymphoma according to stage of thymocyte differentiation: a Pediatric Oncology Group Study. Blood 1988;72:1891–1897.
265. Pui CH, Behm FG, Singh B, et al. Heterogeneity of presenting features and their relation to treatment outcome in 120 children with T-cell acute lymphoblastic leukemia. Blood 1990;75:174–179.
266. Steinherz PG, Gaynon PS, Breneman JC, et al. Treatment of patients with acute lymphoblastic leukemia with bulky extramedullary disease and T-cell phenotype or other poor prognostic features: randomized controlled trial from the Children's Cancer Group. Cancer 1998;82:600–612.
267. Antony R, Roebuck D, Hann IM. Unusual presentations of acute lymphoid malignancy in children. J R Soc Med 2004;97:125–127.
268. Chang CY, Chiou TJ, Hsieh YL, et al. Leukemic infiltration of the urinary bladder presenting as uncontrollable gross hematuria in a child with acute lymphoblastic leukemia. J Pediatr Hematol Oncol 2003;25:735–739.
269. Turker M, Oren H, Yilmaz S, et al. Unusual presentation of childhood acute lymphoblastic leukemia: a case presenting with hypercalcemia symptoms only. J Pediatr Hematol Oncol 2004;26:116–117.
270. Sultan I, Kraveka JM, Lazarchick J. CD19 negative precursor B acute lymphoblastic leukemia presenting with hypercalcemia. Pediatr Blood Cancer 2004;43:66–69.
271. Jonsson OG, Sartain P, Ducore JM, et al. Bone pain as an initial symptom of childhood acute lymphoblastic leukemia: association with nearly normal hematologic indexes. J Pediatr 1990;117:233–237.

272. Nelken RP, Stockman JA III. The hypereosinophilic syndrome in association with acute lymphoblastic leukemia. J Pediatr 1976;89:771–773.
273. Testa JR, Hogge DE, Misawa S, et al. Chromosome 16 rearrangements in acute myelomonocytic leukemia with abnormal eosinophils. N Engl J Med 1984;310:468–469.
274. Bodey GP, Buckley M, Sathe YS, et al. Quantitative relationships between circulating leukocytes and infection in patients with acute leukemia. Ann Intern Med 1966;64: 328–340.
275. Gaydos LA, Freireich EJ, Mantel N. The quantitative relation between platelet count and hemorrhage in patients with acute leukemia. N Engl J Med 1962;266:905–909.
276. Homans AC, Cohen JL, Barker BE, et al. Aplastic presentation of acute lymphoblastic leukemia: evidence for cellular inhibition of normal hematopoietic progenitors. Am J Pediatr Hematol Oncol 1989;11:456–462.
277. Armata J, Grzeskowiak-Melanowska J, Balwierz W, et al. Prognosis in acute lymphoblastic leukemia (ALL) in children preceded by an aplastic phase. Leuk Lymphoma 1994;13:517–518.
278. Kikuchi M, Ohsaka A, Chiba Y, et al. Bone marrow aplasia with prominent atypical plasmacytic proliferation preceding acute lymphoblastic leukemia. Leuk Lymphoma 1999;35:213–217.
279. Ludwig WD, Haferlach T, Schoch C. Classification of acute leukemia: perspective I. In: Pui CH, ed. Treatment of acute leukemias: new directions for clinical research. Totowa, NJ: Humana Press; 2003:3.
280. Pui CH, Relling MV, Lascombes F, et al. Urate oxidase in prevention and treatment of hyperuricemia associated with lymphoid malignancies. Leukemia 1997;11:1813–1816.
281. Bunin NJ, Pui CH. Differing complications of hyperleukocytosis in children with acute lymphoblastic or acute nonlymphoblastic leukemia. J Clin Oncol 1985;3:1590–1595.
282. Kushner DC, Weinstein HJ, Kirkpatrick JA. The radiologic diagnosis of leukemia and lymphoma in children. Semin Roentgenol 1980;15:316–334.
283. Neglia JP, Day DL, Swanson TV, et al. Kidney size at diagnosis of childhood acute lymphocytic leukemia: lack of prognostic significance for outcome. Am J Pediatr Hematol Oncol 1988;10:296–300.
284. Harutsumi M, Akazai A, Kitamura T, et al. A case of acute lymphoblastic leukemia accompanied with the production of parathyroid hormone-related protein. Miner Electrolyte Metab 1995;21:171–176.
285. Masera G, Carnelli V, Ferrari M, et al. Prognostic significance of radiological bone involvement in childhood acute lymphoblastic leukaemia. Arch Dis Child 1977;52: 530–533.
286. Sitarz AL, Berdon WE, Wolff JA, et al. Acute lymphocytic leukemia masquerading as acute osteomyelitis. A report of two cases. Pediatr Radiol 1980;9:33–35.
287. Dowell BL, Borowitz MJ, Boyett JM, et al. Immunologic and clinicopathologic features of common acute lymphoblastic leukemia antigen-positive childhood T-cell leukemia. A Pediatric Oncology Group Study. Cancer 1987;59:2020–2026.
288. Leone G, Gugliotta L, Mazzucconi MG, et al. Evidence of a hypercoagulable state in patients with acute lymphoblastic leukemia treated with low dose of E. coli L-asparaginase: a GIMEMA study. Thromb Haemost 1993;69:12–15.
289. Castaman G, Rodeghiero F. Erwinia- and E. coli-derived L-asparaginase have similar effects on hemostasis. Pilot study in 10 patients with acute lymphoblastic leukemia. Haematologica 1993;78:57–60.
290. Bunin NJ, Pui CH, Hustu HO, et al. Unusual extramedullary relapses in children with acute lymphoblastic leukemia. J Pediatr 1986;109:665–668.
291. Bleyer WA. Central nervous system leukemia. Pediatr Clin North Am 1988;35: 789–814.
292. McIntosh S, Ritchey AK. Diagnostic problems in cerebrospinal fluid of children with lymphoid malignancies. Am J Pediatr Hematol Oncol 1986;8:28–31.
293. Mahmoud HH, Rivera GK, Hancock ML, et al. Low leukocyte counts with blast cells in cerebrospinal fluid of children with newly diagnosed acute lymphoblastic leukemia. N Engl J Med 1993;329:314–319.
294. Gilchrist GS, Tubergen DG, Sather HN, et al. Low numbers of CSF blasts at diagnosis do not predict for the development of CNS leukemia in children with intermediate-risk acute lymphoblastic leukemia: a Childrens Cancer Group report. J Clin Oncol 1994;12: 2594–2600.
295. Tubergen DG, Cullen JW, Boyett JM, et al. Blasts in CSF with a normal cell count do not justify alteration of therapy for acute lymphoblastic leukemia in remission: a Childrens Cancer Group study. J Clin Oncol 1994;12:273–278.
296. Smith M, Arthur D, Camitta B, et al. Uniform approach to risk classification and treatment assignment for children with acute lymphoblastic leukemia. J Clin Oncol 1996; 14:18–24.
297. Hooijkaas H, Hahlen K, Adriaansen HJ, et al. Terminal deoxynucleotidyl transferase (TdT)-positive cells in cerebrospinal fluid and development of overt CNS leukemia: a 5-year follow-up study in 113 children with a TdT-positive leukemia or non-Hodgkin's lymphoma. Blood 1989;74:416–422.
298. Howard SC, Gajjar AJ, Cheng C, et al. Risk factors for traumatic and bloody lumbar puncture in children with acute lymphoblastic leukemia. JAMA 2002;288:2001–2007.
299. Burger B, Zimmermann M, Mann G, et al. Diagnostic cerebrospinal fluid examination in children with acute lymphoblastic leukemia: significance of low leukocyte counts with blasts or traumatic lumbar puncture. J Clin Oncol 2003;21:184–188.
300. Bleyer WA. Biology and pathogenesis of CNS leukemia. Am J Pediatr Hematol Oncol 1989;11:57–63.
301. Evans AE, Gilbert ES, Zandstra R. The increasing incidence of central nervous system leukemia in children. (Children's Cancer Study Group A). Cancer 1970;26:404–409.
302. Sullivan MP, Vietti TJ, Haggard ME, et al. Remission maintenance therapy for meningeal leukemia: intrathecal methotrexate vs. intravenous bis-nitrosourea. Blood 1971;38:680–688.
303. Gribbin MA, Hardisty RM, Chessells JM. Long-term control of central nervous system leukaemia. Arch Dis Child 1977;52:673–678.
304. Kim TH, Hargreaves HK, Brynes RK, et al. Pretreatment testicular biopsy in childhood acute lymphocytic leukaemia. Lancet 1981;2:657–658.
305. Nachman J, Palmer NF, Sather HN, et al. Open-wedge testicular biopsy in childhood acute lymphoblastic leukemia after two years of maintenance therapy: diagnostic accuracy and influence on outcome–a report from Children's Cancer Study Group. Blood 1990;75:1051–1055.
306. Pui CH, Dahl GV, Bowman WP, et al. Elective testicular biopsy during chemotherapy for childhood leukaemia is of no clinical value. Lancet 1985;2:410–412.
307. Kim TH, Hargreaves HK, Chan WC, et al. Sequential testicular biopsies in childhood acute lymphocytic leukemia. Cancer 1986;57:1038–1041.
308. Klein EA, Kay R, Norris DG, et al. Noninvasive testicular screening in childhood leukemia. J Urol 1986;136:864–866.
309. Bowman WP, Aur RJ, Hustu HO, et al. Isolated testicular relapse in acute lymphocytic leukemia of childhood: categories and influence on survival. J Clin Oncol 1984;2: 924–929.
310. Chessells JM. Diagnostic value of testicular biopsy in acute lymphoblastic leukemia. J Pediatr 1986;108:331–332.
311. Chessells JM, Pincott JR, Daniels-Lake W. Terminal transferase positive cells in testicular biopsy specimens from boys with acute lymphoblastic leukaemia. J Clin Pathol 1986;39:1236–1240.
312. Verdi CJ, Hutter J, Grogan TM. Immunophenotyping to detect and characterize acute lymphocytic leukemia in testicular biopsies. Pediatr Pathol 1989;9:117–130.
313. Hustu HO, Aur RJ. Extramedullary leukaemia. Clin Haematol 1978;7:313–337.
314. Miller DR, Leikin SL, Albo VC, et al. The prognostic value of testicular biopsy in childhood acute lymphoblastic leukemia: a report from the Childrens Cancer Study Group. J Clin Oncol 1990;8:57–66.
315. Chessells JM, Veys P, Kempski H, et al. Long-term follow-up of relapsed childhood acute lymphoblastic leukaemia. Br J Haematol 2003;123:396–405.
316. Quaranta BP, Halperin EC, Kurtzberg J, et al. The incidence of testicular recurrence in boys with acute leukemia treated with total body and testicular irradiation and stem cell transplantation. Cancer 2004;101:845–850.
317. Finklestein JZ, Dyment PG, Hammond GD. Leukemic infiltration of the testes during bone marrow remission. Pediatrics 1969;43:1042–1045.
318. Riccardi R, Vigersky RA, Barnes S, et al. Methotrexate levels in the interstitial space and seminiferous tubule of rat testis. Cancer Res 1982;42:1617–1619.
319. Baum E, Heyn R, Nesbit M, et al. Occult abdominal involvement with apparently isolated testicular relapse in children with acute lymphocytic leukemia. Am J Pediatr Hematol Oncol 1984;6:343–346.
320. Kuo TT, Tschang TP, Chu JY. Testicular relapse in childhood acute lymphocytic leukemia during bone marrow remission. Cancer 1976;38:2604–2612.
321. Simone JV, Verzosa MS, Rudy JA. Initial features and prognosis in 363 children with acute lymphocytic leukemia. Cancer 1975;36:2099–2108.
322. Sather HN. Age at diagnosis in childhood acute lymphoblastic leukemia. Med Pediatr Oncol 1986;14:166–172.
323. Reaman G, Zeltzer P, Bleyer WA, et al. Acute lymphoblastic leukemia in infants less than one year of age: a cumulative experience of the Children's Cancer Study Group. J Clin Oncol 1985;3:1513–1521.
324. Kosaka Y, Koh K, Kinukawa N, et al. Infant acute lymphoblastic leukemia with MLL gene rearrangements: outcome following intensive chemotherapy and hematopoietic stem cell transplantation. Blood 2004;104:3527–3536.
325. Pulte D, Gondos A, Brenner H. Trends in survival after diagnosis with hematologic malignancy in adolescence or young adulthood in the United States, 1981–2005. Cancer 2009;115:4957–4979.
326. Crist W, Pullen J, Boyett J, et al. Acute lymphoid leukemia in adolescents: clinical and biologic features predict a poor prognosis–a Pediatric Oncology Group Study. J Clin Oncol 1988;6:34–43.
327. Silverman LB, Gelber RD, Dalton VK, et al. Improved outcome for children with acute lymphoblastic leukemia: results of Dana-Farber Consortium Protocol 91–01. Blood 2001;97:1211–1218.
328. Dinndorf PA, Reaman GH. Acute lymphoblastic leukemia in infants: evidence for B cell origin of disease by use of monoclonal antibody phenotyping. Blood 1986;68:975–978.
329. Peham M, Panzer S, Fasching K, et al. Low frequency of clonotypic Ig and T-cell receptor gene rearrangements in t(4;11) infant acute lymphoblastic leukaemia and its implication for the detection of minimal residual disease. Br J Haematol 2002;117: 315–321.
330. Ludwig WD, Bartram CR, Harbott J, et al. Phenotypic and genotypic heterogeneity in infant acute leukemia. I. Acute lymphoblastic leukemia. Leukemia 1989;3: 431–439.
331. Chowdhury T, Brady HJ. Insights from clinical studies into the role of the MLL gene in infant and childhood leukemia. Blood Cells Mol Dis 2008;40:192–199.
332. Zweidler-McKay PA, Hilden JM. The ABCs of infant leukemia. Curr Probl Pediatr Adolesc Health Care 2008;38:78–94.
333. Lauer SJ, Camitta BM, Leventhal BG, et al. Intensive alternating drug pairs after remission induction for treatment of infants with acute lymphoblastic leukemia: A Pediatric Oncology Group Pilot Study. J Pediatr Hematol Oncol 1998;20:229–233.
334. Murray RA, Thom G, Gardner RV, et al. Infant acute lymphoblastic leukemia: a 20-year children's hospital experience. Fetal Pediatr Pathol 2008;27:197–205.
335. Dordelmann M, Reiter A, Borkhardt A, et al. Prednisone response is the strongest predictor of treatment outcome in infant acute lymphoblastic leukemia. Blood 1999;94: 1209–1217.
336. Whitehead VM, Vuchich MJ, Cooley LD, et al. Accumulation of methotrexate polyglutamates, ploidy and trisomies of both chromosomes 4 and 10 in lymphoblasts from children with B-progenitor cell acute lymphoblastic leukemia: a Pediatric Oncology Group Study. Leuk Lymphoma 1998;31:507–519.
337. Synold TW, Relling MV, Boyett JM, et al. Blast cell methotrexate-polyglutamate accumulation in vivo differs by lineage, ploidy, and methotrexate dose in acute lymphoblastic leukemia. J Clin Invest 1994;94:1996–2001.
338. Pui CH, Boyett JM, Relling MV, et al. Sex differences in prognosis for children with acute lymphoblastic leukemia. J Clin Oncol 1999;17:818–824.
339. Shuster JJ, Wacker P, Pullen J, et al. Prognostic significance of sex in childhood B-precursor acute lymphoblastic leukemia: a Pediatric Oncology Group Study. J Clin Oncol 1998;16:2854–2863.
340. Borowitz MJ, Carroll AJ, Shuster JJ, et al. Use of clinical and laboratory features to define prognostic subgroups in B-precursor acute lymphoblastic leukemia: experience of the Pediatric Oncology Group. Recent Results Cancer Res 1993;131:257–267.
341. Herrera L, Yarbrough S, Ghetie V, et al. Treatment of SCID/human B cell precursor ALL with anti-CD19 and anti-CD22 immunotoxins. Leukemia 2003;17:334–338.
342. Nemecek ER, Matthews DC. Antibody-based therapy of human leukemia. Curr Opin Hematol 2002;9:316–321.
343. Reiter A, Schrappe M, Ludwig WD, et al. Chemotherapy in 998 unselected childhood acute lymphoblastic leukemia patients. Results and conclusions of the multicenter trial ALL-BFM 86. Blood 1994;84:3122–3133.
344. Miller DR, Leikin S, Albo V, et al. Use of prognostic factors in improving the design and efficiency of clinical trials in childhood leukemia: Children's Cancer Study Group Report. Cancer Treat Rep 1980;64:381–392.
345. Arico M, Basso G, Mandelli F, et al. Good steroid response in vivo predicts a favorable outcome in children with T-cell acute lymphoblastic leukemia. The Associazione Italiana Ematologia Oncologia Pediatrica (AIEOP). Cancer 1995;75:1684–1693.
346. Nachman JB, Sather HN, Sensel MG, et al. Augmented post-induction therapy for children with high-risk acute lymphoblastic leukemia and a slow response to initial therapy. N Engl J Med 1998;338:1663–1671.

347. Nachman J, Sather HN, Cherlow JM, et al. Response of children with high-risk acute lymphoblastic leukemia treated with and without cranial irradiation: a report from the Children's Cancer Group. J Clin Oncol 1998;16:920–930.
348. Gaynon PS, Bleyer WA, Steinherz PG, et al. Day 7 marrow response and outcome for children with acute lymphoblastic leukemia and unfavorable presenting features. Med Pediatr Oncol 1990;18:273–279.
349. Steinherz PG, Gaynon PS, Breneman JC, et al. Cytoreduction and prognosis in acute lymphoblastic leukemia–the importance of early marrow response: report from the Childrens Cancer Group. J Clin Oncol 1996;14:389–398.
350. Chessells JM, Harrison CJ, Watson SL, et al. Treatment of infants with lymphoblastic leukaemia: results of the UK Infant Protocols 1987–1999. Br J Haematol 2002;117: 306–314.
351. Gajjar A, Ribeiro R, Hancock ML, et al. Persistence of circulating blasts after 1 week of multiagent chemotherapy confers a poor prognosis in childhood acute lymphoblastic leukemia. Blood 1995;86:1292–1295.
352. Campana D. Minimal residual disease in acute lymphoblastic leukemia. Semin Hematol 2009;46:100–106.
353. Campana D. Status of minimal residual disease testing in childhood haematological malignancies. Br J Haematol 2008;143:481–489.
354. Borowitz MJ, Devidas M, Hunger SP, et al. Clinical significance of minimal residual disease in childhood acute lymphoblastic leukemia and its relationship to other prognostic factors: a Children's Oncology Group study. Blood 2008;111:5477–5485.
355. De Angulo G, Yuen C, Palla SL, et al. Absolute lymphocyte count is a novel prognostic indicator in ALL and AML: implications for risk stratification and future studies. Cancer 2008;112:407–415.
356. Reilly JJ, Odame I, McColl JH, et al. Does weight for height have prognostic significance in children with acute lymphoblastic leukemia? Am J Pediatr Hematol Oncol 1994;16:225–230.
357. Reilly JJ, Weir J, McColl JH, et al. Prevalence of protein-energy malnutrition at diagnosis in children with acute lymphoblastic leukemia. J Pediatr Gastroenterol Nutr 1999; 29:194–197.
358. Mejia-Arangure JM, Fajardo-Gutierrez A, Reyes-Ruiz NI, et al. Malnutrition in childhood lymphoblastic leukemia: a predictor of early mortality during the induction-to-remission phase of the treatment. Arch Med Res 1999;30:150–153.
359. Viana MB, Murao M, Ramos G, et al. Malnutrition as a prognostic factor in lymphoblastic leukaemia: a multivariate analysis. Arch Dis Child 1994;71:304–310.
360. Lobato-Mendizabal E, Ruiz-Arguelles GJ, Marin-Lopez A. Leukaemia and nutrition. I: Malnutrition is an adverse prognostic factor in the outcome of treatment of patients with standard-risk acute lymphoblastic leukaemia. Leuk Res 1989;13:899–906.
361. Antillon F, de Maselli T, Garcia T, et al. Nutritional status of children during treatment for acute lymphoblastic leukemia in the Central American Pediatric Hematology Oncology Association (AHOPCA): preliminary data from Guatemala. Pediatr Blood Cancer 2008;50:502–505; discussion 517.
362. Gupta S, Bonilla M, Fuentes SL, et al. Incidence and predictors of treatment-related mortality in paediatric acute leukaemia in El Salvador. Br J Cancer 2009;100: 1026–1031.
363. Lobato-Mendizabal E, Ruiz-Arguelles GJ. [Leukemia and malnutrition. II. The magnitude of maintenance chemotherapy as a prognostic factor in the survival of patients with standard-risk acute lymphoblastic leukemia]. Rev Invest Clin 1990;42:81–87.
364. Gonzalez A, Cortina L, Gonzalez P, et al. Longitudinal assessment of nutritional status in children treated for acute lymphoblastic leukaemia in Cuba. Eur J Cancer 2004;40: 1031–1034.
365. Corrigan JJ, Feig SA. Guidelines for pediatric cancer centers. Pediatrics 2004;113: 1833–1835.
366. Frei E III, Karon M, Levin RH, et al. The effectiveness of combinations of antileukemic agents in inducing and maintaining remission in children with acute leukemia. Blood 1965;26:642–656.
367. Skipper HE, Perry S. Kinetics of normal and leukemic leukocyte populations and relevance to chemotherapy. Cancer Res 1970;30:1883–1897.
368. Hart JS, Shirakawa S, Trujillo J, et al. The mechanism of induction of complete remission in acute myeloblastic leukemia in man. Cancer Res 1969;29:2300–2307.
369. Schrappe M, Reiter A, Riehm H. Cytoreduction and prognosis in childhood acute lymphoblastic leukemia. J Clin Oncol 1996;14:2403–2406.
370. Ortega JA, Nesbit ME Jr, Donaldson MH, et al. L-Asparaginase, vincristine, and prednisone for induction of first remission in acute lymphocytic leukemia. Cancer Res 1977;37:535–540.
371. Kaspers GJ, Veerman AJ, Popp-Snijders C, et al. Comparison of the antileukemic activity in vitro of dexamethasone and prednisolone in childhood acute lymphoblastic leukemia. Med Pediatr Oncol 1996;27:114–121.
372. Ito C, Evans WE, McNinch L, et al. Comparative cytotoxicity of dexamethasone and prednisolone in childhood acute lymphoblastic leukemia. J Clin Oncol 1996;14:2370–2376.
373. Hurwitz CA, Silverman LB, Schorin MA, et al. Substituting dexamethasone for prednisone complicates remission induction in children with acute lymphoblastic leukemia. Cancer 2000;88:1964–1969.
374. Waber DP, Carpentieri SC, Klar N, et al. Cognitive sequelae in children treated for acute lymphoblastic leukemia with dexamethasone or prednisone. J Pediatr Hematol Oncol 2000;22:206–213.
375. te Winkel ML, Appel IM, Pieters R, et al. Impaired dexamethasone-related increase of anticoagulants is associated with the development of osteonecrosis in childhood acute lymphoblastic leukemia. Haematologica 2008;93:1570–1574.
376. Hinds PS, Hockenberry MJ, Gattuso JS, et al. Dexamethasone alters sleep and fatigue in pediatric patients with acute lymphoblastic leukemia. Cancer 2007;110: 2321–2330.
377. Mauer AM. Treatment of acute leukaemia in children. Clin Haematol 1978;7:245–258.
378. Aur RJ, Simone JV, Verzosa MS, et al. Childhood acute lymphocytic leukemia: study VIII. Cancer 1978;42:2123–2134.
379. Gaynon PS, Bleyer WA, Steinherz PG, et al. Modified BFM therapy for children with previously untreated acute lymphoblastic leukemia and unfavorable prognostic features. Report of Children's Cancer Study Group Study CCG-193P. Am J Pediatr Hematol Oncol 1988;10:42–50.
380. Childhood Acute Lymphoblastic Leukaemia Colaborative Group (CALLCG). Beneficial and harmful effects of anthracyclines in the treatment of childhood acute lymphoblastic leukaemia: a systematic review and meta-analysis. Br J Haematol 2009; 145:376–388.
381. Silverman LB, Gelber RD, Young ML, et al. Induction failure in acute lymphoblastic leukemia of childhood. Cancer 1999;85:1395–1404.
382. Urban C, Benesch M, Lackner H, et al. The influence of maximum supportive care on dose compliance and survival. Single-center analysis of childhood acute lymphoblastic leukemia and non-Hodgkin's-lymphoma treated within 1984–1993. Klin Padiatr 1997;209:235–242.
383. Pui CH, Campana D, Pei D, et al. Treating childhood acute lymphoblastic leukemia without cranial irradiation. N Engl J Med 2009;360:2730–2741.
384. Johnson RE. An experimental therapeutic approach to L1210 leukemia in mice: combined chemotherapy and central nervous system irradiation. J Natl Cancer Inst 1964;32:1333–1341.
385. Aur RJ, Simone JV, Hustu HO, et al. A comparative study of central nervous system irradiation and intensive chemotherapy early in remission of childhood acute lymphocytic leukemia. Cancer 1972;29:381–391.
386. Blatt J, Bercu BB, Gillin JC, et al. Reduced pulsatile growth hormone secretion in children after therapy for acute lymphoblastic leukemia. J Pediatr 1984;104:182–186.
387. Meadows AT, Gordon J, Massari DJ, et al. Declines in IQ scores and cognitive dysfunctions in children with acute lymphocytic leukaemia treated with cranial irradiation. Lancet 1981;2:1015–1018.
388. Pizzo PA, Poplack DG, Bleyer WA. Neurotoxicities of current leukemia therapy. Am J Pediatr Hematol Oncol 1979;1:127–140.
389. Riccardi R, Brouwers P, Di Chiro G, et al. Abnormal computed tomography brain scans in children with acute lymphoblastic leukemia: serial long-term follow-up. J Clin Oncol 1985;3:12–18.
390. Bleyer WA, Poplack DG. Prophylaxis and treatment of leukemia in the central nervous system and other sanctuaries. Semin Oncol 1985;12:131–148.
391. Jankovic M, Brouwers P, Valsecchi MG, et al. Association of 1800 cGy cranial irradiation with intellectual function in children with acute lymphoblastic leukaemia. ISPACC. International Study Group on Psychosocial Aspects of Childhood Cancer. Lancet 1994; 344:224–227.
392. MacLean WE Jr, Noll RB, Stehbens JA, et al. Neuropsychological effects of cranial irradiation in young children with acute lymphoblastic leukemia 9 months after diagnosis. The Children's Cancer Group. Arch Neurol 1995;52:156–160.
393. Waber DP, Silverman LB, Catania L, et al. Outcomes of a randomized trial of hyperfractionated cranial radiation therapy for treatment of high-risk acute lymphoblastic leukemia: therapeutic efficacy and neurotoxicity. J Clin Oncol 2004;22:2701–2707.
394. Tubergen DG, Gilchrist GS, O'Brien RT, et al. Prevention of CNS disease in intermediate-risk acute lymphoblastic leukemia: comparison of cranial radiation and intrathecal methotrexate and the importance of systemic therapy: a Childrens Cancer Group report. J Clin Oncol 1993;11:520–526.
395. Pullen J, Boyett J, Shuster J, et al. Extended triple intrathecal chemotherapy trial for prevention of CNS relapse in good-risk and poor-risk patients with B-progenitor acute lymphoblastic leukemia: a Pediatric Oncology Group study. J Clin Oncol 1993;11:839–849.
396. Conter V, Arico M, Valsecchi MG, et al. Extended intrathecal methotrexate may replace cranial irradiation for prevention of CNS relapse in children with intermediate-risk acute lymphoblastic leukemia treated with Berlin-Frankfurt-Munster-based intensive chemotherapy. The Associazione Italiana di Ematologia ed Oncologia Pediatrica. J Clin Oncol 1995;13:2497–2502.
397. Waber DP, Tarbell NJ. Toxicity of CNS prophylaxis for childhood leukemia. Oncology (Huntingt) 1997;11:259–264.
398. Geiser CF, Bishop Y, Jaffe N, et al. Adverse effects of intrathecal methotrexate in children with acute leukemia in remission. Blood 1975;45:189–195.
399. Bleyer WA, Coccia PF, Sather HN, et al. Reduction in central nervous system leukemia with a pharmacokinetically derived intrathecal methotrexate dosage regimen. J Clin Oncol 1983;1:317–325.
400. Gagliano RG, Costanzi JJ. Paraplegia following intrathecal methotrexate: report of a case and review of the literature. Cancer 1976;37:1663–1668.
401. Mahoney DH Jr, Shuster JJ, Nitschke R, et al. Acute neurotoxicity in children with B-precursor acute lymphoid leukemia: an association with intermediate-dose intravenous methotrexate and intrathecal triple therapy–a Pediatric Oncology Group study. J Clin Oncol 1998;16:1712–1722.
402. Uzal D, Ozyar E, Hayran M, et al. Reduced incidence of the somnolence syndrome after prophylactic cranial irradiation in children with acute lymphoblastic leukemia. Radiother Oncol 1998;48:29–32.
403. Freeman JE, Johnston PG, Voke JM. Somnolence after prophylactic cranial irradiation in children with acute lymphoblastic leukaemia. Br Med J 1973;4:523–525.
404. Harned TM, Gaynon P. Relapsed acute lymphoblastic leukemia: current status and future opportunities. Curr Oncol Rep 2008;10:453–458.
405. Karon M, Freireich EJ, Frei E III, et al. The role of vincristine in the treatment of childhood acute leukemia. Clin Pharmacol Ther 1966;7:332–339.
406. Harris MB, Shuster JJ, Pullen DJ, et al. Consolidation therapy with antimetabolite-based therapy in standard-risk acute lymphocytic leukemia of childhood: a Pediatric Oncology Group Study. J Clin Oncol 1998;16:2840–2847.
407. Rivera GK, Raimondi SC, Hancock ML, et al. Improved outcome in childhood acute lymphoblastic leukaemia with reinforced early treatment and rotational combination chemotherapy. Lancet 1991;337:61–66.
408. Frei E III. Acute leukemia in children. Model for the development of scientific methodology for clinical therapeutic research in cancer. Cancer 1984;53:2013–2025.
409. Bleyer WA, Sather HN, Nickerson HJ, et al. Monthly pulses of vincristine and prednisone prevent bone marrow and testicular relapse in low-risk childhood acute lymphoblastic leukemia: a report of the CCG-161 study by the Childrens Cancer Study Group. J Clin Oncol 1991;9:1012–1021.
410. Conter V, Valsecchi MG, Silvestri D, et al. Pulses of vincristine and dexamethasone in addition to intensive chemotherapy for children with intermediate-risk acute lymphoblastic leukaemia: a multicentre randomised trial. Lancet 2007;369:123–131.
411. Pinkel D. Five-year follow-up of "total therapy" of childhood lymphocytic leukemia. JAMA 1971;216:648–652.
412. Eden OB, Lilleyman JS, Richards S, et al. Results of Medical Research Council Childhood Leukaemia Trial UKALL VIII (report to the Medical Research Council on behalf of the Working Party on Leukaemia in Childhood). Br J Haematol 1991;78:187–196.
413. Dibenedetto SP, Guardabasso V, Ragusa R, et al. 6-Mercaptopurine cumulative dose: a critical factor of maintenance therapy in average risk childhood acute lymphoblastic leukemia. Pediatr Hematol Oncol 1994;11:251–258.
414. Schmiegelow K, Pulczynska MK. Maintenance chemotherapy for childhood acute lymphoblastic leukemia: should dosage be guided by white blood cell counts? Am J Pediatr Hematol Oncol 1990;12:462–467.
415. Pearson AD, Amineddine HA, Yule M, et al. The influence of serum methotrexate concentrations and drug dosage on outcome in childhood acute lymphoblastic leukaemia. Br J Cancer 1991;64:169–173.

416. Koizumi S, Fujimoto T, Takeda T, et al. Comparison of intermittent or continuous methotrexate plus 6-mercaptopurine in regimens for standard-risk acute lymphoblastic leukemia in childhood (JCCLSG-S811). The Japanese Children's Cancer and Leukemia Study Group. Cancer 1988;61:1292–1300.
417. Poplack DG, Balis FM, Zimm S. The pharmacology of orally administered chemotherapy. A reappraisal. Cancer 1986;58:473–480.
418. Chessells JM, Eden OB, Bailey CC, et al. Acute lymphoblastic leukaemia in infancy: experience in MRC UKALL trials. Report from the Medical Research Council Working Party on Childhood Leukaemia. Leukemia 1994;8:1275–1279.
419. Chessells JM, Leiper AD, Tiedemann K, et al. Oral methotrexate is as effective as intramuscular in maintenance therapy of acute lymphoblastic leukaemia. Arch Dis Child 1987;62:172–176.
420. Lilleyman JS, Lennard L. Mercaptopurine metabolism and risk of relapse in childhood lymphoblastic leukaemia. Lancet 1994;343:1188–1190.
421. Matherly LH, Taub JW, Ravindranath Y, et al. Elevated dihydrofolate reductase and impaired methotrexate transport as elements in methotrexate resistance in childhood acute lymphoblastic leukemia. Blood 1995;85:500–509.
422. Nesbit ME Jr, Sather HN, Robison LL, et al. Randomized study of 3 years versus 5 years of chemotherapy in childhood acute lymphoblastic leukemia. J Clin Oncol 1983;1:308–316.
423. Chessells JM, Harrison G, Lilleyman JS, et al. Continuing (maintenance) therapy in lymphoblastic leukaemia: lessons from MRC UKALL X. Medical Research Council Working Party in Childhood Leukaemia. Br J Haematol 1997;98:945–951.
424. Toyoda Y, Manabe A, Tsuchida M, et al. Six months of maintenance chemotherapy after intensified treatment for acute lymphoblastic leukemia of childhood. J Clin Oncol 2000;18:1508–1516.
425. The Medical Research Council's Working Party on Leukaemia in Childhood. Duration of chemotherapy in childhood acute lymphoblastic leukaemia. The Medical Research Council's Working Party on Leukaemia in Childhood. Med Pediatr Oncol 1982;10: 511–520.
426. Riehm H, Gadner H, Henze G, et al. Results and significance of six randomized trials in four consecutive ALL-BFM studies. Haematol Blood Transfus 1990;33:439–450.
427. Slats AM, Egeler RM, van der Does-van den Berg A, et al. Causes of death–other than progressive leukemia–in childhood acute lymphoblastic (ALL) and myeloid leukemia (AML): the Dutch Childhood Oncology Group experience. Leukemia 2005;19:537–544.
428. Guidelines for the use of platelet transfusions. Br J Haematol 2003;122:10–23.
429. Navarro JT, Hernandez JA, Ribera JM, et al. Prophylactic platelet transfusion threshold during therapy for adult acute myeloid leukemia: 10,000/microL versus 20,000/microL. Haematologica 1998;83:998–1000.
430. Wandt H, Frank M, Ehninger G, et al. Safety and cost effectiveness of a 10 × 10(9)/L trigger for prophylactic platelet transfusions compared with the traditional 20 × 10(9)/L trigger: a prospective comparative trial in 105 patients with acute myeloid leukemia. Blood 1998;91:3601–3606.
431. Bailey LC, Reilly AF, Rheingold SR. Infections in pediatric patients with hematologic malignancies. Semin Hematol 2009;46:313–324.
432. Ohno R, Tomonaga M, Kobayashi T, et al. Effect of granulocyte colony-stimulating factor after intensive induction therapy in relapsed or refractory acute leukemia. N Engl J Med 1990;323:871–877.
433. Pui CH, Boyett JM, Hughes WT, et al. Human granulocyte colony-stimulating factor after induction chemotherapy in children with acute lymphoblastic leukemia. N Engl J Med 1997;336:1781–1787.
434. Welte K, Reiter A, Mempel K, et al. A randomized phase-III study of the efficacy of granulocyte colony-stimulating factor in children with high-risk acute lymphoblastic leukemia. Berlin-Frankfurt-Munster Study Group. Blood 1996;87:3143–3150.
435. Inukai T, Sugita K, Iijima K, et al. Leukemic cells with 11q23 translocations express granulocyte colony-stimulating factor (G-CSF) receptor and their proliferation is stimulated with G-CSF. Leukemia 1998;12:382–389.
436. Bennett CL, Stinson TJ, Lane D, et al. Cost analysis of filgrastim for the prevention of neutropenia in pediatric T-cell leukemia and advanced lymphoblastic lymphoma: a case for prospective economic analysis in cooperative group trials. Med Pediatr Oncol 2000;34:92–96.
437. Saarinen-Pihkala UM, Lanning M, Perkkio M, et al. Granulocyte-macrophage colony-stimulating factor support in therapy of high-risk acute lymphoblastic leukemia in children. Med Pediatr Oncol 2000;34:319–327.
438. Wong EC, Perez-Albuerne E, Moscow JA, et al. Transfusion management strategies: a survey of practicing pediatric hematology/oncology specialists. Pediatr Blood Cancer 2005;44:119–127.
439. Steiner I, Aebi C, Ridolfi Luthy A, et al. Fatal adenovirus hepatitis during maintenance therapy for childhood acute lymphoblastic leukemia. Pediatr Blood Cancer 2008;50: 647–649.
440. Kritz A, Sepkowitz K, Weiss M, et al. Pneumocystis carinii pneumonia developing within one month of intensive chemotherapy for treatment of acute lymphoblastic leukemia. N Engl J Med 1991;325:661–662.
441. Weinthal J, Frost JD, Briones G, et al. Successful Pneumocystis carinii pneumonia prophylaxis using aerosolized pentamidine in children with acute leukemia. J Clin Oncol 1994;12:136–140.
442. Ellis RB. Zoster immunoglobulin: an assessment. In: MMWR, 1977:1381.
443. Arbeter AM, Granowetter L, Starr SE, et al. Immunization of children with acute lymphoblastic leukemia with live attenuated varicella vaccine without complete suspension of chemotherapy. Pediatrics 1990;85:338–344.
444. Marin M, Guvis D, Chaves SS, et al. Prevention of varicella. MMWR 2007;56:1–40.
445. Murphy JV, Yunis EJ. Encephalopathy following measles infection in children with chronic illness. J Pediatr 1976;88:937–942.
446. Lobato ME, Ruiz-Arguelles GJ. [Leukemia and malnutrition. III. Effect of chemotherapeutic treatment on the nutritional state and its repercussion on the therapeutic response of patients with acute lymphoblastic leukemia with standard risk]. Sangre (Barc) 1990;35:189–195.
447. Moyer-Mileur LJ, Ransdell L, et al. Fitness of children with standard-risk acute lymphoblastic leukemia during maintenance therapy: response to a home-based exercise and nutrition program. J Pediatr Hematol Oncol 2009;31:259–266.
448. Abshire TC, Buchanan GR, Jackson JF, et al. Morphologic, immunologic and cytogenetic studies in children with acute lymphoblastic leukemia at diagnosis and relapse: a Pediatric Oncology Group study. Leukemia 1992;6:357–362.
449. Borella L, Casper JT, Lauer SJ. Shifts in expression of cell membrane phenotypes in childhood lymphoid malignancies at relapse. Blood 1979;54:64–71.
450. Greaves M, Paxton A, Janossy G, et al. Acute lymphoblastic leukaemia associated antigen. III ALterations in expression during treatment and in relapse. Leuk Res 1980; 4:1–14.
451. Hijiya N, Ness KK, Ribeiro RC, et al. Acute leukemia as a secondary malignancy in children and adolescents: current findings and issues. Cancer 2009;115:23–35.
452. Stass SA, Mirro J Jr. Lineage heterogeneity in acute leukaemia: acute mixed-lineage leukaemia and lineage switch. Clin Haematol 1986;15:811–827.
453. Reaman GH, Ladisch S, Echelberger C, et al. Improved treatment results in the management of single and multiple relapses of acute lymphoblastic leukemia. Cancer 1980;45:3090–3094.
454. Buchanan GR, Rivera GK, Pollock BH, et al. Alternating drug pairs with or without periodic reinduction in children with acute lymphoblastic leukemia in second bone marrow remission: a Pediatric Oncology Group Study. Cancer 2000;88:1166–1174.
455. Bernstein ML, Whitehead VM, Devine S, et al. Ifosfamide with mesna uroprotection and etoposide in recurrent, refractory acute leukemia in childhood. A Pediatric Oncology Group Study. Cancer 1993;72:1790–1794.
456. Bailey LC, Lange BJ, Rheingold SR, et al. Bone-marrow relapse in paediatric acute lymphoblastic leukaemia. Lancet Oncol 2008;9:873–883.
457. Reismuller B, Attarbaschi A, Peters C, et al. Long-term outcome of initially homogenously treated and relapsed childhood acute lymphoblastic leukaemia in Austria–a population-based report of the Austrian Berlin-Frankfurt-Munster (BFM) Study Group. Br J Haematol 2009;144:559–570.
458. Rivera GK, Santana V, Mahmoud H, et al. Acute lymphocytic leukemia of childhood: the problem of relapses. Bone Marrow Transplant 1989;4(Suppl 1):80–85.
459. Buhrer C, Hartmann R, Fengler R, et al. Importance of effective central nervous system therapy in isolated bone marrow relapse of childhood acute lymphoblastic leukemia. BFM (Berlin-Frankfurt-Munster) Relapse Study Group. Blood 1994;83: 3468–3472.
460. Lin WY, Liu HC, Yeh TC, et al. Triple intrathecal therapy without cranial irradiation for central nervous system preventive therapy in childhood acute lymphoblastic leukemia. Pediatr Blood Cancer 2008;50:523–527.
461. Barredo JC, Devidas M, Lauer SJ, et al. Isolated CNS relapse of acute lymphoblastic leukemia treated with intensive systemic chemotherapy and delayed CNS radiation: a pediatric oncology group study. J Clin Oncol 2006;24:3142–3149.
462. Ribeiro RC, Rivera GK, Hudson M, et al. An intensive re-treatment protocol for children with an isolated CNS relapse of acute lymphoblastic leukemia. J Clin Oncol 1995;13:333–338.
463. Thomas ED, Buckner CD, Banaji M, et al. One hundred patients with acute leukemia treated by chemotherapy, total body irradiation, and allogeneic marrow transplantation. Blood 1977;49:511–533.
464. Schroeder H, Gustafsson G, Saarinen-Pihkala UM, et al. Allogeneic bone marrow transplantation in second remission of childhood acute lymphoblastic leukemia: a population-based case control study from the Nordic countries. Bone Marrow Transplant 1999;23:555–560.
465. Davies SM, Ramsay NK, Klein JP, et al. Comparison of preparative regimens in transplants for children with acute lymphoblastic leukemia. J Clin Oncol 2000;18: 340–347.
466. Eapen M, Raetz E, Zhang MJ, et al. Outcomes after HLA-matched sibling transplantation or chemotherapy in children with B-precursor acute lymphoblastic leukemia in a second remission: a collaborative study of the Children's Oncology Group and the Center for International Blood and Marrow Transplant Research. Blood 2006;107:4961–4967.
467. Hongeng S, Krance RA, Bowman LC, et al. Outcomes of transplantation with matched-sibling and unrelated-donor bone marrow in children with leukaemia. Lancet 1997;350:767–771.
468. Eapen M, Rubinstein P, Zhang MJ, et al. Comparable long-term survival after unrelated and HLA-matched sibling donor hematopoietic stem cell transplantations for acute leukemia in children younger than 18 months. J Clin Oncol 2006;24:145–151.
469. Cohen Y, Nagler A. Umbilical cord blood transplantation–how, when and for whom? Blood Rev 2004;18:167–179.
470. Wang Y, Xue MX, Wu XH, et al. Successful treatment of relapsed Philadelphia chromosome-positive acute lymphoblastic leukemia with T315I mutation after haplo-identical hematopoietic stem cell transplantation with donor lymphocyte transfusion and interferon-alpha-2b. Leuk Res 2009;33:e111–e113.
471. Kennedy-Nasser AA, Bollard CM, Myers GD, et al. Comparable outcome of alternative donor and matched sibling donor hematopoietic stem cell transplant for children with acute lymphoblastic leukemia in first or second remission using alemtuzumab in a myeloablative conditioning regimen. Biol Blood Marrow Transplant 2008;14:1245–1252.
472. Dini G, Cornish JM, Gadner H, et al. Bone marrow transplant indications for childhood leukemias: achieving a consensus. The EBMT Pediatric Diseases Working Party. Bone Marrow Transplant 1996;18(Suppl 2):4–7.
473. Butturini A, Rivera GK, Bortin MM, et al. Which treatment for childhood acute lymphoblastic leukaemia in second remission? Lancet 1987;1:429–432.
474. Barrett AJ, Horowitz MM, Pollock BH, et al. Bone marrow transplants from HLA-identical siblings as compared with chemotherapy for children with acute lymphoblastic leukemia in a second remission. N Engl J Med 1994;331:1253–1258.
475. Bostrom B, Woods WG, Nesbit ME, et al. Successful reinduction of patients with acute lymphoblastic leukemia who relapse following bone marrow transplantation. J Clin Oncol 1987;5:376–381.
476. Borowitz MJ, Pullen DJ, Shuster JJ, et al. Minimal residual disease detection in childhood precursor-B-cell acute lymphoblastic leukemia: relation to other risk factors. A Children's Oncology Group study. Leukemia 2003;17:1566–1572.
477. Taube T, Eckert C, Korner G, et al. Real-time quantification of TEL-AML1 fusion transcripts for MRD detection in relapsed childhood acute lymphoblastic leukaemia. Comparison with antigen receptor-based MRD quantification methods. Leuk Res 2004;28: 699–706.
478. Cave H, van der Werff ten B, Suciu S, et al. Clinical significance of minimal residual disease in childhood acute lymphoblastic leukemia. European Organization for Research and Treatment of Cancer–Childhood Leukemia Cooperative Group. N Engl J Med 1998;339:591–598.
479. Yamada M, Wasserman R, Lange B, et al. Minimal residual disease in childhood B-lineage lymphoblastic leukemia. Persistence of leukemic cells during the first 18 months of treatment. N Engl J Med 1990;323:448–455.
480. Neale GA, Coustan-Smith E, Pan Q, et al. Tandem application of flow cytometry and polymerase chain reaction for comprehensive detection of minimal residual disease in childhood acute lymphoblastic leukemia. Leukemia 1999;13:1221–1226.
481. Gehly GB, Bryant EM, Lee AM, et al. Chimeric BCR-abl messenger RNA as a marker for minimal residual disease in patients transplanted for Philadelphia chromosome-positive acute lymphoblastic leukemia. Blood 1991;78:458–465.

482. Lauer SJ, Kirchner PA, Camitta BM. Identification of leukemic cells in the cerebrospinal fluid from children with acute lymphoblastic leukemia: advances and dilemmas. Am J Pediatr Hematol Oncol 1989;11:64–73.
483. Odom LF, Wilson H, Cullen J, et al. Significance of blasts in low-cell-count cerebrospinal fluid specimens from children with acute lymphoblastic leukemia. Cancer 1990;66:1748–1754.
484. Ritchey AK, Pollock BH, Lauer SJ, et al. Improved survival of children with isolated CNS relapse of acute lymphoblastic leukemia: a pediatric oncology group study. J Clin Oncol 1999;17:3745–3752.
485. Raje NS, Vaidya SJ, Kapoor G, et al. Low incidence of CNS relapse with cranial radiotherapy and intrathecal methotrexate in acute lymphoblastic leukemia. Indian Pediatr 1996;33:556–560.
486. Duttera MJ, Bleyer WA, Pomeroy TC, et al. Irradiation, methotrexate toxicity, and the treatment of meningeal leukaemia. Lancet 1973;2:703–707.
487. Kun LE, Camitta BM, Mulhern RK, et al. Treatment of meningeal relapse in childhood acute lymphoblastic leukemia. I. Results of craniospinal irradiation. J Clin Oncol 1984;2:359–364.
488. Willoughby ML. Treatment of overt meningeal leukaemia in children: results of second MRC meningeal leukaemia trial. Br Med J 1976;1:864–867.
489. Blaney SM, Poplack DG. Pharmacologic strategies for the treatment of meningeal malignancy. Invest New Drugs 1996;14:69–85.
490. Bleyer WA, Poplack DG. Intraventricular versus intralumbar methotrexate for central-nervous-system leukemia: prolonged remission with the Ommaya reservoir. Med Pediatr Oncol 1979;6:207–213.
491. Dordelmann M, Reiter A, Zimmermann M, et al. Intermediate dose methotrexate is as effective as high dose methotrexate in preventing isolated testicular relapse in childhood acute lymphoblastic leukemia. J Pediatr Hematol Oncol 1998;20:444–450.
492. Pui CH, Evans WE. Acute lymphoblastic leukemia. N Engl J Med 1998;339:605–615.
493. Steinfeld AD. Radiation therapy in the treatment of leukemic infiltrates of the testes. Radiology 1976;120:681–682.
494. Mirro J Jr, Wharam MD, Kaizer H, et al. Testicular leukemic relapse: rate of regression and persistent disease after radiation therapy. J Pediatr 1981;99:439–440.
495. Speiser B, Rubin P, Casarett G. Aspermia following lower truncal irradiation in Hodgkin's disease. Cancer 1973;32:692–698.
496. Blatt J, Sherins RJ, Niebrugge D, et al. Leydig cell function in boys following treatment for testicular relapse of acute lymphoblastic leukemia. J Clin Oncol 1985;3: 1227–1231.
497. Uderzo C, Grazia ZM, Adamoli L, et al. Treatment of isolated testicular relapse in childhood acute lymphoblastic leukemia: an Italian multicenter study. Associazione Italiana Ematologia ed Oncologia Pediatrica. J Clin Oncol 1990;8:672–677.
498. Finklestein JZ, Miller DR, Feusner J, et al. Treatment of overt isolated testicular relapse in children on therapy for acute lymphoblastic leukemia. A report from the Childrens Cancer Group. Cancer 1994;73:219–223.
499. Heaton DC, Duff GB. Ovarian relapse in a young woman with acute lymphoblastic leukaemia. Am J Hematol 1989;30:42–43.
500. Hinkle AS, Dinndorf PA, Bulas DI, et al. Relapse of acute lymphoblastic leukemia in the inferior rectus muscle of the eye. Cancer 1994;73:1757–1760.
501. Bunin N, Rivera G, Goode F, et al. Ocular relapse in the anterior chamber in childhood acute lymphoblastic leukemia. J Clin Oncol 1987;5:299–303.
502. Mody R, Li S, Dover DC, et al. Twenty-five-year follow-up among survivors of childhood acute lymphoblastic leukemia: a report from the Childhood Cancer Survivor Study. Blood 2008;111:5515–5523.
503. Oeffinger KC, Nathan PC, Kremer LC. Challenges after curative treatment for childhood cancer and long-term follow up of survivors. Pediatr Clin North Am 2008;55: 251–273, xiii.
504. Robison LL, Bhatia S. Late-effects among survivors of leukaemia and lymphoma during childhood and adolescence. Br J Haematol 2003;122:345–359.
505. Ochs J, Mulhern R, Fairclough D, et al. Comparison of neuropsychologic functioning and clinical indicators of neurotoxicity in long-term survivors of childhood leukemia given cranial radiation or parenteral methotrexate: a prospective study. J Clin Oncol 1991;9:145–151.
506. Peylan-Ramu N, Poplack DG, Pizzo PA, et al. Abnormal CT scans of the brain in asymptomatic children with acute lymphocytic leukemia after prophylactic treatment of the central nervous system with radiation and intrathecal chemotherapy. N Engl J Med 1978;298:815–818.
507. Rubinstein LJ, Herman MM, Long TF, et al. Disseminated necrotizing leukoencephalopathy: a complication of treated central nervous system leukemia and lymphoma. Cancer 1975;35:291–305.
508. Gangji D, Reaman GH, Cohen SR, et al. Leukoencephalopathy and elevated levels of myelin basic protein in the cerebrospinal fluid of patients with acute lymphoblastic leukemia. N Engl J Med 1980;303:19–21.
509. Quinn CT, Griener JC, Bottiglieri T, et al. Elevation of homocysteine and excitatory amino acid neurotransmitters in the CSF of children who receive methotrexate for the treatment of cancer. J Clin Oncol 1997;15:2800–2806.
510. Brouwers P, Riccardi R, Fedio P, et al. Long-term neuropsychologic sequelae of childhood leukemia: correlation with CT brain scan abnormalities. J Pediatr 1985;106:723–728.
511. Hill DE, Ciesielski KT, Hart BL, et al. MRI morphometric and neuropsychological correlates of long-term memory in survivors of childhood leukemia. Pediatr Blood Cancer 2004;42:611–617.
512. Oeffinger KC, Hudson MM. Long-term complications following childhood and adolescent cancer: foundations for providing risk-based health care for survivors. CA Cancer J Clin 2004;54:208–236.
513. Rai SN, Hudson MM, McCammon E, et al. Implementing an intervention to improve bone mineral density in survivors of childhood acute lymphoblastic leukemia: BONEII, a prospective placebo-controlled double-blind randomized interventional longitudinal study design. Contemp Clin Trials 2008;29:711–719.
514. Poussaint TY, Siffert J, Barnes PD, et al. Hemorrhagic vasculopathy after treatment of central nervous system neoplasia in childhood: diagnosis and follow-up. AJNR Am J Neuroradiol 1995;16:693–699.
515. Hill JM, Kornblith AB, Jones D, et al. A comparative study of the long term psychosocial functioning of childhood acute lymphoblastic leukemia survivors treated by intrathecal methotrexate with or without cranial radiation. Cancer 1998;82: 208–218.
516. Blatt J, Lee P, Suttner J, et al. Pulsatile growth hormone secretion in children with acute lymphoblastic leukemia after 1800 cGy cranial radiation. Int J Radiat Oncol Biol Phys 1988;15:1001–1006.
517. Mauras N, Sabio H, Rogol AD. Neuroendocrine function in survivors of childhood acute lymphocytic leukemia and non-Hodgkins lymphoma: a study of pulsatile growth hormone and gonadotropin secretions. Am J Pediatr Hematol Oncol 1988; 10:9–17.
518. Sklar CA, Mertens AC, Mitby P, et al. Risk of disease recurrence and second neoplasms in survivors of childhood cancer treated with growth hormone: a report from the Childhood Cancer Survivor Study. J Clin Endocrinol Metab 2002;87:3136–3141.
519. Katz JA, Pollock BH, Jacaruso D, et al. Final attained height in patients successfully treated for childhood acute lymphoblastic leukemia. J Pediatr 1993;123:546–552.
520. Sklar C, Mertens A, Walter A, et al. Final height after treatment for childhood acute lymphoblastic leukemia: comparison of no cranial irradiation with 1800 and 2400 centigrays of cranial irradiation. J Pediatr 1993;123:59–64.
521. Muller HL, Klinkhammer-Schalke M, Kuhl J. Final height and weight of long-term survivors of childhood malignancies. Exp Clin Endocrinol Diabetes 1998;106: 135–139.
522. Fulgoni P, Zoia MC, Corsico A, et al. Lung function in survivors of childhood acute lymphoblastic leukemia. Chest 1999;116:1163–1167.
523. Arikoski P, Kroger H, Riikonen P, et al. Disturbance in bone turnover in children with a malignancy at completion of chemotherapy. Med Pediatr Oncol 1999;33: 455–461.
524. van dSI, de Muinck Keizer-Schrama SM, et al. Bone mineral density in childhood acute lymphoblastic leukemia (ALL) during and after treatment. Pediatr Blood Cancer 2004;43:182–183.
525. Kadan-Lottick N, Marshall JA, Baron AE, et al. Normal bone mineral density after treatment for childhood acute lymphoblastic leukemia diagnosed between 1991 and 1998. J Pediatr 2001;138:898–904.
526. Shaw MP, Bath LE, Duff J, et al. Obesity in leukemia survivors: the familial contribution. Pediatr Hematol Oncol 2000;17:231–237.
527. Asner S, Ammann RA, Ozsahin H, et al. Obesity in long-term survivors of childhood acute lymphoblastic leukemia. Pediatr Blood Cancer 2008;51:118–122.
528. Gofman I, Ducore J. Risk factors for the development of obesity in children surviving ALL and NHL. J Pediatr Hematol Oncol 2009;31:101–107.
529. Butturini AM, Dorey FJ, Lange BJ, et al. Obesity and outcome in pediatric acute lymphoblastic leukemia. J Clin Oncol 2007;25:2063–2069.
530. Bessho F, Kinumaki H, Yokota S, et al. Liver function studies in children with acute lymphocytic leukemia after cessation of therapy. Med Pediatr Oncol 1994;23:111–115.
531. Sorensen K, Levitt G, Bull C, et al. Anthracycline dose in childhood acute lymphoblastic leukemia: issues of early survival versus late cardiotoxicity. J Clin Oncol 1997;15: 61–68.
532. Oeffinger KC. Are survivors of acute lymphoblastic leukemia (ALL) at increased risk of cardiovascular disease? Pediatr Blood Cancer 2008;50:462–467; discussion 468.
533. Lipshultz SE, Colan SD, Gelber RD, et al. Late cardiac effects of doxorubicin therapy for acute lymphoblastic leukemia in childhood. N Engl J Med 1991;324:808–815.
534. Jakacki RI, Larsen RL, Barber G, et al. Comparison of cardiac function tests after anthracycline therapy in childhood. Implications for screening. Cancer 1993;72:2739–2745.
535. Pui CH, Evans WE, Relling MV. Are children with lesser-risk B-lineage acute lymphoblastic leukemia curable with antimetabolite therapy? Nat Clin Pract Oncol 2008;5: 130–131.
536. Wexler LH, Andrich MP, Venzon D, et al. Randomized trial of the cardioprotective agent ICRF-187 in pediatric sarcoma patients treated with doxorubicin. J Clin Oncol 1996;14:362–372.
537. Quigley C, Cowell C, Jimenez M, et al. Normal or early development of puberty despite gonadal damage in children treated for acute lymphoblastic leukemia. N Engl J Med 1989;321:143–151.
538. Nurmio M, Keros V, Lahteenmaki P, et al. Effect of childhood acute lymphoblastic leukemia therapy on spermatogonia populations and future fertility. J Clin Endocrinol Metab 2009;94:2119–2122.
539. Relander T, Cavallin-Stahl E, Garwicz S, et al. Gonadal and sexual function in men treated for childhood cancer. Med Pediatr Oncol 2000;35:52–63.
540. Pasqualini T, Escobar ME, Domene H, et al. Evaluation of gonadal function following long-term treatment for acute lymphoblastic leukemia in girls. Am J Pediatr Hematol Oncol 1987;9:15–22.
541. Blatt J, Poplack DG, Sherins RJ. Testicular function in boys after chemotherapy for acute lymphoblastic leukemia. N Engl J Med 1981;304:1121–1124.
542. Blatt J, Mulvihill JJ, Ziegler JL, et al. Pregnancy outcome following cancer chemotherapy. Am J Med 1980;69:828–832.
543. Kimball DV, Gelber RD, Li F, et al. Second malignancies in patients treated for childhood acute lymphoblastic leukemia. J Clin Oncol 1998;16:2848–2853.
544. Bhatia S, Sklar C. Second cancers in survivors of childhood cancer. Nat Rev Cancer 2002;2:124–132.
545. Nygaard R, Garwicz S, Haldorsen T, et al. Second malignant neoplasms in patients treated for childhood leukemia. A population-based cohort study from the Nordic countries. The Nordic Society of Pediatric Oncology and Hematology (NOPHO). Acta Paediatr Scand 1991;80:1220–1228.
546. Pui CH, Behm FG, Raimondi SC, et al. Secondary acute myeloid leukemia in children treated for acute lymphoid leukemia. N Engl J Med 1989;321:136–142.
547. Weitman SD, Winick NJ, Kamen BA. "Above all do no harm:" horizons in pediatric oncology. Curr Opin Pediatr 1994;6:219–223.
548. Prasannan L, Pu A, Hoff P, et al. Parotid carcinoma as a second malignancy after treatment of childhood acute lymphoblastic leukemia. J Pediatr Hematol Oncol 1999;21: 535–538.
549. Rosso P, Terracini B, Fears TR, et al. Second malignant tumors after elective end of therapy for a first cancer in childhood: a multicenter study in Italy. Int J Cancer 1994; 59:451–456.
550. de Vaan GA, van Munster PJ, Bakkeren JA. Recovery of immune function after cessation of maintenance therapy in acute lymphoblastic leukemia (ALL) of childhood. Eur J Pediatr 1982;139:113–117.
551. Hobbie WL, Stuber M, Meeske K, et al. Symptoms of posttraumatic stress in young adult survivors of childhood cancer. J Clin Oncol 2000;18:4060–4066.
552. Langeveld NE, Grootenhuis MA, Voute PA, et al. Posttraumatic stress symptoms in adult survivors of childhood cancer. Pediatr Blood Cancer 2004;42:604–610.
553. Kingma A, Rammeloo LA, van Der Does-van den B, et al. Academic career after treatment for acute lymphoblastic leukaemia. Arch Dis Child 2000;82:353–357.
554. Pui CH, Schrappe M, Masera G, et al. Ponte di Legno Working Group: statement on the right of children with leukemia to have full access to essential treatment and report on the Sixth International Childhood Acute Lymphoblastic Leukemia Workshop. Leukemia 2004;18:1043–1053.

CHAPTER 20 ■ ACUTE MYELOID LEUKEMIA, MYELOPROLIFERATIVE AND MYELODYSPLASTIC DISORDERS

TODD M. COOPER, HENRIK HASLE, AND FRANKLIN O. SMITH

The term *myeloid* includes all of the cells belonging to the granulocytic (neutrophilic, eosinophilic, basophilic), monocytic/macrophage, erythroid, megakaryocytic, and mast cell lineages. Myeloid neoplasms include myelodysplastic syndrome (MDS), acute myeloid leukemia (AML), and the myeloproliferative neoplasms such as juvenile myelomonocytic leukemia (JMML). Myeloid malignancies result from abnormalities in genes that control cellular proliferation, survival, and differentiation.

Myeloproliferative disorders are characterized by the excessive proliferation of relatively normally differentiated hematopoietic cells. The disorders occur as a result of mutations or gene fusions that exert their effect through aberrant activation of signal transduction pathways, resulting in enhanced proliferation and/or cell survival (Fig. 20.1). One example is the BCR/ABL fusion protein seen in chronic myelogenous leukemia (CML), in which the product oncogene drives proliferation and transformation of myeloid stem cells. When abnormal hematopoietic stem cells (HSCs) possessing these mutations sustain an additional "hit" from mutations conferring abnormal differentiation, subsequent progression to AML occurs.[1,2]

MDSs are clonal disorders arising in progenitor cells restricted to myelopoiesis, erythropoiesis, and megakaryopoiesis. Clinically, they are characterized by progressive cytopenias and bone marrow (BM) failure.[3,4] There are a number of differences between MDS in adults and in children. These differences are reflected in the morphology, cytogenetics, and clinical presentation of the two distinct age groups. For example, adults often present with a more indolent disease course characterized by an isolated anemia and associated with del(5q) chromosome.[5] In contrast, children with MDS are more likely to present with neutropenia and thrombocytopenia, preexisting BM failure or congenital abnormalities, loss of chromosome 7, and more advanced disease.

AML is characterized by abnormal proliferation and differentiation of myeloid precursors. Discovery of a variety of genetic abnormalities linked to leukemogenesis has led to the theory that the development of AML is a multistep process resulting from cooperating mutations. Experiments on murine models and investigations into rare inherited leukemia syndromes such as familial platelet disorder with propensity to develop AML (FPD-AML) demonstrate that these mutations confer a proliferative and survival advantage by affecting differentiation, apoptosis, and self-renewal.[6,7]

INHERITED AND ACQUIRED PREDISPOSITION TO MYELOID NEOPLASMS

Recent advances in molecular genetics have helped to elucidate common mechanisms of leukemogenesis, linking the myeloproliferative disorders as well as identifying molecular abnormalities that lead to their unique clinical and biologic properties. Not surprisingly, myeloid neoplasms share common etiologies, which will be discussed here (Table 20.1).

Primary and Secondary Myeloid Neoplasms

A neoplasm can arise in a previously healthy child and is conformingly named "*de novo*" or "primary." It may also develop in a child with a known predisposing condition and is then referred to as "secondary." Secondary myeloid neoplasms are seen in patients (a) after chemotherapy or radiation therapy, (b) with inherited BM failure disorders, (c) with acquired aplastic anemia (AA), and (d) with familial MDS or AML without any known cause. It is to be recognized, however, that among the children with so-called "primary" neoplasms, some may have an underlying, yet unknown, predisposing genetic defect. Therefore, the distinction between primary and secondary disease may become arbitrary.

Secondary myeloid neoplasia in patients with predisposing conditions often shares the biologic characteristics of MDS regardless of the presenting blast count, and the prognosis appears to depend primarily on the cytogenetic profile. An exception may be families with germline mutations of the transcription factors *CEBPA* or *RUNX1*; they have an increased risk of AML that may share the clinical features and prognosis of *de novo* AML.[8,9] Myeloid leukemias (MLs) occurring in Fanconi anemia and Down syndrome (DS) have very distinct natural histories and need special therapy. There is no solid data documenting whether MLs in patients with other constitutional abnormalities have unique features.

Constitutional Abnormalities

Constitutional abnormalities have been reported in about 30% of patients with MDS,[10–16] compared with 14% in children with AML.[15] However, those studies were from a period when patients with DS were included in series of MDS and AML. It is now recognized that despite a morphologic diagnosis of MDS or AML, the ML in patients with DS is a unique disease. Excluding DS from MDS series significantly changes the distribution of MDS subtypes and halves the proportion of patients with associated abnormalities.[17] ML has been reported in association with a number of constitutional cytogenetic abnormalities other than trisomy 21, but there is only evidence for an increased risk of MDS for trisomy 8 mosaicism.[18] Constitutional trisomy 8 can be found in 15% to 20% of patients with trisomy 8 in the leukemic cells.[19] Reports of MDS and AML in patients with Klinefelter and

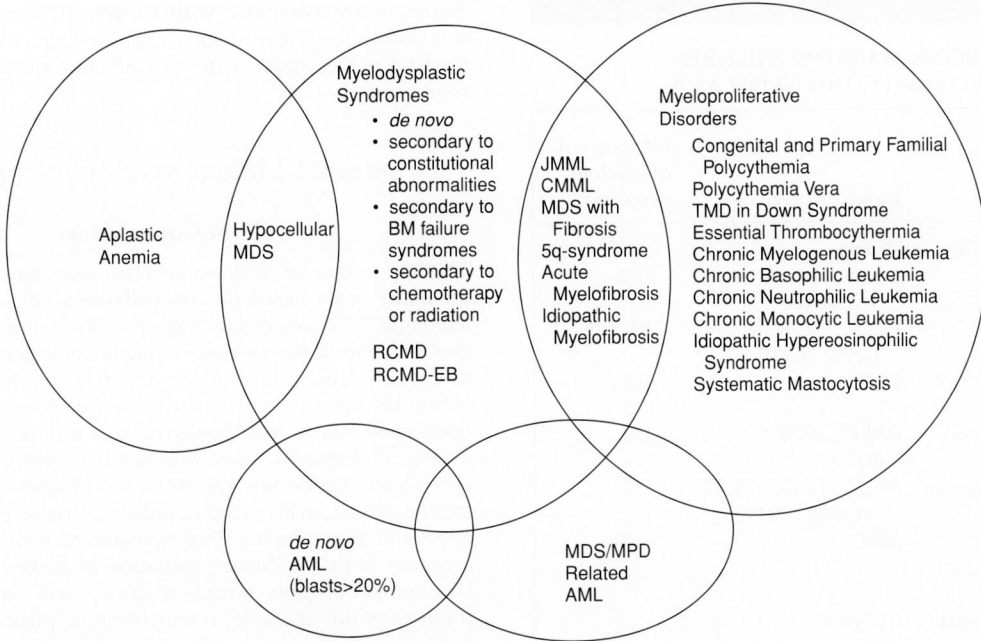

FIGURE 20.1 Conceptual model for the myelodysplastic and myeloproliferative disorders. MDS, myelodysplastic syndrome; RCMD, refractory anemia with multilineage dysplasia; RCMD-EB, RCMD with excess blasts; JMML, juvenile myelomonocytic leukemia; CMML, chronic myelomonocytic leukemia; TMD, transient myeloproliferative disorder; AML, acute myeloid leukemia; BM, bone marrow.

TABLE 20.1

PREDISPOSING CONDITIONS FOR MYELOID NEOPLASMS

Environmental
Ionizing radiation
Chemical exposures
    Pesticides
    Petroleum products
    Cytotoxic chemotherapy (alkylating agents,
        epipodophyllotoxins)
    Prenatal alcohol exposure of fetus
    Prenatal marijuana/tobacco exposure of fetus

Predisposing Conditions
Inherited
    Twinning
    Down syndrome
    Fanconi anemia
    Kostmann syndrome
    Shwachman-Diamond syndrome
    Diamond-Blackfan syndrome
    Neurofibromatosis type I
    Noonan syndrome
    Dyskeratosis congenital
    Familial platelet disorder with a propensity to develop
        acute myelogenous leukemia (FPD/AML)
    Congenital amegakaryocytic thrombocytopenia (CAMT)
    Li-Fraumeni syndrome
    Bloom syndrome
Acquired
    Aplastic anemia
    Myelodysplastic syndrome
    Acquired amegakaryocytic thrombocytopenia (AAMT)
    Paroxysmal nocturnal hemoglobinuria

Turner syndrome have appeared sporadically but no increased risk has been documented in cohort studies.[20] Congenital malformations have been reported in a relatively high number of children with MDS. The multiplicity of reported malformations is considerable although no consistent pattern is evident.

Inherited Bone Marrow Failure

Most inherited BM failure syndromes are associated with an increased risk of malignancy, especially MLs (Table 20.2). The risk of ML is particularly high in Fanconi anemia, developing in up to 50% of patients before 40 years of age. The risk varies according to genetic subgroup and associated abnormalities.[21] The traits associated with Fanconi anemia may be subtle and the diagnosis should always be considered in patients with ML. Diagnosing low-grade MDS in a patient with Fanconi anemia is challenging because cytopenia and dysplasia may be present in the BM. Cytogenetic aberrations may be temporary or reappear as new clones.[22] Gain of 3q material has been reported to be strongly associated with high risk of MDS.[23]

The survival of patients with severe congenital neutropenia (SCN) has improved significantly following the introduction of granulocyte colony-stimulating factor (G-CSF) treatment.[24] Studies from the SCN International Registry have shown a 10-year cumulative risk of ML development of 21%.[25] Partial or complete loss of chromosome 7 is found in more than half of the patients. The development of ML is mostly, but not always, preceded by acquired mutations in the G-CSF receptor gene.[26] Despite considerable concern and anxiety in the medical and lay communities, there is no direct cause-and-effect relationship between the development of myeloid neoplasm and G-CSF therapy, but the risk of leukemia is highest in the less-responsive group of patients (40% at 10 years).[25] Myeloid neoplasms are not seen in cyclic or idiopathic neutropenia treated with G-CSF administered in a similar schedule. For patients with SCN, it is

TABLE 20.2

TABLE 20.2

CONGENITAL BONE MARROW FAILURES
ASSOCIATED WITH MYELOID NEOPLASIA

Constitutional conditions	Genes involved	Lifelong risk of myeloid neoplasia
Bone marrow failure syndromes		
Fanconi anemia	12 Autosomal, 1 X-linked	50%
Severe congenital neutropenia	HAX1, ELA2, GFI1, WASP	20–40%
Shwachman-Diamond syndrome	SBDS	30%
Blackfan-Diamond anemia	RPS19, RPS24, RPS17	2%
Dyskeratosis congenita	DKC1, TERC, TERT, NOP10, NHP2	5%
Amegakaryocytic thrombocytopenia	MPL	<10%
Familial thrombocytopenia	RUNX1	

generally recommended that they have yearly BM examinations to search for morphologic, cytogenetic, or molecular signs of MDS. Early hematopoietic stem cell transplantation (HSCT) before progression seems promising for patients with evidence of MDS.[27,28]

Myeloid neoplasm develops in approximately 30% of children with Shwachman-Diamond syndrome (SDS)[29] and is often associated with chromosome 7 abnormalities. Isochromosome 7q may represent a separate entity with a long stable clinical course. Chromosome abnormalities are more frequent with age and reflect the genetic instability of the syndrome and the risk of progression to ML.[30] Microarray studies have identified several abnormal gene expression patterns in SDS BM mononuclear cells, which might be involved in the evolution of malignant clones.[31] MDS/AML have occasionally been described in patients with Diamond-Blackfan anemia,[15,32,33] dyskeratosis congenita,[34] and congenital amegakaryocytic thrombocytopenia,[35] but no reliable risk estimates are available. ML has also been reported in other types of congenital thrombocytopenia.[9,36,37]

Yearly BM examinations including cytogenetic studies should be performed in all patients with BM failure syndromes and altering cytopenia to ensure early identification of progression toward ML.[38]

Acquired Aplastic Anemia

Myeloid malignancy, most often MDS, develops in 10% to 15% of patients with AA not treated with HSCT.[39,40] Patients diagnosed as nonsevere AA may be overrepresented among those in whom clonal evolution is observed,[41] suggesting that some cases of MDS are misdiagnosed at initial presentation. Myeloid malignancy appears to occur at the same rate in idiopathic and hepatitis-associated AA[42]; however, MDS occurs earlier in children than in adults and is most often diagnosed within the first 3 years after the diagnosis of AA.[39,40] Whether prolonged treatment with the combination of G-CSF and cyclosporine is associated with development of myeloid malignancies is a controversial issue.[39,43] Shorter periods of G-CSF

treatment are associated with a lower incidence of malignant transformation,[44] contrasting with the high risk in patients on long-term treatment with G-CSF and those with a poor response to G-CSF.[45]

Familial-Linked Myeloid Neoplasms

Twin Concordance

The importance of *in utero* genetic events has been suspected for many years based on concordance studies on twins with leukemia.[46,47] Concordance studies on identical twins reveal that an identical twin is twice as likely as the general population to develop leukemia if his or her twin developed the illness before the age of 7 years. If the affected identical twin developed leukemia as an infant, the concordance rate is almost 100%.[47,48] Identical twins who reach 15 years without developing leukemia do not appear to be at higher risk of developing the disease, whereas in nonidentical twins the age cutoff is approximately 6 years. One plausible reason for the age discrepancy is that following initiation of leukemia in one twin fetus, clonal progeny spreads to the co-twin via vascular anastomoses within a single, monochorionic placenta. When this occurs, the leukemia usually arises within weeks to months in the second twin.[49] Molecular markers of clonality, including unique genomic fusion gene sequences, have provided unequivocal evidence that twin pairs of leukemia have a common clonal origin. The analysis of these leukemias has shed light on the natural history of the disease.[47,50,51]

Familial AML/MDS

Families with several members affected with AML/MDS have been described.[52–55] These patients tend to be younger at presentation and have an unusual family history of more than one first-degree relative with AML/MDS. Frequently, affected individuals are syndromic with associated inherited genetic predispositions. A large proportion of the patients have monosomy 7 or deletion 7q. Studies have demonstrated familial MDS in 0% to 10% of childhood MDS associated with monosomy 7.[13,20,32] Familial MDS does also occur without −7 or del(7q).[13,56] Some families show discordance for −7[32] and it is uncertain whether −7 per se increases the risk for familial cases. The putatively inherited predisposing locus in familial MDS with −7/7q− does not seem to be located on chromosome 7,[57] in accordance with the lack of leukemia among persons with constitutional aberrations of chromosome 7[58] and the different parental origin of the remaining chromosome 7 in siblings with monosomy 7.[59] Examinations of families with MDS/AML have identified germline mutations in *RUNX1* and *CEBPA*, but the genetic cause remains obscure in most reported pedigrees.[60] There are no conspicuous clinical characteristics of the familial cases of MDS.[32,54]

Therapy-Related Myeloid Neoplasms

As childhood cancer survival rates increase, so does the incidence of secondary malignancies. The reason for this phenomenon is most likely that the intensification of treatment has led to greater exposure to genotoxic chemotherapy or radiation therapy. The therapy-related myeloid neoplasms (t-AML, t-MDS) are a distinct subgroup in the classification because they encompass a uniform biologic disease with similar genetic features.[61–63] One subset of t-AML or t-MDS is associated with exposure to epipodophyllotoxins such as teniposide and etoposide.[64,65] Many of these therapy-related leukemias are classified as French-American-British (FAB) M4 (monocytic) or M5 (myelomonocytic) and involve rearrangements of the "mixed lineage leukemia" (MLL) gene at chromosome band 11q23.[65] Another subset of therapy-related myeloid neoplasms involves the use of anthracyclines such as doxorubicin, daunorubicin, or mitoxantrone. These myeloid neoplasms also are associated with MLL rearrangements. The common link between epipodophyllotoxins and anthracyclines is that they inhibit DNA topoisomerase II. Inhibition of this enzyme can result in faulty DNA repair, increasing the potential for abnormal gene rearrangement similar to that seen in the 11q23/MLL leukemias.[66] A third subset of t-AML and t-MDS are those associated with exposure to alkylating agents. These patients present less often with MLL rearrangements, but instead have poor-risk cytogenetic features such as 5q− abnormalities and monosomy 7.[67] Most patients who develop therapy-related myeloid neoplasms have received a combination of these genotoxic agents; therefore, classification according to the type of therapy is no longer recommended.[61] The peak incidence of therapy-related MDS and AML occurs 3 to 5 years after initial treatment, but some cases still occur 10 to 12 years later.[68-70] Although historically leukemogenesis correlated with the cumulative dose and schedule of genotoxic drugs such as etoposide, there are published reports of patients who developed secondary leukemia while still on therapy even after minimal doses of causative drugs.[71,72] Patients with therapy-related myeloid neoplasms have significantly worse outcomes than those with *de novo* myeloid disease with the same cytogenetic abnormalities, suggesting a different biologic mechanism of leukemogenesis.[62,73-75]

In addition to the known causative therapeutic agents, individual risk factors exist for therapy-related myeloid neoplasms. A large number of studies demonstrate the importance of individual genetic variation in key genes involved in drug metabolism, cellular protection, and DNA repair. A large number of polymorphisms in genes involved in detoxification of chemotherapeutic agents have been identified. Specifically, polymorphisms in cytochrome p450 and glutathione-S-transferase, genes involved in the detoxification of chemotherapeutic agents, have been linked to the development of t-AML/t-MDS. An additional example is the genetic polymorphism in thiopurine methyltransferase (TPMT). This enzyme catalyzes the S-methylation of thiopurines, including 6-mercaptopurine and 6-thioguanine. There is emerging data that TPMT genotype may influence the risk of developing therapy-related myeloid neoplasms.[68,76]

Environmental Exposures

Environmental leukemogenic factors involve direct damage to DNA or repair mechanisms and may show similarities with the predisposing inherited BM failure syndromes. Several pre- and postnatal factors have been associated with an increased risk of AML, although the etiologic fraction of environmental exposure is very low. Prenatal exposures resulting in increased risk of the development of AML include maternal cigarette use, drug use, and alcohol consumption.[77-81] In addition, significant prenatal exposure to ionizing radiation results in a 10- to 20-fold increase in the incidence of AML. However, the link between the degree of exposure to diagnostic x-ray and the risk of developing AML remains unclear.[82] There is no convincing evidence that leukemogenesis is associated with exposure to nonionizing radiation such as that produced by electromagnetic fields.[83,84] Maternal prenatal diet may affect the risk of AML in children. Maternal ingestion of foods and vegetables with high contents of topoisomerase II inhibitors (e.g., flavinoids such as quercetin, genestein in soy, catechins in green and black tea) during pregnancy has been associated with a higher risk of infant AML, particularly the subtype characterized by MLL gene rearrangements.[77,85,86]

Postnatal exposure to a variety of chemicals, including pesticides, petroleum products, benzenes, and heavy metals, has been confirmed to increase the risk of AML in children.[87] Children are known to be more susceptible to organophosphate accumulation resulting from contact with pesticides.[88] These exposures often occur in farmers and migrant workers.

The rarity of MDS has precluded studies of the etiologic role of exogenous factors in its development.

ACUTE MYELOID LEUKEMIA

Epidemiology

Each year, approximately 10,000 children (ages 0 to 21 years) develop AML worldwide.[89] The incidence of pediatric AML is estimated to be between five to seven cases per million people per year.[90-92] In children younger than 15 years, acute lymphoblastic leukemia (ALL) is approximately five times more common than AML, accounting for 75% of all childhood leukemia diagnoses. AML comprises only 15% to 20% of cases in patients younger than 15 years. The peak incidence of childhood AML occurs in the first year of life and then decreases steadily up to 4 years, at which point it remains relatively constant throughout childhood and early adulthood.[93]

There is no gender-specific difference in incidence; however, racial variation is observed in AML. Although early data demonstrated a higher incidence of AML in whites than in blacks, more recent data show that the incidence is almost equal (6.7 per million in whites and 6.4 per million in blacks). However, Hispanic children have the highest incidence of the racial groups.[94,95] There is evidence of a higher incidence among some Asian populations as well, with 11 cases per million in China and 19 cases per million in South East Asians living in England.[96] A lower incidence exists in India (3.5 cases per million). The frequency of some subtypes of AML may vary according to ethnicity. For example, acute promyelocytic leukemia (APL) occurs at a higher incidence in the Hispanic populations and granulocytic sarcomas are more frequent in children from Africa and Turkey.[97-99]

Biology of AML

AML is characterized by the accumulation of a large number of abnormal cells that fail to differentiate into granulocytes or monocytes. These abnormal cells are the result of a variety of distinct genetic mutations that confer a proliferative and survival advantage due to their effect on differentiation, apoptosis, and self-renewal. These chromosomal abnormalities are heterogeneous and include aberrations such as gains or losses of whole chromosomes, structural abnormalities, or balanced translocations. Many of these genetic rearrangements can be linked to clinical outcomes and will be discussed later in the chapter. New insights into the effect of gene mutations on leukemogenesis have led to improvements in genetic characterization of many cases of cytogenetically normal AML. In fact, up to 45% of patients with a normal karyotype possess genetic abnormalities that are associated with clinical features of the disease and are often powerful prognostic indicators of outcome.[1,6,7,100-107]

The recent discovery of numerous molecular markers has led to a theory of leukemogenesis that revolves around the concept of cooperating mutations and multiple "hits" being required for leukemic transformation. Experiments in murine

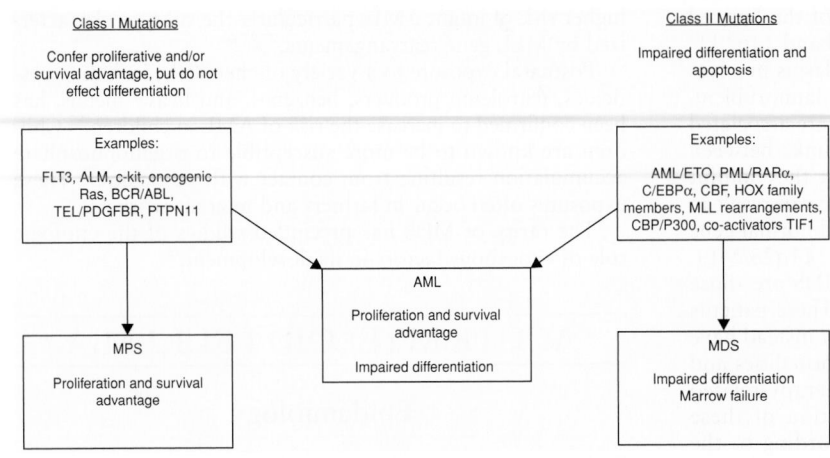

FIGURE 20.2 Cooperating mutations in acute myeloid leukemia. MDS, myelodysplastic syndromes; MPS, myeloproliferative syndromes.

models and investigations into rare inherited leukemia syndromes (FDP-AML) support the theory that multiple steps are required for progression to AML.[7] Analyses of mutations identified in human leukemia suggest that abnormal alleles can be divided into two broad groups: those that confer a proliferative and/or survival advantage (class I mutations), and those that impair differentiation and confer self-renewal properties (class II mutations) (Fig. 20.2). Class I mutant genes exert their effect through aberrant activation of signal transduction pathways. Examples of class I mutations include FLT3/internal tandem duplication (ITD), c-Kit, oncogenic RAS, and PTPN11. Gene fusions included as class I mutations include BCR/ABL and TEL/PDGFRβ. Class II mutations involve abnormalities in transcription factors or transcriptional co-activators that are important for normal hematopoietic differentiation. Examples of class II genetic fusions in AML include AML1/ETO, promyelocytic leukemia/retinoic acid receptor alpha (PML/RARα), and MLL rearrangements. Examples of class II mutations include core binding factor (CBF), HOX family members, C/EPBA, CBP/P300, and co-activators of transcriptional intermediary factor 1 (TIF1).

Data suggest that class I and class II mutations cooperate to induce leukemia. When class I mutations are expressed alone, they induce a CML-like disease characterized by leukocytosis with normal maturation of cells. Likewise, when class II mutations are expressed alone, they confer a phenotype most like MDS. Regardless of the order of acquisition of these mutations, individuals who accrue both class I and class II mutations have a clinical phenotype of AML characterized by excess proliferation and impaired hematopoietic differentiation.[1,2] For example, when FLT3/ITD and PML/RARα are coexpressed, there is invariably progression to AML and the disease may be responsive to agents targeting both molecular abnormalities.[108,109]

There is accumulating evidence that the leukemic stem cell (LSC), also called the "self-renewing leukemia-initiating cell," arises at various stages of differentiation of normal hematopoietic precursors.[102,110,111] In 1994, Dick and colleagues were able to distinguish LSCs from the bulk of AML cells through continued fractionation into subpopulations displaying self-renewal, multipotentiality, and proliferation until a pure population of stem cells was achieved.[110] Further characterization of human AML stem cells defined the immunophenotype as CD34$^+$, CD38$^-$, CD71$^-$, HLA-DR$^-$, CD90$^-$, CD117$^-$, and CD123$^+$.[112] Importantly, CD34$^+$ CD38$^-$ LSCs were able to transmit AML to nonobese diabetic-severe combined immunodeficient mice, whereas the more mature CD34$^+$ CD38$^+$ AML cells did not successfully engraft.[102] These in vivo transplantation studies in immunodeficient mice demonstrated that the self-renewal

capacity of LSCs is significantly higher than that of normal HSCs.[102,110,113,114] These LSCs are quite rare with a frequency range of 0.2 to 200 per 10^6 mononuclear cells.[113,115] From a clinical standpoint, only a small minority of self-renewing LSCs within a functionally heterogeneous population of blasts may be responsible for driving the process of AML and relapsed disease. However, it is not known for certain whether mutations occur in the most primitive hematopoietic stem cells or whether the mutations occur in a more differentiated stem cell, which then acquires the feature of self-renewal. For instance, investigators have reported that the presence of the FLT3/ITD mutation in CD34$^+$/CD33$^-$ precursors is heterogeneous, and detection in the LSC population may be associated with disease resistance.[116]

Classification of AML: Historical Approaches

Although the first published reports of leukemia occurred in 1845 by Bennett and Virchow, the lack of refined diagnostic methodology limited the distinction between myeloid and lymphoid acute leukemia. With the development of refined staining techniques, followed by microscopy and histochemical staining by the mid-20th century, this distinction was possible. The first morphologic classification system for AML was the FAB classification, which was established in 1976 and later revised in 1985. As chemotherapy became increasingly effective, these investigators stressed the importance of a more accurate recording of the distribution of cases entered into clinical trials.[117,118] The FAB classification is based only on morphology and histochemical analysis of malignant cells following staining with Wright, Wright-Giemsa, or May-Grunwald stains, as well as a panel of histochemical markers. Although the classification of neoplasms should take into account all available information—morphology, cytochemistry, immunophenotype, genetics, and clinical features—it has taken a number of years to achieve a comprehensive system.

Evolution of the Current Classification

The FAB classification divided AML into eight subcategories (M0 to M7), which were initially based on staining and histochemical markers only. In 1997, the World Health Organization (WHO) revised the FAB classification to include the percentage, lineage commitment, and differentiation of the cells as determined by morphologic, immunophenotypic, and cytogenetic features. Although the initial classification scheme required 30% BM blasts (with the exception of M6 and M7), the WHO classification lowered the malignant blast percentage required for

AML diagnosis to 20% myeloblasts. As there is little evidence for lowering the blast count to 20%, a pediatric approach has been developed to rely not only on blast count but also to consider clinical features and cytogenetics.[119,120] In 2001, the WHO published a classification that, for the first time, incorporated genetic information along with morphologic, cytochemical, immunophenotypic, and clinical information into diagnostic algorithms for myeloid neoplasms.[121] These changes allowed for the diagnosis of AML to be made regardless of blast count and included entities associated with specific genetic abnormalities. The three abnormalities included in the algorithms involved rearrangements of genes (AML with t(8;21)(q22;q22); RUNX1-RUNX1T1, AML with inv(16)(p13.1q22) or t(16;16)(p13.1; q22); CBFβ-MYH11, and APL with t(15;17)(q22;q12)PML-RARα) that encode transcription factors and are associated with distinct clinical and morphologic features. In 2008, the WHO criteria were revised and included additional entries in the category of AML with recurrent genetic abnormalities. One important revision was to modify "AML with abnormalities of 11q23; MLL" from the previous edition and to change this to t(9;11)(p22;q23);MLLT3-MLL. This was done to reflect that all MLL rearrangements are not identical. In fact, it is recommended that variant MLL translocations also be specified in the diagnosis. Additional chromosomal rearrangements added to the most recent WHO classification include t(6;9)(p23;q34); DEK-NUP21, inv(3)(q21q26.2) or t(3;3)(q26.2);RPN1-EV11, and t(1;22)(p13;q13);RBM15-MKL1 (Table 20.3).

Immunophenotyping

Although the FAB and WHO criteria do not utilize immunophenotyping for classification purposes, its use in initial diagnosis and disease monitoring is considered standard of care and necessary to differentiate AML from ALL[122–124] (Table 20.4). The specificity and sensitivity of distinguishing ALL from AML by cell surface immunophenotyping are quite high.[125,126] Further, flow cytometric detection of leukemic blasts is based on the multiparameter analysis of their aberrant pattern of expression of normal differentiation antigens. Multiparameter analysis by flow cytometry can be used to determine a quantitative measurement of persistent leukemic blasts at levels as low as 1 in 10,000 mononuclear BM cells.[123,127] This level of minimal residual disease (MRD) detection exceeds other methods such as morphology and cytogenetics, which can detect 1 leukemic cell in 100 mononuclear BM cells.[128,129] The prognostic utility of MRD will be discussed in more detail later in the chapter.

Immunophenotyping studies demonstrate significant associations between the expression of cell surface proteins and the WHO classification of AML subtypes. Antigens commonly utilized in the diagnosis of AML include CD11b, CD13, CD14, CD15, CD33, CD34, CD41, CD42, CD56, CD61, CD64, glycophorin A, class II human leukocyte antigens (HLA-DR), myeloperoxidase (MPO), and CD117 (c-kit).[130] CD13, CD33, and c-kit are the most commonly expressed myeloid markers and are present on the blasts of about 90% of patients. The FAB M4 (acute myelomonocytic leukemia) subtype commonly expresses CD14 (73%), CD15 (100%), CD13 (57%), and CD33 (92%), demonstrating differentiation along the monocytic lineage.[131] The M5 subtype (acute monocytic leukemia) shows a similar pattern of expression but loses expression of CD13. CD36 and CD64 are also helpful in identifying cells with monocytic differentiation. In contrast, M1 and M2 blasts often express CD13 (80%), but they express lower levels of CD14 (10% to 20%). Progenitors that differentiate along the erythroid lineage express glycophorin A, which is a helpful marker in the diagnosis of acute erythroblastic leukemia (M6). Expression of platelet-associated cell surface antigens, including

TABLE 20.3

WHO CLASSIFICATION OF ACUTE MYELOID LEUKEMIA AND RELATED MYELOID NEOPLASMS

Acute myeloid leukemia with recurrent genetic abnormalities
  AML with t(8;21)(q22;q22); RUNX1-RUNX1T1
  AML with inv(16)(p13.1;q22) or t(16;16)(p13.1;q22); CBFβ-MYH11
  APL with t(15;17)(q22;q12); PML-RARα
  AML with t(9;11)(p22;q23); MLLT3-MLL
  AML with t(6;9)(p23;q34); DEK-NUP214
  AML with inv(3)(q21;q26.2) or t(3;3)(q21;q26.2); RPN1-EVI1
  AML (megakaryoblastic) with t(1:22)(p13;q13); RBM15-MKL1
  Provisional entity: AML with mutated NPM1
  Provisional entity: AML with mutated CEBPA

Acute myeloid leukemia with myelodysplasia-related changes

Therapy-related myeloid neoplasms

Acute myeloid leukemia, not otherwise specified
  AML with minimal differentiation
  AML without maturation
  AML with maturation
  Acute myelomonocytic leukemia
  Acute monoblastic/monocytic leukemia
  Acute erythroid leukemias
    Pure erythroid leukemia
    Erythroleukemia, erythroid/myeloid
  Acute megakaryoblastic leukemia
  Acute basophilic leukemia
  Acute panmyelosis with myelofibrosis

Myeloid sarcoma

Myeloid proliferations related to Down syndrome
  Transient abnormal myelopoiesis
  Myeloid leukemia associated with Down syndrome

Blastic plasmacytoid dendritic cell neoplasms

AML, acute myeloid leukemia, APL, acute promyelocytic leukemia. Swerdlow SH, Campo E, Harris NL, et al., eds. Tumors of hematopoietic and lymphoid tissues (WHO classification of tumors). Pathology and genetics. Lyon: IARC, 2008 (reproduced with permission).

CD41, CD42, and CD61, indicates differentiation along the megakaryocytic lineage; their expression is helpful in the diagnosis of acute megakaryocytic leukemia (M7). False-positive results using these cell surface proteins can occur when platelets adhere to the surface of blasts. Therefore, detection of intracytoplasmic proteins, such as platelet peroxidase, or immunophenotyping on BM trephine biopsies should be confirmatory.[132]

Leukemia of Ambiguous Lineage

Although immunophenotyping can distinguish AML from ALL in greater than 90% of cases,[125,126] multiparameter flow cytometry has led to the recognition of a greater complexity of antigen expression than previously considered. In particular, flow cytometry may reveal diagnostic criteria strongly indicative of a commitment to one lineage but with aberrant expression of antigens of another lineage. In a retrospective study by the Children's Cancer Group (CCG), 24% of AML cases expressed the B-lineage marker CD19 and 48% expressed one or more T-lineage cell surface antigen.[133] When analyzing

TABLE 20.4

IMMUNOPHENOTYPING OF AML

Marker	M0[a]	M1	M2	M3	M4	M5	M6	M7
Myeloid								
CD11b				+	++	++	−	−
CD13	++	++	+	+	++	++	+	+
CD14	−	−	−	−	++	−	−	−
CD15	+	+	+	++	++	++	−	−
CD33	++	++	++	+++	++	+++	++	++
CD34	++	++	++	+/−	+	+/−	−	+/−
CD65	++	++	++	++	++	++	++	+
Erythroid								
Glycophorin A	−	−	−	−	−	−	++	−
Megakaryocytic								
CD41/61	−	−	−	−	−	−	−	++
CD42	−	−	−	−	−	−	−	++
CD36	+/−	+/−	+/−		++	++		++
B-cell lineage								
CD10	−	−	−	−		−	−	−
CD19	−	−	−	−		−	−	−
CD20	−	−	−	−		−	−	−
T-cell lineage								
CD2	+	+	+	+	+	+	−	++
CD3	−	−	−	−	−	−		
CD4	−	−	−		++	++	−	+
CD7	−	+	+	+	+	+	+	+
CD56	+/−	+/−	+/−	+/−	+	+	−	+
Other								
HLA-DR	++	++	++	+/−	+++	+++	−	+
CD117	++	++	+	+	+	+/−[b]	+/−	+

[a]M0 is negative for myeloperoxidase with light microscopy but may show some positivity at the electron microscopic level.
[b]CD117 expression has been reported to be present on 100% of M5a but negative on M5b.[130]

multicenter trials, up to 60% of AML cases express lymphoid antigens, but without prognostic significance.[134,135] In addition, myeloid antigens may be expressed on ALL blasts in up to 50% of cases.[134,136]

Historically, there has been confusion in the definition, terminology, and criteria used for classifying leukemias expressing mixed phenotypes.[137,138] The third edition of the WHO criteria attempted to categorize these leukemias of ambiguous lineage by utilizing a scoring system proposed by the European Group for the Immunologic Classification of Leukaemia.[121] In this classification scheme, antigenic determinants were given numeric scores based on their degree of lineage specificity. These criteria provided practitioners with a reproducible method of lineage assignment; however, there were flaws in this classification system. Among the drawbacks to this method were controversial "weighting" of some markers and the fact that abnormal molecular genetics were not considered. Ignoring these important diagnostic features often resulted in the arbitrary mixing of biologically distinct leukemias under the same label. The fourth edition of the WHO criteria addressed this confusion by placing acute leukemias of ambiguous lineage in a chapter distinct from those of AML and ALL and altering the criteria used to define them.[139] Leukemia with blasts that coexpress certain antigens of more than one lineage on the same cells or that have separate populations of blasts that are of different lineages are now referred to as mixed phenotype acute

leukemia (MPAL). In the current classification, only a limited number of antigens are used in defining the pattern of lineage involvement. For a blast to be assigned to the myeloid lineage, there must be expression of MPO (by flow cytometry, immunohistochemistry, or cytochemistry) or it must express monocytic differentiation by at least two of the following: nonspecific esterase, CD11c, CD14, CD64, lysosyme, or megakaryoblast markers. Cases of MPAL may be further designated as B/myeloid or T/myeloid based on specific criteria as defined in 2008 WHO classification[61] (Table 20.5).

Cytogenetics

A complete cytogenetic analysis of leukemia cells is essential during initial evaluation to establish the diagnosis and risk classification, and to help to define the biology of the disease[140-143] (Table 20.6). Repeated analyses are recommended as needed after diagnosis for judging the response to therapy or for detecting genetic evolution. The primary approach is conventional karyotyping, which can demonstrate chromosomal number (ploidy) and structural changes such as amplifications, deletions, translocations, or inversions. Additional genetic studies should be guided by the results of the initial karyotype and by the diagnosis suspected based on the clinical, morphologic, and immunophenotypic studies. New technologies have

TABLE 20.5

REQUIREMENTS FOR ASSIGNING MORE THAN ONE LINEAGE TO A SINGLE BLAST POPULATION

Myeloid lineage
Myeloperoxidase (flow cytometry, immunohistochemistry, or cytochemistry)
Or
Monocytic differentiation (at least two of the following: NSE, CD11c, CD14, CD64, lysozyme)

T lineage
Cytoplasmic CD3 (flow cytometry with antibodies to CD3 epsilon chain; immunohistochemistry using polyclonal anti-CD3 antibody may detect CD3 zeta chain, which is not T-cell specific)
Or
Surface CD3 (rare in mixed phenotype acute leukemias)

B lineage (multiple antigens required)
Strong CD19 with at least 1 of the following strongly expressed: CD79a, cytoplasmic CD22, CD10
Or
Weak CD19 with at least two of the following strongly expressed: CD79a, cytoplasmic CD22, CD10

Swerdlow SH, Campo E, Harris NL, et al., eds. Tumors of hematopoietic and lymphoid tissues (WHO classification of tumors). Pathology and genetics. Lyon: IARC, 2008 (reproduced with permission).

---

resulted in a large number of potential methodologies that may have clinical utility.

Florescent *in situ* hybridization (FISH) uses fluorescently labeled nucleic acid probes to detect chromosomal abnormalities in metaphase and interphase cell chromosomes. This technique complements karyotyping through its ability to analyze many more leukemic cells (>500 cells analyzed by FISH) than conventional karyotyping ($\approx$20 to 40 metaphases in routine karyotyping). FISH probes designed specifically for chromosomes and translocations commonly implicated in neoplasms are a useful technique for monitoring for the presence of MRD. Polymerase chain reaction (PCR) techniques allow for selective amplification of defined DNA regions, and thus can be used to identify unique sequences specific to genetic abnormalities such as inversions, deletions, or translocations.[144] When coupled with DNA sequencing, this technique can detect single base pair mutations in DNA and is highly sensitive, identifying a mutation in 100,000 BM cells. Abnormal RNA transcripts, resulting from chromosomal translocations, can be detected at a high level of sensitivity using reverse transcription PCR (RT-PCR). In addition, subclassification using genomic and RNA expression microarray and proteomic technologies will clearly have a major impact on the ability to classify leukemias and determine appropriate molecularly directed therapies in the future.[145]

Subtypes of AML

AML with minimal evidence of myeloid differentiation (AML M0) has no evidence of myeloid differentiation by morphology or light microscopy cytochemistry.[146] These cases comprise less than 3% of pediatric AML. The cytoplasm is agranular with a varying degree of basophilia. The blast cells express one or more myeloid cell surface antigens, including CD13, CD33, and CD117 (c-kit). Often there may be expression of antigens

associated with lymphoid differentiation, including CD2, CD7, or CD19, but at lower intensity than that in lymphoid leukemias.[147,148]

AML without maturation (AML M1) comprises about 20% of pediatric AML and is characterized by a high percentage of BM blasts without significant evidence of maturation to more differentiated neutrophils. Morphologically, myeloblasts are often seen, some with azurophilic granules. In contrast to AML M0, M1 blasts often express MPO. The blasts express at least two myelomonocytic antigens, including CD13, CD33, and CD117, and CD34 is often positive.[147]

AML with maturation (AML M2) comprises about 30% of pediatric AML cases. Blasts with and without azurophilic granules are present. Variable degrees of dysplasia are often present. Cases with increased marrow basophils may have recurrent cytogenetic abnormalities, including deletions and translocations at 12p and t(6;9). The t(8;21) translocation usually occurs in this subtype with a frequency of 10% to 15%.[149]

APL, AML with the t(15;17) (q22;q12) and PML/RARα (AML M3, APL) represents about 5% to 10% of childhood AML. Morphologically, hypergranular and micro- or hypogranular (M3v) types exist. The nuclear size and shape in hypergranular APL are greatly variable and irregular. The cytoplasmic granules may be so large that they totally obscure the nuclear/cytoplasmic margin. Many of these cells contain bundles of Auer rods that are usually larger than that in other types of AML. The hypogranular variant has a paucity or absence of granules and a predominantly bilobed nuclear shape.[150] The MPO reaction is strongly positive. The sensitivity of APL cells to all trans-retinoic acid (ATRA) has led to the discovery that the RARα gene on chromosome 17 fuses with a nuclear regulatory factor on chromosome 15 (PML gene), giving rise to a PML-RARα product.[151] There are three variants involving RARα: t(11;17)(PLZF/RARα), t(11;17)(NuMA/RARα), and t(5;17). These different translocations have prognostic significance, with t(15;17) patients showing excellent response to ATRA and t(11;17) patients being the most resistant.[149,152]

AML M4 accounts for approximately 25% to 30% of pediatric cases of AML, often occurring in children younger than 2 years. The BM usually contains more than 20% blasts, and neutrophilic and monocytic precursors each comprise more than 20% of the marrow cells. This minimal limit of 20% monocytes distinguishes AML M4 from other forms of AML in which monocytes may be present. Another useful tool in the diagnosis is the fact that there are usually a high number ($\geq$5 $\times$ 10^9/L) of peripheral monocytes. The myeloid blasts of AML M4 are usually MPO positive and express characteristic surface antigens such as CD13, CD15, and CD33. The monocytic blasts express typical myeloid surface markers, as well as CD14, CD4, and HLA-DR. A variant of AML M4, called M4Eo, is characterized by an abnormal eosinophil component in the marrow. This variant is strongly associated with alterations of chromosome 16, most commonly inv(16) (16q22). The morphologic appearance of these abnormal eosinophils is most evident at the promyelocyte and myelocyte stages. The granules are often large, purple-violet in color, and often so dense that they obscure the cell morphology. Both inv(16) and t(16;16) result in the fusion of the CBFβ gene at 16q22 to the smooth muscle myosin heavy chain (MYH11) at 16p13. By conventional cytogenetics, the inv(16) is a subtle rearrangement; thus, the use of FISH and RT-PCR may be necessary to find the genetic abnormality.[139]

Acute monoblastic/monocytic leukemia (AML M5) are MLs in which at least 80% of the leukemia cells are of monocytic lineage. This represents approximately 15% of AML in children older than 2 years and about 50% of AML in children

TABLE 20.6

CYTOGENETIC ABNORMALITIES IN CHILDHOOD AML[a]

Chromosome abnormality	AML FAB type	Affected genes	Functions	Frequency (%)	Comments
t(8;21)(q22;q22)	M1, M2	ETO-AML1	Transcription factors	5–15	Auer rods common; chloromas
t(15;17)(q22;q12)	M3, M3v	PML-RARα	Transcription factor, hormone receptor	6–15	Coagulopathy; ATRA responsiveness
t(11;17)(q23;q12)	M3	PLZF-RARα	Transcription factor, hormone receptor	Rare	Coagulopathy; ATRA unresponsiveness
inv (16)(p13;q22); t(16;16)	M4Eo	MYH11-CBFβ	Muscle protein, transcription factor	2–11	CNS leukemia; eosinophilia with basophilic granules
t(8;16)	M5b	MOZ-CBP	Transcription factors	1	Infants or young adults; high WBC count; chloromas; erythrophagocytosis; secondary leukemia after epipodophyllotoxins
t(9;11)(p22;q23)	M4, M5a	AF9-MLL	Homeodomain proteins	5–13	Infants or young adults; high WBC count; chloromas; erythrophagocytosis; secondary leukemia after epipodophyllotoxins
t(10;11)(p12;q23)	M5	AF10-MLL	Homeodomain proteins	Rare	Infants or young adults; high WBC count; chloromas; erythrophagocytosis; secondary leukemia after epipodophyllotoxins
t(11;17)(q23;q21)	M5	MLL-AF17	Homeodomain proteins	Rare	Infants or young adults; high WBC count; chloromas; erythrophagocytosis; secondary leukemia after epipodophyllotoxins
t(11q23)[b]	M4, M5	MLL, other partners	Homeodomain proteins	2–10	Infants; high WBC count, CNS and skin involvement; poor prognosis associated often associated with these, especially t(4;11)
t(1;22)	M7	RBM15-MKL1	RNA binding protein, DNA binding protein	2–3	M7 AML in infants with Down syndrome; myelofibrosis
t(6;9)	M2, M4, MDS	DEK-CAN	Transcription factor, nuclear protein	1	Basophilia
inv(3)(q21;q26) t(3;3) (q21;q26)	M2, M4, MDS	EVI1	Transcription factor	1	Prior MDS; thrombocytosis and abnormal platelets
−7/del(7)(q22-q36)	All subtypes, MDS			2–7	Toxic exposure; prior MDS; more common in older adults; bacterial infections common
−5/del(5)(q11-q35)	All subtypes, MDS			Rare	Toxic exposure; prior MDS; more common in older adults
+8	All subtypes			5–13	Prior MDS; older patients

[a]This table is not a complete list of all chromosomal abnormalities associated with childhood AML but represents some of the more common abnormalities or those with important phenotypic characteristics. See text for references.
[b]11q23 translocations involving the MLL gene have been shown to have many different fusion partners.
AML, acute myeloid leukemia; ATRA, all-trans-retinoic acid; CNS, central nervous system; FAB, French-American-British; MDS, myelodysplastic syndrome; WBC, white blood cell.

younger than 2 years. In infancy, it is frequently associated with the t(9;11) translocation and involves the translocation of the interferon beta 1 gene into the MLL gene locus of 11q23–24.[153] In addition, translocation t(8;16) may be associated with M4 or M5 leukemia, and in the majority of cases it is associated with erythrophagocytosis and coagulopathy. Extramedullary disease and bleeding disorders are also common in AML M5. There are two categories: M5a or monoblastic leukemia, in which more than 80% of BM cells are monoblasts, and M5b or monocytic leukemia, in which 80% of the cells are a mixture of monoblasts, promonocytes, and monocytes. M5a blasts are usually large with multiple nucleoli and do not contain Auer rods. M5b blasts are more differentiated, granular, and Auer rods are often present. These

leukemias variably express myeloid antigens CD13, CD33, and CD117 and usually show markers characteristic of monocytic differentiation such as CD14.

AML with predominant erythroid differentiation (AML M6) is present in 5% of pediatric AML cases.[154] This subtype is diagnosed when more than 50% of the BM cells are erythroblasts and more than 20% of the nonerythroid population are myeloblasts. Pure erythroid leukemia is extremely rare but can occur in childhood. This represents a proliferation of immature cells committed exclusively to the erythroid lineage; these cells comprise more than 80% of marrow cells. The erythroblasts generally lack myeloid-associated markers and are MPO negative but are strongly periodic acid-Schiff and carbonic anhydrase positive. There are no specific chromosomal abnormalities associated with M6 leukemia; however, complex karyotypes are common with chromosomes 5 and 7 being the most affected.

Acute megakaryoblastic leukemia (AMKL) (AML M7) occurs in 5% to 10% of pediatric cases of AML but is the most common type of leukemia in children younger than 2 years with DS.[155,156] Organomegaly is uncommon except in infants with AML M7 associated with the t(1;22) translocation, who often present with large abdominal masses. Morphologically the megakaryoblasts usually have a round, irregular, or indented nucleus, fine chromatin, and one to three nucleoli. The cytoplasm is basophilic, agranular, and shows blebs or pseudopod formation. Occasionally, the blasts are smaller with a low nucleus-to-cytoplasm ratio, resembling L2 lymphoblasts. Often, the blasts present with clusters of platelets surrounding them. In infants expressing the t(1;22) translocation, examination may reveal a stromal pattern of marrow infiltration mimicking a metastatic tumor. These BM examinations may also result in dry "taps" because of a significant amount of fibrosis.[157] Immunophenotyping shows the megakaryoblasts expressing one or more platelet glycoproteins: CD41 (IIb/IIIa), and/or CD61 (IIIa). CD36 is characteristically positive.

Clinical and Laboratory Features

There is a large range of presenting signs and symptoms in children diagnosed with AML. Patients may present with minimal symptoms associated with anemia or with life-threatening complications due to leukemic infiltration resulting in organ dysfunction or failure.

A diagnosis is suggested by a complete blood cell count that demonstrates pancytopenia and peripheral blasts visible on a peripheral smear. The median white blood cell (WBC) count at diagnosis is approximately 20×10^9/L, and about 20% of patients present with a WBC count above $100,000 \times 10^9$/L.[158,159] The hemoglobin count is less than 9 g/dL in more than half of the patients, and platelet counts of less than 100×10^9/L occur in nearly 75% of the patients.[160] Hyperuricemia, hyperkalemia, and hyperphosphatemia may lead to tumor lysis syndrome and require intensive supportive care, although this occurs less frequently in AML than in ALL.[159]

The degree of electrolyte disturbances usually varies depending on the leukemic burden and cell turnover rate and can complicate the initiation of cytoreductive therapy. In particular, hypokalemia, hypophosphatemia, hypocalcemia, and hypoalbunemia can be associated with AML M4/M5. These electrolyte abnormalities are the result of renal tubular dysfunction caused by lysozyme released from leukemic cells.[161] Fever is a common presentation in children with AML, often secondary to pyrogens released by leukemic cells or as an inflammatory response to the blast cells. However, patients are at high risk for bacterial infections because of a low number of functional neutrophils, often less than 1,000 cells/mL. The presence of fever in this patient population should be considered an emergency, blood and urine cultures should be performed and broad-spectrum antibiotic coverage initiated.[162,163] Normocytic, normochromic anemia as a result of marrow infiltration with leukemic blasts is common, with resultant headache, dizziness, pallor, and fatigue.[160] Anemia can also be the result of organ infiltration, blood loss from thrombocytopenia, disseminated intravascular coagulation (DIC) due to infection, or the release of procoagulants from cytoplasmic granules in some AML blasts.[164] Organomegaly is seen in approximately half of the patients with AML due to hepatic and splenic infiltration with leukemic blasts, except in DS patients with AML M7. These patients often present with

hepatomegaly secondary to fibrosis, which can lead to liver failure.[165]

Hyperleukocytosis

Due to the large size of AML blasts and their adhesion properties, children with elevated WBC counts are at risk of complications related to leukostasis. This condition can result in progressive neurologic or respiratory symptoms caused by clumping and sludging of blasts in small blood vessels.[166,167] Death during the first 2 weeks after diagnosis occurs in 2% to 4% of children with AML, mainly due to bleeding and leukostasis.[163] Death occurs in up to 20% of patients with severe leukostasis as a result of intracranial bleeding or pulmonary insufficiency.[168,169] Symptoms of central nervous system (CNS) leukostasis can vary and include confusion, headache, and a somnolence syndrome that can progress to coma. Pulmonary manifestations result from leukemic infiltration of alveoli and pulmonary parenchyma, resulting in pulmonary edema, respiratory failure, and often pulmonary hemorrhage. Although hyperleukocytosis is an important risk factor, an elevated WBC count alone is an inconsistent predictor of leukostasis. In AML, leukostasis occurs at a range of presenting leukocyte counts.[170] Although most children do not develop symptoms of leukostasis with a WBC count above 200×10^9/L, patients with monoblastic leukemia (AML M5) are at high risk even at a WBC count of 100×10^9/L.

Compared with other myeloid blast cells, monoblasts have increased adhesiveness, motility, and potential for tissue invasion.[171] Children with symptomatic leukostasis tend to be younger (<2 years of age) and have an increased incidence of extramedullary involvement, coagulopathy, and a higher incidence of early death.[158] In all patients at risk of leukostasis, rapid lowering of the WBC count is necessary, often using leukapheresis and aggressive hydration.[167] Leukapheresis frequently is initiated in patients with AML who have initial WBC counts above 100 or 200×10^9/L, although the benefit remains untested. The disadvantages of the procedure are the necessity for placement of a central venous catheter, further decrease in the number of platelets as they are removed together with the WBCs, and the finding that the blast counts often rebound quickly after leukapheresis unless additional cytoreductive medications are started immediately.

Coagulopathies

Bleeding and thrombosis are common causes of morbidity and mortality at presentation and as a result of treatment of childhood AML. Patients often present with bruising, petechiae, epistaxis, gingival bleeding, or menorrhagia. More serious hemorrhagic presentations may occur, including overt bleeding from the large or small bowels or CNS hemorrhage. Most patients are thrombocytopenic at diagnosis. Thrombocytopenia is often accompanied by decreased plasma fibrinogen concentrations, prolonged prothrombin time (PT), activated partial thromboplastin (aPTT) time or thrombin time, and elevated levels of plasma fibrinogen.[172,173] Coagulopathy may also occur as a result of DIC due to either infection or the release of procoagulants from the cytoplasmic granules of some AML blasts, particularly in APL but also in AML M4 and M5. APL cells are rich in procoagulants that activate factor VII and factor X. Initiation of chemotherapy may result in the release of these procoagulants and worsen DIC.[158,164,174] Reduction in leukemic cell burden, aggressive clotting factor replacement, and platelet transfusions are frequently necessary to prevent catastrophic bleeding. With the use of ATRA during induction therapy for APL, hemorrhagic complications have been reduced drastically.[175,176] ATRA has provided an alternative to cytotoxic chemotherapy to induce remission by promoting differentiation of promyelocytes, thus inducing apoptosis without acute lysis of leukemic blasts.

Extramedullary Myeloid Disease (EMD)

Myeloid sarcomas (granulocytic sarcoma, chloroma, extramedullary myeloid tumor) consist of myeloblasts or immature myeloid cells at an extramedullary site. Extramedullary involvement (EMD) is observed in 10% to 20% of patients with AML, with gingival hypertrophy, lymphadenopathy, and leukemia cutis being the most common presentations. These tumors should be treated even in the absence of BM involvement. They may occur at diagnosis or relapse and are often found to be associated with t(8;21), inv(16), or 11q23 MLL rearrangements.[177,178] EMD can also be found in the orbit or periorbital areas or may present as a paraspinal mass resulting in cauda equina syndrome or paraparesis.[179] CNS involvement is seen more commonly with the M4 and M5 classifications and often presents with a high WBC count. It can present as either leukemic blasts in the spinal fluid or as chloromas with associated neurologic findings. EMD presenting in the testis is rare, especially when compared with its incidence in children with ALL.[180]

In a retrospective report from the CCG, AML patients were divided into three groups: group 1—EMD involving the skin (with or without other sites), group 2—EMD not involving the skin, and group 3—those without EMD. Group 1 patients tended to be younger, had higher incidence of CNS disease, higher WBC counts, and a higher incidence of AML M4/M5. Nonskin EMD (group 2) was an independent favorable prognostic factor with a 5-year event-free survival (EFS) of 46% compared with groups 1 and 3 with 5-year EFS of 26% and 29%, respectively.[181]

Treatment of Childhood AML

The prognosis for children with AML has improved greatly over the last three decades.[182–189] Complete remission (CR) rates as high as 80% to 90% and overall survival (OS) rates of up to 65% are now reported worldwide[190] (Fig. 20.3A–D). This improvement has been accomplished by a number of factors including enrollment of children into clinical trials, dose intensification, and improved supportive care. These interventions have transformed a disease that was once uniformly fatal into one that is potentially curable. However, despite these advances, the cure rate for children with AML lags behind that for children with ALL, with the main reasons for treatment failure being relapse and treatment-related mortality. Currently, approximately one-third of all deaths due to leukemia in children are attributable to AML.

Chemotherapeutic regimens for AML consist of remission-induction chemotherapy, CNS prophylaxis, and postremission therapy. Initial strategies for AML were based on ALL therapy: intensive induction therapy followed by a prolonged maintenance course, which included cranial irradiation. Development of chemotherapeutic regimens was based on the Goldie-Coldman hypothesis, which stated that the early use of mechanistically rational combinations of non–cross-resistant drugs delivered simultaneously and in sequential rotation would provide a more potent antileukemic effect.[191,192] This therapeutic philosophy led to improvements in 5-year survival estimates from less than 10% prior to 1970 to 25% to 35% in the 1970s and 1980s.

Induction Therapy

Historical Perspective—Introduction of Cytarabine and the Anthracyclines. Aggressive induction therapy is an important treatment principle that improves remission induction rate and leads to improved OS. Historically, the goal of induction chemotherapy has been to achieve complete morphologic remission, defined as less than 5% AML blasts present in the BM in the presence of recovery of trilineage hematopoiesis. In the 1960s, cytarabine (ara-C) and the anthracyclines were used as single agents in the treatment of AML, inducing remission in one-third to one-half of patients.[193] Initially, use of cytarabine as a single agent for 5 to 7 days resulted in CR rates of 25%, and further intensification of cytarabine was found to overcome some resistance mechanisms.[194] Early studies in AML also demonstrated the efficacy of anthracyclines when used as a single agent.[195] The two agents were combined in the 1970s with the introduction of the "7 + 3" regimen, resulting in induction remission rates of 60% to 70% in adults and 75% to 80% in children.[196] This regimen combined a 7-day infusion of cytarabine at a dose of 100 mg/m²/day with 3 days of daunorubicin at a dose of 45 mg/m².[197]

Since the initial single-agent trials utilizing anthracyclines, additional efforts have focused on the development of alternative, non–cross-reactive anthracyclines such as mitoxantrone, idarubicin, and amsacrine.[198–200] Clinical trials from the Medical Research Council (MRC) in the United Kingdom have found daunorubicin and mitoxantrone to be equally efficacious but mitoxantrone to be more myelosuppressive.[186] Compared with daunorubicin, idarubicin enters the cells more quickly, has superior intracellular retention, is associated with less *in vitro* drug resistance, and is converted to active metabolites that have a longer half-life.[201] Berlin-Frankfurt-Munster (BFM) clinical trials have compared the efficacy between idarubicin and daunorubicin in induction therapy. Idarubicin was associated with better early clearance of blast cells in high-risk patients; however, remission rates and EFS were similar between cohorts.[199,200] Additional trials have not achieved higher remission rates using idarubicin[202,203]; however, some argue that the data are not accurate because of the issue of dose equivalency between different anthracyclines.

Since early trials utilizing cytarabine and daunorubicin, improvement of remission induction rates have centered on concepts of dose intensification, prolonged exposure to chemotherapeutic agents, and intensive timing of drug delivery. A series of international trials have been implemented to test all of these concepts of improving remission-induction rates.

Dose Intensification During Induction Chemotherapy. The success of the "7 + 3" combination regimen led to variations that attempted to intensify the 7 + 3 backbone. The CCG 213 trial randomized induction chemotherapy between the 7 + 3 regimen and the "Denver" regimen, which added etoposide, thioguanine, and dexamethasone to the cytarabine/daunorubicin backbone.[204] There was no statistically significant difference in CR rates or OS between the two groups.[197,205]

One focus of Pediatric Oncology Group (POG) studies from 1981 to 2000 was to explore the impact of dose intensification of cytarabine. The POG 8498 study randomized patients to receive either two induction courses of DAT (daunorubicin, cytarabine, thioguanine) or one induction course of DAT followed by a second induction course of high-dose cytarabine. Remission rates were excellent (85%), but similar between the two groups. However, the 3-year EFS was superior for those who received high-dose cytarabine than those who did not (34% vs. 29%).[206] The POG 9421 study advanced this concept by randomizing patients to receive either one course of DAT and high-dose cytarabine during induction or two induction courses

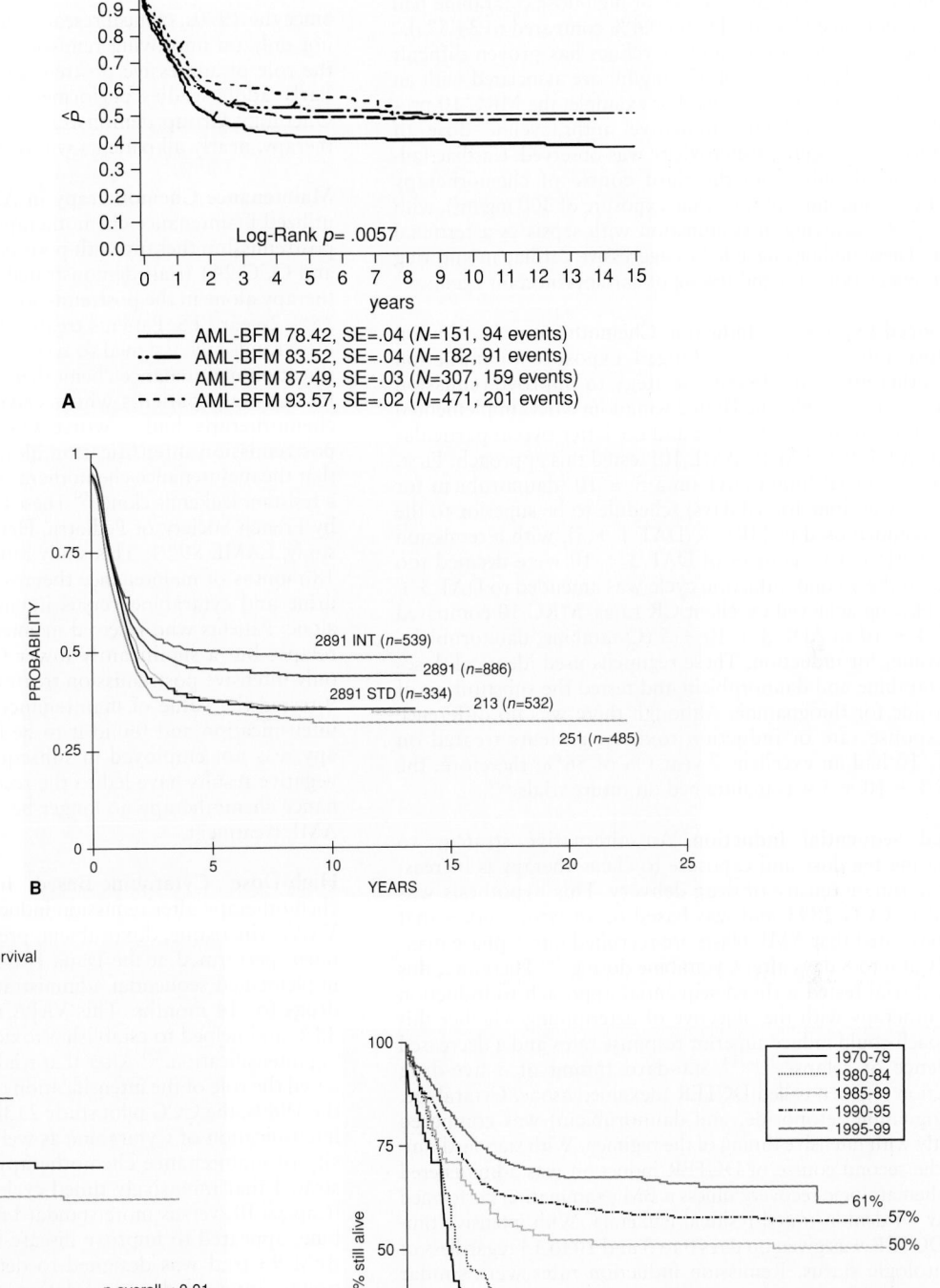

FIGURE 20.3 A: Estimated probability of survival in patients on trials AML-BFM 78–93, 5 year data given. Slash indicates the patient alive with the shortest follow-up. (Creutzig U, Zimmermann M, Ritter J, et al. Leukemia 2005; 19; 2030–42. Reproduced with permission) **B:** Overall survival for CCG 251, CCG 213 and CCG 2891. Standard and intensive timed induction. (Smith FO, Alonzo TA, Gerbing RB, et al. Leukemia 2005; 19; 2054–62. Reproduced with permission) **C:** Estimated probability of survival in patients on studies NOPHO-AML 84/88/93. (Lie SO, Abramsson J, Clausen N,et al. Leukemia 2005; 19:2090–100. Reproduced with permission) **D:** MRC AML trials; overall survival: Age 0–14 years: 1970–1999. (Gibson BES, Wheatley K, Hann IM et al. Leukemia 2005; 19; 2130-38. Reproduced with permission).

of high-dose cytarabine. Remission rates were again similar, but patients who received two courses of high-dose cytarabine had superior outcome (3-year EFS of 40.4% compared to 34.5%).

Dose intensification of anthracyclines has proven difficult because cumulative doses of 375 mg/m² are associated with an increased risk of cardiotoxicity. For example, the MRC 10 protocol delivered a high cumulative anthracycline dose of 550 mg/m² and acute cardiotoxicity was observed. Cardiac failure occurred only from the third course of chemotherapy onwards (minimum anthracycline exposure of 300 mg/m²), with 78% (7/9) occurring in conjunction with sepsis as a terminal event. These findings have led to aggressive cardiac monitoring and investigation into and testing of cardioprotectant agents.[207]

Prolonged Exposure to Induction Chemotherapy. In addition to dose intensification, prolonged exposure to induction chemotherapy is an effective strategy to improve remission rates. As an example, the United Kingdom MRC implemented three trials from 1978 to 1995 and the latter two in particular (MRC AML 9 and MRC AML 10) tested this approach. First, the MRC 9 trial found DAT on a 3 + 10 (daunorubicin for 3 days, cytarabine for 10 days) schedule to be superior to the DAT regimen used in MRC 8 (DAT 1 + 5), with a remission rate of 91%. Two courses of DAT 3 + 10 were deemed too toxic, so the second induction cycle was amended to DAT 3 + 8.[208] Having achieved excellent CR rates, MRC 10 compared DAT 3 + 10 to ADE 3 + 10 + 5 (Cytarabine, daunorubicin, etoposide) for induction. These regimens used identical doses of cytarabine and daunorubicin and tested the substitution of etoposide for thioguanine. Although there was no difference in response rate or induction toxicity, patients treated on MRC 10 had an excellent 7-year OS of 56%; therefore, the ADE 3 + 10 + 5 was maintained on future trials.[209]

Timed Sequential Induction. An alternative strategy to increasing the dose and exposure to chemotherapy is increasing the time-intensity of drug delivery. This hypothesis was tested in CCG-2891 and was based on *in vitro* studies that demonstrated that AML blasts are recruited into S phase maximally at 6 to 8 days after Cytarabine dosing.[210] Therefore, this clinical trial tested a timed sequential approach to induction chemotherapy with the objective of determining whether this approach could induce superior response rates and a decreased incidence of relapse.[211-214] Standard timing of a five-drug induction regimen called DCTER (dexamethasone, Cytarabine, 6-thioguanine, etoposide, and daunorubicin) was compared directly with intensive timing of the regimen. With standard timing, the second course of DCTER induction was administered after hematologic recovery unless a BM examination performed at day 14 demonstrated residual leukemia. With intensive timing, DCTER was given on days 0 to 3 and 10 to 13 regardless of hematologic status. Remission induction rates were similar between the two arms, but a significant survival advantage was observed for the intensified DCTER induction regardless of the type of postremission therapy received (8 year EFS 43% for the intensive arm, and 27% for the standard arm).[211,212] These results demonstrated that intensively timed induction therapy significantly impacts the overall treatment outcome for patients with AML and became the backbone therapy on which the subsequent CCG-2961 trial was tested.[215,216] The Nordic Society of Paediatric Haematology and Oncology (NOPHO) group introduced a time-intensive induction concept in 1988 but the rate of early toxic deaths was too high. The study NOPHO-AML 93 successfully used a time-intensive induction for the one-third of patients who did not experience remission after the first course of induction, whereas those patients with a favorable response were allowed time for regeneration before continuing therapy.[217]

Postremission Therapy

Since the 1970s, clinical research in pediatric AML has focused not only on improving remission induction rates but also on the role of aggressive postremission therapy to improve OS. Early adult studies performed by the Eastern Cooperative Oncology Group demonstrated that without postremission therapy, nearly all patients will relapse.[218,219]

Maintenance Chemotherapy in AML. At first, investigators utilized maintenance chemotherapy as the only component of postremission therapy with poor results. The St. Jude AML 76 and CCG 241 trials demonstrated that extended maintenance therapy alone in the postremission setting resulted in a 20% to 25% 2-year EFS. Patients treated on the CCG 213 pilot study were randomly assigned to receive either 2 years of postintensification maintenance chemotherapy or no further treatment. Interestingly, patients who received additional maintenance chemotherapy had a worse OS than those who received postremission intensification alone. The authors postulated that the maintenance chemotherapy resulted in the selection of a resistant leukemic clone.[204] These findings have been supported by French Society of Pediatric Hematology and Immunology study, LAME 89/91. This study randomized children to receive 18 months of maintenance therapy with low-dose mercaptopurine and cytarabine versus intensive postremission therapy alone. Patients who received maintenance had a similar risk of relapse but a significantly lower OS than patients receiving only intensive postremission treatment.[220] Finally, MRC AML 9 tested the value of maintenance therapy followed by late intensification and found it to be limited. Maintenance therapy was not employed in subsequent MRC trials.[208] These negative results have led to the recommendation that maintenance chemotherapy no longer be a part of pediatric non-M3 AML treatment.

High-Dose Cytarabine-Based Intensification. Multiagent chemotherapy after remission induction was modeled after the VAPA (vincristine, doxorubicin, prednisolone, cytarabine) regimen, performed at the Dana Farber Cancer Institute, which implemented sequential administration of non–cross-resistant drugs for 14 months. This VAPA trial resulted in an EFS of 38% and helped to establish a toxicity profile for HDAC during intensification.[221] After that trial, a number of studies evaluated the role of the intensification of postremission therapy. In the 1980s, the CCG pilot study 213P focused on postremission intensification of Cytarabine as well as determining the necessity of maintenance chemotherapy in AML. It was demonstrated that intensively timed cycles of high-dose cytarabine (Capizzi II), versus more standard timing of high-dose cytarabine, appeared to improve disease-free survival (DFS).[222] The BFM-93 trial was designed to determine whether an additional, intensified consolidation would be of benefit for patients deemed to be "high risk" based on initial morphologic parameters and response to induction therapy. This additional consolidation consisted of HAM (high-dose Cytarabine, mitoxantrone) chemotherapy. In the setting of early blast reduction with daunorubicin, patients who received early and intense consolidation with HAM showed superior 5-year EFS and an acceptable toxicity profile. These results were also supported by other clinical trials, including the SJCRH AML-83, BFM-83, BFM-87, and POG-8498.[206,223,224]

HSCT as Consolidation Therapy for AML

As methods in postremission intensification of chemotherapy continued to evolve, autologous and allogeneic HSCT emerged as a feasible method of improving survival of childhood AML. The benefits of HSCT are its ability to deliver a leukemia-free

TABLE 20.7

TREATMENT OUTCOMES OF HSCT IN PEDIATRIC AML

Trial	No. of Patient	OS% (years)	DFS% (years)	Conclusions from outcome analysis of serial trials
Medical Research Council (MRC12) (1995–2002)	564	66 (5)	61 (5)	No advantage to five courses; four-course therapies sufficient. Allogeneic HSCT only for standard or high-risk AML
AML-97 (St. Jude) (1997–2002)	40	47.5 (5)	58.3 (5)	HSCT was limited to high-risk patients
Pediatric Oncology Group (POG 9421) (1995–1999)	624	55.6 (3) (EFS)	41.2 (3) (EFS)	Patients who had allogeneic HSCT fared better than those who received chemotherapy alone
NOPHO-AML 93 (Nordic) (1993–2001)	243	65 (5)	52 (5)	HSCT not necessary at first remission
AML-BFM 93 (Germany) (1993–1998)	471	57 (5)	61 (5)	HSCT did not provide a survival advantage in first remission
Children's Cancer Group (CCG-2891) (1989–1995)	886	45 (5)	45 (5)	Intensively timed sequential chemotherapy and allogeneic HSCT improved survival
EORTC CLG 58921 (1992–2002)	177	62 (5)	58 (5)	Survival was dependent on prognostic cytogenetic features
LAME 91 (French) (1991–1998)	262	60.6 (5)	52.1 (5)	Allogeneic BMT did not improve outcomes in good-tisk patients
LAM-92 (Italy) (1992–2001)	160	59.5 (5)	60.4 (5)	75% underwent HSCT (auto or allo) following stratification into risk groups; better survival results than previous trials

HSCT, hematopoietic stem cell transplantation, BMT, bone marrow transplant, OS, overall survival, DFS, disease-free survival, EFS, event-free survival.
Shenoy S, Smith FO. Hematopoietic stem cell transplantation for childhood malignancies of myeloid origin. Bone Marrow Transplant 2008;41(2):141–148 (reproduced with permission).

graft and also the production of a strong graft-versus-leukemia effect. However, its potential benefits need to be weighed against the risk of transplant-related mortality and long-term transplant-related morbidity. In addition, the timing of HSCT is controversial. Studies have varied in recommending HSCT in first CR (CR1), second CR (CR2), or for those refractory to chemotherapy.[225] (Table 20.7)

HSCT in CR1. One of the first clinical trials to evaluate allogeneic HSCT was the St. Jude AML 80 trial, which accrued patients from 1980 to 1983.[224] Of the 65 patients who entered CR, 19 received HLA-compatible allogeneic HSCT. The difference in 6-year DFS rates favored the HSCT (43%) cohort over those that received chemotherapy alone (31%), but the results were not statistically significant. However, those that received chemotherapy alone had a higher relapse rate, whereas postremission failures in the HSCT arm were more evenly divided between relapse and transplant-related complications. These results indicated superior leukemia control in those that received HLA-compatible HSCT. Since that clinical study, there have been a series of trials examining the role of autologous and allogeneic transplant versus postremission intensification by chemotherapy alone.

Children's Cancer Group Studies and HSCT. Two sequential studies in the United States, CCG 251 (1979 to 1983) and CCG-213 (1985 to 1989), compared the efficacy of HLA-matched related donor allogeneic HSCT versus chemotherapy alone. In the CCG-251 study, patients receiving an HLA-matched HSCT had a significantly better 5-year EFS than those who received only chemotherapy.[226] Although this advantage was not initially seen in the CCG-213 study, when the results were analyzed by the therapy the patients actually received rather than by intent to treat, a survival advantage was evident for those patients undergoing HLA-matched related donor HSCT.[226]

The CCG-2891 study included analysis of three cohorts of patients: 181 received allogeneic HSCT, 177 received autologous HSCT, and 179 received chemotherapy alone. Allogeneic HSCT was statistically superior to both autologous HSCT and chemotherapy in terms of OS: 60% survival after 8 years for allogeneic HSCT versus 53% and 48% survival for chemotherapy and autologous HSCT, respectively.[215] This benefit for allogeneic transplant was seen in both the standard timing and intensive timing DCTER arms of the study.[215] One result that is consistent among pediatric postremission trials is that autologous BM transplant shows no advantage over intensified chemotherapy.

CCG 2961 incorporated three new agents (idarubicin, fludarabine, and IL-2) into a phase III trial for newly diagnosed AML patients. This trial used intensive-timing remission induction/consolidation based on CCG 2981 and also randomized patients to related donor HSCT versus high-dose cytarabine intensification.[216] For all patients enrolled on this trial, 5-year OS was 52% and EFS was 42%. Five-year DFS for patients with and without a donor was 61% and 50%, respectively ($p = 0.021$), whereas OS between the two groups was not significantly different. Donor availability did not affect DFS or OS for patients with favorable cytogenetic features (inv(16), t(8;21)).[216]

European Clinical Trials and HSCT. "Biologically randomized" studies in the United States, as defined by the presence of an HLA-matched related donor, have consistently demonstrated the benefit of allogeneic HSCT on DFS, EFS, and OS compared to intensive chemotherapy or autologous HSCT.[215,227] In contrast, studies from the MRC, BFM, and NOPHO[217] have not demonstrated the same survival advantage of allogeneic HSCT over chemotherapy alone.[186,199,228,229] MRC AML 10 tested the role of HSCT following four blocks of intensive chemotherapy and found that while both allogeneic HSCT and autologous HSCT significantly reduced the relapse risk, it did not demonstrate a significant improvement in OS. One possibility for this finding could have been the increased number of treatment-related deaths after HSCT. In addition, HSCT did not reduce the risk of relapse among patients with a t(8;21) or inv(16). The lack of benefit for pediatric HSCT in the MRC mirrors the experience in BFM AML[182,230] and NOPHO[217] trials. As a result, most European investigators do not recommend HSCT for patients with low-risk features.

Meta-analysis of Pediatric HSCT Data. A randomized, controlled trial in pediatric patients comparing HSCT with chemotherapy alone is very difficult. Therefore, meta-analysis is an approach that is often utilized to help interpret data from a group of clinical trials. Bleakley et al. performed such an analysis on a group of patients younger than 21 years enrolled in clinical trials from 1985 to 2000. Findings from this analysis were that patients who received an HSCT from a histocompatibility-matched family donor were at reduced risk of relapse and had superior outcomes.[231] Sung et al. performed a decision analysis on pediatric patients by evaluating the outcome of HSCT versus no HSCT for patients without favorable cytogenetics.[232] The results supported that chemotherapy consolidation is a reasonable option for pediatric patients with AML who have favorable cytogenetics, even if a matched-sibling donor is available.[232] Due to the considerable variation in the use and timing of HLA-matched related HSCT for pediatric AML, Horan et al. performed a meta-analysis of four cooperative group clinical trials: POG-8821, CCG-2891, CCG-2961, and MRC-10. Patients were stratified according to cytogenetics and response to the first course of induction therapy into favorable, intermediate, and poor risk disease groups. The results indicate that the antileukemic effect of HSCT is strongly influenced by prognosis and that HLA-matched related donor HSCT is an effective treatment of intermediate-risk AML in first CR[233] (Fig. 20.4). The study suggests that patients with high-risk disease fare poorly even with HSCT, but without statistical significance.

Matched Unrelated Donor Transplantation. The outcomes for children with AML possessing high-risk features are dismal.

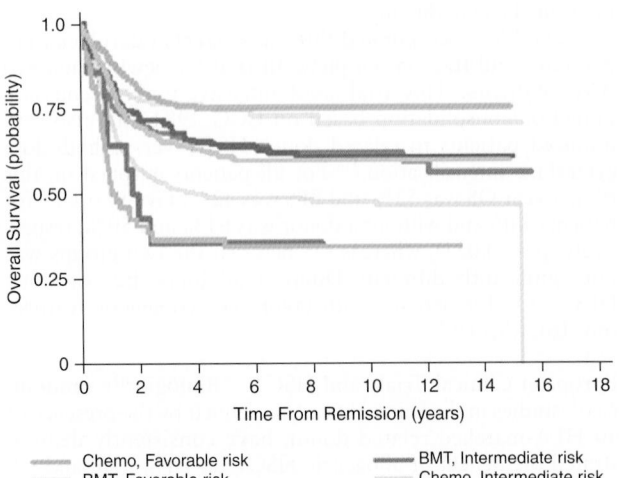

Chemo, Favorable risk
BMT, Favorable risk
BMT, Unknown cytogenetics
Chemo, Unknown cytogenetics
BMT, Intermediate risk
Chemo, Intermediate risk
BMT, High risk
Chemo, High risk

FIGURE 20.4 Estimated overall survival stratified by risk group and postremission treatment (Horan JT, Alonzo TA, Lyman GA, et al. Impact of disease risk on efficacy of matched related bone marrow transplantation for pediatric acute myeloid leukemia: the Children's Oncology Group. J Clin Oncol 2008;26:5797–5801.

These children may include those who never enter remission, those who relapse after chemotherapy or HSCT, or those with therapy-related AML. In addition, those children with high-risk cytogenetic features such as monosomy 5 or 7, del(5q), complex karyotypes, or presence of a high FLT3/ITD allelic ratio have poor survival rates.[234,235]

For those children who do not have an HLA-matched sibling, expanding the search for alternative options is critical. Alternative sources include matched unrelated donor (MUD) HSCs utilizing BM, peripheral blood (PB), or cord blood. Although MUD transplants have demonstrated a potent antileukemic effect, there is an increased risk of acute graft-versus-host disease (aGVHD) and chronic graft-versus-host disease (cGVHD) that can result in an increase in morbidity and mortality.[225,236–238] The degree of GVHD varies depending on the degree of donor mismatch, but estimates of aGHVD and cGVHD range from rates up to 30% and 50%, respectively.[239] Umbilical cord blood transplantation has proven to be a feasible and efficacious approach to HSCT and can result in a lower incidence of severe GVHD.[240,241] Additional advantages include an immediate availability for children with high-risk disease, the need for a lesser degree of HLA match, and an increased donor pool for those with infrequent HLA haplotypes.[225] Disadvantages include an increased graft failure rate, delayed hematopoietic recovery, and lack of additional donor cells in the event of relapse.[242] A Eurocord analysis examined the use of cord blood for the treatment of AML in 95 children (20 in CR1, 47 in CR2, and 28 in a more advanced stage). The 2-year cumulative incidence of relapse was 29% and was associated with disease status. The 2-year DFS was 42% (59% in CR1, 50% in CR2, and 21% for those not in CR).

Another potential alternative donor source is parental HLA haploidentical HSCs. This modality is potentially exciting, particularly because most patients have a donor readily available and can proceed to transplant quickly. However, in spite of good data of haploidentical HSCT in adults, there is less evidence for its role in pediatric AML and therefore it is still considered experimental.[243]

Another potential modality for the treatment of pediatric high-risk AML is the utilization of the antileukemic properties of natural killer (NK) cells. NK cells are a lymphocyte population that have innate cytotoxicity against cells infected with pathogens or cells that have undergone malignant transformation, possibly including AML blasts. The killer cell Ig-like receptors (KIR) on NK cells recognize selected HLA class I major histocompatibility antigens (self-antigens). The binding of the receptors to these class I antigens results in downregulation of NK function. However, when there are mismatches of the class I antigen targets and the respective KIR, then NK cells are able to mediate allogeneic-directed reactions. In HSCT, if there is KIR incompatibility such that inhibitory signals are diminished, donor NK cells could react freely with recipient leukemia cells to induce an NK-mediated graft-versus-leukemia effect.[244–246] This hypothesis is currently being tested in pediatric clinical trials.

In summary, most pediatric cooperative cancer groups worldwide agree that children with good-risk disease should not undergo allogeneic HSCT in CR1, even those with a matched-related donor. There is some evidence of benefit for HSCT in CR1 in those with intermediate-risk disease; however, there is no international consensus on this point. HSCT using any type of donor for high-risk patients is considered experimental and of unknown benefit.

CNS Prophylaxis

Currently, the standard of care in pediatric AML is for all children to receive prophylactic therapy for CNS involvement. Most current AML protocols rely on intrathecal chemotherapy for prophylaxis with either methotrexate or cytarabine; however, some continue to use triple intrathecal therapy (Cytarabine, methotrexate, and hydrocortisone).[206,215,247,248] The BFM 87 study randomized patients to receive either intrathecal Cytarabine or cranial radiation as CNS prophylaxis. Interestingly, while there was a similar CNS relapse rate, the systemic relapse rate was higher in the intrathecal Cytarabine arm.[249] These results remain controversial and most pediatric and adult AML trials do not use cranial irradiation as prophylaxis.

At diagnosis, children with high WBC count, young age, M4 or M5 morphology, or inv(16) are at highest risk of developing CNS disease.[250] For those 5% to 15% of children who do present with CNS disease at diagnosis, an accepted treatment approach is to administer intrathecal therapy weekly until the CSF is clear of leukemic blast cells, and then monthly until the end of therapy.[251] Using these strategies, CNS relapse rates of less than 5% have been achieved.[206,215,247,248] In patients who present with CNS chloromas at diagnosis, there does not appear to be an advantage to local therapy to the site of the chloroma compared with initiation of systemic chemotherapy. Therefore, radiation therapy is not a commonly used modality in the treatment of newly diagnosed AML with CNS chloroma, unless the patient is experiencing significant morbidity due to its location.[181,252]

Prognostic Factors

Much can be learned by observing the successes in the treatment of pediatric ALL. Improved risk assessment has led to intensification of therapy for high-risk patients and de-escalation for those with low-risk features. Despite an improved understanding of the pathogenesis and risk factors in pediatric AML, progress has not been as dramatic over the last two decades. One reason for this is that therapies for AML already incorporate maximally tolerated doses of therapy in concert with intensive supportive measures. Even for those patients who do possess favorable cytogenetics, OS remains approximately 60%, a rate that does not justify dose de-escalation. Therefore, although prognostic factors have been identified in pediatric AML, clinical trials continue to assess the most effective way to implement them (Table 20.8). Currently, prognostic factors include host factors, response to therapy, and disease characteristics.

Host Factors. Host factors such as age, race, and constitutional abnormalities have been demonstrated to have a correlation with outcome in pediatric AML. The data on the association of age with outcome in pediatric AML have been inconsistent. For example, in early CCG studies, infants with monoblastic leukemia had inferior outcomes, with children younger than 1 year having the worst survival.[253] However, the MRC 10 study demonstrated that although infants were treated in the same fashion as other children and even adults, they experienced equal or slightly better outcomes.[254,255] Race, however, consistently influences clinical outcome. In a recent study of approximately 1,600 children treated on CCG-2891 and CCG-2961 clinical trials, Aplenc et al. demonstrated that African American and Hispanic patients had an OS rate of 35%, whereas the OS rate for white patients was 48%.[256]

Children with constitutional syndromes can be classified as high or low risk, depending on the abnormality. Children with DS and AML, particularly those younger than 2 years, have superior outcomes with a remission rate of 90% and an OS rate of 80%.[155,257–261] These superior results appear to be related to their exquisite sensitivity to cytotoxic therapy, particularly Cytarabine.[262–266] In contrast, patients with chromosome instability syndromes such as Fanconi anemia, or inherited genetic defects like Kostmann syndrome, who

develop myeloid neoplasms may display more treatment-related toxicity and may present with poor cytogenetic features such as monosomy 7.

Nutritional status at initial presentation also has an impact on survival. Patients who were either underweight (≤10th percentile) or overweight (≥95th percentile) at diagnosis had inferior OS rates compared to those with intermediate body habitus. CCG 2961 demonstrated that these patients were more susceptible to treatment-related mortality resulting in worse survival.[267] Finally, host genetic alterations involved in drug metabolism pathways have been demonstrated to affect outcome. For example, AML patients with inherited alterations in the detoxification enzyme glutathione-S-transferase theta resulting in the null phenotype show decreased survival secondary to increased toxicity.[268] Despite preliminary findings involving a number of host variables, these factors have not yet been used in risk-group stratification.

Response to Therapy. Response to therapy has always been an important predictor of outcome in both pediatric AML and ALL. Historically, response is assessed using morphology either during or after induction chemotherapy. However, advances in MRD assessment may help identify patients at higher risk of relapse.

Primary induction failure. While morphologic response to induction chemotherapy has been an integral part of risk assessment in ALL, its importance in pediatric AML has only recently been established.[269,270] In the MRC 10 clinical trial, investigators established that patients with a partial remission at end of induction (defined as between 5% and 15% blasts) had a survival rate similar to those with less than 5% blasts. Patients with more than 15% blasts after induction had a poor OS. Therefore, a clinical cutoff was established, and the MRC used the threshold of 15% to define refractory disease.[207,255,271] Currently, the Children's Oncology Group (COG) is using this cutoff to define primary induction failure in their clinical trials. These patients have a dismal prognosis and alternative approaches including unrelated donor HSCT are being evaluated in clinical trials.

Minimal residual disease. Although morphologic response to induction chemotherapy has been established as an important prognostic factor, 30% to 50% of patients that have a CR by BM morphology still relapse. Identification of residual disease in patients in morphologic remission may allow for identification of patients with increased risk of relapse. Several approaches to the detection of MRD have been developed.[272] In order to have clinical utility, it is important that MRD assays fulfill basic criteria: (a) be applicable to all patients with AML, (b) allow for adequate time from detection of MRD to morphologic relapse, (c) be cost-effective, and (d) be reproducible.[272–274]

Molecular MRD. PCR techniques are commonly used to detect unique fusion genes still present during treatment or at relapse.[275–278] The only AML subtype for which PCR is conclusively utilized for MRD detection is APL. Persistence of the t(15;17) fusion product PML-RARα is associated with a high risk of relapse, and therapeutic intervention has been demonstrated to improve outcome.[277] Another example of potential clinical utility of PCR-based MRD is in the detection of t(8;21) fusion transcripts. Initially, qualitative PCR detection of this fusion transcript was questioned because the t(8;21) could remain detectable for a sustained period of time during remission after treatment.[279–281] However, real-time quantitative PCR (RQ-PCR) data show that the abnormal t(8;21) and inv(16) transcripts do disappear during treatment and that the expression level and rate of decline predict clinical outcome

TABLE 20.8

CURRENT RISK GROUP STRATIFICATION IN SEVERAL PEDIATRIC AML COLLABORATIVE GROUP TREATMENT PROTOCOLS (EXCLUDING ACUTE PROMYELOCYTIC LEUKEMIA AND MYELOID LEUKEMIA OF DOWN SYNDROME), AND PERCENTAGES OF THE TOTAL GROUP OF PATIENTS PER RISK-GROUP

Protocol	Standard risk (SR)	% of patients	Medium risk (MR) in SR	% of patients	High risk (HR) in MR	% of patients in HR
AIEOP-LAM 2002/01	t(8;21) or inv(16)/t(16;16)[a]	18	—	—	All other patients	82
BFM-AML 2004	FAB M1/M2 with Auer rods of FAB M4Eo or t(8;21) or inv (16)[b] and blasts on day 15 <5% and absence of FLT3/ITD	30	—	—	All patients with FLT3/ITD, and all patients who are not standard risk	70
COG AAML0531	t(8;21), inv(16), or t(16;16)	25	All others	57	−7, −5, 5q−; bone marrow M3 (>15% of blasts) after course 1, except for those with good risk cytogenetics	18
ELAM 2002	t(8;21)[b] (not eligible for SCT in CR1)	14	All others	81	−7, 5q−, t(9;22), t(6;9)	5
JPLSG AML-05	t(8;21), inv(16), or t(16;16)[c]	40	All others	40	−7, 5q−, t(9;22), t(16;21), FLT3-ITD, no CR after course 1	20
MRC/DCOG AML15	t(8;21) and inv(16)/t(16;16)[b], irrespective of marrow status after first course or the presence of other genetic abnormalities	30	All other patients	55	>15% blasts after the first course, or adverse cytogenetics [−5, −7, del(5q), abn(3q), t(9;22), complex karyotype[d]]	15
NOPHO-AML 2004	<15% blasts after the first and CR after the second course, or t(8;21), inv(16), t(16;16), t(9;11),[b] and CR after the second course	80	—	—	11q23 abnormalities other than t(9;11) or >15% blasts day 15 or lack of remission after two courses of chemotherapy	20
St. Jude AML-2002	t(8;21), inv(16), t(9;11)[b]	35	All other patients	40	Cytogenetic abnormalities [−7, t(6;9), FLT3/ITD], or FAB M7 or M7, or therapy-related AML, or secondary AML after MDS, or lack of remission after two courses	25

[a]As isolated structural abnormality, detected by karyotyping and/or molecular methods.
[b]As detected by karyotyping and/or molecular methods, independent of secondary abnormalities.
[c]As detected by karyotyping, and/or polymerase chain reaction (PCR) but in case of the latter only it must be confirmed by florescent *in situ* hybridization/ French-American-British (FISH/FAB)-classification: morphological classification of acute myeloid leukemia (AML).
[d]Five or more structural karyotypic abnormalities.
SCT, stem cell transplantation; CR, complete remission; MRC, Medical Research Council study group; BFM, Berlin-Frankfurt-Münster study group; NOPHO, Nordic Society for Pediatric Hematology and Oncology; St. Jude, St. Jude Children's Research Hospital, Memphis, USA; AIEOP, Associazione Italiana Ematologia Oncologia Pediatrica; ELAM, Enfant Leucémie Aique Myéloblastique; COG, Childhood Oncology Group; JPLSG, Japanese Pediatric Leukemia/Lymphoma Study Group; DCOG, Dutch Childhood Oncology Group.
Kaspers GJ, Zwaan CM. Pediatric acute myeloid leukemia: towards high-quality cure of all patients. Haematologica 2007;92:1519–1532 (reproduced with permission).

and rate of relapse.[282] Since leukemia-specific fusion genes are found in only about 30% of patients, expression of nonspecific genes like Wilms' tumor 1 (*WT1*) may be useful for MRD monitoring.[283,284]

Immunophenotypic MRD. Immunophenotypic studies utilizing multiparameter flow cytometric (MFC) detection of aber-

rant immunophenotypes are an effective method for determining MRD.[285,286] This method allows for simultaneous analysis of cell size, granularity, and intensity of expression of surface and intracellular molecules. Using these methods, investigators can detect one cell with a leukemic immunophenotype in 1,000 to 10,000 normal cells.[287] The advantage of this method is that it is applicable to most patients with

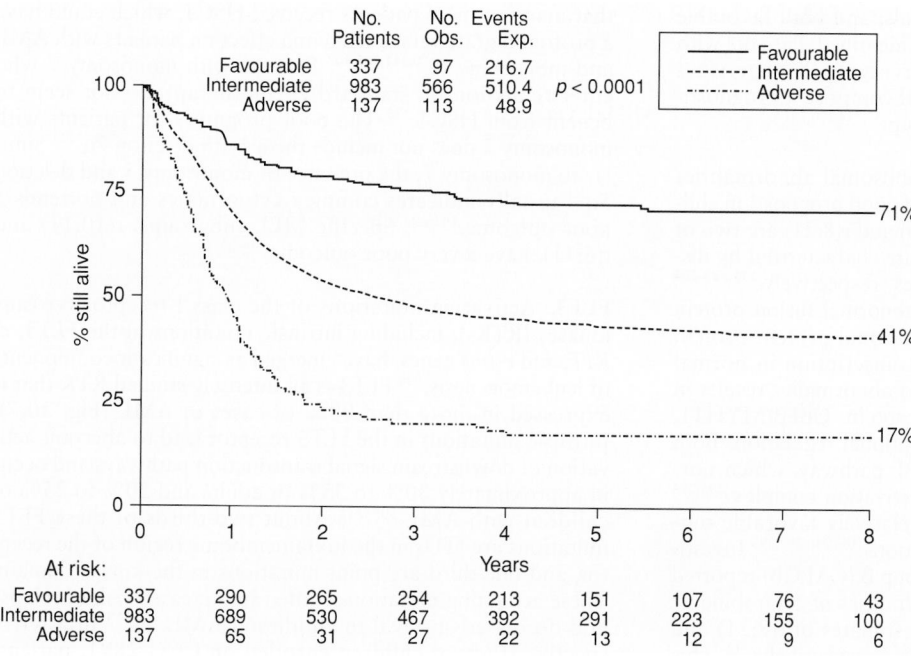

FIGURE 20.5 Clinical significance of diagnostic cytogenetics—MRC 10. (Grimwade D, Walker H, Oliver F. The importance of diagnostic cytogenetics on outcome in AML: analysis of 1,612 patients entered Into the MRC AML 10 trial. The Medical Research Council Adult and Children's Leukaemia Working Parties. Blood 1998;92(7)2322–2333. Reprinted with permission.)

AML, as at least 80% of patients have an aberrant phenotypic signature that can be detected by MFC.[288] A recent prospective study of 252 AML patients enrolled in a CCG study showed that MFC evidence of leukemia after the initiation of therapy was the most powerful independent prognostic factor associated with poor outcome. In a time-dependent multivariate analysis, patients harboring occult leukemia were 4.8 times more likely to relapse and 3.1 times more likely to die than those without detectable leukemia by flow cytometry. OS at 3 years was 41% for patients with occult leukemia versus 69% for those without.[123] Importantly, it was determined that the median time to relapse on this study was 173 days, which allows for adequate time for intervention. Based on these results, current international clinical trials are incorporating MRD testing by MFC to refine the criteria for which intervention would be recommended for a patient with occult disease.

Prognostic Disease Characteristics

Improvements in our classification schemes reflect our improved understanding of the molecular pathogenesis of AML. The current WHO scheme incorporates genetic information into traditional immunophenotypic, cytochemical, morphologic, and clinical methods of determining disease classification. Although all of these disease characteristics may influence prognosis, recurrent cytogenetic alterations and molecular abnormalities currently have the most influence on risk assessment (Figs. 20.5 and 20.6).

Cytogenetics. For patients with AML, karyotypic analysis by diagnostic cytogenetics is one of the most important predictors of outcome. Cytogenetic abnormalities are identified in 70% to 80% of pediatric patients with AML, and clonal abnormalities are identified in almost 80% of those patients.[142,289] The prognostic significance of cytogenetic abnormalities has been

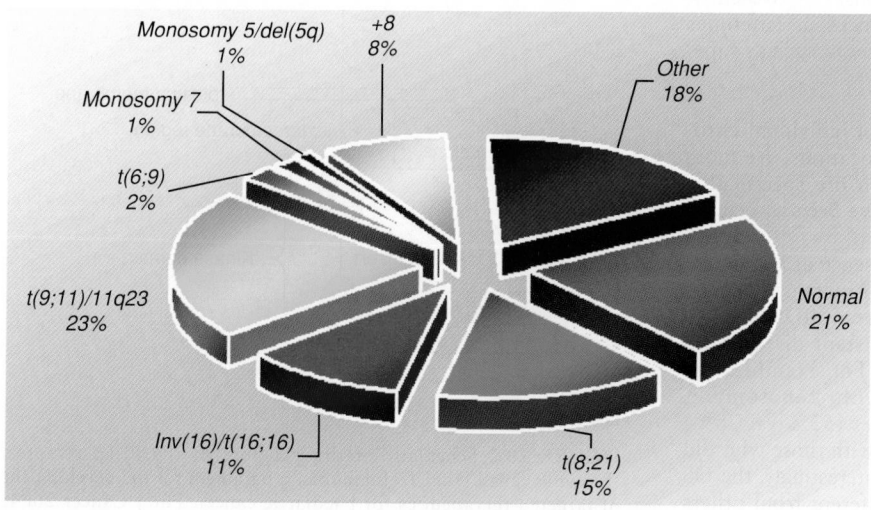

FIGURE 20.6 Cytogenetic makeup in pediatric acute myeloid leukemia (AML). Reprinted with permission from Soheil Meshinchi, 2009.

evaluated retrospectively in several trials, and both favorable and unfavorable risk groups have been identified. Patients with neither favorable nor unfavorable karyotypic characteristics make up about 50% of all patients and comprise a prognostically intermediate or standard risk group.[32,254,290,291]

Favorable cytogenetics. Several chromosomal abnormalities have emerged as favorable predictors of good prognosis in children with AML.[140,255,291,292] The inv(16) and t(8;21) are two of the most common translocations and are characterized by disruption of the CBFβ and AML1 genes, respectively.[255,293,294] The t(8;21) abnormality leads to the abnormal fusion protein AML/ETO. This fusion results in abnormal protein-protein signaling, altering the regulation of transcription in normal hematopoiesis. In addition, the inv(16) abnormality results in the creation of an abnormal fusion protein, CBFβ/MYH11, which results in disruption of transcriptional regulation. Both of these fusion proteins affect the CBF pathway, which normally functions as a transcriptional activation complex.[295,296] Clinical trials have demonstrated a relatively favorable outcome for patients with these translocations.[142,216,297,298] Investigators from Cancer and Leukemia Group B (CALGB) reported that these patients are sensitive to high doses of cytarabine.[297] In the MRC 10 trial, the 5-year OS estimates of t(8;21) and inv(16) patients were 69% and 61%, respectively.[292] This favorable data have led to the recommendation to withhold HSCT in patients with CBFβ AML in CR1.

Prognostically intermediate cytogenetics. There are a limited number of karyotypic abnormalities proven to have a positive or negative impact on outcome in pediatric AML. Patients without prognostically significant genetic abnormalities are deemed to have an intermediate prognosis. Included in this group are those with structural abnormalities involving chromosome band 11q23 on the MLL gene. This is one of the most frequently involved translocations in AML, occurring most commonly in children younger than 2 years.[69,141,142,299–301] In most cases, there is a reciprocal translocation between the amino-terminal portion of the MLL gene and one of nearly 50 partner genes. These abnormal fusion proteins disrupt normal transcriptional regulation of hematopoiesis and result in leukemogenesis. In early studies, the presence of an 11q23 abnormality was associated with an inferior outcome; however, more recent studies do not support these findings.[289,292] Patients with the t(9;11) translocation had initially been thought to have a more favorable outcome.[302,303] In studies from St. Jude Children's Research Hospital and NOPHO, the t(9;11) translocation responded better to therapy and had a superior OS than other 11q23 translocations.[217,301] Recently, larger studies have demonstrated differences in outcomes within 11q23/MLL-rearranged AML subgroups, such as superior survival among those with t(1;11).[304]

Unfavorable cytogenetics. Abnormalities of individual chromosomes, rather than chromosomal translocations, are more likely to be poor prognostic indicators. More specifically, abnormalities of chromosomes 5 and 7 have been associated with poor outcome in pediatric AML.[32,142,234,235,255,292] Monosomy 7 can either occur alone or in the presence of a complex karyotype, defined as the presence of five or more cytogenetic abnormalities. Patients with AML arising from MDS or AML with monosomy 7 tend to have very resistant disease and carry a poor prognosis.[70,140,142,235,305,306] For example, the CCG-2891 study included 40 patients with monosomy 7. These patients had inferior remission rates (53% vs. 78%) and 6-year EFS (19% vs. 39%) compared with those who did not have this chromosomal abnormality. Interestingly, the OS for these patients was not significantly different from others on the study (47% vs. 46%). This survival data could reflect

that many of these patients received HSCT, which could have a profound graft-versus-leukemia effect on patients with AML and monosomy 7.[70,211,215,307] Patients with monosomy 7 who enter remission on standard chemotherapy do not seem to benefit from HSCT.[235] The poor prognosis for patients with monosomy 7 does not include those with deletion 7q.[235] Similar to monosomy 7, the presence of monosomy 5 and deletion 5q− usually indicates complex cytogenetics and portends a poor outcome.[142,292] Specific MLL subgroups, t(10;11) and t(6;11), have a very poor outcome.[304]

FLT3. Activating mutations of the class I receptor tyrosine kinases (RTKs), including intrinsic mutations in the *FLT3*, *c-KIT*, and *c-fms* genes, have emerged as significant components of leukemogenesis.[308] FLT3 is an intensely studied RTK that is expressed in more than 90% of cases of AML (Fig. 20.7). Intrinsic mutations in the FLT3 receptor lead to aberrant activation of downstream signal transduction pathways and occur in approximately 30% to 35% of adults and 20% to 25% of children with AML.[309–311] About two-thirds of these FLT3 mutations are ITDs in the juxtamembrane region of the receptor, and one-third are point mutations in the kinase domain. These activating mutations confer an increased risk of relapse and decreased survival in childhood AML.[312,313] In a retrospective study of children enrolled on CCG-2891, patients with FLT3/ITD had an 8 year OS and EFS of 13% and 7%, respectively, versus 50% and 44% for patients without FLT3/ITD[312] (Fig. 20.8). Further studies in both adult and pediatric AML have demonstrated that in FLT3/ITD+ samples, the ratio of mutant to wild type alleles has additional prognostic significance, such that patients with high ITD allelic ratios have a worse prognosis.[314–316] Taken together, the presence of FLT3/ITD with high allelic ratio appears to be among the strongest prognostic factors in pediatric AML.

Novel Molecular Markers. The discovery of novel gene mutations involved in leukemogenesis has improved our understand-

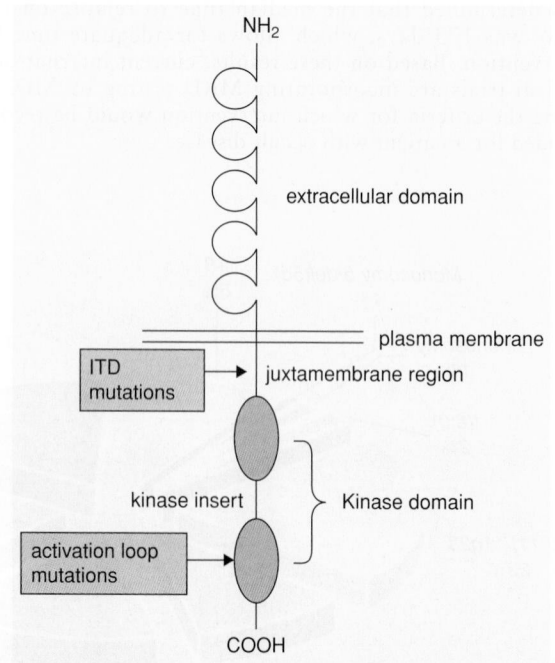

FIGURE 20.7 Schematic of the structure of the FLT3 receptor. (Brown P, Small D. FLT3 Inhibitors: a paradigm for the development of targeted therapeutics for paediatric cancer. Eur J Cancer 2004; 40:707–721. Reprinted with permission.)

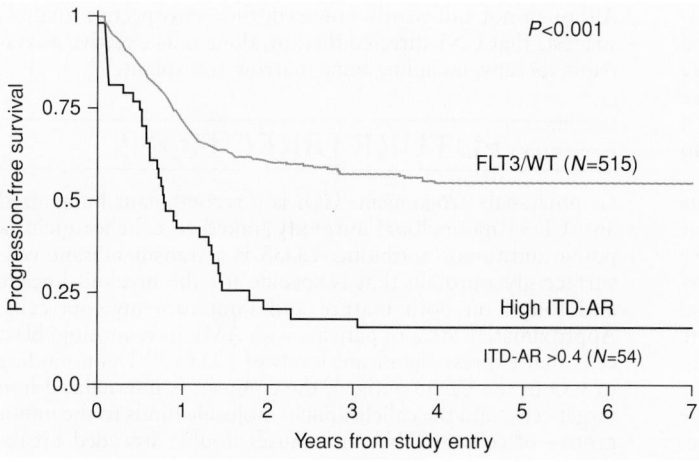

Actuarial progression-free survival from study entry for patients with high ITD-AR(ITD-AR>0.4) compared with those with FLT3/WT

WT = wild type
ITD = internal tandem duplication
AR = allelic ratio

FIGURE 20.8 Survival according to FLT3. (Reprinted with permission. from Meshinchi S, Alonzo TA, Stirewalt DL, et al. Clinical implications of FLT3 mutations in pediatric AML. Blood 2006;108(12):3654–3661.)

ing of cytogenetically normal AML.[104,106,107] The prognostic significance of some of these mutations is currently under study. It has been found that approximately 30% to 50% of adult patients and 10% of children with *de novo* AML possess a mutation in the nucleophosmin (*NPM1*) gene, which encodes a protein regulating the alternative reading frame (ARF)-p53 tumor suppressor pathway.[317] This mutation leads to abnormal cytoplasmic localization of the affected protein.[106] In adults, the presence of this mutation, along with a normal karyotype and absence of FLT3/ITD, confers a favorable outcome.[318,319] Early data indicate that mutations in the *NPM1* gene in children with AML may also be of favorable prognostic significance; however, further data are still under review.[320,321]

The transcription factor C/EPBα modulates granulocytic differentiation and leads to maturational arrest. C/EPBα mutations have been identified in nearly 10% of adult patients with AML, and their expression has been associated with favorable outcome.[322,323] Recently, a retrospective mutation analysis was performed on 847 children with AML treated on CCG-2941, CCG-2961, and COG-AAML03P1. The presence of C/EPBα mutations in these children was an independent prognostic factor for improved outcome.[324] Therefore, future studies will likely include this mutation in risk assessment of newly diagnosed children with AML. Recently, investigations into the clinical relevance of *WT1* mutations demonstrated that they were found in 12% of diagnostic pediatric AML samples. These mutations were associated with a normal karyotype (22%) and FLT3/ITD, and were found to be an independent poor prognostic factor.[325]

Relapsed AML

Despite modest improvements in survival rates in pediatric AML, relapse remains the major cause of treatment failure.[326] Unfortunately, there has not been significant progress in the development of salvage regimens that produce durable second remissions. HSCT remains the best hope for cure in many of these patients; however, the chances of subsequent relapse and transplant-related toxicity remain high. To improve upon dismal outcomes for relapsed patients, it is important that we identify those at highest risk and define the mechanisms responsible for treatment failure.

Resistance to Therapy

Major predictors of relapse in patients with newly diagnosed AML include the karyotype, FLT3 status, and response to induction therapy.[292,327–329] These prognostic features are vital in identifying patients who may avoid relapse through intensification of therapy or the use of novel, targeted agents. Therapeutic resistance is a major factor influencing relapse and can be due to pharmacologic or genetic properties of the leukemia cell. The efficacy of many chemotherapeutic agents depends on the complex interaction of uptake of the metabolite into cells, efflux mechanisms that affect drug toxicity, and metabolism of the drug to its cytotoxic form. The culmination of these events is the initiation of programmed cell death, or apoptosis. Resistance to chemotherapy can occur at any of these levels. For example, nucleoside transporters are essential in mediating the entrance of nucleoside analogs such as Cytarabine into cells. Expression of these transporters, specifically human equilibrative nucleoside transporter 1, correlates with response to therapy.[330–334] Drug resistance has also been associated with overexpression of the multidrug resistance gene 1 (MDR-1) encoding the drug efflux pump P-glycoprotein.[335–337] However, evaluation of MDR genes in pediatric patients has not demonstrated prognostic significance.[338] In addition to influx/efflux mechanisms, recent studies have highlighted the role of programmed cell death pathways in the drug resistance of leukemia.[339,340] Early studies demonstrated that elevated levels of Bcl-2 were associated with a poor response to chemotherapy.[340] Subsequently, it has been demonstrated that the ratio of Bax to Bcl-2 expression (Bax/Bcl-2) is an independent prognostic factor of both OS and time to relapse.[341,342]

Salvage Options in Relapsed AML

Although up to 85% of children diagnosed with AML achieve a first remission, only approximately 50% will be long-term survivors.[183–189,343] For patients who relapse, achieving a second remission is difficult using current salvage regimens. While drug resistance likely mediates the mechanisms of relapse, the most important predictors of response to salvage regimens are karyotype and duration of first remission. The rate of successful reinduction in adult patients whose CR duration is less than 6 months is approximately 10%, compared with 50% if CR1 is greater than 18 to 24 months.[344] These reinduction rates translate into poor OS. Those who achieve CR1 of less than 6 months from diagnosis have a 5-year OS of less than 20% compared with up to 48% for those who achieve a CR1 of greater than 1 year.[326,345]

Cytarabine is one of the most active antileukemic agents and is the backbone of many combination regimens for patients with relapsed AML, showing activity even in those patients who have received high doses during initial therapy.[346,347] The drug requires transport into the cell followed by intracellular phosphorylation to its cytotoxic triphosphate form (ara-CTP). Cytarabine has been used in combination with anthracyclines in the relapsed setting. In CCG-2951, the combination of mitoxantrone and cytarabine was found to be an effective reinduction regimen and is now commonly used. However, exposure to high cumulative doses of these potentially cardiotoxic agents limit the use of repeated cycles.[271,346]

Correlations have been demonstrated between the accumulation of ara-CTP and clinical response in patients with relapsed AML.[348,349] Therefore, strategies focusing on biochemical modulation of ara-CTP with nucleoside analogs such as clofarabine and fludarabine have demonstrated synergistic effects and clinical efficacy.[350-352]

HSCT remains the most important curative strategy in relapsed AML, although a few long-term survivors in nontransplanted patients have been reported.[353] Achieving a second remission prior to HSCT confers a survival benefit when compared with transplantation for patients in relapse. However, about 20% of children transplanted in relapse become long-term survivors.[354,355] It is generally preferred to perform matched-sibling HSCT in relapse, but for those who do not have such a donor, alternative sources include BM, PB, and cord blood donors.[225,356,357]

Some studies have suggested that in patients with standard-risk malignancy, transplantation from HLA-allelically matched donors led to outcomes similar to that of HLA-identical sibling donors.[358] The International Bone Marrow Transplant Registry has shown that approximately 40% of children in CR2 can be rescued by HSCT, regardless of donor source.[359] Factors limiting the success of allogeneic HSCT include the toxicity of the preparative regimen, the absence of a suitable donor, the risk of GVHD, and the high rate of relapse despite an immunologically mediated graft-versus-leukemia effect.[214] For those patients who have primary refractory disease or early relapse and do not have a suitable donor, experimental therapies with haploidentical or KIR incompatible donors are being explored in pediatric patients.

Isolated CNS Relapse

CNS relapse in pediatric AML is infrequent and therefore consensus has not been reached on its management. Johnson et al. reported on 33 patients with isolated CNS relapse after receiving therapy on CCG-2891. The incidence of isolated CNS relapse reported in that study was 4.8%, similar to other studies in which patients received CNS prophylaxis. The authors concluded that risk factors for isolated CNS relapse include CNS disease at diagnosis, M5 FAB subtype, high WBC count, and 11q23 abnormalities. These presenting characteristics are interrelated. Patients with isolated CNS relapse received a variety of treatments including local therapy (intrathecal chemotherapy and/or radiation therapy) and systemic therapy (chemotherapy with or without HSCT). Survival rate in the patients treated with local therapy was only 31.5% compared with 21.4% in patients treated with systemic therapy.

Although not sufficiently powered, this retrospective analysis suggests that CNS-directed therapy alone is as effective as systemic therapy, including bone marrow transplant.[360]

FUTURE DIRECTIONS

Gemtuzumab ozogamicin (GO) is a recombinant humanized anti-CD33 monoclonal antibody linked to calicheamicin, a potent antitumor antibiotic. CD33 is a transmembrane cell-surface glycoprotein that is specific for the myeloid lineage and found on both mature and immature myeloid cells. Approximately 90% of patients with AML have myeloid blast cells that express significant levels of CD33.[361] Upon binding of GO to the CD33 antigen, the complex is internalized into target cells, and the calicheamicin molecule binds to the minor groove of cellular DNA and causes double stranded breaks that lead to apoptosis.[362]

Phase I and phase II studies have demonstrated efficacy of GO both as a single agent and in combination with chemotherapy in adults and children.[343,363-370] Although GO seems to be an effective new agent in the treatment of AML, there has been concern about liver toxicity in adult trials when used in combination with cytotoxic agents at higher doses (6 and 9 mg/m^2). A potential mechanism for the liver toxicity is that GO may target CD33$^+$, CD163$^+$ cells residing in hepatic sinusoids.[371] Subsequent pediatric studies addressed these concerns by reducing the dose of GO, eliminating repeated doses, and not using it with thioguanine.[343,367] Further trials using these strategies revealed that the rate of hepatotoxicity, specifically veno-occlusive disease, did not differ substantially from the rate expected in high-risk MUD-HSCT.[343,372] Of significance is that CD33 is absent on pluripotent HSCs.[373] It is not known if GO exerts its effects by targeting the self-renewing leukemia stem cell or through cytoreduction of all CD33$^+$ cells. The safety and efficacy of GO in combination with conventional AML chemotherapy and transplant is currently being defined in prospective, randomized phase III studies.

Several small molecule kinase inhibitors with activity against FLT3 have been evaluated in AML. In phase I and phase II clinical trials, conducted primarily in relapsed or refractory AML patients, responses were consistently observed, demonstrating that FLT3 inhibition can elicit a therapeutic effect, particularly in FLT3-ITD patients.[374-377] The studies also revealed a relationship between clinical response and the pharmacokinetics/pharmacodynamics of FLT3 inhibition, and highlighted the importance of substantial and sustained inhibition of FLT3.[378,379] Currently, there are active pediatric studies testing FLT3 inhibition in combination with cytotoxic chemotherapy in patients with relapsed AML.

Clofarabine is a purine nucleoside analog that inhibits DNA polymerase and ribonucleotide reductase and also has a direct effect on the mitochondria in inducing apoptosis. It has shown activity in pediatric ALL and AML and is currently being tested in clinical trials for pediatric patients with relapsed AML in combination with cytarabine. This strategy focuses on the biochemical modulation of ara-CTP by clofarabine through its inhibition of ribonucleotide reductase.[352,380,381] Bortezomib is a selective inhibitor of the ubiquitin proteosome pathway and nuclear factor-kappaB (NF-κB). NF-κB is constitutively activated in hematologic malignancies, and its inhibition in these cells promotes apoptosis. In addition, AML "stem cells" demonstrate increased expression of NF-κB and may represent an important therapeutic target for this agent. Currently, clinical trials in the United States are testing the safety and efficacy of bortezomib in combination with standard reinduction chemotherapy for children with relapsed AML.[382-384]

As our understanding of the biology of AML improves, we expect further advances in risk stratification, molecular targeted therapies, HSCT strategies, and supportive care. Novel clinical trial designs testing a large number of new agents will be necessary to test treatment approaches in increasingly small groups of molecularly defined populations of patients.

ACUTE PROMYELOCYTIC LEUKEMIA

APL (AML M3) is characterized by its unique cytogenetic, morphologic, and molecular characteristics. In the United States, it accounts for 4% to 8% of childhood AML, compared with 10% to 15% in adults. Cytogenetically, it is characterized by a balanced translocation between the PML gene on chromosome 15 and the RARα gene on chromosome 17. However, simple or complex variant chromosomal translocations are being more frequently observed. The underlying t(15;17) translocation leads to formation of the PML-RARα transcript and causes maturation arrest in the promyelocyte stage. This maturation arrest is the result of the recruitment of chromatin repressor complexes that involve both histone deacetylases (HDACs) and DNA methyltranferases, which result in the silencing of genes required for normal hematopoiesis.[385–389]

TREATMENT OF APL

In the early 1970s, Bernard et al. demonstrated the sensitivity of APL cells to daunorubicin, leading to a CR rate of 55%.[390] As in other early AML trials, anthracyclines were combined with Cytarabine to improve CR rates in newly diagnosed patients.[391,392] However, treatment was complicated by coagulopathy and severe bleeding diathesis and resulted in a significant mortality rate.[393] In children, coagulopathy and hemorrhage are seen particularly with the M3v subtype.[394] In the early 1980s, with the discovery that ATRA induces the differentiation of leukemic blasts into mature granulocytes, a new era of APL treatment began.[395–397] Following an initial favorable case report, Huang et al. reported the results of 24 patients with APL treated with ATRA alone. Twenty-three of these patients achieved a CR with differentiation of promyelocytes, and the lone nonresponder achieved a CR after the addition of low dose Cytarabine.[398] Although initial ATRA monotherapy studies demonstrated impressive CR rates, the rate of relapse was high (usually within 3 to 6 months) and it was found that ATRA administration could elevate the WBC count and result in a fatal retininoic acid syndrome.[176,399–402] Therefore, in the early 1990s, randomized trials by the European APL group (GIMEMA and PETHEMA) and another by North American Intergroup demonstrated that the sequential combination of ATRA followed by chemotherapy is superior to chemotherapy alone and reduces the risk of retininoic acid syndrome.[277,403–407] In addition, these studies demonstrated the necessity of two to three cycles of anthracycline-based consolidation therapy, sometimes with high-dose Cytarabine.[408,409] In contrast to other subtypes of AML, patients with APL have been shown to benefit from maintenance therapy, as long as it contains further treatment with ATRA.[410] These treatment regimens have led to CR rates of 90% or more and EFS of 70% to 80%.[277,411]

In the largest pediatric clinical trial to date, Testi et al. reported the results on 107 eligible children treated with AIDA (ATRA and idarubicin) induction followed by three courses of consolidation. Ninety-six percentage of patients achieved a CR, with a 10-year OS and EFS of 89% and 76%, respectively.[410] The Programa de Estudio y Tratamiento de las Hemopatías Malignas (PETHEMA) group in Spain reported results on 66 children with APL treated with ATRA/idarubicin

induction therapy, followed by three courses of anthracycline monotherapy consolidation, and maintenance chemotherapy with ATRA, mercaptopurine, and methotrexate. Children treated on this study had comparable results with a CR rate of 92%, 5-year EFS rate of 77%, and a 5-year OS rate of 87%.[412]

Arsenic is one of the oldest remedies in both Western and traditional Chinese medicine. Although the mechanism of action is not completely elucidated, it produces degradation of the PML-RARα fusion protein, induces differentiation of the APL blasts, and induces apoptosis.[413,414] Further work in this area has led to the discovery that arsenic trioxide (ATO) as a single agent has excellent activity in adult patients with relapsed APL, with molecular and morphologic remission obtained in more than 80% of patients.[415,416] As a result, ATO has been studied for remission induction and postremission consolidation therapy for adults with newly diagnosed APL.[417,418] CR rates of 90% or more have been reported.[418,419] Currently, pediatric investigators are evaluating a strategy that implements ATO during consolidation chemotherapy with the goal of decreasing the cumulative dose of potentially cardiotoxic anthracyclines during therapy. Until the safety and efficacy of ATO are established in children, its use remains experimental.

Due to the excellent cure rates in pediatric APL, there is currently no role for HSCT in front-line therapy.[420] However, for the few patients who relapse or have persistent MRD, the prognosis is less favorable and HSCT may be indicated after reinduction chemotherapy. Allogeneic HSCT is the recommended choice for patients with an available HLA-identical donor and who have MRD by PCR after salvage therapy. There is an excellent salvage rate of approximately 70% to 75% with allogeneic HSCT following relapse of APL.[421] For those patients who relapse and do not have an HLA-identical donor, autologo transplant is a viable option. For these patients, achievement of PCR-negativity after salvage therapy is considered mandatory. Those relapsed APL patients who achieve molecular remission and receive autologous HSCT have shown a nearly 80% relapse-free survival and a 7-year OS of approximately 60%.[422]

The favorable treatment outcomes in APL result from understanding its unique biology and the ability to detect the PML-RARα transcript by RQ-PCR. The ability to measure this transcript provides clinicians with an MRD assay to determine molecular remission. Those that achieve molecular remission tend to have a high continuous remission rate, whereas those with detectable disease by quantitative PCR almost uniformly progress.[278,423] The timing of MRD measurement in APL differs from other acute leukemias. Historically, end of induction response evaluations by qualitative PCR, karyotyping, or FISH have demonstrated that evaluation at this time point is not an accurate predictor of outcome.[424] Using RQ-PCR, patients with high risk of relapse can be identified after the first course of consolidation therapy and by testing every 3 months after consolidation is completed.[282,425]

MYELOID LEUKEMIA AND DOWN SYNDROME (ML-DS)

Individuals with DS have a strongly age-related increased risk of leukemia with a more than 50-fold increased risk during the first 5 years of life and a 10-fold increased risk from 5 to 29 years of age. After age 30 years the risk of leukemia is close to that seen in non-DS individuals.[426] The cumulative risk for leukemia by the age of 5 years is 2.1% and by 30 years is 2.7%. Almost half the leukemias are myeloid and most of them occur before 5 years of age.

It is often stated that children with DS have a ~500-fold increased risk of FAB M7 AMKL compared with the general pediatric population.[427] ML-DS is very distinct from AMKL occurring in non-DS children. Children with DS very seldom have normal AML. The types of ML in children with DS and those without DS are so different that it is of little meaning comparing the relative risk of subtypes. It is more meaningful to compare the total risk of ML in children with DS and those without DS. Children with DS below 5 years of age have a 40-fold increased risk of ALL and a 150-fold increased risk of ML.[426] Children with DS who have been cured from leukemia appear to have a reduced risk of secondary malignancies,[428] but the increased risk of both myeloid and lymphoid leukemia may result in both leukemias in the same patient as independent events.[429]

TRANSIENT ABNORMAL MYELOPOIESIS

Increased WBC count with circulating blasts often accompanied by anemia and thrombocytopenia may be seen in 5% of newborns with DS. The blast cells almost invariably have cell surface antigens characteristic of megakaryoblasts.[430] The percentage of blasts is often higher in blood than in BM, and a BM aspiration is of limited additional diagnostic value. Clonal abnormalities are observed in 35%.[431] The condition is referred to as transient abnormal myelopoiesis (TAM), or transient myeloproliferative disorder. The presentation is indistinguishable from leukemia and some have therefore favored the name transient leukemia.[430,431] Transient leukemia may occasionally occur in an infant with normal phenotype and trisomy 21 in the blast cells.[432,433] An unknown portion of these infants may have low-level constitutional trisomy 21 mosaic detectable by FISH only.[434] TAM involves selectively the trisomic cells in individuals with DS mosaic.[435]

Infants with TAM are often asymptomatic presenting with elevated WBC count and hepatomegaly. Life-threatening complications, mainly progressive hepatic dysfunction, may occur in 10% to 20% of patients with TAM, but spontaneous remission appears in the majority within 1 to 3 months.[431,436,437] Generally no chemotherapy is indicated in TAM; however, in those with progressive hepatic or pulmonary problems, WBC count above 100×10^9/L, or bleeding diatheses a short course of low-dose cytarabine (e.g., 1.5 mg/kg/day for 4 to 7 days) may be very effective and improves survival[437,438] (Table 20.9, Fig. 20.9). ML develops 1 to 3 years later in about 25% of the children who have recovered from TAM.[430,431] The development of subsequent ML is associated with acquired clonal cytogenetic abnormalities[431] and persistently elevated WT1 expression.[439]

TABLE 20.9

MULTIVARIATE MODEL OF SIGNIFICANT PROGNOSTIC FACTORS FOR EARLY DEATH IN TAM, BASED UPON DATA FROM KLUSMANN ET AL

Variable	Hazard ratio
Preterm (<37 weeks)	4.1
Ascites	4.6
WBC count $> 100 \times 10^9$/L	5.0
Bleeding diathesis	11.0

Klusmann JH, Creutzig U, Zimmermann M, et al. Treatment and prognostic impact of transient leukemia in neonates with Down syndrome. Blood 2008;111(6):2991–2998. Reprinted with permission.

MYELOID LEUKEMIA

ML in individuals with DS has often been classified as AML[440] despite BM blasts less than 30% in many patients.[15] Of those with a morphological diagnosis of refractory cytopenia (RC), refractory anemia with excess blasts (RAEB), or RAEB in transformation (RAEB-T), 25% have DS.[15,17,441] In contrast to non-DS children, there are no biological or therapeutic differences between MDS and AML in DS. Recognizing the unique biological features, the disease may be best described by the unifying term *myeloid leukemia of Down syndrome*.[120,139] ML-DS is preferred to AMKL because other phenotypes in DS are observed sharing the same biologic and clinical characteristics. It is no longer appropriate to use the terms MDS or AML (AMKL) in young children with DS.

MLs in older children with DS (4 years or older) tend to be *GATA1*-negative and have a higher risk of relapse.[442,443] Such patients may represent spontaneous AML not fulfilling the criteria for ML-DS.

Epidemiology

ML-DS develops in 1% to 2% of children with DS[426] corresponding to an annual incidence of 0.6 to 1.0 per million children[12,15,441] (Table 20.10). The age distribution is very unusual with 50% being 1 year of age at diagnosis, 34% 2 years of age, and only 2% more than 4 years of age.[428] Only very few present before 1 year of age and there appears to be no age-overlap between TAM and ML-DS.[260,440,444,445]

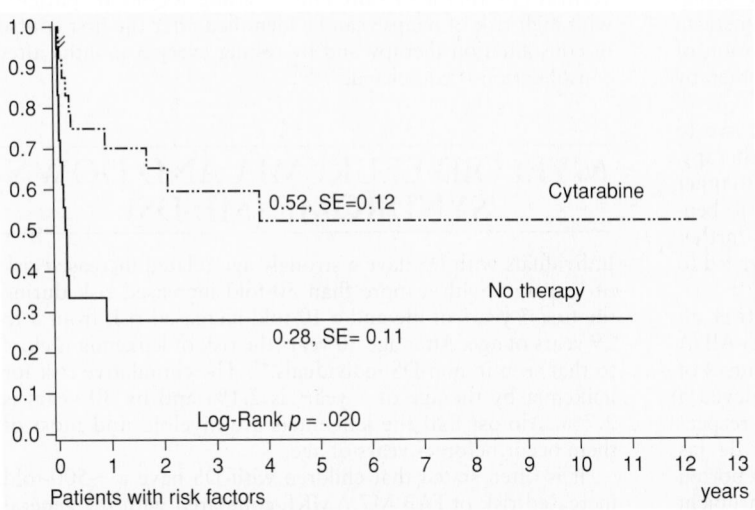

FIGURE 20.9 Survival in high-risk transient abnormal myelopoiesis (TAM) patients according to cytarabine therapy.

ANNUAL INCIDENCE OF HEMATOLOGICAL MALIGNANCIES IN CHILDREN AGED 0 TO 14 YEARS

	Denmark and BC			UK
	N	%	Incidence per million	Incidence per million
ALL	815	79	38.5	Nd
AML[a]	115	11	5.4	5.8
MDS[a]	38	4	1.8	0.8
Myeloid leukemia of DS	19	2	0.9	0.6
JMML	25	2	1.2	0.6
CML	13	1	0.6	0.5
PV/ET	3	0	0.1	Nd
Unclassified	3	0	0.1	
Total	1030	100	48.7	—

[a]Excluding Down syndrome (DS).
ALL, acute lymphoblastic leukemia; AML, acute myeloid leukemia; MDS, myelodysplastic syndrome; JMML, juvenile myelomonocytic leukemia; CML, chronic myelogenous leukemia; PV: polycythemia vera; ET: essential thrombocythemia.
Combined data from Denmark 1980 to 1991 and British Columbia 1982 to 1996 (Hasle H, Kerndrup G, Jacobsen BB. Childhood myelodysplastic syndrome in Denmark: incidence and predisposing conditions. Leukemia 1995;9(9):1569–1572; Hasle H, Wadsworth LD, Massing BG, et al. A population-based study of childhood myelodysplastic syndrome in British Columbia, Canada. Br J Haematol 1999;106(4):1027–1032.) and data from UK 1990 to 1999 (Passmore SJ, Chessells JM, Kempski H, et al. Paediatric myelodysplastic syndromes and juvenile myelomonocytic leukaemia in the UK: a population-based study of incidence and survival. Br J Haematol 2003; 121(5):758–767.)

Pathobiology

Leukemia in children with trisomy 21 mosaicism selectively involves the trisomic cells,[446,447] pointing at the etiological role of the additional chromosome 21 as the first hit in the multistep process leading to leukemia. Trisomy 21 profoundly disturbs fetal liver hematopoiesis, explaining the liver problems and dominant PB and not BM involvement in TAM.[448] Virtually all patients with ML-DS have an acquired mutation in the GATA1 gene.[449] The mutation is not found in AML M7 in non-DS or in other AML patients. The GATA1 mutation is also found in patients with TAM.[450,451] The GATA1 gene encodes a transcription factor essential for normal erythroid and megakaryocytic differentiation in accordance with the selective involvement of these two lineages rather than granulocytic lineage in ML-DS.[452] The studies of GATA1 mutations as well as the unique gene expression profile[453] support the notion of ML-DS as a separate entity.

A model of the pathogenic steps in ML-DS is presented in Figure 20.10. The trisomy 21 is the first event that may predispose the cells to a proliferative advantage or further mutations. GATA1 mutation is found in the majority of patients with TAM and present in 3% to 4% of newborns with DS and normal hematopoiesis.[454] The mechanisms of the regression of TAM remain unexplained but may be associated with the shift of hematopoiesis from the liver to the BM. About 25% of those with TAM and about 1% of DS with normal hematology in the newborn period develop ML-DS.[426]

Clinical and Laboratory Features

Isolated thrombocytopenia is often the presenting feature of ML-DS. At diagnosis, both platelet count and WBC count are lower than that in non-DS patients[440] in contrast to the very high WBC count seen in TAM. Many patients have a relatively indolent course characterized by a period of thrombocytopenia and dysplasia with relatively few blasts in the BM.

Cytogenetics

Numerical aberrations, mainly trisomy 8 and an extra chromosome 21 (tetrasomy 21), are the most common acquired cytogenetic abnormalities.[455] Karyotype is not known to be a prognostic factor in DS. The clonal cells in children with DS are myeloid progenitors with the potential for differentiation along the megakaryocytic and erythroid lineages.[452]

Treatment

In contrast to TAM, ML-DS is fatal if untreated but responds well to AML treatment with a very favorable outcome.[155,259,440] The prognosis of ML in patients with DS was considered very poor before 1990. Then reports from NOPHO[456] and the POG[155] and later the CCG[440] showed a surprisingly high survival rate for DS patients receiving AML treatment. DS was later shown to be the most important prognostic factor in

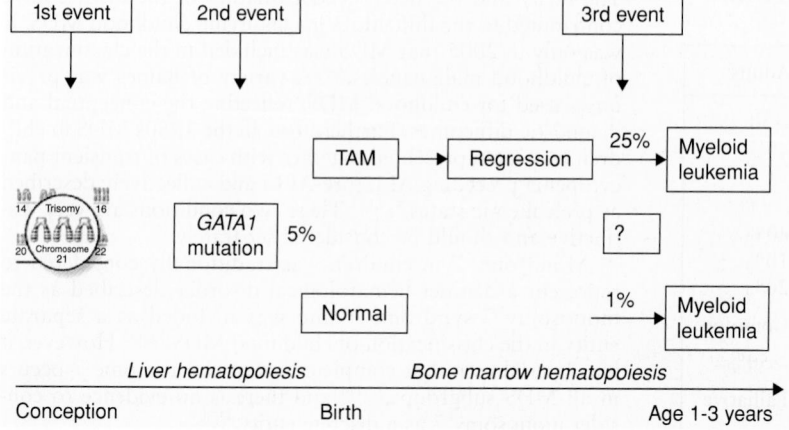

FIGURE 20.10 Pathogenetic model for myeloid leukemia in Down syndrome.

AML.[259] Several groups have reported significantly improved outcome for children with ML-DS during the last 10 to 15 years with long-term survival well above 80%.[261,444,457–459] DS children are at low risk for relapse and due to the high risk for treatment-related toxicity they benefit from less time-intensive therapy, allowing recovery prior to initiation of the next chemotherapeutic course.[440,444,458] HSCT is associated with excess toxicity without therapeutic gain and is not indicated in ML-DS.[257,440]

DS myeloblasts are 10-fold more sensitive to cytarabine than non-DS cells *in vitro*.[264,460,461] The increased sensitivity of DS blasts may be related to the expression of chromosome 21 localized genes like cystathionine-β-synthetase and superoxide dismutase.[461] Elevated cystathionine-β-synthetase activity may modulate cytarabine metabolism by decreasing levels of deoxycytidine triphosphate or decreasing generation of S-adenosylmethionine and hypomethylation of the deoxycytidine kinase gene.[461] The cystathionine-β-synthetase gene polymorphism (844ins68) is more frequently observed in DS myeloblasts than in non-DS myeloblasts; those DS patients with the polymorphism have an increased cytarabine sensitivity compared with those with the wild type gene.[462]

It is remarkable that only the constitutional and not the acquired trisomy 21 is associated with a superior outcome.[440] Further studies of the molecular mechanism of the increased sensitivity to chemotherapy in DS may lead to new approaches in the treatment of AML.

MYELODYSPLASTIC SYNDROME (MDS)

MDS is much rarer in children than in adults and most of the literature on MDS is based upon studies in elderly patients; however, there are significant differences between MDS in children and adults (Table 20.11). The morphologic features and cytogenetic findings at diagnosis differ significantly between children and adults. Many children have associated abnormalities, such as preexisting BM failure or congenital abnormalities. Cure is the therapeutic aim in children with MDS but is often not realistic in adults. The rarity of MDS in children and the lack of an overall accepted classification have contributed to the paucity of MDS in the pediatric literature. However, the publication of large series of childhood MDS patients from the mid-1990s[10–13,15,16,441,463–465] and retrospective studies from the European Working Group on MDS in childhood (EWOG-MDS) gradually increased the awareness of pediatric MDS.[5,32,466]

TABLE 20.11

MAJOR DIFFERENCES BETWEEN MDS IN CHILDREN AND ADULTS

	Children	Adults
Incidence /million	1–2	>30
RA with ringed sideroblasts	2%	25%
Constitutional abnormalities	30%	<5%
Cytogenetic aberrations	50%	40%
−7/del(7q)	30%	10%
−5/del(5q)	1–2%	20%
Mutation of NRAS	Rare	Common
Hypermethylation	>50%	>50%
Main aim of treatment	Curative	Palliative

ML-DS and JMML have often been included under the heading of MDS; there is today consensus that these disorders are distinct from MDS.[120]

Epidemiology

The epidemiological literature on childhood MDS is sparse, mainly because the indolent nature of the disease may not lead to referral to a tertiary center, and many epidemiological data are derived from multi-institutional studies to which MDS patients have been referred only after progression of their disease. Approximately 10% to 20% of childhood AML is preceded by a recognized MDS phase.[212] However, studies underestimate the incidence of MDS because AML does not develop in all cases of MDS and some children die from complications of cytopenia or are treated before progression to AML.

Incidence, Sex, Age, and Subtype Distribution

Combined population-based data from Denmark and British Columbia (BC) in Canada identified 38 cases of MDS, representing 4% of all hematological malignancies in children (Table 20.10); this corresponds to an annual incidence of MDS of 1.8 per million children aged 0 to 14 years.[15,441] MDS and JMML combined constituted 7.7% of childhood leukemia in Japan with a high proportion of therapy-related cases (23%).[10] Data from the United Kingdom suggest a considerably lower annual incidence of MDS of 0.8 per million children (Table 20.10).[12] The U.K. study excluded secondary MDS, which partly explains the lower incidence. The incidence of RC in the United Kingdom, Denmark, and BC is very similar, but the incidence of advanced MDS and JMML differ significantly. Possible differences in classification practice can only explain a small part of the variation, and it is possible that there are genuine regional differences in incidence.[12]

The male/female distribution in pediatric MDS is equal (144/146) with a median age at presentation of 6.8 years.[10,12,15,16,441] Application of the FAB classification in 239 patients showed the following distribution: refractory anemia (RA) 38% (*n* = 90), RA with ringed sideroblasts (RARS) 0% (*n* = 1), RAEB 37% (*n* = 88) and RAEB-T 25% (*n* = 60).[10,12,15,16,441] ML-DS is now considered a separate entity and is no longer considered as MDS.[120] The exclusion of DS from patient series of MDS decreases the number of cases diagnosed as RAEB-T by approximately 50%.[17] The exclusion or inclusion of other constitutional abnormalities contributes to variations in the reported frequency of MDS.[13,52,467,468]

Classification of Childhood MDS

The rarity and the heterogeneous nature of the disease have contributed to the difficulties in classifying childhood MDS. It was only in 2005 that MDS was included in the classification of childhood malignancies.[469] A variety of names was previously used for childhood MDS, reflecting the conceptual and diagnostic difficulties. Furthermore, in the 1980s MDS in children was often presented together with cases of transient pancytopenia preceding ALL (pre-ALL) and collectively described as preleukemic states.[470,471] These two conditions are very distinctive and should be considered separately.[14]

Monosomy 7 in children was traditionally considered to represent a distinct hematological disorder described as the monosomy 7 syndrome[472] and was included as a separate entity in the classification of childhood MDS.[13,473] However, it was later shown that complete loss of chromosome 7 occurs in all MDS subgroups,[32,474] and there is no evidence to consider monosomy 7 as a discrete entity.[32,307]

The FAB group classification from 1982, based upon experiences from adult patients, divided MDS into five subgroups: RA, RARS, RAEB, RAEB-T, and chronic myelomonocytic leukemia (CMML).[475] The FAB classification had prognostic impact in children and facilitated communication about pediatric MDS but did not address the specific disease and morphological features in children and the frequent occurrence of associated anomalies.[13,32]

The WHO classification on neoplastic diseases of the hematopoietic tissues from 2001 incorporated both morphology and cytogenetics.[121] The threshold for distinguishing AML from MDS was lowered from 30% to 20% blasts. Also, the WHO classification was based upon review of adult cases and although JMML was recognized as a separate entity, the classification of MDS did not acknowledge the special features of MDS in children. The WHO subtype RARS is extremely rare in children and the unique 5q− syndrome is absent in pediatrics. Furthermore, the importance of multilineage dysplasia is unknown in children. There is no data to indicate whether a blast threshold of 20% is better than the traditional 30% to distinguish MDS from AML in children. The unique features of DS were not appropriately addressed in the WHO classification.

A pediatric approach to the WHO classification was published in 2003.[120] It separated myeloproliferative disorders in children into three main groups; JMML, MDS, and DS diseases (Table 20.12). MDS was further subdivided into RC, RAEB, and RAEB-T. The classification is used for both *de novo* and secondary MDS. The change in nomenclature from RA to RC reflects that anemia is not a prerequisite for the diagnosis. The RAEB-T entity is retained, but the blast count is insufficient to differentiate AML from MDS (further details under differential diagnoses). ML in children with DS has unique features and is kept separate as a distinct entity. The pediatric modification of the WHO classification allows unambiguous classification of more than 95% of the patients.[120,464]

The Toronto group proposed a descriptive system designed to assess children with MDS according to category, cytology, and cytogenetics (CCC).[476] The system excluded JMML but included patients with DS. The level of dysplasia subdivided both RC and RAEB into three subgroups. The CCC system has an infinite number of possible subgroups, making it difficult to use in clinical practice or research.

The revised WHO classification from 2008 keeps JMML separate and recognizes the ML-DS as a unique group.[139] The classification establishes a separate description of RC of childhood, although for children with more than 2% blasts in the PB or 5% in the BM, application of the same criteria as in adults are recommended (Table 20.12). It should be emphasized that the diagnosis of MDS cannot rely on blast count alone but must include a comprehensive evaluation of clinical features, natural course, morphology, immunophenotype, and cytogenetics.

Pathophysiology

MDS is a clonal disease arising in a progenitor cell restricted to myelopoiesis, erythropoiesis, or megakaryopoiesis.[3,4] The initiating events may infrequently occur in a more immature cell involving the lymphoid cell line resulting in the very rare progression of MDS to ALL.[463,477,478] The initiating events of MDS have remained obscure in children like in adults; however, a recent study identified a tumor-suppressor gene, *TET2*, that is mutated as an early genetic event in about 20% of patients with various myeloid disorders including MDS.[479]

Because MDS is very heterogeneous, different mechanisms of initiation and progression of the disease are likely to exist. Genetic damage in a pluripotent hematopoietic progenitor cell may give rise to genetic instability with subsequent acquisition of numerous molecular and cellular abnormalities.[480] Congenital disorders with DNA repair defects like Fanconi anemia or acquired mutations in genes maintaining genetic stability may result in a mutator phenotype predisposing to MDS.[481,482] About 30% of children with MDS have a known constitutional disorder. It may be speculated that an even higher proportion of the children have a congenital abnormality predisposing them to the acquisition of genetic changes. Subsequent events, such as mutations in proto-oncogenes like *RAS*, *p53*, or *WT1*, or karyotypic changes like monosomy 7, may be part of a final common pathway of disease progression.[54,483,484] Methylation studies in children with RAEB or RAEB-T have demonstrated that at least half the patients had hypermethylation of the *p15* gene[485] or *CALCA* and *CDKN2B* genes,[486] a frequency similar to adult MDS.

Mutations in *TP53* and *FMS* are found in 30% of adult MDS, but the mutations are lacking in children with MDS.[487] Mutations of the *NRAS* proto-oncogene represent the most frequent molecular changes in adult MDS but are rare in children.[483,488]

Mutations in *TERC*, the gene coding for the RNA component of telomerase, result in autosomal dominant dyskeratosis congenita. Two large studies showed *TERC* mutations in only 3 out of 217 children with MDS.[489,490]

TABLE 20.12

DIAGNOSTIC CATEGORIES OF MYELODYSPLASTIC AND MYELOPROLIFERATIVE DISEASES IN CHILDREN ACCORDING TO THE PEDIATRIC APPROACH TO THE WHO CLASSIFICATION[a] AND THE REVISED WHO CLASSIFICATION[b]

Myelodysplastic/Myeloproliferative disease
- Juvenile myelomonocytic leukemia (JMML)

Myeloid proliferations related to Down syndrome (DS)
- Transient abnormal myelopoiesis (TAM)
- Myeloid leukemia of Down syndrome (ML-DS)

Myelodysplastic syndrome (MDS)
- Refractory cytopenia (RC) (PB blasts < 2% and BM blasts < 5%)
- Refractory anemia with excess blasts (RAEB) (PB blasts 2–19% or BM blasts 5–19%)
- RAEB in transformation (RAEB-T) (PB or BM blasts 20–29%)/AML with myelodysplasia-related changes (PB or BM blasts > 20%)

[a]Hasle H, Niemeyer CM, Chessells JM, et al. A pediatric approach to the WHO classification of myelodysplastic and myeloproliferative diseases. Leukemia 2003;17(2):277–282.
[b]Vardiman JW, Thiele J, Arber DA, et al. The 2008 revision of the WHO classification of myeloid neoplasms and acute leukemia: rationale and important changes. Blood 2009;114:937–951.

Using cDNA microarray assays, a clear difference in the gene expression pattern is observed between BM stroma cells obtained from healthy children and from pediatric patients with either MDS or AML. The global gene function profiling analysis indicated that in the pediatric MDS microenvironment the disease stages may be characterized mainly by underexpression of genes associated with biological processes such as transport. Furthermore, a subset of downregulated genes related to endocytosis and protein secretion may be able to discriminate MDS from MDS-AML.[491]

Clinical and Laboratory Features

The presenting features in almost all cases of MDS are those of pancytopenia. Single lineage cytopenia may occasionally be the presenting characteristic. In a few cases, the cytopenia is an incidental finding during a routine work-up. A few patients have been diagnosed during evaluation as a possible sibling stem cell donor. Not all children with RC have anemia, but macrocytosis (elevated mean corpuscular volume [MCV]) is a characteristic finding.[5] Fetal hemoglobin (HbF) is frequently moderately elevated. WBC count is low to normal. Leukocytosis is generally not a feature of MDS and in the case of increased WBC count the diagnosis should be reconsidered. Some patients present with slight hepatosplenomegaly but most have no organomegaly. Extramedullary myeloid tumor may be the presenting feature of MDS[32,492] but blasts are not seen in the cerebrospinal fluid in MDS.

Bone Marrow Features

The BM may be hypo-, normo-, or hypercellular. Decreased cell content has been observed in up to 40% of childhood RC.[5] Both the PB and BM display characteristic dysplastic features with megaloblastic erythropoiesis, bizarre small or unusual large megakaryocytes, and dysgranulopoiesis.[493] The presence of the characteristic dysplastic features is suggestive of MDS but not diagnostic.[120] Interobserver variation in the evaluation of dysplasia exists[494] and centralized review is recommended.[493] The degree of dysplasia and the extent of fibrosis have prognostic relevance in adults with RA,[495,496] but it remains uncertain whether the same is true in children.

Cytogenetics

An abnormal karyotype is found in about 50% of children with MDS.[12,16,497-499] The numerical abnormalities dominate with only 10% showing a translocation, a derivative, or a deletion as the sole abnormality. Structural abnormalities are frequently part of a complex karyotype with numerical abnormalities. This is in contrast to AML where structural abnormalities are by far the most frequent findings.[153,292]

Monosomy 7 is the most common cytogenetic abnormality in childhood MDS, seen in approximately 30% of the patients.[13,497-499] Trisomy 8 and trisomy 21 are the next most common numerical abnormalities. Constitutional trisomy 21 is clinically obvious when present, whereas constitutional trisomy 8 mosaicism may be clinically silent and should be tested for when trisomy 8 is found in the BM.[18]

There are very few data on the prognostic value of cytogenetic abnormalities in children. Monosomy 7 as the only cytogenetic aberration has not been an unfavorable feature in most studies in childhood MDS,[16,32,215,307] whereas complex abnormalities with or without chromosome 7 involvement are

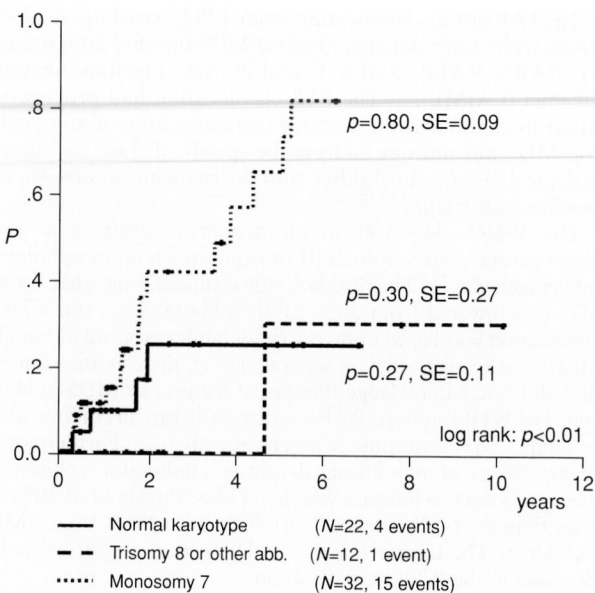

FIGURE 20.11 Risk of progression in RC according to cytogenetics. (Kardos G, Baumann I, Passmore SJ, et al. Refractory anemia in childhood: a retrospective analysis of 67 patients with particular reference to monosomy 7. Blood 2003;102(6):1997–2003. Reprinted with permission)

associated with a poor outcome.[32,499] This is in contrast to adults in whom monosomy 7 is associated with a very poor prognosis. However, monosomy 7 is associated with a shorter time to progression in children with RC[5] (Fig. 20.11). Favorable cytogenetic aberrations have been identified in adults in −Y, 20q−, and 5q−; these aberrations are so infrequent in children that they are of no practical importance.

AML specific translocations, such as t(8;21)(q22;q22), t(15;17)(q22;q12), or inv(16)(p13;q22) may be seen with a low blast cell count but should be considered as AML regardless of the blast count.[139,500]

Immunophenotype

Flow cytometry immunophenotyping does not have the same diagnostic yield in MDS as in acute leukemia but may be of value in the quantitative and qualitative assessment of immature progenitor cells, especially when BM smears are of suboptimal quality. Although no marker-abnormality or abnormal marker profile is specific for MDS, and a normal flow cytometry examination does not preclude MDS, abnormalities may help in discriminating a normal/reactive BM from a clonal myeloid malignancy.[501] Phenotypic abnormalities in MDS may correlate with prognosis. A current disadvantage of flow cytometry in MDS is that there is no generally accepted consensus on uniformly used standard protocols and techniques. Few data on immunophenotype characteristics of MDS in children have been reported.[502]

Differential Diagnosis

The two main diagnostic challenges are to distinguish MDS with a low blast count from AA and other nonclonal disorders and to differentiate MDS with excess of blasts from AML. The traditional classification has been based on pure morphology, but a number of additional factors need to be considered.

Refractory Cytopenia versus Aplastic Anemia

BM cellularity is decreased in 40% of the RC patients.[5] BM fibrosis, dilution, and sampling variation make it difficult to assess the cellularity from an aspirate. A trephine biopsy is therefore essential for the evaluation of a child with suspected AA or MDS. Hypoplastic MDS may be difficult to discriminate from AA. The presenting MCV is higher in MDS than in AA.[503] Careful sequential morphologic studies including BM biopsies will almost always establish a distinction between MDS and AA.[504,505] The biopsy in hypoplastic MDS shows scarcely scattered granulopoietic cells, patchy islands of immature erythropoiesis, and micromegakaryocytes.[139] Marked erythroid hypoplasia may also be a feature of childhood MDS.[506] Clonal hematopoiesis is strongly suggestive of MDS; when standard cytogenetics fail FISH or HUMARA assays may be useful to establish clonality. Immunohistochemcal studies may be helpful showing a high expression of p53 and a low expression of survivin in MDS patients in contrast to nonclonal BM failures.[507]

MDS versus Other Nonclonal Disorders

Dysplasia in the BM may occur in a variety of disorders of very different etiologies, for example, infection, drug therapy, and chronic disease. RC is a diagnosis of exclusion after ruling out infectious diseases like parvovirus,[508,509] herpesvirus 6,[510] HIV,[511] and visceral leishmaniasis.[512] vitamin B_{12} deficiency,[513] copper deficiency,[514,515] drug therapy,[516,517] rheumatoid arthritis,[518] metabolic disorders,[519] and other causes of cytopenia and dysplasia[520–522] should also be considered. Nonclonal chronic disorders with dysplastic features, such as mitochondrial disorders like Pearson syndrome, should not be considered as MDS. RARS is extremely rare in children. The finding of sideroblastic anemia should prompt investigation for possible mitochondrial cytopathy or disorders of heme synthesis.[523,524]

It may be difficult to diagnose MDS in children who have a low blast cell count and no clonal marker. The minimal diagnostic criteria listed in Table 20.13 may help in this case.[120] The WHO classification requires dysplasia in two different cell lineages or exceeding 10% in one single cell lineage.[139] Although dysplasia is essential for the diagnosis, it constitutes only one aspect of the morphological diagnosis. Furthermore, dysplasia may be observed in many reactive conditions in children and MDS may present with very discrete dysplasia. The length of persistent cytopenia should be at least 1 month.

Since hematopoiesis is often dysplastic in patients with congenital BM failure disorders, it is recommended diagnosing MDS in these patients only if the BM blast count is increased, a persistent clonal chromosomal abnormality is present, or the BM becomes hypercellular in the presence of persistent PB cytopenia.[120] A high level of expression of survivin protein in a BM biopsy may be helpful in distinguishing an inherited from an acquired BM failure disorder.[507]

MINIMAL DIAGNOSTIC CRITERIA FOR MDS

At least two of the following:
- Sustained unexplained cytopenia (neutropenia, thrombocytopenia, or anemia)
- At least bilineage morphologic myelodysplasia
- Acquired clonal cytogenetic abnormality in hematopoietic cells
- Increased blasts ($\geq$5%)

MAJOR DIFFERENCES BETWEEN MDS AND AML IN CHILDREN

	MDS	AML
WBC	Low-normal	Low-normal-high
Hepatomegaly	Infrequent	Common
Cytogenetic aberrations	Numerical (-7)	Structural
Dysplasia	Multilineage	Infrequent
Hematopoiesis	Clonal (including CR)	Nonclonal
Cell of origin	Stem cell	Lineage-restricted
Response to chemotherapy	Poor	Moderate
Iatrogenic model	Alkylating agents	Epipodophyllotoxins

Separating MDS from AML

AML is the major differential diagnosis of MDS. There are significant differences in biology, clinical features, cytogenetics, and response to therapy between MDS and AML[525] (Table 20.14). A British study suggested a better outcome following AML therapy in patients with RAEB-T compared with RAEB[526]; however, this was not found in an American study.[307] The conflicting data reflect the fact that the morphologically defined RAEB-T group is heterogeneous and the blast count in a single specimen is insufficient to differentiate MDS from AML. Biological features, rather than any arbitrary cutoff in blast count, may be more important in distinguishing MDS from (chemosensitive) AML.[119] An algorithm to facilitate the distinction between MDS and AML is presented in Figure 20.12. Monosomy 7 is strongly suggestive of MDS,[32] and patients presenting with monosomy 7 and a blast count above 30% may share many features with MDS rather than with true *de novo* AML.[235]

In borderline cases with BM blasts of 20% to 30% and no cytogenetic clues to the diagnosis, it is recommended to repeat the BM examination after 2 weeks. If the blast count has increased to more than 30%, the case should be regarded as AML (Fig. 20.12). Significant organomegaly or increased WBC count is suggestive of a diagnosis of AML. It should be emphasized that most children with myeloid malignancies have clear-cut AML, some have MDS with low blast count and only a few have borderline features. The major diagnostic pitfall may be associated with undue haste in starting therapy.

Prognosis and Natural Course

Progression of MDS to AML with myelodysplasia-related changes may occur at different rates. In some patients, the percentage of blast cells in the BM may increase abruptly after a set of transforming events, whereas other patients show a slow rate of progression, and the 20% or 30% threshold is passed only after a period of months or years. Although any case above the threshold is conventionally defined as AML with myelodysplasia-related changes, most of the biologic characteristics of MDS persist.[527]

Children with RC and RAEB or even RAEB-T may show a long and stable clinical course without treatment. Blood transfusions are only required infrequently and severe infections are rarely seen. The condition may smolder with unchanged cytopenia for months or even years but will eventually progress

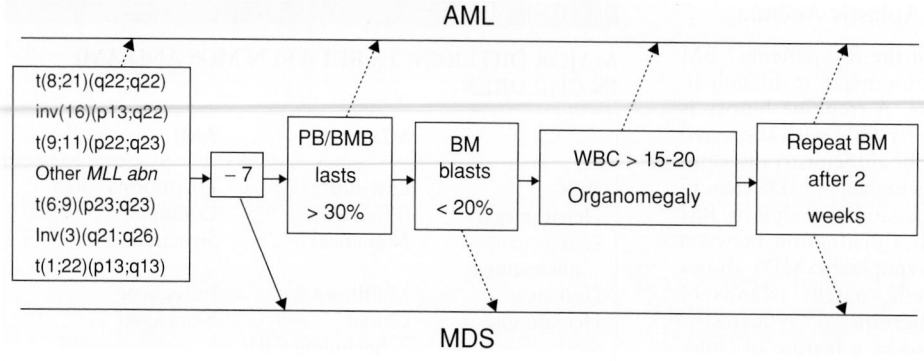

FIGURE 20.12 Algorithm for distinguishing myelodysplastic syndrome (MDS) from acute myeloid leukemia (AML).

in virtually all patients. In a series of 67 children with primary RC, four died from complications of pancytopenia prior to therapy or progression and 20 progressed to more advanced MDS at a median of 1.7 years from presentation.[5] Although RC with monosomy 7 is associated with a higher risk of progression, both RC and RAEB patients with monosomy 7 may show stable disease without treatment for several years.[5,32] Once progression has occurred the outcome is inferior even after HSCT.[5,528]

The International Prognostic Scoring System (IPSS) for MDS weighted data on BM blast count, cytopenia, and cytogenetics and separated patients into four prognostic groups. They noted that children more often have high-risk features compared with adults[466] (Table 20.15). Thrombocytopenia and BM blasts of more than 5% correlated with poor survival in children, whereas 2 to 3 lineage cytopenia and cytogenetics did not provide prognostic information.[466] This contrasts with data from Japan[10] and the United Kingdom[12] showing the cytogenetic component of the IPSS to be significantly associated with outcome due to a poor prognosis in patients with monosomy 7. The Japanese study, like EWOG-MDS, showed a poor outcome in those presenting with BM blasts of more than 5%. Overall, the IPSS provides little diagnostic information in children but identifies a very small group (7%) of patients with low-risk disease and a very favorable outcome.[466]

A pediatric prognostic scoring system (FPC) proposed by the British group assigned one point each for HbF more than 10%, platelets less than 40×10^9/L, and two or more cytogenetic abnormalities.[13] A significantly higher survival was found in children with MDS and a score of zero. Application of the scoring system in other series has been hampered by HbF being available in only a minority of the patients with MDS. Data

from EWOG-MDS were used to evaluate the FPC score in 65 patients with complete data and showed that complex karyotype was the only factor associated with a poor survival[466]; this was also confirmed in a larger series.[499]

Spontaneous regression of MDS has occasionally been reported in the literature.[529–533] The frequency of spontaneous remission is unknown, but estimated to occur in well below 5% of the patients.

Treatment

MDS is a clonal early stem cell disorder with very limited residual nonclonal stem cells. Myeloablative therapy is therefore the only treatment option with a realistic curative potential. A diversity of therapeutic strategies like hematopoietic growth factors, differentiating agents, hormones, amifostine, low-dose cytotoxic drugs, and experimental agents have been investigated in adults and the elderly who were not candidates for HSCT. None of these approaches has been documented to prolong survival and they are generally not indicated in children and adolescents. Given the lack of recurrent molecular abnormalities in MDS, rational drug development for molecular targeted therapy is problematic.

Immunosuppressive therapy has been successful in some adults with MDS and low blast count, especially in patients with BM hypoplasia and HLA-DR15 (DR2).[534] Other studies have been less optimistic, reporting a significant burden of side effects.[535] Immunosuppressive therapy with antithymocyte globulin and cyclosporine in 31 children with hypoplastic RC resulted in a complete or partial response in 22 out of 29 evaluable patients at 6 months. Overall and failure-free survival rates

TABLE 20.15

DISTRIBUTION AND OVERALL SURVIVAL OF CHILDREN[a] AND ADULTS[b] WITH MDS IN THE FOUR GROUPS OF THE INTERNATIONAL PROGNOSTIC SCORING SYSTEM (IPSS)

	Children		Adults	
IPSS group	N = 142 (%)	Median survival (years)	N = 816 (%)	Median survival (years)
Low	7	>10	33	5.7
Intermediate 1	47	9.7	38	3.5
Intermediate 2	25	4.5	22	1.2
High	21	2.2	7	0.4

[a]Hasle H, Baumann I, Bergstrasser E, et al. The International Prognostic Scoring System (IPSS) for childhood myelodysplastic syndrome (MDS) and juvenile myelomonocytic leukemia (JMML). Leukemia 2004; 18(12):2008–2014.
[b]Greenberg P, Cox C, LeBeau MM, et al. International Scoring System for Evaluating Prognosis in Myelodysplastic Syndromes. Blood 1997;89:2079–2088.

at 3 years were 88% and 57%, respectively.[536] The long-term outcome of immunosuppressive therapy in MDS is not known.

DNA methyltransferase inhibitors, azacitidine and decitabine, have shown clinical efficacy in adults with MDS. A recent phase III trial in adult patients with high-risk MDS randomized patients to receive azacitidine or conventional care and showed that treatment with azacitidine increases OS relative to conventional care.[537] Hypermethylation may occur at a similar frequency in children and adults,[485,486] thus making children potential candidates for demethylating therapy; however, so far treatment results from pediatrics are lacking. Children with MDS are at high risk of cytopenia-related complications, and optimal supportive care should be the primary focus during all phases of the disease course.

AML Type Chemotherapy

Conventional intensive chemotherapy without HSCT is unlikely to eradicate the primitive pluripotent cells involved in MDS, rendering the therapy noncurative in most patients, although reported results are somewhat conflicting. Most studies found a significant morbidity and mortality of induction chemotherapy with a CR rate of less than 60%, many relapses, and OS less than 30%.[10,307,525] The treatment-related mortality rate has been between 10% and 30%.[307,525,526] A few studies have reported an outcome in MDS patients not significantly different from that in AML[526] especially in patients with RAEB-T or AML following MDS.[307,526] The results reflect the heterogeneous nature of RAEB-T and emphasize that a single morphological evaluation is insufficient for relevant treatment stratification.[120]

Autologous SCT is often used in younger adults[538] but has been infrequently reported in children. Two studies included eight children receiving autologous SCT with one long-term survivor.[307,526]

Hematopoietic Allogeneic Stem Cell Transplantation

HSCT is the therapy of choice for virtually all forms of MDS in childhood. Studies specifically addressing the question of HSCT in children have indicated a probability of DFS following transplantation with an HLA-matched family donor (MFD) of about 50%.[539-542] Previously, children receiving a graft from an HLA-MUD have suffered a higher transplant-related mortality and lower DFS, but more recent studies have shown survival following MUD-HSCT comparable to that of MFD-HSCT.[543-545]

The European Group for Blood and Marrow Transplantation (EBMT) reported 3-year DFS, treatment-related mortality, and relapse risk of 45%, 30%, and 36%, respectively for MDS patients younger than 20 years who received MFD-HSCT between 1983 and 1998.[546] EWOG-MDS has successfully studied a large number of patients with a preparative regimen of busulfan, cyclophosphamide, and melphalan.[539] The regimen has been studied in a large number of patients under the auspices of EWOG-MDS and EBMT and has shown DFS of 87% in MFD-HSCT and 41% in MUD-HSCT.[547] Other large studies have confirmed a favorable outcome in patients conditioned with a myeloablative busulfan-based regimen.[548] Total body irradiation (TBI) can generally be omitted since it is known to have no superior anti-leukemic efficacy compared with busulfan[528,549] and is associated with more long-term effects in children.

Stage of disease has a significant effect on relapse and outcome following HSCT[546,550-552] with a low relapse rate in RC. HSCT early in the course of the disease has therefore been recommended for all children and adolescents with MDS. However, in children with RC and absence of profound cytopenia, postponement of HSCT with a watch and wait strategy may be justified, especially in patients with a normal karyotype.[5] Following a myeloablative preparative regimen in RC, EWOG-

MDS reported a 5-year DFS of 78% and 76% for children receiving a MFD-HSCT or MUD-HSCT, respectively.[549] Reduced-intensity conditioning regimen showed a promising one-year progression-free survival of 66% in adults.[553] A fludarabine based preparative regimen in 19 children with RC and normal karyotype resulted in an OS and DFS at 3 years of 84% and 74% respectively.[554]

For advanced MDS, intensive GvHD prophylaxis including *in vitro* T-cell-depletion[552] is associated with an increased risk of relapse. It remains unknown whether AML-type induction chemotherapy prior to HSCT for advanced MDS can reduce relapse and thus improve DFS. Data from EWOG-MDS on children with primary advanced MDS showed no benefit of intensive AML-type therapy preceding HSCT.[555] Small series of patients transplanted as first line therapy have shown survival of 65–70%.[525,540] Considering the significant morbidity and mortality of induction chemotherapy and the high rate of TRM following HSCT most children with MDS may benefit from HSCT as first line therapy sparing the toxicity related to induction chemotherapy. Children with progressive disease but without a matched donor should be considered for haploidentical HSCT.[556]

Relapse following HSCT is associated with a very grave outcome. Successful donor leukocyte infusions have occasionally been reported.[557] Especially early relapse detected by increasing mixed chimerism may benefit from withdrawal of immunosuppressive therapy and subsequent donor leukocyte infusion.[558-560] Close analyses of chimerism status post SCT may be indicated to initiate pre-emptive immunotherapy.[561] Increasing *WT1* expression may also be a useful marker to monitor impending relapse post SCT.[562]

Secondary MDS

Children with MDS secondary to chemo- or radiation therapy generally have a very poor survival. AML-type therapy may induce remission but very few patients remain in remission and even HSCT has been reported to offer cure to only 20–30% of patients.[70,542,563-565] The CCG reported a superior, although still poor, outcome using intensive-timing vs. standard-timing induction (32 vs. 0%).[70] The frequency of severe treatment-related toxicity is high,[563] whereas the risk of relapse may be similar to that observed for patients with primary MDS.[546] Recent data documents a significantly improvement over time and survival similar to *de novo* MDS when corrected for cytogenetics.[566]

The few published cases of HSCT in MDS arising from congenital BM failure disorders or acquired AA indicate a poor outcome for this heterogeneous group of patients. Early HSCT before neoplastic transformation or during less advanced MDS may be associated with improved survival.[27,567]

JUVENILE MYELOMONOCYTIC LEUKEMIA (JMML)

JMML is a unique pediatric disorder; it is the pediatric equivalent of what the FAB group termed CMML. JMML was previously named juvenile chronic myeloid leukemia (JCML), recognizing the distinction from CML occurring in older children and adults.[568]

It is considered a separate bridging disorder between MDS and myeloproliferative disorders in the WHO classification.[139]

Epidemiology

In accordance with earlier studies,[568] incidence studies from Denmark and BC[15,441] showed a JMML incidence of 1.2/million children per year, corresponding to 2.4% for all hematologic malignancies (Table 20.10). However, an incidence of only 0.6/million is found in UK.[12]

The median age at presentation is 1.8 years, 35% are below one year of age at presentation and only 4% are more than 5 years of age.[569] JMML displays a male predominance with a male:female ratio of 2:1.[16,569]

Neurofibromatosis type 1 (NF1) is associated with a more than 200-fold increased risk of JMML.[570] NF1 is clinically recognized in 10–15% of the children with JMML and is relatively more frequent in children diagnosed after 5 years of age.[569]

Noonan Syndrome

A JMML-like picture with a strong tendency towards spontaneous regression has been observed in several infants with Noonan syndrome (NS)[571–573] and has resulted in significant insight into the pathogenesis of JMML.[574] This was first reported by Bader-Meunier in 1992[575] followed by several other reports from the same group[571] and others (Table 20.16).[572,573] Only one study has provided an estimate of the incidence of the NS-related myeloproliferative disorder (NS/MPD), showing monocytic proliferation in 4 of 40 (10%) patients with NS; all of them occurred transiently during the neonatal period.[573] This 10% risk of NS/MPD is in contrast to the only 30 cases of NS/MPD reported in the literature as reviewed by Kratz.[576]

Little is known about the clonality of the myeloproliferation in NS; one case tested showed polyclonal hematopoiesis[571] and none of those with transient NS/MPD had any cytogenetic abnormalities. The clinical features of the NS/MPD are indistinguishable from JMML including excessive growth of granulocyte-macrophage colonies *in vitro*.[572,573] However, the activation in STAT5 response to GM-CSF as measured by phosphoflow cytometry may distinguish NS/MPD from JMML.[577]

NS/MPD is diagnosed during the first few months of life. This contrasts to non-NS JMML, in which the median age at diagnosis is 1.8 years and less than 10% are diagnosed before 4 months of age.[569] Most cases resolve spontaneously but fatal progressive disease has been reported in three patients (10% of the approximately 30 patients reported).[573,578,579] Progression to AML occurred in one patient at two years of age.[571] In the majority, the hematological abnormalities gradually resolve but normalization may take several months or even

years, especially the monocytosis and splenomegaly which may persist for more than ten years.[571,580]

The NS/MPD has striking parallels with the transient leukemia of newborns with DS. Unlike the *GATA1* mutation in transient leukemia of DS the NS/MPD has no somatic molecular marker. The MPD disorder in DS patients is very sensitive to low-dose cytarabine. There is no documented effective therapy in those NS patients with an aggressive course. Isotretinoin was tried in one patient without effect[579] whereas low-dose mercaptopurine led to improvement in another patient.[571]

Following the identification of PTPN11 germline mutation in 50% of patients with NS, studies in non-NS JMML showed somatic PTPN11 mutations in 35%.[581] The spectrum of PTPN11 mutations differs between NS without JMML (N308D most common), NS/MPD (N308D most common), and JMML with somatic PTPN11 mutation (E76K substitution most common).[574,582] The PTPN11 mutations found in JMML have a stronger SHP-2 activation than the mutations in NS, whereas the mutations in NS/MPD have an intermediate gain of function effect.[583] It is presumed that the strong activation resulting from the PTPN11 mutation in JMML is incompatible with life when occurring as a germline mutation.

NS with a JMML-like disorder may have a germline KRAS mutation, which was recently shown to be the cause in a few patients with NS,[584] but all other reported patients had a PTPN11 mutation. Interestingly, a few cases of JMML associated with somatic *NRAS* mutations have been reported to regress spontaneously over time.[585,586] Other RAS-MAPK factors such as SOS1 mutations involved in NS and BRAF mutations involved in the cardio-facial-cutaneous (CFC) syndrome, have yet to be implicated in JMML.[587,588]

Clinical and Laboratory Features

Patients with JMML present with pallor, fever, infection, bleeding or symptoms from the organomegaly.[569] Hepatomegaly, splenomegaly, generalized lymphadenopathy, and skin rash may be the first signs leading to medical attention. An elevated WBC with absolute monocytosis, anemia, and thrombocytopenia is almost universal. WBC exceeds 50×10^9/L in 30% of patients at presentation and is above 100×10^9/L in 7%.[569] Increased HbF is characteristic of

TABLE 20.16

CHARACTERISTIC FINDINGS OF JMML-LIKE MYELOPROLIFERATIVE DISORDER (NS/MPD) IN CHILDREN WITH NOONAN SYNDROME AND JMML WITHOUT NOONAN (NON-NS)

	JMML-like Noonan	JMML non-NS
Incidence	~10%	$1.2/10^6$/year
Age at onset	<2 Months	Median age 1.8 years
Leukocytosis	++	++
Monocytosis	++	++
Hepatosplenomegaly	++	++
Myelopoiesis	Polyclonal	Clonal
Cytogenetics	Normal	Abnormal in 35%
PTPN11 mutation	90% (germline)	35% (somatic)
Most common substitution	T73I	E76K
Biological effect	Moderate GoF	Strong GoF
Outcome	Spontaneous regression	Fatal without transplantation

GoF, gain of function.

JMML, with the notable exception of those with monosomy 7 who almost all have normal HbF for age.[569] A macular-papular skin rash is seen in 35% of patients.[569] Diabetes insipidus has been reported as the presenting feature in a few cases with JMML and monosomy 7.[32]

Cytogenetics

Based on standard banding cytogenetics, 25–30% show monosomy 7 (mostly as the sole abnormality), 10% other aberrations (almost half of them with 7q-) and 60% a normal karyotype.[569,589] Data from the EWOG-MDS did not show any major clinical differences between JMML in patients with and without −7[569] and monosomy 7 syndrome is no longer considered a diagnostic entity.[32] However, patients with monosomy 7 tend to have some characteristic hematologic variations. They present with a lower WBC, a higher percentage of monocytes in the blood, a decreased myeloid:erythroid ratio in the BM, a higher MCV, and normal or only moderately elevated HbF.[569]

Differential Diagnoses

JMML may mimic infections or immunodeficiency, delaying the diagnosis. On the other hand, infections, inborn errors of metabolism, and immunodeficiency may cause monocytosis and organomegaly and thus become diagnostic pitfalls. Several viral infections mimicking JMML have been reported, including Epstein-Barr virus,[590] cytomegalovirus,[591] herpes virus-6[592] and parvovirus[593,594] Immunodeficiencies like Wiskott-Aldrich syndrome[595] and leukocyte adhesion defect may mimic JMML as well.[596,597] Therefore, a diagnosis of JMML, especially in infants, should be made with caution.[596] A period of observation is recommended in cases without clear-cut features.

The international consensus on current diagnostic criteria of JMML includes molecular genetics (Table 20.17) as a mandatory part of the work-up as incorporated in the EWOG-MDS 2006 protocol (www.ewog-mds.org). Blood film appearance is characteristic (Fig. 20.13) and often more helpful diagnostically than BM morphology, where monocytosis tends to be more discrete.

Pathophysiology

JMML is a clonal disorder that arises from a pluripotent stem cell.[598–602] Recently, new insights into the understanding of its pathogenesis were gained and could provide prospects for innovative rational therapy approaches. It has been recognized for over 20 years that when JMML mononuclear cells from PB and BM are cultured in semisolid systems, they yield excessive numbers of monocyte-macrophage colonies even without the addition of exogenous growth factors.[603,604] This so-called spontaneous proliferation of JMML myeloid progenitors and GM-CSF hypersensitivity has become the hallmark of the disease and a diagnostic tool.[605] GM-CSF may be mandatory for survival of JMML cells. Diphtheria toxin fused to GM-CSF is toxic to JMML blasts,[606] and treatment with a GM-CSF analogue that acts as a receptor antagonist induced apoptosis.[607,608]

The clinical presentation of JMML has provided crucial clues to the molecular aberrancies underlying this rare disease.[555,609–611] The hypothesis that a specific defect in the GM-CSF signal transduction pathway plays a major role in the pathogenesis of JMML led to studies of the RAS signal trans-

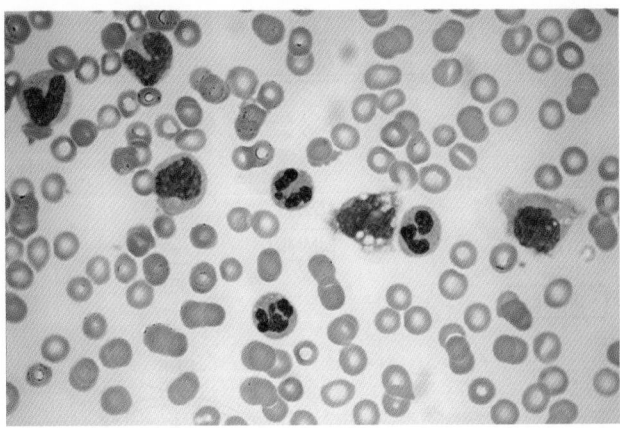

FIGURE 20.13 Juvenile myelomonocytic leukemia-peripheral blood (JMML PB) smear showing leukocytosis with dysplastic neutrophils and monocytes (courtesy of Marit Hellebostad, Oslo).

duction pathway downstream of the receptor (Fig. 20.14). Members of the RAS family of signaling proteins regulate cellular proliferation by cycling between an active guanosine triphosphate (GTP-)-bound state (RAS-GTP) and an inactive guanosine diphosphate (RAS-GDP)-bound state. RAS activation is a crucial component of the proliferative response to growth factors. RAS point mutations that cause high constitutive RAS-GTP levels are noted in up to 25% of JMML patients.[601,612,613]

Children with neurofibromatosis type 1 (NF1), have an increased risk of malignant myeloid disorders, especially

TABLE 20.17

DIAGNOSTIC GUIDELINES FOR JMML ADOPTED FROM THE EWOG-MDS 2006 PROTOCOL AT WWW.EWOG-MDS.ORG

I. Clinical and hematological features (all three features mandatory)
    Peripheral blood monocyte count > 1 × 109/L
    Blast percentage in PB and BM < 20%
    Splenomegaly

II. Oncogenetic studies (1 parameter sufficient)
    Somatic mutation in *PTPN11*[a] or *RAS*
    NF1 mutation or clinical diagnosis of NF1
    Monosomy 7

III. In the absence of one parameter listed under II, the following criteria have to be fulfilled:
    Absence of Philadelphia chromosome (*BCR/ABL* rearrangement) (mandatory)
    And at least two of the following criteria
    Spontaneous growth or GM-CSF hypersensitivity in colony assay
    Hemoglobin F increased for age
    Myeloid precursors on peripheral blood smear
    White blood cell count > 10 × 10⁹/L
    Clonal abnormality besides monosomy 7

[a]In cases with somatic *PTPN11* mutation a germline mutation has to be excluded (Noonan syndrome). JMML-like disorder seen in Noonan syndrome is considered separately.
PB, peripheral blood; BM, bone marrow; GM-CSF, granulocyte-macrophage colony stimulating factor.

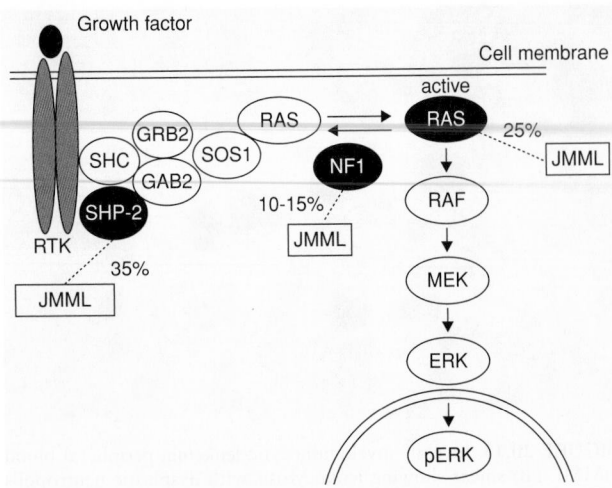

FIGURE 20.14 Simplified RAS signaling pathway. (Niemeyer CM, Kratz CP. Paediatric myelodysplastic syndromes and juvenile myelomonocytic leukaemia: molecular classification and treatment options. Br J Haematol 2008;140:610–624. Reprinted with permission.)

JMML.[570,614] About 15% of children with JMML carry the clinical diagnosis of NF1.[569] In addition, NF1 mutations have been detected in JMML patients in the absence of the clinical diagnosis of NF1,[615,616] suggesting that JMML may be the presenting feature of NF1. The NF1 gene functions as a tumor-suppressor gene, and loss of the normal NF1 allele was noted in leukemic cells of NF-1 patients.[615,617] As expected, leukemic cells showed an elevated percentage of RAS in the GTP-bound state.[618] NF1 and RAS mutations are mutually exclusive in JMML patients, indicating that one abnormality is sufficient to activate RAS.

The evidence that GM-CSF hypersensitivity in JMML is RAS mediated is provided by experiments with homozygous mice lacking the NF1 gene. Hematopoietic cells of these NF1$^{-/-}$ animals are hypersensitive to GM-CSF.[618,619] The NF1$^{-/-}$ progenitor cells showed a constitutive activation of the RAS-RAF-MAP kinase signaling pathway and hyperactivation of MAP kinase after growth factor stimulation.[620] By generating mice whose hematopoietic system was reconstituted with NF1$^{-/-}$ HSCs, it could be demonstrated that loss of the NF1 gene by itself is sufficient to produce myeloproliferation associated with JMML.[619]

Mutually exclusive abnormalities of the RAS signaling pathway are identified in 75% of JMML patients, with PTPN11 mutations in 35%, RAS gene mutations in 25%, and NF1 gene mutations in 15%. A recent study of CBL in a subset of 68 JMML patients without mutations in RAS or PTPN11 identified mutations in 40%, which corresponded to 10–15% of JMML patients overall; in that study no CBL mutations were found in the JMML samples with known mutations in RAS or PTPN11.[621] c-CBL is responsible for the intracellular transport and degradation of a large number of tyrosine kinases. The identification of homozygous CBL mutations in JMML suggests that CBL is a new tumor suppressor gene and indicates that CBL may have a role in deregulating the RAS pathway in JMML.

Natural Course and Prognostic Factors

JMML is often rapidly fatal if left untreated. Low platelet count, age above 2 years, high HbF, and high BM blast count at diagnosis are the main predictors of a short survival.[13,466,569]

Multivariate analysis demonstrates a low platelet count at presentation is the strongest factor predicting a poor survival. Non-transplanted children presenting with a platelet count < 33 × 109/L have an almost 100% mortality within the first year from diagnosis.[569,622] Blastic transformation is infrequent with JMML and most untreated patients die from organ failure due to infiltration of the leukemic cells.

Specific RAS mutations may be associated with spontaneously improving JMML[585,586]; conversely, a poor outcome has been noted in patients with PTPN11 mutations.[623] However, the prognostic value of genetic subtype is not yet established.

Treatment

Patients with Noonan syndrome and a JMML-like disease often regress spontaneously; only supportive care should be given to infants with the Noonan syndrome related myeloproliferative disorder.

Intensive chemotherapy is mostly unsuccessful in JMML because of an increased risk of treatment related death, a low rate of true remissions and long-term survival less than 10%.[525,569,622] Isoretinoin (13-cis retinoic acid) has an inhibitory effect on spontaneous growth *in vitro* and may induce remission in at least a portion of JMML patients.[624] Despite this preliminary success, it is clear that therapy with isoretinoin is not curative. The adjuvant value of retinoic acid is being tested both pre- and post-HSCT in the COG study AAML0122. A number of non-intensive therapies have been tried but with only anecdotal effect.[625,626] The evaluation of the efficacy of JMML therapy is hampered by the lack of uniform criteria for response, often divergent responses in hepatosplenomegaly, white cell, and platelet count, as well as the fact that about 20% of patients observed without therapy show response.[627] Purine analogs, etoposide, and cytarabine as single agents are associated with the best response rates for white cell count and spleen size.[627] For future evaluation of non-HSCT strategies in JMML, an international consensus on the definition of response criteria will be helpful.[611]

The central role of hyperactive RAS in the pathogenesis of JMML has formed the rationale for clinical trials of farnesyltransferase inhibitors, which inhibit the growth of JMML progenitors *in vitro*[628] and partially block GM-CSF induced MAP kinase activation in NF1$^{-/-}$ murine hematopoietic cells.[629] However, the same inhibitor had no effect on the myeloproliferative disorder in irradiated mice reconstituted with NF1$^{-/-}$ progenitor cells.[629] The efficacy and toxicity of the inhibitor tip: farnib (R115777) was tested in a phase II window study as part of COG study AAML0122 in newly diagnosed patients with JMML; in that study 58% showed complete or partial response.[630]

Reduction in methylation and clearance of the cytogenetically abnormal cells was reported in a patient with JMML and monosomy 7 on azacitidine therapy.[631] The potential for demethylating therapy in JMML is unknown.

Allogeneic HSCT is the only curative approach for JMML, resulting in OS in more than half the patients after both family and unrelated donor HSCT[632–635] or cord blood transplant.[636] Generally, HSCT shortly after diagnosis is advocated. Younger age at HSCT and male sex are predictors of improved survival.[634] TBI and cyclophosphamide has often been used as conditioning regimen[637]; however, radiation-induced late effects may be especially deleterious for this group of very young children. Therefore, avoiding TBI is particularly attractive in JMML. Several investigators have reported similar outcome for patients conditioned with TBI as those treated with non-TBI regimens[632,633] and in the retrospective analysis from the EWOG-MDS, busulfan-based myeloablative therapy offered a greater antileukemic efficacy than TBI.[634] The

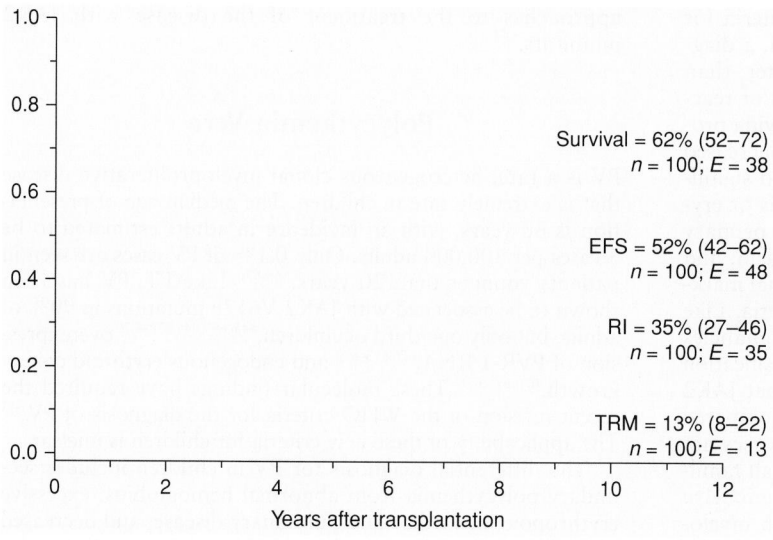

Survival = 62% (52–72)
n = 100; *E* = 38

EFS = 52% (42–62)
n = 100; *E* = 48

RI = 35% (27–46)
n = 100; *E* = 35

TRM = 13% (8–22)
n = 100; *E* = 13

FIGURE 20.15 Overall survival, event-free survival (EFS), relapse incidence (RI), and transplant-related mortality (TRM) of 100 children with juvenile myelomonocytic leukemia (JMML) transplanted after a conditioning regimen including busulfan, cyclophosphamide, and melphalan from a matched related (*n* = 48) or a matched unrelated (*n* = 52) donor. (Locatelli F, Nollke P, Zecca M, et al. Hematopoietic stem cell transplantation (HSCT) in children with juvenile myelomonocytic leukemia (JMML): results of the EWOG-MDS/EBMT trial. Blood 2005;105(1):410–419. Updated figure from Niemeyer CM, Kratz CP. Paediatric myelodysplastic syndromes and juvenile myelomonocytic leukaemia: molecular classification and treatment options. Br J Haematol 2008;140(6):610–624, reproduced with permission).

current EWOG-MDS study uses a preparative regimen with busulfan, cyclophosphamide, and melphalan and has shown EFS around 50%, with no difference between related and unrelated donors.[634]

Disease recurrence remains the major cause of treatment failure (Fig. 20.15). Reduced intensity and duration of GvHD prophylaxis may significantly contribute to successful leukemia control[634] and both acute and chronic GvHD is associated with a lower risk of relapse.[632–634] Older age, female sex, increased percentage of HbF, and blast percentage in the BM above 20% increased the risk of relapse in a univariate analysis. Age above 4 years remained significant in multivariate analysis (Fig. 20.16).[634] Splenectomy before HSCT, as well as spleen

size at time of the allograft, did not appear to have an impact on posttransplantation outcome.[634] Monosomy 7 is associated with an outcome comparable to or even better than that of patients with normal karyotype.[12,634]

Relapse occurs early at a median of 2 to 4 months from transplantation[633,634] and generally within the first year. Early detection of donor cells by increasing mixed chimerism may allow prevention of impending relapse by reducing ongoing immunosuppressive therapy.[638] Donor lymphocyte infusion in JMML relapse is largely unsuccessful.[639] A second or even a third transplantation gives a relatively high chance of survival.[640,641]

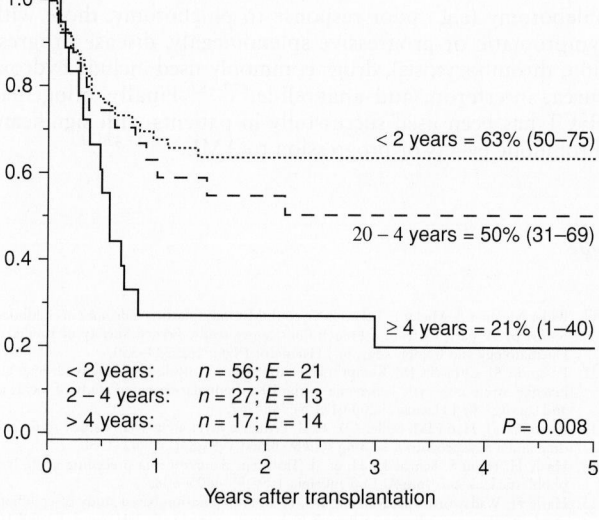

< 2 years = 63% (50–75)

20 – 4 years = 50% (31–69)

≥ 4 years = 21% (1–40)

< 2 years: *n* = 56; *E* = 21
2 – 4 years: *n* = 27; *E* = 13
> 4 years: *n* = 17; *E* = 14   *P* = 0.008

Years after transplantation

FIGURE 20.16 Kaplan-Meier estimate of event-free survival (EFS) in juvenile myelomonocytic leukemia (JMML) after hematopoietic stem cell transplantation (HCST) according to age at diagnosis. (Original figure from Locatelli F, Nollke P, Zecca M, et al. Hematopoietic stem cell transplantation (HSCT) in children with juvenile myelomonocytic leukemia (JMML): results of the EWOG-MDS/EBMT trial. Blood 2005;105(1):410–419. Updated figure from Niemeyer CM, Kratz CP. Paediatric myelodysplastic syndromes and juvenile myelomonocytic leukaemia: molecular classification and treatment options. Br J Haematol 2008;140(6):610–624, reproduced with permission).

OTHER MYELOPROLIFERATIVE DISEASES

Essential Thrombocytopenia

Essential thrombocythemia (ET) is a rare and heterogeneous myeloproliferative disorder characterized by an elevated platelet count and, like other myeloproliferative disorders, also involves changes in other cell lineages. ET is rarely seen in children, with an estimated incidence of 0.09 cases per million for children younger than 14 years,[642] as compared to an incidence of 1 to 1.25 cases per million for adults.[642–644]

Recently, varying percentages of adults and children with ET have been noted to have clonal mutations in V617F in the pseudo-kinase (JH2)-domain of the *JAK2* gene.[645–648] A JAK2 V617F mutation is found in more than 90% of adult patients with polycythemia vera (PV) and in nearly one-half of those with ET, but much less often in children.[649,650] Approximately 1% of adult patients with ET have also been reported to have *MPL515* mutations.[651] In addition, the *PRV-1* gene, a member of the urokinase type plasminogen activator receptor family, has been shown to be overexpressed in patients with ET, but not in patients with other reactive or secondary causes of thrombocytosis.[652] These molecular findings have led to the suggestion that children with sporadic ET be classified into three subgroups: *PRV-1* overexpressed and V617F-positive ET; *PRV-1* overexpressed and V617F-negative ET; and *PRV-1* normal and V617F-negative ET.[648] The clinical implications of these subgroups are currently unclear.

Recently, the WHO proposed new diagnostic criteria for ET and PV.[653] According to the new WHO proposal, a diagnosis of ET includes: a platelet count of greater than 450,000/μL in the absence of other potential causes of reactive or secondary thrombocytosis; BM specimen showing proliferation mainly of the megakaryocytic lineage with increased numbers of enlarged, mature megakaryocytes and no significant increase or left-shift of neutrophil granulopoiesis or erythropoiesis; not meeting WHO criteria for PV, primary myelofibrosis, CML, MDS, or other myeloid neoplasm; and demonstration of JAK2 V617F mutation or other clonal markers. A diagnosis of ET requires meeting all four criteria. Like many classification systems for hematopoietic malignancies designed for adults, the utility of the new WHO classification of ET for children is not clear. For example, given that JAK2 V617F mutations occur less commonly in children compared with adults, a significant proportion of childhood cases are misdiagnosed using the WHO criteria. Furthermore, all familial ETs, including patients with the hereditary *MPL Ser505Asn* activation mutation, are erroneously diagnosed with myeloproliferative disorders, again suggesting that childhood MPDs require specific diagnostic criteria.[654]

The differential diagnosis for sporadic ET includes reactive and secondary forms of thrombocytosis, other myeloproliferative diseases, and familial ET, which is characterized by the dominant-positive activating mutation in c-mpl.

Clinically, ET is characterized by thrombocytosis, hemorrhage, and thrombosis. In adults, severe complications may occur, including cerebral ischemia, deep vein thrombosis, and peripheral vascular ischemia. Evidence suggests that adult patients with JAK2 V617F mutations are at increased risk of thrombosis, and patients who are homozygous for JAK2 V617F are at increased risk of recurrent thrombosis.[655] Median survival in adults is more than 10 years.[656,657] Progression to AML has been reported, usually in ET patients with prior exposure to chemotherapy agents. In contrast to adults, the clinical course in children is typically uncomplicated, with few thrombotic events.[649,658]

Asymptomatic children do not require therapy. Children and adults with thrombosis and hemorrhage have been treated with a variety of agents including hydroxyurea, interferon alpha, and anagrelide.[659-665] HSCT has been used successfully in a very small number of adult patients.[666,667] Finally, a better understanding of the biology of sporadic ET with associated mutations in *JAK2* presents an opportunity for novel approaches to the treatment of the disease with JAK2 inhibitors.[668]

Polycythemia Vera

PV is a rare, heterogeneous clonal myeloproliferative disease that is extremely rare in children. The median age of presentation is 60 years, with an incidence in adults estimated to be 3 cases per 100,000 adults. Only 0.1% of PV cases are seen in patients younger than 20 years.[669,670] Like ET, PV has been shown to be associated with JAK2 V617F mutations in 90% of adults, but only one-third of children,[645-647,649,670-672] overexpression of PVR-1 RNA,[670,673-674] and endogenous erythroid colony growth.[670,675,676] These molecular findings have required the recent revision of the WHO criteria for the diagnosis of PV.[653] The applicability of these new criteria for children is unclear.

The differential diagnosis for PV in children includes secondary polycythemia from abnormal hemoglobins, excessive erythropoietin, cardiac and pulmonary disease, and decreased plasma volume. Also to be considered is familial polycythemia, which is characterized by a specific mutation in the thrombopoietin (*TPO*) gene or Chuvash polycythemia due to a *VHL* gene mutation.

Children with PV have a clinical presentation consistent with an increased red cell mass, with signs and symptoms including headache, dizziness, fatigue, pruritus, night sweats, and a "ruddy" complexion. Hepatosplenomegaly may be present. Although adults can have thrombotic complications from the increased blood viscosity, thrombotic events in children are less common.[649,670]

A number of agents have been used to treat PV in adults; seven randomized clinical trials have tested various drugs.[677] Despite these trials, there remains a lack of clarity around the best approach to the treatment of these patients, especially those who are young. This necessitated the recent development of consensus treatment guidelines.[678] Phlebotomy is generally recommended as the initial intervention for young patients. For patients who require treatment with more than phlebotomy (e.g., poor response to phlebotomy, those with symptomatic or progressive splenomegaly, disease progression, thrombocytosis), drugs commonly used include hydroxyurea, interferon, and anagrelide.[679-682] Finally, allogeneic HSCT has been used successfully in patients with significant thrombotic events or progression to AML.[666,667,670,683]

References

1. Dash A, Gilliland DG. Molecular genetics of acute myeloid leukaemia. Best Pract Res Clin Haematol 2001;14(1):49–64.
2. Kelly LM, Gilliland DG. Genetics of myeloid leukemias. Annu Rev Genomics Hum Genet 2002;3:179–198.
3. Tefferi A, Thibodeau SN, Solberg LA Jr. Clonal studies in the myelodysplastic syndrome using X-linked restriction fragment length polymorphisms. Blood 1990;75(9):1770–1773.
4. Busque L, Gilliland DG. X-inactivation analysis in the 1990s: promise and potential problems. Leukemia 1998;12(2):128–135.
5. Kardos G, Baumann I, Passmore SJ, et al. Refractory anemia in childhood: a retrospective analysis of 67 patients with particular reference to monosomy 7. Blood 2003; 102(6):1997–2003.
6. Gilliland DG. Molecular genetics of human leukemia. Leukemia 1998;12(Suppl 1):S7–S12.
7. Higuchi M, O'Brien D, Kumaravelu P, et al. Expression of a conditional AML1-ETO oncogene bypasses embryonic lethality and establishes a murine model of human t(8;21) acute myeloid leukemia. Cancer Cell 2002;1(1):63–74.
8. Pabst T, Eyholzer M, Haefliger S, et al. Somatic CEBPA mutations are a frequent second event in families with germline CEBPA mutations and familial acute myeloid leukemia. J Clin Oncol 2008;26(31):5088–5093.
9. Shinawi M, Erez A, Shardy DL, et al. Syndromic thrombocytopenia and predisposition to acute myelogenous leukemia caused by constitutional microdeletions on chromosome 21q. Blood 2008;112(4):1042–1047.
10. Sasaki H, Manabe A, Kojima S, et al. Myelodysplastic syndrome in childhood: a retrospective study of 189 patients in Japan. Leukemia 2001;15(11):1713–1720.
11. Bader-Meunier B, Mielot F, Tchernia G, et al. Myelodysplastic syndromes in childhood: report of 49 patients from a French multicentre study. French Society of Paediatric Haematology and Immunology. Br J Haematol 1996;92(2):344–350.
12. Passmore SJ, Chessells JM, Kempski H, et al. Paediatric myelodysplastic syndromes and juvenile myelomonocytic leukaemia in the UK: a population-based study of incidence and survival. Br J Haematol 2003;121(5):758–767.
13. Passmore SJ, Hann IM, Stiller CA, et al. Pediatric myelodysplasia: a study of 68 children and a new prognostic scoring system. Blood 1995;85(7):1742–1750.
14. Hasle H, Heim S, Schroeder H, et al. Transient pancytopenia preceding acute lymphoblastic leukemia (pre-ALL). Leukemia 1995;9(4):605–608.
15. Hasle H, Wadsworth LD, Massing BG, et al. A population-based study of childhood myelodysplastic syndrome in British Columbia, Canada. Br J Haematol 1999;106(4):1027–1032.
16. Luna-Fineman S, Shannon KM, Atwater SK, et al. Myelodysplastic and myeloproliferative disorders of childhood: a study of 167 patients. Blood 1999;93(2):459–466.
17. Stary J, Baumann I, Creutzig U, et al. Getting the numbers straight in pediatric MDS: distribution of subtypes after exclusion of Down syndrome. Pediatr Blood Cancer 2008;50(2):435–436.
18. Hasle H, Clausen N, Pedersen B, et al. Myelodysplastic syndrome in a child with constitutional trisomy 8 mosaicism and normal phenotype. Cancer Genet Cytogenet 1995;79(1):79–81.
19. Maserati E, Aprili F, Vinante F, et al. Trisomy 8 in myelodysplasia and acute leukemia is constitutional in 15–20% of cases. Genes Chromosomes Cancer 2002;33(1):93–97.
20. Hasle H, Olsen JH. Cancer in relatives of children with myelodysplastic syndrome, acute and chronic myeloid leukaemia. Br J Haematol 1997;97(1):127–131.

21. Rosenberg PS, Huang Y, Alter BP. Individualized risks of first adverse events in patients with Fanconi anemia. Blood 2004;104(2):350–355.
22. Alter BP, Caruso JP, Drachtman RA, et al. Fanconi anemia: myelodysplasia as a predictor of outcome. Cancer Genet Cytogenet 2000;117(2):125–131.
23. Tonnies H, Huber S, Kuhl JS, et al. Clonal chromosomal aberrations in bone marrow cells of Fanconi anemia patients: gains of the chromosomal segment 3q26q29 as an adverse risk factor. Blood 2003;101(10):3872–3874.
24. Donadieu J, Leblanc T, Bader Meunier B, et al. Analysis of risk factors for myelodysplasias, leukemias and death from infection among patients with congenital neutropenia. Experience of the French Severe Chronic Neutropenia Study Group. Haematologica 2005;90(1):45–53.
25. Rosenberg PS, Alter BP, Bolyard AA, et al. The incidence of leukemia and mortality from sepsis in patients with severe congenital neutropenia receiving long-term G-CSF therapy. Blood 2006;107(12):4628–4635.
26. Germeshausen M, Ballmaier M, Welte K. Incidence of CSF3R mutations in severe congenital neutropenia and relevance for leukemogenesis: Results of a long-term survey. Blood 2007;109(1):93–99.
27. Zeidler C, Welte K, Barak Y, et al. Stem cell transplantation in patients with severe congenital neutropenia without evidence of leukemic transformation. Blood 2000;95(4):1195–1198.
28. Choi SW, Boxer LA, Pulsipher MA, et al. Stem cell transplantation in patients with severe congenital neutropenia with evidence of leukemic transformation. Bone Marrow Transplant 2005;35(5):473–477.
29. Smith OP. Shwachman-Diamond syndrome. Semin Hematol 2002;39(2):95–102.
30. Maserati E, Pressato B, Valli R, et al. The route to development of myelodysplastic syndrome/acute myeloid leukaemia in Shwachman-Diamond syndrome: the role of ageing, karyotype instability, and acquired chromosome anomalies. Br J Haematol 2009;145(2):190–197.
31. Rujkijyanont P, Beyene J, Wei K, et al. Leukaemia-related gene expression in bone marrow cells from patients with the preleukaemic disorder Shwachman-Diamond syndrome. Br J Haematol 2007;137(6):537–544.
32. Hasle H, Arico M, Basso G, et al. Myelodysplastic syndrome, juvenile myelomonocytic leukemia, and acute myeloid leukemia associated with complete or partial monosomy 7. European Working Group on MDS in Childhood (EWOG-MDS). Leukemia 1999; 13(3):376–385.
33. Vlachos A, Ball S, Dahl N, et al. Diagnosing and treating Diamond Blackfan anaemia: results of an international clinical consensus conference. Br J Haematol 2008;142 (6):859–876.
34. Dokal I. Dyskeratosis congenita in all its forms. Br J Haematol 2000;110(4):768–779.
35. Maserati E, Panarello C, Morerio C, et al. Clonal chromosome anomalies and propensity to myeloid malignancies in congenital amegakaryocytic thrombocytopenia (OMIM 604498). Haematologica 2008;93(8):1271–1273.
36. Ganly P, Walker LC, Morris CM. Familial mutations of the transcription factor RUNX1 (AML1, CBFA2) predispose to acute myeloid leukemia. Leuk Lymphoma 2004;45(1):1–10.
37. Rheingold S. Acute myeloid leukemia in a child with hereditary thrombocytopenia. Pediatr Blood Cancer 2007;48(1):105–107.
38. Gohring G, Karow A, Steinemann D, et al. Chromosomal aberrations in congenital bone marrow failure disorders–an early indicator for leukemogenesis? Ann Hematol 2007;86(10):733–739.
39. Ohara A, Kojima S, Hamajima N, et al. Myelodysplastic syndrome and acute myelogenous leukemia as a late clonal complication in children with acquired aplastic anemia. Blood 1997;90(3):1009–1013.
40. Fuhrer M, Burdach S, Ebell W, et al. Relapse and clonal disease in children with aplastic anemia (AA) after immunosuppressive therapy (IST): the SAA 94 experience. German/Austrian Pediatric Aplastic Anemia Working Group. Klin Padiatr 1998; 210(4):173–179.
41. Fuhrer M, Rampf U, Baumann I, et al. Immunosuppressive therapy for aplastic anemia in children: a more severe disease predicts better survival. Blood 2005;106(6): 2102–2104.
42. Ohara A, Kojima S, Okamura J, et al. Evolution of myelodysplastic syndrome and acute myelogenous leukaemia in children with hepatitis-associated aplastic anaemia. Br J Haematol 2002;116(1):151–154.
43. Locasciulli A, Arcese W, Locatelli F, et al. Treatment of aplastic anaemia with granulocyte-colony stimulating factor and risk of malignancy. Italian Aplastic Anaemia Study Group. Lancet 2001;357(9249):43–44.
44. Kojima S, Hibi S, Kosaka Y, et al. Immunosuppressive therapy using antithymocyte globulin, cyclosporine, and danazol with or without human granulocyte colony-stimulating factor in children with acquired aplastic anemia. Blood 2000;96(6):2049–2054.
45. Kojima S, Ohara A, Tsuchida M, et al. Risk factors for evolution of acquired aplastic anemia into myelodysplastic syndrome and acute myeloid leukemia after immunosuppressive therapy in children. Blood 2002;100(3):786–790.
46. Mahmoud HH, Ridge SA, Behm FG, et al. Intrauterine monoclonal origin of neonatal concordant acute lymphoblastic leukemia in monozygotic twins. Med Pediatr Oncol 1995;24(2):77–81.
47. Greaves MF, Maia AT, Wiemels JL, et al. Leukemia in twins: lessons in natural history. Blood 2003;102(7):2321–2333.
48. Kadan-Lottick NS, Kawashima T, Tomlinson G, et al. The risk of cancer in twins: a report from the childhood cancer survivor study. Pediatr Blood Cancer 2006;46(4): 476–481.
49. Greaves M. Pre-natal origins of childhood leukemia. Rev Clin Exp Hematol 2003;7(3):233–245.
50. Greaves MF, Wiemels J. Origins of chromosome translocations in childhood leukaemia. Nat Rev Cancer 2003;3(9):639–649.
51. Maia AT, Ford AM, Jalali GR, et al. Molecular tracking of leukemogenesis in a triplet pregnancy. Blood 2001;98(2):478–482.
52. Brandwein JM, Horsman DE, Eaves AC, et al. Childhood myelodysplasia: suggested classification as myelodysplastic syndromes based on laboratory and clinical findings. Am J Pediatr Hematol Oncol 1990;12(1):63–70.
53. Gilchrist DM, Friedman JM, Rogers PC, et al. Myelodysplasia and leukemia syndrome with monosomy 7: a genetic perspective. Am J Med Genet 1990;35(3):437–441.
54. Luna-Fineman S, Shannon KM, Lange BJ. Childhood monosomy 7: epidemiology, biology, and mechanistic implications. Blood 1995;85(8):1985–1999.
55. Olopade OI, Roulston D, Baker T, et al. Familial myeloid leukemia associated with loss of the long arm of chromosome 5. Leukemia 1996;10(4):669–674.
56. Mijovic A, Antunovic P, Pagliuca A, et al. Familial myelodysplastic syndromes: a key to understanding leukaemogenesis? Leuk Res 1997;21(Suppl):S6.
57. Shannon KM, Turhan AG, Chang SS, et al. Familial bone marrow monosomy 7. Evidence that the predisposing locus is not on the long arm of chromosome 7. J Clin Invest 1989;84(3):984–989.
58. Hasle H, Olsen JH, Hansen J, et al. Occurrence of cancer in a cohort of 183 persons with constitutional chromosome 7 abnormalities. Cancer Genet Cytogenet 1998; 105(1):39–42.
59. Minelli A, Maserati E, Giudici G, et al. Familial partial monosomy 7 and myelodysplasia: different parental origin of the monosomy 7 suggests action of a mutator gene. Cancer Genet Cytogenet 2001;124(2):147–151.
60. Owen C, Barnett M, Fitzgibbon J. Familial myelodysplasia and acute myeloid leukaemia—a review. Br J Haematol 2008;140(2):123–132.
61. Vardiman JW, Thiele J, Arber DA, et al. The 2008 revision of the WHO classification of myeloid neoplasms and acute leukemia: rationale and important changes. Blood 2009;114:937–951.
62. Smith SM, Le Beau MM, Huo D, et al. Clinical-cytogenetic associations in 306 patients with therapy-related myelodysplasia and myeloid leukemia: the University of Chicago series. Blood 2003;102(1):43–52.
63. Singh ZN, Huo D, Anastasi J, et al. Therapy-related myelodysplastic syndrome: morphologic subclassification may not be clinically relevant. Am J Clin Pathol 2007;127(2): 197–205.
64. Pui CH, Ribeiro RC, Hancock ML, et al. Acute myeloid leukemia in children treated with epipodophyllotoxins for acute lymphoblastic leukemia. N Engl J Med 1991;325 (24):1682–1687.
65. Hawkins MM, Wilson LM, Stovall MA, et al. Epipodophyllotoxins, alkylating agents, and radiation and risk of secondary leukaemia after childhood cancer. BMJ 1992;304(6832):951–958.
66. Ross JA, Potter JD, Reaman GH, et al. Maternal exposure to potential inhibitors of DNA topoisomerase II and infant leukemia (United States): a report from the Children's Cancer Group. Cancer Causes Control 1996;7(6):581–590.
67. Mauritzson N, Albin M, Rylander L, et al. Pooled analysis of clinical and cytogenetic features in treatment-related and de novo adult acute myeloid leukemia and myelodysplastic syndromes based on a consecutive series of 761 patients analyzed 1976–1993 and on 5098 unselected cases reported in the literature 1974–2001. Leukemia 2002; 16(12):2366–2378.
68. Schmiegelow K, Al-Modhwahi I, Andersen MK, et al. Methotrexate/6-mercaptopurine maintenance therapy influences the risk of a second malignant neoplasm after childhood acute lymphoblastic leukemia: results from the NOPHO ALL-92 study. Blood 2009;113(24):6077–6084.
69. Schoch C, Schnittger S, Klaus M, et al. AML with 11q23/MLL abnormalities as defined by the WHO classification: incidence, partner chromosomes, FAB subtype, age distribution, and prognostic impact in an unselected series of 1897 cytogenetically analyzed AML cases. Blood 2003;102(7):2395–2402.
70. Barnard DR, Lange B, Alonzo TA, et al. Acute myeloid leukemia and myelodysplastic syndrome in children treated for cancer: comparison with primary presentation. Blood 2002;100(2):427–434.
71. Pegram LD, Megonigal MD, Lange BJ, et al. t(3;11) translocation in treatment-related acute myeloid leukemia fuses MLL with the GMPS (GUANOSINE 5' MONOPHOSPHATE SYNTHETASE) gene. Blood 2000;96(13):4360–4362.
72. Megonigal MD, Cheung NK, Rappaport EF, et al. Detection of leukemia-associated MLL-GAS7 translocation early during chemotherapy with DNA topoisomerase II inhibitors. Proc Natl Acad Sci U S A 2000;97(6):2814–2819.
73. Bloomfield CD, Archer KJ, Mrozek K, et al. 11q23 balanced chromosome aberrations in treatment-related myelodysplastic syndromes and acute leukemia: report from an international workshop. Genes Chromosomes Cancer 2002;33(4):362–378.
74. Andersen MK, Larson RA, Mauritzson N, et al. Balanced chromosome abnormalities inv(16) and t(15;17) in therapy-related myelodysplastic syndromes and acute leukemia: report from an international workshop. Genes Chromosomes Cancer 2002;33(4): 395–400.
75. Slovak ML, Bedell V, Popplewell L, et al. 21q22 balanced chromosome aberrations in therapy-related hematopoietic disorders: report from an international workshop. Genes Chromosomes Cancer 2002;33(4):379–394.
76. Seedhouse C, Russell N. Advances in the understanding of susceptibility to treatment-related acute myeloid leukaemia. Br J Haematol 2007;137(6):513–529.
77. Alexander FE, Patheal SL, Biondi A, et al. Transplacental chemical exposure and risk of infant leukemia with MLL gene fusion. Cancer Res 2001;61(6):2542–2546.
78. Brondum J, Shu XO, Steinbuch M, et al. Parental cigarette smoking and the risk of acute leukemia in children. Cancer 1999;85(6):1380–1388.
79. Flodin U, Fredriksson M, Persson B, et al. Background radiation, electrical work, and some other exposures associated with acute myeloid leukemia in a case-referent study. Arch Environ Health 1986;41(2):77–84.
80. Severson RK, Buckley JD, Woods WG, et al. Cigarette smoking and alcohol consumption by parents of children with acute myeloid leukemia: an analysis within morphological subgroups–a report from the Childrens Cancer Group. Cancer Epidemiol Biomarkers Prev 1993;2(5):433–439.
81. Shu XO, Ross JA, Pendergrass TW, et al. Parental alcohol consumption, cigarette smoking, and risk of infant leukemia: a Childrens Cancer Group study. J Natl Cancer Inst 1996;88(1):24–31.
82. Shu XO, Reaman GH, Lampkin B, et al. Association of paternal diagnostic X-ray exposure with risk of infant leukemia. Investigators of the Childrens Cancer Group. Cancer Epidemiol Biomarkers Prev 1994;3(8):645–653.
83. Linet MS, Hatch EE, Kleinerman RA, et al. Residential exposure to magnetic fields and acute lymphoblastic leukemia in children. N Engl J Med 1997;337(1):1–7.
84. Mizoue T, Onoe Y, Moritake H, et al. Residential proximity to high-voltage power lines and risk of childhood hematological malignancies. J Epidemiol 2004;14(4): 118–123.
85. Ross JA. Dietary flavonoids and the MLL gene: a pathway to infant leukemia? Proc Natl Acad Sci U S A 2000;97(9):4411–4413.
86. Spector LG, Xie Y, Robison LL, et al. Maternal diet and infant leukemia: the DNA topoisomerase II inhibitor hypothesis: a report from the children's oncology group. Cancer Epidemiol Biomarkers Prev 2005;14(3):651–655.
87. McBride ML. Childhood cancer and environmental contaminants. Can J Public Health 1998;89(Suppl 1):S53–S62, S58–S68.
88. Mills PK, Zahm SH. Organophosphate pesticide residues in urine of farmworkers and their children in Fresno County, California. Am J Ind Med 2001;40(5):571–577.
89. Linet MS, Ries LA, Smith MA, et al. Cancer surveillance series: recent trends in childhood cancer incidence and mortality in the United States. J Natl Cancer Inst 1999; 91(12):1051–1058.

90. Clavel J, Goubin A, Auclerc MF, et al. Incidence of childhood leukaemia and non-Hodgkin's lymphoma in France: National Registry of Childhood Leukaemia and Lymphoma, 1990–1999. Eur J Cancer Prev 2004;13(2):97–103.

91. Hjalgrim LL, Rostgaard K, Schmiegelow K, et al. Age- and sex-specific incidence of childhood leukemia by immunophenotype in the Nordic countries. J Natl Cancer Inst 2003;95(20):1539–1544.

92. Xie Y, Davies SM, Xiang Y, et al. Trends in leukemia incidence and survival in the United States (1973–1998). Cancer 2003;97(9):2229–2235.

93. Weir HK, Thun MJ, Hankey BF, et al. Annual report to the nation on the status of cancer, 1975–2000, featuring the uses of surveillance data for cancer prevention and control. J Natl Cancer Inst 2003;95(17):1276–1299.

94. Parkin DM, Stiller CA, Draper GJ, et al. The international incidence of childhood cancer. Int J Cancer 1988;42(4):511–520.

95. Sandler DP, Ross JA. Epidemiology of acute leukemia in children and adults. Semin Oncol 1997;24(1):3–16.

96. McKinney PA, Feltbower RG, Parslow RC, et al. Patterns of childhood cancer by ethnic group in Bradford, UK 1974–1997. Eur J Cancer 2003;39(1):92–97.

97. Douer D, Preston-Martin S, Chang E, et al. High frequency of acute promyelocytic leukemia among Latinos with acute myeloid leukemia. Blood 1996;87(1):308–313.

98. Zimmerman LE, Font RL. Ophthalmologic manifestations of granulocytic sarcoma (myeloid sarcoma or chloroma). The third Pan American Association of Ophthalmology and American Journal of Ophthalmology Lecture. Am J Ophthalmol 1975;80(6):975–990.

99. Cavdar AO, Babacan E, Gozdasoglu S, et al. High risk subgroup of acute myelomonocytic leukemia (AMML) with orbito-ocular granulocytic sarcoma (OOGS) in Turkish children. Retrospective analysis of clinical, hematological, ultrastructural and therapeutical findings of thirty-three OOGS. Acta Haematol 1989;81(2):80–85.

100. Marcucci G, Mrozek K, Bloomfield CD. Molecular heterogeneity and prognostic biomarkers in adults with acute myeloid leukemia and normal cytogenetics. Curr Opin Hematol 2005;12(1):68–75.

101. Gilliland DG, Tallman MS. Focus on acute leukemias. Cancer Cell 2002;1(5):417–420.

102. Bonnet D, Dick JE. Human acute myeloid leukemia is organized as a hierarchy that originates from a primitive hematopoietic cell. Nat Med 1997;3(7):730–737.

103. Lowenberg B, Downing JR, Burnett A. Acute myeloid leukemia. N Engl J Med 1999;341(14):1051–1062.

104. Mrozek K, Marcucci G, Paschka P, et al. Clinical relevance of mutations and gene-expression changes in adult acute myeloid leukemia with normal cytogenetics: are we ready for a prognostically prioritized molecular classification? Blood 2007;109(2):431–448.

105. Paschka P, Marcucci G, Ruppert AS, et al. Adverse prognostic significance of KIT mutations in adult acute myeloid leukemia with inv(16) and t(8;21): a Cancer and Leukemia Group B Study. J Clin Oncol 2006;24(24):3904–3911.

106. Falini B, Mecucci C, Tiacci E, et al. Cytoplasmic nucleophosmin in acute myelogenous leukemia with a normal karyotype. N Engl J Med 2005;352(3):254–266.

107. Schlenk RF, Dohner K, Krauter J, et al. Mutations and treatment outcome in cytogenetically normal acute myeloid leukemia. N Engl J Med 2008;358(18):1909–1918.

108. Sohal J, Phan VT, Chan PV, et al. A model of APL with FLT3 mutation is responsive to retinoic acid and a receptor tyrosine kinase inhibitor, SU11657. Blood 2003;101(8):3188–3197.

109. Goemans BF, Zwaan CM, Miller M, et al. Mutations in KIT and RAS are frequent events in pediatric core-binding factor acute myeloid leukemia. Leukemia 2005;19(9):1536–1542.

110. Lapidot T, Sirard C, Vormoor J, et al. A cell initiating human acute myeloid leukaemia after transplantation into SCID mice. Nature 1994;367(6464):645–648.

111. Majeti R, Becker MW, Tian Q, et al. Dysregulated gene expression networks in human acute myelogenous leukemia stem cells. Proc Natl Acad Sci U S A 2009;106(9):3396–3401.

112. Guzman ML, Jordan CT. Considerations for targeting malignant stem cells in leukemia. Cancer Control 2004;11(2):97–104.

113. Hope KJ, Jin L, Dick JE. Acute myeloid leukemia originates from a hierarchy of leukemic stem cell classes that differ in self-renewal capacity. Nat Immunol 2004;5(7):738–743.

114. Guan Y, Gerhard B, Hogge DE. Detection, isolation, and stimulation of quiescent primitive leukemic progenitor cells from patients with acute myeloid leukemia (AML). Blood 2003;101(8):3142–3149.

115. Warner JK, Wang JC, Hope KJ, et al. Concepts of human leukemic development. Oncogene 2004;23(43):7164–7177.

116. Pollard JA, Alonzo TA, Gerbing RB, et al. FLT3 internal tandem duplication in CD34+/CD33− precursors predicts poor outcome in acute myeloid leukemia. Blood 2006;108(8):2764–2769.

117. Bennett JM, Catovsky D, Daniel MT, et al. Proposals for the classification of the acute leukaemias. French-American-British (FAB) co-operative group. Br J Haematol 1976;33(4):451–458.

118. Bennett JM, Catovsky D, Daniel MT, et al. Proposed revised criteria for the classification of acute myeloid leukemia. A report of the French-American-British Cooperative Group. Ann Intern Med 1985;103(4):620–625.

119. Vardiman JW, Harris NL, Brunning RD. The World Health Organization (WHO) classification of the myeloid neoplasms. Blood 2002;100(7):2292–2302.

120. Hasle H, Niemeyer CM, Chessells JM, et al. A pediatric approach to the WHO classification of myelodysplastic and myeloproliferative diseases. Leukemia 2003;17(2):277–282.

121. Jaffe ES, Stein H, Vardiman JW, eds. Tumors of haematopoietic and lymphoid tissues (World Health Organization classification of tumours). Lyon: IARC, 2001.

122. Launder TM, Bray RA, Stempora L, et al. Lymphoid-associated antigen expression by acute myeloid leukemia. Am J Clin Pathol 1996;106(2):185–191.

123. Sievers EL, Lange BJ, Alonzo TA, et al. Immunophenotypic evidence of leukemia after induction therapy predicts relapse: results from a prospective Children's Cancer Group study of 252 patients with acute myeloid leukemia. Blood 2003;101(9):3398–3406.

124. Creutzig U, Harbott J, Sperling C, et al. Clinical significance of surface antigen expression in children with acute myeloid leukemia: results of study AML-BFM-87. Blood 1995;86(8):3097–3108.

125. Baumann I, Nenninger R, Harms H, et al. Image analysis detects lineage-specific morphologic markers in leukemic blast cells. Am J Clin Pathol 1996;105(1):23–30.

126. Harada N, Okamura S, Kubota A, et al. Analysis of acute myeloid leukemia cells by flow cytometry, introducing a new light-scattering classification. J Cancer Res Clin Oncol 1994;120(9):553–557.

127. Langebrake C, Brinkmann I, Teigler-Schlegel A, et al. Immunophenotypic differences between diagnosis and relapse in childhood AML: implications for MRD monitoring. Cytometry B Clin Cytom 2005;63(1):1–9.

128. Kern W, Haferlach T, Schoch C, et al. Early blast clearance by remission induction therapy is a major independent prognostic factor for both achievement of complete remission and long-term outcome in acute myeloid leukemia: data from the German AML Cooperative Group (AMLCG) 1992 Trial. Blood 2003;101(1):64–70.

129. Marcucci G, Mrozek K, Ruppert AS, et al. Abnormal cytogenetics at date of morphologic complete remission predicts short overall and disease-free survival, and higher relapse rate in adult acute myeloid leukemia: results from cancer and leukemia group B study 8461. J Clin Oncol 2004;22(12):2410–2418.

130. Cascavilla N, Musto P, D'Arena G, et al. CD117 (c-kit) is a restricted antigen of acute myeloid leukemia and characterizes early differentiative levels of M5 FAB subtype. Haematologica 1998;83(5):392–397.

131. Xu Y, McKenna RW, Wilson KS, et al. Immunophenotypic identification of acute myeloid leukemia with monocytic differentiation. Leukemia 2006;20(7):1321–1324.

132. Betz SA, Foucar K, Head DR, et al. False-positive flow cytometric platelet glycoprotein IIb/IIIa expression in myeloid leukemias secondary to platelet adherence to blasts. Blood 1992;79(9):2399–2403.

133. Smith FO, Lampkin BC, Versteeg C, et al. Expression of lymphoid-associated cell surface antigens by childhood acute myeloid leukemia cells lacks prognostic significance. Blood 1992;79(9):2415–2422.

134. Cheson BD, Cassileth PA, Head DR, et al. Report of the National Cancer Institute-sponsored workshop on definitions of diagnosis and response in acute myeloid leukemia. J Clin Oncol 1990;8(5):813–819.

135. Pui CH, Raimondi SC, Head DR, et al. Characterization of childhood acute leukemia with multiple myeloid and lymphoid markers at diagnosis and at relapse. Blood 1991;78(5):1327–1337.

136. Pui CH, Behm FG, Singh B, et al. Heterogeneity of presenting features and their relation to treatment outcome in 120 children with T-cell acute lymphoblastic leukemia. Blood 1990;75(1):174–179.

137. Matutes E, Morilla R, Farahat N, et al. Definition of acute biphenotypic leukemia. Haematologica 1997;82(1):64–66.

138. Hanson CA, Abaza M, Sheldon S, et al. Acute biphenotypic leukaemia: immunophenotypic and cytogenetic analysis. Br J Haematol 1993;84(1):49–60.

139. Swerdlow SH CE, Harris NL, Jaffe ES, et al., eds. Tumors of hematopoietic and lymphoid tissues (WHO classification of tumors). Lyon: IARC, 2008.

140. Frohling S, Skelin S, Liebisch C, et al. Comparison of cytogenetic and molecular cytogenetic detection of chromosome abnormalities in 240 consecutive adult patients with acute myeloid leukemia. J Clin Oncol 2002;20(10):2480–2485.

141. Hilden JM, Smith FO, Frestedt JL, et al. MLL gene rearrangement, cytogenetic 11q23 abnormalities, and expression of the NG2 molecule in infant acute myeloid leukemia. Blood 1997;89(10):3801–3805.

142. Raimondi SC, Chang MN, Ravindranath Y, et al. Chromosomal abnormalities in 478 children with acute myeloid leukemia: clinical characteristics and treatment outcome in a cooperative Pediatric Oncology Group study-POG 8821. Blood 1999;94(11):3707–3716.

143. Yagi T, Morimoto A, Eguchi M, et al. Identification of a gene expression signature associated with pediatric AML prognosis. Blood 2003;102(5):1849–1856.

144. White TJ, Arnheim N, Erlich HA. The polymerase chain reaction. Trends Genet 1989;5(6):185–189.

145. Virtaneva K, Wright FA, Tanner SM, et al. Expression profiling reveals fundamental biological differences in acute myeloid leukemia with isolated trisomy 8 and normal cytogenetics. Proc Natl Acad Sci U S A 2001;98(3):1124–1129.

146. Venditti A, Del Poeta G, Stasi R, et al. Minimally differentiated acute myeloid leukaemia (AML-M0): cytochemical, immunophenotypic and cytogenetic analysis of 19 cases. Br J Haematol 1994;88(4):784–793.

147. Kotylo PK, Seo IS, Smith FO, et al. Flow cytometric immunophenotypic characterization of pediatric and adult minimally differentiated acute myeloid leukemia (AML-M0). Am J Clin Pathol 2000;113(2):193–200.

148. Barbaric D, Alonzo TA, Gerbing RB, et al. Minimally differentiated acute myeloid leukemia (FAB AML-M0) is associated with an adverse outcome in children: a report from the Children's Oncology Group, studies CCG-2891 and CCG-2961. Blood 2007;109(6):2314–2321.

149. Martinez-Climent JA. Molecular cytogenetics of childhood hematological malignancies. Leukemia 1997;11(12):1999–2021.

150. Golomb HM, Rowley JD, Vardiman JW, et al. "Microgranular" acute promyelocytic leukemia: a distinct clinical, ultrastructural, and cytogenetic entity. Blood 1980;55(2):253–259.

151. Melnick A, Licht JD. Deconstructing a disease: RARalpha, its fusion partners, and their roles in the pathogenesis of acute promyelocytic leukemia. Blood 1999;93(10):3167–3215.

152. Sainty D, Liso V, Cantu-Rajnoldi A, et al. A new morphologic classification system for acute promyelocytic leukemia distinguishes cases with underlying PLZF/RARA gene rearrangements. Group Francais de Cytogenetique Hematologique, UK Cancer Cytogenetics Group and BIOMED 1 European Coomunity-Concerted Acion "Molecular Cytogenetic Diagnosis in Haematological Malignancies." Blood 2000;96(4):1287–1296.

153. Martinez-Climent JA, Garcia-Conde J. Chromosomal rearrangements in childhood acute myeloid leukemia and myelodysplastic syndromes. J Pediatr Hematol Oncol 1999;21(2):91–102.

154. Kowal-Vern A, Mazzella FM, Cotelingam JD, et al. Diagnosis and characterization of acute erythroleukemia subsets by determining the percentages of myeloblasts and proerythroblasts in 69 cases. Am J Hematol 2000;65(1):5–13.

155. Ravindranath Y, Abella E, Krischer JP, et al. Acute myeloid leukemia (AML) in Down's syndrome is highly responsive to chemotherapy: experience on Pediatric Oncology Group AML Study 8498. Blood 1992;80(9):2210–2214.

156. Creutzig U, Ritter J, Ludwig WD, et al. Acute myeloid leukemia in children with Down syndrome. Klin Padiatr 1995;207(4):136–144.

157. Lion T, Haas OA, Harbott J, et al. The translocation t(1;22)(p13;q13) is a nonrandom marker specifically associated with acute megakaryocytic leukemia in young children. Blood 1992;79(12):3325–3330.

158. Creutzig U, Ritter J, Budde M, et al. Early deaths due to hemorrhage and leukostasis in childhood acute myelogenous leukemia. Associations with hyperleukocytosis and acute monocytic leukemia. Cancer 1987;60(12):3071–3079.

159. Bunin NJ, Kunkel K, Callihan TR. Cytoreductive procedures in the early management in cases of leukemia and hyperleukocytosis in children. Med Pediatr Oncol 1987;15(5):232–235.

160. Choi SI, Simone JV. Acute nonlymphocytic leukemia in 171 children. Med Pediatr Oncol 1976;2(2):119–146.
161. Tobelem G, Jacquillat C, Chastang C, et al. Acute monoblastic leukemia: a clinical and biologic study of 74 cases. Blood 1980;55(1):71–76.
162. Sung L, Lange BJ, Gerbing RB, et al. Microbiologically documented infections and infection-related mortality in children with acute myeloid leukemia. Blood 2007;110(10):3532–3539.
163. Creutzig U, Zimmermann M, Reinhardt D, et al. Early deaths and treatment-related mortality in children undergoing therapy for acute myeloid leukemia: analysis of the multicenter clinical trials AML-BFM 93 and AML-BFM 98. J Clin Oncol 2004;22(21):4384–4393.
164. Dixit A, Chatterjee T, Mishra P, et al. Disseminated intravascular coagulation in acute leukemia at presentation and during induction therapy. Clin Appl Thromb Hemost 2007;13(3):292–298.
165. Zipursky A, Poon A, Doyle J. Leukemia in Down syndrome: a review. Pediatr Hematol Oncol 1992;9(2):139–149.
166. Stucki A, Rivier AS, Gikic M, et al. Endothelial cell activation by myeloblasts: molecular mechanisms of leukostasis and leukemic cell dissemination. Blood 2001;97(7):2121–2129.
167. Inaba H, Fan Y, Pounds S, et al. Clinical and biologic features and treatment outcome of children with newly diagnosed acute myeloid leukemia and hyperleukocytosis. Cancer 2008;113(3):522–529.
168. Lowe EJ, Pui CH, Hancock ML, et al. Early complications in children with acute lymphoblastic leukemia presenting with hyperleukocytosis. Pediatr Blood Cancer 2005;45(1):10–15.
169. Bodey GP, Powell RD Jr, Hersh EM, et al. Pulmonary complications of acute leukemia. Cancer 1966;19(6):781–793.
170. Roath S, Davenport P. Leucocyte numbers and quality: their effect on viscosity. Clin Lab Haematol 1991;13(3):255–262.
171. van Furth R, van Zwet TL. Cytochemical, functional, and proliferative characteristics of promonocytes and monocytes from patients with monocytic leukemia. Blood 1983;62(2):298–304.
172. Ribeiro RC, Pui CH. The clinical and biological correlates of coagulopathy in children with acute leukemia. J Clin Oncol 1986;4(8):1212–1218.
173. Wilde JT, Davies JM. Haemostatic problems in acute leukaemia. Blood Rev 1990;4(4):245–251.
174. Ventura GJ, Hester JP, Dixon DO, et al. Analysis of risk factors for fatal hemorrhage during induction therapy of patients with acute promyelocytic leukemia. Hematol Pathol 1989;3(1):23–28.
175. Falanga A, Iacoviello L, Evangelista V, et al. Loss of blast cell procoagulant activity and improvement of hemostatic variables in patients with acute promyelocytic leukemia administered all-trans-retinoic acid. Blood 1995;86(3):1072–1081.
176. Tallman MS, Andersen JW, Schiffer CA, et al. All-trans retinoic acid in acute promyelocytic leukemia: long-term outcome and prognostic factor analysis from the North American Intergroup protocol. Blood 2002;100(13):4298–4302.
177. Tsimberidou AM, Kantarjian HM, Estey E, et al. Outcome in patients with nonleukemic granulocytic sarcoma treated with chemotherapy with or without radiotherapy. Leukemia 2003;17(6):1100–1103.
178. Kobayashi R, Tawa A, Hanada R, et al. Extramedullary infiltration at diagnosis and prognosis in children with acute myelogenous leukemia. Pediatr Blood Cancer 2007;48(4):393–398.
179. Frohna BJ, Quint DJ. Granulocytic sarcoma (chloroma) causing spinal cord compression. Neuroradiology 1993;35(7):509–511.
180. Economopoulos T, Alexopoulos C, Anagnostou D, et al. Primary granulocytic sarcoma of the testis. Leukemia 1994;8(1):199–200.
181. Dusenbery KE, Howells WB, Arthur DC, et al. Extramedullary leukemia in children with newly diagnosed acute myeloid leukemia: a report from the Children's Cancer Group. J Pediatr Hematol Oncol 2003;25(10):760–768.
182. Creutzig U, Zimmermann M, Ritter J, et al. Treatment strategies and long-term results in paediatric patients treated in four consecutive AML-BFM trials. Leukemia 2005;19(12):2030–2042.
183. Smith FO, Alonzo TA, Gerbing RB, et al. Long-term results of children with acute myeloid leukemia: a report of three consecutive Phase III trials by the Children's Cancer Group: CCG 251, CCG 213 and CCG 2891. Leukemia 2005;19(12):2054–2062.
184. Kardos G, Zwaan CM, Kaspers GJ, et al. Treatment strategy and results in children treated on three Dutch Childhood Oncology Group acute myeloid leukemia trials. Leukemia 2005;19(12):2063–2071.
185. Perel Y, Auvrignon A, Leblanc T, et al. Treatment of childhood acute myeloblastic leukemia: dose intensification improves outcome and maintenance therapy is of no benefit–multicenter studies of the French LAME (Leucemie Aigue Myeloblastique Enfant) Cooperative Group. Leukemia 2005;19(12):2082–2089.
186. Gibson BE, Wheatley K, Hann IM, et al. Treatment strategy and long-term results in paediatric patients treated in consecutive UK AML trials. Leukemia 2005;19(12):2130–2138.
187. Ravindranath Y, Chang M, Steuber CP, et al. Pediatric Oncology Group (POG) studies of acute myeloid leukemia (AML): a review of four consecutive childhood AML trials conducted between 1981 and 2000. Leukemia 2005;19(12):2101–2116.
188. Ribeiro RC, Razzouk BI, Pounds S, et al. Successive clinical trials for childhood acute myeloid leukemia at St Jude Children's Research Hospital, from 1980 to 2000. Leukemia 2005;19(12):2125–2129.
189. Lie SO, Abrahamsson J, Clausen N, et al. Long-term results in children with AML: NOPHO-AML Study Group—report of three consecutive trials. Leukemia 2005;19(12):2090–2100.
190. Kaspers GJ, Creutzig U. Pediatric acute myeloid leukemia: international progress and future directions. Leukemia 2005;19(12):2025–2029.
191. Goldie JH, Coldman AJ. A mathematic model for relating the drug sensitivity of tumors to their spontaneous mutation rate. Cancer Treat Rep 1979;63(11–12):1727–1733.
192. Goldie JH, Coldman AJ, Gudauskas GA. Rationale for the use of alternating non-cross-resistant chemotherapy. Cancer Treat Rep 1982;66(3):439–449.
193. Hurwitz CA, Mounce KG, Grier HE. Treatment of patients with acute myelogenous leukemia: review of clinical trials of the past decade. J Pediatr Hematol Oncol 1995;17(3):185–197.
194. Gale RP. Advances in the treatment of acute myelogenous leukemia. N Engl J Med 1979;300(21):1189–1199.
195. Chard RL Jr. Studies with anthracyclines in pediatric acute nonlymphocytic leukemia. Cancer Treat Rep 1981;65(Suppl 4):77–81.
196. Vormoor J, Boos J, Stahnke K, et al. Therapy of childhood acute myelogenous leukemias. Ann Hematol 1996;73(1):11–24.
197. Wells RJ, Woods WG, Lampkin BC, et al. Impact of high-dose cytarabine and asparaginase intensification on childhood acute myeloid leukemia: a report from the Childrens Cancer Group. J Clin Oncol 1993;11(3):538–545.
198. O'Brien TA, Russell SJ, Vowels MR, et al. Results of consecutive trials for children newly diagnosed with acute myeloid leukemia from the Australian and New Zealand Children's Cancer Study Group. Blood 2002;100(8):2708–2716.
199. Creutzig U, Ritter J, Zimmermann M, et al. Improved treatment results in high-risk pediatric acute myeloid leukemia patients after intensification with high-dose cytarabine and mitoxantrone: results of Study Acute Myeloid Leukemia-Berlin-Frankfurt-Munster 93. J Clin Oncol 2001;19(10):2705–2713.
200. Creutzig U, Ritter J, Zimmermann M, et al. Idarubicin improves blast cell clearance during induction therapy in children with AML: results of study AML-BFM 93. AML-BFM Study Group. Leukemia 2001;15(3):348–354.
201. Berman E, McBride M. Comparative cellular pharmacology of daunorubicin and idarubicin in human multidrug-resistant leukemia cells. Blood 1992;79(12):3267–3273.
202. Vogler WR, Velez-Garcia E, Weiner RS, et al. A phase III trial comparing idarubicin and daunorubicin in combination with cytarabine in acute myelogenous leukemia: a Southeastern Cancer Study Group Study. J Clin Oncol 1992;10(7):1103–1111.
203. Creutzig U, Korholz D, Niemeyer CM, et al. Toxicity and effectiveness of high-dose idarubicin during AML induction therapy: results of a pilot study in children. Klin Padiatr 2000;212(4):163–168.
204. Wells RJ, Woods WG, Buckley JD, et al. Treatment of newly diagnosed children and adolescents with acute myeloid leukemia: a Childrens Cancer Group study. J Clin Oncol 1994;12(11):2367–2377.
205. Wells RJ, Arthur DC, Srivastava A, et al. Prognostic variables in newly diagnosed children and adolescents with acute myeloid leukemia: Children's Cancer Group Study 213. Leukemia 2002;16(4):601–607.
206. Ravindranath Y, Steuber CP, Krischer J, et al. High-dose cytarabine for intensification of early therapy of childhood acute myeloid leukemia: a Pediatric Oncology Group study. J Clin Oncol 1991;9(4):572–580.
207. Riley LC, Hann IM, Wheatley K, et al. Treatment-related deaths during induction and first remission of acute myeloid leukaemia in children treated on the Tenth Medical Research Council acute myeloid leukaemia trial (MRC AML10). The MCR Childhood Leukaemia Working Party. Br J Haematol 1999;106(2):436–444.
208. Rees JK, Gray RG, Swirsky D, et al. Principal results of the Medical Research Council's 8th acute myeloid leukaemia trial. Lancet 1986;2(8518):1236–1241.
209. Hann IM, Stevens RF, Goldstone AH, et al. Randomized comparison of DAT versus ADE as induction chemotherapy in children and younger adults with acute myeloid leukemia. Results of the Medical Research Council's 10th AML trial (MRC AML10). Adult and Childhood Leukaemia Working Parties of the Medical Research Council. Blood 1997;89(7):2311–2318.
210. Burke PJ, Karp JE, Vaughan WP. Chemotherapy of leukemia in mice, rats, and humans relating time of humoral stimulation, tumor growth, and clinical response. J Natl Cancer Inst 1981;67(3):529–538.
211. Woods WG, Kobrinsky N, Buckley JD, et al. Timed-sequential induction therapy improves postremission outcome in acute myeloid leukemia: a report from the Children's Cancer Group. Blood 1996;87(12):4979–4989.
212. Woods WG, Kobrinsky N, Buckley J, et al. Intensively timed induction therapy followed by autologous or allogeneic bone marrow transplantation for children with acute myeloid leukemia or myelodysplastic syndrome: a Childrens Cancer Group pilot study. J Clin Oncol 1993;11(8):1448–1457.
213. Wells RJ, Woods WG, Buckley JD, et al. Therapy for acute myeloid leukemia: intensive timing of induction chemotherapy. Curr Oncol Rep 2000;2(6):524–528.
214. Neudorf S, Sanders J, Kobrinsky N, et al. Allogeneic bone marrow transplantation for children with acute myelocytic leukemia in first remission demonstrates a role for graft versus leukemia in the maintenance of disease-free survival. Blood 2004;103(10):3655–3661.
215. Woods WG, Neudorf S, Gold S, et al. A comparison of allogeneic bone marrow transplantation, autologous bone marrow transplantation, and aggressive chemotherapy in children with acute myeloid leukemia in remission. Blood 2001;97(1):56–62.
216. Lange BJ, Smith FO, Feusner J, et al. Outcomes in CCG-2961, a children's oncology group phase 3 trial for untreated pediatric acute myeloid leukemia: a report from the children's oncology group. Blood 2008;111(3):1044–1053.
217. Lie SO, Abrahamsson J, Clausen N, et al. Treatment stratification based on initial in vivo response in acute myeloid leukaemia in children without Down's syndrome: results of NOPHO-AML trials. Br J Haematol 2003;122(2):217–225.
218. van der Does-van den Berg A, Hhlen K, Colly LP, et al. Treatment of childhood acute nonlymphocytic leukemia with high-dose cytosine arabinoside, 6-thioguanine, and doxorubicin without maintenance therapy: pilot study ANLL-80 of the Dutch Childhood Leukemia Study Group (DCLSG). Pediatr Hematol Oncol 1988;5(2):93–102.
219. Cassileth PA, Andersen JW, Bennett JM, et al. Adult acute lymphocytic leukemia: the Eastern Cooperative Oncology Group experience. Leukemia 1992;6(Suppl 2):178–181.
220. Perel Y, Auvrignon A, Leblanc T, et al. Impact of addition of maintenance therapy to intensive induction and consolidation chemotherapy for childhood acute myeloblastic leukemia: results of a prospective randomized trial, LAME 89/91. Leucamie Aique Myeloide Enfant. J Clin Oncol 2002;20(12):2774–2782.
221. Weinstein HJ, Mayer RJ, Rosenthal DS, et al. Treatment of acute myelogenous leukemia in children and adults. N Engl J Med 1980;303(9):473–478.
222. Woods WG, Ruymann FB, Lampkin BC, et al. The role of timing of high-dose cytosine arabinoside intensification and of maintenance therapy in the treatment of children with acute nonlymphocytic leukemia. Cancer 1990;66(6):1106–1113.
223. Ritter J, Creutzig U, Schellong G. Treatment results of three consecutive German childhood AML trials: BFM-78, -83, and -87. AML-BFM-Group. Leukemia 1992;6(Suppl 2):59–62.
224. Dahl GV, Kalwinsky DK, Mirro J Jr, et al. Allogeneic bone marrow transplantation in a program of intensive sequential chemotherapy for children and young adults with acute nonlymphocytic leukemia in first remission. J Clin Oncol 1990;8(2):295–303.
225. MacMillan ML, Davies SM, Nelson GO, et al. Twenty years of unrelated donor bone marrow transplantation for pediatric acute leukemia facilitated by the National Marrow Donor Program. Biol Blood Marrow Transplant 2008;14(9 Suppl):16–22.
226. Nesbit ME Jr, Buckley JD, Feig SA, et al. Chemotherapy for induction of remission of childhood acute myeloid leukemia followed by marrow transplantation or multiagent chemotherapy: a report from the Childrens Cancer Group. J Clin Oncol 1994;12(1):127–135.

227. Michel G, Leverger G, Leblanc T, et al. Allogeneic bone marrow transplantation vs aggressive post-remission chemotherapy for children with acute myeloid leukemia in first complete remission. A prospective study from the French Society of Pediatric Hematology and Immunology (SHIP). Bone Marrow Transplant 1996;17(2):191–196.

228. Creutzig U, Bender-Gotze C, Klingebiel T, et al. Comparison of chemotherapy alone with allogeneic bone marrow transplantation in first full remission in children with acute myeloid leukemia in the AML-BFM-83 and AML-BFM-87 studies–matched pair analysis. Klin Padiatr 1992;204(4):246–252.

229. Burnett AK, Wheatley K, Goldstone AH, et al. The value of allogeneic bone marrow transplant in patients with acute myeloid leukaemia at differing risk of relapse: results of the UK MRC AML 10 trial. Br J Haematol 2002;118(2):385–400.

230. Creutzig U, Reinhardt D, Zimmermann M, et al. Intensive chemotherapy versus bone marrow transplantation in pediatric acute myeloid leukemia: a matter of controversies. Blood 2001;97(11):3671–3672; author reply 3674–3675.

231. Bleakley M, Lau L, Shaw PJ, et al. Bone marrow transplantation for paediatric AML in first remission: a systematic review and meta-analysis. Bone Marrow Transplant 2002;29(10):843–852.

232. Sung L, Buckstein R, Doyle JJ, et al. Treatment options for patients with acute myeloid leukemia with a matched sibling donor: a decision analysis. Cancer 2003;97(3):592–600.

233. Horan JT, Alonzo TA, Lyman GH, et al. Impact of disease risk on efficacy of matched related bone marrow transplantation for pediatric acute myeloid leukemia: the Children's Oncology Group. J Clin Oncol 2008;26(35):5797–5801.

234. Mrozek K, Heinonen K, de la Chapelle A, et al. Clinical significance of cytogenetics in acute myeloid leukemia. Semin Oncol 1997;24(1):17–31.

235. Hasle H, Alonzo TA, Auvrignon A, et al. Monosomy 7 and deletion 7q in children and adolescents with acute myeloid leukemia: an international retrospective study. Blood 2007;109(11):4641–4647.

236. Mickelson EM, Petersdorf EW, Hansen JA. HLA matching and hematopoietic cell transplant outcome. Clin Transpl 2002:263–271.

237. Ottinger HD, Ferencik S, Beelen DW, et al. Hematopoietic stem cell transplantation: contrasting the outcome of transplantations from HLA-identical siblings, partially HLA-mismatched related donors, and HLA-matched unrelated donors. Blood 2003;102(3):1131–1137.

238. Dini G, Cancedda R, Giorgiani G, et al. Unrelated donor marrow transplantation in childhood: a report from the Associazione Italiana Ematologia e Oncologia Pediatrica (AIEOP) and the Gruppo Italiano per il Trapianto Midollo Osseo (GITMO). Haematologica 2002;87(8 Suppl):51–57.

239. Couriel D, Caldera H, Champlin R, et al. Acute graft-versus-host disease: pathophysiology, clinical manifestations, and management. Cancer 2004;101(9):1936–1946.

240. Michel G, Rocha V, Chevret S, et al. Unrelated cord blood transplantation for childhood acute myeloid leukemia: a Eurocord Group analysis. Blood 2003;102 (13):4290–4297.

241. Wagner JE, Barker JN, DeFor TE, et al. Transplantation of unrelated donor umbilical cord blood in 102 patients with malignant and nonmalignant diseases: influence of CD34 cell dose and HLA disparity on treatment-related mortality and survival. Blood 2002;100(5):1611–1618.

242. Barfield RC, Kasow KA, Hale GA. Advances in pediatric hematopoietic stem cell transplantation. Cancer Biol Ther 2008;7(10):1533–1539.

243. Aversa F, Reisner Y, Martelli MF. The haploidentical option for high-risk haematological malignancies. Blood Cells Mol Dis 2008;40(1):8–12.

244. Ruggeri L, Capanni M, Mancusi A, et al. Alloreactive natural killer cells in mismatched hematopoietic stem cell transplantation. Blood Cells Mol Dis 2004;33(3):216–221.

245. Symons HJ, Fuchs EJ. Hematopoietic SCT from partially HLA-mismatched (HLA-haploidentical) related donors. Bone Marrow Transplant 2008;42(6):365–377.

246. Cook MA, Milligan DW, Fegan CD, et al. The impact of donor KIR and patient HLA-C genotypes on outcome following HLA-identical sibling hematopoietic stem cell transplantation for myeloid leukemia. Blood 2004;103(4):1521–1526.

247. Pinkel D, Woo S. Prevention and treatment of meningeal leukemia in children. Blood 1994;84(2):355–366.

248. Abbott BL, Rubnitz JE, Tong X, et al. Clinical significance of central nervous system involvement at diagnosis of pediatric acute myeloid leukemia: a single institution's experience. Leukemia 2003;17(11):2090–2096.

249. Creutzig U, Ritter J, Zimmermann M, et al. Does cranial irradiation reduce the risk for bone marrow relapse in acute myelogenous leukemia? Unexpected results of the Childhood Acute Myelogenous Leukemia Study BFM-87. J Clin Oncol 1993;11(2):279–286.

250. Pui CH, Dahl GV, Kalwinsky DK, et al. Central nervous system leukemia in children with acute nonlymphoblastic leukemia. Blood 1985;66(5):1062–1067.

251. Webb DK, Harrison G, Stevens RF, et al. Relationships between age at diagnosis, clinical features, and outcome of therapy in children treated in the Medical Research Council AML 10 and 12 trials for acute myeloid leukemia. Blood 2001;98(6):1714–1720.

252. Mostafavi H, Lennarson PJ, Traynelis VC. Granulocytic sarcoma of the spine. Neurosurgery 2000;46(1):78–83; discussion 83–74.

253. Lange B, Woods WG, Lampkin BC. Children's Cancer Group transplant trials for acute myeloid leukemia in children: a cross-study analysis of CCG-251, CCG-213, CCG-2861 and CCG-2891. In: Buchner T, Hiddemann W, Wormann B, eds. Leukemias IV: prognostic factors. New York, NY: Springer-Verlag, 1994:724.

254. Webb DK, Wheatley K, Harrison G, et al. Outcome for children with relapsed acute myeloid leukaemia following initial therapy in the Medical Research Council (MRC) AML 10 trial. MRC Childhood Leukaemia Working Party. Leukemia 1999;013(1):25–31.

255. Wheatley K, Burnett AK, Goldstone AH, et al. A simple, robust, validated and highly predictive index for the determination of risk-directed therapy in acute myeloid leukaemia derived from the MRC AML 10 trial. United Kingdom Medical Research Council's Adult and Childhood Leukaemia Working Parties. Br J Haematol 1999;107(1):69–79.

256. Aplenc R, Alonzo TA, Gerbing RB, et al. Ethnicity and survival in childhood acute myeloid leukemia: a report from the Children's Oncology Group. Blood 2006;108(1):74–80.

257. Creutzig U, Ritter J, Vormoor J, et al. Myelodysplasia and acute myelogenous leukemia in Down's syndrome. A report of 40 children of the AML-BFM Study Group. Leukemia 1996;10(11):1677–1686.

258. Stevens RF, Hann IM, Wheatley K, et al. Marked improvements in outcome with chemotherapy alone in paediatric acute myeloid leukemia: results of the United Kingdom Medical Research Council's 10th AML trial. MRC Childhood Leukaemia Working Party. Br J Haematol 1998;101(1):130–140.

259. Lie SO, Jonmundsson G, Mellander L, et al. A population-based study of 272 children with acute myeloid leukaemia treated on two consecutive protocols with different intensity: best outcome in girls, infants, and children with Down's syndrome. Nordic Society of Paediatric Haematology and Oncology (NOPHO). Br J Haematol 1996;94 (1):82–88.

260. Craze JL, Harrison G, Wheatley K, et al. Improved outcome of acute myeloid leukaemia in Down's syndrome. Arch Dis Child 1999;81(1):32–37.

261. Gamis AS, Woods WG, Alonzo TA, et al. Increased age at diagnosis has a significantly negative effect on outcome in children with Down syndrome and acute myeloid leukemia: a report from the Children's Cancer Group Study 2891. J Clin Oncol 2003;21(18):3415–3422.

262. Taub JW, Ge Y. Down syndrome, drug metabolism and chromosome 21. Pediatr Blood Cancer 2005;44(1):33–39.

263. Ge Y, Jensen TL, Stout ML, et al. The role of cytidine deaminase and GATA1 mutations in the increased cytosine arabinoside sensitivity of Down syndrome myeloblasts and leukemia cell lines. Cancer Res 2004;64(2):728–735.

264. Zwaan CM, Kaspers GJ, Pieters R, et al. Different drug sensitivity profiles of acute myeloid and lymphoblastic leukemia and normal peripheral blood mononuclear cells in children with and without Down syndrome. Blood 2002;99(1):245–251.

265. Taub JW, Huang X, Ge Y, et al. Cystathionine-beta-synthase cDNA transfection alters the sensitivity and metabolism of 1-beta-D-arabinofuranosylcytosine in CCRF-CEM leukemia cells in vitro and in vivo: a model of leukemia in Down syndrome. Cancer Res 2000;60(22):6421–6426.

266. Tomizawa D, Tabuchi K, Kinoshita A, et al. Repetitive cycles of high-dose cytarabine are effective for childhood acute myeloid leukemia: long-term outcome of the children with AML treated on two consecutive trials of Tokyo Children's Cancer Study Group. Pediatr Blood Cancer 2007;49(2):127–132.

267. Lange BJ, Gerbing RB, Feusner J, et al. Mortality in overweight and underweight children with acute myeloid leukemia. JAMA 2005;293(2):203–211.

268. Davies SM, Bhatia S, Ross JA, et al. Glutathione S-transferase genotypes, genetic susceptibility, and outcome of therapy in childhood acute lymphoblastic leukemia. Blood 2002;100(1):67–71.

269. Gaynon PS, Desai AA, Bostrom BC, et al. Early response to therapy and outcome in childhood acute lymphoblastic leukemia: a review. Cancer 1997;80(9):1717–1726.

270. Nachman J, Sather HN, Gaynon PS, et al. Augmented Berlin-Frankfurt-Munster therapy abrogates the adverse prognostic significance of slow early response to induction chemotherapy for children and adolescents with acute lymphoblastic leukemia and unfavorable presenting features: a report from the Children's Cancer Group. J Clin Oncol 1997;15(6):2222–2230.

271. Wells RJ, Adams MT, Alonzo TA, et al. Mitoxantrone and cytarabine induction, high-dose cytarabine, and etoposide intensification for pediatric patients with relapsed or refractory acute myeloid leukemia: Children's Cancer Group Study 2951. J Clin Oncol 2003;21(15):2940–2947.

272. Sievers EL, Radich JP. Detection of minimal residual disease in acute leukemia. Curr Opin Hematol 2000;7(4):212–216.

273. Campana D. Status of minimal residual disease testing in childhood haematological malignancies. Br J Haematol 2008;143(4):481–489.

274. Goulden N, Virgo P, Grimwade D. Minimal residual disease directed therapy for childhood acute myeloid leukaemia: the time is now. Br J Haematol 2006;134(3):273–282.

275. Viehmann S, Teigler-Schlegel A, Bruch J, et al. Monitoring of minimal residual disease (MRD) by real-time quantitative reverse transcription PCR (RQ-RT-PCR) in childhood acute myeloid leukemia with AML1/ETO rearrangement. Leukemia 2003;17(6):1130–1136.

276. Buonamici S, Ottaviani E, Testoni N, et al. Real-time quantitation of minimal residual disease in inv(16)-positive acute myeloid leukemia may indicate risk for clinical relapse and may identify patients in a curable state. Blood 2002;99(2):443–449.

277. Mandelli F, Diverio D, Avvisati G, et al. Molecular remission in PML/RAR alpha-positive acute promyelocytic leukemia by combined all-trans retinoic acid and idarubicin (AIDA) therapy. Gruppo Italiano-Malattie Ematologiche Maligne dell'Adulto and Associazione Italiana di Ematologia ed Oncologia Pediatrica Cooperative Groups. Blood 1997;90(3):1014–1021.

278. Grimwade D, Lo Coco F. Acute promyelocytic leukemia: a model for the role of molecular diagnosis and residual disease monitoring in directing treatment approach in acute myeloid leukemia. Leukemia 2002;16(10):1959–1973.

279. Miyamoto T, Nagafuji K, Akashi K, et al. Persistence of multipotent progenitors expressing AML1/ETO transcripts in long-term remission patients with t(8;21) acute myelogenous leukemia. Blood 1996;87(11):4789–4796.

280. Miyamoto T, Nagafuji K, Harada M, et al. Significance of quantitative analysis of AML1/ETO transcripts in peripheral blood stem cells from t(8;21) acute myelogenous leukemia. Leuk Lymphoma 1997;25(1–2):69–75.

281. Jurlander J, Caligiuri MA, Ruutu T, et al. Persistence of the AML1/ETO fusion transcript in patients treated with allogeneic bone marrow transplantation for t(8;21) leukemia. Blood 1996;88(6):2183–2191.

282. Schnittger S, Weisser M, Schoch C, et al. New score predicting for prognosis in PML-RARA+, AML1-ETO+, or CBFBMYH11+ acute myeloid leukemia based on quantification of fusion transcripts. Blood 2003;102(8):2746–2755.

283. Trka J, Kalinova M, Hrusak O, et al. Real-time quantitative PCR detection of WT1 gene expression in children with AML: prognostic significance, correlation with disease status and residual disease detection by flow cytometry. Leukemia 2002;16(7):1381–1389.

284. Ommen HB, Nyvold CG, Braendstrup K, et al. Relapse prediction in acute myeloid leukaemia patients in complete remission using WT1 as a molecular marker: development of a mathematical model to predict time from molecular to clinical relapse and define optimal sampling intervals. Br J Haematol 2008;141(6):782–791.

285. Venditti A, Buccisano F, Del Poeta G, et al. Level of minimal residual disease after consolidation therapy predicts outcome in acute myeloid leukemia. Blood 2000;96 (12):3948–3952.

286. Wormann B, Safford M, Konemann S, et al. Detection of aberrant antigen expression in acute myeloid leukemia by multiparameter flow cytometry. Recent Results Cancer Res 1993;131:185–196.

287. Loken MR, Shah VO, Dattilio KL, et al. Flow cytometric analysis of human bone marrow. II. Normal B lymphocyte development. Blood 1987;70(5):1316–1324.

288. Vidriales MB, San-Miguel JF, Orfao A, et al. Minimal residual disease monitoring by flow cytometry. Best Pract Res Clin Haematol 2003;16(4):599–612.

289. Martinez-Climent JA, Thirman MJ, Espinosa R III, et al. Detection of 11q23/MLL rearrangements in infant leukemias with fluorescence in situ hybridization and molecular analysis. Leukemia 1995;9(8):1299–1304.

290. Creutzig U, Zimmermann M, Ritter J, et al. Definition of a standard-risk group in children with AML. Br J Haematol 1999;104(3):630–639.

291. Chang M, Raimondi SC, Ravindranath Y, et al. Prognostic factors in children and adolescents with acute myeloid leukemia (excluding children with Down syndrome and acute promyelocytic leukemia): univariate and recursive partitioning analysis of patients treated on Pediatric Oncology Group (POG) Study 8821. Leukemia 2000; 14(7):1201–1207.

292. Grimwade D, Walker H, Oliver F, et al. The importance of diagnostic cytogenetics on outcome in AML: analysis of 1,612 patients entered into the MRC AML 10 trial. The Medical Research Council Adult and Children's Leukaemia Working Parties. Blood 1998;92(7):2322–2333.

293. Marcucci G, Caligiuri MA, Bloomfield CD. Molecular and clinical advances in core binding factor primary acute myeloid leukemia: a paradigm for translational research in malignant hematology. Cancer Invest 2000;18(8):768–780.

294. Marcucci G, Caligiuri MA, Bloomfield CD. Core binding factor (CBF) acute myeloid leukemia: is molecular monitoring by RT-PCR useful clinically? Eur J Haematol 2003;71(3):143–154.

295. Mrozek K, Marcucci G, Paschka P, et al. Advances in molecular genetics and treatment of core-binding factor acute myeloid leukemia. Curr Opin Oncol 2008;20(6):711–718.

296. Shigesada K, van de Sluis B, Liu PP. Mechanism of leukemogenesis by the inv(16) chimeric gene CBFB/PEBP2B-MHY11. Oncogene 2004;23(24):4297–4307.

297. Byrd JC, Mrozek K, Dodge RK, et al. Pretreatment cytogenetic abnormalities are predictive of induction success, cumulative incidence of relapse, and overall survival in adult patients with de novo acute myeloid leukemia: results from Cancer and Leukemia Group B (CALGB 8461). Blood 2002;100(13):4325–4336.

298. Delaunay J, Vey N, Leblanc T, et al. Prognosis of inv(16)/t(16;16) acute myeloid leukemia (AML): a survey of 110 cases from the French AML Intergroup. Blood 2003;102(2):462–469.

299. Casillas JN, Woods WG, Hunger SP, et al. Prognostic implications of t(10;11) translocations in childhood acute myelogenous leukemia: a report from the Children's Cancer Group. J Pediatr Hematol Oncol 2003;25(8):594–600.

300. Ernst P, Wang J, Korsmeyer SJ. The role of MLL in hematopoiesis and leukemia. Curr Opin Hematol 2002;9(4):282–287.

301. Rubnitz JE, Raimondi SC, Tong X, et al. Favorable impact of the t(9;11) in childhood acute myeloid leukemia. J Clin Oncol 2002;20(9):2302–2309.

302. Mrozek K, Heinonen K, Lawrence D, et al. Adult patients with de novo acute myeloid leukemia and t(9; 11)(p22; q23) have a superior outcome to patients with other translocations involving band 11q23: a cancer and leukemia group B study. Blood 1997; 90(11):4532–4538.

303. Sandoval C, Head DR, Mirro J Jr, et al. Translocation t(9;11)(p21;q23) in pediatric de novo and secondary acute myeloblastic leukemia. Leukemia 1992;6(6):513–519.

304. Balgobind BV, Raimondi SC, Harbott J, et al. Novel prognostic subgroups in childhood 11q23/MLL-rearranged acute myeloid leukemia: results of an international retrospective study. Blood 2009;114:2489–2496.

305. Chen AR, Alonzo TA, Woods WG, et al. Current controversies: which patients with acute myeloid leukaemia should receive a bone marrow transplantation?—an American view. Br J Haematol 2002;118(2):378–384.

306. Creutzig U, Reinhardt D. Current controversies: which patients with acute myeloid leukaemia should receive a bone marrow transplantation?—a European view. Br J Haematol 2002;118(2):365–377.

307. Woods WG, Barnard DR, Alonzo TA, et al. Prospective study of 90 children requiring treatment for juvenile myelomonocytic leukemia or myelodysplastic syndrome: a report from the Children's Cancer Group. J Clin Oncol 2002;20(2):434–440.

308. Weiner HL, Zagzag D. Growth factor receptor tyrosine kinases: cell adhesion kinase family suggests a novel signaling mechanism in cancer. Cancer Invest 2000;18(6):544–554.

309. Brown P, Small D. FLT3 inhibitors: a paradigm for the development of targeted therapeutics for paediatric cancer. Eur J Cancer 2004;40(5):707–721, discussion 722–704.

310. Levis M, Small D. FLT3: ITDoes matter in leukemia. Leukemia 2003;17(9):1738–1752.

311. Meshinchi S, Appelbaum FR. Structural and functional alterations of FLT3 in acute myeloid leukemia. Clin Cancer Res 2009;15(13):4263–4269.

312. Meshinchi S, Woods WG, Stirewalt DL, et al. Prevalence and prognostic significance of Flt3 internal tandem duplication in pediatric acute myeloid leukemia. Blood 2001;97(1):89–94.

313. Zwaan CM, Meshinchi S, Radich JP, et al. FLT3 internal tandem duplication in 234 children with acute myeloid leukemia: prognostic significance and relation to cellular drug resistance. Blood 2003;102(7):2387–2394.

314. Meshinchi S, Alonzo TA, Stirewalt DL, et al. Clinical implications of FLT3 mutations in pediatric AML. Blood 2006;108(12):3654–3661.

315. Thiede C, Steudel C, Mohr B, et al. Analysis of FLT3-activating mutations in 979 patients with acute myelogenous leukemia: association with FAB subtypes and identification of subgroups with poor prognosis. Blood 2002;99(12):4326–4335.

316. Whitman SP, Archer KJ, Feng L, et al. Absence of the wild-type allele predicts poor prognosis in adult de novo acute myeloid leukemia with normal cytogenetics and the internal tandem duplication of FLT3: a cancer and leukemia group B study. Cancer Res 2001;61(19):7233–7239.

317. Cazzaniga G, Dell'Oro MG, Mecucci C, et al. Nucleophosmin mutations in childhood acute myelogenous leukemia with normal karyotype. Blood 2005;106(4):1419–1422.

318. Schnittger S, Schoch C, Kern W, et al. Nucleophosmin gene mutations are predictors of favorable prognosis in acute myelogenous leukemia with a normal karyotype. Blood 2005;106(12):3733–3739.

319. Thiede C, Koch S, Creutzig E, et al. Prevalence and prognostic impact of NPM1 mutations in 1485 adult patients with acute myeloid leukemia (AML). Blood 2006;107(10):4011–4020.

320. Hollink IH, Zwaan CM, Zimmermann M, et al. Favorable prognostic impact of NPM1 gene mutations in childhood acute myeloid leukemia, with emphasis on cytogenetically normal AML. Leukemia 2009;23(2):262–270.

321. Brown P, McIntyre E, Rau R, et al. The incidence and clinical significance of nucleophosmin mutations in childhood AML. Blood 2007;110(3):979–985.

322. Preudhomme C, Sagot C, Boissel N, et al. Favorable prognostic significance of CEBPA mutations in patients with de novo acute myeloid leukemia: a study from the Acute Leukemia French Association (ALFA). Blood 2002;100(8):2717–2723.

323. Pabst T, Mueller BU, Zhang P, et al. Dominant-negative mutations of CEBPA, encoding CCAAT/enhancer binding protein-alpha (C/EBPalpha), in acute myeloid leukemia. Nat Genet 2001;27(3):263–270.

324. Ho PA, Alonzo TA, Gerbing RB, et al. Prevalence and prognostic implications of CEBPA mutations in pediatric AML: a report from the Children's Oncology Group. Blood 2009;113:6558–6566.

325. Hollink IH, van den Heuvel-Eibrink MM, Zimmermann M, et al. Clinical relevance of Wilms' tumor 1 gene mutations in childhood acute myeloid leukemia. Blood 2009;113:5951–5960.

326. Vignetti M, Orsini E, Petti MC, et al. Probability of long-term disease-free survival for acute myeloid leukemia patients after first relapse: a single-centre experience. Ann Oncol 1996;7(9):933–938.

327. Grimwade D, Walker H, Harrison G, et al. The predictive value of hierarchical cytogenetic classification in older adults with acute myeloid leukemia (AML): analysis of 1065 patients entered into the United Kingdom Medical Research Council AML11 trial. Blood 2001;98(5):1312–1320.

328. Slovak ML, Kopecky KJ, Cassileth PA, et al. Karyotypic analysis predicts outcome of preremission and postremission therapy in adult acute myeloid leukemia: a Southwest Oncology Group/Eastern Cooperative Oncology Group Study. Blood 2000;96(13):4075–4083.

329. Kottaridis PD, Gale RE, Langabeer SE, et al. Studies of FLT3 mutations in paired presentation and relapse samples from patients with acute myeloid leukemia: implications for the role of FLT3 mutations in leukemogenesis, minimal residual disease detection, and possible therapy with FLT3 inhibitors. Blood 2002;100(7):2393–2398.

330. Damaraju VL, Damaraju S, Young JD, et al. Nucleoside anticancer drugs: the role of nucleoside transporters in resistance to cancer chemotherapy. Oncogene 2003;22(47):7524–7536.

331. Mackey JR, Yao SY, Smith KM, et al. Gemcitabine transport in xenopus oocytes expressing recombinant plasma membrane mammalian nucleoside transporters. J Natl Cancer Inst 1999;91(21):1876–1881.

332. Galmarini CM, Thomas X, Calvo F, et al. In vivo mechanisms of resistance to cytarabine in acute myeloid leukaemia. Br J Haematol 2002;117(4):860–868.

333. Stam RW, den Boer ML, Meijerink JP, et al. Differential mRNA expression of Ara-C-metabolizing enzymes explains Ara-C sensitivity in MLL gene-rearranged infant acute lymphoblastic leukemia. Blood 2003;101(4):1270–1276.

334. Molina-Arcas M, Marce S, Villamor N, et al. Equilibrative nucleoside transporter-2 (hENT2) protein expression correlates with ex vivo sensitivity to fludarabine in chronic lymphocytic leukemia (CLL) cells. Leukemia 2005;19(1):64–68.

335. Kim DH, Lee NY, Sung WJ, et al. Multidrug resistance as a potential prognostic indicator in acute myeloid leukemia with normal karyotypes. Acta Haematol 2005;114(2):78–83.

336. Campos L, Guyotat D, Archimbaud E, et al. Clinical significance of multidrug resistance P-glycoprotein expression on acute nonlymphoblastic leukemia cells at diagnosis. Blood 1992;79(2):473–476.

337. Del Poeta G, Stasi R, Aronica G, et al. Clinical relevance of P-glycoprotein expression in de novo acute myeloid leukemia. Blood 1996;87(5):1997–2004.

338. Sievers EL, Smith FO, Woods WG, et al. Cell surface expression of the multidrug resistance P-glycoprotein (P-170) as detected by monoclonal antibody MRK-16 in pediatric acute myeloid leukemia fails to define a poor prognostic group: a report from the Childrens Cancer Group. Leukemia 1995;9(12):2042–2048.

339. Sampath D, Rao VA, Plunkett W. Mechanisms of apoptosis induction by nucleoside analogs. Oncogene 2003;22(56):9063–9074.

340. Kornblau SM, Thall PF, Estrov Z, et al. The prognostic impact of BCL2 protein expression in acute myelogenous leukemia varies with cytogenetics. Clin Cancer Res 1999;5(7):1758–1766.

341. Del Poeta G, Venditti A, Del Principe MI, et al. Amount of spontaneous apoptosis detected by Bax/Bcl-2 ratio predicts outcome in acute myeloid leukemia (AML). Blood 2003;101(6):2125–2131.

342. Schimmer AD, Pedersen IM, Kitada S, et al. Functional blocks in caspase activation pathways are common in leukemia and predict patient response to induction chemotherapy. Cancer Res 2003;63(6):1242–1248.

343. Aplenc R, Alonzo TA, Gerbing RB, et al. Safety and efficacy of gemtuzumab ozogamicin in combination with chemotherapy for pediatric acute myeloid leukemia: a report from the Children's Oncology Group. J Clin Oncol 2008;26(14):2390–3295.

344. Kern W, Schoch C, Haferlach T, et al. Multivariate analysis of prognostic factors in patients with refractory and relapsed acute myeloid leukemia undergoing sequential high-dose cytosine arabinoside and mitoxantrone (S-HAM) salvage therapy: relevance of cytogenetic abnormalities. Leukemia 2000;14(2):226–231.

345. Abrahamsson J, Clausen N, Gustafsson G, et al. Improved outcome after relapse in children with acute myeloid leukaemia. Br J Haematol 2007;136(2):229–236.

346. Wells RJ, Gold SH, Krill CE, et al. Cytosine arabinoside and mitoxantrone induction chemotherapy followed by bone marrow transplantation or chemotherapy for relapsed or refractory pediatric acute myeloid leukemia. Leukemia 1994;8(10):1626–1630.

347. Whitlock JA, Wells RJ, Hord JD, et al. High-dose cytosine arabinoside and etoposide: an effective regimen without anthracyclines for refractory childhood acute non-lymphocytic leukemia. Leukemia 1997;11(2):185–189.

348. Estey EH, Keating MJ, McCredie KB, et al. Cellular ara-CTP pharmacokinetics, response, and karyotype in newly diagnosed acute myelogenous leukemia. Leukemia 1990;4(2):95–99.

349. Kufe D, Spriggs D, Egan EM, et al. Relationships among Ara-CTP pools, formation of (Ara-C)DNA, and cytotoxicity of human leukemic cells. Blood 1984;64(1):54–58.

350. Gandhi V, Estey E, Keating MJ, et al. Fludarabine potentiates metabolism of cytarabine in patients with acute myelogenous leukemia during therapy. J Clin Oncol 1993;11(1):116–124.

351. Faderl S, Gandhi V, O'Brien S, et al. Results of a phase 1–2 study of clofarabine in combination with cytarabine (ara-C) in relapsed and refractory acute leukemias. Blood 2005;105(3):940–947.

352. Cooper T, Ayres M, Nowak B, et al. Biochemical modulation of cytarabine triphosphate by clofarabine. Cancer Chemother Pharmacol 2005;55(4):361–368.

353. Goemans BF, Tamminga RY, Corbijn CM, et al. Outcome for children with relapsed acute myeloid leukemia in the Netherlands following initial treatment between 1980 and 1998: survival after chemotherapy only? Haematologica 2008;93:1418–1420.

354. Bunin NJ, Davies SM, Aplenc R, et al. Unrelated donor bone marrow transplantation for children with acute myeloid leukemia beyond first remission or refractory to chemotherapy. J Clin Oncol 2008;26(26):4326–4332.

355. Ringden O, Labopin M, Frassoni F, et al. Allogeneic bone marrow transplant or second autograft in patients with acute leukemia who relapse after an autograft. Acute Leukaemia Working Party of the European Group for Blood and Marrow Transplantation (EBMT). Bone Marrow Transplant 1999;24(4):389–396.

356. Gluckman E, Rocha V. Cord blood transplantation for children with acute leukaemia: a Eurocord registry analysis. Blood Cells Mol Dis 2004;33(3):271–273.

357. Anasetti C. Transplantation of hematopoietic stem cells from alternate donors in acute myelogenous leukemia. Leukemia 2000;14(3):502–504.

358. Yakoub-Agha I, Mesnil F, Kuentz M, et al. Allogeneic marrow stem-cell transplantation from human leukocyte antigen-identical siblings versus human leukocyte antigen-allelic-matched unrelated donors (10/10) in patients with standard-risk hematologic malignancy: a prospective study from the French Society of Bone Marrow Transplantation and Cell Therapy. J Clin Oncol 2006;24(36):5695–5702.
359. Abella E, Ravindranath Y. Therapy for childhood acute myeloid leukemia: role of allogeneic bone marrow transplantation. Curr Oncol Rep 2000;2(6):529–538.
360. Johnston DL, Alonzo TA, Gerbing RB, et al. Risk factors and therapy for isolated central nervous system relapse of pediatric acute myeloid leukemia. J Clin Oncol 2005; 23(36):9172–9178.
361. Dinndorf PA, Andrews RG, Benjamin D, et al. Expression of normal myeloid-associated antigens by acute leukemia cells. Blood 1986;67(4):1048–1053.
362. Ikemoto N, Kumar RA, Ling TT, et al. Calicheamicin-DNA complexes: warhead alignment and saccharide recognition of the minor groove. Proc Natl Acad Sci U S A 1995; 92(23):10506–10510.
363. Larson RA, Sievers EL, Stadtmauer EA, et al. Final report of the efficacy and safety of gemtuzumab ozogamicin (Mylotarg) in patients with CD33-positive acute myeloid leukemia in first recurrence. Cancer 2005;104(7):1442–1452.
364. Reinhardt D, Diekamp S, Fleischhack G, et al. Gemtuzumab ozogamicin (Mylotarg) in children with refractory or relapsed acute myeloid leukemia. Onkologie 2004;27(3): 269–272.
365. Zwaan CM, Reinhardt D, Corbacioglu S, et al. Gemtuzumab ozogamicin: first clinical experiences in children with relapsed/refractory acute myeloid leukemia treated on compassionate-use basis. Blood 2003;101(10):3868–3871.
366. Zwaan CM, Reinhardt D, Jurgens H, et al. Gemtuzumab ozogamicin in pediatric CD33-positive acute lymphoblastic leukemia: first clinical experiences and relation with cellular sensitivity to single agent calicheamicin. Leukemia 2003;17(2):468–470.
367. Kell WJ, Burnett AK, Chopra R, et al. A feasibility study of simultaneous administration of gemtuzumab ozogamicin with intensive chemotherapy in induction and consolidation in younger patients with acute myeloid leukemia. Blood 2003;102(13): 4277–4283.
368. Piccaluga PP, Martinelli G, Rondoni M, et al. Gemtuzumab ozogamicin for relapsed and refractory acute myeloid leukemia and myeloid sarcomas. Leuk Lymphoma 2004;45(9):1791–1795.
369. Arceci RJ, Sande J, Lange B, et al. Safety and efficacy of gemtuzumab ozogamicin in pediatric patients with advanced CD33+ acute myeloid leukemia. Blood 2005; 106(4):1183–1188.
370. Chevallier P, Delaunay J, Turlure P, et al. Long-term disease-free survival after gemtuzumab, intermediate-dose cytarabine, and mitoxantrone in patients with CD33(+) primary resistant or relapsed acute myeloid leukemia. J Clin Oncol 2008;26(32): 5192–5197.
371. Maniecki MB, Hasle H, Friis-Hansen L, et al. Impaired CD163-mediated hemoglobin-scavenging and severe toxic symptoms in patients treated with gemtuzumab ozogamicin. Blood 2008;112(4):1510–1514.
372. McDonald GB, Hinds MS, Fisher LD, et al. Veno-occlusive disease of the liver and multiorgan failure after bone marrow transplantation: a cohort study of 355 patients. Ann Intern Med 1993;118(4):255–267.
373. Andrews RG, Torok-Storb B, Bernstein ID. Myeloid-associated differentiation antigens on stem cells and their progeny identified by monoclonal antibodies. Blood 1983; 62(1):124–132.
374. Smith BD, Levis M, Beran M, et al. Single-agent CEP-701, a novel FLT3 inhibitor, shows biologic and clinical activity in patients with relapsed or refractory acute myeloid leukemia. Blood 2004;103(10):3669–3676.
375. DeAngelo DJ, Stone RM, Heaney ML, et al. Phase 1 clinical results with tandutinib (MLN518), a novel FLT3 antagonist, in patients with acute myelogenous leukemia or high-risk myelodysplastic syndrome: safety, pharmacokinetics, and pharmacodynamics. Blood 2006;108(12):3674–3681.
376. Safaian NN, Czibere A, Bruns I, et al. Sorafenib (Nexavar) induces molecular remission and regression of extramedullary disease in a patient with FLT3-ITD+ acute myeloid leukemia. Leuk Res 2009;33(2):348–350.
377. Brown P, Levis M, Shurtleff S, et al. FLT3 inhibition selectively kills childhood acute lymphoblastic leukemia cells with high levels of FLT3 expression. Blood 2005;105 (2):812–820.
378. Knapper S, Mills KI, Gilkes AF, et al. The effects of lestaurtinib (CEP701) and PKC412 on primary AML blasts: the induction of cytotoxicity varies with dependence on FLT3 signaling in both FLT3-mutated and wild-type cases. Blood 2006;108(10):3494–3503.
379. Levis M, Brown P, Smith BD, et al. Plasma inhibitory activity (PIA): a pharmacodynamic assay reveals insights into the basis for cytotoxic response to FLT3 inhibitors. Blood 2006;108(10):3477–3483.
380. Jeha S, Razzouk B, Rytting M, et al. Phase II study of clofarabine in pediatric patients with refractory or relapsed acute myeloid leukemia. J Clin Oncol 2009;27(26):4392–4397.
381. Jeha S, Gaynon PS, Razzouk BI, et al. Phase II study of clofarabine in pediatric patients with refractory or relapsed acute lymphoblastic leukemia. J Clin Oncol 2006;24 (12):1917–1923.
382. Bueso-Ramos CE, Rocha FC, Shishodia S, et al. Expression of constitutively active nuclear-kappa B RelA transcription factor in blasts of acute myeloid leukemia. Hum Pathol 2004;35(2):246–253.
383. Gil L, Styczynski J, Dytfeld D, et al. Activity of bortezomib in adult de novo and relapsed acute myeloid leukemia. Anticancer Res 2007;27(6B):4021–4025.
384. Romano MF, Petrella A, Bisogni R, et al. Effect of NF-kappaB/Rel inhibition on spontaneous vs chemotherapy-induced apoptosis in AML and normal cord blood CD34+ cells. Leukemia 2003;17(6):1190–1192.
385. Cote S, Rosenauer A, Bianchini A, et al. Response to histone deacetylase inhibition of novel PML/RARalpha mutants detected in retinoic acid-resistant APL cells. Blood 2002;100(7):2586–2596.
386. Ferrara FF, Fazi F, Bianchini A, et al. Histone deacetylase-targeted treatment restores retinoic acid signaling and differentiation in acute myeloid leukemia. Cancer Res 2001;61(1):2–7.
387. Minucci S, Nervi C, Lo Coco F, et al. Histone deacetylases: a common molecular target for differentiation treatment of acute myeloid leukemias? Oncogene 2001;20(24): 3110–3115.
388. Insinga A, Monestiroli S, Ronzoni S, et al. Inhibitors of histone deacetylases induce tumor-selective apoptosis through activation of the death receptor pathway. Nat Med 2005;11(1):71–76.
389. Mistry AR, Pedersen EW, Solomon E, et al. The molecular pathogenesis of acute promyelocytic leukaemia: implications for the clinical management of the disease. Blood Rev 2003;17(2):71–97.
390. Bernard J, Weil M, Boiron M, et al. Acute promyelocytic leukemia: results of treatment by daunorubicin. Blood 1973;41(4):489–496.
391. Cunningham I, Gee TS, Reich LM, et al. Acute promyelocytic leukemia: treatment results during a decade at Memorial Hospital. Blood 1989;73(5):1116–1122.
392. Sanz MA, Jarque I, Martin G, et al. Acute promyelocytic leukemia. Therapy results and prognostic factors. Cancer 1988;61(1):7–13.
393. Carter M, Kalwinsky DK, Dahl GV, et al. Childhood acute promyelocytic leukemia: a rare variant of nonlymphoid leukemia with distinctive clinical and biologic features. Leukemia 1989;3(4):298–302.
394. Rovelli A, Biondi A, Cantu Rajnoldi A, et al. Microgranular variant of acute promyelocytic leukemia in children. J Clin Oncol 1992;10(9):1413–1418.
395. Calleja EM, Warrell RP Jr. Differentiating agents in pediatric malignancies: all-trans-retinoic acid and arsenic in acute promyelocytic leukemia. Curr Oncol Rep 2000;2(6):519–523.
396. Wolf G, Smas CM. Retinoic acid induces the degradation of the leukemogenic protein encoded by the promyelocytic leukemia gene fused to the retinoic acid receptor alpha gene. Nutr Rev 2000;58(7):211–214.
397. Breitman TR, Selonick SE, Collins SJ. Induction of differentiation of the human promyelocytic leukemia cell line (HL-60) by retinoic acid. Proc Natl Acad Sci U S A 1980;77(5):2936–2940.
398. Huang CH, Chen Y, Reid ME, et al. Rhnull disease: the amorph type results from a novel double mutation in RhCe gene on D-negative background. Blood 1998;92(2): 664–671.
399. Degos L, Chomienne C, Daniel MT, et al. Treatment of first relapse in acute promyelocytic leukaemia with all-trans retinoic acid. Lancet 1990;336(8728):1440–1441.
400. Castaigne S, Chomienne C, Daniel MT, et al. All-trans retinoic acid as a differentiation therapy for acute promyelocytic leukemia. I. Clinical results. Blood 1990;76(9): 1704–1709.
401. Warrell RP Jr, Frankel SR, Miller WH Jr, et al. Differentiation therapy of acute promyelocytic leukemia with tretinoin (all-trans-retinoic acid). N Engl J Med 1991;324(20): 1385–1393.
402. Fenaux P, Le Deley MC, Castaigne S, et al. Effect of all transretinoic acid in newly diagnosed acute promyelocytic leukemia. Results of a multicenter randomized trial. European APL 91 Group. Blood 1993;82(11):3241–3249.
403. Fenaux P, Chastang C, Chevret S, et al. A randomized comparison of all transretinoic acid (ATRA) followed by chemotherapy and ATRA plus chemotherapy and the role of maintenance therapy in newly diagnosed acute promyelocytic leukemia. The European APL Group. Blood 1999;94(4):1192–1200.
404. Sanz MA, Martin G, Gonzalez M, et al. Risk-adapted treatment of acute promyelocytic leukemia with all-trans-retinoic acid and anthracycline monochemotherapy: a multicenter study by the PETHEMA group. Blood 2004;103(4):1237–1243.
405. Burnett AK, Grimwade D, Solomon E, et al. Presenting white blood cell count and kinetics of molecular remission predict prognosis in acute promyelocytic leukemia treated with all-trans retinoic acid: result of the Randomized MRC Trial. Blood 1999;93(12):4131–4143.
406. Lengfelder E, Reichert A, Schoch C, et al. Double induction strategy including high dose cytarabine in combination with all-trans retinoic acid: effects in patients with newly diagnosed acute promyelocytic leukemia. German AML Cooperative Group. Leukemia 2000;14(8):1362–1370.
407. de Botton S, Chevret S, Coiteux V, et al. Early onset of chemotherapy can reduce the incidence of ATRA syndrome in newly diagnosed acute promyelocytic leukemia (APL) with low white blood cell counts: results from APL 93 trial. Leukemia 2003;17(2): 339–342.
408. Ades L, Chevret S, Raffoux E, et al. Is cytarabine useful in the treatment of acute promyelocytic leukemia? Results of a randomized trial from the European Acute Promyelocytic Leukemia Group. J Clin Oncol 2006;24(36):5703–5710.
409. Schlenk RF, Germing U, Hartmann F, et al. High-dose cytarabine and mitoxantrone in consolidation therapy for acute promyelocytic leukemia. Leukemia 2005;19(6): 978–983.
410. Testi AM, Biondi A, Lo Coco F, et al. GIMEMA-AIEOPAIDA protocol for the treatment of newly diagnosed acute promyelocytic leukemia (APL) in children. Blood 2005;106(2):447–453.
411. Fenaux P, Chevret S, Guerci A, et al. Long-term follow-up confirms the benefit of all-trans retinoic acid in acute promyelocytic leukemia. European APL group. Leukemia 2000;14(8):1371–1377.
412. Ortega JJ, Madero L, Martin G, et al. Treatment with all-trans retinoic acid and anthracycline monochemotherapy for children with acute promyelocytic leukemia: a multicenter study by the PETHEMA Group. J Clin Oncol 2005;23(30):7632–7640.
413. Zheng PZ, Wang KK, Zhang QY, et al. Systems analysis of transcriptome and proteome in retinoic acid/arsenic trioxide-induced cell differentiation/apoptosis of promyelocytic leukemia. Proc Natl Acad Sci U S A 2005;102(21):7653–7658.
414. Chen GQ, Zhu J, Shi XG, et al. In vitro studies on cellular and molecular mechanisms of arsenic trioxide (As2O3) in the treatment of acute promyelocytic leukemia: As2O3 induces NB4 cell apoptosis with downregulation of Bcl-2 expression and modulation of PML-RAR alpha/PML proteins. Blood 1996;88(3):1052–1061.
415. Niu C, Yan H, Yu T, et al. Studies on treatment of acute promyelocytic leukemia with arsenic trioxide: remission induction, follow-up, and molecular monitoring in 11 newly diagnosed and 47 relapsed acute promyelocytic leukemia patients. Blood 1999;94 (10):3315–3324.
416. Soignet SL, Maslak P, Wang ZG, et al. Complete remission after treatment of acute promyelocytic leukemia with arsenic trioxide. N Engl J Med 1998;339(19):1341–1348.
417. Mathews V, George B, Lakshmi KM, et al. Single-agent arsenic trioxide in the treatment of newly diagnosed acute promyelocytic leukemia: durable remissions with minimal toxicity. Blood 2006;107(7):2627–2632.
418. Ghavamzadeh A, Alimoghaddam K, Ghaffari SH, et al. Treatment of acute promyelocytic leukemia with arsenic trioxide without ATRA and/or chemotherapy. Ann Oncol 2006;17(1):131–134.
419. Shen ZX, Shi ZZ, Fang J, et al. All-trans retinoic acid/As2O3 combination yields a high quality remission and survival in newly diagnosed acute promyelocytic leukemia. Proc Natl Acad Sci U S A 2004;101(15):5328–5335.
420. Oliansky DM, Rizzo JD, Aplan PD, et al. The role of cytotoxic therapy with hematopoietic stem cell transplantation in the therapy of acute myeloid leukemia in children: an evidence-based review. Biol Blood Marrow Transplant 2007;13(1): 1–25.
421. Bourquin JP, Thornley I, Neuberg D, et al. Favorable outcome of allogeneic hematopoietic stem cell transplantation for relapsed or refractory acute promyelocytic leukemia in childhood. Bone Marrow Transplant 2004;34(9):795–798.

422. de Botton S, Fawaz A, Chevret S, et al. Autologous and allogeneic stem-cell transplantation as salvage treatment of acute promyelocytic leukemia initially treated with all-trans-retinoic acid: a retrospective analysis of the European acute promyelocytic leukemia group. J Clin Oncol 2005;23(1):120–126.
423. Cheson BD, Bennett JM, Kopecky KJ, et al. Revised recommendations of the International Working Group for Diagnosis, Standardization of Response Criteria, Treatment Outcomes, and Reporting Standards for Therapeutic Trials in Acute Myeloid Leukemia. J Clin Oncol 2003;21(24):4642–4649.
424. Sanz MA, Tallman MS, Lo-Coco F. Tricks of the trade for the appropriate management of newly diagnosed acute promyelocytic leukemia. Blood 2005;105(8):3019–3025.
425. Lee S, Kim YJ, Eom KS, et al. The significance of minimal residual disease kinetics in adults with newly diagnosed PML-RARalpha-positive acute promyelocytic leukemia: results of a prospective trial. Haematologica 2006;91(5):671–674.
426. Hasle H, Clemmensen IH, Mikkelsen M. Risks of leukaemia and solid tumours in individuals with Down's syndrome. Lancet 2000;355(9199):165–169.
427. Zipursky A, Thorner P, De Harven E, et al. Myelodysplasia and acute megakaryoblastic leukemia in Down's syndrome. Leuk Res 1994;18(3):163–171.
428. Hasle H. Pattern of malignant disorders in individuals with Down's syndrome. Lancet Oncol 2001;2(7):429–436.
429. Hellebostad M, Carpenter E, Hasle H, et al. GATA1 mutation analysis demonstrates two distinct primary leukemias in a child with Down syndrome; implications for leukemogenesis. J Pediatr Hematol Oncol 2005;27(7):408–409.
430. Zipursky A, Brown E, Christensen H, et al. Leukemia and/or myeloproliferative syndrome in neonates with Down syndrome. Semin Perinatol 1997;21(1):97–101.
431. Massey GV, Zipursky A, Doyle J, et al. A prospective study of the natural history of transient leukemia (TL) in neonates with Down syndrome (DS): a Pediatric Oncology Group (POG) study. Blood 2002;100:87a.
432. Slayton WB, Spangrude GJ, Chen Z, et al. Lineage-specific trisomy 21 in a neonate with resolving transient myeloproliferative syndrome. J Pediatr Hematol Oncol 2002;24(3):224–226.
433. Magalhaes IQ, Splendore A, Emerenciano M, et al. Transient neonatal myeloproliferative disorder without Down syndrome and detection of GATA1 mutation. J Pediatr Hematol Oncol 2005;27(1):50–52.
434. Wu SQ, Loh KT, Chen XR, et al. Transient myeloproliferative disorder in a phenotypically normal infant with i(21q) mosaicism. Cancer Genet Cytogenet 2002;136(2):138–140.
435. Hayashi Y, Eguchi M, Sugita K, et al. Cytogenetic findings and clinical features in acute leukemia and transient myeloproliferative disorder in Down's syndrome. Blood 1988;72(1):15–23.
436. Muramatsu H, Kato K, Watanabe N, et al. Risk factors for early death in neonates with Down syndrome and transient leukaemia. Br J Haematol 2008;142(4):610–615.
437. Klusmann JH, Creutzig U, Zimmermann M, et al. Treatment and prognostic impact of transient leukemia in neonates with Down syndrome. Blood 2008;111(6):2991–2998.
438. Lange B. The management of neoplastic disorders of haematopoiesis in children with Down's syndrome. Br J Haematol 2000;110(3):512–524.
439. Hasle H, Lund B, Nyvold CG, et al. WT1 gene expression in children with Down syndrome and transient myeloproliferative disorder. Leuk Res 2006;30(5):543–546.
440. Lange BJ, Kobrinsky N, Barnard DR, et al. Distinctive demography, biology, and outcome of acute myeloid leukemia and myelodysplastic syndrome in children with Down syndrome: Children's Cancer Group Studies 2861 and 2891. Blood 1998;91(2):608–615.
441. Hasle H, Kerndrup G, Jacobsen BB. Childhood myelodysplastic syndrome in Denmark: incidence and predisposing conditions. Leukemia 1995;9(9):1569–1572.
442. Gamis A, Alonzo T, Lange B, et al. Acute myelogenous leukemia (AML) in Downs Syndrome (DS) patients: Outcome, toxicities, and prognostic factors from the CCG 2891 trial. Blood 2001;98:720a.
443. Hasle H, Abrahamsson J, Arola M, et al. Myeloid leukemia in children 4 years or older with Down syndrome often lacks GATA1 mutation and cytogenetics and risk of relapse are more akin to sporadic AML. Leukemia 2008;22(7):1428–1430.
444. Creutzig U, Reinhardt D, Diekamp S, et al. AML patients with Down syndrome have a high cure rate with AML-BFM therapy with reduced dose intensity. Leukemia 2005;19(8):1355–1360.
445. Zeller B, Gustafsson G, Forestier E, et al. Acute leukaemia in children with Down syndrome: a population-based Nordic study. Br J Haematol 2005;128(6):797–804.
446. Ferster A, Verhest A, Vamos E, et al. Leukemia in a trisomy 21 mosaic: specific involvement of the trisomic cells. Cancer Genet Cytogenet 1986;20(1–2):109–113.
447. Simon JH, Tebbi CK, Freeman AI, et al. Acute megakaryoblastic leukemia associated with mosaic Down's syndrome. Cancer 1987;60(10):2515–2520.
448. Tunstall-Pedoe O, Roy A, Karadimitris A, et al. Abnormalities in the myeloid progenitor compartment in Down syndrome fetal liver precede acquisition of GATA1 mutations. Blood 2008;112(12):4507–4511.
449. Wechsler J, Greene M, McDevitt MA, et al. Acquired mutations in GATA1 in the megakaryoblastic leukemia of Down syndrome. Nat Genet 2002;32(1):148–152.
450. Mundschau G, Gurbuxani S, Gamis AS, et al. Mutagenesis of GATA1 is an initiating event in Down syndrome leukemogenesis. Blood 2003;101(11):4298–4300.
451. Rainis L, Bercovich D, Strehl S, et al. Mutations in exon 2 of GATA1 are early events in megakaryocytic malignancies associated with trisomy 21. Blood 2003;102(3):981–986.
452. Zipursky A, Wang H, Brown EJ, et al. Interphase cytogenetic analysis of in vivo differentiation in the myelodysplasia of Down syndrome. Blood 1994;84(7):2278–2282.
453. Bourquin JP, Subramanian A, Langebrake C, et al. Identification of distinct molecular phenotypes in acute megakaryoblastic leukemia by gene expression profiling. Proc Natl Acad Sci U S A 2006;103(9):3339–3344.
454. Pine SR, Guo Q, Yin C, et al. Incidence and clinical implications of GATA1 mutations in newborns with Down syndrome. Blood 2007;110(6):2128–2131.
455. Forestier E, Izraeli S, Beverloo B, et al. Cytogenetic features of acute lymphoblastic and myeloid leukemias in pediatric patients with Down syndrome: an iBFM-SG study. Blood 2008;111(3):1575–1583.
456. Slordahl SH, Smeland EB, Holte H, et al. Leukemic blasts with markers of four cell lineages in Down's syndrome ("megakaryoblastic leukemia"). Med Pediatr Oncol 1993;21(4):254–258.
457. Rao A, Hills RK, Stiller C, et al. Treatment for myeloid leukaemia of Down syndrome: population-based experience in the UK and results from the Medical Research Council AML 10 and AML 12 trials. Br J Haematol 2006;132(5):576–583.
458. Abildgaard L, Ellebaek E, Gustafsson G, et al. Optimal treatment intensity in children with Down syndrome and myeloid leukaemia: data from 56 children treated on NOPHO-AML protocols and a review of the literature. Ann Hematol 2006;85(5):275–280.
459. Kudo K, Kojima S, Tabuchi K, et al. Prospective study of a pirarubicin, intermediate-dose cytarabine, and etoposide regimen in children with Down syndrome and acute myeloid leukemia: the Japanese Childhood AML Cooperative Study Group. J Clin Oncol 2007;25(34):5442–5447.
460. Frost BM, Gustafsson G, Larsson R, et al. Cellular cytotoxic drug sensitivity in children with acute leukemia and Down's syndrome: an explanation to differences in clinical outcome? Leukemia 2000;14(5):943–944.
461. Taub JW, Huang X, Matherly LH, et al. Expression of chromosome 21-localized genes in acute myeloid leukemia: differences between Down syndrome and non-Down syndrome blast cells and relationship to in vitro sensitivity to cytosine arabinoside and daunorubicin. Blood 1999;94(4):1393–1400.
462. Ge Y, Jensen T, James SJ, et al. High frequency of the 844ins68 cystathionine-beta-synthase gene variant in Down syndrome children with acute myeloid leukemia. Leukemia 2002;16(11):2339–2341.
463. Lopes LF, Lorand-Metze I. Childhood myelodysplastic syndromes in a Brazilian population. Pediatr Hematol Oncol 1999;16(4):347–353.
464. Elghetany MT. Myelodysplastic syndromes in children: a critical review of issues in the diagnosis and classification of 887 cases from 13 published series. Arch Pathol Lab Med 2007;131(7):1110–1116.
465. Polychronopoulou S, Panagiotou JP, Kossiva L, et al. Clinical and morphological features of paediatric myelodysplastic syndromes: a review of 34 cases. Acta Paediatr 2004;93(8):1015–1023.
466. Hasle H, Baumann I, Bergstrasser E, et al. The International Prognostic Scoring System (IPSS) for childhood myelodysplastic syndrome (MDS) and juvenile myelomonocytic leukemia (JMML). Leukemia 2004;18(12):2008–2014.
467. Creutzig U, Cantu-Rajnoldi A, Ritter J, et al. Myelodysplastic syndromes in childhood. Report of 21 patients from Italy and West Germany. Am J Pediatr Hematol Oncol 1987;9(4):324–330.
468. Tuncer MA, Pagliuca A, Hicsonmez G, et al. Primary myelodysplastic syndrome in children: the clinical experience in 33 cases. Br J Haematol 1992;82(2):347–353.
469. Steliarova-Foucher E, Stiller C, Lacour B, et al. International Classification of Childhood Cancer, third edition. Cancer 2005;103(7):1457–1467.
470. Wegelius R. Bone marrow dysfunctions preceding acute leukemia in children: a clinical study. Leuk Res 1992;16(1):71–76.
471. Bernard J, Schaison G. Transitory bone marrow failure. A series of 13 preleukemic cases in children. Am J Pediatr Hematol Oncol 1980;2:141–144.
472. Evans JP, Czepulkowski B, Gibbons B, et al. Childhood monosomy 7 revisited. Br J Haematol 1988;69(1):41–45.
473. Hann IM. Myelodysplastic syndromes. Arch Dis Child 1992;67(7):962–966.
474. Baranger L, Baruchel A, Leverger G, et al. Monosomy-7 in childhood hemopoietic disorders. Leukemia 1990;4(5):345–349.
475. Bennett JM, Catovsky D, Daniel MT, et al. Proposals for the classification of the myelodysplastic syndromes. Br J Haematol 1982;51(2):189–199.
476. Mandel K, Dror Y, Poon A, et al. A practical, comprehensive classification for pediatric myelodysplastic syndromes: the CCC system. J Pediatr Hematol Oncol 2002;24(7):596–605.
477. Aktas D, Tuncbilek E. Myelodysplastic syndrome associated with monosomy 7 in childhood: a retrospective study. Cancer Genet Cytogenet 2006;171(1):72–75.
478. Goel R, Kumar R, Bakhshi S. Transformation of childhood MDS-refractory anemia to acute lymphoblastic leukemia. J Pediatr Hematol Oncol 2007;29(10):725–727.
479. Delhommeau F, Dupont S, Della Valle V, et al. Mutation in TET2 in myeloid cancers. N Engl J Med 2009;360(22):2289–2301.
480. Head DR. Revised classification of acute myeloid leukemia. Leukemia 1996;10(11):1826–1831.
481. Loeb LA. A mutator phenotype in cancer. Cancer Res 2001;61(8):3230–3239.
482. Maserati E, Minelli A, Pressato B, et al. Shwachman syndrome as mutator phenotype responsible for myeloid dysplasia/neoplasia through karyotype instability and chromosomes 7 and 20 anomalies. Genes Chromosomes Cancer 2006;45(4):375–382.
483. Sheng XM, Kawamura M, Ohnishi H, et al. Mutations of the RAS genes in childhood acute myeloid leukemia, myelodysplastic syndrome and juvenile chronic myelocytic leukemia. Leuk Res 1997;21(8):697–701.
484. Tamaki H, Ogawa H, Ohyashiki K, et al. The Wilms' tumor gene WT1 is a good marker for diagnosis of disease progression of myelodysplastic syndromes. Leukemia 1999;13(3):393–399.
485. Hasegawa D, Manabe A, Kubota T, et al. Methylation status of the p15 and p16 genes in paediatric myelodysplastic syndrome and juvenile myelomonocytic leukaemia. Br J Haematol 2005;128(6):805–812.
486. Vidal DO, Paixao VA, Brait M, et al. Aberrant methylation in pediatric myelodysplastic syndrome. Leuk Res 2007;31(2):175–181.
487. Jekic B, Novakovic I, Lukovic L, et al. Lack of TP53 and FMS gene mutations in children with myelodysplastic syndrome. Cancer Genet Cytogenet 2006;166(2):163–165.
488. Jekic B, Novakovic I, Lukovic L, et al. Low frequency of NRAS and KRAS2 gene mutations in childhood myelodysplastic syndromes. Cancer Genet Cytogenet 2004;154(2):180–182.
489. Field JJ, Mason PJ, An P, et al. Low frequency of telomerase RNA mutations among children with aplastic anemia or myelodysplastic syndrome. J Pediatr Hematol Oncol 2006;28(7):450–453.
490. Ortmann CA, Niemeyer CM, Wawer A, et al. TERC mutations in children with refractory cytopenia. Haematologica 2006;91(5):707–708.
491. Roela RA, Carraro DM, Brentani HP, et al. Gene stage-specific expression in the microenvironment of pediatric myelodysplastic syndromes. Leuk Res 2007;31(5):579–589.
492. Hicsonmez G, Cetin M, Yenicesu I, et al. Evaluation of children with myelodysplastic syndrome: importance of extramedullary disease as a presenting symptom. Leuk Lymphoma 2001;42(4):665–674.
493. Cantu Rajnoldi A, Fenu S, Kerndrup G, et al. Evaluation of dysplastic features in myelodysplastic syndromes: experience from the morphology group of the European Working Group of MDS in Childhood (EWOG-MDS). Ann Hematol 2005;84(7):429–433.
494. Barnard DR, Kalousek DK, Wiersma SR, et al. Morphologic, immunologic, and cytogenetic classification of acute myeloid leukemia and myelodysplastic syndrome in childhood: a report from the Childrens Cancer Group. Leukemia 1996;10(1):5–12.
495. Della Porta MG, Malcovati L, Boveri E, et al. Clinical relevance of bone marrow fibrosis and CD34-positive cell clusters in primary myelodysplastic syndromes. J Clin Oncol 2009;27(5):754–762.
496. Rosati S, Anastasi J, Vardiman J. Recurring diagnostic problems in the pathology of the myelodysplastic syndromes. Semin Hematol 1996;33(2):111–126.

497. Hasle H. Myelodysplastic syndromes in childhood—classification, epidemiology, and treatment. Leuk Lymphoma 1994;13(1–2):11–26.
498. Forty-four cases of childhood myelodysplasia with cytogenetics, documented by the Groupe Francais de Cytogenetique Hematologique. Leukemia 1997;11(9):1478–1485.
499. Gohring G, Michalova K, Beverloo B, et al. A complex karyotype but not monosomy 7 is an independent prognostic factor in advanced childhood MDS [abstract 2452]. Blood 2007;110.
500. Latger-Cannard V, Buisine J, Fenneteau O, et al. Dysgranulopoiesis, low blast count and t(8;21): an unusual presentation of t(8;21) AML according to the WHO classification: a pediatric experience. Leuk Res 2001;25(11):1023–1024.
501. Valent P, Horny HP, Bennett JM, et al. Definitions and standards in the diagnosis and treatment of the myelodysplastic syndromes: consensus statements and report from a working conference. Leuk Res 2007;31(6):727–736.
502. Veltroni M, Sainati L, Zecca M, et al. Advanced pediatric myelodysplastic syndromes: can immunophenotypic characterization of blast cells be a diagnostic and prognostic tool? Pediatr Blood Cancer 2009;52(3):357–363.
503. Fuhrer M, Rampf U, Bender-Goetze C. Mean corpuscular volume (MCV) in patients with aplastic anemia does this parameter select patients with clonal disease? A retrospective analysis of data of the SAA 944 study. Leukemia 2000;14:961.
504. Fohlmeister I, Fischer R, Modder B, et al. Aplastic anaemia and the hypocellular myelodysplastic syndrome: histomorphological, diagnostic, and prognostic features. J Clin Pathol 1985;38(11):1218–1224.
505. Elghetany MT, Hudnall SD, Gardner FH. Peripheral blood picture in primary hypocellular refractory anemia and idiopathic acquired aplastic anemia: an additional tool for differential diagnosis. Haematologica 1997;82(1):21–24.
506. Goyal R, Varma N, Marwaha RK. Myelodysplastic syndrome with erythroid hypoplasia. J Clin Pathol 2005;58(3):320–321.
507. Al-Rahawan MM, Alter BP, Bryant BJ, et al. Bone marrow cell cycle markers in inherited bone marrow failure syndromes. Leuk Res 2008;32(12):1793–1799.
508. Hasle H, Kerndrup G, Jacobsen BB, et al. Chronic parvovirus infection mimicking myelodysplastic syndrome in a child with subclinical immunodeficiency. Am J Pediatr Hematol Oncol 1994;16(4):329–333.
509. Yarali N, Duru F, Sipahi T, et al. Parvovirus B19 infection reminiscent of myelodysplastic syndrome in three children with chronic hemolytic anemia. Pediatr Hematol Oncol 2000;17(6):475–482.
510. Kagialis-Girard S, Durand B, Mialou V, et al. Human herpesvirus 6 infection and transient acquired myelodysplasia in children. Pediatr Blood Cancer 2006;47(5):543–548.
511. Mueller BU, Tannenbaum S, Pizzo PA. Bone marrow aspirates and biopsies in children with human immunodeficiency virus infection. J Pediatr Hematol Oncol 1996;18(3): 266–271.
512. Yarali N, Fisgin T, Duru F, et al. Myelodysplastic features in visceral leishmaniasis. Am J Hematol 2002;71(3):191–195.
513. Wollman MR, Penchansky L, Shekhter-Levin S. Transient 7q− in association with megaloblastic anemia due to dietary folate and vitamin B12 deficiency. J Pediatr Hematol Oncol 1996;18(2):162–165.
514. Koca E, Buyukasik Y, Cetiner D, et al. Copper deficiency with increased hematogones mimicking refractory anemia with excess blasts. Leuk Res 2008;32(3):495–499.
515. Angotti LB, Post GR, Robinson NS, et al. Pancytopenia with myelodysplasia due to copper deficiency. Pediatr Blood Cancer 2008;51(5):693–695.
516. Brichard B, Vermylen C, Scheiff JM, et al. Haematological disturbances during long-term valproate therapy. Eur J Pediatr 1994;153(5):378–380.
517. Gesundheit B, Kirby M, Lau W, et al. Thrombocytopenia and megakaryocyte dysplasia: an adverse effect of valproic acid treatment. J Pediatr Hematol Oncol 2002;24(7): 589–590.
518. Yetgin S, Ozen S, Saatci U, et al. Myelodysplastic features in juvenile rheumatoid arthritis. Am J Hematol 1997;54(2):166–169.
519. Hinson DD, Rogers ZR, Hoffmann GF, et al. Hematological abnormalities and cholestatic liver disease in two patients with mevalonate kinase deficiency. Am J Med Genet 1998;78(5):408–412.
520. Bader-Meunier B, Rieux-Laucat F, Croisille L, et al. Dyserythropoiesis associated with a fas-deficient condition in childhood. Br J Haematol 2000;108(2):300–304.
521. Hirose M, Taguchi Y, Makimoto A, et al. New variant of congenital dyserythropoietic anemia with trilineage myelodysplasia. Acta Haematol 1995;94(2):102–104.
522. Kratz CP, Rogge T, Kopp M, et al. Myelodysplastic features in an infant with cystic fibrosis presenting with anaemia, oedema and failure to thrive. Eur J Pediatr 2005;164(1):56–57.
523. Finsterer J. Hematological manifestations of primary mitochondrial disorders. Acta Haematol 2007;118(2):88–98.
524. Atale A, Bonneau-Amati P, Rotig A, et al. Tubulopathy and pancytopaenia with normal pancreatic function: a variant of Pearson syndrome. Eur J Med Genet 2009;52(1): 23–26.
525. Hasle H, Kerndrup G, Yssing M, et al. Intensive chemotherapy in childhood myelodysplastic syndrome. A comparison with results in acute myeloid leukemia. Leukemia 1996;10(8):1269–1273.
526. Webb DK, Passmore SJ, Hann IM, et al. Results of treatment of children with refractory anaemia with excess blasts (RAEB) and RAEB in transformation (RAEBt) in Great Britain 1990–99. Br J Haematol 2002;117(1):33–39.
527. Head DR. Proposed changes in the definitions of acute myeloid leukemia and myelodysplastic syndrome: are they helpful? Curr Opin Oncol 2002;14(1):19–23.
528. Anderson JE, Appelbaum FR, Schoch G, et al. Allogeneic marrow transplantation for refractory anemia: a comparison of two preparative regimens and analysis of prognostic factors. Blood 1996;87(1):51–58.
529. Scheurlen W, Borkhardt A, Ritterbach J, et al. Spontaneous hematological remission in a boy with myelodysplastic syndrome and monosomy 7. Leukemia 1994;8(8): 1435–1438.
530. Benaim E, Hvizdala EV, Papenhausen P, et al. Spontaneous remission in monosomy 7 myelodysplastic syndrome. Br J Haematol 1995;89(4):947–948.
531. Mantadakis E, Shannon KM, Singer DA, et al. Transient monosomy 7: a case series in children and review of the literature. Cancer 1999;85(12):2655–2661.
532. De Simone A, Cantu Rajnoldi A, Sainati L, et al. Spontaneous remission from RAEB in a child. Leukemia 2001;15(5):856–857.
533. Parker TM, Klaassen RJ, Johnston DL. Spontaneous remission of myelodysplastic syndrome with monosomy 7 in a young boy. Cancer Genet Cytogenet 2008;182(2): 122–125.
534. Sauntharajah Y, Nakamura R, Nam JM, et al. HLA-DR15 (DR2) is overrepresented in myelodysplastic syndrome and aplastic anemia and predicts a response to immunosuppression in myelodysplastic syndrome. Blood 2002;100(5):1570–1574.
535. Steensma DP, Dispenzieri A, Moore SB, et al. Antithymocyte globulin has limited efficacy and substantial toxicity in unselected anemic patients with myelodysplastic syndrome. Blood 2003;101(6):2156–2158.
536. Yoshimi A, Baumann I, Fuhrer M, et al. Immunosuppressive therapy with anti-thymocyte globulin and cyclosporine A in selected children with hypoplastic refractory cytopenia. Haematologica 2007;92(3):397–400.
537. Fenaux P, Mufti GJ, Hellstrom-Lindberg E, et al. Efficacy of azacitidine compared with that of conventional care regimens in the treatment of higher-risk myelodysplastic syndromes: a randomised, open-label, phase III study. Lancet Oncol 2009;10(3):223–232.
538. de Witte T, Suciu S, Verhoef G, et al. Intensive chemotherapy followed by allogeneic or autologous stem cell transplantation for patients with myelodysplastic syndromes (MDSs) and acute myeloid leukemia following MDS. Blood 2001;98(8):2326–2331.
539. Locatelli F, Pession A, Bonetti F, et al. Busulfan, cyclophosphamide and melphalan as conditioning regimen for bone marrow transplantation in children with myelodysplastic syndromes. Leukemia 1994;8(5):844–849.
540. Nichols K, Parsons SK, Guinan E. Long-term follow-up of 12 pediatric patients with primary myelodysplastic syndrome treated with HLA-identical sibling donor bone marrow transplantation. Blood 1996;87(9):4020–4022.
541. Rubie H, Attal M, Demur C, et al. Intensified conditioning regimen with busulfan followed by allogeneic BMT in children with myelodysplastic syndromes. Bone Marrow Transplant 1994;13(6):759–762.
542. Leahey AM, Friedman DL, Bunin NJ. Bone marrow transplantation in pediatric patients with therapy-related myelodysplasia and leukemia. Bone Marrow Transplant 1999;23(1):21–25.
543. Davies SM, Wagner JE, Defor T, et al. Unrelated donor bone marrow transplantation for children and adolescents with aplastic anaemia or myelodysplasia. Br J Haematol 1997;96(4):749–756.
544. Hongeng S, Krance RA, Bowman LC, et al. Outcomes of transplantation with matched-sibling and unrelated-donor bone marrow in children with leukaemia. Lancet 1997;350(9080):767–771.
545. Deeg HJ, Storer B, Slattery JT, et al. Conditioning with targeted busulfan and cyclophosphamide for hemopoietic stem cell transplantation from related and unrelated donors in patients with myelodysplastic syndrome. Blood 2002;100(4):1201–1207.
546. de Witte T, Hermans J, Vossen J, et al. Haematopoietic stem cell transplantation for patients with myelo-dysplastic syndromes and secondary acute myeloid leukaemias: a report on behalf of the Chronic Leukaemia Working Party of the European Group for Blood and Marrow Transplantation (EBMT). Br J Haematol 2000;110(3):620–630.
547. Locatelli F, Zecca M, Duffner U, et al. Busulfan, cyclophosphamide and melphalan as pretransplant conditioning regimen for children with MDS and JMML. Interim analysis of the EWOG-MDS/EBMT prospective study. Leukemia 2000;14:971.
548. Castro-Malaspina H, Harris RE, Gajewski J, et al. Unrelated donor marrow transplantation for myelodysplastic syndromes: outcome analysis in 510 transplants facilitated by the National Marrow Donor Program. Blood 2002;99(6):1943–1951.
549. Locatelli F, Noellke P, Fischer A, et al. Hematopoietic stem cell transplantation (HSCT) after a myeloablative conditioning regimen in children with refractory cytopenia (RC): results of a retrospective analysis from the EWOG-MDS group [abstract 251]. Blood 2007:110.
550. Anderson JE, Appelbaum FR, Schoch G, et al. Allogeneic marrow transplantation for myelodysplastic syndrome with advanced disease morphology: a phase II study of busulfan, cyclophosphamide, and total-body irradiation and analysis of prognostic factors. J Clin Oncol 1996;14(1):220–226.
551. Sutton L, Chastang C, Ribaud P, et al. Factors influencing outcome in de novo myelodysplastic syndromes treated by allogeneic bone marrow transplantation: a long-term study of 71 patients Societe Francaise de Greffe de Moelle. Blood 1996;88(1):358–365.
552. Sierra J, Perez WS, Rozman C, et al. Bone marrow transplantation from HLA-identical siblings as treatment for myelodysplasia. Blood 2002;100(6):1997–2004.
553. Martino R, Caballero MD, Perez-Simon JA, et al. Evidence for a graft-versus-leukemia effect after allogeneic peripheral blood stem cell transplantation with reduced-intensity conditioning in acute myelogenous leukemia and myelodysplastic syndromes. Blood 2002;100(6):2243–2245.
554. Strahm B, Locatelli F, Bader P, et al. Reduced intensity conditioning in unrelated donor transplantation for refractory cytopenia in childhood. Bone Marrow Transplant 2007; 40(4):329–333.
555. Niemeyer CM, Kratz CP. Paediatric myelodysplastic syndromes and juvenile myelomonocytic leukaemia: molecular classification and treatment options. Br J Haematol 2008;140(6):610–624.
556. Kalwak K, Wojcik D, Gorczynska E, et al. Allogeneic hematopoietic cell transplantation from alternative donors in children with myelodysplastic syndrome: is that an alternative? Transplant Proc 2004;36(5):1574–1577.
557. Okumura H, Takamatsu H, Yoshida T. Donor leucocyte transfusions for relapse in myelodysplastic syndrome after allogeneic bone marrow transplantation. Br J Haematol 1996;93(2):386–388.
558. Beck JF, Klingebiel T, Kreyenberg H, et al. Relapse of childhood ALL, AML and MDS after allogeneic stem cell transplantation can be prevented by donor lymphocyte infusion in a critical stage of increasing mixed chimerism. Klin Padiatr 2002;214(4): 201–205.
559. Tamura K, Kanazawa T, Suzuki M, et al. Successful rapid discontinuation of immunosuppressive therapy at molecular relapse after allogeneic bone marrow transplantation in a pediatric patient with myelodysplastic syndrome. Am J Hematol 2006;81(2): 139–141.
560. Skinner R, Velangi M, Bown N. Donor lymphocyte infusions for post-transplant relapse of refractory anemia with excess blasts and monosomy 7. Pediatr Blood Cancer 2008;50(3):670–672.
561. Bader P, Niemeyer C, Willasch A, et al. Children with myelodysplastic syndrome (MDS) and increasing mixed chimaerism after allogeneic stem cell transplantation have a poor outcome which can be improved by pre-emptive immunotherapy. Br J Haematol 2005;128(5):649–658.
562. Bader P, Niemeyer C, Weber G, et al. WT1 gene expression: useful marker for minimal residual disease in childhood myelodysplastic syndromes and juvenile myelo-monocytic leukemia? Eur J Haematol 2004;73(1):25–28.
563. Yakoub-Agha I, de La Salmoniere P, Ribaud P, et al. Allogeneic bone marrow transplantation for therapy-related myelodysplastic syndrome and acute myeloid leukemia: a long-term study of 70 patients-report of the French society of bone marrow transplantation. J Clin Oncol 2000;18(5):963–971.
564. Tsurusawa M, Manabe A, Hayashi Y, et al. Therapy-related myelodysplastic syndrome in childhood: a retrospective study of 36 patients in Japan. Leuk Res 2005;29(6): 625–632.

565. Woodard P, Barfield R, Hale G, et al. Outcome of hematopoietic stem cell transplantation for pediatric patients with therapy-related acute myeloid leukemia or myelodysplastic syndrome. Pediatr Blood Cancer 2006;47(7):931–935.
566. Chang C, Storer BE, Scott BL, et al. Hematopoietic cell transplantation in patients with myelodysplastic syndrome or acute myeloid leukemia arising from myelodysplastic syndrome: similar outcomes in patients with de novo disease and disease following prior therapy or antecedent hematologic disorders. Blood 2007;110(4):1379–1387.
567. Cesaro S, Oneto R, Messina C, et al. Haematopoietic stem cell transplantation for Shwachman-Diamond disease: a study from the European Group for Blood and Marrow Transplantation. Br J Haematol 2005;131(2):231–236.
568. Hardisty RM, Speed DE, Till M. Granulocytic leukaemia in childhood. Br J Haematol 1964;10:551–566.
569. Niemeyer CM, Arico M, Basso G, et al. Chronic myelomonocytic leukemia in childhood: a retrospective analysis of 110 cases. European Working Group on Myelodysplastic Syndromes in Childhood (EWOG-MDS). Blood 1997;89(10):3534–3543.
570. Stiller CA, Chessells JM, Fitchett M. Neurofibromatosis and childhood leukaemia/lymphoma: a population-based UKCCSG study. Br J Cancer 1994;70(5):969–972.
571. Bader-Meunier B, Tchernia G, Mielot F, et al. Occurrence of myeloproliferative disorder in patients with Noonan syndrome. J Pediatr 1997;130(6):885–889.
572. Fukuda M, Horibe K, Miyajima Y, et al. Spontaneous remission of juvenile chronic myelomonocytic leukemia in an infant with Noonan syndrome. J Pediatr Hematol Oncol 1997;19(2):177–179.
573. Choong K, Freedman MH, Chitayat D, et al. Juvenile myelomonocytic leukemia and Noonan syndrome. J Pediatr Hematol Oncol 1999;21(6):523–527.
574. Kratz CP, Niemeyer CM, Castleberry RP, et al. The mutational spectrum of PTPN11 in juvenile myelomonocytic leukemia and Noonan syndrome/myeloproliferative disease. Blood 2005;106(6):2183–2185.
575. Bader-Meunier B, Thollot F, Mielot F, et al. Regressive myelodysplastic syndromes in children. Committee on Childhood Myelodysplasia of the Society of Pediatric Hematology and Immunology [in French]. Arch Fr Pediatr 1992;49(10):883–886.
576. Kratz CP, Zampino G, Kriek M, et al. Craniosynostosis in patients with Noonan syndrome caused by germline KRAS mutations. Am J Med Genet A 2009;149A(5):1036–1040.
577. Kotecha N, Flores NJ, Irish JM, et al. Single-cell profiling identifies aberrant STAT5 activation in myeloid malignancies with specific clinical and biologic correlates. Cancer Cell 2008;14(4):335–343.
578. Kratz CP, Nathrath M, Freisinger P, et al. Lethal proliferation of erythroid precursors in a neonate with a germline PTPN11 mutation. Eur J Pediatr 2006;165(3):182–185.
579. Cheong JL, Moorkamp MH. Respiratory failure, juvenile myelomonocytic leukemia, and neonatal Noonan syndrome. J Pediatr Hematol Oncol 2007;29(4):262–264.
580. Niihori T, Aoki Y, Ohashi H, et al. Functional analysis of PTPN11/SHP-2 mutants identified in Noonan syndrome and childhood leukemia. J Hum Genet 2005;50(4):192–202.
581. Tartaglia M, Niemeyer CM, Fragale A, et al. Somatic mutations in PTPN11 in juvenile myelomonocytic leukemia, myelodysplastic syndromes and acute myeloid leukemia. Nat Genet 2003;34(2):148–150.
582. Loh ML, Vattikuti S, Schubbert S, et al. Mutations in PTPN11 implicate the SHP-2 phosphatase in leukemogenesis. Blood 2004;103(6):2325–2331.
583. Kratz CP, Schubbert S, Bollag G, et al. Germline mutations in components of the Ras signaling pathway in Noonan syndrome and related disorders. Cell Cycle 2006;5(15):1607–1611.
584. Schubbert S, Zenker M, Rowe SL, et al. Germline KRAS mutations cause Noonan syndrome. Nat Genet 2006;38(3):331–336.
585. Matsuda K, Shimada A, Yoshida N, et al. Spontaneous improvement of hematologic abnormalities in patients having juvenile myelomonocytic leukemia with specific RAS mutations. Blood 2007;109(12):5477–5480.
586. Flotho C, Kratz CP, Bergstrasser E, et al. Genotype-phenotype correlation in cases of juvenile myelomonocytic leukemia with clonal RAS mutations. Blood 2008;111(2):966–967; author reply 967–968.
587. Kratz CP, Niemeyer CM, Thomas C, et al. Mutation analysis of Son of Sevenless in juvenile myelomonocytic leukemia. Leukemia 2007;21(5):1108–1109.
588. de Vries AC, Stam RW, Kratz CP, et al. Mutation analysis of the BRAF oncogene in juvenile myelomonocytic leukemia. Haematologica 2007;92(11):1574–1575.
589. Harbott J, Haas O, Kerndrup G, et al. Cytogenetic evaluation of children with MDS and JMML. Results of the European working group of childhood MDS (EWOG-MDS). Leukemia 2000;14:961.
590. Herrod HG, Dow LW, Sullivan JL. Persistent epstein-barr virus infection mimicking juvenile chronic myelogenous leukemia: immunologic and hematologic studies. Blood 1983;61(6):1098–1104.
591. Kirby MA, Weitzman S, Freedman MH. Juvenile chronic myelogenous leukemia: differentiation from infantile cytomegalovirus infection. Am J Pediatr Hematol Oncol 1990;12(3):292–296.
592. Lorenzana A, Lyons H, Sawaf H, et al. Human herpes virus-6 (HHV-6) infection in an infant mimicking juvenile chronic myelogenous leukemia. J Pediatr Hematol Oncol 1997;19:370.
593. Gupta N, Gupta R, Bakhshi S. Transient myeloproliferation mimicking JMML associated with parvovirus infection of infancy. Pediatr Blood Cancer 2009;52(3):411–413.
594. Yetgin S, Cetin M, Yenicesu I, et al. Acute parvovirus B19 infection mimicking juvenile myelomonocytic leukemia. Eur J Haematol 2000;65(4):276–278.
595. Watanabe N, Yoshimi A, Kamachi Y, et al. Wiskott-Aldrich syndrome is an important differential diagnosis in male infants with juvenile myelomonocytic leukemialike features. J Pediatr Hematol Oncol 2007;29(12):836–838.
596. Karow A, Baumann I, Niemeyer CM. Morphologic differential diagnosis of juvenile myelomonocytic leukemia—pitfalls apart from viral infection. J Pediatr Hematol Oncol 2009;31(5):380.
597. Kuijpers TW, Van Lier RA, Hamann D, et al. Leukocyte adhesion deficiency type 1 (LAD-1)/variant. A novel immunodeficiency syndrome characterized by dysfunctional beta2 integrins. J Clin Invest 1997;100(7):1725–1733.
598. Busque L, Gilliland DG, Prchal JT, et al. Clonality in juvenile chronic myelogenous leukemia. Blood 1995;85(1):21–30.
599. Lapidot T, Grunberger T, Vormoor J, et al. Identification of human juvenile chronic myelogenous leukemia stem cells capable of initiating the disease in primary and secondary SCID mice. Blood 1996;88(7):2655–2664.
600. Nakazawa T, Koike K, Agematsu K, et al. Cytogenetic clonality analysis in monosomy 7 associated with juvenile myelomonocytic leukemia: clonality in B and NK cells, but not in T cells. Leuk Res 1998;22(10):887–892.
601. Flotho C, Valcamonica S, Mach-Pascual S, et al. RAS mutations and clonality analysis in children with juvenile myelomonocytic leukemia (JMML). Leukemia 1999;13(1):32–37.
602. Cooper LJ, Shannon KM, Loken MR, et al. Evidence that juvenile myelomonocytic leukemia can arise from a pluripotential stem cell. Blood 2000;96(6):2310–2313.
603. Barak Y, Levin S, Vogel R, et al. Juvenile and adult types of chronic granulocytic leukemia of childhood: growth patterns and characteristics of granulocyte-macrophage colony forming cells. Am J Hematol 1981;10(3):269–275.
604. Estrov Z, Zimmerman B, Grunberger T, et al. Characterization of malignant peripheral blood cells of juvenile chronic myelogenous leukemia. Cancer Res 1986;46(12 Pt 1):6456–6461.
605. Emanuel PD, Shannon KM, Castleberry RP. Juvenile myelomonocytic leukemia: molecular understanding and prospects for therapy. Mol Med Today 1996;2(11):468–475.
606. Frankel AE, Lilly M, Kreitman R, et al. Diphtheria toxin fused to granulocyte-macrophage colony-stimulating factor is toxic to blasts from patients with juvenile myelomonocytic leukemia and chronic myelomonocytic leukemia. Blood 1998;92(11):4279–4286.
607. Iversen PO, Rodwell RL, Pitcher L, et al. Inhibition of proliferation and induction of apoptosis in juvenile myelomonocytic leukemic cells by the granulocyte-macrophage colony-stimulating factor analogue E21R. Blood 1996;88(7):2634–2639.
608. Iversen PO, Lewis ID, Turczynowicz S, et al. Inhibition of granulocyte-macrophage colony-stimulating factor prevents dissemination and induces remission of juvenile myelomonocytic leukemia in engrafted immunodeficient mice. Blood 1997;90(12):4910–4917.
609. Koike K, Matsuda K. Recent advances in the pathogenesis and management of juvenile myelomonocytic leukaemia. Br J Haematol 2008;141(5):567–575.
610. Emanuel PD. Juvenile myelomonocytic leukemia and chronic myelomonocytic leukemia. Leukemia 2008;22(7):1335–1342.
611. Chan RJ, Cooper T, Kratz CP, et al. Juvenile myelomonocytic leukemia: a report from the 2nd International JMML Symposium. Leuk Res 2009;33(3):355–362.
612. Miyauchi J, Asada M, Sasaki M, et al. Mutations of the N-ras gene in juvenile chronic myelogenous leukemia. Blood 1994;83(8):2248–2254.
613. Kalra R, Paderanga DC, Olson K, et al. Genetic analysis is consistent with the hypothesis that NF1 limits myeloid cell growth through p21ras. Blood 1994;84(10):3435–3439.
614. Shannon KM, Watterson J, Johnson P, et al. Monosomy 7 myeloproliferative disease in children with neurofibromatosis, type 1: epidemiology and molecular analysis. Blood 1992;79(5):1311–1318.
615. Side LE, Emanuel PD, Taylor B, et al. Mutations of the NF1 gene in children with juvenile myelomonocytic leukemia without clinical evidence of neurofibromatosis, type 1. Blood 1998;92(1):267–272.
616. Watanabe I, Horiuchi T, Hatta N, et al. Analysis of neurofibromatosis type 1 gene mutation in juvenile chronic myelogenous leukemia. Acta Haematol 1998;100(1):22–25.
617. Shannon KM, O'Connell P, Martin GA, et al. Loss of the normal NF1 allele from the bone marrow of children with type 1 neurofibromatosis and malignant myeloid disorders. N Engl J Med 1994;330(9):597–601.
618. Bollag G, Clapp DW, Shih S, et al. Loss of NF1 results in activation of the Ras signaling pathway and leads to aberrant growth in haematopoietic cells. Nat Genet 1996;12(2):144–148.
619. Largaespada DA, Brannan CI, Jenkins NA, et al. Nf1 deficiency causes Ras-mediated granulocyte/macrophage colony stimulating factor hypersensitivity and chronic myeloid leukaemia. Nat Genet 1996;12(2):137–143.
620. Zhang YY, Vik TA, Ryder JW, et al. Nf1 regulates hematopoietic progenitor cell growth and ras signaling in response to multiple cytokines. J Exp Med 1998;187(11):1893–1902.
621. Loh ML, Sakai DS, Flotho C, et al. Mutations in CBL occur frequently in juvenile myelomonocytic leukemia. Blood 2009;114(9):1859–1863.
622. Lutz P, Zix-Kieffer I, Souillet G, et al. Juvenile myelomonocytic leukemia: analyses of treatment results in the EORTC Children's Leukemia Cooperative Group (CLCG). Bone Marrow Transplant 1996;18(6):1111–1116.
623. Yoshida N, Yagasaki H, Xu Y, et al. Correlation of clinical features with the mutational status of GM-CSF signaling pathway-related genes in juvenile myelomonocytic leukemia. Pediatr Res 2009;65(3):334–340.
624. Castleberry RP, Emanuel PD, Zuckerman KS, et al. A pilot study of isotretinoin in the treatment of juvenile chronic myelogenous leukemia. N Engl J Med 1994;331(25):1680–1684.
625. Shimada H, Shima H, Shimasaki N, et al. Little response to zoledronic acid in a child of juvenile myelomonocytic leukemia (JMML) harboring the PTPN11 mutation. Ann Oncol 2005;16(8):1400.
626. Corey SJ, Elopre M, Weitman S, et al. Complete remission following clofarabine treatment in refractory juvenile myelomonocytic leukemia. J Pediatr Hematol Oncol 2005;27(3):166–168.
627. Bergstraesser E, Hasle H, Rogge T, et al. Non-hematopoietic stem cell transplantation treatment of juvenile myelomonocytic leukemia: a retrospective analysis and definition of response criteria. Pediatr Blood Cancer 2007;49(5):629–633.
628. Emanuel PD, Snyder RC, Wiley T, et al. Inhibition of juvenile myelomonocytic leukemia cell growth in vitro by farnesyltransferase inhibitors. Blood 2000;95(2):639–645.
629. Mahgoub N, Taylor BR, Gratiot M, et al. In vitro and in vivo effects of a farnesyltransferase inhibitor on Nf1-deficient hematopoietic cells. Blood 1999;94(7):2469–2476.
630. Castleberry R, Loh ML, Jayaprakash N, et al. Phase II window study of the farnesyltransferase inhibitor R115777 (Zarnestra) in untreated JMML: a COG study. Blood 2005;106:727a–728a.
631. Furlan I, Batz C, Flotho C, et al. Intriguing response to azacitidine in a patient with juvenile myelomonocytic leukemia and monosomy 7. Blood 2009;113(12):2867–2868.
632. Manabe A, Okamura J, Yumura-Yagi K, et al. Allogeneic hematopoietic stem cell transplantation for 27 children with juvenile myelomonocytic leukemia diagnosed based on the criteria of the International JMML Working Group. Leukemia 2002;16(4):645–649.
633. Smith FO, King R, Nelson G, et al. Unrelated donor bone marrow transplantation for children with juvenile myelomonocytic leukaemia. Br J Haematol 2002;116(3):716–724.
634. Locatelli F, Nollke P, Zecca M, et al. Hematopoietic stem cell transplantation (HSCT) in children with juvenile myelomonocytic leukemia (JMML): results of the EWOG-MDS/EBMT trial. Blood 2005;105(1):410–419.
635. Yusuf U, Frangoul HA, Gooley TA, et al. Allogeneic bone marrow transplantation in children with myelodysplastic syndrome or juvenile myelomonocytic leukemia: the Seattle experience. Bone Marrow Transplant 2004;33(8):805–814.

636. de Vries AC, Bredius RG, Lankester AC, et al. HLA-identical umbilical cord blood transplantation from a sibling donor in juvenile myelomonocytic leukemia. Haematologica 2009;94(2):302–304.

637. Locatelli F, Niemeyer C, Angelucci E, et al. Allogeneic bone marrow transplantation for chronic myelomonocytic leukemia in childhood: a report from the European Working Group on Myelodysplastic Syndrome in Childhood. J Clin Oncol 1997;15(2):566–573.

638. Yoshimi A, Niemeyer CM, Bohmer V, et al. Chimaerism analyses and subsequent immunological intervention after stem cell transplantation in patients with juvenile myelomonocytic leukaemia. Br J Haematol 2005;129(4):542–549.

639. Yoshimi A, Bader P, Matthes-Martin S, et al. Donor leukocyte infusion after hematopoietic stem cell transplantation in patients with juvenile myelomonocytic leukemia. Leukemia 2005;19(6):971–977.

640. Yoshimi A, Mohamed M, Bierings M, et al. Second allogeneic hematopoietic stem cell transplantation (HSCT) results in outcome similar to that of first HSCT for patients with juvenile myelomonocytic leukemia. Leukemia 2007;21(3):556–560.

641. Faraci M, Micalizzi C, Lanino E, et al. Three consecutive related bone marrow transplants for juvenile myelomonocytic leukaemia. Pediatr Transplant 2005;9(6):797–800.

642. Hasle H. Incidence of essential thrombocythaemia in children. Br J Haematol 2000;110(3):751.

643. Randi ML, Putti MC, Scapin M, et al. Pediatric patients with essential thrombocythemia are mostly polyclonal and V617FJAK2 negative. Blood 2006;108(10):3600–3602.

644. El-Moneim AA, Kratz CP, Boll S, et al. Essential versus reactive thrombocythemia in children: retrospective analyses of 12 cases. Pediatr Blood Cancer 2007;49(1):52–55.

645. Baxter EJ, Scott LM, Campbell PJ, et al. Acquired mutation of the tyrosine kinase JAK2 in human myeloproliferative disorders. Lancet 2005;365(9464):1054–1061.

646. Levine RL, Wadleigh M, Cools J, et al. Activating mutation in the tyrosine kinase JAK2 in polycythemia vera, essential thrombocythemia, and myeloid metaplasia with myelofibrosis. Cancer Cell 2005;7(4):387–397.

647. Kralovics R, Passamonti F, Buser AS, et al. A gain-of-function mutation of JAK2 in myeloproliferative disorders. N Engl J Med 2005;352(17):1779–1790.

648. Nakatani T, Imamura T, Ishida H, et al. Frequency and clinical features of the JAK2 V617F mutation in pediatric patients with sporadic essential thrombocythemia. Pediatr Blood Cancer 2008;51(6):802–805.

649. Teofili L, Giona F, Martini M, et al. Markers of myeloproliferative diseases in childhood polycythemia vera and essential thrombocythemia. J Clin Oncol 2007;25(9):1048–1053.

650. Veselovska J, Pospisilova D, Pekova S, et al. Most pediatric patients with essential thrombocythemia show hypersensitivity to erythropoietin in vitro, with rare JAK2 V617F-positive erythroid colonies. Leuk Res 2008;32(3):369–377.

651. Pardanani AD, Levine RL, Lasho T, et al. MPL515 mutations in myeloproliferative and other myeloid disorders: a study of 1182 patients. Blood 2006;108(10):3472–3476.

652. Teofili L, Martini M, Luongo M, et al. Overexpression of the polycythemia rubra vera-1 gene in essential thrombocythemia. J Clin Oncol 2002;20(20):4249–4254.

653. Tefferi A, Thiele J, Orazi A, et al. Proposals and rationale for revision of the World Health Organization diagnostic criteria for polycythemia vera, essential thrombocythemia, and primary myelofibrosis: recommendations from an ad hoc international expert panel. Blood 2007;110(4):1092–1097.

654. Teofili L, Giona F, Martini M, et al. The revised WHO diagnostic criteria for Ph-negative myeloproliferative diseases are not appropriate for the diagnostic screening of childhood polycythemia vera and essential thrombocythemia. Blood 2007;110(9):3384–3386.

655. De Stefano V, Za T, Rossi E, et al. Increased risk of recurrent thrombosis in patients with essential thrombocythemia carrying the homozygous JAK2 V617F mutation. Ann Hematol 2010;89:141–146.

656. Tartaglia AP, Goldberg JD, Berk PD, et al. Adverse effects of antiaggregating platelet therapy in the treatment of polycythemia vera. Semin Hematol 1986;23(3):172–176.

657. Rozman C, Giralt M, Feliu E, et al. Life expectancy of patients with chronic nonleukemic myeloproliferative disorders. Cancer 1991;67(10):2658–2663.

658. Hoagland HC, Silverstein MN. Primary thrombocythemia in the young patient. Mayo Clin Proc 1978;53(9):578–580.

659. Giles FJ, Singer CR, Gray AG, et al. Alpha-interferon therapy for essential thrombocythaemia. Lancet 1988;2(8602):70–72.

660. Gilbert HS. Historical perspective on the treatment of essential thrombocythemia and polycythemia vera. Semin Hematol 1999;36(1 Suppl 2):19–22.

661. Pogliani EM, Rossini F, Miccolis I, et al. Alpha interferon as initial treatment of essential thrombocythemia. Analysis after two years of follow-up. Tumori 1995;81(4):245–248.

662. Tornebohm-Roche E, Merup M, Lockner D, et al. Alpha-2a interferon therapy and antibody formation in patients with essential thrombocythemia and polycythemia vera with thrombocytosis. Am J Hematol 1995;48(3):163–167.

663. Spencer CM, Brogden RN. Anagrelide. A review of its pharmacodynamic and pharmacokinetic properties, and therapeutic potential in the treatment of thrombocythaemia. Drugs 1994;47(5):809–822.

664. Chintagumpala MM, Kennedy LL, Steuber CP. Treatment of essential thrombocythemia with anagrelide. J Pediatr 1995;127(3):495–498.

665. Barbui T, Barosi G, Grossi A, et al. Practice guidelines for the therapy of essential thrombocythemia. A statement from the Italian Society of Hematology, the Italian Society of Experimental Hematology and the Italian Group for Bone Marrow Transplantation. Haematologica 2004;89(2):215–232.

666. Anderson JE, Sale G, Appelbaum FR, et al. Allogeneic marrow transplantation for primary myelofibrosis and myelofibrosis secondary to polycythaemia vera or essential thrombocytosis. Br J Haematol 1997;98(4):1010–1016.

667. Kerbauy DM, Gooley TA, Sale GE, et al. Hematopoietic cell transplantation as curative therapy for idiopathic myelofibrosis, advanced polycythemia vera, and essential thrombocythemia. Biol Blood Marrow Transplant 2007;13(4):355–365.

668. Mesa RA, Tefferi A. Emerging drugs for the therapy of primary and post essential thrombocythemia, post polycythemia vera myelofibrosis. Expert Opin Emerg Drugs 2009;14(3):471–479.

669. Osgood EE. Polycythemia Vera: Age relationships and survival. Blood 1965;26:243–256.

670. Cario H, Schwarz K, Herter JM, et al. Clinical and molecular characterisation of a prospectively collected cohort of children and adolescents with polycythemia vera. Br J Haematol 2008;142(4):622–626.

671. Zhao R, Xing S, Li Z, et al. Identification of an acquired JAK2 mutation in polycythemia vera. J Biol Chem 2005;280(24):22788–22792.

672. James C, Ugo V, Le Couedic JP, et al. A unique clonal JAK2 mutation leading to constitutive signalling causes polycythaemia vera. Nature 2005;434(7037):1144–1148.

673. Temerinac S, Klippel S, Strunck E, et al. Cloning of PRV-1, a novel member of the uPAR receptor superfamily, which is overexpressed in polycythemia rubra vera. Blood 2000;95(8):2569–2576.

674. Teofili L, Pierconti F, Di Febo A, et al. The expression pattern of c-mpl in megakaryocytes correlates with thrombotic risk in essential thrombocythemia. Blood 2002;100(2):714–717.

675. Prchal JF, Axelrad AA. Letter: Bone-marrow responses in polycythemia vera. N Engl J Med 1974;290(24):1382.

676. Michiels JJ, Juvonen E. Proposal for revised diagnostic criteria of essential thrombocythemia and polycythemia vera by the Thrombocythemia Vera Study Group. Semin Thromb Hemost 1997;23(4):339–347.

677. McMullin MF. A review of the therapeutic agents used in the management of polycythaemia vera. Hematol Oncol 2007;25(2):58–65.

678. McMullin MF, Bareford D, Campbell P, et al. Guidelines for the diagnosis, investigation and management of polycythaemia/erythrocytosis. Br J Haematol 2005;130(2):174–195.

679. Nand S, Stock W, Godwin J, et al. Leukemogenic risk of hydroxyurea therapy in polycythemia vera, essential thrombocythemia, and myeloid metaplasia with myelofibrosis. Am J Hematol 1996;52(1):42–46.

680. Taylor PC, Dolan G, Ng JP, et al. Efficacy of recombinant interferon-alpha (rIFN-alpha) in polycythaemia vera: a study of 17 patients and an analysis of published data. Br J Haematol 1996;92(1):55–59.

681. Foa P, Massaro P, Ribera S, et al. Role of interferon alpha-2a in the treatment of polycythemia vera. Am J Hematol 1995;48(1):55–57.

682. Petrides PE, Beykirch MK, Trapp OM. Anagrelide, a novel platelet lowering option in essential thrombocythaemia: treatment experience in 48 patients in Germany. Eur J Haematol 1998;61(2):71–76.

683. Stobart K, Rogers PC. Allogeneic bone marrow transplantation for an adolescent with polycythemia vera. Bone Marrow Transplant 1994;13(3):337–339.

CHAPTER 21 ■ CHRONIC LEUKEMIAS OF CHILDHOOD

ARNOLD J. ALTMAN AND CECILIA FU

Chronic leukemias are myeloproliferative disorders characterized by a predominance of relatively mature cells. In contrast to the acute leukemias, these diseases are indolent, with a natural history usually spanning several years. Some subtypes, however, may have a rapidly progressive clinical course.

Chronic leukemias are rare in childhood. The most common type, chronic myelocytic leukemia (CML), accounts for less than 5% of all childhood leukemias, resulting in approximately 100 cases per year in the US pediatric population.[1] Other chronic leukemias discussed in this chapter include juvenile myelomonocytic leukemia (JMML) (formerly known as juvenile CML), familial CML, chronic myelomonocytic leukemia (CMML), and chronic lymphocytic leukemia (CLL).

CHRONIC MYELOCYTIC LEUKEMIA

Chronic myelocytic leukemia is a clonal hematopoietic stem cell disorder involving all the hemic lineages and at least some of the lymphoid lines. It is characterized by myeloid hyperplasia of the bone marrow, extramedullary hematopoiesis, expansion of the total body granulocyte pool, elevation of the leukocyte count (with appearance of the complete range of granulocyte precursor cells in the peripheral blood), and a specific cytogenetic marker, the Philadelphia (Ph[1]) chromosome resulting from the t(9;22)(q34;q11) reciprocal translocation.

Historical Background

CML was the first form of leukemia to be recognized as a distinct clinical entity. Donné[2] described the characteristic hematologic changes in 1844; in 1845, Bennett,[3] Craigie,[4] and Virchow[5] independently described the clinical features and autopsy findings. These early observers were impressed by the marked splenic enlargement and peculiar changes in the color and consistency of the blood. On microscopic examination, the blood contained a predominance of colorless corpuscles similar to those found in small numbers in normal blood and in large numbers in pus. Although he could find no focus of inflammation, Bennett attributed the hematologic findings to "the presence of purulent matter." Virchow, suspecting a neoplastic disorder, used the descriptive term *white blood*, which, translated into Greek, became *leukemia*. Virchow subsequently subdivided leukemia into two categories: splenic and lymphatic.

In 1870, Neumann[6] suggested that the bone marrow, rather than the spleen, was the source of the excess colorless corpuscles in "splenic" leukemia, leading subsequent authors to employ the term *myeloid leukemia*. In 1889, Ebstein[7] recognized the clinical distinction between acute and chronic leukemias, and in 1891, Ehrlich[8] introduced techniques for staining blood cells that permitted the morphologic distinction between myeloid and lymphoid leukemias.

The cytogenetic hallmark of CML, the Ph[1] chromosome, was described by Nowell and Hungerford in 1960.[9] This was the first specific chromosomal abnormality associated with a human malignancy, and its discovery inaugurated the era of cancer cytogenetics. The Ph[1] chromosome was initially thought to be a truncated chromosome 22 resulting from deletion of genetic material; however, in 1973, Janet Rowley demonstrated a reciprocal translocation between chromosomes 9 and 22.[10] The following 25 years defined the pathogenesis of CML by identifying the resultant fusion gene (*BCR-ABL1*) and its protein product, a constitutively activated tyrosine kinase (TK).

The earliest form of therapy for CML was the use of potassium arsenate (Fowler's solution) by Lissauer in 1865[11]; this treatment produced limited and temporary improvement. Radiotherapy, introduced by Pusey in 1902,[12] produced better and more predictable effects with much less toxicity and became the standard therapy until the introduction of busulfan in 1953. Subsequently, hydroxyurea, interferon-α (IFN-α), and cytosine arabinoside replaced busulfan as the initial treatment modalities in chronic phase (CP) CML. However, these agents rarely prevented progression to blast phase and, thus, could not produce sustained cytogenetic or clinical remissions. The introduction of allogeneic stem cell transplantation (SCT) in the mid-1970s can be considered the first approach with significant curative potential. Subsequently, imatinib, a molecularly directed agent targeting the constitutively activated BCR/ABL1 tyrosine kinase, has produced sustained hematologic and cytogenetic remissions with the promise of durable remissions and excellent quality of life; albeit, most patients continue to have low-level persistence of *BCR-ABL* transcripts with risk of relapse after discontinuation of the drug. New TK inhibitors are being developed to deal with resistance to imatinib.

Epidemiology

CML is primarily a disease of middle age; the peak incidence is in the fourth and fifth decades. Its annual incidence is 1 to 2 cases/100,000. Although CML has been diagnosed in infants as young as 3 months (author's personal experience), more than 80% of pediatric cases of CML are diagnosed after age 4 years and 60% after age 6 years.[13,14] No significant racial or sexual predilection exists, and no hereditary component is demonstrable.

The only environmental factor clearly implicated in the etiology of CML is ionizing radiation. An increased incidence of CML has been reported in radiologists, in survivors of atomic bomb explosions, and in persons exposed to therapeutic radiation for treatment of ankylosing spondylitis and other

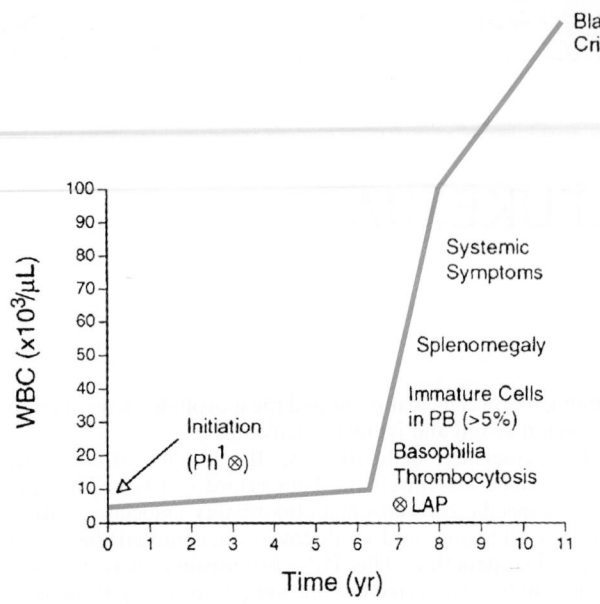

FIGURE 21.1 Timeline for development of clinical symptoms of CML following initial mutational event (atomic bomb irradiation).

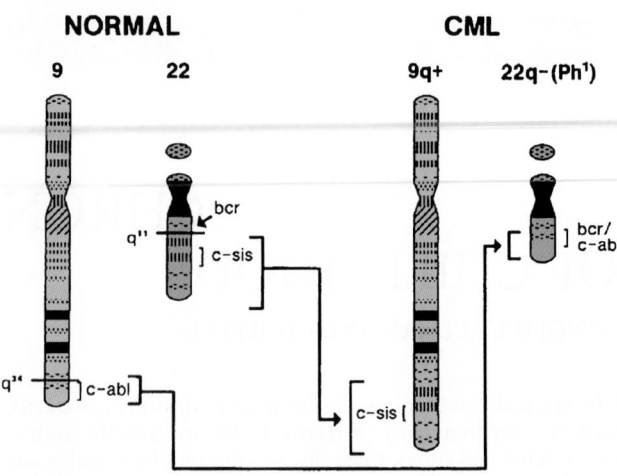

FIGURE 21.2 Anatomy of the (9;22)(q34;q11) translocation with formation of the Philadelphia (Ph^1) chromosome (22q—) containing the hybrid *BCR-ABL1* gene. (See text for further explanation.) CML, chronic myelocytic leukemia.

disorders. In these patients, there is a considerable lag period following exposure, before clinical evidence of CML is detected. Based on epidemiologic data from the atomic bomb data, it would appear that an average of 8 years is required between the original mutational event and the development of clinical symptoms (Fig. 21.1). Obviously, this time line is considerably shortened for CML cases that present in early childhood.

Only 5% to 7% of all patients with CML have documented exposure to excessive radiation, and radiation is rarely implicated in pediatric CML. No infectious agent has been related to the pathogenesis of CML.

Molecular Biology

The cytogenetic hallmark of CML is the Ph^1 chromosome. Initially described as a truncated chromosome 22 (22q-), this anomaly is now recognized to result from the reciprocal translocation t(9;22)(q34;q11) (Fig. 21.2). The molecular

consequence of this event is the production of a chimeric protein (BCR-ABL1) endowed with constitutive kinase activity. Breakpoints on chromosome 9 involve the *ABL* gene and can vary widely (i.e., >100 kilobases [kb] from case to case); on the other hand, breakpoints on chromosome 22 are virtually always restricted to a small (5.8-kb) segment of DNA known as the *major breakpoint cluster region (M-BCR)* (Fig. 21.3). As a result of the reciprocal 9;22 translocation, two hybrid genes are formed: *BCR-ABL1* on 22q- and *ABL1-BCR* on 9q+. Although both of these genes are transcribed, *BCR-ABL1* appears to have the major role in the pathogenesis of CML.

The development of the hybrid *BCR-ABL1* gene may be a more common phenomenon than is commonly recognized. When studied using a very sensitive reverse transcriptase-polymerase chain reaction (RT-PCR) screening technique, 20% of "normal" adult subjects were found to harbor this translocation in a minor subpopulation of cells.[15] The age distribution of these *BCR-ABL1*–positive, but otherwise normal, individuals roughly mirrors the age distribution of CML. The mechanisms preventing these individuals from developing CML are undefined.

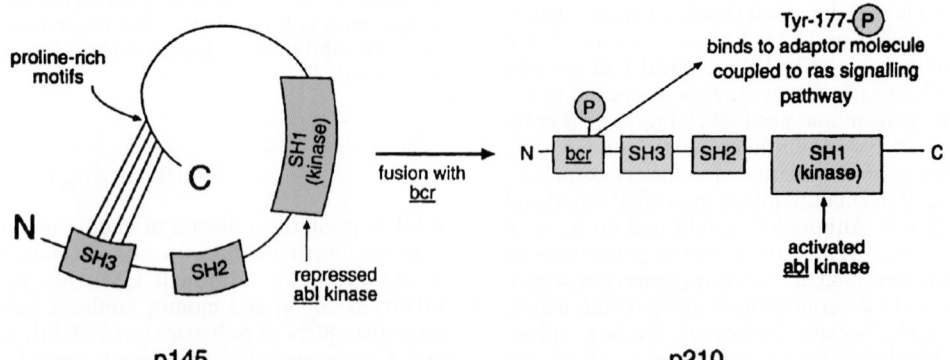

FIGURE 21.3 The normal abl tyrosine kinase (TK) component of P145 is carefully regulated by the SH2 and SH3 domains; genetic alterations that prevent interaction of the SH3 domain with proline-rich motifs within the C terminus result in derepression (constitutive activation) of the TK. In Philadelphia chromosome–positive chronic myelocytic leukemia, fusion with the *bcr* gene leads to production of a chimeric protein (P210) with activated TK and oncogenic properties. Two domains within *bcr* are required for its oncogenic effect: domain I mediates oligomerization of *bcr/abl* and promotes phosphorylation of tyrosine residue 177 within domain II, which, in turn, binds to a signaling adaptor molecule coupling *bcr/abl* with the *ras* signaling pathway. (See text for further explanation.)

Properties of *ABL1* and Its Protein Product (ABL1)

The wild-type *ABL1* gene encodes a 145-kd protein that localizes predominantly in the nucleus and is universally active in hematopoietic cells at all stages of differentiation. It is the human homolog of the Abelson B cell murine leukemia virus oncogene (*v-abl*). The ABL1 protein participates in signal transduction and regulation of gene transcription. One major function is to catalyze the attachment of phosphate groups to the tyrosine residues of various proteins, that is, to act as a TK. Members of the TK family are frequently involved in the pathways that transmit signals from the external milieu to the cytoplasm and nucleus; in this capacity, they may act as growth factors, transmembrane receptors, or submembrane catalytic subunits of surface receptors.

ABL1 protein contains other functional domains in addition to its TK activity (Fig. 21.3; Table 21.1). The carboxy-terminal portion contains a domain involved in binding to F actin as well as a separate domain that can bind to DNA; the DNA-binding activity appears to be cell cycle regulated by the cyclin activated cdc-2 kinase. There are also three nuclear localization signals and one nuclear export signal. At the N-terminal region are three domains known as *src-homology (SH) regions* because of their kinship to the viral *src* oncogene. The first domain (SH1) normally manifests weak TK activity and appears to be tightly regulated by the SH2 and SH3 regions. The presence of SH2 and SH3 regions is significant because these domains play critical roles in intermolecular interactions that specifically mediate protein-protein coupling. The SH2 region can bind to substrates that are tyrosine phosphorylated, whereas the SH3 domain complexes with proline-rich regions involved in coordinating cytoskeletal interactions. The proline-rich SH3 motifs can function as docking sites for the SH3 domains of "adaptor" proteins such as CRK, GRB2 (growth factor receptor-bound protein 2), and NCK. Proteins containing SH2 and SH3 domains are classified as adaptor

molecules because they couple nonreceptor TKs to down-stream signaling cascades regulating gene expression.

The N terminus of *ABL1* consists of a "Cap" region which is covalently linked to a C_{14} myristoyl moiety (Fig. 21.3). This myristoyl modification plays a critical role in controlling the activity of the TK (SH1) domain. By engaging the C-terminal lobe of SH1, it facilitates the docking of the SH2 and SH3 domains onto it, thereby blocking access of ATP and the peptide substrate to the active site and inactivating the TK activity. In contrast, forms of *ABL1* which lack myristoylation (or replace the myristoylated Cap with unmyristoylated BCR) manifest constitutive TK activity.[16]

Properties of *BCR*

The *BCR* region is a component of a much larger gene known as *BCR*, which encodes a 160-kd protein. *BCR* is composed of several regions (Fig. 21.3; Table 21.1) including (a) an N-terminal sequence that contains a coiled-coil oligerimization domain and encodes a serine/threonine kinase; (b) a central portion, which encodes a Rho-guanine nucleotide exchange factor (GEF) that allows the exchange of guanosine triphosphatase (GTP) for guanosine diphosphatase (GDP) and may also activate NF-κB; and (c) a C-terminal portion that codes for a guanosine triphosphatase (GTPase)-activating protein (GAP). A particularly important site is the tyrosine moiety located at position 177 (Tyr177) which can serve as a docking site for GRB2, GRB10, 14-3-3, and the ABL1 protein.[17]

Properties of *BCR/ABL1* and Its Protein Product (BCR-ABL1)

The *BCR/ABL1* gene encodes the tumor-specific BCL-ABL1 molecule, a 210-kd hybrid protein that differs from the normal ABL1 kinase in several respects: (a) it has augmented and constitutive TK activity; (b) it has the ability to autophosphorylate;

TABLE 21.1

FUNCTIONAL DOMAINS OF ABL, BCR, AND BCR-ABL1 PROTEINS

Protein	Chromosome	Domain	Function
p145[ABL]	9q34	N terminal	
		SH1	Tyrosine kinase
		SH2	Interacts with tyrosine-phosphorylated proteins
		SH3	Suppression of tyrosine kinase activity
		Myristoylation site	Localization of p145[ABL1] to nucleus
		C terminal	DNA binding, nuclear localization, actin binding
p160[BCR]	22q11	N terminal	
		Coiled-coil motif	Polymerization with other proteins
		Catalytic domain	Serine-threonine kinase
		Central	
		GEF	GDP-GTP exchange factor
		C terminal	
		GAP	GTPase-activating protein for RAC and RHO (RAS-related proteins)
p210[BCR/ABL]	t(9;22)(q34;q11) (Ph¹ chromosome)	BCR	
		Coiled-coil motif	Increases tyrosine kinase activity of ABL1
		Tyrosine residue 177	Enables binding of F actin by ABL1
		Serine-threonine kinase	Docking site for adaptor proteins
		ABL	Activation of signal-transduction proteins
		SH1 domain	Phosphorylation of signal and adaptor proteins
		Actin-binding domain	Cytoplasmic location. Interference with adhesion.

GAP, guanosine triphosphatase–activating protein; GDP, guanosine diphosphate; GEF, guanine nucleotide exchange factor; GTP, guanosine triphosphatase.

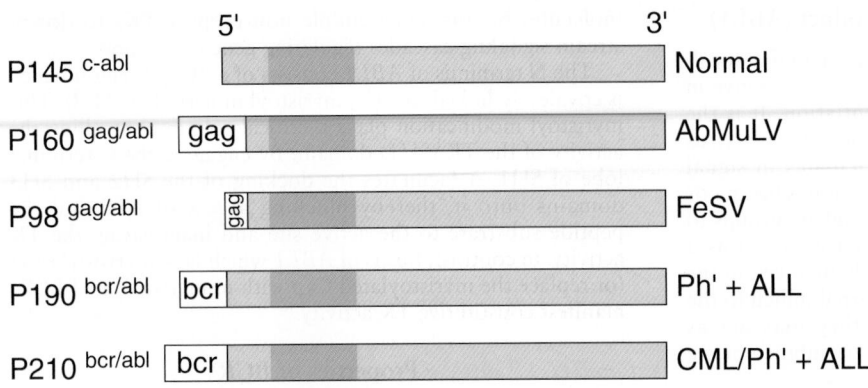

P145 c-abl — Normal
P160 gag/abl — AbMuLV
P98 gag/abl — FeSV
P190 bcr/abl — Ph' + ALL
P210 bcr/abl — CML/Ph' + ALL

FIGURE 21.4 Schematic representation of the normal protein product (P145) of the *ABL1* gene and the modifications associated with leukemogenesis. Note that all variants retain the tyrosine kinase domain (*blue area*) and are altered at the 58 end by insertion of the viral gag component in the case of Abelson murine leukemia virus (AbMuLV) and feline sarcoma virus (FeSV) or with *BCR* segments in the case of Philadelphia chromosome–positive (Ph[1]-positive) acute lymphocytic leukemia (ALL) and chronic myelocytic leukemia (CML).

(c) it is translocated to the cytoplasm, thereby exposing it to a new spectrum of substrates of remarkable diversity; and (d) it binds to bind F-actin. Similar modifications of other ABL proteins have been demonstrated to mediate viral oncogenesis (e.g., v-abl, feline sarcoma virus) and to confer growth-factor independence on various cell lines.[17a] In each of these instances, the critical genetic alteration involves a substitution at the N-terminal end of the *ABL* gene (Fig. 21.4).

As shown in Figure 21.5, the BCR-ABL1 protein is capable of activating multiple downstream signaling pathways. Phosphorylated Tyr177 plays a central role in leukemogenesis by (a) serving as a docking site for GRB2, which, in turn,

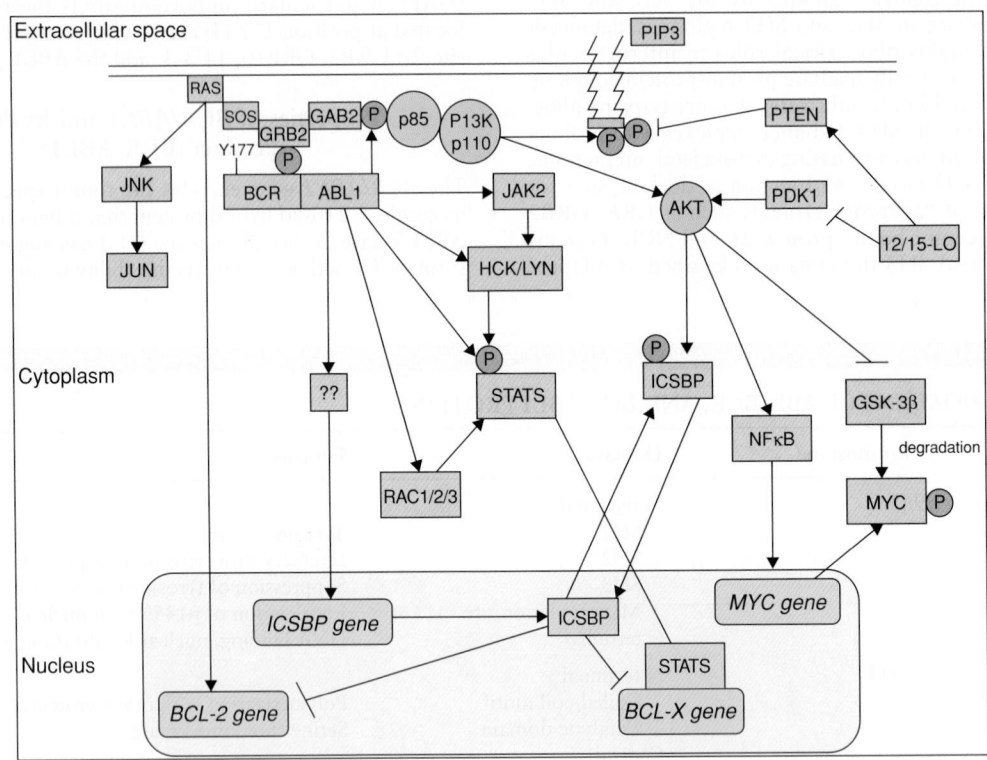

FIGURE 21.5 Molecular signaling in BCR-ABL1–positive myeloid precursors. The phosphorylated Tyr177 residue of BCR serves as a docking site for growth factor receptor-bound protein 2 (GRB2), which binds GRB2-associated binding protein 2 (GAB2), as well as SOS (a guanine-nucleotide exchanger of RAS), resulting in RAS-MAPK activation; this, in turn, promotes transcription of BCL-2 gene. Upon phosphorylation, GAB2 recruits phosphatidylinositol 3-kinase (PI3K), which activates AKT. AKT activation increases transcription of MYC gene and stabilizes MYC protein via inhibition of its degradation by GSK-3β. BCR-ABL-1 also activates STAT5, both directly and indirectly through activation of JAK2 and the SRC kinases HCK and LYN. The end result is the activation of BCL-X gene transcription. In addition, BCR-ABL1 abrogates the transcription of interferon consensus sequence-binding protein (ICSBP), thereby releasing the ISCBP-mediated inhibition of BCL-2 and BCL-X gene transcription, resulting in increased survival of myeloid precursors. Thus, the net effect of BCR-ABL1 kinase activation is the promotion of cell proliferation and survival. Pointed arrows indicate direct interactions and/or activation. Blunt-ended arrows indicate inhibitory effects. GSK-3β, glycogen synthase kinase-3β; PIP₃, phosphatidylinositol-3,4,5 triphosphate. From Quintos-Cardama A, Cortes J. Molecular biology of bcr-abl-positive chronic myeloid leukemia. Blood 2009;113:1619, used with permission.

activates multiple pathways, including those that lead to *RAS* activation and increased transcription of *MYC* and *BCL-X* genes; (b) blocking transcription of interferon consensus sequence-binding protein (ICSBP), thereby preventing its inhibition of *BCL-X* and *BCL-2* gene transcription.[16] BCL-X is a cellular prosurvival protein; its upregulation in CML is thought to inhibit apoptosis[18]; (c) activating the RAC subfamily of GTPases which, in turn, activate downstream signaling molecules such as CRKL, ERK, c-Jun N-terminal kinase (JNK), and p38.[18] The consequence of these events is promotion of cell proliferation and survival.

Alternate Splicing Patterns for *BCR-ABL1*

In the genesis of BCR-ABL1 (P210), the break in *ABL1* typically occurs in the first intron between alternate exons 1a and 1b; the break in *BCR* occurs most often within a 5.8-kb area encompassing exons e12-e16 (Fig. 21.3). There are also at least two other BCR-ABL fusion proteins (P190, P230) that have been associated with neoplastic phenotypes. Since these oncoproteins share the same ABL TK sequences, their different clinical features presumably reflect modulation by the unique protein domains contributed by the various *BCR* breakpoints (Table 21.2).[19]

P190 has been associated with some forms of Ph[1]-positive acute leukemia. Approximately half the adults with this condition have *BCR-ABL1* rearrangements similar to those seen in CML. In the remainder, and in nearly 80% of children with Ph[1]-positive acute leukemia, a different rearrangement occurs, with abl exon 2 spliced to an exon outside the major *BCR* region (known as the *minor BCR region* or *m-BCR*).[20] The resultant protein product (P190) has a molecular weight of 190 kd and has approximately a fivefold higher level of TK activity than does P210. This characteristic appears to correlate with a higher transforming ability of P190. Careful analysis has shown that the p190 transcript, traditionally associated with Ph[1]-positive acute leukemia, can be detected at very low levels (corresponding to approximately 0.02% of the total *BCR-ABL1* transcripts) at diagnosis in virtually all CML patients, apparently arising as a consequence of alternative or missplicing events in the *BCR* gene.[21] As discussed further on, quantitation of p190 transcript can be utilized to assess total tumor burden and as an early indicator of molecular relapse.[22]

A third BCR-ABL fusion protein (P230[BCR-ABL1]) has been associated with a relatively indolent form of chronic leukemia known as chronic neutrophilic leukemia; this translocation involves a third breakpoint cluster region in *BCR* (μ-bcr).[23]

Although the classic t(9;22) is found in approximately 90% of patients with CML, in some instances, other types of translocations may be found.[24–26] Approximately 3% of patients with CML have translocations of 22q11 to regions other than 9q34. Another 3% of patients have complex translocations involving three or more chromosomes; such translocations virtually always involve band 9q34. Other patients may have an undetected or *masked* Ph[1] chromosome (see section "Philadelphia Chromosome–Negative Chronic Myelocytic Leukemia"). A few patients have, in addition to the Ph[1] chromosome, other visible karyotypic abnormalities such as a second Ph[1] chromosome, isochromosome 17, or an extra chromosome 8 or 18; these secondary changes appear to represent a mechanism of tumor progression and are found with increased frequency as the disease evolves to a more aggressive phase.

Philadelphia Chromosome–Negative Chronic Myelocytic Leukemia

Approximately 5% to 10% of patients with otherwise typical CML do not manifest the Ph[1] chromosome. In some of these patients, the Ph[1] chromosome may be masked by translocation of additional genetic material to the 22q11 region.[25] Other patients may have rearrangements or breaks in the 9q34 region without the reciprocal break at 22q11.[26] Molecular biology techniques permit identification of *BCR* rearrangements in Ph[1]-negative patients who have otherwise typical CML.[27,28] In such cases, *ABL1* and *BCR* are presumed to have been juxtaposed on the molecular level by a mechanism other than that producing the typical t(9;22); this phenomenon may result from an interstitial insertion of *ABL1* into *BCR* or a complex translocation with the *BCR-ABL1* fusion gene located on another chromosome.

Patients with a CML-like picture but lacking both Ph[1] and *BCR-ABL1* rearrangement have also been described; such patients appear to have a distinct clinical course characterized by increasing leukocytosis, organomegaly, extramedullary infiltrates, and eventual bone marrow failure.[29] Chromosome abnormalities can be seen in about 30% of Ph[1]-negative CML, with trisomy 8 being the most common. Monosomy 7 and complex karyotypes are rarely seen in Ph[1]-negative CML.[30] In some cases, fusion genes are generated that involve a receptor TK and activate signaling pathways that closely parallel those activated by the BCR-ABL1 fusion molecule.[31,32] The most common such translocations are t(5;12)(q33;p13) and t(8;13)(p11;q12), which involve platelet-derived growth factor receptor (PDGFR) b and fibroblast growth factor receptor 1, respectively. Eosinophilia and monocytosis may be more prominent in these myeloproliferative disorders than in classic CML.[33]

TABLE 21.2

RELATIONSHIP OF *BCR* DOMAINS TO *BCR/ABL1* FUSION GENES

Fusion gene	BCR domains	Clinical phenotype
p185 (or p190)	Dimerization Binding SH2 Serine/threonine kinase	Ph[1]-positive acute leukemia
p210	All of the above plus: Dbl-like Pleckstrin homology	Ph[1]-positive chronic myelocytic leukemia
p230	All of the above plus: Calcium-phospholipid binding 1/3 of GTPase activating gene for p21 rac (racGAP)	Chronic neutrophilic leukemia

PROGNOSTIC CATEGORIZATION OF PH¹-POSITIVE ACUTE LYMPHOCYTIC LEUKEMIA

Prognostic group	Age		Initial WBC	5-year DFS
Favorable	<10		<50,000/mm³	49±5%
Intermediate	>10	And/or	50,000–100,000/mm³	30±5%
Poor prognosis	Any		>100,000/mm³	20±5%

DFS, disease-free survival; WBC, white blood cell count.

Philadelphia Chromosome–Positive Acute Leukemia

Although characteristic of CML, the Ph¹ chromosome is not exclusive to it. This chromosomal abnormality is found in approximately 3% to 10% of childhood acute leukemias, in 2% to 3% of adult acute myeloid leukemias, and in 25% to 33% of adult acute lymphoid leukemias.[34–36] Ph¹-positive acute leukemias have no antecedent CML features and are clinically and hematologically indistinguishable from other acute leukemias except for a relatively poorer prognosis. In a review of 267 patients with Ph¹-positive acute lymphocytic leukemia (ALL), Arico et al.[37] found that complete remission was achieved in 82% of cases. These patients could be subsequently stratified into three prognostic groups based on age and initial white blood cell count (WBC) (Table 21.3). Intensive chemotherapy gave modestly successful results, but only in the most favorable groups; bone marrow transplant from an HLA-matched donor has been the preferred modality for most Ph¹-positive ALL patients. However, improved outcome using imatinib plus intensive chemotherapy was recently reported to achieve 80% 3-year event-free survival in pediatric patients with Ph¹-positive ALL (compared to 35% in historical controls).[37a] Long-term followup studies will needed to determine if these remissions are sustained.

Some Ph¹-positive acute leukemias may represent blastic presentations of CML, whereas others are apparently true *de novo* acute leukemias. Few clinical or hematologic features enable the clinician to distinguish between these two entities, although cases associated with basophilia or marked splenomegaly are more likely to be associated with CML. To confuse the issue further, classic CP CML developed after a period of hematologic and cytogenetic remission in a patient who initially presented with apparent *de novo* Ph¹-positive acute leukemia.[38]

Differences between blastic-phase CML and *de novo* Ph¹-positive acute leukemia are more apparent at the cytogenetic and molecular levels. Ph¹-positive acute leukemias usually do not manifest the specific nonrandom chromosomal aberrations (discussed earlier) that are characteristic of CML as it evolves into blastic phase. Further, the marrow karyotype of the *de novo* acute Ph¹-positive leukemia case usually reverts to normal after therapy, whereas the Ph¹ chromosome persists in the bone marrow of the patient with CML. Patients with CML, regardless of phase, almost universally exhibit typical bcr rearrangements and production of P210. On the other hand, approximately half the patients with *de novo* Ph¹-positive acute leukemias (and virtually all children with this condition) show rearrangements outside the *BCR* region and produce the 190-kd protein.[39,40]

Biology of CML

The cytogenetic changes in the CML precursor cell are expressed in its progeny by a variety of cytologic alterations that, in turn, produce the neoplastic phenotype (Table 21.4).

These biologic features are discussed in the subsequent sections.

Clonality

Independent lines of evidence derived from cytogenetic data and analysis of isoenzyme patterns indicate that CML is an acquired disorder of unicellular origin, and the target of neoplastic transformation is a multilineage stem cell with the potential for generating all the hemic cells (erythrocytes, neutrophils, basophils, eosinophils, monocytes, megakaryocytes) and, in at least some instances, the lymphoid lineages. This multilineage potential accounts for the cytologic heterogeneity of the blastic phase of CML (discussed later in "Natural History" section).

Cytogenetic Evidence of Clonality. The Ph¹ chromosome has proved useful in defining the malignant population in CML. This acquired abnormality arises in a hematopoietic stem cell (CD34+CD38−CD90+Lin−) and can be detected in myeloid, erythroid, and some lymphoid lineages (although rarely in T cells) but not in fibroblasts or other somatic cells.[41] A similar pattern of clonal restriction can be demonstrated for other karyotypic markers, such as that found in CML patients with coincident sexual mosaicism or Down syndrome.[42] The phenomenon of lymphoblastic transformation in some patients with CML suggests that at least some lymphoid lineages are involved in the malignant process. This suggestion is supported by demonstration of the Ph¹ chromosome in a small proportion of B lymphocytes and T lymphocytes when CML

CYTOLOGIC ABNORMALITIES IN CHRONIC MYELOCYTIC LEUKEMIA

Abnormality	Consequence
Reduced adherence to stromal matrix	Decreased stroma/stem cell interaction Abrogation of normal cell surface signal maturation
Discordant nuclear: cytoplasmic maturation	Prolongation of late progenitor proliferative phase Opportunity for further divisions before maturation
Failure of apoptosis program	Prolonged survival/increased accumulation
Production of inhibitory molecules	Suppression of normal hematopoietic stem cells
Insensitivity to regulatory molecules	Selective growth advantage for chronic myelocytic leukemia cells

blood is cultured *in vitro*.[43] Other studies have documented the presence of Ph[1]-positive B and T lymphocytes in multilineage colonies derived from CML precursor cells[44]; furthermore, *BCR-ABL1* transcripts have been detected in T lymphocytes of patients with CML.[45] The small fraction of lymphoid cells with the malignant genotype may be a consequence of the relative longevity of these elements in comparison with myeloid lineages; lymphoid cells are relatively long-lived and, therefore, it might be expected that most lymphocytes present at diagnosis of CML antedate the neoplastic transformation event.

Isoenzyme Pattern Evidence of Clonality. In accordance with the Lyon hypothesis, random inactivation of one X chromosome occurs in each cell during early embryogenesis; the progeny of each of these cells subsequently manifests the same pattern of X chromosome inactivation in a clonal fashion. Because approximately half the cells express one X chromosome and half the other X chromosome, females who are heterozygous for an X-linked enzyme should have roughly equal proportions of the two isoenzymes in each tissue. On the other hand, a neoplastic clone arising from a single cell should manifest only a single isoenzyme pattern. Studies of females with CML who are heterozygous for the X-linked enzyme glucose-6-phosphate dehydrogenase (G6PD) have demonstrated that the normal somatic tissues show the expected double isoenzyme distribution, whereas the Ph[1]-positive hemic lineages contain a single (clonal) isoenzyme phenotype.[46,47] The demonstration that Ph[1]-positive B lymphocytes also manifest a clonal pattern of G6PD distribution confirms that this lineage is also derived from the CML stem cell[48,49]; this finding has important implications with regard to the initial transformation event in CML.

The Initial Transformation Event

Although clearly germane to the pathogenesis of CML, the *BCR-ABL1* translocation may not be the primary event in the neoplastic sequence. In some documented cases, the typical clinical and hematologic abnormalities of CML appear to have antedated the appearance of the Ph[1] chromosome[50,51]; in other cases, the Ph[1] chromosome disappeared during therapy while the clinical and hematologic features of CML persisted.[52] Isoenzyme studies that indicate clonality of some Ph[1]-lymphoid populations also imply a transformation event preceding the (9;22) translocation.[49]

Mechanisms Underlying Growth Advantage of Chronic Myelocytic Leukemia Cells

The expansion of the CML clone from a single transformed cell to predominance in bone marrow and blood is dramatic evidence of its ability to overgrow the normal hemic elements. The mechanisms by which it achieves preeminence have been of great interest to students studying the disease. Some clues have been provided by analysis of proliferative kinetics and *in vitro* colony production.

Cell Kinetics. In CP CML, one sees a 3- to 30-fold increase in peripheral blood band and segmented neutrophils and a 10- to 100-fold increase in the total blood granulocyte pool (TBGP).[53,54] These leukocytes freely exchange between the peripheral blood, bone marrow, and spleen. The average half-life of granulocytes in the blood is 5 to 10 times longer in patients with CML than in healthy persons; this phenomenon is partially a reflection of the large number of immature forms, but even the morphologically mature granulocytes of CML have a peripheral blood half-life two- to fourfold longer than normal.[55] This increased blood transit time contributes to the

expansion of the TBGP. Of greater significance, however, is the increased granulocyte production rate.

The hyperproduction of myeloid cells in CML is not attributable to unregulated or unduly rapid proliferation; indeed, measurements of mitotic activity, DNA synthesis, and generation time indicate that CML progenitor cells divide more slowly than normal hemic precursor cells.[53-55] An overproduction of committed myeloid precursor cells can be demonstrated, however, by assays of the granulocyte-monocyte colony-forming unit (GM-CFU).[55-57] Bone marrow suspensions from patients in CP CML generate 10 to 20 times the number of GM colonies produced by normal marrow. The disparity is even more striking when peripheral blood is studied. Colony growth is qualitatively normal (in CP); mature GM forms are produced, and the process depends on the same colony-stimulating factors (CSFs) that are obligatory for *in vitro* colony formation by normal GM-CFU. After chemotherapy or splenic irradiation, the TBGP and the half-life of circulating granulocytes return to normal values coincident with a reduction in the marrow cellularity, a reduction of the bone marrow and peripheral blood GM-CFU, and disappearance of immature cells from the peripheral blood. This change suggests that most of the kinetic abnormalities found in CP CML do not reflect an intrinsic maturational defect of the neoplastic cells but are a consequence of the premature release of immature cells from the marrow resulting from the mechanical pressure of an increased granulocytic cell mass. The basic defect appears to be discordant maturation with preferential expansion of the progenitor compartment.[54]

As the disease progresses to blast phase, defects in maturation become more conspicuous. Myeloblasts become abundant in the bone marrow and peripheral blood, whereas the relative and absolute numbers of polymorphs decline. An inverse correlation exists between the percentage of myeloblasts in the marrow and the fraction of these cells in DNA synthesis.[57a] This decline in proliferative and maturational potential is reflected in absent or reduced GM colony production *in vitro*.

Abnormalities in Feedback Regulation. Under normal circumstances, myelopoiesis is regulated by at least three negative feedback molecular species: lactoferrin (LF), prostaglandin E (PGE), and acidic isoferritins (AIF). LF, the product of mature polymorphonuclear leukocytes (PMNs), downregulates granulocytopoiesis by reducing monocyte-macrophage production of CSF.[58] PGE and AIF, which are derived from subpopulations of monocytes and macrophages, inhibit proliferation of normal granulocyte-monocyte precursor cells[58,59]; their inhibitory actions appear to be restricted to those cells that express HLA-DR (Ia) antigens.[60,61]

CML cells appear to be relatively insensitive to feedback inhibition by virtue of deficient LF production by the PMN, decreased responsiveness of the monocyte-macrophage to regulation by LF, and decreased sensitivity of progenitor cells to PGE and AIF.[62,63] The PGE and AIF resistance may reflect deficient HLA-DR antigen expression by CML cells or a decreased proportion of sensitive target cells.

CML cells may augment their proliferative advantage by releasing humoral factors to which they are relatively resistant but which suppress normal hematopoietic progenitors. One family of such regulators includes serine proteases such as neutrophil elastase, pro-proteinase C (also known as leukemia-associated inhibitor, or LAI), and cathepsin G. These enzymes are located in the azurophil granules of neutrophils and provide feedback regulation by enzymatically degrading hematopoietic growth factors and/or their receptors.[64,65] The leukocytosis of CML promotes high levels of neutrophil elastase and high levels of other serine proteases (e.g., LAI) which can digest granulocyte colony-stimulating factor (G-CSF) and downregulate Ph[1]-negative granulocytopoiesis.[66,67]

Altered Adhesive Interactions. Under normal conditions, hematopoietic progenitor cells adhere to the extracellular matrix protein fibronectin in bone marrow stroma via fibronectin receptors (integrins). Ph[1]-positive progenitor cells exhibit reduced adhesion to fibronectin. This may result from an acquired functional defect of the fibronectin receptor and/or its downstream signaling pathways. Several cytoskeletal proteins associated with integrin regulation including paxillin, focal adhesion kinase, CKRL, and vinculin are phosphorylated by the bcr/abl TK, and their altered status may contribute to abnormal integrin function.[67a] Defective binding of CML progenitors to marrow stroma may lead to release of immature cells into the circulation and may facilitate hematopoiesis in extramedullary sites. Conversely, this defect in adhesiveness inhibits the survival of CML progenitor cells in long-term culture systems and may be exploited to facilitate selection for normal (Ph[1]-negative) stem cells *in vitro*.

Abnormal Angiogenesis. CML patients manifest abnormal bone marrow vessel production (angiogenesis). Bone marrow vascularity and vascular endothelial growth factor (VEGF) levels have been found to be significantly increased. Overexpression of *BCR-ABL1* upregulates VEGF, leading to phosphorylation of endothelial VEGF regulator, VEGF-R2/KDR, and PKB.Akt, a serine-threonine kinase regulator of endothelial cell activation.[68]

Resistance to Apoptosis. The expansion of a malignant clone reflects an imbalance between the rate of cell proliferation and the rate of cell death. As discussed earlier, studies of the kinetics of CML cells suggest that they are not produced at an increased rate; therefore, the massive accumulation of cells in CML probably results from prolongation of cell survival. Under normal circumstances, hemic cells have a limited life span that is regulated by a genetic program of active autonomous cell death (apoptosis); the presence of the bcr/abl fusion protein appears to render CML cells resistant to the induction of apoptosis.[69,70] The BCR-ABL1 oncoproteins protect cells from apoptosis via several different mechanisms, among which are inhibition of upstream preapoptotic mitochondrial events (e.g., release of cytochrome C or altered fas/fas ligand interaction) and downstream inhibition of caspase 3.[71,72] Many of these effects are mediated by influencing the relative expression levels of apoptosis inhibitors (BCL-2, BCL-X_L) and promoters (BAX, BAD, BCL-X_S) and/or the subcellular localization of these factors. Signal transducers and activators of transcription (STAT) proteins appear to be constitutively phosphorylated by BCR-ABL1. Activation of STAT1 and STAT5 upregulates BCL-X_a and contributes to cellular proliferation and survival.[73,74]

In addition to promoting leukocytosis, suppression of apoptosis may also allow cells to accumulate new genetic changes with consequent neoplastic progression. The BCR/ABL-mediated inhibition of apoptosis is also associated with prolongation of cell cycle arrest at the G_2/M restriction point; this delay may give the cell time to repair chemotherapy-induced damage to DNA rather than proceeding to programmed cell death.[75] Because response to many chemotherapeutic agents depends on activation of the apoptosis program, inhibition of apoptosis may limit the susceptibility of CML cells to standard cytotoxic chemotherapy. Thus, resistance to apoptosis may be implicated in several important features of CML: massive clonal expansion, neoplastic progression, and resistance to chemotherapy.

Acute Transformation

In the course of progression to acute transformation (blast crisis), the CML clone acquires additional genetic (and possibly epigenetic) derangements which inhibit differentiation, resist apoptosis, extend replicative life span, and resist cytotoxic agents. The BCR-ABL1 kinase, while necessary for initiation of leukemogenesis, is not sufficient to account for all of these aspects of further disease evolution. It does appear, however, to have a major role in promoting this process, possibly by increasing genetic instability and allowing genetically damaged cells to survive.

One important feature of acute transformation is the apparent acquisition by granulocyte-macrophage precursors of pluripotent stem cell properties such as self-renewal and resistance to cytotoxic chemotherapy.[76–79] Acute phase CML is associated with a 6- to 10-fold increase of granulocyte-macrophage progenitors, rather than expansion of the hematopoietic stem cell pool.[16] This reversion to stem cell phenotype may be driven by activation of the Wnt/β-catenin signaling pathway (required for hematopoietic stem cell self-renewal and interaction with the bone marrow niche).[76–79]

In the Preisler model of leukemogenesis,[80] the process of acute transformation involves at least two complementary gene families (Table 21.5). Class I genes code for signal transduction proteins that participate in the chain of reactions that transmit signals from the cell surface to the cytoskeletal elements or the nucleus; oncogenic transformation usually produces an abnormal protein that induces abnormalities of proliferation or differentiation. Class II genes code for proteins that interact directly with the genome and regulate the expression of other families of genes; oncogenic transformation usually results in an abnormality in regulation of expression leading to increased proliferative potential or immortalization.

Applying the Preisler model to CML, the CP may be attributed to an abnormal protein (P210) derived from an altered class I proto-oncogene (*ABL1*). Progression to the acute phase does not appear to result from a further change in the BCR-ABL1 gene nor are alterations in other class I genes expected to induce acute transformation. Instead, alteration of a class II gene is more likely to complement the oncogenic potential of the preexisting class I genetic mutation. The low incidence of

TABLE 21.5

CLASSIFICATION OF PROTO-ONCOGENES

Class I (signal transducers)		Class II (signal effectors)	
Gene	Locus of action	Gene	Locus of action
SIS	External milieu (PDGF)	MYC	Nucleus
ERB-B	Cell membrane (EGF-R)	p53	Nucleus
FMS	Cell membrane (CSF-1-R)	RB	Nucleus
RAS	Submembrane (G protein)		
ABL1	Submembrane (tyrosine kinase)		
SRC	Submembrane (tyrosine kinase)		
MOS	Cytoplasm		
RAF	Cytoplasm		
MIL	Cytoplasm		

CSF-1-R, colony-stimulating factor-1 receptor; EGF-R, epidermal growth factor receptor; PDGF, platelet-derived growth factor.

N-*RAS* (class I) mutations and the relatively high incidence (22% to 30%) of p53 (class II) mutations seen in association with blastic transformation of CML are consistent with this model of leukemogenesis.[81,82] The cytogenetic changes associated with blastic crisis are discussed further in section "Cytologic and Cytogenetic Heterogeneity of Blast Phase").

Multistep Pathogenesis

The evolution of CML may be visualized as a multistep process that can be summarized as follows:

1. An initial transformation event (possibly rearrangement of *ABL1*) occurs in a multipotent progenitor cell. This results in production of a clone of *premalignant* hemic (and possibly lymphoid) cells. These cells may be metabolically defective and require a subsequent genetic mutation (e.g., fusion of *BCR-ABL1*) to compensate for the defect and "rescue" them from impending apoptosis.
2. At some point in the evolution of the disease, a recognizable cytogenetic alteration (the Ph[1] chromosome) appears in the transformed clone. The translocation of *ABL1* to chromosome 22 and its fusion with the *BCR* deregulates TK activity, which, in turn, produces novel tyrosine phosphorylated proteins and activates pathways which lead to upregulation of cell survival genes such as *BCL-X* and *MYC*. These genes inhibit apoptosis, and the Ph[1]-positive clone now acquires a growth advantage over normal hemic stem cells. Initially, an overproduction of relatively mature cells occurs, particularly those of the granulocytic series.
3. Genomic instability and spontaneous errors in DNA replication may promote the appearance of progressively more abnormal stem cell clones derived from the original Ph[1]-positive clone; new cytogenetic alterations appear, and an increasing dissociation exists between proliferation and differentiation. The newly evolved clones suppress the proliferation of normal stem cells as well as the cells of the preceding leukemic clones. Eventually, immature (blast) cells predominate, and the process terminates in an acute leukemia.

Natural History

The natural history of CML is divided into **chronic, accelerated,** and **blast** phases. These phases represent the progressive shift in the nature of the disorder from one of hyperproliferation, with production of mainly mature hemic elements, to one characterized by differentiation arrest, with hyperproduction of predominantly immature (blast) cells characterized by reversion to stem cell phenotype, block of apoptosis, and resistance to therapeutic endeavors.

Chronic Phase

CP is characterized by marked expansion of the hematopoietic pools; morphologically mature blood cells are produced that show only subtle functional abnormalities. In general, the neoplastic cells are restricted to the bone marrow, liver, spleen, and peripheral blood. Therefore, symptoms are related to organ infiltration, hyperviscosity, and the metabolic consequences of hyperproliferation, all of which are relatively easy to control. On average, the CP lasts about 3 years.

Symptoms. Patients usually present with nonspecific complaints, such as fever, night sweats, weakness, left upper quadrant pain or fullness, and bone pain. Neurologic dysfunction, respiratory distress, visual difficulties, or priapism may complicate cases characterized by marked hyperleukocytosis.

Physical Findings. The usual physical findings in CP are pallor, low-grade fever, ecchymoses, hepatosplenomegaly, and sternal tenderness. Signs relating to leukostasis (neurologic abnormalities, papilledema, retinal hemorrhages, and tachypnea) are seen in patients with extreme hyperleukocytosis.

Laboratory Findings. A mild normochromic, normocytic anemia, marked leukocytosis with shift to the left and thrombocytosis are common laboratory findings. The mean hematocrit at presentation in children (25 mL/dL) is significantly less than that seen in adults.[13,14] The leukocyte count at diagnosis ranges from approximately 8,000 to 800,000/mm[3]; the median count in children (approximately 250,000/mm[3]) is higher than that seen in adults.[13,83] Extreme hyperleukocytosis (>500,000/mm[3]) is also more common in children. The peripheral blood smear shows myeloid cells at all stages of differentiation; myeloblasts and promyelocytes generally comprise less than 15% of the differential count, and no hiatus leukemicus in maturation occurs (Fig. 21.6A). An absolute increase in the numbers of basophils and eosinophils is noted. Hybrid eosinophilic-basophilic granulocytes may also be seen[84]; because similar chimeric granules may be found in normal immature granulocytes, this phenomenon may reflect incomplete maturation.[53] The mean platelet count in children is approximately 500,000/mm[3], which is not significantly higher than that in adults.[83] Serologic findings include elevation of uric acid, lactate dehydrogenase, vitamin B$_{12}$, and vitamin B$_{12}$-binding protein (transcobalamin 1).

The bone marrow is hypercellular, mainly reflecting granulocytic (and often megakaryocytic) hyperplasia; orderly granulocyte maturation, eosinophilia, and basophilia are present. Myelofibrosis, which occurs in 30% to 40% of patients during the course of the disease, is uncommon in the early CP; however, reticulin fibers can often be demonstrated. The bone marrow and spleen occasionally contain lipid-laden histiocytes that resemble Gaucher cells or sea-blue histiocytes.

The characteristic histochemical abnormality of the granulocyte population is reduction in leukocyte alkaline phosphatase (LAP) activity. Although this abnormality does not appear to affect PMN function adversely, it is of diagnostic utility in distinguishing the leukocytosis of CML from that of inflammation (in which LAP is generally elevated). Low LAP activity is also seen in paroxysmal nocturnal hemoglobinuria, juvenile chronic myelogenous leukemia (JCML), CMML, and Fanconi's anemia. Under normal conditions, LAP activity appears very late in the development of granulocytes and, indeed, may be a terminal marker of granulocyte maturation.[85] In CML, there appears to be no intrinsic defect in the synthesis and translation of LAP mRNA or transport of LAP protein to the plasma membrane; furthermore, LAP activity can be upregulated under a variety of conditions (inflammation, leukoreduction, disease progression, administration of G-CSF). Thus, the low LAP levels in CML cells may result from granulocyte immaturity and/or hypoproduction of G-CSF due to a relative decrease in monocyte mass.[85,86]

LAP activity increases with infection or with a reduction in the granulocyte count after chemotherapy or progression to a more acute phase of the disease. Although subtle functional abnormalities of PMN adherence, chemotaxis, bactericidal activity, and membrane sialylation can be demonstrated in CP CML, the PMNs are sufficiently effective to prevent infectious complications.[87,88] PMN function deteriorates progressively as the disease evolves.

Differential Diagnosis. The differential diagnosis of CP CML includes leukemoid reaction, juvenile myelomonocytic leukemia (JMML), and other myeloproliferative disorders. In the past, assessment of LAP score was pivotal in differentiating CML

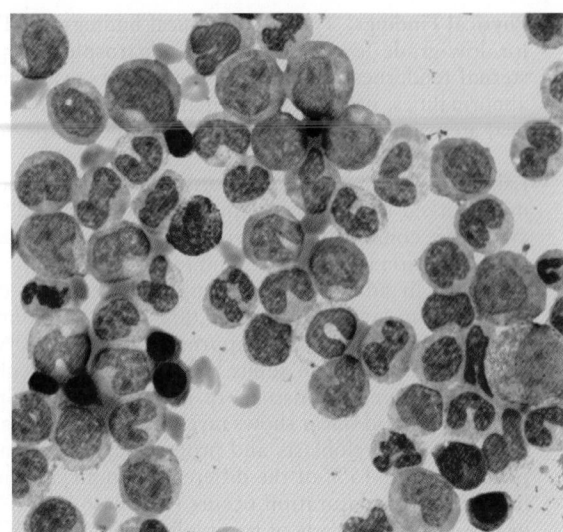
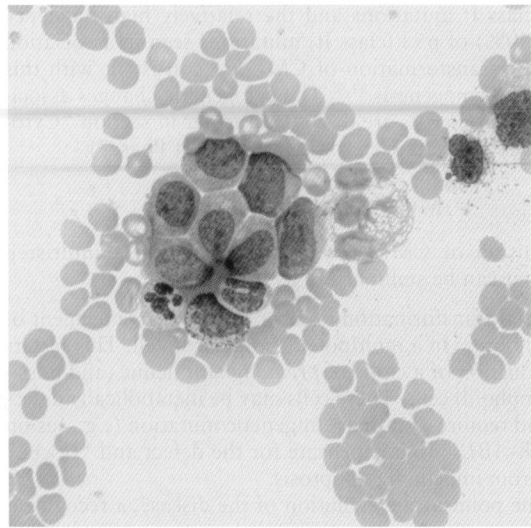

A   B

FIGURE 21.6 Peripheral blood smears of chronic myelocytic leukemia. **A:** Chronic phase—marked leukocytosis showing the entire range of myeloid cells from myeloblast to mature polymorphonuclear leukocytes; a hypergranular eosinophil and basophil are present as well. **B:** Blast phase—blast cells are now more prominent and there is a hiatus in myeloid maturation. (Courtesy of Drs. Hiroko Shinoda and William Rezuke.)

from other causes of neutrophilia. However, with the availability of molecular assays, the diagnosis now rests on demonstration of the Ph[1] chromosome or the *BCR-ABL1* transcript.

In leukemoid reactions, splenomegaly is usually not marked, the LAP score is high, the Ph[1] chromosome is absent, and an inflammatory focus is often demonstrable. In JMML, the LAP may be low, but the Ph[1] chromosome is absent; leukocytosis and splenomegaly are less marked than in CML, and involvement of skin, lymphoid tissue, and the monocytic lineage is more pronounced. CML can be distinguished from other myeloproliferative disorders by the disproportionate involvement of the granulocyte series and the presence of the Ph[1] chromosome and/or *BCR-ABL1* transcripts.

Accelerated Phase

Progression to a more aggressive phase generally proceeds as a gradual multistep evolution. About 50% of patients develop a progressive maturation defect resulting in a hematologic picture similar to that of *de novo* acute leukemia; the remaining 45% have the gradual evolution of a myeloproliferative syndrome. Sudden onset of blastic phase (defined as onset within 3 months from a previously documented complete hematologic response [CHR]) is an unusual event within the first 3 years following diagnosis: the incidence is 0.4% in the first year, 1.8% in the second year, and 2.6% in the third year.[89] Most cases of sudden blastic crisis have lymphoblastic morphology.

The onset of accelerated phase (AP) is characterized by progressive systemic symptoms (fever, night sweats, weight loss), increasing leukocyte counts with a high proportion of immature cells, basophilia, and increasing resistance to chemotherapy. Along with these features is evidence of karyotypic evolution. Mutations in the antioncogene p53 may play a significant role in transformation: p53 mutations are detectable in late CP and may indicate increasing genomic instability and early progression to blast transformation.[90,91] New karyotypic abnormalities (most commonly, duplication of the Ph[1] chromosome, isochromosome 17, or trisomy 8) also begin to appear. Occasionally, the first manifestation of metamorphosis is extramedullary (i.e., meningeal leukemia or a

chloroma arising in soft tissue or bone); such findings usually herald the imminent blast transformation of the marrow.

Blast Phase/Blast Crisis

Blast crisis (BC) is characterized by loss of the leukemic clone's capacity to differentiate. As a consequence, the clinical picture resembles that of an acute leukemia, with anemia, thrombocytopenia, and increased numbers of blast cells in both the peripheral blood (Fig. 21.6B) and the bone marrow. A marrow blast percentage of 20% or more is diagnostic of blast phase. The signs and symptoms are those of a *de novo* acute leukemia; if basophilia is extreme, the patient may also have hyperhistaminemic symptoms (pruritus, cold urticaria, gastric ulceration). As the absolute blast count approaches/exceeds 100,000/mm³, the patient is at progressive risk for hyperleukocytosis syndrome with leukostasis.

Cytologic and Cytogenetic Heterogeneity of Blast Phase. As a reflection of the pluripotent nature of the leukemic stem cells in CML, BC may involve any of the lymphohematopoietic lineages. In approximately 60% to 70% of cases, the blast cell morphology is myeloblastic; unlike *de novo* acute myelocytic leukemia, however, the blast cells are usually peroxidase negative and rarely have Auer rods. Careful analysis using lineage-specific markers such as glycophorin-A, platelet peroxidase, and monoclonal antibodies enables clinicians to identify some of these blast transformations as erythroid, monocytic, or megakaryocytic.[92] Approximately one-third of patients have blast cells with lymphoid morphology. These cells generally express a phenotype corresponding to an early B cell.[92,93] In rare cases, blast cells may express T-lineage markers; these patients usually have marked extramedullary involvement (especially in lymph nodes) and frequently lack a preceding CP.[94] In some patients, the blast cells manifest features of more than one myeloid line or have mixed myeloid-lymphoid features.

BC is frequently associated with new specific molecular and cytogenetic abnormalities. At the molecular level, the most common gene mutations involve the *p53* gene (mutated in 25% to 30% of myeloid conversions) and the INK4A/ARF exon 2 (homozygously deleted in approximately 50% of lymphoid conversions)[95]; other genes potentially involved in phenotypic progression include *JUNB, FOS, PRAME, MXF1, EF1δ,* and *WNT/β-catenin.*[78] These changes may serve to promote genomic instability and or dysregulation of cell cycle progression. The most commonly identifiable karyotypic alterations are duplication of the Ph[1] chromosome (+Ph[1]), trisomy 8 (+8), trisomy 19 (+19), and isochromosome 17q (i17q). A rare consistent chromosomal abnormality, a reciprocal t(3;21)(q26;q22), has been described in patients with CML either before or at the onset of blast transformation.[96–98] In general, these secondary cytogenetic changes are nonspecific and may indicate a generalized genomic instability rather than directly relate to blastic progression; however, other changes clearly mirror the karyotypic features associated with specific subtypes of *de novo* acute leukemia and may be directly related to blastic transformation (Table 21.6).[99] The phenotypic features of blast transformation may be determined by these specific secondary genetic events; for example, rearrangements involving chromosome regions containing Ig genes and T-cell receptor genes have been associated with B-lymphoid and T-lymphoid acute transformations, whereas involvement of region 3q21 may be accompanied by dysmegakaryopoiesis and conversion to acute megakaryoblastic leukemia.[91,97,98]

Differential Diagnosis. Because most instances of BC occur after a well-documented CP, the diagnosis is usually clear-cut. The rare patient who presents in BC without a recognized preceding CP may pose diagnostic difficulty, however. The combination of marked splenomegaly, basophilia, and the Ph[1] chromosome distinguishes BC from most types of *de novo* acute leukemia; the distinction between BC and *de novo* Ph[1]-positive acute leukemia is discussed earlier in this chapter.

TABLE 21.6

ASSOCIATION BETWEEN CHROMOSOME ABNORMALITIES AND ACUTE PHASE CHRONIC MYELOCYTIC LEUKEMIA

	Acute phase	
	Myeloid	Lymphoid
Incidence of abnormalities	80%	30%
Ploidy	Hyper	Hypo, pseudo
Nonrandom chromosome abnormalities		
+Ph[1]	+	+
+21	+	+
±y	+	+
i(17q)	+	−
+8	+	?−
+19	+	−
t(7;11)	+	?−
Specific rearrangements	t(15;17)(q22;q?12)[a] 3q21–3q26(inv. or t)[c]	inv(7)(p15q34)[b] t(14;14)(q11;q32)[d]

[a]Seen in association with acute promyelocytic leukemia.
[b]Seen in association with acute T-cell lymphoblastic leukemia.
[c]Seen in association with acute megakaryoblastic leukemia.
[d]Seen in association with acute B-cell lymphoblastic leukemia.
Modified from Bernstein R, Gale RP. Do chromosome abnormalities determine the type of acute leukemia that develops in CML? Leukemia 1990;4:65.

Prognostic Considerations

Recent advances in the management of CML have improved median survival significantly. Because patients generally die within months of transformation to AP or BC, the major determinant of survival is the duration of the CP, which can be highly variable. For adults, factors at diagnosis that predict early transformation include splenomegaly (>15 cm below costal margin), hepatomegaly (>6 cm below costal margin), thrombocytopenia (<150,000/mm³), thrombocytosis (>500,000/mm³), marked leukocytosis (>100,000/mm³), and high proportions of blast cells (>1%) or immature granulocytes (>20%).[100,101] The role of these factors in the prognosis of pediatric patients with CML is less clear; in one study, only peripheral blood and marrow blast counts at presentation were of prognostic significance.[13]

Once patients have entered BC, the only parameters that correlate with survival are blast cell phenotype and cytogenetic findings. In general, lymphoblastic phenotype and minimal karyotypic evolution augur a more favorable response to therapy.[91]

Therapy

Special Management Problems

Metabolic Disorders. Metabolic consequences of rapid cytolysis (e.g., hyperuricemia, hyperkalemia, hyperphosphatemia) should be anticipated and treated appropriately with hydration, alkalinization, and allopurinol. A detailed discussion of metabolic management is found in Chapter 38.

Hyperleukocytosis. The extremely high leukocyte count associated with some cases of CML can cause leukostatic complications in several organs, especially brain, lung, retina, and penis.[102,103] Because leukocytes are less deformable than erythrocytes, the viscosity of the blood increases dramatically as the fractional volume of leukocytes (leukocrit) increases. Myeloblasts, which are larger and more rigid than other leukocytes, contribute disproportionately to viscosity; thus, the patient with myeloblastic transformation is at particularly high risk. If hyperleukocytosis is symptomatic or extreme (leukocytes, >200,000/mm³ or blast count, >50,000/mm³), it should be treated with the simultaneous use of cytotoxic drugs (e.g., hydroxyurea, 50 to 75 mg/kg/day by intravenous infusion) and leukapheresis (or exchange transfusion); erythrocyte transfusions (which increase blood viscosity) should be avoided if possible until the leukocyte is reduced to a safe level.

Thrombocytosis. Thrombocytosis may be associated with thromboembolic or hemorrhagic complications. If thrombocytosis does not respond to the CML treatment regimen, the use of anagrelide (an agent that prevents megakaryocyte maturation) or thiotepa (75 mg/m² intravenously every 2 to 3 weeks until response occurs) should be considered.[104]

Priapism. Persistent painful penile erection may result from sludging and mechanical obstruction by leukemic cells, coagulation within the corpora cavernosa secondary to thrombocytosis, or impingement by the spleen on abdominal veins and nerves. Treatment includes analgesia, hydration, application of warm compresses, radiotherapy (to penis or spleen), and initiation of high-dose chemotherapy (e.g., hydroxyurea, 50 to 75 mg/kg/day intravenously).[102,103]

Meningeal Leukemia. Meningeal leukemia is almost unknown in CP and is rare in BC. The incidence may increase with improved survival of patients with blast transformation. The usual neurologic signs are cranial nerve palsies and papilledema; the diagnosis is confirmed by demonstrating pleocytosis, with blast cells in the spinal fluid. Intrathecal methotrexate is effective therapy,[105] but most patients eventually die of the hematologic consequences of the blast transformation. The role of prophylactic central nervous system therapy is undefined.[106]

Cytoreduction

The initial goal of treatment for CP has been to ameliorate leukocytosis and organomegaly. Early treatment regimens with busulfan or hydroxyurea achieved this goal but rarely achieved permanent remissions due to failure to eradicate all cells of the CML clone. Interferon was the first agent to achieve a significant rate of cytogenetic remissions. Traditionally, the median survival of patients diagnosed in CP had been 5 to 7 years, with 50% to 60% alive at 5 years and 30% surviving to 10 years. With the advent of BCR-ABL1–targeted therapy with directed tyrosine-kinase inhibitors (TKIs) such as imatinib, complete cytogenetic molecular responses have now been achieved. Currently, TKIs are the frontline therapy for CML and have improved overall survival to 80% to 90% at 6 years.[107] However, SCT remains the only therapy with a long-term track record in producing long-term cure.

Hydroxyurea. Hydroxyurea, an inhibitor of ribonucleoside diphosphate reductase (an enzyme essential for DNA synthesis), is specific for cells in S phase of the cell cycle. The recommended starting dose is 10 to 20 mg/kg/day,[108] and dosages must be adjusted according to the hematologic response.

Interferon-α. In the 1980s, interferon-α (IFN-α) became the standard therapy for CML and is currently used in patients who are intolerant of TKIs. IFN-α appears to exert a direct antiproliferative effect against both normal and CML myeloid precursors, particularly those of the late progenitor compartment, which is preferentially expanded in CML.[109] Other effects include immunomodulation through increase in LFA-3 expression,[110] increase in ability of CML cells to attach to marrow stroma,[111] and modification of expression of HLA-DR antigens.[112]

IFN-α is effective in reversing splenomegaly and normalizing the white blood cell and platelet count in early CP. IFN-α–based protocols can achieve CHR (Table 21.7) in more than 80% of patients; approximately 5% to 30% of these patients will also achieve complete cytogenetic response (CCyR) (Ph¹-negative), while another 10% to 38% show a major cytogenetic response (MCyR) (<35% Ph¹-positive cells). Patients achieving an MCyR have projected 5-year survival approaching 90%. Half of the patients who achieve long-term complete MCyR may achieve molecular remission (PCR-negative for BCR-ABL1).[113] The combination of IFN-α with low-dose cytarabine is superior to IFN-α alone; patients who achieved MCyR or CCyR within 2 years of diagnosis achieved a 7-year survival rate of 85%.[114]

Imatinib Mesylate. An exciting new chapter in the treatment of CML began with the development of imatinib mesylate (STI571, Gleevec, CGP57148B), the first agent designed as a molecularly specific suppressor of the neoplastic clone. Imatinib is a small 2-phenylaminopyrimidine molecule that blocks the activity of BCR-ABL protein by occupying its kinase pocket, thereby blocking the binding of ATP (Fig. 21.7); this prevents the constituent activation of the TK and abrogates its downstream phosphorylation of target proteins responsible for proliferation and for inhibition of apoptosis. It is relatively selective in its activity, with the ability to block all of the abl kinases (including p210, p185, v-abl, and c-abl variants), but relatively few other TKs, with the exception of arg, stem cell factor (cKit), and PDGFR.[122,123]

In comparison with historical controls with IFN regimens, patients treated with imatinib were more likely to achieve a cytogenetic response and have overall better survival outcomes (Table 21.7).[120,124–128] The IRIS (International Randomized Study of Interferon and STI571) study in newly diagnosed adult patients in CP randomly compared imatinib 400 mg daily dose versus interferon plus ara-C.[124] Imatinib achieved higher rates of CHR (95% vs. 56%) and CCyR (76.2% vs. 14.5%) at 18 months. In addition, the rate of progression to AP or BC decreased (3.3% vs. 8.5%). In the 6-year follow-up of patients on the Imatinib arm, the cumulative CCyR was 82% with the estimated 6-year event-free survival, overall survival, and progression-free survival of 83%, 88%, and 93%, respectively.[116] Higher doses of imatinib (800 mg/day) were found to produce higher and more rapid rates of cytogenetic and molecular response in another trial in adult patients with newly diagnosed CP with 90% achieving CCyR compare with 74% in a historical group treated with 400 mg once daily.[125] In the high-dose group, 52% of patients achieved CCyR by 3 months of therapy and 82% by 6 months, whereas the historical group had rates of about 37% and 56%, respectively. Complete molecular response rate was 28% after 12 months of therapy in the high-dose group versus 7% in the standard-dose

TABLE 21.7

RESULTS OF TREATMENT OF CHRONIC PHASE CML

Drug	Dose	Time point	CHR	MCyR	CCyR	OS	PFS
Adult studies							
Interferon (IRIS)[115]		18 mo	56%	34.7%	14.5%	95%	91.5%
Imatinib (IRIS)[115,116]	400 mg daily	18 mo	95%	87.1%	76.2%	97.2%	96.7%
	400 mg daily	6 yr	97%	89%	87%	88%	93%
Imatinib[117]	800 mg daily	15 mo	98	96	90	100%	100%
Dasatinib (START-C)[118]	70 mg BID	24 mo	91%	62%	53%	94%	80%
Nilotinib[119]	400 mg BID	18 mo	77%	57%	41%	91%	67%
Pediatric studies							
Imatinib (COG—phase I)[120]	260–570 mg/m² daily		100%		83%		
Imatinib (AAML0123)[121]	340 mg/m² daily	12 mo	78%*	87%	66%	98%	96%

*CHR, after 2 months of imatinib.
CCyR, complete cytogenetic response; CHR, complete hematological response; MCyR, major cytogenetic response; MMR, major molecular response; OS, overall survival; PFS, progression-free survival.

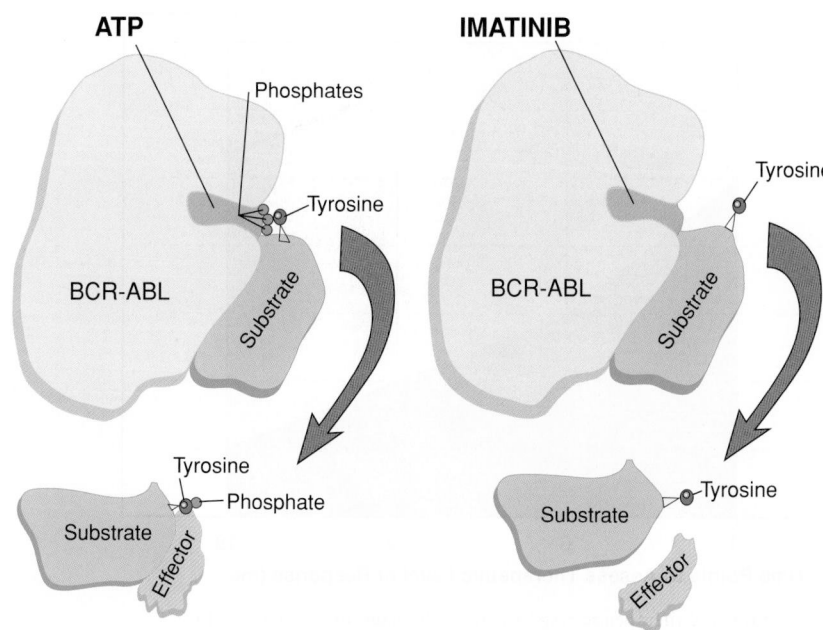

FIGURE 21.7 Mechanism of action of imatinib mesylate. In the untreated state (*left*), BCR-ABL protein has an open pocket accessible to ATP. This facilitates transfer of a phosphate moiety from ATP to a tyrosine residue on a target substrate molecule. The activated molecule is then released to interact with downstream effector molecules, which can promote oncogenesis. Imatinib inhibits this process by competing with ATP for the kinase pocket, thereby preventing phosphorylation of substrate and effector molecules. (Courtesy of Eleanore Rhodes.)

group. However, the high-dose regimen produced greater hematologic toxicity and a higher incidence of fluid retention.

A phase I study of imatinib was conducted by the Children's Oncology Group in pediatric patients with Ph[1]-positive CML refractory to IFN therapy, patients relapsing after SCT, or patients with refractory/relapsed Ph[1]-positive ALL.[120] Doses of 260 to 570 mg/m^2 were well tolerated. The maximum tolerated dose has not yet been determined and dose-limiting toxicity was not seen. CHR was achieved within 30 days in 100% of CP patients presenting with elevated WBC and thrombocytosis. Eighty-three percent obtained a CCyR within 2 to 6 months.[120] The most common side effects were mild nausea, vomiting, and diarrhea. Moderate anemia, thrombocytopenia, and neutropenia were seen in one-third of the patients. Other toxicities included diarrhea, abdominal pain, headaches, fatigue, stomatitis, and bone pain. The adverse effect profile differed slightly from that seen in the adult population, where the most frequently reported toxicities were gastrointestinal, dermatological (rash, edema), and musculoskeletal disturbances.[124]

In the pediatric phase II trial to evaluate the efficacy of imatinib in newly diagnosed children (ages 2 to 19 years) in CP, a daily dose of 340 mg/m^2 was given.[126] This dose is pharmacologically equivalent to the 600 mg dose in adults.[120] CHR was attained by 80% of patients by 2 months of therapy. CCyR was achieved in 36% of patients by 3 months and overall in 66% of patients at a median time of 5.6 months. Ninety-one percent of the patients who achieved CCyR did so by 9 months of therapy. The 1-year event-free survival and overall survival was 96% and 98%, respectively.[126]

Monitoring of response to imatinib therapy. The current National Comprehensive Cancer Network guidelines for adult patients with CML recommend that patients be monitored with complete blood counts, cytogenetic and fluorescent *in situ* hybridization (FISH) analysis, as well as quantitative PCR (QPCR).[129] Cytogenetics should be monitored at months 6, 12, and 18 or until a CcyR is achieved. Although interphase or metaphase FISH can be done using probes for *BCR-ABL1*, routine metaphase cytogenetics should also be performed to detect additional clonal chromosome abnormalities which may occur in Ph1+ cells as well as Ph-negative cells.[130] *BCR-*

ABL1 transcripts levels by QPCR should be obtained every 3 months until patient achieves a CCyR, after which the QPCR can be measured every 3 to 6 months. *BCR-ABL1* studies may be performed on peripheral blood specimens once CCyR is achieved.[129]

The lack of significant cytogenetic response is an unfavorable prognostic factor.[115,131] In a study of adult patients with CP CML who were treated with imatinib after failure of IFN therapy, those who failed to achieve MCyR (<35% Ph[1]) by 6 months were more likely to experience a hematologic relapse than those who did achieve MCyR—27% relapse rate versus 3% relapse rate, respectively.[131] In addition, patients with no cytogenetic response (>95% Ph[1]) by 6 months of therapy were less likely to achieve an MCyR after 15 months of therapy than those who have achieved at least a minimal response (<65% Ph[1])—17% probability of MCyR versus 24%, respectively. The time to achieving an MCyR is also associated with likelihood of achieving a CCyR and survival outcome. In the long-term follow-up of patients treated with imatinib after failure of interferon therapy,[115] among those who achieved an MCyR by 3, 6, or 12 months of therapy, a CCyR was achieved by 85%, 73%, and 71%, respectively. The 4-year survival rate of those patients who achieved an MCyR by 12 months was significantly better than those who had no response—97% versus 74%, respectively. Based on these findings, the following definitions of "suboptimal" response of imatinib therapy in adult patients with CP CML have been proposed by the European LeukemiaNet[116,129]: (a) failure to achieve a CHR following 3 months of therapy; (b) failure to achieve an MCyR following 6 months of therapy; and (c) failure to achieve a CCyR following 12 months of therapy or (d) failure to obtain a 3-log reduction in *BCR-ABL/ABL1* ratios compared with pretreatment levels following 18 months of therapy (Fig. 21.8). For those patients with suboptimal response, a change in therapy may be warranted.

Mechanisms of resistance to imatinib. Resistance to imatinib is categorized as primary (failure to achieve a timely response) or secondary (loss of a previously achieved response). Inability to achieve a primary hematological response is rare in patients with newly diagnosed CML. However, failure to attain an appropriate cytogenetic response occurs in 15% to 25% of patients and

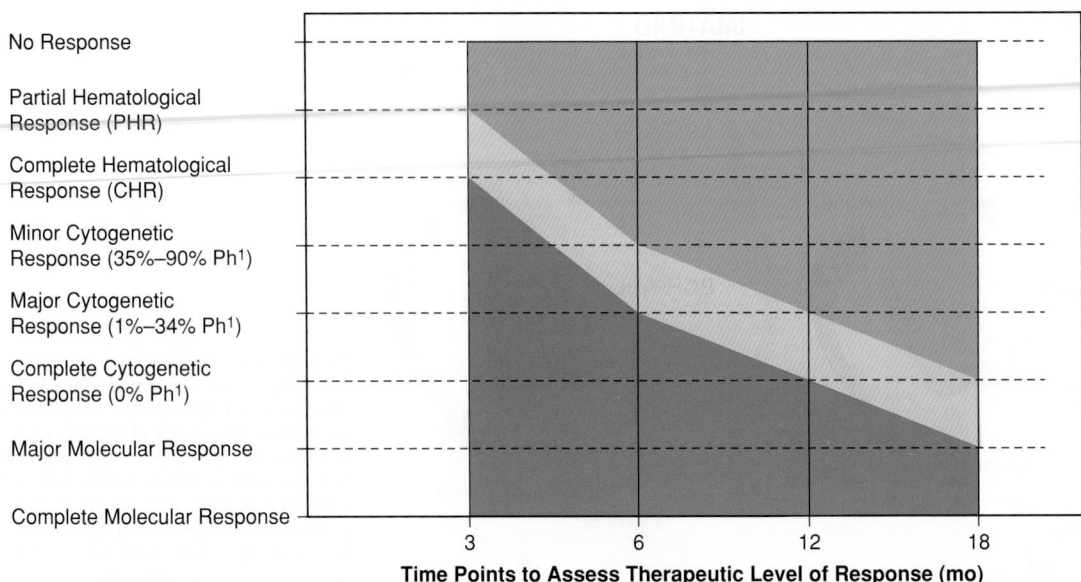

No Response

Partial Hematological
Response (PHR)

Complete Hematological
Response (CHR)

Minor Cytogenetic
Response (35%–90% Ph^1)

Major Cytogenetic
Response (1%–34% Ph^1)

Complete Cytogenetic
Response (0% Ph^1)

Major Molecular Response

Complete Molecular Response

3   6   12   18

Time Points to Assess Therapeutic Level of Response (mo)

FIGURE 21.8 Milestones for initial therapy and therapeutic response in newly diagnosed patients with chronic phase CML. Classification of therapeutic response with CML therapy involves determining the level of response at various time points. When the level of response at a specified time point falls within the *green* shaded region in this graph, this would be considered an "optimal response," while those that fall within the *orange* shaded region would be considered a "suboptimal response" and those levels that fall into the *red* region would be considered "response failure." (For example, at the 3-month time point, a CHR or better would be optimal, a PHR is suboptimal, and less than a PHR or no response would suggest treatment failure.) *Levels of response*: **Partial hematological response (PHR)** = WBC >10,000/mm^3, platelet >450,000/mm^3, but >50% reduction in WBC and platelet, presence of immature cells and splenomegaly; **Complete hematological response (CHR)** = normal CBC/differential with WBC <10,000/mm^3, platelet <450,000/mm^3, absence of immature cells and splenomegaly; **Minor cytogenetic response** = 35%–90% Ph-positive metaphases; **Major cytogenetic response** = 1%–34% Ph-positive metaphases; **Complete cytogenetic response** = no Ph-positive metaphases; **Major molecular response** = ≥ 3-log reduction of BCR-ABL mRNA; **Complete molecular response** = no BCR-ABL mRNA by QPCR. (From Deininger MW. Milestones and monitoring in patients with CML treated with imatinib. Hematology Am Soc Hematol Educ Program 2008:497, copyright the American Society of Hematology, used with permission. Originally published in Blood.)

may be related to pharmacokinetic variability.[117,132] Lower imatinib plasma trough levels were noted in patients who did not achieve CCyR or major molecular response than patients who did.[117] This suggests that higher doses of imatinib may be able to overcome this BCR-ABL–independent resistance. Imatinib is metabolized by the cytochrome p450 isoenzymes, and drugs that interact with this system can affect trough levels. Plasma drug binding and drug transport may also affect availability of drug to the CML cell. Alpha 1 acid glycoprotein 1 is an acute-phase reactant that binds cationic drugs, such as imatinib, and may lead to decreased plasma drug levels and decrease its therapeutic activity.[132] ABCB1 (or MDR1), the adenosine triphosphate-binding cassette (ABC) transporter, is a transmembrane protein that modulates the efflux of chemotherapeutic drugs in some cancer cells. ABCB1 has been found to be overexpressed in cells from patients with CML-BP as well as in patients who did not achieve MCyR.[133] Another drug transporter, hOCT (human organic cation transporter), may regulate the cellular influx of imatinib. Polymorphisms of this carrier resulting in low activity has been associated with suboptimal response to imatinib, whereas high hOCT activity has been associated with good molecular responses.[118]

CML cells may develop resistance to imatinib by a variety of mechanisms.[118,119,134–136] Genetic mechanisms of resistance include (a) overexpression of *BCR-ABL1*; (b) development of point mutations in the *ABL1* kinase domain of *BCR-ABL1*, primarily in the P-loop of the ATP-binding pocket, resulting in steric changes that inhibit the direct binding of imatinib; or (c) mutations in the activation loop of the kinase domain, preventing the closed/inactivated conformation change of ABL1 needed for imatinib binding. Point mutations in the kinase domain (e.g., T3151) have become the most common mechanism of resistance (Fig. 21.9). Patients who develop such mutations have a higher risk of cytogenetic and hematologic relapse as well as progression to BC.[118,119,133–145] Overexpression of src-related kinases has also been found in imatinib-resistant CML cells.[137]

Interleukin-3 (IL-3), a hematopoietic stem cell growth factor, has been shown to have a positive effect on CML cell survival in *in vitro* studies.[138] The IL-3 autocrine loop observed in CML cells may protect the cells from undergoing apoptosis when exposed to imatinib and other bcr-abl TKIs. This IL-3-induced signal transduction pathway may contribute to incomplete cytogenetic responses in patients.

Resistance to imatinib may also reflect the differential sensitivity of CML cells depending on their state of differentiation. CML stem cells may remain viable in a quiescent state in the presence of imatinib and may serve as a source of disease recurrence.[139,140]

In some cases, resistance to conventional doses of imatinib may be overcome by dose increases. Dose escalations to 600 to 800 mg/day from 400 mg/day in patients in CP with hematological or cytogenetic resistance or relapse have resulted in 65% and 56%, respectively, achieving a complete or partial response.[133] Newer approaches to imatinib-resistant CML using dual scr/bcr-abl inhibitors show early promise.[141]

Ba/F3 cellular proliferation IC_{50} values

	imatinib (nM)	nilotinib (nM)	dasatinib (nM)
Native Bcr-Abl	260	13	0.8
M244V	2000	38	1.3
G250E	1350	48	1.8
Q252H	1325	70	3.4
Y253F	3475	125	1.4
Y253H	>6400	450	1.3
E255K	5200	200	5.6
E255V	>6400	430	11
V299L	540†	nd	18†
F311L	480	23	1.3
T315A	971	61	125†
T315I	>6400	>2000	>200
F317L	1050	50	7.4
F317V	350†	nd	53†
F315T	880	15	1.1
F355G	2300†	nd	1.8†
F359V	1825	175	2.2
V379I	1630	51	0.8
L387M	1000	49	2
H396P	850	41	0.6
H396R	1750	41	1.3

Sensitive

Intermediate sensitivity

Insensitive

FIGURE 21.9 Sensitivity of Bcr-Abl kinase domain mutants to Abl kinase inhibitors. *Imatinib*: sensitive (≤1,000 nM), intermediate (≤3,000 nM), insensitive (>3,000 nM); *Nilotinib*: sensitive (≤50 nM), intermediate (≤500 nM), insensitive (>500 nM); *Dasatinib*: sensitive (≤3 nM), intermediate (≤60 nM), insensitive (>60 nM).[a] The IC_{50} value is the concentration of inhibitor resulting in a 50% reduction in cell viability. (From Deininger MW. Milestones and monitoring in patients with CML treated with imatinib. Hematology Am Soc Hematol Educ Program 2008:497, copyright the American Society of Hematology, used with permission. Originally published in Blood.)

Acquired cytogenetic abnormalities following imatinib therapy. An additional concern with imatinib therapy is the potential for emergence of cytogenetic mutations in the normal stem cell population. Acquired chromosome alterations such as aneuploidy, an additional Ph[1] chromosome, trisomy 8, and loss of a p53 allele from aberrations in the short arm of chromosome 17 have been reported. In some patients, multiple changes may occur.[136] In one study, clonal cytogenetic changes were found in the Ph[1]-negative population of 15% of patients treated with imatinib. Imatinib may not directly induce these clonal changes but may allow for emergence of occult abnormal populations due to its molecular specificity. Although nonspecific cytotoxic therapies such as chemotherapy, SCT, and IFN may have broad effects on all stem cells, a targeted agent such as imatinib would only affect those cells with the bcr-abl abnormality; thus, elimination of the Ph[1]-positive population would allow these occult abnormal Ph[1]-negative clones to emerge and dominate hematopoiesis.[142]

Second-generation ABL kinase inhibitors. Two new agents, dasatinib and nilotinib, have emerged in the treatment of CML. Dasatinib (Sprycel™, BMS-354825) is a dual scr-family kinase and ABL kinase inhibitor. In addition, dasatinib also inhibits ephrin receptor kinases, PDGFR, Kit and other tyrosine and serine/threonine kinases. It is more potent than imatinib in inhibiting the growth of resistant cell lines except T315I. Dasatinib binds to both the active and inactive conformation of the ABL kinase domain.[143] In the phase II START trials of dasatinib, 70 mg twice-daily dose was given.[144–146] For patients in CP, CCyR occurred in 53% of patients with major molecular response and progression-free survival seen in 47% and 80%, respectively, of the patients at 24 months.[144] For patients in the AP, Dasatinib produced a 33% MCyR and 76% progression-free survival at 8 months.[145] For patients in lymphoid or myeloid blast crisis, major molecular response

occurred in 50% and 31%, respectively.[146] Recently, a pediatric phase I study of dasatinib has been completed by the Children's Oncology Group.[147] Two complete responses and three partial responses were seen among six patients with CML. The 85-mg/m^2 dose level was well tolerated, and dose-limiting toxicities noted included hypokalemia and diarrhea. Pleural effusions were seen in patients treated at a higher dose level.

Nilotinib (Tasigna™, AMN107) is a second-generation, highly selective, ATP-competitive BCR-ABL inhibitor with 10 to 50 times the potency of imatinib in the inhibition of proliferation and autophosphorylation in imatinib-resistant cell lines (except for those with T315I mutation). The molecule contains a *N*-methylpiperazine moiety and can also inhibit Arg, Kit, and PDGFR.[128] A phase II study of nilotinib at the 400 mg twice-daily dosing in patients resistant to, or intolerant of, imatinib achieve MCyR in 57%, CCyR in 41%, and overall survival of 91% at 18 months.[128] CCyR, MCyR, complete molecular response, and overall survival at 12 months was achieved in 47%, 31%, 19%, and 79%, respectively, in AP patients and 11%, 40%, 29%, and 42%, respectively, in BC patients.[128,148,149] Nilotinib was tolerated well with low incidence of prolonged QTc syndrome, fluid retention, edema, and musculoskeletal discomfort.[128,148,149]

Bosutinib and INNO-406 are new dual ABL kinase inhibitors under investigation. Bosutinib, like Dasatinib, has src inhibitory effect and binds both the active and inactive conformations of bcr-abl.[150] It does not inhibit kit or PDGFR and has overall less toxicity. It is currently in phase II trials in adults with CML. INNO-406 is a dual Abl/Lyn kinase.[151] Overexpression of Lyn kinase has been reported in imatinib-resistant CML, and this drug has more than 55 times the growth inhibitory activity of imatinib.

Splenic Irradiation. Irradiation of the spleen in patients with CP CML reduces splenomegaly, lowers the peripheral leukocyte count, and also reduces the number of immature cells and the mitotic index at sites distant from the spleen (e.g., bone marrow). This distant (abscopal) effect could result from the release of an inhibitor into the plasma or an interruption of the flow of GM-CFU from the splenic parenchyma into the circulation.[152] Splenic irradiation may be considered for transient palliation of the symptoms produced by massive splenomegaly in patients refractory to systemic chemotherapy, but this treatment is generally ineffective and may cause profound myelosuppression.

Splenectomy. The enlarged spleen of the patient with CML contains a substantial burden of leukemic cells, and, in some cases, blast transformation may originate in the spleen.[153] Investigators have proposed that removal of this pool of cells may delay metamorphosis. However, several large controlled trials have failed to demonstrate any benefit from splenectomy in prolonging CP or survival.[154,155] Splenectomy may be of benefit in selected patients with hypersplenism or painful splenomegaly; it may also be useful in reducing the leukemic burden in patients about to undergo SCT. However, these potential benefits must be weighed against the risk of overwhelming postsplenectomy sepsis syndrome and extreme thrombocytosis.

Stem Cell Transplantation. The theoretical and technical aspects of SCT are discussed in Chapter 16. Three sources of hematopoietic stem cells have been used for transplantation in patients with CML: syngeneic (from an identical twin), allogeneic (from an HLA-identical sibling or matched unrelated donor), and autologous (from the patient).

Syngeneic or allogeneic transplantation. Allogeneic SCT remains the only well-documented curative therapy for patients with CML (Table 21.8). Disease status at the time of SCT has been considered to be the most powerful predictor of survival. In early studies, the best results were obtained in patients who had undergone SCT in early first CP (49% to 86% long-term survival); the chances for long-term survival became progressively worse when SCT was performed in second CP (30% to 58%), AP (15% to 35%), or BC (10% to 20%).[156–158] More recent studies have not confirmed that delaying transplant in CP is necessarily an independent adverse prognostic factor.[159,160] Even with ideal transplant candidates whose donors are fully HLA-matched siblings, there is mortality risk by day-100 posttransplant of approximately 15%. However, reduction in the myelotoxicity of the preparative regimen may decrease this risk; one recent study using a reduced-intensity combination of fludarabine-busulfan-antithymocyte globulin achieved a mortality rate of 0% with 21 of 24 patients alive and disease-free after a median follow-up of 42 months.[161]

Some investigators have attempted to ameliorate the morbidity and mortality of graft-versus-host disease (GVHD) by depleting the donor marrow of T cells.[162–165] In general, T-cell depletion has reduced the incidence and severity of GVHD but at the cost of an increase in the leukemia relapse rate, which negates any long-term survival advantage (Table 21.8).[166] Similarly, the use of autologous or syngeneic (identical twin) SCT has been accompanied by virtually no GVHD but a high leukemia recurrence rate. In contrast, development of moderate-to-severe GVHD after administration of an allogeneic or unrelated donor graft appears to confer protection against relapse (Table 21.8). These results indicate that the intense chemotherapy-radiotherapy conditioning regimens used in conjunction with SCT are often inadequate to eradicate the CML clone without augmentation by a graft-versus-leukemia (GVL) effect.

TABLE 21.8

RESULTS OF BONE MARROW TRANSPLANTATION IN CHRONIC MYELOCYTIC LEUKEMIA

Type of transplant	Relapse rate (%)
Autologous	100
T-cell depleted	50–70
Twin (syngeneic)	40–70
Allogeneic	10–20
Without GVHD	11
With GVHD	5
Unrelated	
Matched	3
Mismatched	0
PBSC	11
Pediatrics	
Allogeneic	21–23
First chronic phase	15–17
Other phases	49–52
T-cell depleted	40
Matched unrelated	6–15
First chronic phase	13
Other phases	20
T-cell depleted	18

GVHD, graft-versus-host disease; PBSC, peripheral blood stem cell. Data derived from Clift RA, Appelbaum FR, Thomas ED. Treatment of chronic myeloid leukemia by marrow transplantation [editorial]. Blood 1993;82:1954; Cunningham I, Castro-Malaspina H, Flomenberg N, et al. T-cell depleted bone marrow transplant for chronic myelogenous leukemia. Blood 1988;72:384a; Elmaagacli AH, Basoglu S, Peceny R, et al. Improved disease-free-survival after transplantation of peripheral blood stem cells as compared with bone marrow from HLA-identical unrelated donors in patients with first chronic phase chronic myeloid leukemia. Blood 2002;99:1103–1135; Millot F, Esperou H, Bordigoni P, et al. Allogeneic bone marrow transplantation from chronic myeloid leukemia in childhood: a report from the Societe Francaise de Greffe de Moelle et de Therapie Cellulaire (SFGM-TC). Bone Marrow Transplant 2003;32:993–999; Goldman JM, Gale RP, Horowitz MM, et al. Bone marrow transplantation for chronic myelogenous leukemia in chronic phase: increased risk of relapse associated with T-cell depletion. Ann Intern Med 1988;108:806.

Fewer than 35% of patients with CML have an HLA-identical sibling, with perhaps another 5% having an acceptable, partially histocompatible related donor. For the remaining 60% to 70% of patients, HLA-matched unrelated donors present an alternative source of donor stem cells. Data from the National Marrow Donor Registry[166] indicate a 2-year actuarial disease-free survival (DFS) of 45% for patients who undergo SCT in first CP within 1 year of diagnosis; however, severe problems with GVHD are encountered (Table 21.9). In a recent report of children with CML transplanted in first CP, those with HLA-matched sibling donor had improved 3-year leukemia-free survival (LFS)/overall survival (65%/75%) in comparison with those who had undergone matched unrelated donor SCT (LFS 55%/DFS 66%).[167]

The great debate: SCT versus imatinib for chronic phase CML. The dramatic results achieved by the introduction of imatinib into CML therapy raise the question of whether SCT remains the appropriate first-line therapy for CML, even for those with matched sibling donors. At present, SCT remains the only proven curative therapy for CML. However, this is

TABLE 21.9

RESULTS OF UNRELATED DONOR TRANSPLANT FOR CML (2-YEAR FOLLOW-UP)

Status at time of transplant	Disease-free survival (%)
Chronic phase/1st year	45
Chronic phase/>1 year	36
Accelerated phase	27
Blast crisis	0
Hematologic relapse	11
Severe acute GVHD	54
Extensive chronic GVHD	52
Failure of engraftment	11
Late graft failure	5

CML, chronic myelocytic leukemia; GVHD, graft-versus-host disease. McGlave PB, Bartsch G, Anasetti C, et al. Unrelated donor marrow transplantation for chronic myelogenous leukemia: initial experience of The National Marrow Donor Program. Blood 1993;81:543, with permission.

achieved at the cost of transplant-related morbidity and mortality. On the other hand, imatinib therapy has been associated with a very high rate of hematologic, cytogenetic, and molecular remissions while being relatively nontoxic. However, the long-term survival benefit of imatinib has yet to be demonstrated by a phase III clinical trial. A survey of Children's Oncology Group centers suggests that there is no broad consensus regarding the definitive management of newly diagnosed CML patients—transplant physicians tend to favor SCT, whereas hematologist-oncologists tend to favor imatinib.[168] Guidelines in the management of adult patients with CML currently do not recommend the use of allogeneic SCT as first-line treatment for CML in CP due to the excellent results of the imatinib clinical trials. In addition, adult patients with CML tend to be older (median age in the 60s) and transplant-related mortality may be higher. However, SCT may be a good alternative for those patients with poor prognosticators, such as (a) failure of any cytogenetic response at 6 months; (b) cytogenetic relapse at 12 to 18 months after initially achieving a hematological response; (c) failure of complete CcyR at 18 months; and (d) patients with the T315I mutation who do not respond to imatinib, dasatinib, or nilotinib.[168]

Management of Posttransplant Relapses. Treatment options for patients who relapse after allogeneic BMT include use of IFN-α, TKIs, second SCT, and/or infusion of lymphocytes from the original donor. Remissions may be induced by the use of IFN-α alone, but at least half of these patients ultimately relapse again.[169,170] Imatinib (400 to 1,000 mg/day) has been successful in treating post-SCT relapses of CML.[171] Response was dependent on phase of disease at relapse: CHR rates were 100% for CP, 83% for AP, and 43% for BC, while MCyR/CCyR rates were 63% for CP or AP and 43% for BC. The survival rate following a second BMT is poor and is complicated by increased procedure-related morbidity and mortality.[172,173] Patients with relapsed CML may also be restored to CCyR by administration of IFN-α together with leukocyte transfusions from the donor[174,175] or by the use of donor leukocyte infusions (DLIs) alone.[176] DLI can induce second remission in up to 70% of patients; the probability of success is greater if the DLI is administered before hematologic relapse is evident.[177] The risk of GVHD is minimized if an escalating dose schedule of DLI is followed.[178,179] The durabil-

ity of these remissions (which presumably result from a GVL effect) has not been established.

Detection of Residual Leukemia After Bone Marrow Transplant. Residual leukemic cells may be detected with increasing sensitivity at the morphologic (hematologic or bone marrow changes), cytogenetic (reappearance of the Ph[1] chromosome), or molecular level. Molecular relapses can be detected using qualitative or quantitative RT-PCR analysis for *BCR-ABL1* mRNA transcripts or FISH to assess interphase nuclei at the DNA level. More recently, molecular chimerism in myeloid (CD34+) precursor cells and detection of P190[bcr/abl] have emerged as novel markers of CML evolution that may identify impending cytogenetic relapses after SCT.[21] The National Comprehensive Cancer Center Network[129] has recommended posttransplant follow-up with qualitative RT-PCR every 3 months for 2 years, then every 6 months for 3 years. Because results from peripheral blood analyses tend to correlate well with those using bone marrow, long-term monitoring can utilize peripheral blood.

Quantitative RT-PCR is the most sensitive technique for detecting residual CML, with a sensitivity of $1/10^5$ to $1/10^6$ cells. When performed early (3 to 5 months) posttransplant, this assay has been demonstrated to have a high prognostic value. Three years posttransplant, the cumulative incidence of relapse varied from 16.7% (for patients with no *BCR-ABL1* transcripts detectable) to 86.4% (for patients with high level of residual *BCR-ABL1* transcripts).[180]

Patients may show various karyotypic responses after SCT, including (a) complete eradication of the Ph[1]-positive clone, (b) cytogenetic relapse in the presence or absence of hematologic relapse, (c) transient reappearance of Ph[1]-positive cells in the absence of hematologic relapse, and (d) late (>1 year) disappearance of Ph[1]-positive cells in the absence of further therapy.[181,182]

Approximately 70% of patients are RT-PCR negative at 1 year posttransplant and remain so indefinitely. Ph[1] or PCR positivity up to 6 months after SCT may not have adverse prognostic significance, whereas persistence of cytogenetic or molecular abnormalities in the 6- to 12-month interval posttransplant or in the patient receiving a T-cell–depleted graft identifies those who are at a relatively high risk of relapse.[182–185] Predicting the prognosis for patients who vacillate between PCR-positive and PCR-negative status is more difficult. The transitory nature of Ph[1] or PCR positivity in some patients may reflect the persistence of a few long-living T or B lymphocytes or myeloid cells that lack proliferative potential; alternatively, these PCR-positive patients may have mechanisms (e.g., GVL effect) for continuous suppression of residual clonogenic leukemic cells *in vivo*.[186]

Novel Strategies. The limited success, and excessive toxicity, of conventional chemotherapeutic, immunotherapeutic, and stem cell rescue techniques has stimulated the search for novel therapeutic approaches to the treatment of CML. The most successful of these approaches, blockage of the BCR-ABL1 TK with imatinib, has been discussed earlier. Other new approaches include inhibition of downstream signaling pathways and immunotherapy.

Inhibition of individual signaling pathways downstream of BCR-ABL1. As the specific signal transduction events that contribute to leukemogenesis become elucidated, efforts may be made to develop rational therapeutic interventions designed to block these pathways. One example is the use of imatinib to inhibit the TK activity of BCR-ABL1 (discussed earlier). In addition, molecular strategies may be employed to inhibit individual downstream mediators of the *BCR-ABL1* pathway such as *RAS*,[187] *RAF*,[188] *JUN* kinase,[189] and *MYC*.[190] 17-AAG is a heat shock protein 90 (Hsp90) inhibitor, which binds to the ATP-binding pocket of Hsp90 and inhibits its normal chaperone function with proteins such as raf, Akt, BCR-ABL1 to maintain a stable conformation. This then leads to downregulation of *BCR-ABL1* and apoptosis of CML cells.[191] Activation of the *RAS* pathway plays a central role in the leukemogenesis of CML cells. Farnesyltransferase inhibitors (FTIs), such as Tipifarnib (R115777) and Lonafarnib, target the posttranslational prenylation process of Ras, thereby inhibiting the proliferation of CML cells.[192,193]

Immunotherapy. The junction site of *BCR-ABL1* generates a sequence of amino acids that is unique to the CML cell, thereby presenting a tumor-specific antigen that has the potential of activating an immune response. A BCR-ABL1–derived peptide vaccine has been demonstrated to be well tolerated and to elicit a specific immune response in CP CML patients.[194]

Targeting the T315I mutation. The T315I mutation results in a very resistant phenotype which is unresponsive to imatinib, dasatinib, nilotinib, and many of the newer Abl-kinases.[142,149,150,156] Homoharringtonine (HHT) is a plant alkaloid derived from the *Cephalotaxus* evergreen tree, which inhibits protein synthesis. HHT has been shown *in vitro* to be synergistic with imatinib in inducing apoptosis.[195] Omacetaxine is a semisynthetic HHT and has recently been found to be effective in patients with the T315I mutation, resulting in a decrease in BCR-ABL transcripts in these patients.[196] *In vitro* assays with the aurora kinase inhibitor PHA-739358 has shown strong antiproliferative and proapoptotic activity against imatinib-resistant cell lines, including those with the T315I mutation.[197] Clinical trials to evaluate this compound are in development.

Management of Blast Crisis

BC is generally a treatment-resistant state that terminates fatally within weeks to months. Regimens developed for the treatment of acute myelogenous leukemia have proved disappointing in BC CML (Table 21.10).[92,198–209] Patients with myeloblastic BC have response rates of less than 20% and a median survival of 5 months.[208,209] The subset of patients with lymphoblastic transformation is more sensitive to chemotherapy; approximately two-thirds of such patients revert to CP after treatment with vincristine-prednisone regimens.[92] Unfortunately, the response is of short duration (median, <6 months), and fewer than 20% of patients survive for 1 year.

Imatinib has been reported to produce CHR rate of 15% in BC patients and sustained responses in 8%.[120] MCyRs were observed in 16%, with 7% achieving a CCyR. The second-generation *ABL1* kinase inhibitors have produced slightly better results. Dasatinib has produced MCyR in about 30% of patients in myeloid BC and 50% of patients with lymphoid BC,[145] whereas nilotinib has resulted in MCyR in 40% of patients in BC and CCyR in 29% of those patients.[148] Table 21.11 summarizes the results of more recent trials employing these agents.[145,148,149,211–214]

Decitabine, a hypomethylating agent, has shown some activity in BC, producing a 6% to 10% CHR and 15% to 28% overall objective response rate.[208,215,216] Troxacitabine, a novel L-nucleoside analog, successfully returned 6 out of 16 BC patients to CP in a phase II study.[216a] The functional loss of protein phosphatase 2A (PP2A) activity is relevant to the transformation of CML cells to BC. FTY720, an immunomodulator that activates PP2A, has been shown in *in vitro* and *in vivo* studies to induce apoptosis and decrease proliferation of CML-BC cells.[217]

Intensive chemotherapy regimens incorporating imatinib have shown good response for Ph+ALL and may provide an option for CML in lymphoid BC.[218] Imatinib combined with mitoxantrone and etoposide has produced a high hematological response rate in patients with myeloid blast crisis, but with chemotherapy alone, the median survival remains short.[219]

The results of BMT in BC are uniformly poor; fewer than 15% of patients achieve long-term survival with current regimens. In view of the dismal results achieved with other

---

TABLE 21.10

RESULTS OF TREATMENT OF BLAST-PHASE CHRONIC MYELOCYTIC LEUKEMIA

Regimen	Number of patients	Complete response (%)[a]	Partial response (%)[b]
VCR/pred[92]	10 (myeloid)	0	NR
	11 (lymphoid)	67	NR
TRAMPCOL[198]	19	42	9
HD ara-C[199]	21	24	13
HU/6-MP/pred ±VCR/DNR[200]		12	22
HU/6-MP/VP-16[201]	5	20	NR
L-10/L-10M[202]	15 (lymphoid)	67	NR
5-AZA/VP-16[203]	27	4	6
Mitoxantrone[204–206]	13 (myeloid)	0	31
DATA[207]	30	0	13
Plica/HU[208]	6 (myeloid)	100	NR
	3 (lymphoid)	33	NR
Decitabine[209]	64	28	NR
Imatinib (phase I)[120]	38 (myeloid)	32	24
	20 (lymphoid)	55	15
Imatinib (phase II)[210]	229 (myeloid)	52	

[a]Reversion to chronic phase.
[b]Decline in blast count.
NR, no response.

TREATMENT OF ACCELERATED PHASE AND BLAST CRISIS CML WITH TYROSINE KINASE INHIBITORS

Drug	Dose	CML phase	Time point	CHR (%)	McyR (%)	CcyR (%)	OS (%)	PFS
Imatinib (STI571 0109)[211,212]	600 mg daily	AP	18 mo	81	40	28	79	
	600 mg daily	AP	48 mo	40	27	20	45	
Dasatinib (START-A)[145]	70 mg BID	AP	12 mo	45	39	32	82	66
Nilotinib[148]	400 mg BID	AP	12 mo	11	40	29	42	
Imatinib (STI571 0102)[213]	400–600 mg	BC	12 mo	8	16	7	32	
Dasatinib (START-B)[214]	70 mg BID	BC–myeloid	8 mo	26	31	27	90	88
Dasatinib (START-L)[214]	70 mg BID	BC–lymphoid	8 mo	26	50	43	86	46
Nilotinib[149]	400 mg BID	BC	12 mo	11	40	29	42	

AP, accelerated phase; BC, blast crisis; CcyR, complete cytogenetic response; CHR, complete hematological response; McyR, major cytogenetic response; OS, overall survival; PFS, progression-free survival.

approaches, however, BMT is worth considering in selected cases.

JUVENILE MYELOMONOCYTIC LEUKEMIA

Juvenile myelomonocytic leukemia (JMML) resembles CML in that it is a clonal panmyelopathy, often presenting with leukocytosis and splenomegaly.[220] However, in the late 1990s, a consensus was reached by the International JMML Working Group and the European Working Group of Myelodysplasia (EWOG-MDS) in Childhood to reclassify the condition known previously as JCML as JMML.[221,222] These groups also suggested a group of minimal diagnostic criteria for the diagnosis of JMML (Table 21.12). With the recent identification of certain genetic mutations in JMML, a revised set of diagnostic criteria was proposed by the International JMML Working Group in 2006 (Table 21.13).[223] The World Health Organization has revised the French-American-British classification of myeloid neoplasms to list JMML as a mixed myelodysplastic/myeloproliferative disorder.[224]

Individuals with neurofibromatosis type 1 (NF-1) are at particularly high risk for developing JMML (approximately 200 to 500 times that of the general population).[225–227] Noonan syndrome and constitutional trisomy 8 have also been seen in association with JMML.[228–229] Monosomy 7, another myeloproliferative disorder of childhood, shares many of the features of JMML, but it is usually associated with a lower level of hemoglobin F (Hgb F).[230–232] Although the exact relationship between these two conditions remains unresolved, both the International JMML Working Group and the EWOG-MDS have recommended that they be treated in a similar fashion.[233] It is more important to distinguish JMML from chronic viral infections (especially cytomegalovirus [CMV], Epstein-Barr virus [EBV], and human herpesvirus-6) that can also produce hepatosplenomegaly, lymphadenopathy, leukocytosis, thrombocytopenia, and elevated Hgb F levels. Serologic studies to detect an antibody response to one of these viruses are helpful. Bone marrow examination may be helpful because viral infections may produce hemophagocytosis, which is not a typical feature of JCML but has been described as a rare paraneoplastic phenomenon.[234,235] The distinctive granulocyte-macrophage colony-stimulating factor (GM-CSF) hypersensitivity manifested by JMML marrow

cells in tissue culture (discussed further on) may also be useful in making the distinction.[236]

Biology

Hematologic and cytogenetic evidence confirms that JMML is a clonal stem cell disorder, with the leukemic progenitor cell capable of giving rise to erythroid, myeloid, monocytic, and megakaryocytic lineages[220,232,233,237,238] (and possibly lymphoid lineages as well). The predominant cell in the peripheral blood and the bone marrow appears to be a primitive monocytic

DIAGNOSTIC CRITERIA FOR JUVENILE MYELOMONOCYTIC LEUKEMIA

Categories	Criteria
Suggestive clinical features	Hepatosplenomegaly Lymphadenopathy Pallor Fever Skin rash
Minimal laboratory criteria (must fulfill all three)	Peripheral monocytosis (>1×10⁹/L) Bone marrow blasts >20% Absence of Ph¹ chromosome and bcr/abl rearrangement
Further criteria (minimum of two required)	Elevated Hgb F (corrected for age) WBC >10 × 10⁹/L Immature myeloid cells on peripheral smear Clonal cytogenetic abnormalities (including monosomy 7) Hypersensitivity of myeloid progenitors to GM-CSF (in vitro)

GM-CSF, granulocyte-macrophage colony-stimulating factor; Hgb F, hemoglobin F; WBC, white blood cell count.

TABLE 21.13

REVISED JMML DIAGNOSTIC CRITERIA (PROPOSED)[224]

Category 1 (all of the following required)	Splenomegaly Absolute monocyte count >1,000/μL Blasts in PB/BM <20% Absence of Ph[1] chromosome and BCR/ABL fusion gene Age younger than 13 years
Category 2 (at least one of the following)	Somatic mutations in RAS or PTPN11 Clinical diagnosis of NF1 or NFI gene mutation Monosomy 7
Category 3 (at least two of the following)	Circulating myeloid precursors WBC >10,000/μL Elevated Hgb F (corrected for age) Clonal cytogenetic abnormalities (excluding Monosomy 7)

JMML, juvenile myelomonocytic leukemia; WBC, white blood cell count.

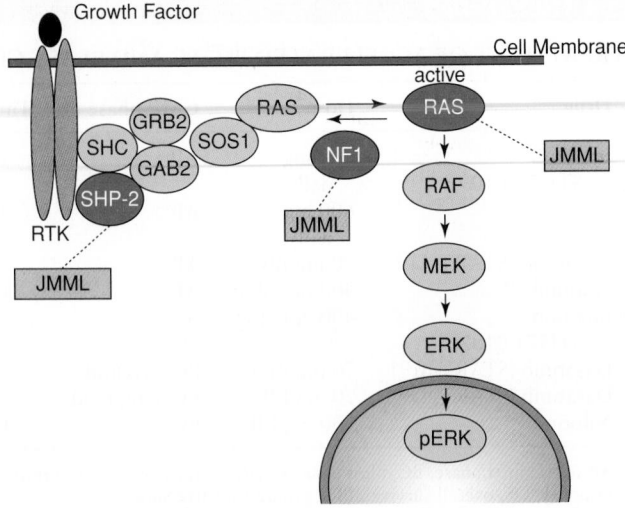

FIGURE 21.10 Simplified *RAS* signaling pathway. Proteins involved in the pathogenesis of juvenile myelomonocytic leukemia (due to biallelic inactivation of *NF1* or somatic mutations of *PTEN11*, *KRAS*, or *NRAS*) are indicated in *black*. JMML, juvenile myelomonocytic leukemia. (From Niemeyer CM, Kratz CP. Paediatric myelodysplastic syndromes and juvenile myelomonocytic leukaemia: molecular classification and treatment options. Br J Haematol 2008;140:610, used with permission.)

precursor, however.[233,237,239,240] The high incidence of *NF-1* and *RAS* mutations in JMML (discussed further on) suggests that deregulation of the *RAS* signal transduction pathway may be a major mechanism in the pathogenesis of JMML. This may occur either via activating mutations of the *RAS* genes or inactivating mutations in genes regulating *RAS* (e.g., *NF-1*), whereby *RAS* remains locked in an activated ATP-bound state, transmitting continuous signals for proliferation. A murine model using homozygous deletions of the *NF-1* gene has confirmed the role of *RAS* deregulation in promoting hypersensitivity to GM-CSF[241] (Fig. 21.10).

A characteristic *in vitro* finding has been the excessive production of monocyte-macrophage colonies without a requirement for exogenous growth factors; this apparent spontaneous proliferation reflects an exquisite sensitivity of the JMML progenitor cells to low concentrations of various endogenous cytokines, including GM-CSF, tumor necrosis factor-α (TNF-α), and interleukin-1b, but normal sensitivity to IL-3 or G-CSF.[242–244] Some evidence suggests that autocrine secretion of TNF-α by the leukemic cells stimulates the production of GM-CSF by target cells, which, in turn, stimulates further proliferation and accumulation of leukemic monocytes and macrophages; IL-1 may represent an important accessory factor that augments the effects of TNF-α and GM-CSF.[243] TNF-α may augment the growth advantage of the malignant clone by inhibiting normal hematopoiesis.[243]

The exquisite sensitivity of the JMML clone to GM-CSF does not appear to result from abnormalities in the GM-CSF molecule or its receptor.[238] Instead, there appear to be aberrations in the *RAS/mitogen-activated protein kinase (MAPK)* pathway by which GM-CSF transmits growth signals to the nucleus.[244] This pathway may be inappropriately amplified either by mutations in *RAS* genes themselves[245] or by defective regulation of *RAS*. Neurofibromin, the protein which is altered in the NF1 gene, a tumor suppressor gene, is normally a GAP and, thereby, a negative regulator of *RAS*; loss of normal neurofibromin control of *RAS* can result in unregulated myeloid proliferation.[225,246] This may account for the

increased incidence of JMML in NF-1 patients, in which 10% to 25% attain a somatic mutation in their wild-type NF1 gene in the hematopoietic cells.[247] In addition, gain of function point mutations of NRAS or KRAS, seen in up to 35% of JMML patients, can affect GTP hydrolysis leading to *RAS* remaining bound in active conformation.[223,247]

About 50% of patients with Noonan syndrome have germline mutations in *PTPN11*, which leads to development of JMML.[229,248] In nonsyndromic patients, 34% of JMML patients have somatic mutations in *PTPN11*.[229] *PTPN11* is a gene on chromosome 12q24 that encodes the protein tyrosine phosphatase SHP2. SHP2 is downstream of growth factors and cytokine receptors and relays growth signals to *RAS*. Mutations in *PTPN11* likely interrupt the autoinhibition of the catalytic phosphatase (PTPase) domain by the N-terminal src homology 2 (N-SH2) domain, resulting in gain of function of SHP2, leading to increase in its phosphatase activity and subsequent prolonged activation of the *RAS* and *ERK2/MAPK1* pathway and cell proliferation.[248,249]

In support of cytogenetic data, functional studies have also implicated the erythroid lineage within the JMML clone. Clonogenic cells of the erythroid series have been demonstrated in large numbers in both the peripheral blood and the bone marrow of patients with JMML.[250] As with myeloid progenitors, these burst-forming unit erythroid cells require minimal concentrations of their poietin (erythropoietin in this instance) for *in vitro* colony production.[232,250,251] Furthermore, constitutive expression of erythroid markers can be demonstrated in clonogenic cells of patients with JMML.[252]

Clinical Features

The incidence of JMML is approximately 1.2 per million persons in the United States with a male predominance of 2.5:1.[253] Most patients are diagnosed before the age of 2 years, commonly between 3 and 12 months of age. It rarely occurs as a congenital leukemia.[222] Presenting physical findings include pallor, cutaneous lesions (eczema, xanthomata, and café-au-lait spots), lymphadenopathy, hepatosplenomegaly, and hemorrhagic manifestations. Respiratory symptoms (chronic tachypnea, cough, expiratory wheezing) may be prominent and diarrhea (secretory or bloody) may occur due to leukemic infiltration into the lungs or intestinal tract, respectively.[233] These findings are relatively nonspecific and may mimic those associated with disseminated microbial infections in infancy, including CMV, toxoplasmosis, EBV, histoplasma, mycobacteria, and human herpes virus 6. Thus, a careful investigation to rule out an infectious etiology is required.

Laboratory Features

The peripheral blood is characterized by leukocytosis with mild-to-moderate monocytosis, anemia, and thrombocytopenia. The leukocytosis is generally not as pronounced as in adult CML (median WBC = 33,000/μL; rarely over 100,000/μL)[253] and is also associated with granulocytic precursors, nucleated RBCs, and dysplastic monocytes. Unlike CML, basophilia in JMML is rare. The bone marrow (Fig. 21.11) shows both erythroid and myeloid hyperplasia; immature cells of the monocytic series are prominent, and megakaryocytes are infrequent.

The erythrocytes show many features characteristic of fetal-type erythropoiesis, including high Hgb F level, fetal glycine-alanine ratio in the c chain of Hgb F, fetal-type glycolytic enzyme pattern, and low I antigen expression.[254,255] The LAP score is low in approximately 40% of patients.[13] Immunologic abnormalities include hypergammaglobulinemia, high incidence of antibodies to nuclear antigen,[256] and possible inability to control EBV infection.[257]

Cytogenetic Features

The cytogenetic pattern of JMML is heterogeneous, the only consistent feature being absence of the Ph[1] chromosome. Abnormalities, when found, most commonly involve chromosomes 7 and 8.[231,257] Monosomy 7 is found in approximately 25% to 33% of patients with features of JMML; however, it is unclear whether the monosomy 7 syndrome is a subset of JMML or a distinct pathogenic entity.[258,259] Trisomy 8 is seen in approximately 4% of patients.[260,261]

At the molecular level, gene changes are found quite frequently in JMML cells. Mutations in *NF-1*, *NRAS*, *KRAS*,

CBL, or *PTPN11* genes are demonstrable in 75% or more of JMML patients.[262] These genes all encode components of *RAS* signaling pathways. Fifteen percent of JMML patients have *NF-1* gene mutations in the absence of other manifestations of neurofibromatosis, while another 15% have clinical features of neurofibromatosis-1 with accompanying *NF-1* mutations[263]; progression to JMML in NF-1 patients may sometimes result from subsequent sequential inactivation of p53 alleles.[264] Approximately 30% of JMML patients will have mutations in the *RAS* genes, usually in codons 12 or 13 of *N-RAS* or *K-RAS*[260]; however, *NF-1* and *RAS* mutations do not occur concurrently in the same patient.[263]

Natural History

The course of JMML is quite variable. Some patients may experience relatively indolent disease with prolonged survival, while the majority will progress to death from infection or other complications of bone marrow failure. Overall median survival time for patients with JMML is less then 9 months. Prognosis varies with age at diagnosis; infants may survive for extended periods (mean 5-year survival, 67%), whereas children older than 1 year have virtually 0% long-term survival.[265] Favorable prognostic factors include a platelet count of more than 33,000/μL and a lower HgF level of less than 15%.[222,261] This subgroup may have a 2- to 4-year survival of 40% to 70% without HSCT. It is unclear whether mutational types correlate with prognosis. Spontaneous resolution has been reported in some young patients with Noonan and PTPN11 mutation and infants with higher platelet counts.[228,229,265] One study showed that PTPN11 mutations are associated with those older than 24 months and HgF of more than 10% at diagnosis, and predictive of relapse following transplant.[266] Transformation to an acute leukemic blast crisis is an unusual event in JMML, occurring in approximately 15% of patients, usually within 2 years of diagnosis. As in adult CML, the blast phase of JMML may be cytologically heterogeneous: cases of B cell and T cell[267,268] as well as stem cell transformation have been reported; JMML may also terminate in a erythroleukemia-like phase, characterized by anemia, erythroblastosis, and megaloblastic erythroid hyperplasia of the bone marrow.[269]

Therapy

In general, chemotherapy has been of limited value in JMML. Oral 6-mercaptopurine, either alone or in combination with subcutaneous cytarabine, has produced symptomatic relief in some patients,[270] but supportive care has been as effective as vigorous chemotherapy in most cases. In some cases, intensive multiagent chemotherapy (as used for treatment of acute nonlymphoid leukemias) has produced clinical remissions lasting as long as 27 months or longer.[271] However, intensive multiagent chemotherapy generally has been associated with high morbidity and short-lived remissions.[272] Thus, the First International Workshop on Myelodysplastic Syndrome (MDS) in Childhood has recommended that such an approach should be utilized only as part of a pretransplant regimen.[233] The combination of hydroxyurea and IFN-α may also show activity in JMML.[273] In 2002, the Children's Cancer Group (CCG) published the first large prospective study of JMML.[274] Children were treated with a five-drug induction regimen, using standard or intensive timing; patients achieving remission then received allogeneic bone marrow transplant if a matched family donor was available. The overall remission rate was 58% with 31% actuarial survival at 6 years. SCT remains the only definitive curative modality for JMML, with recent overall

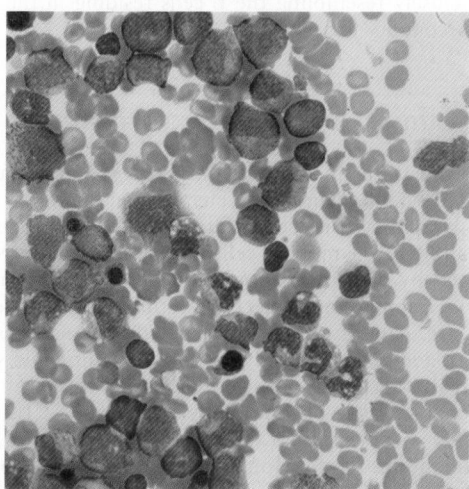

FIGURE 21.11 Juvenile myelomonocytic leukemia. Note immature monocytoid cells. (Courtesy of Drs. Hirako Shinado and William Rezuka).

5-year survival rates of around 50% and transplant-related mortality of 11% to 13%.[274,275] The major barrier to cure with this modality remains the high relapse rate (~50%), with the median time to relapse of 4 to 6 months and very few relapsing more than 1 year after HSCT.[276] Preparative cytoreduction regimens have included busulfan/cyclophosphamide in combination with melphalan or high-dose cytarabine, busulfan/fludarabine/melphalan, and ± total body irradiation. For patients, relapsing after HSCT, successful treatments with donor lymphocyte infusions or reduction of immunosuppressant has been reported, suggestive of a GVL effect.[276,277]

Biologic Approaches to Juvenile Myelomonocytic Leukemia

Isotretinoin. Isotretinoin (13-*cis*-retinoic acid) has been demonstrated to attenuate the *in vitro* spontaneous proliferation of monocyte precursors and their selective hypersensitivity to GM-CSF.[278] An overall response rate of 40% to 50% has been reported in a phase II clinical trial using doses of *cis*-retinoic acid as high as 200 mg/m².[279] However, sustained unmaintained responses are rare.

Inhibitors of RAS Farnesyl Protein Transferase. A critical prerequisite for *RAS* function is localization to the inner leaflet of the plasma membrane; this can only occur if newly synthesized *RAS* undergoes sequential posttranslational enzymatic processing, a process known as prenylation.[280] The initial and rate-limiting step in this sequence is catalyzed by the enzyme farnesyl protein transferase. Inhibitors of farnesyl protein transferase downregulate *RAS* function by preventing proper localization of the ras protein, resulting in an antiproliferative effect.[281] Preclinical studies have indicated that FTIs are well tolerated in laboratory animals and cause regression in some tumors.[282] *Ex vivo* studies of primary cells from patients with JMML treated with FTIs show dose-dependent inhibition of JMML cell growth.[283] An early report of the Children's Oncology Group phase II window study of the FTI R115777 in newly diagnosed JMML patients (AAML0122) show 47% of patients achieving a partial to complete response to the drug. However, response to therapy was not associated with mutational status or the degree of farnesyltransferase activity inhibition.[284]

Other novel biologic approaches specifically designed to target the molecular peculiarities of JMML cells include E21R, an analog of GM-CSF that antagonizes its effect on JMML cells[285] and GM-CSF/diphtheria toxin fusion molecules.[286] Ribozymes, RNA molecules with enzymatic activity, and interleukin-10 have been shown to downregulate the production of GM-CSF and TNF-α in JMML cells, leading to decreased growth and viability of the cells.[287,288] SHIP-1, an inhibitor of cytokine signaling, has been shown to block GM-CSF hypersensitivity in PTPN11 or KRAS mutated JMML cells and lead to decrease in cell proliferation and GM-CSF stimulated colony formation.[289] In *in vitro* studies, the bisphosphonate zoledronic acid, an inhibitor of the RAS pathway, has shown inhibition of the proliferation and differentiation of JMML cells and may be a fresh therapeutic option.[290]

FAMILIAL CHRONIC MYELOCYTIC LEUKEMIA

A familial form of CML has been reported in at least three pairs of infant siblings.[265,291] This disorder is indistinguishable from JCML by standard clinical and laboratory criteria; however, its evolution is less predictable. In each of the families

reported, one sibling died of progressive leukemia and the other had long-term asymptomatic survival.

CHRONIC MYELOMONOCYTIC LEUKEMIA

Chronic myelomonocytic leukemia (CMML) is a rare disorder of childhood characterized by recurrent upper respiratory and pulmonary infections, anemia, unexplained monocytosis, neutropenia, thrombocytopenia, and progressive splenomegaly.[292–294] The World Health Organization has revised the French-American-British classification of myeloid neoplasms to list CMML along with JMML as mixed myelodysplastic/myeloproliferative disorders.[224] Atypical monocytoid cells with unipolar hairy projections are seen in the peripheral smear, and the bone marrow is hypercellular, with a high proportion of young myeloid and monocytoid forms. In some patients, the course of the disease may be relatively indolent, and aggressive chemotherapy may actually shorten survival by producing severe pancytopenia. Low-dose cytarabine has achieved complete remissions in some adults with CMML.[295]

CHRONIC MONOCYTIC LEUKEMIA

Chronic monocytic leukemia (CMOL) is characterized by anemia, neutropenia, and thrombocytopenia in association with an increased number of mature monocytic elements in the blood and bone marrow. Extramedullary tissues, such as skin, gums, and viscera, may also be involved. Only a few cases of childhood CMOL have been reported, and some of these may actually represent cases of acute monocytic leukemia, histiocytosis, or JCML.[296,297]

CHRONIC LYMPHOCYTIC LEUKEMIA

Chronic lymphocytic leukemia (CLL) is a disease primarily of elderly adults; only rare cases have been reported in children.[298–303] The neoplastic cell appears to be a small B lymphocyte closely resembling the B cells residing in the mantle zone of secondary lymphoid follicles.

Clinical and Laboratory Features

Presenting features include pallor, hepatosplenomegaly, and generalized lymphadenopathy. Hematologic findings include anemia, lymphocytosis, and infiltration of the bone marrow with small mature lymphoid cells. Lymph node architecture is obliterated by a diffuse population of small lymphocytes. Functional immunologic defects of both B-cell and T-cell populations are demonstrable. These include hypogammaglobulinemia, inadequate antibody response to antigenic stimuli, and decreased responsiveness to mitogens.

The characteristic phenotypic features of the CLL B lymphocyte are coexpression of CD5 and faint amounts of surface immunoglobulins (sIgs). Monoclonality of the lymphoid population is demonstrable by analysis of membrane sIg and of Ig gene rearrangement. These techniques have been applied to only a handful of pediatric cases.[298,299,301]

Cytogenetics

Common nonrandom cytogenetic abnormalities in adult CLL include trisomy 12, 14q+ translocations, trisomy 3, and abnormalities of chromosome 6.[304,305] In a pediatric case, t(2;14)(p13;q32) with breakpoints at or near the k light chain and heavy chain loci was reported.[298]

Therapy

Because the course of CLL can be quite variable, some patients may have quiescent disease for many years, while others may require urgent therapy. The consensus remains that treatment should be based on severity of symptoms (e.g., bone marrow failure, bulky adenopathy). Traditionally, CLL has been treated in a palliative fashion using alkylating agents (chlorambucil or cyclophosphamide) and sometimes steroids. Only two reported pediatric cases have been treated in this fashion, and both patients responded well.[298,301] At least two others were reported to have stable courses without any chemotherapy.[299,303] The development of chemoimmunotherapy regimens combining monoclonal antibodies (e.g., rituximab, alemtuzumab) with alkylating agents (chlorambucil) or antimetabolites (fludarabine) has achieved complete remission rates of 40% to 70% with durable remissions of 3 to 7 years.[306–309] However, no randomized trial has demonstrated a benefit in terms of survival. Thus, clinical trials utilizing immune modulators, cyclin-dependent kinase inhibitors, BCL-family inhibitors, protein kinase C inhibitors, HSP-90 inhibitors, and other novel agents are in progress.[310]

References

1. SEER Pediatric Cancer Monograph 1975–1995. Bethesda, MD: National Cancer Institute, 1999:19–22.
2. Donnè A. Cours de microscopie complèmentaire des ètudes medicales. Paris: Balliere, 1844.
3. Bennett JH. Two cases of disease and enlargement of the spleen in which death took place from the presence of purulent matter in the blood. Edinb Med Surg J 1845;64: 413.
4. Craigie D. Case of disease of the spleen in which death took place in consequence of the presence of purulent matter in the blood. Edinb Med Surg J 1845;64:400.
5. Virchow R. Weisses blut. Frorleps Notizen 1845;36:151.
6. Neumann E. Ein fall von leukamie mit erkrankung des knochenmarkes. Arch Heilkd 1870;11:1.
7. Ebstein W. Ueber die acute leukamie and pseudoleukamie. Dtsch Arch Klin Med 1888–1889;44:343.
8. Ehrlich P. Farbenanalytisch Untersuchungen zur Klinik une Klinik des Blutes. Berlin, Germany: Hirschwald, 1891.
9. Nowell PC, Hungerford DA. A minute chromosome in human chronic granulocytic leukemia. Science 1960;132:1497.
10. Rowley JD. A new consistent chromosomal abnormality in chronic myelogenous leukemia identified by quinacrine fluorescence and Giemsa staining. Nature 1973;243: 290.
11. Lissauer H. Zwei falle von leucaemie. Berl Klin Wochenschr 1865;2:403.
12. Pusey WA. Report of cases treated with roentgen rays. JAMA 1902;38:911.
13. Castro-Malespina H, Schaison G, Briere J, et al. Philadelphia chromosome-positive chronic myelocytic leukemia in children: survival and prognostic features. Cancer 1983;52:721.
14. Homans AC, Young PC, Dickerman JD, et al. Adult-type CML in childhood: case report and review. Am J Pediatr Hematol Oncol 1984;6:220.
15. Biernaux C, Loos M, Sels A, et al. Detection of major bcr-abl gene expression at a very low level in blood cells of some healthy individual. Blood 1995;36:3118.
16. Quintas-Cardama A, Cortes J. Molecular biology of bcr-abl1-positive chronic myeloid leukemia. Blood 2009;113:1619.
17. Ren R. Mechanisms of BCR-ABL in the pathogenesis of chronic myelogenous leukaemia. Natl Rev Cancer 2005;5:172.
17a. Mathey-Prevot B, Nabel G, Palacios R, et al. Abelson virus abrogation of interleukin-3 dependence in a lymphoid cell line. Mol Cell Biol 1986;6(11):4133–4135.
18. Thomas EK, Cancelas JA, Chae HD, et al. Rac guanosine triphosphatases represent integrating molecular therapeutic targets for BCR-ABL-induced myeloproliferative disease. Cancer Cell 2007;12:467.
19. Quackenbush RC, Reuther GW, Miller JP, et al. Analysis of the biologic properties of p230 Bcr-Abl reveals unique and overlapping properties with the oncogenic p185 and p210 Bcr-Abl tyrosine kinases. Blood 2000;95:2913.
20. Kantarjian H, Talpaz M, Dhingra K, et al. Significance of the P210 versus P190 molecular abnormalities in adults with Philadelphia chromosome-positive acute leukemia. Blood 1991;78:2411.
21. Saglio G, Pane F, Gottardi E, et al. Consistent amounts of acute leukemia-associated p190 BCR/ABL transcript are expressed by chronic myelogenous leukemia patients at diagnosis. Blood 1996;87:1075.
22. Serrano J, Roman J, Sanchez J, et al. Molecular analysis of lineage-specific chimerism and minimal residual disease by RT-PCR of p210$^{BCR-ABL}$ and p190$^{BCR-ABL}$ after allogeneic bone marrow transplantation for chronic myeloid leukemia: increasing mixed myeloid chimerism and p190$^{BCR-ABL}$ detection precede cytogenetic relapse. Blood 2000;95:2659.
23. Pane F, Frigeri F, Sindona M, et al. Neutrophilic chronic myeloid leukemia: a distinct disease with a specific molecular marker (Bcr/Abl with C3/A2 junction). Blood 1996; 88:2410.
24. Sandberg AA. Chromosomes and causation of human cancer and leukemia: XI. The Ph1 and other translocations in CML. Cancer 1986;46:2221.
25. Lessard M, Duval S, Fritz A. Unusual translocation and chronic myelocytic leukemia: masked Philadelphia chromosome (Ph1). Cancer Genet Cytogenet 1981;4:237.
26. Lewis JP, Jenke H, Lazerson J. Philadelphia chromosome-negative chronic myelogenous leukemia in a child with t(8;9) (p11 or 12;q34). Am J Pediatr Hematol Oncol 1983;5:265.
27. Shtalrid M, Talpaz M, Blick M, et al. Philadelphia-negative chronic myelogenous leukemia with breakpoint cluster region rearrangement: molecular analysis, clinical characteristics, and response to therapy. J Clin Oncol 1988;6:1569.
28. van der Plas DC, Hermans ABC, Soekarman D, et al. Cytogentic and molecular analysis in Philadelphia negative CML. Blood 1989;73:1038.
29. Kurzrock R, Kantarjian HM, Shtalrid M, et al. Philadelphia chromosome-negative chronic myelogenous leukemia without breakpoint cluster region rearrangement: a chronic myeloid leukemia with a distinct clinical course. Blood 1990;75:445.
30. Onida F, Ball G, Kantarjian HM, et al. Characteristics and outcome of patients with Philadelphia chromosome negative, bcr/abl negative chronic myelogenous leukemia. Cancer 2002;95(8):1673–1684.
31. Golub TR, Barker GF, Lovett M, et al. Fusion of PDGF receptor beta to a novel ets-like gene, tel, in chronic myelomonocytic leukemia with t(5;12) chromosomal translocation. Cell 1994;77:307.
32. Reiter A, Sohal J, Kulkarni S, et al. Consistent fusion of ZNF198 to the fibroblast growth factor receptor-1 in the t(8;13) (p11;q12) myeloproliferative syndrome. Blood 1998;92:1735.
33. Apperly JF, Gardembas M, Melo JV, et al. Response to imatinib mesylate in patients with chronic myeloproliferative diseases with rearrangement of the platelet-derived growth factor beta. N Engl J Med 2002;347:481.
34. Priest JR, Robison LL, McKenna RW, et al. Philadelphia chromosome positive childhood acute lymphoblastic leukemia. Blood 1980;56:15.
35. Bloomfield CD, Lindquist LL, Brunning RE, et al. The Philadelphia chromosome in acute leukemia. Virchows Arch 1978;29:81.
36. Kurzrock R, Shtalrid M, Kloetzer WS, et al. Expression of c-abl in Philadelphia-positive acute myelogenous leukemia. Blood 1987;70:1584.
37. Arico M, Valsecchi MG, Camitta B, et al. Outcome of treatment in children with Philadelphia chromosome-positive acute lymphoblastic leukemia. N Engl J Med 2000; 342:998.
37a. Schultz KR, Bowman WP, Aledo A, et al. Improved early event-free survival with imatinib in Philadelphia chromosome-positive acute lymphoblastic leukemia: a children's oncology group study. J Clin Oncol 2009;27(31):5175–5181.
38. Beard MEJ, Durrant J, Catovsky D, et al. Blast crisis of chronic myeloid leukemia (CML). I. Presentation simulating acute lymphoid leukaemia (ALL). Br J Haematol 1976;34:167.
39. DeKlein A, Hagemeijer A, Bartram CR, et al. bcr rearrangement and translocation of the c-abl oncogene in Philadelphia chromosome positive acute lymphoblastic leukemia. Blood 1986;68:1369.
40. Heisterkamp N, Jenkins R, Thibodeau S, et al. The bcr gene in Philadelphia chromosome positive acute lymphoblastic leukemia. Blood 1989;73:1307.
41. Kavalerchik E, Goff D, Jamieson CHM. Chronic myeloid leukemia stem cells. J Clin Oncol 2008;26:2911–2915.
42. Fialkow PJ, Gartler SM, Yoshida A. Clonal origin of chronic myelocytic leukemia in man. Proc Natl Acad Sci U S A 1967;58:1468.
43. Bernheim A, Berger R, Preudíhomme JL, et al. Philadelphia chromosome positive blood B lymphocytes in chronic myelocytic leukemia. Leuk Res 1981;5: 331.
44. Fauser AA, Kanz L, Bross KJ, et al. T cells and probably B cells arise from the malignant clone in chronic myelogenous leukemia. J Clin Invest 1985;75:1080.
45. Jonas D, Lübbert M, Kawasaki ES, et al. Clonal analysis of bcr-abl rearrangement in T lymphocytes from patients with chronic myelogenous leukemia. Blood 1992;79(4): 1017–1023.
46. Fialkow PJ, Jacobson RJ, Papayannopoulou T. Chronic myelocytic leukemia: clonal origin in a stem cell common to the granulocyte, erythrocyte, platelet, and monocyte/macrophage. Am J Med 1977;63:125.
47. Barr RD, Fialkow PJ. Clonal origin of chronic myelocytic leukemia. N Engl J Med 1973;289:307.
48. Fialkow PJ, Denman AM, Jacobson RA, et al. Chronic myelocytic leukemia: origin of some lymphocytes from leukemic stem cells. J Clin Invest 1978;62:815.
49. Fialkow PJ, Martin PJ, Najfeld V, et al. Evidence for a multistep pathogenesis of chronic myelogenous leukemia. Blood 1981;58:158.
50. Lisker R, Casas L, Mutchinick O, et al. Late appearing Philadelphia chromosome in two patients with chronic myelogenous leukemia. Blood 1980;56:812.
51. Goldman J, Lu D-P. New approaches in chronic granulocytic leukemia: origin, prognosis and treatment. Semin Hematol 1982;19:241.
52. Hagemeijer A, Smit E, Lowenberg B, et al. Chronic myeloid leukemia with permanent disappearance of the Ph1 chromosome and development of new clonal subpopulation. Blood 1979;53:1.
53. Galbraith PR, Abu-Zahra HT. Granulopoiesis in chronic granulocytic leukaemia. Br J Haematol 1972;22:135.
54. Strife A, Clarkson B. Biology of chronic myelogenous leukemia: is discordant maturation the primary defect? Semin Hematol 1988;25:1.

55. Athens JW, Raab SO, Haab OP, et al. Leukokinetic studies. X. Blood granulocyte kinetics in chronic myelocytic leukemia. J Clin Invest 1965;44:765.
56. Altman AJ, Baehner RL. In vitro colony forming characteristics of chronic granulocytic leukemia in childhood. J Pediatr 1975;86:221.
57. Moore MAS, Mertelsmann R, Pelus LM. Phenotypic evaluation of chronic myeloid leukemia. Blood Cells 1981;7:217.
57a. Gavosto F. Granulopoiesis and cell kinetics in chronic myeloid leukaemia. Cell Tissue Kinet 1974;7:151.
58. Broxmeyer HE, Gentile P, Cooper S, et al. Functional activities of acidic isoferritins and lactoferrin in vitro and in vivo. Blood Cells 1984;10:397.
59. Kurland JI, Broxmeyer HE, Pelus LM, et al. Role for monocyte-macrophage-derived colony-stimulating factor and prostaglandin E in the positive and negative feedback control of myeloid stem cell proliferation. Blood 1978;52:388.
60. Pelus LM, Saletan S, Silver R, et al. Expression of 1a antigens on normal and chronic myeloid leukemic human granulocyte-macrophage colony forming cells is associated with the regulation of cell proliferation by prostaglandin E. Blood 1982;59:284.
61. Cannistra SA, Hermann F, Davis R, et al. Relationship between HLA-Dr expression by normal myeloid progenitor cells and inhibition of colony growth by prostaglandin E: implication for prostaglandin E resistance in chronic myeloid leukemia. J Clin Invest 1986;77:13.
62. Aglietta M, Piacibello W, Gavosto F. Insensitivity of chronic myeloid leukemia cells to inhibition of growth by prostaglandin E. Cancer Res 1980;40:2507.
63. Broxmeyer HE, Frossbard E, Jacobsen N, et al. Evidence for a proliferative advantage of human leukemia colony-forming cells in vitro. J Natl Cancer Inst 1978;60:513.
64. Skold S, Rosberg B, Gulberg U, et al. A secreted proform of neutrophil proteinase 3 regulates the proliferation of granulopoietic progenitor cells. Blood 1999;93:849.
65. Levesque JP, Hendry J, Winkler IG, et al. Granulocyte colony-stimulating factor induces the release in the bone marrow of proteases that cleave c-KIT receptor (CD11&) from the surface of hematopoietic progenitor cells. Exp Hematol 2003;31:109.
66. El Ouriaghli F, Sloand E, Mainwaring L, et al. Clonal dominance of chronic myelogenous leukemia is associated with diminished sensitivity to the antiproliferative effects of neutrophil elastase. Blood 2003;102:3786.
67. Oloffson T, Olsson I. Suppression of normal granulopoiesis in vitro by a leukemia-associated inhibitor (LAI) of acute and chronic leukemia. Blood 1980;55:975.
67a. Salesse S, Verfaille E. Mechanisms underlying abnormal trafficking and expansion of malignant progenitors in CML:BCR/ABL-induced defects in integrin function. Oncogene 2002;21:8605.
68. Ebos JML, Tran J, Master Z, et al. Imatinib mesylate (STI571) reduces bcr-abl-mediated vascular endothelial growth factor secretion in chronic myelogenous leukemia. Mol Cancer Res 2002;(1):89–95.
69. McGahon A, Bissonnette R, Schmitt M, et al. BCR-ABL maintains resistance of chronic myelogenous leukemia cells to apoptotic cell death. Blood 1994;83:1179.
70. Bedi A, Zehnbauer BA, Barber JP, et al. Inhibition of apoptosis by BCR-ABL in chronic myeloid leukaemia. Med Hypotheses 1995;44:301.
71. Aramante-Mendes GP, Naekyung KC, Liu L, et al. Bcr-Abl exerts its anti-apoptotic effect against diverse apoptotic stimuli through blockage of mitochondrial release of cytochrome C and activation of caspase-3. Blood 1998;91:1700.
72. Ravandi F, Kantarjian HM, Talpaz M, et al. Expression of apoptosis proteins in chronic myelogenous leukemia. Associations and significance. Cancer 2001;91:1964.
73. Frank DA, Varticovski L. BCR/abl leads to the constitutive activation of Stat proteins, and shares an epitope with tyrosine phosphorylated Stats. Leukemia 1996;10(11): 1724–1730.
74. Horita M, Andreu EJ, Benito A, et al. Blockade of the bcr-abl kinase activity induces apoptosis of chronic myelogenous leukemia cells by suppressing signal transducer and activator of transcription 5-dependent expression of Bcl-XL. J Exp Med 2000;191(6): 977–984.
75. Bedi A, Barber JP, Bedi G, et al. BCR-ABL-mediated inhibition of apoptosis with delay of G2/M transition after DNA damage: a mechanism of resistance to multiple anticancer agents. Blood 1995;86:1148.
76. Kavalerchik E, Goff D, Jamieson CHM: Chronic myeloid leukemia stem cells. J Clin Oncol 2008;26:2911.
77. Jamieson CH, Ailles LE, Dylla SJ, et al. Granulocyte-macrophage progenitors as candidate leukemic stem cells in blast-crisis CML. N Engl J Med 2004;351:657.
78. Radich JP, Dai H, Mao M, et al. Gene expression changes associated with progression and response in chronic myeloid leukemia. Proc Natl Acad Sci U S A 2006;102:2794.
79. Strathdee GL, Holyoake TL, Sim A, et al. Inactivation of HOXA genes by hypermethylation in myeloid and lymphoid malignancy is frequent and associated with poor prognosis. Clin Cancer Res 2007;13:5048.
80. Preisler HD. A hypothesis regarding the development of acute myeloid leukemia from preleukemic disorders: the role of protooncogenes. Cancer Genet Cytogenet 1988;32:133.
81. LeMaistre A, Lee M-S, Talpaz M, et al. RAS oncogene mutations are rare late stage events in chronic myelogenous leukemia. Blood 1989;73:889.
82. Marshal R, Shtalrid M, Talpaz M, et al. Rearrangement and expression of p53 in the chronic phase and blast crisis of chronic myelogenous leukemia. Blood 1990;75:180.
83. Rowe JM, Lichtman MA. Hyperleukocytosis and leukostasis: common features of childhood chronic myelogenous leukemia. Blood 1984;63:1230.
84. Schmidt U, Mlynek M-L, Leder L-D. Electron-microscopic characterization of mixed granulated (hybridoid) leucocytes of chronic myeloid leukaemia. Br J Haematol 1988; 68:175.
85. Dotti G, Garattini E, Borleri G, et al. Leucocyte alkaline phosphatase identifies terminally differentiated normal neutrophils and its lack in chronic myelogenous leukaemia is not dependent on p210 tyrosine kinase activity. Br J Haematol 1999;105:163.
86. Chikkappa G, Wang GJ, Santella D, et al. Granulocyte colony-stimulating factor (G-CSF) induces synthesis of alkaline phosphatase in neutrophil granulocytes of chronic myelogenous leukemia patients. Leuk Res 1988;12:419.
87. Anklesaria PN, Advani SH, Bhisey AN. Defective chemotaxis and adherence in granulocytes from chronic myeloid leukemia (CML) patients. Leuk Res 1985;9:641.
88. Baker MA, Taub RN, Whelton CH, et al. Aberrant sialylation of granulocyte membranes in chronic myelogenous leukemia. Blood 1984;63:1194.
89. Kantarjian H, O'Brien S, Cortes J, et al. Sudden onset of the blastic phase of chronic myelogenous leukemia. Patterns and implications. Cancer 2003;98:81.
90. Guinn BA, Smith MC, Padua RA, et al. The role of p53 mutations in the switch to blast crisis in chronic myeloid leukemia [abstract]. Br J Haematol 1994;86:49.
91. Bernstein R, Gale RP. Do chromosome abnormalities determine the type of acute leukemia that develops in CML? Leukemia 1990;4:65.
92. Griffin JD, Todd RF III, Ritz J, et al. Differentiation patterns in the blastic phase of chronic myeloid leukemia. Blood 1983;61:85.
93. Bakhshi A, Minowada J, Arnold A, et al. Lymphoid blast crises of chronic myelogenous leukemia represent stages in the development of B-cell precursors. N Engl J Med 1983; 309:826.
94. Akashi K, Mizuno S-I, Harada M, et al. T lymphoid/myeloid bilineal crisis in chronic myelogenous leukemia. Exp Hematol 1993;21:743.
95. Calabretta B, Perrotti D. The biology of CML blast crisis. Blood 2004;103:4010.
96. Nucifora G, Rowley JD. AML1 and the 8;21 and 3;21 translocations in acute and chronic myeloid leukemia. Blood 1995;86:1.
97. Carapeti M, Silly H, Chase A, et al. Expression of the EVI-1 gene in CML blast crisis is associated with dysmegakaryopoiesis [abstract]. Blood 1994;84(suppl 1):2388.
98. Bernstein R, Bagy A, Pinto M, et al. Chromosome 3q21 abnormalities associated with hyperactive thrombopoiesis in acute transformation of chronic myeloid leukemia. Blood 1986;68:652.
99. Anastasi J, Feng J, Le Beau MM, et al. The relationship between secondary chromosomal abnormalities and blast transformation in chronic myelogenous leukemia. Leukemia 1995;9:62.
100. Tura S, Boccarani M, Corbelli G, et al. Staging of chronic myeloid leukaemia. Br J Haematol 1981;47:105.
101. Sokal JE, Cox EB, Baccarani M. Prognostic discrimination in "good-risk" chronic granulocytic leukemia. Blood 1984;63:789.
102. Lichtman MA, Rowe JM. Hyperleukocytic leukemias: rheological, clinical, and therapeutic considerations. Blood 1982;60:279.
103. Graw RG Jr, Skeel RT, Carbone PP. Priapism in a child with chronic granulocytic leukemia. J Pediatr 1969;74:788.
104. Kantarjian HM, Deisseroth A, Kurzrock R, et al. Chronic myelogenous leukemia: a concise update. Blood 1993;82:691.
105. Schwartz JH, Canellos GP, Young RC, et al. Meningeal leukemia in the blastic phase of chronic granulocytic leukemia. Am J Med 1975;59:819.
106. Smith AG, Prentice AG, Lucie NP, et al. Meningeal relapse in Ph1-positive acute lymphoblastic and lymphoid blast crisis of chronic granulocytic leukemia: is CNS prophylaxis indicated? Cancer 1983;51:2031.
107. Hochhaus A, O'Brien SG, Guihot F, et al. Six-year follow-up of patients receiving imatinib for the first-line treatment of chronic myeloid leukemia. Leukemia 2009;23(6): 1054–1061.
108. Schwartz JH, Canellos GP. Hydroxyurea in the management of the hematologic complications of chronic granulocytic leukemia. Blood 1975;46:11.
109. Galvani DW, Cawley JC. Mechanism of action of interferon in chronic granulocytic leukaemia: evidence for preferential inhibition of late progenitors. Br J Haematol 1989; 73:475.
110. Emerson SG, Guba SC, Upadhyaya GH, et al. Chronic myelogenous leukemia progenitor cells are deficient in cell surface LFA-3 and are not recognized by autoregulatory T lymphocytes. Clin Res 1989;37:901A.
111. Dowding C, Guo AP, Osterholz J, et al. Interferon-alpha overrides the deficient adhesion of chronic myeloid leukemia primitive progenitor cells to bone marrow stromal cells. Blood 1991;78:499.
112. Aglietta M, Piacibello W, Stacchini A, et al. Effect of interferon gamma (IFN) on HLA class II antigens and on sensitivity to prostaglandin E by normal and chronic myeloid leukemia progenitors [abstract]. Exp Hematol 1986;14:462.
113. Kloke O, Niederle N, Qiu JY, et al. Impact of interferon alpha-induced cytogenetic improvement on survival in chronic myelogenous leukaemia. Br J Haematol 1993;83:399.
114. Guilhot F, Maloisel F, Guyotat D, et al. Significant survival improvement with a combination of interferon alpha 2b and cytarabine in chronic myeloid leukemia. Update of a randomized trial [abstract 7]. J Clin Oncol 1999;17(suppl).
115. Kantarjian HM, Cortes JE, O'Brien S, et al. Long-term survival benefit and improved complete cytogenetic and molecular response rates with imatinib mesylate in Philadelphia chromosome-positive chronic-phase chronic myeloid leukemia after failure of interferon-alpha. Blood 2004;104:1979.
116. Baccarani M, Saglio G, goldman J, et al. Evolving concepts in the management of chronic myeloid leukemia: recommendations from and expert panel on behalf of the European LeukemiaNet. Blood 2006;108:1809.
117. Picard S, Titier K, Etienne G, et al. Trough imatinib plasma levels are associated with both cytogenetic and molecular responses to standard-dose imatinib in chronic myeloid leukemia. Blood 2007;109:3496.
118. White DL, Saunders VA, Dang P, et al. Most CML patients who have a suboptimal response to imatinib have low OCT-1 activity; higher doses of imatinib may overcome the negative impact of low OCT-1 activity. Blood 2007;110:4064.
119. Chu S, Snyder DS, Sawyers C, et al. Detection of BCR/ABL kinase domain mutations in chronic myelogenous leukemia patients in complete cytogenetic remission on imatinib treatment [abstract 237]. Blood 2003;102:70a.
120. Champagne MA, Capdeville R, Krailo M, et al. Imatinib mesylate (STI571) for treatment of children with Philadelphia chromosome-positive leukemia: results from a Children's Oncology Group phase I study. Blood 2004;104:2655.
121. Galimberti A, Cervetti G, Guerrini F, et al. Quantitative molecular monitoring of BCR-ABL and MDR1 transcripts in patients with chronic myeloid leukemia during imatinib treatment. Cancer Genet Cytogenet 2005;162:57.
122. Carroll M, Ohno-Jones S, Tamura S, et al. CGP 57148, a tyrosine kinase inhibitor. Inhibits the growth of BCR-ABL, TEL-ABL and TEL-PDGFR fusion proteins. Blood 1997;90:4947.
123. Okuda K, Weisberg E, Gilliland DG, et al. ARG tyrosine kinase activity is inhibited by STI571. Blood 2001;97:2440.
124. O'Brien SG, Guihot F, Larson RA, et al. Imatinib compared with interferon and low-dose cytarabine for newly diagnosed chronic-phase chronic myeloid leukemia. N Engl J Med 2003;348:994–1004.
125. Kantarjian H, Talpaz M, O'Brien S, et al. High-dose imatinib mesylate therapy in newly diagnosed Philadelphia chromosome-positive chronic phase chronic myeloid leukemia. Blood 2004;103:2873–2878.
126. Champagne MA, Fu C, Chang M, et al. Imatinib in children with newly diagnosed chronic phase chronic myelogenous leukemia (CP-CML): AAML0123 COG study [abstract 2140]. Blood 2006;108.
127. Mauro MJ, Baccarani M, Cervantes F, et al. Dasatinib 2-year efficacy in patients with chronic phase chronic myelogenous leukemia (CML-CP) with resistance or intolerance to imatinib (START-C) [abstract 7009]. J Clin Oncol 2008;26(15 suppl).
128. Kantarjian HM, Giles FJ, Hochhaus A, et al. Nilotinib in patients with imatinib-resistant or -intolerant chronic myelogenous leukemia in chronic phase (CML-CP): updated phase II results [abstract 7010]. J Clin Oncol 2008;26(15 suppl).
129. O'Brien S, Berman E, Devetten MP, et al. Clinical practice guidelines in oncology: chronic myelogenous leukemia. National Comprehensive Cancer Network 2010;2–5.

130. Jabbour E, Kantarjian HM, Abruzzo LV, et al. Chromosomal abnormalities in Philadelphia chromosome negative metaphases appearing during imatinib mesylate therapy in patients with newly diagnosed chronic myeloid leukemia in chronic phase. Blood 2007; 110:2991.
131. O'Dwyer ME, Mauro MJ, Blasdel C, et al. Clonal evolution and lack of cytogenetic response are adverse prognostic factors for hematologic relapse of chronic phase CML patients treated with imatinib mesylate. Blood 2004;103:451.
132. Gambacorti-Passerini C, Barni R, le Coutre P, et al. Role of alpha 1 acid glycoprotein in the in vivo resistance of human BCR-ABL(+) leukemia cells to the abl inhibitor STI571. J Natl Cancer Inst 2000;92:713.
133. Kantarjian HM, Talpaz M, O'Brien S, et al. Dose escalation of imatinib mesylate can overcome resistance to standard-dose therapy in patients with chronic myelogenous leukemia. Blood 2003;101:473–475.
134. Kreil S, Mueller MC, Hanfstein B, et al. Management and clinical outcome of CML patients after imatinib resistance associated with ABL kinase domain mutations [abstract 238]. Blood 2003;102:71a.
135. Branford S, Rudzki Z, Miller B, et al. Mutations in the catalytic core (P-loop) of the Bcr-ABL kinase domain of imatinib-treated chronic myeloid leukemia patients in chronic phase are strongly associated with imminent progression to blast crisis [abstract 239]. Blood 2003;102:71a.
136. Hochhaus A, Kreil A, Corbin AS, et al. Molecular and chromosomal mechanisms of resistance to imatinib (STI571) therapy. Leukemia 2002;16:2190–2196.
137. Donado D, Wu J, Stapky J, et al. Imatinib mesylate resistance through Bcr-Abl independence in chronic myelogenous leukemia. Cancer Res 2004;64:672.
138. Dorsey JF, Cunnick JM, Lanehart R, et al. Interleukin-3 protects Bcr-Abl-transformed hematopoietic progenitor cells from apoptosis induced by Bcr-Abl tyrosine kinase inhibitors. Leukemia 2002;16:1589–1595.
139. Graham SM, Jorgensen HJ, Allan E, et al. Primitive, quiescent, Philadelphia-positive stem cells from patients with chronic myeloid leukemia are insensitive to STI571 in vitro. Blood 2002;99:319.
140. Bhatia R, Holtz M, Niu N, et al. Persistence of malignant hematopoietic progenitors in chronic myelogenous leukemia patients in complete cytogenetic remission following imatinib mesylate treatment. Blood 2003;101:4701.
141. Kantarjian H. New promising Bcr-Abl tyrosine kinase inhibitors to treat imatinib mesylate (Gleevec) resistant chronic myeloid leukemia (CML). Leuk Insights 2004;9(2):1.
142. Bumm T, Muller C, Al Ali HK, et al. Emergence of clonal cytogenetic abnormalities in Ph-cells in some CML patients in cytogenetic remission to imatinib but restoration of polyclonal hematopoiesis in the majority. Blood 2003;101:1941.
143. Shah NP, Tran C, Lee FY, et al. Overcoming imatinib resistance with a novel ABL kinase inhibitor. Science 2004;305:399.
144. Mauro MJ, Baccarani M, Cervantes F, et al. Dasatinib 2-year efficacy in patients with chronic phase chronic myelogenous leukemia (CML-CP) with resistance or intolerance to imatinib (START-C) [abstract 7009]. J Clin Oncol 2008;26(15 suppl).
145. Guihot F, Apperley J, Kim D-W, et al. Dasatinib induces significant hematologic and cytogenetic responses in patients with imatinib-resistant or -intolerant chronic myeloid leukemia in accelerated phase. Blood 2007;109:4143.
146. Cortes J, Rousselot R, Kim D-W, et al. Dasatinib induces complete hematologic and cytogenetic responses in patients with imatinib-resistant or -intolerant chronic myeloid leukemia in blast crisis. Blood 2007;109:3207.
147. Aplenc R, Strauss LC, Shusterman S, et al. Pediatric Phase I trial and pharmacokinetic (PK) study of dasatinib: a report from the Children's Oncology Group phase I consortium [abstract 14094]. J Clin Oncol 2007;25:(18S suppl).
148. le Coutre P, Ottmann OG, Giles F, et al. Nilotinib (formerly AMN107), a highly selective BCR-abl tyrosine kinase inhibitor, is active in patients with imatinib-resistant or -intolerant accelerated-phase chronic myelogenous leukemia. Blood 2008;111:1834.
149. Giles FJ, Larson RA, Kantarjian HM, et al. Nilotinib in patients with Philadelphia chromosome-positive chronic myelogenous leukemia in blast crisis (CML-BC) who are resistant or intolerant to imatinib [absrtact 7017]. J Clin Oncol 2008;26(15 suppl).
150. Puttini M, Coluccia AM, Boschelli F, et al. In vitro and in vivo activity of SKI-606, a novel scr-abl inhibitor, against imatinib resistant Bcr-Abl+ neoplastic cells. Cancer Res 2006;66:11314.
151. Kimura S, Naito H, Segawa H, et al. NS-187, a potent and selective dual Bcr-Abl/Lyn tyrosine kinase inhibitor, is a novel agent for imatinib-resistant leukemia. Blood 2005; 106:3948.
152. Li JG. The leukocytopenic effect of focal splenic X-irradiation in leukaemic patients. Radiology 1963;80:471.
153. Neiman F, Brandt L, Nilsson PG. Cytogenetic evidence for splenic origin of blastic transformation in chronic myelogenous leukaemia. Scand J Haematol 1973;13: 87.
154. Italian Cooperative Group on Chronic Myeloid Leukemia. Results of a prospective study of early splenectomy in chronic myeloid leukemia. Cancer 1984;54:333.
155. Medical Research Council's Working Party for Therapeutic Trials in Leukaemia. Randomized trial of splenectomy in Ph1-positive chronic granulocytic leukaemia, including an analysis of prognostic factors. Br J Haematol 1983;54:415.
156. Clift RA, Buckner ED, Thomas WI, et al. Marrow transplantation for chronic myeloid leukemia: a randomized study comparing cyclophosphamide and total body irradiation with busulfan and cyclophosphamide. Blood 1994;84:2036.
157. Champlin R. Bone marrow transplantation for chronic leukemias. In Champlin R (moderator). Chronic leukemias: oncogenes, chromosomes, and advances in therapy. Ann Intern Med 1986;104:671.
158. Clift RA, Appelbaum FR, Thomas ED. Treatment of chronic myeloid leukemia by marrow transplantation [editorial]. Blood 1993;82:1954.
159. Giralt S, Szydlo R, Goldman JM, et al. Effect of short-term interferon therapy on the outcome of subsequent HLA-identical sibling bone marrow transplantation for chronic myelogenous leukemia: an analysis from the International Bone Marrow Transplant Registry. Blood 2000;95:410.
160. Kantarjian HM, Giles FJ, O'Brien S, et al. Therapeutic choices in younger patients with chronic myelogenous leukemia. Cancer 2000;89:1647.
161. Or R, Shapira MY, Resnick I, et al. Nonmyeloablative allogeneic stem cell transplantation for the treatment of chronic myeloid leukemia in first chronic phase. Blood 2003; 101:441.
162. Cunningham I, Castro-Malaspina H, Flomenberg N, et al. T-cell depleted bone marrow transplant for chronic myelogenous leukemia. Blood 1988;72:384a.
163. Elmaagacli AH, Basoglu S, Peceny R, et al. Improved disease-free-survival after transplantation of peripheral blood stem cells as compared with bone marrow from HLA-identical unrelated donors in patients with first chronic phase chronic myeloid leukemia. Blood 2002;99:1103–1135.
164. Millot F, Esperou H, Bordigoni P, et al. Allogeneic bone marrow transplantation from chronic myeloid leukemia in childhood: a report from the Societe Francaise de Greffe de Moelle et de Therapie Cellulaire (SFGM-TC). Bone Marrow Transplant 2003;32: 993–999.
165. Goldman JM, Gale RP, Horowitz MM, et al. Bone marrow transplantation for chronic myelogenous leukemia in chronic phase: increased risk of relapse associated with T-cell depletion. Ann Intern Med 1988;108:806.
166. McGlave PB, Bartsch G, Anasetti C, et al. Unrelated donor marrow transplantation for chronic myelogenous leukemia: initial experience of the National Marrow Donor Program. Blood 1993;81:543.
167. Cwynarski K, Roberts IAG, Iacobelli S, et al. Stem cell transplantation for chronic myeloid leukemia in children. Blood 2003;102(4):1224–1231.
168. Thornley I, Perentesis J, Davics SM, et al. Treating children with chronic myeloid leukemia in the imatinib era: a therapeutic dilemma? Med Pediatr Oncol 2003;41: 115.
169. Cortes J, Talpaz M, O'Brien S, et al. Suppression of cytogenetic clonal evolution with interferon alfa therapy in patients with Philadelphia chromosome-positive chronic myelogenous leukemia. J Clin Oncol 1998;16:3279.
170. Higano CS, Raskind WH, Singer JW. Use of a interferon for the treatment of relapse of chronic myelogenous leukemia in chronic phase after allogeneic bone marrow transplantation. Blood 1992;80:1437.
171. Kantarjian HM, O'Brien S, Cortes JE, et al. Imatinib mesylate therapy for relapse after allogeneic stem cell transplantation for chronic myelogenous leukemia. Blood 2002; 100:1590.
172. Mrsic M, Horowitz MM, Atkinson K, et al. Second HLA-identical sibling transplants for leukemia recurrence. Bone Marrow Transplant 1992;9:269.
173. Barrett AJ, Locatelli F, Treleaven JG, et al. Second transplants for leukaemic relapse after bone marrow transplantation: high early mortality but favorable effect on chronic GVHD on continued remission. Br J Haematol 1991;79:567.
174. Kolb HJ, Mittermuller J, Clemm CH, et al. Donor leukocyte transfusions for treatment of recurrent chronic myelogenous leukemia in marrow transplant patients. Blood 1990;76:2462.
175. Porter DL, Roth MS, McGarigle C, et al. Induction of graft-versus-host disease as immunotherapy for relapsed chronic myeloid leukemia. N Engl J Med 1994;330: 100.
176. Bar BM, Schattenberg A, Mensink EJ, et al. Donor leukocyte infusions for chronic myeloid leukemia relapsed after allogeneic bone marrow transplantation. J Clin Oncol 1993;11:513.
177. van Rhee F, Lin F, Cullis JO, et al. Relapse of chronic myeloid leukemia after allogeneic bone marrow transplant: the case for giving donor leukocyte transfusions before the onset of hematologic relapse. Blood 1994;83:3377.
178. Dazzi F, Szydlo RM, Craddock C, et al. A comparison of single dose and escalating dose regimens of donor lymphocyte infusion for patients who relapse after allografting for chronic myeloid leukemia. Blood 2000;95:67.
179. Mackinnon S, Papadopoulos E, Carabesi M, et al. Adoptive immunotherapy evaluating escalating doses of donor leukocytes for relapse of chronic myeloid leukemia after bone marrow transplantation: separation of graft-versus-leukemia effect from graft-versus-host disease. Blood 1995;86:1261.
180. Olavarria E, Kanfer E, Szdlo R, et al. Early detection of BCR-ABL transcripts by quantitative reverse transcriptase-polymerase chain reaction predicts outcome after allogeneic stem cell transplantation for chronic myeloid leukemia. Blood 2001;97: 1560.
181. Arthur CK, Apperly JF, Guo AP, et al. Cytogenetic events after bone marrow transplantation for chronic myeloid leukemia in chronic phase. Blood 1988;71:1179.
182. Offit K, Burns JP, Cunningham I, et al. Cytogenetic analysis of chimerism and leukemia relapse in chronic myelogenous leukemia patients after T-cell depleted bone marrow transplants. Blood 1990;75:1346.
183. Martiat P, Maisin D, Philippe M, et al. Detection of residual BCR/ABL transcripts in chronic myeloid leukaemia patients in complete remission using the polymerase chain reaction and nested primers. Br J Haematol 1990;75:355.
184. Radich JP, Gehly G, Gooley T, et al. Polymerase chain reaction detection of the BCR-ABL fusion transcript after allogeneic bone marrow transplantation for chronic myeloid leukemia: results and implications in 346 patients. Blood 1995;85:2632.
185. Mackinnon S, Barnett L, Heller G. Polymerase chain reaction is highly predictive of relapse in patients following T-cell-depleted allogeneic bone marrow transplantation for chronic myeloid leukemia. Bone Marrow Transplant 1996;17:643.
186. Pichert G, Alyea EP, Soiffer RJ, et al. Persistence of myeloid progenitor cells expressing BCR-ABL mRNA after allogeneic bone marrow transplantation for chronic myelogenous leukemia. Blood 1994;84:2109.
187. Sawyers CL, McLaughlin J, Witte ON. Genetic requirement for Ras in the transformation of fibroblasts and hematopoietic cells by the Bcr-Abl oncogene. Nat Med 1995; 181:307.
188. Skorski T, Nieborowska-Skorska M, Szczylik C, et al. C-RAF-1 serine/threonine kinase is required in BCR/ABL-dependent and normal hematopoiesis. Cancer Res 1995;55: 2275.
189. Dickens M, Rogers FJ, Cavanagh J, et al. A cytoplasmic inhibitor of the JNK signal transduction pathway. Science 1997;277:693.
190. Afar DE, Goga A, McLaughlin J, et al. Differential complementation of Bcr-Abl point mutants with c-Myc. Science 1994;264:424.
191. Nimmanapalli R, O'Bryan E, Bhalla K. Geldanamycin and is analogue 17-allylamino-17-demethoxygeldanamycin lowers Bcr-abl levels and induces apoptosis and differentiation of bcr-abl positive human leukemic blasts. Cancer Res 2001;61: 1799.
192. Cortes J, AlBitar M, Thomas D, et al. Efficacy of the farnesyl transferase inhibitor R115777 in chronic myeloid leukemia and other hematologic malignancies. Blood 2003;101:1692.
193. Hoover RR, Mahon FX, Melo JV, et al. Overcoming STI571 resistance with the farnesyl transferase inhibitor SCH66336. Blood 2002;100:1068.
194. Pinilla-Ibarz J, Cathcart K, Korontsvit T, et al. Vaccination of patients with chronic myelogenous leukemia with bcr-abl oncogene breakpoint fusion peptides generates specific immune responses. Blood 2000;95:1781.
195. Quintas-Cardama A, kantarjian H, Garcia-Manero G, et al. Phase I/II study of subcutaneous homoharringtonine in patients with chronic myeloid leukemia who have failed prior therapy. Cancer 2007;109:248.
196. Legros L, Hayette S, Nicolini FE, et al. BCR-ABL (T315i) transcript disappearance in an imatinib-resistant CML patient treated with homoharringtonine: a new therapeutic challenge? Leukemia 2007;21:2204.

197. Gontarewicz A, Balabanov S, Keller G, et al. Simultaneous targeting of Aurora kinases and Bcr-abl kinase by the small molecule inhibitor PHA-739358 is effective against imatinib-resistant Bcr-Abl mutations including T315I. Blood 2008;111:4355.
198. Spiers ASD, Goldman JM, Catovsky D, et al. Multiple-drug chemotherapy for acute leukemia: the TRAMPCOL regimen: results in 86 patients. Cancer 1977;40:20.
199. Lacoboni SJ, Plunkett W, Kantarjian HM, et al. High-dose cytosine arabinoside: treatment and cellular pharmacology of chronic myelogenous leukemia blast crisis. J Clin Oncol 1986;4:1079.
200. Coleman M, Silver RT, Pajek TF, et al. Combination chemotherapy for terminal-phase chronic granulocytic leukemia: Cancer and Leukemia Group B studies. Blood 1980;55:29.
201. Donadio D, Marty M, Navarro M, et al. Hydroxyurea, 6MP and VP-16 in the accelerated phase or in blastic transformation of CML. In: Mandelli F, ed. Proceedings of the 3rd International Symposium on therapy for acute leukemia. Rome, Italy: University of Rome, 1982:333.
202. Jain K, Arlin A, Mertelsmann R, et al. Philadelphia chromosome and terminal transferase positive acute leukemia: similarity of terminal phase of chronic myelogenous leukemia and de novo acute leukemia. J Clin Oncol 1983;1:669.
203. Schiffer CA, deBellis R, Kasdorf H, et al. Treatment of blast crisis of chronic myelogenous leukemia with 5-azacytidine and VP16–213. Cancer Treat Rep 1982;66:267.
204. Schulman P, van Echo D, Budman D, et al. Phase II trial of mitoxantrone (DHAD NSC 301739) in blastic phase in chronic myelogenous leukemia (B-CML) [abstract]. Blood 1982;60(suppl 1):558.
205. Hulhoven R, Prentice G, Michaux JL, et al. A phase I/II study of mitoxantrone in acute myelogenous leukemia. In: Mandelli F, ed. Proceedings of the 3rd International Symposium for therapy of acute leukemia. Rome, Italy: University of Rome, 1982:383.
206. Paciucci P, Ohnuma T, Cuttner J, et al. Phase I/II evaluation of mitoxantrone inn patients with refractory leukemia. In: Proceedings of the 3rd International Symposium for Therapy of Acute Leukemia. University of Rome, Rome, Italy. 1982:382.
207. Winton EF, Miller D, Vogler WR. Intensive chemotherapy with daunorubicin, 5-azacytidine, 6-thioguanine, and cytarabine (DATA) for the blastic transformation of chronic granulocytic leukemia. Cancer Treat Rep 1981;65:389.
208. Koller CA, Miller DM. Preliminary observations on the therapy of the myeloid blast phase of chronic granulocytic leukemia with plicamycin and hydroxyurea. N Engl J Med 1986;315:1433.
209. Kantarjian HM, O'Brien S, Cortes J, et al. Results of decitabine (5-aza-2′deoxycytidine) therapy in 130 patients with chronic myelogenous leukemia. Cancer 2003;98: 522–528.
210. Sawyers CL, Hochhaus A, Feldman E, et al. Imatinib induces hematologic and cytogenetic responses in patients with chronic myelogenous leukemia in myeloid blast crisis: results of a phase II study. Blood 2003;99:3530–3539.
211. Silver RT, Cortes J, Waltzman R, et al. Sustained durability of responses and improved progression-free and overall survival with imatinib treatment for accelerated phase and blast crisis chronic myeloid leukemia: long-term followup of the STI571 0102 and 0109 trials. Haematologica 2009;94:743.
212. Druker BJ, Sawyers CL, Kantarjian H, et al. Activity of a specific inhibitor of the bcr-abl tyrosine kinase in the blast crisis of chronic myeloid leukemia and acute lymphoblastic leukemia with the Philadelphia chromosome. N Engl J Med 2001;344: 1038–1042.
213. Sawyers CL, Hochhaus A, Feldman E, et al. Imatinib induces hematologic and cytogenetic responses in patients with chronic myelogenous leukemia in myeloid blast crisis blast crisis: results of a phase II study. Blood 2002;99:3530.
214. Cortes J, Rousselot R, Kim D-W, et al. Dasatinib induces complete hematologic and cytogenetic responses in patients with imatinib-resistant or -intolerant chronic myeloid leukemia in blast crisis. Blood 2007;109:3207.
215. Kantarjian HM, O'Brien SM, Keating M, et al. Results of decitabine therapy in the accelerated and blastic phases of chronic myelogenous leukemia. Leukemia 1997;11:1617.
216. Sacchi S, Kantarjian JM, O'Brien S, et al. Chronic myelogenous leukemia in nonlymphoid blastic phase. Analysis of the results of first salvage therapy with three different treatment approaches for 163 patients. Cancer 1999;86:2632.
216a. Giles FA, Garcia-Manero G, Cortes JE, et al. Phase II study of troxacitabine, a novel dioxolane nucleoside analog in patients with refractory leukemia. J Clin Oncol 2002; 20:656.
217. Neviani P, Santhanam R, Oaks JJ, et al. FYT720, a new alternative for treating blast crisis chronic myelogenous leukemia and Philadelphia chromosome-positive acute lymphocytic leukemia. J Clin Invest 2007:117:2408.
218. Schultz KR, Bowman WP, Slayton W, et al. Improved early event free survival (EFS) in children with Philadelphia chromosome-positive (Ph+) acute lymphoblastic leukemia (ALL) with intensive imatinib in combination with high dose chemotherapy: Children's Oncology Group (COG) Study AALL0031 [meeting abstract]. Blood 2007;110:4.
219. Fruehauf S, Topaly J, Buss EC, et al. Imatinib combined with mitoxantrone/etoposide and cytarabine is an effective induction therapy for patients with chronic myeloid leukemia in myeloid blast crisis. Cancer 2007;109:1543.
220. Altman AJ, Palmer CG, Baehner RL. Juvenile "chronic granulocytic" leukemia: a panmyelopathy with prominent monocytic involvement and circulating monocyte colony-forming cells. Blood 1974;43:341.
221. Arico M, Biondi A, Pui C-H. Juvenile myelomonocytic leukemia. Blood 1997;90:479.
222. Niemeyer C, Arico M, Basso G, et al. Chronic myelomonocytic leukemia in childhood: a retrospective analysis of 110 cases. Blood 1997;89:3534.
223. Chan RJ, Cooper T, Kratz CP, et al. Juvenile myelomonocytic leukemia: a report from the 2nd International JMML Symposium. Leuk Res 2009;33:355.
224. Vardiman JW, Thiele J, Arber DA, et al. The 2008 revision of the World Health Organization classification of myeloid neoplasms and acute leukemia: rationale and important changes. Blood 2009;112:45.
225. Shannon KM, O'Connell P, Martin GA, et al. Loss of the normal NF1 allele from the bone marrow of children with type 1 neurofibromatosis and malignant myeloid disorders. N Engl J Med 1994;330:597.
226. Bader JL, Miller RW. Neurofibromatosis and childhood leukemia. J Pediatr 1978;92: 925.
227. Side L, Taylor B, Cavouette M, et al. Homozygous inactivation of the NF1 gene in bone marrow cells from children with neurofibromatosis type 1 and malignant myeloid disorders. N Engl J Med 1997;336:1713.
228. Choong K, Freedman MH, Chitayat D, et al. Juvenile myelomonocytic leukemia and Noonan syndrome. J Pediatr Hematol Oncol 1999;21:523–527.
229. Tartaglia M, Niemeyer CM, Fragale A, et al. Somatic mutations in PTPN11 in juvenile myelomonocytic leukemia, myelodysplastic syndromes and acute myeloid leukemia. Nat Genet 2003;34:148–150.
230. Sieff CA, Chessels JM, Harvey BAM, et al. Monosomy 7 in childhood: a myeloproliferative disorder. Br J Haematol 1981;49:235.
231. Luna-Fineman S, Shannon KM, Lange BJ. Childhood monosomy 7: epidemiology, biology, and mechanistic implications. Blood 1995;85(8):1985–1999.
232. Kojima S, Mimaya J, Tonouchi T, et al. Erythropoiesis during an erythroblastic phase of chronic myeloproliferative disorder associated with monosomy 7. Br J Haematol 1987;65:391.
233. Emanuel PD. Myelodysplasia and myeloproliferative disorders in childhood: an update. Br J Haematol 1999;105:852.
234. Gerritsen A, Lam K, Schneider EM, et al. An exclusive case of juvenile myelomonocytic leukemia in association with Kikuchi's disease and hemophagocytic lymphohistiocytosis and a review of the literature. Leuk Res 2006;30:1299.
235. Shin HT, Haris MB, Orlow SL. Juvenile myelomonocytic leukemia presenting with features of hemophagocytic lymphohistiocytosis in association with neurofibromatosis and juvenile xanthogranulomas. J Pediatr Hematol Oncol 2004;26:591.
236. Kirby MA, Weitzman S, Freedman MH. Juvenile chronic myelogenous leukemia: differentiation from infantile cytomegalovirus infection. Am J Pediatr Hematol Oncol 1990; 12:292.
237. Shannon K, Nunez G, Dow LW, et al. Juvenile chronic myelogenous leukemia: surface antigen phenotyping by monoclonal antibodies and cytogenetic studies. Pediatrics 1986;77:330.
238. Busque L, Gilliland DG, Prchal JT, et al. Clonality in juvenile chronic myelogenous leukemia. Blood 1995;85:21.
239. Estrov Z, Grunberger T, Chan HSL, et al. Juvenile chronic myelogenous leukemia: characteristics of the disease using cell cultures. Blood 1986;67:1382.
240. Suda T, Miura Y, Mizoguchi H, et al. Characterization of hemopoietic precursor cells in juvenile-type chronic myelocytic leukemia. Leuk Res 1982;6:43.
241. Largaespada DA, Brannan CI, Jenkins NA, et al. Nf1 deficiency causes Ras mediated granulocyte/macrophage colony stimulating factor hypersensitivity and chronic myeloid leukaemia. Nat Genet 1996;12:137.
242. Emanuel PD, Bates LJ, Castelberry RP, et al. Selective hypersensitivity to granulocyte-macrophage colony-stimulating factor by juvenile chronic myeloid leukemia hematopoietic precursors. Blood 1991;77:925.
243. Freedman MH, Cohen A, Grunberger T, et al. Central role of tumor necrosis factor, GM-CSF, and interleukin 1 in the pathogenesis of juvenile chronic myelogenous leukaemia. Br J Haematol 1992;80:40.
244. Satoh T, Nakafu M, Miyajima A, et al. Involvement of ras21 protein in signal-transduction pathways from interleukin 2, interleukin 3, and granulocyte/macrophage colony-stimulating factor, but not from interleukin-4. Proc Natl Acad Sci U S A 1991;88:3314.
245. Miyauchi J, Asada M, Sasaki M, et al. Mutations of the N-ras gene in juvenile chronic myelogenous leukemia. Blood 1994;83:2248.
246. Hess JL, Zutter MM, Castleberry RP, et al. Juvenile chronic myelogenous leukemia. Am J Clin Pathol 1996;105:238.
247. Lauchle JO, Braun BS, Loh ML, et al. Inherited predispositions and hyperactive Ras in myeloid leukemogenesis. Pediatr Blood Cancer 2006;46:579.
248. Fragale A, Tartaglia M, Wu J, et al. Noonan syndrome-associated SHP2/PTPN11 mutants cause EGF-dependent prolonged GAB1-binding and sustained ERK2/MAPK1 activation. Hum Mutat 2004;23:267–277.
249. Loh M, Vattikuti S, Schubberts S, et al. Mutations in PTPN11 implicate the SHP-2 phosphatase in leukemogenesis. Blood 2004;103:2325–2331.
250. Papayannoupoulou T, Nakamoto B, Anagnou NP, et al. Expression of embryonic globins by erythroid cells in juvenile chronic myelocytic leukemia. Blood 1991;12:2569.
251. Symann M, de Montpellier C, Niname J, et al. Spontaneous erythroid progenitor cells in the circulation and monosomy 7 in juvenile chronic myelogenous leukemia. Cancer Genet Cytogenet 1982;6:183.
252. Privitera E, Schiro R, Longoni D, et al. Constitutive expression of GATA-1m, EPOR, a-globin and c-globin genes in myeloid clonogenic cells from juvenile chronic granulocytic leukemia. Blood 1995;86:323.
253. Niemeyer CM, Locatelli F. Chronic myeloproliferative disorders in childhood—an update. In: Pui C-H, ed. Childhood leukemias. New York, NY: Cambridge University Press, 2006:571–598.
254. Maurer HC, Vida LN, Honig GR. Similarities of the erythrocytes in juvenile chronic myelogenous leukemia to fetal erythrocytes. Blood 1972;39:778.
255. Travis SF. Fetal erythropoiesis in juvenile chronic myelocytic leukemia. Blood 1983; 62:602.
256. Cannat A, Seligmann M. Immunological abnormalities in juvenile myelomonocytic leukaemia. Br Med J 1973;1:71.
257. Ghione F, Merucci C, Symann M. Cytogenetic investigation in childhood chronic myelocytic leukemia. Cancer Genet Cytogenet 1986;20:317.
258. Butcher M, Frenck R, Emperor J, et al. Molecular evidence that childhood monosomy 7 syndrome is distinct from juvenile chronic myelogenous leukemia and other childhood myeloproliferative disorders. Genes Chromosomes Cancer 1995;12:50.
259. Woods WG, Barnard DR, Alonzo TA, et al. Prospective study of 90 children requiring treatment for juvenile myelomonocytic leukemia or myelodysplastic syndrome: a report from the Children's Cancer Group. J Clin Oncol 2002;20:434.
260. Luna-Fineman S, Shannon KM, Atwater SK, et al. Myelodysplastic and myeloproliferative disorders of childhood: a study of 167 patients. Blood 1999;93:459.
261. Passmore SJ, Chessells JM, Kempski H, et al. Paediatric myelodysplastic syndromes and juvenile myelomonocytic leukaemia in the UK: a population-based study of incidence and survival. Br J Haematol 2003;121:758–767.
262. Loh ML, Sakai DS, Flotho C, et al. Mutations in *CBL* occur frequently in juvenile myelomonocytic leukemia. Blood 2009;124:1859.
263. Side LE, Emanuel PD, Taylor B, et al. Mutations of the NF1 gene in children with juvenile myelomonocytic leukemia without clinical evidence of neurofibromatosis, type 1. Blood 1998;92:267.
264. Luri D, Avigad S, Cohen IJ, et al. p53 mutation as the second event in juvenile chronic myelogenous leukemia in a patient with neurofibromatosis type 1. Cancer 1997;80: 2013.
265. Castro-Malaspina H, Schaison G, Passe S, et al. Subacute and chronic myelomonocytic leukemia in children (juvenile CML). Clinical and hematologic observations, and identifications of prognostic factors. Cancer 1984;54:675.
266. Yoshida N, Yagasaki H, Yoshimi A, et al. Correlation of clinical features with the mutational status of GM-CSG signaling pathway-related genes in children with juvenile myelomonocytic leukemia. Blood 2007;110:457a.
267. Lau RC, Squire J, Brisson L, et al. Lymphoid blast crisis of B-lineage phenotype with monosomy 7 in a patient with juvenile chronic granulocytic leukemia (JCML). Leukemia 1994;8:903.

268. Cooper LJN, Shannon KM, Loken MR, et al. Evidence that juvenile myelomonocytic leukemia can arise from a pluripotential stem cell. Blood 2000;96:2310.

269. Hoffman R, Zanjani ED. Erythropoietin-dependent erythropoiesis during the erythroblastic phase of juvenile chronic granulocytic leukaemia. Br J Haematol 1978;38:511.

270. Lilleyman JS, Harrison JF, Black JA. Treatment of juvenile chronic myeloid leukemia with sequential subcutaneous cytarabine and oral mercaptopurine. Blood 1977;49:559.

271. Chan HS, Estrov Z, Weitzman SS, et al. The value of intensive combination chemotherapy for juvenile chronic myelogenous leukemia. J Clin Oncol 1987;5:1960.

272. Woods WG, Buckley JD, Lange BJ, et al. The treatment of children with myelodysplastic syndrome (MDS): the Children's Cancer Group (CCG) experience. J Pediatr Hematol Oncol 1997;97:356a.

273. Suttorp M, Rister M, Schmitz N. Interferon-alpha-2 (IFN) plus hydroxyurea for treatment of juvenile chronic myelogenous leukemia [letter]. Med Pediatr Oncol 1994;22:359.

274. Manabe A, Okamura J, Yumura-Yagi K, et al. Allogeneic hematopoietic stem cell transplantation for 27 children with juvenile myelomonocytic leukemia diagnosed based on the criteria of the International JMML Working Group. Blood 2002;16:645.

275. Locatell F, Nollke P, Zecca M, et al. Hematopoietic stem cell transplantation (HSCT) in children with juvenile myelomonocytic leukemia (JMML): results of the EWOG-MDS/EBMT trial. Blood 2005;105:410.

276. Yoshimi A, Bader P, Matthes-Martin S, et al. Donor leukocyte infusion after hematopoietic stem cell transplantation in patients with juvenile myelomonocytic leukemia. Leukemia 2005;19:971.

277. Tanoshima R, Goto H, Yanagimachi M, et al. Graft versus leukemia effect against juvenile myelomonocytic leukemia after unrelated cord blood transplantation. Pediatr Blood Cancer 2008;50:665.

278. Emanuel PD, Zuckerman KS, Wimmer R, et al. In vivo 13-cis retinoic acid therapy decreases the in-vitro GM-CSF hypersensitivity in juvenile chronic myelogenous leukemia (JCML) [abstract]. Blood 1991;78(suppl 1):170a.

279. Castleberry RP, Chang M, Maybee D, et al. A phase II study of 13-cis retinoic acid (CRA) in juvenile myelomonocytic leukemia (JMML): a Pediatric Oncology Group (POG) study. Blood 1997;90(suppl 1):346a.

280. Rebollo A, Martinez AC. Ras proteins: recent advances and new functions. Blood 1999;94:2971.

281. Zujewski J, Horak ID, Bol CJ, et al. Phase I and pharmacologic study of farnesyl protein transferase inhibitor R115777 in advanced cancer. J Clin Oncol 2000;18:927.

282. Rowinski EK, Windle JJ, von Hoff DD. Ras protein farnesyltransferase: a strategic target for anticancer therapeutic development. J Clin Oncol 1999;17:3631.

283. Emanuel PD, Synder RC, Wiley T, et al. Inhibition of juvenile myelomonocytic leukemia cell growth in vitro by farnesyltransferase inhibitors. Blood 2000;95:639–645.

284. Castlebery RP, Loh ML, Jayaprakash N, et al. Phase II window study of the farnesyl-transferase inhibitor RII5777 (Zarnestra®) in untreated juvenile myelomonocytic leukemia (JMML): a children's oncology group study. Blood 2005;106:727a.

285. Bernard F, Thomas C, Emile JF, et al. Transient hematologic and clinical effect of E21R in a child with end-stage juvenile myelomonocytic leukemia. Blood 2001;99:2615.

286. Frankel AE, Lilly M, Kreitman R, et al. Diphtheria toxin fused to granulocyte-macrophage colony-stimulating factor is toxic to blasts from patients with juvenile myelomonocytic leukemia and chronic myelomonocytic leukemia. Blood 1998;92:4279.

287. Iverson PO, Sioud M. Modulation of granulocyte-macrophage colony-stimulating factor gene expression by a tumor necrosis factor specific ribozyme in juvenile myelomonocytic leukemic cells. Blood 1998;92:4263–4268.

288. Iverson PO, Hart PH, Bonder CS, et al. Interleukin (IL)-10, but not IL-4 or IL-3, inhibits cytokine production and growth in juvenile myelomonocytic leukemia cells. Cancer Res 1997;57:476–480.

289. Metzner A, Horstmann MA, Fehse B, et al. Gene transfer of SHIP-1 inhibits proliferation of juvenile myelomonocytic leukemia cells carrying KRAS or PTPN11 mutations. Gene Ther 2007;14:699.

290. Ohtsuka Y, Manabe A, Kawasaki H, et al. RAS-blocking bisphosphonate zoledronic acid inhibits the abnormal proliferation and differentiation of juvenile myelomonocytic leukemia cells in vitro. Blood 2005;106:3134.

291. Holton CP, Johnson WW. Chronic myelocytic leukemia in infant siblings. J Pediatr 1968;72:377.

292. Thomas WJ, North RB, Poplack DG, et al. Chronic myelomonocytic leukemia in childhood. Am J Hematol 1981;10:181.

293. Stockley RJ, Eden OB. Chronic myelomonocytic leukaemia in infancy: a case report. Med Pediatr Oncol 1983;11:284.

294. Weisgerber G, Schaison G, Chavelet F, et al. Les leucemies myelo-mono-cytaires de l'enfant. Arch Fr Pediatr 1972;29:11.

295. Solal-Celigny P, Desaint B, Herrara A, et al. Chronic myelomonocytic leukemia according to FAB classification: analysis of 35 cases. Blood 1984;63:634.

296. Pearson HA, Diamond LK. Chronic monocytic leukemia in childhood. J Pediatr 1958;53:259.

297. Orchard NP. Letterer-Siwe's syndrome: review of a case with unusual peripheral blood changes. Arch Dis Child 1950;25:151.

298. Sonnier JA, Buchanan GR, Howard-Peebles PN, et al. Chromosomal translocation involving the immunoglobulin kappa-chain and heavy-chain loci in a child with chronic lymphocytic leukemia. N Engl J Med 1983;309:590.

299. Rewald R, Estevez ME, Sen L. Monoclonal B-cell lymphocytosis in early childhood: a case report. Am J Pediatr Hematol Oncol 1985;7:331.

300. Sardemann H. Chronic lymphocytic leukemia in an infant. Acta Paediatr Scand 1972;61:213.

301. Behm FL, McWilliams NB, Westin EH, et al. Chronic lymphocytic leukemia in a child [abstract 883]. Proceedings APS/SPR 1985;19:258A.

302. Casey TP. Chronic lymphocytic leukaemia in a child presenting at the age of two years and eight months. Aust Ann Med 1968;17:70.

303. Darte JMM, McClure PD, Saunders EF, et al. Congenital lymphoid hyperplasia with persistent hyperlymphocytosis. N Engl J Med 1971;284:431.

304. Gahrton G, Robert KH. Chromosomal aberrations in chronic B-cell lymphocytic leukemia. Cancer Genet Cytogenet 1982;6:171.

305. Han T, Ozer H, Sadamori H, et al. Cytogenetic abnormalities in chronic lymphocytic leukemia (CLL): a clinical correlation [abstract]. Blood 1982;60(suppl 1):127a.

306. Ferrajoli A, O'Brien SM. Treatment of chronic lymphocytic leukemia. Semin Oncol 2004;31(suppl 4):60.

307. Keating MJ, O'Brien S, Albitar M, et al. Early results of a chemoimmunotherapy regimen of fludarabine, cyclophosphamide, and rituximab as initial therapy for chronic lymphocytic leukemia. J Clin Oncol 2005;23:4079.

308. Byrd JC, Peterson BL, Morrison VA, et al. Randomized phase 2 study of fludarabine with concurrent versus sequential treatment with rituximab in symptomatic, untreated patients with B-cell chronic lymphocytic leukemia: results from Cancer and Leukemia Group B 9712 (CALGB 9712). Blood 2003;101:6.

309. Kay NE, Geyer SM, Call TG, et al. Combination chemotherapy with pentostatin, cyclophosphamide, and rituximab shows significant clinical activity with low accompanying toxicity in previously untreated B chronic lymphocytic leukemia. Blood 2007;109(2):405–411.

310. O'Brien, S. New agents in the treatment of CLL. In: Hematology. American Society of Hematology Education Book, 2008:457.

CHAPTER 22 ■ HODGKIN LYMPHOMA

MONIKA METZGER, MATTHEW J. KRASIN, MELISSA M. HUDSON, AND MIHAELA ONCIU

The original paper by Hodgkin in 1832 was entitled "On Some Morbid Appearances of the Absorbent Glands and Spleen."[1] In that era of anatomic description of disease, investigators were concerned with differentiating inflammatory disease from infection or idiopathic hypertrophy of the lymphoid organs. Not until the second half of the nineteenth century, as the criteria for making diagnoses came to depend more on microscopic morphology, did investigators recognize that abnormal giant cells were present in Hodgkin material. Sternberg in 1898[2] and Reed[3] in 1902 are generally credited with the first definitive and thorough descriptions of the histopathology of Hodgkin lymphoma (HL). Reed in particular gave a precise description of the multinucleated giant cells in this disease, which led her finally to refute the idea that it was an unusual form of tuberculosis despite the frequent association of the two diseases in the same patient. After the histologic definition of the disease was established, Fox,[4] in 1926, reexamined the histologic features of Hodgkin original seven patients and concluded that three of them, one of whom was a pediatric patient, met the new criteria for definition of the disease.

In the ensuing years, although HL was recognized as a possible malignancy, the potential of an infectious or autoimmune etiology was still considered.[5] The pleomorphic nature of the cellular infiltrate in HL made investigators uncomfortable with the idea that this was a clonal proliferation of a single malignant cell. However, the successful cultivation of Reed-Sternberg cells[6] permitted the demonstration of the cells' malignant nature and reinforced the idea that HL was truly a malignant disorder.

Initial attempts with radiotherapy for this disease were disappointing; dramatic regression was followed by recurrence and, inevitably, death.[7] Improvements in radiation therapy technology eventually resulted in the cure of early stage disease with radiotherapy alone. In 1940, as a by-product of wartime work on compounds related to the mustard gases, nitrogen mustard's powerful lymphocytolytic effects were discovered.[8] Experimental studies indicating the advantage of using combinations of non–cross-resistant antineoplastic agents with nonoverlapping toxicities led to the introduction in 1964 of the four-drug MOPP regimen (mechlorethamine [nitrogen mustard], Oncovin [vincristine], procarbazine, prednisone).[9] MOPP was the first effective systemic therapy for HL. Trials using MOPP in adult patients produced prolonged disease-free survival in approximately 50% of patients when MOPP was administered at full doses.[10] Subsequently, pediatric trials demonstrated similar or better outcomes after MOPP chemotherapy.[11–15] With improved survival after MOPP, investigators appreciated that both adults and children were vulnerable to its adverse effects, which consist of an increased risk of treatment related acute myeloid leukemia (AML) and infertility. The development of the non–cross-resistant ABVD regimen (Adriamycin [doxorubicin], bleomycin, vinblastine, dacarbazine) in the 1970s provided effective systemic therapy for HL that was not associated with an excess risk of secondary AML or infertility.[16] ABVD was initially used in adult trials to salvage patients who did not respond to MOPP chemotherapy.[17] The lack of leukemogenesis and permanent gonadal toxicity and superior treatment outcomes has led to the standard use of ABVD in adults with newly diagnosed HL. However, the sole use of ABVD therapy in children has been less popular because of concerns about potential cardiopulmonary toxicity.

With greater appreciation of treatment sequelae after standard-dose radiotherapy and non–cross-resistant chemotherapy, pediatric investigators modified treatment strategies in the 1980s to address the specific needs of children. Combined-modality therapy regimens evolved in which cycles of chemotherapy replaced a portion of the radiation therapy in laparotomy-staged children with HL.[11,18,19] The success of this approach coupled with advances in diagnostic imaging technology ultimately resulted in the abandonment of surgical staging in the 1990s. This decade also saw the evolution of risk-adapted trials in which patients with favorable clinical presentations received combined-modality treatment prescribing fewer cycles of multiagent chemotherapy and lower radiation doses and treatment volumes.[20–22] Currently under investigation are novel approaches using compacted dose-intensive multiagent chemotherapy for patients with advanced and unfavorable disease. Advances in functional imaging have led to new studies investigating therapy reductions, or complete radiation omission, in patients that achieve early complete responses to initial chemotherapy.

EPIDEMIOLOGY

HL has a unique bimodal age distribution that differs geographically and ethnically. In industrialized countries, the early peak occurs in the middle to late 20s and the second peak after the age of 50 years. In developing countries, the early peak occurs before adolescence. Epidemiologic studies demonstrate three distinct forms of HL: a childhood form (in patients aged 14 years or younger), a young adult form (in patients aged 15 to 34 years), and an older adult form (most commonly presenting in patients aged 55 to 74 years).[23] HL is rarely diagnosed in children younger than 5 years. There is a slight overall male predominance in the childhood form.[24] Among adolescents, the gender distribution is roughly equal. In the United States, the incidence of HL among Whites is slightly higher than among Blacks, and is the lowest for Asian Americans.[25]

The childhood form of HL tends to increase with increasing family size and decreasing socioeconomic status. In contrast, the young adult form is associated with a higher socioeconomic status in industrialized countries. The risk for young adult HL decreases significantly with increased sibship size and birth order.[26] Swedish investigators recently observed a lower risk of HL in young adults with multiple older, but not younger siblings, a finding consistent with the hypothesis that early exposure to viral infection (which the siblings bring home from school) may play a role in the pathogenesis of the disease.[27] Likewise, early exposure to common infections in preschool appears to decrease the risk of HL, most likely by promoting maturation of cellular immunity.[27] Furthermore, a British case-control study found HL patients to have excess visits to their primary care provider for random infections in the years preceding their diagnosis, possibly reflecting an underlying immune abnormality.[28] Histologic subtypes also show variability related to age at diagnosis. Mixed cellularity (MC) HL is more common at younger ages, whereas nodular sclerosing HL has a higher incidence in more affluent societies.

Familial Hodgkin Lymphoma

Clustering of cases of HL within families or races may suggest a genetic predisposition to the disease or a common exposure to an etiologic agent. Studies of affected families have suggested an increased association of HL with specific human leukocyte antigens.[29] The concordance of HL in first-degree relatives, especially monozygotc twins, but also siblings, and parent-child pairs has been noted in numerous reports.[5,30] In the Swedish Family-Cancer Database, elevated risk of HL ranges from threefold among parent-offspring pairs to fivefold among siblings (eightfold among brothers and elevenfold among sisters), and the familial risk being greater in index cases younger than 35 years.[31,32] The repeated observation of gender concordance in sibling-pairs of different populations could be explained by a gene in a pseudoautosomal region of the sex chromosomes.[33] A genome-wide screen of families with HL found a potential recessive susceptibility gene on chromosome 4.[34]

Reports of HL in both marriage partners are extremely rare, as are data suggestive of transplacental transmission. HL is diagnosed more commonly in person whose immune system is abnormal, a finding that may reflect the slight increase in familial incidence.[35] The etiologic factors underlying the immune deficiency include genetic (e.g., ataxia telangiectasia), infectious (e.g., human immunodeficiency virus, HIV), and iatrogenic agents.[35]

Epstein-Barr Virus and Hodgkin Lymphoma

The epidemiologic characteristics of HL suggest that its etiology may vary by age at presentation.[5] In the young adult form, delayed exposure to an infectious agent has been proposed as a risk factor for the development of HL because its epidemiologic features are similar to that seen with paralytic poliomyelitis. Early and intense exposure to an infectious agent might increase the risk for the childhood form of HL. Epstein-Barr virus (EBV) has been implicated in the causation of HL. The large proportion of patients with HL who have high EBV antibody titers suggests that enhanced activation of EBV may precede the development of HL. This hypothesis is also supported by *in situ* hybridization evidence of EBV genomes in Hodgkin Reed-Sternberg (HRS) cells[36] and of EBV early RNA (EBER1 and EBER2) sequences.[37] In cases associated with EBV, the virus is localized to the Reed-Sternberg cell, EBV latent gene products are expressed, and the EBV infection is clonal. HL that is EBV positive at initial diagnosis is usually also positive for EBV at relapse with persistence of the same EBV strain.[38] EBV-associated antigens have been demonstrated in Hodgkin tissues.[39] EBV-infected HRS cells and their variants consistently express the latent membrane protein 1 (LMP1), LMP2A, and the Epstein-Barr nuclear antigen 1 (EBNA-1), but not Epstein-Barr nuclear antigen 2, viral capsid antigen, or early antigen.[39–41] This expression pattern is associated with the latency type II pattern of EBV infection.[42] EBV LMP1 expression varies among the histo-

logic subtypes of classical HL (cHL) (virtually 100% of the HIV-associated lymphocyte depleted [LD] HL, 75% of the MC HL, 40% to 45% of the lymphocyte-rich classical HL, and 10% to 40% of nodular sclerosis HL). Only rare cases of nodular lymphocyte-predominant HL have been found to contain EBV.[43,44]

EBV strain subtypes identified within HRS and HL also vary geographically. EBV strain type 1 is predominant in the United Kingdom, South Africa, Australia, and Greece, whereas EBV type 2 is predominant in Egypt. The presence of infection by both EBV strains in 21% of cases supports the possibility of an underlying immune deficiency in these cases. EBV-positive tumor genomes are more frequently observed in children aged 10 years or younger and in children living in developing countries. The incidence of EBV-associated HL also varies by ethnic background, as evidenced by its presence in 93% of Asian, 86% of Hispanic, 46% of Caucasian, and 17% of African American children with HL in one series. The precise role of EBV in the pathogenesis and biology of HL is not entirely clear. Clonality studies indicate that EBV infection precedes expansion of the tumor cell population. Infected Hodgkin and HRS cells express high levels of LMP1, a viral protein that resembles a constitutively activated member of the tumor necrosis factor receptor (TNFR) superfamily. As such, its effects result from the activation of a variety of signaling apoptotic and growth pathways, including the transcription factor NF-κB.[45,46] Interestingly, NF-κB is constitutively activated in the HRS cells.[47] Furthermore, experimental data suggest that in the EBV-negative cases, this mechanism of NF-κB activation is substituted by inactivating mutations in members of the IκB family which are known negative regulators of NF-κB.[47–50] LMP1 expression is also associated with upregulation of cellular bcl2, interleukin-10 (IL-10), and major histocompatibility complex (MHC) class I proteins in some but not all cell lines. EBV-positive cases of HL have higher levels of IL-10 and EBV-specific cytotoxic T-cells and express higher levels of MHC class I molecules than EBV-negative cases.[51] In addition, experimental data indicate that LMP2A, another EBV-related protein strongly expressed by HRS cells, interferes with normal B-cell development by blocking B-cell receptor signaling.[46] Association of EBV with cHL is therefore provocative, since, as further detailed below, the HRS cells are B-lineage lymphocytes with an aberrant pattern of differentiation. All of these data have led to the speculation that EBV is directly involved in the pathogenesis of some cases of HL either alone or with other carcinogens. The disease may represent a common result of multiple pathologic processes that include viral infection and exposure of a genetically susceptible host to a sensitizing agent.

BIOLOGY

HL is a B-lineage lymphoma characterized by a small number of clonal tumor cells (HRS cells, lymphocytic and histiocytic [L & H] cells, and their morphologic variants), surrounded by rosettes of T lymphocytes and a polymorphous inflammatory cell population which constitutes the bulk of the tumoral tissue. Consequently, the true origin of the neoplastic cells in this disease has remained uncertain until recently, when techniques such as microdissection and single-cell polymerase chain reaction (PCR) have made it possible to analyze enriched populations of tumor cells removed from their benign polyclonal inflammatory background. These studies have shown that the malignant cells of HL are clonal cells with at least three distinct origins. In the nodular lymphocyte predominant HL, the tumor cells (L & H) derive from germinal center (GC) or post-GC B-cells, showing rearranged immunoglobulin variable

(IgV) genes. The presence of intraclonal IgV gene diversity further indicates an origin in mutated and antigen-selected GC B-cells. These neoplastic cells retain expression of all B-cell specific molecules, such as CD19, CD20, CD79a, J chain, PAX5, Ig (with light chain restriction), Oct-2, BOB.1, and PU-1, although at reduced levels of expression. In cHL, the tumor cells (HRS) are also GC B-cells, but they additionally show crippling mutations that destroy the coding capacity of their previously functional IgV gene rearrangements. In the normal GC, such cells are typically targeted for apoptosis. This suggests that HRS cells may originate in preapoptotic GC B-cells that escape apoptosis through various mechanisms. The inhibition of apoptosis in these cells has been attributed to a variety of molecular and genetic alterations found in these cells, including constitutive activation of the NF-κB pathway, activation of NOTCH-1, aberrant activities of multiple receptor tyrosine kinases, and activation of STAT (STAT 3, 5 and 6) and AP-1 transcription factors. The CD30 molecule, highly expressed by HRS cells, appears to play an important role in at least two of these altered signaling pathways, including NF-κB and AP-1. The HRS cells show an aberrant differentiation program that includes the profound down-regulation of most B-cell–specific genes (including those for CD19, CD20, CD79a, Ig, and the transcription factors Oct-2, BOB.1, and PU-1), although they retain weak expression of PAX-5/BSAP, a B-lineage commitment and maintenance factor. They also retain molecules important in B-T cell interactions, such as CD80, CD86, and MHC class II, and often express molecules typically upregulated in plasma cells (CD138 and MUM-1).[52,53] Last, in a minority (2%) of cHL cases, the HRS cells show a cytotoxic T-lymphoid immunophenotype that may be associated with a B-cell genotype or harbor T-cell receptor beta gene rearrangements.[52,54,55] Thus, HL is a unique type of B-cell neoplasm and hence the current World Health Organization (WHO) classifications[56,57] have abandoned the term "Hodgkin disease" thought to reflect the lack of knowledge regarding the true origin of the HRS cells.

Two clinically distinct subtypes of HL are currently recognized at the morphologic and immunophenotypic level, based on the distinct characteristics of the neoplastic cells, their inflammatory background, and the overall tumor growth pattern (Table 22.1).

In the *cHL* of all histologic subtypes, the HRS cells and their mononuclear (Hodgkin cells) and multinucleated variants most commonly lack immunophenotypic evidence of B-lineage differentiation. As a result of the molecular alterations described previously, the HRS cells are negative for leukocyte common antigen (CD45), B-lineage antigens (such as CD20, CD79a, and J chain), and BCL6. They characteristically coexpress the CD15 (LeuM1) and CD30 (Ki-1) antigens. In a limited number of cases (10% to 20%), the classical Reed-Sternberg cells may express CD20 with variable intensity. The inflammatory background of cHL typically includes a mixture of T and B lymphocytes, histiocytes, and granulocytes, most commonly eosinophils, and often necrotizing granulomata. In some of the subtypes (e.g. nodular sclerosis), there is significant associated fibrosis. A subset of cHL contains EBV (see earlier).

In the *nodular lymphocyte predominant HL*, the L & H (popcorn) cells consistently show molecular and immunophenotypic evidence of B-lineage differentiation. The L & H cells show immunophenotypic evidence of B-lymphoid differentiation, including expression of CD45, CD20, CD79a, J chain, and BCL6 and usually lack expression of CD15 and CD30. Most of these tumors show at least partially a nodular growth pattern. The neoplastic nodules are related to normal GCs by a predominance of small CD20-positive lymphocytes and an underlying follicular dendritic cell meshwork that can be highlighted with staining for CD21 and CD35 characteristic for the latter cells. Fibrosis is uncommon in nodular lymphocyte predominance HL (nodular LP HL). EBV has only rarely been identified in this type of HL.

The CD30 antigen was initially recognized on the HRS cells using the Ki-1 monoclonal antibody.[58] It was subsequently found to be expressed and/or upregulated on a variety of normal lymphoid cells of T lineage and B lineage and it appears to be a key modulator for the T-cell activity. In addition, CD30 is expressed in a variety of T-cell non-HL subtypes, including anaplastic large cell lymphoma[58] and peripheral T-cell lymphoma. The CD30 molecule is a membrane glycoprotein that belongs to the TNFR superfamily. The extracellular domain of this receptor molecule binds the CD30 ligand, while its intracellular portion signals through the TNFR-associated factor pathways, to modulate the transcription of a variety of cytokines either directly (interleukin-13) or through activation of the NF-κB transcription factor (interleukin-6).[59] The precise role of CD30 expression in cHL is not clear. The serum levels of soluble CD30 have been found to correlate with outcome in advanced stage HL. Elevated serum levels of CD30 and CD25 (IL-2 receptor, another molecule highly expressed by HRS cells) have been associated with advanced stage, constitutional (B) symptoms, and poor outcome.[60,61] In addition, CD30 and CD25 have been proposed as a suitable molecular targets in the immunotherapy of HL and other CD30-positive lymphomas, and the use of an anti-CD30 and anti-CD25 antibody-immunotoxin conjugates has already been reported in phase I studies.[62–64]

HL is associated with the production of a variety of cytokines by the neoplastic cells and by the recruited inflam-

TABLE 22.1

IMMUNOPHENOTYPE OF THE NEOPLASTIC CELLS AND PATHOLOGIC FEATURES IN HODGKIN LYMPHOMAS AND NON-HODGKIN LYMPHOMAS

Tumor type	LCA (CD45)	CD15 (LeuM1)	CD30 (Ki-1)	CD20	EMA	ALK	Growth pattern
HL, classical type (HRS cell)	−	+	+	−/+	−	−	Nodular, diffuse
HL, nodular LP (L & H cell)	+	−	−	+	+/−	−	Nodular +/− diffuse
T-cell rich large B-cell lymphoma	+	−	−	+	+/−	−	Diffuse
Anaplastic large cell lymphoma, T/null cell	+	−	+	−	+	+/−	Diffuse, interfollicular, sinusoidal

TABLE 22.2

CLINICAL AND PATHOLOGIC FEATURES OF HODGKIN LYMPHOMA RELATED
TO CYTOKINE PRODUCTION

Clinical and pathologic features of Hodgkin lymphoma	Cytokines
Constitutional (B) symptoms	TNF, LT-α, IL-1, IL-6
Polykaryon formation	Interferon-γ, IL-4
Sclerosis	TGF-β, LIF, PDGF, IL-1, TNF
Acute phase reactions	IL-1, IL-6, IL-11, LIF
Eosinophilia	IL-5, granulocyte M-CSF, IL-2, IL-3
Plasmacytosis	IL-6, IL-11
Mild thrombocytosis	IL-6, IL-11, LIF
T-cell and Hodgkin and Reed-Sternberg cell interaction	IL-1, IL-2, IL-6, IL-7, IL-9, TNF, LT-α, CD30L, CD40L, B7 ligands (CD80 and CD86)
Immune deficiency	TGF-β, IL-10
Autocrine growth factors (?)	IL-6, IL-9, TNF, LT-α, CD30L, M-CSF
Increased alkaline phosphatase	M-CSF
Neutrophil accumulation/activation	IL-8, TNF, TGF-β

IL, interleukin; LIF, leukemia inhibitory factor; LT, lymphotoxin; M-CSF, macrophage colony-stimulating factor; PDGF, platelet-derived growth factor; TGF, transforming growth factor; TNF, tumor necrosis factor.
Adapted from Kadin ME, Liebowitz DN. Cytokines and cytokine receptors in Hodgkin disease. In: Mauch PM, Armitage JO, Diehl V, et al., eds. Hodgkin disease. Philadelphia, PA: Lippincott Williams & Wilkins, 1999:139.

matory cells. Distinct patterns of cytokine production are associated with the two main subtypes of HL, resulting in a distinct histologic appearance and spectrum of clinical features in each of these types. The high levels of expression of CD30 and CD40 by the HRS cells may result in activation of NF-κB and c-Jun N-terminal kinase pathways, which regulate HRS cell proliferation, expression of adhesion molecules, and secretion of cytokines.[59,65] The histopathologic features of cHL, such as eosinophilia and collagen sclerosis, have been attributed to the production of cytokines such as IL-4, IL-5, eotaxin, IL-6, IL-7, IL-13, TNF, lymphotoxin, transforming growth factor-β (TGF-β), and basic fibroblast growth factor.[65] Adhesion molecules regulated by cytokines are thought to influence the interaction of HRS cells with the neighboring T lymphocytes, as well as the metastatic capacity of the disease. Systemic symptoms have been best correlated with elevated serum levels of IL-6 and immunosuppression in untreated patients with TGF-β.[65] Table 22.2 summarizes the relationship among cytokine production and common clinical and pathologic features of HL.

PATHOLOGY

HL is characterized by a minority of malignant cells which account for 0.1% to 10% of the total cell population of the tumor.[56] The majority of the tumor is composed of an infiltrate of inflammatory cells (e.g., histiocytes, plasma cells, lymphocytes, eosinophils, neutrophils) and fibrosis, which develops as a result of cytokine release. In its most typical forms, HL must therefore be differentiated from several subtypes of non-HL with similar morphologic characteristics (i.e., T-cell–rich large B-cell lymphoma and anaplastic large cell lymphoma) and from benign lymphoid hyperplasias with a similar cellular composition (e.g. infectious mononucleosis, progressive trans-

formation of GCs).[66–68] In addition, less common variants of HL (e.g. LD and syncytial variants) may overlap morphologically with nonhematopoietic malignancies, such as carcinomas and sarcomas. With the advent of widely available immunohistochemical staining, the latter entities are usually easy to exclude. However, the differential diagnosis with certain non-HLs of B-cell lineage may still represent a challenge especially in tumors that show overlapping features of HL and diffuse large B-cell lymphoma (so called grey-zone lymphomas).[69,70]

Table 22.1 summarizes the main immunophenotypic features of the neoplastic cells in the two main HL subtypes and the non-HLs most commonly employed in the differential diagnosis of HL. The neoplastic cells of cHL (designated here as HRS cells) are the classic Reed-Sternberg cells and their variants, including mononuclear variants (Hodgkin cells) and multinucleated variants. The classic Reed-Sternberg cell is large (≥15 to 45 μm in diameter), with abundant slightly basophilic cytoplasm and two nuclei or two nuclear lobes. These cells have a thick nuclear membrane, pale chromatin, and two large eosinophilic nucleoli (one in each nuclear lobe). The nucleoli are characteristically large (macronucleoli), often equal in size to the neighboring lymphocytes (Fig. 22.1a). Additional variants of the Reed-Sternberg cell characteristically seen in nodular sclerosing HL subtype include the lacunar cell and the mummified cell. The lacunar cell is a mononuclear HRS cell that appears to sit in a space (lacuna) due to a membrane retraction artifact induced by formalin fixation. The mummified cells have condensed cytoplasm and dark pyknotic nuclei. In some patients, Hodgkin cells may be highly pleomorphic raising the differential diagnosis with high-grade sarcomas and diffuse large cell lymphomas with anaplastic features. The neoplastic cells of nodular LP HL are the L & H cells (Fig. 22.1b). These are typically mononuclear cells with markedly convoluted and lobated nucleus (popcorn cells), thin nuclear membrane, pale chromatin, and one-to-several small basophilic nucleoli.

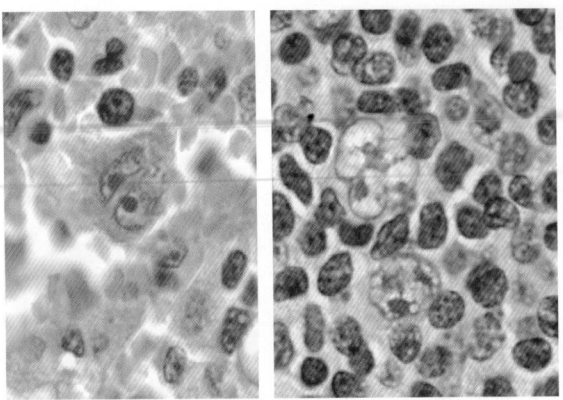

FIGURE 22.1 Morphologic features of the neoplastic cells in Hodgkin lymphoma. **A:** Reed-Sternberg cell seen in classical HL. **B:** L & H cells seen in nodular lymphocyte predominant HL (hematoxylin and eosin stain; original magnification 600×, oil immersion).

Definition of Histologic Subtypes

The current WHO histologic classification of HL is largely based on the Rye modification of the Lukes and Butler classification schema.[71] The WHO classification[57] recognizes two major subtypes of HL, cHL and nodular LP HL, based on their biological and clinical features (Table 22.3). The cHL contains HRS cells with the classical morphology and immunophenotype. Four histologic subtypes are further included in this category based on tissue architecture, the presence of fibrosis, and the features of the associated inflammatory infiltrate. Historically, prognosis for some of the categories of HL was linked to the ratio of lymphocytes to abnormal cells. Since the development of highly curative treatment regimens, however, all histologic subtypes of HL are equally responsive to treatment.

In the nodular LP HL, the tumor has at least partially a nodular architecture. The neoplastic nodules contain classic L & H cells and only rare classic HRS cells, along with many small benign B lymphocytes, histiocytes, and epithelioid histiocytes. The presence of nodularity is essential in the differential diagnosis with T-cell–rich B-cell lymphoma, which has an exclusively diffuse growth pattern. The cellular composition and the immunophenotypic features differentiate between nodular LP HL and progressive transformation GCs, a pattern of benign lymphoid hyperplasia that may precede, coexist with, or follow this type of HL.[66] Nodular LP Hodgkin disease affects 10% to 15% of patients, is more common among male and younger patients, and usually presents as clinically localized disease.

Affecting approximately 40% of younger patients and 70% of adolescents, nodular sclerosis cHL is the most common

TABLE 22.3

HISTOLOGICAL CLASSIFICATION OF HL ACCORDING TO THE WHO CLASSIFICATION

Nodular lymphocyte predominant HL
Classical HL
Nodular sclerosis subtype
Mixed cellularity subtype
Lymphocyte-rich subtype
Lymphocyte-depleted subtype

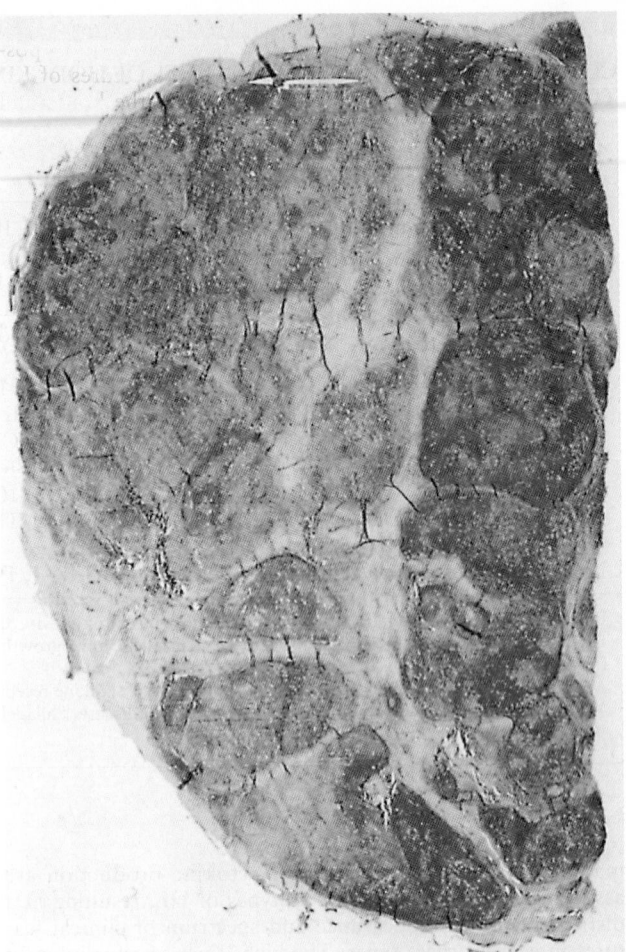

FIGURE 22.2 Lymph node, nodular sclerosing HL. Cellular nodules are surrounded by dense fibrous bands (hematoxylin and eosin; 8×).

subtype.[72] It is characterized by nodules of neoplastic and inflammatory cells (including HRS cells and their lacunar variant), a markedly thickened lymph node capsule, and thick sclerotic collagenous bands that surround completely at least one cellular nodule. In its most characteristic form, the sclerosis is so pronounced that the nodular architecture of the tumor can be readily appreciated on gross examination of the involved lymph node (Fig. 22.2). This process has a striking propensity to involve the lower cervical, supraclavicular, and mediastinal lymph nodes. Because of the abundance of collagen, the radiographic appearance of these lesions (particularly in the mediastinum) may only slowly return to normal, even when the patient is responding to therapy.

In the MC subtype of cHL, HRS cells and their variants are often numerous (5 to 15 per high-power field). The tumor usually has a diffuse or a vaguely nodular growth pattern and lacks significant associated fibrosis. The inflammatory background consists of lymphocytes, plasma cells, eosinophils, and histiocytes. Fine interstitial fibrosis may be seen, and focal necrosis may be present but usually is not marked. This subtype is observed in approximately 30% of patients, is more common in children aged 10 years or younger,[73,74] and frequently presents as advanced disease with extranodal involvement.[72]

LD HL is rare in children, but it is common in HIV-infected patients. The presence of numerous, large, bizarre, malignant cells, many Reed-Sternberg cells, and few lymphocytes characterizes this subtype. Diffuse fibrosis and necrosis are common. This subtype of cHL is often EBV positive in the HIV-positive patients.[75] Clinical features of LD HL include widespread disease that involves the bones and bone marrow.

The lymphocyte-rich variant of cHL is characterized by classical HRS cells and a cellular background that consists mostly of small B lymphocytes. The tumor may have a nodular or less commonly diffuse growth pattern. Immunophenotypic studies are often necessary to differentiate this rare form of cHL from the nodular LP subtype.[76] This subtype comprises approximately 5% of all HL and closely overlaps with the nodular LP subtype in presenting clinical features and prognosis. The median age at presentation is, however, higher than for the latter (32 years) and there is a slightly higher incidence of a mediastinal mass and stage III disease at presentation.[77]

CLINICAL PRESENTATION

Lymphadenopathy

Usually, patients present with painless supraclavicular or cervical adenopathy. Affected lymph nodes are firmer than inflammatory nodes, they feel rubbery, and may be sensitive to palpation if they have grown rapidly. At least two-thirds of patients present with some degree of mediastinal involvement (Fig. 22.3), which may cause a nonproductive cough or other symptoms of tracheal or bronchial compression. Posteroanterior and lateral thoracic radiographs should be performed as soon as HL becomes part of the differential diagnosis and to assess airway patency. In younger children, mediastinal lymphadenopathy may be difficult to distinguish from a large, normal thymus. Infrequently, axillary or inguinal lymphadenopathy is the first presenting sign. Primary disease presenting in a subdiaphragmatic site is rare and occurs in only approximately 3% of cases.[78]

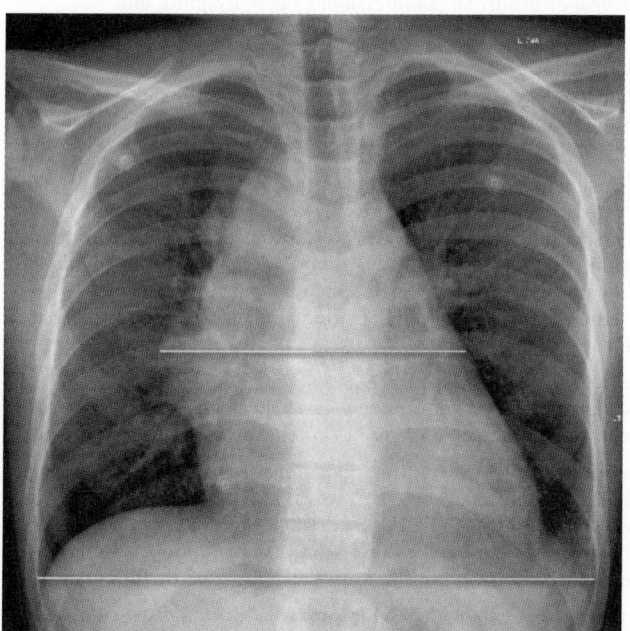

FIGURE 22.3 Anteroposterior chest film of a patient with bulky mediastinal mass.

Systemic Symptoms

Nonspecific systemic symptoms may include fatigue, anorexia, and slight weight loss. Three specific constitutional (B) symptoms correlate with prognosis: unexplained fever with temperatures above 38.0°C orally, unexplained weight loss of 10% within 6 months preceding diagnosis, and drenching night sweats.[79]

Pruritus, which may be mild or severe enough that scratching can cause excoriations, is another systemic symptom commonly observed in patients with HL. Although it is not considered one of the classic "B" symptoms, some studies suggest that it has a similar prognostic significance and confers a poor prognosis.[79,80] It occurs more frequently in patients with advanced-stage disease, may accompany other systemic symptoms, is more common in women, and is usually generalized.[81,82] Proposed mechanism include cholestatic liver disease and peripheral sensory neuropathy and it typically resolves when the HL is treated.[83]

Another unusual syndrome associated with HL is alcohol-induced pain.[82] The pain usually occurs in areas of nodal enlargement and begins within minutes of drinking alcohol. Pain may also develop in the chest and radiate to the extremities or back. Alcohol-induced pain resolves with treatment of HL; its mechanism is unknown.

Laboratory Profile

Hematologic and chemical blood parameters show nonspecific changes that may correlate with disease extent. Abnormalities of peripheral blood counts may include neutrophilic leukocytosis, lymphopenia, eosinophilia, and monocytosis. At the onset of disease, the absolute lymphocyte count is usually normal in children,[84] although adults with extensive disease commonly have lymphopenia. Anemia may indicate the presence of advanced disease and usually results from impaired mobilization of iron stores.[85] Hemolytic anemia associated with HL may be Coombs' positive and is accompanied by a reticulocytosis and normoblastic hyperplasia of the bone marrow.[86]

Several autoimmune disorders have been observed in association with HL, including nephrotic syndrome, autoimmune hemolytic anemia, autoimmune neutropenia, and immune thrombocytopenia (ITP). ITP has been reported in 1% to 2% of cases of HL and may occur in association with autoimmune hemolytic anemia.[87–89] Thrombocytopenia may develop before, at the same time, or after the diagnosis of HL.[87,89] ITP frequently occurs in patients in remission after completion of therapy for HL and is not usually associated with relapse. The treatment approach recommended for ITP in patients with HL is similar to that in patients without malignancy. Response to ITP therapy is also similar.

The erythrocyte sedimentation rate, serum copper, and ferritin levels may be elevated, reflecting activation of the reticuloendothelial system.[90] C-reactive protein is another acute phase reactant produced in the liver that holds promise as a diagnostic and prognostic index for both HL and cardiovascular disease.[91] These nonspecific tests, if abnormal at diagnosis, may be useful in follow-up evaluation.

Immunologic Status

Patients with HL exhibit a variety of immune system abnormalities at diagnosis that may persist during and after therapy.[92] Natural killer cell cytotoxicity may be reduced in untreated patients.[84,92] Typically, enhanced sensitivity to suppressor T lymphocytes present at diagnosis results in abnormal cellular immunity. After treatment, humoral immunity may be transiently depressed. *In vitro* studies have provided insights regarding the mechanism of immune dysregulation in HL.[93] Several cytokine interactions have been proposed to explain the paradoxical presence of extensive inflammatory infiltrate, ineffective host antitumor response, and generalized cellular immune deficiency.[65]

DIFFERENTIAL DIAGNOSIS

HL must be differentiated from other malignant lymphomas that can have similar presentations (lymphoblastic lymphoma and primary mediastinal large B-cell lymphomas presenting with a large anterior mediastinal mass) or similar histologic appearance (CD30-positive anaplastic large cell lymphomas). In general, however, the growth rate of these affected lymph nodes is often more rapid than in HL and are accompanied of elevated uric acid or lactic dehydrogenase levels (see Chapter 23). Furthermore, soft tissue sarcomas and germ cell tumors can present in the neck or mediastinum, as can metastatic adenopathy from other primary tumors (e.g., nasopharyngeal carcinoma and soft tissue sarcoma); infectious causes of lymphadenopathy, particularly those with an indolent course (e.g., EBV, atypical mycobacterium, histoplasmosis, and toxoplas-

mosis), need to be considered. Another benign entity that can sometimes be difficult to differentiate from HL is progressive transformation of GCs.[94] Occasionally, biopsy of recurrent or persistent lymphadenopathy originally attributed to infectious mononucleosis or reactive hyperplasia yields the diagnosis of lymphoma. A more difficult problem is that of a mediastinal mass that must be differentiated from normal thymus in an otherwise asymptomatic patient. The thymus is maximal in size in children aged approximately 10 years and may be differentiated from tumor on thoracic computed tomographic (CT) scans by its texture.[95] Ultimately, however, only biopsy can definitively confirm a diagnosis.

DIAGNOSTIC WORKUP

Table 22.4 shows the recommended steps in the diagnostic workup of a child with HL. An excisional lymph node biopsy is the preferred procedure to establish the diagnosis, as it permits evaluation of the malignant HRS cells within the background of characteristic architectural changes associated with the specific histologic subtypes. A careful physical examination with assessment of all node-bearing areas, including Waldeyer ring, is essential, with measurement of enlarged nodes so changes can later be quantified. Evaluation by an ear nose and throat specialist can sometimes be necessary, and a CT of the neck is always recommended.

TABLE 22.4

DIAGNOSTIC EVALUATION FOR CHILDREN WITH HL

Diagnostic evaluation	Important elements	Comments
Medical history	"B" symptoms	Unexplained fever with temperatures above 38.0°C orally, unexplained weight loss ≥ 10% within 6 months preceding diagnosis, and drenching night sweats.
	Symptoms of a large mediastinal mass	*Superior Vena Cava syndrome*: Dyspnea, facial swelling, cough, orthopena, and headache *Tracheal or bronchial compression*: Cough, dyspnea, and orthopnea
Physical examination	Lymph nodes Tonsils Lung auscultation Abdomen	Location and size Symmetry, size and nodularity Stridor and wheezing Hepatomegaly and splenomegaly
Laboratory tests	Complete blood count Biochemistry profile	Anemia, leukocytosis, and lymphopenia Elevated lactate dehydrogenase and low albumin. Renal and hepatic function studies prior to starting chemotherapy to determine need for dose adjustments and tolerability. Elevated alkaline phosphatase is associated with bone involvement.
	Erythrocyte sedimentation rate, C-reactive protein, serum ferritin	Elevation of markers of inflammation at diagnosis can be followed for response to therapy.
Diagnostic imaging, anatomic	Chest radiograph CT of neck, chest CT or MRI of abdomen and pelvis	Mediastinal to thoracic ratio Location and size of lymph nodes to evaluate pulmonary involvement. Location and size of lymph nodes and hepatosplenic involvement.
Diagnostic imaging, functional	FDG-PET	Metabolic activity of involved nodes and organs. High sensitivity but low specificity.
	Gallium-67 scintigraphy	Metabolic activity of involved nodes and organs. Low sensitivity, being mostly replaced by PET scan.
	Technetium-99 bone scintigraphy	Metabolic activity in bone lesions. Being replaced by PET scan.
Biopsy	Bone marrow	Limited to patients with B symptoms or advanced disease (Stages III and IV).
	Lymph node	Histologic confirmation

The chest radiograph provides preliminary information about mediastinal involvement and intrathoracic structures. Patients are considered to have "bulky" mediastinal lymphadenopathy if it measures greater than or equal to 33% of the maximum intrathoracic cavity. The pulmonary parenchyma, chest wall, pleura, and pericardium are the most commonly involved extranodal sites of disease and should be further assessed by CT.

The presence of infradiaphragmatic disease is most frequently evaluated by CT with both oral and intravenous contrast agents to accurately delineate lymphadenopathy from other infradiaphragmatic structures. Evaluation of the extent of abdominal and pelvic disease by CT scan is further complicated in children by the lack of retroperitoneal fat.

Splenic involvement occurs in 30% to 40% of patients with HL, and the size of the spleen may not correlate with the degree of disease involvement. Liver size and liver function studies are also unreliable indicators of hepatic disease. Organ size and degree of involvement do not strictly correlate because tumor deposits may be less than 1 cm in diameter and not visualized by diagnostic imaging modalities. Both CT and MRI scans may suggest splenic or hepatic involvement when these organs appear enlarged with areas of abnormal density.[96] Occasional characterization of the visualized lesions by ultrasound may also be useful; however, only histologic assessment can provide definitive evaluation of the spleen and liver.

Functional nuclear imaging studies are now routinely used in patients with HL as a diagnostic and monitoring modality. Positron emission tomography (PET) has mostly replaced gallium as the preferred functional imaging modality for lymphoma staging and follow-up.[97–104] The integration of functional and anatomic tumor characteristics provided by PET-CT imaging has popularized its use for staging and monitoring of pediatric patients with lymphoma because it is both an accurate and cost-effective modality. In PET scanning, uptake of the radioactive glucose analogue 18-fluoro-2-deoxyglucose (FDG) correlates with proliferative activity in tumors undergoing anaerobic glycolysis. PET-CT combinations can be very helpful in determining whether residual mass-like opacities on CT represent active disease or areas of fibrosis.[105] Residual or persistent FDG avidity appears to be useful in predicting prognosis and the need for additional therapy in posttreatment evaluation.[97–99] However, FDG-PET also has limitations in the pediatric setting.[100] Tracer avidity may be seen in a variety of nonmalignant conditions including thymic rebound commonly observed after completion of lymphoma therapy. FDG avidity in normal tissues, for example, brown fat of cervical musculature, may confound interpretation of the presence of nodal involvement by lymphoma. Lastly, tumor activity cannot be correlated with FDG in patients with diabetes who do not have well-controlled blood glucose levels.

Primary bone involvement in HL is rare; however, it may occur in 5% to 20% of patients during the course of disease.[106] In a child who has bone pain, elevated serum alkaline phosphatase concentration beyond that expected for age or extranodal disease identified by other staging studies should prompt evaluation of bony sites. Traditionally, a technetium-99 bone scan with corresponding plain radiographs of abnormal areas is used for characterization of bony disease sites; however, studies in adults suggest that FDG PET may be more sensitive and specific for the detection of osseous involvement.[107]

Bone marrow involvement at the time of initial presentation of HL is uncommon and rarely occurs as an isolated site of extranodal disease. The pattern of infiltration in the bone marrow may be diffuse or focal and is often accompanied by reversible marrow fibrosis. A bone marrow aspirate alone is not adequate to assess the marrow for disease. A bone marrow biopsy is typically performed in any patient with clinical

TABLE 22.5

ANN ARBOR STAGING CLASSIFICATION FOR HL

Stage	Definition
I	Involvement of a single lymph node region (I) or of a single extralymphatic organ or site (I_E)
II	Involvement of two or more lymph node regions on the same side of the diaphragm (II) or localized involvement of an extralymphatic organ or site and one or more lymph node regions on the same side of the diaphragm (II_E)
III	Involvement of lymph node regions on both sides of the diaphragm (III), which may be accompanied by involvement of the spleen (III_S) or by localized involvement of an extralymphatic organ or site (III_E) or both (III_{SE})
IV	Diffuse or disseminated involvement of one or more extralymphatic organs or tissues with or without associated lymph node involvement

Note: The absence or presence of fever higher than 38°C for 3 consecutive days, drenching night sweats, or unexplained loss of 10% or more of body weight in the 6 months preceding admission are to be denoted in all cases by the suffix letters A or B, respectively.

stage III to IV disease or B symptoms, or in any patient at the time of disease recurrence. The exceedingly low yield of an abnormal bone marrow in a patient with newly diagnosed clinical stage IA or IIA disease does not support its routine use during staging.

STAGING

HL appears to spread along contiguous lymph nodes until late in the course of disease.[82] The currently used Ann Arbor staging system, adopted in 1971, is based on this observation (Table 22.5).[108] The anatomic locations of lymph node chains designated as regions for the purpose of staging are illustrated in Figure 22.4.[109] The substage classifications A, B, and E amend each stage based on defined clinical features. Substage A indicates "asymptomatic" disease. B symptoms include fever exceeding 38°C for 3 consecutive days, drenching night sweats, and an unexplained loss of at least 10% of body weight over 6 months. Substage E denotes minimal extralymphatic extension from contiguous nodal disease. Disease involving the spleen is designated a substage S.

TREATMENT

Principles of Radiotherapy

Incorporation of radiation therapy in the management of pediatric HL has evolved over the past 30 years from single modality approaches incorporating high-dose extensive nodal irradiation or aggressive multiagent systemic chemotherapy to combined-modality therapy. This shift has taken place because standard-dose irradiation and alkylator-based chemotherapy have significant treatment effects, which can often be attenuated by combined-modality approaches incorporating more limited chemotherapy with reduced dose limited volume radiation therapy. Multiple clinical trials have addressed the additive value of involved-field radiation to multiagent chemotherapy,

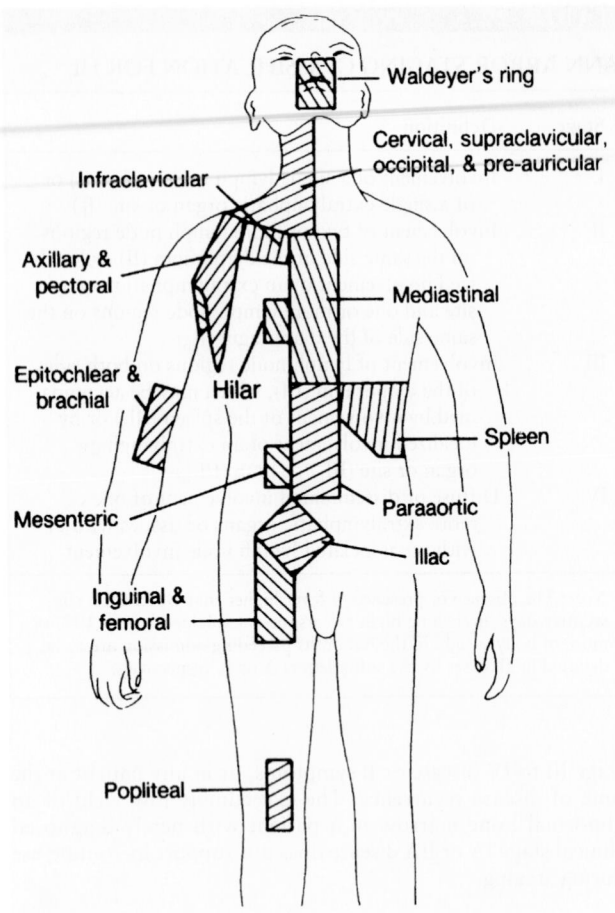

FIGURE 22.4 Anatomic definition of separate lymph node regions used for staging purposes. (Adapted from Kaplan HS, Rosenberg SA. The treatment of Hodgkin disease. Med Clin North Am 1966; 50:1591.)

suggesting a benefit for the population of HL patients as a whole.[110–113] Based, in part, on these studies, a risk-adapted approach has been developed that attempts to tailor the amount and intensity of therapy, both chemotherapy and particularly radiation, to the severity of disease.[112,114,115] Because of this evolution, the majority of pediatric patients with HL are currently managed with a combined-modality, risk-adapted therapeutic approach. Several important questions remain in the integration of radiation for HL occurring in children and adolescents. Selection of patients for radiation avoidance, integration of modern radiotherapeutic approaches for improved conformal delivery of dose, and further reduction in the volume of treatment remain important questions for study in the context of the excellent disease control rates already achieved with traditional radiation techniques. Understanding the principles and approaches of radiation therapy employed in existing and published studies as well as the opportunities for improvement in the delivery of this modality will be important for pediatric oncologists and radiation oncologists as we continue to make progress in this highly curable disease.

Selection of Dose and Volume

Dose Selection

Selection of radiation dose in the modern era tends to be trial and group specific though the dose ranges are similar, as noted earlier. Clinical trials have employed 20, 21, and 25.5 Gy,[110,113,114] using daily doses of 2, 1.75, and 1.5 Gy, respectively. Local control rates remain high, 89% to 95%, despite the lower radiation dose and reduced intensity of systemic therapy.[113,116] Modifications to these doses are made based on the response to systemic therapy, employing specific time points and methods for response assessment. Dose elimination, dose reduction, and dose escalation are all used in modern clinical trials, but the approach from one trial is not transferable to another. It is important to understand the methods and timing of response assessments as one compares each clinical trial or treats with its specific approach (Table 22.6). Despite the

TABLE 22.6

RADIATION DOSE MODIFICATIONS IN MODERN TRIALS FOR PEDIATRIC HL

Study/group	Standard dose	Response time	Imaging response method	Modified dose
Hodgkin Collaborators	25.5 Gy/1.5 Gy fxn	8 weeks	CT FDG-PET Product of perpendicular diameter CR = >75% reduction	If CR: 0 Gy—stage I–IIa (<3 nodal sites) 15 Gy—all other sites except bulky mediastinal disease
German Pediatric Hodgkin Studies	20 Gy/2 Gy fxn	8 weeks 16 weeks 24 weeks (Stage dependent)	CT US MR 3D measurement CR = 100% reduction PR = 75–<100% <PR = <75%	If CR: 0 Gy If PR: 20 Gy If <PR: 30 Gy
Children's Oncology Group	21 Gy/1.5 Gy fxn	6 weeks	CT Product of *perpendicular* diameter CR = >80% reduction VGPR = >60%	If CR/VGPR: Randomize 0 or 21 Gy If PR: 21 Gy

CR, complete response; Fxn, daily radiation fraction size; PR, partial response; VGPR, very good partial response.

differences in radiation therapy across the studies, several prognostic factors emerge. Bulky mediastinal disease predicts a higher risk of local failure, 21.6% versus 6%, at 5 years.[116] Higher stage patients experienced greater failure rates, particularly in the absence of radiation therapy, despite favorable responses.[112] Based on this greater understanding of response to risk-adapted therapy, current clinical trials in all studies are looking to better select patients for radiation avoidance, maintaining high nodal control rates while continuing to reduce therapy.

Volume Selection

Significantly less investigated is the role of volume reduction in radiation therapy treatment fields. The "standard" involved field grew out of the components of the classic mantle field, used for treatment of HL with radiation therapy alone. In the combined-modality era, treatment volumes no longer need to account for the potential spread of all microscopic disease, focusing more on areas of large volume disease or poor response. The definition of a standard involved field is not standard at all, but attempts have been made to standardize it.[117] Definitions of involved fields in pediatric trials for HL have varied and must be understood by the radiation oncologist in the context of the specific chemotherapy being delivered. Figure 22.5 shows a typical involved field defined in the HL collaborators' trials.[114] The German Pediatric Hodgkin Study group was the first to deliver less than standard involved fields in a clinical trial for children with HL.[118] Radiation planning was developed in conjunction with a centralized review of imaging resulting in a standardized radiotherapeutic approach across many institutions and disease presentations. The importance in moving beyond standard involved fields is not to improve the local control rates (which already exceed 90%) but to further reduce late effects from radiation therapy. The simplest method for reduction in end organ toxicity such as hypothyroidism or secondary breast cancer is to avoid treating the organ at risk. The implementation of more tailored fields is progress toward this goal, treating only the individual lymph

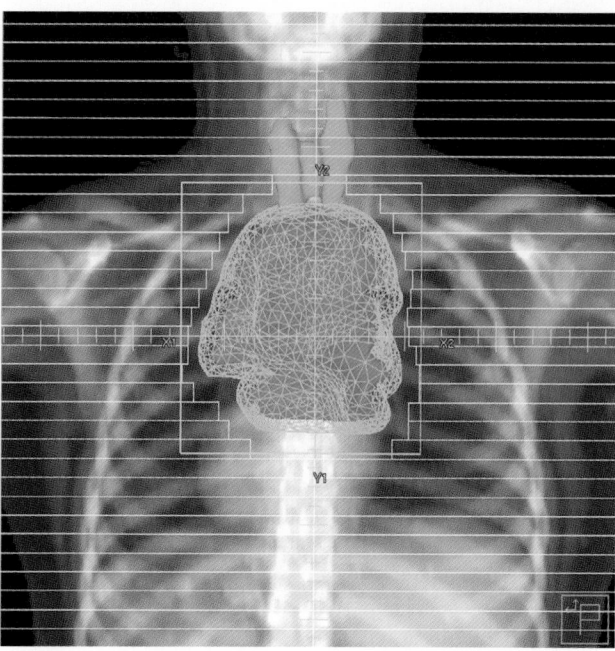

FIGURE 22.6 Tailored treatment field for a patient with clinical stage IB Hodgkin lymphoma. The CTV (*blue*), PTV (*yellow*) and thyroid (*orange*) are displayed on the beams eye view with multi-leaf collimator shaped around the PTV.

nodes with a margin for microscopic disease (Fig. 22.6). This in conjunction with modern imaging will continue to reduce exposure of normal tissue to radiation while maintaining equivalent local disease control rates.[119] Current clinical trials are ongoing testing this approach.

Radiotherapy Techniques

Radiation simulation is the process of positioning the patient in a consistent, comfortable, and reproducible position for daily therapy. Simulation in the modern era is accomplished on a CT-based simulator, often with intravenous contrast administered to allow definition of the vasculature next to which the lymphatics reside. CT simulation allows a 3-dimensional or volumetric rendering of the patient for mapping of the regions to be radiated as well as adjacent normal tissues. CT simulation and subsequent volumetric treatment planning require dose calculation for the imaged patient volume and can yield dose information for any point or volume in the patient's image (Fig. 22.7). Two advantages come from this technique: (a) doses can be homogenized to a greater degree across the patients treated volume compared with prior 2-dimensional techniques resulting in less dose variation from the prescribed dose and potentially less toxicity and (b) dose can be assessed for any target or normal tissue that is delineated (contoured) on CT. This improved knowledge of specific doses to an organ may help better understand end organ toxicities that result from radiation as well as allowing for avoidance when possible. When the chest or abdomen is part of the treatment volume, it may be appropriate to obtain a CT simulation to assess motion of the mediastinum, hila, diaphragm, and spleen. This study, called a 4D-CT (describing the 4th dimension of time during which targets and organs move), is obtained at the same time as the CT simulation.

Targeting for treatment occurs in a "virtual" or simulated computer environment. Nodal regions and other tissues that need treatment as well as normal tissues for avoidance or dose

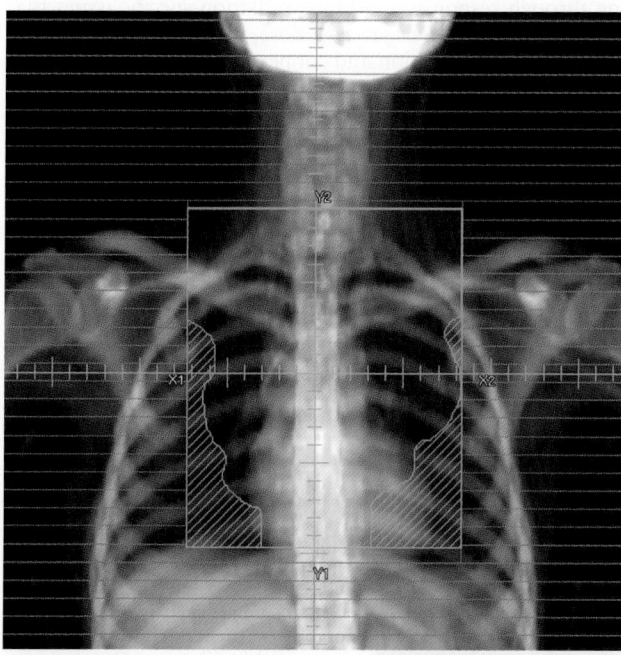

FIGURE 22.5 Classic involved treatment field for a patient with clinical stage IB Hodgkin lymphoma.

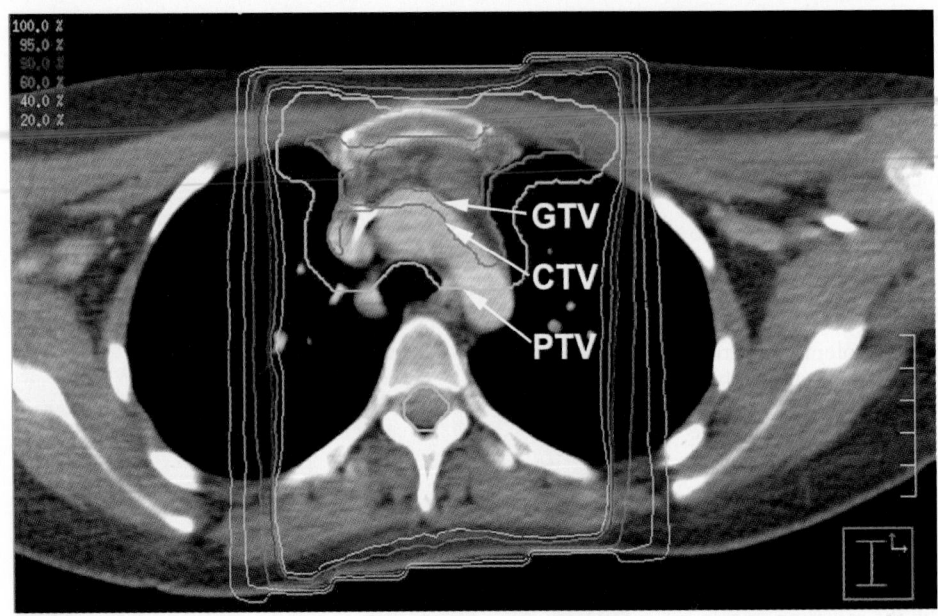

FIGURE 22.7 Treatment volumes with target volumes defined for gross nodal disease (gross target volume or GTV), microscopic disease (clinical target volume or CTV), and setup uncertainty (planning target volume or PTV). Treatment radiation dose levels are shown as a percent of the total prescribed dose.

calculation are mapped on each CT image slice. These targets and normal tissues (referred to as contours) are then rendered as 3-dimensional shapes. Treatment beams are then created with the aid of the medical physicist in the computer environment to treat the areas at risk and avoid adjacent normal tissues. Beam arrangements are often from the anterior and posterior but are not limited to these orientations; current clinical trials are investigating the safety and benefit of more complex beam arrangements. Before treatment of disease in the pelvic region, it may be necessary to transpose the ovaries medially or use a testicular shield to maintain hormone production and fertility.

Modern radiation therapy is delivered with a linear accelerator with a typical beam energy of 6 MV. Higher energies may be desired when treating the abdominal region in particularly thick patients. Setup on a daily basis is aided by imaging obtained on the treatment machine, either of the treatment portals or with a cone-beam CT (Fig. 22.8). Both localizations prior to treatment may be done as often as daily if needed. All beams are treated daily for a site or region of treatment (i.e.

chest including neck and mediastinal lymphatics, abdomen including para-aortic lymphatics and spleen). Treatment regions may need to be separated by a 1- to 2-week break to ensure bone marrow recovery.

Integration of Radiation Therapy

Radiation therapy remains an integral component of therapy for pediatric HL of all stages. Its integration in the combined-modality therapy approach continues to evolve and also continues to become more complex. Pediatric HL is a rare entity compared with its adult counterpart and the approaches to radiation differ considerably. It is important to include the radiation oncologist as part of the treatment team from staging through response to address radiation-specific issues that will alter the treatment process, dose, and volumes. Only with this degree of integration and cooperation will patients receive the full benefit of risk-adapted therapy.

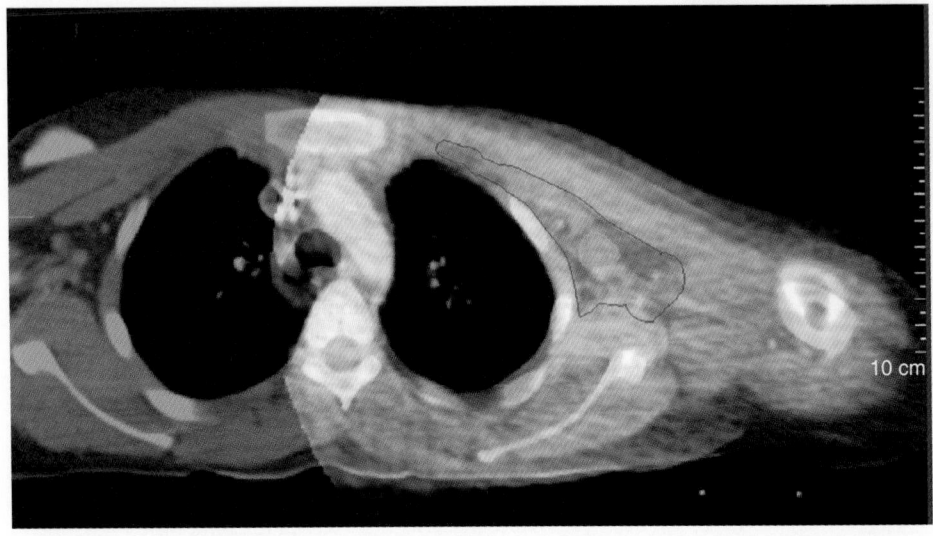

FIGURE 22.8 Cone-beam CT (CBCT) obtained immediately prior to treatment on the linear accelerator for patient setup and localization. *Orange* image is the CBCT overlaid on the simulation CT (*grey*) to localize patient.

Combination Chemotherapy

Current effective multidrug regimens for HL and other pediatric malignancies combine non–cross-resistant agents with the following properties:

- Each agent should be individually active against the tumor.
- The agents should differ in the mechanism of antineoplastic activity, thereby targeting different cellular or biochemical events and preventing development of resistance.
- Toxicities of the agents should not overlap, so that each drug can be administered at full single-agent dose. Table 22.7 lists some of the regimens used in HL.

The MOPP combination, with agents delivered at full doses, produces long-term disease-free survival in approximately 50% of adult patients with advanced disease.[9,10] Additional maintenance therapy does not extend remission but rather predisposes to excess morbidity from higher cumulative exposures of agents with dose-related toxicity. Children with HL have similar or better treatment outcomes after MOPP therapy compared with adult patients,[11–15] but are also at risk for adverse MOPP-related effects which are correlated with the cumulative doses of alkylating agent chemotherapy. The recognized risk of secondary AML has been dramatically reduced by restricting cumulative doses of alkylating agent chemotherapy and substituting other, less leukemogenic alkylating agents (e.g., cyclophosphamide for mechlorethamine).[120] Similarly, the risk of infertility, which is almost universal in boys following six to eight cycles of MOPP therapy, may be reduced when treatment with gonadotoxic alkylating drugs, especially procarbazine, is limited to three cycles.[121,122]

The development of the ABVD in the 1970s provided another effective non–cross-resistant chemotherapy regimen that did not produce an excess risk of secondary AML or infertility.[123] However, dose-related toxicity attributed to agents in the ABVD combination includes cardiomyopathy and pulmonary fibrosis, resulting from the doxorubicin and bleomycin, respectively. ABVD was initially used as salvage therapy for adults with MOPP-resistant disease, and later alternated with MOPP in an effort to enhance antineoplastic activity.[124] Subsequent studies in adult patients demonstrated that ABVD was superior to MOPP alone and had comparable efficacy to MOPP alternating with ABVD.[17] Superior treatment

TABLE 22.7

CHEMOTHERAPY REGIMENS FOR HL (REPEAT CYCLE EVERY 28 DAYS)

Name	Drugs	Dosage	Route	Days
MOPP	Mechlorethamine (nitrogen mustard)	6.0 mg/m^2	IV	1, 8
	Vincristine (Oncovin)	1.4 mg/m^2	IV	1, 8
	Procarbazine	100 mg/m^2	PO	1–15
	Prednisone	40 mg/m^2	PO	1–15
COPP	Cyclophosphamide substituted for mechlorethamine in MOPP	600 mg/m^2	IV	1, 8
OPPA	Vincristine (Oncovin)	1.5 mg/m^2	IV	1, 8, 15
	Procarbazine	100 mg/m^2	PO	1–15
	Prednisone	60 mg/m^2	PO	1–15
	Doxorubicin (Adriamycin)	40 mg/m^2	IV	1, 15
OEPA	Etoposide substituted for procarbazine in OPPA	125 mg/m^2	IV	3–6
ABVD	Doxorubicin (Adriamycin)	25 mg/m^2	IV	1, 15
	Bleomycin	10 U/m^2	IV	1, 15
	Vinblastine	6 mg/m^2	IV	1, 15
	Dacarbazine	375 mg/m^2	IV	1, 15
COPP/ABV	Cyclophosphamide	600 mg/m^2	IV	0
	Vincristine (Oncovin)	1.4 mg/m^2	IV	0
	Procarbazine	100 mg/m^2	PO	0–6
	Prednisone	40 mg/m^2	PO	0–13
	Doxorubicin (Adriamycin)	35 mg/m^2	IV	7
	Bleomycin	10 U/m^2	IV	7
	Vinblastine	6 mg/m^2	IV	7
VAMP	Vinblastine	6 mg/m^2	IV	1, 15
	Doxorubicin (Adriamycin)	25 mg/m^2	IV	1, 15
	Methotrexate	20 mg/m^2	IV	1, 15
	Prednisone	40 mg/m^2	PO	1–14
DBVE	Doxorubicin	25 mg/m^2	IV	1, 15
	Bleomycin	10 U/m^2	IV	1, 15
	Vincristine (Oncovin)	1.5 mg/m^2	IV	1, 15
	Etoposide	100 mg/m^2	IV	1–5
DBVE-PC	Doxorubicin	30 mg/m^2	IV	0, 1
	Bleomycin	10 U/m^2	IV	0, 7
	Vincristine (Oncovin)	1.4 mg/m^2	IV	0, 7
	Etoposide	75 mg/m^2	IV	0–4
	Prednisone	40 mg/m^2	PO	0–9
	Cyclophosphamide	800 mg/m^2	IV	0

results and absence of leukemogenesis and permanent gonadal toxicity have made ABVD the preferred frontline regimen for adults with HL. However, concerns regarding potential cardiopulmonary sequelae have restricted its use as the sole regimen in pediatric patients. Currently, ABVD, or similar hybrid combinations, are incorporated into risk-adapted treatment regimens prescribing fewer cycles of chemotherapy for children with localized, favorable HL. In patients with advanced and unfavorable HL, ABVD is more likely to be supplemented with other agents with differing toxicities to improve disease control and reduce dose-related toxicity related to the alkylating agent, anthracycline, and bleomycin chemotherapy.

Treatment Results

Optimal therapy involves a multidisciplinary approach from the time of diagnosis. This is particularly important, as treatment decisions are currently based on risk features present at diagnosis, including the presence of B symptoms, stage, peripheral nodal and/or mediastinal bulk, and number of involved nodal regions. Assignment of stage and treatment are best determined after the pediatric and radiation oncologists have had the opportunity to examine the patient and review staging study results, preferably with simultaneous input from a diagnostic imager. In this way, a consistent plan for chemotherapy and radiation therapy can be presented to the family by all health care providers and reviewed periodically after response evaluations.

Combined-Modality Therapy

From the 1960s to 1980s, standard-dose (35 to 44 Gy), extended-volume radiation therapy was commonly used in conjunction with combination chemotherapy to enhance local tumor control. The observation of substantial late effects in children who received high-dose radiotherapy provided the impetus for studies evaluating combined-modality treatments prescribing low-dose (15.0 to 25.5 Gy), involved-field radiation therapy.[11,125] As more trials established that local disease control was maintained with reduced radiation, six cycles of non–cross-resistant combination chemotherapy evolved as the standard pediatric approach in combined-modality regimens. Tables 22.8 and 22.9 summarize the results of major pediatric trials organized from the 1970s through the 1990s that established the efficacy of combined-modality therapy.[11–14,18,20–22,111,126–130]

Combined-Modality Therapy versus Chemotherapy Alone

Multiple trials have established the efficacy of treatment with non–cross-resistant chemotherapy alone for pediatric HL (Table 22.10).[15,19,130–140] This treatment approach is selected for children managed in centers without access to radiation facilities, trained personnel, and diagnostic imaging modalities needed for clinical staging. Systemic chemotherapy also avoids the potential long-term musculoskeletal complications, organ dysfunction, and solid tumor malignancies associated with high-dose, extended-field radiation therapy.

Earlier chemotherapy-alone trials prescribed 6 to 12 cycles of MOPP or hybrid therapies containing alkylating agents (ChlVPP [chlorambucil, vinblastine, procarbazine, and prednisone] and CVPP [cyclophosphamide, vinblastine, procarbazine, and prednisone]) in clinically staged children.[15,132,141,142] While acute hematologic and infectious toxicities associated with these treatments were acceptable, follow-up data regarding long-term toxicity have not been reported, although preliminary reports suggest a high frequency of gonadal toxicity in boys.[15,143]

TABLE 22.8

TREATMENT RESULTS OF NORTH AMERICAN PEDIATRIC COMBINED-MODALITY TRIALS

Chemotherapy	Radiation therapy	Stage	No. of patients	Outcome (year)			
				Event-free survival	Disease-free survival	Relapse-free survival	Survival
Stanford[11,128]							
3 MOPP/3 ABVD	15.0–25.5 Gy, IF	CS/PS I–IV	57	96 (6.7)	—	—	93 (6.7)
6 MOPP	15.0–25.5 Gy, IF	PS I–IV	55	—	—	90 (15)	89 (15)
St. Jude[127]							
4–5 COP(P)/3–4 ABVD	20 Gy, IF	CS II–IV	85	—	93 (5)	—	93 (5)
Pediatric Oncology Group[19,111]							
4 MOPP/4 ABVD	21 Gy, EF	CS/PS IIB, IIIA$_2$, IIIB–IV	80	80 (5)	—	—	87 (5)
4 MOPP/4 ABVD	21 Gy, TLI	CS/PS IIB, IIIA$_2$, IIIB, IV	62	77 (3)	—	—	91 (3)
Toronto[12]							
6 MOPP	20–30 Gy, EF	CS I–IIIA	57	—	—	80 (10)	85 (10)
	25–30 Gy, EF	CS IIIB, IV					
Children's Cancer Group[18]							
6 ABVD	21 Gy, EF	PS III–IV	54	87 (4)	—	—	90 (4)
12 ABVD	21 Gy, regional	PS III–IV	64	87 (3)	—	—	89 (3)
Intergroup Hodgkin[14]							
6 MOPP	35 Gy, IF	PS I–II	97	—	—	95 (5)	90 (5)

ABVD, doxorubicin (Adriamycin), bleomycin, vinblastine, dacarbazine; COP(P), cyclophosphamide, vincristine (Oncovin), procarbazine, prednisone; CS, clinical stage; EF, extended field; IF, involved field; MOPP, mechlorethamine (Mustargen), vincristine (Oncovin), procarbazine, prednisone; PS, pathologic stage; TLI, total lymphoid irradiation.

TABLE 22.9

TREATMENT RESULTS OF EUROPEAN AND SOUTH AMERICAN PEDIATRIC COMBINED-MODALITY TRIALS

Chemotherapy	Radiation therapy	Stage	No. of patients	Outcome (year)		
				Event-free survival	Disease-free survival	Survival
French						
Gustave-Roussy[13]						
3 MOPP	40 Gy, IF	All stages	40	86% (15)	—	93 (15)
6 MOPP	40 Gy, IF		20	86% (15)	—	93 (15)
SFOP MDH-82[20]						
4 ABVD	20–40 Gy, IF	I–IIA	79	—	90 (6)	92 (6)
2 MOPP/2 ABVD	20–40 Gy, IF	I–IIA	67	—	87 (6)	
3 MOPP/3 ABVD	20–40 Gy, EF	I–II	31	—	89 (6)	
3 MOPP/3 ABVD	20–40 Gy, EF	III	40	—	82 (6)	
3 MOPP/3 ABVD	20–40 Gy, EF	IV	21	—	62 (6)	
Associazione Italiana di Ematologia ed Oncologia Pediatrica-MH-83[22]						
3 ABVD	20–40 Gy, IF	IA	83	—	95 (7)	86 (7)
3 ABVD	20–40 Gy, R	IIA (M/T <0.33)	—	—		
3 MOPP/3 ABVD	20–40 Gy, R	IIA (M/T ≥0.33)	132	—	81	
3 MOPP/3 ABVD	20–40 Gy, EF	IIIA	—	—		
5 MOPP/5 ABVD	20–40 Gy, EF	IIIB–IV	—	—	60	
German-Austria[21]						
HD-82						
2 OPPA	35 Gy, IF	IA/IB–IIA	100	98 (9)	—	100 (9)
2 OPPA/2 COPP	30 Gy, IF	IIB–IIIA	53	94	—	96
2 OPPA/4 COPP	25 Gy, IF	IIIB–IV	50	86	—	85
HD-85[154]						
2 OPA	35 Gy, IF	IA/IB–IIA	53	85 (6)	—	98 (6)
2 OPA/2 COMP	30 Gy, IF	IIB–IIIA	21	55	—	95
2 OPA/4 COMP	25 Gy, IF	IIIB–IV	24	49	—	100
HD-90[121]						
2 OEPA/OPPA	25 Gy, IF	IA/IB–IIA	275	94/95 (5)	—	99 (5)
2 OEPA/OPPA + 2 COPP	25 Gy, IF	IIB–IIIA	124	90/96	—	97
2 OEPA/OPPA + 4 COPP	20 Gy, IF	IIIB–IV	179	84/89	—	94
United Kingdom Children's Cancer Study Group[129]						
6–10 ChlVPP	35 Gy, IF	I	99	—	70 (10)	92 (10)
6–10 ChlVPP	35 Gy, IF	II	125	—	85	92
6–10 ChlVPP	35 Gy, IF	III	80	—	73	84
6–10 ChlVPP	35 Gy, IF	IV	27	—	38	71
Grupo Argentino de Tratamiento de Leucemia Aguda[131]						
6 CVPP	30–40 Gy, IF	I–IV	64	—	87 (5)	—
6 AOPE	30–40 Gy, IF	IPR[a]		—	67 (5)	—

[a]IPR, intermediate prognostic group determined on the basis of age, symptoms, stage, and number of nodal regions.
ABVD, doxorubicin (Adriamycin), bleomycin, vinblastine, dacarbazine; AOPE, doxorubicin (Adriamycin), vincristine (Oncovin), prednisone, etoposide; ChlVPP, chlorambucil, vinblastine, procarbazine, prednisone; COMP, cyclophosphamide, vincristine (Oncovin), methotrexate, prednisone; COPP, cyclophosphamide, vincristine (Oncovin), procarbazine, prednisone; CVPP, cyclophosphamide, vincristine, prednisone, procarbazine; EF, extended field; IF, involved field; MOPP, mechlorethamine (Mustargen), vincristine (Oncovin), procarbazine, prednisone; M/T, mediastinal mass/thoracic ratio; OEPA, vincristine (Oncovin), etoposide, prednisone, doxorubicin (Adriamycin); OPA, vincristine (Oncovin), prednisone, doxorubicin (Adriamycin); OPPA, vincristine (Oncovin), prednisone, procarbazine, doxorubicin (Adriamycin); R, regional.

Contemporary chemotherapy-only trials have used alternating non–cross-resistant regimens (MOPP/ABVD, COPP [cyclophosphamide, vincristine (Oncovin), procarbazine, prednisone]/ABV hybrid, CVPP/EBO [etoposide, bleomycin, and vincristine]) or combinations without alkylating agent chemotherapy (ABVD, EVAP [etoposide, vinblastine, cytarabine, and cisplatin]/ABV).[131,133–137,144] Early results from these studies demonstrate treatment outcomes similar to those achieved with combined-modality therapy. Acute hematologic and infectious toxicities related to these regimens appear acceptable, but long-term cardiopulmonary sequelae have not been evaluated.

Evaluation of the efficacy of chemotherapy-only treatment regimens has been difficult because most reports describe outcome after nonrandom treatment assignments in small clinically staged cohorts. Several trials specifically exclude patients with

TABLE 22.10

TREATMENT RESULTS OF PEDIATRIC CHEMOTHERAPY-ALONE TRIALS

Chemotherapy	Stage	No. of patients	Outcome (year) Event-free survival	Outcome (year) Disease-free survival	Outcome (year) Survival
Children's Cancer Group[130]					
6 MOPP/6 ABVD	PS III–IV	57	77 (4)	—	84 (4)
Pediatric Oncology Group[111,140]					
4 MOPP/4 ABVD	CS IIB, IIIA$_2$, IIB, IV	81	79 (5)	—	96 (5)
3 MOPP/3 ABVD	PS I, IIA, IIIA	79	83 (8)	—	94 (8)
Grupo Argentino de Tratamiento de Leucemia Aguda[131]					
3 CVPP	CS IA, IIA	10	86 (6.7)	—	—
6 CVPP	CS IB, IIB	16	87 (6.7)	—	—
The Netherlands[135,137,139,142]					
6 MOPP	CS I–IV (lymph nodes <4 cm)	21	91 (10)	—	100 (10)
6 ABVD	CS I–IV (lymph nodes <4 cm)	17	70 (10)	—	94
6 ABVD/MOPP	CS I–IV	21	91 (10)	—	91
6 ABVD	CS I–IV	17	—	71 (8)	92 (8)
6 EBVD	CS I–IIA	23	96 (10)	—	100 (10)
3–5 EBVD/MOPP	CS IIB–IV	23	87 (10)	—	91 (10)
6 MOPP (<4 cm lymph node)	CS I–II	21	—	100 (5)	100 (5)
6 MOPP (≥4 cm lymph node)	CS I–II	16	—	92 (5)	
Nicaragua[134]					
6 COPP	CS I, IIA	14	100 (3)	—	100 (3)
8–10 COPP-ABV	CS IIB, III, IV	34	75 (3)	—	—
Madras, India[144]					
6 COPP/ABV	CS I–IIA	10	89 (5)	—	—
6 COPP/ABV	CS IIB–IVB	43	90 (5)	—	—
Australia/New Zealand[132,136,156]					
5–6 VEEP	All stages	53	—	78 (5)	92 (5)
3 EVAP/ABV	CS IA–IVA	25	—	60 (3.5)	100
6–8 MOPP or 6 ChlVPP	CS I–IIB	38	—	92 (4)	94 (4)
Uganda[15]					
6 MOPP	CS I–IIIA	38	—	75 (5)	—
	CS IIIB–IV	10	—	60 (5)	—

ABVD, doxorubicin (Adriamycin), bleomycin, vinblastine, dacarbazine; ChlVPP, chlorambucil, vinblastine, procarbazine, prednisone; COPP, cyclophosphamide, vincristine (Oncovin), procarbazine, prednisone; CS, clinical stage; CVPP, cyclophosphamide, vincristine, procarbazine, prednisone; EBO, epirubicin, bleomycin, vincristine (Oncovin); EBVD, epirubicin, bleomycin, vinblastine, dacarbazine; EVAP, etoposide, vinblastine, cytosine arabinoside, cisplatin; MOPP, mechlorethamine (Mustargen), vincristine (Oncovin), procarbazine, prednisone; PS, pathologic stage; VEEP, vincristine, etoposide, epirubicin, prednisone.

unfavorable risk features based on bulk and number of involved nodal sites. Only a few randomized pediatric trials have compared treatment outcome after chemotherapy alone with combined-modality therapy. The Grupo Argentino de Tratamiento de Leucemia Aguda prospectively evaluated CVPP chemotherapy alone to CVPP plus involved-field radiotherapy.[145] Treatment outcomes after both regimens were comparable in stage I to II patients. Combined-modality therapy with CVPP plus radiation compared with CVPP chemotherapy alone, however, resulted in better disease-free survival in patients with localized unfavorable (more than two involved nodal areas, bulky peripheral [greater than 5 cm] and bulky mediastinal lymphadenopathy) and advanced stage disease. The next Grupo Argentino de Tratamiento de Leucemia Aguda trial demonstrated comparable event-free survival among patients with favorable disease presentations (as defined by a prognostic factor index based on age, presence of B symptoms, stage, and number of involved nodal regions) randomly assigned to three or six cycles of CVPP.[131]

North American pediatric cooperative group randomized trials have also prospectively compared treatment with combined-modality therapy to chemotherapy alone. A Children's Cancer Group trial showed equivalent efficacy of 12 cycles of alternating MOPP/ABVD and six cycles of ABVD plus low-dose (21 Gy) involved-, extended-, or total-lymphoid radiation fields in children with pathologic stage III to IV HL.[130] Although event-free and overall survival were not statistically different between the two groups, children randomized to combined-modality therapy showed higher 4-year event-free and overall survival rates (87% and 90%, respectively) compared with those who received chemotherapy alone (77% and 90%, respectively). A randomized Pediatric Oncology Group trial comparing chemotherapy (six cycles of MOPP/ABVD) with chemoradiotherapy (four cycles of MOPP/ABVD followed by 2,550 cGy of involved-field radiotherapy) in children with stages I, IIA, and IIIA showed no significant difference in overall and event-free survival at 8 years between both arms.[140] Of interest, however, was the difference in event-free survival for early responders compared with those that were not early responders (93% vs. 77%; $p = 0.006$), a difference that did not hold significance in overall survival (98% vs. 91%; $p = 0.07$). In advanced stage HL, low-dose radiation therapy added to eight cycles of alternating MOPP-ABVD was compared with chemotherapy alone.[111] Analysis of results based on treatment intent failed to show an advantage for combined-modality therapy. However, analysis based on treatment actually delivered showed a superior outcome in patients treated with chemotherapy and radiation therapy.

Children's Cancer Group investigators reported their early results of a randomized controlled trial comparing survival outcomes in children treated with COPP/ABV hybrid chemotherapy alone with those treated with COPP/ABV hybrid chemotherapy plus low-dose, involved-field radiation.[110] Treatment assignment was based on clinical features including the presence of "B" symptoms, hilar adenopathy, mediastinal and peripheral lymph node bulk, and the number of involved nodal regions. Patients achieving a complete response to chemotherapy were eligible for randomization to receive low-dose, involved-field radiation or no further therapy. A significantly higher number of relapses among patients treated with chemotherapy alone resulted in early closure of the study. The difference in 3-year event-free survival was most marked for stage IV patients who had a 90% event-free survival if randomized to receive combined-modality therapy with involved-field radiation compared with 81% in those randomized to receive chemotherapy alone. Estimates for overall survival are not different between the randomized groups due to successful salvage therapy after relapse, but follow-up of the cohort is early.

German-Austrian pediatric oncology investigators also observed superior disease-free survival for patients who received radiation consolidation following combination chemotherapy in the GPOG-HD 95 trial.[112] In this study, radiation was omitted for patients completely responding to risk- and gender-based OEPA or OPPA/COPP chemotherapy. The estimated 5-year disease-free survival was significantly lower in the 222 patients treated with chemotherapy alone compared with the 758 patients treated with combined-modality therapy (88% vs. 92%; $p = 0.049$).[112] The event-free survival advantage was most pronounced for intermediate- (TG 2) and high-risk (TG 3) irradiated patients compared with nonirradiated patients (91% vs. 79%); there was no difference in disease-free survival among irradiated and nonirradiated patients assigned to the favorable-risk (TG 1) group. Again, overall survival was not significantly reduced due to the effectiveness of retrieval therapy. These results prompted a recommendation for omission of radiation therapy only for early stage favorable risk patients.

In summary, several studies have demonstrated that chemotherapy alone is effective therapy for pediatric HL. The advantage of this approach is the elimination of radiation-associated adverse sequelae including musculoskeletal underdevelopment, cardiac dysfunction, and solid tumor induction. Chemotherapy-alone treatment protocols rely on higher cumulative doses of agents with established dose-related toxicity, however, especially alkylating agent chemotherapy, which may contribute to acute and late treatment morbidity. The results of controlled randomized trials suggest that the addition of radiation therapy improves outcome in children with unfavorable and advanced-stage HL.[110] Especially, patients who do not achieve an early complete response to chemotherapy may benefit the most from further radiation consolidation. Current studies in Europe and North America are evaluating the role of FDG-PET scan early-on during therapy to better characterize patients in whom radiotherapy can safely be omitted.

Risk-Adapted Therapy

Favorable Clinical Presentations. In the 1990s, pediatric HL trials confirmed that disease-free survival was not compromised by reducing the number of multiagent chemotherapy cycles, radiation doses, and treatment volumes in clinically staged patients with "favorable" clinical presentations.[20–22,110,121,146–148] The favorable designation has varied among the individual studies but is typically characterized by localized nodal involvement in the absence of B symptoms and bulky disease. *Bulky* mediastinal lymphadenopathy is designated when the ratio of the maximum measurement of mediastinal lymphadenopathy to intrathoracic cavity on an upright chest radiograph equals or exceeds 33%. Risk factors considered in other studies include the number of involved nodal regions, the presence of hilar adenopathy, the size of peripheral lymphadenopathy, and extranodal extension. Multiagent regimens that have been effective for favorable risk HL include MOPP/ABVD, OPPA or OEPA/COPP, COPP/ABV hybrid, and a variety of nonalkylating agent containing regimens such as ABVD, OEPA, VAMP, and VBVP.[20,110,121,147,148] Treatment for patients with a favorable clinical presentation typically consists of two to four cycles of chemotherapy and low-dose, involved-field radiation. Several trials have reduced the dose of radiation in patients achieving a favorable response to chemotherapy.[110,112,115,147] Treatment results of selected risk-adapted trials are summarized in Table 22.11.

Unfavorable Clinical Presentations. Clinical presentations are designated *unfavorable* when associated with the presence of B symptoms, bulky mediastinal or peripheral lymphadenopathy, extranodal extension of disease, and advanced (stage IIIB to IV) disease. Localized disease (stage I/II and IIIA) with unfavorable features may be treated similarly to advanced stage disease in some treatment protocols or given a therapy of intermediate intensity.[112,113] Chemotherapy used for this group includes derivative combination of MOPP and ABVD. COPP has replaced MOPP because cyclophosphamide is less myelosuppressive and leukemogenic than mechlorethamine.[120] Etoposide is frequently added to enhance treatment response and reduce cumulative doses of alkylating and anthracycline chemotherapy.[149] Two standard treatment approaches have been used for pediatric patients with unfavorable clinical presentations. Conventional therapy prescribes non–cross-resistant chemotherapy on a twice-monthly schedule for a total of 6 months. Low-dose (15.0 to 25.5 Gy), involved-field radiation therapy may be delivered between treatment cycles or, more commonly, following completion of chemotherapy to consolidate remission. Treatment results for unfavorable pediatric HL using combined-modality therapy with conventional chemotherapy regimens (e.g., MOPP/ABVD, COPP/ABVD, OPPA [vincristine (Oncovin), procarbazine, prednisone, doxorubicin (Adriamycin)]/COPP) are summarized in Tables 22.8 and 22.9.

The second treatment approach uses the strategy of abbreviated dose-intensive multiagent chemotherapy featured in adult trials, such as the MOPP/ABV hybrid combination and the Stanford V regimen.[150,151] Advantages of these regimens include reduced therapy duration and cumulative chemotherapy doses. Chemotherapy is administered at weekly intervals for a period of 3 to 5 months during which myelosuppressive agents are alternated with nonmyelosuppressive agents. Consolidative radiation therapy, usually standard-dose in the adult setting, is administered to sites of bulky or residual disease. Preliminary results of North American pediatric cooperative groups support the feasibility of this approach combined with low-dose radiation therapy.[110,152,153] Long-term follow-up is not yet available to evaluate efficacy and treatment sequelae.

TABLE 22.11

RESULTS OF SELECTED RECENT RISK-ADAPTED TRIALS FOR PEDIATRIC HL

Chemotherapy	Radiation	Stage	No. of patients	Event-free survival	Survival
Stanford, St. Jude, Dana Farber Consortium[115,147,155]					
4 VAMP	15–25.5, IF	CS I/II[a]	110	89 (10)	96 (10)
6 VEPA	15–25.5, IF	CS I/II bulky, III/IV	56	68 (5)	82 (5)
6 VAMP/COP	15–25.5, IF	CS I/II bulky or B, III/IV	159	76 (5)	93 (5)
USA-CCG[110]					
4 COPP/ABV	21, IF/none	CS IA/B, IIA[b]	294	97/91(3)	100/100 (3)
6 COPP/ABV	21, IF/none	CS I/II,[a] CS IIB, CS III	394	87/83 (3)	100/95 (3)
Ara-C/VP-16+COPP/ ABV+CHOP	21, IF/none	CS IV	141	90/81 (3)	100/94 (3)
German Multicenter GPOH HD 95[112]					
2 OEPA/OPPA	20–35, IF/none	I, IIA	281/113	94/97 (5)	
2 OEPA/OPPA + 2 COPP	20–35, IF/none	II$_E$A, IIB, IIIA	212/52	92/78 (5)	
2 OEPA/OPPA + 4 COPP	20–35, IF/none	II$_E$B, III$_E$A/B, IIIB, IVA/B	265/57	91/80 (5)	
SFOP MDH-90[148]					
4 VBVP, good responders	20, IF	I–II	171	91 (5)	98 (5)
4VBVP + 1–2 OPPA, poor responders	20, IF	I–II	27	78 (5)	
UKCCSG[138]					
6–8 ChlVPP	None[c]	CS IV	67	55 (5)	81 (5)
6 ChlVPP/EVA	30, IF	I/II (bulk/B), III, IV	144	78 (5)	89 (5)
VAPEC-B	30, IF	I/II (bulk/B), III, IV	138	58 (5)	79 (5)

Ara-C/VP-, cytarabine/etoposide; CCG, Children's Cancer Group; CS, clinical stage; EFS, event-free survival; IF, involved field; **ChlVPP**, chlorambucil, vinblastine, procarbazine and prednisolone; **EVA**, etoposide, vinblastine, doxorubicin (Adriamycin); **COPP**, cyclophosphamide, vincristine (Oncovin), prednisone and procarbazine; **ABV**, doxorubicin (Adriamycin), bleomycin, vinblastine; **CHOP**, cyclophosphamide, doxorubicin (Adriamycin), vincristine and prednisone; **OEPA**, vincristine (Oncovin), etoposide, prednisone, doxorubicin (Adriamycin); **OPPA**, vincristine (Oncovin), procarbazine, prednisolone and doxorubicin (Adriamycin); UKCCSG, United Kingdom Children Cancer Study Group; **VAMP**, vinblastine, doxorubicin (Adriamycin), methotrexate and prednisone; **VAPEC-B**, vincristine, doxorubicin (Adriamycin), prednisolone, etoposide, cyclophosphamide, bleomycin; **VBVP**, vinblastine, bleomycin, etoposide, and prednisone; **VEPA**, vinblastine, etoposide, prednisone, doxorubicin (Adriamycin).

Recent trials evaluating the substitution of nonalkylating agent chemotherapy (e.g., methotrexate or etoposide) as an alternative to alkylating agent chemotherapy demonstrated an inferior event-free survival among patients with unfavorable clinical presentations (Table 22.11).[154–156] The results of several studies support the designation of an intermediate-risk group, however, which includes patients with clinically localized disease (stages I to IIIA) with unfavorable presentation, including bulky lymphadenopathy or extranodal extension. Long-term results of the German Pediatric Oncology Group trials indicate that event-free survival has not been compromised with reduction from six to four chemotherapy cycles in children with these "intermediate" risk features.[157] Investigators from Stanford, St Jude Children's Research Hospital, and the Dana Farber Cancer Institute identified several factors (male gender; stage IIB, IIIB, or IV diseases; bulky mediastinal disease; high WBC; and low hemoglobin) that were associated with inferior disease-free survival. The presence of four to five of these pretreatment factors correlated with a particularly poor 5-year disease-free survival and survival of only 49% and 72%, respectively.[158] This prognostic index is useful in risk-adapted therapy to assign patients in the highest risk category to the most aggressive therapy.

Relapsed Disease

Most relapses in patients with HL occur within the first 3 years, although some patients may relapse as long as 10 years after initial diagnosis. The excellent outcome for the majority of children with HL has limited opportunities for pediatric investigators to evaluate salvage therapy programs in large patient cohorts. Treatment and ultimate prognosis after relapse is largely dependent on the initial therapy type and time of relapse. As many as 50% to 80% of patients who relapse after radiation therapy alone can be salvaged with chemotherapy or combined-modality therapy. Standard multiagent chemotherapy and radiation therapy may salvage 40% to 50% of children with 1-year or longer initial remissions, but subsequent treatment sequelae, including second malignancies, may reduce ultimate survival.[159] Patients who develop refractory disease during or within 1 year of completing therapy respond poorly to conventional salvage therapy, as do patients with multiple relapses. For these high-risk patients, consolidation with myeloablative therapy followed by hematopoietic stem cell transplantation (HSCT) provides the best opportunity for a durable remission. Several studies support the feasibility and efficacy of this approach, which produce overall survival rates ranging from 30% to 60% in children and adolescents with relapsed HL.[159–162] Recognized risk factors for failure are early relapse and refractory disease at the time of autologous HSCT.[163] The acute morbidity and mortality associated with HSCT may be substantial and are influenced by previous therapy exposures in the often extensively pretreated patients. Transplant-associated mortality occurs in approximately 10% of patients and most commonly results from infectious, cardiopulmonary, or neoplastic complications.[159] Patients have been reported to be at risk for relapse as late as 5 years after HSCT, emphasizing the need for heightened surveillance to assure continued remission status and monitor for late treatment sequelae.

The use of HSCT as initial therapy remains controversial because of the overall excellent prognosis of children with advanced and unfavorable HL. Consensus has not been established among investigators regarding prognostic features that justify the risks of this aggressive approach. Until these issues are further clarified, HSCT should be reserved for patients after relapse or for those who are refractory to primary conventional therapy, including alkylating agents. Cooperative group investigations are required to address the issues of prognostic factors, optimal conditioning regimens, and timing of stem cell transplantation in children.

Autologous HSCT has been preferred for patients with relapsed HL because of the historically high transplant-related mortality associated with allogeneic transplantation.[164] However, recent investigations of reduced intensity allogeneic transplantation have demonstrated acceptable rates of transplant-related mortality.[165–167] Nonmyeloablative conditioning regimens most often use fludarabine or low-dose total body irradiation to provide a nontoxic immunosuppression. The aim is to establish a graft-versus-lymphoma effect that provides a platform for adoptive cellular immunotherapy. Relapse within 6 months of a prior autologous HSCT, chemorefractory disease and poor performance status are associated with a lower progression-free survival.[168] Relapse remains the most important treatment failure after allogeneic HSCT, and donor lymphocyte infusions are being used with increased frequency to induce a graft-versus-host effect and therefore also graft-versus-lymphoma effect.[168,169]

Other novel therapeutic approaches for relapsed HL are currently under investigation. Immunotoxin therapy targeting antigens expressed by HRS cells include CD25 (the IL-2 receptor) and CD30 (the Ki-1 antigen). Clinical trials to date have included only small numbers of patients.[62,64] The feasibility of adoptive immunotherapy with cytotoxic clones of T lymphocytes specific for EBV LMP1 continues to be explored for patients with EBV-associated HL.[170,171]

Acute Toxicity

Acute Radiation Effects

The short-term side effects of irradiation are generally not serious (see Chapter 11). They are a function of the total dose delivered and the volume irradiated, with the most acute toxicity reported after high-dose, large-volume, radiation-only programs, which today are seldom used in children. Low-dose, involved-field radiation as used in combined-modality treatment programs is well tolerated. Potential toxicity from the radiation component of the combined-modality program may include mild erythema or hyperpigmentation of the irradiation skin. There may be transient partial hair thinning at the occiput from a high neck radiation field. Mild dysphagia may occur and possible alteration in taste or xerostomia if a large Waldeyer ring field is required to a moderately high dose. Granulocytopenia and thrombocytopenia may occur but usually reflect bone marrow suppression from prior chemotherapy. Lhermitte syndrome, a sensation of an electric shock radiating down the back and into the extremities on flexion of the neck, is rare, self-limited, and does not represent a prodrome of later neurologic dysfunction. In general, acute radiation effects are self-limited and reversible.

Immediate Effects of Chemotherapy

Multiagent chemotherapy programs can cause nausea and vomiting. The efficacy of serotonin receptor antagonist antiemetics, such as ondansetron, greatly improves tolerance to chemotherapy. Anticipatory nausea, which commonly occurs in teenagers, often responds to premedication with benzodiazepines. Nitrogen mustard, vincristine, and doxorubicin may cause severe local tissue damage if infiltrated into the subcutaneous tissues. Vinblastine and dacarbazine may cause a local burning sensation as they are injected. Many chemotherapy programs produce some degree of reversible alopecia. The neurotoxicity of vincristine, the cardiac toxicity of doxorubicin, and the pulmonary toxicity of bleomycin, as well as other side effects, are discussed in Chapter 10. A thorough review of the toxicities of individual chemotherapy agents should be made before administered, either alone or in combination.

Infection

The most common dose-limiting acute toxicity of multiagent chemotherapy is myelosuppression. Courses of treatment may need to be delayed because of low blood counts. It is preferable to give therapy on schedule at full doses and thus the use of transfusion or simulating factors may be needed for patients receiving aggressive therapy for advanced disease. Some patients may require hospitalization for antibiotic therapy if they develop fever during a period of neutropenia.

The risk of serious bacterial infection, once attributable to splenectomy associated with staging laparotomy,[172] is less frequently observed now that surgical staging is no longer performed. Patients who have undergone a prior splenectomy or splenic radiation, however, should be given a prophylactic antibiotic regimen and guidelines to follow during febrile illnesses. In addition, vaccines available against pneumococcus, *Haemophilus influenzae*, and meningococcus may further decrease the risk of serious bacterial infection for these patients, although sustained antibody titers have not been achieved in patients with HL.[173]

Herpes zoster and varicella infections are seen in 35% of children with HL. The frequency is directly related to the intensity of treatment.[174] Prompt administration of antiviral therapy has reduced the severity and morbidity of these infections. The management of immunosuppression with these and other infections is discussed in Chapter 40.

Late Effects

Soft Tissue and Bone Growth Alterations

Early reports described a disproportionate alteration in sitting height compared with standing height among a group of children who received axial skeletal radiation.[175] A follow-up study demonstrated that prepubertal children who received high-dose radiotherapy (>33 Gy) to the entire spine experienced a significant height loss.[176] Pubertal and postpubertal children given similar treatment and prepubertal children given less than 33 Gy to more restricted radiation volumes did not show clinically significant height impairment.[176] A measurable bone growth abnormality has been observed by plain film analysis in fully and partially irradiated clavicles following 15 Gy and chemotherapy, but this is generally not detectable by inspection.[177] Other investigators have confirmed that lower doses of involved-field radiation used with chemotherapy are not associated with clinically significant bone growth retardation.[178]

Other musculoskeletal abnormalities observed after high-dose radiation may include narrowing of the thoracic apex, intraclavicular narrowing with symmetric shortening of the clavicles, and atrophy of the soft tissues of the neck. Rare sequelae include retroperitoneal fibrosis and brachial plexopathy.

Avascular necrosis of the femoral head has been seen with corticosteroid use, but high-dose radiation may also be a contributing factor.[179] The current treatment protocols with lower dose and smaller volumes of radiation are expected to lessen or eliminate the marked changes observed in long-term survivors of high-dose radiotherapy as delivered in the past. Contemporary risk-adapted therapy with lower cumulative doses of corticosteroids appear to predispose to negligible risk of bone density deficits.[180]

Pulmonary Sequelae

Acute and chronic pulmonary complications reported after high dose therapy for HL may include radiation pneumonitis, pulmonary fibrosis, and spontaneous pneumothorax, although these sequelae are uncommon and are a result of therapy given years ago.[125] However, more current pediatric HL therapy using radiation therapy and ABVD have shown a significant incidence of asymptomatic pulmonary dysfunction after treatment, which appears to improve with time.[127,128] However, grade 3 and 4 pulmonary toxicity has been reported in 9% of children receiving 12 cycles of ABVD followed by 21-Gy radiation.[130] In addition, ABVD-related pulmonary toxicity may result from fibrosis induced by bleomycin or "radiation recall" pneumonitis related to administration of doxorubicin. Pulmonary veno-occlusive disease has been observed rarely and has been attributed to bleomycin chemotherapy.[181] This incidence of veno-occlusive disease may be underreported, as some cases have been misdiagnosed as pulmonary fibrosis.

Cardiovascular Sequelae

Both radiation therapy and chemotherapy used in the treatment of HL may have toxic effects on the heart and blood vessels, although symptomatic sequelae are uncommon. They include cardiomyopathy with congestive heart failure, acute pericarditis, pericardial effusion, chronic constrictive pericarditis, coronary artery disease with myocardial infarction, conducting system abnormalities with arrhythmia, and valvular dysfunction.[182] Also peripheral vascular disease has been observed with vascular narrowing and cerebral vascular accidents from embolic disease or vascular occlusion.[183,184] Reduction of anthracycline chemotherapy doses and radiation doses and volumes in contemporary pediatric regimens have diminished the frequency of acute toxicity. However, delayed subclinical cardiovascular injury and its effect on the progression of degenerative cardiovascular disease is just now becoming apparent as survivors of pediatric HL enter their third and fourth decades of live.

Cardiac injury from radiation is also related to dose, volume, and fraction size. The pericardium, myocardium, conducting system, valves, and arterial vessels may be affected. The spectrum of cardiac dysfunction ranges from asymptomatic radiographic abnormalities to life-threatening illness. The incidence of cardiac injury after high-dose mantle/heart irradiation (>40 Gy) is at least 10% to 15% in both children and adults.[125,184] General risk factors for cardiovascular disease include anthracycline cumulative dose and type, radiation therapy technique, age, obesity, hypertension, family history, abnormal lipoprotein levels, and smoking.[182] The relevance of these atherosclerotic risk factors in children is being evaluated. It appears that increased body fat, hypertension, abnormal cholesterol levels, left ventricular systolic performance, and wall thickness are particularly important among childhood cancer survivors 5 years or more following treatment.[182] Clinically apparent cardiovascular disease occurs infrequently in survivors of HL treated during childhood or adolescence with modern radiotherapy techniques. Attention to the relative weighting of the radiation beams, limiting the volume of heart

treated as well as total dose and fraction size has greatly reduced the risk of long-term sequelae observed with older techniques and practice. However, longitudinal follow-up to determine the lifetime incidence of clinically significant cardiovascular disease is essential.[185]

In a series of survivors of childhood HL from Stanford, the actuarial risk of cardiac disease requiring pericardiectomy was 4% at 17 years.[186] Patients with severe pericardial complications received little or no cardiac blocking, and most were irradiated before the introduction of subcarinal blocking. The recognition of radiation-induced pericardial disease described in this and other series has resulted in the modification of irradiation techniques to reduce the dose of radiation to the heart.[187] The rates of acute pericarditis and effusion have declined in later cohorts in which patients received partial cardiac shielding and subcarinal blocking,[188] confirming that risks for radiation-related significant pericardial disease are attributed to the total cardiac dose and volume.

Premature coronary artery disease and acute myocardial infarction have also been reported in pediatric HL survivors.[186,189] Young age at diagnosis increases the risk. In the Stanford series, there is a 45-fold excess mortality risk from acute myocardial infarction in patients who received mediastinal irradiation in doses exceeding 30 Gy before age 20 years.[186] With lower volumes of radiation and protective cardiac shielding, the risk of radiation-related cardiac injury is greatly diminished. The Stanford cohort of 192 children treated with combined-modality treatment using lower doses and volumes of radiation reveal no death from myocardial infarction. Other cardiovascular sequelae, including arterial vascular injury, underdevelopment of the great vessels, coronary artery disease with coronary fibrosis, and accelerated atherogenesis, have been observed in long-term survivors of HL treated with high-dose mantle irradiation.[125,190] The true incidence after modern treatment may be difficult to determine, as appropriate radiation treatment plans now prescribe low doses and volumes of mediastinal radiation and protective cardiac shielding.

The most common chemotherapeutic agents implicated in the development of cardiovascular complications in patients with HL include the vinca alkaloids, alkylating agents, and anthracyclines. Raynaud's disease is an uncommon toxicity observed in some patients. This phenomenon appears to be caused by irreversible microvascular injury in patients treated with combination of vinblastine and bleomycin.[191] Rarely, myocardial infarction in HL patients has been attributed to vinca alkaloid therapy.[189] Proposed mechanisms for this complication include ischemia resulting from coronary artery spasm or hypercoagulability. Although high cumulative doses of cyclophosphamide have resulted in adverse effects on the myocardium, these have largely been observed in the setting of HSCT in both adults and children.[192,193] Conventional doses of cyclophosphamide may exacerbate either anthracycline- or radiation-induced cardiac injury.

The cardiac dysfunction most commonly occurring after chemotherapy is related to anthracycline therapy, particularly with doxorubicin. Acute toxicities include sinus and supraventricular tachycardias and premature ventricular complexes. More serious arrhythmias, such as complete heart block, ventricular tachycardias, and sudden death, are uncommon. These abnormalities bear no relationship to chronic cardiomyopathy. Congestive heart failure with pericardial effusion and diffuse myocardial injury may occur acutely or as a chronic event with progressive failure associated with early mortality. The incidence of congestive heart failure increases with the cumulative doxorubicin doses greater than 550 mg/m^2 in adults. Young children may be more sensitive to anthracycline injury because of its adverse effect on cardiac myocyte growth.[194] In addition, children have a high frequency of anomalies of afterload and contractility.[194] Mediastinal radiation and other chemotherapies are thought to lower the threshold cumulative doses to the range of 350 to 400 mg/m^2. The risk of cardiotoxicity may also be impacted by the schedule of administration of doxorubicin. Schedules using smaller weekly doses or continuous infusion are associated with a lower incidence of congestive heart failure than are large doses given every 3 weeks. Factors associated with late cardiac decompensation include childbirth, viral infections, isometric exercises, alcohol and drug ingestion, and growth hormone–induced growth spurts. With current protocols using three to four cycles of ABVD and total cumulative doxorubicin doses of 150 to 200 mg/m^2 and low-dose radiation, the incidence of clinically symptomatic cardiac disease is low.[115,127,128] Nevertheless, all patients treated with doxorubicin-containing chemotherapy and cardiac radiotherapy should be followed systematically for potential cardiac injury.

Endocrine Sequelae

Using an elevated thyroid-stimulating hormone (TSH) level to define hypothyroidism, the incidence of thyroid dysfunction in irradiated patients has ranged from 4% to 79%.[195,196] The sensitivity of the preadolescent thyroid may be higher than that of the adult gland. The dose of radiation is important; only 17% of children who received neck irradiation of less than 26 Gy developed thyroid abnormalities compared with 78% in children who receive 26 Gy or more. In one series, investigators noted improvement in 36% of biochemically compensated hypothyroid children with time.[195] Thyroid nodules, hyperthyroidism, and thyroid cancer have been observed in patients treated for HL. Female sex and increasing dose of radiation are predisposing factors for the development of hypothyroidism and thyroid nodules; older age at diagnosis of HL is also associated with an increased risk of hypothyroidism.[196] TSH and free thyroxine levels should be checked annually in patients who have received radiotherapy to the neck, and children who have elevated TSH levels should receive thyroid replacement therapy to reduce stimulation from prolonged TSH elevation. Periodic withdrawal of hormonal therapy in asymptomatic patients should be considered to assess recovery of gland function. Persistent and enlarging thyroid nodules should be monitored by ultrasound and periodic fine needle aspiration.

Sterility, alterations in fertility, and potential gonadal injury after staging and treatment are important issues that should be addressed at the time of diagnosis and before therapy is instituted. Pelvic radiation carries a high likelihood of ablation of ovarian function. The technique of oophoropexy, with transfer of the ovaries to a midline location, has allowed the preservation of ovarian function in young women with HL.[197]

The younger the woman at the time of therapy, the higher the probability of maintenance of regular menses after therapy.[198] When chemotherapy and radiation are used, the potential exists for increased risk of ovarian failure,[198] although in the Stanford series, 87% of girls with HL had normal menstrual function at long-term follow-up.[199] Normal pregnancies can occur after oophoropexy and pelvic radiation with no increased risk of fetal wastage or spontaneous abortion.[199,200] Of the pregnancies carried to term, no increase in birth defects was observed when compared with the offspring of sibling controls.

Treatment for HL may carry a considerable risk of premature menopause related to the specific treatment modality and age at the time of therapy. Childhood Cancer Survivor Study investigators observed a significantly higher cumulative incidence of nonsurgical premature menopause in survivors than compared with a sibling cohort (8% vs. 0.8%; RR = 13.21, 95% confidence interval [CI] = 3.26 to 53.51; $p < 0.001$).

Risk factors for nonsurgical premature menopause included attained age, exposure to increasing doses of radiation to the ovaries, increasing alkylating agent score (based on number of alkylating agents and cumulative dose), and a diagnosis of HL. For survivors who were treated with alkylating agents plus abdominopelvic radiation, the cumulative incidence of nonsurgical premature menopause approached 30%.[201]

Male patients are much more susceptible to treatment-induced germ cell failure, which underscores the importance of discussing sperm cryopreservation with older patients if gonadal toxic treatment is planned. Primary gonadal dysfunction may exist at the time of diagnosis of HL in 30% to 40% of patients.[202] Six to eight cycles of MOPP, ChlVPP, and COPP chemotherapy are associated with azoospermia in 80% to 90% of adult or pediatric males.[203–206] A high and dose-related incidence of testicular dysfunction has also been reported in pediatric patients treated with OPPA or OPPA/COPP, a result of the gonadotoxic agent procarbazine.[207] Anthracycline-based regimens, such as ABVD, are associated with a lower incidence of testicular damage: approximately 30% of males.[16,206] This azoospermia is transient with full recovery of spermatogenesis. Recovery of spermatogenesis has also been reported 10 to 15 years after documented azoospermia in boys after six cycles of MOPP in childhood[199] and in 50% of adult males after two to three cycles of MOPP.[122] Etoposide has been incorporated into some treatment regimens in an effort to reduce cumulative doses of alkylating agent chemotherapy. A report from the German-Austrian Hodgkin trials using the etoposide-based regimen of OEPA (vincristine [Oncovin], etoposide, prednisone, and doxorubicin) indicates that this strategy is helpful in preserving testicular function in boys with more favorable presentations of HL.[149] Since the hormone-producing cells of the testes are more resistant to the effects of treatment than are the spermatogonia, boys retain normal growth and development. Current treatment approaches are risk adapted so to spare those with favorable, early-stage disease from the gonadotoxic sequelae, occurring with the chemotherapy programs needed to cure more advanced, unfavorable stage disease.

Second Malignant Tumors

The development of a second malignant neoplasm is a distressing late complication observed in HL survivors treated with chemotherapy, radiation therapy, and combined-modality therapy. Risk for secondary cancers are multifactorial and include host- (age, gender, genetics) and cancer-related (tumor location, tumor biology/response, treatment modality) factors. Disease and treatment-induced immune defects may predispose to carcinogenesis. Behavioral risk factors (tobacco use, sun exposure, sedentary lifestyle, and dietary practices) likely contribute but have not been well studied in pediatric survivor cohorts. The relationship of genetic predisposition and secondary carcinogenesis in HL survivors also requires further investigation. The limited reports of predominantly adult cohorts with secondary breast cancer have not identified an association with cancer-predisposing genetic mutations like *TP53*, *BRCA1*, *BRCA2*, or *ATM*.[208–210] Finally, as in the general population, aging enhances cancer risk as is apparent from numerous studies demonstrating an increasing incidence of radiation-associated solid tumors with extended follow-up after childhood HL.[211–214] Although much is known about the association between second malignancy and Hodgkin treatment, knowledge deficits in other areas underscore the need for future investigation to characterize high-risk groups and implement risk-reducing interventions.

Secondary acute myeloid leukemia (s-AML) and its precursor—a pancytopenic myelodysplastic syndrome—represents the most common hematologic malignancy seen in these patients. A standardized incidence ratio (SIR) (calculated as the ratio of observed to expected cases, or relative risk) for leukemia of 174.8 (95% CI, 115.1 to 254.3) has been reported from the Late Effects Study Group (LESG) for children younger than 16 years treated with chemotherapy with a plateau in cumulative incidence at 2.1% (95% CI, 1.3% to 2.9%) after 14 years.[211] Alkylating agents do not have equivalent leukemogenicity, as indicated by German-Austrian investigators who observed a decline in secondary hematologic malignancy risk (SIR of 122 [95% CI, 36 to 254]; 15-year cumulative incidence of 1.1% [95% CI, 0.0% to 2.2%]) following the substitution of cyclophosphamide for mechlorethamine in their treatment regimens.[120]

The use of ABVD in lieu of MOPP and its derivatives greatly reduces the leukemia risk.[215] However, the epipodophyllotoxins and nitrosoureas are associated with s-AML.[216] The leukemia risk after radiation alone is extremely low (zero probability in LESG experience). The peak frequency for secondary leukemia is within the first 5 to 10 years after treatment.[211] Some investigators have described a higher frequency of s-AML in splenectomized adults with HL and have suggested that the spleen has a protective role,[216,217] whereas other investigators have found no such effect in adults[218,219] or in children younger than 16 years when treated.[220]

The risk for non-Hodgkin lymphoma (NHL) is also increased with an SIR of 11.7 (95% CI, 4.7 to 24.2) in the LESG experience and an estimated 20- and 30-year cumulative incidence of 1.5%.[211] An SIR of 15 (95% CI, 4.9 to 35.0) is reported for children younger than 20 years from five Nordic countries.[221] The risk of NHL may be related to overall immunosuppression associated with the disease as well as its treatment.

A variety of secondary solid tumors have been observed in patients treated for HL. The risk of a secondary solid tumor escalates with the passage of time after diagnosis of HL, with a latency of 20 years or more. The SIR of a solid tumor after treatment for HL in the LESG data is 18.5 (95% CI, 15.2 to 22.3).[211] The most common solid tumors observed involved the breast (SIR, 56.7; CI, 40.5 to 77.3), thyroid (SIR, 36.4; CI, 21.9 to 56.8), bone (SIR, 37.1; CI, 15.9 to 73.1), colon/rectum

(SIR, 36.4; CI, 15.7 to 71.8), stomach (SIR, 63.9; CI, 12.9 to 186.9), and lung (SIR 27.3; CI, 7.4 to 69.9).[211] Several institutions have reported a comparable distribution of second cancer histologies in pediatric Hodgkin survivor cohorts.[212–214,221–223] Breast, thyroid, and nonmelanoma skin cancers consistently comprise the most commonly reported second cancers; in older cohorts, gastrointestinal and lung cancers are beginning to appear with increasing frequency.

Age at treatment appears to have a major effect on risk of second malignant tumors in survivors of pediatric HL; the increased risk of solid tumors in adolescent and young adults decreases as these individuals grow older.[213,214,224] The risks of secondary solid tumors vary by treatment and are largely related to radiation and radiation plus chemotherapy.[213,214,224] Notably, alkylating agent chemotherapy may enhance radiation-induced carcinogenesis of respiratory and gastrointestinal tissues.[213,214] The risks of solid tumors greatly increase after relapse of HL in association with higher cumulative doses of chemotherapy and radiation.[214,222]

Much attention has been given to the significant risk of secondary breast cancers in young women treated with thoracic radiation.[211,223,225–228] The risk becomes elevated some 5 to 9 years after radiation, is highest for girls who received radiation at age 10 years or older, and declines with increasing age.[211] There is no excess risk in women older than 30 years at the time of radiotherapy.[229] A high dose of radiation is a risk factor, with most breast cancers arising after 40 to 46 Gy of mantle irradiation, which includes treatment to the axilla.[229] Recent investigations demonstrate a substantial reduction in breast cancer risk in women with treatment-induced ovarian damage, suggesting a role for hormonal stimulation in the development of breast cancer.[227,228]

The quantitative estimate of risk of secondary cancers after pediatric HL varies, depending on the length and completeness of follow-up. The updated LESG experience of secondary cancers is especially valuable, as it contains a large number of patients with consistent and thorough long-term follow-up, with a median of 17 years as shown in Table 22.12.[211] This

TABLE 22.12

OBSERVED AND EXPECTED RATE OF SUBSEQUENT MALIGNANCIES IN LATE EFFECTS STUDY GROUP, ACCORDING TO CANCER DIAGNOSIS

Cancer diagnosis	No. of observed/ expected cases	Standardized incidence ratio with 95% CI	Absolute rate per 10^3 person-years	20-Year cumulative incidence, %, with 95% CI	30-Year cumulative incidence, %, with 95% CI
All cancers[a,b]	143/7.8	18.5 (15.6–21.7)	6.5	10.6 (8.6–12.7)	26.3 (20.8–31.8)
Leukemia[b]	27/0.2	174.8 (115.1–254.3)	1.3	2.1 (1.3–2.9)	2.1 (1.3–2.9)
Non-HL	7/0.6	11.7 (4.7–24.2)	0.3	1.5 (0.1–1.1)	1.5 (0–3.3)
Solid tumors[c]	109/5.9	18.5 (15.2–22.3)	5.1	7.3 (5.5–9.1)	23.5 (18.2–28.9)
Breast, all[d]	40/0.7	56.7 (40.5–77.3)	1.9	2.0 (1.0–2.9)	7.2 (3.7–10.6)
Breast, females[d]	39/0.7	55.5 (39.5–75.9)	5.3	5.6 (2.8–8.3)	16.9 (9.4–24.5)
Thyroid	19/0.5	36.4 (21.9–56.8)	0.9	1.9 (0.9–2.8)	4.4 (1.3–7.8)
Bone	8/0.2	37.1 (15.9–73.1)	0.4	0.5 (0.1–0.9)	0.8 (0.1–0.4)
Colorectal	8/0.2	36.4 (15.7–71.8)	0.4	0.4 (0–0.8)	2.4 (0.1–4.7)
Gastric	3/0.1	63.9 (12.9–186.9)	0.2	0.3 (0–0.7)	0.6 (0–1.2)
Lung	4/0.2	27.3 (7.4–69.9)	0.2	0.1 (0–0.3)	2.1 (0–4.4)

[a]Excludes nonmelanoma skin cancers, including squamous cell cancer ($n = 1$), basal cell cancer ($n = 24$); meningioma ($n = 1$); breast cancer (ductal carcinoma *in situ*; $n = 2$); benign tumors ($n = 40$); and patients with missing information ($n = 1$).
[b]Date of birth not available for one patient.
[c]Excludes lymphatic ($n = 7$) and hematopoietic tumors ($n = 27$), benign tumors ($n = 40$), and patients with missing information ($n = 1$).
[d]Excludes ductal carcinoma *in situ*; $n = 2$.
From Bhatia S, Yasui Y, Robison L, et al. High risk of subsequent neoplasms continues with extended follow-up of childhood Hodgkin disease: report from the Late Effects Study Group. J Clin Oncol 2003;21(23):4386–4394, with permission.

experience reviews 1,380 pediatric patients with 212 malignancies occurring in 173 patients. The risk of developing a second malignancy was 18.5-fold in excess of that expected in the general population (SIR, 18.5; 95% CI, 15.6 to 21.7). The cumulative incidence of any second malignancy was 10.6% at 20 years, increasing to 26.3% at 30 years and of solid malignancies was 7.3% at 20 years, increasing to 23.5% at 30 years.[211] The excess risk of breast cancer among females in the cohort was 55.5-fold (SIR, 55.5; 95% CI, 39.5 to 75.9). The cumulative incidence of breast cancer was 5.6% (95% CI, 2.8 to 8.3) at 20 years and increased to 16.9% (95% CI, 9.4 to 24.5).[211] These data highlight the importance of long-term monitoring of these patients, as the highest reported risks appear in series with the longest follow-up.

As successfully treated children and adolescents with HL have a substantial risk for subsequent neoplasm, many of which are readily detected by physical examination and available screening procedures (breast, thyroid, and skin cancers), patients and physicians must be alerted to the importance of routine examinations and screening procedures.[230] Importantly, the risk of second malignant tumors comes from treatment given many years ago and does not reflect contemporary therapy. Thus, with the current recommended treatment of risk-adapted multiagent chemotherapy and low-dose, involved-field radiotherapy, the risk of second cancers is expected to be substantially lower than that reported in the past. Many groups have shown that the highest risk of complications of treatment is relapse of the HL itself.[223,231] Similarly, death from primary disease is consistently reported as the most common cause of death in series evaluating long-term outcomes after pediatric HL.[223,231] Thus, the goal for pediatric HL must continue to be curative treatment with initial therapy, resulting in the overall treatment that carries with it minimal morbidity and the highest quality of life.

FUTURE CONSIDERATIONS

Refinement of risk-adapted therapy approaches that optimize disease control and reduce treatment-related complications will continue to be a focus of future pediatric investigations in the next decade. Making progress in this initiative is challenging due to the overall success rate of contemporary treatment regimens, which produce long-term survival for the vast majority of patients. Until novel agents and modalities with safer toxicity profiles are available, refinements in treatment strategies must proceed cautiously to assure that disease-free survival is not compromised. Discretion must also be used in efforts to introduce innovative biologic agents and small molecules of undetermined efficacy and long-term toxicity based on *in vitro* studies of cellular behavior. Progress in the future will require large-scale cooperative group collaboration to obtain sufficient numbers of patients to demonstrate improvement in disease-free survival. National and international consensus regarding prognostic factors used for risk categorization will facilitate comparison of treatment regimens and evaluation of new agents and modalities. Considering currently used chemotherapy and radiation approaches, priority questions include determination of the minimal number of chemotherapy cycles required to maintain remission and identification of patients who require radiation to optimize event-free survival. Early tumor response, as demonstrated by functional imaging modalities like PET scanning, may facilitate the identification of patients who may safely have therapy truncated or who require therapy intensification to enhance disease control. Evaluation and integration of targeted therapy with biologic agents and small molecules represents a difficult, but important, objective that should be pursued because of its potential to provide an effective alternative to cytotoxic therapy. Identification of biologic factors that correlate with tumor response and host predisposition to treatment toxicity will be critical to more accurately guide risk-adapted therapeutic recommendations.

References

1. Hodgkin T. On some morbid appearances of the absorbent gland and spleen. Med Chir Trans 1832;17:68–114.
2. Sternberg C. Uber eine Eigenartige unter dem Bilde der Pseudoleukmie verlaufende Tuberculose des lymphatischen. Apparates Z Heilkd 1898;19:21.
3. Reed DM. On the pathological changes in Hodgkin's disease, with special reference to its relation to tuberculosis. Johns Hopkins Hosp Rep 1902;10:133.
4. Fox H. Remarks on microscopic preparations made from some of the original tissue described by Thomas Hodgkin, 1832. Ann Med Hist 1926;8:370.
5. Glaser SL, Jarrett RF. The epidemiology of Hodgkin's disease. Baillieres Clin Haematol 1996;9(3):401–416.
6. Kaplan HS, Gartner S. "Sternberg-reed" giant cells of Hodgkin's Disease: cultivation in vitro, heterotransplantation, and characterization as neoplastic macrophages. Int J Cancer 1977;19(4):511–525.
7. Pusey W. Cases of sarcomas and of Hodgkin's disease treated by exposures to X rays: a preliminary report. JAMA 1902;38:166–170.
8. Goodman LS, Wintrobe MM, Dameshek W, et al. Use of methyl-bis (beta-chloroethyl) amine hydrochloride and tris (beta-chloroethyl) amine hydrochloride for Hodgkin's disease, lymphosarcoma, leukemia and certain allied and miscellaneous disorders. JAMA 1946;251(17):2255–2261.
9. Devita VT Jr, Serpick AA, Carbone PP. Combination chemotherapy in the treatment of advanced Hodgkin's disease. Ann Intern Med 1970;73(6):881–895.
10. Longo DL, Young RC, Wesley M, et al. Twenty years of MOPP therapy for Hodgkin's disease. J Clin Oncol 1986;4(9):1295–1306.
11. Donaldson SS, Link MP. Combined modality treatment with low-dose radiation and MOPP chemotherapy for children with Hodgkin's disease. J Clin Oncol 1987;5(5):742–749.
12. Jenkin D, Doyle J, Berry M, et al. Hodgkin's disease in children: treatment with MOPP and low-dose, extended field irradiation without laparotomy. Late results and toxicity. Med Pediatr Oncol 1990;18(4):265–272.
13. Oberlin O, Boilletot A, Leverger G, et al. Clinical staging, primary chemotherapy and involved field radiotherapy in childhood Hodgkin's disease. Eur Paediatr Haematol Oncol 1985;2:65–70.
14. Gehan EA, Sullivan MP, Fuller LM, et al. The intergroup Hodgkin's disease in children. A study of stages I and II. Cancer 1990;65(6):1429–1437.
15. Olweny CL, Katongole-Mbidde E, Kiire C, et al. Childhood Hodgkin's disease in Uganda: a ten year experience. Cancer 1978;42(2):787–792.
16. Santoro A, Bonadonna G, Valagussa P, et al. Long-term results of combined chemotherapy-radiotherapy approach in Hodgkin's disease: superiority of ABVD plus radiotherapy versus MOPP plus radiotherapy. J Clin Oncol 1987;5(1):27–37.
17. Canellos GP, Anderson JR, Propert KJ, et al. Chemotherapy of advanced Hodgkin's disease with MOPP, ABVD, or MOPP alternating with ABVD. N Engl J Med 1992;327(21):1478–1484.
18. Fryer CJ, Hutchinson RJ, Krailo M, et al. Efficacy and toxicity of 12 courses of ABVD chemotherapy followed by low-dose regional radiation in advanced Hodgkin's disease in children: a report from the Children's Cancer Study Group. J Clin Oncol 1990;8(12):1971–1980.
19. Weiner MA, Leventhal BG, Marcus R, et al. Intensive chemotherapy and low-dose radiotherapy for the treatment of advanced-stage Hodgkin's disease in pediatric patients: a Pediatric Oncology Group study. J Clin Oncol 1991;9(9):1591–1598.
20. Oberlin O, Leverger G, Pacquement H, et al. Low-dose radiation therapy and reduced chemotherapy in childhood Hodgkin's disease: the experience of the French Society of Pediatric Oncology. J Clin Oncol 1992;10(10):1602–1608.
21. Schellong G, Bramswig JH, Hornig-Franz I. Treatment of children with Hodgkin's disease—results of the German Pediatric Oncology Group. Ann Oncol 1992;3(suppl 4):73–76.
22. Vecchi V, Pileri S, Burnelli R, et al. Treatment of pediatric Hodgkin disease tailored to stage, mediastinal mass, and age. An Italian (AIEOP) multicenter study on 215 patients. Cancer 1993;72(6):2049–2057.
23. Grufferman S, Delzell E. Epidemiology of Hodgkin's disease. Epidemiol Rev 1984;6:76–106.
24. Spitz MR, Sider JG, Johnson CC, et al. Ethnic patterns of Hodgkin's disease incidence among children and adolescents in the United States, 1973–82. J Natl Cancer Inst 1986;76(2):235–239.
25. Morton LM, Wang SS, Devesa SS, et al. Lymphoma incidence patterns by WHO subtype in the United States, 1992–2001. Blood 2006;107(1):265–276.
26. Westergaard T, Melbye M, Pedersen JB, et al. Birth order, sibship size and risk of Hodgkin's disease in children and young adults: a population-based study of 31 million person-years. Int J Cancer 1997;72(6):977–981.
27. Chang ET, Montgomery SM, Richiardi L, et al. Number of siblings and risk of Hodgkin's lymphoma. Cancer Epidemiol Biomarkers Prev 2004;13(7):1236–1243.
28. Newton R, Crouch S, Ansell P, et al. Hodgkin's lymphoma and infection: findings from a UK case-control study. Br J Cancer 2007;97(1):1310–1314.
29. Robertson SJ, Lowman JT, Grufferman S, et al. Familial Hodgkin's disease. A clinical and laboratory investigation. Cancer 1987;59(7):1314–1319.

30. Mack TM, Cozen W, Shibata DK, et al. Concordance for Hodgkin's disease in identical twins suggesting genetic susceptibility to the young-adult form of the disease. N Engl J Med 1995;332(7):413–418.
31. Altieri A, Hemminki K. The familial risk of Hodgkin's lymphoma ranks among the highest in the Swedish Family-Cancer Database. Leukemia 2006;20(11):2062–2063.
32. Goldin LR, Bjorkholm M, Kristinsson SY, et al. Highly increased familial risks for specific lymphoma subtypes. Br J Haematol 2009;146(1):91–94.
33. Horwitz MS, Mealiffe ME. Further evidence for a pseudoautosomal gene for Hodgkin's lymphoma: reply to 'The familial risk of Hodgkin's lymphoma ranks among the highest in the Swedish Family-Cancer Database' by Altieri A and Hemminki K. Leukemia 2007;21(2):351.
34. Goldin LR, McMaster ML, Ter-Minassian M, et al. A genome screen of families at high risk for Hodgkin lymphoma: evidence for a susceptibility gene on chromosome 4. J Med Genet 2005;42(7):595–601.
35. Riggs S, Hagemeister FB. Immunodeficiency states: a predisposition to lymphoma. In: Fuller LM, ed. Hodgkin's disease and non-Hodgkin's lymphomas in adults and children. New York, NY: Raven Press, 1988:451.
36. Weiss LM, Movahed LA, Warnke RA, et al. Detection of Epstein-Barr viral genomes in Reed-Sternberg cells of Hodgkin's disease. N Engl J Med 1989;320(8):502–506.
37. Wu TC, Mann RB, Charache P, et al. Detection of EBV gene expression in Reed-Sternberg cells of Hodgkin's disease. Int J Cancer 1990;46(5):801–804.
38. Brousset P, Schlaifer D, Meggetto F, et al. Persistence of the same viral strain in early and late relapses of Epstein-Barr virus-associated Hodgkin's disease. Blood 1994;84(8):2447–2451.
39. Haluska FG, Brufsky AM, Canellos GP. The cellular biology of the Reed-Sternberg cell. Blood 1994;84(4):1005–1019.
40. Pallesen G, Hamilton-Dutoit SJ, Rowe M, et al. Expression of Epstein-Barr virus latent gene products in tumour cells of Hodgkin's disease. Lancet 1991;337(8737):320–322.
41. Khan G, Coates PJ. The role of Epstein-Barr virus in the pathogenesis of Hodgkin's disease. J Pathol 1994;174(3):141–149.
42. Rowe M, Rowe DT, Gregory CD, et al. Differences in B cell growth phenotype reflect novel patterns of Epstein-Barr virus latent gene expression in Burkitt's lymphoma cells. Embo J 1987;6(9):2743–2751.
43. Andriko JA, Aguilera NS, Nandedkar MA, et al. Childhood Hodgkin's disease in the United States: an analysis of histologic subtypes and association with Epstein-Barr virus. Mod Pathol 1997;10(4):366–371.
44. Khalidi HS, Lones MA, Zhou Y, et al. Detection of Epstein-Barr virus in the L & H cells of nodular lymphocyte predominance Hodgkin's disease: report of a case documented by immunohistochemical, in situ hybridization, and polymerase chain reaction methods. Am J Clin Pathol 1997;108(6):687–692.
45. Henderson S, Rowe M, Gregory C, et al. Induction of bcl-2 expression by Epstein-Barr virus latent membrane protein 1 protects infected B cells from programmed cell death. Cell 1991;65(7):1107–1115.
46. Portis T, Dyck P, Longnecker R. Epstein-Barr virus (EBV) LMP2A induces alterations in gene transcription similar to those observed in Reed-Sternberg cells of Hodgkin lymphoma. Blood 2003;102(12):4166–4178.
47. Bargou RC, Emmerich F, Krappmann D, et al. Constitutive nuclear factor-kappaB-RelA activation is required for proliferation and survival of Hodgkin's disease tumor cells. J Clin Invest 1997;100(12):2961–2969.
48. Jungnickel B, Staratschek-Jox A, Brauninger A, et al. Clonal deleterious mutations in the IkappaBalpha gene in the malignant cells in Hodgkin's lymphoma. J Exp Med 2000;191(2):395–402.
49. Emmerich F, Meiser M, Hummel M, et al. Overexpression of I kappa B alpha without inhibition of NF-kappaB activity and mutations in the I kappa B alpha gene in Reed-Sternberg cells. Blood 1999;94(9):3129–3134.
50. Cabannes E, Khan G, Aillet F, et al. Mutations in the IkBa gene in Hodgkin's disease suggest a tumour suppressor role for IkappaBalpha. Oncogene 1999;18(20):3063–3070.
51. Flavell KJ, Murray PG. Hodgkin's disease and the Epstein-Barr virus. Mol Pathol 2000;53(5):262–269.
52. Kuppers R, Schmitz R, Distler V, et al. Pathogenesis of Hodgkin's lymphoma. Eur J Haematol Suppl 2005(66):26–33.
53. Stein H, Marafioti T, Foss HD, et al. Down-regulation of BOB.1/OBF.1 and Oct2 in classical Hodgkin disease but not in lymphocyte predominant Hodgkin disease correlates with immunoglobulin transcription. Blood 2001;97(2):496–501.
54. Seitz V, Hummel M, Anagnostopoulos I, et al. Analysis of BCL-6 mutations in classic Hodgkin disease of the B- and T-cell type. Blood 2001;97(8):2401–2405.
55. Muschen M, Rajewsky K, Brauninger A, et al. Rare occurrence of classical Hodgkin's disease as a T cell lymphoma. J Exp Med 2000;191(2):387–394.
56. Stein H, Delsol G, Pileri S, et al. Hodgkin lymphoma. In: Jaffe ES, Harris NL, Stein H, et al., eds. World Health Organization classification of tumors: tumors of hematopoietic and lymphoid tissues. Lyon, France: IARC Press, 2001:237–253.
57. Swerdlow S, Campo E, Harris N, et al. WHO classification of tumours of haematopoietic and lymphoid tissues. 4th ed. Lyon, France: IARC Press, 2008:321–334.
58. Stein H, Mason DY, Gerdes J, et al. The expression of the Hodgkin's disease associated antigen Ki-1 in reactive and neoplastic lymphoid tissue: evidence that Reed-Sternberg cells and histiocytic malignancies are derived from activated lymphoid cells. Blood 1985;66(4):848–858.
59. Tarkowski M. Expression and a role of CD30 in regulation of T-cell activity. Curr Opin Hematol 2003;10(4):267–271.
60. Zanotti R, Trolese A, Ambrosetti A, et al. Serum levels of soluble CD30 improve International Prognostic Score in predicting the outcome of advanced Hodgkin's lymphoma. Ann Oncol 2002;13(12):1908–1914.
61. Pui CH, Ip SH, Thompson E, et al. High serum interleukin-2 receptor levels correlate with a poor prognosis in children with Hodgkin's disease. Leukemia 1989;3(7):481–484.
62. Hartmann F, Renner C, Jung W, et al. Treatment of refractory Hodgkin's disease with an anti-CD16/CD30 bispecific antibody. Blood 1997;89(6):2042–2047.
63. Schnell R, Staak O, Borchmann P, et al. A Phase I study with an anti-CD30 ricin A-chain immunotoxin (Ki-4.dgA) in patients with refractory CD30+ Hodgkin's and non-Hodgkin's lymphoma. Clin Cancer Res 2002;8(6):1779–1786.
64. Engert A, Diehl V, Schnell R, et al. A phase-I study of an anti-CD25 ricin A-chain immunotoxin (RFT5-SMPT-dgA) in patients with refractory Hodgkin's lymphoma. Blood 1997;89(2):403–410.
65. Kadin ME, Liebowitz DN. Cytokine and cytokine receptors in Hodgkin's disease. In: Mauch PM, Armitage JO, Diehl V, et al., eds. Hodgkin's disease. Philadelphia, PA: Lippincott Williams & Wilkins, 1999:139–157.
66. Nguyen PL, Ferry JA, Harris NL. Progressive transformation of germinal centers and nodular lymphocyte predominance Hodgkin's disease: a comparative immunohistochemical study. Am J Surg Pathol 1999;23(1):27–33.
67. Lukes RJ, Tindle BH, Parker JW. Reed-Sternberg-like cells in infectious mononucleosis. Lancet 1969;2(7628):1003–1004.
68. Isaacson PG, Schmid C, Pan L, et al. Epstein-Barr virus latent membrane protein expression by Hodgkin and Reed-Sternberg-like cells in acute infectious mononucleosis. J Pathol 1992;167(3):267–271.
69. Rudiger T, Jaffe ES, Delsol G, et al. Workshop report on Hodgkin's disease and related diseases ('grey zone' lymphoma). Ann Oncol 1998;9(suppl 5):S31–S38.
70. Lim MS, Beaty M, Sorbara L, et al. T-cell/histiocyte-rich large B-cell lymphoma: a heterogeneous entity with derivation from germinal center B cells. Am J Surg Pathol 2002;26(11):1458–1466.
71. Lukes RJ, Butler JJ. The pathology and nomenclature of Hodgkin's disease. Cancer Res 1966;26(6):1063–1083.
72. Donaldson SS, Hudson M, Oberlin O, et al. Pediatric Hodgkin's disease. In: Mauch PM, Armitage JO, Diehl V, et al., eds. Hodgkin's disease. Philadelphia, PA: Lippincott Williams & Wilkins, 1999:531–605.
73. Macfarlane GJ, Evstifeeva T, Boyle P, et al. International patterns in the occurrence of Hodgkin's disease in children and young adult males. Int J Cancer 1995;61(2):165–169.
74. Belgaumi A, Al-Kofide A, Joseph N, et al. Hodgkin lymphoma in very young children: clinical characteristics and outcome of treatment. Leuk Lymphoma 2008;49(5):910–916.
75. Uccini S, Monardo F, Stoppacciaro A, et al. High frequency of Epstein-Barr virus genome detection in Hodgkin's disease of HIV-positive patients. Int J Cancer 1990;46(4):581–585.
76. Anagnostopoulos I, Hansmann ML, Franssila K, et al. European Task Force on Lymphoma project on lymphocyte predominance Hodgkin disease: histologic and immunohistologic analysis of submitted cases reveals 2 types of Hodgkin disease with a nodular growth pattern and abundant lymphocytes. Blood 2000;96(5):1889–1899.
77. Diehl V, Sextro M, Franklin J, et al. Clinical presentation, course, and prognostic factors in lymphocyte-predominant Hodgkin's disease and lymphocyte-rich classical Hodgkin's disease: report from the European Task Force on Lymphoma Project on Lymphocyte-Predominant Hodgkin's Disease. J Clin Oncol 1999;17(3):776–783.
78. Krikorian JG, Portlock CS, Mauch PM. Hodgkin's disease presenting below the diaphragm: a review. J Clin Oncol 1986;4(10):1551–1562.
79. Gobbi PG, Cavalli C, Gendarini A, et al. Reevaluation of prognostic significance of symptoms in Hodgkin's disease. Cancer 1985;56(12):2874–2880.
80. Feiner AS, Mahmood T, Wallner SF. Prognostic importance of pruritus in Hodgkin's disease. JAMA 1978;240(25):2738–2740.
81. Seymour JF. Splenomegaly, eosinophilia, and pruritus: Hodgkin's disease, or . . .? Blood 1997;90(4):1719–1720.
82. Kaplan H. Hodgkin's disease. Cambridge, MA: Harvard University Press, 1980.
83. Olsson H, Brandt L. Relief of pruritus as an early sign of spinal cord compression in Hodgkin's disease. Acta Med Scand 1979;206(4):319–320.
84. Tan CT, De Sousa M, Good RA. Distinguishing features of the immunology of Hodgkin's disease in children. Cancer Treat Rep 1982;66(4):969–975.
85. Ratkin GA, Presant CA, Weinerman B, et al. Correlation of anemia with infradiaphragmatic involvement in Hodgkin's disease and other malignant lymphomas. Can Med Assoc J 1974;111(9):924–927.
86. Cline MJ, Berlin NI. Anemia in Hodgkin's disease. Cancer 1963;16:526–532.
87. Xiros N, Binder T, Anger B, et al. Idiopathic thrombocytopenic purpura and autoimmune hemolytic anemia in Hodgkin's disease. Eur J Haematol 1988;40(5):437–441.
88. Sonnenblick M, Kramer R, Hershko C. Corticosteroid responsive immune thrombocytopenia in Hodgkin's disease. Oncology 1986;43(6):349–353.
89. Bradley SJ, Hudson GV, Linch DC. Idiopathic thrombocytopenic purpura in Hodgkin's disease: a report of eight cases. Clin Oncol (R Coll Radiol) 1993;5(6):355–357.
90. Hrgovcic M, Tessmer CF, Minckler TM, et al. Serum copper levels in lymphoma and leukemia. Special reference to Hodgkin's disease. Cancer 1968;21(4):743–755.
91. Wieland A, Kerbl R, Berghold A, et al. C-reactive protein (CRP) as tumor marker in pediatric and adolescent patients with Hodgkin disease. Med Pediatr Oncol 2003;41(1):21–25.
92. Slivnick DJ, Nawrocki JF, Fisher RI. Immunology and cellular biology of Hodgkin's disease. Hematol Oncol Clin North Am 1989;3(2):205–220.
93. Klein S, Jucker M, Diehl V, et al. Production of multiple cytokines by Hodgkin's disease derived cell lines. Hematol Oncol 1992;10(6):319–329.
94. Licup AT, Campisi P, Ngan BY, et al. Progressive transformation of germinal centers: an uncommon cause of pediatric cervical lymphadenopathy. Arch Otolaryngol Head Neck Surg 2006;132(7):797–801.
95. Heiberg E, Wolverson MK, Sundaram M, et al. Normal thymus: CT characteristics in subjects under age 20. AJR Am J Roentgenol 1982;138(3):491–494.
96. Leite NP, Kased N, Hanna RF, et al. Cross-sectional imaging of extranodal involvement in abdominopelvic lymphoproliferative malignancies. Radiographics 2007;27(6):1613–1634.
97. Jerusalem G, Beguin Y, Fassotte MF, et al. Whole-body positron emission tomography using 18F-fluorodeoxyglucose for posttreatment evaluation in Hodgkin's disease and non-Hodgkin's lymphoma has higher diagnostic and prognostic value than classical computed tomography scan imaging. Blood 1999;94(2):429–433.
98. Friedberg JW, Fischman A, Neuberg D, et al. FDG-PET is superior to gallium scintigraphy in staging and more sensitive in the follow-up of patients with de novo Hodgkin lymphoma: a blinded comparison. Leuk Lymphoma 2004;45(1):85–92.
99. Spaepen K, Stroobants S, Dupont P, et al. Prognostic value of positron emission tomography (PET) with fluorine-18 fluorodeoxyglucose ([18F]FDG) after first-line chemotherapy in non-Hodgkin's lymphoma: is [18F]FDG-PET a valid alternative to conventional diagnostic methods? J Clin Oncol 2001;19(2):414–419.
100. Hudson MM, Krasin MJ, Kaste SC. PET imaging in pediatric Hodgkin's lymphoma. Pediatr Radiol 2004;34(3):190–198.
101. Rini JN, Nunez R, Nichols K, et al. Coincidence-detection FDG-PET versus gallium in children and young adults with newly diagnosed Hodgkin's disease. Pediatr Radiol 2005;35(2):169–178.
102. Depas G, De Barsy C, Jerusalem G, et al. 18F-FDG PET in children with lymphomas. Eur J Nucl Med Mol Imaging 2005;32(1):31–38.
103. Miller E, Metser U, Avrahami G, et al. Role of 18F-FDG PET/CT in staging and follow-up of lymphoma in pediatric and young adult patients. J Comput Assist Tomogr 2006;30(4):689–694.
104. Hines-Thomas M, Kaste SC, Hudson MM, et al. Comparison of gallium and PET scans at diagnosis and follow-up of pediatric patients with Hodgkin lymphoma. Pediatr Blood Cancer 2008;51(2):198–203.
105. Abramson SJ, Price AP. Imaging of pediatric lymphomas. Radiol Clin North Am 2008;46(2):313–338, ix.
106. Guermazi A, Brice P, de Kerviler EE, et al. Extranodal Hodgkin disease: spectrum of disease. Radiographics 2001;21(1):161–179.

107. Moog F, Kotzerke J, Reske SN. FDG PET can replace bone scintigraphy in primary staging of malignant lymphoma. J Nucl Med 1999;40(9):1407–1413.
108. Carbone PP, Kaplan HS, Musshoff K, et al. Report of the Committee on Hodgkin's Disease Staging Classification. Cancer Res 1971;31(11):1860–1861.
109. Kaplan HS, Rosenberg SA. The treatment of Hodgkin's disease. Med Clin North Am 1966;50(6):1591–1610.
110. Nachman JB, Sposto R, Herzog P, et al. Randomized comparison of low-dose involved-field radiotherapy and no radiotherapy for children with Hodgkin's disease who achieve a complete response to chemotherapy. J Clin Oncol 2002;20(18):3765–3771.
111. Weiner MA, Leventhal B, Brecher ML, et al. Randomized study of intensive MOPP-ABVD with or without low-dose total-nodal radiation therapy in the treatment of stages IIB, IIIA2, IIIB, and IV Hodgkin's disease in pediatric patients: a Pediatric Oncology Group study. J Clin Oncol 1997;15(8):2769–2779.
112. Dorffel W, Luders H, Ruhl U, et al. Preliminary results of the multicenter trial GPOH-HD 95 for the treatment of Hodgkin's disease in children and adolescents: analysis and outlook. Klin Padiatr 2003;215(3):139–145.
113. Ruhl U, Albrecht M, Dieckmann K, et al. Response-adapted radiotherapy in the treatment of pediatric Hodgkin's disease: an interim report at 5 years of the German GPOH-HD 95 trial. Int J Radiat Oncol Biol Phys 2001;51(5):1209–1218.
114. Hudson MM, Krasin M, Link MP, et al. Risk-adapted, combined-modality therapy with VAMP/COP and response-based, involved-field radiation for unfavorable pediatric Hodgkin's disease. J Clin Oncol 2004;22(22):4541–4550.
115. Donaldson SS, Link MP, Weinstein HJ, et al. Final results of a prospective clinical trial with VAMP and low-dose involved-field radiation for children with low-risk Hodgkin's disease. J Clin Oncol 2007;25(3):332–337.
116. Krasin MJ, Rai SN, Kun LE, et al. Patterns of treatment failure in pediatric and young adult patients with Hodgkin's disease: local disease control with combined-modality therapy. J Clin Oncol 2005;23(33):8406–8413.
117. Yahalom J, Mauch P. The involved field is back: issues in delineating the radiation field in Hodgkin's disease. Ann Oncol 2002;13(suppl 1):79–83.
118. Dieckmann K, Potter R, Wagner W, et al. Up-front centralized data review and individualized treatment proposals in a multicenter pediatric Hodgkin's disease trial with 71 participating hospitals: the experience of the German-Austrian pediatric multicenter trial DAL-HD-90. Radiother Oncol 2002;62(2):191–200.
119. Krasin MJ, Hudson MM, Kaste SC. Positron emission tomography in pediatric radiation oncology: integration in the treatment-planning process. Pediatr Radiol 2004;34 (3):214–221.
120. Schellong G, Riepenhausen M, Creutzig U, et al. Low risk of secondary leukemias after chemotherapy without mechlorethamine in childhood Hodgkin's disease. German-Austrian Pediatric Hodgkin's Disease Group. J Clin Oncol 1997;15(6):2247–2253.
121. Schellong G, Potter R, Bramswig J, et al. High cure rates and reduced long-term toxicity in pediatric Hodgkin's disease: the German-Austrian multicenter trial DAL-HD-90. The German-Austrian Pediatric Hodgkin's Disease Study Group. J Clin Oncol 1999; 17(12):3736–3744.
122. da Cunha MF, Meistrich ML, Fuller LM, et al. Recovery of spermatogenesis after treatment for Hodgkin's disease: limiting dose of MOPP chemotherapy. J Clin Oncol 1984;2(6):571–577.
123. Bonadonna G, Zucali R, Monfardini S, et al. Combination chemotherapy of Hodgkin's disease with adriamycin, bleomycin, vinblastine, and imidazole carboxamide versus MOPP. Cancer 1975;36(1):252–259.
124. Bonadonna G, Valagussa P, Santoro A. Alternating non-cross-resistant combination chemotherapy or MOPP in stage IV Hodgkin's disease. A report of 8-year results. Ann Intern Med 1986;104(6):739–746.
125. Donaldson SS, Kaplan HS. Complications of treatment of Hodgkin's disease in children. Cancer Treat Rep 1982;66(4):977–989.
126. Weiner M, Leventhal B, Cantor A, et al. Gallium-67 scans as an adjunct to computed tomography scans for the assessment of a residual mediastinal mass in pediatric patients with Hodgkin's disease. A Pediatric Oncology Group study. Cancer 1991;68(11): 2478–2480.
127. Hudson MM, Greenwald C, Thompson E, et al. Efficacy and toxicity of multiagent chemotherapy and low-dose involved-field radiotherapy in children and adolescents with Hodgkin's disease. J Clin Oncol 1993;11(1):100–108.
128. Hunger SP, Link MP, Donaldson SS. ABVD/MOPP and low-dose involved-field radiotherapy in pediatric Hodgkin's disease: the Stanford experience. J Clin Oncol 1994; 12(10):2160–2166.
129. Shankar AG, Ashley S, Radford M, et al. Does histology influence outcome in childhood Hodgkin's disease? Results from the United Kingdom Children's Cancer Study Group. J Clin Oncol 1997;15(7):2622–2630.
130. Hutchinson RJ, Fryer CJ, Davis PC, et al. MOPP or radiation in addition to ABVD in the treatment of pathologically staged advanced Hodgkin's disease in children: results of the Children's Cancer Group Phase III Trial. J Clin Oncol 1998;16(3):897–906.
131. Sackmann-Muriel F, Zubizarreta P, Gallo G, et al. Hodgkin disease in children: results of a prospective randomized trial in a single institution in Argentina. Med Pediatr Oncol 1997;29(6):544–552.
132. Ekert H, Waters KD, Smith PJ, et al. Treatment with MOPP or ChlVPP chemotherapy only for all stages of childhood Hodgkin's disease. J Clin Oncol 1988;6(12): 1845–1850.
133. Lobo-Sanahuja F, Garcia I, Barrantes JC, et al. Pediatric Hodgkin's disease in Costa Rica: twelve years' experience of primary treatment by chemotherapy alone, without staging laparotomy. Med Pediatr Oncol 1994;22(6):398–403.
134. Baez F, Ocampo E, Conter V, et al. Treatment of childhood Hodgkin's disease with COPP or COPP-ABV (hybrid) without radiotherapy in Nicaragua. Ann Oncol 1997;8(3):247–250.
135. Behrendt H, Brinkhuis M, Van Leeuwen EF. Treatment of childhood Hodgkin's disease with ABVD without radiotherapy. Med Pediatr Oncol 1996;26(4):244–248.
136. Ekert H, Fok T, Dalla-Pozza L, et al. A pilot study of EVAP/ABV chemotherapy in 25 newly diagnosed children with Hodgkin's disease. Br J Cancer 1993;67(1):159–162.
137. van den Berg H, Zsiros J, Behrendt H. Treatment of childhood Hodgkin's disease without radiotherapy. Ann Oncol 1997;8(suppl 1):15–17.
138. Atra A, Higgs E, Capra M, et al. ChlVPP chemotherapy in children with stage IV Hodgkin's disease: results of the UKCCSG HD 8201 and HD 9201 studies. Br J Haematol 2002;119(3):647–651.
139. Hakvoort-Cammel FG, Buitendijk S, van den Heuvel-Eibrink M, et al. Treatment of pediatric Hodgkin disease avoiding radiotherapy: excellent outcome with the Rotterdam-HD-84-protocol. Pediatr Blood Cancer 2004;43(1):8–16.
140. Kung FH, Schwartz CL, Ferree CR, et al. POG 8625: a randomized trial comparing chemotherapy with chemoradiotherapy for children and adolescents with Stages I, IIA, IIIA1 Hodgkin disease: a report from the Children's Oncology Group. J Pediatr Hematol Oncol 2006;28(6):362–368.
141. Jacobs P, King HS, Karabus C, et al. Hodgkin's disease in children. A ten-year experience in South Africa. Cancer 1984;53(2):210–213.
142. Behrendt H, Van Bunningen BN, Van Leeuwen EF. Treatment of Hodgkin's disease in children with or without radiotherapy. Cancer 1987;59(11):1870–1873.
143. Ekert H, Waters KD. Results of treatment of 18 children with Hodgkin disease with MOPP chemotherapy as the only treatment modality. Med Pediatr Oncol 1983;11 (5):322–326.
144. Sripada PV, Tenali SG, Vasudevan M, et al. Hybrid (COPP/ABV) therapy in childhood Hodgkin's disease: a study of 53 cases during 1989–1993 at the Cancer Institute, Madras. Pediatr Hematol Oncol 1995;12(4):333–341.
145. Sackmann-Muriel F, Bonesana AC, Pavlovsky S, et al. Hodgkin's disease in childhood: therapy results in Argentina. Am J Pediatr Hematol Oncol 1981;3(3):247–254.
146. Vecchi V. Childhood Hodgkin's disease: results of the Italian Multicentric Study AIEOP-MH'89-CNR. Med Pediatr Oncol 1997;29:434.
147. Donaldson SS, Hudson MM, Lamborn KR, et al. VAMP and low-dose, involved-field radiation for children and adolescents with favorable, early-stage Hodgkin's disease: results of a prospective clinical trial. J Clin Oncol 2002;20(14):3081–3087.
148. Landman-Parker J, Pacquement H, Leblanc T, et al. Localized childhood Hodgkin's disease: response-adapted chemotherapy with etoposide, bleomycin, vinblastine, and prednisone before low-dose radiation therapy-results of the French Society of Pediatric Oncology Study MDH90. J Clin Oncol 2000;18(7):1500–1507.
149. Gerres L, Bramswig JH, Schlegel W, et al. The effects of etoposide on testicular function in boys treated for Hodgkin's disease. Cancer 1998;83(10):2217–2222.
150. Klimo P, Connors JM. MOPP/ABV hybrid program: combination chemotherapy based on early introduction of seven effective drugs for advanced Hodgkin's disease. J Clin Oncol 1985;3(9):1174–1182.
151. Horning SJ, Williams J, Bartlett NL, et al. Assessment of the stanford V regimen and consolidative radiotherapy for bulky and advanced Hodgkin's disease: Eastern Cooperative Oncology Group pilot study E1492. J Clin Oncol 2000;18(5):972–980.
152. Schwartz CL. The management of Hodgkin disease in the young child. Curr Opin Pediatr 2003;15(1):10–16.
153. Kelly KM, Hutchinson RJ, Sposto R, et al. Feasibility of upfront dose-intensive chemotherapy in children with advanced-stage Hodgkin's lymphoma: preliminary results from the Children's Cancer Group Study CCG-59704. Ann Oncol 2002;13 (suppl 1):107–111.
154. Schellong G. The balance between cure and late effects in childhood Hodgkin's lymphoma: the experience of the German-Austrian Study-Group since 1978. German-Austrian Pediatric Hodgkin's Disease Study Group. Ann Oncol 1996;7(suppl 4):67–72.
155. Friedmann AM, Hudson MM, Weinstein HJ, et al. Treatment of unfavorable childhood Hodgkin's disease with VEPA and low-dose, involved-field radiation. J Clin Oncol 2002;20(14):3088–3094.
156. Ekert H, Toogood I, Downie P, et al. High incidence of treatment failure with vincristine, etoposide, epirubicin, and prednisolone chemotherapy with successful salvage in childhood Hodgkin disease. Med Pediatr Oncol 1999;32(4):255–258.
157. Schellong G. Treatment of children and adolescents with Hodgkin's disease: the experience of the German-Austrian Paediatric Study Group. Baillieres Clin Haematol 1996;9(3):619–634.
158. Smith RS, Chen Q, Hudson MM, et al. Prognostic factors for children with Hodgkin's disease treated with combined-modality therapy. J Clin Oncol 2003;21(10):2026–2033.
159. Baker KS, Gordon BG, Gross TG, et al. Autologous hematopoietic stem-cell transplantation for relapsed or refractory Hodgkin's disease in children and adolescents. J Clin Oncol 1999;17(3):825–831.
160. Williams CD, Goldstone AH, Pearce R, et al. Autologous bone marrow transplantation for pediatric Hodgkin's disease: a case-matched comparison with adult patients by the European Bone Marrow Transplant Group Lymphoma Registry. J Clin Oncol 1993; 11(11):2243–2249.
161. Lieskovsky YE, Donaldson SS, Torres MA, et al. High-dose therapy and autologous hematopoietic stem-cell transplantation for recurrent or refractory pediatric Hodgkin's disease: results and prognostic indices. J Clin Oncol 2004;22(22):4532–4540.
162. Verdeguer A, Pardo N, Madero L, et al. Autologous stem cell transplantation for advanced Hodgkin's disease in children. Spanish group for BMT in children (GET-MON), Spain. Bone Marrow Transplant 2000;25(1):31–34.
163. Claviez A, Sureda A, Schmitz N. Haematopoietic SCT for children and adolescents with relapsed and refractory Hodgkin's lymphoma. Bone Marrow Transplant 2008;42 (suppl 2):S16–S24.
164. Anderson JE, Litzow MR, Appelbaum FR, et al. Allogeneic, syngeneic, and autologous marrow transplantation for Hodgkin's disease: the 21-year Seattle experience. J Clin Oncol 1993;11(12):2342–2350.
165. Carella AM, Cavaliere M, Lerma E, et al. Autografting followed by nonmyeloablative immunosuppressive chemotherapy and allogeneic peripheral-blood hematopoietic stem-cell transplantation as treatment of resistant Hodgkin's disease and non-Hodgkin's lymphoma. J Clin Oncol 2000;18(23):3918–3924.
166. Robinson SP, Goldstone AH, Mackinnon S, et al. Chemoresistant or aggressive lymphoma predicts for a poor outcome following reduced-intensity allogeneic progenitor cell transplantation: an analysis from the Lymphoma Working Party of the European Group for Blood and Bone Marrow Transplantation. Blood 2002;100(13):4310–4316.
167. Devetten MP, Hari PN, Carreras J, et al. Unrelated donor reduced-intensity allogeneic hematopoietic stem cell transplantation for relapsed and refractory Hodgkin lymphoma. Biol Blood Marrow Transplant 2009;15(1):109–117.
168. Robinson SP, Sureda A, Canals C, et al. Reduced intensity conditioning allogeneic stem cell transplantation for Hodgkin's lymphoma: identification of prognostic factors predicting outcome. Haematologica 2009;94(2):230–238.
169. Moskowitz AJ, Perales MA, Kewalramani T, et al. Outcomes for patients who fail high dose chemoradiotherapy and autologous stem cell rescue for relapsed and primary refractory Hodgkin lymphoma. Br J Haematol 2009;146(2):158–163.
170. Lucas KG, Salzman D, Garcia A, et al. Adoptive immunotherapy with allogeneic Epstein-Barr virus (EBV)-specific cytotoxic T-lymphocytes for recurrent, EBV-positive Hodgkin disease. Cancer 2004;100(9):1892–1901.
171. Rooney CM, Smith CA, Ng CY, et al. Use of gene-modified virus-specific T lymphocytes to control Epstein-Barr-virus-related lymphoproliferation. Lancet 1995;345(8941):9–13.
172. Hays DM, Ternberg JL, Chen TT, et al. Postsplenectomy sepsis and other complications following staging laparotomy for Hodgkin's disease in childhood. J Pediatr Surg 1986;21(7):628–632.
173. Donaldson SS, Vosti KL, Berberich FR, et al. Response to pneumococcal vaccine among children with Hodgkin's disease. Rev Infect Dis 1981;3(suppl):S133–S143.

174. Reboul F, Donaldson SS, Kaplan HS. Herpes zoster and varicella infections in children with Hodgkin's disease: an analysis of contributing factors. Cancer 1978;41(1):95–99.

175. Papadakis V, Tan C, Heller G, et al. Growth and final height after treatment for childhood Hodgkin disease. J Pediatr Hematol Oncol 1996;18(3):272–276.

176. Willman KY, Cox RS, Donaldson SS. Radiation induced height impairment in pediatric Hodgkin's disease. Int J Radiat Oncol Biol Phys 1994;28(1):85–92.

177. Merchant TE, Nguyen L, Nguyen D, et al. Differential attenuation of clavicle growth after asymmetric mantle radiotherapy. Int J Radiat Oncol Biol Phys 2004;59(2):556–561.

178. Donaldson S, Hudson M, Oberlin O, et al. Pediatric Hodgkin's disease. In: Mauch PM, Armitage JO, Diehl, V, et al., eds. Hodgkin's disease. Philadelphia, PA: Lippincott Williams & Wilkins, 1999:531–605.

179. Kadan-Lottick NS, Dinu I, Wasilewski-Masker K, et al. Osteonecrosis in adult survivors of childhood cancer: a report from the childhood cancer survivor study. J Clin Oncol 2008;26(18):3038–3045.

180. Kaste SC, Metzger ML, Minhas A, et al. Pediatric Hodgkin lymphoma survivors at negligible risk for significant bone mineral density deficits. Pediatr Blood Cancer 2009;52(4):516–521.

181. Polliack A. Late therapy-induced cardiac and pulmonary complications in cured patients with Hodgkin's disease treated with conventional combination chemoradiotherapy. Leuk Lymphoma 1995;15(suppl 1):7–10.

182. Adams MJ, Lipshultz SE, Schwartz C, et al. Radiation-associated cardiovascular disease: manifestations and management. Semin Radiat Oncol 2003;13(3):346–356.

183. Bowers DC, McNeil DE, Liu Y, et al. Stroke as a late treatment effect of Hodgkin's disease: a report from the Childhood Cancer Survivor Study. J Clin Oncol 2005;23(27):6508–6515.

184. Hull MC, Morris CG, Pepine CJ, et al. Valvular dysfunction and carotid, subclavian, and coronary artery disease in survivors of Hodgkin lymphoma treated with radiation therapy. JAMA 2003;290(21):2831–2837.

185. Kadota RP, Burgert EO Jr, Driscoll DJ, et al. Cardiopulmonary function in long-term survivors of childhood Hodgkin's lymphoma: a pilot study. Mayo Clin Proc 1988;63(4):362–367.

186. Hancock SL, Tucker MA, Hoppe RT. Factors affecting late mortality from heart disease after treatment of Hodgkin's disease. JAMA 1993;270(16):1949–1955.

187. Greenwood RD, Rosenthal A, Cassady R, et al. Constrictive pericarditis in childhood due to mediastinal irradiation. Circulation 1974;50(5):1033–1039.

188. Carmel RJ, Kaplan HS. Mantle irradiation in Hodgkin's disease. An analysis of technique, tumor eradication, and complications. Cancer 1976;37(6):2813–2825.

189. Scholz KH, Herrmann C, Tebbe U, et al. Myocardial infarction in young patients with Hodgkin's disease—potential pathogenic role of radiotherapy, chemotherapy, and splenectomy. Clin Investig 1993;71(1):57–64.

190. Constine LS, Schwartz RG, Savage DE, et al. Cardiac function, perfusion, and morbidity in irradiated long-term survivors of Hodgkin's disease. Int J Radiat Oncol Biol Phys 1997;39(4):897–906.

191. Doll DC, Ringenberg QS, Yarbro JW. Vascular toxicity associated with antineoplastic agents. J Clin Oncol 1986;4(9):1405–1417.

192. Pihkala J, Saarinen UM, Lundstrom U, et al. Effects of bone marrow transplantation on myocardial function in children. Bone Marrow Transplant 1994;13(2):149–155.

193. Eames GM, Crosson J, Steinberger J, et al. Cardiovascular function in children following bone marrow transplant: a cross-sectional study. Bone Marrow Transplant 1997;19(1):61–66.

194. Lipshultz SE, Colan SD, Gelber RD, et al. Late cardiac effects of doxorubicin therapy for acute lymphoblastic leukemia in childhood. N Engl J Med 1991;324(12):808–815.

195. Constine LS, Donaldson SS, McDougall IR, et al. Thyroid dysfunction after radiotherapy in children with Hodgkin's disease. Cancer 1984;53(4):878–883.

196. Sklar C, Whitton J, Mertens A, et al. Abnormalities of the thyroid in survivors of Hodgkin's disease: data from the Childhood Cancer Survivor Study. J Clin Endocrinol Metab 2000;85(9):3227–3232.

197. Le Floch O, Donaldson SS, Kaplan HS. Pregnancy following oophoropexy and total nodal irradiation in women with Hodgkin's disease. Cancer 1976;38(6):2263–2268.

198. Chemaitilly W, Mertens AC, Mitby P, et al. Acute ovarian failure in the childhood cancer survivor study. J Clin Endocrinol Metab 2006;91(5):1723–1728.

199. Ortin TT, Shostak CA, Donaldson SS. Gonadal status and reproductive function following treatment for Hodgkin's disease in childhood: the Stanford experience. Int J Radiat Oncol Biol Phys 1990;19(4):873–880.

200. Horning SJ, Hoppe RT, Kaplan HS, et al. Female reproductive potential after treatment for Hodgkin's disease. N Engl J Med 1981;304(23):1377–1382.

201. Sklar CA, Mertens AC, Mitby P, et al. Premature menopause in survivors of childhood cancer: a report from the childhood cancer survivor study. J Natl Cancer Inst 2006;98(13):890–896.

202. Chapman RM, Sutcliffe SB, Malpas JS. Male gonadal dysfunction in Hodgkin's disease. A prospective study. JAMA 1981;245(13):1323–1328.

203. Anselmo AP, Cartoni C, Bellantuono P, et al. Risk of infertility in patients with Hodgkin's disease treated with ABVD vs MOPP vs ABVD/MOPP. Haematologica 1990;75(2):155–158.

204. Hobbie WL, Ginsberg JP, Ogle SK, et al. Fertility in males treated for Hodgkin's disease with COPP/ABV hybrid. Pediatr Blood Cancer 2005;44(2):193–196.

205. Mackie EJ, Radford M, Shalet SM. Gonadal function following chemotherapy for childhood Hodgkin's disease. Med Pediatr Oncol 1996;27(2):74–78.

206. Viviani S, Santoro A, Ragni G, et al. Gonadal toxicity after combination chemotherapy for Hodgkin's disease. Comparative results of MOPP vs ABVD. Eur J Cancer Clin Oncol 1985;21(5):601–605.

207. Bramswig JH, Heimes U, Heiermann E, et al. The effects of different cumulative doses of chemotherapy on testicular function. Results in 75 patients treated for Hodgkin's disease during childhood or adolescence. Cancer 1990;65(6):1298–1302.

208. Gaffney DK, Hemmersmeier J, Holden J, et al. Breast cancer after mantle irradiation for Hodgkin's disease: correlation of clinical, pathologic, and molecular features including loss of heterozygosity at BRCA1 and BRCA2. Int J Radiat Oncol Biol Phys 2001;49(2):539–546.

209. Nichols KE, Heath JA, Friedman D, et al. TP53, BRCA1, and BRCA2 tumor suppressor genes are not commonly mutated in survivors of Hodgkin's disease with second primary neoplasms. J Clin Oncol 2003;21(24):4505–4509.

210. Offit K, Gilad S, Paglin S, et al. Rare variants of ATM and risk for Hodgkin's disease and radiation-associated breast cancers. Clin Cancer Res 2002;8(12):3813–3819.

211. Bhatia S, Yasui Y, Robison LL, et al. High risk of subsequent neoplasms continues with extended follow-up of childhood Hodgkin's disease: report from the Late Effects Study Group. J Clin Oncol 2003;21(23):4386–4394.

212. Constine LS, Tarbell N, Hudson MM, et al. Subsequent malignancies in children treated for Hodgkin's disease: associations with gender and radiation dose. Int J Radiat Oncol Biol Phys 2008;72(1):24–33.

213. Swerdlow AJ, Barber JA, Hudson GV, et al. Risk of second malignancy after Hodgkin's disease in a collaborative British cohort: the relation to age at treatment. J Clin Oncol 2000;18(3):498–509.

214. van Leeuwen FE, Klokman WJ, Veer MB, et al. Long-term risk of second malignancy in survivors of Hodgkin's disease treated during adolescence or young adulthood. J Clin Oncol 2000;18(3):487–497.

215. Valagussa P, Santoro A, Fossati-Bellani F, et al. Second acute leukemia and other malignancies following treatment for Hodgkin's disease. J Clin Oncol 1986;4(6):830–837.

216. Van Leeuwen FE, Klokman W, Hagenbeek A. Second cancer risk following Hodgkin's disease: a 20-year follow-up study. J Clin Oncol 1994;12(2):312–325.

217. Tura S, Fiacchini M, Zinzani PL, et al. Splenectomy and the increasing risk of secondary acute leukemia in Hodgkin's disease. J Clin Oncol 1993;11(5):925–930.

218. Andrieu JM, Ifrah N, Payen C, et al. Increased risk of secondary acute nonlymphocytic leukemia after extended-field radiation therapy combined with MOPP chemotherapy for Hodgkin's disease. J Clin Oncol 1990;8(7):1148–1154.

219. Rodriguez MA, Fuller LM, Zimmerman SO, et al. Hodgkin's disease: study of treatment intensities and incidences of second malignancies. Ann Oncol 1993;4(2):125–131.

220. Meadows AT, Obringer AC, Marrero O, et al. Second malignant neoplasms following childhood Hodgkin's disease: treatment and splenectomy as risk factors. Med Pediatr Oncol 1989;17(6):477–484.

221. Sankila R, Garwicz S, Olsen JH, et al. Risk of subsequent malignant neoplasms among 1,641 Hodgkin's disease patients diagnosed in childhood and adolescence: a population-based cohort study in the five Nordic countries. Association of the Nordic Cancer Registries and the Nordic Society of Pediatric Hematology and Oncology. J Clin Oncol 1996;14(5):1442–1446.

222. Green DM, Hyland A, Barcos MP, et al. Second malignant neoplasms after treatment for Hodgkin's disease in childhood or adolescence. J Clin Oncol 2000;18(7):1492–1499.

223. Wolden SL, Lamborn KR, Cleary SF, et al. Second cancers following pediatric Hodgkin's disease. J Clin Oncol 1998;16(2):536–544.

224. Metayer C, Lynch CF, Clarke EA, et al. Second cancers among long-term survivors of Hodgkin's disease diagnosed in childhood and adolescence. J Clin Oncol 2000;18(12):2435–2443.

225. Bhatia S, Robison LL, Oberlin O, et al. Breast cancer and other second neoplasms after childhood Hodgkin's disease. N Engl J Med 1996;334(12):745–751.

226. Basu SK, Schwartz C, Fisher SG, et al. Unilateral and bilateral breast cancer in women surviving pediatric Hodgkin's disease. Int J Radiat Oncol Biol Phys 2008;72(1):34–40.

227. Travis LB, Hill DA, Dores GM, et al. Breast cancer following radiotherapy and chemotherapy among young women with Hodgkin disease. JAMA 2003;290(4):465–475.

228. van Leeuwen FE, Klokman WJ, Stovall M, et al. Roles of radiation dose, chemotherapy, and hormonal factors in breast cancer following Hodgkin's disease. J Natl Cancer Inst 2003;95(13):971–980.

229. Hancock SL, Tucker MA, Hoppe RT. Breast cancer after treatment of Hodgkin's disease. J Natl Cancer Inst 1993;85(1):25–31.

230. Oeffinger KC, Ford JS, Moskowitz CS, et al. Breast cancer surveillance practices among women previously treated with chest radiation for a childhood cancer. JAMA 2009;301(4):404–414.

231. Hudson MM, Poquette CA, Lee J, et al. Increased mortality after successful treatment for Hodgkin's disease. J Clin Oncol 1998;16(11):3592–3600.

CHAPTER 23 ■ MALIGNANT NON-HODGKIN LYMPHOMAS IN CHILDREN

THOMAS G. GROSS AND SHERRIE L. PERKINS

INTRODUCTION

Non-Hodgkin lymphoma (NHL) of childhood is a diverse collection of different lymphomas that includes all of the malignant lymphomas that are not classified as Hodgkin lymphoma (HL). Advances in histopathology, immunology, cytogenetics, and molecular biology have resulted in enormous progress in our understanding of the biology of the NHL, which, consequently, has led to more rational classification of these diseases. The study of malignant lymphomas has, in turn, contributed substantially to our comprehension of normal lymphocyte development.

Clinically, it has been recognized for many years that childhood NHL is a much more systemic disease than HL, with hematologic dissemination that is more akin to what is observed in leukemia. Studies to detect minimal disease have now demonstrated that NHL in children involves cells that usually traffic throughout the body and tends to be systemic diseases from the outset. This systemic nature of childhood NHL has led to a different clinical staging system for childhood NHL, and treatment strategies that differ from HL and NHL observed in adult patients. As recently as the 1970s, fewer than 20% of children with NHL were projected to survive their disease, and the majority of affected children died within 2 years of diagnosis. Virtually all of the survivors were patients who presented with localized disease. Progress in therapy of childhood NHL is one of the stunning success stories of the past two decades. In developed countries, more than 80% of children with NHL can now be cured with modern therapy, even patients with widely disseminated disease. It is notable, however, that these extraordinary advances in treatment have not come from the development of new more effective agents, as all of the drugs featured in modern treatment protocols were available in the early 1970s. Rather, more rational classification systems; improvements in clinical risk stratifications; advances in supportive care to reduce the life-threatening complications of NHL and of therapy; and more rational application of chemotherapy with the empirical development of intensive regimens for children presenting with advanced-stage disease have all contributed to improvements in outcome for children with NHL. However, the future requires that new approaches and novel agents be developed to not only improve outcome but also to reduce acute and long-term consequences of treatment.

INCIDENCE AND EPIDEMIOLOGY

The incidence of lymphoma in children varies by age and varies considerably in different world regions.[1] In the United States and in developed countries, malignant lymphoma (including NHL and HL) comprise the third most common group of malignancies in children after leukemias and brain tumors and account for 15% of all childhood malignancies in children younger than 20 years.[2] NHL is more common than HL in children younger than 10 years, but the relative incidence of HL increases rapidly in children older than 10 years, making the incidence of HL almost twice that of NHL in children between the ages of 15 and 19.[2] Approximately 750 to 800 new cases of childhood NHL are diagnosed in the United States each year.[2] There is a marked male predominance in all age groups, but particularly in children younger than 15 years in whom three-fourths of the cases occur in males.[2] The incidence of NHL varies considerably by age; NHL is uncommon in children younger than 5 years and accounting for only 3% of cancers, but the incidence of NHL increases steadily throughout life, accounting for 8% to 9% of cancers in children older than 10 years.[2] Furthermore, the age-specific incidence of NHL varies according to the histologic subtype of NHL. Burkitt lymphoma (BL) characteristically occurs in children between the ages of 5 and 15 years, whereas the incidence of lymphoblastic lymphoma (LL) is reasonably constant across all age groups. Large cell lymphoma, diffuse large B-cell lymphoma (DLBCL), and anaplastic large cell lymphoma (ALCL) occur more frequently in older children and adolescents, demonstrating a steady increase in incidence throughout childhood and peaking in the 15- to 19-year age group.[2] Both the incidence and relative frequency of the different subtypes of NHL also vary considerably in different parts of the world; in equatorial Africa, lymphomas account for almost one-half of the childhood cancers, reflecting the very high incidence of BL and the relative paucity of LL in this region.[3,4] In adults, the overall incidence of NHL has increased over time, a trend that is also noted in the 15- to 19-year age group and in young adults older than 20 years; however, the incidence has remained relatively stable in younger children.[2]

The etiology of NHL is largely unknown. Epidemiologic studies evaluating prenatal and postnatal exposures have not been fruitful for the most part, and exposures studied to date have not been associated with increased risk of lymphoma.[5] The use of pesticides in the home has been linked to the risk of NHL, although no specific agent has been identified.[6] Exposure to drugs and radiation have not been demonstrated to be major risk factors for NHL (except for immunosuppressive drugs; see Chapter 24). Therapy-related secondary NHL in children is rare and is primarily LL or DLBCL.[7] Phenytoin has been associated with "pseudolymphoma," which usually regresses when the drug is discontinued.[8] Immunodeficiency, whether inherited or acquired, is clearly related to the development of NHL, increasing the incidence of NHL more than 100-fold compared with age-matched controls[9,10] (more details provided in Chapter 24).

The relationship between Epstein-Barr virus (EBV) and the pathogenesis of NHL began with the elegant investigations into the epidemiology of a lymphoma of children of equatorial Africa conducted by Denis Burkitt. Dr. Burkitt demonstrated that the disease was associated with climate, occurring most frequently in areas of equatorial Africa, where the rainfall exceeded 20 inches annually and where the mean temperature exceeded 60°F during the coolest months—in short, the regions where malaria is holoendemic.[11] This observation lead to a collaboration with a young virologist named Anthony Epstein, who was searching for human oncogenetic viruses and resulted in the discovery of a herpesvirus from cultures of endemic BL tissue.[12] Subsequent serologic studies demonstrated that EBV is the causative agent for infectious mononucleosis.[13] Since that time, it has been demonstrated that EBV can very efficiently transform human B cells into immortal cell lines *in vitro* and is associated with numerous human malignancies, especially lymphoproliferative disease of the immunocompromised host[14] (see Chapter 24). The role of EBV in the pathogenesis of NHL in immunocompetent individuals is less clear. Presence of EBV is found in only 10% to 20% of BL cases from North America and Europe,[15,16] suggesting that factors other than EBV are important in the pathogenesis of BL.

PATHOLOGY AND MOLECULAR BIOLOGY

NHL of childhood is a diverse collection of malignant neoplasms derived from both mature and immature (blastic precursor) lymphoid cells of either B-cell or T-cell origin (Table 23.1). Although nearly all subtypes of NHL have been reported in children, the majority of cases are limited to a few subtypes, including LL, BL, DLBCL, and ALCL.[2,17] NHL in children is typically intermediate- to high-grade (clinically aggressive) tumors, in contrast to adults where more than two-thirds of the tumors are indolent, low-grade malignancies.[17,18] Indolent lymphomas seen in children (<5% of all cases)[17] appear to have unique clinical and pathologic features, and both pediatric follicular lymphoma (FL) and pediatric nodal marginal zone lymphoma (NMZL) have been recognized as provisional distinct diagnostic entities in the most current WHO classification.[19,20] Pediatric NHL also appears very different from adult lymphomas in that nearly all of the tumors are morphologically diffuse neoplasms, while follicular (nodular) lymphomas are exceedingly rare. Pediatric NHL is nearly evenly split between

B-cell and T-cell lineages, whereas in adults, nearly 80% are of B-cell phenotype. And finally, while precursor (lymphoblastic) lymphomas are relatively common, accounting for 15% to 20% of all pediatric lymphomas,[2] more than 95% of adult lymphomas have a mature lymphocyte phenotype.[17,20]

The classification of NHL by the World Health Organization (WHO) has been recently updated.[20] The WHO classification is based on principles of defining disease entities so that they may be reproducibly identified using a combination of clinical features, morphology, immunophenotyping, and molecular or cytogenetic features. It is well recognized that there is wide variation in the amount of information available for each disease. Some entities are defined primarily on clinical and morphologic features, while others are defined by molecular or genetic characteristics (in addition to clinical and morphologic characteristics).[20]

As pediatric NHLs are usually aggressive, highly proliferative neoplasms, efficient and appropriate handling of pathologic materials is essential to ensure that all necessary ancillary testing can be carried out so that a timely diagnosis can be made (Table 23.2). Morphology and immunophenotype (immunostaining of fixed tissue or flow cytometry) provide the cornerstones of diagnosis, with some problematic cases requiring additional diagnostic ancillary testing, including cytogenetics (to identify specific recurrent cytogenetic abnormalities) or molecular studies (to determine clonality or specific translocations).[18] To obtain sufficient tissue to allow for morphologic analysis and appropriate ancillary testing, an open tissue biopsy is usually required. In some cases, cytologic preparations may be sufficient to make a diagnosis, particularly if sufficient for immunophenotypic studies by flow cytometry. Many ancillary studies, including flow cytometry, and cytogenetic studies require fresh tissue. Immunophenotypic analysis, molecular studies, and limited cytogenetic analysis by fluorescent *in situ* hybridization (FISH) studies may be performed on fixed tissues if no fresh tissue is available. Communication between surgeon, pathologist, and oncologist is imperative to obtain necessary material and information so that clinical, morphologic, immunophenotypic, cytogenetic, and molecular data can be integrated to come to an accurate final diagnosis.

Precursor Lymphomas

LL is part of the spectrum of the precursor blast cell neoplasms seen in children and accounts for 15% to 20% of all pediatric NHL (Table 23.1). These neoplasms may present as disseminated bone marrow disease, that is, more than 25% blasts, which is by convention defined as acute lymphoblastic leukemia (ALL) or as tissue masses (LL). This definition is arbitrary; therefore, the current WHO classification, recognizing that this entity represents a spectrum of precursor lymphoid cell disease, has developed the diagnostic category of lymphoblastic leukemia/lymphoma.[20] It should be noted that while ALL and LL show significant clinical and pathologic overlap, small molecular profiling studies and genomic heterozygosity studies have demonstrated differential gene expression profiles and loss of heterozygosity at the 6q locus, suggesting that there may be underlying biologic differences between these entities.[21,22] Cytologically, the neoplastic cells of LL are indistinguishable from the blasts seen in ALL. It should be noted that cytoplasmic vacuoles may occasionally be seen in precursor lymphoblastic lesions and are not specific for BL. Characteristically, LL shows diffuse or partial effacement of nodal architecture. Particularly in T-cell LL, the small- to intermediate-sized neoplastic cells may infiltrate in an interfollicular pattern with sparing of benign, reactive follicles. LLs are often rapidly dividing neoplasms with a high mitotic rate, and there may be numerous

---

TABLE 23.1

MAIN SUBTYPES OF PEDIATRIC NHL (2008 WHO CLASSIFICATION)

Subtype of lymphoma	Frequency
Precursor lymphoid neoplasms	
T-lymphoblastic lymphoma	15%–20%
B-lymphoblastic lymphoma	3%
Mature B-cell neoplasms	
Burkitt lymphoma	35%–40%
Diffuse large B-cell lymphoma	15%–20%
Primary mediastinal B-cell lymphoma	1%–2%
Pediatric follicular lymphoma	Rare
Pediatric nodal marginal zone lymphoma	Rare
Mature T-cell neoplasms	
Anaplastic large cell lymphoma, ALK positive	15%–20%
Peripheral T-cell lymphoma (NOS)	Rare

ALK, anaplastic lymphoma kinase; NHL, non-Hodgkin lymphoma; NOS, not otherwise specified.

TABLE 23.2

WORKUP OF PEDIATRIC NON-HODGKIN LYMPHOMA

Approach	Utility	Tissue requirement
Morphology	Required for diagnosis	Fixed
Immunophenotypic analysis	Very helpful, usually required	Fixed, fresh
Cytogenetics	May provide diagnostic or prognostic information	Fresh
Molecular analysis	May provide diagnostic or prognostic information	Fresh, fixed
FISH for specific translocation	May provide diagnostic or prognostic information	Fresh, fixed
Immunoglobulin gene arrangements	May help in diagnosis	Fresh frozen, fixed

reactive macrophages present creating a "starry-sky" appearance similar to that seen in BL.

In LL, cell surface immunoglobulin is absent or weakly expressed, but cytoplasmic immunoglobulin may be detected. TdT will be seen in the majority of cases of precursor B- or T-LL and may be detected by flow cytometric, immunohistochemical, or cytochemical methods.[18] T-LL will typically display a cortical thymocyte immunophenotype, usually reflecting middle to late stages of T-cell differentiation. Antigenic deletion is common; however, most neoplasms will express some combination of CD1a, CD2, CD5, and CD7 along with co-expression of CD4 and/or CD8. Occasionally, both CD4 and CD8 are absent. Cell surface CD3 and T-cell receptor (TCR) antigens are usually not expressed but CD3 may be seen in the cytoplasm. CD10 is expressed in 15% to 40% of cases. B-LL most often displays an early pre-B or pre-B phenotype, with expression of CD19, CD10, and TdT and variable expression of CD20, CD22, and HLA-DR.

LL and ALL appear to be characterized by the many of the same underlying cytogenetic abnormalities, although very limited data regarding LL separately from ALL is available. Chromosomal translocations are the most frequent cytogenetic abnormalities that occur in T-LL and typically juxtapose promoter and enhancer elements from TCR genes next to transcription factor genes such as HOX11, TAL1, and LYL1[23,24] (Table 23.3). Precursor T-LL will display early TCR gene rearrangements by molecular studies, although some very immature cells may not demonstrate a rearrangement. Cytogenetic and molecular abnormalities in B-LL are substantially less well characterized than T-LL. Classical chromosomal translocations that occur in pre-B-ALL, such as hyperdiploidy, t(12;21), t(1;19), and t(9;22), appear to occur less frequently in B-LL.[23,24] B-LL will usually show monoclonal immunoglobulin gene rearrangements.

Mature B-Cell Lymphomas

Mature B-cell NHLs in children are most typically BL (including atypical Burkitt lymphoma [aBL]) and DLBCL. BL is relatively common in children (about 40% of all pediatric NHL) but much more rarely seen in adults, particularly in immunocompetent adults. Although rare in children, the new WHO classification now recognizes two low-grade B-cell neoplasms with features that are sufficiently different from adult disease to designate them as separate entities, that is, pediatric FL and pediatric NMZL.[20]

One feature of pediatric mature B-cell NHL is the relatively high proportion of germinal center cell derived neoplasms compared with adults where there is more of a split between germinal center and postgerminal center neoplasms.[25,26] This may, in part, be due to the developing immune system and primary responses to antigens in the pediatric age group. Pediatric mature B-cell NHL tends to have a high proliferation rate and overexpression of pro-proliferative proteins (such as cMYC),[26] suggesting that the mechanism of lymphomagenesis is due to abnormal proliferation rather than defective apoptosis seen as many adult B-cell lymphomas.

Several of the mature B-cell NHLs seen in the pediatric age group are associated with specific cytogenetic and molecular characteristics (Table 23.3). Translocations of the cMYC oncogene have been used to define BL, but it should be noted that abnormalities in the cMYC locus are also seen in many cases of DLBCL.[27] Conversely, the t(14;18) translocation (IgH-BCL2) seen in many adult DLBCL is not seen in pediatric DLBCL and is usually not seen in the rare cases of pediatric FL.[27,28]

Molecular approaches will usually identify B-cell immunoglobulin gene rearrangements in most cases of pediatric B-NHL.[29] In some cases, translocations result in a fusion protein resulting in expression of a protein that possesses oncogenic capabilities. Another mechanism is whereby translocations deregulate gene function resulting in the overexpression of the gene product, that is, juxtaposing genes with one of the immunoglobulin gene loci. Many of these translocations and fusion proteins are unique to lymphoma, allowing FISH or reverse transcriptase polymerase chain reaction (RT-PCR) to be used for detection.[29] Overexpression of the gene may lead to increased protein expression, detectable by immunohistochemical methods as well.[18]

Burkitt Lymphoma

Classic morphologic, immunophenotypic, and genetic features have been described for Burkitt lymphoma (BL). However, no single parameter can be used as a diagnostic standard and a combination of diagnostic techniques is required for diagnosis.[20] Morphologically, BL is characterized by intermediate-sized homogeneous cells with round to oval nuclei containing multiple, variably prominent basophilic nucleoli with a modest amount of somewhat basophilic cytoplasm, which will appear vacuolated, due to lipid droplets, on cytologic preparations (Fig. 23.1A). These tumors have very high mitotic activity, and tissue sections will often show a "starry-sky" appearance that results from reactive macrophages scattered among the malignant lymphoid cells that are engulfing apoptotic debris from the rapidly dividing tumor cells[20] (Fig. 23.1B). As noted

TABLE 23.3

CORRELATION OF HISTOPATHOLOGY, IMMUNOPHENOTYPE, CLINICAL FEATURES, CYTOGENETICS, AND MOLECULAR FEATURES IN CHILDHOOD NON-HODGKIN LYMPHOMA

Histology	Immunology	Clinical features	Cytogenetics	Genes involved
Burkitt and Burkitt-like	B cell (sIg+)	Abdominal masses, gastrointestinal tract tumors, involvement of Waldeyer's ring	t(8;14)(q24;q32) t(2;8)(p11;q24) t(8;22)(q24;q11)	IgH-cMYC Igκ-cMYC Igλ-cMYC
Diffuse large B cell	B cells of germinal center or postgerminal center	Nodes, abdominal masses, bone		
Mediastinal large B cell	B cells of medullary thymus	Mediastinum		
Anaplastic large cell	T cell (mostly), null cell, or NK cell (CD30+)	Skin, nodes, bone	t(2;5)(p23;q35) t(1;2)(q21;p23) t(2;3)(p23;q21) t(2;17)(p23;q23) t(X;2)(q11–12;p23) inv 2(p23;q35)	NPM-ALK TPM3-ALK TFG-ALK CLTC-ALK MSN-ALK ATIC-ALK
Precursor T lymphoblastic	T cell (thymocyte phenotype)	Anterior mediastinal mass with upper torso adenopathy	t(1;14)(p32;q11) t(11;14)(p13;q11) t(11;14)(p15;q11) t(10;14)(q24;q11) t(7;19)(q35;p13) t(8;14)(q24;q11) t(1;7)(p34;q34)	TCRαδ-TAL1 TCRαδ-RHOMB2 TCRαδ-RHOMB1 TCRαδ-HOX11 TCRβ-LYL1 TCRαδ-MYC TCRβ-LCK
Precursor B lymphoblastic	B-cell precursors	Cutaneous masses, isolated lymph node masses, primary bone lymphoma		

NK, natural killer.

previously, the "starry-sky" appearance is not specific for BL but can be seen in any rapidly dividing NHL.[18,20]

BL also includes a related histologic subtype that has previously been termed *non-Burkitt*, *Burkitt-like lymphoma*, *high-grade mature B-cell lymphomas*, or atypical Burkitt or *aBL*. The ability to reproducibly distinguish BL from aBL strictly on the basis of morphology has been very unreliable. The use of aBL as a distinct diagnostic category has fallen into disfavor, and some degree of morphologic diversity is now acceptable in a diagnosis of BL. The WHO classification advocates placing tumors with features intermediate between DLBCL and BL into the category of B-cell lymphoma, unclassifiable,[20] though this is also not very helpful for pathologist or clinicians. This distinction is less of a concern clinically for pediatric oncologist, as BL and DLBCL are treated with the same regimens. Studies have shown that independent of morphologic features, BL has a distinct molecular signature by molecular profiling and may provide the most reproducible means to diagnose BL.[30]

Immunophenotypic features of BL demonstrate a population of mature B cells that express cell surface CD19, CD20, CD22, and CD10 and monoclonal surface immunoglobulin. Usually, the immunoglobulin is IgM heavy chain with light chain restriction.[18] The immunophenotype expression profile of a mature B cell, that is, CD20, immunoglobulin expression, and co-expression of CD10, suggests that BL has a germinal center origin.[20] A characteristic finding of BL is lack of expression of significant levels of the antiapoptotic protein BCL2. This may be very helpful in distinguishing BL from DLBCL, where BCL2 expression is more commonly seen.[31] However,

BCL2 expression is observed less frequently in pediatric DLBCL than disease seen in adults.[26] Immunohistochemical staining for cMYC protein is positive in BL but may also be seen in DLBCL, especially in pediatric disease.[26,31] Since BL is one of the most rapidly proliferating human tumors, with a doubling time of approximately 12 to 24 hours, immunohistochemical staining with proliferation markers, such as Ki-67 or MIB-1, will usually show staining in 99% of the tumor cells, and this has been used as a defining immunophenotypic feature in the WHO classification.[20]

The WHO classification requires demonstration of a translocation involving the cMYC oncogene locus at chromosome 8q24 to make a definitive diagnosis of BL.[20] Roughly 80% of BL contain a t(8;14)(q24;q32) rearrangement in which translocation of one allele of the transcription factor gene cMYC, on chromosome 8, to the immunoglobulin heavy chain gene locus on chromosome 14 occurs. The remaining cases have either a t(2;8)(p12;q24) (15% of cases) or a t(8;22)(q24;q11) (5% of cases) involving cMYC and either the κ or λ immunoglobulin light chain gene loci on chromosomes 2 or 22, respectively.[29,32] Differences in the chromosome 8 breakpoint location also exist between endemic and sporadic BL. Most endemic BL possess breakpoints upstream of cMYC, whereas sporadic tumors almost always have breakpoints within or very near to the cMYC locus, but the significance of this observation remains unclear[32] (Table 23.4). cMYC translocations are most reliably identified by karyotyping of metaphase chromosomes or FISH on either metaphase or interphase nuclei in intact cells or paraffin sections.[29] In addition to cMYC translocations, more

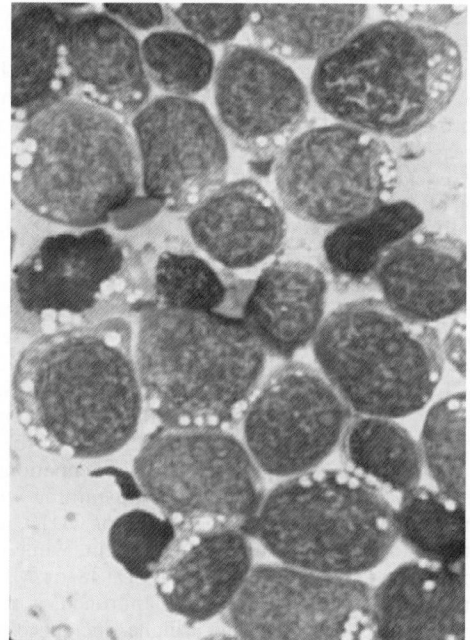
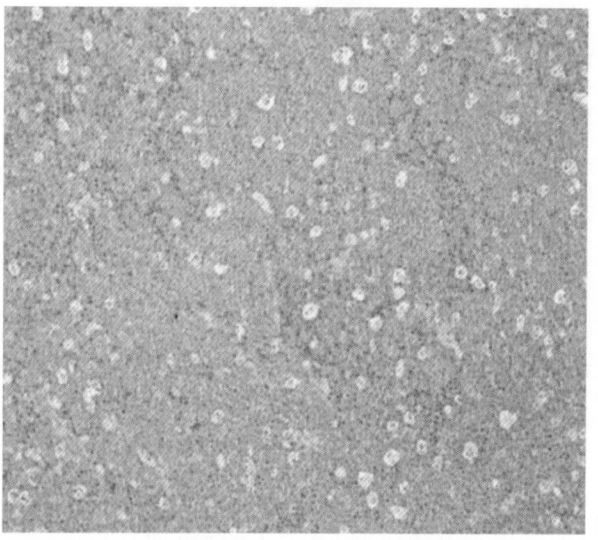

FIGURE 23.1 Burkitt lymphoma (BL). **A:** Wright-Giemsa stain cytologic preparation of Burkitt leukemia demonstrating the uniform cells with basophilic cytoplasm and cytoplasmic vacuoles. Wright-Giemsa stain, 100×. **B:** A low power view of BL demonstrating the starry-sky pattern imparted by admixed tingible body macrophages that have ingested apoptotic debris. There is diffuse effacement of the lymph node architecture by a monomorphous infiltrate. Hematoxylin and eosin stain 4×.

than half of children with BL will have additional cytogenetic abnormalities. The most commonly seen additional chromosomal changes include deletion 13q, duplication 1q, and deletion 6q and may impact upon prognosis.[27]

Diffuse Large B-Cell Lymphoma

DLBCL will diffusely efface lymph node architecture and may display a variety of morphologic and cytologic appearances. There are numerous morphologic subtypes of DLBCL (cen-

troblastic, immunoblastic, anaplastic, and T cell/histiocyte rich), but all are considered to be of similar clinical aggressiveness.[20] The neoplastic lymphoid cells are large and have a nucleus that is at least the size of a tissue histiocyte or twice the size of a small, reactive lymphocyte (Fig. 23.2). The cytoplasm in DLBCL is variable in appearance and may range from pale to plasmacytoid or granular appearing. The cytoplasm may also vary in volume but is always significantly more abundant than that seen in BL. The overall growth pattern is diffuse, although tissue components such as vessels or fibrosis may impart a vaguely nodular appearance in some cases.

TABLE 23.4

COMPARISON OF ENDEMIC AND SPORADIC BURKITT LYMPHOMA

Feature	Endemic	Sporadic
Clinical features	5–10 years Males > females	6–12 years Males > females
Most common distribution of disease	Equatorial Africa, New Guinea, Amazonian Brazil, Turkey	North America, Europe most common
Annual incidence	10 in 100,000	0.2 in 100,000
Common tumor sites	Jaw, abdomen, central nervous system, cerebrospinal fluid	Abdomen, marrow, lymph nodes, ovaries
Histopathologic features	Diffuse growth pattern, monomorphic intermediate-sized cell, starry-sky pattern	Same
Immunologic features	CD20+, usually IgM, κ or λ CD10+, BCL2−	CD10+, usually IgM, κ or λ CD10+, BCL2−
Presence of Epstein-Barr virus DNA in tumor cells	95%	15%
Presence of t(8;14), t(2;8), or t(8;22)	Yes	Yes
Chromosome 8 breakpoints	Upstream of cMYC	Within cMYC

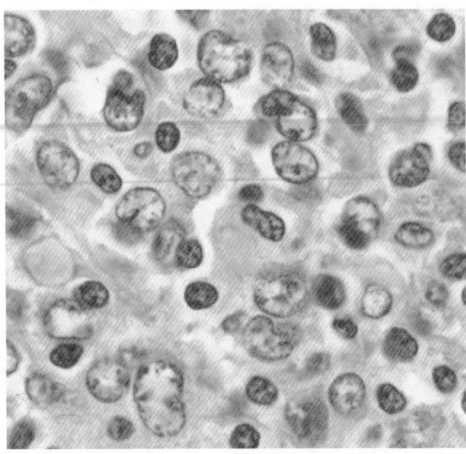

FIGURE 23.2 Diffuse large B-cell lymphoma (DLBCL). Medium power view of DLBCL demonstrating diffuse effacement of lymph node architecture by large noncleaved cells that are admixed with occasional reactive smaller lymphocytes. Hematoxylin and eosin stain, 20×.

Immunophenotypic characterization of DLBCL demonstrates a mature B-cell phenotype with expression of cell surface immunoglobulin and B-cell–specific lineage markers such as CD19, CD20, CD22, CD79a, and PAX-5.[20] Most DLBCL will express monoclonal cell surface immunoglobulin light chains. CD30 expression may be seen in some cases of DLBCL, where it represents a nonspecific activation marker and may create a differential diagnostic consideration of HL or ALCL. However, HL should also express CD15 (Leu M1) and lack expression of most B-cell markers such as CD79a and PAX-5. Approximately 20% to 30% of HL may express variable levels of CD20, although usually less uniform and not as strong expression typically seen in DLBCL. There exists a rare variant, anaplastic lymphoma kinase (ALK)-positive DLBCL, but true ALCL is a T-cell neoplasm and inclusion of appropriate T- and B-cell markers should allow for proper diagnosis.[20]

Pediatric DLBCL tends to have a high mitotic rate as determined by Ki-67 or MIB-1, although this is usually lower than that seen in BL, that is, less than 90%.[20] In contrast to adult DLBCL, pediatric cases tend to have high expression of cMYC protein and lower expression levels of BCL2.[26,31] Pediatric DLBCL has high levels of expression of the germinal center markers BCL6 and CD10. Expression of CD10 is variable but can be seen in approximately half of the cases, while BCL-6 expression may be seen in 50% to 80% of pediatric DLBCL.[25,26] As opposed to adult DLBCL, CD5 co-expression is not commonly seen in pediatric cases.

There are no specific or recurrent characteristic cytogenetic abnormalities associated with DLBCL in children and adolescents.[27] Most cases contain three or more cytogenetic aberrations, typically creating more complex karyotypes than observed in BL.[27,33] Unlike adults, where 20% to 40% of cases will demonstrate a BCL2 translocation, this is rarely seen in pediatric DLBCL.[25,27] However, translocations associated with the cMYC are much more frequently seen in pediatric DLBCL, being reported in as many as 30% to 40% of cases in some studies.[25,27] The prominence of cMYC abnormalities in contrast to BCL2 abnormalities suggests that stimulation of proliferation may be an important pathogenetic mechanism for development of DLBCL in children and adolescents, in contrast to the BCL2 abnormalities that function to inhibit apoptosis seen most commonly in adults.

Several gene expression profiling (microarray) studies have addressed the biological and clinical heterogeneity of adult and pediatric DLBCL.[34–36] Genes that define the germinal center stage of B-cell differentiation are used to define two prominent DLBCL subgroups. The "germinal center B-cell–like" DLBCL subgroup (GCB DLBCL) expresses genes characteristic of normal germinal center B cells (e.g., CD10, BCL6, A-myb), whereas the "activated B-cell–like" DLBCL subgroup (ABC DLBCL) expresses genes that are induced during mitogenic activation of peripheral blood B cells (e.g., BCL2, IRF-4, cyclin D2). In adult studies using CHOP-based therapy, it has been shown that the GCB DLBCL has a favorable outcome compared with ABC DLBCL in adult patients.[36] A larger gene expression profiling study of DLBCL cases confirmed the existence of these two DLBCL subgroups and also identified another set of cases, termed "*Type 3*" DLBCLs, that do not resemble GCB or ABC DLBCL and may represent an additional molecular subgroup of DLBCL.[35] These studies suggest that the DLBCL subgroups represent pathogenetically distinct entities that are derived from cells at different stages of B-lymphoid differentiation.

It has been suggested that immunostaining with specific germinal center markers, such as BCL6 or CD10, may help to identify DLBCL of germinal center origin, while other post-germinal center proteins, such as CD138 or MUM-1, will identify ABC tumors.[37] Using this approach, it appears that the pediatric cases have a much higher incidence of germinal center (GCB) phenotype than is seen in adult populations, with more than 85% to 90% of DLBCLs in two large pediatric studies displaying a GCB phenotype.[25,26] Together, these findings suggest that the majority of DLBCL observed in children and adolescents is different from the DLBCL observed in the majority of adults. It appears that a substantial percentage of DLBCL in pediatrics more closely resembles BL than DLCBL seen in older patients.[34]

Primary Mediastinal Large B-Cell Lymphoma

In the pediatric population, primary mediastinal (thymic) large B-cell lymphoma (PMBL) is seen predominantly in older adolescents.[38] These tumors account for 1% to 2% of all pediatric NHL, and is almost exclusively seen in adolescents.[2] These tumors arise in the mediastinum from thymic B-cells and show a diffuse large cell proliferation with compartmentalizing sclerosis that compartmentalizes neoplastic cells[20] (Fig. 23.3). This type of lymphoma may be difficult to clinically and morphologically distinguish from HL in small mediastinal biopsies because of extensive sclerosis and necrosis, although immunophenotypic analysis will usually reliably separate these entities.[39] In the current WHO classification, PMBL is defined as a clinically and pathologically distinct diagnostic entity.[20] Cell surface markers are similar to that seen in DLBCL such as CD19, CD20, CD22, CD79a, and PAX-5; however, PMBL often lacks cell surface immunoglobulin expression but may display cytoplasmic immunoglobulins and CD30 expression is commonly present.[20] PMBL often shows gains in chromosome 9p with amplification of the cREL gene, which can help distinguish it from other subtypes of DLBCL.[40] Gene expression profiling studies of PMBL have shown significant overlap of the gene expression profiles with classical HL, suggesting that the pathogenesis of PBML may be more akin to HL than to DLBCL.[35]

Pediatric Follicular Lymphoma

Follicular lymphoma (FL) is rare in children and adolescents in contrast to older adults, where they comprise approximately 25% to 30% of all adult NHL.[17,41] Pediatric FL has mostly been described in several small series of patients and

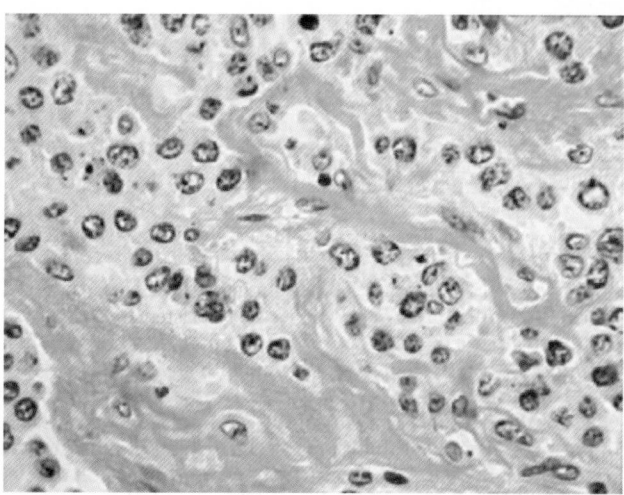

FIGURE 23.3 Primary mediastinal B-cell lymphoma (PMBL). PMBL demonstrating the large neoplastic B cells with abundant clear cytoplasm and surrounding compartmentalizing sclerosis. Hematoxylin and eosin stain, 100×.

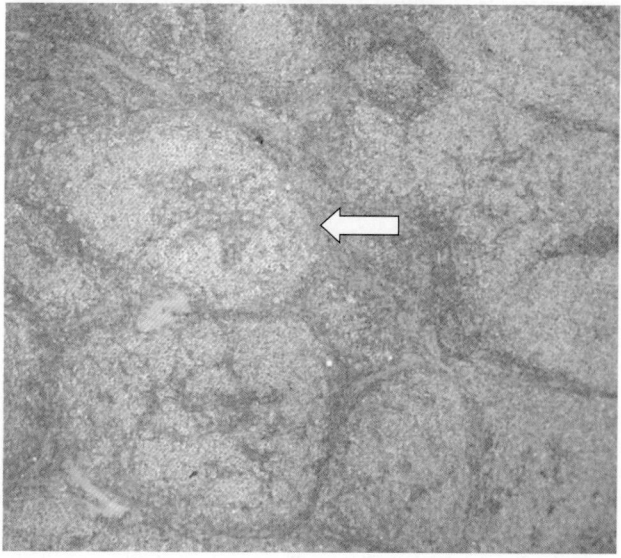

FIGURE 23.4 Pediatric follicular lymphoma. Low power magnification of pediatric FL demonstrating high density, back-to-back follicles with relatively homogeneous composition within the neoplastic follicles. This is a grade 3 (predominantly large cell) follicular lymphoma. (*Arrow*) Several large sized follicles are present. Hematoxylin and eosin stain, 4×.

overall appears to comprise less than 3% of pediatric NHL.[28,41] Studies suggest a male predominance (male:female ratio between 2:1 and 4:1) and broad age range of 3 years to adolescence.[28] Most cases of FL in children appear to differ from adult FL in several important features, leading to its inclusion as a separate provisional diagnosis in the newest WHO classification.[20] However, older adolescents may present with more typical adult features.[41]

Clinically, pediatric FL is more likely to be localized disease[28,41] in contrast to adults where FL often presents as disseminated disease. Cervical lymph nodes and tonsils are common sites, but disease in extranodal sites such as testis, kidney, gastrointestinal tract, and parotid has also been reported.[28,41]

In adults, FL is characterized by overexpression of BCL2 protein in germinal centers allowing it to be distinguished from follicular hyperplasia. In contrast, most pediatric FL do not have overexpression of BCL2.[19,28,41] Virtually all cases of adult FL will have cytogenetic abnormalities. The most common abnormality seen in adults is the rearrangement of the BCL2 gene associated with the t(14;18)(q32;q21) rearrangement which is seen in 70% to 95% of cases.[20] Pediatric cases are much less likely to have BCL2 rearrangements or overexpression of BCL2 protein, suggesting an alternative mechanism of lymphomagenesis in children and adolescents, perhaps involving the BCL6 gene.[19,41] Abnormalities including BCL6 rearrangements and isochromosome (17q) have been described in pediatric FL.[19]

The morphologic features seen in pediatric FL are identical to those seen in adults. FL is characterized by effacement of lymph node architecture by a nodular proliferation of neoplastic lymphocytes that recapitulates the normal follicle structure.[20] However, most pediatric FL displays a primarily follicular growth pattern, although mixed follicular and diffuse patterns have been noted.[20] A higher proportion of pediatric FL have a grade 3 (follicular large cell lymphoma) component (Fig. 23.4) than observed in adults.[19,28] Often the differential diagnostic consideration in pediatric cases of FL is with reactive follicular hyperplasia.[19] Pediatric FL is derived from follicular center cells and are mature B-cell monoclonal processes. Specific B-cell antibodies available (CD20, CD45RA, CD79a, CD22, PAX-5) stain both reactive and neoplastic follicles similarly and may not be helpful in distinguishing between these processes.[20] Both reactive and

neoplastic follicles may also have interspersed T cells. FL in adults will overexpress the BCL2 protein, although this feature is often lacking in pediatric cases, and when present is associated with more disseminated disease.[28,41] However, CD10 and BCL6 staining will be seen in both FL as well as reactive germinal centers and is not helpful in distinguishing between these two processes. Molecular genetic analysis of FL by Southern blot analysis or RT-PCR will demonstrate immunoglobulin heavy and light chain rearrangements, confirming the monoclonality of FL. Monoclonality can be detected by flow cytometry but may be difficult to demonstrate in by immunohistochemistry on fixed tissue.

Pediatric Nodal Marginal Zone Lymphoma

Pediatric nodal marginal zone lymphoma (NMZL) also appears to have distinct clinical and morphologic features, leading to recognition as a provisional diagnostic entity in the WHO classification.[20] There is a striking male predominance (male:female ratio of 20:1) in pediatric NMZL. More than 90% of disease presents with localized lymphadenopathy (usually clinical stage I).[42] Morphologically and immunophenotypically pediatric NMZL appears similar to adult cases.[20] NMZL is characterized by morphologic diversity with the neoplastic cellular component consisting of small to medium lymphocytes and irregular nuclear contours that resemble small cleaved lymphocytes (termed *centrocyte-like cells*), small lymphocytes, large centroblasts, monocytoid B-cells, and monotypic plasma cells[20,42] (Fig. 23.5). Often there are reactive components admixed with the neoplasm, including germinal centers and reactive (polyclonal) plasma cells.[19,20] In pediatric NMZL, follicles resembling progressively transformed germinal centers are frequently seen, and this feature has not been described in adult NMZL.[19,42]

NMZL is a mature B-cell neoplasm that will express pan-B-cell markers such as CD20, CD19, CD22, CD79a, and PAX-5 often with expression of CD43.[20] Molecular analysis of NMZL demonstrates the presence of both heavy and light

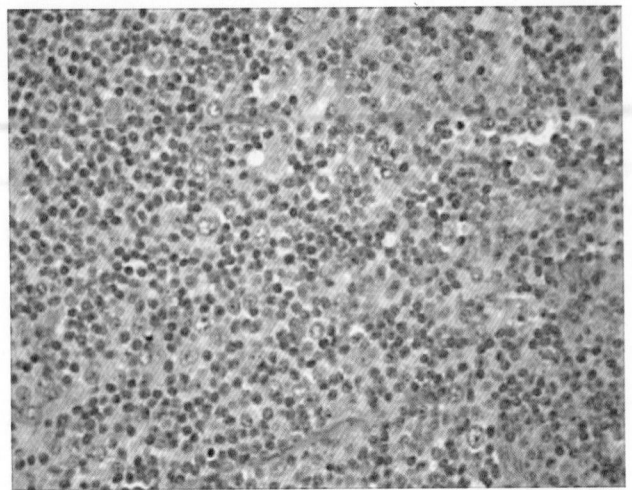

FIGURE 23.5 Pediatric nodal marginal zone lymphoma (NMZL). High power view of an NMZL demonstrating the diversity of cell types in the neoplastic infiltrate. The neoplastic infiltrate includes small cells, small cleaved cells, large admixed large cells, rare plasma cells, and monocytoid B-cells. Hematoxylin and eosin stain, 40×.

chain immunoglobulin rearrangements by both Southern blot and PCR analysis.[20] Often gene rearrangements are required to distinguish pediatric NMZL from reactive conditions. There is no available information on cytogenetic abnormalities in pediatric NMZL.

Extranodal marginal zone B-cell lymphomas arising in mucosa-associated lymphoid tissue (MALT) have been reported in children and usually present as localized disease and are associated with *Helicobacter pylori* and require no more than local therapy of surgery and/or radiation therapy to cure.[43]

Other Pediatric Mature B-Cell Lymphoma

Other subtypes of pediatric mature B-cell lymphoma are extremely rare and appear mostly as individual case reports in the literature when children or adolescents are affected. These appear to represent very young presentations of typical adult diseases in most cases.

Mature T-Cell Lymphoma or Peripheral T-Cell Lymphoma

Mature T-cell lymphoma or peripheral T-cell lymphoma (PTCL) in children and adolescents comprise about 20% to 25% of NHL cases in Western countries, although the incidence is higher in Asia and Latin America.[20] Unlike adults where there is a broad spectrum of T-cell neoplasms, the vast majority of mature T-cell disease in pediatrics is ALCL with other subtypes of PTCL being much more rarely observed[44,45] (Table 23.1). Mature T- and NK-cell lymphomas tend to present with a broad spectrum of clinical disease including nodal, extranodal, and leukemic diseases and are frequently associated with paraneoplastic phenomena such as hemophagocytosis, fevers, rashes, and other manifestations that may be, in part, attributable to cytokines produced by the neoplastic cells.[45,46] PTCL in children has a higher proportion of T/NK-cell tumors that are derived from cytotoxic T cells, including NK cells and γδ T cells.[45] It appears that the innate immune system is more susceptible to development of lymphoma in children, whereas

lymphomas arising from the more mature, antigen-driven, or adaptive immune system are very rare in the pediatric population and more common in adults.[45,47]

Anaplastic Large Cell Lymphoma (Anaplastic Lymphoma Kinase Positive)

ALK-positive ALCL is a PTCL in the WHO classification.[20] The majority of ALCL will express T-cell markers (80%), but 20% may fail to demonstrate staining with either T- or B-cell markers (null cell).[20] However, ALK-positive ALCL will demonstrate TCR gene rearrangements, even when immunophenotypic analysis fails to demonstrate expression of T-cell antigens.[20] ALCL is characterized by expression of CD30 and contains a translocation leading to overexpression of the ALK gene[48] (Table 23.3). Related lymphomas include primary cutaneous ALCL (C-ALCL), and a provisional category of ALK-negative ALCL has similar morphologic features but slightly different clinical and molecular features.[49,50]

The first pathologic descriptions of ALCL were based on identification of large neoplastic cells with significant anaplasia and cytologic atypia with strong expression of the CD30 (Ki-1) antigen in a golgi and membranous staining pattern.[51] However, there is a broad morphologic spectrum and several morphologic variants have been recognized that contain at least some proportion of the characteristic large, pleomorphic, multinucleated cells or horseshoe-like "hallmark" cells[52,53] (Fig. 23.6A). The most common ALCL morphologic subtype is the common (anaplastic) or classic variant (>75% of ALCL, ALK positive) composed primarily of large anaplastic cells and hallmark cells.[20,52] The lymphohistiocytic variant (10% of ALCL) is more rarely seen in children and is characterized by a large number of benign histiocytes that may obscure the relatively fewer, larger neoplastic cells. This may be confused with a reactive disorder or classical HL.[53] The small cell variant (5% to 10% of ALCL) is characterized by a predominance of small neoplastic cells and only scattered hallmark cells.[54] This small cell variant is more commonly associated with high-stage disease, blood, and central nervous system (CNS) involvement.[55] More than one morphologic pattern may be seen, giving rise to a composite pattern in as many as 15% of cases.[20]

Despite the relatively broad morphologic diversity, all subtypes of ALK-positive ALCL have similar immunophenotypic features including consistent expression of CD30.[20] It should be noted that expression of CD30 is not diagnostic of ALCL, as CD30 is also expressed in classical HLs, in a subset of diffuse B-large cell lymphoma, in other subtypes of mature T-cell lymphoma, as well as in benign lymphocytes (in its role as an activation marker).[56] CD45 expression may vary from strong to weak or absent, and may be focally expressed which should be kept in mind when considering the differential diagnosis of classic HL, where Reed-Sternberg cells are typically CD45 negative and CD30 positive.[49] A somewhat unique feature of ALCL is the frequent expression of epithelial membrane antigen (EMA).[20]

This lymphoma is characterized by expression of ALK via chromosomal translocation. Classically, this is a t(2;5)(p23;q35) translocation (70% to 80% of cases) that produces a fusion gene, nucleophosmin (NPM)-ALK.[56–58] As a result of the t(2;5), transcription of the ALK kinase domain is driven by the strong NPM gene promoter, leading to its inappropriate overexpression in lymphoid cells.[57] Less common or variant translocations, comprise the remaining 20% to 30% of cases, include translocations of ALK to partner genes on chromosomes 1, 2, 3, 17, and X also resulting in upregulation of ALK expression[57,58] (Table 23.3). ALK translocations may be detected by conven-

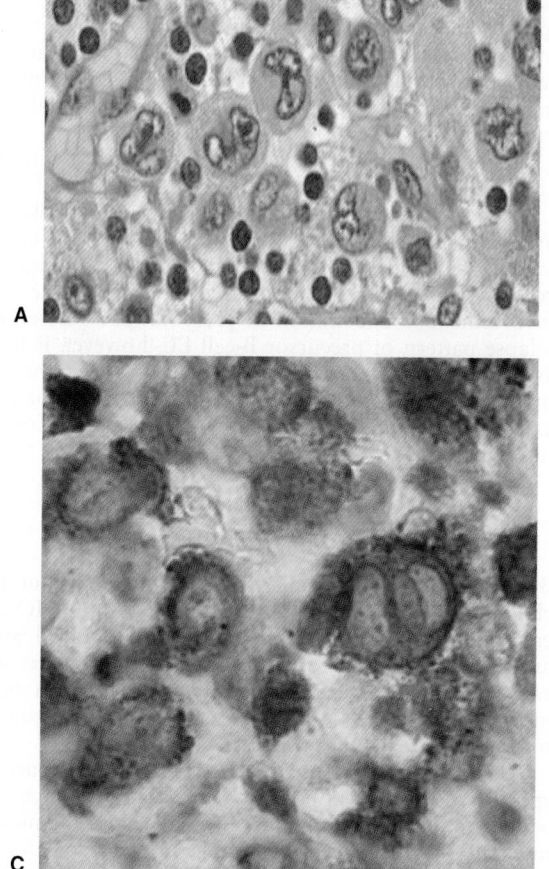

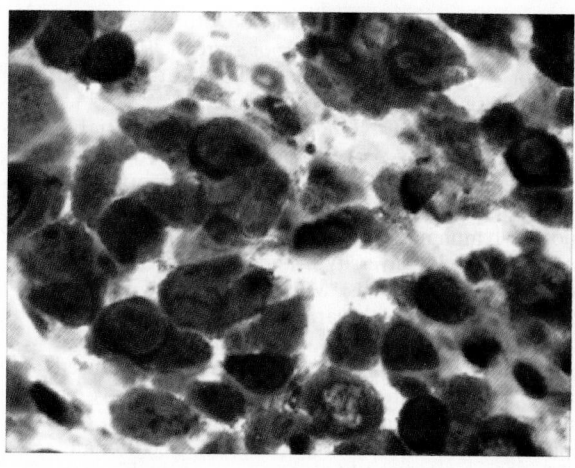

FIGURE 23.6 Anaplastic large cell lymphoma (ALCL). **A:** Common type of ALCL demonstrating characteristic hallmark cells which are large and pleomorphic with eccentric horseshoe-shaped nuclei and abundant clear to slightly basophilic cytoplasm. Occasional hallmark cells are multinucleated. Hematoxylin and eosin stain, 100×. **B:** ALK-1 immunostain of ALCL. **Panel B** shows the characteristic nuclear and cytoplasmic staining that is associated with the t(2;5) translocation in ALCL. **C:** Cytoplasmic ALK staining that is associated with the less common, alternative translocations in ALCL. ALK immunostain, 100×.

tional cytogenetics, RT-PCR, or FISH using ALK-specific probes.[59–61] There does not appear to be a strong correlation with disease presentation, clinical outcome, or morphologic subtype of ALCL and specific translocations in most studies.[49,52] ALK translocations are typically absent in C-ALCL and seen less frequently in adults resulting in a much higher incidence of ALK-negative ALCL (23% to 30% of cases).[20,50,62] The presence of an ALK translocation or ALK protein expression appears to be associated with a better prognosis in adults[63,64]; although this association has not been observed in pediatric patients, this might be a reflection of the small numbers of ALK-negative cases available for study.[65]

ALK antibodies detect the fusion protein generated by translocations associated with ALCL and are used to define the ALK-positive diagnosis. ALK staining is very specific for ALCL with the translocation and is otherwise only noted in brain cells, some rhabdomyosarcomas, and inflammatory myofibroblastic tumors.[60] ALK staining is characteristically absent or very rarely seen in C-ALCL, and if observed in a skin presentation, indicates the likelihood that systemic disease is present.[20] Anti-ALK immunohistochemical staining usually shows a typical staining pattern in both the cytoplasm and the nucleus of the tumor cells and is associated with the most frequently observed NPM translocation partner[57] (Fig. 23.6B). However, 20% to 25% of ALCLs exhibit anti-ALK staining in the cytoplasm only and this represents variant chromosomal translocations involving the ALK gene locus

2p23 but not the NPM gene, such as partner genes on chromosomes 1, 2, 3, 17, 19, 22, and X[57,60] (Fig. 23.6C). Detection bone marrow involvement of ALCL morphologically can be problematic, sometimes necessitating immunostaining with CD30 and/or ALK to identify rare tumor cells.[66]

Peripheral T-Cell Lymphoma Not Otherwise Specified

Peripheral T-cell lymphoma not otherwise specified (PTCL-NOS) is relatively infrequent in pediatrics, although it represents the most common subtype of T-cell lymphoma in adults.[44,46,64] Most series of large cell lymphomas in pediatric populations describe 1% to 5% PTCL-NOS or about 1% to 2% of all NHL in pediatrics. Many of the cases reported in the older literature have been classified as large cell lymphoma, most likely as ALCL, but with appropriate immunophenotyping and molecular analysis may be better subclassified under the WHO classification as PTCL-NOS.[20] Most pediatric PTCL-NOS present as mediastinal masses or nodal disease, although extranodal disease (including skin, organs, bone, bone marrow, and blood) may occur. The diagnosis of PTCL-NOS is one of exclusion such that they do not have characteristics that would place them in any of the other, better defined subtypes of T/NK-cell lymphoma described in the

WHO classification.[20] Many of the patients with PTCL-NOS will present with advanced stage disease or systemic (B) symptoms of fever or weight loss, or paraneoplastic features, such as hemophagocytosis, pruritus, or eosinophilia.[44,67]

Morphologically, PTCL-NOS has somewhat variable tumor cells which typically efface normal lymph node architecture or show infiltration into normal structures, but some cases will present with expansion of the interfollicular (T-zone) area of the lymph node with preservation of reactive follicles. There may be wide diversity in tumor cell size, ranging from small to large sized cells. Most tumors will show a medium to large cell size with variably prominent nucleoli, variably irregular nuclear contours, and variable amounts of clear to basophilic cytoplasm. Some cases may be confused with reactive T-cell infiltrates. It is also common to have an inflammatory background of plasma cells, eosinophils, and small lymphocytes associated with PTCL-NOS. Occasionally, clusters of benign epithelioid histiocytes may also be present.[44,68]

Ancillary testing is often essential in making a diagnosis of PTCL-NOS. The immunophenotype, as determined by either flow cytometric analysis or immunoperoxidase staining, will usually show deletion or aberrant expression levels of one or more of the normally observed T-cell antigens (CD2, CD3, CD5, or CD7). The cells will typically express either CD4 or CD8, though expression of both or neither can also be observed. PTCL-NOS will express cytotoxic granule proteins, for example, granzyme A or B, perforin or TIA-1, in about 50% to 60% of cases. It is important to exclude precursor lymphomas which will express marker of immaturity (CD1a and TdT). CD30 may be expressed in some cases of PTCL-NOS, but CD30 expression is weaker and less consistent than seen in ALCL.[20] Distinction of ALK-negative ALCL from CD30-positive PTCL-NOS is often problematic and based on somewhat subjective criteria such as lack of anaplasia in tumor cells and/or expression of cytotoxic proteins (TIA-1 and granzyme A) being more consistent with PTCL-NOS.[20] CD56 may be expressed in some cases, and EBV has been reported in some pediatric cases.[45,67] Molecular analysis of PTCL-NOS will detect TCR gene rearrangements by either RT-PCR or Southern blot analysis, but it must be kept in mind that T-cell clonality detected by RT-PCR is not specific for malignant processes. Cytogenetic abnormalities are common and usually are complex in nature, but no recurrent cytogenetic abnormalities are described for PTC-NOS.

Although extremely rare, other types of PTCL such as angioimmunoblastic T-cell lymphoma, enteropathy-associated T-cell lymphoma (associated with celiac disease), panniculitis-like T-cell lymphoma, mycosis fungoides, and hepatosplenic T-cell lymphoma (which has been associated with Crohn's disease)[69] have been reported in pediatrics.[44,45]

CLINICAL PRESENTATION

Childhood NHL may present very heterogeneously. The classic clinical manifestations of the different subtypes are summarized in Table 23.3.

Precursor Lymphoblastic Lymphoma

LL accounts for 15% to 20% of childhood NHL[2] and share many clinical and biologic features with ALL. As previously discussed, more than 90% of LL has a precursor T immunophenotype. The majority (50% to 70%) of children with precursor T-LL present with rapidly enlarging neck and mediastinal lymphadenopathy, although subdiaphragmatic

nodal presentations are occasionally seen (Table 23.3).[17,70,71] Symptoms often include cough, wheezing, shortness of breath, and orthopnea, though swelling of the neck, face, and upper extremities from superior vena cava (SVC) obstruction can occur. Hemodynamic compromise due to pericardial effusions may also occur. Subdiaphragmatic disease is often present and may include hepatosplenomegaly, kidney infiltration, and retroperitoneal nodal disease.[70] Fewer than 2% of males will have overt testicular disease manifest as painless enlargement of one or both testes.[70]

In contrast to the clinical features associated with precursor T-cell LL, children and adolescents with precursor B-cell LL tend to have limited disease in sites including skin, bone, and peripheral lymph nodes[72,73] (Table 23.3). The cutaneous lesions are typically in the scalp and appear as enlarging, discolored masses. Morphologically detectable bone marrow involvement is uncommon at presentation.[77] Based on the relapse pattern of precursor B-cell LL, however, it has been assumed that submicroscopic disease is present in the marrow in most patients. Highly sensitive diagnostic techniques such as PCR or multidimensional flow cytometry are confirming this hypothesis.[75]

Burkitt Lymphoma/Leukemia

Burkitt lymphoma/leukemia (BL) accounts for about 40% of childhood NHL.[2] As previously discussed, the WHO classification recognizes both Burkitt and atypical Burkitt lymphoma as BL. In children, there are no consistent differences in clinical presentation, biology, or natural history between these two morphologic types of BL; therefore, they are considered together for treatment purposes.

The predominant sites of involvement and patterns of spread are different in patients with sporadic compared with endemic BL (Table 23.4). Jaw involvement is the most common site of disease in endemic BL. In endemic cases of BL, lesions in multiple quadrants of the jaw are observed in the majority of children, especially those younger than 5 years.[3] These children may also have orbital tumors with or without maxillary disease. Abdominal disease is also very common but interestingly involves the mesentery and omentum more often than the ileum and cecum. Tumor masses of one or both ovaries are also common but overt testicular disease is rare.[76] In contrast to sporadic BL, bone marrow infiltration at diagnosis and at relapse is uncommon, but CNS disease occurs in almost one-third of patients.[3] CNS disease may present as headache and increased intracranial pressure from meningeal infiltration, cranial nerve palsies, or an isolated epidural tumor and paraplegia.[78]

The most common site of disease in sporadic cases of BL is the abdomen (Table 23.4).[70,79,80] These children are often boys between 5 and 10 years of age, who present with abdominal pain or distention, nausea and vomiting, gastrointestinal bleeding, or rarely intestinal perforation. Approximately 25% to 30% of children present with a right lower quadrant mass or acute abdominal pain caused by an ileocecal intussusception.[3] This presentation is often confused with acute appendicitis. An exploratory laparotomy is indicated for diagnostic purposes and in some patients, leads to complete resection of the tumor. Lymphomas involving the ileocecal region in children are all invariably Burkitt or aBL. Complete resection of the involved segment of gut with its associated mesentery, followed by an end-to-end anastomosis, is the recommended surgical approach. Children with completely resected BL of the intestinal tract (stage II in the St. Jude staging system) have an excellent prognosis after treatment with a limited course of chemotherapy. However, the majority of patients with abdominal BL have massive disease that involves the mesentery, retroperitoneum, kidneys, ovaries, and peritoneal surfaces (often associated with malignant ascites). Surgical debulking is neither feasible nor appropriate in these patients.[81]

The head and neck region is the second most common site of disease in sporadic BL. Affected children may have disease in pharyngeal or nasopharyngeal sites, as well as the paranasal sinuses or tonsils. In contrast to patients with endemic BL, jaw involvement is observed in fewer than 10% of cases of sporadic disease. Other unusual sites of disease include testes, breasts, thyroid gland, skin, epidural space, bone, and pancreas; however, mediastinal primaries are more rarely seen than in other pediatric NHL. Bone marrow involvement occurs in approximately 20% of cases of sporadic BL.[82] Almost 20% of patients present without lymphomatous masses but with fever, pallor, and/or bleeding secondary to pancytopenia from extensive marrow replacement by tumor cells (>25% blasts).[83,84] These children may also have peripheral lymphadenopathy and hepatosplenomegaly. By staging criteria, these children have Burkitt leukemia or mature B-cell ALL (L3 morphology by the French-American-British [FAB] convention).[70]

Of interest, the breakpoint involved in the chromosome translocations and the structural alterations of the c-myc locus differ between endemic and sporadic variants of BL.[85,86] The immunoglobulin heavy chain switch region is involved in the translocations in sporadic cases, whereas the heavy chain joining region is involved in endemic cases, suggesting that an early B cell is the target of transformation in these cases, whereas, in sporadic cases, the translocation occurs in a cell further along in B-cell development.[85,86] The occurrence of malignant transformation in different target cells might help explain the clinical and other differences observed between endemic and sporadic cases.

Diffuse Large B-Cell Lymphoma

DLBCL accounts for 15% to 20% of all childhood NHL.[2] Children with DLBCL have a more heterogeneous range of clinical presentations compared with patients with BL (Table 23.4).[87,88] In contrast to BL, the bone marrow and CNS are unusual sites of disease. DLBCL usually presents with nodal disease, though bone (single or multiple sites) is relatively common (Table 23.4). In immunocompromised individuals, extranodal disease is common and primary DLBCL of the brain is not uncommon[89] (see Chapter 24).

As mentioned previously, PMBL is a distinct entity. It is typically diagnosed in young adult females in the third to fourth decades of life.[38] The tumor is locally invasive (e.g., pericardial and lung extension), often associated with the SVC syndrome, and extrathoracic involvement often involves the kidney.

Anaplastic Large Cell Lymphoma

ALCL accounts for 15% to 20% of childhood NHL.[2] ALCL tends to present in lymph nodes and extranodal sites, especially the skin, soft tissues, and bone (Table 23.4).[90] ALCL includes primary cutaneous (C-ALCL) and systemic ALCL. Primary C-ALCL can be difficult to distinguish from lymphoid papulosis (LyP), and both are quite rare in children.[91] There are reports of coexistence of LyP and ALCL in some patients and this has led to the view by some that these cutaneous lesions are a spectrum of the same disorder. LyP is defined as a chronic, recurrent, self-healing papulonecrotic or papulonodular skin disease. The lesions are usually smaller than 2 cm and are red-brown papules and nodules that may develop cen-

tral hemorrhage, necrosis, crusting, and subsequently disappear spontaneously within 3 to 8 weeks. As these lesions resolve, patients may have residual hypo- or hyperpigmented macules. In primary C-ALCL, the nodules are usually larger than 2 cm and may be single or multiple and show ulceration. This entity is distinguishable from the systemic form of ALCL because the neoplastic cells in C-ALCL do not express EMA or ALK. Distinguishing LyP from C-ALCL presents a substantial diagnostic challenge, because of clinical, histologic, and immunologic overlap with C-ALCL.[20,91] Children presenting with cutaneous lesions (ALK negative) without deeper tissue involvement can probably be safely observed without specific therapy unless disease develops in extracutaneous sites. Similarly, great care is required before diagnosing solely cutaneous relapse of systemic ALCL.

The clinical presenting features of ALCL in children are quite variable but often include constitutional symptoms of fever and weight loss. About two-third of the cases present with disseminated disease. The most frequent sites of involvement in systemic ALCL are peripheral nodes; mediastinal adenopathy; and extranodal sites including skin, soft tissue, and bone.[92] Skin involvement is much more frequent than in other childhood lymphomas and is a most common site of extranodal disease in ALCL.[90] Spontaneous regression or waxing and waning of skin disease has been observed in systemic ALCL, albeit less frequently than in primary C-ALCL. Bone disease is also common and it is multifocal in as many as 10% of patients. The CNS and bone marrow are occasionally involved, and in several cases, a leukemic presentation has been described.[93] As mentioned previously, sometimes marrow involvement requires immunostaining with CD30 and/or ALK to identify rare tumor cells.[66]

Rare Non-Hodgkin Lymphoma in Pediatrics

As mentioned previously, indolent mature B-cell NHLs in children are rare but include FL which tends to present with cervical lymph node involvement (although primary tumors of the testis have been reported).[28,94,95] Marginal zone lymphoma is an indolent B-cell lymphoma and can present as nodal or extranodal disease MALT.[42,43]

Mature (peripheral) T-cell and NK-cell lymphomas are a heterogeneous group of aggressive lymphomas that tend to follow an aggressive course and respond poorly to therapy.[64,68] Among these, the NK-cell lymphoma and NK-like T-cell lymphomas usually involve the upper aerodigestive tract (midline lethal granuloma, angiocentric T-cell lymphoma) but can present in the skin as well.[96–98] Mycosis fungoides is the most common form of cutaneous T-cell lymphoma occurring in adults, and approximately 4% to 5% of cases are diagnosed in patients younger than 20 years. Children and adolescents with mycosis fungoides have been reported to have several differences in clinical presentation from adults.[99–101] Pediatric patients tend to have hypopigmented lesions, particularly located on the buttocks, early-stage disease, and often a long interval from onset of symptoms until diagnosis (3 months to 10 years). Most children have been treated with psoralen plus ultraviolet A and have done well, but there are anecdotal cases of aggressive disease.

STAGING AND PROGNOSTIC FACTORS

The goal of staging studies should be to assess rapidly the extent of disease to determine prognosis and to assign appropriate therapy. Developing a prognostically useful staging system for children with NHL has been challenging because of the unique biology and differing patterns of spread and response to therapy of the four major subtypes of NHL seen in children and adolescents.[102] The Ann Arbor staging classification,[103] which is used for pediatric HL and NHL in adults, does not adequately reflect prognosis in childhood NHL for several reasons. The progression of disease in childhood NHL does not follow an orderly and predictable pattern of lymphatic spread, as in HL. Extensive extranodal disease is more common in children with NHL limiting the usefulness of Ann Arbor staging. The clinical staging system proposed at the St. Jude Children's Research Hospital[102] (Table 23.5) has been widely accepted. It relies on noninvasive procedures that can be carried out expeditiously. Like other staging systems that have been found to be more appropriate, primary site as well as disease extent is considered in assigning clinical stage. The primary differences between St. Jude staging system and the Ann Arbor staging system are as follows. In the St. Jude stage I disease, localized thoracic and abdominal diseases are excluded, other localize extranodal disease, however, is included. In St. Jude stage II disease, localized (resected) abdominal disease is included, but again any thoracic disease is excluded. St. Jude stage III disease includes any thoracic disease and paraspinal disease or facial nerve palsy. And the only disease included in St. Jude stage IV is marrow or CNS disease, other than paraspinal or facial nerve palsy. Using the St. Jude staging system, almost 40% of children with NHL present with stage I and II and the remainder with more advanced stage III and IV disease.[102] The distinction between lymphoma and leukemia is arbitrary and is based simply on the percentage of a bone marrow aspirate that is infiltrated by malignant cells. If the bone marrow has more than 25% blasts or malignant cells, the patient is considered to have acute leukemia rather than NHL. Children with between 5% and 25% marrow involvement are considered to have stage IV NHL, whereas less than 5% blasts in the marrow is considered to be normal.

As opposed to many leukemia criteria, any identifiable tumor cell in the CSF constitutes CNS disease.

The French Society of Pediatric Oncology (SFOP) and Berlin-Frankfurt-Munster (BFM) groups have adapted the St. Jude staging system for treatment assignment for children with B-cell lymphomas[104,105] (Table 23.6). The French risk stratification identifies the very best risk patients (Group A) and worst risk patients (Group C) and has a very heterogeneous Group B, consisting of patients with all clinical stages I to IV.[104] The BFM risk stratification subdivides the group based on clinical stage, as well as lactic dehydrogenase (LDH) at diagnosis, a surrogate marker for total disease burden.[105] For LL patients, studies have shown that all patients, regardless of stage, have better outcome when treated like ALL.[105-108] For ALCL, the European Intergroup for Childhood NHL (EICNHL) has stratified patients into low risk versus high risk based on clinical factors.[109] Patients with one of the following risk factors are considered high risk—visceral (lung, liver, or spleen), skin, or mediastinal involvement.[65] However, a Children's Oncology Group study could confirm only bone marrow involvement as poor prognostic clinical factor.[110]

With more sensitivity techniques, such as flow cytometry or PCR, several groups have now demonstrated that systemic disease in marrow and blood is much more frequent than would be predicted by clinical staging systems.[75,111-113] Early reports suggest that minimal disseminated disease or minimal residual disease detection in all the major subtypes of pediatric NHL may have prognostic value.[111-114]

DIAGNOSTIC WORKUP

The most expeditious and least invasive procedure should be used to establish the diagnosis, and the staging evaluation should be expedited because many children with NHL have rapidly growing tumor masses that can cause life-threatening

---

TABLE 23.5

ST. JUDE STAGING SYSTEM FOR NON-HODGKIN LYMPHOMA

Stage I
   A single tumor (extranodal) or single anatomic area (nodal) with the exclusion of thoracic or abdomen

Stage II
   A single tumor (extranodal) with regional node involvement
   Two or more nodal areas on the same side of the diaphragm
   Two single (extranodal) tumors with or without regional node involvement on the same side of the diaphragm
   A primary gastrointestinal tract tumor that is resectable, usually in the ileocecal area, with or without involvement of associated mesenteric nodes

Stage III
   Two single tumors (extranodal) on opposite sides of the diaphragm
   Two or more nodal areas above and below the diaphragm
   All the primary intrathoracic tumors (mediastinal, pleural, and thymic)
   All extensive primary intraabdominal disease
   All paraspinal or epidural tumors, regardless of other tumor site(s)

Stage IV
   Any of the above with initial central nervous system and/or bone marrow involvement

---

Note: >25% blasts in the marrow is considered leukemic disease. Any identifiable tumor cell in the CSF constitutes CNS disease.
Modified from Murphy SB. Classification, staging and end results of treatment of childhood non-Hodgkin lymphomas: dissimilarities from lymphomas in adults. Semin Oncol 1980;7:332–339.

TABLE 23.6

RISK STRATIFICATION SCHEMA

B-cell NHL (FAB/LMB)	
Stratum	Disease manifestations
A	Completely resected stage I and abdominal stage II
B	Multiple extra-abdominal sites. Nonresected stage I and II, III, IV (marrow <25% blasts, no CNS disease)
C	Mature B ALL (>25% blasts in marrow) and/or CNS disease
B-cell NHL (BFM)	
Stratum	Disease manifestations
R1	Completely resected stage I and abdominal stage II
R2	Nonresected stage I/II and stage III with LDH <500
R3	Stage III with LDH 500–999
	Stage IV, B-ALL (>25% blasts), no CNS disease and LDH <1,000
R4	Stage III, IV, B-ALL, and LDH ≥1,000 Any CNS disease

ALL, acute lymphoblastic leukemia; BFM, Berlin-Frankfurt-Munster; CNS, central nervous system; FAB, French-American-British; LDH, lactic dehydrogenase; NHL, non-Hodgkin lymphoma.

complications. Essentially all types of pediatric NHL may present as an anterior mediastinal mass, which may result in significant respiratory distress or SVC syndrome; epidural lesions may result in spinal cord compression and life-threatening metabolic disturbances with renal insufficiency may result from tumor lysis syndrome (TLS) even before therapy is initiated. A close examination of the peripheral blood and a bone marrow aspirate/biopsy should be undertaken in all patients. A bone marrow or pleural fluid examination may be diagnostic in the evaluation of a child with a mediastinal mass and the risks of anesthesia may be avoided. Similarly, examination of marrow or ascites may provide a diagnosis in a child with unresectable abdominal tumors. A lack of anemia, neutropenia, or thrombocytopenia does not rule out marrow involvement. All fluid, bone marrow, and tissue biopsy specimens should be adequate in quantity and appropriately prepared for special studies including karyotyping, molecular genetic studies, and immunophenotyping.

Radiologic studies should include computed tomography (CT) or magnetic resonance imaging of the primary site. A neck and chest CT scan should be obtained before any invasive procedure is undertaken in a child with a mediastinal mass to assess the major airways. Biopsy under general anesthesia should be avoided if at all possible, especially with significant airway narrowing or symptoms of respiratory distress.[115,116] The prebiopsy use of irradiation or steroids for respiratory distress may result in rapid shrinkage of the mediastinal mass but may jeopardize establishing a tissue diagnosis.[117,118] However, prednisone given up to 48 hours (40 to 60 mg/m^2/day) may result in rapid clinical improvement and preservation of diagnostic tissue. However, the use of steroids can make it difficult to determine if CNS disease was present at diagnosis. The role of routine bone scans is controversial, though other functional imaging such as gallium scans or positron emission tomography (PET) scans are usually performed at diagnostic workup. PET may be more

sensitive than gallium and is becoming the preferred study in patients with malignant lymphomas. At present, there are no data that upstaging a patient based solely on PET scanning is prognostic in childhood NHL. Data in HL and adult large cell lymphoma patients suggest that PET scanning to assess rapidity of response may be prognostic.[119] However, numerous studies have demonstrated that PET scanning has poor predictive value for detecting recurrence for pediatric lymphoma.[120–122] The remainder of the workup should include a complete serum metabolic profile and a lumbar puncture with examination of a cytocentrifuge specimen of cerebrospinal fluid.

CLINICAL MANAGEMENT

NHL in children and adolescents is a diverse group of aggressive neoplasms often requiring prompt intervention.[17] Therapy for children with NHL is best delivered by an experienced multidisciplinary team of pediatric subspecialists in oncology, surgery, radiotherapy, nursing, psychology, social work, nutrition, and physical therapy. Clinical trials are available for most types of NHL in children, and the opportunity to participate in these studies is offered to the majority of patients/families at tertiary care pediatric centers. Chemotherapy is the main component of treatment for NHL in children.

Prior to 1975, the prognosis for children with NHL was dismal.[17] Most of the children who survived had surgical removal of early-stage disease with or without radiation therapy. The addition of single cytotoxic agents only slightly improved the results with the exception of African children with BL.[3] The original studies of African BL included single-agent chemotherapy because radiation was not readily available. Surprisingly, treatment with one or more doses of cyclophosphamide resulted in some cures.[123] Even today, about 50% of African BL can be cured with a 28-day course of low-dose cyclophosphamide and prednisone and four intrathecal injections costing less than $50 (USD).[124]

The morphologic similarity between NHL and ALL and the invariable progression of LL to a leukemic phase led investigators at St. Jude in the early 1970s to treat NHL with chemotherapy regimens known to be effective in ALL.[125,126] This novel approach proved to be successful, especially for children with early-stage NHL. However, children with NHL involving the mediastinum had only transient remissions. More intensive ALL regimens such as the Memorial Sloan-Kettering LSA2L2 protocol[127] and the adriamycin (doxorubicin), prednisone, and vincristine (APO) regimen[128,129] developed at the Dana Farber Cancer Institute proved to be more successful in children with advanced-stage NHL. During this same time period, Ziegler[130] reported long-term disease control in both American and African patients with BL using a four-drug regimen of cyclophosphamide, methotrexate, vincristine, and prednisone, and Djerassi and Kim[131] demonstrated remissions in children with NHL after moderate-dose methotrexate infusions with citrovorum rescue. The results paved the way for prospective randomized clinical trials comparing leukemia versus lymphoma therapy for NHL in children.[132,133] These studies provided principles that still hold true today. Leukemia regimens proved to be superior to the lymphoma regimens for LL and the converse was noted for BL. However, results were roughly equivalent in children with advanced-stage large cell lymphoma.

During the next decade, there was continued progress due to refinements in chemotherapy and advances in supportive care.[17,134] The 5-year event-free survival (EFS) rates improved to 85% to 95% for children with early-stage NHL and to 70% to 90% for advanced-stage disease. CNS-directed therapy was recognized as an important component of these successful regimens, especially for children with lymphoblastic and BLs.[135,136] The addition of radiation therapy to chemotherapy for both early- and advanced-stage NHL was shown not to improve survival.[106,108,137,138] Since long-term follow-up studies have shown that the most significant factor for late death following treatment of pediatric NHL is radiation therapy,[139] it is currently recommended only for select patients, that is, treating CNS disease in LL patients and life-threatening emergencies at diagnosis such as airway compression from a mediastinal mass. The role of surgery in the treatment of children with NHL is mostly limited to diagnostic biopsies, placement of central venous access devices, and treatment of complications of therapy. However, in children presenting with localized disease, for example, ileocecal intussusception secondary to BL, complete resection of the involved segment of intestine and associated mesentery is recommended. Otherwise, there is no role for performing major tumor resection or debulking procedures in children with NHL.

Another major advancement is the decrease in early death due to TLS. Particular attention to kidney function and to serum levels of uric acid, potassium, calcium, and phosphorus is critical in these children. These patients, particularly BL and LL, are at high risk for TLS and uric acid nephropathy.[140] Measures should be instituted emergently to reduce the likelihood of uric acid nephropathy, including vigorous intravenous hydration, alkalinization of urine with sodium bicarbonate, administration of allopurinol, and careful monitoring of serum electrolytes. Rasburicase, a recombinant urate oxidase, has been shown in recent clinical trials to rapidly lower serum uric acid levels and prevent the metabolic problems associated with tumor lysis, including hyperphosphatemia and renal failure.[141-143] It is not necessary to alkalinize the urine when using rasburicase. Rasburicase should be used in place of allopurinol for children with NHL who have hyperuricemia or who are at high risk for TLS.[143] For the most part, this includes patients with stage III and IV BL, mature B-cell ALL, and select patients with bulky LL and DLBCL. The use of rasburicase has dramatically reduced the requirement for dialysis in this population.[141,143] In addition, a cytoreduction prophase has been added to many regimens, which also helps achieve tumor control without increasing the risk of clinical deterioration during initiation of therapy,[138,144,145,152] though this does not obviate the need for hydration and uric acid nephropathy prophylaxis.

Precursor Lymphoblastic Lymphoma

As previously discussed, the use of ALL regimens for children with LL proved to be a successful strategy.[125] The results of the early St. Jude trials demonstrated that the strategy was most effective in children with early-stage LL, whereas patients with mediastinal disease experienced a good initial response to therapy, but this remission was invariably followed by rapid progression of disease to involve the bone marrow and/or CNS within several months after diagnosis.[70,125] The use of intensive protocols designed for children with ALL, such as the BFM regimens, have been shown to be more effective in advanced-stage disease.[73,107,144] Irradiation of primary sites was a component of many of the early protocols, but it has subsequently shown not to improve outcome when added to chemotherapy. As in the management of ALL, CNS-directed therapy (intrathecal methotrexate and/or high-dose methotrexate as CNS consolidation therapy) was shown to be important to prevent CNS relapse even without the use of prophylactic CNS irradiation.[108]

The results of a Children's Cancer Group (CCG) trial that randomized children with NHL to cyclophosphamide, vincristine, intermediate-dose methotrexate, and prednisone (COMP) or to a modified LSA2L2 regimen (multiagent chemotherapy regimen pioneered at Memorial Sloan-Kettering Cancer Center) led to the paradigm of using regimens effective in ALL for advanced-stage LL.[132,133] In the CCG study, EFS for patients with localized NHL was 84% at 5 years, and no difference was seen between the two treatment regimens. Based on the results of this study, both CCG and the Pediatric Oncology Group (POG) began a series of studies using lymphoma protocols (cyclophosphamide, doxorubicin, vincristine, and prednisone [CHOP] or COMP) in early-stage lymphoma.[106,132,133,146] The POG demonstrated that CHOP followed by maintenance chemotherapy with mercaptopurine and methotrexate resulted in long-term EFS for approximately 65% of patients with early-stage LL.[106] These studies did not show a survival benefit for children who received involved field irradiation. Although the EFS was only 65%, the overall survival at 20 years was more than 90% because of the successful salvage of relapsed patients with the use of conventional ALL therapy. Although survival was excellent for these children, the EFS was inferior to the results achieved by investigators using the BFM ALL regimen (EFS, 90%).[107] Based on these findings, an ALL treatment approach rather than lymphoma-like therapy should be use for children even with early-stage LL (Table 23.7).

The mainstay of therapy for children with advanced-stage LL continues to be chemotherapy protocols designed for children with either high-risk ALL or T-cell ALL.[107,108] Therapeutic components common to all of these regimens include at least a four-drug induction with intrathecal therapy, intensification/consolidation incorporating high-dose methotrexate and leucovorin rescue, for CNS prophylaxis and maintenance. Studies from POG demonstrated the benefit of intensive L-asparaginase during the consolidation phase of therapy.[147] Until recently, CNS prophylaxis included the combined use of cranial irradiation and intrathecal chemotherapy. However, recent studies have demonstrated that cranial irradiation can be safely omitted if systemic high-dose methotrexate combined with intrathecal chemotherapy is administered.[108] However, cranial irradiation may be necessary for children who

TABLE 23.7

RECOMMENDED THERAPY FOR LOCALIZED NHL

WHO classification	Regimen	EFS (%)
Burkitt	CHOP[106] FAB/LMB[151,152] (Group A, B) BFM 90/95[145] (R1, R2)	90–95
Lymphoblastic (mostly precursor B)	BFM 90/95[107]	85–90
DLBCL	CHOP[106] FAB/LMB (Group A, B)[151,152] BFM 90/95 (R1, R2)[107]	90–95
ALCL	CHOP[106] BFM 90[168]	90

ALCL, anaplastic large cell lymphoma; BFM, Berlin-Frankfurt-Munster; CHOP, cyclophosphamide, doxorubicin, vincristine, and prednisone; DLBCL, diffuse large B-cell lymphoma; EFS, event-free survival; FAB, French-American-British; WHO, World Health Organization.

present with CNS disease (fewer than 5% of children with LL).[108]

Refractory disease or relapse at any site is a significant obstacle to long-term survival for children with advanced-stage LL with overall survival of less than 20%, with the only survivors achieving second CR and allogeneic blood or marrow transplant (BMT).[148,149] Most of the relapses occur within 2 years of diagnosis, but an occasional late relapse can be observed. In contrast to relapse for early-stage disease, the outcome after a second course of chemotherapy is poor for children with advanced-stage disease at initial presentation. If a remission can be achieved and approximately 30% to 50% can obtain long-term remissions following allogeneic BMT.[148,149]

Burkitt Lymphoma

Historically, cyclophosphamide was the single most active agent for the treatment of African children with BL.[3,123,130] Patients with facial tumors (early stage) had sustained remissions with single- or multiple-dose cyclophosphamide, whereas the majority of children with abdominal tumors relapsed with widespread disease that often included the CNS. Successor protocols incorporated cyclophosphamide in combination with other agents and included intrathecal methotrexate.[124] The combination of cyclophosphamide and vincristine with methotrexate or cytarabine was associated with higher remission rates and more durable remissions compared with outcomes after single-agent therapy.[130]

An EFS of 98% can achieved using as little as 6 weeks of cyclophosphamide, vincristine, prednisone, and doxorubicin (COPAD) chemotherapy for selected patients with completely resected stage I and stage II B-cell lymphoma (Table 23.6).[151] For localized, unresected disease, 95% EFS can be achieved with four cycles of multiagent chemotherapy using either the FAB/LMB or BFM 90/95 regimen (Table 23.6).[144,145,151]

More intensive chemotherapy is required for patients with advanced-stage BL and mature B-cell ALL. Several groups began to evaluate dose-intensified systemic and intrathecal chemotherapy for these higher risk patients.[79,80,104] Cyclophosphamide, methotrexate, and cytarabine were administered in high doses with or without anthracyclines and the epipodophyllotoxins. Treatment courses were repeated at early signs of bone marrow recovery in an attempt to prevent regrowth of lymphoma between cycles of chemotherapy. Growth factors such as filgrastim (G-CSF) were given in some protocols to speed bone marrow recovery. CNS prophylaxis included systemic chemotherapy that penetrated the CNS (high-dose methotrexate and cytarabine) and intensive intrathecal chemotherapy. The duration of treatment ranged from 2 months to 1 year. With this approach, EFS increased from 50% to 90% for stage III and for stage IV or mature B-cell ALL, the EFS rose from less than 20% to 85% to 90% for patients with stage IV (Table 23.6).[138,144,152] Patients with CNS disease fare less well but still achieved 70% EFS and do not benefit from CNS irradiation.[138,145] Adverse prognostic factors identified in these studies include high LDH, CNS disease at diagnosis, and slow response to the early phase of chemotherapy (days 1 to 7).[138,145] Further, chromosome abnormalities in addition to c-myc translocations involving deletion of 13q and duplication of 7q appear to be associated with an adverse outcome.[27]

The management of patients with BL who have refractory or relapsed disease presents even more of a challenge than for relapsed LL patients. Relapse tends to occur early, within 2 years of diagnosis, many while the patient is still receiving chemotherapy, and drug resistance is a major obstacle to successful therapy.[138] Salvage rates have remained at less than 20% for many years.[149,153] Allogeneic or autologous BMT offers the best chance of long-term survival after relapse.[149,154,155]

A remarkable improvement in outcome has been seen in adults with DLBCL by the addition of the anti-CD20 monoclonal antibody, rituximab to CHOP-like regimens.[156,157] It has become the standard of care for adults with DLBCL. There is not much experience with adding rituximab to regimens used to treat BL; however, MD Anderson Cancer Center has data that suggest an improved outcome in adult patients with BL adding rituximab to the hyper-CVAD regimen in a small cohort of patients compared with a historical cohort.[166] There currently exist no data to support the addition of rituximab to current aggressive regimens used in pediatric BL. A recent study from COG demonstrated safety and efficacy of adding rituximab to ifosfamide, carboplatin, and etoposide (ICE) for relapsed or refractory BL and DLBCL patients in a small cohort of patients.[158] The risk of increased immunosuppression is of particular concern as prolonged B-cell recovery and hypogammaglobulinemia has occurred with rituximab. Serious viral infections have occurred with rituximab use, including fatal progressive leukoencephalopathy associated with JC virus.[159,160] There is at present investigational studies combining current chemotherapy with rituximab in pediatric B-cell NHL.

Diffuse Large B-Cell Lymphoma

Most children with DLBCL have been treated on protocols designed for BL[138,144,145,152,153] (Table 23.6). Current molecular data seem to support this strategy, as it appears that much of the DLBCL observed in pediatrics is a more aggressive, highly proliferative disease with many tumors molecularly more resembling BL than DLBCL seen in adults.[25,26,30,34] The adult CHOP regimen was modified by POG investigators to include an induction phase of weekly vincristine, 1 month of prednisone, and a total therapy duration of 9 weeks. Children with stage I and II DLBCL in the POG studies achieved long-term survival exceeding 90%.[106] Results with LMB/FAB or BFM therapy for localized DLBCL are the same as for BL, that is, 98% EFS for completely resected disease with two cycles of chemotherapy and 95% EFS for stage I/II disease not resected with four cycles of chemotherapy.[145,151,152] In the past, children with primary bone disease received combined modality therapy including high-dose irradiation and were at risk for secondary malignancies in the field of irradiation.[161] The recent studies demonstrated that such irradiation may be safely omitted from therapy of children with NHL of bone.[145,151,152]

Patients with disseminated disease (stage III or IV) again have similar outcomes, for example, EFS 85% to 90%, as BL patients on current regimens.[138,144,145,152] Protocols for children with DLBCL have empirically included CNS-directed therapy. However, the risk of CNS involvement for patients with DLBCL (3%) and PBML (<1%) is much lower than for those with BL (9%) patients,[162] so it may be that patients with DLBCL may not require CNS-directed therapy, but this has yet to be demonstrated in children. Future studies will address this issue. Of interest, patients with PBML treated on these pediatric regimens had an inferior EFS of 65% to 70%, compared with DLBCL.[144,152] These results are very similar to the results observed for adult patients with PBML with regimen such as MACOP-B or VACOP-B[163] or dose-adjusted EPOCH.[164] It appears as in DLBCL of adults that rituximab may improve outcome in PBML.[165]

Children with DLBCL who develop relapse are often treated with salvage chemotherapy regimens based on the adult experience. The addition of rituximab to the ICE

RECOMMENDED THERAPY FOR DISSEMINATED NHL

WHO classification	Regimen	EFS (%)
Burkitt	FAB/LMB (Group B, C)[138,152] BFM 90/95[144,145] No craniospinal irradiation	70–90
Lymphoblastic (mostly precursor T)	BFM–NHL 90/95[107,108] Craniospinal irradiation for CNS (+) only	80–90
DLBCL	FAB/LMB (Group B, C)[138,155] BFM 90/95[144,145] No craniospinal irradiation	85–90
ALCL	APO[170], NHL BFM 90[168] ALCL 99[109] No craniospinal irradiation	70–75

ALCL, anaplastic large cell lymphoma; APO, Adriamycin (doxorubicin), prednisone, and vincristine; BFM, Berlin-Frankfurt-Munster; DLBCL, diffuse large B-cell lymphoma; EFS, event-free survival; FAB, French-American-British; WHO, World Health Organization.

regimen resulted in 50% complete responses.[158] If patient's disease remains chemosensitive then outcome with autologous BMT is better than with LL and BL, that is, 50% to 60% EFS.[149,154] Based on the results of recent trials for adults with DLBCL, which demonstrate an improved outcome when rituximab is added to standard chemotherapy,[156,157] future pediatric trials are planned to evaluate whether the favorable outcomes achieved with current regimens can be improved by the addition of rituximab (Table 23.8).

Anaplastic Large Cell Lymphoma

Patients with primary C-ALCL have not been treated in a uniform fashion. Despite the lack of controlled clinical trials, recommendations for treating primary C-ALCL include surgical removal and close observation. It is, therefore, very important to distinguish systemic ALCL with secondary involvement of skin from C-ALCL. One of the most helpful differentiating features is that primary C-ALCL usually fails to express ALK, whereas systemic ALCL in children is ALK+. Five-year survival exceeds 90% for C-ALCL.

Therapy for systemic ALCL varies considerably. Stage I and II disease is very effectively treated, that is, more than 90% EFS with CHOP for three cycles without radiation therapy.[106] Strategies for treating children with more advanced ALCL have included short-pulse chemotherapy proven effective in B-cell lymphomas, or modifications of high-risk ALL or T-cell protocols.[109,168,169] In the BFM B-NHL studies, children with stage II unresected and stage III ALCL received six courses of chemotherapy, and patients with stage IV or multifocal bone disease received six intensified courses.[168] The chemotherapy includes moderate or high-dose methotrexate, dexamethasone, ifosfamide, cyclophosphamide, etoposide, cytarabine, doxorubicin, and intrathecal chemotherapy. The EFS was about 75% for patients with stage II, III, and IV diseases. A follow-up study using this backbone of chemotherapy demonstrated that

intrathecal chemotherapy could be eliminated if high-dose methotrexate was given.[109] The POG conducted two randomized trials for children with large cell lymphoma that included systemic ALCL.[169,170] The standard arm of each protocol was based on the APO regimen. The first study tested whether the addition of cyclophosphamide to APO would improve EFS,[170] and the second protocol tested whether the addition of consolidation cycles of intermediate-dose methotrexate and cytarabine[169] would improve EFS. All patients received CNS prophylaxis with intrathecal chemotherapy and total duration of therapy was 1 year. Neither study demonstrated a benefit for the experimental arms, and the EFS was approximately 70% for the subgroup of patients with stage III and IV ALCL.

An observation in several studies has been the favorable outcome for survival after relapse of ALCL.[109,149,170,171] This is in contrast to the less optimistic outcome for children with relapsed advanced-stage LL and BL. Interestingly, in a French study of relapsed ALCL, there was an excellent response to single-agent vinblastine followed by some very durable second remissions.[171] The potential benefit of vinblastine combined with either an APO or BFM-like regimen is currently under investigation.

Rare Non-Hodgkin Lymphoma in Pediatrics

FL in children tends to be early stage. The overall prognosis has been excellent for all sites of FL in children with survivals exceeding 90%. Therapy has ranged from excisional biopsy alone to radiation therapy with or without chemotherapy. The chemotherapy has varied but often includes CHOP usually three to four cycles.[28] Given the unknown natural history of FLs in children, conservative management seems prudent.[172] Rituximab is used extensively in adult FL, but there are no data for its use in pediatric FL.

In the pediatric population, NMZL is more common than extranodal disease. Most children have localized disease involving nodes in the head and neck region and an excellent prognosis. Extranodal sites of disease have included the ocular adnexal structures and occasionally the stomach. Local treatment with surgery with or without local irradiation is recommended, but there are insufficient data to support any definitive treatment approaches.

All the PTCLs, excluding ALCL, are rare in children. Two retrospective studies have recently been published treating a variety of histologies. The POG experience reported on 20 patients treated on large cell lymphoma protocols.[44] Eight of 10 patients with localized disease had durable remissions, while only 4 of 10 with disseminated disease survived. The UKCCSG reported on 25 patients with a 5-year overall survival of 50%.[173] They also felt that the outcome was better for patients treated on T-cell ALL regimens as opposed to B-NHL regimens. A common strategy for adult patients with PTCL (other than ALCL) is to attempt to induce a remission, usually using CHOP-like therapy, followed by consolidation with BMT and with allogeneic BMT if a suitable donor is available. A couple of very rare forms of PTCL include subcutaneous panniculitic T-cell lymphoma and hepatosplenic T-cell lymphoma. Subcutaneous panniculitic T-cell lymphoma typical presents as subcutaneous nodules on the trunk and lower extremities but occasionally on the face. The most common differential diagnosis includes panniculitis, especially erythema nodosum, and cellulitis. The presence of hemophagocytic syndrome is a poor prognostic sign. Treatment has included steroids, multiagent chemotherapy, cyclosporine, and BMT. Hepatosplenic T-cell lymphoma is another rare lymphoma in both children and adults. Patients tend to be young males with marked splenomegaly, hepatomegaly, fever, and anemia, but without lymphadenopathy or association with

EBV. The diagnosis can be very difficult to make, as tumor cells tend not to grow in aggregates but within sinusoids of the spleen, liver, and bone marrow and can look like reactive T cells unless immunostaining is performed.[174] The prognosis is very poor. Hepatosplenic T-cell lymphoma has also been associated with hemophagocytic syndrome, and in some patients, cytogenetics have revealed isochromosome 7q and trisomy 8.[175] There have been anecdotal reports of survival following allogeneic BMT.[177] Hepatosplenic T-cell lymphoma has been associated with Crohn's disease and the anti-TNF antibody as therapy.[69] It is unclear if the anti-TNF antibody is part of the etiology, as this entity has not been observed in other types of patients receiving this agent. It more likely reflects a predisposition in patients with Crohn's disease. To date, more than 12 patients with Crohn's disease have developed hepatosplenic T-cell lymphoma but none have survived despite aggressive therapy including allogeneic BMT.[69]

Primary CNS lymphoma (PCNSL) represents 3% to 5% of all extranodal lymphomas.[17,89] It is estimated that about 1% of all PCNSL occur in people younger than 19 years. The majority of primary CNS lymphomas are of B-cell lineage (usually DLBCL) and many occur at a younger age in the setting of immunodeficiency. A few patients with PCNSL have been treated on the aggressive, CNS-directed regimens used of BL and DLBCL and appear to have 60% to 70% EFS without the use of radiation therapy.[138,145,176]

FUTURE CONSIDERATIONS

Refinements in systemic chemotherapy based largely on patterns of spread, risk of relapse, and the immunophenotype of the NHL in children have led to cure rates in approximately 80% to 85% of all patients. The emphasis for the near future is on further identification of children destined to do poorly and the development of new therapeutic approaches for these individuals. New targets for therapy will emerge as the molecular pathogenesis of the malignant lymphomas are elucidated using gene expression arrays. This information will also be valuable for developing more sensitive diagnostic tools, measurement of submicroscopic disease, and early response to therapy and for identifying new prognostic subgroups.

The use of monoclonal antibodies directed to B-cell antigens, particularly CD20, has been shown to improve the initial response rates and durations of remission when added to CHOP chemotherapy for adults with B-cell lymphoma. Similar approaches are being explored in the B-cell lymphomas of childhood. Similarly, antibodies to the CD30 antigen present on ALCL and HL are currently in early-phase clinical trials. Radioimmunoconjugates and drug conjugates to more specifically deliver cytotoxic therapy have considerable promise in the treatment of lymphomas. There are now small molecule inhibitors, such as ALK inhibitors in early-phase trials. It is likely that targeted therapy will substitute for some of the dose-intensive chemotherapy that is currently necessary for cure of children with advanced-stage NHL and thereby minimize the acute and long-term complications of therapy.

The future of improving outcome for children and adolescents with NHL is not in more randomized trials of empirically adding agents or dosages or schedules of currently available agents. The future must be biology driven focusing on specific molecule/pathway targeting.

References

1. International incidence of childhood cancer. Vol. II. Lyons, France: IARC Scientific Publication, 1998:1–391.
2. Percy CL, Smith MA, Linet M, et al. Lymphomas and reticuloendothelial neoplasms. In: Ries LAG, Smith MA, Gurney JG, et al., eds. Cancer incidence and survival among children and adolescents. United States SEER Program 1975–1995. Bethesda, MD: National Cancer Institute, SEER Program, 1999:35–49. NIH Pub. No. 99–4649.
3. Magrath IT. African Burkitt's lymphoma. History, biology, clinical features, and treatment. Am J Pediatr Hematol Oncol 1991;13:222–246.
4. Williams CK. Some biological and epidemiological characteristics of human leukaemia in Africans. Lyons, France: IARC Scientific Publication, 1984:687–712.
5. Adami J, Glimelius B, Cnattingius S, et al. Maternal and perinatal factors associated with non-Hodgkin's lymphoma among children. Int J Cancer 1996;65:774–777.
6. Buckley JD, Meadows AT, Kadin ME, et al. Pesticide exposures in children with non-Hodgkin lymphoma. Cancer 2000;89:2315–2321.
7. Landmann E, Oschlies I, Zimmermann M, et al. Secondary non-Hodgkin lymphoma (NHL) in children and adolescents after childhood cancer other than NHL. Br J Hematol 2008;143:387–394.
8. Dethloff LA, Graziano MJ, Goldenthal E, et al. Perspective on the carcinogenic potential of phenytoin based on rodent tumor bioassays and human epidemiological data. Hum Exp Toxicol 1996;15:335–348.
9. Gatti RA, Good RA. Occurrence of malignancy in immunodeficiency diseases. A literature review. Cancer 1971;28:89–98.
10. Kersey JH, Spector BD, Good RA. Cancer in children with primary immunodeficiency diseases. J Pediatr 1974;84:263–264.
11. Burkitt D. Determining the climatic limitations of a children's cancer common in Africa. Br Med J 1962;5311:1019–1023.
12. Epstein MA, Achong BG, Barr YM. Virus particles in cultured lymphoblasts from Burkitt's lymphoma. Lancet 1964;15:702–703.
13. Henle G, Henle W, Clifford P, et al. Antibodies to Epstein-Barr virus in Burkitt's lymphoma and control groups. J Natl Cancer Inst 1969;43:1147–1157.
14. Cohen JI. Epstein-Barr virus infection. N Engl J Med 2000;343:481–492.
15. Pagano JS, Huang CH, Levine P. Absence of Epstein-Barr viral DNA in American Burkitt's lymphoma. N Engl J Med 1973;289:1395–1399.
16. Karajannis MA, Hummel M, Oschlies I, et al. Epstein-Barr virus infection in Western European pediatric non-Hodgkin lymphomas. Blood 2003;102:4244.
17. Sandlund JT, Downing JR, Crist WM, et al. Non-Hodgkin's lymphoma in childhood. N Engl J Med 1996;334:1238–1248.
18. Perkins, SL. Work-up and diagnosis of pediatric non-Hodgkin's lymphomas. Pediatr Dev Pathol 2000;3:374–90.
19. Swerdlow, SH. Pediatric follicular lymphomas, marginal zone lymphomas, and marginal zone hyperplasia. Am J Clin Pathol 2004;122(suppl):S98–S109.
20. WHO classification of tumours of haematopoietic and lymphoid tissues. Lyon, France: IARC, 2008.
21. Raetz EA, Perkins SL, Bhojwani D, et al. Gene expression profiling reveals intrinsic differences between T-cell acute lymphoblastic leukemia and T-cell lymphoblastic lymphoma. Pediatr Blood Cancer 2006;47:130–140.
22. Burkhardt B, Moericke A, Klapper W, et al. Pediatric precursor T lymphoblastic leukemia and lymphoblastic lymphoma: differences in the common regions with loss of heterozygosity at chromosome 6q and their prognostic impact. Leuk Lymphoma 2008;49:451–461.
23. Mrozek K, Heerema NA, Bloomfield CD, et al. Cytogenetics in acute leukemia. Blood Rev 2004;18:115–136.
24. Harrison, CJ. Cytogenetics of paediatric and adolescent acute lymphoblastic leukaemia. Br J Haematol 2009;144:147–156.
25. Oschlies I, Klapper W, Zimmermann M, et al. Diffuse large B-cell lymphoma in pediatric patients belongs predominantly to the germinal-center type B-cell lymphomas: a clinicopathologic analysis of cases included in the German BFM (Berlin-Frankfurt-Munster) Multicenter Trial. Blood 2006;107:4047–4052.
26. Miles RR, Raphael M, McCarthy K, et al. Pediatric diffuse large B-cell lymphoma demonstrates a high proliferation index, frequent c-Myc protein expression, and a high incidence of germinal center subtype: report of the French-American-British (FAB) international study group. Pediatr Blood Cancer 2008;5:369–374.
27. Poirel HA, Cairo MS, Heerma NA, et al. Specific cytogenetic abnormalities are associated with a inferior outcome in children and adolescents with mature B-cell non-Hodgkin lymphoma: results of the FAB/LMB 96 international study. Leukemia 2009;23:323–331.
28. Lorsbach RB, Shay-Seymore D, Moore J, et al. Clinicopathologic analysis of follicular lymphoma occurring in children. Blood 2002;99:1959–1964.
29. Hartmann EM, Ott G, Rosenwald A, et al. Molecular biology and genetics of lymphomas. Hematol Oncol Clin North Am 2008;22:807–823.
30. Dave SS, Fu K, Wright GW, et al. Molecular diagnosis of Burkitt's lymphoma. N Engl J Med 2006;354:2431–2442.
31. Frost M, Newell JO, et al. Comparative immunohistochemical analysis of pediatric Burkitt lymphoma and diffuse large B-cell lymphoma. Am J Clin Pathol 2004;121:384–392.
32. Yustein JT, Dang CV. Biology and treatment of Burkitt's lymphoma. Curr Opin Hematol 2007;14:375–381.
33. Reiter A, Klapper W. Recent advances in the understanding and management of diffuse large B-cell lymphoma in children. Br J Hematol 2008;142:329–347.
34. Klapper W, Szczepanowski M, Burkhardt B, et al. Molecular profiling of pediatric mature B-cell lymphoma treated in population-based prospective clinical trials. Blood 2008;112:1374–1381.
35. Rosenwald A, Wright G, Leroy K, et al. Molecular diagnosis of primary mediastinal B cell lymphoma identifies a clinically favorable subgroup of diffuse large B cell lymphoma related to Hodgkin lymphoma. J Exp Med 2003;198(6):851–862.

36. Alizadeh AA, Eisen MB, Davis RE, et al. Distinct types of diffuse large B-cell lymphoma identified by gene expression profiling. Nature 2000;403:503–511.
37. Hans CP, Weisenburger DD, Greiner TC, et al. Confirmation of the molecular classification of diffuse large B-cell lymphoma by immunohistochemistry using a tissue microarray. Blood 2004;103:275–282.
38. Seidemann K, Tiemann M, Lauterbach I, et al. Primary mediastinal large B-cell lymphoma with sclerosis in pediatric and adolescent patients: treatment and results from three therapeutic studies of the Berlin-Frankfurt-Münster Group. J Clin Oncol 2003; 21:1782–1789.
39. Chadburn A, Frizzera G. Mediastinal large B-cell lymphoma versus classic Hodgkin lymphoma. Am J Clin Pathol 1999;112:155–158.
40. Joos S, Otano-Joos MI, Ziegler S, et al. Primary mediastinal (thymic) B-cell lymphoma is characterized by gains of chromosome material including 9p and amplification of the REL gene. Blood 1996;87:1571–1578.
41. Agrawal R, Wang J. Pediatric follicular lymphoma: a rare clinicopathologic entity. Arch Pathol Lab Med 2009;133:142–146.
42. Taddesse-Heath L, Pittaluga S, et al. Marginal zone B-cell lymphoma in children and young adults. Am J Surg Pathol 2003;27:522–531.
43. Claviez A, Meyer U, Dominick C, Sorbara L, et al. MALT lymphoma in children: a report from the NHL-BFM Study Group. Pediatr Blood Cancer 2006;47:210–214.
44. Hutchison RE, Laver JH, Chang M, et al. Non-anaplastic peripheral t-cell lymphoma in childhood and adolescence: a Children's Oncology Group study. Pediatr Blood Cancer 2008;51:29–33.
45. Jaffe ES. Mature T-cell and NK-cell lymphomas in the pediatric age group. Am J Clin Pathol 2004;122(suppl):S110–S121.
46. Savage KJ. Peripheral T-cell lymphomas. Blood Rev 2007;21:201–216.
47. Jones D, Dorfman DM. Phenotypic characterization of subsets of T cell lymphoma: towards a functional classification of T cell lymphoma. Leuk Lymphoma 2001;40: 449–459.
48. Amin HM, Lai R. Pathobiology of ALK+ anaplastic large-cell lymphoma. Blood 2007; 110:2259–2267.
49. Medeiros LJ, Elenitoba-Johnson KS. Anaplastic large cell lymphoma. Am J Clin Pathol 2007;127:707–722.
50. Querfeld C, Kunzel TM, Guitart J, Rosen ST. Primary cutaneous CD30+ lymphoproliferative disorders: new insights into biology and therapy. Oncology 2007;21:689–696.
51. Stein H, Mason DY, Gerdes J, et al. The expression of the Hodgkin's disease associated antigen Ki-1 in reactive and neoplastic lymphoid tissue: evidence that Reed-Sternberg cells and histiocytic malignancies are derived from activated lymphoid cells. Blood 1985;66:848–858.
52. Stein H, Foss HD, Dürkop H, et al. CD30(+) anaplastic large cell lymphoma: a review of its histopathologic, genetic, and clinical features. Blood 2000;96:3681–3695.
53. Kadin M. Anaplastic large cell lymphoma and its morphologic variants. Cancer Surv 1997;30:77–86.
54. Kinney M, Collins R, Greer JP, et al. A small-cell-predominant variant of primary Ki-1 (CD30)+ T-cell lymphoma. Am J Surg Pathol 1993;17:859–868.
55. Kinney MC, Kadin ME. The pathologic and clinical spectrum of anaplastic large cell lymphoma and correlation with ALK gene dysregulation. Am J Clin Pathol 1999;111 (1, suppl 1):S56–S67.
56. Chiarle R, Podda A, Prolla G, et al. CD30 in normal and neoplastic cells. Clin Immunol 1999;90:157–164.
57. Morris SW, Kirstein MN, Valentine MB, et al. Fusion of a kinase gene, ALK, to a nucleolar protein gene, NPM, in non-Hodgkin's lymphoma. Science 1994;26:1281–1284.
58. Duyster J, Bai RY, Morris SW. Translocations involving anaplastic lymphoma kinase (ALK). Oncogene 2001;20:5623–5637.
59. Mathew P, Sanger WG, Weisenburger DD, et al. Detection of the t(2;5)(p23;q35) and NPM-ALK fusion in non-Hodgkin's lymphoma by two-color fluorescence in situ hybridization. Blood 1997;89:1678–1685.
60. Pulford K, Morris SW, Mason DY. Anaplastic lymphoma kinase proteins and malignancy. Curr Opin Hematol 2001;8:231–236.
61. Perkins SL, Pickering D, Lowe EJ, et al. Childhood anaplastic large cell lymphoma has a high incidence of ALK gene rearrangement as determined by immunohistochemical staining and fluorescent in situ hybridisation: a genetic and pathological correlation. Br J Haematol 2005;131(5):624–627.
62. Cataldo KA, Jalal SM, Law ME, et al. Detection of t(2;5) in anaplastic large cell lymphoma: comparison of immunohistochemical studies, FISH, and RT-PCR in paraffin-embedded tissue. Am J Surg Pathol 1999;23:1386–1392.
63. Gascoyne RD, Aoun P, Wu D, et al. Prognostic significance of anaplastic lymphoma kinase (ALK) protein expression in adults with anaplastic large cell lymphoma. Blood 1999;93(11):3913–3921.
64. International T-cell Lymphoma Project. International peripheral T-cell and natural killer/T-cell lymphoma study: pathology findings and clinical outcomes. J Clin Oncol 2008;26:4124–4130.
65. Le Deley M-C, Reiter A, Williams D, et al. Prognostic factors in childhood anaplastic large cell lymphoma: results of a large European intergroup study. Blood 2008;111: 1560–1566.
66. Fraga M, Brousset P, Schlaifer D, et al. Bone marrow involvement in anaplastic large cell lymphoma. Am J Clin Pathol 1995;103:82–89.
67. Gordon BG, Weisenburger DD, Warkentin PI, et al. Peripheral T-cell lymphoma in childhood and adolescence. A clinicopathologic study of 22 patients. Cancer 1993;71:257–263.
68. Agnarsson B, Kadin M. Peripheral T-cell lymphomas in children. Semin Diagn Pathol 1995;12:314–324.
69. Rosh JR, Gross T, Mamula P, et al. Hepatosplenic T-cell lymphoma in adolescents and young adults with Crohn's disease: a cautionary tale. Inflamm Bowel Dis 2007;13: 1024–1030.
70. Bennett JM, Catovsky D, Daniel MT, et al. Proposals for the classification of the acute leukaemias. French-American-British (FAB) co-operative group. Br J Haematol 1976; 33:451–458.
71. Cohen MH, Bennett JM, Berard CW, et al. Burkitt's tumor in the United States. Cancer 1969;23:1259–1272.
72. Link MP, Roper M, Dorfman RF, et al. Cutaneous lymphoblastic lymphoma with pre-B markers. Blood 1983;61:838–841.
73. Neth O, Seidemann K, Jansen P, et al. Precursor B-cell lymphoblastic lymphoma in childhood and adolescence: clinical features, treatment, and results in trials NHL-BFM 86 and 90. Med Pediatr Oncol 2000;35:20–27.
74. Stein H, Foss HD, Durkop H, et al. CD30(+) anaplastic large cell lymphoma: a review of its histopathologic, genetic, and clinical features. Blood 2000;96:3681–3695.
75. Sabesean V, Cairo MS, Lones M, et al. Assessment of minimal residual disease in childhood non-Hodgkin's Lymphoma by polymerase chain reaction using patient-specific primers. J Pediatr Hematol Oncol 2003;25:109–113.
76. Dalle JH, Mechinaud F, Michon J, et al. Testicular disease in childhood b-cell non-Hodgkin's lymphoma: the French Society of Pediatric Oncology experience. J Clin Oncol 2001;19:2397–2403.
77. Lin P, Jones D, Dorfman DM, et al. Precursor B-cell lymphoblastic lymphoma: a predominantly extranodal tumor with low propensity for leukemic involvement. Am J Surg Pathol 2000;24:1480–1490.
78. Haddy TB, Adde MA, Magrath IT. CNS involvement in small noncleaved-cell lymphoma: is CNS disease per se a poor prognostic sign? J Clin Oncol 1991;9:1973–1982.
79. Magrath IT, Janus C, Edwards BK, et al. An effective therapy for both undifferentiated (including Burkitt's) lymphomas and lymphoblastic lymphomas in children and young adults. Blood 1984;63:1102–1111.
80. Murphy SB, Bowman WP, Abromowitch M, et al. Results of treatment of advanced-stage Burkitt's lymphoma and B cell (SIg+) acute lymphoblastic leukemia with high-dose fractionated cyclophosphamide and coordinated high-dose methotrexate and cytarabine. J Clin Oncol 1986;4:1732–1739.
81. Reiter A, Zimmermann W, Zimmermann M, et al. The role of initial laparotomy and second-look surgery in the treatment of abdominal B-cell non-Hodgkin's lymphoma of childhood. A report of the BFM Group. Eur J Pediatr Surg 1994;4:74–81.
82. Magrath IT, Ziegler JL. Bone marrow involvement in Burkitt's lymphoma and its relationship to acute B-cell leukemia. Leuk Res 1980;4:33–59.
83. Patte C, Auperin A, Michon J, et al. The Societe Francaise d'Oncologie Pediatrique LMB89 protocol: highly effective multiagent chemotherapy tailored to the tumor burden and initial response in 561 unselected children with B-cell lymphomas and L3 leukemia. Blood 2001;97:3370–3379.
84. Reiter A, Schrappe M, Ludwig WD, et al. Favorable outcome of B-cell acute lymphoblastic leukemia in childhood: a report of three consecutive studies of the BFM group. Blood 1992;80:2471–2478.
85. Pelicci PG, Knowles DM, Magrath I, et al. Chromosomal breakpoints and structural alterations of the c-myc locus differ in endemic and sporadic forms of Burkitt lymphoma. Proc Natl Acad Sci U S A 1986;83:2984–2988.
86. Shiramizu B, Barriga F, Neequaye J, et al. Patterns of chromosomal breakpoint locations in Burkitt's lymphoma: relevance to geography and Epstein-Barr virus association. Blood 1991;77:1516–1526.
87. Sandlund JT, Santana V, Abromowitch M, et al. Large cell non-Hodgkin lymphoma of childhood: clinical characteristics and outcome. Leukemia 1994;8:30–34.
88. Cairo MS, Sposto R, Hoover-Regan M, et al. Childhood and adolescent large-cell lymphoma (LCL): a review of the Children's Cancer Group experience. Am J Hematol 2003;72:53–63.
89. Eby NL, Grufferman S, Flannelly CM, et al. Increasing incidence of primary brain lymphoma in the US. Cancer 1988;62:2461–2465.
90. Kadin ME, Sako D, Berliner N, et al. Childhood Ki-1 lymphoma presenting with skin lesions and peripheral lymphadenopathy. Blood 1986;68:1042–1049.
91. LeBoit PE. Lymphomatoid papulosis and cutaneous CD30+ lymphoma. Am J Dermatopathol 1996;18:221–235.
92. Sandlund JT, Pui CH, Santana VM, et al. Clinical features and treatment outcome for children with CD30+ large-cell non-Hodgkin's lymphoma. J Clin Oncol 1994;12: 895–898.
93. Onciu M, Behm FG, Raimondi SC, et al. ALK-positive anaplastic large cell lymphoma with leukemic peripheral blood involvement is a clinicopathologic entity with an unfavorable prognosis. Report of three cases and review of the literature. Am J Clin Pathol 2003;120:617–625.
94. Finn LS, Viswanatha DS, Belasco JB, et al. Primary follicular lymphoma of the testis in childhood. Cancer 1999;85:1626–1635.
95. Lu D, Medeiros J, Eskenazi AE, et al. Primary follicular large cell lymphoma of the testis in a child. Arch Pathol Lab Med 2001;125:551–554.
96. Shaw PH, Cohn SL, Morgan ER, et al. Natural killer cell lymphoma: report of two pediatric cases, therapeutic options, and review of the literature. Cancer 2001;91:642–646.
97. Mraz-Gernhard S, Natkunam Y, Hoppe RT, et al. Natural killer/natural killer-like T-Cell lymphoma, CD56+, presenting in the skin: an increasingly recognized entity with an aggressive course. J Clin Oncol 2001;19:2179–2188.
98. Natkunam Y, Smoller BR, Zehnder JL, et al. Aggressive cutaneous NK and NK-like T-cell lymphomas: clinicopathologic, immunohistochemical, and molecular analyses of 12 cases. Am J Surg Pathol 1999;23:571–581.
99. Wain EM, Orchard GE, Whittaker SJ, et al. Outcome in 34 patients with juvenile-onset mycosis fungoides: a clinical, immunophenotypic, and molecular study. Cancer 2003;98:2282–2290.
100. Zackheim HS, McCalmont TH, Deanovic FW, et al. Mycosis fungoides with onset before 20 years of age. J Am Acad Dermatol 1997;36:557–562.
101. Quaglino P, Zaccagna A, Verrone A, et al. Mycosis fungoides in patients under 20 years of age: report of 7 cases, review of the literature and study of the clinical course. Dermatology 1999;199:8–14.
102. Murphy SB. Classification, staging and end results of treatment of childhood non-Hodgkin's lymphomas: dissimilarities from lymphomas in adults. Semin Oncol 1980; 7:332–339.
103. Carbone PP, Kaplan HS, Musshoff K, et al. Report of the Committee on Hodgkin's Disease Staging Classification. Cancer Res 1971;31:1860–1861.
104. Patte C, Philip T, Rodary C, et al. Improved survival rate in children with stage III and IV B cell non-Hodgkin's lymphoma and leukemia using multi-agent chemotherapy: results of a study of 114 children from the French Pediatric Oncology Society. J Clin Oncol 1986;4:1219–1226.
105. Reiter A, Schrappe M, Parwaresch R, et al. Non-Hodgkin's lymphomas of childhood and adolescence: results of a treatment stratified for biologic subtypes and stage—a report of the Berlin-Frankfurt-Munster Group. J Clin Oncol 1995;13:359–372.
106. Link MP, Shuster JJ, Donaldson SS, et al. Treatment of children and young adults with early-stage non-Hodgkin's lymphoma. N Engl J Med 1997;337:1259–1266.
107. Reiter A, Schrappe M, Ludwig WD, et al. Intensive ALL-type therapy without local radiotherapy provides a 90% event-free survival for children with T-cell lymphoblastic lymphoma: a BFM group report. Blood 2000;95:416–421.
108. Burkhardt B, Woessmann W, Zimmermann M, et al. Impact of cranial radiotherapy on central nervous system prophylaxis in children and adolescents with central nervous system-negative stage III or IV lymphoblastic lymphoma. J Clin Oncol 2006;24: 491–499.

109. Brugieres L, Le Deley M-C, Rosolen A, et al. Impact of the methotrexate administration dose on the need for intrathecal treatment in children and adolescents with anaplastic large cell lymphoma: results of a randomized trial of the EICNHL group. J Clin Oncol 2009;27:897–903.
110. Lowe EJ, Sposto R, Perkins SL, et al. Intensive, compressed chemotherapy for nonlocalized anaplastic large cell lymphoma in children and adolescents: a Children's Cancer Group study. Pediatr Blood Cancer 2009;52:335–339.
111. Damm-Welk C, Busch K, Burkhardt B, et al. Prognostic significance of circulating tumor cells in bone marrow or peripheral blood as detected by qualitative and quantitative PCR in pediatric NPM-ALK-positive anaplastic large-cell lymphoma. Blood 2007;110:670–677.
112. Mussolin K, Pillon M, d'Amore ES, et al. Prevalence and clinical implications of bone marrow involvement in pediatric anaplastic large cell lymphoma. Leukemia 2005;19: 1643–1647.
113. Coustan-Smith E, Sandlund JT, Perkins SL, et al. Minimal disseminated disease in childhood T-cell lymphoblastic lymphoma: a report from the Children's Oncology Group. J Clin Oncol 2009;27:3533–3539.
114. Mussolin L, Pillon M, Conter V, et al. Prognostic role of minimal residual disease in mature B-cell acute lymphoblastic leukemia of childhood. J Clin Oncol 2007;25: 5254–5261.
115. King DR, Patrick LE, Ginn-Pease ME, et al. Pulmonary function is compromised in children with mediastinal lymphoma. J Pediatr Surg 1997;32:294–299; discussion 299–300.
116. Shamberger RC, Holzman RS, Griscom NT, et al. Prospective evaluation by computed tomography and pulmonary function tests of children with mediastinal masses. Surgery 1995;118:468–471.
117. Loeffler JS, Leopold KA, Recht A, et al. Emergency prebiopsy radiation for mediastinal masses: impact on subsequent pathologic diagnosis and outcome. J Clin Oncol 1986; 4:716–721.
118. Borenstein SH, Gerstle T, Malkin D, et al. The effects of prebiopsy corticosteroid treatment on the diagnosis of mediastinal lymphoma. J Pediatr Surg 2000;35:973–976.
119. Cheson BD, Pfistner B, Juweid ME, et al. Revised response criteria for malignant lymphoma. J Clin Oncol 2007;25:579–586.
120. Levine JM, Weiner M, Kelly KM. Routine use of PET scans after completion of therapy in pediatric Hodgkin disease results in a high false positive rate. J Pediatr Hematol Oncol 2006;28:711–714.
121. Rhodes MM, Delbeke D, Whitlock JA, et al. Utility of FDG-PET/CT in follow-up of children treated for Hodgkin and non-Hodgkin lymphoma. J Pediatr Hematol Oncol 2006;28:300–306.
122. Meany HJ, Gidvani VK, Minniti CP. Utility of PET scans to predict disease relapse in pediatric patients with Hodgkin lymphoma. Pediatr Blood Cancer 2007;48:399–402.
123. Burkitt D. Long-term remissions following one and two-dose chemotherapy for African lymphoma. Cancer 1967;20:756–759.
124. Hesseling P, Molyneux E, Kamiza S, et al. Endemic Burkitt lymphoma; a 28 day treatment schedule with cyclophosphamide and intrathecal methotrexate. Ann Trop Paediatr 2009;29:29–34.
125. Pinkel D, Johnson W, Aur RJ. Non-Hodgkin's lymphoma in children. Br J Cancer 1975;31(suppl 2):298–323.
126. Lemerle M, Gerard-Marchant R, Sancho H, et al. Natural history of non-Hodgkin's malignant lymphomata in children. A retrospective study of 190 cases. Br J Cancer 1975;31(suppl 2):324–331.
127. Wollner N, Exelby PR, Lieberman PH. Non-Hodgkin's lymphoma in children: a progress report on the original patients treated with the LSA2-L2 protocol. Cancer 1979;44:1990–1999.
128. Weinstein HJ, Vance ZB, Jaffe N, et al. Improved prognosis for patients with mediastinal lymphoblastic lymphoma. Blood 1979;53:687–694.
129. Weinstein HJ, Cassady JR, Levey R. Long-term results of the APO protocol (vincristine, doxorubicin [adriamycin], and prednisone) for treatment of mediastinal lymphoblastic lymphoma. J Clin Oncol 1983;1:537–541.
130. Ziegler JL. Treatment results of 54 American patients with Burkitt's lymphoma are similar to the African experience. N Engl J Med 1977;297:75–80.
131. Djerassi I, Kim JS. Methotrexate and citrovorum factor rescue in the management of childhood lymphosarcoma and reticulum cell sarcoma (non-Hodgkin's lymphomas): prolonged unmaintained remissions. Cancer 1976;38:1043–1051.
132. Anderson JR, Wilson JF, Jenkin DT, et al. Childhood non-Hodgkin's lymphoma. The results of a randomized therapeutic trial comparing a 4-drug regimen (COMP) with a 10-drug regimen (LSA2-L2). N Engl J Med 1983;308:559–565.
133. Anderson JR, Jenkin RD, Wilson JF, et al. Long-term follow-up of patients treated with COMP or LSA2L2 therapy for childhood non-Hodgkin's lymphoma: a report of CCG-551 from the Childrens Cancer Group. J Clin Oncol 1993;11:1024–1032.
134. Pinkerton CR. The continuing challenge of treatment for non-Hodgkin's lymphoma in children. Br J Haematol 1999;107:220–234.
135. Mandell LR, Wollner N, Fuks Z. Is cranial radiation necessary for CNS prophylaxis in pediatric NHL? Int J Radiat Oncol Biol Phys 1987;13:359–363.
136. Murphy SB, Bleyer WA. Cranial irradiation is not necessary for central-nervous-system prophylaxis in pediatric non-Hodgkin's lymphoma. Int J Radiat Oncol Biol Phys 1987;13:467–468.
137. Murphy SB, Hustu HO. A randomized trial of combined modality therapy of childhood non-Hodgkin's lymphoma. Cancer 1980;45:630–637.
138. Cairo MS, Gerrard M, Sposto R, et al. Results of a randomized international study of high-risk central nervous system B non-Hodgkin lymphoma and B acute lymphoblastic leukemia in children and adolescents. Blood 2007;109:2736–2743.
139. Bluhm EC, Ronckers C, Hayashi RJ, et al. Cause-specific mortality and second cancer incidence after non-Hodgkin lymphoma: a report from the Childhood Cancer Survivor Study. Blood 2008;111:4014–4021.
140. Tsokos GC, Balow JE, Spiegel RJ, et al. Renal and metabolic complications of undifferentiated and lymphoblastic lymphomas. Medicine (Baltimore) 1981;60:218–229.
141. Pui CH, Mahmoud HH, Wiley JM, et al. Recombinant urate oxidase for the prophylaxis or treatment of hyperuricemia in patients with leukemia or lymphoma. J Clin Oncol 2001;19:697–704.
142. Pui CH, Relling MV, Lascombes F, et al. Urate oxidase in prevention and treatment of hyperuricemia associated with lymphoid malignancies. Leukemia 1997;11:1813–1816.
143. Goldman SC, Holcenberg JS, Finklestein JZ, et al. A randomized comparison between rasburicase and allopurinol in children with lymphoma or leukemia at high risk for tumor lysis. Blood 2001;97:2998–3003.
144. Reiter A, Schrappe M, Tiemann M, et al. Improved treatment results in childhood B-cell neoplasms with tailored intensification of therapy: a report of the Berlin-Frankfurt-Münster Group Trial NHL-BFM 90. Blood 1999;94:3294–3306.
145. Woessmann W, Seidemann K, Mann G, et al. The impact of the methotrexate administration schedule and dose in the treatment of children and adolescents with B-cell neoplasms: a report of the BFM Group Study NHL-BFM95. Blood 2005;105:948–958.
146. Meadows AT, Sposto R, Jenkin RD, et al. Similar efficacy of 6 and 18 months of therapy with four drugs (COMP) for localized non-Hodgkin's lymphoma of children: a report from the Childrens Cancer Study Group. J Clin Oncol 1989;7:92–99.
147. Amylon MD, Shuster J, Pullen J, et al. Intensive high-dose asparaginase consolidation improves survival for pediatric patients with T cell acute lymphoblastic leukemia and advanced stage lymphoblastic lymphoma: a Pediatric Oncology Group study. Leukemia 1999;13:335–342.
148. Abromowitch M, Sposto R, Perkins S, et al. Shortened intensified multi-agent chemotherapy and non-cross resistant maintenance therapy for advanced lymphoblastic lymphoma in children and adolescents: report from the Children's Oncology Group. Br J Haematol 2008;143:261–267.
149. Attarbaschi A, Dworzak M, Steiner M, et al. Outcome of children with primary resistant or relapsed non-Hodgkin lymphoma and mature B-cell leukemia after intensive first-line treatment: a population-based analysis of the Austrian Cooperative Study Group. Pediatr Blood Cancer 2005;44:70–76.
150. Burkhardt B, Reiter A, Landmann E, et al. Poor outcome for children and adolescents with progressive disease or relapse of lymphoblastic lymphoma: a report from the Berlin-Frankfurt-Munster group. J Clin Oncol 2009;27:3363–3369.
151. Gerrard M, Cairo MS, Weston C, et al. Excellent survival following two courses of COPAD chemotherapy in children and adolescents with resected localized B-cell non-Hodgkin's lymphoma: results of the FAB/LMB 96 international study. Br J Haematol 2008;141:840–847.
152. Patte C, Auperin A, Gerrard M, et al. Results of the randomized international FAB/LMB96 trial for intermediate risk B-cell non-Hodgkin lymphoma in children and adolescents: it is possible to reduce treatment for the early responding patients. Blood 2007;109:2773–2780.
153. Cairo MS, Sposto R, Perkins SL, et al. Burkitt's and Burkitt-like lymphoma in children and adolescents: a review of the Children's Cancer Group experience. Br J Haematol 2003;120:660–670.
154. Sandlund JT, Bowman L, Heslop HE, et al. Intensive chemotherapy with hematopoietic stem-cell support for children with recurrent or refractory NHL. Cytotherapy 2002; 4:253–258.
155. Ladenstein R, Pearce R, Hartmann O, et al. High-dose chemotherapy with autologous bone marrow rescue in children with poor-risk Burkitt's lymphoma: a report from the European Lymphoma Bone Marrow Transplantation Registry. Blood 1997;90: 2921–2930.
156. Coiffier B, Lepage E, Briere J, et al. CHOP chemotherapy plus rituximab compared with CHOP alone in elderly patients with diffuse large-B-cell lymphoma. N Engl J Med 2002;346:235–242.
157. Pfreundschuh M, Trümper L, Osterborg A, et al. CHOP-like chemotherapy plus rituximab versus CHOP-like chemotherapy alone in young patients with good-prognosis diffuse large-B-cell lymphoma: a randomised controlled trial by the MabThera International Trial (MInT) Group. Lancet Oncol 2006;7:379–391.
158. Griffin TC, Weitzman S, Weinstein H, et al. A study of rituximab and ifosfamide, carboplatin, and etoposide chemotherapy in children with recurrent/refractory B-cell (CD20+) non-Hodgkin lymphoma and mature B-cell acute lymphoblastic leukemia: a report from the Children's Oncology Group. Pediatr Blood Cancer 2009;52:177–181.
159. Askoy S, Harputluoglu H, Kilckap S, et al. Rituximab-related viral infections in lymphoma patients. Leuk Lymphoma 2007;48:1307–1312.
160. Carson KR, Evens AM, Richey EA, et al. Progressive multifocal leukoencephalopathy after rituximab therapy in HIV-negative patients: a report of 57 cases from the Research on Adverse Drug Events and Reports project. Blood 2009;113:4834–4840.
161. Loeffler JS, Tarbell NJ, Kozakewich H, et al. Primary lymphoma of bone in children: analysis of treatment results with adriamycin, prednisone, Oncovin (APO), and local radiation therapy. J Clin Oncol 1986;4:496–501.
162. Salzburg J, Burkhardt B, Zimmermann M, et al. Prevalence, clinical pattern, and outcome of CNS involvement in childhood and adolescent non-Hodgkin's lymphoma differ by non-Hodgkin's lymphoma subtype: a Berlin-Frankfurt-Munster Group Report. J Clin Oncol 2007;25:3915–3922.
163. Todeschini G, Secchi S, Mora E, et al. Primary mediastinal large B-cell lymphoma (PMLBCL): long term results from a retrospective multicentre Italian experience in 138 patients treated with CHOP or MACOP-B/VACOP-B. Br J Cancer 2004;90: 372–376.
164. Wilson WH, Grossbard ML, Pittaluga S, et al. Dose-adjusted EPOCH chemotherapy for untreated large B-cell lymphomas: a pharmacodynamic approach with high efficacy. Blood 2002;99:2685–2693.
165. Dunleavy K, Pittaluga S, janik J, et al. Primary mediastinal large B-cell lymphoma (PMBL) outcome may be significantly improved by the addition of rituximab to dose-adjusted (DA)-EPOCH and obviates the need for radiation: results from a prospective study of 44 patients [abstract]. Blood 2006;108:209.
166. Thomas DA, Fadel S, O'Brien S, et al. Chemoimmunotherapy with hyper-CVAD plus rituximab for the treatment of adult Burkitt and Burkitt-type lymphoma or acute lymphoblastic leukemia. Cancer 2006;106:1569–1580.
167. Kobrinsky NL, Sposto R, Shah NR, et al. Outcomes of treatment of children and adolescents with recurrent non-Hodgkin's lymphoma and Hodgkin's disease with dexamethasone, etoposide, cisplatin, cytarabine, and l-asparaginase, maintenance chemotherapy, and transplantation: Children's Cancer Group Study CCG-5912. J Clin Oncol 2001;19:2390–2396.
168. Seidemann K, Tiemann M, Schrappe M, et al. Short-pulse B-non-Hodgkin lymphoma-type chemotherapy is efficacious treatment for pediatric anaplastic large cell lymphoma: a report of the Berlin-Frankfurt-Munster Group Trial NHL-BFM 90. Blood 2001; 97:3699–3706.
169. Laver JH, Kraveka JM, Hutchinson RE, et al. Advanced-stage large-cell lymphoma in children and adolescents: results of a randomized trial incorporating intermediate dose methotrexate and high dose ARA-C in the maintenance phase of the APO regimen. A Pediatric Oncology Group phase III trial. J Clin Oncol 2005;23:541–547.
170. Laver JH, Mahmoud H, Pick TE, et al. Results of a randomized phase III trial in children and adolescents with advanced stage diffuse large cell non-Hodgkin's lymphoma: a Pediatric Oncology Group study. Leuk Lymphoma 2001;42:399–405.

171. Brugieres L, Quartier P, Le Deley MC, et al. Relapses of childhood anaplastic large-cell lymphoma: treatment results in a series of 41 children—a report from the French Society of Pediatric Oncology. Ann Oncol 2000;11:53–58.

172. Atra A, Meller ST, Stevens RS, et al. Conservative management of follicular non-Hodgkin's lymphoma in childhood. Br J Haematol 1998;103:220–223.

173. Windsor R, Stiller C, Webb D. Peripheral T-cell lymphoma in childhood: population-based experience in the United Kingdom over 20 years. Pediatr Blood Cancer 2008;50:784–787.

174. Farcet J, Gaulard P, Marolleau JP, et al. Hepatosplenic T-cell lymphoma: sinusoidal/sinusoidal localization of malignant cells expressing the T-cell receptor gamma delta. Blood 1990;75:2213–2219.

175. Chin M, Mugishima H, Takamura M, et al. Hemophagocytic syndrome and hepatosplenic gammadelta T-cell lymphoma with isochromosome 7q and 8 trisomy. J Pediatr Hematol Oncol 2004;26:375–378.

176. Abla O, Sandlund JT, Sung L, et al. A case series of pediatric primary central nervous system lymphoma: favorable outcome without cranial irradiation. Pediatr Blood Cancer 2006;47:880–855.

177. Domm JA, Thompson M, Kuttesch JF, et al. Allogeneic bone marrow transplantation for chemotherapy-refractory hepatosplenic gd T-cell lymphoma. J Pediatr Hematol Oncol 2005;27:607–610.

CHAPTER 24 ■ LYMPHOPROLIFERATIVE DISORDERS AND MALIGNANCIES RELATED TO IMMUNODEFICIENCIES

BRUCE SHIRAMIZU, ROBERT WILKINSON, AND ROBERT HAYASHI

INTRODUCTION

In 1959, Thomas conceptualized that the immune system played a role in oncogenesis.[1] He hypothesized that immune surveillance was an active process that controlled the emergence of malignant clones from somatic cells in an immunocompetent individual. Data to support this hypothesis were drawn from reports of increased malignancies in patients with immunodeficiencies, both primary and secondary, compared with the general population.[2,3] Primary immunodeficiencies result from genetic defects, while secondary immunodeficiencies are acquired from human immunodeficiency virus (HIV) type 1 infection or immunosuppression following solid organ transplantation (SOT) or hematopoietic blood or marrow transplantation (BMT).

Children and adolescents with primary and secondary immunodeficiencies are at risk for developing unique types of cancers. In the majority of primary and secondary immunodeficiency conditions, reactivated or chronic infections play a pivotal role in the development of lymphomas and carcinomas. Patients with primary or secondary immunodeficiencies affecting T-cell function are at increased risk of developing lymphomas, often associated with Epstein-Barr virus (EBV). Prolonged immune-suppressed states, as a result of HIV infection or iatrogenic immunosuppression used in transplantation, also increases the risk for solid tumors that are linked to infection with other viruses such as human herpesvirus-8 (HHV-8)–associated Kaposi's sarcoma (KS) or human papillomavirus (HPV)–associated squamous cell carcinoma (skin, cervical, and anal cancers).[4-8] Alternatively, individuals with inherited defects of DNA repair and genomic instability, for example, Bloom syndrome and ataxia telangiectasia (AT), have a propensity to develop tumors of hematopoietic and epithelial origin.[9] In fact, many cancers diagnosed in immunocompromised patients are not specifically associated with an infectious agent. Therefore, the defect in immune surveillance may involve more than just the inability to properly control infections but also the inability to identify and/or eliminate cells with abnormalities in proliferation, function, and/or apoptosis.

The malignancies diagnosed in children with immunodeficiencies may be cancers not typically encountered in pediatric oncology; and the therapeutic response to standard treatment may be compromised due to the underlying immunodeficiency. In general, if baseline immunity can be restored or enhanced, that is, reduction of immunosuppression in transplant recipients, effective antiviral therapy for HIV-infected patients, or immune replacement with hematopoietic stem cell transplant in primary immunodeficient patients, the risk of cancer or recurrence can be greatly reduced or eliminated.

Regardless of the etiology of the immune defect, immunodeficient patients with cancer have increased morbidity and mortality than the general population with histologically similar malignancies. However, the malignancies associated with immunodeficiencies are not necessarily more resistant to conventional therapies. These patients usually tolerate cytotoxic therapy poorly due to an increased risk of infectious complications. This chapter will focus on advances made in understanding the pathogenesis and progress in the treatment of malignancies and lymphoproliferative disorders (LPDs) related to immunodeficiencies in children.

EPSTEIN-BARR VIRUS AND MALIGNANCIES

Lymphoproliferative disease associated with EBV (EBV-LPD) is the most common "malignancy" seen in patients with T-cell defects, either inherited or acquired. EBV-LPD represents a spectrum of clinically and morphologically heterogeneous lymphoid proliferative processes. Primarily due to the growing number of SOT and BMT, it is estimated that more than 150 cases of EBV-LPD are diagnosed in children in the United States each year.[10] This compares with the approximately 750 cases of childhood and adolescent non-Hodgkin lymphoma (NHL) diagnosed per year in the United States consisting of 300 Burkitt lymphoma (BL), 200 lymphoblastic lymphoma, 100 anaplastic large cell lymphoma, 100 diffuse large B-cell lymphoma (DLBCL), and 50 cases of other NHL.[11,12]

Pathophysiology of Epstein-Barr Virus Infection

EBV is a gamma herpesvirus and one of eight known HHVs. Human beings are the only host that EBV infects naturally where B lymphocytes and the epithelium of the oronasopharynx provide natural cell targets for the virus. EBV initially infects B lymphocytes in lymphoid tissue of Waldeyer's ring where B cells may remain latently infected.[13,14] The latently infected B lymphocytes circulate as resting memory B cells to secondary lymphatic organs, that is, lymph nodes, spleen, and bone marrow,[15] and become the reservoir for EBV infection.[16] The number of latently infected B lymphocytes is approximately 10^{-5} to 10^{-6} of all B lymphocytes and this number remains stable for a lifetime.[16,17] During viral reactivation and replication, cell lysis occurs with viral shedding into the saliva. Salivary EBV can subsequently be transmitted horizontally or result in infection of host epithelium, and during virus replication can infect other B cells.

During latent infection, nine viral-encoded proteins (EBNA-1, EBNA-2, EBNA-3A, EBNA-3B, EBNA-3C, leader protein, latent membrane protein 1 [LMP-1], LMP-2A, and LMP-2B) are expressed.[18] Over the last few years, studies have provided insight into understanding the role of EBV-encoded RNAs (EBERs), EBER-1 and EBER-2, in latently infected cells.[19-23] In addition, the Bam HI-A rightward transcripts (BARTs) are generally found in infected cells and expressed in EBV-associated tumors with their function not entirely clear.[24,25] Expression of EBV genes varies among the spectrum of EBV-associated diseases and often differs from in vitro immortalized lymphoblastoid B-cell lines (LCLs) or normal human resting B cells infected by EBV.[26] Briefly, EBV-positive Burkitt lymphoma cells commonly express only EBNA-1, EBER-1, and EBER-2 that define type I latency. Type I latency is also observed in a portion of EBV-positive gastric carcinoma. Type II latency, as defined by EBNA-1, LMP-1, LMP-2, EBER1, and EBER2 expression, is found in EBV-positive nasopharyngeal carcinoma, T-cell NHL, and the Reed-Sternberg cells of some Hodgkin lymphoma. The EBV-LPD–infected cells observed in immunodeficient patients resemble in vitro immortalized LCL and generally express all nine of EBV-related latent proteins (type III latency). It has been shown that peripheral resting CD23+ B cells are the source of EBV latency in seropositive healthy individuals. These EBV-infected resting B cells express only LMP-2, EBER1, and EBER2 together with BART (type IV latency).[27]

Virus reactivation and replication is characterized by expression of EBV BZLF1 gene product or ZEBRA (ZEBV replication activator) protein, an immediate early gene product that triggers viral replication in these cells.[18,28] This protein also transactivates other immediate early genes that results in upregulation and expression of early gene products essential for viral replication, including viral DNA polymerase and viral thymidine kinase. Expression of late viral gene products follows, including VCA (viral capsid antigen), the major envelope glycoprotein (gp350), and the viral protein BCRF1.[18] It is important to keep in mind that viral replication always results in lysis and death of the host T cell, so when discussing therapies for EBV-associated B-cell proliferation, inhibition of viral replication would appear to be counterproductive.

Immune Response to Epstein-Barr Virus Infection

Understanding the immune response to EBV infection is essential to understand the pathogenesis of EBV-related disease. EBV is a very potent immune stimulus. The immune system controls lymphoproliferation in the normal host and maintains a host/virus symbiosis. Figure 24.1 illustrates the delicate balance between the host T-cell immune response and control of B-cell proliferation of latently infected B cells. In a healthy individual, while only 10^{-5} to 10^{-6} B cells are latently infected with EBV, approximately 1% to 5% of all circulating CD8+ T cells are capable of reacting against EBV.[18,29] Initially, B-cell proliferation results in production of EBV-specific and nonspecific antibodies. The quantity of virus-containing B cells rises during the acute phase but never exceeds 0.03% to 0.1% of the circulating mononuclear cells.[30] Subsequently, a cellular immune response occurs, composed primarily of cytotoxic T lymphocytes (CTLs) that are EBV specific and nonspecific. Figure 24.1 illustrates the pathologic consequences of an abnormal CTL response to EBV infection. A deficient CTL response, either quantitative or qualitative, results in an EBV-driven B-cell proliferative process. The lack of an appropriate CTL response can also result in an aggressive, predominantly T-cell and histiocytic reaction that is not EBV specific. This reaction is characterized by extensive infiltration of lymphoid and parenchymal organs with hemophagocytosis and tissue destruction that can be rapidly progressive and usually fatal.[31,32]

The humoral response to EBV is well characterized.[33-36] VCA antibodies appear initially, IgM followed by IgG. IgM antibodies probably arise during the incubation period, peak with symptoms, and then decline rapidly. IgG anti-VCA antibodies reach a peak 2 to 3 weeks after IgM and persist for life. The majority of patients also have a transient response to the EBV early antigen (EA), peaking usually within a month of infection. Antibodies to EBNA may appear several weeks after the onset of the illness in some patients, but in general, take several months to appear with titers, rises slowly over 1 to 2 years, and persist for life. The majority of normal individuals will have detectable IgG to EBNA by 6 months following

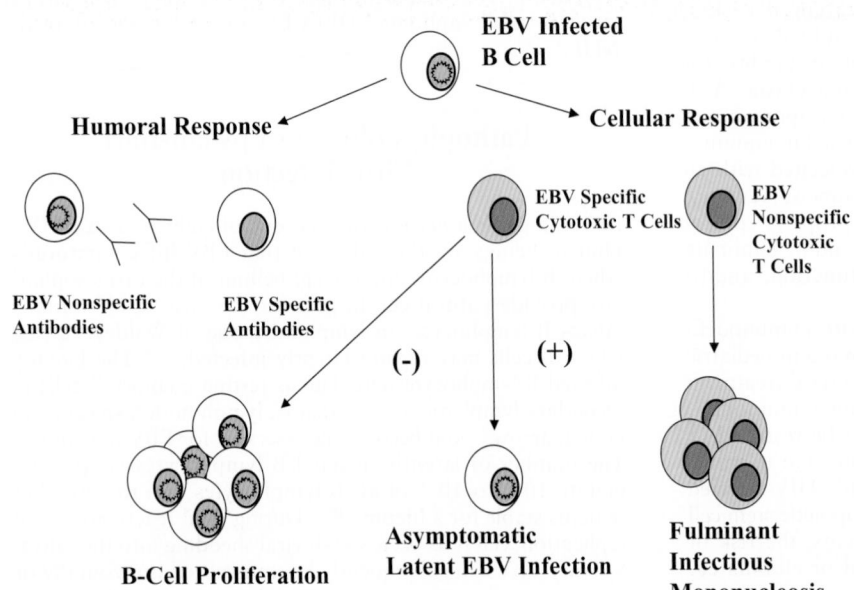

FIGURE 24.1 Immune response to EBV infection. EBV, Epstein-Barr virus. (From Gross TG. Infectious mononucleosis and other EBV-related disorders. In: Greer JP, Foerster J, Lukens JN, et al., eds. Wintrobe's clinical hematology. 11th ed. Philadelphia, PA: Lippincott Williams & Wilkins, 2004.)

EBV infection, though it may take years to develop detectable anti-EBNA titers. In young children, the anti-VCA and -EA responses may be much less intense and anti-EBNA may take much longer to appear.[37] An EBV nonspecific humoral response also occurs with EBV infection. This phenomenon was first described in 1932 by Paul and associates when they reported that the sera of patients with infectious mononucleosis (IM) contain heterophil antibodies against sheep erythrocytes in concentrations far above normal.[38] The "monospot" test is the detection of these heterophil antibodies, and hence this test is not specific for EBV infection. There can be many other EBV nonspecific antibodies produced with primary EBV infection and some may function as autoantibodies.[39-41]

Although neutralizing antibodies produced following primary infection may play a role in thwarting the spread to additional B cells, it is the cellular response that is critical for controlling EBV infections. Natural killer (NK) cells and CD4+ T cells have been shown to play some role, but it is the CD8+ memory cytotoxic T cells (EBV-CTL) that are the primary defense against EBV infections and B-cell proliferation.[42-46] Initially, cytotoxic T cells are polyclonal and are neither EBV specific nor HLA restricted as evidenced by their ability to readily kill EBV-negative and MHC-incompatible targets.[44] They resemble activated killer cells induced *in vitro* by exposure of T cells to nonspecific mitogens or IL-2.[44] These CD8+ lymphocytes account for the majority of the cells during the classic lymphocytosis characteristic of IM and are the large, pleomorphic, atypical lymphocytes or "Downey cells" commonly observed.[46,47] The quantity of circulating CD8+ T cells correlates with IM symptoms, not the number of EBV-infected B cells or viral load.[48] These CD8+ lymphocytes disappear during convalescence[44] and are replaced by EBV-specific CTL that maintain a latent viral infection and control EBV-driven B-cell proliferation.[42-45] This symbiosis of EBV and the infected host is preserved by interactions between viral gene expression in latently infected B cells and host EBV-CTL surveillance.

The diagnosis of EBV infection is not trivial, especially in the immunodeficient patient. The "gold standard" test for EBV exposure has been serology consistent with a primary infection. Serology for EBV infection has limited value in many immunocompromised patients, as they may not have the ability to respond normally. In addition, many of these patients may have detectable anti-EBV antibodies but acquired the antibodies from intravenous gammaglobulin or blood products. The detection of EBV DNA in peripheral blood or serum by polymerase chain reaction (PCR) provides good evidence that the patient has been infected with EBV. Increased levels of EBV DNA detected by PCR have been associated with EBV-associated disease. However, interpretation of quantitative EBV DNA PCR or "viral loads" results can be problematic (discussed in detail in section "Posttransplant Lymphoproliferative Disease"), especially in the immunodeficient patient. Immunocompromised patients tend to have higher levels of EBV DNA compared with healthy individuals with latent EBV infection. Also different laboratories use different methods of detection, different specimens (blood vs. serum vs. mononuclear cells), and different measurements (copies per micrograms DNA vs. cells vs. milliliter of serum/blood). The best method to diagnosis EBV as an etiologic agent is tissue biopsy and *in situ* hybridization.

MALIGNANCIES IN PRIMARY IMMUNODEFICIENCIES

Advances in prevention and treatment of opportunistic infections have improved morbidity and mortality for patients with primary immunodeficiencies. However, neoplastic disorders, particularly lymphoproliferative complications, remain the second most common cause of premature mortality behind infectious etiologies.[49,50] The incidence of tumors in immunodeficiency diseases such as Wiskott-Aldrich syndrome (WAS), ataxia telangiectasia (AT), and common variable immunodeficiency (CVID) is estimated to be 15% to 25% with the risk increasing with age and possibly in subgroups amongst the disease categories.[51-54] Following observations by Drs. Good and Gatti in the early 1970s, the International Immunodeficiency Cancer Registry (ICR) was established and maintained at the University of Minnesota.[55] This voluntary registry has been pivotal in the description of tumors observed in primary immunodeficiencies. Table 24.1 is a summary of earlier publications of the ICR data listing tumor types reported for the various primary immunodeficiency diseases.

TABLE 24.1

IMMUNODEFICIENCY CANCER REGISTRY CASES: DISTRIBUTION OF TUMORS AND IMMUNODEFICIENCIES

Immunodeficiency	Adeno carcinoma	Lymphoma	Hodgkin disease	Leukemia	Other tumors	Total (per immunodeficiency)
Severe combined immunodeficiency	1 (2.4%)	31 (73.8%)	4 (9.5%)	5 (11.9%)	1 (2.4%)	42
X-linked agammaglobulinemia	3 (14.3%)	7 (33.3%)	3 (14.3%)	7 (33.3%)	1 (4.8%)	21
Common variable immunodeficiency	20 (16.7%)	55 (45.8%)	8 (6.7%)	8 (6.7%)	29 (24.2%)	120
IgA deficiency	8 (21.1%)	6 (15.8%)	3 (7.9%)	0 (0%)	21 (55.3%)	38
Hyper-IgM syndrome	0 (0%)	9 (56.3%)	4 (25.0%)	0 (0%)	3 (18.8%)	16
Wiskott-Aldrich syndrome	0 (0%)	59 (75.6%)	3 (3.8%)	7 (9.0%)	9 (11.5%)	78
Ataxia telangiectasia	13 (8.7%)	69 (46.0%)	16 (10.7%)	32 (21.3%)	20 (13.3%)	150
Other immunodeficiencies	1 (4.0%)	12 (48.0%)	1 (4.0%)	4 (16.0%)	7 (28.0%)	25
Total (in each category)	46	248	42	63	91	500

From Filipovich AH, Gross TG. Immunodeficiency and cancer. In: Martin D, Abeloff MD, et al. eds, Clinical oncology. 3rd ed. Portland OR: Book News, Inc., 2004.

With better understanding of molecular defects and more accurate diagnoses, it is clear that improvements in the original cataloguing have been achieved over the last few decades. For example, it is likely that a significant proportion of the boys originally diagnosed with hypogammaglobulinemia who developed lymphomas may have had X-linked severe combined immunodeficiency (XSCID). Similarly, current pathologic and immunohistochemistry review of "leukemia" in patients with SCID, hypogammaglobulinemia, and WAS suggests that these may have actually been disseminated LPDs or lymphoma with mature B-cell phenotype. Nonetheless the general outline of tumor types and their proportional distribution in various immunodeficiencies provided by the ICR has withstood the test of time.

Non-Hodgkin Lymphoma

Non-Hodgkin lymphomas (NHLs) observed in primary immunodeficiency have the following characteristics: (a) male predominance, even in autosomal recessive disorders such as AT; (b) young median age at diagnosis; and (c) high frequency of extranodal presentation, particularly the gastrointestinal tract and central nervous system (CNS). Although EBV has been identified as a common cofactor predominantly in the B-cell phenotypes, EBV DNA and latent viral proteins have also been found in Hodgkin disease (HD) as well as T-cell NHL. However, not all NHLs, including B-cell NHL, are EBV associated. Even in X-linked lymphoproliferative disease (XLP), where affected boys have a very aberrant immune response to EBV infection, many of the NHLs have been found to be EBV negative.[56,57] In addition, lymphoproliferative disease, lymphoma or leukemia, in AT is often EBV negative. This is consistent with the hypothesis that the genetic predisposition to cancer in AT occurs directly from mutations arising from the chromosomal repair defect.

Limited data are available on treatment and prognosis of primary immunodeficiency-associated NHL given the rarity, wide variety of predisposing immunodeficiencies, and ineligibility for enrolment in clinical trial.[58] In the absence of randomized clinical trials, treatment is usually tailored according to histological subtype.[58] Historically, NHL treatment with conventional doses of chemotherapy and radiation has met with limited success in primary immunodeficient patients.[59] This is primarily due to opportunistic infections and increase in treatment-related mortality due to end-organ dysfunction. In the current era, improved antiviral and antifungal therapies have allowed patients with primary immunodeficiency-associated NHL to be treated more aggressively.[60] Replacement immunoglobulin is indicated for hypogammaglobulinemia, as is early and aggressive treatment for infections with special consideration for *Pneumocystis jirovecii* pneumonia antibiotic prophylaxis.[58] Patients who respond well initially to treatment are at risk for relapse. It remains unclear if recurrence is a true recurrence of the same clonal process or if a "new" disease with different clonal origin has developed.[61] Because the primary risk factor for cancer is the underlying immunodeficiency, immune system replacement with allogeneic hematopoietic stem cell transplantation may be the only means of durable disease-free survival.

Hodgkin Disease

Based on ICR reporting, HD accounts for approximately 10% of tumors arising in patients with primary immunodeficiencies and occurs at an early median age.[49,62] A case control study performed by the ICR in the late 1980s compared the immun-

odeficiency HD cases with other pediatric HD cases from a multi-institutional international cooperative study group.[62] Patients with immunodeficiency were diagnosed with HD earlier in life (mean 7.8 years vs. 11.5 years), were significantly less likely to achieve remission, and if remission was achieved the 5-year probability of survival was inferior (53% vs. 86%). There is some speculation whether the majority of HD diagnosed in this population is truly HD. Histologies other than nodular sclerosing, that is, mixed cellularity, lymphocyte predominate, and lymphocyte depleted are more common in patients with primary immunodeficiency.[62] HD in patients with immunodeficiencies is often associated with EBV and may reflect a spectrum of B-cell lymphoproliferation with a mixture of cells that reflect an abnormal or inadequate immune response.[63] Patients with primary immunodeficiency-related HD who achieve remission may benefit from allogeneic hematopoietic stem cell transplantation.[64–66]

SPECIFIC IMMUNODEFICIENCY STATES AND ASSOCIATED MALIGNANT LYMPHOPROLIFERATIVE CONDITIONS

Severe Combined Immunodeficiencies

SCIDs are a group of monogenic diseases that profoundly affect lymphocyte development and function. Affected individuals are prone to life-threatening infections and without treatment do not survive beyond the first year of life.[67] NHL is typically the cancer diagnosed in patients with SCIDs.[67–69] In general, only patients with SCIDs who retain the ability to make B cells are felt to be at risk for developing NHL including patients with (a) X-linked SCIDs in which loss of function through mutations in the X-linked common gamma chain gene of multiple interleukin receptors blocks T-cell development, but maintain adequate B-cell numbers; (b) purine nucleoside phosphorylase deficiency in which T-cell expansion and function are impaired by accumulation of toxic intracellular metabolites, with lesser effects on B cells; and (c) Omenn syndrome, caused by mutations in RAG1 genes predominantly that severely restricts both B- and T-cell repertoire development, and results in marked skewing toward a type 2 cytokine production that is suppressive of T-cell cytotoxic functions, but enhance T-cell help for B-cell proliferation.[70–72] Although the majority of adenosine deaminase–deficient SCID patients lack B cells, cases of NHL have been reported.[73,74] Challenges remain for optimal therapy NHL in these patients who are generally resistant to therapy.[74]

Wiskott-Aldrich Syndrome

WAS is an X-linked disorder of broad ranging and variable immunodeficiency and characterized by microthrombocytopenia, resulting from mutations in the Wiskott-Aldrich syndrome protein (WASP) gene.[75,76] The WASP gene encodes a large intracellular protein with several functional domains involved with cytoskeletal integrity and signal transduction. Several molecules reported to be associated with WASP are involved in normal progression through the cell cycle. WASP is expressed in cells of hematopoietic origin and in the thymus. Experimental evidence suggests that WASP-negative B cells are relatively resistant to apoptosis. Recent advances in understanding the role of the WASP gene and proteins provides evidence as a regulator of actin polymerization in hematopoietic cells with functional domains involved in cell signaling and cell locomotion, immune synapse formation, and apoptosis.[77–82] Mutations in the WASP protein impairs its interaction with the WIPF1 protein, thus making patients diagnosed with WAS at risk for leukemia and lymphoma.[83] Patients with WAS-associated malignancies are typically related to EBV.[54,76] Although rare, there are reports of EBV-negative B-cell lymphomas in WAS and these appear to be more frequently seen in adult males with clinically milder forms of WAS or what has been referred to in the past as X-linked thrombocytopenia.[77]

X-Linked Lymphoproliferative Syndrome

Males affected with XLP were originally recognized for fatal complications of EBV infection and high risk of lymphoma.[42] The defective gene has been identified as SH2D1 A or SAP (signaling lymphocytic activation molecule (SLAM)-associated protein).[84] SAP is a small adaptor protein of only a SH2 binding domain and short C and N terminus. Although the function of SAP is still being delineated, it has been shown to bind to at least four regulatory molecules known to alter T and NK cell functions by both activation and suppression, and it is thought to be involved in T-B cell interactions through cytokine regulation.[85–92]

Clinical features of XLP include an excessive immune reaction to EBV associated with hemophagocytosis and liver failure that is clinically indistinguishable from other forms of hemophagocytic syndromes and has been called fulminant infectious mononucleosis (FIM) or EBV-associated hemophagocytic lymphohistiocytosis (EBV-HLH).[93–96] Both FIM and EBV-HLH can be seen in patients without XLP. XLP patients may also present with lymphoproliferative disease, hypogammaglobulinemia, or hematologic cytopenias.[56,57] Patients who develop FIM/EBV-HLH may initially present with the usual signs and symptoms of IM, but these symptoms are often more severe. The course and progression of the disease are variable ranging from presentation in multiorgan failure developing over hours to persistent or recurring symptoms of IM for months. An atypical lymphocytosis is usually present at early stages of the disease, but patients subsequently develop severe, persistent pancytopenia, hepatic dysfunction resulting in fulminant hepatitis, meningoencephalitis, and varying degrees of myocarditis.[32,56] The development of hepatic dysfunction, often with coagulation abnormalities secondary to liver failure or disseminated intravascular coagulation, and pancytopenia are ominous signs, as are other signs and symptoms of hemophagocytic syndromes, such as hypofibrinogenemia and elevated triglycerides.[31,32,56]

As mentioned previously, EBV is a potent stimulus to the immune system, resulting in a massive EBV-specific and nonspecific response of both the humoral and cellular immune system. Here, the EBV nonspecific response, primarily the cellular immune response, is uncontrolled and is characterized by extensive infiltration of parenchymal organs by lymphoid cells, primarily CD8+ cells in varying degrees of transformation and histiocytes with surprisingly few B cells. If this aggressive immune reaction goes unabated, ultimately all organs and even vessels will sustain extensive damage. This reaction culminates in the phagocytosis, tissue destruction, and cellular depletion with death usually following shortly thereafter due to multisystem organ failure. Once this develops, therapy is difficult and usually unsuccessful, with a median survival time of approximately 4 weeks.[57] Antiviral drugs, immunoglobulins, IL-2, IFN-α, IFN-γ, plasmapheresis,

corticosteroids, and most cytotoxic drugs have been ineffective.[32,56] The most consistent success in treatment is early use of etoposide and immunosuppression with corticosteroids and cyclosporin A or tacrolimus (FK506).[97] Therapy may be required for 6 to 12 months. These patients are profoundly immunocompromised from their disease and the therapy. Therefore, a successful outcome is dependent on control of FIM/EBV-HLH symptoms while preventing and treating life-threatening infectious complications. Even with remission of symptoms, recurrences are common and tend to be more difficult to control resulting in an extremely poor prognosis. When control of symptoms can be achieved, allogeneic BMT is recommended and is felt to be the only curative therapy.[98]

LPDs develop in approximately one-fourth of patients with XLP.[50,56,57] Most lymphomas are of B-cell phenotype, but approximately 10% of LPD are of a non–B-cell phenotype.[88,90,91,95] Non–B-cell lymphoproliferative diseases include HD, T-cell NHL, lymphomatoid granulomatosis, or angiocentric immunoproliferative lesions.[31,56] As in other immunodeficiencies, the role of EBV in LPD remains unclear with approximately 50% of patients with LPD showing no evidence of prior EBV infection and EBV found in only 25% of tumor specimens.[57] Treatment options are relatively limited but allogeneic hematopoietic stem cell transplantations have had some success in patients achieving remission.[61,98,99]

Chediak-Higashi Syndrome

Chediak-Higashi syndrome (CHS) is an autosomal recessive disorder characterized by recurrent bacterial infections, oculocutaneous albinism, abnormal platelets, varied neurologic dysfunction, and a 90% probability prior to the age of 20 years of developing a lethal hemophagocytic complication associated with EBV infection (referred to as the accelerated phase, again clinically indistinguishable from other forms of hemophagocytic syndromes and should be treated similarly).[100] CHS is caused by mutations in the LYST gene (lysosomal trafficking regulator), and giant lysosomes are the characteristic findings in leukocytes on blood smear. Because lysosomes are the key storage compartments for cytolytic proteins including perforin and Granzyme B, cytotoxic effector function of NK and T cells is typically impaired in CHS that are felt to be the reasons for recurrent infections and inability to respond appropriately to EBV infection.[101] A transport defect inhibiting peptide loading and antigen presentation by HLA class II molecules on EBV-transformed B lymphocytes from CHS patients has also been proposed as a mechanism contributing to the pathogenesis of EBV-LPD in CHS patients. Other hematopoietic malignancies such as leukemias have also been reported in CHS.[102–104] Treatment for lymphoproliferative disease and/or hematophagocytic lymphohistiocytosis in CHS consists of immunosuppressive treatment with possible cure achieved after bone marrow transplantation.[56,105,106]

X-Linked Hyper-IgM Syndrome

X-linked hyper-IgM syndrome, also known as X-linked CD40 ligand deficiency, results in a failure of immunoglobulin switching by B cells that requires signaling through CD40 and in decreased development and maintenance of type 1 cell-mediated responses (including NK cell function) due to impaired responsiveness of CD40 expressing monocyte-derived antigen presenting cells.[107] Patients with X-linked hyper-IgM syndrome have an increased risk of lymphomas, including HD associated with EBV infection, as well as adenocarcinoma of the gastrointestinal tract.[66,108] Presumably, depressed cell-mediated function required for control of EBV is the mechanism. Patients at increased risk for biliary carcinomas also present with sclerosing cholangitis with a history of chronic cryptosporidiosis.[109] For hematopoietic malignancies, bone marrow transplantation is an option,[66] while those with adenocarcinoma, liver transplants and/or chemotherapy have been attempted with poor prognosis.[109]

Autoimmune Lymphoproliferative Syndrome

Autoimmune lymphoproliferative syndrome is a constellation of genetic apoptosis defects associated with mutations in FAS, Fas ligand and Caspase 8 genes.[110] Most of the cases described have heterozygous, dominant negative mutations involving FAS. Characteristic clinical features present in early childhood or even at birth. These include chronic multifocal lymphadenopathy, splenomegaly, and autoimmune hemolytic anemia (and often other immune cytopenias), with increased proportions of circulating senescent T cells (CD3+, CD4−, CD8−), so-called double-negative T cells. The majority of patients experience symptomatic improvement with steroid therapy, and generally, the autoimmune complications lessen in severity with age. However, the estimated risk of lymphoma in such patients is around 30%, with some patients diagnosed with multiple-lymphoid tumors over time. Nearly half of patients with Evan syndrome meet the criteria for the syndrome.[111] Patients with the most severe forms should be considered for correction with allogeneic hematopoietic stem cell transplantation. Patients who develop NHL or HD may respond to chemotherapy.[58,112–115] Rituximab and sulfadoxine/pyrimethamine,[116] agents that induce apoptosis in the senescent lymphocytes bypassing the FAS/FAS ligand signal, have been shown to reduce lymphadenopathy and autoimmune symptoms. Whether such strategies will ultimately reduce risk of lymphomas remains to be determined.

OTHER MALIGNANCIES WITH PRIMARY IMMUNODEFICIENCIES

Gastric Carcinomas and Mucosa-Associated Lymphoid Tissue Lymphomas

A relationship between gastric atrophy, long-standing dyspepsia and gastric ulcer disease and the development of gastric carcinomas in adults with CVID was observed decades before the discovery of a causal link to chronic *Helicobacter pylori* infestation.[117,118] A retrospective study of banked sera from a group of presumed nonimmunodeficient adult patients diagnosed with gastric carcinoma revealed an increased incidence of IgA deficiency in cancer-bearing subjects (1 in 20) compared with the general blood donor pool (1 in 400), further implicating defective humoral immunity as a contributing factor to this unusual tumor type.[119] It is now recognized that *H. pylori* infection is the most common cofactor for gastric carcinoma and is associated with mucosa-associated lymphoid tissue (MALT) lymphomas in nonimmunodeficient Caucasians.[120–127] MALT is not present in healthy gastric mucosa, yet can develop in sites of long-persisting inflammation.[128] MALT lymphomas are generally monoclonal and can take on the appearance of aggressive large B-cell lymphomas. These tumors are reported not only in adults with primary immunodeficiency but also in immunosuppressed organ transplant recipients, thought rarely seen in children. Organ transplant recipients also carry an increased risk of gastric carcinoma, and diagnostic endoscopy is now recommended as part of the posttransplant follow-up in symptomatic individuals.[129–132] Surgery and/or chemotherapy are therapeutic options available for organ transplant recipients diagnosed with gastric carcinoma.[130,133] Fortunately, effective eradication of *H. pylori* with antibiotics,[133] antacid therapy, and occasionally surgical excision is highly curative for both gastric carcinomas and MALT lymphomas. Presumably, surveillance for *H. pylori* infection and antibiotic suppression can prevent these tumors in immunodeficient populations.

Immunodeficiency and Cancer in Genetic Disorders of DNA Repair

Several rare genetic disorders of DNA repair in which resultant immunodeficiency and intrinsic susceptibility to carcinomas have been identified (Table 24.2). DNA is constantly exposed to potentially damaging insults, both external (e.g., environmental radiation) and intrinsic (e.g., by-products of cellular metabolism). A number of molecular strategies exist to maintain genomic stability. Mechanisms utilized in eukaryotes include those involved in (a) recognition and direct repair of DNA damage, (b) cell cycle checkpoints that pause cell cycle progression in the presence of DNA damage allowing the time needed for repair, and (c) mechanisms for removal of irreversibly damaged cells such as the triggering of apoptosis. DNA double-strand breaks represent the most potentially serious damage to the genome. Two major pathways exist to

TABLE 24.2

GENETIC DISORDERS ASSOCIATED WITH CHROMOSOMAL INSTABILITY THAT RESULT IN IMMUNODEFICIENCY AND PREDISPOSITION TO CANCER

Disorder	Gene defect[Ref]	Immune defects	Cancers reported
Ataxia telangiectasia	ATM[136]	IgA deficiency, ↓ T cells	Lymphoma, leukemia, hepatocarcinoma, genitourinary carcinoma, skin cancer
Nijmegen breakage syndrome	NBS1[72]	Hypogammaglobulinemia, lymphopenia	Myeloid leukemia, lymphoma
Bloom syndrome	BLM[147]	Hypogammaglobulinemia NK-cell deficiency	Lymphoma, epithelial cancer
Werner syndrome	WRN[153]	Antibody deficiency?	Lymphoma

From Filipovich AH, Gross TG. Immunodeficiency and cancer. In: Abeloff MD, et al., eds. Clinical oncology. 3rd ed. Portland OR: Book News, Inc., 2004.

repair such damage: homologous recombination repair and nonhomologous end joining. Defects in either of these pathways can result in chromosomal rearrangements, loss of heterozygosity, and gene mutations leading to cancers. Generation of immunologic diversity among both B and T cells requires a well-orchestrated "creation" of DNA breaks followed by rearrangement of immunoglobulin and T-cell receptor gene sequences and repair to stabilize the final genetic product. In this process of gene rearrangement, mutations and additions that contribute to the desired diversity of new coding regions frequently occur. Mechanisms creating this immunologic diversity likely include helicases, polymerases, and DNA ligases. Several of the known genetic defects associated with immunodeficiency and predisposition to cancers are described later. Many other rare cases with immunodeficiency and cancers have been identified, but the specific molecular defects are still unknown.

Ataxia Telangiectasia

AT is an autosomal disorder with cancer predisposition that has variable and profound immunologic and other systemic manifestations, principally cerebellar degeneration.[134,135] For some time, it has been recognized that AT cells fail to normally activate cell cycle checkpoints after exposure to γ-irradiation or radiomimetic agents. The mutant gene in AT (ATM) is a member of the phosphatidyl inositol kinase family of molecules involved in signal transduction and has also been implicated in meiotic recombination.[136] ATM appears to act as a sensor of double-stranded DNA breakage, for example, in response to oxidative stress, activating numerous damage repair pathways including cell cycle checkpoint control, p53 activation, and DNA repair. Mutations in ATM lead to accelerated telomere loss and premature aging.[137] In the context of normal lymphopoiesis, ATM is clearly involved in control of productive gene rearrangements of the B- and T-cell immune receptor molecules, since AT lymphocytes demonstrate a 25-fold increase in nonrandom rearrangements of immunoglobulin and TCR genes compared with lymphocytes from normal individuals.[138] Thymic output in AT is greatly reduced and subsequent restricted T-cell repertoire resulting in oligoclonal postthymic expansion.[139] Some of the nonrandom rearrangements involve translocation of Ig chains with *c-myc* reflecting, in magnified proportion, commonly seen cytogenetic rearrangements in lymphomagenesis. Although lymphoid tumors (both lymphomas and leukemias) predominate, patients with AT also experience high rates of epithelial cancers involving the skin, gastrointestinal tract, genitourinary tract, CNS, and breast cancer.[60,135,140–142] Multiple tumors can be present simultaneously or develop sequentially. Early reports from the ICR discussed concordance of histologies in tumors affecting AT siblings from the same family—an intriguing but still mysterious observation. The extent of response of tumors in AT patients to conventional chemotherapy remains controversial; however, the frequent development of chronic lung disease in AT and inability to maintain chemotherapy intensity may contribute to poorer outcomes.

Nijmegen Breakage Syndrome

Nijmegen breakage syndrome is another rare autosomal recessive syndrome that is associated with both humoral and T-cell defects, clinical radiosensitivity, chromosomal instability and predisposition to lymphoid, epithelial cancers, and sarcomas.[143–145] Other characteristics of patients with NBS are growth retardation, microcephaly, and "birdlike" facies. The protein defective in NBS—NBS1, nibrin, or p95—appears to function together with ATM to "sense" DNA double-strand breaks and activate a diversity of corrective actions. As in AT, frequent chromosomal aberrations at the sites of TCR and IgH rearrangement are observed in lymphocytes of patients with NBS. Standard chemotherapy regimen for HD has successfully been used in one case.[146]

Bloom Syndrome

Bloom syndrome has an autosomal recessive inheritance pattern involving mutations in the BLM gene.[147] In addition to immunodeficiency, especially humoral defects and predisposition to cancer, patients with Bloom syndrome experience growth retardation, progeria, impaired fertility, sun-sensitive erythema of the face, and chronic lung disease (similar to patients with AT). The defective protein is a member of the RecQ helicase family and appears to function during DNA replication or in the postreplication process to resolve aberrancies incurred during replication. The BLM protein colocalizes with a gene, hMLH1, that is linked to DNA mismatch repair. A propensity for colonic adenomas, epidermal carcinomas, and acute myeloid leukemia has been reported in these patients.[148–152]

Werner Syndrome

Werner syndrome is an autosomal recessive disorder with features of progeria and multiple endocrine neoplasias result from loss of function mutations in the WRN gene that encodes a helicase/exonuclease.[153] Reports of immunodeficiency are not well substantiated, but predilection to sinopulmonary infections is noted. Genomic instability in these patients is typified by elevated illegitimate recombination events and accelerated loss of telomerase sequences. Cancer susceptibility appears increased with aging and noted with carcinomas.[154–156]

HUMAN IMMUNODEFICIENCY VIRUS–RELATED MALIGNANCIES

The morbidity and mortality associated with the HIV type 1 continues to increase globally with similar dire consequences seen in North America. With name-based HIV reporting fully implemented since April 2008, an estimated 1.1 million adults and adolescents (447.8 per 100,000 population) were living with HIV or acquired immunodeficiency syndrome (AIDS) in the United States by 2006.[157] In a similar time frame, between 9,000 and 10,000 children younger than 13 years were diagnosed with AIDS in the United States.[158] One of the impacts of the HIV/AIDS epidemic is the increased incidence of cancers in individuals infected with HIV, both AIDS-defining and non–AIDS-defining cancers.[159–164] For many pediatric and adolescent AIDS cases with hemophilia, malignancy was the first indication of HIV infection.[165] Children infected with HIV by other means (perinatal) are similarly at increased risk for malignancies.[162,166–170] In a survey of Children's Cancer Group institutions, an estimated 100-fold increased risk of NHL or KS as AIDS-defining malignancies was seen in HIV-infected children.[171] In a separate study from a US surveillance cohort of 4,954 children with AIDS, 124 children (2.5%) were identified as having a malignancy with an estimated relative risk (RR) of 651 for children who were 2 or more years beyond their AIDS diagnosis.[167]

As patients live longer with HIV infection, risks for malignancies increase.[172] The epidemiology of HIV-related malignancies (HRM), which includes KS and HIV-associated non-Hodgkin lymphoma (H-NHL), has changed as improvements in antiretroviral therapies have evolved in the United States as well as globally.[161-164,170,173-175] Even though a decrease in the incidence of HRM with the introduction of highly active antiretroviral therapy (HAART) in resource-rich countries occurred, the incidence of some specific types of cancers is still relatively higher than in non–HIV-infected individuals both in adults and in children.[164,170,173,175] The risk of lymphoma in an HIV-infected individual is 100 times that of an uninfected person with similar trends seen in outside the United States.[164,170,174-176] Lymphomas associated with HIV are usually aggressive, with the majority occurring in extra-lymphatic sites.[177] Diagnosis of a second H-NHL was reported in a pediatric patient.[178] Although, the use of HAART is correlated with a significant decline in KS, the decrease in H-NHL cases appears to be less dramatic.[172] The increased risks for KS and H-NHL have been particularly noted in adults, but children are at risk as well.[162,163,169,171,179,180] In contrast to adults, there is also an apparent increased risk for leiomyosarcoma seen in HIV-infected children as well as other malignancies.[165,168,169,171,179,181-185]

Specific risk factors associated with the development of malignancies in HIV-infected children were studied in a large multicenter cohort study and identified high viral burden with EBV as being associated with HRM, although the effect was modified by CD4 cell count.[169] In contrast, route of HIV infection, demographic characteristics, and zidovudine use were not associated with the development of malignancy. However, specific pathogenic mechanisms of pediatric HRM remain unclear in the setting of immune dysfunction associated with HIV infection.[169] The immunocompromised state induced by HIV leads to a lack of surveillance of proliferative cells and/or incomplete control of other viral infections. One of the consequences of this process results in virus-induced or virus-associated cancers as is seen with EBV (B-cell lymphoma, nasopharyngeal carcinoma, leiomyosarcoma), HHV-8/KSHV (KS, body cavity-based lymphoma), HPV (cervical and anal neoplasm, skin cancer), or even HIV itself (large cell NHL, Burkitt NHL).[176,186-190] The malignant pathways involving viral agents in HIV infection is likely multifactorial ranging from cellular transformation, dysregulation of the immune system, to chromosomal abnormalities. Thus, in HRM, the pathological heterogeneity is reflected in the different abnormalities observed amongst the various types of malignancies.

Kaposi Sarcoma

KS was, and still is, an extremely rare condition in immuno-competent individuals, but its association in the setting of HIV infection is well documented.[159,169,191,192] The incidence of KS in adults, which had been as high as 30% of newly diagnosed AIDS cases in resource-rich countries, has dramatically declined with the introduction of HAART.[179,193-195] However, in resource-poor countries, the incidence of KS continues to rise, both in adults and children.[192,193,195-202] KS in HIV-infected children typically occurs several years after AIDS diagnosis.[167] In a review of the Tanzania cancer registry data of pediatric KS, 150 histologically confirmed pediatric KS cases were reported from 126 male and 24 female children with little difference in the gender ratio pre- and post-AIDS epidemic, 5.1:1 and 5.4:1, respectively.[196] The majority of children were infected by HIV vertically, accounting for the highest occurrence of KS observed in the 0 to 5 years age group. The study further demonstrated a statistically significant increase in disseminated childhood KS cases during the AIDS epidemic.

The pathogenic pathways leading to KS are still unknown, but the histological appearance of KS has been described as lesions composed of endothelial cells and spindle cells mixed with mononuclear immune and red blood cells.[203] About a decade ago, HHV-8/KSHV was reported as a highly associated pathogenic agent responsible for KS.[204] It was subsequently postulated that the inability of a patient with AIDS to control HHV-8/KSHV infection leads to the development of KS, suggesting that KS is an opportunistic malignancy.[192,203] The fact that younger HIV-infected children (<5 years) are at high risk for developing KS supports the hypothesis that a dysfunctional immune system may lead to low resistance to HHV-8/KSHV infection.[196] HHV-8/KSHV incorporates several eukaryotic cellular protein genes that may contribute to tumor formation, including G-protein homologs, cyclin D, interleukin 6, bcl-2, latent nuclear antigen-1, viral cyclin, and interferon regulatory factor.[173,204] The tumor microenvironment has been shown to be an essential aspect of KS progression.[173] The cross talk of cytokines and chemokines between host T cells and cancer cells can lead to further proliferation and survival of circulating malignant T cells.

Clinically, HIV-associated KS presents as mucocutaneous lesions and/or a disseminated lymphadenopathic form.[192,196,205] The spindle cell proliferation surrounded by reticulum and collagen fibers with extensive vascularization can present as purple/brown cutaneous macular, plaque-like or nodular lesions (Fig. 24.2). On the skin, the lesions can be present on any surface including the palms and soles, scalp, and auditory canals associated with edema or venous congestion.[192,205] The lymphadenopathic form, predominant in Africa, has been characterized in the oro-facial, inguinal-genital, or ano-genital regions.[166,205] The pathology of the vascular spindle cell proliferation is consistent with a monoclonal origin of multicentric KS lesions.[203] The KS cells stain positive for markers including α-actin (smooth muscle), vimentin, von Willebrand factor, CD68, and CD14.[206]

A recommended staging system, evaluating extent of tumor involvement, CD4 cell count, and systemic symptoms categorizes adult patients in risk groups, but the validity of the same staging system for children has not been shown.[207] Similarly, recommended standard treatment of childhood KS is lacking due to limited clinical trials in children.[166,168,205] In some cases, institution of HAART, thus reconstituting the immune system, resulted in resolution of KS lesions.[192,194,196,206] If KS occurs while on effective HAART for their HIV infection, other treatment modalities including local/systemic chemotherapy and immune modulators have had variable success.[208-213]

Non-Hodgkin Lymphoma and Hodgkin Disease

NHL of B-cell origin is a recognized AIDS-associated malignancy, but other lymphoproliferative diseases, including HD, are increasingly being reported.[168,169,174,178,179,197,202,214] H-NHL can be broadly grouped into three subcategories: systemic (nodal and extranodal), primary central nervous system lymphoma (PCNSL), and body cavity-based lymphoma, or also referred to as primary effusion lymphoma (PEL) (Table 24.3). Approximately 80% of all H-NHLs are considered to be systemic, defined as not being limited to the CNS (PCNSL) or other anatomic regions (PEL).[215] In children, within the first 2 years after AIDS diagnosis, the incidence of H-NHL was 510 per 100,000 person-years with the median time for developing H-NHL after AIDS diagnosis being 14 months.[167] The RR for

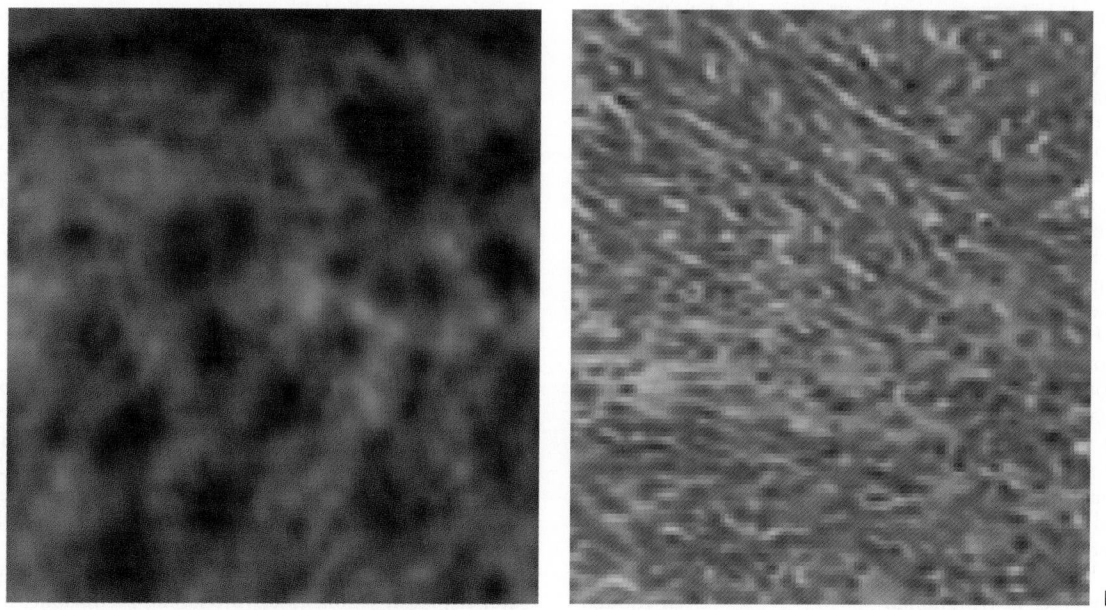

FIGURE 24.2 A: Cutaneous Kaposi's sarcoma lesions on the extremity. **B:** Monomorphic spindle-shaped cells of Kaposi's sarcoma (H & E stain).

developing H-NHL, with the most common type being Burkitt lymphoma, was 651. In contrast, the risk of PCNSL (91 per 100,000 person-years) was particularly high with a RR of 7,143.[167] PEL, a unique lymphomatous effusion associated with HHV-8/KSHV, is primarily observed in adults infected with HIV and rarely in children.[216,217] HD also appears to be increased in HIV-infected individuals, including children.[167,197,214] The explanation for an increase in HD in HIV-infected children is still unknown; however, EBV has been speculated in playing a role.[214,218] The introduction of HAART has lowered the incidence of systemic lymphomas; however, the decrease has not been as successful as noted with the incidence of KS. Globally, H-NHL remains one of the most common HRM with a high morbidity and mortality rate.[159,219-222] Similarly, in children, H-NHL is also one of the most common HRM with over 80% in one study being H-NHL.[168] Others report similar findings with H-NHL, either systemic or PCNSL being predominantly represented.[167,169,171,179,191,195,197] The pathology of childhood H-NHL is typically B cell in origin.[191] The pathological spectrum seen in

childhood H-NHL ranges from MALT, small non-cleaved cell lymphoma (Burkitt lymphoma), to diffuse large cell lymphoma (DLCL).[168,170,192,195,214,223,224] In limited molecular studies, abnormalities in known specific B-cell–associated neoplastic genes have been found in pediatric cases: *c-myc* oncogene mutations, immunoglobulin gene mutations, as well as the presence of EBV in tumor tissue.[169,214,225] Other coinfections that may synergistically promote lymphomagenesis in HIV-infected individuals have been hypothesized including EBV and KSHV/HHV-8. These pathogenic agents probably act in concert during the differentiation and transformation processes leading to the various histological subtypes of H-NHL. The histological characterization of H-NHL can provide some clues as to the pathways involved in development.[173] Naive B cells evolve into memory B cells and plasma cells that produce immunoglobulin. Upon entering the germinal center (GC), these naive B cells become proliferating centroblasts and progress toward maturation into nonproliferating centrocytes. At the same time, this process is associated with somatic hypermutation of the immunoglobulin

TABLE 24.3

FEATURES OF HIV-ASSOCIATED LYMPHOMA

H-NHL[a]	Cells	Clonality	Characteristics	Coinfection	Location
Systemic	B cells	Monoclonal and polyclonal	Lack genetic mutations associated with most malignancies (p53, Ras, RB1); Burkitt's and diffuse large-cell lymphomas: express BCL6 and c-myc translocations	Not typically associated with oncoviruses	80% extranodal involvement
PCNSL	B cells	Mostly monoclonal	Large cell lymphomas lacking *c-myc* translocations; low CD4 cell counts	Most EBV associated	CNS
PEL	B cells	Monoclonal and polyclonal	Lack B-cell antigens (CD19 and/or CD20) or *c-myc* translocations; CD45, MUM1, CD38, and Syndecan-1	HHV-8, 100% EBV, 70%	Body cavities (pleural, peritoneal, pericardial)

[a]H-NHL, HIV-associated non-Hodgkin lymphoma; PCNSL, primary central nervous system lymphoma; PEL, primary effusion lymphoma; Systemic, H-NHL not localized to PCNSL or body cavity (PEL).

variable genes and BCL6 mutations. The immunoglobulin heavy and light chains accumulate point mutations as rearranged genes. At various stages during differentiation, B cells undergo transformation resulting in various types of NHL. Markers such as BCL6, multiple myeloma oncogene (MUM1), or syndecan-1 are used to identify histological subtypes. H-NHL BL and DLCL express BCL6+ but are MUM1− and syndecan-1− as GC centroblasts and early centrocytes. In contrast, as post-GC B cells, PEL express MUM1+ and syndecan-1+ but not BCL6−. Both EBV and KSHV/HHV-8 interact with the immunological picture along the way and ultimately, the presence of either or both of the viruses is characteristic of the histological subtypes. Systemic H-NHL is characterized by 30% of the cases being positive for EBV. In contrast, PEL is characterized by the presence of both viruses, 100% are positive for KSHV/HHV-8 and approximately 70% are also positive for EBV. Although there are some similarities between the EBV and KSHV/HHV-8, there are significant differences between the two infectious agents that may account for the different disease patterns associated with each. Factors such as EBV and c-myc oncogene rearrangement are known entities and are well established as being closely associated with H-NHL, particularly with primary CNS lymphoma.[159,178,215,218,226,227] Even though EBV is detected in the majority of primary CNS H-NHL, only approximately 50% to 60% of large cell H-NHL have detectable EBV and frequently express EBV latency type III antigens, that is, EBNA-1, 2, 3 and LMP-1 and LMP-2.[228-231] In contrast, the association of EBV with BL is slightly less (30%) and typically express only EBNA-1 (latency type I) that is different compared with almost 100% of posttransplantation NHL.[204,230-234] Worldwide, most individuals have been exposed to EBV with B lymphocytes acting as the reservoir for latent infection. Immunosuppression as a result of HIV infection promotes the development of EBV-infected and immortalized B-cell clones. A second hit resulting in genetic changes can lead to an EBV-containing monoclonal proliferation. Because EBV genome can only be detected in 60% of large cell H-NHL, other factors have been implicated in the etiology, including impairment of T-cell immunosurveillance and polyclonal B-cell expansion that may result in gene rearrangements.

Gene rearrangements involving oncogenes and immunoglobulin genes have been extensively studied amongst H-NHL. Although the exact role of c-myc is still unclear, rearrangements of the oncogene have been clearly documented in H-NHL.[226,230,231,235-237] Study of the molecular genetics of H-NHL has provided some insight into the pathogenesis of the malignancies. In part, our understanding of the molecular events leading to H-NHL has been strengthened by analyses of the immunoglobulin region, c-myc, p53, bcl-6 regions.[235,238-241] Marked B-cell proliferation in the setting of HIV-associated immunosuppression may be an important factor in the pathogenesis of H-NHL.[242-246] The proliferation may lead to patterns of translocation of part of the c-myc gene on chromosome 8 and the immunoglobulin heavy chain gene on chromosome 14 with defective recombination during isotype class switching of the constant region with preferential V_H immunoglobulin usage.[236,246-251] The vast majority of studies demonstrate evidence for monoclonality based on immunoglobulin rearrangements or by other means such as EBV or light chain analysis, but there are unique cases in which monoclonality cannot be established.[214,221,225,252,253] These so-called polyclonal H-NHL cases appear to be unique and more studies are necessary to confirm the significance of the H-NHL subtype.[178,214,215]

Although still rare, the incidence of HD appears to be slightly higher than in HIV seronegative children.[169,254] Lymphocyte depletion and mixed cellularity histologies are the most common in adults, and there is some information to support the same histology subtypes in children.[254,255]

The clinical presentation of H-NHL in children can vary depending on the age, CD4 cell count, and sites of involvement.[169,223] Symptoms range from vague complaints (fatigue, loss of appetite) to those related to specific organ involvement (hepatosplenomegaly, pleural effusion). HIV-infected children diagnosed with HD also present similarly to non–HIV-infected children with HD. Prior to instituting treatment, careful and complete staging of H-NHL is necessary to assess tumor burden and organ involvement as noted for NHL (Chapter 23) and HD (Chapter 22).

Therapeutic options for pediatric H-NHL have primarily been based on the adult experience.[168,172,191,195,224,225,256-263] Like adult HRM, cancer-directed treatment is recommended for children who have a reasonable chance of survival with concurrent HAART.[168,191,264] Optimal treatment strategies and recommendations continue to evolve for childhood HRM as treatment for HIV improves, allowing for better tolerability of chemotherapy regimens. HIV-infected children with H-NHL have been treated with combination chemotherapy consisting of different regimens including cyclophosphamide, methotrexate, cisplatin, vinblastine, vincristine, prednisone, mercaptopurine, and intrathecal chemotherapy.[168,178,258-260,262,265] Although the prognosis is not as good as seen in pediatric non–HIV-NHL, improvements are being seen with 5-year event-free survival approaching 50%.[168] In some cases, bone marrow or stem cell transplantation improves prognosis.[178,260] The experience in HD for HIV-infected children is similarly limited with respect to chemotherapy strategies. From the successful treatment regimens used for HD in immunocompetent adult patients, the same drug combinations and doses have been tried in HIV-infected cases with limited success.[254,266,267] Although still responsive to therapy for localized and systemic HD, the need for prompt diagnosis and intervention is recommended to improve prognosis.[168,191,223]

Smooth Muscle Tumors

Since the observation that the incidence of leiomyoma and leiomyosarcoma were increased in children infected with HIV, leiomyosarcoma has been included as part of the clinical case definition for Category B (Moderately Symptomatic) children who have a symptomatic condition.[268] These smooth muscle tumors have been reported to occur later in the course of HIV infection, again suggesting a strong role for prolonged or advanced immunosuppression.[167,269-271] Leiomyoma and leiomyosarcoma in HIV-infected children constituted from 3% to as high as 17% of all cancers in HIV-infected children, the difference probably reflecting lack of data collection on benign soft tissue sarcoma in cancer registries.[167,223] For reasons that are not clear, leiomyomas and leiomyosarcomas do not appear to be increased in HIV-infected adults. They can be found in the lung, brain, adrenal glands, and spleen.[270,272,273] The presence of EBV appears to be unique to smooth tumors in immunocompromised children, but its pathogenic role is unclear.[270] The clinical course is highly variable with aggressive treatment with HAART including primary excision followed by chemotherapy and/or radiation recommended based on the experience in non–HIV-infected children.[274]

Cervical and Anal Neoplasms

With the increase in cervical cancer among HIV-infected women, the Centers for Disease Control and Prevention (CDC) 1993 Revised Classification of AIDS Case Definition included invasive cervical cancer.[275] Particularly for adolescent females, the risk of lower genital tract neoplasia, such as cervical cancer, is increased in women infected with HIV.[179,189,194,219] HPV infection of the lower genital tract is associated with cervical cancer that accounts for much of the increase. Therefore, the significance for sexually active HIV-infected adolescents is magnified because they are approximately four times more likely to be infected with HPV (including infection with high oncogenic risk HPV types: 16, 18, 31, 33, 35, 39, 45, 51, 52, 56, and 58) than are HIV-uninfected women.[276] In addition, HPV infections are likely to be persistent and the associated lesions may be more difficult to treat in HIV-infected women.[276] In sexually active males, anal neoplasms due to HPV is also of concern due to increasing prevalence of HPV association with anal squamous intraepithelial lesions and association with anal cancer.[8,160,277]

Although HPV vaccines are currently available and recommended for non–HIV-infected females aged 11 to 12 years with catch-up vaccination recommended for females aged 13 to 26 years, the recommendations for HIV-infected women await the results of ongoing clinical trials.[278,279] Similarly, the efficacy of the vaccine in HIV-infected males remains unknown.[279–281] Therapy for cervical cancer in HIV-infected females requires consultation with experienced oncology gynecologists.[282–285] Similarly, anal dysplasia and anal cancer in HIV-infected individuals (males and females) require experience clinicians in diagnoses and therapy.[286–289]

Other Malignancies

Other cancers that have been noted and described in the pediatric HIV-infected population include B-cell acute lymphoblastic leukemia, liver tumors, schwannoma/neuronal tumors, MALT lymphomas, malignant histiocytosis, fibrous histiocytoma, neurofibrosarcoma, Wilms' tumor, sarcomas, and retinoblastoma.[167–169,171,191,195,264,290,291] The importance of recognizing the malignancies in HIV-infected children and adolescents is that overall, the incidence is low for some of the tumor types in the HIV-seronegative population; thus, more information is needed to determine if HIV plays a role in increasing the risk as a HRM. The prognosis and treatment recommendations for these malignancies in HIV-infected children are variable. There is little experience, due to the low numbers, in the setting of AIDS for the pediatric population.

MALIGNANCIES IN THE POSTTRANSPLANT PATIENT

The risks of developing cancer after following a transplant procedure is about 5- to 10-fold higher than the general population. The cumulative risk of cancer in SOT recipients rises to more than 50% at 20 years.[292] Cancer is now one of the most frequent causes of death in this population.[293,294] The cumulative incidence of a new malignancy following BMT is about 5% to 12%.[295,296] Age appears to be a significant risk factor for malignancy particularly for SOT patients. Excluding nonmelanoma skin cancer, transplant recipients younger than 25 years carry as high as a 50-fold increased risk of cancer compared with the general population in the same age group. This is in contrast to older patients whose risk is only increased fourfold.[297] The cumulative incidence of cancer following transplantation increases with age, making children receiving transplants at very high risk to develop a malignancy throughout their lifetime.[298] Table 24.4 demonstrates the types of cancers observed in recipients of transplantation. The scope of malignancies is similar to those in other immunodeficient populations. In addition to the defect in immune surveillance, this population may be at increased risk of cancer from exposure to potential carcinogenic agents, such as alkylator chemotherapy agents, irradiation, or antimetabolite agents administered for immunosuppression, for example, azathioprine or methotrexate.

Viral-associated cancers are the most common malignancies seen in this population, that is, posttransplant lymphoproliferative disease (PTLD) and smooth muscle tumors (EBV), KS (HHV-8/KSHV), and squamous cell carcinoma of skin, cervical, and anus (HPV). Other tumors observed include those that are thought to be responsive to a cellular immune response, such as renal cell carcinoma, melanoma, and lymphoma and thus may emerge in the context of chronic immunosuppression. Excluding PTLD, squamous cell and basal cell carcinoma are the most common malignancy reported (Table 24.4). These patients appear to be exquisitely sensitive to the carcinogenic effects of sun exposure.[299] Thus, the immune system may play a role in surveillance and elimination of cells of epithelial origin with sun-induced DNA damage.

Disease that is localized to one site and that can be readily controlled with surgery and/or radiation has an excellent outcome, but for nonlocalized disease requiring more intensive therapy, the outcome has been dismal due to infection- and treatment-related mortality. Following BMT, the median survival for patients with a new cancer is less than 2 years.[295] Analysis of data from the Israel Penn International Transplant Tumor Registry (IPITTR) revealed that for all patients with posttransplant malignancies, excluding PTLD, only those with complete surgical resection survived.[300]

Posttransplant Lymphoproliferative Disease

PTLD represents a spectrum of clinically and morphologically heterogeneous lymphoid proliferations and is the most common neoplasm for children posttransplant (Table 24.4). Most cases of PTLD following BMT are associated with EBV.[301,302] As discussed previously, a delicate balance exists between the host T-cell immune response and EBV latently infected B cells. Intensive immunosuppressive therapy or prolonged states of chronic immunosuppression invariably disrupt this balance and can lead to lymphoproliferation. EBV-associated PTLD may initially present in many ways, such as isolated hepatitis, lymphoid interstitial pneumonitis, meningoencephalitis, or as an IM-like syndrome. Frequently, PTLD presents as lymphomatous lesions (localized or diffuse) that are often extranodal, frequently in the allograft. Although less common, PTLD may present as a rapidly progressive, disseminated disease that clinically resembles septic shock and almost always results in death.[301,303]

Pathology and Molecular Biology of Posttransplant Lymphoproliferative Disease

In 2001, the World Health Organization published the classification of lymphomas and leukemias[304] that included recommendations for classification of PTLD from a 1997 Society for Hematopathology workshop.[302] PTLD has been divided into three subtypes: early lesions, polymorphous, and monomorphic PTLD. The presence of infiltrating T cells and lack of necrosis are major criteria for classifying polymorphic PTLD. However, depending upon the status of the immune system, the number of T cells and the amount of necrosis in the lesions will vary in the polymorphous subtype. Multiple clones of proliferating B cells may emerge within a single patient and

TABLE 24.4

DE NOVO MALIGNANCIES IN CHILDREN FOLLOWING BMT AND SOT

Malignancies following SOT	Malignancies following BMT
Data from IPITTR (n = 363)	Data from University of Minnesota[295] (n = 53)
PTLD (80%)	PTLD 45%
Skin (12%)	Skin (9.5%)
• Squamous cell CA (9%)	• Squamous cell CA (6.5%)
• Basal cell CA (1%)	• Basal cell CA (3%)
• Basal and squamous (2%)	
Kaposi sarcoma (3.2%)	Leukemia/MDS (9.5%)
	• MDS (6.5%)
	• ALL (1.5%)
	• JMML (1.5%)
Leiomyosarcoma (1.6%)	Sarcoma (9.5%)
	• Osteosarcoma (6.5%)
	• Rhabdomyosarcoma (1.5%)
	• Fibrosarcoma (1.5%)
Liver (1.2%)	Melanoma (7.5%)
• Hepatoblastoma (0.8%)	
• Hepatocellular CA (0.4%)	
Leukemia (1.2%)	Lymphoma (5.5%)
	• Hodgkin disease (4%)
	• Non-Hodgkin lymphoma (1.5%)
Melanoma (0.6%)	Brain tumor (5.5%)
Renal cell CA (0.6%)	Renal cell CA (2%)
Breast CA (0.6%)	Breast CA (2%)
Non-Hodgkin lymphoma (0.6%)	Hepatocellular CA (2%)
Thyroid (0.6%)	Head/neck CA (2%)
Adenocarcinoma NOS (0.6%)	
Bladder CA (0.6%)	

ALL, acute lymphoblastic leukemia; BMT, blood or marrow transplantation; IPITTR, Israel Penn International Transplant Tumor Registry; JMML, juvenile myelomonocytic leukemia; MDS, myelodysplasia syndrome; NOS, not otherwise specified; PTLD, posttransplant lymphoproliferative disease; SOT, solid organ transplantation.

thus both polymorphous and monomorphous forms may be present within the same PTLD lesion.[305] Thus, histology of a single biopsied site may not be representative of the entire disease process. Monomorphic histology is similar to *de novo* NHL, with DLBCL the most common histology observed and less frequently, BL or Burkitt-like.[306] This is in contrast to what is observed in NHL in children outside the transplant setting, where Burkitt or lymphoblastic lymphoma predominate.[12] A rare monomorphous B-cell subtype of PTLD is multiple myeloma or plasmacytoma.[302] In PTLD, as opposed to *de novo* NHL, there appears to be no difference in the histologies observed between pediatric and adult cases.

Not all forms of PTLD are of the B-cell phenotype. T-cell PTLD tends to occur late, often more than 10 years after transplantation.[307] Approximately 25% of T-cell PTLD is EBV positive.[308] PTLD with an HD phenotype also tends to occur late, long after the transplant procedure and is also generally EBV positive.[309] Some investigators have questioned whether the HD phenotype truly exists as a form of PTLD, and they have suggested that this condition may be simply a variant of polymorphic B-cell PTLD.[63] Data supporting this view include (a) Reed-Sternberg (RS) cells can often be seen in lymph nodes from patients with IM[310] and (b) RS in PTLD are

usually CD20(+), CD15(−) in contrast to RS in HD in non-transplant patients.[63] The reason for the long latency in non–B-cell PTLD is unknown. B-cell PTLD can also occur later after transplant, but it tends to be EBV negative.[311,312]

Evaluation of the biopsied specimen by *in situ* hybridization with EBERS probes for EBV sequences is important in making the diagnosis of PTLD. Reliance upon immunohistochemical staining for the LMP-1 is inadequate, as LMP-1 is positive in only 75% of EBERS-positive cases.[313] Careful evaluation must be taken in making a diagnosis of PTLD, as there are typically an increased number of EBV-positive cells in lymphoid tissue in the posttransplant period.[314] Perhaps, the greatest challenge in making the diagnosis of PTLD occurs in clinical scenarios that do not produce a mass lesion but have disseminated or infiltrative disease in solid organs. The diagnosis can sometimes be suspected upon examination of the peripheral blood, bone marrow, cerebrospinal fluid, or other body fluids for the presence of plasmacytoid cells or large B cells. Elusive cases as these are often first discovered at autopsy. An autopsy study of pediatric PTLD revealed that the diagnosis can be missed in widely disseminated cases leading to death.[295,315,316] The study reported that a third of the cases of PTLD following BMT were found at autopsy with the antemortem cause of death originally felt to be severe graft-versus-host disease (GVHD) and/or infection.[295,316]

It is important to understand that the phenotype of the B cells in PTLD can be highly variable. Because of the propensity for PTLD to exhibit plasmacytoid differentiation, the expression of CD20 can be different compared with *de novo* lymphomas. In some instances, CD20 expression is absent, whereas other B-cell antigens such as CD79a and/or CD22 may be present. Approximately two-thirds of PTLD cases had diffuse expression of CD20, while the remaining cases expressed only focal or undetectable CD20 expression.[317] Typically, CD10 and bcl-6 expression are absent, with MUM-1 positivity in the majority of cases. This suggests that most PTLD is derived from post-GC derived B cells.[318]

There is no unifying cytogenetic abnormality in PTLD. Published small series or case reports have identified translocations and deletions that are seen in other lymphomas, but finding cytogenetic abnormalities in PTLD is rare. Reported cytogenetic abnormalities include translocations such as the t(14;18), t(13;14), t(8;14), and t(3;22); trisomy 3 and 12; amplifications of n-myc; and other complex abnormalities.[319,320] Using comparative genomic hybridization, approximately half of the PTLD cases had amplifications or deletions in chromosomes 3q and 8q, or 17p, 1p, and 4q, respectively.[321] Clonality as defined by immunoglobulin gene rearrangements occurs with a greater frequency in the monomorphous subtype of PTLD compared with the polymorphous subtype. Mutations in known tumor suppressor genes and oncogenes such as p53, c-myc, and ras genes have been identified in rare cases.[232,322] The most common mutations have been found in bcl-6, consistent with the view that most PTLD appear to be derived from post-GC B cells. Mutations in bcl-6 have been reported in 40% overall and up to 90% of monomorphous PTLD.[318,322] The significance of this finding in the pathogenesis or prognosis of PTLD remains unclear.[323–326] Analysis of somatic hypermutation in immunoglobulin genes confirm that most monomorphous PTLD (>90%) have been differentiated post the GC stage.[318]

Previous investigations of EBV substrains suggested that a "super tumorigenetic" EBV strain exists. A characteristic 30 base pair deletion in the LMP-1 oncogene was present in about 30% of PTLD cases but not predictive of outcome.[327,328] Similar nonpredictive findings were shown with EBNA-1 substrain analysis. Thus, it is most likely that the distribution of substrains of EBV in PTLD is reflective of the geographic and ethnic distribution of EBV and does not play a role in tumorigenesis.[232,328]

Analysis by microarray was prognostic for DLBCL in the nontransplant population.[329,330] Studies of PTLD tissue found that the mRNA gene expression profiles of polymorphous PTLD clustered with lesions from IM cases. As expected, IM and polymorphic PTLD lesions express numerous T cell and macrophage-associated genes, whereas monomorphous PTLD expresses more abnormalities in cell cycle regulation genes. However, when T cell and macrophage genes are excluded, PTLD cases segregate into two large clusters. One cluster is composed entirely of monomorphous PTLD (about 50% of all monomorphic lesions) and the second cluster contains the cases of IM, all polymorphous disease, and the remaining monomorphous PTLD cases.[10] Further investigation is necessary to establish the value of gene profiling in the diagnosis and prognosis of this disease.

Posttransplant Lymphoproliferative Disease Following Blood or Marrow Transplantation

The incidence of PTLD in patients following BMT is between 1.0% and 1.6%.[295,316,331–333] Any factor(s) that either stimu-late B-cell proliferation and/or decrease or delay T-cell immunity will increase the risk of PTLD. For allogeneic BMT recipients, the risk of PTLD has consistently been found to be strongly associated with HLA disparity, T-cell depletion (TCD) of the stem cell graft, and use of antithymocyte globulin.[295,316,331–333] Data from the University of Minnesota that included 43 cases of PTLD found that patients were diagnosed at a median of 0.3 years post-SCT (range 0.1 to 7.3 years) and that the incidence plateaued by 5 years post-BMT.[295] All but one case was diagnosed in patients receiving an allogeneic BMT. Only 9 of the 43 patients diagnosed with PTLD survived, and in 15 patients, the diagnosis was made postmortem. Median survival was 36 days and the 1-year survival rate was 25%.

TCD methods that specifically remove T cells, for example, sheep red blood cell rosetting and the use of anti–T-cell monoclonal antibodies, conferred a higher risk of PTLD compared with "pan-lymphocyte"–depleted stem cell grafts, for example, CAMPATH-1 monoclonal antibodies or elutriation.[332] Since "pan-lymphocyte" depletion methods decrease the number of EBV-infected B cells as well as T cells, this may delay B-cell proliferation until EBV-CTL function recovers. The use of CD34-positive selection has become a popular method for TCD of allogeneic PBSC. Early results suggest that the incidence of PTLD is similar to other "pan-lymphocyte" depletion methods. However, PTLD has been reported following the use of highly immunosuppressive therapy with CD34-selected autologous peripheral blood stem cells rescue to treat autoimmune disease or malignancy.[334,335]

Despite the degree of HLA mismatching and relatively low T cell numbers contained within the graft, umbilical cord blood transplants are associated with a relatively low incidence of PTLD. Review of 272 umbilical cord blood procedures from two institutions revealed only a 2% incidence of PTLD.[336] A subsequent study suggested that patients receiving umbilical cord bloods within the context of nonmyeloablative preparative regimens were at increased risk, particularly if antithymocyte globulin was used in the pretransplant conditioning.[337]

The diagnosis of PTLD in the BMT setting is not always obvious, since approximately a third of cases have been diagnosed from postmortem examinations.[295] PTLD in the BMT setting may frequently present with a disseminated or fulminant form of the disease that lacks a well-defined tumor mass or adenopathy. For this reason, semiquantitative viral load determination by PCR on peripheral blood has been used to identify high-risk patients before they develop disease. There are many reports that correlate increased viral load with the development of PTLD.[338–340] However, there are no blinded, prospective studies to determine the predictive value of quantitative PCR for the development of PTLD. Limitations in interpreting EBV viral load results stem from variability between different methods.[341] High viral loads with symptoms, such as fever and adenopathy, may predict development of PTLD, but in an asymptomatic patient, a single elevated EBV level does not correlate with the development of disease. Recipients of T-cell–depleted grafts who have high viral loads may develop disease even when asymptomatic.[340] Further investigations are needed to better define the role of viral load determinations in clinical practice.

Preemptive therapeutic approaches, using anti-CD20 monoclonal antibody rituximab, have been used to reduce B-cell proliferation until EBV-CTL activity recovers in patients with persistently increased EBV viral loads to reduce the risk of PTLD.[316] For some patients, a simple reduction in immunosuppressive therapy, if possible, may result in improvement of EBV viral load levels, although this has rarely been successful in treating established PTLD after BMT.[316] Once the disease is clinically evident, a variety of treatments have been tried. Currently, there are no standardized treatment approaches for BMT recipients who have developed PTLD and frequently a combination of methods are used. Surgical resection and/or radiotherapy can be effective for localized PTLD, but disease following BMT is typically extensive. Success has been reported in a very small number of patients treated with interferon-α.[316] Cytotoxic chemotherapy has been frequently utilized in SOT patients with PTLD, but its usefulness after BMT has been limited due to concerns regarding toxicity when administered early after the transplant procedure. Several reports demonstrated that a majority of patients treated with rituximab will respond and complete remission (CR) has been achieved in many patients.[342–350] The use of donor leukocyte infusion (DLI) successfully treated BLPD in post-BMT cases.[339,351] However, severe GVHD has occurred, and DLI is not always successful at controlling the disease.[338] To circumvent the GVHD problem, investigators inserted a suicide gene, herpes thymidine kinase, into donor lymphocytes,[352] or produced *ex vivo* EBV-specific CTL.[339] These strategies were successful in treating some cases, but these approaches are not feasible for most centers due to the cost and regulatory oversight.

Posttransplant Lymphoproliferative Disease following Solid Organ Transplantation

The risk factors for PTLD in the SOT recipients are well described. The primary risk factor appears to be patients who are EBV seronegative at the time of transplant.[353] Therefore, it is not surprising that recipients of younger age have the highest risk of PTLD.[354,355] The type of organ transplanted has also been identified as a risk factor with an incidence of 1% to 5% in "low-risk" patients, for example, renal, heart, and liver, to 10% to 30% in the "high-risk" patients, for example, lung, small bowel, and multiple organ grafts. The more T-cell specific the immunosuppression, the higher is the associated incidence of PTLD for a particular population. Thus, the use of T-cell antibodies results in the highest incidence.[356] Calcineurin inhibitors also increase the risk of PTLD, and there is some evidence that tacrolimus predisposes a higher risk than cyclosporin.[354,356–358] Subsequent studies demonstrated that if serum levels are monitored closely, there is no increased risk of using FK506 as compared with cyclosporin.[359] Finally, hepatitis C infection was reported in early studies to be a possible risk factor for the development of certain forms of PTLD, particularly multiple myeloma.[360] However, a registry study examining more than 200,000 transplant recipients failed to demonstrate that hepatitis was significantly associated with PTLD.[360]

Prognostic factors for affected patients are difficult to ascertain, since most studies contain small numbers of patients and uniformity in therapy is rare. Some studies suggested that monomorphic subtypes have a worse prognosis than polymorphic subtypes,[306,311,361] but this has not been found in other series.[312] Some studies suggested that clonality is a poor prognostic factor,[312] while others failed to confirm this.[311] The combination of monomorphic histology, clonal immunoglobulin gene rearrangement, and/or abnormal karyotype may predict a poor prognosis. The stage of disease can also adversely affect prognosis. Classical NHL staging classifications have limited value in PTLD due to the high predilection for extranodal involvement, but multiple (>2) sites of disease appears to identify patient with poorer prognosis, and CNS involvement portends a dismal outcome.[312,362] PTLD associated with primary EBV infection appears to have a superior prognosis.[312,363,364] Although PTLD observed greater than 1-year posttransplant, non–B-cell phenotype and/or tumor

that is EBV negative has a very poor prognosis.[307,311,312] The exception to this rule is HD that is associated with EBV in the majority of cases and responds well to standard therapy for HD.[309]

Prophylaxis and preemptive strategies to reduce the incidence of PTLD in SOT have been largely unsuccessful. Viral load monitoring has not been as helpful in predicting patients at risk in recipients of SOT as compared with BMT.[365–369] The treatment of PTLD patients presents several therapeutic challenges. As other immunodeficient patients with cancer, these patients are very susceptible to regimen-related toxicity, including infections and end-organ toxicity. Furthermore, they are at risk of rejecting the transplanted allograft. Therefore, the ideal therapy for PTLD would be minimally toxic, yet cytotoxic to the B cells, prevent allograft rejection, and minimize the inhibition of immune responses required to control EBV-driven B-cell proliferation.

The approach most widely used as initial therapy is reduction of immunosuppression.[370–377] This may be sufficient to control disease, especially in localized disease, polyclonal lesions, or cases that present like IM. In studies of pediatric PTLD cases, response to immunosuppression reduction favored patients with polymorphic histology compared with patients with monomorphic histology.[306,378] Antiviral agents (acyclovir or ganciclovir) and/or intravenous immunoglobulin have been used extensively for prophylaxis and treatment of PTLD. This approach may be useful in prophylaxis or delaying primary EBV infection or reactivation, but the efficacy of antivirals in treating PTLD is uncertain. It has been difficult to ascertain the role of antiviral agents in treating PTLD, since they are seldom used without other interventions, for example, reduction of immunosuppression.[303,379,380] A prospective trial using ganciclovir prophylaxis failed to influence viral load or the incidence of PTLD.[380] Local control with surgery and/or radiotherapy is very effective in curing localized disease, but this represents only a small percentage of patients.[379,381] Even monomorphic, monoclonal, or aggressive histology, such as Burkitt histology, can be cured by local therapy alone if truly localized.

Complete responses have been achieved with interferon-α, but rejection, relapses, and death from infection have been high.[377,382] Given these results, IFN should no longer be considered an option for the treatment of PTLD. The use of anti-B-cell antibodies to treat PTLD is an attractive approach. Using anti-CD20, the observed response rate was 65%, with an 18% relapse rate, 4% death due to allograft rejection, and 12% infectious deaths as confirmed by others.[344,383] However, subsequent reports using anti-CD20 to treat patients following SOT with monomorphic disease, who failed reduction of immunosuppression, showed only 27% CR rates.[384] Treatment with rituximab, either alone or in combination with other treatment for PTLD, is showing promise as an effective approach.[347,349,374,376,378] This may be particularly true for EBV-associated PTLD.[385]

For patients who fail reduction of immunosuppression, cytotoxic chemotherapy has become an attractive option because it will treat the disease and maintain an immunosuppressive state to protect the allograft. In adult patients with PTLD, the use of conventional dosed chemotherapy used to treat NHL has been complicated by toxicity and infection, with regimen related mortality as high as 50%.[311,312] Small studies using conventional dosing of chemotherapy to treat childhood NHL found less treatment-related mortality compared with adults.[306,386] A low-dose chemotherapy regimen of cyclophosphamide and prednisone was used to treat children with PTLD who were refractory to reduction of immunosuppression, antiviral therapy, interferon, and/or rituximab.[387] This treatment regimen resulted in a 77% CR rate, 18% relapse rate, 5% regimen-related mortality, and 9% of patients lost their allograft to rejection. The 2-year failure-free survival defined as alive, in continuous CR, and with original functioning allograft was 67%. Others have similar responses with low-dose chemotherapy.[388,389] Rituximab was added to this chemotherapy backbone to increase efficacy without added toxicity.[390] The use of rituximab may be associated with a lower requirement for alkylating agents and anthracyclines and thus decreased toxicity from these agents.[388] Rituximab-based regimens are currently under investigation in the Children's Oncology Group (COG) and in other groups including the use of the agent in CNS disease.[345,349,388,391] Use of similar regimens with rituximab in PTLD post–heart transplant patients has resulted in excellent response and survival.[376]

Utilizing adoptive T-cell therapy, that is, DLI, in organ transplant recipients is complex. Because cadaveric organs are universally utilized, donor leukocytes are often not available. Second, in contrast to BMT, PTLD following organ transplant is derived from recipient cells, so the immunologic recognition, specificity, and efficacy of donor leukocytes are uncertain. Finally, the use of closely matched relatives' leukocytes runs the risk of both rejection and GVHD.[392] The *ex vivo* generation of EBV-specific CTL is a possible alternative approach and several groups have investigations underway.[393–397] A major obstacle, as opposed to BMT, has been the lack of persistence of the transferred EBV-CTL in the host. Although very exciting, this approach remains prohibitive for most centers due to the high level of technology, regulatory issues, and cost.

SUMMARY

Increasing numbers of pediatric oncologists are now being faced with the difficult task of caring for immunodeficient children with malignancies. These patients present numerous challenges. First, the types of tumors observed in this population are not typical of cancers seen in the immunocompetent pediatric oncology population. Second, regardless of the etiology of the immune defect, immunodeficient patients with cancer fare worse than the general population even histologically similar malignancies. With advances in supportive care, particularly prevention and treatment of opportunistic infections, patients with cancer associated with immunodeficiencies now enjoy longer lives than ever before, but cancer remains a major cause of morbidity and mortality in the immunodeficient child. Despite the therapeutic challenges, these patients present a remarkable opportunity to study and explore how the immune system functions to prevent cancer. Although many malignancies observed in immunocompromised patients are associated with infectious agents, a substantial number are not. Therefore, anticancer immune surveillance must be more than just an inability to control infections. Immune surveillance must also protect against the development of neoplasia by the identification and/or elimination of cells with abnormalities in proliferation, function, and/or apoptosis.

References

1. Thomas L. Cellular and humoral aspects of hypersensitivity states. New York, NY: Hoeber, 1959.
2. Filipovich A. Malignancies in the immunocompromised human. New York, NY: Elsevier, 1980.
3. Filipovich AH, Mathur A, Kamat D, et al. Lymphoproliferative disorders and other tumors complicating immunodeficiencies. Immunodeficiency 1994;5:91–112.
4. Lefrere JJ, Meyohas MC, Mariotti M, et al. Detection of human herpesvirus 8 DNA sequences before the appearance of Kaposi's sarcoma in human immunodeficiency virus (HIV)-positive subjects with a known date of HIV seroconversion. J Infect Dis 1996;174:283–287.
5. Orenstein JM, Alkan S, Blauvelt A, et al. Visualization of human herpesvirus type 8 in Kaposi's sarcoma by light and transmission electron microscopy. AIDS 1997;11:F35–F45.
6. Beckmann AM, Daling JR, Sherman KJ, et al. Human papillomavirus infection and anal cancer. Int J Cancer 1989;43:1042–1049.
7. Kiyabu MT, Shibata D, Arnheim N, et al. Detection of human papillomavirus in formalin-fixed, invasive squamous carcinomas using the polymerase chain reaction. Am J Surg Pathol 1989;13:221–224.
8. Palefsky J. Human papillomavirus infection among HIV-infected individuals. Implications for development of malignant tumors. Hematol Oncol Clin North Am 1991;5:357–370.
9. Gennery AR, Cant AJ, Jeggo PA. Immunodeficiency associated with DNA repair defects. Clin Exp Immunol 2000;121:1–7.
10. Greiner TC, Baker KS, Gross TG. Posttransplant lymphoproliferative disease in children. In: American Society of Clinical Oncology Annual Meeting, Alexandria, VA, 2004.
11. Smith MA, Ries LA. Childhood cancer: incidence, survival, and mortality. In: Pizzo PA, Poplack DG, eds. Principles and practice of pediatric oncology. Philadelphia, PA: Lippincott-Raven, 1997:1–20.
12. Sandlund JT. Malignant lymphomas in childhood. In: Hoffman R, ed. Hematology basic principles and practice. New York, NY: Churchill Livingstone, 2000:1339–1349.
13. Anagnostopoulos I, Hummel M, Kreschel C, et al. Morphology, immunophenotype, and distribution of latently and/or productively Epstein-Barr virus-infected cells in acute infectious mononucleosis: implications for the interindividual infection route of Epstein-Barr virus. Blood 1995;85:744–750.
14. Li QX, Young LS, Niedobitek G, et al. Epstein-Barr virus infection and replication in a human epithelial cell system. Nature 1992;356:347–350.
15. Masucci MG, Ernberg I. Epstein-Barr virus: adaptation to a life within the immune system. Trends Microbiol 1994;2:125–130.
16. Babcock GJ, Decker LL, Volk M, et al. EBV persistence in memory B cells in vivo. Immunity 1998;9:395–404.
17. Yang J, Tao Q, Flinn IW, et al. Characterization of Epstein-Barr virus-infected B cells in patients with posttransplantation lymphoproliferative disease: disappearance after rituximab therapy does not predict clinical response. Blood 2000;96:4055–4063.
18. Kieff E. Epstein Barr virus and its replication. In: Fields BN, Knipe DM, Howley PM, eds. Fields virology. 3rd ed. Philadelphia, PA: Lippincott-Raven, 1996.
19. Felton-Edkins ZA, Kondrashov A, Karali D, et al. Epstein-Barr virus induces cellular transcription factors to allow active expression of EBER genes by RNA polymerase III. J Biol Chem 2006;281:33871–33880.
20. Samanta M, Iwakiri D, Kanda T, et al. EB virus-encoded RNAs are recognized by RIG-I and activate signaling to induce type I IFN. EMBO J 2006;25:4207–4214.
21. Wu Y, Maruo S, Yajima M, et al. Epstein-Barr virus (EBV)-encoded RNA 2 (EBER2) but not EBER1 plays a critical role in EBV-induced B-cell growth transformation. J Virol 2007;81:11236–11245.
22. Yoshizaki T, Endo K, Ren Q, et al. Oncogenic role of Epstein-Barr virus-encoded small RNAs (EBERs) in nasopharyngeal carcinoma. Auris Nasus Larynx 2007;34:73–78.
23. Yajima M, Kanda T, Takada K. Critical role of Epstein-Barr virus (EBV)-encoded RNA in efficient EBV-induced B-lymphocyte growth transformation. J Virol 2005;79:4298–4307.
24. Edwards RH, Marquitz AR, Raab-Traub N. Epstein-Barr virus BART microRNAs are produced from a large intron prior to splicing. J Virol 2008;82:9094–9106.
25. Zhang J, Chen H, Weinmaster G, et al. Epstein-Barr virus BamHi-a rightward transcript-encoded RPMS protein interacts with the CBF1-associated corepressor CIR to negatively regulate the activity of EBNA2 and NotchIC. J Virol 2001;75:2946–2956.
26. Cohen JI. Epstein-Barr virus infection. N Engl J Med 2000;343:481–492.
27. Chen H, Smith P, Ambinder RF, et al. Expression of Epstein-Barr virus BamHI-A rightward transcripts in latently infected B cells from peripheral blood. Blood 1999;93:3026–3032.
28. Miller G. The switch between latency and replication of Epstein-Barr virus. J Infect Dis 1990;161:833–844.
29. Brooks LA, Lear AL, Young LS, et al. Transcripts from the Epstein-Barr virus BamHI A fragment are detectable in all three forms of virus latency. J Virol 1993;67:3182–3190.
30. Thorley-Lawson DA. Basic virological aspects of Epstein-Barr virus infection. Semin Hematol 1988;25:247–260.
31. Okano M, Gross TG. Epstein-Barr virus-associated hemophagocytic syndrome and fatal infectious mononucleosis. Am J Hematol 1996;53:111–115.
32. Greiner T, Gross T. Atypical immune lymphoproliferations. In: Hoffman R, ed. Hematology basic principles and practice. 3rd ed. New York, NY: Churchill Livingstone, 2000.
33. Evans AS, Niederman JC, Cenabre LC, et al. A prospective evaluation of heterophile and Epstein-Barr virus-specific IgM antibody tests in clinical and subclinical infectious mononucleosis: specificity and sensitivity of the tests and persistence of antibody. J Infect Dis 1975;132:546–554.
34. Henle W, Henle GE, Horwitz CA. Epstein-Barr virus specific diagnostic tests in infectious mononucleosis. Hum Pathol 1974;5:551–565.
35. Horwitz CA, Henle W, Henle G, et al. Long-term serological follow-up of patients for Epstein-Barr virus after recovery from infectious mononucleosis. J Infect Dis 1985;151:1150–1153.
36. Pearson G. Infectious mononucleosis: the humoral response. In: Schlossberg D, ed. Infectious mononucleosis. 2nd ed. New York, NY: Springer-Verlag, 1989.
37. Durbin WA, Sullivan JL. Epstein-Barr virus infection. Pediatr Rev 1994;15:63–68; quiz 68.
38. Paul JR, Bunnell WW. The presence of heterophile antibodies in infectious mononucleosis. Am J Med Sci 1974;267:178–188.
39. Frishman W, Kraus ME, Zabkar J, et al. Infectious mononucleosis and fatal myocarditis. Chest 1977;72:535–538.
40. Garzelli C, Taub FE, Scharff JE, et al. Epstein-Barr virus-transformed lymphocytes produce monoclonal autoantibodies that react with antigens in multiple organs. J Virol 1984;52:722–725.
41. Ritter K, Brestrich H, Thomssen R. IgM autoantibodies against two cellular antigens always appear in acute Epstein-Barr virus infection. Scand J Infect Dis 1990;22:135–143.
42. Appay V, Dunbar PR, Callan M, et al. Memory CD8+ T cells vary in differentiation phenotype in different persistent virus infections. Nat Med 2002;8:379–385.
43. Callan MF, Tan L, Annels N, et al. Direct visualization of antigen-specific CD8+ T cells during the primary immune response to Epstein-Barr virus In vivo. J Exp Med 1998;187:1395–1402.

44. Rickinson AB, Moss DJ. Human cytotoxic T lymphocyte responses to Epstein-Barr virus infection. Annu Rev Immunol 1997;15:405–431.
45. Tan LC, Gudgeon N, Annels NE, et al. A re-evaluation of the frequency of CD8+ T cells specific for EBV in healthy virus carriers. J Immunol 1999;162:1827–1835.
46. Tomkinson BE, Wagner DK, Nelson DL, et al. Activated lymphocytes during acute Epstein-Barr virus infection. J Immunol 1987;139:3802–3807.
47. McKenna RW, Parkin J, Gajl-Peczalska KJ, et al. Ultrastructural, cytochemical, and membrane surface marker characteristics of the atypical lymphocytes in infectious mononucleosis. Blood 1977;50:505–515.
48. Silins SL, Sherritt MA, Silleri JM, et al. Asymptomatic primary Epstein-Barr virus infection occurs in the absence of blood T-cell repertoire perturbations despite high levels of systemic viral load. Blood 2001;98:3739–3744.
49. Filipovich AH, Heinitz KJ, Robison LL, et al. The immunodeficiency cancer registry. A research resource. Am J Pediatr Hematol Oncol 1987;9:183–184.
50. Elenitoba-Johnson KS, Jaffe ES. Lymphoproliferative disorders associated with congenital immunodeficiencies. Semin Diagn Pathol 1997;14:35–47.
51. Aghamohammadi A, Parvaneh N, Tirgari F, et al. Lymphoma of mucosa-associated lymphoid tissue in common variable immunodeficiency. Leuk Lymphoma 2006;47:343–346.
52. Chua I, Quinti I, Grimbacher B. Lymphoma in common variable immunodeficiency: interplay between immune dysregulation, infection and genetics. Curr Opin Hematol 2008;15:368–374.
53. Salavoura K, Kolialexi A, Tsangaris G, et al. Development of cancer in patients with primary immunodeficiencies. Anticancer Res 2008;28:1263–1269.
54. Shcherbina A, Candotti F, Rosen FS, et al. High incidence of lymphomas in a subgroup of Wiskott-Aldrich syndrome patients. Br J Haematol 2003;121:529–530.
55. Gatti RA, Good RA. Occurrence of malignancy in immunodeficiency diseases. A literature review. Cancer 1971;28:89–98.
56. Seemayer TA, Gross TG, Egeler RM, et al. X-linked lymphoproliferative disease: twenty-five years after the discovery. Pediatr Res 1995;38:471–478.
57. Sumegi J, Huang D, Lanyi A, et al. Correlation of mutations of the SH2D1A gene and epstein-barr virus infection with clinical phenotype and outcome in X-linked lymphoproliferative disease. Blood 2000;96:3118–3125.
58. Tran H, Nourse J, Hall S, et al. Immunodeficiency-associated lymphomas. Blood Rev 2008;22:261–281.
59. Seidemann K, Tiemann M, Henze G, et al. Therapy for non-Hodgkin lymphoma in children with primary immunodeficiency: analysis of 19 patients from the BFM trials. Med Pediatr Oncol 1999;33:536–544.
60. Sandoval C, Swift M. Treatment of lymphoid malignancies in patients with ataxia-telangiectasia. Med Pediatr Oncol 1998;31:491–497.
61. Hoffmann T, Heilmann C, Madsen HO, et al. Matched unrelated allogeneic bone marrow transplantation for recurrent malignant lymphoma in a patient with X-linked lymphoproliferative disease (XLP). Bone Marrow Transplant 1998;22:603–604.
62. Robison LL, Stoker V, Frizzera G, et al. Hodgkin's disease in pediatric patients with naturally occurring immunodeficiency. Am J Pediatr Hematol Oncol 1987;9:189–192.
63. Ranganathan S, Jaffe R. Is there a difference between Hodgkin's disease and a Hodgkin's-like post-transplant lymphoproliferative disorder, and why should that be of any interest? Pediatr Transplant 2004;8:6–8.
64. Ambinder RF. Epstein-Barr virus-associated lymphoproliferative disorders. Rev Clin Exp Hematol 2003;7:362–374.
65. Comito MA, Sun Q, Lucas KG. Immunotherapy for Epstein-Barr virus-associated tumors. Leuk Lymphoma 2004;45:1981–1987.
66. Isam H, Al-Wahadneh A. Successful bone marrow transplantation in a child with X-linked hyper-IgM syndrome. Saudi J Kidney Dis Transpl 2004;15:489–493.
67. Fischer A. Primary immunodeficiency diseases: an experimental model for molecular medicine. Lancet 2001;357:1863–1869.
68. Kohn DB, Sadelain M, Glorioso JC. Occurrence of leukaemia following gene therapy of X-linked SCID. Nat Rev Cancer 2003;3:477–488.
69. Monforte-Munoz H, Kapoor N, et al. Epstein-Barr virus-associated leiomyomatosis and posttransplant lymphoproliferative disorder in a child with severe combined immunodeficiency: case report and review of the literature. Pediatr Dev Pathol 2003; 6:449–457.
70. Furman RR, Hoelzer D. Purine nucleoside phosphorylase inhibition as a novel therapeutic approach for B-cell lymphoid malignancies. Semin Oncol 2007;34:S29–S34.
71. Ravandi F, Gandhi V. Novel purine nucleoside analogues for T-cell-lineage acute lymphoblastic leukaemia and lymphoma. Expert Opin Investig Drugs 2006;15:1601–1613.
72. Varon R, Schoch C, Reis A, et al. Mutation analysis of the Nijmegen breakage syndrome gene (NBS1) in nineteen patients with acute myeloid leukemia with complex karyotypes. Leuk Lymphoma 2003;44:1931–1934.
73. Husain M, Grunebaum E, Naqvi A, et al. Burkitt's lymphoma in a patient with adenosine deaminase deficiency-severe combined immunodeficiency treated with polyethylene glycol-adenosine deaminase. J Pediatr 2007;151:93–95.
74. Kaufman DA, Hershfield MS, Bocchini JA, et al. Cerebral lymphoma in an adenosine deaminase-deficient patient with severe combined immunodeficiency receiving polyethylene glycol-conjugated adenosine deaminase. Pediatrics 2005;116:e876–e879.
75. Derry JM, Ochs HD, Francke U. Isolation of a novel gene mutated in Wiskott-Aldrich syndrome. Cell 1994;79(5):following 922.
76. Perry GS III, Spector BD, Schuman LM, et al. The Wiskott-Aldrich syndrome in the United States and Canada (1892–1979). J Pediatr 1980;97:72–78.
77. Bosticardo M, Marangoni F, Aiuti A, et al. Recent advances in understanding the pathophysiology of Wiskott-Aldrich syndrome. Blood 2009;113(25):6288–6295.
78. Fernando HS, Kynaston HG, Jiang WG. WASP and WAVE proteins: vital intrinsic regulators of cell motility and their role in cancer (review). Int J Mol Med 2009;23:141–148.
79. Lee PP, Chen TX, Jiang LP, et al. Clinical and Molecular Characteristics of 35 Chinese Children with Wiskott-Aldrich Syndrome. J Clin Immunol 2009;29(4):490–500.
80. Locci M, Draghici E, Marangoni F, et al. The Wiskott-Aldrich syndrome protein is required for iNKT cell maturation and function. J Exp Med 2009;206:735–742.
81. Ochs HD. Mutations of the Wiskott-Aldrich syndrome protein affect protein expression and dictate the clinical phenotypes. Immunol Res 2009;44(1–3):84–88.
82. Ochs HD, Filipovich AH, Veys P, et al. Wiskott-Aldrich syndrome: diagnosis, clinical and laboratory manifestations, and treatment. Biol Blood Marrow Transplant 2008; 15:84–90.
83. Staub E, Groene J, Heinze M, et al. An expression module of WIPF1-coexpressed genes identifies patients with favorable prognosis in three tumor types. J Mol Med 2009;87 (6):633–644.
84. Coffey AJ, Brooksbank RA, Brandau O, et al. Host response to EBV infection in X-linked lymphoproliferative disease results from mutations in an SH2-domain encoding gene. Nat Genet 1998;20:129–135.

85. Sayos J, Wu C, Morra M, et al. The X-linked lymphoproliferative-disease gene product SAP regulates signals induced through the co-receptor SLAM. Nature 1998;395:462–469.
86. Bassiri H, Janice Yeo WC, Rothman J, et al. X-linked lymphoproliferative disease (XLP): a model of impaired anti-viral, anti-tumor and humoral immune responses. Immunol Res 2008;42:145–159.
87. Engel P, Eck MJ, Terhorst C. The SAP and SLAM families in immune responses and X-linked lymphoproliferative disease. Nat Rev Immunol 2003;3:813–821.
88. Gilmour KC, Gaspar HB. Pathogenesis and diagnosis of X-linked lymphoproliferative disease. Expert Rev Mol Diagn 2003;3:549–561.
89. Latour S. Natural killer T cells and X-linked lymphoproliferative syndrome. Curr Opin Allergy Clin Immunol 2007;7:510–514.
90. Miyawaki T. Primary immunodeficiencies inducing EBV-associated severe illnesses. Iran J Allergy Asthma Immunol 2004;3:51–57.
91. Nichols KE, Ma CS, Cannons JL, et al. Molecular and cellular pathogenesis of X-linked lymphoproliferative disease. Immunol Rev 2005;203:180–199.
92. Veillette A. Immune regulation by SLAM family receptors and SAP-related adaptors. Nat Rev Immunol 2006;6:56–66.
93. Yang J, Lemas VM, Flinn IW, et al. Application of the ELISPOT assay to the characterization of CD8(+) responses to Epstein-Barr virus antigens. Blood 2000;95:241–248.
94. Hoshino T, Kanegane H, Doki N, et al. X-linked lymphoproliferative disease in an adult. Int J Hematol 2005;82:55–58.
95. Hugle B, Astigarraga I, Henter JI, et al. Simultaneous manifestation of fulminant infectious mononucleosis with haemophagocytic syndrome and B-cell lymphoma in X-linked lymphoproliferative disease. Eur J Pediatr 2007;166:589–593.
96. Kanegane H, Ito Y, Ohshima K, et al. X-linked lymphoproliferative syndrome presenting with systemic lymphocytic vasculitis. Am J Hematol 2005;78:130–133.
97. Imashuku S, Kuriyama K, Teramura T, et al. Requirement for etoposide in the treatment of Epstein-Barr virus-associated hemophagocytic lymphohistiocytosis. J Clin Oncol 2001;19:2665–2673.
98. Gross TG, Filipovich AH, Conley ME, et al. Cure of X-linked lymphoproliferative disease (XLP) with allogeneic hematopoietic stem cell transplantation (HSCT): report from the XLP registry. Bone Marrow Transplant 1996;17:741–744.
99. Trottestam H, Beutel K, Meeths M, et al. Treatment of the X-linked lymphoproliferative, Griscelli and Chediak-Higashi syndromes by HLH directed therapy. Pediatr Blood Cancer 2009;52:268–272.
100. Barbosa MD, Nguyen QA, Tchernev VT, et al. Identification of the homologous beige and Chediak-Higashi syndrome genes. Nature 1996;382:262–265.
101. Ward DM, Shiflett SL, Kaplan J. Chediak-Higashi syndrome: a clinical and molecular view of a rare lysosomal storage disorder. Curr Mol Med 2002;2:469–477.
102. Premalata C, Devi L, Madhumathi DS, et al. Chediak-Higashi syndrome masquerading as acute leukemia: the significance of lymphocyte inclusions. J Clin Oncol 2006;24: 3505–3507.
103. Chang H, Yi QL. Acute myeloid leukemia with pseudo-Chediak-Higashi anomaly exhibits a specific immunophenotype with CD2 expression. Am J Clin Pathol 2006; 125:791–794.
104. Ghavamzadeh A, Alimogaddam K, Jahani M, et al. Stem cell transplantation; Iranian experience. Arch Iran Med 2009;12:69–72.
105. Henter JI, Arico M, Egeler RM, et al. HLH-94: a treatment protocol for hemophagocytic lymphohistiocytosis. HLH study group of the Histiocyte Society. Med Pediatr Oncol 1997;28:342–347.
106. Pasic S, Micic D, Kuzmanovic M. Epstein-Barr virus-associated haemophagocytic lymphohistiocytosis in Wiskott-Aldrich syndrome. Acta Paediatr 2003;92:859–861.
107. Notarangelo LD, Duse M, Ugazio AG. Immunodeficiency with hyper-IgM (HIM). Immunodefic Rev 1992;3:101–121.
108. Malhotra RK, Li W. Poorly differentiated gastroenteropancreatic neuroendocrine carcinoma associated with X-linked hyperimmunoglobulin M syndrome. Arch Pathol Lab Med 2008;132:847–850.
109. Hayward AR, Levy J, Facchetti F, et al. Cholangiopathy and tumors of the pancreas, liver, and biliary tree in boys with X-linked immunodeficiency with hyper-IgM. J Immunol 1997;158:977–983.
110. Rieux-Laucat F, Le Deist F, Hivroz C, et al. Mutations in Fas associated with human lymphoproliferative syndrome and autoimmunity. Science 1995;268:1347–1349.
111. Teachey DT, Manno CS, Axsom KM, et al. Unmasking Evans syndrome: T-cell phenotype and apoptotic response reveal autoimmune lymphoproliferative syndrome (ALPS). Blood 2005;105:2443–2448.
112. Bleesing JJ. Autoimmune lymphoproliferative syndrome (ALPS). Curr Pharm Des 2003;9:265–278.
113. Clementi R, Dagna L, Dianzani U, et al. Inherited perforin and Fas mutations in a patient with autoimmune lymphoproliferative syndrome and lymphoma. N Engl J Med 2004;351:1419–1424.
114. Poppema S, Maggio E, van den Berg A. Development of lymphoma in autoimmune lymphoproliferative syndrome (ALPS) and its relationship to Fas gene mutations. Leuk Lymphoma 2004;45:423–431.
115. Rao VK, Straus SE. Causes and consequences of the autoimmune lymphoproliferative syndrome. Hematology 2006;11:15–23.
116. van der Werff Ten Bosch J, Schotte P, Ferster A, et al. Reversion of autoimmune lymphoproliferative syndrome with an antimalarial drug: preliminary results of a clinical cohort study and molecular observations. Br J Haematol 2002;117:176–188.
117. Battle WM, Brooks FP. Adenocarcinoma of the stomach with common variable immunodeficiency syndrome. Arch Intern Med 1978;138:1682–1684.
118. Cox JE, Ott DJ. Gastric adenocarcinoma in a patient with common variable immunodeficiency. Abdom Imaging 1994;19:501–502.
119. den Hartog G, van der Meer JW, Jansen JB, et al. Decreased gastrin secretion in patients with late-onset hypogammaglobulinemia. N Engl J Med 1988;318:1563–1567.
120. Atherton JC. The pathogenesis of Helicobacter pylori-induced gastro-duodenal diseases. Annu Rev Pathol 2006;1:63–96.
121. Capelle LG, de Vries AC, Looman CW, et al. Gastric MALT lymphoma: epidemiology and high adenocarcinoma risk in a nation-wide study. Eur J Cancer 2008;44:2470–2476.
122. Iida T, Iwahashi M, Nakamura M, et al. Primary hepatic low-grade B-cell lymphoma of MALT-type associated with Helicobacter pylori infection. Hepatogastroenterology 2007;54:1898–1901.
123. Kandulski A, Selgrad M, Malfertheiner P. Helicobacter pylori infection: a clinical overview. Dig Liver Dis 2008;40:619–626.
124. Lee SY, Kim JJ, Lee JH, et al. Synchronous adenocarcinoma and mucosa-associated lymphoid tissue (MALT) lymphoma in a single stomach. Jpn J Clin Oncol 2005;35:591–594.
125. Lochhead P, El-Omar EM. Helicobacter pylori infection and gastric cancer. Best Pract Res Clin Gastroenterol 2007;21:281–297.

126. Nakamura T, Seto M, Tajika M, et al. Clinical features and prognosis of gastric MALT lymphoma with special reference to responsiveness to *H. pylori* eradication and API2-MALT1 status. Am J Gastroenterol 2008;103:62–70.
127. Seo DB, Kwon KS, Park HS, et al. Metachronous gastric MALT lymphoma and early gastric cancer: a case report. Korean J Gastroenterol 2007;49:245–250.
128. Kusic B, Gasparov S, Katicic M, et al. Monoclonality in *Helicobacter pylori*-positive gastric biopsies: an early detection of mucosa-associated lymphoid tissue lymphoma. Exp Mol Pathol 2003;74:61–67.
129. Hung YM, Chou KJ, Hung SY, et al. De novo malignancies after kidney transplantation. Urology 2007;69:1041–1044.
130. Nagata Y, Eguchi S, Takatsuki M, et al. Experience of gastric cancer in a patient who had received a living-donor liver transplantation. Gastric Cancer 2007;10:187–190.
131. Odashima M, Otaka M, Jin M, et al. Rapid regression of multiple gastric carcinoid tumors with hypergastrinemia and atrophic gastritis after renal transplantation. Dig Dis Sci 2008;53:865–866.
132. Sanchez-Fructuoso A, Conesa J, Perez Flores I, et al. Conversion to sirolimus in renal transplant patients with tumors. Transplant Proc 2006;38:2451–2452.
133. Aull MJ, Buell JF, Peddi VR, et al. MALToma: a *Helicobacter pylori*-associated malignancy in transplant patients: a report from the Israel Penn International Transplant Tumor Registry with a review of published literature. Transplantation 2003;75:225–228.
134. Shiloh Y, Rotman G. Ataxia-telangiectasia and the ATM gene: linking neurodegeneration, immunodeficiency, and cancer to cell cycle checkpoints. J Clin Immunol 1996;16:254–260.
135. Lavin MF. Ataxia-telangiectasia: from a rare disorder to a paradigm for cell signalling and cancer. Nat Rev Mol Cell Biol 2008;9:759–769.
136. Shiloh Y. ATM and related protein kinases: safeguarding genome integrity. Nat Rev Cancer 2003;3:155–168.
137. Wong KK, Maser RS, Bachoo RM, et al. Telomere dysfunction and Atm deficiency compromises organ homeostasis and accelerates ageing. Nature 2003;421:643–648.
138. Hecht F, Hecht BK. Chromosome changes connect immunodeficiency and cancer in ataxia-telangiectasia. Am J Pediatr Hematol Oncol 1987;9:185–188.
139. Giovannetti A, Mazzetta F, Caprini E, et al. Skewed T-cell receptor repertoire, decreased thymic output, and predominance of terminally differentiated T cells in ataxia telangiectasia. Blood 2002;100:4082–4089.
140. Hall J. The ataxia-telangiectasia mutated gene and breast cancer: gene expression profiles and sequence variants. Cancer Lett 2005;227:105–114.
141. Hoglund P. DNA damage and tumor surveillance: one trigger for two pathways. Sci STKE 2006;2006:pe2.
142. Prokopcova J, Kleibl Z, Banwell CM, et al. The role of ATM in breast cancer development. Breast Cancer Res Treat 2007;104:121–128.
143. Kruger L, Demuth I, Neitzel H, et al. Cancer incidence in Nijmegen breakage syndrome is modulated by the amount of a variant NBS protein. Carcinogenesis 2007;28:107–111.
144. Meyer S, Kingston H, Taylor AM, et al. Rhabdomyosarcoma in Nijmegen breakage syndrome: strong association with perianal primary site. Cancer Genet Cytogenet 2004;154:169–174.
145. Gladkowska-Dura M, Dzierzanowska-Fangrat K, Dura WT, et al. Unique morphological spectrum of lymphomas in Nijmegen breakage syndrome (NBS) patients with high frequency of consecutive lymphoma formation. J Pathol 2008;216:337–344.
146. Jovanovic A, Minic P, Scekic-Guc M, et al. Successful treatment of Hodgkin lymphoma in Nijmegen breakage syndrome. J Pediatr Hematol Oncol 2009;31:49–52.
147. Langland G, Elliott J, Li Y, et al. The BLM helicase is necessary for normal DNA double-strand break repair. Cancer Res 2002;62:2766–2770.
148. Amor-Gueret M. Bloom syndrome, genomic instability and cancer: the SOS-like hypothesis. Cancer Lett 2006;236:1–12.
149. Baris HN, Kedar I, Halpern GJ, et al. Prevalence of breast and colorectal cancer in Ashkenazi Jewish carriers of Fanconi anemia and Bloom syndrome. Isr Med Assoc J 2007;9:847–850.
150. Thomas ER, Shanley S, Walker L, et al. Surveillance and treatment of malignancy in Bloom syndrome. Clin Oncol (R Coll Radiol) 2008;20:375–379.
151. Ding SL, Yu JC, Chen ST, et al. Genetic variants of BLM interact with RAD51 to increase breast cancer susceptibility. Carcinogenesis 2009;30:43–49.
152. Draznin M, Robles DT, Nguyen V, et al. An unusual case of Bloom syndrome presenting with basal cell carcinoma. Dermatol Surg 2009;35:131–134.
153. Orren DK, Theodore S, Machwe A. The Werner syndrome helicase/exonuclease (WRN) disrupts and degrades D-loops in vitro. Biochemistry 2002;41:13483–13488.
154. Dotto J, Nose V. Familial thyroid carcinoma: a diagnostic algorithm. Adv Anat Pathol 2008;15:332–349.
155. Tsurubuchi T, Yamamoto T, Tsukada Y, et al. Meningioma associated with Werner syndrome—case report. Neurol Med Chir (Tokyo) 2008;48:470–473.
156. Wang Z, Xu Y, Tang J, et al. A polymorphism in Werner syndrome gene is associated with breast cancer susceptibility in Chinese women. Breast Cancer Res Treat 2009; 118(1):169–175.
157. Campsmith ML, Rhodes P, Hall HI, Green T. Centers for disease control and prevention. HIV prevalence estimates—2006. MMWR 2008;57:1073–1076.
158. Prevention CfDCa, Cases of HIV infection and AIDS in the United States and dependent areas. Health Surveillance Report, 2007.
159. Scadden DT. AIDS-related malignancies. Annu Rev Med 2003;54:285–303.
160. Chiao EY, Krown SE. Update on non-acquired immunodeficiency syndrome-defining malignancies. Curr Opin Oncol 2003;15:389–397.
161. Sriplung H, Parkin DM. Trends in the incidence of acquired immunodeficiency syndrome-related malignancies in Thailand. Cancer 2004;101:2660–2666.
162. Kest H, Brogly S, McSherry G, et al. Malignancy in perinatally human immunodeficiency virus-infected children in the United States. Pediatr Infect Dis J 2005;24:237–242.
163. Chiappini E, Galli L, Tovo PA, et al. Cancer rates after year 2000 significantly decrease in children with perinatal HIV infection: a study by the Italian Register for HIV Infection in Children. J Clin Oncol 2007;25:97–101.
164. Engels EA, Biggar RJ, Hall HI, et al. Cancer risk in people infected with human immunodeficiency virus in the United States. Int J Cancer 2008;123:187–194.
165. Rabkin CS, Hilgartner MW, Hedberg KW, et al. Incidence of lymphomas and other cancers in HIV-infected and HIV-uninfected patients with hemophilia. JAMA 1992;267: 1090–1094.
166. Ziegler JL, Katongole-Mbidde E. Kaposi's sarcoma in childhood: an analysis of 100 cases from Uganda and relationship to HIV infection. Int J Cancer 1996;65:200–203.
167. Biggar RJ, Frisch M, Goedert JJ. Risk of cancer in children with AIDS. AIDS-Cancer Match Registry Study Group. JAMA 2000;284:205–209.
168. Caselli D, Klersy C, de Martino M, et al. Human immunodeficiency virus-related cancer in children: incidence and treatment outcome—report of the Italian Register. J Clin Oncol 2000;18:3854–3861.
169. Pollock BH, Jenson HB, Leach CT, et al. Risk factors for pediatric human immunodeficiency virus-related malignancy. JAMA 2003;289:2393–2399.
170. Mbulaiteye SM, Katabira ET, Wabinga H, et al. Spectrum of cancers among HIV-infected persons in Africa: the Uganda AIDS-Cancer Registry Match Study. Int J Cancer 2006;118:985–990.
171. Mueller BU. HIV-associated malignancies in children. AIDS Patient Care STDS 1999;13:527–533.
172. Levine AM. Acquired immunodeficiency syndrome-related lymphoma: clinical aspects. Semin Oncol 2000;27:442–453.
173. Boshoff C, Weiss R. AIDS-related malignancies. Nat Rev Cancer 2002;2:373–382.
174. Silverberg MJ, Neuhaus J, Bower M, et al. Risk of cancers during interrupted antiretroviral therapy in the SMART study. AIDS 2007;21:1957–1963.
175. Dhir AA, Sawant S, Dikshit RP, et al. Spectrum of HIV/AIDS related cancers in India. Cancer Causes Control 2008;19:147–153.
176. Sparano JA. Human immunodeficiency virus associated lymphoma. Curr Opin Oncol 2003;15:372–378.
177. Levine AM. AIDS-related malignancies: the emerging epidemic. J Natl Cancer Inst 1993;85:1382–1397.
178. Cabalo E, Wilkinson R, Lu NT, et al. Molecular analysis and pathology of a second pediatric HIV-associated Burkitt lymphoma. Pediatr Pathol Mol Med 2002;21: 525–530.
179. Goedert JJ. The epidemiology of acquired immunodeficiency syndrome malignancies. Semin Oncol 2000;27:390–401.
180. Kincaid L. Modern HAART decreases cancers in children with HIV. Lancet Oncol 2007;8:103.
181. Mo JQ, Dimashkieh H, Mallery SR, et al. MALT lymphoma in children: case report and review of the literature. Pediatr Dev Pathol 2004;7:407–413.
182. Moore SW, Davidson A, Hadley GP, et al. Malignant liver tumors in South African children: a national audit. World J Surg 2008;32:1389–1395.
183. Mwanda OW, Rochford R, Moormann AM, et al. Burkitt's lymphoma in Kenya: geographical, age, gender and ethnic distribution. East Afr Med J 2004;S68–S77.
184. Parkin DM, Sitas F, Chirenje M, et al. Part I: Cancer in indigenous Africans—burden, distribution, and trends. Lancet Oncol 2008;9:683–692.
185. Paul T, Challa S, Tandon A, et al. Primary central nervous system lymphomas: Indian experience, and review of literature. Indian J Cancer 2008;45:112–118.
186. Baumforth KR, Young LS, Flavell KJ, et al. The Epstein-Barr virus and its association with human cancers. Mol Pathol 1999;52:307–322.
187. Cesarman E, Chang Y, Moore PS, et al. Kaposi's sarcoma-associated herpesvirus-like DNA sequences in AIDS-related body-cavity-based lymphomas. N Engl J Med 1995;332:1186–1191.
188. Chang Y, Cesarman E, Pessin MS, et al. Identification of herpesvirus-like DNA sequences in AIDS-associated Kaposi's sarcoma. Science 1994;266:1865–1869.
189. Kuhn L, Sun XW, Wright TC Jr. Human immunodeficiency virus infection and female lower genital tract malignancy. Curr Opin Obstet Gynecol 1999;11:35–39.
190. Shiramizu B, Herndier BG, McGrath MS. Identification of a common clonal human immunodeficiency virus integration site in human immunodeficiency virus-associated lymphomas. Cancer Res 1994;54:2069–2072.
191. Mueller BU. Cancers in children infected with the human immunodeficiency virus. Oncologist 1999;4:309–317.
192. Serraino D, Franceschi S. Kaposi's sarcoma and non-Hodgkin's lymphomas in children and adolescents with AIDS. AIDS 1996;10:643–647.
193. Chokunonga E, Levy LM, Bassett MT, et al. Aids and cancer in Africa: the evolving epidemic in Zimbabwe. AIDS 1999;13:2583–2588.
194. Gates AE, Kaplan LD. AIDS malignancies in the era of highly active antiretroviral therapy. Oncology (Williston Park) 2002;16:657–665; discussion 665, 668–670.
195. Sanpakit K, Veerakul G, Kriengsuntornkij W, et al. Malignancies in HIV-infected children at Siriraj Hospital. J Med Assoc Thai 2002;85(suppl 2):S542–S548.
196. Amir H, Kaaya EE, Manji KP, et al. Kaposi's sarcoma before and during a human immunodeficiency virus epidemic in Tanzanian children. Pediatr Infect Dis J 2001;20: 518–521.
197. Newton R, Ziegler J, Beral V, et al. A case-control study of human immunodeficiency virus infection and cancer in adults and children residing in Kampala, Uganda. Int J Cancer 2001;92:622–627.
198. Feller L, Anagnostopoulos C, Wood NH, et al. Human immunodeficiency virus-associated Kaposi sarcoma as an immune reconstitution inflammatory syndrome: a literature review and case report. J Periodontol 2008;79:362–368.
199. Mbah N, Abdulkareem IH, Panti A. AIDS-associated Kaposi's sarcoma in Sokoto, Nigeria. Niger J Clin Pract 2008;11:181–184.
200. Sullivan RJ, Pantanowitz L, Casper C, et al. HIV/AIDS: epidemiology, pathophysiology, and treatment of Kaposi sarcoma-associated herpesvirus disease: Kaposi sarcoma, primary effusion lymphoma, and multicentric Castleman disease. Clin Infect Dis 2008;47:1209–1215.
201. Biggar RJ, Chaturvedi AK, Bhatia K, et al. Cancer risk in persons with HIV/AIDS in India: a review and future directions for research. Infect Agent Cancer 2009;4:4.
202. Bowa K, Wood C, Chao A, et al. A review of the epidemiology of cancers at the University Teaching Hospital, Lusaka, Zambia. Trop Doct 2009;39:5–7.
203. Rabkin CS, Janz S, Lash A, et al. Monoclonal origin of multicentric Kaposi's sarcoma lesions. N Engl J Med 1997;336:988–993.
204. Bower M, Fife K. Current issues in the biology of AIDS-related lymphoma. HIV Med 2001;2:141–145.
205. Balarezo FS, Joshi VV. Proliferative and neoplastic disorders in children with acquired immunodeficiency syndrome. Adv Anat Pathol 2002;9:360–370.
206. Antman K, Chang Y. Kaposi's sarcoma. N Engl J Med 2000;342:1027–1038.
207. Krown SE, Testa MA, Huang J. AIDS-related Kaposi's sarcoma: prospective validation of the AIDS Clinical Trials Group staging classification. AIDS Clinical Trials Group Oncology Committee. J Clin Oncol 1997;15:3085–3092.
208. Clayton G, Omasta-Martin A, Bower M. The effects of HAART on AIDS-related Kaposi's sarcoma and non-Hodgkin's lymphoma. J HIV Ther 2006;11:51–53.
209. Dittmer DP, Krown SE. Targeted therapy for Kaposi's sarcoma and Kaposi's sarcoma-associated herpesvirus. Curr Opin Oncol 2007;19:452–457.
210. Potthoff A, Brockmeyer NH. HIV-associated Kaposi sarcoma: pathogenesis and therapy. J Dtsch Dermatol Ges 2007;5:1091–1094.
211. Udhrain A, Skubitz KM, Northfelt DW. Pegylated liposomal doxorubicin in the treatment of AIDS-related Kaposi's sarcoma. Int J Nanomedicine 2007;2:345–352.
212. Yarchoan R, Pluda JM, Wyvill KM, et al. Treatment of AIDS-related Kaposi's sarcoma with interleukin-12: rationale and preliminary evidence of clinical activity. Crit Rev Immunol 2007;27:401–414.

213. Martin-Carbonero L, Palacios R, Valencia E, et al. Long-term prognosis of HIV-infected patients with Kaposi sarcoma treated with pegylated liposomal doxorubicin. Clin Infect Dis 2008;47:410–417.
214. McClain KL, Leach CT, Jenson HB, et al. Molecular and virologic characteristics of lymphoid malignancies in children with AIDS. J Acquir Immune Defic Syndr 2000;23:152–159.
215. Nador RG, Chadburn A, Gundappa G, et al. Human immunodeficiency virus (HIV)-associated polymorphic lymphoproliferative disorders. Am J Surg Pathol 2003;27:293–302.
216. Gessain A, Briere J, Angelin-Duclos C, et al. Human herpes virus 8 (Kaposi's sarcoma herpes virus) and malignant lymphoproliferations in France: a molecular study of 250 cases including two AIDS-associated body cavity based lymphomas. Leukemia 1997; 11:266–272.
217. Jaffe ES. Primary body cavity-based AIDS-related lymphomas. Evolution of a new disease entity. Am J Clin Pathol 1996;105:141–143.
218. Ambinder RF. Epstein-Barr virus associated lymphoproliferations in the AIDS setting. Eur J Cancer 2001;37:1209–1216.
219. International Collaboration on HIV and Cancer. Highly active antiretroviral therapy and incidence of cancer in human immunodeficiency virus-infected adults. J Natl Cancer Inst 2000;92:1823–1830.
220. Dal Maso L, Franceschi S. Epidemiology of non-Hodgkin lymphomas and other haemolymphopoietic neoplasms in people with AIDS. Lancet Oncol 2003;4:110–119.
221. Knowles DM, Pirog EC. Pathology of AIDS-related lymphomas and other AIDS-defining neoplasms. Eur J Cancer 2001;37:1236–1250.
222. Tirelli U, Bernardi D, Spina M, et al. AIDS-related tumors: integrating antiviral and anticancer therapy. Crit Rev Oncol Hematol 2002;41:299–315.
223. Granovsky MO, Mueller BU, Nicholson HS, et al. Cancer in human immunodeficiency virus-infected children: a case series from the Children's Cancer Group and the National Cancer Institute. J Clin Oncol 1998;16:1729–1735.
224. Orem J, Maganda A, Mbidde EK, et al. Clinical characteristics and outcome of children with Burkitt lymphoma in Uganda according to HIV infection. Pediatr Blood Cancer 2009;52:455–458.
225. Pinkerton CR, Hann I, Weston CL, et al. Immunodeficiency-related lymphoproliferative disorders: prospective data from the United Kingdom Children's Cancer Study Group Registry. Br J Haematol 2002;118:456–461.
226. Gaidano G, Pastore C, Lanza C, et al. Molecular pathology of AIDS-related lymphomas. Biologic aspects and clinicopathologic heterogeneity. Ann Hematol 1994;69:281–290.
227. Klein U, Gloghini A, Gaidano G, et al. Gene expression profile analysis of AIDS-related primary effusion lymphoma (PEL) suggests a plasmablastic derivation and identifies PEL-specific transcripts. Blood 2003;101:4115–4121.
228. Antinori A, Ammassari A, De Luca A, et al. Diagnosis of AIDS-related focal brain lesions: a decision-making analysis based on clinical and neuroradiologic characteristics combined with polymerase chain reaction assays in CSF. Neurology 1997;48:687–694.
229. Auperin I, Mikolt J, Oksenhendler E, et al. Primary central nervous system malignant non-Hodgkin's lymphomas from HIV-infected and non-infected patients: expression of cellular surface proteins and Epstein-Barr viral markers. Neuropathol Appl Neurobiol 1994;20:243–252.
230. Knowles DM. Etiology and pathogenesis of AIDS-related non–Hodgkin's lymphoma. Hematol Oncol Clin North Am 1996;10:1081–1109.
231. Meeker TC, Shiramizu B, Kaplan L, et al. Evidence for molecular subtypes of HIV-associated lymphoma: division into peripheral monoclonal, polyclonal and central nervous system lymphoma. AIDS 1991;5:669–674.
232. Greiner TC, Abou-Elella AA, Smir BN, et al. Molecular epidemiology of EBNA-1 substrains of Epstein-Barr virus in posttransplant lymphoproliferative disorders which have infrequent p53 mutations. Leuk Lymphoma 2000;38:563–576.
233. Gross TG, Loechelt BJ. Epstein-Barr virus associated disease following blood or marrow transplant. Pediatr Transplant 2003;7(suppl 3):44–50.
234. Okano M, Gross TG. A review of Epstein-Barr virus infection in patients with immunodeficiency disorders. Am J Med Sci 2000;319:392–396.
235. Ballerini P, Gaidano G, Gong J, et al. Molecular pathogenesis of HIV-associated lymphomas. AIDS Res Hum Retroviruses 1992;8:731–735.
236. Ng VL, McGrath MS. The immunology of AIDS-associated lymphomas. Immunol Rev 1998;162:293–298.
237. Pelicci PG, Knowles DM, Arlin ZA, et al. Multiple monoclonal B cell expansions and c-myc oncogene rearrangements in acquired immune deficiency syndrome-related lymphoproliferative disorders. Implications for lymphomagenesis. J Exp Med 1986;164: 2049–2060.
238. De Re V, Carbone A, De Vita S, et al. p53 protein over-expression and p53 gene abnormalities in HIV-1-related non-Hodgkin's lymphomas. Int J Cancer 1994;56:662–667.
239. Knowles DM. Molecular pathology of acquired immunodeficiency syndrome-related non-Hodgkin's lymphoma. Semin Diagn Pathol 1997;14:67–82.
240. Nador RG, Cesarman E, Chadburn A, et al. Primary effusion lymphoma: a distinct clinicopathologic entity associated with the Kaposi's sarcoma-associated herpes virus. Blood 1996;88:645–656.
241. Nakamura H, Said JW, Miller CW, et al. Mutation and protein expression of p53 in acquired immunodeficiency syndrome-related lymphomas. Blood 1993;82:920–926.
242. Davi F, Delecluse HJ, Guiet P, et al. Burkitt-like lymphomas in AIDS patients: characterization within a series of 103 human immunodeficiency virus-associated non-Hodgkin's lymphomas. Burkitt's Lymphoma Study Group. J Clin Oncol 1998;16:3788–3795.
243. Delecluse HJ, Hummel M, Marafioti T, et al. Common and HIV-related diffuse large B-cell lymphomas differ in their immunoglobulin gene mutation pattern. J Pathol 1999;188:133–138.
244. Herndier BG, Kaplan LD, McGrath MS. Pathogenesis of AIDS lymphomas. AIDS 1994;8:1025–1049.
245. Martinez-Maza O, Breen EC. B-cell activation and lymphoma in patients with HIV. Curr Opin Oncol 2002;14:528–532.
246. Tarantul V, Nikolaev A, Hannig H, et al. Detection of abundantly transcribed genes and gene translocation in human immunodeficiency virus-associated non-Hodgkin's lymphoma. Neoplasia 2001;3:132–142.
247. Bessudo A, Cherepakhin V, Johnson TA, et al. Favored use of immunoglobulin V(H)4 genes in AIDS-associated B-cell lymphoma. Blood 1996;88:252–260.
248. Grulich AE, Wan X, Law MG, et al. B-cell stimulation and prolonged immune deficiency are risk factors for non-Hodgkin's lymphoma in people with AIDS. AIDS 2000; 14:133–140.
249. Muller JR, Janz S, Goedert JJ, et al. Persistence of immunoglobulin heavy chain/c-myc recombination-positive lymphocyte clones in the blood of human immunodeficiency virus-infected homosexual men. Proc Natl Acad Sci U S A 1995;92:6577–6581.
250. Ng VL, Hurt MH, Herndier BG, et al. VH gene use by CD5+ AIDS-associated B-cell lymphoproliferations. Ann N Y Acad Sci 1995;764:507–508.
251. Przybylski GK, Goldman J, Ng VL, et al. Evidence for early B-cell activation preceding the development of Epstein-Barr virus-negative acquired immunodeficiency syndrome-related lymphoma. Blood 1996;88:4620–4629.
252. Ng VL, Hurt MH, Herndier BG, et al. VH gene use by HIV type 1-associated lymphoproliferations. AIDS Res Hum Retroviruses 1997;13:135–149.
253. Rodriguez-Alfageme C, Chen Z, Sonoda G, et al. B cells malignantly transformed by human immunodeficiency virus are polyclonal. Virology 1998;252:34–38.
254. Preciado MV, De Matteo E, Fallo A, et al. EBV-associated Hodgkin's disease in an HIV-infected child presenting with a hemophagocytic syndrome. Leuk Lymphoma 2001;42: 231–234.
255. Preciado MV, Fallo A, Chabay P, et al. Epstein Barr virus-associated lymphoma in HIV-infected children. Pathol Res Pract 2002;198:327–332.
256. Kaplan LD, Straus DJ, Testa MA, et al. Low-dose compared with standard-dose m-BACOD chemotherapy for non-Hodgkin's lymphoma associated with human immunodeficiency virus infection. National Institute of Allergy and Infectious Diseases AIDS Clinical Trials Group. N Engl J Med 1997;336:1641–1648.
257. Sandler AS, Kaplan LD. Diagnosis and management of systemic non-Hodgkin's lymphoma in HIV disease. Hematol Oncol Clin North Am 1996;10:1111–1124.
258. Crosswell HE, Bergsagel DJ, Yost R, et al. Successful treatment with modified CHOP-rituximab in pediatric AIDS-related advanced stage Burkitt lymphoma. Pediatr Blood Cancer 2008;50:883–885.
259. Fedorova A, Mlyavaya T, Alexeichik A, et al. Successful treatment of the HIV-associated Burkitt lymphoma in a three-year-old child. Pediatr Blood Cancer 2006;47:92–93.
260. Fluri S, Ammann R, Luthy AR, et al. High-dose therapy and autologous stem cell transplantation for children with HIV-associated non-Hodgkin lymphoma. Pediatr Blood Cancer 2007;49:984–987.
261. Galli L, Chiappini E, Lippi A, et al. Immune recovery following antineoplastic chemotherapy and highly active antiretroviral therapy (HAART) in a child with HIV-1 infection previously unresponsive to HAART. Int J Immunopathol Pharmacol 2006;19: 919–922.
262. Simonelli C, Zanussi S, Cinelli R, et al. Impact of concomitant antiblastic chemotherapy and highly active antiretroviral therapy on human immunodeficiency virus (HIV) viremia and genotyping in HIV-infected patients with non-Hodgkin lymphoma. Clin Infect Dis 2003;37:820–827.
263. Neumann Y, Toren A, Mandel M, et al. Favorable response of pediatric AIDS-related Burkitt's lymphoma treated by aggressive chemotherapy. Med Pediatr Oncol 1993;21:661–664.
264. McClain KL, Joshi VV, Murphy SB. Cancers in children with HIV infection. Hematol Oncol Clin North Am 1996;10:1189–1201.
265. Kawabata KC, Hagiwara S, Takenouchi A, et al. Autologous stem cell transplantation using MEAM regimen for relapsed AIDS-related lymphoma patients who received highly active anti-retroviral therapy: a report of three cases. Intern Med 2009;48:111–114.
266. Errante D, Gabarre J, Ridolfo AL, et al. Hodgkin's disease in 35 patients with HIV infection: an experience with epirubicin, bleomycin, vinblastine and prednisone chemotherapy in combination with antiretroviral therapy and primary use of G-CSF. Ann Oncol 1999;10:189–195.
267. Levine AM. Hodgkin's disease in the setting of human immunodeficiency virus infection. J Natl Cancer Inst Monogr 1998;23:37–42.
268. Caldwell MB, Oxtoby MJ, Simonds RJ. 1994 revised classification system for human immunodeficiency virus infection in children less than 13 years of age. MMWR Recomm Rep 1994;43:1–10.
269. Barbashina V, Heller DS, Hameed M, et al. Splenic smooth-muscle tumors in children with acquired immunodeficiency syndrome: report of two cases of this unusual location with evidence of an association with Epstein-Barr virus. Virchows Arch 2000;436:138–139.
270. Jenson HB, Leach CT, McClain KL, et al. Benign and malignant smooth muscle tumors containing Epstein-Barr virus in children with AIDS. Leuk Lymphoma 1997;27:303–314.
271. Tulvatana W, Pancharoen C, Mekmullica J, et al. Epstein-Barr virus-associated leiomyosarcoma of the iris in a child infected with human immunodeficiency virus. Arch Ophthalmol 2003;121:1478–1481.
272. Chadwick EG, Connor EJ, Hanson IC, et al. Tumors of smooth-muscle origin in HIV-infected children. JAMA 1990;263:3182–3184.
273. Sabatino D, Martinez S, Young R, et al. Simultaneous pulmonary leiomyosarcoma and leiomyoma in pediatric HIV infection. Pediatr Hematol Oncol 1991;8:355–359.
274. Ferrari A, Bisogno G, Casanova M, et al. Childhood leiomyosarcoma: a report from the soft tissue sarcoma Italian Cooperative Group. Ann Oncol 2001;12:1163–1168.
275. Castro KG, Ward JW, Slutsker L, Buehler JW, Jaffe HW, Berkelman RL, Curran JW. 1993 revised classification system for HIV infection and expanded surveillance case definition for AIDS among adolescents and adults. MMWR Recomm Rep 1992;41(RR-17):1–19.
276. Moscicki AB, Ellenberg JH, Vermund SH, et al. Prevalence of and risks for cervical human papillomavirus infection and squamous intraepithelial lesions in adolescent girls: impact of infection with human immunodeficiency virus. Arch Pediatr Adolesc Med 2000;154:127–134.
277. Piketty C, Darragh TM, Heard I, et al. High prevalence of anal squamous intraepithelial lesions in HIV-positive men despite the use of highly active antiretroviral therapy. Sex Transm Dis 2004;31:96–99.
278. Markowitz LE, Dunne EF, Saraiya M, et al. Quadrivalent human papillomavirus vaccine: recommendations of the Advisory Committee on Immunization Practices (ACIP). MMWR Recomm Rep 2007;56:1–24.
279. Palefsky JM, Gillison ML, Strickler HD. Chapter 16: HPV vaccines in immunocompromised women and men. Vaccine 2006;24(suppl 3):S3/140–146.
280. Franceschi S, De Vuyst H. Human papillomavirus vaccines and anal carcinoma. Curr Opin HIV/AIDS 2009;4:57–63.
281. Palefsky J. Human papillomavirus and anal neoplasia. Curr HIV/AIDS Rep 2008;5: 78–85.
282. Lehtovirta P, Paavonen J, Heikinheimo O. Risk factors, diagnosis and prognosis of cervical intraepithelial neoplasia among HIV-infected women. Int J STD AIDS 2008;19: 37–41.
283. Lillo FB, Lodini S, Ferrari D, et al. Determination of human papillomavirus (HPV) load and type in high-grade cervical lesions surgically resected from HIV-infected women during follow-up of HPV infection. Clin Infect Dis 2005;40:451–457.
284. Massad LS, Fazzari MJ, Anastos K, et al. Outcomes after treatment of cervical intraepithelial neoplasia among women with HIV. J Low Genit Tract Dis 2007;11:90–97.
285. Ramos MC, Pizarro De Lorenzo BH, et al. High-grade cervical intraepithelial neoplasia, human papillomavirus and factors connected with recurrence following surgical treatment. Clin Exp Obstet Gynecol 2008;35:242–247.

286. Hessol NA, Holly EA, Efird JT, et al. Anal intraepithelial neoplasia in a multisite study of HIV-infected and high-risk HIV-uninfected women. AIDS 2009;23:59–70.
287. Kreuter A, Wieland U. Human papillomavirus-associated diseases in HIV-infected men who have sex with men. Curr Opin Infect Dis 2009;22:109–114.
288. Nathan M, Hickey N, Mayuranathan L, et al. Treatment of anal human papillomavirus-associated disease: a long term outcome study. Int J STD AIDS 2008;19: 445–449.
289. Palefsky J. Human papillomavirus-related disease in people with HIV. Curr Opin HIV AIDS 2009;4:52–56.
290. Chitsike I, Siziya S. Seroprevalence of human immunodeficiency virus type 1 infection in childhood malignancy in Zimbabwe. Cent Afr J Med 1998;44:242–245.
291. Mueller BU, Pizzo PA. Malignancies in pediatric AIDS. Curr Opin Pediatr 1996;8: 45–49.
292. Sheil AG, Disney AP, Mathew TH, et al. De novo malignancy emerges as a major cause of morbidity and late failure in renal transplantation. Transplant Proc 1993;25: 1383–1384.
293. Howard RJ, Patton PR, Reed AI, et al. The changing causes of graft loss and death after kidney transplantation. Transplantation 2002;73:1923–1928.
294. System URD, USRDS 1998 annual data report, N.I.o.D. National Institutes of Health, Digestive, and Kidney Diseases, Editor, 1998.
295. Baker KS, DeFor TE, Burns LJ, et al. New malignancies after blood or marrow stem-cell transplantation in children and adults: incidence and risk factors. J Clin Oncol 2003;21:1352–1358.
296. Kolb HJ, Socie G, Duell T, et al. Malignant neoplasms in long-term survivors of bone marrow transplantation. Late Effects Working Party of the European Cooperative Group for Blood and Marrow Transplantation and the European Late Effect Project Group. Ann Intern Med 1999;131:738–744.
297. Abu-Elmagd KM, Zak M, Stamos JM, et al. De novo malignancies after intestinal and multivisceral transplantation. Transplantation 2004;77:1719–1725.
298. Bustami RT, Ojo AO, Wolfe RA, et al. Immunosuppression and the risk of post-transplant malignancy among cadaveric first kidney transplant recipients. Am J Transplant 2004;4:87–93.
299. Euvrard S, Kanitakis J, Claudy A. Skin cancers after organ transplantation. N Engl J Med 2003;348:1681–1691.
300. Buell JF, Gross TG, Thomas MJ, et al. Malignancy in pediatric transplant recipients. Semin Pediatr Surg 2006;15:179–187.
301. Greiner T, Armitage JO, Gross T. Atypical lymphoproliferative diseases. In: American Society of Hematology Education Program. Washington, DC, 2000.
302. Harris NL, Ferry JA, Swerdlow SH. Posttransplant lymphoproliferative disorders: summary of Society for Hematopathology Workshop. Semin Diagn Pathol 1997;14: 8–14.
303. Gross TG. Treatment of Epstein-Barr virus-associated posttransplant lymphoproliferative disorders. J Pediatr Hematol Oncol 2001;23:7–9.
304. Jaffe ES, Harris NL. Pathology and genetics of tumours of haematopoietic and lymphoid tissues. Lyon, France: IARC Press, 2001.
305. Chadburn A, Cesarman E, Liu YF, et al. Molecular genetic analysis demonstrates that multiple posttransplantation lymphoproliferative disorders occurring in one anatomic site in a single patient represent distinct primary lymphoid neoplasms. Cancer 1995;75: 2747–2756.
306. Hayashi RJ, Kraus MD, Patel AL, et al. Posttransplant lymphoproliferative disease in children: correlation of histology to clinical behavior. J Pediatr Hematol Oncol 2001; 23:14–18.
307. Hanson MN, Morrison VA, Peterson BA, et al. Posttransplant T-cell lymphoproliferative disorders—an aggressive, late complication of solid-organ transplantation. Blood 1996;88:3626–3633.
308. Rajakariar R, Bhattacharyya M, Norton A, et al. Post transplant T-cell lymphoma: a case series of four patients from a single unit and review of the literature. Am J Transplant 2004;4:1534–1538.
309. Bierman PJ, Vose JM, Langnas AN, et al. Hodgkin's disease following solid organ transplantation. Ann Oncol 1996;7:265–270.
310. Childs CC, Parham DM, Berard CW. Infectious mononucleosis. The spectrum of morphologic changes simulating lymphoma in lymph nodes and tonsils. Am J Surg Pathol 1987;11:122–132.
311. Dotti G, Fiocchi R, Motta T, et al. Lymphomas occurring late after solid-organ transplantation: influence of treatment on the clinical outcome. Transplantation 2002;74: 1095–1102.
312. Leblond V, Dhedin N, Mamzer Bruneel MF, et al. Identification of prognostic factors in 61 patients with posttransplantation lymphoproliferative disorders. J Clin Oncol 2001;19:772–778.
313. Dhir RK, Nalesnik MA, Demetris AJ. Latent membrane protein expression in post-transplant lymphoproliferative diseases. Appl Immunohistochem 1995;3:123–126.
314. Finn L, Reyes J, Bueno J, et al. Epstein-Barr virus infections in children after transplantation of the small intestine. Am J Surg Pathol 1998;22:299–309.
315. Collins MH, Montone KT, Leahey AM, et al. Autopsy pathology of pediatric posttransplant lymphoproliferative disorder. Pediatrics 2001;107:E89.
316. Gross TG, Steinbuch M, DeFor T, et al. B cell lymphoproliferative disorders following hematopoietic stem cell transplantation: risk factors, treatment and outcome. Bone Marrow Transplant 1999;23:251–258.
317. Gulley ML, Swinnen LJ, Plaisance KT Jr, et al. Tumor origin and CD20 expression in posttransplant lymphoproliferative disorder occurring in solid organ transplant recipients: implications for immune-based therapy. Transplantation 2003;76:959–964.
318. Capello D, Cerri M, Muti G, et al. Molecular histogenesis of posttransplantation lymphoproliferative disorders. Blood 2003;102:3775–3785.
319. Delecluse HJ, Rouault JP, Ffrench M, et al. Post-transplant lymphoproliferative disorders with genetic abnormalities commonly found in malignant tumours. Br J Haematol 1995;89:90–97.
320. Gallego MS, Bernasconi A, Davila MT, et al. Trisomy 3 in two paediatric post-transplant lymphomas. Br J Haematol 2002;117:558–562.
321. Poirel HA, Bernheim A, Schneider A, et al. Characteristic pattern of chromosomal imbalances in posttransplantation lymphoproliferative disorders: correlation with histopathological subcategories and EBV status. Transplantation 2005;80:176–184.
322. Knowles DM, Cesarman E, Chadburn A, et al. Correlative morphologic and molecular genetic analysis demonstrates three distinct categories of posttransplantation lymphoproliferative disorders. Blood 1995;85:552–565.
323. Cesarman E, Chadburn A, Liu YF, et al. BCL-6 gene mutations in posttransplantation lymphoproliferative disorders predict response to therapy and clinical outcome. Blood 1998;92:2294–2302.
324. Capello D, Rasi S, Oreste P, et al. Molecular characterization of post-transplant lymphoproliferative disorders of donor origin occurring in liver transplant recipients. J Pathol 2009;218(4):478–486.
325. Johnson LR, Nalesnik MA, Swerdlow SH. Impact of Epstein-Barr virus in monomorphic B-cell posttransplant lymphoproliferative disorders: a histogenetic study. Am J Surg Pathol 2006;30:1604–1612.
326. Novoa-Takara L, Perkins SL, Qi D, et al. Histogenetic phenotypes of B cells in posttransplant lymphoproliferative disorders by immunohistochemical analysis correlate with transplant type: solid organ vs hematopoietic stem cell transplantation. Am J Clin Pathol 2005;123:104–112.
327. Scheinfeld AG, Nador RG, Cesarman E, et al. Epstein-Barr virus latent membrane protein-1 oncogene deletion in post-transplantation lymphoproliferative disorders. Am J Pathol 1997;151:805–812.
328. Smir BN, Hauke RJ, Bierman PJ, et al. Molecular epidemiology of deletions and mutations of the latent membrane protein 1 oncogene of the Epstein-Barr virus in posttransplant lymphoproliferative disorders. Lab Invest 1996;75:575–588.
329. Alizadeh AA, Eisen MB, Davis RE, et al. Distinct types of diffuse large B-cell lymphoma identified by gene expression profiling. Nature 2000;403:503–511.
330. Shipp MA, Ross KN, Tamayo P, et al. Diffuse large B-cell lymphoma outcome prediction by gene-expression profiling and supervised machine learning. Nat Med 2002;8:68–74.
331. Bhatia S, Ramsay NK, Steinbuch M, et al. Malignant neoplasms following bone marrow transplantation. Blood 1996;87:3633–3639.
332. Curtis RE, Travis LB, Rowlings PA, et al. Risk of lymphoproliferative disorders after bone marrow transplantation: a multi-institutional study. Blood 1999;94:2208–2216.
333. Socie G, Curtis RE, Deeg HJ, et al. New malignant diseases after allogeneic marrow transplantation for childhood acute leukemia. J Clin Oncol 2000;18:348–357.
334. Nash RA, Dansey R, Storek J, et al. Epstein-Barr virus-associated posttransplantation lymphoproliferative disorder after high-dose immunosuppressive therapy and autologous CD34-selected hematopoietic stem cell transplantation for severe autoimmune diseases. Biol Blood Marrow Transplant 2003;9:583–591.
335. Powell JL, Bunin NJ, Callahan C, et al. An unexpectedly high incidence of Epstein-Barr virus lymphoproliferative disease after CD34+ selected autologous peripheral blood stem cell transplant in neuroblastoma. Bone Marrow Transplant 2004;33:651–657.
336. Barker JN, Martin PL, Coad JE, et al. Low incidence of Epstein-Barr virus-associated posttransplantation lymphoproliferative disorders in 272 unrelated-donor umbilical cord blood transplant recipients. Biol Blood Marrow Transplant 2001;7:395–399.
337. Brunstein CG, Weisdorf DJ, DeFor T, et al. Marked increased risk of Epstein-Barr virus-related complications with the addition of antithymocyte globulin to a nonmyeloablative conditioning prior to unrelated umbilical cord blood transplantation. Blood 2006;108:2874–2880.
338. Lucas KG, Filo F, Heilman DK, et al. Semiquantitative Epstein-Barr virus polymerase chain reaction analysis of peripheral blood from organ transplant patients and risk for the development of lymphoproliferative disease. Blood 1998;92:3977–3978.
339. Rooney CM, Smith CA, Ng CY, et al. Infusion of cytotoxic T cells for the prevention and treatment of Epstein-Barr virus-induced lymphoma in allogeneic transplant recipients. Blood 1998;92:1549–1555.
340. van Esser JW, van der Holt B, Meijer E, et al. Epstein-Barr virus (EBV) reactivation is a frequent event after allogeneic stem cell transplantation (SCT) and quantitatively predicts EBV-lymphoproliferative disease following T-cell–depleted SCT. Blood 2001;98:972–978.
341. Rowe DT, Webber S, Schauer EM, et al. Epstein-Barr virus load monitoring: its role in the prevention and management of post-transplant lymphoproliferative disease. Transpl Infect Dis 2001;3:79–87.
342. Faye A, Quartier P, Reguerre Y, et al. Chimaeric anti-CD20 monoclonal antibody (rituximab) in post-transplant B-lymphoproliferative disorder following stem cell transplantation in children. Br J Haematol 2001;115:112–118.
343. Kuehnle I, Huls MH, Liu Z, et al. CD20 monoclonal antibody (rituximab) for therapy of Epstein-Barr virus lymphoma after hemopoietic stem-cell transplantation. Blood 2000;95:1502–1505.
344. Milpied N, Vasseur B, Parquet N, et al. Humanized anti-CD20 monoclonal antibody (Rituximab) in post transplant B-lymphoproliferative disorder: a retrospective analysis on 32 patients. Ann Oncol 2000;11(suppl 1):113–116.
345. Al-Akash SI, Al Makadma AS, Al Omari MG. Rapid response to rituximab in a pediatric liver transplant recipient with post-transplant lymphoproliferative disease and maintenance with sirolimus monotherapy. Pediatr Transplant 2005;9:249–253.
346. Berney T, Delis S, Kato T, et al. Successful treatment of posttransplant lymphoproliferative disease with prolonged rituximab treatment in intestinal transplant recipients. Transplantation 2002;74:1000–1006.
347. Bueno J, Ramil C, Somoza I, et al. Treatment of monomorphic B-cell lymphoma with rituximab after liver transplantation in a child. Pediatr Transplant 2003;7:153–156.
348. Comoli P, Basso S, Zecca M, et al. Preemptive therapy of EBV-related lymphoproliferative disease after pediatric haploidentical stem cell transplantation. Am J Transplant 2007;7:1648–1655.
349. Hayashida M, Ogita K, Matsuura T, et al. Successful prolonged rituximab treatment for post-transplant lymphoproliferative disorder following living donor liver transplantation in a child. Pediatr Transplant 2007;11:671–675.
350. Herman J, Vandenberghe P, van den Heuvel I, et al. Successful treatment with rituximab of lymphoproliferative disorder in a child after cardiac transplantation. J Heart Lung Transplant 2002;21:1304–1309.
351. Papadopoulos EB, Ladanyi M, Emanuel D, et al. Infusions of donor leukocytes to treat Epstein-Barr virus-associated lymphoproliferative disorders after allogeneic bone marrow transplantation. N Engl J Med 1994;330:1185–1191.
352. Bonini C, Ferrari G, Verzeletti S, et al. HSV-TK gene transfer into donor lymphocytes for control of allogeneic graft-versus-leukemia. Science 1997;276:1719–1724.
353. Ho M, Jaffe R, Miller G, et al. The frequency of Epstein-Barr virus infection and associated lymphoproliferative syndrome after transplantation and its manifestations in children. Transplantation 1988;45:719–727.
354. Cox KL, Lawrence-Miyasaki LS, Garcia-Kennedy R, et al. An increased incidence of Epstein-Barr virus infection and lymphoproliferative disorder in young children on FK506 after liver transplantation. Transplantation 1995;59:524–529.
355. Swinnen LJ, Mullen GM, Carr TJ, et al. Aggressive treatment for postcardiac transplant lymphoproliferation. Blood 1995;86:3333–3340.
356. Newell KA, Alonso EM, Whitington PF, et al. Posttransplant lymphoproliferative disease in pediatric liver transplantation. Interplay between primary Epstein-Barr virus infection and immunosuppression. Transplantation 1996;62:370–375.
357. Guthery SL, Heubi JE, Bucuvalas JC, et al. Determination of risk factors for Epstein-Barr virus-associated posttransplant lymphoproliferative disorder in pediatric liver transplant recipients using objective case ascertainment. Transplantation 2003;75:987–993.

358. McDonald RA, Smith JM, Ho M, et al. Incidence of PTLD in pediatric renal transplant recipients receiving basiliximab, calcineurin inhibitor, sirolimus and steroids. Am J Transplant 2008;8:984–989.

359. McDiarmid SV, Jordan S, Kim GS, et al. Prevention and preemptive therapy of post-transplant lymphoproliferative disease in pediatric liver recipients. Transplantation 1998;66:1604–1611.

360. Caillard S, Agodoa LY, Bohen EM, et al. Myeloma, Hodgkin disease, and lymphoid leukemia after renal transplantation: characteristics, risk factors and prognosis. Transplantation 2006;81:888–895.

361. Dror Y, Greenberg M, Taylor G, et al. Lymphoproliferative disorders after organ transplantation in children. Transplantation 1999;67:990–998.

362. Ghobrial IM, Habermann TM, Maurer MJ, et al. Prognostic analysis for survival in adult solid organ transplant recipients with post-transplantation lymphoproliferative disorders. J Clin Oncol 2005;23:7574–7582.

363. Kullberg-Lindh C, Ascher H, Saalman R, et al. Epstein-Barr viremia levels after pediatric liver transplantation as measured by real-time polymerase chain reaction. Pediatr Transplant 2006;10:83–89.

364. Roque J, Rios G, Humeres R, et al. Early posttransplant lymphoproliferative disease in pediatric liver transplant recipients. Transplant Proc 2006;38:930–931.

365. Green M, Webber SA. EBV viral load monitoring: unanswered questions. Am J Transplant 2002;2:894–895.

366. Gartner BC, Fischinger J, Schafer H, et al. Epstein-Barr viral load as a tool to diagnose and monitor post-transplant lymphoproliferative disease. Recent Results Cancer Res 2002;159:49–54.

367. Gartner BC, Schafer H, Marggraff K, et al. Evaluation of use of Epstein-Barr viral load in patients after allogeneic stem cell transplantation to diagnose and monitor posttransplant lymphoproliferative disease. J Clin Microbiol 2002;40:351–358.

368. Merlino C, Cavallo R, Bergallo M, et al. Epstein Barr viral load monitoring by quantitative PCR in renal transplant patients. New Microbiol 2003;26:141–149.

369. Riddler SA, Breinig MC, McKnight JL. Increased levels of circulating Epstein-Barr virus (EBV)-infected lymphocytes and decreased EBV nuclear antigen antibody responses are associated with the development of posttransplant lymphoproliferative disease in solid-organ transplant recipients. Blood 1994;84:972–984.

370. Starzl TE, Nalesnik MA, Porter KA, et al. Reversibility of lymphomas and lymphoproliferative lesions developing under cyclosporin-steroid therapy. Lancet 1984;1:583–587.

371. Aversa SM, Stragliotto S, Marino D, et al. Post-transplant lymphoproliferative disorders after heart or kidney transplantation at a single centre: presentation and response to treatment. Acta Haematol 2008;120:36–46.

372. Faye A, Vilmer E. Post-transplant lymphoproliferative disorder in children: incidence, prognosis, and treatment options. Paediatr Drugs 2005;7:55–65.

373. Frey NV, Tsai DE. The management of posttransplant lymphoproliferative disorder. Med Oncol 2007;24:125–136.

374. Gross TG. Treatment for Epstein-Barr virus-associated PTLD. Herpes 2009;15:64–67.

375. Markert E, Siebolts U, Habbig S, et al. Evolution of PTLD following renal transplantation in a child. Pediatr Transplant 2009;13:379–383.

376. Schubert S, Abdul-Khaliq H, Lehmkuhl HB, et al. Diagnosis and treatment of posttransplantation lymphoproliferative disorder in pediatric heart transplant patients. Pediatr Transplant 2009;13:54–62.

377. Swinnen LJ, LeBlanc M, Grogan TM, et al. Prospective study of sequential reduction in immunosuppression, interferon alpha-2B, and chemotherapy for posttransplantation lymphoproliferative disorder. Transplantation 2008;86:215–222.

378. Gong JZ, Bayerl MG, Sandhaus LM, et al. Posttransplant lymphoproliferative disorder after umbilical cord blood transplantation in children. Am J Surg Pathol 2006;30:328–336.

379. Cohen JI. Epstein-Barr virus lymphoproliferative disease associated with acquired immunodeficiency. Medicine (Baltimore) 1991;70:137–160.

380. Humar A, Hebert D, Davies HD, et al. A randomized trial of ganciclovir versus ganciclovir plus immune globulin for prophylaxis against Epstein-Barr virus related post-transplant lymphoproliferative disorder. Transplantation 2006;81:856–861.

381. Buadi FK, Heyman MR, Gocke CD, et al. Treatment and outcomes of post-transplant lymphoproliferative disease: a single institution study. Am J Hematol 2007;82:208–214.

382. Davis CL, Wood BL, Sabath DE, et al. Interferon-alpha treatment of posttransplant lymphoproliferative disorder in recipients of solid organ transplants. Transplantation 1998;66:1770–1779.

383. Oertel SH, Verschuuren E, Reinke P, et al. Effect of anti-CD 20 antibody rituximab in patients with post-transplant lymphoproliferative disorder (PTLD). Am J Transplant 2005;5:2901–2906.

384. Suryanarayan K, Natkunam Y, Berry G, et al. Modified cyclophosphamide, hydroxydaunorubicin, vincristine, and prednisone therapy for posttransplantation lymphoproliferative disease in pediatric patients undergoing solid organ transplantation. J Pediatr Hematol Oncol 2001;23:452–455.

385. Elstrom RL, Andreadis C, Aqui NA, et al. Treatment of PTLD with rituximab or chemotherapy. Am J Transplant 2006;6:569–576.

386. Gross TG. Low-dose chemotherapy for children with post-transplant lymphoproliferative disease. Recent Results Cancer Res 2002;159:96–103.

387. Orjuela M, Gross TG, Cheung YK, et al. A pilot study of chemoimmunotherapy (cyclophosphamide, prednisone, and rituximab) in patients with post-transplant lymphoproliferative disorder following solid organ transplantation. Clin Cancer Res 2003;9:3945S–3952S.

388. Gallego S, Llort A, Gros L, et al. Post-transplant lymphoproliferative disorders in children: the role of chemotherapy in the era of rituximab. Pediatr Transplant 2010; 14(1):61–66.

389. Gross TG, Bucuvalas JC, Park JR, et al. Low-dose chemotherapy for Epstein-Barr virus-positive post-transplantation lymphoproliferative disease in children after solid organ transplantation. J Clin Oncol 2005;23:6481–6488.

390. Emanuel DJ, Lucas KG, Mallory GB Jr, et al. Treatment of posttransplant lymphoproliferative disease in the central nervous system of a lung transplant recipient using allogeneic leukocytes. Transplantation 1997;63:1691–1694.

391. van de Glind G, de Graaf S, Klein C, et al. Intrathecal rituximab treatment for pediatric post-transplant lymphoproliferative disorder of the central nervous system. Pediatr Blood Cancer 2008;50:886–888.

392. Sherritt MA, Bharadwaj M, Burrows JM, et al. Reconstitution of the latent T-lymphocyte response to Epstein-Barr virus is coincident with long-term recovery from posttransplant lymphoma after adoptive immunotherapy. Transplantation 2003;75:1556–1560.

393. Haque T, Taylor C, Wilkie GM, et al. Complete regression of posttransplant lymphoproliferative disease using partially HLA-matched Epstein Barr virus-specific cytotoxic T cells. Transplantation 2001;72:1399–1402.

394. Savoldo B, Goss J, Liu Z, et al. Generation of autologous Epstein-Barr virus-specific cytotoxic T cells for adoptive immunotherapy in solid organ transplant recipients. Transplantation 2001;72:1078–1086.

395. Haque T, Wilkie GM, Jones MM, et al. Allogeneic cytotoxic T-cell therapy for EBV-positive posttransplantation lymphoproliferative disease: results of a phase 2 multicenter clinical trial. Blood 2007;110:1123–1131.

396. Merlo A, Turrini R, Dolcetti R, et al. Adoptive cell therapy against EBV-related malignancies: a survey of clinical results. Expert Opin Biol Ther 2008;8:1265–1294.

397. Savoldo B, Goss JA, Hammer MM, et al. Treatment of solid organ transplant recipients with autologous Epstein Barr virus-specific cytotoxic T lymphocytes (CTLs). Blood 2006;108:2942–2949.

CHAPTER 25 ■ HISTIOCYTIC DISEASES

KENNETH L. MCCLAIN, CARL E. ALLEN, AND JOHN HICKS

INTRODUCTION

The *histiocytoses* represent a broad spectrum of diseases defined by pathologic involvement of cells with specific functions in phagocytosis and antigen presentation. There are many similarities between monocytes, macrophages, histiocytes, and dendritic cells (DCs), making a morphologic distinction difficult. The use of immunophenotyping by immunocytochemistry or cell surface flow cytometry to define Cluster Designation (CD) types on the surface of these cells aids in differentiating the cell types, but clinical factors as well as cytological atypia, or cytogenetic or molecular tools, may be needed to arrive at a final diagnosis.[1] (Table 25.1) The origin of cells responsible for the various histiocytic diseases is illustrated in Figure 25.1.

Langerhans cells (LCs) are the most avid antigen presenting cells of the immune system and are found in the skin and several other locations. In other organs, except the cornea and the brain, the *interdigitating dendritic cells* serve as antigen gathering/presenting cells, similar to LCs. When either of these cells obtains an antigen and is migrating toward a lymph node, their morphology changes and they are identified as *veiled or indeterminate cells*. During this stage, these cells have the same surface markers as LCs, but lack Birbeck granules and complex interdigitating cellular junctions. *Follicular dendritic cells* are found in the germinal center (B-cell region) of lymph nodes and have the characteristic immunophenotype of CD21+, CD35+, CD1a− and S100+/−.

Favara and Jaffe et al. have published classifications of the histiocytic disorders based upon whether these disorders are DC-related, monocyte/macrophage-related, or true malignancies[2,5] (Table 25.1). The DC-related disorders include Langerhans cell histiocytosis (LCH) that has classically been thought to be derived from the LCs found at the dermal/epidermal junction in the skin, as well as in the lungs, lymph nodes, spleen, or bone marrow. The unique staining of these cells with anti-CD207 (anti-langerin) has provided a specific tool to identify the protein composing Birbeck granules, as seen by electron microscopy.[3] However Allen et al. have shown that the histiocytes in LCH originate from myeloid dendritic cells not the skin Langerhans cell.[4a] Immunocytochemical staining with anti-CD207 and anti-CD1a is considered the gold standard for making the diagnosis of LCH. Other antigens, such as S-100 or HLA-DR are characteristic, but not specific for LCs. True malignant histiocytosis has evolved as a specific diagnostic entity after excluding cases of anaplastic large cell lymphoma and other large cell lymphomas with unique immunophenotypes. The third group of DC disorders derived from the dermal/interstitial dendrocyte that stains with antibodies to CD68, fascin, and Factor XIIIa and are found in patients with Erdheim-Chester disease (ECD) and juvenile xanthogranuloma (JXG). These cells lack CD1a and CD207 expression. Abnormal exuberant macrophage function is central to the pathophysiology of hemophagocytic lymphohistiocytosis (HLH). The other macrophage disease discussed here is Rosai-Dorfman disease (RDD) also known as *sinus histiocytosis with*

massive lymphadenopathy (SHML). The key histopathologic finding in RDD is the presence of intact lymphocytes in the cytoplasm of macrophages (emperipolesis) that must be found to diagnose this disorder. RDD progresses slowly, but patients with HLH can become acutely ill in a few hours.

LANGERHANS CELL HISTIOCYTOSIS

Definition and History

Paul Langerhans first described the epidermal cells with multiple cell surface branching pseudopodia that have become known as Langerhans cells in 1868 after staining skin with gold colloid. He originally believed these cells to be neurons due to the appearance of branching dendrites.[6] In 1973, Christian Nezelof and colleagues used electron microscopy to evaluate biopsies from a disease then known as histiocytosis X (HX).[7] They found pentalaminar Birbeck granules in the HX cells that were identical to those previously described in epidermal LCs and therefore suggested re-classifying HX as LCH. Staining with the Birbeck granule-associated antigen CD207 (langerin) is now considered diagnostic of LCH (Fig. 25.2). The Langerhans cell was believed to be central to a common condition that has been described with various names including histiocytosis-X, eosinophilic granuloma, Abt-Letterer-Siwe disease, Hand-Sch?ller-Christian disease and diffuse reticuloendotheliosis.[7–9] LCH is currently the appropriate nomenclature for pathologic conditions characterized by CD207+ LCs. Until further delineation of the myeloid dendritic cell or origin is published.[4a]

LCH is thought to result from the proliferation of immunophenotypically and functionally immature, rounded Langerhans cells along with eosinophils, macrophages, lymphocytes, and sometimes multinucleated giant cells. A controversy exists as to whether LCH arises due to malignant transformation or immune dysregulation of the Langerhans cell.[10] In either case, clinical outcomes have improved with chemotherapeutic agents with activity against malignant and activated immune cells.

Epidemiology

The incidence of LCH has been estimated to be 2 to 10 cases per million children under the age of 15 years.[11] The male to female ratio is close to 1, with the median age at presentation being 30 months, although patients may present from birth through the ninth decade. A few identical and fraternal twins with early onset of LCH have been reported. There are rare case reports of non-twin siblings or multiple cases in one family.[12] Evidence of a single gene defect in LCH is lacking. Solvent exposure in parents and perinatal infections has a weak association with LCH[13] An increased frequency of family members with thyroid disease has been reported.[14]

TABLE 25.1

IMMUNOPHENOTYPES OF HISTIOCYTIC DISORDERS

Disease	LCH	Malignant histiocytosis	ECD/JXG	HLH	RDD
Cell of origin	MD	IDC/FDC	DD/IDC	M/M	M/M
HLA-DR	++	+	−	+	+
CD1a	++	−	−	−	−
CD14	−	−	++	++	++
CD68	+/−	+/−	++	++	++
CD163	−	−	+	++	++
CD 207 (Langerin)	+++	+	−	−	−
Factor XIIIa	−	−	++	−	−
Fascin	−	++	++	+/−	+
Birbeck granules	+	−	−	−	−
Hemophagocytosis	+/−	−/+	−	+/−	−
Emperiopolesis	−	−	−	−	+

LCH, Langerhans cell histiocytosis; ECD, Erdheim Chester disease; JXG, juvenile xanthogranuloma; HLH, hemophagocytic lymphohistiocytosis; RDD, Rosai-Dorfman disease; IDC, interstitial dendritic cell; DD, dermal dendritic cell; M/M, monocyte/macrophage; FDC, follicular dendritic cell; MD, myeloid dendritic cell.
Adapted from Jaffe,[2] Chikwava and Jaffe,[3] and Lau.[4], Allen.[4a]

Etiology and Pathogenesis

LCH has features of malignant transformation as well as immune dysregulation, leading to ongoing debate regarding the etiology of LCH.

Dysplasia/Malignancy

Studies showing clonality in LCH were published in 1994 using polymorphisms of methylation-specific restriction enzyme sites on the X-chromosome regions coding for the human androgen receptor assay (HUMARA), as well as polymorphism for three other loci.[15,16] Biopsies of lesions from both single system or multisystem disease were found to have a proliferation of LCs from a single clone. Pulmonary LCH in adults is nonclonal.[17] Loss of heterozygosity at loci of possible tumor suppressor genes has been reported by two studies, but

a more recent study using CGH arrays failed to identify any amplifications or deletions in the DNA from CD207 cells.[18] Markedly elevated levels of FLT3-ligand and M-CSF have been found in the plasma of LCH patients with good correlation to the extent of disease, as well as response to treatment and increased circulating immature myeloid DCs.[19] This latter finding was not confirmed by a later study; although there was a trend toward higher myeloid DC levels in LCH patients.[20]

Immune Dysregulation

LCH CD207+ cells have some features of immature DCs as well as some features of activated DCs. Antibody staining for the DC markers, CD80, CD86, and class II antigens, has shown that in LCH, the abnormal cells are phenotypically similar to immature DCs and, like immature DCs, present antigen poorly to T cells.[21,22] Transforming growth factor-beta (TGF-beta), as well as IL-10, are purportedly responsible for

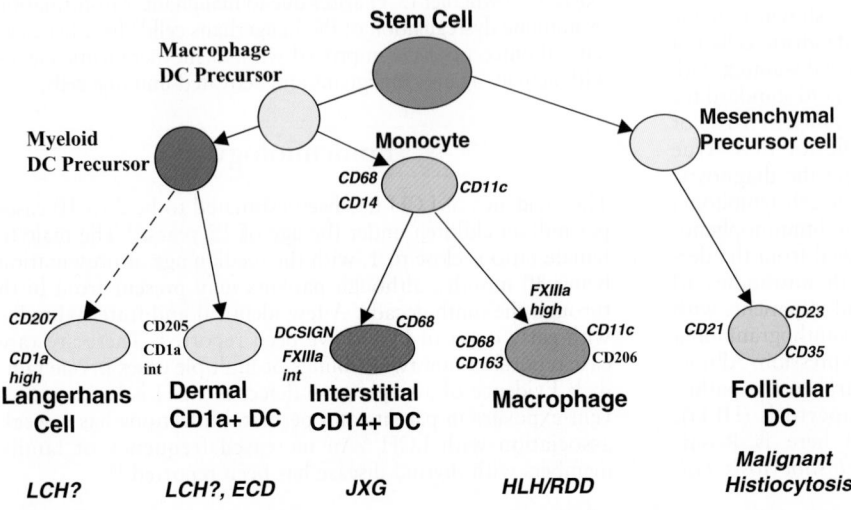

CELL ORIGINS OF HISTIOCYTIC DISEASES

FIGURE 25.1 Schematic representation of the cells from which the various histiocytic diseases originate. The interrupted arrow from the myeloid dendritic cell precursor to the Langerhans cells represents the embryonal origin of the Langerhans cells. Question marks after LCH convey uncertainty of the cellular origin based upon work in the authors' laboratory.[4a] Abbreviations: DC, dendritic cell; LCH, Langerhans cell histiocytosis; JXG, juvenile xanthogranuloma; ECD, Erdheim Chester disease; RDD, Rosai-Dorfman disease; HLH, hemophagocytic lymphohistiocytosis; int, intermediate.

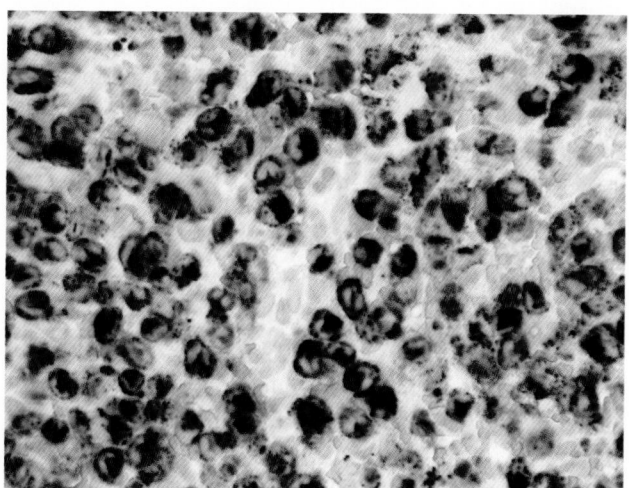

FIGURE 25.2 Langerhans cell histiocytosis: Langerhan cell histiocytes demonstrating typical grooved and reniform nuclei with moderate amount of eosinophilic cytoplasm and immunocytochemistry staining with CD207 (Langerin) (original magnification 400×).

preventing LC maturation in LCH.[22] While LCH CD207+ cells may appear phenotypically immature, they are associated with production of proinflammatory cytokines and migration, features typical of activated immature myeloid DCs.[4a]

No immune stimulus has been defined in LCH. Efforts to define a viral cause have been unsuccessful.[23,24] There is enrichment of regulatory T cells in LCH lesions as well as expansion of these inhibitory immune cells in peripheral blood of patients with active disease, though the etiology and significance of these observations is not clear.[20] Elevated levels of another regulator of the immune system and bone metabolism, osteoprotegerin (OPG), are present in the plasma of patients with active LCH.[25,26] OPG levels were highest in patients with multisystem disease and decreased with response to therapy.

Clinical Features

The most frequent presenting signs of LCH are skin rash or painful bone lesion. Patients may also have fever, weight loss, diarrhea, edema, dyspnea, polydipsia, and polyuria.

LCH patients are divided into *high-risk* or *low-risk* categories based upon specific organ involvement. High-risk organs include liver, spleen, lungs, and bone marrow. Low-risk organs include skin, bones, lymph nodes, and pituitary gland. Patients may present with disease at one site (single site or single system), or at multiple sites (multisystem). Treatment decisions for patients are based upon whether or not *high-risk* or *low-risk* organs are involved, and if LCH presents as a single site or multisystem disease. Patients may have LCH of the skin, bone, lymph nodes, and pituitary in any combination, and still be considered *low risk*.

Pathologic Features

The typical LCH lesion is comprised of an admixture of LC histiocytes, intermediate cells, and interdigitating cells of a DC lineage, T-cell lymphocytes, eosinophils, and macrophages (Fig. 25.2). The hallmark cell is the LC histiocyte. This cell has abundant eosinophilic to amphophilic cytoplasm, and a nucleus which is reniform, deeply indented or grooved. The presence of eosinophils is quite variable. Occasional giant

cells representing fusion of either macrophages or LC histiocytes may be seen. LCH can be distinguished from other DC disorders by cytoplasmic and cell surface markers (Table 25.1). CD1a is expressed by LC histiocytes, cortical thymocytes, and interdigitating DCs within the dermis and lymph nodes. LC histiocytes demonstrate a membranous to cytoplasmic pattern with CD1a. A highly specific and sensitive antibody against LCs and LC histiocytes is CD207 (langerin, Fig. 25.2). CD207 detects a type II transmembrane protein expressed with LCs and LC histiocytes. Langerin is located on the cell surface and induces membrane superimposition, leading to pentalaminar Birbeck granule formation. These granules capture antigen and are rapidly internalized into the cells for antigen processing. Electron microscopic identification of Birbeck granules is necessary with difficult-to-characterize histiocytic disorders, or when aberrant immunocytochemical results are obtained. Birbeck granules have a *tennis racket with handle* appearance with a bulbous and rod-shaped component. Birbeck granules tend to be rare when LC histiocytosis involves the liver, spleen, and gastrointestinal tract. Differentiation of LCH from other histiocytic and DC disorders is important. The immunophenotypes of histiocytic and DC disorders are presented in Table 25.1.[27]

Specific Organ Involvement

Skin

Infants may have a seborrheic scalp rash, often mistaken for *cradle cap*. Children and adults may develop red papular lesions in the scalp, groin, abdomen, back, or chest that resemble a diffuse candida rash. (Fig. 25.3) Seborrhea-like involvement of the scalp may be mistaken for a severe case of

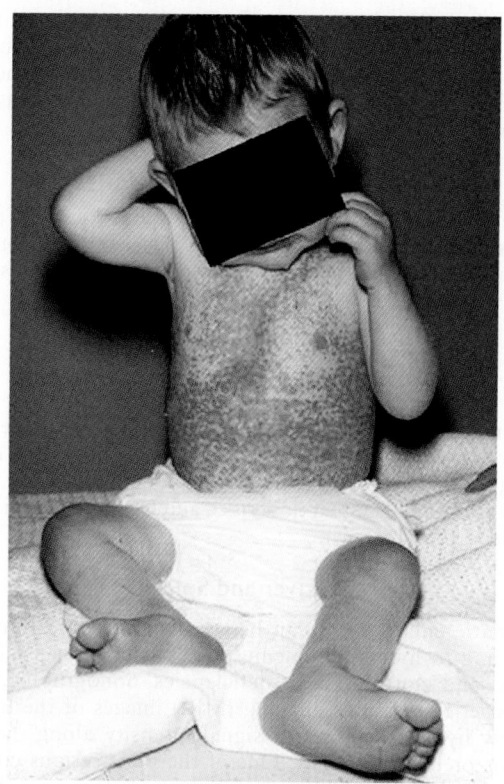

FIGURE 25.3 Cutaneous Langerhans cell histiocytosis. An erythematous, popular rash resembling a *candida* diaper rash.

dandruff. Ulcerative lesions behind the ears, or involving the scalp, genitalia, or perianal region are often misdiagnosed as bacterial or fungal infections. Patients may also present with brown to purplish papules over any part of their body (Hashimoto-Pritzker disease).[28] This manifestation may be self-limited as the lesions often disappear during the first year of life with no therapy. However, such patients should be monitored frequently for systemic disease.[29,30] In a report of 61 neonatal LCH cases from 1069 patients in the Histiocyte Society database, almost 60% of neonates had multisystem disease and 72% had risk organ involvement.[31]

Oral Mucosa

In the mouth, presenting symptoms include gingival hypertrophy, ulcers of the soft or hard palate, buccal mucosa, or on the tongue and lips. Lesions of the oral mucosa may precede evidence of LCH elsewhere.[27,32]

Bone

The most frequent site of LCH in children is a lytic lesion of the skull, which may be asymptomatic or painful.[33] Other sites are skull, femur, ribs, vertebra, and humerus. Spine lesions are most often located in the cervical vertebrae. Proptosis from a LCH mass in the orbit mimics rhabdomyosarcoma, leukemia, neuroblastoma, inflammatory pseudotumors, and benign fatty tumors of the eye. Some skull lesions are not only lytic, but may have an accompanying soft tissue mass that impinges on the dura. Lesions of the facial bones or anterior or middle cranial fossae (e.g., temporal, sphenoid, ethmoid, or zygomatic) with intracranial tumor extension constitute part of a *CNS-risk* group. These patients have a threefold increased risk for developing diabetes insipidus and an increased risk of other central nervous system (CNS) disease (described later).

Lymph Nodes and Thymus

The cervical nodes are most frequently involved and may be soft or hard-matted groups with accompanying lymphedema. An enlarged thymus or mediastinal node involvement can mimic lymphoma or an infectious process and may cause asthma-like symptoms.

Pituitary Gland

The posterior pituitary gland can be affected in LCH patients causing central diabetes insipidus (DI) (see section "Endocrine System"). Anterior pituitary involvement often results in failure of growth and sexual maturation.

Multisystem Disease Presentation

In multisystem LCH, the disease presents in multiple organs or body systems, including liver, spleen, lungs, bone marrow (high risk), or bones, skin, lymph nodes, endocrine system, gastrointestinal system (low risk), and CNS (intermediate risk, depending on extent).

Liver and Spleen

Hepatic enlargement can be accompanied by dysfunction, leading to hypoalbuminemia with ascites, hyperbilirubinemia, and clotting factor deficiencies. Sonographic, CT, or magnetic resonance imaging (MRI) images of the liver will show hypoechoic or low signal intensity along the portal veins or biliary tracts.[34] One of the most serious complications of hepatic LCH is cholestasis and sclerosing cholangitis.[35] In the case of sclerosing cholangitis, biopsies show no LC histiocytes, but periportal lymphocyte infiltrates instead.

It is thought that cytokines elaborated by periportal lymphocytes may damage the bile ducts. Seventy-five percent of children with sclerosing cholangitis will not respond to chemotherapy, and all of these patients require liver transplantation.[35] Massive splenomegaly may lead to cytopenias, because of hypersplenism and respiratory compromise, though splenectomy is rarely indicated.

Lung

The lung is also considered a high-risk organ, but is less frequently involved in children than in adults, in whom smoking is a key etiologic factor.[36] Chest x-rays may show a nonspecific interstitial infiltrate. A high resolution CT of the chest is needed to visualize the cystic/nodular pattern of LCH that leads to the destruction of lung tissue. A *spontaneous* pneumothorax often may be the first sign of LCH in the lung, although patients may present with tachypnea or dyspnea from widespread fibrosis and destruction of lung tissue. Children with pulmonary LCH plus low-risk organs have a 5-year survival of 83% compared with 94% for those with only *low-risk* organ involvement.[37] Declining diffusion capacity may also herald the onset of pulmonary hypertension.[38] In young children with diffuse disease, therapy can halt tissue destruction, and repair mechanisms may restore some function.

Bone Marrow

Bone marrow involvement occurs most frequently in young children who have diffuse disease involving the liver, spleen, lymph nodes, and skin, and significant thrombocytopenia or neutropenia.[39] Others have only mild cytopenias and are found to have marrow involvement with LCH by sensitive immunohistochemical or flow cytometric analysis of the bone marrow.[40] LCH patients with very high-risk disease may present with marrow hemophagocytosis.[41] The cytokine milieu driving LCH is probably responsible for this epiphenomenon of macrophage activation. These patients may be confusing as to which histiocytic syndrome is primary: HLH or LCH.

Endocrine System

Diabetes insipidus (DI) is the most frequent endocrine manifestation of LCH. Some patients present with an apparent *idiopathic* presentation of DI before other lesions are identified. A review of such patients found that 51% would have other lesions diagnostic of LCH within a year of identifying DI.[42] A study of 589 LCH patients in France revealed that the 10-year risk of pituitary involvement was 24%.[43] These investigators did not see a decreased incidence of DI in chemotherapy-treated patients. However, Grois et al. reported a decline in the incidence of DI from 40% to 20% with 6 months of treatment that included velban and prednisone for CNS-risk patients.[44]

Gastrointestinal System

A few patients with diarrhea, hematochezia, perianal fistulas, diarrhea, or malabsorption have been reported.[45,46] Diagnosing gastrointestinal lesions in LCH is difficult because of patchy involvement. Careful endoscopic evaluation, including multiple biopsies, is needed.

Central Nervous System—Diabetes Insipidus

Acute Manifestations of Diabetes Insipidus. DI caused by damage to the posterior pituitary is the most frequent initial sign of LCH (4%) in the CNS.[47] Ultimately DI occurred in 12% of patients in the Deutsche Arbeitsgemeinschaft für Leukaemieforschung und therapie im Kindesalter (DAL) studies.[44] Pituitary biopsies are rarely done, usually when the stalk is >6.5 mm or when there is a hypothalamic mass. Most often, the diagnosis is established by biopsy of skin, bone, or lymph node of a patient who also has the pituitary abnormalities noted.

Chronic Manifestations of Diabetes Insipidus. Fifty-six percent of LCH patients with DI will develop anterior pituitary hormone deficiencies (growth, thyroid, or gonadal-stimulating hormones) within 10 years of the onset of DI.[44,48]

Other Chronic CNS Disease Manifestations

LCH patients may develop mass lesions of the choroid plexus, grey, or white matter.[49] These lesions contain CD1a-positive LCs as well as CD8+ lymphocytes.[50] In 1% to 4% of LCH patients a chronic neurodegenerative syndrome that is manifested by dysarthria, ataxia, dysmetria, and sometimes behavior changes has been reported.[49] MRI shows hyperintensity of the dentate nucleus and white matter of the cerebellum on T2-weighted images, or hyperintense lesions of the basal ganglia on T1-weighted images, and atrophy of the cerebellum.[51] (Fig. 25.4) The diagnostic imaging findings may precede the onset of symptoms by many years or be coincident. A study of 83 LCH patients, with at least two brain MRIs for evaluation of craniofacial lesions, diabetes insipidus, and/or other endocrine deficiencies or neuropsychological symptoms, was recently published.[52] Forty-seven of 83 patients (57%) had radiological neurodegenerative changes at a median time of 34 months from diagnosis. Of the 47 patients, 12 (25%) had clinical neurological deficits that presented 3 to 15 years after LCH diagnosis.

Laboratory Features

Patients with high-risk disease may present with anemia and thrombocytopenia if the marrow is involved.[39,40] An elevated erythrocyte sedimentation rate and thrombocytosis may correlate with active LCH.[53] When the liver is involved, hypoalbuminemia, elevated liver enzymes, and elevated bilirubin are present. Intestinal involvement may also cause hypoalbuminemia. Lytic lesions of the bone are found by plain films, CT, MRI, bone scan, or positron emission tomography (PET) scan. PET scans are useful for detecting lesions not found by bone scan or plain films, and comparison PET scans are particularly good for providing evidence of healing after 6 to 12 weeks of therapy.[54] A biopsy of an affected organ is necessary to make the diagnosis of LCH with staining of the LC histiocytes by CD1a or CD207 (Fig. 25.2).[2]

Treatment

The optimal treatment of LCH patients is with enrollment on clinical trials sponsored by the Histiocyte Society (http://www.histiocytesociety.org/). Patients with skin-only LCH, some single-bone lesions (non–CNS-risk), and isolated diabetes insipidus have not been included in these trials in the past, but will be on the LCH-IV study.

Single System

Patients with LCH limited to skin may be observed to determine if the lesions resolve spontaneously. If they do not, a variety of treatments including topical steroids,[30] oral methotrexate,[55] oral thalidomide,[56] topical application of nitrogen mustard,[57] and psoralen with UV light have been used.[58]

A single skull lesion involving the frontal, parietal, or occipital bones, or single lesion of any other bone may be treated with curettage only, or curettage plus injection of methylprednisolone.[59] Skull lesions in the mastoid, temporal, or orbital bones (*CNS-risk* lesions) need to be treated with 6 to 12 months of vinblastine and prednisone to decrease the risk of developing DI.[44]

Bone

Multiple bone lesions, or combinations of skin, lymph node, or pituitary gland with or without bone lesions, should be treated with 12 months of vinblastine and prednisone. (Readers should look for publication of the LCH-III trial, completed in early 2009, which may clarify issues on the length of treatment for low-risk patients who were randomized to receive 6 or 12 months of velban/prednisone.) A short (<6 months) treatment course with only a single agent (e.g., prednisone) results in a higher number of relapses than one with combination chemotherapy: 18% LCH reactivation rate with a 2-drug regimen has been reported versus 50% to 80% with only surgery or single-drug treatments.[60–62]

Treatment of LCH in the spleen, liver, bone marrow, or lung (with or without the low-risk sites) is based upon LCH-I, LCH-II, and the DAL-HX 83 studies. Treatment time in these studies varies from 6 months (LCH-I and LCH-II) to 1 year (DAL-HX-83 and LCH-III).[63,64] The LCH-II study was a randomized trial to compare treatment of patients with velban/prednisone/mercaptopurine to that with velban/etoposide/prednisone/mercaptopurine.[65] The outcomes of response at 6 weeks, 5-year probability of survival, relapses, and permanent consequences showed no statistical difference between the two treatment arms. Etoposide has not been used in subsequent Histiocyte Society trials. However, in comparison with historical data, use of etoposide may result in reduced mortality of patients with risk organ involvement. Although controversial, this comparison of patients in the LCH-I to LCH-II trials suggested that increased treatment intensity promoted additional early responses and reduced mortality.

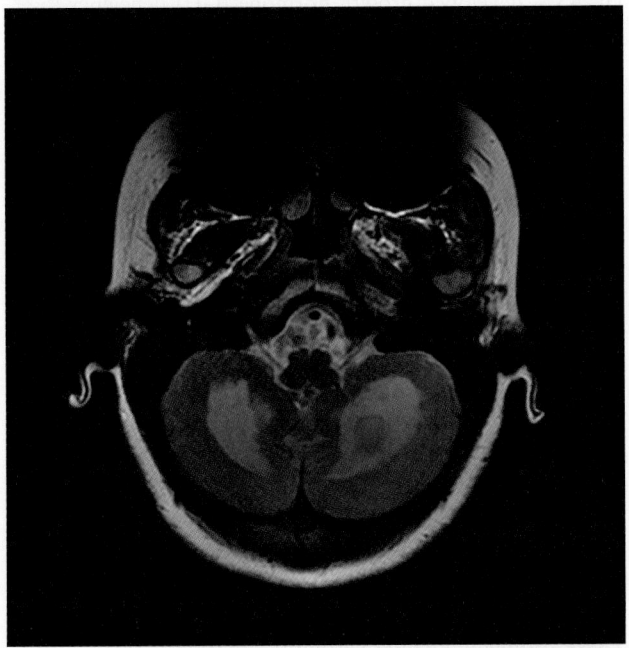

FIGURE 25.4 MRI image illustrating CNS LCH. T2-weighted flair image with hyperintense signal in the cerebellum.

Another more intensive regimen has been reported, which included cytarabine, vincristine, prednisolone, and methotrexate for good responders, or a salvage therapy with daunorubicin, cyclophosphamide, vincristine, and prednisolone for poor responders.[66] Both treatments lasted 7.5 months.

Vertebral or Femoral Bone Lesions at Risk for Collapse. Isolated radiation therapy is indicated for patients with single-bone lesions of only the vertebrae or femoral neck which are at risk of collapse.[67,68] When instability of the cervical vertebrae and neurologic symptoms are present, bracing or spinal fusion may be needed.[69] Certain skull lesions, not in the CNS-risk region, could also be considered for radiation therapy.

CNS

Treatment of mass lesions with cladribine has been effective in 13 reported cases.[70–72] Mass lesions included enlargement of the hypothalamic-pituitary axis, parenchymal mass lesions, and leptomeningeal involvement. Doses of cladribine ranged from 5 to 13 mg/m^2, given at varying frequencies.[72]

For treatment of the LCH-CNS neurodegenerative syndrome with clinical signs, use of dexamethasone, cladribine, retinoic acid, and intravenous immunoglobulin has been reported.[73,74] MRI findings were stable, but clinical efficacy was difficult to judge because patients were reported to have no progression in their neurologic symptoms or MRIs. The authors have published a study showing efficacy of vincristine/cytosine arabinoside in these patients with improvement in clinical symptoms and MRI images in five of eight patients.[75]

Refractory or Progressive Childhood Langerhans Cell Histiocytosis

Recurrent *Low-Risk* Organ Involvement. The optimal therapy for patients with relapsed or recurrent disease has not been determined and several treatment options are effective. Patients with bone disease which recurs more than 6 months after terminating vinblastine and prednisone can benefit from treatment with *reinduction* of vinblastine and prednisone with the addition of oral methotrexate weekly and mercaptopurine nightly for 1 year. Cladribine is also an effective agent for patients with recurrent bone disease.[76] An alternative treatment regimen employs vincristine and cytosine arabinoside.[77]

A phase II trial of thalidomide for LCH patients (10 low-risk patients, 6 high-risk patients) who failed primary and at least one secondary regimen demonstrated complete (4/10) and partial (3/10) responses for the low-risk patients.[56]

Recurrent *High-Risk* Organ Involvement. A new treatment plan is indicated when a patient with multisystem high-risk involvement shows progressive disease after 6 weeks of standard treatment, or has not had a partial response by 12 weeks. Data from the DAL studies have shown that these children have only a 10% chance of surviving.[63] Results of the LCH-II study revealed that patients treated with vinblastine/prednisone who did not respond well by 6 weeks had a 27% chance of survival.[65] Those treated with vinblastine/prednisone/etoposide and showing poor response at 6 weeks had a 52% chance of survival. Use of cladribine and 2'-deoxycoformycin as salvage therapies for LCH has also been published.[78] These drugs were more often effective for patients with bone, skin, or lymph node involvement. Only one-third of the patients with LCH of the liver, bone marrow, spleen, or lung responded.

The current Histiocyte Society clinical trial for patients with refractory *high-risk* organ (liver, spleen, or bone marrow) involvement is an intensive *acute myeloid leukemia (AML)-like* protocol, using cladribine and cytosine arabinoside, and appears to provide improved overall survival with 7 of 10 patients achieving a complete remission, though responses are often slow.[79]

Stem cell transplantation (SCT) has been done for patients with multisystem high-risk organ involvement that is refractory to salvage chemotherapy. Reduced-intensity conditioning regimens are curative and associated with less toxicity.[80–82]

Course and Prognosis

LCH patients with low-risk disease treated with vinblastine and prednisone have a 99% chance of being cured of their disease, but up to 46% have relapsed when treated for only 6 months or with just those two drugs.[64,66,83] Almost all of these patients are ultimately cured of LCH, but they may experience two to four relapses and require multiple regimens to effect the cure.[83] Other therapies including pamidronate, cyclosporine, and interferon have been reported, but have not become standard treatments.[84]

Late Effects

Permanent consequences or late effects in LCH patients related to their disease and therapy remain a challenging issue. Children with low-risk organ involvement (skin, bones, lymph nodes, or pituitary gland) have a 24% chance of developing long-term sequelae.[85] Patients with multisystem involvement have a 71% incidence of long-term problems.[86]

Endocrine

Those with DI are at risk for panhypopituitarism and should be monitored carefully for adequacy of growth and development. In a retrospective review of 141 patients with LCH and DI, 43% developed growth hormone (GH) deficiency.[48,86,87] The 5- and 10-year risks of GH deficiency among children with LCH and DI were 35% and 54%, respectively. There was no increase in LCH reactivation in patients who received GH compared with those who did not.[48]

Neurologic

Neurologic symptoms secondary to vertebral compression of cervical lesions have been reported in LCH patients with spinal lesions.[88] CNS-LCH occurs most often in children with LCH of the pituitary or of CNS-risk skull bones (mastoid, orbit, and temporal bone). Significant cognitive defects, as well as MRI abnormalities, may develop in some long-term survivors with CNS-risk skull lesions.[88] Some patients have markedly abnormal cerebellar function and behavior abnormalities, while others have subtle deficits in short-term memory and brain-stem–evoked potentials.[89] Hearing loss has been found in 13% of children treated for LCH.[86]

Orthopedic

Orthopedic problems from lesions involving the spine, femur, tibia, or humerus may be seen in 20% of patients. These problems include vertebral collapse or instability of the spine that may lead to scoliosis and facial or limb asymmetry.

Dental Problems

Dental problems characterized by loss of teeth have been significant for some patients, usually related to bone loss or overly aggressive dental surgery.[85]

Pulmonary

Diffuse pulmonary disease may result in poor lung function with higher risk for infections and decreased exercise tolerance. These patients should be followed with pulmonary function testing, including the diffusing capacity of carbon monoxide (DLCO) and ratio of residual volume to total lung capacity.[38]

Hematologic

Marrow failure secondary to LCH or from therapy is rare, and is associated with a higher risk of malignancy. Patients with LCH have a higher than normal risk of developing secondary cancers.[90] Leukemia (usually acute myeloid) occurs after treatment, as does lymphoblastic lymphoma. Concurrent LCH and other malignancies have been reported in a few patients, and some patients have had their non-LCH malignancy first, followed by development of LCH. Three patients with T-cell acute lymphoblastic leukemia (T-ALL) and aggressive LCH, which shared markers of clonality, have been reported.[91,92]

HEMOPHAGOCYTIC LYMPHOHISTIOCYTOSIS

Definition and History

Farquhar and Claireux first described siblings with this disease in 1952.[93] Although many case reports using several eponyms ensued, Henter and Elinder provided a logical organization of the multiple presentations.[94] Hemophagocytic lymphohistiocytosis (HLH) is an aggressive and potentially fatal syndrome that results from inappropriate prolonged activation of lymphocytes and macrophages. The name describes the characteristic, but not diagnostic, histopathologic finding of macrophages engulfing all types of blood cells in bone marrow, lymph nodes, spleen, or liver biopsies (Fig. 25.5). HLH is

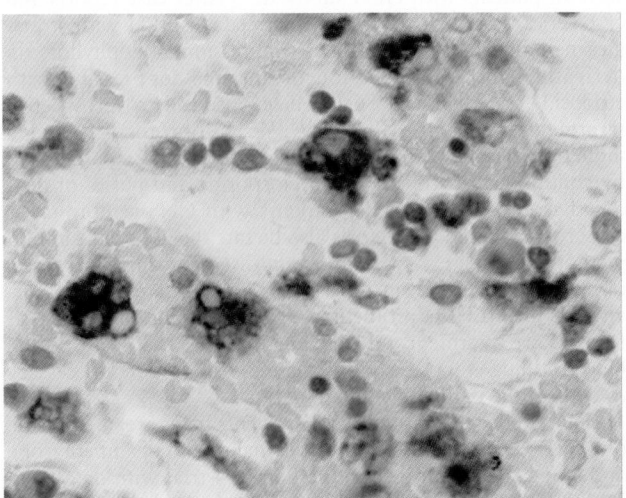

FIGURE 25.5 Hemophagocytic lymphohistiocytosis: CD68 immunostain highlights frequent histiocytes engorged with red blood cells (CD68 immunocytochemistry, original magnification 600×).

also known as autosomal recessive familial hemophagocytic lymphohistiocytosis, familial erythrophagocytic lymphohistiocytosis, viral-associated hemophagocytic syndrome, or infection-associated hemophagocytosis. Young children with HLH and known gene mutations, or a family history of HLH, are described as *primary* HLH. Older children with HLH, or children without identifiable mutations are sometimes described as having *secondary'* or *acquired* HLH, with the assumption that the condition is due to infection or other stimulus and not genetic predisposition. The same mutations may be present in both situations, and there is no rapid and definitive gene testing strategy to define these two groups. In general, presentation and outcome are the same for primary and acquired HLH. Thus, this distinction is not clinically useful in the acute setting, as they both must be diagnosed promptly and treated aggressively.

Epidemiology

The incidence of HLH in Sweden was estimated at 1.2 children per million per year, or 1 in 50,000 live births with equal sex distribution.[94] At the authors' institution, HLH was diagnosed in 1 of 3,000 inpatient admissions over a 2-year period.[95]

Etiology and Pathogenesis

Defects in the function of natural killer (NK) cells and cytotoxic T cells have been found in HLH patients. This results in the pathological activation of T cells and macrophages, which produce proinflammatory cytokines, including interferon gamma, tumor necrosis factor alpha, interleukin (IL)-6, IL-10, IL-12, and soluble IL-2 receptor alpha (sCD25).[96,97] Hypercytokinemia generated by activated T cells and macrophages results in multiorgan dysfunction that can rapidly lead to death.

Perforin Expression

Perforin was identified as a candidate HLH gene by gene mapping and was confirmed by low expression of perforin in NK cells and cytotoxic T lymphocytes from some HLH patients.[98] Perforin is secreted from NK cells and cytotoxic T cells upon activation by target cells. Perforin induces pore formation in the target cell's membrane, allowing granzyme to enter and trigger apoptosis.[99] Some HLH characteristics were reproducible in *PRF1* knockout mice.[100]

Other Gene Defects Causing HLH

Mutations in other genes encoding proteins involved in NK and cytotoxic T-cell–mediated killing of target cells have also been discovered in patients with HLH, including *granzyme B*, *UNC13D*, and *syntaxin 11*.[101]

Immune Deficiencies Associated with HLH

Patients with other immune deficiencies associated with lysosomal trafficking defects (e.g., Chediak-Higashi syndrome, Hermansky-Pudlack syndrome type II) also have a high frequency of developing HLH.[101] HLH associated with Epstein-Barr infection is the most common fatal complication of X-linked lymphoproliferative disease.[102] Mutations in *RAB27A*, which encodes protein that controls secretion of lytic granules, have been identified in patients with Griscelli syndrome who develop HLH.[101]

Clinical Features

One of the major challenges to effective management of HLH is appropriate and swift diagnosis and treatment of this disorder. Initial signs and symptoms of HLH mimic more common problems.[103] Confounding diagnoses, such as infection, autoimmune disease, hepatitis, multisystem organ failure, encephalitis, and malignancy, do not exclude a diagnosis of HLH. A family history of consanguinity, recurrent spontaneous abortions, or HLH in siblings (or symptoms suggesting undiagnosed HLH) should prompt a full evaluation for HLH.

Prominent early clinical signs include fever (91%), hepatomegaly (90%), splenomegaly (84%), neurological symptoms (47%), rash (43%), and lymphadenopathy (42%).[104] HLH patients develop liver failure with markedly elevated bilirubins, pancytopenia, coagulopathy; renal failure heralded by hyponatremia; and pulmonary failure similar to acute respiratory distress syndrome (ARDS) with interstitial infiltrates on chest x-ray. In addition, 75% of patients with HLH have CNS symptoms that may mimic encephalitis.[105]

Diagnostic Criteria

The cumulative experiences from the first prospective international treatment protocol of the Histiocyte Society, HLH-94, as well as other observations and studies, have led to HLH-2004, which includes diagnostic guidelines (Table 25.2).[106] Evidence of mutations in *PRF1* (encodes perforin),[107] *UNC13D* (encodes MUNC13–4),[108] or *syntaxin 11* genes[109] are diagnostic of HLH. Gene mutation studies are rarely helpful in the acute setting, because it may take months to complete the genetic testing. In the absence of a known gene mutation, a diagnosis of HLH can be made when at least five of eight criteria are identified

Tissue hemophagocytosis is sometimes misunderstood as pathognomonic for HLH. Marrow aspirates or biopsies fail to demonstrate hemophagocytosis in 20% or more HLH

TABLE 25.2

CLINICAL CRITERIA FOR DIAGNOSIS OF HLH

HLH diagnosis is established with at least five of the following:
- Fever
- Splenomegaly
- Cytopenias in at least two cell lines:
  Hemoglobin <90 g/L
  Platelets <100 × 10⁹/L
  Neutrophils <1 × 10⁹/L
- Hypertriglyceridemia and/or hypofibrinogenemia:
  Fasting triglycerides >3 mmol/L (>265 mg/dL)
  Fibrinogen <1.5 g/L
- Hemophagocytosis in bone marrow or spleen or lymph nodes
- Low or absent activity of natural killer cells (specialized laboratory test)
- Ferritin >500 μg/L
- Soluble cD25 (soluble interleukin-2 receptor) >2400 units/mL

patients.[110] Repeat testing, as well as lymph node or liver biopsies, may be necessary. Finding hemophagocytosis is highly suggestive of HLH, but is neither necessary nor sufficient to make the diagnosis. Cerebrospinal fluid should be tested in patients with signs of CNS abnormalities; pleocytosis and hyperproteinemia support HLH with CNS involvement. The clonal proliferation of lymphocytes in lymph nodes may be confused with a lymphomatous infiltrate.[111]

Laboratory Features

Ferritin

Although no one diagnostic criterion is sufficient to make the diagnosis of HLH, a highly elevated serum ferritin along with four other criteria can be very helpful. The Histiocyte Society included a ferritin concentration of >500 μg/L in the eight diagnostic criteria. Ferritin concentrations >500 μg/L were 100% sensitive for HLH in a retrospective review over a 2-year period at the authors' institution.[95] However, at this modest level, there is considerable overlap with many other diagnoses. Ferritin concentrations more than 10,000 μg/L were 90% sensitive and 96% specific for HLH with very minimal overlap with sepsis, infections, and liver failure.

It is recommended that the following tests be performed with a previously healthy patient who presents with persistent fevers, hepatosplenomegaly, and cytopenia of at least two cell lines: serum ferritin, AST/ALT, lactate dehydrogenase, bilirubin, coagulation studies, fibrinogen, and triglycerides. A bone marrow biopsy and aspirate is needed, as well as a lumbar puncture and brain MRI if lumbar puncture is contraindicated. NK-cell function, perforin expression of T cells and NK cells, and sCD25 concentrations should be evaluated if four or more of the HLH diagnostic criteria are met.[112] Following daily serum ferritin levels is useful because rapidly rising ferritin is a strong indicator of HLH. Other conditions should be evaluated and treated, because sepsis, viral infection, autoimmune disease, and malignancy do not exclude a concurrent diagnosis of HLH.

Therapy

Before treatment with immune-modulating therapy fewer than 10% of patients with HLH survived.[104] After case reports and case series described successful treatment of HLH with strategies including aggressive immune suppression, podophyllotoxin derivatives, or a combination of immune suppression with etoposide, the Histiocyte Society developed the first prospective treatment protocol, HLH-94.[113,114] This protocol included induction therapy with dexamethasone and etoposide, followed by continuous treatment with cyclosporine and pulses of dexamethasone and etoposide. Patients with CNS symptoms or cerebrospinal fluid pleocytosis also dictate the use of intrathecal methotrexate. Patients with resistant disease, recurrent disease, or familial HLH received SCT. The overall estimated 3-year survival on the HLH-94 protocol was 55%.[115] Some clinicians prefer to start treatment with dexamethasone and cyclosporine before adding etoposide. However, etoposide is often necessary to control the pathologic inflammation.

The standard of care for HLH patients being treated outside of a therapeutic research trial is treatment with dexamethasone and etoposide as outlined in the HLH-94 trial with data from HLH-2004 pending. Cyclosporine may be added, but benefit during induction therapy is not proven and has been associated with posterior reversible encephalopathy syndrome (PRES).[116] HLH patients require multiple transfusions of red blood cells, platelets, and fresh frozen plasma. Prophylactic protection against *Pneumocystis* jiroveci infection with sulfamethoxazole and fungi with fluconazole is necessary. Newly diagnosed HLH patients should be referred to a SCT service early to begin evaluation for potential donors. Sibling donor should be evaluated for occult immune dysfunction (perforin expression, NK-cell function) due to the potential of transplanting a new graft with the same HLH predisposition. Patients with systemic juvenile rheumatoid arthritis or systemic lupus erythematosus with macrophage activation syndrome (MAS; described later) may be adequately treated with dexamethasone and cyclosporine.

Antithymocyte globulin (ATG) has been used as a primary treatment of 38 cases of familial HLH.[117] It was the intent that all of these patients have SCT, which ultimately cured 16 of 19 cases. ATG was not effective for patients previously treated with etoposide/dexamethasone/cyclosporine who had relapsed while on therapy.

SCT is needed for all patients with familial HLH or gene defects, CNS disease, or who relapse. Survival ranges from 45% to 60% in several series, which included use of matched related and matched unrelated donors with conventional or reduced intensity conditioning.[118–120]

Macrophage Activation Syndrome

Macrophage activation syndrome (MAS) describes patients with symptoms of HLH in the setting of juvenile rheumatoid arthritis or systemic lupus erythematosus. Similar to classic HLH, MAS is characterized by proliferation of macrophages and T cells. Patients present with continuous fever, purpura, hepatosplenomegaly, mental status changes, cytopenias, coagulopathy, and hypofibrinogenemia. Laboratory findings may include defective NK-cell function and low perforin expression, as seen in HLH.[121] Unlike classic HLH, patients with MAS may be successfully treated with cyclosporine and corticosteroids without etoposide.[122] However, chemotherapy including etoposide is recommended if the patient fails to improve after 2 days of corticosteroid/cyclosporine alone.

Course and Prognosis

Patients with HLH are critically ill and need highly toxic chemotherapy. They should be treated at institutions familiar with the complications of chemotherapy and immune suppression. Some patients have an initial good response to therapy with etoposide, dexamethasone, and cyclosporine, but then have progressive disease as evidenced by elevation of the serum ferritin, worsening coagulopathy, or need for increased respiratory, blood pressure, or renal support. Despite being profoundly toxic to the bone marrow, it is important to continue etoposide because it is the only medication that will cause apoptosis of the activated macrophages. Treatment of active EBV infection with rituximab[123] or addition of anti-TNFa agents, such as infliximab or etanercept, has also proven useful.[124–126]

SINUS HISTIOCYTOSIS WITH MASSIVE LYMPHADENOPATHY (ROSAI-DORFMAN DISEASE)

Definition and History

Rosai and Dorfman recognized this nonmalignant proliferation of histiocytes as a unique histopathologic entity included in the differential diagnosis for massive lymphadenopathy.[127] RDD is self-limited in some patients, but others experience airway obstruction, orbital tumors, or brain tumors that may require therapy.[128]

Epidemiology

RDD occurs in children and young adults (mean age: 20.6 years) with no gender, ethnic, or socioeconomic predilection. However, digestive system RDD occurs more commonly in males and blacks.[129] Intracranial disease is found in patients with a mean age of 37.5 years.[130] RDD may be associated with rheumatologic disorders and hemolytic anemia.[131]

Etiology and Pathogenesis

There is no consistent evidence of an infectious etiology for RDD, although infectious causes may stimulate lymphocyte phagocytosis by the macrophages. The cells in RDD lesions are polyclonal as determined by restriction fragment polymorphisms of the human androgen receptor gene (the HUMARA assay).[132]

Clinical Features

Massive, painless bilateral cervical adenopathy is the presenting finding in 87% of patients. Some affected persons have fever, night sweats, malaise, weight loss, polyarthralgia, rheumatoid arthritis, glomerulonephritis, asthma, and diabetes mellitus. Sixteen percent have painless maculopapular eruptions, sometimes being red, blue, or yellow xanthomatous rashes. Subcutaneous nodules can be found anywhere on the body. Other presentations include nasal cavity and paranasal sinus involvement with obstruction of the airways, epistaxis, septal displacement, and mass lesions infiltrating the sinuses. A variety of other sites have been documented.[133]

Pathologic Features

Lymph nodes in RDD are markedly enlarged with a thickened fibrous capsule. The characteristic feature of RDD is dramatically expanded sinusoids and interfollicular regions by histiocytic cells with abundant amphophilic cytoplasm (Fig. 25.6). The lymph nodes have occasional residual hyperplastic follicles. The histiocytes in RDD demonstrate emperipolesis, with intact viable lymphocytes and plasma cells within cytoplasmic vacuoles passing through the histiocytes cytoplasm. RDD histiocytes are CD1a negative, but express CD68, CD14, CD15, lysozyme, transferrin receptor, interleukin-2 receptor, and CD163.[128] RDD is usually not a diagnostic problem, but can be separated from other histiocytic and dendritic disorders by immunocytochemical and flow cytometric phenotyping (Table 25.1).

Laboratory Features

Patients may have hemolytic anemia, anemia of chronic disease, elevated erythrocyte sedimentation rate, and immunoglobulins. Elevated liver enzymes and other laboratory abnormalities depend on the organs involved.[134]

Therapy

Many cases are self-limited and do not require therapy. Surgery may be useful for symptomatic treatment of large

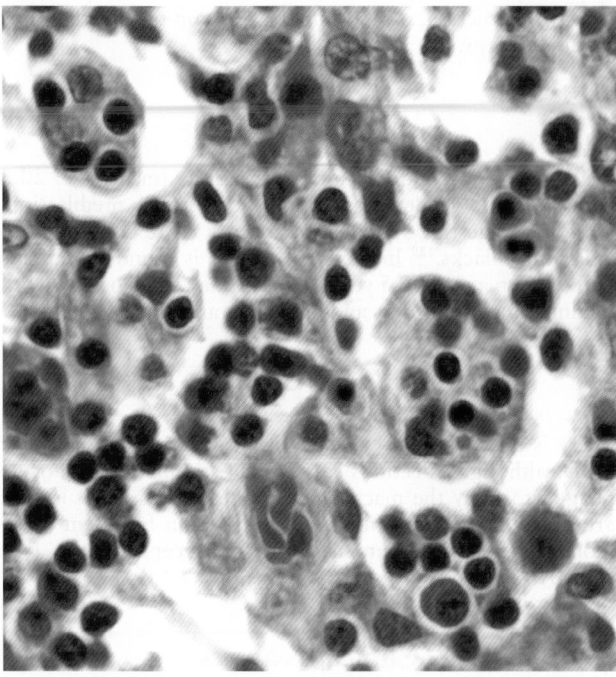

FIGURE 25.6 Rosai-Dorfman disease (sinus histiocytosis with massive lymphadenopathy): lymph node with sinusoids markedly distended by histocytes showing emperipolesis (lymphocytes in the cytoplasm) (H & E, original magnification 100×).

lymph nodes. However, multiorgan involvement or dysfunction, and association with immune dysfunction are poor prognostic indicators and indicate the necessity of treatment.[135] A variety of therapies have been used, including steroids and chemotherapy, with success in some cases. Several case reports have described improvement or cure of RDD patients with dexamethasone, methotrexate/mercaptopurine, 2-chlorodeoxyadenosine, and vinorelbine/methotrexate.[136–139]

Course and Prognosis

The literature suggests that most patients will have a slow but steady decrease in the size of their lymph nodes over months to years. For those patients requiring treatment because of impingement on vital organs, responses are variable. Because clinical trials have not been done, treatment recommendation is based upon anecdotal reports.

JUVENILE XANTHOGRANULOMA

Definition and History

JXG is histiocytic disorder that affects the skin with multiple nodules in the head, neck, and trunk primarily in children, although adults may also be affected. Other organ systems are rarely affected. The lesional cells are derived from the dermal dendrocyte.[140]

Epidemiology

Children with single lesions are affected at a median age of 2 years with a male/female ratio of 1.5:1. Those with multiple

lesions average 5 months of age and have a male/female ratio of 12:1. No epidemiologic study of JXG has been done, so the true incidence is unknown. A review of JXG from the Kiel Pediatric Tumor Registry recorded 129 (0.52%) cases of JXG and 800 (3.25%) cases of LCH among 24,600 cases over a 36-year period.[141]

Etiology and Pathogenesis

There is no known inciting etiology for JXG. Patients with JXG and neurofibromatosis (NF) Types 1 and 2 as well as a triad with juvenile chronic myelogenous leukemia (JCML) have been reported.[142–144] These and other cases have led to discussion of apparent increased risk of the leukemia in NF patients with JXG, but there is no rigorous proof for this concept.[145]

Clinical Features

The majority (80% to 90%) of patients are children less than two years of age who have solitary skin nodules on their head, neck, or trunk.[140,141] The lesion is most often the same color as the surrounding skin, but may be erythematous or yellow (xanthomatous). Rarely nodules may be in the subcutaneous fat, deep soft tissue, or in skeletal muscle. Organ involvement is very rare and has been reported in soft tissue, central nervous system, bone, lung, liver, spleen, pancreas, adrenal, intestines, kidneys, lymph nodes, marrow, and heart.[140,141,146] Systemic signs and symptoms occur only if these organ systems are involved.

Pathologic Features

JXG lesions are typically relatively well-demarcated nodules composed of a mixture of small oval to slightly spindled histiocytes with bland nuclei, and giant cells with the nuclei typically organized in a peripheral wreath-like pattern (Touton giant cells). Touton giant cells with variably foamy cytoplasm are characteristic for JXG. Early lesions tend to have vacuolated histiocytes with foamy cytoplasm (xanthoma cells) intermingled with a few lymphocytes and eosinophils. Mononuclear JXG with no foam cells or Touton giant cells may occur and not be recognized as this entity and mistaken on routine histopathologic examination for LCH or other histiocytic disorder. Mature JXG lesions tend to have a *granulomatous* morphology with foam cells, Touton giant cells, foreign-body giant cells, histiocytes, lymphocytes, and eosinophils. Regressing lesions may demonstrate fibroblasts and fibrosis replacing a portion of the histiocytic infiltrate, and have S100-negative fusiform macrophages. Typical LCs may be seen at the periphery of the lesion. Immunophenotyping is not usually necessary. However, when xanthoma (foam) cells and/or Touton giant cells are not present, immunocytochemical evaluation is helpful in providing an accurate diagnosis (Table 25.1). JXG histiocytes express Factor XIIIa, Fascin, CD14 and CD163, and lack expression CD207. The tumor cells also are positive for CD68 (Ki-M1P), vimentin, and often anti-CD4.[1,141,147]

Laboratory Features

If the marrow is involved, patients may have cytopenias and liver infiltration that may cause elevation of liver enzymes, hypoalbuminemia, and an elevated erythrocyte sedimentation rate. Pituitary involvement may lead to diabetes insipidus. Hypercalcemia has been reported.

Therapy

Patients with a single or only a few lesions need no therapy or only an excisional biopsy if desired for cosmetic reasons. For the rare patients who have systemic disease and require treatment, a wide variety of chemotherapy and radiotherapy regimens have been reported.[146,148] Inclusion of a vinca alkaloid and steroid is associated with better overall response rates. A child with CNS JXG who failed to respond to vinblastine was successfully treated with cladribine.[149]

Course and Prognosis

All patients with only skin or soft tissue involvement survive and the lesions spontaneously disappear over time in a majority of cases. Infants with large retroperitoneal masses, liver, bone marrow, or central nervous system involvement usually survive with chemotherapy treatment. Two of 17 patients with multisystem JXG reported in the literature died despite multiagent chemotherapy.[148]

MALIGNANT HISTIOCYTIC DISEASES

Definition and History

Scott and Robb-Smith first reported cases of a rapidly fatal disease with jaundice, lymphadenopathy, anemia, leukopenia, and hepatosplenomegaly that they termed *histiocytic medullary reticulosis*.[150] It was believed that the malignant cell was a histiocyte based upon morphologic criteria. There has been considerable debate about the identity of true malignancies of LC histiocytes. By excluding patients with anaplastic large cell lymphomas and other T- or B-lineage large cell lymphomas, the number with true histiocytic malignancies becomes very small. Favara et al. suggested that such diseases be considered sarcomas of histiocytic or macrophage-related lineage.[5] Cases of malignant histiocytes and accessory DCs have been subdivided by a panel of cell surface markers.[151] Table 25.1 illustrates the differential expression of various cell surface markers in malignant histiocytic diseases versus the nonmalignant types. Monocytic leukemias (FAB M4 and M5) represent the other group of true malignant disorders of the monocyte/macrophage cells and are discussed in Chapter 20.

Epidemiology

Although malignant dendritic/histiocytic cell tumors affect all age groups, the median age is at least 33 years.[151] Males are affected more often than females. One review of over 2,000 lymphoma cases found only eight patients with histiocytic sarcomas (4/1000).[152]

Clinical Features

Systemic symptoms of fever, headache, malaise, weight loss, dyspnea, and sweating occur in patients with diffuse disease.[151–153] Infiltration of the marrow is found in approximately one quarter of the patients.

Dendritic or Langerhans cell sarcoma patients may have systemic symptoms of fever, pain, or weight loss. They usually present with erythematous nodules or skin rash, but may also have involvement of bone, lymph nodes in any location, lung, liver, or brain.[154,155] A series of histiocytic/DC sarcomas in patients with follicular lymphomas showed a clonal evolution from B-cell lymphoma to myeloid-derived sarcomas.[156]

Interdigitating dendritic cell sarcomas (IDCS) may occur as extranodal tumors in children and primarily lymph node tumors in adults.[157] A series of four pediatric cases of IDCS with chest wall, vertebral, lymph node/bone marrow, and a pelvic mass were reported.[157] Extranodal presentations include intestinal or mediastinal tumors which can be very aggressive.[158,159]

Pathologic Features

Malignant histiocytosis lesions are composed of a diffuse proliferation of discohesive large cells that may occupy the sinusoidal spaces of the spleen, liver, and lymph nodes. The cells are typically large pleomorphic, oval to round cells with oval to irregularly grooved and indented nuclei. There is relatively abundant eosinophilic cytoplasm with some vacuolization. Hemophagocytosis may be seen on occasion. Focal areas of spindled tumor cells may be present. Immunocytochemical evaluation (Table 25.1) is helpful in eliminating anaplastic large cell lymphoma, B- and T-cell large cell lymphoma, carcinoma, melanoma, and other large cell tumors from consideration. Electron microscopy confirms the absence of Birbeck granules and intercellular junctions, and demonstrates frequent lysosomes within the abundant cytoplasm of the tumor cells.[1,158,160,161]

Laboratory Findings

Patients with diffuse disease may have pancytopenia, although leukocytosis occurs in some with an inflammatory response. Hemophagocytosis is occasionally seen in the bone marrow aspirate of biopsy. As with lymphomas, an elevated lactate dehydrogenase and erythrocyte sedimentation rate may be found.

Treatment, Course, and Prognosis

Therapy for DC/LC sarcomas has usually been unsuccessful.[156] However, case reports of long-term remissions with thalidomide[162] or MESNA, doxorubicin, ifosfamide, and dacarbazine have been published.[163] In some instances, surgical resection of a localized mass with radiotherapy has been adequate.

SUMMARY

Disorders of DCs and macrophages include as diverse a spectrum of diseases as their cells of origin. Patients with *high-risk* LCH, malignant histiocytosis, or HLH have a poor prognosis unless they have an early response to therapy. *Low-risk* LCH, JXG, and RDD have excellent prognoses, but may be chronic conditions. Clinical trials for LCH and HLH have markedly improved the outcome of patients with these disorders. Enrollment of all these patients on clinical trials or registries through the Histiocyte Society is the only way to improve knowledge of these rare diseases.

References

1. Jaffe R, Pileri SA, Facchetti F, et al. Histocytic and dendritic cell neoplasms. In: Swerdlow SH, Campo E, Harris NL et al. eds. WHO classification of tumours of haematopoietic and lymphoid tissues. Lyon, France: IARC Press, 2008;353–357.

2. Jaffe R. The diagnostic histopathology of Langerhans cell histiocytosis. In: Weitzman S, Egeler RM, eds. Histiocytic disorders of children and adults. Basic science clinical features, and therapy. Cambridge, UK: Cambridge University Press, 2005:14–39.

3. Chikwava K, Jaffe R. Langerin (CD207) staining in normal pediatric tissues, reactive lymph nodes, and childhood histiocytic disorders. Pediatr Dev Pathol 2004;7(6): 607–614.

4. Lau SK, Chu PG, Weiss LM. Immunohistochemical expression of Langerin in Langerhans cell histiocytosis and non-Langerhans cell histiocytic disorders. Am J Surg Pathol 2008;32(4):615–619.

4a. Allen CE, Leung HCE, Yu A, et al. Cell-specific gene expression in Langerhans cell histiocytosis lesions reveals a distinct profile compared to epidermal Langerhans cells. J Immunology 2010;184(8):4557–4567.

5. Favara BE, Feller AC, Pauli M, et al. Contemporary classification of histiocytic disorders. The WHO Committee On Histiocytic/Reticulum Cell Proliferations. Reclassification Working Group of the Histiocyte Society. Med Pediatr Oncol 1997;29(3):157–166.

6. Langerhans P. Ueber die nerven der menschlichen Haut. Virchows Arch 1868; A(44):325.

7. Nezelof C, Basset F, Rousseau MF. Histiocytosis X histogenetic arguments for a Langerhans cell origin. Biomedicine 1973;18(5):365–371.

8. Coppes-Zantinga A, Egeler RM. The Langerhans cell histiocytosis X files revealed. Br J Haematol 2002;116(1):3–9.

9. Arceci R. Langerhans cell histiocytosis in children and adults: pathogenesis, clinical manifestations, and treatment. Hematology Am Soc Hematol Educ Program 2002; 297–314.

10. Laman JD, Leenen PJ, Annels NE, et al. Langerhans-cell histiocytosis 'insight into DC biology'. Trends Immunol 2003;24(4):190–196.

11. Carstensen H, Ornvold K. The epidemiology of LCH in children in Denmark, 1975–89. Med Pediatr Oncol 1993;21387–21388.

12. Arico M, Nichols K, Whitlock JA, et al. Familial clustering of Langerhans cell histiocytosis. Br J Haematol 1999;107(4):883–888.

13. Nicholson HS, Egeler RM, Nesbit ME. The epidemiology of Langerhans cell histiocytosis. Hematol Oncol Clin North Am 1998;12(2):379–384.

14. Bhatia S, Nesbit ME Jr, Egeler RM, et al. Epidemiologic study of Langerhans cell histiocytosis in children. J Pediatr 1997;130(5):774–784.

15. Willman CL, Busque L, Griffith BB, et al. Langerhans'-cell histiocytosis (histiocytosis X)—a clonal proliferative disease. N Engl J Med 1994;331(3):154–160.

16. Yu RC, Chu C, Buluwela L, et al. Clonal proliferation of Langerhans cells in Langerhans cell histiocytosis. Lancet 1994;343(8900):767–768.

17. Yousem SA, Colby TV, Chen YY, et al. Pulmonary Langerhans' cell histiocytosis: molecular analysis of clonality. Am J Surg Pathol 2001;25(5):630–636.

18. Da Costa CE, Szuhai K, van ER, et al. No genomic aberrations in Langerhans cell histiocytosis as assessed by diverse molecular technologies. Genes Chromosomes Cancer 2009;48(3):239–249.

19. Rolland A, Guyon L, Gill M, et al. Increased blood myeloid dendritic cells and dendritic cell-poietins in Langerhans cell histiocytosis. J Immunol 2005;174(5):3067–3071.

20. Senechal B, Elain G, Jeziorski E, et al. Expansion of regulatory T cells in patients with Langerhans cell histiocytosis. PLoS Med 2007;4(8):e253.

21. Yu RC, Morris JF, Pritchard J, et al. Defective alloantigen-presenting capacity of 'Langerhans cell histiocytosis cells'. Arch Dis Child 1992;67(11):1370–1372.

22. Geissmann F, Lepelletier Y, Fraitag S, et al. Differentiation of Langerhans cells in Langerhans cell histiocytosis. Blood 2001;97(5):1241–1248.

23. McClain K, Jin H, Gresik V, et al. Langerhans cell histiocytosis: lack of a viral etiology. Am J Hematol 1994;47(1):16–20.

24. Jeziorski E, Senechal B, Molina TJ, et al. Herpes-virus infection in patients with Langerhans cell histiocytosis: a case-controlled sero-epidemiological study, and in situ analysis. PLoS One 2008;3(9):e3262.

25. Ishii R, Morimoto A, Ikushima S, et al. High serum values of soluble CD154, IL-2 receptor, RANKL and osteoprotegerin in Langerhans cell histiocytosis. Pediatr Blood Cancer 2006;47(2):194–199.

26. Rosso DA, Karis J, Braier JL, et al. Elevated serum levels of the decoy receptor osteoprotegerin in children with langerhans cell histiocytosis. Pediatr Res 2006;59(2): 281–286.

27. Hicks J, Flaitz CM. Langerhans cell histiocytosis: current insights in a molecular age with emphasis on clinical oral and maxillofacial pathology practice. Oral Surg Oral Med Oral Pathol Oral Radiol Endod 2005;100(2 suppl):S42–S66.

28. Munn S, Chu AC. Langerhans cell histiocytosis of the skin. Hematol Oncol Clin North Am 1998;12(2):269–286.

29. Stein SL, Paller AS, Haut PR, et al. Langerhans cell histiocytosis presenting in the neonatal period: a retrospective case series. Arch Pediatr Adolesc Med 2001;155(7): 778–783.

30. Lau L, Krafchik B, Trebo MM, et al. Cutaneous Langerhans cell histiocytosis in children under one year. Pediatr Blood Cancer 2006;46(1):66–71.

31. Minkov M, Prosch H, Steiner M, et al. Langerhans cell histiocytosis in neonates. Pediatr Blood Cancer 2005;45(6):802–807.

32. Mortellaro C, Pucci A, Palmeri A, et al. Oral manifestations of langerhans cell histiocytosis in a pediatric population: a clinical and histological study of 8 patients. J Craniofac Surg 2006;17(3):552–556.

33. Slater JM, Swarm OJ. Eosinophilic granuloma of bone. Med Pediatr Oncol 1980; 8(2):151–164.

34. Wong A, Ortiz-Neira CL, Reslan WA, et al. Liver involvement in Langerhans cell histiocytosis. Pediatr Radiol 2006;36(10):1105–1107.

35. Braier J, Ciocca M, Latella A, et al. Cholestasis, sclerosing cholangitis, and liver transplantation in Langerhans cell Histiocytosis. Med Pediatr Oncol 2002;38(3):178–182.

36. Vassallo R, Ryu JH, Colby TV, et al. Pulmonary Langerhans'-cell histiocytosis. N Engl J Med 2000;342(26):1969–1978.

37. Braier J, Latella A, Balancini B, et al. Outcome in children with pulmonary Langerhans cell Histiocytosis. Pediatr Blood Cancer 2004;43(7):765–769.

38. Bernstrand C, Cederlund K, Henter JI. Pulmonary function testing and pulmonary Langerhans cell histiocytosis. Pediatr Blood Cancer 2007;49(3):323–328.

39. McClain K, Ramsay NK, Robison L, et al. Bone marrow involvement in histiocytosis X. Med Pediatr Oncol 1983;11(3):167–171.

40. Minkov M, Potschger U, Grois N, et al. Bone marrow assessment in Langerhans cell histiocytosis. Pediatr Blood Cancer 2007;49(5):694–698.

41. Favara BE, Jaffe R, Egeler RM. Macrophage activation and hemophagocytic syndrome in langerhans cell histiocytosis: report of 30 cases. Pediatr Dev Pathol 2002;5(2): 130–140.

42. Prosch H, Grois N, Prayer D, et al. Central diabetes insipidus as presenting symptom of Langerhans cell histiocytosis. Pediatr Blood Cancer 2004;43(5):594–599.

43. Donadieu J, Rolon MA, Thomas C, et al. Endocrine involvement in pediatric-onset Langerhans' cell histiocytosis: a population-based study. J Pediatr 2004;144(3): 344–350.

44. Grois N, Potschger U, Prosch H, et al. Risk factors for diabetes insipidus in langerhans cell histiocytosis. Pediatr Blood Cancer 2006;46(2):228–233.

45. Hait E, Liang M, Degar B, et al. Gastrointestinal tract involvement in Langerhans cell histiocytosis: case report and literature review. Pediatrics 2006;118(5):e1593–e1599.

46. Geissmann F, Thomas C, Emile JF, et al. Digestive tract involvement in Langerhans cell histiocytosis. The French Langerhans Cell Histiocytosis Study Group. J Pediatr 1996; 129(6):836–845.

47. Dunger DB, Broadbent V, Yeoman E, et al. The frequency and natural history of diabetes insipidus in children with Langerhans-cell histiocytosis. N Engl J Med 1989; 321(17):1157–1162.

48. Donadieu J, Rolon MA, Pion I, et al. Incidence of growth hormone deficiency in pediatric-onset Langerhans cell histiocytosis: efficacy and safety of growth hormone treatment. J Clin Endocrinol Metab 2004;89(2):604–609.

49. Grois NG, Favara BE, Mostbeck GH, et al. Central nervous system disease in Langerhans cell histiocytosis. Hematol Oncol Clin North Am 1998;12(2):287–305.

50. Grois N, Prayer D, Prosch H, et al. Neuropathology of CNS disease in Langerhans cell histiocytosis. Brain 2005;128(Pt 4):829–838.

51. Prayer D, Grois N, Prosch H, et al. MR imaging presentation of intracranial disease associated with Langerhans cell histiocytosis. AJNR Am J Neuroradiol 2004;25(5): 880–891.

52. Wnorowski M, Prosch H, Prayer D, et al. Pattern and course of neurodegeneration in Langerhans cell histiocytosis. J Pediatr 2008;153(1):127–132.

53. Calming U, Henter JI. Elevated erythrocyte sedimentation rate and thrombocytosis as possible indicators of active disease in Langerhans' cell histiocytosis. Acta Paediatr 1998;87(10):1085–1087.

54. Phillips M, Allen C, Gerson P, et al. Comparison of FDG-PET scans to conventional radiography and bone scans in management of Langerhans cell histiocytosis. Pediatr Blood Cancer 2009;52(1):97–101.

55. Steen AE, Steen KH, Bauer R, et al. Successful treatment of cutaneous Langerhans cell histiocytosis with low-dose methotrexate. Br J Dermatol 2001;145(1):137–140.

56. McClain K, Li L, Kozinetz C. A phase II trial using thalidomide for Langerhans cell histiocytosis. Pediatr Blood Cancer 2007;48:44–49.

57. Hoeger PH, Nanduri VR, Harper JI, et al. Long term follow up of topical mustine treatment for cutaneous langerhans cell histiocytosis. Arch Dis Child 2000;82(6):483–487.

58. Kwon OS, Cho KH, Song KY. Primary cutaneous Langerhans cell histiocytosis treated with photochemotherapy. J Dermatol 1997;24(1):54–56.

59. Nauert C, Zornoza J, Ayala A, et al. Eosinophilic granuloma of bone: diagnosis and management. Skeletal Radiol 1983;10(4):227–235.

60. Titgemeyer C, Grois N, Minkov M, et al. Pattern and course of single-system disease in Langerhans cell histiocytosis data from the DAL-HX 83- and 90-study. Med Pediatr Oncol 2001;37(2):108–114.

61. McCullough C. Eosinophilic granuloma of bone. Acta Orthop Scand 1980;(51):389–398.

62. Raney RB Jr, D'Angio GJ. Langerhans' cell histiocytosis (histiocytosis X): experience at the Children's Hospital of Philadelphia, 1970–1984. Med Pediatr Oncol 1989;17(1): 20–28.

63. Gadner H, Grois N, Arico M, et al. A randomized trial of treatment for multisystem Langerhans' cell histiocytosis. J Pediatr 2001;138(5):728–734.

64. Gadner H, Heitger A, Grois N, et al. Treatment strategy for disseminated Langerhans cell histiocytosis. DAL HX-83 Study Group. Med Pediatr Oncol 1994;23(2):72–80.

65. Gadner H, Grois N, Potschger U, et al. Improved outcome in multisystem Langerhans cell histiocytosis is associated with therapy intensification. Blood 2008;111(5):2556–2562.

66. Morimoto A, Ikushima S, Kinugawa N, et al. Improved outcome in the treatment of pediatric multifocal Langerhans cell histiocytosis: Results from the Japan Langerhans Cell Histiocytosis Study Group-96 protocol study. Cancer 2006;107(3):613–619.

67. Nesbit ME, Kieffer S, D'Angio GJ. Reconstitution of vertebral height in histiocytosis X: a long-term follow-up. J Bone Joint Surg Am 1969;51(7):1360–1368.

68. Womer RB, Raney RB Jr, D'Angio GJ. Healing rates of treated and untreated bone lesions in histiocytosis X. Pediatrics 1985;76(2):286–288.

69. Mammano S, Candiotto S, Balsano M. Cast and brace treatment of eosinophilic granuloma of the spine: long-term follow-up. J Pediatr Orthop 1997;17(6):821–827.

70. Buchler T, Cervinek L, Belohlavek O, et al. Langerhans cell histiocytosis with central nervous system involvement: follow-up by FDG-PET during treatment with cladribine. Pediatr Blood Cancer 2005;44(3):286–288.

71. Watts J, Files B. Langerhans cell histiocytosis: central nervous system involvement treated successfully with 2-chlorodeoxyadenosine. Pediatr Hematol Oncol 2001; 18(3):199–204.

72. Dhall G, Finlay JL, Dunkel IJ, et al. Analysis of outcome for patients with mass lesions of the central nervous system due to Langerhans cell histiocytosis treated with 2-chlorodeoxyadenosine. Pediatr Blood Cancer 2008;50:72–79.

73. Imashuku S, Ishida S, Koike K, et al. Cerebellar ataxia in pediatric patients with Langerhans cell histiocytosis. J Pediatr Hematol Oncol 2004;26(11):735–739.

74. Idbaih A, Donadieu J, Barthez MA, et al. Retinoic acid therapy in "degenerative-like" neuro-langerhans cell histiocytosis: a prospective pilot study. Pediatr Blood Cancer 2004;43(1):55–58.

75. Allen CE, Flores R, RauchR, et al. Neurodegenerative central nervous system Langerhans cell histiocytosis and coincident hydrocephalus: treated with vincristine/cytosine arabinoside. Pediatr Blood Cancer 2010;54:416–423.

76. Stine KC, Saylors RL, Saccente S, et al. Efficacy of continuous infusion 2-CDA (cladribine) in pediatric patients with Langerhans cell histiocytosis. Pediatr Blood Cancer 2004;43(1):81–84.

77. Egeler RM, de KJ, Voute PA. Cytosine-arabinoside, vincristine, and prednisolone in the treatment of children with disseminated Langerhans cell histiocytosis with organ dysfunction: experience at a single institution. Med Pediatr Oncol 1993;21(4):265–270.
78. Weitzman S, Braier J, Donadieu J, et al. 2′-chlorodeoxyadenosine (2-CdA) as salvage therapy for Langerhans cell histiocytosis (LCH). Results of the LCH-S-98 protocol of the histiocyte society. Pediatr Blood Cancer 2009;53:1271–1276.
79. Bernard F, Thomas C, Bertrand Y, et al. Multi-centre pilot study of 2-chlorodeoxyadenosine and cytosine arabinoside combined chemotherapy in refractory Langerhans cell histiocytosis with haematological dysfunction. Eur. J Cancer 2005; 41(17):2682–2689.
80. Akkari V, Donadieu J, Piguet C, et al. Hematopoietic stem cell transplantation in patients with severe Langerhans cell histiocytosis and hematological dysfunction: experience of the French Langerhans Cell Study Group. Bone Marrow Transplant 2003; 31(12):1097–1103.
81. Nagarajan R, Neglia J, Ramsay N, et al. Successful treatment of refractory Langerhans cell histiocytosis with unrelated cord blood transplantation. J Pediatr Hematol Oncol 2001;23(9):629–632.
82. Cooper N, Rao K, Goulden N, et al. The use of reduced-intensity stem cell transplantation in haemophagocytic lymphohistiocytosis and Langerhans cell histiocytosis. Bone Marrow Transplant. 2008;42(Suppl 2)S47–S50.
83. Minkov M, Steiner M, Potschger U, et al. Reactivations in multisystem Langerhans cell histiocytosis: data of the international LCH registry. J Pediatr 2008;153(5):700–705, 705.e1–e2.
84. Allen CE, McClain KL. Langerhans cell histiocytosis: a review of past, current and future therapies. Drugs Today (Barc.) 2007;43(9):627–643.
85. Haupt R, Nanduri V, Calevo MG, et al. Permanent consequences in Langerhans cell histiocytosis patients: a pilot study from the Histiocyte Society-Late Effects Study Group. Pediatr Blood Cancer 2004;42(5):438–444.
86. Willis B, Ablin A, Weinberg V, et al. Disease course and late sequelae of Langerhans' cell histiocytosis: 25-year experience at the University of California, San Francisco. J Clin Oncol 1996;14(7):2073–2082.
87. Komp DM. Long-term sequelae of histiocytosis X. Am J Pediatr Hematol Oncol 1981;3(2):163–168.
88. Nanduri VR, Lillywhite L, Chapman C, et al. Cognitive outcome of long-term survivors of multisystem langerhans cell histiocytosis: a single-institution, cross-sectional study. J Clin Oncol 2003;21(15):2961–2967.
89. Mittheisz E, Seidl R, Prayer D, et al. Central nervous system-related permanent consequences in patients with Langerhans cell histiocytosis. Pediatr Blood Cancer 2007;48(1):50–56.
90. Egeler RM, Neglia JP, Puccetti DM, et al. Association of Langerhans cell histiocytosis with malignant neoplasms. Cancer 1993;71(3):865–873.
91. Feldman AL, Berthold F, Arceci RJ, et al. Clonal relationship between precursor T-lymphoblastic leukaemia/lymphoma and Langerhans-cell histiocytosis. Lancet Oncol 2005;6(6):435–437.
92. Rodig SJ, Payne EG, Degar BA, et al. Aggressive Langerhans cell histiocytosis following T-ALL: Clonally related neoplasms with persistent expression of constitutively active NOTCH1. Am J Hematol 2007;83(2):116–121.
93. Farquhar JW, Claireaux AE. Familial haemophagocytic reticulosis. Arch Dis Child 1952;27(136):519–525.
94. Henter JI, Elinder G, Soder O, et al. Incidence in Sweden and clinical features of familial hemophagocytic lymphohistiocytosis. Acta Paediatr Scand 1991;80(4):428–435.
95. Allen CE, Yu X, Kozinetz CA, et al. Highly elevated ferritin levels and the diagnosis of hemophagocytic lymphohistiocytosis. Pediatr Blood Cancer 2008;50(6):1227–1235.
96. Henter JI, Elinder G, Soder O, et al. Hypercytokinemia in familial hemophagocytic lymphohistiocytosis. Blood 1991;78(11):2918–2922.
97. Imashuku S, Hibi S, Sako M, et al. Heterogeneity of immune markers in hemophagocytic lymphohistiocytosis: comparative study of 9 familial and 14 familial inheritance-unproved cases. J Pediatr Hematol Oncol 1998;20(3):207–214.
98. Stepp SE, Dufourcq-Lagelouse R, Le DF, et al. Perforin gene defects in familial hemophagocytic lymphohistiocytosis. Science 1999;286(5446):1957–1959.
99. Stepp SE, Mathew PA, Bennett M, et al. Perforin: more than just an effector molecule. Immunol Today 2000;21(6):254–256.
100. Jordan MB, Hildeman D, Kappler J, et al. An animal model of hemophagocytic lymphohistiocytosis (HLH): CD8+ T cells and interferon gamma are essential for the disorder. Blood 2004;104(3):735–743.
101. Filipovich AH. Hemophagocytic lymphohistiocytosis and related disorders. Curr Opin Allergy Clin Immunol 2006;6(6):410–415.
102. Arico M, Imashuku S, Clementi R, et al. Hemophagocytic lymphohistiocytosis due to germline mutations in SH2D1A, the X-linked lymphoproliferative disease gene. Blood 2001;97(4):1131–1133.
103. Palazzi DL, McClain KL, Kaplan SL. Hemophagocytic syndrome in children: an important diagnostic consideration in fever of unknown origin. Clin Infect Dis 2003; 36(3):306–312.
104. Janka GE. Familial hemophagocytic lymphohistiocytosis. Eur J Pediatr 1983;140(3): 221–230.
105. Haddad E, Sulis ML, Jabado N, et al. Frequency and severity of central nervous system lesions in hemophagocytic lymphohistiocytosis. Blood 1997;89(3):794–800.
106. Henter JI, Horne A, Arico M, et al. HLH-2004: Diagnostic and therapeutic guidelines for hemophagocytic lymphohistiocytosis. Pediatr.Blood Cancer 2007;48(2):124–131.
107. Molleran Lee S, Villanueva J, Sumegi J, et al. Characterisation of diverse PRF1 mutations leading to decreased natural killer cell activity in North American families with haemophagocytic lymphohistiocytosis. J Med Genet 2004;(41):137–144.
108. Ueda I, Ishii E, Morimoto A, et al. Correlation between phenotypic heterogeneity and gene mutational characteristics in familial hemophagocytic lymphohistiocytosis (FHL). Pediatr Blood Cancer 2006;46(4):482–488.
109. Bryceson YT, Rudd E, Zheng C, et al. Defective cytotoxic lymphocyte degranulation in syntaxin-11 deficient familial hemophagocytic lymphohistiocytosis 4 (FHL4) patients. Blood 2007;110(6):1906–1915.
110. Gupta A, Weitzman S, Abdelhaleem M. The role of hemophagocytosis in bone marrow aspirates in the diagnosis of hemophagocytic lymphohistiocytosis. Pediatr.Blood Cancer 2008;50(2):192–194.
111. Nagano M, Kimura N, Ishii E, et al. Clonal expansion of alphabeta-T lymphocytes with inverted Jbeta1 bias in familial hemophagocytic lymphohistiocytosis. Blood 1999; 94(7):2374–2382.
112. Kogawa K, Lee SM, Villanueva J, et al. Perforin expression in cytotoxic lymphocytes from patients with hemophagocytic lymphohistiocytosis and their family members. Blood 2002;99(1):61–66.
113. Ambruso DR, Hays T, Zwartjes WJ, et al. Successful treatment of lymphohistiocytic reticulosis with phagocytosis with epipodophyllotoxin VP 16–213. Cancer 1980; 45(10):2516–2520.
114. Henter JI, Elinder G, Finkel Y, et al. Successful induction with chemotherapy including teniposide in familial erythrophagocytic lymphohistiocytosis. Lancet 1986;2(8520): 1402.
115. Henter JI, Samuelsson-Horne A, Arico M, et al. Treatment of hemophagocytic lymphohistiocytosis with HLH-94 immunochemotherapy and bone marrow transplantation. Blood 2002;100(7):2367–2373.
116. Thompson PA, Allen CE, Horton T, et al. Severe neurologic side effects in patients being treated for hemophagocytic lymphohistiocytosis. Pediatr Blood Cancer 2009;52:621–625.
117. Mahlaoui N, Ouachee-Chardin M, de Saint BG, et al. Immunotherapy of familial hemophagocytic lymphohistiocytosis with antithymocyte globulins: a single-center retrospective report of 38 patients. Pediatrics 2007;120(3):e622–e628.
118. Baker KS, Filipovich AH, Gross TG, et al. Unrelated donor hematopoietic cell transplantation for hemophagocytic lymphohistiocytosis. Bone Marrow Transplant 2008; 42(3):175–180.
119. Baker KS, DeLaat CA, Steinbuch M, et al. Successful correction of hemophagocytic lymphohistiocytosis with related or unrelated bone marrow transplantation. Blood 1997;89(10):3857–3863.
120. Cooper N, Rao K, Gilmour K, et al. Stem cell transplantation with reduced-intensity conditioning for hemophagocytic lymphohistiocytosis. Blood 2006;107(3):1233–1236.
121. Grom AA, Villanueva J, Lee S, et al. Natural killer cell dysfunction in patients with systemic-onset juvenile rheumatoid arthritis and macrophage activation syndrome. J Pediatr 2003;142(3):292–296.
122. Mouy R, Stephan JL, Pillet P, et al. Efficacy of cyclosporine A in the treatment of macrophage activation syndrome in juvenile arthritis: report of five cases. J Pediatr 1996;129(5):750–754.
123. Balamuth NJ, Nichols KE, Paessler M, et al. Use of rituximab in conjunction with immunosuppressive chemotherapy as a novel therapy for Epstein Barr virus-associated hemophagocytic lymphohistiocytosis. J Pediatr Hematol Oncol 2007;29(8):569–573.
124. Mischler M, Fleming GM, Shanley TP, et al. Epstein-Barr virus-induced hemophagocytic lymphohistiocytosis and X-linked lymphoproliferative disease: a mimicker of sepsis in the pediatric intensive care unit. Pediatrics 2007;119(5):e1212–e1218.
125. Henzan T, Nagafuji K, Tsukamoto H, et al. Success with infliximab in treating refractory hemophagocytic lymphohistiocytosis. Am J Hematol 2006;81(1):59–61.
126. Makay B, Yilmaz S, Turkyilmaz Z, et al. Etanercept for therapy-resistant macrophage activation syndrome. Pediatr Blood Cancer 2008;50(2):419–421.
127. Rosai J, Dorfman RF. Sinus histiocytosis with massive lymphadenopathy. A newly recognized benign clinicopathological entity. Arch Pathol 1969;87(1):63–70.
128. Natkunam Y. Sinus histiocytosis with massive lymphadenopathy (Rosai-Dorfman disease): an update. Hematology 2004;287–291.
129. Lauwers GY, Perez-Atayde A, Dorfman RF, et al. The digestive system manifestations of Rosai-Dorfman disease (sinus histiocytosis with massive lymphadenopathy): review of 11 cases. Hum Pathol 2000;31(3):380–385.
130. Deodhare SS, Ang LC, Bilbao JM. Isolated intracranial involvement in Rosai-Dorfman disease: a report of two cases and review of the literature. Arch Pathol Lab Med 1998;122(2):161–165.
131. Grabczynska SA, Toh CT, Francis N, et al. Rosai-Dorfman disease complicated by autoimmune haemolytic anaemia: case report and review of a multisystem disease with cutaneous infiltrates. Br J Dermatol 2001;145(2):323–326.
132. Paulli M, Bergamaschi G, Tonon L, et al. Evidence for a polyclonal nature of the cell infiltrate in sinus histiocytosis with massive lymphadenopathy (Rosai-Dorfman disease). Br J Haematol 1995;91(2):415–418.
133. Foucar E, Rosai J, Dorfman R. Sinus histiocytosis with massive lymphadenopathy (Rosai-Dorfman disease): review of the entity. Semin Diagn Pathol 1990;7(1):19–73.
134. Chow CP, Ho HK, Chan GC, et al. Congenital Rosai-Dorfman disease presenting with anemia, thrombocytopenia, and hepatomegaly. Pediatr Blood Cancer 2009;52(3):415–417.
135. Pulsoni A, Anghel G, Falcucci P, et al. Treatment of sinus histiocytosis with massive lymphadenopathy (Rosai-Dorfman disease): report of a case and literature review. Am J Hematol 2002;69(1):67–71.
136. Horneff G, Jurgens H, Hort W, et al. Sinus histiocytosis with massive lymphadenopathy (Rosai-Dorfman disease): response to methotrexate and mercaptopurine. Med.Pediatr Oncol 1996;27(3):187–192.
137. Stine KC, Westfall C. Sinus histiocytosis with massive lymphadenopathy (SHML) prednisone resistant but dexamethasone sensitive. Pediatr Blood Cancer 2005;44(1):92–94.
138. Rodriguez-Galindo C, Helton KJ, Sanchez ND, et al. Extranodal Rosai-Dorfman disease in children. J Pediatr Hematol Oncol 2004;26(1):19–24.
139. Perry R, Penk J, Kapoor N, et al. Venorelbine and methotrexate for the treatment of Rosai-Dorfman Disease in children. Pediatr Blood Cancer 2005;(45):84–85.
140. Dehner LP. Juvenile xanthogranulomas in the first two decades of life: a clinicopathologic study of 174 cases with cutaneous and extracutaneous manifestations. Am J Surg Pathol 2003;27(5):579–593.
141. Janssen D, Harms D. Juvenile xanthogranuloma in childhood and adolescence: a clinicopathologic study of 129 patients from the kiel pediatric tumor registry. Am J Surg Pathol 2005;29(1):21–28.
142. Tan HH, Tay YK. Juvenile xanthogranuloma and neurofibromatosis 1. Dermatology 1998;197(1):43–44.
143. Iyengar V, Golumb CA, Schachner L. Neurilemmomatosis, NF2, and juvenile xanthogranuloma. J Am Acad Dermatol 1998;39(5 pt 2):831–834.
144. van Leeuwen RL, Berretty PJ, Knots E, et al. Triad of juvenile xanthogranuloma, von Recklinghausen's neurofibromatosis and trisomy 21 in a young girl. Clin Exp Dermatol 1996;21(3):248–249.
145. Gutmann DH, Gurney JG, Shannon KM. Juvenile xanthogranuloma, neurofibromatosis 1, and juvenile chronic myeloid leukemia. Arch Dermatol 1996;132(11):1390–1391.
146. Freyer DR, Kennedy R, Bostrom BC, et al. Juvenile xanthogranuloma: forms of systemic disease and their clinical implications. J Pediatr 1996;129(2):227–237.
147. Flaitz C, Allen C, Neville B, et al. Juvenile xanthogranuloma of the oral cavity in children: a clinicopathologic study. Oral Surg.Oral Med Oral Pathol Oral Radiol Endod 2002;94(3):345–352.
148. Stover DG, Alapati S, Regueira O, et al. Treatment of juvenile xanthogranuloma. Pediatr Blood Cancer 2008;51(1):130–133.
149. Rajendra B, Duncan A, Parslew R, et al. Successful treatment of central nervous system juvenile xanthogranulomatosis with cladribine. Pediatr Blood Cancer 2009;52(3): 413–415.

150. Scott R, Robb-Smith AHT. Histiocytic Medullary Reticulosis. Lancet 1939;(2):194–198.
151. Pileri SA, Grogan TM, Harris NL, et al. Tumours of histiocytes and accessory dendritic cells: an immunohistochemical approach to classification from the International Lymphoma Study Group based on 61 cases. Histopathology 2002;41(1):1–29.
152. Lauritzen AF, Delsol G, Hansen NE, et al. Histiocytic sarcomas and monoblastic leukemias. A clinical, histologic, and immunophenotypical study. Am J Clin Pathol 1994;102(1):45–54.
153. Kamel OW, Gocke CD, Kell DL, et al. True histiocytic lymphoma: a study of 12 cases based on current definition. Leuk Lymphoma 1995;18(1–2):81–86.
154. Newman B, Hu W, Nigro K, et al. Aggressive histiocytic disorders that can involve the skin. J Am Acad Dermatol 2007;56(2):302–316.
155. Julg BD, Weidner S, Mayr D. Pulmonary manifestation of a Langerhans cell sarcoma: case report and review of the literature. Virchows Arch 2006;448(3):369–374.
156. Feldman AL, Arber DA, Pittaluga S, et al. Clonally related follicular lymphomas and histiocytic/dendritic cell sarcomas: evidence for transdifferentiation of the follicular lymphoma clone. Blood 2008;111(12):5433–5439.
157. Pillay K, Solomon R, Daubenton JD, et al. Interdigitating dendritic cell sarcoma: a report of four paediatric cases and review of the literature. Histopathology 2004;44(3):283–291.
158. Kairouz S, Hashash J, Kabbara W, et al. Dendritic cell neoplasms: an overview. Am J Hematol 2007;82(10):924–928.
159. Porter DW, Gupte GL, Brown RM, et al. Histiocytic sarcoma with interdigitating dendritic cell differentiation. J Pediatr Hematol Oncol 2004;26(12):827–830.
160. Skoog L, Tani E. Histiocytic and dendritic neoplasms. Monogr Clin Cytol 2009;18:1856–1859.
161. Soriano AO, Thompson MA, Admirand JH, et al. Follicular dendritic cell sarcoma: a report of 14 cases and a review of the literature. Am J Hematol 2007;82(8):725–728.
162. Abidi MH, Tove I, Ibrahim RB, et al. Thalidomide for the treatment of histiocytic sarcoma after hematopoietic stem cell transplant. Am J Hematol 2007;82(10):932–933.
163. Uchida K, Kobayashi S, Inukai T, et al. Langerhans cell sarcoma emanating from the upper arm skin: successful treatment by MAID regimen. J Orthop Sci 2008;13(1):89–93.

CHAPTER 26A ■ GLIOMAS, EPENDYMOMAS, AND OTHER NONEMBRYONAL TUMORS OF THE CENTRAL NERVOUS SYSTEM

SUSAN M. BLANEY, DAPHNE HAAS-KOGAN, TINA YOUNG POUSSAINT, MARIARITA SANTI, RICHARD GILBERTSON, DONALD "WILL" PARSONS, AND IAN POLLACK

Tumors of the central nervous system (CNS) constitute the second most common pediatric cancer diagnosed in the United States each year, comprising approximately 25% of childhood cancers.[1] Depending on the upper age chosen, the number of children, adolescents, and young adults who received diagnoses of a CNS tumor in 2007 was predicted to range between 2,820 (for ages 0 to 14 years) and 3,750 (for ages 0 to 20 years).[2] The approximate incidence of the common pediatric and CNS tumors is shown in Figure 26A.1.[3]

Unfortunately, the morbidity associated with CNS tumors and their therapy may be significant in terms of physical deficits as well as neuropsychological and neuroendocrine sequelae. Although not quantifiable, the long-term morbidity of childhood CNS tumors likely exceeds that associated with other pediatric malignancies. Deaths caused by CNS tumors are among the highest for pediatric cancers. Nevertheless, there has been a 17% survival rate increase for children with CNS tumors between 1975–1979 and 1996–2003 such that the overall survival is now approximately 74%.[4] Despite these modest increases in survival, the optimal treatment of childhood CNS tumors continues to pose a tremendous challenge that requires a multidisciplinary approach involving many pediatric specialists and subspecialists including neurosurgeons, neuropathologists, neuro-oncologists, neuroradiologists, radiation oncologists, neurologists, ophthalmologists, and physiatrists. In addition, the contributions of molecular biologists, pharmacologists, nurses, neuropsychologists, social workers, audiologists, nutritional experts, child-life specialists, and physical, occupational, and speech therapists are invaluable.

In the next two chapters, we review the current understanding of the biology of brain tumors and the principles associated with each of the diagnostic and treatment modalities. We then provide an overview of the clinical management and associated long-term sequelae of the more frequently encountered CNS tumors. This chapter includes information about gliomas, ependymomas, and other nonembryonal CNS tumors of childhood and Chapter 26B includes information about embryonal (e.g., medulloblastoma, supratentorial primitive neuroectodermal tumor [sPNET], atypical teratoid rhabdoid tumor) and pineal region tumors.

EPIDEMIOLOGY

In the early 1990s, there appeared to be an increase in the incidence of CNS tumors from 2.7 cases per 100,000 children during the years 1977–1981 to 3.3 cases per 100,000 children from 1990–1994.[5] This higher incidence was primarily attributed to the greater utilization of magnetic resonance imaging (MRI) for evaluating children with neurologic conditions, although this has not been definitively proven.[6] Another contributing factor to the apparent increased incidence of pediatric brain tumors was the increasingly widespread use of stereotactic biopsies to document tumor histologies at nonbrainstem sites in tumors that previously would not have been subject to biopsy. In addition, during this time, the World Health Organization (WHO) classification of malignant gliomas changed, resulting in a shift of some diagnoses from benign to malignant. These combined factors affected the detection and reporting of brain tumors.[6] Ongoing observation is required to determine whether there was truly a rise in the incidence of childhood CNS tumors or whether the changes in the detection and reporting of brain tumors resulted in the observed increase.

The incidence of brain tumors peaks in the first decade of life, then decreases until a second peak in older adulthood. The first peak is characterized by a predominance of males and by equal incidence rates for whites and blacks, except for the first 2 to 3 years of life, when a greater percentage of whites than nonwhites are affected.[7] The male predominance is primarily explained by a disproportionate incidence of both medulloblastoma and ependymoma in males. For other tumor types, the genders are equally affected. During the first 2 years of life, supratentorial tumors predominate, whereas infratentorial lesions are more common through the rest of the first decade. Supratentorial tumors again predominate during late adolescence and through adulthood. Tumors of embryonal histology such as medulloblastoma, sPNETs, and pineoblastomas occur almost exclusively in children and young adults and primarily occur during the first decade. High-grade gliomas, including glioblastoma multiforme, are much less common in children than in adults.

Only two factors are consistently known to place a child at increased risk for a CNS malignancy: various genetic disorders and exposure to ionizing radiation.

ASSOCIATIONS WITH INHERITED SYNDROMES

Fewer than 10% of children with brain tumors have a genetic disorder that places them at increased risk for developing a brain tumor. Although rare, these syndromes (Table 26A.1) place affected children at a markedly higher risk for developing other tumors as well. All of the currently known syndromes associated with a predisposition for developing brain tumors have an autosomal dominant pattern of inheritance, and somatic mutations have been demonstrated in specific genes for each (Table 26A.1).

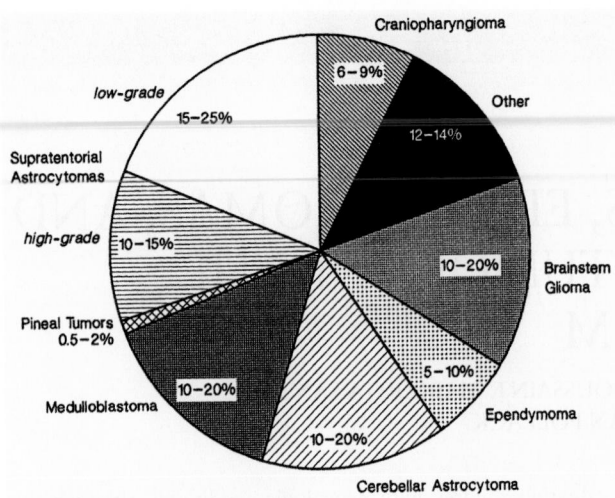

FIGURE 26A.1 Approximate incidence of common central nervous system tumors in children.

Children with Turcot syndrome have an autosomal dominant disorder in which a patient with a primary brain tumor also develops colorectal adenomas and/or colorectal adenocarcinoma.[8] Two subgroups of Turcot syndrome appear to exist. In the first, which is due to mutation of the adenomatosis polyposis coli (APC) gene, patients have an increased risk of medulloblastoma, extensive colorectal adenomas, and extracolonic manifestations such as osteomas, desmoid tumors, jaw cysts, and supernumerary teeth.[8] Patients in the second subgroup, which is associated with mutations in DNA mismatch repair genes (hPMS2 and hMLH1), develop gliomas and colorectal adenocarcinoma.[8]

Children with Li-Fraumeni syndrome, which is caused by germline mutations in the TP53 gene, may develop multiple cancer types.[9] The protein encoded by this gene is multifunctional, having a role in cell cycle control, in ensuring DNA integrity and repair and, in some circumstances, in inducing apoptotic cell death. Children with inherited mutations of the TP53 gene most commonly develop low- or high-grade gliomas that may be multifocal. They may also develop medulloblastomas, primitive neuroectodermal tumors (PNETs), or choroid plexus tumors as well as tumors outside the CNS such as sarcomas, leukemias, and adrenocortical carcinomas.

Children with neurofibromatosis type 1 (NF1), due to mutation of the NF-1 gene, are at risk for developing dermal and plexiform neurofibromas and have a markedly increased risk for astrocytomas. The astrocytomas are typically low-grade neoplasms that occur within the optic pathway and involve optic nerves, the chiasm, and the optic radiations. Low-grade gliomas may also occur within the cerebral hemispheres, the brainstem, or the cerebellum. Gliomas and plexiform neurofibromas may undergo malignant transformation. Other cancers that occur in association with NF1 include myelogenous leukemia, rhabdomyosarcoma, and pheochromocytoma.

Neurofibromatosis type 2, resulting from mutations in the NF-2 gene, is associated with meningiomas within the brain and spine and schwannomas of the cranial nerves, spinal nerves, and peripheral nervous system. Bilateral acoustic nerve schwannomas are highly associated with neurofibromatosis type 2. Gliomas and ependymomas also occur with increased frequency and tend to be located in the spinal cord.

Finally, several rare tumor types occur most frequently in association with specific inherited disorders. Subependymal giant-cell astrocytomas, which occur in the anteromedial aspect of the brain near the foramina of Monro, most often occur in children with tuberous sclerosis. Cerebellar gangliocytoma (Lhermitte-Duclos) occurs in the context of Cowden syndrome, owing to mutation of the PTEN gene that encodes a dual specificity phosphatase.[10] Hemangioblastomas, typically

TABLE 26A.1

INHERITED DISORDERS ASSOCIATED WITH BRAIN TUMORS

Syndrome	Gene(s)	CNS tumor type(s)	Non-CNS tumors
Cowden	PTEN	Dysplastic gangliocytoma of the cerebellum (Lhermitte-Duclos)	
Hereditary retinoblastoma	Rb	Pineoblastoma, glioma, meningioma	Retinoblastoma, osteosarcoma, malignant melanoma
Li-Fraumeni	TP53	Multiple brain tumor types, most commonly supratentorial PNET, medulloblastomas and astrocytoma	Sarcoma, adrenocortical tumor, acute leukemia, premenopausal breast cancer
Neurofibromatosis type 1	NF-1	Neurofibroma, optic nerve glioma, astrocytoma	
Neurofibromatosis type 2	NF-2	Acoustic and peripheral schwannoma, meningioma, spinal ependymoma	
Nevoid basal cell carcinoma (Gorlin syndrome)	PTCH	Medulloblastoma, meningiomas	Basal cell carcinomas
Rubenstein-Taybi	CBP	Medulloblastoma, oligodendroglioma, meningioma	
Tuberous sclerosis	TSC1, TSC2	Subependymal giant-cell astrocytoma	
Turcot	APC	Medulloblastoma (most common)	Colorectal adenomas
	hMLH1, hPMS2	Astrocytoma and ependymoma (less common)	Colorectal adenocarcinoma
von Hippel-Lindau	VHL	Hemangioblastoma	

PNET, primitive neuroectodermal tumor.

in the cerebellum, spinal cord, or retinas, occur in association with von Hippel-Lindau syndrome, which arises from mutation of the *VHL* gene that appears to have a role in DNA replication.

OTHER ASSOCIATIONS WITH CENTRAL NERVOUS SYSTEM TUMORS

Ionizing Radiation

Exposure to ionizing radiation is a well-documented cause of brain tumors. Children treated with radiation therapy for tinea capitis during the 1940s and 1950s were found to have increased risk for the development of meningiomas, gliomas, and nerve sheath tumors 22 to 34 years later.[11] In more recent decades, brain tumors after cranial irradiation for acute lymphoblastic leukemia or intracranial embolization have been reported.[12–16]

Other Cancers

Brain tumors may be seen in association with other cancers or as a result of their treatment. Pituitary tumors occur in patients with various forms of the multiple endocrine adenomatosis syndrome (see Chapter 36). Finally, brain tumors, particularly high-grade astrocytomas or meningiomas, may occur in patients who previously received CNS radiation therapy, particularly in childhood cancer patients with inherited cancer syndromes who have an increased genetic susceptibility to multiple primary malignancies that is enhanced by sensitivity to ionizing radiation. For example, patients with retinoblastoma, NF1 and optic glioma, Li Fraumeni syndrome, or nevoid basal cell carcinoma syndrome are at substantial risk of developing radiation-related cancers,[17] many of which are CNS tumors as a result of the location of the radiation field for the primary tumor.

Immunosuppression

CNS lymphomas occur with increased frequency in patients with a variety of underlying primary or secondary disorders of the immune system, including the Wiskott-Aldrich syndrome, ataxia-telangiectasia, acquired immunodeficiency syndrome, and after solid-organ transplantation.[18]

Familial Conditions

Data are inconclusive regarding less completely understood familial factors outside of known Li-Fraumeni families. Some studies show no influence of family history on the occurrence of brain tumors, whereas others report an increased risk of brain tumors with a family history of bone cancer, leukemia, and lymphoma. The children or siblings of persons with brain tumors may be at higher risk for developing brain tumors themselves.[19–21] Reports of familial clustering of embryonal tumors, gliomas, and choroid plexus papillomas (CPPs) also exist.[22–26] Since a family history of glioma has been observed in approximately 5% of cases, an international consortium known as GLIOGENE, consisting of 15 research groups from North America, Europe, and Israel, has been formed to understand the inherited risk factors associated with this devastating disease.[27] The goal of this consortium is to characterize genes in glioma families using a genome-wide single-nucleotide polymorphism approach with linkage analyses to see if new genomic regions or loci with genes critical to the development of glioma can be identified.[27]

Environmental Exposures

The effect of environmental exposures, including diet, on the occurrence of childhood brain tumors has been studied by numerous investigators without conclusive evidence for an association.[28–30] Studies of the effect of cellular telephones on the occurrence of childhood brain tumors have not been performed. Although studies with regard to mobile phone use and brain tumor development have been performed in adults, they are associated with a variety of limitations including small subject number, lack of appropriate controls, and short follow-up duration. The results of these studies are variable: some suggest there is no conclusive evidence for association, some are inconclusive, and others suggest a slight to significant increase risk of CNS tumor development.[31] An association of polyomavirus (e.g., JC and SV-40 viruses) with certain types of pediatric brain tumors such as medulloblastoma, ependymoma, and choroid plexus tumors has been reported[32]; however, there is no definitive evidence that such viruses are directly involved in the pathogenesis of these tumors.[33,34]

Several factors confound the epidemiologic study of pediatric brain tumors. First, until recently, etiologic studies considered pediatric cancer a single entity, and brain tumors were not examined separately. Second, the etiology of brain tumors is most likely multifactorial, and these factors may influence distinct histological types of tumors to variable degrees. Finally, pediatric brain tumors are rare, and this rarity affects research methodology. Nearly all studies of pediatric brain tumors are case-control studies in which individuals with and without brain tumors are compared with respect to past exposures. Inaccuracies and disparities in patient or parent recall may limit observations of disease and their associations.[28] Should a link with environmental exposures truly exist, it may be difficult to establish.

CENTRAL NERVOUS SYSTEM TUMOR BIOLOGY: TUMOR ORIGINS AND GENETICS

Cancers arise as a result of mutations in genes that regulate cell proliferation and death. Gene mutations may originate within the germline or may occur as somatic mutations exclusively within tumor cells. As previously noted, only a small fraction of children with brain tumors have germline mutations either acquired from their parents (giving them an inherited predisposition to cancer) or as new mutations. Although the causes of the somatic mutations underlying the vast majority of all brain tumors are unknown, the ongoing prospective characterization of genetic abnormalities typically associated with childhood brain tumors is important as it may have implications for tailoring treatment.

Fluorescence-activated cell sorting and direct chromosomal preparations from biopsy specimens have demonstrated that low-grade gliomas, meningiomas, and pituitary adenomas almost universally possess a unimodal diploid DNA content.[33] In contrast, direct biopsy preparations from more aggressive and malignant tumors, such as anaplastic astrocytoma and glioblastoma multiforme, frequently show bizarre chromosomal aberrations and a dominance of triploid and tetraploid cells in the cell lines derived from these tumors. These findings are in agreement with the genetic analyses of cancers arising in other sites, which generally have demonstrated increasingly abnormal genetic content as cancers evolve into high-grade malignancies. Conversely, fluorescence-activated cell sorting and karyotyping performed on freshly prepared tumor cell populations show near-diploid genetic content, possibly as a result of tumor contamination with normal diploid stromal cells. Alternatively, small diploid or near-diploid anaplastic cells may harbor specific mutations that render them both drug and radiation resistant, such that their malignant characteristics are not caused by overt loss or gain of chromatin.[35–42]

Chromosomal abnormalities have been further defined using technologies that determine DNA copy number and loss of heterozygosity, on a genome-wide scale (e.g., single nucleotide polymorphism mapping arrays and array comparative genomic hybridization [CGH]). These techniques have largely superseded older technologies including spectral karyotyping, although fluorescence *in situ* hybridization (FISH) is still useful for confirming focal changes.

The chromosomal alterations that accumulate in ependymomas vary with the site of the primary tumor.[43] Gain of 1q and 9q with or without amplification of the *NOTCH1* locus at 9q34.3 has been reported in aggressive posterior fossa tumors, while loss of 22q occurs most commonly in spinal tumors and a subset of cerebral ependymomas. Deletion of 9p21 including the *INK4A/ARF* locus is also limited to cerebral tumors. A variety of genetic events have been associated with the progression of low-grade gliomas to high-grade glioblastomas in adults: nonrandom loss of chromosome 10 or of portions of 9p, 17p, and others; gene amplifications of epidermal growth factor receptor (EGFR) or MDM2; and mutations of genes such as PTEN and TP53.[35,44–46] These observations suggest that, as in colon carcinoma, malignant progression of CNS tumors may be a multistep process involving the accumulation of genetic abnormalities that promote activation of multiple dominant oncogenes and inactivation of recessive tumor suppressor genes. However, there are apparent differences between pediatric and adult malignant gliomas in their patterns of genetic alterations, specifically a much lower incidence of EGFR amplification in glioblastoma,[47] a paucity of TP53 mutations in malignant gliomas arising in infants,[48] and an association between TP53 mutations and outcome in older children.[47] These observations call attention to the need for studies specifically targeted to childhood gliomas to address issues of genetic progression and age-specific molecular contributors to tumor growth. Chromosomal alterations in embryonal CNS tumors are addressed in Chapter 26B.

Although chromosomal studies can provide lists of the genetic events that contribute to the expansion of malignant clones, they do not inform us regarding the chronology or relative importance of each of these alterations in the cancer process. A more comprehensive understanding of cancer that spans the life of the disease from the birth of the first malignant cell to clinical presentation would be invaluable in the hunt for more effective treatments of cancer. With this in mind, considerable excitement has surrounded the recent discovery of cancer stem cells (CSCs).[50] CSCs make up just a small fraction of the total population of the malignant cells in many solid tumors and leukemias. However, evidence indicates that these self-renewing and multipotent stem cell-like cells generate all of the phenotypically diverse cells that populate tumors. The discovery of CSC has therefore provided researchers with a practical point of focus for studying the natal cellular and molecular events of tumorigenesis. The identification of CSC is likely to have important implications

for the treatment of cancer. If tumors are derived entirely from CSC, then it would follow that to be curative, cancer treatments should disable or destroy these cells. Indeed, drugs that are designed to kill CSC could prove highly effective treatments of cancer. On the other hand, evidence that CSCs are remarkably similar to normal stem cells predicts that such treatments may also possess significant toxicities. For example, brain CSCs express the neural stem cell markers Nestin and CD133,[43,51–53] whereas acute myeloid leukemic CSCs display the CD34+/CD38− immunophenotype of hematopoietic stem cells.[54,55] Thus, the development of safe and effective therapies for all cancers is likely to require understanding of the similarities and differences between normal and malignant stem cells in tissues. Recent evidence that gliomas, medulloblastomas, and ependymomas contain CSC has opened up new important avenues of research for these tumors.

PATHOLOGIC CLASSIFICATION OF CENTRAL NERVOUS SYSTEM TUMORS

Background

Classification of CNS tumors has been a challenge as several different histological classifications have coexisted, reflecting a lack of consensus among neuropathologists. All classification schemes are basically arbitrary; however, they ideally change with progress in knowledge. Classification of CNS tumors became clinically important after successful establishment of neurosurgery as a specialty and received major impetus from Harvey Cushing during the 1920s and 1930s. The classification system proposed by Cushing's student, Percival Bailey, in 1926 has served as the prototype system for CNS tumors. That scheme, which was based on the cell-of-origin notion introduced by German pathologists, suggested that tumors developed from cells arrested at various stages of development; for each putative developmental stage of a cell, a corresponding tumor was identified. Figure 26A.2 outlines Bailey and Cushing's basic schema, denoting the different cell types, the developmental stages through which they were said to pass before reaching maturity, and the corresponding tumor types presumed to arise from them (noted in parentheses in the figure). This classification was embraced immediately because it reflected some aspects of clinical behavior and prognosis, corresponding to Cushing's experience, and because of the esteem that Cushing enjoyed.

Methods of Classification

Morphologic and Histogenetic Classification

In addition to their cell-of-origin concept, Bailey and Cushing recognized that tumors were composed of heterogeneous cells. They decided to classify tumors on the basis of the morphology and presumed histogenesis of the predominant cell type. Hence, if the majority of cells resembled astrocytes, the tumor was called an astrocytoma, even though a small number of other cells (e.g., oligodendrocytes) also were present. Most classifications in current use are based on this concept.

Approximately 60 years ago, Kernohan et al.[56] introduced a grading system based on the concept that glial cells of all types become progressively more malignant over time. Criteria were advanced for grading glial tumors on a scale from 1 (most benign) to 4 (most malignant), and this scheme was to be applied to astrocytomas, oligodendrogliomas, and ependymomas.

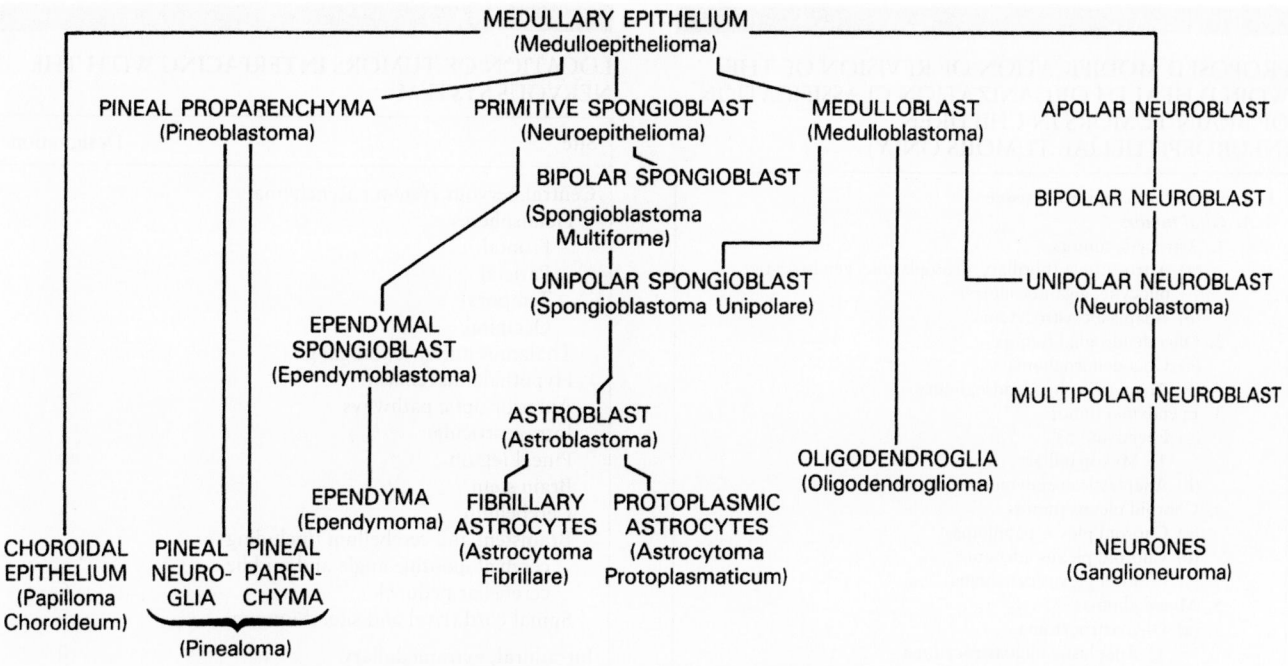

FIGURE 26A.2 Bailey and Cushing schema of normal developing cells and neuroepithelial tumors derived from them.

Based on histologic features, it has been readily adopted and is used commonly for astrocytomas for which clinical correlations exist. For oligodendrogliomas and ependymomas, the scheme has been an awkward fit, resulting in inconsistent use. Revision of the Kernohan grading system for astrocytomas was proposed by Daumas-Duport et al.[57] An international panel of neuropathologists, working under the aegis of the WHO, expanded the concept of grading all CNS tumors, using the 1-to-4 scale to indicate biologic malignancy.[58]

Although it is generally accepted that CNS tumors in children differ in many respects from those in adults, there had been no separate classification system for pediatric tumors until an adaptation of the 1979 WHO scheme was published in 1985[57] and later modified as shown in Table 26A.2. This scheme for pediatric CNS tumors not only includes morphologic entities of neoplasia but also tumor location as shown in Table 26A.3. Consideration of location acknowledges the importance of site of origin as a factor in determining clinical outcome. An obvious example is the pilocytic astrocytoma: a child with a lesion in the cerebellum generally has a better prognosis than one whose lesion is in the diencephalon.

Pitfalls of Morphologic and Histogenetic Classification. It is important to recognize that the histogenetic concepts underlying the morphologic classification schemes are not fully tenable in light of current knowledge. Cancer is a genetic disease in which the genotypic instability of neoplastic cells may change the histologic features consequent to both time and treatment, although a remarkably large proportion of tumors exhibit relatively characteristic features, allowing easy diagnosis to the trained eye. It is no longer appropriate to seriously consider the cell-of-origin hypothesis advanced by Bailey and Cushing, because it has been established that cell populations displaying similar, or even identical, patterns of differentiation may not have a common embryogenesis. Hence, it is not possible to determine either ancestry or progeny of a tumor cell or cells. In addition, such theorizing is largely irrelevant because the behavior of the tumor is dependent on the intrinsic nature of the component cells and other factors.

Phenotypic Classification

An alternative to classification based on histogenetic concepts is the phenotypic approach. Essentially, this involves evaluation of the tumor by identification of cell types comprising it.[60–62] Beyond examination of sections stained by routine hematoxylin and eosin (H & E), other special stains, immunohistochemistry, ultrastructural study, and cytogenetics can now be used to determine the cell types comprising the tumor with greater precision than was possible a decade ago. Use of monoclonal antibodies to identify specific antigens, such as cytoskeletal and membrane proteins, hormonal polypeptides, and neurotransmitter substances, has been especially useful in classifying, on routine light microscopy, tumors with unusual morphologic features that previously were relegated to the "unknown" category. Use of this phenotypic approach, coupled with increasing information of the cytogenetics and microarray analyses of CNS tumors, has forced changes in the historic classification schemes.

Technical Handling of Tissues

For optimal study, tumor tissues removed at biopsy and postmortem require special handling. If a tumor is in an accessible location, the surgeon should be encouraged to remove and submit as much tissue as is safely possible; postmortem, generally no limitations apply. Some of the specimen should be placed in formalin for paraffin embedding and histological analysis. A tiny fragment may be fixed in glutaraldehyde in the event that ultrastructural study is required. The discovery of CSC has increased interest in the study of stem-like cells in tumors. Isolation of these cells requires that fresh, unprocessed tumor be placed in special serum-free medium in the operating room. All genomic studies of microRNAs

TABLE 26A.2

PROPOSED MODIFICATION OF REVISION OF THE WORLD HEALTH ORGANIZATION CLASSIFICATION OF BRAIN TUMORS IN CHILDREN (NEUROEPITHELIAL TUMORS ONLY)

I. Tumors of neuroepithelial tissue
  A. *Glial tumors*
    1. Astrocytic tumors
      (a) Astrocytoma (fibrillary, protoplasmic, gemistocytic, pilocytic, gigantocellular)
      (b) Anaplastic astrocytoma
    2. Oligodendroglial tumors
      (a) Oligodendroglioma
      (b) Anaplastic oligodendroglioma
    3. Ependymal tumors
      (a) Ependymoma
        1) Myxopapillary
      (b) Anaplastic ependymoma
    4. Choroid plexus tumors
      (a) Choroid plexus papilloma
      (b) Choroid plexus adenoma
      (c) Choroid plexus carcinoma
    5. Mixed gliomas
      (a) Oligoastrocytoma
        1) Anaplastic oligoastrocytoma
      (b) Ependymoastrocytoma
        1) Anaplastic ependymoastrocytoma
      (c) Oligoastroependymoma
        1) Anaplastic oligoastroependymoma
      (d) Gliofibroma
    6. Glioblastomatous tumors
      (a) Glioblastoma multiforme
      (b) Giant-cell glioblastoma
      (c) Gliosarcoma
    7. Gliomatosis cerebri
  B. *Mixed glial-neuronal tumors*
    1. Ganglioglioma
      (a) Dysembryoplastic neuroepithelial tumor
    2. Superficial cerebral astrocytoma–desmoplastic infantile ganglioglioma
    3. Pleomorphic xanthoastrocytoma
    4. Subependymal giant-cell tumor (of tuberous sclerosis)
    5. Anaplastic ganglioglioma
      (a) Anaplastic superficial cerebral astrocytoma–desmoplastic infantile ganglioglioma
      (b) Anaplastic pleomorphic xanthoastrocytoma
  C. *Neural tumors*
    1. Gangliocytoma
      (a) Anaplastic gangliocytoma
    2. Neurocytoma
      (a) Anaplastic neurocytoma
  D. *Embryonal tumors*
    1. Primitive neuroectodermal tumor (PNET)
      (a) PNET, not otherwise specified
      (b) PNET with glial differentiation
      (c) PNET with ependymal differentiation
      (d) PNET with neuronal differentiation
      (e) PNET with retinal differentiation
      (f) PNET with mesenchymal differentiation
      (g) PNET with melanocytic differentiation
      (h) PNET with differentiation along multiple lines
    2. Medulloepithelioma
      (a) Medulloepithelioma with differentiation along divergent lines as above (1.b–h)
    3. Atypical teratoid-rhabdoid tumor
  E. *Pineal cell tumors*
    1. Pineocytoma

From Rorke LB, Gilles FH, Davis RL, et al. Revision of the World Health Organization classification of brain tumors for childhood brain tumors. Cancer 1985;56:1869–1886, with permission.

TABLE 26A.3

LOCATION OF TUMORS INTERFACING WITH THE NERVOUS SYSTEM

Site	Designation
Central nervous system parenchyma	I
Hemispheres	a
Frontal	
Parietal	
Temporal	
Occipital	
Thalamus and/or basal ganglia	b
Hypothalamus/chiasm	c
Anterior optic pathways	d
Intraventricular	e
Pineal region	f
Brain stem	g
Cerebellum	h
Brainstem and cerebellum (including cerebellopontine angle and middle cerebellar peduncle)	i
Spinal cord (level and site, if known)	j
Intradural, extramedullary	jl
Meninges	II
Intradural	a
Extradural	b
Parasellar region	III
Skull and/or vertebral column	IV
Orbit (eye)	V
Peripheral nervous system	VI

(miRNAs), total RNA, and DNA can be performed using frozen tumor material.

High-quality technical preparations are of utmost importance to establish a diagnosis. Use of the microwave enhancement technique for certain antigens is recommended.[63,64] Even under the most optimal circumstances, however, classification based on phenotypes may be problematic.

Table 26A.4 contains a listing of the widely available markers that are used most commonly and their utility in the differential diagnosis of tumors arising in the CNS. These tumors include primary neuroepithelial tumors, those arising from meningeal covering, and germ cell tumors.

CLINICAL PRESENTATION: NEUROLOGY OF CENTRAL NERVOUS SYSTEM TUMORS

No single clinical finding is pathognomonic for the diagnosis of a childhood brain tumor. At the onset of illness, the nature of neurologic and systemic dysfunction is varied. Signs and symptoms may be a direct result of tumor infiltration into adjacent brain and/or spinal cord or a consequence of CSF flow obstruction with resultant increased intracranial pressure (ICP). The clinical presentation primarily reflects the site of tumor origin, the age and developmental level of the affected child, and, occasionally, the tumor type. Clinical prodromes may include features of increased ICP, symptoms and signs of a localizing nature, or symptoms and signs without a localizing quality.

COMMON MARKERS FOR DIAGNOSIS OF CENTRAL NERVOUS SYSTEM TUMORS

Marker	Tumor types containing positive cells
Glial fibrillary acidic protein	Astrocytoma, ependymoma, mixed glioma, gliosarcoma, ganglioglioma, glioblastoma multiforme, gliofibroma; positive cells occasionally may be found in oligodendroglioma, capillary hemangioblastoma, choroid plexus papilloma, PNET, AT/RT
Neurofilament	Ganglioglioma, gangliocytoma, PNET, neurocytoma, subependymal giant-cell tumor, AT/RT
Vimentin	Mesenchymal tumors, meningiomas, sarcoma, melanoma, lymphoma, ependymoma, astrocytoma, gliofibroma, chordoma, schwannoma, hemangioblastoma, carcinoma, PNETs, AT/RT
S100 and neuron-specific enolase	Positive in a variety of normal and neoplastic cells of neural and nonneural origin; of questionable utility for diagnostic purposes
Desmin	Tumors containing muscle (rhabdomyosarcoma, teratoma, etc.), PNET
Cytokeratin	Chordoma, choroid plexus tumors, meningioma, certain anaplastic gliomas, nongerminomatous germ-cell tumors, PNET, AT/RT
Epithelial membrane antigen	Meningioma, ependymoma, epithelial areas of teratomas, rhabdoid tumor (AT/RT)
Synaptophysin	PNET, ganglioglioma, gangliocytoma, central neurocytoma, neuroendocrine tumors
Smooth muscle actin	Tumors containing muscle, AT/RT
Retinal S-antigen	Pineal parenchymal tumors, PNETs, retinoblastoma
Alpha-fetoprotein	Embryonal carcinoma, endodermal sinus (yolk sac) tumor
Human chorionic gonadotrophin	Germinoma, choriocarcinoma
Placental alkaline phosphatase	Germ cell tumors

AT/RT, atypical teratoid-rhabdoid tumor; PNET, primitive neuroectodermal tumor.

Increased Intracranial Pressure

Brain tumors cause increased ICP directly by infiltrating or compressing normal CNS structures or indirectly by causing obstruction of cerebrospinal fluid (CSF) pathways, resulting in noncommunicating hydrocephalus. Initial features of elevated ICP are typically insidious, nonspecific, and nonlocalizing. Among school-aged children, declining academic performance, fatigue, personality changes, and vague intermittent headaches are common. Over time, morning headaches, vomiting, and lethargy ensue. Papilledema may develop if the pressure is longstanding. Rapid progression of symptoms secondary to increased ICP is infrequent. However, when such occurs, a quickly growing midline or posterior fossa tumor requiring immediate intervention should be suspected.

Headaches resulting from brain tumors may have ominous features distinct from tension headaches or migraines. When children with a tumor are recumbent, increased ICP may worsen, resulting in a headache that wakens them at night or is present on waking in the morning. On arising, vomiting may occur along with some relief of pain. Once such patients are upright, the headache may diminish over the course of the day. Over time, headaches gradually increase in severity and frequency and clearly differ from any previous pain. The pain, which usually is frontal or occipital rather than temporal, may be further exacerbated with Valsalva maneuvers. The clinical suspicion for tumor should be greatest in those children with recent and continuing complaints of headache, and such should prompt a careful history and evaluation for related symptoms and signs. In fact, by 6 months from headache onset, nearly 100% of children have associated neurologic signs, such as papilledema, strabismus, ataxia, or weakness.[65]

Signs and symptoms of elevated ICP in infants and young children, whose skulls may more easily accommodate the growth of a mass lesion, may be quite different and may include irritability, anorexia, failure to thrive, and developmental delay or regression. Chronically increased pressure may lead to macrocephaly and separation of the cranial sutures. Infants may develop a tense or bulging anterior fontanelle associated with a shrill, neurogenic cry. Funduscopic evaluation of these patients may reveal only optic pallor but no evidence of papilledema. The setting-sun sign, a seemingly forced downward deviation of the eyes and part of Parinaud syndrome, may also be seen.

Parinaud syndrome is a collection of ophthalmologic findings stemming from increased ICP at the dorsal midbrain. In addition to the impaired upward gaze seen in infants, older children also display large pupils with impaired reflex constriction to light but not with accommodation. Convergence of gaze may evoke repetitive, bilateral, adducting nystagmus with retraction of the globes in the orbit. Cranial nerve IV palsy, with the affected eye deviated upward and laterally, may also occur. Affected children often compensate for the trochlear nerve palsy by tilting their heads toward the shoulder of the unaffected eye.

A head tilt may occur also with increased ICP because of a stiff neck and cervical root irritation from incipient cerebellar herniation of a posterior fossa mass. Other signs of increased ICP include listlessness and horizontal diplopia from pressure on the long, free intracranial course of the abducens nerve.

Localizing Symptoms and Signs

Children with supratentorial tumors (i.e., of the cerebrum, basal ganglia, thalamus, hypothalamus, and optic chiasm) may demonstrate various localizing symptoms and signs that precede those of increased ICP. The most common of these signs and symptoms include hemiparesis, hemisensory loss, hyperreflexia, seizures, and visual complaints.

Vision loss may localize to any location in the optic pathway. Complaints occasionally start insidiously with such events as a failed school eye examination or a need for eyeglasses. Tumors confined to the optic nerve produce monocular vision loss. Chiasmatic tumors present often with a complex visual field loss and decrement in acuity, whereas lesions located more posteriorly, in the optic tract, lateral geniculate nucleus, optic radiations, or occipital cortex, demonstrate some aspect of hemianopsia. A paradoxical increase in pupillary size to light when moving the source from one eye to the other indicates a relative afferent pupillary defect (the Marcus-Gunn pupil), a potential sign of tumor at the optic nerve or chiasm. Among infants, chiasmatic tumors may result in unilateral or bilateral pendular nystagmus, with head nodding and head tilt, a triad known as spasmus nutans.

In contrast to the experience in adults, seizures are seldom the *sine qua non* of a supratentorial mass in children. Nevertheless, all/simple and complex partial (i.e., focal) seizures and most unexplained generalized (grand mal) seizures mandate computed tomography (CT) or MRI of the brain. After a first seizure and subsequent neuroimaging, fewer than 1% of patients are given diagnoses of a tumor.[66] Examples of seizure features that are associated with an increased risk of a tumor include a change in the character of preexisting seizures, status epilepticus as the first seizure, prolonged postictal paralysis, resistance to medical control, and the presence of focal symptoms or deficits. An initially normal CT scan in patients with any of these seizure characteristics or with persistent epilepsy does not rule out the possibility of a tumor, and repeat imaging with MRI may be indicated.

Other localizing signs of a supratentorial tumor may be more subtle. For example, children with frontal lobe tumors may have a long history of behavioral problems. Likewise, hypothalamic tumors in infants may cause failure to thrive and emaciation with a paradoxical euphoric mood and increased appetite, the so-called diencephalic syndrome, rather than motor or visual symptoms.

For infratentorial tumors—those arising from the cerebellum and brainstem—localizing features may include ataxia, long-tract signs, or cranial neuropathies. Initial cerebellar dysfunction may be insidious, with clumsiness, worsening handwriting, difficulty with hopping or running, or slow or halting speech. Tumors arising in the cerebellar hemispheres more commonly cause lateralizing signs, such as appendicular dysmetria and nystagmus, whereas midline cerebellar masses lead to truncal unsteadiness or increased ICP.

Cranial neuropathies often suggest brainstem pathology. Diplopia, with images seen side by side, is common from invasion of the abducens nerve within the pons. Inability to abduct one or both eyes (abducens palsy), however, can be a false localizing sign, because it may result also from increased ICP trapping the abducens nerve against the edge of the tentorium. Inability to deviate both eyes conjugately (gaze palsy) or the inability to adduct one eye properly on attempted lateral gaze implies an intrinsic brainstem disorder. These latter findings alone or, more likely, in combination with deficits of the trigeminal, facial, or auditory nerve strongly suggest tumor involving the brainstem. Masses involving the cerebellopontine angle may result in facial weakness, absent corneal reflex, and hearing loss. Weakness of an entire half of the face (peripheral seventh nerve palsy) suggests a posterior fossa tumor; weakness of the lower face on one side, with spared eyelid closure and forehead movement (central seventh nerve palsy), suggests involvement anywhere superior to the pons. Drooling and swallowing difficulties may arise from involvement of the medulla. A partial Horner syndrome (ipsilateral ptosis, miosis, and anhidrosis) may also be present in some patients with hypothalamic, brainstem, or upper cervical cord disease as a result of compromise of the descending sympathetic tracts.

Nonlocalizing Symptoms and Signs

Some symptoms are characteristic of a brain tumor but not specifically localizing. Affected children may display changes in affect, energy level, motivation, or behavior. They may exhibit weight gain or loss with anorexia. Sexual precocity or delayed puberty, growth failure, somnolence, or symptoms of an autonomic nature may suggest hypothalamic or pituitary dysfunction or may be nonspecific. Vomiting can occur with irritation of the area postrema in the floor of the fourth ventricle from a generalized increase in ICP or from direct irritation by a mass.

As many as 15% of primary CNS tumors, particularly medulloblastoma, germ cell tumors, ependymoma, and high-grade gliomas, have disseminated to other CNS sites by the time of diagnosis.[67] Although such dissemination usually is asymptomatic, neurologic dysfunction from such lesions sometimes overshadows the symptoms of the primary tumor, confusing the localization of tumor origin. For example, spinal cord and cauda equina involvement may cause back or radicular pain, bowel or bladder dysfunction, or long-tract symptoms. Thus, examination at the time of diagnosis should include a search for local tenderness of the spine, focal extremity weakness, or sensory loss.

Syndromes Specific to Tumor Types

Although a pathologic brain tumor diagnosis requires tissue biopsy, certain patterns of symptoms and signs are particularly suggestive of specific tumor histologies. In the suprasellar region, pilocytic astrocytomas of the optic pathway and hypothalamus may cause visual field loss, nystagmus, and diencephalic syndrome. Craniopharyngiomas also occur in the suprasellar and sellar regions, but these neoplasms present more often with visual deficits and endocrinopathies, particularly short stature and diabetes insipidus. Endocrinopathies may be obscured, however, if increased ICP and hydrocephalus from obstruction of the third ventricle and foramen of Monro are present.

Germ cell tumors may occur in the anterior hypothalamus or the pineal region (See Chapter 26B). Hypothalamic tumors frequently cause endocrinologic abnormalities such as growth failure and diabetes insipidus that precede the diagnosis by several years. Emotional and behavioral disturbances also can occur.

Pineal region tumors, including germ cell tumors and pineal parenchymal tumors, pineoblastoma and pineocytoma, are apt to be associated with Parinaud syndrome. Focal motor deficits appear more commonly with infiltrating glial tumors in the pineal region (See Chapter 26B).[68]

In the posterior fossa, brainstem glioma, medulloblastoma, ependymoma, and pilocytic astrocytoma form the oncologic differential diagnosis. Medulloblastoma and ependymoma often compress the fourth ventricle, leading to signs and symptoms of increased ICP. Vomiting may be extreme with ependymoma because of invasion of the area postrema, an emetic chemoreceptor on the dorsal medulla that protrudes into the fourth ventricle. The classic brainstem glioma, a diffusely infiltrative pontine glioma, presents with a prodrome of less than 6 months consisting of a triad of long-tract signs, ataxia, and cranial neuropathies, particularly an abducens palsy. The atypical, focal brainstem glioma presents with a longer prodrome, often without abducens palsy. Cerebellar pilocytic astrocytomas frequently present first with vague symptoms and then with ataxia of long duration, usually a period of 18 months. In the rare cerebellar hemangioblastoma, an elevated hemoglobin level may be noted, secondary to extramedullary hematopoiesis.[69]

Although a single seizure seldom is the presenting symptom for histologically malignant cerebral tumors, long-standing epilepsy may be associated with low-grade neoplasms. In children with long-standing epilepsy found to harbor a tumor, the most common diagnoses are ganglioglioma, dysembryoplastic neuroepithelial tumor (DNET), oligodendroglioma, and low-grade gliomas.[57,70] Tumors are found in 12% to 33% of children who undergo surgery for intractable seizures.[71]

Among infants with brain tumors, seizures may occur in conjunction with macrocephaly as the harbinger of desmoplastic infantile ganglioglioma (DIG), a massive, cystic, and malignant-appearing tumor with a favorable prognosis.[72] CPP presents during infancy with hydrocephalus in nearly all cases. In congenital brain tumors, the most common diagnoses are malignant astrocytoma, teratoma, embryonal tumors, and CPP.[73] For those tumors diagnosed within 2 months of birth, the mass occupies more than one-third of the intracranial volume in 75% of patients.

NEUROIMAGING IN PEDIATRIC CENTRAL NERVOUS SYSTEM TUMORS: CURRENT STATUS AND FUTURE DIRECTIONS

Magnetic Resonance Imaging

Preoperative assessment of tumor type and extent, by imaging, is based on the combination of anatomic location, tissue characterization, and enhancement pattern coupled with the clinical history. Since its introduction into clinical practice, MRI has superseded CT as the diagnostic tool of choice for pediatric brain and spinal cord tumors. Advantages of MRI include the ease of imaging in multiple planes without the need to move the patient, imaging without the use of x-irradiation, and improved anatomic detail as well as superior resolution. Nevertheless, the clinical presentation of children with brain tumors most frequently leads to initial evaluation by unenhanced CT. Whenever MRI is readily available in a timely fashion, CT with iodinated contrast is not recommended because of its inferiority in delineating tumor extent as compared with gadolinium-enhanced MRI.

Routine MRI sequences include T1-weighted imaging (T1WI) before and after gadolinium, T2-weighted, and FLAIR (fluid-attenuated inversion recovery) imaging. Postgadolinium imaging may be performed with magnetization transfer suppression, which amplifies contrast enhancement by suppressing the signal intensity of normal background brain tissue. As a result, the detection of contrast enhancement is increased by a factor of two to three.[74] This can be useful in demonstrating enhancement within a tumor, extension of the tumor along white matter pathways, and the subarachnoid spread of tumor. Notable is that contrast enhancement is a reflection not of vascularity but of breakdown of the blood-brain barrier (BBB) and, given this factor, neither CT nor MRI defines the true extent of tumor spread.

MRI offers other advantages over CT scanning such as FLAIR sequences and fast-echo planar imaging. In addition, the availability of higher field strengths allows for faster scan acquisition and improved resolution. The penumbra of edema surrounding a tumor, which may contain metastatic foci, can be delineated with a FLAIR sequence. This sequence may be useful to the radiation oncologist for targeting focal therapy, although it tends to overestimate the extent of tumor. Fast-echo planar imaging has enabled the development of diffusion, perfusion, and gradient echo (GE) techniques, which are discussed later in this section. Finally, with the advent of frameless stereotaxy, MRI has superseded CT for preoperative planning since the resultant three-dimensional (3D) volumetric data can be reformatted in any plane in the operating room, allowing for tumor localization in relation to markers placed on the skin.

Because it has been replaced by magnetic resonance (MR) angiography, conventional angiography is rarely performed in pediatric CNS tumors. Digital subtraction angiography may still be indicated, however, in those cases displaying a mass with blood and a differential diagnosis of vascular malformation versus hemorrhagic tumor. In addition, if a highly vascular tumor is suspected, diagnostic angiography may be performed as part of a neurointerventional procedure before resection to minimize blood loss.

Assessment of pediatric brain tumors has historically focused on morphology. However, with the introduction of higher field strengths, faster gradients, parallel imaging, and new sequence design, together with new contrast agents, the ability to combine parameters of function with anatomy may provide meaningful insights into tumor physiology.[75] For example, T1WI as well as T2*-weighted (T2*-W) dynamic gadolinium enhanced imaging can be used to assess vascularity, permeability, and microcirculation of brain neoplasms. In the future, arterial spin labeling (ASL) perfusion techniques that do not use an intravenous contrast agent may play a role in pediatric brain tumor imaging. Characterization of cerebral blood flow is possible using dynamic MR angiography, and activation functional MRI (fMRI) enables visualization of alterations in cortical blood flow secondary to selective cortical stimulation. Diffusion-weighted imaging can be used to better delineate and even differentiate tumors. Spectroscopic chemical shift imaging allows for metabolic mapping both within and around tumors and helps to differentiate tumor recurrence from radiation necrosis and can potentially be used to assess response to therapy. The combined use of these new techniques enables us to learn more about the pathophysiology of CNS lesions *in vivo* and may ultimately lead to improvements in the planning of therapy as well as prognostication.

It has been shown that repeated follow-up at appropriate time intervals is the best method for detecting early recurrence. To this end, techniques for re-localizing whole brain acquisitions, so that they are more strictly comparable over time for the radiologist to read and compare, may improve the accuracy of interpretation and allow for earlier intervention, when required. Perhaps, the single most important and highest impact factor will be the establishment and implementation of rigorous imaging protocols that will result in strictly comparable images with the exact same order and timing of image acquisition.

Magnetic Resonance Spectroscopy

Magnetic resonance spectroscopy (MRS) is a noninvasive *in vivo* technique that provides measurement of metabolites within the tissue under investigation. For example, proton MRS (HMRS) determines in both a qualitative and a quantitative fashion the chemical environment of the hydrogen nuclei within the tissues targeted. Frequency-domain spectra, which reflect the distribution of resonance frequency of the particular nuclei in the sample, form the data for analysis.

Spectra are represented by a series of peaks with positions expressed in parts per million (ppm); the result can be considered a histogram of nuclei with different precession frequencies.

Spectra can be acquired using a single- or multivoxel techniques, with short (10 to 30 ms) or long (135 to 280 ms) echo times. In using a short echo time, more peaks are captured, but the spectrum is superimposed by a complicated baseline, and its analysis is more difficult. With longer echo times, fewer peaks are captured, but the measurement precision is improved. In pediatric brain tumors, the three most important metabolic peaks (reading from right to left) are N-acetyl aspartate (NAA), 2.02 ppm; creatine-phosphocreatine (Cr/PCr), 3.02 ppm; and choline (Cho), 3.22 ppm (Fig. 26A.3).

NAA is a marker of neuronal and axonal integrity. Cr is a marker for energy metabolism. Cho is a marker for cell membrane turnover and, as such, is elevated in tumors, demyelination, and inflammation; it is decreased in liver disease. The relative ratios of different metabolites vary, depending on the location of the voxel in the brain and on the age of the child. Normal age-matched control data from the same brain region are useful for interpreting the spectra from young children. As a general rule, the NAA increases over time, especially during the first 18 months of life, whereas the Cho slightly decreases over the same period. Cr/PCr tends to remain rather stable over time; for this reason, it has historically been used as an internal control when metabolic data are expressed as ratios.

The finding of a lipid-lactate peak usually indicates the presence of ischemia or necrosis. Lactate is a marker of anaerobic metabolism in hypoxic regions. Lactate peaks have been found to be more prominent in malignant gliomas than in low-grade gliomas.[76]

Single-voxel MRS can be used to interrogate new tumors having a volume greater than 1 mL³. However, a multivoxel technique, such as two-dimensional chemical shift imaging, in which several subcentimeter voxels can be examined simultaneously, can be very helpful in distinguishing recurrent tumor from radiation necrosis, which can be the great mimicker, having both mass effect and enhancing following Gd administration.[77]

With higher field strength magnets that provide improved spectral resolution with shorter acquisition times, 3D spectroscopic evaluation of tumors can readily be performed.[78,79]

Single-voxel long TE MRS data obtained by plotting Cr:Cho against NAA:Cho ratios has been used with benefit in separating posterior fossa medulloblastoma from pilocytic astrocytoma and ependymoma and in predicting disease progression.[80] It has also been used in the presurgical diagnosis of large suprasellar tumors, successfully separating craniopharyngioma from pituitary adenoma and hypothalamic region astrocytoma using single-voxel short or long TE stimulated echo acquisition mode (STEAM) or point resolved spectroscopy (PRESS) acquisis.[81] In other series, MRS findings have been shown to have prognostic information for supratentorial tumors as evidence by low NAA:Cho and Cr:Cho ratios in patients who died versus high ratios in survivor.[82] MRS also appears to be useful in monitoring the response of histologically proven pediatric glioma to adjuvant chemotherapy or radiation therapy as demonstrated by correlations between the ratio of tumor Cho to brain Cho versus tumor volume or clinical response.[83] In patients with recurrent brain tumors, the Cho:NAA ratio also appears to have prognostic significance; children with a maximum Cho:NAA ratio of less than or equal to 4.5 had a projected survival of more than 50% at 63 weeks.[84] Increasing Cho/NAA ratio has been associated with tumor progression and nonprogressing or stable tumors exhibited a decrease in the Cho/NAA ratio.[85]

Gradient Echo Imaging

T_2* GE imaging has been used with good effect in detecting the presence of altered blood and blood products within tumors. There is some evidence for its lack of sensitivity and it may be replaced by susceptibility-weighted imaging (SWI), which is a high spatial resolution 3D GE MR imaging technique that uses phase processing to accentuate the paramagnetic properties of blood products.[86] SWI has already proven itself superior to conventional GE imaging in the detection of hemorrhage in traumatic brain injury, coagulopathic or other hemorrhagic disorders, in vascular malformations, in the demonstration of venous thrombosis, and in delineating neoplasms that have hemorrhage, increased vascularity, or calcification.[87] An example of a hemorrhage within a tumor demonstrated on SWI is shown in Figure 26A.4.

Diffusion-Weighted Imaging

MR diffusion images reflect the molecular translational motion (Brownian motion) of water within the section of the brain studied. Restriction of the water molecule motion can be observed in normal white matter tracts. This is called anisotropy; water molecules are restricted orthogonal to the white matter tracts. The motion of the molecules between the applications of the diffusion gradients leads to attenuation of the signal within each image voxel. From these images, a diffusion coefficient termed the *apparent diffusion coefficient* (ADC) can be calculated. MR diffusion using predominately echoplanar techniques has been useful in the characterization of tissue, tumor cellularity, tumor grading, tumor response to treatment, and distinction of tissue types. Numerous studies have confirmed that diffusion MRI is a biomarker for treatment response.[88,89]

Diffusion tensor imaging provides visualization of fiber bundle integrity and direction with *in vivo* characterization of the rate and direction of white matter diffusion. This imaging is based on the diffusion tensor, a 3×3 matrix of vectors, which a mathematical model of the 3D pattern of diffusion anisotropy of white matter tracts.[90] It is used for presurgical

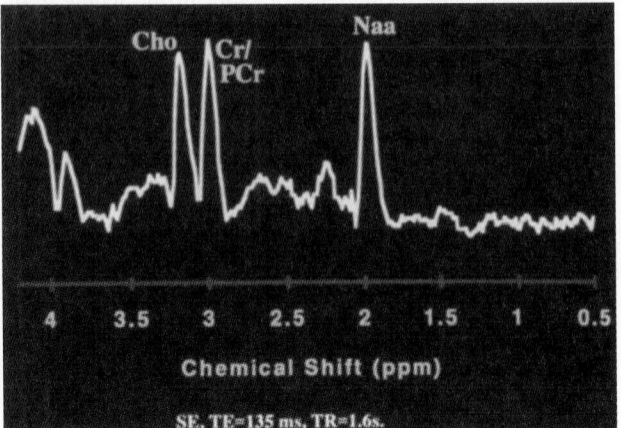

FIGURE 26A.3 Normal long-echo single-voxel spectrum from the cerebellum of an age-matched control for a patient with a posterior fossa brain tumor. Reading from right to left, note normal peaks of N-acetyl aspartate (NAA), creatine-phosphocreatine (CR/PCr), and choline (Cho).

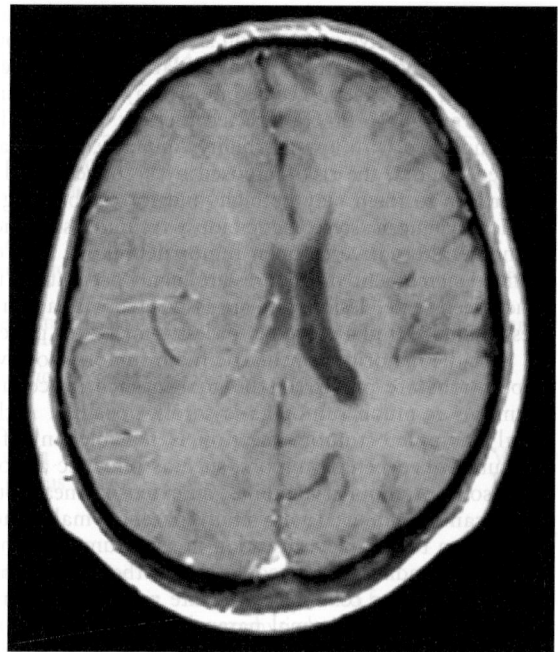
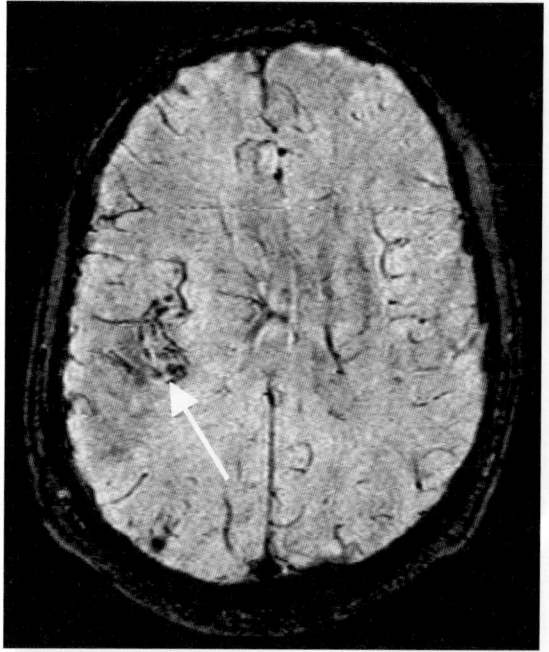

A   B

FIGURE 26A.4 A: T1-weighted MRI with contrast. **B:** Susceptibility-weighted image (SWI) showing hemorrhage in a glioma (*arrow*). (Courtesy of Mark Haacke Ph.D., The Magnetic Resonance Imaging Institute for Biomedical Research, Detroit, Michigan.)

planning or coregistration of tractography data with radio-surgical planning and functional MR data.[91]

Magnetic Resonance Perfusion Imaging

MR perfusion imaging is used to evaluate cerebral perfusion dynamics by analysis of the hemodynamic parameters of relative cerebral blood volume, relative cerebral blood flow, and mean transit time. The techniques used to perform perfusion imaging include T2*W dynamic susceptibility techniques, ASL techniques, and T1WI dynamic contrast-enhanced perfusion techniques. These techniques use either exogenous tracer agents, such as paramagnetic contrast material, or endogenous tracer agents, such as magnetically labeled blood (arterial water).[92]

The development of fast-echo planar imaging has made possible an assessment of the vascularity of tumors using a gadolinium first-pass bolus technique. Imaging is performed dynamically, (rapid imaging over time during a bolus injection) using echoplanar imaging-based spin echo or gradient echo sequences. This relies on changes in the T2 signal of gadolinium-laden blood as it passes through the region of interest.[93] Resulting data, reflected in maps of relative cerebral blood volume, provide some semiquantitative analysis of the blood flow to a particular region. Early work has suggested a positive correlation between relative cerebral blood volume and tumor grade.[94] Perfusion imaging may be helpful in targeting a lesion for biopsy. Application of perfusion imaging may be particularly useful for the study of neovascularization and angiogenesis inhibition particularly using the T1WI technique. A 3D dynamic sequence is used with short TR and short TE employed. Kinetic modeling of the dynamic signal changes can yield estimates of regional fractional blood volume and microvascular permeability (Kps), which is an indicator of BBB disruption and correlates with angiogenesis.[95]

ASL is an MR perfusion technique that does not use an intravenous contrast agent. The perfusion contrast in the image results from the subtraction of two successively acquired images; one with and one without proximal labeling of arterial water spins with a magnetic gradient used to invert the magnetization of inflowing blood.[80,96]

Activation Functional Magnetic Resonance Imaging

After the use of a stimulation paradigm or task designed to activate a specific functional area of the brain, the target can be located anatomically by an increase in blood flow to that area. fMRI uses the BOLD (blood oxygen level dependent) technique to generate differential signals based on the relative hemoglobin-oxyhemoglobin content of the blood flowing away from activated brain during an appropriate stimulus. Repetition of the task improves the robustness of the data, and subtraction of rest from activity reduces background signal. Data are presented on maps that outline the activated area of interest in relation to the lesion, and these may be useful in preoperative planning. An example involving finger-thumb opposition and the motor cortex of the hand is shown in Figure 26A.5. Different activation tasks can be designed to stimulate other eloquent areas of the brain for vision, hearing, and language.

Positron Emission Tomography

PET can serve as an imaging biomarker that enables early detection of response and can be correlated with outcome and/or progression-free survival in children with brain tumors. The most commonly used tracer in the evaluation of brain tumors has been fluorodeoxyglucose. However, molecular imaging researchers are evaluating new markers of tumor physiology through novel F18-labeled agents such as

postoperatively, careful attention to fluid replacement and cautious administration of synthetic vasopressin, where indicated, are essential to avoid potentially deleterious swings in electrolyte levels and fluid balance.

Children with cerebral cortical tumors and those in whom cortical retraction is required in the approach to a deep-seated lesion may be at risk for seizures during the perioperative period. Preoperatively, such patients often are started on an anticonvulsant medication (e.g., phenytoin) that is continued during the postoperative period, even if they have not experienced previous seizures. Patients generally are maintained on anticonvulsants for at least 1 week postoperatively; the decision to continue such therapy in patients without documented seizures is of uncertain benefit. In patients who experience a preoperative seizure disorder from the tumor and have been rendered seizure free by tumor resection, anticonvulsants often can be stopped within several months after surgery.

Intraoperative Considerations and Surgical Technique

Multiple studies have demonstrated that the extent of surgical resection has a major impact on the likelihood of long-term survival for children with many types of pediatric brain tumors, particularly ependymomas,[101–103] high-grade gliomas,[104–106] medulloblastomas (See Chapter 26B), low-grade gliomas,[107] and choroid plexus tumors.[108–109] Accordingly, with the exceptions noted earlier, in which surgical resection is not indicated or in which stereotactic biopsy may be a preferable initial step, extensive resection is the goal for many types of pediatric brain tumors.

A major limitation to the widespread incorporation of extensive surgical resections in the management of childhood brain tumors has been the fact that aggressive resections may increase the risk of immediate- and long-term morbidity, particularly for tumors in functionally critical locations. Although morbidity generally is less than 10% for polar supratentorial gliomas and less than 20% for cerebellar astrocytomas, more deep-seated lesions, such as ependymomas and craniopharyngiomas, carry morbidity rates in excess of 40% with extensive resection.[110] Although some studies have observed that morbidity is lower if operations are performed by neurosurgeons who do such operations frequently,[111,112] other studies show that pediatric neurosurgeons are more likely to attempt extensive removals, on the basis of their recognition that this influences prognosis, and therefore may have overall rates of management morbidity comparable with those of general neurosurgeons, albeit with a higher frequency of complete or nearly complete tumor resections.[113]

During the last 10 to 20 years, a number of intraoperative modalities have been developed or refined to allow tumor resection to be performed more safely and efficiently. Foremost among these are the progressive improvements in operative microscopy, which facilitates illumination and visualization of the interface between neoplasm and normal brain. Localization techniques, such as frame-based and frameless stereotactic guidance systems, allow preoperative targeting of the tumor so that the surgical approach can be tailored precisely to minimize manipulation of normal brain structures and to maximize the extent of resection of deep-seated subcortical lesions.[114,115]

Ultrasonographic guidance also is useful in this regard. Intraoperative MRI units have become available in a limited number of centers and may help to refine further the accuracy of intraoperative decision making,[116] provided that issues of cost and the difficulties involved in operating in or adjacent to a high field-strength magnet can be resolved effectively.

In children whose tumors are in and around functionally critical brain regions, intraoperative monitoring of visual, auditory, and somatosensory pathways and direct assessment of motor and speech pathways often are used in an attempt to improve the safety of the tumor resection. In addition, areas of essential cortex overlying a deep-seated tumor may be delineated using cortical stimulation techniques to plan an approach to the tumor that avoids traversing important structures. Functional MRI and diffusion tensor imaging also provide a noninvasive way of delineating localizing important cortical and subcortical areas[117] to identify a safe trajectory to an underlying lesion. Finally, in children with intractable seizures from cerebral neoplasms, intraoperative or extraoperative electrocorticography (ECOG) may be used to define areas of epileptogenic cortex in and around the tumor to increase the likelihood that seizure control will be obtained postoperatively.[118]

For supratentorial craniotomies, children generally are placed in the supine or lateral position or prone for occipital lesions. For infratentorial craniotomies, the prone or lateral position is used more often than the "sitting" position because of concern over potential venous air embolism. Intraoperatively, the head of an infant often is positioned on a soft headrest, rather than being held by pins that can perforate the skull or cause a depressed fracture. For cortical and many subcortical tumors, the surgical approach follows the most direct trajectory to the lesion. However, for deep-seated lesions that are subjacent to functionally critical regions of the brain, alternate approaches often are required. Details of the operative approaches for specific tumor types are provided in subsequent tumor-specific sections of this Chapter and Chapter 26B.

The actual tumor resection often is aided by the use of ultrasonic aspiration, which provides a relatively atraumatic way to debulk many pediatric brain tumors. The surgical laser also may be used, depending on the consistency and location of the tumor. In general, tumors are resected "from the inside out." With many extra-axial tumors and a small percentage of intraparenchymal lesions, a clearly defined peritumoral plane is encountered through which the tumor may be dissected carefully from the surrounding brain, cranial nerves, and vessels after the central portion of the mass has been debulked. However, for most intraparenchymal tumors, a well-defined tumor capsule is not present, and the resection must proceed via gradual internal debulking until the boundary between tumor and normal brain is reached.

Because the extent of resection is so important in defining prognosis and choice of subsequent therapy for many tumor types, objective confirmation of the volume of residual tumor, if any, is essential before embarking on further therapy. Because a surgeon's impression of the extent of tumor resection is subject to error, postoperative confirmation of the extent of resection generally is established by CT or, preferably, by MRI. This imaging typically is performed within the first 24 to 72 hours postoperatively to minimize the impact of postoperative inflammation on the delineation of areas of residual tumor.

A trend over the last decade in the surgical management of selected types of brain tumors has been the concept of second-look surgery. For large, relatively vascular tumors in which an initial complete resection cannot be obtained, the patient is treated with several courses of postoperative chemotherapy in the hope of making the tumor amenable to complete resection at a second procedure. This approach has been applied anecdotally in ependymomas, a tumor type in which the extent of residual disease before initiation of radiation therapy has a substantial impact on long-term outcome.[119] What remains to be determined is whether patients who undergo a second-stage complete resection have as good a prognosis as those who were amenable to complete resection initially; this issue is being examined systematically in studies of the Children's Oncology Group (COG).

Surgical resection has been used increasingly as a component of the management of recurrent disease, particularly in children without evidence of tumor dissemination. For children with malignant lesions, this relieves mass effect in preparation for additional investigational chemotherapy on phase I or II clinical trials. Some recurrent tumors, such as JPAs and craniopharyngiomas, can be treated with reoperation alone, without the need for additional adjuvant therapy, if a gross total resection (GTR) can be achieved. For children with recurrence of other, more malignant tumors that may also be subject to dissemination, data are lacking for a survival benefit from re-resection.

Postoperative Considerations

The postoperative recovery of patients who undergo a complete or partial resection of a posterior fossa tumor, particularly a tumor in or around the cerebellar vermis, may be complicated by posterior fossa syndrome. Posterior fossa syndrome, also known as "cerebellar mutism," may range from a mild to severe disorder that is characterized by mutism, ataxia, hemiparesis, cognitive impairment, behavioral changes, cranial nerve palsies, bulbar palsy, and tremor.[120] The onset is typically within the first week after surgery and appears to occur more commonly with medulloblastoma than with other posterior fossa tumors.[121,122]

The etiology of the posterior fossa syndrome is unknown but appears to be associated with edema in the brachium pontis or with decreased blood flow during surgery. Previously reported as a rare complication of posterior fossa surgery, for unclear reasons, this syndrome is now observed in 10% to 25% of patients following tumor resection in the posterior fossa.[121] Although recovery may be complete, particularly for the mutism, there are patients in whom it is incomplete with long-term neurologic sequelae.[121,123,124]

RADIATION THERAPY

Radiation therapy is a central component of curative as well as palliative therapy for a majority of children with CNS tumors. The potential efficacy of irradiation in pediatric CNS tumors has been apparent since the middle of the 20th century. During the last 25 years, the potential detrimental effects of irradiation in the developing and mature CNS have also been quantified. Recognition of the unique CNS vulnerabilities in children and the concurrent demonstration of brain tumor responsiveness to chemotherapy introduced a paradigm of delaying or avoiding irradiation in children. With the introduction of sophisticated, 3D image-guided radiation techniques capable of relative sparing of the normal brain structures, the focus of pediatric brain tumor trials has shifted to investigating broader indications for irradiation as a key element in achieving disease control. Current studies are addressing ways to optimize the risk-to-benefit ratio of accurate, limited-volume radiation delivery, sometimes in the setting of reduced radiation dose as well.

The rational application of radiation therapy in pediatric brain tumors requires an understanding of brain development, biologic effects of ionizing radiation on the brain of a child, the behavior and natural history of various brain tumors, radiobiology and physics, techniques and technology

of radiation therapy, and the interactions of radiation with other treatment modalities, such as chemotherapy.

Indications for Radiation Therapy

The indications for radiation therapy depend on tumor histology. Pretreatment histological diagnosis is required except in cases of diffusely infiltrating pontine gliomas and visual pathway gliomas, both diagnosed on the basis of neuroimaging and neurologic findings. For ependymomas and many of the astroglial tumors, the use and timing of irradiation also depend on anatomic site of involvement and degree of resection. Specific indications for radiation therapy and controversies concerning its use are discussed later under the individual tumor type headings.

Radiation Volume

The radiation target volume is determined by tumor histiotype, anatomic extent, and known patterns of spread and failure. Advances in neuroimaging (particularly MRI, with current treatment planning often based on fusion of MRI and CT imaging and the use of fMRI and PET imaging currently under exploration)[125,126] have made tumor localization more accurate.

Local target volumes are used for tumors that are typically confined to a single anatomic location (e.g., ependymomas, craniopharyngiomas, and most astroglial tumors). Determining the target volume requires a complex integration of preoperative and postoperative/preirradiation imaging (accounting for reconfiguration of the brain following surgery and, in clearly defined settings, response to chemotherapy) to identify the "tumor" or "tumor bed" as the gross target volume (GTV). Depending on the tumor type, a margin for potential microscopic infiltration (the clinical target volume or CTV) is identified by a 3D expansion of the GTV by approximately 1 cm (e.g., discrete JPAs, craniopharyngioma, ependymomas), 1 to 2 cm (e.g., medulloblastomas when boosting only the tumor bed region [See Chapter 26B]), or 2 cm (e.g., high-grade gliomas, diffuse infiltrating brainstem gliomas, or infiltrating WHO grade II astrocytomas). Finally, a volumetric expansion of the CTV (typically by 0.5 cm) defines the planning target volume (PTV), recognizing some variability in daily setup or patient positioning despite considerable attention to immobilization and reproducibility (see Fig. 13.2).

Craniospinal irradiation is a technically demanding technique that provides homogeneous irradiation to the cranium and spine, targeting the entire subarachnoid space in tumors with known potential for (or established) intracranial and/or spinal leptomeningeal metastasis (e.g., medulloblastoma or disseminated ependymoma).

Radiobiological Considerations

The biology of radiation cell lethality for tumors and normal tissues is outlined in Chapter 13. There are differences in inherent tumor cell radiosensitivity; for instance, medulloblastoma cell lines show significantly greater cell death after 2-Gy exposure than glioblastoma multiforme cell lines.[127] Fractionation (the principle of multiple, relatively small doses of irradiation protracted over time) is particularly important in the normal tissue tolerances seen in the brain, spinal cord, and several other critical organs. Most data have been derived from radiation effects following conventional fractionation (i.e., use of a single daily fraction of 1.8 to 2.0 Gy, typically on a 5 days per week schedule). Hyperfractionated delivery (delivering two daily fraction of 1.0 to 1.2 Gy each to total doses up to 20% to 30% higher than "tolerance levels" defined following conventional fractionation) was purported to show a significant benefit in childhood brainstem gliomas.[128] The therapeutic ratio (i.e., risk-to-benefit ratio) was felt to be improved after high-dose hyperfractionated irradiation. The primary theoretical benefit of hyperfractionated radiation is the opportunity to escalate the total radiation dose without increasing damage to normal structures. In theory, benefit from hyperfractionation should result because the antitumor effects from irradiation are primarily related to the total dose rather than the dose per fraction, whereas the side effects of irradiation correlate more often with dose per fraction.[129]

Radiation effects on brain generally are characterized as delayed reactions, reflecting slow turnover times of normal brain parenchymal cells or indirect effects on the cerebrovascular. Prospective data from a number of cooperative group and single institution experiences show no clear benefit in tumor response or outcome following hyperfractionated irradiation in brainstem gliomas.[130] Details about hyperfractionation in medulloblastoma are outlined in Chapter 26B.

Techniques in Radiation Therapy

Conventional External-Beam Radiation Therapy

Conventional radiotherapeutic techniques are appropriate for pediatric brain tumors only when large volumes are treated (e.g., craniospinal or full cranial irradiation). Simple geometric field arrangements (typically two or three per radiation volume) with customized blocking provide relatively homogeneous irradiation within the defined target volume.

Three-Dimensional Conformal Radiation Therapy

Advances in neuroimaging and sophisticated 3D computerized treatment planning systems have greatly improved the ability to target the tumor while significantly sparing the surrounding normal tissues. Three-dimensional conformal radiation therapy (3D-CRT) typically involves multiple, individually shaped (or collimated) fields, arranged in coplanar, nonaxial, and noncoplanar orientation delivered in either static or dynamic modes. Compared with conventional radiation therapy, 3D-CRT more accurately targets the chosen CTV while significantly reducing the volume of normal brain exposed to high-dose irradiation.

Intensity-Modulated Radiation Therapy

Intensity-modulated radiation therapy (IMRT) is a more complex form of 3D-CRT, combining two advanced concepts with 3D-CRT: (a) inverse treatment planning (in which both the target volume and the adjacent or subtended normal tissues are assigned specific dose levels), allowing optimization of beam trajectories and weights in an overall plan and (b) computer-controlled intensity modulation of the radiation beam during treatment. IMRT allows a high degree of flexibility in reducing the dose to the surrounding normal tissues by the creation of so-called avoidance areas during the treatment planning process. Most IMRT programs prioritize dose avoidance over target volume homogeneity; the latter is a potential consideration in intrinsic brain tumors.[131]

Some have hypothesized that IMRT may increase the risk of second malignancies because of the use of multiple fields and higher leakage doses, a hypothesis that rests on the assumption that second malignancy risk is heavily influenced by low dose exposure. However, a comprehensive review of 22 large cohort and case-control studies with IMRT led to the conclusion that IMRT and multi-beam plans do not significantly increase the risk of second malignancy and that risk increases with dose.[132]

Stereotactic Radiosurgery

Radiosurgery is generally administered by a Gamma-Knife unit (based on a highly collimated dose array using 192–201 fixed cobalt-60 sources), CyberKnife or modified linear accelerator unit. Radiosurgery systems are designed to deliver a high radiation dose to a small intracranial target in one fraction by focusing multiple small radiation beams from different directions to the target, resulting in a steep dose gradient just outside the edge of the target. The application of radiosurgery usually is limited to tumors measuring 3 cm or less in maximum diameter, to minimize the risk of toxicity to normal tissue surrounding the target. Lesions within or immediately adjacent to critical structures (optic nerve/chiasm, brainstem) may be treated, though the size limitation may be stricter. Radiosurgery commonly is used for the management of brain metastases, acoustic neuroma, arteriovenous malformations (AVMs), vestibular schwannomas, meningiomas, and a variety of other tumors. In children and adolescents, radiosurgery has been used quite selectively in well-circumscribed, intrinsic low-grade gliomas (e.g., JPAs in the midbrain) not amenable to complete resection and in focal areas of residual craniopharyngiomas.[133,134] Note that subacute reactions (intralesional necrosis, often associated with transient expansion of a space-occupying lesion) limit enthusiasm for this approach in treating lesions intrinsic to the brainstem.[135,136]

Particle Beam Irradiation

There is considerable current interest in the use of particle beams (most often protons) in radiation therapy for children with CNS tumors. Proton beam irradiation provides an advantage over conventional or photon irradiation in that the proton energy can be modulated to provide irradiation to a selected depth, nearly obviating exposure of underlying tissue (compared with photon beams that pass through the target region with gradually diminishing dose intensity). Current explorations focus primarily on medulloblastoma, providing a potential advantage in dose distribution when targeting the primary tumor bed (especially with regard to cochlear and temporal lobe sparing) and the neuraxis (sparing exit from the spinal field, especially for thyroid and breast tissues).[137,138] Retrospective results of clinical outcome in children with ependymoma treated with proton radiotherapy also appear favorable.[139]

The physical advantages of proton beam radiotherapy must be weighed against proton beam contamination by neutrons that may theoretically increase the risk of second malignancies, particularly in children. Such increased risk may be mitigated as passive scatter techniques are replaced by active scanning approaches.[140] In passive scanning, protons are scattered by a foil to cover the target, which leads to production of neutrons and, in turn, increases the total-body dose up to 10-fold compared with IMRT. Conversely, active scanning techniques offer better conformity of highest doses, potentially lower doses to normal structures, and reduced beam contamination by neutrons. Extensive simulations evaluating proton versus IMRT suggest that both passively scattered and scanned-beam proton therapies confer lower risks of second cancers than conventional and intensity-modulated photon therapies.[141]

Brachytherapy

Brachytherapy, or interstitial irradiation, involves the implantation of radioactive sources directly into brain tumors. Iodine-125 and iridium-192 are radioisotopes that have been used for either permanent or temporary implants. Brachytherapy has been used for patients with glioblastoma as an additional boost after external-beam radiotherapy and for selected patients with recurrent high-grade glioma. Anecdotal favorable results have also been reported in patients with low-grade gliomas.[142] Dose homogeneity and ready availability of 3D-CRT or IMRT have supplanted much of the enthusiasm for technically demanding implant procedures in CNS tumors. Intralesional brachytherapy (typically phosphorus-32) has been utilized with some success in cystic neoplasms, most often craniopharyngioma cysts.[143,145]

Radiation and the Developing Brain

Brain development is most rapid during the first 3 years of life. Axonal growth and synaptogenesis are most active during the growth phase. The rate of growth and development decrease after 6 years of age. However, maturation of the brain, judged by degree of myelinization, is not complete until puberty.[136] For infants and young children, white matter alterations after irradiation appear to mediate the functional and neurocognitive changes most concerning with regard to functional integrity.[146] Younger children are more vulnerable to white matter changes that may be localized within or adjacent to the high-dose PTV or may extend, presumably by axonal degeneration, along white matter tracts remote from the primary tumor and PTV.[147]

Radiation Effects on the Brain

CNS responses following irradiation are classically divided temporally as (a) acute reactions, occurring during treatment; (b) subacute or early delayed reactions, occurring a few weeks to 2 months after irradiation; and (c) late reactions, occurring several months to years after treatment.[148] The pathogenesis of early and, more often, subacute radiation-induced brain injury includes inflammatory-like changes with associated intra- or perilesional edema; direct damage to oligodendrogliocytes resulting in inhibition of myelin synthesis and consequent white matter degeneration/loss; and damage to the vascular endothelium, resulting in areas of hypoxia or release of necrosis factors with attendant white matter necrosis.[149–152] Immediate peritumoral edema or intralesional necrosis is uncommon with conventional fraction sizes (i.e., 1 to 3 Gy per fraction).

Subacute reactions include imaging and clinical findings that may mimic the primary tumor or results in constitutional symptoms (e.g., lassitude, low-grade fever, less often alterations in recent memory; diffuse white matter changes identified as leukoencephalopathy); these reactions are typically time-limited, resolving within several weeks to a few months.

Late reactions are more clearly dose and volume dependent, occurring beyond 6 to 12 months after irradiation; these effects are typically permanent. Late reactions include focal radiation necrosis, a more diffuse pattern of radiation- and/or chemotherapy-induced leukoencephalopathy, neuropsychological effects, cerebrovascular effects, and secondary neoplasms (both benign and malignant). Late effects can be progressive, irreversible, and sometimes fatal. Late neuropsychological effects are particularly concerning in younger children and include intellectual impairment, memory deficits, and limited

ability to acquire new knowledge.[152] Impairment in cognition is most pronounced in children younger than 4 to 7 years.[153] Deterioration in IQ is more prevalent in children following whole-brain or "focal" supratentorial irradiation than after treatment confined to the posterior fossa.[152]

The presence and severity of radiation reactions depend on (a) irradiation treatment factors, including total dose, fraction size, interfractional interval, and treatment volume; (b) patient factors, such as age, presence of preexisting brain injury by tumor or surgery, infection, and vascular diseases; and (c) other treatment modalities, most commonly surgery and chemotherapy. The influence of certain factors, such as fraction size, treatment volume, and dose homogeneity, can be modified or optimized to limit the incidence and severity of brain injury.[148]

Radiosensitivity of Specific Structures in the Central Nervous System

Brainstem

In the modern radiotherapy era, incidental brainstem necrosis is quite rare; there are no data suggesting the brainstem is more sensitive to irradiation than other normal brain structures. Subacute radiation effects, such as those that occur in the management of diffusely infiltrating brainstem gliomas or large, focal intrinsic JPAs, can be problematic. For example, imaging changes can be difficult to differentiate from tumor progression and clinical signs may be quite pronounced, particularly focal intrinsic brainstem reactions. With 3D-CRT to "tolerance" levels of 54 to 60 Gy, one can see subacute white matter changes on MRI several months after irradiation; changes are often asymptomatic and transitory but may progress to frank necrosis.[154,155]

Spinal Cord

In view of its location, the tolerance of spinal cord to irradiation is a major dose-limiting factor in delivering high-dose irradiation to tumors of the head and neck region, the thorax, and the upper abdomen; cord tolerance is more problematic in general adult radiation oncology than in pediatrics, in which tolerance levels are often approached only in intrinsic spinal cord tumors or with sizable metastatic subarachnoid foci. In pediatric radiation oncology, the spinal cord is more often the targeted tumor volume than an unintended critical structure. Craniospinal irradiation is common although dose levels to the entire spine rarely approach or exceed the 44-Gy level identified as "safe" in the United States using conventional fractionation.[148,156] More limited spinal volumes are often treated to dose levels approximately 45 to 50 Gy or, occasionally, 54 Gy.[148,157] With contemporary 3D, image-guided irradiation for low-lying posterior fossa lesions (e.g., fourth ventricular ependymomas), subacute white matter lesions, as described previously for the brainstem, can occur in the cervicomedullary or upper cervical cord regions.[154] Although most subacute effects are transitory (white matter on MRI, Lhermitte syndrome of a shock-like sensation radiating down the extremities associated with neck flexion), such changes can be associated with significant neurologic signs and symptoms.

Frank postirradiation myelopathy can occur from 1 year to several years after treatment.[157] The traditional dogma concerning the pathogenesis of radiation myelopathy rests on postmitotic cell death in the endothelial cells or oligodendrocytes (or both).[148] Current concepts view radiation as producing cell death that, in turn, induces a complex pathophysiologic reaction in which the response of surviving cells may contribute to the impact of radiation on tissue integrity and functions. Cytokines, such as tumor necrosis factor and interleukin-6 (IL-6), appear to play important roles.[158] Also, some researchers suggest that the tolerance of the spinal cord is 5% to 10% lower in children than in adults.[158] Large fraction sizes (≥ 25 Gy) are disproportionately associated with untoward biologic effect on the spinal cord. An apparent volume relationship suggests that the dose to the spinal cord should be reduced when the irradiated length is large.[148] Results of primate studies indicated that an increase in treatment volume reduces the threshold and steepens the slope of the sigmoid dose-response curve for myelopathy.[158]

Cranial Nerves

Most cranial nerves are relatively resistant to radiation-induced damage. Two cranial nerves, the second (optic) and eighth (vestibulocochlear), are particularly worth mentioning in the radiation treatment of pediatric cancers. The optic nerve and visual pathway can be damaged during the delivery of therapeutic radiation to periorbital tumors (e.g., orbital rhabdomyosarcoma, optic glioma, paranasal, and nasopharyngeal tumors) and suprasellar tumors (e.g., craniopharyngioma, pituitary adenoma, germ cell tumor, hypothalamic-chiasmatic glioma).[159] The risk of radiation-induced optic neuropathy is related to total radiation dose, fraction size, and irradiated volume. No injuries were observed in 106 optic nerves that received a total dose of less than 59 Gy. The 15-year actuarial risk of optic neuropathy after a dose of greater than 60 Gy was 11% when treatment was administered in fraction sizes of less than 1.9 Gy, as compared with 47% when given in fraction sizes of greater than 1.9 Gy.[160]

The vestibular cochlear nerve and auditory apparatus must be considered in the delivery of high-dose radiation to posterior fossa tumors, such as medulloblastoma, ependymoma, and astrocytoma. Although the incidence of early ototoxicity is typically related to cisplatin delivery (and potentially enhanced when administered with or after irradiation), radiation exposure to more than 40 to 50 Gy is associated with a small but finite incidence of late radiation-induced ototoxicity, presumably as a late effect on vestibular nerves.[161,162] The combination of irradiation and cis-platinum may be associated with a greater incidence of ototoxicity, highlighting the importance of prospective audiologic studies in children with CNS tumors receiving both therapies.[163] To minimize the risk of hearing loss, some recommend a cumulative cochlear dose of less than 35 Gy for patients planned to receive 54 to 59.4 Gy in 30 to 33 treatment fractions.[162]

Retina

The retina, a specialized neural end organ supplied by an end-arterial system, is sensitive to vascular injury and has little ability for repair.[156] It is sensitive to radiation as well. Deterioration of vision, resulting from radiation-induced progressive obliteration of small retinal vessels, can occur 1.5 to 6.0 years after irradiation. The dose-response curve is steep (with increasing incidence at dose levels between 50 and 60 Gy), and 45 Gy produces a 5% risk of visual injury within 5 years.[147] Again, as the fraction size increases up to 2.5 Gy or more, the frequency of injury increases.[164]

Lens

The lens is one of the most radiosensitive organs, even to very low doses of radiation. For example, 1 Gy can lead to cataract formation. From total body irradiation data, the risk of developing a cataract requiring surgery was 20% for fractionated doses of 12 to 16 Gy.[165] The dose that could produce a 5% risk of damage to the lens within 5 years is 10 Gy.

Hypothalamic-Pituitary Axis

Irradiation of the region of the hypothalamus and pituitary gland can result in significant neuroendocrine abnormalities and long-term sequelae. This is especially important in children. The hormones affected include growth hormone (GH), thyroid-stimulating hormone, adrenocorticotropic hormone, and follicle-stimulating hormone and luteinizing hormone. The largest volume of data concerns the effect of cranial irradiation on GH production and release. Impaired serum GH response with provocative testing is apparent in 60% to 80% of children who have survived brain tumors.[129,166] A dose-response relationship is seen with a threshold of 18 to 25 Gy. The higher the dose of radiation, the earlier the GH deficiency occurs.

Deficiencies of other hypothalamic-pituitary hormones have also been described. The responsible irradiated site can be the hypothalamus, the pituitary, or both. Constine et al. have described non-GH abnormalities (thyroidal, gonadal, prolactin, and adrenal) in 20 children with brain tumors not involving the hypothalamic-pituitary region and treated with either cranial or craniospinal irradiation.[167] In patients receiving only cranial irradiation, the hypothalamic-pituitary region is estimated to receive a mean dose of 53.6 Gy (40 to 70 Gy).[167]

PRINCIPLES OF CHEMOTHERAPY

The role of chemotherapy in the treatment of childhood brain tumors has become increasingly important over the past several decades particularly for some of the embryonal (Chapter 26B) and low-grade glial neoplasms. The specific indications for chemotherapy in childhood CNS tumors are described in the respective tumor-specific sections.

Factors Influencing Drug Exposure in the Central Nervous System

The BBB and blood-CSF barrier are natural membrane barriers in the CNS that profoundly influence the penetration of most substances into the CNS. The BBB is located at the level of the endothelial lining of brain capillaries, whereas the blood-CSF barrier is located in the epithelium of the organs (e.g., choroid plexus, median eminence, and area postrema) that surround the ventricles. Metabolic enzymes and transporters such as P-glycoprotein, multidrug resistance-associated proteins (MRP1 and MRP3), and organic acid transporters that influence drug transport are not present in normal endothelial cells but are present in the endothelial cells of brain capillaries and may also be present in the epithelial cells at the level of the blood-CSF barrier.[168-172] Factors that influence CNS tumor penetration of an agent across the BBB include the physiochemical properties of the agent, the degree of protein binding, and the affinity of the agent for carriers that facilitate transport of endogenous compounds into the CNS. Characteristics that negatively impact BBB penetration include poor lipid solubility, significant ionization, and high protein or tissue binding.[173,174] The blood-tumor barrier is another important variable that may restrict the delivery of systemically administered chemotherapy to tumor tissue.[175-177]

These barriers to CNS drug delivery are not uniformly intact in brain tumors, as reflected by the intra- and intertumoral variability in the degree and the amount of tumor enhancement following administration of water-soluble contrast agents such as gadolinium. Thus, the commonly held notion that water-soluble chemotherapeutic agents are unlikely to be useful in the treatment of CNS tumors is not entirely correct. In fact, a number of compounds, such as the classic alkylators and the platinum analogues, are of clinical value in the treatment of some CNS tumors. Thus, there is controversy regarding the magnitude of the role of the BBB in the resistance of CNS tumors to chemotherapy.

Administration of drugs that increase the systemic clearance of those chemotherapeutic agents that are substrates for cytochrome P450 isoenzymes is another important variable that may negatively impact delivery of systemically administered agents to the CNS. Particularly relevant to patients with CNS tumors are the use of the enzyme-inducing anticonvulsants such as phenytoin or phenobarbital and the concomitant use of dexamethasone. For example, phenytoin has been shown to dramatically decrease the systemic exposure, and therefore equivalently decrease the CSF exposure, of agents such as topotecan and irinotecan.[178,179] Corticosteroids may also decrease CNS drug exposure both through induction of CYP3A4-mediated drug clearance and reduction in the transcapillary transport of various compounds. Another clinical variable that may impact CNS drug exposure is concomitant radiation therapy, which at higher doses may enhance drug exposure through increased transcapillary transport.[180,181] Increased drug exposure may result in enhanced cytotoxicity but also has the potential to increase neurotoxicity.

Drug Delivery Strategies

A variety of approaches have been employed to either disrupt or circumvent the BBB in an attempt to enhance drug delivery to the target tumor site(s) within the CNS. Some of these approaches include (a) BBB disruption with osmotic agents such as mannitol or vasoactive compounds such as the bradykinin analog labradimil (Cereport, RMP-7); (b) administration of very high-dose systemic chemotherapy; and (c) regional chemotherapy approaches (e.g., intrathecal therapy, intra-arterial therapy, intratumoral therapy using biodegradable polymers or convection enhanced delivery). Strategies using nanoparticles to circumvent the BBB are in development.

Blood-Brain Barrier Disruption

Osmotic opening of the BBB using infusions of hypertonic arabinose or mannitol can enhance the penetration of different agents into the CNS. Exposure of capillary endothelial cells to the hyperosmolar solution leads to cell shrinkage and stress on the tight junctions. This pulls the junctions apart, allowing increased capillary permeability. Although the effect is brief (generally reversible within 10 minutes), increases in CNS and CSF drug levels have been documented and correlated favorably with clinical responses in some but not all instances.[182–184] Although BBB disruption is feasible, the actual effectiveness remains uncertain. This approach has many drawbacks including the need for general anesthesia and intra-BBB catheterization. It may also be associated with profound and unpredictable side effects such as pulmonary embolus, stroke, visual loss, hearing loss, and seizures.[183] In addition, because the effects are nonspecific, that is, not limited to the tumor, this approach may be associated with an increased potential for neurotoxicity. Pediatric experience with osmotic BBB disruption is very limited and cannot be recommended outside of a clinical trial setting.

High-Dose Systemic Therapy

Tumors of the CNS may fail to respond to standard-dose chemotherapy as a result of inherent or acquired drug resistance or because of limited and/or heterogeneous drug exposure in the tumor tissue. In an attempt to overpower these resistance mechanisms and maximize the therapeutic potential for agents with a steep-dose response cure, the use of high-dose chemotherapy with autologous bone marrow or peripheral blood stem cell rescue has been explored by a number of investigators. The nitrosoureas, which are extremely lipophilic, were among the first agents to be studied using this approach. However, substantial dose escalations were not feasible owing to unacceptable neurologic toxicity.[185] Subsequent trials have used classic (cyclophosphamide, melphalan, and thiotepa) and nonclassic (carboplatin) alkylating agents, often combined with etoposide.

High-dose systemic chemotherapy approaches in children with CNS tumors have been most widely evaluated in infants, for whom postponement of radiation therapy is desirable because of its potential late neurologic toxicities, and in patients with recurrent tumors. Feasibility has been clearly demonstrated and encouraging results have been seen in patients with medulloblastoma,[186,187] supratentorial PNET,[188,189] and germ cell tumors, as well as in infants with embryonal tumors (see Chapter 26B). Clinical trials wherein these regimens are compared prospectively with those using standard-dose chemotherapy have not been performed. The high-dose chemotherapy experience in children with gliomas, including those of the brainstem, has been less promising.[190–191] Patients who appear most likely to benefit from this approach are those with minimal disease at entry into myeloablative therapy, those whose tumors have shown response to standard-dose chemotherapy, and those with little prior exposure to chemotherapy.[194] The optimal timing of this approach, either as a consolidative or a salvage treatment, remains uncertain, particularly as primary chemotherapy regimens are intensified. There are no prospectively established indications for this approach, which at the present time should continue to be limited to clinical trial settings.

Regional Chemotherapy

Intrathecal Chemotherapy. Delivery of drug directly into the intrathecal space, through either a lumbar puncture or a ventricular reservoir, is a form of regional chemotherapy designed to circumvent the limited penetration of most systemically administered agents across the blood-brain and blood-CSF barriers. This approach has been successfully utilized in the frontline treatment of childhood CNS leukemias and lymphomas. The primary advantage of intrathecal chemotherapy is that very high drug exposures can be attained in the CSF using a relatively small drug dose because the initial volume of distribution in the CSF is very small relative to that of plasma. As a result, total drug exposure is lower, minimizing the potential for systemic toxicity. A primary limitation to this approach is that drug penetration into the brain parenchyma or tumor is only a few millimeters, which limits the utility for patients with either parenchymal or bulky leptomeningeal disease.[195] Another limitation to intrathecal therapy, particularly in patients with CNS tumors, include the fact that distribution throughout the neuraxis is uneven.[196] This is particularly problematic for patients with hydrocephalus, ventriculoperitoneal shunts, or bulky leptomeningeal disease. Intrathecal therapy should not be administered to patients with abnormal CSF flow dynamics because of the potential for increased neurotoxicity and/or decreased efficacy.

Unfortunately, there are a limited number of anticancer drugs, specifically methotrexate, cytarabine, and hydrocortisone, that are specifically available for intrathecal use. Although these agents utilized are routinely used for hematologic malignancies, they have historically played a role in the treatment of childhood CNS tumors. Results of a trial of postoperative chemotherapy, including intraventricular methotrexate, showed excellent overall survival for children with desmoplastic medulloblastoma,[197] the role for that the intrathecal component of that therapy played in this outcome has not been defined. The U.S. Pediatric Brain Tumor Consortium (PBTC) has completed a trail to evaluate feasibility of intrathecal drug delivery in infants with newly diagnosed embryonal CNS tumors using intrathecal mafosfamide, a preactivated cyclophosphamide derivative, as one component of the frontline therapy of infants with newly diagnosed embryonal tumors.[198] Results of this trial are forthcoming.

Intratumoral Chemotherapy. Another strategy to enhance intratumoral delivery of therapeutic agents involves direct administration of the agent into the tumor bed. This approach has been extensively evaluated in adults with recurrent high-grade gliomas using microencapsulated, drug-loaded, biodegradable polymers that are implanted into the tumor tissue or tumor cavity at the time of surgery. The agent Gliadel™, a polymeric "wafer" impregnated with BCNU (carmustine), passively diffuses from the polymer over a period of several weeks, thereby providing high drug concentrations to the tumor tissue or tumor bed while minimizing systemic drug exposure. This approach has resulted in a modest prolongation of survival in adults with recurrent or newly diagnosed (median increase from 11.6 to 13.9 months) high-grade gliomas.[199] Trials in adults that evaluated the use of surgically implanted BCNU wafers administered in conjunction with radiotherapy[200] or systemic O[6]-benzylguanine, to counteract one of the primary mechanisms of BCNU-mediated drug resistance, specifically increased alkylguanyl alkyl-transferase activity, showed the therapy was well tolerated.[201,202] In one retrospective series in which newly diagnosed patients received Gliadel™, temozolomide, and radiation following surgery, the median survival was 21 months.[203] This approach has not been prospectively evaluated in children.

An alternate approach to intratumoral therapy, which is better suited for the delivery of larger molecules, involves the direct infusion of a soluble agent into the tumor using an implanted catheter connected to an external infusion pump. High concentrations of a therapeutic agent are provided to the tumor and peritumoral brain tissue as a result of bulk flow of the agent through the interstitial spaces of the brain. Interstitial drug delivery (also known as convection-enhanced delivery or intracerebral clysis) has been anecdotally applied to the delivery of conventional chemotherapeutic agents, such as BCNU or carmustine and docetaxel,[204] or to mutated toxin genes conjugated to ligands that target receptors (e.g., EGFR, transferrin receptor, IL-13 receptor) expressed at levels higher within the brain tumor than in the surrounding normal brain.[205,206] The toxin component of the conjugate, such as diphtheria toxin and *Pseudomonas* exotoxin, contains mutations within the domains necessary for cell internalization, which restricts toxin entry to those cells that express the receptor for the ligand conjugate.[207] Because each of the receptors that have been targeted to date is expressed also on cells outside the CNS, the infusion approach to delivery minimizes the concentration of toxin that reaches other "vulnerable" cells while maximizing the amounts that are delivered to the tumor. Most recently, investigators have reported the use of interstitial photodynamic therapy with stereotactically implanted light diffusers in patients with recurrent nonresectable malignant gliomas.[208]

Interarterial Therapy. In theory, intra-arterial delivery of chemotherapy for CNS tumors offers the potential for achieving higher drug concentrations in the tumor bed without a concomitant increase in systemic exposure and toxicity. The best candidates for this approach are agents that are rapidly cleared after systemic administration or that are metabolized or inactivated after their first pass through the liver. Although the use of intra-arterial nitrosoureas and cisplatin has resulted in a modest number of clinical responses, there is not yet a demonstrated clinical benefit to routine intra-arterial drug delivery.[209–211] A potential disadvantage to this approach is that drug penetration into normal brain tissue appears to increase as well, resulting in focal neurologic toxicity, particularly to the retina.[212,213] Some of the other observed toxicities may have been due to nonuniform mixing of drug and blood at the infusion site, resulting in "streaming" during arterial delivery and to exposure of the brain to alcohol-containing diluents.[213,214]

Novel Agents and Approaches

Differentiating Agents

The potential utility of differentiating agents, such as retinoic acid and inhibitors of histone deacetylase (phenylbutyrate, valproic acid, depsipeptide, and suberoylanilide hydroxamic acid [SAHA]), in the treatment of pediatric brain tumors, has been demonstrated preclinically.[215–218] *In vitro* studies suggested, in addition to inducing differentiation and suppressing tumor growth,[215,219–223] that these agents may also cause a direct apoptotic effect.[224] Current or recently completed investigations with histone deacetylase inhibitors include a phase I studies of valproic acid, which has also been shown to enhance nuclear receptor activity through mitogen-activated protein kinase (MAPK) activation,[225,226] and phase I and II trials of newer generation histone deacetylase inhibitors such as depsipeptide[227] and SAHA with and without *cis*-retinoic acid.[228] Phase II trials that incorporated valproic acid or SAHA either alone or in combination with retinoic acid are in development for children with newly diagnosed high-grade gliomas, including brainstem gliomas.

Antiangiogenic Agents

Abnormal angiogenesis has been implicated in the development of many tumor types including brain tumors and presents an attractive strategy for the targeted development of new anticancer agents. Antiangiogenic agents have been evaluated in adults with high-grade glioma. Bevacizumab is the most promising to date with demonstrated antitumor activity in adults with recurrent high-grade gliomas when administered with or without irinotecan.[229,230] The U.S. Food and Drug Administration granted accelerative approval for bevacizumab as a single agent in adults with progressive glioblastoma multiforme in 2009. Studies evaluating the antitumor activity of bevacizumab in children with recurrent[231] or newly diagnosed high-grade gliomas and other CNS tumors are ongoing. Among the other antiangiogenic agents that have been studied in children with brain tumors are SU5416, a small molecule inhibitor of vascular endothelial growth factor (VEGF),[232] and thalidomide.[233] Phase I or II trials of lenalidomide,[234] cediranib, and enzastaurin are ongoing. Although antiangiogenesis represents an exciting area of new drug development, it is too early to know whether any of these antiangiogenic agents will ultimately have a place in the treatment of childhood brain tumors. Some investigators have suggested that antiangiogenic therapy targeted against the VEGF pathway elicits tumor cell adaptation with resultant increased local invasion and distant metastasis.[235]

Small Molecule Inhibitors

There is increasing knowledge about the underlying molecular biology of pediatric CNS tumors, particularly with respect to aberrant signal transduction pathways. A number of small molecule inhibitors for abnormal signaling pathways are currently in various stages of preclinical and clinical development, particularly agents that inhibit receptor tyrosine kinase pathways. Some of the agents that have recently been evaluated in cooperative groups are briefly discussed.

Imatinib, which competitively inhibits the bcr-abl tyrosine kinase that results from the Philadelphia (9,22) chromosome translocation in chronic myelogenous leukemia, also inhibits platelet-derived growth factor receptor (PDGF-R), stem cell factor receptor, and *c-kit*-mediated signaling.[236] Because aberrant PDGF-mediated signaling may play a role in brain tumors, particularly gliomas,[237] trials with imatinib were pursued in children with newly diagnosed brainstem gliomas. In the PBTC phase I trial of imatinib, commencing approximately 4 weeks after completion of XRT, drug was well tolerated. However, intratumoral hemorrhages, primarily asymptomatic, were observed in 3 of 16 children with brainstem glioma.[238] The role of imatinib in the development of intratumoral hemorrhage is unknown.

ERBB is another receptor tyrosine kinase family that has been shown to play a role in critical cell cycle functions involved in proliferation, apoptosis, migration, survival, and differentiation.[239-243] ERBB1 amplification and overexpression have been demonstrated in pediatric high-grade gliomas and brainstem gliomas.[47,244] Likewise coexpression of ERB2 and ERB4 plus a high proliferative index as determined by the Ki-67 labeling index are associated with an aggressive tumor phenotype in pediatric ependymomas.[245] Pediatric phase I and II clinical trials of a number of ERBB inhibitors have recently been completed or are being developed, including trials of gefitinib (ZD-1839), erlotinib (OSI-774), and lapatinib.[246-248]

Farnesyltransferase inhibitors (FTIs) such as tipifarnib have also been recently evaluated in glial tumors. FTIs impede Ras functions such as promotion of oncogenesis and radiation resistance either through direct blockade of Ras function or by interrupting the effects of tyrosine kinase receptors that signal through Ras.[249] Glioma cells that overexpress EGFR have shown enhanced sensitivity to FTI treatment and can sensitize glioma cells to irradiation.[250] A phase I trial of tipifarnib plus radiation was performed by the PBTC[251] and a subsequent phase II trial in children with brainstem gliomas was recently completed.

Immunotherapy

The CNS is a relatively immunologically privileged site. The brain lacks defined lymphatic drainage,[252] the expression of major histocompatibility complex antigens is low,[253] and the BBB limits the interaction of the peripheral host immune system and the brain.[254] Nevertheless, the privilege is not absolute. For example, patterns of allogeneic and xenogeneic tissue transplant rejection from immunologically naive[255] and non-naive brains[256] suggest that peripheral T-cell activity may be carried into the CNS.[257]

Immunotherapy of CNS tumors is based on the hypothesis that stimulation of the immune system, or blocking of the immunosuppressive effects of tumors, might enhance an antitumor response. Immunotherapy has been studied primarily in the preclinical setting and some preliminary adult phase I studies of patients with malignant gliomas have been performed.[258]

Pediatric data are in their very early stages. Strategies of immunotherapy are based on eliciting systemic antitumor immune responses that are carried into the CNS and on inducing a primary immune response in the brain itself. Adults with malignant gliomas are known to have, to some degree, altered immunity, owing to effects on T-cell proliferation, natural killer cell activity, and immunoglobulin production. The current thought is that these effects most likely are due to production of transforming growth factor β. These observations form the basis for another immunotherapy strategy that of decreasing tumorigenicity of malignant gliomas by blocking the immunosuppressive effects of transforming growth factor β. A variety of approaches have been studied: administration of cytokines, such as interleukins and interferons; delivery of monoclonal antibodies; and the use of cancer vaccines.

The majority of CNS tumor vaccines are currently being developed for high-grade glial tumors. Strategies for vaccination include the use of cytokine-transfected tumor cells, adoptive transfer of tumor-activated T-cells, and antigen-pulsed dendritic cell vaccines. A randomized trial that incorporates a vaccine against the EGFR variant III (EGFRIII) mutation commonly found in adult glioblastomas is ongoing in adults; however, this is not a widely identified mutation in high-grade gliomas of childhood. An approach that utilizes adoptive transfer of HER2-specific T cells has shown marked activity in preclinical studies of both gliomas and medulloblastomas and will soon enter early phase clinical trials.[259]

Interferons show cytostatic and cytotoxic effects on human glioma cell lines. However, phase I and phase II clinical trials of interferon-α and interferon-β to boost systemic immune responses against intracranial tumors have yielded clinical responses in only a minority of patients.[260-262] In addition, clinical trials of interferon-γ, which is a much more potent inducer of major histocompatibility complex class I and II antigen expression, have demonstrated unacceptable toxicities with little clinical benefit.[263,264] Although the interferons appear to have anti-CNS tumor properties, their clinical potential has not yet been realized.

IL-2, a cytokine that can increase the antitumor activity of T cells and natural killer cells, has been used in the treatment of melanoma and renal cell carcinoma. Systemic and intratumoral administration of IL-2 to boost the antitumor cellular immune response of patients with malignant gliomas has resulted in significant neurotoxicity, primarily from cerebral edema, and in little clinical benefit.[254] Adoptive immunotherapy using IL-2 and lymphokine-activated killer cells has resulted in inconsistent clinical and neurotoxic effects.[265,266] IL-2 and tumor-infiltrating lymphocytes appear to have activity against CNS tumors *in vitro* and in extracerebral sites but not in the brain.[265,266] In yet another adoptive approach, stable disease and prolonged survival, albeit with disease, were demonstrated in an adult phase I clinical trial of cytotoxic T-lymphocyte therapy for patients with primary or recurrent malignant gliomas.[267] Taken together, these data indicate an *in vitro* antitumor potential of adoptive immunotherapy of CNS tumors that has yet to be fully realized in the clinical setting.

A potential role for monoclonal antibodies in the diagnosis and treatment of brain tumors also has been investigated. Systemically administered radionuclide-conjugated antibodies have prolonged survival in mice with human glioma xenografts, but human applications of these products have shown only limited efficacy. Although disrupted by tumor, the BBB may be sufficiently intact as to block penetration of large-molecular-weight antibodies. The application of these products currently is limited by tumor heterogeneity and rapid immune antibody clearance and, for radioconjugated antibody therapy, by dehalogenation and loss of radionuclides and excessive radiation to nontarget tissues.[268] Intrathecal or intraventricular delivery of monoclonal products may bypass some of the limitations of systemic administration. Such studies are limited but promising.[269,270]

Gene Transfer

Gene transfer therapy, the process through which genetic material is transferred into cells for the purpose of eliciting a therapeutic response, is a new and innovative approach to the treatment of brain tumors and of other malignancies and disease processes (see Chapter 14). The gene of interest generally is transferred to the target brain or tumor cell using a virus-mediated delivery system. The postmitotic environment of the CNS tissue may offer an advantage over other tissues in that it may allow more specific targeting of the viral vectors to only mitotically active tumor. Cell killing by transferred genes may occur directly through cellular toxins or indirectly through the expression of drug-mediating enzymes.[271] The therapeutic response of gene therapy can be through immunomodulation or antiangiogenesis as well.[257]

The herpes simplex virus thymidine kinase type 1 (HSV-Tk1) gene is a type of suicide gene that can be transferred to tumor cells. When exposed to systemically administered ganciclovir, the gene product causes phosphorylation of the drug that results in death not only of transfected tumor cells but of surrounding tumor cells.[257] Packer et al. demonstrated the feasibility of HSV-Tk1 gene therapy in children with recurrent supratentorial malignant brain tumors, although significant toxicities including seizures, headache, lethargy, weakness, cerebral edema, and symptoms of increased ICP occurred in 4 of 12 patients.[272] All of these toxicities resolved spontaneously or with a short course of glucocorticoid therapy.

Although preclinical and early clinical data support a potential role for gene therapy against CNS tumors, the majority of work at the present time is focused on the vaccine approaches outlined earlier.

Clinical Trials Groups

The use of chemotherapy for CNS tumors now is commonplace and, for specific tumors, is considered the standard of care (as discussed in later sections). The COG, consisting of pediatric cancer programs from North America, Europe, and Australia, conducts numerous clinical trials of chemotherapy for nearly every brain tumor type and for children of all ages. New agents, or new schedules of established agents, are studied in clinical trials for the primary therapy of newly diagnosed disease or as treatment for recurrent disease. Extensive correlative biologic and genomic studies are being conducted by COG investigators in several tumor types. Similar national and international cooperative groups exist worldwide. In 1999, the National Cancer Institute also established the PBTC, which is composed of eight member institutions that collectively diagnose disease and treat a large proportion of U.S. children with primary brain tumors. The objectives of the PBTC are to rapidly evaluate new therapeutic agents and treatment strategies for children with high-risk CNS tumors. The PBTC has a dedicated neuroimaging consortium to pilot new imaging techniques for CNS tumors. Results from PBTC studies are made available to the COG and other international cooperative groups for confirmatory testing in larger phase II and phase III studies.

Physicians and interested families can learn more about investigational chemotherapy protocols by contacting any of these cooperative groups or by contacting foundations that support pediatric brain tumor research. Details are presented at the end of this chapter in section "Information on Clinical Trials."

EPENDYMOMA

Demography

Ependymomas, which constitute approximately 10% of all primary CNS tumors in children, usually arise within or adjacent to the ependymal lining of the ventricular system or the central canal of the spinal cord. Ninety percent of the tumors are intracranial, and up to two-thirds of these occur in the posterior fossa. In children younger than 3 years, more than 85% of tumors may occur in the posterior fossa.[273] The highest incidence of ependymoma in children occurs in the first 7 years of life, with a second peak in the third to fifth decades of life.[274] Although in the past, the ratio of male to female patients was reported to be near unity, contemporary series report a male-to-female ratio of between 1.3 and 2.0.[275–277]

Imaging

Ependymomas may be supratentorial or infratentorial in location. Within the posterior fossa, they are the fourth most common posterior fossa tumor in children, following medulloblastoma, cerebellar astrocytoma, and brainstem glioma. Ependymomas arise from ependymal cells lining the ventricles; they grow out of the fourth ventricle via the foramina of Luschka and Magendie into the cisterna magna, basilar cisterns, cerebellopontine angles, and through the foramen magnum into the upper cervical canal around the spinal cord. On CT scans, the tumor has a mixed density, with punctate calcification in 50% of cases, and variable enhancement. These tumors are heterogeneous on MR reflecting a combination of solid component, cyst, calcification, necrosis, edema, or hemorrhage. On T1-weighted images, ependymomas are usually hypointense, and on T2-weighted images, the mass is often isointense to gray matter with foci of dark T2 signal related to calcification or blood and foci of bright T2 signal related to cyst or necrosis within the tumor. Following contrast administration, there is heterogeneous enhancement in the tumor.

CT scans of supratentorial ependymomas tumors reveal a heterogeneous mass with calcification and cyst formation. On MR imaging, these tumors are heterogeneous containing cysts, calcification, and occasional hemorrhage as well as irregular, heterogeneous enhancement with gadolinium.

Pathology and Patterns of Spread

Ependymomas are typically soft, tan masses with well-demarcated borders that may have areas of calcification, hemorrhage, and cysts. Microscopically, the classical pattern is a monomorphic nuclear morphology with round to oval nuclei. A key histological feature is the perivascular pseudorosette, which is characterized by tumor cell processes converging on vessels, creating a perivascular fibrillary zone (Fig. 26A.6). Less commonly, the true ependymal rosette, composed of radially aligned columnar cells about a central lumen, is present. The following histopathological variants of ependymoma can be distinguished: cellular, papillary, clear cells, and tanycytic. There is also a myxopapillary variant, which is a slowly growing tumor almost exclusively located in the region of the conus medullaris and filum terminale of the spinal cord.[278]

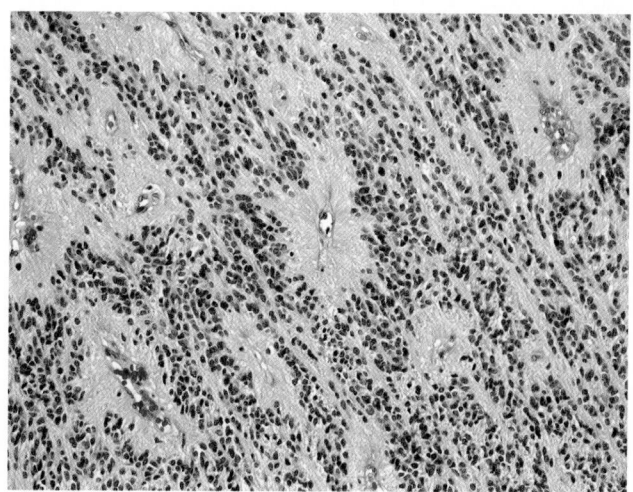

FIGURE 26A.6 Section from a fourth ventricular ependymoma displaying typical perivascular pseudorosettes. (H&E, ×200, ×.)

Ependymomas vary from well-differentiated tumors with no anaplasia, rare or absent mitoses and little polymorphism to highly cellular lesions with brisk mitotic activity, anaplasia, microvascular proliferation, and pseudopalisading necrosis. The former are low-grade tumors (WHO grade II) and the latter are high-grade, anaplastic tumors (WHO grade III).[58] Although the impact of histology on disease behavior and outcome has been debated for two decades, some contemporary reviews suggest a significant correlation between anaplastic histology and a higher rate of disease recurrence.[279,280]

Ependymomas are locally invasive tumors that spread contiguously into adjacent brain. Tumors arising in the posterior fossa frequently infiltrate the brainstem. In as many as one-third of these cases, tumor may project through the foramina of Luschka and/or Magendie to involve the cerebellopontine angle and upper spinal canal.[281] The incidence of spinal subarachnoid dissemination has been estimated to be 7% to 12%, most commonly occurring in high-grade and posterior fossa tumors.[274,282] Systemic metastases are rare and, when present, show a predilection for liver, lung, and bone.

Biology

By comparing the gene expression profiles of developing tissues and ependymoma subsets, Taylor et al. identified populations of cells in the CNS that might act as the cells of origin of ependymomas.[41] In an analysis of more than 100 ependymomas, they found that tumor subsets exhibit distinct patterns of gene expression and regions of chromosome gain and loss that correlate with the anatomic location of the tumor (supratentorial region, posterior fossa, or spine). Gene expression signatures that most discriminated supratentorial, posterior fossa, and spinal ependymoma included many genes that are known regulators of neural precursor cells in the corresponding region of the CNS. For example, supratentorial ependymomas express markedly elevated levels of members of the EPHB-EPHRIN and NOTCH cell signal systems that play key roles in maintaining normal neural stem cells in the cerebral subventricular zone.[283,284]

Conversely, spinal ependymomas expressed multiple Homeobox (HOX) family members that coordinate anteroposterior tissue patterning and development of the spine.[285]

In situ hybridization and immunofluorescence mapped the site of expression of ependymoma signature genes in the developing mouse to embryonic radial glia (RG) that are neural progenitor cells and the source of adult neural stem cells.[286,287] Importantly, this same study showed that self-renewing and multipotent CSCs isolated from fresh samples of ependymoma are bipolar RG-like cells that express the CD133+/Nestin+/RC2+/BLBP+ immunophenotype of RG and are both required and sufficient to generate tumors *in vivo*. These data suggest a new hypothesis for the origin of ependymoma, that is, that RG in different parts of the CNS are predisposed to acquire distinct genetic abnormalities that transform these cells into CSC of supratentorial, posterior fossa, and spinal ependymoma.

Prognostic Considerations

The single most important prognostic factor that emerges from review of single- and multi-institutional experience with ependymoma is the extent of tumor resection. Whether gauged by the surgeon's estimate or measured by postoperative MRI, the survival rate is higher following a gross total (66% to 75%) versus a less complete resection (0% to 11%). Perhaps related to degree of resection has been the finding in some series that location of primary intracranial tumor and patient age are prognostic.[288,289] However, these data are inconsistent with the exception of ependymomas of the spinal cord, which are associated with the best outcome. Younger children are more likely to have tumors arising from the posterior fossa, and in this location, tumors tend to be more invasive, making a GTR more difficult. However, when lower age (<2 to 4 years) has been found to have a negative impact on survival, it appears to be confounded by the fact that lower radiations doses were typically administered to these younger patients. Finally, histologic subtype, particularly anaplastic ependymoma, has inconsistently been associated with a worse prognosis versus that for patients with a well-differentiated ependymoma. Because this factor has seemed to be an important prognostic variable in larger studies, especially those with consistent central neuropathology review, it is being examined prospectively as a therapeutic stratification variable in the ongoing COG ACNS0121 study.

Emerging genomic data suggest that chromosomal alterations might help in the classification of ependymomas and provide leads concerning their initiation and progression.[290,291] A recent array CGH analysis revealed a significant increase in genomic imbalances in relapsed versus primary ependymomas, such as gain of 9qter and 1q and loss of 6q.[291] Gain of 9qter (including the *NOTCH1* locus) was associated with tumor recurrence, age older than 3 years, and posterior fossa location. Interestingly, overexpression of NOTCH1 ligands and *NOTCH1* missense mutations were also observed in posterior fossa tumors, and this study suggested that inhibition of the NOTCH pathway might impair ependymoma CSC proliferation.

Treatment

Surgery

Techniques for the resection of posterior fossa ependymomas are similar to those used for resecting medulloblastoma (Chapter 26B), although the rationale for intraoperative monitoring of evoked potentials and cranial electromyography may be even greater because of the higher frequency of brainstem infiltration. Supratentorial ependymomas, often located subcortically, are resected in a fashion similar to that used in other deep-seated gliomas (described further on).

The prognostic benefit of complete tumor resection has been stated. However, such a result has been feasible in only approximately 50% to 66% of ependymomas in most series. GTRs generally are more difficult for posterior fossa ependymomas than for supratentorial ependymomas because of the propensity for infratentorial lesions to infiltrate the brainstem and to surround cranial nerves and vessels lateral and ventral to the brainstem, precluding complete removal without unacceptable neurologic morbidity. Infants are particularly likely to have large infratentorial ependymomas with significant ventrolateral extension, which in part accounts for their less favorable prognosis in most series.[292–294] In such patients, multiple lower cranial nerve palsies as a result of both tumor and surgery often necessitate a tracheostomy and gastric feeding device. Resolution (if any) of neurologic impairment may be delayed for several weeks to months.[294] Because the prognosis in children with incompletely resected ependymomas is so poor, several recent treatment protocols have selectively incorporated second-look surgery in children with objective evidence of residual disease after an initial procedure. This generally has been attempted after a short course of neoadjuvant chemotherapy, administered in the hope of reducing the vascularity and invasiveness of the residual disease. A multi-institutional study, designed to examine the ability of this approach to improve outcome in such children without an unacceptable trade-off of morbidity, was recently conducted in the COG ACNS0121, and those results should be forthcoming in the near future.

Radiation Therapy

Local postoperative radiation therapy has increased the overall survival rates of patients with ependymoma from 50% to 73% at 5 years to 85%.[295] The indications for radiation therapy are strongly supported in the literature; only among differentiated supratentorial ependymomas[296,297] and intramedullary spinal cord or cauda equina ependymomas[298,299] is there suggestive data indicating that patients with a GTR may not require postoperative irradiation.

Posterior fossa tumors are frequently intertwined with cranial nerves or adherent to the pontomedullary region and/or the cerebellopontine angle. Thus, resection is typically followed by local irradiation to include the tumor bed. In addition, attention to potential extension into the foramina of Luschka or below the foramen magnum along the cervical spinal cord is critical in targeting ependymomas.

Long-standing debate regarding the appropriate volume for radiation therapy has shifted from identifying cases that might require craniospinal irradiation to diminishing the target volume from cranial compartments to the tumor/operative bed.[300–301] An image-guided approach using 3D-CRT (with narrow [1 cm] margins around the tumor/operative bed defining the CTV) to 59.6 Gy has shown excellent tolerance and disease control.[161]

A large prospective study of 153 children with localized ependymomas (56% anaplastic) highlights the benefit of gross-total resection and conformal, high-dose, postoperative radiation (59.4 Gy with a 10 mm margin around the target volume).[295] Seven-year local control, event-free survival, and overall survival rates were 87.3%, 69.1%, and 81.0%, respectively. Of note is the very favorable 85% 5-year event-free survival rate for children with gross-total resection and immediate postoperative radiation, without chemotherapy. Of note, this trial included children younger than 3 years. The authors suggest that consideration be given to higher doses of radiation since, despite promising results, cumulative incidence of local failure was nevertheless high at 16%. This study also sheds light on the proportion of local versus metastatic failures. As local control has improved, the percentage of metastatic recurrences increased and was influenced by anaplastic histology only. Thus, systemic therapy or extended radiation fields may be considered in the future if those with higher risk of metastatic recurrence are identified.

Chemotherapy

Single- and multiagent chemotherapeutic regimens have been used in ependymoma therapy; however, despite the demonstrated activity of various multiagent regimens, the use of chemotherapy has not improved the overall survival for older children with either completely or incompletely resected ependymoma.[302,303] Similarly, chemotherapy does not have a demonstrated role for children with recurrent ependymoma.[304,305] In contrast, Fouladi and colleagues recently reported that infants with localized ependymoma who had a GTR followed by a carboplatin-based chemotherapy regimen had a 5-year progression-free survival of 57 ± 17%.[306] The contribution of the chemotherapy to survival is not known. Thus, for older children, chemotherapy is recommended only as part of a clinical trial. The recently completed COG ACNS0121 trial will provide data as to whether two cycles of multiagent chemotherapy in patients with subtotal resections will make their tumors more amenable to a GTR prior to the initiation of CRT.

LOW-GRADE GLIOMAS

Low-grade glial neoplasms are a diverse group of tumors that include JPA, fibrillary (also called protoplasmic or diffuse) astrocytoma, oligodendroglioma, ganglioglioma, and such mixed tumors as oligoastrocytoma. Their unifying features are their generally slowly evolving, clinical behavior, and relatively benign histological appearance. In general, high rates of long-term survival are characteristic as well, despite low but steady rates of disease progression even 10 years from diagnosis.[307] Optic pathway tumors (OPTs) are generally low-grade glial neoplasms that are not routinely biopsied. As a result of their unique location and association with NF1, these tumors will be discussed in a separate section.

Demography

Cerebellar astrocytomas are the most prevalent, representing 15% to 25% of all CNS tumors, followed in prevalence by cerebral hemispheric astrocytomas and tumors of deep midline structures (each representing 10% to 15% of all CNS tumors) and tumors of the optic pathway (accounting for approximately 5% of all CNS tumors).[308] Seventy to 75% of cerebellar astrocytomas occur in childhood.[309,310] The average age at diagnosis ranges from 6.5 to 9.0 years.[311–313] Boys are affected more commonly than are girls.[314] Neuraxis dissemination of low-grade gliomas from any location in the brain is distinctly uncommon, occurring in only approximately 5% of cases.[315,316] Tumors arising from the hypothalamus and periventricular areas may be more likely to disseminate.

Imaging

Pilocytic Astrocytoma

Pilocytic astrocytomas in the infratentorium can occur in the midline or in the cerebellar hemispheres. These tumors may be associated with hydrocephalus due to compression of the aqueduct or fourth ventricle. They classically appear as a cerebellar mass consisting of a large cyst with a solid tumor nodule. However, on imaging, they may present with a wide spectrum of appearances including cystic, solid, or a mix of cystic and solid. The solid, enhancing component of cerebellar pilocytic astrocytomas has greater ADC values than other pediatric cerebellar tumors such as ependymoma, rhabdoid tumor, and medulloblastoma.[317]

MRS of these tumors has demonstrated high lactate concentrations and consistently high Cho content and Cho/NAA and Cho/Cr ratios despite the benign clinical course of this tumor type.[318]

Supratentorial pilocytic astrocytomas within the cerebral hemispheres are typically well demarcated with the T2 signal abnormality matching the amount of gadolinium enhancement, occasionally presenting with an associated cyst; however, solid enhancement can occur.

Ganglioglioma

The temporal lobe is by the far the most common location of these tumors, followed by the parietal lobe, frontal lobe, occipital lobe, third ventricle, and hypothalamus. The cerebellum, brainstem, and spinal cord can also be affected.

On standard CT scans, these tumors tend have low attenuation (38%), followed in decreasing order of frequency as mixed attenuation (32%), isodense (15%), or hyperdense (15%).[319] Calcification is seen in approximately 35% to 50% of the time. Contrast enhancement can be seen in the solid component of the lesion. When located peripherally, erosion of the adjacent of inner table of calvarium may be present. On standard MR examinations, these tumors tend to have a variable and nonspecific appearance. In general, they typically appear hypointense to isointense relative to gray matter on short TR images and hyperintense to gray matter on long TR images. They also tend to be solid or mixed solid and cystic in nature, and the solid elements usually, but not always, enhance. It is interesting to also note that gangliogliomas demonstrate high cerebral blood volume, which helps to differentiate them from other low-grade gliomas.[320]

Oligodendroglioma

Oligodendrogliomas account for approximately 2% to 5% of all brain neoplasms and less than 1% of all pediatric CNS neoplasms. These lesions are primarily supratentorial in the frontal or temporal lobes. On standard CT scans, these tumors typically appear as either hypodense or isodense masses with the majority containing coarse calcifications. Cystic degeneration, hemorrhage, and remodeling of the adjacent calvarium may all be seen. Enhancement is variable with up to 50% showing enhancement. On standard MRI examinations, oligodendrogliomas typically are heterogenous in nature and are mostly hypointense on T1-weighted images and hyperintense on T2-weighted images compared with gray matter. As on CT, heterogenous enhancement may be seen. The presence of enhancement tends to be seen in more aggressive oligodendrogliomas, but this is not significantly sensitive. Recent studies have shown that increased cerebral blood volume seen on perfusion imaging in combination with elevated Cho/Cr ratios on MR spectroscopy yields a higher accuracy in differentiating high-grade and low-grade oligodendrogliomas.[321]

Dysembryoplastic Neuroepithelial Tumors

DNETs commonly present with partial complex seizures in young adults and children. These tumors present in a supratentorial location with the majority found in the temporal lobe followed by the frontal lobe. On standard CT scans, they typically appear as well-demarcated, lobulated cortical masses that are hypodense compared with white matter without associated edema. Occasionally, there are areas of calcification (~20%), and if peripherally located, remodeling of the adjacent inner table of the skull may be seen.[322]

On standard MR examinations, DNETs tumors typically appear as cortical masses that are hypointense on T1-weighted images and hyperintense on T2-weighted images without associated surrounding vasogenic edema. They will enhance in approximately one-third of cases, usually in a nodular pattern.

Desmoplastic Infantile Ganglioglioma

Desmoplastic infantile gangliogliomas (DIGs), rare intracranial tumors that contain abnormal ganglion and glial cells, occur supratentorially with a predilection for the frontal and parietal lobes.[323] On standard CT scans, these tumors typically appear as a large cystic lesion with a superficial solid component that is slightly hyperdense and enhances strongly after contrast administration. Calcification and hemorrhage are uncommon. On standard MRI examinations, these tumors typically present with a large cystic component that is hypointense on T1-weighted images and hyperintense on T2-weighted images, and a smaller peripheral solid component which is generally isointense to gray matter on T1- and T2-weighted images. As on CT, the solid component intensely enhances after contrast administration and this enhancement usually involves the leptomeninges.

Pathology and Patterns of Spread

Classifications, such as that of Kernohan, St. Anne/Mayo, and WHO, identify low-grade glial tumors primarily on the basis of their cellularity or degree of anaplasia rather than on histological type. Neoplasms that are only modestly cellular and contain few or none of the histological criteria of malignancy are designated as low-grade or grade I and grade II lesions in these classifications. The WHO brain tumor classification uses the grade I designation for pilocytic astrocytomas and grade I or grade II for the neuronal and mixed neuronal-glial tumors. The diffuse astrocytomas (fibrillary, gemistocytic, or protoplasmic) that make up most adult low-grade lesions are designated as grade II as are oligodendrogliomas and oligoastrocytomas.[58] Grade III and IV tumors are high-grade lesions characterized by aggressive clinical behavior and malignant histology (considered separately in section "Supratentorial High-Grade Gliomas"). Although the utility of such grading systems has been questioned because of their subjective nature and their reliance on often small biopsies from tumors that may be heterogeneous, these systems remain popular because applying and understanding them is simple and because they have some prognostic value.

Supratentorial Low-Grade Gliomas

Most supratentorial low-grade gliomas are astrocytomas, a diverse group of neoplasms generally composed of GFAP-positive bipolar or stellate cells. Such designations as fibrillary, protoplasmic, gemistocytic, xanthomatous, and pilocytic often are used to describe the appearance of the astrocytes and their various histological patterns.[324,325] Only the pilocytic and fibrillary astrocytoma are seen commonly in children.

Pilomyxoid astrocytomas (PMAs) are closely related to pilocytic astrocytomas. In contrast to the typical biphasic pattern of pilocytic astrocytomas, PMAs have an angiocentric arrangement of monomorphous bipolar cells in a loose fibrillary and mucoid background. Rosenthal fibers or eosinophilic granular bodies, which are characteristic of pilocytic astrocytomas, are not found.[326,327] PMAs appear to have a more aggressive course than typical pilocytic astrocytomas and typically occur as hypothalamic/chiasmatic tumors in a younger children.[326] Anaplastic transformation of low-grade astrocytomas to more malignant-appearing and clinically aggressive entities, such as anaplastic astrocytoma and glioblastoma multiforme, is a common event in adults that seldom occurs in children and young adults.[328]

Oligodendrogliomas, a separate category of glial neoplasms, are characterized by a generally monotonous collection of uniform, round cells with more homogenous nuclei than are seen in the fibrillary astrocytoma, the tumor that represents the principal diagnostic alternative. An abundant clear cytoplasm surrounding a dark nucleus produces the appearance of a perinuclear halo that gives a distinctive fried-egg appearance. As in astrocytomas, grading of oligodendrogliomas appears to identify groups with differing prognoses. Most investigators reserve the use of the terms high-grade or anaplastic oligodendroglioma for tumors with increased cellularity, marked cytological atypia, high mitotic activity, microvascular proliferation, and necrosis.[329] These tumors have a predilection for the frontal and temporal lobes.[330]

Mixed neuronal-glial cell neoplasms, such as ganglioglioma, gangliocytoma, DNET, and DIG, are grouped for convenience with the low-grade gliomas. Gangliogliomas are the predominant type of mixed tumors, and they are composed of glial elements and a disorderly array of ganglion cells, some of which may be binucleate, that must be distinguished from entrapped neurons in the area involved. The glial component most commonly is astrocytic, but it may be oligodendroglial. Although anaplastic gangliogliomas are uncommon, when they do occur, they usually involve anaplasia within the glial component; anaplastic involvement of the neuronal component is unusual.[331]

Low-Grade Cerebellar Tumors

Low-grade gliomas occurring in the cerebellum typically are astrocytomas. Two principal histological variants have been described. The classic, or pilocytic, astrocytoma that accounts for 80% to 85% of these tumors (Fig. 26A.7) is composed of fusiform astrocytes loosely interwoven with a fine fibrillary background and no (or rare) mitoses. A frequent microcystic component and the presence of Rosenthal fibers, thought to represent degenerative changes in astrocytes, also are common.

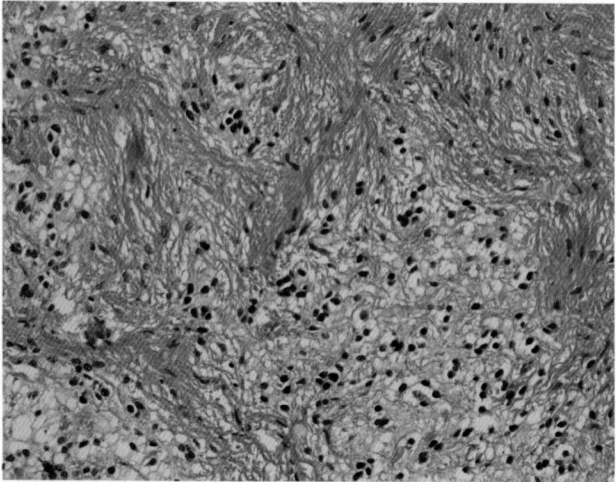

FIGURE 26A.7 Typical biphasic pattern of a pilocytic astrocytoma. Note the dense, relatively anuclear fibrillar areas alternating with looser honeycombed fields. (H&E, ×200.)

Large macrocystic structures filled with proteinaceous fluid and containing a mural nodule are seen in as many as 50% of patients. The walls of these cysts may be highly vascular, leading to occasional instances of spontaneous hemorrhage. Although this tumor often displays features otherwise associated with malignant behavior, such as nuclear atypia and focal leptomeningeal invasion, it rarely behaves in other than a benign fashion.[322,333] Although most tumors remain confined to the cerebellum, direct extension through the cerebellar peduncles to involve the brainstem may occur. As noted earlier, pilocytic cerebral astrocytomas have occasionally demonstrated either neuraxis dissemination or late malignant transformation, a behavior that belies their typically low-grade histological features.

The second variety of cerebellar astrocytoma is the diffuse or fibrillary astrocytoma, which accounts for 15% of cerebellar astrocytomas and is similar to the diffuse fibrillary, low-grade astrocytoma of the cerebral hemispheres. This tumor is more densely cellular, lacks the microcysts and Rosenthal fibers common to the pilocytic tumors, is more widely infiltrative, and is more likely to undergo anaplastic change than is its counterpart.[332]

Biology

Although the constellation of molecular alterations occurring in pediatric low-grade gliomas has not been comprehensively determined, several key genetic events in the pathogenesis of these tumors have been identified. Most notably, activation of the RAS/RAF (MAPK) signaling cascade, a critical pathway for regulation of cell growth and proliferation, has been found to occur in the vast majority of JPAs and a minority of grade II astrocytomas.[334-338] Activation of the MAPK pathway occurs most often via duplication events affecting the BRAF locus on 7q34 that produce constitutive kinase activity of the BRAF protein,[334-336] but also through less common mechanisms including point mutation of BRAF,[334,337,338] point mutation or duplication of RAF1,[337,338] and point mutation of KRAS.[338-340] In NF1-associated pilocytic astrocytomas, activation of the RAS/RAF (MAPK) signaling pathway occurs through homozygous inactivation of the NF1 gene.[341-343]

Several of the most common genetic alterations of adult low-grade gliomas are much less frequent in the corresponding pediatric tumors, indicating that the biology of pediatric low-grade gliomas differs significantly from their adult counterparts. Loss of 1p and 19q has been identified in the majority of adult oligodendrogliomas[344] and is due to a translocation between these loci[345,346]; in pediatric oligodendrogliomas, these alterations are relatively uncommon.[347,348] Similarly, mutation of IDH1, which occurs in greater than 70% of adult grade II astrocytomas, oligodendrogliomas, and oligoastrocytomas,[349,350] is found in a minority of these tumors in children,[350-352] predominantly in adolescent patients. Further research efforts will be required to identify the common alterations, other than MAPK pathway activation, occurring in pediatric lower grade gliomas.

Prognostic Considerations

Published reports of the management of low-grade glial tumors in children are complex, and the identification of consistent prognostic factors is difficult. Most reports include adult and pediatric cases, tumors from all sites, and patients treated over several decades, during which time diagnostic and therapeutic techniques have changed. The very good outcome reported by most authors and the indolent natural history of these tumors confounds analysis as well. Even so, certain factors consistently emerge in analyses but with inconsistent results. Complete resection of tumor seems most important for achieving prolonged disease-free survival in most, but not all, series. After a radical resection (i.e., >90% of tumor resected), 5-year PFS rates for cerebral astrocytomas exceed 75%[353–355] (Table 26A.6) versus less than 50% after incomplete resections.[355,356] However, the amenability of these tumors to second surgical explorations results in survival rates that may not differ from tumors completely resected at diagnosis.

The independent influence of the histology of tumors—generally pilocytic versus nonpilocytic—is controversial. Some reports support superior survival rates with pilocytic histology,[357–361] and others report equivalent outcomes for pilocytic and nonpilocytic tumors.[314,356,362,363] Within the histologic category of pilocytic astrocytomas, some retrospective reports suggest that tumors with a higher proliferative fraction, measured by either a MIB-1 labeling index or a bromodeoxyuridine (BrdU) labeling index, are associated with a shortened PFS or outcome, respectively.[364,365] PMAs, which in retrospective series were previously classified as pilocytic astrocytomas, appear to have more aggressive biologic behavior with a predilection for the hypothalamic/chiasmatic region, a tendency to occur among young children, and a greater potential for leptomeningeal dissemination, compared with pilocytic astrocytomas.[326] Other factors that are somewhat related to histology and to the degree of resection include the invasiveness of the tumor into surrounding structures and the amount of residual tumor. For example, pilocytic and oligodendroglial tumors, which often are well circumscribed, appear more often to be amenable to extensive resection are more likely than fibrillary astrocytomas to have a favorable prognosis.[330,353,356,366,367] The tendency toward invasiveness among nonpilocytic astrocytomas is in keeping with the less favorable prognosis that some have reported for these tumors.[358,360] However, separating the effects of histology and the extent of resection is difficult. Invasion into the brainstem is a primary factor limiting complete resection of cerebellar low-grade gliomas[309,357,368] and is an independent prognostic factor in one of these series.[368] Volume of tumor residual emerged in another series as the most important predictor of cerebellar low-grade glioma progression, emphasizing the importance of maximal tumor resection.[357]

Although the long-term benefit of radiation therapy is not entirely clear, higher-dose radiation (i.e., >53 Gy) significantly improved length of survival in Shaw's series.[366,367] Young age is noted consistently to be associated with an increased risk of progressive disease, but this may, in large part, reflect that low-grade gliomas in young children tend to involve the mid-line structures, which may limit their amenability to extensive resections.[309,314,369] The CCG9891/POG9031 natural history study, which accumulated more than 700 cases of low-grade gliomas with centrally reviewed pathologic material and radiologic studies, confirmed the strong association between resection extent and outcome and may help to address more conclusively the independent contributions to prognosis of histology and tumor location.[107]

Treatment

Surgery

The goals of surgery for low-grade gliomas are to obtain tissue for diagnosis and to remove as much tumor as is safely feasible. Operative mortality rates are less than 1%; morbidity depends largely on tumor location and is highest in diencephalic tumors, in which the incidence of hemiparesis or visual field deficits may be 10% to 20%. Gross total excisions are possible in the majority of hemispheric tumors, but a minority of diencephalic tumors. Although, the use of microsurgical techniques has led to high rates of resection in selected diencephalic tumors, the efficacy of chemotherapy for deep-seated low-grade gliomas in young children has tempered enthusiasm for aggressive resections of such tumors in view of the potential for substantial morbidity.[370]

Cerebral Hemisphere Gliomas

Although complete resection usually is the operative goal for cerebral hemisphere low-grade gliomas, its achievement may be difficult for nonpilocytic tumors, which rarely have a distinct tumor-brain interface. Because malignant degeneration of nonirradiated cerebral low-grade gliomas is uncommon, lesions that progress after an initial operation often are amenable to repeat resection. This possibility contrasts with the situation in adults, in which low-grade gliomas often exhibit malignant features at the time of progression.[371]

For cortical and many subcortical tumors, the surgical approach follows the most direct trajectory to the lesion. A variety of physiologic monitoring tools have been implemented to facilitate extensive resection of gliomas in "eloquent" regions of the brain. These include fMRI, diffusion tensor imaging, and direct cortical mapping using strip, grid, and bipolar contact electrodes. Although it is difficult to prove that any of these modalities are essential to achieving tumor resection, they clearly increase the comfort level of a surgeon attempting resection of a tumor in, or adjacent to, a functionally critical region of the cortex. Similarly, investigators have

SURVIVAL RATE ACCORDING TO THERAPY IN LOW-GRADE ASTROCYTOMAS

Treatment	Survival in year (%)			References
	5	7	10	
Complete resection	76–100	86 60 (d)	69–100	353, 366, 439
Incomplete resection	62	—	67–87	366, 642
Incomplete resection plus irradiation	58–93 (d)	— 77 (d)	67 (d)	366, 642

d, diencephalic.

debated the need for intraoperative ECOG (direct cortical electroencephalographic monitoring) in children with tumor-associated epilepsy; 75% of patients whose tumor resections are performed without ECOG are free of seizures postoperatively versus 85% of those with ECOG.[372,373] If used, ECOG is likely to be of most value in treating those patients with long-standing or severe seizure disorders.

For deep or poorly circumscribed superficial lesions, imaging-based neuronavigation and intraoperative imaging using ultrasonography and MRI guidance are helpful for planning an approach to the tumor that avoids traversing critical regions and for monitoring the progress of the resection. These strategies are particularly valuable for lesions that arise from or extend into the thalamus and basal ganglia.

The approach to deep subcortical lesions also is influenced substantially by the predominant direction of tumor growth. Lesions deep within the temporal lobe or temporal horn of the lateral ventricle are approached through a corticotomy in the middle temporal gyrus or sulcus. Lesions that grow medially and encroach on or expand within the lateral ventricle can be approached transcallosally or transfrontally, through the middle frontal gyrus, whereas tumors that extend laterally in the nondominant hemisphere may be approached through the insula after the sylvian fissure has been opened. Laterally extending lesions within the dominant hemisphere and tumors that arise more posteriorly within the thalamus may be reached using a posterior parietal approach situated behind the sensorimotor cortex and above the angular gyrus or through a posterior incision in the middle temporal gyrus. Such lesions can be reached also via an occipital transtentorial trajectory via an opening in the pulvinar or suboccipital subtemporal approach above the tentorium. Finally, tumors that project anteriorly and laterally can be reached from a paramedian frontal trajectory, provided that care is taken to avoid injury to the motor pathways.

Cerebellar Gliomas. As with supratentorial hemispheric gliomas, a close correlation exists between the extent of resection and outcome in cerebellar gliomas; complete tumor excision is associated with improved long-term and disease-free survival. Because the long-term survival of patients with GTRs is as high as 90%, attempts at aggressive extensive resection are warranted, except when the tumor has invaded the cerebellar peduncles or brainstem. The operative approach is similar to that described earlier for resection of a medulloblastoma, with the caveat that a bilateral suboccipital exposure is typically required for a vermian or large paramedian lesion, whereas a unilateral suboccipital craniectomy or craniotomy may be preferable for a glioma centered in the cerebellar hemisphere. Data suggest that as few as 36% of patients with subtotal resections remain free of relapse at 6 years, and progression-free survival percentages may decline further with longer follow-up times of 10 to 20 years.[374,375] Thus, the appearance of resectable residual tumor on a postoperative scan frequently is an indication for reoperation.

Most pilocytic astrocytomas have a distinct margin and can be separated from adjacent cerebellum with reasonable safety; currently, as many as 90% of patients have GTRs with an operative mortality rate of less than 1%.[376] Although complete resection is also feasible for the majority of nonpilocytic astrocytomas, its achievement is more difficult because these lesions rarely are as well circumscribed as the pilocytic tumors.

Gangliogliomas and Other Low-Grade Neuroepithelial Tumors. The approach to gangliogliomas is similar to that for other low-grade gliomas. Complete resection of cerebral gangliogliomas may be associated with survival rates in excess of 90% at 10 years. The recurrence rate is substantially higher for deep-seated lesions, such as those within the diencephalon, because of the difficulties in achieving a GTR. However, even after partial resection, long-term progression-free intervals may ensue. The response of the desmoplastic mixed neuronal-glial tumors appears similar; GTRs generally are curative, whereas incomplete removals have been associated with local recurrence or tumor progression.[72,377,378]

Radiation Therapy

The role of radiation therapy in patients with low-grade gliomas depends on the anatomic location and tumor extent, age of the child, and the degree of resection. With current neuroimaging, children with completely resected tumors or small amounts of apparent residual are followed without further intervention.[107,273,314,379,380] For unresectable tumors (e.g., midbrain, many thalamic or large temporal lobe lesions), radiation therapy has been shown to be effective as gauged by disease response and durable disease control.[273,381–383] In most recent series, local irradiation has been quite narrowly applied for discrete JPAs or focal astrocytomas that are not histologically characterized. Margins in several instances are ≤1 cm beyond the enhancing tumor, allowing truly conformal techniques for many of the focal presentations. The use of conformal irradiation for recurrent and high-risk newly diagnosed children older than 10 years with low-grade gliomas will be evaluated prospectively in the COG ACNS0221 study.

A major retrospective review of childhood astrocytomas confirmed the improvement in long-term event-free survival following irradiation for incompletely resected astrocytomas, while showing no apparent benefit in overall survival.[310] However, a more recent study of 90 children older than 3 years with WHO grade II low-grade gliomas showed that administration of early radiation did not appear to influence PFS or OS ($p = 0.98$ and 0.40, respectively; log-rank test). In this series, patients who underwent GTRs had significantly longer PFS ($p = 0.02$) but did not have significantly improved OS.[384]

There are specific histologic subtypes of the low-grade gliomas that are associated with more aggressive biology (e.g., PMAs and pilocytic tumors with high MIB-1); the potential role of early postoperative irradiation in these settings has yet to be fully explored.[327]

The role of radiation therapy in incompletely resected cerebellar tumors is unclear. All reported comparisons involve retrospective reviews of patients accumulated over periods as long as 40 years, in most instances following patients after incomplete resection or with inconsistent indications for and techniques of irradiation. As suggested for other low-grade gliomas, patients with incomplete resections of cerebellar tumors should be considered for further surgery, and radiation therapy should be reserved for progressive residual or unresectable recurrent tumors. Radiosurgery has been utilized for highly focal recurrences in difficult to resect locations, such as the cerebellar peduncles or brainstem.[385,386]

Irradiation has been proposed for patients who have gangliogliomas and have undergone incomplete resections or disease recurrence. However, the reported numbers of patients treated with radiation therapy are insufficient to estimate reliably the long-term utility of such treatment. Long periods free of tumor progression may follow incomplete resection alone.

A few investigators have suggested that irradiation may be associated with late anaplastic transformation of low-grade tumors.[387] The phenomenon has not been suggested in other major institutional series with long-term follow-up of astrocytic tumors after irradiation; it is difficult to be categorical regarding an etiologic relationship between tumor dedifferentiation and radiation exposure in childhood astrocytomas.[380,381]

Chemotherapy

Low-grade glioma within the cerebral hemispheres and cerebellum is primarily a surgical disease. If tumors recur after complete or incomplete resection, subsequent resection may lead again to prolonged disease-free status. However, as outlined earlier, aggressive primary or secondary surgery may be unsafe for tumors in deep locations or eloquent structures. In such situations, particularly in young children in whom a delay in radiation therapy may be desirable, or for children whose tumor has progressed after irradiation, chemotherapy has been explored. Numerous single-agent and combination chemotherapy regimens, which generally include classic and/or nonclassic alkylators, nitrosoureas, and/or platinum analogues, have been explored in children from infancy through adolescence with low-grade gliomas of all sites.[388–400] More recent studies have evaluated temozolomide, weekly vinblastine, and the combination of irinotecan plus bevacizumab.[401–404] The usual benefit of chemotherapy is disease stabilization, although partial responses may occur. Complete tumor regression is rare for both single-agent and combination chemotherapy regimens although stable disease may in some instances be prolonged.

The most promising chemotherapy data for children with low-grade gliomas come from two reports. In the first, carboplatin and vincristine (CV) were administered to 73 children (mean age, 3 years) with newly diagnosed, progressive, low-grade gliomas that were primarily diencephalic. Radiographic responses were seen in 56% of patients and the 3-year PFS rates were 68%. There were no correlations among tumor histology, location, or maximum response to chemotherapy and duration of disease control. However, children 5 years old and younger had a significantly higher rate of 3-year PFS (74%) as compared with children older than 5 years (39%; $p < 0.01$).[392] Similarly, another chemotherapeutic regimen consisting of 6-thioguanine, procarbazine, dibromodulcitol, CCNU, and vincristine (TPCV) resulted in tumor reduction in 36% of patients, stable disease in 59%, and a 5-year survival of 78%.[397] In contrast to the CV data, older age was the only factor that improved survival significantly. These two regimens formed the basis for a randomized study within the COG A9952, for patients with progressive low-grade glioma.[405] This trial enrolled 401 children (52% female, 60% <5 years, and 83% hypothalamic/optic pathway or JPAs in other sites). Five-year overall survival rates were 57% and 61% for the CV in non-NF patients and NF patients, respectively, and 58% for the TCPV arm. As anticipated, both regimens showed efficacy in controlling low-grade gliomas allowing for a delay in treatment with radiotherapy. Although there was not a statistically significant difference in the 5-year event-free survival for randomized subjects (35 ± 4.7% for CV vs. 48 ± 4.8% for TPCV [$p = 0.11$]), the median time to progression was shorter for CV versus TCPN (3.2 vs. 4.9 years).[405] Further analysis of data from this trial is ongoing.

Although chemotherapy appears to be a viable treatment option for children in whom either aggressive surgery or radiation therapy is inadvisable, the natural history of low-grade gliomas, characterized by recurrence or progression rates many years after diagnosis or after irradiation, will require up to 20 years of follow-up to determine its long-term benefit. In the shorter run, comparative activity of various agents will be determined. Biologic factors may guide chemotherapy further in the future.

TUMORS OF THE OPTIC PATHWAY

Optic pathway tumors (OPTs) are low-grade glial tumors. However, because of the particular challenges posed by their location, they are generally considered as a separate entity.

Demography

OPTs generally arise in the optic nerves, chiasm, and hypothalamus and may extend from these sites to adjacent brain structures. They comprise approximately 3% to 5% of pediatric intracranial tumors.[406] Nearly two-thirds of OPTs are diagnosed in the first 5 years of life.[407] Seventy-five percent of OPTs will become symptomatic in the first decade of life, and 90% will become so before the age of 20.[408] Boys and girls are affected equally.

OPTs are prevalent in patients with NF1. The incidence of NF1 in reported series of OPT ranges from 11% to 30%,[406,408] whereas as many as 70% of OPTs may be associated with NF1.[409] The sites of OPT involvement appear to differ in patients with and without NF1. Unilateral or bilateral optic nerve involvement alone is seen almost exclusively in patients with NF1, whereas chiasmal involvement is significantly more common in patients without NF1.

Imaging

OPTs may involve any portion of the optic pathway including one or both optic nerves, the chiasm tracts, the lateral geniculate bodies, or the optic radiations. These lesions are usually T1-hypointense and T2-hyperintense with typically homogeneous gadolinium enhancement, and in large tumors, heterogenous enhancement. MRI with fat suppression leads to optimal visualization of the optic pathways.

Cranial and intracranial manifestations inherent in NF-1 include vacuolization of the myelin (NF spots), plexiform neurofibromas, and optic pathway gliomas as well as other astrocytomas, vascular dysplasias (e.g., stenoses, occlusions, moyamoya disease, aneurysms internal carotid dolichoectasia, AVM, and fistula), calvarial and orbital abnormalities (i.e., defects along the sphenoid wing and lambdoid suture), and neurofibromas and plexiform neurofibromas. The regions of vacuolization of the myelin sheaths can be seen in children with NF1 and consist of foci of hyperintense T2 signal intensity that represent spongiotic intramyelinic vacuolization.[410] These foci are not space occupying and are typically located in the basal ganglia, internal capsule, brainstem, and cerebellum; they appear by 3 years of age, increasing in number and size until about 10 to 12 years of age, followed by a decrease during adolescence.[411] Three-dimensional multivoxel proton MRS has been used in children with NF1 to interrogate these areas of focal signal abnormality. Proton MRS indicated that these areas of myelin vacuolization (a) are characterized by significantly elevated Cho, reduced Cr, a Cho:Cr ratio greater than 1.3, and near-normal NAA levels; (b) are different from tumors that exhibit Cho:Cr greater than 2 and no NAA; (c) have no lipid or lactate signal; and (d) correlate in spatial extent but are more extensive than indicated by conventional MRI sequences.[412] Use of 3D CSI, as opposed to single-voxel imaging spectroscopy, to delineate metabolically the extent and volume of the lesion, may be useful for following the effects of treatment (Fig. 26A.8).

One small series suggests that the clinical behavior of OPTs in children may be differentiated by diffusion-weighted and

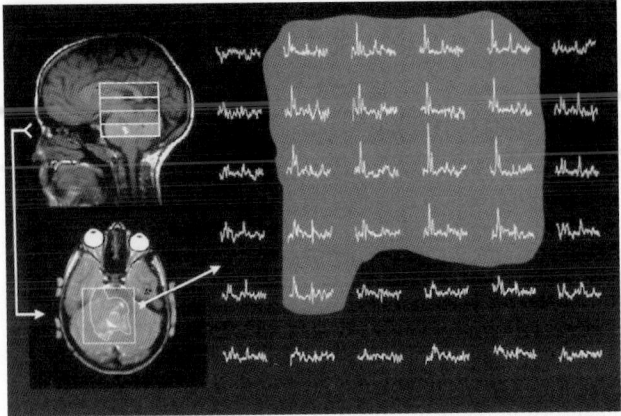

FIGURE 26A.8 Composite image demonstrating a setup for three-dimensional chemical shift imaging (stack of two-dimensional slabs), in a patient with neurofibromatosis type 1 complicated by a brainstem glioma. The tumor is outlined from the spectroscopy grid by the extent of the abnormal N-acetyl aspartate–choline pattern.

dynamic contrast-enhanced MRI. Clinically aggressive OPTs had higher mean permeability values ($p = 0.05$) than clinically stable tumors.[413] Further studies evaluating the role of this imaging modality in OPTs are required.

Pathology and Patterns of Spread

Histologically, OPTs are usually low-grade astrocytoma; the majority are pilocytic although fibrillary astrocytomas are reported.[406] Although these tumors usually are confined to the structures of the visual pathways and extend in contiguity along them (Fig. 26A.9), they may extend also into the frontal lobes, hypothalamus, thalamus, and other midline structures. Such events are more frequent in chiasmal tumors. Overall, tumor growth is slow, although alternating periods of clinical progression and stability suggest an erratic growth pattern. Malignant degeneration is rare.

PMAs, which were once classified with pilocytic astrocytomas, have also been described in the optic pathway,

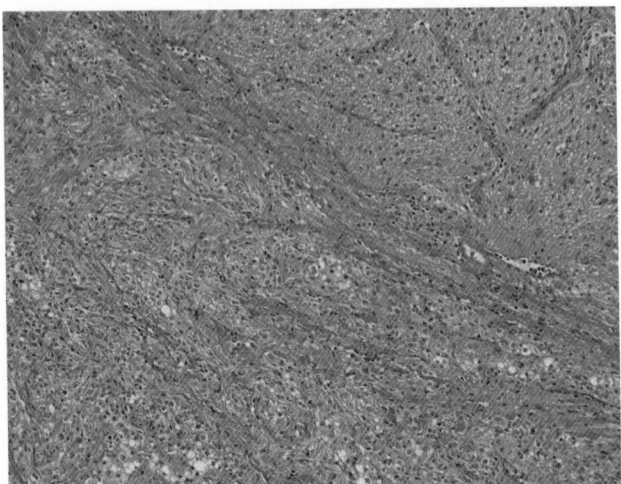

FIGURE 26A.9 Microscopic features of an optic nerve glioma composed of swirling piloid processes of astrocytes (H&E, ×100×).

albeit rarely. They typically occur in younger children (<18 months of age) and have a much more aggressive behavior.[326,406] PMAs infiltrate and enlarge the septated nerve and expand and may disseminate within the leptomeninges and CSF.[278]

Biology

As for low-grade gliomas occurring elsewhere in the CNS, activation of the RAS/RAF (MAPK) signaling cascade has been implicated as a critical event in the pathogenesis of both sporadic and NF1-associated optic pathway gliomas. In NF1-associated optic pathway gliomas, this is caused by homozygous inactivation of the *NF1* gene, which is relatively uncommon in the sporadic tumors.[341–343] For sporadic optic pathway gliomas, the current data suggest that MAPK pathway activation occurs predominantly through duplication or mutation of *BRAF* in the same manner as for sporadic nonoptic pathway pilocytic astrocytomas.[336]

Biologically relevant mouse models have been created for the study of NF1-associated optic pathway gliomas. Interestingly, the development of optic pathway gliomas in these systems requires both complete loss of neurofibromin in the astroglial cells as well as heterozygous neurofibromin loss in the remainder of the mouse, indicating that signals derived from the microenvironment of the optic pathway may play a critical role in tumor development.[414–418] Mice heterozygous for constitutional loss of NF1 with astrocyte-specific activation of *KRAS* also develop optic pathway gliomas.[419] Candidate stromal factors contributing to the pathogenesis of NF1-associated optic pathway gliomas include regulation of CXCL12 expression[420] and microglia-derived JNK signaling.[421] These mouse models appear promising for use in the preclinical evaluation of potential therapies for NF1-associated optic pathway gliomas.[417]

Prognostic Considerations

The three factors that appear to have prognostic importance for the outcome of patients with OPTs include NF1 status, tumor location, and age. The presence of NF1 generally is associated with more indolent disease, reflected in longer times to disease progression and higher rates of PFS and survival. For example, 15-year relapse-free survival in Jenkin's report[422] was 84% for patients with NF1 and 47% for those without NF1 ($p = 0.0007$). In Imes's series,[423] patients with NF1 survived their OPT better than did those without NF1 but died of other causes, including other intracranial tumors and complications of NF1 resulting in a survival not different from non-neurofibromatosis patients. However, in other series, NF1 does not offer a protective effect.[381,424,425] Tumors involving the chiasm and hypothalamus have a worse prognosis in most (but not all) series.[422,426–429] Finally, as with most other CNS tumors, the youngest children, generally younger than 3 to 5 years, do worse than do their older counterparts.[424,427,430,431]

The role of radiographic screening for optic pathway gliomas in children with NF1 and the impact of screening have been debated in the literature. The 1997 Optic Pathway Glioma Task Force did not find conclusive evidence that early detection of tumors would reduce the rate of vision loss.[432] Moreover, it was felt that identification of asymptomatic OPGs would increase parental anxiety and result in exposure to the risks of repeated sedation for neuroimaging studies.[433] Nevertheless, some institutions screen young children with NF1 using systematic neuroimaging.[434]

Treatment

Surgery

Because of the variability in the growth properties of OPTs, diverse approaches to management have been advocated in different clinical situations and in different institutions. In children with NF1, the etiology of the lesion rarely is in question. Because the tumor usually exhibits diffuse involvement of the chiasm and nerves, it is not amenable to extensive resection. If the tumor is behaving in a biologically indolent fashion, resection generally is not pursued,[382,435–437] and adjuvant therapy, if needed, is initiated empirically.

Lesions that seem particularly well suited to radical excision are those that involve only a single optic nerve and produce progressive, disfiguring proptosis or blindness (or both) and those that grow exophytically from the optic chiasm and produce significant mass effect or hydrocephalus.[438] For isolated optic nerve gliomas, which are fairly uncommon, the tumor can be removed with preservation of the globe. In such cases, the resected segment of the optic nerve should be as long as possible, preferably extending close to the chiasm, to diminish the risk of local tumor recurrence. Ruling out the diagnosis of NF1 before embarking on surgery is essential, because such children commonly exhibit widespread involvement of the optic pathways and may have long-term stabilization of vision without aggressive intervention. For exophytic chiasmatic-hypothalamic tumors, resection often is pursued to relieve obstructive hydrocephalus, to reduce local mass effect, and to establish a tissue diagnosis. For lesions amenable to resection, the tumor is usually approached via a subfrontal, transsylvian, or transcallosal exposure, depending on the pattern of tumor growth. Although a complete resection is not feasible because these lesions infiltrate the optic chiasm or hypothalamus (or both), substantial symptomatic improvement sometimes can be achieved.[382,430] In occasional cases, removal of a significant portion of the tumor may stabilize the disease and delay the need for additional therapy.[430]

Open biopsy also is pursued sometimes for lesions involving the chiasm in which the histologic diagnosis is uncertain, before instituting further therapy. This is especially the case in children without neurofibromatosis or those with isolated chiasmatic-hypothalamic lesions without contiguous optic nerve or optic tract involvement. However, this procedure may further compromise vision in a significant percentage of patients. Alternatively, some neurosurgeons prefer to perform a stereotactic biopsy and treat with chemotherapy, reserving open resection for lesions that fail to respond or subsequently progress. Although aggressive surgery may be of potential benefit in some patients with large, progressive lesions, it may be associated with significant morbidity, particularly in the youngest patients, and does not convincingly improve survival in comparison with more limited open or stereotactic or endoscopic biopsy and adjuvant therapy.[430,439]

Radiation Therapy

Radiation therapy is effective in stabilizing or improving chiasmatic/hypothalamic gliomas. Response is apparent in objective reduction in tumor size and long-term stabilization. Functionally, irradiation typically results in stable visual acuity; vision has been documented to improve in 20% to 25% of instances and to deteriorate in an equal percentage.[379–381,440,441] Deterioration is often associated with enlargement of tumor-associated cysts or a postirradiation phenomenon of transient increase in tumor size seen in a significant minority of children within 3 to 9 months after irradiation.[381]

In older children (institutionally defined over a broad range of older than 4 to 5 years to after puberty), irradiation is the standard intervention when disease progression or significant visual compromise prompts therapy. For relatively younger children, particularly those younger than 4 to 5 years, radiation therapy is often employed after chemotherapy, reserving the more durable efficacy of irradiation for children with documented progression postchemotherapy.[380,440,442]

Delaying irradiation is appropriate in view of age-related toxicities, particularly vascular effects (vascular compromise believed to result from cicatricial reduction of the major arteries in the circle of Willis, either focally or globally, resulting in moyamoya syndrome, essentially complete loss of the major intracranial vessels in the suprasellar region), neuroendocrine and neurocognitive deterioration.[379,433,442–444] These adverse events are of particular concern for children with NF1.

Radiation therapy for OPTs should be highly conformed to the chiasm/hypothalamus for lesions localized to that region, using 3D-CRT, IMRT, stereotactic radiation therapy (i.e., fractionated radiosurgery), or proton beam.[273,445,446] In more extensive tumors extending into the optic tracts, margins are somewhat greater for the tumor components outside the suprasellar region. Dose levels have been established at 50 to 54 Gy using fraction sizes approximating 180 cGy.

Although chemotherapy effectively delays the initiation of chemotherapy in children with hypothalamic/chiasmatic gliomas, many will progress after chemotherapy and ultimately require radiation therapy. Mishra et al. recently reported 15-year follow-up data of a phase II study ($n = 33$) designed to evaluate the efficacy of upfront chemotherapy (6-thioguanine, procarbazine, dibromodulcitol, 1-(2-chloroethyl)-3-cyclohexyl-1-nitrosourea [CCNU], and vincristine) for the treatment of hypothalamic/chiasmatic low-grade gliomas. Seventeen of the 25 patients who progressed underwent subsequent radiation as part of their salvage therapy and seven remain disease free.[447]

Chemotherapy

The optic glioma chemotherapy experience is greatest for children who are younger than 3 years and for whom delay of radiation therapy is desirable for avoidance of long-term neuropsychological and neuroendocrine effects. Packer's regimen of vincristine and actinomycin-D was the first to successfully defer radiation therapy for children who were younger than 5 years with progressive chiasmatic and hypothalamic gliomas. At a median of 4 years of follow-up, 62.5% of the patients remained free of progressive disease and had not received radiation therapy.[436] By 7 years, however, only one-third of patients were free from progression. Packer also tested a CV regimen described for low-grade gliomas.[392] A POG phase II study of children who were younger than 5 years with progressive OPT evaluated single agent carboplatin (560 mg/m^2) every 4 weeks. After two courses, patients were evaluated, and those with stable disease or better were continued on therapy for 18 months or until disease progression. Of 50 eligible children, including 21 with NF1, 39 (78%) had stable disease or better, and 34 completed 18 months of therapy.[448]

Petronio et al.[449] reported improvement or stable disease in 15 of 18 patients with progressive OPT, a five-drug regimen consisting of 6-thioguanine, procarbazine, dibromodulcitol, CCNU, and vincristine. Of 15 patients, 11 had a greater than 50% decrease in their tumor mass. Those children whose tumors progressed on or after completion of chemotherapy were successfully treated with radiation therapy. Using chemotherapy, vision was stabilized in 14 of 18 patients and improved in two.

Results of the randomized phase III trial (carboplatin-vincristine vs. 6-thioguanine, procarbazine, cisplatin, and vincristine) for children with progressive low-grade gliomas, including those with OPTs, are presented in the low-grade glioma section. Other reports of limited numbers of patients have identified cisplatin and vincristine, tamoxifen and carboplatin, oral etoposide, velban, and temozolomide as having activity against progressive OPTs.[450-454] Most reports of chemotherapy for low-grade gliomas include patients whose tumors arose from the optic pathway (see section "Low-Grade Gliomas" for additional chemotherapy data).

SUPRATENTORIAL HIGH-GRADE GLIOMAS

Demography

Anaplastic astrocytoma, glioblastoma multiforme, and mixed glial tumors with a preponderance of malignant astrocytic elements collectively compose malignant or high-grade astrocytic tumors in children. These tumors represent 7% to 11% of childhood CNS tumors. When primary brainstem tumors are excluded, combined series suggest that approximately 25% of malignant or high-grade astrocytic tumors occur in deep midline structures of the cerebrum, not more than 15% occur in the posterior fossa, and the majority occur in the cerebral hemispheres.[106,455,456] The median age at diagnosis is 9 to 10 years, and the male-to-female ratio is near unity.[457]

Imaging

Supratentorial high-grade gliomas are heterogeneous on CT and MR with areas that have ill-defined margins, edema, hemorrhage, necrosis, mass effect, and irregular enhancement. High-grade glial tumors (Fig. 26A.13) demonstrate a pattern of marked enhancement with evidence for restricted diffusion on ADC maps. MRS of these tumors demonstrates a marked elevation in Cho with a reduction in NAA.[458] On perfusion imaging, these tumors tend to have high relative cerebral blood volume values.[459]

Pathology and Patterns of Spread

High-grade lesions, unlike their low-grade counterparts, generally are characterized by the presence of several histologic features of malignancy including hypercellularity, cytologic and nuclear atypia, mitoses, necrosis, and vascular proliferation with endothelial hyperplasia. Tumors with these features may be termed *malignant* or *high grade*. The most common

malignant glial neoplasms are the high-grade astrocytomas, such as anaplastic astrocytoma (Fig. 26A.10) and glioblastoma multiforme (Fig. 26A.11), which may alternatively be termed *grade III* and *grade IV astrocytomas*, respectively. Similarly, the term *high grade* or anaplastic may be used to describe other, less common glial neoplasms, such as oligodendroglioma, ganglioglioma, or mixed astrocytic-oligodendroglial neoplasms.

The high-grade astrocytomas are clinically aggressive, regionally invasive, and capable of extraneural dissemination to lung, lymph nodes, liver, and bone, particularly in adults. In children, these and the other malignant gliomas occur most commonly in the cerebral hemispheres, in contrast to the more frequent cerebellar and deep midline locations for low-grade tumors. Although the rapid growth and effacement of normal tissue produced by high-grade tumors may produce what appears to be a well-demarcated tumor, microscopic study frequently demonstrates extension for up to several centimeters beyond this margin. Distant neuraxial dissemination, once considered unusual, has been demonstrated in as many as 25% to 50% of high-grade astrocytomas, both at diagnosis and postmortem led in carefully evaluated series of patients.[460-462]

High-grade gliomas may have a histologically heterogeneous nature in that areas of low-grade histology commonly are noted in many high-grade tumors, particularly in small biopsies taken from the more superficial areas of tumor. Diagnostic confusion may be reduced by more generous sampling and by directing stereotactic biopsies toward the contrast-enhancing or more central portions of the tumor.

Biology

A number of genes are known to be frequently altered in high-grade gliomas, including *TP53*, *PTEN*, *CDKN2A*, *EGFR*, *RB1*, *NF1*, and *PIK3CA*.[463-470] Recent large-scale initiatives to categorize the molecular alterations occurring in glioblastomas have confirmed the involvement of these known genes[471,472] and led to discoveries of novel glioma genes, most prominently the identification of *IDH1*.[471] These studies have predominantly focused on adult glioblastomas, however, making generalization of the results to high-grade gliomas in children problematic. Although pediatric high-grade gliomas have not been as extensively studied, a number of genetic differences between pediatric and adult high-grade glioma (HGG) have been reported, including lower frequencies of EGFR amplification,[47,473-475] PTEN alteration,[473,474,476] and CDKN2A/ARF deletion[443] in children. The frequency of *TP53* mutations is similar in high-grade gliomas of older children and adults but lower in infants.[48,475]

It has become clear from these genetic studies that distinct molecular subtypes of glioblastomas exist. Historically,

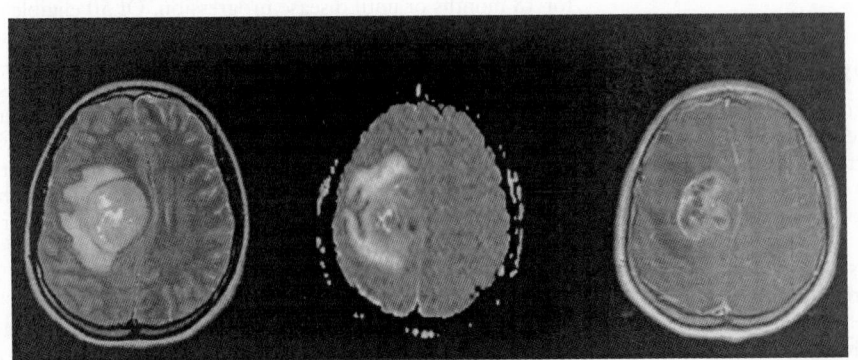

A,B   **C**

FIGURE 26A.10 A: Axial T2-weighted image demonstrating a well-defined mixed signal intensity mass with marked surrounding edema. **B:** Axial apparent diffusion coefficient map demonstrates a medial focus of restricted diffusion suspicious for an aggressive tumor. **C:** Axial T1-weighted postgadolinium magnetization transfer contrast, image through the tumor demonstrates marked rim enhancement. Histopathology revealed a glioblastoma multiforme.

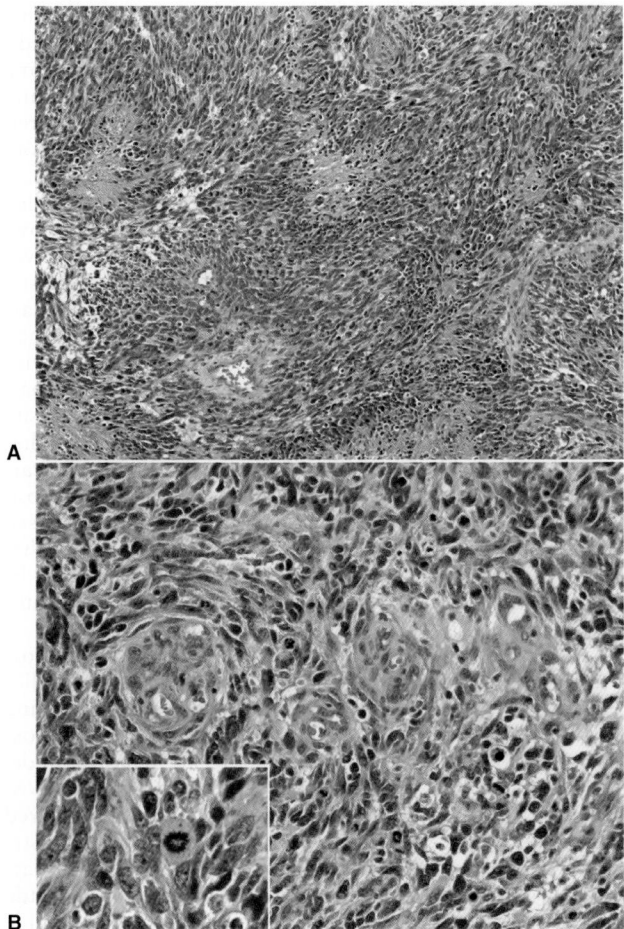

FIGURE 26A.11 Panel A: Typical field in a glioblastoma showing hypercellularity and several areas of pseudopalisading necrosis (H&E, ×100). **Panel B:** Higher magnification of a different field from the same tumor revealing nuclear atypia, numerous mitoses, and microvascular proliferation (H&E, ×200). In the inset, the anaplastic features of the neoplastic astrocytes and the bizarre mitoses are highlighted (H&E, ×400).

glioblastomas have been categorized into two groups ("primary" and "secondary") on the basis of clinical presentation. Secondary glioblastoma multiformes (GBMs) are defined as cancers that are known to have progressed from a preexisting lower grade tumor, whereas primary GBMs have no such history and present at diagnosis as advanced cancers.[58] Secondary GBMs occur in younger adults, are associated with a less dismal prognosis, nearly always have *IDH1* mutations, have a higher frequency of *TP53* mutations, and are less commonly associated with alterations of *PTEN*, *EGFR*, *RB1*, and *CDKN2A*.[350,471,477,478] Pediatric glioblastomas are distinct from either of these groups, however: although they exhibit some molecular similarities to secondary glioblastomas, the characteristic *IDH1* mutations of these tumors are less frequent in children.[350–352] The genetic heterogeneity between pediatric and adult high-grade gliomas is reflected in the clinical observation that low-grade gliomas in children are much less likely to transform to high-grade gliomas than the equivalent tumors in adults.[371,479,480] Studies designed to comprehensively examine the genetic alterations occurring in high-grade gliomas of childhood remain needed to further clarify the unique molecular basis of these tumors.

Prognostic Considerations

The extent of surgical resection, regardless of the primary tumor site, is the most important clinical prognostic factor for children with high-grade astrocytomas as demonstrated by institutional and cooperative group series.[104,106,455,456,481] Outcome is better for patients with a complete or near-complete resection of primary disease. For example, in the CCG-945 study, children with greater than a 90% tumor resection had a median PFS; this was significantly longer than patients with more limited resections. The difference was more pronounced for patients with anaplastic astrocytomas (31 vs. 12 months) than for those with glioblastoma multiforme (12 vs. 8 months) but was statistically significant for both groups.[104,456] The relationship may be surprising, given the fact that tumor often extends well beyond the identified central component of tumor and that, even after a radiologically confirmed GTR of all contrast-enhancing tumor, extensive residual tumor is known to remain. A caveat worth emphasizing is that factors specific to the tumor, such as the pattern of growth and degree of infiltration, may determine which tumors are amenable to extensive resection. Thus, tumors that are amenable to resection may constitute a group biologically more favorable than those that infiltrate extensively into the surrounding brain.[482] Insights from genomic analyses of these tumors may provide better understanding of these issues.[471,483]

In several series, site of disease is independently prognostic of outcome as well, with deep midline tumors showing a survival poorer than that of cerebral hemispheric tumors. However, hemispheric tumors are more amenable to radical resection than midline tumors. The impact of histology—anaplastic astrocytoma versus glioblastoma multiforme—on outcome is debated. Anaplastic astrocytoma may be favorably prognostic for subsets of patients,[104,456] although this association has not been uniformly confirmed, possibly reflecting challenges in the reliable classification of these tumors in historical series.[484] The prognosis of biologic markers in children with supratentorial high-grade gliomas is not well defined. Factors that have been associated with outcome, independent of histology, include the presence of *TP53* overexpression,[49] MIB-1 proliferation index,[485] and expression of methylguanine DNA methyltransferase.[486] *PTEN* mutations have been associated with an unfavorable outcome, and overexpression of basic fibroblast growth factor has also been associated with an unfavorable outcome.[473,487] In addition, recent studies have suggested that Akt activation, the downstream consequence of PTEN mutation, may be enhanced by factors other than PTEN mutation in pediatric malignant gliomas[471,486] and may constitute an adverse prognostic factor.[483,489]

Treatment

Surgery

The surgical techniques employed for tumor resection are similar to those used for supratentorial low-grade gliomas. As with the latter tumors, malignant gliomas often are amenable to reoperation at the time of disease progression, because most lesions recur at the primary site. Although the majority of children succumb to further disease progression despite additional intervention, attempted re-resection may be warranted in tumors that are amenable to gross total or radical subtotal removal, in view of reports of long-term survival after extensive resection followed by high-dose chemotherapy.[490] In addition, a host of novel molecularly targeted therapeutic agents have advanced to clinical trials for these tumors, in some cases incorporating repeat tumor resection as a way of assessing molecular phenotype at progression and facilitating reduction of disease burden prior to additional therapy.

Radiation Therapy

Radiation therapy is a standard component of postoperative management for children with malignant gliomas. Although rarely curative, the addition of radiation alone had shown improved survival intervals in adults, and pediatric series demonstrating higher rates of 1- to 3-year disease control and survival have been based on a combination of radiation and chemotherapy.[106,455,456]

Except in infants and children younger than 3 to 4 years, postoperative therapy incorporates wide local irradiation. Volumes are MRI derived, typically from both the enhancing tumor on T1 (preoperatively and as modified by surgical resection) and the extent of perilesional infiltration best estimated by findings on T2 or FLAIR sequences. There is evolving experience using other imaging modalities, such as PET or multinuclear MRS, to improve the targeting of subclinical disease.[491,492]

Dose levels are typically 56 to 60 Gy in pediatrics, often incorporating volume reductions after 45 to 50 Gy. The use of concurrent radiation and temozolomide followed by temozolomide and lomustine for pediatric high-grade gliomas has been evaluated in a COG trial (ACNS0423). This study closed in October 2007 and results are pending. In addition, the COG trial ACNS0126 combined radiation therapy with temozolomide, 90 mg/m^2/day, daily for 42 days, followed by 10 cycles of adjuvant temozolomide, 200 mg/m^2/day × 5 days given every 28 days. Event-free survival for 99 eligible high-grade glioma patients on ACNS0126 was compared with a similar cohort of 122 patients from CCG-945, which was open to accrual between 1985 and 1992. Outcome for ACNS0126 did not significantly differ from historical control, with 1-year event-free survival of 39 ± 5% for ACNS0126 compared with 42 ± 4.5% for CCG-945 (logrank $p = 0.14$). In addition, there was no significant difference in overall survival between the two cohorts; 1-year overall survival rates were 71 ± 5% for ACNS01 and 68 ± 4% for CCG-945 (logrank $p = 0.68$). Thus, the benefit of adding chemotherapy to radiation for children with high-grade gliomas is dubious at best, based on currently available studies.[493]

Chemotherapy

The role of chemotherapy for treatment of high-grade gliomas is evolving; the best results to date were observed in CCG-945, a prospective randomized trial performed between 1976 and 1981. Children with high-grade astrocytomas (excluding lesions of the brainstem or spinal cord) between 2 and 21 years of age were randomized to receive radiation therapy with or without adjuvant chemotherapy consisting of prednisone, CCNU, and vincristine (PCV). The PFS for children receiving postradiation chemotherapy was significantly higher (46%) than for those receiving radiation therapy alone (16%; $p = 0.026$).[494] However, other studies in children and adults have not shown a similar benefit. For example, a follow-up CCG study randomized patients to receive adjuvant chemotherapy with 8-in-1 or PCV. No difference was observed between the two chemotherapy arms, and 5-year PFS rates were 33% and 36% for 8-in-1 chemotherapy and PCV, respectively.[456] Taken together, these studies suggest that the benefit from addition of chemotherapy, when compared with surgery and radiation therapy alone, is modest at best. As noted earlier in section "Radiation Therapy," the results of COG trial ACNS0423 are pending.

In contrast to this experience with anaplastic astrocytoma and glioblastoma multiforme, children in the CCG-945 study, with eligible diagnoses other than anaplastic astrocytoma and glioblastoma multiforme, fared well. Their 5-year PFS and survival rates were 64% and 71%, respectively. Although retrospective neuropathology review of this cohort using contemporary WHO classification guidelines demonstrated a high frequency of discordance among these "other eligible" patients with inclusion of a substantial percentage of low-grade tumors,[495] the survival of the remaining subgroup was still more favorable than that of children with anaplastic astrocytoma or glioblastoma. Chemotherapy with procarbazine, CCNU, and vincristine has resulted in greater than 50% partial and complete responses in adult patients with anaplastic oligodendrogliomas and anaplastic mixed gliomas, particularly in those tumors that exhibit loss of heterozygosity in chromosomes 1p and 19q.[496–498] These data suggest that CCNU and vincristine, combined with prednisone or procarbazine and in addition to radiation therapy, may have a positive impact on outcome for children with newly diagnosed high-grade gliomas. However, it is important to point out that anaplastic oligodendroglial tumors of childhood may not be molecularly identical to their adult counterparts[499] and, thus, may warrant distinct management approaches.

As a result of the poor outcome for children with most high-grade gliomas, numerous single-agent phase II studies have been conducted using a variety of agents, including cisplatin, carboplatin, CCNU, procarbazine, cyclophosphamide, ifosfamide, etoposide, topotecan, temozolomide, irinotecan, as well as interferon-γ and low dose cyclophosphamide.[394,484,500–508] Although temozolomide was approved for use in adults with recurrent or progressive anaplastic gliomas, the response rate following temozolomide treatment in children with recurrent or refractory high-grade gliomas is low.[505,509] However, the activity of temozolomide may be higher in newly diagnosed patients; a strategy that as noted earlier is being evaluated in the ACNS0126 study. Theoretically, overcoming temozolomide resistance mediated by the DNA repair protein O^6-alkylguanine alkyltransferase with an agent such as O^{6}BG should benefit patients with high-grade glioma. However, this approach is not specific to the tumor cells and the resultant myelosuppression limits the dose of the concomitantly administered cytotoxic agent as has now been observed with both nitrosoureas as well as temozolomide.[510–512] Results of a phase II PBTC trial (PBTC 015) of temozolomide and O^{6}BG are pending.

Another approach to circumventing temozolomide resistance is through inhibition of PARP (poly-ADP ribose polymerase), a critical nuclear enzyme that activates proteins in the base excision repair and other DNA repair pathways.[513,514] Inhibition of this enzymatic activity with a PARP inhibitor such as ABT-888 may overcome temozolomide resistance. The PBTC has recently activated a phase I trial evaluating ABT-888 plus temozolomide.

Combination regimens of BCNU with cisplatin and cyclophosphamide with etoposide were evaluated by the POG. Although activity was demonstrated, superiority over CCNU and vincristine has not been demonstrated.[515] Myeloablative chemotherapeutic regimens have shown activity against bulk residual disease but have not demonstrated convincing superiority over standard therapy.[105,490,516–518] Both procarbazine and topotecan were inactive when evaluated as single agents in patients with newly diagnosed high-grade glioma and measurable disease after diagnostic surgery.[519]

Clearly, new agents and new approaches to therapy are needed and this is an active area of clinical investigation. The PBTC and COG are conducting a phase I and II studies of novel small molecule inhibitors, including signaling mediators that are putatively involved in glioma growth, such as PDGF-R, EGFR, and Ras. Trials targeting angiogenesis with agents such as cilengitide and bevacizumab (± irinotecan) and histone deacetylase are also in progress. Results of these trials should be forthcoming in the immediate future.

BRAINSTEM GLIOMAS

Demography

Tumors arising in the midbrain, pons, and medulla oblongata now account for approximately 20% of all CNS tumors among children younger than 15 years.[6] This apparent rise from 10% in the late 1970s does not reflect a truly increased incidence. Instead, this jump stems from the advent of MRI and increased detection of focal brainstem tumors, subsequently confirmed microscopically as low-grade gliomas. The median age of occurrence for all brainstem gliomas is 6 to 7 years.[520] The male-to-female ratio is near unity. Brainstem tumors are noted to be increasingly frequent among patients with NF1.[521,522]

Imaging

Brainstem gliomas can be classified as diffuse or focal and can be categorized by location as diffuse intrinsic pontine, focal pontine, medullary, and midbrain. The imaging characteristics for brainstem tumors in each location are described later.

Diffuse Intrinsic Pontine Gliomas

Typically, these tumors cause the pons to expand by more than 50% and may infiltrate into the medulla or midbrain. Diagnosis is based on the characteristic changes on MR imaging of diffuse, T2-weighted, hyperintense expansion of the brainstem. On CT, these tumors are of low density or isodense. On MR, they are typically isointense to hypointense on T1-weighted images and are hyperintense on T2 images. Enhancement is usually absent or minimal. Calcification and hemorrhage within the tumor is rare at diagnosis. MR spectroscopy has potential utility to determine tumor response or failure to therapy and to guide biopsy. Using multivoxel MR spectroscopy, Laprie et al. followed eight patients with diffuse pontine glioma after radiotherapy. Spectroscopy in these tumors was evaluated before RT, at response, and at recurrence. Cho:NAA and Cho:Cr values within the imaging abnormalities were significantly higher than the mean values in normal-appearing regions. Cho:NAA values decreased in studies performed from diagnosis to the time of response to RT followed by an increase at the time of relapse.[523–525] In some circumstances, PET imaging has been used to guide biopsy of these tumors.[526,527]

Focal Pontine Gliomas

These tumors are uncommon and usually demonstrate marked enhancement after gadolinium and are low-grade in pathology.

Medullary Tumors

Cervicomedullary astrocytomas are a unique group of brainstem tumors with a good prognosis when compared with the diffuse pontine group of brainstem gliomas. On CT, these tumors are isodense; on MR, these tumors are isointense on T1-weighted images and are hyperintense on T2-weighted images. They are typically well circumscribed, often demonstrate enhancement.

Midbrain Tumors

Tumors of the midbrain include focal and diffuse midbrain tumors as well as tectal tumors. The focal midbrain tumor has a better prognosis than the diffuse pontine glioma. Tectal tumors are a unique subset of tumors of the brainstem. They are typically low-grade pilocytic astrocytomas that present with obstructive hydrocephalus and usually do not require treatment beyond CSF diversion such as third ventriculostomy. Before the advent of MR, patients with tectal tumors were frequently misdiagnosed as having aqueductal stenosis on CT. On MR, the lesions are usually isointense on T1-weighted images and hyperintense on T2-weighted images without enhancement. Tumors larger than 2.5 cm in diameter with enhancement are significant radiologic predictors of those patients who will need further treatment beyond CSF diversion.[528] In a study of 40 children with tectal tumors, the only factor predictive of tumor enlargement was lesion volume at presentation ($p = 0.002$). Lesions with a volume less than 4 cm^3 were likely to follow a benign course. All large lesions defined as a volume greater than 10 cm^3 at presentation eventually required treatment.[529]

Pathology and Classification

The term *brainstem glioma* is an imprecise descriptor suggesting that all these tumors behave in the same way. As a result of advances in neuroimaging over the last 2 decades, a plethora of terms emerged to subclassify brainstem gliomas (sometimes confusingly) by site of origin or imaging features. Terms used have included midbrain tumor, tectal glioma, pontine glioma, focal medullary tumor, cervicomedullary tumor, diffuse glioma, intrinsic glioma, pencil glioma, dorsal exophytic brainstem tumor, focal glioma, and cystic glioma. Brainstem tumors are sometimes also subcategorized by pathology, as either low-grade or high-grade (malignant) gliomas. As an alternative, brainstem gliomas can be better biologically classified as diffusely infiltrative brainstem gliomas and focal gliomas, categories that combine tumor location and histology.

Diffusely infiltrative brainstem gliomas have an extremely poor prognosis. Most arise in the pons, and cause diffuse enlargement of that structure (Fig. 26A.12). Engulfment of the basilar artery by tumor is specific for the diagnosis of diffusely infiltrative brainstem glioma but is not seen in all cases (Fig. 26A.12B).[520] A component of exophytic growth is commonly seen.[530] Neoplastic infiltration extending into the midbrain, cerebral peduncle, cerebellum, or medulla is exceedingly common. These tumors may be low-grade, diffuse, fibrillary-type, WHO grade II, or, more often, high-grade anaplastic astrocytoma (WHO grade III) or glioblastoma multiforme (WHO grade IV).[520] These diffuse gliomas may occasionally show disseminated neuraxis spread.[531,532]

Focal brainstem tumors are discrete, well-circumscribed tumors without evidence of infiltration. These tumors may occur in any level in the brainstem but are most frequently seen in the midbrain or medulla rather than the pons (Fig. 26A.13). More often, focal tumors are dorsally exophytic to the brainstem, sometimes effacing the fourth ventricle. Histopathology reveals that these tumors are most commonly pilocytic astrocytomas or, rarely, gangliogliomas, both WHO grade I.[520,533] Sometimes they are cystic.[533]

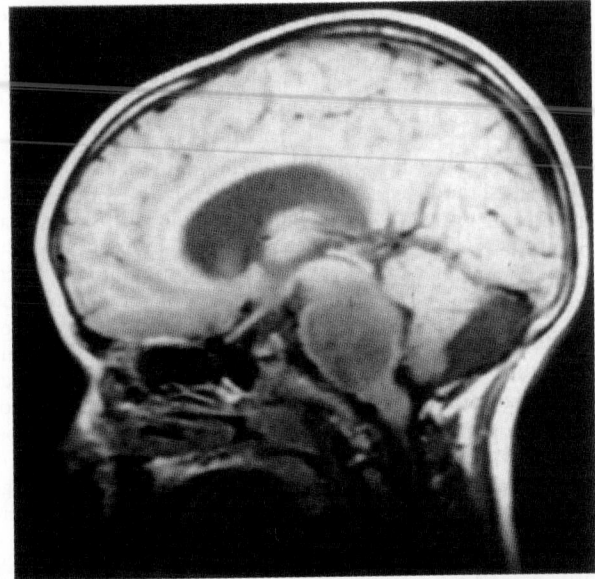

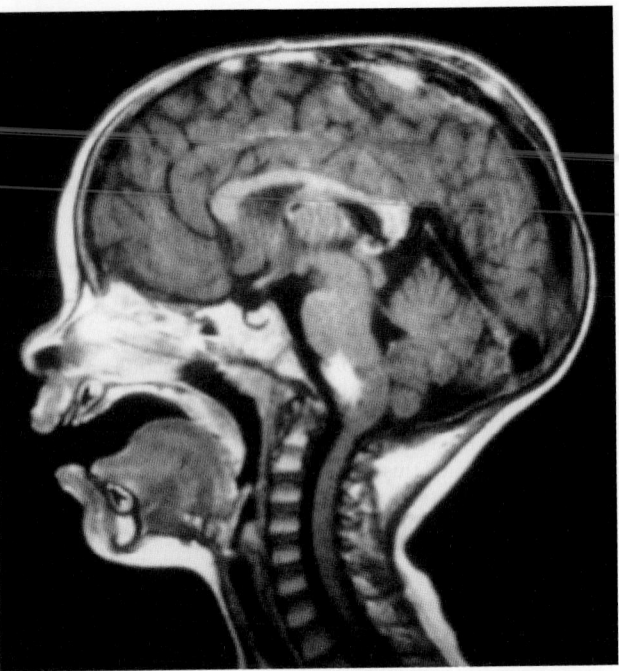

FIGURE 26A.13 T1-weighted transverse magnetic resonance imaging with gadolinium shows a focal brainstem tumor with avidß enhancement at the medulla. Biopsy demonstrated the tumor to be a pilocytic astrocytoma.

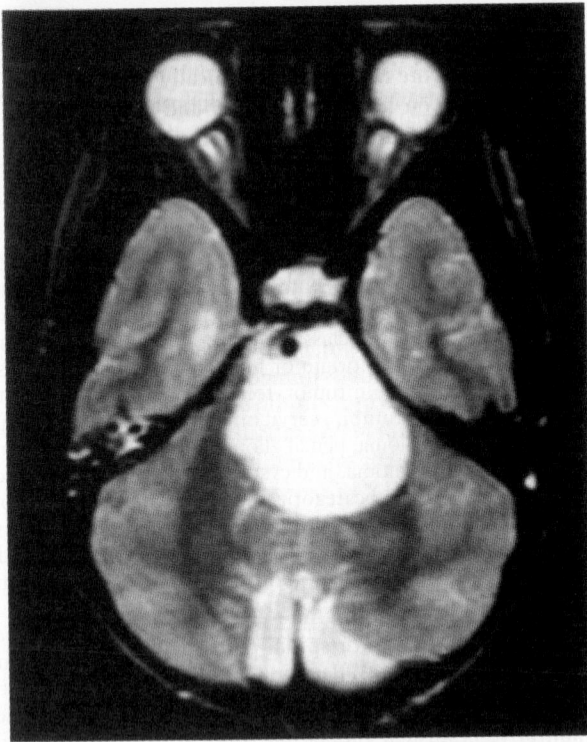

FIGURE 26A.12 Typical magnetic resonance imaging findings in a diffusely infiltrating brainstem glioma. A: T1-weighted sagittal view shows diffuse, fusiform enlargement of the pons with tumor spread superiorly and inferiorly. B: T2-weighted transverse view shows engulfment of the basilar artery.

Biology

There is a paucity of information about the biology of brainstem lesions, since intrinsic lesions are not amenable to surgical resection and biopsies are infrequently performed. Since intrinsic brainstem lesions are typically high-grade glial tumors, investigators have typically extrapolated information from histologically similar tumors outside the brainstem. A retrospective evaluation of IL-13Rα2 expression as assessed by immunohistochemistry in archived brainstem tumor samples obtained either at diagnoses or postmortem revealed that there was differential expression of IL-13Rα2 protein in brainstem tumors versus normal brain.[536] This suggests that the IL-13Rα2 receptor is a potential therapeutic target. Other recent studies have noted some similarity in antigen expression profiles between brainstem and nonbrainstem malignant gliomas, although further brainstem studies are required to assess whether or not the biology of high-grade gliomas in the brainstem is comparable with those arising in other locations in the brain.[537] Efforts are underway at a number of centers to collect this information from tumor specimens obtained in the immediate postmortem period.

Prognostic Considerations

Prognosis depends principally on the tumor type but is also influenced by whether or not the patient has NF1. Patients with diffusely infiltrative gliomas fare dismally, regardless of therapy. In most series, median survival is less than 1 year, and survival rates at 2 years are lower than 10% to 20%.[538,539] In contrast, the prognosis for patients with focal brainstem tumors is relatively good if the tumor is accessible. Survival

Rarely, tumors of histologic types other than gliomas are found in the brainstem. Among infants, the highly malignant AT/RT can arise in the brainstem.[534] Embryonal tumors, including PNETs, can also occur in very young children as localized pontine tumors with an exophytic component and extension beyond the pons. Such tumors may have a predilection for leptomeningeal dissemination at diagnosis.[535] Hemangioblastoma may arise at the brainstem also, although more commonly during adolescence or adulthood.

for these patients is reported to be between 50% and 100%.[521,530,540,541] Many patients with small focal tumors in the midbrain, particularly the tectum, may do extremely well after shunting or third ventriculostomy alone and can demonstrate PFSs of up to 10 years or more.[512–514]

Among patients with NF1, brainstem gliomas, whether diffuse or focal, display a generally indolent biologic behavior.[521,522] The tumor may stabilize in size or regress without intervention and survival approximates 90% at 5 years. Thus, intervention should be limited to those lesions that exhibit rapid or unrelenting growth on serial neuroimaging or lesions that produce significant clinical deterioration.

Treatment

The choice of treatment depends largely on whether the tumor is a diffusely infiltrative brainstem glioma or a focal brainstem tumor. Even among focal lesions, the site of the tumor affects selection of therapy.

Surgery

A major advance in the surgical management of brainstem gliomas followed the recognition that this broad category of tumors encompasses biologically distinct groups that demand individualized therapeutic strategies. At one extreme are the diffuse intrinsic gliomas, which are biologically malignant, highly infiltrative, and not amenable to resection. Although biopsy usually is associated with low morbidity, it no longer is considered necessary because, in the context of a typical clinical presentation and characteristic MRI findings, histologic results do not currently influence treatment.[545] However, with the increasing adoption of molecularly targeted therapeutic strategies, stereotactic needle biopsy may in the future play a role in guiding protocol-directed therapy, provided it can be accomplished with low morbidity.[526,546] At the other extreme are the benign intrinsic tectal gliomas, which also are not appropriate for resection because these lesions are extremely indolent and are best treated symptomatically with CSF diversion and observation (Fig. 26A.14).[542,543,547]

In contrast to the preceding groups, and because of improvements in neurosurgical techniques and postoperative care, surgical resection is a reasonable option for focal gliomas that arise at the cervicomedullary junction and for dorsally exophytic gliomas. These lesions are histologically and biologically benign but, unlike tectal gliomas, commonly show gradual enlargement over time. In particular, extensive resection of exophytic tumors, leaving a thin rim of tumor on the surface of the brainstem, frequently achieves long-term PFS without further treatment.[383,533,541] Some focal intrinsic, cystic, and solid brainstem lesions are likewise surgically resectable, and several authors have suggested that even after only partial resection, many patients require no further postoperative treatment. Although good survival rates have been achieved with surgical resection of symptomatic focal midbrain and medullary lesions, it remains to be determined whether these results represent an improvement over those obtained with stereotactic biopsy and local irradiation,[547,548] particularly in view of the potential for significant surgical morbidity from aggressive attempts at resection.

Radiation Therapy

Radiation therapy is the mainstay of treatment for children with diffusely infiltrative brainstem gliomas. Improvement in symptoms, signs, and neuroimaging occurs in a majority of children,

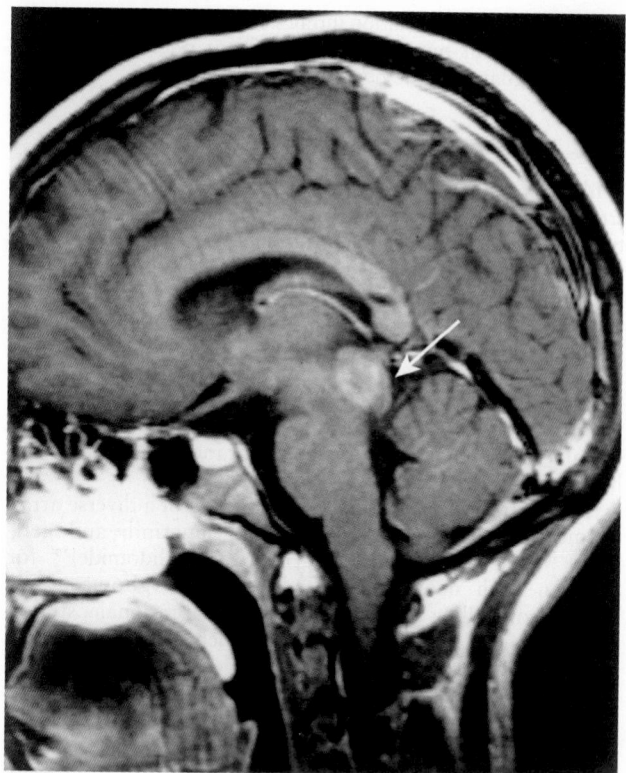

FIGURE 26A.14 T1-weighted sagittal magnetic resonance imaging with gadolinium of a tectal glioma with minimal contrast enhancement.

although the duration of benefit is measured in months, with few long-term survivors.[549,550] Attempts to improve outcome in the diffusely infiltrating pontine gliomas focused on altered radiation fractionation in the 1980s and 1990s; hyperfractionated delivery consisting of twice-daily irradiation with fractions of 100 to 125 cGy to doses ranging from 64.8 to 78.0 Gy showed no significant improvement.[550–554] A randomized trial comparing hyperfractionated irradiation at the "apparently best" dose level of 70.2 Gy with conventional fractionation (180 cGy once daily to 55.8 Gy) showed no difference, leading North American centers to consider conventional fractionation as the standard for current management and trials.[130]

Attempts at radiosensitization using *cis*-platinum concurrently with irradiation seemed to show similar or marginally inferior outcome for children with brainstem tumors when compared with irradiation alone.[538] A trial of tipifarnib plus radiotherapy in brainstem glioma was recently completed[251] and results of the phase II trial are pending. The PBTC is currently conducting a trial with capecitabine plus radiotherapy. Radiation therapy is a potent inducer of thymidine phosphorylase (TP), which is the key enzyme for intratumoral conversion of capecitabine to 5-fluorouracil.[555] Capecitabine antitumor activity is correlated with intratumoral TP; therefore, this combination may be more effective than radiotherapy alone for brainstem gliomas.

For dorsally exophytic brainstem tumors, radiation therapy is typically utilized when progression is apparent after initial surgery. Durable control after irradiation has been recorded in the majority of cases so managed.[383,533] Similarly, focal intrinsic brainstem gliomas, which are often pilocytic lesions, respond well to fractionated focal irradiation, usually with long-term disease control.[556–558] The low-grade brainstem lesions are treated with minimal margins circumscribing the immediate tumor region; dose levels are 50 to 54 Gy by conventional fractionation. Postirradiation intralesional necrosis or "swelling" is an infrequent but clinically significant phenomenon that requires vigilance in the postirradiation interval.[559]

Chemotherapy

A role has yet to be established for chemotherapy as standard treatment in the management of patients with brainstem tumors. With focal brainstem gliomas, weekly carboplatin with vincristine has shown activity in a very limited number of patients younger than 5 years.[392] For diffusely infiltrative pontine gliomas, response rates to various single-agent and multi-agent regimens have been disappointingly low, even when chemotherapy is given as first treatment, before radiation therapy.[560–564] Adjuvant chemotherapy using PCV did not improve survival when compared with conventional radiation therapy alone in the only prospective, randomized study that has tested this question.[565]

Recent trials have evaluated the addition of a diverse array of molecularly targeted agents (e.g., imatinib and gefitinib)[238,566] or antiangiogenic agents (e.g., thalidomide)[567] for children with newly diagnosed brainstem gliomas.[238,566] Despite compelling scientific and preclinical rationale, studies evaluating radiosensitizers, cytotoxic chemotherapy, or "targeted" therapies have to date failed to significantly prolong survival for children with diffuse brainstem gliomas.

A series of radiosensitizing strategies, such as the use of concurrent gadolinium texaphyrin or vorinostat, are being examined in the COG. As patients with progressive, diffusely infiltrative pontine gliomas survive, on average, at least 3 months after their first relapse, they can be candidates for further treatment in clinical trials. Such efforts may delay further disease progression and are requisite for improving the outcome in this disease group.

CRANIOPHARYNGIOMA

Demography

Craniopharyngiomas account for between 6% and 9% of all primary CNS tumors in children. These lesions exhibit a bimodal age distribution, with one peak during childhood at approximately 8 to 10 years of age and a second peak in middle age.[568] This tumor rarely occurs in infants. No gender predilection has been noted. Although these lesions are predominantly suprasellar tumors, which involve the pituitary stalk and hypothalamus, they may occur within the sella turcica or third ventricle as well.

Imaging

MRI defines the solid and cystic nature of the tumor, its extent, and its relation to adjacent structures better than does any other modality (Fig. 26A.15).

Pathology and Patterns of Spread

Craniopharyngiomas in children are thought to arise predominantly from pharyngeal cell rests left from the embryonic hypophyseal-pharyngeal duct that connects the infundibular bud with the stomodeum. Although, in adults, these tumors may result from neoplastic transformation of cell rests within the pituitary gland that have undergone squamous metaplasia,[569] this mechanism is less likely in children.[309] Grossly, these tumors are smooth, lobulated masses with both solid and cystic components. The cyst contents may range from gelatinous to viscous oily fluid rich in cholesterol crystals. Rupture of a cyst into the CSF may cause an intense chemical meningitis. Calcification is frequently apparent. Both the cystic lining and the solid portions of the tumor are characterized by squamous epithelium, usually with some evidence of keratinization (Fig. 26A.16). Nodules of "wet keratin," representing remnants of pale nuclei embedded within an eosinophilic keratinous mass, may be found throughout the tumor.[58]

Although craniopharyngioma is a histologically benign tumor composed of well-differentiated tissue, it may have a malignant clinical course because of its location and its propensity to infiltrate surrounding normal structures. A thick glial layer may encase the tumor, and small islands of epithelial tumor arising within this gliotic scar can extend into adjacent tissues. The tight adherence of this layer to surrounding tissue can make complete resection difficult and hazardous.

Clinical Presentation

Childhood craniopharyngiomas often manifest with short stature, symptoms of increased ICP, delayed puberty, vision loss, and neurobehavioral abnormalities. Hydrocephalus is observed

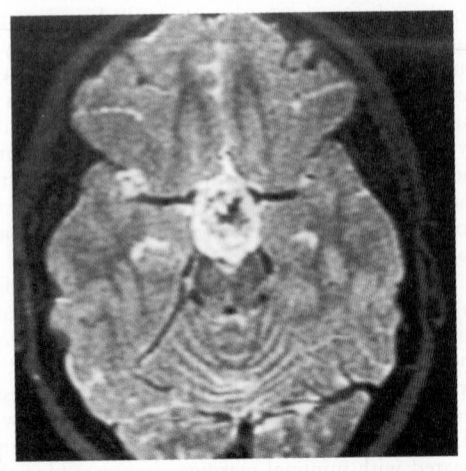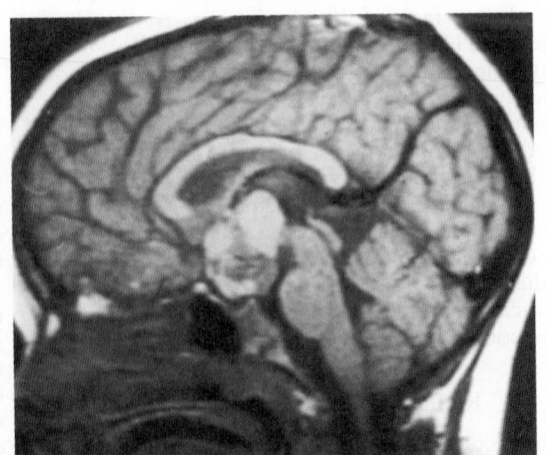

A **B**

FIGURE 26A.15 Axial (**A**) and sagittal (**B**) T2-weighted MR image show of mixed-density cranio-pharyngioma with foci of calcification (*black*).

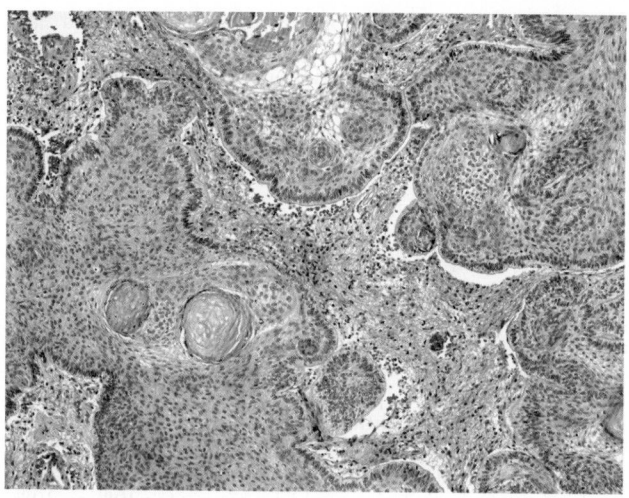

FIGURE 26A.16 Photomicrograph of craniopharyngioma revealing lobules of squamous epithelium with honeycombed character, bordered by palisaded columnar epithelium. Nodules of "wet" keratin are present (H&E, ×100).

in approximately 50% of children as a result of obstruction of the third ventricle and the foramen of Monro by superior tumor extension. Because of slow tumor growth, papilledema is less common than optic pallor. Visual field defects of various degrees of severity occur in 50% to 90% of patients, homonymous hemianopsia and bitemporal hemianopsia being the most frequent defects encountered. Despite the fact that many children show evidence of vision loss on examination, only approximately 25% present with complaints of visual deterioration.[570]

Various neuroendocrine deficits are present in as many as 90% of patients at diagnosis, decreases in GH, and resultant growth delay being the most common findings.[571] Diabetes insipidus is seen in fewer than 10% of children in whom craniopharyngiomas are diagnosed in the modern era and, if present in a child with a suprasellar lesion, should raise concern about the possibility of a germ cell tumor or histiocytosis.

Differential Diagnosis and Evaluation

The differential diagnosis of craniopharyngioma includes intrinsic hypothalamic gliomas, large chiasmal gliomas, Rathke's cleft cyst, and suprasellar germ cell tumors or teratomas. Plain skull radiographs, commonly used before the advent of CT and MRI, often show an enlarged or distorted sella with suprasellar tumor calcification. The CT scan characteristically demonstrates a partially cystic, low-density, contrast-enhancing lesion with calcification.

Owing to the high incidence of clinical and subclinical neuroendocrine deficits at diagnosis, a thorough evaluation of the hypothalamic-pituitary axis should be undertaken preoperatively. Secondary abnormalities of adrenal function and of the regulation of fluid and electrolyte balance, in particular, can lead to serious perioperative problems if not anticipated. Neuroendocrine evaluations should be repeated postoperatively and periodically thereafter for at least 1 year, because hormonal deficits often increase postoperatively and may take several months to stabilize fully.[572]

Prognostic Considerations

The extent of tumor resection has been an important factor in series in which the initial treatment has consisted of surgery

alone. Patients with totally excised tumors have had considerably better survival rates than those managed by biopsy alone or by subtotal resection.[573] However, several studies have shown that the combination of subtotal resection and radiation therapy achieves survival results that rival those obtained with attempted GTR.[112] The purported prognostic significance of tumor size probably is not an independent variable but rather is related to the ease and extent of resection. Although the data show only a trend, patients with purely cystic lesions appear to survive longer than those with solid or mixed solid and cystic tumors; in addition, children older than 5 years seem to have a better prognosis than do younger patients.[543,544]

Treatment

Surgery

Preoperative and perioperative considerations for operation on tumors in the region of the pituitary gland are reviewed in Chapter 26B. Those considerations specific to craniopharyngioma are discussed here.

Because tumor resection may cause or exacerbate endocrine deficiencies, the management of these problems must begin preoperatively and continue through the postoperative period. Stress doses of hydroxycorticosteroids (e.g., hydrocortisone, 100 mg/m² intravenously followed by 25 mg/m² every 6 hours) are administered before, during, and immediately after the surgical procedure, often in addition to dexamethasone, which is used to reduce peritumoral edema. Doses then are tapered but, if postoperative endocrine testing demonstrates a need for long-term steroid hormone replacement, then hydrocortisone is continued at maintenance levels. Following extensive tumor removal, many children will also require supplementation of other anterior pituitary hormones, including thyroid and GH, and ongoing endocrine monitoring is typically warranted.

Tumor removal can also lead to diabetes insipidus, particularly if the pituitary stalk is transected or manipulated extensively during the course of the resection. This risk necessitates vigilant monitoring of electrolytes in the intraoperative and postoperative period, since many children will manifest a triphasic response, characterized by an initial interval of diabetes insipidus beginning shortly after stalk interruption, followed several days later by an interval of inappropriate antidiuretic hormone release (SIADH), followed by return of diabetes insipidus. Because of the potential for rapid swings in serum sodium levels, careful monitoring of urine output and specific gravity, and serum electrolytes is needed to guide fluid replacement and the timing of institution of antidiuretic hormone replacement (e.g., with desmopressin).

In contrast to endocrine issues, which are often exacerbated by the tumor removal, hydrocephalus in patients with craniopharyngiomas generally resolves after the tumor has been resected. If the hydrocephalus is severe, a ventriculostomy can be inserted before the tumor resection is begun and can be removed within several days of surgery if the operative procedure opens the CSF pathways. If the hydrocephalus persists, a ventriculoperitoneal shunt is inserted.

The extent of surgical removal to be attempted is a matter of intense debate. Some authors strongly recommend radical surgery in all cases,[575,576] whereas others suggest partial resection followed by local irradiation.[112] The debate centers on the prognostic advantage gained by complete resection balanced by the morbidity associated with such a procedure. With the use of microsurgical techniques, a radiologically complete resection can be achieved in 60% to 90% of children.[570,575–578] Under these circumstances, the likelihood of long-term PFS is 80% to 90%. However, significant neurologic morbidity, memory and cognitive dysfunction, and appetite and neurobehavioral disturbances are encountered in 10% to 30% of patients; mortality ranges from 0% to 5%; and panhypopituitarism develops in 80% to 90% of patients.[575,576,579–581] The operative morbidity is lower in children operated on by neurosurgeons who perform such procedures frequently.[112] Although morbidity may also be lessened somewhat by more limited resections, the likelihood of long-term disease control is substantially lower than with complete resection. Without radiation therapy, the vast majority of subtotally resected tumors progress within 2 to 5 years.[582,583] The recurrence rate is diminished significantly with the use of postoperative external irradiation,[112,584] although some studies indicate that the results, in terms of PFS, remain inferior to those achieved with total resection.[582] Although repeat microsurgical resection is feasible in patients with recurrent tumor, morbidity and mortality may be substantially higher than at the primary operation.[575] The primary cause of death in these patients is either recurrent tumor or chronic neuroendocrine problems.[585]

Craniopharyngiomas are extra-axial tumors, tenaciously attached to surrounding structures, such as the optic chiasm, hypothalamus, and vessels of the circle of Willis. These characteristics impose practical limits on a surgeon's attempt at tumor resection. Regardless of the degree of surgical resection intended at the outset, most cases have historically been approached via a subfrontal or transsylvian exposure, working between the optic nerves, carotid arteries, and third nerves, or through the lamina terminalis. Large tumors extending to the roof of the third ventricle can also be approached through the corpus callosum. A recent advance in the management of these lesions has been the use of extended endonasal approaches, which has broadened the potential indications for subcranial removal of these tumors.[586] An appeal of this approach is the reduced need for brain retraction and the direct visualization of the attachment of the tumor to the hypothalamus, pituitary stalk, and optic apparatus,[587] although longer-term follow-up will be needed to determine whether the results in terms of morbidity and disease control compare favorably to conventional management strategies. In some cases, a combination of therapeutic approaches is required. Other approaches may be used, depending on tumor extent and location and a growing trend is to tailor the treatment strategy based on tumor size and composition. Tumors with a sizable solid component (>3 cm) are treated microsurgically. Thin-walled cystic lesions can be treated using intracavitary techniques; if small residual solid components of the tumor subsequently enlarge, stereotactic radiosurgery or microsurgical techniques can be used. The management of small, solid tumors (<3 cm in diameter) remains particularly controversial, with most groups favoring microsurgical resection and others employing stereotactic techniques.

Radiation Therapy

There is considerable controversy regarding primary irradiation versus primary surgery for craniopharyngiomas. Long-term results with limited surgery (biopsy, limited decompression, or planned subtotal resection) followed by external beam irradiation approximate the same 80% to more than 90% rate of disease control reported after imaging-confirmed complete surgical resection.[112,588–593] Similar results are reported following irradiation for disease residual after attempted total resection.[581,589,590,594,595] Although most institutions stress initial irradiation for documented disease residual, there is limited experience suggesting adequate outcome when irradiation is deferred until documented postoperative progression.[596,597]

Contemporary irradiation requires image-guided approaches, using either 3D-CRT or IMRT to target volumes closely approximating visible tumor. The role for limited surgical resection to decompress cystic components or remove peripheral tumor resulting in more limited radiation target volumes is yet under study.[590] The target volume dose is 54 to 56 Gy.

Although a controlled trial has not been done, multiple comparisons strongly suggest that patients treated with incomplete tumor resection followed by irradiation have less neuroendocrine dysfunction and fewer serious sensory, motor, and visual deficits than do those who have undergone aggressive attempts at complete tumor resection. These patients may also have an improved level of function and better quality of life than patients treated with radical surgery alone.[579,581,590,591] In addition, neuropsychological function is reportedly better preserved in the combined-therapy group despite the known detrimental effect of irradiation.[581,584,592] Predominantly cystic lesions, which account for 20% to 30% of tumors, may be treated with intracystic instillation of yttrium-90 or phosphorus-32 to deliver high-dose intralesional therapy.[135,136,598,599] Involution of the cyst is achieved in more than 80% of patients,[598–600] morbidity and mortality are lower than with microsurgical resection, and the recurrence rate is comparable with that achieved with attempted total microsurgical removal.[598,600] Because of the limited tissue penetration of the radiation from these β-emitting isotopes, radiation exposure to the adjacent hypothalamus and optic nerves is often minimized; focal high-dose regions adjacent to the chiasm can result in visual complications.[590] After intracavitary therapy, small, residual solid-tumor components can be treated with stereotactic radiosurgery.[444,598]

Chemotherapy

Chemotherapy has no established role in the treatment of craniopharyngiomas. An anecdotal response to a vincristine, BCNU, and procarbazine combination has been described in one patient.[601] Intracystic administration of bleomycin has also led to response and significant second remissions in some patients with recurrent disease,[602] but concerns have been raised regarding local toxicity. The use of systemic interferon-α has also been evaluated in a phase II study, with some favorable responses.[603]

CHOROID PLEXUS NEOPLASMS

Demography

Choroid plexus neoplasms constitute between 1% and 4% of brain tumors in children. Seventy percent of these occur during the first 2 years of life; the median age at diagnosis ranges from 10 to 32 months.[604–606] CPPs, benign tumors treated only surgically, outnumber the malignant counterpart, choroid plexus carcinoma (CPC), by nearly four to one.[607] Tumors arise from the lateral ventricles approximately 75% of the time, from the fourth ventricle and cerebellopontine angle in 15% of cases (Fig. 26A.17), and from the third ventricle in 10% of affected children.[608]

Imaging

CPPs are intraventricular tumors that are well circumscribed. In children, these tumors arise in the lateral ventricle, often the trigone, whereas, in adults, they are found in the fourth ventricle. CPPs are lobulated in appearance and are associated with

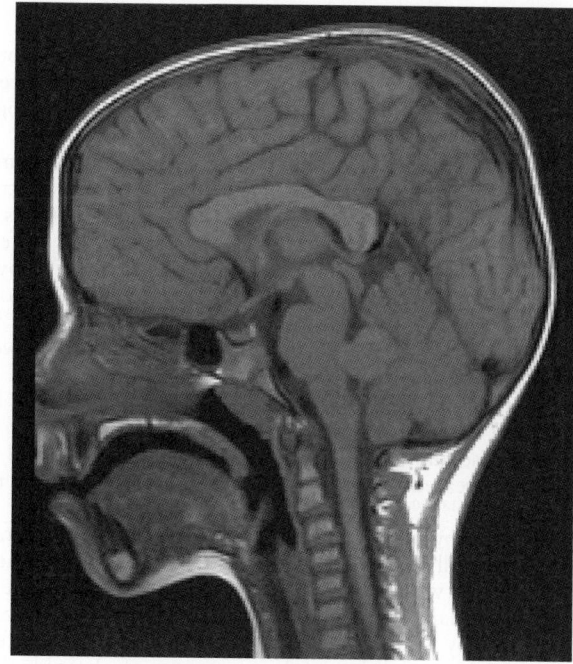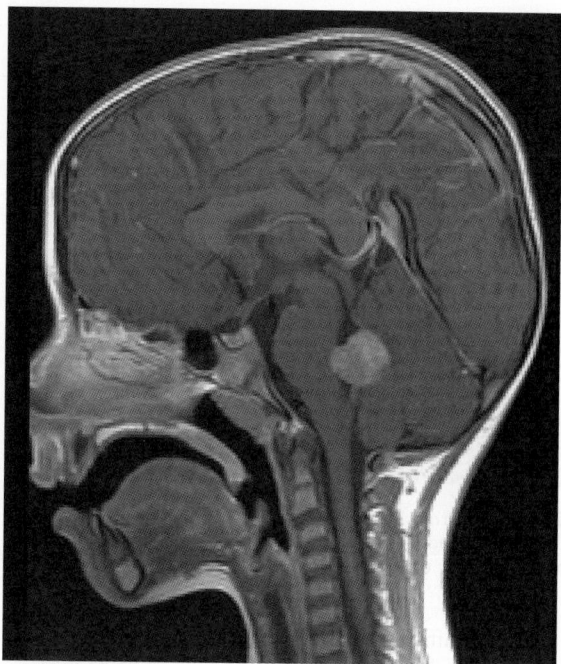

A   **B**

FIGURE 26A.17 A: Sagittal T1-weighted pre- and post-Gd imaging of a well-defined posterior fossa mass within the fourth ventricle. **B:** It demonstrates avid enhancement following the administration of contrast, typical for a choroid plexus papilloma, which in this case was not causing hydrocephalus.

hydrocephalus often containing punctate regions of calcification, hemorrhage, and vascular flow voids. The hydrocephalus may arise from CSF overproduction and/or obstruction. Imaging features on CT include a lobulated intraventricular mass with calcification and homogenously intense enhancement. MR features include T1 isointense to hypointense signal with T2 hypointensity and intense contrast enhancement. On MR spectroscopy, these tumors exhibited a significantly higher level of the metabolite, myoinositol; low Cr; and decreased Cho when compared with CPCs.[609]

CPCs are heterogeneous on MR with regions of necrosis and hemorrhage, extend beyond the margin of the ventricle, and are associated with edema and mass effect. Both CPPs and CPCs can seed the CSF pathways. These tumors have elevated Cho levels compared with CPPs.[610]

Pathology and Patterns of Spread

CPPs generally arise as functioning intraventricular papillomas capable of secreting CSF. Grossly, CPPs resemble a soft coral, with fronds of tumor attached to a pedicle that floats in the CSF. Microscopically, these tumors are similar to normal choroid plexus and have cuboidal or columnar epithelium and a well-preserved epithelial-stromal border overlying fibrovascular septa (Fig. 26A.18). Their neoplastic nature is reflected in the heaping and redundancy of the epithelial component. These tumors tend to be slow growing and, because of their intraventricular location, often reach a size of 60 to 70 g before they are diagnosed. Fewer than 5% are bilateral. CPPs can invade adjacent brain parenchyma, typically with a benign cellular appearance. One retrospective series suggested that local invasion does not adversely impact prognosis.[611]

The CPC, a more aggressive and anaplastic tumor, accounts for up to 40% of choroid plexus neoplasms. This tumor has lost the well-differentiated papillary structure and the epithelial-stromal border of the CPP (Fig. 26A.19). It is a hypercellular tumor with pleomorphic cells, frequent mitoses, and foci of necrosis.[612] Both papillomas and carcinomas are capable of

leptomeningeal dissemination. In CPPs, the clinical behavior and histology of the isolated and frequently noted deposits are benign, and symptoms are uncommon. Conversely, CPCs may have frank metastases along CSF pathways.[58]

Prognostic Considerations

Tumor histology and degree of resection are the primary prognostic factors for choroid plexus neoplasms. The long-term recurrence-free survival after complete resection of CPP approaches 100%.[608,613] Even less-than-complete resection is associated with long periods of PFS. The outcome is less favorable in patients with CPC,[614] because these lesions invade the brain parenchyma and are extremely vascular, making

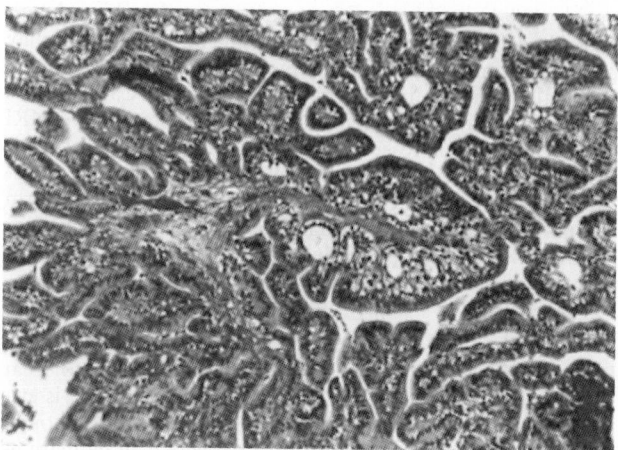

FIGURE 26A.18 Choroid plexus carcinoma. The papillary pattern is only partially retained by the tumor (field on the right) while the large majority demonstrates diffuse and solid growth (field on the left) (H & E, 200×).

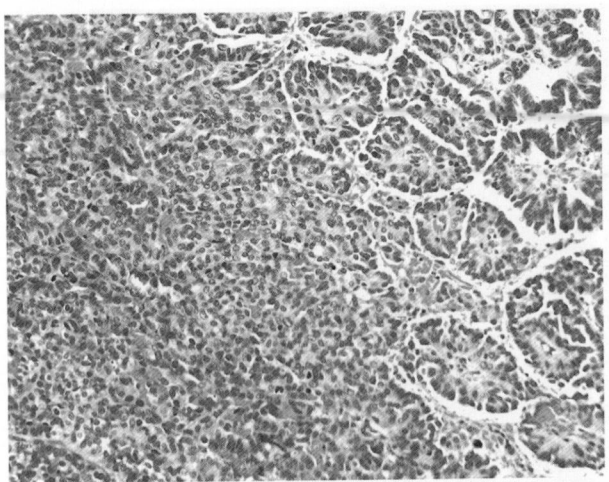

FIGURE 26A.19 Choroid plexus papilloma. The photograph illustrates the papillary structures composed of loose fibrovascular cores lined by a single layer of cuboidal-columnar epithelium (H & E, 100×).

complete resection difficult. In addition, these tumors often disseminate within the CSF. Nevertheless, in reviews of experience with CPC, complete resection of disease appears to be the single variable that most affects long-term survival. In fact, GTR of CPC may be curative by itself in a proportion of children.[615]

Treatment

Surgery

Surgical excision is the primary mode of therapy for both CPP and CPC. These lesions most commonly arise in the trigone; tumors in this location usually are approached through a posterior temporoparietal craniotomy, through a cortical sulcus. Tumors of the anterior third ventricle and the body and frontal horn of the lateral ventricle may be approached transcallosally or transcortically through the middle frontal gyrus. Fourth ventricular tumors are approached by the suboccipital route. Intraventricular tumors outside the posterior fossa may be more easily removed if the ventricles are large; for this reason, preoperative shunts usually are not inserted in patients who are otherwise clinically stable. Contemporary surgical morbidity and mortality rates are less than 20% and 5%, respectively. Complete resections are possible in approximately 80% of patients and is much more easily achieved with CPPs than CPCs, in which brain invasion and vascularity may preclude tumor removal.[608] Even after complete tumor removal, persistent hydrocephalus requiring a CSF shunt is present in up to 60% of patients.[616] If the postoperative MRI scan demonstrates resectable residual tumor, reoperation is indicated. Appreciation for the importance of complete surgical resection has provided an impetus for efforts to perform second-look surgery with initially unresectable CPCs in those children whose incompletely resected tumors persist but decrease in size after a trial of neoadjuvant chemotherapy.

Radiation Therapy

Postoperative radiation therapy frequently is used to treat CPC, especially if the resection is incomplete or if there is evidence of leptomeningeal dissemination of disease. Although the survival times of some irradiated patients may be marginally better than those of nonirradiated patients, such results are not entirely separable from results with surgery alone. No randomized trial has yet tested the benefit of radiation therapy.

Chemotherapy

Surgery alone is usually sufficient for cure of CPP; chemotherapy has no role in the treatment of this tumor. Tumor recurrence after GTR in CPP is rare; however, malignant progression to CPC can occur, albeit rarely.[617]

As with other uncommon malignant pediatric CNS tumors, the role of chemotherapy is difficult to define in the treatment of CPC. Numerous reports of small numbers of patients collectively demonstrate that CPC can respond to different chemotherapeutic regimens at initial diagnosis or following relapse. The regimens given to the highest number of patients were based on a platinum-containing regimen,[608,618,619] cyclophosphamide[615] or included multiple agents.[614] However, whereas most patients with CPC treated with GTR and chemotherapy appear to be long-term survivors, cure has been achieved with GTR alone. Furthermore, the majority of children whose tumors are less than completely resected and who also are treated with chemotherapy ultimately die of their disease.[614,618,620] Anecdotal reports, however, suggest that chemotherapy may render CPC less vascular and infiltrative and potentially amenable to complete removal, even if the initial attempt was unsuccessful.[614,619,621] Thus, chemotherapy may potentially contribute to higher chances of survival as suggested by a meta-analysis evaluating the role of different therapeutic modalities in the treatment of choroid plexus neoplasms.[622] Because the number of children with choroid plexus neoplasms is too low, international collaborative clinical trials will be needed to test hypotheses related to outcome of therapy.

INTRAMEDULLARY SPINAL CORD TUMORS

Demography

Intrinsic tumors of the spinal cord make up 1% to 10% of pediatric CNS tumors.[623–627] These tumors occur throughout childhood, and the median age at diagnosis is 10 years. Male patients are slightly more commonly affected than female patients, in a 1.3:1.0 ratio. Patients with neurofibromatosis appear to have a higher incidence of spinal cord tumors, as they do with other astrocytic neoplasms.

Imaging

Intrinsic tumors of the spinal cord, such as primary gliomas and ependymomas, are best imaged with MRI. It is also the imaging modality of choice for leptomeningeal spinal seeding. The spine should be scanned preoperatively, however when such a scan cannot be performed, a baseline study should be performed approximately 3 weeks into the postoperative period to avoid the problems of interpreting the appearances of postsurgical subdural blood. CSF cytology is complementary to spinal imaging in detecting subarachnoid disease.

Sagittal T1 images of the entire spine with gadolinium are obtained with axial T1 images obtained as needed.

Pathology and Patterns of Spread

In children, up to 70% of intramedullary tumors are astrocytomas, primarily diffuse rather than pilocytic astrocytomas. The remaining 30% are ependymomas, other glial neoplasms such as oligodendrogliomas, gangliogliomas, and malignant gliomas. Histologically, these tumors are indistinguishable from their intracranial counterparts. Large cysts, both within the tumor and at the superior and inferior margins, are common. In as many as 60% of cases, extensive involvement by tumor and cysts may be present. Slow and contiguous extension across several vertebral segments, with compression and effacement of normal tissues, is the usual mode of growth.[628-630] Leptomeningeal dissemination has been reported in as many as 58% of patients with high-grade tumors, but it is uncommon in patients with low-grade tumors.[630,631] The presence of multiple discrete tumors is associated with neurofibromatosis. Tumor location in the spinal cord appears to be random, with the incidence in each anatomic region (cervical, thoracic, lumbar) roughly proportional to the length of that region. The only exception is the myxopapillary ependymoma, which has a predilection for the conus medullaris and filum terminale.

Prognostic Considerations

Spinal cord tumors in children are rare occurrences. The low number of patients and relative lack of inclusion in clinical trials with prescribed treatment approaches make the identification of published prognostic factors difficult. Bouffet et al.[627] reviewed the experience of 13 French treatment centers with spinal cord astrocytoma and found high-grade histology and short duration of presenting symptoms to be associated with poorer survival.[627] From review of other series, low-grade lesions are compatible with long-term survival, whereas this appears not to be the case with high-grade lesions. Although investigators have suggested that complete tumor removal may be associated with longer survival and less frequent local recurrences, the degree of resection has not been associated with outcome in several studies. However, such a determination is problematic in view of the small sizes of the study cohorts.[627,632-634] Ependymomas may be an exception to this generalization, in that patients who undergo total tumor resection have fewer recurrences than do those who undergo incomplete tumor resections.[635]

Treatment

Surgery

Complete surgical resection is difficult for astrocytoma because a distinct tumor-cord interface often is absent, but extensive subtotal resections may be performed in most instances. Ependymomas are associated with a clearer cleavage plane and can usually be resected completely. Intramedullary tumors usually are approached by an osteoplastic laminectomy, removing as a single unit all laminae covering the solid portion of the tumor. Replacement of the lamina after surgery not only helps to protect the spinal cord but also may diminish the risk of subsequent spinal deformity. Operative morbidity and the amount of neurologic recovery are generally related to the severity of preoperative dysfunction and to the definition of the tumor-cord interface. In one report of 69 patients undergoing operations for intramedullary tumors, at a mean follow-up of 54 months, 17% were better than they had been preoperatively, 56% were unchanged, and 31% were worse.[636] Postoperative orthopedic follow-up and monitoring for spinal deformity are important. In 25% to 40% of children, the development or progression of such deformity occurs within a mean of 3 years.

Radiation Therapy

No controlled trial of radiation therapy has been conducted in patients with intramedullary tumors, and evidence for its util-

ity is inferred from the treatment of similar tumors in other CNS locations. As with low-grade lesions in the cerebrum, irradiation may be deferred for incompletely resected low-grade tumors in very young children or when there is expectation that subsequent surgery might be truly extirpative. With significant disease residual, common practice often includes local postoperative irradiation to dose levels of 50 Gy.[298,637-639]

Data on spinal ependymomas are sparse, and prognostic factors remain controversial. A study of a historical cohort, with large patient numbers and long follow-up, provides estimates of time to progression, survival after progression, and influence of potential prognostic variables. At 5, 10, and 15 years, percentages of patients who were progression free were 75%, 50%, and 46%, respectively. Local relapse rates for spinal ependymomas were higher than previously cited, with a large proportion of failures occurring more than 5 years after diagnosis. Extensive surgical resection correlated with longer time to recurrence supporting the recommendation of maximal excision while avoiding surgical morbidity. The overall high rate of recurrence led these investigators to recommend radiation to doses of 45 to 54 Gy for all patients who do not have GTRs and long, close follow-up.[640] Some series indicate that in intramedullary spinal cord or cauda equina ependymomas, postoperative radiation therapy may be withheld if a microscopically complete surgical excision is documented.[298,299]

For malignant gliomas, postoperative irradiation is standard therapy. Target volumes typically extend 2 to 5 cm beyond the lesion identified by T1 imaging; dose levels to the primary tumor site are often in the 50- to 54-Gy range.[635,641]

The overall survival rates for low-grade gliomas with various degrees of resection and postoperative radiation therapy are 66% to 70% at 5 years, 55% to 73% at 10 years, and 67% at 20 years.[298,632,634,635,638,641,642] Durable control of anaplastic astrocytoma or glioblastoma has been elusive. For patients with ependymomas, survival rates of 50% to 100% at 5 years and 50% to 70% at 10 years are reported, and local recurrences are relatively high in patients with subtotally resected tumors.[298,628,632,637-639]

Chemotherapy

Tumors of the spinal cord have been treated as their histologic counterparts in other parts of the brain. Chemotherapy has been employed for high-grade lesions at diagnosis, for recurrent low-grade lesions, and in very young children in whom the avoidance of radical surgery or radiation therapy has been desired.[623,625,643] The largest of these series involved 13 children with high-grade astrocytoma of the spine who were treated with 8-in-1 chemotherapy along with radiation therapy, postoperatively. The response to preradiation chemotherapy was not measurable in three patients, complete in one patient, partial in two, stable in four, mixed in two, and progressive in one. After completion of therapy, with the time of median follow-up not stated, 2 of the 13 patients were alive without disease at the report, and 5 were alive with disease. Five-year PFS and survival rates were 46% and 54%, respectively.[625]

Until biologic factors or other clinical trial results indicate otherwise, it seems rational to use chemotherapy for tumors of the spinal cord only as would be used for tumors of like histologies in other areas of the brain.

SEQUELAE OF TREATMENT

Mortality rates for children with brain tumors have declined less rapidly than those of other cancers.[644] Nevertheless, the 5-year overall survival for children with brain tumors, aside from the favorable low-grade gliomas, has improved to 60%.[645] Despite successful therapy, children with CNS tumors may have physical, cognitive, neurologic, endocrinologic, or other deficits as direct sequelae of their tumor or as a result of therapy. As a whole, these patients function at lower intellectual, social, and physical levels than their peers, which in turn leads to a diminished quality of life. The eventual magnitude of these problems may be greatest in patients who are the youngest at diagnosis (see Chapters 13, 15, and 47).

The acute and late effects amongst pediatric brain tumor patients arise from several sources. Before diagnosis, the tumor mass distorts and even destroys normal brain tissue and increases ICP, which may be associated with hydrocephalus. Surgical trauma, postoperative meningitis, shunt infection, or repeat surgery can cause some degree of irreversible neurologic damage. Likewise, chemotherapy may be capable of producing encephalopathy. Radiation therapy has been implicated as the chief cause of many adverse sequelae, which are listed in Table 26A.7.

The subacute effects of irradiation, apparent 2 to 6 months or more after therapy, include intralesional necrosis or edema, perilesional white matter changes, or alterations in adjacent white matter or cerebral nuclei (e.g., basal ganglia) that may be silent or accompanied by site-specific symptomatology.[148]

Cognitive impairment is among the most devastating problems of the child treated with radiation therapy.[152,646-649] Neurocognitive deficits are inversely related to age at the time of irradiation and correlate directly with both site (supratentorial irradiation >> posterior fossa irradiation) and radiation dose.[153,153,646,649] Detailed prospective studies indicate that radiation-related cognitive problems include relative difficulty with selective attending and acquisition of new knowledge; over time, the relatively mild difference in intellectual development equates to significant declines in IQ for children younger than 5 to 8 years when treated, with more subtle changes in older children.[152,650-652]

Full-brain irradiation to dose levels of more than 30 to 36 Gy in infants and very young children has been associated with severe intellectual deficits; such children have median IQ scores of 60 to 65 at 5 to 7 years posttherapy, indicating little likelihood of ultimate independent function as adults.[653] Sophisticated local radiation techniques, particularly when tumors are confined to the posterior fossa, have shown rather stable neurocognitive function even in children averaging only 2.8 years of age.[152] Detailed assessment of neuropsychological function usually identifies multiple areas of damage in information processing. Some studies have found specific neurocognitive deficits in attention, memory, coordination, fine motor speed, visual motor processing, mathematics, and spatial relations.[153,646,653]

Treatment of neurocognitive deficits with pharmacologic and/or rehabilitative interventions may ameliorate the learning and memory difficulties associated with declines in IQ.[152] Methylphenidate has been shown to reverse attentional problems and improve memory/learning at least in time-limited measures.[654] Ongoing studies are being performed to address prospective interventions during and immediately after irradiation.

As another consequence of radiation therapy to whole brain, hypothalamic-pituitary region, or spine, growth failure occurs commonly among brain tumor patients. Irradiation along the spinal axis retards the growth of the vertebral column and spinal cord, leading to a child with a short trunk and disproportionately longer extremities. Spinal irradiation alone has been associated with a decrease in eventual height of 9, 7, and 5.5 cm when administered at ages 1, 5, and 10 years, respectively.[655] A larger contribution to decreased stature

stems from impaired GH secretion. Noted in up to 25% of brain tumor children even before irradiation, deficits appear in almost all children within 1 to 2 years after irradiation that includes the hypothalamic-pituitary axis.[166,656] The use of concomitant chemotherapy may increase further the severity of growth retardation.[657] The effect of precocious puberty prematurely fusing bony epiphyses also can contribute to short stature.

Hormone replacement therapy should be considered in patients whose growth velocity has declined and who do not respond to provocative GH testing. The decision regarding whether and when to initiate replacement remains emotional and controversial for parents and physicians, most North American neurooncology groups recommend initiation of GH after 1 or more years of disease control or stabilization.[658]

Although the hormone is mitogenic, it does not appear to produce any increased risk for tumor recurrence.[658,669] Other neuroendocrine deficits may also be seen. Primary, or less commonly secondary or tertiary, hypothyroidism may occur in more than half of patients as a result of irradiation to the thyroid gland or the hypothalamic-pituitary axis, respectively.[661,662] Puberty may occur prematurely or at normal onset but only seldom is delayed. Abnormalities of gonadotropin or corticotropin secretion may be less common.[661] Male patients appear to be less at risk than female patients for gonadal dysfunction secondary to spinal irradiation, but the synergistic effect from commonly used drugs such as cyclophosphamide and nitrosoureas, known to affect oogenesis and spermatogenesis, has not been estimated.[662]

High-frequency, sensorineural hearing loss is another complication that is frequent among brain tumor survivors, most commonly caused by repeated administration of cisplatin. Cisplatin results in rather immediate, dose-dependent reduction in high frequency hearing; if continued, more pronounced hearing deficits occur into the speech range. Irradiation is associated with a relatively late, pronounced, typically unilateral sensorineural hearing loss that occurs in 10% to 15% of children after doses of more than 50 to 54 Gy. Highly CRT may reduce the risk of ototoxicity.[161]

The optimal management of the potential acute and long-term needs of children with tumors of the CNS requires a multidisciplinary team. This team should include physicians (oncologists, neurologists, neurosurgeons, radiation oncologists, ophthalmologists, endocrinologists, cancer geneticists, physiatrists) and nurses as well as an occupational therapist, physical therapist, child life worker, educational psychologist, audiologist, and social worker. The team and family must remember that the effects resulting from the tumor or its treatment may not occur or become fully manifest until several years after completion of therapy. Consequently, yearly physical examinations and neuropsychological evaluations should be performed for at least the first 5 years after therapy. Children who have intellectual impairments require further evaluation so that proper educational intervention can begin, if not already implemented. Educational interventions have been associated with improvements in spelling and reading, particularly when written feedback was provided to parents and schools, even years after therapy.[647]

Other routine evaluations should be tailored to the patient's tumor and prior therapy. An evaluation by an occupational therapist may be indicated to assess fine motor and visual skills. Endocrinologic evaluation should be based on the tumor location and treatment. For the majority of patients, this will include an annual thyroid function studies (for a minimum of 5 years) to monitor for subclinical manifestations of hypothyroidism. Appropriate thyroid replacement is critical to growth, learning, and prevention of thyroid

SYNDROMES OF POSTRADIATION SEQUELAE WITH CHILDHOOD BRAIN TUMORS

Syndrome	Onset	Cause	Clinical manifestation	Treatment and outcome
Somnolence syndrome	4–8 wk after RT	Whole-brain or large-field supratentorial RT	7–14 days of lethargy, malaise, nausea, vomiting, and anorexia	Can respond to dexamethasone; usually self-limited
Radiation necrosis	Usually 3 mo–3 yr after RT	Idiosyncratic, 0.1%–1.0% with conventional RT; increased with higher dose per fraction or total dosage, usually after ≥5,500 cGy	Focal neurologic dysfunction, seizures, symptoms of increased intracranial pressure, coma, or death	Focal areas resectable; dexamethasone if unresectable or small
Mineralizing microangiopathy with dystrophic calcification	Unknown; 9 mo–several years after RT	≥2,000 cGy; perhaps potentiated by intrathecal methotrexate or cytarabine	None or possible headaches, seizures, strokes	Unclear (often an autopsy finding)
Moyamoya disease	6 mo–15 yr after RT, particularly in children ≤3 yr	Arterial occlusion after ≥4,000 cGy RT; associated with neurofibromatosis type 1	Headaches, seizures, transient ischemic attacks, strokes, progressive mental deterioration	Some stabilize from spontaneous collateral vessel formation; arterial bypass surgery may improve outcome
Endocrinologic dysfunction	Biphasic; early dysfunction and then fixed damage 1–5 yr after RT	RT to hypothalamus, pituitary gland, thyroid gland, or gonads	Growth failure, thyroid deficiency, gonadotropin deficiency	Requires hormonal replacement; static damage
Neuropsychological damage	Increases with time from RT; unclear whether plateaus	Any brain RT; increases with larger total dosage or volume or younger age; also complicated by the effects of the tumor itself, surgery, and chemotherapy	Cognitive deficits, learning disabilities, and behavioral abnormalities	Requires remediation and special education; may progress over time
Secondary brain tumor	5–25 yr after RT	≥1,800 cGy RT, perhaps potentiated by chemotherapy and genetic predisposition	Meningioma, high-grade astrocytoma, or sarcoma	Often poor prognosis

RT, radiation therapy.

tumors from persistently elevated thyroid-stimulating hormone. Longitudinal audiometry should also be considered for at least several years, particularly in patients who received platinum analogues or radiation to the posterior fossa.

Long-term management of the child with a brain tumor also includes surveillance for disease relapse. Surveillance of brain tumor patients, unlike patients with other childhood cancers, is indeed a chronic issue. Progression or recurrence of tumors such as ependymoma or the low-grade gliomas frequently does not occur until 3 to 5 or more years from diagnosis. The ideal surveillance modalities and schedule for all the diverse tumor pathologies is unclear. Despite fair agreement that serial clinical examination is important not only to detect signs suggestive of relapse but also to monitor for the already mentioned sequelae of treatment, controversy surrounds the timing and need for surveillance MRI. For malignant brain tumors, the COG has recommended surveillance MRI every 3 months during the first year after diagnosis, every 4 months during the second year, biannually during years 3 and 4 from diagnosis, and, finally, annual to biennial scanning until 12 years after diagnosis.[663] Most recommendations today are based on retrospective analyses. Prospective evaluation of neuroimaging surveillance schedules appropriate to the heterogeneous CNS tumor pathologies is needed.

Although prevention of these deleterious sequelae is beginning to receive attention, judging the efficacy of current interventions is difficult. Reduction of radiation effects on the CNS can be achieved by diminishing radiation volume (through use of image-guided 3D-CRT or IMRT), dose, or the use of irradiation (particularly in infants and very young children who require large treatment volumes). Several factors other than radiation therapy can influence neurocognitive and neuroendocrine function, and chemotherapy itself may have deleterious effects on the developing nervous system. Furthermore, prolonged chemotherapy with alkylators and etoposide among infants with brain tumors has been associated with an excess risk of second malignancies.[664] Other new strategies to mitigate damage have yet to be tested. Conformal techniques can better focus the radiation delivered, such as in the posterior fossa where, in the past, local field treatment still exposed the hypothalamus and hippocampus just beyond the posterior clinoid processes. The chemoprotectant amifostine has yet to be widely studied with cisplatin administration.

Because most patients with neurocognitive deficits do not have observable histopathologic changes, the location and pathogenesis of their problems are not well established. Thus, understanding the ways in which radiation and chemotherapy alter axonal growth, dendritic arborization and pruning, synaptogenesis, and myelination, all of which occur in childhood and adolescence, is presumably critical to understanding the development of these problems and remains largely unknown. Evidence suggests that MRI is capable of demonstrating areas of treatment-related white matter abnormalities not visible on CT that may correlate with the degree of clinical neurologic compromise, particularly in IQ, factual knowledge, and verbal and nonverbal thinking.[615] Prospective evaluation with new MRI techniques and other novel neuroimaging modalities may improve understanding of the location and dynamics of damage associated with various therapies.

Imprecise methods, small patient numbers, and limited funding for studying patients with CNS tumors have been barriers to our knowledge of late effects. Closer collaboration with schools for assessment and intervention might help. In the future, comprehensive batteries that take the entire child into account are needed. Given that executive function, memory, pragmatic language, and other cognitive functions change over time, such evaluations should steer assessment away from IQ and toward developmental neuropsychological models. More precise definitions of disability and quality of life are needed. Newly validated instruments that measure quality of life should be implemented. Assessments will also have to consider practical outcomes, such as the ability to hold a job, drive a car, manage finances, or live independently. Interventional trials of medications that improve arousal, attention, and memory, such as modafinil, methylphenidate, or donepezil, are also needed.

INFORMATION ON CLINICAL TRIALS

For more information about clinical trials or other support services for children with brain tumors, a list of resources is provided in Table 26A.8.

TABLE 26A.8

RESOURCES FOR INFORMATION REGARDING CLINICAL TRIALS OR SUPPORT SERVICES FOR CHILDREN WITH CNS TUMORS

Organization	Phone number	Website
American Brain Tumor Association	800.886.2282	www.abta.org
Brain Tumor Foundation of Canada		http://www.braintumour.ca/braintumour.nsf/eng/home
Children's Cause for Cancer Advocacy	301.562.2765	www.childrenscause.org/about
Children's Oncology Group	800.458.6223	www.childrensoncologygroup.org
Childhood Brain Tumor Foundation	301.515.2900	www.childhoodbraintumor.org
Children's Brain Tumor Foundation	212.448.9494	http://cbtf.org/cms
	866.228.4673	
National Brain Tumor Foundation	800.934.CURE	www.braintumor.org
National Cancer Institute	301.496.6641	www.cancer.gov/clinicaltrials
Musella Foundation for Brain Tumor Research	516.295.4740	www.virtualtrials.com/musella.cfm
Pediatric Brain Tumor Consortium	301.496.6641	www.pbtc.org
Pediatric Brain Tumor Foundation of the United States	800.253.6530	www.pbtfus.org
The Brain Tumor Society	800.770.8287	www.tbts.org
United Kingdom Children's Cancer Study Group		www.ukccsg.org

References

1. Arora RS, Alston RD, Eden TO, et al. Age-incidence patterns of primary CNS tumors in children, adolescents, and adults in England. Neuro Oncol 2008;11(4):403–413.
2. Central Brain Tumor Registry of the United States. Fact Sheet. Stromberg Allen Company, 2009.
3. Fisher PG, Jenab J, Goldthwaite PT, et al. Outcomes and failure patterns in childhood craniopharyngiomas. Childs Nerv Syst 1998;14:558–563.
4. Jemal A, Siegel R, Ward E, et al. Cancer statistics, 2008. CA Cancer J Clin 2008; 58:71–96.
5. Ries LA, Kosary CL, Hankey BF, et al. SEER cancer statistics review, 1973–1994. NIH Pub No. 97-2789. Bethesda, MD: National Cancer Institute, SEER Program, 1997.
6. Smith MA, Freidlin B, Ries LA, et al. Trends in reported incidence of primary malignant brain tumors in children in the United States. J Natl Cancer Inst 1998;90:1269–1277.
7. Bleyer WA. Epidemiologic impact of children with brain tumors. Childs Nerv Syst 1999;15:758–763.
8. Taylor MD, Mainprize TG, Rutka JT. Molecular insight into medulloblastoma and central nervous system primitive neuroectodermal tumor biology from hereditary syndromes: a review. Neurosurgery 2000;47:888–901.
9. Malkin D, Li FP, Strong LC, et al. Germ line p53 mutations in a familial syndrome of breast cancer, sarcomas, and other neoplasms. Science 1990;250:1233–1238.
10. Liaw D, Marsh DJ, Li J, et al. Germline mutations of the PTEN gene in Cowden disease, an inherited breast and thyroid cancer syndrome. Nat Genet 1997;16:64–67.
11. Ron E, Modan B, Boice JD Jr., et al. Tumors of the brain and nervous system after radiotherapy in childhood. N Engl J Med 1988;319:1033–1039.
12. Kimball Dalton VM, Gelber RD, Li F, et al. Second malignancies in patients treated for childhood acute lymphoblastic leukemia. J Clin Oncol 1998;16:2848–2853.
13. Loning L, Zimmermann M, Reiter A, et al. Secondary neoplasms subsequent to Berlin-Frankfurt-Munster therapy of acute lymphoblastic leukemia in childhood: significantly lower risk without cranial radiotherapy. Blood 2000;95:2770–2775.
14. Rimm IJ, Li FC, Tarbell NJ, et al. Brain tumors after cranial irradiation for childhood acute lymphoblastic leukemia. A 13-year experience from the Dana-Farber Cancer Institute and the Children's Hospital. Cancer 1987;59:1506–1508.
15. Neglia JP, Meadows AT, Robison LL, et al. Second neoplasms after acute lymphoblastic leukemia in childhood. N Engl J Med 1991;325:1330–1336.
16. Thierry-Chef I, Simon SL, Land CE, et al. Radiation dose to the brain and subsequent risk of developing brain tumors in pediatric patients undergoing interventional neuroradiology procedures. Radiat Res 2008;170:553–565.
17. Kleinerman RA. Radiation-sensitive genetically susceptible pediatric sub-populations. Pediatr Radiol 2009;39(suppl 1):S27–S31.
18. Penn I. De novo malignances in pediatric organ transplant recipients. Pediatr Transplant 1998;2:56–63.
19. Kuijten RR, Bunin GR. Risk factors for childhood brain tumors. Cancer Epidemiol Biomarkers Prev 1993;2:277–288.
20. Farwell J, Flannery JT. Cancer in relatives of children with central-nervous-system neoplasms. N Engl J Med 1984;311:749–753.
21. Kuijten RR, Strom SS, Rorke LB, et al. Family history of cancer and seizures in young children with brain tumors: a report from the Children's Cancer Group (United States and Canada). Cancer Causes Control 1993;4:455–464.
22. Taylor MD, Gokgoz N, Andrulis IL, et al. Familial posterior fossa brain tumors of infancy secondary to germline mutation of the hSNF5 gene. Am J Hum Genet 2000;66:1403–1406.
23. Moschovi M, Sotiris Y, Prodromou N, et al. Familial medulloblastoma. Pediatr Hematol Oncol 1998;15:421–424.
24. Zwetsloot CP, Kros JM, Gueze HD. Familial occurrence of tumours of the choroid plexus. J Med Genet 1991;28:492–494.
25. Fitzgerald LF. Familial brainstem glioma. Clin Neurol Neurosurg 2000;102:106–108.
26. Dirven CM, Tuerlings J, Molenaar WM, et al. Glioblastoma multiforme in four siblings: a cytogenetic and molecular genetic study. J Neurooncol 1995;24:251–258.
27. Malmer B, Adatto P, Armstrong G, et al. GLIOGENE an International Consortium to Understand Familial Glioma. Cancer Epidemiol Biomarkers Prev 2007;16:1730–1734.
28. Bunin G. What causes childhood brain tumors? Limited knowledge, many clues. Pediatr Neurosurg 2000;32:321–326.
29. Robison LL, Buckley JD, Bunin G. Assessment of environmental and genetic factors in the etiology of childhood cancers: the Children's Cancer Group epidemiology program. Environ Health Perspect 1995;103(suppl 6):111–116.
30. Connelly JM, Malkin MG. Environmental risk factors for brain tumors. Curr Neurol Neurosci Rep 2007;7:208–214.
31. Croft RJ, McKenzie RJ, Inyang I, et al. Mobile phones and brain tumours: a review of epidemiological research. Australas Phys Eng Sci Med 2008;31:255–267.
32. Khalili K, Del Valle L, Otte J, et al. Human neurotropic polyomavirus, JCV, and its role in carcinogenesis. Oncogene 2003;22:5181–191.
33. Fine HA. Polyomavirus and medulloblastoma: a smoking gun or guilt by association? J Natl Cancer Inst 2002;94:240–241.
34. Kim JY, Koralnik IJ, LeFave M, et al. Medulloblastomas and primitive neuroectodermal tumors rarely contain polyomavirus DNA sequences. Neuro Oncol 2002;4:165–170.
35. Bigner SH, Bjerkvig R, Laerum OD. DNA content and chromosomal composition of malignant human gliomas. Neurol Clin 1985;3:769–784.
36. Mork SJ, Laerum OD. Modal DNA content of human intracranial neoplasms studied by flow cytometry. J Neurosurg 1980;53:198–204.
37. Christov K, Zapryanov Z. Flow cytometry in brain tumors. I. Ploidy abnormalities. Neoplasma 1986;33:49–55.
38. Giangaspero F, Burger PC. Correlations between cytologic composition and biologic behavior in the glioblastoma multiforme. A postmortem study of 50 cases. Cancer 1983;52:2320–2333.
39. Shapiro JR, Mehta BM, Fiola MR. Intrinsically chemo- and radio-resistant subpopulations identified in freshly resected human gliomas become the dominant population in recurrent tumor samples. Neurology 1990;40:395.
40. Raffel C, Gilles FE, Weinberg KI. Reduction to homozygosity and gene amplification in central nervous system primitive neuroectodermal tumors of childhood. Cancer Res 1990;50:587–591.
41. Douglass EC, Look AT, Kun LE. Cellular DNA content is predictive of early relapse in medulloblastoma. Pediatr Neurosci 1990;15:140.
42. Yasue M, Tomita T, Engelhard H, et al. Prognostic importance of DNA ploidy in medulloblastoma of childhood. J Neurosurg 1989;70:385–391.
43. Taylor MD, Poppleton H, Fuller C, et al. Radial glia cells are candidate stem cells of ependymoma. Cancer Cell 2005;8:323–335.
44. Lang FF, Miller DC, Koslow M, et al. Pathways leading to glioblastoma multiforme: a molecular analysis of genetic alterations in 65 astrocytic tumors. J Neurosurg 1994; 81:427–436.
45. Coons SW, Johnson PC, Shapiro JR. Cytogenetic and flow cytometry DNA analysis of regional heterogeneity in a low grade human glioma. Cancer Res 1995;55:1569–1577.
46. Pollack IF, Hamilton RL, Finkelstein SD, et al. The relationship between TP53 mutations and overexpression of p53 and prognosis in malignant gliomas of childhood. Cancer Res 1997;57:304–309.
47. Bredel M, Pollack IF, Hamilton RL, et al. Epidermal growth factor receptor expression and gene amplification in high-grade non-brainstem gliomas of childhood. Clin Cancer Res 1999;5:1786–1792.
48. Pollack IF, Finkelstein SD, Burnham J, et al. Age and TP53 mutation frequency in childhood malignant gliomas: results in a multi-institutional cohort. Cancer Res 2001;61:7404–7407.
49. Pollack IF, Finkelstein SD, Woods J, et al. Expression of p53 and prognosis in children with malignant gliomas. N Engl J Med 2002;346:420–427.
50. Clarke MF, Fuller M. Stem cells and cancer: two faces of eve. Cell 2006;124:1111–1115.
51. Hemmati HD, Nakano I, Lazareff JA, et al. Cancerous stem cells can arise from pediatric brain tumors. Proc Natl Acad Sci U S A 2003;100:15178–15183.
52. Galli R, Binda E, Orfanelli U, et al. Isolation and characterization of tumorigenic, stem-like neural precursors from human glioblastoma. Cancer Res 2004;64:7011–7021.
53. Singh SK, Clarke ID, Hide T, et al. Cancer stem cells in nervous system tumors. Oncogene 2004;23:7267–7273.
54. Lapidot T, Sirard C, Vormoor J, et al. A cell initiating human acute myeloid leukaemia after transplantation into SCID mice. Nature 1994;367:645–648.
55. Bonnet D, Dick JE. Human acute myeloid leukemia is organized as a hierarchy that originates from a primitive hematopoietic cell. Nat Med 1997;3:730–737.
56. Kernohan JW, Mabon RF, Svien HJ, et al. A simplified classification of the gliomas Proc Staff Meet Mayo Clinic 1949;24:71–75.
57. Daumas-Duport C, Scheithauer B, O'Fallon J, et al. Grading of astrocytomas. A simple and reproducible method. Cancer 1988;62:2152–2165.
58. Louis D, Ohgaki H, Wiestler O, et al. WHO classification of tumors of the central nervous system. Lyon, France: IARC, 2007.
59. Rorke L, Gilles FH, Davis RL, et al. Pathology of brain and spinal cord tumors. London, England: Churchill Livingstone, 1999.
60. Clark HB. Immunohistochemistry of nervous system antigens: diagnostic applications in surgical neuropathology. Semin Diagn Pathol 1984;1:309–316.
61. Coakham HB, Brownell B. Monoclonal antibodies in the diagnosis of cerebral tumors and cerebrospinal fluid neoplasia. In: Cavanaugh JB, ed. Recent advances in neuropathology. Edinburgh: Churchill Livingstone, 1986:25–53.
62. Perentes E, Rubinstein LJ. Recent applications of immunoperoxidase histochemistry in human neuro-oncology. An update. Arch Pathol Lab Med 1987;111:796–812.
63. Shi SR, Key ME, Kalra KL. Antigen retrieval in formalin-fixed, paraffin-embedded tissues: an enhancement method for immunohistochemical staining based on microwave oven heating of tissue sections. J Histochem Cytochem 1991;39:741–748.
64. Yachnis AT, Trojanowski JQ. Studies of childhood brain tumors using immunohistochemistry and microwave technology: methodological considerations. J Neurosci Methods 1994;55:191–200.
65. Honig PJ, Charney EB. Children with brain tumor headaches. Distinguishing features. Am J Dis Child 1982;136:121–124.
66. Glaser JS, Hoyt WF, Corbett J. Visual morbidity with chiasmal glioma. Long-term studies of visual fields in untreated and irradiated cases. Arch Ophthalmol 1971;85:3–12.
67. Packer RJ, Siegel KR, Sutton LN, et al. Leptomeningeal dissemination of primary central nervous system tumors of childhood. Ann Neurol 1985;18:217–221.
68. Packer RJ, Sutton LN, Rosenstock JG, et al. Pineal region tumors of childhood. Pediatrics 1984;74:97–102.
69. Zec N, Cera P, Towfighi J. Extramedullary hematopoiesis in cerebellar hemangioblastoma. Neurosurgery 1991;29:34–37.
70. Ettinger AB. Structural causes of epilepsy. Tumors, cysts, stroke, and vascular malformations. Neurol Clin 1994;12:41–56.
71. Drake J, Hoffman HJ, Kobayashi J, et al. Surgical management of children with temporal lobe epilepsy and mass lesions. Neurosurgery 1987;21:792–797.
72. Duffner PK, Burger PC, Cohen ME, et al. Desmoplastic infantile gangliogliomas: an approach to therapy. Neurosurgery 1994;34:583–589.
73. Buetow PC, Smirniotopoulos JG, Done S. Congenital brain tumors: a review of 45 cases. Am J Neuroradiol 1990;11:793–799.
74. Zimmerman RA, Haselgrove JC, Bilaniuk LT, et al. Magnetization transfer suppression in gadolinium enhancement of the child's brain. In: Proceedings of the XV Symposium Neuroradiologicum, 1994:267–269.
75. Poussaint TY, Rodriguez D. Advanced neuroimaging of pediatric brain tumors: MR diffusion, MR perfusion, and MR spectroscopy. Neuroimaging Clin N Am 2006;16:169–192, ix.
76. Astrakas LG, Zurakowski D, Tzika AA, et al. Noninvasive magnetic resonance spectroscopic imaging biomarkers to predict the clinical grade of pediatric brain tumors. Clin Cancer Res 2004;10:8220–8228.
77. Rock JP, Hearshen D, Scarpace L, et al. Correlations between magnetic resonance spectroscopy and image-guided histopathology, with special attention to radiation necrosis. Neurosurgery 2002;51:912–919; discussion 919–920.
78. Jeun SS, Kim MC, Kim BS, et al. Assessment of malignancy in gliomas by 3T 1H MR spectroscopy. Clin Imaging 2005;29:10–15.
79. Vigneron D, Bollen A, McDermott M, et al. Three-dimensional magnetic resonance spectroscopic imaging of histologically confirmed brain tumors. Magn Reson Imaging 2001;19:89–101.
80. Wang J, Licht DJ. Pediatric perfusion MR imaging using arterial spin labeling. Neuroimaging Clin N Am 2006;16:149–167, ix.
81. Sutton LN, Wang ZJ, Wehrli SL, et al. Proton spectroscopy of suprasellar tumors in pediatric patients. Neurosurgery 1997;41:388–394; discussion 394–395.

82. Girard N, Wang ZJ, Erbetta A, et al. Prognostic value of proton MR spectroscopy of cerebral hemisphere tumors in children. Neuroradiology 1998;40:121–125.
83. Lazareff JA, Gupta RK, Alger J. Variation of post-treatment H-MRSI choline intensity in pediatric gliomas. J Neurooncol 1999;41:291–298.
84. Warren KE, Frank JA, Black JL, et al. Proton magnetic resonance spectroscopic imaging in children with recurrent primary brain tumors. J Clin Oncol 2000;18:1020–1026.
85. Tzika AA, Astrakas LG, Zarifi MK, et al. Spectroscopic and perfusion magnetic resonance imaging predictors of progression in pediatric brain tumors. Cancer 2004;100: 1246–1256.
86. Haacke EM, Xu Y, Cheng YC, et al. Susceptibility weighted imaging (SWI). Magn Reson Med 2004;52:612–618.
87. Tong KA, Ashwal S, Obenaus A, et al. Susceptibility-weighted MR imaging: a review of clinical applications in children. AJNR Am J Neuroradiol 2008;29:9–17.
88. Hamstra DA, Galban CJ, Meyer CR, et al. Functional diffusion map as an early imaging biomarker for high-grade glioma: correlation with conventional radiologic response and overall survival. J Clin Oncol 2008;26:3387–3394.
89. Moffat BA, Chenevert TL, Lawrence TS, et al. Functional diffusion map: a noninvasive MRI biomarker for early stratification of clinical brain tumor response. Proc Natl Acad Sci U S A 2005;102:5524–5529.
90. Mukherjee P, Berman JI, Chung SW, et al. Diffusion tensor MR imaging and fiber tractography: theoretic underpinnings. AJNR Am J Neuroradiol 2008;29:632–641.
91. Witwer BP, Moftakhar R, Hasan KM, et al. Diffusion-tensor imaging of white matter tracts in patients with cerebral neoplasm. J Neurosurg 2002;97:568–575.
92. Sorensen AG, Reimer P. Cerebral MR perfusion imaging. New York, NY: Thieme, 2000:10–27.
93. Knopp EA, Cha S, Johnson G, et al. Glial neoplasms: dynamic contrast-enhanced T2*-weighted MR imaging. Radiology 1999;211:791–798.
94. Aronen HJ, Gazit IE, Louis DN, et al. Cerebral blood volume maps of gliomas: comparison with tumor grade and histologic findings. Radiology 1994;191:41–51.
95. Kassner A, Roberts TP. Beyond perfusion: cerebral vascular reactivity and assessment of microvascular permeability. Top Magn Reson Imaging 2004;15:58–65.
96. Golay X, Hendrikse J, Lim TC. Perfusion imaging using arterial spin labeling. Top Magn Reson Imaging 2004;15:10–27.
97. Chen W, Delaloye S, Silverman DH, et al. Predicting treatment response of malignant gliomas to bevacizumab and irinotecan by imaging proliferation with [18F] fluorothymidine positron emission tomography: a pilot study. J Clin Oncol 2007;25:4714–4721.
98. Lunsford LD. Diagnosis of mass lesions using the Leksell system. In: Lunsford LD, ed. Modern stereotactic surgery. Boston, MA: Martinus Nijhoff, 1987.
99. Broggi G, Franzini A, Migliavacca F, et al. Stereotactic biopsy of deep brain tumors in infancy and childhood. Childs Brain 1983;10:92–98.
100. Dias MS, Albright AL. Management of hydrocephalus complicating childhood posterior fossa tumors. Pediatr Neurosci 1989;15:283–289.
101. Pollack IF, Gerszten PC, Martinez AJ, et al. Intracranial ependymomas of childhood: long-term outcome and prognostic factors. Neurosurgery 1995;37:655–666.
102. Robertson PL, Zeltzer PM, Boyett JM, et al. Survival and prognostic factors following radiation therapy and chemotherapy for ependymomas in children: a report of the Children's Cancer Group. J Neurosurg 1998;88:695–703.
103. Rousseau P, Habrand JL, Sarrazin D, et al. Treatment of intracranial ependymomas of children: review of a 15-year experience. Int J Rad Biol Oncol Biol Phys 1994;28:381–386.
104. Wisoff JH, Boyett JM, Berger MS, et al. Current neurosurgical management and the impact of the extent of resection in the treatment of malignant gliomas of childhood: a report of the Children's Cancer Group trial no. CCG-945. J Neurosurg 1998;89: 52–59.
105. Mason WP, Grovas A, Halpern S, et al. Intensive chemotherapy and bone marrow rescue for young children with newly diagnosed malignant brain tumors. J Clin Oncol 1998;16:210–221.
106. Campbell JW, Pollack IF, Martinez AJ, et al. High-grade astrocytomas in children: radiologically complete resection is associated with an excellent long-term prognosis. Neurosurgery 1996;38:258–264.
107. Shaw EG, Wisoff JH. Prospective clinical trials of intracranial low-grade glioma in adults and children. Neuro Oncol 2003;5:153–160.
108. Berger C, Thiesse P, Lellouch-Tubiana A, et al. Choroid plexus carcinomas in childhood: clinical features and prognostic factors. Neurosurgery 1998;42:470–475.
109. Pencalet P, Sainte-Rose C, Lellouch-Tubiana A, et al. Papillomas and carcinomas of the choroid plexus in children. J Neurosurg 1998;88:521–528.
110. Cochrane DD, Gustavsson B, Poskitt KP, et al. The surgical and natural morbidity of aggressive resection for posterior fossa tumors in childhood. Pediatr Neurosurg 1994; 20:19–29.
111. Albright AL, Wisoff JH, Zeltzer PM, et al. Current neurosurgical treatment of medulloblastomas in children. A report from the Children's Cancer Study Group. Pediatr Neurosurg 1989;15:276–282.
112. Sanford RA. Craniopharyngioma: results of survey of the American Society of Pediatric Neurosurgery. Pediatr Neurosurg 1994;21(suppl 1):39–43.
113. Albright AL, Sposto R, Holmes E, et al. Correlation of neurosurgical subspecialization with outcomes in children with malignant brain tumors. Neurosurgery 2000;47: 879–885.
114. Kelly PJ. Stereotactic craniotomy. Neurosurg Clin N Am 1990;1:781–799.
115. Barnett GH, Kormos DW, Steiner CP, et al. Use of a frameless, armless stereotactic wand for brain tumor localization with two-dimensional and three-dimensional neuroimaging. Neurosurgery 1993;33:674–678.
116. Martin AJ, Hall WA, Liu H, et al. Brain tumor resection: intraoperative monitoring with high-field-strength MR imaging-initial results. Radiology 2000;215:221–228.
117. Schneider W, Noll DC, Cohen JD. Functional topographic mapping of the cortical ribbon in human vision with conventional MRI scanners. Nature 1993;365: 150–153.
118. Berger MS, Ojemann GA, Lettich E. Neurophysiological monitoring during astrocytoma surgery. Neurosurg Clin N Am 1990;1:65–80.
119. Merchant TE, Boop FA, Kun LE, et al. A retrospective study of surgery and reirradiation for recurrent ependymoma. Int J Radiat Oncol Biol Phys 2008;71:87–97.
120. Pollack IF. Posterior fossa syndrome. Int Rev Neurobiol 1997;41:411–432.
121. Gajjar A, Sanford RA, Bhargava R, et al. Medulloblastoma with brain stem involvement: the impact of gross total resection on outcome. Pediatr Neurosurg 1996;25: 182–187.
122. Pollack IF. Infratentorial primitive neuroectodermal tumors. New York, NY: Thieme, 2001.
123. Steinbok P, Cochrane DD, Perrin R, et al. Mutism after posterior fossa tumour resection in children: incomplete recovery on long-term follow-up. Pediatr Neurosurg 2003; 39:179–183.
124. Gelabert-Gonzalez M, Fernandez-Villa J. Mutism after posterior fossa surgery. Review of the literature. Clin Neurol Neurosurg 2001;103:111–114.
125. Ciernik IF, Dizendorf E, Baumert BG, et al. Radiation treatment planning with an integrated positron emission and computer tomography (PET/CT): a feasibility study. Int J Radiat Oncol Biol Phys 2003;57:853–863.
126. Nelson SJ, Graves E, Pirzkall A, et al. In vivo molecular imaging for planning radiation therapy of gliomas: an application of 1H MRSI. J Magn Reson Imaging 2002;16: 464–476.
127. Taghian A, DuBois W, Budach W, et al. In vivo radiation sensitivity of glioblastoma multiforme. Int J Radiat Oncol Biol Phys 1995;32:99–104.
128. Freeman CR. Hyperfractionated radiotherapy for diffuse intrinsic brain stem tumors in children. Pediatr Neurosurg 1996;24:103–110.
129. Halperin EC, Constine LS, Tarbell NJ, et al. Late effects of cancer treatment. In: Halperin EC, Constine LS, Tarbell NJ, et al., eds. Pediatric radiation oncology. New York, NY: Raven Press, 1994:485–554.
130. Mandell LR, Kadota R, Freeman C, et al. There is no role for hyperfractionated radiotherapy in the management of children with newly diagnosed diffuse intrinsic brainstem tumors: results of a Pediatric Oncology Group phase III trial comparing conventional vs. hyperfractionated radiotherapy. Int J Radiat Oncol Biol Phys 1999;43:959–964.
131. Kirsch DG, Tarbell NJ. Conformal radiation therapy for childhood CNS tumors. Oncologist 2004;9:442–450.
132. Olch A. Evidence against the increased risk of second malignancy with IMRT. Montreal, Canada: Pediatric Radiation Oncology Society, 2009. Abstract FP6.
133. Hadjipanayis CG, Kondziolka D, Gardner P, et al. Stereotactic radiosurgery for pilocytic astrocytomas when multimodal therapy is necessary. J Neurosurg 2002;97:56–64.
134. Boethius J, Ulfarsson E, Rahn T, et al. Gamma knife radiosurgery for pilocytic astrocytomas. J Neurosurg 2002;97:677–680.
135. Chiou SM, Lunsford LD, Niranjan A, et al. Stereotactic radiosurgery of residual or recurrent craniopharyngioma, after surgery, with or without radiation therapy. Neuro Oncol 2001;3:159–166.
136. Plowman PN, Wraith C, Royle N, et al. Stereotactic radiosurgery. IX. Craniopharyngioma: durable complete imaging responses and indications for treatment. Br J Neurosurg 1999;13:352–358.
137. Miralbell R, Bleher A, Huguenin P, et al. Pediatric medulloblastoma: radiation treatment technique and patterns of failure. Int J Radiat Oncol Biol Phys 1997;37:523–529.
138. Hug EB, Muenter MW, Archambeau JO, et al. Conformal proton radiation therapy for pediatric low-grade astrocytomas. Strahlenther Onkol 2002;178:10–7.
139. MacDonald SM, Safai S, Trofimov A, et al. Proton radiotherapy for childhood ependymoma: initial clinical outcomes and dose comparisons. Int J Radiat Oncol Biol Phys 2008;71:979–986.
140. Hall EJ. Intensity-modulated radiation therapy, protons, and the risk of second cancers. Int J Radiat Oncol Biol Phys 2006;65:1–7.
141. Newhauser WD, Fontenot JD, Mahajan A, et al. The risk of developing a second cancer after receiving craniospinal proton irradiation. Phys Med Biol 2009;54:2277–2291.
142. Kortmann RD, Kuhl J, Timmermann B, et al. Postoperative neoadjuvant chemotherapy before radiotherapy as compared to immediate radiotherapy followed by maintenance chemotherapy in the treatment of medulloblastoma in childhood: results of the German prospective randomized trial HIT '91. Int J Radiat Biol Oncol Biol Phys 2000;46: 269–279.
143. Hasegawa T, Kondziolka D, Hadjipanayis CG, et al. Management of cystic craniopharyngiomas with phosphorus-32 intracavitary irradiation. Neurosurgery 2004;54: 813–820; discussion 820–822.
144. Backlund EO, Axelsson B, Bergstrand CG, et al. Treatment of craniopharyngiomas—the stereotactic approach in a ten to twenty-three years' perspective. I. Surgical, radiological and ophthalmological aspects. Acta Neurochir (Wien) 1989;99:11–19.
145. Dobbing J, Sands J. Quantitative growth and development of human brain. Arch Dis Child 1973;48:757–767.
146. Mulhern RK, White HA, Glass JO, et al. Attentional functioning and white matter integrity among survivors of malignant brain tumors of childhood. J Int Neuropsychol Soc 2004;10(2):180–189.
147. Reddick WE, Glass JO, Langston JW, et al. Quantitative MRI assessment of leukoencephalopathy. Magn Reson Med 2002;47:912–920.
148. Schultheiss TE, Kun LE, Ang KK, et al. Radiation response of the central nervous system. Int J Radiat Oncol Biol Phys 1995;31:1093–1112.
149. Tofilon PJ, Fike JR. The radioresponse of the central nervous system: a dynamic process. Radiat Res 2000;153:357–370.
150. Yuan H, Gaber MW, McColgan T, et al. Radiation-induced permeability and leukocyte adhesion in the rat blood-brain barrier: modulation with anti-ICAM-1 antibodies. Brain Res 2003;969:59–69.
151. Gaber MW, Yuan H, Killmar JT, et al. An intravital microscopy study of radiation-induced changes in permeability and leukocyte-endothelial cell interactions in the microvessels of the rat pia mater and cremaster muscle. Brain Res Brain Res Protoc 2004;13:1–10.
152. Mulhern RK, Merchant TE, Gajjar A, et al. Late neurocognitive sequelae in survivors of brain tumours in childhood. Lancet Oncol 2004;5:399–408.
153. Mulhern RK, Palmer SL, Reddick WE, et al. Risks of young age for selected neurocognitive deficits in medulloblastoma are associated with white matter loss. J Clin Oncol 2001;19:472–479.
154. Fouladi M, Chintagumpala M, Laningham FH, et al. White matter lesions detected by magnetic resonance imaging following radiotherapy and high dose chemotherapy in children with medulloblastoma/PNET. J Clin Oncol 2005.
155. Helton K, Edwards M, Steen RG, et al. Late transient MRI findings associated with treatment in pediatric brain tumor patients. J Neurosurg 2005;102(2 suppl):179–186.
156. Emami B, Lyman J, Brown A, et al. Tolerance of normal tissue to therapeutic irradiation. Int J Radiat Biol Oncol Biol Phys 1991;21:109–122.
157. Leibel S, Sheline GE. Tolerance of the central and peripheral nervous system to therapeutic irradiation. Adv Radiat Biol 1987;12:257–288.
158. Ang KK, Stephens LC. Prevention and management of radiation myelopathy. Oncology (Huntingt) 1994;8:71–76.
159. Jiang GL, Tucker SL, Guttenberger R, et al. Radiation-induced injury to the visual pathway. Radiother Oncol 1994;30:17–25.
160. Parsons JT, Bova FJ, Fitzgerald CR, et al. Radiation optic neuropathy after megavoltage external-beam irradiation: analysis of time-dose factors. Int J Radiat Biol Oncol Biol Phys 1994;30:755–763.

161. Merchant TE, Gould CJ, Xiong X, et al. Early neuro-otologic effects of three-dimensional irradiation in children with primary brain tumors. Int J Radiat Oncol Biol Phys 2004;58:1194–1207.
162. Hua C, Bass JK, Khan R, et al. Hearing loss after radiotherapy for pediatric brain tumors: effect of cochlear dose. Int J Radiat Oncol Biol Phys 2008;72:892–899.
163. Miettinen S, Laurikainen E, Johansson R, et al. Radiotherapy enhances ototoxicity of cisplatin in children. Acta Otolarngol Suppl 1997;529:90–94.
164. Wara WM, Irvine AR, Neger RE, et al. Radiation retinopathy. Int J Radiat Biol Oncol Biol Phys 1979;5:81–83.
165. Deeg HJ, Flournoy N, Sullivan KM, et al. Cataracts after total body irradiation and marrow transplantation: a sparing effect of dose fractionation. Int J Radiat Biol Oncol Biol Phys 1984;10:957–964.
166. Merchant TE, Goloubeva O, Pritchard DL, et al. Radiation dose-volume effects on growth hormone secretion. Int J Radiat Oncol Biol Phys 2002;52:1264–1270.
167. Constine LS, Woolf PD, Cann D, et al. Hypothalamic-pituitary dysfunction after radiation for brain tumors. N Engl J Med 1993;328:87–94.
168. Wijnholds J, deLange EC, Scheffer GL, et al. Multidrug resistance protein 1 protects the choroid plexus epithelium and contributes to the blood-cerebrospinal fluid barrier. J Clin Invest 2000;105:279–285.
169. Bart J, Groen HJ, Hendrikse N, et al. The blood-brain barrier and oncology: new insights into function and modulation. Cancer Treat Rev 2000;26:449–462.
170. Rao VV, Dahlheimer JL, Bardgett ME, et al. Choroid plexus epithelial expression of MDR1 P glycoprotein and multidrug resistance-associated protein contribute to the blood-cerebrospinal-fluid drug-permeability barrier. Proc Natl Acad Sci U S A 1999; 96:3900–3905.
171. Angeletti RH, Novikoff PM, Juvvadi SR, et al. The choroid plexus epithelium is the site of the organic anion transport protein in the brain. Proc Natl Acad Sci U S A 1997; 94:283–286.
172. Schinkel AH. P-Glycoprotein, a gatekeeper in the blood-brain barrier. Adv Drug Deliv Rev 1999;36:179–194.
173. Mellett LB. Physicochemical considerations and pharmacokinetic behavior in delivery of drugs to the central nervous system. Cancer Treat Rep 1977;61:527–531.
174. Koch-Weser J, Sellers E. Binding of drugs to serum albumin. N Engl J Med 1976; 294:311–316.
175. Rao VV, Dahlheimer JL, Bardgett ME, et al. Choroid plexus epithelial expression of MDR1 P glycoprotein and multidrug resistance-associated protein contribute to the blood-cerebrospinal-fluid drug-permeability barrier. Proc Natl Acad Sci U S A 1999;96: 3900–3905.
176. Angeletti RH, Novikoff PM, Juvvadi SR, et al. The choroid plexus epithelium is the site of the organic anion transport protein in the brain. Proc Natl Acad Sci U S A 1997; 94:283–286.
177. Wijnholds J, deLange EC, Scheffer GL, et al. Multidrug resistance protein 1 protects the choroid plexus epithelium and contributes to the blood-cerebrospinal fluid barrier. J Clin Invest 2000;105:279–285.
178. Murry DJ, Cherrick I, Salama V, et al. Influence of phenytoin on the disposition of irinotecan: a case report. J Pediatr Hematol Oncol 2002;24:130–133.
179. Zamboni WC, Gajjar AJ, Heideman RL, et al. Phenytoin alters the disposition of topotecan and *N*-desmethyl topotecan in a patient with medulloblastoma. Clin Cancer Res 1998;4:783–789.
180. Jarden JO, Dhawan V, Moeller JR, et al. The time course of steroid action on blood-to-brain and blood-to-tumor transport of 82Rb: a positron emission tomographic study. Ann Neurol 1989;25:239–245.
181. Nakagawa H, Groothuis DR, Owens ES, et al. Dexamethasone effects on [125I]albumin distribution in experimental RG-2 gliomas and adjacent brain. J Cereb Blood Flow Metab 1987;7:687–701.
182. Neuwelt EA, Balaban E, Diehl J, et al. Successful treatment of primary central nervous system lymphomas with chemotherapy after osmotic blood-brain barrier opening. Neurosurgery 1983;12:662–671.
183. Doolittle ND, Miner ME, Hall WA, et al. Safety and efficacy of a multicenter study using intraarterial chemotherapy in conjunction with osmotic opening of the blood-brain barrier for the treatment of patients with malignant brain tumors. Cancer 2000;88:637–647.
184. Iwadate Y, Namba H, Saegusa T, et al. Intra-arterial mannitol infusion in the chemotherapy for malignant brain tumors. J Neurooncol 1993;15:185–193.
185. Hochberg FH, Parker LM, Takvorian T, et al. High-dose BCNU with autologous bone marrow rescue for recurrent glioblastoma multiforme. J Neurosurg 1981;54:455–460.
186. Ridola V, Grill J, Doz F, et al. High-dose chemotherapy with autologous stem cell rescue followed by posterior fossa irradiation for local medulloblastoma recurrence or progression after conventional chemotherapy. Cancer 2007;110:156–163.
187. Gajjar A, Chintagumpala M, Ashley D, et al. Risk-adapted craniospinal radiotherapy followed by high-dose chemotherapy and stem-cell rescue in children with newly diagnosed medulloblastoma (St Jude Medulloblastoma-96): long-term results from a prospective, multicentre trial. Lancet Oncol 2006;7:813–820.
188. Chintagumpala M, Hassall T, Palmer S, et al. A pilot study of risk-adapted radiotherapy and chemotherapy in patients with supratentorial PNET. Neuro Oncol 2009;11: 33–40.
189. Sung KW, Yoo KH, Cho EJ, et al. High-dose chemotherapy and autologous stem cell rescue in children with newly diagnosed high-risk or relapsed medulloblastoma or supratentorial primitive neuroectodermal tumor. Pediatr Blood Cancer 2007;48: 408–415.
190. Finlay JL, August C, Packer R, et al. High-dose multi-agent chemotherapy followed by bone marrow 'rescue' for malignant astrocytomas of childhood and adolescence. J Neurooncol 1990;9:239–248.
191. Jakacki RI, Siffert J, Jamison C, et al. Dose-intensive, time-compressed procarbazine, CCNU, vincristine (PCV) with peripheral blood stem cell support and concurrent radiation in patients with newly diagnosed high-grade gliomas. J Neurooncol 1999;44: 77–83.
192. Kedar A, Maria BL, Graham-Pole J, et al. High-dose chemotherapy with marrow reinfusion and hyperfractionated irradiation for children with high-risk brain tumors. Med Pediatr Oncol 1994;23:428–436.
193. Shih CS, Hale GA, Gronewold L, et al. High-dose chemotherapy with autologous stem cell rescue for children with recurrent malignant brain tumors. Cancer 2008;112: 1345–1353.
194. Finlay JL, Dhall G, Boyett JM, et al. Myeloablative chemotherapy with autologous bone marrow rescue in children and adolescents with recurrent malignant astrocytoma: outcome compared with conventional chemotherapy: a report from the Children's Oncology Group. Pediatr Blood Cancer 2008;51:806–811.
195. Blasberg RG, Patlak C, Fenstermacher JD. Intrathecal chemotherapy: brain tissue profiles after ventriculocisternal perfusion. J Pharmacol Exp Ther 1975;195:73–83.
196. Blaney S, Poplack D, Godwin K, et al. The effect of body position on ventricular cerebrospinal fluid methotrexate concentration following intralumbar administration. J Clin Oncol 1995;13:177–179.
197. Rutkowski S, Bode U, Deinlein F, et al. Treatment of early childhood medulloblastoma by postoperative chemotherapy alone. N Engl J Med 2005;352:978–986.
198. Blaney SM, Boyett J, Friedman H, et al. Phase I clinical trial of mafosfamide in infants and children aged 3 years or younger with newly diagnosed embryonal tumors: a pediatric brain tumor consortium study (PBTC-001). J Clin Oncol 2005;23:525–531.
199. Westphal M, Hilt DC, Bortey E, et al. A phase 3 trial of local chemotherapy with biodegradable carmustine (BCNU) wafers (Gliadel wafers) in patients with primary malignant glioma. Neuro Oncol 2003;5:79–88.
200. Ewend MG, Brem S, Gilbert M, et al. Treatment of single brain metastasis with resection, intracavity carmustine polymer wafers, and radiation therapy is safe and provides excellent local control. Clin Cancer Res 2007;13:3637–3641.
201. Weingart J, Grossman SA, Carson KA, et al. Phase I trial of polifeprosan 20 with carmustine implant plus continuous infusion of intravenous O6-benzylguanine in adults with recurrent malignant glioma: new approaches to brain tumor therapy CNS consortium trial. J Clin Oncol 2007;25:399–404.
202. Quinn JA, Jiang SX, Carter J, et al. Phase II trial of Gliadel plus O6-benzylguanine in adults with recurrent glioblastoma multiforme. Clin Cancer Res 2009;15:1064–1068.
203. McGirt MJ, Than KD, Weingart JD, et al. Gliadel (BCNU) wafer plus concomitant temozolomide therapy after primary resection of glioblastoma multiforme. J Neurosurg 2009;110:583–588.
204. Kaiser MG, Parsa AT, Fine RL, et al. Tissue distribution and antitumor activity of topotecan delivered by intracerebral clysis in a rat glioma model. Neurosurgery 2000;47:1391–1398; discussion 1398–1399.
205. Weber FW, Floeth F, Asher A, et al. Local convection enhanced delivery of IL4-Pseudomonas exotoxin (NBI-3001) for treatment of patients with recurrent malignant glioma. Acta Neurochir Suppl 2003;88:93–103.
206. Kunwar S, Pai LH, Pastan I. Cytotoxicity and antitumor effects of growth factor-toxin fusion proteins on human glioblastoma multiforme cells. J Neurosurg 1993;79:569–576.
207. Rand RW, Kreitman RJ, Patronas N, et al. Intratumoral administration of recombinant circularly permuted interleukin-4-Pseudomonas exotoxin in patients with high-grade glioma. Clin Cancer Res 2000;6:2157–2165.
208. Beck TJ, Kreth FW, Beyer W, et al. Interstitial photodynamic therapy of nonresectable malignant glioma recurrences using 5-aminolevulinic acid induced protoporphyrin IX. Lasers Surg Med 2007;39:386–393.
209. Bashir R, Hochberg FH, Linggood RM, et al. Pre-irradiation internal carotid artery BCNU in treatment of glioblastoma multiforme. J Neurosurg 1988;68:917–919.
210. Mahaley MS Jr., Hipp SW, Dropcho EJ, et al. Intracarotid cisplatin chemotherapy for recurrent gliomas. J Neurosurg 1989;70:371–378.
211. Newton HB, Page MA, Junck L, et al. Intra-arterial cisplatin for the treatment of malignant gliomas. J Neurooncol 1989;7:39–45.
212. Kapp J, Vance R, Parker JL, et al. Limitations of high dose intra-arterial 1,3-bis (2-chloroethyl)-1-nitrosourea (BCNU) chemotherapy for malignant gliomas. Neurosurgery 1982;10:715–719.
213. Blacklock JB, Wright DC, Dedrick RL, et al. Drug streaming during intra-arterial chemotherapy. J Neurosurg 1986;64:284–291.
214. Ross RL, Kapp JP, Hochberg F, et al. Solvent systems for intracarotid 1,3-bis (2-chloroethyl)-1-nitrosourea (BCNU) infusion. Neurosurgery 1983;12:512–514.
215. Li XN, Parikh S, Shu Q, et al. Phenylbutyrate and phenylacetate induce differentiation and inhibit proliferation of human medulloblastoma cells. Clin Cancer Res 2004;10: 1150–1159.
216. Spiller SE, Ditzler SH, Pullar BJ, et al. Response of preclinical medulloblastoma models to combination therapy with 13-cis retinoic acid and suberoylanilide hydroxamic acid (SAHA). J Neurooncol 2008;87:133–141.
217. Shu Q, Antalffy B, Su JM, et al. Valproic acid prolongs survival time of severe combined immunodeficient mice bearing intracerebellar orthotopic medulloblastoma xenografts. Clin Cancer Res 2006;12:4687–4694.
218. Graham C, Tucker C, Creech J, et al. Evaluation of the antitumor efficacy, pharmacokinetics, and pharmacodynamics of the histone deacetylase inhibitor depsipeptide in childhood cancer models in vivo. Clin Cancer Res 2006;12:223–234.
219. Mukherjee P, Das SK. Antiproliferative action of retinoic acid in cultured human brain tumour cells Gl-As-14(S). Cancer Lett 1990;52:83–89.
220. Agrawal A, Martell LA, Ross DA, et al. Retinoic acid modulation of proliferation and differentiation in brain tumors. Proc Am Assoc Cancer Res 1993;20.
221. Rodts GE Jr., Black KL. Trans retinoic acid inhibits in vivo tumour growth of C6 glioma in rats: effect negatively influenced by nerve growth factor. Neurol Res 1994;16:184–186.
222. Stockhammer G, Manley GT, Johnson R, et al. Inhibition of proliferation and induction of differentiation in medulloblastoma- and astrocytoma-derived cell lines with phenylacetate. J Neurosurg 1995;83:672–681.
223. Samid D, Ram Z, Hudgins WR, et al. Selective activity of phenylacetate against malignant gliomas: resemblance to fetal brain damage in phenylketonuria. Cancer Res 1994;54:891–895.
224. Gumireddy K, Sutton LN, Phillips PC, et al. All-trans-retinoic acid-induced apoptosis in human medulloblastoma: activation of caspase-3/poly(ADP-ribose) polymerase 1 pathway. Clin Cancer Res 2003;9:4052–4059.
225. Hao Y, Creson T, Zhang L, et al. Mood stabilizer valproate promotes ERK pathway-dependent cortical neuronal growth and neurogenesis. J Neurosci 2004;24: 6590–6599.
226. Jansen MS, Nagel SC, Miranda PJ, et al. Short-chain fatty acids enhance nuclear receptor activity through mitogen-activated protein kinase activation and histone deacetylase inhibition. Proc Natl Acad Sci U S A 2004;101:7199–7204.
227. Fouladi M, Furman WL, Chin T, et al. Phase I study of depsipeptide in pediatric patients with refractory solid tumors: a Children's Oncology Group report. J Clin Oncol 2006; 24:3678–3685.
228. Fouladi M, Park JR, Sun J, et al. A phase I trial and pharmacokinetic (PK) study of vorinostat (SAHA) in combination with 13 cis-retinoic acid (13cRA) in children with refractory neuroblastomas, medulloblastomas, primitive neuroectodermal tumors (PNETs), and atypical teratoid rhabdoid tumor [ASCO abstract 10012]. J Clin Oncol 2008.
229. Friedman HS, Prados MD, Wen PY, et al. Bevacizumab alone and in combination with irinotecan in recurrent glioblastoma. J Clin Oncol 2009;27:4733–4740.

230. Vredenburgh JJ, Desjardins A, Herndon JE II, et al. Phase II trial of bevacizumab and irinotecan in recurrent malignant glioma. Clin Cancer Res 2007;13:1253–1259.
231. Gururangan S, Chi S, Onar A, et al. Phase II study of bevacizumab plus irinotecan in children with recurrent malignant glioma and diffuse brainstem glioma—a Pediatric Brain Tumor Consortium study (PBTC-022). Neuro Oncol 2008;10:833.
232. Kieran MW, Supko JG, Wallace D, et al. Phase I study of SU5416, a small molecule inhibitor of the vascular endothelial growth factor receptor (VEGFR) in refractory pediatric central nervous system tumors. Pediatr Blood Cancer 2009;52:169–176.
233. Chintagumpala M, Blaney SM, Bomgaars LR, et al. Phase I and pharmacokinetic study of thalidomide with carboplatin in children with cancer. J Clin Oncol 2004;22:4394–4400.
234. Warren K, Goldman S, Stewart C, et al. Phase I trial of CC-5013 (lenalidomide) in pediatric patients with recurrent or refractory primary CNS tumors. Neuro Oncol 2008;10:835.
235. Paez-Ribes M, Allen E, Hudock J, et al. Antiangiogenic therapy elicits malignant progression of tumors to increased local invasion and distant metastasis. Cancer Cell 2009;15:220–231.
236. Carroll M, Ohno-Jones S, Tamura S, et al. CGP 57148, a tyrosine kinase inhibitor, inhibits the growth of cells expressing BCR-ABL, TEL-ABL, and TEL-PDGFR fusion proteins. Blood 1997;90:4947–4952.
237. Nistér M, Claesson-Welch L, Eriksson A, et al. Differential expression of platelet-derived growth factor receptors in human malignant glioma cell lines. J Biol Chem 1991;266:16755–16763.
238. Pollack IF, Jakacki RI, Blaney SM, et al. Phase I trial of imatinib in children with newly diagnosed brainstem and recurrent malignant gliomas: a Pediatric Brain Tumor Consortium report. Neuro Oncol 2007;9:145–160.
239. Yarden Y, Sliwkowski MX. Untangling the ErbB signalling network. Nat Rev Mol Cell Biol 2001;2:127–137.
240. Sartor CI, Zhou H, Kozlowska E, et al. Her4 mediates ligand-dependent antiproliferative and differentiation responses in human breast cancer cells. Mol Cell Biol 2001;21:4265–4275.
241. Adam L, Vadlamudi R, Kondapaka SB, et al. Heregulin regulates cytoskeletal reorganization and cell migration through the p21-activated kinase-1 via phosphatidylinositol-3 kinase. J Biol Chem 1998;273:28238–28246.
242. Zhou BP, Hu MC, Miller SA, et al. HER-2/neu blocks tumor necrosis factor-induced apoptosis via the Akt/NF-kappaB pathway. J Biol Chem 2000;275:8027–8031.
243. Yang HY, Zhou BP, Hung MC, et al. Oncogenic signals of HER-2/neu in regulating the stability of the cyclin-dependent kinase inhibitor p27. J Biol Chem 2000;275:24735–24739.
244. Gilbertson RJ, Hill DA, Hernan R, et al. ERBB1 is amplified and overexpressed in high-grade diffusely infiltrative pediatric brain stem glioma. Clin Cancer Res 2003;9:3620–3624.
245. Gilbertson RJ, Bentley L, Hernan R, et al. ERBB receptor signaling promotes ependymoma cell proliferation and represents a potential novel therapeutic target for this disease. Clin Cancer Res 2002;8:3054–3064.
246. Fouladi M, Blaney SM, Onar A, et al. A phase 1 trial of lapatinib in children with refractory CNS malignancies: a Pediatric Brain Tumor Consortium study. Chicago, IL: International Society of Pediatric Neuro-Oncology, 2008.
247. Jakacki RI, Hamilton M, Gilbertson RJ, et al. Pediatric phase I and pharmacokinetic study of erlotinib followed by the combination of erlotinib and temozolomide: a Children's Oncology Group Phase I Consortium Study. J Clin Oncol 2008;26:4921–4927.
248. Daw NC, Furman WL, Stewart CF, et al. Phase I and pharmacokinetic study of gefitinib in children with refractory solid tumors: a Children's Oncology Group Study. J Clin Oncol 2005;23:6172–6180.
249. Prendergast GC. Farnesyltransferase inhibitors: antineoplastic mechanism and clinical prospects. Curr Opin Cell Biol 2000;12:166–173.
250. Jones HA, Hahn SM, Bernhard E, et al. Ras inhibitors and radiation therapy. Semin Radiat Oncol 2001;11:328–337.
251. Haas-Kogan DA, Banerjee A, Kocak M, et al. Phase I trial of tipifarnib in children with newly diagnosed intrinsic diffuse brainstem glioma. Neuro Oncol 2008;10:341–347.
252. Yoffey JM, Courtice FC. Lymphatics, lymph and the lymphomyeloid complex. New York, NY: Academic Press, Inc., 1970.
253. Daar AS, Fuggle SV, Fabre JW, et al. The detailed distribution of MHC Class II antigens in normal human organs. Transplantation 1984;38:293–298.
254. Pollack IF, Okada H, Chambers WH. Exploitation of immune mechanisms in the treatment of central nervous system cancer. Semin Pediatr Neurol 2000;7:131–143.
255. Barker CF, Billingham RE. Immunologically privileged sites. Adv Immunol 1977;25:1–54.
256. Medawar PB. Immunity to homologous grafted skin; the fate of skin homografts transplanted to the brain, to subcutaneous tissue, and to the anterior chamber of the eye. Br J Exp Pathol 1948;29:58–69.
257. Fathallah-Shaykh H. New molecular strategies to cure brain tumors. Arch Neurol 1999;56:449–453.
258. Plautz GE, Miller DW, Barnett GH, et al. T cell adoptive immunotherapy of newly diagnosed gliomas. Clin Cancer Res 2000;6:2209–2218.
259. Ahmed N, Ratnayake M, Savoldo B, et al. Regression of experimental medulloblastoma following transfer of HER2-specific T cells. Cancer Res 2007;67:5957–5964.
260. Mahaley MS Jr., Dropcho EJ, Bertsch L, et al. Systemic beta-interferon therapy for recurrent gliomas: a brief report. J Neurosurg 1989;71:639–641.
261. Nagai M, Arai T. Clinical effect of interferon in malignant brain tumours. Neurosurg Rev 1984;7:55–64.
262. Olson JJ, James CD, Lawson D, et al. Correlation of the response of recurrent malignant gliomas treated with interferon alpha with tumor interferon alpha gene content. Int J Oncol 2004;25:419–427.
263. Mahaley MS Jr., Bertsch L, Cush S, et al Systemic gamma-interferon therapy for recurrent gliomas. J Neurosurg 1988;69:826–829.
264. Farkkila M, Jaaskelainen J, Kallio M, et al. Randomised, controlled study of intratumoral recombinant gamma-interferon treatment in newly diagnosed glioblastoma. Br J Cancer 1994;70:138–141.
265. Barba D, Saris SC, Holder C, et al. Intratumoral LAK cell and interleukin-2 therapy of human gliomas. J Neurosurg 1989;70:175–182.
266. Yoshida S, Tanaka R, Takai N, et al. Local administration of autologous lymphokine-activated killer cells and recombinant interleukin 2 to patients with malignant brain tumors. Cancer Res 1988;48:5011–506.
267. Plautz GE, Barnett GH, Miller DW, et al. Systemic T cell adoptive immunotherapy of malignant gliomas. J Neurosurg 1998;89:42–51.
268. Colapinto EV, Zalutsky MR, Archer GE, et al. Radioimmunotherapy of intracerebral human glioma xenografts with 131I-labeled F(ab')2 fragments of monoclonal antibody Mel-14. Cancer Res 1990;50:1822–1827.
269. Lashford LS, Davies AG, Richardson RB, et al. A pilot study of 131I monoclonal antibodies in the therapy of leptomeningeal tumors. Cancer 1988;61:857–868.
270. Johnson VG, Wrobel C, Wilson D, et al. Improved tumor-specific immunotoxins in the treatment of CNS and leptomeningeal neoplasia. J Neurosurg 1989;70:240–248.
271. Lowenstein PR, Cowen R, Thomas C, et al. The basic science of brain-tumour gene therapy. Biochem Soc Trans 1999;27:873–881.
272. Packer RJ, Raffel C, Villablanca JG, et al. Treatment of progressive or recurrent pediatric malignant supratentorial brain tumors with herpes simplex virus thymidine kinase gene vector-producer cells followed by intravenous ganciclovir administration. J Neurosurg 2000;92:249–254.
273. Merchant TE, Zhu Y, Thompson SJ, et al. Preliminary results from a Phase II trail of conformal radiation therapy for pediatric patients with localised low-grade astrocytoma and ependymoma. Int J Radiat Oncol Biol Phys 2002;52:325–332.
274. Kun LE, Kovnar EH, Sanford RA. Ependymomas in children. Pediatr Neurosci 1988;14:57–63.
275. Rousseau P, Habrand JL, Sarrazin D, et al. Treatment of intracranial ependymomas of children: review of a 15-year experience. Int J Radiat Biol Oncol Biol Phys 1994;28:381–386.
276. Horn B, Heideman R, Geyer R, et al. A multi-institutional retrospective study of intracranial ependymoma in children: identification of risk factors. J Pediatr Hematol Oncol 1999;21:203–211.
277. Bouffet E, Perilongo G, Canete A, et al. Intracranial ependymomas in children: a critical review of prognostic factors and a plea for cooperation. Med Pediatr Oncol 1998;30:319–329.
278. Burger P, Scheithauer B. AFIP atlas of tumor pathology. Washington, DC: American Registry of Pathology, 2007.
279. Tihan T, Zhou T, Holmes E, et al. The prognostic value of histological grading of posterior fossa ependymomas in children: a Children's Oncology Group study and a review of prognostic factors. Mod Pathol 2008;21:165–177.
280. Merchant TE, Jenkins JJ, Burger PC, et al. Influence of tumor grade on time to progression after irradiation for localized ependymoma in children. Int J Radiat Oncol Biol Phys 2002;53:52–57.
281. Goldwein JW, Leahy JM, Packer RJ, et al. Intracranial ependymomas in children. Int J Radiat Oncol Biol Phys 1990;19:1497–1502.
282. Vanuytsel L, Brada M. The role of prophylactic spinal irradiation in localized intracranial ependymoma. Int J Radiat Biol Oncol Biol Phys 1991;21:825–830.
283. Conover JC, Doetsch F, Garcia-Verdugo JM, et al. Disruption of Eph/ephrin signaling affects migration and proliferation in the adult subventricular zone. Nat Neurosci 2000;3:1091–1097.
284. Hitoshi S, Tropepe V, Ekker M, et al. Neural stem cell lineages are regionally specified, but not committed, within distinct compartments of the developing brain. Development 2002;129:233–244.
285. Dasen JS, Liu JP, Jessell TM. Motor neuron columnar fate imposed by sequential phases of Hox-c activity. Nature 2003;425:926–933.
286. Merkle FT, Tramontin AD, Garcia-Verdugo JM, et al. Radial glia give rise to adult neural stem cells in the subventricular zone. Proc Natl Acad Sci U S A 2004;101:17528–17532.
287. Barry D, McDermott K. Differentiation of radial glia from radial precursor cells and transformation into astrocytes in the developing rat spinal cord. Glia 2005;50:187–197.
288. McLaughlin MP, Marcus RB Jr., Buatti JM, et al. Ependymoma: results, prognostic factors and treatment recommendations. Int J Radiat Biol Oncol Biol Phys 1998;40:845–850.
289. Needle MN, Goldwein JW, Grass J, et al. Adjuvant chemotherapy for the treatment of intracranial ependymoma of childhood. Cancer 1997;80:341–347.
290. Hirose Y, Aldape K, Bollen A, et al. Chromosomal abnormalities subdivide ependymal tumors into clinically relevant groups. Am J Pathol 2001;158:1137–1143.
291. Puget S, Grill J, Valent A, et al. Candidate genes on chromosome 9q33–34 involved in the progression of childhood ependymomas. J Clin Oncol 2009;27:1884–1892.
292. Duffner PK, Horowitz ME, Krischer JP, et al. The treatment of malignant brain tumors in infants and very young children: an update of the Pediatric Oncology Group experience. Neuro Oncol 1999;1:152–161.
293. Nagib MG, O'Fallon MT. Posterior fossa lateral ependymoma in childhood. Pediatr Neurosurg 1996;24:299–305.
294. Sanford RA, Kun LE, Heideman RL, et al. Cerebellar pontine angle ependymoma in infants. Pediatr Neurosurg 1997;27:84–91.
295. Merchant TE, Li C, Xiong X, et al. Conformal radiotherapy after surgery for paediatric ependymoma: a prospective study. Lancet Oncol 2009;10:258–266.
296. Hukin J, Epstein F, Lefton D, et al. Treatment of intracranial ependymoma by surgery alone. Pediatr Neurosurg 1998;29:40–45.
297. Wallner KE, Wara WM, Sheline GE, et al. Intracranial ependymomas: results of treatment with partial or whole brain irradiation without spinal irradiation. Int J Radiat Biol Oncol Biol Phys 1986;12:1937–1941.
298. Merchant TE, Kiehna EN, Thompson SJ, et al. Pediatric low-grade and ependymal spinal cord tumors. Pediatr Neurosurg 2000;32:30–36.
299. Nadkarni TD, Rekate HL. Pediatric intramedullary spinal cord tumors. Critical review of the literature. Childs Nerv Syst 1999;15:17–28.
300. Goldwein JW, Leahy JM, Packer RJ, et al. Intracranial ependymomas in children. Int J Radiat Oncol Biol Phys 1990;19:1497–1502.
301. Wallner KE, Wara WM, Sheline GE, et al. Intracranial ependymomas: results of treatment with partial or whole brain irradiation without spinal irradiation. Int J Rad Biol Oncol Biol Phys 1986;12:1937–1941.
302. Evans AE, Anderson JR, Lefkowitz-Boudreaux IB, et al. Adjuvant chemotherapy of childhood posterior fossa ependymoma: cranio-spinal irradiation with or without adjuvant CCNU, vincristine, and prednisone: a Childrens Cancer Group study. Med Pediatr Oncol 1996;27:8–14.
303. Wright KD, Gajjar A. New chemotherapy strategies and biological agents in the treatment of childhood ependymoma. Childs Nerv Syst 2009.
304. Bouffet E, Capra M, Bartels U. Salvage chemotherapy for metastatic and recurrent ependymoma of childhood. Childs Nerv Syst 2009.
305. Sangra M, Thorp N, May P, et al. Management strategies for recurrent ependymoma in the paediatric population. Childs Nerv Syst 2009.
306. Fouladi M, Gururangan S, Moghrabi A, et al. Carboplatin-based primary chemotherapy for infants and young children with CNS tumors. Cancer 2009;115:3243–3253.

307. Burkhard C, Di Patre PL, Schuler D, et al. A population-based study of the incidence and survival rates in patients with pilocytic astrocytoma. J Neurosurg 2003;98:1170–1174.
308. Freeman CR, Farmer JP, Montes J. Low-grade astrocytomas in children: evolving management strategies. Int J Radiat Oncol Biol Phys 1998;41:979–987.
309. Campbell JW, Pollack IF. Cerebellar astrocytomas in children. J Neuro Oncol 1996;28:223–231.
310. Wallner KE, Gonzales MF, Edwards MS, et al. Treatment results of juvenile pilocytic astrocytoma. J Neurosurg 1988;69:171–176.
311. Campbell JW, Pollack IF. Cerebellar astrocytomas in children. J Neurooncol 1996;28:223–231.
312. Wallner KE, Gonzales MF, Edwards MS, et al. Treatment results of juvenile pilocytic astrocytoma. J Neurosurg 1988;69:171–176.
313. Farwell JR, Dohrmann GJ, Flannery JT. Central nervous system tumors in children. Cancer 1977;40:3123--3132, 1977.
314. Gajjar A, Sanford RA, Heideman R, et al. Low-grade astrocytoma: a decade of experience at St. Jude Children's Research Hospital. J Clin Oncol 1997;15:2792–2799.
315. Gajjar A, Bhargava R, Jenkins JJ, et al. Low-grade astrocytoma with neuraxis dissemination at diagnosis. J Neurosurg 1995;83:67–71.
316. Civitello LA, Packer RJ, Rorke LB, et al. Leptomeningeal dissemination of low-grade gliomas in childhood. Neurology 1988;38:562–566.
317. Rumboldt Z, Camacho DL, Lake D, et al. Apparent diffusion coefficients for differentiation of cerebellar tumors in children. AJNR Am J Neuroradiol 2006;27:1362–1369.
318. Hwang JH, Egnaczyk GF, Ballard E, et al. Proton MR spectroscopic characteristics of pediatric pilocytic astrocytomas. AJNR Am J Neuroradiol 1998;19:535–540.
319. Castillo M, Davis PC, Takei Y, et al. Intracranial ganglioglioma: MR, CT, and clinical findings in 18 patients. AJR Am J Roentgenol 1990;154:607–612.
320. Law M, Meltzer DE, Wetzel SG, et al. Conventional MR imaging with simultaneous measurements of cerebral blood volume and vascular permeability in ganglioglioma. Magn Reson Imaging 2004;22:599–606.
321. Spampinato MV, Smith JK, Kwock L, et al. Cerebral blood volume measurements and proton MR spectroscopy in grading of oligodendroglial tumors. AJR Am J Roentgenol 2007;188:204–212.
322. Ostertun B, Wolf HK, Campos MG, et al. Dysembryoplastic neuroepithelial tumors: MR and CT evaluation. AJNR Am J Neuroradiol 1996;17:419–430.
323. Tamburrini G, Colosimo C Jr., Giangaspero F, et al. Desmoplastic infantile ganglioglioma. Childs Nerv Syst 2003;19:292–297.
324. Kleihues P, Burger PC, Scheithauer B, et al. Histological typing of tumors of the central nervous system. Berlin, Germany: Springer-Verlag, 1993.
325. Kepes JJ, Rubinstein LJ, Eng LF. Pleomorphic xanthoastrocytoma: a distinctive meningocerebral glioma of young subjects with relatively favorable prognosis. A study of 12 cases. Cancer 1979;44:1839–1852.
326. Komotar RJ, Burger PC, Carson BS, et al. Pilocytic and pilomyxoid hypothalamic/chiasmatic astrocytomas. Neurosurgery 2004;54:72–79; discussion 79–80.
327. Tihan T, Fisher PG, Kepner JL, et al. Pediatric astrocytomas with monomorphous pilomyxoid features and a less favorable outcome. J Neuropathol Exp Neurol 1999;58:1061–1068.
328. Broniscer A, Baker SJ, West AN, et al. Clinical and molecular characteristics of malignant transformation of low-grade glioma in children. J Clin Oncol 2007;25:682–689.
329. Burger P. Atlas of tumor pathology: tumors of the central nervous system. Washington, DC: Armed Forces Institute of Pathology, 1993.
330. Tice H, Barnes PD, Goumnerova L, et al. Pediatric and adolescent oligodendrogliomas. Am J Neuroradiol 1993;14:1293–1300.
331. Jay V, Squire J, Becker LE, et al. Malignant transformation in a ganglioglioma with anaplastic neuronal and astrocytic components. Report of a case with flow cytometric and cytogenetic analysis. Cancer 1994;73:2862–2868.
332. Russell DS, Rubenstein LJ. Pathology of tumors of the nervous system. 5th ed. Baltimore, MD: Williams & Wilkins, 1989.
333. Gol A, McKissock W. The cerebellar astrocytomas: a report on 98 verified cases. J Neurosurg 1959;16:287–296.
334. Pfister S, Janzarik WG, Remke M, et al. BRAF gene duplication constitutes a mechanism of MAPK pathway activation in low-grade astrocytomas. J Clin Invest 2008;118:1739–1749.
335. Bar EE, Lin A, Tihan T, et al. Frequent gains at chromosome 7q34 involving BRAF in pilocytic astrocytoma. J Neuropathol Exp Neurol 2008;67:878–887.
336. Jones DT, Kocialkowski S, Liu L, et al. Tandem duplication producing a novel oncogenic BRAF fusion gene defines the majority of pilocytic astrocytomas. Cancer Res 2008;68:8673–8677.
337. Jones DT, Kocialkowski S, Liu L, et al. Oncogenic RAF1 rearrangement and a novel BRAF mutation as alternatives to KIAA1549:BRAF fusion in activating the MAPK pathway in pilocytic astrocytoma. Oncogene 2009;28:2119–2123.
338. Forshew T, Tatevossian RG, Lawson AR, et al. Activation of the ERK/MAPK pathway: a signature genetic defect in posterior fossa pilocytic astrocytomas. J Pathol 2009;218:172–181.
339. Sharma MK, Zehnbauer BA, Watson MA, et al. RAS pathway activation and an oncogenic RAS mutation in sporadic pilocytic astrocytoma. Neurology 2005;65:1335–1336.
340. Janzarik WG, Kratz CP, Loges NT, et al. Further evidence for a somatic KRAS mutation in a pilocytic astrocytoma. Neuropediatrics 2007;38:61–63.
341. Gutmann DH, Donahoe J, Brown T, et al. Loss of neurofibromatosis 1 (NF1) gene expression in NF1-associated pilocytic astrocytomas. Neuropathol Appl Neurobiol 2000;26:361–367.
342. Kluwe L, Hagel C, Tatagiba M, et al. Loss of NF1 alleles distinguish sporadic from NF1-associated pilocytic astrocytomas. J Neuropathol Exp Neurol 2001;60:917–920.
343. Wimmer K, Eckart M, Meyer-Puttlitz B, et al. Mutational and expression analysis of the NF1 gene argues against a role as tumor suppressor in sporadic pilocytic astrocytomas. J Neuropathol Exp Neurol 2002;61:896–902.
344. Reifenberger J, Reifenberger G, Liu L, et al. Molecular genetic analysis of oligodendroglial tumors shows preferential allelic deletions on 19q and 1p. Am J Pathol 1994;145:1175–1190.
345. Griffin CA, Burger P, Morsberger L, et al. Identification of der(1;19)(q10;p10) in five oligodendrogliomas suggests mechanism of concurrent 1p and 19q loss. J Neuropathol Exp Neurol 2006;65:988–994.
346. Jenkins RB, Blair H, Ballman KV, et al. A t(1;19)(q10;p10) mediates the combined deletions of 1p and 19q and predicts a better prognosis of patients with oligodendroglioma. Cancer Res 2006;66:9852–9861.
347. Raghavan R, Balani J, Perry A, et al. Pediatric oligodendrogliomas: a study of molecular alterations on 1p and 19q using fluorescence in situ hybridization. J Neuropathol Exp Neurol 2003;62:530–537.
348. Kreiger PA, Okada Y, Simon S, et al. Losses of chromosomes 1p and 19q are rare in pediatric oligodendrogliomas. Acta Neuropathol 2005;109:387–392.
349. Balss J, Meyer J, Mueller W, et al. Analysis of the IDH1 codon 132 mutation in brain tumors. Acta Neuropathol 2008;116:597–602.
350. Yan H, Parsons DW, Jin G, et al. IDH1 and IDH2 mutations in gliomas. N Engl J Med 2009;360:765–773.
351. Hartmann C, Meyer J, Balss J, et al. Type and frequency of IDH1 and IDH2 mutations are related to astrocytic and oligodendroglial differentiation and age: a study of 1,010 diffuse gliomas. Acta Neuropathol 2009;118(4):469–474.
352. De Carli E, Wang X, Puget S. IDH1 and IDH2 mutations in gliomas. N Engl J Med 2009;360:2248; author reply 2249.
353. Hirsch JF, Sainte RC, Pierre-Kahn A, et al. Benign astrocytic and oligodendrocytic tumors of the cerebral hemispheres in children. J Neurosurg 1989;70:568–572.
354. Laws ER Jr., Taylor WF, Clifton MB, et al. Neurosurgical management of low-grade astrocytoma of the cerebral hemispheres. J Neurosurg 1984;61:665–673.
355. Mercuri S, Russo A, Palma L. Hemispheric supratentorial astrocytomas in children. Long-term results in 29 cases. J Neurosurg 1981;55:170–173.
356. Palma L, Guidetti B. Cystic pilocytic astrocytomas of the cerebral hemispheres. Surgical experience with 51 cases and long-term results. J Neurosurg 1985;62:811–815.
357. Smoots DW, Geyer JR, Lieberman DM, et al. Predicting disease progression in childhood cerebellar astrocytoma. Childs Nerv Syst 1998;14:636–648.
358. Winston K, Gilles FH, Leviton A, et al. Cerebellar gliomas in children. J Natl Cancer Inst 1977;58:833–838.
359. Conway PD, Oechler HW, Kun LE, et al. Importance of histologic condition and treatment of pediatric cerebellar astrocytoma. Cancer 1991;67:2772–2775.
360. Gjerris F, Klinken L. Long-term prognosis in children with benign cerebellar astrocytoma. J Neurosurg 1978;49:179–184.
361. Hayostek CJ, Shaw EG, Scheithauer B, et al. Astrocytomas of the cerebellum. A comparative clinicopathologic study of pilocytic and diffuse astrocytomas. Cancer 1993;72:856–869.
362. Schneider JH Jr., Raffel C, McComb JG. Benign cerebellar astrocytomas of childhood. Neurosurgery 1992;30:58–62.
363. Pollack IF, Hurtt M, Pang D, et al. Dissemination of low grade intracranial astrocytomas in children. Cancer 1994;73:2869–2878.
364. Bowers DC, Gargan L, Kapur P, et al. Study of the MIB-1 labeling index as a predictor of tumor progression in pilocytic astrocytomas in children and adolescents. J Clin Oncol 2003;21:2968–2973.
365. Prados MD, Krouwer HG, Edwards MS, et al. Proliferative potential and outcome in pediatric astrocytic tumors. J Neuro Oncol 1992;13:277–282.
366. Pollack IF, Claassen D, al Shboul Q, et al. Low-grade gliomas of the cerebral hemispheres in children: an analysis of 71 cases. J Neurosurg 1995;82:536–547.
367. Shaw EG, Daumas-Duport C, Scheithauer BW, et al. Radiation therapy in the management of low-grade supratentorial astrocytomas. J Neurosurg 1989;70:853–861.
368. Pencalet P, Maixner W, Sainte-Rose C, et al. Benign cerebellar astrocytomas in children. J Neurosurg 1999;90:265–273.
369. Garcia DM, Latifi HR, Simpson JR, et al. Astrocytomas of the cerebellum in children. J Neurosurg 1989;71:661–664.
370. Albright AL, Price RA, Guthkelch AN. Diencephalic gliomas of children. A clinicopathologic study. Cancer 1985;55:2789–2793.
371. Vertosick FT Jr., Selker RG, Arena VC. Survival of patients with well-differentiated astrocytomas diagnosed in the era of computed tomography. Neurosurgery 1991;28:496–501.
372. Packer RJ, Sutton LN, Patel KM, et al. Seizure control following tumor surgery for childhood cortical low-grade gliomas. J Neurosurg 1994;80:998–1003.
373. Berger MS, Ghatan S, Haglund MM, et al. Low-grade gliomas associated with intractable epilepsy: seizure outcome utilizing electrocorticography during tumor resection. J Neurosurg , 1993;79:62–69.
374. Schneider JH, Jr., Raffel C, McComb JG: Benign cerebellar astrocytomas of childhood. Neurosurgery 1992;30:58–62.
375. Garcia DM, Latifi HR, Simpson JR, et al. Astrocytomas of the cerebellum in children. J Neurosurg 1989;71:661–664.
376. Sutton LN, Schut L. Cerebellar astrocytomas. In: McLaurin RL, Vennes JL, Schut L (eds), Pediatric neurosurgery: surgery of the developing nervous system. (ed 2nd). Philadelphia: WB Saunders, 1989:338.
377. VandenBerg SR. Desmoplastic infantile ganglioglioma and desmoplastic cerebral astrocytoma of infancy. Brain Pathol 1993;3:275–281.
378. Chintagumpala MM, Armstrong D, Miki S, et al. Mixed neuronal-glial tumors (gangliogliomas) in children. Pediatr Neurosurg 1996;24:306–313.
379. Cappelli C, Grill J, Raquin M, et al. Long-term follow up of 69 patients treated for optic pathway tumours before the chemotherapy era. Arch Dis Child 1998;79:334–338.
380. Fouladi M, Wallace D, Langston JW, et al. Survival and functional outcome of children with hypothalamic/chiasmatic tumors. Cancer 2003;15:1084–1092.
381. Tao ML, Barnes PD, Billett AL, et al. Childhood optic chiasm gliomas: radiographic response following radiotherapy and long-term clinical outcome. Int J Radiat Oncol Biol Phys 1997;39:579–587.
382. Hoffman HJ, Humphreys RP, Drake JM, et al. Optic pathway/hypothalamic gliomas: a dilemma in management. Pediatr Neurosurg 1993;19:186–195.
383. Pollack IF, Hoffman HJ, Humphreys RP, et al. The long-term outcome after surgical treatment of dorsally exophytic brain-stem gliomas. J Neurosurg 1993;78:859–863.
384. Mishra KK, Puri DR, Missett BT, et al. The role of up-front radiation therapy for incompletely resected pediatric WHO grade II low-grade gliomas. Neuro Oncol 2006;8:166–174.
385. Hadjipanayis CG, Kondziolka D, Gardner P, et al. Stereotactic radiosurgery for pilocytic astrocytomas when multimodal therapy is necessary. J Neurosurg 2002;97:56–64.
386. Boethius J, Ulfarsson E, Rahn T, et al. Gamma knife radiosurgery for pilocytic astrocytomas. J Neurosurg 2002;97:677–680.
387. Dirks PB, Jay V, Becker LE, et al. Development of anaplastic changes in low-grade astrocytomas of childhood. Neurosurgery 1994;34:68–78.

388. Friedman HS, Krischer JP, Burger P, et al. Treatment of children with progressive or recurrent brain tumors with carboplatin or iproplatin: a Pediatric Oncology Group randomized phase II study. J Clin Oncol 1992;10:249–256.
389. Castello MA, Schiavetti A, Varrasso G, et al. Chemotherapy in low-grade astrocytoma management. Childs Nerv Syst 1998;14:6–9.
390. McCowage G, Tien R, McLendon R, et al. Successful treatment of childhood pilocytic astrocytomas metastatic to the leptomeninges with high-dose cyclophosphamide. Med Pediatr Oncol 1996;27:32–39.
391. Gajjar A, Heideman RL, Kovnar EH, et al. Response of pediatric low grade gliomas to chemotherapy. Pediatr Neurosurg 1993;19:113–118.
392. Packer RJ, Lange B, Ater J, et al. Carboplatin and vincristine for recurrent and newly diagnosed low-grade gliomas of childhood. J Clin Oncol 1993;11:850–856.
393. Pons MA, Finlay JL, Walker RW, et al. Chemotherapy with vincristine (VCR) and etoposide (VP-16) in children with low-grade astrocytoma. J Neuro Oncol 1992;14:151–158.
394. Longee DC, Friedman HS, Albright RE Jr., et al. Treatment of patients with recurrent gliomas with cyclophosphamide and vincristine. J Neurosurg 1990;72:583–588.
395. Brown MT, Friedman HS, Oakes WJ, et al. Chemotherapy for pilocytic astrocytomas. Cancer 1993;71:3165–3172.
396. Chamberlain MC. Recurrent cerebellar gliomas: salvage therapy with oral etoposide. J Child Neurol 1997;12:200–204.
397. Prados MD, Edwards MS, Rabbitt J, et al. Treatment of pediatric low-grade gliomas with a nitrosourea-based multiagent chemotherapy regimen. J Neurooncol 1997;32:235–241.
398. Kuo DJ, Weiner HL, Wisoff J, et al. Temozolomide is active in childhood, progressive, unresectable, low-grade gliomas. J Pediatr Hematol Oncol 2003;25:372–378.
399. Quinn JA, Reardon DA, Friedman AH, et al. Phase II trial of temozolomide in patients with progressive low-grade glioma. J Clin Oncol 2003;21:646–651.
400. Moghrabi A, Friedman HS, Ashley DM, et al. Phase II study of carboplatin (CBDCA) in progressive low-grade gliomas. Neurosurg Focus 1998;4:e3.
401. Bouffet E, Jakacki R, Goldman S, et al. Phase II study of weekly vinblastine in recurrent/refractory pediatric low-grade gliomas, Thirteenth International Symposium on Pediatric Neuro-Oncology. Chicago, IL: Neuro-Oncology, 2008:450.
402. Gururangan S, Fisher MJ, Allen JC, et al. Temozolomide in children with progressive low-grade glioma. Neuro Oncol 2007;9:161–168.
403. Khaw SL, Coleman LT, Downie PA, et al. Temozolomide in pediatric low-grade glioma. Pediatr Blood Cancer 2007;49:808–811.
404. Packer RJ, Jakacki R, Horn M, et al. Objective response of multiply recurrent low-grade gliomas to bevacizumab and irinotecan. Pediatr Blood Cancer 2009;52:791–795.
405. Ater J, Holmes E, Zhou T, et al. Results of COG protocol A9952: a randomized phase 3 study of two chemotherapy regimens for incompletely resected low-grade glioma in young children, International Symposium on Pediatric Neuro-Oncology. Chicago, IL: Neuro-Oncology, 2008:451–452.
406. Binning MJ, Liu JK, Kestle JR, et al. Optic pathway gliomas: a review. Neurosurg Focus 2007;23:E2.
407. Alshail E, Rutka JT, Becker LE, et al. Optic chiasmatic-hypothalamic glioma. Brain Pathol 1997;7:799–806.
408. Lewis RA, Gerson LP, Axelson KA, et al. von Recklinghausen neurofibromatosis. II. Incidence of optic gliomata. Ophthalmology 1984;91:929–935.
409. Gonen O, Viswanathan AK, Catalaa I, et al. Total brain *N*-acetylaspartate concentration in normal, age-grouped females: quantitation with non-echo proton NMR spectroscopy. Magn Reson Med 1998;40:684–689.
410. DiPaolo DP, Zimmerman RA, Rorke LB, et al. Neurofibromatosis type 1: pathologic substrate of high-signal-intensity foci in the brain. Radiology 1995;195:721–724.
411. Sevick RJ, Barkovich AJ, Edwards MS, et al. Evolution of white matter lesions in neurofibromatosis type 1: MR findings. AJR Am J Roentgenol 1992;159:171–175.
412. Gonen O, Wang ZJ, Viswanathan AK, et al. Three-dimensional multivoxel proton MR spectroscopy of the brain in children with neurofibromatosis type 1. Am J Neuroradiol 1999;20:1333–1341.
413. Jost SC, Ackerman JW, Garbow JR, et al. Diffusion-weighted and dynamic contrast-enhanced imaging as markers of clinical behavior in children with optic pathway glioma. Pediatr Radiol 2008;38:1293–1299.
414. Jacks T, Shih TS, Schmitt EM, et al. Tumour predisposition in mice heterozygous for a targeted mutation in Nf1. Nat Genet 1994;7:353–361.
415. Brannan CI, Perkins AS, Vogel KS, et al. Targeted disruption of the neurofibromatosis type-1 gene leads to developmental abnormalities in heart and various neural crest-derived tissues. Genes Dev 1994;8:1019–1029.
416. Bajenaru ML, Hernandez MR, Perry A, et al. Optic nerve glioma in mice requires astrocyte Nf1 gene inactivation and Nf1 brain heterozygosity. Cancer Res 2003;63:8573–8577.
417. Bajenaru ML, Garbow JR, Perry A, et al. Natural history of neurofibromatosis 1-associated optic nerve glioma in mice. Ann Neurol 2005;57:119–127.
418. Zhu Y, Harada T, Liu L, et al. Inactivation of NF1 in CNS causes increased glial progenitor proliferation and optic glioma formation. Development 2005;132:5577–5588.
419. Dasgupta B, Li W, Perry A, et al. Glioma formation in neurofibromatosis 1 reflects preferential activation of K-RAS in astrocytes. Cancer Res 2005;65:236–245.
420. Warrington NM, Woerner BM, Daginakatte GC, et al. Spatiotemporal differences in CXCL12 expression and cyclic AMP underlie the unique pattern of optic glioma growth in neurofibromatosis type 1. Cancer Res 2007;67:8588–8595.
421. Daginakatte GC, Gianino SM, Zhao NW, et al. Increased c-Jun-NH2-kinase signaling in neurofibromatosis-1 heterozygous microglia drives microglia activation and promotes optic glioma proliferation. Cancer Res 2008;68:10358–10366.
422. Jenkin D, Angyalfi S, Becker L, et al. Optic glioma in children: surveillance, resection, or irradiation? Int J Radiat Oncol Biol Phys 1993;25:215–225.
423. Imes RK, Hoyt WF. Childhood chiasmal gliomas: update on the fate of patients in the 1969 San Francisco Study. Br J Ophthalmol 1986;70:179–182.
424. Medlock MD, Madsen JR, Barnes PD, et al. Optic chiasm astrocytomas of childhood. 1. Long-term follow-up. Pediatr Neurosurg 1997;27:121–128.
425. Thiagalingam S, Flaherty M, Billson F, et al. Neurofibromatosis type 1 and optic pathway gliomas: follow-up of 54 patients. Ophthalmology 2004;111:568–577.
426. Rush JA, Younge BR, Campbell RJ, et al. Optic glioma. Long-term follow-up of 85 histopathologically verified cases. Ophthalmology 1982;89:1213–1219.
427. Chan MY, Foong AP, Heisey DM, et al. Potential prognostic factors of relapse-free survival in childhood optic pathway glioma: a multivariate analysis. Pediatr Neurosurg 1998;29:23–28.
428. Wong JY, Uhl V, Wara WM, et al. Optic gliomas. A reanalysis of the University of California, San Francisco experience. Cancer 1987;60:1847–1855.
429. Allen JC. Initial management of children with hypothalamic and thalamic tumors and the modifying role of neurofibromatosis-1. Pediatr Neurosurg 2000;32:154–162.
430. Wisoff JH, Abbott R, Epstein F. Surgical management of exophytic chiasmatic-hypothalamic tumors of childhood. J Neurosurg 1990;73:661–667.
431. Khafaga Y, Hassounah M, Kandil A, et al. Optic gliomas: a retrospective analysis of 50 cases. Int J Radiat Oncol Biol Phys 2003;56:807–812.
432. Listernick R, Louis DN, Packer RJ, et al. Optic pathway gliomas in children with neurofibromatosis 1: consensus statement from the NF1 Optic Pathway Glioma Task Force. Ann Neurol 1997;41:143–149.
433. Listernick R, Ferner RE, Liu GT, et al. Optic pathway gliomas in neurofibromatosis-1: controversies and recommendations. Ann Neurol 2007;61:189–198.
434. Blazo MA, Lewis RA, Chintagumpala MM, et al. Outcomes of systematic screening for optic pathway tumors in children with Neurofibromatosis Type 1. Am J Med Genet A 2004;127A:224–229.
435. Listernick R, Charrow J, Gutmann DH. Intracranial gliomas in neurofibromatosis type 1. Am J Med Genet 1999;89:38–44.
436. Packer RJ, Bilaniuk LT, Cohen BH, et al. Intracranial visual pathway gliomas in children with neurofibromatosis. Neurofibromatosis 1988;1:212–222.
437. Sawamura Y, Kamada K, Kamoshima Y, et al. Role of surgery for optic pathway/hypothalamic astrocytomas in children. Neuro Oncol 2008;10:725–733.
438. Wisoff JH, Abbott R, Epstein F. Surgical management of exophytic chiasmatic-hypothalamic tumors of childhood. J Neurosurg 1990;73:661–667.
439. Sutton LN, Molloy PT, Sernyak H, et al. Long-term outcome of hypothalamic/chiasmatic astrocytomas in children treated with conservative surgery. J Neurosurg 1995;83:583–589.
440. Janss AJ, Grundy R, Cnaan A, et al. Optic pathway and hypothalamic/chiasmatic gliomas in children younger than age 5 years with a 6-year follow-up. Cancer 1995;75:1051–1059.
441. Bataini JP, Delanian S, Ponvert D. Chiasmal gliomas: results of irradiation management in 57 patients and review of literature. Int J Radiat Oncol Biol Phys 1991;21:615–623.
442. Packer RJ. Chemotherapy: low-grade gliomas of the hypothalamus and thalamus. Pediatr Neurosurg 2000;32:259–263.
443. Kestle JR, Hoffman HJ, Mock AR. Moyamoya phenomenon after radiation for optic glioma. J Neurosurg 1993;79:32–35.
444. Wilhelm H. Primary optic nerve tumours. Curr Opin Neurol 2009;22:11–18.
445. Dunbar SF, Tarbell NJ, Kooy HM, et al. Stereotactic radiotherapy for pediatric and adult brain tumors: preliminary report. Int J Radiat Oncol Biol Phys 1994;30:531–539.
446. Loeffler JS, Smith AR, Suit HD. The potential role of proton beams in radiation oncology. Semin Oncol 1997;24:686–695.
447. Mishra KK, Squire S, Lamborn KR, et al. Long-term outcomes for pediatric low-grade hypothalamic/chiasmatic gliomas treated on phase I chemotherapy trial, ASTRO. Int J Radiat Oncol Biol Phys 2008:S35.
448. Mahoney DH Jr., Cohen ME, Friedman HS, et al. Carboplatin is effective therapy for young children with progressive optic pathway tumors: a Pediatric Oncology Group phase II study. Neuro Oncol 2000;2:213–220.
449. Petronio J, Edwards MS, Prados M, et al. Management of chiasmal and hypothalamic gliomas of infancy and childhood with chemotherapy. J Neurosurg 1991;74:701–708.
450. Kato T, Sawamura Y, Tada M, et al. Cisplatin/vincristine chemotherapy for hypothalamic/visual pathway astrocytomas in young children. J Neuro Oncol 1998;37:263–270.
451. Walter AW, Gajjar A, Reardon DA, et al. Tamoxifen and carboplatin for children with low-grade gliomas: a pilot study at St. Jude Children's Research Hospital. J Pediatr Hematol Oncol 2000;22:247–251.
452. Chamberlain MC, Grafe MR. Recurrent chiasmatic-hypothalamic glioma treated with oral etoposide. J Clin Onol 1995;13:2072–2076.
453. Oxenhandler DC, Sayers MP. The dilemma of childhood optic gliomas. J Neurosurg 1978;48:34–41.
454. Packer RJ, Savino PJ, Bilaniuk LT, et al. Chiasmatic gliomas of childhood. A reappraisal of natural history and effectiveness of cranial irradiation. Childs Brain 1983;10:393–403.
455. Heideman RL, Kuttesch J Jr., Gajjar AJ, et al. Supratentorial malignant gliomas in childhood: a single institution perspective. Cancer 1997;80:497–504.
456. Finlay JL, Boyett JM, Yates AJ, et al. Randomized phase III trial in childhood high-grade astrocytoma comparing vincristine, lomustine, and prednisone with the eight-drugs-in-1-day regimen. Childrens Cancer Group. J Clin Oncol 1995;13:112–123.
457. Finlay JL, Boyett JM, Yates AJ, et al. Randomized phase III trial in childhood high-grade astrocytoma comparing vincristine, lomustine, and prednisone with the eight-drugs-in-1-day regimen. Childrens Cancer Group. J Clin Oncol 1995;13:112–123.
458. Fayed N, Modrego PJ. The contribution of magnetic resonance spectroscopy and echo-planar perfusion-weighted MRI in the initial assessment of brain tumours. J Neurooncol 2005;72:261–265.
459. Magalhaes A, Godfrey W, Shen Y, et al. Proton magnetic resonance spectroscopy of brain tumors correlated with pathology. Acad Radiol 2005;12:51–57.
460. Dropcho EJ, Wisoff JH, Walker RW, et al. Supratentorial malignant gliomas in childhood: a review of fifty cases. Ann Neurol 1987;22:355–364.
461. Marchese MJ, Chang CH. Malignant astrocytic gliomas in children. Cancer 1990;65:2771–2778.
462. Kandt RS, Shinnar S, D'Souza BJ, et al. Cerebrospinal metastases in malignant childhood astrocytomas. J Neurooncol 1984;2:123–128.
463. Nigro JM, Baker SJ, Preisinger AC, et al. Mutations in the p53 gene occur in diverse human tumour types. Nature 1989;342:705–708.
464. Li J, Yen C, Liaw D, et al. PTEN, a putative protein tyrosine phosphatase gene mutated in human brain, breast, and prostate cancer. Science 1997;275:1943–1947.
465. Ueki K, Ono Y, Henson JW, et al. CDKN2/p16 or RB alterations occur in the majority of glioblastomas and are inversely correlated. Cancer Res 1996;56:150–153.
466. Wong AJ, Bigner SH, Bigner DD, et al. Increased expression of the epidermal growth factor receptor gene in malignant gliomas is invariably associated with gene amplification. Proc Natl Acad Sci U S A 1987;84:6899–6903.
467. Li Y, Bollag G, Clark R, et al. Somatic mutations in the neurofibromatosis 1 gene in human tumors. Cell 1992;69:275–281.
468. Thiel G, Marczinek K, Neumann R, et al. Somatic mutations in the neurofibromatosis 1 gene in gliomas and primitive neuroectodermal tumours. Anticancer Res 1995;15:2495–2499.

469. Samuels Y, Wang Z, Bardelli A, et al. High frequency of mutations of the PIK3CA gene in human cancers. Science 2004;304:554.
470. Broderick DK, Di C, Parrett TJ, et al. Mutations of PIK3CA in anaplastic oligodendrogliomas, high-grade astrocytomas, and medulloblastomas. Cancer Res 2004;64: 5048–5050.
471. Parsons DW, Jones S, Zhang X, et al. An integrated genomic analysis of human glioblastoma multiforme. Science 2008;321:1807–1812.
472. The Cancer Genome Atlas Research Network. Comprehensive genomic characterization defines human glioblastoma genes and core pathways. Nature 2008;455:1061–1068.
473. Raffel C, Frederick L, O'Fallon JR, et al. Analysis of oncogene and tumor suppressor gene alterations in pediatric malignant astrocytomas reveals reduced survival for patients with PTEN mutations. Clin Cancer Res 1999;5:4085–4090.
474. Pollack IF, Hamilton RL, James CD, et al. Rarity of PTEN deletions and EGFR amplification in malignant gliomas of childhood: results from the Children's Cancer Group 945 cohort. J Neurosurg 2006;105:418–424.
475. Nakamura M, Shimada K, Ishida E, et al. Molecular pathogenesis of pediatric astrocytic tumors. Neuro Oncol 2007;9:113–123.
476. Rasheed BK, McLendon RE, Herndon JE, et al. Alterations of the TP53 gene in human gliomas. Cancer Res 1994;54:1324–1330.
477. Ohgaki H, Dessen P, Jourde B, et al. Genetic pathways to glioblastoma: a population-based study. Cancer Res 2004;64:6892–6899.
478. Ohgaki H, Kleihues P. Genetic pathways to primary and secondary glioblastoma. Am J Pathol 2007;170:1445–1453.
479. Broniscer A, Baker SJ, West AN, et al. Clinical and molecular characteristics of malignant transformation of low-grade glioma in children. J Clin Oncol 2007;25:682–689.
480. McCormack BM, Miller DC, Budzilovich GN, et al. Treatment and survival of low-grade astrocytoma in adults—1977–1988. Neurosurgery 1992;31:636–642; discussion 642.
481. Wood JR, Green SB, Shapiro WR. The prognostic importance of tumor size in malignant gliomas: a computed tomographic scan study by the Brain Tumor Cooperative Group. J Clin Oncol 1988;6:338–343.
482. Curran WJ Jr., Scott CB, Horton J, et al. Does extent of surgery influence outcome for astrocytoma with atypical or anaplastic foci (AAF)? A report from three Radiation Therapy Oncology Group (RTOG) trials. J Neuro Oncol 1992;12:219–227.
483. Faury D, Nantel A, Dunn SE, et al. Molecular profiling identifies prognostic subgroups of pediatric glioblastoma and shows increased YB-1 expression in tumors. J Clin Oncol 2007;25:1196–1208.
484. Phuphanich S, Edwards MS, Levin VA, et al. Supratentorial malignant gliomas of childhood. Results of treatment with radiation therapy and chemotherapy. J Neurosurg 1984;60:495–499.
485. Pollack IF, Hamilton RL, Burnham J, et al. Impact of proliferation index on outcome in childhood malignant gliomas: results in a multi-institutional cohort. Neurosurgery 2002;50:1238–1244; discussion 1244–1245.
486. Pollack IF, Hamilton RL, Sobol RW, et al. O6-methylguanine-DNA methyltransferase expression strongly correlates with outcome in childhood malignant gliomas: results from the CCG-945 cohort. J Clin Oncol 2006;24:3431–3437.
487. Bredel M, Pollack IF, Campbell JW, et al. Basic fibroblast growth factor expression as a predictor of prognosis in pediatric high-grade gliomas. Clin Cancer Res 1997;3: 2157–2164.
488. Gallia GL, Rand V, Siu IM, et al. PIK3CA gene mutations in pediatric and adult glioblastoma multiforme. Mol Cancer Res 2006;4:709–714.
489. Thorarinsdottir HK, Santi M, McCarter R, et al. Protein expression of platelet-derived growth factor receptor correlates with malignant histology and PTEN with survival in childhood gliomas. Clin Cancer Res 2008;14:3386–3394.
490. Finlay JL, Goldman S, Wong MC, et al. Pilot study of high-dose thiotepa and etoposide with autologous bone marrow rescue in children and young adults with recurrent CNS tumors. The Children's Cancer Group. J Clin Oncol 1996;14:2495–2503.
491. Pirzkall A, Li X, Oh J, et al. 3D MRSI for resected high-grade gliomas before RT: tumor extent according to metabolic activity in relation to MRI. Int J Radiat Oncol Biol Phys 2004;59:126–137.
492. Tralins KS, Douglas JG, Stelzer KJ, et al. Volumetric analysis of 18F-FDG PET in glioblastoma multiforme: prognostic information and possible role in definition of target volumes in radiation dose escalation. J Nucl Med 2002;43:1667–1673.
493. Cohen K. The treatment of high-grade gliomas in pediatrics: where have we been? Where are we going? International Symposium on Pediatric Neuro-Oncology. Chicago, IL: Neuro-Oncology, 2008:427.
494. Sposto R, Ertel IJ, Jenkin RD, et al. The effectiveness of chemotherapy for treatment of high grade astrocytoma in children: results of a randomized trial. A report from the Childrens Cancer Study Group. J Neurooncol 1989;7:165–177.
495. Pollack IF, Boyett JM, Yates AJ, et al. The influence of central review on outcome associations in childhood malignant gliomas: results from the CCG-945 experience. Neuro Oncol 2003;5:197–207.
496. Cairncross JG, Macdonald DR, Ramsay DA. Aggressive oligodendroglioma: a chemosensitive tumor. Neurosurgery 1992;31:78–82.
497. Kyritsis AP, Yung WK, Bruner J, et al. The treatment of anaplastic oligodendrogliomas and mixed gliomas. Neurosurgery 1993;32:365–370.
498. Ino Y, Betensky RA, Zlatescu MC, et al. Molecular subtypes of anaplastic oligodendroglioma: implications for patient management at diagnosis. Clin Cancer Res 2001;7: 839–845.
499. Pollack IF, Finkelstein SD, Burnham J, et al. Association between chromosome 1p and 19q loss and outcome in pediatric malignant gliomas: results from the CCG-945 cohort. Pediatr Neurosurg 2003;39:114–121.
500. Blaney SM, Phillips PC, Packer RJ, et al. Phase II evaluation of topotecan for pediatric central nervous system tumors. Cancer 1996;78:527–531.
501. Prados MD, Warnick RE, Mack EE, et al. Intravenous carboplatin for recurrent gliomas. A dose-escalating phase II trial. Am J Clin Oncol 1996;19:609–612.
502. Heideman RL, Douglass EC, Langston JA, et al. A phase II study of every other day high-dose ifosfamide in pediatric brain tumors: a Pediatric Oncology Group Study. J Neurooncol 1995;25:77–84.
503. Chastagner P, Sommelet-Olive D, Kalifa C, et al. Phase II study of ifosfamide in childhood brain tumors: a report by the French Society of Pediatric Oncology (SFOP). Med Pediatr Oncol 1993;21:49–53.
504. Walker MD, Alexander E Jr., Hunt WE, et al. Evaluation of BCNU and/or radiotherapy in the treatment of anaplastic gliomas. A cooperative clinical trial. J Neurosurg 1978; 49:333–343.
505. Lashford LS, Thiesse P, Jouvet A, et al. Temozolomide in malignant gliomas of childhood: a United Kingdom Children's Cancer Study Group and French Society for Pediatric Oncology Intergroup Study. J Clin Oncol 2002;20:4684–4691.
506. Wagner S, Erdlenbruch B, Langler A, et al. Oral topotecan in children with recurrent or progressive high-grade glioma: a Phase I/II study by the German Society for Pediatric Oncology and Hematology. Cancer 2004;100:1750–1757.
507. Gajjar A, Chintagumpala MM, Bowers DC, et al. Effect of intrapatient dosage escalation of irinotecan on its pharmacokinetics in pediatric patients who have high-grade gliomas and receive enzyme-inducing anticonvulsant therapy. Cancer 2003;97:2374–2380.
508. Wolff JE, Wagner S, Reinert C, et al. Maintenance treatment with interferon-gamma and low-dose cyclophosphamide for pediatric high-grade glioma. J Neurooncol 2006; 79:315–321.
509. Nicholson HS, Kretschmar CS, Krailo M, et al. Phase 2 study of temozolomide in children and adolescents with recurrent central nervous system tumors: a report from the Children's Oncology Group. Cancer 2007;110:1542–1550.
510. Broniscer A, Gururangan S, MacDonald TJ, et al. Phase I trial of single-dose temozolomide and continuous administration of 06-benzylguanine in children with brain tumors: a pediatric brain tumor consortium report. Clin Cancer Res 2007;13:6712–6718.
511. Adams DM, Zhou T, Berg SL, et al. Phase 1 trial of O6-benzylguanine and BCNU in children with CNS tumors: a Children's Oncology Group study. Pediatr Blood Cancer 2008;50:549–553.
512. Warren KE, Aikin AA, Libucha M, et al. Phase I study of O6-benzylguanine and temozolomide administered daily for 5 days to pediatric patients with solid tumors. J Clin Oncol 2005;23:7646–653.
513. Schreiber V, Ame JC, Dolle P, et al. Poly(ADP-ribose) polymerase-2 (PARP-2) is required for efficient base excision DNA repair in association with PARP-1 and XRCC1. J Biol Chem 2002;277:23028–23036.
514. Jagtap P, Szabo C. Poly(ADP-ribose) polymerase and the therapeutic effects of its inhibitors. Nat Rev Drug Discov 2005;4:421–440.
515. Pollack IF, Boyett JM, Finlay JL. Chemotherapy for high-grade gliomas of childhood. Childs Nerv Syst 1999;15:529–544.
516. Grovas A, Fremgen A, Rauck A, et al. The National Cancer Data Base report on patterns of childhood cancers in the United States. Cancer 1997;80:2321–2332.
517. Bouffet E, Mottolese C, Jouvet A, et al. Etoposide and thiotepa followed by ABMT (autologous bone marrow transplantation) in children and young adults with high-grade gliomas. Eur J Cancer 1997;33:91–95.
518. Heideman RL, Douglass EC, Krance RA, et al. High-dose chemotherapy and autologous bone marrow rescue followed by interstitial and external-beam radiotherapy in newly diagnosed pediatric malignant gliomas. J Clin Oncol 1993;11:1458–1465.
519. Chintagumpala MM, Friedman HS, Stewart CF, et al. A phase II window trial of procarbazine and topotecan in children with high-grade glioma: a report from the children's oncology group. J Neurooncol 2006;77:193–198.
520. Fisher PG, Breiter SN, Carson BS, et al. A clinicopathologic reappraisal of brain stem tumor classification. Identification of pilocytic astrocytoma and fibrillary astrocytoma as distinct entities. Cancer 2000;89:1569–1576.
521. Pollack IF, Shultz B, Mulvihill JJ. The management of brainstem gliomas in patients with neurofibromatosis 1. Neurology 1996;46:1652–1660.
522. Molloy PT, Bilaniuk LT, Vaughan SN, et al. Brainstem tumors in patients with neurofibromatosis type 1: a distinct clinical entity. Neurology 1995;45:1897–1902.
523. Laprie A, Pirzkall A, Haas-Kogan DA, et al. Longitudinal multivoxel MR spectroscopy study of pediatric diffuse brainstem gliomas treated with radiotherapy. Int J Radiat Oncol Biol Phys 2005;62:20–31.
524. Helton KJ, Weeks JK, Phillips NS, et al. Diffusion tensor imaging of brainstem tumors: axonal degeneration of motor and sensory tracts. J Neurosurg Pediatr 2008;1:270–276.
525. Lui YW, Law M, Chacko-Mathew J, et al. Brainstem corticospinal tract diffusion tensor imaging in patients with primary posterior fossa neoplasms stratified by tumor type: a study of association with motor weakness and outcome. Neurosurgery 2007;61: 1199–1207; discussion 1207–1208.
526. Pirotte BJ, Lubansu A, Massager N, et al. Results of positron emission tomography guidance and reassessment of the utility of and indications for stereotactic biopsy in children with infiltrative brainstem tumors. J Neurosurg 2007;107:392–399.
527. Kwon JW, Kim IO, Cheon JE, et al. Paediatric brain-stem gliomas: MRI, FDG-PET and histological grading correlation. Pediatr Radiol 2006;36:959–964.
528. Poussaint TY, Kowal JR, Barnes PD, et al. Tectal tumors of childhood: clinical and imaging follow-up. AJNR Am J Neuroradiol 1998;19:977–983.
529. Ternier J, Wray A, Puget S, et al. Tectal plate lesions in children. J Neurosurg 2006; 104:369–376.
530. Barkovich AJ, Krischer J, Kun LE, et al. Brain stem gliomas: a classification system based on magnetic resonance imaging. Pediatr Neurosurg 1990;16:73–83.
531. Silbergeld D, Berger M, Griffin B, et al. Brainstem glioma with multiple intraspinal metastases during life: case report and review of the literature. Pediatr Neurosci 1988;14:103–107.
532. Packer RJ, Allen J, Nielsen S, et al. Brainstem glioma: clinical manifestations of meningeal gliomatosis. Ann Neurol 1983;14:177–182.
533. Khatib ZA, Heideman RL, Kovnar EH, et al. Predominance of pilocytic histology in dorsally exophytic brain stem tumors. Pediatr Neurosurg 1994;20:2–10.
534. Burger PC, Yu IT, Tihan T, et al. Atypical teratoid/rhabdoid tumor of the central nervous system: a highly malignant tumor of infancy and childhood frequently mistaken for medulloblastoma: a Pediatric Oncology Group study. Am J Surg Pathol 1998;22: 1083–1092.
535. Zagzag D, Miller DC, Knopp E, et al. Primitive neuroectodermal tumors of the brainstem: investigation of seven cases. Pediatrics 2000;106:1045–1053.
536. Joshi BH, Puri RA, Leland P, et al. Identification of interleukin-13 receptor alpha2 chain overexpression in situ in high-grade diffusely infiltrative pediatric brainstem glioma. Neuro Oncol 2008;10:265–274.
537. Okada H, Low KL, Kohanbash G, et al. Expression of glioma-associated antigens in pediatric brain stem and non-brain stem gliomas. J Neuro Oncol 2008;88:245–250.
538. Freeman CR, Kepner J, Kun LE, et al. A detrimental effect of a combined chemotherapy-radiotherapy approach in children with diffuse intrinsic brain stem gliomas? Int J Radiat Biol Oncol Biol Phys 2000;47:561–564.
539. Packer RJ, Prados M, Phillips P, et al. Treatment of children with newly diagnosed brain stem gliomas with intravenous recombinant beta-interferon and hyperfractionated radiation therapy: a Childrens Cancer Group phase I/II study. Cancer 1996;77:2150–2156.
540. Lesniak MS, Klem JM, Weingart J, et al. Surgical outcome following resection of contrast-enhanced pediatric brainstem gliomas. Pediatr Neurosurg 2003;39:314–322.

541. Pierre-Kahn A, Hirsch JF, Vinchon M, et al. Surgical management of brain-stem tumors in children: results and statistical analysis of 75 cases. J Neurosurg 1993;79:845–852.
542. May PL, Blaser SI, Hoffman HJ, et al. Benign intrinsic tectal "tumors" in children. J Neurosurg 1991;74:867–871.
543. Pollack IF, Pang D, Albright AL. The long-term outcome in children with late-onset aqueductal stenosis resulting from benign intrinsic tectal tumors. J Neurosurg 1994; 80:681–688.
544. Squires LA, Allen JC, Abbott R, et al. Focal tectal tumors: management and prognosis. Neurology 1994;44:953–956.
545. Albright AL, Packer RJ, Zimmerman R, et al. Magnetic resonance scans should replace biopsies for the diagnosis of diffuse brain stem gliomas: a report from the Children's Cancer Group. Neurosurgery 1993;33:1026–1029.
546. Roujeau T, Machado G, Garnett MR, et al. Stereotactic biopsy of diffuse pontine lesions in children. J Neurosurg 2007;107:1–4.
547. Vandertop WP, Hoffman HJ, Drake JM, et al. Focal midbrain tumors in children. Neurosurgery 1992;31:186–194.
548. Epstein F, Wisoff J. Intra-axial tumors of the cervicomedullary junction. J Neurosurg 1987;67:483–487.
549. Freeman CR, Farmer JP. Pediatric brain stem gliomas: a review. Int J Radiat Biol Oncol Biol Phys 1998;40:265–271.
550. Packer RJ, Boyett JM, Zimmerman RA, et al. Hyperfractionated radiation therapy (72 Gy) for children with brain stem gliomas. A Childrens Cancer Group Phase I/II Trial. Cancer 1993;72:1414–1421.
551. Freeman CR, Krischer JP, Sanford RA, et al. Final results of a study of escalating doses of hyperfractionated radiotherapy in brain stem tumors in children: a Pediatric Oncology Group study. Int J Radiat Biol Oncol Biol Phys 1993;27:197–206.
552. Shrieve DC, Wara WM, Edwards MS, et al. Hyperfractionated radiation therapy for gliomas of the brainstem in children and in adults. Int J Radiat Biol Oncol Biol Phys 1992;24:599–610.
553. Packer RJ, Boyett JM, Zimmerman RA, et al. Outcome of children with brain stem gliomas after treatment with 7800 cGy of hyperfractionated radiotherapy. A Childrens Cancer Group Phase I/II Trial. Cancer 1994;74:1827–1834.
554. Prados MD, Wara WM, Edwards MS, et al. The treatment of brain stem and thalamic gliomas with 78 Gy of hyperfractionated radiation therapy. Int J Radiat Oncol Biol Phys 1995;32:85–91.
555. Sawada N, Ishikawa T, Sekiguchi F, et al. X-ray irradiation induces thymidine phosphorylase and enhances the efficacy of capecitabine (Xeloda) in human cancer xenografts. Clin Cancer Res 1999;5:2948–2953.
556. Boydston WR, Sanford RA, Muhlbauer MS, et al. Gliomas of the tectum and periaqueductal region of the mesencephalon. Pediatr Neurosurg 1991;17:234–238.
557. Edwards MS, Wara WM, Ciricillo SF, et al. Focal brain-stem astrocytomas causing symptoms of involvement of the facial nerve nucleus: long-term survival in six pediatric cases. J Neurosurg 1994;80:20–25.
558. Farmer JP, Montes JL, Freeman CR, et al. Brainstem gliomas. A 10-year institutional review. Pediatr Neurosurg 2001;34:206–214.
559. Kun LE. Tumors of the posterior fossa and the spinal canal. In: Halperin EC, Constine LS, Tarbell NJ, et al., eds. Pediatric radiation oncology. Philadelphia: Lippincott, Williams & Wilkins, 2004:89.
560. Fulton DS, Levin VA, Wara WM, et al. Chemotherapy of pediatric brain-stem tumors. J Neurosurg 1981;54:721–725.
561. Levin VA, Edwards MS, Wara WM, et al. 5-Fluorouracil and 1-(2-chloroethyl)-3-cyclohexyl-1-nitrosourea (CCNU) followed by hydroxyurea, misonidazole, and irradiation for brain stem gliomas: a pilot study of the Brain Tumor Research Center and the Childrens Cancer Group. Neurosurgery 1984;14:679–681.
562. Jennings MT, Sposto R, Boyett JM, et al. Preradiation chemotherapy in primary high-risk brainstem tumors: phase II study CCG-9941 of the Children's Cancer Group. J Clin Oncol 2002;20:3431–3437.
563. Kretschmar CS, Tarbell NJ, Barnes PD, et al. Pre-irradiation chemotherapy and hyperfractionated radiation therapy 66 Gy for children with brain stem tumors. A phase II study of the Pediatric Oncology Group, Protocol 8833. Cancer 1993;72:1404–1413.
564. Pendergrass TW, Milstein JM, Geyer JR, et al. Eight drugs in one day chemotherapy for brain tumors: experience in 107 children and rationale for preradiation chemotherapy. J Clin Oncol 1987;5:1221–1231.
565. Jenkin RD, Boesel C, Ertel I, et al. Brain-stem tumors in childhood: a prospective randomized trial of irradiation with and without adjuvant CCNU, VCR, and prednisone. A report of the Childrens Cancer Study Group. J Neurosurg 1987;66:227–233.
566. Geyer R, Stewart CF, Kocak M, et al. A phase I trial of gefitinib and radiation in pediatric patients newly diagnosed with brain stem tumors or incompletely resected supratentorial malignant high grade gliomas provides evidence of amplified epidermal factor receptor in STMG: a Pediatric Brain Tumor Consortium study (PBTC-007). Submitted, 2010.
567. Turner CD, Chi S, Marcus KJ, et al. Phase II study of thalidomide and radiation in children with newly diagnosed brain stem gliomas and glioblastoma multiforme. J Neurooncol 2007;82:95–101.
568. Bunin GR, Surawicz TS, Witman PA, et al. The descriptive epidemiology of craniopharyngioma. J Neurosurg 1998;89:547–551.
569. Luse SA, Kerhnohan JW. Squamous-cell nests of the pituitary gland. Cancer 1955;8:623–628.
570. Pang D. Surgical management of craniopharyngiomas. New York, NY: Raven Press, 1993.
571. Sklar CA. Craniopharyngioma: endocrine abnormalities at presentation. Pediatr Neurosurg 1994;21(suppl 1):18–20.
572. Curtis J, Daneman D, Hoffman HJ, et al. The endocrine outcome after surgical removal of craniopharyngiomas. Pediatr Neurosurg 1994;21(suppl 1):24–27.
573. Richmond IL, Wara WM, Wilson CB. Role of radiation therapy in the management of craniopharyngiomas in children. Neurosurgery 1980;6:513–517.
574. Danoff BF, Cowchock FS, Kramer S. Childhood craniopharyngioma: survival, local control, endocrine and neurologic function following radiotherapy. Int J Radiat Biol Oncol Biol Phys 1983;9:171–175.
575. Yasargil MG, Curcic M, Kis M, et al. Total removal of craniopharyngiomas. Approaches and long-term results in 144 patients. J Neurosurg 1990;73:3–11.
576. Hoffman HJ, De Silva M, Humphreys RP, et al. Aggressive surgical management of craniopharyngiomas in children. J Neurosurg 1992;76:47–52.
577. Duff JM, Meyer FB, Ilstrup DM. Long-term outcomes for surgically resected craniopharyngiomas. Neurosurgery 2000;46:291–305.
578. Carmel PW: Radical removal of craniopharyngioma: 1971 to 1991. J Neurosurg 1993: 351a.
579. Weiss M, Sutton L, Marcial V, et al. The role of radiation therapy in the management of childhood craniopharyngioma. Int J Radiat Biol Oncol Biol Phys 1989;17:1313–1321.
580. Baskin DS, Wilson CB. Surgical management of craniopharyngiomas. A review of 74 cases. J Neurosurg 1986;65:22–27.
581. Hetelekidis S, Barnes PD, Tao ML, et al. 20-year experience in childhood craniopharyngioma. Int J Radiat Biol Oncol Biol Phys 1993;27:189–195.
582. Manaka S, Teramoto A, Takakura K. The efficacy of radiotherapy for craniopharyngioma. J Neurosurg 1985;62:648–656.
583. Cabezudo JM, Vaquero J, Areitio E, et al. Craniopharyngiomas: a critical approach to treatment. J Neurosurg 1981;55:371–375.
584. Fischer EG, Welch K, Shillito J Jr., et al. Craniopharyngiomas in children. Long-term effects of conservative surgical procedures combined with radiation therapy. J Neurosurg 1990;73:534–540.
585. Lyen KR, Grant DB. Endocrine function, morbidity, and mortality after surgery for craniopharyngioma. Arch Dis Child 1982;57:837–841.
586. Kassam A, Thomas AJ, Snyderman C, et al. Fully endoscopic expanded endonasal approach treating skull base lesions in pediatric patients. J Neurosurg 2007;106:75–86.
587. Kassam A, Thomas AJ, Snyderman C, et al. Fully endoscopic expanded endonasal approach treating skull base lesions in pediatric patients. J Neurosurg 2007;106:75–86.
588. Bloom HJ, Glees J, Bell J, et al. The treatment and long-term prognosis of children with intracranial tumors: a study of 610 cases, 1950–1981. Int J Radiat Biol Oncol Biol Phys 1990;18:723–745.
589. Rajan B, Ashley S, Gorman C, et al. Craniopharyngioma—a long-term results following limited surgery and radiotherapy. Radiother Oncol 1993;26:1–10.
590. Merchant TE, Kiehna EN, Sanford RA, et al. Craniopharyngioma: the St. Jude Children's Research Hospital experience 1984–2001. Int J Radiat Oncol Biol Phys 2002;53: 533–542.
591. Regine WF, Kramer S. Pediatric craniopharyngiomas: long term results of combined treatment with surgery and radiation. Int J Radiat Biol Oncol Biol Phys 1992;24: 611–617.
592. Scott RM, Hetelekidis S, Barnes PD, et al. Surgery, radiation, and combination therapy in the treatment of childhood craniopharyngioma—a 20-year experience. Pediatr Neurosurg 1994;21(suppl 1):75–81.
593. Habrand JL, Ganry O, Couanet D, et al. The role of radiation therapy in the management of craniopharyngioma: a 25-year experience and review of the literature. Int J Radiat Oncol Biol Phys 1999;44:255–263.
594. Brada M, Thomas DG. Craniopharyngioma revisited. Int J Radiat Oncol Biol Phys 1993;27:471–475.
595. Varlotto JM, Flickinger JC, Kondziolka D, et al. External beam irradiation of craniopharyngiomas: long-term analysis of tumor control and morbidity. Int J Radiat Oncol Biol Phys 2002;54:492–499.
596. Kalapurakal JA, Goldman S, Hsieh YC, et al. Clinical outcome in children with craniopharyngioma treated with primary surgery and radiotherapy deferred until relapse. Med Pediatr Oncol 2003;40:214–218.
597. Kalapurakal JA, Goldman S, Hsieh YC, et al. Clinical outcome in children with recurrent craniopharyngioma after primary surgery. Cancer J 2000;6:388–393.
598. Backlund EO. Treatment of craniopharyngiomas: the multimodality approach. Pediatr Neurosurg 1994;21(suppl 1):82–89.
599. Pollack IF, Lunsford LD, Slamovits TL, et al. Stereotaxic intracavitary irradiation for cystic craniopharyngiomas. J Neurosurg 1988;68:227–233.
600. Lunsford LD, Pollock BE, Kondziolka DS, et al. Stereotactic options in the management of craniopharyngioma. Pediatr Neurosurg 1994;21(suppl 1):90–97.
601. Bremer AM, Nguyen TQ, Balsys R. Therapeutic benefits of combination chemotherapy with vincristine, BCNU, and procarbazine on recurrent cystic craniopharyngioma. A case report. J Neuro Oncol 1984;2:47–51.
602. Takahashi H, Nakazawa S, Shimura T. Evaluation of postoperative intratumoral injection of bleomycin for craniopharyngioma in children. J Neurosurg 1985;62:120–127.
603. Jakacki RI, Cohen BH, Jamison C, et al. Phase II evaluation of interferon-alpha-2a for progressive or recurrent craniopharyngiomas. J Neurosurg 2000;92:255–260.
604. Ellenbogen RG, Winston KR, Kupsky WJ. Tumors of the choroid plexus in children. Neurosurgery 1989;25:327–335.
605. Chow E, Reardon DA, Shah AB, et al. Pediatric choroid plexus neoplasms. Int J Rad Biol Oncol Biol Phys 1999;44:249–254.
606. Pierga JY, Kalifa C, Terrier-Lacombe MJ, et al. Carcinoma of the choroid plexus: a pediatric experience. Med Pediatr Oncol 1993;21:480–487.
607. Packer RJ, Perilongo G, Johnson D, et al. Choroid plexus carcinoma of childhood. Cancer 1992;69:580–585.
608. Ellenbogen RG, Winston KR, Kupsky WJ. Tumors of the choroid plexus in children. Neurosurgery 1989;25:327–335.
609. Panigrahy A, Krieger MD, Gonzalez-Gomez I, et al. Quantitative short echo time 1H-MR spectroscopy of untreated pediatric brain tumors: preoperative diagnosis and characterization. AJNR Am J Neuroradiol 2006;27:560–572.
610. Krieger MD, Panigrahy A, McComb JG, et al. Differentiation of choroid plexus tumors by advanced magnetic resonance spectroscopy. Neurosurg Focus 2005;18:E4.
611. Levy ML, Goldfarb A, Hyder DJ, et al. Choroid plexus tumors in children: significance of stromal invasion. Neurosurgery 2001;48:303–309.
612. Carpenter DB, Michelsen WJ, Hays AP. Carcinoma of the choroid plexus. Case report. J Neurosurg 1982;56:722–727.
613. McGirr SJ, Ebersold MJ, Scheithauer BW, et al. Choroid plexus papillomas: long-term follow-up results in a surgically treated series. J Neurosurg 1988;69:843–849.
614. Berger C, Thiesse P, Lellouch-Tubiana A, et al. Choroid plexus carcinomas in childhood: clinical features and prognostic factors. Neurosurgery 1998;42:470–475.
615. Duffner PK, Horowitz ME, Krischer JP, et al. Postoperative chemotherapy and delayed radiation in children less than three years of age with malignant brain tumors. N Engl J Med 1993;328:1725–1731.
616. Milhorat TH, Hammock MK, Davis DA, et al. Choroid plexus papilloma. I. Proof of cerebrospinal fluid overproduction. Childs Brain 1976;2:273–289.
617. Jeibmann A, Wrede B, Peters O, et al. Malignant progression in choroid plexus papillomas. J Neurosurg 2007;107:199–202.
618. Packer RJ, Perilongo G, Johnson D, et al. Choroid plexus carcinoma of childhood. Cancer 1992;69:580–585.
619. Allen J, Wisoff J, Helson L, et al. Choroid plexus carcinoma—responses to chemotherapy alone in newly diagnosed young children. J Neurooncol 1992;12:69–74.

620. Pierga JY, Kalifa C, Terrier-Lacombe MJ, et al. Carcinoma of the choroid plexus: a pediatric experience. Med Pediatr Oncol 1993;21:480–487.

621. St Clair SK, Humphreys RP, Pillay PK, et al. Current management of choroid plexus carcinoma in children. Pediatr Neurosurg 1991;17:225–233.

622. Wrede B, Liu P, Wolff JE. Chemotherapy improves the survival of patients with choroid plexus carcinoma: a meta-analysis of individual cases with choroid plexus tumors. J Neuro Oncol 2007;85:345–51.

623. Lowis SP, Pizer BL, Coakham H, et al. Chemotherapy for spinal cord astrocytoma: can natural history be modified? Childs Nerv Syst 1998;14:317–321.

624. Lonjon M, Goh KY, Epstein FJ. Intramedullary spinal cord ependymomas in children: treatment, results and follow-up. Pediatr Neurosurg 1998;29:178–183.

625. Allen JC, Aviner S, Yates AJ, et al. Treatment of high-grade spinal cord astrocytoma of childhood with "8-in-1" chemotherapy and radiotherapy: a pilot study of CCG-945. Children's Cancer Group. J Neurosurg 1998;88:215–220.

626. Mottl H, Koutecky J. Treatment of spinal cord tumors in children. Med Pediatr Oncol 1997;29:293–295.

627. Bouffet E, Pierre-Kahn A, Marchal JC, et al. Prognostic factors in pediatric spinal cord astrocytoma. Cancer 1998;83:2391–2399.

628. Peschel RE, Kapp DS, Cardinale F, et al. Ependymomas of the spinal cord. Int J Radiat Biol Oncol Biol Phys 1983;9:1093–1096.

629. Reimer R, Onofrio BM. Astrocytomas of the spinal cord in children and adolescents. J Neurosurg 1985;63:669–675.

630. Hardison HH, Packer RJ, Rorke LB, et al. Outcome of children with primary intramedullary spinal cord tumors. Childs Nerv Syst 1987;3:89–92.

631. Cohen AR, Wisoff JH, Allen JC, et al. Malignant astrocytomas of the spinal cord. J Neurosurg 1989;70:50–54.

632. Cooper PR. Outcome after operative treatment of intramedullary spinal cord tumors in adults: intermediate and long-term results in 51 patients. Neurosurgery 1989;25:855–859.

633. Epstein F, Epstein N. Surgical treatment of spinal cord astrocytomas of childhood. A series of 19 patients. J Neurosurg 1982;57:685–689.

634. O'Sullivan C, Jenkin RD, Doherty MA, et al. Spinal cord tumors in children: long-term results of combined surgical and radiation treatment. J Neurosurg 1994;81:507–512.

635. Muszynski CA, Constantini S, Epstein FJ. Intraspinal intramedullary neoplasms. In: Albright LA, Pollack IF, Adelson PD, eds. Principles and practice of pediatric neurosurgery. New York, NY: Thieme, 1999:697–709.

636. Cristante L, Herrmann HD. Surgical management of intramedullary spinal cord tumors: functional outcome and sources of morbidity. Neurosurgery 1994;35:69–74.

637. Albright AL. Pediatric intramedullary spinal cord tumors. Childs Nerv Syst 1999;15:436–438.

638. Linstadt DE, Wara WM, Leibel SA, et al. Postoperative radiotherapy of primary spinal cord tumors. Int J Radiat Biol Oncol Biol Phys 1989;16:1397–1403.

639. Chun HC, Schmidt-Ullrich RK, Wolfson A, et al. External beam radiotherapy for primary spinal cord tumors. J Neuro Oncol 1990;9:211–217.

640. Gomez DR, Missett BT, Wara WM, et al. High failure rate in spinal ependymomas with long-term follow-up. Neuro Oncol 2005;7:254–259.

641. Merchant TE, Nguyen D, Thompson SJ, et al. High-grade pediatric spinal cord tumors. Pediatr Neurosurg 1999;30:1–5.

642. Leibel SA, Sheline GE, Wara WM, et al. The role of radiation therapy in the treatment of astrocytomas. Cancer 1975;35:1551–1557.

643. Doireau V, Grill J, Zerah M, et al. Chemotherapy for unresectable and recurrent intramedullary glial tumours in children. Brain Tumours Subcommittee of the French Society of Paediatric Oncology (SFOP). Br J Cancer 1999;81:835–840.

644. Linet MS, Ries LA, Smith MA, et al. Cancer surveillance series: recent trends in childhood cancer incidence and mortality in the United States. J Natl Cancer Inst 1999;91:1051–1058.

645. Jemal A, Clegg LX, Ward E, et al. Annual report to the nation on the status of cancer, 1975–2001, with a special feature regarding survival. Cancer 2004;101:3–27.

646. Packer RJ, Sutton LN, Atkins TE, et al. A prospective study of cognitive function in children receiving whole-brain radiotherapy and chemotherapy: 2-year results. J Neurosurg 1989;70:707–713.

647. Anderson VA, Godber T, Smibert E, et al. Cognitive and academic outcome following cranial irradiation and chemotherapy in children: a longitudinal study. Br J Cancer 2000;82:255–262.

648. Jannoun L, Bloom HJ. Long-term psychological effects in children treated for intracranial tumors. Int J Radiat Biol Oncol Biol Phys 1990;18:747–753.

649. Silber JH, Radcliffe J, Peckham V, et al. Whole-brain irradiation and decline in intelligence: the influence of dose and age on IQ score. J Clin Oncol 1992;10:1390–1396.

650. Mulhern RK, Kepner JL, Thomas PR, et al. Neuropsychologic functioning of survivors of childhood medulloblastoma randomized to receive conventional or reduced-dose craniospinal irradiation: a Pediatric Oncology Group study. J Clin Oncol 1998;16:1723–1728.

651. Palmer SL, Gajjar A, Reddick WE, et al. Predicting intellectual outcome among children treated with 35–40 Gy craniospinal irradiation for medulloblastoma. Neuropsychology 2003;17:548–555.

652. Palmer SL, Goloubeva O, Reddick WE, et al. Patterns of intellectual development among survivors of pediatric medulloblastoma: a longitudinal analysis. J Clin Oncol 2001;19:2302–2308.

653. Johnson DL, McCabe MA, Nicholson HS, et al. Quality of long-term survival in young children with medulloblastoma. J Neurosurg 1994;80:1004–1010.

654. Thompson SJ, Leigh L, Christensen R, et al. Immediate neurocognitive effects of methylphenidate on learning-impaired survivors of childhood cancer. J Clin Oncol 2001;19:1802–1808.

655. Shalet SM. Growth and hormonal status of children treated for brain tumours. Childs Brain 1982;9:284–293.

656. Duffner PK, Cohen ME, Thomas PR, et al. The long-term effects of cranial irradiation on the central nervous system. Cancer 1985;56:1841–1846.

657. Olshan JS, Gubernick J, Packer RJ, et al. The effects of adjuvant chemotherapy on growth in children with medulloblastoma. Cancer 1992;70:2013–2017.

658. Packer RJ, Boyett JM, Janss AJ, et al. Growth hormone replacement therapy in children with medulloblastoma: use and effect on tumor control. J Clin Oncol 2001;19:480–487.

659. Moshang T Jr., Rundle AC, Graves DA, et al. Brain tumor recurrence in children treated with growth hormone: the National Cooperative Growth Study experience. J Pediatr 1996;128:S4–S7.

660. Swerdlow AJ, Reddingius RE, Higgins CD, et al. Growth hormone treatment of children with brain tumors and risk of tumor recurrence. J Clin Endocrinol Metab 2000;85:4444–4449.

661. Livesey EA, Hindmarsh PC, Brook CG, et al. Endocrine disorders following treatment of childhood brain tumours. Br J Cancer 1990;61:622–625.

662. Duffner PK, Cohen ME. Long-term consequences of CNS treatment for childhood cancer, Part II: Clinical consequences. Pediatr Neurol 1991;7:237–242.

663. Kramer ED, Vezina LG, Packer RJ, et al. Staging and surveillance of children with central nervous system neoplasms: recommendations of the Neurology and Tumor Imaging Committees of the Children's Cancer Group. Pediatr Neurosurg 1994;20:254–262.

664. Duffner PK, Krischer JP, Sanford RA, et al. Prognostic factors in infants and very young children with intracranial ependymomas. Pediatr Neurosurg 1998;28:215–222.

CHAPTER 26B ■ EMBRYONAL AND PINEAL REGION TUMORS

ROGER J. PACKER, LUCY B. RORKE-ADAMS, CHING C. LAU, MICHAEL D. TAYLOR, GILBERT VEZINA, AND LARRY E. KUN

EMBRYONAL TUMORS

Embryonal tumors constitute approximately 25% of all primary central nervous system (CNS) tumors occurring in patients 18 years or younger at the time of diagnosis.[1-3] They comprise nearly 40% of all malignant neoplasms, and frequent transient and permanent morbidity is associated with their diagnosis and treatment.[1,4] Although these neoplasms occur all along the pediatric age spectrum, they often arise early in life, with one-fifth or more of tumors being diagnosed in the first 3 years of life, making diagnosis and management even more difficult.[1-4] In the World Health Organization (WHO) classification of CNS tumors, embryonal tumors constitute a collection of biologically heterogeneous lesions that are malignant and share the tendency to disseminate the nervous system via cerebrospinal fluid (CSF) pathways early in the course of illness.[1] The most common embryonal tumor is the medulloblastoma, of which the WHO recognizes five subtypes (see Table 26B.1).[1] Central nervous system primitive neuroectodermal tumors (PNETs) are lesions which arise in the cerebral hemispheres, brainstem and spinal cord, and also have five recognized subtypes (see Table 26B.1). Since the late 1980s, another highly aggressive form of malignant CNS tumor, the atypical teratoid/rhabdoid tumor, has been increasingly diagnosed and has characteristic histologic, immunohistochemical, and molecular genetic features.[1,5,6]

Tumors of the pineal region are considered a distinct subset of neoplasms in the WHO classification, although they are composed of biologically and clinically different tumor types, including the pineoblastoma that histologically most closely resembles embryonal tumors, such as medulloblastoma[1,7] (see Table 26B.2). Although primary CNS germ cell tumors may occur anywhere within the neuroaxis, they most commonly arise in the pineal region, and for this reason the subgroup of germ cell tumors will also be discussed in this chapter. Once again, there are multiple subtypes of germ cell tumors, classified on the basis of histology and secretion pattern, with variable prognosis.[1,8]

General considerations of the diagnosis and treatment of CNS tumors will be covered in Chapter 26B. Discussions, primarily germane to embryonal, pineal region, and germ cell tumors, will be included in this chapter.

Medulloblastoma

Introduction

Medulloblastoma is the most common malignant brain tumor of childhood.[3,4,9] By definition, it is an embryonal tumor that occurs in the posterior fossa and, as other embryonal tumors, may metastasize either early or late in diagnosis. Multiple subtypes of medulloblastoma have been recognized, as noted in Table 26B.1 The classical medulloblastoma makes up the majority of cases, and the diagnosis of other subtypes, such as the anaplastic or desmoplastic form, is often subjective, as tumors may share overlapping histological features or only focally display a specific histologic feature.[10-12] The biology of medulloblastomas has been extensively studied and much has been learned about their origins and molecular pathogenesis over the past decade.[12-19] Institutional and consortium studies have demonstrated an increasing survival rate for medulloblastoma, although some of this apparent improvement in outcome may be related to reclassification or alterations in disease stratification.[3,4,20-22] Tumor and treatment-related morbidity remains a major issue, especially in young children with this disease.[23,24]

Demographics

Medulloblastomas constitute approximately 20% of all primary CNS tumors in children between the ages of 0 and 14 years.[1,2] They are less common in patients between 15 and 19 years of age, constituting 6% of brain tumors in this age group. Medulloblastomas do arise in adulthood; however, they comprise less than 2% of all adult brain tumors.[25-27] Medulloblastomas have a bimodal distribution peaking at 3 to 4 years of age, and then again between 8 and 10 years of age. Fifteen percent or more of tumors are diagnosed in infancy.

Medulloblastomas are more likely to occur in Caucasians, as compared with other ethnic groups, at a ratio of 1.75/1. In most epidemiologic studies in the United States, nearly 80% of all medulloblastomas have been diagnosed in non-Hispanic White children.[1,28-30] This ethnic pattern is even more marked in cooperative group trials raising issues concerning disparity of access or utilization of health care.[28-30] However, the relative ratio of medulloblastoma to other childhood brain tumors is similar in other ethnic groups.[31-34]

Etiology

The etiology of medulloblastoma is unknown for the majority of patients. Several familial syndromes have been associated with an increased risk of developing medulloblastoma, including Turcot syndrome, Gorlin syndrome, ataxia telangiectasia, and Li Fraumeni syndrome.[35-41] The associations with Gorlin syndrome and Turcot syndrome have stimulated research into possible molecular pathways active in medulloblastoma.

Gorlin syndrome, also known as the nevoid basal cell carcinoma syndrome, is diagnosed by characteristic dermatological and skeletal features, including multiple basal cell carcinomas and odontogenic keratocysts of the jaw.[35,36] However, some stigmata may be present only later in life. This association accounts for less than 2% of all patients with medulloblastoma but has led to a better understanding of the molecular underpinnings of a subset of medulloblastomas. Gorlin syndrome is caused by an inherited germ line mutation of the PATCHED1 gene on chromosome 9, which encodes the sonic hedgehog (SHH) receptor PATCHED1 (PTCH1) and normally suppresses SHH signaling.[36,37,42–45] Mutations of PTCH1 have been demonstrated in up to 40% of medulloblastomas and have been found more frequently in the desmoplastic variant.[43–45] Another important factor in the association of medulloblastoma with Gorlin syndrome is that these children are predisposed to development of basal cell carcinoma years after treatment, especially in the fields of radiation utilized to treat medulloblastoma.[35,36] This makes the use of craniospinal radiotherapy problematic in children with the syndrome. Diagnosis of Gorlin syndrome early in life is quite difficult, although the presence of skeletal abnormalities, including bifid or fused ribs, macrocephaly, or early calcification of the falx cerebri, should raise concerns. Overall, 3% to 5% of patients with Gorlin syndrome will develop medulloblastoma.

Turcot syndrome is an autosomal dominant disorder in which patients not only have a proclivity to develop primary brain tumors but also colorectal adenomas and/or colorectal adenocarcinomas. Turcot syndrome may be due to mutations of the adenomatous polyposis coli gene (type 2), which is associated with extensive colorectal adenomas and extra colonic manifestations such as osteomas, desmoid tumors, jaw cysts, and supernumerary teeth, or secondary to mutations in DNA mismatch repair genes HPS2 and MLH1 (type 1).[17,38,45,46] Patients with the latter mutation are more prone to developing colorectal adenocarcinomas and gliomas. Patients with type 2 disease are at increased risk of developing medulloblastomas. Abnormalities in the WNT molecular pathway, which is aberrant in Turcot syndrome, have been identified in up to 15% of patients older than 3 years of age with medulloblastoma and may constitute a different form of the disease, with a favorable prognosis.

Patients with Li-Fraumeni syndrome, caused by germ line mutations in the TP53 gene, may develop multiple CNS cancer types, including medulloblastoma, although gliomas are more common.[40,41,45] This syndrome is caused by a germ in the TP53 gene, which is multifunctional.

Epidemiologic studies have not demonstrated a clear link between environmental exposures and the development of medulloblastomas.[47,48] Factors that had been found to be associated with a higher incidence of the development of medulloblastomas, in some but not all studies, include farm residence of the mother during pregnancy and pesticide exposure.[47–49] Multivitamin use and fruit consumption by mothers during pregnancy has been found to be potentially protective of development. Exposure to ionizing radiation has been associated with the increased risk of developing all types of childhood brain tumors, including medulloblastoma.[37,47–53] Viral exposure has been extensively evaluated in patients with medulloblastoma and although preliminary studies described a relationship with SV40 virus exposure, subsequent studies have not confirmed this association.[54–56] Medulloblastomas have also been reported in children with congenital anomalies and syndromes, such as Rubenstein-Taybi and Fanconi's; however, it is unclear whether this is a chance occurrence or is related to increased predisposition.[57–65]

Clinical Presentation

Medulloblastoma, by definition, arises in the posterior fossa, predominantly in the region of the roof of the fourth ventricle, and causes signs and symptoms by obstruction of CSF pathways or direct damage to the cerebellum or other brainstem structures.[3,4,32,33] The most common presentation of medulloblastoma is vomiting and headache, occurring in nearly 80% of patients by the time of diagnosis, usually associated with obstruction of cerebrospinal CSF flow at the outlet of the third or fourth ventricle and secondary hydrocephalus. Symptom duration is usually 1 to 3 months before diagnosis, and the majority of children are diagnosed within 45 and 60 days after onset of symptoms. There is overlap between symptoms caused by medulloblastoma and other posterior fossa tumors, such as ependymomas, cerebellar astrocytomas, and atypical teratoid/rhabdoid tumors (see Table 26B.3). Patients with metastatic disease are likely to be diagnosed earlier after onset of symptoms, raising the possibility that this is due to greater biological aggressivity of their tumors and associated increased early neurologic impairment.[3,4,32,33,66]

The headache pattern in children with medulloblastoma is often nonspecific early in the course of illness. Later in the course of disease, especially when hydrocephalus is present, the headaches are more likely to be those classically associated with increased intracranial pressure, occurring upon wakening, with accompanying morning nausea and vomiting. Unsteadiness is noted in 50% to 80% of children by the time of diagnosis. Because of the tumor's primary midline location, unsteadiness is more frequently truncal than lateralized. Sixth nerve palsies, manifest by turning in of one or both eyes, occur in 90% of children with medulloblastoma. Other ophthalmologic findings such as nystagmus are less well characterized in reports but are also frequent. Papilledema is present in approximately three-fourths of patients at time of diagnosis. Nonspecific findings such as head tilt, stiff neck, and weight loss may also occur.[4]

Medulloblastomas may present acutely, especially when there is hemorrhage within the tumor.[67] This characteristically results in acute alternations of consciousness, including coma, probably secondary to both acute hydrocephalus and direct brainstem compression.

Diagnosis in infants and very young children may be more difficult and delayed. Symptoms and signs in infants include

TABLE 26B.3

CLINICAL PRESENTATION OF POSTERIOR FOSSA TUMORS

Tumor type	Peak age (yr)	Duration of symptoms (mo)	Early signs/symptoms
Medulloblastoma	Two peaks: 3–5; 7–10	1–3	Headaches, vomiting; truncal unsteadiness and gait disturbance
Cerebellar astrocytoma	6–10	2–5	Dysmetria; gait disturbance; later headaches
Brain stem glioma	5–15	1–6	Diplopia, facial weakness, swallowing difficulties, unsteadiness; cranial neuropathies, crossed hemiparesis
Ependymoma	5–9, though 40% less than 3	2–4	Ataxia, diplopia, headaches, nausea; cerebellopontine (sixth, seventh, eighth) neuropathies
AT/RT	Less than 2	1–3	Vomiting, cranial neuropathies, ataxia

AT/RT, atypical teratoid/rhabdoid tumor.

macrocephaly, unexplained intermittent lethargy, head tilt, and poorly characterized ophthalmologic findings.[4,66] The classical "setting sun" sign, manifest by downward deviation of the eyes due to tectal pressure and loss of upgaze may occur but is documented in less than 10% of infants at diagnosis.

Presentation in older children and adults does not differ dramatically from that seen in younger patients. In adult series, the time to diagnosis has been slightly longer than in series reporting children alone. The majority of older patients do have headaches, nausea, and ataxia. Cerebellopontine involvement due to laterally placed lesions with resultant sixth, seventh, and possibly eighth nerve paresis are somewhat more common in older patients, including adults.[68–70]

Neuroimaging

Medulloblastomas are characteristically relatively well-defined mass lesions that arise in the inferior medullary velum/roof of the fourth ventricle, and grow anteriorly into the fourth ventricle; they can invade the middle cerebellar peduncle or the dorsal brain stem (Fig. 26B.1). In older children and adolescents, medulloblastomas have the tendency to present either in the lateral cerebellar hemisphere or near the cerebellopontine angle cistern (Fig. 26B.2). Ninety percent of tumors demonstrate some hyperattenuation compared with normal cerebellar attenuation on computed tomography (CT), a reliable imaging feature that distinguishes medulloblastomas from juvenile pilocytic astrocytomas.[71] Calcifications are present in 10% to 20% of cases.

On magnetic resonance imaging (MRI), medulloblastomas are usually homogeneous with iso- to hypointense signal on T1-weighted images, and generally hypointense signal (between gray matter and white matter) on T2-weighted images; signal is often isointense to gray matter on FLAIR images and hyperintense on diffusion-weighted images.[72] Although most medulloblastomas show moderate to intense contrast enhancement, approximately 5% to 10% of tumors do not enhance, and another 10% to 15% show only minimal (<25%) contrast enhancement (Fig. 26B.1). In infancy, "medulloblastomas with extensive nodularity" may occur. This entity displays multiple, discrete, contrast-enhancing masses in almost a grape-like cluster.

Both diffusion imaging and MR spectroscopy are helpful in differentiation of medulloblastomas from other posterior fossa tumors, namely, juvenile pilocytic astrocytomas and ependymomas. The apparent diffusion coefficient values of medulloblastoma are significantly lower than those of ependymoma and juvenile pilocytic astrocytomas, a reflection of the high cellularity and large nuclear areas of medulloblastoma.[73–75] Using a discriminant analysis, single-voxel magnetic resonance spectroscopy of pediatric cerebellar tumors has been proven capable of separating medulloblastomas from juvenile pilocytic astrocytomas and ependymomas and from normal cerebellar tissue based on a plot of creatine-choline (Cr:Cho) ratios against N-acetyl aspartate (NAA):Cho ratios[76] (Fig. 26B.3). Medulloblastomas have very high levels of choline and very low, lower, or absent NAA peak (decreased NAA to creatine ratio). High choline levels indicate a high degree of membrane metabolism, which usually takes place in rapidly proliferating malignant tumors (Fig. 26B.4). Lactate and lipid peaks can also be identified as a result of metabolic acidosis and tissue breakdown.

Other tumors also occur in the posterior fossa. Atypical teratoid/rhabdoid tumors most closely mimic medulloblastomas but have a greater propensity to present with hemorrhagic components. In the posterior fossa, atypical teratoid/rhabdoid tumors (AT/RTs) are often located in the cerebellopontine angle, as opposed to the medulloblastomas, which favor the midline (vermis, fourth ventricle) in the first decade. Leptomeningeal invasion, surrounding edema, and enhancement from breakdown of the blood-brain barrier are also common. Ependymomas may be distinguished by their different anatomic location and pattern of spread through the foramina of Luschka and Magendie, and their characteristic appearance of speckled calcification on CT. MRs can give additional support to the diagnosis, especially in those cases in which the size and extent of the mass render difficult the identification of its point of origin. Solitary cerebellar hemangioblastoma usually will demonstrate serpiginous flow voids, reflecting the vascularity of the lesion, in addition to intense enhancement after intravenous contrast.[77]

PATHOLOGIC CLASSIFICATION OF MEDULLOBLASTOMA

From the time that the prototypic CNS embryonal tumor—medulloblastoma—was described by Bailey and Cushing, controversy has swirled around its nature, origin, and name.[78] The essential issue at the heart of the controversy is whether the medulloblastoma is a tumor unique to the cerebellum. If tumors of their histology and biologic behavior occurred only in the cerebellum, no problem would exist. In reality, however, histologically identical tumors may arise in cerebrum, pineal and suprasellar regions, spinal cord, and brainstem. Such

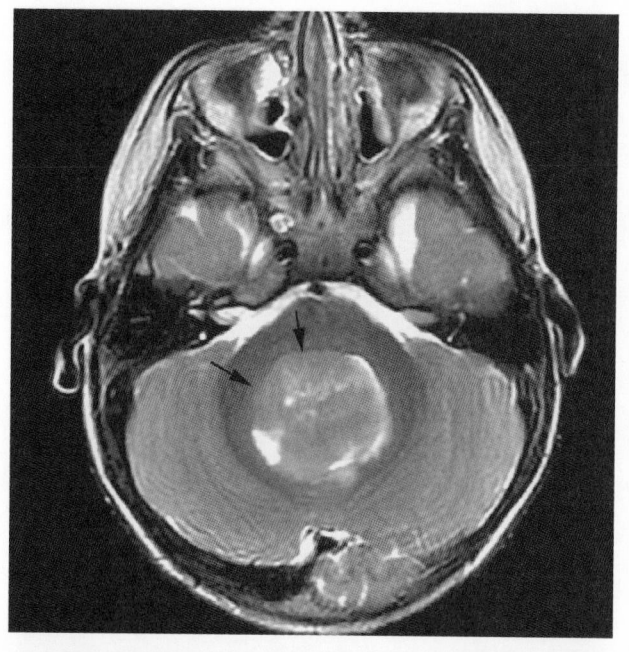

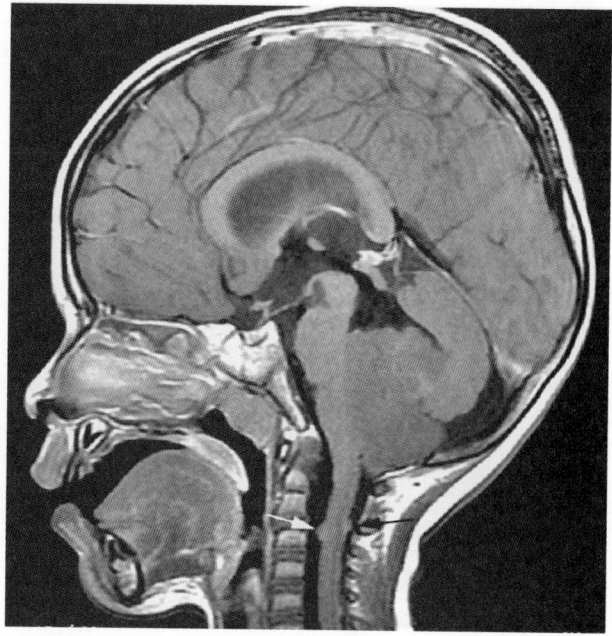

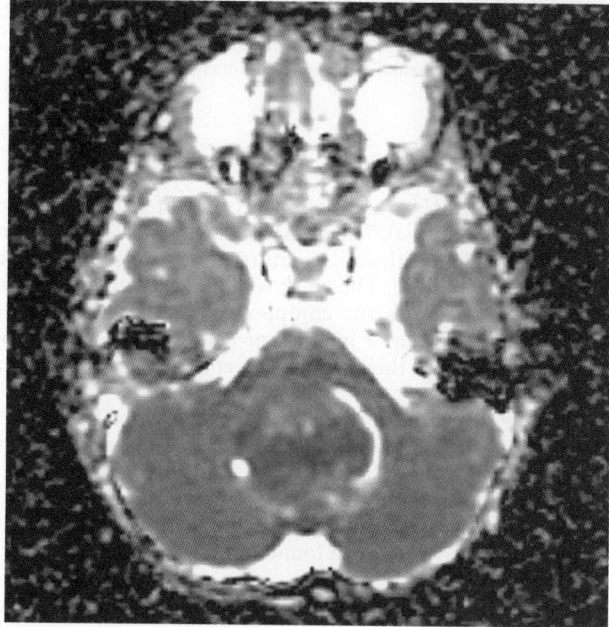

FIGURE 26B.1 Typical medulloblastoma in a 3-year-old child. Axial T2 (**A**) and postcontrast sagittal T1 (**B**) images show a midline tumor filling the fourth ventricle, with suspect invasion of the right middle cerebellar peduncle and the dorsal right hemipons (*arrow*, **A**). T2 signal is hypointense (**A**); the mass does not enhance, though small weakly enhancing metastatic nodules are evident in the upper cervical canal (*arrows*, **B**). The tumor shows reduced apparent diffusion coefficient (ADC) with low signal on the ABC map (**C**).

tumors were well known to Bailey and Cushing who, however, remained ambivalent in regard to what name should be given to the extracerebellar tumors resembling medulloblastomas.[79] As a consequence, a large number of diagnostic terms have been applied to medulloblastoma-like tumors that arise outside the cerebellum.

A proposal to resolve the problem in 1983 seemed, instead, to stimulate further controversy.[80] Specifically, it was proposed that tumors composed primarily of apparently undifferentiated neuroepithelial cells be considered a unique diagnostic group regardless of site of origin in the CNS, recognizing that the majority of such tumors do, in fact, arise in the cerebellum. Introduced by Hart and Earle, the diagnostic term *PNET* was suggested as appropriate for this group, with the addition of modifiers specifying differentiation along one or more lines (e.g., neuronal, glial) if such were identified by the use of phenotypic markers (i.e., antibodies for NFP, GFAP).[81] This

proposal was criticized as a "simplistic" approach that would foster intellectual languor among pathologists who would use the diagnosis of PNET as a catchall term for all difficult-to-diagnose tumors primarily composed of poorly differentiated neuroepithelial cells.[81] In addition, many were reluctant to abandon the diagnostic term medulloblastoma because of its familiarity and association with an enormous body of medical literature.

Studies yielding conflicting data relative to the question of whether the medulloblastoma was a tumor specific to the cerebellum accounted for some of the controversy. More than 60 years ago, it was claimed that the tumor arose from embryonic cells of the granular layer.[82–84] This assertion was challenged by later investigators,[85–87] but a considerable number of recent studies provide evidence that at least some medulloblastomas likely result from malignant transformation of external granular cells and, hence by necessity, can be found

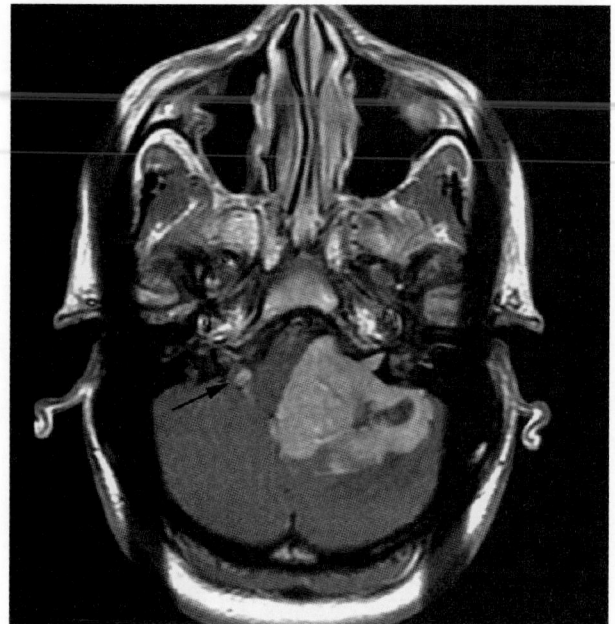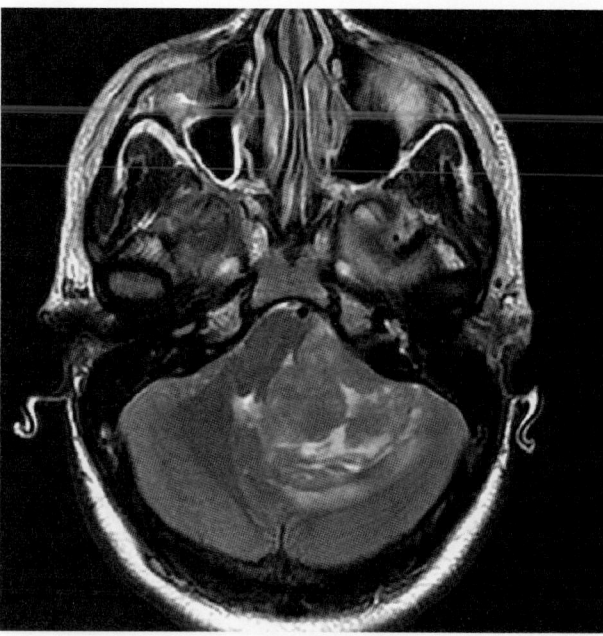

A   **B**

FIGURE 26B.2 Teenage boy with a medulloblastoma in the left cerebellopontine angle. Axial T2 (**A**) and postcontrast axial T1 (**B**) images reveal a predominately T2 isointense mass in the CP angle cistern, with a mild amount of surrounding cerebellar edema, and fairly homogeneous, intense enhancement following gadolinium (**B**). Enhancement in the right foramen of Luschka represents normal choroid, not metastatic disease (*arrow*, **B**).

only in the cerebellum.[88–90] The best candidate in this category is the desmoplastic medulloblastoma.[91–95] This histologic subtype is almost never seen in PNETs that occur in other CNS sites, although such tumors elsewhere may exhibit other patterns of desmoplasia.

Evidence in support of the desmoplastic medulloblastoma as a uniquely cerebellar tumor derived from granular neurons has come from identification of allelic losses of the tumor suppressor locus, PTCH, located on the long arm of chromosome 9. PTCH inhibits the Hedgehog signaling pathway, which is important in development of cerebellar granular cells.

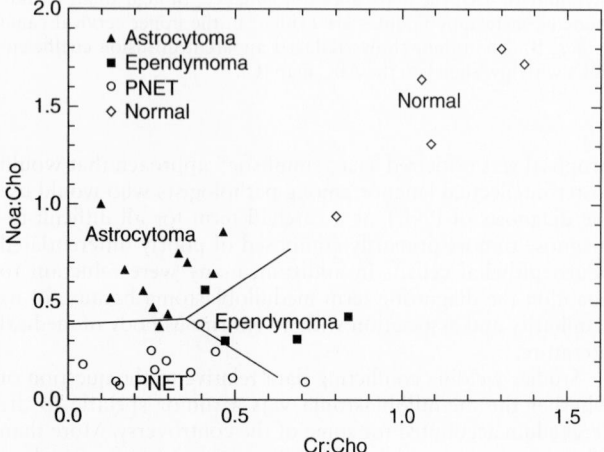

FIGURE 26B.3 *N*-acetyl aspartate-choline (NAA:Cho) versus creatine-choline (Cr:Cho) scattergram for astrocytoma, ependymoma, medulloblastoma, and normal cerebellar tissue. The straight lines are boundaries between the three tumor types found by discriminant analysis. PNET, primitive neuroectodermal tumor.

Study of mRNA expression profiles of 62 medulloblastomas by Kool et al.[96] identified five subtypes with distinct genetic profiles, pathway signatures, and clinicopathological features (Fig. 26B.4). The work is of clinical significance, as it not only establishes the complexity of this most common embryonal CNS tumor but also provides insight into biological subgroups and their unique susceptibility to various treatment regimens.

The cytogenetics of medulloblastomas differ from PNETs elsewhere in the CNS. In particular, an i(17)q abnormality has been identified in 30% to 50% of medulloblastomas but, to date, has been found in only one cerebral PNET.[94,97,98] In addition, other cytogenetic abnormalities that occur in medulloblastomas have not been found in PNETs elsewhere and vice versa.[93,94]

Studies of cell signaling systems and transcription factors associated with normal cerebellar development and possible dysregulation as a factor in the pathogenesis of medulloblastomas also contribute to emerging information regarding the medulloblastoma.[92,94,99,100]

Neurodevelopmental studies in fact offer evidence that primitive neuroepithelial cells, although histologically similar, are genetically programmed differently depending on location.[101–107] Hence, it is conceivable that the behavior of transformed cells in different locations in the CNS would reflect biologic heterogeneity as well. Such a concept is in keeping with observations, already noted previously, that the site of origin of histologically similar tumors is of significance in governing biology and prognosis and lends credence to the suggestion by Rorke et al.[108] that tumor location should be indicated, along with histologic diagnosis.

Until further insight is gained relative to these complex issues, it seems prudent, at least as a start, to base a classification scheme on phenotypic features of a tumor or group of tumors. These characteristics may be determined by utilization of immunohistochemical techniques, ultrastructural

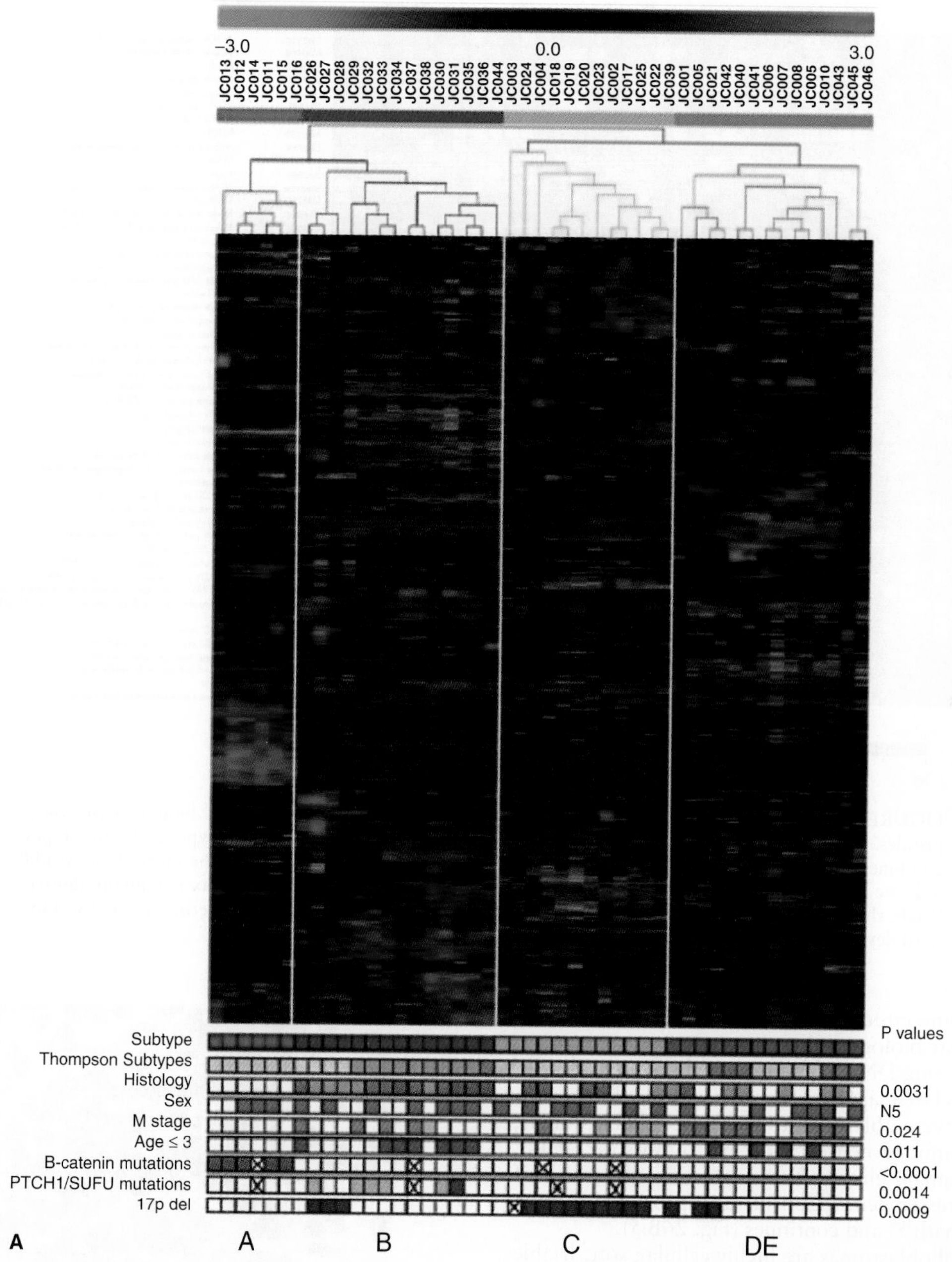

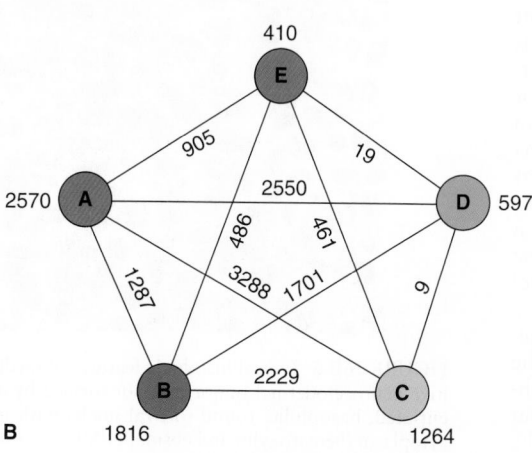

	P values
Subtype	
Thompson Subtypes	
Histology	0.0031
Sex	N5
M stage	0.024
Age ≤ 3	0.011
B-catenin mutations	<0.0001
PTCH1/SUFU mutations	0.0014
17p del	0.0009

A   A   B   C   DE

FIGURE 26B.4 Identification of molecular subtypes in medulloblastoma. **A:** Unsupervised two-way hierarchical cluster analysis of 62 medulloblastoma samples and expression data of 1,300 most differentially expressed genes identified five distinct clusters indicated as **A, B, C, D,** and **E.** Clinical annotations are at the bottom. Histology: grey = desmoplastic, orange = large cell/anaplastic, white = classic; sex: pink = female, white = male; metastatic disease at diagnosis indicated with M stage: yellow = M1, orange = M2, white = M0; age: purple = age 3 years, white = age 3 years; β-catenin mutations: brown = mutations, white = wild type; PTCH1 mutations: blue = mutations, white = wild type. A cross means not analyzed. **B:** Schematic pentagram showing the correlations between the five molecular subtypes of medulloblastoma. Numbers at the outside near each subtype indicate number of genes that are significantly differently expressed between that subtype and all other subtypes.

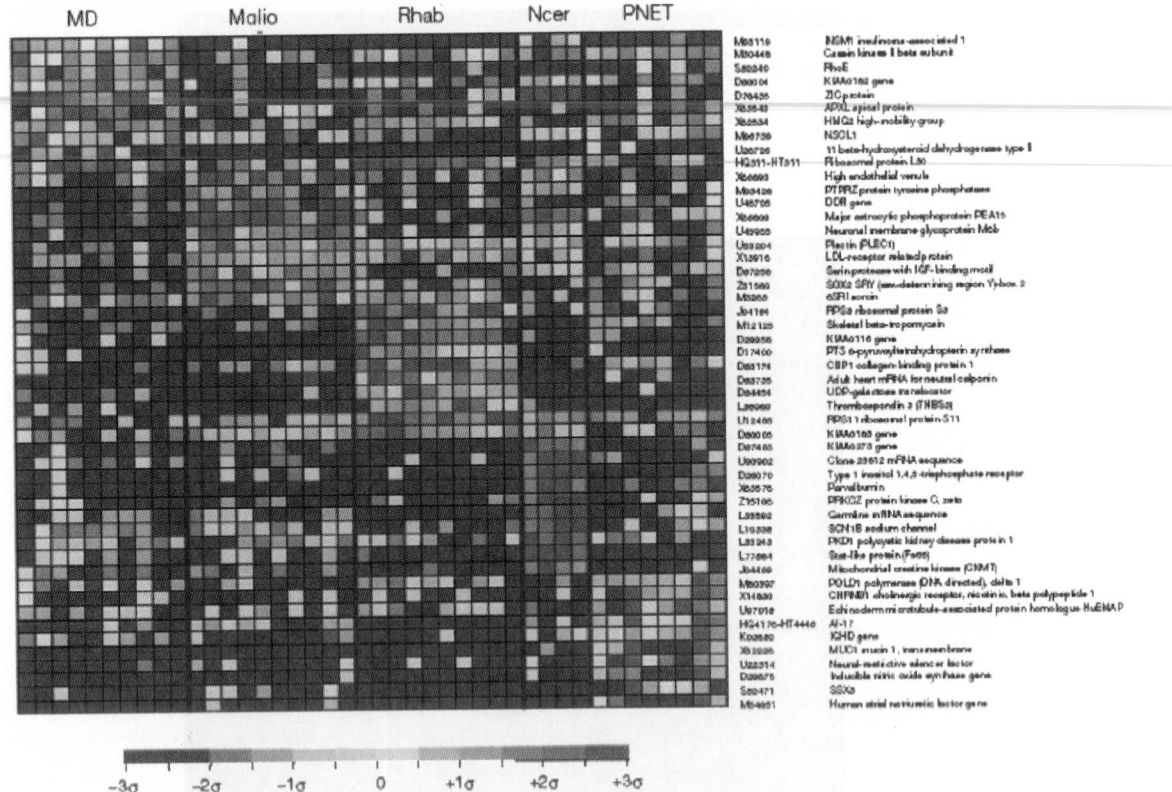

FIGURE 26B.5 Classification of childhood central nervous system (CNS) tumors by gene expression profiles. This figure shows signal-to-noise rankings of genes comparing each tumor type to all other types combined. For each gene, red would indicate a high level of expression relative to the mean; blue would indicate a low level of expression relative to the mean. MD, medulloblastoma; Mglio, malignant glioma; Rhab, rhabdoid; Ncer, normal cerebella; PNET, supratentorial primitive neuroectodermal tumor; s, standard deviation from the mean.

evaluation (in some circumstances), cytogenetic study, and available molecular biology techniques.

For example, using DNA microarray technology to screen the expression level of a large number of genes simultaneously, Pomeroy et al.[93] were able to distinguish medulloblastomas, supratentorial primitive neuroectodermal tumors (sPNETs), AT/RTs, and malignant gliomas based on a limited number of differentially expressed genes. Considerable progress has been made along this path[109] and continues (Fig. 26B.5).

Classical medulloblastomas are highly cellular, soft, friable tumors composed of cells with deeply basophilic nuclei of variable size and shape, little discernible cytoplasm, and, often, abundant mitoses (Fig. 26B.6) although they may exhibit surprising histologic heterogeneity. Homer Wright rosettes and pseudorosettes are variably present. Various degrees of glial or neuronal differentiation are noted, suggesting that the primitive cell of origin possesses the capacity for bipotential differentiation.[110,111] A histologic variant with an abundant stromal component, desmoplastic medulloblastoma (Fig. 26B.7), occurs dominantly in the lateral cerebellar areas of adolescents and adults and in the setting of Gorlin syndrome in infants and young children.[35,36] These may have a nodular appearance. A second somewhat different histologic subtype containing nodules is the so-called cerebellar (or cerebral) neuroblastoma.

An aggressive variant of medulloblastoma, termed *large-cell* and *large-cell anaplastic*, has been described.[112,113] As the names imply, the histologic features that distinguish this subset of medulloblastoma are large round nuclei with prominent nucleoli, frequent mitoses, abundant apoptosis, and, in the

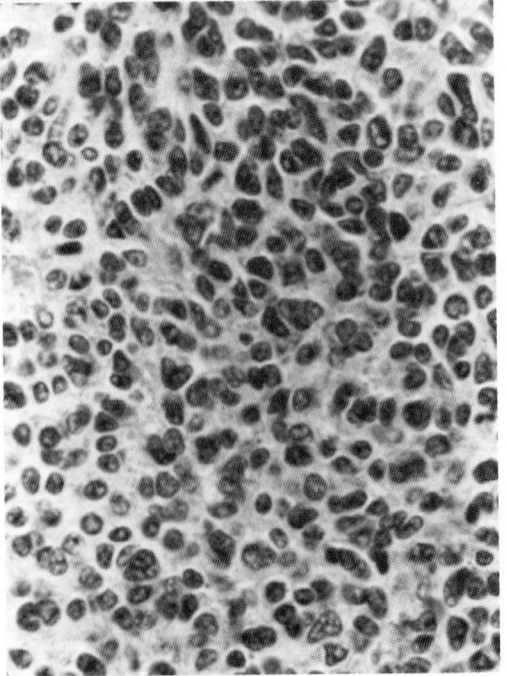

FIGURE 26B.6 Typical histologic features of medulloblastoma (primitive neuroectodermal tumor). Tumor formed by apparently undifferentiated, basophilic, round-to-oval nuclei with minimal perceptible cytoplasm (hematoxylin and eosin, 3,400).

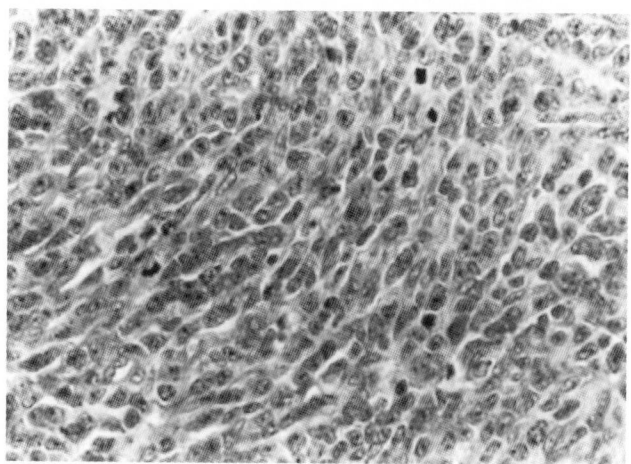

FIGURE 26B.7 Desmoplastic medulloblastoma showing linear arrangement of cells along delicate background fibers (hematoxylin and eosin, 3,400).

anaplastic subset, nuclear pleomorphism. These tumors typically express synaptophysin and chromogranin. Monosomy 22 has not been seen in the cases described, but it tends to be associated with MYC or MCYN amplification.[114] The large-cell anaplastic variant represented 4% of the nearly 500 cases of medulloblastoma reviewed by Brown et al.[115]

Medulloblastomas often grow to several centimeters and may fill the posterior fossa, invading surrounding CNS structures as they occupy the regional subarachnoid and ventricular spaces. As with other CNS tumors of presumed primitive neuroepithelial origin, widespread seeding of the subarachnoid space may occur (Fig. 26B.17). The reported frequency of CNS spread outside the area of the primary tumor at diagnosis is 11% to 43%, and such spread eventually occurs in as many as 93% of patients who come to necropsy.[116,117]

Of all pediatric CNS neoplasms, the medulloblastoma has the greatest propensity for extraneural spread. Although this has been observed in 20% to 35% of patients in smaller institutional studies, more recent larger series suggest that the rate of such events is less than 4%.[118–121] Bone and bone marrow are the most common extraneural sites, accounting for more than 80% of metastases; lymph nodes, liver, and lung are other reported sites.[122]

Biology

Consistent genetic abnormalities have been found in medulloblastomas using a number of genomic technologies, such as chromosomal banding, multicolor spectral karyotyping (SKY/m- fluorescence in situ hybridization [FISH]), comparative genomic hybridization (CGH), array based-CGH, and FISH) Deletions of the short arm of chromosome 17 (17p) distal to the TP53 locus occur in 30% to 50% of medulloblastomas.[123,124] Loss of 17p frequently occurs in association with duplication of 17q, which is characteristic of isochromosome 17q (i17q), the most common cytogenetic abnormality of medulloblastomas.[123–125] However, no single candidate gene either as a tumor suppressor gene or as oncogene on chromosome 17 has been identified. TP53 is not considered a major target of 17p loss, since the minimal deleted region is distal to TP53 and the incidence of mutation is low (5% to 10%).[126,127] Trisomy 7 is the second most common cytogenetic abnormality and tends to be associated with i17q.[123,128] A novel amplicon at 7q21.2 containing only the cyclin-dependent kinase

6 gene was recently identified by array CGH.[129] The cyclin-dependent kinase 6 gene can phosphorylate retinoblastoma 1, and its overexpression is associated with poor prognosis in medulloblastomas. Deletions or mutations of chromosome 9q involving the Sonic hedgehog receptor PTCH1 have been found in association with approximately 10% to 15% of sporadic medulloblastomas.[130–133] Loss of chromosome 6 occurs independently of i17q and is associated with WNT pathway activation.[43,134] A variety of other chromosomal deletions or additions have been found less consistently.[135,136] The nonrandom occurrence of monosomy 22 is common in several neural tumors, including medulloblastomas, ependymomas, meningiomas, acoustic neuromas, and AT/RTs.[137,138]

During the past decade, several signaling pathways were identified to be involved in the pathogenesis and possibly the prognosis of medulloblastoma including those of SHH/PTCH1/SMO, WNT, NOTCH, and ERBB2. The SHH and WNT signaling pathways interact with each other, but also with other signaling pathways including NOTCH and ERBB2, Not only that Patched knockout mice spontaneously develop medulloblastomas, but smoothened inhibitors could inhibit the proliferation of these tumors in the ptc+/− mice.[139,140] Likewise, medulloblastomas from both experimental animal models and patients showed upregulating the NOTCHED pathway and gamma secretase inhibitors against the NOTCHED receptors could also suppress the growth of medulloblastoma cell lines both in vitro and in xenografts.[141] In addition, gamma secretase inhibitor treatment also depleted the CD133+ stem-like cells in medulloblastoma cell lines. Overexpression of ERBB2 is associated with worse prognosis and increases the migration of medulloblastoma cells in vitro, and prometastatic genes involved in cell adhesion and invasion are up-regulated by ERBB2.[142]

A number of developmentally active genes are found to be aberrantly expressed in medulloblastoma. For example, OTX2 on chromosome 14q22 was originally found to be amplified in medulloblastoma cell line by digital karyotyping and subsequently discovered to be also overexpressed in a significant portion of clinical cases.[14,142] Apoptosis is induced when the OTX gene is knocked down in medulloblastoma cells, either by RNAi or by treatment with all-trans-retinoic acid in vitro.

Another area of genetic alterations in medulloblastoma involves epigenetic changes, which include both histone modifications (acetylation, methylation, and phosphorylation) and hypermethylation of CpG islands that could lead to transcriptional silencing of tumor suppressor genes. Several putative tumor suppressor genes are aberrantly methylated in subgroups of medulloblastoma such as RASSF1A.[143]

Staging and Risk Stratification

Staging and risk stratification are critical in the management of medulloblastoma and is a cornerstone of treatment.[4] Staging remains predominantly based on determination of the extent of tumor at the time of diagnosis and the degree of surgical resection. Retrospective studies have shown the potential importance of histologic and biologic parameters in determination of the likelihood of disease relapse, and studies are underway attempting to integrate these parameters into staging schema.[14,15] Complete staging requires pre- or postoperative MRI of the entire brain and spine, postoperative MRI of the tumor site, and CSF analysis.[14]

Historically, the Chang staging system, utilizing preoperative imaging studies, the surgeon's intraoperative impression, and CSF cytology, was used to assign stages of primary (T stage) and metastatic (M stage) disease[14] (see Table 26B.4), This system has been significantly modified and the assessment

TABLE 26B.4

CHANG STAGING SYSTEM FOR POSTERIOR-FOSSA MEDULLOBLASTOMA

Stage	Definition
Tumor	
T1	Tumor, 3 cm in diameter and limited to the midline position in the vermis, the roof of the fourth ventricle, and, less frequently, to the cerebellar hemispheres
T2	Tumor, 3 cm in diameter, further invading one adjacent structure or partially filling the fourth ventricle
T3	Divided into T3a and T3b
T3a	Tumor invading two adjacent structures or completely filling the fourth ventricle with extension into the aqueduct of Sylvius, foramen of Magendie, or foramen of Luschka, thus producing marked internal hydrocephalus
T3b	Tumor arising from the floor of the fourth ventricle or brainstem and filling the fourth ventricle
T4	Tumor further spreading through the aqueduct of Sylvius to involve the third ventricle or midbrain, or tumor extending to the upper cervical cord
Metastases	
M0	No evidence of gross subarachnoid or hematogenous metastasis
M1	Microscopic tumor cells found in cerebrospinal fluid
M2	Gross nodule seedings demonstrated in the cerebellar-cerebral subarachnoid space or in the third or lateral ventricles
M3	Gross nodule seedings in the spinal subarachnoid space
M4	Extraneuraxial metastasis

of the preoperative size of the tumor (T stage) has been supplanted by a postoperative evaluation of the extent of resection or, more specifically, the amount of postoperative residual disease, at times, modified by the impression of the surgeon at the time of diagnosis (see Table 26B.5).

The M stage of the disease remains the single, most prognostic clinical parameter.[144,145] The prognostic significance of M1 disease, indicating positive CSF cytology, without radiographic evidence of disseminated disease, has been debated and has been found to be predictive in some, but not all, studies. Part of this difference may be due to the means to assess the presence of free-floating tumor cells. Lumbar CSF cytology has been shown to be the most sensitive, but in some studies,

TABLE 26B.5

STRATIFICATION OF MEDULLOBLASTOMA

	Standard risk	High risk
Age at diagnosis	>3 yr	≤3 yr
Extent surgical resection	>1.5 cm² residual tumor	≤1.5 cm² residual tumor
Extent of disease	Stage M0	Stage M1–M4

either ventricular and/or spinal fluid have been used for assessment. Gajjar and colleagues found lumbar CSF to be more sensitive in the detection of disseminated disease than ventricular fluid and found cytological assessment to be complementary to neuroaxis neuroimaging.[146] In the German HIT 1991 study, 13% of patients had M1 disease and their overall survival (OS) rate of 65% did not differ from those with M0 disease.[144] A similar nonsignificant finding was noted for a small number of patients with M1 disease in the French M7 study.[147] In contradistinction, the Children's Cancer Group (CCG)-921 study found that 18% of patients had M1 disease, utilizing almost exclusively lumbar CSF, and found a 5-year and a progression-free survival of 57% for those patients with positive cytology, a rate lower than that for those with M0 disease, and higher than that for patients with M2 or M3 disease, although differences were of borderline significance.[145]

Cerebrospinal fluid for staging is most predictive if obtained 2 weeks or greater following tumor resection.[4,146] Preoperative lumbar puncture may be contraindicated if there is postoperative mass effect of the tumor and the potential for cerebellar herniation. Cisternal fluid, obtained at the time of diagnosis, has been variably related to outcome. Arachnoid biopsy, at the time of surgery, is presently being evaluated as a possible independent prognostic factor.

Neuroradiographically confirmed metastatic disease (M2 or M3) has been prognostic in all series.[144–147] Extraneural spread at diagnosis (M4 disease) is rare outside of infancy, and assessment for extraneural disease by bone scans and bone marrow analysis is now not recommended, in most prospective studies, as a part of initial staging. The sensitivity of MRI for the detection of metastatic disease is much greater than that of CT or myelography. Because of this, no doubt, patients who in the past would have been diagnosed as nonmetastatic, or with M1 disease, are now being classified as having M2 disease. This results in the inclusion of possibly lower-risk patients into high-risk protocols, and the exclusion of patients with minor amounts of disease from low-risk protocols. Such a change in determination of classification has likely resulted in making results seem better in newer treatment trials, as patients with less extensive disease are included in the high-risk studies and the low-risk studies have become more pristine.

Despite the accepted use of MRI for staging, performance and interpretation of neuroimaging studies for the evaluation of disease dissemination at the time of diagnosis remains imperfect. In a recent Children's Oncology Group (COG) study and French prospective studies, upon central review, inadequate imaging studies, due to patient movement or incomplete staging, were noted in up to 10% of patients.[20,147] Another 5% to 10% of patients, upon central neuroimaging review, were found to have significant residual postoperative disease or evidence of dissemination not appreciated by the treating institutions. Patients with evidence of dissemination, upon central review, had a particularly poor prognosis if treated on reduced-radiotherapy protocols. Patients with inadequate imaging had intermediary outcomes between those with evidence of disease dissemination and those with no evidence of disseminated disease upon central review. Determination of extent of disease on neuroimaging studies is particularly challenging in those with nonenhancing tumors, as spinal metastasis can be quite difficult to appreciate. Similarly, spread to the third ventricle and cisterns around the brainstem was problematic to appreciate.

Extent of Resection

A near-total (arbitrarily defined as more than a 90% resection) or a total resection is now achieved in approximately

80% of children with medulloblastoma, utilizing contemporary microsurgical techniques, entered on cooperative group studies.[148] Evidence suggesting that the extent of resection correlates with outcome has been provided by several single institutions and by multi-institutional studies.[149,150] For example, in the series reported by Jenkin, a 93%, 5-year progression-free survival rate was noted in children undergoing gross total resection as compared with only 45% in those undergoing a partial resection.[151] However, in some recent series and other multi-institutional trials, the impact of the degree of resection on outcome is not as clear. In one CCG study, a clear relationship was found between the degree of resection and outcome, but only in the subset of patients with no evidence of tumor dissemination.[146,150] This study also found, regardless of the surgeon's estimate of the disease of resection, that the presence of greater than 1.5 cm^2 residual disease on postoperative imaging was associated with a significantly lower progression-free survival rate in patients with nonmetastatic disease. Arbitrarily, most cooperative group studies have continued to utilize some measure of the extent of residual disease after surgery as a staging criteria, as children with less than 1.5 cm^2 of postoperative residual disease have been included in the average-risk category, while those with a greater amount of disease are classified as high-risk. It is widely accepted that patients who undergo only a minimal degree of resection fare poorly.

Brainstem involvement at the time of diagnosis was found in older studies, in which patients were predominantly treated with radiation therapy alone, to be predictive of poor outcome.[9,146] However, in most studies that have coupled chemotherapy with radiation therapy, the presence of brainstem involvement has not been found to be a significant prognostic variable.[20,144,152] Similarly, there is little evidence to support improved outcome in patients with "gross total" resection as compared with those with "near total" resections. This is an important issue, as medulloblastomas often infiltrate the floor of the fourth ventricle and attempts at "total" removal may result in increased morbidity. There is also concern that the increasingly reported "posterior fossa mutism" syndrome may be related to a trend for more aggressive surgical approaches.

Age at Diagnosis

Younger children, predominantly those 3 years of age or less at the time of diagnosis, have been shown to have poorer outcome than older patients with medulloblastoma.[9,152–154] Determining the influence of age as an independent prognostic factor is difficult for a variety of reasons, including younger age at diagnosis, which has been associated with a higher rate of disease dissemination at diagnosis and an overall lower rate of complete tumor resection.[116,118] In past reports, younger children with medulloblastoma, in general, have received lower doses of both craniospinal and local radiotherapy or were more likely to receive chemotherapy prior to the initiation of radiation therapy, confounding comparisons to series of older children with the disease. The inclusion of the atypical teratoid/rhabdoid tumor, which tends to arise in children younger than 3, within the medulloblastoma subgroup may have also skewed outcome, as this tumor type has a very poor prognosis. Despite all these caveats, there is evidence that there are biologic differences between medulloblastomas arising in different ages and these differences, at least partially, underlie the poorer prognosis of infants.[13,14,15,19] Although series have demonstrated inferior survival rates for children younger than 3, there is no specific relationship between age in the first 2 years of life and the likelihood of relapse. When

standard doses of craniospinal and local boost radiotherapy have been utilized for children younger than 3 years, especially those between 2 and 3 years of age, outcome has been poorer in some, but not in all, series.[144,145,152,153,155,156] Once again, the timing of radiation seems to be of importance, as in some reports radiation therapy has been delayed for weeks to months by the use of postsurgical chemotherapy.

Histology

The significance of different histological patterns on survival has been variable. In infants, the desmoplastic variant of medulloblastoma has been related to improved survival.[11,12] Some studies have demonstrated that the degree of apparent histological differentiation is predictive of outcome, with tumors that are more differentiated along histologically identifiable cellular lineages portending a poorer prognosis.[111] More recently, the anaplastic or large cell variant had been linked with more extensive and/or disseminated tumors and, even in cases without dissemination, poorer prognosis.[12,22,44] This latter finding has been demonstrated predominantly by retrospective reviews, and in the most recent COG prospective national studies, patients with extensive or "diffuse" anaplasia have been included on high-risk protocols. The significance of anaplasia as an outcome measure has been confounded by its subjectivity and relationship to biologic markers (such as higher myc expression) that have been related to poorer prognosis.[22]

Biologic Markers

Extensive laboratory research efforts are directed at identifying molecular markers that will reliably predict the outcome of children with medulloblastoma (see Table 26B.6). Early flow cytometry studies indicated an association between aneuploidy and a more favorable prognosis.[157] Later cytogenetic studies further refined the link between genomic mutations and tumor behavior, demonstrating that deletions of chromosome 17p were associated with poor outcome.[158] However, more recent studies demonstrated that loss of heterozygosity on 17p may not be a significant predictor of prognosis in medulloblastoma.[159] Amplification of c-myc was linked strongly to poor prognosis but was found to occur in fewer than 20% of all medulloblastomas.[160,161]

Several recent investigations have focused on gene expression as a marker of medulloblastoma prognosis (see Table 26B.6). Expression of the neurotrophin-3 receptor TrkC has

TABLE 26B.6

BIOLOGIC PROGNOSTIC PARAMETERS

Neurotrophin-3 receptor[92]	Increased expression associated with improved survival
ERBB2[14]	Increased expression associated with poorer survival and metastasis
PDGFRA[162]	Overexpression associated with metastasis
RAS/MAPK pathway[162]	Overexpression associated with increased metastasis
MYCC/MYCN	Amplification and expression associated with poorer survival
γ- and β-catenin[17]	Expression associated with better survival
p53[19]	Immunopositivity associated with poorer survival

been found to be associated with a favorable prognosis.[163–165] The majority of medulloblastomas express both TrkC and neurotrophin-3, suggesting an autocrine or paracrine receptor activation of the TrkC receptor tyrosine kinase.[165] Moreover, TrkC activation induces medulloblastoma apoptosis that possibly may contribute to the more favorable prognosis of tumors with high TrkC expression.[165] In contrast, a poorer prognosis has been linked to increased expression of the neuregulin receptors ErbB-2 and ErbB-4 and of c-myc or loss of caspase-8 protein expression.[14,166] ErbB2, in particular, has been strongly linked to outcome and appears to provide prognostic information that supplements information available from clinical risk factors.[14] Genome-wide profiling based on RNA expression,[96,167] DNA copy number, and microRNA expression[167,168] provide even more powerful tools for identifying molecular prognostic features, which also appears to provide prognostic information that supplements rather than duplicates information provided by clinical features.[16,168–170] In view of the strong association between the above molecular factors and outcome, their evaluation has been incorporated into the new phase III prospective standard- and high-risk medulloblastoma studies of the COG, ACNS0331, and ACNS0332, respectively.

These discoveries suggest that inherent biologic differences, reflected in the divergent expression of genes that regulate tumor growth and response to therapy, determine the clinical outcome of morphologically similar-appearing medulloblastomas.[163,166,162] Efforts now are under way, through multi-institutional therapeutic trials, to test prospectively molecular markers that might be used for the stratification of patients in future clinical investigations. Furthermore, the molecules identified by these investigations might serve as targets for future, biologically based therapies specifically designed on the basis of molecular mechanisms regulating tumor growth.

Risk Groups Combining Clinical and Biologic Information

Retrospective analyses utilizing both clinical and biological information have been shown to be predictive of patient survival and have been proposed as more informative stratification schemas. In a single institution study, at Hospital for Sick Children, of 119 children with medulloblastoma, M stage, p53 immunoreactivity, ErbB2 expression and p53 immunopositivity were associated with outcome and by combining biologic parameters and clinical features, a prognostic index was obtained that was valid for both patients treated with and without radiotherapy.[19] deHaas and coworkers evaluated 124 tissue samples accrued from multiple institutions.[171] Protein expression analysis disclosed that low myc expression identified patients with a better outcome. In contrast, concomitant expression of LDHB and CCNBI characterized tumors with poorer outcome and multivariate analysis disclosed that expression of both myc and LDHB/CCNBI was a strong prognostic predictor, independent of clinical parameters, including metastasis and residual disease. In a study of 133 children between 3 and 18 years of age with medulloblastoma treated on a prospective HIT '91 randomized multi-center trial, formaline and fixed paraffin sections were analyzed for DNA amplification of C-myc and M-myc and mRNA expression of C-myc and TrkC.[13] The investigators identified three prognostic groups: (1) those with elevated TrkC and reduced myc expression had the best survival; (2) patients with metastatic disease and high C-myc and low TrkC expression had the highest risk of relapse; and (3) the group of remaining patients formed the largest group and had intermediate risk of relapse with an OS rate of 65%. In a study of 86 patients, Gajjar and colleagues combined clinical characteristics and

molecular findings to determine risk.[14] ErbB2 protein and C-myc, N-myc, and Trkc mRNA levels were measured. The investigators identified an extremely good risk group of patients who were clinically of average risk and had ErbB2-negative disease. TrkC, C-myc, and N-myc expression and histopathological subtype were not associated with prognosis.

In an overlapping group of patients, the gene expression profile of 46 snap-frozen medulloblastoma specimens were analyzed and validated with reverse transcriptase polymerase chain reaction and in situ hybridization.[43] Five subgroups were identified including those with mutations in the WNT pathways and deletions in chromosome 6 and mutations in the SHH pathway. Utilizing a gene profile expression classification coupled with clinical parameters, Pfister and colleagues also demonstrated that gene expression profiling could provide prognostic information that could not be obtained from histological criteria.[16] They found that all patients with 6q-deleted tumors survived, thought to be representative of activating β-catenin mutations and WNT pathway activation. In contrast, gain of 6q portended a poor outcome. Using a hierarchical molecular classification system, utilizing MYC/MYCN amplification, 6q gain, 6q and 17q balanced, and 6q deletion, risk of disease relapse and death could be assessed.

As noted earlier, although utilizing biologic data to supplement clinical information is potentially a great advance, there is no uniformity on which parameters should be assessed or how they are best measured. For these staging systems to become clinically applicable, molecular studies on tumor tissue must become available in real time and this will most likely require centralized laboratories evaluating similar molecular markers. In addition, these stratification systems must be evaluated in the context of the treatment received. Although parameters may be valid in patients homogenously treated with radiation therapy and/or chemotherapy, if the doses and volume of radiotherapy employed are altered, or if the type or sequencing of chemotherapy is changed, specific parameters may lose their predictive value.

A separate stratification system will probably be employed for infants and younger children. The presence of desmoplasia or potentially evidence of activation of specific signaling pathways, such as the SHH pathway, may dramatically alter risk and therapy.[172,173]

In adults with medulloblastoma, the same staging system of degree of resection and extent of metastasis is often utilized. Biologic predictors have not been widely explored in adult tumors.

Treatment

General Aspects

Current therapy for medulloblastoma in older children (generally older than 3 years) consists of maximal surgical resection, craniospinal radiation therapy, and chemotherapy.[4] Current treatment challenges include a determination of the optimal dose of radiation therapy; the optimal timing, dose, and combination of chemotherapy agents; and the identification of prognostic factors to identify patients who require less intensive therapy.

Surgery

A fundamental decision in evaluating a child with a posterior fossa tumor is determining whether the tumor is a mass lesion arising from the cerebellar hemisphere, vermis, or fourth ventricular floor or is an intrinsic tumor of the brainstem. Children with the former lesion types (e.g., medulloblastomas, ependymomas, cerebellar astrocytomas) undergo surgical intervention to allow for diagnosis, unblock CSF pathways, remove pressure on critical posterior fossa structures, and achieve cytoreduction.

In children with a resectable lesion, such as a medulloblastoma, the timing of surgery is determined by the clinical status of the child. If they are alert, high-dose corticosteroids are administered and a spinal MRI scan is obtained to determine the presence of evidence of leptomeningeal dissemination; the craniotomy then is performed on the following day.[174] This approach is reasonable also if such children are lethargic but become alert after administration of corticosteroids. However, in the rare situations in which such children are extremely somnolent, urgent surgical intervention is preferred.

A ventriculostomy is placed in most cases for temporary CSF diversion, and this is "weaned" by gradual elevation of the drip chamber during the postoperative period. If affected children need CSF drainage for more than 7 days after tumor removal, permanent CSF diversion usually is performed. Some centers are now advocating endoscopic third ventriculostomy at the time of presentation as a tool to avoid CSF shunting.[175,176] Whether an endoscopic third ventriculostomy can prevent post-tumor removal shunting and its inherent risks is yet to be properly defined.

The tumor usually is approached through a suboccipital craniotomy or craniectomy, with the patient in a prone or modified prone (Concorde) position. The dura is opened in a Y-shaped fashion. Cerebellar hemispheric lesions, which are encountered most commonly in older children, are exposed fully by a transverse or vertical incision in the cerebellar hemisphere. The more common vermian and fourth ventricular lesions may be visible within the foramen of Magendie but, if not, are exposed by dividing the caudal 1 to 2 cm of the inferior vermis. Because approximately 20% of patients develop a postoperative syndrome of pseudobulbar symptoms and mutism (the "posterior fossa syndrome") after vermian tumor resections,[177–181] which may be related in part to the extent of the vermis incision, an attempt is made to incise only as much vermis as is needed to provide adequate exposure of the tumor. Some authors have advocated the "telo-velar" approach in which the Foramen of Luschka is opened up to allow retraction of the cerebellum superiorly, and thereby decrease the amount of resection of the inferior cerebellar vermis. The central portion of the lesion is then debulked using the ultrasonic aspirator.[180,181] The plane between the tumor and the vermis is followed rostrally until the roof of the fourth ventricle is reached. There is usually a very discrete plane between the purplish medulloblastoma and the grayish cerebellum. Once the tumor has been partially de-bulked, a cottonoid patty is inserted under the caudal aspect of the tumor along the floor of the fourth ventricle to minimize the risk of injury to the brainstem as additional tumor is removed from within the fourth ventricle. Some surgeons monitor electromyograms of the lateral rectus and facial muscles during the resection to reduce the risk of abducens and facial nerve palsies. Next, tumor extending laterally within the foramina of Luschka or the cerebellar peduncles is removed. Finally, tumor adherent to the floor of the fourth ventricle is carefully removed. The aggressiveness of the resection in this region is guided by the frozen-section diagnosis. For medulloblastomas, the tumor can be shaved down to just above the floor of the fourth ventricle, but removal of tumor below the floor is unnecessary, as it does not appear to improve outcome and clearly increases the potential for morbidity.

Once the tumor has been removed, the dura is closed, generally with a graft. Because a CSF examination is an important component of the postoperative staging of children with medulloblastomas and because blood and debris can settle in the lumbar thecal sac within several hours of surgery, complicating

interpretation of the cytology for several weeks, many groups delay the puncture until the third postoperative week. A postoperative MRI is performed, preferably within 24 to 72 hours after surgery, to confirm the extent of resection.

Postoperative Considerations

The postoperative recovery of patients who undergo a complete or partial resection of a posterior fossa tumor, particularly a tumor in or around the cerebellar vermis, may be complicated by posterior fossa syndrome. Posterior fossa syndrome, also known as "cerebellar mutism," may range from a mild to severe disorder that is characterized by mutism, ataxia, hemiparesis, cognitive impairment, behavioral changes, cranial nerve palsies, bulbar palsy, and tremor.[177–181] The onset is typically within the first week after surgery[182–184] and appears to occur more commonly with medulloblastoma than with other posterior fossa tumors.

The etiology of the posterior fossa syndrome is unknown but has been suggested to be secondary to damage to the cerebellar vermis, the floor of the fourth ventricle, the deep cerebellar nuclei, the middle cerebellar peduncle, and the superior cerebellar peduncle. None of the suggested etiologies accounts very well for the delayed onset of symptoms. Previously reported as a rare complication of posterior fossa surgery, for unclear reasons this syndrome is now observed in greater than 25% of children following tumor resection in the posterior fossa.[177–181] Although recovery may be complete, particularly for the mutism, there are patients in whom it is incomplete with long-term neurologic sequelae.[178,179,185]

Radiation Therapy

Medulloblastoma is a radiosensitive, radiocurable CNS tumor; for decades, the standard therapy for medulloblastoma has been postoperative irradiation to the entire subarachnoid space (the "neuraxis,"), termed *craniospinal irradiation* (CSI), along with a "boost" to the posterior fossa primary site. Attempts at not irradiating the entire neuraxis or omitting radiation therapy altogether have resulted in compromised survival.[186] Conversely, CSI is associated with dose-related effects on cognition, growth, and endocrine function; long-term functional changes are most marked in younger patients.[187] The emphasis of recent trials has been to identify cohorts of children in whom one can reduce CSI dose levels without compromising disease control. A prospective Pediatric Oncology Group (POG)-CCG study in the late 1980s compared standard-dose CSI (36 Gy) with reduced-dose CSI (23.4 Gy) in children with favorable presenting signs. The study showed an excess of subarachnoid failures in the reduced-dose arm, with a marginal benefit following standard-dose (23.4 Gy) CSI.[188] The companion POG neuropsychologic study showed superior cognitive function following the lower CSI dose, significant for those younger than 8 years.[189] Treatment regimens using postoperative irradiation alone require standard (36 Gy) CSI dose even with M0 disease.[188] Further experience in North America has built upon an encouraging single-arm pilot CCG study in the 1990s documenting disease control in excess of 80% following the same reduced-dose CSI (23.4 Gy/13 fractions) followed by local posterior fossa boost (54 Gy) but in conjunction with postirradiation chemotherapy, cisplatin, vincristine, and CCNU.[190] The subsequent COG protocol for standard risk medulloblastoma used 23.4 Gy CSI with one of two different chemotherapeutic regimens. Disease control at 3.5 years is in excess of 80% for both treatment arms, confirming the outcome noted in the earlier CCG pilot. Similar results were seen in a multicenter study utilizing cyclophosphamide-base high-dose postradiotherapy chemotherapy supported by peripheral stem cell rescue. In this study, the exposure to cisplatin was 50% less, although the alkylator dose was significantly higher.[191] The feasibility of further reduction in the CSI dose (18 Gy) is being evaluated for children 3 to 8 years old in the current COG trial. Whether the 18 Gy CSI dose is adequate in an identifiable cohort has been questioned, the phase III COG trial is ongoing, with power to detect a significant reduction in disease control or a change in the pattern of failure.[192,193] It is of note that recent trials show a reversal of earlier findings of predominant posterior fossa failures, now systematically indicating leptomeningeal dissemination to be the most common mode of failure in standard risk medulloblastoma.[20,191–195]

For children and adolescents with leptomeningeal metastasis at diagnosis, the accepted CSI dose is 36 Gy.[196] One of the most positive results in treating advanced stage disease was recently reported from St. Jude, where 70% long-term event-free survival (EFS) followed a regimen using CSI at 36 Gy (for positive CSF cytology without imaging evidence of metastasis, M1) and 39.6 Gy (for imaging-positive metastatic disease, M2–3).[193–195] Other recent series approach 65% to 70% disease control with overt metastasis with CSI doses of 36 to 40 Gy.

The time-dose relationship for radiation therapy correlates significantly with outcome. Prolonged interruptions in radiation therapy have consistently been associated with reduced likelihood of disease control.[196,197] Several series have assessed hyperfractionated radiation schedules (using 100 to 150 cGy twice daily to cumulative levels of 32 to 40 Gy dependent upon M status); no obvious benefit in disease control or later toxicities has been demonstrated.[194,195,198] The technique of CSI is well known. However, ensuring at least a 5-mm margin of coverage of the cribriform plate is important, as inadequate irradiation of that area can lead to an increase in recurrence at this location.[199–201] Spinal MRI is key to determining the inferior border of the thecal sac.

The radiation dose to the posterior fossa or tumor bed is based upon earlier observations defining a "threshold" dose of more than 50 Gy, in practice indicating near-tolerance levels of 54.0 to 55.8 Gy. The potential benefit of "boost" irradiation (>55.8 Gy) in cases with overt primary disease residual, either by reduced-volume fractionated radiation therapy (often to 59.4 Gy) or radiosurgery, has not been demonstrated. Several studies over the past 15 years indicate one can effectively control medulloblastoma with smaller boost volumes, targeting the tumor bed and any imaging-visible residual with a 2-cm margin rather than the entire posterior fossa.[187,193] Ongoing trials include a prospective comparison of posterior fossa versus local tumor bed irradiation and, independently, further reduction in the volumetric margin defining the clinical target from a 2-cm expansion to 1 or 1.5 cm beyond the tumor bed itself. The use of three-dimensional (3-D), image-based conformal techniques (including 3-D conformal—3DCRT, intensity modulated—IMRT, or proton beam irradiation—PBRT) provide greater restriction of the high-dose region to the targeted tumor volume, while selectively reducing the radiation dose to the cochlea and the hypothalamic-pituitary axis.[187,202–206] Current planning parameters also seek to relatively reduce radiation dose levels to the temporal lobe(s) and, in sophisticated settings, to the hippocampus region (in attempts to reduce cognitive deficits.)[205,207] The potential advantage of PBRT has been summarized, based upon modeling of dosimetry and clinically derived dose:volume:anatomic correlations.[206,208]

Chemotherapy

Chemotherapy is presently an integral component of treatment for all infants and children with medulloblastoma.[4,20,26]

It is also used extensively in adults with the disease, although proof of its efficacy for adults is less compelling. At the time of disease relapse, multiple single agents and drug combinations have resulted in objective responses, although cure with chemotherapy alone has been infrequent.[4,209–215] Objective response rates, ranging between 40% and 60%, have been documented with cisplatin, etoposide, and a variety of different alkylators, with the best responses being seen with multidrug regimens.[4,20,211–215]

Because of its chemosensitivity, medulloblastoma was one of the first pediatric brain tumors to have chemotherapy extensively evaluated in newly diagnosed patients. Prospective randomized studies performed as early as the late 1970s by the CCG and the International Society of Pediatric Oncology, which compared progression-free and OS in children treated with radiotherapy alone to those receiving radiotherapy plus chemotherapy given during and after radiation, demonstrated a statistically significant 15% to 20% survival advantage for patients with poorer risk disease, defined as those with disseminated disease, larger, more infiltrative tumors, and/or significant amounts of tumor left after surgery, as determined by the operating neurosurgeon.[152,154] Neither group demonstrated a statistically significant survival advantage for children with nondisseminated disease. These results were the basis of a series of trials performed over the ensuing two decades evaluating the efficacy of chemotherapy given at higher dose, coupled with other agents, or given in various sequences with radiotherapy, in children with high-risk medulloblastoma (see Table 26B.7). Also, because of the encouraging survival rates seen in children with poor-risk disease, chemotherapy was added to radiation therapy in children with nondisseminated (average-risk disease) in attempts to both improve survival and allow a reduction in the dose of craniospinal radiation.[4,9,20] Chemotherapy was also widely utilized for infants and young children with medulloblastoma to delay, if not obviate, the need for radiation therapy.

For children with average risk disease, 5-year survival rates of 80% to 85% have been seen after radiotherapy and a variety of chemotherapeutic agents used during and after radiotherapy (see Table 26B.7).

Treatment results, with different chemotherapy regimens used for variable intervals of time prior to radiotherapy, have been mixed.[149,216,217] Treatment with preradiation chemotherapy was associated with poorer survival in children with average-risk disease, especially when the dose of CSI therapy was reduced in a study performed by SIOP and the German Society of Pediatric Oncology, as only a 41% ± 8% 5-year, EFS was seen in 36 children treated with sandwich chemotherapy and delayed, reduced-dose radiotherapy.[149] In a French Society of Pediatric Oncology trial, 5-year recurrence-free survival was 65% ± 8%, utilizing a more aggressive proirradiation regimen of eight-drug-in-1-day plus carboplatin and also etoposide, followed by reduced-dose (2,500 cGy) CSI.[147] A poorer survival rate was also found in a CCG trial utilizing preradiation chemotherapy with the eight-drug-in-1-day regimen, as compared with chemotherapy during and after radiation. In a prospective, randomized, multi-agent German trial of combination chemotherapy prior to radiation, compared with postradiotherapy CCNU, vincristine, and cisplatin, survival was found to be inferior in those who received preradiation chemotherapy.[146]

For children with high-risk disease, primarily those with disseminated disease at the time of diagnosis, chemotherapy has been utilized prior to, during, and after radiotherapy[20,193,218,219] (see Table 26B.8). Once again, studies to date utilizing chemotherapy prior to radiotherapy have not shown benefit and possibly may have demonstrated inferior overall disease control rates.[149,218] In a report from the SFOP, in

TABLE 26B.7

TABLE 26B.7

MEDULLOBLASTOMA: SELECTED COOPERATIVE GROUP STUDIES FOR NONDISSEMINATED DISEASE

Study	N	Treatment	Outcome	Primary conclusion
SIOP II [149] (1984–1989)	293	3,500 cGy CSRT vs. 2,500 cGy CSRT +/− sandwich chemoRx	5-yr EFS; Standard RT: 60% ± 7.8% Reduced RT: 69% ± 7.8% Standard RT plus chemoRx: 75% ± 7.2% Reduced RT plus chemoRx: 41.7% ± 8.2%	Pre-RT chemoRx plus reduced CSRT poorer outcome
CCG-POG [188] (1986–1990)	126	3,600 cGy CSRT vs. 2,340 cGy CSRT	8-yr EFS, 3,600 CSRT: 67% ± 8.8% 2,340 CSRT: 52% ± 11%	Increased early subarachnoid failure in reduced-arm; marginal difference in EFS
HIT 1991 [144] (1991–1997)	130	Pre-RT CHT vs. immediate RT plus chemoRx	Pre-RT chemoRx 3-yr PFS: 62% ± 1% RT plus chemoRx: 84% ± 1%	Use of pre-RT chemoRx poorer PFS
SIOP/UKCCSG [197] PNET-3	179	3,500 cGy CSRT vs. 3,500 cGy plus pre-RT chemoRx	5-yr PFS RT: 59% ± 8% 5-yr PFS RT + chemoRx: 74% ± 2%	Addition of chemoRx improved PFS
FSOP [147] (1991–1998)	136	ChemoRx followed by CSRT (2,500)	5-yr PFS: 65% ± 8%	Can reduce CSRT if chemoRx is given
CCG-POG [20] A 9961	379	2,340 cGy plus one of two chemoRx during and post-RT	5-yr PFS: 86% ± 9% (no difference between chemoRx arms)	Excellent PFS in reduced RT plus chemoRx

CSRT, craniospinal RT; chemoRx, chemotherapy; RT, radiotherapy; PFS, progression-free survival.

115 patients older than 3 years with high-risk medulloblastoma, 5-year, EFS was 49% and OS was 61% in children treated with preradiation, eight-drug-in-1-day chemotherapy, and etoposide and carboplatin prior to and after radiation therapy.[220] In a SIOP/UKCCSG trial, the use of preradiation chemotherapy also resulted in a relatively disappointing disease control rate of approximately 50% in children with high-risk disease.[218]

In a prospective, single-arm study by Packer and colleagues, the use of radiotherapy with concomitant vincristine and postradiation therapy, CCNU and vincristine, and cisplatin resulted in approximately a 65% progression-free survival rate in patients with metastatic disease.[9] A 70% 5-year progression-free survival rate was reported in the St. Jude prospective study utilizing postradiotherapy high-dose chemotherapy and stem cell rescue in a similar group of high-risk patients.[193] This is similar to the survival rate noted by a recently completed, unpublished, POG trial that utilized a cyclophosphamide adjuvant approach.[196,221] In a study recently completed by the COG, the feasibility of using carboplatin during radiation

TABLE 26B.8

TABLE 26B.8

MEDULLOBLASTOMA: SELECTED COOPERATIVE GROUP STUDIES FOR "HIGH-RISK" DISEASE

Study	N	Treatment	Outcome	Primary conclusion
CCG 921 [146] (1986–1992)	188	8-in-1 pre-RT vs. RT plus chemoRx	5-yr PFS: pre-RT chemoRx 45% ± 5% RT plus chemoRx 63% ± 5%	Inferior survival if preRT chemoRx
SIOP/UKCCSG [216] PNET-3 (1992–2000)	68	Pre-RT chemoRx	At 7.2 yr OS 50.0%	Overall disappointing survival
HIT '97 [218] (1991–1997)	19	Pre-RT chemoRx vs. RT plus chemoRx for M2/M3	3-yr PFS: 30% ± 15%	Poor survival in M2/M3; too small to assess benefit of chemoRx
CCG-9931 [195] (1994–1997)	124	Pre-RT (2 regimens) chemoRx and hyperfract RT	5-yr PFS: 43% ± 5%	No advantage for pre-RT chemoRx

ChemoRx, chemotherapy; RT, radiotherapy; OS, overall survival; PFS, progression-free survival.

therapy, as both an antineoplastic agent and a radiosensitizer was studied; the drug was found to be tolerable and treatment in high-risk patients with carboplatin during radiotherapy and postradiation therapy multi-agent chemotherapy resulted in a 3-year survival rate of more than 80%.[222] Randomized studies are presently underway within the COG prospectively comparing the efficacy of carboplatin during radiotherapy to radiotherapy without concomitant chemotherapy; patients in both arms of the study are to receive somewhat intensified postradiotherapy chemotherapy. In this COG study, a second randomization is being performed to determine the additive benefit of a maturation agent, retinoic acid. Other studies are attempting to determine whether higher-dose chemotherapy supplemented with peripheral stem cell rescue or the addition of methotrexate to multi-agent chemotherapeutic regimens will improve survival for patients with "high-risk" disease.

The benefits of chemotherapy have also been widely explored in infants with medulloblastoma (see Table 26B.9). As early as the 1970s, small single institution studies suggested that some children with medulloblastoma were responsive to chemotherapy and might be cured with chemotherapy alone utilizing drug regimens such as mechlorethamine, vincristine, procarbazine, and prednisone (MOPP).[223]

A multi-agent chemotherapy regimen using cyclophosphamide, cisplatin, etoposide, and vincristine was utilized by the POG study in attempts to delay the need for radiotherapy in young children with a variety of different tumors, including medulloblastoma, for 1 year or until the child reached 3 years of age.[224] A subgroup of children with medulloblastoma, primarily those with nondisseminated disease at the time of diagnosis, had their radiation therapy successfully delayed; however, in that study, all patients were to receive craniospinal radiation therapy at the end of treatment. In a subsequent study, the COG utilized similar drugs with an intensification of cyclophosphamide or replacement of the cyclophosphamide with ifosfamide for children younger than 3 years with disseminated and nondisseminated medulloblastoma. Thirty-two percent ± 5% of patients with medulloblastoma in this study had long-term disease control without the use of

postchemotherapy radiation therapy.[225] The use of intravenous and intrathecal methotrexate coupled with multi-agent chemotherapy was explored by the German Oncology Group, with 58% ± 9% of patients experiencing long-term control with chemotherapy alone. This study demonstrated that a subgroup of patients, primarily those with desmoplastic tumors and/or tumors that were localized at the time of diagnosis, could be treated with chemotherapy alone, with a disease-free survival rate of more than 80% for those with desmoplastic tumors.[173] The incorporation of methotrexate remains problematic as, although it may improve survival for a subset of patients, its use has been reported to result in a high incidence of leukoencephalopathy (19 of 23 patients in the German study), the significance of which regards long-term neurologic and neurocognitive outcome is unclear. Similarly, high-dose chemotherapy regimens utilizing stem cell rescue or autologous bone marrow rescue, including the "head-start" studies, those done by the French Society of Pediatric Oncology, and a recently completed COG study, have demonstrated a possible improvement in survival over treatment with multi-agent chemotherapy regimens, not utilizing high-dose chemotherapy consolidation.[155]

Studies that have been just recently completed, or are actively accruing patients, or are soon to open are determining the relative benefits of intrathecal and intravenous methotrexate, the utility of an intrathecal cyclophosphamide derivative—mafosfamide, or the higher-dose chemotherapy regimens on survival in randomized trials. These will be especially crucial in children with disseminated medulloblastoma as, to date, studies have not demonstrated a significant improvement in long-term survival for children in this patient population.

Relapsed Medulloblastoma

Treatment of children with relapsed medulloblastoma remains an extremely problematic, unsettled therapeutic issue. Objective responses have been noted after treatment with a variety of different agents, such as cisplatin, carboplatin, cyclophosphamide,

---

TABLE 26B.9

CONSORTIUM TRIALS FOR INFANTS AND YOUNG CHILDREN WITH MEDULLOBLASTOMA

Trial	Age range	Number of subjects	Treatment	Outcome	Major conclusions
POG[224]	Less than 36 mo	62	Cyclo/VCR; CPDD/VP16 for 24 mo (12 mo for those 24–36 mo of age); post-chemoRx 3,520 CSRT, 5,400 local	2-yr PFS: 34% ± 8%; 2-yr OS: 46 ± 7%	ChemoRx can delay time to RT in 30%–50%
CCG[225]	Less than 36 mo	92	Cyclo/CPDD/VCR/VP16 vs. Ifos/Carbo/VCR/VP16	5-yr EFS: 32% ± 5%; 5-yr OS 45% ± 5%	Approximately 30% of patients can be Rx with chemoRx alone
SFOP[155]	Less than 60 mo	79	Carbo/Procarbazine; VP16/CPDD; Cyclo/VCR for seven cycles	5-yr PFS: 29% in ROMO; 6% in R1, M1; 13% in M+	ChemoRx can cure in non metastatic, totally resected disease
German Pediatric Brain Tumor Study Group[173]	Less than 36 mo	43	IV MTX/Cyclo/VCR; HDMTX/IV MTX/VCR; IVMTX/Carbo/VP16	5-yr PFS: 58% ± 9%; 5-yr OS: 66% ± 7%; no residual; 5-yr PFS 82% ± 9% and 5-yr OS: 93% ± 6%	Excellent survival w/o RT in totally resected, nonmetastatic and desmoplastic tumors

Carbo, carboplatin; chemoRx, chemotherapy; CPDD, cisplatin; CSRT, craniospinal radiotherapy; Cyclo, cyclophosphamide; HDMTX, high-dose methotrexate; Ifos, ifosfamide; IV MTX, intraventricular methotrexate; M, metastasis; OS, overall survival; PFS, progression-free survival; RO, totally resected; R1, partially resected; RT, radiotherapy; VCR, vincristine; VP16, etoposide.

and etoposide.[4,212,226–230] Temozolomide has been used with mixed results, with some studies suggesting only minimal activity and one trial reporting an objective response in the majority of those with leptomeningeal disease.[231] When these drugs have been used in combination, between 50% and 80% of patients have been noted to have objective radiographic response, raising the hope that patients with relapsed disease could be cured.[4,212,226–230] However, after treatment with standard doses of chemotherapy, the vast majority of relapsed patients will relapse again within a few months of initiation of salvage therapy.[4,226–230] For this reason, there has been an interest in utilizing further therapies to consolidate response, including high-dose chemotherapy supported by either autologous bone marrow transplant or stem cell rescue, and radiation therapy. Mephalan, cyclophosphamide, busulphan, and thiotepa, with or without carboplatin and/or etoposide, have been most widely used in high-dose consolidation chemotherapy regimens, possibly with the best disease control rates being reported for thiotepa-based approaches.[231–233]

Long-term survival and possibly cure have been noted predominantly in patients with localized relapse, who with further surgery and/or induction chemotherapy can be shown to have no measurable residual disease at time of consolidation. Even in these situations, long-term disease control has been seen predominantly in children who have not received radiotherapy previously and are treated with primary site irradiation or in those who are re-irradiated.[233,234] In a French study in children initially treated on chemotherapy alone , survival rates of greater than 50% have been documented after retreatment with surgery, high-dose thiotepa-based chemotherapy with peripheral stem cell rescue, and localized radiotherapy to the primary tumor site.[235] Those children with relapsed disseminated disease are rarely cured even if craniospinal radiotherapy is used at recurrence.

Most newly diagnosed patients older than 3 years will have already been treated with radiation therapy and chemotherapy, and in this patient population long-term disease control, at relapse, is much less likely, ranging from between 0% and 30%, with most studies suggesting that only those patients with localized recurrence amenable to re-resection and who receive primary site radiotherapy will survive.[231–233] Recent prospective studies in both average- and poor-risk medulloblastoma demonstrate that nearly two-thirds of patients who relapse will have some component of disease outside the primary tumor site, and the group of patients with relapse medulloblastoma who are likely to have long-term benefit from current means of salvage is small.[20,216] An initial approach to determine who might benefit from high-dose chemotherapy was to utilize chemotherapy, such as cyclophosphamide, as the initial treatment in those with evaluable disease to determine chemosensitivity.[231–233] More recent studies have not shown better survival for responders and suggest that re-operation with the objective of obtaining a complete resection of the recurrent disease should be the first step in treatment in patients with isolated primary disease relapse. Biologic agents, such as epidermal growth factor receptor inhibitors and anti-angiogenesis drugs, are being actively explored in patients with relapsed disease, as is the use of maintenance therapy with maturation agents, such as retinoic acid or low-dose chemotherapy (possibly anti-angiogenic regimens known as metronomic treatment). However, the long-term benefits of such maintenance approaches are unclear.

Outcome

It has been clearly shown that children surviving medulloblastoma are at high risk for long-term sequelae believed to be due, in great part, to the dose of craniospinal radiation therapy received, but also related to preoperative neurologic status, the presence of hydrocephalus at the time of diagnosis, perioperative complications including posterior fossa mutism, and possibly the use of adjuvant chemotherapy.[236] Neurocognitive sequelae are frequently seen, especially in children treated between the ages of 3 and 7 years, who have received craniospinal radiation therapy.[236–246] With 3,600 cGy of craniospinal radiation, patients younger than 8 years are likely to experience a 20 to 30 or more point I.Q. drop within 3 to 5 years of diagnosis. This drop in intelligence can be seen as early as 1-year posttreatment, is progressive, and may not plateau over time. Reduction of radiotherapy to 2,400 cGy has resulted in a somewhat lesser drop in overall intelligence but still severe sequelae in many patients, with younger patients having a 10- to 20-point I.Q. drop.[246] General intelligence is a crude estimate of intellectual function and patients have also been noted to have a variety of different types of intellectual deficits including memory difficulties, processing dysfunction, executive functioning abnormalities, visual-spatial difficulties, and attention deficit disorders. These all result in children being at significant risk for learning problems as they enter and proceed in school.[245,246]

Intellectual declines are intensified by the damage patients may have suffered prior to receiving definitive treatment and 70% or more of children who are older than 3 years at the time of diagnosis with medulloblastomas function at an overall intelligence level of 100 or below at the time of initiation of postsurgery treatment.[233,246] Older children are somewhat more resistant to the detrimental neurocognitive effects of radiotherapy, but there is interpatient variability in their vulnerability to radiation sequelae and selective learning deficits and executive dysfunction are common. The situation is possibly even more complex in children younger than 3 years, especially infants, with medulloblastoma.[247] The vast majority are significantly developmentally delayed at diagnosis, due to the tumor or associated hydrocephalus, and they may be significantly impaired postoperatively. Obtaining reliable baseline data concerning cognitive function is difficult. Frank mental retardation has been documented in 70% of infants treated with craniospinal radiotherapy and 30% or more of those who received chemotherapy alone or chemotherapy plus local radiotherapy. It is unclear how the addition of methotrexate to infant chemotherapy-alone approaches will affect neurocognitive outcome.

Chemotherapy may also play an additive role in the intellectual deterioration and complications seen, although this has not been conclusively shown.[248] Cisplatin may result in significant ototoxicity in patients with medulloblastoma, which complicates schooling and probably further intensifies intellectual compromise. The effects of many drugs on the developing nervous system are poorly documented.

Endocrinologic sequelae are also common, with growth hormone insufficiency being the most common sequelae seen.[249–252] This occurs predominantly in patients who have received greater than 2,400 cGy (?2,900 cGy) of craniospinal radiation to the hypothalamic area. Other hormonal deficiencies that may occur include gonadotrophin abnormalities, thyroid dysfunction, and less frequently adrenocortical deficiency. The timing and safety of growth hormone replacement therapy in children with medulloblastoma remains somewhat controversial.[253–255] In a large retrospective review of more than 500 patients, the use of growth hormone replacement therapy was not associated with an increased likelihood of disease relapse.[253] This review also demonstrated that there was no uniformity in initiation of hormone replacement therapy and most centers delayed growth hormone therapy for at least 2 years following the completion of treatment.

Secondary tumors, including malignant brain tumors, are an increasing concern in long-term survivors of medulloblastoma.[20,182–184] In a recent prospective COG study of 379 children, within 8 years of treatment, 13 secondary malignancies were identified, including malignant gliomas and leukemia.[20] More than 8 years from diagnosis, patients in this study were more likely to suffer a secondary malignancy than tumor relapse.[20] As this patient population ages, it is likely that more tumors will be diagnosed, as meningiomas become more common 10 years or greater after diagnosis.

These sequelae are probably only the tip of the iceberg as regards disabilities for medulloblastoma long-term survivors. Reports from the Children's Cancer Survivor Study and others have demonstrated that children with medulloblastoma receiving therapy given before 1990 were at high risk for neurologic (including strokes), neuropsychological, and psychosocial deficits, sequelae that occur or are at least recognized by patients or their families 5 years or greater from their time of diagnosis.[256–259] Survivors' abilities to live independently, have families, and be gainfully employed is also far below that of their peers. In patients treated between 1992 and 2000, health status was noted to be poor in patients surviving medulloblastoma in many domains. There was also the suggestion in the latter study that treatment with chemotherapy may have intensified the difficulties encountered. These worrisome results are a prime reason for the ongoing studies attempting to further reduce the dose of craniospinal radiation therapy and possibly alter the type of chemotherapy given. In addition, they are used as a major rationale for the incorporation of biologic agents with possible less long-term detrimental sequelae, as a means to reduce the dose of radiotherapy or alter the type of chemotherapy required for disease control.

SUPRATENTORIAL PRIMITIVE NEUROECTODERMAL TUMORS

Supratentorial primitive neuroectodermal tumors (sPNETs) are the second most common form of childhood embryonal tumor.[1,3] In the past, sPNETs have also been classified as cerebral or central neuroblastomas, cerebral medulloblastomas, and pineoblastomas. Pineoblastomas are now considered a subtype of pineal region tumor.[2] Molecular genetic investigations have shown that these tumors are biologically different from medulloblastomas and from the pineoblastoma.[92]

Demographics

Because of the different nomenclatures employed for sPNETs, their incidence has been poorly defined. They probably account for 2.5% or less of childhood brain tumors and most commonly arise during the first decade of life, especially in infancy.[260–263] In a questionnaire study of 50 patients, performed by the Canadian Pediatric Brain Tumor Consortium, the median age at time of diagnosis was found to be 49.5 months and ranged from 0 to 214 months.[264] In this study, the male to female ratio was 1:1, although other studies have suggested a male predominance, as high as 2:1. The etiology of these tumors is unknown.

Clinical Presentation

Nausea, vomiting, and headaches remain the most common initial symptomats, occurring in 50% or greater of patients; however, early age at diagnosis makes headaches a difficult symptom to discern.[260–264] Duration of symptoms prior to diagnosis tend to be relatively short, with the majority of patients being diagnosed within 1 month of onset of illness. Approximately one-quarter to one-third of patients will present with seizures. At the time of presentation, focal neurologic deficits, including hemiparesis and visual difficulties, are noted in approximately 50% of patients. In infancy, these tumors may be notoriously large and time to diagnosis is often delayed in infancy.

Neuroimaging

Imaging studies typically reveal a large mass with well-defined borders, most often located in the frontoparietal region; supratentorial primitive neuro-ectodermal tumors can arise either cortically or in the deep periventricular white matter. MR and CT features are heterogeneous; two-third demonstrate cystic and/or necrotic foci.[264] The solid portions are hyperdense on CT; calcifications are seen in 50% of cases, hemorrhage in 20%. On MRI, solid tumor tissue is often isointense to gray matter on FLAIR images, hyperintense on diffusion-weighted images (and a reduction in apparent diffusion coefficient) (Fig. 26B.8). Contrast enhancement is seen in most of cases. Peritumoral edema is commonly mild or absent—a useful differentiator from gill tumors of similar size.[265] As in the posterior fossa, the lesion that most closely resembles the sPNET is the AT/RT; anaplastic gliomas and glioblastoma multiformes are more infiltrative with greater amount of peritumoral edema.

Pathology

Despite the presence of considerable microscopic extension, sPNETs generally appear as well-circumscribed masses.[80,101,108,110] Grossly, they are lobulated, soft, hemorrhagic, often cystic masses. Microscopically, sheets of uniform embryonal-appearing, small, round cells with hyperchromatic oval nuclei and frequent mitoses are noted (Fig. 26B.9). Homer Wright rosettes and perivascular pseudorosettes and areas of necrosis are common. Although foci with various degrees of glial, neuronal, or ependymal differentiation are seen in 70% of tumors, light microscopy and ultrastructural evaluation generally reveal most individual cells to be primitive and undifferentiated. They may contain a prominent connective tissue component or display the nodular pattern that has been called "neuroblastoma."

Biology

Although histologically similar, sPNETs are genetically heterogenous from medulloblastomas. In early studies of medulloblastomas and sPNETs using conventional CGH, the most common CNA in medulloblastomas was gain of chromosome 17q in 37% while none of the sPNETs had gain of 17q.[266] Loss of 14q and 19q was detected in 40% of sPNETs but hardly in medulloblastomas. Losses at chromosome 16p and 19p were more frequent in sPNET, whereas losses at chromosome 10 were detected only in medulloblastoma.[267] The 1q gain was more frequent in sPNET, whereas gains at 17q and chromosome 7 were more frequent in medulloblastoma.[267]

Genome-wide screening for DNA-copy number aberrations by high-resolution array-based CGH demonstrated that gain of 17q was significantly more common in medulloblastomas than in sPNETs. Loss of the telomeric end of 13q was more common in sPNETs than in medulloblastomas. However, sPNETs were significantly more likely than

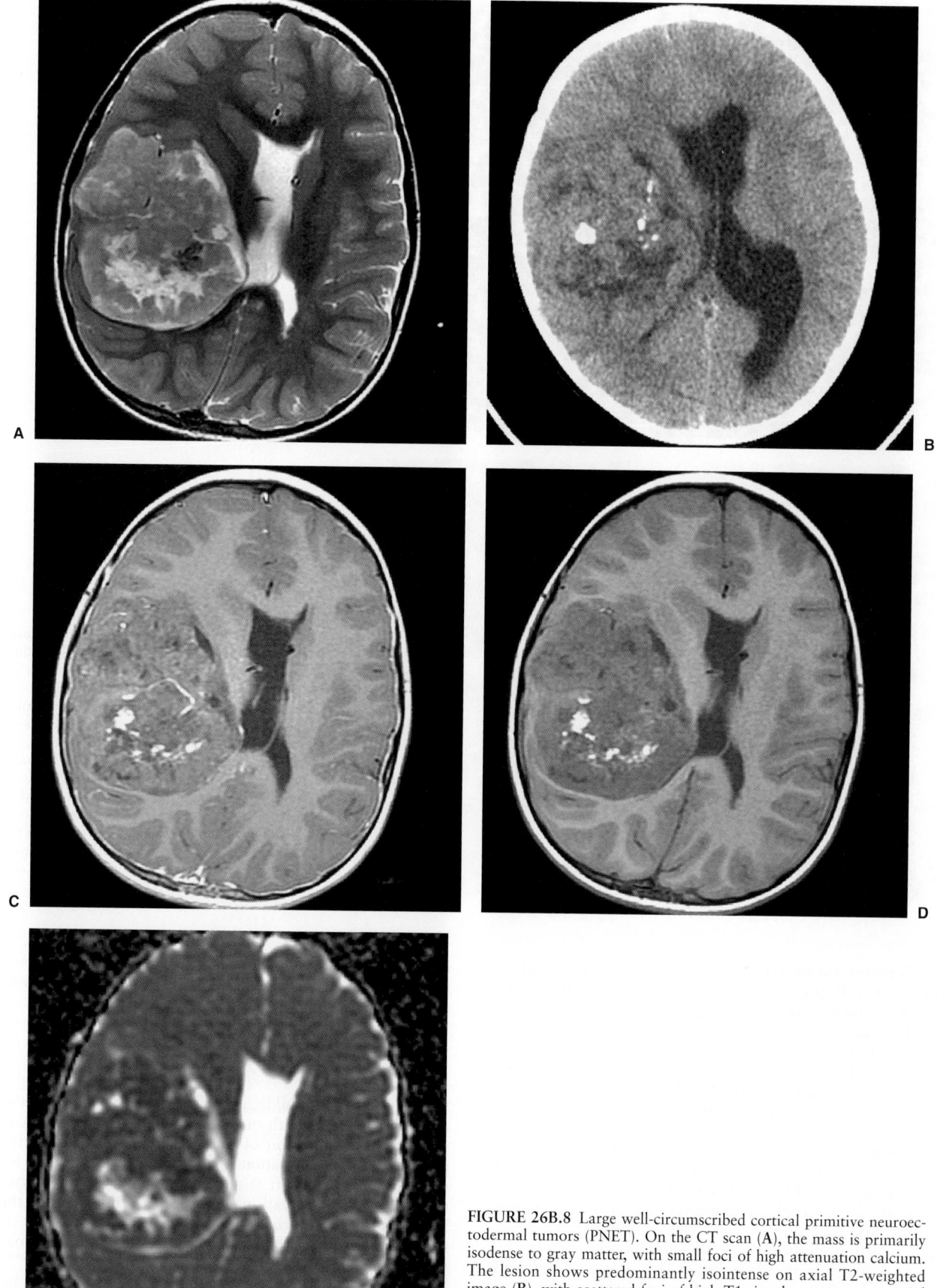

FIGURE 26B.8 Large well-circumscribed cortical primitive neuroectodermal tumors (PNET). On the CT scan (A), the mass is primarily isodense to gray matter, with small foci of high attenuation calcium. The lesion shows predominantly isointense on axial T2-weighted image (B), with scattered foci of high T1 signal on precontrast axial T1 sequence (C), representing either hemorrhage or calcium. Only minimal enhancement seen on postcontrast axial T1 (D), and reduced diffusion on apparent diffusion coefficient (ADC) map compared with surrounding gray matter (E).

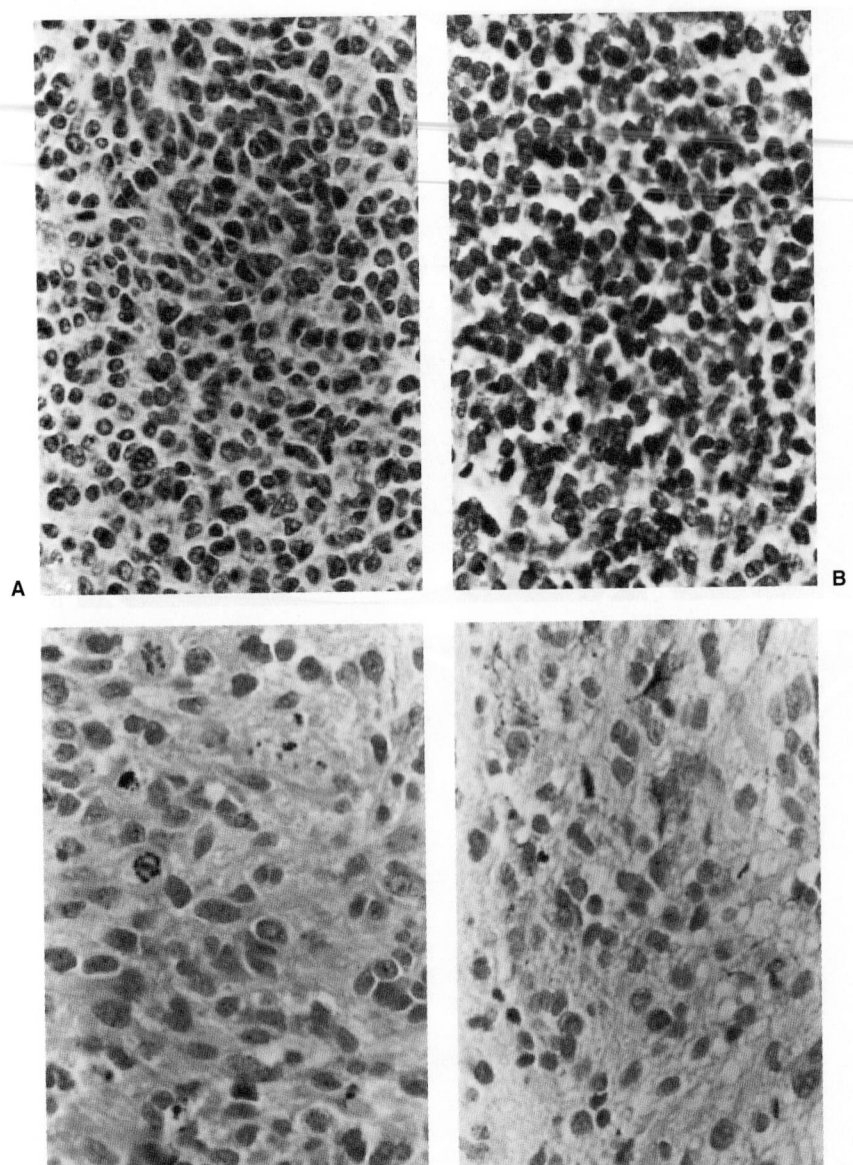

FIGURE 26B.9 A: Typical field of medulloblastoma. Tumor is formed by apparently undifferentiated, basophilic, round-to-oval nuclei with minimal perceptible cytoplasm. (Hematoxylin and eosin, 3,400.) **B:** Typical field of pineoblastoma. Note the similarity to the photomicrograph in **A**. (Hematoxylin and eosin, 3,400.) **C:** One of several nests of malignant astrocytes in supratentorial primitive neuroectodermal tumor, displaying mild pleomorphism and several mitotic figures. (Hematoxylin and eosin, 3,400.) **D:** Another similar field from the same tumor shown in C stained with glial fibrillary acidic protein (GFAP) showing a few cells staining for GFAP (GFAP, 3,400).

medulloblastomas to have amplifications. In another study comparing pediatric sPNETs with medulloblastomas, deletions of 1p and 9p and gains of 19p were all more frequent in sPNETs; aberrations involving chromosome 17 tend to be more frequent in medulloblastomas.[129,268] To validate these findings, FISH with probes from 1p36, 9p21, and 17q21 were applied to an independent set of pediatric sPNETs.[268] Losses of 1p in 3/11, heterozygous deletions of 9p21 in ~18%, and homozygous deletions of 9p21 in ~27% were detected.[268] All 9p21 deletions were associated with loss of CDKN2A protein expression. Altogether, CDKN2A deletions were detected more commonly in sPNETs than in medulloblastomas.[268]

On the RNA level, gene expression profiling studies demonstrated the expression of external granular cell genes only in medulloblastoma not in sPNETs, supporting the hypothesis of different cell origins.[129] The molecular signature of sPNET was distinctly different from medulloblastoma.

Summarizing, common CNA in sPNETs include 1p, 13q, 14q, 19q, 16p, 19p loss, 1p, 9p deletion, and 19p gain. CN losses are generally more common. Medulloblastomas demon-strate different CNA in contrast to sPNET. Gene expression profiling shows that sPNET has a different molecular signature from medulloblastoma at the RNA level.[92]

Staging

Staging studies for children with sPNETs are similar to those utilized in patients with medulloblastoma. However, because of the cortical location of these lesions and the associated potential risk of herniation if these tumors are causing local pressure and brain shift at diagnosis, at times CSF analysis is inadvisable. The overall incidence of dissemination of these lesions is not well documented and seems somewhat less than that reported in medulloblastoma, occurring at the time of diagnosis in approximately 10% to 15% of children.[260–264] The degree of tumor extent at the time of diagnosis has been found to be predictive of survival, as patients with metastatic disease have a poorer prognosis. The degree of surgical resection has been variably related to outcome.

Treatment

Surgery

Gross-total and near-total tumor resection are less frequent for sPNETs than for medulloblastomas because sPNETs are usually large, fairly vascular tumors that invade functionally important cortex.[269] Accordingly, the surgical management for sPNETs is similar to that for other cerebral malignant tumors, such as high-grade glioma, in which the primary goal is to make a diagnosis, relieve mass effect, and achieve safe cytoreduction. However, gross-total resection may be associated with better survival and is a goal whenever possible.

Radiation Therapy

Radiation therapy is central to the treatment of sPNETs. Contemporary data in children older than 3 years show a survival benefit following irradiation in two recent single-institution retrospective reports.[270,271] Outcome following postsurgical irradiation alone is not optimal; the most favorable survival data reflect the SIOP-UKCCSG PNET3 trial documenting 5-year EFS and OS of 47% in a prospective trial (1992–2000).[272] The European trial included postoperative CSI (35 Gy) with boost to the tumor residual/bed (55 Gy cumulative dose). Patterns of failure analysis showed that 60% of failures occurred as isolated local recurrence/progression at the original tumor site.[272,273] Superior data have been reported from the St. Jude-centered SJMB 96 trial, reporting 68% 5-year EFS and 73% OS with "risk-adapted" radiation therapy followed by four cycles of CDDP-based dose-intensive chemotherapy (with stem cell reconstitution), using the same criteria and treatment regimen documented in medulloblastoma.[273,274] While most clinical studies have included sPNETs as "high risk" by definition and utilized standard-dose CSI (36 Gy), the SJMB 96 trial has shown 75% 5-year EFS and 88% OS with reduced CSI dose (23.4 Gy) for M0 disease after gross-total or near-total resection followed by local boost to 55.8 Gy.[92,274] With irradiation alone, primary (local) disease control appears to be the limiting factor, especially with tumors greater than 5 cm in diameter or following incomplete resection; with the addition of effective chemotherapy and target definitions requiring a 1- or 2-cm margin (for microscopic extension) beyond the initial tumor bed (and including any residual tumor identifiable postsurgery), failures appear to equally involve the primary site and/or the neuraxis.[270,272–275] The most important principles in radiation therapy for sPNET now appear to be use of CSI, consideration of attenuated CSI dose if given in conjunction with aggressive surgery and chemotherapy, and detailed, 3-D treatment planning for the "boost" volume (primary or local tumor site) to include the initial tumor extent and postoperative signs of potentially infiltrating residual disease.[273,274]

Chemotherapy

Chemotherapy has been extensively utilized for children with sPNETs and, in general, has been the same type of chemotherapy utilized for patients with high-risk medulloblastoma.[260,263,275] Many studies have combined sPNETs and pineoblastomas in treatment trials, making determinations of the relative benefits of chemotherapy for children with sPNETs difficult. There is some suggestion that combination chemotherapy with radiation is more effective in older children than radiation therapy alone, as noted above.[260,263,275] Similar to medulloblastomas, infants with sPNETs are often treated, postoperatively, with chemotherapy in an attempt to delay, if not obviate, the need for radiotherapy.

Outcome

The reported outcomes for patients with sPNETs are not as favorable as those reported for medulloblastoma.[260,271–275] With the use of combined treatment with radiation and chemotherapy, older children with such lesions have approximately a 50%, 5-year progression-free survival. The survival rate for infants with sPNETs is, overall, somewhat less favorable than that reported with medulloblastomas, with survival rates ranging between 20% and 40% with the use of chemotherapy alone or chemotherapy followed by local or craniospinal radiation therapy.[260,271–275] Given the relative rarity of these tumors, the quality of life of survivors and their associated neurologic, neurocognitive, and endocrinologic sequelae have been poorly delineated.

PINEOBLASTOMAS

Pineoblastomas, although classified with the pineal region tumors by the WHO, are clinically usually grouped with other embryonal tumors in treatment trials because of their similar histological appearance and proclivity to disseminate the CNS.[1,3,7] There is biologic evidence that they differ from both medulloblastomas and sPNETs.[92]

Demographics

Pineoblastomas are rare supratentorial tumors, probably comprising no more than 1% of cases of childhood brain tumors.[276–278] In most studies, they are approximately 50% less frequent than sPNETs. They may occur in children of all ages, but they are most likely to arise early in life. Numbers are small, but there does seem to be a suggestion of a male predominance.

Clinical Presentation

Signs and symptoms of pineoblastomas may be quite nonspecific, especially in very young children. Pineoblastomas usually cause compression of the third ventricle with resultant hydrocephalus, vomiting, headaches, and somnolence.[276,277] As the tumor enlarges, it may also compress or infiltrate the tectum of the midbrain and result in upward gaze palsy, retraction or convergence nystagmus, pupils that react better to accommodation than light, and the lid retraction (Parinaud syndrome). Pineoblastomas may also infiltrate the thalamic area and result in hemiplegia or sensory abnormalities early in illness.

Neuroimaging

Pineoblastomas are large, lobulated, heterogeneous tumors. They are usually hyperdense on CT; calcifications are seen in about a third of cases. The tumors are often isointense on T1-weighted images; on T2-weighted images, lesions are heterogeneous due to the presence of calcifications, cysts (seen in 20% of cases), and necrosis; the solid components tend to be hypointense, a reflection of the hypercellular nature of the tumors (Fig. 26B.10). Enhancing characteristics are mixed, homogeneous in half of cases, heterogeneous in the other half.[279]

Pathology

Pineoblastomas are indistinguishable from medulloblastomas (Fig. 26B.9).[80,101,108,110,280] The tumor consists of densely

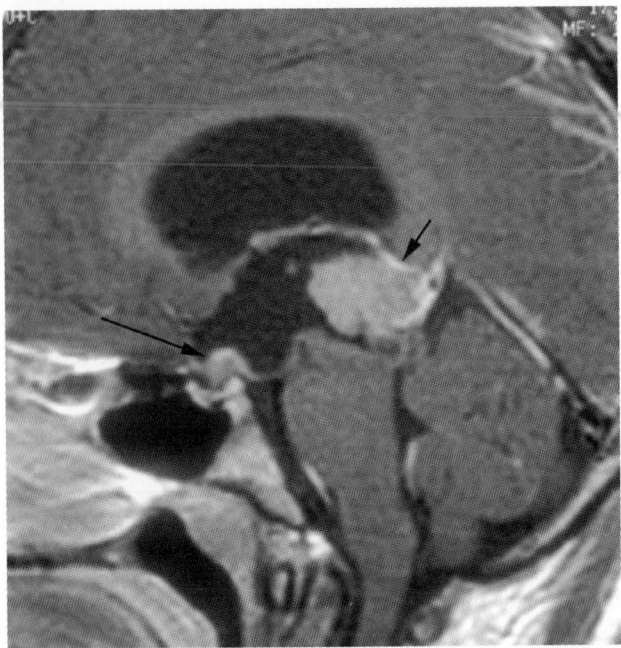

FIGURE 26B.10 Pineoblastoma with metastasis to the anterior tear third ventricle in an 18-year-old male. Sagittal contrast-enhanced T1-weighted image reveals a mass lesion in the pineal region/posterior third ventricle (*short arrow*) and a metastatic lesion in the infundibular recess of the third ventricle (*long arrow*). A similar appearance and presentation could be seen in the case of disseminated pineal germinoma.

packed small round nuclei with abundant chromatin, but minimal perceptible cytoplasm. Mitoses are typically abundant. They may contain Flexner-Wintersteiner rosettes and fleurettes, two features suggesting differentiation toward retinoblastoma. In fact, tumors of this type occasionally arise in children with retinoblastoma, in which event this is regarded as trilateral retinoblastoma.[281] The tumors may exhibit evidence of astrocytic, neuronal, or even ganglion cell differentiation.[80,108,101,110,280] They are often hemorrhagic and may contain necrotic foci.

Staging

Pineoblastomas are usually similarly staged as medulloblastomas.[276–278] Tumor dissemination at the time of diagnosis occurs in approximately 15% to 30% of patients. Extent of resection can be very difficult to determine, due to the high vascularity of the pineal region and the difficulty of neuroradiographically confirming the degree of tumor removal, especially documenting "total" resection. In most series, the majority of patients have been biopsied or subtotally resected, although total resection has been reported.

Biology

Cytogenetics of pineoblastomas have shown deletions of 11 qc, isochromosome 17 qd, der (10) + (10;17), and der (16)+(1:16).[282] The most frequent DNA copy number changes among pineoblastoma (in series that also included pineal parenchymal tumors of intermediate differentiation) were gains in 12q, 4q, 5p, and 5q and losses of 22, 9q, and 16q. Whether these genetic alterations are responsible for

tumorgenesis or are of prognostic significance remains to be seen in larger cohorts. A genetic susceptibility has been found for pineoblastomatous pineal tumors in the setting of familial bilateral retinoblastoma, an occurrence termed *trilateral retinoblastoma syndrome*.[283] So far, there is no convincing evidence in favor of a particular gene involved in the tumorigenesis of pineal parenchymal tumors.

Treatment

Surgery

The surgical approach to a pineoblastoma can be either endoscopic or open. Endoscopic approaches allow for treatment of the hydrocephalus (endoscopic third ventriculostomy) and possible endoscopic tissue biopsy. Notably, endoscopic procedures do not currently allow for cytoreduction, and the biopsy provided is small. Open approaches to the pineal region include superior routes and posterior routes. Examples would include an interhemispheric, transcallosal, interforniceal approach (superior) and the occipital transtentorial route (posterior). Choice of the open surgical approach is based on the location of the tumor (more anterior vs. more posterior), the degree of hydrocephalus, and probably most important, surgeon familiarity. Pineoblastomas are often very stuck to the deep venous system (internal cerebral veins, vein of Galen), which can limit their resection. Because of the well-known poor prognosis of children with metastatic pineoblastoma, efforts at complete resection should be tempered with wisdom in these children.

Radiation Therapy

There is relatively little radiation therapy data specifically addressing pineoblastoma. Earlier experience from CCG has suggested that postoperative irradiation (CSI at 36 Gy with localized "boost" to the initial and residual tumor volume to 54 Gy) with adjuvant chemotherapy has been relatively successful, certainly in comparison to experience in infants and young children where radiation therapy has been delayed or obviated.[226,284] The use of immediate postoperative CSI may be advantageous in comparison to initial or preirradiation chemotherapy in children older than 3 years.[285,286] Details of radiation dose and volume are similar to those noted earlier for supratentorial PNETs in general.

Chemotherapy

The chemotherapy utilized for children with pineoblastomas has been similar to that used for high-risk medulloblastomas.[276–278] As is the case for infants with medulloblastomas, chemotherapy for young children is often utilized in attempts to delay, of not completely avoid, the need for radiotherapy. Given the small number of patients usually reported in studies, the relative efficacy of different chemotherapeutic regimens is essentially impossible to determine. In the CCG study, survival and progression-free survival rates for patients with pineoblastomas were reported to be significantly higher than those for children with sPNETs.[278] The reverse was found in a multi-centered study that utilized chemotherapy followed by consolidated myeloablative chemotherapy, with or without radiotherapy.[276] Other studies have suggested that older children with pineoblastoma have prolonged tumor control after combined modality treatment.[276–278,284–286]

Outcome

Outcome for children with pineoblastomas has been quite variable between studies. Some have reported survival rates as high as 70% when both radiation therapy and chemotherapy are utilized. Other reports have not been nearly as favorable, with OS rates of well less than 40% at 5 years.[276–278,284,285] There is little data concerning the long-term sequelae survivors face.

Atypical Teratoid/Rhabdoid Tumor

Atypical teratoid/rhabdoid tumors (AT/RTs) were first clearly described as a distinct entity in 1987 by Rorke and colleagues.[5,287] Over the past two decades, this tumor has engendered significant interest due to its histological and immunohistochemical features, its proclivity to arise in infancy, its molecular-genetic uniqueness, and its aggressivity.[5,287–290]

Demographics

The exact incidence of AT/RTs is still unclear.[286–290] Initial information about the tumor was obtained from tumor registries and single-institution reports from centers acting as referral sites for the diagnosis or treatment of such tumors. These reports suggested that AT/RTs comprise less than 2% of all childhood brain tumors and less than 1% of those occurring in patients older than 3 years.[286–289] Retrospective analyses of studies that treated infants and children younger than 3 years found that between 10% and 20% of tumors that were classified as medulloblastomas or sPNETs were AT/RTs.[225] Median age at diagnosis has been approximately 1 to 2 years of age and dependent on series, 70% to 80% of patients have been younger than 3 years at the time of diagnosis.[286–289] The ratio of infratentorial to supratentorial tumors has varied between series, with the overall incidence of AT/RTs being approximately equal in the supratentorial and infratentorial space; infratentorial tumors are more frequently diagnosed in younger patients. Leptomeningeal dissemination is present in 20% to 25% of patients at diagnosis. There is male predominance, the male-to-female ratio being 2:1.[286–289]

The largest single study of 1,351 neuroepithelial tumors in children younger than 18 years, diagnosed at The Children's Hospital of Philadelphia from 1979 to 2005, which included a large number of patients referred for histological second opinion, disclosed an overall incidence of 22.4% in the embryonal group that included medulloblastoma, sPNETs, pineoblastomas, AT/RTs, and medulloepithelioma.[109] If only infants 1 year of age or less were considered, this figure jumps to 38%. Site of origin in this study differed according to age. Tumors in the infants were located primarily in the posterior fossa and pineal, only one was both supra and infratentorial, and no tumor was found only supratentorially. In contrast, only 52% of the tumors in patients aged 13 months to 18 years arose in the posterior fossa, whereas 36% were cerebral and only 8% pineal. No cerebral AT/RTs were found in infants younger than 1 year.

The etiology of AT/RTs is unknown and the simultaneous rhabdoid tumors of the kidneys occur but are infrequent. Germ line mutations were initially noted in the minority of patients; subsequent studies have found that as high as 10% of patients may have such mutations. In a consensus workshop, it was recommended that the presence of an hSNF5/INI1 gene mutation in a tumor with features suggestive of a medulloblastoma or a supratentorial PNET was sufficient to make the diagnosis of an AT/RT.[288]

Clinical Presentation

AT/RTs have presentations similar to other embryonal tumors occurring in infants and young children.[109,286–290] Time between onset of symptoms and diagnosis is short, usually approximately 1 month in most patients. In some series, it has been suggested that posterior fossa tumors are more likely to involve the cerebellopontine angle and cause multiple cranial nerve palsies, especially sixth and seventh nerve palsies, early in the course of illness, than are medulloblastomas.

Neuroimaging

Radiological features of AT/RTs are heterogeneous due to the frequent presence of cystic and necrotic areas, calcifications, and hemorrhage. The CT findings of AT/RTs are relatively characteristic but not diagnostic; the tumors are usually hyperdense and enhance intensely (Fig. 26B.11). Calcifications may occur but are not as common as in sPNETs.

On MRI, T1-weighted images often feature hyperintense foci within the lesion, due to the hemorrhagic components. On T2-weighted images, the lesions are often heterogeneous; the solid components are iso- to hypointense on T2-weighted images, hemorrhagic, and have hypertense necrotic foci. Most AT/RTs enhance avidly with gadolinium (Fig. 26B.11).[288]

Within the posterior fossa, 20% to 50% of AR/RTs presents in the cerebellopontine angle (Fig. 26B.11); much fewer medulloblastomas present in this location (10% of all medulloblastomas, but rarely in the first decade of life). Intratumoral hemorrhage is seen in about 50% of AT/RTs versus 5% of medulloblastomas.[288] Lack of enhancement (or minimal enhancement) is evident in 10% of AT/RTs versus 20% to 25% of medulloblastomas.[289] The distinction between sPNET and AT/RTs is more difficult due to their shared propensity to display necrotic and hemorrhagic foci (Fig. 26B.12).[288]

Pathology

Definitive diagnosis of AT/RTs is based upon a combination of histologic and cytogenetic features. Although these tumors exhibit considerable morphologic variability, the most common findings consist of a combination of rhabdoid cells and areas resembling primitive neuroectodermal tumors with little or no evidence of differentiation (Fig. 26B.13). However, in some instances Homer Wright, Flexner-Wintersteiner, and ependymal rosettes or primitive neural tube-like structures are present. Some tumors are composed entirely of rhabdoid cells, whereas other features that may be found in these neoplasms consist of epithelium of various types and/or mesenchymal tissue.[109,286,287] Typically, the rhabdoid cells express epithelial membrane antigen (EMA) and vimentin, and less often smooth muscle actin (SMA). Remarkably, they may also express NFP, GFAP, and keratin. An antibody raised to INI1 and used with immunohistochemical techniques shows lack of expression as a characteristic feature of AT/RTs. Cytogenetic studies have demonstrated deletion of chromosome 22 and alterations of the hSNF5/INI1 gene in these tumors.[291,292]

Biology

CGH of pediatric AT/RTs demonstrated losses from chromosome 22q, 19, 8p, and 1p.[291,292] Some tumors presented with normal karyotypes, whereas in others, a normal chromosome 22 but other structural arrangements in chromosomes 6 and 11 had been reported.[293]

Cerebral and extracerebral AT/RTs are characterized by monosomy 22 or partial deletion of 22q11.2[294,295] which contains the INI1/hSNF5 (SMARCB1) gene that encodes a component of the SWI/SNF chromatin remodeling complex.[296–301] This gene has been suggested to be a tumor suppressor gene and is inactivated by truncating mutations or by partial or total deletion of the gene. Inactivating mutations of the hSNF5/INI-1 gene or absence of its RNA and protein (in the absence of genomic alterations) are present in approximately 85% of the cases.[294,296] INI1 protein is a component of the SWI/SNF complex, interacting with sequence-specific DNA

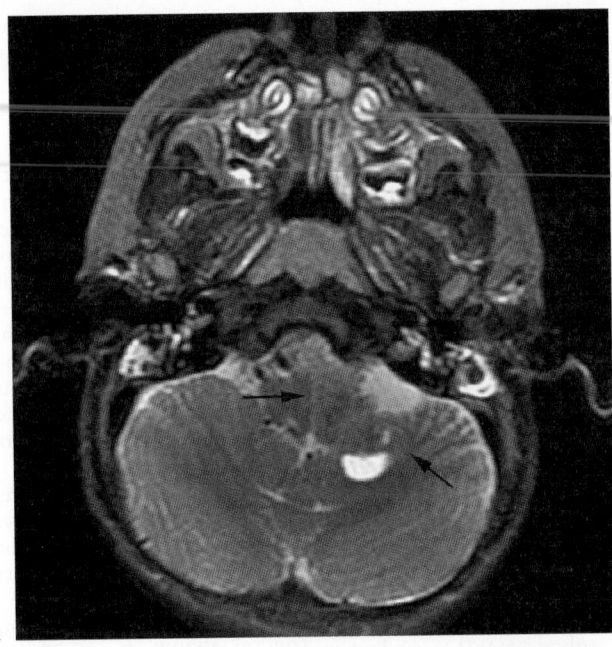
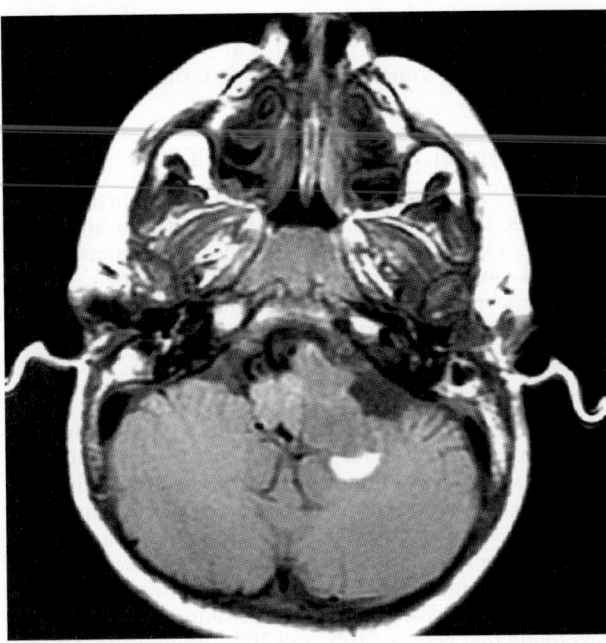

FIGURE 26B.11 Atypical teratoid/rhabdoid tumor (AT/RT) in a 2-year-old child. A mass is evident in the left cerebellopontine angle, showing predominantly isointense signal on axial T2-weighted image (*arrows*, **A**), a hemorrhagic T1 bright component on axial T1-weighted image (**B**), fairly diffuse enhancement (**C**, axial T1 postcontrast) and mostly reduced diffusion of the solid elements on apparent diffusion coefficient (ADC) map (**D**).

binding proteins such as MYC, EBNA-2, and GADD34.[294] It has been hypothesized that INI1 can modify the transcription of many cellular genes implicated in tumorigenesis by this mechanism. Targeted deletion of INI1 gene causes rhabdoid tumors in a subgroup of mice, which demonstrates its crucial role in the pathogenesis of rhabdoid tumors.[302]

In humans, germline inactivation of the hSNF5/INI1 gene causes, in children, multiple rhabdoid neoplasms including cerebral AT/RTs.[294,303–305] Predisposition to the development of cerebral and extracerebral rhabdoid tumors indicates that INI1 acts as a tumor suppressor gene, following Knudson's 2 hit model. Sevenet et al.[303] therefore proposed the designation

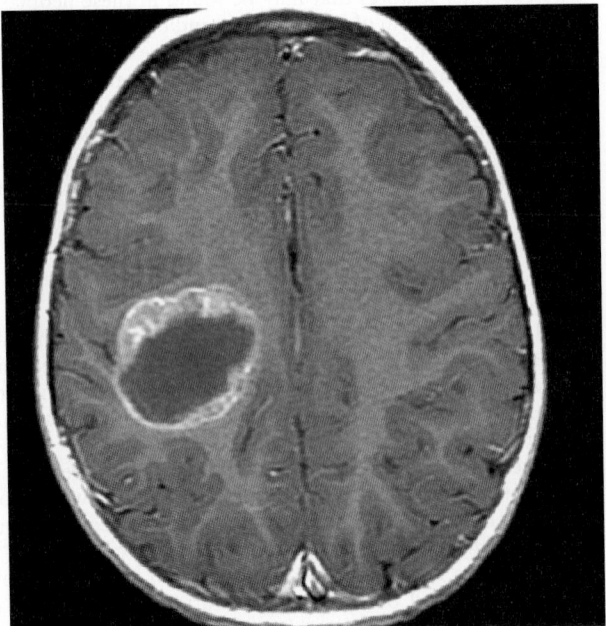
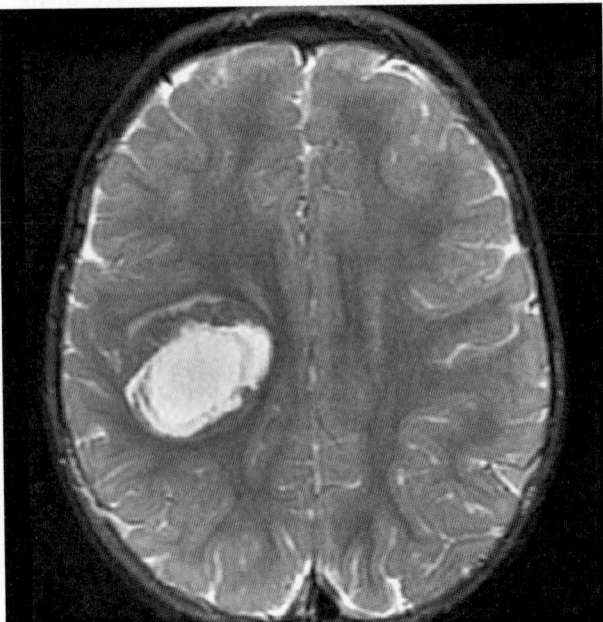

FIGURE 26B.12 Subcortical atypical teratoid/rhabdoid tumor (AT/RT). Axial T2-weighted (**A**) and contrast-enhanced axial T1 (**B**) images reveal a rim enhancing mass with a central necrotic component; the solid component is hypointense to gray matter on T2-weighted image (**A**) and shows a moderate diffuse enhancement (**B**).

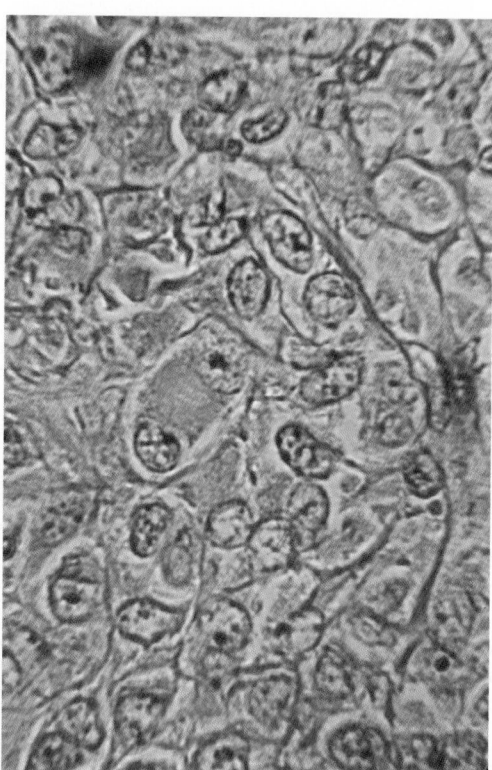

FIGURE 26B.13 Field of rhabdoid cells illustrating characteristic features consisting of cells with finely granular cytoplasm, eccentrically placed nuclei containing prominent nucleolus and distinct cell membranes. Note binucleated cell in center. Hematoxylin and eosin 400×.

of rhabdoid predisposition syndrome. However in such families, other brain tumor entities have been diagnosed, including medulloblastomas and choroid plexus carcinomas.[303,305] Several reports in the literature have demonstrated familial cases of rhabdoid tumors indicating an inherited trait.[306–308] In each of the published familial cases, mutations of either the locus in 22q or the gene SMARCB1 have been detected. A more recent report demonstrated a family with rhabdoid tumor predisposition syndrome without linkage to SMARCB1, indicating that a second locus other than SMARCB1 is involved in the origin of these tumors.[309]

Staging

AT/RTs are usually staged as other embryonal tumors. Fifteen to 20% of patients will have evidence of disseminated disease at the time of diagnosis.[286–290]

Treatment

The optimal treatment for AT/RTs is not known, but reported survival rates are slowly improving over time.[288,310]

Surgery

As AT/RTs can be found throughout the CNS, the specifics of their resection are highly related to the location or origin and are similar to other entities discussed in this chapter. Similar to metastatic pineoblastoma and sPNETs, aggressive surgical approaches to children with metastatic AT/RTs should be tempered in keeping with the child's prognosis.

Radiation Therapy

The literature for AT/RTs suggests a role for radiation therapy that is difficult to prove for a relatively uncommon tumor occurring predominantly in very young children. Single-institution studies and a national registry showed similarly poor results in AT/RTs in younger children.[288,311,312] The overwhelming pattern of failure (both early progression and later recurrence) has been at the primary tumor site, suggesting a role for at least local postoperative irradiation.[226] Positive experience with AT/RTs has been reported only in a few relatively small cohort analyses of children older than 3 years, where results as high as 5-year EFS of 78% have been documented following immediate postoperative irradiation (CSI to 23.4 to 36 Gy, with local "boost" to 54 to 55.8 Gy) and adjuvant chemotherapy.[310–313] The current approach to AT/RTs utilizes postoperative irradiation for older (greater than 3 or 4) children; for children younger than 3 to 4 years old, current recommendations include irradiation to the primary tumor site following a limited number of chemotherapy cycles, with radiation targeting a 1- to –2-cm margin for microscopic disease and a dose level of 50 to 54 Gy.[314]

Chemotherapy

Because of their initial recognition in infants, the earliest therapeutic experience with AT/RTs involved predominantly postsurgical chemotherapy. Chemotherapeutic protocols utilized for infants with embryonal tumors, especially medulloblastoma, were used with limited success, with 20% or less of patients surviving in most series.[288–290] However, some degree of chemosensitivity was reported in children receiving platinum-based and/or alkylator-based regimens. In addition to the more standard chemotherapeutic regimens utilized for embryonal tumors, subsequent series have suggested that rhabdomyosarcoma protocols that also included the use of anthracyclines may be somewhat more effective.[315] Similarly, there is some suggestion that higher-dose chemotherapy protocols supported by peripheral stem cell rescue may result in a higher response and long-term tumor control rate.[316]

For older children, chemotherapy has been used in combination with radiotherapy. There is no consensus on which adjuvant chemotherapeutic approach is best.[310,312–314,317] Approaches have included standard medulloblastoma regimens, higher-dose medulloblastoma regimens supplemented by peripheral stem cell rescue, and sarcoma regimens.[221,310–313,316]

Outcome

Although, as a group, outcome is poor in children with AT/RTs, with early reports suggesting that less than 20% of children survive, recently somewhat more encouraging survival results have been noted.[288,289,310,316,318,319] Two-year, EFS of 70% or higher have been noted in patients who have undergone a total resection followed by craniospinal radiation therapy and chemotherapy.[310] Survival rates are lower for infants, but in those children younger than 3 years whose tumors can be totally resected or in those with residual disease following surgery who obtain a complete response to induction chemotherapy, survival rates of above 50% have been noted at 2 to 3 years.[310] EFS remains less than 20% for those patients with metastatic disease or for those whose tumors are not fully responsive to chemotherapy.[310,313,314,316–320] The COG has developed a prospective cooperative group trial to prospectively evaluate a multimodality approach for AT/RTs.

Medulloepitheliomas

Medulloepitheliomas are a rare embryonal tumor that is highly aggressive and tends to arise in young children.[321] The tumor is characterized by an histologic appearance that mimics the embryonal neural tube.

Demographics

Medulloepitheliomas comprise less than one percent of childhood brain tumors.[321,322] They are usually diagnosed prior to 6 years of age, with a mean age of diagnosis of 3 to 4 years. Congenital medulloepitheliomas have been reported. This rare tumor seems to occur equally in males and females. Medulloepitheliomas may arise both in the supratentorial and in the infratentorial compartments of the brain, and they seem to have a predilection for the cerebral hemispheres, especially periventricularly. They have been rarely noted to involve the orbit. Medulloepitheliomas may also arise in the cauda equina and the sciatic nerve, presumably due to their primitive neural tube and medullary plate origin.

Clinical Presentation

Clinical diagnosis is as for any highly aggressive malignant brain tumor that occurs early in life.[321] Medulloepitheliomas may present with symptoms of increased intracranial pressure or with focal neurologic deficits.

Neuroimaging

Lesions are usually mildly heterogeneous—hypointense on T1-weighted images, hyperintense on T2-weighted images—and show restricted signal on diffusion. Enhancement is variable. They tend to be of moderate to large size with relatively well-circumscribed margins and lobulations. Hemorrhage is rare at presentation but is observed with progressive tumors.[226,322] Partly cystic cases have been reported. On CT, the lesions are iso- or hypodense; most do not demonstrate contrast enhancement.

Pathology

Medulloepitheliomas are large, relatively discrete tumors with regions of hemorrhage and calcifications; cystic changes may also be present.[321,322] The tumor histopathologically mimics the embryonal neural tube and is characterized by papillary or tubular neoplastic neuroepithelium with an external limiting membrane. This epithelial arrangement is the hallmark of the disease and is intermixed with other highly cellular, undifferentiated areas. Mitotic figures are abundant and in some areas, mitotic activity is greater than 50%. In addition, there may be areas of more mature neurons and astrocytes. In the neuroepithelial areas, immunohistochemical studies demonstrate staining for both nestin and vimentin; other areas may show expression of neurofilament protein, cytokeratin, and epithelial membrane antigen. In more differentiated areas, neuronal and glial markers may be seen.

Biology

There is very limited knowledge about the underlying biology of medulloepithelioma because of its low incidence. In a series of 50 embryonal brain tumors evaluated for hTERT gene copy number and expression level, two were medulloepitheliomas that had both copy number gain and overexpression of hTERT.[323] One of these medulloepitheliomas actually had the highest hTERT expression compared with the other medulloblastomas. In another single case report of an ocular medulloepithelioma, G banding karyotype showed der(16)t(1;16) and other chromosomal abnormalities.[323]

Staging

There is very little information concerning the staging of medulloepitheliomas or the incidence to disseminate to other areas of other parts of the nervous system early in illness.[321] However, the tumor may be disseminated at the time of diagnosis and for this reason probably staged as other embryonal tumors.

Treatment

Surgery

Surgery for medulloepithelioma is similar to that for other embryonal nervous systems when located intracranially. Intraorbital involvement may also require involvement of an ophthalmologist.

Radiation Therapy

Lacking any specific guidelines or data for this rare tumor type, indications for radiation therapy and radiation parameters are the same as those for medulloblastoma or cortical PNETs.

Chemotherapy

Data concerning the relative sensitivity of medulloepitheliomas to chemotherapy are essentially nonexistent.[321,322]

Outcome

Because of its rarity, the exact rate of survival for medulloepitheliomas is difficult to determine.[321–323] The tumor tends to be aggressive and the majority of patients die of their disease within 1 year of diagnosis. Survival has been noted primarily in those amenable to a gross total resection, followed by some form of adjuvant therapy that includes radiation therapy and, possibly, chemotherapy.

Ependymoblastomas

Ependymoblastomas are a rare form of pediatric brain tumor that are often included in series reporting medulloblastomas or other primitive embryonal tumors. First described by Bailey and Cushing, their existence as a specific diagnostic entity has been questioned, but these remain in the most recent WHO classification.[324]

Demographics

Ependymoblastomas usually arise in the first 2 years of life and congenital tumors have been noted; most are diagnosed before 4 years of age.[324–327] There is no clear-cut sexual predilection, but a male preponderance has been suggested. Ependymoblastomas are more common in the supratentorial space but may occur infratentorially or in the spine. Congenital sacrococcygeal ependymoblastomas have also been reported.

Clinical Presentation

Ependymoblastomas usually present explosively with focal neurologic deficits and symptoms of increased intracranial pressure.[324,327]

Neuroimaging

The lesions are radiographically indistinguishable from medulloblastomas, sPNETs, or AT/RTs.[328] They tend to be large in size (especially in younger patients), yet well circumscribed, with occasional cystic change; calcifications, necrosis, and hemorrhage are common, giving the lesion a heterogeneous appearance on T1- and T2- weighted images. Most show contrast-enhancement and surrounding edema.

Pathology

Ependymoblastomas tend to be well-circumscribed and vascular. They are histologically characterized by regions of ependymoblastic multilayered rosettes with sheets of small, hyperchromatic cells. The lumens of the rosettes may be round or slit-like.[324,327,329] The cells comprising the rosettes are highly mitotic and the outer layer of the rosettes merges with the surrounding undifferentiated cells. Histologic features overlap with other brain tumors, especially "pediatric tumor with abundant neuropil and true rosettes."[324,330]

Biology

There is little biologic data. In four children with ependymoblastomas, comparative genomic hybridization demonstrated gains of chromosome 2, as well as loss of 6q and 13q. These tumors showed a mean of 3.25 DNA copy number changes, with gains being less frequent than losses.[331]

Staging

Ependymoblastomas are staged as other embryonal tumors. Widespread leptomeningeal invasion and less commonly extraneural metastases have been noted.

Treatment

Surgery

The tumors are often quite large at diagnosis and most have been biopsied or subtotally resected. It is unclear whether the degree of resection affects outcome, as overall prognosis has been so poor.

Radiotherapy

Ependymoblastoma is treated similarly to supratentorial PNET; indications for local irradiation (in a tumor type overwhelmingly occurring in infants) and radiation parameters are discussed in the "Supratentorial Primitive Neuroectodermal Tumor" section earlier.

Chemotherapy

There is little, if any, information concerning the chemosensitivity of ependymoblastomas. Usually those treatment protocols utilized for high-risk medulloblastomas have been used.

Outcome

The outcome of children with ependymoblastomas is poor and there is some suggestion that those tumors that are totally resected may have a more favorable prognosis.[324,327] However, it has been difficult to determine whether ependymoblastomas have a distinct pattern of outcome as these are often included in series of other embryonal tumors, such as medulloblastomas and sPNETs. In the past, ependymoblastomas were also included in series of patients with ependymomas.

PINEAL REGION TUMORS

Tumors of the pineal area account for 0.4% to 2.0% of all primary CNS tumors in children.[1,7,8] Three principal groups of tumors—germ cell tumors, pineal parenchymal tumors, and astrocytomas—account for most tumors in this location.[1,7,8] The most recent WHO classification of CNS tumors recognized four major types of pineal tumors.[1] Pineoblastomas have previously been discussed within the embryonal tumor section. Papillary tumors of the pineal region are a rare neuro-epithelial tumor, predominantly of adults, with immunopositivity for cytokeratin and ultrastructural features suggesting ependymal differentiation. The two major types of pineal parenchymal tumors that occur in children are the pineocytoma, classified as a grade 1 tumor, and pineal parenchymal tumor of intermediate differentiation, classified as a grade 2 or 3 tumor. In combined clinical series, astrocytomas constitute 15%, the pineal parenchymal tumors 17%, and germ cell tumors 40% to 65% of all neoplasms in this area.[1,315,332–337] Of CNS germ cell tumors, two-thirds occur in the pineal region and the remaining one-third in the suprasellar region.[315,331–337]

Demographics

Pineal parenchymal tumors are more frequent in the first decade of life and have a male-to-female ratio near unity. Germ cell tumors are most common in the second decade of life or later, have a peak incidence at between 10 and 14 years of age, and are associated with a male-to-female ratio of at least 2:1 and as high as 9:1. Astrocytomas tend to occur in two separate age groups, 2- to 6-year-old children and 12- to 18-year-old teens, and each group has a 2:1 male-to-female incidence, characteristic of astrocytomas elsewhere in the CNS.[315,332–337]

Diagnosis

Because of the diversity in the biologic behavior and response to treatment of different types of pineal area tumors, biopsy is recommended whenever possible to establish a tissue diagnosis, which guides subsequent therapy.[315,332–337] One exception is patients with benign intrinsic tectal tumors. A second exception is patients with malignant germ cell tumors where elevated levels of a-fetoprotein or beta-human chorionic gonadotrophin (or both) can be detected within the CSF and, at times, blood. Appropriate elevations can be considered diagnostic and negate the need for biopsy.

Current neurosurgical techniques include stereotactic, endoscopic, or open biopsies in most patients, with morbidity generally limited to transient worsening of prior visual symptoms, although new or permanent losses may occur. The mortality rate is generally less than 2%. Direct visually guided biopsy is preferred by many neurosurgeons because of concern that stereotactic biopsies may injure adjacent deep veins. However, recent reports have demonstrated that stereotactic biopsy can be performed with acceptable morbidity, provided that a low frontal entry point is used to allow access to the tumor below the internal cerebral veins.[338] This approach also provides CSF for analysis of a-fetoprotein and b-human chorionic gonadotrophin, because the biopsy trajectory often traverses the lateral ventricle. Often, it is feasible to achieve CSF diversion using endoscopic third ventriculostomy while the patient is under the same anesthetic. With advances in endoscopic techniques, many surgeons opt to biopsy the tumor endoscopically under direct visualization, rather than stereotactically, at the same setting as the third ventriculostomy. Although these minimally invasive approaches have significant appeal and appear to carry a lower morbidity than conventional open craniotomy approaches, a major concern is the issue of sampling error. As many as 15% of germ cell tumors have mixed histology, which calls attention to the importance of adequate biopsy and of performing CSF and blood marker studies in such patients.[335,339]

If a stereotactic or endoscopic biopsy is nondiagnostic or equivocal, or if the histology of the lesion suggests that an open surgical resection is likely to be of benefit, as in the case of benign teratoma, tumor removal can be accomplished using one of a variety of operative approaches. An infratentorial supracerebellar approach is used for lesions that exhibit predominant growth below the level of the vein of Galen and basal veins of Rosenthal. A suboccipital transtentorial approach is preferred for larger lesions that extend above the basal veins or down into the rostral fourth ventricle. Both approaches can be accomplished using a prone or modified prone position, which is generally preferred to the sitting position, to minimize the risk of air embolism. After division of the precentral cerebellar vein and surrounding arachnoid, the lesion is subjected to biopsy and then debulked using the ultrasonic aspirator. Great care is taken to avoid injury to the deep veins.

Except for well-encapsulated teratomas, few pineal region tumors are amenable to complete resection, generally because of extensive local or regional disease. Even though subtotal resections are possible for many patients with localized tumors, no evidence indicates that such resections improve outcome. Because many tumors in this area are sensitive to both radiation therapy and chemotherapy, and because aggressive surgery may cause significant morbidity, biopsy alone or limited tumor debulking to relieve hydrocephalus often is the most prudent approach initially, particularly for patients with germinomas. In addition, a variety of current treatment protocols for nongerminomatous germ cell tumors are employing intensive neoadjuvant chemotherapy after an initial open or stereotactic biopsy, followed by second-look surgery to perform a biopsy or remove areas of residual enhancement.[340–342] In some cases, such reoperations indicate only scar tissue without evidence of viable tumor. In other cases, tumor recurrence or progression can be difficult to separate neuroradiographically from transformation of a nongerminomatous germ cell tumor to a mature teratoma (the "growing teratoma syndrome"), requiring surgery to confirm diagnosis and, at times, improve symptoms.

Pineocytomas

Demographics

Pineocytomas and pineal parenchymal tumors of intermediate differentiation are rare, accounting for less than 1 % of all intracranial neoplasms in childhood and comprising 25% or less of pineal tumors.[334,335,337,343,344] Although pineocytomas are reported most frequently in adults, they can occur in children. There is no clear-cut sexual predilection.

Pineal parenchymal tumors of intermediate differentiation are even rarer and have probably been underreported because of the relative subjectivity of diagnosis.[1] Another term that has been utilized to describe this tumor has been the atypical pineocytoma. Because, by definition, these tumors may also have evidence of pineoblastoma-like histological features, the tumor has also been classified within the pineoblastoma grouping.

Clinical Presentation

Pineocytomas present as other pineal region tumors with pressure on the tectum resulting in Parinaud syndrome. The tumor may also present acutely with intratumoral hemorrhage.[335,343,344] Accompanying hydrocephalus is frequent with associated headaches and mental status changes. In other patients, the tumor can present insidiously, suggesting that the tumor has been present for many years.

Neuroimaging

Pineocytomas are well marginated and frequently harbor large cysts and heterogeneous calcifications (Fig. 26B.14). The lesions

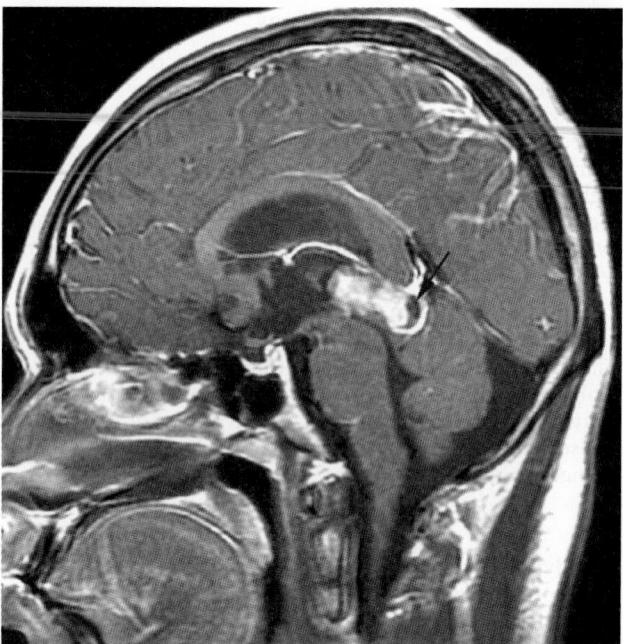

FIGURE 26B.14 Intermediate grade pineocytomas. Postcontrast sagittal T1 image reveals a large, primarily solid tumor, with a small nonenhancing cystic component posteriorly (*arrow*).

are usually rounded, sometimes slightly lobulated; their margins are clear, without infiltration of adjacent structures.[345,346] Pineocytomas tend to have low signal on T1-weighted sequences and are hyperintense on T2 images. Contrast enhancement is intense and more homogeneous than in pineoblastoma. The aggressive forms have soft-tissue components that may show significant, heterogeneous signal intensity and contrast enhancement.

Pathology

Pineocytoma bears a strong resemblance to normal pineal, which may present a diagnostic challenge, especially if the biopsy is small (Fig. 26B.15). The cells are larger and obviously more mature than those forming pineoblastoma, although there may be a mixture of both types in some tumors. Such

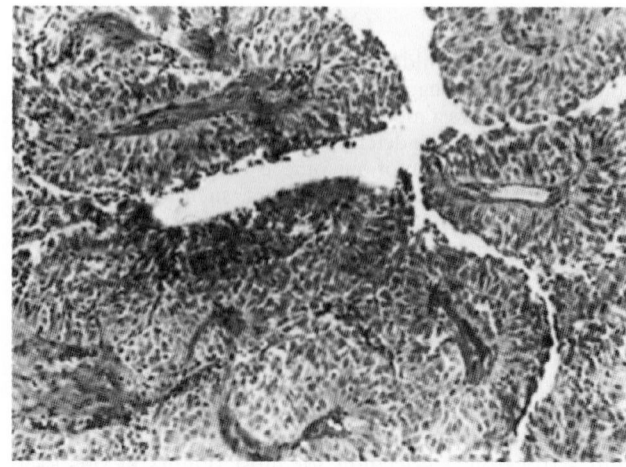

FIGURE 26B.15 Primary pineal tumor displaying prominent perivascular growth of neoplastic cells characteristic of pineocytoma. Note the papillary pattern (hematoxylin and eosin, 3,250).

tumors have been given a separate diagnostic term, namely "pineal parenchymal tumor of intermediate differentiation."[347] Tumor cells have a relation to blood vessels, but true rosettes are rarely seen. A rare histological subtype of pineocytoma exhibits a papillary pattern.[348]

Biology

Cytogenetic analyses of two cases of pineocytomas have revealed losses of chromosomes 11 and 22, as well as deletions of distal 12q in both.[349,350] CGH data[351] on pineal parenchymal tumors show that pineal parenchymal tumors of intermediate differentiation are cytogenetically more similar to pineoblastomas and prognostically more similar to pineocytomas. Pineal parenchymal tumors have also been investigated for mutations of the TP53 tumor suppressor gene; however, no mutations were detected in the pineocytomas that were examined.[352–354]

Staging

There is no clear evidence that staging for pineocytomas is of clinical use as the majority are localized at the time of diagnosis. For patients with atypical features or coexisting pineoblastoma-like histology, staging is indicated. In one series, a high incidence of tumor dissemination was noted; this occurred in very young children with pineocytomas, the majority being younger than 10 years at the time of diagnosis and questions have been raised whether this is truly a series of pineocytomas or a mixed series including atypical pineocytomas or pineoblastomas.[343,344]

Treatment

Surgery

Surgical resection of pineocytomas is similar to that of other pineal region neoplasms.

Radiotherapy

Pineocytomas are typically considered localized, low-grade tumors occurring infrequently in children. In cases where complete resection is not feasible, local irradiation is indicated for residual or progressive tumor (either highly conformal 3-D or IMRT, including potential use of stereotactic radiosurgery or fractionated stereotactic radiotherapy).

Chemotherapy

Since the majority of patients with pineocytomas are treated with surgery or surgery plus radiation therapy, there is little data concerning the efficacy of chemotherapy.

Outcome

After treatment with observation, surgery, and, at times, radiation therapy, 5-year survival rates of up to 100% have been noted, especially after gross-total resections.[334,343,344] The 5-year survival rate for pineal parenchymal tumors of intermediate differentiation is difficult to determine, given the tumor's rarity, its variability of diagnosis, and overlap with pineoblastomas. In general, the survival rates have been lower than for pineocytomas, although numbers are quite small.[334,343,344]

Germ Cell Tumors

Primary CNS germ cell tumors are a confusing subset of brain tumors classified on the basis of histological and immunohistochemical features supplemented by determination of protein

TABLE 26B.10

WHO CLASSIFICATION OF GERM CELL TUMORS

Germinoma
Embryonal carcinoma
Yolk sac tumor
Choriocarcinoma
Teratoma
Mature
Immature
Teratoma with malignant transformation
Mixed germ cell tumor

markers secreted or produced by the tumors into the CSF and blood. The WHO recognizes multiple different types of germ cell tumors, ranging from mature teratomas to a variety of highly aggressive nongerminomatous germ cell tumors[1] (see Table 26B.10). For management purposes, these tumors are usually conceptualized as being teratomas (at times with immature elements), pure germinomas, or mixed germ cell tumors (nongerminomatous germ cell tumors).[332,355–357] Even with this simplified classification, there are important subtleties, such as the syncytiotrophoblastic variant of germinoma, which may portend a poorer prognosis.[355] Separation of so-called secreting pure germinomas with small components of presumed syncytiotrophoblastic giant cells, the syncytiotrophoblastic variant of germinoma and choriocarcinomas is somewhat arbitrary, being based on CSF levels of beta human chorionic gonadotrophin. Secretion or production of alpha-fetoprotein is used as a marker for the mixed germ variant, as well as for embryonal carcinoma, endodermal sinus tumor, and, at times, teratomas with immature elements.

The classification of germ cell tumors is primarily a derivation of that first outlined by Teilum, suggesting that all germ cell tumors were derived from a primordial germ cell that may either differentiate into a germinoma or be the origin of totipotential cells that give rise to other types of germ cell tumors.[332,358] In this schema, the embryonal carcinoma is a tumor of totipotential cells that ultimately may give risk to other types of germ cell neoplasm. If the neoplastic process involves differentiated embryonic tissues, such as ectoderm, mesoderm, or endoderm, the tumor will become a teratocarcinoma or malignant teratoma. The tumor, likewise, can differentiate into one that develops into a choriocarcinoma derived from the trophoblastic tissue or from yolk cell elements, becoming an endodermal sinus tumor. An alternative theory, proposed by Takei and Pearl, suggests that the fetal yolk sack was the origin of the primordial germ cell tumor that then can develop along multiple different pathways. In this conceptual framework, the embryonal carcinoma is considered a relative end-stage tumor.[359] Another concept suggested by Sano et al. is that the germinoma is the only neoplasm purely arising from the germ cell, while other tumors are dysembryogenic and become misinvolved-misenfolded into the lateral mesoderm and carried into the future brain regions of the developing embryo.[360]

Demographics

Between 80% and 90% of CNS germ cell tumors arise in patients younger than 25 years, with incidence peaking in 10- to 14-year-olds.[315,332–337] Teratomas, however, are more likely to be diagnosed early in life, especially infancy. Nongerminomatous germ cell tumors are more frequently diagnosed between birth and 9 years of age than are germinomas.

For unknown reasons, there is a marked geographic variation in CNS germ cell tumors, with the tumor being much more prevalent in Far East Asia as compared with North America. In tumor registries in the United States, germ cell tumors account for approximately 2% to 3% of all primary intracranial neoplasms, as compared with 8% to 15% of pediatric series from Japan, Taiwan, and Korea.[315,332-337]

In most studies, males more frequently develop germ cell tumors than do females, in a ratio of approximately 2:1, but this male excess is limited to those tumors arising in the pineal region.[315,332-337] This is most striking in Japanese tumor registries, which suggest that greater than 75% of germ cell tumors arise in males, including teratomas, pure germ cell tumors, and mixed germ cell tumors. In contradistinction, females are at higher risk of developing suprasellar germinomas and choriocarcinomas.

Central nervous system germ cell tumors preferentially are found in the midline, with the majority being found in the pineal region. Approximately 20% will originate in the suprasellar area.[315,332-337] Other locations, which may be more commonly found in patients of the Far East, include intraventricular, diffuse periventricular, basal ganglionic, and thalamic regions. In the suprasellar compartment, pure germinomas are the most common tumor type. Nongerminomatous germ cell tumors are more likely to be found in the basal ganglionic and thalamic region or other nonpineal/nonsuprasellar locations. Germinomas also are notoriously present in both suprasellar and pineal region at the time of diagnosis. This multifocal, apparent simultaneous presentation, may occur in up to 10% of patients and diagnosis is often dependent on a high level of suspicion of second site involvement.

Clinical Presentation

The diagnosis of germ cell tumors can be difficult.[315,332-337,361,362] Despite the histologically apparent malignant nature of germinomas and nongerminomatous germ cell tumors, symptoms may be present for many months or, at times, years prior to diagnosis. This is especially true for those tumors that arise in the suprasellar region causing diabetes insipidus or those that are more widely infiltrated in the brain resulting in nonspecific findings such as school failure and psychomotor retardation.

Tumors that arise in the pineal region most commonly present with hydrocephalus, Parinaud syndrome, and obduntation, at times with motor weakness and unsteadiness.[361,362] Parinaud syndrome is the classical neurologic complex of findings related to pineal region tumors, manifest by failure of upgaze, pupils that react better to accommodation than light, lid retraction, and convergence or retraction nystagmus. Patients with pure germinomas are almost equally likely to present with hydrocephalus, and obduntation, or Parinaud syndrome. In contradistinction, patients with nongerminomatous germ cell tumors, such as the mixed germ cell tumors or malignant teratomas, tend to have more neurologic compromise and focal deficits at the time of diagnosis. In general, symptom duration for patients with pineal germ cell tumors is somewhat shorter than those with suprasellar lesions.

Endocrinologic sequelae seen are frequent in patients with suprasellar germ cell tumors, including diabetes insipidus, delayed sexual development, panhypopituitarism, diabetes insipidus, and isolated growth failure.[315,332-337,361,362] Up to 35% of suprasellar tumors may be symptomatic for greater than 6 months and occasionally symptoms may be present for well over 1 year. Precocious puberty has been reported in children with suprasellar and pineal region tumors, and the cause of precocious puberty in patients with pineal region tumors has been speculated for many years. Although this finding

may be caused by secretion of human chorionotic gonadotrophin, a stimulant of testosterone production that is secreted by the neoplastic syncytiotrophoblast, it does not explain all of the cases of precocious puberty, especially in girls. It is conceivable that many of the patients diagnosed with pineal region tumors who had precocious puberty had undiagnosed suprasellar or hypothalamic involvement in addition. As stated previously, CSF analysis is critical in the diagnosis of mixed germ cell tumors and secreting germinomas. Without such analysis, diagnosis would be delayed even more in many patients.

Teratomas, with or without immature elements, can arise in very young children and are likely congenital in many affected young children.[315,332-337,361,362] In congenital cases, these teratomatous tumors are often extremely large at the time of diagnosis with resultant hydrocephalus, macrocephaly, and marked neurologic impairments.

Neuroimaging

Germinomas are relatively homogeneous; however, small cysts are seen in almost 50% of lesions. On CT, tumors are iso- to hyperdense; almost all are associated with calcification of the pineal gland, which appears "engulfed."[363] The solid parts are nearly isointense with grey matter on T1-weighted images, and hypo to isointense on T2-weighted images; calcifications may appear as T2 hypointense foci. Intense enhancement is usually demonstrated on both MR and CT (Fig. 26B.16).

Nongerminomatous germ cell tumors are more heterogeneous, and more invasive than germinomas, with an increased frequency of cysts and hemorrhage; enhancement is more heterogeneous.[363] Mixed germ cell tumors commonly invade the midbrain and thalamus. Appearance on T2 images is heterogeneous. On CT, they are hyperdense, with or without calcifications and most enhance. Teratomas tend to be heterogeneous, with multilocular mixed cystic and solid elements; lipomatous elements within the tumors (characterized by signal identical to fat on T1 and T2 sequences, low/fatty attenuation on CT) are pathognomonic. Choriocarcinoma are hypervascular and often hemorrhagic. Foci of subacute hemorrhage are typically demonstrated on MR imaging and are a clue to the diagnosis. Local infiltration is common.[346]

Pathology

Germinomas have a typical two-cell appearance indistinguishable from that of gonadal germinomas and are composed of large, primitive-appearing cells intermixed with smaller lymphoid cells[7,112,364] (Fig. 26B.17).

Teratomas and mixed germ cell tumors harbor various mature and immature elements. The histologic appearance of these tumors is identical to that of similar tumors occurring outside the CNS. Teratomas generally remain local, well encapsulated, and noninvasive. However, areas with more primitive germ cell elements may be present and are associated with a more aggressive clinical course that may include neuroaxis dissemination.[7,112,364]

Biology

Our current knowledge and understanding of the biology of intracranial germ cell tumors are extremely limited. The etiology or pathogenesis of these tumors remains elusive. Cytogenetic and molecular data of intracranial germ cell tumors are sparse with only a handful of reports on the cytogenetic analysis available. Among various chromosomal abnormalities, extranumerary X chromosome, gains of 12p including isochromosome 12p and 1q were commonly observed. A recent study of CNS germ cell tumors (germinomas, malignant nongerminomatous germ cell tumors) using chromosomal

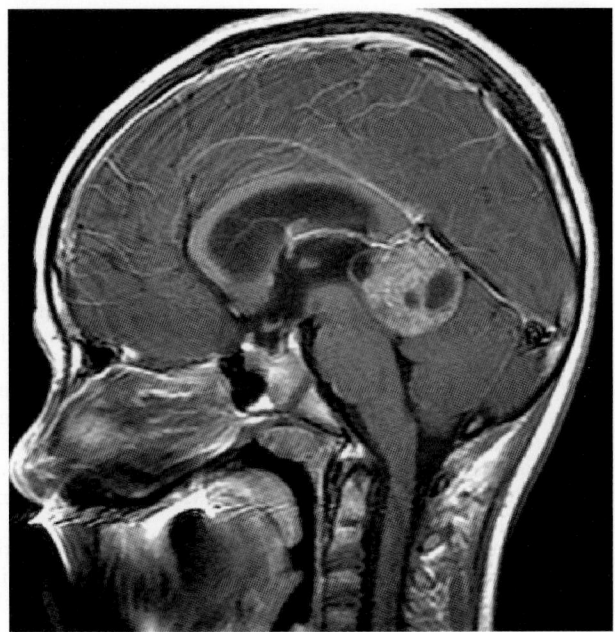 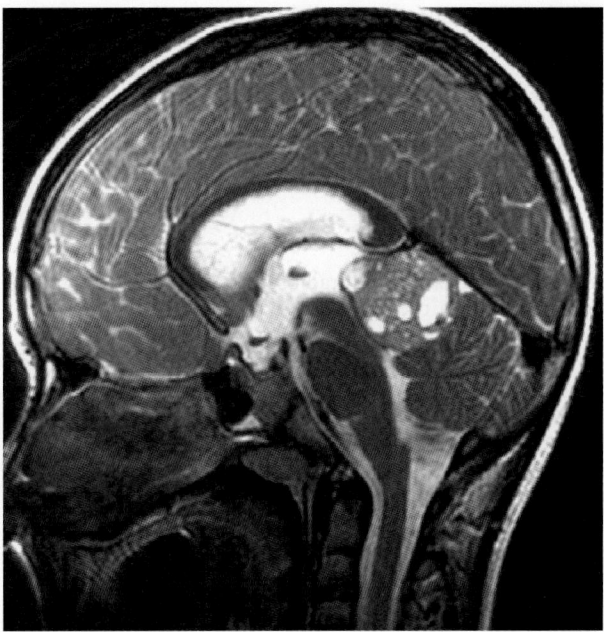

A

B

FIGURE 26B.16 Typical pineal germinoma in a 12-year-old. Sagittal T2 (A) and contrast enhanced T1 (B) images reveal a large predominantly cystic mass of the pineal region, with multiple small cysts (and a few larger cysts). The solid aspects of the tumor show homogeneous enhancement (B) and isointense T2 signal compared with cerebral cortical signal (A).

CGH demonstrated multiple chromosomal imbalances in all malignant germ cell tumors and some teratomas.[365] Chromosomal gains were observed more frequently than losses. 12p gain (which is considered characteristic for germ cell tumors of adult testis) was detected in 58% of tumors and 67% of malignant CNS germ cell tumors. Other common gains were found on 1q and 8q. Among chromosomal losses, parts of chromosome 11, 18, and 13 were deleted most frequently. Notably, there was no observed difference in genetic profiles of germinomas and nongerminomatous germ cell tumors; however, the average number of imbalances was higher in nongerminomatous germ cell tumors. A meta-analysis[365] comparing 116 malignant gonadal and extragonadal germ cell tumors revealed that the genomic alterations in CNS germ cell tumors are virtually indistinguishable from those found in their gonadal or other extragonadal counterparts. This strongly argues in favor of common pathogenesis in gonadal and extragonadal germ cell tumors.

In another study,[366] the most frequent imbalances were gains on 12p (40%), 8q (27%), and 1q (20%) as well as losses on 13q (47%), 18q (33%), 9q (20%), and 11q (20%). Among germinomas, the most common chromosomal changes were −13q (38%) and −18q (38%) and in mixed teratomas-germinomas, +8q (100%), +12p (75%), and −9q (50%). Gains of hypomethylated, active X chromosomes occur in nearly all intracranial germ cell tumors, regardless of histological subtype.[367] Along with the observed male predominance of intracranial germ cell tumors and the predisposition for these lesions in Klinefelter syndrome, sex chromosome aberrations may be integral to the pathogenesis of intracranial germ cell tumors.

Staging

Staging is an accepted component of the management of patients with germ cell tumors. Evidence of tumor spread outside the primary site has been noted in between 10% and 30% of patients, even higher in some selected series.[315,332–337,364] Endoscopic evaluation also may disclose intraventricular seeding not demonstrable on neuroradiographic studies. Systemic metastases have been reported but are rare. As more localized forms of radiotherapy are increasingly being utilized for germ cell tumors, detailed staging by means of MRI imaging of the entire neuroaxis and CSF cytologic examination becomes even more important.

Treatment

Surgery

FIGURE 26B.17 Typical field of germinoma displaying large cells with large nucleoli and focus of lymphocytes (right half of field) (hematoxylin and eosin, × 400).

Most germ cell tumors do not require cytoreduction, but rather tissue sampling (biopsy) and CSF diversion. Mature teratomas are an exception to this rule and can be completely removed without undue morbidity, and with a long-term disease free outcome in most cases. In a minority of cases of mixed germ cell tumor, there is an element of the tumor that does not respond to therapy, or which regrows after therapy. Biopsy and subsequent resection in these cases often reveals a large component of mature teratomas (growing-teratoma syndrome).

Radiotherapy

Germinomas are exquisitely radiosensitive tumors; outcome following radiation therapy alone typically results in greater than 90% disease control.[337,339,368-374] For children older than 10 to 13 years, radiation therapy is the standard of care; the use of combined chemotherapy and reduced radiation volume and dose has increasingly been utilized, especially in children presenting prior to puberty. The relative lack of consensus on radiation parameters (particularly the appropriate volume, ranging from targeting only the local tumor to full craniospinal irradiation), limited data regarding long-term disease control for children/adolescents treated with combined chemoradiation, and positive functional outcomes in series reporting intelligence and quality of life following management with irradiation alone (or in conjunction with chemotherapy) all combine to make it difficult to be dogmatic to one therapeutic approach, recognizing generally excellent rates of disease control. The major controversy concerning radiation therapy is the appropriate volume. There has been ongoing debate whether germinomas require CSI, cranial irradiation (i.e., whole brain but without spinal irradiation), treatment to the ventricular system (lateral and third ventricles), the third ventricle only, or only the local tumor volume.[369-392] For localized pineal germinomas, series utilizing wide local volumes (defined as "local" or including only the third ventricle) achieve durable disease control (or cure) in 75% to 90% of instances.[368,373,378,379] Patterns of failure analyses show a number of intracranial recurrences following less than full cranial (or CSI) therapy.[368,380,381] Series utilizing low-dose CSI as the initial "wide field" volume have reported few, if any, failures, with long-term EFS at 95% to 100%.[336,369-371,376] At the time the COG study noted earlier was planned, there was preliminary experience from European trials showing subependymal failures within the ventricular system following radiation volumes limited to the primary tumor (with a 1.5- to –2-cm margin).[382-385] Both North American and European strategies have subsequently identified whole ventricular irradiation as the "minimal" wide field component of therapy when irradiation alone is utilized.[368] The ability to target the two lateral ventricles and the central third ventricle (with or without the fourth ventricle) using intensity modulated radiation therapy (IMRT) allows one to relatively protect much of the cerebral cortex during this initial component of radiation therapy.[368,387,388]

The role of spinal irradiation, as distinct from full cranial coverage, is even more controversial, with several large series showing a small to negligible incidence of spinal failures following ventricular or cranial irradiation for disease localized at diagnosis (i.e., M0).[368,372,373,378,389]

Most contemporary protocols utilize 21 to 27 Gy to the wider field (CSI, cranial, or ventricular); experience with 24 Gy at 150 cGy/fraction has been uniformly successful at St. Jude.[368,371,373,377,386] The primary tumor is typically targeted with a 1.5- to –2-cm margin; total dose to the primary site is 40 to 45 Gy.[368,371,373,379,390] Adolescent males present not uncommonly with "multiple midline germinoma," most often disease at both ends of the third ventricle (suprasellar and pineal sites). Such presentations have been uniformly controlled using CSI with intermediate "boost" or full therapeutic dose levels to the third ventricular region.[369,378] There is

some recent data suggesting multiple midline presentations may be treated with full ventricular rather than full cranial irradiation or CSI.[374]

Leptomeningeal metastasis at diagnosis[368,382] occurs in 10% to 30% of cases; patients are curable with primary irradiation using doses of 30 to 36 Gy CSI with subsequent "boost" to the primary site or areas of significant infiltration to 40 to 45 Gy.[393-395]

When combined chemoradiation is utilized in germinomas, tumors demonstrating complete or near complete response to "induction" chemotherapy are typically treated to local volumes (essentially incorporating only the regions identified as boost volumes with primary radiation strategies) with postchemotherapy doses of 30 to 35 Gy or lower doses of whole-ventricular or CSI.[385,391,382] There is data regarding "salvage" irradiation after chemotherapy alone as management for germinomas; excellent secondary disease control has been documented after high-dose cyclophosphamide and irradiation (25 to 36 Gy CSI with boost to 45 to 54 Gy to the primary site).[396]

Radiation therapy is required for disease control in the higher-grade malignant CNS germ cell tumor histotypes.[394,397-399] In North American studies, CSI has been the standard of care for nongerminomatous germ cell tumors in conjunction with chemotherapy.[372,395,397-400] There is limited data suggesting more localized radiation volumes may be adequate in conjunction with aggressive chemotherapy for the malignant CNS germ cell tumors.[383,401,402] Dose levels recommended for these histotypes include 36 Gy CSI (typically in 180-cGy fractions) and 54 Gy to the primary tumor volume.[395,397,402] The use of conformal techniques to boost the primary site has been reported with both fractionated stereotactic radiotherapy and single-fraction stereotactic radiosurgery.[403,404]

Chemotherapy

Germ cell tumors of the CNS, like germ cell tumors in other sites of the body, are chemosensitive.[340,405-411] This chemosensitivity, seen both in pure germinomas and in nongerminomatous germ cell tumors, has resulted in the utilization of chemotherapy in attempts to reduce the amount or volume of radiation therapy required for germinomas and to improve OS in patients with nongerminomatous germ cell tumors. Chemotherapeutic agents that have shown activity include cyclophosphamide, ifosfamide, etoposide, cisplatin, carboplatin, and possibly bleomycin.[400,405-412] Both cyclophosphamide and carboplatin, used individually, resulted in tumor response in newly diagnosed patients with germinomas and allowed for a reduction of the dose and volume of radiotherapy required for long-term disease control.[405,406] In these two studies, radiotherapy was given to all patients after induction chemotherapy, although the volume and dose of radiotherapy varied dependent on response. Cisplatin has been shown to be effective but was considered less desirable because of concerns of ototoxicity, nephrotoxicity, and electrolyte derangements.[405-408] In a chemotherapy-alone study, patients with newly diagnosed germinomas were treated with four cycles of carboplatin, etoposide, and bleomycin, and for those patients who achieved a complete response, further chemotherapy was given, but no radiation therapy was used.[340] Seventy-eight percent of the 45 patients with a germinoma were noted to have a complete response; however, 20 of the 45 patients with germinomas ultimately relapsed. In a SIOP germinoma protocol, patients received two courses of carboplatin and etoposide alternating with two cycles of etoposide and ifosfamide, followed by focal radiation or craniospinal radiation for those patients with localized disease and craniospinal radiation for those patients with disseminated disease.[410] EFS of patients with localized disease treated with chemotherapy and focal radiation therapy was 85% at 40 months, compared with 96% for those treated with craniospinal radiation, although OS did not differ between the two groups. EFS in patients with metastatic disease was 98% at 44 months.[413] The Japanese experience, utilizing carboplatin and etoposide followed by focal radiation therapy, demonstrated an OS rate of 98%, but within this study, a significant number of patients recurred and required retreatment. Given these results and the pattern of relapse, the investigators suggested the use of whole ventricular irradiation instead of local radiation therapy for further studies.

For patients with nongerminomatous germ cell tumors, platinum-based chemotherapeutic regimens have been most widely employed, often used in combination with drugs including vinblastine, etoposide, and/or bleomycin.[400,405-412,414,415] In a German cooperative group study, two cycles of cisplatin, etoposide, and bleomycin were given to patients with nongerminomatous germ cell tumors followed by radiation and ifosfamide, cisplatin, and vinblastine, and resulted in an 80% 5-year survival rate.[416] In the French Society of Pediatric Oncology study, carboplatin and etoposide were alternated with ifosfamide and etoposide, followed by focal or craniospinal radiation therapy dependent on the extent of disease at the time of diagnosis.[414] At 53 months, 74% of patients (20 of 27) were alive. The SIOP nongerminomatous germ cell protocol utilized four cycles of cisplatin, etoposide, and ifosfamide followed by focal radiotherapy for those patients with undisseminated tumor and CSI therapy for those with tumor dissemination at the time of diagnosis. Progression-free survival in this study, at a median follow up of 39 months, was 67% for those patients with localized disease and 72% for those with disseminated disease.[417] Recently, the COG completed a prospective study evaluating the efficacy of carboplatin and etoposide alternating with ifosfamide and etoposide for children with nongerminomatous germ cell tumors. In this study, patients who went into a complete response after chemotherapy were treated with craniospinal (3,600 cGy) and local boost radiotherapy, while those with a response that was less than a complete response were randomized to treatment with either craniospinal and local boost radiotherapy or thiotepa and etoposide supported by peripheral stem cell rescue and radiation therapy. Preliminary results of this study also encouraging but are early in analysis.

Outcome

Overall, the studies utilizing radiotherapy alone or chemotherapy followed by radiation therapy for children with germinomas are encouraging, with greater than a 90% survival rate being noted in most studies.[378-395,418] Improving survival rates have also been noted for nongerminomatous germ cell tumors treated with combination therapy. The relative toxicities of radiotherapy alone, including craniospinal radiation therapy, compared with chemotherapy with reduced dose or volume of radiotherapy have never been demonstrated.[372,397-400,405,406,418]

References

1. Louis DN, Ohgaki H, Wiestler OD, et al., eds. WHO classification of tumors of the central nervous system. Lyon, France: IARC, 2007.
2. CBTRUS. Statistical report, primary brain tumors in the United States, 2000–2004. Published by the Central Brain Tumor Registry of the United States, 2008.
3. Burger PC, Scheithauer BW. Embryonal tumors. In: Tumors of the central nervous system, AFIP atlas of tumor pathology. Series 4. Washington, DC: American Registry of Pathology, 2007:251–295.
4. Packer RJ, Cogen P, Vezina G, et al. Medulloblastoma: clinical and biologic aspects. Neuro-Oncol 1999;1:232–259.
5. Rorke LB, Packer R, Biegel J. Central nervous system atypical teratoid/rhabdoid tumors of infancy and childhood. J Neuro-Oncol 1995;24:21–28.
6. Haberler C, Laggner U, Slavc I, et al. Immunohistochemical analysis of INI1 protein in malignant pediatric CNS tumors: lack of INI1 in atypical teratoid/rhabdoid tumors and in a fraction of primitive neuroectodermal tumors without rhabdoid phenotype. Am J Surg Pathol 2006;30:1462–1468.
7. Burger PC, Scheithauer BW. Tumors of the pineal region. In: AFIP atlas of tumor pathology. Series 4. Washington, DC: American Registry of Pathology, 2007:295–304.
8. Burger PC, Scheithauer BW. Germ cell tumors. In: Tumors of the central nervous system, AFIP atlas of tumor pathology. Series 4. Washington, DC: American Registry of Pathology, 2007:321–327.
9. Packer RJ, Sutton LN, Elterman R, et al. Outcome for children with medulloblastoma treated with radiation and cisplatin, CCNU, and vincristine chemotherapy. J Neurosurg 1994;81(5):690–698.
10. Burger PC, Grahmann FC, Bliestle A, et al. Differentiation in the medulloblastoma. A histological and immunohistochemical study. Acta Neuropathol (Berl) 1987;73(2):115–123.
11. Giangaspero F, Perilongo G, Fondelli MP, et al. Medulloblastoma with extensive nodularity: a variant with favorable prognosis. J Neurosurg 1999;91(6):971–977.
12. Giangaspero F, Wellek S, Masuoka J, et al. Stratification of medulloblastoma on the basis of histopathological grading. Acta Neuropathol 2006;112:5–12.
13. Grotzer MA, von Hoff K, von Bueren AO, et al. Which clinical and biological tumor markers proved predictive in the prospective multicenter trial HIT '91—implications for investigating childhood medulloblastoma. Klin Padiatr 2007;219:312–317.
14. Gajjar A, Hernan R, Kocak M, et al. Clinical, histopathologic, and molecular markers of prognosis: toward a new disease risk stratification system for medulloblastoma. J Clin Oncol 2004;22(6):984–993.
15. Fernandez-Teijeiro Ana, Betensky RB, Sturla LM, et al. Combining gene expression profiles and clinical parameters for risk stratification in medulloblastomas. J Clin Oncol 2004;22:994–998.
16. Pfister S, Remke M, Benner A, et al. Outcome prediction in pediatric medulloblastoma based on DNA copy-number aberrations of chromosomes 6q and 17q and the MYC and MYCN loc. J Clin Oncol 2009;27:1–10.
17. Ellison DW, Onilude OE, Lindsey M, et al. β-catenin status predicts a favorable outcome in childhood medulloblastoma: the United Kingdom Children's Cancer Study Group Brain Tumour Committee. J Clin Oncol 2005;23:7951–7957.
18. Read T-A, Hegedus B, Wechsler-Reya R, et al. The neurobiology of neuro-oncology. Ann Neurol 2006;6:3–11.
19. Ray A, Ho M, Ma J, et al. A clinicobiological model predicting survival in medulloblastoma. Clin Cancer Res 2004;10:7613–7620.
20. Packer RJ, Gajjar A, Vezina G, et al. Phase III study of craniospinal radiation therapy followed by adjuvant chemotherapy for newly diagnosed average-risk medulloblastoma. J Clin Oncol 2006;24(25):4202–4208.
21. Grotzer MA, von Hoff K, von Bueren AD, et al. Which clinical and biological tumor markers proved predictive in the prospective multicenter trial HIT'91—implications for investigating childhood medulloblastoma. Klin Padiatr 2007;219:312–317.
22. Eberhart CG, Kratz J, Wang Y, et al. Histopathological and molecular prognostic markers in medulloblastoma: c-myc, N-myc, TrkC, and anaplasia. J Neuropathol Exp Neurol 2004;63(5):441–449.
23. Ris MD, Packer R, Goldwein J, et al. Intellectual outcome after reduced-dose radiation therapy plus adjuvant chemotherapy for medulloblastoma: a Children's Cancer Group study. J Clin Oncol 2001;19:3470–3476.
24. Mulhern RK, Kepner JL, Thomas PR, et al. Neuropsychologic functioning of survivors of childhood medulloblastoma randomized to receive conventional or reduced-dose craniospinal irradiation: a Pediatric Oncology Group study. J Clin Oncol 1998;16:1723–1728.
25. Sheikh BY, Kanaan IN. Medulloblastoma in adults. J Neurosurg Sci 1994;38:229–234.
26. Prados MD, Warnick RE, Wara WM, et al. Medulloblastoma in adults. Int J Radiat Oncol Biol Phys 1994;32(4):1145–1152.
27. Herrlinger U, Steinbrecher A, Rieger J, et al. Adult medulloblastoma: prognostic factors and response to therapy at diagnosis and at relapse. J Neurol 2005;252:291–299.
28. Halperin EC, Miranda ML, Watson DM, et al. Medulloblastoma and birth date: evaluation of 3 US datasets. Arch Environ Health 2004;59:26–30.
29. Barnholtz-Sloan JS, Severson RK, Stanton B, et al. Pediatric brain tumors in non-Hispanics, Hispanics, African Americans and Asians: differences in survival after diagnosis. Cancer Causes Control 2005;16:587–592.
30. McNeill DE, Coté TR, Clegg L, et al. Incidence and trends in pediatric malignancies medulloblastoma/primitive neuroectodermal tumor: a SEER update. Med Pediatr Oncol 2002;39:190–194.
31. Suh Y-L, Koo H, Kim TS, et al. Tumors of the central nervous system in Korea. J Neurooncol 2002;56:251–259.
32. Kadri H, Mawla AA, Murad L. Incidence of childhood brain tumors in Syria (1993–2002). Pediatr Neurosurg 2005;41:173–177.
33. López-Aguilar E, Sepúlveda-Vildósola AC, Rivera-Márquez HR, et al. Clinical and molecular parameters for risk stratification in Mexican children with medulloblastoma. Arch Med Res 2007;38:769–773.
34. Dreifaldt AC, Carlberg M, Hardell L. Increasing incidence rates of childhood malignant diseases in Sweden during the period 1960–1998. Eur J Cancer 2004;40:1351–1360.
35. Stavrou T, Bromley CM, Nicholson HS, et al. Prognostic factors and secondary malignancies in childhood medulloblastoma. J Pediatr Hematol Oncol 2001;23:431–436.
36. Amlash SFA, Riffaud L, Brassier G, et al. Nevoid basal cell carcinoma syndrome: relation with desmoplastic medulloblastoma in infancy. Cancer 2003;98:618–624.
37. Bakhshi S, Cerosaletti KM, Concannon P, et al. Medulloblastoma with adverse reaction to radiation therapy in Nijmegen breakage syndrome. J Pediatr Hematol Oncol 2003;25:248–251.
38. Attard TM, Giglio P, Koppula S, et al. Brain tumors in individuals with familial adenomatous polyposis. Cancer 2007;109:761–766.
39. Ng D, Stavrou T, Liu L, et al. Retrospective family study of childhood medulloblastoma. Am J Med Genet 2005;134A:399–403.

40. Evans G, Burnell L, Campbell R, et al. Congenital anomalies and genetic syndromes in 173 cases of medulloblastoma. Med Pediatr Oncol 1993;21:433–434.
41. Srivastava S, Zou ZQ, Pirollo K, et al. Germ-line transmission of a mutated p53 gene in a cancer-prone family with Li-Fraumeni syndrome. Nature 1990;348:747–749.
42. de Bont J, Packer R, Michiels E, et al. Biologic background of pediatric medulloblastoma and ependymoma: a review from a translational research standpoint. Neuro-Oncol 2008;10:1040–1060.
43. Thompson MC, Fuller C, Hogg TL, et al. Genomics identifies medulloblastoma subgroups that are enriched for specific genetic alterations. J Clin Oncol 2006;24:924–1931.
44. Eberhart CG, Kepner JL, Goldthwaite PT, et al. Histopathologic grading of medulloblastomas: a Pediatric Oncology Group study. Cancer 2002;94:552–560.
45. Taylor MD, Mainprize TG, Rutka JT, et al. Molecular insight into medulloblastoma and central nervous system primitive neuroectodermal tumor biology from hereditary syndromes: a review. Neurosurgery 2000;47:888–901.
46. Clifford SB, Lusher MR, Lindsey JC, et al. Wnt/wingless pathway activation and chromosome 6 loss characterize a distinct molecular sub-group of medulloblastomas associated with a favorable prognosis. Cell Cycle 2006;5:2666–2670.
47. Bunin G. What causes childhood brain tumors? Limited knowledge, many clues. Pediatr Neurosurg 2000;32:321–326.
48. Preston-Martin S. Epidemiology of primary CNS neoplasms. Neurol Clin 1996;14: 273–290.
49. Bunin GR, Kushi LH, Gallagher PR, et al. Maternal diet during pregnancy and its association with medulloblastoma in children: a Children's Oncology Group study. Cancer Causes Control 2005;16:877–891.
50. Ron E, Modan B, Boice JD Jr, et al. Tumors of the brain and nervous system after radiotherapy in childhood. N Engl J Med 1988;319:1033–1039.
51. Kimball DV, Gelber RD, Li F, et al. Second malignancies in patients treated for childhood acute lymphoblastic leukemia. J Clin Oncol 1998;16:2848–2853.
52. Rimm IJ, Li FC, Tarbell NJ, et al. Brain tumors after cranial irradiation for childhood acute lymphoblastic leukemia. A 13-year experience from the Dana-Farber Cancer Institute and the Children's Hospital. Cancer 1987;59:1506–1508.
53. Neglia JP, Meadows AT, Robison LL, et al. Second neoplasms after acute lymphoblastic leukemia in childhood. N Engl J Med 1991;325:1330–1336.
54. Hoffman S, Schellinger KA, Propp JM, et al. Seasonal variation in incidence of pediatric medulloblastoma in the United States, 1995–2001. Neuroepidemiology 2007;29: 89–95.
55. Farwell JR, Dohrmann GJ, Glannery JT. Medulloblastoma in childhood: an epidemiological study. J Neurosurg 1984;61:657–664.
56. Fine HA. Polyomavirus and medulloblastoma: a smoking gun or guilt by association? J Natl Cancer Inst 2002;94:240–241.
57. Khalili K, Del Valle L, Otte J, et al. Human neurotropic polyomavirus, JCV, and its role in carcinogenesis. Oncogene 2003;22:5181–5191.
58. Kim JY, Koralnik IJ, LeFave M, et al. Medulloblastomas and primitive neuroectodermal tumors rarely contain polyomavirus DNA sequences. Neuro-Oncol 2002;4:165–170.
59. Ruud E, Wesenberg F. Microcephalus, medulloblastoma and excessive toxicity from chemotherapy: an unusual presentation of Fanconi anaemia. Acta Paediatr 2001;90: 580–583.
60. Taylor MD, Mainprize TG, Rutka JT, et al. Medulloblastoma in a child with Rubenstein-Taybi syndrome: case report and review of the literature. Pediatr Neurosurg 2001;35: 235–238.
61. Bisson E, Florman J, Wald S, et al. Primitive neuroectodermal tumor arising in long-standing cerebellar atrophy. Pediatr Neurosurg 2003;38:76–78.
62. Erman T, Sasmaz I, Göcer AI, et al. Turner syndrome and medulloblastoma. Neurosurg Q 2004;14:17–184.
63. Tischkowitz MD, Chisholm J, Gaze M, et al. Medulloblastoma as a first presentation of Fanconi anemia. J Pediatr Hematol Oncol 2004;26:52–55.
64. Palmer L, Nordborg C, Steneryd K, et al. Large-cell medulloblastoma in Aicardi syndrome. Neuropediatrics 2004;35:307–311.
65. Monteith SJ, Heppner PA, Woodfield MJ, et al. Paediatric central nervous system tumours in a New Zealand population: a 10-year experience of epidemiology, management strategies and outcomes. J Clin Neurosci 2006;13:722–729.
66. MacDonald TJ, Rood B, Santi MR, et al. Advances in the diagnosis, molecular genetics, and treatment of pediatric embryonal CNS tumors. Oncologist 2003;8:174–186.
67. Elgamal EA, Richards PG, Patel UJ. Fatal haemorrhage in medulloblastoma following ventricular drainage. Pediatr Neurosurg 2006;42:45–48.
68. Akay KM, Erdogan E, Izci Y, et al. Medulloblastoma of the cerebellopontine angle. Neurol Med Chir (Tokyo) 2003;3:555–558.
69. Jaiswal AK, Mahapatra AK, Sharma MC. Cerebellopointine angle medulloblastoma. J Clin Neurosci 2004;11:42–45.
70. Malheiros SMF, Franco CMR, Stávale JN, et al. Medulloblastoma in adults: a series from Brazil. J Neuro-Oncol 2002;60:247–253.
71. Koeller KK, Rushing EJ. From the archives of the AFIP: medulloblastoma: a comprehensive review with radiologic-pathologic correlation. Radiographics 2003;23(6): 1613–1637.
72. Zimmerman RA, Haselgrove JC, Bilaniuk LT, et al. Diffusion-weighted imaging and fluid attenuated inversion recovery imaging in the evaluation of primitive neuroectodermal tumors. Neuroradiology 2001;43:927–933.
73. Rumboldt Z, Camacho DL, Lake D, et al. Apparent diffusion coefficients for differentiation of cerebellar tumors in children. AJNR Am J Neuroradiol 2006;27(6):1362–1369.
74. Sugahara T, Korogi Y, Kochi M, et al. Usefulness of diffusion-weighted MRI with echo-planar technique in the evaluation of cellularity in gliomas. J Magn Reson Imaging 1999;9:53–60.
75. Erdem E, Zimmerman RA, Haselgrove JC, et al. Diffusion-weighted imaging and fluid attenuated inversion recovery imaging in the evaluation of primitive neuroectodermal tumors. Neuroimaging Clin N Am 2001;43:927–933.
76. Wang Z, Sutton LN, Cnaan A, et al. Proton MR spectroscopy of pediatric cerebellar tumors. Am J Neuroradiol 1995;16:1821–1833.
77. Sutton LN, Lasner T, Hunter J, et al. Thirteen-year-old female with hemangioblastomas. Pediatr Neurosurg 1997;27:50–55.
78. Bailey P, Cushing H. Medulloblastoma cerebelli: a common type of cerebellar glioma of childhood. Arch Neurol Psychiatry 1925;14:192–225.
79. Cushing H. Experiences with the cerebellar medulloblastoma: a critical review. Acta Pathol Microbiol Scand 1930;7:1–86.
80. Rorke LB. The cerebellar medulloblastoma and its relationship to primitive neuroectodermal tumors. J Neuropathol Exp Neurol 1983;42:1–15.
81. Hart MN, Earle KM. Primitive neuroectodermal tumors of the brain in children. Cancer 1973;32:890–897.
82. Kershman J. The medulloblast and medulloblastoma. A study of human embryos. Arch Neurol Psychiat 1938;40:937–967.
83. Fujita S. Quantitative analysis of cell proliferation and differentiation in the cortex of the postnatal mouse cerebellum. J Cell Biol 1967;32:277–287.
84. Fujita S, Shimada M, Nakamura T. H3-thymidine autoradiographic studies on the cell proliferation and differentiation in the external and the internal granular layers of the mouse cerebellum. J Comp Neurol 1966;128:191–208.
85. Swarz JR, Del Cerro M. Lack of evidence for glial cells originating from the external granular layer in mouse cerebellum. J Neurocytol 1977;6:241–250.
86. Fulop Z, Lakos I, Basco E, et al. Identification of early glial elements as the precursors of Bergmann-glia: a Golgi-analysis of the developing rat cerebellar cortex. Acta Morphol Acad Sci Hung 1979;27:273–280.
87. Ghandour MS, Labourdette G, Vincendon G, et al. A biochemical and immunohistological study of S100 protein in developing rat cerebellum. Dev Neurosci 1981;4: 98–109.
88. Wechsler-Reya RJ, Scott MP. Control of neuronal precursor proliferation in the cerebellum by Sonic Hedgehog. Neuron 1999;22:103–114.
89. Kenney AM, Cole MD, Rowitch DH. Nmyc upregulation by sonic hedgehog signaling promotes proliferation in developing cerebellar granule neuron precursors. Development 2003;130:15–28.
90. Wetmore C. Sonic hedgehog in normal and neoplastic proliferation: insight gained from human tumors and animal models. Curr Opin Genet Dev 2003;13:34–42.
91. Marino S, Vooijs M, van Der Gulden H, et al. Induction of medulloblastomas in p53-null mutant mice by somatic inactivation of Rb in the external granular layer cells of the cerebellum. Genes Dev 2000;14:994–1004.
92. Pomeroy SL, Tamayo P, Gaasenbeek M, et al. Prediction of central nervous system embryonal tumour outcome based on gene expression. Nature 2002;415:436–442.
93. Pomeroy SL, Sturla LM. Molecular biology of medulloblastoma therapy. Pediatr Neurosurg 2003;39:299–304.
94. Ellison D. Classifying the medulloblastoma: insights from morphology and molecular genetics. Neuropathol Appl Neurobiol 2002;28:257–282.
95. Giangaspero F, Eberhart CG, Haapasalo H, et al. Medulloblastoma. In: Louis DN, Ohgaki H, Wiestler OD, et al., eds. WHO classification of tumours of the central nervous system. Lyon, France: Intl Agency Research Cancer, 2007:132–146.
96. Kool M, Koster J, Bunt J, et al. Integrated genomics identifies five medulloblastoma subtypes with distinct genetic profiles, pathway signatures and clinicopathological features. PLoS One 2008;3(8):e3088.
97. Taylor MD, Liu L, Raffel C, et al. Mutations in SUFU predispose to medulloblastoma. Nat Genet 2002;31:306–310.
98. Aldosari N, Rasheed BK, McLendon RE, et al. Characterization of chromosome 17 abnormalities in medulloblastomas. Acta Neuropathol (Berl) 2000;99:345–351.
99. deHaas T, Oussoren E, Grajkowska W, et al. OTX 1 and OTX 2 expression correlates with the clinicopathologic classification of medulloblastoma. J Neuropath Exp Neurol 2006;65:176–186.
100. Briggs KJ, Corcoran-Schwaratz IM, Zhang W, et al. Cooperation between the Hic 1 and Ptch 1 tumor suppressors in medulloblastoma. Genes Dev 2008;22:770–785.
101. Rorke L, Hart M, McLendon RE. Supratentorial primitive neuroectodermal tumor (PNET). Lyon, France: IARC Press, 2000.
102. Shapira E, Marom K, Yelin R, et al. A role for the homeobox gene Xvex-1 as part of the BMP-4 ventral signaling pathway. Mech Dev 1999;86:99–111.
103. Tarabykin V, Britanova O, Fradkov A, et al. Expression of PTTG and prc1 genes during telencephalic neurogenesis. Mech Dev 2000;92:301–304.
104. Boquet I, Hitier R, Dumas M, et al. Central brain postembryonic development in Drosophila: implication of genes expressed at the interhemispheric junction. J Neurobiol 2000;42:33–48.
105. Ho KS, Scott MP. Sonic hedgehog in the nervous system: functions, modifications and mechanisms. Curr Opin Neurobiol 2002;12:57–63.
106. Schuurmans C, Guillemot F. Molecular mechanisms underlying cell fate specification in the developing telencephalon. Curr Opin Neurobiol 2002;12:26–34.
107. Rubenstien J, Puelles L. Development of the nervous system. New York: Oxford University Press, 2004.
108. Rorke LB. Pathology of brain and spinal cord tumors. In: Chous M, Di Rocco C, Hockley AD, et al., eds. Pediatric neurosurgery. London: Churchill Livingstone, 1999.
109. Rorke-Adams L. Tumors. In: Gilbert-Barness E, ed. Potter's pathology of the fetus, infant and child. 2nd ed. Philadelphia, PA: Mosby-Elsevier, 2007:2077–2092.
110. Gould VE, Jansson DS, Molenaar WM, et al. Primitive neuroectodermal tumors of the central nervous system. Patterns of expression of neuroendocrine markers, and all classes of intermediate filament proteins. Lab Invest 1990;62:498–509.
111. Molenaar WM, Jansson DS, Gould VE, et al. Molecular markers of primitive neuroectodermal tumors and other pediatric central nervous system tumors. Monoclonal antibodies to neuronal and glial antigens distinguish subsets of primitive neuroectodermal tumors. Lab Invest 1989;61:635–643.
112. Russell DS, Rubinstein LJ. Pathology of tumors of the nervous system. 5th ed. Baltimore, MD: Williams & Wilkins, 1989.
113. Giangaspero F, Rigobello L, Badiali M, et al. Large-cell medulloblastomas. A distinct variant with highly aggressive behavior. Am J Surg Pathol 1992;16:687–693.
114. Eberhart C, Kratz J, Schuster A, et al. Comparative genomic hybridization detects an increased number of chromosomal alterations in large cell/anaplastic medulloblastomas. Brain Pathol 2002;12:36–44.
115. Brown HG, Kepner JL, Perlman EJ, et al. "Large cell/anaplastic" medulloblastomas: a Pediatric Oncology Group Study. J Neuropathol Exp Neurol 2000;59:857–865.
116. Allen JC, Epstein F. Medulloblastoma and other primary malignant neuroectodermal tumors of the CNS. The effect of patients' age and extent of disease on prognosis. J Neurosurg 1982;57:446–451.
117. Deutsch M, Reigel DH. The value of myelography in the management of childhood medulloblastoma. Cancer 1980;45:2194–2197.
118. Berry MP, Jenkin RD, Keen CW, et al. Radiation treatment for medulloblastoma. A 21-year review. J Neurosurg 1981;55:43–51.
119. Kleinman GM, Hochberg FH, Richardson EP Jr. Systemic metastases from medulloblastoma: report of two cases and review of the literature. Cancer 1981;48: 2296–2309.
120. Campbell AN, Chan HS, Becker LE, et al. Extracranial metastases in childhood primary intracranial tumors. A report of 21 cases and review of the literature. Cancer 1984; 53:974–981.

121. Tarbell NJ, Loeffler JS, Silver B, et al. The change in patterns of relapse in medulloblastoma. Cancer 1991;68:1600–1604.
122. Eberhart CG, Cohen KJ, Tihan T, et al. Medulloblastomas with systemic metastases: evaluation of tumor histopathology and clinical behavior in 23 patients. J Pediatr Hematol Oncol 2003;25:198–203.
123. Biegel JA, Burk CD, Barr FG, et al. Evidence for a 17p tumor related locus distinct from p53 in pediatric primitive neuroectodermal tumors. Cancer Res 1992;52:3391–3395.
124. Thomas GA, Raffel C. Loss of heterozygosity on 6q, 16q, and 17p in human central nervous system primitive neuroectodermal tumors. Cancer Res 1991;51:639–643.
125. Bigner SH, Mark J, Friedman HS, et al. Structural chromosomal abnormalities in human medulloblastoma. Cancer Genet Cytogenet 1988;30:91–101.
126. McDonald JD, Daneshvar L, Willert JR, et al. Physical mapping of chromosome 17p13.3 in the region of a putative tumor suppressor gene important in medulloblastoma. Genomics 1994;23:229–232.
127. Adesina AM, Nalbantoglu J, Cavenee WK. p53 gene mutation and mdm2 gene amplification are uncommon in medulloblastoma. Cancer Res 1994;54:5649–5651.
128. Griffin CA, Hawkins AL, Packer RJ, et al. Chromosome abnormalities in pediatric brain tumors. Cancer Res 1988;48:175–180.
129. Mendrzyk F, Radlwimmer B, Joos S, et al. Genomic and protein expression profiling identifies CDK6 as novel independent prognostic marker in medulloblastoma. J Clin Oncol 2005;23(34):8853–8862.
130. Pietsch T, Waha A, Koch A, et al. Medulloblastomas of the desmoplastic variant carry mutations of the human homologue of Drosophila patched. Cancer Res 1997;57: 2085–2088.
131. Raffel C, Jenkins RB, Frederick L, et al. Sporadic medulloblastomas contain PTCH mutations. Cancer Res 1997;57:842–845.
132. Xie J, Johnson RL, Zhang X, et al. Mutations of the PATCHED gene in several types of sporadic extracutaneous tumors. Cancer Res 1997;57:2369–2372.
133. Dong J, Gailani MR, Pomeroy SL, et al. Identification of PATCHED mutations in medulloblastomas by direct sequencing. Hum Mutat 2000;16:89–90.
134. Gilbertson R. Paediatric embryonic brain tumours: biological and clinical relevance of molecular genetic abnormalities. Eur J Cancer 2002;38:675–685.
135. Reardon DA, Michalkiewicz E, Boyett JM, et al. Extensive genomic abnormalities in childhood medulloblastoma by comparative genomic hybridization. Cancer Res 1997;57:4042–4047.
136. Biegel JA, Zhou JY, Rorke LB, et al. Germ-line and acquired mutations of INI1 in atypical teratoid and rhabdoid tumors. Cancer Res 1999;59:74–79.
137. Raffel C, Gilles FE, Weinberg KI. Reduction to homozygosity and gene amplification in central nervous system primitive neuroectodermal tumors of childhood. Cancer Res 1990;50:587–591.
138. Seizinger BR, Martuza RL, Gusella JF. Loss of genes on chromosome 22 in tumorigenesis of human acoustic neuroma. Nature 1986;322:644–647.
139. Goodrich LV, Milenkovic L, Higgins KM, et al. Altered neural cell fates and medulloblastoma in mouse patched mutants. Science 1997;227(22):1109–1112.
140. Berman DM, Karhadkar SS, Hallahan AR, et al. Medulloblastoma growth inhibition by hedgehog pathway blockade. Science 2002,297:1550–1561.
141. Fan X, Matsui W, Khaki L, et al. Notch pathway inhibition depletes stem-like cells and blocks engraftment in embryonal brain tumors. Cancer Res 2006;66:7445–7452.
142. Hernan R, Fasheh R, Calabrese C, et al. ERBB2 up-regulates S100A4 and several other prometastatic genes in medulloblastoma. Cancer Res 2003;63:140–148.
143. Lusher ME, Lindsey JC, Latif F, et al. Biallelic epigenetic inactivation of the RASSF1. A tumor suppressor gene in medulloblastoma development. Cancer Res 2001;62:5906–5911.
144. Kortmann RD, Kuhl J, Timmermann B, et al. Postoperative neoadjuvant chemotherapy before radiotherapy as compared to immediate radiotherapy followed by maintenance chemotherapy in the treatment of medulloblastoma in childhood: results of the German prospective randomized trial HIT '91. Int J Radiat Oncol Biol Phys 2000;46:269–279.
145. Bouffet E, Gentet JC, Doz F, et al. Metastatic medulloblastoma: the experience of the French Cooperative M7 Group. Eur J Cancer 1994;30A:1478–1483.
146. Zeltzer PM, Boyett JM, Finlay JL, et al. Metastasis stage, adjuvant treatment, and residual tumor are prognostic factors for medulloblastoma in children: conclusions from the Children's Cancer group 921 randomized phase III study. J Clin Oncol 1999;17: 8322–8345.
147. Oyharcabal-Bourden V, Kalifa C, Gentet JC, et al. Standard-risk medulloblastoma treated by adjuvant chemotherapy followed by reduced-dose craniospinal radiation therapy: a French Society of Pediatric Oncology study. J Clin Oncol 2005;23:4726–4734.
148. Albright AL, Sposto R, Holmes E, et al. Correlation of neurosurgical subspecialization with outcomes in children with malignant brain tumors. Neurosurgery 2000;47:879–885.
149. Bailey CC, Gnekow A, Wellek S, et al. Prospective randomized trial of chemotherapy given before radiotherapy in childhood medulloblastoma. International Society of Paediatric Oncology (SIOP) and the (German) Society of Paediatric Oncology (GPO): SIOP II. Med Pediatr Oncol 1995;25:166–178.
150. Albright AL, Wisoff JH, Zeltzer PM, et al. Effects of medulloblastoma resections on outcome in children: a report from the Children's Cancer Group. Neurosurgery 1996;38:265–271.
151. Jenkin D, Goddard K, Armstrong D, et al. Posterior fossa medulloblastoma in childhood: treatment results and a proposal for a new staging system. Int J Radiat Oncol Biol Phys 1990;19:265–274.
152. Evans AE, Jenkin RD, Sposto R, et al. The treatment of medulloblastoma. Results of a prospective randomized trial of radiation therapy with and without CCNU, vincristine, and prednisone. J Neurosurg 1990;72:572–582.
153. Hughes EN, Shillito J, Sallan SE, et al. Medulloblastoma at the joint center for radiation therapy between 1968 and 1984. The influence of radiation dose on the patterns of failure and survival. Cancer 1988;61:1992–1998.
154. Tait DM, Thornton-Jones H, Bloom HJ, et al. Adjuvant chemotherapy for medulloblastoma: the first multi-centre control trial of the International Society of Paediatric Oncology (SIOP I). Eur J Cancer 1990;26:464–469.
155. Grill J, Sainte-Rose C, Jouvet A, et al. Treatment of medulloblastoma with postoperative chemotherapy alone: an SFOP prospective trial in young children. Lancet 2005;6: 573–579.
156. Dhall G, Grodman H, Ji L, et al. Outcome of children less than three years old at diagnosis with non-metastatic medulloblastoma treated with chemotherapy on the "Head Start" I and II protocols. Pediatr Blood Cancer 2008;50:1169–1175.
157. Tomita T, Yasue M, Engelhard HH, et al. Flow cytometric DNA analysis of medulloblastoma. Prognostic implication of aneuploidy. Cancer 1988;61:744–749.
158. Batra SK, McLendon RE, Koo JS, et al. Prognostic implications of chromosome 17p deletions in human medulloblastomas. J Neurooncol 1995;24:39–45.
159. Jung HL, Wang KC, Kim SK, et al. Loss of heterozygosity analysis of chromosome 17p13.1–13.3 and its correlation with clinical outcome in medulloblastomas. J Neuro Oncol 2004;67:41–46.
160. Scheurlen WG, Schwabe GC, Joos S, et al. Molecular analysis of childhood primitive neuroectodermal tumors defines markers associated with poor outcome. J Clin Oncol 1998;16:2478–2485.
161. Rasmussen T. Surgical aspects of temporal lobe epilepsy. Results and problems. Acta Neurochir Suppl (Wien) 1980;30:13–24.
162. MacDonald TJ, Brown KM, LaFleur B, et al. Expression profiling of medulloblastoma: PDGFRA and the RAS/MAPK pathway as therapeutic targets for metastatic disease. Nat Genet 2001;29:143–149.
163. Segal RA, Goumnerova LC, Kwon YK, et al. Expression of the neurotrophin receptor TrkC is linked to a favorable outcome in medulloblastoma. Proc Natl Acad Sci U S A 1994;91:12867–12871.
164. Grotzer MA, Janss AJ, Fung K, et al. TrkC expression predicts good clinical outcome in primitive neuroectodermal brain tumors. J Clin Oncol 2000;18:1027–1035.
165. Kim JY, Sutton ME, Lu DJ, et al. Activation of neurotrophin-3 receptor TrkC induces apoptosis in medulloblastomas. Cancer Res 1999;59:711–719.
166. Pingoud-Meier C, Lang D, Janss AJ, et al. Loss of caspase-8 protein expression correlates with unfavorable survival outcome in childhood medulloblastoma. Clin Cancer Res 2003;9:6401–6409.
167. Gilbertson R, Wickramashinghe C, Hernan R, et al. Clinical and molecular stratification of disease risk in medulloblastoma. Br J Cancer 2001;85:705–712.
168. Lamont JM, McManamy CS, Pearson AD, et al. Combined histopathological and molecular cytogenetic stratification of medulloblastoma patients. Clin Cancer Res 1004;20:5482–5493.
169. Northcott PA, Nakahara Y, Wu X, et al. Multiple recurrent genetic events converge on control of histone lysine methylation in medulloblastoma. Nat Genet 2009;41(4): 465–472.
170. Garzia L, Andolfo I, Cusanelli E, et al. MicroRNA-199b-5p impairs cancer stem cells through negative regulation of HES1 in medulloblastoma. PLoS One 2009;4(3): e4998.
171. De Haas T, Hasselt N, Troost D, et al. Molecular risk stratification of medulloblastoma patients based on immunohistochemical analysis of MYC, LDHB, and CCNB1 expression. Clin Cancer Res 2008;14:4154–4160.
172. Takei H, Nguyen Y, Mehta V, et al. Low-level copy gain versus amplification of myc oncogenes in medulloblastoma: utility in predicting prognosis and survival. J Neurosurg Pediatr 2009;3:61–65.
173. Rutkowski S, Bode U, Deinlein F, et al. Treatment of early childhood medulloblastoma by postoperative chemotherapy alone. N Engl J Med 2005;352:978–986.
174. Dias MS, Albright AL. Management of hydrocephalus complicating childhood posterior fossa tumors. Pediatr Neurosci 1989;15:283–289.
175. Jones RF, Stening WA, Brydon M. Endoscopic third ventriculostomy. Neurosurgery 1990;26:86–91.
176. Hopf NJ, Grunert P, Fries G, et al. Endoscopic third ventriculostomy: outcome analysis of 100 consecutive procedures. Neurosurgery 1999;44:795–804.
177. Wisoff JH, Epstein FJ. Pseudobulbar palsy after posterior fossa operation in children. Neurosurgery 1984;15:707–709.
178. Wells EM, Waalsh KS, Khademian ZP, et al. The cerebellar mutism syndrome and its relation to cerebellar cognitive function and the cerebellar cognitive affective disorder. Deve Disabil Res Rev 2008;14:221–228.
179. Robertson PL, Muraszko KM, Holmes EJ, et al. Incidence and severity of postoperative cerebellar mutism syndrome in children with medulloblastoma: a prospective study by the Children's Oncology Group. J Neurosurg 2006;105(6 suppl):444–451.
180. Ozgur BM, Berberian J, Aryan HE. The pathophysiologic mechanism of cerebellar mutism. Surg Neurol 2006;66:18–25.
181. Turgut M. Transient "cerebellar" mutism. Childs Nerv Syst 1998;14:161–166.
182. Belza MG, Donaldson SS, Steinberg GK, et al. Medulloblastoma: freedom from relapse longer than 8 years—a therapeutic cure? J Neurosurg 1991;75:575–582.
183. Shaw DW, Geyer JR, Berger MS, et al. Asymptomatic recurrence detection with surveillance scanning in children with medulloblastoma. J Clin Oncol 1997;15:1811–1813.
184. Neglia JP, Robison LL, Stovall M, et al. New primary neoplasms of the central nervous system in survivors of childhood cancer: a report from the Childhood Cancer Survivor Study. J Natl Cancer Inst 2006;98:1528–1537.
185. Siffert J, Poussaint TY, Goumnerova LC, et al. Neurological dysfunction associated with postoperative cerebellar mutism. J Neuro-Oncol 2000;48:75–81.
186. Bouffet E, Bernard JL, Frappaz D, et al. M4 protocol for cerebellar medulloblastoma: supratentorial radiotherapy may not be avoided. Int J Radiat Oncol Biol Phys 1992; 24:79–85.
187. Merchant TE, Kun LE, Krasin MJ, et al. Multi-institution prospective trial of reduced-dose craniospinal irradiation (23.4 Gy) followed by conformal posterior fossa (36 Gy) and primary site irradiation (55.8 Gy) and dose-intensive chemotherapy for average-risk medulloblastoma. Int J Radiat Oncol Biol Phys 2008;70(3):782–787.
188. Thomas PR, Deutsch M, Kepner JL, et al. Low-stage medulloblastoma: final analysis of trial comparing standard-dose with reduced-dose neuraxis irradiation. J Clin Oncol 2000;18:3004–3011.
189. Butler RW, Haser JK. Neurocognitive effects of treatment for childhood cancer. Mental retardation and developmental disabilities research reviews. 2006;12:184–191.
190. Packer RJ, Goldwein J, Nicholson HS, et al. Treatment of children with medulloblastomas with reduced-dose craniospinal radiation therapy and adjuvant chemotherapy: a Children's Cancer Group Study. J Clin Oncol 1999;17:2127–2136.
191. Goldwein JW, Radcliffe J, Johnson J, et al. Updated results of a pilot study of low dose craniospinal irradiation plus chemotherapy for children under five with cerebellar primitive neuroectodermal tumors (medulloblastoma). Int J Radiat Oncol Biol Phys 1996; 34:899–904.
192. Jakacki RI, Feldman H, Jamison C, et al. A pilot study of preirradiation chemotherapy and 1800 cGy craniospinal irradiation in young children with medulloblastoma. Int J Radiat Oncol Biol Phys 2004;60(2):531–536.
193. Gajjar A, Chintagumpala M, Ashley D, et al. Risk-adapted craniospinal radiotherapy followed by high-dose chemotherapy and stem-cell rescue in children with newly diagnosed medulloblastoma (St Jude Medulloblastoma-96): long-term results from a prospective, multicentre trial. Lancet Oncol 2006;7(10):813–820.
194. Gandola L, Massimino M, Cefalo G, et al. Hyperfractionated accelerated radiotherapy in the Milan strategy for metastatic medulloblastoma. J Clin Oncol 2009;27(4): 566–571.

195. Allen J, Donahue B, Mehta M, et al. A phase II study of preradiotherapy chemotherapy followed by hyperfractionated radiotherapy for newly diagnosed high-risk medulloblastoma/primitive neuroectodermal tumor: a report from the Children's Oncology Group (CCG 9931). Int J Radiat Oncol Biol Phys 2009;74(4):1006–1011.
196. Miralbell R, Fitzgerald TJ, Laurie F, et al. Radiotherapy in pediatric medulloblastoma: quality assessment of Pediatric Oncology Group Trial 9031. Int J Radiat Oncol Biol Phys 2006;64(5):1325–1330.
197. Taylor RE, Bailey CC, Robinson KJ, et al. Impact of radiotherapy parameters on outcome in the International Society of Paediatric Oncology/United Kingdom Children's Cancer Study Group PNET-3 study of preradiotherapy chemotherapy for M0-M1 medulloblastoma. Int J Radiat Oncol Biol Phys 2004;58(4):1184–1193.
198. Carrie C, Muracciole X, Gomez F, et al. Conformal radiotherapy, reduced boost volume, hyperfractionated radiotherapy, and online quality control in standard-risk medulloblastoma without chemotherapy: results of the French M-SFOP 98 protocol. Int J Radiat Oncol Biol Phys 2005;63(3):711–716.
199. Miralbell R, Lomax A, Bortfeld T, et al. Potential role of proton therapy in the treatment of pediatric medulloblastoma/primitive neuroectodermal tumors: reduction of the supratentorial target volume. Int J Radiat Oncol Biol Phys 1997;38:477–484.
200. Gripp S, Kambergs J, Wittkamp M, et al. Coverage of anterior fossa in whole-brain irradiation. Int J Radiat Oncol Biol Phys 2004;59(2):515–520.
201. Wilson VC, McDonough J, Tochner Z. Proton beam irradiation in pediatric oncology: an overview. J Pediatr Hematol Oncol 2005;27(8):444–448.
202. Wolden SL, Dunkel IJ, Souweidane MM, et al. Patterns of failure using a conformal radiation therapy tumor bed boost for medulloblastoma. J Clin Oncol 2003;21:3079–3083.
203. Muscal JA, Jones JY, Paulino AC, et al. Changes mimicking new leptomeningeal disease after intensity-modulated radiotherapy for medulloblastoma. Int J Radiat Oncol Biol Phys 2009;73(1):214–221.
204. Breen SL, Kehagioglou P, Usher C, et al. A comparison of conventional, conformal and intensity-modulated coplanar radiotherapy plans for posterior fossa treatment. Br J Radiol 2004;77(921):768–774.
205. Huang E, Teh BS, Strother DR, et al. Intensity-modulated radiation therapy for pediatric medulloblastoma: early report on the reduction of ototoxicity. Int J Radiat Oncol Biol Phys 2002;52(3):599–605.
206. St Clair WH, Adams JA, Bues M, et al. Advantage of protons compared to conventional X-ray or IMRT in the treatment of a pediatric patient with medulloblastoma. Int J Radiat Oncol Biol Phys 2004;58(3):727–734.
207. Merchant TE, Boop FA, Kun LE, et al. A retrospective study of surgery and reirradiation for recurrent ependymoma. Int J Radiat Oncol Biol Phys 2008;71(1):87–97.
208. Merchant TE, Hua CH, Shukla H, et al. Proton versus photon radiotherapy for common pediatric brain tumors: comparison of models of dose characteristics and their relationship to cognitive function. Pediatr Blood Cancer 2008;51(1):110–117.
209. Bertolone SJ, Baum ES, Krivit W, et al. A phase II study of cisplatin therapy in recurrent childhood brain tumors: a report from the Children's Cancer Group. J Neuro-Oncol 1989;7:5–11.
210. Packer RJ. Childhood medulloblastoma: Progress and future challenges. Brain Dev 1999;21:75–81.
211. Allen JC, Helson L, Jereb B. Preradiation chemotherapy for newly diagnosed childhood brain tumors. A modified Phase II trial. Cancer 1983;52:2001–2006.
212. Pendergrass TW, Milstein JM, Geyer JR, et al. Eight drugs in one day chemotherapy for brain tumors: experience in 107 children and rationale for preradiation chemotherapy. J Clin Oncol 1987;5:1221–1231.
213. Kovnar EH, Kellie SJ, Horowitz ME, et al. Preirradiation cisplatin and etoposide in the treatment of high-risk medulloblastoma and other malignant embryonal tumors of the central nervous system: a phase II study. J Clin Oncol 1990;8:330–336.
214. Mosijczuk AD, Nigro MA, Thomas PR, et al. Preradiation chemotherapy in advanced medulloblastoma. A Pediatric Oncology Group pilot study. Cancer 1993;72:2755–2762.
215. Heideman RL, Kovnar EH, Kellie SJ, et al. Preirradiation chemotherapy with carboplatin and etoposide in newly diagnosed embryonal pediatric CNS tumors. J Clin Oncol 1995;13:2247–2254.
216. Taylor RE, Bailey CC, Robinson K, et al. Results of a randomized study of preradiation chemotherapy versus radiotherapy alone for nonmetastatic medulloblastoma: The International Society of Paediatric Oncology/United Kingdom Children's Cancer Study Group PNET-3 Study. J Clin Oncol 2003;21:1581–1591.
217. Loeffler JS, Kretschmar CS, Sallan SE, et al. Pre-radiation chemotherapy for infants and poor prognosis children with medulloblastoma. Int J Radiat Oncol Biol Phys 1988;15:177–181.
218. Taylor RE, Bailey CC, Robinson KJ, et al. Outcome for outpatients with metastatic (2–3) medulloblastoma treated with SIOP/KCCSG PNET-3 chemotherapy. Eur J Cancer 2005;41:727–734.
219. Di C, Liao S, Adamson DC, et al. Identification of OTX2 as a medulloblastoma oncogene whose product can be targeted by all-trans retinoic acid. Cancer Res 2005;65(3):919–24.
220. Gentet JC, Bouffet E, Doz F, et al. Preirradiation chemotherapy including "eight drugs in 1 day" regimen and high dose methotrexate in childhood medulloblastoma: results of the M7 French cooperative study. J Neurosurg 1995;82:608–14.
221. McIntosh S, Chen M, Sartain PA, et al. Adjuvant chemotherapy for medulloblastoma. Cancer 1985;56:1316–1319.
222. Jakacki R, Zhou T, Holmes E, et al. PNET/MED 31. Outcome for patients with nonpineal supratentorial PNET treated with carboplatin as a radiosensitizer during radiotherapy (RT) followed by adjuvant cyclophosphamide (CPM) and vincristine (VCR): preliminary results of COG 99701. Neuro-Oncology 2009;10:485.
223. Ater JL, van Eys J, Woo SY, et al. MOPP chemotherapy without irradiation as primary postsurgical therapy for brain tumors in infants and young children. J Neuro-Oncol 1997;32:243–252.
224. Duffner PK, Horowitz ME, Krischer JP, et al. Postoperative chemotherapy and delayed radiation in children less than three years of age with malignant brain tumors. N Engl J Med 1993;328(24):1725–1731.
225. Geyer JR, Jennings M, Sposto R, et al. Multiagent chemotherapy and deferred radiotherapy in infants with malignant brain tumors: a report from the Children's Cancer Group. J Clin Oncol 2005;23:7621–7631.
226. Gaynon PS, Ettinger LJ, Baum ES, et al. Carboplatin in childhood brain tumors. A Children's Cancer Study Group phase II trial. Cancer 1990;66:2465–2469.
227. Lefkowitz IB, Packer RJ, Siegel KR, et al. Results of treatment of children with recurrent medulloblastoma/primitive neuroectodermal tumors with lomustine, cisplatin, and vincristine. Cancer 1990;65:412–417.
228. Mooghrabi A, Fuchs H, Brown M, et al. Cyclophosphamide in combination with sargramostim for treatment of recurrent medulloblastoma. Med Pediatr Oncol 1995;25:190–196.
229. Friedman HS, Mahaley S, Schold SC, et al. Efficacy of vincristine and cyclophosphamide in the therapy of recurrent medulloblastoma. Neurosurgery 1986;18:335–340.
230. Allen JC, Walker R, Luks E, et al. Carboplatin and recurrent childhood brain tumors. J Clin Oncol 1987;5:459–463.
231. Dunkel IJ, Finlay J. High dose chemotherapy with autologous stem cell rescue for patients with medulloblastoma. J Neuro-Oncol 1996;29:69–74.
232. Gururangan S, McLaughliln C, Quinn J, et al. High-dose chemotherapy with autologous stem-cell rescue in children and adults with newly diagnosed pineoblastomas. J Clin Oncol 2003;21(11):2187–2191.
233. Mason WP, Grovas A, Halpern S, et al. Intensive chemotherapy and bone marrow rescue for young children with newly diagnosed malignant brain tumors. J Clin Oncol 1998;16:210–221.
234. Fisher PG, Needle MN, Cnaan A, et al. Salvage therapy after postoperative chemotherapy for primary brain tumors in infants and very young children. Cancer 1998;83(3):566–574.
235. Dupuis-Girod S, Hartmann O, Benhamou E, et al. Will high dose chemotherapy followed by autologous bone marrow transplantation supplant cranio-spinal irradiation in young children treated for medulloblastoma? J Neurooncol 1996;27:87–98.
236. Mulhern RK, Horowitz ME, Kovnar EH, et al. Neurodevelopmental status of infants and young children treated for brain tumors with preirradiation chemotherapy. J Clin Oncol 1989;7:1660–1666.
237. Kao GD, Goldwein JW, Schultz DJ, et al. The impact of perioperative factors on subsequent intelligence quotient deficits in children treated for medulloblastoma/posterior fossa primitive neuroectodermal tumors. Cancer 1994;74:965–971.
238. Packer RJ, Sutton LN, Atkins TE, et al. A prospective study of cognitive function in children receiving whole-brain radiotherapy and chemotherapy: 2-year results. J Neurosurg 1989;70:707–713.
239. Anderson VA, Godber T, Smibert E, et al. Cognitive and academic outcome following cranial irradiation and chemotherapy in children: a longitudinal study. Br J Cancer 2000;82:255–262.
240. Johnson DL, McCabe MA, Nicholson HS, et al. Quality of long-term survival in young children with medulloblastoma. J Neurosurg 1994;80:1004–1010.
241. Silber JH, Radcliffe J, Peckham V, et al. Whole-brain irradiation and decline in intelligence: the influence of dose and age on IQ score. J Clin Oncol 1992;10:1390–1396.
242. Palmer SL, Goloubeva O, Reddick WE, et al. Patterns of intellectual development among survivors of pediatric medulloblastoma: a longitudinal analysis. J Clin Oncol 2001;19:2302–2308.
243. Palmer SL, Gajjar A, Reddick WE, et al. Predicting intellectual outcome among children treated with 35–40 Gy craniospinal irradiation for medulloblastoma. Neuropsychology 2003;17:548–555.
244. Hoppe-Hirsch E, Renier D, Lellouch-Tubiana A, et al. Medulloblastoma in childhood: progressive intellectual deterioration. Childs Nerv Syst 1990;6:60–65.
245. Dennis M, Spiegler BJ, Hoffman HJ, et al. Brain tumors in children and adolescents—I. Effects on working, associative and serial-order memory of IQ, age at tumor onset and age of tumor. Neuropsychologia 1991;29:813–827.
246. Mulhern RK, Merchant TE, Gajjar A, et al. Late neurocognitive sequelae in survivors of brain tumours in childhood. Lancet Oncol 2004;5:399–408.
247. Duffner PK, Cohen ME, Thomas PRM, et al. The long-term effects of cranial irradiation on the central nervous system. Cancer 1985;56:1841–1846.
248. Bull KS, Spoudeas HA, Yadegarfar G, et al. Reduction of health status 7 years after addition of chemotherapy to craniospinal irradiation for medulloblastoma: a follow-up study in PNET 3 trial survivors—on behalf of the CCLG (formerly UKCCSG). J Clin Oncol 2007;25(27):4239–4245.
249. Shalet SM, Gibson B, Swindell R, et al. Effect of spinal irradiation on growth. Arch Dis Child 1987;62:461–464.
250. Packer RJ, Gurney JG, Punyko JA, et al. Long-term neurologic and neurosensory sequelae in adult survivors of a childhood brain tumor. Childhood Cancer Survivor Study. J Clin Oncol 2003;21(17):3255–3261.
251. Olshan JS, Gubernick J, Packer RJ, et al. The effects of adjuvant chemotherapy on growth in children with medulloblastoma. Cancer 1992;70:2013–2017.
252. Gurney J, Ness KK, Stoval M, et al. Final height and body mass index among adult survivors of childhood brain cancer: Childhood Cancer Survivor Study. J Clin Endocrinol Metab 2003;88:4371–4379.
253. Packer RJ, Boyett JM, Janss AJ, et al. Growth hormone replacement therapy in children with medulloblastoma: use and effect on tumor control. J Clin Oncol 2001;19:480–487.
254. Moshang T Jr, Rundle AC, Graves DA, et al. Brain tumor recurrence in children treated with growth hormone: the National Cooperative Growth Study experience. J Pediatr 1996;128:S4–S7.
255. Swerdlow AJ, Reddingius RE, Higgins CD, et al. Growth hormone treatment of children with brain tumors and risk of tumor recurrence. J Clin Endocrinol Metab 2000;85:4444–4449.
256. Bowers DC, Liu Y, Leisenring W, et al. Late-occurring stroke among long-term survivors of childhood leukemia and brain tumors: a report from the Childhood Cancer Survival Study. J Clin Oncol 2006;24:5277–5282.
257. Robison LL, Green DM, Hudson M, et al. Long-term outcomes of adult survivors of childhood cancer: results from the Childhood Cancer Survivor Study 2005;104(S11):2557–25564.
258. Diller L, Chow RJ, Gurney JG, et al. Chronic disease in the childhood cancer survivor study cohort: a review of published findings. J Clin Oncol 2009;27:2339–2355.
259. Armstrong GT, Liu Q, Yasui Y, et al. Long-term outcome among adult survivors of childhood central nervous system malignancies: a report from the Childhood Cancer Survivor Study. J Natl Cancer Inst 2009;101:1–12.
260. Gaffney CC, Sloane JP, Bradley NJ, et al. Primitive neuroectodermal tumours of the cerebrum. Pathology and treatment. J Neurooncol 1985;3:23–33.
261. Yang HJ, Nam DH, Wang KC, et al. Supratentorial primitive neuroectodermal tumor in children: clinical features, treatment outcome and prognostic factors. Childs Nerv Syst 1999;15:377–383.
262. Dirks PB, Harris L, Hoffman HJ, et al. Supratentorial primitive neuroectodermal tumors in children. J Neuro Oncol 1996;29:75–84.
263. Cohen BH, Zeltzer PM, Boyett JM, et al. Prognostic factors and treatment results for supratentorial primitive neuroectodermal tumors in children using radiation and chemotherapy: a Children's Cancer Group randomized trial. J Clin Oncol 1995;13:1687–1696.

264. Johnston DL, Keene DL, Lafay-Cousin L, et al. Supratentorial primitive neuroectodermal tumors: a Canadian pediatric brain tumor consortium report. N Neurooncol 2008;86:101–108.
265. Al D, Backstrom JW, Burger PC, et al. Supratentorial primitive neuroectodermal tumors of infancy: clinical and radiologic findings. Pediatr Neurol 2003;29(5):430–434.
266. Russo C, Pellarin M, Tingby O, et al. Comparative genomic hybridization in patients with supratentorial and infratentorial primitive neuroectodermal tumors. Cancer 1999; 86:331–339.
267. Inda MM, Perot C, Guillaud-Battaille M, et al. Genetic heterogeneity in supratentorial and infratentorial primitive neuroectodermal tumors of the central nervous system. Histopathology 2005;47:631–637.
268. Pfister S, Remke M, Toedt G, et al. Supratentorial primitive neuroectodermal tumors of the central nervous system frequently harbor deletions of the CDKN2A locus and other genomic aberrations distinct from medulloblastomas. Genes, chromosomes and cancer 20007;46:839–851.
269. Albright AL, Wisoff JH, Zeltzer P, et al. Prognostic factors in children with supratentorial (nonpineal) primitive neuroectodermal tumors. A neurosurgical perspective from the Children's Cancer Group. Pediatr Neurosurg 1994;22:1–7.
270. McBride SM, Daganzo SM, Banerjee A, et al. Radiation is an important component of multimodality therapy for pediatric non-pineal supratentorial primitive neuroectodermal tumors. Int J Radiat Oncol Biol Phys 2008;72(5):1319–1323.
271. Albright AL, Wisoff JH, Zeltzer P, et al. Prognostic factors in children with supratentorial (nonpineal) primitive neuroectodermal tumors. Pediatr Neurosurg 1995;22:1–7.
272. Pizer BL, Weston CL, Robinson KJ, et al. Analysis of patients with supratentorial primitive neuro-ectodermal tumours entered into the SIOP/UKCCSG PNET 3 study. Eur J Cancer 2006;42(8):1120–1128.
273. Taylor RE, Donachie PH, Weston CL, et al. Impact of radiotherapy parameters on outcome for patients with supratentorial primitive neuro-ectodermal tumours entered into the SIOP/UKCCSG PNET 3 study. Radiother Oncol 2009;92(1):83–88.
274. Chintagumpala M, Hassall T, Palmer S, et al. A pilot study of risk-adapted radiotherapy and chemotherapy in patients with supratentorial PNET. Neuro Oncol 2009;11(1): 33–40.
275. Massimino M, Gandola L, Spreafico F, et al. Supratentorial primitive neuroectodermal tumors (S-PNET) in children: a prospective experience with adjuvant intensive chemotherapy and hyperfractionated accelerated radiotherapy. Int J Radiat Oncol Biol Phys 2006;64(4):1031–1037.
276. Hinkes BG, von Hoff K, Deinlein F, et al. Childhood pineoblastoma: experiences from the prospective multicenter trials HIT-SKK87, HIT-SKK92 and HIT91. J Neurooncol 2007;81(2):217–223.
277. Jakacki R. Pineal and nonpineal supratentorial primitive neuroectodermal tumors. Child Nerv Syst 1999;15:586–591.
278. Jakacki R, Zeltzer PM, Boyett JM, et al. Survival and prognostic factors following radiation and/or chemotherapy for primitive neuroectodermal tumors of the pineal region in infants and children: a report of the Childrens Cancer Group. J Clin Oncol 1995; 13(6):1377–1383.
279. Cuccia V, Rodriguez F, Palma F, et al. Pinealoblastoma in children. Childs Nerv Syst 2006;22(6):577–585.
280. DeGirolami U, Fevre-Montague M, Seilhean D, et al. Pathology of tumors of the pineal region. Rev Neurol 2008;164:882–895.
281. Bader JL, Meadows AT, Zimmerman LE, et al. Bilateral retinoblastoma with ectopic intracranial retinoblastoma: trilateral retinoblastoma. Cancer Genet Cytogenet 1982; 5:203–213.
282. Kees UR, Spagnolo D, Hallam et al. A new pineoblastoma cell line, PER 480, with der(10)t(10;17), der(16)t(1;16) and enhanced MYC expression in the absence of gene amplification. Cancer Genet Cytogenet 1998;100:159–164.
283. Mena H, Nakazato Y, Jouvet A, et al. Pineoblastoma. Pineocytoma. Pineal parenchymal tumor of intermediate differentiation. In: Kleihues P, Cavenee WK, eds. Tumors of the nervous system. 2nd ed. Lyon, France: IARC, 2000, 116–121.
284. Gilheeney SW, Saad A, Chi S, et al. Outcome of pediatric pineoblastoma after surgery, radiation and chemotherapy. J Neurooncol 2008;89(1):89–95.
285. Reddy AT, Janss AJ, Phillips PC, et al. Outcome for children with supratentorial primitive neuroectodermal tumors treated with surgery, radiation and chemotherapy. Cancer 2000;88:2189–2193.
286. Horton BC, Rubinstein LJ. Primary cerebral neuroblastoma, a clinicopathological study of 35 cases. Brain 1976;99:735–756.
287. Burger PC, Yu IT, Tihan T, et al. Atypical teratoid/rhabdoid tumor of the central nervous system: a highly malignant tumor of infancy and childhood frequently mistaken for medulloblastoma: a Pediatric Oncology Group study. Am J Surg Pathol 1998;22: 1083–1092.
288. Packer RJ, Biegel JA, Blaney S, et al. Atypical teratoid/rhabdoid tumor of the central nervous system: report on workshop. J Pediatr Hematol Oncol 2002;24:337–342.
289. Hilden JM, Meerbaum S, Burger P, et al. Central nervous system atypical teratoid/rhabdoid tumor: results of therapy in children enrolled in a registry. J Clin Oncol 2004;22: 2877–2884.
290. Meyers SP, Khademian ZP, Biegel JA, et al. Primary intracranial atypical teratoid/rhabdoid tumors of infancy. Am J Neuroradiol 2006;27:962–971.
291. Wharton SB, Wardle C, Ironside JW, et al. Comparative genomic hybridization and pathological findings in atypical teratoid/rhabdoid tumour of the central nervous system. Neuropathol Appl Neurobiol 2003;29:254–261.
292. Rickert CH, Paulus W. Chromosomal imbalances detected by comparative genomic hybridization in atypical teratoid/rhabdoid tumours. Childs Nerv Syst 2004;20: 221–224.
293. Lopez-Gines C, CerdaNicolas M, Kepes J, et al. Complex rearrangement of chromosomes 6 and 11 as the sole anomaly in atypical teratoid/rhabdoid tumors of the central nervous system. Cancer Genet Cytogenet 2000;122:149–152.
294. Gessi M, Giangaspero F, Pietsch T. Atypical teratoid/rhabdoid tumors and choroid plexus tumors: when genetics "surprise" pathology. Brain Pathol 2003;13:409–414.
295. Biegel JA, Kalpana G, Knudsen ES, et al. The role of INI1 and the SWI/SNF complex in the development of rhabdoid tumors: meeting summary from the Workshop on Childhood Atypical Teratoid/Rhabdoid Tumors. Cancer Res 2002;62:223–328.
296. Rousseau-Merck M-F, Versteege I, Legrand I, et al. hSNF5/INI1 inactivation is mainly associated with homozygous deletions and mitotic recombinations in rhabdoid tumors. Cancer Res 1999;59:3152–3156.
297. Judkins AR, Mauger J, Rorke LB, et al. Immunohistochemical analysis of hSNF5/INI1 in pediatric CNS neoplasms. Am J Surg Pathol 2004;28(5),644–650.
298. Versteege I, Sevenet N, Lange J, et al. Truncating mutations of hSNF5/INI1 in aggressive paediatric cancer. Nature 1998;394:203–206.
299. Schnitzler G, Sif S, Kingston RE. Human SWI/SNF interconverts a nucleosome between its base state and a stable remodeled state. Cell 1998;94:17–27.
300. Biggar SR, Crabtree GR. Continuous and widespread roles of SWI/SNF complex in transcription. EMBO J 1999;18:2254–2264.
301. Biegel JA, Fogelgren B, Wainwright LM, et al. Germline INI1 mutation in a patient with a central nervous system atypical teratoid tumor and renal rhabdoid tumor. Genes Chromosomes Cancer 2000;28(1):31–37.
302. Roberts CW, Galusha SA, McMenamin ME, et al. Haploinsufficiency of Snf5 predisposes to malignant rhabdoid tumors in mice. Proc Natl Acad Sci U S A 1997;97:13796–13780.
303. Sevenet N, Lellouch-Tubiana A, Schofield D, et al. Spectrum of hSNF5/INI1 somatic mutations in human cancer and genotype-phenotype correlations. Hum Mol Genet 1999;8:2359–2368.
304. Savla J, Chen TT, Schneider NR, et al. Mutations of hSNF5/INI gene in renal rhabdoid tumors with secondary primary brain tumors. J Natl Cancer Inst 2000;92:648–650.
305. Taylor MD, Gokgoz N, Andrulis IL, et al. Familial posterior fossa brain tumors of infancy secondary to germline mutations of hSNF5 gene. Am J Human Genet 2000;66: 1403–1406.
306. Lynch HT, Shurin SB, Dahms BB, et al. Paravertebral malignant rhabdoid tumor in infancy. In vitro studies of a familial tumor. Cancer 1983;52:290–296.
307. Proust F, Laquerriere A, Constantin B, et al. Simultaneous presentation of atypical teratoid/rhabdoid tumor in siblings. J Neuro Oncol 1999;43:63–70.
308. Sevenet N, Sheridan E, Amram D, et al. Constitutional mutations of the hSNF5/INI gene predispose to a variety of cancers. Am J Hum Genet 1999;65:1342–1348.
309. Fruhwald MC, Hasselblatt M, Wirth S, et al. Non-linkage of familial rhabdoid tumors to SMARCB1 implies a second locus for the rhabdoid tumor predisposition syndrome. Pediatr Blood Cancer 2006;47:273–278.
310. Chi SN, Zimmerman MA, Yao X, et al. Intensive multimodality treatment for children with newly diagnosed CNS atypical teratoid rhabdoid tumor. J Clin Oncol 2009;27 (3):385.
311. Chen YW, Wong TT, Ho DM, et al. Impact of radiotherapy for pediatric CNS atypical teratoid/rhabdoid tumor (single institute experience). Int J Radiat Oncol Biol Phys 2006;64(4):1038–1043.
312. Fouladi M, Gururangan S, Moghrabi A, et al. Carboplatin-based primary chemotherapy for infants and young children with CNS tumors. Cancer 2009;115(14):3243–3253.
313. Tekautz TM, Fuller CE, Blaney S, et al. Atypical teratoid/rhabdoid tumors (ATRT): improved survival in children 3 years of age and older with radiation therapy and high-dose alkylator-based chemotherapy. J Clin Oncol 2005;23(7):1491–1499.
314. Squire SE, Chan MD, Marcus KJ. Atypical teratoid/rhabdoid tumor: the controversy behind radiation therapy. J Neurooncol 2007;81(1):97–111.
315. Jennings MT, Gelman R, Hochberg F. Intracranial germ-cell tumors: natural history and pathogenesis. J Neurosurg 1985;63:155–167.
316. Strother D. Atypical teratoid rhabdoid tumors of childhood: diagnosis, treatment and challenges. Expert Rev Anticancer Ther 2005;5(5):907–915.
317. Olson TA, Bayar E, Kosnik E, et al. Successful treatment of disseminated central nervous system malignant rhabdoid tumor. J Pediatr Hematol Oncol 1994;17:71–75.
318. Lefkowitz I, Rorke LB, Packer RJ, et al. Atypical teratoid tumor of infancy: definition of an entity. Ann Neurol 1987;22:448–449.
319. Peters O, Marienhagen J, Stadler P, et al. Combined multimodality therapy for pediatric central nervous system atypical teratoid/rhabdoid tumor: an interim analysis of the German ATRT/CNS pilot study [abstract 148]. Neuro Oncol 2007;9:200.
320. Ronghe MD, Moss TH, Lowis S. Treatment of CNS malignant rhabdoid tumors. Pediatr Blood Cancer 2004;42(3):254–260.
321. Molloy PT, Yachris AT, Rorke LB, et al. Central nervous system medulloepitheliomas: a series of eight cases including two arising in the pons. J Neurosurg 1996;84:430–436.
322. Sharma MC, Mahapatra AK, Gailwad S, et al. Pigmented medulloepitheliomas: report of a case and review of the literature. Childs Nerv Syst 1998;14:74–78.
323. Norris LS, Snodgrass S, Miller DC, et al. Recurrent central nervous system medulloepitheliomas: response and outcome following marrow-ablative chemotherapy with stem cell rescue. J Pediatr Hematol Oncol 2005;27:264–266.
324. Judkins AR, Ellison DW. Ependymoblastoma: dear, damned, distracting diagnosis, farewell! Journal compilation: International Society of Neuropathology. Brain Pathol 2008;SSN: 1015–6305.
325. Becker LE, Hinton D. Primitive neuroectodermal tumors of the central nervous system. Hum Pathol 1983;14:538–550.
326. Mork SJ, Rubinstein LJ. Ependymoblastomas. A reappraisal of a rare embryonal tumor. Cancer 1985;55:1536–1542.
327. Rubinstein LJ. The definition of the ependymoblastomas. Arch Pathol 1970;90:35–45.
328. Dorsay TA, Rovira MJ, Ho VB, et al. Ependymoblastoma: MR presentation. A case report and review of the literature. Pediatr Radiol 1995;25(6):433–435.
329. Rubinstein LJ. Presidential address. Cytogenesis and differentiation of primitive central neuroepithelial tumors. J Neuropathol Exp Neurol 1972;31:7–26.
330. Eberhart CG, Brat DJ, Cohen KJ, et al. Pediatric neuroblastic brain tumors containing abundant neuropil and true rosettes. Pediatr Dev Pathol 2000;3:346–352.
331. Rickert CH, Hasselblatt M. Cytogenetic features of ependymoblastomas. Acta Neuropathol 2006;111:559–562.
332. Packer RJ, Cohen BH, Cooney K. Intracranial germ cell tumors. Oncologist 2000; 5:312–320.
333. Kretschmar CS. Germ cell tumors of the brain in children: a review of current literature and new advances in therapy. Cancer Invest 1997;15:187–198.
334. Wara WM, Jenkin RD, Evans A, et al. Tumors of the pineal and suprasellar region: Childrens Cancer Study Group treatment results 1960–1975: a report from Childrens Cancer Study Group. Cancer 1979;43:698–701.
335. Edwards MS, Hudgins RJ, Wilson CB, et al. Pineal region tumors in children. J Neurosurg 1988;68:689–697.
336. Jenkin D, Berry M, Chan H, et al. Pineal region germinomas in childhood treatment considerations. Int Radiat Oncol Biol Phys 1990;18:541–545.
337. Abay EO, Laws ER Jr, Grado GL, et al. Pineal tumors in children and adolescents. Treatment by CSF shunting and radiotherapy. J Neurosurg 1981;55:889–895.
338. Regis J, Bouillot P, Rouby-Volot F, et al. Pineal region tumors and the role of stereotactic biopsy: review of the mortality, morbidity, and diagnostic rates in 370 cases. Neurosurgery 1996;39:907–912.
339. Matsutani M, Sano K, Takakura K, et al. Primary intracranial germ cell tumors: a clinical analysis of 153 histologically verified cases. J Neurosurg 1997;86:446–455.
340. Balmaceda C, Heller G, Rosenblum M, et al. Chemotherapy without irradiation—a novel approach for newly diagnosed CNS germ cell tumors: results of an international

cooperative trial. The First International Central Nervous System Germ Cell Tumor Study. J Clin Oncol 1996;14:2908–2915.
341. Ushio Y, Kochi M, Kuratsu J, et al. Preliminary observations for a new treatment in children with primary intracranial yolk sac tumor or embryonal carcinoma. Report of five cases. J Neurosurg 1999;90:133–137.
342. Yoshida J, Sugita K, Kobayashi T, et al. Prognosis of intracranial germ cell tumours: effectiveness of chemotherapy with cisplatin and etoposide (CDDP and VP-16). Acta Neurochir (Wien) 1993;120:111–117.
343. D'Andrea AD, Packer RJ, Rorke LB, et al. Pineocytomas of childhood. A reappraisal of natural history and response to therapy. Cancer 1987;59:1353–1357.
344. Disclafani A, Hudgins RJ, Edwards MS, et al. Pineocytomas. Cancer 1989;63:302–304.
345. Nakamura M, Saeki N, Iwadate Y, et al. Neuroradiological characteristics of pineocytoma and pineoblastoma. Neuroradiology 2000;42(7):509–514.
346. Smirniotopoulos JG, Rushing EJ, Mena H. Pineal region masses: differential diagnosis. Radiographics 1992;12:577–596.
347. Schild SE, Scheithauer BW, Schomberg PJ, et al. Pineal parenchymal tumors. Clinical, pathologic, and therapeutic aspects. Cancer 1993;72:870–880.
348. Trojanowski JQ, Tascos NA, Rorke LB. Malignant pineocytomas with prominent papillary features, Cancer 1982;50:1789–1793.
349. Rainho CA, Rogatto SR, de Moraes LC, et al. Cytogenetic study of a pineocytoma. Cancer Genet Cytogenet 1992:64:127–132.
350. Bello MJ, Rey JA, de Campos JM, et al. Chromosomal abnormalities in a pineocytomas. Cancer Genet Cytogenet 1993;72:185–186.
351. Rickert CH, Simon R, Bergmann M, et al. Comparative genomic hybridization in pineal parenchymal tumors. Genes, Chromosomes and Cancer 2001;30:99–104.
352. Tsumanuma I, Sato M, Okazaki H, et al. The analysis of p53 tumor suppressor gene in pineal parenchymal tumors. Noshuyo Byori 1995;12:39–43.
353. Nozaki M, Tada M, Matsumoto R, et al. Rare occurrence of inactivating p53 gene mutation in primary non-astrocytic tumors of the central nervous system: reappraisal by yeast functional assay. Acta Neuropathol 1998;95:291–296.
354. Brockmeyer DL, Walker ML, Thompson G, et al. Astrocytoma and pineoblastoma arising sequentially in the fourth ventricle of the same patient. Case report and molecular analysis. Pediatr Neurosurg 1997;26:36–40.
355. Paulino AC, Wen BC, Mohideen MN. Controversies in the management of intracranial germinomas. Oncology (Huntingt) 1999;13:513–521; discussion 521–522, 528–533.
356. Matsutani M, Sano K, Takakura K, et al. Combined treatment with chemotherapy and radiation therapy for intracranial germ cell tumors. Childs Nerv Syst 1990;14:59–62.
357. Calaminus G, Bambert M, Harams D, et al. AFP/β-HcG secreting CNS germ cell tumors: long-term outcome with respect to initial symptoms and primary tumor resection. Results of the Cooperative Trial MAKEI 89. Neuropediatrics 2005;36:71–77.
358. Teilum G. Special tumors of the ovary and testis and related extragonadal lesions. Philadelphia, PA: J.B. Lippincott, 1976.
359. Takei Y, Pearl GS. Ultrastructure study of intracranial yolk sac tumor: with special reference to the oncologic phylogeny of germ-cell tumors. Cancer 1981;48:2038–2046.
360. Sano K, Matsutani M. Pinealoma (germinoma) treated by direct surgery and postoperative irradiation. Childs Brain 1981;8:81–97.
361. Crawford J, Vezina LG, Packer RJ. Central nervous system germ cell tumors of childhood, presentation and delay in diagnosis. Neurology 2007;68:1668–1673.
362. Rushing EJ, Sandberg GD, Judkins AR, et al. Germinoma: unusual imaging and pathological characteristics. Report of 2 cases. J Neurosurg 2006;104(S2):143–148.
363. Liang L, Korogi Y, Sugahara T, et al. MRI of intracranial germ-cell tumors. Neuroradiology 2002;44:382–388.
364. Packer RJ, Sutton LN, Rosenstock JG, et al. Pineal region tumors of childhood. Pediatrics 1984;74:97–102.
365. Schneider DT, Zahn S, Sievers S, et al. Molecular genetic analysis of central nervous system germ cell tumors with comparative genomic hybridization. Mod Pathol 2006; 19:864–873.
366. Rikert CH, Simon R, Bergmann M, et al. Comparative genomic hybridization in pineal germ cell tumors. J Neuropathol Exp Neurol 2000;59:815–821.
367. Okada Y, Nighikawa R, Matsutani M, et al. Hypomethylated X chromosome gain and rare isochromosome 12p in diverse intracranial germ cell tumors. J Neuropathol Exp Neurol 2002;61:531–538.
368. Haas-Kogan DA, Missett BT, Wara WM, et al. Radiation therapy for intracranial germ cell tumors. Int J Radiat Oncol Biol Phys 2003;56:511–518.
369. Rich TA, Cassady JR, Strand RD, et al. Radiation therapy for pineal and suprasellar germ cell tumors. Cancer 1985;55(5):932–940.
370. Sung DI, Harisliadis L, Chang CH. Midline pineal tumors and suprasellar germinomas: highly curable by irradiation. Radiology 1978;128(3):745–751.
371. Shirato H, Nishio M, Sawamura Y, et al. Analysis of long-term treatment of intracranial germinoma. Int J Radiat Oncol boil Phys 1997;37(3):511–515.
372. Wolden SL, Wara WM, Larson DA, et al. Radiation therapy for primary intracranial germ-cell tumors. Int J Radiat Oncol Biol Phys 1995;32(4):943–949.
373. Ogawa K, Yoshii Y, Shikama N, et al. Spinal recurrence from intracranial germinoma: risk factors and treatment outcome for spinal recurrence. Int J Radiat Oncol Biol Phys 2008;72(5):1347–1354.
374. Lafay-Cousin L, Millar BA, Mabbott D, et al. Limited-field radiation for bifocal germinoma. Int J Radiat Oncol Biol Phys 2006;65(2):486–492.
375. Shirato H, Aoyama H, Ikeda J, et al. Impact of margin for target volume in low-dose involved field radiotherapy after induction chemotherapy for intracranial germinoma. Int J Radiat Oncol Biol Phys 2004;60(1):217–217.
376. Maity A, Shu HK, Janss A, et al. Craniospinal radiation in the treatment of biopsy-proven intracranial germinomas: twenty-five years' experience in a single center. Int J Radiat Oncol Biol Phys 2004;58(4):1165–1170.
377. Merchant TE, Sherwood SH, Mulhern RK, et al. CNS germinoma: disease control and long-term functional outcome for 12 children treated with craniospinal irradiation. Int J Radiat Oncol Biol Phys 2000;46(5):1171–1176.
378. Linstadt D, Wara WM, Edwards MS, et al. Radiotherapy of primary intracranial germinomas: the case against routine craniospinal irradiation. Int J Radiat Oncol Biol Phys 1988;15(2):291–297.
379. Shibamoto Y, Sasai K, Oya N, et al. Intracranial germinoma: radiation therapy with tumor volume-based dose selection. Radiology 2001;218(2):452–456.
380. Nguyen QN, Chang EL, Allen PK, et al. Focal and craniospinal irradiation for patients with intracranial germinoma and patterns of failure. Cancer 2006;107(9):2228–2236.
381. Ogawa K, Shikama N, Toita T, et al. Long-term results of radiotherapy for intracranial germinoma: a multi-institutional retrospective review of 126 patients. Int J Radiat Oncol Biol Phys 2004;58(3):705–713.
382. Bamberg M, Kortmann RD, Calaminus G, et al. Radiation therapy for intracranial germinoma: results of the German cooperative prospective trials MAKEI 83/86/89. J Clin Oncol 1999;17:2585–2592.
383. Baranzelli MC, Patte C, Bouffet E, et al. Nonmetastatic intracranial germinoma: the experience of the French Society of Pediatric Oncology. Cancer 1997;80:1792–1797.
384. Shibamoto Y, Oda Y, Yamashita J, et al. The role of cerebrospinal fluid cytology in radiotherapy planning for intracranial germinoma. Int J Radiat Oncol Biol Phys 1994;29:1089–1094.
385. Bouffet E, Baranzelli MC, Patte C, et al. Combined treatment modality for intracranial germinomas: results of a multicentre SFOP experience. Societe Francaise d'Oncologie Pediatrique. Br J Cancer 1999;79:1199–1204.
386. Schoenfeld GO, Amdur RJ, Schmalfuss IM, et al. Low-dose prophylactic craniospinal radiotherapy for intracranial germinoma. Int J Radiat Oncol Biol Phys 2006;65(2): 481–485.
387. Raggi E, Mosleh-Shirazi MA, Saran FH. An evaluation of conformal and intensity-modulated radiotherapy in whole ventricular radiotherapy for localised primary intracranial germinomas. Clin Oncol (R Coll Radiol) 2008;20(3):253–260.
388. Roberge D, Kun LE, Freeman CR. Intracranial germinoma: on whole-ventricular irradiation. Pediatr Blood Cancer 2005;44(4):358–362.
389. Shikama N, Ogawa K, Tanaka S, et al. Lack of benefit of spinal irradiation in the primary treatment of intracranial germinoma: a multiinstitutional, retrospective review of 180 patients. Cancer 2005;104(1):126–134.
390. Hardenbergh PH, Golden J, Billet A, et al. Intracranial germinoma: the case for lower dose radiation therapy. Int J Radiat Oncol Biol Phys 1997;39(2):419–426.
391. Alapetite C, Ricardi U, Saran F, et al. Whole ventricular irradiation in combination with chemotherapy in intracranial germinoma: the consensus of the SIOP CNS GCT Study Group [abstract]. Med Pediatr Oncol 2002;39(4):248.
392. Aoyama H, Shirato H, Ikeda J, et al. Induction chemotherapy followed by low-dose involved-field radiotherapy for intracranial germ cell tumors. J Clin Oncol 2002;20(3): 857–865.
393. Shibamoto Y, Abe M, Yamashita J, et al. Treatment results of intracranial germinoma as a function of the irradiated volume. Int J Radiat Oncol Biol Phys 1988;15;285–290.
394. Fouladi M, Grant R, Baruchel S, et al. Comparison of survival outcome in patients with intracranial germinomas treated with radiation alone versus reduced dose radiation and chemotherapy. Childs Nerv Syst 1998;14:596–601.
395. Aoyama H, Shirato H, Kakuto Y, et al. Pathologically-proven intracranial germinoma treated with radiation therapy. Radiother Oncol 1998;47:201–205.
396. Merchant TE, Davis BJ, Sheldon JM, et al. Radiation therapy for relapsed CNS germinoma after primary chemotherapy. J Clin Oncol 1998;16(1):204–209.
397. Robertson PL, DaRosso RC, Allen JC. Improved prognosis of intracranial non-germinoma germ cell tumors with multimodality therapy. J Neuro Oncol 1997;32:71–80.
398. Villano JL, Propp JM, Porter KR, et al. Malignant pineal germ-cell tumors: an analysis of cases from three tumor registries. Neuro Oncol 2008;10(2):121–130.
399. Calaminus G, Bamberg M, Jurgens H, et al. Impact of surgery, chemotherapy and irradiation on long term outcome of intracranial malignant non-germinomatous germ cell tumors: results of the German Cooperative Trial MAKEI 89. Klin Padiatr 2004; 216(3):141–149.
400. Kobayashi T, Yoshida J, Ishiyama J, et al. Combination chemotherapy with cisplatin and etoposide for malignant intracranial germ-cell tumors. An experimental and clinical study. J Neurosurg 1989;70:676–681.
401. Shibamoto Y, Takahashi M, Abe M. Reduction of the radiation dose for intracranial germinoma: a prospective study. Br J Cancer 1994;70:984–989.
402. Schild SE, Haddock MG, Scheithauer BW, et al. Nongerminomatous germ cell tumors of the brain. Int J Radiat Oncol Biol Phys 1996;36:557–563.
403. Zissiadis Y, Dutton S, Kieran M, et al. Stereotactic radiotherapy for pediatric intracranial germ cell tumors. Int J Radiat Oncol Biol Phys 2001;51(1):108–112.
404. Hasegawa T, Kondziolka D, Hadjipanayis CG, et al. Stereotactic radiosurgery for CNS nongerminomatous germ cell tumors. Report of four cases. Pediatr Neurosurg 2003; 38(6):329–33.
405. Allen JC, Kim JH, Packer RJ. Neoadjuvant chemotherapy for newly diagnosed germ-cell tumors of the central nervous system. J Neurosurg 1987;67:65–70.
406. Allen JC, DaRosso RC, Donahue B, et al. A phase II trial of preirradiation carboplatin in newly diagnosed germinoma of the central nervous system. Cancer 1994;74:940–944.
407. Buckner JC, Peethambaram PP, Smthson WA, et al. Phase II trial of primary chemotherapy followed by reduced-dose radiation for CNS germ cell tumors. J Clin Oncol 1999; 17:933–940.
408. Allen JC, Bosl G, Walker R. Chemotherapy trials in recurrent primary intracranial germ cell tumors. J Neuro Oncol 1985;3:147–152.
409. Pinkerton CR, Broadbent V, Horwich A, et al. 'JEB'—a carboplatin based regimen for malignant germ cell tumours in children. Br J Cancer 1990;62:257–262.
410. Calaminus G, Alapetite C, Frappaz D, et al. Outcome of localized and metastatic germinoma treated according to SIOP CNS GCT 96. Abstract from 13th International Symposium on Pediatric Neuro-Oncology (ISPNO). Neuro-Oncol 2008;10:420.
411. Patel SR, Buckner JC, Smithson WA, et al. Cisplatin-based chemotherapy in primary central nervous system germ cell tumors. J Neuro Oncol 1992;12:47–52.
412. Hooda BS, Finlay J. Recent advances in the diagnosis and treatment of central nervous system germ-cell tumours. Curr Opin Neurol 1999;12:693–696.
413. Matsutani M. Treatment of intracranial germ cell tumors: the second phase II study of Japanese GCT Study Group. Neuro-Oncol 2008;10:420–421.
414. Baranzelli MC, Patte C, Bouffet E, et al. Carboplatin-based chemotherapy (CT) and focal irradiation (RT) in primary cerebral germ cell tumors (GCT): a French Society of Pediatric Oncology (SFOP) experience [abstract 140]. Proc ASCO 1999;18:538.
415. Motzer RJ, Mazumdar M, Bosl GJ, et al. High-dose carboplatin, etoposide and cyclophosphamide with autologous bone marrow transplantation in first-line therapy for patients with poor-risk germ cell tumors. J Clin Oncol 1997;15:2546–2552.
416. Claminus G, Bamberg M, Branzellii MC, et al. Intracranial germ cell tumors: a comprehensive update of the European data. Neuropediatrics 1994;25(1):26–31.
417. Calaminus G, Frappaz D, Kortmann R-D, et al. Localized and metastatic nongerminoma treated according to the SIOP CNS GCT 96 protocol: update on risk profiles and outcome. Neuro-Oncol 2008;10:418.
418. Sawamura Y, Shirato H, Ikeda J, et al. Induction chemotherapy followed by reduced-volume radiation therapy for newly diagnosed central nervous system germinoma. J Neurosurg 1998;88:66–72.
419. McCabe MG, Ichimura K, Liu L, et al. High-resolution array-based comparative genomic hybridization of medulloblastomas and supratentorial primitive neuroectodermal tumors. J Neuropathol Exp Neurol 2006;65(6):549–561.

CHAPTER 27 ■ RETINOBLASTOMA

RICHARD L. HURWITZ, CAROL L. SHIELDS, JERRY A. SHIELDS, PATRICIA CHÉVEZ-BARRIOS,
DAN GOMBOS, MARY Y. HURWITZ, AND MURALI M. CHINTAGUMPALA

INTRODUCTION

Retinoblastoma, a malignant tumor of the embryonic neural retina, is the most common intraocular malignancy in children. Although usually not recognized at birth, retinoblastoma predominantly affects young children. The tumor has a variable growth rate, can originate from single or multiple foci in one or both eyes, and, in bilateral cases, may be manifest in one eye many months before it is evident in the other. Retinoblastoma is caused by a mutation in a gene that expresses a protein central to the control of the cell cycle and may occur sporadically or be inherited. Children with the hereditary type of retinoblastoma have a particular susceptibility to developing other malignant tumors. This disease serves as a model for understanding the genetics and heredity of childhood cancer.

The term *retinoblastoma* was first adopted by the American Ophthalmological Society in 1926.[1] The cellular origin of retinoblastoma had been a topic of debate since 1809 when, based only on gross pathological findings, the Scottish surgeon Wardrop first recognized that retinoblastoma is a discrete tumor arising from the retina.[2,3] After this was published, other pathologists, including Robin and Langenbeck, confirmed the observations at a microscopic level. Virchow, however, thought that the cell of origin was glial and named it "glioma of the retina." In the late 1800s, the term *neuroepithelioma* was proposed by Flexner and supported later by Wintersteiner because they believed that the tumor originated from the neuroepithelium and that the typical rosettes that now bear their names were attempts to form photoreceptors. In the early 1900s, Verhoeff concluded that the tumor was derived from undifferentiated embryonic retinal cells called retinoblasts and proposed the term *retinoblastoma*.[1] Zimmerman proposed the term *retinocytoma* for the well-differentiated tumor that displays benign features.[4] For this same tumor, Gallie et al. described the clinical features and proposed the term *retinoma*.[5] The histopathological, ultrastructural, immunohistochemical, and molecular characteristics of retinoblastoma support the concept that this tumor originates from a multipotent precursor cell. This cell could develop into almost any type of inner or outer retina cell, including photoreceptors.[6–21] Alternatively, investigations have supported the concept that a differentiated cell could be the precursor cell by de-differentiating into a malignant cell.[22,23] That the benign retinoma is a precursor to the malignant retinoblastoma has also been proposed.[24]

EPIDEMIOLOGY

The Third National Cancer Survey predicts an average incidence of 11 new cases of retinoblastoma per million population less than 5 years of age, or 1 in 18,000 live births in the United States,[25] and this rate has proven stable over time.[26] Although data from developing countries is less complete,

oncologists in Central and South America, the Middle East and India generally feel that the incidence may be greater in these regions.[27,28] A multicenter report from Mexico concluded that retinoblastoma is the second most frequent solid malignancy after Central nervous system (CNS) tumors in children.[29] The estimated frequency of bilateral retinoblastoma ranges from 25% to 35%.[26,30] Thus, in the United States, an estimated 200 children per year develop retinoblastoma; 40 to 60 of these cases are bilateral. There are no racial or gender predilections.

Retinoblastoma is often present at birth and is almost entirely restricted to early childhood. About 80% of cases are diagnosed before 3 to 4 years of age, with a median age at diagnosis of 2 years.[26,27,30,31] The discovery of retinoblastoma beyond the age of 6 years is rare. Bilateral disease is diagnosed earlier than unilateral disease. Sporadic bilateral retinoblastoma has been associated with advanced parental age[32] but a recent analysis shows no increase in incidence of retinoblastoma with advancing maternal age.[33]

Multiple congenital anomalies associated with retinoblastoma have been reported in approximately 0.05% of U.S. patients with retinoblastoma.[34] The reported anomalies include congenital cardiovascular defects, cleft palate, infantile cortical hyperostosis, dentinogenesis imperfecta, familial congenital cataracts, and incontinentia pigmenti or Bloch-Sulzberger syndrome (an X-linked inherited disease that is lethal in males but affects females with pigmentary retinopathy, corneal opacities, cataracts, nystagmus, blue sclerae, myopia, pseudoglioma, dental abnormalities, abnormal skin pigmentation, and mental deficiency).[31] An association with mental retardation has been suggested in children with the D-deletion syndrome; however, most patients with retinoblastoma have no intellectual impairment.

GENETICS

The majority of retinoblastomas appear sporadically; however, an inherited form of the disease has been documented[35] and is transmitted with few exceptions as a typical Mendelian autosomal dominant trait with high but incomplete penetrance. Of all cases, about 60% are nonhereditary and unilateral, 15% are hereditary and unilateral, and 25% are hereditary and bilateral.[36,37]

A *two-hit* model has been proposed to explain the observations that familial cases are generally multifocal and bilateral whereas sporadic cases typically present with unilateral unifocal disease at a later age.[36,38] According to the model, as few as two stochastic mutational events are required for tumor initiation, the first of which can be inherited through the germline (in heritable cases) or can occur somatically in individual retinal cells (in non-heritable cases). The second event occurs somatically in either case and leads to tumor formation from each doubly defective retinal cell.

The presence of a microscopically visible deletion in one chromosome 13 homologue in constitutional cells of a small number of retinoblastoma patients was the first evidence that supported an inherited mechanism for retinoblastoma development.[39–42] Although the deletions varied between families, each deletion minimally encompassed chromosome 13, band q14.[43,44] This chromosomal locus contains the *RB1* retinoblastoma gene. In the *two-hit* model, such deletions in the germline could act as the first hit and confer the risk of tumor formation as an autosomal dominant trait. The increasing resolution of cytogenetic technology and the development of DNA probes for loci in the immediate vicinity of the *RB1* gene locus have allowed the detection of more subtle genomic rearrangements. These techniques can be used to identify people who carry nonpenetrant mutations in the retinoblastoma susceptibility locus.[45]

Patients without a gross 13th chromosomal deletion but who have bilateral or familial retinoblastoma have submicroscopic mutations at the *RB1* locus similar to mutations that have been found in the tumor cells of patients with nonhereditary retinoblastoma. The second step in tumorigenesis in both heritable and nonhereditary retinoblastoma involves somatic alteration of the normal allele at the *RB1* locus in such a way that the mutant allele is unmasked. Thus, the first mutation in this process, although it may be inherited as an autosomal dominant trait in the child, is in fact a recessive defect in the individual retinal cell. Elimination of the chromosome containing the wild-type allele followed by reduplication of the remaining mutant chromosome may be one mechanism by which the affected *RB1* locus becomes homozygous within the cell.[46,47] Other mechanisms of mutagenesis, including the generation of point mutations, deletions, and silencing of the promoter by methylation, are frequently encountered in the second allele. The result is that the potential tumor cell becomes functionally recessive for the mutant allele.

Although the unmasking of predisposing mutations at the *RB1* locus occurs in mechanistically similar ways in sporadic and heritable retinoblastoma, only the latter carries the initial mutation in each cell. Patients with heritable disease also seem to be at greatly increased risk for the development of second primary tumors, particularly osteosarcoma.[48] This high propensity is genetically determined by the predisposing *RB1* mutation. The notion of a pathogenetic association between these two rare tumor types was tested by determining the constitutional and osteosarcoma genotypes at restriction fragment length polymorphism (RFLP) loci on chromosome 13. The data indicated that osteosarcomas arising in patients with retinoblastoma had become homozygous specifically around the chromosomal region carrying the *RB1* locus.[49] Furthermore, these same chromosomal mechanisms eliciting losses of constitutional heterozygosity were observed in sporadic osteosarcomas, suggesting a genetic similarity in pathogenetic causality.

These studies provided data useful for the molecular isolation of the *RB1* gene.[50] The 200 Kb *RB1* locus contains 27 exons that are transcribed into a 4.7-Kb transcript in normal human and rat tissues, including brain, kidney, ovary, spleen, liver, placenta, and retina.[51] Although the number of different types of tumors that occur as a result of inherited mutations in the *RB1* locus is small, the broad tissue expression and species conservation of this gene suggest a common and potentially important role in the growth or differentiation of many cell types.[52–55] Introduction of the wild-type gene into retinoblastoma and osteosarcoma cell lines using recombinant retroviral vector transfer resulted in a partial reversal of the tumorigenic phenotype.[56,57] Further characterization of the complete *RB1* genomic sequence[58] allowed a rigorous cataloging of the different mutations affecting the gene in retinoblastoma tumors.

Over 200 disease-causing mutations have been identified in the retinoblastoma genes of patients.[45,59–68]

The examination of sporadic cases of bilateral retinoblastoma showed that disease frequently arises subsequent to a new germline mutation in the paternal allele, followed by somatic alteration or loss of the maternally derived wild-type allele.[69,70] This finding suggests either that mutations in the *RB1* locus occur more commonly during spermatogenesis or that the paternal chromosome in the early embryo is at a higher risk of mutation. Analyses of sporadic osteosarcomas also showed preferential mutation of the paternal allele.[71]

Investigations of *RB1* gene alterations at both the DNA and the RNA levels cumulatively reveal a strong correlative relationship between the lack of *RB1* gene product RB protein and the appearance of retinoblastoma tumors. In addition to osteosarcomas, other tumor types contain mutations involving the retinoblastoma gene. Molecular analyses of small cell lung carcinomas have revealed *RB1* structural abnormalities in approximately 15% of cases.[72] Loss of heterozygosity for chromosome 13 has been detected in about 25% of breast cancers and related breast cancer–derived cell lines.[73,74] However, a more detailed analysis of the effects of chromosome 13 mutations in tumors has been compiled and clearly shows that not all tumors are either a direct or an indirect result of loss of heterozygosity of the *RB1* locus.[75] The cumulative data suggest that only subsets of tumors may share a common pathogenetic mechanism that results from unmasking mutations affecting the tumor suppressing function of the RB protein.

The RB protein is comprised of 928 amino acids and has an estimated molecular mass of 110 Kd. The expressed protein has been shown to be primarily localized in the cell nucleus.[76] Post-translational phosphorylation of the RB protein in quiescent cells overrides growth suppression and allows cell division to occur.[77] The RB protein also has a role in the regulation of the cell cycle of actively dividing cells. The unphosphorylated RB protein (p110RB) has been shown to bind E2F1, a transcription factor, and a cell cycle regulator during the G1 stage of the cell cycle. The RB/E2F1 complex masks the E2F1 transactivation domain and inhibits surrounding enhancer elements, thereby causing transcription of E2F1-regulated genes to cease. The RB protein accomplishes this by physically associating with a histone deacetylase (HDAC1). This recruitment of the deacetylase to the E2F1 regulating domain by RB allows deacetylation of histone, thereby modulating the local structure of the chromatin.[78,79] Phosphorylation of the RB protein at the G1/S boundary results in the release of these transcriptional factors, allowing them to become positive transcriptional elements. Additional cell cycle–specific kinases become activated and facilitate the progression of the cells through G2 and M. At the completion of the cell cycle, phosphatases dephosphorylate the RB protein, allowing the protein to again sequester E2F1 and form an inactive complex. Thus, positive and negative regulation of transcription and, therefore, cell proliferation are linked to the phosphorylation cycle of the RB protein. In tumors in which the RB protein is mutated or absent, these intracellular transcriptional elements are dissociated and free to promote consistent and uncontrolled progression through the cell cycle. Such behavior results in unchecked cell proliferation consistent with a malignant phenotype.

The viral oncoproteins of polyomaviruses (SV40), adenoviruses (Ad-2 and Ad-5), and papillomaviruses (HPV-16) have also been shown to complex with the RB protein.[80–82] Because one function of these viral oncoproteins appears to be the creation of a cellular environment that is permissive for DNA synthesis, one of their modes of action may involve sequestration of the antiproliferative unphosphorylated RB protein. Releasing the cell from its negative regulation by RB might allow the cell to enter S phase and synthesize DNA. Taken together, the data support a model in which the unphosphorylated form of RB is the species active in growth suppression.

The understanding of the complex interrelationships of the RB proteins, mutations in the RB proteins that lead to disease, and the metabolic consequences of these events in the cell have lead to the investigation of novel therapies to treat a variety of cancers, including retinoblastoma.[83,84]

Genetic Counseling

Approximately 40% of patients with retinoblastoma have the inherited form of the disease. Since the inherited form of retinoblastoma is transmitted as an autosomal dominant trait with high but incomplete penetrance, there is a 45% chance that any given child of the patient will inherit the disease. In addition, although there is high penetrance of the retinoblastoma phenotype, the possibility exists that one of the patient's siblings could also develop retinoblastoma due to germline mosaicism and low penetrant alleles even if neither of the parents was affected by the disease (see Chapter 2).[85–87] All children with a family history of retinoblastoma should be screened shortly after birth by a qualified ophthalmologist to permit early detection of the disease and increase the chance of ocular and vision salvage. These increased familial risks support the need for expert genetic counseling.

To effectively counsel patients and families of retinoblastoma patients, the underlying cause of the disease must be determined. Patients who present with bilateral disease can be assumed to have a germline mutation in the *RB1* gene. Patients with unilateral disease at presentation may also have an underlying germline mutation. If a mutation in the *RB1* gene is detected in the tumor, somatic cells should also be screened. A mutation initially detected in the somatic cells is presumptive evidence of a mutation in the germline. Genetic testing for the presence of this specific mutation in siblings or offspring should be pursued. These children can then be aggressively surveyed for the presence of emerging tumors. If genetic testing is not pursued, then tumor surveillance is recommended for all siblings of the affected patient. Current recommendations suggest examination at birth and after every 4 months until the child attains 4 years of age. For children with unilateral disease, genetic screening for *RB1* mutations can now be offered to families at the time of enucleation. Testing for patients with unilateral disease requires a sample of tumor and peripheral blood.[45] Testing for patients with bilateral disease requires only a blood sample. This topic has been further discussed in Chapter 2.

CLINICAL PRESENTATION

Most cases of retinoblastoma in the United States are diagnosed while the tumor remains contained within the eye (intraocular) without local invasion or distant metastases. In developing countries, however, the diagnosis is frequently made only after an enlarged eye (buphthalmos) or gross orbital extension is apparent. These patients more commonly present with local invasion.

The signs and symptoms of an intraocular tumor depend on its size and position. The most common presenting sign is leukocoria of one or both eyes (Fig. 27.1). Leukocoria, white papillary reflex instead of the normal red reflex, is manifest when the tumor is large or has caused a total retinal detachment leading to a retrolental mass visible through the pupil. In some cases, a small tumor centered in the macula (central portion of the retina) can produce leukocoria. If vitreous

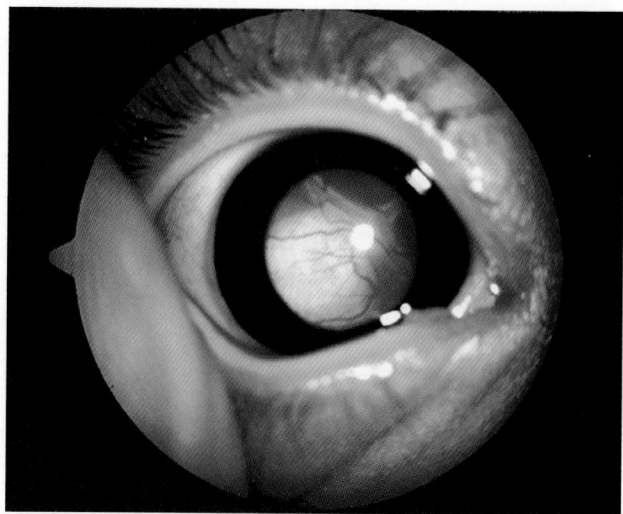

FIGURE 27.1 Photograph of an eye from a patient with retinoblastoma who presented with leukocoria.

hemorrhage occurs because of bleeding from the retinoblastoma vessels (Fig. 27.2), the pupil can appear to have a dark red reflex (hemocoria) or black reflex (nigrocoria) instead of the white reflex typically seen in retinoblastoma.[18,88,89] The second most common presenting sign is strabismus. Loss of central vision from a tumor in the macula can result in a disruption of fusional ability and cause the affected eye to drift.

Other ophthalmic features accompany some cases of retinoblastoma and may indicate the necessity for immediate enucleation. Heterochromia (different color for each iris) can present as an initial sign of retinoblastoma secondary to iris neovascularization. The diagnosis of retinoblastoma should be excluded in children that present with this condition.[20] Rubeosis iridis (neovascularization of the surface of the iris) occurs in approximately 17% of patients with retinoblastoma and in more than 50% of patients with advanced retinoblastoma requiring enucleation[20,90–93] (Fig. 27.2). Extensive necrosis of the tumor and liberated angiogenic factors may be responsible for this neovascularization of the iris.

Spontaneous bleeding from rubeosis iridis can also cause hyphema (blood in the anterior chamber) and the potential diagnosis of retinoblastoma should be investigated in a child presenting with spontaneous hyphema without history of trauma.[18,20,88,89] Glaucoma can be secondary to neovascularization of the anterior chamber angle and/or anterior synechia as a result of rubeosis iridis. Closed-angle glaucoma can also be secondary to mechanical obstruction of the anterior chamber angle by the iris and lens that has been pushed forward by a large intravitreal tumor. Most children with these presentations undergo enucleation.[18,88,89] Anterior chamber seeding from endophytic tumors or diffuse infiltrating tumors may produce pseudohypopyon (cells in the anterior chamber)[94] (Fig. 27.2). Intraocular tumors are not associated with pain unless secondary glaucoma or inflammation is present.

DIAGNOSIS

Most commonly, a parent or relative of an affected child notes an abnormality of the eye that prompts a pediatrician to look for leukocoria using an ophthalmoscope. The gross appearance of a creamy pink to snow white mass projecting into the vitreous (Fig. 27.1) may suggest retinoblastoma; however, associated findings of retinal detachment, vitreous hemorrhage, or

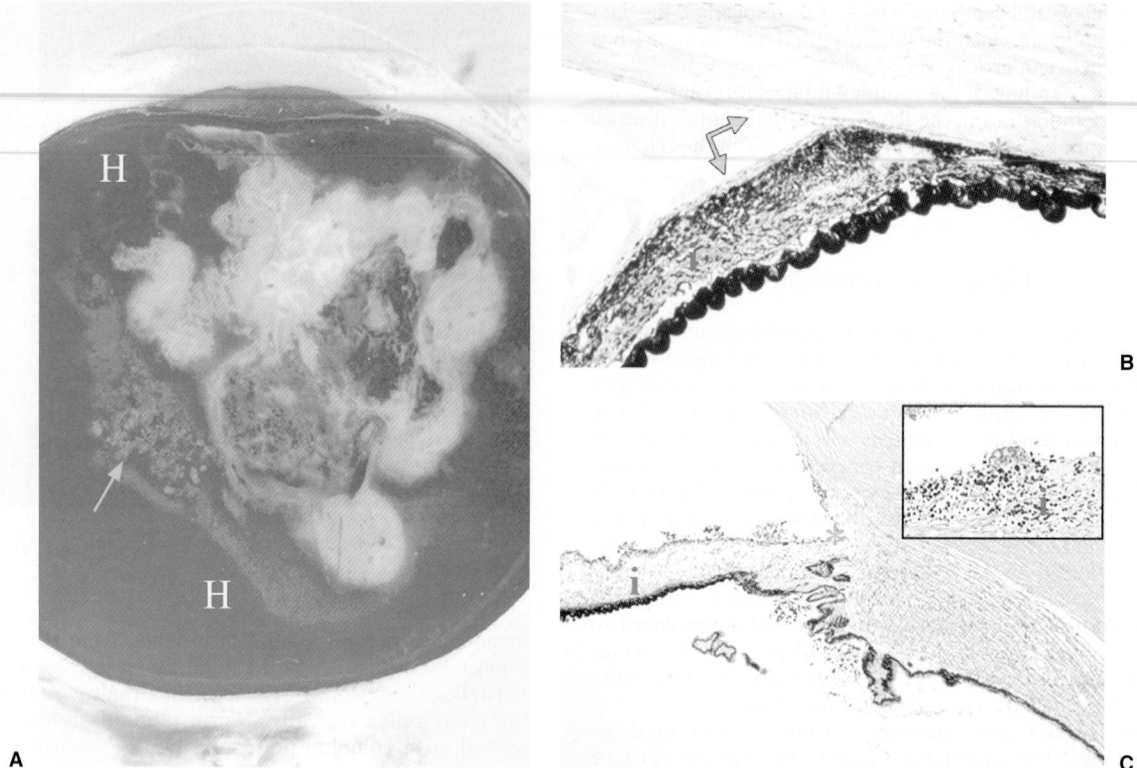

FIGURE 27.2 A: Gross photograph of an eye with retinoblastoma (white membranous tissue at center of the eye) with subretinal tumor seeds (*arrow*), and vitreous and subretinal hemorrhages (H). Neovascularization of the anterior chamber and partial closure of the anterior angle (*) are also present. **B**: Histologic picture of rubeosis iridis showing neovascularization (*arrows*) of the anterior portion of the iris (i) and focally on the endothelial surface of the cornea (*arrow*). Contraction of the neovascular membrane produces closure of the anterior chamber angle (*). Hematoxylin and eosin, original magnification 20×. **C**: Histologic picture of the anterior segment of an eye with retinoblastoma seeds on the surface of the iris (i) with focal rosette formation (insert). The anterior chamber angle (*) is opened. Hematoxylin and eosin, original magnification 20×.

opaque media often make inspection difficult. Pupillary dilation and examination with the patient under anesthesia are essential to fully evaluate the retina. Characteristically, the diagnosis is made by the ophthalmoscopic and ultrasonographic appearance, and pathologic confirmation is unnecessary. When the tumor is at an advanced stage, distinguishing vitreous seeding from multifocal tumors can be difficult; however, this distinction has important ramifications for the prognosis for the patient and for genetic counseling for the family. Earlier detection of the tumor would benefit the patient both by decreasing the chance of a child presenting with metastatic disease and by increasing the chance of being able to salvage the affected eye. A suggestion has been made to include dilation of the pupil prior to examination at the first well-child visit. An additional benefit of screening would be the earlier detection and treatment of congenital and infantile cataracts. Whether routine screening would be practical is controversial because diseases such as retinoblastoma and congenital cataracts are rare (congenital cataracts affect approximately 1 in 2,000 live births) and because pediatricians may not be adequately trained to recognize these conditions.

Ultrasonography, magnetic resonance imaging (MRI), and computed tomography (CT) (Fig. 27.3) of the orbit are the imaging studies most frequently used to confirm the diagnosis of retinoblastoma and to detect ectopic disease in the pineal gland.[95] MRI of the orbit is a more useful technique to detect soft-tissue tumor extension into the optic nerve and orbital coats.[96] CT is better for detecting intraocular calcification that could provide confirmation of retinoblastoma. However, in recent years, CT of children has fallen into disfavor due to the long-term risks for radiation-induced second malignancies.[97]

The pretreatment evaluation must be individualized for each patient. For patients who present with small tumors, careful scleral depressed examination in the office and later under anesthesia as well as office ultrasonography is necessary to make the diagnosis. A more extensive metastatic work-up is not necessary for these patients unless there is a question of optic nerve extension or extensive choroidal invasion. A lumbar puncture to obtain cerebral spinal fluid cytology and MRI or CT of the brain to rule out brain metastases can be performed for those patients. Because of the rarity of distant metastases in patients with retinoblastoma, a bone marrow examination or bone scan is usually not warranted unless the physician has suspicions of systemic involvement.

Differential Diagnosis

A number of benign conditions (pseudoretinoblastomas) can clinically simulate retinoblastoma and sometimes create considerable diagnostic difficulty for the ophthalmologist. Clinical definition is mandatory because the management of these entities differs considerably from the radical treatment of

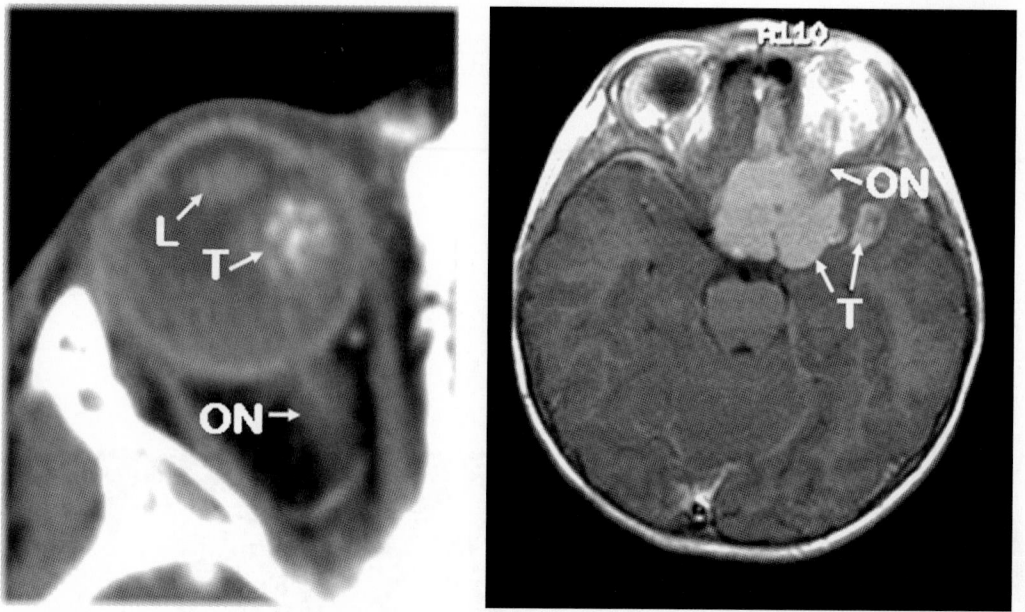

FIGURE 27.3 Diagnostic imaging of children with retinoblastoma. **A:** CT scan of the orbit. Axial view showing a partially calcified mass (T) consistent with retinoblastoma, a normal lens (L) and normal optic nerve (ON). The globe is intact and shows no evidence of extraocular invasion by tumor. **B:** MRI of the orbits and brain. Contrast-enhanced coronal T1-weighted image showing parasellar and left middle fossa spread of retinoblastoma (T) with extension along the sylvian fissure. The eye on the left is normal. The orbit on the right contains a prosthesis.

retinoblastoma. Early reports of the frequency of enucleations performed for suspected retinoblastomas when an alternative final pathological diagnosis is made varied from 30% to 16% according to the degree of oncologic experience of, and the type of referrals received by, the group reporting the series.[18,89,98,99] Most clinicians are now more familiar with pseudoretinoblastomas and the frequency of erroneous enucleation is currently much lower.[20]

Other conditions that might be confused clinically also produce or simulate a mass in the vitreous or the retina. With the exception of medulloepithelioma, these lesions have in common a variety of histopathologic features distinct from retinoblastoma that create a difficult differential diagnosis for the pathologist.[91,100–112]

Approximately 60% of pseudoretinoblastomas include the differential diagnosis of three non-neoplastic entities: *Toxocara canis* endophthalmitis, persistent hyperplastic primary vitreous (PHPV), or Coats' disease.[18] All of these entities might present with retinal detachment and may have retrolenticular fibrosis. *Toxocara canis* endophthalmitis is caused by the larvae of the nematode *Toxocara canis* and presents almost always in children, although never at birth. Clinical history and serology are important for the diagnosis. Usually there are no signs of ocular inflammation as the live larvae do not elicit an inflammatory response. Dead larvae elicit the formation of a localized eosinophilic abscess surrounding the microorganism. Condensed vitreous with gliosis and fibrosis may be present at the site of infection. Because these organisms are very small and degenerate, histological confirmation is very difficult.

Persistent hyperplastic primary vitreous (PHPV, or Persistent Fetal Vasculature [PFV]) is a congenital anomaly of the primary vitreous where embryonal vessels do not regress and may pull the retina, resulting in an anterior retinal detachment. A posterior subcapsular cataract forms if the posterior capsule of the lens is ruptured by the traction of the vessels

and fibrous membrane. Some cases of PHPV are associated with a wide band to the optic nerve and with retinal dysplasia. There are rare cases reported when PHPV has been associated with retinoblastoma.[113–117]

In contrast to toxocariasis and PHPV, Coats' disease lacks the fibrosis and vascularization of vitreous. Coats' disease is characterized by peripheral retinal vascular telangiectasia. These abnormal vessels leak and create an exudative retinal detachment rich in lipids with subretinal foamy macrophages and cholesterol clefts. Toxocariasis and PHPV simulate endophytic retinoblastoma and Coats' disease mimics the exophytic type (see Pathology).[98,102,118–122] Ultrasound, CT scans, MRI, and other ancillary imaging technology have greatly helped in the differential diagnosis of these lesions.[113,122–127]

The Use of Cytology in the Diagnosis of Retinoblastoma

Retinoblastoma is one of the only human tumors radically treated without tissue biopsy confirmation. The clinical presentation and the ancillary radiologic and ultrasonic findings are typical for retinoblastoma in the majority of patients. Usually the correct diagnosis does not represent a diagnostic dilemma for the experienced pediatric/oncologic ophthalmologist. The resistance to biopsy confirmation of the tumor arises from the dramatic difference between survivals for patients with contained intraocular tumors versus those with extraocular seeding of the tumor. The bias against biopsy is also aggravated by reports of cases where the tumor was misdiagnosed as *uveitis* or obscured by cataract, and patients developed orbital extensions of retinoblastoma after vitrectomy.[128] Aggressive post-vitrectomy therapy has resulted in prevention of metastasis in most patients with unsuspected retinoblastoma.[129]

Recently, the development of more refined techniques of fine-needle aspiration biopsy (FNAB) and the increased

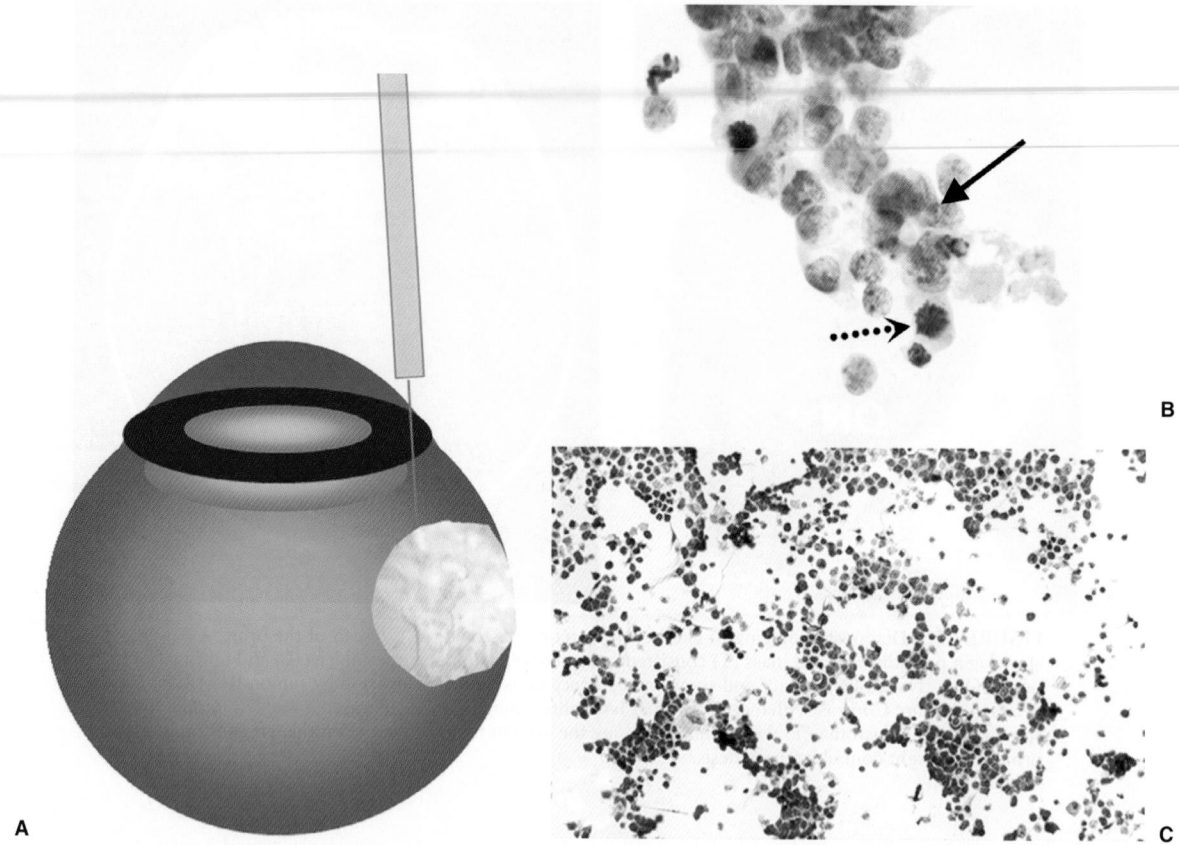

FIGURE 27.4 A: Drawing of an eye with retinoblastoma indicating the entrance of the needle through the peripheral cornea, peripheral iris, then, between the ciliary body and the lens into the tumor. The technique avoids vascularized conjunctiva of the limbus and the orbit, sclera and pars plana preventing possible spreading of tumor cells via the needle tract. **B:** Cytologic preparation of a retinoblastoma showing cohesive groups of neoplastic cells with high nuclear: cytoplasmic ratio, increased mitotic activity (*dotted arrow*) and focal rosette formation (*solid arrow*). Papanicolaou stain, original magnification 100×. **C:** Cytologic preparation of cerebrospinal fluid in a patient with retinoblastoma metastatic to the brain. Notice the cohesive groups of neoplastic cells with high nuclear: cytoplasmic ratio. Hematoxylin and eosin stain. Original magnification 20×.

knowledge of the biological behavior of retinoblastoma has allowed some patients to benefit from pretreatment biopsy.[118,130–137] The technique of FNAB for retinoblastoma involves a transcorneal approach rather than the typical *trans pars plana* approach. The transcorneal technique is more difficult to perform; it is, however, safer for the patient because the needle penetrates several tissue layers before it enters the tumor, reducing the risk for extraocular spread. The 30-gauge needle passes through the peripheral cornea, anterior chamber, peripheral iris, lens zonules (avoiding puncture of the lens), vitreous, and penetrates the tumor (Fig. 27.4). The cytological findings are small- to medium-size basophilic cells with scanty cytoplasm that tend to group together (rosette-like). Mitoses may be easy to find and necrosis is frequently encountered (Fig. 27.4). Similar features can be seen in cytologic CSF specimens in children with intracranial metastases (Fig. 27.4). There have been no reports of extraocular tumor spread through the needle tract after transcorneal FNAB, but FNAB is recommended only in selected cases where the diagnosis is ambiguous and when adequate steps are taken to prevent extraocular seeding of tumor cells.[138] In one series of FNAB of pediatric intraocular tumors, the overall accuracy of FNAB was 95% and the accuracy of cytologic interpretation was 100%. FNAB is, therefore, a reliable and accurate diagnostic tool for the assessment of selected pediatric ophthalmic diseases when the diagnosis is in question.[139,140]

PATHOLOGY

Guidelines for Processing Eyes with Retinoblastoma

To obtain an adequate specimen for evaluation of tumor characteristics, histopathologic risk features (described later), and genetic evaluation, it is necessary to process the freshly enucleated eye and obtain tumor without excessive contamination of the intraocular structures. Sections of the eye should include the structures to evaluate (choroid, tumor, all levels of the optic nerve, and anterior chamber structures).[141] In summary, there are three recommended techniques to obtain fresh tumor: a) creation of a chorioscleral window with a blade (Fig. 27.5), b) creation of a chorioscleral window with a corneal trephine, or c) by aspiration of tumor with a wide bore syringe. Any of these techniques should be performed immediately after enucleation, with awareness of the anatomic orientation and taking care to avoid collapsing the eye or excessively contaminating

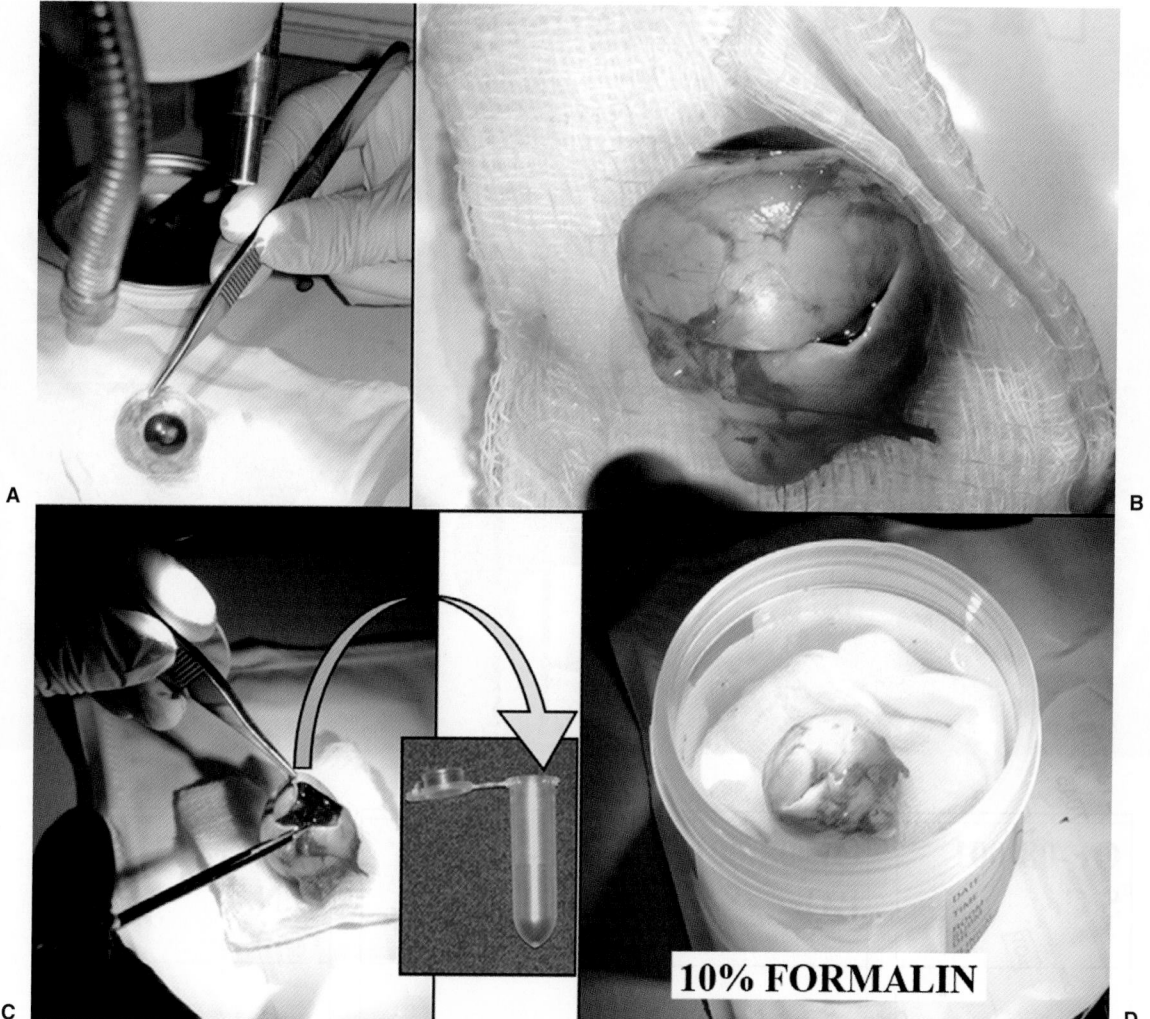

FIGURE 27.5 Handling of the enucleated eye with retinoblastoma for tumor retrieval. **A:** Preferably under a stereoscopic microscope the eye is examined to select the area in which most of the tumor is present. This is achieved by retroillumination to identify the area of the tumor by the denser shadow. Before sectioning the eye one must obtain the cross-section of the optic nerve margin for histologic examination. The scleral window should be created perpendicular to this site to obtained tumor at the edge of the larger mass. **B:** The opening of the eye is made with a sharp blade or by using a corneal trephine (not shown here), to obtain a scleral window. **C:** Under the microscope, select the areas of least necrosis and calcification without disturbing intraocular structures such as retina and optic nerve head. Retrieve tumor and placed in cryoresistant tubes to immediately freeze and store until needed for genetic studies or research. **D:** Place the eye in 10% formalin gently reforming the round shape of the eye and fix for at least 24 hours.

ocular structures with the tumor. Before opening the eye, a cross-section of the optic nerve should be obtained and submitted for histopathologic examination to avoid contamination by the tumor. Tumor for genetic analysis is then retrieved and immediately frozen at −70 to −80 degrees centigrade in cryoresistant tubes (Fig. 27.5). The eye is then placed in 10% formalin and, after adequate fixation, the eye is grossed to obtain a central section including the optic nerve, tumor, and pupil (P.O. pupil-optic nerve section), and two calottes (remainder of eye). The calottes should be further sectioned into anterior and posterior segments, and submitted on edge for histopathologic examination of the choroid. In total, there should be four blocks: one with the optic nerve surgical margin cross-section, one with the PO section, and one for each calotte in segments (Fig. 27.6). Several levels of each block should be reviewed for diagnosis.

Gross Features

Primary retinoblastomas originate in the sensory retina and occupy the retina and vitreous cavity. Retinoblastoma tumors are usually white-gray with a chalky appearance and a soft, friable consistency. Bright white speckles corresponding to calcifications are present throughout the tumor. The gross features of retinoblastoma depend on the growth pattern of the tumor.[18,88,142] Some of these patterns correlate with clinical presentations and differences in biological behavior, especially as they relate to intraocular and extraocular types of tumor spread.

The endophytic growth pattern is represented by tumors arising from the retina and growing into the vitreous cavity (Fig. 27.7). These tumors tend to entirely fill the cavity and produce floating tumor spheres called vitreous seeds. A tumor

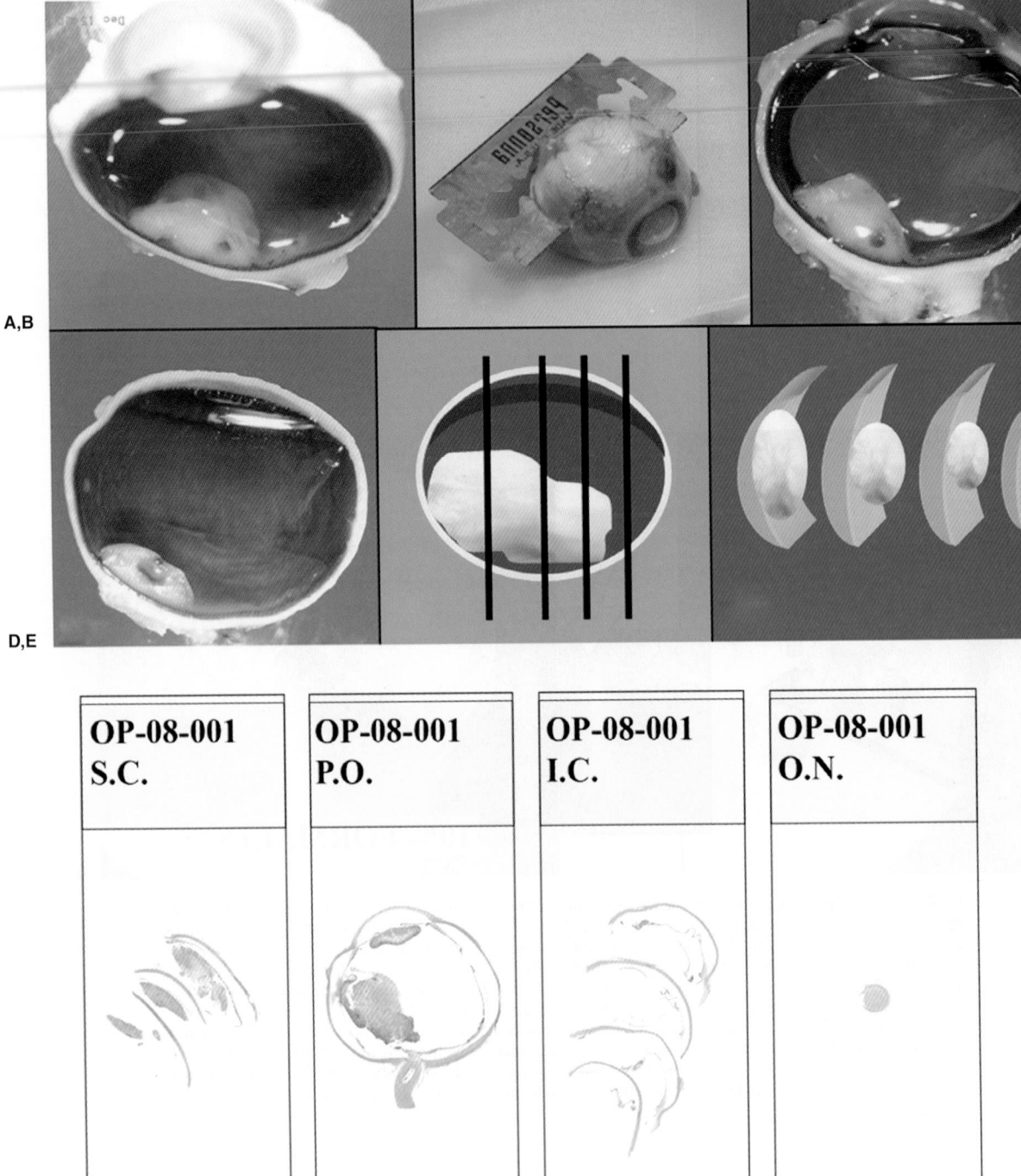

FIGURE 27.6 Grossing of the eye with retinoblastoma. **A:** After adequate fixation remove the calotte where the window to obtain fresh tumor was created by cutting nearer to the optic nerve (without transecting it) and to avoid the opened area of the sclera. **B:** Cut and remove the opposite calotte to obtain the central pupil optic nerve section (P.O.). **C:** Central P.O. section showing anterior chamber, pupil, lens, tumor and optic nerve in one section. **D:** Calotte with some tumor. **E:** Schematic representation of the anterior-posterior sections of the calottes. **F:** Schematic representation of the sections already cut from the calottes to submit for processing into paraffin blocks and slides. **G:** At the end of the process there should be 4 blocks that give rise to slides with sections of the calottes (2), the PO sections (1) and the cross-section of the optic nerve margin (1).

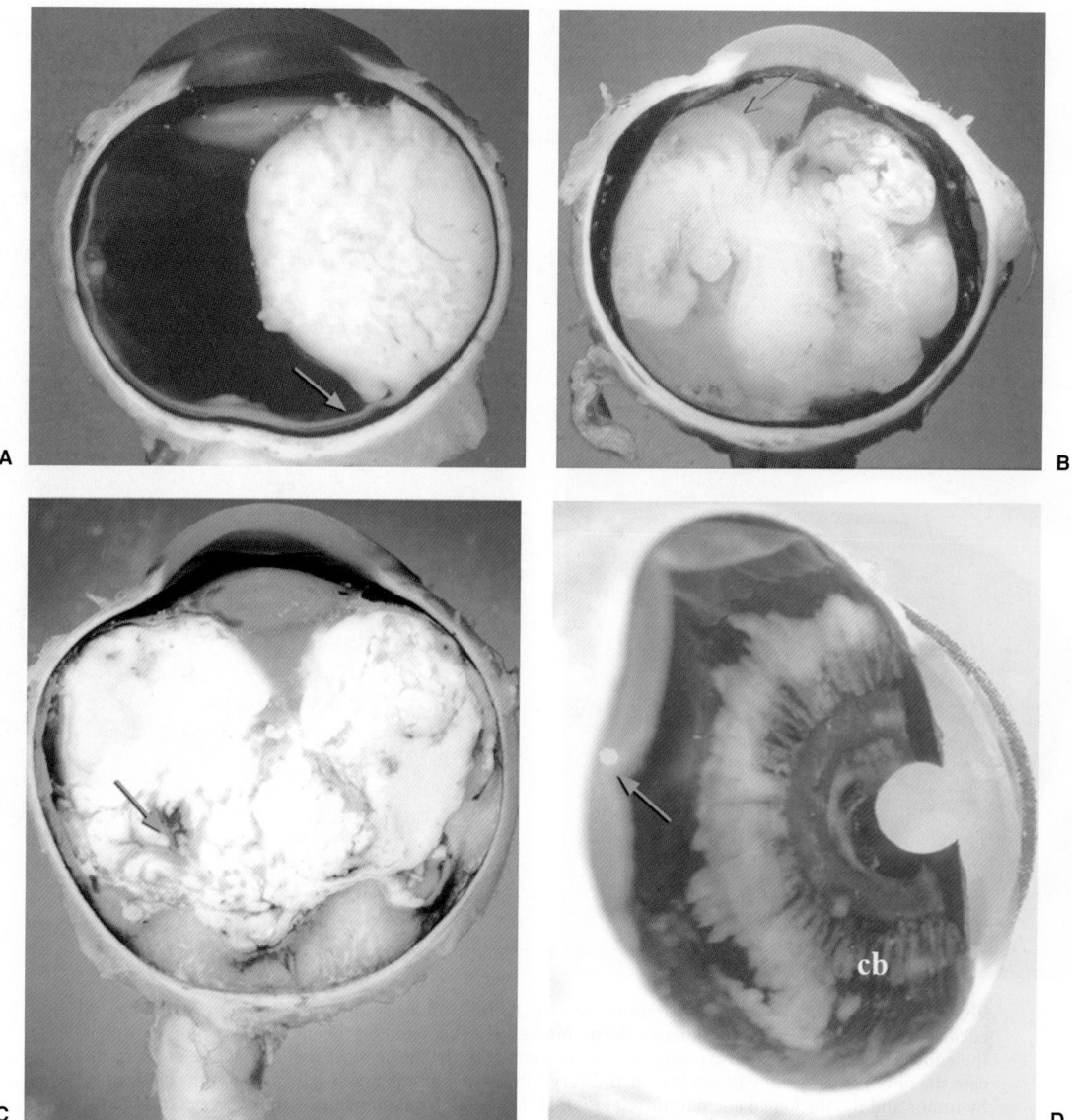

FIGURE 27.7 A: Gross photograph of an eye with a retinoblastoma showing an endophytic growth pattern. Notice that the tumor mass is growing from the retina (*arrow*) into the vitreal cavity. **B:** Gross photograph of an eye with a retinoblastoma showing an exophytic growth pattern. Notice that the tumor is growing from the retina (*arrow*) into the subretinal space with associated retinal detachment. **C:** Gross photograph of an eye with a retinoblastoma showing a mixed growth pattern, the most frequent type. Notice that the tumor grows both into the vitreous cavity and into the subretinal space with the retina (*arrow*) entrapped in the middle. The tumor has massively invaded the choroid (**C**). **D:** Gross photograph of an eye with a diffuse retinoblastoma. Notice the absence of a well-formed mass; instead there are white seeds of tumor cells along the retina (*arrow*) and ciliary body (cb).

left untreated eventually invades the anterior portion of the eye, reaching the aqueous venous channels and the conjunctiva. From there, the tumor can permeate the lymphatic vessels and metastasize to regional lymph nodes.[18,142–145]

Exophytic tumors grow from the retina into the subretinal space and often cause serous detachments of the retina (Fig. 27.7). These tumors may invade the choroid through Bruch's membrane.[18,142,146,147] Mixed endophytic and exophytic tumor growth is the most common pattern encountered[18,20,142] (Fig. 27.7).

Diffuse infiltrating retinoblastoma is the least common tumor growth pattern, but is the most diagnostically challenging because there is no predominant mass (Fig. 27.7). This presentation of retinoblastoma is seen in children with an average age of 6 years. The tumor cells grow throughout the retina while single cells and vitreous seeds invade the anterior portions of the retina, the ciliary body, and, eventually, the anterior chamber. Clinically, this type of tumor resembles an inflammatory process presenting as pseudohypopyon mimicking inflammatory cell accumulation (hypopyon) in the anterior chamber and vitreous seeds simulating the inflammatory cellular reaction seen in uveitis. Because this type of retinoblastoma resembles an inflammatory process, the diagnosis is often delayed until cytological examination of the aqueous humor or, in rare cases, of the vitreous. Almost all reported cases have a unilateral, sporadic presentation without family history. Although the diagnosis is difficult, children with diffuse infiltrating retinoblastoma have a good prognosis after enucleation.[115,145,148–157] Any child,

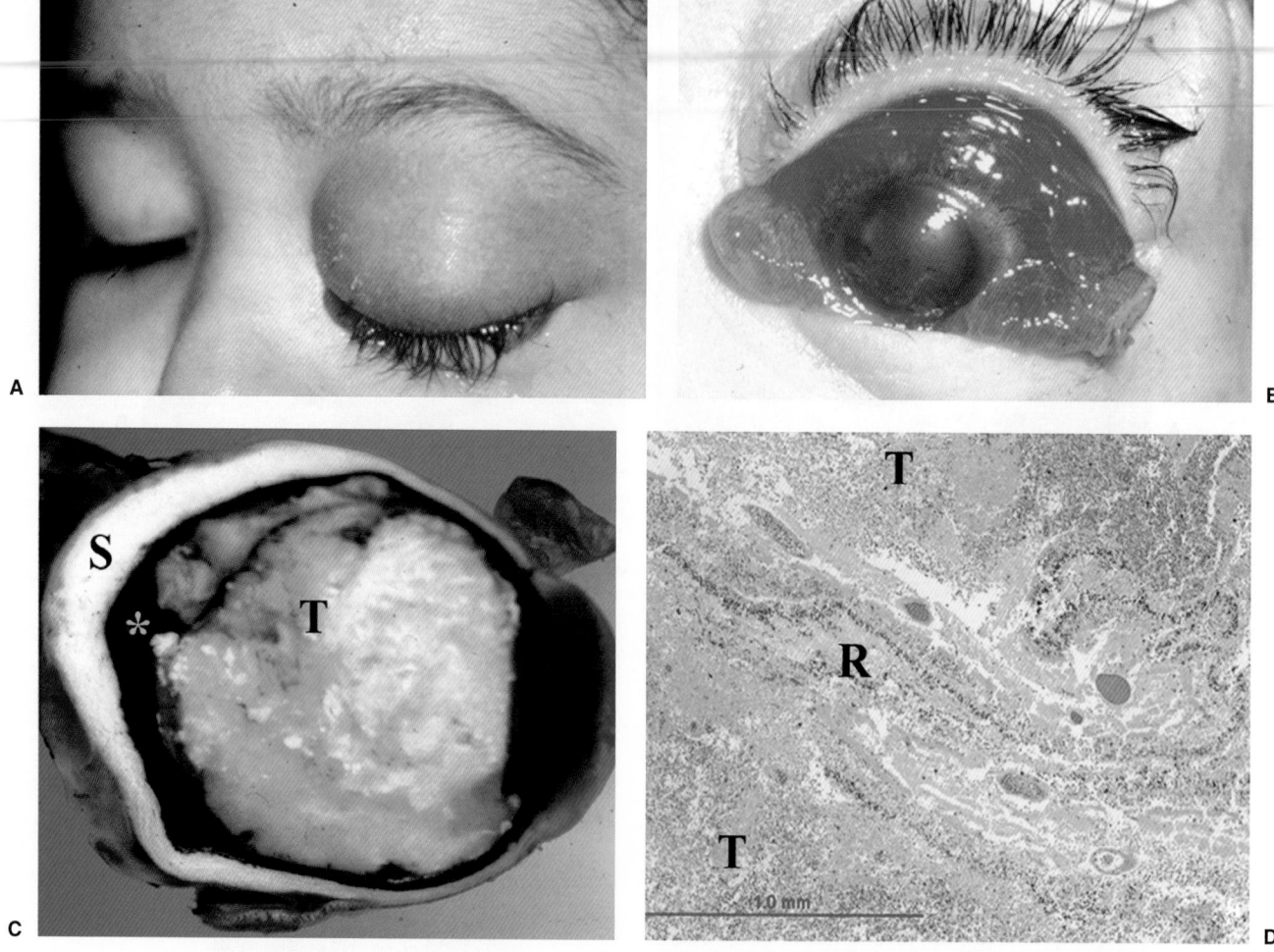

FIGURE 27.8 Extensively necrotic retinoblastoma. **A:** Inflammatory presentation with erythema and edema of the eyelids. **B:** The conjunctiva shows marked chemosis and erythema. **C:** Gross photograph of the enucleated eye with extensive necrosis of the tumor (T) that instead of the even white color in this case the tumor is tan yellow to tan brown and very soft. Also note the massive invasion of the choroid (*) by tumor and the thickened edematous sclera (s). **D:** Microphotograph of the extensively necrotic tumor (T) that surrounds necrotic retina (R) (original magnification 4×, H & E stain).

regardless of age, who presents with signs of endophthalmitis should be considered to have diffuse infiltrating retinoblastoma until proven otherwise.[155]

Another unusual presentation is the extensively necrotic retinoblastoma that presents as severe inflammatory reaction with massive necrosis of the tumor (more than 95%) and with necrosis of the intraocular structures. If the eye is left untreated, this may be followed by phthisis bulbi (complete atrophy of the eye).[158–170] If the eye is enucleated at the time of acute necrosis, the gross findings are those of massive tumor necrosis, intraocular tissue necrosis with dispersion of pigment, and edema of the conjunctiva[166,171] (Fig. 27.8). Extensively necrotic retinoblastoma is associated with statistically significant increase in histopathologic risk factors such as choroidal invasion and optic nerve invasion.[172] Through unknown mechanisms, complete spontaneous tumor regression occurs more commonly in retinoblastoma than in any other malignant tumor. In most of these cases, complete occlusion of the central retinal artery is found; however, it is not known whether this is a primary event or the result of tumor necrosis.[166,167] If the eye is examined after complete atrophy has occurred, the findings are those of a small shrunken eye with mostly necrotic calcified tumor and a disorganized retina.

Histologic Features

Microscopic examination of the affected eye displays one or more tumors with large areas of necrosis and multifocal calcifications replacing portions of the retina (Fig. 27.9). The majority of the tumor is formed by small- to medium-size hyperchromatic cells with a high nuclear to cytoplasmic ratio. The tumor cells are mitotically active but frequently exhibit apoptosis[18,20,88,109,142,173–177] (Fig. 27.9). Viable cells surround blood vessels in a range of 90–110 μm forming a collarette (pseudorosettes) (Fig. 27.9). Viability of the tumor cells depends on the intrinsic tumor blood supply. Areas of coagulative necrosis contain multiple foci of dystrophic calcification. Tumor-cell necrosis liberates DNA from the nuclei of the cells. The released DNA forms deposits on the basement membranes of the vessels, the lens (capsule), the retina (internal limiting membrane), and the choroid (Bruch's membrane)[178] (Fig. 27.9).

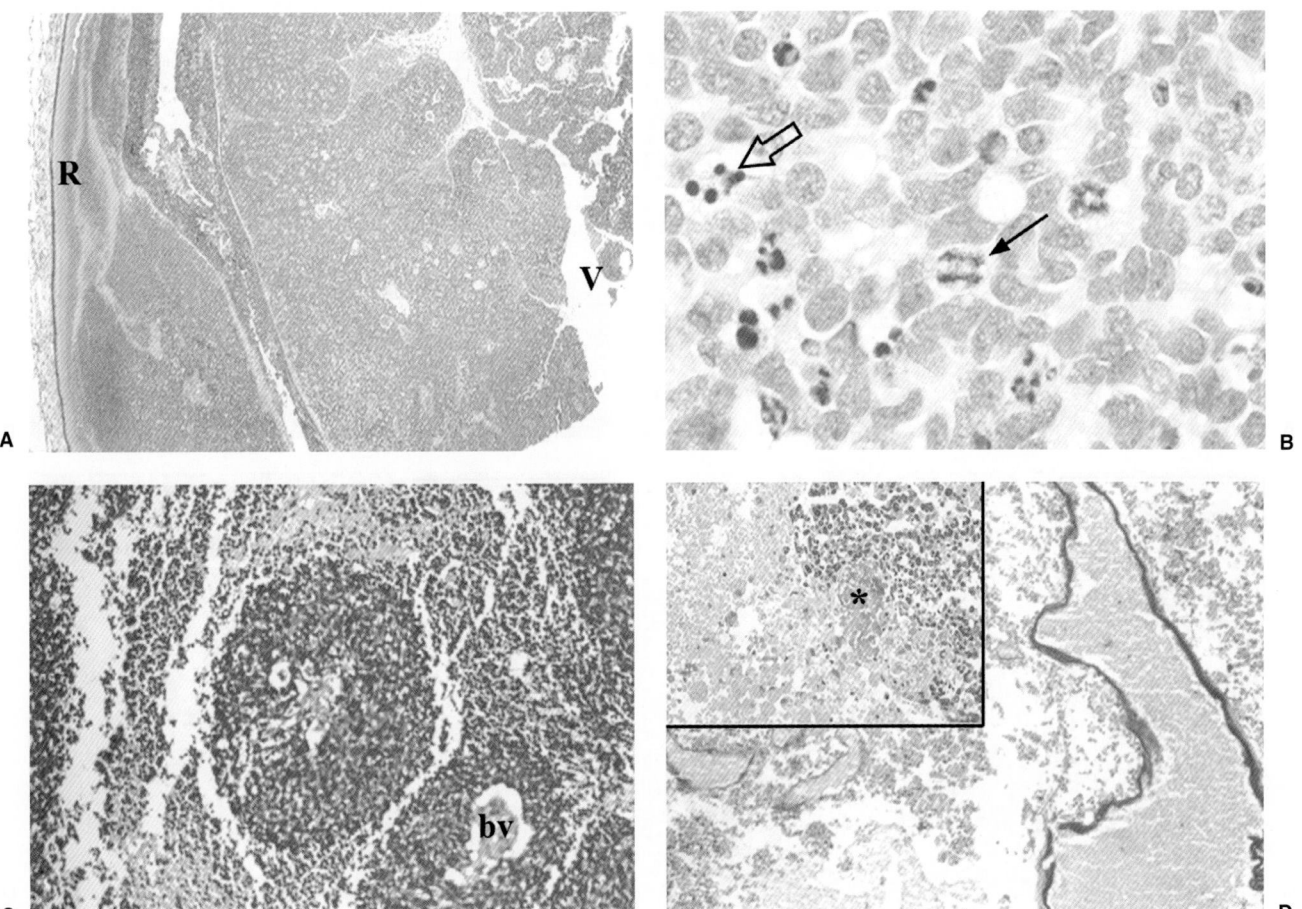

FIGURE 27.9 A: Histologic picture of a retinoblastoma growing from the retina (R) into the vitreous cavity (V). Hematoxylin and eosin stain. Original magnification 4×. **B:** Histologic photograph showing poorly differentiated retinoblastoma cells with high nuclear: cytoplasmic ratio, increased mitotic activity (*solid arrow*), and increased apoptosis (*hollow arrow*). Hematoxylin and eosin stain. Original magnification 100×. **C:** Microphotograph showing viable tumor cells surrounding blood vessels (bv) with necrotic cells beyond a rim of approximately 110 μm. Hematoxylin and eosin stain. Original magnification 20×. **D:** Microphotograph of retinoblastoma with extensive necrosis (insert) with foci of calcification (*). Notice the large vessel darkly stained with hematoxylin (basophilic) secondary to DNA deposits in the vascular basement membrane as a result of extensive tumor cell necrosis that liberates nuclear DNA. Hematoxylin and eosin stain. Original magnification 10×.

Some retinoblastomas show large areas of undifferentiated or poorly differentiated tumor (Fig. 27.10); other retinoblastomas show a certain degree of differentiation represented by formation of rosettes. It has been reported that the degree of differentiation decreases with age at enucleation.[179] Flexner-Wintersteiner rosettes are highly characteristic of retinoblastoma, although they are also seen in pinealoblastomas and medulloepitheliomas. Flexner-Wintersteiner rosettes are lined by tall cuboidal cells that circumscribe an apical lumen. The apical ends attach to each other by terminal bars and the cells may have apical cytoplasmic projections into the lumen of the rosette (Fig. 27.10). Electron microscopy has demonstrated that these projections represent inner and outer segments of photoreceptors.[107,180,181] This and several other observations support the idea that retinoblastomas arise from undifferentiated retinal cells that may differentiate into photoreceptors,[107,180–187] usually of the cone-cell lineage.[6,7] An explanation for this observation may have been found in the mouse where RB protein expression is required for retinal progenitor cells to exit the cell cycle and for rod photoreceptor differentiation to occur.[188] Homer Wright rosettes are less common than Flexner-Wintersteiner rosettes and are found in a variety of neuroblastic tumors in addition to retinoblastoma. These rosettes do not surround a lumen but rather extend cytoplasmic processes that fill the center of the rosette. Homer Wright rosettes may be incomplete and admixed with well-formed Flexner-Wintersteiner rosettes (Fig. 27.10).

Approximately 6% to 20% of tumors show benign photoreceptor differentiation into groups of cells with short cytoplasmic processes, abundant cytoplasm, and small round nuclei similar to photoreceptors.[179] These groups of cells which resemble a bouquet of flowers are called *fleurettes*.[16,189,190] Neither significant mitotic activity nor necrosis is observed within the fleurettes[191–193] (Fig. 27.10).

Retinocytoma

A benign counterpart to retinoblastoma called *retinocytoma* (also *retinoma*) that solely contains well-differentiated glial

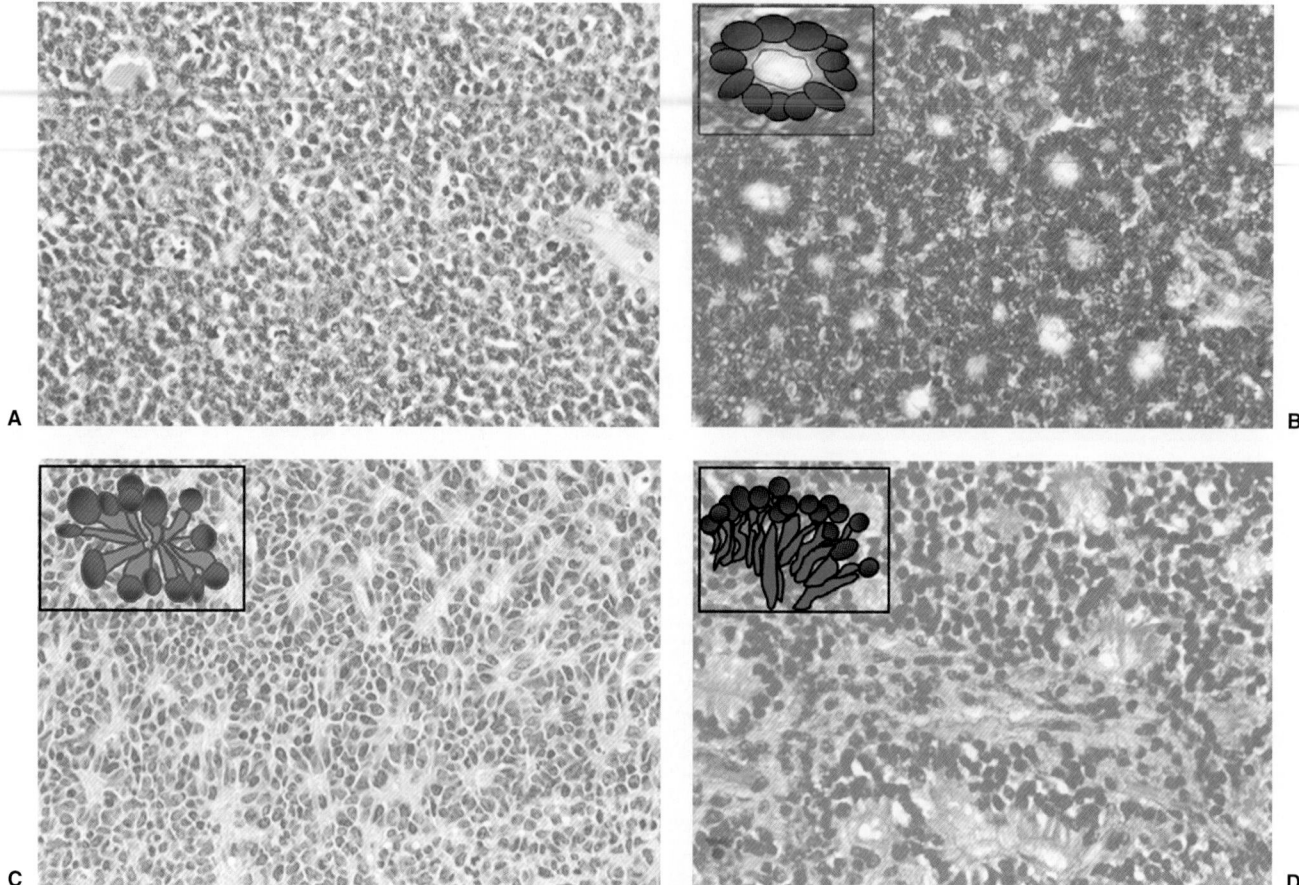

FIGURE 27.10 A: Microphotograph of a poorly differentiated retinoblastoma showing sheets of neoplastic cells without rosette formation. Hematoxylin and eosin stain. Original magnification 40×. **B**: Microphotograph of a retinoblastoma showing Flexner-Wintersteiner rosette formation (insert). Notice that these rosettes have a center partially filled by cytoplasmic prolongations with apical terminal bars. Hematoxylin and eosin stain. Original magnification 40×. **C**: Microphotograph of a retinoblastoma showing Homer Wright rosette formation (insert). The lumen of the rosette is filled by cytoplasmic prolongations. Hematoxylin and eosin stain. Original magnification 40×. **D**: Microphotograph of a well-differentiated retinoblastoma showing fleurettes (insert). Fleurettes are groups of well-differentiated cells similar to photoreceptors joined by cytoplasmic junctions and forming a figure similar to a bouquet of flowers. Hematoxylin and eosin stain. Original magnification 40×.

cells and fleurettes has been described. These benign tumors contain large areas of abrupt calcification associated with retinal pigment epithelium proliferation (Fig. 27.11). They exhibit specific features that allow experienced clinicians to follow the behavior of the tumor without radical treatment.[4,9,88,194,195] Singh et al.[194] described the characteristic ophthalmoscopic features of 24 retinocytomas, including the presence of a translucent retinal mass in 21 (88%), calcification in 15 (63%), and retinal pigment epithelial alteration in 13 (54%) of the tumors. A combination of all three features was observed in 8 (33%) of the 24 tumors. In 13 (54%) of the tumors, a zone of chorioretinal atrophy could be observed. Although the majority of these tumors behave as benign lesions, close follow-up is suggested because a few tumors have been reported to have undergone malignant transformation into retinoblastomas that eventually required enucleation.[189,194] Recently, it has been shown that both copies of the *RB1* gene are deleted or inactive in retinocytomas, suggesting that these lesions are precursors of retinoblastoma and that this double deletion of the *RB1* gene is not enough for malignant transformation, for which additional events are necessary.[24]

In retinoblastoma (malignant) tumors that have undergone complete regression, either spontaneously or secondary to treatment, mummified calcified tumor cells and large areas of dystrophic calcification are observed. Exuberant reactive retinal pigment epithelial proliferation and glial cells with occasional ossification accompany this process which mimics the findings seen in retinocytoma.[88]

METASTASIS AND RECURRENCE

If left untreated, retinoblastoma usually fills the eye and completely destroys the internal architecture of the globe. The most common route of spread is by invasion through the optic nerve. Once in the optic nerve, the tumor spreads directly along the nerve fiber bundles towards the optic chiasm or infiltrates through the pia into the subarachnoid space. From the subarachnoid space, the retinoblastoma can involve the CSF, the brain, and the spine. The second major route of spread is through massive involvement of the choroid into the orbit via either scleral canals (areas within the sclera

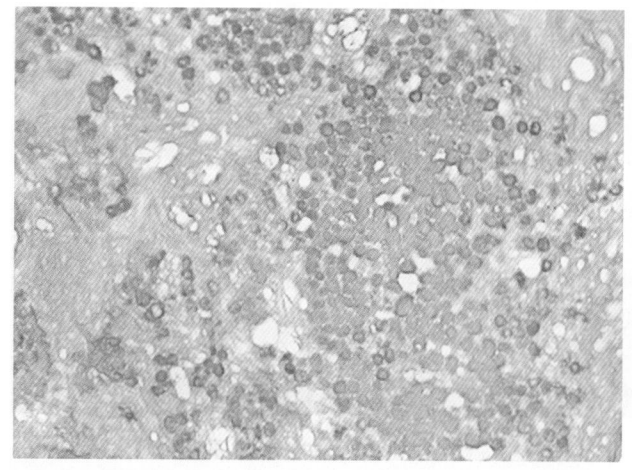

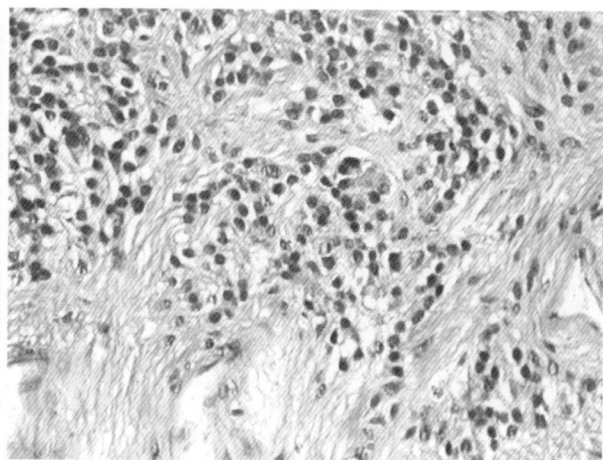

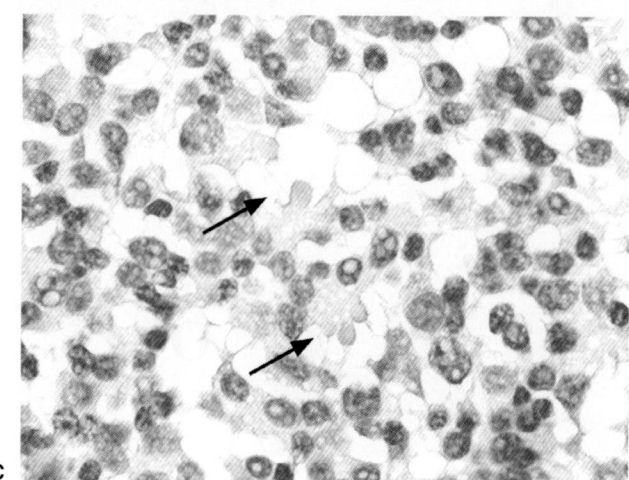

FIGURE 27.11 **A:** Histologic picture of abrupt cell calcification in a retinocytoma. Hematoxylin and eosin stain. Original magnification 40×. **B:** Histologic picture of a well-differentiated area of a retinocytoma showing glial and neural differentiation (*). Hematoxylin and eosin stain. Original magnification 40×. **C:** Histologic picture of a well-differentiated area of a retinocytoma showing fleurettes (*arrows*). Hematoxylin and eosin stain. Original magnification 40×.

where ciliary vessels, nerves, and vortex veins enter or exit the eye) or by direct extension through the sclera[196] (Fig. 27.12). Although not in every patient, extraocular extension generally occurs within 6 months if intraocular tumors are left untreated.

Extraocular extension dramatically increases the chances of hematogenous and lymphatic spread. There are four routes for metastatic spread of retinoblastoma:[18,88]

1. By direct infiltration either through the optic nerve into the brain, or through the choroid into the orbit soft tissues and bones.
2. By dispersion of the tumor cells through the subarachnoid space of the optic nerve into the opposite optic nerve, or through the CSF into the brain and spine, which can occur without detectable presence of retinoblastoma at the surgical margin of the optic nerve.
3. By hematogenous dissemination secondary to orbital and bone invasion, or when lymphatic invasion reaches the lymph nodes. Among other sites, wide-spread metastasis can present in lung, bone, and brain.
4. Via lymphatic dissemination in tumors that spread anteriorly into the conjunctiva and eyelids, or extend into extraocular tissues. Lymphatic vessels and lymphoid tissue are absent in the orbit and intraocular tissues. In the ocular region, only conjunctiva and skin have lymphatic channels. Tumors must first reach these areas to permeate the lymphatic vessels and then spread into regional lymph nodes.

Histologically, retinoblastoma metastases appear less differentiated than intraocular tumors. Rosettes are rarely encountered and fleurettes have never been described. When very well-differentiated extraocular tumors appear outside of the orbit, a differential diagnosis of a primary primitive neuroectodermal tumor (PNET) must be considered.

TRILATERAL RETINOBLASTOMA AND OTHER TUMORS

Primary retinoblastomas of the pineal and parasellar sites have been called pinealoblastoma and are usually present as single tumors. Trilateral retinoblastoma presenting with tumors in both eyes and the pineal is a well recognized, although rare, syndrome.[197] The majority of the reported cases have involved patients with a family history of retinoblastoma and the disease is usually fatal. There are recent observations that newer chemoreduction treatments can minimize the risk for the development of pinealoblastoma.[198] These pineal tumors can appear several years after successful treatment of intraocular retinoblastoma. They can be far more differentiated than the primary tumor and may contain numerous rosettes, fleurettes, and individual cells showing photoreceptor differentiation. The presentation of trilateral retinoblastoma contrasts with metastatic retinoblastoma since metastatic retinoblastoma presents as

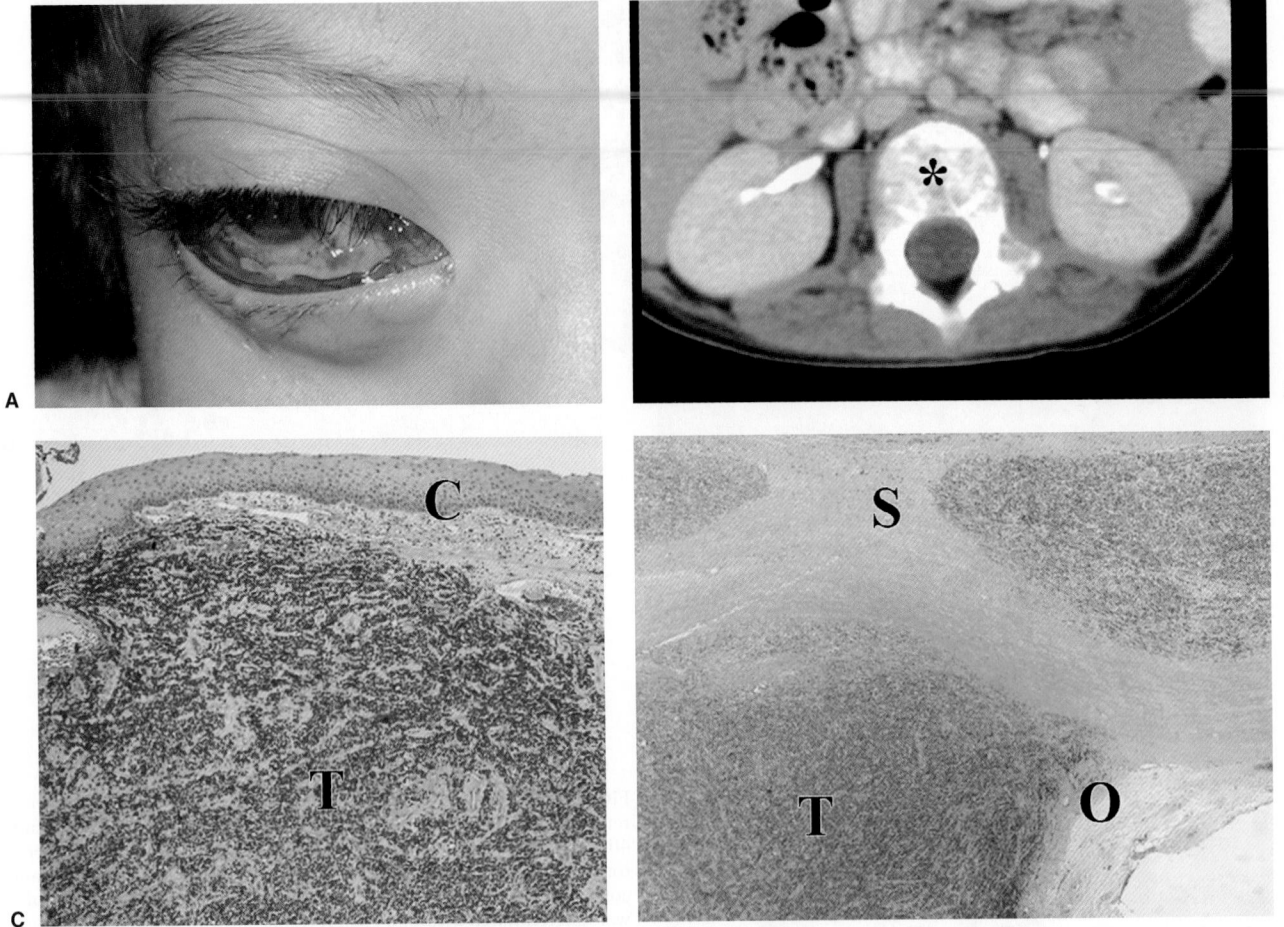

FIGURE 27.12 Metastatic retinoblastoma in a child with extraocular extension of tumor. **A:** Buphthalmus and nodularity of the inferior eyelid produced by extraocular extension of tumor. Please also note the pale color of the skin and conjunctiva secondary to involvement of bone marrow by tumor causing severe anemia. **B:** CT scan with contrast showing extensive lytic lesion of the vertebra (*). **C:** Histologic section of the bulbar conjunctiva showing massive tumor (T) infiltrate of the stroma underlying the conjunctival epithelium (C) Hematoxylin and eosin stain. Original magnification 10×. **D:** Histologic section of the sclera (S) demonstrating extraocular extension of the tumor (T) into the orbital tissues (O). Hematoxylin and eosin stain. Original magnification 4×.

multiple, undifferentiated tumors within 2 years of initial treatment.

STAGING

Different classifications have been introduced as guidelines for predicting prognosis for vision, for globe salvage, and for survival. The Reese-Ellsworth classification[199] (Table 27.1A) relates to eyes treated by methods other than enucleation, specifically by radiotherapy. This classification, devised prior to the development of current ophthalmologic methodologies for diagnosis and treatment, has often been used to imply prognosis for life rather than for vision. Although the Reese-Ellsworth classification is not necessarily prognostic for outcomes using modern treatment modalities, it is still the classification used most often to compare therapeutic results. The American Joint Committee on Cancer (AJCC) has proposed a clinical and pathologic staging classification for retinoblastoma where complete spontaneous regression of the tumor has not occurred. Using these criteria for cases of bilat-

eral retinoblastoma, each eye is staged separately. Histologic verification of the disease in an enucleated eye is required and any unconfirmed cases must be reported separately. The extent of retinal involvement is indicated as a percentage of the total retinal area. For the pathologic staging, all of the clinical and pathologic data from the resected specimen are to be used. A revised staging classification was adopted in 2003 and is called the International Classification of Retinoblastoma (ICRB)[200–202] (Table 27.1B).

Prognostic Factors

Prognosis for vision in children with unilateral retinoblastoma is excellent for the uninvolved eye. The development of tumors in the contralateral eye after 3 years is very rare. A primary tumor with vitreous, subretinal, and retinal seeds can be mistaken as a multifocal primary tumor. Primary tumors arise from the sensory retina in contrast to retinal seedings, which sit on top of the retina (Fig. 27.13) or on the inner subretinal surface of the photoreceptors.

TABLE 27A.1

REESE-ELLSWORTH CLASSIFICATION FOR CONSERVATIVE TREATMENT OF RETINOBLASTOMA[a]

Group I: Very favorable
  a) Solitary tumor, less than 4 disc diameters in size, at or behind the equator
  b) Multiple tumors, none over 4 disc diameters in size, all at or behind the equator

Group II: Favorable
  a) Solitary tumor, 4 to 10 disc diameters in size, at or behind the equator
  b) Multiple tumors, 4 to 10 disc diameters in size, behind the equator

Group III: Doubtful
  a) Any lesion anterior to the equator
  b) Solitary tumors larger than 10 disc diameters behind the equator

Group IV: Unfavorable
  a) Multiple tumors, some larger than 10 disc diameters
  b) Any lesion extending anteriorly to the ora serrata

Group V: Very unfavorable
  a) Massive tumors involving over half the retina
  b) Vitreous seeding

[a]Refers to chances of salvaging the affected eye and not systemic prognosis.

The presence of multiple primary tumors or the emergence of tumors in both eyes (bilateral retinoblastoma) supports a diagnosis of inherited retinoblastoma. The prognosis for vision in bilateral retinoblastoma depends on the extent of tumor involvement and the effectiveness of treatment modalities. If the tumors are small and away from the fovea (central portion of the retina with best visual acuity), one may anticipate a good prognosis for vision after successful treatment.[18,88,142]

The survival rate for retinoblastoma patients has improved dramatically over the last century. One of the first retinoblastoma survival studies was reported in 1897 by Wintersteiner.[203] The 13% survival rate reported then is in sharp contrast to the 90% overall 5-year survival reported by many centers today.[204–207] The main reasons for this improvement are the improved ability to detect retinoblastoma prior to the onset of metastatic disease and the development of alternative treatment strategies (see section "Therapeutic Options").

TABLE 27.1B

INTERNATIONAL CLASSIFICATION OF RETINOBLASTOMA (ICRB), LONG FORM

Group	Subgroup	Quick reference	Specific features
A	A	Small tumor	Rb ≤3 mm in size[a]
B	B	Larger tumor Macula Juxtapapillary Subretinal fluid	Rb >3 mm in size[a] or • Macular Rb location (≤3 mm to foveola) • Juxtapapillary Rb location (≤1.5 mm to disc) • Clear subretinal fluid (≤3 mm from margin)
C		Focal seeds	Rb with
	C1		• Subretinal seeds (≤3 mm from Rb)
	C2		• Vitreous seeds (≤3 mm from Rb)
	C3		• Both subretinal and vitreous seeds (≤3 mm from Rb)
D		Diffuse seeds	Rb with
	D1		• Subretinal seeds (>3 mm from Rb)
	D2		• Vitreous seeds (>3 mm from Rb)
	D3		• Both subretinal and vitreous seeds (>3 mm from Rb)
E	E	Extensive Rb	Extensive Rb occupying >50% globe or • Neovascular glaucoma • Opaque media from hemorrhage in anterior chamber, vitreous or subretinal space • Invasion of postlaminar optic nerve, choroid (>2 mm), sclera, orbit, anterior chamber

Rb, retinoblastoma.
[a]Refers to 3 mm in basal dimension or thickness.

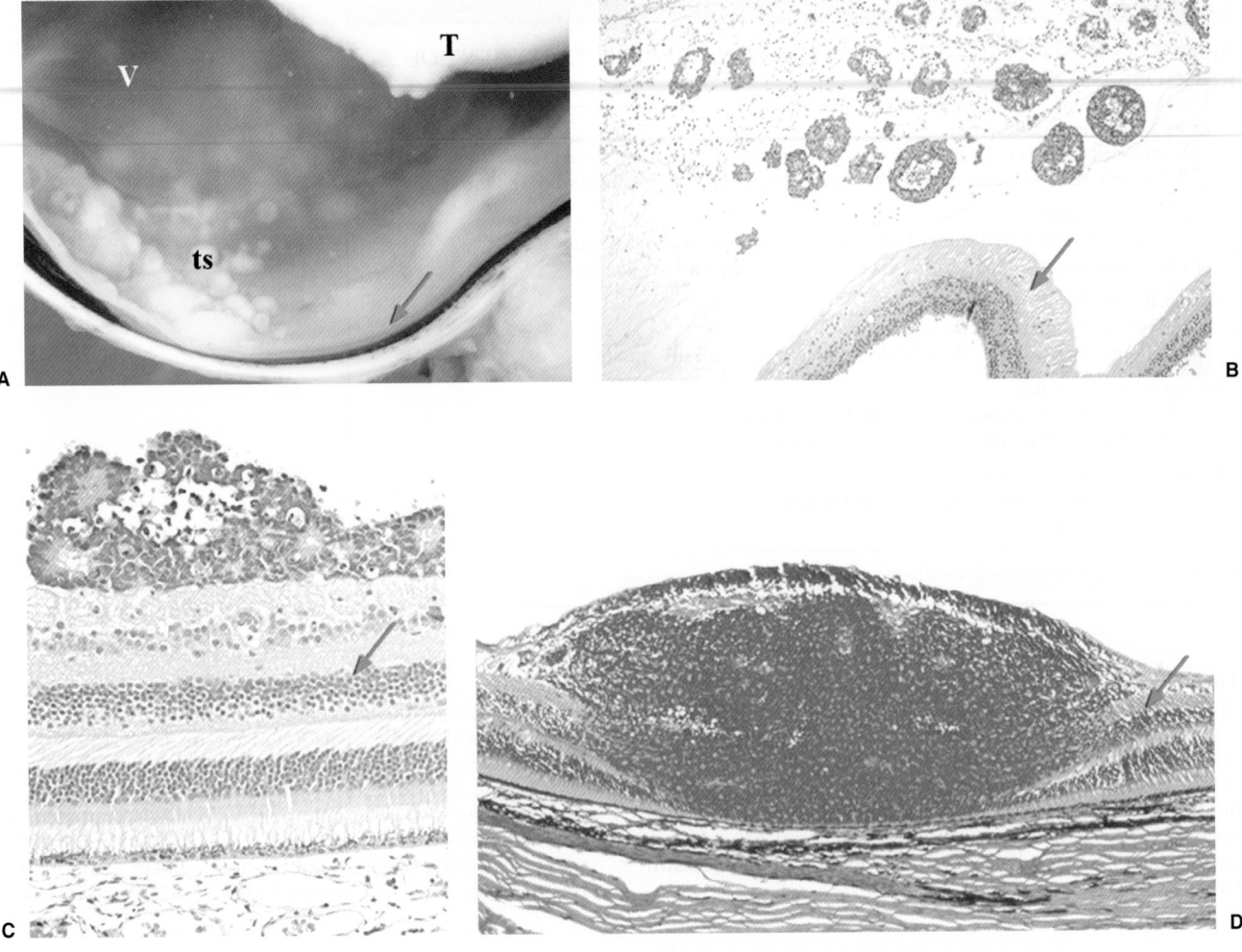

FIGURE 27.13 **A:** Gross photograph showing a primary retinoblastoma tumor (T) with tumor seeds (ts) on the inner retina (*arrow*) and in the vitreous (v). **B:** Microphotograph of an area of vitreous tumor seeds. Notice the hollow center of the retinoblastoma seeds. The retina (*arrow*) is without tumor. Hematoxylin and eosin stain. Original magnification 10×. **C:** Microphotograph of a retinoblastoma seed on the inner surface of the retina. Notice the rosette formation of the tumor and the intact architecture of the retina (*arrow*). Hematoxylin and eosin stain. Original magnification 40×. **D:** Microphotograph of a retinoblastoma arising from the retina (*arrow*). Notice the tumor replacing the normal architecture of the retina. Hematoxylin and eosin stain. Original magnification 20×.

Histopathologic Risk Factors

Metastatic disease is still associated with a poor prognosis. Most clinical findings are not useful in predicting the occurrence of metastasis in children with retinoblastoma, although histopathologic data provide a fair estimate of its risk. Recently, a retrospective study showed that patients presenting with glaucoma and/or buphthalmia have a significantly higher risk for histopathologic risk factors, including those resulting in microscopically residual disease.[208] Multivariate statistical analysis has suggested the correlation of certain histopathologic findings and prognostic risk factors.[206,209–213] The most important prognostic indicators for the development of metastasis are the presence of tumor in the optic nerve posterior to the lamina cribrosa at the site of surgical transection and extrascleral extension of tumor into the orbit.[118,143,144,146,196,206,210,213–220] Two retrospective studies on histopathologic high-risk features, one from a developed country and the other from a developing country, were pub-lished recently and showed that high risk features were present in 20.4% of children in the developed country and in 54.2% of the children in the developing country.[179,221] The results suggest that this increased risk seen in the developing countries may be due to a delay in diagnosis and treatment, but the possibility of different biological behavior cannot be excluded.

The Children's Oncology Group (COG), through the prospective protocol ARET0332 "A study of unilateral retinoblastoma with and without histopathologic risk factors and the role of adjuvant chemotherapy," as well as the consensus meetings from the International Retinoblastoma Staging Working Group (IRSWG) on the pathology guidelines for the examination of enucleated eyes and evaluation of prognostic risk factors in retinoblastoma[141] address the inconsistency in previous reports of definitions for histopathologic risk factors. Both groups specifically address the definition of massive versus focal choroidal invasion and the necessity for objective measurement of invasive tumor in the ocular coats and optic nerve (Table 27.2).

TABLE 27.2

HISTOPATHOLOGIC RISK FEATURES BASED ON TUMOR INVASION OF OCULAR STRUCTURES

Choroid:	Massive invasion 3 mm or more	Focal invasion Less than 3 mm
Optic nerve:	No increased risk a. Prelaminar b. Lamina cribrosa	Increased risk a. Postlaminar b. At surgical margin c. Subarachnoid
Other:	Anterior segment invasion Neovascularization of iris with glaucoma Extensively necrotic retinoblastoma Buphthalmus	

Optic Nerve Invasion

The extent of tumor invasion in the optic nerve correlates with prognosis (Fig. 27.14). Superficial invasion of the optic disc is associated with a mortality rate of 10%, a rate similar to that seen when the optic nerve is not involved. The presence of tumor up to the lamina cribrosa is associated with a mortality rate of 29%. Invasion of tumor posterior to the lamina cribrosa is associated with a mortality rate of 42%, while the presence of tumor at the transected surgical margin is associated with a mortality of 80%.[143,196,206,210,213,222] The importance of obtaining a large portion of optic nerve at the time of enucleation is underscored by these results. Specific studies related to the length of the optic nerve stump alone show that patients with the optic nerve measuring <5 mm attached to the enucleated eye have a worse prognosis than those having >5 mm stumps.[206,217,223–225] Thus, histopathology reports should include the level of invasion of the optic nerve (prelaminar, laminar, postlaminar, at cut margin, or/and subarachnoid space of optic nerve), and adequate histology is imperative to evaluate these structures. The amount of tumor is also required in these prospective studies and should be measured from the inner limiting membrane of the optic nerve head or from the level of Bruch's membrane when the tumor obliterates the optic nerve head to the deepest point of invasion (Fig. 27.14).

Uveal Tract Invasion

Several retrospective studies have shown that massive, but not focal, invasion of the choroid by tumor increases the possibility for hematogenous spread, either through vascular permeation of choroidal vessels or, more frequently, by extension through the sclera into the orbital tissues[143,206,212,214] (Fig. 27.14). Both COG and IRSWG have proposed the objective definitions for massive versus focal uveal invasion.[141] Massive choroidal invasion is defined as a tumor ≥3 mm in any dimension and the IRSWG also adds that the tumor should reach the inner layer of the sclera. Focal choroidal invasion is any tumor in the choroid that measures <3 mm in maximum diameter (Table 27.2). MRI studies may be helpful in evaluating the extent of involvement of choroid or optic nerve by tumor only when there is massive invasion.[127]

Extensively necrotic retinoblastoma presents clinically with orbital cellulitis or with severe chemosis and histopathologically shows that more than 95% of the tumor is necrotic and accompanied by intraocular structure necrosis, often with cataract. This presentation has been associated with a statistically significant increase in histopathologic risk factors, such as choroidal and optic nerve invasion[172] (Fig. 27.14).

Retinoblastomas that are poorly differentiated tend to behave more aggressively and are associated with a worse prognosis. Other factors associated with some risk for metastatic behavior, especially in conjunction with the major factors cited above, are tumor invasion into the anterior chamber, large tumor size with vitreous seeding, rubeosis iridis, and glaucoma.

THERAPEUTIC OPTIONS

The management of retinoblastoma is complex. The diagnosis and treatment of patients with retinoblastoma involves a team approach requiring pediatric oncologists, ophthalmologists, and radiologists skilled in the treatment of patients with retinoblastoma. Child psychologists, social workers, nurses, and genetic counselors who can support families dealing with the difficulties of caring for a child who not only has cancer but also may lose an eye and vision also fill important team roles. The goals of treatment are most importantly to save the child's life and, secondly, to salvage the eye and/or vision. Therapy is tailored to each individual case and is based on the overall situation, including threat of metastatic disease, risks for second cancers, systemic status, laterality of the disease, size and location of the tumor(s), and visual prognosis. There are several medical and surgical options for treatment of retinoblastoma and the ocular oncologist should be thoroughly familiar with the indications, techniques, and expected outcomes as well as the associated systemic and visual problems of all treatment methods.[226] The treatment options currently available for retinoblastoma include enucleation, external beam radiotherapy, plaque radiotherapy, laser photocoagulation, cryotherapy, thermotherapy, chemothermotherapy, intravenous chemoreduction, subconjunctival chemoreduction, intra-arterial chemotherapy, systemic chemotherapy for possible metastatic disease, and orbital exenteration.

Enucleation

Enucleation is still the treatment of choice for advanced retinoblastoma with concern of tumor invasion into the optic nerve, choroid or orbit, and no hope for salvage of useful vision in the affected eye. Those eyes with secondary glaucoma, *pars plana* seeding, or anterior chamber invasion are also generally best managed with enucleation.

In the past, most children with unilateral retinoblastoma were managed with enucleation. Those patients with bilateral retinoblastoma usually had the more advanced eye enucleated and the less advanced eye treated with external beam radiotherapy.[20] This management philosophy has been gradually modified with the advent of newer, more conservative but effective methods.[225,227,228] There has been a substantial decrease in the frequency of enucleation over recent decades.[229] In a review of 324 consecutive cases of retinoblastoma managed on the Oncology Service at Wills Eye Institute from 1974 to 1988, Shields and coworkers found that unilateral retinoblastoma was managed with enucleation in 96% of the cases from 1974 to 1978, in 86% of the cases from 1979 to 1983, and in 75% of the cases from 1984 to 1988.[229] A similar decreasing trend was found with bilateral retinoblastoma.[229] The frequency of enucleation is even less today.

Enucleation involves the gentle removal of the intact eye without seeding the malignancy into the orbit. Special care must be taken to perform all steps in a controlled fashion to avoid globe perforation or compression. Shields et al. have

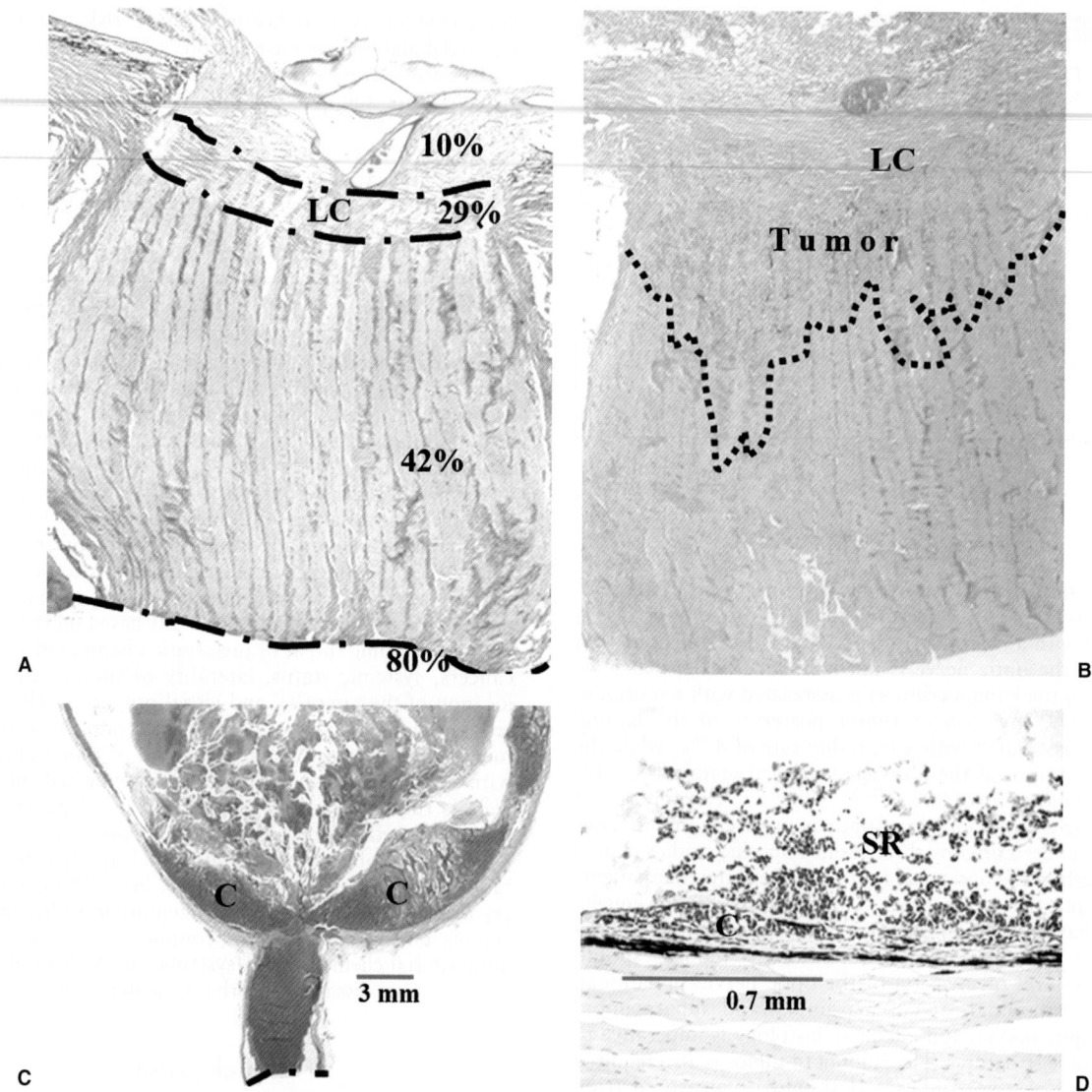

FIGURE 27.14 A: Microphotograph of a normal optic nerve showing the prognostic percentages of survival of patients with invasion of the optic nerve by anatomic portions of the nerve. Patients with tumors invading the pre-lamina cribrosa have a 10% mortality rate similar to that seen without invasion of the nerve. Invasion into the lamina cribrosa (LC – between the two dotted lines) carries a 29% mortality rate and invasion beyond the lamina cribrosa carries a 42% mortality rate. Patients with tumors that are present at the surgical margin of resection (*single dotted line*) have an 80% mortality rate. Myelin stain. Original magnification 10×. **B:** Microphotograph of an optic nerve showing tumor invasion beyond the lamina cribrosa (LC) but not at the surgical margin of resection. Hematoxylin and eosin stain. Original magnification 10×. **C:** Microphotograph of the posterior pole and optic nerve of an eye with massive involvement of the choroid (C) and optic nerve by tumor. Notice that retinoblastoma tumor is present at the surgical margin of resection of the optic nerve (single dotted line). Hematoxylin and eosin stain. Original magnification 4×. **D:** Microphotograph of the subretinal space (SR) and choroid (C) of an eye with retinoblastoma with focal involvement of the subretinal space and minimal involvement of the choroid. Hematoxylin and eosin stain. Original magnification 20×.

described the surgical technique for enucleation of an eye with retinoblastoma.[20,230,231] Because the underlying sclera is thin at the site of muscle insertions, the rectus muscles are handled delicately when the hook is placed flat along the sclera. At the time of optic nerve cutting, scleral or muscle insertion traction sutures are avoided to prevent inadvertent globe perforation. Mild traction with a hemostat on the medial rectus muscle stump is used to lift the globe cautiously to avoid inadvertent lamellar tear of the sclera and cornea which could threaten the integrity of the eye. Optic nerve snares or clamps should be avoided because they induce more vigorous trauma to the eye

and can produce crush artifact in the optic nerve. This artifact can cause difficulty for the pathologist assessing the possibility of retinoblastoma invasion of the optic nerve. The use of minimally curved enucleation scissors is preferred to achieve a long optic nerve section (Fig. 27.15).

Historically, an orbital implant was not usually placed after enucleation for retinoblastoma because of potential interference with palpation of the socket and clinical detection of orbital tumor recurrence. More recently, with improved knowledge of the behavior of retinoblastoma and the risks of local orbital recurrence, there is less hesitation for placing an orbital

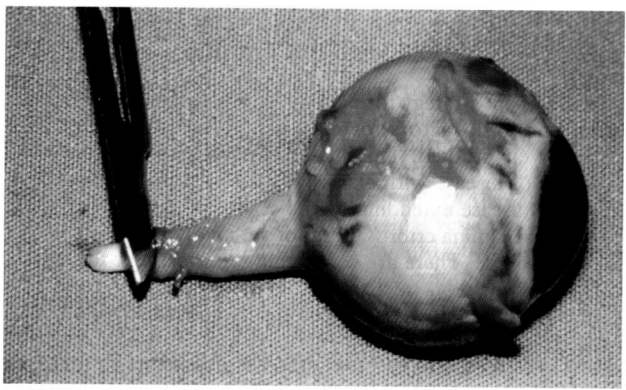

FIGURE 27.15 Enucleation and fresh tissue harvesting. A long section of optic nerve is obtained with the globe at enucleation of an eye with retinoblastoma. The posterior aspect of the optic nerve is cut and submitted to pathology separately for analysis of optic nerve invasion.

implant. Available orbital imaging modalities, including CT and MRI, allow detailed orbital analysis despite the presence of an implant. The orbital implant provides a more natural cosmetic appearance of the patient's artificial eye, minimizes sinking of the prosthesis, and enables motility of the prosthesis. Orbital implants made of polymethylmethacrylate sphere, coralline hydroxyapatite, or coralline hydroxyapatite with polymer coating (coated implant) or polyethylene are commonly used.[230,232] A tissue wrap is usually provided to these implants so that the four rectus muscles can be anatomically reattached to the implant and provide implant mobility with little resistance in the orbit. Available tissue wraps are many and include povidone iodine–treated human sclera, irradiated human sclera, bovine pericardium, fascia lata, and vicryl mesh. More recently, the polymer-coated hydroxyapatite implant has been developed so that a tissue wrap is not necessary and the extraocular muscles can be sutured directly to the prepared implant. This implant has been found safe and effective for children and allows for excellent motility of the prosthesis.[233] Orbital implants, when properly placed surgically, have been shown to be well tolerated by children and adults.[230,231,234]

Laser Photocoagulation

Laser photocoagulation can be used to treat small posterior retinoblastomas using argon laser, diode laser, or xenon arc photocoagulation. Since the tumor size is important to the successful use of this treatment, tumors ≤4.5 mm in base and ≤2.5 mm in thickness with no evidence of vitreous seeds are usually selected.[235,236] The treatment is directed to delimit the tumor and specifically coagulate all blood supply to the tumor. Two or three sessions at 1-month intervals are usually adequate to control most tumors. Use of the indirect ophthalmoscope laser photocoagulation system has greatly improved the facility of laser delivery.[237] With laser treatment of properly selected cases of retinoblastoma, a 70% tumor control rate can be achieved. Recurrences are often treated with plaque radiotherapy. Complications of treatment include transient serous retinal detachment, visually significant retinal vascular occlusion, retinal traction, retinal hole, and preretinal fibrosis.

Cryotherapy

Cryotherapy is useful for managing equatorial and peripheral small retinoblastomas and is most successful if limited to

tumors measuring ≤3.5 mm in diameter and ≤2 mm in thickness.[238] Tumor destruction is usually achieved with one or two sessions of triple freeze-thaw cryotherapy at 1-month intervals. Cryotherapy will usually fail if there are overlying vitreous seeds. In these failed cases, plaque radiotherapy is usually employed. Complications of cryotherapy include transient serous retinal detachment, retinal tear, localized preretinal fibrosis, and rhegmatogenous retinal detachment.[239]

Chemotherapy

Intravenous Chemoreduction for Intraocular Retinoblastoma

Until the mid-1990s, chemotherapy played only a minor role in the treatment of retinoblastoma. Chemotherapy was only used for patients in whom the disease had spread into the choroid, optic nerve, orbit, or to distant extraocular sites. Since 1994, considerable experience has been gained in the use of chemotherapy for patients with intraocular retinoblastoma involving only the retina. The main objective of ongoing clinical trials using chemotherapy in localized intraocular retinoblastoma has been to reduce the size of the tumors to an extent that would allow a variety of local surgical modalities such as laser photocoagulation, cryotherapy, or thermotherapy to control the residual disease. Successful management using chemotherapy in combination with local surgical methods can eliminate the use of external beam radiotherapy and, therefore, significantly reduce the risk of development of secondary malignancies and abnormalities of growth of orbital and facial bones associated with radiotherapy.[240-243]

Chemoreduction is employed for unilateral or bilateral retinoblastoma. It is effective for all stages of disease, but very advanced disease shows the highest failure rate. The goal of chemoreduction is to preserve the patient's life, globe, and vision. A pilot study involving 40 eyes in 31 patients with bilateral disease who were treated with vincristine, teniposide, and carboplatin combined with cyclosporine resulted in a relapse-free rate of 89% in patients who were not previously treated.[244] Relapse in this study was defined as tumor progression requiring either radiotherapy or enucleation. The median follow-up at the time of this report was 2 to 8 years. In another study of 20 patients who had 54 tumors in 31 eyes, a 2-month chemoreduction program with vincristine, carboplatin, and etoposide was followed by local treatment methods.[245] Enucleation was avoided in all and external beam radiation therapy was necessary in only nine eyes because of diffuse vitreous seeds. Prior to therapy the mean tumor base was 12 mm and the thickness 7 mm. Vitreous seeds were present in 14 eyes. After the 2-month chemotherapy regimen, there was no evidence of residual viable tumor in 25 of 54 tumors. There was a mean decrease of 35% in tumor base and nearly 50% decrease in tumor thickness with resolution of subretinal fluid in 76% of the cases. However, of the 14 eyes that had vitreous seeds, only 5 showed 90% to 100% calcification, indicating that different therapeutic modalities must be developed for the treatment of vitreous seeds. Careful follow-up of patients treated with chemoreduction is very important. Young patients with large tumors are at risk for recurrence of subretinal seeds. There is an increased risk for recurrence of retinal tumor and vitreous seeds in eyes with subretinal seeds at initial evaluation. These recurrences typically appear within 3 years of follow-up.[246] In addition, new retinoblastomas develop at a mean interval of 5 months from initiation of chemoreduction and affect 24% of patients by 5 years of follow-up. These new intraretinal tumors develop most commonly in patients who had developed the disease as young

Advances in lateral lens sparing techniques were successful in reducing some of these side affects. At the same time Stallard, a British ocular oncologist, expanded the role of episcleral brachytherapy with cobalt for select patients. Although only applicable to certain cases with single isolated tumor foci, this approach lacked many of the toxicities associated with external beam. Cobalt however could not be shielded and exposed the patient and surgeon to additional radiation.

External beam radiotherapy is a method of delivering whole eye irradiation to treat advanced retinoblastoma particularly when there is diffuse vitreous seeding. The whole eye and lens sparing techniques used currently have been shown to improve the eye preservation rate as compared to reported older techniques. The rate of ocular salvage depends on the Reese-Ellsworth stage of the disease at the time of treatment as well as on the availability of focal therapy for limited recurrences.[268,269] Recurrence of retinoblastoma after external beam radiotherapy continues to be a problem and can develop within the first 1 to 4 years after treatment.[270] Tumor recurrence in other studies has also been found to be related to the stage of the disease and to the size of the largest tumor at the time of treatment.[270-273] Prophylactic radiotherapy to a normal contralateral eye is almost never indicated today.[274]

Little has been written on the visual outcome after external beam radiotherapy for retinoblastoma. Radiation damage to the retina, optic nerve, and lens can be challenging to manage.[275] Patients with macular retinoblastoma have visual outcomes that are dependent on the size of the tumor and the degree of involvement of the fovea.[276] Superimposed amblyopia can pose a problem and patching therapy should be employed if hope for vision remains.

External beam radiotherapy may induce a second cancer in the field of irradiation. The 30-year cumulative incidence for second cancers in bilateral retinoblastoma has been reported to be 35% for patients who received radiation therapy compared to 6% for those who did not receive radiation.[277] Overall, the cumulative probability of death from second primary neoplasms was reported at 26% at 40 years after bilateral retinoblastoma diagnosis, and external beam radiotherapy has been reported to further increase the risk of mortality from second neoplasms.[48] Abramson and Frank found that external beam radiotherapy increased the incidence of second cancers in the field of radiation but did not stimulate second cancers outside the field of irradiation.[243] In their series, patients under 12 months of age were more likely to develop second malignancies following external beam radiotherapy than patients over 12 months of age.[243] Survivors of these second malignancies had a very high rate of developing subsequent tumors particularly if they had been treated with radiation therapy.[278] Fletcher and his colleagues have shown that second malignancies found in patients with bilateral retinoblastoma treated before the use of this modality were usually late-onset epithelial tumors whereas second malignancies in patients following radiation therapy were usually earlier-onset sarcomas.[279] Although there is much data describing the increased risk of second nonocular tumors following radiation in patients with retinoblastoma, it must be noted that many of these cases were treated with less precise orthovoltage techniques. Today many centers use intensity modulated radiation therapy (IMRT) to administer more focused therapy to the eye with reduced scatter to the adjacent orbital bones and CNS. An emerging technique is the role of proton beam radiation. This modality, limited to a handful of centers world wide, has been demonstrated to administer radiation plans with the least exposure to nearby structures. In theory, more focused radiation should be associated with lower rates of radiation-induced tumor, but this has yet to be demonstrated. The ideal dose for adjuvant and salvage radiation therapy following primary chemotherapy is under investigation with centers utilizing doses ranging from 20 Gy to 45 Gy.

The long-term secondary tumor risk associated with external beam radiation was a major factor in promoting systemic chemotherapy as a primary modality. This development during the 1990s led many clinicians to utilize external radiation in one of two methods. Some administered it as a salvage technique for those failing primary chemotherapy. Others used it as planned adjuvant, administered after systemic chemotherapy. With this approach, external radiation could be delayed and administered at an older age, when the risk of radiation-induced tumors was thought to be lower (particularly after 12 months).

While no longer a primary modality, the sensitivity of retinoblastoma to radiation makes it an important treatment option for resistant and challenging cases; it must remain a critical option for any center managing patients with retinoblastoma.

Plaque Radiotherapy

Plaque radiotherapy is a form of brachytherapy in which a radioactive implant is placed on the sclera over the base of a retinoblastoma with the intent of irradiating the tumor transsclerally. The use of plaque radiotherapy is limited to tumors ≤16 mm in base and ≤8 mm in thickness. Effective treatment requires an average of 2 to 4 days of treatment time to deliver the total dose of 4,000 cGy to the apex of the tumor. Plaque radiotherapy can be used as either a primary treatment or a secondary treatment (Fig. 27.17).[280-283] In 70% of cases, plaque radiotherapy is used as a secondary treatment to salvage a globe after failure of prior treatment, usually failed external beam radiotherapy or chemotherapy.[280-283] In one series, solitary plaque radiotherapy was used in 91 cases of recurrent or residual retinoblastoma in which the only other option was enucleation.[283] Tumor control and globe salvage was achieved in nearly 90% of these eyes.[283] In another series of 84 eyes that showed individual tumor recurrence following chemoreduction, plaque radiotherapy was employed and led to permanent tumor control in 95% of the cases at 10 years. The few that recurred were always detected within 1 year of plaque treatment.[284]

Overall, there is nearly a 90% tumor control rate with one application of plaque radiotherapy.[285] Carefully selected retinoblastomas, even juxtapapillary and macular tumors, can be successfully treated with plaque radiotherapy. The visual outcome for the patient varies with tumor size and location as well as associated radiation toxicity, which can include retinopathy or papillopathy. Positive visual outcomes have been reported in 62% of patients; the measured vision was 20/20 to 20/30 in over half the cases.[280] Radiation retinopathy and papillopathy become clinically manifest at approximately 18 months after irradiation, and these complications are more prominent in children who have been exposed to systemic chemotherapy. In an effort to avoid these problems with chemotherapy-treated patients, the tumor apex dose has been decreased to 3,500 cGy and radiation plaque therapy is delayed for at least 1 month after the child has discontinued chemotherapy. Innovations with custom design of plaques, especially those for small tumor recurrences, have also assisted in avoiding radiation retinopathy. Because of the use of focal, shielded radiation fields, plaque radiotherapy has not yet been found to be associated with induction of second cancers.

Advances in episcleral brachytherapy have also improved outcomes for children with retinoblastoma. Shielded plaques using sources such as iodine and ruthenium have largely replaced cobalt and are not thought to harbor the same second tumor risk as external radiation. Ruthenium, in particular, has

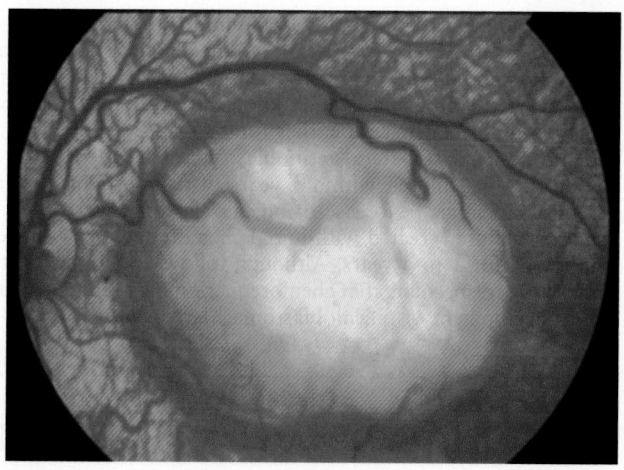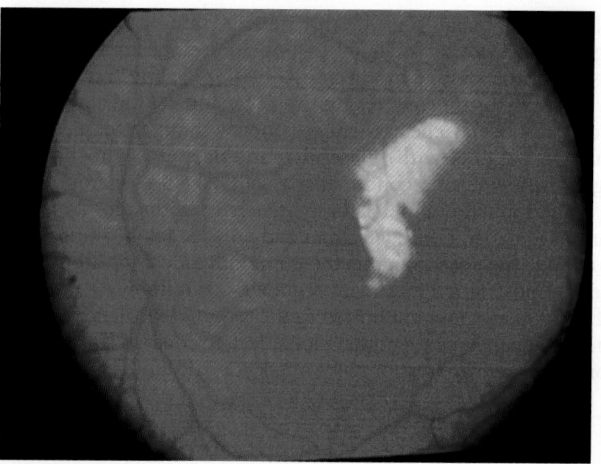

FIGURE 27.17 Plaque radiotherapy. **A:** Macular retinoblastoma before plaque radiotherapy. **B:** Regressed retinoblastoma after plaque radiotherapy.

limited scatter with less radiation to adjacent sensitive ocular structures including the lens, macula, and optic nerve.

Combined Radiotherapy and Chemotherapy

In three separate studies, patients presenting with Reese-Ellsworth eye group V retinoblastoma treated with radiotherapy alone have had 10%, 29%, and 66% of their eyes salvaged.[268,273,286] For patients with bilateral retinoblastoma Reese-Ellsworth eye group V, Kingston et al have shown that 2 cycles of chemotherapy in addition to external beam radiation therapy can preserve 70% of the eyes treated (14/20 eyes) with a median follow-up of 60 months.[287] The study reporting a 66% salvage rate with radiotherapy alone and the study using chemotherapy in addition to radiotherapy were performed at the same institution, however, the patients in the latter study were reportedly more severely affected. Taken together these data suggest that, for patients with retinoblastoma group V disease, the combination of chemotherapy with external beam radiotherapy may result in a superior salvage rate than with radiotherapy alone. In a recent study with a median follow-up of 13 months chemotherapy alone (six cycles of carboplatin, vincristine and etoposide) resulted in the salvage of only 50% of the eyes with groups IV and V disease without requiring external beam radiotherapy or enucleation.[256] In the same study, chemotherapy eliminated the need for external beam radiotherapy or enucleation in all 39 eyes with groups I, II, and III disease (Table 27.4).

From the above data it is clear that chemoreduction is an effective initial measure for selected children with intraocular retinoblastoma. Retinal tumor and seed recurrence remain a worrisome problem with chemoreduction.[228] Seeds in the vitreous or subretinal space can recur in about 30% of eyes and

TABLE 27.4

PERCENTAGE OF GLOBES SALVAGED USING EXTERNAL BEAM RADIOTHERAPY ALONE, EXTERNAL BEAM RADIOTHERAPY AND SALVAGE TREATMENT, AND CHEMOREDUCTION AND FOCAL ADJUVANT TREATMENT

Reese-Ellsworth Group	EBRT alone Ellsworth[273] (1965–1972)	EBRT + Salvage Rxb Hungerford[268] (1970–1985)	CRDc + ATd Shields[228] (1994–1996)
I	91%	100%	100%
II	83%	84%	100%
III	82%	82%	100%
IV	62%	43%	100%
V	29%	66%	78%

EBRT, external beam radiotherapy; Rx, treatment; CRD, chemoreduction using vincristine, etoposide, and carboplatin; AT, adjuvant treatment (laser photocoagulation, cryotherapy, thermotherapy, chemothermotherapy, plaque radiotherapy, external beam radiotherapy).

CHEMOREDUCTION REGIMEN (6 CYCLES) FOR INTRAOCULAR RETINOBLASTOMA

Day	Vincristine	Etoposide	Carboplatin
0	X	X	X
1		X	

Vincristine, 1.5 mg/m², 0.05 mg/kg for children ≤36 months of age and maximum dose ≤2 mg; etoposide, 150 mg/m², 5 mg/kg for children ≤36 months of age; carboplatin, 560 mg/m², 18.6 mg/kg for children ≤36 months of age.

enlarge to a visual- and life-threatening state. Chemotherapy regimens previously included carboplatin, etoposide, and vincristine. Cyclosporine has been used with the above regimen in an attempt to improve results by reversing multidrug resistance.[288,289] Use of chemotherapy is not without concern, especially in patients with bilateral retinoblastoma who have a higher incidence of second malignancies. The use of etoposide, an epipodophyllotoxin, has been associated with second malignancies in patients with leukemia and non-Hodgkin lymphoma. However, the schedule and the cumulative dose of etoposide used in most of the treatment regimens for retinoblastoma are different from those implicated in the reported incidence of second malignancies.[290] Another side effect of concern is transient bone marrow suppression with a risk for infection.

Treatment of Systemic Retinoblastoma

Treatment of extraocular retinoblastoma requires a combined therapeutic approach using both chemotherapy and radiotherapy. Scleral involvement, orbital or bony involvement, involvement beyond the cut end of the optic nerve, metastatic disease involving brain or other sites, and trilateral retinoblastoma—all these require an aggressive combined therapeutic approach. CNS involvement generally carries a poor prognosis.

Many different agents have been employed to treat systemic retinoblastoma. One regimen is the three-drug regimen including vincristine, carboplatin, and etoposide, similar to the chemoreduction regimen mentioned above but with a much longer course of 6 to 18 months depending on the clinical response.[228,245] Others have found favorable results with similar chemotherapy regimens along with external beam radiation therapy for regional extraocular retinoblastoma (involvement of the orbit and/or pre-auricular nodes, tumor at the cut end of the optic nerve).[291–296] White has recently advocated cyclophosphamide, etoposide, and vincristine as well as the support of peripheral stem-cell rescue in multiple sequential courses for metastatic retinoblastoma.[297] High-dose chemotherapy with autologous bone-marrow or stem-cell rescue appears to benefit patients with metastatic disease without CNS involvement.[298–301]

A prospective study is underway within COG with participation including international institutions to estimate the proportion of patients with extraocular regional disease and systemic disease (with and without CNS involvement) who can be cured with a combination of chemotherapy, external beam radiation therapy, and high-dose chemotherapy and stem-cell rescue.

Orbital Exenteration

Orbital exenteration is rarely used for retinoblastoma management in the United States as most retinoblastoma patients present with no evidence of extraocular invasion.[302] Exenteration is most often used for orbital recurrence after the child has received a maximum acceptable dose of irradiation and chemotherapy. In other countries, patients may present with more advanced retinoblastoma, including orbital involvement. For these patients, exenteration, chemotherapy, and external beam radiotherapy are crucial for survival. Use of more advanced exenteration techniques, such as the eyelid-sparing exenteration, allows for rapid healing of the wound.[303]

Trilateral Retinoblastoma

Trilateral retinoblastoma, the association of bilateral retinoblastoma and neuroblastic tumor in the pineal gland or other midline structures, occurs in children 4 years of age or younger.[304] MRI or CT is essential to the diagnosis. The disease is highly fatal despite aggressive treatment with chemotherapy, radiation therapy, and gamma knife therapy. Longer survival has been correlated with earlier tumor diagnosis in asymptomatic patients. Trilateral retinoblastoma is a major cause of mortality in children within 5 years of diagnosis of bilateral retinoblastoma.[305] No case of pinealoblastoma was observed in 147 children treated with initial chemoreduction who were followed for 1 to 4 years. Although follow-up is limited, it is tempting to speculate that chemoreduction may reduce the risk for development of pinealoblastoma.[198,306]

HISTOPATHOLOGIC CHANGES ASSOCIATED WITH TREATMENT

Enucleation of eyes from patients with retinoblastoma treated with different modalities that either fail to eradicate the tumor or result in major treatment complications allow the study of effects of therapy on the tumor and the ocular structures. Clinically, three types of regression patterns have been described in tumors that have undergone treatment: type 1 (cottage cheese), type 2 (fish flesh), or type 3 (combined).

In one study, five patients with sporadic bilateral retinoblastoma underwent planned enucleation of their functionally blind eye after two, three (in two patients), four, or six courses of primary chemotherapy with carboplatin, etoposide, cyclophosphamide, and vincristine. The eyes were examined histopathologically using light microscopy and immunohistochemical analysis with proliferation markers. One patient had a type 1 (cottage cheese) regression and four patients had either a type 2 (fish flesh) or a type 3 (combined) regression pattern. Histopathologic examination revealed complete tumor necrosis with calcification (Fig. 27.18) in one patient with type 1 regression after three courses of chemotherapy and in one patient with type 3 regression after four courses of chemotherapy. The remaining three patients with type 2 or type 3 regressions had histological evidence of actively proliferating tumor cells after two, three, or six courses of chemotherapy. This report confirms histopathologically the clinically described efficacy of primary chemotherapy in the treatment of retinoblastoma. The necessity of careful observation and the use of ancillary treatment whenever there is incomplete tumor regression (type 2 and 3 regression patterns) is, however, underscored.[307] In another study, photoreceptor differentiation was observed in 17 of 42 enucleated eyes containing viable tumor following radiotherapy. Complications of external beam radiation include massive necrosis of the retina with associated hemorrhage (Fig. 27.18). Patients with retinoblastoma that have undergone chemotherapy and radiotherapy sometimes are left with tumors with large areas of fossilized cells and calcification, with areas of photoreceptor differentiation similar to retinocytoma. Whether these cases represent a focus of chemotherapy- or radiotherapy-resistant retinocytoma or treatment-induced differentiation of retinoblastoma has not been elucidated.[308]

FUTURE DIRECTIONS

Subconjunctival Chemoreduction for Intraocular Retinoblastoma

To avoid the toxicity of systemic administration of chemotherapy, there is increasing interest in local delivery of these drugs

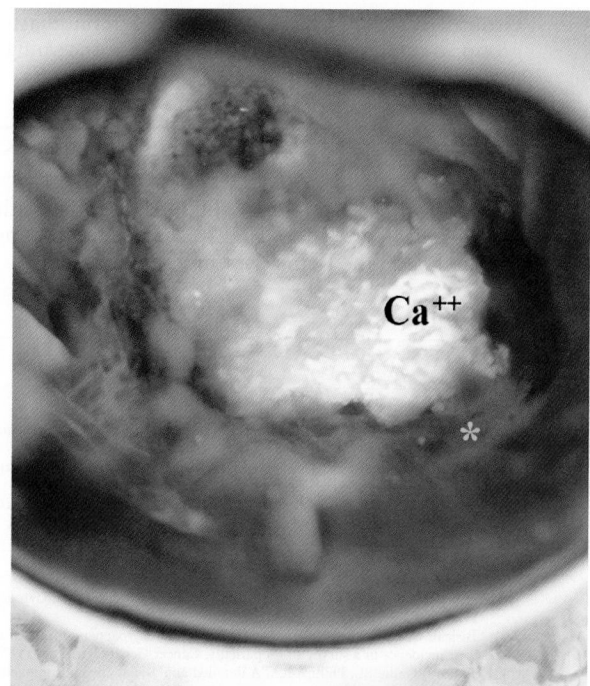

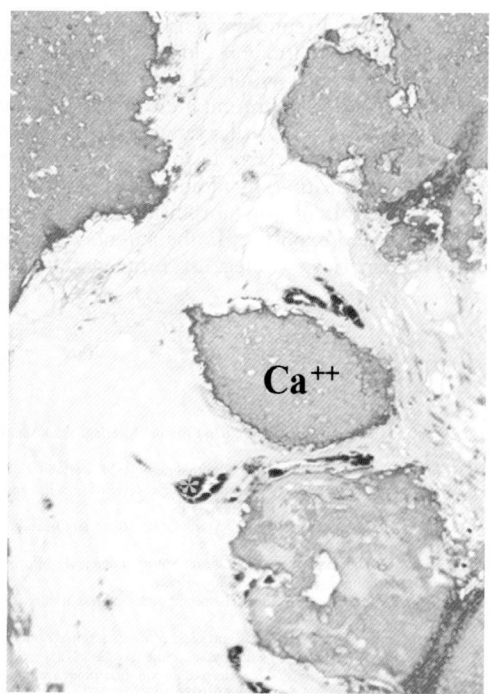

FIGURE 27.18 A: Gross photograph of an autopsy eye in a patient with regressed retinoblastoma for more than 6 years after chemotherapy and radiotherapy. The patient died of complications of chemotherapy (cardiomyopathy). Notice the cottage cheese appearance (type 1 regression pattern) of the calcified (Ca++) tumor associated with proliferation of retinal pigment epithelium (*). **B:** Microscopic photograph of the same eye showing the calcified tumor (Ca++), proliferation of retinal pigment epithelium (*) and admixed glial tissue. Hematoxylin and eosin stain. Original magnification 20×.

to achieve chemoreduction for intraocular retinoblastoma. Studies in animal models show that carboplatin penetrates the sclera into the vitreous cavity, allowing for effective dosages within the eye with minimal toxicity.[309–311] Local subconjunctival injection of carboplatin in humans as both a secondary treatment and a primary treatment have been used.[312] The current usage of subconjunctival delivery is generally limited to those children on systemic chemotherapy protocols so the local boost of chemotherapy works jointly with the systemic dose. A phase I trial of periocular topotecan was recently completed.[313]

Intra-arterial chemotherapy is another local delivery option being studied for retinoblastoma. The femoral artery is catheterized to the internal carotid and then into the ophthalmic artery. A bolus of chemotherapy using melphalan, carboplatin, topotecan, or other drugs is injected with the dose being 10% of the usual systemic dose. This technique is difficult and requires collaboration with neurosurgery or interventional neuro-radiology. Early results show remarkable tumor control; long-term assessment has, however, not been determined.

A screening of 2,640 approved drugs and compounds identified several medications, such as cardenolides like digitalis and ouabain, which have activity toward retinoblastoma cell lines *in vitro*.[314] These older drugs are being revisited for potential intra-arterial injection and are being tested using xenograft mice.

Animal Models

The development of innovative modalities for the treatment of retinoblastoma has been hampered by the lack of suitable animal models of this uniquely human disease. Murine models of

retinoblastoma using human xenografts in the vitreal space that mimic both metastatic and nonmetastatic disease[315] as well as transgenic mouse models of retinoblastoma[316] have been developed. These newer animal models will aid the testing of new therapeutic approaches to retinoblastoma.

Gene Therapy

An alternative approach to local chemoreduction without the side effects of systemic chemotherapy is gene therapy. One form of gene therapy, *suicide gene therapy*, uses a replication-defective adenoviral vector to deliver the herpes simplex thymidine kinase gene. The vector is injected directly into the tumor. Ganciclovir, a nucleoside analog, is then administered intravenously. The expressed thymidine kinase phosphorylates the ganciclovir within the tumor cells, resulting in a nucleotide analog that is a potent inhibitor of DNA synthesis and causes the death of the dividing tumor cells. Non-dividing cells are left unaffected. Effective reduction of retinoblastoma tumors in a mouse model of the disease has been demonstrated.[317] The safety of this form of suicide gene therapy has been demonstrated in patients with brain tumors[318] and a phase I clinical trial for children with retinoblastoma has been completed. This treatment was shown to be safe and possibly effective for the treatment of children with retinoblastoma complicated by vitreous seeds.[319]

International Cooperative Studies

COG has a long and extensive experience in the conduct of clinical trials for children with cancer, resulting in remarkable strides in improving the prognosis for children with many types of cancer. In 2001, a retinoblastoma committee consisting of ophthalmologists, radiation oncologists, pediatric oncologists, and others was formed within COG and, shortly thereafter, four clinical protocols were initiated for patients with group B, C, and D disease, extraocular retinoblastoma, and for patients with unilateral disease with histopathologic high-risk features noted after enucleation. In addition, an epidemiologic study to evaluate the role of polymorphisms in DNA repair genes and environmental exposures in the parents of patients is underway. The American College of Surgeons Oncology Group (ACOSOG) has also formed a retinoblastoma study group to address therapeutic questions concerning the treatment of retinoblastoma.

ACKNOWLEDGEMENTS

Support for this chapter was obtained from the National Institutes of Health (NCI and NEI), the Clayton Foundation for Research, and the Retina Research Foundation.

References

1. Verhoeff F, Jackson E. Minutes of Proceedings, 62nd Annual Meeting. Trans Am Ophthalmol Soc 1926;24:38.
2. Albert DM. Historic review of retinoblastoma. Ophthalmology 1987;94:654–662.
3. Albert DM. Wardrop Lecture, 1974. James Wardrop: a brief review of his life and contributions. Trans Ophthalmol Soc UK 1974;94:892–908.
4. Margo C, Hidayet A, Kopelman A, et al. Retinocytoma: a benign variant of retinoblastoma. Arch Ophthalmol 1983;101:1519–1531.
5. Gallie BL, Phillips RA, Ellsworth RM, et al. Significance of retinoma and phthisis bulbi for retinoblastoma. Ophthalmology 1982;89:1393–1399.
6. Bogenmann E, Lochrie MA, Simon MI. Cone cell-specific genes expressed in retinoblastoma. Science 1988;240:76–78.
7. Hurwitz RL, Bogenmann E, Font RL, et al. Expression of the functional cone phototransduction cascade in retinoblastoma. J Clin Invest 1990;85:1872–1878.
8. Donoso LA, Folberg R, Arbizo V. Retinal S antigen and retinoblastoma: a monoclonal antibody histopathologic study. Arch Ophthalmol 1985;103:855–857.
9. Nork TM, Millecchia LL, de Venecia GB, et al. Immunocytochemical features of retinoblastoma in an adult. Arch Ophthalmol 1996;114:1402–1406.
10. Nork TM, Schwartz TL, Doshi HM, et al. Retinoblastoma: cell of origin. Arch Ophthalmol 1995;113:791–802.
11. Ohira A, Yamamoto M, Honda O, et al. Glial-, neuronal- and photoreceptor-specific cell markers in rosettes of retinoblastoma and retinal dysplasia. Curr Eye Res 1994;13:799–804.
12. Munier FL, Balmer A, Van Melle G, et al. Radial asymmetry in the topography of retinoblastoma: clues to the cell of origin. Ophthalmic Genet 1994;15:101–106.
13. Yi YZ, Yang WZ, Zhen HL. [Retinoblastoma: cell origin and differentiation]. Chung Hua Yen Ko Tsa Chih 1994;30:214–217.
14. Rajagopalan S, Rodrigues MM, Wiggert B, et al. Retinoblastoma. Interphotoreceptor retinoid binding protein mRNA analysis by polymerase chain reaction. Ophthalmic Paediatr Genet 1993;14:117–125.
15. Chévez P, Font RL. Practical applications of some antibodies labelling the human retina. Histol Histopathol 1993;8:437–442.
16. Gonzalez-Fernandez F, Lopes MB, Garcia-Fernandez JM, et al. Expression of developmentally defined retinal phenotypes in the histogenesis of retinoblastoma. Am J Pathol 1992;141:363–375.
17. Kivela T. Parvalbumin, a horizontal cell-associated calcium-binding protein in retinoblastoma eyes. Invest Ophthalmol Vis Sci 1998;39:1044–1048.
18. McLean IW, Burnier M, Zimmerman L, et al. Tumors of the retina. In: McLean IW, Burnier MN, Zimmerman LE, Jakobiec FA, eds. Atlas of tumor pathology. tumors of the eye and ocular adnexa. Washington, D.C.: Armed Forced Institute of Pathology, 1994:100–135.
19. Petersen RA. Retinoblastoma. In: Albert D, Jakobiec F, eds. Principles and practice of ophthalmology: clinical practice. Philadelphia, PA: Saunders, 1994:3279–3284.
20. Shields JA, Shields CL. Management and prognosis of retinoblastoma. In: Intraocular tumors: a text and atlas. Philadelphia, PA: WB Suanders, 1992:377–392.
21. McLean IW. Retinoblastoma, retinocytomas, and pseudoretinoblastomas. In: Spencer WH, ed. Ophthalmic pathology. an atlas and textbook. Philadelphia, PA: American Academy of Ophthalmology, WB Saunders Company, 1990:1332–1438.
22. Ajioka I, Martins RA, Bayazitov IT, et al. Differentiated horizontal interneurons clonally expand to form metastatic retinoblastoma in mice. Cell 2007;131:378–390.
23. Xu XL, Fang Y, Lee TC, et al. Retinoblastoma has properties of a cone precursor tumor and depends upon cone-specific MDM2 signaling. Cell 2009;137:1018–1031.
24. Dimaras H, Khetan V, Halliday W, et al. Loss of RB1 induces non-proliferative retinoma: increasing genomic instability correlates with progression to retinoblastoma. Hum Mol Genet 2008;17:1363–1372.
25. Devesa S. The incidence of retinoblastoma. Am J Ophthalmol 1975;80:263–265.
26. Broaddus E, Topham A, Singh AD. Incidence of retinoblastoma in the USA: 1975–2004. Br J Ophthalmol 2009;93:21–23.
27. de Camargo B, de Oliveira AM, Rebelo MS, et al. Cancer incidence among children and adolescents in Brazil: First report of 14 population-based cancer registries. Int J Cancer 2010;126:715–720.
28. Agboola AO, Adekanmbi FA, Musa AA, et al. Pattern of childhood malignant tumours in a teaching hospital in south-western Nigeria. Med J Aust 2009;190:12–14.
29. Leal-Leal C, Flores-Rojo M, Medina-Sanson A, et al. A multicentre report from the Mexican Retinoblastoma Group. Br J Ophthalmol 2004;88:1074–1077.
30. MacCarthy A, Birch JM, Draper GJ, et al. Retinoblastoma in Great Britain 1963–2002. Br J Ophthalmol 2009;93:33–37.
31. Greene DM. Retinoblastoma. Diagnosis and management of malignant solid tumors in infants and children. Boston: Martinus Nijhoff, 1985:90.
32. Francois J, Matton M, deBie S, et al. Genesis and genetics of retinoblastoma. Ophthalmologica 1970;405.
33. Johnson KJ, Carozza SE, Chow EJ, et al. Parental age and risk of childhood cancer: a pooled analysis. Epidemiology 2009;20:475–483.
34. Jensen RD, Miller RW. Retinoblastoma: epidemiologic characteristics. N Engl J Med 1971;285:307–311.
35. Schappert-Kimmiiser J, Hemmes GD, Nijiland R. The heredity of retinoblastoma. Ophthalmologica 1966;151:197–213.
36. Knudson AG Jr. Mutation and cancer: statistical study of retinoblastoma. Proc Natl Acad Sci U S A 1971;68:820–823.
37. Bonaiti-Pellie C, Briard-Guillemot ML. Segregation analysis in hereditary retinoblastoma. Hum Genet 1981;57:411–419.
38. Hethcote HW, Knudson AG Jr. Model for the incidence of embryonal cancers: application to retinoblastoma. Proc Natl Acad Sci U S A 1978;75:2453–2457.
39. Lele KP, Penrose LS, Stallard HB. Chromosome deletion in a case of retinoblastoma. Ann Hum Genet 1963;27:171–174.
40. Chaum E, Ellsworth RM, Abramson DH, et al. Cytogenetic analysis of retinoblastoma: evidence for multifocal origin and in vivo gene amplification. Cytogenet Cell Genet 1984;38:82–91.
41. Turleau C, de Grouchy J, Chavin-Colin F, et al. Cytogenetic forms of retinoblastoma: their incidence in a survey of 66 patients. Cancer Genet Cytogenet 1985;16:321–334.
42. Squire J, Gallie BL, Phillips RA. A detailed analysis of chromosomal changes in heritable and non-heritable retinoblastoma. Hum Genet 1985;70:291–301.
43. Francke U. Retinoblastoma and chromosome 13. Cytogenet Cell Genet 1976;16:131–134.
44. Ward P, Packman S, Loughman W, et al. Location of the retinoblastoma susceptibility gene(s) and the human esterase D locus. J Med Genet 1984;21:92–95.
45. Harbour JW. Overview of RB gene mutations in patients with retinoblastoma. Implications for clinical genetic screening. Ophthalmology 1998;105:1442–1447.
46. Dryja TP, Cavenee W, White R, et al. Homozygosity of chromosome 13 in retinoblastoma. N Engl J Med 1984;310:550–553.
47. Godbout R, Dryja TP, Squire J, et al. Somatic inactivation of genes on chromosome 13 is a common event in retinoblastoma. Nature 1983;304:451–453.
48. Eng C, Li FP, Abramson DH, et al. Mortality from second tumors among long-term survivors of retinoblastoma [comments]. J Natl Cancer Inst 1993;85:1121–1128.
49. Hansen MF, Koufos A, Gallie BL, et al. Osteosarcoma and retinoblastoma: a shared chromosomal mechanism revealing recessive predisposition. Proc Natl Acad Sci U S A 1985;82:6216–6220.
50. Dryja TP, Friend S, Weinberg RA. Genetic sequences that predispose to retinoblastoma and osteosarcoma. Symp Fundam Cancer Res 1986;39:115–119.
51. Lee W-H, Bookstein R, Hong F, et al. Human retinoblastoma susceptibility gene: cloning, identification, and sequence. Science 1987;235:1394–1399.
52. De Falco G, Giordano A. pRb2/p130: a new candidate for retinoblastoma tumor formation. Oncogene 2006;25:5333–5340.
53. Khidr L, Chen PL. RB: the conductor that orchestrates life, death and differentiation. Oncogene 2006;25:5210–5219.
54. van den HS, Dyson NJ. Conserved functions of the pRB and E2F families. Nat Rev Mol Cell Biol 2008;9:713–724.
55. Burkhart DL, Sage J. Cellular mechanisms of tumour suppression by the retinoblastoma gene. Nat Rev Cancer 2008;8:671–682.
56. Huang HJ, Yee JK, Shew JY, et al. Suppression of the neoplastic phenotype by replacement of the RB gene in human cancer cells. Science 1988;242:1563–1566.
57. Takahashi R, Hashimoto T, Xu HJ, et al. The retinoblastoma gene functions as a growth and tumor suppressor in human bladder carcinoma cells. Proc Natl Acad Sci U S A 1991;88:5257–5261.
58. Bookstein R, Lee EY, To H, et al. Human retinoblastoma susceptibility gene: genomic organization and analysis of heterozygous intragenic deletion mutants. Proc Natl Acad Sci U S A 1988;85:2210–2214.
59. Dryja TP, Rapaport JM, Epstein J, et al. Chromosome 13 homozygosity in osteosarcoma without retinoblastoma. Am J Hum Genet 1986;38:59–66.
60. Friend SH, Bernards R, Rogelj S, et al. A human DNA segment with properties of the gene that predisposes to retinoblastoma and osteosarcoma. Nature 1986;323:643–646.
61. Fung YK, Murphree AL, T'Ang A, et al. Structual evidence for the authenticity of the human retinoblastoma gene. Science 1987;236:1657–1661.
62. Dunn JM, Phillips RA, Zhu X, et al. Mutations in the RB1 gene and their effects on transcription. Mol Cell Biol 1989;9:4596–4604.
63. Yandell DW, Campbell TA, Dayton SH, et al. Oncogenic point mutations in the human retinoblastoma gene: Their application to genetic counseling. N Engl J Med 1989;321:1689–1695.
64. Lohmann DR, Brandt B, Hopping W, et al. The spectrum of RB1 germ-line mutations in hereditary retinoblastoma. Am J Hum Genet 1996;58:940–949.
65. Yilmaz S, Horsthemke B, Lohmann DR. Twelve novel RB1 gene mutations in patients with hereditary retinoblastoma: mutations in brief no. 206. Online. Hum Mutat 1998;12:434.
66. Blanquet V, Turleau C, Gross-Morand MS, et al. Spectrum of germline mutations in the RB1 gene: a study of 232 patients with hereditary and non hereditary retinoblastoma. Hum Mol Genet 1995;4:383–388.
67. Cowell JK, Jaju R, Kempski H. Isolation and characterisation of a panel of cosmids which allows unequivocal identification of chromosome deletions involving the RB1 gene using fluorescence in situ hybridisation. J Med Genet 1994;31:334–337.
68. Szijan I, Lohmann DR, Parma DL, et al. Identification of RB1 germline mutations in Argentinian families with sporadic bilateral retinoblastoma. J Med Genet 1995;32:475–479.

69. Dryja TP, Mukai S, Petersen R, et al. Parental origin of mutations of the retinoblastoma gene. Nature 1989;339:556–558.
70. Zhu XP, Dunn JM, Phillips RA, et al. Preferential germline mutation of the paternal allele in retinoblastoma. Nature 1989;340:312–313.
71. Toguchida J, Ishizaki K, Sasaki MS, et al. Preferential mutation of paternally derived RB gene as the initial event in sporadic osteosarcoma. Nature 1989;338:156–158.
72. Harbour JW, Lai S-L, Whang-Peng J, et al. Abnormalities in structure and expression of the human retinoblastoma gene in SCLC. Science 1988;241:353–357.
73. T'Ang A, Varley JM, Chakraborty S, et al. Structural rearrangement of the retinoblastoma gene in human breast carcinoma. Science 1988;242:263–266.
74. Bookstein R, Lee EY, Peccei A, et al. Human retinoblastoma gene: long-range mapping and analysis of its deletion in a breast cancer cell line. Mol Cell Biol 1989;9:1628–1634.
75. Seizinger BR, Klinger HP, Junien C, et al. Report of the committee on chromosome and gene loss in human neoplasia. Cytogenet Cell Genet 1991;58:1080–1096.
76. Lee WH, Shew JY, Hong FD, et al. The retinoblastoma susceptibility gene encodes a nuclear phosphoprotein associated with DNA binding activity. Nature 1987;329: 642–645.
77. Buchkovich K, Duffy LA, Harlow E. The retinoblastoma protein is phosphorylated during specific phases of the cell cycle. Cell 1989;58:1097–1105.
78. Magnaghi-Jaulin L, Groisman R, Naguibneva I, et al. Retinoblastoma protein represses transcription by recruiting a histone deacetylase [comments]. Nature 1998;391:601–605.
79. Brehm A, Miska EA, McCance DJ, et al. Retinoblastoma protein recruits histone deacetylase to repress transcription [comments]. Nature 1998;391:597–601.
80. Whyte P, Buchkovich KJ, Horowitz JM, et al. Association between an oncogene and an anti-oncogene: the adenovirus E1A proteins bind to the retinoblastoma gene product. Nature 1988;334:124–129.
81. DeCaprio JA, Ludlow JW, Figge J, et al. SV40 large tumor antigen forms a specific complex with the product of the retinoblastoma susceptibility gene. Cell 1988;54:275–283.
82. Dyson N, Howley PM, Münger K, et al. The human papilloma virus-16 E7 oncoprotein is able to bind to the retinoblastoma gene product. Science 1989;243:934–937.
83. Elison JR, Cobrinik D, Claros N, et al. Small molecule inhibition of HDM2 leads to p53-mediated cell death in retinoblastoma cells. Arch Ophthalmol 2006;124:1269–1275.
84. Marine JC, Dyer MA, Jochemsen AG. MDMX: from bench to bedside. J Cell Sci 2007; 120:371–378.
85. Vogel F. Genetics of retinoblastoma. Hum Genet 1979;52:1–54.
86. Bremner R, Du DC, Connolly-Wilson MJ, et al. Deletion of RB exons 24 and 25 causes low-penetrance retinoblastoma. Am J Hum Genet 1997;61:556–570.
87. Sippel KC, Fraioli RE, Smith GD, et al. Frequency of somatic and germ-line mosaicism in retinoblastoma: implications for genetic counseling. Am J Hum Genet 1998;62: 610–619.
88. Zimmerman L. Retinoblastoma and retinocytoma. In: Spencer WH, ed. Ophthalmic pathology. An Atlas and Textbook. Philadelphia: American Academy of Ophthalmology, WB Saunders Company, 1985:1292–1351.
89. Margo CE, Zimmerman LE. Retinoblastoma: the accuracy of clinical diagnosis in children treated by enucleation. J Pediatr Ophthalmol Strabismus 1983;20:227–229.
90. Shields CL, Shields JA, Shields MB, et al. Prevalence and mechanisms of secondary intraocular pressure elevation in eyes with intraocular tumors. Ophthalmology 1987;94:839–846.
91. Shields JA, Shields CL, Parsons HM. Differential diagnosis of retinoblastoma. Retina 1991;11:232–243.
92. Shields JA, Augsburger JJ. Current approaches to the diagnosis and management of retinoblastoma. Surv Ophthalmol 1981;25:347–372.
93. Yoshizumi MO, Thomas JV, Smith TR. Glaucoma-inducing mechanisms in eyes with retinoblastoma. Arch Ophthalmol 1978;96:105–110.
94. Shields CL, Ghassemi F, Tuncer S, et al. Clinical spectrum of diffuse infiltrating retinoblastoma in 34 consecutive eyes. Ophthalmology 2008;115:2253–2258.
95. Arrigg PG, Hedges TR III, Char DH. Computed tomography in the diagnosis of retinoblastoma. Br J Ophthalmol 1983;67:588–591.
96. Smith EV, Gragoudas ES, Kolodny NH, et al. Magnetic resonance imaging: an emerging technique for the diagnosis of ocular disorders. Int Ophthalmol 1990;14:119–124.
97. Mills DM, Tsai S, Meyer DR, et al. Pediatric ophthalmic computed tomographic scanning and associated cancer risk. Am J Ophthalmol 2006;142:1046–1053.
98. Chang MM, McLean IW, Merritt JC. Coats' disease: a study of 62 histologically confirmed cases. J Pediatr Ophthalmol Strabismus 1984;21:163–168.
99. Morgan KS, McLean IW. Retinoblastoma and persistent hyperplastic vitreous occurring in the same patient. Ophthalmology 1981;88:1087–1089.
100. Gassleı ᐟᐟ Lommatzsch PK. [Clinicopathologic study of 817 enucleations]. Klin Monatsbl Augenheilkd 1995;207:295–301.
101. Wieckowska A, Napierala A, Pytlarz E, et al. [Persistent hyperplastic primary vitreous–diagnosis and differentiation]. Klin Oczna 1995;97:234–238.
102. Steidl SM, Hirose T, Sang D, et al. Difficulties in excluding the diagnosis of retinoblastoma in cases of advanced Coats' disease: a clinicopathologic report. Ophthalmologica 1996:210:336–340.
103. Ells A, Clarke WN, Noel LP. Pseudohypopyon in acute myelogeneous leukemia. J Pediatr Ophthalmol Strabismus 1995;32:123–124.
104. Riss JM, Girard NJ, Proust H, et al. Diffuse choroidal hemangioma: report of a clinicopathological study in a 4-year-old boy. Ophthalmologica 1995;209:284–288.
105. Hanssens M, Meire F. Pseudoglioma: a clinico-pathological report [clinical conference]. Bull Soc Belge Ophtalmol 1995;255:99–105.
106. Smirniotopoulos JG, Bargallo N, Mafee MF. Differential diagnosis of leukokoria: radiologic-pathologic correlation. Radiographics 1994;14:1059–1079.
107. Tajima Y, Nakajima T, Sugano I, et al. Cytodiagnostic clues to primary retinoblastoma based on cytologic and histologic correlates of 39 enucleated eyes. Acta Cytol 1994;38: 151–157.
108. Caruso J, Miller KB, Pietrantonio JJ. Combined hamartoma of the retina and retinal pigment epithelium. Optom Vis Sci 1993;70:860–862.
109. Scott MH, Richard JM. Retinoblastoma in the state of Oklahoma: a clinicopathologic review. J Okla State Med Assoc 1993;86:111–118.
110. Minoda K, Hirose Y, Sugano I, et al. Occurrence of sequential intraocular tumors: malignant medulloepithelioma subsequent to retinoblastoma. Jpn J Ophthalmol 1993;37:293–300.
111. Sharma A, Ram J, Gupta A. Solitary retinal astrocytoma. Acta Ophthalmol (Copenh) 1991;69:113–116.
112. Hausmann N, Stefani FH. Medulloepithelioma of the ciliary body. Acta Ophthalmol (Copenh) 1991;69:398–401.
113. Kuker W, Ramaekers V. Persistent hyperplastic primary vitreous: MRI. Neuroradiology 1999;41:520–522.
114. Kaste SC, Jenkins JJ III, Meyer D, et al. Persistent hyperplastic primary vitreous of the eye: imaging findings with pathologic correlation. AJR Am J Roentgenol 1994;162: 437–440.
115. Liang JC, Augsburger JJ, Shields JA. Diffuse infiltrating retinoblastoma associated with persistent primary vitreous. J Pediatr Ophthalmol Strabismus 1985;22:31–33.
116. Haddad R, Font RL, Reeser F. Persistent hyperplastic primary vitreous: a clinicopathologic study of 62 cases and review of the literature. Surv Ophthalmol 1978;23: 123–134.
117. Irvine AR, Albert DM, Sang DN. Retinal neoplasia and dysplasia. II. Retinoblastoma occurring with persistence and hyperplasia of the primary vitreous. Invest Ophthalmol Vis Sci 1977;16:403–407.
118. Gunalp I, Gunduz K, Arslan Y. Retinoblastoma in Turkey: treatment and prognosis. Jpn J Ophthalmol 1996;40:95–102.
119. Stewart J, Halliwell T, Gupta RK. Cytodiagnosis of Coats' disease from an ocular aspirate: a case report. Acta Cytol 1993;37:717–720.
120. Kremer I, Nissenkorn I, Ben-Sira I. Cytologic and biochemical examination of the subretinal fluid in diagnosis of Coats' disease. Acta Ophthalmol (Copenh) 1989;67: 342–346.
121. Haik BG, Koizumi J, Smith ME, et al. Fresh preparation of subretinal fluid aspirations in Coats' disease. Am J Ophthalmol 1985;100:327–328.
122. Manschot WA, de Bruijn WC. Coats's disease: definition and pathogenesis. Br J Ophthalmol 1967;51:145–157.
123. Sherman JL, McLean IW, Brallier DR. Coats' disease: CT-pathologic correlation in two cases. Radiology 1983;146:77–78.
124. Katz NN, Margo CE, Dorwart RH. Computed tomography with histopathologic correlation in children with leukokoria. J Pediatr Ophthalmol Strabismus 1984;21:50–56.
125. Potter PD, Shields CL, Shields JA, et al. The role of magnetic resonance imaging in children with intraocular tumors and simulating lesions. Ophthalmology 1996;103:1774–1783.
126. Edward DP, Mafee MF, Garcia-Valenzuela E, et al. Coats' disease and persistent hyperplastic primary vitreous. Role of MR imaging and CT. Radiol Clin North Am 1998;36: 1119–1131, x.
127. Wycliffe ND, Mafee MF. Magnetic resonance imaging in ocular pathology. Top Magn Reson Imaging 1999;10:384–400.
128. Roth AM. Retinoblastoma seen after surgery for traumatic cataract. Ann Ophthalmol 1978;10:1561–1564.
129. Shields CL, Honavar S, Shields JA, et al. Vitrectomy in eyes with unsuspected retinoblastoma. Ophthalmology 2000;107:2250–2255.
130. Char DH, Miller TR. Fine needle biopsy in retinoblastoma. Am J Ophthalmol 1984;97: 686–690.
131. Akhtar M, Ali MA, Sabbah R, et al. Fine-needle aspiration biopsy diagnosis of round cell malignant tumors of childhood. A combined light and electron microscopic approach. Cancer 1985;55:1805–1817.
132. Alio J, Ludena M, Millan A, et al. Ultrastructural study of a retinoma by intraocular fine-needle aspiration biopsy. Ophthalmologica 1988;196:192–199.
133. Akhtar M, Ali MA, Sabbah R, et al. Aspiration cytology of retinoblastoma: light and electron microscopic correlations. Diagn Cytopathol 1988;4:306–311.
134. Das DK, Das J, Chachra KL, et al. Diagnosis of retinoblastoma by fine-needle aspiration and aqueous cytology. Diagn Cytopathol 1989;5:203–206.
135. Shields JA, Shields CL, Ehya H, et al. Fine-needle aspiration biopsy of suspected intraocular tumors. The 1992 Urwick Lecture. Ophthalmology 1993;100:1677–1684.
136. Robertson DM. Fine-needle biopsy and retinoblastoma [letter; comment]. Ophthalmology 1997;104:567–568.
137. Decaussin M, Boran MD, Salle M, et al. Cytological aspiration of intraocular retinoblastoma in an 11-year-old boy. Diagn Cytopathol 1998;19:190–193.
138. Karcioglu ZA. Fine needle aspiration biopsy (FNAB) for retinoblastoma. Retina 2002;22:707–710.
139. O'hara BJ, Ehya H, Shields JA, et al. Fine needle aspiration biopsy in pediatric ophthalmic tumors and pseudotumors. Acta Cytol 1993;37:125–130.
140. Augsburger JJ, Shields JA, Folberg R, et al. Fine needle aspiration biopsy in the diagnosis of intraocular cancer. Cytologic-histologic correlations. Ophthalmology 1985;92: 39–49.
141. Sastre X, Chantada GL, Doz F, et al. Proceedings of the consensus meetings from the International Retinoblastoma Staging Working Group on the pathology guidelines for the examination of enucleated eyes and evaluation of prognostic risk factors in retinoblastoma. Arch Pathol Lab Med 2009;133:1199–1202.
142. Spencer WH. Optic nerve extension of intraocular neoplasms. Am J Ophthalmol 1975;80:465–471.
143. Karcioglu ZA, al Mesfer SA, Abboud E, et al. Workup for metastatic retinoblastoma: a review of 261 patients. Ophthalmology 1997;104:307–312.
144. Tosi P, Cintorino M, Toti P, et al. Histopathological evaluation for the prognosis of retinoblastoma. Ophthalmic Paediatr Genet 1989;10:173–177.
145. Croxatto JO, Fernandez Meijide R, Malbran ES. Retinoblastoma masquerading as ocular inflammation. Ophthalmologica 1983;186:48–53.
146. Kopelman JE, McLean IW, Rosenberg SH. Multivariate analysis of risk factors for metastasis in retinoblastoma treated by enucleation. Ophthalmology 1987;94:371–377.
147. Donaldson SS, Smith LM. Retinoblastoma: biology, presentation, and current management. Oncology (Huntingt) 1989;3:45–51.
148. Grossniklaus HE, Dhaliwal RS, Martin DF. Diffuse anterior retinoblastoma. Retina 1998;18:238–241.
149. Moll AC, Koten JW, Lindenmayer DA, et al. Three histopathological types of retinoblastoma and their relation to heredity and age of enucleation. J Med Genet 1996;33:923–927.
150. Zilelioglu G, Gunduz K. Ultrasonic findings in intraocular retinoblastoma and correlation with histopathologic diagnosis. Int Ophthalmol 1995;19:71–75.
151. Nemeth J, Szabo A, Vegh M. Unusual echographic form of retinoblastoma. Acta Ophthalmol Suppl 1992;204:107–109.
152. Bhatnagar R, Vine AK. Diffuse infiltrating retinoblastoma. Ophthalmology 1991;98: 1657–1661.
153. Mansour AM, Greenwald MJ, O'Grady R. Diffuse infiltrating retinoblastoma. J Pediatr Ophthalmol Strabismus 1989;26:152–154.
154. Girard B, Le Hoang P, D'Hermies F, et al. [Diffuse infiltrating retinoblastoma]. J Fr Ophtalmol 1989;12:369–381.
155. Shields JA, Shields CL, Eagle RC, et al. Spontaneous pseudohypopyon secondary to diffuse infiltrating retinoblastoma. Arch Ophthalmol 1988;106:1301–1302.

156. Nicholson DH, Norton EW. Diffuse infiltrating retinoblastoma. Trans Am Ophthalmol Soc 1980;78:265–289.
157. Morgan G. Diffuse infiltrating retinoblastoma. Br J Ophthalmol 1971;55:600–606.
158. Galimova RZ, Zuikova TP, Buriakova ZA. [Clinico-morphological features of retinoblastoma with spontaneous regression]. Vestn Oftalmol 1990;106:56–59.
159. Greger V, Passarge E, Hopping W, et al. Epigenetic changes may contribute to the formation and spontaneous regression of retinoblastoma. Hum Genet 1989;83:155–158.
160. Krasnovid TA. [Spontaneous regression of bilateral retinoblastoma]. Oftalmol Zh 1987;4:248–249.
161. Assaf AA, Phillips CI. Spontaneous regression of unilateral retinoblastoma in a father of three sons with bilateral retinoblastoma. Ophthalmic Paediatr Genet 1985;6:179–182.
162. Gangwar DN, Jain IS, Gupta A, et al. Bilateral spontaneous regression of retinoblastoma with dominant transmission. Ann Ophthalmol 1982;14:479–480.
163. Brodwall J. Spontaneous regression of a retinoblastoma: a case report. Acta Ophthalmol (Copenh) 1981;59:430–434.
164. Khodadoust AA, Roozitalab HM, Smith RE, et al. Spontaneous regression of retinoblastoma. Surv Ophthalmol 1977;21:467–478.
165. Nehen JH. Spontaneous regression of retinoblastoma. Acta Ophthalmol (Copenh) 1975;53:647–651.
166. Lindley J, Smith S. Histology and spontaneous regression of retinoblastoma. Trans Ophthalmol Soc U.K. 1974;94:953–967.
167. Andersen SR, Jensen OA. Retinoblastoma with necrosis of central retinal artery and vein and partial spontaneous regression. Acta Ophthalmol 1974;52:183–193.
168. Pearce WG, Gillan JG. Bilateral spontaneous regression of retinoblastoma. Can J Ophthalmol 1972;7:234–239.
169. Karsgaard AT. Spontaneous regression of retinoblastoma. A report of two cases. Can J Ophthalmol 1971;6:218–222.
170. Boniuk M, Bishop DW. Oligodendroglioma of the retina. Surv Ophthalmol 1969;13:284–289.
171. Mullaney PB, Karcioglu ZA, Huaman AM, et al. Retinoblastoma associated orbital cellulitis. Br J Ophthalmol 1998;82:517–521.
172. Chong EM, Coffee RE, Chintagumpala M, et al. Extensively necrotic retinoblastoma is associated with high-risk prognostic factors. Arch Pathol Lab Med 2006;130:1669–1672.
173. Salazar-Flores M, Ambrosius-Diener K. [Retinoblastoma: anatomical study of 406 cases]. Bol Med Hosp Infant Mex 1986;43:106–112.
174. Shuangshoti S, Chaiwun B, Kasantikul V. A study of 39 retinoblastomas with particular reference to morphology, cellular differentiation and tumour origin. Histopathology 1989;15:113–124.
175. Lamping KA, Albert DM, Snyder C, et al. The Harrower collection and its place in the history of ophthalmic pathology. Surv Ophthalmol 1983;27:374–380.
176. Sang DN, Albert DM. Retinoblastoma: clinical and histopathologic features. Hum Pathol 1982;13:133–147.
177. Bierring F, Egeberg J, Jensen OA. A contribution to the ultrastructural study of retinoblastomas. Acta Ophthalmol 1967;45:424–428.
178. Datta BN. DNA coating of blood vessels in retinoblastomas. Am J Clin Pathol 1974;62:94–96.
179. Eagle RC Jr. High-risk features and tumor differentiation in retinoblastoma: a retrospective histopathologic study. Arch Pathol Lab Med 2009;133:1203–1209.
180. Radnot M. Scanning electron microscopy of retinoblastoma. J Pediatr Ophthalmol Strabismus 1978;15:36–39.
181. Ts'o MO, Fine BS, Zimmerman LE. The Flexner-Wintersteiner rosettes in retinoblastoma. Arch Pathol 1969;88:664–671.
182. Vrabec T, Arbizo V, Adamus G, et al. Rod cell-specific antigens in retinoblastoma. Arch Ophthalmol 1989;107:1061–1063.
183. Abramson DH, Greenfield DS, Ellsworth RM, et al. Neuron-specific enolase and retinoblastoma. Clinicopathologic correlations. Retina 1989;9:148–152.
184. Bardenstein DS, Rodrigues MM, Alroy J, et al. Lectin binding in retinoblastoma. Curr Eye Res 1987;6:1141–1150.
185. Kivela T, Tarkkanen A. S-100 protein in retinoblastoma revisited: an immunohistochemical study. Acta Ophthalmol (Copenh) 1986;64:664–673.
186. Rodrigues MM, Wilson ME, Wiggert B, et al. Retinoblastoma: a clinical, immunohistochemical, and electron microscopic case report. Ophthalmology 1986;93:1010–1015.
187. Donoso LA, Felberg NT, Augsburger JJ, et al. Retinal S-antigen and retinoblastoma: a monoclonal antibody and flow cytometric study. Invest Ophthalmol Vis Sci 1985;26:568–571.
188. Zhang J, Gray J, Wu L, et al. Rb regulates proliferation and rod photoreceptor development in the mouse retina. Nat Genet 2004;36:351–360.
189. Eagle RC Jr, Shields JA, Donoso L, et al. Malignant transformation of spontaneously regressed retinoblastoma, retinoma/retinocytoma variant. Ophthalmology 1989;96:1389–1395.
190. Spraul CW, Lim JI, Lambert SR, et al. Retinoblastoma recurrence after iodine 125 plaque application. Retina 1996;16:135–138.
191. Ts'o MO, Fine BS, Zimmerman LE. The nature of retinoblastoma. II. Photoreceptor differentiation: an electron microscopic study. Am J Ophthalmol 1970;69:350–359.
192. Ts'o MO, Zimmerman LE, Fine BS. The nature of retinoblastoma. I. Photoreceptor differentiation: a clinical and histopathologic study. Am J Ophthalmol 1970;69:339–349.
193. Ts'o MO, Zimmerman LE, Fine BS, et al. A cause of radioresistance in retinoblastoma: photoreceptor differentiation. Trans Am Acad Ophthalmol Otolaryngol 1970;74:959–969.
194. Singh AD, Santos CM, Shields CL, et al. Observations on 17 patients with retinocytoma. Arch Ophthalmol 2000;118:199–205.
195. Benhamou E, Borges J, Tso MO. Magnetic resonance imaging in retinoblastoma and retinocytoma: a case report. J Pediatr Ophthalmol Strabismus 1989;26:276–280.
196. Khelfaoui F, Validire P, Auperin A, et al. Histopathologic risk factors in retinoblastoma: a retrospective study of 172 patients treated in a single institution. Cancer 1996;77:1206–1213.
197. Kivela T. Trilateral retinoblastoma: a meta-analysis of hereditary retinoblastoma associated with primary ectopic intracranial retinoblastoma [comments]. J Clin Oncol 1999;17:1829–1837.
198. Shields CL, Meadows AT, Shields JA, et al. Chemoreduction for retinoblastoma may prevent intracranial neuroblastic malignancy (trilateral retinoblastoma). Arch Ophthalmol 2001;119:1269–1272.
199. Reese AB, Ellsworth RM. Management of retinoblastoma. Ann N Y Acad Sci 1964;114:958–962.
200. Shields CL, Mashayekhi A, Demirci H, et al. Practical approach to management of retinoblastoma. Arch Ophthalmol 2004;122:729–735.
201. Murphree AL. Intraocular retinoblastoma: The case for a new group classification. Ophthalmol Clin North Am 2005;18:41–53.
202. Shields CL, Shields JA. Basic understanding of current classification and management of retinoblastoma. Curr Opin Ophthalmol 2006;17:228–234.
203. Wintersteiner H. Das Neuroepithelioma Retinae. Leipzig und Wien: Franz Doeticke, 1897.
204. Magramm I, Abramson DH, Ellsworth RM. Optic nerve involvement in retinoblastoma. Ophthalmology 1989;96:217–222.
205. Mustafa MM, Jamshed A, Khafaga Y, et al. Adjuvant chemotherapy with vincristine, doxorubicin, and cyclophosphamide in the treatment of postenucleation high risk retinoblastoma. J Pediatr Hematol Oncol 1999;21:364–369.
206. Chantada GL, Fandino A, Mato G, et al. Phase II window of idarubicin in children with extraocular retinoblastoma. J Clin Oncol 1999;17:1847–1850.
207. Gunduz K, Shields CL, Shields JA, et al. The outcome of chemoreduction treatment in patients with Reese-Ellsworth group V retinoblastoma. Arch Ophthalmol 1998;116:1613–1617.
208. Chantada GL, Gonzalez A, Fandino A, et al. Some clinical findings at presentation can predict high-risk pathology features in unilateral retinoblastoma. J Pediatr Hematol Oncol 2009;31:325–329.
209. Messmer EP, Heinrich T, Hopping W, et al. Risk factors for metastases in patients with retinoblastoma. Ophthalmology 1991;98:136–141.
210. Messmer EP, Fritze H, Mohr C, et al. Long-term treatment effects in patients with bilateral retinoblastoma: ocular and mid-facial findings. Graefes Arch Clin Exp Ophthalmol 1991;229:309–314.
211. Margo C, Hidayat AA, Marshall CF, et al. Cryotherapy and photocoagulation in the management of retinoblastoma: treatment failure and unusual complication. Ophthalmic Surg 1983;14:336–342.
212. Shields CL, Shields JA, Baez KA, et al. Choroidal invasion of retinoblastoma: metastatic potential and clinical risk factors [comments]. Br J Ophthalmol 1993;77:544–548.
213. Shields CL, Shields JA, Baez K, et al. Optic nerve invasion of retinoblastoma: metastatic potential and clinical risk factors. Cancer 1994;73:692–698.
214. Mohney BG, Robertson DM. Ancillary testing for metastasis in patients with newly diagnosed retinoblastoma. Am J Ophthalmol 1994;118:707–711.
215. The Committee for the National Registry of Retinoblastoma. Survival rate and risk factors for patients with retinoblastoma in Japan. Jpn J Ophthalmol 1992;36:121–31.
216. Erwenne CM, Franco EL. Age and lateness of referral as determinants of extra-ocular retinoblastoma. Ophthalmic Paediatr Genet 1989;10:179–184.
217. Rubin CM, Robison LL, Cameron JD, et al. Intraocular retinoblastoma Group V: an analysis of prognostic factors. J Clin Oncol 1985;3:680–685.
218. MacKay CJ, Abramson DH, Ellsworth RM. Metastatic patterns of retinoblastoma. Arch Ophthalmol 1984;102:391–396.
219. Rootman J, Ellsworth RM, Hofbauer J, et al. Orbital extension of retinoblastoma: a clinicopathological study. Can J Ophthalmol 1978;13:72–80.
220. de Buen S, Gonzalez-Almaraz G, Cruz-Perez R. [Retinoblastoma. Considerations on its biological behavior]. Gac Med Mex 1974;108:177–186.
221. Gupta R, Vemuganti GK, Reddy VA, et al. Histopathologic risk factors in retinoblastoma in India. Arch Pathol Lab Med 2009;133:1210–1214.
222. Stannard C, Lipper S, Sealy R, et al. Retinoblastoma: correlation of invasion of the optic nerve and choroid with prognosis and metastases. Br J Ophthalmol 1979;63:560–570.
223. Shields CL, Shields JA. Recent developments in the management of retinoblastoma. J Pediatr Ophthalmol Strabismus 1999;36:8–18.
224. Augsburger JJ, Oehlschlager U, Manzitti JE. Multinational clinical and pathologic registry of retinoblastoma. Retinoblastoma International Collaborative Study report 2. Graefes Arch Clin Exp Ophthalmol 1995;233:469–475.
225. Shields JA, Shields CL. Current management of retinoblastoma. Mayo Clin Proc 1994;69:50–56.
226. Shields JA. Misconceptions and techniques in the management of retinoblastoma. The 1992 Paul Henkind Memorial Lecture. Retina 1992;12:320–330.
227. Dudgeon J. Retinoblastoma: trends in conservative management [editorial comment]. Br J Ophthalmol 1995;79:104.
228. Shields CL, Shields JA, Needle M, et al. Combined chemoreduction and adjuvant treatment for intraocular retinoblastoma [comments]. Ophthalmology 1997;104:2101–2111.
229. Shields JA, Shields CL, Sivalingam V. Decreasing frequency of enucleation in patients with retinoblastoma. Am J Ophthalmol 1989;108:185–188.
230. Shields JA, Shields CL, Eagle RC, et al. Calcified intraocular abscess simulating retinoblastoma [letter]. Am J Ophthalmol 1992;114:227–229.
231. Shields JA, Shields CL, de Potter P. Enucleation technique for children with retinoblastoma. J Pediatr Ophthalmol Strabismus 1992;29:213–215.
232. Karcioglu ZA, al Mesfer SA, Mullaney PB. Porous polyethylene orbital implant in patients with retinoblastoma. Ophthalmology 1998;105:1311–1316.
233. Shields CL, Uysal Y, Marr BP, et al. Experience with the polymer-coated hydroxyapatite implant after enucleation in 126 patients. Ophthalmology 2007;114:367–373.
234. Shields CL, Shields JA, de Potter P, et al. Lack of complications of the hydroxyapatite orbital implant in 250 consecutive cases. Trans Am Ophthalmol Soc 1993;91:177–189.
235. Shields JA. The expanding role of laser photocoagulation for intraocular tumors. 1993 H. Christian Zweng Memorial Lecture. Retina 1994;14:310–322.
236. Shields JA, Shields CL, Parsons H, et al. The role of photocoagulation in the management of retinoblastoma. Arch Ophthalmol 1990;108:205–208.
237. Shields CL, Shields JA, Kiratli H, et al. Treatment of retinoblastoma with indirect ophthalmoscope laser photocoagulation. J Pediatr Ophthalmol Strabismus 1995;32:317–322.
238. Shields JA, Parsons H, Shields CL, et al. The role of cryotherapy in the management of retinoblastoma. Am J Ophthalmol 1989;106:260–264.
239. Baumal CR, Shields CL, Shields JA, et al. Surgical repair of rhegmatogenous retinal detachment after treatment for retinoblastoma. Ophthalmology 1998;105:2134–2139.
240. Tucker MA, D'Angio GJ, Boice JD, et al. Bone sarcomas linked to radiotherapy and chemotherapy in children. N Engl J Med 1987;317:588–593.
241. Wong FL, Boice JD Jr, Abramson DH, et al. Cancer incidence after retinoblastoma:radiation dose and sarcoma risk. JAMA 1997;278:1262–1267.
242. Abramson DH, Ellsworth RM, Kitchin FD, et al. Second nonocular tumors in retinoblastoma survivors: are they radiation-induced? Ophthalmology 1984;91:1351–1355.
243. Abramson DH, Frank CM. Second nonocular tumors in survivors of bilateral retinoblastoma: a possible age effect on radiation-related risk [comments]. Ophthalmology 1998;105:573–579.

244. Gallie BL, Budning A, DeBoer G, et al. Chemotherapy with focal therapy can cure intraocular retinoblastoma without radiotherapy [published erratum appears in Arch Ophthalmol 1997 Apr;115(4):525] [comments]. Arch Ophthalmol 1996;114:1321–1328.
245. Shields CL, de Potter P, Himelstein BP, et al. Chemoreduction in the initial management of intraocular retinoblastoma. Arch Ophthalmol 1996;114:1330–1338.
246. Shields CL, Honavar SG, Shields JA, et al. Factors predictive of recurrence of retinal tumors, vitreous seeds, and subretinal seeds following chemoreduction for retinoblastoma. Arch Ophthalmol 2002;120:460–464.
247. Shields CL, Shelil A, Cater J, et al. Development of new retinoblastomas after 6 cycles of chemoreduction for retinoblastoma in 162 eyes of 106 consecutive patients. Arch Ophthalmol 2003;121:1571–1576.
248. Shields CL, Mashayekhi A, Au AK, et al. The International Classification of Retinoblastoma predicts chemoreduction success. Ophthalmology 2006;113:2276–2280.
249. Shields CL, Ramasubramanian A, Thangappan A, et al. Chemoreduction for group E retinoblastoma: comparison of chemoreduction alone versus chemoreduction plus low-dose external radiotherapy in 76 eyes. Ophthalmology 2009;116:544–551.
250. Yamane T, Kaneko A, Mohri M. The technique of ophthalmic arterial infusion therapy for patients with intraocular retinoblastoma. Int J Clin Oncol 2004;9:69–73.
251. Abramson DH, Dunkel IJ, Brodie SE, et al. A phase I/II study of direct intraarterial (ophthalmic artery) chemotherapy with melphalan for intraocular retinoblastoma initial results. Ophthalmology 2008;115:1398–1404, 1404.
252. Redler LD, Ellsworth RM. Prognostic importance of choroidal invasion in retinoblastoma. Arch Ophthalmol 1973;90:294–296.
253. Chantada GL, Doz F, Orjuela M, et al. World disparities in risk definition and management of retinoblastoma: a report from the International Retinoblastoma Staging Working Group. Pediatr Blood Cancer 2008;50:692–694.
254. Chantada GL, Dunkel IJ, Antoneli CB, et al. Risk factors for extraocular relapse following enucleation after failure of chemoreduction in retinoblastoma. Pediatr Blood Cancer 2007;49:256–260.
255. Pratt CB, Kun LE. Response of orbital and central nervous system metastases of retinoblastoma following treatment with cyclophosphamide/doxorubicin. Pediatr Hematol Oncol 1987;4:125–130.
256. Friedman DL, Himelstein B, Shields CL, et al. Chemoreduction and local ophthalmic therapy for intraocular retinoblastoma. J Clin Oncol 2000;18:12–17.
257. Uusitalo MS, Van Quill KR, Scott IU, et al. Evaluation of chemoprophylaxis in patients with unilateral retinoblastoma with high-risk features on histopathologic examination. Arch Ophthalmol 2001;119:41–48.
258. Honavar SG, Singh AD, Shields CL, et al. Postenucleation adjuvant therapy in high-risk retinoblastoma. Arch Ophthalmol 2002;120:923–931.
259. Chantada G, Fandino A, Davila MT, et al. Results of a prospective study for the treatment of retinoblastoma. Cancer 2004;100:834–842.
260. Lagendijk JJ. A microwave heating technique for the hyperthermic treatment of tumours in the eye, especially retinoblastoma. Phys Med Biol 1982;27:1313–1324.
261. Shields CL, Santos MC, Diniz W, et al. Thermotherapy for retinoblastoma. Arch Ophthalmol 1999;117:885–893.
262. Murray TG, Cicciarelli N, McCabe CM, et al. In vitro efficacy of carboplatin and hyperthermia in a murine retinoblastoma cell line. Invest Ophthalmol Vis Sci 1997;38: 2516–2522.
263. Kaneko A. [Malignant ophthalmic tumors]. Nippon Rinsho 1993;51(Suppl):1013–1020.
264. Murphree AL, Munier FL. Retinoblastoma. In: Ryan SJ, ed. Retina. St. Louis: Mosby, 1994:605–606.
265. Shields CL. Turning up the heat on retinoblastoma. Rev Ophthalmol 1997;4:116–118.
266. Shields JA, Shields CL. Atlas of intraocular tumors. Philadelphia, PA: Lippincott Williams & Wilkins, 1999.
267. Shields JA, Shields CL, de Potter P, et al. Bilateral macular retinoblastoma managed by chemoreduction and chemothermotherapy. Arch Ophthalmol 1996;114:1426–1427.
268. Hungerford JL, Toma NM, Plowman PN, et al. External beam radiotherapy for retinoblastoma: I. Whole eye technique [comments]. Br J Ophthalmol 1995;79: 109–111.
269. Toma NM, Hungerford JL, Plowman PN, et al. External beam radiotherapy for retinoblastoma: II Lens sparing technique [comments]. Br J Ophthalmol 1995;79: 112–117.
270. Singh AD, Garway-Heath D, Love S, et al. Relationship of regression pattern to recurrence in retinoblastoma. Br J Ophthalmol 1993;77:12–16.
271. Abramson DH, Servodidio CA, De Lillo AR, et al. Recurrence of unilateral retinoblastoma following radiation therapy. Ophthalmic Genet 1994;15:107–113.
272. Fontanesi J, Pratt CB, Hustu HO, et al. Use of irradiation for therapy of retinoblastoma in children more than 1 year old: the St. Jude Children's Research Hospital experience and review of literature. Med Pediatr Oncol 1995;24:321–326.
273. Ellsworth RM. Retinoblastoma. Mod Probl Ophthalmol 1977;18:94–100.
274. Plowman PN, Kingston JE, Hungerford JL. Prophylactic retinal radiotherapy has an exceptional place in the management of familial retinoblastoma [comments]. Br J Cancer 1993;68:743–745.
275. Brooks HL Jr, Meyer D, Shields JA, et al. Removal of radiation-induced cataracts in patients treated for retinoblastoma. Arch Ophthalmol 1990;108:1701–1708.
276. Weiss AH, Karr DJ, Kalina RE, et al. Visual outcomes of macular retinoblastoma after external beam radiation therapy. Ophthalmology 1994;101:1244–1249.
277. Roarty JD, McLean IW, Zimmerman LE. Incidence of second neoplasms in patients with bilateral retinoblastoma. Ophthalmology 1988;95:1583–1587.
278. Abramson DH, Melson MR, Dunkel IJ, et al. Third (fourth and fifth) nonocular tumors in survivors of retinoblastoma. Ophthalmology 2001;108:1868–1876.
279. Fletcher O, Easton D, Anderson K, et al. Lifetime risks of common cancers among retinoblastoma survivors. J Natl Cancer Inst 2004;96:357–363.
280. Shields CL, Shields JA, de Potter P, et al. Plaque radiotherapy in the management of retinoblastoma: use as a primary and secondary treatment [comments]. Ophthalmology 1993;100:216–224.
281. Hernandez JC, Brady LW, Shields CL, et al. Conservative treatment of retinoblastoma: the use of plaque brachytherapy. Am J Clin Oncol 1993;16:397–401.
282. Desjardins L, Levy C, Labib A, et al. An experience of the use of radioactive plaques after failure of external beam radiation in the treatment of retinoblastoma. Ophthalmic Paediatr Genet 1993;14:39–42.
283. Shields JA, Shields CL, de Potter P, et al. Plaque radiotherapy for residual or recurrent retinoblastoma in 91 cases. J Pediatr Ophthalmol Strabismus 1994;31:242–245.
284. Shields CL, Mashayekhi A, Sun H, et al. Iodine 125 plaque radiotherapy as salvage treatment for retinoblastoma recurrence after chemoreduction in 84 tumors. Ophthalmology 2006;113:2087–2092.
285. Shields CL, Shields JA, Minelli S, et al. Regression of retinoblastoma after plaque radiotherapy [comments]. Am J Ophthalmol 1993;115:181–187.
286. Abramson DH, Ellsworth RM, Tretter P, et al. Simultaneous bilateral radiation for advanced bilateral retinoblastoma. Arch Ophthalmol 1981;99:1763–1766.
287. Kingston JE, Hungerford JL, Madreperla SA. Results of combined chemotherapy and radiotherapy for advanced intraocular retinoblastoma. Arch Ophthalmol 1996;114: 1339–1343.
288. Chan HS, Thorner PS, Haddad G, et al. Multidrug-resistant phenotype in retinoblastoma correlates with P-glycoprotein expression. Ophthalmology 1991;98:1425–1431.
289. Chan HS, Lu Y, Grogan TM, et al. Multidrug resistance protein (MRP) expression in retinoblastoma correlates with the rare failure of chemotherapy despite cyclosporine for reversal of P-glycoprotein. Cancer Res 1997;57:2325–2330.
290. Smith MA, Rubinstein L, Anderson JR, et al. Secondary leukemia or myelodysplastic syndrome after treatment with epipodophyllotoxins. J Clin Oncol 1999;17:569–577.
291. Doz F, Neuenschwander S, Plantaz D, et al. Etoposide and carboplatin in extraocular retinoblastoma: a study by the Societe Francaise d'Oncologie Pediatrique. J Clin Oncol 1995;13:902–909.
292. Kiratli H, Bilgic S, Ozerdem U. Management of massive orbital involvement of intraocular retinoblastoma. Ophthalmology 1998;105:322–326.
293. Pratt CB, Fontanesi J, Chenaille P, et al. Chemotherapy for extraocular retinoblastoma. Pediatr Hematol Oncol 1994;11:301–309.
294. Goble RR, McKenzie J, Kingston JE, et al. Orbital recurrence of retinoblastoma successfully treated by combined therapy. Br J Ophthalmol 1990;74:97–98.
295. Kingston JE, Hungerford JL, Plowman PN. Chemotherapy in metastatic retinoblastoma. Ophthalmic Paediatr Genet 1987;8:69–72.
296. Chantada G, Fandino A, Casak S, et al. Treatment of overt extraocular retinoblastoma. Med Pediatr Oncol 2003;40:158–161.
297. White L. Chemotherapy for retinoblastoma [letter; comment]. Med Pediatr Oncol 1995;24:341–342.
298. Saleh RA, Gross S, Cassano W, et al. Metastatic retinoblastoma successfully treated with immunomagnetic purged autologous bone marrow transplantation. Cancer 1988; 62:2301–2303.
299. Saarinen UM, Sariola H, Hovi L. Recurrent disseminated retinoblastoma treated by high-dose chemotherapy, total body irradiation, and autologous bone marrow rescue. Am J Pediatr Hematol Oncol 1991;13:315–319.
300. Namouni F, Doz F, Tanguy ML, et al. High-dose chemotherapy with carboplatin, etoposide and cyclophosphamide followed by a haematopoietic stem cell rescue in patients with high-risk retinoblastoma: a SFOP and SFGM study. Eur J Cancer 1997; 33:2368–2375.
301. Dunkel IJ, Aledo A, Kernan NA, et al. Successful treatment of metastatic retinoblastoma. Cancer 2000;89:2117–2121.
302. Shields JA. Secondary orbital tumors: diagnosis and management of orbital tumors. Philadelphia, PA: WB Saunders, 1989:341–347.
303. Shields JA, Shields CL, Suvarnamani C, et al. Orbital exenteration with eyelid sparing: indications, technique, and results. Ophthalmic Surg 1991;22:292–297.
304. de Potter P, Shields CL, Shields JA. Clinical variations of trilateral retinoblastoma: a report of 13 cases. J Pediatr Ophthalmol Strabismus 1994;31:26–31.
305. Blach LE, McCormick B, Abramson DH, et al. Trilateral retinoblastoma—incidence and outcome: a decade of experience. Int J Radiat Oncol Biol Phys 1994;29:729–733.
306. Shields CL, Shields JA, Meadows AT. Chemoreduction for retinoblastoma may prevent trilateral retinoblastoma [letter; comment]. J Clin Oncol 2000;18:236–237.
307. Bechrakis NE, Bornfeld N, Schueler A, et al. Clinicopathologic features of retinoblastoma after primary chemoreduction. Arch Ophthalmol 1998;116:887–893.
308. Dithmar S, Rusciano D, Grossniklaus HE. A new technique for implantation of tissue culture melanoma cells in a murine model of metastatic ocular melanoma. Melanoma Res 2000;10:2–8.
309. Mendelsohn ME, Abramson DH, Madden T, et al. Intraocular concentrations of chemotherapeutic agents after systemic or local administration. Arch Ophthalmol 1998;116:1209–1212.
310. Murray TG, Cicciarelli N, O'Brien JM, et al. Subconjunctival carboplatin therapy and cryotherapy in the treatment of transgenic murine retinoblastoma. Arch Ophthalmol 1997;115:1286–1290.
311. Harbour JW, Murray TG, Hamasaki D, et al. Local carboplatin therapy in transgenic murine retinoblastoma. Invest Ophthalmol Vis Sci 1996;37:1892–1898.
312. Abramson DH, Frank CM, Dunkel IJ. A phase I/II study of subconjunctival carboplatin for intraocular retinoblastoma. Ophthalmology 1999;106:1947–1950.
313. Chantada GL, Fandino AC, Carcaboso AM, et al. A phase I study of periocular topotecan in children with intraocular retinoblastoma. Invest Ophthalmol Vis Sci 2009; 50:1492–1496.
314. Antczak C, Kloepping C, Radu C, et al. Revisiting old drugs as novel agents for retinoblastoma: *in vitro* and *in vivo* antitumor activity of cardenolides. Invest Ophthalmol Vis Sci 2009;50:3065–3073.
315. Chévez-Barrios P, Wiseman AL, Rojas E, et al. Cataract development in gamma-glutamyl transpeptidase-deficient mice. Exp Eye Res 2000;71:575–582.
316. Mills MD, Windle JJ, Albert DM. Retinoblastoma in transgenic mice: models of hereditary retinoblastoma. Surv Ophthalmol 1999;43:508–518.
317. Hurwitz MY, Marcus KT, Chévez-Barrios P, et al. Suicide gene therapy for treatment of retinoblastoma in a murine model. Hum Gene Ther 1999;10:441–448.
318. Trask TW, Trask RP, Aguilar-Cordova E, et al. Phase I study of adenoviral delivery of the HSV-tk gene and ganciclovir administration in patients with current malignant brain tumors. Mol Ther 2000;1:195–203.
319. Chévez-Barrios P, Chintagumpala M, Mieler W, et al. Response of retinoblastoma with vitreous tumor seeding to adenovirus-mediated delivery of thymidine kinase followed by ganciclovir. J Clin Oncol 2005;23:7927–7935.

CHAPTER 28 ■ PEDIATRIC LIVER TUMORS

REBECKA L. MEYERS, DANIEL C. ARONSON, DIETRICH VON SCHWEINITZ,
ARTHUR ZIMMERMANN, MARCIO H. MALOGOLOWKIN

HISTORICAL CONTEXT

One hundred and ten years ago, the first case report of a hepatoblastoma (HB) was published in the English literature in 1898 by Misick in Prague.[1] Under the title "A case of Teratoma Hepatis," a 6-week-old boy was described who died of respiratory problems. Autopsy showed a large tumor that occupied the lower half of the right liver lobe. Cysts, cartilaginous, and bony deposits were seen, as well as venous tumor infiltration. It was therefore not surprising that the tumor was described as a teratoma, with tissue representatives of the three embryonic germ-cell layers. More than 60 years later in 1962, Willis introduced the term *Hepatoblastoma* for this type of tumor that he defined as "an embryonic tumor that contains hepatic epithelial parenchyma."[2] At that time, usually HB was not distinguished from hepatocellular carcinoma (HCC). Through the work of Ishak and Glunz in 1967, morphologic criteria were defined for HB and HCC that were refined in the decennia that followed.[3,4]

In 1975, Exelby published the landmark paper that has been cited in most recent reviews dealing with liver tumors in children, in which he reported results of a survey of the American Academy of Pediatrics Surgical Section—1974.[5] Through questionnaires sent to the members of the Surgical Section of the Academy of Pediatrics, data on liver tumors in children operated upon during the previous 10 years were requested. From 110 replies, 375 liver tumors were reported of which 252 were malignant (HB = 129, HCC = 98) and 123 were benign. In 15% of the HB patients, the tumor was multicentric in origin. In HCC, both lobes were involved in almost 45% of the patients, and in 30%, the tumor was multicentric. All patients with HB underwent primary surgical exploration with an attempt at definitive resection in 86, and biopsy only in 43. Seventy-eight patients had complete excision of the tumor for cure and 45 (60% of those resected) survived. In two-thirds of the patients, the tumor was never able to be excised completely and there were no survivors in this group. Excessive blood loss was the most common complication during and immediately after operation, after which cardiac arrest occurred in nine patients. There were eight deaths in the operating room and 17 deaths in the immediate postoperative period attributable to the operation. Fifteen HB patients had irradiation of the liver, 53 patients had chemotherapy utilizing a wide variety of agents. It was apparent that no cures were obtained from irradiation and/or chemotherapy in the absence of complete surgical resection. There were three survivors with HB who were originally thought to have inoperable tumor and became operable after preoperative radiation and chemotherapy (vincristine, actinomycin, and cyclophosphamide). Eight of the 11 patients who were given postoperative chemotherapy survived.

In Exelby's landmark 1975 survey, the overall survival for HB was 35% and for HCC was 13%. With incomplete surgical excision no patient survived. There was no evidence that radiation therapy or chemotherapy controlled disease which could not be completely excised surgically. At this time, before the introduction of cisplatin-based chemotherapy and modern surgical techniques, it seemed that complete operative excision carried a high risk of morbidity, even mortality, but offered the only chance of cure.

DIAGNOSIS

Clinical Presentation

Most liver tumors present with an asymptomatic abdominal mass palpated either by a parent or pediatrician.[6] In the youngest children (infants and toddlers), most malignant tumors are HB and present with an asymptomatic right upper quadrant or epigastric abdominal mass. Some children may have fatigue, fever, pain, anorexia, and weight loss. Rarely HB may present with abdominal pain and hemorrhage after posttraumatic or "spontaneous" rupture of a previously occult tumor. HCC and hepatic sarcomas are more likely to present at an advanced stage. Nonspecific symptoms of inanition or respiratory failure may appear insidiously. As the cancer grows, the pain in the abdomen may progress to shoulder or back pain and become more pronounced. The child may develop progressive anorexia and vomiting and appear thin and sickly. Tumor growth may compress or obstruct the normal hepatic architecture causing (a) ascites secondary to occlusion of the portal or hepatic veins; (b) gastrointestinal (GI) bleeding or splenomegaly from the portal hypertension of portal vein occlusion; or (c) jaundice, scleral icterus, and pruritus from obstruction of the biliary tree. Symptoms of biliary obstruction are most common with biliary rhabdomyosarcoma.[7,8]

Differential Diagnosis

Differential diagnosis of a pediatric liver mass includes malignant tumors, benign tumors, and a wide assortment of congenital and acquired lesions of the liver, listed as "other masses" in Table 28.1. For many of the "other masses" listed in Table 28.1, the key to the diagnosis might lie in the underlying medical condition. For example, one might expect to see a bacterial hepatic abscess in a child with chronic granulomatous disease, a fatty deposit in the liver of a child with hyperlipidemia, or perhaps an inspissated bile lake in a child with biliary atresia as shown in Figure 28.1. Organizing intrahepatic hematoma should be suspected in any child with a history of hepatic trauma or in newborns with sepsis and coagulopathy, especially if there is a history of perinatal birth trauma or hemodynamic collapse requiring cardiopulmonary resuscitation. Congenital liver cysts are rare and represent a spectrum ranging from large simple cysts, intrahepatic choledochal cyst, and ciliated hepatic foregut cyst. Acquired cysts might be

TABLE 28.1

DIFFERENTIAL DIAGNOSIS OF PEDIATRIC LIVER MASSES

- **Malignant tumors**
  - Hepatoblastoma (HB)
  - Hepatocellular carcinoma (HCC)
  - Sarcoma
    - Biliary rhabdomyosarcoma
    - Angiosarcoma
    - Rhabdoid
    - Undifferentiated
  - Metastatic/other
    - Wilms' tumor
    - Neuroblastoma
    - Colorectal
    - Carcinoid tumor
    - Kaposiform hemangioendothelioma
    - Hemophagocytic lymphohistiocytosis (HLH)
    - Langerhans' cell histiocytosis
    - Megakaryoblastic leukemia
- **Benign tumors**
  - Mesenchymal hamartoma
  - Focal nodular hyperplasia
  - Infantile hemangioma
  - Hepatic adenoma
  - Nodular regenerative hyperplasia
  - Teratoma
  - Inflammatory myofibroblastic tumor
  - Biliary cystadenoma
- **Other masses**
  - Vascular malformations
    - AV malformation
    - Blue rubber nevus syndrome
  - Congenital/acquired cysts
    - Simple
    - Ciliated foregut cyst
    - Polycystic liver disease
    - Choledochal cyst
    - Inspissated bile lake/biliary atresia
  - Parasitic cysts
    - Amoebic
  - Abscess
    - Bacterial
    - Fungal
    - Chronic granulomatous disease
  - Hematoma
  - Fatty liver

bacterial, hydatid, or amoebic abscess. A simple, asymptomatic congenital liver cyst may be safely observed.[9] If infectious or large and symptomatic (Fig. 28.2), cyst drainage, marsupialization, or excision may be needed to relieve pain and prevent risk of rupture. Recent literature suggests a risk of squamous cell carcinoma arising later in life in those congenital hepatic cysts with a ciliated epithelial lining (ciliated hepatic foregut cyst), and therefore these should probably be excised rather than observed or marsupialized.[10,11]

Neoplastic liver masses, including benign and malignant tumors, account for about 1.0% to 1.5% of all pediatric tumors.[12] Age at presentation is often the key to differential diagnosis (Table 28.2). In newborns, the most common tumor is infantile hepatic hemangioma.[13] Infantile hepatic hemangioma is to be distinguished from the much rarer kaposiform hemangioendothelioma which may present in the extremities, chest, or retroperitoneum. Kaposiform hemangioendothelioma of the retroperitoneum may present with Kasabach Merritt phenomenon and progress to obstruct the porta hepatis.[14] HB is most commonly diagnosed between 4 months and 4 years of age. Benign tumors in toddlers are mesenchymal hamartoma and focal nodular hyperplasia (FNH). HCC and hepatic adenoma are seen in older children. The other tumors listed in Table 28.2 are more rare. Although the most common benign tumors often show classic distinguishing features on computed tomography (CT), imaging is *not* usually a reliable way to differentiate benign from malignant tumors.[15]

Laboratory Evaluation

Routine laboratory investigation should include complete blood count; many children with a malignant liver tumor will exhibit some degree of anemia and thrombocytosis.[17] In HB, the thrombocytosis is thought to be caused by tumor production of thrombopoietin, interleukin-6, and interleukin 1B.[18-20] Additional labs include a liver panel (albumin, transaminases, glutamyl transferase, alkaline phosphatase, and total and conjugated bilirubin), lactate dehydrogenase, tumor markers (alpha-fetoprotein [AFP], beta-human choriogonadotropin [B-HCG], ferritin, and carcinoembryonic antigen [CEA], catecholamines), and viral titers (hepatitis A, B, and C and Ebstein-Barr virus).[16]

The most important tumor marker is the serum AFP. AFP will be elevated in 90% if children with HB, and 50% of children with HCC.[21] Although AFP is elevated in most children with HB, increased AFP is *not* pathognomonic for a malignant liver tumor. European, German, and American multicenter trials have all concluded that HB tumors that fail to express AFP at diagnosis (diagnosis AFP level <100) are biologically more aggressive with a worse prognosis.[22-26] Rarely, the opposite

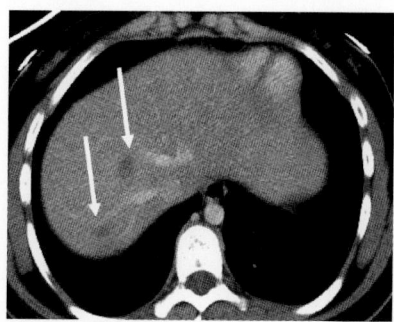
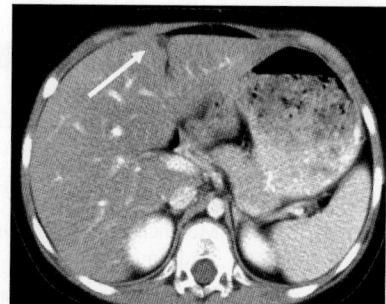
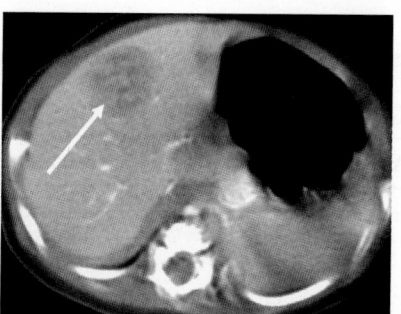

A,B   **C**

FIGURE 28.1 Examples of non-neoplastic liver masses. **A:** Bacterial abscess in chronic granulomatous disease. **B:** Fatty deposit in hyperlipidemia. **C:** Inspissated bile lake in biliary atresia.

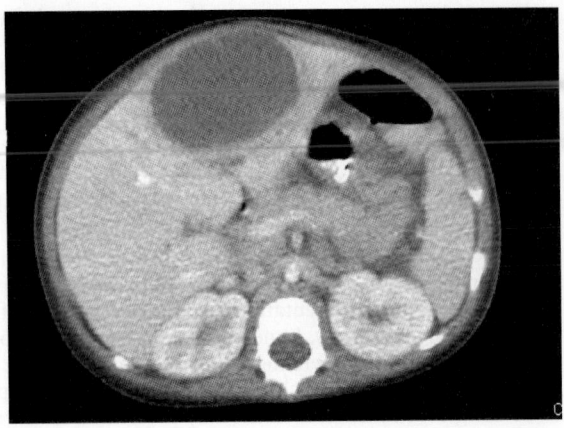 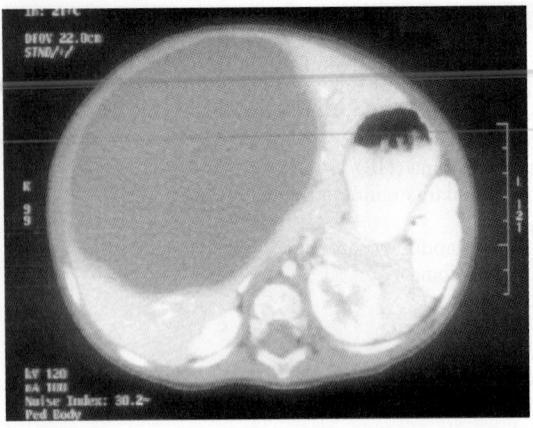

FIGURE 28.2 Acquired and congenital hepatic cysts. **A:** Acquired cyst, amoebic abscess. **B:** Congenital cyst so large that it causes symptoms (pain, compression of stomach and duodenum, and upward pressure on diaphragm).

has been reported with a case of well-differentiated, fetal-type, favorable prognosis HB that did not express AFP.[27] AFP levels must be interpreted with caution in neonates because AFP is the major protein produced by the fetal liver and is thus produced in high amounts in the normal newborn. AFP may be especially high in neonates after hepatic damage and during regeneration of liver parenchyma. The half-life of AFP is 5 to 7 days and levels fall throughout the first several months of life so that by one year of age, the AFP should be less than 10 ng/mL.[28] Moreover, there are many reports of benign tumors, especially infantile hemangioma and mesenchymal hamartoma, in children presenting high AFP levels.[29–31]

The other tumor markers may be useful in differential diagnosis as follows: B-HCG elevated in germ cell tumors; ferritin elevated in HCC and metastatic neuroblastoma; CEA elevated in HCC and metastatic colorectal; lactate dehydrogenase elevated in many malignant tumors; catecholamines elevated in metastatic neuroblastoma; Hepatitis C in HCC; and Ebstein-Barr viral titers in lymphoproliferative disease or lymphoma.

Radiology

HB appears as a large multinodular expansile mass, usually unifocal, but occasionally multifocal. The tumor is generally well demarcated from the normal liver but not encapsulated. HB may invade hepatic veins, disseminate to the lungs, or penetrate the liver capsule to reach contiguous tissues. An initial ultrasound will identify the liver as the organ of origin; additional testing, usually a contrast-enhanced abdominal CT scan, is aimed at determining the extent of involved parenchyma and the presence or absence of macrovascular compression,

displacement, or invasion. The characteristic radiographic appearances of the three most common benign liver tumors in the differential diagnosis are shown in Figure 28.3. Mesenchymal hamartoma is classically multicystic with the complex cysts separated by thick vascular septae. FNH is generally well demarcated with a characteristic central stellate scar. Infantile hemangioma classically will demonstrate bright peripheral contrast enhancement. Metastatic liver tumors compared with primary malignant liver tumors have been reported to be more hypoechogenic on ultrasound and have less vessel invasion and contrast enhancement on abdominal CT.[32]

In HB and HCC, the contrast-enhanced abdominal CT or magnetic resonance imaging (MRI) outlines the anatomic extent of the tumor, clarifies its relationship to the central venous structures, and evaluates for multicentricity.[33] The radiographic appearance of the tumor at diagnosis is used to assign the tumor **Pret**reatment **Ext**ent of tumor (PRETEXT). The radiographic appearance of the tumor after preoperative (neoadjuvant) chemotherapy has been called **Post-t**reatment **Ext**ent of tumor (POSTTEXT).[33] Chest CT scan is an essential part of the initial radiographic evaluation to rule out metastatic pulmonary disease. In children with HB, about 20% will present with metastatic disease in the lungs. In HCC, the number of children who present with advanced disease is quite high and pulmonary metastases at diagnosis has been reported as high as 50% in some series (Fig. 28.4).[34]

MALIGNANT LIVER TUMORS

After neuroblastoma and Wilms' tumor, primary tumors of the liver are the third most common intra-abdominal neoplasms in

---

AGE AT PRESENTATION, PRIMARY LIVER TUMORS OF CHILDHOOD[16]

Age group	Malignant	Benign
Infant/toddler	Hepatoblastoma 43% Rhabdoid tumor 1% Malignant germ cell 1%	Hemangioma/vascular 14% Mesenchymal hamartoma 6% Teratoma 1%
School age/adolescent	Hepatocellular (and transitional cell tumors) 23% Sarcomas 7%	Focal nodular hyperplasia 3% Hepatic adenoma 1%

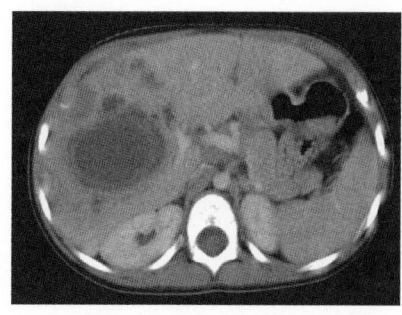
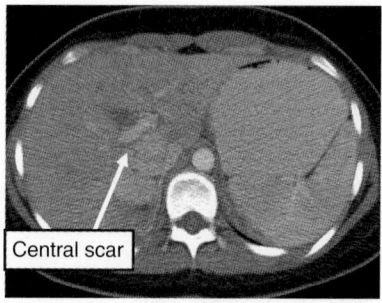
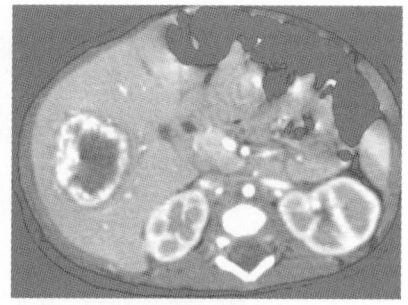

FIGURE 28.3 Characteristic radiographic findings of the three most common benign liver tumors in children. **A:** Mesenchymal hamartoma: *complex multicystic* mass with solid septae. **B:** Focal nodular hyperplasia: contrast hyperenhancing lesion with *central scar*. **C:** Infantile hepatic hemangioma: very bright *peripheral contrast enhancement* with a central area of water attenuation.

children.[35] HB is the most frequent liver tumor in children in Western countries, whereas in Asia and Africa, HCC occurs more frequently than HB, probably a consequence of the higher prevalence of hepatitis B infection on those continents.[36,37] Other less common malignant pediatric liver tumors are listed in Table 28.1.

PRETEXT and Staging

"Risk group" stratification determines treatment for HB in current trials run by the Children's Oncology Group (COG) and the Liver Tumor Strategy Group of the Societe Internationale d'Oncologie Pediatrique (SIOPEL): COG has a low-, intermediate-, and high-risk groups; SIOPEL a standard and high-risk group. COG uses traditional COG (Evans) stage I–IV, and prognostic factors (pure fetal and small cell undifferentiated (SCU) histology and AFP <100) to assign risk groups. COG uses PRETEXT to define whether or not a tumor should be resected at diagnosis ... timing of resection will determine the tumor stage for all nonmetastatic tumors. SIOPEL uses PRETEXT and prognostic factors to define risk groups.

PRETEXT was devised by the Liver Tumor Strategy Group (SIOPEL) of the International Society of Pediatric Oncology (SIOP) for their first trial—SIOPEL 1.[38] Subsequent SIOPEL trials (SIOPEL 2 and SIOPEL 3) have used PRETEXT as a tool to stratify treatment, define risk categories, and report outcomes in HB. Although the risk stratification schema differ somewhat between groups, the three other major multicenter pediatric liver tumor study groups, COG, German Pediatric Oncology Hematology (GPOH), and the Japanese Pediatric Liver Tumor (JPLT), have all chosen to adopt PRETEXT in their current and future protocols (Fig. 28.5). Although

PRETEXT has been found to have a slight tendency to overstage patients, it shows good interobserver agreement (reproducibility) and offers an opportunity to monitor the effect of preoperative therapy when it is applied serially to assess tumor response to neoadjuvant chemotherapy.[23] In America, COG uses PRETEXT to define surgical resectability (i.e., surgical resection guidelines) in its current HB protocol (AHEP 0731). American pediatric oncologists, radiologists, and surgeons will need to become familiar and fluent with the PRETEXT system ... it has become the international language of pediatric malignant liver tumors. Building upon the Couinaud 8-segment anatomic structure of the liver, the PRETEXT system divides the liver into four parts, called "sections" (Fig. 28.6). The left lobe of the liver consists of a lateral (Couinaud segments 2 and 3) and medial section (segment 4), whereas the right lobe is divided into an anterior (segments 5 and 8) and posterior section (segments 6 and 7). Couinaud segment 1 is the caudate lobe and when involved is shown with the annotation "C."

As shown by the examples in Figure 28.7, the tumor is classified into one of the following four PRETEXT groups depending on the number of liver sections that are free of tumor: PRETEXT I, three adjacent sections free of tumor; PRETEXT II, two adjacent sections free of tumor (or one section in each hemi-liver); PRETEXT III, one section free of tumor (or two sections in one hemi-liver and one nonadjacent section in the other hemi-liver); and PRETEXT IV, no tumor-free sections. Extrahepatic growth and macrovascular involvement is indicated by adding one or more of the following: V, vena cava or all three hepatic veins involved; P, main portal or *both* portal branches involved; C, involvement of the caudate lobe; E, extrahepatic contiguous growth (e.g., diaphragm or stomach), and M, distant metastases (mostly lungs, otherwise specify).[39]

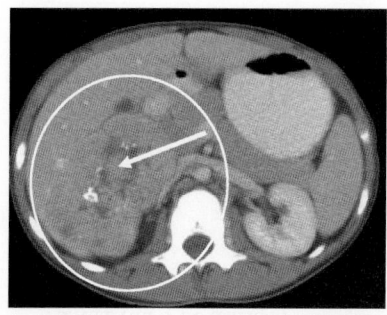
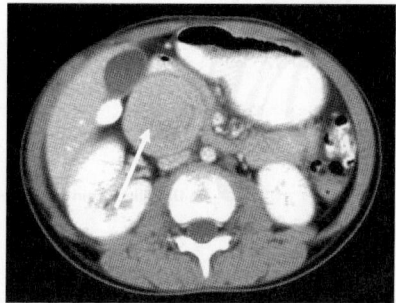
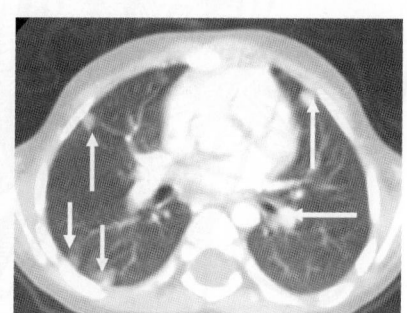

FIGURE 28.4 Hepatocellular carcinoma (HCC) is often advanced at diagnosis. **A:** Primary tumor is PRETEXT II (involves right posterior and right anterior sections). **B:** Large metastatic retroperitoneal lymph node obstructing duodenum. **C:** Multiple metastatic lung nodules bilaterally.

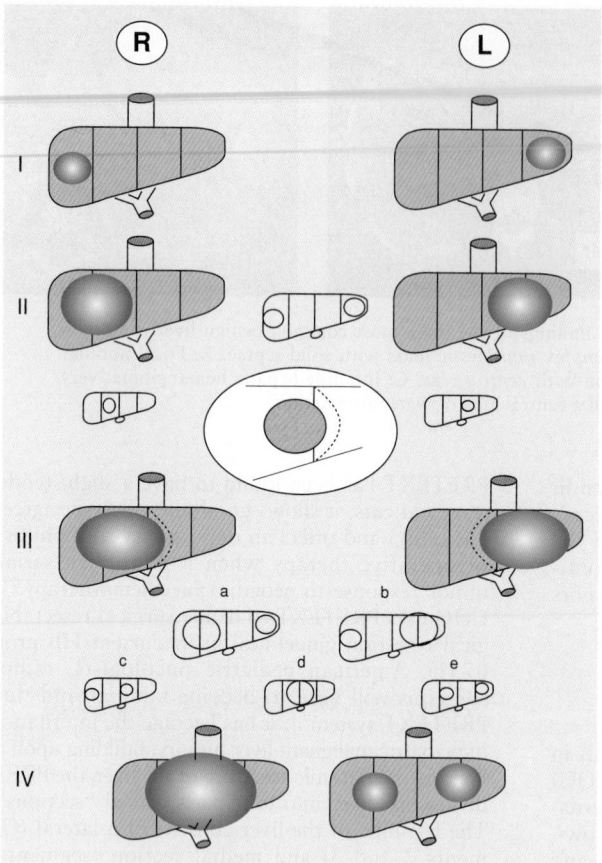

I ... 3 contiguous sections tumor free
II ... 2 contiguous sections tumor free
III ... 1 contiguous sections tumor free
IV ... no contiguous sections tumor free

**In addition, any group
may have:**

+ V ... ingrowth vena cava, all 3 hepatic veins
+ P ... ingrowth portal vein, portal bifurcation
+ E ... extrahepatic contiguous tumor
+C ... caudate lobe involved
+ M ... distant metastasis

FIGURE 28.5 PRETEXT (pretreatment extent of disease), anatomic extent of tumor to define resectability.

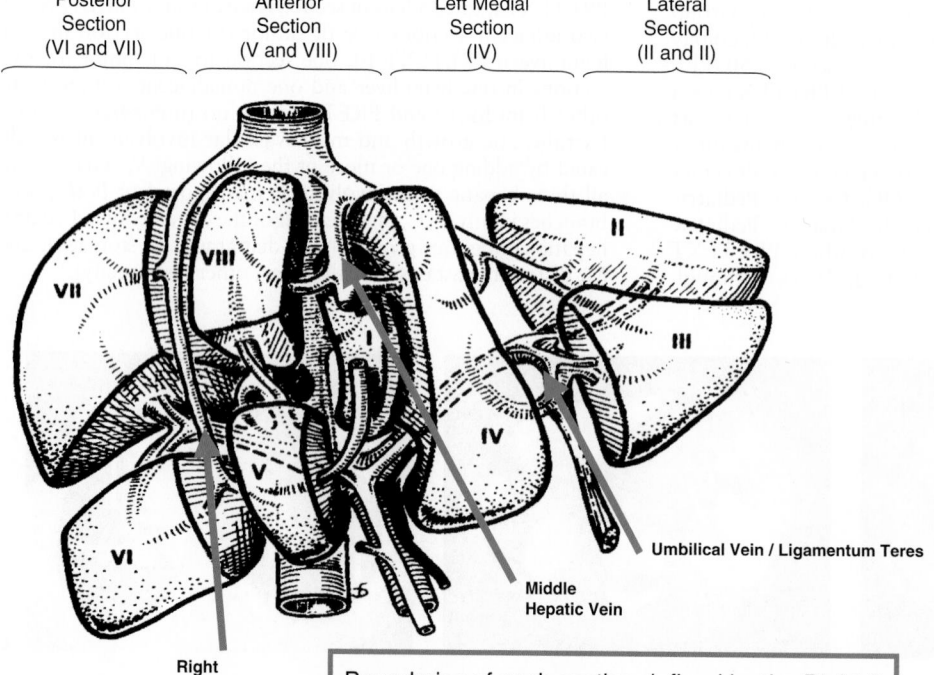

Right
Posterior
Section
(VI and VII)

Right
Anterior
Section
(V and VIII)

Left Medial
Section
(IV)

Left
Lateral
Section
(II and II)

Right
Hepatic Vein

Boundaries of each section defined by the Right &
Middle Hepatic Veins, and Umbilical Vein

Middle
Hepatic Vein

Umbilical Vein / Ligamentum Teres

FIGURE 28.6 PRETEXT is an extension of the Couinaud 8-segment anatomic division of the liver. PRETEXT defines four "sections."

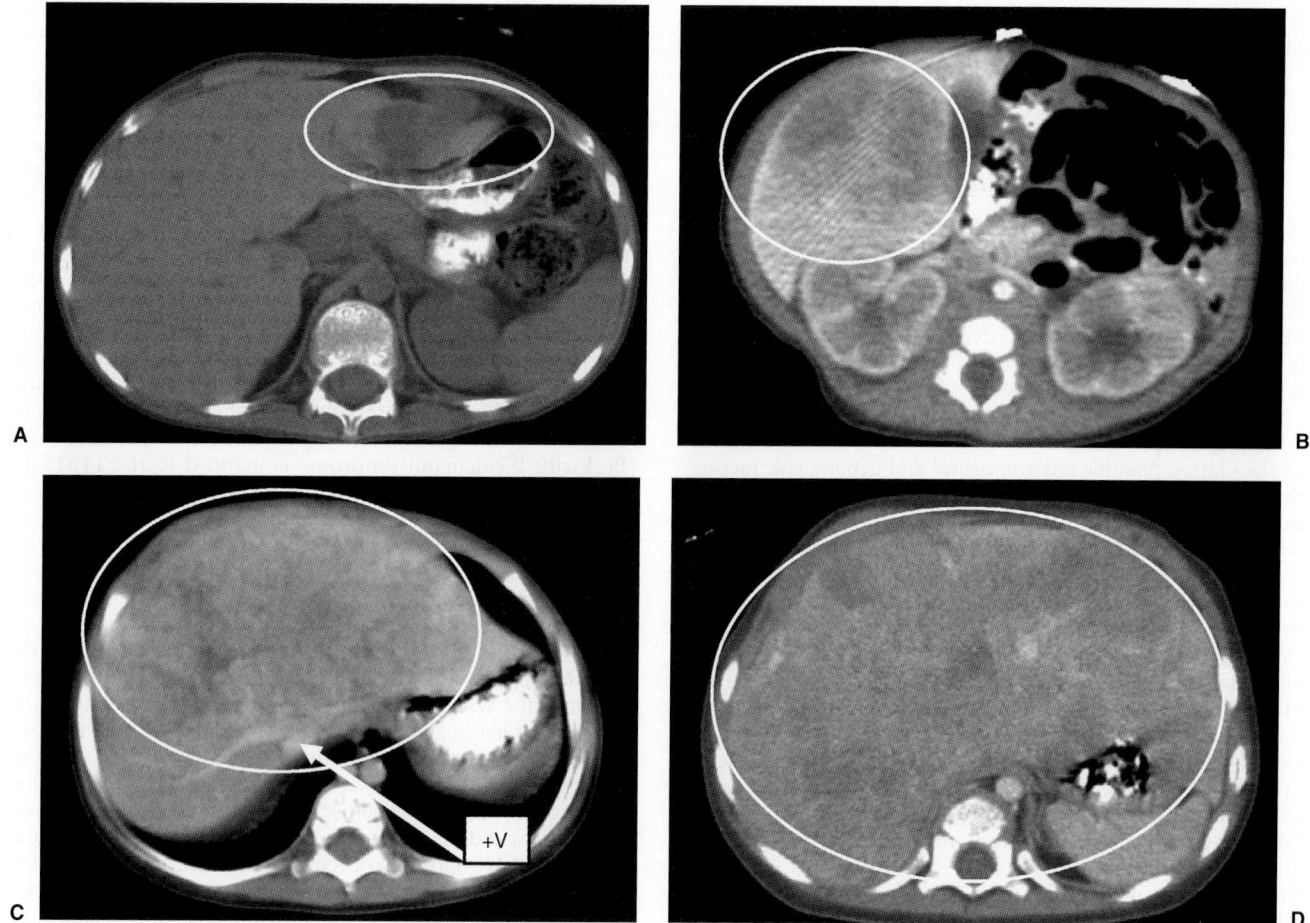

FIGURE 28.7 Examples of PRETEXT grouping for risk stratification of pediatric hepatoblastoma (HB). **A:** PRETEXT I: left lateral section. **B:** PRETEXT II: right anterior and posterior sections. **C:** PRETEXT III, +V: left lateral section, left medial section, and right anterior section with invasion of all three hepatic veins (+V). **D:** PRETEXT IV, +V, +P: tumor involves all four sections and invades vena cava and portal bifurcation.

A universally accepted staging system for childhood liver tumors still does not exist. Through the various staging systems used, the different approaches to treatment adopted by the dominant multicenter study groups are reflected.[40] The North American Cooperative Study Groups, historically Children's Cancer Group (CCG) and Pediatric Oncology Group (POG), now COG, have favored primary surgery when feasible and have used a postsurgical staging system based on the results of the initial surgical treatment of the tumor (Table 28.3) Going back to the early work of Evans in the 1970s,[41] COG defines four stages: stage 1 complete resection at diagnosis; stage II resection at diagnosis with microscopic residual; stage III biopsy (not resection) at diagnosis, attempted resection with gross residual, or preoperative spontaneous tumor rupture; and stage IV distant metastases at diagnosis (usually lung). This surgical staging system is in contrast to the risk stratification system that was developed and used by the Liver Tumour Study Group (SIOPEL) of the SIOP, whose therapeutic strategy is based on preoperative (neoadjuvant) chemotherapy for *all* patients. SIOPEL divides patients into two main treatment strata: (a) SIOPEL Standard Risk HB includes PRETEXT I, II, and III and 2) SIOPEL high-risk HB includes PRETEXT IV, AFP <100, metastatic disease, and SCU histology. COG has recently elected to follow the trend toward risk stratification, and the current COG study, AHEP0731, bases treatment on risk groups, low, intermediate, and high as follows: (a) COG

low-risk HB includes traditional COG stage I (resection at diagnosis PRETEXT I and II); (b) COG intermediate risk includes traditional COG stages II and III and stages I, II, and III with SCU histology; and finally (c) COG high-risk traditional stage IV patients with metastatic disease, or AFP <100 at diagnosis.[42]

COG staging for HCC does not use risk stratification and simply follows the traditional COG stage I, II, III, and IV shown in Table 28.3. Nevertheless, discussions with colleagues

---

TABLE 28.3

TRADITIONAL (EVANS)[a] COG STAGING SYSTEM[41]

Stage I: complete gross resection at diagnosis with clear margins
Stage II: complete gross resection at diagnosis with microscopic residual disease at the margins of resection
Stage III: biopsy only at diagnosis, or gross total resection with nodal involvement or tumor spill or incomplete resection with gross intrahepatic disease
Stage IV: metastatic disease at diagnosis

[a]A modification of this postsurgical staging system has also been used in some German Cooperative Trials (GPOH).[16]

describing the extent of tumor involvement of the liver are based upon PRETEXT.

Hepatoblastoma

Epidemiology, Biology, and Genetics

Hepatoblastoma (HB) accounts for about 80% of the malignant liver tumors in children.[12,43] In the United States, the incidence of HB has increased from 0.6 to 1.2 cases per million population in the last two decades.[43] It comprises 1% of all pediatric malignancies and affects mostly young children between 6 months and 3 years, but cases in neonates and school age children are also seen.

Researchers at the University of Minnesota are conducting a large epidemiologic study termed the "HOPE study" aimed at elucidating possible environmental and genetic risk factors that might account for the increasing incidence of HB seen in the United States over the past two decades. The HOPE study (Hepatoblastoma Origins and Pediatric Epidemiology) can be reached at http://www.cancer.umn.edu/hopestudy. A leading theory is that the increased incidence is due to the growing prevalence of premature birth and very low-birth-weight (VLBW) babies. Both prematurity and VLBW have been associated with an increased risk for HB. The association between HB and prematurity or VLBW was first shown in Japan and has since been confirmed in multiple studies.[44-48] No association has yet been found between prematurity as a risk factor and the age at which the tumor diagnosis is eventually made or the histologic subtype of the tumor. Unproven, but postulated, environmental risk factors include occupational exposure of the father to metals such as welding and soldering fumes, petroleum products, and paint.[49] The list of possible iatrogenic exposures of the premature or VLBW baby in the neonatal care unit include light, oxygen, irradiation, electromagnetic fields, plasticizers, medications, and total parenteral nutrition.[50]

HB is also associated with fetal alcohol syndrome and hemihyperplasia (formerly termed hemihypertrophy).[51] Hemihyperplasia increases the risk of embryonal tumors, primarily Wilms' tumor and HB. Curiously, although there is clinical overlap between hemihyperplasia and Beckwith-Weidemann syndrome, the genetic abnormalities seen in HB patients with Beckwith-Weidemann syndrome are not seen in those with hemihyperplasia.[52] In addition to Beckwith-Weidemann syndrome, a number of other genetic syndromes have been associated with an increased risk of HB including familial adenomatous polyposis (FAP), Li-Fraumeni syndrome, trisomy 18, and others as shown in Table 28.4.[53-68] Familial case reports of HB with FAP are striking and suggest a role in the pathogenesis of HB for chromosomes 5 and 11.[56,69] Additional screening for cases in FAP kindred families is recommended by testing for germline mutations in the APC tumor suppressor gene.[55,70] Germline APC mutations are not commonly seen in children with sporadic HB.[71] The association between Beckwith-Weidemann syndrome and HB is so strong that experts recommend that children with Beckwith-Weidemann syndrome be screened with abdominal ultrasound and AFP at regular intervals until they reach the age of 7 years.[72] The genetic abnormality in HB patients with Beckwith-Weidemann syndrome is mapped to the 11p15.15 locus and suggests the presence of a tumor suppressor gene at this location.[73] Additional biologic markers may include trisomy 2, 8, 18, 20 and translocation of the NOTCH2 gene on chromosome 1q12–21.[61] Upregulation of insulin-like growth factor 2 may be mediated by overexpression of PLGA1 oncogene, a transcriptional activator on the 8q chromosome.[74]

One of the most provocative genetic findings has been the association between HB and mutations of beta-catenin and activation of the Wnt/beta-catenin signaling.[75-77] Microarray analysis of Wnt/beta-catenin and myc signaling has defined two tumor subclasses resembling distinct phases of liver development and characterized by a discriminating 16 gene signature. The highly proliferating tumor subclass showed gains of chromosome 8q and 2p and upregulated myc signaling.[29] Histologic subtypes of HB have also been characterized by different patterns of Wnt and Notch pathway activation in DLK+ precursors.[78] In these studies, the SCU pathologic subtype appeared genetically distinct and was the only subtype with negative GLUL expression. HES1 expression and HES1/AXIN2 used to measure Notch versus Wnt activation ratio were particularly elevated in the pure fetal histologic subtype and lowest in SCU pathologic histologic subtype. Hepatocyte nuclear factor 4 alpha was relatively elevated only in embryonal HB, whereas DLK1, DLK, AXIN2, IGF2, and epidermal growth factor receptor were elevated in all subtypes. The authors speculate that HB may arise from proliferating bipotential precursors

TABLE 28.4

GENETIC SYNDROMES ASSOCIATED WITH PEDIATRIC LIVER TUMORS[53]

Disease	Tumor	Chromosome	Gene	Reference
Familial adenomatous polyposis (FAP)	HB, HCC, adenoma	5q21.22	APC	(54,55)
Beckwith-Wiedemann syndrome (BWS)	HB, infantile hemangioma	11p15.5	P57KiP2, Wnt, others	(56,57)
Li-Fraumeni syndrome	HB, undifferentiated sarcoma	17p13	TP53, others	(58)
Trisomy 18	HB	18	—	(59,60)
Other trisomies	HB	2, 8, 20	—	(61)
Glycogen storage disease type I–IV	HB, HCC, adenoma	Several	—	(62)
Hereditary tyrosinemia	HCC	15q23–25	Fumarylacetoacetate hydrolase	(63)
Alagille syndrome	HCC	20p12	Jagged-1	(64)
Progressive familial intrahepatic cholestasis (PFIC)	HCC	18q21–22, 2q24	F1C1, BSEP	(65)
Neurofibromatosis	HCC, Schwannoma, angiosarcoma	17q11.2	NF-1	(66)
Ataxia telangiectasia	HCC	11q22–23	ATM	(67)
Fanconi's anemia	HCC, adenoma	1q42, 3p, 20q13	FAA, FAC	(68)

with Wnt activation most prevalent in embryonal and mixed histologic subtypes and Notch activation more prevalent in the more differentiated pure fetal subtype.[78] In addition, deregulation of MAPK signaling pathway and antiapoptotic signaling is preferentially upregulated in aggressive epithelial HB with an SCU component.[79] These gene expression signatures may provide prognostic and diagnostic markers, perhaps even therapeutic targets, in the future.[78,79]

Other genetic markers which have been associated with biologic behavior include multidrug-resistance genes and the hedgehog pathway.[80–83] Hedgehog signaling is known to contribute to tumor growth in adult HCC. Recent study has shown a similar association in HB with the hedgehog target genes GLI1 and PTCH1 overexpressed and increased methylation of the HHIP promoter indicating a key role for hedgehog signaling activation in the malignant transformation of embryonal liver cells.[83] Increased expression of multidrug-resistance genes is seen in response to chemotherapy in many childhood tumors, and this seems to be particularly true in HB.[80] Chemotherapy has been shown to induce overexpression of the multidrug-resistance gene MDR1, MDR-associated protein MRP1, and lung-related protein.[82]

Pathology

According to the WHO tumor classification, HB is defined as a malignant tumor with divergent patterns of differentiation, ranging from cells resembling fetal epithelial hepatocytes to embryonal cells, and with differentiated tissues including osteoid-like material, fibrous connective tissue, and striated muscle fibers. In fact, the morphology of HB seems to reflect distinctive phases of hepatogenesis, recapitulating cell lineages derived from endoderm and fated to become mature liver cells.[84] The neoplastic offspring of these cell systems is present in HB in a variety of proportions, used as the baseline of HB classifications, of which the current SIOPEL classification is shown in Table 28.5. Untreated HB presents as a lobulated mass up to more than 20 cm in diameter, being solitary tumors in 80% of the patients, and located to the right liver lobe in about 60%. The lesions usually show an expanding growth pattern, but conglomerated masses with satellite nodules are also observed. The color of the cut surfaces are variegated in many HB, partly caused by necrosis and hemorrhage, with the exception of fetal HB, which has the tan color of normal liver. The gross presentation of HB postchemotherapy is characterized by firm and well-delineated and sometimes multinodular masses with whitish fibrotic areas and calcifications.

TABLE 28.5

CLASSIFICATION OF HEPATOBLASTOMA HISTOLOGIC SUBTYPE[a]

Hepatoblastoma, wholly epithelial type
Fetal
Embryonal/mixed fetal and embryonal
Macrotrabecular (MT)
Small cell undifferentiated (SCU; formerly anaplastic)
Hepatoblastoma mixed epithelial and mesenchymal type (HB-MEM)
Without teratoid features
With teratoid features
Hepatoblastoma, not otherwise specified (HB-NOS)

[a]This is the classification used by the SIOPEL liver tumor study group.

Histologically, the epithelial components range in their differentiation from an undifferentiated (previously anaplastic) phenotype, resembling other cellular blue tumors, to cells that are close to mature hepatocytes (the fetal phenotype). The current, histology-based classification is not consistent in regard to cellular differentiation, because one subtype (macrotrabecular) reflects a growth pattern rather than a distinct differentiation step. The fetal subtype, occurring in a purely fetal and a so-called crowded fetal variant, displays the highest level of differentiation. Pure fetal histology (PFH) HB is associated with both a diploid DNA complement and a low proliferative activity. Around 20% of epithelial HB shows a mixture of fetal and less differentiated, embryonal-type cells, with a more pronounced mitotic activity. The macrotrabecular subtype (<5% of the tumors) reveals a growth pattern with large cell plates consisting either of fetal-embryonal or hepatocyte-like cells. The latter variant, macrotrabecular type 1 (MT-1), is difficult to distinguish from HCC and may have an unfavorable biology.[20] Undifferentiated HB (formerly termed *anaplastic*) mostly occurs as a small-cell neoplasm not associated with elevated serum AFP (SCU HB), but variants with larger cells also occur. SCU HB form a complex group of tumors in that at least part of the lesions seem to have a relation to rhabdoid tumors and are INI1 negative.[85,86]

A large proportion of HB (around 45% when examined after chemotherapy) reveal a mixed epithelial and mesenchymal phenotype (HB mixed epithelial and mesenchymal type [HB-MEM]; Table 28.5). Among diverse mesenchymal (heterologous) components, osteoid-like bone tissue is a common feature. The same epithelial components as found in the wholly epithelial HB subtypes occur in variable expression. The relative proportions of the components in HB-MEM undergo marked changes subsequent to chemotherapy. After exposure to chemotherapy, often the osteoid dominates the histologic pattern. A small proportion of HB-MEM exhibits unusual tissues such as glioneuronal, enteric, or melanocytic tissues. These tumors are termed *HB-MEM* with teratoid features. It has to be emphasized that this term is descriptive and does not imply that these neoplasms are germ cell tumors. The prognostic significance of these histologic types and subtypes is currently under study in large trials.

So far, a prognostic relevance has been worked out for the fetal subtype (favorable)[87] and for HB-SCU (unfavorable).[25,26,88] An unfavorable histology of HB-SCU is also present in cases where the SCU feature is expressed in a focal pattern only.[89] In addition to the lesions listed in Table 28.5, an increased number of variants of HB or lesions thought to be related to HB have been described, leading to the concept of *tumor families*.[4] They are listed in Table 28.6 and are not discussed in more detail here.

Treatment Strategy, Chemotherapy and Surgery

In the treatment of HB, complete surgical resection remains the cornerstone of curative therapy. And yet, as has become increasingly clear in recent large multicenter trials, surgery alone cannot cure patients who present with advanced disease. More than half of the patients present with either an initial unresectable tumor or with distant metastases. In the early years when these children were treated with surgery alone, there was a 30% relapse rate in those patients whose tumor could be completely resected. Evidence that HB is a chemosensitive tumour began to accumulate in the early 1970s when responses were seen to combinations of cyclophosphamide, vincristine, 5-fluorouracil, and actinomycin-D,[41] but not until the introduction of cisplatin- and doxorubicin-containing regimens in the 1980s was there a major impact of chemotherapy on survival.[90] Twenty years later, cisplatin remains the

TABLE 28.6

REVISED AND EXTENDED CLASSIFICATION OF
EPITHELIAL LIVER TUMOR "FAMILIES" WITH AN
HEPATOCYTE LINEAGE[4]

Hepatoblastoma, wholly epithelial type
- Fetal subtype
  - Purely fetal
  - Crowded fetal
- Mixed embryonal and fetal subtype
- Macrotrabecular subtype
  - MT-1
  - MT-2
- Undifferentiated subtypes
  - Small cell undifferentiated (SCU)
    - Focal
    - Diffuse
  - Intermediate/large cell undifferentiated
  - SCU with rhabdoid features (INI1-negative)
- Multilineage
- Unusual HB variants
  - Myxoid
  - Papillary
  - Organoid
  - Hamartoma-like

*Hepatoblastoma mixed epithelial and mesenchymal type
(HB-MEM)*
- Without teratoid features
- With teratoid features

Tumors with a cholangiocellular component
- Cholangioblastic hepatoblastoma
- Ductal plate tumors

Stromal-epithelial and stromal tumors
- Nested stromal-epithelial tumor
- Pediatric hepatic stromal tumors

backbone of current chemotherapy regimen. In fact in the most recent study of standard risk HB by SIOPEL, SIOPEL 3, treatment results with cisplatin monotherapy were comparable with those achieved with cisplatin/doxorubicin combination chemotherapy (PLADO).[91] Chemotherapy may reduce tumour volume making the tumor resectable and may lead to the complete disappearance of lung metastases. The tumor response rate to the present cisplatin-containing chemotherapy regimens varies from 70% to 90% according to the different series.[26,90-95] Neoadjuvant (preoperative) chemotherapy not only makes the tumor "smaller" and consequently more likely to be completely resected but also more solid, less prone to bleeding, and more demarcated from the remaining healthy liver parenchyma.[96] Also when chemotherapy is given as soon as possible at diagnosis, occult (micro)metastases in the lung have no delay in treatment. For all these reasons, many clinicians recommend starting treatment with neoadjuvant chemotherapy immediately upon diagnosis in *all* patients, deferring definitive surgical resection of the primary tumor until after 2 to 3 months of neoadjuvant chemotherapy. This treatment philosophy was adopted by the SIOPEL starting with SIOPEL 1 in the 1980s.[97] The role of a tumor biopsy at diagnosis has been debated in SIOPEL, and biopsy was not mandatory in early SIOPEL studies. However, with the advent of simple percutaneous techniques, diagnostic biopsy has become more prevalent. SIOPEL adopted the philosophy of delayed surgery following neoadjuvant chemotherapy with the following objectives: to increase the number of patients for

whom complete surgical resection will be feasible; to reduce the surgical morbidity; and to provide more time for making definitive surgical plans including liver transplantation when indicated.[98] Because of the large number of countries participating in the SIOPEL studies, standardization of both sophisticated surgical approaches and supportive care measures has been difficult; therefore, the use of preoperative chemotherapy in everyone has permitted patients from countries with limited resources to participate in these studies.

In contrast to the SIOPEL approach, the North American "legacy groups" CCG and POG, now COG, and the German Study Groups (GPOH) have historically recommended primary surgery, *whenever prudently possible*, as the initial treatment. The decision about which tumors are "resectable," and which ones are not, has been subjectively made by the treating surgeon and is highly variable. Since traditional Evans staging depends on the surgical resection decision at diagnosis, and since this is a subjective decision, the stage has often depended more on the surgeon than on the tumor. Nevertheless, the American strategy continues to believe that surgical resection at diagnosis is desirable for smaller easily resectable tumors (PRETEXT I and II). This recommendation has been based on several different factors: Gross total resection of the tumor continues to be the most important favorable factor predictive of cure; approximately one-third of HB patients can successfully achieve a gross total resection of tumor at diagnosis, and among them, it is possible to identify some that require minimal or no chemotherapy. Although it has been debated, postsurgical complications do *not* appear to be more frequent with this approach in the modern era[25,99]; although it is nearly impossible to ferret out the confounding factor that those tumors resected up-front are the smaller, most easily resected tumors. The potential to reduce cumulative chemotherapy exposure is important given the ability of HB to develop resistance to standard chemotherapy agents by increasing the expression of multidrug-resistance genes in response to prolonged exposure to chemotherapy.[81,82] Recent data on magnitude of AFP response actually suggest that the majority of chemotherapy tumor kill probably occurs in the first two cycles.[100]

The strategy in the German trials HB-89 and HB-94 was similar to that previously used in America—that is, resection at diagnosis, when feasible, at the discretion of the operating surgeon. In a review of these studies, 30% of children with primary tumor resection had macro or microscopic residual tumor.[26] Despite the larger number of advanced HB in the neoadjuvant chemotherapy group, an incomplete tumor resection was performed in only 18%. Based upon this statistically significant difference, GPOH adopted neoadjuvant chemotherapy for all patients in their latest trial, HB-99, and recommends against any surgical consideration of atypical, nonanatomic, or wedge resection.[20]

Contrary to these earlier American and German trials, surgical guidelines in the current COG trial, AHEP-0731, *do not* leave the decision about surgical resection at diagnosis up to the discretion of the individual surgeon. Resection attempt at diagnosis determines tumor stage, and PRETEXT is used to define which tumors should be resected at diagnosis (Fig. 28.8). Resection at diagnosis, stage I/II, is recommended only when segmentectomy or facile, nonextended lobectomy will predictably yield a complete resection—that is, PRETEXT I or II tumors with at least 1 cm of clear margin anticipated upon review of diagnostic radiographic imaging PRETEXT is also used by the surgical guidelines to determine the potential need for extreme resection or liver transplant so that arrangements and any needed referrals or treatments necessary for transplant cadaveric organ donor (United Network of Organ Sharing UNOS) listing can be made early in the course of treatment (see discussion on liver

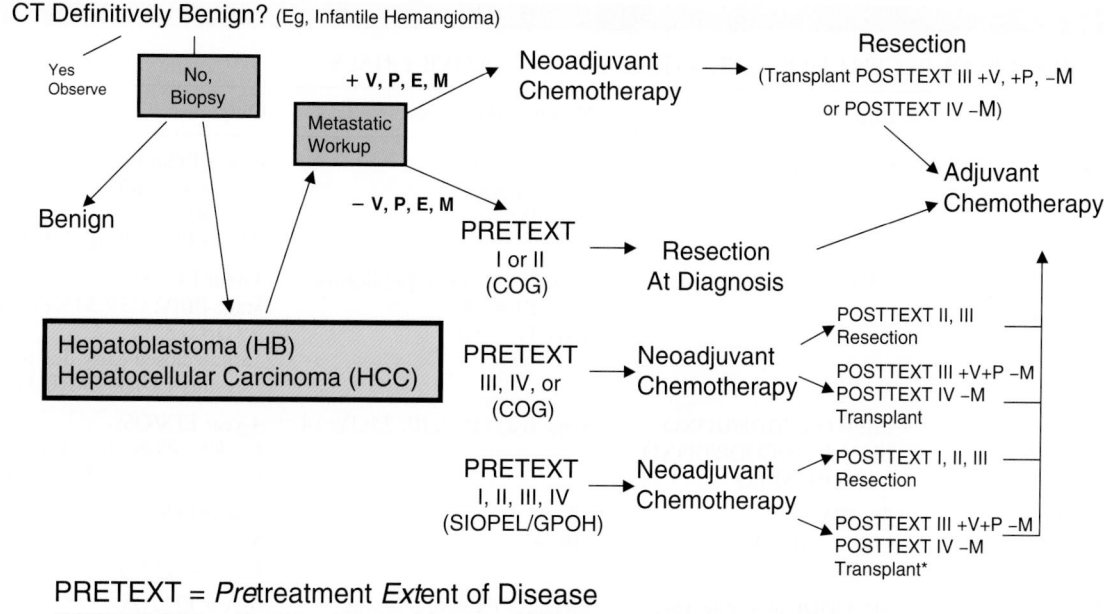

PRETEXT = *Pre*treatment *Ext*ent of Disease

POSTTEXT = *Post*treatment *Ext*ent of Disease after chemotherapy

FIGURE 28.8 Pediatric malignant liver tumor ... *simplified treatment algorithm.*

transplant later). Accuracy of PRETEXT is moderate (due to difficulty to differentiated tumor vessel compression from vessel in growth) with a slight tendency to overstage.[40] Nevertheless, good interobserver agreement has been reported and comparing PRETEXT to POSTTEXT allows for an objective analysis of tumor response to chemotherapy.[23] The predictive value for survival using PRETEXT is excellent and combining PRETEXT with traditional COG staging yields additional predictive value.[25,40]

Postoperative (adjuvant) chemotherapy has been much less controversial, it is currently recommended by *all* study groups, for *all* patients with one small exception. Stage I PFH in INT-0098 and COG P9645 received reduced or no chemotherapy[89,99,101] and have a 5-year event-free survival (EFS) and overall survival (OS) of 100%, and 100%, respectively. Thus, no chemotherapy is recommended for PFH patients, very low-risk treatment stratum, in COG AHEP-0731. Cisplatin remains the backbone of the chemotherapy regimen in all the cooperative study groups, but the drug combinations differ somewhat. Although most use some form of doxorubicin, COG currently uses cisplatin/5FU/vincristine (C5V) for low-risk tumors, C5V + doxorubicin for intermediate risk, and will investigate new agents (irinotecan) with up-front window therapy in high-risk tumors.[42] SIOPEL-3 compared cisplatin monotherapy with PLADO for standard risk[91] and used SUPERPLADO for high risk.[102] The current SIOPEL-4 high-risk study uses an intensified platinum regimen.[103] The recent GPOH trial HB-94 used IPA (ifosfamide/cisplatin/doxorubicin)[26] and the ongoing GPOH trial HB-99 uses IPA for standard risk and carboplatin-VP-16 for high risk.[104] The recent Japanese trial JPLT-2 has used CITA (cisplatin/THP-ADR) for standard risk and ITEC (ifosfamide/carboplatin/doxorubicin/etoposide) + HACE (hepatic arterial chemoembolization) for high risk.[105] Irinotecan, with or without doxorubicin, has been used in both America and Europe for patients with relapse.[93]

So far, no controlled comparison has been done between the two therapeutic strategies, primary chemotherapy for all versus primary surgery for some. In terms of OS rates, however, the results of the different study groups are more or less comparable, projecting 3-year OS rates, regardless of the first

therapeutic modality used of 62% to 70%[26,92,99,101,102,104,105] (Table 28.7). The improved results in the high-risk group achieved in SIOPEL 3 highlight some important lessons learned over the past two decades. (a) With standard treatment, only about 25% of patients who present with metastatic disease are ultimately cured and alternative chemotherapy and surgical resection of pulmonary metastatic disease should be considered in patients who do not show an excellent early response to chemotherapy. (b) The presence of a positive microscopic margin may not portend a poor prognosis in patients who have had an excellent response to chemotherapy. (c) Liver transplant or extreme resection (i.e., mesohepatectomy and major venous resection and reconstruction) should be considered in every child with unresectable HB (about 15% of cases).[106–109]

The current COG trial, AHEP-0731, is a risk-stratified therapy study that seeks to diminish toxicity in the approximately 30% of low-risk patients, increase survival in intermediate-risk patients, and identify new agents(s) that may be used in high-risk and recurrent patients.[42] In this study, all patients with stage I PFH HB will be classified as very low risk and will be treated with surgery only, while stage I non-PFH, non-SCU HB or with stage II non-SCU HB will be classified as low risk and will be treated with two adjuvant cycles of cisplatin, 5-fluorouracil, and vincristine (C5V), a reduction from the standard four cycles of chemotherapy used in previous COG trials. To improve the resection and survival rates for the intermediate-risk patients with stage I SCU, stage II SCU, or any stage III HB, the chemotherapy regimen will incorporate doxorubicin to the C5V therapy (C5VD). To identify potential new agents in high-risk patients with metastatic stage IV or initial AFP <100 ng/mL, patients will be treated with an up-front window of a novel agent (irinotecan) in addition to therapy with C5VD.

New Treatment Modalities

Liver Transplant and Extreme Surgical Resection. A growing experience with liver transplantation has shown that liver transplant is a good treatment option in children with

TABLE 28.7

SUMMARY RESULTS OF RECENT HEPATOBLASTOMA COOPERATIVE TRIALS

Study	Chemotherapy	Number of patients	Outcomes
INT0098 (CCSG, POG)[99]	C5V vs. CDDP/DOXO	Stage I/II: 50 Stage III: 83 Stage IV: 40	4-year EFS/OS: I/II = 88%/100% vs. 96%/96% III = 60%/68% vs. 68%/71% IV = 14%/33% vs. 37%/42%

P9645 (COG)[101]	C5V vs. CDDP/CARBO	Stage I/II: pending publication
		Stage III = 38
		Stage IV = 50
			1-year EFS*:
			Stage III/IV: C5V 51%; CDDP/
			  Carbo 37%
			*Study closed early due to inferior
			  results CDDP/CARBO arm

HB-94 (GPOH)[26]	I/II: IFOS/CDDP/DOXO III/IV: IFOS/CDDP/DOXO + VP/CARBO	Stage I: 27; II: 3; III: 25; IV: 14	4-year EFS/OS: I = 89%/96%; II = 100%/100%; III = 68%/76%; IV = 21%/36%
HB-99 (GPOH)[104]	SR: IPA HR: CARBO/VP16	SR: 58 HR: 42	3-year EFS/OS: SR: 90%/88% HR: 52%/55%
SIOPEL 2[92]	SR: CDDP monotherapy HR: CDDP/CARBO/DOXO	PRETEXT I = 6; II = 36; III = 25; IV = 21; Mets: 25	3-year EFS/OS: SR: 73%/91% HR: IV = 48%/61% HR Mets: 36%/44%

SIOPEL 3[91,102]	SR: CDDP vs. PLADO
	HR: SUPERPLADO
		SR: PRETEXT I = 18;
		  II = 133; III = 104
		HR: PRETEXT IV = 74;
		  +VPE = 70; mets = 70;
		  AFP < 100 = 12
			3-year EFS/OS:
			SR: CDDP 83%/95%; PLADO
			  85%/93%
			HR: overall 65%/69%;
			  mets 57%/63%

JPLT1[105]	I/II: CDDP(30)/THPA-
	  DOXO
	III/IV: CDDP(60)/
	  THPA-DOXO
		Stage:
		I: 9; II: 32; IIIa: 48, IIIb 25;
		IV: 20
			5-year EFS/OS:
			I = ? /100%; II = ? /76%;
			IIa = ? /50%; IIIb = ? /64%;
			IV = ?/ 77%

CARBO, carboplatin; C5V, cisplatin, fluorouracil, and vincristine; CDDP, cisplatin; DOXO, doxorubicin; EFS, event-free survival; HR, high risk; IFOS, ifosfamide; IPA, ifosfamide, cisplatin, adriamycin; PRETEXT, pretreatment extent of disease staging system; SR, standard risk; SUPERPLADO, CDDP/CARBO/DOXO; +VPE Mets, metastatic disease; OS, overall survival; VP, etoposide.

unresectable primary tumors and without demonstrable metastatic disease (after neoadjuvant chemotherapy and pulmonary metastasectomy if necessary). In PRETEXT IV HB, especially multifocal tumors invading all four sectors of the liver, transplantation has resulted in long-term disease-free survival in up to 80% of children.[106,107] Results are not as good when transplant is performed as a "rescue" procedure after an initial inadequate resection or relapse.[110] Although most agree that "extreme" resection of tumors will avoid the need for transplantation in some children, hazardous attempts at incomplete tumor resection in children with major venous involvement or with extensive multifocal tumors should be discouraged.[107,109–111] Extensive hepatic surgery in children should be carried out in centers that have a facility for liver transplant, where surgical expertise, as well as willingness to embark on more radical surgery with a transplant "safety net," is likely to be greater.[112]

The criteria set forth in SIOPEL 3 and COG AHEP0731 for early referral to a specialty liver center with transplant capability are as follows[42,89,107,109]: (a) Multifocal PRETEXT IV HB is a clear and undisputed indication for liver transplantation, whatever the result of chemotherapy. Apparent clearance of one liver section should not distract from this guideline because of the high probability of persistent microscopic viable neoplastic cells. Clinicians should resist the temptation to intensify chemotherapy in a vain effort to avoid transplantation. These patients should be treated within the same protocol as patients with localized tumors amenable to partial hepatectomy, with the same number of pre- and postoperative cycles of chemotherapy. (b) Liver transplantation for solitary PRETEXT IV HB, involving all four sections of the liver, unless neoadjuvant chemotherapy results in a clear downstaging to POSTTEXT III. (c) Unifocal, centrally located PRETEXT II and III tumors involving main hilar structures (+P) or all three main hepatic veins (+V). A decision to make an heroic attempt at extreme resection in these cases should not be done unless the surgeon is confident that a complete resection is safe and feasible, and should only be done by an experienced liver surgeon with the availability of transplant as a safety net. The liver transplantation should not be delayed in excess of a few weeks after the fourth course of chemotherapy as per protocol. An expeditious access to organ donors is required to meet this necessity. It this is not possible with a cadaveric donor, a live donor should be considered.

At present, the SIOPEL study group together with support from COG, GPOH, and SPLIT has established a worldwide electronic registry for liver transplant in childhood liver tumors (HB, HCC, and diffuse infantile hemangioma). The PLUTO registry (PLUTO, pediatric liver unresectable tumor observatory) can be reached at http://pluto.cineca.org.[111]

Hepatic Arterial Chemoembolization, Transarterial Chemoembolization. HACE and TACE are different acronyms for the same interventional radiologic procedure also sometimes referred to as transcatheter arterial chemoembolization. This technique continues to be quite popular in China where recent experience in infants and children showed a mean tumor shrinkage of 59%, mean decrease in AFP of 60%, and mean tumor necrosis in the surgical specimens of 87%.[113] Widespread use has been somewhat limited by toxicity which includes fever, pain, nausea, vomiting, transient coagulopathy, and, most worrisome, pulmonary oil (lipiodol) embolism.[113–115] Pulmonary oil embolism is infrequent and although fatalities have been reported, the clinical course is usually self-limited oxygen desaturation for 24 to 48 hours and pulmonary infiltrate for about a week.[116] Chemotherapeutic cocktails have included various combinations of cisplatin, doxorubicin, vincristine, pirarubicin, mitomycin, and lipiodol followed by gelatin foam particles or stainless steel coils.[112–115] There are scattered case reports of complete cure without the need for surgical resection,[117] although it is most often used as a definitive treatment as palliation tool for large unresectable tumors in the presence of uncontrolled metastatic disease.[113]

Ototoxicity. Both SIOPEL and COG have put considerable effort in trying to decrease the significant ototoxicity induced by the use of cisplatin-based chemotherapy in young patients, especially infants. The risk of cisplatin causing bilateral moderate-to-sever high-frequency hearing loss is significantly increased in children younger than 5 years with higher cumulative doses of cisplatin received.[118] The COG 9645 trial failed to reduce ototoxicity with the agent amifostine.[119] The recently opened SIOPEL-6 study will investigate sodium thiosulfate[120] as an agent to decrease the cisplatin-induced ototoxicity. The current COG trial, AHEP0731, attempts to reduce ototoxicity by limiting the extended use of cisplatin in the low-risk patients.

Risk Stratification, International Collaboration, and the CHIC Project. Current data suggest that PFH and PRETEXT I and II tumors have a favorable prognosis.[23,25] Risk factors that seem to portend a worse outcome include metastatic disease at diagnosis (COG stage IV, PRETEXT +M), PRETEXT IV, AFP <100 at diagnosis, SCU histology, and possibly macrotrabecular and/or extensive multifocal histology.[20,25,88,121] In 2007, SIOPEL, GPOH, and COG decided to embark on a mutual project that was called the Childhood *Hepatic* tumors *International* Collaboration (CHIC). The complete databases of these groups are in the process of being united to be able to address mutual questions. To identify these common data points for prognostication and risk stratification, data regarding prognostic factors (i.e., histology AFP, stage, multi-focality, biologic markers) can thus be studied in much larger patient groups in which the clinical outcome is known. These developments show the starting point of a new transatlantic converging cooperation on a large intercontinental scale that will be of eventual benefit for children with liver tumors.

New Agents, Tumor Relapse. The prognosis for a patient with recurrent or progressive HB depends on many factors, including the site of recurrence, prior treatment, and individual patient considerations. It was recently shown that in patients who initially received only cisplatin/5FU/vincristine cure may be possible with a relapse multidrug regimen including doxorubicin.[93] Surgical resection of pulmonary relapse is possible, and has been reported to produce long-term cure, but does not carry as good a prognosis as resection of pulmonary metastatic lesions present at diagnosis that simply fail to completely resolve on chemotherapy.[122–124] If possible,

isolated metastases should be resected completely in patients whose primary tumor is controlled.[111,125] Success with autologous peripheral blood stem cell transplantation with a double conditioning regimen has been reported in a child with pulmonary relapse after liver transplant.[126] Irinotecan has been used in chemotherapy relapse regimens with some success.[127] In recurrent refractory disease, phase I and II clinical trials may be appropriate and should be considered. Multidrug chemotherapy resistance is a key factor for the poor outcome of relapsed HB. Novel gene directed treatment approaches such as adenovirus-mediated cytosine deaminase/5-fluorocytosine suicide gene therapy may offer hope for treatment of these chemotherapy-resistant cell lines in the future.[80,128] Recent COG phase I trials for which HB patients have been eligible include the studies of oxaliplatin, docetaxel, irinotecan, sunitinib, vascular endothelial growth factor (VEGF) trap, aurora kinase inhibitor MLN 8237, and IGF1R antibody IMCA12. Information on current COG trials can be found at http://www.childrensoncologygroup.org.

Hepatocellular Carcinoma

Epidemiology, Biology, and Genetics

In Western countries, hepatocellular carcinoma (HCC) occurs approximately half as often as HB or in 23% of all primary pediatric liver tumor cases, most often in school-age children and adolescents. Although described earlier, it was not until 1967 that childhood HCC was identified by Ishak and Glunz[3] as an entity to be separated from HB. In 1974, Exelby et al.[5] analyzed the clinical course of childhood HCC and found an overall dismal outcome.

HCC occurs predominantly in the setting of underlying liver disease and cirrhosis. Compared with adults, in children cirrhosis is less commonly part of the antecedent process, while congenital or acquired disorders of the liver, such as metabolic disease, are common.[12] Table 28.8 shows the conditions that are associated with HCC in children.[37,66,129–144] Patients with tyrosinemia seem to be a particularly high risk and should be vigilantly screened with serial AFP and imaging.[143] In East Asia

TABLE 28.8

CONDITIONS ASSOCIATED WITH HEPATOCELLULAR CARCINOMA (HCC) IN CHILDREN

α_1-Antitrypsin deficiency[129]
Anomalous abdominal venous drainage[130]
Alagille syndrome[131]
Biliary atresia[132]
Congenital hepatic fibrosis[133]
Familial polyposis/Gardner syndrome[134]
Focal nodular hyperplasia[135]
Hemochromatosis[136]
Hepatic adenoma[137]
Hepatitis B and C[37]
Glycogen storage disease (type I and III)[138]
Methotrexate therapy[135]
Neurofibromatosis[66]
Oral contraceptives[139]
Parenteral nutrition-associated liver disease (PNALD); TPN cholestatic liver failure[140]
Progressive familial intrahepatic cholestasis (PFIC)[141,142]
Tyrosinemia[143]
Wilms' tumor/Bloom syndrome[144]

TABLE 28.9

HEPATOCELLULAR CARCINOMA TUMOR FAMILY[4]

Hepatocellular carcinoma, adult type
　Cirrhotic liver (more common in adults)
　Noncirrhotic liver (more common in children)

Fibrolamellar hepatocellular carcinoma (FL-HCC)

Transitional liver cell tumor (TCLT)

and Africa, HCC is more common than HB due to the widespread prevalence of hepatitis B and C.[37] In Taiwan, where HCC is most often seen in carriers of the hepatitis B virus, vaccination programs targeted against hepatitis have led to a significant decrease in the incidence of HCC.[36] In contrast to hepatitis B, the cirrhosis and the subsequent development of HCC in the hepatitis C population usually takes several decades to develop.[145] The genetic syndromes associated with HCC are shown in Table 28.4.[63–68]

Pathology

In the pediatric age group, more than two-thirds of HCC occur in children older than 10 years, but only 0.5% to 1% of all HCC manifest before 20 years of age, and very few HCCs are diagnosed in children younger than 5 years. About 20% to 35% of children with HCC have underlying chronic liver disease. It is still disputed whether classic (adult-type) HCC in the pediatric age group is the same or a different disease with respect to HCC in adult patients. It is currently suggested that HCC forms a tumor family (Table 28.9), consisting of adult-type HCC and its variants, fibrolamellar HCC, and a novel entity occurring in older children and young adolescents, transitional liver cell tumor (TLCT).[4]

The gross presentation is in the form of solitary or multiple (multifocal) lesions. Solitary tumors display four main growth patterns, that is, expanding (or pushing) mass lesions, pedunculated (or hanging) lesions, invading tumors with poor delineation, and multifocal tumors resembling metastatic disease. These growth patterns exert a considerable influence on the surgical resectability of the tumors. The color of the cut surfaces of HCCs depends, apart from bleeding and necrosis, on differentiation features of the tumor cells, for example, bile synthesis and accumulation.

The microscopic features of pediatric classical HCC are similar to or the same as that in adult patients. Many tumors exhibit a trabecular growth pattern with intervening sinusoid-like vascular channels and a reduced reticulin network. In regard to grading, Edmondson and Steiner developed a system comprising a scale of I to IV.[146]

Fibrolamellar Hepatocellular Carcinoma. This tumor usually arises in noncirrhotic livers of adolescents or young adult patients and is encountered more frequently in Western countries.[147] Overall, fibrolamellar hepatocellular carcinoma (FL-HCC) accounts for less than 10% of all HCCs. Recent data show that FL-HCC has a biology similar to that of adult-type HCC. FL-HCC shows vascular invasion in up to 35% of cases, frequently metastasizes into locoregional lymph nodes (about 50% of cases), and tends to show unusual spreading patterns, including intraperitoneal spread. FL-HCC is typically a solitary lesion, which has a predilection for the left liver lobe (two-thirds; unusual for hepatic primary tumors). It reveals well-defined margins and a central scar in 70%. The cut surface often shows a firm and tan-to-brown tissue with radiating septa, sometimes closely resembling FNH. The leading cell is a large and polygonal, hepatocyte-like cell with a granular cytoplasm of large vesicular nuclei. These cells form strands embedded in the typical fibrosclerotic stroma which may form a central stellate scar. A considerable proportion of the tumor cells contain large, ground glass-like inclusions, the so-called pale bodies, which are helpful in bioptic diagnosis. PAS-positive globular inclusions in part contain alpha-1-antitrypsin and other glycoproteins. Typically, cells of FL-HCC show marked immunostaining for cytokeratin 7.

Transitional Liver Cell Tumor. TLCT is a recently identified liver neoplasm that occurs in older children and young adolescents. The term, transitional, had been proposed to denote a putative intermediate position of the tumor cells between hepatoblasts and more mature hepatocyte-like cells. TLCT are highly aggressive lesions that have a treatment response pattern clearly different from HB.[148] The usual presentation is that of a large or very large solitary hepatic tumor (mostly in the right liver lobe), commonly associated with very high serum AFP levels. Grossly, the tumors display an expanding growth pattern and sometimes exhibit a large central necrosis. Histologically, the tumor cells vary between HCC-type cell and cells found in HB, sometimes with formation of multinuclear giant cells. The lesions markedly express beta-catenin, typically in a mixed nuclear and cytoplasmic pattern.[149]

Treatment Strategies

HCC is relatively chemoresistant and therefore carries a poor prognosis with a dismal cure rate.[150,151] Complete surgical resection or transplantation of tumor localized to the liver is often the only hope. Even with aggressive attempts at surgical resection, tumor relapse is common and tumor-free survival rates of not more than 25% to 30% can be achieved. These mostly depend on the extent of disease, and the main prognostic factor for childhood HCC is resectability. The first multicenter clinical trials on pediatric liver tumors were conducted in the United States by the CCG and POG, some of which included HCC in addition to HB.[151] These confirmed the poor response of HCC to chemotherapy and radiation and the dismal cure rates of less than 25% of the patients (Table 28.8).

The North American cooperative study (INT-0098) as well as SIOPEL 1[150,151] utilized preoperative chemotherapy in an attempt to increase surgical respectability for the children and adolescents with HCC, since this is the foundation for curative therapy of liver tumors. Of the 46 patients entered into INT-0098, only 8 had completely resected tumors (stage I) at study entry, 25 had unresectable tumors (stage III), and 13 presented with metastatic disease (stage IV). Patients were randomized to receive cisplatin with either doxorubicin or 5-fluorouracil and vincristine. There were no differences regarding response or survival rates between the two treatment regimens. Seven of the eight stage I patients (88%) with complete tumor excision at the time of diagnosis followed by adjuvant cisplatin-based chemotherapy survived. This is a significant improvement when compared with only 12 of 33 patients (36%) treated before the consistent use of adjuvant chemotherapy. This result suggests that adjuvant chemotherapy may be of benefit for patients with completely resected HCC. However, since one-third of these initially resected patients have faired well without any additional chemotherapy, the question of the necessity for adjuvant chemotherapy will only be answered in a randomized trial. In contrast, outcome was uniformly poor for patients with advanced-stage disease. The 5-year EFS for stage III and IV patients was 23% and 10%, respectively (Table 28.10).

HCC patients have been treated in three consecutive studies of the German Society for Pediatric Oncology and

TABLE 28.10

SUMMARY RESULTS OF HEPATOCELLULAR CARCINOMA (HCC) COOPERATIVE TRIALS

Study	Chemotherapy	Number of patients	Outcomes
INT0098 (CCSG, POG)[151]	CDDP/DOXO	Stage I: 8 Stage II: 0 Stage III: 25 Stage IV: 13	5-year EFS/OS: I/II = 88%/88% III = 8%/23% IV = 19%/34%
HB-89 (GPOH)[21]	IPA	Stage I/II/IIIa: 6 Stage IIIb, IV: 6	5-year DFS: I/II/IIIa = 50% Stage IIIb, IV = 17%
HB-94 (GPOH)[21]	IPA + CARBO + VP	Stage I/II/IIIa: 5 Stage IIIb, IV: 20	5-year DFS: Stage I/II/IIIa = 60% Stage IIIb, IV = 25%
HB-99 (GPOH)[21]	CDDP/CARBO	Stage I/II/IIIa: 14 Stage IIIb, IV: 27	5-year DFS: Stage I/II/IIIa = 71% Stage IIIb, IV = 15%
SIOPEL 1[150]	PLADO	PRETEXT: I = 1; II = 14; III = 11; IV = 13; +VPEM = 8	5-year EFS/OS: 17%/28%
SIOPEL 2[150]	SUPERPLADO CDDP/DOXO/CARBO	PRETEXT: I = 1; II = 3; III = 1; IV = 7; +VPEM = 5	5-year EFS/OS: 23%/23%
SIOPEL 3[151]	SUPERPLADO CDDP/DOXO/CARBO	PRETEXT: I = 4; II = 22; III = 14; IV = 21; +VPEM = ?	3-year EFS/OS: 10%/16%

CARBO, carboplatin; CDDP, cisplatin; DFS, disease-free survival; DOXO, doxorubicin; EFS, event-free survival; IFOS, ifosfamide; IPA, ifosfamide, cisplatin, adriamycin; PRETEXT, pretreatment extent of disease staging system; +VPEM, vena cava, portal vein, extrahepatic, metastatic disease; OS, overall survival; VP, etoposide.

Hematology (Table 28.10).[21] In the first study, HB-89 neo-adjuvant and adjuvant chemotherapy consisted of conventional dosed ifosfamide, cisplatin, and doxorubicin (IPA), which did not show any substantial benefit.[21] Thus, of the registered 12 patients, only 4 with resectable tumor survived. In the second study, HB-94 patients with nonresectable HCC received conventionally dosed carboplatin and etoposide in addition to IPA, which seemed to produce at least short-term partial benefit.[21] Of the registered 25 patients, 9 had locally unresectable and 11 metastatic HCC. Three of the nine and one of the eleven patients survived free of disease in addition to four of five patients with resectable tumor (total 8 of 25 = 32%).

Results of SIOPEL 1, 2, and 3 are shown in Table 28.10.[150,151] Only 2 of the 39 patients entered into the SIOPEL-1 study underwent complete resection of the tumor at diagnosis followed by chemotherapy, while the remaining 37 patients had preoperative chemotherapy with cisplatin and doxorubicin. Metastases were identified in 31% of the patients, and extrahepatic tumor extension, vascular invasion, or both in 39%. Although partial tumor response to chemotherapy was observed in 49% (18 of 37) of the patients, complete tumor resection was achieved in only 36% (14 of 39) of the patients. Outcome of patients in this study was also unsatisfactory, with a 5-year EFS of 17%. All long-term survivors had complete surgical excision of their tumor. Twenty-one patients were enrolled on the subsequent study SIOPEL 2. Data were available for 17 of these. One patient died 17 days after diagnosis from massive GI bleeding, and never received treatment. Thirteen of the 16 treated patients received preoperative chemotherapy with cisplatin, carboplatin, and doxorubicin. Partial response to preoperative chemotherapy was observed in 6 of 13 cases (46%). Gross total tumor resection was achieved in eight patients (47%), three at the time of diagnosis, and one through liver transplantation. Nine tumors

(53%) never became operable. One patient was lost to follow-up just before planned surgery. Four of the resected patients were alive at a median follow-up time of 53 months (range of 35 to 73 months). Twelve patients died due to progressive disease and one from surgical complications. The 3-year OS for this study was 22%.

In comparing the results of these studies, the outcome for patients with HCC has shown no significant improvement, despite the progress in surgical techniques, chemotherapy delivery, and patient support. It seems obvious that a new treatment approach is needed to increase the cure rate of childhood HCC.

In adults, fibrolamellar type of HCC has been traditionally associated with a higher resection rate and better survival when compared with the typical pathological variant of HCC both in adolescents and young adults.[152,153] The higher resection rate for patients with the fibrolamellar variant of HCC was not supported by the studies reported by Katzenstein[151] and Czauderna.[150] Patients with the fibrolamellar variant did not have a better outcome when compared with those with typical HCC, the 5-year EFS was 30% compared with 14%, respectively ($p = 0.18$), although the median survival was longer for patients with the fibrolamellar variant.

Concerning the poor response of HCC to chemotherapy and radiation, the mainstay of treatment is surgery. This means that in contrast to HB, a primary radical tumor resection has to be attempted whenever possible using all available techniques to reach this goal.[21] Therefore, in school-age children and adolescents with a primary liver tumor, the surgeon has to be prepared to perform highly sophisticated liver surgery after confirmation of the diagnosis by pathological investigation of intraoperative frozen sections. Patients with the clinical constellation for advanced HCC should always be treated in consultation with a specialized center with experience in childhood liver surgery.

New Agents and Treatment Modalities

Antiangiogenesis, Sorafanib. New treatment modalities including metronomic chemotherapy[154] and adjuvant antiangiogenic therapy[155] are the target of investigation based upon some early promising results. Most promising has been the recent adult experience with sorafenib, an antiangiogenic tyrosine kinase inhibitor, where a survival advantage has clearly been shown in prospective trials of sorafenib in the treatment of HCC in adults with unresectable tumors.[156] Interestingly, this seems to be also the case in some preliminary investigation in childhood HCC.[157]

Chemoembolization and Theraspheres. HACE and TACE refers to the intra-arterial administration of chemotherapeutic and vascular occlusive agents (generally gelatin or lipiodol) along with cytotoxic drugs. The drugs most frequently used for chemoembolization are doxorubicin, mitomycin, and cisplatin. Intra-arterial injection of cytotoxic agents results in higher local concentration of drugs with reduced systemic side effects, while the intra-arterial embolization causes ischemic necrosis of the tumor. This therapeutic strategy has been used in small number of children and adolescents with recurrent HCC while awaiting the availability of a liver donor, or as adjuvant therapy in an attempt to facilitate tumor resection.[113,158] There are no large trials in children, however, in an adult study of adult HCC patients without liver failure or cirrhosis; although TACE successfully reduced tumor growth, it frequently caused acute liver failure, and did not improve survival.[159] A related approach that combines radiation therapy with angiographic embolization has been the intra-arterial injection of 90Yttrium radioactive microspheres, called Theraspheres.[160]

Portal Venous Embolization. Portal venous embolization has been used in adults with liver disease to induce hypertrophy of the remaining liver remnant[161] and reported experimentally in children.[162] The portal venous branch on the side of the tumor is cannulated percutaneously and polyvinyl alcohol and coils are inserted to induce portal vein occlusion under fluoroscopic control. This has a dual effect of alcohol thrombosis of the embolized tumor and compensatory hypertrophy of the unharmed opposite liver lobe increasing the potential hepatic functional reserve in patients with cirrhosis and underlying liver dysfunction in preparation for hepatic resection of the tumor.

Percutaneous Ablative Therapies. Ablative percutaneous methods of local control may be considered, especially in recurrent tumors. They include percutaneous radiofrequency ablation (RFA) and percutaneous ethanol injection (PEI) and cryotherapy. Cryotherapy refers to cold injury produced by cryoprobe delivery of liquid nitrogen and although once popular in adults, it has now fallen out of favor due to superior results achieved with RFA and PEI. In most cases, these treatment approaches are palliative and are suitable for smaller size tumors only, generally below 3 to 4 cm maximum diameter. Percutaneous ablation is most often used in adults with underlying cirrhotic liver disease. Percutaneous ablation is fairly low risk, is repeatable, and should not damage nonneoplastic tissue, which is especially important in cirrhotic patients. RFA provides slightly better tumor kill than PEI (90% *vs.* 80% complete tumor necrosis) with less sessions (mean of 1.2 *vs.* 4.8).[163] It is also associated with fewer side effects; thus, in many centers, RFA is now preferred over PEI;

however, RFA is contraindicated in lesions located adjacent to the major biliary ducts or to bowel loops. The presence of immediately adjacent tumor satellite lesions is also a relative contraindication to RFA. Local recurrence is common (>60%) and may be related to growth of a previously occult microscopic satellite lesion rather than recurrence in the treated nodule. Complications of these ablative techniques occur in about 8% to 9% of cases, mainly in the form of pain, fever, bleeding, tumor seeding, and GI perforation.[164] Percutaneous ablation has not been well studied in children.

Liver Transplant and Milan Criteria. Metastatic relapse is more common after transplantation for HCC than after transplantation for HB, and therefore liver transplant is restricted to patients whose tumor has *always* been completely localized to the liver. Guidelines for the use of liver transplant for HCC are mainly derived from experience in adults using tumor size and number of nodules to determine outcome. The most conventional criteria are the Milan criteria.[165] Yet, the biology of HCC in children without cirrhotic liver disease in distinct, and the Milan criteria for liver transplant in cirrhotic adults with HCC (<3 nodules, largest nodule <5 cm) may *not* apply to children.[166] Similarly, the criteria are often appropriately expanded in noncirrhotic adults.[167] Survival after liver transplantation for HCC in children has been reported to be about 60%.[168-170] The transplant criteria used in SIOPEL 5, a study of noncirrhotic HCC in patients younger than 30 years, are as follows: (a) nonresectable unifocal tumors (independent of their upper size limit); (b) nonresectable multifocal tumors provided their number is below 5 and the biggest is <5 cm; and (c) no transplant in the presence of metastases, even if they clear after neoadjuvant chemotherapy. Any history of, or continuing presence of, extrahepatic disease, hilar lymph nodes, and/or macroscopic vascular invasion is an absolute contraindication to liver transplantation for HCC. The PLUTO registry may shed further light on the role of transplantation for HCC in children. The registry can be reached at http://www.pluto.cineca.org.

Other Malignant Tumors

Hepatic Sarcomas

Primary hepatic sarcomas are a rare. Outcome depends primarily on tumor histology, sensitivity to chemotherapy and/or radiotherapy, and the ability to achieve complete tumor resection.[171]

Biliary Rhabdomyosarcoma. The classic presentation of biliary rhabdomyosarcoma is in young children (average 3½ years) with jaundice and abdominal pain, and is often associated with distension, vomiting, and fever.[8] Histology is exclusively either embryonal or botryoid, both histologic subtypes that are known to have a favorable prognosis. Gross total resection is rare, but the tumor is often both chemotherapy and radiation sensitive and long-term survival is seen in 60% to 70% of patients. Surgical intervention has two goals: to establish an accurate diagnosis and to determine the localregional extent of disease. Although chemotherapy is generally effective at relief of the associated biliary obstruction, it is sometimes too late. Patients remain at high risk of death from biliary sepsis during the first 2 months of their disease and empiric broad-spectrum antibiotic coverage is of paramount importance in febrile patients.

Angiosarcoma. We have personal experience with cases that support the case reports in the literature of malignant transformation of infantile hemangioma to angiosarcoma.[172,173] Histologic verification of malignancy may be difficult and this rare entity must be suspected if the biologic behavior of an infantile hemangioma shows unusual progression or recurrence after a period or relative quiescence. Relatively chemoresistant, prognosis is generally poor.

Rhabdoid Tumor. Malignant rhabdoid tumor of the liver is a rare and aggressive tumor of toddlers and school-age children which may present with spontaneous rupture.[174,175] These rare tumors are often chemoresistant and fatal,[174] although a recent case report documents potential for cure with multimodal therapy including ifosfamide, vincristine, and actinomycin D.[175]

Undifferentiated Sarcomas. Undifferentiated (embryonal) sarcoma of the liver is a rare childhood hepatic tumor and has historically been considered an aggressive neoplasm with an unfavorable prognosis. These tumors may arise in a solitary liver cyst.[176] Survival has improved in recent multimodal approaches, designed for patients with soft tissue sarcomas at other sites, including conservative surgery at diagnosis, multi-agent chemotherapy, and second-look operation in cases of residual disease. Using these techniques, several small series have reported survival in up to 70% of children.[177-179]

Metastatic Liver Tumors

Unlike the large body of literature concerning liver resection for metastatic colorectal tumors in adults, there is little published data that addresses the treatment of metastatic tumors in the liver from abdominal solid tumors in childhood. A recent series from a large metropolitan children's cancer center reported only 15 such patients over a 17-year period including neuroblastoma (7); Wilms' tumor (3); osteogenic sarcoma (2); gastric epithelial (1); and desmoplastic small round cell tumor (2).[180] Eleven of the 15 patients died of progressive disease; 4 had a local recurrence. These results lead the authors to conclude that the overall prognosis in these patients remains poor and the decision to perform hepatic metastasectomy should be made with caution. The treatment approach should not, however, be uniformly nihilistic, because not all liver lesions in children with abdominal solid tumors turn out to be metastatic disease. Both nodular regenerative hyperplasia (NRH) and FNH have been reported to mimic hepatic metastasis in children[181]; definitive diagnosis requires biopsy and/or resection.

Hemophagocytic Lymphohistiocytosis

Hemophagocytic lymphohistiocytosis (HLH) may occasionally present as an abnormal liver mass in a newborn with coagulopathy. Predisposing factors include familial, herpes simplex virus, and severe combined immunodeficiency.[182] Diagnostic criteria according to HLH-2004 include fever, splenomegaly, bicytopenia, hypotriglyceridemia, hypofibrinogenemia, hemophagocytosis, low NK cell activity, hyperferritinemia, and high IL-2 receptor levels.[183] Treatment is with combination chemoimmunotherapy, including etoposide, dexamethasone, and cyclosporine A, and anticipated mortality of about 40% is increased if the diagnosis or appropriate therapy is delayed.

BENIGN LIVER TUMORS

Differential Diagnosis

The characteristic radiographic appearances of the three most common benign liver tumors in children are shown in Figure 28.3. We see mesenchymal hamartoma with complex cysts that are separated by thick vascular septae; FNH hyperenhancing with well-demarcated borders and its characteristic central stellate scar; and infantile hemangioma showing bright peripheral enhancement. Other less common benign tumors include kaposiform hemangioendothelioma, hepatic adenoma, NRH, teratoma, inflammatory myofibroblastic tumor, hemophagocytic lymphohistiocytosis, biliary cystadenoma, and the nonneoplastic "other masses" listed in Table 28.1.

Infantile Hepatic Hemangioma

Infantile hemangioma is the most common benign tumor of the liver in infancy.[13] Figure 28.9 illustrates the striking variability of the three subtypes of infantile hemangioma: focal, multinodular, and diffuse. Many focal lesions are often discovered incidentally and are localized and small enough to be of little clinical significance. Symptoms seen with larger lesions may include abdominal distention, hepatomegaly, congestive heart failure, vomiting, anemia, thrombocytopenia and consumptive coagulopathy, jaundice secondary to biliary obstruction, and associated cutaneous or visceral hemangiomas.[6] The diagnosis of infantile hepatic hemangioma is usually straightforward and based on the combination of clinical symptoms and radiographic appearance on ultrasound and CT scan. Contrast-enhanced CT scan shows an area of diminished density, and after bolus injection of intravenous contrast, there is contrast enhancement from the periphery toward the center of the lesion, and, after a short delay, there essentially is complete isodense filling of the lesion and liver. MRA has been used in complex cases to identify atypical radiographic features that may portend a poor prognosis.[184] Unfavorable radiographic features include central varix with arteriovenous shunt, central necrosis or thrombosis, and diffuse hemangiomatous

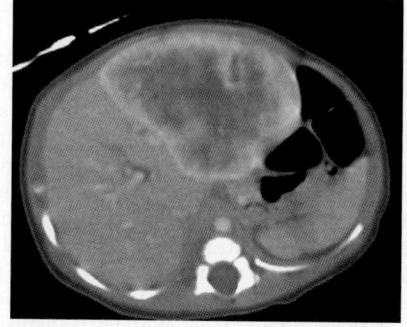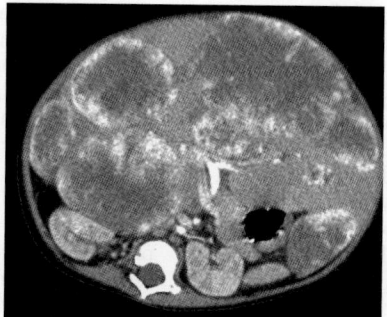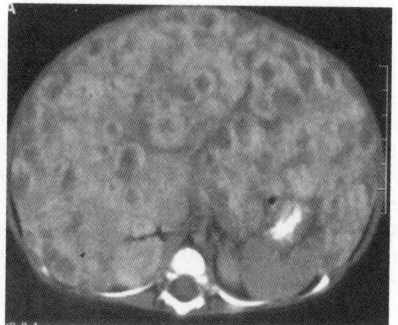

A,B   C

FIGURE 28.9 Three types of infantile hepatic hemangioma, most common benign tumor of infancy. A: Focal. B: Multinodular. C: Diffuse.

involvement of the liver with abdominal vascular compression.[184] Arterial angiography may be used in infants with refractory symptoms in whom either hepatic artery ligation or embolization is considered.

If a definitive diagnosis of simple infantile hepatic hemangioma can be made radiographically, management can be noninvasive because spontaneous regression occurs in most cases—especially those with focal tumors. The terminology is confusing, however, with different authors often using the terms *hepatic hemangioma, infantile hepatic hemangioma, hepatic hemangioendothelioma,* or *kaposiform hemangioendothelioma* interchangeably.[185] True kaposiform hemangioendothelioma presents with Kasabach-Merritt phenomenon and is discussed in more detail below.

Sometimes, a large rapidly growing infantile hepatic hemangioma can be life-threatening with intractable high-output cardiac failure from intralesional arteriovenous shunting, intraperitoneal hemorrhage, respiratory distress as a result of pulmonary congestion, and massive hepatomegaly compressing abdominal vasculature and producing abdominal compartment syndrome. Historically, the initial medical intervention for symptomatic tumors has been corticosteroids. Many other medical treatment options exist, although no single treatment has been shown to be universally effective. Congestive heart failure is treated with supportive care, digitalis, and diuretics. Anemia and coagulopathy are treated with corrective blood product replacement therapy. Both success and complete failure have been reported variously with many other treatments including epsilon-aminocaproic acid, tranexamic acid, low-molecular-weight heparin, vincristine, cyclophosphamide, interferon 2-alpha, AGM-1470, and newer generation antiangiogenic drugs.[186-189] The angiogenesis inhibitor interferon-alpha may be clinically efficacious; however, it must be avoided or used with great caution in children younger than 1 year because of the risk of producing an irreversible spastic diplegia[190] Recent studies have shown that the large tumors may produce antibodies to TSH, and screening to rule out secondary hypothyroidism is recommended.[191] Treatment is with thyroid hormone replacement therapy, and reports demonstrate resolution of the hypothyroidism after liver transplantation in cases that fail medical management.[192] Most recently, propranolol has been shown to inhibit the growth of infantile hemangioma.[193] Potential explanations for the therapeutic effect of propranolol, a nonselective β-blocker, include vasoconstriction, decreased expression of VEGF and bFGF genes through downregulation of the RAF-mitogen activated protein kinase pathway, and the triggering of apoptosis of capillary endothelial cells.[193] Although rare, malignant transformation to angiosarcoma has been reported and close follow-up is recommended.[172,173,194,195]

In infants who fail medical management, symptomatic solitary tumors may be treated by excision, hepatic arterial ligation, or selective angiographic embolization. Although potentially hazardous, hepatic arterial embolization can be especially helpful in tumors causing high output cardiac failure due to arteriovenous shunts within the tumor.[196] A treatment algorithms may stratify treatment based upon whether or not the tumor is solitary, multifocal, or diffuse (Fig. 28.9).[197,198] About 65% of tumors are solitary or unifocal with a survival of 86% and death usually not caused by the tumor but by a comorbidities.[13] Thirty-five percent of tumors are multifocal or diffuse with a survival somewhere between 60% and 100% with death usually secondary to cardiorespiratory compromise caused tumors refractory to medical and interventional management.[13,196,198] Orthotopic liver transplantation may be lifesaving for cases with diffuse angiomatous change in which the lesion is progressive with intractable high-output cardiac failure, abdominal

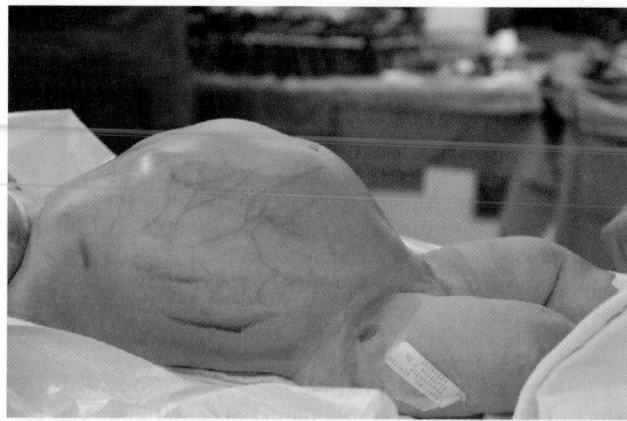

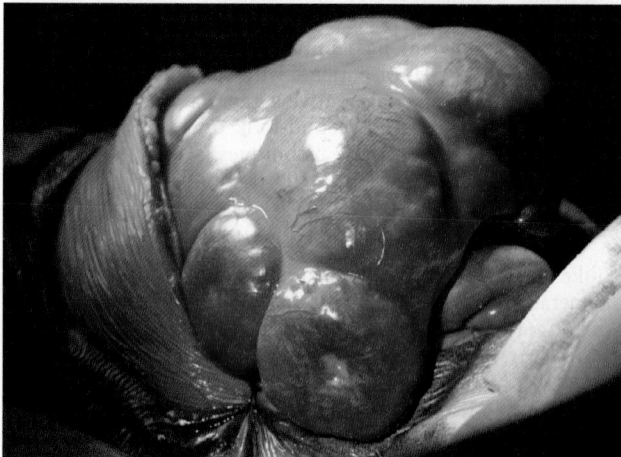

FIGURE 28.10 Exceptionally large multinodular infantile hemangioma refractory to medical management.

compartment syndrome, and failure of lesser treatment options (Fig. 28.10).

Kaposiform Hemangioendothelioma

Kaposiform hemangioendothelioma is a rare benign tumor that behaves in a biologically aggressive fashion. The tumor may occur in the extremities, cervicofacial, thoracic, or retroperitoneal locations. Retroperitoneal tumors may extend to involve the liver, porta hepatis, pancreas, and mesentery. The literature is quite confusing regarding the use of the term "hemangioendothelioma" and there are many literature reports using the term "hepatic hemangioendothelioma" to describe a patient with a severe progressive "infantile hemangioma" associated with high-output heart failure and consumptive coagulopathy. The distinction is often difficult, but we prefer to restrict the use of the term "hemangioendothelioma" specifically to the more rare group of kaposiform invasive tumors that present with Kasabach-Merritt syndrome.[199,200] True Kasabach Merritt phenomenon refers to a life-threatening hemorrhage due to coagulopathy and thrombocytopenia. Platelets are consumed by the tumor with a half-life of 1 to 24 hours, and platelet transfusions may actually promote tumor growth through intralesional clotting and the release of proangiogenic proteins with increased vascular permeability by VEGFs such as platelet-derived growth factor (PDGF). Because of these phenomena, platelet transfusions should only be given when the patient is actively bleeding or as a preparation for surgery.[201] Tumor growth can be so rapid

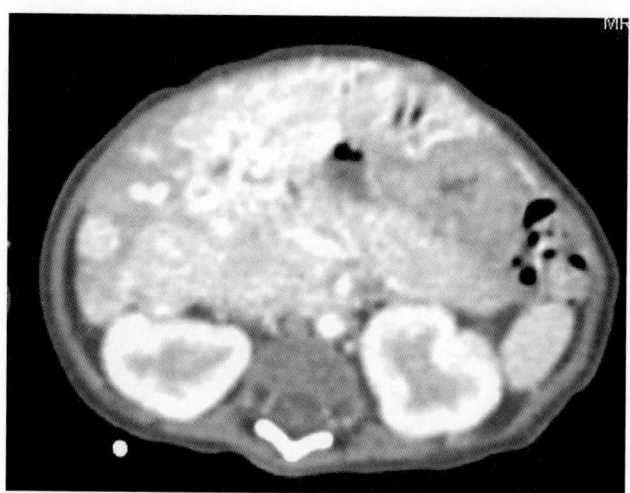

FIGURE 28.11 Retroperitoneal kaposiform hemangioendothelioma infant with invasive vascular tumor involving liver, retroperitoneum, pancreas, and base of mesentery. Tumor presented in infant with abdominal distension, heart failure, profound thrombocytopenia of Kasabach-Merritt phenomenon, and biliary and portal venous obstruction.

that it causes fibrosis and destruction of the neighboring tissues and mortality ranges from 12% to 24% for tumors at all sites,[199,202] but may be as high as 60% for those tumors involving the retroperitoneum.[199] Successful treatment of retroperitoneal kaposiform hemangioendothelioma has been reported with alpha-interferon[203]; however, in tumors refractory to antiangiogenic therapy, multidrug chemotherapy regimens may be required and success has been reported with vincristine combined with cyclophosphamide, actinomycin D, and methotrexate[203] The radiographic appearance of an extensive retroperitoneal kaposiform hemangioendothelioma involving liver, retroperitoneum, pancreas, mesentery, colon, and encasing the porta hepatis is shown in Figure 28.11.

Mesenchymal Hamartoma

Although mesenchymal hamartoma of the liver is the second most common benign liver tumor in children, its biology and pathogenesis are poorly understood.[204] Historically, mesenchymal hamartoma has been described in the literature by various names including pseudocystic mesenchymal tumor, hepatic and giant cell lymphangioma, cystic hamartoma, bile cell fibroadenoma, hamartoma, and cavernous lymphangiomatoid tumor. Edmondson recognized these to be similar lesions and described them as mesenchymal hamartoma in 1956. Mesenchymal hamartoma typically presents before 2 years of age with abdominal swelling as the initial symptom. Before sophisticated diagnostic imaging became so readily accessible, many of these tumors became very large, eventually presenting with mass effect such as vena cava compression, feeding difficulties, and respiratory distress. With the widespread use of ultrasound and CT, these tumors are now usually detected early as a palpable mass in an otherwise asymptomatic child. The AFP may be variably elevated in this tumor confounding the differentiation from HB. The pathogenesis of mesenchymal hamartoma is unclear. The three leading theories postulate (a) abnormal embryologic development of the mesenchyme producing obstruction of the developing biliary tree that results in cystic, anaplastic, and proliferating bile ducts with most of the proliferative growth just before or after birth, because no mesenchymal mitotic activity in seen histologically[135]; (b) abnormal development of blood supply with

ischemic necrosis and reactive cystic changes[205]; (c) abnormal proliferation of embryologic hepatic mesenchyme with increased expression of fibroblast growth factor-2 (FGF-2).[206] Microscopically, the tissue consists of a mixture of bile ducts, liver cell cysts, and mesenchyme. The cysts may simply be dilated bile ducts, dilated lymphatics, or amorphous fluid surrounded by mesenchyme. Elongated or tortuous bile ducts surrounded by connective tissue are unevenly distributed with the bile ducts at the periphery often exhibiting active proliferation.[135]

Mesenchymal hamartoma is more common in the right lobe of the liver, although any lobe may be involved. On ultrasonography, one sees multiple echogenic cysts although, if the cysts are small, the entire tumor may appear as an echogenic mass. The typical CT scan shows a well-circumscribed, multilocular, multicystic mass that contains low-density cysts separated by solid septae and stroma (Fig. 28.3). The stroma and septae may be vascular and occasionally show contrast enhancement on CT scan similar to that seen in infantile hemangioma. When the cysts are small, the tumor may appear solid rather than cystic and biopsy is required to rule out malignancy. Occasionally, a highly vascular tumor in a neonate may present with hydrops, high-output heart failure, and respiratory distress.[207] More commonly, the tumor tends to increase in size during the first several months of life and subsequently may either stabilize, continue to grow, or undergo spontaneous regression.

Traditionally, the surgical treatment has been complete tumor excision, either nonanatomically with a rim of normal tissue or as an anatomic hepatic lobectomy. The gross appearance of a mesenchymal hamartoma can be strikingly similar to that of a focal infantile hemangioma with which this tumor is sometimes confused (Fig. 28.12). If the tumor is considered unresectable, the surgical options include enucleation and marsupialization. Although facile, marsupialization may result in tumor recurrence.[208] Management continues to evolve, however, with debate in the literature regarding the feasibility of nonoperative management in the asymptomatic patient.[209] Caution is warranted if a path of expectant management is chosen due to reports of malignant transformation or association with undifferentiated (embryonal) sarcoma.[204,210–212]

Focal Nodular Hyperplasia

Focal nodular hyperplasia (FNH) may be diagnosed at any age, from newborns to the elderly. In children, it usually is diagnosed between 2 and 5 years of age.[213] It is a benign epithelial tumor that has been referred to by various names in the literature including benign hepatoma, solitary hyperplastic nodule, focal cirrhosis, cholangiohepatoma, and even mixed adenoma. FNH has been seen in association with a variety of different conditions and situations including previous trauma to the liver,[214] other liver tumors,[51] hemochromatosis,[215] Klinefelter syndrome,[216] itraconazole,[217] smoking,[218] oral contraceptives,[218] congenital absence of the portal vein (Abernathy syndrome),[219] and a history of pediatric treatment with chemotherapy for a Wilms' tumor or neuroblastoma.[220,221] FNH is a well-circumscribed, lobulated lesion whose typical architecture on gross examination consists of bile ducts and a central stellate scar containing blood vessels that supply the hyperplastic process. Usually, there is no real capsule, but often the fibrous tissue surrounds the liver in lesions varying in size from a few millimeters to more than 20 cm in diameter and may be single or multiple. Microscopically, the proliferating cells are practically identical to the surrounding hepatocytes.

Like other benign liver tumors, small lesions may be asymptomatic incidental findings. Larger lesions eventually

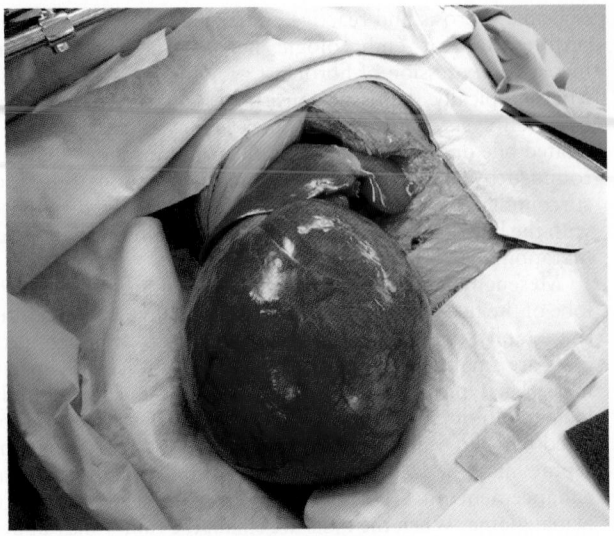
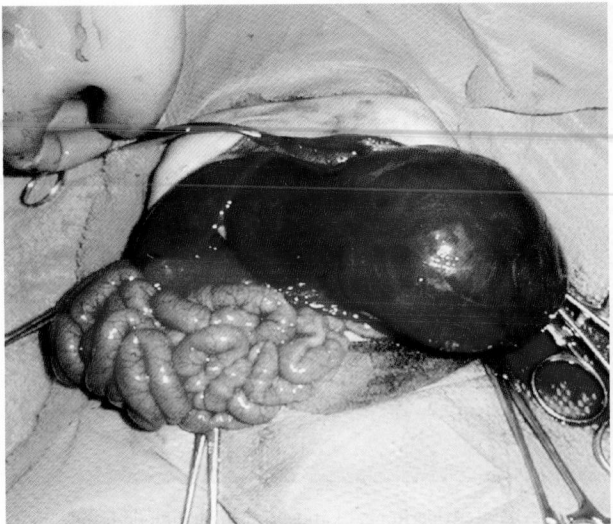

FIGURE 28.12 Gross appearance of mesenchymal hamartoma and infantile hemangioma can be very similar. **A:** Mesenchymal hamartoma. **B:** Infantile hemangioma.

will present with mass symptoms, usually abdominal pain. The diagnosis of FNH is suggested by the ultrasonographic appearance of a well-demarcated, hyperechoic, and homogenous lesion; the tumor may be much more evident on CT angiography or MR angiography after intravenous contrast enhancement, and usually has normal accumulation of ^{99m}Tc sulfur colloid on liver scintigraphy. Although approximately 50% of tumors will have normal accumulation of ^{9m}Tc sulfur colloid, this finding is not universally specific, and there have been case reports of scintigraphic findings suggestive of FNH in children who turned out to have HB[222] or HCC.[223] In fact, FNH can be a radiographic chameleon and although a radiographic "central stellate scar" is a characteristic finding, the radiographic appearance can be quite variable as shown in Figure 28.13. If biopsy does not definitively confirm the diagnosis, excision may be necessary.

Complete surgical resection of biopsy-proven FNH is not mandatory in asymptomatic patients. Spontaneous regression is rare although it may be seen after cessation of oral contraceptives. Symptomatic patients in whom the diagnosis of malignancy has not been definitively ruled out will require surgical excision. Symptomatic patients in whom the benign diagnosis has been confirmed may be candidates for ablative therapy with transcatheter arterial embolization.[224]

Hepatic (Hepatocellular) Adenoma

Rare in children, hepatic adenoma, sometimes called hepatocellular adenoma, is most common in young women in their twenties, especially in response to birth control hormonal therapy. The differential diagnosis from FNH remains a challenge. Other associations have been reported with glycogen storage disease types 1 and 3, galactosemia, hyperthyroidism, polycythemia, diabetes, Fanconi's anemia, polycystic ovary syndrome, and anabolic steroids.[51] When associated with oral contraceptives or anabolic steroids, the tumor may regress with cessation of the hormonal therapy.[225] Persistent or progressive adenomas are at risk of rupture and bleeding and surgical excision is often recommended. Alternative contemporary management may include percutaneous RFA.[226]

In patients with glycogen storage disease type 1A multiple adenomas may develop progressively in about 50% of patients. In these patients, there is a risk of HCC in up to 18% of patients and HCC has been reported as early as 6 years of age. These patients need to be monitored very closely with serial AFP, radiographic imaging, and biopsy if any question of HCC is raised.[227] In patients in whom the adenomas are multiple and progressive, liver transplant not only corrects the underlying metabolic disorder but also eliminates the risk of tumor rupture and bleeding and eliminates the risk of HCC.

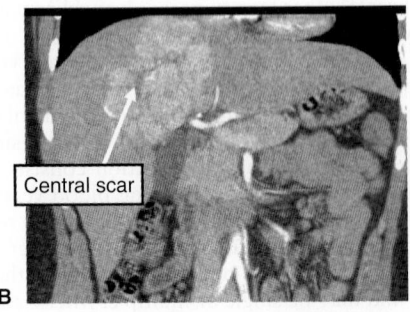
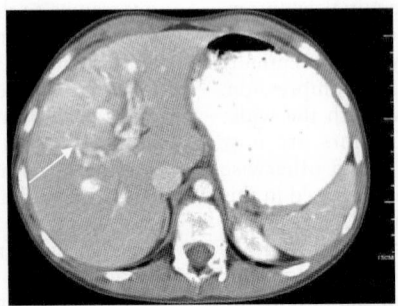
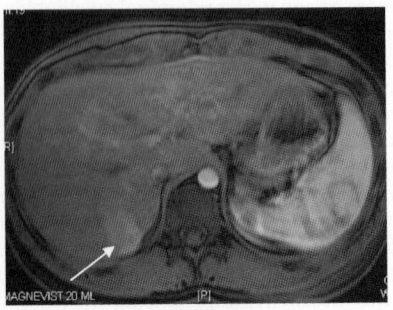

Figure 28.13 Three examples of focal nodular hyperplasia (FNH). **A:** FNH with classic findings ... well demarcated, hyperenhancing, with central stellate scar. **B:** Hypervascular with unusual nest of dilated vessels encasing the tumor. **C:** Tumor was isodense with liver on MRI T1 and T2 ... seen here only after gadolinium contrast enhancement.

Hepatic Teratoma

True hepatic teratoma is extremely rare. Twenty-four cases have been reported in the literature, 18 of which were in children younger than 3 years.[228] About half of these tumors have been malignant, about half benign. The characteristic histological finding is the predominance of hepatic tissue in the resected specimen.

Nodular Regenerative Hyperplasia

Nodular regenerative hyperplasia (NRH) of the liver is a multiacinar regenerative nodular lesion in a noncirrhotic liver. It is a rare entity of unknown etiology but has been associated in children with a variety of other diseases and drugs. In about half of the children, there is some component of associated portal hypertension. NRH has been reported in children with portal hypertension and hepatopulmonary syndrome, celiac disease,[229] mimicking metastatic nodules in children with prior treatment of Wilms' tumor or neuroblastoma,[181,230] azathioprine treatment of inflammatory bowel disease,[231] intrahepatic occlusive venopathy in children treated with 6 thioguanine for acute lymphoblastic leukemia,[232] Budd-Chiari syndrome,[233] pulmonary arterial hypertension and connective tissue disorders,[234] chronic granulomatous disease,[235] and a spectrum of other disorders many of which involve some sort of perturbation of the hepatic vasculature. Radiologically, its nodular appearance may look like neoplasia and open wedge biopsy is often required to definitively rule out malignancy.[236] Prognosis in the absence of portal hypertension is good and complications are rare.

Inflammatory Myofibroblastic Tumor

Inflammatory myofibroblastic tumor is a rare benign entity formerly known as inflammatory pseudotumor. These tumors occur throughout the body and tumors isolated to the liver appear as scattered case reports in both children and adults. This rare tumor has been associated with underlying chronic infections such as mycobacterium avium intracellular,[237] immunodeficiency, biliary obstruction, and autoimmune sclerosing cholangitis.[238] Treatment of symptomatic lesions is with surgical excision.

References

1. Misick OS. A case of teratoma hepatis. J Pathol Bacteriol 1898;5:128–137.
2. Willis RA. In: Cameron R, Payling Wright G, eds. The pathology of the tumours of children. Springfield: Charles C. Thomas, 1962:57–61.
3. Ishak KG, Glunz PR. Hepatoblastoma and hepatocarcinoma in infancy and childhood: report of 47 cases. Cancer 1967;20:396–422.
4. Zimmermann A. Hepatoblastoma with cholangioblastic features ('cholangioblastic hepatoblastoma') and other liver tumors with bimodal differentiation in young patients. Med Pediatr Oncol 2002;39:487–491.
5. Exelby PR, Filler RM, Grosfeld IL. Liver tumors in children in particular reference to hepatoblastoma and hepatocellular carcinoma; American Academy of Pediatrics Surgical Section Survey—1974. J Pediatr Surg 1975;10:329–337.
6. Stringer MD. Liver tumors. Semin Pediatr Surg 2000;9:196–208.
7. Meyers RL. Malignant liver tumors in children. Pediatr Health 2008;2:617–629.
8. Spunt SL, Lobe TE, Pappo A, et al. Aggressive surgery is unwarranted for biliary tract rhabdomyosarcoma. J Pediatr Surg 2000;35:309–316.
9. Rogers TN, Woodley H, Ramsden W, et al. Solitary liver cysts in children: not always so simple. J Pediatr Surg 2007;42:333–339.
10. Rygl M, Snajdauf J, Petru O, et al. Congenital solitary liver cysts. Eur J Pediatr Surg 2006;16:443–448.
11. Guerin F, Hadhri R, Fabre M, et al. Ciliated hepatic foregut cyst in infants: benign in appearance but malignant in adulthood. In: SIOP Abstract Book 2008 pp 219, 40th Congress of the International Society of Pediatric Oncology, Berlin Germany, October 2008.
12. Darbari A, Sabin KM, Shapiro CN, et al. Epidemiology of primary hepatic malignancies in US children. Hepatology 2003;38:560–566.
13. Isaacs H Jr. Fetal and neonatal hepatic tumors J Pediatr Surg 2007;42:1797–1803.
14. Sakar M, Mulliken JB, Kozakewich HP, et al. Thrombocytopenic coagulopathy (Kasabach-Merritt phenomenon) is associated with kaposiform hemangioendothelioma and not with common infantile hemangioma. Plast Reconstr Surg 1997;100:1377–1386.
15. Meyers RL. Tumors of the liver in children. Surg Oncol 2007;16:195–203.
16. Von Schweinitz D. Management of liver tumors in childhood. Semin Pediatr Surg 2006;15:17–24.
17. Jung SE. Clinical characteristics and prognosis of patients with hepatoblastoma. World J Surg 2001;25:126–130.
18. Nickerson HJ, Bilberman TL, McDonald TP. Hepatoblastoma thrombocytosis and increased thrombopoietin. Cancer 1980;45:315–320.
19. Von Schweinitz D, Hadam MR, Welte K, et al. Production of interleukin-1 beta and interleukin-6 in hepatoblastoma. Int J Cancer 1993;53:728–734.
20. Oda H, Imai Y, Nakatsuru Y, et al Somatic mutations of the APC gene in sporadic hepatoblastoma. Cancer Res 1996;56:3320–3323.
21. Von Schweinitz D. Treatment of liver tumors in children. In: Clavien PA, Fong Y, Lyerly K, et al., eds. Malignant liver tumors: current and emerging therapies. 2nd ed. Boston, MA: Jones and Bartlett, 2004:406–426.
22. Von Schweinitz D, Byrd DJ, Hecker H, et al. Efficiency and toxicity of ifosfamide, cisplatin, and doxorubicin in the treatment of childhood hepatoblastoma. Study committee of the Cooperative Paediatric Liver Tumour Study HB89 of the German Society of Paediatric Oncology and Haematology. Eur J Cancer 1997;33:1243–1249.
23. Aronson DC, Schnater JM, Staalman CR, et al. Predictive value of the pretreatment extent of disease system in hepatoblastoma: results from the international society of pediatric oncology liver tumor study group SIOPEL-1 study. J Clin Oncol 2005;23:1245–1252.
24. Deloris M, Brugieres L, Zimmerman A, et al. Hepatoblastoma with a low serum alphafetoprotein at diagnosis: the SIOPEL group experience. Eur J Cancer 2008;44:545–550.
25. Meyers RL, Rowland JH, Krailo M, et al. Pretreatment prognostic factors in hepatoblastoma: a report of the Children's Oncology Group. Pediatr Blood Cancer 2009;53:1016–1022.
26. Fuchs J, Rydzynski J, vonSchweinitz D, et al. Pretreatment prognostic factors and treatment results in children with hepatoblastoma: a report from the German Cooperative Pediatric Liver Tumor Study HB94. Cancer 2002;95:172–182.
27. Von Schweinitz D, Hecker H, Harms D, et al. Complete resection before development of drug resistance is essential for survival from advanced hepatoblastoma—a report from the German Cooperative Pediatric Liver Tumor study HB-89. J Pediatr Surg 1995;30:845–852.
28. Schneider DT, Calaminus G, Gobel U. Diagnostic value of alpha-fetoprotein and beta-human chorionic gonadotropin in infancy and childhood. Pediatr Hematol Oncol 2001;18:11–26.
29. Sari N, Yalcin B, Akyuz C, et al. Infantile hepatic hemangioendothelioma with very elevated serum alpha-fetoprotein. Pediatr Hematol Oncol 2006;23:639–647.
30. Cajalba MM, Sarita-Reyes C, Zambrano E, et al. Mesenchymal hamartoma of the liver associated with Beckwith-Weidemann syndrome and high serum alpha-fetoprotein levels. Pediatr Dev Pathol 2007;10:233–238.
31. Boman F, Bossard C, Fabre M, et al. Mesenchymal hamartomas of the liver may be associated with increased serum alpha-fetoprotein concentrations and mimic hepatoblastoma. Eur J Pediatr Surg 2004;14:63–66.
32. Wang JD, Chang TK, Chen HC, et al. Pediatric liver tumors: initial presentation, image finding, outcome. Pediatr Int 2007;49:491–496.
33. Roebuck DJ, Perilongo G. Hepatoblastoma: an oncological review. Pediatr Radiol 2006;36:183–186.
34. Saar B, Kellner-Weldon F. Radiologic diagnosis of hepatocellular carcinoma. Liver Int 2008;28:189–199.
35. Clatworthy HW, Schiller M, Grosfeld JL. Primary liver tumors in infancy and childhood. 41 cases variously treated. Arch Surg 1974;109:143–147.
36. Chang MH, Chen CJ, Lai MS, et al. Universal hepatitis B vaccination in Taiwan and the incidence of hepatocellular carcinoma in children. N Engl J Med 1997;336:1855–1859.
37. Chen DS. Hepatitis B vaccination: the key toward eradication of hepatitis B. J Hepatol 2009;50:805–816.
38. Plaschkes J, Perilongo G, Shafford EA, et al. SIOP trial report—overall preliminary results of SIOPEL-I for the treatment of hepatoblastoma (HB) with preoperative chemotherapy–continuous infusion cisplatin and doxorubicin (PLADO). Med Pediatr Oncol 1994;23:170.
39. Roebuck DJ, Aronson DC, Clayput P, et al. 2005 PRETEXT: a revised staging system for primary malignant liver tumors of childhood developed by the SIOPEL group. Pediatr Radiol 2007;37:123–132.
40. Aronson DC. Liver tumours and the SIOPEL story. In: SIOP education book 2008. Berlin, Germany: International Society of Pediatric Oncology, 2008:68–75.
41. Evans AE, Land VJ, Newton WA, et al. Combination chemotherapy (vincristine, adriamycin, cyclophosphamide, and 5-fluorouracil) in the treatment of children with malignant hepatoma. Cancer 1982;50:821–826.
42. Katzenstein HM. Biology and treatment of children with all stages of hepatoblastoma: COG protocol AHEP-0731. Approved by CTEP and NCI 2008, open for enrollment September 2009. http://www.childrensoncologygroup.org, accessed June 2010.
43. McLaughlin C, Baptiste MS, Schymura MJ, et al. Maternal and infant birth characteristics and hepatoblastoma. Am J Epidemiol 2006;163:818–828.
44. Ikeda H, Matsuyama S, Tanimura M. Association between hepatoblastoma and very low birth weight: a trend or a chance [see comments]? J Pediatr 1997;130:557–560. Comments in: J Pediatr 1997;130:516–517; J Pediatr 1998;132:750; J Pediatr 1998; 133:585–586.
45. Feusner J, Plaschkes J. Hepatoblastoma and low birth weight: a trend or chance observation? Med Pediatr Oncol 2002;39:508–509.
46. Reynolds P, Urayama KY, Von Behren J, et al. Birth characteristics and hepatoblastoma risk in young children. Cancer 2004;100:1070–1076.
47. Oue T, Kubota A, Okuyama H, et al. Hepatoblastoma in children of extremely low birth weight: a report from a single prenatal center. J Pediatr Surg 2003;38:134–137.
48. Spector LG, Puumala SE, Carozza SE, et al. Cancer risk among children with very low birth weights. Pediatrics 2009;124:96–104.
49. Satge D, Sasco AJ, Little J. Antenatal therapeutic drug exposure and fetal/neonatal tumors: Review of 89 cases. Paediatr Perinat Epidemiol 1998;12:84–117.
50. Lai TT, Bearer CF. Iatrogenic environmental hazards in the neonatal intensive care unit. Clin Perinatol 2008;35:163–181.

51. Andrews WS. Lesions of the liver. In: Ashcroft KW, Holcomb GW, Murphy JP, eds. Pediatric surgery. 4th ed. Philadelphia, PA: Elsevier Saunders, 2005:950–971.
52. Clericuzio CL, Martin RA. Diagnostic criteria and tumor screening for individuals with isolated hemihyperplasia. Genet Med 2009;11:220–222.
53. Mueller BU, Lopez-Terrada D, Finegold MJ. Tumors of the liver. In: Pizzo PA, Poplack DG, eds. Principles and practices of pediatric oncology. 5th ed. Baltimore, MD: Lippincott Williams & Wilkins, 2006:887–904.
54. Thomas D, Pritchard J, Davidson R, et al. Familial hepatoblastoma and APC gene mutations: renewed call for molecular research. Eur J Cancer 2003;39:2200–2204.
55. Hirschman BA, Pollock BH, Tomlinson GE. The spectrum of APC mutations in children with hepatoblastoma from familial adenomatous polyposis kindreds. J Pediatr 2005; 147:263–266.
56. Steenman M, Westerveld A, Mannens M. Genetics of Beckwith–Wiedemann syndrome-associated tumors: common genetic pathways. Genes Chromosomes Cancer 2000;28: 1–13.
57. Fukuzawa R, Hata J, Hayaski Y, et al. Beckwith-Wiedemann syndrome associated hepatoblastoma: wnt signal activation occurs later in tumorigenesis in patients with 11p15.5 uniparental disomy. Pediatr Dev Pathol 2003;6:299–306.
58. Fraumeni JF, Rosen PJ, Hull EW, et al. Hepatoblastoma in infant sisters. Cancer 1969;24:1086–1090.
59. Bove KE, Soukup S, Ballard Et, et al. Hepatoblastoma in a child with trisomy 18: cytogenetics, liver anomalies, and literature review. Pediatr Pathol Lab Med 1996;16: 253–262.
60. Maruyama K, Ikeda H, Koizumi T. Hepatoblastoma associated with trisomy 18 syndrome: case report and review of the literature. Pediatr Int 2001;43:302–305.
61. Tomlinson GE, Douglass EC, Pollock BH, et al. Cytogenetic analysis of a large series of hepatoblastoma: numerical aberrations with recurring translocations involving 1q12–21. Genes Chromosomes Cancer 2006;44:177–187.
62. Siliano M, de Candia E, Ballarin S, et al. Hepatocellular carcinoma complicating liver cirrhosis in type IIIa glycogen storage disease. J Clin Gastroenterol 2000;31:80–82.
63. Demers SI, Russo P, Lettre F, et al. Frequent mutation reversion inversely correlates with clinical severity in a genetic liver disease, hereditary tyrosinemia. Hum Pathol 2003; 34:1313–1320.
64. Keefe FB, Pinson CW, Ragsdale J, et al. Hepatocellular carcinoma in arteriohepatic dysplasia. Am J Gastroenterol 1993;88:1446–1449.
65. Alonso EM, Snover DC, Montag A, et al. Histologic pathology of the liver in progressive familial intrahepatic cholestasis. J Pediatr Gastroenterol Nutr 1994;18:128–133.
66. Kanai Y, Tsuda H, Oda T, et al. Analysis of the neurofibromatosis 2 gene in human breast and hepatocellular carcinoma. Jpn J Clin Oncol 1995;25:1–4.
67. Geoffroy-Perez B, Janin N, Ossian K, et al. Cancer risk in heterozygotes for ataxia-telangiectasia. Int J Cancer 2001;93:288–293.
68. Touraine RL, Bertrand Y, Foray P, et al. Hepatic tumors during androgen therapy in Fanconi anemia. Eur J Pediatr 1993;152:691–693.
69. Haas OA, Zoubek A, Grumayer ER, et al. Constitutional interstitial deletion of 11p11 and pericentric inversion of chromosome 9 in a patient with Wiedemann–Beckwith syndrome and hepatoblastoma. Cancer Genet Cytogenet 1986;23:95–104.
70. Aretz S, Koch A, Uhlhaas S, et al. Should children at risk for familial adenomatous polyposis be screened for hepatoblastoma and children with apparantly sporadic hepatoblastoma be screened for APC germline mutations? Pediatr Blood Cancer 2006;47: 811–818.
71. Harvey J, Clark S, Hyer W, et al. Germline APC mutations are not commonly seen in children with sporadic hepatoblastoma. J Pediatr Gastroenterol Nutr 2008;47:675–677.
72. McNeil DE, Brown M, Ching A, et al. Screening for Wilms' tumor and hepatoblastoma in children with Beckwith Wiedemann syndrome: a cost effective model. Med Pediatr Oncol 2001;37:349–356.
73. Koufos A, Grundy P, Morgan K, et al. Familial Beckwith Wiedemann syndrome and a second Wilms' tumor locus both map to 11p15.5. Am J Hum Genet 1989;44:711–719.
74. Zatkova A, Rouillard JM, Hartmann W, et al. Amplification and overexpression of the IGF2 regulator PLAG1 in hepatoblastoma. Genes Chromosomes Cancer 2004;39: 126–137.
75. Buendia MA. Genetic alterations in hepatoblastoma and hepatocellular carcinoma: common and distinctive aspects. Med Pediatr Oncol 2002;39:530–535.
76. Koch A, Waha A, Hartmann W, et al. Elevated expression of Wnt antagonists is a common event in HB. Clin Cancer Res 2005; 11:4295–4304.
77. Yamaoka H, Ohtsu K, Sueda T, et al. Diagnostic and prognostic impact of beta-catenin alterations in pediatric liver tumors. Oncol Res 2006;15:551–556.
78. Lopez-Terrada D, Gunarathe PH, Adesina AM, et al. Hepatoblastoma histologic heterogeneity may correlate with molecular heterogeneity. Hem Pathol 2009;40:783–794.
79. Adesina AM, Lopez-Terrado D, Wong KK, et al. Gene expression profiling reveals signatures characterizing histologic subtypes of hepatoblastoma and global deregulation in cell growth and survival pathways. Hum Pathol 2009;40:843–853.
80. Warman SW, Armeau S, Heigolt H, et al. Adenovirus-mediated cytosine deaminase/5 flurocysteine suicide gene therapy of human hepatoblastoma in vitro. Pediatr Blood Cancer 2009;53:145–151.
81. Warman SW, Fuchs J. Drug resistance in hepatoblastoma. Curr Pharm Biotechnol 2007;8:93–97.
82. Oue T, Yoneda A, Uehara S, et al. Increased expression of multidrug resistance associated genes after chemotherapy in pediatric solid malignancies. J Pediatr Surg 2009;44:377–380.
83. Eichenmuller M, Gruner I, Hagl B, et al. Blocking the hedgehog pathway inhibits hepatoblastoma growth. Hepatology 2009;49:482–490.
84. Rowland JM. Hepatoblastoma: assessment of criteria for histologic classification. Med Pediatr Oncol 2002;39:478–483.
85. Trobaugh-Lotrario AD, Tomlinson GE, Finegold MJ, et al. Small cell undifferentiated variant of hepatoblastoma: adverse clinical and molecular features similar to rhabdoid tumors. Pediatr Blood Cancer 2009;52:328–334.
86. Yuri T, Danbara N, Shikata N, et al. Malignant rhabdoid tumor of the liver: case report and literature review. Pathol Int 2004;54:623–629.
87. Malogolowkin MH, et al. Pure fetal histology: is chemotherapy necessary. J Clin Oncol In press.
88. Haas JE, Feusner JH, Ringegold MJ. Small cell undifferentiated histology in hepatoblastoma may be unfavorable. Cancer 2001;92:3130–3134.
89. Finegold MJ, Egler RA, Goss JA, et al. Liver tumors: pediatric population. Liver Transpl 2008;14:1545–1556.
90. Perilongo G, Shafford E, Maibach R, et al. Risk adapted treatment for childhood hepatoblastoma: final report of the second study of the internal society of pediatric oncology, SIOPEL 2. Eur J Cancer 2004;40:411–421.
91. Perilongo G, Maibach R, Shafford E, et al. Cisplatin versus cisplatin plus doxorubicin for standard risk hepatoblastoma. N Engl J Med 2009;361:1662–1670.
92. Ortega JA, Kralio MD, Haas JE, et al. Effective treatment of unresectable or metastatic hepatoblastoma with cisplatin and continuous infusion doxorubicin. A report from the Children's Cancer Study Group. J Clin Oncol 1991;9:2167–2176.
93. Malogolowkin MH, Katzenstein HM, Krailo M, et al. Redefining the role of doxorubicin for the treatment of children with hepatoblastoma. J Clin Oncol 2008;26:2379–2383.
94. Douglass EC, Reynolds M, Finegold M, et al. Cisplatin, vincristine and fluorouracil therapy for hepatoblastoma: a Pediatric Oncology Group Study. Clin Oncol 1993;11: 96–99.
95. Plaschkes J, Perilongo G, Shafford E, et al. Pre-operative chemotherapy cisplatin (PLA) and doxorubicin (DO) PLADO for the treatment of hepatoblastoma and hepatocellular carcinoma results after 2 years' follow-up. Med Pediatr Oncol 1996;27:256.
96. Schnater JM, Aronson DC, Plaschkes J, et al. Surgical view of the treatment of patients with hepatoblastoma. Cancer 2002; 94:1111–1120.
97. Pritchard J, Plaschkes J, Shafford EA, et al. SIOPEL I: the first SIOP hepatoblastoma (HB) and hepatocellular carcinoma (HCC) study. Preliminary results. Med Pediatr Oncol 1992;20:389.
98. Pritchard J, Brown J, Shafford E, et al. Cisplatin, doxorubicin, and delayed surgery for childhood hepatoblastoma: a successful approach—results of the First Prospective Study of the International Society of Pediatric Oncology. J Clin Oncol 2000;18:3819–3828.
99. Ortega JA, Douglass, EC, Feusner, JH, et al. Randomized comparison of cisplatin/vincristine/5-fluorouracil and cisplatin/doxorubicin for the treatment of pediatric hepatoblastoma (HB): a report from the Children's Cancer Group and the Pediatric Oncology Group. J Clin Oncol 2000;18:2665–2675.
100. Lovvorn HN, Hilmes M, Ayres D, et al. Defining hepatoblastoma responsiveness to neoadjuvant therapy as measured by tumor volume and serum alpha-fetoprotein kinetics. In: 40th Annual Meeting American Pediatric Surgical Association, Fajardo, Puerto Rico, May 2009.
101. Malogolowkin MH, Katzenstein HM, Krailo M, et al. Intensified platinum therapy is an ineffective strategy for improving outcome in pediatric patients with advanced hepatoblastoma. J Clin Oncol 2006;24:2879–2884.
102. Casanova M, Zsiros J, Brock P, et al. Metastatic hepatoblastoma—results of the SIOPEL 3 study from the International childhood liver tumour strategy group—SIOPEL. 41st Annual Conference of the International Society of Paediatric Oncology, SIOP 2009. Pediatr Blood Cancer 2009;53:744.
103. Perilongo G. State of the art: treatment of childhood liver tumors. In: 38th Annual Meeting of SIOP, Geneva, Switzerland, 2006.
104. Von Schweinitz D, Haberle B. German liver tumor study: HB 99. In: First International Symposium Childhood Hepatoblastoma. Gdansk, Poland, March 2007.
105. Sasaki F, Matsunaga T, Iwafuchi M, et al. Outcome of hepatoblastoma treatment with JPLT-1 protocol-1: a report from the Japanese study group for pediatric liver tumor. J Pediatr Surg 2002;37:851–856.
106. Tiao GM, Bobey N, Allen S, et al. The current management of hepatoblastoma: a combination of chemotherapy, conventional resection, and liver transplant. J Pediatr 2005;146:204–211.
107. Otte JB, deVille de Goyet J, Reding R. Liver transplantation for hepatoblastoma: indications and contraindications in the modern era. Pediatr Transplant 2005;9:557–656.
108. Chardot C, Sant Martin C, Gilles A, et al. Living related liver transplantation and vena cava reconstruction after total hepatectomy including the vena cava for hepatoblastoma. Transplantation 2002;73:90–92.
109. Czauderna P, Otte JB, Aronson DC, et al. Guidelines for surgical treatment of hepatoblastoma in the modern era: recommendations from the childhood Liver Tumour Strategy Group of the International Society of Paediatric Oncology (SIOPEL). Eur J Cancer 2005;41:1031–1036.
110. Otte JB, Pritchard J, Aronson DC, et al. Liver transplantation for hepatoblastoma: results from the International Society of Pediatric Oncology (SIOP) study SIOPEL-1 and review of the World Experience. Pediatr Blood Cancer 2004;42:74–83.
111. Otte JB, Meyers RL. Liver transplantation. J Pediatr Surg 2006;41:607–608.
112. Dantiga L, Vallortigara F, Cillou et al. Features predicting unresectability in hepatoblastoma. Cancer 2007;110:1050–1058.
113. Li JP, Chu JP, Yand JY, et al. Preoperative transcatheter selective arterial chemoembolization in treatment of unresectable hepatoblastoma in infants and children. Cardiovasc Intervent Radiol 2008;31:1117–1123.
114. Malogolowkin MH, Stanley P, Steele DA, et al. Feasibility and toxicity of chemoembolization in children with liver tumors. J Clin Oncol 2000;18:1279–1284.
115. Czauderna P, Zbrzeniak G, Narozanski W, et al. Preliminary experience with arterial chemoembolization for hepatoblastoma and hepatocellular carcinoma in children. Pediatr Blood Cancer 2006;46:825–828.
116. Ohtsuka Y, Matsunaga T, Yoshida H, et al. Optimal strategy of preop transcatheter arterial chemoembolization for hepatoblastoma. Surg Today 2004;34:127–133.
117. Xianliang H, Jianhong L, Xuewe J, et al Cure of hepatoblastoma with transcatheter arterial chemoembolization. J Pediatr Hematol Oncol 2004;26:60–63.
118. Li Y, Womer RB, Silber JH. Predicting cisplatin ototoxicity in children: the influence of age and cumulative dose. Eur J Cancer 2004;40:2445–2451.
119. Katzenstein HM, Chang KW, Krailo M, et al. Amifostine does not prevent platinum-induced hearing loss associated with treatment of children with hepatoblastoma: a report of the Intergroup Hepatoblastoma Study P9645 as part of childrens oncology group. Cancer 2009;115:5828–35.
120. Muldoon LL, Pagel MA, Kroll RA, et al. Delayed administration of sodium thiosulfate in animal models reduces platinum ototoxicity without reduction of antitumor activity. Clin Cancer Res 2000;6:309–315.
121. Brown J, Perilongo G, Shafford E, et al. Pretreatment prognostic factors for children with Hepatoblastoma—results from the International Society of Pediatric Oncology (SIOP) study SIOPEL 1. Eur J Cancer 2000;36:1418–1425.
122. Feusner JH, Krailo MD, Haas JE, et al. Treatment of pulmonary metastases of initial stage I hepatoblastoma in childhood: report from the Childrens Cancer Group. Cancer 1993;71:859–864.
123. Matsunaga T, Sasaki F, Ohira M, et al. Analysis of treatment outcome for children with recurrent or metastatic hepatoblastoma. Pediatr Surg Int 2003;19:142–146.
124. Meyers RL, Katzenstein HM, Krailo M, et al. Surgical resection of pulmonary metastatic lesions in hepatoblastoma. J Pediatr Surg 2007;42:2050–2056.
125. Fuchs J, Seitz G, Euerkamp V, et al. Analysis of sternotomy as treatment option for resection of bilateral pulmonary metastasis in pediatric solid tumors. Surg Oncol 2008:17:323–330.

126. Perilongo G, Otte JB. Autologous peripheral blood stem cell transplantation with a double conditioning regimen for recurrent hepatoblastoma after liver transplant: a valid therapeutic option or just too much? Pediatr Transplant 2009;13:148–149.
127. Ijichi O, Ishikawa S, Shikoda Y, et al. Response of heavily treated and relapsed hepatoblastoma in the transplanted liver to single agent therapy with Irinotecan. Pediatr Transplant 2006;10:635–638.
128. Warman SW, Frank H, Heitmann H, et al. BU-2 silencing in pediatric epithelial liver tumors. J Surg Res 2008;144:43–48.
129. Hadzic N, Quaglia A, Mieli-Vergani G. Hepatocellular carcinoma in a 12 year old child with PiZZ alpha-1-antitrypsin deficiency. Hepatology 2006;43:194–196.
130. Pichon N, Maisonette F, Pichon-Lefievre F, et al. Hepatocellular carcinoma with congenital agenesis of the portal vein. Jpn J Clin Oncol 2003;33:314–316.
131. Bhadri VA, Storman MO, Arbuckle S, et al. Hepatocellular carcinoma in children with Allagille's syndrome. J Pediatr Gastroenterol Nutr 2005;51:676–678.
132. Hol L, VandenBos IC, Hussain SM, et al. Hepatocellular carcinoma complicating biliary atresia after Kasai portoenterostomy. Eur J Gastroenterol Hepatol 2008;20:227–231.
133. Moore L, Bourne AJ, Preston H, et al. Hepatocellular carcinoma following neonatal hepatitis. Pediatr Pathol Lab Med 1997;17:601–610.
134. Gruner BA, DeNapoli TS, Andrews W, et al. Hepatocellular carcinoma in children associated with Gardner's syndrome or familial adenomatous polyposis. J Pediatr Hematol Oncol 2000;22:90–91.
135. Stocker J, Ishak K. mesenchymal hamartoma of the liver: report of 30 cases and a review of the literature. Pediatr Pathol 1983;1:245–267.
136. Grosfeld JL, Otte JB. Liver tumors in children. In: Carachi R, Grosfeld J, Azmy AF, eds. The surgery of children's tumors. London: Springer, 2008:227–260.
137. Ghaferi AA, Hutchins GM. Progression of liver pathology in patients undergoing the Fontan procedure: chronic passive congestion, cardiac cirrhosis, hepatic adenoma and hepatocellular carcinoma. J Thorac Cardiovasc Surg 2005;129:1348–1352.
138. Franco LM, Krishnamurthy V, Bali D, et al. Hepatocellular carcinoma in glycogen storage disease type 1a. J Inherit Metab Dis 2005;28:153–162.
139. Mays ET, Christopherson W. Hepatic tumors induced by sex steroids. Semin Liver Dis 1984;4:147–157.
140. Vileisi RA, Sorenson K, Bonzalez-Crussi F. Liver malignancy after parenteral nutrition. J Pediatr 1982;100:88–90.
141. Whitington PF, Freese DK, Alonso EM, et al. Clinical and biochemical findings in progressive familial intrahepatic cholestasis. J Pediatr Gastroenterol Nutr 1994;18: 134–141.
142. Knisely AS, Strautnieks SS, Meier Y. Hepatocellular carcinoma in children with bile salt export pump deficiency. Hepatology 2006;44:478–486.
143. Van spronson FJ, Bijleveldem M, van Maldegem BT, et al. Hepatocellular carcinoma in hereditary tyrosinemia type 1. J Pediatr Gastroenterol Nutr 2005;40:90–93.
144. Jain D, Hui P, McNamara J, et al. Bloom syndrome in siblings: Hepatocellular carcinoma and Wilms' tumor with documented anaplasia and nephrogenic rests. Pediatr Dev Pathol 2001;4:585–589.
145. Strickland DK, Jenkins JJ, Hudson MN. Hepatitis C infection and hepatocellular carcinoma after treatment of childhood cancer. J Pediatr Hematol Oncol 2001;23:527–529.
146. Zhou L, Rui JA, Ye DX, et al. Edmondson-Steiner grading increases the predictive efficacy of TNM staging for long-term survival of patients with hepatocellular carcinoma after curative resection. World J Surg 2008;32:1748–1756.
147. Katzenstein HM, Krailo MD, Malogolowkin MH, et al. Fibrolamellar hepatocellular carcinoma in children and adolescents. Cancer 2003;97:2006–2012.
148. Prokurat A, Kluge P, Kosciesza A, et al. Transitional liver cell tumors (TLCT) in older children and adolescents: a novel group of aggressive hepatic tumors expressing beta-catenin. Med Pediatr Oncol 2002;39:510–518.
149. Peng SY Chin WJ, Lai PL, et al. High AFP correlates with high stage, early recurrence, poor prognosis of hepatocellular carcinoma: significance of hepatitis virus infection, age, p53, and B-catenin mutations. Int J Cancer 2005;112:44–50.
150. Czauderna P, MacKinley G, Perilongo G, et al. Hepatocellular carcinoma in children: results of the first prospective study of the international society of pediatric oncology group. J Clin Oncol 2002;20:2798–2804.
151. Katzenstein HM, Krailo MD, Malogolowkin MH, et al. Hepatocellular carcinoma in children and adolescents: results from the Pediatric Oncology Group and the Children's Cancer Group Study. J Clin Oncol 2002;29:2980–2897.
152. Epstein BE, Pajak TF, Haulk TL, et al. Metastatic nonresectable fibrolamellar hepatocellular carcinoma: prognostic features and natural history. Am J Clin Path 1999;22:22–28.
153. Saab S, Yao F. Fibrolamellar hepatocellular carcinoma: case reports and a review of the literature. Dig Dis Sci 1996;41:1981–1985.
154. Gille J, Spieth K, Kaufmann R. Metronomic low-dose chemotherapy as antiangiogenic therapeutic strategy for cancer. J Dtsch Dermatol Ges 2005;3:26–32.
155. Pang R, Poon RT. Angiogenesis and antiangiogenic therapy in hepatocellular carcinoma. Cancer Lett 2006;242:151–167.
156. Llovet JM, Ricci S, Mazzaferro V, et al. Sorafenib in advanced hepatocellular carcinoma. N Engl J Med 2008;359:378–390.
157. Schmid I, Albert MH, Haeberle B, et al. First experience with sorafenib and cisplatin/doxorubicin for pediatric hepatocellular carcinoma [abstract]. Pediatr Blood Cancer 2009;53:745.
158. Rose DM, Chapman WC, Brockenbrough AT, et al. Transcatheter arterial chemoembolization as a primary treatment for hepatocellular carcinoma. Am J Surg 1999;177:405–410.
159. Groupe etude hepatocellulaire. A comparison of lipiodol chemoembolization and conservative treatment for unresectable hepatocellular carcinoma. N Engl J Med 1995;332: 1256–1261.
160. Salem R, Lewandowski RJ, Atassi B, et al. Treatment of unresectable hepatocellular carcinoma with 90Y microspheres (Theraspheres): safety, tumor response, survival. J Vasc Interv Radiol 2005;16:1627–1639.
161. Farges O, Belgheti J, Kianmanesen R, et al. Portal vein embolization before hepatectomy: Prospective clinical trial. Ann Surg 2003;237:208–217.
162. Ghandour K, Masarweh M, Ali H, et al. Portal vein branch ligation: an adjunct to trisegmentectomy PRETEXT III hepatoblastoma. SIOP Abstract Book 2008 pp 221, 40th Congress of the International Society of Pediatric Oncology. Berlin, Germany, October 2008.
163. Chen MS, Li SQ, Zheng V, et al. A prospective randomized trial comparing local ablative therapy and partial hepatectomy for smaller hepatocellular carcinoma. Ann Surg 2006;243:321–328.
164. Curley SA, Marra P, Beaty K, et al. Early and late complications after radiofrequency ablation of malignant liver tumors in 608 patients. Ann Surg 2004;239:430–468.
165. Mazzaferro V, Regalia E, Doci R, et al. Liver transplant for the treatment of hepatocellular carcinoma in patients with cirrhosis. N Eng J Med 1996;334:696–699.
166. Otte JB. Should the selection of children with hepatocellular carcinoma be based on Milan criteria? Pediatr Transplant 2008;12:1–3.
167. Roayaie S, Frischer JS, Emre SH, et al. Long term results with multimodal therapy and liver transplant for the treatment of hepatocellular carcinoma larger than 5 cm. Ann Surg 2002;235:533–539.
168. Austin MT, Leys CM, Feusner ID, et al. Liver transplant for childhood hepatic malignancy: a review of the United Network of Organ Sharing (UNOS) database. J Pediatr Surg 2006;41:182–186.
169. Reyes JD, Carr B, Dvorchik I, et al. Liver transplant and chemotherapy for hepatoblastoma and hepatocellular carcinoma in childhood and adolescence. J Pediatr 2000; 136:795–804.
170. Beaunoyer M, Vanetta JM, Ogihara M, et al. Outcomes of transplantation in children with primary hepatic malignancy. Pediatr Transplant 2007;12:1–3.
171. Weitz J, Klimstra DS, Cymes K, et al. Management of primary liver sarcomas. Cancer 2007;109:1391–1396.
172. Awan S, Davenport M, Portmann B, et al. Angiosarcoma of the liver in children. J Pediatr Surg 31:1729–1732.
173. Nazir Z, Pervez S. Malignant vascular tumors of liver in neonates. J Pediatr Surg 2006;41:e49–e51.
174. Clairotte A, Ringenbach R, Laithier V, et al. Malignant rhabdoid tumor of the liver with spontaneous rupture: a case report. Ann Pathol 2006;26:122–125.
175. Ravindra KV, Cullinane C, Lewis IJ, et al. Long-term survival after spontaneous rupture of a malignant rhabdoid tumor of the liver. J Pediatr Surg 2002;37:1488–1490.
176. Chowdhary SK, Trehan A, Das A, et al. Undifferentiated embryonal sarcoma in children: beware of the solitary liver cyst. J Pediatr Surg 2004;39:9–12.
177. Bisogno G, Pilz T, Perilongo G, et al. Undifferentiated sarcoma of the liver in childhood: a curable disease. Cancer 2002;94:252–257.
178. Kim DY, Kim KH, Jung SE, et al. Undifferentiated (embryonal) sarcoma of the liver: combination treatment by surgery and chemotherapy. J Pediatr Surg 2002;37:1419–1423.
179. Baron PW, Majiessipour F, Bedros AA, et al. Undifferentiated embryonal sarcoma of the liver successfully treated with chemotherapy and liver resection. J Gastrointest Surg 2007;11:73–75.
180. Su WT, Rutigilano DN, Ghollizadeh M, et al. Hepatic metastasectomy in children. Cancer 2007;109:2089–2092.
181. Citak EC, Karadenia C, Oquz A, et al. Nodular regenerative hyperplasia and focal nodular hyperplasia of the liver mimicking hepatic metastasis in children with solid tumors and a review of the literature. Pediatr Hematol Oncol 2007;24: 281–289.
182. Susuki N, Morimoto A, Ohga S, et al. Characteristics of hemophagocytic lymphohistiocytosis in neonates: a nationwide survey in Japan. J Pediatr 2009;155:235–238.
183. Henter JI, Horne A, Aricom, et al. HLH-2004 diagnostic and therapeutic guidelines for hemophagocytic lymphohistiocytosis. Pediatr Blood Cancer 2007;48:124–131.
184. Kassarjian A, Zurakowski D, Dubois J, et al. Infantile hepatic hemangioma: clinical and imaging findings and their correlation with therapy. AJR Am J Roentgenol 2004;18: 785–789.
185. Davenport M, Hansen L, Heaton N, et al. Hemangioendothelioma of the liver in infants. J Pediatr Surg 1995;30:44–48.
186. Meyers RL, Scaife ER. Benign liver and biliary tract masses in infants and toddlers. Semin Pediatr Surg 2000;9:145–146.
187. Morad A, McClain K, Ogden A. The role of tranexamic acid in the treatment of giant hemangiomas in newborns. J Pediatr Hematol Oncol 1993;15:383–385.
188. Perez-Payarols J, Pardo-Masferrer J, Gomea-Bellvert C. Treatment of life threatening hemangiomas with vincristine. N Engl J Med 1985;333:69.
189. Warrell R, Kemping J. Treatment of severe coagulopathy in Kasabach Merritt syndrome with amino-caproic acid and cryoprecipitate. N Engl J Med 1985;313:309–312.
190. Michaud AP, Burman NB, Burke DK, et al. Spastic diplegia and other motor disturbances in infants receiving interferon alpha. Laryngoscope 2004;114:1231–1236.
191. Huang SA, Tu HM, Harney JW, et al. Severe hypothyroidism caused by type 3 iodothyronine deiodinase in infantile hemangioma. N Engl J Med 2000;343:185–189.
192. Lee TC, Barshes NR, Agee EE, et al. Resolution of medically resistant hypothyroidism after liver transplantation for hepatic hemangioendothelioma. J Pediatr Surg 2006;41: 1783–1785.
193. Leaute-Labreze L, Dumas del la Rogue, Hubich T, et al. Propranolol for severe hemangiomas of infancy. N Engl J Med 2008;358:2649–2651.
194. Bien E, Stachowicz-Stencel T, Balcerska A, et al. Angiosarcoma in children: still uncontrollable oncologic problem. Report of Polish Pediatric Rare tumor Study. Eur J Cancer Care 2009;18:411–420.
195. Daller J, Bueno J, Guitierrez J, et al. Hepatic hemangioendothelioma: clinical experience and management strategy. J Pediatr Surg 1999;34:98–106.
196. Draper H, Diamond IR, Temple M, et al. Multimodal management of endangering hepatic hemangioma. J Pediatr Surg 2008;43:120–125.
197. Christison-Lagay ER, Burrows PE, Alomari A, et al. Hepatic hemangiomas: subtype classification and development of a clinical practice algorithm and registry. J Pediatr Surg 2007;42:62–68.
198. Dickie B, Dasgupta R, Nair R, et al. Spectrum of hepatic hemangiomas: management and outcome. J Pediatr Surg 2009;44:125–133.
199. Sarkar M, Mulliken JB, Kozakewich HP, et al. Thrombocytopenic coagulopathy (Kasabach-Merritt phenomenon) is associated with kaposiform Hemangioendothelioma and not with common infantile hemangioma. Plastic Reconstruct Surg 1997;100: 1377–1386.
200. Mulliken J, Fishman SJ, Burrows PE. Vascular anomalies. Curr Probl Surg 2000;37: 517–584.
201. Hauer J, Graubner U, Konstantopoulos N, et al. Effective treatment of kaposiform hemangioendothelioma associated with Kasabach-Merritt phenomenon using four drug regimen. Pediatr Blood Cancer 2007;49:852–854.
202. Drolet BA, Esterly NB, Frieden IJ, et al. Hemangiomas in children. N Engl J Med 1999;34:173–181.
203. Harper L, Michel JL, Enjolras O, et al. Successful management of a retroperitoneal kaposiform hemangioendothelioma with Kasaback-Merritt phenomenon using alpha interferon. Eur J Pediatr Surg 2006;16:369–372.
204. Stringer MD, Alizai NK. Mesenchymal hamartoma of the liver: a systematic review. J Pediatr Surg 2005;40:1681–1690.
205. Helal A, Nolan M, Bower R, et al. Pathologic case of the month. Arch Pediatr Adolesc Med 1995;149:315–316.

206. Von Schweinitz D, Dammeier BG, Gluer S. Mesenchymal hamartoma of the liver: new insights into histogenesis. J Pediatr Surg 1999;34:1269–1271.

207. Kamata S, Nose K, Sawai T, et al. Fetal mesenchymal hamartoma of the liver: report of a case. J Pediatr Surg 2003;38:639–641.

208. Meinders AJ, Simons MP, Heij A. Mesenchymal hamartoma of the liver: failed management by marsupialization. J Pediatr Gastroenterol Nutr 1998;26:353–355.

209. Barnhart D, Hirschl R, Garver K, et al. Conservative management of mesenchymal hamartoma of the liver. J Pediatr Surg 1997;32:1495–1498.

210. Dechadarevian JP, Pawei BR, Faeber EN, et al. Undifferentiated embryonal sarcoma arising in conjunction with mesenchymal hamartoma of the liver. Mod Pathol 1994;7;490–494.

211. O'sullivan MJ, Swanson PE, Knool J, et al. Undifferentiated embryonal sarcoma with unusual features arising within mesenchymal hamartoma of the liver. Pediatr Dev Pathol 2001;4:482–489.

212. Ramanujam, TM, Ramesh JC, Goh DW, et al. Malignant transformation of mesenchymal hamartoma of the liver: case report and review of the literature. J Pediatr Surg 1999;43:1684–1686.

213. Reymond D, Plaschkes J, Ridolfi-Luthy A, et al. Focal nodular hyperplasia of the liver in children: review of follow-up and outcome. J Pediatr Surg 1995;30:1590–1593.

214. Savoye-Collet C, Herve S, Koning E, et al. Focal nodular hyperplasia occurring after blunt abdominal trauma. Eur J Gastroenterol Hepatol 2002;14:329–330.

215. Hohler T, Lohse A, Schiemacher P. Progressive focal nodular hyperplasia of the liver in a patient with genetic hemochromatosis. Dig Dis Sci 2000;45:587–590.

216. Santarelli L, Gabrielli M, Orefice R, et al. Association between Klinefelter syndrome and focal nodular hyperplasia. J Clin Gastroenterol 2003;37:189–191.

217. Wolf R, Wolf D, Kuperman S, et al. Focal nodular hyperplasia of the liver after itraconazole treatment. J Clin Gastroenterol 2001;33:418–420.

218. Scalori A, Tavani A, Gallus S, et al. Risk factors for focal nodular hyperplasia of the liver: an Italian case-control study. Am J Gastroenterol 2002;97:2371–2373.

219. Tanaka Y, Takayanagi M, Shiratori Y, et al. congenital absence of portal vein with multiple hyperplastic nodular lesions in the liver. J Gastroenterol 2003;38:288–294.

220. Icher-de Bouyn C, Leclere J, Raimondo G, et al. Hepatic focal nodular hyperplasia in children previously treated for a solid tumor: Incidence, risk factors and outcome. Cancer 2003;97:3017–3113.

221. Gutweiler JR, Yu DC, Kim HB, et al. Hepatoblastoma presenting as focal nodular hyperplasia after treatment of neuroblastoma. J Pediatr Surg 2008;43:2297–2300.

222. Tanasecu D, Hurwitz C, Waxman A. Scintigraphic findings mimicking focal nodular hyperplasia in a case of hepatoblastoma. Clin Nucl Med 1991;16:236–238.

223. Belghiti J, Paterson D, Panis Y, et al. Resection of presumed benign liver tumors. Br J Surg 1993;80:380–283.

224. Geschwind JFH, Degli M, Morris J, Choti M. Treatment of focal nodular hyperplasia with selective transcatheter arterial embolization using iodized oil and polyvinyl alcohol [editorial]. Cardiovasc Intervent Radiol 2002;24:340–341.

225. Aseni P, Sansalone CV, Sammartino C, et al. Rapid disappearance of hepatic adenoma after contraceptive withdrawal. J Clin Gastroenterol 2001;33:234–236.

226. Rocourt DV, Shiels WE, Hammond S, et al. Contemporary management of benign hepatic adenoma using percutaneous radiofrequency ablation. J Pediatr Surg 2006;41:1149–1152.

227. Labrune P, Trioche P, duvaltier I, et al. Hepatocellular adenoma in glycogen storage disease type 1 and 3: a series of 43 patients and review of the literature. J Pediatr Gastroenterol Nutr 1997;24:276–279.

228. Todani T, Tabuchi K, Watanabe Y, et al. True hepatic teratoma with high serum alpha-fetoprotein in serum. J Pediatr Surg 1997;32:591–592.

229. Cancado El, Medeiros DM, Dequiti MM, et al. Celiac disease associated with nodular regenerative hyperplasia pulmonary abnormalities and IGA anticardiolipin antibodies. J Clin Gastroenterol 2006;40:135–139.

230. Chu WC, Roebuck DJ. Nodular regenerative hyperplasia of the liver simulating metastasis following treatment for bilateral Wilms tumor. Med Pediatr Oncol 2003;41:85–87.

231. Vernier-Masouille G, Cosnes J, Lemann M, et al. Nodular regenerative hyperplasia in patients with inflammatory bowel disease treated with azothioprine. Gut 2007;56:1404–1409.

232. DeBruyne R, Portmann B, Samyn M, et al. Chronic liver disease related to 6 thioguanine in children with acute lymphoblastic leukemia. J Hepatol 2006;44:407–410.

233. Rha SE, Lee MG, Lee YS, et al. Nodular regenerative hyperplasia of the liver in Budd-Chiari syndrome: CT and MR features. Abdom Imaging 2000;25:255–258.

234. Watube H, Akahoski T, Okada J. Coexistence of nodular regenerative hyperplasia of the liver and pulmonary arterial hypertension in patient with connective tissue disorders Mod Rheumatol 2006;16:389–394.

235. Hussein N, Feld JJ, Kleiner DE, et al. Hepatic abnormalities in patient with chronic granulomatous disease. Hepatology 2007;45:675–683.

236. Trenschel GM, Schubert A, Dries V, et al. Nodular regenerative hyperplasia of the liver: case report of a 13 year old girl and review of the literature. Pediatr Radiol 2000;30:64–68.

237. Manolaki N, Vaos G, Zavras N, et al. Inflammatory myofibroblastic tumor of the liver due to mycobacterium tuberculosis. Ped Surg Int 2009;25:451–454.

238. Schnelldorfer T, Chavin KD, Lin A, et al. Inflammatory myofibroblastic tumor of the liver. J Hepatobil Pancreat Surg 2007;14:421–423.

CHAPTER 29 ■ RENAL TUMORS

CONRAD FERNANDEZ, JAMES I. GELLER, PETER F. EHRLICH, D. ASHLEY HILL,
JOHN A. KALAPURAKAL, PAUL E. GRUNDY, AND JEFFREY S. DOME

The kidney is the site of approximately 7% of childhood malignancies including nephroblastoma (Wilms' tumor), clear cell sarcoma of the kidney, malignant rhabdoid tumor, renal cell carcinoma (RCC), and congenital mesoblastic nephroma. Wilms' tumor is a paradigm for the multimodal treatment of pediatric solid tumors. Improvements in surgical techniques and postoperative care, recognition of the sensitivity of Wilms' tumor to irradiation, and the availability of active chemotherapeutic agents have led to a dramatic change in the prognosis for this, once uniformly lethal, malignancy. This chapter reviews the epidemiology, molecular biology, pathology, treatment and prognosis of children with Wilms' tumor and other pediatric renal cancers.

EPIDEMIOLOGY

The incidence of renal tumors in the United States is 7.1 cases per million children younger than 15 years. The total national incidence has been estimated at 500 cases per year. The vast majority of pediatric renal tumors are Wilms' tumors, but RCC surpasses Wilms' tumor as the most common renal malignancy in the 15- to 19-year age group.[1]

The incidence rate for Wilms' tumor is slightly higher for black populations, but substantially lower in Asians, both nationally and internationally.[2] Wilms' tumor in the United States is slightly less frequent in boys than in girls. The male:female ratio is 0.92:1.00 for those with unilateral disease and 0.60:1.00 for those with bilateral disease.[2] The tumor presents at an earlier age among boys, with the mean age at diagnosis for those with unilateral disease being 41.5 months compared with 46.9 months among girls. The mean age at diagnosis for those who present with bilateral disease is 29.5 months for boys and 32.6 months for girls.[2]

Approximately 10% of children with Wilms' tumor have congenital anomalies, either isolated or as part of a congenital malformation syndrome. Table 29.1 lists syndromes that are convincingly associated with Wilms' tumor.[3,4] Wilms' tumor has also been reported in other syndromes such as neurofibromatosis type I, Down syndrome, and Marfan syndrome, but these are likely to be chance associations without increased Wilms' tumor risk compared with the general population.[4]

Stimulated by an early report of an excess of Wilms' tumor among children whose fathers worked in occupations having the potential for contact with hydrocarbons or lead, a series of epidemiologic studies investigated the potential role of parental occupational and environmental exposures as risk factors for Wilms' tumor.[5-8] These were mostly small case-control studies that suffered from methodological weaknesses, including inaccurate exposure assessment and unavoidable bias in the selection of the control series. While several studies noted an excess of fathers who worked as machinists or vehicle mechanics, no consistent positive findings have emerged. Previously reported associations between maternal smoking, tea consumption, and hypertension during pregnancy likewise have not been confirmed. On balance, the inconsistent findings from case-control studies suggest that genetic risk factors are likely to be of greater consequence for Wilms' tumor initiation than environmental risk factors.

GENETICS AND MOLECULAR BIOLOGY

Although Wilms' tumor was initially presented as one of the paradigms for Knudson's two-hit hypothesis,[9] it is now clear that the development of Wilms' tumor is more complex than the loss of function of a single gene. Not only do Wilms' tumors harbor alterations to several genes, but they are also genetically heterogeneous.

WT1

The first gene identified in the development of Wilms' tumor was named *WT1*. Its discovery resulted directly from the observation that individuals with the syndrome of aniridia, genitourinary anomalies, and mental retardation (WAGR syndrome) are at high risk (>30%) for developing Wilms' tumor. Children with the WAGR syndrome were shown to have heterozygous germline deletions at chromosome 11p13,[10] which were later found to encompass a contiguous set of genes including *PAX6*, the gene responsible for aniridia and *WT1*.[11,12] Clinically of importance, patients with sporadic aniridia (*PAX6* defect with normal *WT1*) are not at increased risk for developing Wilms' tumor. The mental retardation seen in WAGR syndrome may result from deletion of yet other genes, possibly *SLC1A2* or *BDNF* (brain-derived neurotrophic factor).[13]

The WT1 protein is a transcription factor with a carboxyl terminus that contains four zinc fingers, a motif involved with sequence-specific binding to DNA.[14] WT1 regulates the transcription of growth factors, growth factor receptors, and other transcription factors, many of which are involved in cell growth, differentiation, and apoptosis.[14] However, it has remained unclear which putative targets are functionally important for Wilms' tumorigenesis. In most respects, *WT1* is a classic tumor suppressor gene, requiring the loss of both alleles for tumor development, but specific alterations to only one allele may contribute to abnormal cell growth. Patients with the Denys-Drash syndrome, which is defined by pseudohermaphroditism, early renal failure with diffuse mesangial sclerosis, and Wilms' tumor harbor constitutional point mutations in only one *WT1* allele.[15] Most Denys-Drash mutations are single-base-pair mutations. The abnormal protein product is thought to disrupt the function of the normal gene product (from the remaining normal allele) through the formation of protein complexes or through abnormal interactions with

TABLE 29.1

SYNDROMES ASSOCIATED WITH WILMS' TUMOR

Syndrome	Locus	Genetic lesion	Phenotype	Estimated Wilms' tumor risk
WAGR	11p13	Deletion of *WT1* gene	Aniridia, genitourinary anomalies, delayed-onset renal failure	30%
Denys-Drash	11p13	Point mutation in zinc-finger region of *WT1* gene	Ambiguous genitalia, diffuse mesangial sclerosis	>90%
Frasier	11p13	Point mutation in *WT1* intron 9 donor splice site	Ambiguous genitalia, streak gonads, focal segmental glomerulosclerosis	8%
Beckwith-Wiedemann	11p15	Dysregulation of imprinted genes including *IGF2* and *H19*	Organomegaly, large birth weight, macroglossia, omphalocele, hemihypertrophy, ear pits and creases, neonatal hypoglycemia	5%
Simpson-Golabi-Behmel	Xq26	Mutations/deletions of GPC3 gene	Overgrowth, course facial features	10%
Li-Fraumeni	17p13	Heterozygous p53 mutations	Familial predisposition to cancer	Low, but several cases reported
Mosaic variegated aneuploidy	15q15	Biallelic BUB1B mutations	Microcephaly, growth retardation, developmental delay, cataracts, heart defects	25%
Fanconi anemia D1	13q12	Biallalic BRCA2 mutations	Short stature, radial ray defects, bone marrow failure	20%
Hyperparathyroid-jaw tumor	1q25–q31	Heterozygous HRPT2 mutations	Fibro-osseous lesions of jaw, parathyroid tumors	Low, but several cases reported
Bloom	15q26	Biallelic BLM mutations	Short stature, photosensitivity, characteristic facial features	3%
Perlman	?	?	Prenatal overgrowth, facial dysmorphism, developmental delay, cryptorchidism, renal dysplasia	33%
Mulibrey nanism	17q22–23	Mutations of *TRIM37*	Short stature, distinct facial appearance, pericardial constriction, yellow dots in retina, hepatomegaly	<3%
Trisomy 18	18	?	Multiple congenital anomalies	Low, but several cases reported
Trisomy 13	13	?	Multiple congenital anomalies	Low, but two cases reported
2q37 deletion	2q37	Possible miR-562 deletion	Developmental delay, dysmorphic facies, skeletal abnormalities, heart defects	3%

DNA targets. Thus, loss of *WT1* function may result from a dysfunctional mutation in only one allele (a dominant effect). The phenotypic effects of the constitutional *WT1* mutations found in Denys-Drash syndrome are in fact far more severe than those resulting from complete deletion of *WT1*, seen in patients with the WAGR syndrome.

Since approximately 30% to 40% of Wilms' tumors manifest loss of heterozygosity (LOH) for the region encompassing *WT1*, a similar incidence of tumors with underlying *WT1* mutations was expected. Surprisingly, though the incidence of *WT1* mutations in seemingly sporadic, Wilms' tumors remain low, approximately 10% to 20%.[16] About 2% of nonsyndromic Wilms' tumor patients harbor a constitutional *WT1* mutation, usually a truncating mutation, yet have no obvious genitourinary anomalies.[17]

WTX

The *WTX* gene (Wilms' tumor gene on X chromosome) was first reported in 2007 by Haber's group when they observed 15 of 51 Wilms' tumors with inactivation of *WTX*.[18] The mechanism of inactivation mainly involved whole gene deletion or truncating mutations on the only allele present in males and on the active allele in females. All deletions reported in Wilms' tumors have been somatic. In contrast, constitutional *WTX* mutations are the cause of the rare familial condition osteopathia striata congenita with cranial sclerosis, a condition in which Wilms' tumor is not a feature.[19]

WTX inhibits the WNT signal transduction pathway[20] by interacting directly with β-catenin to promote ubiquitination and degradation.[21] In the absence of WTX, β-catenin fails to be phosphorylated, is subsequently stabilized, and accumulates in the nucleus,[22] where it forms a complex with the Lef-1/TCF family of transcription factors to promote expression of growth-related genes such as *c-myc* and *cyclin D1* among others. Lending importance to this finding, activation of the WNT signal pathway through mutation of proteins involved in the degradation of β-catenin such as APC is seen in many diseases such as colon cancer and melanoma.[21]

CTNNB1

Activating mutations of the cadherin-associated protein β1 gene (*CTNNB1*), coding for the β-catenin protein, the central effector of the WNT pathway,[23] were first identified in about 15% of Wilms' tumors.[24] Initially, it was thought that *CTNNB1* mutations occurred only in *WT1* mutant tumors,[21] but it now appears that mutations in exon 3 of *CTNNB1* are usually seen in *WT1* mutant tumors while exon 7 or 8 mutations are more common in *WTX* mutant tumors.[25] Considering that *CTNNB1* mutations are rarely found in the absence of *WT1* or *WTX* mutation, it is suggested that activation of β-catenin in the presence of intact WT1 protein must be inadequate for tumor promotion.[21]

WT2

The existence of a second Wilms' tumor gene on chromosome 11p (termed "*WT2*") was first appreciated by the fact that a subset of Wilms' tumors undergoes LOH for markers telomeric to 11p13, not including *WT1*. Linkage analysis first suggested that the locus for the familial form of Beckwith-Wiedemann syndrome, a syndrome characterized by overgrowth (hemihypertrophy, visceromegaly, macroglossia) and a predisposition to embryonal tumors including Wilms' tumor and hepatoblastoma, also mapped to chromosome 11p15.[26,27] While most BWS cases are sporadic, approximately 15% are familial or associated with chromosomal abnormalities. In tumors with LOH, it is invariably the maternal copy of chromosome 11p15 which is lost,[28] suggesting that the two copies of *WT2* are not functionally equivalent. It is now understood that this phenomenon is due to genomic imprinting, a process whereby one allele is marked, or imprinted, in a parental-specific manner to be functionally inactive.

BWS seems to result from aberrations at one of several different loci within 11p15, which may be divided into two clusters of imprinted genes, imprinting center 1 (IC1) and imprinting center 2 (IC2). Recent evidence indicates that Wilms' tumors are initiated by changes confined to IC1 and the target gene insulin-like growth factor 2 (*IGF2*).[29,30] *IGF2* encodes an embryonal growth factor that is highly expressed in fetal kidney and Wilms' tumors. In humans only the paternal *IGF2* allele is normally expressed.[31]

IC1 is a methylation-sensitive chromatin insulator that is normally methylated on the paternally derived chromosome and controls the expression of *IGF2* and H19, an untranslated RNA. The nonmethylated allele (normally the maternal) is bound by a protein called CTCF, which maintains the hypomethylation at IC1, which in turn prevents the activation of *IGF2* and causes activation of *H19* instead. Mutations at the IC1 locus itself, uniparental paternal isodisomy for 11p15 (two copies of the same paternally derived chromosome), and somatic LOH of maternal 11p15 (the somatic equivalent of constitutional uniparental isodisomy) all have been demonstrated in Wilms' tumors and all result in an approximate doubling of the expression of *IGF2* with a concomitant loss of *H19*. What is most common though is a loss of imprinting (LOI) whereby hypermethylation of the IC1 is observed without an accompanying change in the DNA itself or in the CTCF gene/protein leading to the same consequence, that is, increased *IGF2* expression[32] and loss of *H19*.[30,33] Although *H19* codes for an untranslated RNA, it may have tumor suppressor activity.[34]

Consistent with the high frequency of amplified *IGF2* expression is the finding that some Wilms' tumors also have amplification of the *IGF1* receptor, which is the cell surface receptor through which IGF2 imparts its mitogenic activity.[35] Preliminary evidence suggests that patients whose tumors harbor increased copy number of this region may have an increased risk of relapse.[35]

Most recently, a new technique called methylation-specific multiplex ligation-dependent probe amplification (MS-MLPA) was optimized to detect all known epigenetic and IC1 mutations at 11p15. With this technique, it was demonstrated that 13 of 437 cases with nonsyndromic Wilms' tumor had 11p15 constitutional abnormalities.[36] Although this group of 13 patients had a higher than expected proportion of bilateral tumors and perilobar nephrogenic rests, none had any other features of BWS.

No incidences of IC2 alteration were identified in the cases with WT alone, without BWS, although IC2 hypermethylation is the most common cause of BWS. This suggests that surveillance for Wilms' tumor may not need to be performed in patients with BWS caused by isolated IC2 methylation abnormalities, though these individuals are at risk for other embryonal tumors such as neuroblastoma and hepatoblastoma.[37]

Genotype/Phenotype Relationships in Wilms' Tumor

It has been recognized for some time that although Wilms' tumors are classically triphasic, containing blastemal, stromal, and epithelial cell types, many tumors are stromal predominant or express ectopic mesenchymal elements; while another group shows predominant epithelial differentiation without ectopic mesenchyma. The former group is often associated with intralobar nephrogenic rests and the latter with perilobar rests. The molecular basis for these categories of tumors is becoming apparent.

Tumors in the stromal-predominant group tend to have inactivating mutations or decreased expression of *WT1* and nuclear accumulation of β-catenin whether or not *CTNNB1* is mutated.[25,38–41] *WT1* mutation appears to be the initiating event, with *CTNNB1* mutation occurring later, since *WT1* mutations are detected in the precursor lesions, intralobar rests, while *CTNNB1* mutations are found only in the tumor.[42] Further, multiple different *CTNNB1* mutations are observed in multifocal cases with constitutional *WT1* mutation.[43] In these tumors, activation of the WNT pathway appears to be the central theme. *WTX* mutations are seen in some of these tumors, with or without mutation of *WT1* or *CTNNB1*.

In the epithelial-predominant tumors, there is a distinct absence of *WT1* and *CTNNB1* mutations and a lack of nuclear β-catenin, but *WTX* mutations are present at about the same frequency as in the previous group.[25,40] Since one central theme for this group of tumors seems to be the absence of WNT pathway activation, this implies that *WTX* must have functions other than those recognized as part of the canonical WNT pathway, at least in these cell types.[40] Alternatively, there may be WNT targets not previously recognized, which might be impacted by *WTX* or other genes.[39] The other theme is that the epithelial-predominant, perilobar rest-associated tumors have upregulation of the *IGF2* pathway.[32] Current thinking would suggest that alteration of *IGF2* may cause early proliferation but that subsequent changes occur that result in actual tumorigenesis.[44] Interestingly, it has been shown that in Japan, where the incidence of Wilms' tumor is lower than in white populations, there is a paucity of tumors arising from loss of imprinting at the *IGF2* locus.[45]

Familial Wilms' Tumor

Familial predisposition to Wilms' tumor is rare and accounts for only 1% to 2% of all cases.[46] In view of the absence of parental consanguinity in such families, the mode of inheritance is generally thought to be autosomal dominant, with variable penetrance and expressivity.[47] Only one-tenth of the kindreds reported involve affected parents.[46] More often, the disease occurs in siblings, cousins, or other relatives. A survey of 191 children of 99 patients with unilateral Wilms' tumor did not identify a single case of cancer.[48,49] True estimates of the risks in offspring of Wilms' tumor patients will await follow-up of offspring from survivors of the NWTSG and other large patient populations.

Although constitutional mutations of the WT1 gene have been implicated in a few Wilms' tumor families,[17] genetic linkage analysis excluded 11p13 as the predisposing locus in many other affected families.[50,51] Analysis of two families revealed linkage with chromosome 17q, and the putative Wilms' tumor gene at this locus has been named FWT1.[52,53] Interestingly, neither familial nor sporadic Wilms' tumors have undergone LOH for this region, as would be expected if FWT1 were a tumor suppressor locus.[52] A second locus, FWT2, has been mapped to chromosome 19q13.3-q13.4.[47] The specific genes at the FWT1 and FWT2 loci have yet to be identified. As some families exhibit evidence against linkage to WT1, FWT1, and FWT2, the existence of yet additional Wilms' tumor loci must be assumed.[47,53,54]

Rare families have been described with biallelic BRCA2 mutations without the expected Fanconi's anemia phenotype,[55] and Wilms' tumor is an infrequent but definite feature of the multicancer Li-Fraumeni syndrome.[56]

Chromosomes 16q, 1p, and 7p

Loss of heterozygosity (LOH) for markers on the distal long arm of chromosome 16 has been found in 17% of Wilms' tumors, and loss of the short arm of chromosome 1 has been found in approximately 10% of cases, although constitutional changes at these loci have not been observed in Wilms' tumor patients.[57] Loss of either locus has been associated with adverse prognosis, independent of tumor stage and histology.[57,58] The fifth National Wilms Tumor Study (NWTS-5) demonstrated a two- to threefold increased risk of relapse in stage I/II patients with LOH of 1p or 16q while a similar increased risk of relapse was observed in stage III/IV patients whose tumors had LOH for both loci.[57] The fact that there seemed to be less impact of LOH in those treated with doxorubicin (in addition to dactinomycin and vincristine) suggested that intensification of therapy may have overcome the adverse effect on prognosis. Current Children's Oncology Group (COG) studies are testing this premise.

These results were not duplicated by a very similar study of patients in United Kingdom (UK) trials 1 to 3 in which a comparable incidence of LOH for 16q (14%) and 1p (10%) was found, but no association with 1p LOH and outcome was observed.[59] No obvious reason for this difference in findings is apparent, although perhaps the larger doses of doxorubicin used in the UK studies served to eliminate part of the adverse impact on prognosis.

Analyses of karyotypes from Wilms' tumors and from patients with Wilms' tumor have also identified recurrent deletions and translocations involving the short arm of chromosome 7.[60–62] Studies suggest a locus of interest between 7p13 and 7p21,[63,64] perhaps the POU6F2 gene at 7p14.[65] Clinical correlates of 7p LOH have not been published and so the exact role of this possible Wilms' locus, if any, has yet to be determined.

TP53

Constitutional p53 mutations are associated with the multicancer predisposition syndrome named after Li and Fraumeni.[66]

Although uncommon, Wilms' tumor is a rare component of the Li-Fraumeni syndrome.[56] The incidence of p53 mutations in sporadic Wilms' tumors, unlike that observed in many other malignancies, is relatively low in tumors with favorable histology, but these mutations are detected in approximately 75% of tumors with anaplastic histology.[67–69] Microdissection analysis of tumors containing both histologic subtypes has indicated that p53 mutations were restricted to areas of anaplasia, suggesting that acquisition of p53 mutations is inherent to the process of anaplastic progression.[70] The precise incidence and association between the anaplastic histology and p53 mutation is being examined in the current COG trial.

PATHOLOGY

Gross Appearances and Patterns of Extension

Wilms' tumors are typically solitary lesions with no predilection for the left or right kidney or sites within the kidney. Approximately 10% arise multifocally within a single kidney and 7% involve both kidneys either at presentation or subsequently.[2] Extrarenal Wilms' tumors are rare and generally occur in the retroperitoneum adjacent to, but unconnected with, the kidney. Others have been found in the pelvis, inguinal region, and thorax and are thought to arise in displaced metanephric elements and mesonephric remnants.

Wilms' tumor tissue is typically pale tan, soft and friable, and easily spread upon capsular rupture or during gross dissection. Hemorrhage and necrosis frequently impart a variegated appearance. Cysts are commonly encountered and may be a dominant feature. Not uncommonly, especially in infants, a polypoid extension into the pyelocalyceal lumen may resemble the growth pattern seen in botryoid rhabdomyosarcoma.[71] Wilms' tumors are usually sharply demarcated from the adjacent renal parenchyma, separated by a fibrous pseudocapsule. This fibrous pseudocapsule may be the only feature to distinguish Wilms' tumor from a hyperplastic nephrogenic rest. In addition, because mesoblastic nephroma, clear cell sarcoma, rhabdoid tumor, and renal lymphoma all demonstrate infiltrative borders, the presence of a fibrous pseudocapsule can indicate the correct diagnosis on gross examination. Wilms' tumors not infrequently involve the renal vein, and may extend up the inferior vena cava to reach the right atrium.

Histology

The most distinctive microscopic feature of Wilms' tumor is its diversity. The classic nephroblastoma is made up of varying proportions of three patterns, blastemal, stromal, and epithelial, often recapitulating various stages of normal renal development (Fig. 29.1). Blastemal cells are undifferentiated small blue cells that may be arranged in diffuse or organoid patterns.[72] Epithelial structures such as glomeruli and tubules simulating the normal nephrogenic zone are commonly seen. Less commonly, papillary formations or heterologous squamous or mucinous epithelium unlike any in the normal developing kidney are identified. Stromal differentiation is usually manifest as immature spindled cells, heterologous skeletal muscle, cartilage, osteoid, or fat.[73] Tumors that exhibit exclusively one pattern can present diagnostic difficulties. Monophasic blastemal Wilms' tumors are often highly invasive and may raise the differential diagnosis of other small round blue cell tumors, such as primitive neuroectodermal tumor, neuroblastoma, and

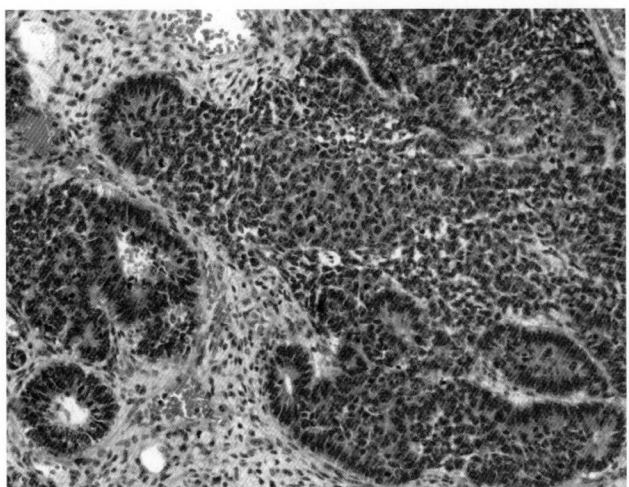

FIGURE 29.1 Triphasic Wilms' tumor, with well-defined tubules emerging from dense clusters of cohesive blastemal cells. Zones of pink-staining stromal differentiation separate blastemal nodules (H & E 100×).

lymphoma. Similarly, monophasic undifferentiated stromal Wilms' tumors may simulate primary sarcomas such as clear cell sarcoma of the kidney, congenital mesoblastic nephroma, or synovial sarcoma. Other stromal Wilms' tumors show a predominance of skeletal muscle differentiation varying from well differentiated (rhabdomyomatous) to poorly differentiated skeletal muscle (rhabdomyoblastic). The distinction of a pure rhabdomyoblastic Wilms' tumor (which is quite rare) from a primary renal rhabdomyosarcoma is often impossible on morphologic grounds. Finally, purely tubular and papillary Wilms' tumor may at times be difficult to distinguish from metanephric adenoma and papillary RCC.[72] In fact, it has been suggested that there may be a biologic link between nephroblastic lesions and some RCCs.[72]

Wilms' tumors often contain scattered cysts and, not uncommonly, tumors may be predominantly or purely cystic. Those that have grossly identifiable solid nodules of tumor are best classified as cystic Wilms' tumors. Tumors that are devoid of any solid nodular growth but contain immature nephrogenic elements within their septa are designated cystic partially differentiated nephroblastoma (CPDN). Others contain only mature cell types and are classified as cystic nephroma (CN). CPDN and CN are both curable by surgery alone, and are thought to represent the most favorable end of the Wilms' spectrum in children.[74] Either lesion can recur if ruptured or incompletely excised, so the distinction of CN from CPDN is of little clinical significance.[75] A familial association between cystic nephroma and the often cystic pleuropulmonary blastoma has been reported.[76]

A correlation between the histologic pattern and the clinical behavior of Wilms' tumor has long been sought. The most significant correlation that has been reported is the distinction of "favorable" from "unfavorable" histology Wilms' tumor. When anaplastic nuclear changes, as described below, are not present, the histology is termed "favorable" because of the generally good outcome for these patients.[73] Other more limited correlations between behavior and histology have been reported. Blastemal-rich tumors tend to be extremely invasive and present at a high stage; however, these tumors often respond well to chemotherapy. In contrast, predominantly epithelial and rhabdomyomatous Wilms' tumors more frequently present at a low stage, reflecting less aggressiveness, yet are often resistant to chemotherapy.[77]

The International Society of Pediatric Oncology (SIOP) protocols administer 4 weeks of chemotherapy before the primary Wilms' tumor is resected, allowing pathologists to develop a histologic grading system that reflects postchemotherapy changes (Table 29.2). In the SIOP classification system, completely necrotic tumors have an outstanding prognosis and blastemal-predominant tumors have a high risk of recurrence.[78,79] The adverse prognostic significance of blastemal cells is greater in Wilms' tumors exposed to chemotherapy compared with untreated tumors.

Anaplastic Wilms' Tumor

Anaplasia is defined by the presence of markedly enlarged polyploid nuclei within the tumor sample (Fig. 29.2). The criteria for the diagnosis of anaplasia include the following: (1) the identification of nuclei with a diameter at least three times those of adjacent cells; (2) hyperchromasia of the

---

TABLE 29.2

THE REVISED SIOP WORKING CLASSIFICATION OF RENAL TUMORS

Risk category	With preoperative chemotherapy	With primary nephrectomy
Low-risk tumors	• Mesoblastic nephroma • Cystic partially differentiated nephroblastoma • Complete necrosis—nephroblastoma	• Mesoblastic nephroma • Cystic partially differentiated nephroblastoma
Intermediate-risk tumors	• Nephroblastoma—epithelial • Nephroblastoma—stromal • Nephroblastoma—mixed • Nephroblastoma—regressive • Nephroblastoma—focal anaplasia	• Nonanaplastic nephroblastoma and its variants • Nephroblastoma-focal anaplasia
High-risk tumors	• Nephroblastoma—blastemal type • Nephroblastoma—diffuse anaplasia • Clear cell sarcoma kidney • Rhabdoid tumor kidney	• Nephroblastoma—diffuse anaplasia • Clear cell sarcoma of the kidney • Rhabdoid tumor of the kidney

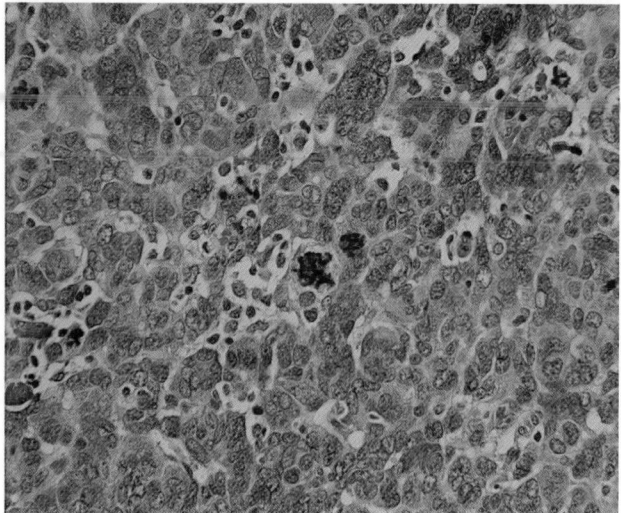

FIGURE 29.2 Anaplastic Wilms' tumor with a large, darkly stained multipolar mitotic figure, near the center, and a markedly enlarged interphase nucleus to its left. Nuclei throughout this field exhibit increased variation in size and shape (H & E 600×).

enlarged cells providing evidence for increased chromatin content; and (3) the presence of multipolar or otherwise recognizably polyploid mitotic figures.[77] All of these features must be identified for the diagnosis of anaplasia, although occasionally, when only a small biopsy is available, the presence of a single multipolar mitotic figure or an unequivocally gigantic tumor cell nucleus will suffice to establish the diagnosis. The frequency of anaplasia is approximately 8% and correlates with patient age. It is rare in the first 2 years of life (2%), and then increases to a relatively stable rate of about 13% in patients older than 5 years. It is significantly more frequent in African-American than in Caucasian patients and more frequent in girls than in boys.[77,80]

Anaplasia is subcategorized into diffuse and focal subtypes, on the basis of the distribution of anaplastic changes within the tumor. The diagnosis of focal anaplasia requires that cells with anaplastic nuclear changes be confined to sharply circumscribed regions within the primary tumor, and that these cells are not present in any site outside the kidney parenchyma. The diagnostic criteria for diffuse anaplasia include any one of the following: (1) the presence of anaplasia in any extrarenal site, including vessels of the renal sinus, extracapsular infiltrates, or nodal or distant metastases; (2) the presence of anaplasia in a random biopsy specimen; (3) unequivocal anaplasia in one region of the tumor, coupled with extreme nuclear pleomorphism approaching the criteria of anaplasia (extreme nuclear unrest) elsewhere in the lesion; (4) the presence of anaplasia in more than one tumor slide, unless (a) it is

known that every slide showing anaplasia came from the same region of the tumor or (b) anaplastic foci on the various slides are minute and surrounded on all sides by nonanaplastic tumor. The distinction between focal and diffuse anaplasia has been demonstrated to be prognostically significant.[81]

It has been suggested that anaplasia is a marker of resistance to therapy rather than tumor aggressiveness.[77] This supposition was based largely on early National Wilms Tumor Studies (NWTS) showing that stage I anaplastic Wilms' tumors had a similar prognosis to stage I favorable-histology Wilms' tumors. However, the results of NWTS-5 demonstrated that stage I anaplastic Wilms' tumors were significantly more likely to recur than stage I favorable-histology Wilms' tumors.[80] Moreover, on the whole, anaplastic tumors presented at a more advanced stage (III/IV) than favorable-histology tumors. Collectively, the current data indicate that anaplasia portends both resistance to therapy and tumor aggressiveness.

Nephrogenic Rests

The existence of precursor lesions to Wilms' tumor has been recognized for many years.[81,82] These nephrogenic rests are found in almost 1% of unselected pediatric autopsies, in 35% of kidneys with unilateral Wilms' tumors, and in nearly 100% of kidneys with bilateral Wilms' tumors. They are composed of abnormally persistent embryonal nephroblastic tissue with small clusters of blastemal cells, tubules, or stromal cells. Nephrogenic rests are classified by their position within the kidney. Intralobar nephrogenic rests (ILNR) are randomly distributed but tend to be situated deep within the renal lobe, likely reflecting an earlier developmental insult to the kidney. These lesions are commonly stroma rich and intermingle with the adjacent renal parenchyma. Perilobar nephrogenic rests (PLNR) are located at the periphery, are usually subcortical, sharply demarcated, and contain predominantly blastema and tubules. These presumably reflect later developmental disturbances in nephrogenesis. Morphologic distinction of the two types of rests is of interest because they have different clinical and pathologic associations (Table 29.3). The term nephroblastomatosis is used to refer to the presence of multiple nephrogenic rests. Diffuse overgrowth of perilobar nephrogenic rests may produce a thick "rind" of blastemal or tubular cells that enlarge the kidney but preserve its original shape (Fig. 29.3). Only a small number of nephrogenic rests develop a clonal transformation into Wilms' tumor. When this happens, the Wilms' tumor is typically spherical and develops a pseudocapsule separating it from the nephrogenic rest. Some rests may become hyperplastic, with dramatic enlargement that preserves the shape of the preceding rest. Such lesions may be histologically indistinguishable from Wilms' tumor on biopsy unless the interface between the rest and the adjacent normal kidney is present within the sample. Hyperplastic nephrogenic rests may completely regress or differentiate following the administration of chemotherapy. The majority of nephrogenic rests become

TABLE 29.3

CHARACTERISTICS OF PERILOBAR VERSUS INTRALOBAR NEPHROGENIC RESTS

	Intralobar	Perilobar
Associated syndromes	WAGR, Denys-Drash	Beckwith-Wiedemann
Location within renal lobe	Random, often central	Peripheral
Interface with kidney	Intermingling	Distinct
Dominant histologic component	Stroma	Blastema or tubules
Number	Usually single	Often multiple

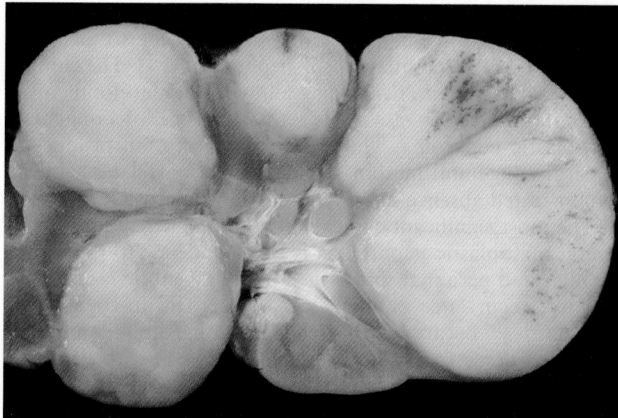

FIGURE 29.3 Perilobar nephrogenic rests. Grossly, these perilobar nephrogenic rests are roughly wedge shaped following the contours of the renal lobule. The nephrogenic rest tissue is homogeneous and paler than the normal surrounding renal parenchyma.

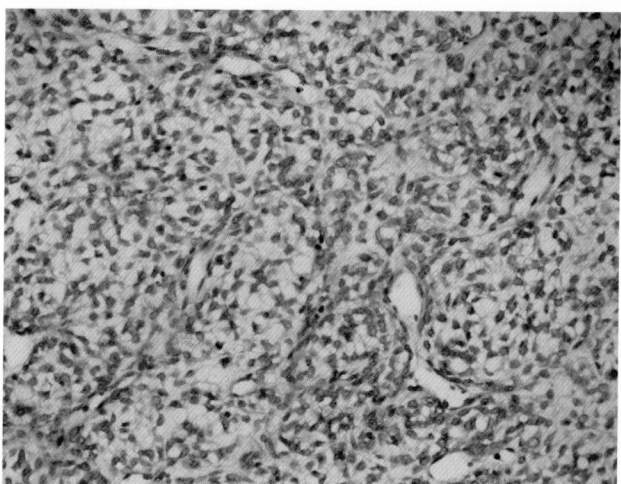

FIGURE 29.4 Clear cell sarcoma of the kidney, classical pattern. Nests of pale-stained tumor cells are separated by a delicate but distinct network of fine vascular septa. Nuclei are vesicular, with poorly stained chromatin and inconspicuous nucleoli (H & E 200×).

dormant or involute spontaneously. The presence of nephrogenic rests within a kidney resected for a Wilms' tumor indicates the need for monitoring the contralateral kidney for tumor development, particularly in young infants.[83]

Clear Cell Sarcoma of the Kidney

Clear cell sarcoma of the kidney is the second most common pediatric renal neoplasm, and is a tumor associated with a significantly higher rate of relapse and death than favorable-histology Wilms' tumor unless treated more aggressively. This variant was described in detail in 1978.[73] The descriptive term "clear cell sarcoma of the kidney" is based on the staining characteristics of the predominant cell type; others have been referred to as "bone-metastasizing renal tumor of childhood" because bone is a common metastatic site. Clear cell sarcoma of the kidney has a far wider distribution of metastases than favorable-histology Wilms' tumor; both tumors spread to the lungs, but clear cell sarcoma of the kidney has a strikingly increased number of brain, bone, and soft tissue metastases.[84]

Most clear cell sarcoma of the kidney specimens have a distinct histologic appearance, but a number of variant patterns, such as epithelioid, spindling, myxoid, and cystic, invite confusion with Wilms' tumor or other tumor types.[84–86] As a result, clear cell sarcoma of kidney remains the pediatric renal tumor most frequently misdiagnosed. The classic morphologic pattern of clear cell sarcoma is biphasic, composed of nests of plump cord cells containing abundant extracellular matrix separated by a network of capillary vascular arcades that are often surrounded by more spindled septal cells (Fig. 29.4). Finally, clear cell sarcoma can show anaplastic nuclear features identical to those of anaplastic Wilms' tumor. Immunohistochemical studies are useful in the exclusion of other tumors, but no positive diagnostically useful immunohistochemical or genetic markers have been identified to date.[86]

Rhabdoid Tumor of Kidney

A distinctive and highly malignant tumor, rhabdoid tumor of the kidney was identified in 1978 by National Wilms Tumor Study Group (NWTSG) pathologists.[73] Rhabdoid tumor of the kidney occurs most frequently in infants and toddlers, with 85% of cases occurring within the first 2 years of life and

a sharp decline thereafter. The diagnosis should be considered highly suspect over the age of 5 years.[87] The tumor is commonly widely metastatic at presentation, and in both NWTSG and SIOP studies, over 80% of children die within 1 year of diagnosis.[87,88]

Renal rhabdoid tumors are usually bulky masses centered in the renal hilum with a grossly indistinct tumor border reflecting aggressive invasion. Prominent intrarenal vascular invasion leads to frequent satellite nodules that may be seen grossly. The tumor characteristically grows as sheets of discohesive cells characterized by vesicular nuclei, prominent macronucleoli, and eosinophilic cytoplasmic inclusions (Fig. 29.5). However, these cytologic features may be variably present, and diligent search may be required before diagnostic foci are

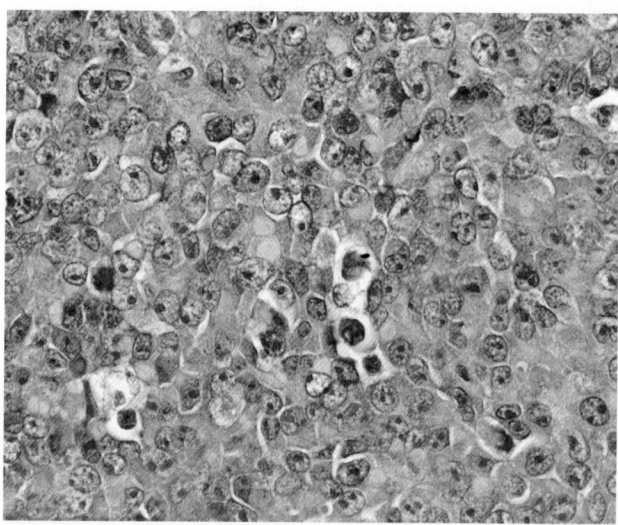

FIGURE 29.5 Rhabdoid tumor. Most nuclei have dispersed chromatin and a large single nucleolus, imparting an "owl's eye" appearance to the nucleus. Several cells, including one near the center, have hyaline globular cytoplasmic inclusions. Ultrastructurally, the latter inclusions consist of whorled masses of intermediate filaments, usually composed of vimentin (H & E 600×).

encountered. In addition, a large number of variant patterns have been described, including sclerosing, epithelioid, spindled, vascular, and lymphomatoid, all of which can simulate other neoplasms.[89] Rhabdoid tumor received its name because of the prominent acidophilic cytoplasm, resembling rhabdomyoblasts. However, rhabdoid tumors do not show immunohistochemical or ultrastructural features of skeletal muscle. The cell of origin for this distinctive tumor remains unknown.[89–91] It is not a variant of Wilms' tumor and has not been encountered as a focal change in a conventional Wilms' tumor. Rhabdoid tumors are not limited to the kidney. They occur in the central nervous system where they are referred to as atypical teratoid/rhabdoid tumor, soft tissue, liver, and other sites.[92,93]

Genetic analysis of malignant rhabdoid tumors shows loss of function mutations or deletions in the *hSNF5/INI1* gene on chromosome 22q11–12.[94–96] Germline mutations have been demonstrated in some children and familial association of rhabdoid tumors has been described.[97] The mechanism of tumor development resulting from loss of *INI1* is unknown but may involve dysregulation of cell cycle genes.[98,99]

Rhabdoid tumors characteristically show a polyphenotypic immunohistochemical staining pattern, with focal strong positivity for a variety of markers. Vimentin is diffusely positive in rhabdoid tumors and characteristically shows a dot-like pattern corresponding to the eosinophilic inclusions, which actually represent bundles of intermediate filaments. The presence of scattered clusters of intensely EMA or cytokeratin positive cells in a background of negative staining is a characteristic. Other markers including smooth muscle actin, neurofilament, and CD99 are positive in a proportion of tumors. One of the most helpful stains in the diagnosis of rhabdoid tumors is for the protein product of *INI1*, the gene most commonly deleted/mutated in this tumor. The nuclei of rhabdoid tumor cells are negative for INI1.[92] Since this protein is ubiquitously expressed, positive nuclear staining in nonneoplastic tissue within the tumor (vessels, lymphocytes, normal kidney) serves as an internal control for staining.

A variety of renal and nonrenal tumors can show rhabdoid histologic features.[100,101] The majority of such tumors in patients older than 5 years represent other neoplasms. Many of these "pseudorhabdoid" lesions have been identified by immunohistochemistry or other techniques to be carcinomas, melanomas, histiocytic tumors, or sarcomas.

Congenital Mesoblastic Nephroma

This term was applied by Bolande and colleagues in 1967 to a distinctive renal neoplasm of infancy.[102] Congenital mesoblastic nephroma occurs predominantly in infants, with a median age of 2 months.[102] Three histologic subtypes have been defined: the classic type (24% of cases), the more frequent cellular type (66% of cases), and mixed type (10% of cases) showing both classic and cellular patterns.[103] The classic subtype of congenital mesoblastic nephroma grows as intersecting fascicles of bland spindle cells with tapered nuclei and pink cytoplasm and is histologically similar to infantile fibromatosis. Mitoses are usually infrequent and necrosis is absent. The cellular subtype of congenital mesoblastic nephroma has a solid, cellular, sheet-like growth pattern of oval or round cells with little cytoplasm, and frequent mitoses and necrosis. The mixed type of congenital mesoblastic nephroma features areas resembling both classical and cellular morphologies. While classic congenital mesoblastic nephroma histologically resembles infantile myofibromatosis, the cellular congenital mesoblastic nephroma resembles infantile fibrosarcoma. Recently, a genetic linkage between infantile fibrosarcoma and cellular congenital mesoblastic nephroma was established

when the chromosome translocation, t(12;15)(p13;q25), initially discovered in infantile fibrosarcoma, was also identified in cellular congenital mesoblastic nephroma.[104–106] The cloning of the resulting gene fusion has allowed the development of molecular detection assays for this subtype of congenital mesoblastic nephroma. The absence of the fusion product in classical congenital mesoblastic nephroma correlates with its demonstrated absence in infantile myofibromatosis.

The most significant clinical and pathologic feature of congenital mesoblastic nephromas is their tendency to grow into the hilar and perirenal soft tissue, often in a subtle fashion. As a result, recurrence or metastasis is seen in up to 20% of patients.[107–109] Because of this tendency, congenital mesoblastic nephroma deserves a radical surgical approach, with efforts to secure a margin of uninvolved tissue on all aspects of the specimen, but particularly the medial aspect. Following surgery, any residual tumor may recur with astonishing rapidity; therefore, close radiographic follow-up is indicated for the first year.

Renal Cell Carcinoma

Renal cell carcinomas (RCCs) represent 8% of the malignant neoplasms occurring in kidneys of children and adolescents. Of the common adult types, papillary RCC appears more frequently than classic clear cell, chromophobe, or collecting duct types, and some of these occur in the setting of genetic predisposition.[110] Over the past several years, it has become clear that there is a unique subtype of RCC that preferentially presents in adolescents and young adults. Accounting for nearly one-third of all RCC in children, these predominantly clear cell neoplasms are genetically unique and are characterized by chromosomal translocations involving the *TFE3* gene on Xp11.2 (so-called Xp11 translocation RCC)[111–113] or the *TFEB* gene on 6p21.[114,115] Similar to other translocation-associated neoplasms, the abnormal gene fusions result in dysregulation of one of the fusion gene partners. In translocation RCC, each gene fusion results in overexpression of either TFE3 or TFEB transcription factors, which contribute to the pathogenesis. Immunohistochemistry can detect aberrant expression for TFE3 or TFEB and, thus, can be useful in establishing the diagnosis.[115,116]

Clinically, translocation-positive RCC have been described as second malignancies following previous chemotherapy.[117] Histologically, these may show a great resemblance to clear cell RCC; cells are in a nested arrangement and have copious clear cytoplasm. Papillary architecture and psammomatous calcifications provide some clues to the diagnosis. Translocation-positive tumors have a distinctive immunohistochemical profile from adult-type clear cell RCC. In addition to the unique expression of fusion-specific proteins detectable by immunohistochemistry, these tumors appear to lack immunoreactivity for epithelial markers and vimentin, which is in sharp contrast to other RCCs. Some translocation-positive RCCs stain with melanocytic markers.[114,118] Early outcome studies indicate that translocation-positive RCCs are a heterogeneous group. While some tumors appear to have an indolent course, others present with advanced stage disease and are rapidly progressive.[119–121] Clinical trials now underway may help shed light on the clinical heterogeneity of this group of tumors.

CLINICAL PRESENTATION AND DIAGNOSTIC WORKUP

The majority of children with Wilms' tumor present with an asymptomatic abdominal mass that is incidentally noted while bathing or dressing the child.[122] Pain is seen in approximately 40% of patients, although this symptom is not well correlated with tumor rupture.[122,123] Fever is less commonly observed. Gross (18%) or microscopic (24%) hematuria may occur on an intermittent basis in children with Wilms' tumor,[123] but finding Wilms' tumor as a cause of gross hematuria in childhood is rare. Hypertension occurs in over a quarter of patients and is caused by increased renin secretion and, thus, a logical strategy for its management has been shown to be angiotensin-converting enzyme inhibitors.[124] The hypertension may be severe, resulting in encephalopathy and retinal hemorrhage, but usually resolves quickly following nephrectomy. Signs or symptoms of hypercalcemia are very uncommon in Wilms but may be seen in renal rhabdoid tumors.[123] The physical examination will demonstrate a mass that is typically smooth and eccentrically located in the abdomen towards the flank. It should be distinguished from a palpable spleen that moves with respiration, and other abdominal masses such as neuroblastoma that are more frequently centrally located and are typically immobile. Features related to the Wilms' tumor mass and its effects on normal structures may include pulmonary insufficiency secondary to lung metastases, congestive heart failure, prominent abdominal wall vessels, varicocele related to obstruction of the inferior vena cava and consequent spermatic vein thrombosis, and rarely pulmonary embolus.

As up to 7% of children with Wilms have a known syndromic association such as Denys-Drash, WAGR, or Beckwith-Wiedemann syndromes, careful assessment for clinical features such as aniridia, urogenital anomalies (hypospadias, cryptorchidism, pseudohermaphrodism), developmental delay, overgrowth, and hemihypertrophy should be undertaken. A French study demonstrated a significant excess of congenital heart defects,[125] as did a study in Great Britain at 1.8% of the study participants.[126]

Differential Diagnosis

The clinical approach to a child with a renal mass begins with the assumption that the most likely diagnosis is Wilms' tumor. However, other benign and malignant intrarenal masses may mimic clinical and radiological features of Wilms' tumor. Leukemia, Burkitt lymphoma, rhabdomyosarcoma, sarcoma, and non-Wilms' primary renal tumors may be mistaken on diagnostic imaging for Wilms' tumor. Benign conditions that may mimic Wilms' tumor include polycystic kidney disease, abscess, and hydronephrosis. Results from early SIOP and NWTSG trials demonstrated that 7% to 10% of patients with a preoperative diagnosis of Wilms' tumor turned out to have a different condition,[127,128] although with current imaging techniques the figure ranges between 2% and 5%.[129] The primary extrarenal tumor that may be mistaken for Wilms' tumor is neuroblastoma, but the latter can usually be distinguished on diagnostic imaging by the absence of a claw sign (Fig. 29.6), adrenal or paravertebral sympathetic ganglion origin, and a propensity for invasion rather than capsule formation.

Laboratory Workup

Laboratory evaluations that should be performed preoperatively include a complete blood count with differential, liver function tests, renal function including urinalysis, electrolytes, and serum calcium. Acquired von Willebrand's disease can occur in approximately 1% to 2% of patients with Wilms' tumor, so some clinicians recommend preoperative measurement of coagulation parameters (PT, PTT, von Willebrand's factor antigen, ristocetin cofactor, and factor VIII levels).[130,131]

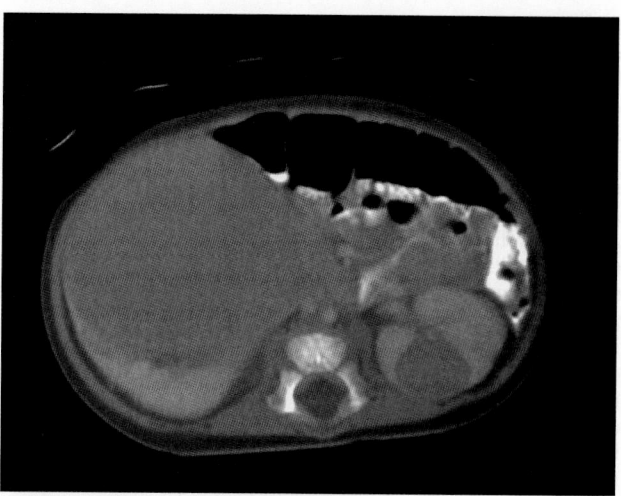

FIGURE 29.6 Axial computed tomography scan of the abdomen demonstrating bilateral Wilms' tumors. The larger right kidney tumor demonstrates the "claw" sign, in which the renal parenchyma is stretched around and cupping the tumor suggesting the organ of origin.

Perioperative management has included DDAVP, von Willebrand's factor concentrates, IVIG, and plasmapheresis, although the most effective strategy to resolve this acquired condition is surgical resection of the tumor.[132]

IMAGING STUDIES

Initial imaging studies should fulfill five goals. They should establish confirmation that the mass arises from the kidney, ascertain if there is contiguous spread outside of the kidney including regional lymph nodes and inferior vena cava, determine if the urinary tract anatomy is normal (looking for single, horseshoe, or ectopic kidneys), provide evidence as to the involvement of the opposite kidney (Fig. 29.6), and provide preliminary evidence of whether or not there is metastatic involvement, most typically lung or liver. With current imaging techniques, the chance of missing synchronous Wilms' tumor is low enough (0.3%) that routine surgical exploration of the opposite kidney is no longer recommended.[133]

Ultrasonography

Ultrasound is typically rapidly available and usually requires no sedation. The echo pattern is typically heterogeneous and not specific to Wilms' tumor. Calcifications are uncommon in Wilms' tumor. Involvement of the renal vein or IVC occurs in 4% to 10% of Wilms patients[134] and color Doppler ultrasound has a good level of positive predictive value in assisting in identifying if there is intravascular tumor thrombus and its extent.[135] Ultrasound is, however, a modality that is operator dependent, limited by intra-abdominal gas and obesity, and not easily amenable to central review.[136]

Computed Tomography

Contrast enhanced computed tomography (CT) scanning is the modality that provides the most accurate assessment in detecting metastatic lung nodules and may be of utility in further defining intra-abdominal anatomy. Chest x-ray alone misses significant numbers of small lesions (termed CT-only lung lesions); in one study 10% were missed and recent evidence suggests that these patients fare worse if treatment is administered according to local primary tumor stage only.[137] There is, however, controversy with respect to the utility of identifying lung nodules in guiding treatment and subsequent impact upon outcome. There is significant interobserver variability in reliably identifying CT nodules.[138] A significant portion of small lung nodules represent nonmalignant conditions such as fibrosis, atelectasis, or infection, and this may be quite prominent in areas with endemic histoplasmosis.[139] In assessing renal masses, the portal venous phase of contrast enhanced CT is typically sufficient to address tumor anatomy including vascular extension. CT does play a role in determining the likelihood of preoperative rupture and distinguishing it from local and intraperitoneal locations and, thus, is useful in jurisdictions where preoperative chemotherapy is used routinely.[140] It is also very sensitive in identifying nephrogenic rests in the contralateral kidney.

Magnetic Resonance Imaging

MRI plays an increasingly important role in Wilms' tumor staging and management and in some areas has replaced CT scanning as a primary means of baseline abdominal imaging.[141] MRI has the advantage of decreasing exposure to ionizing radiation. It has the disadvantage of usually requiring general anesthesia in this age group and is not adequate for lung assessment. An emerging concern is the occurrence of gadolinium-related nephrogenic systemic fibrosis; individuals with a calculated GFR of less than 60 mL/min/1.73 m² appear to be most at risk for this devastating complication.[141,142] MRI will typically show low signal intensity on T1-weighted images and hypo- or isointensity on T2-weighted data capture.[136] Brisse et al. have proposed an MR protocol for baseline imaging of Wilms patients at diagnosis.[143] An attempt has been made to correlate MRI signals with active nephrogenic rests or Wilms' tumor but this has not been widely adopted.[144] It is the modality of choice for detecting intracranial metastases and should be routinely undertaken before treatment, if the histological diagnosis is rhabdoid tumor or clear cell tumor of the kidney.[89,145]

Positron Emission Tomography/CT Scan

Studies with limited numbers of patients have demonstrated mixed reports that PET/CT does not appear to routinely add to conventional imaging techniques for the initial diagnostic work up, response to therapy in which a preoperative chemotherapy strategy is used, or clinical outcome.[146,147] However, it may provide superior information with respect to residual disease at end of therapy and extent of disease at relapse and in distinguishing anaplastic Wilms from favorable histology.[147] There is no current published evidence whether PET is valuable in distinguishing Wilms' tumor from nephrogenic rests.[136] The role of PET/CT in clinical decision-making should be further evaluated in clinical trials.

Screening in Predisposition Syndromes

Recommendations for Wilms' tumor surveillance screening in predisposition syndromes is limited to expert opinion and cohort reports.[148] The evidence for efficacy is imperfect although it is plausible that early detection in high-risk patients will result in lower stage Wilms' tumor, the opportunity to consider renal-sparing surgical techniques, the avoidance of radiotherapy, and the provision of less intensive chemotherapy. Scott et al. recently conducted an extensive literature review of Wilms' tumor predisposition syndromes and developed recommendations for screening these patients.[149] When screening is indicated, the recommended modality is abdominal ultrasound performed every 3 to 4 months. It is important to remember that screening and disease recurrence surveillance is not without costs. There are economic costs to regular imaging studies, medical and surgical costs of investigating false-positive findings, and psychological costs inherent in counseling families and children with respect to cancer risks. Further research is warranted to understand the risks and benefits related to frequency, duration, and modalities of screening.

STAGING

There are two main staging systems in use for Wilms' tumor. The COG classification is based on the NWTSG approach of immediate nephrectomy and takes into account surgical-pathological findings with imaging for distant metastasis (Table 29.4). SIOP utilizes a preoperative chemotherapy approach and staging criteria are based on a combination of prechemotherapeutic imaging to define metastatic disease and local operative findings following chemotherapy. Although the stage definitions are similar, the prechemotherapy stage does not have equivalent clinical significance to the postchemotherapy stage, hence confounding head-to-head comparisons of SIOP and NWTSG/COG trial results.

Patterns of Spread

Wilms' tumor may spread locally or hematogenously. Locally, the tumor may extend directly through the renal capsule and most typically develops an inflammatory pseudocapsule during its growth. The tumor may grow directly into the renal sinus or ureter.[177] Wilms' tumor may also grow by contiguous spread through the renal vein into the inferior vena cava IVC (4% to 10%), with rare direct extension into the right atrium.[150] Wilms' tumor spreads to regional lymph nodes in approximately 15% to 20% of cases.[151]

Hematogenous metastases in Wilms' tumor are uncommon at baseline diagnosis (12%),[152] and when present most frequently involve the lung (80%), liver (15%), and, rarely, bone, bone marrow, or brain.[152] Rhabdoid tumor and clear cell sarcoma of the kidney have a greater propensity for bone and brain metastases and baseline imaging and follow-up should examine these potential sites of spread.[84,123]

Approximately 5% to 7% of Wilms' tumor will have bilateral disease.[153,154] The majority will present with synchronous disease at diagnosis and 1.2% of children will develop metachronous involvement of the kidney with the majority occurring by 4 years postdiagnosis.[155] This metachronous occurrence is more common in infants younger than 12 months with perilobar nephrogenic rests in the nephrectomy specimen at the time of presentation.

PROGNOSTIC CONSIDERATIONS

The prognosis of children with renal tumors is related to multifactorial considerations including histology at diagnosis, histological response to preoperative chemotherapy, tumor

TABLE 29.4

CHILDREN'S ONCOLOGY GROUP STAGING SYSTEM FOR WILMS' TUMOR

Stage I	Tumor limited to kidney, completely resected. The renal capsule is intact. The tumor was not ruptured or biopsied prior to removal. The vessels of the renal sinus are not involved. There is no evidence of tumor at or beyond the margins of resection. *Note:* For a tumor to qualify for certain therapeutic protocols as stage I, regional lymph nodes must be examined microscopically.
Stage II	The tumor is completely resected and there is no evidence of tumor at or beyond the margins of resection. The tumor extends beyond kidney, as is evidenced by any one of the following criteria: • There is regional extension of the tumor (i.e., penetration of the renal capsule or extensive invasion of the soft tissue of the renal sinus, as discussed later). • Blood vessels within the nephrectomy specimen outside the renal parenchyma, including those of the renal sinus, contain tumor. *Note:* Rupture of spillage confined to the flank, including biopsy of the tumor, is no longer included in stage II and is now included in stage III.
Stage III	**Residual nonhematogenous tumor present following surgery, and confined to abdomen. Any one of the following may occur:** • Lymph nodes within the abdomen or pelvis are involved by tumor. (Lymph node involvement in the thorax or other extra-abdominal sites is a criterion for stage IV.) • The tumor has penetrated through the peritoneal surface. • Tumor implants are found on the peritoneal surface. • Gross or microscopic tumor remains postoperatively (e.g., tumor cells are found at the margin of surgical resection on microscopic examination). • The tumor is not completely resectable because of local infiltration into vital structures. • Tumor spillage occurring either before or during surgery. • The tumor is treated with preoperative chemotherapy (with or without a biopsy regardless of type tru-cut, open, or fine needle aspiration) before removal. • Tumor is removed in greater than one piece (e.g., tumor cells are found in a separately excised adrenal gland; a tumor thrombus within the renal vein is removed separately from the nephrectomy specimen). Extension of the primary tumor within vena cava into thoracic vena cava and heart is considered stage III, rather than stage IV even though outside the abdomen.
Stage IV	Hematogenous metastases (lung, liver, bone, brain, etc.) or lymph node metastases outside the abdomino-pelvic region are present. (The presence of tumor within the adrenal gland is not interpreted as metastasis and staging depends on all other staging parameters present.)
Stage V	Bilateral renal involvement by tumor is present at diagnosis. An attempt should be made to stage each side according to the above criteria on the basis of the extent of disease.

weight, stage, age at diagnosis, rapidity of response to therapy, and increasingly identified molecular markers.

Histopathological Features

Histology remains the most powerful prognostic factor for pediatric renal tumors. The COG classification system has been adopted from findings of the NWTSG and divides Wilms' tumors into two broad histologic types: favorable and anaplastic histology (see pathology section for descriptions and definitions). The anaplastic histology tumors are further divided into diffuse and focal, on the basis of the distribution of anaplastic cells throughout the tumor. The histologic subtype has prognostic significance such that favorable-histology tumors have the best outcomes, diffuse anaplastic tumors have the worst outcomes, and focal anaplastic tumors have intermediate prognosis.[80,156] Other histologic types including clear cell sarcoma of the kidney (CCSK) and rhabdoid tumor were traditionally grouped into the "unfavorable" histology category of Wilms' tumor, but it is now recognized that these are distinct biologic entities. The prognosis for CCSK has improved greatly with the incorporation of doxorubicin into treatment regimens, whereas the prognosis for rhabdoid tumor remains poor despite intensive chemotherapy.[84,89,157]

The SIOP classification schema is more complex than the COG schema because it takes into account the histologic response to chemotherapy. SIOP has demonstrated three prognostic groups termed low, intermediate, and high risk (Table 29.2).[79]

Stage

Adequate staging is crucial to risk-stratified therapy in Wilms' tumor. Current COG trials continue to use stage as the starting point for a stratification algorithm. In general, lower stage patients (I and II) are managed with two-drug chemotherapy (vincristine and dactinomycin), whereas higher stage patients (III and IV) receive at least three drugs (vincristine, dactinomycin, and doxorubicin) and are treated with radiotherapy.[57,158]

Age

Age has long been known to correlate with prognosis in Wilms' tumor, with older age associated with adverse prognosis. There are several factors that explain this association. First, there is a subset of very young patients whose Wilms'

tumor capsule during operative removal whether accidental, unavoidable, or by design. Spill is also considered to have occurred if a preoperative or intraoperative needle/open biopsy from the anterior or posterior approach, or if the renal vein or ureter was transected when they contain tumor. "Rupture" refers to either the spontaneous or posttraumatic rupture of the tumor preoperatively with the result that tumor cells are disseminated throughout the peritoneum or retroperitoneal space. Bloody peritoneal fluid is considered a sign of soilage, whether or not gross or microscopic tumor is identified in the fluid. Rupture is also considered to have occurred if the tumor penetrates the kidney capsule, with open raw neoplastic tissue surface being in free communication with the peritoneal cavity. All of these situations must be carefully documented in the operative note.

Lung Metastasis

Lungs metastasis is the most common site of stage IV disease in children with Wilms' tumor. Lung metastasis, however, does not necessarily imply that the abdominal tumor is unresectable. A common surgical pitfall is not to attempt upfront resection of the abdominal tumor just because lung metastases are visualized. The abdominal tumor should be removed and staged locally if possible. There are three situations when a surgeon may be asked to intervene in a child with a pulmonary lesion. The first is at diagnosis if the diagnosis of metastatic disease is in doubt. In the case of small lesions seen on CT scan but not chest x-ray (so-called "CT-only" nodules), there is a 70% to 80% chance that the nodules are tumors.[139] The second indication is if lung lesions shrink but do not go away completely after chemotherapy. It is then important to discern whether the residual lesions contain viable tumors. The third situation is if tumor remains after both chemotherapy and radiotherapy, requiring surgical resection for cure. Most WT metastases are peripheral and superficial and many of these lesions can now be fully excised by video-assisted thoracic surgery.

Bilateral Wilms' Tumor

Bilateral Wilms' tumors (BWT) occur in 4% to 13% of patients and may be synchronous or metachronous.[2,179] Despite 35 years of clinical trials by cooperative groups, patients with BWT have not been formally studied in a prospective manner. On NWTS-5, the 4-year event-free and overall survival rates for BWT were only 61% and 80%, respectively. BWT presents the paradoxical challenge of resecting the malignancy while preserving renal parenchyma.

Breslow reported 20-year end-stage renal disease (ESRD) outcomes in children treated for Wilms' tumor.[180] For unilateral tumors, 55 of 5,526 patients (0.99%) developed renal failure at 20 years. By contrast, for BWT, 55 of 379 patients (14.5%) developed ESRD at 20 years. Renal failure was most commonly associated with progressive disease, necessitating resection with inadequate remaining renal parenchyma. Some cases of renal failure were related to genetic predisposition (WAGR or Denys-Drash syndromes), nephrotoxic effects of chemotherapy and radiation therapy, and hyperfiltration injury to the remaining renal parenchyma.[180,181] Thus, preservation of renal tissue without sacrificing long-term survival is of particular importance for those with BWT.

Initial management of a child with bilateral renal lesions can present a conundrum for the surgeon. The primary reasons to perform a biopsy are to confirm the diagnosis of Wilms' tumor and to detect anaplasia. Of all the reports on

BWT from NWTSG, SIOP, GPOH (German Society for Pediatric Oncology & Hematology), and UKCCSG (United Kingdom Children's Cancer Study Group), there have been no patients with bilateral lesions who did not have Wilms' tumor or nephrogenic rests. Hence, there is limited rationale to perform biopsy solely to confirm the diagnosis of Wilms' tumor. A patient with BWT may have disparate histology in each kidney, but biopsy sampling rarely identifies anaplasia.[80,182] Hence, the current BWT protocol from the COG does not recommend obtaining a biopsy prior to starting therapy. After 6 weeks of therapy, nonresponsive disease mandates generous open biopsies from both kidneys to define tumor histology.

Nephron-sparing surgery for children should be considered for all patients with BWT with the exception of those with extensive tumor thrombus that does not respond to therapy and patients with anaplastic histology where clear margins cannot be obtained. In patients with anaplastic histology where clear margins cannot be obtained with a partial nephrectomy, a complete nephrectomy is mandated. There are several practical considerations to remember with nephron-sparing surgery. Preoperative imaging is very useful to help plan the operation. Furthermore, the size of the renal lesion(s) does not appear to influence resectability. Large lesions compress adjacent normal kidney parenchyma such that more viable renal parenchyma exists than may have been anticipated by the preoperative imaging studies.[183,184] Once the tumor is removed, the kidney volume can appear remarkably normal as these patients are followed over time. This argues for an attempt at nephron-sparing surgery for all lesions.

RADIOTHERAPY CONSIDERATIONS

Wilms' tumor is a very radiosensitive tumor. In 1950, Gross and Neuhauser published encouraging results in children treated with nephrectomy and postoperative irradiation. The first dose of irradiation was administered immediately after nephrectomy while the child was still under general anesthesia. By using this approach, the survival was 47% in children of all ages. No child in this report received chemotherapy.[185] The discovery of effective chemotherapeutic agents and their incorporation into clinical protocols for the treatment of Wilms' tumor had a profound impact not only on the general management of these children but also on the indications for the administration of postnephrectomy abdominal irradiation.

Abdominal Irradiation

The NWTSG trials 1 through 3 greatly refined the indications for and dosages of abdominal irradiation for children with Wilms' tumor. The major radiotherapy conclusions of these studies were that (1) the majority of children with Wilms' tumor who have either stage I or II tumors do not require any irradiation, (2) those who need irradiation (stage III tumors) require only 10 Gy with vincristine/dactinomycin/doxorubicin therapy, and (3) no dose-response association was detected for doses ranging from 18 Gy in younger children to 40 Gy in older children.[186–188]

Lung Metastases

Whole-lung irradiation (WLI) has long been recommended by the NWTSG for patients with pulmonary metastases visible on plain chest radiographs. However, a study conducted by

SIOP withheld WLI for lung metastases that resolved with chemotherapy and/or surgical resection. This approach produced similar outcomes to those of the NWTSG, but patients received substantially higher doses of doxorubicin than were used in the NWTSG protocols.[189] The UKCCSG, using a similar approach as SIOP, reported results that were inferior to those of the NWTSG in this group of patients.[190] In the subsequent UKCCSG Wilms' tumor study (UKWT2), the majority of children with lung metastases received WLI and the 4-year survival rate improved to 75%.[191] Another UKCCSG report revealed that children with stage IV lung metastases detected on chest x-ray had a significantly worse outcome when treated with 3 drugs alone (doxorubicin dose of 360 mg/m²) without WLI compared with those who received WLI and lower dose of doxorubicin (300 mg/m²). The event-free survival was 53.3% versus 79.2%. However there was no significant difference in overall survival (73.2% vs. 84.7%).[192]

A recent report suggested that children with favorable-histology Wilms' tumor and CT-only lung metastases registered on NWTS-4 and NWTS-5 had inferior relapse-free survival rates with two-drug chemotherapy with or without WLI compared with those who received doxorubicin. There were no additional benefits to WLI when doxorubicin was added to two-drug chemotherapy.[193] A report from the UKCCSG also showed a significantly higher pulmonary relapse rate (43%) in children with CT positive disease compared with 10% with normal CT scans among patients with stage I tumors and small pulmonary metastases treated with single agent vincristine alone.[137]

The COG study AREN0533 is evaluating the use of chemotherapy response rate to predict for the need of WLI. Those patients with stage IV favorable-histology Wilms' tumor with pulmonary metastases who have complete resolution of the pulmonary lesions after 6 weeks of vincristine/dactinomycin/doxorubicin chemotherapy will continue the same chemotherapy without WLI. However, those who do not have resolution of pulmonary metastases by week 6 will have addition of cyclophosphamide and etoposide to the other three drugs and WLI.

Tumor Spillage and Peritoneal Implants

The NWTSG evaluated the frequency with which spilled tumor cells of favorable-histology produced intra-abdominal disease recurrence in NWTS-3 and NWTS-4. Surgical tumor spillage was identified in 22% of patients analyzed. Flank irradiation, but not doxorubicin, reduced abdominal relapse rates. The odds ratio for the risk of recurrence relative to no radiation was 0.35 for 10 Gy and 0.08 for 20 Gy. Tumor spillage resulted in a higher relapse rate and significantly lower survival rates among stage II patients.[174]

In a report from NWTS-4 and NWTS-5, children with favorable-histology tumors and peritoneal implants were shown to have excellent survival after treatment with DD4 A chemotherapy and whole-abdomen irradiation. The whole-abdomen irradiation dose was 10.5 Gy in 88% of patients. The overall abdominal and systemic tumor control rates were 97% and 93%, respectively, and the 5-year event-free survival was 90%.[174]

Anaplastic Wilms' Tumor

The optimal irradiation dose for anaplastic Wilms' tumor remains unknown. Although diffuse anaplastic tumors are thought to be resistant to chemotherapy, these tumors have not shown a radiation dose response between 10 and 40 Gy.[156] Therefore, in NWTS-5, it was decided to treat patients with stage II and III abdominal tumors with 10 Gy. The 4-year event-free survival in stage II and III diffuse anaplastic tumors after immediate nephrectomy, irradiation, and regimen I chemotherapy was 82.6% and 64.7%, respectively.[80] Half the recurrences in stage III disease were local, suggesting that the dose of 10 Gy was not adequate for this group of patients. Patients with stage I focal or diffuse anaplasia were treated without abdominal irradiation in NWTS-5, with resulting 4-year event-free and overall survival estimates of only 69.5% and 82.6%. These results form the basis for the current COG study that recommends addition of irradiation for patients with stage I focal or diffuse anaplasia and augmentation of irradiation for patients with stage III diffuse anaplasia.[80]

Treatment Recommendations

Megavoltage x-rays (4 to 6 MV) are recommended. The recommended daily dose per fraction is 1.8 Gy. However, the fraction size may be reduced to 1.5 Gy when large volumes, such as the whole abdomen or the whole lungs, are irradiated. The use of immobilization devices and CT simulation is essential for accurate treatment delivery.

NWTS-1 and NWTS-2 have shown that although irradiation does not need to be given immediately after surgery, a delay of 10 days or more after surgery was associated with a significantly higher abdominal relapse, particularly among patients with unfavorable-histology tumors.[186,188,194] However, in a recent analysis of patients with favorable-histology tumors in NWTS-3 and NWTS-4, a delay of 10 or more days did not demonstrably influence abdominal tumor recurrence rates.[195] Thus, in the COG protocols it is recommended that abdominal irradiation be delivered as soon as practical after nephrectomy and not later than 14 days after surgery.

The COG radiation indications and dosages for Wilms' tumor, clear cell sarcoma, and rhabdoid tumor are summarized in Table 29.5. The tumor bed is defined as the kidney and its associated lesion as they are visualized on preoperative imaging studies. A planning margin of 1 cm is advised all around the tumor bed. The portal is always extended medially to include the entire vertebral column at the implicated levels. The field is extended as needed to include the para-aortic chains when para-aortic nodes are found to be involved (Fig. 29.9). The portal for whole-abdominal irradiation includes all the peritoneal surfaces and extends from the domes of the diaphragm to the inferior margins of the obturator foramina. External beam blocks are introduced to shield the femoral heads. For stage IV disease, abdominal irradiation is given only to patients whose primary tumor is classified as abdominal stage III.

For whole-lung irradiation, the entire thoracic cavity is irradiated without shielding, except for the humeral heads. The field extends from the apex of the lung to the posterior inferior recesses of the costophrenic sulci inferiorly with a margin of at least 1 cm. The inferior border of the whole-lung portal may extend to the bottom of T12 or lower (Fig. 29.10). If the lungs and either flank or abdomen have to be treated simultaneously, it is preferable to include them in one irradiation portal.

For liver metastases, only those that are unresectable at diagnosis are irradiated. The treatment portal includes that portion of the liver known to be involved as identified by CT or MRI studies. The whole liver is treated in children with diffuse metastases.

CHEMOTHERAPY

Historically, the largest clinical trials for Wilms' tumor and other renal malignancies of childhood have been conducted by

TABLE 29.5

RADIATION THERAPY GUIDELINES IN CHILDREN'S ONCOLOGY GROUP STUDIES

Treatment site	Clinical presentation and dose	
Flank irradiation	Stage III FH	
Patients with residual tumor will receive supplemental irradiation with 10.8 Gy.	Stage I–III FA Stage I–II DA Stage I–III CCSK	10.8 Gy
	Stage III DA Stage I–III MRT	19.8 Gy (10.8 Gy for patients ≤12 mo)
Whole-abdomen irradiation (WAI)	Stage III FH, FA, CCSK	
Patients with residual tumor will receive supplemental irradiation with 10.5 Gy.	(a) Cytology-positive ascites (b) Any preoperative tumor rupture (c) Diffuse surgical spillage (d) Peritoneal seeding	10.5 Gy
	Stage III DA, MRT (a) Cytology-positive ascites (b) Any preoperative tumor rupture (c) Diffuse surgical spillage (d) Peritoneal seeding	21.0 Gy (10.5 Gy for patients ≤12 mo)
Whole-lung irradiation (WLI)	Lung metastases	10.5 Gy; age <12 mo 12 Gy; age ≥12 mo
Whole-brain irradiation	Brain metastases	21.6 Gy + 10.8 Gy boost; age <16 yr 30.6 Gy; age ≥16 yr
Liver irradiation	Focal metastases Diffuse metastases	19.8 Gy 19.8 Gy
Bone irradiation	Bone metastases	25.2 Gy; age <16 yr 30.6 Gy; age ≥16 yr
Lymph node irradiation	Resected LN metastases Unresected LN metastases	10.8 Gy 19.8 Gy

CCSK, clear cell sarcoma of kidney; CR, complete response; DA, diffuse anaplasia; FA, focal anaplasia; FH, favorable histology; Gy, gray; MRT, malignant rhabdoid tumor; WT, Wilms' tumor.

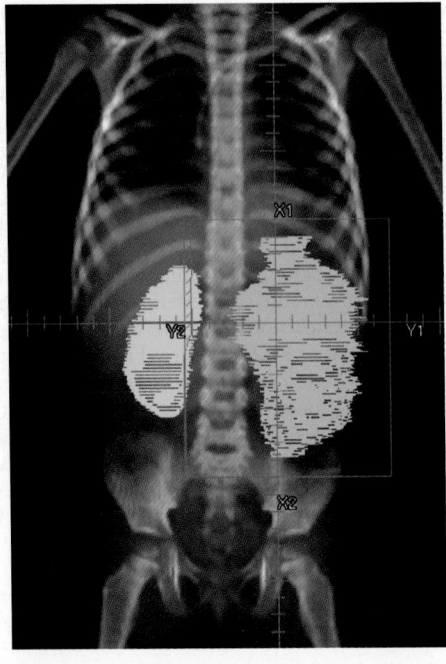

FIGURE 29.9 A typical flank irradiation field in a child with left-sided Wilms' tumor. The preoperative CT scan–based tumor volume is shown in *blue* and the right kidney is shown in *yellow*.

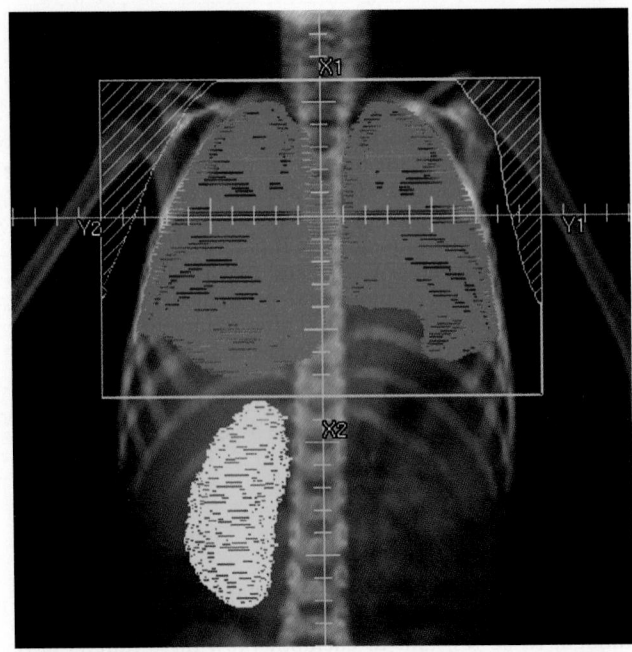

FIGURE 29.10 A typical whole-lung irradiation field in a child with left-sided Wilms' tumor and lung metastases. The total lung volume is shown in *red* and the right kidney is shown in *yellow*.

TABLE 29.6

OUTCOMES FOR PEDIATRIC RENAL TUMORS

Stage	Relapse-free survival (%)	Overall survival (%)
Favorable-histology Wilms' tumor without LOH[a]		
I (≥24 mo/tumor weight ≥550 g)	94.2	98.4
II	86.2	97.7
III	86.5	94.4
IV	76.4	86.1
Diffuse anaplastic Wilms' tumor[b]		
I	68.4	78.9
II	82.6	81.5
III	64.7	66.7
IV	33.3	33.3
V	25.1	41.6
Clear cell sarcoma[c]		
I	100	100
II	86.8	97.3
III	73.8	86.9
IV	35.6	45.0
Rhabdoid tumor[d]		
I	—	33.3
II	—	46.9
III	—	21.8
IV	—	8.4
Renal cell carcinoma[e]		
I	—	92.4
II	—	84.6
III	—	72.7
IV	—	13.9

[a]Figures represent 4-yr survival estimates.[57]
[b]Figures represent 4-yr survival estimates.[80]
[c]Figures represent 5-yr survival estimates.[201]
[d]Figures represent survival estimates for patients treated on NWTS-1–5.[157]
[e]Figures represent percentage of patients alive from an extensive literature review.[202]

the National Wilms Tumor Study Group (NWTSG), based in North America, and the International Society of Pediatric Oncology (SIOP), based in Europe. Although these two cooperative groups have generally used similar chemotherapeutic agents, their treatment approaches are fundamentally different in that the NWTSG recommends upfront nephrectomy whereas SIOP advocates preoperative chemotherapy. Both approaches yield excellent outcomes for patients with favorable-histology Wilms' tumor,[57,158,190,196–200] whereas outcomes for the other renal malignancies are suboptimal (Table 29.6).

In 2002, the NWTSG joined the COG, and shortly thereafter, the first COG Renal Tumor Committee protocols were launched internationally at participating COG sites. The following discussion focuses on the treatment regimens developed by the COG, treatment of relapsed Wilms' tumor, and an update of novel therapy initiatives.

Favorable-Histology Wilms' Tumor

The use of dactinomycin for the adjuvant treatment of children with Wilms' tumor was pioneered by Farber et al.[203] Subsequently, other agents with activity against Wilms'

tumor were identified, including vincristine, doxorubicin, and cyclophosphamide.[122] On the basis of the activity of these drugs as single agents, the NWTSG initiated a series of clinical trials (NWTS-1–4) to evaluate the efficacy of different chemotherapy combinations and treatment schedules.[186,187,197,198,204–206]

By the end of NWTS-4, survival for favorable-histology Wilms' tumor approximated 90%, so the primary goal of NWTS-5 (1995–2002) was to identify novel biologic prognostic markers for favorable-histology Wilms' tumor. LOH at chromosomes 1p and 16q, DNA ploidy, telomerase expression, and expression of multidrug-resistance proteins were evaluated. Patients with stage II disease received vincristine and dactinomycin (Regimen EE-4 A), and patients with stages III and IV disease received vincristine, dactinomycin, and doxorubicin (Regimen DD-4 A). Concurrent LOH for chromosomes 1p and 16q, found in approximately 5% of favorable-histology Wilms' tumors, was demonstrated to be statistically significantly associated with a relative risk of relapse and death of 2.9 ($p = 0.001$) and 4.3 ($p = 0.01$), respectively, for patients with stage I/II disease combined, and 2.4 ($p = 0.01$) and 2.7 ($p = 0.04$), respectively, for patients with stage III/IV disease combined.[57] These findings form the basis of molecular stratification of patients on the current COG favorable-histology Wilms' tumor treatment protocols.

A second objective of NWTS-5 tested the hypothesis that young patients (younger than 24 months) with 'small' stage I favorable-histology Wilms' tumors [nephrectomy specimens (combined tumor and kidney) weighing less than 550 grams] could be treated with surgery alone without adjuvant chemotherapy.[207] Eight of 75 such patients experienced recurrence to the lung ($n = 5$) or operative bed ($n = 3$) and three patients developed metachronous contralateral Wilms' tumor, resulting in a 2-year disease-free survival estimate of 86.5%.[159] On the basis of predefined stopping rules, this arm of the study was closed early with a recommendation that future patients fulfilling this category receive Regimen EE-4 A as adjuvant chemotherapy. However, additional analysis revealed a 2-year overall survival rate of 100%.

The successes of NWTS-1–5 in both improving treatment outcomes and in identifying molecular tumor markers predictive of adverse outcomes form the basis of the current COG favorable-histology Wilms' tumor studies. The objectives of these studies are to (1) reassess whether omitting adjuvant therapy is okay for patients with very low risk favorable-histology Wilms' tumors (stage I, age <2 years, nephrectomy specimen plus tumor weight <550 grams) and to evaluate biological markers for this very low risk group, (2) evaluate whether augmentation of therapy improves outcomes for patients with LOH at 1p and 16q, (3) evaluate whether patients with stage IV disease based on pulmonary lesions only (no other sites of metastases) whose lung disease disappears by CT imaging after 6 weeks of DD-4 A therapy have good outcomes without lung radiation, and (4) evaluate whether patients with stage IV disease whose lung nodules do not disappear after 6 weeks of chemotherapy have improved outcomes with a new regimen containing cyclophosphamide/etoposide (Regimen M). Results for AREN0532 and AREN0533 are not available at the time of this publication, and as such, the NWTS-5 treatment approach listed in Figure 29.11 remains a reasonable standard of care for the treatment of patients with favorable-histology Wilms' tumor.

Anaplastic Wilms' Tumor

NWTS-3 and NWTS-4 were the first studies to prospectively evaluate the benefit of additional therapy for patients with anaplastic Wilms' tumor. On these randomized studies, patients

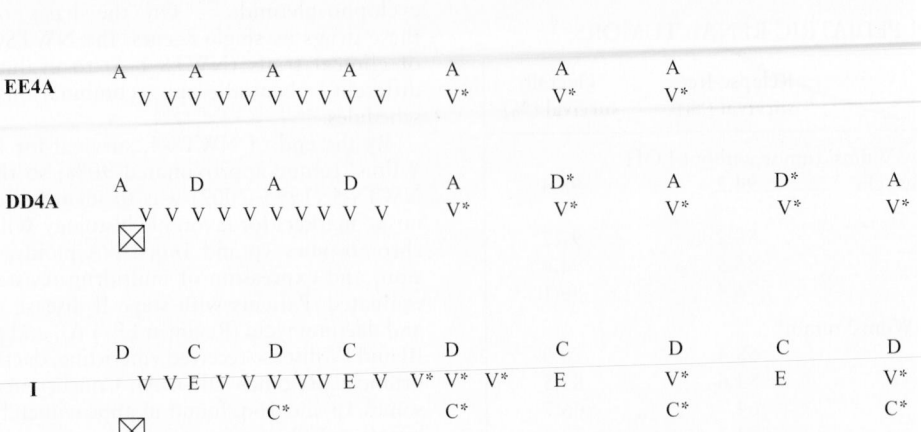

FIGURE 29.11 Treatment regimens used on National Wilms Tumor Study-5: A—dactinomycin (0.045 mg/kg/day × 1; 1.35 mg/m²/day × 1 day for weight >30 kg, max 2.3 mg); V—vincristine (0.05 mg/kg/day × 1; 1.5 mg/m²/day × 1 for weight >30 kg, max 2 mg); V*—vincristine (0.067 mg/kg/day × 1; 2 mg/m²/day × 1 for weight >30 kg, max, 2 mg); D—doxorubicin (1.5 mg/kg/day × 1; 45 mg/m²/day × 1 for weight >30 kg); D*—doxorubicin (1 mg/kg/day × 1; 30 mg/m²/day × 1 for weight >30 kg); C—cyclophosphamide (14.7 mg/kg/day × 5; 440 mg/m²/day × 5 for weight >30 kg); C*—cyclophosphamide (14.7 mg/kg/day × 3; 440 mg/m²/day × 3 for weight >30 kg); E—etoposide (3.3 mg/kg/day × 5; 100 mg/m²/day × 5 for weight >30 kg); X—radiation therapy. All doses decreased by 50% for infants <12 months old.

received 15 months of vincristine, dactinomycin, and doxorubicin, with or without cyclophosphamide. For patients with stages II to IV diffuse anaplastic histology, the addition of cyclophosphamide revealed an increase in the 4-year relapse-free survival estimate from 27.2% when treated without cyclophosphamide to 54.8% when treated with cyclophosphamide (*p* = 0.02).[156]

Of the 2,596 patients enrolled on NWTS-5, 281 (10.8%) were found to have anaplastic histology on central review.[80] On NWTS-5, patients with stage I diffuse anaplastic Wilms' tumor were treated with regimen EE-4 A based on the excellent outcomes for this patient group on previous studies. The 4-year event-free and overall survival estimates for stage I diffuse anaplastic Wilms' tumor were 69.5% and 82.6%, respectively, suggesting that regimen EE-4 A is inadequate for these patients. Patients with stage II to IV diffuse anaplastic Wilms' tumor were treated with vincristine, doxorubicin, and cyclophosphamide (VDC) alternating with cyclophosphamide and etoposide (CyE) (Regimen I). The 4-year event-free survival estimates for stages II to IV diffuse anaplastic Wilms' tumor on NWTS-5 were 82.6%, 64.7%, and 33.3%, respectively, with similar overall survival. Patients on NWTS-5 with bilateral Wilms' tumor and anaplastic features had a 4-year event-free and overall survival of 43.8% and 55.2%, respectively.[80] These findings, along with the preclinical and clinical evidence showing that protracted therapy with camptothecin chemotherapeutic agents is active against highly resistant Wilms' tumor,[208] form the basis for the current COG AREN0321 study for very high-risk renal tumors. This new protocol is testing the efficacy of a new carboplatin-containing regimen (Regimen UH-1) as well as the activity of vincristine/irinotecan in a phase II window study for patients with stage IV diffuse anaplastic Wilms' tumor.

Clear Cell Sarcoma of the Kidney

Data from NWTS-1 to NWTS-3 suggested that the addition of doxorubicin to the combination of vincristine and dactinomycin improved the 6-year relapse-free survival percentage for patients with clear cell sarcoma of the kidney (CCSK), although the improvement did not achieve conventional levels of statistical significance.[209] The beneficial effect of doxorubicin therapy was confirmed in a retrospective review of 351 cases including 182 cases from NWTS-1 through NWTS-4.[84] Hence, doxorubicin has become a standard component of therapy for CCSK. NWTS-4 randomized patients with CCSK to receive 6 or 15 months of therapy with vincristine, dactinomycin, and doxorubicin. Eight-year relapse-free survival estimates were superior in the patients who received the longer duration of therapy (60.6% vs. 87.8%); however, overall survival was similar.[210] With the knowledge that the combination of ifosfamide and etoposide (IE) demonstrated activity against other sarcomas[211,212] NWTS-5 tested the effectiveness of regimen I, which uses cyclophosphamide and etoposide (CyE), against CCSK. Preliminary results from NWTS-5 revealed that among 79 patients treated with CCSK, 12 relapsed (77.6% 4-year relapse-free survival). Six of the relapses occurred in the 9 patients presenting with stage IV disease. Thus, regimen I appears to compare favorably to the prolonged regimen of vincristine, dactinomycin, and doxorubicin used in NWTS-4 and is recommended as an appropriate treatment regimen for patients with stage I to III CCSK in the absence of a clinical trial.

A recent report of 8 children with recurrent CCSK and brain metastases demonstrated that there may be a trend for a shift in relapse patterns to predominantly include the brain. Ifosfamide, carboplatin, and etoposide (ICE) chemotherapy in combination with surgery and radiation proved highly effective for the majority of these patients with recurrent CCSK, as 6 of the 8 reported have maintained a second remission for a median follow-up of 30 months.[213]

Rhabdoid Tumor of the Kidney

Patients with rhabdoid tumor of the kidney (RTK) were historically treated in NWTS trials with regimens used for the treatment of Wilms' tumor, including vincristine, dactinomycin, and doxorubicin, with or without cyclophosphamide.

The outcomes attained with these regimens were poor.[90] NWTS-5 adopted a different treatment strategy consisting of carboplatin and etoposide alternating with cyclophosphamide (Regimen RTK). Preliminary analysis of patients treated with regimen RTK revealed that this regimen was unlikely to demonstrate an improvement compared with previous studies, and this treatment arm was closed. Case reports have demonstrated that ifosfamide-carboplatin-etoposide (ICE) or ifosfamide-etoposide (IE) chemotherapy alternating with vincristine-doxorubicin-cyclophosphamide is effective against metastatic rhabdoid tumor of the kidney.[214,215] As such, patients with malignant rhabdoid tumor (MRT) (of the kidney or any other nonintracranial primary site) who enroll on the current COG AREN0321 study are treated with Regimen UH-1 (VDC/CyCE). Novel agents are desperately needed for patients with MRT.

Renal Cell Carcinoma

The NWTSG historically did not study pediatric renal cell carcinoma (RCC), although Surveillance, Epidemiology, and End Results (SEER) data indicate that RCC represents 5.9% of pediatric renal malignancies. A systematic review of the literature revealed that like adult RCC, survival rates for pediatric RCC decrease with advancing stage: I (90%), II (80%), III (70%), and IV (15%), though children and adolescents with RCC and local lymph node involvement appear to have a more favorable outcome compared with adult RCC patients with a similar presentation.[202] The clinical differences between adult and pediatric RCC may be explained, at least in part, by the recent acknowledgment that a majority of pediatric RCC is of the translocation morphology subtype, with elevated expression of the TFE3 or TFEB transcription factors.[111,120]

The optimal treatment for pediatric or translocation RCC is unknown. Most reported patients received some form of chemotherapy (typically Wilms' tumor therapy), although the consensus from adult studies is that traditional chemotherapy agents are not highly effective. Several children with RCC received interleukin-2 (IL-2) or interferon-alfa, with case reports of responses.[216,217] However, it is not clear which histologic subtype of RCC responded to immunotherapy. Recent preclinical investigation has demonstrated that translocation RCC demonstrates a genomic signature more similar to alveolar soft part sarcoma (ASPS) rather than adult-type clear cell RCC.[218] Published experience in adults with 'sarcomatoid' RCC suggests a possible treatment effect with gemcitabine/doxorubicin-based therapy,[219] and anecdotal evidence from the authors suggests that a subset of pediatric/translocation RCCs may respond to such therapy. In addition, like the fusion product found in ASPS, TFE3 fusion products bind to the c-Met promoter causing pathway activation, and providing one reasonable molecular target for this disease.[220] A phase II study of c-Met inhibition is currently underway for the treatment of translocation RCC for patients aged 13 years and older. Clinical efficacy data of anti-VEGF or anti-mTOR therapies for pediatric or translocation RCC are not yet available.

On the basis of the favorable outcomes for most children with localized and completely resected RCC, including those with completely resected involved local lymph nodes,[120,202] the COG AREN0321 study is not providing adjuvant therapy to prospectively accrued patients. By contrast, the poor outcomes associated with stage IV disease warrant the use of medical therapies.

Recurrent Wilms' Tumor

Approximately 15% of patients with favorable-histology Wilms' tumor and 50% of patients with anaplastic Wilms'

tumor experience recurrence. Most recurrences occur within 2 years of diagnosis and the most common sites of recurrence are the lungs and pleura, tumor bed, and liver.[221] Less frequently, recurrences can occur in the bone, brain, and distant lymph nodes. Most "recurrences" in the contralateral kidney likely represent second primary tumors rather than true relapses.

Children with relapsed Wilms' tumor have a variable prognosis that depends upon their initial stage, histology, site of relapse, time from initial diagnosis to relapse, and previous therapy. Favorable prognostic factors include favorable histology, no prior treatment with doxorubicin, relapse more than 6 to 12 months after diagnosis, and subdiaphragmatic relapse in a patient not previously given abdominal irradiation.[221,222]

Treatment regimens for recurrent Wilms' tumor are designed to include chemotherapy agents that were not used during primary therapy. Several highly effective chemotherapy combinations, including ifosfamide-carboplatin-etoposide (ICE), cyclophosphamide-etoposide, and carboplatin-etoposide, are considered first-line treatment for recurrent disease. Although surgical excision of pulmonary metastases does not improve outcome, surgical biopsy or excision of recurrence should nonetheless be performed to histologically confirm the presence of recurrent disease, and particularly in the case of intra-abdominal recurrence, to reduce the tumor burden prior to the initiation of radiation therapy and combination chemotherapy.[223]

Whereas the salvage rate for patients with recurrent favorable-histology Wilms' tumor was historically 25% to 40%,[221,224] modern treatment combinations have improved the survival rate postrecurrence.[222,225-227] For patients who have relapsed after initial treatment with vincristine and dactinomycin treated on the NWTS-5 stratum B protocol (surgical resection, radiation therapy, and alternating courses of vincristine/doxorubicin/cyclophosphamide and etoposide/cyclophosphamide), the 4-year event-free and overall survival were 71.1% and 81.8%, respectively.[225] For patients who have relapsed after initial treatment with vincristine, dactinomycin, and doxorubicin treated on the NWTS-5 stratum C protocol (surgical resection, radiation therapy, and alternating courses of cyclophosphamide/etoposide and carboplatin/etoposide), the 4-year event-free and overall survival were only 42.3% and 48%, respectively, suggesting the need for novel agents for the treatment of relapsed Wilms' tumor.[226]

The effective use of high-dose therapy with stem cell rescue for the treatment of recurrent Wilms' tumor has been reported by several groups, with event-free or disease-free survival rates of 36% to 60%,[228-232] comparable to that achieved with conventional chemotherapy. There is a suggestion that patients most likely to achieve long-term disease control following high-dose therapy with stem cell rescue are those with chemotherapy-sensitive disease, preferably in complete remission at the time of high-dose consolidative therapy.[232] Given the limitations inherent in small retrospective series, a larger prospective randomized study will be necessary to determine whether stem cell transplant provides any advantage over standard chemotherapy with regard to efficacy, in balance of likely increased morbidity, for relapsed Wilms' tumor.

Novel Agents for the Treatment of Pediatric Renal Tumors

The prognosis for patients with relapsed Wilms' tumor, anaplastic Wilms' tumor, malignant rhabdoid tumor, and advanced stage clear cell sarcoma of the kidney and RCC remains unsatisfactory. Further medical advance for the treatment of such patients depends on the discovery and early phase development of novel agents.

Phase II investigations of novel agents for patients with relapsed Wilms' tumor have been informative. Low signal activity was noted in relapsed Wilms' tumor patients treated with paclitaxel on the Pediatric Oncology Group study POG 9262 where among 15 patients, 2 responded and 4 showed disease stabilization for a response rate and clinical benefit rate of 13% and 40%, respectively.[233] The development of dactinomycin in combination with recombinant tumor necrosis factor-alpha for Wilms' tumor was halted because of the unavailability of rTNF, though a 15% complete response rate (3/19) was noted in relapsed Wilms' tumor patients treated with this combination.[234] Recently, protracted topotecan (daily × 5 × 2 consecutive weeks) has been shown to be active in relapsed Wilms' tumor, with 12 partial remissions and 6 with stable disease out of the 25 assessable patients with relapsed favorable-histology Wilms' tumor (response rate = 48%), and 2 partial remissions and 1 stable disease among the 11 assessable patients with relapsed anaplastic histology Wilms' tumor, providing the rationale for further study of camptothecin agents in the high-risk Wilms' tumors.[208]

LONG-TERM TOXICITIES

Cardiac

Higher stage patients (III and IV) have been receiving anthracyclines since the 1970s. The cumulative dose of anthracyclines on current front-line high-risk COG protocols for stage III and IV FH WT is 150 mg/m^2, which is much lower than earlier NWTS protocols, where total anthracycline doses exceeded 300 mg/m^2 in the majority of patients. The cumulative frequency of congestive heart failure in patients treated on NWTS-1–4 was 4.4% at 20 years for patients treated initially with doxorubicin, but that figure is expected to be lower with current cumulative doses.[235] The risk of late cardiac toxicity is exacerbated by left flank radiotherapy, lung radiation, and female sex of the patient.[236,237] It appears that the risk of cardiotoxicity caused by currently used lower doses of radiation is much less, but emerging evidence demonstrates an increased life-time risk of developing cardiac dysfunction including vascular abnormalities.[236,238]

Lung

Radiation therapy is particularly injurious to very young children with respect to growth and development. Acute lung injury is relatively uncommon, occurring in a minority of children.[239] However, chronic late effects are more worrisome. Whole-lung radiation may cause a small thoracic cage, lower gas transfer per unit lung volume, and restrictive lung disease.[240,241] Even flank radiation is associated with capture of part of the lungs and thus lower mean percent predicted for forced expiratory volume in one second, residual volume, and total lung capacity.[242] Some of these patients may be symptomatic with exercise although this is uncommonly described at rest.

Renal

The incidence of end-stage renal failure in nonsyndromic unilateral Wilms' tumor is <1% at 20 years.[181,243] However, patients with Denys-Drash syndrome (75%), WAGR syndrome (36% to 90%), and those males with cryptorchidism or hypospadias (7%) all had significant rates of renal failure, some contributing to late mortality.[244] Similarly, patients with bilateral disease had an overall incidence of end-stage renal

disease (ESRD) of at least 14%.[180] Additional renal toxicity can be expected from exposure to ifosfamide, as cumulative doses of greater than 72 mg/m^2 are associated with the possibility of a permanent Fanconi syndrome. Lifelong nephrological follow-up for patients at significant risk of ESRD (syndromic unilateral patients and all bilateral patients) should be provided and proactive counseling discussed for renal protection in all those with just one kidney.[245]

Fertility

Male fertility is generally not at risk for compromise in Wilms' tumor therapy unless alkylators are used. On the other hand, female fertility may be impacted in several ways. In addition to the toxicity of alkylator therapy, radiation therapy to the abdomen may encompass the pelvic structures resulting in absent ovaries or a small uterus.[246] Abnormal ovarian function is very common, as are higher than expected spontaneous abortion rates, small-for-gestational-age infants, and prematurity in those who have received abdomino-pelvic radiation.[247–250] Premature menopause has also been documented to occur more frequently. All girls with a history of abdominal radiation should be considered as higher risk for pregnancy complications and have appropriate referrals for fertility and obstetrical care.

Second Malignancy

Pediatric patients with cancer have a well-recognized increased risk of second malignancy. The cumulative risk of 0.6% to 1.5% at 15 years following diagnosis is in part attributable to known carcinogens such as alkylating agents and radiotherapy.[238,251,252] Longer term studies suggest much higher rates of 12% at 50 years, but these risks are difficult to extrapolate to modern radiotherapy techniques and chemotherapy dosing.[253] Second malignancies include bone and soft tissue sarcomas, breast carcinoma, non-Hodgkin lymphoma, basal cell carcinoma, melanoma, gastrointestinal tract cancer, and acute leukemia, with an overall standardized incidence ratio of 4–8.[238] The majority of solid tumors occur within radiation fields, with an increased frequency seen with concurrent use of doxorubicin.

SURVEILLANCE AFTER THERAPY

The intensity and modality of imaging in follow-up for relapse vary between the COG and the SIOP.[136] The former uses more monitoring with CT scans for early detection of small recurrences, while the latter group tends to use more chest x-rays and abdominal ultrasounds. Each strategy has its theoretical merits. CT scans are associated with higher doses of ionizing radiation and detection of very small lesions of uncertain significance, while allowing for early intervention, perhaps before metastatic spread of isolated recurrences. On the other hand, less invasive monitoring is reasonably sensitive, requires no sedation, and no evidence exists that early detection of relapse impacts upon ultimate outcome.[136,254] Recommendations for surveillance after completion of therapy are shown in Table 29.7.

Renal tumors with anaplasia, RCC, and rhabdoid tumors all have a propensity for relatively early relapse in the first 2 to 4 years following treatment. Rhabdoid tumors and clear cell sarcoma of the kidney may have metastasis to the brain or bone, and thus, neuroimaging and bone scanning should be considered.[157,213] Unlike most renal tumors, CCSK has a

TABLE 29.7

RECOMMENDED IMAGING STUDIES FOR FOLLOW-UP

Patient characteristics	Imaging study	Schedule
Favorable-histology Wilms' tumor	Chest x-ray or CT chest Abdominal ultrasound[a]	Every 6 weeks until complete remission is documented; every 3 mo × 8, then every 6 mo × 4 Postoperatively after 6 weeks and 3 mo then every 3 mo × 8, then every 6 mo × 4
Anaplastic Wilms' tumor; Rhabdoid tumor	CT chest CT abdomen/pelvis Abdominal ultrasound/ Chest x-ray MRI brain (for rhabdoid tumor only)	Every 6 weeks until complete remission is documented; every 3 mo × 8 Postoperatively after 6 weeks and 3 mo then every 3 mo × 8 Starting 2 yr from end of therapy: every 6 mo × 4 Every 3 mo × 4, then every 6 mo × 2
Clear cell sarcoma; Renal cell carcinoma	Chest x-ray or CT chest Abdominal ultrasound or CT abdomen Bone scan MRI brain	Every 6 weeks until complete remission is documented; every 3 mo × 8, then every 6 mo × 6 Every 6 weeks until complete remission is documented; every 3 mo × 8, then every 6 mo × 6 Every 6 mo × 6 Every 6 mo × 6

[a]*Note:* Abdominal ultrasounds should be performed every 3 months until age 8 years for patients with bilateral Wilms' tumor or nephrogenic rests.

prolonged period of 10 years after diagnosis at risk for relapse, and thus, a higher index of suspicion and surveillance should be undertaken for these patients.[84]

Long-Term Follow-up

A recent study found that the standardized mortality ratio for Wilms' tumor survivors remained elevated beyond 10 years postdiagnosis and that an important contributor to this ratio was second malignant neoplasms.[238] This and other studies highlight the essential notion that patients must be informed of these risks, and made aware of life-style strategies to reduce risk. Appropriate surveillance should be undertaken such as breast screening for girls with thoracic radiation, endocrine screening for thyroid cancer, cardiac and lung function for those with thoracic radiation, and ovarian function in those with abdominal radiation.

While long-term toxicity of chemotherapy, surgery, and radiation in the setting of Wilms' tumor may have very significant impact upon some long-term survivors, these are in the minority (<20%).[255] The majority of children with Wilms' tumor are cured and have few, if any, late effects. Careful monitoring and education are key to supporting long-term survivors who are at higher risk or who have suffered complications. Reduction of personal life-style risks such as smoking, obesity, lack of exercise, and unsafe sun exposure are all discussions that should routinely occur with childhood cancer survivors.[256] Continuing refinement of risk categories should assist in reducing therapeutic burdens, both acute and chronic, with disease destined to be cured by less intense therapies.

ACKNOWLEDGMENTS

The authors thank the investigators of the Children's Oncology Group and the National Wilms' Tumor Study Group and the many professionals who managed the children entered on cooperative group renal tumor studies. The authors are indebted to the following individuals for their enduring contributions to pediatric renal tumor research and for authoring previous editions of this chapter: Drs. Bruce Beckwith, Norman Breslow, Max Coppes, Dan D'Angio, Daniel Green, Roger Macklis, Elizabeth Perlman, and Michael Ritchey. This work was supported in part by a grant to the Children's Oncology Group, NIH CA-42326.

References

1. Horner MJ, Ries LAG, Krapcho M, et al. SEER Cancer Statistics Review, 1975–2006. Bethesda, Maryland: National Cancer Institute, 2009. http://seer.cancer.gov
2. Breslow N, Olshan A, Beckwith JB, et al. Epidemiology of Wilms tumor. Med Pediatr Oncol 1993;21:172–181.
3. Dome JS, Coppes MJ. Recent advances in Wilms tumor genetics. Curr Opin Pediatr 2002;14:5–11.
4. Scott RH, Stiller CA, Walker L, et al. Syndromes and constitutional chromosomal abnormalities associated with Wilms tumour. J Med Genet 2006;43:705–715.
5. Kantor AF, Curnen MG, Meigs JW, et al. Occupations of fathers of patients with Wilms's tumour. J Epidemiol Community Health 1979;33:253–256.
6. Wilkins JR III, Sinks TH Jr. Paternal occupation and Wilms' tumour in offspring. J Epidemiol Community Health 1984;38:7–11.
7. Bunin GR, Nass CC, Kramer S, et al. Parental occupation and Wilms' tumor: results of a case-control study. Cancer Res 1989;49:725–729.
8. Olshan A, Breslow N, Faletta JM, et al. Risk factors for Wilms tumor: report from the National Wilms Tumor Study. Cancer 1993;72:938–944.
9. Knudson AG, Strong LC. Mutation and cancer: a model for Wilms' tumor of the kidney. J Nat Cancer Inst 1972;48:313–324.
10. Riccardi VM, Sujansky E, Smith AC, et al. Chromosomal imbalance in the Aniridia-Wilms' tumor association: 11p interstitial deletion. Pediatrics 1978;61:604–610.
11. Bonetta L, Kuehn SE, Huang A, et al. Wilms tumor locus on 11p13 defined by multiple CpG island-associated transcripts. Science 1990;250:994–997.
12. Gessler M, Poustka A, Cavenee W, et al. Homozygous deletion in Wilms tumours of a zinc-finger gene identified by chromosome jumping. Nature 1990;343:774–778.
13. Xu S, Han JC, Morales A, et al. Characterization of 11p14-p12 deletion in WAGR syndrome by array CGH for identifying genes contributing to mental retardation and autism. Cytogenet Genome Res 2008;122:181–187.
14. Discenza MT, Pelletier J. Insights into the physiological role of WT1 from studies of genetically modified mice. Physiol Genomics 2004;16:287–300.

15. Pelletier J, Bruening W, Kashtan CE, et al. Germline mutations in the Wilms' tumor suppressor gene are associated with abnormal urogenital development in Denys–Drash syndrome. Cell 1991;67:437–447.
16. Huff V. Wilms tumor genetics. Am J Med Genet 1998;79:260–267.
17. Little SE, Hanks SP, King-Underwood L, et al. Frequency and heritability of WT1 mutations in nonsyndromic Wilms' tumor patients: a UK Children's Cancer Study Group Study. J Clin Oncol 2004;22:4140–4146.
18. Rivera MN, Kim WJ, Wells J, et al. An X chromosome gene, WTX, is commonly inactivated in Wilms tumor. Science 2007;315:642–645.
19. Jenkins ZA, van KM, Morgan T, et al. Germline mutations in WTX cause a sclerosing skeletal dysplasia but do not predispose to tumorigenesis. Nat Genet 2009;41:95–100.
20. Rivera MN, Kim WJ, Wells J, et al. The tumor suppressor WTX shuttles to the nucleus and modulates WT1 activity. Proc Natl Acad Sci U S A 2009;106:8338–8343.
21. Major MB, Camp ND, Berndt JD, et al. Wilms tumor suppressor WTX negatively regulates WNT/beta-catenin signaling. Science 2007;316:1043–1046.
22. Su MC, Huang WC, Lien HC. Beta-catenin expression and mutation in adult and pediatric Wilms' tumors. APMIS 2008;116:771–778.
23. Nusse R. Cancer. Converging on beta-catenin in Wilms tumor. Science 2007;316: 988–989.
24. Koesters R, Ridder R, Kopp-Schneider A, et al. Mutational activation of the β-catenin proto-oncogene is a common event in the development of Wilms tumors. Cancer Res 1999;59:3880–3882.
25. Ruteshouser EC, Robinson SM, Huff V. Wilms tumor genetics: mutations in WT1, WTX, and CTNNB1 account for only about one-third of tumors. Genes Chromosomes Cancer 2008;47:461–470.
26. Koufos A, Grundy P, Morgan K, et al. Familial Wiedemann-Beckwith syndrome and a second Wilms tumor locus both map to 11p15.5. Am J Hum Genet 1989;44: 711–719.
27. Ping AJ, Reeve AE, Law DJ, et al. Genetic linkage of Beckwith-Wiedemann syndrome to 11p15. Am J Hum Genet 1989;44:720–723.
28. Schroeder WT, Chao LY, Dao DD, et al. Nonrandom loss of maternal chromosome 11 alleles in Wilms tumors. Am J Hum Genet 1987;40:413–420.
29. DeBaun MR, Niemitz EL, McNeil DE, et al. Epigenetic alterations of H19 and LIT1 distinguish patients with Beckwith-Wiedemann syndrome with cancer and birth defects. Am J Hum Genet 2002;70:604–611.
30. Riccio A, Sparago A, Verde G, et al. Inherited and sporadic epimutations at the IGF2-H19 locus in Beckwith-Wiedemann syndrome and Wilms' tumor. Endocr Dev 2009; 14:1–9.
31. Rainier S, Johnson LA, Dobry CJ, et al. Relaxation of imprinted genes in human cancer. Nature 1993;362:747–749.
32. Ravenel JD, Broman KW, Perlman EJ, et al. Loss of imprinting of insulin-like growth factor-II (IGF2) gene in distinguishing specific biologic subtypes of Wilms tumor. J Natl Cancer Inst 2001;93:1698–1703.
33. Cui H, Niemitz EL, Ravenel JD, et al. Loss of imprinting of insulin-like growth factor-II in Wilms' tumor commonly involves altered methylation but not mutations of CTCF or its binding site. Cancer Res 2001;61:4947–4950.
34. Hao Y, Crenshaw T, Moulton T, et al. Tumour-suppressor activity of H19 RNA. Nature 1993;365:764–767.
35. Natrajan R, Little SE, Reis-Filho JS, et al. Amplification and overexpression of CACNA1E correlates with relapse in favorable histology Wilms' tumors. Clin Cancer Res 2006;12(24):7284–7293.
36. Scott RH, Douglas J, Baskcomb L, et al. Constitutional 11p15 abnormalities, including heritable imprinting center mutations, cause nonsyndromic Wilms tumor. Nat Genet 2008;40:1329–1334.
37. Weksberg R, Nishikawa J, Caluseriu O, et al. Tumor development in the Beckwith–Wiedemann syndrome is associated with a variety of constitutional molecular 11p15 alterations including imprinting defects of KCNQ1OT1. Hum Mol Genet 2001;10:2989–3000.
38. Fukuzawa R, Heathcott RW, Sano M, et al. Myogenesis in Wilms' tumors is associated with mutations of the WT1 gene and activation of Bcl-2 and the Wnt signaling pathway. Pediatr Dev Pathol 2004;7:125–137.
39. Corbin M, de RA, Rickman DS, et al. WNT/beta-catenin pathway activation in Wilms tumors: a unifying mechanism with multiple entries? Genes Chromosomes Cancer 2009;48:816–827.
40. Fukuzawa R, Anaka MR, Weeks RJ, et al. Canonical WNT signalling determines lineage specificity in Wilms tumour. Oncogene 2009;28:1063–1075.
41. Schumacher V, Schuhen S, Sonner S, et al. Two molecular subgroups of Wilms' tumors with or without WT1 mutations. Clin Cancer Res 2003;9:2005–2014.
42. Fukuzawa R, Heathcott RW, More HE, et al. Sequential WT1 and CTNNB1 mutations and alterations of beta-catenin localisation in intralobar nephrogenic rests and associated Wilms tumours: two case studies. J Clin Pathol 2007;60:1013–1016.
43. Royer-Pokora B, Weirich A, Schumacher V, et al. Clinical relevance of mutations in the Wilms tumor suppressor 1 gene WT1 and the cadherin-associated protein beta1 gene CTNNB1 for patients with Wilms tumors: results of long-term surveillance of 71 patients from International Society of Pediatric Oncology Study 9/Society for Pediatric Oncology. Cancer 2008;113:1080–1089.
44. Vuononvirta R, Sebire NJ, Dallosso AR, et al. Perilobar nephrogenic rests are nonobligate molecular genetic precursor lesions of insulin-like growth factor-II-associated Wilms tumors. Clin Cancer Res 2008;14:7635–7644.
45. Fukuzawa R, Breslow NE, Morison IM, et al. Epigenetic differences between Wilms' tumours in white and east-Asian children. Lancet 2004;363:446–451.
46. Breslow NE, Olson J, Moksness J, et al. Familial Wilms' tumor: a descriptive study. Med Pediatr Oncol 1996;27:398–403.
47. McDonald JM, Douglass EC, Fisher R, et al. Linkage of familial Wilms' tumor predisposition to chromosome 19 and a two-locus model for the etiology of familial tumors. Cancer Res 1998;58:1387–1390.
48. Li FP, Gimbrere K, Gelber RD, et al. Outcome of pregnancy in survivors of Wilms' tumor. JAMA 1987;257:216–219.
49. Hawkins MM, Winter DL, Burton HS, et al. Heritability of Wilms' tumor. J Natl Cancer Inst 1995;87:1323–1324.
50. Grundy P, Koufos A, Morgan K, et al. Familial predisposition to Wilms' tumour does not map to the short arm of chromosome 11. Nature 1988;336:374–376.
51. Huff V, Compton DA, Chao L-Y, et al. Lack of linkage of familial Wilms' tumour to chromosomal band 11p13. Nature 1988;336:377–378.
52. Rahman N, Arbour L, Tonin P, et al. Evidence for a familial Wilms' tumour gene (FWT1) on chromosome 17q12-q21. Nat Genet 1996;13:461–463.
53. Rahman N, Abidi F, Ford D, et al. Confirmation of FWT1 as a Wilms' tumour susceptibility gene and phenotypic characteristics of Wilms' tumour attributable to FWT1. Hum Genet 1998;103:547–556.
54. Huff V, Amos CI, Douglass EC, et al. Evidence for genetic heterogeneity in familial Wilms' tumor. Cancer Res 1997;57:1859–1862.
55. Reid S, Renwick A, Seal S, et al. Biallelic BRCA2 mutations are associated with multiple malignancies in childhood including familial Wilms tumour. J Med Genet 2005; 42:147–151.
56. Hartley AL, Birch JM, Tricker K, et al. Wilms' tumor in the Li–Fraumeni cancer family syndrome. Cancer Genet Cytogenet 1993;67:133–135.
57. Grundy PE, Breslow NE, Li S, et al. Loss of heterozygosity for chromosomes 1p and 16q is an adverse prognostic factor in favorable-histology Wilms tumor: a report from the National Wilms Tumor Study Group. J Clin Oncol 2005;23:7312–7321.
58. Grundy RG, Pritchard J, Scambler P, et al. Loss of heterozygosity on chromosome 16 in sporadic Wilms' tumour. Br J Cancer 1998;78:1181–1187.
59. Messahel B, Williams R, Ridolfi A, et al. Allele loss at 16q defines poorer prognosis Wilms tumour irrespective of treatment approach in the UKW1–3 clinical trials: a Children's Cancer and Leukaemia Group (CCLG) Study. Eur J Cancer 2009;45:819–826.
60. Wilmore HP, White GFJ, Howell RT, et al. Germline and somatic abnormalities of chromosome 7 in Wilms' tumor. Cancer Genet Cytogenet 1994;77:93–98.
61. Rivera H. Constitutional and acquired rearrangements of chromosome 7 in Wilms tumor. Cancer Genet Cytogenet 1995;81:97–98.
62. Miozzo M, Perotti D, Minoletti F, et al. Mapping of a putative tumor suppressor locus to proximal 7p in Wilms tumors. Genomics 1996;37:310–315.
63. Perotti D, Testi MA, Mondini P, et al. Refinement within single yeast artificial chromosome clones of a minimal region commonly deleted on the short arm of chromosome 7 in Wilms tumours. Genes Chromosomes Cancer 2001;31:42–47.
64. Reynolds PA, Powlesland RM, Keen RJ, et al. Localization of a novel t(1;7) translocation associated with Wilms' tumor predisposition and skeletal abnormalities. Genes Chromosomes Cancer 1996;17:151–155.
65. Perotti D, De VG, Testi MA, et al. Germline mutations of the POU6F2 gene in Wilms tumors with loss of heterozygosity on chromosome 7p14. Hum Mutat 2004;24: 400–407.
66. Malkin D, Li FP, Strong LC, et al. Germ line p53 mutations in a familial syndrome of breast cancer, sarcomas, and other neoplasms. Science 1990;250:1233–1238.
67. Bardeesy N, Falkoff D, Petruzzi MJ, et al. Anaplastic Wilms' tumour, a subtype displaying poor prognosis, harbours p53 gene mutations. Nat Genet 1994;7:91–97.
68. Malkin D, Sexsmith E, Yeger H, et al. Mutations of the p53 tumor suppressor gene occur infrequently in Wilms' tumor. Cancer Res 1994;54:2077–2079.
69. Hill DA, Shear TD, Liu T, et al. Clinical and biologic significance of nuclear unrest in Wilms tumor. Cancer 2003;97:2318–2326.
70. Bardeesy N, Beckwith JB, Pelletier J. Clonal expansion and attenuated apoptosis in Wilms' tumors are associated with p53 gene mutations. Cancer Res 1995;55:215–219.
71. Mahoney JP, Saffos RO. Fetal rhabdomyomatous nephroblastoma with a renal pelvic mass simulating sarcoma botryoides. Am J Surg Pathol 1981;5:297–306.
72. Beckwith JB. Wilms' tumor and other renal tumors of childhood: a selective review from the National Wilms' Tumor Study Pathology Center. Hum Pathol 1983;14: 481–492.
73. Beckwith JB, Palmer NF. Histopathology and prognosis of Wilms tumor. Cancer 1978;41:1937–1948.
74. Shao L, Hill DA, Perlman EJ. Expression of WT-1, Bcl-2, and CD34 by primary renal spindle cell tumors in children. Pediatr Dev Pathol 2004;7:577–582.
75. Blakely ML, Shamberger RC, Norkool P, et al. Outcome of children with cystic partially differentiated nephroblastoma treated with or without chemotherapy. J Pediatr Surg 2003;38:897–900.
76. Boman F, Hill DA, Williams GM, et al. Familial association of pleuropulmonary blastoma with cystic nephroma and other renal tumors: a report from the International Pleuropulmonary Blastoma Registry. J Pediatr 2006;149:850–854.
77. Beckwith JB, Zuppan CE, Browning NG, et al. Histological analysis of aggressiveness and responsiveness in Wilms' tumor. Med Pediatr Oncol 1996;27:422–428.
78. Vujanic GM, Sandstedt B, Harms D, et al. Revised International Society of Paediatric Oncology (SIOP) working classification of renal tumors of childhood. Med Pediatr Oncol 2002;38:79–82.
79. Weirich A, Leuschner I, Harms D, et al. Clinical impact of histologic subtypes in localized non-anaplastic nephroblastoma treated according to the trial and study SIOP-9/GPOH. Ann Oncol 2001;12:311–319.
80. Dome JS, Cotton CA, Perlman EJ, et al. Treatment of anaplastic histology Wilms' tumor: results from the fifth National Wilms' Tumor Study. J Clin Oncol 2006;24: 2352–2358.
81. Faria P, Beckwith B, Mishra K, et al. Focal versus diffuse anaplasia in Wilms tumor-new definitions with prognostic significance. Am J Surg Pathol 1996;20:909–920.
82. Beckwith JB. New developments in the pathology of Wilms tumor. Cancer Invest 1997;15:153–162.
83. Beckwith JB. Precursor lesions of Wilms tumor: clinical and biological implications. Med Pediatr Oncol 1993;21:158–168.
84. Argani P, Perlman EJ, Breslow NE, et al. Clear cell sarcoma of the kidney: a review of 351 cases from the National Wilms Tumor Study Group Pathology Center. Am J Surg Pathol 2000;24:4–18.
85. Beckwith JB, Larson E. Case 7. Clear cell sarcoma of kidney. Pediatr Pathol 1989; 9:211–218.
86. Marsden HB, Lawler W, Kumar PM. Bone metastasizing renal tumor of childhood: morphological and clinical features, and differences from Wilms' tumor. Cancer 1978; 42:1922–1928.
87. Schuster AE, Schneider DT, Fritsch MK, et al. Genetic and genetic expression analyses of clear cell sarcoma of the kidney. Lab Invest 2003;83:1293–1299.
88. Palmer NF, Sutow W. Clinical aspects of the rhabdoid tumor of the kidney: a report of the National Wilms' Tumor Study Group. Med Pediatr Oncol 1983;11:242–245.
89. Vujanic GM, Sandstedt B, Harms D, et al. Rhabdoid tumour of the kidney: a clinicopathological study of 22 patients from the International Society of Paediatric Oncology (SIOP) nephroblastoma file. Histopathology 1996;28:333–340.
90. Weeks DA, Beckwith JB, Mierau GW, et al. Rhabdoid tumor of kidney. A report of 111 cases from the National Wilms' Tumor Study Pathology Center. Am J Surg Pathol 1989; 13:439–458.
91. Vogel AM, Gown AM, Caughlan J, et al. Rhabdoid tumors of the kidney contain mesenchymal specific and epithelial specific intermediate filament proteins. Lab Invest 1984;50:232–238.

92. Hoot AC, Russo P, Judkins AR, et al. Immunohistochemical analysis of hSNF5/INI1 distinguishes renal and extra-renal malignant rhabdoid tumors from other pediatric soft tissue tumors. Am J Surg Pathol 2004;28:1485–1491.

93. Bonnin JM, Rubinstein LJ, Palmer NF, et al. The association of embryonal tumors originating in the kidney and in the brain. A report of seven cases. Cancer 1984;54:2137–2146.

94. Biegel JA, Rorke LB, Emanuel BS. Monosomy 22 in rhabdoid or atypical teratoid tumors of the brain. N Engl J Med 1989;321:906.

95. Schofield DE, Beckwith JB, Sklar J. Loss of heterozygosity at chromosome regions 22q11–12 and 11p15.5 in renal rhabdoid tumors. Genes Chromosomes Cancer 1996;15:10–17.

96. Versteege I, Sevenet N, Lange J, et al. Truncating mutations of hSNF5/INI1 in aggressive paediatric cancer. Nature 1998;394:203–206.

97. Biegel JA, Zhou JY, Rorke LB, et al. Germ-line and acquired mutations of INI1 in atypical teratoid and rhabdoid tumors. Cancer Res 1999;59:74–79.

98. Zhang ZK, Davies KP, Allen J, et al. Cell cycle arrest and repression of cyclin D1 transcription by INI1/hSNF5. Mol Cell Biol 2002;22:5975–5988.

99. Isakoff MS, Sansam CG, Tamayo P, et al. Inactivation of the Snf5 tumor suppressor stimulates cell cycle progression and cooperates with p53 loss in oncogenic transformation. Proc Natl Acad Sci U S A 2005;102:17745–17750.

100. Weeks DA, Beckwith JB, Mierau GW, et al. Renal neoplasms mimicking rhabdoid tumor of kidney. A report from the National Wilms' Tumor Study Pathology Center. Am J Surg Pathol 1991;15:1042–1054.

101. Parham DM, Weeks DA, Beckwith JB. The clinicopathologic spectrum of putative extrarenal rhabdoid tumors. An analysis of 42 cases studied with immunohistochemistry or electron microscopy. Am J Surg Pathol 1994;18:1010–1029.

102. Bolande RP, Brough AJ, Izant RJ Jr. Congenital mesoblastic nephroma of infancy. A report of eight cases and the relationship to Wilms' tumor. Pediatrics 1967;40:272–278.

103. Pettinato G, Manivel JC, Wick MR, et al. Classical and cellular (atypical) congenital mesoblastic nephroma: a clinicopathologic, ultrastructural, immunohistochemical, and flow cytometric study. Hum Pathol 1989;20:682–690.

104. Knezevich SR, McFadden DE, Tao W, et al. A novel ETV6-NTRK3 gene fusion in congenital fibrosarcoma. Nat Genet 1998;18:184–187.

105. Lowery M, Issa B, Pysher T, et al. Cytogenetic findings in a case of congenital mesoblastic nephroma. Cancer Genet Cytogenet 1995;84:113–115.

106. Knezevich SR, Garnett MJ, Pysher TJ, et al. ETV6-NTRK3 gene fusions and trisomy 11 establish a histogenetic link between mesoblastic nephroma and congenital fibrosarcoma. Cancer Res 1998;58:5046–5048.

107. Argani P, Fritsch M, Kadkol SS, et al. Detection of the ETV6-NTRK3 chimeric RNA of infantile fibrosarcoma/cellular congenital mesoblastic nephroma in paraffin-embedded tissue: application to challenging pediatric renal stromal tumors. Mod Pathol 2000;13:29–36.

108. Beckwith JB, Weeks DA. Congenital mesoblastic nephroma. When should we worry? Arch Pathol Lab Med 1986;110:98–99.

109. Vujanic GM, Delemarre JF, Moeslichan S, et al. Mesoblastic nephroma metastatic to the lungs and heart—another face of this peculiar lesion: case report and review of the literature. Pediatr Pathol 1993;13:143–153.

110. Raney RBJ, Palmer N, Sutow WW, et al. Renal cell carcinoma in children. Med Pediatr Oncol 1983;11:91–98.

111. Bruder E, Passera O, Harms D, et al. Morphologic and molecular characterization of renal cell carcinoma in children and young adults. Am J Surg Pathol 2004;28:1117–1132.

112. Argani P, Antonescu CR, Couturier J, et al. PRCC-TFE3 renal carcinomas: morphologic, immunohistochemical, ultrastructural, and molecular analysis of an entity associated with the t(X;1)(p11.2;q21). Am J Surg Pathol 2002;26:1553–1566.

113. Argani P, Antonescu CR, Illei PB, et al. Primary renal neoplasms with the ASPL-TFE3 gene fusion of alveolar soft part sarcoma: a distinctive tumor entity previously included among renal cell carcinomas of children and adolescents. Am J Pathol 2001;159:179–192.

114. Argani P, Hawkins A, Griffin CA, et al. A distinctive pediatric renal neoplasm characterized by epithelioid morphology, basement membrane production, focal HMB45 immunoreactivity, and t(6;11)(p21.1;q12) chromosome translocation. Am J Pathol 2001;158:2089–2096.

115. Argani P, Lae M, Hutchinson B, et al. Renal carcinomas with the t(6;11)(p21;q12): clinicopathologic features and demonstration of the specific alpha-TFEB gene fusion by immunohistochemistry, RT-PCR, and DNA PCR. Am J Surg Pathol 2005;29:230–240.

116. Argani P, Lal P, Hutchinson B, et al. Aberrant nuclear immunoreactivity for TFE3 in neoplasms with TFE3 gene fusions: a sensitive and specific immunohistochemical assay. Am J Surg Pathol 2003;27:750–761.

117. Argani P, Lae M, Ballard ET, et al. Translocation carcinomas of the kidney after chemotherapy in childhood. J Clin Oncol 2006;24:1529–1534.

118. Argani P, Aulmann S, Karanjawala Z, et al. Melanotic Xp11 translocation renal cancers: a distinctive neoplasm with overlapping features of PEComa, carcinoma, and melanoma. Am J Surg Pathol 2009;33:609–619.

119. Argani P. The evolving story of renal translocation carcinomas. Am J Clin Pathol 2006;126:332–334.

120. Geller JI, Argani P, Adeniran A, et al. Translocation renal cell carcinoma: lack of negative impact due to lymph node spread. Cancer 2008;112:1607–1616.

121. Argani P, Olgac S, Tickoo SK, et al. Xp11 translocation renal cell carcinoma in adults: expanded clinical, pathologic, and genetic spectrum. Am J Surg Pathol 2007;31:1149–1160.

122. Green DM. Diagnosis and management of malignant solid tumors in infants and children. Boston, MA: Martinus Nijhoff Publishing, 1985:129–186.

123. Amar AM, Tomlinson G, Green DM, et al. Clinical presentation of rhabdoid tumors of the kidney. J Pediatr Hematol Oncol 2001;23:105–108.

124. Maas MH, Cransberg K, Van GM, et al. Renin-induced hypertension in Wilms tumor patients. Pediatr Blood Cancer 2007;48:500–503.

125. Bonaiti-Pellie C, Chompret A, Tournade MF, et al. Genetics and epidemiology of Wilms' tumor: the French Wilms' tumor study. Med Pediatr Oncol 1992;20:284–291.

126. Stiller CA, Lennox EL, Wilson LM. Incidence of cardiac septal defects in children with Wilms' tumour and other malignant diseases. Carcinogenesis 1987;8:129–132.

127. D'Angio GJ. Pre- or postoperative therapy for Wilms' tumor? J Clin Oncol 2008;26:4055–4057.

128. Lemerle J, Voute PA, Tournade MF, et al. Preoperative versus postoperative radiotherapy, single versus multiple courses of actinomycin D, in the treatment of Wilms' tumor. Preliminary results of a controlled clinical trial conducted by the International Society of Paediatric Oncology (S.I.O.P.). Cancer 1976;38:647–654.

129. Green DM. Controversies in the management of Wilms tumour—immediate nephrectomy or delayed nephrectomy? Eur J Cancer 2007;43:2453–2456.

130. Scott JP, Montgomery RR, Tubergen DG, et al. Acquired von Willebrand's disease in association with Wilms' tumor: regression following treatment. Blood 1981;58:665–669.

131. Blanchette V, Coppes MJ. Routine bleeding history and laboratory tests in children presenting with a renal mass. Pediatr Blood Cancer 2009;52:314–315.

132. Baxter PA, Nuchtern JG, Guillerman RP, et al. Acquired von Willebrand syndrome and Wilms tumor: not always benign. Pediatr Blood Cancer 2009;52:392–394.

133. Ritchey ML, Shamberger RC, Hamilton T, et al. Fate of bilateral renal lesions missed on preoperative imaging: a report from the National Wilms Tumor Study Group. J Urol 2005;174:1519–1521.

134. Ritchey ML, Kelalis PP, Breslow N, et al. Intracaval and atrial involvement with nephroblastoma: review of National Wilms Tumor Study-3. J Urol 1988;140:1113–1118.

135. Solwa Y, Sanyika C, Hadley GP, et al. Colour Doppler ultrasound assessment of the inferior vena cava in patients with Wilms' tumour. Clin Radiol 1999;54:811–814.

136. Brisse HJ, Smets AM, Kaste SC, et al. Imaging in unilateral Wilms tumour. Pediatr Radiol 2008;38:18–29.

137. Owens CM, Veys PA, Pritchard J, et al. Role of chest computed tomography at diagnosis in the management of Wilms' tumor: a study by the United Kingdom Children's Cancer Study Group. J Clin Oncol 2002;20:2768–2773.

138. Wilimas JA, Douglass EC, Magill HL, et al. Significance of pulmonary computed tomography at diagnosis in Wilms' tumor. J Clin Oncol 1988;6:1144–1146.

139. Ehrlich PF, Hamilton TE, Grundy P, et al. The value of surgery in directing therapy for patients with Wilms' tumor with pulmonary disease. A report from the National Wilms' Tumor Study Group (National Wilms' Tumor Study 5). J Pediatr Surg 2006;41:162–167.

140. Brisse HJ, Schleiermacher G, Sarnacki S, et al. Preoperative Wilms tumor rupture: a retrospective study of 57 patients. Cancer 2008;113:202–213.

141. Schenk JP, Graf N, Gunther P, et al. Role of MRI in the management of patients with nephroblastoma. Eur Radiol 2008;18:683–691.

142. Kribben A, Witzke O, Hillen U, et al. Nephrogenic systemic fibrosis: pathogenesis, diagnosis, and therapy. J Am Coll Cardiol 2009;53:1621–1628.

143. Brisse H. The radiologic contribution to surgical aspects of kidney tumors in children. JBR-BTR 2005;88:250–253.

144. Gylys-Morin V, Hoffer FA, Kozakewich H, et al. Wilms tumor and nephroblastomatosis: imaging characteristics at gadolinium-enhanced MR imaging. Radiology 1993;188:517–521.

145. van den Heuvel-Eibrink MM, Grundy P, Graf N, et al. Characteristics and survival of 750 children diagnosed with a renal tumor in the first seven months of life: A collaborative study by the SIOP/GPOH/SFOP, NWTSG, and UKCCSG Wilms tumor study groups. Pediatr Blood Cancer 2008;50:1130–1134.

146. Shulkin BL, Chang E, Strouse PJ, et al. PET FDG studies of Wilms tumors. J Pediatr Hematol Oncol 1997;19:334–338.

147. Misch D, Steffen IG, Schonberger S, et al. Use of positron emission tomography for staging, preoperative response assessment and posttherapeutic evaluation in children with Wilms tumour. Eur J Nucl Med Mol Imaging 2008;35:1642–1650.

148. Choyke PL, Siegel MJ, Craft AW, et al. Screening for Wilms tumor in children with Beckwith-Wiedemann syndrome or idiopathic hemihypertrophy. Med Pediatr Oncol 1999;32:196–200.

149. Scott RH, Walker L, Olsen OE, et al. Surveillance for Wilms tumour in at-risk children: pragmatic recommendations for best practice. Arch Dis Child 2006;91:995–999.

150. Shamberger RC, Ritchey ML, Haase GM, et al. Intravascular extension of Wilms tumor. Ann Surg 2001;234:116–121.

151. Breslow N, Sharples K, Beckwith JB, et al. Prognostic factors for Wilms' tumor patients with nonmetastatic disease at diagnosis-results of the third National Wilms' Tumor Study. Cancer 1991;68:2345–2353.

152. Breslow N, Churchill G, Nesmith B, et al. Clinicopathologic features and prognosis for Wilms' tumor patients with metastases at diagnosis. Cancer 1986;58:2501–2511.

153. Owens CM, Brisse HJ, Olsen OE, et al. Bilateral disease and new trends in Wilms tumour. Pediatr Radiol 2008;38:30–39.

154. Montgomery BT, Kelalis PP, Blute ML, et al. Extended followup of bilateral Wilms tumor: results of the National Wilms Tumor Study. J Urol 1991;146:514–518.

155. Coppes MJ, Arnold M, Beckwith JB, et al. Factors affecting the risk of contralateral Wilms tumor development: a report from the National Wilms Tumor Study Group. Cancer 1999;85:1616–1625.

156. Green DM, Beckwith JB, Breslow NE, et al. Treatment of children with stages II to IV anaplastic Wilms' tumor: a report from the National Wilms' Tumor Study Group. J Clin Oncol 1994;12:2126–2131.

157. Tomlinson GE, Breslow NE, Dome J, et al. Rhabdoid tumor of the kidney in the National Wilms' Tumor Study: age at diagnosis as a prognostic factor. J Clin Oncol 2005;23:7641–7645.

158. Reinhard H, Semler O, Burger D, et al. Results of the SIOP 93–01/GPOH trial and study for the treatment of patients with unilateral nonmetastatic Wilms Tumor. Klin Padiatr 2004;216:132–140.

159. Green DM, Breslow NE, Beckwith JB, et al. Treatment with nephrectomy only for small, stage I/favorable histology Wilms' tumor: a report from the National Wilms' Tumor Study Group. J Clin Oncol 2001;19:3719–3724.

160. Pritchard-Jones K, Kelsey A, Vujanic G, et al. Older age is an adverse prognostic factor in stage I, favorable histology Wilms' tumor treated with vincristine monochemotherapy: a study by the United Kingdom Children's Cancer Study Group, Wilms' Tumor Working Group. J Clin Oncol 2003;21:3269–3275.

161. Bonadio JF, Storer B, Norkool P, et al. Anaplastic Wilms' tumor: clinical and pathologic studies. J Clin Oncol 1985;3:513–520.

162. Izawa JI, Al-Omar M, Winquist E, et al. Prognostic variables in adult Wilms tumour. Can J Surg 2008;51:252–256.

163. Reinhard H, Aliani S, Ruebe C, et al. Wilms' tumor in adults: results of the Society of Pediatric Oncology (SIOP) 93–01/Society for Pediatric Oncology and Hematology (GPOH) Study. J Clin Oncol 2004;22:4500–4506.

164. Kalapurakal JA, Nan B, Norkool P, et al. Treatment outcomes in adults with favorable histologic type Wilms tumor-an update from the National Wilms Tumor Study Group. Int J Radiat Oncol Biol Phys 2004;60:1379–1384.

165. Grundy PE, Telzerow PE, Breslow N, et al. Loss of heterozygosity for chromosomes 16q and 1p in Wilms' tumors predicts an adverse outcome. Cancer Res 1994;54:2331–2333.

166. Hing S, Lu YJ, Summersgill B, et al. Gain of 1q is associated with adverse outcome in favorable histology Wilms' tumors. Am J Pathol 2001;158:393–398.
167. Natrajan R, Little SE, Sodha N, et al. Analysis by array CGH of genomic changes associated with the progression or relapse of Wilms' tumour. J Pathol 2007;211:52–59.
168. Dome JS, Bockhold CA, Li SM, et al. High telomerase RNA expression level is an adverse prognostic factor for favorable-histology Wilms' tumor. J Clin Oncol 2005;23: 9138–9145.
169. Huang CC, Gadd S, Breslow N, et al. Predicting relapse in favorable histology Wilms tumor using gene expression analysis: a report from the Renal Tumor Committee of the Children's Oncology Group. Clin Cancer Res 2009;15:1770–1778.
170. Ehrlich PF, Ritchey ML, Hamilton TE, et al. Quality assessment for Wilms' tumor: a report from the National Wilms' Tumor Study-5. J Pediatr Surg 2005;40:208–212.
171. Shamberger RC, Guthrie KA, Ritchey ML, et al. Surgery-related factors and local recurrence of Wilms tumor in National Wilms Tumor Study-4. Ann Surg 1999;229: 292–297.
172. Ritchey ML, Shamberger RC, Haase G, et al. Surgical complications after primary nephrectomy for Wilms' tumor: report from the National Wilms' Tumor Study Group. J Am Coll Surg 2001;192:63–68.
173. Fuchs J, Kienecker K, Furtwangler R, et al. Surgical aspects in the treatment of patients with unilateral Wilms tumor: a report from the SIOP 93–01/German Society of Pediatric Oncology and Hematology. Ann Surg 2009;249:666–671.
174. Kalapurakal JA, Li SM, Breslow NE, et al. Intraoperative spillage of favorable histology Wilms tumor cells: influence of irradiation and chemotherapy regimens on abdominal recurrence. A Report from the National Wilms Tumor Study Group. Int J Radiat Oncol Biol Phys 2010;76(1):201–206.
175. Othersen HB Jr, DeLorimer A, Hrabovsky E, et al. Surgical evaluation of lymph node metastases in Wilms' tumor. J Pediatr Surg 1990;25:330–331.
176. Ehrlich PF, Ferrer FA, Ritchey ML, et al. Hepatic metastasis at diagnosis in patients with Wilms tumor is not an independent adverse prognostic factor for stage IV Wilms tumor: a report from the Children's Oncology Group/National Wilms Tumor Study Group. Ann Surg 2009.
177. Ritchey M, Daley S, Shamberger RC, et al. Ureteral extension in Wilms' tumor: a report from the National Wilms' Tumor Study Group (NWTSG). J Pediatr Surg 2008; 43(9):1625–1629.
178. Ehrlich PF. Re: Intracaval and intracardiac extension of Wilms' tumor. The influence of preoperative chemotherapy on surgical morbidity. Int Braz J Urol 2007;33:847–848.
179. Coppes MJ, de Kraker J, van Dijken PJ, et al. Bilateral Wilms' tumor: long-term survival and some epidemiological features. J Clin Oncol 1989;7:310–315.
180. Breslow NE, Collins AJ, Ritchey ML, et al. End stage renal disease in patients with Wilms tumor: results from the National Wilms Tumor Study Group and the United States Renal Data System. J Urol 2005;174:1972–1975.
181. Ritchey ML, Green DM, Thomas PR, et al. Renal failure in Wilms' tumor patients: a report from the National Wilms' Tumor Study Group. Med Pediatr Oncol 1996;26: 75–80.
182. Hamilton TE, Green DM, Perlman EJ, et al. Bilateral Wilms' tumor with anaplasia: lessons from the National Wilms' Tumor Study. J Pediatr Surg 2006;41:1641–1644.
183. Cozzi DA, Zani A. Nephron-sparing surgery in children with primary renal tumor: indications and results. Semin Pediatr Surg 2006;15:3–9.
184. Davidoff AM, Giel DW, Jones DP, et al. The feasibility and outcome of nephron-sparing surgery for children with bilateral Wilms tumor. The St Jude Children's Research Hospital experience: 1999–2006. Cancer 2008;112:2060–2070.
185. Gross RE, Nehhauser EB. Treatment of mixed tumors of the kidney in childhood. Pediatrics 1950;6:843–852.
186. D'Angio GJ, Evans AE, Breslow N, et al. The treatment of Wilms' tumor: results of the national Wilms' tumor study. Cancer 1976;38:633–646.
187. D'Angio GJ, Evans A, Breslow N, et al. The treatment of Wilms' tumor: results of the second national Wilms' tumor study. Cancer 1981;47:2302–2311.
188. D'Angio GJ, Tefft M, Breslow N, et al. Radiation therapy of Wilms' tumor: results according to dose, field, post-operative timing and histology. Int J Radiat Oncol Biol Phys 1978;4:769–780.
189. de Kraker J, Lemerle J, Voute PA, et al. Wilms' tumor with pulmonary metastases at diagnosis: the significance of primary chemotherapy. International Society of Pediatric Oncology Nephroblastoma Trial and Study Committee. J Clin Oncol 1990;8:1187–1190.
190. Pritchard J, Imeson J, Barnes J, et al. Results of the United Kingdom children's cancer study group first Wilms' tumor study. J Clin Oncol 1995;13:124–133.
191. Mitchell C, Jones PM, Kelsey A, et al. The treatment of Wilms' tumour: results of the United Kingdom Children's Cancer Study Group (UKCCSG) second Wilms' tumour study. Br J Cancer 2000;83:602–608.
192. Nicolin G, Taylor R, Baughan C, et al. Outcome after pulmonary radiotherapy in Wilms' tumor patients with pulmonary metastases at diagnosis: a UK Children's Cancer Study Group, Wilms' Tumour Working Group Study. Int J Radiat Oncol Biol Phys 2008;70:175–180.
193. Dirks A, Li S, Breslow N, et al. Outcome of patients with lung metastases on NWTS 4 and 5 [abstract]. Med Pediatr Oncol 2003;41(4):251–252.
194. Thomas PR, Tefft M, Farewell VT, et al. Abdominal relapses in irradiated second National Wilms' Tumor Study patients. J Clin Oncol 1984;2:1098–1101.
195. Kalapurakal JA, Li SM, Breslow NE, et al. Influence of radiation therapy delay on abdominal tumor recurrence in patients with favorable histology Wilms' tumor treated on NWTS-3 and NWTS-4: a report from the National Wilms' Tumor Study Group. Int J Radiat Oncol Biol Phys 2003;57:495–499.
196. Tournade MF, Com-Nougue C, Voute PA, et al. Results of the sixth international society of pediatric oncology Wilms' tumor trial and study: a risk-adapted therapeutic approach in Wilms' tumor. J Clin Oncol 1993;11:1014–1023.
197. Green DM, Breslow NE, Beckwith JB, et al. Comparison between single-dose and divided-dose administration of dactinomycin and doxorubicin for patients with Wilms' tumor: a report from the National Wilms' Tumor Study Group. J Clin Oncol 1998;16:237–245.
198. Green DM, Breslow NE, Beckwith JB, et al. Effect of duration of treatment on treatment outcome and cost of treatment for Wilms' tumor: a report from the National Wilms' Tumor Study Group. J Clin Oncol 1998;16:3744–3751.
199. Tournade MF, Com-Nougue C, de Kraker J, et al. Optimal duration of preoperative therapy in unilateral and nonmetastatic Wilms' tumor in children older than 6 months: results of the Ninth International Society of Pediatric Oncology Wilms' Tumor Trial and Study. J Clin Oncol 2001;19:488–500.
200. de Kraker J, Graf N, van TH, et al. Reduction of postoperative chemotherapy in children with stage I intermediate-risk and anaplastic Wilms' tumour (SIOP 93–01 trial): a randomised controlled trial. Lancet 2004;364:1229–1235.
201. Seibel NL, Sun J, Anderson JR, et al. Outcome of clear cell sarcoma of the kidney (CCSK) treated on the National Wilms Tumor Study-5 (NWTS). Proc Am Soc Clin Oncol 2006;24(18S):502S.
202. Geller JI, Dome JS. Local lymph node involvement does not predict poor outcome in pediatric renal cell carcinoma. Cancer 2004;101:1575–1583.
203. Farber S. Chemotherapy in the treatment of leukemia and Wilms' tumor. JAMA 1966;198:826–836.
204. D'Angio GJ, Breslow N, Beckwith JB, et al. Treatment of Wilms' tumor. Results of the Third National Wilms' Tumor Study. Cancer 1989;64:349–360.
205. Thomas PR, Tefft M, Compaan PJ, et al. Results of two radiation therapy randomizations in the third National Wilms' Tumor Study. Cancer 1991;68:1703–1707.
206. Green DM, Breslow NE, Evans I, et al. The effect of chemotherapy dose intensity on the hematological toxicity of the treatment for Wilms' tumor. A report from the National Wilms' Tumor Study. Am J Pediatr Hematol Oncol 1994;16:207–212.
207. Green DM, Breslow NE, Beckwith JB, et al. Treatment outcomes in patients less than 2 years of age with small, stage I, favorable-histology Wilms' tumors: a report from the National Wilms' Tumor Study. J Clin Oncol 1993;11:91–95.
208. Metzger ML, Stewart CF, Freeman BB III, et al. Topotecan is active against Wilms' tumor: results of a multi-institutional phase II study. J Clin Oncol 2007;25:3130–3136.
209. Green DM, Breslow NE, Beckwith JB, et al. Treatment of children with clear-cell sarcoma of the kidney: a report from the National Wilms' Tumor Study Group. J Clin Oncol 1994;12:2132–2137.
210. Seibel NL, Li S, Breslow NE, et al. Effect of duration of treatment on treatment outcome for patients with clear-cell sarcoma of the kidney: a report from the National Wilms' Tumor Study Group. J Clin Oncol 2004;22:468–473.
211. Miser J, Krailo M, Hammond GD. A very active regimen in the treatment of recurrent Wilms tumor [abstract]. Proc Am Soc Clin Oncol 1993;12:417.
212. Kung FH, Pratt CB, Vega RA, et al. Ifosfamide/etoposide combination in the treatment of recurrent malignant solid tumors of childhood. A Pediatric Oncology Group Phase II study. Cancer 1993;71:1898–1903.
213. Radulescu VC, Gerrard M, Moertel C, et al. Treatment of recurrent clear cell sarcoma of the kidney with brain metastasis. Pediatr Blood Cancer 2008;50(2):246–249.
214. Gururangan S, Bowman LC, Parham DM, et al. Primary extracranial rhabdoid tumors. Clinicopathologic features and response to ifosfamide. Cancer 1993;71:2653–2659.
215. Wagner L, Hill DA, Fuller C, et al. Treatment of metastatic rhabdoid tumor of the kidney. J Pediatr Hematol Oncol 2002;24:385–388.
216. MacArthur CA, Isaacs H Jr, Miller JH, et al. Pediatric renal cell carcinoma: a complete response to recombinant interleukin-2 in a child with metastatic disease at diagnosis. Med Pediatr Oncol 1994;23:365–371.
217. Bauer M, Reaman GH, Hank JA, et al. A phase II trial of human recombinant interleukin-2 administered as a 4-day continuous infusion for children with refractory neuroblastoma, non-Hodgkin's lymphoma, sarcoma, renal cell carcinoma, and malignant melanoma. Cancer 1995;75:2959–2964.
218. Lae M, Argani P, Olshen AB, et al. Global gene expression profiles of renal carcinomas with Xp11 translocations (TFE3 gene fusions) suggest a closer relationship to alveolar soft part sarcoma tan to adult type renal cell carcinomas. Mod Pathol 2004;17 (suppl 1):163A.
219. Nanus DM, Garino A, Milowsky MI, et al. Active chemotherapy for sarcomatoid and rapidly progressing renal cell carcinoma. Cancer 2004;101:1545–1551.
220. Tsuda M, Davis IJ, Argani P, et al. TFE3 fusions activate MET signaling by transcriptional up-regulation, defining another class of tumors as candidates for therapeutic MET inhibition. Cancer Res 2007;67:919–929.
221. Grundy P, Breslow N, Green DM, et al. Prognostic factors for children with recurrent Wilms' tumor: results from the Second and Third National Wilms' Tumor Study. J Clin Oncol 1989;7:638–647.
222. Dome JS, Liu T, Krasin M, et al. Improved survival for patients with recurrent Wilms tumor: the experience at St. Jude Children's Research Hospital. J Pediatr Hematol Oncol 2002;24:192–198.
223. Green DM, Breslow NE, Li Y, et al. The role of surgical excision in the management of relapsed Wilms' tumor patients with pulmonary metastases: a report from the National Wilms' Tumor Study. J Pediatr Surg 1991;26:728–733.
224. Wilimas JA, Douglas EC, Hammond E, et al. Relapsed Wilms' tumor. Am J Clin Oncol 1985;8:324–328.
225. Green DM, Cotton CA, Malogolowkin M, et al. Treatment of Wilms tumor relapsing after initial treatment with vincristine and actinomycin D: a report from the National Wilms Tumor Study Group. Pediatr Blood Cancer 2007;48:493–499.
226. Malogolowkin M, Cotton CA, Green DM, et al. Treatment of Wilms tumor relapsing after initial treatment with vincristine, actinomycin D, and doxorubicin. A report from the National Wilms Tumor Study Group. Pediatr Blood Cancer 2008;50:236–241.
227. Reinhard H, Schmidt A, Furtwangler R, et al. Outcome of relapses of nephroblastoma in patients registered in the SIOP/GPOH trials and studies. Oncol Rep 2008;20: 463–467.
228. Pein F, Michon J, Valteau-Couanet D, et al. High-dose melphalan, etoposide, and carboplatin followed by autologous stem-cell rescue in pediatric high-risk recurrent Wilms' tumor: a French Society of Pediatric Oncology study. J Clin Oncol 1998;16:3295–3301.
229. Garaventa A, Hartmann O, Bernard JL, et al. Autologous bone marrow transplantation for pediatric Wilms' tumor: the experience of the European Bone Marrow Transplantation Solid Tumor Registry. Med Pediatr Oncol 1994;22:11–14.
230. Kremens B, Gruhn B, Klingebiel T, et al. High-dose chemotherapy with autologous stem cell rescue in children with nephroblastoma. Bone Marrow Transplant 2002;30: 893–898.
231. Campbell AD, Cohn SL, Reynolds M, et al. Treatment of relapsed Wilms' tumor with high-dose therapy and autologous hematopoietic stem-cell rescue: the experience at Children's Memorial Hospital. J Clin Oncol 2004;22:2885–2890.
232. Spreafico F, Bisogno G, Collini P, et al. Treatment of high-risk relapsed Wilms tumor with dose-intensive chemotherapy, marrow-ablative chemotherapy, and autologous hematopoietic stem cell support: experience by the Italian Association of Pediatric Hematology and Oncology. Pediatr Blood Cancer 2008;51:23–28.
233. Harris MB, Hurwitz C, Sullivan JG, et al. Taxol in pediatric solid tumors: a Pediatric Oncology Group (POG) phase II study (POG #9262). Proc Am Soc Clin Oncol 1999;18:563.
234. Meany HJ, Seibel NL, Sun J, et al. Phase 2 trial of recombinant tumor necrosis factor-alpha in combination with dactinomycin in children with recurrent Wilms tumor. J Immunother 2008;31:679–683.
235. Green DM, Grigoriev YA, Nan B, et al. Congestive heart failure after treatment for Wilms' tumor: a report from the National Wilms' Tumor Study group. J Clin Oncol 2001;19:1926–1934.

236. Pein F, Sakiroglu O, Dahan M, et al. Cardiac abnormalities 15 years and more after adriamycin therapy in 229 childhood survivors of a solid tumour at the Institut Gustave Roussy. Br J Cancer 2004;91:37–44.

237. Green DM, Grigoriev YA, Nan B, et al. Correction to "congestive heart failure after treatment for Wilms' tumor". J Clin Oncol 2003;21:2447–2448.

238. Cotton CA, Peterson S, Norkool PA, et al. Early and late mortality after diagnosis of Wilms tumor. J Clin Oncol 2009;27:1304–1309.

239. Green DM, Finklestein JZ, Tefft ME, et al. Diffuse interstitial pneumonitis after pulmonary irradiation for metastatic Wilms' tumor. A report from the National Wilms' Tumor Study. Cancer 1989;63:450–453.

240. Benoist MR, Lemerle J, Jean R, et al. Effects of pulmonary function of whole lung irradiation for Wilms' tumour in children. Thorax 1982;37:175–180.

241. Attard-Montalto SP, Kingston JE, Eden OB, et al. Late follow-up of lung function after whole lung irradiation for Wilms' tumour. Br J Radiol 1992;65:1114–1118.

242. Shaw NJ, Eden OB, Jenney ME, et al. Pulmonary function in survivors of Wilms' tumor. Pediatr Hematol Oncol 1991;8:131–137.

243. Weirich A, Ludwig R, Graf N, et al. Survival in nephroblastoma treated according to the trial and study SIOP-9/GPOH with respect to relapse and morbidity. Ann Oncol 2004;15:808–820.

244. Breslow NE, Takashima JR, Ritchey ML, et al. Renal failure in the Denys–Drash and Wilms' tumor-aniridia syndromes. Cancer Res 2000;60:4030–4032.

245. Sonn G, Shortliffe LM. Management of Wilms tumor: current standard of care. Nat Clin Pract Urol 2008;5:551–560.

246. Nussbaum RH, Kohnlein W. Radiation and childhood cancer. Environ Health Perspect 1996;104:353–354.

247. Kalapurakal JA, Peterson S, Peabody EM, et al. Pregnancy outcomes after abdominal irradiation that included or excluded the pelvis in childhood Wilms tumor survivors: a report from the National Wilms Tumor Study. Int J Radiat Oncol Biol Phys 2004;58: 1364–1368.

248. Hawkins MM, Smith RA. Pregnancy outcomes in childhood cancer survivors: probable effects of abdominal irradiation. Int J Cancer 1989;43:399–402.

249. Green DM, Peabody EM, Nan B, et al. Pregnancy outcome after treatment for Wilms tumor: a report from the national Wilms tumor study group. J Clin Oncol 2002;20: 2506–2513.

250. Wallace WH, Shalet SM, Hendry JH, et al. Ovarian failure following abdominal irradiation in childhood: the radiosensitivity of the human oocyte. Br J Radiol 1989;62: 995–998.

251. Breslow NE, Takashima JR, Whitton JA, et al. Second malignant neoplasms following treatment for Wilms' tumor: a report from the National Wilms' tumor study group. J Clin Oncol 1995;13:1851–1859.

252. Carli M, Frascella E, Tournade MF, et al. Second malignant neoplasms in patients treated on SIOP Wilms tumour studies and trials 1, 2, 5, and 6. Med Pediatr Oncol 1997;29:239–244.

253. Breslow NE, Ou SS, Beckwith JB, et al. Doxorubicin for favorable histology, Stage II-III Wilms tumor: results from the National Wilms Tumor Studies. Cancer 2004;101: 1072–1080.

254. Kaste SC, McCarville MB. Imaging pediatric abdominal tumors. Semin Roentgenol 2008;43:50–59.

255. Oeffinger KC, Mertens AC, Sklar CA, et al. Chronic health conditions in adult survivors of childhood cancer. N Engl J Med 2006;355:1572–1582.

256. Robison LL, Green DM, Hudson M, et al. Long-term outcomes of adult survivors of childhood cancer. Cancer 2005;104:2557–2564.

CHAPTER 30 ■ NEUROBLASTOMA

GARRETT M. BRODEUR, MICHAEL D. HOGARTY, YAEL P. MOSSE, AND JOHN M. MARIS

Few tumors have engendered as much fascination and frustration for clinical and laboratory investigators as neuroblastoma, the most common and deadly solid tumor of childhood. These tumors may regress spontaneously, particularly in infants, or they may mature into a benign ganglioneuroma. In contrast, most older children have unresectable or metastatic disease at the time of diagnosis, and their overall prognosis has been poor. However, molecular genetic and biological analysis of tumor tissue has shed considerable light on these disparate clinical behaviors.

Many genetic features of neuroblastomas have now been identified that correlate with clinical outcome. Indeed, specific genetic gains (or losses), as well as discrete patterns of gene expression, are linked with tumor behavior and prognosis. Recently, mutations in two genes have been identified that are responsible for almost all cases of hereditary neuroblastoma, and other genes have been found that may also contribute to neuroblastoma susceptibility. These and other observations have given us tremendous insight into mechanisms of malignant transformation and progression, as well as spontaneous differentiation and regression.

Patterns of genetic change allow neuroblastomas to be classified into subsets with distinct biological features and clinical behavior. Indeed, certain genetic abnormalities are very powerful predictors of response to therapy and outcome, and they have become essential components of tumor characterization at diagnosis. Thus, neuroblastoma serves as a model tumor in which the genetic and biological analyses of tumor cells provide important information that guides optimal patient management. The challenge for the next decade is to translate this information into more effective and less toxic therapy for these patients. This chapter reviews the current understanding of various clinical and biological features of neuroblastoma and relates these characteristics to trends in predicting outcome as well as future strategies for treatment. It also reviews the current approach to the diagnosis, staging, and management of patients with neuroblastoma.

EPIDEMIOLOGY

Neuroblastoma is the most common extracranial solid tumor in children, accounting for 8% to 10% of all childhood cancers. The prevalence is about 1 case per 7,000 live births, and there are about 800 new cases of neuroblastoma per year in the United States.[1,2] This corresponds to an incidence of 10.4 per million per year in white children and 8.3 per million per year in black children younger than 15 years. Evidence indicates that this incidence is fairly uniform throughout the world, at least for industrialized nations. Neuroblastoma is slightly more common in boys than in girls, with a male-to-female sex ratio of 1.1 to 1 in most large studies.

Neuroblastoma is a pediatric neoplasm that is the most common cancer diagnosed during infancy.[3] Review of 3,666 neuroblastoma patients registered on cooperative group studies at POG and CCG institutions from 1986 to 2001 showed

a median age at diagnosis of about 19 months. In this cohort, 36% were infants, 89% were younger than 5 years, and 98% were diagnosed by 10 years of age (Fig. 30.1). The distribution of cases by age clearly shows that this is a disease of infancy and early childhood, with the highest number of cases diagnosed in the first month of life.

The etiology of neuroblastoma is unknown, and to date there are no data supporting a major role for environmental exposures. There have been one or a few reports associating a variety of parental occupations or drug exposures with an increased risk of neuroblastoma.[4-9] However, no particular prenatal or postnatal exposure to drugs, chemicals, viruses, or radiation has been associated strongly, consistently, or unequivocally with an increased incidence of neuroblastoma. This does not preclude a possible role of environment in the pathogenesis of neuroblastomas, but to date no strong environmental exposure or factor has been identified. Likewise, some have been associated with a protective effect, such as maternal vitamin use, as well as early childhood infections and allergies.[10-12] Finally, there has been a positive association between congenital anomalies, especially urogenital cardiac anomalies, and neuroblastoma.[13-15] These cases may reflect some underlying genetic abnormality that contribute to both, but no consistent pattern has been identified.

Neuroblastomas frequently produce increased levels of catecholamines with metabolites (VMA, HVA) that are detectable in the urine. Also, the outcome of infants was substantially better than older children with this disease; therefore, mass screening of infants for neuroblastoma was initiated in Japan, and the early results were very promising.[16,17] This led to similar efforts in North America (principally in Quebec, Canada) and in Europe (mainly France and Germany) to answer questions concerning the feasibility and utility of mass screening for neuroblastoma.[18-22] Current results indicate that mass screening has resulted in a substantial increase in the prevalence of neuroblastoma in screened compared with unscreened populations, but without a significant decrease in the prevalence or mortality of neuroblastoma in patients older than 1 year.[23-28] Thus, mass screening efforts have essentially stopped throughout the world.

Despite the fact that mass screening was not successful in reducing the overall mortality for neuroblastoma, it was extremely valuable for providing additional insight into the pathogenesis and clinical behavior of biologically favorable tumors. For example, the increased prevalence of neuroblastoma that has been observed consistently in screened populations suggests that spontaneous regression of neuroblastoma (without clinical detection) is at least as prevalent as clinically detected neuroblastoma. In addition, the studies that have been performed on screened tumors show that virtually all of the tumors are biologically favorable, in contrast to the higher prevalence of unfavorable biological features found in older children that are detected clinically.[29-31] There have also been several reports of the incidental prenatal detection of neuroblastoma by maternal ultrasound.[32-35] These cases are similar both clinically and biologically to those identified by screening,

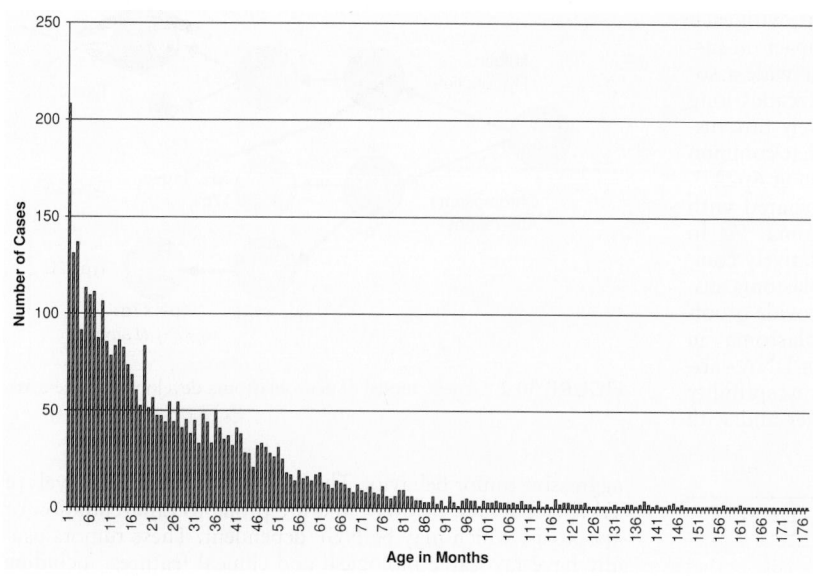

FIGURE 30.1 Distribution of age at diagnosis for 3,666 neuroblastoma patients. Shown is the age at diagnosis in months (x-axis) and the number of patients at that age (y-axis). (Courtesy of W.B. London, COG Statistical Office.)

and the vast majority do well with little or no therapy. Although mass screening studies are no longer being performed, recent advances in identifying neuroblastoma predisposition and susceptibility genes may lead to the identification of individuals who are at increased risk, and future screening efforts could be focused on them.

GENETIC PREDISPOSITION

Like most human cancers, a subset of patients with neuroblastoma exhibits a predisposition to develop this disease, and this predisposition follows an autosomal dominant pattern of inheritance, with a penetrance of about 65% to 70%.[36] A family history of the disease is found in about 1% to 2% of newly diagnosed cases, with a standardized incidence ratio of 9.7 for siblings of index cases.[37] Neuroblastoma pedigrees show notable heterogeneity in the type of tumors that arise, with both benign and malignant forms occurring in the same family.[38] Patients with hereditary neuroblastoma differ from those with sporadic disease in that they are diagnosed at an earlier age and/or with more than one primary tumor; clinical characteristics that are hallmarks of cancer predisposition syndromes. Knudson and Strong predicted in 1972 that neuroblastoma fit the two-mutation model of oncogenesis developed for retinoblastoma.[36] Because of the lethality of neuroblastoma before reproductive age, previous genetic linkage scans have been underpowered, and results have been difficult to replicate.[39–41] However, Mosse et al., and others,[42,43] recently used a genome-wide scan to discover activating mutations in the tyrosine kinase domain of the ALK oncogene in most cases of hereditary neuroblastoma. These germline mutations encode for single-base substitutions in key regions of the kinase domain that result in constitutive activation of the kinase and a premalignant state. Indeed, to date, all mutations have been found in the kinase domain. It is likely that ALK is further activated either through somatically acquired duplication or amplification of the mutant allele, which could represent the second hit. Interestingly, similar activating mutations are also somatically acquired in 5% to 15% of sporadic neuroblastomas.[42–45]

Notably, neuroblastoma can occur in association with disorders related to abnormal development of neural-crest–derived tissues, including CCHS and Hirschsprung disease.[46,47] In addition, there have been reports of the coexistence of neuroblastoma and NF1, including the coincidence of these disorders in familial neuroblastoma.[40] Indeed, homozygous inactivation of the NF1 gene has been described in primary neuroblastomas,[48,49] although the overall prevalence of NF1 mutations in neuroblastomas is very low. Overall, these data suggest that the genes implicated in the genesis of Hirschsprung disease (RET, EDNRB, EDN3, GDNF, ECE1, and ZFHX1B), central hypoventilation (RET, GDNF, EDN3, BDNF and PHOX2B), and/or NF1 may be causally involved in the initiation or progression of human neuroblastoma, especially in the context of these syndromes. Missense or nonsense mutations in PHOX2B, a homeobox gene that is a master regulator of normal autonomic nervous system development, were recently shown to predispose to this rare field defect of the sympathoadrenal lineage tissues.[50] However, PHOX2B mutations explain only a small subset of hereditary neuroblastoma, are restricted to the cases with associated disorders of neural-crest–derived tissues, and are not somatically acquired in tumors.[51–53] Coupled with the discovery that gain of function mutations in the ALK oncogene explains the majority of cases of hereditary neuroblastoma, it appears that the majority, if not all, of the mutated genes that lead to familial neuroblastoma have been discovered. Therefore, genetic testing for mutations in these two genes should be considered whenever a patient has a family history of the disease or other clinical factors such as bilateral adrenal primary tumors suspicious for a highly penetrant transmissible mutation.

Constitutional chromosome abnormalities are rare in patients with neuroblastoma, but these rare cases may help localize genes critical to tumor initiation.[54] Patients frequently show associated congenital disorders, and these may be quite severe. Although no common constitutional chromosomal aberration has been discovered, germline hemizygous deletions at chromosome bands 1p36 and 11q14–23 have been reported most frequently.[54–58] Interestingly, these genomic regions are frequently deleted somatically during the malignant evolution of a large number of sporadic neuroblastomas (see later). These rare cases further emphasize the complex underlying genetics of neuroblastoma and suggest that aberrant expression or regulation of multiple genes may work together to initiate malignant transformation of undifferentiated sympathoadrenal neuroblasts.

In the vast majority of neuroblastoma cases that occur sporadically, malignant transformation likely arises from a synergistic interaction of common DNA variations, with each individual variation having a relatively modest impact on susceptibility. The COG has mounted a large genome-wide association study of neuroblastoma, leveraging a decades-long commitment to specimen banking for this relatively rare disease. So far, this ongoing study has discovered that common SNP variations within the putative gene FLJ22536 at 6p22.3, and the BARD1 gene at 2q35, are highly associated with increased likelihood of developing neuroblastoma.[59,60] In addition, this study has recently shown that a relatively common CNV at 1q21 is also associated with neuroblastoma susceptibility.[61] Taken together, these observations provide proof-of-concept that the development of neuroblastoma in individual patients may be influenced by common DNA variations. Future work will define the remaining susceptibility loci, as well as how they interact with each other and with environmental exposures.

MOLECULAR PATHOGENESIS

Although germline *ALK* or *PHOX2B* mutations predispose to neuroblastoma with high penetrance, the overwhelming majority of children presenting with this tumor do not have a strong genetic predisposition or family history of neuroblastoma. Tumor initiation in these sporadic cases is a consequence of somatically acquired genomic changes. Many such changes have been identified and correlated with tumor behavior, and are summarized below. More recently, the inheritance of common DNA variants (or polymorphisms) has been shown to contribute to tumor susceptibility (see above). Particular polymorphisms may modestly enhance or reduce one's risk, and individuals harboring a sufficient number of risk alleles may have a higher likelihood to develop neuroblastoma. However, it remains that somatic acquired genomic changes are paramount in neuroblastoma initiation and progression.

Somatic Genomic Changes

Early karyotype analyses revealed most neuroblastomas to be aneuploid, with recurring nonrandom alterations including genomic amplifications and unbalanced translocations, as well as chromosome losses and gains. Subsequent studies using molecular techniques such as FISH and PCR-based LOH assays have validated and extended these findings for specific genomic sites. Alterations with prognostic value have been identified and are used by groups worldwide in risk classification and therapy planning, and these are described below. More recently, robust whole-genome technologies have been applied to further characterize the patterns of genetic change that are correlated with distinct tumor behaviors.[62-65] This accumulated research on the genomics and biology of neuroblastoma provides for an evolutionary model, which proposes that all neuroblastomas arise from a common precursor cell, but that different types of genomic instabilities lead to different patterns of alterations, and therefore tumors with very divergent clinical behaviors.[62-66] This model suggests that tumors that are genomically and biologically unfavorable do not evolve from favorable tumors, and vice versa. These data also predict at least two distinct neuroblastoma subtypes[66-68] (Fig. 30.2).

Type 1. The first type is characterized by gains and losses of whole chromosomes, with few if any segmental (or partial) chromosome aberrations.[63,66] Defective mitotic segregation likely contributes, although the causative mechanisms remain poorly understood. The resulting tumors have a hyperdiploid (often near-triploid) modal karyotype, and lack *MYCN* amplification or other specific genetic changes associated with

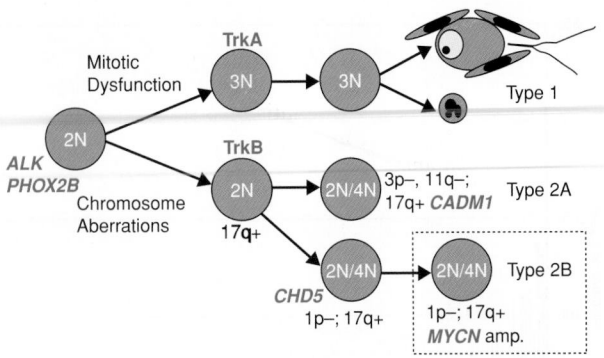

FIGURE 30.2 Genetic model of neuroblastoma development (see text).

aggressive tumor behavior. These tumors express high levels of TrkA (see RTKs, below)[69] and are prone to differentiation or apoptosis, which may be NGF dependent. These tumors usually have favorable biological and clinical features, including lower stage and younger age at diagnosis (<18 months). The prognosis for such children is excellent.

Type 2. The second type is characterized by segmental CNAs, often arising from unbalanced translocations, with or without additional whole chromosome changes.[63,66] There are nonrandom segmental alterations of chromosome arms 1p, 1q, 3p, 11q, and 17q, although segmental CNAs may be found at many other sites. Tumors in this group tend to have a near-diploid (or near-tetraploid) karyotype as well as additional unfavorable biological and clinical characteristics, such as unbalanced 17q gain. Within this type, two further subtypes can be distinguished: (2A) The first subtype is characterized by segmental deletions at 3p, 11q, and other sites, but these tumors usually do not have *MYCN* amplification or 1p deletion. (2B) The second subtype, comprising the most aggressive subset, has amplification of the *MYCN* oncogene, usually accompanied by 1p deletion and additional CNAs, but usually without loss of 11q or 3p. These tumors frequently express the TrkB receptor plus BDNF ligand, which presumably activates an autocrine survival pathway to confers a selective advantage.[70]

Although full genomic characterization of all tumors at presentation may be the goal, it is clear that the detection of a subset of prognostic CNAs can be integrated with traditional clinical factors to refine neuroblastoma risk classes. A number of such molecular features are discussed individually below. Until recently (with the exception of *MYCN* amplification), genomic aberrations were only surrogates for the genes and biopathways altered during tumorigenesis. However, one or several candidate genes have been identified on 1p36 (CHD5, miR34, KIF1BB), 11q23 (CADM1), and 17q25 (BIRC5/Survivin) that are likely targets of these genetic alterations.[71-80]

Tumor Cell DNA Content (Ploidy)

The DNA index, as determined by flow cytometry, measures tumor DNA content relative to a diploid reference to determine the ploidy of a tumor specimen. The DNA index for neuroblastomas falls into two main groups: near-diploid/near-tetraploid (DNA index ~1.0 or ~2.0) or hyperdiploid (often near triploid with a DNA index ~1.5). Tumor ploidy is used by the COG to stratify therapy for infants younger than 18 months with stage 4 or 4S disease, as it is most predictive of disease outcome for these subgroups.[81-84] It may also have prognostic value for localized tumors with *MYCN* amplification.[85] In each of these settings, hyperdiploid DNA content is associated with a more favorable outcome. Detection of tumor cell ploidy predated genome-wide tumor assessments, but it is now accepted that hyperdiploidy largely reflects tumors with whole chromosome alterations (with predominant chromosome gains), whereas near diploidy reflects segmental CNAs that do not substantially alter total cellular DNA content. Thus, the DNA index provides a simple method to define the global aneuploidy of a tumor, although it does not characterize the specific genomic alterations that contribute to this change. Furthermore, tumor cell ploidy loses its prognostic significance in older patients (older than 18 months), as hyperdiploidy in these tumors is usually associated with segmental chromosome gains and losses.[81,84]

Amplification of the *MYCN* Oncogene

Neuroblastoma karyotypes frequently reveal the cytogenetic hallmarks of gene amplification, namely, DMs or HSRs. Schwab et al.[86] originally identified the *MYC*-related oncogene *MYCN* as the target of this amplification event. *MYCN* is located on the distal short arm of chromosome 2 (2p24), but in cells with *MYCN* amplification, the extra copies reside within these DMs or HSRs.[87,88] DMs are more common in primary tumors, whereas HSRs are seen in more common in cell lines and may represent concatemerization and reintegration of amplicons. Additional genes may be coamplified with *MYCN* in a subset of cases, but *MYCN* is the only gene consistently amplified from this locus.[89,90] Genomic amplification of additional genomic loci independent of *MYCN* is rare.[91–94]

MYCN amplification can be detected by a variety of molecular techniques. Most laboratories consider interphase FISH the technique of choice because morphologic verification of the *MYCN* signal affords outstanding quality control, while also allowing low level amplification and intratumor heterogeneity to be detected[95,96] (Fig. 30.3). The clinical relevance of these less common findings is unclear currently and is being evaluated prospectively. The degree of increased copy number required to constitute "amplification" remains somewhat arbitrary, but most cooperative groups define genomic amplification as more than 4 times the normal number of *MYCN* copies (FISH signals), as compared with a control 2p probe. Fortunately, in most tumors with *MYCN* amplification, the *MYCN* copy number grossly exceeds this threshold, with most tumors averaging 50 to 400 copies/cell.

Amplification of *MYCN* is associated with advanced stages of disease, unfavorable biological features, and a poor outcome (Table 30.1). Yet it is also associated with poor outcome in otherwise favorable patient groups (such as infants and patients with lower stages of disease), underscoring its biological importance.[82,97–100] Therefore, the status of the *MYCN* gene is routinely determined from neuroblastoma samples obtained at diagnosis to assist in therapy planning. The overall prevalence

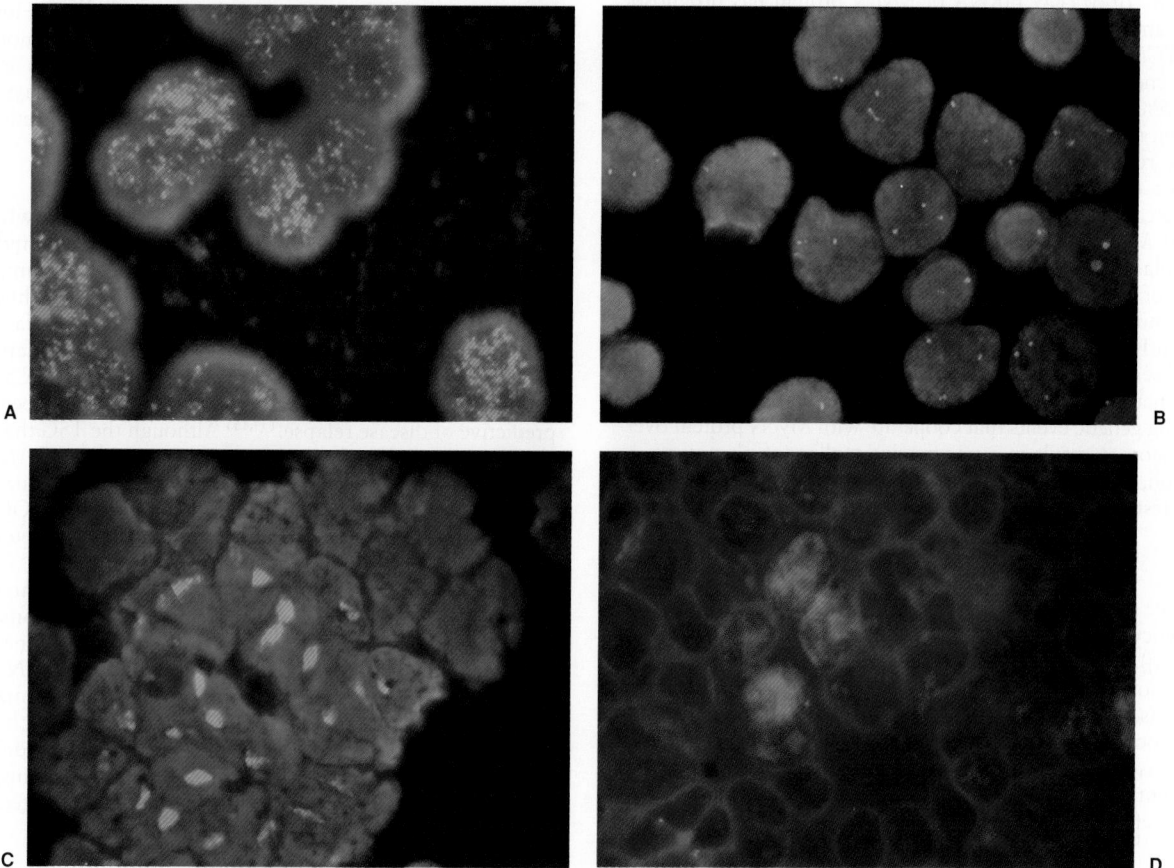

FIGURE 30.3 Detection of *MYCN* amplification by FISH in human neuroblastomas. Shown are four panels of neuroblastoma cells hybridized with a fluorescent *MYCN* probe, and the nuclei are counterstained with DAPI. **A:** Neuroblastoma cells without *MYCN* amplification, showing two to three discrete copies per cell. **B:** Neuroblastoma cells with *MYCN* amplification in the form of extrachromosomal DMs. The copy number is variable from cell to cell, and the extra copies are dispersed throughout the nucleus. **C:** Neuroblastoma cells with *MYCN* amplification in the form of chromosomally integrated homogeneously staining regions. The extra *MYCN* signal is more uniform from cell to cell, and the signal is localized to a discrete region of the nucleus. **D:** Focal *MYCN* amplification in a subset of the neuroblastoma cells, demonstrating heterogeneity in this cell population. (Courtesy of Lisa Moreau and A. Thomas Look at the Dana Farber Cancer Institute, Boston, MA.)

TABLE 30.1

RELATIONSHIP OF *MYCN* AMPLIFICATION WITH EXTENT OF DISEASE AT DIAGNOSIS

INSS stage at diagnosis	*MYCN* amplification N (%)	3-yr EFS rate ± standard error
1	15/545 (3)	91 ± 1
2a/2b	19/505 (4)	86 ± 2
3	114/464 (25)	72 ± 2
4	350/1,110 (32)	36 ± 1
4s	17/201 (8)	78 ± 3
Overall	520/2,877 (18)	60 ± 1

Courtesy of Wendy London, PhD, Children's Oncology Group Statistical Office.

of *MYCN* amplification is about 20%,[101] with near-complete concordance when multiple sites are assessed, or between samples obtained at diagnosis and relapse.[102] Therefore, it is an inherent feature of a subset of aggressive tumors at diagnosis, rather than a genomic event acquired during tumor progression. In general, levels of *MYCN* expression in tumors with amplification are much higher than in tumors without amplification.[103] However, it is controversial whether or not "overexpression" of *MYCN* mRNA or MycN protein has prognostic significance independent of *MYCN* amplification.[98,104–107]

MYCN is a member of the *MYC* proto-oncogene family, which encodes transcription factors that govern the expression of ~15% of all human genes, such that deregulated overexpression markedly impacts cell behavior.[108,109] *MYC* genes play a large role in regulating metabolism and cellular biomass in support of proliferation and are commonly deregulated in diverse cancers. The most compelling evidence that deregulation of *MYCN* is a fundamental event in a subset of human neuroblastomas comes from a genetically engineered murine model of the disease. Weiss et al.[110] directed *MYCN* expression to the murine neural crest using a TH promoter. These animals frequently develop tumors of the sympathetic nervous system that resemble human neuroblastomas both morphologically and genetically.[111] This mouse model is a useful tool for understanding genetic events that cooperate with MycN protein overexpression to result in an aggressive malignant phenotype. In addition, this genetically engineered mouse model may be useful to test new therapeutic strategies in the preclinical setting.

Unbalanced Gain of 17q

Another specific CNA that has been detected with substantial frequency is unbalanced gain of the long arm of chromosome 17 (17q). Allelotyping and CGH studies have suggested that this genomic aberration may occur in over half of all neuroblastomas.[112,113] Although gain of 17q can occur independently, it also occurs as part of an unbalanced translocation between chromosomes 1 and 17.[114] The 17q breakpoints vary, but preferential gain of a region from 17q22-qter suggests that a dosage effect of one or more genes provides a selective advantage.[115,116] Indeed, unbalanced 17q trisomy is one of the most common changes in all of neoplasia, so it is common in neuroblastomas, but not specific for these tumors. The genes responsible for the selective advantage are unknown, but *BIRC5* (survivin, an inhibitor of apoptosis), *PPM1D*, and *NME1* (NM23, which plays a critical role in the synthesis of nucleoside triphosphates) have been suggested as possible targets of this gain of genomic material.[78,117,118] Unbalanced gain of 17q is clearly associated with more aggressive neuroblastomas, although its prognostic significance relative to other

genetic and biological markers awaits a large prospective trial and multivariate analysis. It should be noted that although a segmental gain of 17q is predictive of a poor outcome, gain of whole chromosome 17 is characteristic of the hyperdiploid favorable subtype.[63,93]

Deletion of 1p36

Deletion of the short arm of chromosome 1 (1p) is identifiable in about 35% of primary neuroblastomas at diagnosis.[58,119–122] Deletion of 1p is found more commonly in patients with advanced stages of disease, and 1p allelic loss is highly associated with *MYCN* amplification.[121–123] The independent prognostic significance of 1p LOH has been controversial, but current evidence suggests that allelic loss at 1p36 predicts for an increased risk of disease relapse in patients with localized tumors, and tumors lacking *MYCN* amplification.[124–126] A number of laboratories have tried to identify one or more TSGs deleted from this region by looking for homozygous deletion, but such events are extremely rare.[92,127–129] Brodeur and coworkers defined a <2 Mb region of consistent deletion after examining over 1,200 neuroblastomas using a panel of DNA-based polymorphisms.[130] They have identified *CHD5*, a chromatin remodeling gene, as a bona fide TSG that is deleted from this region. Low expression of *CHD5* is highly correlated with unfavorable clinical and biological features as well as outcome.[71] At least two other potential TSGs (miR34a, KIF1BB) have been identified on 1p36 by other groups.[72,73,79,80] However, none of these genes are located in the region of common deletion defined above. Nevertheless, most 1p36 deletions are relatively large, so it is likely that more than one TSG plays a role in neuroblastoma pathogenesis in tumors with 1p deletions.

Deletion of 11q and Other Sites

Allelic loss of 11q is present in 35% to 40% of newly diagnosed primary tumors.[131–133] Interestingly, this genomic aberration is almost never seen in tumors with *MYCN* amplification, but it is still highly associated with other high-risk features such as advanced stage, older age, and unfavorable pathology. Therefore, deletion of 11q is a great candidate prognostic marker in the subset of tumors without *MYCN* amplification, and recent data strongly suggest that it is independently predictive of disease relapse.[134,135] Although the TSG that is the presumptive target of 11q deletions is not certain, *CADM1* at 11q23 has been proposed as a good candidate.[75] Evaluation of 11q and 1p status will be incorporated into future COG clinical trials for further risk stratification and therapy determination for patients with intermediate-risk disease.

Allelic loss has been reported at multiple other chromosomal loci. Recent evidence suggests that 3p deletions often occur coincidentally with 11q deletions and help define a subset of patients with aggressive disease who lack *MYCN* amplification.[134,136] Other genomic regions showing hemizygous deletions that have potential biological relevance include 4p, 9p, 14q, and 19q.[129,137–139] However, homozygous deletions are rarely identified in this disease,[129] thus complicating traditional approaches for identifying the TSGs postulated to be targeted by the hemizygous deletions noted above.

Gene Expression and Molecular Signatures in Neuroblastomas

Molecular Signatures in Neuroblastoma

Just as improved genomic technologies have led to new insights into the DNA alterations occurring in neuroblastoma, robust gene expression platforms have led to insights into neuroblastoma biology. Transcriptome datasets have identified relevant biopathways associated with specific tumor subtypes.[64,140–145] Examples include identification of polyamine metabolism as a tractable therapeutic target downstream of *MYCN* amplification,[146–148] and enrichment in sympathoadrenal developmental genes in favorable low-risk disease.[149–151] Importantly, independent datasets have implicated *MYC* signaling in neuroblastomas with poor outcome that do not have *MYCN* gene amplification,[149,152,153] suggesting that deregulated *MYC* is essential to the high-risk phenotype. Pathway discovery is also facilitated by integrating transcriptome datasets with DNA profiles. Since identified CNAs in neuroblastoma are large and without demonstrable biallelic inactivation of regional candidate genes, these approaches may help implicate the important gene or genes from these regions.

Molecular signatures have also been sought to improve upon current risk classification schemes, which currently rely on clinical features and genomic changes in the tumor. Numerous gene-lists have been identified and validated to identify risk class for all neuroblastomas at diagnosis,[141,144,145,154] or provide prognostic information for specific subsets, such as older children with stage 4 non-*MYCN* amplified disease.[142] Their utility in patient management awaits robust validation in prospective clinical trials and will require efforts to increase the percentage of patients from whom high-quality tumor RNA can be obtained in a timely manner for these purposes. Finally, molecular signatures have been used to identify possible novel therapeutics. Gene signatures that define specific neuroblastoma subtypes (compared with nontransformed neuroblasts) were matched to gene signatures downstream of pharmacologic perturbations. A small number of compound classes were identified that are plausible therapeutics.[155]

Expression of RTKs

The factors responsible for regulating the malignant transformation of sympathetic neuroblasts to neuroblastoma cells are incompletely understood, but evidence supports a role for RTKs in this process. The neurotrophin receptors (*NTRK1*, *NTRK2* and *NTRK3* encoding TrkA, TrkB and TrkC) and their ligands (NGF, BDNF and NT-3, respectively) are important regulators of survival, growth, and differentiation of neural cells.[156–159] Their temporospatial expression plays a critical role in the normal development of the sympathetic nervous system, and their co-opted signaling correlates with neuroblastoma phenotype.

High TrkA expression correlates with younger age at diagnosis, lower tumor stage, favorable biological features, and good outcome.[69,160,161] Both normal sympathetic neurons and explanted neuroblastoma cells with high TrkA expression differentiate when exposed to NGF or undergo apoptosis in the absence of NGF,[69] suggesting a possible role for this receptor in neuroblastoma differentiation or regression.[69,162] Activation of TrkA by NGF present in the tumor microenvironment would promote survival and differentiation into ganglion cells, whereas NGF deprivation would initiate apoptosis, with TrkA functioning as a dependence receptor.[69,162,163] Thus, the regression seen particularly in TrkA-expressing neuroblastomas in infants may be due, at least in part, to delayed activation of developmentally programmed cell death resulting from NGF deprivation. Recently, a neurodevelopmentally regulated oncogenic splice variant of TrkA (TrkA-III) has been identified that is constitutively activated, ligand independent, antagonizes the anti-oncogenic NGF/TrkA-I signaling, and promotes neuroblastoma tumor growth.[164]

In contrast to TrkA, expression of TrkB is strongly associated with aggressive tumor behavior and unfavorable biological features, such as *MYCN* amplification.[70] These tumors also commonly express the cognate TrkB ligand BDNF,[165,166] which may represent an autocrine or paracrine survival pathway. Constitutive activation of the TrkB/BDNF pathway also contributes to chemotherapeutic drug resistance and metastasis, perhaps through suppression of anoikis.[167–169] These characteristics make targeted inhibition of this pathway an attractive therapeutic goal. The independent role of TrkC expression remains to be elucidated, as TrkC expression occurs in a subset of tumors that also express TrkA[170,171] and may cooperate to facilitate TrkA-mediated functions. Another transmembrane neurotrophin receptor called p75 (p75NTR; *TNFRSF16*) binds all the NGF family of neurotrophins with low affinity. Expression of p75 in neuroblastomas has generally been associated with a favorable outcome,[69,160,161] but its biological and prognostic significance independent of Trk receptor expression is unclear.[172]

Several other RTKs involved in normal neuronal development have been implicated in NB biology. RET is an RTK that is preferentially expressed in neural-crest–derived cell lineages, and RET has also been implicated in regulating growth and differentiation of neuroblastomas.[173–176] Expression of ALK, another RTK, is restricted to the developing nervous system, and it is postulated to play a role in the regulation of neuronal differentiation. As discussed above, activation of *ALK* by mutation, amplification, or other mechanisms has been implicated in the pathogenesis of both familial and sporadic neuroblastomas.[42–45] Several other RTKs have been implicated in the pathogenesis of neuroblastoma, including *IGF1R* and the *EGFR* family,[177–179] and some of these may also play a role in the clinical behavior of this tumor. Furthermore, all of these RTKs represent potential therapeutic targets.

Common Cancer Pathways in Neuroblastomas

The cancer genes most commonly altered in adult carcinogenesis (e.g., *TP53*, *CDKN2A*, *RAS*) are rarely deleted or mutated in neuroblastoma. The *TP53* gene, encoding the p53 protein, is one of the most commonly mutated genes in human neoplasia, yet mutations are rarely found in primary neuroblastomas,[180,181] although they have been documented in cell lines at relapse.[182–184] Alternative mechanisms for p53 dysfunction, including *HDM2* amplification, cytoplasmic sequestration, or *TWIST1*-mediated suppression have been proposed, but their contribution to p53 pathway inactivation in primary tumors remains limited.[185–187] The *CDKN2A* (INK4A/p16) gene is deleted or mutated in many types of adult cancers, especially in established cell lines, as there is strong selective pressure to lose p16 function in adaptation to long-term propagation *in vitro*. Homozygous deletion of *CDKN2A* (INK4A/p16) has been identified in a subset of neuroblastoma cell lines,[129] but there is no consistent evidence for inactivation of this locus, or the related *CDKN2B* (KIP1/p27) and *CDKN2C* (INK4C/p18) genes, in primary tumors.[129,188–191] Finally, though persuasive evidence supports *RAS* and *MYC* gene cooperation in tumorigenesis,[192–194] activation of *RAS* does not appear to constitute a preferred secondary pathway for neuroblastomas, even for tumors with *MYCN* amplification.[195] The only other examples of biallelic gene inactivation documented in neuroblastoma are in the *NF1* gene in two neuroblastoma cell lines and two primary tumors,[48,49,196,197] though the overall prevalence of *NF1* mutations appears to be very low.

PATHOLOGY

Neuroblastoma is one of the "small, round blue-cell" neoplasms of childhood; also included are Ewing sarcoma, non-Hodgkin lymphoma, peripheral primitive neuroectodermal

Neuroblastoma can metastasize by lymphatic and hematogenous dissemination. Regional lymph node metastases are noted in up to 35% of patients with apparently localized tumors (INSS stage 2 and 3), and 30% of patients with INSS stage 4 and 4S disease also have regional lymph node involvement.[204] Spread of tumor to lymph nodes outside the cavity of origin is considered to be INSS stage 4 disease, but these patients may have a better outlook if there is no bone marrow, cortical bone, or other parenchymal organ involvement. Hematogenous spread occurs most frequently to bone marrow, cortical bone, liver, and skin (subcutaneous tissue). Rarely, disease may spread to lungs or the central nervous system at diagnosis,[205] but this is more commonly a manifestation of recurrent or end-stage disease. Neuroblastoma can disseminate to the central nervous system by inward compression on the brain from cranial metastases or by meningeal involvement.[204,206-210] The route of spread may be hematogenous or via the cerebral spinal fluid. The proportion of patients presenting with localized, regional, or metastatic disease is age dependent (Table 30.2).

The signs and symptoms of neuroblastoma reflect the location of primary, regional, and metastatic disease. Abdominal disease results in complaints of fullness or discomfort, but biologically favorable disease can present as an asymptomatic mass or even be identified incidentally. Physical examination commonly reveals a fixed, hard abdominal mass in which the borders are difficult to define due to the retroperitoneal origin. If primary tumors arise from the organ of Zuckerkandl, bladder and bowel symptoms may occur as a result of direct compression. Massive involvement of the liver with metastatic disease is particularly frequent in infants with stage 4S and may result in respiratory compromise. Occasionally, the size of primary or metastatic abdominal tumors can result in compression of venous and lymphatic drainage from the lower extremities, leading to scrotal and lower extremity edema. Rarely, patients will experience renin-mediated hypertension because of compromise of renal vasculature. Hypertension, tachycardia, flushing, and sweating are uncommon symptoms because epinephrine is rarely released from most neuroblastomas, since they lack the enzyme necessary for synthesis.

Primary thoracic tumors present as symptomatic masses or can be discovered incidentally when chest radiographs are obtained to evaluate patients for other reasons. High thoracic and cervical masses can be associated with Horner syndrome, which consists of unilateral ptosis, myosis, and anhydrosis. Occasionally, large thoracic tumors are associated with mechanical obstruction and resultant superior vena cava syndrome. Cervical masses from primary or metastatic neuroblastoma may be confused with infection and are correctly diagnosed only at the time of attempted incision and drainage. Paraspinal tumors in the thoracic, abdominal, and pelvic regions may extend into the neural foramina of the vertebral bodies and cause symptoms related to compression of nerve roots and spinal cord. The range of symptomatology includes subacute or acute paraplegia, bladder or bowel dysfunction, or less commonly radicular pain. This situation can be a medical emergency (see Chapter 38), and there is controversy as to the optimal approach to managing spinal cord compression (see later).

Several classical signs and symptoms have been associated with metastatic neuroblastoma. Proptosis and periorbital ecchymoses are frequent and result from tumor infiltration of periorbital bones. The reason for the predilection of bony metastases to the bones of the skull and orbits remains obscure. Widespread bone and bone marrow disease causes bone pain, which can lead to limping, or irritability in a younger child. In addition, there may be bone marrow replacement and symptoms such as anemia, bleeding, or infection.[211,212] Skin involvement is seen almost exclusively in infants with INSS stage 4S tumors and is characterized by a variable number of nontender, bluish subcutaneous nodules.[213] Constitutional symptoms associated with disseminated disease may include failure to thrive and fever, the latter observed most often in the presence of extensive bone metastases.

Although rare, neuroblastoma does occur in adolescents and adults. In general, the distribution of primary sites is similar to that seen in children. The course of the disease is somewhat more indolent, but it is frequently fatal.[214-216] Neuroblastomas in these older patients represent a difficult challenge, because even localized tumors can be recurrent and ultimately fatal over a long period of time.

Paraneoplastic Syndromes

OMAS is a unique paraneoplastic syndrome that is observed in 2% to 4% of newly diagnosed neuroblastoma patients.[217-219] OMAS is manifested by rapid and chaotic eye movements, ataxia, and myoclonia. Most children with this syndrome have a favorable outcome with respect to their tumor, as this syndrome is correlated with an immune-mediated antitumor host response.[220,221] However, 70% to 80% of these children appear to have long-term neurologic deficits, including cognitive and motor delays, language deficits, and behavioral abnormalities.[217-219] These are presumably due to antineural antibodies directed against the tumor that cross-react with neural cells in the cerebellum or elsewhere in the brain,[222] but the pathogenesis of the early and late neurologic manifestations of OMAS are incompletely understood. Treatment of OMAS remains controversial. Tumor removal may result in at least temporary improvement of neurologic symptomatology, but recurrence of OMAS symptoms are common. It was recently noted in a retrospective review of cases registered in the POG that OMAS patients that happened to be treated with chemotherapy had a better neurologic outcome than those patients not exposed to cytotoxic treatment.[223] However, this was not observed in a similar CCG study.[219] About half the cases of OMAS occur without associated neuroblastoma, although some of these cases may be due to tumors that spontaneously regressed. All children with OMAS should have a complete diagnostic workup for neuroblastoma including ^{123}I-MIBG scintigraphy.[224] Glucocorticoids and intravenous immunoglobulin (IVIG) have been used with varying degrees of success.[225-227] Ongoing clinical trials are exploring the role of IVIG, glucocorticoids, Rituximab, and other agents in managing this syndrome.[228]

Intractable watery diarrhea associated with abdominal distension, hypokalemia, and dehydration is a manifestation of

TABLE 30.2

EXTENT OF DISEASE AT DIAGNOSIS ACCORDING TO AGE

INSS stage at diagnosis	<1 yr N (%)	≥1 yr N (%)	Overall N (%)
1	333 (26)	255 (12)	588 (17)
2A/2B	276 (22)	264 (12)	540 (16)
3	184 (14)	354 (16)	538 (16)
4	258 (20)	1264 (59)	1522 (44)
4s	233 (18)	11 (1)	244 (7)
Overall	1284	2148	3432

Courtesy of Wendy London, PhD, Children's Oncology Group Statistical Office.

the VIP syndrome.[229–231] Most tumors associated with this syndrome secrete VIP and are mature histologically (ganglioneuroblastomas or ganglioneuroma), and these patients almost always have a favorable tumor outcome.[232] Unlike the OMAS, surgical removal of the tumor usually results in complete resolution of symptoms, because tumor secretion of VIP is responsible for the syndrome, and tumor removal eliminates this.

CLINICAL AND LABORATORY EVALUATION

Physical examination should include detailed evaluation for an abdominal mass and estimation of location and size. Hepatomegaly is also an important finding that may be apparent on general physical examination. Detailed evaluation of all lymph node structures should be performed, with note made of any enlarged, discolored, or nontender nodes. An enlarged left supraclavicular node may be seen in high-risk neuroblastoma patients with intraabdominal disease and extensive dissemination. Detailed head-and-neck evaluation for proptosis, Horner's syndrome, or skull-based metastases should be performed. Detailed neurologic examination is required, and this is especially critical in young patients with paraspinal masses to ensure that evolving paralysis is not missed.

To confirm this diagnosis, histological evidence is required that demonstrates neural origin or differentiation by light microscopy or immunohistochemistry. Alternatively, because the bone marrow is frequently involved, some patients can be diagnosed with neuroblastoma on the basis of the presence of "unequivocal" neuroblastic cells involving the bone marrow, accompanied by increased urinary catecholamine metabolites. Because tumor-specific genetic markers and histopathological evaluation are critical determinants of treatment planning, especially for younger children, sufficient material for *MYCN* amplification, CNAs, ploidy, histology, and other studies should be obtained for the majority of patients. Because a clearly involved marrow specimen is often adequate for genetic studies, children older than 2 years with extensive marrow involvement may not require a primary tumor biopsy. Nevertheless, treatment planning for infants, and perhaps children between 1 and 2 years of age (see later), can vary greatly depending on genetic features, so a primary tumor biopsy should be performed if adequate tumor tissue cannot be obtained by other means.

The goal of diagnostic testing is to definitively establish the diagnosis and precisely define the extent of disease. CT is the preferred method for evaluation of the primary tumor in the abdomen, pelvis, or posterior mediastinum (Fig. 30.6). MRI evaluation may be superior for paraspinal lesions and is essential when evaluating intraforaminal extension with the potential for cord compression. Either modality can be used to evaluate primary tumors arising in the neck. Practically speaking, for the majority of patients a CT of the chest, abdomen, and pelvis should be performed, with CT and/or MRI of the head, neck, and/or spine performed on the basis of physical findings and clinical suspicion. Patients should also have evaluation for metastatic lesions. Although the trend for patients with localized tumors with favorable biological characteristics has been

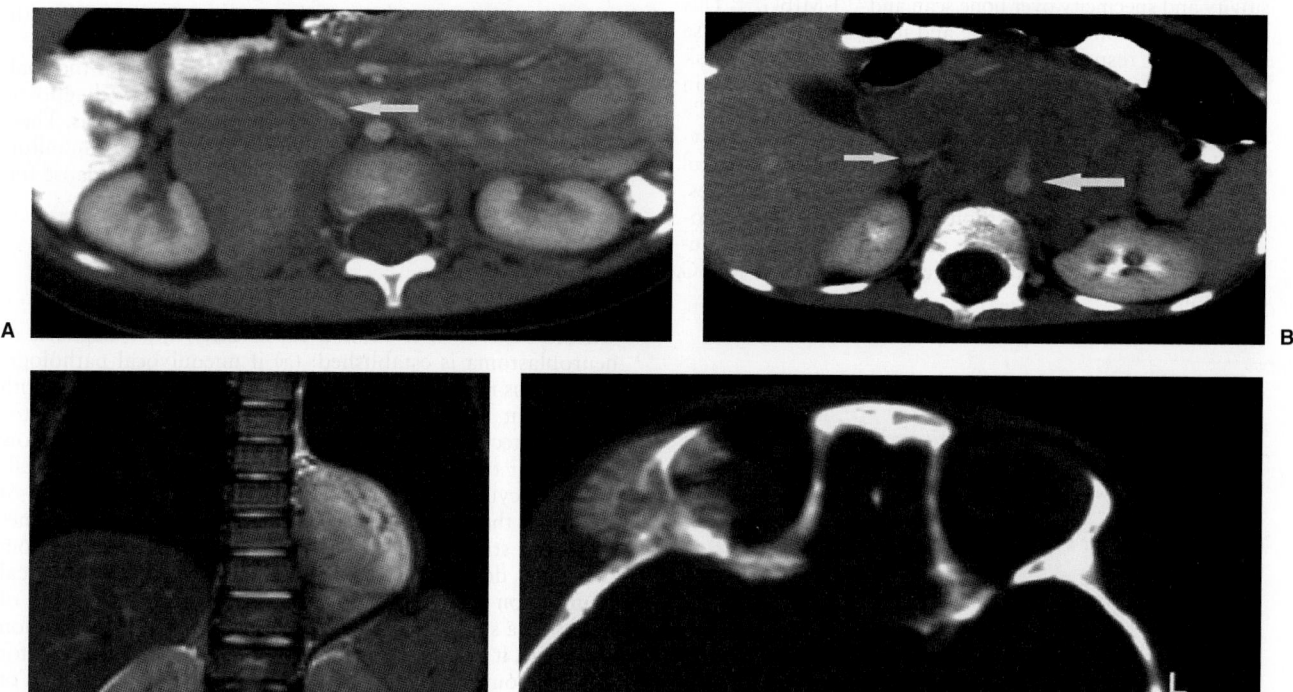

FIGURE 30.6 Anatomic imaging of neuroblastoma. **A:** Contrast-enhanced CT scan of a 2-year-old girl with right-sided localized retroperitoneal neuroblastoma elevating the inferior vena cava (IVC) (*arrow*). **B:** Contrast-enhanced CT scan in a 3-year-old boy with stage 4 neuroblastoma encircling the aorta (*small arrow*) and partially surrounding the IVC (*large arrow*). **C:** Coronal T2-weighted MR image of a 6-year-old girl with left paraspinal ganglioneuroblastoma. **D:** Bone windows from orbital CT with "hair on end" appearance due to periosteal reaction from neuroblastoma metastasis. (Courtesy of James Meyer and Avrum Pollock, Children's Hospital of Philadelphia Department of Radiology.)

to minimize diagnostic testing, most patients should have an evaluation of the bone marrow and bony skeleton for metastatic disease. Exclusion of the tests recommended later may be considered in some settings (e.g., perinatal detection of a small adrenal mass) but only in a setting in which careful follow-up is ensured.

▪ *Evaluation of the bone marrow compartment.* Patients should have bilateral bone marrow aspirates and trephine biopsies. Aspirate amounts should be sufficient for both standard histology and histochemical stains, as well as for immunocytology. Although light microscopy is generally considered sensitive to the level of 1 neuroblastic cell per 100 nucleated cells, immunohistochemical staining with neural-specific antibodies increases the sensitivity to at least 1 in 100,000 cells.[233,234] Currently, panels of anti-GD2 monoclonal antibodies (as well as antibodies against other neural-specific proteins such as NSE, NCAM, synaptophysin) are used routinely for immunocytochemical detection of neuroblastoma. The clinical significance of not clearing readily detectable marrow disease has been demonstrated,[233,234] but the clinical relevance of finding rare positive cells, especially in otherwise low-risk patients, is not clear. There have been a number of studies utilizing PCR-based technologies to detect "neuroblastoma-specific" transcripts such as TH, GD2 synthase, PgP9.5, or others in marrow or blood samples,[235] but the clinical utility of these assays is not yet of proven.

▪ *Evaluation of the bony skeleton.* Classically, evaluation for bone metastases has relied on Tc-99-diphosphonate scintigraphy (bone scan). Plain radiographs may still be useful in infants or to confirm questionable bone metastases. Bone scans are a rapid and reliable technique to evaluate for osteolytic lesions. ^{123}I-MIBG is a radionuclide with superior sensitivity and specificity over bone scan and ^{131}I-MIBG.[236] This modality is becoming a routine and integral part of disease staging and response evaluation, especially in high-risk patients (Fig. 30.7).[216,237] It is common practice to obtain both MIBG and bone scan at diagnosis, because up to 10% of patients may have tumors that are not MIBG avid. However, because discordance is sometimes seen, the most useful single modality should be used for subsequent evaluations. Positron emission tomography with fluorine-18 fluorodeoxyglucose may play a role in metastatic disease evaluation in the future but may be less sensitive than MIBG scintigraphy.[238,239]

The exact type of surgical procedure that should be recommended for any newly diagnosed neuroblastoma patient who has an unresectable primary tumor is controversial. The clinician must recognize the value of having adequate tissues to establish the diagnosis and analyze for all available prognostic factors, while being cognizant of avoiding hemorrhagic or other surgical complications that may lead to patient injury or delay in instituting chemotherapy. In the United States, most investigators have recommended limited open biopsy because it is easier to ensure hemostasis, the biopsy specimens are larger, and the COG has relied on Shimada histopathology for risk classification that is difficult to assess in a specimen derived from a needle biopsy.[200,201] Several centers elsewhere have been using CT-guided needle biopsies more frequently and have reported that this can be performed safely with adequate materials for molecular studies, even if fine needle aspirates are used.[240] Although the care of the patient is paramount, most investigators also recognize the critical importance of submitting residual biological materials (beyond those required for diagnosis) to tumor banks that support translational research.

Catecholamine Metabolism

Because of their noradrenergic derivation, neuroblastomas typically express essential enzymes involved in catecholamine synthesis, affording a technique for noninvasive detection of tumor markers. A simplified diagram of catecholamine synthesis and metabolism is depicted in Figure 30.8. Because monamine oxidase and catechol-O-methyltransferase enzymes are typically expressed in neuroblastomas, and most do not express phenylethanolamine-N-methyltransferase, HVA and VMA are the metabolites that show the highest sensitivity and specificity for tumor detection. Using sensitive HPLC technology, the sensitivity and specificity can approach 100% without significant influence from diet or adrenergic drive.[241] Screening for HVA and VMA in spot urine samples (normalized per mg creatinine) should be part of every diagnostic workup if neuroblastoma is in the differential diagnosis. These markers also provide a relatively reliable method for monitoring response to therapy and surveying for disease relapse following completion of therapy.

Diagnostic Criteria

On the basis of international consensus,[242,243] a diagnosis of neuroblastoma is established: (a) if unequivocal pathologic diagnosis is made from tumor tissue by light microscopy, with or without immunohistology, EM, or increased urine (or serum) catecholamines or metabolites; or (b) if bone marrow aspirate or trephine biopsy contains unequivocal tumor cells (e.g., syncytia or immunocytologically positive clumps of cells) and there are increased urine or serum catecholamines molecular studies. The COG currently excludes infants from the latter definition because the tumor-specific biological information is so important for risk assignment. Because of recent data suggesting a later age cut-off for risk classification (see later), it may be warranted to encourage tumor biopsy for children younger than 18 years of age to ensure acquisition of adequate tumor material for histology and molecular studies.

A Anterior Posterior   Anterior Posterior **B**

FIGURE 30.7 ^{123}I-MIBG imaging of neuroblastoma. **A:** ^{123}I-MIBG scintigraphy shows normal biodistribution to liver and heart. Free ^{123}I concentrated in salivary glands. Other areas of uptake in axial and appendicular skeleton are abnormal in this scan (anterior and posterior views shown) obtained at diagnosis. **B:** Same patient with resolution of all abnormal uptake after induction chemotherapy.

Differential Diagnosis

Because of the many different clinical presentations, neuroblastoma may be confused with a variety of other neoplasms as well as nonneoplastic conditions. This is a problem particularly in

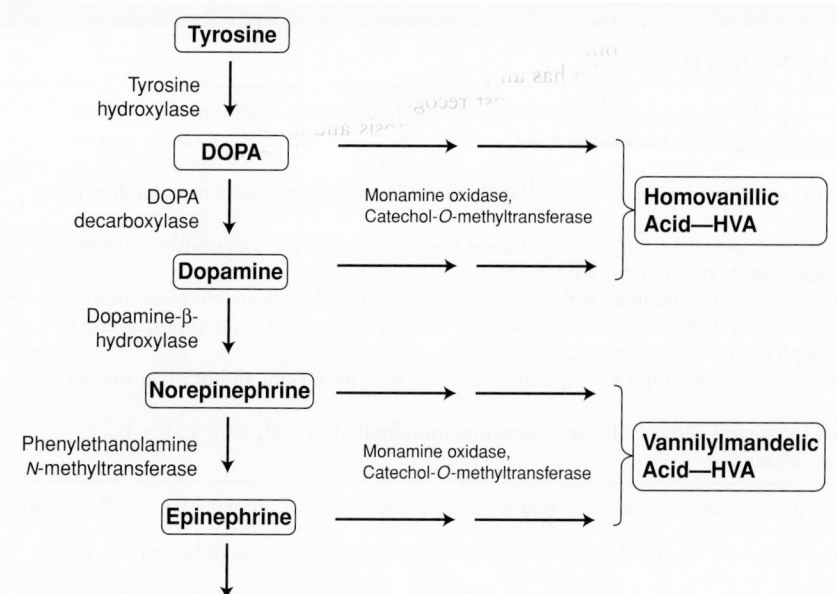

FIGURE 30.8 Pathway of catecholamine metabolism. Shown is a simplified diagram of catecholamine synthesis and metabolism. HVA and VMA are the urinary catecholamine metabolites usually measured for diagnostic purposes and to follow response to therapy.

the 5% to 10% of tumors that do not produce catecholamines and/or show MIBG avidity, as well as in the rare patients who do not have an obvious primary tumor. Alternatively, neuroblastoma should be considered in the differential diagnosis of a variety of nonneoplastic conditions. Patients with disseminated bone disease may resemble those with systemic infections or inflammatory diseases, such as osteomyelitis or rheumatoid arthritis. The VIP syndrome can be confused with infectious or inflammatory bowel disease, and the OMAS can resemble primary neurologic condition. Neuroblastoma may be confused with a calcified adrenal gland following adrenal hemorrhage. Patients with hepatomegaly must have multicystic or storage diseases considered.

Histologically, neuroblastoma tissue from primary or metastatic sites may be undifferentiated, and may be confused with other small, round blue-cell tumors (see the Pathology section). Differential diagnosis of metastatic disease involving the marrow must include rhabdomyosarcoma, Ewing sarcoma/neuroepithelioma/PNET, lymphoma, or leukemia (especially megakaryoblastic leukemia). A battery of monoclonal antibodies or histochemical stains, as well as molecular studies looking for characteristic genetic changes (such as translocations), should allow reliable diagnosis of these various disease entities.[244-247]

STAGING AND TREATMENT RESPONSE

Staging of neuroblastoma has evolved considerably since the first neuroblastoma-specific staging system was introduced by Evans et al. in 1971.[248] Other staging systems were developed in the United States (POG),[249] Japan[250] and elsewhere, and all were highly predictive of outcome in earlier studies. However, some of the differences between these and other staging systems are substantial, particularly as applied to patients with intermediate stages, and the results of one group could not be compared readily with another. Therefore, a broadly representative international group met to formulate and then refine an INSS that would lead to uniformity in staging of patients with neuroblastoma for clinical trials and biological studies

around the world[242,243] (Table 30.3). Stage of disease by the INSS replaced these other systems but retained their most useful aspects. The INSS system is most similar to the system utilized by the POG in that it is surgically based. The INSS gained acceptance worldwide and has been utilized by essentially all major cooperative groups and countries.

However, because the skill and aggressiveness of the local surgeon could substantially change the stage of individual patients (e.g., from an INSS-3 to an INSS-1), an alternative approach was needed for presurgical staging that was based on clinical assessment and imaging.[251] Again, an international group was convened that represented every major group, country, and discipline to develop a consensus for neuroblastoma risk groups (utilizing clinical features as well as biological features of the tumor), as well as a presurgical staging system (using image-defined "risk factors"). This has led to an INRG classification system[203] (see below) and an INRG staging system[252] (Table 30.4). Currently, the INRGSS is being evaluated prospectively, and the INSS is still being used for clinical staging. Once utility and consistency of the INRGSS are validated, it will likely replace the INSS as the primary approach to neuroblastoma staging throughout the world. This should make it easier to compare studies conducted by different groups and countries to assess therapeutic protocols and biological classification schemes. However, at the present time, the INSS is still used as the primary staging system in the United States, Europe and Japan, so this will be reviewed in more detail below.

Stage 1 is a localized tumor that is surgically resected. Microscopic residual tumor at the margins is allowed. Stage 2 represents localized tumors with gross residual disease (2A) or localized tumors with ipsilateral lymph node involvement, regardless of resectability (2B). At the present time, it does not appear that there is a substantial difference in outcome between 2A and 2B, so this distinction may be dropped.[164] Patients with a unilateral tumor and ipsilateral pleural effusion are considered to have stage 2. Stage 3 tumors show invasion across the midline, either on the basis of direct extension or by lymph node involvement. Most stage 3 tumors arise in the abdomen, because tumors crossing the midline by contiguous infiltration or by lymph node involvement are less common in the thorax. Infiltration is meant to indicate

TABLE 30.3

INTERNATIONAL NEUROBLASTOMA STAGING SYSTEM

Stage 1	Localized tumor with complete gross excision, with or without microscopic residual disease; representative ipsilateral lymph nodes negative for tumor microscopically (nodes attached to and removed with the primary tumor may be positive).
Stage 2A	Localized tumor with incomplete gross excision; representative ipsilateral nonadherent lymph nodes negative for tumor microscopically.
Stage 2B	Localized tumor with or without complete gross excision, with ipsilateral nonadherent lymph nodes positive for tumor. Enlarged contralateral lymph nodes must be negative microscopically.
Stage 3	Unresectable unilateral tumor infiltrating across the midline,[a] with or without regional lymph node involvement; *or* localized unilateral tumor with contralateral regional lymph node involvement; *or* midline tumor with bilateral extension by infiltration (unresectable) or by lymph node involvement.
Stage 4	Any primary tumor with dissemination to distant lymph nodes, bone, bone marrow, liver, skin, and/or other organs (except as defined for stage 4S).
Stage 4S	Localized primary tumor (as defined for stage 1, 2A, or 2B), with dissemination limited to skin, liver, and/or bone marrow[b] (limited to infants, 1 year of age).

Note: Multifocal primary tumors (e.g., bilateral adrenal primary tumors) should be staged according to the greatest extent of disease, as defined previously, followed by a subscript "M" (e.g., 3_M).
[a]The midline is defined as the vertebral column. Tumors originating on one side and "crossing the midline" must infiltrate to or beyond the opposite side of the vertebral column.
[b]Marrow involvement in stage 4S should be minimal, that is, less than 10% of total nucleated cells identified as malignant on bone marrow biopsy or on marrow aspirate. More extensive marrow involvement would be considered to be stage 4. The MIBG scan (if done) should be negative in the marrow.
From Brodeur GM, Seeger RC, Barrett A, et al. International criteria for diagnosis, staging and response to treatment in patients with neuroblastoma. J Clin Oncol 1988;6:1874–1881; and Brodeur GM, Pritchard J, Berthold F, et al. Revisions in the international criteria for neuroblastoma diagnosis, staging, and response to treatment. J Clin Oncol 1993;11:1466–1477.

contiguous invasion of tumor across the midline (defined as the vertebral column), rather than a pedunculated tumor that hangs over the midline.

Patients with disseminated disease involving distant lymph nodes, bone, bone marrow, liver, and/or other organs are categorized as having stage 4 disease (except as defined in stage 4S). There is some evidence that patients who have stage 4 on the basis of distant lymph node, liver, or marrow involvement (excluding 4S), especially patients younger than 2 years, do better than those who have stage 4 on the basis of cortical bone involvement.[250,253] Because these distinctions may affect prognosis or choice of therapy, the criteria by which patients are considered to have stage 4 should be recorded. However, such distinctions may also be affected or obliterated by improvements in treatment.

TABLE 30.4

INTERNATIONAL NEUROBLASTOMA RISK GROUP STAGING SYSTEM

L1	Localized tumor not involving vital structures as defined by the list of image-defined risk factors and confined to one body compartment
L2	Locoregional tumor with the presence of one or more image-defined risk factors
M	Distant metastatic disease (except stage MS)
MS	Metastatic disease in children younger than 18 months with metastases confined to skin, liver, and/or bone marrow

Note: See primary reference for detailed criteria and image-defined risk factors. Patients with multifocal primary tumors should be staged according to the greatest extent of disease, as defined in the table. From Monclair T, Brodeur GM, Ambros PF, et al. The International Neuroblastoma Risk Group (INRG) Staging System: An INRG Task Force Report. J Clin Oncol 2008;27:298–303.

Stage 4S has been retained as a distinct stage, based on the favorable outcome generally experienced with these patients,[213,254–256] and because of recent biological evidence distinguishing these patients from infants with conventional stage 4 disease. For example, the majority of stage 4S tumors have a hyperdiploid DI and less than 10% have *MYCN* amplification, in contrast to tumors from stage 4 infants, in which the DI is more often diploid and *MYCN* is amplified in about one-third.[84] Bone marrow involvement is allowed if less than 10% of nucleated marrow cells are malignant cells.[242,243] Patients with more extensive marrow involvement should be classified as stage 4. Patients with multifocal primary tumors are staged on the basis of the greatest tumor extent, and the multifocal nature of the primary is noted with a subscript (e.g., stage 3M).[242]

The POG and CCG evaluated the efficacy of these staging definitions to define prognostic subsets of patients by applying the INSS criteria to prospectively collected surgicopathological data.[257,258] This experience with the INSS suggests that these new criteria clearly provide prognostic information that is at least equivalent or superior to the staging systems used previously. This is an important step toward furnishing a stable clinical background on which multivariate analyses can be performed to identify biologically based risk groups (see later). However, the INSS will likely be replaced by the INRGSS in the future, once this image-based presurgical staging system is validated prospectively in ongoing clinical trials.

The same tests that are used for determining extent of disease should be used to assess response of primary and metastatic sites to treatment. Table 30.5 lists internationally proposed criteria to determine response to therapy in patients with neuroblastoma.[242,243] These definitions are consistent with recently proposed standards for definitions of treatment response in solid tumors.[259] It is important to note that a given level of overall response involves thorough assessment of both primary and metastatic sites. For example, a CR overall requires that the primary tumor and all metastatic sites fulfill CR criteria. A CR in metastatic sites and a PR in the primary

TABLE 30.5

DEFINITIONS OF RESPONSE TO TREATMENT

Response[a]	Primary	Metastases	Markers
CR	No tumor	No tumor (chest, abdomen, liver, bone, bone marrow, nodes, etc.)	HVA/VMA normal
VGPR	Reduction >90% but <100%	No tumor (as above except bone); no new bone lesions, all preexisting lesions improved	HVA/VMA decreased >90%
PR	Reduction 50%–90%	No new lesions; 50%–90% reduction in measurable sites; 0–1 bone marrow samples with tumor; bone lesions same as VGPR	HVA/VMA decreased 50%–90%
MR	No new lesions; >50% reduction of any measurable lesion (primary or metastases) with <50% reduction in any other; <25% increase in any existing lesion[b]		
NR	No new lesions; <50% reduction but <25% increase in any existing lesion[b]		
PD	Any new lesion; increase of any measurable lesion by >25%; previous negative marrow positive for tumor		

[a]CR, complete response; MR, mixed response; NR, no response; PD, progressive disease; PR, partial response; VGPR, very good partial response.
[b]Quantitative assessment does not apply to marrow disease.
From Brodeur GM, Seeger RC, Barrett A, et al. International criteria for diagnosis, staging and response to treatment in patients with neuroblastoma. J Clin Oncol 1988;6:1874–1881; and Brodeur GM, Pritchard J, Berthold F, et al. Revisions in the international criteria for neuroblastoma diagnosis, staging, and response to treatment. J Clin Oncol 1993;11:1466–1477.

tumor would be considered a PR overall. For high-risk patients, response is typically evaluated prior to second-look surgery, at the end of induction chemotherapy, recovery from stem cell rescue and local radiotherapy, and at the end of maintenance biotherapy.

Neuroblastoma is unique in that scintigraphic and bone marrow evaluations play such an important role in response evaluation. Because it is difficult to measure disease in these sites, objective scoring systems have been proposed for MIBG,[237,260] and quantification of marrow disease has been attempted using immunocytochemistry and/or RT-PCR,[233,234,261] but these systems are not currently employed outside of the research setting. The response system proposed in Table 30.5 is adequate for measuring response to front-line treatment, although the increasing quality of MIBG scans makes comparisons to past studies difficult. This system is rather inadequate in evaluating response in high-risk patients following relapse, as many of these patients only have evaluable disease in bone and bone marrow. Thus, current clinical trials have incorporated objective measures of MIBG and bone marrow response in an attempt to more precisely and accurately define response rates in phase 1 and 2 clinical trials.

PROGNOSTIC CONSIDERATIONS

Neuroblastoma has served as a paradigm for the incorporation of both clinical and tumor-specific biological variables into risk prediction algorithms. The major prognostic variables in current use, or being considered, are discussed later. All cooperative groups use at least a subset of the major variables. The prognostic criteria currently used by COG to define risk groups are shown in Table 30.6. The impact of the five most commonly used prognostic variables, as well as a risk grouping based on these variables, is shown in Figure 30.9. The recently proposed INRG classification schema is shown in Table 30.7.

Disease Stage

Stage of disease by the INSS[242,243] is clearly correlated with patient outcome and is used by all cooperative groups to stratify therapy (Fig. 30.9A). Most patients with INSS stage 1 are cured by surgery alone, whereas most patients with INSS stage 4 require either moderate or highly intensive multimodality therapy. The most appropriate therapy for patients with INSS stages 2 and 3 disease is more dependent on other factors. Currently, the COG is testing for 1p and 11q allelic loss to stratify patients who are at higher risk of relapse, and who, therefore, may benefit from additional courses of moderate-dose chemotherapy. As the genetic and biological characterization of neuroblastomas becomes more comprehensive, it is likely that we will rely more on biological characteristics and less on the subtle distinctions in disease stage to make therapeutic decisions. In the coming years, the INRGSS will replace the INSS, as this system is implemented and validated worldwide.

Age at Diagnosis

Breslow and McCann[261] first reported the relationship between age at diagnosis with patient outcome in 1971 (Table 30.2). Traditionally, age has been analyzed as a binary function, with a cut point at the first year of life being used by most groups, and this has proven clinical utility (Fig. 30.9B). However, because age is a continuous variable, alternative ages have recently been explored as surrogates for tumor behavior. Recent reviews by the CCG and POG reached similar conclusions that 18 months of age more clearly discriminated outcome in patients, such as those with INSS stage 4 disease and no MYCN amplification.[263–265] It is important to recognize that the children aged 12 to 18 months in the studies cited here were all treated with significant chemotherapeutic dose intensity, and many received myeloablative chemotherapy. Whether therapy can be safely reduced in children between 1 and 2 years of age with INSS stage 3 or 4 is being explored in a controlled research setting.

Tumor Pathology

Like the evolution of neuroblastoma staging systems over time, a variety of histopathological grading systems have been proposed and utilized by different investigators.[198,266] As mentioned previously, an international consensus on a histopathological grading system was agreed upon and is being evaluated prospectively. The INPC again places tumors into two broad categories of "favorable" and "unfavorable" on the basis of analysis of the stromal component, degree of differentiation, MKI, and patient age[199–201,267] (Fig. 30.9C). This system clearly defines nodular ganglioneuroblastomas as an unfavorable histopathological subtype. The critical component of age as a covariate in the INPC complicates the independent value of this system for prognostication in any risk stratification system that also uses age. The new INRG classification system[203] will include tumor grade and differentiation as independent variables for risk stratification, at least in subsets of patients, but patient age will no longer be linked to histological features.

Tumor Cell Ploidy

The tumor cell DNA index (DI, or ploidy) is also a powerful prognostic marker for patients younger than 2 years at diagnosis with disseminated disease and especially for patients with INSS stage 4S disease.[82,84,85,263,268–272] Of the major variables used by COG to stratify therapy, ploidy appears to have the most restricted utility because the univariate impact

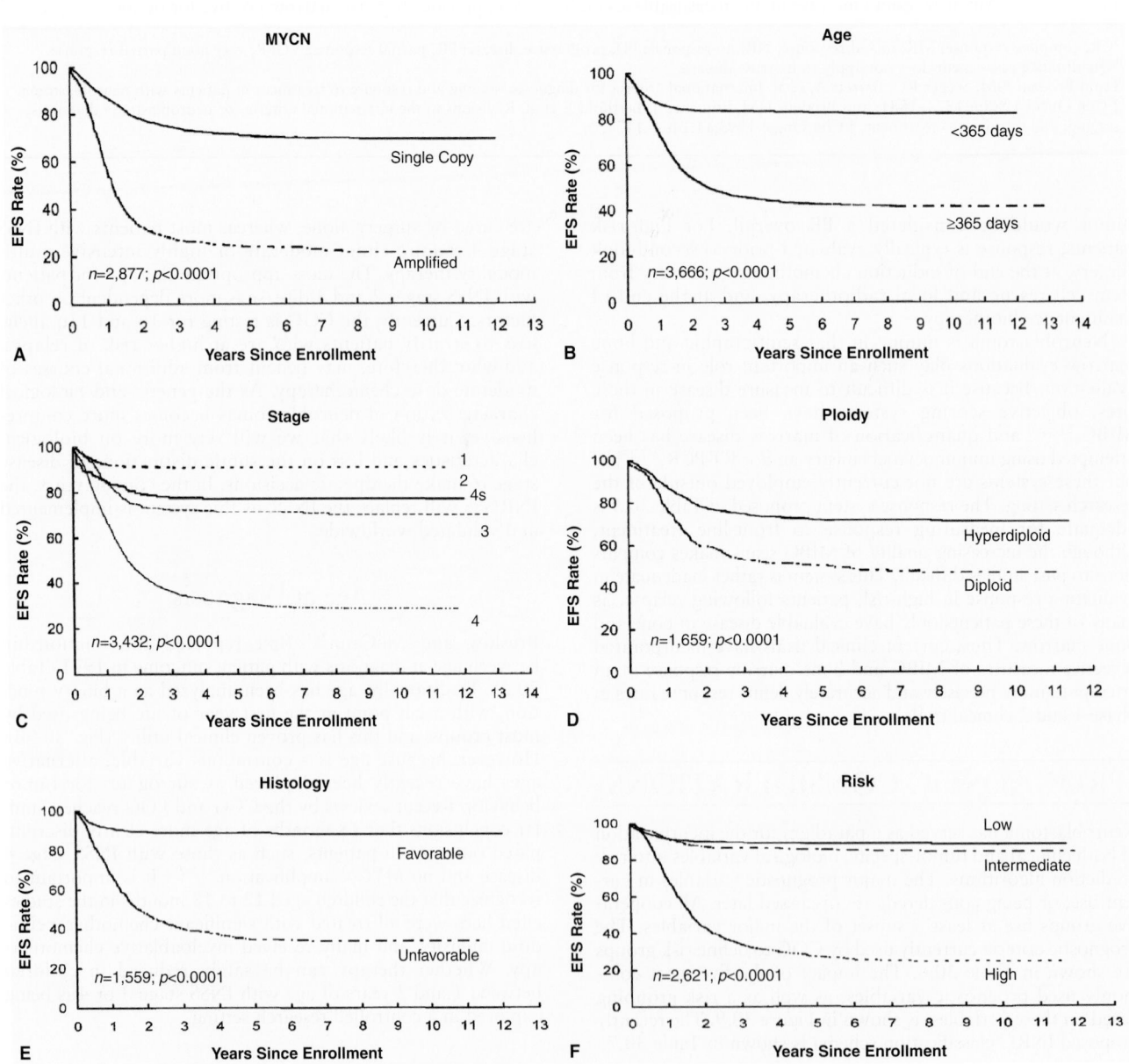

FIGURE 30.9 Analysis of EFS by risk factors. A cohort of 3666 neuroblastoma patients was analyzed for EFS by individual risk factors. The number for each indicates the number of patients for whom information about that variable was available. **A:** INSS stage. **B:** Patient age. **C:** Shimada/INPC histopathology classification. **D:** Tumor cell DNA index (ploidy). **E:** MYCN amplification status. **F:** COG risk group (see Table 30.6). (From Maris JM. The biological basis for neuroblastoma heterogeneity and risk stratification. Curr Opin Pediatr 2005;17:7–13.)

TABLE 30.6

COG RISK GROUP AND PROTOCOL ASSIGNMENT SCHEMA

INSS stage	Age	MYCN status	Shimada histology	DNA ploidy	Risk group
1	0–21 yr	Any[a]	Any[b]	Any[c]	Low
2A/2B	<365 d	Any[a]	Any[b]	Any[c]	Low
	>365 d–21 yr	Non-amp	Any[b]	—	Low
	>365 d–21 yr	Amp	Fav	—	Low
	>365 d–21 yr	Amp	Unfav	—	High
3	<365 d	Non-amp	Any[b]	Any[c]	Intermediate
	<365 d	Amp	Any[b]	Any[c]	High
	>365 d–21 yr	Non-amp	Fav	—	Intermediate
	>365 d–21 yr	Non-amp	Unfav	—	High
	>365 d–21 yr	Amp	Any	—	High
4	<365 d	Non-amp	Any[b]	Any[c]	Intermediate
	<365 d	Amp	Any	Any	High
	>365 d–21 yr	Any	Any	—	High
4S	<365 d	Non-amp	Fav	.1	Low
	<365 d	Non-amp	Any[b]	51	Intermediate
	<365 d	Non-amp	Unfav	Any[c]	Intermediate
	<365 d	Amp	Any	Any	High

Biology defined by *MYCN* status: amplified (Amp) vs. non-amplified (non-amp); Shimada histopathology: favorable (Fav) vs. unfavorable (Unfav); DNA ploidy: DNA index (DI) >1 or = 1; hypodiploid tumors (with DI <1) will be treated as a tumor with a DI >1.
[a]Must be "not amplified" or "amplified" cannot be unsatisfactory.
[b]Must be "favorable" or "unfavorable" cannot be inadequate.
[c]Must be >1 or = 1 (for patients <365 d) cannot be unsatisfactory.

TABLE 30.7

INTERNATIONAL NEUROBLASTOMA RISK GROUP (INRG) CONSENSUS PRETREATMENT CLASSIFICATION SCHEMA

INRG stage	Age (mo)	Histologic category	Grade of tumor differentiation	MYCN	11q Aberration	Ploidy		Pretreatment risk group
L1/L2		GN maturing; GNB intermixed					A	Very low
L1		Any, except GN maturing or GNB intermixed		NA			B	Very low
				Amp			K	High
L2	<18	Any, except GN maturing or GNB intermixed		NA	No		D	Low
					Yes		G	Intermediate
	≥18	GNB nodular; neuroblastoma	Differentiating	NA	No		E	Low
					Yes		H	Intermediate
			Poorly differentiated or undifferentiated	NA				
				Amp			N	High
M	<18			NA		Hyperdiploid	F	Low
	<12			NA		Diploid	I	Intermediate
	12 to <18			NA		Diploid	J	Intermediate
	<18			Amp			O	High
	≥18						P	High
MS	<18			NA	No		C	Very low
				Amp	Yes		Q	High
							R	High

Pretreatment risk group H has two entries. 12 months 365 days; 18 months 547 days; blank field "any"; diploid (DNA index 1.0); hyperdiploid (DNA index 1.0 and includes near-triploid and near-tetraploid tumors); very low risk (5-yr EFS 85%); low risk (5-yr EFS 75% to 85%); intermediate risk (5-yr EFS 50% to 75%); high risk (5-yr EFS 50%).
GN, ganglioneuroma; GNB, ganglioneuroblastoma; Amp, amplified; NA, not amplified; L1, localized tumor confined to one body compartment and with the absence of image-defined risk factors; L2, locoregional tumor with the presence of one or more image-defined risk factors; M, distant metastatic disease (except stage MS); MS, metastatic disease confined to skin, liver, and/or bone marrow in children younger than 18 months [for staging details, see text and Monclair et al. (ref 251)].

on outcome is least dramatic (Fig. 30.9D) and it loses prognostic significance in older patients and in multivariate analyses.

MYCN Amplification Status

Molecular diagnostic detection of *MYCN* amplification provided the seminal example of the clinical utility of tumor-specific genetic information[99,100] (Fig. 30.9E). The prognostic impact of this genomic aberration is currently most important in patients who otherwise would be judged to be at low or intermediate risk, such as infants with INSS stage 4 disease[97] (Fig. 30.10A). The likelihood of detecting *MYCN* amplification in a tumor specimen is highly correlated with other prognostic variables, such as advanced stage, older age, near diploidy, and unfavorable histology (Table 30.1). On the other hand, in INSS stage 4 disease, the distribution of *MYCN* amplification is unimodal with a peak at over 65% of cases in patients 18 to 24 months of age (Fig. 30.10B). Although the prognostic relevance of *MYCN* amplification within the group of patients older than 1 year with metastatic disease is diluted by the generally poor outcome observed currently,[272] it is possible that the prognostic relevance will emerge even in this group as OS improves.

Specific Regions of Allelic Gain or Loss

A variety of genetic changes in neuroblastoma cells have been proposed as useful prognostic markers. Of all of the markers

discussed previously, deletions of chromosome 1p and 11q are the only ones currently being integrated into risk stratification algorithms in the United States and Europe.[124,125,133,134]

Other Proposed Prognostic Markers

Several serum markers have been proposed either to predict outcome or to follow disease activity, including serum ferritin, NSK, LDH, and circulating GD2.[274–277] Although all of these markers have prognostic significance in univariate analyses, most or all lose their predictive value in multivariable analyses. Thus, none of these markers are being used currently by major groups or countries to predict outcome or select therapy.

PRINCIPLES OF INITIAL THERAPY

The treatment modalities traditionally employed in the management of neuroblastoma are surgery, chemotherapy, and radiotherapy. Recently, immunotherapy has been established as an important component of advanced neuroblastoma treatment. The role of each modality is determined by the anticipated clinical behavior of the tumor in individual cases, considering both clinical and tumor genomic features. As targeted therapy for neuroblastoma becomes more established in the therapeutic arsenal, assessment of tumor cells for target expression will need to be considered.

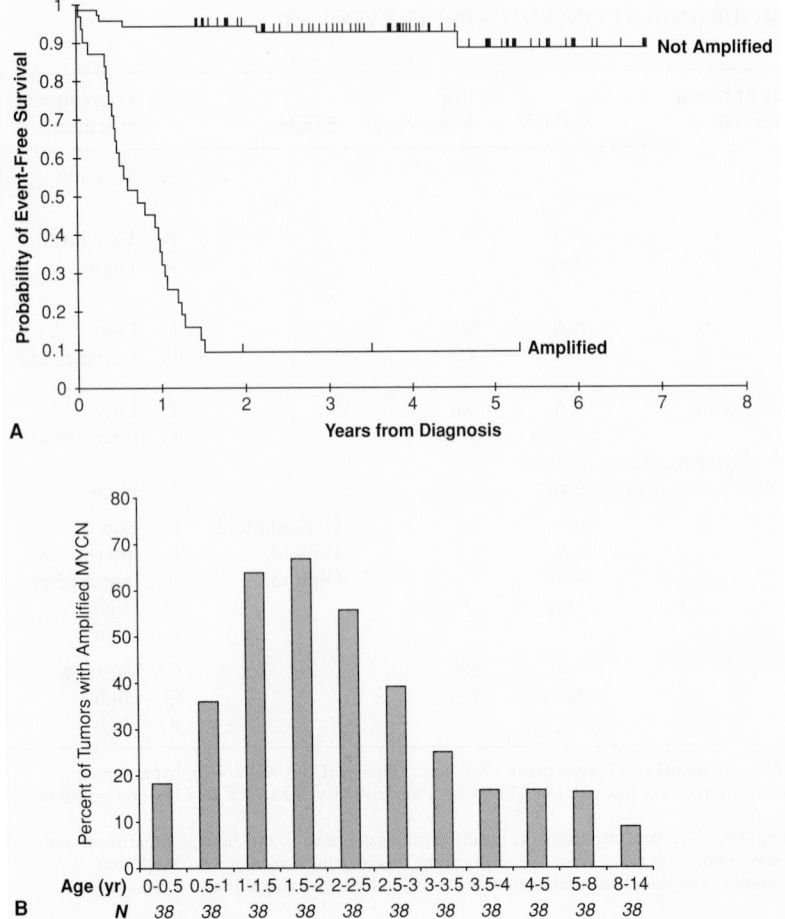

FIGURE 30.10 A: EFS for 102 infants with stage 4 neuroblastoma, stratified by *MYCN* gene status.[176] Not amplified, N = 71; amplified, N = 31; *p* < 0.0001. (Figure redrawn with permission from Dr. Mary Lou Schmidt, University of Illinois, Chicago, IL.) **B:** Percent of neuroblastoma patients at various age intervals whose tumors had *MYCN* amplification.

Surgery

Surgery plays a pivotal role in the management of neuroblastoma, both for diagnosis and for treatment.[278] The goals of primary surgical procedures performed prior to any therapy are to establish the diagnosis, to provide tissue for genetic studies, to determine if regional dissemination has occurred, and to excise the tumor if possible without injury to vital structures. In delayed primary (or "second-look") surgery for high-risk patients, the surgeon would determine response to therapy and remove residual disease when possible. Surgery is not the primary modality of treatment for children with high-risk neuroblastoma. However, it is likely that biopsies in the diagnosis or relapse setting will become more common because of the increasing focus on molecular biomarkers for treatment stratification, and the resultant data will be used to select appropriate clinical trials and/or established therapies.

For newly diagnosed patients, the surgeon has played a central role in the initial diagnostic staging as the INSS system, which was designed as a surgical staging system.[242] As mentioned above, a new INRG system has been proposed, and although surgery remains a critical aspect of patient care, the presurgical staging will be defined by radiographic imaging in the future.[251] We will be in a transition phase at least for the next several years, as the INRG needs to be validated, so operative protocol for surgicopathological staging as recommended by INSS criteria remains relevant. The major points are detailed here:

- The resectability of primary or metastatic tumor should be determined by tumor location, mobility, relationship to major vessels and nerves, ability to control blood supply, the presence of distant metastases, and overall patient prognosis. With the efficacy of modern chemotherapy to reduce the size of large primary tumors and metastases, sacrifice of vital structures to achieve resection at diagnosis should be avoided.
- Nonadherent, intracavitary lymph nodes should be sampled. Gross examination during surgery may be inaccurate for detecting or ruling out lymph node metastases in up to 25% of cases. The status of lymph nodes adherent to and removed *en bloc* with the primary tumor seems to have little relevance in predicting outcome of the patient.[279] Ideally, lymph nodes superior and inferior to the primary tumor should be sought and sampled, with documentation of location. Problematic situations for lymph node sampling include patients with cervical, high thoracic, or large abdominal primary tumors that are unresectable. In these cases, access to lymph nodes may be difficult. Because there are other prognostic factors that may be assessed in these cases, the value of additional information regarding lymph node involvement is questionable. There is no indication for random liver biopsies to rule out occult hepatic metastases.[280]

The importance of gross total resection in the management of disseminated neuroblastoma remains controversial. Haase et al.[281] noted improved EFS in 39 children with complete resection versus the 23 undergoing partial resection. Neither the timing of the surgery nor the tumor *MYCN* copy number predicted resectability of primary tumors. In a retrospective review of 141 cases at Memorial Sloan-Kettering Cancer Center by LaQuaglia et al.,[282] gross total resection of the primary tumor correlated with improved survival ($p < 0.01$). Chamberlain et al.[283] noted superior rates of survival at 3 years (40% vs. 15%) in patients undergoing complete versus partial surgical resection. In contrast, the experience at Great Ormond Street showed that gross total resection did not provide a survival advantage.[284,285] Nakagawara et al.[286] noted that the degree of surgical resection of the primary tumor was directly related to improved survival in patients with Evans stages III and IV *MYCN* amplified tumors, but not in tumors with a normal *MYCN* copy number. Further examination of this area is needed, but it is likely that resectability is a surrogate for tumor biology, and that gross total resection should be the goal, but not at the risk of damage to vital structures or significant postoperative morbidity. It is important to recognize that gross total resection in high-risk patients is generally attempted during or at the end of induction chemotherapy, and so long postoperative recovery will just delay the institution of cytotoxic therapy.

Surgical complications in neuroblastoma have been reported at rates from 5% to 25%.[282,287–289] Cecchetto et al.[290] have defined surgical risk factors that were associated with surgical morbidity and validated these in the setting of localized disease. These form the basis of the new INRGSS, and they are being studied in the COG prospectively, along with INSS staging. The incidence of surgical morbidity is highest with aggressive attempts to resect abdominal tumors at diagnosis. Commonly encountered problems include nephrectomy, operative hemorrhage, postoperative intussusception or adhesions, injury to renal vessels with subsequent renal failure, and neurologic deficits such as Horner syndrome. Because complications are more frequent in infants, who have a substantially better survival, avoidance of surgical risk is particularly important. This is especially challenging in infants 0 to 2 months of age with INSS stage 4S disease and rapidly expanding abdominal distension. Complications generally are lower for delayed or second-look procedures after tumor shrinkage by chemotherapy,[288] but the surgical management of high-risk tumors that are difficult to resect even after cytotoxic therapy remains controversial.

There has been extensive discourse on the proper diagnostic surgical procedure that should be performed when gross total resection is not possible. The general principle is to perform the least invasive procedure possible, but to assure that there is adequate collection of tissues for diagnosis, molecular analysis of prognostically relevant variables, and tumor banking. In the past, open biopsies were preferred mainly due to the relative ease of dealing with tumor hemorrhage, and because the Shimada histopathological grading system required larger tissue specimens for optimal assessment of tumor differentiation status and MKI.[198] However, there has been an increasing trend toward percutaneous fine or true-cut needle biopsies for diagnosis and molecular classification of high-risk neuroblastomas. The optimal intervention must be individualized for a given patient, but it must be emphasized that adequate tissue sampling is of paramount importance both for proper molecular characterization and for advancing the field through innovative research on banked tissue specimens.

Radiation Therapy

High-risk neuroblastoma is generally considered a radiosensitive but not a radiocurable tumor, because of the prevalence of metastatic disease.[291,292] Accepted tumoricidal doses of ionizing radiation range from 15 to 30 Gy, depending on patient age, tumor volume, and tumor location.[293,294] Fractional radiation doses range from 150 to 300 cGy, again depending on tumor volume. Historically, radiation has been used in the multimodality management of residual neuroblastoma, bulky unresectable tumors, and disseminated disease. More recently, the role of external beam radiotherapy in neuroblastoma continues to be refined with the improvement in multiagent chemotherapy and the increasing trend toward reduction of therapy in patients with low- and intermediate-risk disease.

The role of radiation therapy for patients with locoregional disease has evolved. From a randomized trial in children with regional lymph node metastases (INSS stages 2B, 3), Castleberry et al.[280] reported statistically superior rates of CR (76% vs. 46%, $p = 0.013$), EFS (59% vs. 32%, $p = 0.009$), and OS (73% vs. 41%, $p = 0.008$) in patients receiving low-dose, sequential cyclophosphamide and doxorubicin[294] in combination with local radiation (24 to 30 Gy) compared with the same chemotherapy alone. However, in the context of more dose-intensive chemotherapy, and accounting for the status of *MYCN* copy number, this may no longer be true. Strother et al. from the POG[296] reported a study in which INSS stage 2B/3 tumors were treated with high-dose cisplatin and etoposide alternated with low-dose sequential cyclophosphamide plus doxorubicin. Radiation was given only if a CR was not achieved after 15 weeks of treatment plus second-look surgery. Sixteen of 21 patients without *MYCN*-amplified tumors remain free of disease, most without radiotherapy, compared with only 1 of 11 who had tumors with *MYCN* amplification. De Bernardi[297] found no advantage for radiotherapy in a randomized trial (chemotherapy ± radiotherapy) in nonmetastatic patients with residual tumor or positive lymph nodes (INSS stages 2 and 3) following initial surgery. Also, nonrandomized addition of radiation therapy for patients with gross residual disease following second surgery for Evans stage III disease had no apparent influence on disease outcome.[298] Currently, most cooperative groups are withholding radiation therapy for the majority of intermediate-risk patients, except for the patients with disease progression despite surgery and chemotherapy, or patients with unresectable primary tumors at the end of chemotherapy that have unfavorable biological features.[299]

One indication for emergent radiation therapy is the neonate with INSS stage 4S neuroblastoma who develops respiratory distress secondary to hepatomegaly, and treatment with chemotherapy is ineffective.[213,255,300–302] Effective doses are 3 to 6 Gy in single or multiple fractions.[293] However, considering the potential long-term side effects, chemotherapy alone should remain the initial approach in these patients.

Emergent radiation alone or in combination with laminectomy has been employed in the past for children with dumbbell extension of neuroblastoma and symptoms of spinal cord compression. Radiation doses employed range from 7.5 to 30 Gy.[303] Although effective, these modalities are associated with a significant incidence of vertebral body damage or growth arrest and spinal instability leading to scoliosis. In newly diagnosed patients, the use of chemotherapy alone has been reported to be an efficacious alternative associated with fewer long-term side effects,[304–307] and is, thus, the preferred primary intervention for symptomatic patients with paraspinal neuroblastoma.

TBI has been used in myeloablative conditioning regimens followed by stem cell rescue.[308–312] Doses of 7.5 to 12 Gy given in three to five fractions have traditionally been employed. Most cooperative groups are currently using non-TBI containing conditioning regimens currently, because of the late effects associated with this therapy in young children,[312] and the increased experience with chemotherapy-only conditioning regimens in the autologous setting.

In patients with high-risk disease, radiation therapy has been used for both local control of primary tumor and refractory metastatic sites. Doses of 10 to 21 Gy are typically given,[311,312] and most centers deliver this in single daily fractions of 180 to 200 cGy. Because no randomized trial involving a radiotherapy question in high-risk neuroblastoma has ever been performed, it is very difficult to judge its impact on outcome. Review of the CCG experience, in which patients either received 10-Gy local external beam radiotherapy or 10 Gy plus the dose received by 10 Gy TBI in the context of myeloablative consolidation chemotherapy (CCG-3891, see later), showed increased local control rates for the patients receiving the equivalent of 20 Gy.[311] Although these data strongly suggest a role, and perhaps a dose-response effect, for external beam radiotherapy in high-risk neuroblastoma, the results must be viewed with caution because of the different consolidation approaches (myeloablative vs. continuation chemotherapy) received in these patients. The COG is currently studying whether or not 36 Gy to the tumor bed for patients achieving less than a VGPR at the primary tumor site might decrease local failure rates in the context of an ongoing high-risk clinical trial.

Finally, external beam radiation therapy remains a mainstay for palliation of painful end-stage disease. Higher fractional doses may be used in this setting, and pain relief from bony expansion of metastatic deposits can often be observed in a matter of days. In addition, targeted radiotherapy with ^{131}I-MIBG has been studied extensively in the relapse setting (see later), and several groups are making plans to further investigate this active agent at the end of chemotherapy induction for patients with high-risk disease.

Chemotherapy

Chemotherapy is the predominant modality of management in neuroblastoma patients who have intermediate- or high-risk disease, and it is also used in low-risk patients with symptomatic involvement of vital organs. Single-agent or combination phase 2 trials conducted in patients with recurrent or advanced neuroblastoma have identified a number of active agents that form the backbone of current induction chemotherapy regimens. In particular, these data have established the activity of alkylating agents, anthracyclines, platinum analogs, and the camptothecins in this disease. Many years ago, phase 2 window studies in children with newly diagnosed neuroblastoma established cyclophosphamide, cisplatin, doxorubicin, and the epipodophyllotoxins as active agents, with response rates ranging from 34% to 45%[314–316] (Table 30.8). More recently, the camptothecin analogs topotecan and irinotecan have shown activity in the relapse setting when combined with the alkylating agents cyclophosphamide[317] or temozolomide,[318] respectively, and these are considered active combination therapies against neuroblastoma.

Treatment of Low-Risk Disease

Treatment of low-risk neuroblastoma consists of surgical removal of the primary tumor. Unique to neuroblastoma, a complete resection is not necessary in the setting of localized disease and favorable biological features. Patients with localized and completely resected neuroblastomas have an EFS probability of greater than 90%, regardless of age.[319–323] Perez et al.[322] reported a 93% EFS rate for 141 Evans stage I patients treated with surgery alone. Six of the 10 disease recurrences occurred at distant sites, but two of these occurred in patients with *MYCN*-amplified tumors (see later). The OS rate for this cohort of patients was 99%. Similar data were reported in a study of 329 POG stage A patients, with EFS and OS rates of 91% and 96%, respectively.[324] These data strongly support surgery alone as effective initial therapy of INSS stage 1 neuroblastomas. Local recurrences can be managed with second surgeries, but even metastatic recurrences are often salvageable with chemotherapy.[325]

Surgery alone is also the initial treatment of choice for the majority of patients with INSS stage 2 neuroblastoma.

TABLE 30.8

ACTIVITY OF AGENTS STUDIED IN PHASE 2 WINDOWS FOR NEWLY DIAGNOSED HIGH-RISK NEUROBLASTOMA PATIENTS

Study	Reference	Drug and schedule	N	CR + PR (%)
POG 8741	223	Carboplatin 560 mg/m^2	49	54
		Ifosfamide 2 g/m^2/d × 4	52	45
		Iproplatin 325 mg/m^2	54	40
		Epirubicin 90 mg/m^2	23	14
ENSG 3A	222	Ifosfamide 3 g/m^2/d × 2	18	44
POG 9341	224	Topotecan 2 mg/m^2/d × 5	33	38
		Topotecan 2 mg/m^2/d × 5 and Cyclophosphamide 250 mg/m^2/d × 5	36	29
		Taxol 350 mg/m^2	33	18

ENSG, European Neuroblastoma Study Group; POG, Pediatric Oncology Group.

Historically, many of these patients were treated with chemotherapy, and survival results were excellent.[326] However, several individual institutions and cooperative groups have reported results of treatment with surgery only, and survival does not appear to be compromised.[319,321,323,327,328] In a prospective CCG study, 233 Evans stage II patients (56% INSS stage 2) with single-copy MYCN were managed with surgery alone.[323] Although the 4-year EFS rate was 81%, the majority of patients who experienced recurrence were salvaged, as the 4-year OS rate was 98%. Thus, even in the setting of macroscopic residual disease, adjuvant chemotherapy or radiotherapy does not seem warranted for the vast majority of INSS stage 2 patients.

Although there appears to be no significant prognostic distinction between INSS stages 2A and 2B,[257] it may be that INSS stage 2 disease that undergoes biopsy only has a significant chance for local tumor progression. There are no clear data for this situation because traditionally patients with localized disease who have biopsy only received adjuvant therapy. The COG currently recommends four cycles of intermediate-risk chemotherapy (see later) for INSS stage 2 patients with less than 50% tumor resection. However, recent experience with observation alone for a number of patients with biologically favorable nonmetastatic neuroblastoma suggests that at least a subset of these patients may be safely observed, or perhaps treated with less chemotherapy.

The COG has recently completed a large observational clinical trial accrued over 900 patients with biologically favorable neuroblastomas (INSS Stages 1, 2 and 4S without symptoms). The primary goal was to determine if children with localized and incompletely resected tumors could be cured with surgery alone. Preliminary results show a 3-year EFS rate of 85%, but a 3-year OS rate of 97%, suggesting that the majority of events were salvaged.[329] These results highlight the importance of assessing tumor biological features in order to identify the rare patient with occult malignant neuroblastoma masquerading as low-risk disease.

It remains controversial how best to manage the rare patients with INSS stage 1 or 2 neuroblastomas and MYCN amplification. Cohn et al.[330] reported that five of six patients with MYCN amplified INSS stage 1 (N = 3) or stage 2A (N = 3) tumors survived without evidence of disease at 71 to 381 months. On the other hand, Perez et al.[323] recently reported that four of seven INSS stage 1 (N = 4, all infants) and stage 2b (N = 3, two infants) cases with MYCN amplification had metastatic relapse at 2 to 22 months from surgery, and three of these patients died from disease progression.[323]

Likewise, a French cooperative group reported that three of four patients with INSS stage 1 or 2 neuroblastoma and MYCN amplification relapsed and died from disease progression. More recently, Bagatell et al.[85] reviewed 2,660 low-stage neuroblastoma patients with known MYCN status with 87 tumors showing amplification (3%). The EFS and OS rates were 53% and 72%, respectively, for those with MYCN amplification, compared with 90% and 98% for those with normal MYCN status. They discovered that the DNA index was an independent prognostic variable in this cohort, but this retrospective study was not able to conclude whether these patients should be observed closely following surgery, or if intensive chemoradiotherapy should be recommended. Currently, the COG recommends observation for patients with a gross total resection, but treatment as a high-risk patient if gross residual tumor remains after surgery. Further international cooperation to study this relatively rare clinical situation is required.

Taken together, it appears that a large proportion of neuroblastomas will behave in a relatively benign fashion. Although spontaneous regression is most classically described as part of stage 4S disease, the experience with newborn screening of urinary catecholamines for neuroblastoma strongly suggests that the vast majority of localized cases will regress as well (see above). Indeed, a recent German study followed 93 patients with biologically favorable neuroblastoma and gross residual disease after surgery only, and spontaneous regression was documented in 47% at anywhere from 1 to 18 months after diagnosis.[331] This "wait-and-see" approach has been extended to adrenal masses discovered incidentally in the perinatal period, where an ongoing COG study (and a planned SIOPEN study) recommends close observation with serial ultrasonography for select tumors (small and uncomplicated masses) without biopsy or any surgical intervention.[332]

Treatment of Intermediate-Risk Disease

This is a heterogeneous group of patients consisting mainly of very young patients with metastatic disease, or patients of all ages with large, unresectable primary tumors. Patients currently defined as INSS stage 3 have been treated in a heterogeneous fashion in part because of protocol differences used by the major groups and countries around the world. In addition, INSS-3 patients are somewhat heterogeneous, because the aggressiveness of the surgical approach can affect the INSS stage. Therefore, treatment results have been difficult to compare. International acceptance of the INRG system should allow for easier comparison of treatment approaches and outcome in this subset of patients.

Matthay et al.[298] reported the CCG experience with Evans stage III disease, and, because 92% of their patients were INSS stage 3, results can be extrapolated to the current risk stratification system. Of 228 Evans stage III patients prospectively evaluated for risk status by analysis of age, stage, *MYCN* amplification status, Shimada pathology,[333] and serum ferritin,[274] 143 met the current criteria for intermediate-risk disease. These 143 patients were treated with moderately dose-intensive chemotherapy including cyclophosphamide, doxorubicin, cisplatin, and etoposide, as well as local radiation for any gross residual disease following delayed surgery. Patients with Evans stage III disease and normal *MYCN*, favorable Shimada, and low serum ferritin had a 4-year EFS of 100%. Infants with Evans stage III disease and at least one unfavorable biological feature had 4-year EFS and OS rates of 90% and 93%, respectively. In contrast, patients with Evans stage III disease older than 1 year at diagnosis with at least one unfavorable biological feature had 4-year EFS and OS rates of 75% and 65%, respectively, despite a much more dose-intensive treatment regimen. In multivariate analysis, age at diagnosis and *MYCN* status were the only factors that were independently prognostic in this group of patients.

The majority of infants with INSS stage 4 neuroblastoma are currently categorized as intermediate risk. It is now clear that infants with metastatic neuroblastoma that is *MYCN* amplified uniformly have a highly aggressive clinical course[97,270,273,334] and, therefore, should be categorized as high risk. However, infants with neuroblastomas that do not have amplified *MYCN* typically have a much less aggressive clinical course and respond to moderate intensity chemotherapy. Schmidt et al.[97] reviewed the CCG experience and reported a 3-year EFS rate of 93% for infants with *MYCN* single-copy neuroblastomas treated with moderately intensive chemotherapy. This is in contrast to the 10% EFS noted for those infants with *MYCN*-amplified tumors, many of whom were treated with much more intensive therapy (Fig. 30.10). These data compare favorably to previous reports from the POG,[326,335] perhaps because of the fact that the CCG study used a somewhat more intensive chemotherapy induction regimen.

The COG recently completed a study focused on maintaining outstanding survival rates in children with intermediate-risk neuroblastoma while reducing chemotherapy and eliminating radiotherapy for local control. This study further attempted to refine therapy by prescribing 4 or 8 cycles of chemotherapy on the basis of biological features of the tumor. The 3-year EFS and OS rates were 88% and 96%, respectively, so this study showed that substantial reduction of therapy could be achieved safely in this heterogeneous group of patients.[336] The ongoing COG intermediate-risk study is attempting to further reduce chemotherapy by using a response-based algorithm to guide duration of therapy, and also using 1p36 and 11q23 deletion status to identify the cases with the highest risk of treatment failure. These patients are assigned to a longer treatment plan, with the hope of further improving their cure rate.

Treatment of High-Risk Disease

Historically, high-risk neuroblastoma patients have had long-term survival probabilities of less than 15%.[295,337–347] With the advent of comprehensive treatment approaches that include (a) intensive induction chemotherapy, (b) myeloablative consolidation therapy with stem cell rescue, and (c) targeted therapy for MRD, OS rates have improved (Fig. 30.11). However, the current survival rates remain unacceptable and have come

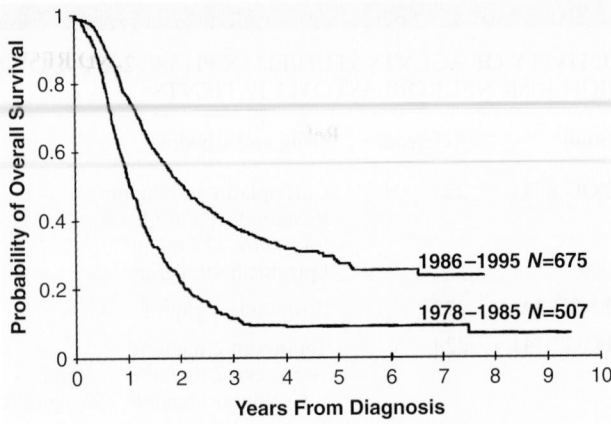

FIGURE 30.11 Improving survival for high-risk neuroblastoma patients. Survival by interval treated. Comparison of 1,182 consecutive patients with stage 4 neuroblastoma diagnosed after 1 year of age and treated at CCG institutions. (Figure redrawn with permission from Dr. Katherine Matthay, University of San Francisco, California.)

at the expense of substantial immediate and long-term morbidity.[313,348–354] The current therapeutic regimens used for high-risk patients throughout the world generally have three phases: induction therapy, consolidation therapy, and maintenance aimed at MRD.

Induction Therapy. The goal of this phase of therapy is to induce maximum reduction in tumor bulk at primary and metastatic sites. Neuroblastoma is typically sensitive to initial chemotherapy, even in the cases with amplified *MYCN*. Retrospective analyses have shown an association of chemotherapy dose intensity with response and survival rates.[355,356] In particular, the dose intensity of the platinum compounds appears to correlate most significantly with disease outcome.[355] The appropriate duration of induction therapy is currently not known, although it is generally agreed that it should be accomplished in as rapid a time frame as possible, before the acquisition of drug resistance.

The efficacy of induction chemotherapy regimens is assessed by the response rate, usually a combined measure of complete and partial responses, and typically determined after a second surgical procedure. There is a substantial body of evidence suggesting that the quality of remission at the end of induction chemotherapy is associated with long-term survival probability.[310,355,357–362] In a multivariate analysis performed with 549 high-risk neuroblastoma patients registered on the European Bone Marrow Transplantation Solid Tumor Registry, Ladenstein et al.[360] showed that persistent cortical bone lesions ($p < 0.004$) and bone marrow involvement ($p < 0.03$) were the only independent adverse prognostic factors. More recently, MIBG scintigraphy has become an important component of response evaluation, and the quality of MIBG response to induction chemotherapy is also highly correlated with outcome.[237,363–365] Thus, patients who achieve a CR or VGPR with induction chemotherapy have a better chance of cure, although some patients with a PR can be converted to CR with high-dose myeloablative therapy.[273,366]

Table 30.9 reviews the induction chemotherapy regimens used in the most recent cooperative group studies in the United States. It can be concluded from this experience that induction chemotherapy response rates were greatest in the regimens that contained higher overall dose intensities, especially in those with higher intensity of the platinum agents. For example, in POG 8742, regimen 1 contained almost twice

TABLE 30.9

INDUCTION CHEMOTHERAPY REGIMENS AND RESPONSE RATES FROM RECENT POG AND CCG COOPERATIVE GROUP TRIALS

Study	Reference	Years	N	Regimen	CR + PR (%)
POG-8104 (Regimen A)	433	1981–1984	70	Day 1–7, cyclophosphamide 150 mg/m²/d (p.o.) Day 8, doxorubicin 35 mg/m² Repeat every 21 d × 5	59
POG-8104 (Regimen B)	433	1981–1984	64	Day 1, cisplatin 90 mg/m² Day 3, teniposide 100 mg/m² Repeat every 21 d × 5	64
CCG-321P2	293	1985–1989	207	Day 1, cisplatin 60 mg/m² Day 3, doxorubicin 30 mg/m² Day 3 and 6, etoposide 100 mg/m² Day 4 and 5, cyclophosphamide 900 mg/m² Repeat every 28 d × 5–7	76[c]
POG-8742 (Regimen 1)	223	1987–1991	111	Day 1–5, cisplatin 40 mg/m²/d Day 2–4, etoposide 100 mg/m²/d Alternate every 21 d with: Day 1–7, cyclophosphamide 150 mg/m²/d (p.o.) Day 8, doxorubicin 35 mg/m² Total of 5 cycles	77
POG-8742 (Regimen 2)	223	1987–1991	115	Day 1, cisplatin 90 mg/m² Day 2, etoposide 100 mg/m² Day 3–10, cyclophosphamide 150 mg/m²/d (p.o.) Day 11, doxorubicin 35 mg/m² Repeat every 21 d × 5	68
CCG-3891	177	1991–1996	539	Day 1, cisplatin 60 mg/m² Day 3, doxorubicin 30 mg/m² Day 3 and 6, etoposide 100 mg/m² Day 4 and 5, cyclophosphamide 900 mg/m² Repeat every 28 d × 5	78
COG-A3973	279	2001–		Cycles 1, 2, 4, 6 Days 1, 2, cyclophosphamide 2.1 g/m² Days 1–3, doxorubicin 25 mg/m² Days 1–3, vincristine 0.67 mg/m² Cycles 3, 5 Days 1–4, cisplatin 50 mg/m² Days 1–3, etoposide 200 mg/m²	?

the dose intensity of cisplatin and had nearly a 10% better induction response rate.[314] The most recent US phase 3 trial (COG-A3973) has an induction regimen based on the Memorial Sloan Kettering experience,[367] and utilized further dose intensification of the platinum and alkylator components compared with prior cooperative group experience. However, the induction response rate was similar to prior studies.[368,369] Although increasingly sensitive radiographic techniques may partly explain this result (more patients with minimal disease burden at the end of induction may now have it detected by 123I-MIBG compared with past studies), it is also likely that we have maximized the dose-response effect with the core chemotherapy agents used. In addition, there is increasing concern that this regimen with significant alkylator exposure may be associated with an unacceptable risk of treatment-related leukemia,[348] especially after prolonged cycles of therapy.[370]

The Study Group of Japan for Advanced Neuroblastoma has reported a 92% CR + PR rate with six cycles of conventional doses of cyclophosphamide, vincristine, pirarubicin,

and cisplatin, although some of these patients may have progressed before consolidation therapy.[359] The French cooperative group was not able to validate the outstanding results originally reported from MSKCC,[367] with a *metastatic site* complete remission rate of only 43%.[371] More recently the European-based SIOPEN group directly tested the hypothesis that an increased dose intensity of induction chemotherapy would improve the response rate and survival. The investigators nearly doubled the dose intensity of induction chemotherapy by shortening the chemotherapy interval substantially, but showed no significant difference in OS, with an overall induction response rate (CR + PR) of 78%.[372] Finally, the COG has piloted the incorporation of topotecan and cyclophosphamide into induction chemotherapy,[373] with an ongoing phase 3 trial designed to define the induction response rate, impact on stem cell collection quantity and quality, and effect on patient outcome (COG ANBL0532).

Consolidation Therapy. The concept of eliminating resistant tumor clones that survive induction therapy with supralethal doses of chemotherapy supported by autologous bone marrow infusion has been actively investigated in neuroblastoma since the early 1980s. The first published trial of myeloablative consolidation therapy used high-dose melphalan alone,[373] but since then multiple single arm trials and registry reviews have been reported in the literature.[308–310,312,359,360,375–391] These studies are difficult to compare due to the heterogeneity of induction and consolidation regimens, as well as varying strategies for stem cell harvesting and reinfusion. However, the majority of studies reported at least a trend toward improved survival probabilities compared with nonrandomized control groups and historical controls lacking consolidation with stem cell rescue. Recent consolidation regimens and their success are shown in Table 30.10.

Three randomized controlled studies of myeloablative chemotherapy with autologous hematopoietic stem cell rescue for patients with high-risk neuroblastoma have been completed, and two additional studies are ongoing. The ENSG reported a trial of either high-dose melphalan myeloablation with autologous, unpurged bone marrow rescue versus no further therapy for patients who achieved a CR with induction chemotherapy.[41] Of 140 infants and children with disseminated disease, 95 achieved CR and 65 were randomized. The projected EFS strongly favored the transplanted group compared with the group stopping treatment (50% vs. 27%, at

2 years; $p < 0.03$). Recent long-term follow-up of this cohort confirmed a trend toward improved outcome in the melphalan cohort with 5-year EFS of 38% (CI, 21% to 54%) compared with 27% (CI, 12% to 42%) in the subjects not receiving melphalan myeloablation ($p = 0.08$).[392]

Matthay et al.[273] reported the results of a 5-year CCG study in which high-risk patients were randomized to consolidation with myeloablative chemotherapy followed by purged autologous bone marrow rescue or to continuation chemotherapy that was fairly intense, but nonmyeloablative. A total of 539 eligible patients were enrolled onto this clinical trial designed with two sequential randomizations (±autologous marrow rescue, and ±13-cRA, see later). A total of 379 patients were randomly assigned to autologous marrow rescue ($N = 189$) or continuation chemotherapy ($N = 190$). An intent-to-treat analysis showed a significant improvement in 3-year, EFS probability for the patients assigned to myeloablative therapy ($34 \pm 4\%$ vs. $22 \pm 4\%$; $p = 0.034$; Fig. 30.11A). Importantly, autologous transplantation appeared to have the largest impact on survival for the ultra-high–risk subset of patients, such as those with *MYCN* amplification and metastatic disease diagnosed after age 2 years. The follow-up for this study was relatively short, but a recent long-term follow-up of this cohort confirmed improved 5-year EFS and OS for the subjects randomized to transplant.[393]

TABLE 30.10

CONSOLIDATION REGIMENS AND 3-YEAR EVENT-FREE SURVIVAL RATES FROM TIME OF AUTOLOGOUS STEM CELL TRANSPLANTATION FROM RECENT POG AND CCG COOPERATIVE GROUP TRIALS

Study	Reference	N	Regimen[a]	3-yr EFS[b]
POG-8340[c]	213	81	Melphalan TBI	38
CCG-321P3 (Regimen 1)	293	45	Cisplatin Teniposide Doxorubicin Melphalan TBI	42
CCG-321P3 (Regimen 2)	293	54	Cisplatin Etoposide Melphalan TBI	50
CCG-321P3 (Regimen 3)	293	48	Carboplatin Etoposide Melphalan TBI	41
CCG-3891	177	129	Carboplatin Etoposide Melphalan TBI	43
CCG-LA-6[d]	434	77	Carboplatin Etoposide Melphalan Local radiation	62

[a]All studies used purged autologous bone marrow unless otherwise noted. TBI, total body irradiation.
[b]Three-year EFS rate from time of autologous marrow infusion.
[c]Ten percent of these patients received allogeneic bone marrow.
[d]This study was a CCG sanctioned single institution pilot study.
Modified from Matthay KK, Castleberry RP. Treatment of advanced neuroblastoma: the U.S. experience. In: Brodeur GM, Sawada T, Tsuchida Y, et al., eds. Neuroblastoma. Amsterdam, The Netherlands: Elsevier Science BV, 2000:417–436, with permission of Drs. Katherine Matthay and Robert Castleberry.

The German cooperative group compared a non-TBI containing carboplatin, etoposide, and melphalan (CEM) myeloablative chemotherapy regimen to oral maintenance chemotherapy with low-dose cyclophosphamide. Like the other studies, there was a significantly improved 3-year EFS rate, but only a trend toward improved OS.[394] There are many potential explanations for the general observation of improved EFS, but not OS, including extending, but not eliminating, EFS duration on the one hand, or perhaps improved salvage probability in patients who suffer relapse but have not had myeloablative therapy on the other. A fourth randomized controlled trial involving myeloablative consolidation regimens is an ongoing comparison of CEM with busulfan and melphalan by the SIOPEN group. This is based on an extensive experience in Europe that suggests that the busulfan and melphalan regimen will lead to improved cure rates compared with others.[395] Finally, the COG is currently comparing tandem myeloablative consolidation with a thiotepa and cyclophosphamide regimen followed by a slightly attenuated CEM regimen to a single conventional CEM regimen, on the basis of extensive pilot experience suggesting that the tandem transplant may improve EFS.[396,397]

Over the past decade, the field has moved from the use of autologous bone marrow to support myeloablative consolidation to autologous PBSCs. PBSCs provide superior engraftment kinetics compared with conventional bone marrow grafts, and this technique might abrogate some transplant-related morbidity.[395,397,398] PBSC products are also less likely to contain contaminating tumor cells. To address the potential impact of occult clonogenic tumor cells that may contaminate PBSC harvests, the COG performed a randomized controlled trial of unmanipulated PBSCs compared with products that were subjected to immunomagnetic bead based purging of pheresates with a panel of neuroblastoma-specific monoclonal antibodies.[235,399] This recently closed COG A3973 trial clearly demonstrated no impact on EFS or OS for patients whose PBSCs were subject to purging in a centralized laboratory,[368] suggesting that tumor cell contamination is either rare and clinically unimportant, and/or that posttransplant therapy is effective in eradicating MRD. Thus, the COG will not pursue *ex vivo* purging in future trials, but instead will focus on improving *in vivo* purging with more effective induction therapy.

Continued controversy exists regarding the optimal timing of collection and whether or not "positive selection" with CD34+ purification plays any role in optimizing the stem cell product. Regardless, it is clear that multiple aliquots of PBSCs should be stored either to support tandem myeloablative consolidations (as discussed above) and/or to be available for a variety of therapies that may be used in the setting of recurrent or refractory disease.[400] Related to these efforts, there is also a critical need to determine if detection of rare residual neuroblastoma cells using RT-PCR directed at neuroblastoma-specific transcripts (e.g., TH or PHOX2B) in patient blood, PBSC product, and/or bone marrow is predictive of disease outcome. There has been extensive effort in developing the methodology for these assays,[261] but as yet there has been no definitive study to show if detection of MRD has clinical importance in neuroblastomas, as seen in the pediatric hematopoietic cancers.

There remains interest in allogeneic transplant as a mechanism to potentially induce a graft versus tumor effect. A nonrandomized study was conducted by CCG comparing 20 patients receiving allogeneic marrows to 36 children undergoing autologous transplantation following marrow purging.[385] The estimated EFS at 4 years was 25% for the allogeneic group versus 49% for the autologous group ($p = 0.51$). In a similar study from the European Group for Bone Marrow Transplantation,[384] the 2-year EFS for 17 allogeneic transplants (35%) was not significantly different from that of 34 autologous transplants (41%). However, several groups are still investigating the utility of allogeneic transplant with a reduced intensity/submyeloablative conditioning regimen, for high-risk neuroblastoma patients in second response.[401]

Maintenance Therapy Focused on MRD. The goal of this phase of therapy is to eradicate any residual tumor cells using agents that are theoretically active against highly chemoresistant MRD. Despite the improvements in induction chemotherapy response rates and efficacy of myeloablative consolidation procedures, a large number of high-risk neuroblastoma patients will experience disease relapse. This is often despite the fact that many patients reach the end of consolidation therapy with no disease detectable by conventional methodologies. Therefore, it is assumed that microscopic residual disease is often present following myeloablative consolidation, and further emphasizes the need for sensitive and specific assays to detect rare residual tumor cells, as described above.[261] In addition, cell lines derived from relapse specimens have been shown to be highly chemoresistant,[402] suggesting that acquired drug resistance is an important mechanism by which these tumor cells survive intensive induction and consolidation therapies.

Several novel agents specifically targeted to the unique biology of neuroblastoma may be effective for eliminating MRD. The retinoids are a class of compounds that have been known for over two decades to induce cellular differentiation and decrease in proliferation of neuroblastoma cells *in vitro*.[403] A phase 1 trial of 13-cRA in neuroblastoma patients with any disease status following myeloablative consolidation defined a maximum tolerated dose of 160 mg/m^2 per day given on bid schedule for 2 weeks per month.[404] Of 10 patients with measurable disease at study entry, 3 had complete clearing of bone marrow metastases. The efficacy of 13-cRA was then tested in a randomized trial using a factorial design following a randomization to myeloablative or continuation chemotherapy (Fig. 30.12).[273] A total of 130 patients were randomized to receive either six cycles of 13-cRA (given as above) or no further therapy. The cohort of patients assigned to receive posttransplant therapy with 13-cRA had a significantly improved EFS probability (46% vs. 29% from second randomization; $p = 0.027$; Fig. 30.11B). The synthetic retinoid fenretinide has shown impressive evidence for activity against neuroblastoma in preclinical models, and a variety of formulations are currently being tested in phase 1 and 2 clinical trials. This agent could complement or even replace 13-cRA in the setting of posttransplant therapy.

Immunotherapy targeting neuroblastoma-specific antigens is an alternative strategy that recently has been proven to be effective during the MRD phase of therapy. Murine, chimeric, and humanized antibodies specific to the cell surface ganglioside GD2, either alone or with cytokines, have shown activity in preclinical models[405–409] as well as phase 1[410–416] and phase 2[417,418] clinical trials. The murine monoclonal antibodies 3F8[406] and GD2a[412] and the human-mouse chimeric monoclonal antibody ch14.18[415] have been tested most extensively in clinical trials. Measurable responses have been observed in refractory neuroblastoma patients,[411,416,417] and ch14.18 has been shown to be safe with concomitant cytokine administration.[419] Neuropathic pain during and following administration is nearly universal, and this toxicity can be dose limiting.[411,413,416,417,419] The ch14.18 antibody was used in both the German NB90 and NB97 studies at the end of conventional therapy in a nonrandomized fashion without concomitant cytokines.[420] These investigators concluded that the acute toxicities were substantial but manageable. However,

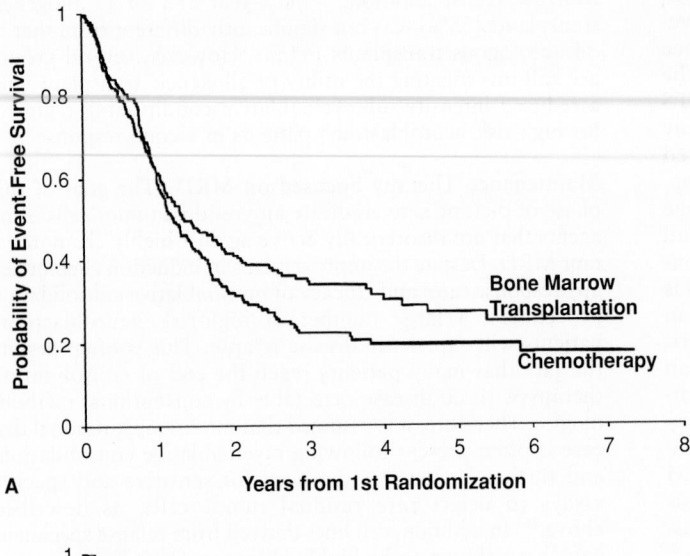

A   Years from 1st Randomization

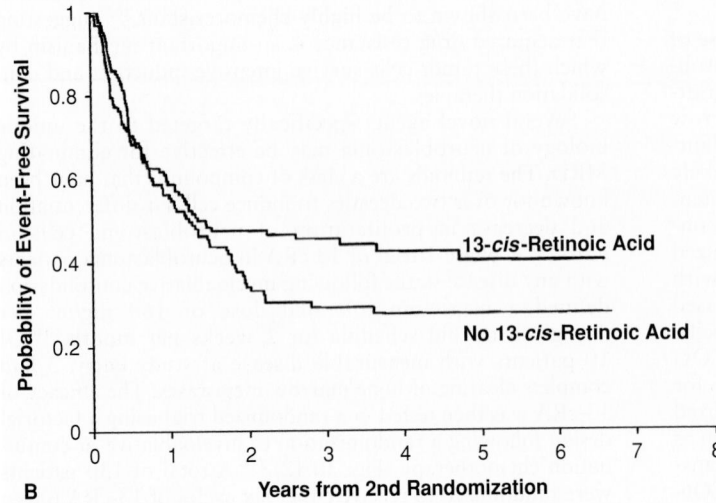

B   Years from 2nd Randomization

FIGURE 30.12 Autologous bone marrow transplantation and 13-cRA improve EFS for high-risk neuroblastoma patients—results of CCG study 3891.[177] All patients were treated with identical induction chemotherapy and were first randomized to either purged, autologous bone marrow transplantation (ABMT) or continuation chemotherapy, and then to either 13-cRA or no further therapy. **A:** EFS for patients randomized to ABMT ($N = 189$) or intensive but nonmyeloablative continuation chemotherapy ($N = 190$) ($p = 0.034$). **B:** EFS from time of randomization to 13-cRA ($N = 130$) or no further therapy ($N = 128$) ($p = 0.027$). (Figures redrawn with permission from Dr. Katherine Matthay, University of San Francisco, California.)

they detected no clear impact on outcome when compared with historical or nonrandomized control patients who received no further therapy, or 12 months of maintenance chemotherapy.

Yu et al. in the COG recently completed a randomized clinical trial designed to test the efficacy of ch14.18 with IL-2, GM-CSF, and 13-cRA ($N = 113$) compared with 13-*cis*-retinoic alone ($N = 113$) following myeloablative chemotherapy. Toxicities of this immunotherapy regimen were manageable, with grade 3 or greater pain in 21% of therapy cycles, and significant vascular leak syndromes or allergic reactions in about 7% of cycles. There was a significant improvement in survival for the experimental (immunotherapy-containing) arm compared with standard treatment (retinoid only), with 2-year EFS estimates of 66% ± 5% versus 46% ± 5% ($p = 0.012$) and 2-year OS estimates of 86% ± 4% versus 75% ± 5% ($p = 0.022$) (Fig. 30.13).[421] This study strongly supports the inclusion of immunotherapy as a critical modality in the treatment of high-risk neuroblastoma. It is important to emphasize that the COG study was done as an immunotherapy package with three agents (ch14.18, IL2, GM-CSF) in addition to 13-cRA, and it is unclear at this time which of these components are essential for the clinical activity observed. Future studies will focus on limiting the known toxicity of this immunotherapy regimen, and perhaps determining if a humanized

anti-GD2 antibody, with or without molecular fusion to a cytokine, can improve upon these impressive results and/or lessen the acute toxicity experienced with anti-GD2 immunotherapy.

Treatment of Stage 4S Disease

Retrospective analyses have shown OS rates ranging from 57% to 97% for stage 4S patients overall.[300,302,327,335,422–427] Recent prospective analyses have confirmed these observations, with OS probabilities of 85% to 92%.[82,256] However, it has become clear that some infants with this unique pattern of disease are at much higher risk for life-threatening complications. First, the subset of patients diagnosed in the first 2 months of life appear particularly vulnerable to respiratory compromise secondary to rapidly progressive hepatomegaly.[82,256,424] In addition, there is a subset of stage 4S patients with unfavorable biological features such as *MYCN* amplification that often show rapid tumor progression or eventual disease relapse, similar to stage 4 disease.[82,256,428] These data emphasize the importance of biological assessment of tumor tissue in patients with stage 4S.

The indications for intervening and the methods of managing infants with stage 4S neuroblastoma are becoming increasingly standardized. Symptomatic patients need emergent medical intervention, and limited cycles of moderate intensity

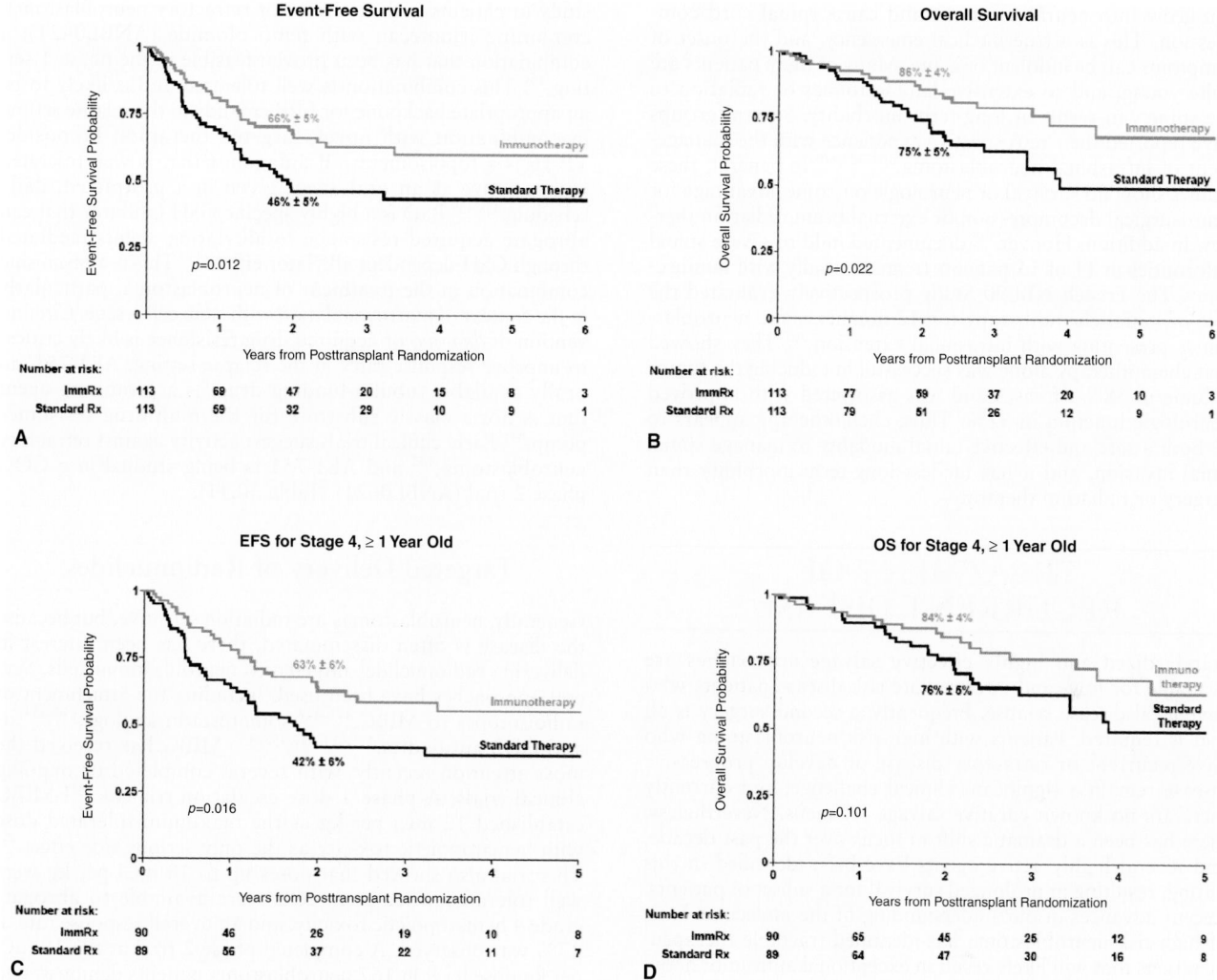

FIGURE 30.13 Kaplan-Meier curves by treatment group for the COG ANBL0032 trial of immunotherapy for high-risk neuroblastoma patients in first response. Standard treatment ($n = 113$) versus immunotherapy ($n = 113$). Survival rates at the 2-year time point are presented on each plot. **A:** Event-free survival for all randomized patients ($p = 0.012$). **B:** Overall survival for all randomized patients ($p = 0.022$). **C:** Event-free survival for randomized stage 4 patients ≥1 year of age ($p = 0.016$). **D:** Overall survival for randomized stage 4 patients ≥1 year of age ($p = 0.101$).

chemotherapy are typically prescribed, such as that currently recommended for intermediate-risk disease.[82,256,300,301,429] A diagnostic biopsy is indicated for evaluation of tumor biological features, as these can dramatically alter the therapeutic strategy, but resection of the primary tumor does not appear to influence outcome.[82,256] Thus, the safest surgical procedure, such as removal of a subcutaneous nodule, should be performed. Patients with a 4S pattern of disease whose tumors show *MYCN* amplification have a high likelihood of treatment failure, and thus, are typically treated according to high-risk regimens, regardless of symptomatology. It remains controversial how best to manage patients with the 4S pattern of disease and no evidence for *MYCN* amplification, but with other adverse prognostic features such as diploidy, unfavorable histopathology, or segmental chromosomal aberrations such as 1p and 11q deletion. The INRG analyses support 11q deletions in this population as indicating a very poor outcome and, thus, warranting high-risk categorization, but this is based on relatively few observations and requires additional validation.[203] The COG currently assigns patients with unfavorable INPC

pathology and/or diploidy to the intermediate-risk protocol that is exploring 4 to 8 cycles of moderate intensity chemotherapy, with the longer duration prescribed for those showing 1p or 11q LOH in the diagnostic biopsy specimen.

Asymptomatic patients with 4S disease and favorable tumor biological features should be observed closely, especially in the first ~3 months of life. If respiratory compromise or other signs of organ dysfunction (e.g., cord compression or renal compromise) become evident, moderately intensive chemotherapy is indicated, as noted above. Radiation therapy should be reserved for those patients with life-threatening complications who progress despite chemotherapy. If necessary, a minimal dose of radiation, such as 450 to 600 cGy in three to four fractions, is generally sufficient to halt tumor progression and will often induce regression.

Treatment of Paraspinal Neuroblastoma

Because of the anatomic location of paraspinal sympathetic ganglia, primary neuroblastomas arising in these structures can grow into neural foramina and cause spinal cord compression. This is a true medical emergency, and the onset of symptoms can be indolent or acute. Many of these patients are quite young, and so extensive laminectomies or radiation to the spine can result in long-term morbidity. Several groups have reported their retrospective experience with the management of intraspinal neuroblastoma.[304–307,430] In general, these studies show no survival or neurologic outcome advantage for neurosurgical decompression or external beam radiation therapy. In addition, Hoover[306] documented mild to severe spinal deformities in 11 of 15 patients treated initially with laminectomy. The French NBL90 Study prospectively evaluated the role of initial chemotherapy for 42 nonmetastatic neuroblastomas presenting with intraspinal extension.[307] They showed that chemotherapy alone was successful in reducing the tumor volume in 58% of cases and was associated with improved neurologic function in 92%. Thus, chemotherapy appears to be both a safe and effective initial modality to manage spinal canal invasion, and it has far less long-term morbidity than surgery or radiation therapy.

TREATMENT OF RECURRENT DISEASE

Standardized and highly effective salvage approaches are available for low- and intermediate-risk disease patients who have local disease relapse. Frequently, a second surgery is all that is required. Patients with high-risk neuroblastoma who have recurrent or refractory disease or develop progressive disease remain a significant clinical challenge, and currently there are no known curative salvage regimens. Nevertheless, there has been a dramatic shift in focus over the past decade, and several highly active agents have been identified in this setting, resulting in prolonged survival for a subset of patients. Recent advances in our understanding of the molecular basis of high-risk neuroblastoma has identified tractable therapeutic targets that will likely result in exceptional antitumor activity when studied in the clinic. This section highlights recent advances in the treatment of recurrent or refractory high-risk neuroblastoma.

Novel Conventional Chemotherapeutic Agents

The camptothecin analogs topotecan and irinotecan are topoisomerase I antagonists that have proven activity against refractory neuroblastoma.[431–435] Combining topotecan with low-dose cyclophosphamide on a 5-day schedule was shown to be superior to topotecan alone in a randomized clinical trial, with response rates (CR 1 PR) of 31% and 19%, respectively.[317] Disease stabilization was seen in many cases, and because this regimen is well tolerated in other independent trials,[316,433] many have considered it as front-line therapy for high-risk neuroblastoma patients in first relapse. Garaventa[436] reported a 64% response rate with higher dose topotecan for 5 days followed by a 48-hour infusion of vincristine and doxorubicin. A dose-intensive topotecan-containing regimen is now being used in induction of high-risk patients on ANBL0532. Two cycles of dose-intensive cyclophosphamide and topotecan are substituted for the initial two cycles of induction utilized on the prior COG A3973 protocol. Irinotecan has been studied intensively in recent years because of the relatively mild hematologic toxicity and potential for abrogation of diarrheal complications by concomitant administration of oral antibiotics.[437] The COG has completed a phase 2

study in patients with recurrent or refractory neuroblastoma, combining irinotecan with temozolomide (ANBL0421); a combination that has been proven feasible in the phase 1 setting.[435] This combination is well tolerated and is likely to be an appropriate backbone for further study in the relapse setting in combination with novel, targeted therapies. Etoposide/VP-16 is a topoisomerase II antagonist that is well tolerated and is active as an oral agent given in a protracted, daily schedule.[438,439] BSO is a highly specific GSH inhibitor that can abrogate acquired resistance to alkylating agents mediated through GSH-dependent alkylator efflux.[440] This is a promising combination in the treatment of neuroblastoma, particularly in the context of marrow ablation with stem cell rescue. Circumvention of de novo or acquired drug resistance is likely critical to improve response rates in the relapse setting. ABT-751, an orally available tubulin-binding drug, is a promising agent that is not a classic substrate for the multidrug resistance pump.[441] Early clinical trials suggest activity against refractory neuroblastoma,[442] and ABT-751 is being studied in a COG phase 2 trial (ANBL0621) (Table 30.11).

Targeted Delivery of Radionuclides

Generally, neuroblastomas are radiation sensitive, but because the disease is often disseminated, there has been interest in delivering radionuclides targeted to neuroblastoma cells. Several approaches have been used, including the attachment of radioisotopes to MIBG,[443–449] somatostatin analogs,[450–454] or anti-GD2 antibodies.[411,414–417,455–457] MIBG has received the most attention recently, with several completed or ongoing clinical trials. A phase 1 dose escalation trial of ^{131}I-MIBG established 12 mCi per kg as the maximum tolerated dose with hematopoietic toxicity as the only serious side effect.[447] This trial also showed that doses up to 18 mCi per kg were well tolerated when stem cells were available to abrogate grade 4 hematopoietic toxicity, and an overall response rate of 37% was observed. A completed phase 2 trial at the 18 mCi per kg dose level in 167 neuroblastoma patients demonstrated acceptable toxicity and objective response rates of 45% to 50% in a heavily pretreated patient population.[458] Single-agent ^{131}I-MIBG is currently being used as initial therapy for newly diagnosed high-risk patients in the Netherlands.[459] Pilot clinical trials have been completed that are designed to capitalize on the minimal nonhematopoietic toxicity observed with single-agent ^{131}I-MIBG administration by combining it with conventional low-dose or myeloablative chemotherapy,[460] and larger studies are in progress that are designed to measure response rates. The NANT consortium is leading an ongoing phase 1 trial of irinotecan/vincristine and ^{131}I-MIBG to determine if the activity of ^{131}I-MIBG could be potentiated using these radiosensitizing agents. The European experience combining topotecan and ^{131}I-MIBG has excellent preclinical activity in mouse xenograft models of neuroblastoma, and there have been no unexpected toxicities in a pilot clinical study. Current clinical investigation with ^{131}I-MIBG is directed toward integration of this active single agent into initial treatment strategies. A prospective phase 1 study of ^{131}I-MIBG plus myeloablative chemotherapy (CEM) and stem cell support in patients with primary refractory neuroblastoma showed that concurrent administration of ^{131}I-MIBG with myeloablative chemotherapy was feasible, and all patients engrafted successfully. Currently, there is an ongoing phase 2 trial of ^{131}I-MIBG with CEM and stem cell rescue in patients who have not received prior myeloablative therapy, and this study has shown tolerable toxicity. A pilot study for children with newly diagnosed high-risk neuroblastoma will open soon to assess the feasibility of a topotecan-containing induction regimen

TABLE 30.11

NEW AGENTS IN PHASE 1 AND PHASE 2 CLINICAL TRIALS

Agent	Mechanism of action/target	Phase	Reference
ABT-751	Tubulin binding	1	(442)
Beta-D-glucan	Immune response enhancer/iC3b leukocyte receptor	1	(469)
Buthionine Sulfoximime	Depletes glutathione (GSH)	1	(440)
CEP-701	Trk tyrosine kinase inhibitor	1	(486)
Decitabine	Demethylation	1	(500)
Depsipeptide	Histone deacetylase inhibitor	1	(514)
Genasense	BCL2 antisense	1	(515)
IL12	Immune modulator	1	(408, 516)
MAb1A7	Anti-anti-GD2 (anti-id antibody)	1	(468)
MS-27–275	Histone deacetylase inhibitor	1	(501, 502)
Pyrazoloacridine	DNA intercalator	1	(517, 518)
Safingol	Ceramide modulator	1	(462, 519)
SAHA	Histone deacetylase inhibitor	1	(501)
ZD1839 (Iressa)	EGFR tyrosine kinase inhibitor	1	(177)
Zoledronic acid	Bisphosphonate	1	(520)
131I-MIBG	Norepinephrine receptor/targeted radiotherapeutic	2	(445, 447, 460, 521)
3F8	Murine-derived anti-GD2	2	(522)
Fenretinide	Increases reactive oxygen species and *de novo* ceramides	2	(463)
Hu14.18-IL2	Humanized anti-GD2 and IL2 fusion protein	2	(523)
Imatinib mesylate	c-kit, PDGFR	2	(487, 488)
Ch14.18	Chimeric anti-GD2	3	(416, 419)

combined with ^{131}I-MIBG+CEM intensified consolidation with autologous stem cell rescue (ANBL07P1) (Table 30.11).

Molecularly Targeted Agents

Retinoid Compounds

On the basis of the results from the randomized trial of 13-cRA following myeloablative chemotherapy,[273] most investigators now consider this agent as standard of care for high-risk patients in CR or VGPR, typically after myeloablative chemotherapy and stem cell rescue. Current preclinical and clinical studies are focused on determining which naturally occurring retinoid or synthetic derivative gives optimal systemic exposure allowing for maximum tumor differentiation (or kill) without excessive toxicity.[235] Fenretinide is currently the lead retinoid compound being developed because of its ability to induce multilog cellular cytotoxicity *in vitro* through induction of apoptosis and necrosis via ceramide up-regulation, even in cells that may be retinoic acid resistant.[461–463] Phase 1 clinical trials of an oral formulation completed in the United States and Italy[464] have shown that the drug is generally well tolerated and have established recommended doses for phase 2 trials. However, because of relatively poor oral bioavailability of the formulation studied, a very large number of capsules were required to deliver the maximum tolerated dose. This demonstrated the need for an improved oral or intravenous formulation. Indeed, the NANT consortium is conducting two phase 1 trials testing both an oral powder and an IV formulation of fenretinide to circumvent this issue (Table 30.11).

Immunotherapy

Immunotherapeutic strategies for treating neuroblastoma were originally postulated on the basis of the hypothesis that spontaneous regression might result from a host immune response to neuroblastoma. This hypothesis was further supported by the detection of tumor infiltrating lymphocytes in some favorable neuroblastomas, particularly in patients with the OMAS.[221] This has resulted in a strategy to employ monoclonal antibodies directed against neuroblastoma-specific cellular antigens for the MRD phase of therapy. Antibodies or antibody conjugates directed against the neuroblastoma-specific cell surface ganglioside GD2 have received the most attention. Anti-GD2 antibody therapy has shown a clear survival advantage in a recent phase 3 clinical trial when administered with GM-CSF, IL-2 and 13-cRA in high-risk neuroblastoma patients following myeloablative therapy.[421] This pivotal study from Yu and colleagues establishes a new paradigm for neuroblastoma, and the field of cancer immunotherapy, as this was the first study to prove a survival advantage for an antibody targeting a glycolipid, and also for a strategy that presumably enhances ADCC via combination therapy with cytokines. Future efforts will build on these results, firstly via a humanized anti-GD2 immunocytokine that is engineered to target delivery of IL-2 to the tumor microenvironment. This approach has been shown to have activity and manageable toxicity in a recent phase 2 study.[465] Additional immunotherapeutic strategies in development include cellular,[466] DNA[467] and anti-idiotypic[468] vaccination strategies; enhancing ADCC with immune modulators such as beta-glucan[469]; and engineered cytolytic T lymphocytes for cellular immunotherapy.[470] Recent work has shown that EBV-specific cytotoxic T lymphocytes that express a chimeric antigen receptor directed to GD2 can be modified to function as tumor-directed effector cells, enhancing survival and antitumor activity.[471]

Antiangiogenesis Agents

Neuroblastomas are often heavily vascularized tumors, and the degree of vascularity correlates with biological features such as *MYCN* amplification.[472,473] In addition, proangiogenic molecules appear to be aberrantly overexpressed in high-risk tumors,[474–476] and low-risk tumors are characterized by a rich stromal compartment that secretes antiangiogenic molecules in the microenvironment.[477] Thus, several groups have examined a variety of antiangiogenic agents in preclinical studies that have had varying degrees of success,[478–484] but translation to the clinic has been slow. Several strategies focused on neutralization of circulating VEGF are planned or ongoing, including a phase 2 trial of AZD2171 (Cediranib). However, neovascular inhibition strategies are challenging in young children with developing organs and tissues, and this needs to be considered during the preclinical and clinical development of this class of drugs.

Kinase Inhibitor Therapies

Paradigm shifting advances in cancer require discovering the key oncogenic drivers of the malignant process, understanding the detailed molecular mechanisms, and exploiting this transdisciplinary knowledge therapeutically. For example, *ALK* encodes an RTK and has been identified as the major neuroblastoma predisposition gene. Furthermore, *ALK* activation by somatic mutation or gene amplification has been found in up to 15% of sporadic neuroblastomas. Accumulating preclinical data show that targeted inhibition of *ALK* in cell models harboring *ALK* mutation or amplification is highly effective, and this strategy is currently being translated into early phase clinical trials. ADVL0912 is a phase 1/2 COG trial of PF-02341066 (ADVL0912); a dual MET/ALK inhibitor that has shown dramatic activity in adult malignancies with *ALK* activation. This will represent the first therapy for neuroblastoma specifically developed for a mutated oncogenic driver. If the preclinical models are predictive of success in the planned clinical trials, and activity is restricted to patients with tumors that have aberrant ALK signaling, it will be imperative to obtain tumor tissue at the time of relapse to identify the patients most likely to benefit from ALK-targeted therapy.

Although mutations in the neurotrophin receptors have not been seen, there is evidence that aberrant Trk receptor expression contributes to aggressive clinical behavior in neuroblastomas and may be a good therapeutic target. Evans et al.[484,485] showed a significant growth inhibitory effect on several human neuroblastoma xenografts when targeting the BDNF-TrkB autocrine pathway with small molecule inhibitors (CEP-701/Lestaurtinib and related compounds), providing the preclinical rationale for the now completed phase 1 clinical trial. Other tyrosine kinase inhibitors have entered clinical trials, such as the EGF receptor inhibitor Iressa (AstraZeneca), and this may also have efficacy in some neuroblastomas.[177] Imatinib mesylate is also being studied in neuroblastoma because some tumors express c-kit and/or PDGFR,[487,488] but activating mutations in these receptors have not been reported. Screens of the neuroblastoma "kinome" for other potential drug targets, especially those in late-stage clinical development for adult malignancies, are ongoing.

Chromosome instability is a prevalent finding in pediatric and adult cancers, and functional abnormalities of centrosomes have been strongly associated with aneuploidy in cancer cells.[489–492] The Aurora family of serine/threonine protein kinases plays a critical role in the regulation of chromosomal segregation and cytokinesis during mitotic progression. The Aurora A kinase gene is amplified and/or overexpressed in many adult cancers,[493–497] and its overexpression results in the transformation of normal cells, thus supporting its role as an oncogene. Preliminary data suggest that the Aurora A kinase gene is overexpressed in neuroblastoma cells,[498,499] and that selective small molecule inhibition of this kinase has potential application in this disease. Strategies focused on Aurora Kinase A inhibition are currently in phase 1/2 trials (ADVL0812) in the COG.

Other Strategies

Because epigenetic silencing of genes such as caspase 8, which are critical for inducing programmed cell death, appears to occur frequently in neuroblastomas,[500] use of demethylating agents such as decitabine are being explored. Inhibitors of histone deacetylation are being developed for multiple cancers and have demonstrated preclinical activity against neuroblastoma.[501,502] At least three are currently in clinical trials for patients with refractory solid tumors. Moreover, there is an expanding portfolio of potential drugs to be tested in pediatric phase 1 clinical trials, so it is becoming increasingly important to have firm biological rationale and evidence for efficacy in appropriate preclinical models in order to prioritize drug development and guide their use in the patients most likely to benefit.

LATE EFFECTS

A variety of complications of neuroblastoma and its treatment may occur that are not unique to this tumor. These include late effects of chemotherapy, radiation therapy, and surgery.[264] Patients in the low-risk category will likely experience only the consequences of surgery, and because their prognosis is excellent, aggressive surgery should be minimized. Indeed, there is a trend toward observation for patients with localized and biologically favorable tumors, but the consequences of not removing large tumors will have to be followed carefully. Patients in the intermediate-risk category are exposed to surgery as well as moderately intensive chemotherapy. However, recent approaches have been directed toward overall reduction in therapy to avoid treatment-related morbidity for these patients, and this trend will likely continue as we improve our ability to more precisely define patient risk using biological markers.

High-risk patients are at the greatest risk of experiencing treatment-related complications. Survivors often have significant long-term health issues that can affect multiple organ systems, and these can be partly anticipated based on the treatment delivered.[349] Severe sensorineural hearing loss has become a particularly difficult problem because of the use of dose-intensive platinum-containing regimens to treat very young children.[503] The extensive use of alkylating agents and topoisomerase II inhibitors results in a higher prevalence of sterility as well as second malignancies, particularly myelodysplastic syndromes and acute nonlymphoblastic leukemias.[348,349] However, this latter problem may be regimen and schedule dependent.

A number of different second neoplasms have been reported in patients with neuroblastoma following treatment, such as thyroid cancer, pheochromocytoma, brain tumors, acute leukemia, osteosarcoma, breast cancer, and renal cell carcinoma.[504–512] None of these second cancers have occurred with sufficient frequency to indicate a specific relationship between neuroblastoma and any other neoplasm.[513] Therefore, the risk of developing second malignancies in patients with neuroblastoma is probably related to the risk associated with the chemotherapeutic agents or radiation therapy they received, rather than an underlying predisposition.

FUTURE CONSIDERATIONS

In the short term, improvements in outcome for neuroblastoma patients are likely to come from more effective use of existing treatment modalities. Integration of newer cytotoxic agents with proven activity in the relapse setting into front-line strategies remains a challenge but is ongoing for topotecan and ^{131}I-MIBG. Continued improvements in risk stratification based on evolving knowledge of neuroblastoma biology should allow the most appropriate intensity of therapy to be selected, minimizing the likelihood of either undertreatment or overtreatment. Longer term improvements in cure rates are likely only to come from a more precise understanding of the biological basis of neuroblastoma. The ability to survey the entire cancer genome, transcriptome, or proteome is in hand, and many investigators are applying these technologies to neuroblastoma. Ongoing experiments will very likely identify additional tumor-specific molecules and/or pathways that are aberrant in neuroblastoma, such as those recently discovered in *ALK*, that are critical for sustenance of the malignant phenotype.

Translation of these findings to the clinic will include further refinement of risk stratification so that treatment can be individually tailored. Perhaps more important, these data will allow for the identification of rational targets for drug development. The major cooperative groups will need to adopt more facile early phase clinical trial designs to efficiently evaluate candidate drugs with a longer term focus on where these agents will fit into the current multimodal high-risk neuroblastoma therapy backbone.

ACKNOWLEDGMENTS

Some of this material has been published previously.[3,38,66,101] This work was supported in part by NIH grants CA039771 and CA094194 (GMB), CA078545 and CA087847 (JMM), CA097323 (GMB, MDH, JMM, YPM), the Audrey E. Evans Endowed Chair (GMB), the Richard and Sheila Sanford Endowment (MDH), the Abramson Family Cancer Research Institute and the Neuroblastoma Research Endowed Chair (JMM), K08CA111733 and the Hillman Fund (YPM).

ABBREVIATIONS

13-cRA	13-*cis*-retinoic acid	HSRs	Homogeneously staining regions	PBSC	Peripheral blood stem cell
ADCC	Antibody-dependent cellular cytotoxicity	HVA	Homovanillic acid	PCR	Polymerase chain reaction
BDNF	Brain-derived neurotrophic factor	IL-2	Interleukin-2	PD	Progressive disease
BSO	Buthionine sulfoxime	INPC	International Neuroblastoma Pathology Classification	PDGFR	Platelet-derived growth factor receptor
CCG	Children's Cancer Group	INRG	International Neuroblastoma Risk Groups	PNET	Primitive neuroectodermal tumor
CGH	Comparative genomic hybridization	INRGSS	International Neuroblastoma Risk Group Staging System	POG	Pediatric Oncology Group
CCHS	Central hypoventilation syndrome			PR	Partial response
CEM	Cyclophosphamide, etoposide and melphalan	INSS	International Neuroblastoma Staging System	RT-PCR	Reverse transcriptase polymerase chain reaction
CNA	Copy number aberration	LDH	Lactate dehydrogenase	RTKs	Receptor tyrosine kinases
CNV	Copy number variation	LOH	Loss of heterozygosity	SD	Stable disease
COG	Children's Oncology Group	MIBG	Meta-iodo-benzylguanidine	SIOPEN	International Society of Pediatric Oncology European Neuroblastoma
CR	Complete response	MKI	Mitosis-karyorrhexis index		
CT	Computerized tomography	MR	Mixed response		
DI	DNA index	MRD	Minimal residual disease	TBI	Total body irradiation
DMs	Double-minute chromosomes	MRI	Magnetic resonance imaging	TH	Tyrosine hydroxylase
DOPA	3,4-dihydroxyphenylalanine	NANT	New Approaches to Neuroblastoma Therapy	TrkA	Nerve growth factor receptor
EFS	Event-free survival			TrkB	Brain-derived neurotrophin receptor
EGFR	Epidermal growth factor receptor	NCAM	Neural cell adhesion molecule		
EM	Electron microscopy	NF1	Neurofibromatosis type 1	TrkC	Neurotrophin-3 receptor
ENSG	European Neuroblastoma Study Group	NGF	Nerve growth factor	TSG	Tumor suppressor gene
		NSE	Neuron-specific enolase	VEGF	Vascular endothelial growth factor
FISH	Fluorescence in situ hybridization	NT-3	Neurotrophin-3		
GM-CSF	Granulocyte-macrophage colony stimulating factor	OMAS	Opsoclonus-myoclonus ataxia syndrome	VGPR	Very good partial response
				VIP	Vasoactive intestinal peptide
GSH	Glutathione synthetase	OS	Overall survival	VMA	Vanillylmandelic acid
HPLC	High-pressure liquid chromatography				

References

1. Gurney JG, Davis S, Severson RK, et al. Trends in cancer incidence among children in the U.S. Cancer 1996;78:532–541.
2. Gurney JG, Ross JA, Wall DA, et al. Infant cancer in the U.S.: histology-specific incidence and trends, 1973 to 1992. J Pediatr Hematol Oncol 1997;19:428–432.
3. Brodeur GM, Maris JM. Neuroblastoma. In: Pizzo PA, Poplack DG, eds. Principles and practice of pediatric oncology. 5th ed. Philadelphia PA: Lippincott Williams & Wilkins, 2006:933–970.
4. Olshan AF, Bunin GR. Epidemiology of neuroblastoma. In: Brodeur GM, Sawada T, Tsuchida Y, et al., eds. Neuroblastoma. Amsterdam, The Netherlands: Elsevier Science B.V., 2000:33–39.
5. Olshan AF, De Roos AJ, Teschke K, et al. Neuroblastoma and parental occupation. Cancer Causes Control 1999;10:539–549.
6. Heck JE, Ritz B, Hung RJ, et al. The epidemiology of neuroblastoma: a review. Paediatr Perinat Epidemiol 2009;23:125–143.
7. Cook MN, Olshan AF, Guess HA, et al. Maternal medication use and neuroblastoma in offspring. Am J Epidemiol 2004;159:721–731.
8. De Roos AJ, Olshan AF, Teschke K, et al. Parental occupational exposures to chemicals and incidence of neuroblastoma in offspring. Am J Epidemiol 2001;154:106–114.
9. De Roos AJ, Teschke K, Savitz DA, et al. Parental occupational exposures to electromagnetic fields and radiation and the incidence of neuroblastoma in offspring. Epidemiology 2001;12:508–517.
10. Menegaux F, Olshan AF, Neglia JP, et al. Day care, childhood infections, and risk of neuroblastoma. Am J Epidemiol 2004;159:843–851.
11. Daniels JL, Olshan AF, Pollock BH, et al. Breast-feeding and neuroblastoma, USA and Canada. Cancer Causes Control 2002;13:401–405.
12. Olshan AF, Smith JC, Bondy ML, et al. Maternal vitamin use and reduced risk of neuroblastoma. Epidemiology 2002;13:575–580.
13. Menegaux F, Olshan AF, Reitnauer PJ, et al. Positive association between congenital anomalies and risk of neuroblastoma. Pediatr Blood Cancer 2005;45:649–655.
14. Chow EJ, Friedman DL, Mueller BA. Maternal and perinatal characteristics in relation to neuroblastoma. Cancer 2007;109:983–992.

15. George RE, Lipshultz SE, Lipsitz SR, et al. Association between congenital cardiovascular malformations and neuroblastoma. J Pediatr 2004;144:444–448.
16. Sawada T, Kidowaki T, Sakamoto I, et al. Neuroblastoma. Mass screening for early detection and its prognosis. Cancer 1984;53:2731–2735.
17. Takeda T, Hatae Y, Nakadate H, et al. Japanese experience of screening. Med Pediatr Oncol 1989;17:368–372.
18. Bergeron C, Tafese T, Kerbl R, et al. European Experience with screening for neuroblastoma before the age of 12 months. Med Pediatr Oncol 1998;31:442–449.
19. Erttmann R, Tafese T, Berthold F, et al. 10 years' neuroblastoma screening in Europe: preliminary results of a clinical and biological review from the Study Group for Evaluation of Neuroblastoma Screening in Europe (SENSE). Eur J Cancer 1998;34:1391–1397.
20. Schilling FH, Spix C, Berthold FE, et al. German neuroblastoma mass screening study at 12 months of age: statistical aspects and preliminary results. Med Pediatr Oncol 1998;31:435–441.
21. Woods WG, Tuchman M, Bernstein M, et al. Screening infants for neuroblastoma does not reduce the incidence of poor-prognosis disease. Med Pediatr Oncol 1998;31:450–454.
22. Woods WG, Tuchman M, Robison LL, et al. A population-based study of the usefulness of screening for neuroblastoma. Lancet 1996;348:1682–1687.
23. Bessho F. Comparison of the incidences of neuroblastoma for screened and unscreened cohorts. Acta Paediatr 1999;88:404–406.
24. Schilling FH, Spix C, Berthold F, et al. Neuroblastoma screening at one year of age. N Engl J Med 2002;346:1047–1053.
25. Suita S, Tajiri T, Akazawa K, et al. Mass screening for neuroblastoma at 6 months of age: difficult to justify. J Pediatr Surg 1998;33:1674–1678.
26. Tsubono Y, Hisamichi S. A halt to neuroblastoma screening in Japan. N Engl J Med 2004;350:2010–2011.
27. Woods WG, Gao RN, Shuster JJ, et al. Screening of infants and mortality due to neuroblastoma. N Engl J Med 2002;346:1041–1046.
28. Yamamoto K, Ohta S, Ito E, et al. Marginal decrease in mortality and marked increase in incidence as a result of neuroblastoma screening at 6 months of age: cohort study in seven prefectures in Japan. J Clin Oncol 2002;20:1209–1214.
29. Brodeur GM, Ambros PF, Favrot MC. Biological aspects of neuroblastoma screening. Med Pediatr Oncol 1998;31:394–400.
30. Hayashi Y, Hanada R, Yamamoto K. Biology of neuroblastomas in Japan found by screening. Am J Pediatr Hematol Oncol 1992;14:342–347.
31. Kaneko Y, Kanda N, Maseki N, et al. Current urinary mass screening for catecholamine metabolites at 6 months of age may be detecting only a small portion of high-risk neuroblastomas: a chromosome and *N*-myc amplification study. J Clin Oncol 1990;8:2005–2013.
32. Acharya S, Jayabose S, Kogan SJ, et al. Prenatally diagnosed neuroblastoma. Cancer 1997;80:304–310.
33. Granata C, Fagnani AM, Gambini C, et al. Features and outcome of neuroblastoma detected before birth. J Pediatr Surg 2000;35:88–91.
34. Ho PTC, Estroff JA, Kozakewich H, et al. Prenatal detection of neuroblastoma: a ten-year experience from the Dana-Farber Cancer Institute and Children's Hospital. Pediatrics 1993;92:358–364.
35. Saylors RLI, Cohn SL, Morgan ER, et al. Prenatal detection of neuroblastoma by fetal ultrasonography. Am J Pediatr Hematol Oncol 1994;16:356–360.
36. Knudson AGJ, Strong LC. Mutation and cancer: neuroblastoma and pheochromocytoma. Am J Hum Genet 1972;24:514–522.
37. Friedman DL, Kadan-Lottick NS, Whitton J, et al. Increased risk of cancer among siblings of long-term childhood cancer survivors: a report from the childhood cancer survivor study. Cancer Epidemiol Biomarkers Prev 2005;14:1922–1927.
38. Maris JM, Brodeur GM. Genetics. In: Cheung NKV, Cohn SL, eds. Neuroblastoma. New York: John Wiley & Sons, 2005:21–26.
39. Longo L, Panza E, Schena F, et al. Genetic predisposition to familial neuroblastoma: identification of two novel genomic regions at 2p and 12p. Hum Hered 2007;63: 205–211.
40. Maris JM, Weiss MJ, Mosse Y, et al. Evidence for a hereditary neuroblastoma predisposition locus at chromosome 16p12–13. Cancer Res 2002;62:6651–6658.
41. Pinkerton CR. ENSG 1-randomised study of high-dose melphalan in neuroblastoma. Bone Marrow Transplant 1991;7:112–113.
42. Janoueix-Lerosey I, Lequin D, Brugieres L, et al. Somatic and germline activating mutations of the ALK kinase receptor in neuroblastoma. Nature 2008;455:967–970.
43. Mosse YP, Laudenslager M, Longo L, et al. Identification of ALK as a major familial neuroblastoma predisposition gene. Nature 2008;455:930–935.
44. Chen Y, Takita J, Choi YL, et al. Oncogenic mutations of ALK kinase in neuroblastoma. Nature 2008;455:971–974.
45. George RE, Sanda T, Hanna M, et al. Activating mutations in ALK provide a therapeutic target in neuroblastoma. Nature 2008;455:975–978.
46. Maris JM, Tonini GP. Genetics of familial neuroblastoma. In: Brodeur GM, Sawada T, Tsuchida Y, et al., eds. Neuroblastoma. Amsterdam, The Netherlands: Elsevier Science B.V., 2000:125–135.
47. Verloes A, Elmer C, Lacombe D, et al. Ondine-Hirschsprung syndrome (Haddad syndrome). Further delineation in two cases and review of the literature. Eur J Pediatr 1993;152:75–77.
48. Martinsson T, Sjoberg RM, Hedborg F, et al. Homozygous deletion of the neurofibromatosis-1 gene in the tumor of a patient with neuroblastoma. Cancer Genet Cytogenet 1997;95:183–189.
49. Origone P, Defferrari R, Mazzocco K, et al. Homozygous inactivation of NF1 gene in a patient with familial NF1 and disseminated neuroblastoma. Am J Med Genet 2003; 118A:309–313.
50. Trochet D, Bourdeaut F, Janoueix-Lerosey I, et al. Germline mutations of the paired-like homeobox 2B (PHOX2B) gene in neuroblastoma. Am J Hum Genet 2004;74:761–764.
51. Mosse YP, Laudenslager M, Khazi D, et al. Germline PHOX2B mutation in hereditary neuroblastoma. Am J Hum Genet 2004;75:727–730.
52. Raabe EH, Laudenslager M, Winter C, et al. Prevalence and functional consequence of PHOX2B mutations in neuroblastoma. Oncogene 2008;27:469–476.
53. van Limpt V, Schramm A, van Lakeman A, et al. The Phox2B homeobox gene is mutated in sporadic neuroblastomas. Oncogene 2004;23:9280–9288.
54. Satge D, Moore SW, Stiller CA, et al. Abnormal constitutional karyotypes in patients with neuroblastoma: a report of four new cases and review of 47 others in the literature. Cancer Genet Cytogenet 2003;147:89–98.
55. Biegel JA, White PS, Marshall HN, et al. Constitutional 1p36 deletion in a child with neuroblastoma. Am J Hum Genet 1993;52:176–182.
56. Laureys G, Speleman F, Versteeg R, et al. Constitutional translocation t(1;17)(p36.31-p36.13;q11.2-q12.1) in a neuroblastoma patient. Establishment of somatic cell hybrids and identification of PND/A12M2 on chromosome 1 and NF1/SCYA7 on chromosome 17 as breakpoint flanking single copy markers. Oncogene 1995;10:1087–1093.
57. Mosse Y, Greshock J, King A, et al. Identification and high-resolution mapping of a constitutional 11q deletion in an infant with multifocal neuroblastoma. Lancet Oncol 2003;4:769–771.
58. White PS, Thompson PM, Seifried BA, et al. Detailed molecular analysis of 1p36 in neuroblastoma. Med Pediatr Oncol 2001;36:37–41.
59. Capasso M, Devoto M, Hou C, et al. Common variations in BARD1 influence susceptibility to high-risk neuroblastoma. Nat Genet 2009;41:718–723.
60. Maris JM, Mosse YP, Bradfield JP, et al. Chromosome 6p22 locus associated with clinically aggressive neuroblastoma. N Engl J Med 2008;358:2585–2593.
61. Diskin SJ, Hou C, Glessner JT, et al. Copy number variation at 1q21.1 associated with neuroblastoma. Nature 2009;459:987–991.
62. Janoueix-Lerosey I, Schleiermacher G, Michels E, et al. Overall genomic pattern is a predictor of outcome in neuroblastoma. J Clin Oncol 2009;27:1026–1033.
63. Mosse YP, Diskin SJ, Wasserman N, et al. Neuroblastomas have distinct genomic DNA profiles that predict clinical phenotype and regional gene expression. Genes Chromosomes Cancer 2007;46:936–949.
64. Tomioka N, Oba S, Ohira M, et al. Novel risk stratification of patients with neuroblastoma by genomic signature, which is independent of molecular signature. Oncogene 2008;27:441–449.
65. Vandesompele J, Baudis M, De Preter K, et al. Unequivocal delineation of clinicogenetic subgroups and development of a new model for improved outcome prediction in neuroblastoma. J Clin Oncol 2005;23:2280–2299.
66. Brodeur GM. Neuroblastoma: biological insights into a clinical enigma. Nat Rev Cancer 2003;3:203–216.
67. Brodeur GM, Maris JM, Yamashiro DJ, et al. Biology and genetics of human neuroblastomas. J Pediatr Hematol Oncol 1997;19:93–101.
68. Brodeur GM, Nakagawara A. Molecular basis of clinical heterogeneity in neuroblastoma. Am J Pediatr Hematol Oncol 1992;14:111–116.
69. Nakagawara A, Arima-Nakagawara M, Scavarda NJ, et al. Association between high levels of expression of the TRK gene and favorable outcome in human neuroblastoma. N Engl J Med 1993;328:847–854.
70. Nakagawara A, Azar CG, Scavarda NJ, et al. Expression and function of TRK-B and BDNF in human neuroblastomas. Mol Cell Biol 1994;14:759–767.
71. Fujita T, Igarashi J, Okawa ER, et al. CHD5, a tumor suppressor gene deleted from 1p36.31 in neuroblastomas. J Natl Cancer Inst 2008;100:940–949.
72. Cole KA, Attiyeh EF, Mosse YP, et al. A functional screen identifies miR-34a as a candidate neuroblastoma tumor suppressor gene. Mol Cancer Res 2008;6:735–742.
73. Schlisio S, Kenchappa RS, Vredeveld LC, et al. The kinesin KIF1Bbeta acts downstream from EglN3 to induce apoptosis and is a potential 1p36 tumor suppressor. Genes Dev 2008;22:884–893.
74. Michels E, Hoebeeck J, De Preter K, et al. CADM1 is a strong neuroblastoma candidate gene that maps within a 3.72 Mb critical region of loss on 11q23. BMC Cancer 2008; 8:173.
75. Nowacki S, Skowron M, Oberthuer A, et al. Expression of the tumour suppressor gene CADM1 is associated with favourable outcome and inhibits cell survival in neuroblastoma. Oncogene 2008;27:3329–3338.
76. Miller MA, Ohashi K, Zhu X, et al. Survivin mRNA levels are associated with biology of disease and patient survival in neuroblastoma: a report from the children's oncology group. J Pediatr Hematol Oncol 2006;28:412–417.
77. Ito R, Asami S, Motohashi S, et al. Significance of survivin mRNA expression in prognosis of neuroblastoma. Biol Pharm Bull 2005;28:565–568.
78. Islam A, Kageyama H, Takada N, et al. High expression of Survivin, mapped to 17q25, is significantly associated with poor prognostic factors and promotes cell survival in human neuroblastoma. Oncogene 2000;19:617–623.
79. Wei JS, Song YK, Durinck S, et al. The MYCN oncogene is a direct target of miR-34a. Oncogene 2008;27:5204–5213.
80. Welch C, Chen Y, Stallings RL. MicroRNA-34a functions as a potential tumor suppressor by inducing apoptosis in neuroblastoma cells. Oncogene 2007;26:5017–5022.
81. Kaneko Y, Cohn SL. Ploidy and cytogenetics of neuroblastoma. In: Brodeur GM, Sawada T, Tsuchida Y, et al., eds. Neuroblastoma. Amsterdam, The Netherlands: Elsevier Science B.V., 2000:41–56.
82. Katzenstein H, Bowman LC, Brodeur GM, et al. Prognostic significance of age, MYCN oncogene amplification, tumor cell ploidy, and histology in 110 infants with stage D(S) neuroblastoma: the pediatric oncology group experience—a Pediatric Oncology Group study. J Clin Oncol 1998;16:2007–2017.
83. Look AT, Hayes FA, Nitschke R, et al. Cellular DNA content as a predictor of response to chemotherapy in infants with unresectable neuroblastoma. N Engl J Med 1984;311: 231–235.
84. Look AT, Hayes FA, Shuster JJ, et al. Clinical relevance of tumor cell ploidy and N-myc gene amplification in childhood neuroblastoma. A Pediatric Oncology Group Study. J Clin Oncol 1991;9:581–591.
85. Bagatell R, Beck-Popovic M, London WB, et al. Significance of MYCN amplification in international neuroblastoma staging system stage 1 and 2 neuroblastoma: a report from the International Neuroblastoma Risk Group database. J Clin Oncol 2009;27:365–370.
86. Schwab M, Alitalo K, Klempnauer KH, et al. Amplified DNA with limited homology to myc cellular oncogene is shared by human neuroblastoma cell lines and a neuroblastoma tumour. Nature 1983;305:245–248.
87. Corvi R, Amler LC, Savelyeva L, et al. MYCN is retained in single copy at chromosome 2 band p23–24 during amplification in human neuroblastoma cells. Proc Natl Acad Sci U S A 1994;91:5523–5527.
88. Schwab M, Ellison J, Busch M, et al. Enhanced expression of the human gene N-myc consequent to amplification of DNA may contribute to malignant progression of neuroblastoma. Proc Natl Acad Sci U S A 1984;81:4940–4944.
89. Reiter JL, Brodeur GM. High-resolution mapping of a 130-kb core region of the MYCN amplicon in neuroblastomas. Genomics 1996;32:97–103.
90. Reiter JL, Brodeur GM. MYCN is the only highly expressed gene from the core amplified domain in human neuroblastomas. Genes Chromosomes Cancer 1998;23:134–140.
91. Brinkschmidt C, Christiansen H, Terpe HJ, et al. Comparative genomic hybridization (CGH) analysis of neuroblastomas-an important methodological approach in paediatric tumour pathology. J Pathol 1997;181:394–400.
92. Mosse YP, Greshock J, Margolin A, et al. High-resolution detection and mapping of genomic DNA alterations in neuroblastoma. Genes Chromosomes Cancer 2005;43: 390–403.

93. Plantaz D, Mohapatra G, Matthay KK, et al. Gain of chromosome 17 is the most frequent abnormality detected in neuroblastoma by comparative genomic hybridization. Am J Pathol 1997;150:81–89.
94. Vandesompele J, Van Roy N, Van Gele M, et al. Genetic heterogeneity of neuroblastoma studied by comparative genomic hybridization. Genes Chromosomes Cancer 1998;23:141–152.
95. Ambros PF, Ambros IM, Kerbl R, et al. Intratumoural heterogeneity of 1p deletions and MYCN amplification in neuroblastomas. Med Pediatr Oncol 2001;36:1–4.
96. Mathew P, Valentine MB, Bowman LC, et al. Detection of MYCN gene amplification in neuroblastoma by fluorescence in situ hybridization: a pediatric oncology group study. Neoplasia 2001;3:105–109.
97. Schmidt ML, Lukens JN, Seeger RC, et al. Biologic factors determine prognosis in infants with stage IV neuroblastoma: a prospective Children's Cancer Group study. J Clin Oncol 2000;18:1260–1268.
98. Bordow SB, Norris MD, Haber PS, et al. Prognostic significance of MYCN oncogene expression in childhood neuroblastoma. J Clin Oncol 1998;16:3286–3294.
99. Seeger RC, Brodeur GM, Sather H, et al. Association of multiple copies of the N-myc oncogene with rapid progression of neuroblastomas. N Engl J Med 1985;313:1111–1116.
100. Brodeur GM, Seeger RC, Schwab M, et al. Amplification of N-myc in untreated human neuroblastomas correlates with advanced disease stage. Science 1984;224:1121–1124.
101. Brodeur GM. Clinical and biological aspects of neuroblastoma. In: Vogelstein B, Kinzler KW, eds. The genetic basis of human cancer. 2nd ed. New York: McGraw-Hill, Inc., 2002:751–772.
102. Brodeur GM, Hayes FA, Green AA, et al. Consistent N-myc copy number in simultaneous or consecutive neuroblastoma samples from sixty individual patients. Cancer Res 1987;47:4248–4253.
103. Nakagawara A, Arima M, Azar CG, et al. Inverse relationship between trk expression and N-myc amplification in human neuroblastomas. Cancer Res 1992;52:1364–1368.
104. Chan HS, Gallie BL, DeBoer G, et al. MYCN protein expression as a predictor of neuroblastoma prognosis. Clin Cancer Res 1997;3:1699–706.
105. Cohn SL, London WB, Huang D, et al. MYCN expression is not prognostic of adverse outcome in advanced-stage neuroblastoma with nonamplified MYCN. J Clin Oncol 2000;18:3604–3613.
106. Seeger RC, Wada R, Brodeur GM, et al. Expression of N-myc by neuroblastomas with one or multiple copies of the oncogene. Prog Clin Biol Res 1988;271:41–49.
107. Wada RK, Seeger RC, Brodeur GM, et al. Human neuroblastoma cell lines that express N-myc without gene amplification. Cancer 1993;72:3346–3354.
108. Fernandez PC, Frank SR, Wang L, et al. Genomic targets of the human c-Myc protein. Genes Dev 2003;17:1115–1129.
109. O'Connell BC, Cheung AF, Simkevich CP, et al. A large scale genetic analysis of c-Myc-regulated gene expression patterns. J Biol Chem 2003;278:12563–12573.
110. Weiss WA, Aldape K, Mohapatra G, et al. Targeted expression of MYCN causes neuroblastoma in transgenic mice. Embo J 1997;16:2985–2995.
111. Hackett CS, Hodgson JG, Law ME, et al. Genome-wide array CGH analysis of murine neuroblastoma reveals distinct genomic aberrations which parallel those in human tumors. Cancer Res 2003;63:5266–5273.
112. Bown N, Cotterill S, Lastowska M, et al. Gain of chromosome arm 17q and adverse outcome in patients with neuroblastoma. N Engl J Med 1999;340:1954–1961.
113. Caron H. Allelic loss of chromosome 1 and additional chromosome 17 material are both unfavourable prognostic markers in neuroblastoma. Med Pediatr Oncol 1995;24:215–221.
114. Van Roy N, Laureys G, Van Gele M, et al. Analysis of 1;17 translocation breakpoints in neuroblastoma: implications for mapping of neuroblastoma genes. Eur J Cancer 1997;33:1974–1978.
115. Lastowska M, Cotterill S, Bown N, et al. Breakpoint position on 17q identifies the most aggressive neuroblastoma tumors. Genes Chromosomes Cancer 2002;34:428–436.
116. Schleiermacher G, Raynal V, Janoueix-Lerosey I, et al. Variety and complexity of chromosome 17 translocations in neuroblastoma. Genes Chromosomes Cancer 2004;39:143–150.
117. Godfried MB, Veenstra M, v Sluis P, et al. The N-myc and c-myc downstream pathways include the chromosome 17q genes nm23-H1 and nm23-H2. Oncogene 2002;21:2097–2101.
118. Saito-Ohara F, Imoto I, Inoue J, et al. PPM1D is a potential target for 17q gain in neuroblastoma. Cancer Res 2003;63:1876–1883.
119. Gehring M, Berthold F, Edler L, et al. The 1p deletion is not a reliable marker for the prognosis of patients with neuroblastoma. Cancer Res 1995;55:5366–5369.
120. Martinsson T, Sjoberg RM, Hedborg F, et al. Deletion of chromosome 1p loci and microsatellite instability in neuroblastomas analyzed with short-tandem repeat polymorphisms. Cancer Res 1995;55:5681–5686.
121. White PS, Maris JM, Beltinger C, et al. A region of consistent deletion in neuroblastoma maps within 1p36.2-.3. Proc Natl Acad Sci U S A 1995;92:5520–5524.
122. White PS, Thompson PM, Gotoh T, et al. Definition and characterization of a region of 1p36.3 consistently deleted in neuroblastoma. Oncogene 2005;24:2684–2694.
123. Fong CT, Dracopoli NC, White PS, et al. Loss of heterozygosity for the short arm of chromosome 1 in human neuroblastomas: correlation with N-myc amplification. Proc Natl Acad Sci U S A 1989;86:3753–3757.
124. Caron H, van Sluis P, de Kraker J, et al. Allelic loss of chromosome 1p as a predictor of unfavorable outcome in patients with neuroblastoma. N Engl J Med 1996;334:225–230.
125. Maris JM, Weiss MJ, Guo C, et al. Loss of heterozygosity at 1p36 independently predicts for disease progression but not decreased overall survival probability in neuroblastoma patients: a Children's Cancer Group study. J Clin Oncol 2000;18:1888–1899.
126. Spitz R, Hero B, Westermann F, et al. Fluorescence in situ hybridization analyses of chromosome band 1p36 in neuroblastoma detect two classes of alterations. Genes Chromosomes Cancer 2002;34:299–305.
127. Chen YZ, Soeda E, Yang HW, et al. Homozygous deletion in a neuroblastoma cell line defined by a high-density STS map spanning human chromosome band 1p36. Genes Chromosomes Cancer 2001;31:326–332.
128. Ohira M, Kageyama H, Mihara M, et al. Identification and characterization of a 500-kb homozygously deleted region at 1p36.2-p36.3 in a neuroblastoma cell line. Oncogene 2000;19:4302–4307.
129. Thompson PM, Maris JM, Hogarty MD, et al. Homozygous deletion of CDKN2A (p16INK4a/p14ARF) but not within 1p36 or at other tumor suppressor loci in neuroblastoma. Cancer Res 2001;61:679–686.
130. Okawa ER, Gotoh T, Manne J, et al. Expression and sequence analysis of candidates for the 1p36.31 tumor suppressor gene deleted in neuroblastomas. Oncogene 2008;27:803–810.
131. Guo C, White PS, Weiss MJ, et al. Allelic deletion at 11q23 is common in MYCN single copy neuroblastomas. Oncogene 1999;18:4948–4957.
132. Plantaz D, Vandesompele J, Van Roy N, et al. Comparative genomic hybridization (CGH) analysis of stage 4 neuroblastoma reveals high frequency of 11q deletion in tumors lacking MYCN amplification. Int J Cancer 2001;91:680–686.
133. Spitz R, Hero B, Ernestus K, et al. Deletions in chromosome arms 3p and 11q are new prognostic markers in localized and 4s neuroblastoma. Clin Cancer Res 2003;9:52–58.
134. Attiyeh EF, London WB, Mosse YP, et al. Chromosome 1p and 11q deletions and outcome in neuroblastoma. N Engl J Med 2005;353:2243–2253.
135. Spitz R, Hero B, Ernestus K, et al. FISH analyses for alterations in chromosomes 1, 2, 3, and 11 define high-risk groups in neuroblastoma. Med Pediatr Oncol 2003;41:30–35.
136. Breen CJ, O'Meara A, McDermott M, et al. Coordinate deletion of chromosome 3p and 11q in neuroblastoma detected by comparative genomic hybridization. Cancer Genet Cytogenet 2000;120:44–49.
137. Caron H, van Sluis P, Buschman R, et al. Allelic loss of the short arm of chromosome 4 in neuroblastoma suggests a novel tumour suppressor gene locus. Hum Genet 1996;97:834–837.
138. Mora J, Cheung NK, Chen L, et al. Loss of heterozygosity at 19q13.3 is associated with locally aggressive neuroblastoma. Clin Cancer Res 2001;7:1358–1361.
139. Thompson PM, Seifried BA, Kyemba SK, et al. Loss of heterozygosity for chromosome 14q in neuroblastoma. Med Pediatr Oncol 2001;36:28–31.
140. Warnat P, Oberthuer A, Fischer M, et al. Cross-study analysis of gene expression data for intermediate neuroblastoma identifies two biological subtypes. BMC Cancer 2007;7:89.
141. Oberthuer A, Berthold F, Warnat P, et al. Customized oligonucleotide microarray gene expression-based classification of neuroblastoma patients outperforms current clinical risk stratification. J Clin Oncol 2006;24:5070–5078.
142. Asgharzadeh S, Pique-Regi R, Sposto R, et al. Prognostic significance of gene expression profiles of metastatic neuroblastomas lacking MYCN gene amplification. J Natl Cancer Inst 2006;98:1193–1203.
143. Schulte JH, Schramm A, Klein-Hitpass L, et al. Microarray analysis reveals differential gene expression patterns and regulation of single target genes contributing to the opposing phenotype of TrkA- and TrkB-expressing neuroblastomas. Oncogene 2005;24:165–177.
144. Schramm A, Schulte JH, Klein-Hitpass L, et al. Prediction of clinical outcome and biological characterization of neuroblastoma by expression profiling. Oncogene 2005;24:7902–7912.
145. Wei JS, Greer BT, Westermann F, et al. Prediction of clinical outcome using gene expression profiling and artificial neural networks for patients with neuroblastoma. Cancer Res 2004;64:6883–6891.
146. Rounbehler RJ, Li W, Hall MA, et al. Targeting ornithine decarboxylase impairs development of MYCN-amplified neuroblastoma. Cancer Res 2009;69:547–553.
147. Hogarty MD, Norris MD, Davis K, et al. ODC1 is a critical determinant of MYCN oncogenesis and a therapeutic target in neuroblastoma. Cancer Res 2008;68:9735–9745.
148. Mo H, Vita M, Crespin M, et al. Myc overexpression enhances apoptosis induced by small molecules. Cell Cycle 2006;5:2191–2194.
149. Fredlund E, Ringner M, Maris JM, et al. High Myc pathway activity and low stage of neuronal differentiation associate with poor outcome in neuroblastoma. Proc Natl Acad Sci U S A 2008;105:14094–14099.
150. Ohira M, Morohashi A, Inuzuka H, et al. Expression profiling and characterization of 4200 genes cloned from primary neuroblastomas: identification of 305 genes differentially expressed between favorable and unfavorable subsets. Oncogene 2003;22:5525–5536.
151. Wang Q, Diskin S, Rappaport E, et al. Integrative genomics identifies distinct molecular classes of neuroblastoma and demonstrates that multiple genes are targeted by regional alterations in DNA copy number. Cancer Res 2006;66:6050–6062.
152. Liu X, Mazanek P, Dam V, et al. Deregulated Wnt/B-catenin program in high-risk neuroblastomas without MYCN amplification. Oncogene 2008;27:1478–1488.
153. Westermann F, Muth D, Benner A, et al. Distinct transcriptional MYCN/c-MYC activities are associated with spontaneous regression or malignant progression in neuroblastomas. Genome Biol 2008;9:R150.
154. Vermeulen J, De Preter K, Naranjo A, et al. Predicting outcomes for children with neuroblastoma using a multigene-expression signature: a retrospective SIOPEN/COG/GPOH study. Lancet Oncol 2009;10:663–671.
155. De Preter K, De Brouwer S, Van Maerken T, et al. Meta-mining of neuroblastoma and neuroblast gene expression profiles reveals candidate therapeutic compounds. Clin Cancer Res 2009;15:3690–3696.
156. Huang EJ, Reichardt LF. Trk receptors: roles in neuronal signal transduction. Annu Rev Biochem 2003;72:609–642.
157. Nakagawara A. Trk receptor tyrosine kinases: a bridge between cancer and neural development. Cancer Lett 2001;169:107–114.
158. Patapoutian A, Reichardt LF. Trk receptors: mediators of neurotrophin action. Curr Opin Neurobiol 2001;11:272–280.
159. Yano H, Chao MV. Neurotrophin receptor structure and interactions. Pharm Acta Helv 2000;74:253–260.
160. Kogner P, Barbany G, Dominici C, et al. Coexpression of messenger RNA for TRK protooncogene and low affinity nerve growth factor receptor in neuroblastoma with favorable prognosis. Cancer Res 1993;53:2044–2050.
161. Suzuki T, Bogenmann E, Shimada H, et al. Lack of high-affinity nerve growth factor receptors in aggressive neuroblastomas. J Natl Cancer Inst 1993;85:377–384.
162. Nakagawara A, Brodeur GM. Role of neurotrophins and their receptors in human neuroblastomas: a primary culture study. Eur J Cancer 1997;33:2050–2053.
163. Ambros IM, Zellner A, Roald B, et al. Role of ploidy, chromosome 1p, and Schwann cells in the maturation of neuroblastoma. N Engl J Med 1996;334:1505–1511.
164. Tacconelli A, Farina AR, Cappabianca L, et al. TrkA alternative splicing: a regulated tumor-promoting switch in human neuroblastoma. Cancer Cell 2004;6:347–360.
165. Acheson A, Conover JC, Fandi JP, et al. A BDNF autocrine loop in adult sensory neurons prevents cell death. Nature 1995;374:450–453.
166. Matsumoto K, Wada RK, Yamashiro JM, et al. Expression of brain-derived neurotrophic factor and p145TrkB affects survival, differentiation, and invasiveness of human neuroblastoma cells. Cancer Res 1995;55:1798–1806.
167. Douma S, Van Laar T, Zevenhoven J, et al. Suppression of anoikis and induction of metastasis by the neurotrophic receptor TrkB. Nature 2004;430:1034–1039.
168. Ho R, Eggert A, Hishiki T, et al. Resistance to chemotherapy mediated by TrkB in neuroblastomas. Cancer Res 2002;62:6462–6466.

169. Jaboin J, Hong A, Kim CJ, et al. Cisplatin-induced cytotoxicity is blocked by brain-derived neurotrophic factor activation of TrkB signal transduction path in neuroblastoma. Cancer Lett 2003;193:109–114.
170. Ryden M, Sehgal R, Dominici C, et al. Expression of mRNA for the neurotrophin receptor trkC in neuroblastomas with favourable tumour stage and good prognosis. Br J Cancer 1996;74:773–779.
171. Yamashiro DJ, Nakagawara A, Ikegaki N, et al. Expression of TrkC in favorable human neuroblastomas. Oncogene 1996;12:37–41.
172. Ho R, Minturn JE, Simpson A, et al. Differential effect of P75 coexpression on TrkA and TrkB response to ligands in neuroblastoma. Proc Am Assoc Cancer Res 2005; 46:687.
173. Borrello MG, Bongarzone I, Pierotti MA, et al. TRK and RET protooncogene expression in human neuroblastoma specimens: high-frequency of TRK expression in non-advanced stages. Int J Cancer 1993;54:540–545.
174. Ikeda I, Ishizaka Y, Tahira T, et al. Specific expression of the ret proto-oncogene in human neuroblastoma cell lines. Oncogene 1990;5:1291–1296.
175. Tahira T, Ishizaka Y, Itoh F, et al. Expression of the ret proto-oncogene in human neuroblastoma cell lines and its increase during neuronal differentiation induced by retinoic acid. Oncogene 1991;6:2333–2338.
176. Tahira T, Ishizaka Y, Itoh F, et al. Characterization of ret proto-oncogene mRNAs encoding two isoforms of the protein product in a human neuroblastoma cell line. Oncogene 1990;5:97–102.
177. Ho R, Minturn JE, Hishiki T, et al. Proliferation of human neuroblastomas mediated by the epidermal growth factor receptor. Cancer Res 2005;65:9868–9875.
178. Layfield LJ, Thompson JK, Dodge RK, et al. Prognostic indicators for neuroblastoma: stage, grade, DNA ploidy, MIB-1-proliferation index, p53, HER-2/neu and EGFr—a survival study. J Surg Oncol 1995;59:21–27.
179. Tamura S, Hosoi H, Kuwahara Y, et al. Induction of apoptosis by an inhibitor of EGFR in neuroblastoma cells. Biochem Biophys Res Commun 2007;358:226–232.
180. Hosoi G, Hara J, Okamura T, et al. Low frequency of the p53 gene mutations in neuroblastoma. Cancer 1994;73:3087–3093.
181. Vogan K, Bernstein M, Brisson L, et al. Absence of p53 gene mutations in primary neuroblastomas. Cancer Res 1993;53:5269–5273.
182. Keshelava N, Zuo JJ, Chen P, et al. Loss of p53 function confers high-level multidrug resistance in neuroblastoma cell lines. Cancer Res 2001;61:6185–6193.
183. Tweddle DA, Malcolm AJ, Bown N, et al. Evidence for the development of p53 mutations after cytotoxic therapy in a neuroblastoma cell line. Cancer Res 2001;61: 8–13.
184. Carr J, Bell E, Pearson AD, et al. Increased frequency of aberrations in the p53/MDM2/p14(ARF) pathway in neuroblastoma cell lines established at relapse. Cancer Res 2006;66:2138–2145.
185. Moll UM, LaQuaglia M, Benard J, et al. Wild-type p53 protein undergoes cytoplasmic sequestration in undifferentiated neuroblastomas but not in differentiated tumors. Proc Natl Acad Sci U S A 1995;92:4407–4411.
186. Corvi R, Savelyeva L, Breit S, et al. Non-syntenic amplification of *MDM2* and *MYCN* in human neuroblastoma. Oncogene 1995;10:1081–1086.
187. Valsesia-Wittmann S, Magdeleine M, Dupasquier S, et al. Oncogenic cooperation between H-Twist and N-Myc overrides fail safe programs in cancer cells. Cancer Cell 2004;6:625–630.
188. Beltinger CP, White PS, Sulman EP, et al. No CDKN2 mutations in neuroblastomas. Cancer Res 1995;55:2053–2055.
189. Iolascon A, Giordani L, Moretti A, et al. Structural and functional analysis of cyclin-dependent kinase inhibitor genes (CDKN2A, CDKN2B, and CDKN2C) in neuroblastoma. Pediatr Res 1998;43:139–144.
190. Kawamata N, Seriu T, Koeffler HP, et al. Molecular analysis of the cyclin-dependent kinase inhibitor family: p16(CDKN2/MTS1/INK4A), p18(INK4C) and p27(Kip1) genes in neuroblastomas. Cancer 1996;77:570–575.
191. Takita J, Hayashi Y, Kohno T, et al. Deletion map of chromosome 9 and p16 (CDKN2A) gene alterations in neuroblastoma. Cancer Res 1997;57:907–912.
192. Sears RC, Nevins JR. Signaling networks that link cell proliferation and cell fate. J Biol Chem 2002;277:11617–11620.
193. Sears R, Nuckolls F, Haura E, et al. Multiple Ras-dependent phosphorylation pathways regulate Myc protein stability. Genes Dev 2000;14:2501–2514.
194. Yaari S, Jacob-Hirsch J, Amariglio N, et al. Disruption of cooperation between Ras and MycN in human neuroblastoma cells promotes growth arrest. Clin Cancer Res 2005; 11:4321–4330.
195. Dam V, Morgan BT, Mazanek P, et al. Mutations in PIK3CA are infrequent in neuroblastoma. BMC Cancer 2006;6:177.
196. Johnson M, Look A, DeClue J, et al. Inactivation of the NF1 gene in human melanoma and neuroblastoma cell lines without impaired regulation of GTP-Ras. Proc Natl Acad Sci U S A 1993;90:5539–5543.
197. The I, Murthy A, Hannigan G, et al. Neurofibromatosis type 1 gene mutations in neuroblastoma. Nat Genet 1993;3:62–66.
198. Shimada H, Chatten J, Newton WA Jr, et al. Histopathological prognostic factors in neuroblastic tumors: definition of subtypes of ganglioneuroblastoma and an age-linked classification of neuroblastomas. J Natl Cancer Inst 1984;73:405–413.
199. Shimada H, Umehara S, Monobe Y, et al. International neuroblastoma pathology classification for prognostic evaluation of patients with peripheral neuroblastic tumors: a report from the Children's Cancer Group. Cancer 2001;92:2451–2461.
200. Shimada H, Ambros IM, Dehner LP, et al. Terminology and morphologic criteria of neuroblastic tumors: recommendations by the International Neuroblastoma Pathology Committee. Cancer 1999;86:349–363.
201. Shimada H, Ambros IM, Dehner LP, et al. The International Neuroblastoma Pathology classification (the Shimada system). Cancer 1999;86:364–372.
202. Maris JM. The biologic basis for neuroblastoma heterogeneity and risk stratification. Curr Opin Pediatr 2005;17:7–13.
203. Cohn SL, Pearson AD, London WB, et al. The International Neuroblastoma Risk Group (INRG) classification system: an INRG Task Force report. J Clin Oncol 2009; 27:289–297.
204. DuBois SG, Kalika Y, Lukens JN, et al. Metastatic sites in stage IV and IVS neuroblastoma correlate with age, tumor biology, and survival [see comments]. J Pediatr Hematol Oncol 1999;21:181–189.
205. Dubois SG, London WB, Zhang Y, et al. Lung metastases in neuroblastoma at initial diagnosis: a report from the International Neuroblastoma Risk Group (INRG) project. Pediatr Blood Cancer 2008;51:589–592.
206. de la Monte SM, Moore GW, Hutchins GM. Nonrandom distribution of metastases in neuroblastic tumors. Cancer 1983;52:915–925.
207. Feldges AJ, Stanisic M, Morger R, et al. Neuroblastoma with meningeal involvement causing increased intracranial pressure and coma in two children. Am J Pediatr Hematol Oncol 1986;8:355–357.
208. Kellie SJ, Hayes FA, Bowman L, et al. Primary extracranial neuroblastoma with central nervous system metastases. Characterization by clinicopathologic findings and neuroimaging. Cancer 1991;68:1999–2006.
209. Rohrlich P, Hartmann O, Couanet D, et al. Secondary metastatic neuromeningeal localization of neuroblastoma in children. Arch Fr Pediatr 1989;46:5–10.
210. Shaw PJ, Eden T. Neuroblastoma with intracranial involvement: an ENSG study. Med Pediatr Oncol 1992;20:149–155.
211. Quinn JJ, Altman AJ. The multiple hematologic manifestations of neuroblastoma. Am J Pediatr Hematol Oncol 1979;1:201–205.
212. Scott JP, Morgan E. Coagulopathy of disseminated neuroblastoma. J Pediatr 1983; 103:219–222.
213. Evans AE, Chatten J, D'Angio GJ, et al. A review of 17 IV-S neuroblastoma patients at the children's hospital of Philadelphia. Cancer 1980;45:833–839.
214. Conte M, Parodi S, De Bernardi B, et al. Neuroblastoma in adolescents: the Italian experience. Cancer 2006;106:1409–1417.
215. Franks LM, Bollen A, Seeger RC, et al. Neuroblastoma in adults and adolescents: an indolent course with poor survival. Cancer 1997;79:2028–2035.
216. Kushner BH, Kramer K, LaQuaglia MP, et al. Neuroblastoma in adolescents and adults: the Memorial Sloan-Kettering experience. Med Pediatr Oncol 2003;41:508–515.
217. Hayward K, Jeremy RJ, Jenkins S, et al. Long-term neurobehavioral outcomes in children with neuroblastoma and opsoclonus-myoclonus-ataxia syndrome: relationship to MRI findings and anti-neuronal antibodies. J Pediatr 2001;139:552–559.
218. Mitchell WG, Davalos-Gonzalez Y, Brumm VL, et al. Opsoclonus-ataxia caused by childhood neuroblastoma: developmental and neurologic sequelae. Pediatrics 2002; 109:86–98.
219. Rudnick E, Khakoo Y, Antunes NL, et al. Opsoclonus-myoclonus-ataxia syndrome in neuroblastoma: clinical outcome and antineuronal antibodies—a report from the Children's Cancer Group Study. Med Pediatr Oncol 2001;36:612–622.
220. Antunes NL, Khakoo Y, Matthay KK, et al. Antineuronal antibodies in patients with neuroblastoma and paraneoplastic opsoclonus-myoclonus. J Pediatr Hematol Oncol 2000;22:315–320.
221. Cooper R, Khakoo Y, Matthay KK, et al. Opsoclonus-myoclonus-ataxia syndrome in neuroblastoma: histopathological features—a report from the Children's Cancer Group. Med Pediatr Oncol 2001;36:623–629.
222. Pranzatelli MR, Travelstead AL, Tate ED, et al. B- and T-cell markers in opsoclonus-myoclonus syndrome: immunophenotyping of CSF lymphocytes. Neurology 2004; 62:1526–1532.
223. Russo C, Cohn SL, Petruzzi MJ, et al. Long-term neurologic outcome in children with opsoclonus-myoclonus associated with neuroblastoma: a report from the Pediatric Oncology Group. Med Pediatr Oncol 1997;28:284–288.
224. Swart JF, de Kraker J, van der Lely N. Metaiodobenzylguanidine total-body scintigraphy required for revealing occult neuroblastoma in opsoclonus-myoclonus syndrome. Eur J Pediatr 2002;161:255–258.
225. Borgna-Pignatti C, Balter R, Marradi P, et al. Treatment with intravenously administered immunoglobulins of the neuroblastoma-associated opsoclonus-myoclonus. J Pediatr 1996;129:179–180.
226. Petruzzi MJ, de Alarcon PA. Neuroblastoma-associated opsoclonus-myoclonus treated with intravenously administered immune globulin G. J Pediatr 1995;127:328–329.
227. Veneselli E, Conte M, Biancheri R, et al. Effect of steroid and high-dose immunoglobulin therapy on opsoclonus-myoclonus syndrome occurring in neuroblastoma. Med Pediatr Oncol 1998;30:15–17.
228. Pranzatelli MR, Tate ED, Travelstead AL, et al. Rituximab (anti-CD20) adjunctive therapy for opsoclonus-myoclonus syndrome. J Pediatr Hematol Oncol 2006;28:585–593.
229. El Shafie M, Samuel D, Klippel CH, et al. Intractable diarrhea in children with VIP-secreting ganglioneuroblastomas. J Pediatr Surg 1983;18:34–36.
230. Kaplan S, Holbrook C, McDaniel H, et al. Vasoactive intestinal peptide secreting tumors of childhood. Am J Dis Child 1980;134:21–24.
231. Muller JM, Philippe M, Chevrier L, et al. The VIP-receptor system in neuroblastoma cells. Regul Pept 2006;137:34–41.
232. Qualman SJ, O'Dorisio MS, Fleshman DJ, et al. Neuroblastoma. Correlation of neuropeptide expression in tumor tissue with other prognostic factors. Cancer 1992;70: 2005–2012.
233. Cheung IY, Barber D, Cheung NK. Detection of microscopic neuroblastoma in marrow by histology, immunocytology, and reverse transcription-PCR of multiple molecular markers. Clin Cancer Res 1998;4:2801–2805.
234. Seeger RC, Reynolds CP, Gallego R, et al. Quantitative tumor cell content of bone marrow and blood as a predictor of outcome in stage IV neuroblastoma: a Children's Cancer Group Study. J Clin Oncol 2000;18:4067–4076.
235. Reynolds CP. Detection and treatment of minimal residual disease in high-risk neuroblastoma. Pediatr Transplant 2004;8(suppl 5):56–66.
236. Shulkin BL, Shapiro B. Current concepts on the diagnostic use of MIBG in children. J Nucl Med 1998;39:679–688.
237. Matthay KK, Edeline V, Lumbroso J, et al. Correlation of early metastatic response by 123I-metaiodobenzylguanidine scintigraphy with overall response and event-free survival in stage IV neuroblastoma. J Clin Oncol 2003;21:2486–2491.
238. Kushner BH, Yeung HW, Larson SM, et al. Extending positron emission tomography scan utility to high-risk neuroblastoma: fluorine-18 fluorodeoxyglucose positron emission tomography as sole imaging modality in follow-up of patients. J Clin Oncol 2001; 19:3397–3405.
239. Scanga DR, Martin WH, Delbeke D. Value of FDG PET imaging in the management of patients with thyroid, neuroendocrine, and neural crest tumors. Clin Nucl Med 2004; 29:86–90.
240. Frostad B, Martinsson T, Tani E, et al. The use of fine-needle aspiration cytology in the molecular characterization of neuroblastoma in children. Cancer 1999;87:60–68.
241. Monsaingeon M, Perel Y, Simonnet G, et al. Comparative values of catecholamines and metabolites for the diagnosis of neuroblastoma. Eur J Pediatr 2003;162:397–402.
242. Brodeur GM, Pritchard J, Berthold F, et al. Revisions in the international criteria for neuroblastoma diagnosis, staging, and response to treatment. J Clin Oncol 1993;11: 1466–1477.
243. Brodeur GM, Seeger RC, Barrett A, et al. International criteria for diagnosis, staging and response to treatment in patients with neuroblastoma. J Clin Oncol 1988;6:1874–1881.
244. Donner K, Triche TJ, Israel MA, et al. A panel of monoclonal antibodies which discriminate neuroblastoma from Ewing's sarcoma, rhabdomyosarcoma, neuroepithelioma, and hematopoietic malignancies. Prog Clin Biol Res 1985;175:367–378.

245. Kemshead JT, Goldman A, Fritschy J, et al. Use of panels of monoclonal antibodies in the differential diagnosis of neuroblastoma and lymphoblastic disorders. Lancet 1983;1:12–15.

246. Sugimoto T, Sawada T, Arakawa S, et al. Possible differential diagnosis of neuroblastoma from rhabdomyosarcoma and Ewing's sarcoma by using a panel of monoclonal antibodies. Jpn J Cancer Res 1985;76:301–307.

247. Triche TJ, Askin FB, Kissane JM. Neuroblastoma, Ewing's sarcoma, and the differential diagnosis of small-, round-, blue-cell tumors. In: Finegold M, ed. Pathology of neoplasia in children and adolescents. Philadelphia, PA: W.B. Saunders Co., 1986:145–195.

248. Evans AE, D'Angio GJ, Randolph JA. A proposed staging for children with neuroblastoma. Children's Cancer Study Group A. Cancer 1971;27:374–378.

249. Hayes FA, Green AA, Hustu HO, et al. Surgicopathologic staging of neuroblastoma: prognostic significance of regional lymph node metastases. J Pediatr 1983;102:59–62.

250. Nakagawara A, Morita K, Okabe I, et al. Proposal and assessment of Japanese Tumor Node Metastasis postsurgical histopathological staging system for neuroblastoma based on an analysis of 495 cases. Jpn J Clin Oncol 1990;21:1–7.

251. Monclair T, Brodeur GM, Ambros PF, et al. The International Neuroblastoma Risk Group (INRG) staging system: an INRG Task Force report. J Clin Oncol 2009;27:298–303.

252. Monclair T, Brodeur GM, Ambros PF, et al. The International Neuroblastoma Risk Group (INRG) staging system: an INRG Task Force report. J Clin Oncol 2009;27:298–303.

253. Sawaguchi S, Suganuma Y, Watanabe I, et al. Studies of the biological and clinical characteristics of neuroblastoma. III. Evaluation of the survival rate in relation to 17 factors. Nippon Shoni Geka Gakkai Zasshi 1980;16:51–66.

254. D'Angio GJ, Evans AE, Koop CE. Special pattern of widespread neuroblastoma with a favorable prognosis. Lancet 1971;1:1046–1049.

255. Evans AE, Baum E, Chard R. Do infants with stage IV-S neuroblastoma need treatment? Arch Dis Child 1981;56:271–274.

256. Nickerson HJ, Matthay KK, Seeger RC, et al. Favorable biology and outcome of stage IV-S neuroblastoma with supportive care or minimal therapy: a Children's Cancer Group study. J Clin Oncol 2000;18:477–486.

257. Castleberry RP, Shuster JJ, Smith EI. The POG experience with the International Staging System. J Clin Oncol 1994;12:2378–2381.

258. Haase GM, Atkinson JB, Stram DO, et al. Surgical management and outcome of locoregional neuroblastoma: comparison of the Childrens Cancer Group and the International Staging systems. J Pediatr Surg 1995;30:289–294.

259. Therasse P, Arbuck SG, Eisenhauer EA, et al. New guidelines to evaluate the response to treatment in solid tumors. J Natl Cancer Inst 2000;92(3):205–216.

260. Ady N, Zucker JM, Asselain B, et al. A new 123I-MIBG whole body scan scoring method—application to the prediction of the response of metastases to induction chemotherapy in stage IV neuroblastoma. Eur J Cancer 1995;31A:256–261.

261. Beiske K, Burchill SA, Cheung IY, et al. Consensus criteria for sensitive detection of minimal neuroblastoma cells in bone marrow, blood and stem cell preparations by immunocytology and QRT-PCR: recommendations by the International Neuroblastoma Risk Group Task Force. Br J Cancer 2009;100:1627–1637.

262. Breslow N, McCann B. Statistical estimation of prognosis for children with neuroblastoma. Cancer Res 1971;31:2098–2103.

263. George RE, London WB, Cohn SL, et al. Hyperdiploidy plus nonamplified MYCN confers a favorable prognosis in children 12 to 18 months old with disseminated neuroblastoma: a Pediatric Oncology Group study. J Clin Oncol 2005;23:6466–6473.

264. London WB, Castleberry RP, Matthay KK, et al. Evidence for an age cutoff greater than 365 days for neuroblastoma risk group stratification in the Children's Oncology Group. J Clin Oncol 2005;23:6459–6465.

265. Schmidt ML, Lal A, Seeger RC, et al. Favorable prognosis for patients 12 to 18 months of age with stage 4 nonamplified MYCN neuroblastoma: a Children's Cancer Group Study. J Clin Oncol 2005;23:6474–6480.

266. Joshi VV, Cantor AB, Altshuler G, et al. Age-linked prognostic categorization based on a new histologic grading system of neuroblastomas. A clinicopathologic study of 211 cases from the Pediatric Oncology Group. Cancer 1992;69:2197–2211.

267. Peuchmaur M, d'Amore ES, Joshi VV, et al. Revision of the International Neuroblastoma Pathology Classification: confirmation of favorable and unfavorable prognostic subsets in ganglioneuroblastoma, nodular. Cancer 2003;98:2274–2281.

268. Bourhis J, De Vathaire F, Wilson GD, et al. Combined analysis of DNA ploidy index and N-myc genomic content in neuroblastoma. Cancer Res 1991;51:33–36.

269. Bowman LC, Castleberry RP, Altshuler G, et al. Therapy based on DNA index (DI) for infants with unresectable and disseminated neuroblastoma (NB): preliminary results of the Pediatric Oncology Group "Better Risk" study [abstract]. Med Pediatr Oncol 1990;18:364.

270. Bowman LC, Castleberry RP, Cantor A, et al. Genetic staging of unresectable or metastatic neuroblastoma in infants: a Pediatric Oncology Group study. J Natl Cancer Inst 1997;89:373–380.

271. Cohn SL, Rademaker AW, Salwen HR, et al. Analysis of DNA ploidy and proliferative activity in relation to histology and N-myc amplification in neuroblastoma. Am J Pathol 1990;136:1043–1052.

272. Oppedal BR, Storm-Mathisen I, Lie SO, et al. Prognostic factors in neuroblastoma. Clinical, histopathological immunohistochemical features and DNA ploidy in relation to prognosis. Cancer 1988;72:772–779.

273. Matthay KK, Villablanca JG, Seeger RC, et al. Treatment of high-risk neuroblastoma with intensive chemotherapy, radiotherapy, autologous bone marrow transplantation, and 13-cis-retinoic acid. Children's Cancer Group. N Engl J Med 1999;341:1165–1173.

274. Hann HWL, Evans AE, Siegel SE, et al. Prognostic importance of serum ferritin in patients with stages III and IV neuroblastoma. The Children's Cancer Study Group Experience. Cancer Res 1985;45:2843–2848.

275. Quinn JJ, Altman AJ, Frantz CN. Serum lactic dehydrogenase, an indicator of tumor activity in neuroblastoma. J Pediatr 1980;97:89–91.

276. Shuster JJ, McWilliams NB, Castleberry R, et al. Serum lactate dehydrogenase in childhood neuroblastoma. A Pediatric Oncology Group recursive partitioning study. Am J Clin Oncol 1992;15:295–303.

277. Zeltzer PM, Marangos PJ, Evans AE, et al. Serum neuron-specific enolase in children with neuroblastoma. Relationship to stage and disease course. Cancer 1986;57:1230–1234.

278. Smith EI, Castleberry RP. Neuroblastoma. In: Wells SA Jr, ed. Current problems in pediatric surgery. St. Louis, MO: C.V. Mosby, 1990:577–620.

279. Contador MP, Johnston S, Smith EI, et al. Lymph node sampling in localized neuroblastoma: a Pediatric Oncology Group study. J Pediatr Surg 1999;34:967–974.

280. Castleberry RP, Kun L, Shuster JJ, et al. Radiotherapy improves the outlook for children older than one year with POG stage C neuroblastoma. J Clin Oncol 1991;9:789–795.

281. Haase GM, O'Leary MC, Ramsay NK, et al. Aggressive surgery combined with intensive chemotherapy improves survival in poor-risk neuroblastoma. J Pediatr Surg 1991; 26:1119–1123.

282. La Quaglia MP, Kushner BH, Su W, et al. The impact of gross total resection on local control and survival in high-risk neuroblastoma. J Pediatr Surg 2004;39:412–417; discussion 412–417.

283. Chamberlain RS, Quinones R, Dinndorf P, et al. Complete surgical resection combined with aggressive adjuvant chemotherapy and bone marrow transplantation prolongs survival in children with advanced neuroblastoma. Ann Surg Oncol 1995;2:93–100.

284. Kiely EM. Radical surgery for abdominal neuroblastoma. Semin Surg Oncol 1993; 9:489–492.

285. Kiely EM. The surgical challenge of neuroblastoma. J Pediatr Surg 1994;29:128–133.

286. Nakagawara A, Ikeda K, Yokoyama T, et al. Surgical aspects of N-myc oncogene amplification of neuroblastoma. Surgery 1988;104:34–40.

287. Azizkjan RG, Shaw A, Chandler JG. Surgical complications of neuroblastoma resection. Surgery 1985;97:514–517.

288. Berthold F, Utsch S, Holschneider AM. The impact of preoperative chemotherapy on resectability of primary tumor and complication rate in metastatic neuroblastoma. Z Kinderchir 1989;44:21–24.

289. Nitschke R, Smith EI, Shochat S, et al. Localized neuroblastoma treated by surgery—a Pediatric Oncology Group Study. J Clin Oncol 1988;6:1271–1279.

290. Cecchetto G, Mosseri V, De Bernardi B, et al. Surgical risk factors in primary surgery for localized neuroblastoma: the LNESG1 study of the European International Society of Pediatric Oncology Neuroblastoma Group. J Clin Oncol 2005;23:8483–8489.

291. Habrand JL, D'Angio GJ. Radiotherapy in neuroblastoma. In: Brodeur GM, Sawada T, Tsuchida Y, et al., eds. Neuroblastoma. Amsterdam, The Netherlands: Elsevier, 2000: 479–496.

292. Weichselbaum RR, Epstein J, Little JB. In vitro cellular radiosensitivity of human malignant tumors. Eur J Cancer 1976;36:47.

293. Halperin EC, Cox EB. Radiation therapy in the management of neuroblastoma: the Duke University Medical Center experience 1967–1984. Int J Radiat Oncol Biol Phys 1986;12:1829–1837.

294. Jacobson GM, Sause WT, O'Brien RT. Dose response analysis of pediatric neuroblastoma to megavoltage radiation. Am J Clin Oncol 1984;7:693–697.

295. Green AA, Hustu HO, Kumar M. Sequential cyclophosphamide and doxorubicin for induction of complete remission in children with disseminated neuroblastoma. Cancer 1981;48:2310–2317.

296. Strother D, Cantor A, Halperin E, et al. Treatment of Pediatric Oncology Group stage C neuroblastoma: a preliminary POG report [abstract]. Proc Am Soc Clin Oncol 1993;12: 1422.

297. de Bernardi B, Rogers D, Carli M, et al. Localized neuroblastoma. Surgical and pathologic staging. Cancer 1987;60:1066–1072.

298. Matthay KK, Perez C, Seeger RC, et al. Successful treatment of stage III neuroblastoma based on prospective biologic staging: a Children's Cancer Group study. J Clin Oncol 1998;16:1256–1264.

299. Simon T, Hero B, Bongartz R, et al. Intensified external-beam radiation therapy improves the outcome of stage 4 neuroblastoma in children >1 year with residual local disease. Strahlenther Onkol 2006;182:389–394.

300. McWilliams NB. Stage IV-S neuroblastoma: treatment controversy revisited. Med Pediatr Oncol 1986;14:41–44.

301. McWilliams NB. Neuroblastoma in infancy. In: Pochedly C, ed. Neuroblastoma: tumor biology and therapy. Boca Raton: CRC Press, 1990:229–243.

302. Nickersen HJ, Nesbit ME, Grosfeld JL, et al. Comparison of stage IV and IV-S neuroblastoma in the first year of life. Med Pediatr Oncol 1985;13:261–268.

303. Punt N, Pritchard J, Pincott J, et al. Neuroblastoma: a review of 21 cases presenting with spinal cord compression. Cancer 1980;45:3095.

304. Hayes FA, Green AA, O'Connor DM. Chemotherapeutic management of epidural neuroblastoma. Med Pediatr Oncol 1989;17:6–8.

305. Hayes FA, Thompson E, Hvizdala E, et al. Chemotherapy as an alternative to laminectomy and radiation in the management of epidural tumor. J Pediatr 1984;104:221–224.

306. Hoover M, Bowman LC, Crawford SE, et al. Long-term outcome of patients with intraspinal neuroblastoma. Med Pediatr Oncol 1999;32:353–359.

307. Plantaz D, Rubie H, Michon J, et al. The treatment of neuroblastoma with intraspinal extension with chemotherapy followed by surgical removal of residual disease. A prospective study of 42 patients—results of the NBL 90 Study of the French Society of Pediatric Oncology. Cancer 1996;78:311–319.

308. August CS, Serota FT, Koch PA, et al. Treatment of advanced neuroblastoma with supralethal chemotherapy, radiation and allogeneic or autologous marrow reconstitution. J Clin Oncol 1984;2:609–616.

309. Graham-Pole J, Casper J, Elfenbein G, et al. High-dose chemoradiotherapy supported by marrow infusions for advanced neuroblastoma: a Pediatric Oncology Group study. J Clin Oncol 1991;9:152–158.

310. Philip T, Zucker JM, Bernard JL, et al. Improved survival at 2 and 5 years in the LMCE1 unselected group of 72 children with stage IV neuroblastoma older than 1 year of age at diagnosis: is cure possible in a small subgroup? J Clin Oncol 1991;9:1037–1044.

311. Haas-Kogan DA, Swift PS, Selch M, et al. Impact of radiotherapy for high-risk neuroblastoma: a Children's Cancer Group study. Int J Radiat Oncol Biol Phys 2003;56:28–39.

312. Kushner BH, O'Reilly RJ, Mandell LR, et al. Myeloablative combination chemotherapy without total body irradiation for neuroblastoma. J Clin Oncol 1991;9:274–279.

313. Hobbie WL, Moshang T, Carlson CA, et al. Late effects in survivors of tandem peripheral blood stem cell transplant for high-risk neuroblastoma. Pediatr Blood Cancer 2008;51:679–683.

314. Castleberry RP, Cantor AB, Green AA, et al. Phase II investigational window using carboplatin, iproplatin, ifosfamide, and epirubicin in children with untreated disseminated neuroblastoma: a Pediatric Oncology Group Study. J Clin Oncol 1994;12:1616–1620.

315. Kellie SJ, DeKraker J, Lilleyman JS, et al. Ifosfamide in previously untreated disseminated neuroblastoma. Results of Study 3A of the European Neuroblastoma Study Group. Eur J Cancer Clin Oncol 1988;24:903.

316. Kretschmar CS, Kletzel M, Murray K, et al. Response to paclitaxel, topotecan, and topotecan-cyclophosphamide in children with untreated disseminated neuroblastoma treated in an upfront phase II investigational window: a Pediatric Oncology Group study. J Clin Oncol 2004;22:4119–4126.

317. Frantz CN, London WB, Diller L, et al. Recurrent neuroblastoma: randomized treatment with topotecan + cyclophosphamide (T+C) vs. topotecan alone(T). A POG/CCG Intergroup Study. 2004 ASCO Annual Meeting, 2004. Abstract no. 8512.

318. Bagatell R, Wagner LM, Cohn SL, et al. Irinotecan plus temozolomide in children with recurrent or refractory neuroblastoma: a phase II Children's Oncology Group study. J Clin Oncol 2009;27:10011.

319. Evans AE, Silber JH, Shpilsky A, et al. Successful management of low-stage neuroblastoma without adjuvant therapies: a comparison of two decades, 1972 through 1981 and 1982 through 1992, in a single institution. J Clin Oncol 1996;14:2504–2510.
320. Kushner BH, Cheung NK, LaQuaglia MP, et al. International neuroblastoma staging system stage 1 neuroblastoma: a prospective study and literature review. J Clin Oncol 1996;14:2174–2180.
321. Matthay KK, Sather HN, Seeger RC, et al. Excellent outcome of stage II neuroblastoma is independent of residual disease and radiation therapy. J Clin Oncol 1989;7:236–244.
322. Nitschke R, Smith EI, Altshuler G, et al. Treatment of grossly unresectable localized neuroblastoma. A Pediatric Oncology Group study. J Clin Oncol 1991;9:1181–1188.
323. Perez CA, Matthay KK, Atkinson JB, et al. Biologic variables in the outcome of stages I and II neuroblastoma treated with surgery as primary therapy: a Children's Cancer Group study. J Clin Oncol 2000;18:18–26.
324. Alvarado CS, London WB, Look AT, et al. Natural history and biology of stage A neuroblastoma: a Pediatric Oncology Group Study. J Pediatr Hematol Oncol 2000;22: 197–205.
325. Kushner BH, Kramer K, LaQuaglia MP, et al. Curability of recurrent disseminated disease after surgery alone for local-regional neuroblastoma using intensive chemotherapy and anti-G(D2) immunotherapy. J Pediatr Hematol Oncol 2003;25:515–519.
326. Castleberry RP, Shuster JJ, Altshuler G, et al. Infants with neuroblastoma and regional lymph node metastases have a favorable outlook after limited postoperative chemotherapy: a Pediatric Oncology Group study. J Clin Oncol 1992;10:1299–1304.
327. Kushner BH, Cheung NK, LaQuaglia MP, et al. Survival from locally invasive or widespread neuroblastoma without cytotoxic therapy. J Clin Oncol 1996;14:373–381.
328. Rubie H, Hartmann O, Michon J, et al. N-Myc gene amplification is a major prognostic factor in localized neuroblastoma: results of the French NBL 90 study. Neuroblastoma Study Group of the Societe Francaise d'Oncologie Pediatrique. J Clin Oncol 1997;15:1171–1182.
329. Strother DR, London WB, Schmidt ML, et al. Surgery alone or followed by chemotherapy for patients with stages 2A and 2B neuroblastoma: results of Children's Oncology Group Study. Advances in Neuroblastoma Research—2006. Los Angeles, 2006.
330. Cohn SL, Brodeur GM, Holbrook T, et al. N-myc gene amplification in localized neuroblastoma. A Pediatric Oncology Group Study. Cancer Res 1995;55:721–726.
331. Hero B, Simon T, Spitz R, et al. Localized infant neuroblastomas often show spontaneous regression: results of the prospective trials NB95-S and NB97. J Clin Oncol 2008; 26:1504–1510.
332. Nuchtern JG. Perinatal neuroblastoma. Semin Pediatr Surg 2006;15:10–16.
333. Shimada H, Stram DO, Chatten J, et al. Identification of subsets of neuroblastomas by combined histopathological and N-myc analysis. J Natl Cancer Inst 1995;87:1470–1476.
334. Kawa K, Ohnuma N, Kaneko M, et al. Long-term survivors of advanced neuroblastoma with MYCN amplification: a report of 19 patients surviving disease-free for more than 66 months. J Clin Oncol 1999;17:3216–3220.
335. Strother D, Shuster JJ, McWilliams N, et al. Results of Pediatric Oncology Group protocol 8104 for infants with stages D and DS neuroblastoma. J Pediatr Hematol Oncol 1995;17:254–259.
336. Baker DL, Schmidt M, Cohn S, et al. A phase III trial of biologically-based therapy reduction for intermediate risk neuroblastoma. J Clin Oncol 2007;25:9504.
337. Bernard JL, Philip T, Zucker JM, et al. Sequential cisplatin/VM26 and vincristine/cyclophosphamide/doxorubicin in metastatic neuroblastoma: an effective alternating non-cross resistant regimen? J Clin Oncol 1987;5:1952–1959.
338. Berthold F, Treuner J, Brandeis WE, et al. Neuroblastoma study NBL-79 of the German Society for Pediatric Oncology: report after 2 years. Klin Pediatr 1982;194:262–269.
339. Finklestein JZ, Klemperer MR, Evans A, et al. Multiagent chemotherapy for children with metastatic neuroblastoma; a Report from Children's Cancer Study Group. Med Pediatr Oncol 1979;6:179–188.
340. Gasparini M, Bellani FF, Musumeci R, et al. Response and survival of patients with metastatic neuroblastoma after combination chemotherapy with adriamycin (NSC-123127, cyclophosphamide (NSC-26271) and vincristine (NSC-67574). Cancer Chemother Rep 1974;58:365–370.
341. Hayes FA, Green AA, Casper J, et al. Clinical evaluation of sequentially scheduled cisplatin and VM26 in neuroblastoma: response and toxicity. Cancer 1981;48:1715–1718.
342. Helson L, Vanichayangkul P, Tan C, et al. Combination intermittent chemotherapy for patients with disseminated neuroblastoma. Cancer Chemother Rep 1972;56:499–503.
343. Nitschke R, Cangir A, Crist W, et al. Intensive chemotherapy for metastatic neuroblastoma: a Southwest Oncology Group study. Med Pediatr Oncol 1980;8:281–288.
344. Nitschke R, Starling K, Lui VKS, et al. Doxorubicin and cisplatin therapy in children with neuroblastoma resistant to conventional therapy: a Southwest Oncology Group study. Cancer Treat Rep 1981;65:1105–1108.
345. Rosen EM, Cassady JR, Frantz CN, et al. Neuroblastoma: the Joint Center for Radiation Therapy/Dana-Farber Cancer Institute/Children's Hospital experience. J Clin Oncol 1984;2:714–732.
346. Shafford EA, Rogers DW, Pritchard J. Advanced neuroblastoma: improved response rate using a multi-agent regimen (OPEC) including sequential cisplatin and VM-26. J Clin Oncol 1984;2:742–747.
347. Shuster JJ, Land VJ, Nitschke R, et al. Phase II study for four-drug chemotherapy for metastatic neuroblastoma: Pediatric Oncology Group study. Cancer Treat Rep 1983; 67:187–188.
348. Kushner BH, Cheung NK, Kramer K, et al. Neuroblastoma and treatment-related myelodysplasia/leukemia: the Memorial Sloan-Kettering experience and a literature review. J Clin Oncol 1998;16:3880–3889.
349. Meadows AT, Tsunematsu Y. Late effects of treatment for neuroblastoma. In: Brodeur GM, Sawada T, Tsuchida Y, et al., eds. Neuroblastoma. Amsterdam, The Netherlands: Elsevier Science B.V., 2000:561–570.
350. Zeltzer LK, Recklitis C, Buchbinder D, et al. Psychological status in childhood cancer survivors: a report from the Childhood Cancer Survivor Study. J Clin Oncol 2009;27: 2396–2404.
351. Gurney JG, Tersak JM, Ness KK, et al. Hearing loss, quality of life, and academic problems in long-term neuroblastoma survivors: a report from the Children's Oncology Group. Pediatrics 2007;120:e1229–e1236.
352. Escobar MA, Grosfeld JL, Powell RL, et al. Long-term outcomes in patients with stage IV neuroblastoma. J Pediatr Surg 2006;41:377–381.
353. Bassal M, Mertens AC, Taylor L, et al. Risk of selected subsequent carcinomas in survivors of childhood cancer: a report from the Childhood Cancer Survivor Study. J Clin Oncol 2006;24:476–483.
354. Oeffinger KC, Mertens AC, Sklar CA, et al. Chronic health conditions in adult survivors of childhood cancer. N Engl J Med 2006;355:1572–1582.
355. Cheung NV, Heller G. Chemotherapy dose intensity correlates strongly with response, median survival, and median progression-free survival in metastatic neuroblastoma [see comments]. J Clin Oncol 1991;9:1050–1058.
356. Helson L, Helson C, Peterson RF, et al. A rationale for the treatment of metastatic neuroblastoma. J Natl Cancer Inst 1976;57:727–729.
357. Hartmann O, Berthold F. Treatment of advanced neuroblastoma: the European experience. In: Brodeur GM, Sawada T, Tsuchida Y, et al., eds. Neuroblastoma. Amsterdam, The Netherlands: Elsevier Science B.V., 2000:437–452.
358. Hartmann O, Valteau-Couanet D, Vassal G, et al. Prognostic factors in metastatic neuroblastoma in patients over 1 year of age treated with high-dose chemotherapy and stem cell transplantation: a multivariate analysis in 218 patients treated in a single institution. Bone Marrow Transplant 1999;23:789–795.
359. Kaneko M, Tsuchida Y, Uchino J, et al. Treatment results of advanced neuroblastoma with the first Japanese study group protocol. Study Group of Japan for Treatment of Advanced Neuroblastoma [see comments]. J Pediatr Hematol Oncol 1999;21:190–197.
360. Ladenstein R, Philip T, Lasset C, et al. Multivariate analysis of risk factors in stage 4 neuroblastoma patients over the age of one year treated with megatherapy and stem-cell transplantation: a report from the European Bone Marrow Transplantation Solid Tumor Registry. J Clin Oncol 1998;16:953–965.
361. Pinkerton R, Philip T, Bouffet E, et al. Autologous bone marrow transplantation in paediatric solid tumours. Clin Haematol 1986;15:187–203.
362. Saarinen UM, Wikstrom S, Makipernaa A, et al. In vivo purging of bone marrow in children with poor-risk neuroblastoma for marrow collection and autologous bone marrow transplantation. J Clin Oncol 1996;14:2791–2802.
363. Katzenstein HM, Cohn SL, Shore RM, et al. Scintigraphic response by 123I-metaiodobenzylguanidine scan correlates with event-free survival in high-risk neuroblastoma. J Clin Oncol 2004;22:3909–3915.
364. Kushner BH, Yeh SD, Kramer K, et al. Impact of metaiodobenzylguanidine scintigraphy on assessing response of high-risk neuroblastoma to dose-intensive induction chemotherapy. J Clin Oncol 2003;21:1082–1086.
365. Schmidt M, Simon T, Hero B, et al. The prognostic impact of functional imaging with (123)I-mIBG in patients with stage 4 neuroblastoma >1 year of age on a high-risk treatment protocol: results of the German Neuroblastoma Trial NB97. Eur J Cancer 2008; 44:1552–1558.
366. Matthay KK, Castleberry RP. Treatment of advanced neuroblastoma: the U.S. experience. In: Brodeur GM, Sawada T, Tsuchida Y, et al., eds. Neuroblastoma. Amsterdam, The Netherlands: Elsevier Science B.V., 2000:417–436.
367. Kushner BH, LaQuaglia MP, Bonilla MA, et al. Highly effective induction therapy for stage 4 neuroblastoma in children over 1 year of age. J Clin Oncol 1994;12:2607–2613.
368. Kreissman SG, Villablanca JG, Seeger RC, et al. A randomized phase III trial of myeloablative autologous peripheral blood stem cell (PBSC) transplant (ASCT) for high-risk neuroblastoma (HR-NB) employing immunomagnetic purged (P) versus unpurged (UP) PBSC: a Children's Oncology Group study. J Clin Oncol 2008;26:abstract 10011.
369. Kreissman SG, Villablanca JG, Diller L, et al. Response and toxicity to a dose-intensive multi-agent chemotherapy induction regimen for high risk neuroblastoma (HR-NB): a Children's Oncology Group (COG A3973) study. J Clin Oncol 2007;25:abstract 9505.
370. Kushner BH, Kramer K, Modak S, et al. Reduced risk of secondary leukemia with fewer cycles of dose-intensive induction chemotherapy in patients with neuroblastoma. Pediatr Blood Cancer 2009;53:17–22.
371. Valteau-Couanet D, Michon J, Boneu A, et al. Results of induction chemotherapy in children older than 1 year with a stage 4 neuroblastoma treated with the NB 97 French Society of Pediatric Oncology (SFOP) protocol. J Clin Oncol 2005;23:532–540.
372. Pearson AD, Pinkerton CR, Lewis IJ, et al. High-dose rapid and standard induction chemotherapy for patients aged over 1 year with stage 4 neuroblastoma: a randomised trial. Lancet Oncol 2008;9:247–256.
373. Park JR, Stewart CF, London WB, et al. A topotecan-containing induction regimen for treatment of high risk neuroblastoma. J Clin Oncol 2006;24:67.
374. Pritchard J, McElwain TJ, Graham-Pole J. High dose melphalan with autologous marrow for treatment of advanced neuroblastoma. Br J Cancer 1982;45:86–94.
375. Cohn SL, Moss TJ, Hoover M, et al. Treatment of poor-risk neuroblastoma patients with high-dose chemotherapy and autologous peripheral stem cell rescue. Bone Marrow Transplant 1997;20:543–551.
376. Dini G, Lanino E, Garaventa A, et al. Myeloablative therapy and unpurged autologous bone marrow transplantation for poor-prognosis neuroblastoma: report of 34 cases. J Clin Oncol 1991;9:962–969.
377. Dini G, Philip T, Hartmann O, et al. Bone marrow transplantation for neuroblastoma: a review of 509 cases. EBMT Group. Bone Marrow Transplant 1989;4:42–46.
378. Evans AE, August CS, Kamani N, et al. Bone marrow transplantation for high risk neuroblastoma at the Children's Hospital of Philadelphia: an update. Med Pediatr Oncol 1994;23:323–327.
379. Garaventa A, Rondelli R, Lanino E, et al. Myeloablative therapy and bone marrow rescue in advanced neuroblastoma. Report from the Italian Bone Marrow Transplant Registry. Italian Association of Pediatric Hematology-Oncology, BMT Group. Bone Marrow Transplant 1996;18:125–130.
380. Gee AP, Graham Pole J. Use of bone marrow purging and bone marrow transplantation for neuroblastoma. In: Pochedly C, ed. Neuroblastoma: tumor biology and therapy. Boca Raton, FL: CRC Press, 1990:317–332.
381. Hartmann O, Kalifa C, Benhamou E, et al. Treatment of advanced neuroblastoma with high-dose melphalan and autologous bone marrow transplantation. Cancer Chemother Pharmacol 1986;16:165–169.
382. Kamani N, August CS, Bunin N, et al. A study of thiotepa, etoposide and fractionated total body irradiation as a preparative regimen prior to bone marrow transplantation for poor prognosis patients with neuroblastoma. Bone Marrow Transplant 1996;17: 911–916.
383. Kletzel M, Abella EM, Sandler ES, et al. Thiotepa and cyclophosphamide with stem cell rescue for consolidation therapy for children with high-risk neuroblastoma: a phase I/II study of the Pediatric Blood and Marrow Transplant Consortium. J Pediatr Hematol Oncol 1998;20:49–54.
384. Ladenstein R, Lasset C, Hartmann O, et al. Comparison of auto versus allografting as consolidation of primary treatments in advanced neuroblastoma over one year of age at diagnosis. Report from the European Group for Bone Marrow Transplantation. Bone Marrow Transplantation 1994;14:37–46.
385. Matthay KK, Seeger RC, Reynolds CP, et al. Allogeneic versus autologous purged bone marrow transplantation for neuroblastoma: a report from the Childrens Cancer Group. J Clin Oncol 1994;12:2382–2389.

386. McCowage GB, Vowels MR, Shaw PJ, et al. Autologous bone marrow transplantation for advanced neuroblastoma using teniposide, doxorubicin, melphalan, cisplatin, and total-body irradiation. J Clin Oncol 1995;13:2789–2795.
387. Ohnuma N, Takahashi H, Kaneko M, et al. Treatment combined with bone marrow transplantation for advanced neuroblastoma: an analysis of patients who were pretreated intensively with the protocol of the Study Group of Japan. Med Pediatr Oncol 1995;24:181–187.
388. Philip T, Ladenstein R, Lasset C, et al. 1070 myeloablative megatherapy procedures followed by stem cell rescue for neuroblastoma: 17 years of European experience and conclusions. European Group for Blood and Marrow Transplant Registry Solid Tumour Working Party. Eur J Cancer 1997;33:2130–2135.
389. Philip T, Ladenstein R, Zucker JM, et al. Double megatherapy and autologous bone marrow transplantation for advanced neuroblastoma: the LMCE2 study. Br J Cancer 1993;67:119–127.
390. Shuster JJ. The role of autologous bone marrow transplantation in advanced neuroblastoma. J Clin Oncol 1996;14:2413–2414.
391. Stram DO, Matthay KK, O'Leary M, et al. Consolidation chemoradiotherapy and autologous bone marrow transplantation versus continued chemotherapy for metastatic neuroblastoma: a report of two concurrent Children's Cancer Group studies. J Clin Oncol 1996;14:2417–2426.
392. Pritchard J, Cotterill SJ, Germond SM, et al. High dose melphalan in the treatment of advanced neuroblastoma: results of a randomised trial (ENSG-1) by the European Neuroblastoma Study Group. Pediatr Blood Cancer 2005;44:348–357.
393. Matthay KK, Reynolds CP, Seeger RC, et al. Long-term results for children with high-risk neuroblastoma treated on a randomized trial of myeloablative therapy followed by 13-cis-retinoic acid: a children's oncology group study. J Clin Oncol 2009;27:1007–1013.
394. Berthold F, Boos J, Burdach S, et al. Myeloablative megatherapy with autologous stem-cell rescue versus oral maintenance chemotherapy as consolidation treatment in patients with high-risk neuroblastoma: a randomised controlled trial. Lancet Oncol 2005;6: 649–658.
395. Ladenstein R, Potschger U, Hartman O, et al. 28 years of high-dose therapy and SCT for neuroblastoma in Europe: lessons from more than 4000 procedures. Bone Marrow Transplant 2008;41(suppl 2):S118–S127.
396. George RE, Li S, Medeiros-Nancarrow C, et al. High-risk neuroblastoma treated with tandem autologous peripheral-blood stem cell-supported transplantation: long-term survival update. J Clin Oncol 2006;24:2891–2896.
397. Grupp SA, Stern JW, Bunin N, et al. Tandem high-dose therapy in rapid sequence for children with high-risk neuroblastoma. J Clin Oncol 2000;18:2567–2575.
398. Kletzel M, Katzenstein HM, Haut PR, et al. Treatment of high-risk neuroblastoma with triple-tandem high-dose therapy and stem-cell rescue: results of the Chicago Pilot II Study. J Clin Oncol 2002;20:2284–2292.
399. Reynolds CP, Seeger RC, Vo DD, et al. Model system for removing neuroblastoma cells from bone marrow using monoclonal antibodies and magnetic immunobeads. Cancer Res 1986;46:5882–5886.
400. Grupp SA, Cohn SL, Wall D, et al. Collection, storage, and infusion of stem cells in children with high-risk neuroblastoma: saving for a rainy day. Pediatr Blood Cancer 2006;46:719–722.
401. Kanold J, Paillard C, Tchirkov A, et al. Allogeneic or haploidentical HSCT for refractory or relapsed solid tumors in children: toward a neuroblastoma model. Bone Marrow Transplant 2008;42(suppl 2):S25–S30.
402. Keshelava N, Seeger RC, Groshen S, et al. Drug resistance patterns of human neuroblastoma cell lines derived from patients at different phases of therapy. Cancer Res 1998;58:5396–5405.
403. Sidell N. Retinoic acid-induced growth inhibition and morphologic differentiation of human neuroblastoma cells in vitro. J Natl Cancer Inst 1982;68:589–596.
404. Villablanca JG, Khan AA, Avramis VI, et al. Phase I trial of 13-cis-retinoic acid in children with neuroblastoma following bone marrow transplantation. J Clin Oncol 1995; 13:894–901.
405. Barker E, Mueller BM, Handgretinger R, et al. Effect of a chimeric anti-ganglioside GD2 antibody on cell-mediated lysis of human neuroblastoma cells. Cancer Res 1991;51:144–149.
406. Cheung NK, Landmeier B, Neely J, et al. Complete tumor ablation with iodine 131-radiolabeled disialoganglioside GD2-specific monoclonal antibody against human neuroblastoma xenografted in nude mice. J Natl Cancer Inst 1986;77:739–745.
407. Kushner BH, Cheung NK. GM-CSF enhances 3F8 monoclonal antibody-dependent cellular cytotoxicity against human melanoma and neuroblastoma. Blood 1989;73:1936–1941.
408. Lode HN, Xiang R, Duncan SR, et al. Tumor-targeted IL-2 amplifies T cell-mediated immune response induced by gene therapy with single-chain IL-12. Proc Natl Acad Sci U S A 1999;96:8591–8596.
409. Saarinen UM, Coccia PF, Gerson SL, et al. Eradication of neuroblastoma cells in vitro by monoclonal antibody and human complement: method for purging autologous bone marrow. Cancer Res 1985;45:5969–5975.
410. Cheung NK, Lazarus H, Miraldi FD, et al. Ganglioside GD2 specific monoclonal antibody 3F8: a phase I study in patients with neuroblastoma and malignant melanoma [see comments]. J Clin Oncol 1987;5:1430–1440.
411. Frost JD, Hank JA, Reaman GH, et al. A phase I/IB trial of murine monoclonal anti-GD2 antibody 14.G2a plus interleukin-2 in children with refractory neuroblastoma: a report of the Children's Cancer Group. Cancer 1997;80:317–333.
412. Handgretinger R, Baader P, Dopfer R, et al. A phase I study of neuroblastoma with the anti-ganglioside GD2 antibody 14.G2a. Cancer Immunol Immunother 1992;35:199–204.
413. Murray JL, Cunningham JE, Brewer H, et al. Phase I trial of murine monoclonal antibody 14G2a administered by prolonged intravenous infusion in patients with neuroectodermal tumors. J Clin Oncol 1994;12:184–193.
414. Uttenreuther-Fischer MM, Huang CS, Reisfeld RA, et al. Pharmacokinetics of anti-ganglioside GD2 mAb 14G2a in a phase I trial in pediatric cancer patients. Cancer Immunol Immunother 1995;41:29–36.
415. Uttenreuther-Fischer MM, Huang CS, Yu AL. Pharmacokinetics of human-mouse chimeric anti-GD2 mAb ch14.18 in a phase I trial in neuroblastoma patients. Cancer Immunol Immunother 1995;41:331–338.
416. Yu AL, Uttenreuther-Fischer MM, Huang CS, et al. Phase I trial of a human-mouse chimeric anti-disialoganglioside monoclonal antibody ch14.18 in patients with refractory neuroblastoma and osteosarcoma. J Clin Oncol 1998;16:2169–2180.
417. Cheung NK, Kushner BH, Yeh SD, et al. 3F8 monoclonal antibody treatment of patients with stage 4 neuroblastoma: a phase II study. Int J Oncol 1998;12:1299–1306.
418. Yu AL, Batova A, Alvarado C, et al. Usefulness of a chimeric anti-GD2 (ch 14.18) and GM-CSF for refractory neuroblastoma: a POG Phase II study. Proc Am Soc Clin Oncol 1997;16:513a.
419. Ozkaynak MF, Sondel PM, Krailo MD, et al. Phase I study of chimeric human/murine anti-ganglioside G(D2) monoclonal antibody (ch14.18) with granulocyte-macrophage colony-stimulating factor in children with neuroblastoma immediately after hematopoietic stem-cell transplantation: a Children's Cancer Group Study. J Clin Oncol 2000;18: 4077–4085.
420. Simon T, Hero B, Faldum A, et al. Consolidation treatment with chimeric anti-GD2-antibody ch14.18 in children older than 1 year with metastatic neuroblastoma. J Clin Oncol 2004;22:3549–3557.
421. Yu A, Gilman A, Ozkaynak F, et al. Anti-GD2 Antibody with GM-CSF, IL2 and Isotretinoin for Neuroblastoma New Engl J Med. 2010 (in press).
422. Altman AJ, Schwartz AD. Tumors of the sympathetic nervous system. Malignant diseases of infancy, childhood and adolescence. Philadelphia, PA: W.B. Saunders, Co., 1983:368–388.
423. De Bernardi B, Pianca C, Boni L, et al. Disseminated neuroblastoma (stage IV and IV-S) in the first year of life. Outcome related to age and stage. Italian Cooperative Group on Neuroblastoma. Cancer 1992;70:1625–1633.
424. Hsu LL, Evans AE, D'Angio GJ. Hepatomegaly in neuroblastoma stage 4s: criteria for treatment of the vulnerable neonate. Med Pediatr Oncol 1996;27:521–528.
425. Mancini AF, Rosito P, Vitelli A, et al. IV-S neuroblastoma: a cooperative study of 30 children. Med Pediatr Oncol 1984;12:155–161.
426. Martinez DA, King DR, Ginn-Pease ME, et al. Resection of the primary tumor is appropriate for children with stage IV-S neuroblastoma: an analysis of 37 patients. J Pediatr Surg 1992;27:1016–1020.
427. Suarez A, Hartmann O, Vassal G, et al. Treatment of stage IV-S neuroblastoma: a study of 34 cases treated between 1982 and 1987. Med Pediatr Oncol 1991;19:473–477.
428. Nakagawara A, Sasazuki T, Akiyama H, et al. N-myc oncogene and stage IV-S neuroblastoma. Preliminary observations on 10 cases. Cancer 1990;65:1960–1967.
429. Stephenson SR, Cook BA, Mease AD, et al. The prognostic significance of age and pattern of metastases in stage IV-S neuroblastoma. Cancer 1986;58:372.
430. Rubie H, Hartmann O, Giron A, et al. Nonmetastatic thoracic neuroblastomas: a review of 40 cases. Med Pediatr Oncol 1991;19:253–257.
431. Furman WL, Stewart CF, Poquette CA, et al. Direct translation of a protracted irinotecan schedule from a xenograft model to a phase I trial in children. J Clin Oncol 1999;17:1815–1824.
432. Langler A, Christaras A, Abshagen K, et al. Topotecan in the treatment of refractory neuroblastoma and other malignant tumors in childhood—a phase-II-study. Klin Padiatr 2002;214:153–156.
433. Saylors RL III, Stine KC, Sullivan J, et al. Cyclophosphamide plus topotecan in children with recurrent or refractory solid tumors: a Pediatric Oncology Group phase II study. J Clin Oncol 2001;19:3463–3469.
434. Vassal G, Doz F, Frappaz D, et al. A phase I study of irinotecan as a 3-week schedule in children with refractory or recurrent solid tumors. J Clin Oncol 2003;21:3844–3852.
435. Wagner LM, Crews KR, Iacono LC, et al. Phase I trial of temozolomide and protracted irinotecan in pediatric patients with refractory solid tumors. Clin Cancer Res 2004; 10:840–848.
436. Garaventa A, Luksch R, Biasotti S, et al. A phase II study of topotecan with vincristine and doxorubicin in children with recurrent/refractory neuroblastoma. Cancer 2003; 98:2488–2494.
437. Alimonti A, Satta F, Pavese I, et al. Prevention of irinotecan plus 5-fluorouracil/leucovorin-induced diarrhoea by oral administration of neomycin plus bacitracin in first-line treatment of advanced colorectal cancer. Ann Oncol 2003;14:805–806.
438. Davidson A, Gowing R, Lowis S, et al. Phase II study of 21 day schedule oral etoposide in children. New Agents Group of the United Kingdom Children's Cancer Study Group (UKCCSG). Eur J Cancer 1997;33:1816–1822.
439. Kushner BH, Kramer K, Cheung NK. Oral etoposide for refractory and relapsed neuroblastoma. J Clin Oncol 1999;17:3221–3225.
440. Anderson CP, Reynolds CP. Synergistic cytotoxicity of buthionine sulfoximine (BSO) and intensive melphalan (L-PAM) for neuroblastoma cell lines established at relapse after myeloablative therapy. Bone Marrow Transplant 2002;30:135–140.
441. Segreti JA, Polakowski JS, Koch KA, et al. Tumor selective antivascular effects of the novel antimitotic compound ABT-751: an in vivo rat regional hemodynamic study. Cancer Chemother Pharmacol 2004;54:273–281.
442. Cho SY, Adamson PC, Hagey AE, et al. Phase I trial and pharmacokinetic (PK) study of ABT-751, an orally bioavailable tubulin binding agent, in pediatric patients with refractory solid tumors [ASCO Annual Meeting Proceedings 2004]. J Clin Oncol 2004; 22:2080.
443. Garaventa A, Bellagamba O, Lo Piccolo MS, et al. 131I-metaiodobenzylguanidine (131I-MIBG) therapy for residual neuroblastoma: a mono-institutional experience with 43 patients. Br J Cancer 1999;81:1378–1384.
444. Goldberg SS, DeSantes K, Huberty JP, et al. Engraftment after myeloablative doses of 131I-metaiodobenzylguanidine followed by autologous bone marrow transplantation for treatment of refractory neuroblastoma. Med Pediatr Oncol 1998;30:339–346.
445. Kang TI, Brophy P, Hickeson M, et al. Targeted radiotherapy with submyeloablative doses of 131I-MIBG is effective for disease palliation in highly refractory neuroblastoma. J Pediatr Hematol Oncol 2003;25:769–773.
446. Mastrangelo R, Tornesello A, Mastrangelo S. Role of 131I-metaiodobenzylguanidine in the treatment of neuroblastoma. Med Pediatr Oncol 1998;31:22–26.
447. Matthay KK, DeSantes K, Hasegawa B, et al. Phase I dose escalation of 131I-metaiodobenzylguanidine with autologous bone marrow support in refractory neuroblastoma. J Clin Oncol 1998;16:229–236.
448. Sisson JC, Shapiro B, Hutchinson RJ, et al. Survival of patients with neuroblastoma treated with 125-I MIBG. Am J Clin Oncol 1996;19:144–148.
449. Tepmongkol S, Heyman S. 131I MIBG therapy in neuroblastoma: mechanisms, rationale, and current status. Med Pediatr Oncol 1999;32:427–431; discussion 432.
450. Albers AR, O'Dorisio MS. Clinical use of somatostatin analogues in paediatric oncology. Digestion 1996;57:38–41.
451. Borgstrom P, Hassan M, Wassberg E, et al. The somatostatin analogue octreotide inhibits neuroblastoma growth in vivo. Pediatr Res 1999;46:328–332.
452. Kogner P, Borgstrom P, Bjellerup P, et al. Somatostatin in neuroblastoma and ganglioneuroma. Eur J Cancer 1997;33:2804–2809.
453. O'Dorisio MS, Chen F, O'Dorisio TM, et al. Characterization of somatostatin receptors on human neuroblastoma tumors. Cell Growth Differ 1994;5:1–8.
454. Wiseman GA, Kvols LK. Therapy of neuroendocrine tumors with radiolabeled MIBG and somatostatin analogues. Semin Nucl Med 1995;25:272–278.

455. Cheung NK, Kushner BH, Cheung IY, et al. Anti-G(D2) antibody treatment of minimal residual stage 4 neuroblastoma diagnosed at more than 1 year of age. J Clin Oncol 1998;16:3053–3060.
456. Cheung NK, Kushner BH, Yeh SJ, et al. 3F8 monoclonal antibody treatment of patients with stage IV neuroblastoma: a phase II study. Prog Clin Biol Res 1994;385:319–328.
457. Handgretinger R, Anderson K, Lang P, et al. A phase I study of human/mouse chimeric antiganglioside GD2 antibody ch14.18 in patients with neuroblastoma. Eur J Cancer 1995;31A:261–267.
458. Matthay KK, Yanik G, Messina J, et al. Phase II study on the effect of disease sites, age, and prior therapy on response to iodine-131-metaiodobenzylguanidine therapy in refractory neuroblastoma. J Clin Oncol 2007;25:1054–1060.
459. Hoefnagel CA, De Kraker J, Valdes Olmos RA, et al. [131I]MIBG as a first line treatment in advanced neuroblastoma. Q J Nucl Med 1995;39:61–64.
460. Yanik GA, Levine JE, Matthay KK, et al. Pilot study of iodine-131-metaiodobenzylguanidine in combination with myeloablative chemotherapy and autologous stem-cell support for the treatment of neuroblastoma. J Clin Oncol 2002;20:2142–2149.
461. Lovat PE, Ranalli M, Annichiarrico-Petruzzelli M, et al. Effector mechanisms of fenretinide-induced apoptosis in neuroblastoma. Exp Cell Res 2000;260:50–60.
462. Maurer BJ, Melton L, Billups C, et al. Synergistic cytotoxicity in solid tumor cell lines between *N*-(4-hydroxyphenyl)retinamide and modulators of ceramide metabolism. J Natl Cancer Inst 2000;92:1897–1909.
463. Maurer BJ, Metelitsa LS, Seeger RC, et al. Increase of ceramide and induction of mixed apoptosis/necrosis by *N*-(4-hydroxyphenyl)-retinamide in neuroblastoma cell lines [see comments]. J Natl Cancer Inst 1999;91:1138–1146.
464. Garaventa A, Luksch R, Lo Piccolo MS, et al. Phase I trial and pharmacokinetics of fenretinide in children with neuroblastoma. Clin Cancer Res 2003;9:2032–2039.
465. Osenga KL, Hank JA, Albertini MR, et al. A phase I clinical trial of the hu14.18-IL2 (EMD 273063) as a treatment for children with refractory or recurrent neuroblastoma and melanoma: a study of the Children's Oncology Group. Clin Cancer Res 2006;12:1750–1759.
466. Rousseau RF, Haight AE, Hirschmann-Jax C, et al. Local and systemic effects of an allogeneic tumor cell vaccine combining transgenic human lymphotactin with interleukin-2 in patients with advanced or refractory neuroblastoma. Blood 2003;101:1718–1726.
467. Pertl U, Wodrich H, Ruehlmann JM, et al. Immunotherapy with a posttranscriptionally modified DNA vaccine induces complete protection against metastatic neuroblastoma. Blood 2003;101:649–654.
468. Cheung NKC, Sondel PM. Immunology and immunotherapy. In: Cheung NKC, Cohn SL, eds. Neuroblastoma. Berlin, Germany: Springer-Verlag, 2005:223–242.
469. Cheung NK, Modak S. Oral (1->3),(1->4)-beta-D-glucan synergizes with antiganglioside GD2 monoclonal antibody 3F8 in the therapy of neuroblastoma. Clin Cancer Res 2002;8:1217–1223.
470. Gonzalez S, Naranjo A, Serrano LM, et al. Genetic engineering of cytolytic T lymphocytes for adoptive T-cell therapy of neuroblastoma. J Gene Med 2004;6:704–711.
471. Pule MA, Savoldo B, Myers GD, et al. Virus-specific T cells engineered to coexpress tumor-specific receptors: persistence and antitumor activity in individuals with neuroblastoma. Nat Med 2008;14:1264–1270.
472. Canete A, Navarro S, Bermudez J, et al. Angiogenesis in neuroblastoma: relationship to survival and other prognostic factors in a cohort of neuroblastoma patients. J Clin Oncol 2000;18:27–34.
473. Meitar D, Crawford SE, Rademaker AW, et al. Tumor angiogenesis correlates with metastatic disease, N-myc amplification, and poor outcome in human neuroblastoma. J Clin Oncol 1996;14:405–414.
474. Eggert A, Ikegaki N, Kwiatkowski J, et al. High-level expression of angiogenic factors is associated with advanced tumor stage in human neuroblastomas. Clin Cancer Res 2000;6:1900–1908.
475. Fotsis T, Breit S, Lutz W, et al. Down-regulation of endothelial cell growth inhibitors by enhanced MYCN oncogene expression in human neuroblastoma cells. Eur J Biochem 1999;263:757–764.
476. Rossler J, Breit S, Havers W, et al. Vascular endothelial growth factor expression in human neuroblastoma: up-regulation by hypoxia. Int J Cancer 1999;81:113–117.
477. Chlenski A, Liu S, Crawford SE, et al. SPARC is a key Schwannian-derived inhibitor controlling neuroblastoma tumor angiogenesis. Cancer Res 2002;62:7357–7363.
478. Erdreich-Epstein A, Shimada H, Groshen S, et al. Integrins alpha(v)beta3 and alpha(v)beta5 are expressed by endothelium of high-risk neuroblastoma and their inhibition is associated with increased endogenous ceramide. Cancer Res 2000;60:712–721.
479. Katzenstein HM, Rademaker AW, Senger C, et al. Effectiveness of the angiogenesis inhibitor TNP-470 in reducing the growth of human neuroblastoma in nude mice inversely correlates with tumor burden. Clin Cancer Res 1999;5:4273–4278.
480. Klement G, Baruchel S, Rak J, et al. Continuous low-dose therapy with vinblastine and VEGF receptor-2 antibody induces sustained tumor regression without overt toxicity [In Process Citation]. J Clin Invest 2000;105:R15–R24.
481. Lode HN, Moehler T, Xiang R, et al. Synergy between an antiangiogenic integrin alpha-v antagonist and an antibody-cytokine fusion protein eradicates spontaneous tumor metastases. Proc Natl Acad Sci U S A 1999;96:1591–1596.
482. Nagabuchi E, VanderKolk WE, Une Y, et al. TNP-470 antiangiogenic therapy for advanced murine neuroblastoma. J Pediatr Surg 1997;32:287–293.
483. Shusterman S, Grupp SA, Maris JM. Inhibition of tumor growth in a human neuroblastoma xenograft model with TNP-470. Med Pediatr Oncol 2000;35:673–676.
484. Wassberg E, Pahlman S, Westlin JE, et al. The angiogenesis inhibitor TNP-470 reduces the growth rate of human neuroblastoma in nude rats. Pediatr Res 1997;41:327–333.
485. Evans AE, Kisselbach KD, Liu X, et al. Effect of CEP-751 (KT-6587) on neuroblastoma xenografts expressing TrkB. Med Pediatr Oncol 2001;36:181–184.
486. Evans AE, Kisselbach KD, Yamashiro DJ, et al. Antitumor activity of CEP-751 (KT-6587) on human neuroblastoma and medulloblastoma xenografts. Clin Cancer Res 1999;5:3594–3602.
487. Beppu K, Jaboine J, Merchant MS, et al. Effect of imatinib mesylate on neuroblastoma tumorigenesis and vascular endothelial growth factor expression. J Natl Cancer Inst 2004;96:46–55.
488. Vitali R, Cesi V, Nicotra MR, et al. c-Kit is preferentially expressed in MYCN-amplified neuroblastoma and its effect on cell proliferation is inhibited in vitro by STI-571. Int J Cancer 2003;106:147–152.
489. D'Assoro AB, Lingle WL, Salisbury JL. Centrosome amplification and the development of cancer. Oncogene 2002;21:6146–6153.
490. Fukasawa K. Oncogenes and tumour suppressors take on centrosomes. Nat Rev Cancer 2007;7:911–924.
491. Shinmura K, Bennett RA, Tarapore P, et al. Direct evidence for the role of centrosomally localized p53 in the regulation of centrosome duplication. Oncogene 2007;26:2939–2944.
492. Sugihara E, Kanai M, Saito S, et al. Suppression of centrosome amplification after DNA damage depends on p27 accumulation. Cancer Res 2006;66:4020–4029.
493. Li JJ, Weroha SJ, Lingle WL, et al. Estrogen mediates Aurora-A overexpression, centrosome amplification, chromosomal instability, and breast cancer in female ACI rats. Proc Natl Acad Sci U S A 2004;101:18123–18128.
494. Tanaka T, Kimura M, Matsunaga K, et al. Centrosomal kinase AIK1 is overexpressed in invasive ductal carcinoma of the breast. Cancer Res 1999;59:2041–2044.
495. Warner SL, Munoz RM, Stafford P, et al. Comparing Aurora A and Aurora B as molecular targets for growth inhibition of pancreatic cancer cells. Mol Cancer Ther 2006;5:2450–2458.
496. Rojanala S, Han H, Munoz RM, et al. The mitotic serine threonine kinase, Aurora-2, is a potential target for drug development in human pancreatic cancer. Mol Cancer Ther 2004;3:451–457.
497. Li D, Zhu J, Firozi PF, et al. Overexpression of oncogenic STK15/BTAK/Aurora A kinase in human pancreatic cancer. Clin Cancer Res 2003;9:991–997.
498. Shang X, Burlingame SM, Okcu MF, et al. Aurora A is a negative prognostic factor and a new therapeutic target in human neuroblastoma. Mol Cancer Ther 2009;8:2461–2469.
499. Otto T, Horn S, Brockmann M, et al. Stabilization of N-Myc is a critical function of Aurora A in human neuroblastoma. Cancer Cell 2009;15:67–78.
500. Teitz T, Wei T, Valentine MB, et al. Caspase 8 is deleted or silenced preferentially in childhood neuroblastomas with amplification of MYCN. Nat Med 2000;6:529–535.
501. Coffey DC, Kutko MC, Glick RD, et al. The histone deacetylase inhibitor, CBHA, inhibits growth of human neuroblastoma xenografts in vivo, alone and synergistically with all-trans retinoic acid. Cancer Res 2001;61:3591–3594.
502. Jaboin J, Wild J, Hamidi H, et al. MS-27-275, an inhibitor of histone deacetylase, has marked in vitro and in vivo antitumor activity against pediatric solid tumors. Cancer Res 2002;62:6108–6115.
503. Parsons SK, Neault MW, Lehmann LE, et al. Severe ototoxicity following carboplatin-containing conditioning regimen for autologous marrow transplantation for neuroblastoma. Bone Marrow Transplant 1998;22:669–674.
504. Ben-Arush MW, Doron Y, Braun J,et al. Brain tumor as a second malignant neoplasm following neuroblastoma stage IVS. Med Pediatr Oncol 1990;18:240–245.
505. Fairchild RS, Kyner JL, Hermreck A, et al. Neuroblastoma, pheochromocytoma and renal cell carcinoma. Occurrence in a single patient. J Am Med Assoc 1979;242:2210–2211.
506. Kato K, Ijiri R, Tanaka Y,et al. Metachronous renal cell carcinoma in a child cured of neuroblastoma [letter]. Med Pediatr Oncol 1999;33:432–433.
507. Kriss VM, Stelling CB. Osteosarcoma after chemotherapy for neuroblastoma. Skeletal Radiol 1995;24:633–635.
508. Kuefer MU, Moinuddin M, Heideman RL, et al. Papillary thyroid carcinoma: demographics, treatment, and outcome in eleven pediatric patients treated at a single institution. Med Pediatr Oncol 1997;28:433–440.
509. Rogers DA, Lobe TE, Rao BN, et al. Breast malignancy in children. J Pediatr Surg 1994;29:48–51.
510. Secker-Walker LM, Stewart EL, Todd A. Acute lymphoblastic leukaemia with t(4;11) follows neuroblastoma: a late effect of treatment? Med Pediatr Oncol 1985;13:48–50.
511. Shah NR, Miller DR, Steinherz PG, et al. Acute monoblastic leukemia as a second malignant neoplasm in metastatic neuroblastoma. Am J Pediatr Hematol Oncol 1983;7:309–314.
512. Weh HJ, Kabisch H, Landbeck G, et al. Translocation (9;11)(p21;q23) in a child with acute monoblastic leukemia following 2 1/2 years after successful chemotherapy for neuroblastoma. J Clin Oncol 1986;4:1518–1520.
513. Meadows AT, Baum E, Fossati-Bellani F, et al. Second malignant neoplasms in children: an update from the Late Effects Study Group. J Clin Oncol 1985;3:532–538.
514. Marks PA, Richon VM, Breslow R, et al. Histone deacetylase inhibitors as new cancer drugs. Curr Opin Oncol 2001;13:477–483.
515. Banerjee D. Genasense (Genta Inc). Curr Opin Investig Drugs 2001;2:574–580.
516. Siapati KE, Barker S, Kinnon C, et al. Improved antitumour immunity in murine neuroblastoma using a combination of IL-2 and IL-12. Br J Cancer 2003;88:1641–1648.
517. Berg SL, Blaney SM, Sullivan J, et al. Phase II trial of pyrazoloacridine in children with solid tumors: a Pediatric Oncology Group phase II study. J Pediatr Hematol Oncol 2000;22:506–509.
518. Keshelava N, Tsao-Wei D, Reynolds CP. Pyrazoloacridine is active in multidrug-resistant neuroblastoma cell lines with nonfunctional p53. Clin Cancer Res 2003;9:3492–3502.
519. Reynolds CP, Maurer BJ, Kolesnick RN. Ceramide synthesis and metabolism as a target for cancer therapy. Cancer Lett 2004;206:169–180.
520. Sohara Y, Shimada H, Scadeng M, et al. Lytic bone lesions in human neuroblastoma xenograft involve osteoclast recruitment and are inhibited by bisphosphonate. Cancer Res 2003;63:3026–3031.
521. DuBois SG, Messina J, Maris JM, et al. Hematologic toxicity of high-dose iodine-131-metaiodobenzylguanidine therapy for advanced neuroblastoma. J Clin Oncol 2004;22:2452–2460.
522. Kushner BH, Kramer K, Cheung NK. Phase II trial of the anti-GD2 monoclonal antibody 3F8 and granulocyte-macrophage colony-stimulating factor for neuroblastoma. J Clin Oncol 2001;19:4189–4194.
523. Neal ZC, Yang JC, Rakhmilevich AL, et al. Enhanced activity of hu14.18-IL2 immunocytokine against murine NXS2 neuroblastoma when combined with interleukin 2 therapy. Clin Cancer Res 2004;10:4839–4847.

CHAPTER 31 ■ RHABDOMYOSARCOMA

LEONARD H. WEXLER, WILLIAM H. MEYER, AND LEE J. HELMAN

A malignant tumor of mesenchymal cell origin is called a *sarcoma*. Mesenchymal cells normally mature into skeletal muscle, smooth muscle, fat, fibrous tissue, bone, and cartilage. *Rhabdomyosarcoma* (RMS) is thought to arise from immature mesenchymal cells that are committed to skeletal muscle lineage, but these tumors can also arise in tissues in which striated muscle is not normally found, such as in the urinary bladder. *Undifferentiated* sarcomas are mesenchymally derived tumors that cannot be ascribed to any specific lineage. Some tumors may also display multilineage markers; examples include ectomesenchymomas, which are tumors with evidence of both skeletal muscle and neuronal lineage,[1] and malignant Triton tumors, which are malignant peripheral nerve sheath tumors (schwannomas) with evidence of rhabdomyoblastic elements. These tumors are discussed in greater detail elsewhere.

The incidence of RMS is slightly less than half that of all other forms of non-RMS soft tissue sarcomas (NRSTSs) combined. Important epidemiologic, biologic, and treatment differences exist both within the family of RMS and between RMS and NRSTS. Although RMS was originally staged by a unique surgicopathologic staging system, the Clinical Group (CG) system, present cooperative group studies also use a modified (site-based) tumor-nodes-metastasis (TNM) staging system comparable to what has been used for adult NRSTS. The development of increasingly intensive, large-scale, international collaborative multimodality therapeutic protocols for treating these tumors, particularly the prior Intergroup Rhabdomyosarcoma Studies (IRS) and now those conducted by the Soft Tissue Sarcoma Committee of the Children's Oncology Group (COG), was instrumental in leading to dramatic improvements in the curability of these neoplasms, especially for patients with locally extensive but unresectable tumors. Over the past two decades, however, outcome has plateaued for the majority of patients with locoregional disease and improvements in outcome for patients with metastatic or recurrent tumors have proven elusive. As treatments have become more effective at prolonging survival for nearly all patients, and producing cures in the majority, there has been an increased awareness of, and focus on reducing, the short- and long-term sequelae of therapy.

EPIDEMIOLOGY AND GENETICS

The annual incidence of RMS in children 20 years of age or younger is 4.3 cases per million children, with approximately 350 new cases diagnosed in the United States each year.[2] Among the extracranial solid tumors of childhood, RMS is the third most common neoplasm after neuroblastoma and Wilms' tumor. Almost two-thirds of cases of RMS are diagnosed in children aged 6 years or younger, with a smaller incidence peak in early mid-adolescence. The tumor is slightly more common in males (11.8 per million) than in females (10.3 per million).[2] A recent analysis compared 2,600 cases of adult (20 years of age and older) and pediatric RMS captured over 22 years in the Surveillance, Epidemiology and End Results (SEER) Program.[3] Although the incidence of RMS in adult was substantially lower than that in younger children, particularly those during the first decade of life, approximately 40% of the total number of cases were in adults. Although a higher proportion of adults had one or more "unfavorable" prognostic features, and potentially important differences in treatment could not be ruled out as a contributing factor, pediatric patients had a consistently better outcome than adult patients. A separate analysis of SEER data between 1975 and 2005 for nearly 1,000 children and adolescents aged 19 years and younger revealed a stable incidence of embryonal RMS (ERMS) over this time period, but a significant increase in the incidence of alveolar RMS (ARMS), possibly the result of shifting diagnostic criteria.[4] This analysis confirmed a bimodal age peak for ERMS, though the second peak during adolescence was noted for males only; in this analysis, ARMS incidence did not vary by age or gender. Improved survival over this period was seen only for cases of ERMS.

An international study confirmed previous reports of racial and gender differences in the incidence of RMS.[5] In the United States, the incidence of RMS for African American females was found to be only half that for Caucasian females, whereas the rate for males was similar in both ethnic groups. The incidence of RMS appears to be lower in most of Asia than in the white populations of the Western industrialized countries, confirming an earlier finding of a lower relative frequency of RMS in children of South Asian ethnic origin residing in Britain.[6]

Although these tumors may arise virtually anywhere in the body, there are certain distinctive clusters of features regarding age at diagnosis, site of primary tumor, and histology. For example, head and neck tumors are most common in children younger than 8 years and, if arising in the orbit, are almost always of the embryonal variety. On the other hand, extremity tumors are more commonly seen in adolescents and are more frequently of the alveolar subtype. A unique form of RMS arising from the bladder or vagina, the botryoid variant (so named because of its resemblance to a protruding cluster of grapes), is seen almost exclusively in younger children.

Until recently, published studies of potential etiologic factors related to the development of RMS were composed of relatively small series. Although the overwhelming majority of cases of RMS occur sporadically, the development of RMS has been associated with certain familial syndromes, such as neurofibromatosis and the Li-Fraumeni syndrome (LFS), which includes familial clustering of RMS and other soft tissue tumors in children, with adrenocortical carcinoma and early-onset breast carcinoma in adult relatives.[7,8] The LFS has been associated with germline mutations of the *p53* tumor suppressor gene.[9] In a study of 33 cases of sporadic RMS, 3 out of 13 children younger than 3 years at diagnosis (compared with none of the 20 children older than 3 years) were found to have germline mutations in their *p53* gene.[10]

The overall risk of a genetic predisposition to cancer has been estimated to be 7% to 33%, on the basis of the patterns of cancer in the families of 151 children with soft tissue sarcomas.[11] These included syndromes that appeared to be independent of *p53* abnormalities. Of further interest, RMS has been observed in association with Beckwith-Wiedemann syndrome, a fetal overgrowth syndrome associated with abnormalities on 11p15, where the insulinlike growth factor 2 (*IGF-2*) gene is located[12] (also see Chapter 2). Some of the factors that may play a role in these phenomena are discussed later in this chapter.

In a study of fetal loss and infant deaths in families of children with soft tissue sarcomas (two-thirds of which were RMS), 50 out of the 157 families were classified as being genetically predisposed to cancer; one-third of these families had either classic LFS or a variant of LFS.[13] Studies of children with Costello syndrome, a rare congenital disorder characterized by postnatal growth retardation, typical coarse facies, loose skin, and developmental delay, have noted an increased risk for development of solid tumors, most commonly RMS. Costello syndrome is caused by heterozygous *de novo* point mutations in Harvey rat sarcoma (H-*ras*), resulting in increased activation of the mitogen-activated protein kinase pathway.[14,15] Out of about 100 known Costello syndrome patients, 10 RMSs have been reported.[16,17] A review of IRS cases reported five cases of RMS patients with neurofibromatosis type 1(NF-1) out of the 1,025 cases enrolled in IRS-IV.[18] Results of a large national case-control study were reported in 1993; this study involved 322 RMS patients younger than 20 years who were enrolled on IRS-III and an equal number of randomly selected age-, sex-, and race-matched controls.[19] Use of marijuana by the mother in the year before the child's birth was associated with a threefold increased risk of RMS in the child, and maternal cocaine use was associated with a fivefold increased risk. Use of marijuana, cocaine, or any recreational drug by the father was also associated with an approximately twofold increased risk. Consistent with a potential interaction between genetic susceptibility (e.g., germline *p53* mutations) and environmental factors in the development of some cases of RMS, use of cocaine by the mother and use of marijuana by both parents were associated with a significantly earlier age at diagnosis of RMS (compared with all children on IRS-III). A more recent case-control study conducted by the COG involving more than 300 RMS cases and an equal number of matched controls confirmed an association between prenatal x-ray exposure and the subsequent development of RMS, with the strongest association seen between first-trimester exposure and the subsequent development of ERMS (relative risk [RR] 10.5; 95% confidence interval [CI], 1.5 to 458.4).[20]

MOLECULAR BIOLOGY

It appears likely that multiple molecular genetic alterations involving both muscle differentiation pathways as well as cell proliferation pathways lead to the development of RMS. As the details of these pathways become better defined, lesions at any point within a given pathway will likely have similar consequences and thus an entire pathway will need to be evaluated rather than looking at an isolated genetic alteration. For example, if alterations in the pRB pathway were common in RMSs, one would need to consider *p16*, *pRB*, and *CDK4* all as targets within this pathway. Much has been learned in the past decade regarding the specific molecular genetic alterations that are associated with the development of this tumor. In this section, known genetic alterations that occur in RMS are reviewed, as well as the alterations in growth factors, oncogenes, and tumor suppressor genes that have been described in these tumors.

The two major histologic subtypes of RMS, namely ERMS and ARMS, have been found to have characteristic but distinct genetic alterations that are presumed to play a role in the pathogenesis of these tumors. ARMS has been demonstrated to have a characteristic translocation between the long arm of chromosome 2 and the long arm of chromosome 13, referred to in shorthand notation as t(2;13)(q35;q14).[21,22] This translocation has been molecularly cloned and shown to involve the juxtaposition of the *PAX3* gene on chromosome 2q35 (or, rarely, the *PAX7* gene located at chromosome 1p36 leading to a t(1;13)(p36;q14)), believed to regulate transcription during early neuromuscular development, and the *FKHR* gene, also known as *FOXO1 A*, a member of the forkhead family of transcription factors.[23,24] It is presumed that the consequence of this fusion transcription factor (*PAX3-FOXO1 A* [PF]) is the abnormal activation of transcription from a gene or genes that contribute to the transformed phenotype. Although the precise consequence of this tumor-specific translocation remains to be elucidated, several independent investigations now suggest a common final mechanism of transformation in ARMS. The PF fusion transcription factor appears to work in concert with loss of the *CDKN2* locus, which encodes for both *p16INK4a*, regulating the RB pathway, and *p16ARF*, regulating the p53 pathway. In addition, ARMS tumors commonly have overexpression/amplification of *MYCN* and this combination of alterations appears to be a common underlying feature of these tumors.[25,26] The PF fusion transcription factor has also been found to upregulate c-MET expression, a receptor tyrosine kinase that has been implicated in transformation.[27]

The other major histologic subtype, ERMS, is known to have loss of heterozygosity (LOH) at the 11p15 locus.[28,29] It has been shown that this LOH involves loss of maternal genetic information with duplication of paternal genetic material at this locus.[30] This region is of particular interest because it is the location of the *IGF-2* gene, which codes for a growth factor believed to play a role in the pathogenesis of RMS (see later discussion). *IGF-2* has been demonstrated to be imprinted with only the paternal allele being transcriptionally active.[31,32] It is therefore conceivable that in this tumor, LOH with paternal disomy may lead to overexpression of *IGF-2*. However, it is also possible that LOH at 11p15 may reflect the loss of a tumor suppressor activity that has not been identified, or that both activation of *IGF-2* and loss of tumor suppressor activity result from LOH at 11p15 in ERMS.[33] Recently, the fibroblast growth factor receptor 1 was noted to be highly expressed in ERMS tumors along with *c-myc*, in contradistinction to the *MYCN* overexpression found in ARMS.[34]

The most frequently observed oncogene abnormalities seen in RMS are *ras* mutations. Activated forms of both neuroblastoma *ras* (N-*ras*) and Kirsten-*ras* (K-*ras*) have been isolated from both RMS cell lines as well as from tumor specimens.[35,36] A survey of ERMS tumor specimens found a 35% incidence of either activated N-*ras* or K-*ras*.[37] As with the *p53* tumor suppressor gene, it is not known whether these alterations are primarily involved in the pathogenesis of these tumors or reflect secondary abnormalities that occur during progression events. The finding of *ras* activation has recently been confirmed by investigators who created a *ras*-induced zebrafish model of RMS (see the section on Animal Models) and noted a "*ras*-induced gene signature" that was evident in human ERMS as well.[38]

The discovery of the myogenic basic helix-loop-helix (bHLH) MyoD family of proteins (including MyoD, myogenin, Myf5, and MRF4) has greatly enhanced understanding of normal skeletal muscle differentiation.[39] These proteins function to commit mesenchymal cells to a skeletal muscle lineage and to activate their terminal differentiation program by inducing transcription of skeletal muscle-specific proteins such as myosin and creatine kinase. The almost universal expression of MyoD family proteins in RMS provides further strong evidence of the skeletal muscle lineage of these tumors and has allowed for further refinement in the classification of pediatric sarcomas. For example, some cases that would previously have been called undifferentiated sarcomas can be classified as RMS on the basis of the expression of these lineage-specific transcription factors.

The failure of RMS cells to terminally differentiate and growth arrest despite the expression of these bHLH proteins has raised the question of what is altered in this pathway compared with normal skeletal muscle cells. A recent report suggests the alteration could be with microRNAs (miRNAs) a recently discovered novel class of gene regulators that are transcribed by RNA pol II but do not encode for proteins. In this report, investigators found that miR-29 is normally repressed by an NF-κB pathway in proliferating myoblasts, but is derepressed during normal skeletal muscle differentiation. However, in RMS cell lines, miR-29 appears to be epigenetically silenced leading to a block in differentiation.[40]

ANIMAL MODELS

A mouse model of ARMS driven by the PF fusion gene has been established.[41] The model used a PF knock-in allele targeted to Myf6 expressing, differentiating myofibers in a background of either p53 or CDKN2A deficiency. This mouse model has been shown to recapitulate many features of human ARMS and is currently being used to help identify potential downstream targets that might be amenable to novel therapeutic intervention.[42] This is currently the only animal model of ARMS.

In contrast, several models of ERMS have been established, including the two mouse models and a zebrafish model mentioned previously. A heterozygous knockout mouse lacking the PTC gene was shown to develop RMSs at high frequency.[43] This is of interest because the PTC gene is known to function as the receptor for Sonic Hedgehog, a known mediator of early skeletal muscle development.[44] A combined transgenic-knockout mouse model where HGF is the transgene and INK4A locus is knocked out also has been found to lead to a high frequency of RMS.[45] This model is of interest since INK4A knock-down has also been required for mouse models of ARMS and because the receptor for HGF, c-Met is known to play a critical role in normal myogenesis and suggests a role for muscle satellite cells in rhabdomyogenesis.[46] Most recently, as noted previously, a ras-driven zebrafish model of ERMS has been established.[38] Using microarray analysis and cross-species comparisons, a ras-induced gene signature was found to be common in human ERMS, which is clearly of interest since activated N-ras or K-ras has been reported in up to 35% of human ERMS tumors (see above). It was also noted in this zebrafish model that the cancer stem cells shared similar characteristics to human satellite cells. Taken together, these mouse and zebrafish models of RMS suggest involvement of CDKN2 (Rb and p53 pathways), ras, altered skeletal muscle differentiation as common features involved in the development of these tumors. Furthermore, it is hoped that these models may provide a new approach for rational search for novel targeted therapy.

PATHOLOGY

RMS falls into the broader category of small round blue cell tumors of childhood. The role of the pathologist is to identify characteristic features, both by conventional light microscopic techniques and by newer immunohistochemical, electron microscopic, and molecular genetic techniques that allow a tumor to be classified as an RMS. The characteristic feature that permits such classification is the identification of skeletal myogenic lineage. Typically, this consists of the light microscopic identification of cross-striations characteristic of skeletal muscle, or characteristic rhabdomyoblasts. Immunohistochemical staining is a useful and reliable adjunctive means of identifying skeletal muscle and muscle-specific proteins or genes and remains the method of choice for evaluating small round blue cell tumors and confirming cases of suspected RMS.[47] These proteins include muscle-specific actin and myosin, desmin, myoglobin, Z-band protein, and MyoD.[48–50] Myogenin expression was demonstrated to be present in 22 out of 26 RMS specimens; however, it appeared that expression is significantly higher in ARMS than in ERMS.[51] These findings, confirmed by other groups looking at larger numbers of patients, emphasized both the utility and prognostic significance of both the pattern and intensity of myogenin immunostaining in cases of suspected RMS.[52–56] Electron microscopy can provide additional information if light microscopy and immunohistochemistry results are ambiguous. The finding of actin-myosin bundles or Z-band material on electron microscopic analysis provides strong support for the diagnosis of RMS.

There have been a series of modifications and refinements to the histologic classification of RMS since the establishment of the original RMS classification system of Horn and Enterline (embryonal, botryoid [a subtype of embryonal], alveolar, and pleomorphic).[57] The two major variants of RMS, ERMS and ARMS, have relatively characteristic histologic appearances and have specific and distinctive molecular genetic abnormalities, as described previously (Fig. 31.1). Histologic appearance, which is based on the identification of typical cytologic and architectural features, is usually sufficiently distinctive to permit straightforward categorization of the two subtypes. An international pathology study, carried out to assess agreement within and between groups of pathologists specializing in the classification of RMS, highlighted the proliferation of subtle differences in diagnostic criteria that had developed since the publication of the Horn and Enterline schema.[58–60] This prompted the development of the International Classification of Rhabdomyosarcoma schema.[61] Four broad subtypes of RMS were established: (a) botryoid and spindle cell RMS (both less common variants of ERMS), generally having a superior prognosis; (b) ERMS, generally having an intermediate prognosis; (c) ARMS (including the solid alveolar variant), generally having a poorer prognosis; and (d) undifferentiated sarcoma, also generally having a poorer prognosis. Finally, a category of sarcoma not otherwise specified was created for tumors that could not otherwise be classified into a specific subtype.

Under this new classification schema, embryonal tumors are diagnosed if the tumor has a stroma-rich, less dense, spindle cell appearance, and there is no evidence of an alveolar pattern. Variant forms of ERMS include the botryoid and leiomyomatous (spindle cell) subtypes. The botryoid tumors have a particularly favorable prognosis and tend to arise almost exclusively from the bladder or vagina in infants and young children or from the nasopharynx in slightly older children.[62] Microscopically, they present as a polypoid mass growing under an epithelial surface and have as their characteristic feature the presence of a dense tumor cell layer under the epithelium (the cambium layer). The spindle cell variants tend to arise disproportionately in the paratesticular region but may also be seen in the head and neck, extremities, and orbit.[63] These cells have a characteristic elongated, spindle

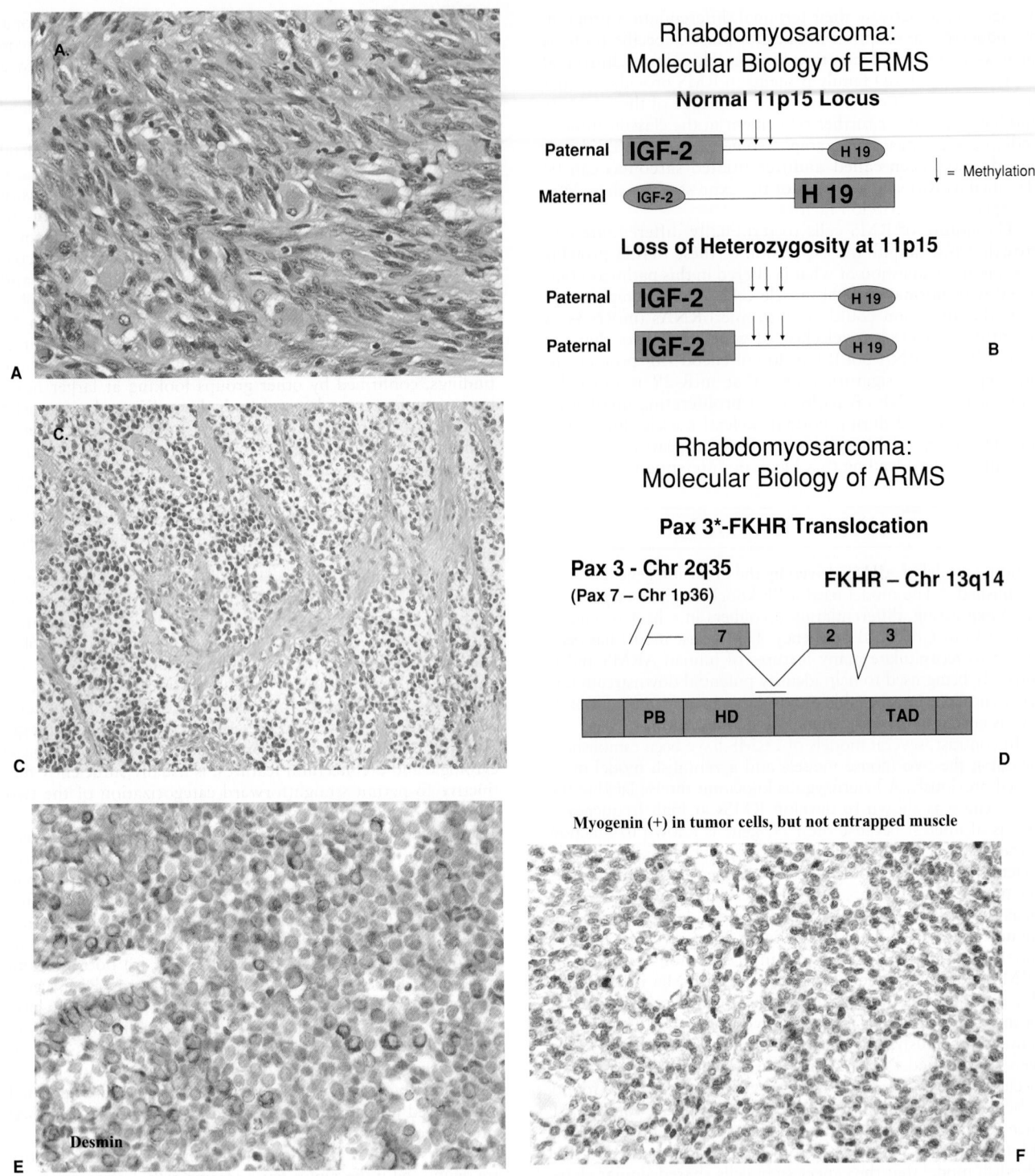

FIGURE 31.1 Light microscopic appearance and genetic alterations indicative of embryonal (**panels A, B**) and alveolar (**panels C, D**) rhabdomyosarcoma (RMS), and characteristic immunohistochemical staining for desmin (**panel E**) and myogenin (**panel F**). Embryonal RMS (ERMS) (**panel A**): Typical spindle-shaped cells with stromal-rich appearance and scattered large rhabdomyoblasts, characterized by loss of the maternal allele (loss of heterozygosity [LOH]) at 11p15 with duplication of the paternal allele (**panel B**). Note the paternal allele is characterized by expression of "proliferation-stimulating" insulin-like growth factor 2 (IGF-2), whereas the maternal allele is characterized by expression of the "antiproliferative" H19 gene. Thus, LOH with paternal duplication leads to an "overdose" of IGF-2 from bi-allelic expression. Alveolar RMS (**panel C**): Typical small round cells with dense appearance, lined up along spaces resembling pulmonary alveoli. These tumors are associated with a characteristic reciprocal chromosomal translocation between the long arms of chromosomes 2 (or, less commonly, chromosome 1) and 13. This translocation fuses the paired-box (PB) and homeodomain (HD) binding regions of the *PAX3* gene (or *PAX7* gene when chromosome 1 is involved) with the *FKHR* gene. *Horizontal line* indicates fusion region of messenger RNA. Immunohistochemical staining of RMS tumors typically demonstrates diffuse desmin positivity (**panel E**). Myogenin immunoreactivity (**panel F**) is more variable, tending to be relatively stronger and more diffuse in cases of ARMS and more focal in cases of ERMS.

appearance and grow either in a storiform pattern with abundant collagen between the tumor cells or in bundles with a low to moderate amount of collagen. They are almost always associated with limited disease; they appear to have a less aggressive pattern of behavior than the classic embryonal tumors and an extremely good prognosis. Approximately two-thirds of newly diagnosed cases of RMS are of the embryonal subtype.

Under this system, the presence of any alveolar pattern is sufficient to categorize the tumor as an alveolar subtype. Typically, these tumors are composed of densely packed, small, round cells lining septations that appear histologically reminiscent of pulmonary alveoli. A variant form, known as solid ARMS, has been identified in tumors that lack the characteristic architectural appearance (i.e., the alveolar septations) but have cells that are small, round, and densely packed.[59] The clinical behavior of the solid alveolar variant appears to be identical to that of the conventional alveolar subtype. More recently, the COG has required that the majority of a tumor have an alveolar appearance to be classified as ARMS. Depending on the diagnostic criteria utilized, 20% to 35% of newly diagnosed cases of RMS are of the alveolar subtype, with a higher proportion (nearly 50%) in cases of metastatic RMS. Undifferentiated sarcomas are generally lacking in any defining cytologic or architectural features and fail to express antigenic markers that would otherwise allow their more precise classification. This subtype appears to have a prognosis somewhere between that of ERMS and ARMS, although these tumors are no longer treated on front-line COG RMS therapeutic trials and are addressed in more detail elsewhere[64] (see also Chapter 32). Pleomorphic RMS is only rarely diagnosed today; the finding of anaplastic cells in large aggregates or diffuse sheets is of uncertain prognostic significance.[65] The COG prospectively evaluated the prevalence and clinical impact of anaplasia in nearly 550 cases of RMS treated between 1995 and 1998.[66] Cases were defined as focal or diffuse according to the method of Kodet in his analysis of 3,000 RMS cases registered in the first three IRS.[65] Thirteen percentage (71 out of 546) of samples had anaplasia, with slightly more cases having focal (40) anaplasia. Anaplasia was equally common among cases of ERMS and ARMS and seemed to be predictive of inferior outcome, on univariate but not multivariate analysis, for patients with intermediate-risk ERMS.

Sclerosing RMS, first described in three adult patients in 2000, and first described in a pediatric patient by Folpe et al. in 2002, is a more recently characterized and quite rare histologic subtype that appears to be associated with more aggressive clinical behavior and poor prognosis.[67–71] To date, fewer than 2 dozen pediatric cases have been described; a whole genome analysis of a left deltoid tumor from a 7-year-old boy revealed an aneuploid profile with amplification of the MDM2-HMGA2 locus at 12q13–15.[72] It remains unclear if sclerosing RMS is a variant of ERMS or ARMS, or an entity unto itself.[73,74]

When the diagnosis of RMS is uncertain or in need of further support, the application of molecular diagnostic approaches is helpful. The characteristic t(2;13)(q35;q14) abnormality can be determined by reverse transcriptase polymerase chain reaction (RT-PCR) techniques and, when present, defines the alveolar subtype. However, approximately 20% of centrally reviewed alveolar histology tumors lack this translocation or any of its variants with the use of standard RT-PCR techniques. Approximately 10% of cases of seemingly translocation-negative ARMS contain a "cryptic" fusion transcript that can be found with the use of high-sensitivity RT-PCR techniques, including cases with an FKHR "variant" partner gene (e.g., AFX, NCOA1).[75] This approach often requires the availability of fresh frozen tumor tissue for RNA

extraction but increasingly can be carried out on material obtained from paraffin blocks. A commercially available FKHR dual-color, break-apart rearrangement probe has demonstrated excellent performance on fluorescence in situ hybridization (FISH) testing of paraffin-embedded RMS specimens for detecting FKHR gene rearrangements; however, the identity of the potentially prognostically significant partner gene (i.e., PAX3 or PAX7) cannot be determined with this assay.[76] With ERMS, the availability of highly polymorphic markers at the 11p15 locus allows for the application of PCR technology for rapid identification of LOH of 11p15 in paraffin sections.[77]

There has been conflicting evidence concerning the prognostic significance of histology.[59,78] Although histology was found to be an important prognostic variable in IRS-II, histology was not prognostically significant in the subsequent more intensive, risk-based therapy of IRS-III (see later discussion).[79–83] Previous analyses of the prognostic significance of histologic subtype in noncontemporaneously treated patients may have suffered from differences in diagnostic criteria.[62,84–88] More recent data, however, strongly support the independent prognostic significance of histology. Investigators from the National Cancer Institute (NCI) and St. Jude Children's Research Hospital evaluated a group of 159 patients with RMS treated at the two institutions over a 15-year period.[59] Among patients with nonmetastatic tumors, histology was found to be an independent prognostic variable, with embryonal tumors having a better outcome than the identically behaving alveolar or solid alveolar tumor variants (6-year survival rate, 60% vs. 25%, $p = 0.001$). In a study of outcome among 264 patients with orbital RMS treated on IRS I-III, and IRS-IV pilot, the 5-year survival for the 221 patients with ERMS (and variant subtypes) was 94% versus 74% for the 24 children with ARMS ($p < 0.001$).[89] Finally, in the IRS-IV study (where, unlike in IRS-III, treatment was identical regardless of histology) alveolar histology truly did define a population of patients with more aggressive and poorer prognosis tumors.[90] One important caveat is the need to perform multivariate analyses to account for the clustering of histologic subtype with site and tumor size and invasiveness. For example, a report of outcome among 139 patients with extremity RMS (more than two-thirds of whom had ARMS) treated on IRS-IV identified group (extent of initial surgical resection) and stage (tumor size and/or regional lymph node positivity)—but not histologic subtype—as the variables most predictive of outcome.[91] Nonetheless, the current and most recent COG trials do require the "upstaging" of patients with what would otherwise be "favorable" or "low-risk" disease to "intermediate" risk therapy if a diagnosis of ARMS is confirmed on central pathology review.

The application of molecular pathology and gene expression profiling to classification of RMS subtypes may help in the future to resolve some of these controversies by the use of more objective criteria based on genetic differences between alveolar and embryonal tumors. It may also address questions regarding the pathogenesis of these tumors and prove useful at defining distinct prognostic subgroups within categories of histologic subtype. The COG conducted a genomic-based classification analysis of 148 centrally reviewed RMS tumors.[92] This study found that gene expression profiles and patterns of LOH of ARMS tumors lacking a PAX-FKHR translocation are indistinguishable from cases of ERMS. A distinctive expression signature was not found for either the spindle cell or botryoidal variants of ERMS. This important study highlights the potential power of molecular classification of RMS tumor into genetically distinct entities. Similar findings were reported in a study exploring the diagnostic and prognostic utility of a gene expression–based immunohistochemistry panel for testing

252 RMS tumors; using as few as two markers (AP2β and p-Cadherin for ARMS, and epidermal growth factor receptor and fibrillin-2 for ERMS, proved both highly sensitive and specific for subgroup determination, and appeared to be useful for stratifying patients into prognostically distinct groups.[93]

The significance of fusion subtype in ARMS is uncertain. For example, a relatively small study suggested that patients with the variant *PAX7-FKHR* translocation have a more favorable prognosis than do those with the more common *PAX3-FKHR* translocation.[94] However, in the cooperative group experience patients with metastatic disease and variant-translocation positive ARMS had an improved outcome (estimated 4-year overall survival 75% vs. 8% for patients with *PAX3-FKHR* positive ARMS, $p = 0.0015$), although this difference was not detected in those without metastatic disease.[95] It is possible that other, secondary genetic changes may be linked to the specific fusion type to drive partially transformed myoblasts into a fully tumorigenic state.[25,96]

Because of the increasing significance of central pathology review and the need to have tumor specimens available for molecular analysis, a standardized protocol has been developed for handling tissue specimens from those suspected of having RMS.[97] This protocol, developed in collaboration between the Soft Tissue Sarcoma Committee of the Children's Oncology Group, and the Members of the Cancer Committee, College of American Pathologists, includes a description of how to process tumor specimens from patients with suspected RMS, and a detailed checklist for describing both the surgical specimen as well as key microscopic features including histologic subtype, margin status, presence of anaplasia, and percent necrosis.

PATTERNS OF SPREAD AND CLINICAL PRESENTATION

With the completion of five generations of cooperative group clinical trials over the past three-plus decades, the biologic behavior of RMS is now well understood. In the early, prechemotherapy era, RMS had a uniformly high rate of eventual metastasis after local control measures alone,[98–100] with almost all patients with alveolar histology tumors eventually dying of disease.[101] In the current era of combined modality therapy, the development of effective adjuvant chemotherapy regimens has led to a clearer picture of the patterns of metastatic spread after treatment failure.[102–104] Between 15% and 25% of newly diagnosed patients have distant metastases, and almost half of those patients have only a single site of involvement (most commonly consisting of one or more pulmonary metastases). The lung is the most frequent site of metastasis (40% to 50%); less common sites, either isolated or in conjunction with multimetastatic disease, are bone marrow (20% to 30%), bone (10%), and, depending on the site of the primary tumor, lymph node (up to 20%).[105–109] Visceral organ metastases are rare in newly diagnosed patients. These findings, confirmed in a recent international study of 788 patients with newly diagnosed RMS, when combined with other risk factors including age, site, histologic subtype, and regional nodal spread, define groups of "high-risk" patients with a fourfold difference in prognosis.[110] These same sites are common locations for distant failure in patients who relapse after receiving systemic therapy; however, preterminally, visceral metastases (e.g., brain, liver) may be seen in up to 25% of patients.[79] RMS produces clinically evident signs and symptoms in two main ways: the appearance of a mass lesion in a body region without the history of temporally associated trauma and the disturbance of a normal body function by an otherwise unsuspected, critically located enlarging tumor (or enlarging regional or distant lymph nodes).[108,109] Typical signs, symptoms, and patterns of spread are discussed in terms of the primary tumor and are summarized here. In the first four IRS trials, approximately 35% to 40% of all tumors arose from a site in the head or neck region (orbit, parameningeal, other head and neck), slightly less than 25% from the genitourinary tract (bladder and prostate, vagina and uterus, paratesticular), approximately 20% from an extremity, and the remainder from truncal primaries and other miscellaneous sites (approximately 10% each)[81–83] (Fig. 31.2).

Head and Neck Region

Of the nearly 40% of RMS tumors that arise in head and neck structures, approximately one-quarter arise in the orbit or conjunctivae; 50% arise in parameningeal sites (often referred to as "skull base" and including the nasal cavity and paranasal sinuses, pterygopalatine/infratemporal fossa, nasopharynx, and middle ear); and 25% in nonorbital, nonparameningeal locations such as the scalp, face, buccal mucosa, oropharynx, larynx, and neck[111] (Fig. 31.3). The sex ratio is almost equal, and the median age at diagnosis is approximately 6 years. At times, it can be difficult to distinguish between orbit/eyelid tumors and parameningeal tumors since tumors arising in both locations can produce proptosis and occasionally ophthalmoplegia; nasal, aural, or sinus "congestion," and/or obstruction, with or without mucopurulent or sometimes sanguinous discharge are seen primarily with parameningeal tumors as are cranial nerve palsies, sometimes multiple, as a result of direct extension of tumor through the skull base toward the meninges.[112–115] Headache, vomiting, and systemic hypertension may result from intracranial growth of tumor after erosion of contiguous bone at the cranial base.[115,116] Autopsy studies show diffuse involvement of the cranial and spinal meninges reminiscent of central nervous system leukemia.[114] These tumors can also spread distantly, primarily to lungs or bones.[117] Although relatively more common for parameningeal primary tumors, regional nodal spread is uncommonly seen in orbital and nonparameningeal head and neck sarcomas where tumors typically present as painless, progressively enlarging growths and tend to remain localized.[118–122]

GENITOURINARY TRACT

Genitourinary tract sarcomas are most frequently seen in the bladder and prostate[123] (Fig. 31.4). Bladder tumors tend to grow intraluminally, in or near the trigone, and have a polypoid appearance on gross or endoscopic examination. Hematuria, urinary obstruction, and occasionally the extrusion of mucosanguineous tissue can occur, particularly if the tumor is botryoid. Affected children are usually younger than 4 years. Prostate tumors usually produce large pelvic masses with or without urethral strangury; constipation may occur. These tumors can occur in infants or older children; even adults may be affected.[124] Bladder tumors tend to remain localized, but prostate tumors often disseminate early to lungs and sometimes to bone marrow or bone.[125,126]

Male and female genital tracts can harbor sarcoma.[127] Vaginal tumors are commonly botryoid and are almost exclusively found in very young children who may have a mucosanguineous discharge reminiscent of that seen with a foreign body.[128] Cervical and uterine sarcomas are diagnosed more

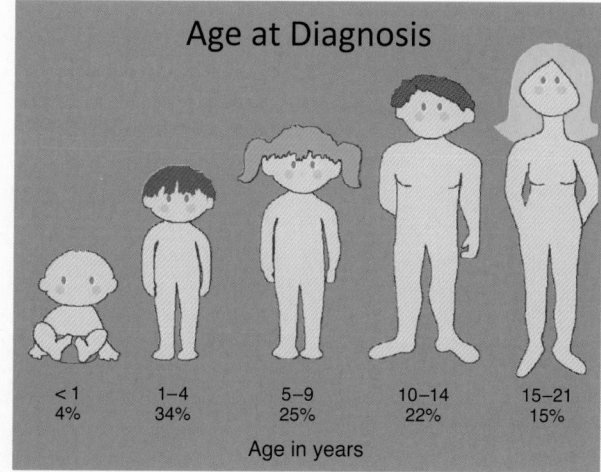

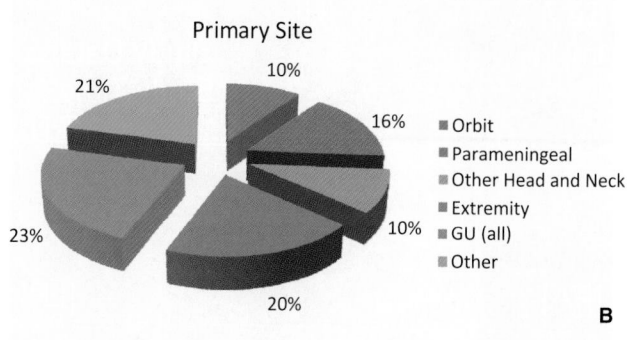

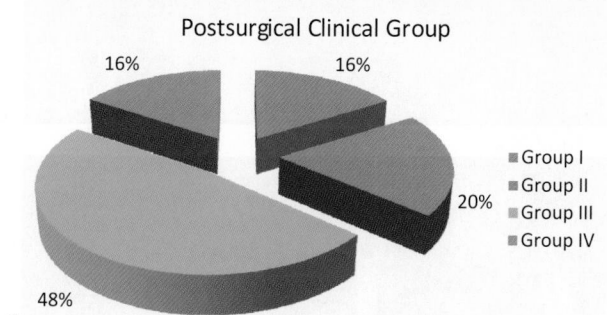

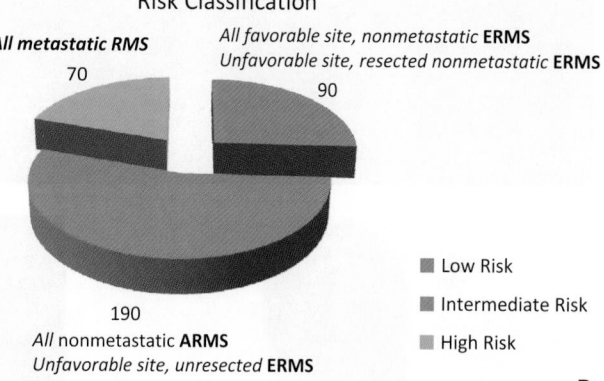

FIGURE 31.2 Clinical features of rhabdomyosarcoma. **A:** Age at diagnosis. The median age at diagnosis is 5 years, and two-thirds of patients are diagnosed before 6 years of age. **B:** Site of primary tumor. Slightly more than one-third of tumors arise in the head and neck [orbit (10%), parameningeal sites (16%), other head and neck structures (10%)]; next most common are genitourinary tumors (bladder, prostate, para-testis, female GU structures), followed by tumors of the extremities. **C:** Clinical Group. Approximately half of all patients have unresected tumors (Clinical group III) at presentation, while nearly one-third of patients have completely (Clinical group I) or gross totally resected tumors with microscopic residual disease (Clinical group II). **D:** Risk classification. Out of approximately 350 patients with RMS diagnosed each year in the United States, more than half (190) will have "intermediate-risk" disease (all nonmetastatic ARMS, and all nonmetastatic unfavorable-site, unresected ERMS [stage II/III, group III]), and approximately one-quarter (90) will have "low-risk" disease (nonmetastatic ERMS only, either arising in favorable sites (stage I, groups I-III) OR arising in unfavorable sites but resected (stage II or III, groups I or II).

commonly in older girls than in infants and present with a mass, with or without vaginal discharge. Regional nodal involvement (NI) is uncommon.[108,109] Paratesticular tumors usually produce painless, unilateral scrotal or inguinal enlargement in prepubertal or postpubertal males. The risk of tumor dissemination to regional retroperitoneal lymph nodes appears to be closely linked to age at diagnosis, being distinctly uncommon in boys younger than 10 years, and being present in 50% or more of older boys.[129,130] Alveolar histology is distinctly unusual in sarcomas of the genitourinary tract.[123] Several recent analyses have raised the question of whether select patients with group I alveolar histology in this location may have a favorable outcome with more limited therapy.[131,132]

Extremities

Sarcomas of the extremity are characterized by swelling in the affected body part (Fig. 31.5). The male to female ratio is approximately 1:1. Pain, tenderness, and redness may occur.

Between half and three quarters of these tumors are alveolar.[91,133] Regional lymph node spread may be found in up to half of patients undergoing surgical exploration and is more likely if the primary tumor is an ARMS than an ERMS or undifferentiated sarcoma.[91,133–135] The tumors can be extensive because of their propensity to spread along fascial planes. The fact that injuries are frequent and expected on the extremities of school-aged children may lead to a delay in diagnosis.

Trunk

Truncal sarcomas are similar in evolution to those of the extremities in that they exhibit all histologic types and have a tendency for local recurrence despite wide local excision and for distant spread. They are of relatively large diameter compared with tumors of the head and neck or of the bladder.[136,137] Contiguous involvement of the thoracolumbar spine may exist, depending on the location of the primary lesion, but regional lymph node spread is unusual.

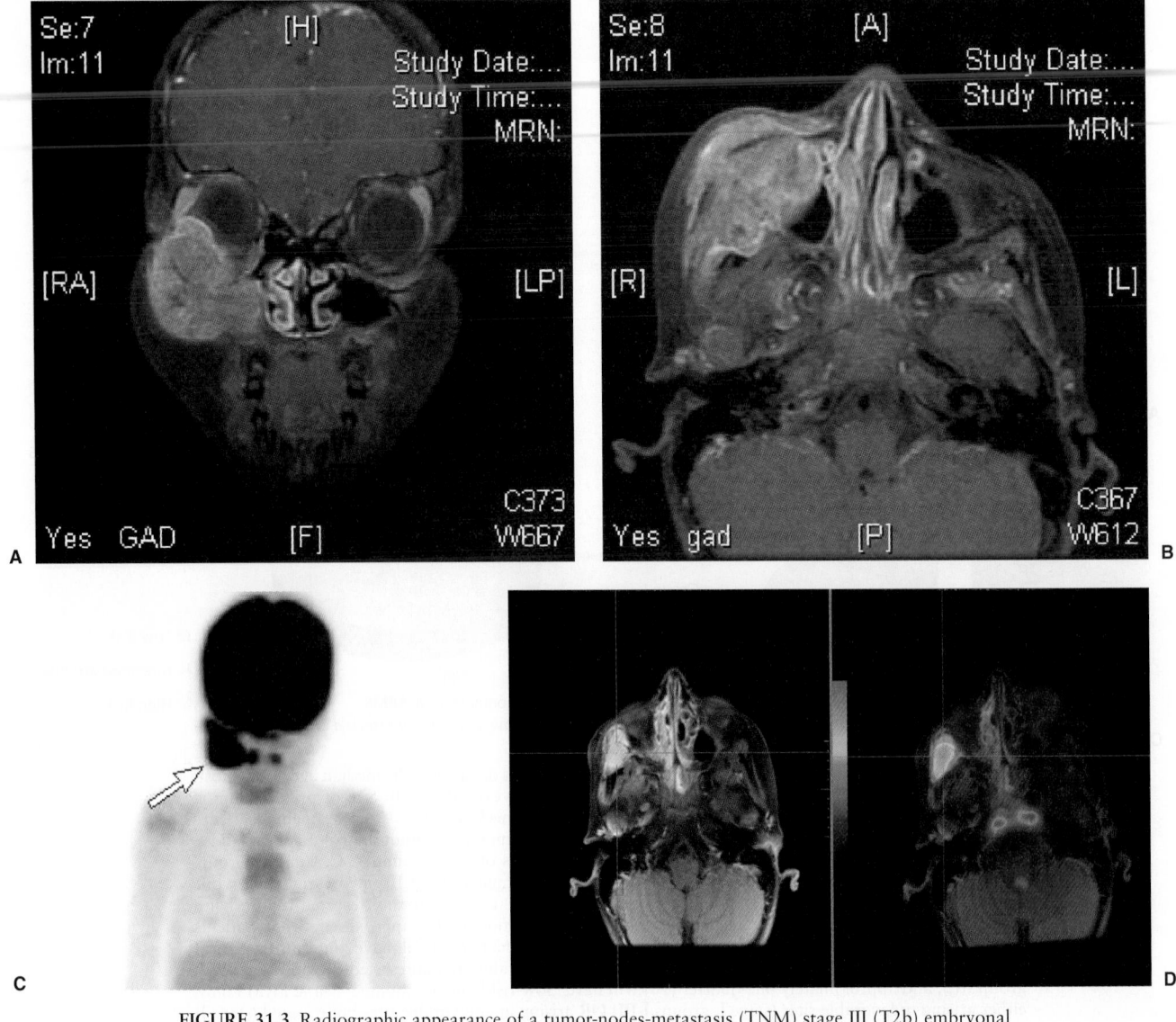

FIGURE 31.3 Radiographic appearance of a tumor-nodes-metastasis (TNM) stage III (T2b) embryonal RMS of the head and neck (parameningeal) region in a 7-year-old girl treated with 2 months of antibiotics for "sinusitis" prior to the development of a proptotic right eye. **A, B:** Coronal T1 fat saturated postcontrast (**A**) and axial T1 fat-saturated postcontrast magnetic resonance imaging (MRI) demonstrating a large tumor (>5 cm maximum diameter) originating in the right maxillary sinus invading into the inferior and lateral aspect of the right orbit. This tumor was intensely hypermetabolic (SUV 8.5) on baseline PET scan (**C**) but normalized following treatment with chemotherapy and radiation therapy, concurrent with disappearance of the soft tissue mass (not shown). **D:** Fifteen months following completion of treatment, routine surveillance PET scan showed marked interval increase in FDG accumulation (SUV 6.4) in the right zygoma (right panel) and follow-up MRI confirmed the interval progression of a previously stable and nonenhancing lesion centered in the right zygoma now with an associated extraosseous soft tissue mass and was biopsy confirmed recurrent RMS (left panel).

Other Sites

Intrathoracic and Retroperitoneal-Pelvic Regions

Intrathoracic and retroperitoneal-pelvic tumors can become large before the diagnosis is made because they are deep within the body.[138] They are often incompletely accessible to the surgeon, because vital vessels are usually surrounded, and wide infiltration is the rule; however, more recent data fail to support the notion that differences in outcome for patients with thoracic tumors are accounted for by a higher proportion of patients with unresectable disease.[139] Patients with tumors in these locations have a higher-than-expected risk of local recurrence despite combined-modality treatment. Aggressive attempts at initial or delayed surgical resection, combined with appropriate postoperative radiotherapy, may improve prognosis.[140]

Perineal-Perianal Region

Lesions in the perineal-perianal region are unusual.[141] They can mimic abscesses or polyps and are often alveolar.[142] A relatively high incidence of regional lymph node involvement was reported for the first series of these patients from the IRS.[143]

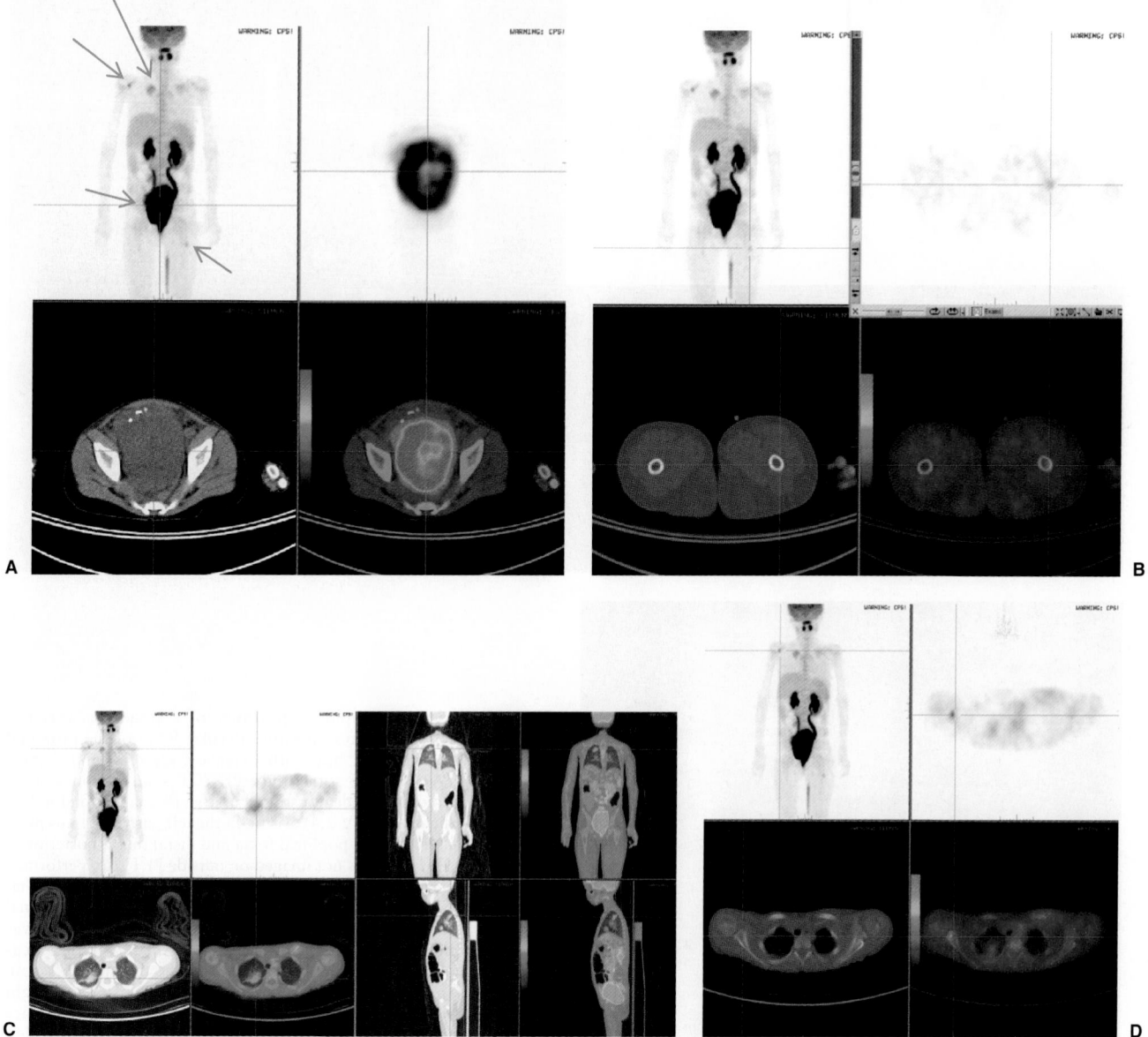

FIGURE 31.4 Radiographic appearance of a stage IV translocation-negative alveolar rhabdomyosarcoma of the bladder-prostate/pelvic region in a 6-year-old girl with a 2-week history of abdominal pain and constipation. **A:** Large, intensely hypermetabolic (SUV 12.7) pelvic mass with central necrosis displacing the bladder and compressing the ureters and bowel. Dedicated chest CT and technetium bone scan did not demonstrate lung or osseous metastases. Baseline PET scan demonstrated multiple osseous metastases including the left proximal femur (**B**), and right glenoid (**D**), as well as an area of low-grade uptake in the right upper lobe with an associated patchy opacity consistent with infection/inflammation (**C**). These osseous lesions were confirmed to be metastases on total body MRI (not shown).

Biliary Tract

Biliary tract tumors are even rarer than perineal-perianal tumors. They often produce obstructive jaundice, spread within the liver, and then spread to the retroperitoneum or lungs.[144–146] Aggressive surgical resection appears to be less important to good outcome for tumors in this location.[147]

Less Common Sites

Occasionally, the liver, brain, trachea, heart, breast, or ovary may harbor a primary sarcoma.[148–153] In some cases, no definite primary site can be determined.[154]

METHODS OF DIAGNOSIS

The differential diagnosis of RMS includes other oncologic entities and an assortment of nononcologic conditions. Trauma may produce an enlarging soft tissue mass, especially over the extremities, face, or trunk. Usually, a history of an accident is available, and an associated hematoma is tender and discolored. Sarcomas are usually nontender and impart no unusual hue to the overlying skin or subcutaneous tissue. Growth of a nontender mass, especially without a clear-cut history of trauma, should always alert the examiner to consider biopsy, especially if expansion is confirmed by repeated

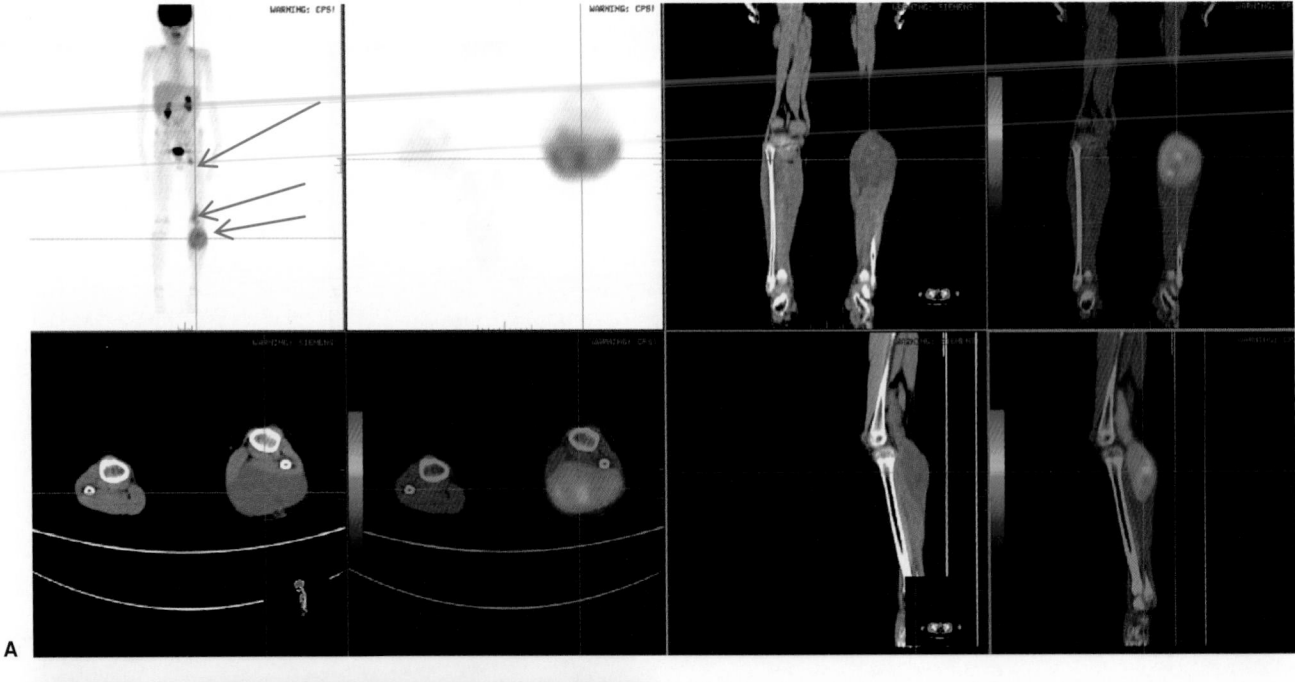

A

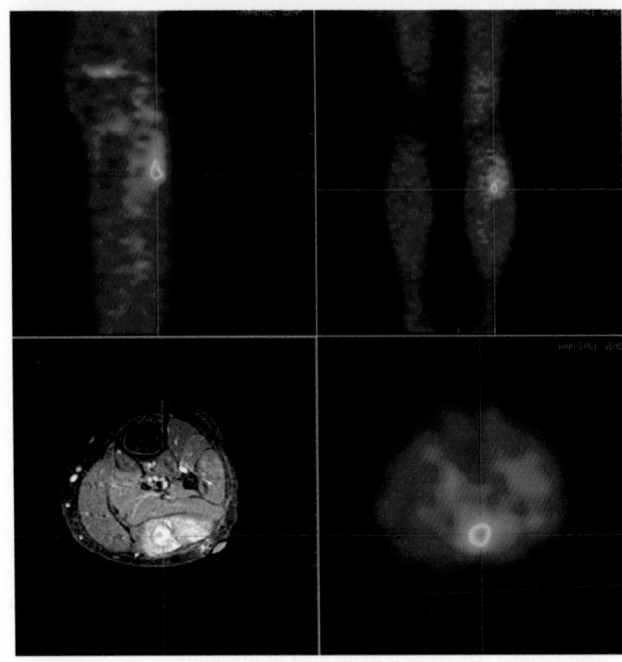

B

FIGURE 31.5 Radiographic appearance of a stage IV "variant" (PAX7-FKHR) translocation positive alveolar RMS of the proximal left calf in a 5-year-old boy with extensive regional and distant adenopathy. A: Baseline total body PET/CT scan obtained after 1 week of chemotherapy demonstrated a large (8.2 cm) round mildly hypermetabolic mass (SUV 2.4) arising in the left gastrocnemius muscle extending into the left popliteal fossa and distal thigh (posterior to the femur). (This area was not imaged on outside PET scan performed prior to the start of therapy [that only imaged to the mid-thigh] that demonstrated intensely hypermetabolic left inguina-femoral, external iliac, and para-aortic adenopathy.) A faint hypermetabolic focus was also seen in the left inguinal region (*indicated by arrow*). Other areas of hypermetabolic lymphadenopathy seen on the baseline PET scan done 1 week prior had resolved on this first follow-up study. B: Eight weeks following the completion of radiation therapy to the primary tumor in the left calf and all sites of initially involved lymph nodes, follow-up MRI (lower left corner) and PET scan demonstrated a small residual mass with a focal area of enhancement and a corresponding area of focally increased FDG accumulation. Resection of the residual mass demonstrated viable tumor mapping to this area of radiographic abnormality. Long-term control of disease at the primary site and elsewhere was achieved.

observations over 1 to 2 weeks. A mass within a body cavity can produce obstruction or discharge; both mandate a biopsy.

On rare occasions, cystitis may produce imaging and cystoscopic findings that mimic the appearance of RMS of the bladder; however, follow-up imaging almost always shows a return to normal over the course of 1 to 2 weeks, precluding the need for biopsy under those circumstances.[155] Occasionally, a histologically benign lesion such as a lipoma, rhabdomyoma, or neurofibroma may be diagnosed; if so, complete surgical removal should be performed if mutilation can be avoided. Rarely, an unusual condition such as myositis ossificans, pyogenic myositis, or inflammatory myofibrohistiocytic proliferation (also known as pseudosarcomatous myofibroblastic tumor or inflammatory pseudotumor of the bladder) may be discovered.[156–160] This last condition is a rare, benign lesion that may be difficult to differentiate from RMS by conventional diagnostic techniques.[161] It may present as an ulcerated, hemorrhagic, polypoid growth with intraluminal invasion that is found during routine radiologic evaluation of hematuria and dysuria (not uniformly associated with documented cystitis).

Biopsy should also be considered if a young person has a mass and is failing to thrive, even if the affected region is tender and the patient is febrile (if appropriate studies for infection have been nonproductive), because a treatable neoplasm may be the underlying disorder. Other childhood malignancies can mimic RMS or undifferentiated sarcoma. Non-Hodgkin lymphoma, neuroblastoma, and Ewing's sarcoma can simulate RMS at the light microscopic level, and special stains, electron microscopic ultrastructure studies, monoclonal antibody assays, and collection of urine for catecholamine excretion studies may be necessary to differentiate these entities. Occasionally, a leukemic chloroma or collection of histiocytes (e.g., Langerhans' cell histiocytosis) can produce unilateral proptosis or a mass in another body region, which should be biopsied to establish the correct diagnosis.[162,163]

After the diagnosis of RMS has been entertained and even without confirmatory pathologic material, several clinical and radiographic studies may be done to define the limits of the lesion and to look for evidence of spread. A complete physical examination should be performed, with particular attention to regional lymphatic structures and to the surrounding tissues. Laboratory studies that should be simultaneously obtained include a complete blood cell count with differential, serum electrolytes, blood urea nitrogen and creatinine, liver function tests, serum calcium and phosphorus and magnesium, and a uric acid level, in anticipation of chemotherapy. Patients with bone marrow metastases from a primary sarcoma may have altered peripheral blood values; however, counts may be normal even with bone marrow metastases. Traditionally, bilateral bone marrow aspirations and core needle biopsies have been recommended as part of the routine pretreatment assessment even in the absence of altered blood counts or other sites of obvious metastases. In IRS-I, however, only 3 out of 500 patients presented with isolated bone marrow metastases.[107] Similarly, of the slightly more than 1,000 patients treated on IRS-IV, only 12 out of 901 patients with no other sites of metastatic disease were found to have isolated bone marrow metastases.[164] Thus, in the absence of other metastatic lesions, the likelihood of finding isolated bone marrow metastases is less than 2%. Although disseminated intravascular coagulation (DIC) is uncommon, even among patients with bone marrow involvement, baseline coagulation studies (prothrombin time, activated partial thromboplastin time, fibrinogen) should be performed in all patients and appropriate supportive care measures initiated if evidence of the condition is found.[123] Metastatic bone involvement can rarely be complicated by DIC and/or hypercalcemia.[165,166]

Radiographic studies should include plain films of the affected part, if appropriate. Nuclear medicine scans using technetium-99 m diphosphonate are required to evaluate for osseous metastases.[167] 99mTc bone scans are highly sensitive and relatively specific for detecting osseous metastases and are probably more reliable than a routine skeletal survey.[168] Gallium-67 can be concentrated in the bowel and in areas of inflammation, and it is not usually a routine part of the diagnostic workup.[169] The role of positron emission tomography (PET) scans in determining initial extent of disease and response to treatment, or for radiation treatment-planning purposes, has been the subject of a number of recent reports and continues to be defined (see Fig. 31.3).[170–174] In a report from Memorial Sloan-Kettering Cancer Center, however, radiation treatment planning was modified to include regional nodes in 3 out of 21 patients with pretreatment PET scans with nodal disease detected only on whole-body PET or computed tomography (CT) scan.[171]

CT scans, with or without contrast enhancement, have long been the standard imaging modality. Preoperative scanning is critical to enable the radiation therapist to assess the volume at risk for subclinical tumor invasion and to plan treatment fields.[175] Imaging of the abdomen and pelvis may also be useful for detecting clinically occult abnormalities of the genitourinary tract. Ultrasound examinations may be especially useful as an adjunct to CT in serial assessment of tumors of the pelvis (including the bladder, prostate, and retroperitoneum), because the characteristic water-density of the urine-filled bladder helps in localization.[176] Ultrasonography does not use radiation, and dye injection is unnecessary. Magnetic resonance imaging (MRI) is the imaging modality of choice in several anatomic regions, especially for head and neck, extremity, and pelvic tumors, because of its multiplanar capability, its ability to attenuate bone artifact, and the superior soft tissue contrast that it provides.[177–180] However, there is no value for routine brain imaging for tumors arising outside of the head and neck region.[181]

STAGING

Assessing the extent of the tumor in every patient is critical because therapy and prognosis depend on the degree to which the mass has spread beyond the primary site. Patients with localized, surgically removable tumors have a better prognosis than do those whose disease has produced clinically detectable metastatic deposits. Two major staging systems are currently employed in combination: the Children's Cancer Group (CCG) surgicopathologic staging system (CG), developed by the Intergroup Rhabdomyosarcoma Study Group (IRSG) in 1972 (Table 31.1), and the pretreatment, site-modified TNM staging system (stage), developed by the IRSG (Table 31.2).[87,182] CG

TABLE 31.1

CLINICAL GROUP STAGE SYSTEM EMPLOYED IN INTERGROUP RHABDOMYOSARCOMA STUDIES I THROUGH III

Clinical group	Extent of disease and surgical result
IA	Localized tumor, confined to site of origin, completely resected
B	Localized tumor, infiltrating beyond the site of origin, completely resected
IIA	Localized tumor, gross total resection, but with microscopic residual disease
B	Locally "extensive" tumor (spread to regional lymph nodes), completely resected
C	Extensive tumor (spread to regional lymph nodes), gross total resection, but with microscopic residual disease
IIIA	Localized or locally extensive tumor, gross residual disease after biopsy only
B	Localized or locally extensive tumor, gross residual disease after "major" resection (≥50% debulking)
IV	Any size primary tumor, with or without regional lymph node involvement, with distant metastases, irrespective of surgical approach to primary tumor

TABLE 31.2

TNM STAGING OF RHABDOMYOSARCOMA: TNM PRETREATMENT STAGING
CLASSIFICATION FOR IRS-IV

Stage	Sites	T-invasiveness	T-size	N	M
I	Orbit	T1 or T2	a or b	N0 N1 or Nx	M0
	Head and neck[a]	T1 or T2	a or b	N0 N1 or Nx	
	Genitourinary[b]	T1 or T2	a or b	N0 N1 or Nx	
II	Bladder/prostate	T1 or T2	a	N0 or Nx	
	Extremity	T1 or T2	a	N0 or Nx	
	Cranial parameningeal	T1 or T2	a	N0 or Nx	
	Other[c]	T1 or T2	a	N0 or Nx	
III	Bladder/prostate	T1 or T2	a	N1	
	Extremity	T1 or T2	b	N0 N1 or Nx	
	Cranial parameningeal	T1 or T2	b	N0 N1 or Nx	
	Other[c]	T1 or T2	b	N0 N1 or Nx	
IV	All	T1 or T2	a or b	N0 or Nx	M1

TNM, tumor-nodes-metastasis; T (tumor): T1, confined to anatomic site of origin; T2, extension; a,
≤5 cm in diameter; b, >5 cm in diameter. N (regional nodes): N0, not clinically involved; N1, clinically
involved; Nx, clinical status unknown. M (metastases): M0, no distant metastases; M1, distant metastasis
present.
[a]Excluding parameningeal.
[b]Nonbladder-nonprostate.
[c]Includes trunk, retroperitoneum, etc.

defines patients by the extent of their initial surgery, with sub-classification of patients with microscopic residual disease (group II) with (II B, C) or without (II A) regional NI. The TNM system, which was retrospectively evaluated by numerous investigators and shown to be highly predictive of outcome, divides patients into favorable and unfavorable sites, and requires "upstaging" of patients with unfavorable site tumors that are large (0.5 cm) and/or have clinical evidence of regional NI.[86–88,182] Favorable sites include the orbit and eyelid, and other nonparameningeal head and neck structures, as well as nonbladder, nonprostate genitourinary locations (paratesticular, vulva-vagina-uterus). All other primary sites are considered unfavorable sites and include the extremities (including the buttocks and perineum), urinary bladder and prostate, cranial parameningeal sites, and the trunk and retroperitoneum.

The likelihood of infiltration of regional lymph nodes or adjacent structures varies with the site of the primary tumor, ranging from as low as 5% for head and neck tumors to as high as 50% for extremity and paratesticular tumors (in older boys).[91,108,109] Imaging studies and physical examination findings are usually adequate for establishing the presence of regional NI. If staging or local or systemic treatment options will be affected, consideration should be given to surgical removal of palpably or radiographically enlarged regional lymph nodes. Routine surgical sampling of radiographically "benign" regional nodes is unwarranted with two important exceptions: all cases of extremity RMS should undergo aggressive sampling of regional nodal basins, and older boys (10 years of age and older) with paratesticular tumors should undergo ipsilateral lymph node dissection. Radiation therapy (RT) is delivered to the region if tumor involvement of nodes is found on pathologic examination. Radiographic studies and bone marrow examination are used to ascertain whether distant metastases are present; histologic verification of radiographic abnormalities is not required, however, where treatment issues will be determined by the presence or absence of metastatic disease, surgical evaluation of an equivocal radiographic abnormality may be warranted. Histologic subtype does not affect either the stage or CG, although it may impact systemic and/or local treatment choices (e.g., the use of local irradiation in completely resected (group I), low stage (I and II) ARMS.[183] The classification system and assignment to treatment protocol can seem complicated (see Table 31.3); a Web-based decision support tool can aid in the process of appropriate treatment assignment.[184]

PROGNOSTIC CONSIDERATIONS

The identification of prognostic variables is of major importance in understanding the behavior of sarcomas and developing careful clinical trials, the goals of which are to improve survival for all patients with RMS and undifferentiated sarcoma and to reduce morbidity. Several key prognostic variables have been identified and are currently being used in cooperative group studies to define risk-adapted therapy (Table 31.3). These variables, which define distinct groups of patients with excellent, very good, intermediate, and poor prognoses, include the presence or absence of distant metastases; site (favorable vs. unfavorable, with the most favorable site being the orbit); surgical resectability [groups I and II vs. group III (excluding the orbit)]; histology (ERMS and variants vs. ARMS); and age (see discussion under Treatment Results).[185] Recent data clearly show that age is an independent prognostic factor, with those younger than 1 year or older than 10 years having a less favorable outcome.[110,186] As previously discussed, recent data suggest that the specific type of molecular abnormality present in ARMS may be prognostically significant, particularly for patients with metastases.

Patients with no detectable metastases at diagnosis fare much better than those with widespread disease (Fig. 31.6).[81–83,187] Among patients with localized sarcoma, those with completely excised tumors (CG I) have a better survival rate than those with microscopic residual tumor or with excised but regionally extensive lesions (CG II). Among patients with

TABLE 31.3

PROGNOSTIC STRATIFICATION FOR RHABDOMYOSARCOMA

Prognosis (event-free survival)	Stage	Group	Site[a]	Size	Age (yr)	Histology	Metastasis	Regional lymph nodes
Excellent (≥85%) (Low risk)	1	I	Favorable	a or b	<21	ERMS	M0	N0
	1	II	Favorable	a or b	<21	ERMS	M0	N0
	1	III	Orbit only	a or b	<21	ERMS	M0	N0
	2	I	Unfavorable	a	<21	ERMS	M0	N0 or Nx
Very good (70%–85%) (Low risk)	1	II	Favorable	a or b	<21	ERMS	M0	N1
	1	III	Orbit only	a or b	<21	ERMS	M0	N1
	1	III	Favorable (excluding orbit)	a or b	<21	ERMS	M0	N0 or N1 or Nx
	2	II	Unfavorable	a	<21	ERMS	M0	N0 or Nx
	3	I or II	Unfavorable	a	<21	ERMS	M0	N1
	3	I or II	Unfavorable	b	<21	ERMS	M0	N0 or N1 or Nx
Good (50%–70%) (Intermediate risk)	2	III	Unfavorable	a	<21	ERMS	M0	N0 or Nx
	3	III	Unfavorable	a	<21	ERMS	M0	N1
	3	III	Unfavorable	a	<21	ERMS	M0	N0 or N1 or Nx
	1 or 2 or 3	I or II or III	Favorable or unfavorable	a or b	<21	ARMS	M0	N0 or N1 or Nx
Poor (≤30%) (High risk)	4	IV	Favorable or unfavorable	a or b	Any	ERMS	M1	N0 or N1
	4	IV	Favorable or unfavorable	a or b	Any	ARMS[b]	M1	N0 or N1

a, tumor size ≤5 cm in diameter; ARMS, alveolar rhabdomyosarcoma; ERMS, embryonal rhabdomyosarcoma (or botryoid or leiomyomatous variant); b, tumor size >5 cm in diameter; M0, no distant metastasis(es); M1, distant metastasis(es); N0, regional nodes not clinically involved; N1, regional nodes clinically involved; Nx, node status unknown.
[a]Favorable sites are orbit and eyelid, nonparameningeal head and neck, biliary tract and nonbladder and nonprostate genitourinary tract. Unfavorable sites are bladder, prostate, extremity, parameningeal, and other (trunk, retroperitoneum, etc.).
[b]Preliminary data suggest that variant-translocation (PAX7-FKHR) positive metastatic ARMS may have a more favorable prognosis, with estimated 4-year survival of 75% (see text).

microscopic residual disease, those without regional NI (IIA) or with completely resected regional nodes (IIB) fare better than those with both (IIC) [5-year failure-free survival (FFS) 75% vs. 74% vs. 58% for patients with IIA, IIB, and IIC, respectively, $p = 0.0037$], with improvement noted during more recent IRS trials.[188] For the first time, an improved outcome was seen for patients treated on IRS-IV with CG II tumors compared to those with CGI tumors, presumably due to the uniform administration of radiation in the former group (Fig. 31.6). Patients with gross residual disease (CG III) fare less well; however, for patients with ERMS, outcome within this group varies by whether the tumor originates in a favorable (92% 3-year FFS) or an unfavorable (75% 3-year FFS) site.[189] Although not specifically limited to patients with RMS, an analysis of 553 consecutively treated patients with previously untreated, localized soft tissue sarcomas, demonstrated that tumor size, particularly when "normalized" for body surface area, may be more prognostically significant than tumor size alone.[190] An analysis of 1,164 patients with localized RMS treated on sequential CWS studies (CWS-81, CWS-86, CWS-91, and CWS-96) confirmed that the combination of age 10 years and older (RR 1.6), ARMS histologic subtype (RR 2.2), tumor size of more than 5 cm (RR 1.3) and unfavorable site (RR 1.3), gross-residual disease (CG III, RR 2.1), and omission of radiotherapy (RR 1.6) were factors associated with inferior outcome.[191] Although young patients (younger than 10 years) with metastatic ERMS[192] and those with variant-translocation (PAX7-FKHR)-positive metastatic ARMS[95] may have an

intermediate prognosis (40% to 50%), the prognosis for most patients with metastatic RMS remains grim. Patients with two or fewer metastatic sites and embryonal histology tumors did somewhat better than those with more extensive metastatic disease in IRS-IV and similar results were seen in a pooled analysis of data from the Unites States and European Cooperative Groups.[110,164] The relatively more favorable prognosis of age between 1 and 9 years and a limited number of metastatic sites of disease, but not embryonal histology, were confirmed to be associated with relatively more favorable outcome in the two most recent European Intergroup Studies (MMT4-89 and MMT4-91).[193] Those patients whose tumors progress during initial therapy have a poor outcome. Although early response to treatment appears to correlate with a better outcome[190] and is used to define further therapy in European studies, a recent analysis of early response in IRS-IV patients found no difference in outcome by response.[194]

The impact of p53 mutations, MDM2 alterations, CDK4 amplification, INK4 mutation, or pRB mutation on prognosis remains to be determined. Prospective molecular characterization gene expression profiling of tumors will serve to delineate further the impact of these changes on overall prognosis.

TREATMENT

The three currently recognized modalities of treating children with sarcomas are surgical removal (if feasible), RT for control

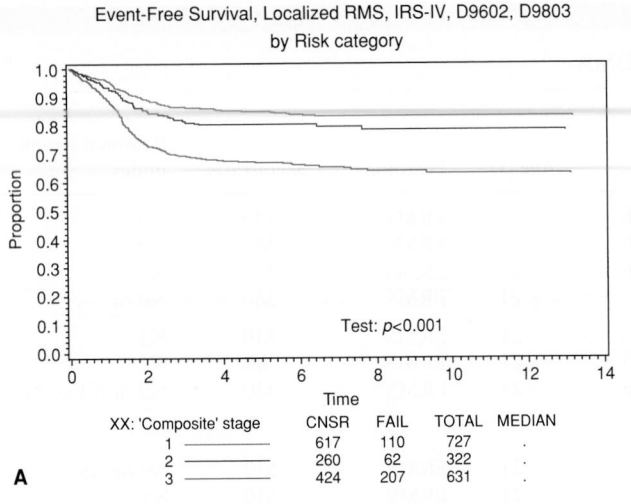

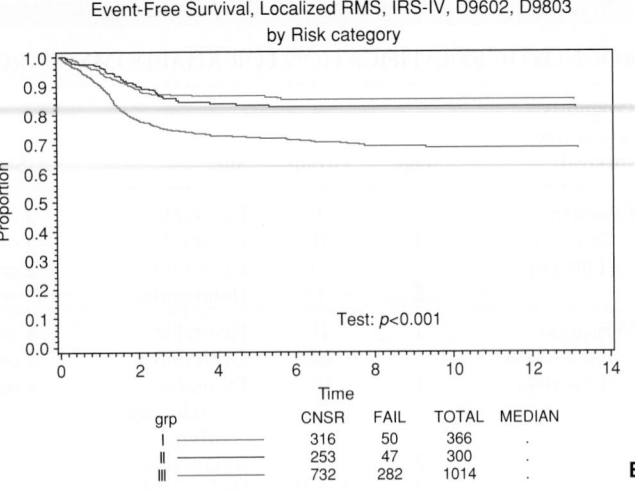

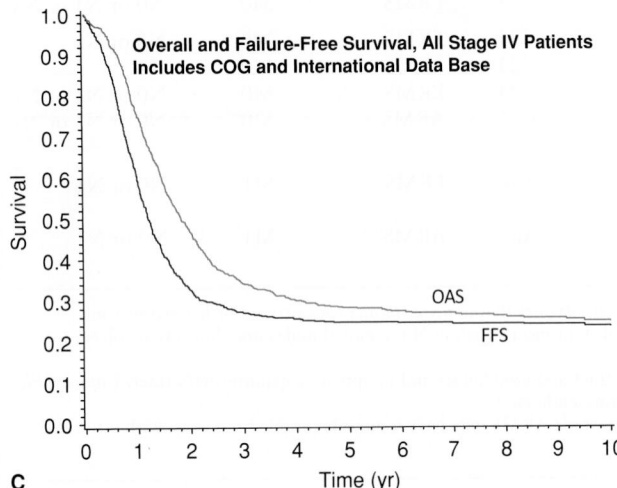

FIGURE 31.6 Outcome of patients by extent of disease at diagnosis. **A:** Event-free survival of patients with localized tumors treated on IRS-IV, D9602 (low-risk "IRS-V"), and D9803 (intermediate-risk "IRS-V") by STAGE. Patients with stage III tumors (unfavorable site more than 5 cm and/or regional node involvement) had inferior outcome compared to patients with stage I or II tumors. (Anderson JR, personal communication). **B:** Event-free survival of patients with localized tumors treated on IRS-IV, D9602 (low-risk "IRS-V"), and D9803 (intermediate-risk "IRS-V") by Clinical Group. Patients with group III tumors (unresected) had inferior outcome compared to patients with group I or II tumors; there was no difference in outcome between patients with group I and group II tumors. (Anderson JR, personal communication). **C:** Failure-free survival and overall survival for patients with metastatic rhabdomyosarcoma. The outcome for this group of patients from an International RMS data analysis remains extremely poor, with less than one patient in three alive at 10 years from diagnosis. (Oberlin O, personal communication).

of residual bulk or microscopic tumor, and systemic chemotherapy (for primary cytoreduction and eradication of gross and micrometastases). Much of the information regarding current use of these modalities derives from therapeutic programs developed initially by the IRSG and subsequently by the COG.

Principles of Surgical Management

Surgery is the most rapid way to ablate the disease, and it should always be used if subsequent function or cosmesis will not be greatly impaired. In some sites, such as the vagina and female genital tract, the urinary bladder, the orbit, and the biliary tract, aggressive surgical treatment is unwarranted. In other sites, such as the head and neck, a diagnostic incisional biopsy may be the only feasible surgical procedure because of proximity to vital blood vessels and nerves, cosmetic considerations, or both. If microscopic residual disease is found after an initial excision, or if the initial operation was carried out without knowledge of the type of neoplasm involved, re-excision of the area may be indicated. In localized lesions of the trunk and extremities, improvement in survival time can be produced by primary surgical re-excision of all residual tumor before the initiation of chemotherapy.[139,195] Occasionally, debulking surgery is used to reduce the volume of residual tumor beyond that which would remain after incisional biopsy alone. Carefully reviewed data in support of this

theoretically reasonable maneuver for children with RMS are not available.

Second-look surgical procedures have been evaluated in three clinical circumstances: (a) to pathologically verify the completeness of an apparently complete clinical (radiographic) remission for the purpose of eliminating further local control measures such as radiotherapy; (b) to resect any residual viable tumor cells that have survived after induction chemotherapy and local irradiation; and (c) to permit a reduction in the dose of radiation in patients who initially present with group III tumors.

The International Society of Pediatric Oncology (SIOP) enrolled 425 patients on their 1984 Malignant Mesenchymal Tumors Study, which consisted of nonradical surgery or biopsy followed by three to six cycles of induction chemotherapy with vincristine, actinomycin D, and ifosfamide (VAI).[196] Definitive local treatment (surgery or radiotherapy) depended on the response to chemotherapy. Additional local therapy was not given to patients having no evidence of residual tumor after induction therapy. Out of 237 patients with initially incompletely resected, nonparameningeal, localized tumors, 140 patients (including 92 with RMS) achieved a complete clinical response to induction chemotherapy. Approximately half of these patients, who received no further local therapy, ultimately had local recurrence, and there was no difference in the local recurrence rate between patients undergoing biopsy confirmation of complete remission status (26 out of 52) and those followed clinically (18 out of 39). Therefore, as a strategy to permit the withholding of definitive local therapy after the achievement of a complete clinical response, biopsy confirmation is inappropriate because of the high rate of false-negative results and the unacceptable local relapse rate when such an approach is followed.

Data regarding the role of secondary (second-look) operations to resect residual viable tumor after the administration of definitive local therapy were collected in CG III patients enrolled in IRS-III, for whom a delayed resection of the residual primary tumor was recommended, whenever possible, after the first 20 weeks of treatment (i.e., after the completion of induction chemotherapy and local radiotherapy). Second-look operations were found to produce complete responses by removing residual tumor after primary chemoradiotherapy and to improve the accuracy of clinical and radiologic assessment of response by providing tissue for pathologic examination.[83,197] Sixty-four percentage of CG III patients who underwent secondary operations in radiographic partial remission were found to be in complete remission, and, more important, 52% of those who underwent secondary operations after achieving only a minor response (<50% regression in cross-sectional tumor diameter) were converted to complete remission status by the procedure. These findings formed the basis of the IRS Committee's cautious endorsement of the role of second-look surgery for CG III patients in partial remission after induction chemoradiotherapy. The Committee acknowledged, however, that the contribution of second-look surgery to the improvement in long-term survival of these patients could not adequately be assessed because of the frequent concomitant use of alternative induction therapy in those same persons.[83]

Finally, investigators at St. Jude Children's Research Hospital reported maintenance of local control in 22 out of 28 patients with initially group III tumors treated with lower-than-standard dose radiation after being rendered free of gross disease with chemotherapy alone ($n = 16$) or plus surgery ($n = 12$).[198] There was a trend toward improved local control within this group among patients receiving ≥40 Gy versus those receiving <40 Gy (15 out of 17 vs. 7 out of 11, $p < 0.14$). These preliminary results form the basis for a more formal evaluation of the role of second-look surgery in reducing the risk of local recurrence (as well as the dose of local irradiation) in patients with initially unresectable tumors being treated on present COG studies.

Tumors of the Head and Neck

Head and neck tumors, with the exception of those arising in relatively superficial locations, are rarely amenable to wide local excision. Incisional biopsy for diagnostic purposes is usually all that is feasible, and in the case of orbital tumors, biopsy is all that is necessary given the excellent results achieved with chemoradiotherapy regimens. Tumors arising in the orbit have an excellent prognosis, and as noted the orbit is considered a favorable site. Paramemeningeal sites are unfavorable, although with modern therapy approaches the outcome for parameningeal, including middle ear tumors, without base of skull involvement or intracranial extension, has dramatically improved.[120,199] Other nonorbital, nonparameningeal head and neck sites also do well with 80% cure rates.[200] A recent review of 62 tumors from studies IRS I to IV arising in the parotid region show that most were group III, and with appropriate multimodality therapy and without aggressive surgery, the 5-year survival was 84%.[201] Unless clinically suspicious nodes are present, routine cervical lymph node sampling is unnecessary, because the incidence of regional lymph node involvement is quite low. However, nodal disease in this site was correlated with a poorer outcome.[200] In a single institutional series from Memorial Sloan-Kettering Cancer Center of 28 patients with head and neck tumors, most of which arose in one of the parameningeal locations, alveolar histology tumors were associated with an elevated risk of regional NI.[202] The availability of highly skilled otolaryngology and craniofacial reconstruction teams at select institutions may permit the resection of some tumors that would otherwise be unresectable, particularly if surgical resection can be performed without cosmetically mutilating effects and would result in down-staging that would lead to lower-dose RT, less intensive systemic chemotherapy, or both.[203,204]

Tumors of the Genitourinary Tract

Paratesticular Tumors

Paratesticular tumors should be removed by radical inguinal orchiectomy with resection of the entire spermatic cord. An inguinal approach is used to avoid scrotal contamination, which is likely if a transscrotal biopsy is performed. The necessity of subsequent retroperitoneal lymph node dissection (RPLND), which is done to determine whether regional retroperitoneal lymph nodes harbor tumor deposits, has been controversial. Although at least one European study had advised avoidance of RPLND if radical inguinal orchiectomy resulted in complete microscopic excision and if radiographic imaging studies were normal,[205] the IRS Committee continued to recommend it in IRS-III. RPLND was performed in 121 patients with nonmetastatic paratesticular RMS treated on IRS-III.[206] Only 14% of patients without radiographic evidence of lymph node involvement were found to have pathologically involved nodes, whereas 94% of those with radiographically enlarged nodes were confirmed to have NI. Only patients with pathologically confirmed positive nodes received RT in addition to postoperative adjuvant chemotherapy. The 5-year survival rate was significantly better for those patients with clinically negative lymph nodes than for those with clinically positive nodes (96% vs. 69%, $p < 0.001$); however, treatment failures were usually caused by distant, not locoregional, lymph node disease recurrence. Routine RPLND was not, therefore, recommended in the IRS-IV trial for patients with completely resected localized tumors and negative imaging studies, although systematic retroperitoneal lymph node sampling was recommended, including ipsilateral high and low infrarenal (caval, interaortocaval, and aortic) and bilateral iliac nodes. A preliminary analysis of IRS-IV data suggested that this approach resulted in a dramatic "down-staging" of patients (from group II to group I) and was associated with a worse outcome, particularly for boys aged 10 years and older who were treated with two-drug VA (vincristine, actinomycin-D) chemotherapy.[130] These findings form the basis of the current COG recommendation to perform ipsilateral RPLND (iRPLND) in all boys aged 10 years and older at diagnosis. Whether noninvasive imaging modalities such as PET scan, or more limited surgical procedures such as sentinel lymph node mapping can be used in lieu of iRPLND is uncertain. Surgical resection of enlarged lymph nodes in younger boys is also warranted to convert them from group III to group II. Given the inferior outcome of older boys treated on IRS-III (where surgical exploration was required),[206] an alternative approach to iRPLND in such patients is the routine administration of more intensive 3-drug (VA plus cyclophosphamide or ifosfamide) chemotherapy.[207] Similarly, the necessity of postoperative irradiation in such patients with intensively treated resected retroperitoneal nodes has been called into question.[207] The small number of patients with known nodal tumor makes execution of a controlled study difficult.[208,209]

Vulvar, Vaginal, and Uterine Tumors

Wide local excision of vulvar and vaginal tumors is rarely indicated before the commencement of primary chemotherapy. These tumors usually respond sufficiently well to induction chemotherapy to render them easily resectable, often with histologically negative margins. Tumors of the proximal vagina may require hysterectomy with partial or complete vaginectomy. Uterine tumors are usually managed without oophorectomy in the absence of overt ovarian involvement. Most patients are not initially managed with hysterectomy, but for those in whom hysterectomy is performed, distal vaginal preservation is possible. Second-look surgery and radical resection of lesions in these areas are usually reserved for patients with gross residual disease after the initial surgical resection when these patients have either failed to achieve a complete radiographic response within 6 months after the completion of induction chemotherapy and radiotherapy, or have had early disease progression after the commencement of chemotherapy and radiotherapy. High cure rates can be achieved with conservative surgery in many of these children, with only selected use of local irradiation.[210–212]

Bladder and Prostate Tumors

Management of tumors arising in the bladder or the prostate has evolved from a primary surgical approach (pelvic exenteration and total cystectomy) to a multimodal approach at present.[213–216] Radical surgical methods resulted in excellent rates of local control, but the morbidity of these operations was considered unacceptable. Current guidelines recommend complete resection reserved only for those patients in whom preservation of bladder and urethral function can be assured.[217,218] Partial cystectomy, which is usually reserved for tumors arising in the dome of the bladder, can be performed either before the onset of chemoradiotherapy or after induction chemotherapy with or without RT. This approach results in no compromise in the survival rate but a comparable or perhaps even higher rate of preservation of bladder function than with other treatment modalities.[213,214] Total cystectomy and anterior pelvic exenteration are reserved for patients who do not achieve local control with the combination of chemotherapy and RT and have been reported to result in survival rates higher than 80% if they are performed in the absence of distant dissemination.[215,216] However, local therapy continues to be suboptimal for this site, with many children having substantial long-term bladder dysfunction.[219]

Tumors of the Extremities

Initial complete surgical removal of extremity sarcomas should be attempted, provided that limb function will not be greatly impaired, because the prognosis is considerably worse if grossly visible tumor is left behind.[195,196] Because up to half of patients with extremity tumors have regional lymph node involvement,[91] sampling of clinically negative regional lymph nodes was recommended in IRS-IV and was required in IRS-V and the current generation of COG clinical trials. Biopsy of clinically suspicious lymph nodes should commence with the most proximal nodes before proceeding to dissection or aggressive nodal sampling. Involvement of the ipsilateral supraclavicular lymph nodes for upper extremity tumors and iliac or paraaortic lymph nodes, or both, for lower extremity tumors is considered evidence of distant spread (stage IV). As with paratesticular tumors in

older boys, the role of noninvasive imaging modalities such as PET scan, or less aggressive surgical sampling with the use of sentinel lymph node mapping, to assess regional nodal spread is the subject of intense interest. Amputation is usually not necessary, although it may be considered for patients with extensive lesions involving the bone or major neurovascular structures and for patients for whom radiotherapy will probably result in significant impairment of limb function.

Tumors Arising in Other Sites

Surgical removal should be attempted for truncal lesions.[220] Tumors arising in the pelvis, retroperitoneum, or intrathoracic area often cannot be removed completely because of infiltration or encirclement of major blood vessels or nerves or because of the surgeon's unwillingness to perform exenteration for pelvic-retroperitoneal tumors. Wide local resection of chest wall tumors consists of removal of the entire soft tissue mass and en bloc resection of uninvolved tissue extending at least one rib above and below the lesion.[140] An analysis of outcome among 84 IRS-II and III patients with thoracic sarcomas demonstrated inferior outcome among group I patients (7 out of 13 suffered local recurrence), suggesting that microscopic residual disease is present in some patients and supporting the more routine application of primary re-excision, particularly if there is a question about the adequacy of margins.[139] Similarly, tumors arising in the diaphragm are usually not resectable and require a similar approach to therapy.[221]

Surgical Management of Metastatic Disease

The role of surgical metastectomy in improving the outcome of patients with distant tumor spread is unclear. In a retrospective study of outcome after resection of pulmonary metastases in 152 patients with childhood sarcomas (Ewing's sarcoma, osteosarcoma, RMS, and other high-grade NRSTS) treated at the NCI, Temeck et al. found a uniformly poor outcome among patients with RMS.[222] Nonetheless, given the poor outcome of such patients with conventional chemotherapy alone, removal of metastatic deposits (e.g., pulmonary nodules) may be of benefit in selected patients who have otherwise responded well to induction chemotherapy, particularly if potentially active chemotherapeutic agents or radiotherapy approaches are still available.

Complications of Surgery

Complications of operative management are related to the tumor site. Any procedure involving the skin and subcutaneous tissue produces a scar and loss of tissue in the region from which bulk tumor is removed. The surgeon's experience is critical in executing the proper operation. Radical regional lymph node dissections are discouraged because of subsequent scarring and lymphedema and because there are no convincing data that radical node dissection is therapeutic in pediatric RMS. Similarly, surgical resection of involved regional nodes rarely results in the ability to administer biologically meaningfully lower doses of postoperative radiation. Skill is especially important in the surgical exploration of lesions arising in the head and neck, where major blood vessels and important nerves are so closely apposed. In the genitourinary region, total cystectomy for bladder or prostate tumors is currently generally deferred until it is clear that viable malignant cells have persisted despite chemotherapy and radiotherapy. In infants and toddlers, for whom the effects of full-dose RT may be particularly devastating, combined modality therapy with preirradiation surgical resection followed by reduced dose (or, rarely, no) postoperative RT, may be appropriate in selected cases after a full assessment of the potential risks associated with both modalities. In patients with paratesticular sarcoma, bilateral RPLND can produce retrograde ejaculation and is therefore discouraged.

Principles of Radiation Therapy

RT is a major tool in the treatment of children with RMS in the United States and the treatment modality for which the greatest philosophical differences of opinion and practice exist between the COG and other North American investigators and many European cooperative groups where RT is less uniformly applied, particularly in younger children and for tumors that regress completely after a period of neoadjuvant chemotherapy.[223] This "agreement to disagree" is clearly associated with differences in local control rates, late effects, and in some instances overall survival, with most series from the United States consistently demonstrating both higher rates of local control and greater number and types of long-term complications with the more uniform administration of RT; less clear, however, is the impact on survival, at least for some sites.[224] Whether individual patients with initially gross totally resected or unresected tumors can be identified for whom radiation can be safely withheld remains unclear. RT can eradicate residual tumor cells from sites where surgical therapy alone cannot ablate the mass, especially in the head, neck, and pelvis. Soft tissue sarcomas infiltrate so widely that after simple excision or enucleation, without wide excision, RT, or chemotherapy, local recurrence rates approximate 75%.[225] Soft tissue sarcomas were considered insensitive to RT before 1960, when Dritschilo et al. first reported a local control rate of 96% for 27 children younger than 16 years with RMS or undifferentiated sarcoma who received 5,500 to 6,500 cGy, delivered by a 4- or 8-mV accelerator.[226]

Current RT guidelines have evolved over time from the logical and stepwise approach of the sequential intergroup studies.[227-233] Daily fractions of between 180 and 200 cGy are standard; smaller daily fractions of 150 cGy may be used when large fields (e.g., whole abdomen) must be treated. A cumulative dose of between 36 and 41.4 Gy is generally sufficient to control microscopic residual disease, whereas higher cumulative RT doses of between 50.4 and 54 Gy (45 Gy for orbital tumors) are utilized to control gross residual disease. It is important that accurate pretreatment images be obtained and that the treatment field encompasses the initial pretreatment tumor volume as well as a margin (usually 2 cm) of normal surrounding tissue. The use of a "cone-down" or "shrinking-field" technique may be utilized at doses in excess of 36 to 41 Gy for patients whose initially unresectable tumors have responded to neoadjuvant therapy. Most patients can have treatment safely delayed until 3 to 12 weeks after diagnosis, after a period of neoadjuvant chemotherapy, during which tumor regression is the norm.

The approach to parameningeal tumors has evolved dramatically in the last several decades. Although utilized in early IRS studies, in the absence of overt meningeal involvement, whole-brain irradiation is now unwarranted for cranial parameningeal tumors, in part because modern imaging provides excellent delineation of tumor extent and assures better quality control for local RT.[120] A retrospective analysis of 595 patients treated on IRS II through IV found that initiation of RT within 2 weeks of diagnosis was associated with a marked improvement in local control (but not FFS) in patients with signs of meningeal impingement (18% local failure rate vs. 33% local failure rate when RT started more than 2 weeks from diagnosis).[234] Several pilot studies have, however, demonstrated excellent local-control rates and survival with "delayed" local radiation even in "high-risk" patients with

parameningeal tumors and intracranial extension. [235-238] Two recent reports have suggested that traditional volumetric considerations may be reduced without compromising the efficacy of radiation for parameningeal tumors.[234,239]

The role of RT in the local management of patients with initially completely resected tumors (CG I) was elucidated in a report from the IRSG looking at outcome in 439 patients treated on IRS I through III.[183] Pretreatment factors that were identified as being associated with inferior outcome were tumor size greater than 5 cm, sites other than the genitourinary tract, and alveolar or undifferentiated histology. Patients with ARMS who received RT had a significantly improved outcome compared with those who did not. Current COG treatment guidelines, therefore, recommend that all patients with completely resected ARMS receive postoperative radiotherapy to a dose of at least 36 Gy. An analysis of local treatment failure among patients with CG III tumors treated on IRS-II reported an overall local control rate of 78%; a subset of patients with bulky (size 10 cm) tumors or tumors originating in unfavorable sites (chest, pelvis, extremity, trunk) was identified as being at especially high risk of local treatment failure.[240] Local control continued to be the predominant type of relapse in IRS-III, group III patients, with a local failure rate of 19%, and distant failure of 11%. There was no significant effect of radiotherapy dose over the prescribed range of 41.4 to 50.4 Gy.[241]

One of the major therapeutic objectives of IRS-IV, therefore, was to evaluate the effect on local control of conventional fractionation (CF)-RT (using daily fractions of 180 cGy to a cumulative dose of 50.4 Gy) versus hyperfractionated (HF) RT (using twice-daily fractions of 110 cGy, separated by at least 6 hours, to a cumulative dose of 59.4 Gy) for patients with group III tumors.[242] Investigators at St. Jude Children's Research Hospital piloted this approach and demonstrated an absolute 2-year continuous local tumor control rate of 75% with minimal late radiation morbidity in 14 patients with CG III and IV tumors and persistent gross residual disease after induction chemotherapy.[243] A pilot study (IRS-IV-P) of HF-RT confirmed that it was feasible to administer concurrent HF-RT and intensive chemotherapy and suggested that the acute toxicities of hyperfractionated radiation were less severe than those seen with CF-RT protocols.[242] Similar to other published reports noting the failure of HF-RT to improve local disease control,[91,189] the IRS-IV study showed no improvement in outcome for those receiving HF-RT.[244]

Although there were no primary radiation questions addressed in the most recently completed COG studies, a major goal of the current COG intermediate-risk study, ARST 0531, is to nonrandomly assess the impact on local control and failure-free and overall survival of the "early" administration of local RT (at week 4) after only one course of chemotherapy.

Sequelae of treatment are numerous. RT can produce an acute reaction characterized by erythema and swelling of the irradiated volume, which can lead to desquamation if extreme. The later effects of radiation are loss of function or growth, chiefly because of fibrosis, which increases with increasing dose and volume and diminishes with increasing age of the patient.[245,246] Fully 70% of patients with orbital RMS have impaired vision; many have abnormal dentofacial development; and almost half of patients with nonorbital RMS fail to maintain their initial height velocity, and treatment with supplemental growth hormone is not uncommon.[247-251]

Other controversies in the area of RT for the local control of RMS include the role of primary RT for patients with orbital tumors,[252-254] the problem of poor local control (and overall survival) in patients with cranial parameningeal tumors and extensive bony erosion,[116,120,255] the issue of the optimal timing of local irradiation relative to the initiation of postoperative systemic chemotherapy,[256] and the related questions of what constitutes the minimally acceptable dose of RT that can be administered without compromising local control and under what circumstances can such reduced-dose radiation be safely administered.[257-259] Although differences in practice continue within the international community, there are convincing data that local RT improves outcome for patients with parameningeal RMS.[260] The role of whole-lung RT (generally to a cumulative dose of 1,440 cGy) for patients who present with overt pulmonary metastases is unclear; however, some treatment protocols continue to recommend it—a not unreasonable practice, if a state of minimal residual disease can be achieved—given the radiosensitivity of RMS. Techniques other than traditional external-beam megavoltage RT may sometimes be considered. One technique employs radiation implants, especially for children with small, critically located tumors of the head and neck, bladder, prostate, vagina, or extremity.[261-264] Because the dose is delivered to a carefully restricted volume, adjacent normal structures receive less scatter radiation and may be expected to have less fibrosis. Another newer approach for large, deeply seated tumors is treatment of the tumor by the radiation therapist under direct vision while it is exposed in the operating room (intraoperative RT). More data are needed in pediatric patients to assess the utility of this method.[265]

Advances in the ability to incorporate three-dimensional (3-D) imaging into radiation treatment planning have led to the growing use of 3-D conformal radiotherapy and intensity-modulated RT (IMRT) as particularly promising approaches to maximize the dose of radiation delivered to tumor-bearing tissue while minimizing the dose received by normal surrounding structures.[266-269] Although still limited, there is a growing body of data to suggest that these newer techniques produce excellent rates of local control.[202,269-272] Still newer "biologically functional" imaging techniques, such as PET and nuclear MRI and spectroscopy, may be combined with the "dose-sculpting" ability of IMRT to generate highly precise delivered dose distributions.[273] More recently, due to the theoretically superior normal tissue sparing achieved with its use, there has been a growing interest in the role of proton beam radiotherapy, particularly in the management of patients with parameningeal tumors; to date, however, there are no clinical data to suggest that local control rates or long-term radiation-related complications can be marginally improved compared to what is possible with IMRT.[274]

Principles of Chemotherapy

Early clinical trials evaluated the activity of single chemotherapeutic agents in children with recurrent or metastatic tumors. Few patients were cured with such an approach. The most active single agents that were identified in this manner were dactinomycin, cyclophosphamide, vincristine, and doxorubicin.[275-282] Combinations of these agents led to improvements in response rates.[283-285] Wilbur et al. pioneered the administration of repetitive doses of vincristine, actinomycin D (dactinomycin), and cyclophosphamide (VAC regimen) to children with advanced RMS. Out of 24 children with inoperable localized tumors (16 patients) or metastatic deposits at diagnosis (8 patients), 16 (67%) were alive and well at a median follow-up approaching 2 years.[286] The benefit of systemic therapy on prolonging and improving overall survival was confirmed in numerous studies involving limited numbers of patients.[287-292] Multicenter studies evaluating larger numbers of patients were subsequently initiated to ascertain better methods of treatment and to learn more about potential prognostic factors. In 1972, members of the Children's Cancer Study Group and the Pediatric Divisions of the Southwest Oncology Group and the Cancer and Acute Leukemia Group B banded together to form the IRS group. More than 4,500 patients with RMS and undifferentiated sarcoma have been treated on the IRS (and subsequently COG) investigations that have been completed since then.[81-83,189] With the creation of the COG, the IRSG investigations became the responsibility of the Soft Tissue Sarcoma Committee. The "mainstay" of chemotherapy over the past two-plus decades of IRSG and now COG RMS studies has been the combination of vincristine and dactinomycin with cyclophosphamide. The selection of "secondary" regimens for inclusion into randomized front line studies has been based on activity in a series of "phase II window" studies in patients with newly diagnosed metastatic RMS.[293] One obvious problem with treating patients with recurrent tumors is that an agent's true activity may be grossly underestimated because such tumors are likely to have developed complex mechanisms of resistance to a broad spectrum of agents[294] and such patients are less likely to tolerate treatment with sufficiently high doses of potentially active agents. In conjunction with a highly predictive murine xenograft model of RMS,[295-297] phase II window studies have been utilized to identify several agents with moderate-to-high activity, including melphalan,[298] methotrexate,[299] topotecan,[300] and topotecan-cyclophosphamide[301] that were mostly "inactive" in previously treated patients,[302,303] although the combination of topotecan-cyclophosphamide had some activity in the relapse setting.[304] Although a follow-up study by this same group failed to show a similarly improved response rate after dacarbazine (DTIC) and doxorubicin were administered to newly diagnosed patients,[305] the concept of alternative induction therapy, consisting of the early introduction of pairs of active drugs, was incorporated into the design of IRS-III for patients who had failed to achieve a complete response by week 20. The results of the three 2-drug phase II window studies that were conducted in IRS-IV identified the combinations of ifosfamide plus doxorubicin (ID), ifosfamide plus etoposide (IE), and vincristine plus melphalan (VM) as potentially significant drug pairs for improving outcome in patients with metastatic RMS.[306-308]

These studies have been instrumental in improving outcome, identifying important prognostic variables, and developing risk-based therapies for patients with RMS (Fig. 31.7). Children from ethnic minorities have benefited equally from improvements in therapy.[309]

The goal of identifying additional active agents is to be able to incorporate as many active agents as possible, ideally without overlapping toxicities, into the front-line management of newly diagnosed patients to avoid the development of multidrug resistance (MDR).[312,313] Cisplatin (CDDP), and more recently carboplatin, etoposide (VP-16), and DTIC have been shown to be active, singly and in various combinations, over the past two-plus decades.[314-320]

Ifosfamide, alone and in combination with etoposide or doxorubicin, has been shown to be highly active in both newly diagnosed and recurrent RMS.[306,317,321-323] These observations formed the rationale for the basic experimental design of IRS-IV in which the efficacy of equitoxic doses[324] of cyclophosphamide versus ifosfamide (VAC versus VAI versus vincristine, ifosfamide, and etoposide [VIE]) was evaluated. More recently, the camptothecin analogs, topotecan and irinotecan, were identified as particularly promising new agents. These compounds poison the DNA repair enzyme topoisomerase I, and have both striking activity in the murine xenograft model,[297] as well as encouraging responses in phase I and phase II window testing.[300,301,325,326] The IRS window study

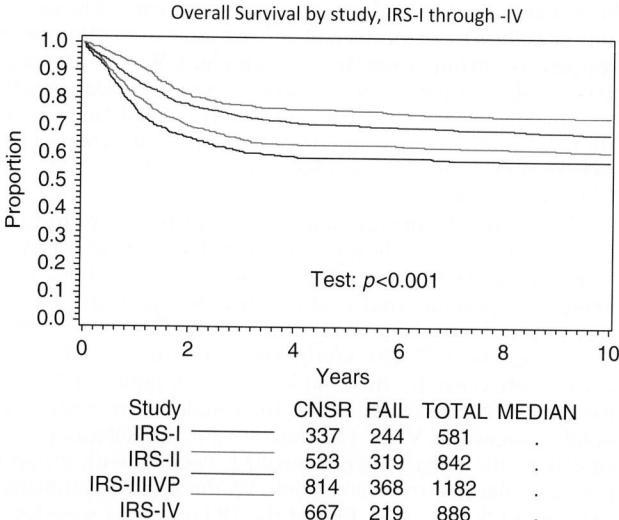

Overall Survival by study, IRS-I through -IV

Test: *p*<0.001

Study		CNSR	FAIL	TOTAL	MEDIAN
IRS-I	——	337	244	581	.
IRS-II	——	523	319	842	.
IRS-IIIVP	——	814	368	1182	.
IRS-IV	——	667	219	886	.

FIGURE 31.7 Overall survival by Study, IRS-I through -IV. After marked improvement in outcome over the course of the first three IRS studies (IRS-I 1972–1978; IRS-II 1978–1984; IRS-III 1984–1991), there has been relatively little subsequent improvement in outcome beginning with IRS-IV (1991–1997). Results of two of the three "IRS-V" series of studies (D9803 for patients with "intermediate-risk" tumors, D9802 for patients with "high-risk" tumors) have now been published, and the remaining results for patients with "low-risk" tumors (D9602) are expected in 2010.[310,311]

evaluating topotecan-cyclophosphamide showed substantial activity[301] and complemented the activity noted in relapse patients,[304] forming the rationale for the most recently completed COG intermediate-risk study, D9803.

Unfortunately, as was also true for the randomized interventions of IRS-IV, D9803 failed to demonstrate an improvement in outcome with the replacement of six cycles of VAC with VTC; and, in patients with stage II/III, group II/III ARMS, outcome in the VAC/VTC arm was inferior (4-year FFS 52% vs. 68% with VAC, *p* = 0.05).[310] The observation that survival was comparable between the two arms for the entire group of patients with intermediate-risk tumors was a compelling justification for the reduction of the cyclophosphamide dosage from 2,200 mg/m² per course to 1,200 mg/m²/course in the current generation of COG trials.

Irinotecan, alone or in combination with vincristine, proved to be a highly active drug, both singly and in combination, in patients younger than 21 years with newly diagnosed metastatic RMS treated on D9802 and D9802R. Although 42% of patients (*n* = 19) treated with single agent irinotecan achieved an objective response to two cycles of therapy, the high disease progression rate of 32% prompted the closure of the single-agent window and its replacement with the combination of vincristine plus irinotecan; the response rate of 50 patients treated on this successor version of the study was 70% with only 8% of patients progressing.[311] This striking response rate to this generally well-tolerated drug combination with nonoverlapping toxicities formed the basis for the current chemotherapy question in ARST-0531 in which newly diagnosed patients with intermediate-risk disease are randomly assigned to receive 14 cycles of VAC chemotherapy or 7 cycles of VAC in combination with 7 cycles of vincristine + irinotecan; randomized patients are all treated with early local RT at week 4.

Paclitaxel (Taxol) and its semisynthetic analog docetaxel (Taxotere) are unique tubulin-binding compounds that produce cytotoxicity by blocking dividing cells at either the G2 or

M phase of the cell cycle and have demonstrated antitumor activity against a variety of neoplasms.[327] Although there were reports of antitumor responses in phase I studies in pediatric patients with recurrent solid tumors,[328,329] including those with RMS, these agents have little activity in traditional phase II testing in RMS. Vinorelbine, a semisynthetic vinca alkaloid with unique pharmacologic principles, has also demonstrated activity in refractory and recurrent RMS or soft tissue sarcomas,[330,331] and is being evaluated in the current European high-risk RMS study.

Combined-Modality Therapy

The general principle of complete surgical removal of tumor, if feasible, should be emphasized. Patients whose tumors are removed at the outset continue to fare better than those with gross residual sarcoma, especially with primary tumors of an extremity. Operative removal of residual tumor may be performed from weeks to months after completion of chemotherapy and RT and may help to eradicate resistant cells that may otherwise contribute to relapse.[332]

The timing of RT in relation to chemotherapy has been somewhat variable. RT was historically begun at the same time as chemotherapy for patients with group I or II sarcomas but was delayed until week 6 for those with group III or IV tumors to assess the response to chemotherapy, to potentially exploit the booster effect of certain drugs (e.g., dactinomycin), and to minimize mucositis or other damage.[333,334] Currently, in the COG studies, RT commences immediately for selected "high-risk" patients with locally advanced cranial parameningeal tumors. However, in several single institution studies, carefully selected patients with parameningeal primary tumors had local irradiation delayed.[235,239] In the most recently completed low-risk COG trial, RT was initiated at week 3. For most other patients, the recently completed COG trials delayed RT until at least week 12. For the subset of female genitourinary primary tumors, local irradiation could be delayed until week 25. In the present COG studies, local RT is planned to begin at week 12 for most patients. As noted above, a goal of the current COG intermediate risk study is to evaluate the role of early-timing RT (3 weeks from initiation of chemotherapy) as a strategy to improve local control in patients with intermediate-risk tumors.

Because most relapses occur within 2 or 3 years of diagnosis, two to five chemotherapeutic agents have historically been administered for 12 to 24 months with a trend toward decreased total length of therapy in the newer studies. IRS-IV planned therapy for slightly less than 1 year for most risk groups. The recently completed low-risk COG trial (D9602) used either VA or VAC therapy for 44 weeks of total therapy. Recent European studies have demonstrated similar overall survival with less intensive therapy. The current low-risk COG trial utilizes marked dose reduction of cyclophosphamide and only 22 weeks of therapy for those patients with embryonal histology tumors that are stage I or II, group I or II or the subset of orbit group III tumors. Other low-risk embryonal patients receive the same initial four cycles of VAC followed by VA therapy for a total length of therapy of 45 weeks. Optimal therapy for patients with unresectable ERMS in unfavorable sites, and for patients with ARMS considered to be intermediate risk for present COG studies continues to be refined. Although VAC has continued to be the "gold standard," the absence of any improvement in outcome for this group of patients over now two decades gives pause for concern.[90] Most patients with metastatic RMS continue to have a poor outcome, although those with embryonal histology tumors who are younger than 10 years may fare somewhat better (nonetheless, even this group of patients with relatively more favorable outcome is still treated on current high-risk protocols). Results are not yet available for the now-completed ARST-0431, a more intensive seven-drug regimen that incorporated the highly active vincristine + irinotecan drug pair into an interval-compressed, alkylator-intensive "core" utilizing alternating cycles of ifosfamide-etoposide and vincristine-doxorubicin-cyclophosphamide (or vincristine-dactinomycin-cyclophosphamide after reaching the maximum cumulative doxorubicin dosage). It remains unclear what direction the next COG high-risk RMS study will take; however, encouraging results with a "low-dose, maintenance" strategy have been achieved by the German-led CWS group, and is being explored further in the ongoing CWS-2007-HR study.[189] Similarly, the combination of low-dose oral cyclophosphamide and weekly vinorelbine as maintenance therapy is being evaluated by the European Paediatric Soft tissue Sarcoma Study Group (EpSSG RMS 2005).[335,336]

Treatment Results

The results of the last two generations of IRS studies, IRS-III and IRS-IV, have now been published, and publication of the next generation of studies ("IRS-V" replaced henceforth by COG terminology "D" series studies, the subsequently revised "ARST" studies) will occur in late 2009 or early 2010. The sixth generation of these studies, ARST-0331 and ARST-0531, continue to accrue patients with low- and intermediate-risk tumors, respectively. Preliminary results have been published of at least some parts of the relapsed RMS protocol ARST-0121, for which accrual was completed in late 2007.[337,338] Results are not likely to be available before 2010 for the high-risk study, ARST-0431, which completed accrual in the mid-2008. The results of the more recently completed IRSG/COG studies confirmed the major findings of most other single- and limited-institution studies, as well as the earlier IRS series, concerning the relation between outcome and the extent of initial surgical resection and site of the primary tumor.[81,82,288,289,292,339–341] Even after the difference in the distribution of patients by CG is taken into account, the overall outcome for patients treated on IRS-III was significantly better than that in IRS-II (5-year progression-free survival [PFS], 65% ± 2% vs. 55% ± 2%, $p < 0.001$; Fig. 31.7) and the overall outcome for IRS-IV is slightly improved, compared with IRS-III. Most of the improvement in outcome was accounted for by the significantly improved results among selected groups of higher-risk patients, specifically those with CG III special pelvic tumors (5-year PFS, 74% ± 4% vs. 58% ± 5% in IRS-II, $p = 0.01$); unfavorable histology CG I and II (71% ± 6% vs. 59% ± 5% in IRS-II, $p = 0.002$); and CG III tumors excluding special pelvic, orbit, and selected head sites (61% ± 3% vs. 52% ± 3% in IRS-II, $p = 0.01$. Compared with earlier series, outcome was improved for patients with localized tumors at virtually all sites, but no improvement in outcome was seen among patients with metastatic tumors. Outcome was best among patients with primary tumors of the orbit or nonbladder, nonprostate genitourinary tract; intermediate among patients with tumors arising in other head and neck sites and in the bladder or prostate; and worst among patients with extremity, cranial parameningeal, and other (trunk, pelvis-perineum, retroperitoneal, and paravertebral) sites.

One major question left unanswered by IRS-III is what role, if any, doxorubicin has in the front-line management of selected patients with RMS. Compared with the standard VAC regimen, the inclusion of cisplatin and etoposide did not appear to improve the complete response rate or PFS; however, differences in outcome among patients receiving doxoru-

bicin were seen in two distinct groups of patients. The use of anthracyclines has continued in at least some of the European cooperative group studies: for example, CWS-91 prospectively evaluated the impact of doxorubicin. No clear benefit on outcome for patients with comparably defined "intermediate-risk" tumors was seen compared with that achieved on contemporaneous COG studies using "standard" VAC- or VAC-like regimens.[342]

The major therapeutic objectives of IRS-IV were to randomly compare the efficacy of three 3-drug regimens (VAC, VAI, VIE) as well as two schedules of RT (CF and HF). This prospective, randomized trial enrolled 838 patients. Three-year FFS and overall survival figures for RMS were 77% and 86%, respectively.[90] This study demonstrated that VAC was equally effective to ifosfamide-based therapies. Fifty-six patients with preexisting renal abnormalities were nonrandomly assigned to VAC. The outcome for this subgroup was similar to the other patients enrolled. Patients with group I paratesticular tumors received only VA therapy. The estimated FFS was 81% at 3 years. Out of the 19 failures 13 were local or regional, with a high recurrence rate in those older than 10 years, indicating the necessity of lymph node sampling in this group.[130] Overall FFS for patients enrolled on IRS-IV did not differ from that seen in IRS-III. FFS was improved for patients with embryonal histology tumors ($p = 0.02$), but not for those with ARMS. The improvement was restricted to those with certain subsets of embryonal histology tumors, including those that were resectable, node positive, those with group III head and neck tumors, those with genitourinary nonbladder-nonprostate tumors, and those that were group I or II at unfavorable sites.[189] Subsequently, the IRS performed a pilot trial of increased alkylator dose intensity. This trial showed no benefit to higher cyclophosphamide doses.[343]

Three-year FFS was similarly unchanged among patients with metastatic disease at diagnosis treated on the IRS-IV series of studies, for whom one of three phase II windows were employed (VM, IE, ID), although treatment on the VM arm appeared to be associated with a somewhat worse outcome than treatment on either of the other two arms, perhaps due to cumulative hematologic toxicity following early treatment with melphalan.[306,308]

The major objectives of the now-completed IRS-V series of studies (D9602 for "low-risk" RMS, D9803 for "intermediate-risk" RMS, and D9802 for "high-risk") RMS was to maintain excellent outcome for patients with low-risk tumors through the selective reduction of therapy amongst a subset of patients with especially favorable prognoses, and to assess the role of the camptothecins, topotecan, and irinotecan, in the front-line management of newly diagnosed patients (See Fig. 31.8).

D9803, as described above, randomized patients to receive 14 cycles of "standard" VAC (with a cyclophosphamide dose fraction of 2.2 g/m^2/cycle given as a 30-minute infusion on day 1) versus 8 cycles of VAC alternating with 6 cycles of fractionated topotecan (0.75 mg/m^2/day × 5 days) + cyclophosphamide (250 mg/m^2/day × 5 days, for a total of 1250 mg/m^2 per course). Radiation guidelines were similar to those used in the standard arm of IRS-IV. No difference in outcome was seen between the two chemotherapy arms and, as in IRS-IV, outcome was again inferior for patients with ARMS.

As has been true with COG cooperative group trials originating in the United States, the results of other international collaborative studies published in the last several years have proved similarly disappointing regarding improving outcome for any group of patients with newly diagnosed RMS. The SIOP treated 186 newly diagnosed patients with nonmetastatic RMS on its MMT-84 study.[344] Treatment consisted of 3 courses of ifosfamide, vincristine, and actinomycin (IVA) for patients with completely resected tumors, and 6 to 10 courses

EFS, by IRS Risk Category, IRS-IV, D9602, D9803 Localized Disease
Event-Free Survival, Localized RMS, IRS-IV, D9602, D9803
by Risk category

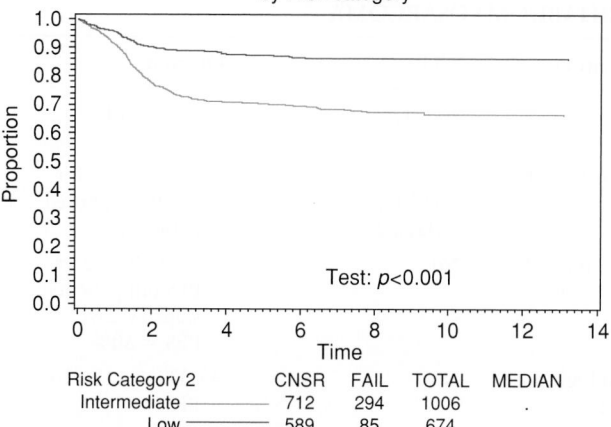

Risk Category 2		CNSR	FAIL	TOTAL	MEDIAN
Intermediate		712	294	1006	.
Low		589	85	674	.

FIGURE 31.8 Outcome of patients by risk-category at diagnosis, for patients with nonmetastatic disease treated on IRS-IV and IRS-V (D9602 and D9803). Event-free survival is significantly greater for patients with low-risk tumors (nonmetastatic tumors of embryonal histology arising in favorable sites regardless of the extent of upfront resection, or arising in unfavorable sites but with complete or gross total upfront resection) compared to patients with intermediate-risk tumors (all nonmetastatic alveolar tumors, and unresected unfavorable site embryonal tumors without metastases). Therapy for low-risk patients is increasingly focused on reducing the short-and long-term burdens of treatment while maintaining the same excellent outcome. (Anderson JR, personal communication).

of IVA for those with incompletely resected tumors. The major difference in therapeutic approach between the MMT-84 study and the IRSG studies was the omission of radiotherapy (or second-look surgery) for patients achieving a complete remission with chemotherapy alone (radiation was, however, given to patients older than 5 years with parameningeal tumors, reflecting the recommendations of an international workshop on the management of such tumors[252] and to patients older than 12 years with tumors in any site). With a median duration of follow-up of 8 years, the 5-year event-free survival (EFS) was 53% and overall survival was 68%. With the exception of the excellent outcome (5-year EFS of 85% vs. 12%) among the small number of patients (27) with completely resected tumors receiving three cycles of IVA over 2 months, EFS in all other groups was inferior to that of similar-risk patients treated on IRS-III and IV, largely due to a significantly greater risk of local relapse. Nearly one-third of patients (54 local only, 7 local plus distant) experienced an isolated local relapse and most did not subsequently achieve long-term disease-free status even after the application of aggressive local RT and/or surgery. As in the IRSG studies, factors associated with improved prognosis included embryonal histology (56% 5-year EFS vs. 33% for patients with ARMS, $p = 0.001$) and favorable site (orbit and genitourinary [nonbladder-nonprostate] sites). Although the intent of avoiding the late effects of potentially "unnecessary" RT was laudable, the inability to salvage the majority of the large number of patients who relapse with this approach suggests that it represents a suboptimal strategy for the vast majority of patients with newly diagnosed RMS. Similar findings were achieved, again without any overall improvement in outcome, in the MMT-89 trial that treated 503 newly diagnosed patients with nonmetastatic RMS between 1989 and 1995; this study, however, continued to build upon the results of the earlier study in

demonstrating that nearly half of the survivors were cured without significant local therapy (i.e., radiation).[223]

The German Soft Tissue Sarcoma Study (CWS-86) treated 286 RMS patients, including 251 with localized disease, with four-drug chemotherapy (vincristine, doxorubicin, ifosfamide, actinomycin [VAIA]), for varying durations of time (ranging from 16 to 40 weeks) based upon the initial extent of disease.[345] The use of local RT was stratified by stage of disease, primary tumor site, response to neoadjuvant chemotherapy, and the results of second-look surgery ("good responders" received 32 Gy, while "poor responders" received 54.5 Gy in split courses of accelerated hyperfractionation). Children younger than 2 years did not receive RT, and those between the ages of 2 and 3 years did so on a case-by-case basis. More than half of all patients had tumors that were unresectable and/or metastatic at diagnosis. Five-year EFS for all RMS patients was 60% ± 3%, and for those without metastases, it was 68%. As in the IRSG and SIOP studies, outcome was closely related to stage of the disease at diagnosis, ranging from 83% in patients with stage I disease ($n = 46$) to 67% in patients with stage II disease ($n = 56$) to 63% in patients with stage III disease ($n = 149$). The risk of local relapse was clearly related to failure to administer consolidative local RT in patients with either positive margins or gross residual disease. Better outcome was seen among the patients with ERMS than ARMS (67% ± 4% vs. 41% ± 6%, $p = 0.01$) and among patients with genitourinary (nonbladder-nonprostate) tumors. Other factors that were found to correlate with improved outcome differed according to stage at diagnosis: among patients with stage I disease, only tumor size ≥5 cm was associated with an adverse outcome, whereas for patients with stage III tumors, female gender, tumor size ≥5 cm, alveolar histology, and all sites other than genitourinary (nonbladder-nonprostate) were associated with poorer outcome. The results of the successor CWS-91 study involving 441 patients younger than 21 years with newly diagnosed localized soft tissue sarcomas (of whom 326 had RMS) have been recently published.[191] This study's primary objective was to stratify therapy for patients on the basis of postsurgical "IRS" clinical group, histology, and site; intensification of therapy with a five-drug regimen consisting of etoposide, vincristine, dactinomycin, ifosfamide, and doxorubicin (EVAIA) plus hyperfractionated accelerated radiotherapy (HART) to either 32 or 48 Gy was administered to 210 "high-risk" group C RMS patients, whereas cumulative chemotherapy dosages and treatment duration were reduced (compared with CWS-86) for the remaining 38 "favorable-risk" and 77 "intermediate-risk" RMS patients. Unfortunately, as has been the case with the IRS/COG and SIOP/MMT studies, no improvement in outcome compared with CSW-86 was seen with 5-year EFS rates of 64% (95% CI = 12%) versus 83% (95% CI = 12%); 62% (95% CI = 13%) versus 67% (95% CI = 14%); and, 59% (95% CI = 6%) versus 62% (95% CI = 8%), for groups A, B, and C, respectively.

Smaller, single and limited institution pilot studies, primarily in patients with intermediate-risk RMS, have achieved encouraging results utilizing five-drug chemotherapy consisting of alternating cycles of vincristine, doxorubicin, cyclophosphamide (VAdriaC) and IE. Arndt et al. treated 30 patients with intermediate risk tumors (14 with parameningeal primaries, 6 with extremity primaries, 5 with bladder-prostate, 12 with ARMS, 2 with undifferentiated sarcoma) with 14 cycles of alternating VAdriaC and IE; most patients received 5,040 cGy for local control beginning immediately following week 12/cycle 5 chemotherapy.[346] Three-year EFS in this group of "high-risk" patients with nonmetastatic tumors was 85% (95% CI 72% to 99%). Similar encouraging results were seen in 15 patients with "intermediate-risk" RMS treated on granulocyte colony-stimulating

TABLE 31.4

SUMMARY OF RESULTS OF MEGATHERAPY CONSOLIDATION WITH AUTOLOGOUS HEMATOPOIETIC BONE MARROW AND STEM CELL SUPPORT FOR PATIENTS WITH RHABDOMYOSARCOMA

Study	Group	No. of patients	Chemoablation	±TBI	Outcome
Horowitz[340]	NCI-PB	25 (some without metastases)	VAdrC	800 cGy/2 Fx	24% 6-yr EFS
Koscielniak[348]	G/A PBMTG	36 (27 stage IV; 9 postrelapse; 5 alloBMT)	Varied (most CME)	Varied [11 FTBI (12 Gy; 2 × 1.5 Gy/day); 2 TLI]	19% survival (for newly diagnosed patients)
Boulad[349]	MSKCC	26 (12 nonmetastatic; 7 no transplant)	ME (4-HC purged bone marrow)	No	53% ± 20% 2-yr PFS (all patients); stage IV 2-yr PFS = 50%
Bisogno[350]	AIEOP RMS4.99	70 (8 no transplant; PBSCT used)	Sequential high-dose therapy: $TT+PAM_1$ $C+TT_2$ PAM_3	No	35.3% ± 11% 3-yr PFS
Carli[351]	IES MMT4–91	52	Varied—42 M; 10 M + E ± C ± TT/Bu	No	30% ± 14% 3-yr EFS
Malogolowkin[335]	CCG	34 (23 with RMS; PBSCT used)	CME	No	44% ± 12% 2-yr EFS

AIEOP, Associazione Italiana di Ematologia e Oncologia Pediatria; alloBMT, allogeneic bone marrow transplantation; CCG, Children's Cancer Group; CCMH, Chicago Children's Memorial Hospital; C, carboplatin; $C+TT_2$, cyclophosphamide, thiotepa (cycle 2); CME, carboplatin, melphalan, etoposide; CTC, carboplatin, thiotepa, and cyclophosphamide; E, etoposide; EFS, event-free survival; (F)TBI (fractionated) total-body irradiation; G/A PBMTG, German/Austrian Pediatric Bone Marrow Transplantation Group; 4-HC, 4-hydroperoxycyclophosphamide; IES MMT4–91, Intergroup European Studies Malignant Mesenchymal Tumors Study 4–91; M, melphalan; MSKCC, Memorial Sloan-Kettering Cancer Center; NCI-PB, National Cancer Institute–Pediatric Branch; PAM_3, melphalan (cycle 3); PBSCT, peripheral blood stem cell transplantation; PFS, progression-free survival; RMS, rhabdomyosarcoma; TBI, total-body irradiation; TLI, total lymphoid irradiation; T T/Bu, thiotepa and busulfan; $TT+PAM_1$, thiotepa, melphalan (cycle 1); VAdrC, vincristine, Adriamycin, and cyclophosphamide.

factor (G-CSF)-supported "interval compression" variation of the same basic five-drug regimen.[347] The results of these small, nonrandomized pilot studies cannot be directly compared with those seen on cooperative group studies because often the patient population is highly selected and is not representative of the overall population with RMS. For patients at high risk of treatment failure, primarily those with metastatic disease at diagnosis, consolidation with high-dose chemotherapy with autologous bone marrow or peripheral blood stem cell rescue ("bone marrow or stem cell transplant") has been studied as a way of improving outcome by overcoming intrinsic or acquired drug resistance by delivering what would otherwise be "lethal" doses of chemotherapy (generally including one or more alkylating agents)—with or without total body irradiation—and then "rescuing" the patient by infusing previously cryopreserved hematopoietic progenitor cells. A series of small studies, with differing eligibility criteria, different myeloablative regimens, and different subsets of patients with metastatic disease, have failed to demonstrate any significant benefit of "transplant" in this setting[340,348–353] (Table 31.4). Thus, this strategy, though still being pursued, must be considered of no proven benefit and highly experimental.

Complications of Therapy

Complications of therapy include residual effects of operative management, RT, and chemotherapy (see also Chapters 10, 12, and 49). Clearly, the extent of surgical treatment has a bearing on the functional outcome. Extremity amputations and extensive formal lymph node dissections are rarely performed for that reason. Infection, anemia, and bleeding can result from intensive drug combinations. Infants may develop more toxicity than do older children.[354] Leukoencephalopathy, which is very uncommon, can be seen in patients with cranial parameningeal sarcoma given intensive chemotherapy and RT, including repeated doses of intrathecal methotrexate, hydrocortisone, and cytosine arabinoside.[355] Ascending myelitis of the cervical-thoracic region has been observed in 5 out of 149 children treated between 1972 and 1984 with intensive chemotherapy and irradiation for high-risk cranial parameningeal sarcoma.[356] Fibrosis, diminished growth of underlying or surrounding structures, cataracts, disturbed dentition, and growth hormone deficiency have all been reported in children receiving multimodality therapy for tumors arising in the head and neck.[357,358] Combined therapy with drugs and radiation can produce severe fibrosis and limitation of function in irradiated sites. For orbital tumors, the severity of radiation-related complications may be reduced by the avoidance of simultaneous administration of radiation and sensitizing chemotherapy (e.g., actinomycin D or doxorubicin).[253]

With modern therapy, a minority of patients with tumors of the bladder or prostate require total or partial cystectomy.[83,359] Nonetheless, a substantial proportion of those who do retain their bladders suffer from significant bladder dysfunction (incontinence, frequency, nocturia), and all patients with bladder or prostate tumors are at risk for hematuria, structural renal abnormalities, and delayed growth and pubertal development requiring sex hormone replacement therapy.[360,361] A recent review of the IRSG experience with bladder and prostate tumors reported an EFS of 77% and overall 6-year survival of 82%; however, only 40% (36 out of 88) who entered on study and survive event-free have normal functioning bladders.[219] The incidence of hematuria after cyclophosphamide therapy can increase as much as fourfold if pelvic irradiation is used, but the use of the bladder-protectant mesna has all but eliminated this potentially life-threatening complication.[362,363] Infertility can result from gonadal effects of cyclophosphamide or RT or from surgical interruption of nerves conveying impulses for antegrade ejaculation, as in boys with pelvic or paratesticular sarcoma.[364]

Several reports have described a broad spectrum of late complications, including small bowel obstruction, esophageal and common bile duct strictures, inguinal nerve entrapment syndrome, and lymphedema of the leg in patients treated with multimodality therapy for paratesticular RMS.[365,366] Among the newer active agents, ifosfamide can cause renal tubular dysfunction, which may be severe, with aminoaciduria, glycosuria, cation leakage, increased serum creatinine, and acidosis with growth failure.[367] Renal toxicity data were recently reported for 194 previously untreated patients enrolled on one of two ifosfamide-containing pilot regimens in IRS-IV.[368] The overall incidence of any nephrotoxicity was 14% (28 patients), with the most frequent toxicities being renal tubular dysfunction and decreased glomerular function. Preexisting renal abnormalities (primarily hydronephrosis), and age younger than 3 years (especially for those who received a cumulative ifosfamide dose of 72 g/m^2) greatly increased the risk of renal tubular dysfunction.

The most devastating late complication of therapy is the development of a second malignant neoplasm (SMN). Twenty-two of these neoplasms developed among 1,770 patients entered onto IRS-I and IRS-II, including 11 radiation-related bone sarcomas and 5 cases of acute nonlymphoblastic leukemia, at a median of 7 years after therapy.[369] The observation that three of the affected patients had neurofibromatosis and that the families of seven of the affected patients had histories compatible with LFS, raises the possibility that genetic susceptibility plays a significant role in the development of an SMN after treatment for RMS. Early results from IRS-III described the early occurrence of five cases of acute myeloid leukemia (AML) in children, as well as one case of osteosarcoma and one case of myelodysplastic syndrome (MDS).[370] A preliminary report of SMN in 1,040 patients enrolled in IRS-IV found 14 cases in 13 patients at a median of 3.2 years from diagnosis.[371] The 7.2% risk of secondary leukemia (MDS/AML and acute lymphoblastic leukemia) in patients treated with melphalan (as part of the phase II window strategy for patients with metastatic disease) was significantly greater than that for all other treatment arms. Early concerns about an increased risk of AML/MDS in patients receiving etoposide did not appear to be substantiated; however, prospective monitoring of the contribution of a strong family history of cancer to the risk of developing a treatment-related SMN is prudent.[372] A more recent update of the IRS experience noted 67 SMN and two-third malignancies in 4,367 patients enrolled on IRS studies from 1972 through 1997. Only seven had a recognized genetic predisposition syndrome. The estimated cumulative incidence for SMN at 20 years was 3.5%.[373]

The development of risk-based therapies is clearly the most important strategy to minimize the risk of late treatment-related complications. As was demonstrated in IRS-III and IV, and is being further evaluated in IRS-V and in studies in several European countries, selected groups of patients with favorable prognosis can be identified for whom the elimination of one or more chemotherapy agents appears to not adversely affect ultimate outcome. Although this approach does not appear to have been successful for pelvic tumors, it is possible that individual components of the multimodality treatment regimens can be withheld from the front-line man-

agement of patients without compromising ultimate outcome. Such an approach has been tried for patients with orbital RMS, and despite a local recurrence rate of 45% in patients not receiving initial radiotherapy, long-term survival does not appear to have been compromised.[252]

Patients with adverse prognostic features are increasingly being treated with more intensive and complex therapies. As therapy for even high-risk patients becomes more successful, it is increasingly important to monitor these patients for the development of other, potentially life-threatening, late treatment-related adverse events and to better understand the relation between genetic susceptibility and the development of SMNs. It may be possible to identify people for whom the selective elimination of one category of antineoplastic agents (e.g., epipodophyllotoxins, alkylating agents) is appropriate because of the presence of high-risk genetic markers. Improvements in evaluation of the presence or absence of microscopic (residual) disease, for example, with the use of molecular genetic markers unique to the tumor cell, may permit individualization of the duration of therapy. The goal of all these therapeutic maneuvers is the identification of better treatments, that is, treatments that achieve maximum long-term survival with minimum short- and long-term morbidity.

Treatment of Recurrent Disease

The management of patients with recurrent or unresponsive sarcoma is problematic. Although it is rare after 3 or 4 years from diagnosis, recurrence can take place many years after apparently successful treatment.[374-376] Reports of recurrences occurring in the second or subsequent decade of off-therapy follow-up are extremely rare.[376,377] Out of the 2,534 patients enrolled in IRS-III, IV-pilot, and IV, 48 "late" events developed in 1,160 patients who were still event-free 5 years from diagnosis; approximately half of those late events were relapses, with the remainder being SMNs or late-onset organ failure.[378] Recurrence connotes relative or absolute resistance to the chemotherapy or irradiation used in initial therapy. Among the various molecular mechanisms that may play a role in the development of drug resistance are overexpression of *P*-glycoprotein (the mediator of the MDR phenotype), hypermethylation of the tumor cells' DNA, elevated levels of DNA polymerase-alpha and -beta and topoisomerase II, overexpression of O6-methylguanine-DNA methyltransferase, and constitutive expression of the c-H-*ras* oncogene.[379-386]

The optimal treatment of patients with recurrent tumor is, at best, imprecisely defined. Patients with suspected recurrent disease should be fully evaluated and staged before the formulation of a treatment plan. Strong consideration should always be given to documenting suspected recurrence by biopsy or fine-needle aspiration. At a minimum, imaging studies (plain films, CT, and/or MRI) should be performed to evaluate the lungs, site of primary tumor, and any sites suggested by the history and physical examination. Hematologic abnormalities, if present, should be followed up with a bone marrow biopsy. After pathologic verification of recurrent disease, factors that should be considered in the formulation of a treatment plan include the timing of the recurrence relative to the completion of therapy (i.e., progression or recurrence while on therapy, within the first 6 to 12 months off therapy, or after more than 12 months off therapy), the extent of disease at recurrence (localized vs. disseminated), the extent of disease at diagnosis, and the nature of prior therapy (extent and intensity of chemotherapy, sites and doses of previous irradiation). Long-term survival is particularly difficult to achieve in patients who progress on therapy or shortly after completing treatment and in patients who initially had unresectable or metastatic sarcoma.[333] The 3-year postrelapse survival rates for patients treated on IRS-III were 48% vs. 12%, 12% vs. 9%, 11% vs. 5%, and 8% vs. 4%, for patients with CG I, II, III, and IV, respectively ($p < 0.001$ in favor of CG I).[83]

Several recent reports have better defined the risk of death from disease following relapse. Postrelapse survival was analyzed in 605 children who had previously been treated on IRS-III, IRS-IV pilot, and IRS-IV (1984 to 1997).[387] Ninety-five percentage of all relapses occurred within 3 years of diagnosis; the latest reported recurrence was at 9 years. The median survival time from first recurrence was 0.8 years; fewer than 20% of patients were projected to be alive 5 years from relapse. Postrelapse treatment was nonuniform. Subset analyses were able to identify groups with different prognoses. Approximately one patient in five, primarily those with ERMS who initially presented with stage I or group I disease, had a relatively "favorable" 5-year survival rate of approximately 50%, and the likelihood of subsequent survival appeared to correlate with whether the relapse was local (72%) or regional (50%) or distant (30%). The estimated 5-year postrelapse survival for patients with stage II or 3-group II or III tumors was 20%, and for those with group IV disease it was 12%. For this latter group of patients, the type of relapse (local vs. regional vs. distant) was not prognostically relevant. Patients with recurrent ARMS had a worse prognosis, with only those who initially had group I disease enjoying a relatively favorable prognosis (40% 5-year survival vs. 3% for groups II through IV). Although potentially important treatment variables existed, similar findings were reported by the CWS group.[388] Forty-four patients (17 with ERMS, 13 with ARMS) with relapsed soft tissue sarcomas were treated with multiagent chemotherapy; 5-year EFS appeared to be better in patients with ERMS (41% vs. 12%) versus those with ARMS (23% vs. 12%). The administration of postrelapse radiation (presumably given to those who had not previously been irradiated and, therefore, at greater risk of locoregional relapse after presenting with limited stage disease) was associated with improved outcome.

A more recent European retrospective analysis of postrelapse survival among 234 patients with RMS treated on CWS-86, CWS-91, and CWS-96 identified time-to-relapse as an important predictor of postrelapse survival for patients with both ERMS and ARMS, with "early" recurrences within 6 months of the completion of primary therapy having a particularly poor 4-year postrelapse survival (12%), "late" recurrences of more than 12 months following the completion of therapy having a relatively more favorable 4-year postrelapse survival (41%), and "intermediate" recurrences having a 4-year postrelapse survival of 21%.[389]

To better address postrelapse outcome in uniformly treated patients, the COG enrolled 138 patients with recurrent or progressive RMS on ARST-0121, a prospective therapeutic trial exploring the efficacy of intensified therapy with vincristine, doxorubicin, cyclophosphamide, etoposide, ifosfamide, the radiosensitizer tirapazamine, and two-schedules of irinotecan (50 mg/m²/day × 5 days per cycle vs. 20 mg/m²/day × 10 days per cycle) from June 2002 through October 2006. Preliminary results of this study showed no difference in initial response rate among the 92 patients randomized to either irinotecan schedule, thus forming the basis for the selection of the daily × 5 irinotecan scheduled in the current generation of COG STS studies (ARST-0431 and ARST-0531, for patients with high- and intermediate-risk tumors, respectively).[337] Tirapazamine use in combination with cyclophosphamide and doxorubicin appeared safe, but no further plans are in place for this agent's subsequent development in RMS.[338] It is not yet known what impact, if any, this intensified multiagent regimen will have on postrelapse survival.

Localized Recurrence

An aggressive multimodality approach should be considered for the patient with an isolated site of recurrent disease. The best chance for long-term survival is the situation in which a complete surgical resection can be accomplished, potentially followed by adjuvant postoperative irradiation and chemotherapy, in a patient with an initially stage I-group I ERMS tumor. For example, for patients with vaginal and paratesticular localized recurrences, long-term survival can still be achieved with this aggressive approach.[215] The choice of a salvage chemotherapeutic regimen depends on the previous chemotherapy and the timing of the relapse. There are well-described examples of durable responses achieved in patients with recurrence of therapy using the same drugs as previously administered.[390] For patients who have not previously received known active agents such as ifosfamide, doxorubicin, or etoposide, or newer agents such as topotecan or irinotecan, these agents should be strongly considered when choosing a regimen, although the tolerability and activity of these agents is likely to be reduced in heavily pretreated patients.[391] In patients who have already received all known active agents and who have recurrence during or shortly after completion of therapy, investigational phase I and II agents should be considered.

Disseminated Recurrence

In contrast to localized recurrence, in which the chance of long-term survival is a small but real possibility, patients in whom recurrence develops with metastatic disease are essentially incurable. Surgical resection of metastatic lesions, even if complete, is unlikely to be of benefit regarding curative potential, although low-morbidity procedures may be useful for palliative purposes.[222,392–394] Chemotherapy is the primary therapeutic modality, with palliative radiotherapy usually reserved to treat painful lesions or to prevent spinal cord compression. The choice of chemotherapeutic agents should be guided by the same principles listed previously.

Although high-dose chemotherapy with autologous bone marrow or peripheral blood progenitor cell support has not been demonstrated to be efficacious in patients with newly diagnosed metastatic disease, the efficacy of programs incorporating these strategies for children with recurrent soft tissue sarcoma is unclear because few studies have been undertaken and, with rare exceptions, only short-term results are available.[395–397] Because soft tissue sarcomas are usually less sensitive to irradiation than are leukemia or neuroblastoma cells, total-body irradiation may be less effective in eradicating recurrent sarcoma.[340] Further investigation of consolidation with high-dose chemotherapy and bone marrow or peripheral blood stem cell rescue for select patients with recurrent RMS is not unreasonable given the current lack of good therapeutic options. One possible advantage of such an approach, particularly in heavily pretreated patients who are relatively intolerant of additional myelosuppressive chemotherapy, is to utilize growth factor–supported autologous peripheral blood progenitor cell transfusions to permit repetitive monthly cycles of myeloablative chemotherapy.[398]

Immunotherapy and Other Targeted Interventions

Recent advances in understanding the basic biology of RMS have led to the possibility of novel therapeutic interventions, including specific antitumor immune responses as well as targeted disruption of critical signaling pathways. These approaches are still in the earliest stages are summarized in this section.

The recognition that intracellular proteins can be processed and presented as peptides on the cell surface by major histocompatibility complex class I molecules has suggested the possibility that tumor-specific mutant gene products may be targets for cytotoxic T cells (CTL).[399,400] For example, investigators have shown that a peptide derived from a mutant p53 protein is specifically recognized by CTLs.[401,402] In a similar way, translocation-specific fusion proteins could also potentially be targeted by CTL. Specifically, the PF fusion protein generated by the t(2;13)(q35;q14) translocation in ARMS is a potential target for CTL therapeutic approaches. A pilot clinical study using PF-specific peptide pulsed dendritic cell vaccination in metastatic patients following standard chemotherapy was recently reported.[403] This study demonstrated the ability of patients to generate immune responses to a control influenza peptide, immune responses directed against the PF were generated sporadically. The success of immune-based approaches in RMS thus will likely depend on the identification of more potent antigens in RMS tumors. If such antigens are identified, multiple approaches could then be taken to overcome potential deficits that allowed the tumor to initially escape cellular immunity.[404,405]

Because an *IGF-2* autocrine pathway has been demonstrated to play a role in the growth of RMS,[406,407] disruption of this pathway offers another potential therapeutic target. Blockade of the IGF-1 receptor, a ligand-inducible tyrosine kinase receptor that mediates the IGF-2 mitogenic signal, has been shown to inhibit the growth of established human RMS tumors in nude mouse xenografts.[406,408,409] There are now several fully human IGFIR monoclonal antibodies in clinical trials, including in patients with RMS but results are not yet available. Clearly the use of such antibodies in combination with other therapies will be required, as is the case with several antibodies now in routine clinical practice, including Herceptin and Rituxan.[410,411] In addition to the development of targeted humanized monoclonal antibodies, there is an ever increasing number of tyrosine kinase inhibitors at varying stages of clinical development. Of particular interest for RMS would be kinase inhibitors of the *ras* pathway due to its likely involvement in ERMS and MET inhibitors as discussed earlier. A number of such inhibitors are currently making their way through early clinical development and are worth considering for experimental approaches in RMS. In addition, several other targets have been suggested from the mouse model of ARMS, including the PDGFR-A receptor[412] and Aurora B kinase and several polo-like kinases.[41]

Another approach to treatment of many solid tumors that has shown great promise is the use of angiogenic inhibitors. A humanized vascular endothelial growth factor (VEGF) monoclonal antibody, bevacizumab, has been approved for the treatment of metastatic colon and breast cancer, as well as for non-small cell lung cancer and glioblastoma. Although bevacizumab has not been directly tested against RMS, it has been previously reported that other antiangiogenic compounds have activity against RMS xenografts.[413] Currently, several small molecule kinase inhibitors of the VEGF receptor tyrosine kinase family are also in clinical trials and may warrant evaluation similar to bevacizumab. Finally, camptothecin (irinotecan) and topotecan agents currently in clinical trial in patients with RMS have been demonstrated to have significant antiangiogenic activity, raising the possibility of achieving an "accidental" inhibitory effect, particularly with protracted low-dose drug administration.[414] In summary, both antibodies and small molecule kinase inhibitors that target signaling pathways that seem to play a role in the biology of RMS are in active clinical development and these newer agents should

be rationally considered in future clinical trials for patients with advanced stage RMS.

PERSPECTIVES

The "fifth generation" of IRSG/COG cooperative group trials have completed accrual and published results are imminent. The current low-risk trial is evaluating whether decreased therapy can maintain excellent cure rates. The current intermediate-risk trial is exploring whether early timing radiation (at week 4, after one cycle of chemotherapy) can improve outcome for patients randomly assigned to receive VAC alone or VAC plus irinotecan. An intensified, seven-drug chemotherapy regimen incorporating irinotecan into an anthracycline-containing, alkylator-intensive core has been completed and plans for a successor "high-risk" study are in development. Although great progress has been made in the treatment of RMS, and most patients with nonmetastatic tumors are now cured, most of this progress occurred during the course of the first two decades of cooperative group studies. These improvements have been largely based on a foundation of empiric observations achieved in the setting of well-designed clinical studies rather than basic insights resulting from epidemiologic and laboratory studies of the underlying biology of RMS. Little subsequent improvement in outcome has been achieved since the completion of IRS-III in 1991. Although important clues are now being discovered correlating distinct molecular abnormalities with both pathogenesis and prognosis, a plateau has been reached for the majority of patients who present with unresectable ERMS in unfavorable sites and for those with ARMS of any site. Improvements in both local and systemic disease control are still needed for these groups of patients. Local and locoregional recurrences continue to represent an unacceptably high proportion of all treatment failures. Whether newer radiation techniques such as IMRT, the use of hypoxic cell sensitizers, or the use of "radiosensitizing" chemotherapy[415] can improve local control rates remains to be seen. Although better ways of preserving the bladder and female genitourinary structures have become the norm, many of these patients still have significant organ dysfunction. Newer treatment modalities are needed to lessen the late adverse effects on structures in the head and neck. As new agents with antisarcoma activity become available, it is possible that RT can be reduced still further (e.g., in patients with orbital lesions). Given the constraints of study design and the relatively small differences that may be expected for patients with localized, favorable-prognosis tumors, future clinical studies will continue to focus on questions of therapeutic equivalence: that is, treatments that maintain excellent outcome while reducing the short- and long-term complications of therapy. For patients with intermediate-risk tumors, including the majority of those with unresectable ERMS arising in unfavorable locations and patients with ARMS, the current COG strategy to improve outcome continues to evaluate the efficacy of adding a topoisomerase I poison in combination with one or more other active agents which demonstrate synergy in preclinical xenograft model systems, as well as to evaluate the role of more aggressive use of delayed surgical resection in patients with initially unresected tumors.

Single investigational drugs or drug pairs are increasingly being assessed in the setting of a phase II window before introduction of standard therapy in newly diagnosed patients with metastases. This approach continued in the now completed high-risk arm of IRS-V in which the activity of the low-dose, protracted-schedule of administration of irinotecan, singly and in combination with vincristine, was evaluated. Although this strategy has been shown to be useful in identifying highly active compounds, the addition of conventionally dosed supplemental agents with similar mechanisms of action has thus far failed to significantly improve the outlook for patients with metastases at diagnosis. For these patients, it is hoped that the use of newer "molecularly targeted" agents will offer new hope for cure.

References

1. Boue DR, Parham DM, Webber B, et al. Clinicopathologic study of ectomesenchymomas from Intergroup Rhabdomyosarcoma Study Groups III and IV. Pediatr Dev Pathol 2000;3:290–300.
2. Gurney JG, Young JL Jr, Roffers SD, et al. Soft tissue sarcomas. In: Ries LAG, Smith MA, Gurney JG, et al. eds. Cancer incidence and survival among children and adolescents: United States SEER Program 1975–1995. NIH Pub. No. 99-4649. Bethesda, MD: National Cancer Institute, SEER Program, 1999:111.
3. Sultan I, Qaddoumi I, Yaser S, et al. Comparing adult and pediatric rhabdomyosarcoma in the Surveillance, Epidemiology and End Results Program, 1973–2005: an analysis of 2600 patients. J Clin Oncol 2009;27:3391–3397.
4. Ognjanovic S, Linabery AM, Charbonneau B, et al. Trends in childhood rhabdomyosarcoma incidence and survival in the United States, 1975–2005. Cancer 2009;115:4218–4226.
5. Stiller CA, Parkin DM. International variations in the incidence of childhood soft tissue sarcomas. Paediatr Perinat Epidemiol 1994;8:107–119.
6. Stiller CA, McKinney PA, Bunch KJ, et al. Childhood cancer and ethnic groups in Britain: a United Kingdom Children's Cancer Study Group (UKCCSG) study. Br J Cancer 1991;64:543–548.
7. Li FP, Fraumeni JF Jr. Soft-tissue sarcoma, breast cancer, and other neoplasms: a familial syndrome. Ann Intern Med 1969;71:747–752.
8. Li FP, Fraumeni JF Jr, Mulvihill JJ, et al. A cancer family syndrome in twenty-four kindreds. Cancer Res 1988;48:5358–5362.
9. Malkin D, Li FP, Strong LC, et al. Germ line p53 mutations in a familial syndrome of breast cancer, sarcomas, and other neoplasms. Science 1990;250:1233–1238.
10. Diller L, Sexsmith E, Gottlieb A, et al. Germline p53 mutations are frequently detected in young children with rhabdomyosarcoma. J Clin Invest 1995;95:1606–1611.
11. Hartley AL, Birch JM, Blair V, et al. Patterns of cancer in the families of children with soft tissue sarcoma. Cancer 1993;72:923–930.
12. Steenman M, Westerveld A, Mannens M. Genetics of Beckwith-Wiedemann syndrome-associated tumors: common genetic pathways. Genes Chromosomes Cancer 2000;28: 1–13.
13. Hartley AL, Birch JM, Blari V, et al. Foetal loss and infant deaths in families of children with soft-tissue sarcoma. Int J Cancer 1994;56:646–649.
14. Quezada E, Gripp KW. Costello syndrome and related disorders. Curr Opin Pediatr 2007;19:636–644.
15. Estep AL, Tidyman WE, Teitell MA, et al. HRAS mutations in Costello syndrome: detection of constitutional activating mutations in codon 12 and 13 and loss of wild-type allele in malignancy. Am J Med Genetics 2006;140A:8–16.
16. Hennekam RC. Costello syndrome: an overview. Am J Med Genet 2003;117C:42–48.
17. Gripp KW, Scott CIJ, Nicholson L, et al. Five additional Costello syndrome patients with rhabdomyosarcoma: proposal for a tumor screening protocol. Am J Med Genet 2002;108:80–87.
18. Sung L, Anderson JR, Arndt C, et al. Neurofibromatosis in children with Rhabdomyosarcoma: a report from the Intergroup Rhabdomyosarcoma study IV. J Pediatr 2004;144:666–668.
19. Grufferman S, Schwartz AG, Ruymann FM, et al. Parents use of cocaine and marijuana and increased risk of rhabdomyosarcoma in their children. Cancer Causes Control 1993;4:217–224.
20. Grufferman S, Ruymann F, Ognjanovic S, et al. Prenatal x-ray exposure and rhabdomyosarcoma in children: a report from the Children's Oncology Group. Cancer Epidemiol Biomarkers Prev 2009;18:1271–1276.
21. Turc-Carel C, Lizard-Nacol S, Justrabo E, et al. Consistent chromosomal translocation in alveolar rhabdomyosarcoma. Cancer Genet Cytogenet 1986;19:361–362.
22. Douglass EC, Valentine M, Etcubanas E, et al. A specific chromosomal abnormality in rhabdomyosarcoma [published erratum appears in Cytogenet Cell Genet 1988;47(4): following 232]. Cytogenet Cell Genet 1987;45:148–155.
23. Shapiro DN, Sublett JE, Li B, et al. Fusion of PAX3 to a member of the forkhead family of transcription factors in human alveolar rhabdomyosarcoma. Cancer Res 1993;53: 5108–5112.
24. Davis RJ, D'cruz CM, Lovell MA, et al. Fusion of PAX7 to FKHR by the variant t(1;13)(p36;q14) translocation in alveolar rhabdomyosarcoma. Cancer Res 1994;54: 2869–2872.
25. Naini S, Etheridge KT, Adam SJ, et al. Defining the cooperative genetic changes that temporally drive alveolar rhabdomyosarcoma. Cancer Res 2008;68:9583–9588.
26. Mercado GE, Xia SJ, Zhang C, et al. Identification of PAX3-FKHR-regulated genes differentially expressed between alveolar and embryonal rhabdomyosarcoma: focus on MYCN as a biologically relevant target. Genes Chromosomes Cancer 2008;47:510–520.
27. Ginsberg JP, Davis RJ, Bennicelli JL, et al. Up-regulation of MET but not neural cell adhesion molecule expression by the Pax-3-FKHR fusion protein in alveolar rhabdomyosarcoma. Cancer Res 1998;58:3542–3546.
28. Scrable H, Witte D, Lampkin B, et al. Chromosomal localization of the human rhabdomyosarcoma locus by mitotic recombination mapping. Nature 1987;329:645–647.
29. Scrable H, Witte D, Shimada H, et al. Molecular differential pathology of rhabdomyosarcoma. Genes Chromosomes Cancer 1989;1:23–35.
30. Scrable H, Cavenee W, Ghavimi F, et al. A model for embryonal rhabdomyosarcoma tumorigenesis that involves genome imprinting. Proc Natl Acad Sci U S A 1989;86: 7480–7484.
31. Rainier S, Johnson LA, Dobry CJ, et al. Relaxation of imprinted genes in human cancer. Nature 1993;362:747–749.
32. Ogawa O, Eccles MR, Szeto J, et al. Relaxation of insulin-like growth factor II gene imprinting implicated in Wilms' tumour. Nature 1993;362:749–751.
33. Feinberg AP. Genomic imprinting and gene activation in cancer. Nat Genet 1993; 4:110–113.
34. Taylor JG IV, Cheuk AT, Tsang PS, et al. FGFR4 is a mutationally activated oncogene that promotes metastasis in rhabdomyosarcoma. J Clin Invest 2009;119:3395–3407.
35. Pulciani S, Santos E, Lauver AV, et al. Oncogenes in solid human tumours. Nature 1982;300:539–542.
36. Chardin P, Yeramian P, Madaule P, et al. N-ras gene activation in the RD human rhabdomyosarcoma cell line. Int J Cancer 1985;35:647–652.
37. Stratton MR, Fisher C, Gusterson BA, et al. Detection of point mutations in N-ras and K-ras genes of human embryonal rhabdomyosarcomas using oligonucleotide probes and the polymerase chain reaction. Cancer Res 1989;49:6324–6327.
38. Langenau DM, Keefe MD, Storer NY, et al. Effects of RAS on the genesis of embryonal rhabdomyosarcoma. Genes Dev 2007;21:1382–1395.
39. Edmondson DG, Olson EN. Helix-loop-helix proteins as regulators of muscle-specific transcription. J Biol Chem 1993;268:755–758.
40. Wang H, Garzon R, Sun H, et al. NF-kappaB-YY1-miR-29 regulatory circuitry in skeletal myogenesis and rhabdomyosarcoma. Cancer Cells 2008;14:369–381.
41. Keller C, Arenkiel BR, Coffin CM, et al. Alveolar rhabdomyosarcomas in conditional Pax3:Fkhr mice: cooperativity of Ink4a/ARF and Trp53 loss of function. Genes Dev 2004;18:2614–2626.
42. Nishijo K, Chen QR, Zhang L, et al. Credentialing a preclinical mouse model of alveolar rhabdomyosarcoma. Cancer Res 2009;69:2902–2911.
43. Hahn H, Wojnowski L, Zimmer AM, et al. Rhabdomyosarcomas and radiation hypersensitivity in a mouse model of Gorlin syndrome [see comments]. Nat Med 1998;4: 619–622.
44. Munsterberg AE, Kitajewski J, Bumcrot DA, et al. Combinatorial signaling by Sonic hedgehog and Wnt family members induces myogenic bHLH gene expression in the somite. Genes Dev 1995;9:2911–2922.
45. Sharp R, Recio JA, Chamell J, et al. Synergism between INK4a/ARF inactivation and aberrant HGF/SF signaling in rhabdomyosarcomagenesis. Nat Med 2002;8:1276–1280.
46. Tiffin N, Williams RD, Shipley J, et al. PAX7 expression in embryonal rhabdomyosarcoma suggests an origin in muscle satellite cells. Br J Cancer 2003;89:327–332.
47. Morotti R, Nicol KK, Parham DM, et al. An immunohistochemical algorithm to facilitate diagnosis and subtyping of rhabdomyosarcoma: the Children's Oncology Group experience. Am J Surg Pathol 2006;30:962–968.
48. Parham DM, Webber B, Holt H, et al. Immunohistochemical study of childhood rhabdomyosarcomas and related neoplasms. Cancer 1991;67:3072–3080.
49. Dodd S, Malone M, McCulloch W. Rhabdomyosarcoma in children: a histological and immunohistological study of 59 cases. J Pathol 1989;158:13–18.
50. Dias P, Parham DM, Shapiro DN, et al. Myogenic regulatory protein (MyoD1) expression in childhood solid tumors: diagnostic utility in rhabdomyosarcoma. Am J Pathol 1990;137:1283–1291.
51. Dias P, Chen B, Dilday B, et al. Strong immunostaining for myogenin in rhabdomyosarcoma is significantly associated with tumors of the alveolar subclass. Am J Pathol 2000;156:399–408.
52. Kumar S, Perlman E, Harris CA, et al. Myogenin is a specific marker for rhabdomyosarcoma: an immunohistochemical study in paraffin-embedded tissues. Mod Pathol 2000;13:988–993.
53. Cessna MH, Zhou H, Perkins SL, et al. Are myogenin and MyoD1 expression specific for rhabdomyosarcoma? A study of 150 cases with emphasis on spindle cell mimics. Am J Surg Pathol 2001;25:1150–1157.
54. Hostein I, Andraud-Fregeville M, Guillou L, et al. Rhabdomyosarcoma: value of myogenin expression analysis and molecular testing in diagnosing the alveolar subtype. An analysis of 109 paraffin-embedded specimens. Cancer 2004;101:2817–2824.
55. Morgenstern DA, Rees H, Sebire NJ, et al. Rhabdomyosarcoma subtyping by immunohistochemical assessment of myogenin: tissue array study and review of the literature. Pathol Oncol Res 2008;14:233–238.
56. Heerema-McKenney A, Wijnaendts LCD, Pulliam JF, et al. Diffuse myogenin expression by immunohistochemistry is an independent marker of poor survival in pediatric rhabdomyosarcoma. A tissue microarray study of 71 primary tumors including correlation with molecular phenotype. Am J Surg Pathol 2008;32:1513–1522.
57. Horn RC Jr, Enterline HT. Rhabdomyosarcoma: a clinicopathological study and classification of 39 cases. Cancer 1958;1:181–199.
58. Asmar L, Gehan EA, Newton WA, et al. Agreement among and within groups of pathologists in the classification of rhabdomyosarcoma and related childhood sarcomas: report of an international study of four pathology classifications. Cancer 1994;74:2579–2588.
59. Tsokos M, Webber BL, Parham DM, et al. Rhabdomyosarcoma: a new classification scheme related to prognosis. Arch Pathol Lab Med 1992;116:847–855.
60. Tsokos M. The diagnosis and classification of childhood rhabdomyosarcoma. Semin Diagn Pathol 1994;11:26–38.
61. Newton WA Jr, Gehan EA, Webber BL, et al. Classification of rhabdomyosarcoma and related sarcomas: pathologic aspects and proposal for a new classification. An Intergroup Rhabdomyosarcoma Study. Cancer 1995;76:1073–1085.
62. Newton WA Jr, Soule EH, Hamoudi AB, et al. Histopathology of childhood sarcomas, Intergroup Rhabdomyosarcoma Studies I and II: clinicopathologic correlation. J Clin Oncol 1988;6:67–75.
63. Leuschner I, Newton WA Jr, Schmidt D, et al. Spindle cell variants of embryonal rhabdomyosarcoma in the paratesticular region. A report of the Intergroup Rhabdomyosarcoma Study. Am J Surg Pathol 1993;17:221–230.
64. Pawel BR, Hamoudi AB, Asmar L, et al. Undifferentiated sarcomas of children: pathology and clinical behavior. An Intergroup Rhabdomyosarcoma Study. Med Pediatr Oncol 1997;29:170–180.
65. Kodet R, Newton WA Jr, Hamoudi AB, et al. Childhood rhabdomyosarcoma with anaplastic (pleomorphic) features. A report of the Intergroup Rhabdomyosarcoma Study. Am J Surg Pathol 1993;17:443–453.
66. Qualman S, Lynch J, Bridge J, et al. Prevalence and clinical impact of anaplasia in childhood rhabdomyosarcoma. A report from the Soft Tissue Sarcoma Committee of the Children's Oncology Group. Cancer 2008;113:3242–3427.

67. Mentzel T, Katenkamp D. Sclerosing, pseudovascular rhabdomyosarcoma in adults. Clinicopathological and immunohistochemical analysis of three cases. Virchows Arch 2000;436:305–311.
68. Folpe AL, McKenney JK, Bridge JA, et al. Sclerosing rhabdomyosarcoma in adults. Report of four cases of a hyalinizing, matrix-rich variant of rhabdomyosarcoma that may be confused with osteosarcoma, chondrosarcoma, or angiosarcoma. Am J Surg Pathol 2002;26:1175–1183.
69. Vadgama B, Sebire NJ, Malone M, et al. Sclerosing rhabdomyosarcoma in childhood: case report and review of the literature. Pediatr Dev Pathol 2004;7:391–396.
70. Chiles MC, Parham DM, Qualman SJ, et al. Sclerosing rhabdomyosarcoma in children and adolescents: a clinicopathologic review of 13 cases from the Intergroup Rhabdomyosarcoma Study Group and Children's Oncology Group. Pediatr Dev Pathol 2004;7:583–594.
71. Wang J, Tu X, Sheng W. Sclerosing rhabdomyosarcoma. A clinicopathologic and immunohistochemical study of five cases. Am J Clin Pathol 2008;129:410–415.
72. Soglio DB-D, Rougemont A-L, Absi R, et al. SNP genotyping of a sclerosing rhabdomyosarcoma reveals highly aneuploid profile and specific MDM2/HMGA2 amplification. Hum Pathol 2009;40:1347–1352.
73. Kuhnen C, Herter P, Leuschner I, et al. Sclerosing pseudovascular rhabdomyosarcoma—immunohistochemical, ultrastructural, and genetic findings indicating a distinct subtype of rhabdomyosarcoma. Virchows Arch 2006;449:572–578.
74. Parham DM, Ellison DA. Rhabdomyosarcoma in adults and children: an update. Arch Pathol Lab Med 2006;130:1454–1465.
75. Barr FG, Qualman SJ, Macris MH, et al. Genetic heterogeneity in the alveolar rhabdomyosarcoma subset without typical gene fusions. Cancer Res 2002;62:4704–4710.
76. Matsumura T, Yamaguchi T, Seki K, et al. Advantage of FISH analysis using FKHR probes for an adjunct to diagnosis of rhabdomyosarcoma. Virchows Arch 2008;452: 251–258.
77. Mao L, Lee DJ, Tockman MS, et al. Microsatellite alterations as clonal markers for the detection of human cancer. Proc Natl Acad Sci U S A 1994;91:9871–9875.
78. Newton WA. Classification of rhabdomyosarcoma. In: Harms D, Schmidt D, eds. Current topics in pathology. Berlin: Springer-Verlag, 1995:241.
79. Shimada H, Newton WA Jr, Soule EH, et al. Pathology of fatal rhabdomyosarcoma. Report from Intergroup Rhabdomyosarcoma Study (IRS-I and IRS-II). Cancer 1987;59: 459–465.
80. Crist WM, Garnsey L, Beltangady MS, et al. Prognosis in children with rhabdomyosarcoma: a report of the Intergroup Rhabdomyosarcoma Studies I and II. J Clin Oncol 1990;8:443–452.
81. Maurer HM, Beltangady M, Gehan EA, et al. The Intergroup Rhabdomyosarcoma Study-I: a final report. Cancer 1988;61:209–220.
82. Maurer HM, Gehan EA, Beltangady M, et al. The Intergroup Rhabdomyosarcoma Study-II. Cancer 1993;71:1904–1922.
83. Crist W, Gehan EA, Ragab AH, et al. The Third Intergroup Rhabdomyosarcoma Study. J Clin Oncol 1995;13:610–630.
84. Rodary C, Flamant F, Donaldson SS. An attempt to use a common staging system in rhabdomyosarcoma: a report of an international workshop initiated by the International Society of Pediatric Oncology (SIOP). Med Pediatr Oncol 1989;17:210–215.
85. LaQuaglia MP, Heller G, Ghavimi F, et al. The effect of age at diagnosis on outcome in rhabdomyosarcoma. Cancer 1994;73:109–117.
86. Pedrick TJ, Donaldson SS, Cox RS. Rhabdomyosarcoma: the Stanford experience using a TNM staging system. J Clin Oncol 1986;4:370–378.
87. Lawrence W Jr, Gehan EA, Hays DM, et al. Prognostic significance of staging factors of the UICC staging system in childhood rhabdomyosarcoma: a report from the Intergroup Rhabdomyosarcoma Study (IRS-II). J Clin Oncol 1987;5:46–54.
88. Rodary C, Gehan EA, Flamant F, et al. Prognostic factors in 951 nonmetastatic rhabdomyosarcoma in children: a report from the International Rhabdomyosarcoma workshop. Med Pediatr Oncol 1991;19:89–95.
89. Kodet R, Newton WA Jr, Hamoudi AB, et al. Orbital rhabdomyosarcoma and related tumors in childhood: relationship of morphology to prognosis. An Intergroup Rhabdomyosarcoma Study. Med Pediatr Oncol 1997;29:51–60.
90. Crist WM, Anderson JR, Meza JL, et al. Intergroup rhabdomyosarcoma study-IV: results for patients with nonmetastatic disease. J Clin Oncol 2001;19:3091–3102.
91. Neville HL, Andrassy RJ, Lobe TE, et al. Preoperative staging, prognostic factors, and outcome for extremity rhabdomyosarcoma: a preliminary report from the Intergroup Rhabdomyosarcoma Study IV (1991–1997). J Pediatr Surg 2000;35:317–321.
92. Davicioni E, Anderson MJ, Finckenstein FG, et al. Molecular classification of rhabdomyosarcoma—genotypic and phenotypic determinants of diagnosis. A report from the Children's Oncology Group. Am J Pathol 2009;174:550–564.
93. Wachtel M, Runge T, Leuschner I, et al. Subtype and prognostic classification of rhabdomyosarcoma by immunohistochemistry. J Clin Oncol 2006;24:816–822.
94. Kelly KM, Womer RB, Sorensen PH, et al. Common and variant gene fusions predict distinct clinical phenotypes in rhabdomyosarcoma. J Clin Oncol 1997;15:1831–1836.
95. Sorensen PH, Lynch JC, Qualman SJ, et al. PAX3-FKHR and PAX7-FKHR gene fusions are prognostic indicators in alveolar rhabdomyosarcoma: a report from the Children's Oncology Group. J Clin Oncol 2002;20:2672–2679.
96. Barr FG, Duan F, Smith LM, et al. Genomic and clinical analyses of 2p24 and 12q13-q14 amplification in alveolar rhabdomyosarcoma: a report from the Children's Oncology Group. Genes Chromosomes Cancer 2009;48:661–672.
97. Qualman SJ, Bowen J, Parham DM, et al. Protocol for the examination of specimens from patients (children and young adults) with rhabdomyosarcoma. Arch Pathol Lab Med 2003;127:1290–1297.
98. Soule EH, Mahour GH, Mills SD, et al. Soft-tissue sarcomas of infants and children: a clinicopathologic study of 135 cases. Mayo Clin Proc 1968;43:313–326.
99. Ehrlich FE, Hass JE, Kiesewetter WB. Rhabdomyosarcoma in infants and children: factors affecting long-term survival. J Pediatr Surg 1971;6:571–577.
100. Sutow WW, Sullivan MP, Ried HL, et al. Prognosis in childhood rhabdomyosarcoma. Cancer 1970;25:1384–1390.
101. Enzinger FM, Shiraki M. Alveolar rhabdomyosarcoma. An analysis of 110 cases. Cancer 1969;24:18–31.
102. Ghavimi F, Exelby PR, DíAngio GJ, et al. Multidisciplinary treatment of embryonal rhabdomyosarcoma in children. Cancer 1975;35:677–686.
103. Ortega JA, Rivard GE, Isaacs H, et al. The influence of chemotherapy on the prognosis of rhabdomyosarcoma. Med Pediatr Oncol 1975;1:227–234.
104. Flamant F, Hill C. The improvement in survival associated with combined chemotherapy in childhood rhabdomyosarcoma: a historical comparison of 345 patients in the same center. Cancer 1984;3:2417–2421.
105. Raney RB Jr, Tefft M, Maurer HM, et al. Disease patterns and survival rate in children with metastatic soft-tissue sarcoma. Cancer 1988;62:1257–1266.
106. Koscielniak E, Rodary C, Flamant F, et al. Metastatic rhabdomyosarcoma and histologically similar tumors in childhood: a retrospective European multi-center analysis. Med Pediatr Oncol 1992;20:209–214.
107. Ruymann FB, Newton WA, Ragab AH, et al. Bone marrow metastases at diagnosis in children and adolescents with rhabdomyosarcoma: a report from the Intergroup Rhabdomyosarcoma Study. Cancer 1984;53:368–373.
108. Lawrence W Jr, Hays DM, Moon TE. Lymphatic metastasis with childhood rhabdomyosarcoma. Cancer 1977;39:556–559.
109. Lawrence W Jr, Hays DM, Heyn R, et al. Lymphatic metastases with childhood rhabdomyosarcoma. A report from the Intergroup Rhabdomyosarcoma Study. Cancer 1987; 60:910–915.
110. Oberlin O, Rey A, Lyden E, et al. Prognostic factors in metastatic rhabdomyosarcomas: results of pooled analysis from United States and European Cooperative Groups. J Clin Oncol 2008;26:2384–2389.
111. Months SR, Raney RB. Rhabdomyosarcoma of the head and neck in children: the experience at the Children's Hospital of Philadelphia. Med Pediatr Oncol 1986;14:288–292.
112. Tefft M, Fernandez C, Donaldson M, et al. Incidence of meningeal involvement by rhabdomyosarcoma of the head and neck in children. Cancer 1978;42:253–258.
113. Leviton A, Davidson R, Gilles F. Neurological manifestations of embryonal rhabdomyosarcoma of the middle ear cleft. J Pediatr 1972;80:596–602.
114. Gasparini M, Lombardi F, Gianni C, et al. Childhood rhabdomyosarcoma with meningeal extension: results of combined therapy including central nervous system prophylaxis. Am J Clin Oncol 1983;6:393–398.
115. Raney RB. Spinal cord "drop metastases" from head and neck rhabdomyosarcoma: proceedings of the Tumor Board of the Children's Hospital of Philadelphia. Med Pediatr Oncol 1978;4:3–9.
116. Mandell LR, Massey V, Ghavani F. The influence of extensive bone erosion on local control in nonorbital rhabdomyosarcoma of the head and neck. Int J Radiat Oncol Biol Phys 1989;17:649–653.
117. Raney RB Jr, Tefft M, Newton WA, et al. Improved prognosis with intensive treatment of children with cranial soft tissue sarcomas arising in nonorbital parameningeal sites: a report from the Intergroup Rhabdomyosarcoma Study. Cancer 1987;59:147–155.
118. Wharam MD Jr, Foulkes MA, Lawrence W Jr, et al. Soft tissue sarcoma of the head and neck in childhood: non-orbital and non-parameningeal sites. A report of the Intergroup Rhabdomyosarcoma Study (IRS)-I. Cancer 1984;53:1016–1019.
119. Wharam MD, Beltangady MS, Heyn RM, et al. Pediatric orofacial and laryngopharyngeal rhabdomyosarcoma. An Intergroup Rhabdomyosarcoma Study report. Arch Otolaryngol Head Neck Surg 1987;113:1225–1227.
120. Raney RB, Meza J, Anderson JR, et al. Treatment of children and adolescents with localized parameningeal sarcoma: experience of the Intergroup Rhabdomyosarcoma Study Group protocols IRS-II through -IV, 1978–1997. Med Pediatr Oncol 2002;38: 22–32.
121. Defachelles A-S, Rey A, Oberlin O, et al. Treatment of nonmetastatic cranial parameningeal rhabdomyosarcoma in children younger than 3 years old: results from International Society of Pediatric Oncology Studies MMT 89 and 95. J Clin Oncol 2009;27: 1310–1315.
122. Raney B, Anderson J, Breneman J, et al. Results in patients with cranial parameningeal sarcoma and metastases (Stage 4) treated on Intergroup Rhabdomyosarcoma Study Group (IRSG) protocols II-IV, 1978–1997: report from the Children's Oncology Group. Pediatr Blood Cancer 2008;51:17–22.
123. Shapiro E, Strother D. Pediatric genitourinary rhabdomyosarcoma. J Urol 1992;148: 1761–1768.
124. Waring PM, Newland RC. Prostatic embryonal rhabdomyosarcoma in adults: a clinicopathologic review. Cancer 1992;69:755–762.
125. Hays DM, Raney RB Jr, Lawrence W Jr, et al. Bladder and prostatic tumors in the Intergroup Rhabdomyosarcoma Study (IRS)-I. Cancer 1982;50:1472–1482.
126. LaQuaglia MP, Ghavimi F, Herr H, et al. Prognostic factors in bladder and bladder-prostate rhabdomyosarcoma. J Pediatr Surg 1990;25:1066–1072.
127. Raney RB Jr, Gehan EA, Hays DM, et al. Primary chemotherapy with or without radiation therapy, and/or surgery for children with localized sarcoma of the bladder, prostate, vagina, uterus, and cervix: a comparison of the results in IRS-I and -II. Cancer 1990;66: 2072–2081.
128. Hays DM, Shimada H, Raney RB Jr, et al. Clinical staging and treatment results in rhabdomyosarcoma of the female genital tract among children and adolescents. Cancer 1988;61:1893–1903.
129. Raney RB Jr, Tefft M, Lawrence W Jr, et al. Paratesticular sarcoma in childhood and adolescence: a report from the Intergroup Rhabdomyosarcoma Studies I and II, 1973–1983. Cancer 1987;60:2337–2343.
130. Wiener ES, Anderson JR, Ojimba JI, et al. Controversies in the management of paratesticular rhabdomyosarcoma: is staging retroperitoneal lymph node dissection necessary for adolescents with resected paratesticular rhabdomyosarcoma? Semin Pediatr Surg 2001;10:146–152.
131. Ferrari A, Bisogno G, Casanova M, et al. Is alveolar histotype a prognostic factor in paratesticular rhabdomyosarcoma? The experience of Italian and German Soft Tissue Sarcoma Cooperative Group. Pediatr Blood Cancer 2004;42:134–138.
132. Anderson J, Meyer W, Wiener E. Favorable outcome for children with paratesticular alveolar history rhabdomyosarcoma [letter]. Pediatric Blood Cancer 2004;43:180.
133. Hays DM, Soule EH, Lawrence W Jr, et al. Extremity lesions in the Intergroup Rhabdomyosarcoma Study (IRS-I): a preliminary report. Cancer 1982;49:1–8.
134. Heyn R, Beltangady M, Hays D, et al. Results of intensive therapy in children with localized alveolar extremity rhabdomyosarcoma: a report from the Intergroup Rhabdomyosarcoma Study. J Clin Oncol 1989;7:200–207.
135. Mandell L, Ghavimi F, LaQuaglia M, et al. Prognostic significance of regional lymph node involvement in childhood extremity rhabdomyosarcoma. Med Pediatr Oncol 1990;18:466–471.
136. Raney RB Jr, Ragab AH, Ruymann FB, et al. Soft-tissue sarcoma of the trunk in childhood: results of the Intergroup Rhabdomyosarcoma Study. Cancer 1982;49:2612–2616.
137. Ortega JA, Wharam M, Gehan EA, et al. Clinical features and results of therapy for children with paraspinal soft tissue sarcoma: a report of the Intergroup Rhabdomyosarcoma Study. J Clin Oncol 1991;9:796–801.
138. Crist WM, Raney RB, Tefft M, et al. Soft tissue sarcomas arising in the retroperitoneal space in children: a report from the Intergroup Rhabdomyosarcoma Study (IRS) Committee. Cancer 1985;56:2125–2132.

139. Andrassy RJ, Wiener ES, Raney RB, et al. Thoracic sarcomas in children. Ann Surg 1998;227:170–173.
140. Saenz NC, Ghavimi F, Gerald W, et al. Chest wall rhabdomyosarcoma. Cancer 1997;80: 1513–1517.
141. Blakely ML, Andrassy RJ, Raney RB, et al. Prognostic factors and surgical treatment guidelines for children with rhabdomyosarcoma of the perineum or anus: a report of intergroup rhabdomyosarcoma studies I through IV, 1972 through 1997. J Pediatr Surg 2003;38:347–353.
142. Srouji MN, Donaldson MH, Chatten J, et al. Perianal rhabdomyosarcoma in childhood. Cancer 1976;38:1008–1012.
143. Raney RB, Crist W, Hays D, et al. Soft tissue sarcoma of the perineal region in childhood. Cancer 1990;65:2787–2792.
144. Ruymann FB, Raney RB Jr, Crist WM, et al. Rhabdomyosarcoma of the biliary tree in childhood: a report from the Intergroup Rhabdomyosarcoma Study. Cancer 1985;56: 575–581.
145. Isaacson C. Embryonal rhabdomyosarcoma of the ampulla of Vater. Cancer 1978; 41:365–368.
146. Mihara S, Matsumoto H, Tokunaga F, et al. Botryoid rhabdomyosarcoma of the gallbladder in a child. Cancer 1982;49:812–818.
147. Spunt SL, Lobe TE, Pappo AS, et al. Aggressive surgery is unwarranted for biliary tract rhabdomyosarcoma. J Pediatr Surg 2000;35:309–316.
148. Leuschner I, Schmidt D, Harms D. Undifferentiated sarcoma of the liver in childhood: morphology, flow cytometry, and literature review. Hum Pathol 1990;21:68–76.
149. Dropcho EJ, Allen JC. Primary intracranial rhabdomyosarcoma: case report and review of the literature. J Neurooncol 1987;5:139–150.
150. Kedar A, Cantrel G, Rosen G. Rhabdomyosarcoma of the trachea. J Laryngol Otol 1988;102:735–736.
151. Schmaltz AA, Apitz J. Primary rhabdomyosarcoma of the heart. Pediatr Cardiol 1982;2:73–75.
152. Nunez C, Abboud SL, Lemon NC, et al. Ovarian rhabdomyosarcoma presenting as leukemia. Cancer 1983;52:297–300.
153. Rogers DA, Lobe TE, Rao BN, et al. Breast malignancy in children. J Pediatr Surg 1994;29:48–51.
154. Etcubanas E, Peiper S, Stass S, et al. Rhabdomyosarcoma presenting as disseminated malignancy from an unknown primary site: a retrospective study of ten pediatric cases. Med Pediatr Oncol 1989;17:39–44.
155. Rosenberg HK, Eggli KD, Zerin JM, et al. Benign cystitis in children mimicking rhabdomyosarcoma. J Ultrasound Med 1994;13:921–932.
156. Ferlito A, Barion U, Nicolai P. Myositis ossificans of the head and neck: review of the literature and report of a case. Eur Arch Otorhinolaryngol 1983;237:103–113.
157. Reid SE Jr, Nambisan R, Karakousis CP. Pyomyositis: a differential diagnosis from sarcoma. J Surg Oncol 1985;29:143–146.
158. Tang TT, Segura AD, Oechler HW, et al. Inflammatory myofibrohistiocytic proliferation simulating sarcoma in children. Cancer 1990;65:1626–1634.
159. Jones EC, Clement PB, Young RH. Inflammatory pseudotumor of the urinary bladder: a clinicopathological, immunohistochemical, ultrastructural, and flow cytometric study of 13 cases. Am J Surg Pathol 1993;17:264–274.
160. Hojo H, Newton WA Jr, Hamoudi AB, et al. Pseudosarcomatous myofibroblastic tumor of the urinary bladder in children: a study of 11 cases with review of the literature. An Intergroup Rhabdomyosarcoma Study. Am J Surg Pathol 1995;19:1224–1236.
161. Netto JMB, Perez LM, Kelly DR, et al. Pediatric inflammatory bladder tumors: myofibroblastic and eosinophilic subtypes. J Urol 1999;162:1424–1429.
162. Lusher JM. Chloroma as a presenting feature of acute leukemia: a report of two cases in children. Am J Dis Child 1964;108:62–66.
163. Matus-Ridley M, Raney RB Jr, Thawerani H, et al. Histiocytosis X in children: patterns of disease and results of treatment. Med Pediatr Oncol 1983;11:99–105.
164. Breneman JC, Lyden E, Pappo AS, et al. Prognostic factors and clinical outcomes in children and adolescents with metastatic rhabdomyosarcoma: a report from the Intergroup Rhabdomyosarcoma Study IV. J Clin Oncol 2003;21:78–84.
165. Ruymann FB, Thomas P. Disseminated intravascular coagulopathy, hypercalcemia, and hyperuricemia in rhabdomyosarcoma. In: Maurer HM, Ruymann FB, Pochedly C, eds. Rhabdomyosarcoma and related tumors in children and adolescents. Boca Raton, FL: CRC Press, 1991:215.
166. De la Serna FJ, Martinez MA, Valdes MD, et al. Rhabdomyosarcoma presenting with diffuse bone marrow involvement, hypercalcemia and renal failure. Med Pediatr Oncol 1988;16:123–127.
167. Podoloff DA. The role of radionuclide scans in sarcoma. Hematol Oncol Clin North Am 1995;9:605–626.
168. Quddus FF, Espinola D, Kramer SS, et al. Comparison between x-ray and bone scan detection of bone metastases in patients with rhabdomyosarcoma. Med Pediatr Oncol 1983;11:125–129.
169. Cogswell A, Howman-Giles R, Bergin M. Bone and gallium scintigraphy in children with rhabdomyosarcoma: a 10-year review. Med Pediatr Oncol 1994;22:15–21.
170. McCarville MB, Christie R, Daw NC, et al. PET/CT in the evaluation of childhood sarcomas. Am J Radiol 2005;184:1293–1304.
171. Klem ML, Grewal RK, Wexler LH, et al. PET for staging in rhabdomyosarcoma: an evaluation of PET as an adjunct to current staging tools. J Pediatr Hematol Oncol 2007;29:9–14.
172. Tateishi U, Hosono A, Makimoto A, et al. Accuracy of 18 F fluorodeoxyglucose positron emission tomography/computed tomography in staging of pediatric sarcomas. J Pediatr Hematol Oncol 2007;29:608–612.
173. Völker T, Denecke T, Steffen I, et al. Positron emission tomography for staging of pediatric sarcoma patients: results of a prospective multicenter trial. J Clin Oncol 2007; 25:5435–5441.
174. Tateishi U, Hosono A, Makimoto A, et al. Comparative study of FDG PET/CT and conventional imaging in staging of rhabdomyosarcoma. Ann Nucl Med 2009;23:155–161.
175. Raney RB Jr, Zimmerman RA, Bilaniuk LT, et al. Management of craniofacial sarcoma in childhood assisted by computed tomography. Int J Radiat Oncol Biol Phys 1979;5: 529–534.
176. Bahnson RR, Zaontz MR, Maizels M, et al. Ultrasonography and diagnosis of pediatric genitourinary rhabdomyosarcoma. Urology 1989;33:64–68.
177. Cohen MD, DeRosa GP, Kleiman M, et al. Magnetic resonance evaluation of disease of the soft tissues in children. Pediatrics 1987;79:696–701.
178. Kent DL, Haynor Dr, Longstreth WT Jr, et al. The clinical efficacy of magnetic resonance imaging in neuroimaging. Ann Intern Med 1994;120:856–871.
179. Massengill AD, Seeger LL, Eckardt JJ. The role of plain radiography, computed tomography, and magnetic resonance imaging in sarcoma evaluation. Hematol Oncol Clin North Am 1995;9:571–604.
180. Finelli A, Babyn P, McLorie GA, et al. The use of magnetic resonance imaging in the diagnosis and follow-up of pediatric pelvic rhabdomyosarcoma. J Urol 2000;163: 1952–1953.
181. Spunt SL, Anderson JR, Teot LA, et al. Routine brain imaging is unwarranted in asymptomatic patients with rhabdomyosarcoma arising outside of the head and neck region that is metastatic at diagnosis: a report from the Intergroup Rhabdomyosarcoma Study Group. Cancer 2001;92:121–125.
182. Lawrence W Jr, Anderson JR, Gehan EA, et al. Pretreatment TNM staging of childhood rhabdomyosarcoma. A report of the Intergroup Rhabdomyosarcoma Study Group. Cancer 1997;80:1165–1170.
183. Wolden SL, Anderson JR, Crist WM, et al. Indications for radiotherapy and chemotherapy after complete resection in rhabdomyosarcoma: a report from the Intergroup Rhabdomyosarcoma Studies I to III. J Clin Oncol 1999;17:3468–3475.
184. Breitfeld PP, Ullrich F, Anderson J, et al. Web-based decision support for clinical trial eligibility determination in an international clinical trials network. Control Clin Trials 2003;24:702–710.
185. Gehan EA, Glover FN, Maurer HM, et al. Prognostic factors in children with rhabdomyosarcoma. Natl Cancer Inst Monogr 1981;56:83–92.
186. Joshi D, Anderson JR, Paidas C, et al. Age is an independent prognostic factor in rhabdomyosarcoma: a report from the Soft Tissue Sarcoma Committee of the Children's Oncology Group. Pediatr Blood Cancer 2004;42:64–73.
187. Okamura J, Sutow WW, Moon TE. Prognosis in children with metastatic sarcoma. Med Pediatr Oncol 1977;3:243–251.
188. Smith LM, Anderson JR, Qualman SJ, et al. Which patients with microscopic disease and rhabdomyosarcoma experience relapse after therapy? A report from the soft tissue sarcoma committee of the children's oncology group. J Clin Oncol 2001;19:4058–4064.
189. Baker KS, Anderson JR, Link MP, et al. Benefit of intensified therapy for patients with local or regional embryonal rhabdomyosarcoma: results from the Intergroup Rhabdomyosarcoma Study IV. J Clin Oncol 2000;18:2427–2434.
190. Ferrari A, Miceli R, Meazza C, et al. Soft tissue sarcomas of childhood and adolescence: the prognostic role of tumor size in relation to patient body size. J Clin Oncol 2009;27: 371–376.
191. Dantonello TM, Int-Veen C, Harms D, et al. Cooperative Trial CWS-91 for localized soft tissue sarcoma in children, adolescents, and young adults. J Clin Oncol 2009;27: 1446–1455.
192. Anderson JR, Ruby E, Link M, et al. Identification of a favorable subset of patients (pts) with metastatic (MET) rhabdomyosarcoma (RMS): a report from the Intergroup Rhabdomyosarcoma Study Group (IRSG) [abstract]. Proc Am Soc Clin Oncol 1997;16:510.
193. Carli M, Colombatti R, Oberlin O, et al. European Intergroup Studies (MMT4–89 and MMT4–91) on childhood metastatic rhabdomyosarcoma: final results and analysis of prognostic factors. J Clin Oncol 2004;23:4735–4742.
194. Rodeberg DA, Stoner JA, Hayes-Jordan A, et al. Prognostic significance of tumor response at the end of therapy in group III rhabdomyosarcoma: a report from the Children's Oncology Group. J Clin Oncol 2009;27:3705–3711.
195. Hays DM, Lawrence W Jr, Wharam M, et al. Primary reexcision for patients with "microscopic residual" tumor following initial excision of sarcomas of trunk and extremity sites. J Pediatr Surg 1989;24:5–10.
196. Godzinski J, Flamant F, Rey A, et al. Value of postchemotherapy bioptical verification of complete clinical remission in previously incompletely resected (Stage I and II pT3) malignant mesenchymal tumors in children: International Society of Pediatric Oncology 1984 Malignant Mesenchymal Tumors Study. Med Pediatr Oncol 1994;22:22–26.
197. Hays DM, Raney RB, Crist WM, et al. Secondary surgical procedures to evaluate primary tumor status in patients with chemotherapy-responsive stage III and IV sarcomas: a report from the Intergroup Rhabdomyosarcoma Study. J Pediatr Surg 1990;25: 1100–1105.
198. Regine WF, Fontanesi J, Kumar P, et al. Local tumor control in rhabdomyosarcoma following low-dose irradiation: comparison of group II and select group III patients. Int J Radiat Oncol Biol Phys 1995;31:485–491.
199. Hawkins DS, Anderson JR, Paidas CN, et al. Improved outcome for patients with middle ear rhabdomyosarcoma: a children's oncology group study. J Clin Oncol 2001;19: 3073–3079.
200. Pappo AS, Meza JL, Donaldson SS, et al. Treatment of localized nonorbital, nonparameningeal head and neck rhabdomyosarcoma: lessons learned from intergroup rhabdomyosarcoma studies III and IV. J Clin Oncol 2003;21:638–645.
201. Walterhouse DO, Pappo AS, Baker KS, et al. Rhabdomyosarcoma of the parotid region occurring in childhood and adolescence. A report from the Intergroup Rhabdomyosarcoma Study Group. Cancer 2001;92:3135–3146.
202. Wolden SL, Wexler LH, Kraus DH, et al. Intensity-modulated radiotherapy for head-and-neck rhabdomyosarcoma. Int J Radiat Oncol Biol Phys 2005;61:1432–1438.
203. Daya H, Chan HSL, Sirkin W, et al. Pediatric rhabdomyosarcoma of the head and neck. Is there a place for surgical management. Arch Otolaryngol Head Neck Surg 2000;126: 468–472.
204. Buwalda J, Schouwenburg PF, Blank LE, et al. A novel local treatment strategy for advanced stage head and neck rhabdomyosarcomas in children: results of the AMORE protocol. Eur J Cancer 2003;39:1594–1602.
205. Olive D, Flamant F, Zucker JM, et al. Paraaortic lymphadenectomy is not necessary in the treatment of localized paratesticular rhabdomyosarcoma. Cancer 1984;54:1283–1287.
206. Wiener ES, Lawrence W, Hays D, et al. Retroperitoneal node biopsy in paratesticular rhabdomyosarcoma. J Pediatr Surg 1994;29:171–177.
207. Hermans BP, Foster RS, Bihrle R, et al. Is retroperitoneal lymph node dissection necessary for adult paratesticular rhabdomyosarcoma? J Urol 1998;160:2074–2077.
208. Goldfarb B, Khoury AE, Greenberg ML, et al. The role of retroperitoneal lymphadenectomy in localized paratesticular rhabdomyosarcoma. J Urol 1994;152:785–787.
209. Gamba PG, Cecchetto G, Katende M, et al. Paratesticular rhabdomyosarcoma (RMS) and paraaortic lymphadenectomy. Eur J Paediatr Surg 1994;4:158–160.
210. Martelli H, Oberlin O, Rey A, et al. Conservative treatment for girls with nonmetastatic rhabdomyosarcoma of the genital tract: a report from the Study Committee of the International Society of Pediatric Oncology. J Clin Oncol 1999;17:2117–2122.
211. Andrassy RJ, Wiener ES, Raney RB, et al. Progress in the surgical management of vaginal rhabdomyosarcoma: a 25-year review from the Intergroup Rhabdomyosarcoma Study Group. J Pediatr Surg 1999;34:731–734.
212. Arndt CA, Donaldson SS, Anderson JR, et al. What constitutes optimal therapy for patients with rhabdomyosarcoma of the female genital tract? Cancer 2001;91:2454–2468.
213. Hays DM, Lawrence W Jr, Crist WM, et al. Partial cystectomy in the management of rhabdomyosarcoma of the bladder: a report from the Intergroup Rhabdomyosarcoma Study. J Pediatr Surg 1990;25:719–723.

214. Hays DM, Raney RB, Wharam MD, et al. Children with vesical rhabdomyosarcoma (RMS) treated by partial cystectomy with neoadjuvant or adjuvant chemotherapy, with or without radiotherapy. J Pediatr Hematol Oncol 1995;17:46–52.
215. Hays DM. Bladder/prostate rhabdomyosarcoma: results of the multi-institutional trials of the Intergroup Rhabdomyosarcoma Study. Semin Surg Oncol 1993;9:520–523.
216. Fryer CJH. Pelvic rhabdomyosarcoma: paying the price of bladder preservation [editorial]. Lancet 1995;345:141–142.
217. Lobe TE, Wiener E, Andrassy RJ, et al. The argument for conservative, delayed surgery in the management of prostatic rhabdomyosarcoma. J Pediatr Surg 1996;31:1084–1087.
218. Heyn R, Newton WA, Raney RB, et al. Preservation of the bladder in patients with rhabdomyosarcoma. J Clin Oncol 1997;15:69–75.
219. Arndt C, Rodeberg D, Breitfeld PP, et al. Does bladder preservation (as a surgical principle) lead to retaining bladder function in bladder/prostate rhabdomyosarcoma? Results from Intergroup Rhabdomyosarcoma Study IV. J Urol 2004;171:2396–2403.
220. Beech TR, Moss RL, Anderson JA, et al. What comprises appropriate therapy for children/adolescents with rhabdomyosarcoma arising in the abdominal wall? A report from the Intergroup Rhabdomyosarcoma Study Group. J Pediatr Surg 1999;34:668–671.
221. Raney RB, Anderson JR, Andrassy RJ, et al. Soft-tissue sarcomas of the diaphragm: a report from the Intergroup Rhabdomyosarcoma Study Group from 1972 to 1997. J Pediatr Hematol Oncol 2000;22:510–514.
222. Temeck BK, Wexler LH, Steinberg SM, et al. Metastectomy for sarcomatous pediatric histologies: results and prognostic factors. Ann Thorac Surg 1995;59:1385–1390.
223. Stevens MCG, Rey A, Bouver N, et al. Treatment of nonmetastatic rhabdomyosarcoma in childhood and adolescence: Third Study of the International Society of Paediatric Oncology—SIOP Malignant Mesenchyma Tumor 89. J Clin Oncol 2005;23:2618–2628.
224. Donaldson SS, Anderson JR. Rhabdomyosarcoma: many similarities, a few philosophical differences. J Clin Oncol 2005;23:2586–2587.
225. Suit HD, Russell WO, Martin RG. Management of patients with sarcoma of soft tissue in an extremity. Cancer 1973;31:1247–1255.
226. Dritschilo A, Weichselbaum R, Cassady JR, et al. The role of radiation therapy in the treatment of soft tissue sarcomas of childhood. Cancer 1978;42:1192–1203.
227. Heyn RM, Holland R, Newton WA Jr, et al. The role of combined chemotherapy in the treatment of rhabdomyosarcoma in children. Cancer 1974;34:2128–2142.
228. Tefft M, Lindberg RD, Gehan EA. Radiation therapy combined with systemic chemotherapy of rhabdomyosarcoma in children: local control in patients enrolled in the Intergroup Rhabdomyosarcoma Study. Natl Cancer Inst Monogr 1981;56:75–81.
229. Tefft M, Wharam M, Ruymann F, et al. Radiotherapy (RT) for rhabdomyosarcoma in children: a report from the Intergroup Rhabdomyosarcoma Study 2 (IRS-2) [abstract]. Proc Am Soc Clin Oncol 1985;4:234.
230. Tefft M, Wharam M, Gehan E. Radiation therapy in embryonal rhabdomyosarcoma (ERS): local control (LC) in children less than one year of age and in children with tumors of the orbit [abstract]. Proc Am Soc Clin Oncol 1986;5:205.
231. Raney RB Jr, Crist WM, Maurer HM, et al. Prognosis of children with soft tissue sarcoma who relapse after achieving a complete response. A report from the Intergroup Rhabdomyosarcoma Study I. Cancer 1983;52:44–50.
232. Tefft M, Wharam M, Gehan E. Local and regional control by radiation of rhabdomyosarcoma in IRS [abstract]. Proc Am Soc Clin Oncol 1988;7:259.
233. Tefft M, Wharam M, Gehan E. Local and regional control by radiation of rhabdomyosarcoma in IRS II [abstract]. Int J Radiat Oncol Biol Phys 1988;15(suppl 1):159.
234. Michalski JM, Meza J, Breneman JC, et al. Influence of radiation therapy parameters on outcome in children treated with radiation therapy for localized parameningeal rhabdomyosarcoma in Intergroup Rhabdomyosarcoma Study Group Trials II Through IV. Int J Radiat Oncol Biol Phys 2004;59:1027–1038.
235. Smith SC, Lindsley SK, Felgenhauer J, et al. Intensive induction chemotherapy and delayed irradiation in the management of parameningeal rhabdomyosarcoma. J Pediatr Hematol Oncol 2003;25:774–779.
236. Puri DR, Wexler LH, Meyers PA, et al. The challenging role of radiation therapy for very young children with rhabdomyosarcoma. Int J Radiat Oncol Biol Phys 2006;65:1177–1184.
237. Klingebiel T, Boos J, Beske F, et al. Treatment of children with metastatic soft tissue sarcoma with oral maintenance compared to high dose chemotherapy: report of the HD CWS-96 trial. Pediatr Blood Cancer 2008;50:739–745.
238. McDonald MW, Esiashvili N, George BA, et al. Intensity-modulated radiation therapy with use of cone-down boost for pediatric head-and-neck rhabdomyosarcoma. Int J Radiat Oncol Biol Phys 2008;72:884–891.
239. Chen C, Shu HK, Goldwein JW, et al. Volumetric considerations in radiotherapy for pediatric parameningeal rhabdomyosarcomas. Int J Radiat Oncol Biol Phys 2003;55:1294–1299.
240. Wharam MD, Hanfelt JJ, Tefft MC, et al. Radiation therapy for rhabdomyosarcoma: local failure risk for Clinical Group III patients on Intergroup Rhabdomyosarcoma Study II. Int J Radiation Oncol Biol Phys 1997;38:797–804.
241. Wharam MD, Meza J, Anderson J, et al. Failure pattern and factors predictive of local failure in rhabdomyosarcoma: a report of group III patients on the third Intergroup Rhabdomyosarcoma Study. J Clin Oncol 2004;22:1902–1908.
242. Donaldson SS, Asmar L, Breneman J, et al. Hyperfractionated radiation in children with rhabdomyosarcoma: results of an Intergroup Rhabdomyosarcoma Pilot Study. Int J Radiat Oncol Biol Phys 1995;32:903–911.
243. Regine WF, Fontanesi J, Kumar P, et al. A phase II trial evaluating selective use of altered radiation dose and fractionation in patients with unresectable rhabdomyosarcoma. Int J Radiat Oncol Biol Phys 1995;31:799–805.
244. Donaldson SS, Meza J, Breneman JC, et al. Results from the IRS-IV randomized trial of hyperfractionated radiotherapy in children with rhabdomyosarcoma: a report from the IRSG. Int J Radiat Oncol Biol Phys 2001;51:718–728.
245. Tefft M, Lattin PB, Jereb B, et al. Acute and late effects on normal tissues following combined chemo- and radiotherapy for childhood rhabdomyosarcoma and Ewing's sarcoma. Cancer 1976;37(2 suppl):1201–1217.
246. Wohl ME, Griscom NT, Traggis DG, et al. Effects of therapeutic irradiation delivered in early childhood upon subsequent lung function. Pediatrics 1975;55:507–516.
247. Abramson DH, Notis CM. Visual acuity after radiation for orbital rhabdomyosarcoma. Am J Ophthalmol 1994;118:808–809.
248. Raney RB, Asmar L, Vassilopoulou-Sellin R, et al. Late complications of therapy in 213 children with localized, nonorbital soft-tissue sarcoma of the head and neck: a descriptive report from the Intergroup Rhabdomyosarcoma Studies (IRS)-II and -III. Med Pediatr Oncol 1999;33:362–371.
249. Raney RB, Anderson JR, Kollath J, et al. Late effects of therapy in 94 patients with localized rhabdomyosarcoma of the orbit: report from the Intergroup Rhabdomyosarcoma Study (IRS)-III, 1984–1991. Med Pediatr Oncol 2000;34:413–420.
250. Fiorillo A, Migliorati R, Vassallo P, et al. Radiation late effects in children treated for orbital rhabdomyosarcoma. Radiother Oncol 1999;53:143–148.
251. Estilo CL, Huryn JM, Kraus DH, et al. Effects of therapy on dentofacial development in long-term survivors of head and neck rhabdomyosarcoma: the Memorial Sloan-Kettering Cancer Center experience. J Pediatr Hematol Oncol 2003;25:215–222.
252. Rousseau P, Flamant F, Quintana E, et al. Primary chemotherapy in rhabdomyosarcoma and other malignant mesenchymal tumors of the orbit: results of the International Society of Pediatric Oncology MMT 84 Study. J Clin Oncol 1994;12:516–521.
253. Plowman PN, Mannor G, Kingston J, et al. Optimal management of localized orbital rhabdomyosarcoma [abstract]. Proc Am Soc Clin Oncol 1995;14:450.
254. Oberlin O, Rey A, Anderson J, et al. Treatment of orbital rhabdomyosarcoma: survival and late effects of treatment–results of an international workshop. J Clin Oncol 2001;19:197–204.
255. Howard S, Marcus K, Grier H, et al. The effects of extensive bone erosion on prognosis in children with non-orbital rhabdomyosarcoma of the head and neck [abstract]. Int J Radiat Oncol Biol Phys 1994;29:205.
256. Jaffe N, Rott J, Woo S, et al. Is there a safe therapeutic window for the delivery of chemotherapy (CT) prior to initiation of radiation therapy (XRT) and/or surgery (S) for treatment of the primary tumor in children with rhabdomyosarcoma (RMS)? [abstract]. Proc Am Assoc Cancer Res 1992;33:209.
257. Cassady JR. How much is enough? The continuing evolution of therapy in childhood rhabdomyosarcoma and its refinement [editorial]. Int J Radiat Oncol Biol Phys 1995;31:675–676.
258. Mandell L, Ghavimi F, Peretz T, et al. Radiocurability of microscopic disease in childhood rhabdomyosarcoma with radiation doses less than 4000 cGy. J Clin Oncol 1990;8:1536–1542.
259. Koscielniak E, Herbst Niethammer D, et al. Improvement of local tumor control in primary nonresectable rhabdomyosarcoma by early, risk-adapted radiotherapy: report of the German Cooperative Soft Tissue Sarcoma Studies CSW-81 and 86. Klin Padiatr 1994;206:269–276.
260. Benk V, Rodary C, Donaldson SS, et al. Parameningeal rhabdomyosarcoma: results of an international workshop. Int J Radiat Oncol Biol Phys 1996;36:533–540.
261. Stowe SM, Littman P, Wara W, et al. The use of implantation in childhood tumors: the experience of the Children's Cancer Study Group member institutions [abstract]. Am J Clin Oncol 1982;5:129.
262. Novaes PE. Interstitial therapy in the management of soft-tissue sarcomas in childhood. Med Pediatr Oncol 1985;13:221–224.
263. Nag S, Grecula J, Ruymann FB. Aggressive chemotherapy, organ-preserving surgery, and high-dose-rate remote brachytherapy in the treatment of rhabdomyosarcoma in infants and children. Cancer 1993;72:2769–2776.
264. Fontanesi J, Rao BN, Fleming ID, et al. Pediatric brachytherapy: the St. Jude Children's Research Hospital experience. Cancer 1994;74:733–739.
265. Kaufman BH, Gunderson LL, Evans RG, et al. Intraoperative irradiation: a new technique in pediatric oncology. J Pediatr Surg 1984;19:861–862.
266. Teh BS, Woo SY, Butler EB. Intensity modulated radiation therapy (IMRT): a new promising technology in radiation oncology. Oncologist 1999;4:433–442.
267. Purdy JA. Future directions in 3-D treatment planning and deliver: a physicist's perspective [editorial]. Int J Radiat Oncol Biol Phys 2000;46:3–6.
268. Wu Q, Manning M, Schmidt-Ullrich R, et al. The potential for sparing of parotids and escalation of biologically effective dose with intensity-modulated radiation treatments of head and neck cancers: a treatment design study. Int J Radiat Oncol Biol Phys 2000;46:195–205.
269. Wolden SL, La TH, LaQuaglia MP, et al. Long-term results of three-dimensional conformal radiation therapy for patients with rhabdomyosarcoma. Cancer 2003;97:179–185.
270. Michalski JM, Sur RK, Harms WB, et al. Three-dimensional conformal radiation therapy in pediatric parameningeal rhabdomyosarcomas. Int J Radiat Oncol Biol Phys 1995;33:985–991.
271. Miralbell R, Cella L, Weber D, et al. Optimizing radiotherapy of orbital and paraorbital tumors: intensity-modulate x-ray beams vs. intensity-modulated proton beams. Int J Radiat Oncol Biol Phys 2000;47:1111–1119.
272. Hug EB, Adams J, Fitzek M, et al. Fractionated, three-dimensional, planning-assisted proton-radiation therapy for orbital rhabdomyosarcoma: a novel technique. Int J Radiat Oncol Biol Phys 2000;47:979–984.
273. Ling CC, Humm J, Larson S, et al. Towards multidimensional radiotherapy (MD-CRT): biological imaging and biological conformity. Int J Radiat Oncol Biol Phys 2000;47:551–560.
274. Kozak KR, Adams J, Krejcarek SJ, et al. A dosimetric comparison of proton and intensity-modulated photon radiotherapy for pediatric parameningeal rhabdomyosarcomas. Int J Radiat Oncol Biol Phys 2009;74:179–186.
275. Pinkel D. Actinomycin D in childhood cancer: a preliminary report. Pediatrics 1959;23:342–347.
276. Tan CTC, Dargeon HW, Burcheral JH. The effect of actinomycin-D on cancer in childhood. Pediatrics 1959;24:544–561.
277. Haddy TB, Nora AH, Sutow WW, et al. Cyclophosphamide treatment for metastatic soft tissue sarcoma: intermittent large doses in the treatment of children. Am J Dis Child 1967;114:301–308.
278. Sutow WW, Berry DH, Haddy TB, et al. Vincristine sulfate therapy in children with metastatic soft tissue sarcoma. Pediatrics 1966;38:465–472.
279. Sutow WW. Vincristine (NSC-67574) therapy for malignant solid tumors in children (except Wilms' tumor). Cancer Chemother Rep 1968;52:485–487.
280. Bonadonna G, Monfardini S, DeLena M, et al. Phase I and preliminary phase II evaluation of Adriamycin (NSC-123127). Cancer Res 1970;30:2572–2582.
281. Tan C, Etcubanas E, Wollner N, et al. Adriamycin: an antitumor antibiotic in the treatment of neoplastic diseases. Cancer 1973;32:9–17.
282. Sutow WW, Vietti TJ, Lonsdale D, et al. Daunomycin in the treatment of metastatic soft tissue sarcoma in children. Cancer 1972;29:1293–1297.
283. Fisher BK, Elliott GB. Triple drug therapy with actinomycin D (NSC-3053), chlorambucil (NSC-3088), and methotrexate (NSC-740) in metastatic solid tumors in children. Cancer Chemother Rep 1965;45:45–51.
284. Green DM. Evaluation of single-dose vincristine, actinomycin D, and cyclophosphamide in childhood solid tumors. Cancer Treat Rep 1978;62:1517–1520.
285. Gottlieb JA, Baker LH, Quagliana JM, et al. Chemotherapy of sarcomas with a combination of Adriamycin and dimethyl triazeno imidazole carboxamide. Cancer 1972;30:1632–1638.

286. Wilbur JR. Combination chemotherapy for embryonal rhabdomyosarcoma. Cancer Chemother Rep 1974;58:281–284.
287. James DH, Hustu O, Wrenn EL, et al. Childhood malignant tumors: concurrent chemotherapy with dactinomycin and vincristine sulfate. JAMA 1966;197:1043–1045.
288. Holton CP, Chapman KE, Lackey RW, et al. Extended combination therapy of childhood rhabdomyosarcoma. Cancer 1973;32:1310–1316.
289. Razek AA, Perez CA, Lee FA, et al. Combined treatment modalities of rhabdomyosarcoma in children. Cancer 1977;39:2415–2421.
290. Pratt CB, Hustu HO, Mahesh-Kumar AP, et al. Treatment of childhood rhabdomyosarcoma at St. Jude Children's Research Hospital, 1962–1978. Natl Cancer Inst Monogr 1981;56:93–101.
291. Kingston JE, McElwain TJ, Malpas JS. Childhood rhabdomyosarcoma: experience of the Children's Solid Tumor Group. Br J Cancer 1983;48:195–207.
292. Ghavimi F, Exelby PR, Lieberman PH, et al. Multidisciplinary treatment of embryonal rhabdomyosarcoma in children: a progress report. Natl Cancer Inst Monogr 1981;56: 111–120.
293. Lager JJ, Lyden ER, Anderson JR, et al. Pooled analysis for phase II window studies in children with contemporary high-risk metastatic rhabdomyosarcoma: a report from the Soft Tissue Sarcoma Committee of the Children's Oncology Group. J Clin Oncol 2006;24:3415–3422.
294. Chan HSL, DeBoer G, Haddad G, et al. Multidrug resistance in pediatric malignancies. Hematol Oncol Clin North Am 1995;9:275–318.
295. Houghton JA, Cook RL, Lutz PJ, et al. Childhood rhabdomyosarcoma xenografts: responses to DNA-interacting agents and agents used in current clinical therapy. Eur J Cancer Clin Oncol 1984;20:955–960.
296. Houghton JA, Cook RL, Lutz PJ, et al. Melphalan: a potential new agent in the treatment of childhood rhabdomyosarcoma. Cancer Treat Rep 1985;69:91–96.
297. Houghton P, Cheshire P, Myers L, et al. Evaluation of 9-dimethylaminomethyl-10-hydroxy camptothecin against xenografts derived from adult and childhood tumors. Cancer Chemother Pharmacol 1992;31:229–239.
298. Horowitz ME, Etcubanas E, Christensen ML, et al. Phase II testing of melphalan in children with newly diagnosed rhabdomyosarcoma: a model for anticancer drug development. J Clin Oncol 1988;6:308–314.
299. Pappo AS, Bowman LC, Furman WL, et al. A phase II trial of high-dose methotrexate in previously untreated children and adolescents with high-risk unresectable or metastatic rhabdomyosarcoma. J Pediatr Hematol Oncol 1997;19:438–442.
300. Pappo AS, Lyden E, Breneman J, et al. Up-front window trial of topotecan in previously untreated children and adolescents with metastatic rhabdomyosarcoma: an intergroup rhabdomyosarcoma study. J Clin Oncol 2001;19:213–219.
301. Walterhouse DO, Lyden ER, Breitfeld PP, et al. Efficacy of topotecan and cyclophosphamide given as a phase II window in children with newly diagnosed metastatic rhabdomyosarcoma: a report from the Soft Tissue Sarcoma Committee of the Children's Oncology Group. J Clin Oncol 2004;22:1398–1403.
302. Bode U. Methotrexate as relapse therapy for rhabdomyosarcoma. Am J Pediatr Hematol Oncol 1986;8:70–72.
303. Blaney SM, Needle MN, Gillespie A, et al. Phase II trial of topotecan administered as a 72-hour continuous infusion in children with refractory solid tumors: a collaborative Pediatric Branch, National Cancer Institute, and Children's Cancer Group Study. Clin Cancer Res 1998;4:357–360.
304. Saylors RL, Stine KC, Sullivan J, et al. Cyclophosphamide plus topotecan in children with recurrent or refractory solid tumors: a Pediatric Oncology Group Phase II Study. J Clin Oncol 2001;19:3463–3469.
305. Etcubanas E, Horowtiz M, Vogel R. Combination of dacarbazine and doxorubicin in the treatment of childhood rhabdomyosarcoma. Cancer Treat Rep 1985;69:999–1000.
306. Breitfeld PP, Lyden E, Beverly RR, et al. Ifosfamide and etoposide are superior to vincristine and melphalan for pediatric metastatic rhabdomyosarcoma when administered with irradiation and combination chemotherapy: a report from the Intergroup Rhabdomyosarcoma Study Group. Am J Pediatr Hematol Oncol 2001;23:225–233.
307. Ruymann FB, Grovas AC. Progress in the diagnosis and treatment of rhabdomyosarcoma and related soft tissue sarcomas. Cancer Invest 2000;18:223–241.
308. Sandler E, Lyden E, Ruymann F, et al. Efficacy of ifosfamide and doxorubicin given as a phase II "window" in children with newly diagnosed metastatic rhabdomyosarcoma: a report from the Intergroup Rhabdomyosarcoma Study Group. Med Pediatr Oncol 2001;37:442–448.
309. Baker KS, Anderson JR, Lobe TE, et al. Children from ethnic minorities have benefited equally as other children from contemporary therapy for rhabdomyosarcoma: a report from the Intergroup Rhabdomyosarcoma Study Group. J Clin Oncol 2002;20:4428–4433.
310. Arndt CAS, Stoner JA, Hawkins DS, et al. Vincristine/actinomycin/cyclophosphamide (VAC) versus VAC alternating with vincristine/topotecan/cyclophosphamide for intermediate risk rhabdomyosarcoma. Results of COG D9803. A report from the Children's Oncology Group. J Clin Oncol 2009;27:5182–5186.
311. Pappo AS, Lyden E, Breitfeld P, et al. Two consecutive phase II window trials of irinotecan alone or in combination with vincristine for the treatment of metastatic rhabdomyosarcoma: the Children's Oncology Group. J Clin Oncol 2007;25:362–369.
312. Goldie JH, Coldman AJ. The genetic origin of drug resistance in neoplasms: implications for systemic therapy. Cancer Res 1984;4:3643–3653.
313. Pastan I, Gottesman M. Multiple-drug resistance in human cancer. N Engl J Med 1987; 316:1388–1393.
314. Baum ES, Gaynon P, Greenberg L, et al. Phase II trial of cisplatin in refractory childhood cancer: Children's Cancer Study Group Report. Cancer Treat Rep 1981;65:815–822.
315. Chard RL Jr, Krivit W, Bleyer WA, et al. Phase II study of VP-16–213 in childhood malignant disease: a Children's Cancer Study Group report. Cancer Treat Rep 1979;63: 1755–1759.
316. Finkelstein JZ, Albo V, Ertel I, et al. 5-(3,3-Dimethyl-triazeno) imidazole-4-carboxamide (NSC-45388) in the treatment of solid tumors in children. Cancer Chemother Rep 1975;59:351–357.
317. Miser JS, Kinsella TJ, Triche TJ, et al. Ifosfamide with mesna uroprotection and etoposide: an effective regimen in the treatment of recurrent sarcomas and other tumors of children and young adults. J Clin Oncol 1987;5:1191–1198.
318. Raney RB Jr. Inefficacy of cisplatin and etoposide as salvage therapy for children with recurrent or unresponsive soft issue sarcoma. Cancer Treat Rep 1987;71:407–408.
319. Crist W, Raney RB, Ragab A, et al. Intensive chemotherapy including cisplatin with or without etoposide for children with soft-tissue sarcomas. Med Pediatr Oncol 1987;15: 51–57.
320. Chisholm JC, Machin D, McDowell H, et al. Efficacy of carboplatin given in a phase II window study to children and adolescents with newly diagnosed metastatic soft tissue sarcoma. Eur J Cancer 2007;43:2537–2544.
321. Kung FH, Pratt CB, Bernstein M, et al. Ifosfamide/VP-16 combination in the treatment of recurrent malignant solid tumors of childhood: a POG phase II study [abstract]. Proc Am Soc Clin Oncol 1991;10:307.
322. Carli M, Treuner J, Koscileniak E, et al. Ifosfamide (IFO) more is better? 6 vs. 10 gr/m^2 in VAIA may influence the tumor response rate in childhood rhabdomyosarcoma (RMS)? The experience of the German (CWS-86) and the Italian (ICS-RMS 88) Cooperative Studies [abstract]. Proc Am Soc Clin Oncol 1991;10:319.
323. Pappo AS, Etcubanas E, Santana VM, et al. A phase II trial of ifosfamide in previously untreated children and adolescents with unresectable rhabdomyosarcoma. Cancer 1993;71:2119–2125.
324. Kamen BA, Frenkel E, Colvin OM. Ifosfamide: should the honeymoon be over? [editorial]. J Clin Oncol 1995;13:307–309.
325. Furman WL, Steward CF, Poquette CA, et al. Direct translation of a protracted irinotecan schedule from a xenograft model to a phase I trial in children. J Clin Oncol 1999; 17:1815–1824.
326. Pappo AS, Lyden E, Breitfeld PP, et al. Irinotecan (CPT-11) is active against pediatric rhabdomyosarcoma (RMS): a phase II window trial from the Soft Tissue Sarcoma Committee (STS) of the Children's Oncology Group (COG) [abstract]. Proc Am Soc Clin Oncol 2002;21.
327. Huizing MT, Sewberath Misser VH, Pieters RC, et al. Taxanes: a new class of antitumor agents. Cancer Invest 1995;13:381–404.
328. Blaney SM, Seibel NL, O'Brien M, et al. Phase I trial of docetaxel administered as a 1-hour infusion in children with refractory solid tumors: a collaborative Pediatric Branch, National Cancer Institute and Children's Cancer Group Trial. J Clin Oncol 1997;15:1538–1543.
329. Hurwitz CA, Relling MV, Weitman SD, et al. Phase I trial of paclitaxel in children with refractory solid tumors: a Pediatric Oncology Group study. J Clin Oncol 1993;11: 2324–2329.
330. Epelman S, Aguiar S, Melaragno R, et al. High response rate of vinorelbine (VNR) in children and adolescents with refractory or recurrent rhabdomiosarcomas (RMS) or other sarcomas (STS) [abstract]. Med Pediatr Oncol 1999;33:227.
331. Casanova M, Ferrari A, Spreafico F, et al. Vinorelbine in previously treated advanced childhood sarcomas: evidence of activity in rhabdomyosarcoma. Cancer 2002;94: 3263–3268.
332. Etcubanas E, Rao BN, Kun LE, et al. The impact of delayed surgery on radiotherapy dose and local control of rhabdomyosarcoma. Arch Surg 1987;122:1451–1454.
333. Tefft M, Fernandez CH, Moon TE. Rhabdomyosarcoma: response to chemotherapy prior to radiation in patients with gross residual disease. Cancer 1977;39:665–670.
334. Phillips TL, Fu KK. Quantification of combined radiation therapy and chemotherapy effects on critical normal tissues. Cancer 1976;37(2 suppl):1186–1200.
335. Casanova M, Ferrari A, Bisogno G, et al. Vinorelbine and low-dose cyclophosphamide in the treatment of pediatric sarcomas. Pilot study for the upcoming European rhabdomyosarcoma protocol. Cancer 2004;101:1664–1671.
336. Stevens MCG. Treatment for childhood rhabdomyosarcoma: the cost for cure. Lancet Oncol 2005;6:77–84.
337. Mascarenhas L, Lyden ER, Breitfeld PP, et al. Randomized phase II window study of two schedules of irinotecan (CPT-11) and vincristine (VCR) in rhabdomyosarcoma (RMS) at first relapse/disease progression. Proc Am Soc Clin Oncol 2008;26:10013.
338. Breitfeld PP, Mascarenhas L, Lyden ER, et al. Safety and efficacy of tirapazamine (TPZ) combined with cyclophosphamide (C) and doxorubicin (D) in rhabdomyosarcoma (RMS) at first relapse/disease progression. Proc Am Soc Clin Oncol 2008;26:10035.
339. Treuner J, Kuehl J, Beck J, et al. New aspects in the treatment of childhood rhabdomyosarcoma: results of the German Cooperative Soft-Tissue Sarcoma Study (CWS-81). Prog Pediatr Surg 1989;22:162–173.
340. Horowitz ME, Kinsella TJ, Wexler LH, et al. Total-body irradiation and autologous bone marrow transplant in the treatment of high-risk Ewing's sarcoma and rhabdomyosarcoma. J Clin Oncol 1993;11:1911–1918.
341. Ghavimi F, Mandell LR, Heller G, et al. Prognosis in childhood rhabdomyosarcoma of the extremity. Cancer 1989;64:2233–2337.
342. Dantonello TM, Int-Veen C, Winkler P, et al. Initial patient characteristics can predict pattern and risk of relapse in localized rhabdomyosarcoma. J Clin Oncol 2008;26: 406–413.
343. Spunt SL, Smith LM, Ruymann FB, et al. Cyclophosphamide dose intensification during induction therapy for intermediate-risk pediatric rhabdomyosarcoma is feasible but does not improve outcome: a report from the Soft Tissue Sarcoma Committee of the Children's Oncology Group. Clin Cancer Res 2004;10:6072–6079.
344. Flamant F, Rodary C, Rey A, et al. Treatment of non-metastatic rhabdomyosarcomas in childhood and adolescence. Results of the second study of the International Society of Paediatric Oncology: MMT84. Eur J Cancer 1998;34:1050–1062.
345. Koscielniak E, Harms D, Henze G, et al. Results of treatment for soft tissue sarcoma in childhood and adolescence: a final report of the German Cooperative Soft Tissue Sarcoma Study CWS-86. J Clin Oncol 1999;17:3706–3719.
346. Arndt CAS, Nascimento AG, Schroeder G, et al. Treatment of intermediate risk rhabdomyosarcoma and undifferentiated sarcoma with alternating cycles of vincristine/ doxorubicin/cyclophosphamide and etoposide/ifosfamide. Eur J Cancer 1998;34:1224–1229.
347. Womer RB, Daller RE, Gallagher Fenton J, et al. Granulocyte colony stimulating factor permits dose intensification by interval compression in the treatment of Ewing's sarcomas and soft tissue sarcomas in children. Eur J Cancer 2000;36:87–94.
348. Koscielniak E, Klingebiel TH, Peters C, et al. Do patients with metastatic and recurrent rhabdomyosarcoma benefit from high-dose therapy with hematopoietic rescue? Report of the German/Austrian Pediatric Bone Marrow Transplantation Group. Bone Marrow Transplant 1997;19:227–231.
349. Boulad F, Kernan NA, LaQuaglia MP, et al. High-dose induction chemoradiotherapy followed by autologous bone marrow transplantation as consolidation therapy in rhabdomyosarcoma, extraosseous Ewing's sarcoma, and undifferentiated sarcoma. J Clin Oncol 1998;16:1697–1706.
350. Bisogno G, Ferrari A, Prete A, et al. Sequential high-dose chemotherapy for children with metastatic rhabdomyosarcoma. Eur J Cancer 2009;45:3035–3041. doi:10.1016/ j.ejca.2009.08.019.
351. Carli M, Colombatti R, Oberlin O, et al. High-dose melphalan with autologous stem-cell rescue in metastatic rhabdomyosarcoma. J Clin Oncol 1999;17:2796–2803.
352. Malogolowkin MH, Sposto R, Grovas L, et al. Lack of improvement in survival of children with metastatic rhabdomyosarcoma (RMS) treated with intensive therapy

followed by stem cell transplant (SCT) for control of minimal residual disease [abstract]. Proc Am Soc Clin Oncol 1999;18:555.

353. Weigel BJ, Breitfeld PP, Hawkins D, et al. Role of high-dose chemotherapy with hematopoietic stem cell rescue in the treatment of metastatic or recurrent rhabdomyosarcoma. J Pediatr Hematol Oncol 2001;23:272–276.

354. Lobe TE, Wiener ES, Hays DM, et al. Neonatal rhabdomyosarcoma: the IRS experience. J Pediatr Surg 1994;29:1167–1170.

355. Fusner JE, Poplack DG, Pizzo PA, et al. Leukoencephalopathy following chemotherapy for rhabdomyosarcoma: reversibility of cerebral changes demonstrated by computed tomography. J Pediatr 1977;91:77–79.

356. Raney B, Tefft M, Heyn R, et al. Ascending myelitis in children with cranial parameningeal sarcoma. Cancer 1992;60:1498–1506.

357. Heyn RM. Late effects of therapy in rhabdomyosarcoma. Clin Oncol 1985;4:287–297.

358. Raney RB, Asmar L, Vassilopoulou-Sellin R, et al. Late sequelae in 162 patients with non-orbital soft-tissue sarcoma of the head and neck: report from Intergroup Rhabdomyosarcoma Studies (IRS)-II and -III [abstract]. Proc Am Soc Clin Oncol 1995;14:454.

359. Atra A, Ward HC, Aitken K, et al. Conservative surgery in multimodal therapy for pelvic rhabdomyosarcoma in children. Br J Cancer 1994;70:1004–1008.

360. Raney B Jr, Heyn R, Hays DM, et al. Sequelae of treatment in 109 patients followed for 5 to 15 years after diagnosis of sarcoma of the bladder and prostate. A report from the Intergroup Rhabdomyosarcoma Study Committee. Cancer 1993;71:2387–2394.

361. Yeung CK, Ward HC, Ransley PG, et al. Bladder and kidney function after cure of pelvic rhabdomyosarcoma in childhood. Br J Cancer 1994;70:1000–1003.

362. Jayalakshmamma B, Pinkel D. Urinary-bladder toxicity following pelvic irradiation and simultaneous cyclophosphamide therapy. Cancer 1976;38:701–707.

363. Andriole GL, Sandlund JT, Miser JS, et al. The efficacy of mesna (2-mercaptoethane sodium sulfonate) as a uroprotectant in patients with hemorrhagic cystitis receiving further oxazaphosphorine chemotherapy. J Clin Oncol 1987;5:799–803.

364. Lentz RD, Bergstein J, Steffes MW, et al. Postpubertal evaluation of gonadal function following cyclophosphamide therapy before and during puberty. J Pediatr 1977;91:385–394.

365. Heyn R, Raney RB, Hays DM, et al. Late effects of therapy in patients with paratesticular rhabdomyosarcoma. J Clin Oncol 1992;10:614–623.

366. Hughes LL, Baruzzi MJ, Ribeiro RC, et al. Paratesticular rhabdomyosarcoma: delayed effects of multimodality therapy and implications for current management. Cancer 1994;73:476–482.

367. Skinner R, Pearson ADJ, Price L, et al. Nephrotoxicity after ifosfamide. Arch Dis Child 1990;65:732–738.

368. Raney B, Ensign LG, Foreman J, et al. Renal toxicity of ifosfamide in pilot regimens of the Intergroup Rhabdomyosarcoma Study for patients with gross residual tumor. Am J Pediatr Hematol Oncol 1994;16:286–295.

369. Heyn R, Haeberlen V, Newton WA, et al. Second malignant neoplasms in children treated for rhabdomyosarcoma. J Clin Oncol 1993;11:262–270.

370. Heyn R, Khan F, Ensign LG, et al. Acute myeloid leukemia in patients treated for rhabdomyosarcoma with cyclophosphamide and low-dose etoposide on Intergroup Rhabdomyosarcoma Study III: an interim report. Med Pediatr Oncol 1994;23:99–106.

371. Pappo A, Anderson J, Qualman S, et al. Second malignant neoplasms in IRSG-IV: a preliminary report from the Intergroup Rhabdomyosarcoma Study Group [abstract]. Proc Am Soc Clin Oncol 2000;19:584.

372. Smith MA, Rubinstein L, Ungerleider RS. Therapy-related acute myeloid leukemia following treatment with epipodophyllotoxins: establishing the risks. Med Pediatr Oncol 1994;23:86–98.

373. Spunt SL, Meza JL, Anderson JR. Second malignant neoplasms (SMN) in children treated for rhabdomyosarcoma: a report from the Intergroup Rhabdomyosarcoma Studies (IRS) I-IV [abstract]. Proc Annu Meet Am Soc Clin Oncol 2001;20:2173.

374. Chestler RJ, Dortzbach RK, Kronish JW. Late recurrence in primary orbital rhabdomyosarcoma. Am J Ophthalmol 1988;106:92–93.

375. Wight RG, Harris SC, Shortland JR, et al. Rhabdomyosarcoma of the nasopharynx, a case with recurrence of tumour after 20 years. J Laryngol Otolaryngol 1988;102:1182–1184.

376. Zacharin M, Waters K, Chow CW, et al. Recurrent rhabdomyosarcoma after 25 years: a possible association with estrogen and progestogen therapy. J Pediatr Hematol Oncol 1997;19:477–481.

377. Sivanandan R, Kong C, Kaplan MJ, et al. Laryngeal embryonal rhabdomyosarcoma: a case of cervical metastases 13 years after treatment and a 25-year review of existing literature. Arch Otolaryngol Head Neck Surg 2004;130:1217–1222.

378. Sung L, Anderson JR, Donaldson SS, et al. Late events occurring five years or more after successful therapy for childhood rhabdomyosarcoma: a report from the Soft Tissue Sarcoma Committee of the Children's Oncology Group. Eur J Cancer 2004;40:1878–1885.

379. Gerlach JH, Bell DR, Karakousis C, et al. P-Glycoprotein in human sarcoma: evidence for multidrug resistance. J Clin Oncol 1987;5:1452–1460.

380. Chan HSL, Thorner PS, Haddad G, et al. Immunohistochemical detection of P-glycoprotein: prognostic correlation in soft tissue sarcoma of childhood. J Clin Oncol 1990;8:689–704.

381. Kuttesch J, Parham D, Luo X, et al. P-glycoprotein (PGP) expression at diagnosis is not predictive of worse outcome in pediatric rhabdomyosarcoma [abstract]. Proc Am Soc Clin Oncol 1994;13:413.

382. McDowell H, Peuchmaur M, Dominici C, et al. Multidrug resistance gene transcript level, and P-glycoprotein expression in paediatric malignant mesenchymal tumours. Anticancer Res 1993;13:1863–1866.

383. Nyce J. Drug-induced DNA hypermethylation and drug resistance in human tumors. Cancer Res 1989;49:5829–5836.

384. Friedman HS, Dolan ME, Kaufmann SH, et al. Elevated DNA polymerase a, DNA polymerase b, and DNA topoisomerase II in a melphalan-resistant rhabdomyosarcoma xenograft that is cross-resistant to nitrosoureas and topotecan. Cancer Res 1994;54:3487–3493.

385. Brent TP, von Wronski MA, Edwards CC, et al. Identification of nitrosourea-resistant human rhabdomyosarcomas by in situ immunostaining of O6-methylguanine-DNA methyltransferase. Oncol Res 1993;5:83–86.

386. Nooter K, Boersma AWM, Oostrum RG, et al. Constitutive expression of the c-H-ras oncogene inhibits doxorubicin-induced apoptosis and promotes cell survival in a rhabdomyosarcoma cell line. Br J Cancer 1995;71:556–561.

387. Pappo AS, Anderson JR, Crist WM, et al. Survival after relapse in children and adolescents with rhabdomyosarcoma: a report from the Intergroup Rhabdomyosarcoma Study Group. J Clin Oncol 1999;17:3487–3493.

388. Klingebiel T, Pertl U, Hess CF, et al. Treatment of children with relapsed soft tissue sarcoma: report of the German CESS/CWS REZ 91 trial. Med Pediatr Oncol 1998;30:269–275.

389. Mattke AC, Bailey EJ, Schuck A, et al. Does the time-point of relapse influence outcome in pediatric rhabdomyosarcomas? Pediatr Blood Cancer 2009;52:772–776.

390. Hayes FA, Thompson EI, Kumar M, et al. Long-term survival in patients with Ewing's sarcoma relapsing after completing therapy. Med Pediatr Oncol 1987;15:254–256.

391. Schiavetti A, Castello MA, Gauthier F, et al. Long-lasting complete remission after prolonged administration of etoposide in a child with a second recurrence of alveolar rhabdomyosarcoma. Med Pediatr Oncol 1997;28:144–146.

392. Rizzoni WE, Pass HI, Wesley MN, et al. Resection of recurrent pulmonary metastases in patients with soft-tissue sarcomas. Arch Surg 1986;121:1248–1252.

393. Pastorino U, Valente M, Gasparini M, et al. Lung resection for metastatic sarcomas: total survival from primary treatment. J Surg Oncol 1989;40:275–280.

394. Jablons D, Steinberg SM, Roth J, et al. Metastasectomy for soft tissue sarcoma. J Thorac Cardiovasc Surg 1989;97:695–705.

395. Seeger RC, Reynolds PC. Treatment of high-risk solid tumors of childhood with intensive therapy and autologous bone marrow transplantation. Pediatr Clin North Am 1991;38:393–424.

396. Pinkerton CR, Philip T, Hartmann O, et al. High-dose chemo-radiotherapy with autologous bone marrow rescue in pediatric solid sarcomas. In: Dicke KA, Spitzer G, Jagannath S, et al, eds. Autologous bone marrow transplantation. Houston, TX: University of Texas MD Anderson Cancer Center, 1989:617.

397. Lucidarme N, Couanet-Valteau D, Oberlin O, et al. Phase II study of high-dose thiotepa and hematopoietic stem cell transplantation in children with solid tumors. Bone Marrow Transplant 1998;22:535–540.

398. Wexler LH, Leitman SF, Carter CS, et al. Peripheral blood progenitor cell (PBPC) transfusions permit repetitive cycles of myeloablative chemotherapy for pediatric sarcoma patients [abstract]. Proc Am Soc Clin Oncol 1995;14:454.

399. Townsend A, Bodmer H. Antigen recognition by class I-restricted T lymphocytes. Annu Rev Immunol 1989;7:601–624.

400. Berke G. The CTL's kiss of death. Cell 1995;81:9–12.

401. Yanuck M, Carbone DP, Pendleton CD, et al. A mutant p53 tumor suppressor protein is a target for peptide-induced CD8+ cytotoxic T-cells. Cancer Res 1993;53:3257–3261.

402. Wiedenfeld EA, Fernandez-Vina M, Berzofsky JA, et al. Evidence for selection against human lung cancers bearing p53 missense mutations which occur within the HLA A*0201 peptide consensus motif. Cancer Res 1994;54:1175–1177.

403. Mackall CL, Rhee EH, Read EJ, et al. A pilot study of consolidative immunotherapy in patients with high-risk pediatric sarcomas. Clin Cancer Res 2008;14:4850–4858.

404. Guinan EC, Gribben JG, Boussiotis VA, et al. Pivotal role of the B7:CD28 pathway in transplantation tolerance and tumor immunity. Blood 1994;84:3261–3282.

405. Schmidt W, Schweighoffer T, Herbst E, et al. Cancer vaccines: the interleukin 2 dosage effect. Proc Natl Acad Sci U S A 1995;92:4711–4714.

406. Kalebic T, Tsokos M, Helman LJ. In vivo treatment with antibody against IGF-1 receptor suppresses growth of human rhabdomyosarcoma and down-regulates p34cdc2. Cancer Res 1994;54:5531–5534.

407. Zhan S, Shapiro DN, Helman LJ. Activation of an imprinted allele of the insulin-like growth factor II gene implicated in rhabdomyosarcoma. J Clin Invest 1994;94:445–448.

408. Cao L, Yu Y, Darko I, et al. Addiction to elevated insulin-like growth factor I receptor and initial modulation of the AKT pathway define the responsiveness of rhabdomyosarcoma to the targeting antibody. Cancer Res 2008;68:8039–8048.

409. Wan X, Harkavy B, Shen N, et al. Rapamycin induces feedback activation of Akt signaling through an IGF-1R-dependent mechanism. Oncogene 2007;26:1932–1940.

410. Pegram MD, Slamon DJ. Combination therapy with trastuzumab (Herceptin) and cisplatin for chemoresistant metastatic breast cancer: evidence for receptor-enhanced chemosensitivity. Semin Oncol 1999;26:89–95.

411. Davis TA, White CA, Grillo-Lopez AJ, et al. Single-agent monoclonal antibody efficacy in bulky non-Hodgkin's lymphoma: results of a phase II trial of rituximab. J Clin Oncol 1999;17:1851–1857.

412. Taniguchi E, Nishijo K, Mccleish AT, et al. PDGFR-A is a therapeutic target in alveolar rhabdomyosarcoma. Oncogene 2008;27:6550–6560.

413. Kalebic T, Tsokos M, Helman LJ. Suppression of rhabdomyosarcoma growth by fumagillin analog TNP-470. Int J Cancer 1996;68:596–599.

414. Kerbel RS, Viloria-Petit A, Klement G, et al. 'Accidental' anti-angiogenic drugs. anti-oncogene directed signal transduction inhibitors and conventional chemotherapeutic agents as examples. Eur J Cancer 2000;36:1248–1257.

415. Chastagner P, Merlin JL, Marchal C, et al. In vivo potentiation of radiation response by topotecan in human rhabdomyosarcoma xenografted into nude mice. Clin Cancer Res 2000;6:3327–3333.

CHAPTER 32 ■ THE NONRHABDOMYOSARCOMA SOFT TISSUE SARCOMAS

M. FATIH OKCU, ALBERTO S. PAPPO, JOHN HICKS, LYNN MILLION, RICHARD J. ANDRASSY, AND SHERI L. SPUNT

The clinician's decision-making skill can be exercised to its maximum when developing a therapeutic approach to a soft tissue sarcoma (STS) other than rhabdomyosarcoma (RMS). The rarity and heterogeneity of these diseases and their variable biologic potential have, for the most part, precluded the conduct of prospective clinical trials in pediatrics that could provide the necessary guidance to develop a unified treatment approach. The aim of this chapter is to frame the current state of our knowledge of these diseases and to elucidate the general therapeutic principles that will assist the clinician in developing a logical treatment strategy.

Although STSs account for less than 1% of all cancer diagnoses in the general population, they are considerably more common in children, representing approximately 7% of all cancers in patients younger than 20 years.[1] Rhabdomyosarcoma is the most common STS in children, comprising approximately half of pediatric STSs,[1] and is discussed in Chapter 31. The remaining diseases, collectively known as nonrhabdomyosarcoma soft tissue sarcomas (NRSTSs), are a heterogeneous group of neoplasms of presumed mesenchymal origin. In the first section of this chapter, we describe the general features common to all NRSTSs. In the second section, the common subtypes are discussed in more detail with an emphasis on their distinguishing features. We recommend that a reader of this chapter with an interest in a particular histologic subtype first read the general section and then the specific subsection of interest.

The information presented in this chapter is drawn from both the adult and pediatric published data. Because NRSTSs are significantly more numerous in adults, there is more information available about their natural history and treatment in adult populations. Caution is needed when extrapolating findings in adults to pediatric populations, however. The distribution of histologic subtypes differs in adults and children[2] (Table 32.1); thus, analyses of prognostic factors and therapies must be interpreted within the context of these observations. In certain NRSTS subtypes, infants and young children are known to have biologically less aggressive disease.[3,4] Treatment considerations also differ in children because certain therapeutic interventions may affect normal growth and development or may lead to greater late effects when administered in childhood.

EPIDEMIOLOGY

In 2008, 10,390 new cases of STS were diagnosed in the United States and about 10% of these cases were seen in patients younger than 20 years.[5] The incidence of specific STS histologies varies by age (Table 32.1). For example, RMS accounts for 60% of STS in children younger than 5 years but for only 23% of STSs in patients 15 to 19 years of age.[1] In contrast, NRSTS account for more than 75% of STSs in the 15- to 19-year-old age group. (Fig. 32.1).[1] Fibrosarcoma is the most common histologic subtype of NRSTS in infants, whereas dermatofibrosarcoma protuberans, synovial sarcoma, malignant peripheral nerve sheath tumor (MPNST), and malignant fibrous histiocytoma (MFH) are the most frequently encountered histologies in older children and adolescents.[1,6] There is a slight male predominance of STS (male-to-female ratio, 1.2:1) in both adults and children.[1] Black children may have a slightly higher incidence rate than white children (rate ratio, 1.17:1), with the largest difference observed in 15- to 19-year-olds (rate ratio, 1.33:1).[1] From 1975 to 2000, the incidence of non-Kaposi STSs increased at a statistically significant rate in patients 10 to 29 years of age and in patients older than 60 years.[7]

Few patients with NRSTS are found to have an underlying genetic predisposition. Patients with Li-Fraumeni syndrome, a rare autosomal dominant cancer predisposition syndrome characterized by germline mutations of the *p53* gene has an increased risk for the development of STS.[8,9] Germline mutation of the *RB* gene, seen in children with hereditary retinoblastoma, is a risk factor for the development of STSs, especially leiomyosarcoma (LMS).[10,11] An excess of various STSs has also been observed in patients with Werner syndrome.[12] Patients with neurofibromatosis type 1 have a significantly increased risk of developing MPNST, with a lifetime risk estimated to be in the 6% to 13% range.[13,14] Leiomyosarcoma is the second most common malignancy in children with acquired immunodeficiency syndrome (AIDS), and Epstein-Barr viral infection is thought to play a causal role in the development of this malignancy.[15] Desmoid fibromatosis has been reported to develop in up to 28% of patients with familial adenomatous polyposis (FAP); the risk appears to be increased for those with *APC* gene mutations that occur after codon 1444 and for those who undergo abdominal surgery.[16,17]

Secondary sarcomas of both soft tissue and bone have been well documented in adults following radiation therapy (RT).[18,19] The risk of developing a secondary sarcoma (including soft tissue and bone sarcomas) among 14,374 participants in the Childhood Cancer Survivor Study was more than ninefold higher than in the general population.[20] Multivariate analysis indicated that a primary diagnosis of sarcoma, a history of other secondary neoplasms, and treatment with radiotherapy or higher doses of anthracyclines or alkylating agents were associated with an increased risk of developing secondary sarcoma. In adults, exposure to vinyl chloride is causally related to angiosarcoma of the liver,[21,22] and chronic lymphedema has been identified as a risk factor for lymphangiosarcoma.[23] Less certain etiologic associations include exposure to phenoxyacetic herbicides, chlorophenols, and their contaminants (dioxin).[24,25]

TABLE 32.1

DISTRIBUTION OF HISTOLOGIC SUBTYPES OF SOFT TISSUE SARCOMAS DERIVED FROM THE SURVEILLANCE, EPIDEMIOLOGY, AND END RESULTS DATABASE IN CHILDREN AND ADULTS IN THE UNITED STATES, 1993–2002

Rank	Pediatric (age < 20 yr) Subtype	%	Adult (age ≥ 20 yr) Subtype	%
1	Rhabdomyosarcoma	41.3	Kaposi sarcoma	27.0
2	Dermatofibrosarcoma protuberans	8.4	Leiomyosarcoma	13.7
3	Synovial sarcoma	7.7	Malignant fibrous histiocytoma	10.1
4	Sarcoma, NOS	5.4	Liposarcoma	8.0
5	Malignant fibrous histiocytoma	4.9	Dermatofibrosarcoma protuberans	6.5
6	Fibrosarcoma	4.5	Sarcoma, NOS	5.5
7	Malignant peripheral nerve sheath tumor	3.4	Carcinosarcoma	4.9
8	Liposarcoma	2.8	Gastrointestinal stromal tumor	3.7
9	Epithelioid sarcoma	2.0	Hemangiosarcoma	2.5
10	Leiomyosarcoma	1.8	Spindle cell sarcoma	2.3

NOS, not otherwise specified.
From Spunt SL, Pappo AS. Childhood nonrhabdomyosarcoma soft tissue sarcomas are not adult-type tumors. J Clin Oncol 2006;24:1958–1959.

BIOPATHOLOGY

The pathologist's role in the management of the child with an NRSTS is to make the appropriate diagnosis, define the biologically important prognostic features of the tumor, determine whether the margins of resection are adequate, and, in some cases, assign a tumor grade. Please see the specific disease subsections for detailed descriptions of the histopathology of the various entities.

The accurate diagnosis of the NRSTS is complex requiring information from biologic studies in addition to more traditional histopathologic techniques. Many of the current treatment protocols are based on the clinical, pathologic, and molecular studies of specific tumor types. Therefore, it is essential that tissue be triaged appropriately (Table 32.2). The optimal biopathologic evaluation includes the morphologic, immunocytochemical, ultrastructural, cytogenetic, molecular, and biochemical factors that influence response to oncologic management and overall survival (Tables 32.3 to 32.6). A general schema for triaging tissue from pediatric tumors is presented in Table 32.2. Adequate tissue must be available for intraoperative interpretation and final diagnosis. The pathologist may elect to perform a frozen section and/or cytologic imprints to formulate an initial opinion. Once the pathologist determines that adequate tissue has been obtained for histologic tumor diagnosis, assessment of the amount of residual tissue available for cytogenetics, molecular analysis, and biologic study is necessary. If tissue is inadequate, the surgeon may be able to provide additional tissue to meet the needs for studies. In the event that the surgeon is not able to obtain adequate tumor tissue, the pathologist will need to determine the priority of various components of the tumor protocol and submit the tissue accordingly.

Submission of tissue for cytogenetics and retention of the frozen section tissue block at −70°C for molecular, reverse transcriptase polymerase chain reaction (RT-PCR), biochemical, and microarray gene product analyses will aid in diagnosis. The preparation of cytologic imprints from fresh tissue can be performed before submitting the tissue for other protocol studies. Cytologic imprints allow for fluorescent *in situ* hybridization (FISH) evaluation of mutated genes, tumor-defining translocations, and other cytogenetic abnormalities. Specific chromosomal translocations define several STSs in children (Table 32.3).[26] For example, t(X;18)(p11;q11) occurs in about 90% of synovial sarcomas. Molecular studies identified two novel genes that are rearranged in synovial sarcoma: SS18 (formerly SYT) at 18q11 and SSX at Xp11.[27] In addition, two predominant forms of the SS18-SSX fusion transcript, SS18-SSX1 and SS18-SSX2, have been described and

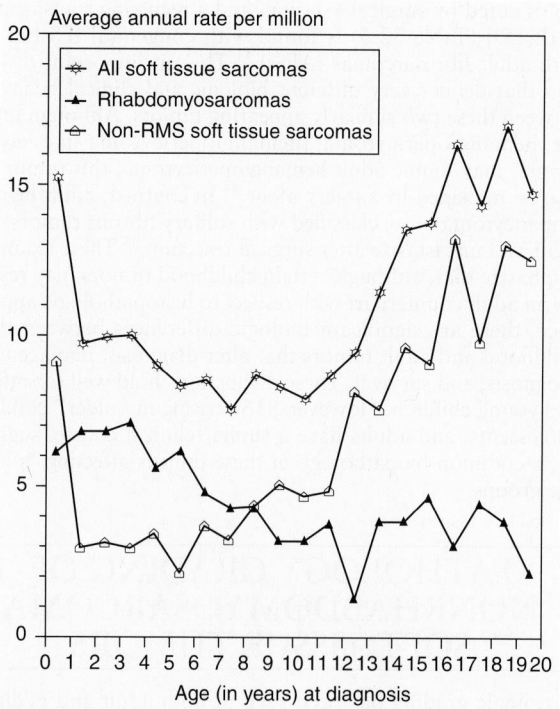

FIGURE 32.1 Graph shows the annual incidence of soft tissue sarcomas by year of age. Rhabdomyosarcoma (RMS) is more common from 1 to 7 years of age, whereas NRSTS is more common in infants younger than 1 year and in children older than 8 years. (From Gurney JG, Young JL, Roffers SD, et al. Soft tissue sarcomas. In: Gloeckler Ries LA, Smith MA, Gurney JG, et al, eds. SEER Pediatric Monograph: cancer incidence and survival among children and adolescents, United States SEER program 1975–1995. Bethesda, MD: National Cancer Institute, 1999:111–124.)

TABLE 32.2

TRIAGING OF SOFT TISSUE TUMORS FOR DIAGNOSIS, TREATMENT, AND PROGNOSIS

Soft tissue tumors of childhood

- Frozen tissue with cryopreservative for intraoperative diagnosis
- Cytologic, scrape, and squash imprints for intraoperative diagnosis
- Formalin-fixed tissue for routine histopathology, immunocytochemistry, *in situ* hybridization, and reverse transcriptase polymerase chain reaction (RT-PCR) evaluation
- Glutaraldehyde-fixed tissue for electron microscopy
- Fresh tissue in tissue culture media for cytogenetics and molecular studies and tissue cultures
- Frozen tissue without cryopreservative for molecular studies, gene rearrangement, and microarray gene analysis
- Fresh tissue for flow cytometric analysis for DNA ploidy or cell surface markers
- Fresh tissue for biochemical analyses of tumor-specific products
- Cytologic imprints of neoplastic tissue
- Cytogenetic interphase studies
- Fluorescent *in situ* hybridization for cytogenetics
- Special stains and immunocytochemical phenotyping
- Alcohol-fixed tissue for improved cytoplasmic glycogen preservation, immunocytochemistry (requiring such fixation), and microarray gene analysis

Tissue with inflammatory and/or infectious histopathologic features

- Fresh tissue for microbiologic studies
- Bacterial (aerobic and anaerobic) cultures
- Mycologic cultures
- Acid-fast bacillus culture and RT-PCR
- Fresh tissue for virology studies
- Viral cultures
- RT-PCR for rapid viral identification or for viruses that cannot be cultured
- Molecular virology studies
- Frozen tissue without cryopreservative for molecular microbiology and virology studies, including the RT-PCR study

are related to histopathologic and clinical features. SSX1 is associated with both biphasic and monophasic tumors, whereas SSX2 is identified with monophasic tumors exclusively.[28] This suggests that the two altered genes affect epithelial differentiation in this tumor.[29] More important, the SSX1 transcript is associated with a higher proliferation rate, metastatic disease occurrence, and shortened survival than the SSX2 transcript.[28,29]

Myxoid liposarcoma, which is most commonly seen in children and adolescents, is similarly characterized by tumor-defining translocations t(12;16)(q13;p11) (FUS/TLS-CHOP) and t(12;22)(q13;q12) (EWS-CHOP) (Table 32.3). These translocations lead to fusion of transcription factors participating in adipocytic differentiation.[30,31] The *EWS* gene is also fused with other genes associated with several childhood sarcomas, including Ewing's sarcoma, desmoplastic small round cell tumor (DSRCT), clear cell sarcoma (malignant melanoma of soft parts), and extraskeletal myxoid chondrosarcoma.[32,33]

Many NRSTSs are associated with loss of heterozygosity (LOH) of tumor suppressor genes (Table 32.3). The role of LOH of the tumor suppressor gene *p53* in tumor development with the familial cancer syndrome was first described by Li and Fraumeni.[34,35] As many as 10% of STSs in children may be associated with the autosomal dominant Li-Fraumeni syndrome. Further supporting this LOH effect is the strong association between MPNST and NF1, a common autosomal dominant disorder associated with chromosomal abnormalities at 17q11.2 (NF1 tumor suppressor gene locus) (Tables 32.3 and 32.4).[36] These MPNSTs may also possess p53 point mutations at 17p13 near the *NF1* gene locus, implicating an additional tumor suppressor gene in tumorigenesis. Homozygous gene deletions on both the long and short arms of chromosome 17 have been noted in MPNST in individuals with neurofibromatosis.[36] A somatic NF1 deletion may occur in nonsyndromatic MPNST as well.[37] Interestingly, MPNSTs tend to arise in NF1 patients with neurofibromatosis at an earlier age than in patients without neurofibromatosis, emphasizing the importance of LOH of tumor suppressor genes, secondary to somatic mutations in sarcoma development.[38–41] Other sarcomas such as RMS have also been associated with neurofibromatosis.[42] These examples highlight only two of the numerous tumor suppressor genes that participate in tumorigenesis in children (Table 32.4). In addition, there are many other tumor suppressor genes, protooncogenes, growth factors, and even viral agents that have been implicated in pediatric soft tissue tumors (Table 32.4).

There are considerable differences in the biology and natural history of STS in infants and young children when compared with those in adults. In contrast to its adult counterpart, congenital infantile fibrosarcoma (IFS) rarely metastasizes and usually is cured by surgical excision, and a recurring translocation [t(12;15)] (Table 32.3) is found with congenital IFS but not with adult fibrosarcomas (AFSs).[43] This an important distinction that defines very different biologic and clinical behaviors between these two similarly appearing tumors. Although infantile hemangiopericytoma (hemangiopericytoma-like myofibroma) may mimic adult hemangiopericytoma, this tumor can also be managed by surgery alone.[44] In contrast, adult hemangiopericytoma (now classified with solitary fibrous tumors) can recur and metastasize after surgical resection.[45] These examples emphasize that, although certain childhood tumors may resemble an adult counterpart with respect to histopathologic appearance, there are significant biologic differences between these childhood and adult tumors that alter diagnosis, management, prognosis, and survival. These distinctions hold well for infants and young children. However, STSs arising in "older" children, adolescents, and adults have a similar clinical course, suggesting a common biopathology of these tumors affecting "older" age groups.

PATHOLOGY GRADING OF NONRHABDOMYOSARCOMA SOFT TISSUE TUMORS

Histologic grading has been used in both adult and pediatric studies as an adjunct to clinical staging because it is highly predictive of clinical outcome.[46–48] The system developed by the National Cancer Institute of the United States (NCI) by Costa and colleagues stratifies STS into three different grades based on histologic subtype and a composite of histopathologic parameters that includes tumor necrosis, cellularity, pleomorphism, and mitotic activity.[46] The grading system used by the French Federation of Cancer Centers Sarcoma Group is

TABLE 32.3

MALIGNANT AND BENIGN CHILDHOOD TUMORS: CYTOGENETIC ABNORMALITIES

Tumor	Abnormality	Affected gene or fusion product
Alveolar soft part sarcoma	t(X;17)(p11.2;q25) Gains 1q, 8q, 12q, 16p	TFE3-ASPL
Angiomatoid fibrous histiocytoma	t(2;22)(q33;q12) t(12;22)(q13;q22) t(12;16)(q13;p11) Complex rearrangements 2, 12, 16, 17 deletion 11q24	EWSR1-CREB1 EWSR1-ATF1 FUS-ATF1
Congenital infantile fibrosarcoma and mesoblastic nephroma	t(12;15)(p13;q25) Trisomy 8, 11, 17, 20	ETV6-NTRK3
Dermatofibrosarcoma protuberans and giant cell fibroblastoma	t(17;22)(q22;q13)	COL1A1-PDGFB
Desmoid	5q21 Trisomy 8, 20	APC β-catenin
Desmoplastic small round cell tumor	t(11;22)(p13;q12)	EWS-WT1
Fibrosarcoma, adult	2q14-22 Complex rearrangements	Unknown
Inflammatory myofibroblastic tumor	2p23 Chromosome 12	TPM3-ALK; TPM4-ALK CTLC-ALK HMGIC (HMGA2)

Leiomyosarcoma	Rearrangement 12q t(12;14)(q14-15;q23-24)
	Loss 1p, 3p21-23, 6q, 8p21-pter, 11p,
	  13q12-13, 13q32-pter, 22q
	Amplification 1q21, 5p14-pter, 12q13-15,
	  13q31, 17p11, 20q13
	Loss of heterozygosity chromosomes 11 and 13
		Not known
		Not known
		Not known

Liposarcoma (myxoid and round cell)	t(12;16)(q13;p11) t(12;22)(q13;q12) t(12;22;20)(q13;q12;q11)	FUS (TLS)-DDIT3 (CHOP) EWS-DDIT3 EWS-DDIT3
Malignant peripheral nerve sheath tumor	17q11.2 Loss or rearrangement 10p, 11q, 17q, 22q	NF1
Melanoma of soft tissue (clear cell sarcoma of soft tissue)	t(12;22)(q13;q22) Trisomy 7, 8	EWS-ATF1
Myofibroma	Chromosome 8 Deletions 16p, 16p13.3	Not known TSC2 (mTOR dysregulation)
PEComa (perivascular endothelial cell tumors)	Loss of heterozygosity 9q34 Loss 19, 16p, 17p, 1p, 18p Gains X, 12q, 3q, 5, 2q Microsatellite instability t(3;10)(p13;q23)	TSC1
Pericytoma with t(7;12)	t(7;12)(p21-22;q13-15)	GLI-ACTB
Solitary fibrous tumor/hemangiopericytoma (adult form), extrapleural	t(12;19)(q13;q13) t(13;22)(q22;q13.3) Loss 3p, 12q, 13q, **17p**, 17q, 19q, 10 (entire) Gain 5q	Not known Not known Not known
Synovial Sarcoma	t(X;18)(p11.23;q11) t(X;18)(p11.21;q11) t(X;20)(p11.2;q13.3) t(5;18)(q11;q11) Trisomy 7, 8, 12 Loss 3	SS18-SSX1, SS18-SSX4 SS18-SSX2 SS18L-SSX1 SS18-Not known
Undifferentiated embryonal sarcoma of liver	t(11;19)(q13;q13.4) Gain 1q, 5p, 6q, 8p, 12q Loss 9p, 11p, 14	MALAT1-MHLB1 Gain 12q: MDM2, CDK4

TABLE 32.4

FACTORS IMPLICATED IN NONRHABDOMYOSARCOMA SOFT TISSUE SARCOMAS

Tumor suppressor genes
Retinoblastoma gene (RB1, 13q14)
Tumor protein p53 gene (TP53, 17p13.1)
Checkpoint kinase 2 gene (CHEK2, 22q12)
Cyclin-dependent kinase inhibitor-2A gene (CDKN2A, 9p21)
Wilms tumor gene (WT1, 11p13)
SMARCB1 (hSNF5/INI1, 22q11.2)
Neurofibromatosis type 1 gene (NF1, 17q11.2)
Neurofibromatosis type 2 gene (NF2, 22q12.2)
Adenomatous polyposis coli gene (APC, 5q21)
β-Catenin gene (CTNNB1, 5q21)

Growth factor and signaling pathways
Insulin-like growth factor 1-receptor pathway (IGF1)
Platelet-derived growth factor pathway (PDGF)
c-KIT receptor pathway
c-MET receptor pathway
GLI (12q13)
HDM2 (12q13-14)
SAS (12q13-14)
CDK4
P16
Epidermal growth factor

Congenital syndromes
Beckwith-Wiedemann syndrome (11p15, CDKN1C, IGF2, myxomas, fibromas, hamartomas, rhabdomyosarcoma, Wilms tumor, pancreatoblastoma, hepatoblastoma)
Carney complex (17q23-4, PRKAR1AK, 2p16, cardiac and other myxomas, melanocytic schwannomas, gastrointestinal stromal tumos)
Diaphyseal medullary stenosis (9q21-2, pleomorphic undifferentiated sarcoma [MFH])
Familial adenomatous polyposis and familial infiltrative fibromatosis (5q21, APC, desmoids, colon cancer)
Myofibromatosis (autosomal recessive, myofibromas)
Neurofibromatosis type 1 (17q11, NF1, neurofibroma, malignant peripheral nerve sheath tumor, pheochromocytoma)
Neurofibromatosis type 2 (22q12, NF2, schwannoma auditory neuroma)
Retinoblastoma (13q14, RB1, retinoblastoma, osteosarcoma, soft tissue sarcomas)
Rhabdoid predilection syndrome (22q11, SMARCB1, rhabdoid tumor, atypical teratoid/rhabdoid tumor)
Rubinstein-Taybi syndrome (myogenic sarcomas)
Werner syndrome (8p11-12, WRN, bone and soft tissue sarcomas)

Viral infection
Epstein-Barr virus
Human herpes virus type 8

---

based on tumor differentiation, mitotic count, and necrosis and appears to better predict the risk of developing metastases and mortality than the NCI grading system.[49]

The Pediatric Oncology Group (POG) developed and prospectively tested a pediatric grading system for NRSTS[47] (Table 32.7) based on the histopathologic system developed by Costa et al. This grading system identified three different grades of tumors based on the histopathologic subtype, the amount of necrosis, number of mitoses, and cellular pleomorphism. Infantile fibrosarcoma is considered grade 1 in this classification, given its relatively benign clinical course despite its aggressive appearance on histologic examination. The Children's Oncology Group (COG) is conducting a prospective trial for the treatment of NRSTS and is comparing the predictive value of histologic grade by the POG and French Federation of Cancer Centers grading systems (COG protocol ARST 0332).

CLINICAL PRESENTATION

Because of their rarity, NRSTS may not be suspected by the treating clinician. In a retrospective study of children with cancer, those with STSs experienced a median lag time of 9.5 weeks between symptom onset and establishment of the diagnosis.[50] A painless mass is the most common clinical presentation, although impingement on normal structures may produce pain or other symptoms. NRSTS may arise in any part of the body, but the extremities and trunk are the most common sites (Fig. 32.2). Systemic symptoms such as fever, night sweats, and weight loss are rare, although occasionally they are seen in patients with widely metastatic disease. Non–islet cell tumor-induced hypoglycemia, a rare paraneoplastic phenomenon, has been reported in a variety of NRSTS, including hemangiopericytoma, solitary fibrous tumor,

TABLE 32.5

IMMUNOCYTOCHEMISTRY WITH NONRHABDOMYOSARCOMA SOFT TISSUE TUMORS

Alveolar soft part sarcoma	TFE3, MCT1, CD147, desmin, MyoD1 cytoplasmic, muscle-specific actin, sarcomeric actin, β-enolase, S100 protein, neuron-specific enolase
Angiomatoid fibrous histiocytoma	Desmin, epithelial membrane antigen, muscle-specific actin, laminin, type IV collagen, CD68, CD99
Congenital infantile fibrosarcoma and mesoblastic nephroma	Vimentin, neuron-specific enolase, alpha-smooth muscle, HHF35 actin, muscle-specific actin, desmin, S100 protein, CD34, CD57 (Leu 7), CD68, factor XIIIa, CAM5.2 cytokeratin
Dermatofibrosarcoma protuberans and giant cell fibroblastoma	CD34, vimentin, p75, p53
Desmoid	Vimentin, muscle-specific actin, smooth muscle actin, β-catenin (nuclear)
Desmoplastic small round cell tumor	Cytokeratins, epithelial membrane antigen, vimentin, desmin, neuron-specific enolase, WT1, placental alkaline phosphatase, CD99
Fibrosarcoma, adult	Vimentin, smooth muscle actin
Inflammatory myofibroblastic tumor	ALK (metastatic tumors Alk negative, vimentin, smooth muscle actin, muscle-specific actin, cytokeratin
Leiomyosarcoma	Smooth muscle actin, desmin, H-caldesmon, cytokeratin, epithelial membrane antigen, S100 protein, CD34, Epstein-Barr virus latent membrane protein 1 (LMP1), EBER-1 (Epstein-Barr virus)
Liposarcoma, myxoid	S100 protein, aP2
Malignant peripheral nerve sheath tumor	S100 protein (<50% of tumors), keratins 8 and 18, glial fibrillary acidic protein, collagen type IV, CD57 (Leu 7), PGP 9.5, myelin basic protein, EMA, topoisomerase-II-alpha
Melanoma of soft tissue (clear cell sarcoma of soft tissue)	HMB-45, Melan-A, MART1, tyrosine kinase, S100 protein, neuron-specific enolase, synatophysin, CD57 (Leu7), cytokeratin, actin, microphthalmic transcription factor, MelCAM
Myofibroma	Vimentin, Smooth Muscle Actin. HHF-35 Actin, β-catenin
PEComa (perivascular endothelial cell tumor)	HMB-45, HMB-50, Melan-A, MART1, CD63, tyrosine, microphthalmia transcription factor, smooth muscle actin, calponin, muscle-specific actin, myosin, desmin, CD117, S100 protein, TFE3
Pericytoma with t(7;12)	Smooth muscle actin, laminin, collagen IV
Solitary fibrous tumor/hemangiopericytoma (adult-type), extrapleural	CD34, CD99, epithelial membrane antigen, cytokeratin, bcl-2, β-catenin, smooth muscle actin
Synovial sarcoma	TLE1, epithelial membrane antigen, cytokeratin (including 7, 8, 18, 19), bcl-2, CD99, S100 protein, calponin, vimentin, collagen type IV, E-cadherin
Undifferentiated embryonal sarcoma of liver	CD68, bcl2, alpha-1-antitrypsin, antichymotrypsin, desmin, keratin, CD10, p53, calponin

LMS/gastrointestinal stromal tumor (GIST), and fibrosarcoma.[51] Elevated levels of high-molecular-weight forms of insulin growth factor-II have been implicated in the pathogenesis of this complication.[52] Hypophosphatemic rickets has been reported in hemangiopericytoma.[53] Only a small proportion of patients have metastatic disease at the time of diagnosis, and the lung is mot commonly involved.[54,55] Regional lymph node involvement is unusual except in certain histologic subtypes such as epithelioid sarcoma (ES) and clear cell sarcoma.[55–57] Bone, liver, subcutaneous, and brain metastases have been reported in a small proportion of children with metastatic NRSTS; bone marrow involvement is exceedingly rare.[54,55,58]

PROGNOSTIC FACTORS

Because few prospective studies have been conducted in children with NRSTS, most information about predictors of outcome in childhood NRSTS is derived from retrospective,

single-institution analyses.[55,59,60] The factors that most clearly influence survival in pediatric NRSTS are as follows:

1. Extent of disease (nonmetastatic vs. metastatic)
2. Histologic grade (low vs. high)
3. Size of the primary tumor (≤5 cm vs. >5 cm)
4. Extent of surgical resection (resected vs. unresected).

These factors are also key predictors of survival in adults with STSs.[48,61] On the basis of these four factors, patients may be grouped into high-, intermediate-, and low-risk groups (Fig. 32.3). Those in the high-risk category have metastatic disease. These patients have a dismal survival rate of 15% at best, and most die of progressive metastatic disease. Those in the intermediate-risk category include patients with nonmetastatic but unresectable tumors and those with nonmetastatic tumors that are both high grade and more than 5 cm in maximal diameter. Survival in this patient cohort is approximately 50%. Patients with unresectable tumors, regardless of histologic grade, usually die of local tumor

TABLE 32.6

ULTRASTRUCTURAL FEATURES IN NONRHABDOMYOSARCOMA SOFT TISSUE TUMORS

Alveolar soft part sarcoma	Rhomboid crystals with 10-nm periodicity, 6-nm noncrystallized, dense granules, glycogen, well-developed Golgi, abnormal mitochondria
Angiomatoid fibrous histiocytoma	Fibroblastic/myofibroblastic features, actin filaments, dilated rough endoplasmic reticulum, lipid, iron pigment (hemosiderin)
Congenital infantile fibrosarcoma and mesoblastic nephroma	Fibroblastic/myofibroblastic features, intermediate filaments, dilated rough endoplasmic reticulum, focal basement membrane–like material, actin filaments, well-developed Golgi, amorphous matrix, infrequent collagen
Dermatofibrosarcoma protuberans and giant cell fibroblastoma	Dermal Fibroblastic features, elaborate cell processes, desmosomes (moderate), focal basal lamina, convoluted nuclei
Desmoid	Fibroblastic features, abundant mature collagen, intranuclear collagen inclusions
Desmoplastic small round cell tumor	Mesenchymal, rhabdoid, epithelial, neuroblastic/neural features, intermediate filament whirls, neurosecretory dense core granules, small glycogen lakes, focal basal lamina, cell junctions
Fibrosarcoma, adult	Elongated fibroblasts, indented nuclei, infrequent nucleoli, rough endoplasmic reticulum, intermediate filaments (up to 60-nm bundles), variable collagen
Inflammatory myofibroblastic tumor	Fibroblastic and myofibroblastic features, poorly developed Golgi, rough endoplasmic reticulum, collagen, thin myofilaments, and dense bodies
Leiomyosarcoma	Smooth muscle cell features, elongated nuclei with deeply grooved nuclei, actin filaments (6–8 nm) with dense body attachment plaques, pinocytotic vesicles, basal lamina, cell junctions
Liposarcoma, myxoid	Lipogenic features, primitive mesenchymal cells to lipoblasts with univesicular and multivesicular lipid, polyribosomes
Malignant peripheral nerve sheath tumor	Spindled to polygonal cells, tapered nonbranching processes in parallel arrangement with other cells, microtubules, neurofilaments, basal lamina, collagen
Melanoma of soft tissue (clear cell sarcoma of soft tissue)	Oval to fusiform cells, round nucleus with prominent, large, central nucleolus, premelanosomes, numerous mitochondria, polyribosomes
Myofibroma	Myofibroblastic/fibroblastic features: collagen, infrequent actin filaments
PEComa (perivascular endothelial cell tumor)	Melanocytic features: premelanosomes in epithelioid cells Smooth muscle features: actin filaments, dense bodies in spindled cells
Pericytoma with t(7;12)	Pericytic features: incomplete basal lamina, subplasmalemmal thickenings, thin filaments with focal dense bodies
Solitary fibrous tumor/ hemangiopericytoma (adult-type), extrapleural	Myofibroblastic/fibroblastic/pericytic features, rough endoplasmic reticulum, primitive junctions
Synovial sarcoma	Epithelial cell differentiation: well-defined ovoid nuclei, abundant cytoplasm, paranuclear, intermediate filaments, rare tonofilaments, gland-like clusters with microvilli, villous filopodia Spindle cell differentiation: fibroblastic-like, irregular nuclei, prominent Golgi, rough endoplasmic reticulum, continuous basal lamina
Undifferentiated embryonal sarcoma of liver	Dilated rough endoplasmic reticulum, secondary lysosomes with dense precipitates, dilated mitochondria and mitochondrial-RER complexes, fat droplets, scant actin filaments, focal glycogen pools

progression, whereas those with large, high-grade tumors tend to develop fatal distant disease dissemination. Patients in the low-risk category includes those with nonmetastatic, resectable tumors that are either high grade and less than 5 cm in maximal diameter or low grade (any size). These patients have a long-term survival estimate of approximately 90%. Recently, a relationship between body size and tumor size has been documented in pediatric patients, arguing in favor of considering the relative tumor size as it relates to body size when analyzing prognostic factors in children with NRSTS.[62] Other factors that may contribute to survival outcomes but that are not known to be independent of the other prognostic features include micro-

scopic surgical margin (in resected tumors), primary site (visceral sites seem to have a worse outcome), and older age (age ≥ 10 years has been reported to be an adverse prognostic factor in unresected tumors). Other predictors of survival in adults with STS including anatomic location (upper extremity vs. lower extremity), tumor depth (superficial vs. deep), and histologic subtype have not been shown to be prognostically important in pediatric NRSTS.

Prognostic factors for local tumor control in pediatric NRSTS are not well delineated. However, the extent of surgical resection seems to play a key role. Patients who undergo a gross total tumor resection have a cumulative incidence of

TABLE 32.7

PEDIATRIC ONCOLOGY GROUP HISTOLOGIC GRADING SYSTEM

Grade	Description
1 (Low)	Myxoid and well-differentiated liposarcoma Well-differentiated or infantile (age ≤ 4 yr) fibrosarcoma Well-differentiated or infantile (age ≤ 4 yr) hemangiopericytoma Well-differentiated malignant peripheral nerve sheath tumor Angiomatoid malignant fibrous histiocytoma Deep-seated dermatofibrosarcoma protuberans Myxoid chondrosarcoma
2 (Intermediate)	Soft tissue sarcomas in which: <15% of the surface area shows necrosis The mitotic count is ≤5/10 high-power fields by using a 40× objective Nuclear atypia is not marked The tumor is not markedly cellular[a]
3 (High)	Tumors with the following diagnosis: Pleomorphic or round cell liposarcoma Mesenchymal chondrosarcoma Extraskeletal osteogenic sarcoma Malignant triton tumor Alveolar soft part sarcoma Any other sarcoma not in grade 1 with >15% necrosis or ≥5 mitoses/10 high-power fields by using a 40× objective

[a]Necrosis and mitotic count are by far the most important parameters in making this assessment. The other parameters are of borderline significance and may be helpful in a case that is difficult to place by necrosis and mitotic count alone. Specific diagnoses included in grades 1 or 3 are excluded from grade 2. From Parham DM, Webber BL, Jenkins JJ III, et al. Nonrhabdomyosarcomatous soft tissue sarcomas of childhood: formulation of a simplified system for grading. Mod Pathol 1995;8:705–710. Used with permission.

local recurrence in the 15% range, whereas those who present with unresectable tumors experience local tumor recurrence or progression in about 45% of cases.[55,59,60] The data on other predictors of local tumor control are contradictory, most likely due to inadequate numbers of patients available for analysis. However, in patients with resected NRSTS, large tumor size, invasiveness, intra-abdominal primary site, the presence of microscopic residual tumor, and avoidance of radiotherapy have been associated with poorer local control in univariate analyses.[55,60] In patients with initially unresected tumors, univariate analyses have identified female sex, age more than 10 years, a diagnosis of MPNST, and lower doses of radiotherapy to be correlated with the risk of local recurrence.[55,59]

STAGING

Despite the fact that NRSTS is as common as RMS in pediatric patients, no staging system has been prospectively validated for this patient population. Pediatric NRSTS have traditionally been staged according to the Intergroup Rhabdomyosarcoma Study Group surgicopathologic grouping system and the International Union Against Cancer staging systems.[63]

For adults with NRSTS, the most commonly employed system is the one developed by the American Joint Committee on Cancer (AJCC), which dates to 1977.[64] This system is used for all STSs, with the exception of dermatofibrosarcoma, Kaposi sarcoma, IFS, and angiosarcoma, as well as sarcomas arising within the confines of the dura mater, in parenchymatous organs, and in hollow viscera. This system recognizes four distinct histologic grades, and this attribute in

combination with size, depth, and extent of nodal and distant metastatic disease are the primary determinants of clinical stage (Table 32.8).

Alternate staging systems for adults have been proposed by Memorial Sloan-Kettering Cancer Center and the Musculoskeletal Tumor Society. The Memorial Sloan-Kettering Cancer Center system assigns stage based on the number of adverse prognostic factors, including large tumor size, deep location, and high histologic grade.[65] The Surgical Staging System of the Musculoskeletal Tumor Society is based on tumor grade and tumor compartment status only.[66] In 2000, these two staging systems, and the fourth and fifth editions of the AJCC staging system were compared in 300 adults with newly diagnosed nonmetastatic STS of the lower extremity.[67] This report concluded that grade, depth, and size were the most important predictors of clinical outcome. The Memorial Sloan-Kettering Cancer Center staging system proved to be superior to the other two systems for predicting metastasis-free survival. In this staging system, adults with no adverse prognostic factors as defined by histologic grade, depth, and size had an estimated 5-year metastasis-free survival of 100% whereas those with three adverse factors had a 49% 5-year metastases-free survival.

A nomogram that estimates the likelihood of 12-year sarcoma-specific death has been developed by Memorial Sloan-Kettering Cancer Center based on an analysis of 2,136 adult patients prospectively followed at that institution (Fig. 32.4).[68] This nomogram utilizes histologic grade, tumor size, depth, site, histology, and age to predict outcome. An effort to validate this nomogram in pediatric patients has been undertaken.[69] Although the prognostic factors seen in adults were

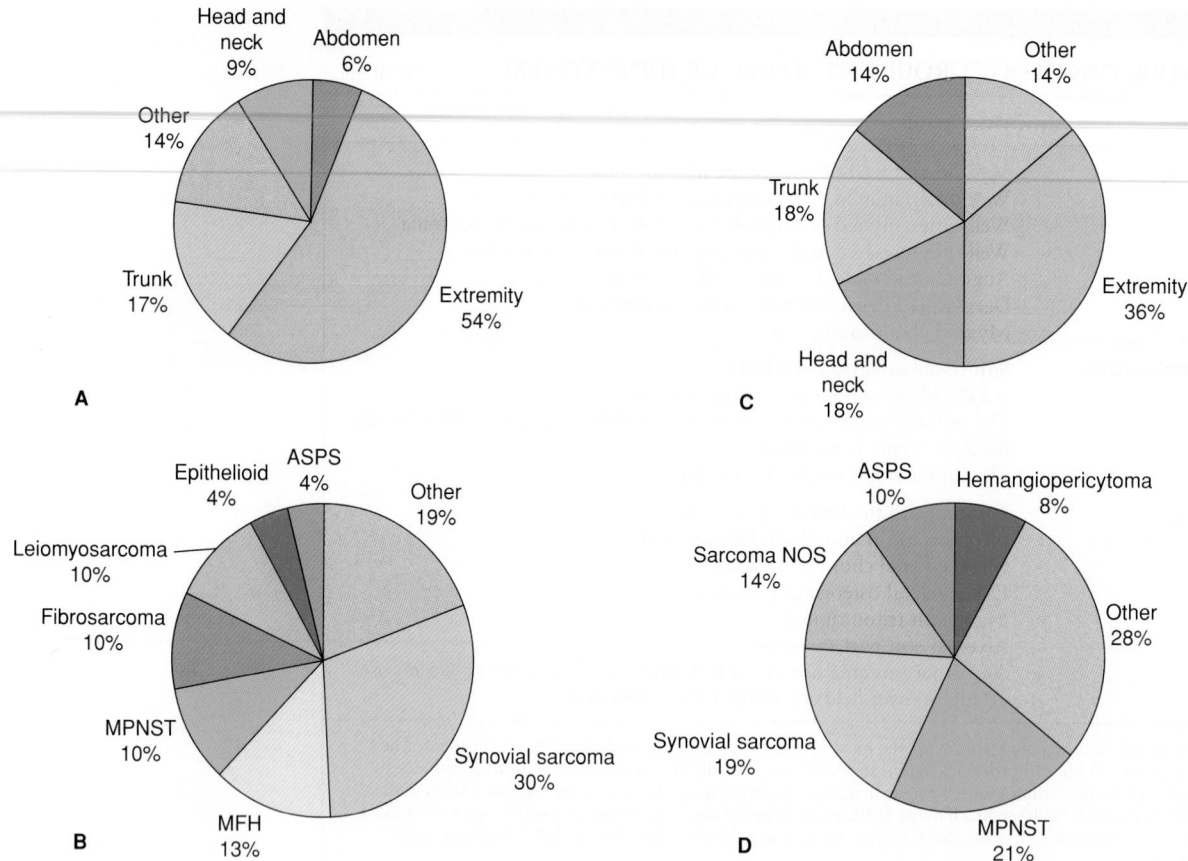

FIGURE 32.2 Distribution by primary tumor site (**A**) and histologic subtype (**B**) in children with surgically resected (groups I and II) nonrhabdomyosarcomatous soft tissue sarcoma. ASPS, alveolar soft part sarcoma; MFH, malignant fibrous histiocytoma; MPNST, malignant peripheral nerve sheath tumor; NOS, not otherwise specified. (From Spunt SL, Poquette CA, Hurt YS, et al. Prognostic factors for children and adolescents with surgically resected nonrhabdomyosarcoma soft tissue sarcoma: an analysis of 121 patients treated at St. Jude Children's Research Hospital. J Clin Oncol 1999;17:3697–3705; and Pratt CB, Pappo AS, Gieser P, et al. Role of adjuvant chemotherapy in the treatment of surgically resected pediatric nonrhabdomyosarcomatous soft tissue sarcomas: a Pediatric Oncology Group study. J Clin Oncol 1999;17:1219, with permission.) Distribution by primary tumor site (**C**) and histologic subtype (**D**) among children with unresected (group III) or metastatic (group IV) nonrhabdomyosarcomatous soft tissue sarcomas. ASPS, alveolar soft part sarcoma; HPC, hemangiopericytoma; MFH, malignant fibrous histiocytoma; MPNST, malignant peripheral nerve sheath tumor; NOS, not otherwise specified. (From Pappo AS, Rao BN, Jenkins JJ, et al. Metastatic nonrhabdomyosarcomatous soft-tissue sarcomas in children and adolescents: the St. Jude Children's Research Hospital experience. Med Pediatr Oncol 1999;33:76; and Spunt SL, Hill DA, Motosue AM, et al. Clinical features and outcome of children with unresected non-rhabdomyosarcoma soft tissue sarcoma (NRSTS). J Clin Oncol 2002;20:3225.)

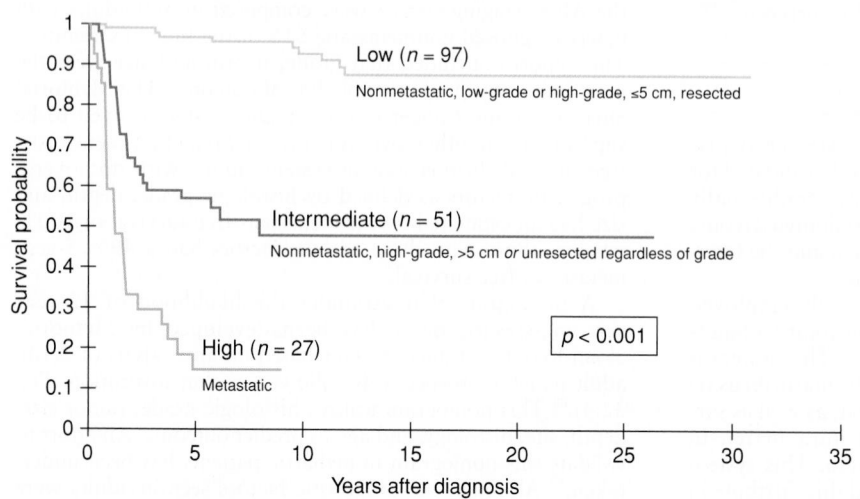

FIGURE 32.3 Kaplan-Meier survival distributions of patients treated at St. Jude Children's Research Hospital according to risk group. (From Spunt SL, Poquette CA, Hurt YS, et al. Prognostic factors for children and adolescents with surgically resected nonrhabdomyosarcoma soft tissue sarcoma: an analysis of 121 patients treated at St. Jude Children's Research Hospital. J Clin Oncol 1999;17:3697–3705; Spunt SL, Hill DA, Motosue AM, et al. Clinical features and outcome of children with unresected non-rhabdomyosarcoma soft tissue sarcoma (NRSTS.). J Clin Oncol 2002;20:3225; and Pappo AS, Rao BN, Jenkins JJ, et al. Metastatic nonrhabdomyosarcomatous soft-tissue sarcomas in children and adolescents: the St. Jude Children's Research Hospital experience. Med Pediatr Oncol 1999;33:76.)

TABLE 32.8

AJCC STAGING OF SOFT TISSUE SARCOMAS

Stage I

Stage I tumor is defined as nonmetastatic, low-grade, superficial or deep, and ≤5 or >5 cm in largest dimension

- G1-2 T1a, N0, M0
- G1-2, T1b, N0, M0
- G1-2, T2a, N0, M0
- G1-2, T2b, N0, M0

Stage II

Stage II tumor is defined as nonmetastatic, high-grade, and either ≤5 cm in largest dimension and superficial or deep or >5 cm in largest dimension and superficial

- G3-4, T1a, N0, M0
- G3-4, T1b, N0, M0
- G3-4, T2a, N0, M0

Stage III

Stage III tumor is defined as nonmetastatic, high grade, >5 cm in largest dimension, and deep

- G3-4, T2b, N0, M0

Stage IV

Stage IV is defined as metastatic involvement of lymph nodes or distant sites

- Any G, any T, N1, M0
- Any G, any T, N0, M1

---

[a]T1, tumor ≤5 cm in largest dimension; T2, tumor > 5 cm in largest dimension; a, superficial tumor; b, deep tumor; N0, no regional nodes; N1, regional nodes involved; M0, no distant metastases; M1, presence of distant metastases, G1 well differentiated, G2, moderately differentiated, G3, poorly differentiated, G4, poorly differentiated or undifferentiated (four-tiered systems only).
From Greene FL, Page DL, Fleming ID, et al. AJCC cancer staging handbook. New York: Springer-Verlag, 2002.

---

mostly applicable to children, differences in age and tumor size made interpretation of results difficult.

GENERAL TREATMENT CONSIDERATIONS

Optimally, children with NRSTS should be cared for by a multidisciplinary team of experts that include a pediatric surgeon or surgical subspecialist with expertise in cancer surgery, a radiation oncologist, and a pediatric oncologist. Key support services should include pathology, diagnostic imaging, rehabilitation (physical/occupational/speech therapy), nutrition, and psychosocial services (social work, child life, psychology, chaplain).

Although the general approach to children with these tumors is often similar to that for adults, important differences exist.[70–72] For example, the distribution of histologic subtypes of STS differs in adults and children (Table 32.1),[2] and caution must be exercised when extrapolating treatment recommendations from adult to children. Although some histologic subtypes appear to have a similar behavior than adult tumors, some, such as IFS, behave differently.[3,73] Local control measures such as surgery and radiotherapy pose unique challenges in children due to their incomplete growth and development. Primary tumor resections might be complicated

by the small amount of surrounding normal anatomic structures and may result in deformity or disability that is lifelong. Limb-sparing procedures in younger children are more difficult to perform, but newer techniques and expandable prostheses may allow for a greater number of these procedures.[74] The morbidity of RT in children is often much greater than that in adults because the doses required to treat NRSTS usually impair normal tissue growth. Chemotherapy carries risks, including infertility, cardiomyopathy, renal dysfunction, and secondary neoplasia, that may be of greater concern in children. Late effects are of particular concern in young children, whose potential survival after successful therapy is much longer. The goal of therapy is to achieve long-term disease control with minimum morbidity in both the short and long term. Patients should be entered on prospective clinical trials whenever possible.

The first therapeutic consideration is to determine how to best achieve local control. When feasible, a complete surgical resection should be performed with the goal of excising the primary tumor with margins sufficient to prevent local recurrence. If, at diagnosis, the tumor cannot be widely resected with acceptable morbidity, other strategies should be considered. Adjuvant radiotherapy produces adequate local tumor control after a marginal tumor resection.[75] For tumors that are unresectable, the use of preoperative chemotherapy, radiotherapy, or a combination of both modalities, may facilitate tumor resection.[76,77] The importance of achieving a complete resection of tumor at diagnosis cannot be overemphasized. In a retrospective review of 121 surgically completely resected cases of childhood NRSTS from St. Jude Children's Research Hospital, the estimated 5-year survival was 89%, with 12.8% of patients experiencing a local failure and 11.8% a distant failure.[60] In contrast, only half of patients with unresected disease and 34% of those with metastatic disease were alive at 5 and 2 years, respectively.[54,59] Similar results were documented by the Instituto Nazionale Tumori in Milan, where patients with resected, unresected, and metastatic disease had estimated 5-year survival rates of 86%, 52%, and 17%, respectively.[55]

Strategies for managing patients with localized unresectable tumor that cannot be rendered resectable with preoperative chemotherapy or irradiation and those with metastatic disease at diagnosis rely heavily on the use of chemotherapy and radiotherapy. These treatment modalities are discussed in more detail in the sections that follow.

Surgical Evaluation and Treatment Approaches

The surgeon plays a key role in the initial diagnosis and staging. The surgeon must first ensure that the local diagnostic imaging staging of the tumor is complete prior to biopsy. The appropriate biopsy technique and management of tissue are very important. The biopsy should be carefully planned to avoid complications that interfere with wide local excision (WLE) or a limb salvage procedure. When possible, the surgeon who will perform the definitive surgical approach should evaluate the patient prior to the biopsy to assist in determining the appropriate approach. The biopsy incision or track will need to be excised at the time of definitive surgery.

The biopsy may be performed in the operating room, clinic, or the radiology suite under computed tomographic (CT) guidance. Histologic diagnosis can often be made by fine needle aspiration (FNA) or core needle biopsy.[78] The decision

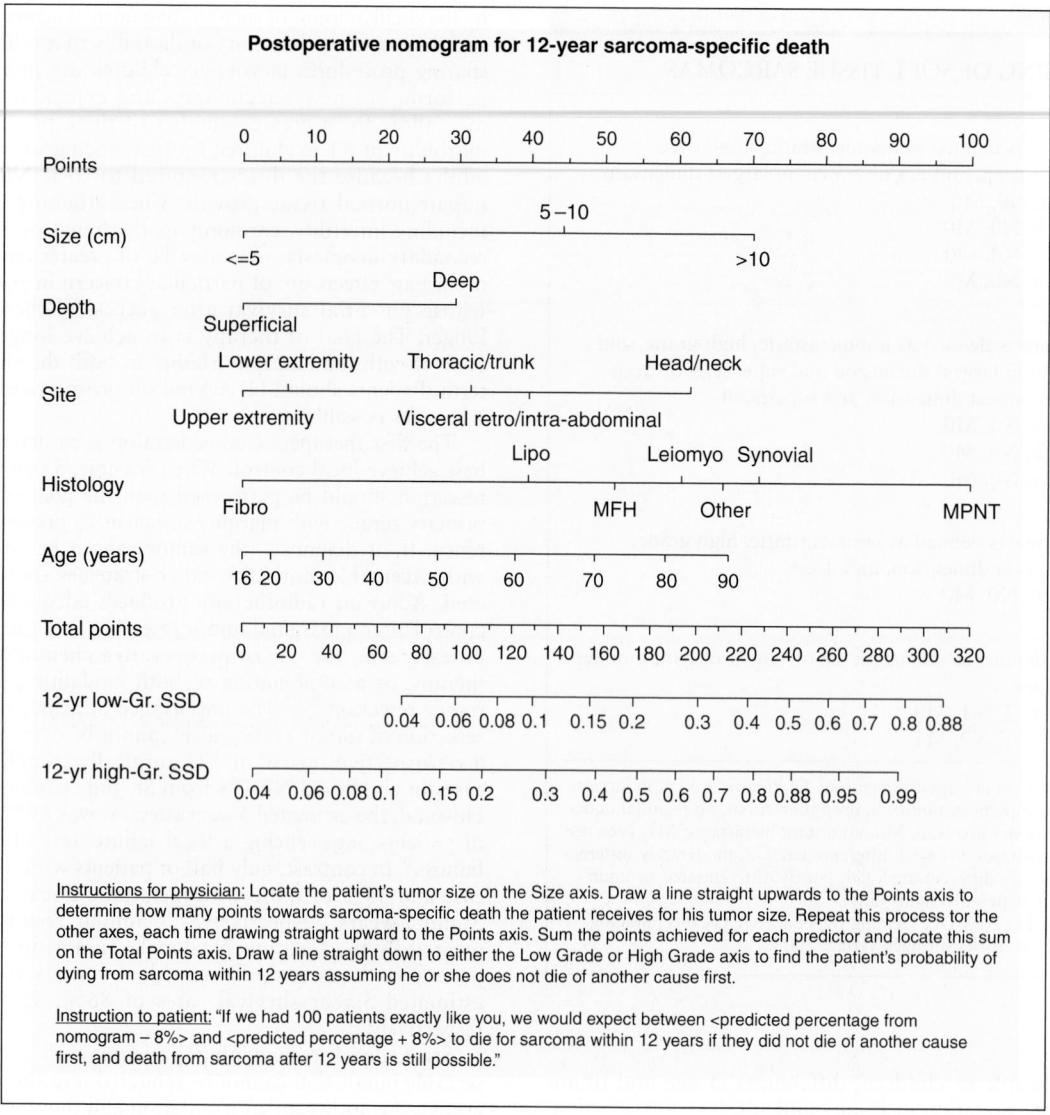

FIGURE 32.4 Nomogram that estimates the death rate at 12 years for sarcoma has been developed by Memorial Sloan-Kettering Cancer Center. Fibro, fibrosarcoma; Gr, grade; Leiomyo, leiomyosarcoma; Lipo, liposarcoma; MFH, malignant fibrous histiocytoma; MPNT, malignant peripheral nerve tumor; SSD, sarcoma-specific death. (From Kattan MW, Leung DH, Brennan MF. Postoperative nomogram for 12-year sarcoma-specific death. J Clin Oncol 2002;20:791. Reprinted with permission from the American Society of Clinical Oncology.)

to use these techniques depends, in part, on the experience of the institution's pathologists in diagnosing these rare tumors on very small samples of tumor. In one study, the experience with FNA biopsy in children has been quite good, making a diagnosis in more than 90% of the patients.[78] However, the classification of NRSTS is now heavily dependent on cytogenetic and molecular studies. It is essential that sufficient diagnostic material be obtained for these biologic studies. This is more reliably achieved with a core or open biopsy. An FNA with insufficient material for diagnosis should be followed by a core or open biopsy when clinical suspicion of malignancy is high. FNA or core biopsy has the advantage that it can be performed under local anesthesia in many patients. In addition, the use of CT or ultrasound guidance may enable biopsy of deeply located lesions that would require laparotomy or thoracotomy for open biopsy. Depending on local expertise, the surgeon, radiologist, or pathologist may perform the biopsy. The presence of an experienced cytopathologist nearby when

the biopsy is being performed is also important. A well-trained cytopathologist can direct the FNA biopsy and may be able to increase the yield. Core needle biopsies may be performed in many of the same situations as FNA biopsies and may provide tissue with intact architecture that is helpful to the pathologist. The biopsy procedure should also be planned to obtain adequate tissue for cytogenetic and molecular studies since they play an integral part of the diagnosis of NRSTS.

Open Biopsy

In most instances, an open biopsy is performed by an incisional technique. Excisional biopsies are reserved for very small superficial lesions. Longitudinal incisions are frequently better than horizontal incisions in such areas as the extremity. The definitive surgery for these malignancies requires that the biopsy tract be excised at the time of definitive operation. If the biopsy site is inappropriately placed, this excision may require much larger incisions or resections than otherwise would have been necessary. Inappropriately placed incisions on the trunk, head, neck, or other areas may make closure more difficult. Flaps should not be reconstructed during incisional biopsies because this may contaminate a larger area. Careful hemostasis is also important to not allow the spread of malignant cells in a hematoma. Ideally, excisional biopsies are planned to achieve negative margins. If an excisional biopsy would result in too large a resection, then performing an incisional biopsy and planned resection is a more appropriate approach. Incisional biopsy margins should be carefully marked to aid the surgeon in subsequently obtaining negative margins.

Definitive Surgery

What constitutes an adequate margin for local control remains controversial. Many adult studies suggest the necessity of achieving a 2-cm margin. This would be impractical or impossible in the pediatric age group. It appears that narrow margins near neurovascular structures may not be as significant as narrow or thin margins in muscular planes. Recurrence is less common nearer the neurovascular bundle than in other tissue planes. In one study by Blakely et al.,[79] a margin less than 1 cm had a higher local recurrence rate. An adequate wide resection includes the tumor, its pseudocapsule, and a margin of normal tissue removed in all directions en bloc. Cure can be obtained without removal of the entire muscle compartment, and proper resection may obviate the need for postoperative radiation or at least decrease the intensity. Because some sarcomas have a pseudocapsule, they may be inappropriately shelled out with the operating surgeon believing that he or she has completely removed the tumor, although microscopic, if not gross disease, was left behind. Local recurrence rates are extremely high in these instances. High-grade tumors that are larger than 5 cm or extend beneath the fascia may require a much more aggressive approach, because their potential for local recurrence is significant.[80] Pathologic examination or postoperative imaging studies suggesting that there is residual tumor or very thin margins should prompt the surgeon to recommend reexcision of the primary site to ensure local control. Overall, the most important surgical aspect for local control and decreasing recurrence is a WLE with clear margins.

Lymph Node Sampling and Dissection

In general, because lymph node involvement for most NRSTS is rare, evaluation has not been routine. However, regional lymph node involvement may be present in as many as 15% of patients with synovial sarcoma and other high-grade lesions such as angiosarcoma, clear cell sarcoma, and ES.[56,81] Therefore, some centers routinely perform sentinel lymph node mapping and biopsy in these histologic subtypes of STSs of the extremity or trunk.[82] This may best be accomplished at the time of initial WLE and is performed with the injection of a combination of technetium-labeled sulfur colloid and isosulfan blue dye (Lymphazurin).[83] A radioisotope detector is used to localize the sentinel node, and an incision is made over the localized area to then identify the blue nodes with high radioisotope count that represent the nodal basin. Formal lymph node dissection is not performed for node positivity, but radiation is considered. Recent clinical experience at Memorial Sloan-Kettering Cancer Center[84] and Italy[85] confirms the validity of this procedure in the pediatric patient. Since many of these tumors are rare, a prospective multicenter trial of sentinel node mapping should be encouraged. Sentinel lymph node mapping allows for minimal dissection and a very accurate means of assessing regional lymph node status. The low incidence of lymph node metastases in NRSTSs may allow withholding regional therapy in these patients.

Surgical Reresection

It is not infrequent for a patient with an NRSTS to be referred to the treatment center after an excisional biopsy elsewhere. The initial surgical procedure may not have been performed anticipating a malignancy. In this case, the quality of resection and the adequacy of margins are questionable. In some series, as many as half of re-resections demonstrate microscopic or gross residual disease despite the initial surgeon reporting that clear margins were obtained initially.[86,87] The importance of the completeness of surgical resection for the cure of this disease cannot be overemphasized. With this as a guiding principle, it is important for an experienced oncology surgeon to consider a re-resection when the adequacy of the initial procedure cannot be confirmed. In a recent study by Cecchetto et al. from Italy,[88] achievement of complete surgical resection was particularly important in the outcome of 29 patients with nonchemosensitive sarcomas. Sixteen of 19 (84%) patients with complete excision were alive without disease, whereas only 6 of 10 patients with incomplete or no surgery were alive. Among chemosensitive sarcomas, the completeness of excision did not improve the outcome. Ten of 12 (83%) patients with complete and 7 of 8 (87%) patients with incomplete excision are alive without disease.

Surgery for Extremity Tumors

Amputation, once the mainstay of therapy for NRSTS of the extremity, is now rarely used for primary management. Primary surgical approach for extremity tumors begins with ascertaining the diagnosis, extent of disease, and tumor biology. This is followed by wide local resections with adequate margins. Although the 2-cm margin as mentioned previously is frequently mentioned in the adult NRSTS literature, there are no prospective, randomized trials that have conclusively demonstrated that 2 cm is better than 2 to 3 mm in the pediatric age group. As previously emphasized, it is important to reexcise the biopsy wound and any area of possible tumor spill. Amputation is generally used only in the following situations: locally recurrent disease not associated with metastases; persistent, unresectable tumor after attempted complete resection; or in the case of extensive disease involving the neurovascular bundle when negative margins cannot be achieved.

On rare occasion, resection of the vessels and reconstruction may be in order. We have routinely stripped the periosteum when the tumor extends close to bone. Margins close to the perineural or perivascular sheath are frequently thin and may benefit from RT. External beam radiation or a brachytherapy (BRT) may be used to enhance local control. As mentioned earlier, amputation is generally used only in recurrent or persistent disease or for very distal lesions of the toes or fingers.

Surgery for Trunk Primary Tumors

Incisional biopsies of chest wall and trunk lesions are often best performed in conjunction with magnetic resonance imaging (MRI) or CT scan guidance. It is important to make a chest wall biopsy incision in the line of the ribs so that resection of the biopsy site, along with the ribs, may be performed at the time of definitive resection. Frequently, chest wall lesions have pleural involvement or even attachment to the lung surface, which must be factored into the resection. Very large defects can be closed with synthetic material such as Gore-Tex and then muscle flaps over the deficit.

Other Sites

Other sites such as abdominal wall tumors, visceral tumors, and retroperitoneal tumors are rare in children. Primary resection remains the treatment of choice. Unfortunately, this is quite difficult in the pediatric age group. Sites such as the head and neck require coordination with plastic surgeons or reconstructive techniques including regional rotation flaps or vascularized flaps.

Resection of Pulmonary Metastatic Disease

Approximately 20% of patients with NRSTS will develop evidence of metastatic disease, and the lung is the site that is most commonly affected. A review of 1,643 cases of pulmonary metastases treated at Memorial Sloan Kettering reveled that the most common histologic subtypes were MFH, synovial sarcoma, and LMS.[89] Complete surgical resection of all visible disease is required for cure, but even when this is performed, long-term cures are seen in less than 10% of patients.[90]

RADIATION THERAPY

There are no standardized RT guidelines for pediatric NRSTS. Although similar treatment strategies are used in the management of pediatric RMS, NRSTSs typically require higher radiation doses and are less sensitive to chemotherapy. A current COG trial (ARST 0332) is attempting to provide a framework for therapeutic approaches, including defining radiation dose and volume and timing with respect to surgery and chemotherapy, in this diverse group of tumors. Until such outcome data are available, recommendations have been based on retrospective data primarily from the adult STS experience.[91-93] Radiation therapy is considered for most cases of pediatric NRSTS; however, specific factors at initial diagnosis influence the decision for RT in the therapeutic plan and include extent of surgical resection (resected vs. unresectable), pathologic grade (low grade vs. high grade), tumor size, location of the primary tumor, and stage of disease (local vs. metastatic).[60,94,95]

Indications for RT

The extent of resection at the time of diagnosis is one of the most important factors determining the need for RT. If negative surgical margins are achieved after WLE, postoperative RT is not required for low-grade tumors and may be avoided in high-grade tumors that measure 5 cm or less.[96,97] The supporting data for this strategy come from single-institution retrospective series in adult sarcomas that report low local recurrence rates (15%) in small, high-grade tumors when treated with WLE only.[98-100] Some series argue that larger tumor size is associated with a greater risk for local recurrence, and postoperative radiation may play a role in optimizing local control; however, the use of this modality has not been proven to increase survival.[75,97,101]

In adults, the definition of a negative surgical margin varies according to the reporting institution (usually 1–2 cm) and the indications for radiotherapy vary accordingly.[86,96,102-104] In pediatric NRSTS, there is no standard definition of a negative surgical margin and the indications for radiotherapy within this setting have not been prospectively studied. In one single-institution study, radiotherapy improved local control in patients with high-grade tumors and pathological margins of less than 1 cm.[79] The current COG NRSTS protocol defines a negative surgical margin as at least 0.5 cm of nonmalignant tissue around the surgical specimen. When tumor abuts the periosteum or fascia and is removed in continuity with the tumor specimen, the margin can be considered negative.

Postoperative RT should also be considered if the surgical resection entails less than a WLE, if the surgeon did not expect a sarcoma at initial diagnosis and no preoperative imaging is obtained, if there were multiple attempts at resection and the surgical margins are unknown, or if attempts at tumor excision were not performed by a skilled oncology team that would place the patient at high risk for local failure.

Resectable tumors that have been totally excised grossly with microscopically positive margins benefit from the administration of postoperative RT.[75,104,105] An exception to this recommendation is for low-grade tumors that can be observed without postoperative RT. In these patients, reexcision is often successful and RT can be avoided, limiting the growth and functional impairment that is often associated with this treatment modality.[106,107]

Sarcomas that are unresectable outside of a mutilating procedure, such as an amputation, may benefit from a course of preoperative RT or chemoradiotherapy.[76,108,109] Even if the tumor mass does not decrease in size after preoperative therapy, pathology may show necrotic debris with little viable tumor and additional RT in the form of BRT, intraoperative radiotherapy, or external beam radiation therapy (EBRT) can be administered in the event of positive surgical margins.

RT Technical Factors

External beam radiation therapy is the most commonly used type of RT to treat pediatric sarcomas. Photons from a linear accelerator can target tumors below the skin surface with a variety of delivery techniques. The primary goal is to choose a method that delivers the most precise coverage of the tumor volume while protecting the adjacent tissues and organs critical for normal development. Conformal radiation therapy relies on acquiring three-dimensional (3-D) images, such as with CT, while the patient is in the treatment position. Once the tumor volume and surrounding organs are identified on sophisticated computer planning systems, multiple radiation beams are shaped to encompass the target volume. Intensity-modulated radiation therapy is a conformal technique that relies on modulating the intensity of multiple pencil-thin radiation beams. To ensure that the treatment plan is accurately reproduced newer methods such as image-guided radiation therapy can capture 3-D images of the patient's organs during radiation treatment, enabling physicians to make precise adjustments in the radiation field in relation to the patient position, These technologic advances work in concert to achieve improved tumor localization and meet the critical objective of protecting normal tissues from unnecessary irradiation.

Proton therapy is a type of EBRT that requires a specialized particle accelerator to generate the proton beam. Proton facilities are located at a small number of specialized facilities around the country. The advantage of protons compared with photons is less scatter radiation dose in the tissues and very little radiation dose beyond the desired depth of penetration. High target accuracy and tighter control of radiation deposition may lead to fewer normal tissue side effects including secondary cancers. Further studies are needed to determine whether these theoretical advantages translate to superior local control and functional outcome in pediatric tumors.[110]

Brachytherapy is frequently given as a boost after EBRT in an effort to deliver high doses of radiation to a focal area within the operative bed when clear surgical margins are difficult to achieve, such as an extremity neurovascular bundle. At the time of surgery, removable catheters are placed in the operative bed and 5 to 6 days after surgery loaded with high-dose rate or low-dose rate radioactive sources.[111]

TABLE 32.9

RADIATION THERAPY GUIDELINES FOR THE CHILDREN'S ONCOLOGY GROUP NRST TRIAL ARST 0332

Primary tumor	Tumor grade	Tumor size	Margin status at enrollment	Preoperative RT	Postoperative RT
Resected	Low	Any	Negative or positive	None	None
	High	≤5 cm	Negative	None	None
	High	≤5 cm	Positive	None	55.8 Gy
	High	>5 cm	Negative or positive	None	55.8 Gy
Unresected	Low or high	Any	Not applicable	45 Gy	No boost for negative margins
					10.8 Gy boost for microscopic margins
					19.8 Gy boost for macroscopic margins

Intraoperative radiation therapy is the delivery of RT to a target volume while the operative bed is exposed. The major advantage of this technique is that critical structures, such as small intestine, can be positioned to allow direct high-dose, single-fraction RT to be delivered to the tumor bed with minimal toxicity.[112]

Radiation Dose and Volumes

For resectable tumors, postoperative radiation doses in the range of 45 of 50 Gy are delivered to an initial radiation field (PTV1) defined by the tumor volume on preoperative MRI or CT imaging, the tumor bed defined by operative report and surgical clips, and any potential occult tumor spread encompassed by at least a 2-cm margin. If the surgical margins are positive, an additional 10 to 20 Gy is delivered to a reduced field (PTV2) targeting microscopic or gross disease. In the case of very young children, lower doses may be considered; however, there is no evidence that NRSTSs are more sensitive to RT in younger children than in adolescents or adults.

For unresected tumors, preoperative RT is delivered in the range of 45 to 50 Gy to the initial target volume (PTV1) defined by preoperative imaging and should include potential occult tumor spread and biopsy site encompassed by at least a 2-cm margin. If the surgeon is able to perform a surgical resection after a course of preoperative radiation, the surgical margins determine whether additional radiation is necessary. In general, 10 to 20 Gy is delivered for microscopic or gross disease, respectively. Brachytherapy is an excellent method to deliver radiation after a surgical resection if residual disease is anticipated. The surgeon can help to define the volume to be implanted and place surgical clips to delineate the appropriate volume for radiation treatment planning. If postoperative EBRT is used for a boost, the radiation doses are similar and the PTV2 is defined by the pathology and surgeons report, surgical clips, and postoperative imaging.

Table 32.9 shows the RT guidelines for the current COG NRSTS trial (ARST 0332). The doses are lower than those used for adults, as are the margins encompassing the tumor volume and have been chosen on the basis of concerns regarding side effects of RT, combined modality therapy, including neoadjuvant chemotherapy, and the broad range of ages for patients who might be enrolled on the study.

CHEMOTHERAPY

Although guidelines for surgery and radiotherapy in pediatric NRSTS are fairly well established, the role of systemic therapy has not been well studied. Since 1986, only three prospective

pediatric clinical trials that have accrued 182 patients have been completed and published in North America.[113–115] European STS studies have routinely included certain subtypes of NRSTS in their upfront STS studies, but the treatment guidelines for these tumors have been extrapolated in large part from the management guidelines used to treat RMS.[88,116]

The clearest indication for chemotherapy in pediatric NRSTS is unresectable tumor, since few patients are cured in the setting of gross residual disease.[117] Chemotherapy may also have a role in patients with resected tumors who are at high risk for metastatic tumor recurrence, that is, those with large, high-grade tumors. To date, only two agents have been shown to have clinical benefit by eliciting objective responses in a wide variety of NRSTS subtypes: doxorubicin and ifosfamide.[118–121] In pediatrics, objective responses to these agents have been reported in some histologic subtypes such as synovial sarcoma.[113] Unfortunately, the absolute survival benefit conferred by chemotherapy in the presence of unresected or metastatic disease is modest at best. Certain histologic subtypes (i.e., desmoid fibromatosis) respond to other drugs and are discussed further in the following sections.

Adjuvant Therapy—Adult Trials

The role of adjuvant chemotherapy for adults with resectable STS is controversial. Table 32.10 depicts 15 randomized, controlled clinical trials of adjuvant chemotherapy that have been published over the past 25 years. Among the 13 trials conducted in the 1970s and 1980s, the addition of chemotherapy improved overall survival in only 2. To address the concern that modest benefit from chemotherapy may have been overlooked because of the small size of many of these studies, the Sarcoma Meta-Analysis Collaboration (SMAC) conducted a meta-analysis of outcome for more than 1,500 adults included in 14 randomized controlled clinical trials comparing local therapy alone to local therapy plus chemotherapy.[142] This study showed that although chemotherapy significantly lengthened the local, distant, and overall recurrence-free interval ($p = 0.016$, $p = 0.0003$, $p = 0.0001$, respectively), the hazard ratio for overall survival was not significantly affected (hazard ratio [HR], 0.89; 95% confidence interval [CI], 0.76–1.03; $p = 0.12$). Various disease features, including primary site, histology, grade, and size, did not appear to influence the likelihood of survival benefit from chemotherapy. There was also no evidence that the addition of other agents to doxorubicin produced a different outcome than doxorubicin alone. This meta-analysis has been criticized for including tumors at all anatomic locations and of all histologic grades, which may have diluted the observed benefits of chemotherapy.[143] Furthermore, only one of the trial chemotherapy regimens

TABLE 32.10

PUBLISHED RANDOMIZED, CONTROLLED CLINICAL TRIALS OF ADJUVANT CHEMOTHERAPY IN ADULT SOFT TISSUE SARCOMAS

Study	Year	Number of evaluable patients	Eligibility	Drug(s)	Doxorubicin/epirubicin dose per cycle (mg/m²)	Cumulative doxorubicin dose (mg/m²)	Ifosfamide dose per cycle (g/m²)	Cumulative ifosfamide dose (g/m²)	Outcome
GOG (Omura)[122]	1973	156	Uterus only, any grade	Dox	60 q3wk	480	N/A	N/A	No difference in PFS or OS
MDACC (Benjamin)[123]	1973	43	Intermediate/high-grade, extremity	Dox, Vcr, Cyc, Act	60 q4wk	420	N/A	N/A	5-yr DFS benefit (60% vs. 35%, $p = 0.05$); OS not significantly different
Mayo (Edmonson)[124,125]	1975	61	Any grade, trunk or extremity	Dox, Vcr, Cyc, Act, DTIC	50 q6wk	200	N/A	N/A	No difference in OS; time to development of metastases longer in patients receiving chemotherapy
NCI (Rosenberg/Chang)[126,127]	1977	65	Intermediate/high-grade, extremity only	Dox, Cyc, Mtx	50–70 q4wk	550 maximum	N/A	N/A	5-yr DFS benefit (75% vs. 54%, $p = 0.37$), no 5-yr OS benefit (83% vs. 60%, $p = 0.124$)
NCI (Glenn)[128,129]	1977	31	Intermediate/high-grade, head/neck/breast/trunk/retroperitoneum	Dox, Cyc, Mtx	50–70 q4wk	550 maximum	N/A	N/A	3-yr actuarial DFS benefit (79% vs. 52%, $p = 0.018$), no 3-yr actuarial OS benefit ($p = 0.46$) for head/neck/breast/trunk sites; no DFS or OS benefit for retroperitoneal sites
EORTC (Bramwell)[130]	1977	317	Any grade, any site	Dox, Cyc, Vcr, DTIC	50 q4wk	400	N/A	N/A	7-yr actuarial RFS benefit (56% vs. 43%, $p = 0.007$), no difference in OS
DFCI/MGH (Antman)[131]	1978	42	Intermediate/high-grade, any site	Dox	90 q3wk	450	N/A	N/A	No difference in DFS or OS
ECOG (Lerner)[132]	1978	30	Intermediate/high-grade, any site	Dox	70 q3wk	490	N/A	N/A	No difference in DFS or OS
Bergonie (Ravaud)[133]	1980	59	Intermediate/high-grade, nonvisceral sites only	Dox, Cyc, Vcr, DTIC	50 q3wk	400–500	N/A	N/A	Metastasis-free survival and OS benefit ($p = 0.003$ and $p = 0.002$, respectively)
SSG (Alvegard)[134]	1981	181	High-grade, any site	Dox	60 q4wk	540	N/A	N/A	No difference in DFS or OS
Rizzoli (Gherlinzoni/Picci)[135,136]	1981	77	High-grade, extremity only	Dox	75 q3wk	450	N/A	N/A	5-yr DFS (68% vs. 42%) and OS (88% vs. 68%) benefit
ISSG (Baker/Antman)[137,138]	1983	86	Intermediate/high-grade, any site	Dox	70–90 q3wk	420	N/A	N/A	Reported only in aggregate with other trials
Siena (Petrioli)[139]	1985	88	Intermediate/high-grade, any site	Epi, Ifo	75 q3wk alone or 75 q4wk with ifosfamide	300	6	24	5-yr DFS benefit (69% vs. 44%, $p = 0.01$), no OS benefit
Vienna (Brodowicz)[140]	1992	59	Intermediate/high-grade, any site	Dox, Ifo, DTIC	50 q2wk	300	6	36	No RFS or OS benefit
Italian National Council for Research (Frustaci)[141]	1992	104	>5 cm, deep, high-grade, extremity	Epi, Ifo	120 q3wk	600	9	45	DFS and OS benefit ($p = 0.001$ and $p = 0.03$, respectively)

Act, actinomycin D; Cyc, cyclophosphamide; DFS, disease-free survival; Dox, doxorubicin; DTIC, imidazole carboxamide; Epi, epirubicin; Ifo, ifosfamide; Mtx, methotrexate; OS, overall survival; PFS, progression-free survival; RFS, relapse-free survival; VCR, vincristine.

included ifosfamide, which is widely acknowledged to be among the most active agents in adult STS. A more recent update included the 14 trials in the SMAC analysis as well as 4 additional studies that incorporated ifosfamide.[144] Included were six studies that used single-agent doxorubicin, five studies that used ifosfamide and an anthracycline (with or without dacarbazine), and seven that used doxorubicin in combination with agents other than ifosfamide. Patients receiving adjuvant chemotherapy had a small but statistically significant reduction in the risk of local recurrence, distant recurrence, and overall recurrence, and a slight but statistically significant improvement in survival. The absolute risk reduction was 4% for local recurrence, 9% for distant recurrence, and 10% for overall recurrence. Adjuvant chemotherapy significantly reduced the risk of death, with an HR of 0.77 (95% CI, 0.64–0.93; $p = 0.01$). This translated to an absolute risk reduction of 6%, or a 40% versus 46% risk of death. There was some evidence that ifosfamide-containing regimens were superior to those without ifosfamide. The absolute reduction in risk of death was 11% for ifosfamide-containing regimens ($p = 0.01$) but only 5% for doxorubicin alone ($p = 0.07$).

Interpreting the findings of adjuvant chemotherapy studies in adult STS for a pediatric patient population is difficult. The distribution of histologic subtypes of STS differs in children,[2] so outcomes after chemotherapy in children may not reflect the adult experience. Indeed, some data suggest that synovial sarcoma, one of the most common pediatric NRSTS, may respond better to ifosfamide than other types of STS more common in adults.[145] Children have a potentially longer life span than adults, so minor improvements in overall survival in a pediatric patient population may lead to substantially more years of life saved. However, children may also be more likely to experience long-term complications from chemotherapy exposure than adults because their growth and development are incomplete and because they have a longer life span. Whenever possible, adjuvant chemotherapy for pediatric NRSTS should be administered in the context of a clinical trial so that further data can be collected about its risks and benefits in these young patients.

Adjuvant Therapy—Pediatric Trials

In children, there has only been one prospective randomized trial of adjuvant chemotherapy for NRSTS. From June 1986 through May 1991, the POG evaluated the benefit of adjuvant chemotherapy (vincristine, doxorubicin, cyclophosphamide, and dactinomycin) compared with observation in surgically resected pediatric NRSTS.[115] Of the 81 eligible patients, only 30 accepted randomization and no evidence of improved outcome was observed in the subgroup that received adjuvant chemotherapy (Fig. 32.5A and B). Five-year survival and event-free survival estimates were significantly worse for patients who received adjuvant chemotherapy; however, this is likely the result of an excess of patients with high-grade lesions who received adjuvant chemotherapy.

In 2007, the COG opened a clinical trial to evaluate a risk-based treatment approach for patients younger than 30 years with all stages of NRSTS. The risk stratification treatment plan is illustrated in Figure 32.6 In this study, adjuvant chemotherapy is administered only to patients with high-grade tumors larger than 5 cm in maximal diameter who have undergone an upfront gross tumor resection. Other patients at high risk for distant disease dissemination (i.e., those with unresected, high-grade tumors > 5 cm in maximal diameter and those with metastases at the time of diagnosis) receive neoadjuvant combined chemotherapy and radiotherapy. The chemotherapy regimen being tested in this clinical trial is doxorubicin (75 mg/m²/cycle) and ifosfamide (9 g/m²/cycle). A similar clinical trial in Europe, sponsored by the European Pediatric Soft Tissue Sarcoma Study Group, utilizes a virtually identical ifosfamide/doxorubicin regimen but slightly different criteria for patient selection. These two trials, which should be completed in the early part of the next decade, will provide much additional information about outcomes in pediatric patients following local therapy in combination with adjuvant chemotherapy.

Therapy for Advanced Disease—Adult Trials

Because chemotherapy is relatively ineffective for STS, it is often difficult to judge which patients with advanced disease will benefit from systemic therapy. The clearest indication for chemotherapy in advanced disease is the presence of an unresectable tumor that may become resectable with chemotherapy-induced shrinkage. A retrospective analysis of 488 adults with unresectable or metastatic STS showed that 45% derived clinical benefit (defined as an objective response or ≥6 months of stable disease) from chemotherapy.[146] The median time to progression of the entire cohort was 3 months. However, the median duration of response in those who responded to chemotherapy was 9 months and the median duration of stable disease among those for whom this was the best response was 6 months. Combination chemotherapy produced a better response rate than single-agent chemotherapy (47% vs. 25%, $p < 0.001$). On multivariate analysis, favorable prognostic factors for survival included age less than 40 years, synovial sarcoma or liposarcoma histology, the absence of bone metastases, and the use of combination chemotherapy.

Doxorubicin has been a mainstay of STS chemotherapy since the 1970s.[147] More recent studies have confirmed the modest activity of doxorubicin as a single agent, with response rates in the 25% range.[148,149] Dose intensification of doxorubicin does not seem to improve the rate of response or the likelihood of long-term survival significantly.[150] Dacarbazine has also been used for STS since the 1970s when a single-agent response rate of 17% was seen in adult patients.[151] Temozolomide, an oral prodrug of the active metabolite of dacarbazine, has demonstrated response rates below 15%.[152–154] The rate of response to single-agent cyclophosphamide approaches 10%.[118] Ifosfamide has produced responses in approximately 20% to 30% of newly diagnosed adults with STS.[118,155] There is some evidence of an ifosfamide dose-response relationship,[156,157] although ifosfamide dose escalation in combination with doxorubicin did not improve the rate of response or disease-free survival.[158] A randomized comparison of single-agent doxorubicin to two different schedules of single-agent ifosfamide showed no difference in progression-free survival, but toxicity was greater on the ifosfamide arms.[159] Gemcitabine has limited efficacy overall in STS in adults[160,161] but appears to be particularly effective in LMS.[162]

Combination chemotherapy for STS in adults dates back to the 1970s. In general, combination chemotherapy regimens have demonstrated higher response rates, although these have been accompanied by greater toxicity and, in most cases, no clear survival advantage. The earliest combination, doxorubicin and dacarbazine, demonstrated response rates that exceeded those observed with single-agent doxorubicin therapy.[151,163,164] Cyclophosphamide and vincristine were added to doxorubicin and dacarbazine in CYVADIC.[165] However, this regimen failed to produce a higher response rate, a longer duration of response, or a longer median survival than single-agent doxorubicin.[149] MAID (mesna, doxorubicin,

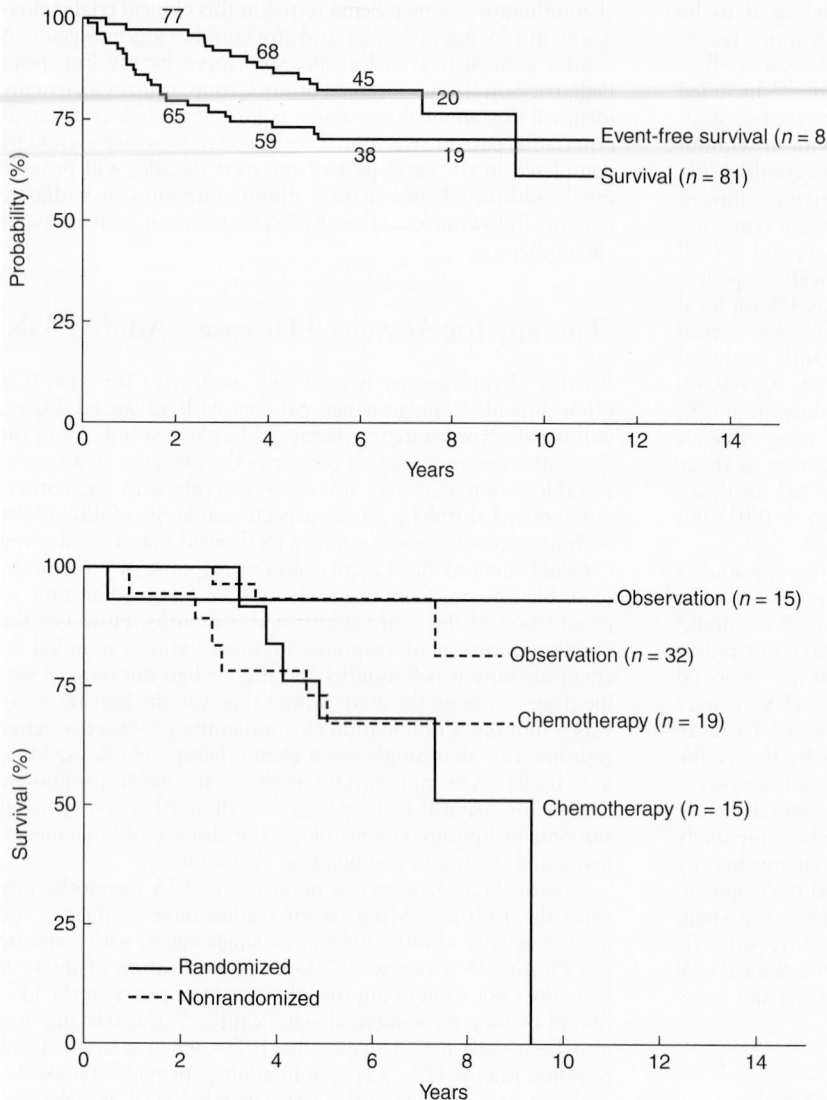

FIGURE 32.5 A: Event-free and overall survival curve of 81 children and adolescents treated with POG8653 protocol. (From Pratt CB, Pappo AS, Gieser P, et al. Role of adjuvant chemotherapy in the treatment of surgically resected pediatric nonrhabdomyosarcomatous soft tissue sarcomas: a Pediatric Oncology Group Study. J Clin Oncol 1999;17:1219, with permission.) **B:** Overall survival curve of 81 children and adolescents treated with POG8653 protocol based on the randomization and treatment status. (From Pratt CB, Pappo AS, Gieser P, et al. Role of adjuvant chemotherapy in the treatment of surgically resected pediatric nonrhabdomyosarcomatous soft tissue sarcomas: a Pediatric Oncology Group Study. J Clin Oncol 1999;17:1219, with permission.)

ifosfamide, and dacarbazine) chemotherapy[119,166] proved superior to doxorubicin/dacarbazine in terms of response rate and time to progression.[121] Dacarbazine was omitted from MAID to permit dose intensification of ifosfamide and doxorubicin.[167] This two-drug combination produced responses in about two-thirds of patients. However, a randomized study of doxorubicin in combination with 6 or 12 g/m^2/cycle of ifosfamide showed no benefit of the higher dose of ifosfamide in terms of disease-free or overall survival.[158] Finally, the combination of gemcitabine and docetaxel has produced modest rates of response in STSs.[168]

Therapy for Advanced Disease—Pediatric Trials

Pediatric studies in advanced NRSTS are limited. In the 1980s, the POG evaluated the role of dacarbazine in the context of multiagent chemotherapy with vincristine, doxorubicin, cyclophosphamide, and dactinomycin for patients with unresected or metastatic NRSTS.[114] The addition of dacarbazine did not improve the response rate (44% with vs. 56% without, $p = 0.4$), or 4-year event-free survival (26.4% with vs. 36% without). A subsequent POG phase II study of vin-

cristine, ifosfamide (9 g/m^2/cycle), and doxorubicin (60 mg/m^2/cycle) for unresectable or metastatic NRSTS demonstrated similar findings.[113] Forty-one percent of patients experienced a complete or partial response and the 3-year progression-free survival was 60% ± 10% for unresectable disease and 14.3% ± 9% for metastatic disease. In 2007, the COG opened a clinical trial for patients younger than 30 years with newly diagnosed NRSTS (Fig. 32.6). In this study, patients with intermediate- and high-risk disease (defined as a high-grade tumor > 5 cm, unresectable disease, or metastatic disease) are receiving dose-intensive chemotherapy (ifosfamide 9 g/m^2/cycle and doxorubicin 75 mg/m^2/cycle) and those whose primary tumor has not been resected also receive 45 Gy of neoadjuvant radiotherapy. After a delayed surgical resection, a radiotherapy boost is given on the basis of the margin status. This study is expected to complete accrual in 2013.

Towards Targeted Therapies in NRSTS

The discovery of specific genetic changes and unique pathways involved in the pathogenesis of various STSs is rapidly changing the therapeutic landscape of these diseases. For example, the use of mTOR inhibitors and PI3K inhibitors might hold

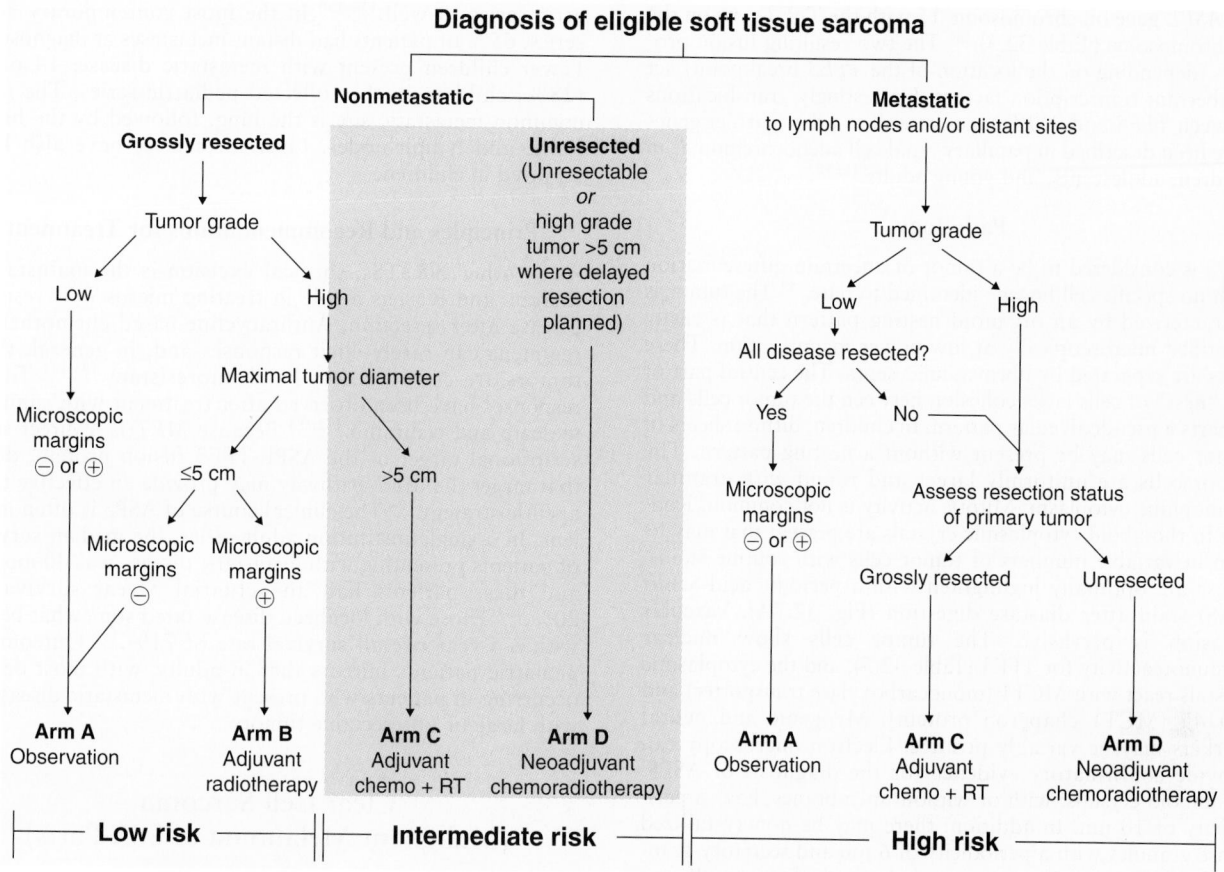

FIGURE 32.6 Risk group and treatment assignment algorithm for Children's Oncology Group protocol ARST 0332, "Risk-Based Treatment for Non-Rhabdomyosarcoma Soft Tissue Sarcomas (NRSTS) in Patients Under 30 Years of Age."

promise for the treatment of MPNSTs.[169] The use of trabectedin has been shown to be active in myxoid liposarcomas, and recent evidence suggests that this agent causes adipocyte differentiation by targeting the FUS/CHOP-mediated transcriptional block.[170,171] Sunitinib has shown promising activity in alveolar soft part sarcoma and DSRCTs,[172,173] sorafenib has shown preliminary activity in angiosarcoma.[174] Imatinib mesylate has been successfully used to treat dermatofibrosarcoma protuberans. This low-grade malignancy that affects the skin and subcutaneous tissue is characterized by a translocation t(17;22)(q22;q13) that fuses the *COL1A1* and *PDGFRB* genes.[175] Upregulation of MET has been documented in alveolar soft part sarcoma and clear cell sarcoma, suggesting that these tumors might benefit from the administration of c-MET inhibitors.[176]

Conclusions

On the basis of existing data in adults and children, the role of adjuvant chemotherapy continues to be controversial. Chemotherapy appears to have a modest effect on the risk of local and distant tumor recurrence, and there is some evidence that it may slightly improve overall survival. However, the degree of benefit is quite small and the toxicity of therapy is substantial. For patients with unresectable disease, chemotherapy plays an important role in facilitating tumor resection, which greatly increases the likelihood of cure. Less clear is whether the use of chemotherapy lengthens the quan-

tity and/or quality of life for patients with metastatic disease for which prognosis remains dismal.

SELECTED SPECIFIC DISEASES (LISTED IN ALPHABETICAL ORDER)

Alveolar Soft Part Sarcoma

Epidemiology

Alveolar soft part sarcoma (ASPS) is a rare STS that accounts for less than 1% of cases. Data from the SEER registries indicate a peak incidence in the third decade of life.[177] A female predominance has been well documented and evidence suggests that the increased risk in females is due to their possession of an extra X chromosome and the *ASPL-TFE3* fusion gene not being subject to X-inactivation.[177] Three pediatric case series have been published.[178–180] These series confirm that ASPS can occur in children younger than 5 years, although no cases in infants were described. Among the 50 patients in these 3 case series, 29 (58%) patients were female.

Biology and Genetics

ASPS is characterized by an unbalanced chromosomal translocation der(17)t(X;17)(p11;q25) that results in the fusion of the *ASPL* gene on chromosome 17 with the *TFE3* gene on the X chromosome (Table 32.3).[181] The two resulting fusion proteins (depending on the location of the *TFE3* breakpoint) act as aberrant transcription factors. Interestingly, translocations between *TFE3* and *ASPL* genes as well as other partner genes have been described in papillary renal cell adenocarcinomas in children, adolescents, and young adults.[182,183]

Pathology

ASPS is considered to be a tumor of uncertain differentiation with no specific cell lineage identified to date.[184] The tumor is characterized by an organoid nesting pattern that is easily identified microscopically at low-power magnification. These nests are separated by fibrovascular septa. The central part of the "nest" of cells lacks cohesion between the tumor cells and imparts a pseudoalveolar pattern. In children, diffuse sheets of tumor cells may be present without a nesting pattern. The tumor cells are uniformly larger and round with granular eosinophilic cytoplasm. Mitotic activity is not common. Rod-like to rhomboid cytoplasmic crystals are present that may be seen in variable numbers of tumor cells with routine stains. These are optimally highlighted with a periodic acid-Schiff (PAS) stain after diastase digestion (Fig. 32.7A). Vascular invasion is pervasive. The tumor cells show nuclear immunoreactivity for TFE3 (Table 32.5), and the cytoplasmic crystals react with MCT1 (monocarboxylase transporter) and CD147 (MCT1 chaperon protein). Myogenic and neural markers may be variably positive. Electron microscopy can provide confirmatory evidence for the diagnosis of ASPS. Rhomboid crystals, with or without membranes, have a periodicity of 10 nm. In addition, there may be noncrystallized dense granules with a periodicity of 6 nm and secretory granules with homogeneous material that may have small foci undergoing crystallization.

Clinical Presentation

In adults, about half of the patients present with an extremity mass, the thigh being the most common location.[185,186] Extremity tumors account for about half of the cases in pedi-atric series as well.[178–180] In the most contemporary adult series, 65% of patients had distant metastases at diagnosis.[185] Fewer children present with metastatic disease: 14 of 50 (28%) children in the collected pediatric series. The most common metastatic site is the lung, followed by the brain, bone, and lymph nodes. Liver metastases have also been reported in children.

Principles and Recommendations for Treatment

As in other NRSTSs, surgical excision is the mainstay of therapy and RT has a role in treating microscopic residual disease after resection. Anthracycline-based chemotherapy regimens can rarely elicit responses and, in general, these tumors are considered to be chemoresistant.[185,187] Tumor responses have been observed after treatment with sunitinib maleate and cediranib.[172,188] Because *MET* is a direct transcriptional target of the ASPL-TFE3 fusion protein, drugs that target the *MET* pathway may provide an effective therapeutic strategy.[176] The clinical course of ASPS is often indolent. In a single-institution adult series, the median survival of patients presenting with metastatic disease was 40 months and these patients had an actuarial 5-year survival of 20%.[185] Those with localized disease fared somewhat better, with a 5-year overall survival rate of 71%.[185] Outcome in pediatric patients mirrors that in adults, with most deaths occurring in patients who present with metastatic disease or with large or unresectable tumors.

Clear Cell Sarcoma (Malignant Melanoma of Soft Parts)

Epidemiology

Clear cell sarcoma is a rare aggressive STS usually affecting young adults.[189,190] There does not seem to be any gender predilection. The largest pediatric case series included 28 patients ranging in age from 2 to 21 years, and the ratio of males to females was approximately 2:1.[191]

FIGURE 32.7 Differentiated soft tissue sarcomas other than rhabdomyosarcoma. **A:** Alveolar soft part sarcoma. This problematic tumor is easily differentiated from all other sarcomas. The glandular or alveolar pattern is always prominent; tumor cells appear to rest on a basement membrane. As shown here, spaces within are variably present. The tumor cells possess abundant pink cytoplasm that by light microscopy resembles muscle. However, periodic acid-Schiff-positive, diastase-resistant cytoplasmic crystalloids (*center*) are present in tumor cells. These crystals are diagnostic by electron microscopy (EM) (*inset*). Evidence favors a myogenous origin of this tumor, although myogenous differentiation has never been identified using EM [hematoxylin and eosin (H&E), 250×]. **B:** Fibrosarcoma. This tumor is rare in adults and uncommon in older children, but it is one of the most common nonmyogenous soft tissue sarcomas in the first decade. Interlacing fascicles of spindle cells appear either elongate (*left*) or round (*right*), depending on the plane of section. The cells are closely packed and homogeneous and resemble normal fibroblasts. Mitoses, pleomorphism, and nuclear hyperchromatism are rare (H&E stain, 250×). **C:** Leiomyosarcoma. Smooth muscle tumors in children are rare but do occur. Leiomyosarcoma in children and adults is characterized by spindle cells that resemble fibroblasts but stain intensely with eosin because of their content of smooth muscle actin-myosin bundles. Some degree of pleomorphism (*bottom center*) and mitosis (*upper center*) are often found (H&E, 250×). **D:** Liposarcoma. All liposarcomas are rare in children, and of the four types commonly seen in adults, only the myxoid type is common in children. This relatively low-grade sarcoma resembles fetal lipoblasts, often interspersed among more differentiated adipocytes (large clear cells). The vasculature (*left*) is routinely prominent in liposarcomas and helps to differentiate this tumor from lipoblastoma and related benign fatty tumors (H&E, 3,400×). **E:** Neurofibrosarcoma. The light microscopic appearance of this tumor may be indistinguishable from that of fibrosarcoma. Electron microscopy reveals evidence of nerve sheath differentiation, although not often as well developed as seen here, in which some tumor cells envelop neurites (*upper center*), mimicking Schwann cells. More often, only fragmented basal lamina and slender cell processes are present (EM, 2,00×0): **F:** Synovial sarcoma. Classic biphasic synovial sarcoma is an unmistakable entity. Distinct epithelial, glandular differentiation (*center*) alternates with fibrosarcomatous stroma (*right*). Islands of tumor cells separated by hyaline stroma are sometimes seen (*left*), and staghorn vasculature (not illustrated) is often conspicuous (H&E, 100×).

Biology and Genetics

Clear cell tumors of soft tissues possess a tumor-defining translocation [t(12;22)(q13;q12), EWS-ATF1] that is present in more than 90% of cases and has not been identified in other malignancies.[192] This translocation is not present in cutaneous, mucosal, or visceral malignant melanoma. The resulting EWS-ATF fusion protein is involved in repression of p53/CBP-mediated transactivation. These tumors also overexpress a melanocytic specific form of microphthalmia transcription factor. These tumors are of neural crest derivation, often attached to tendons and aponeuroses, and may be derived from the spindle apparatus in these structures. Trisomy

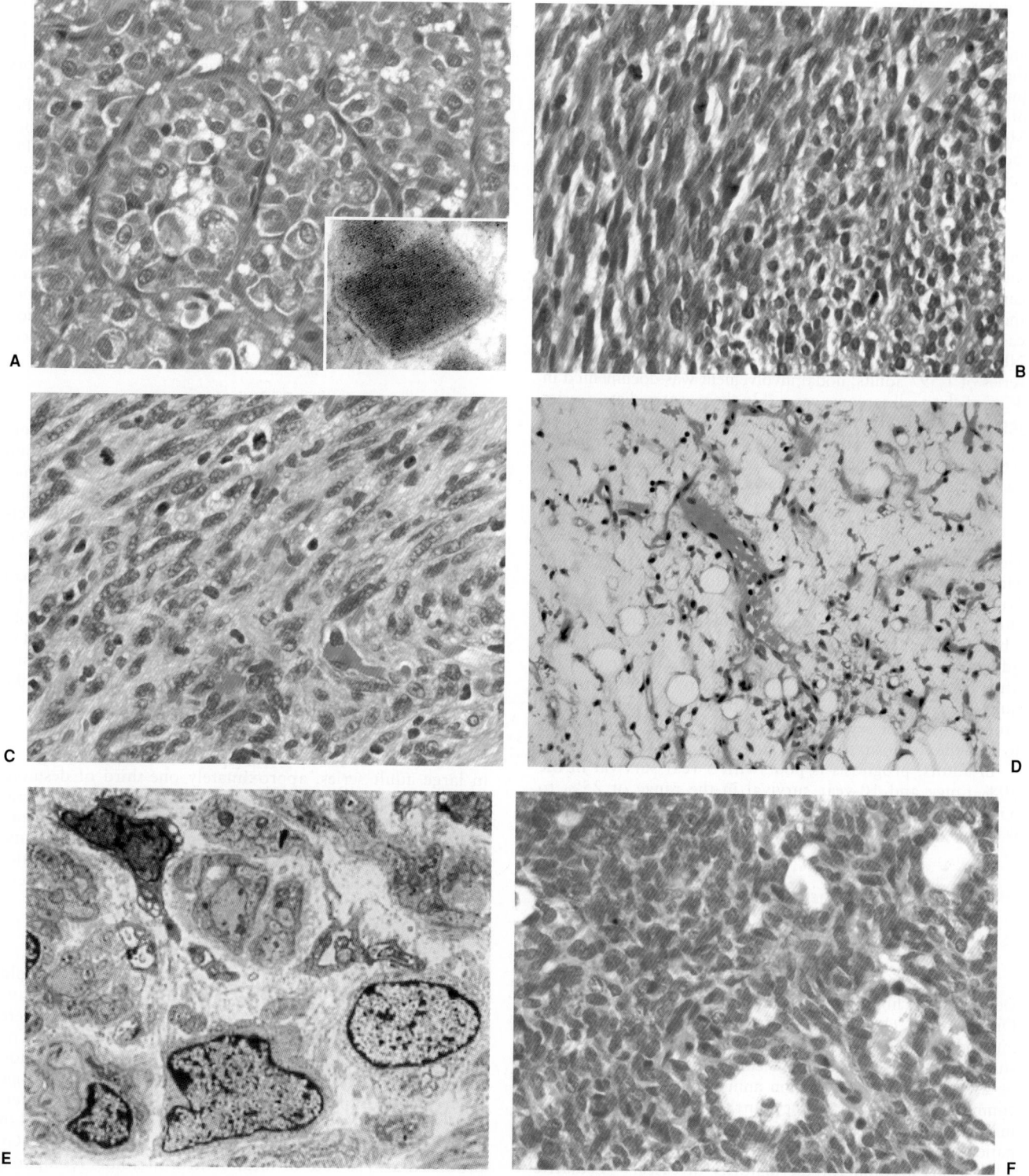

of chromosomes 7 and 8 may also be found on cytogenetic karyotypes.

Pathology

The majority of these tumors appear identical to malignant melanoma of skin. The tumor cells are arranged in nests or fascicles separated by fibrous septa. The cells are polygonal to spindled, with abundant eosinophilic cytoplasm, infrequent melanin pigment, and nuclei with large prominent nucleoli. Occasional wreath-like tumor giant cells may be present. Mitotic activity and pleomorphism are usually quite low. The cellular morphology may vary in a small proportion of cases from a spindle cell arrangement, with marked pleomorphism and mitotic activity to a solid round cell pattern. Infrequently, the stroma may have a microcystic or myxoid character. Immunocytochemical staining reveals the melanocytic nature of the tumor cells with immunoreactivity for HMB-45, Melan-A, MART1, S100 protein, and other markers for melanoma. On ultrastructural examination, melanosomes of various stages can be appreciated.

Clinical Presentation

In adults, almost all patients present with extremity tumors involving tendons and aponeuroses.[193] Slow growing masses can be present weeks to years and are painful in up to half of the cases. Foot and ankle region tumors compose 40% of all cases. Clear cell sarcoma (along with ES) is unique among NRSTS in having a propensity for regional nodal spread. In a series of 1,597 adults, nodal involvement was documented in 17% of clear cell sarcoma cases.[81] In the recent pediatric series reported by the Italian and German Soft Tissue Sarcoma Cooperative Group, 20 (71%) of the 28 patients presented with extremity primaries. Five patients had lymph node, and two patients had distant metastases.[191]

Principles and Recommendations for Treatment

General NRSTS therapy principles apply for this tumor. However, because of the propensity of this tumor to involve lymph nodes, sentinel lymph node biopsy or lymph node sampling is indicated at the time of initial presentation. The ultimate surgical goal should be wide excision, with adjuvant radiotherapy if the margins are close or positive after maximal surgery. The chemotherapy response rate is quite low,[189,191] so a trial of chemotherapy is probably warranted only in the setting of unresectable disease in an effort to facilitate tumor resection.

In adults, prognosis is poor with 5-year survival in the 50% range and 10-year survival in the range of 25% to 35%.[189,190] In one pediatric series, the overall 5-year survival was 66.4% at a median follow-up of 102 months.[191]

Desmoid Tumor (Desmoid-Type Fibromatosis, Aggressive Fibromatosis)

Epidemiology

Desmoid-type fibromatosis is classified by the World Health Organization classification of soft tissue tumors as an intermediate (locally aggressive) tumor.[194] A population-based study in Finland estimated the incidence of desmoid tumors to be 2.4 to 4.3 cases per million annually.[195] The tumor most commonly occurs during the fourth decade of life, and the male:female ratio is approximately 1:1.5.[196–198] In pediatric patients, desmoid tumors have been described in infancy but adolescents account for the majority of cases.[199] Pediatric

desmoid fibromatosis does not seem to have a sex predominance.[199] Desmoid tumors usually occur sporadically, although they are seen in about 10% of patients with FAP.[200,201] The risk of developing a desmoid tumor increases to 25% in individuals with FAP who have a family member with a desmoid tumor.[200]

Biology and Genetics

The cytogenetic findings in desmoid tumors vary from a normal karyotype to trisomy of chromosomes 8 and 20 in about 30% of cases to mutation of the APC gene (5q21). The significance of trisomies is not known but is seen in many soft tissue tumors. There has been a suggestion that trisomy may be seen in "more advanced" disease; however, this may simply be a late event in the course of tumorigenesis. Desmoid tumors are known to occur in FAP syndrome (APC mutation at 5q21) but may also occur in sporadic cases (with or without APC mutation) or as familial desmoid tumor syndromes without evidence of colon polyps (APC mutation). Wild-type APC interacts with and inhibits β-catenin, a cell signaling protein, also located at 5q21, in the Wnt pathway. When APC is mutated, the inhibitory effect of β-catenin is removed and allows for cell proliferation. Some sporadic desmoid tumors have β-catenin–activating mutations, which allow for overriding the inhibitory effect of wild-type APC. Mutations in exon 3 of the β-catenin gene have been documented in 85% of sporadic desmoids tumors, and the presence of a 45 F mutation in the tumor has been associated with an inferior, recurrence-free survival.[202]

Pathology

These diffusely infiltrative and poorly circumscribed tumors are composed of elongated fibroblastic cells embedded in an usually abundant collagen matrix. The collagen matrix may have areas with broad, thick bands of collagen fibers with a keloid appearance. There are regularly distributed vessels with perivascular edema. The fibroblasts are spindled to stellate with bland nuclear features and lack cytologic atypia. Mitotic activity is sparse. The cells may be arranged in broad sweeping fascicles. The tumor cells express vimentin, muscle-specific actin, and smooth muscle actin, indicative of fibroblastic and myofibroblastic differentiation (Table 32.5). On electron microscopy, the majority of cells have a fibroblastic character (Table 32.6), with the minority appearing more like myofibroblasts.

Clinical Presentation

In large adult series, approximately one-third of desmoid tumors originate in the extremities, one-third in the viscera, 10% in the head and neck region, and the remainder in trunk wall.[196–198] In a retrospective series of 63 pediatric patients, desmoids tumors more commonly occurred in the extremities (61%), head and neck (18%), and trunk (13%). Eight percent of the tumors in this series were multicentric.[199]

Principles and Recommendations for Treatment

Surgical excision is the mainstay of treatment of desmoid fibromatosis; local recurrence rates of 15% to 30% have been reported after surgery in which negative margins were achieved, with or without adjuvant radiotherapy.[203] The reported risk of local recurrence after marginal excision ranges from 22% to 68%, although rates in the 25% range are typical for patients who receive adjuvant radiotherapy.[196,203,204] Radiotherapy may be less effective for control of gross disease; however, the use of doses higher than 50 Gy produced a 77% rate of local control in adults (compared with a 40% rate of local control when the dose was ≤50 Gy).[196] Radiotherapy appears to be less effective in pediatric patients.[205] In recent years, the benefits of systemic therapy in desmoid fibromatosis have led to an increase in its use.[197] The combination of vinblastine and methotrexate was documented to produce a tumor response or stabilization in all 30 patients in an adult phase II study;[206] similar findings were documented in pediatric patients.[207] Imatinib, a selective tyrosine kinase inhibitor that targets c-kit, PDGFR-α, and PDGFR-β, has shown some activity (16% partial response, 21% stable disease) in desmoid fibromatosis that appears to be mediated by PDGFR-β kinase activity.[208] In a Japanese study, the administration of meloxicam, doxorubicin, and DTIC produced significant objective responses in seven adults with desmoids tumors associated with FAP.[209]

Desmoplastic Small Round Cell Tumor

Epidemiology

Desmoplastic small round cell tumor is a rare aggressive sarcoma that is most commonly seen in adolescents and young adults.[210] There is a striking male predominance, with 82% to 96% of patients being male in relatively large single-institution series.[210–212]

Biology and Genetics

This malignant tumor of serosa lining body cavities has a specific tumor-defining translocation that involves fusion of the *EWS* (Ewing's sarcoma) gene with the *WT1* (Wilms tumor) gene [t(11;22)(p13;q12)].[210] *WT1* is expressed in a high degree in intermediate mesoderm tissue that undergoes differentiation from mesoderm to epithelium during development. The fact that this tumor appears to arise from body cavity serosal linings, and the "mesothelial nature" of this tumor raises a question as to whether this tumor should be considered a mesothelioblastoma. The *EWS-WT1* gene can be identified both by karyotyping and by RT-PCR and allows for a definitive diagnosis in suspect or questionable cases.

Pathology

"Desmoplastic small round cell tumor" provides a description of the histopathologic pattern for this malignant tumor. There is an abundant, dense fibrotic stroma with small round cells embedded within this desmoplastic stroma. The small round cells may be arranged in variably sized nests or large sheets of tumor cells. There are frequent mitotic figures and central necrosis of the tumor nests with cystic degeneration. Glandular, rosette, and glomeruloid structures may be noted. Rhabdoid cells with eccentric eosinophilic cytoplasm inclusions displacing the nuclei may be found in up to 50% of cases. Within a single tumor, there may be cytologic features suggesting epithelial, neuroendocrine, neuroblastic, rhabdomyoblastic, and rhabdoid differentiation of the tumor cells. This impression is borne out by the diversity in immunophenotype (Table 32.5). The tumor cells express epithelial (cytokeratins, epithelial membrane antigen), myogenic (desmin in unique dot-like pattern), mesenchymal (vimentin), and neural (neuron-specific enolase). The tumor cells also immunoreact with the WT1 antibody. Electron microscopy reveals the polyphenotypic nature of this tumor, with infrequent to rare neurosecretory dense core granules, occasional desmosomes, and abundant intermediate filaments, with some arranged in a whirling pattern (Table 32.6). Thick and thin filaments and Z-band material typical of myogenic differentiation are not identified. The rhabdoid cell character of the tumor cells is most prominent.

Clinical Presentation

The vast majority of patients with DSRCT present with an abdominal and/or pelvic primary tumor, often with infiltration into other organs (liver, pancreas, spleen) and serosal dissemination.[210–213] Primary renal DSRCT has been described in young children (<10 years of age).[214] Thoracic, head and neck, extremity, and intracranial presentations are less common. Metastases of serosal surfaces, regional lymph nodes, liver, and lung are frequent[210,212]; metastatic involvement of the spleen, kidneys, bone, and bone marrow has been reported.[211,212,215]

Principles and Recommendations for Treatment

DSRCT typically responds favorably to sarcoma-directed chemotherapy,[212,215] but the ultimate outcome is very poor despite multimodal therapy. In a series reported by investigators at M.D. Anderson Cancer Center, 25 of the 35 patients for whom follow-up information was available were dead of widespread metastases 8 to 50 months (mean, 25.2 months) after diagnosis and the remaining 10 were alive with disease.[213] Investigators at Memorial Sloan-Kettering Hospital used induction chemotherapy, aggressive surgical resection, radiotherapy, and myeloablative chemotherapy with stem-cell rescue, with an overall survival at 5 years of only 15%.[216] Long-term, disease-free survival has been reported in pediatric patients with extra-abdominal tumors treated with chemotherapy and gross resection ± radiotherapy.[212]

Epithelioid Sarcoma

Epidemiology

Epithelioid sarcoma is quite rare in adults; a retrospective analysis at Memorial Sloan-Kettering Cancer Center identified only 16 cases among 2,678 patients with STS (0.6%).[217] In childhood, ES is somewhat more common, accounting for approximately 2% of pediatric STS in the United States.[2] A striking male predominance has been noted in both adult and pediatric series.[217–221] The mean age at presentation in adult populations is approximately 30 years.[217,219,221] Epithelioid sarcoma has been described in infancy and throughout childhood.[218,220]

Biology and Genetics

The few cytogenetic studies of conventional type ES that have been conducted to date have documented that most have complex karyotypes with various deletions and gains but without recurring rearrangements.[222] In proximal type ES, the most common site of structural rearrangement is 22q and recurring rearrangements involving 22q11 have been observed.[222] The *SMARCB1/INI1* gene, located within the 22q11 breakpoint region, has been found to be disrupted in a significant proportion of proximal type ESs, suggesting a role for this gene in the genesis and/or progression of the disease.[223] c-Met receptor and hepatocyte growth factor (scatter factor) overexpression have been detected in ES, indicating a role for this signaling pathway in its pathogenesis.[224]

Pathology

This sarcoma of unknown histogenesis occurs in two separate forms: distal (conventional) and proximal types. The distal ES often occurs as a small, poorly circumscribed firm dermal or subcutaneous mass of less than 5 cm, or a larger somewhat necrotic tendinous or fascial mass up to 15 cm in size. Microscopically, the distal type has a nodular growth pattern with the tumor consisting of epithelioid and spindled cells. This tumor may be confused with a granulomatous process, resembling granuloma annulare or pseudorheumatoid nodule. Other features that may be present include discohesive cells, dystrophic calcifications, metaplastic bone formation, and chronic inflammation. The tumors may have a pseudoangiosarcomatous appearance (angiomatoid pattern). Perineural and perivascular involvement is common. There is also a fibroma-like pattern that may occur with spindle cells and abundant collagen stroma. Proximal (conventional) ES is the more recently described form and has features that are similar to extrarenal rhabdoid tumors. These tend to occur in older adults and are deep-seated tumors. The growth pattern tends to be multinodular, with large epithelioid cells that resemble poorly differentiated carcinoma, and have densely eosinophilic cytoplasm, vesicular nuclei, and prominent nucleoli. Rhabdoid features are frequent and may be the dominant component. Tumor necrosis is a common finding and often results in a granulomatous pattern. The typical immunohistochemical profile includes uniform vimentin reactivity and pankeratin AE1/AE3 and epithelial membrane antigen positivity; CD34 is positive in about half of cases, and S-100 protein is focally positive in a minority of cases.[225,226] Loss of expression of SMARCB1/INI1 protein is evident in most cases of both the conventional and proximal type variants.[225,227,228]

Clinical Presentation

Epithelioid sarcoma may present as a mass or as an ulcerated skin lesion. The mean duration of symptoms preceding the initial surgical intervention ranged from 18 to 29 months in several adult series.[217] In a review of 241 cases submitted to the Armed Forces Institute of Pathology (AFIP), the distal upper extremities were most frequently involved (58%), particularly the hands and forearms. Epithelioid sarcoma is characterized by a tendency to metastasize to regional lymph nodes, so regional lymph node sampling is recommended. In most adult series, the proportion of patients with nodal involvement at the time of initial presentation exceeds 15% whereas the incidence of lymph node metastases in STSs overall is 2% to 3%.[56,81,229] The most common sites of first metastasis are lymph nodes (48%), lung (25%), and skin (16%).[219] The pattern of metastatic spread in pediatric patients appears to be similar,[218] although an unusual pattern including liver, kidney, and bone metastases has been described in an infant with a distal forearm primary tumor.[230]

Principles and Recommendations for Treatment

The treatment of ES is similar to that of other NRSTSs. Surgery is clearly the mainstay of therapy and wide excision of the tumor is optimal if achievable. Because these tumors frequently arise in the distal extremities, ray resections and other amputative procedures are commonly required. When microscopic residual tumor remains after maximal surgical resection, adjuvant radiotherapy can increase the likelihood of local tumor control.[231] Grossly involved lymph nodes should be excised and radiotherapy delivered to the remainder of the involved lymph node bed. For unresectable disease, neoadjuvant chemotherapy and/or radiotherapy may be used. Data on the responsiveness of ES to chemotherapy are scant, but the largest published pediatric series documented responses in three of seven children, all of whom received ifosfamide- and doxorubicin-containing chemotherapy.[218]

Infantile Fibrosarcoma and Adult-Type Fibrosarcoma

Epidemiology

Fibrosarcoma accounts for about 5% of pediatric NRSTS and for approximately 25% to 30% of soft tissue malignancies in children younger than 1 year.[2,232,233] In adults, fibrosarcoma is estimated to comprise at most 2% of all STSs.[2] Because fibrosarcoma in young children is considerably less aggressive and more curable than the variety seen in older children and adults, it is labeled "infantile fibrosarcoma."[73] According to the POG staging system for NRSTS, a fibrosarcoma is considered IFS if it occurs in a child 4 years or younger.[47] However, there is some evidence that the age cutoff should be lower.[234]

Biology and Genetics

Despite the name fibrosarcoma, in infants, this unique tumor does not commonly metastasize, even though there may be local recurrences.[235] The AFIP series documented a metastatic rate of only 10%. The low metastatic potential, combined with failure of xenograft tumor formation in murine models, and a near-diploid karyotype have raised questions regarding the use of the term *fibrosarcoma*.[236,237] More recently, karyotypic studies have documented a recurring t(12;15) translocation leading to a novel gene fusion between ETV6 (TEL) and the high-affinity nerve growth factor NTRK3 (TRKC). This abnormality is not found in infantile myofibromatosis, other early childhood fibromatoses, or AFS occurring in older children.[43] This unique translocation distinguishes this tumor from other, similar appearing tumors such as infantile myofibromatosis and infantile hemangiopericytoma (hemangiopericytoma-like myofibroma). Infantile fibrosarcoma shares a tumor-defining translocation (ETV6-NTRK3) with cellular mesoblastic nephroma (Table 32.2). In addition, it may have other cytogenetic abnormalities, such as trisomy of certain chromosomes.

Adult fibrosarcomas typically have complex chromosomal abnormalities, as well as a recurring 2q14-22 aberration (Table 32.3). Other recurrent genetic abnormalities have also been noted,[234] but none are capable of distinguishing between high-grade and low-grade lesions. Because p53 mutations occur at high frequency in many STSs[238] and are associated with poor prognosis, p53 mutational analysis may provide a means to discriminate true fibrosarcoma from other fibroblastic tumors.[239]

Pathology

For IFS, the tumor is a highly cellular neoplasm with a herringbone pattern. The cells are spindled in outline but have a high nuclear to cytoplasm ratio. There is considerable nuclear hyperchromasia, tumor necrosis, and frequent mitoses scattered throughout the tumor. The tumor cells are closely packed and overlap one another. Focal hemangiopericytoma-like areas with increased vascularity may be seen. These tumors typically are diffusely positive for vimentin and focally reactive for actin (Table 32.5). Electron microscopy provides evidence for fibroblastic differentiation (Table 32.6). The ultrastructural features of lack of extremely rare extracellular banded collagen, rare to absent basal lamina, branching and markedly dilated rough endoplasmic reticulum, irregular nuclear membranes, and extracellular fibrillogranular material are helpful in separating this malignant fibroblastic tumor from myofibromas. These features are also more characteristic of origin from a primitive mesenchymal spindle cell, representing a precursor cell in the fibroblastic/myofibroblastic cell line. Electron microscopy plays a critical role in distinguishing this malignant tumor from spindle cell RMS, infantile RMS, undifferentiated pleomorphic sarcoma, and benign fibroblastic/myofibroblastic neoplasms. Ultrastructural examination is particularly important with the approximately 20% to 30% of IFS that immunoreact with desmin and/or muscle-specific actin (Table 32.3) and may result in confusion with a spindle cell RMS. An extensive search for striated muscle differentiation (well-formed external lamina, monoparticulate glycogen, myofilaments, and Z-band material) should be undertaken with a spindle cell tumor possessing a predominance of banded collagen and absence of extracellular matrix fibrillogranular material. In addition, the herringbone pattern, nuclear hyperchromasia, necrosis, and cystic degeneration distinguish this tumor from a benign myofibromatous tumor. An unusual childhood tumor that may be confused with IFS is the infantile rhabdofibrosarcoma. The identification of rhabdomyoblasts by immunocytochemistry, or more likely by electron microscopy, and chromosome 19 monosomy define the high-grade infantile rhabdofibrosarcoma. IFS must also be distinguished from primitive myxoid mesenchymal tumor of infancy, which is characterized by primitive mesenchymal cells in a myxoid background with mild cytologic atypia and absence of the *ETV6-NTRK3* gene fusion.[240]

Adult fibrosarcoma is an overtly malignant spindle cell tumor with a characteristic herringbone pattern consisting of interweaving fascicles of tumor cells in parallel arrays (Fig. 32.7B). The tumor cells typically demonstrate abnormal mitoses, nuclear pleomorphism, increased cytoplasmic basophilia, and occasional anaplastic features. The cells are closely packed, but reticulin staining reveals stromal collagen fibers are not easily appreciated on routine staining. It is critical that one distinguishes this tumor from tumors that are benign or of intermediate behavior, such as aggressive fibromatosis, nodular fasciitis, myositis ossificans, and inflammatory myofibroblastic tumor, and other spindle cell malignant tumors, including MPNST, poorly differentiated embryonal RMS, and monophasic synovial sarcoma. Differentiation may require immunocytochemical, ultrastructural, and cytogenetic studies (Tables 32.3 through 32.6). The pathologist also needs to correlate the findings with clinical information such as age, site, history, and duration of the lesion.

Clinical Presentation

The clinical presentation of IFS differs somewhat from that of adult-type fibrosarcoma in children.[73,234] Most published series of IFS indicate that extremity sites predominate. In adult-type fibrosarcoma, the distribution of axial and extremity sites is relatively even. Tumor growth in IFS may be quite rapid, whereas the tumor typically grows more slowly in adult-type fibrosarcoma. Metastases are uncommon at the time of initial presentation; the lung is a common site of tumor recurrence and bone metastases have been reported.[241]

Principles and Recommendations for Treatment

Infantile fibrosarcoma is unlike most NRSTS in that it often grows quite rapidly, may spontaneously regress, and may be cured with chemotherapy in the absence of surgical resection.[4,73,242,243] The vast majority of children with IFS become long-term survivors. When IFS is resectable with minimal impact on function or cosmesis, the treatment of choice is surgical excision. Although the surgical goal should be to achieve wide margins if possible, long-term survival has been documented after marginal and even subtotal resection.[4] Therefore, aggressive efforts to achieve wide margins are unnecessary. Patients who experience local recurrence after initial surgery

are usually curable with further surgery, with or without chemotherapy and/or radiotherapy. When IFS is unresectable, it responds well to sarcoma-based chemotherapy and some patients can be cured with chemotherapy alone if surgical resection is not possible.[4] The most common chemotherapeutic approach in IFS is vincristine and actinomycin D (VA), with or without cyclophosphamide.[244] Regimens that include doxorubicin, ifosfamide, and etoposide have also been used, although these drugs may be more toxic, particularly to young children.[73,244] Because patients with IFS are quite young and the disease is usually successfully treated with surgery, with or without chemotherapy, radiotherapy is usually avoided except in the setting of multiple local recurrences not controlled with surgery and chemotherapy.

The approach to treatment of adult-type fibrosarcoma is similar to that of other NRSTSs.[73] Wide local excision should be the goal of surgical intervention, with adjuvant radiotherapy prescribed for microscopic residual disease. Chemotherapy, with or without radiotherapy, is used for the treatment of patients with unresectable tumors. As in other NRSTSs, the use of chemotherapy in an adjuvant setting is somewhat controversial.

Infantile Myofibromatosis (Myofibromatosis, Myofibroma)

Epidemiology

Myofibroma and *myofibromatosis* are terms used to describe solitary and multifocal presentations of soft tissue tumors characterized by benign neoplastic myofibroblast proliferation. Although these tumors can be seen in elderly people, most are diagnosed in the first year of life and many at birth.[245] They are more common in males with no race predilection.[246] The relative frequency of solitary versus multicentric forms is unclear from the literature. Etiology is unknown; however, rare familial cases have been reported.[247,248]

Biology and Genetics

Cytogenetic analyses of myofibromas have shown nonspecific findings (Table 32.3) with chromosome 8 abnormalities. A small number of reports of familial myofibromatosis have implicated an autosomal dominant inheritance pattern. It must be emphasized that the vast majority of myofibromas are sporadic, isolated occurrences. Most important, these tumors lack the tumor-defining translocation (ETV6-NTRK3) found in IFS and cellular mesoblastic nephroma. In particularly troublesome cases, RT-PCR or FISH for the ETV6-NTRK3 translocation should be performed to eliminate the possibility of IFS.

Pathology

Myofibromas are characterized by nodular or multinodular proliferation with a zoning phenomenon, characterized by peripheral spindle-shaped cells organized into fascicles. These tend to merge and blend with centrally placed sheets of less-differentiated ovoid to polygonal shaped cells. A prominent hemangiopericytoma architecture may be seen throughout the tumor but more prominently within the center of the tumor. The recognition of this pattern has resulted in inclusion of the tumor previously considered to be infantile hemangiopericytoma into the infantile myofibromatosis category. This is appropriate because these tumors lack the cytogenetics features and other features of true adult hemangiopericytoma (solitary fibrous tumor). Myofibromas with this pattern are often referred to as hemangiopericytoma-like myofibromas. Myofibromas may have a relatively high mitotic rate without atypical mitotic figures, areas of necrosis and calcifications, stromal hyalinization, nuclear atypia, and even subendothelial "intravascular" tumor growth. These histopathologic features have no bearing on the clinical outcome of myofibromas. Immunocytochemical staining of the tumor cells reveals vimentin and alpha-smooth muscle actin reactivity, with lack of immunoreactivity with S100 protein, epithelial membrane antigen, keratin, and desmin (Table 32.4). Ultrastructural examination shows myofibroblastic differentiation with prominent dilated rough endoplasmic reticulum, longitudinal filaments with dense bodies, and focal basal lamina (Table 32.6).

Certain tumors may have features of both infantile myofibromatosis and IFS and may thus be called "composite infantile myofibromatosis."[249] Molecular analysis for the *ETV6-NTRK3* gene fusion can identify the subset of these tumors more appropriately classified as IFS. The remainder that lack the characteristic IFS gene fusion seem to be morphologic variants of classic infantile myofibromatosis.

Clinical Presentation

In a series of 61 cases, approximately one-third of cases occurred in the head and neck and another third in the trunk, followed by the extremities.[246] In the multicentric form, visceral involvement occurs in up to 25% of patients.[246,250] The lesions appear as vascular neoplasms with painless purplish macules. Visceral lesions can involve any organ and cause associated symptoms. Radiologic appearance is variable; however, calcification is common.

Principles and Recommendations for Treatment

Spontaneous regression has been reported in both the solitary and multicentric forms in up to one-third of patients.[246,251] Therefore, aggressive surgical interventions may not be necessary in tumors located in favorable locations. Survival is greater than 90% with surgical excision or observation; however, progressive disease and deaths have been reported in patients with visceral involvement.[246,251] In such patients, tumor regression or stabilization has been induced with vincristine/actinomycin D and vinblastine/methotrexate.[250,252]

Leiomyosarcoma

Epidemiology

Although LMSs account for approximately 14% of all STSs in adults, this tumor is rare in children, accounting for less than 2% of cases.[2] Because GIST was only recently recognized to be a distinct clinical entity, most published pediatric case series of "LMS" include patients with both diseases.[253-255] A retrospective analysis that included CD117 (KIT) staining of 11 pediatric tumors that had an original diagnosis of LMS or GIST identified 7 GIST (including 1 that arose outside the gastrointestinal tract) and 4 LMS.[256] Children with AIDS have an increased susceptibility to LMS, which seems to be related to underlying Epstein-Barr virus (EBV) infection of smooth muscle cells.[15] When LMS occurs in children with human immunodeficiency virus (HIV) infection, it typically occurs late in the course of the infection, implying a role for prolonged or severe immunosuppression.[257] LMS has also been observed in pediatric patients who have undergone liver transplantation, in whom it also appears to be EBV related.[258] EBV appears not to play a role in the development of LMS in patients without underlying immunosuppression from HIV infection or organ transplantation.[259]

Leiomyosarcoma has been reported as a second malignant neoplasm following the treatment of childhood cancer.[260] It was the most common subtype of secondary STS in a cohort of 963 survivors of hereditary retinoblastoma, with 78% of cases having a diagnosis 30 or more years after the retinoblastoma diagnosis.[11] In this study, LMS was found more frequently outside the prior radiation field than within it, suggesting an etiologic role for the underlying germline *RB1* gene mutation.

Biology and Genetics

Although smooth muscle tumors have been rare in children, the appearance of HIV infection in adult and pediatric populations has altered the normal incidence of both smooth muscle and vascular tumors in both age groups in some populations.[261] This is the first example of EBV associated with an STS, although it is well known to be associated with Hodgkin lymphoma and lymphoproliferative syndromes. These tumors have also been reported after the treatment of acute lymphocytic leukemia and during immunosuppression to prevent renal allograft rejection.[262,263] A t(12;14) translocation has been reported in an LMS arising in a child. The same translocation has been found in LMSs arising in adults and in uterine LMSs. This suggests that genes arising near the breakpoint of t(12;14)(q14-15;q23-24) are probably important in the pathogenesis of benign and malignant smooth muscle tumors.[264,265] Other authors have suggested three patterns of cytogenetic abnormalities: (a) hypodiploid; (b) pseudodiploid, associated with reciprocal translocations; and (c) heterogeneous karyotypic findings (Table 32.2).[266]

Pathology

Leiomyomas and LMSs have prominent clumped eosinophilia into their cytoplasm because of cytoplasmic myofilaments (Fig. 32.7C). Tumors associated with immune compromise or suppression are described as being less differentiated with decreased amounts of cytoplasm. The nuclei are elongated with blunt ends (cigar-shaped) and typically have a small perinuclear cytoplasmic clearing at one tip of the nucleus. The cells are closely adapted to one another with minimal intercellular space and organized in longitudinal intersecting fascicles. Although leiomyomas have features that distinguish them from LMSs, cellular leiomyomas closely resemble LMS but lack cytologic atypia. The diagnosis of LMS in peripheral soft tissues is based solely on mitotic activity (1 in 10 high-power fields, 5 in 50 high-power fields). Fewer mitotic figures are necessary with retroperitoneal and intraabdominal LMSs (2 in 10 high-power fields). The tumors react with antibodies against smooth muscle actin, desmin, h-caldesmon, and cytokeratin (Table 32.5). In the pediatric population, EBV can be detected by *in situ* hybridization for EBER-1, as well as by EBV-PCR (Table 32.3). Entry of EBV into smooth muscle cells occurs via a CD21 receptor present on smooth muscle cell membranes. Ultrastructural features include longitudinally oriented actin myofilaments with dense bodies and cell membrane attachment plaques (Table 32.6). The nuclei are typically deeply indented owing to artifactual contraction of the actin myofilaments during fixation. Rarely will viral particles resembling herpes be noted within the nuclei or cytoplasm of the tumor cells.

Clinical Presentation

Because most pediatric case series of LMS include patients with both GIST and LMS, it is difficult to clarify the most commonly affected anatomic sites. However, confirmed pediatric LMS has been reported in the extremity, head and neck, retroperitoneum, and uterus.[256] In adults, LMS accounts for less than 10% of extremity STS.[61] When it occurs within the abdomen, it is most commonly located in the retroperitoneum or uterus.[267]

Principles and Recommendations for Treatment

The limited data available suggest that the predictors of outcome in LMS are similar to those of other STS and include tumor size and extent of disease.[268] Wide local excision or marginal excision with adjuvant radiotherapy can be curative.[256] The role of chemotherapy is unclear. In adults, about one-third of patients respond to ifosfamide/doxorubicin/dacarbazine chemotherapy.[166] The combination of gemcitabine and docetaxel had produced high response rates in women with uterine LMS, although it is less clear how well this finding translates to extrauterine LMS.[269] A phase II study of trabectedin in adults with recurrent advanced STS demonstrated arrest of tumor growth (PR and SD) in 56% of patients with LMS.[270] A pediatric phase I study of trabectedin has been completed, and a phase II study including a stratum for NRSTS has been recently completed by COG.

Liposarcoma

Epidemiology

According to SEER data, liposarcoma accounts for 8% of STS in adults and 2.8% of STS in children. The largest series of pediatric cases (82 cases) demonstrates a female predominance (1.9:1) and tendency toward its occurrence during the adolescent years (median age at presentation 15.5 years).[271]

Biology and Genetics

As is the case with many soft tissue tumors, recurrent genetic abnormalities of probable etiologic and diagnostic value have been discovered. Three unique and tumor-defining translocations occur in myxoid and round cell liposarcoma—t(12;16)(q13;p11) associated with FUS (TLS)-DDIT3(CHOP), t(12;22)(q13;q12) associated with EWS-DDIT3, and t(12;22;20)(q13;q12;q11) associated with EWS-DDIT3.[30,272] The locus at chromosome 12q13 plays an important role in the pathogenesis of these liposarcomatous tumors. Specifically, fusion of a transcription factor (DDIT3/CHOP) that is essential for adipocytic differentiation to FUS/TLS or EWS appears to play a critical role in transformation to myxoid and round cell liposarcomas.[30,31,273] Lipomas also have structural changes in chromosome 12q13-q14, suggesting that the degree of abnormality at this locus may be related to the growth of lipogenic tumors.[264,274]

Pathology

The majority of adipocytic tumors in young children represent lipoblastomas, maturing lipoblastomas, or lipomas. There is a certain degree of overlap between histologic features of lipoblastoma and myxoid liposarcoma; however, these are easily placed into the appropriate category by pediatric pathologists. In pediatric patients, myxoid liposarcoma is most common, representing 68% of the cases in one large series.[271] Myxoid liposarcoma is considerably less common in adults, accounting for roughly one-third of all cases.[275] The typical myxoid liposarcoma is organized in a nodular fashion, with the highest cellularity at the peripheries of the nodules. The tumor comprises a mixture of round to oval nonlipogenic mesenchymal cells, with occasional to rare signet ring cell lipoblasts. These cells are embedded in a myxoid stroma with a prominent capillary network, resembling chicken wire (Fig.

32.7D). The lack of obvious lipoblasts may require the use of either immunocytochemistry (Table 32.5) for S100 protein and aP2 or electron microscopy (Table 32.6) to identify lipid droplets in tumor cells to confirm the diagnosis. About 15% of pediatric liposarcomas are described as pleomorphic myxoid liposarcoma because they include components of both pleomorphic and myxoid liposarcomas. These tumors have a predilection for the mediastinum and have a poor outcome.[271]

Clinical Presentation

In children, approximately half of liposarcomas arise in the lower extremity.[271,276,277] The remainder arise in the body wall, visceral sites (mediastinum, pelvis, retroperitoneum), upper extremity, and head and neck region. Lymph node involvement is rare (0.3% in a large adult series).[81] Although metastases are uncommon at the time of initial presentation, the most frequent site is the lung.[277] Extrapulmonary sites, including bone, breast, liver, meninges, and soft tissues, account for a significant proportion of metastases that develop after initial therapy in adults.[278]

Principles and Recommendations for Treatment

Because these tumors rarely metastasize but can be locally invasive, the treatment of choice for localized liposarcoma is WLE.[271,276,277] Adjuvant radiotherapy appears to be effective in the control of microscopic disease in adults[279,280]; its role in the treatment of children is less well defined, but its use is certainly indicated for control of microscopic residual disease after maximal surgery. The role of adjuvant chemotherapy in the treatment of childhood liposarcoma is unclear. However, the long-term prognosis for children with this rare tumor is very good with surgery alone as long as the tumor can be locally controlled with surgery, with or without radiotherapy.[276,277] Therefore, chemotherapy is best reserved for those with unresectable or metastatic disease, or in the context of a clinical trial. Phase I and II clinical trials have documented excellent responses to trabectedin in adults with liposarcoma[270,281]; a phase II study in pediatric patients that includes a stratum for NRSTS has been recently completed by COG.

According to a population-based Scandinavian study, about two-thirds of adults with liposarcoma become long-term survivors.[280] The histologic subtype and location of initial surgery (at a specialized sarcoma center or not) influenced the likelihood of local tumor recurrence, whereas histologic subtype, patient age, tumor size, and histologic grade predicted metastatic recurrence. In pediatric patients, outcome for myxoid liposarcoma is excellent (no deaths among 58 patients in one series) but less favorable outcomes have been documented for other histologic subtypes.[271,276,277]

Malignant Peripheral Nerve Sheath Tumor (Malignant Schwannoma, Neurofibrosarcoma)

Epidemiology

According to SEER data, MPNST account for 3.4% of STSs in children.[2,282] They are less common in adults.[2,61] There is no clear gender or race predilection. MPNSTs occur in association with neurofibromatosis 1 (NF1) in a substantial proportion of cases, so children presenting with MPNST should be examined carefully for evidence of NF1. The average age at presentation with MPNST is lower in patients with NF1 than those with sporadic disease (29 years vs. 40 years).[283] Approximately 10% of patients with NF1 develop MPNST during their lifetime.[13]

However, even relatively low doses of doxorubicin can lead to long-term cardiac compromise. Alkylating agents cause infertility, acute gonadal failure, and premature menopause.[319-321] Male patients seem to be at greater risk than do females,[322,323] and cyclophosphamide appears to be more gonadotoxic than ifosfamide.[324] Although improvements in supportive care have decreased the risk of hemorrhagic cystitis, alkylating agents can cause chronic or recurrent hemorrhagic cystitis that leads to bladder fibrosis and dysfunctional voiding.[325,326] Ifosfamide, but not cyclophosphamide, can cause permanent glomerular and tubular nephrotoxicity and associated metabolic bone disease.[327-329] Overlapping toxicities of different treatment modalities may lead to even greater long-term toxicity. For example, nephrotoxicity may be heightened by the combination of ifosfamide-containing chemotherapy and radiotherapy following nephrectomy for resection of retroperitoneal NRSTS. Cardiotoxicity may be worsened by the combination of doxorubicin-containing chemotherapy and radiotherapy to the heart, such as might occur in a chest wall tumor.

Because the long-term toxicities of NRSTS therapy may be substantial, the pediatric oncologist overseeing the treatment of the patient with NRSTS must carefully consider these potential side effects before selecting a treatment approach. Further studies are needed to define the degree of risk associated with each of the treatment modalities utilized in patients with NRSTS and to clarify the optimal treatment strategy to achieve a cure with a minimum of late effects.

FUTURE DIRECTIONS

There are a number of important issues to address in the treatment of children with NRSTS. More effective chemotherapy regimens and incorporation of targeted therapies in selected histologies must be developed to prevent recurrences for patients with completely resected localized tumors and for the treatment of patients with advanced disease. Patients should be enrolled in phase I and II drug studies, whenever appropriate. Agents that have shown activity in adult should be tested in children. The rapidly evolving biologic understanding of these myriad tumors is improving the accuracy of diagnosis as detailed in this chapter. It will be important to identify factors that predict local or distant recurrence in prospective clinical trials. Further refinements in risk assessment will be useful to tailor therapy. The rarity of these tumors dictates the enrollment of patients on collaborative group trials, which is the only means through which progress can be made. Multinational collaborative group trials should be designed.

References

1. Ries LA, Smith MA, Gurney J, et al. Cancer incidence and survival among children and adolescents: United States SEER Program 1975–1995. Bethesda, MD: National Cancer Institute, 1999. SEER Program Pub No. 99-4649.
2. Spunt S, Pappo A. Childhood nonrhabdomyosarcoma soft tissue sarcomas are not adult-type tumors. J Clin Oncol 2006;24:1958–1959.
3. Ferrari A, Casanova M, Bisogno G, et al. Hemangiopericytoma in pediatric ages: a report from the Italian and German Soft Tissue Sarcoma Cooperative Group. Cancer 2001;92:2692–2698.
4. Loh ML, Ahn P, Perez-Atayde AR, et al. Treatment of infantile fibrosarcoma with chemotherapy and surgery: results from the Dana-Farber Cancer Institute and Children's Hospital, Boston. J Pediatr Hematol Oncol 2002;24:722–726.
5. Jemal A, Siegel R, Ward E, et al. Cancer statistics, 2008. CA Cancer J Clin 2008;58:71–96.
6. Hayes-Jordan AA, Spunt SL, Poquette CA, et al. Nonrhabdomyosarcoma soft tissue sarcomas in children: is age at diagnosis an important variable? J Pediatr Surg 2000;35:948–953.
7. Bleyer A, O'Leary M, Barr R, et al. Cancer epidemiology in older adolescents and young adults 15 to 29 years of age, including SEER incidence and survival: 1975–2000. Bethesda, MD: National Cancer Institute, 2006. NIH Pub. No. 06-5767.
8. Malkin D, Li FP, Strong LC. Germ line p53 mutations in a familial syndrome of breast cancer, sarcomas, and other neoplasms. Science 1990;250:1233–1238.
9. Nichols KE, Malkin D, Garber JE, et al. Germ-line p53 mutations predispose to a wide spectrum of early-onset cancers. Cancer Epidemiol Biomarkers Prev 2001;10:83–87.
10. Eng C, Li FP, Abramson DH, et al. Mortality from second tumors among long-term survivors of retinoblastoma. J Natl Cancer Inst 1993;85:1121–1128.
11. Kleinerman RA, Tucker MA, Abramson DH, et al. Risk of soft tissue sarcomas by individual subtype in survivors of hereditary retinoblastoma. J Natl Cancer Inst 2007;99:24–31.
12. Goto M, Miller RW, Ishikawa Y, et al. Excess of rare cancers in Werner syndrome (adult progeria). Cancer Epidemiol Biomarkers Prev 1996;5:239–246.
13. Evans DG, Baser ME, McGaughran J, et al. Malignant peripheral nerve sheath tumours in neurofibromatosis type 1. J Med Genet 2002;39:311–314.
14. McCaughan JA, Holloway SM, Davidson R, et al. Further evidence of the increased risk for malignant peripheral nerve sheath tumour from a Scottish cohort of patients with neurofibromatosis type 1. J Med Genet 2007;44:463–466.
15. McClain KL, Leach CT, Jenson HB, et al. Association of Epstein-Barr virus with leiomyosarcomas in children with AIDS. N Engl J Med 1995;332:12–18.
16. Lefevre JH, Parc Y, Kerneis S, et al. Risk factors for development of desmoid tumours in familial adenomatous polyposis. Br J Surg 2008;95:1136–1139.
17. Speake D, Evans DG, Lalloo F, et al. Desmoid tumours in patients with familial adenomatous polyposis and desmoid region adenomatous polyposis coli mutations. Br J Surg 2007;94:1009–1013.
18. Brady MS, Gaynor JJ, Brennan MF. Radiation-associated sarcoma of bone and soft tissue. Arch Surg 1992;127:1379–1385.
19. Robinson E, Neugut AI, Wylie P. Clinical aspects of postirradiation sarcomas. J Natl Cancer Inst 1988;80:233–240.
20. Henderson TO, Whitton J, Stovall M, et al. Secondary sarcomas in childhood cancer survivors: a report from the Childhood Cancer Survivor Study. J Natl Cancer Inst 2007;99:300–308.
21. Bosetti C, La Vecchia C, Lipworth L, et al. Occupational exposure to vinyl chloride and cancer risk: a review of the epidemiologic literature. Eur J Cancer Prev 2003;12:427–430.
22. Boffetta P, Matisane L, Mundt KA, et al. Meta-analysis of studies of occupational exposure to vinyl chloride in relation to cancer mortality. Scand J Work Environ Health 2003;29:220–229.
23. Stewart FW, Treves N. Lymphangiosarcoma in postmastectomy lymphedema; a report of six cases in elephantiasis chirurgica. Cancer 1948;1:64–81.
24. Hansen ES, Lander F, Lauritsen JM. Time trends in cancer risk and pesticide exposure, a long-term follow-up of Danish gardeners. Scand J Work Environ Health 2007;33:465–469.
25. Eriksson M, Hardell L, Adami HO. Exposure to dioxins as a risk factor for soft tissue sarcoma: a population-based case-control study. J Natl Cancer Inst 1990;82:486–490.
26. Fletcher JA. Molecular biology and cytogenetics of soft tissue sarcomas: relevance for targeted therapies. Cancer Treat Res 2004;120:99–116.
27. Clark J, Rocques PJ, Crew AJ, et al. Identification of novel genes, SYT and SSX, involved in the t(X;18)(p11.2;q11.2) translocation found in human synovial sarcoma. Nat Genet 1994;7:502–508.
28. Kawai A, Woodruff J, Healey JH, et al. SYT-SSX gene fusion as a determinant of morphology and prognosis in synovial sarcoma. N Engl J Med 1998;338:153–160.
29. Nilsson G, Skytting B, Xie Y, et al. The SYT-SSX1 variant of synovial sarcoma is associated with a high rate of tumor cell proliferation and poor clinical outcome. Cancer Res 1999;59:3180–3184.
30. Aman P, Ron D, Mandahl N, et al. Rearrangement of the transcription factor gene CHOP in myxoid liposarcomas with t(12;16)(q13;p11). Genes Chromosomes Cancer 1992;5:278–285.
31. Crozat A, Aman P, Mandahl N, et al. Fusion of CHOP to a novel RNA-binding protein in human myxoid liposarcoma. Nature 1993;363:640–644.
32. Ohno T, Ouchida M, Lee L, et al. The EWS gene, involved in Ewing family of tumors, malignant melanoma of soft parts and desmoplastic small round cell tumors, codes for an RNA binding protein with novel regulatory domains. Oncogene 1994;9:3087–3097.
33. Panagopoulos I, Mertens F, Isaksson M, et al. Molecular genetic characterization of the EWS/CHN and RBP56/CHN fusion genes in extraskeletal myxoid chondrosarcoma. Genes Chromosomes Cancer 2002;35:340–352.
34. Li FP, Fraumeni JF Jr. Prospective study of a family cancer syndrome. JAMA 1982;247:2692–2694.
35. Malkin D. p53 and the Li-Fraumeni syndrome. Cancer Genet Cytogenet 1993;66:83–92.
36. Glover TW, Stein CK, Legius E, et al. Molecular and cytogenetic analysis of tumors in von Recklinghausen neurofibromatosis. Genes Chromosomes Cancer 1991;3:62–70.
37. Legius E, Marchuk DA, Collins FS, et al. Somatic deletion of the neurofibromatosis type 1 gene in a neurofibrosarcoma supports a tumour suppressor gene hypothesis. Nat Genet 1993;3:122–126.
38. D'Agostino AN, Soule EH, Miller RH. Sarcomas of the peripheral nerves and somatic soft tissues associated with multiple neurofibromatosis (von Recklinghausen's disease). Cancer 1963;16:1015–1027.
39. Fienman NL, Yakovac WC. Neurofibromatosis in childhood. J Pediatr 1970;76:339–346.
40. Guccion JG, Enzinger FM. Malignant schwannoma associated with von Recklinghausen's neurofibromatosis. Virchows Arch A Pathol Anat Histol 1979;383:43–57.
41. Angelov L, Davis A, O'Sullivan B, et al. Neurogenic sarcomas: experience at the University of Toronto. Neurosurgery 1998;43:56–64; discussion 64–65.
42. Sung L, Anderson JR, Arndt C, et al. Neurofibromatosis in children with rhabdomyosarcoma: a report from the intergroup Rhabdomyosarcoma study IV. J Pediatr 2004;144:666–668.
43. Knezevich SR, McFadden DE, Tao W, et al. A novel ETV6-NTRK3 gene fusion in congenital fibrosarcoma. Nat Genet 1998;18:184–187.
44. Rodriguez-Galindo C, Ramsey K, Jenkins JJ, et al. Hemangiopericytoma in children and infants. Cancer 2000;88:198–204.
45. Park MS, Araujo DM. New insights into the hemangiopericytoma/solitary fibrous tumor spectrum of tumors. Curr Opin Oncol 2009;21:327–331.

46. Costa J, Wesley RA, Glatstein E, et al. The grading of soft tissue sarcomas. Results of a clinicohistopathologic correlation in a series of 163 cases. Cancer 1984;53:530–541.
47. Parham DM, Webber BL, Jenkins JJ III, et al. Nonrhabdomyosarcomatous soft tissue sarcomas of childhood: formulation of a simplified system for grading. Mod Pathol 1995;8:705–710.
48. Coindre JM, Terrier P, Guillou L, et al. Predictive value of grade for metastasis development in the main histologic types of adult soft tissue sarcomas: a study of 1240 patients from the French Federation of Cancer Centers Sarcoma Group. Cancer 2001;91: 1914–1926.
49. Guillou L, Coindre JM, Bonichon F, et al. Comparative study of the National Cancer Institute and French Federation of Cancer Centers Sarcoma Group grading systems in a population of 410 adult patients with soft tissue sarcoma. J Clin Oncol 1997;15:350–362.
50. Haimi M, Peretz Nahum M, Ben Arush MW. Delay in diagnosis of children with cancer: a retrospective study of 315 children. Pediatr Hematol Oncol 2004;21:37–48.
51. Rikhof B, de Jong S, Suurmeijer AJ, et al. The insulin-like growth factor system and sarcomas. J Pathol 2009;217:469–482.
52. de Groot JW, Rikhof B, van Doorn J, et al. Non-islet cell tumour-induced hypoglycaemia: a review of the literature including two new cases. Endocr Relat Cancer 2007;14:979–993.
53. Hanukoglu A, Chalew SA, Sun CJ, et al. Surgically curable hypophosphatemic rickets. Diagnosis and management. Clin Pediatr (Phila) 1989;28:321–325.
54. Pappo AS, Rao BN, Jenkins JJ, et al. Metastatic nonrhabdomyosarcomatous soft-tissue sarcomas in children and adolescents: the St. Jude Children's Research Hospital experience. Med Pediatr Oncol 1999;33:76–82.
55. Ferrari A, Casanova M, Collini P, et al. Adult-type soft tissue sarcomas in pediatric-age patients: experience at the Istituto Nazionale Tumori in Milan. J Clin Oncol 2005;23: 4021–4030.
56. Fong Y, Coit DG, Woodruff JM, et al. Lymph node metastasis from soft tissue sarcoma in adults. Analysis of data from a prospective database of 1772 sarcoma patients. Ann Surg 1993;217:72–77.
57. Mazeron JJ, Suit HD. Lymph nodes as sites of metastases from sarcomas of soft tissue. Cancer 1987;60:1800–1808.
58. Bramwell VH, Littley MB, Chang J, et al. Bone marrow involvement in adult soft tissue sarcomas. Eur J Cancer Clin Oncol 1982;18:1099–1106.
59. Spunt SL, Hill DA, Motosue AM, et al. Clinical features and outcome of initially unresected nonmetastatic pediatric nonrhabdomyosarcoma soft tissue sarcoma. J Clin Oncol 2002;20:3225–3235.
60. Spunt SL, Poquette CA, Hurt YS, et al. Prognostic factors for children and adolescents with surgically resected nonrhabdomyosarcoma soft tissue sarcoma: an analysis of 121 patients treated at St Jude Children's Research Hospital. J Clin Oncol 1999;17: 3697–3705.
61. Pisters PW, Leung DH, Woodruff J, et al. Analysis of prognostic factors in 1,041 patients with localized soft tissue sarcomas of the extremities. J Clin Oncol 1996; 14:1679–1689.
62. Ferrari A, Miceli R, Meazza C, et al. Soft tissue sarcomas of childhood and adolescence: the prognostic role of tumor size in relation to patient body size. J Clin Oncol 2009; 27:371–376.
63. Lawrence W Jr, Anderson JR, Gehan EA, et al. Pretreatment TNM staging of childhood rhabdomyosarcoma: a report of the Intergroup Rhabdomyosarcoma Study Group, Children's Cancer Study Group, Pediatric Oncology Group. Cancer 1997;80:1165–1170.
64. AJCC cancer staging handbook. New York: Springer-Verlag, 2002.
65. Hajdu SI, Shiu MH, Brennan MF. The role of the pathologist in the management of soft tissue sarcomas. World J Surg 1988;12:326–331.
66. Enneking WF, Spanier SS, Goodman MA. A system for the surgical staging of musculoskeletal sarcoma. Clin Orthop Relat Res 1980;153:106–120.
67. Wunder JS, Healey JH, Davis AM, et al. A comparison of staging systems for localized extremity soft tissue sarcoma. Cancer 2000;88:2721–2730.
68. Kattan MW, Leung DH, Brennan MF. Postoperative nomogram for 12-year sarcoma-specific death. J Clin Oncol 2002;20:791–796.
69. Ferrari A, Miceli R, Casanova M, et al. Adult-type soft tissue sarcomas in paediatric age: a nomogram-based prognostic comparison with adult sarcoma. Eur J Cancer 2007; 43:2691–2697.
70. Skene AI, Barr L, Robinson M, et al. Adult type (nonembryonal) soft tissue sarcomas in childhood. Med Pediatr Oncol 1993;21:645–648.
71. Salloum E, Flamant F, Caillaud JM, et al. Diagnostic and therapeutic problems of soft tissue tumors other than rhabdomyosarcoma in infants under 1 year of age: a clinicopathological study of 34 cases treated at the Institut Gustave-Roussy. Med Pediatr Oncol 1990;18:37–43.
72. Horowitz ME, Pratt CB, Webber BL, et al. Therapy for childhood soft-tissue sarcomas other than rhabdomyosarcoma: a review of 62 cases treated at a single institution. J Clin Oncol 1986;4:559–564.
73. Cecchetto G, Carli M, Alaggio R, et al. Fibrosarcoma in pediatric patients: results of the Italian Cooperative Group studies (1979–1995). J Surg Oncol 2001;78:225–231.
74. Neel MD, Wilkins RM, Rao BN, et al. Early multicenter experience with a noninvasive expandable prosthesis. Clin Orthop Relat Res 2003;415:72–81.
75. Yang JC, Chang AE, Baker AR, et al. Randomized prospective study of the benefit of adjuvant radiation therapy in the treatment of soft tissue sarcomas of the extremity. J Clin Oncol 1998;16:197–203.
76. O'Sullivan B, Davis AM, Turcotte R, et al. Preoperative versus postoperative radiotherapy in soft-tissue sarcoma of the limbs: a randomised trial. Lancet 2002;359:2235–2241.
77. DeLaney TF, Spiro IJ, Suit HD, et al. Neoadjuvant chemotherapy and radiotherapy for large extremity soft-tissue sarcomas. Int J Radiat Oncol Biol Phys 2003;56:1117–1127.
78. Smith MB, Katz R, Black CT, et al. A rational approach to the use of fine-needle aspiration biopsy in the evaluation of primary and recurrent neoplasms in children. J Pediatr Surg 1993;28:1245–1247.
79. Blakely ML, Spurbeck WW, Pappo AS, et al. The impact of margin of resection on outcome in pediatric nonrhabdomyosarcoma soft tissue sarcoma. J Pediatr Surg 1999;34: 672–675.
80. Gustafson P. Soft tissue sarcoma. Epidemiology and prognosis in 508 patients. Acta Orthop Scand Suppl 1994;259:1–31.
81. Daigeler A, Kuhnen C, Moritz R, et al. Lymph node metastases in soft tissue sarcomas: a single center analysis of 1,597 patients. Langenbecks Arch Surg 2009;394:321–329.
82. Maduekwe UN, Hornicek FJ, Springfield DS, et al. Role of sentinel lymph node biopsy in the staging of synovial, epithelioid, and clear cell sarcomas. Ann Surg Oncol 2009;16:1356–1363.
83. Neville HL, Andrassy RJ, Lally KP, et al. Lymphatic mapping with sentinel node biopsy in pediatric patients. J Pediatr Surg 2000;35:961–964.
84. Kayton ML, Delgado R, Busam K, et al. Experience with 31 sentinel lymph node biopsies for sarcomas and carcinomas in pediatric patients. Cancer 2008;112:2052–2059.
85. De Corti F, Dall'Igna P, Bisogno G, et al. Sentinel node biopsy in pediatric soft tissue sarcomas of extremities. Pediatr Blood Cancer 2009;52:51–54.
86. Zagars GK, Ballo MT, Pisters PW, et al. Surgical margins and reresection in the management of patients with soft tissue sarcoma using conservative surgery and radiation therapy. Cancer 2003;97:2544–2553.
87. Giuliano AE, Eilber FR. The rationale for planned reoperation after unplanned total excision of soft-tissue sarcomas. J Clin Oncol 1985;3:1344–1348.
88. Cecchetto G, Alaggio R, Dall'Igna P, et al. Localized unresectable non-rhabdo soft tissue sarcomas of the extremities in pediatric age: results from the Italian studies. Cancer 2005;104:2006–2012.
89. Temple LK, Brennan MF. The role of pulmonary metastasectomy in soft tissue sarcoma. Semin Thorac Cardiovasc Surg 2002;14:35–44.
90. Billingsley KG, Burt ME, Jara E, et al. Pulmonary metastases from soft tissue sarcoma: analysis of patterns of diseases and postmetastasis survival. Ann Surg 1999;229:602–610; discussion 610–612.
91. Lindberg RD, Martin RG, Romsdahl MM, et al. Conservative surgery and postoperative radiotherapy in 300 adults with soft-tissue sarcomas. Cancer 1981;47:2391–2397.
92. Rosenberg SA, Kent H, Costa J, et al. Prospective randomized evaluation of the role of limb-sparing surgery, radiation therapy, and adjuvant chemoimmunotherapy in the treatment of adult soft-tissue sarcomas. Surgery 1978;84:62–69.
93. Suit H, Spiro I. Radiation as a therapeutic modality in sarcomas of the soft tissue. Hematol Oncol Clin N Am 1995;9:733–746.
94. Kaytan E, Yaman F, Cosar R, et al. Prognostic factors in localized soft-tissue sarcomas. Am J Clin Oncol 2003;26:411–415.
95. Rao BN, Rodriguez-Galindo C. Local control in childhood extremity sarcomas: salvaging limbs and sparing function. Med Pediatr Oncol 2003;41:584–587.
96. Pisters PW, O'Sullivan B, Maki RG. Evidence-based recommendations for local therapy for soft tissue sarcomas. J Clin Oncol 2007;25:1003–1008.
97. Paulino AC, Ritchie J, Wen BC. The value of postoperative radiotherapy in childhood nonrhabdomyosarcoma soft tissue sarcoma. Pediatr Blood Cancer 2004;43:587–593.
98. Baldini EH, Goldberg J, Jenner C, et al. Long-term outcomes after function-sparing surgery without radiotherapy for soft tissue sarcoma of the extremities and trunk. J Clin Oncol 1999;17:3252–3259.
99. Rydholm A, Gustafson P, Rooser B, et al. Limb-sparing surgery without radiotherapy based on anatomic location of soft tissue sarcoma. J Clin Oncol 1991;9:1757–1765.
100. Fabrizio PL, Stafford SL, Pritchard DJ. Extremity soft-tissue sarcomas selectively treated with surgery alone. Int J Radiat Oncol Biol Phys 2000;48:227–232.
101. Zagars GK, Ballo MT, Pisters PW, et al. Prognostic factors for patients with localized soft-tissue sarcoma treated with conservation surgery and radiation therapy: an analysis of 225 patients. Cancer 2003;97:2530–2543.
102. McKee MD, Liu DF, Brooks JJ, et al. The prognostic significance of margin width for extremity and trunk sarcoma. J Surg Oncol 2004;85:68–76.
103. Dickinson IC, Whitwell DJ, Battistuta D, et al. Surgical margin and its influence on survival in soft tissue sarcoma. ANZ J Surg 2006;76:104–109.
104. Alektiar KM, Velasco J, Zelefsky MJ, et al. Adjuvant radiotherapy for margin-positive high-grade soft tissue sarcoma of the extremity. Int J Radiat Oncol Biol Phys 2000; 48:1051–1058.
105. Pisters PW, Harrison LB, Leung DH, et al. Long-term results of a prospective randomized trial of adjuvant brachytherapy in soft tissue sarcoma. J Clin Oncol 1996;14:859–868.
106. Marcus SG, Merino MJ, Glatstein E, et al. Long-term outcome in 87 patients with low-grade soft-tissue sarcoma. Arch Surg 1993;128:1336–1343.
107. Canter RJ, Qin LX, Ferrone CR, et al. Why do patients with low-grade soft tissue sarcoma die? Ann Surg Oncol 2008;15:3550–3560.
108. Kraybill WG, Harris J, Spiro IJ, et al. Phase II study of neoadjuvant chemotherapy and radiation therapy in the management of high-risk, high-grade, soft tissue sarcomas of the extremities and body wall: Radiation Therapy Oncology Group Trial 9514. J Clin Oncol 2006;24:619–625.
109. Mack LA, Crowe PJ, Yang JL, et al. Preoperative chemoradiotherapy (modified Eilber protocol) provides maximum local control and minimal morbidity in patients with soft tissue sarcoma. Ann Surg Oncol 2005;12:646–653.
110. Hall EJ. Intensity-modulated radiation therapy, protons, and the risk of second cancers. Int J Radiat Oncol Biol Phys 2006;65:1–7.
111. Merchant TE, Parsh N, del Valle PL, et al. Brachytherapy for pediatric soft-tissue sarcoma. Int J Radiat Oncol Biol Phys 2000;46:427–432.
112. Ellis RJ, Kim E, Kinsella TJ, et al. Intraoperative radiotherapy in the multimodality approach to bone and soft tissue cancers. Surg Oncol Clin N Am 2003;12:1015–1029.
113. Pappo AS, Devidas M, Jenkins J, et al. Phase II trial of neoadjuvant vincristine, ifosfamide, and doxorubicin with granulocyte colony-stimulating factor support in children and adolescents with advanced-stage nonrhabdomyosarcomatous soft tissue sarcomas: a Pediatric Oncology Group Study. J Clin Oncol 2005;23:4031–4038.
114. Pratt CB, Maurer HM, Gieser P, et al. Treatment of unresectable or metastatic pediatric soft tissue sarcomas with surgery, irradiation, and chemotherapy: a Pediatric Oncology Group study. Med Pediatr Oncol 1998;30:201–209.
115. Pratt CB, Pappo AS, Gieser P, et al. Role of adjuvant chemotherapy in the treatment of surgically resected pediatric nonrhabdomyosarcomatous soft tissue sarcomas: a Pediatric Oncology Group Study. J Clin Oncol 1999;17:1219.
116. Dantonello TM, Int-Veen C, Harms D, et al. Cooperative trial CWS-91 for localized soft tissue sarcoma in children, adolescents, and young adults. J Clin Oncol 2009;27: 1446–1455.
117. Kepka L, DeLaney TF, Suit HD, et al. Results of radiation therapy for unresected soft-tissue sarcomas. Int J Radiat Oncol Biol Phys 2005;63:852–859.
118. Bramwell VH, Mouridsen HT, Santoro A, et al. Cyclophosphamide versus ifosfamide: a randomized phase II trial in adult soft-tissue sarcomas. The European Organization for Research and Treatment of Cancer [EORTC], Soft Tissue and Bone Sarcoma Group. Cancer Chemother Pharmacol 1993;31(Suppl 2):S180–S184.
119. Bramwell V, Quirt I, Warr D, et al. Combination chemotherapy with doxorubicin, dacarbazine, and ifosfamide in advanced adult soft tissue sarcoma. Canadian Sarcoma Group—National Cancer Institute of Canada Clinical Trials Group. J Natl Cancer Inst 1989;81:1496–1499.
120. Edmonson JH, Ryan LM, Blum RH, et al. Randomized comparison of doxorubicin alone versus ifosfamide plus doxorubicin or mitomycin, doxorubicin, and cisplatin against advanced soft tissue sarcomas. J Clin Oncol 1993;11:1269–1275.

121. Antman K, Crawley J, Balcerzak SP, et al. An intergroup phase III randomized study of doxorubicin and dacarbazine with or without ifosfamide and mesna in advanced soft tissue and bone sarcomas. J Clin Oncol 1993;11:1276–1285.
122. Omura GA, Blessing JA, Major F, et al. A randomized clinical trial of adjuvant Adriamycin in uterine sarcomas: a Gynecologic Oncology Group Study. J Clin Oncol 1985;3:1240–1245.
123. Benjamin RS, Terjanian TO, Fenoglio CJ, et al. The importance of combination chemotherapy for adjuvant treatment of high-risk patients with soft-tissue sarcomas of the extremities. In: Salmon SE, ed. Adjuvant therapy of cancer V. Orlando, FL: Grune & Stratton, 1987:735–744.
124. Edmonson JH. Systemic chemotherapy following complete excision of nonosseous sarcomas: Mayo Clinic experience. Cancer Treat Symp 1985;3:89–97.
125. Edmonson JH, Fleming TR, Ivins JC, et al. Randomized study of systemic chemotherapy following complete excision of nonosseous sarcomas. J Clin Oncol 1984;2:1390–1396.
126. Chang AE, Kinsella T, Glatstein E, et al. Adjuvant chemotherapy for patients with high-grade soft-tissue sarcomas of the extremity. J Clin Oncol 1988;6:1491–1500.
127. Rosenberg SA, Tepper J, Glatstein E, et al. Prospective randomized evaluation of adjuvant chemotherapy in adults with soft tissue sarcomas of the extremities. Cancer 1983;52:424–434.
128. Glenn J, Kinsella T, Glatstein E, et al. A randomized, prospective trial of adjuvant chemotherapy in adults with soft tissue sarcomas of the head and neck, breast, and trunk. Cancer 1985;55:1206–1214.
129. Glenn J, Sindelar WF, Kinsella T, et al. Results of multimodality therapy of resectable soft-tissue sarcomas of the retroperitoneum. Surgery 1985;97:316–325.
130. Bramwell V, Rouesse J, Steward W, et al. Adjuvant CYVADIC chemotherapy for adult soft tissue sarcoma—reduced local recurrence but no improvement in survival: a study of the European Organization for Research and Treatment of Cancer Soft Tissue and Bone Sarcoma Group. J Clin Oncol 1994;12:1137–1149.
131. Antman K, Suit H, Amato D, et al. Preliminary results of a randomized trial of adjuvant doxorubicin for sarcomas: lack of apparent difference between treatment groups. J Clin Oncol 1984;2:601–608.
132. Lerner HJ, Amato DA, Savlov ED, et al. Eastern Cooperative Oncology Group: a comparison of adjuvant doxorubicin and observation for patients with localized soft tissue sarcoma. J Clin Oncol 1987;5:613–617.
133. Ravaud A, Bui NB, Coindre J-M, et al. Adjuvant chemotherapy with CYVADIC in high risk soft tissue sarcoma: a randomized prospective trial. In: Salmon SE, ed. Adjuvant therapy of cancer VI. Philadelphia, PA: WB Saunders, 1990:556–566.
134. Alvegard TA, Sigurdsson H, Mouridsen H, et al. Adjuvant chemotherapy with doxorubicin in high-grade soft tissue sarcoma: a randomized trial of the Scandinavian Sarcoma Group. J Clin Oncol 1989;7:1504–1513.
135. Gherlinzoni F, Bacci G, Picci P, et al. A randomized trial for the treatment of high-grade soft-tissue sarcomas of the extremities: preliminary observations. J Clin Oncol 1986;4:552–558.
136. Picci P, Bacci G, Gherlinzoni F, et al. Results of a randomized trial for the treatment of localized soft tissue tumors (STS) of the extremities in adult patients. In: Ryan JR, Baker LO, eds. Recent concepts in sarcoma treatment. Dordrecht, the Netherlands: Kluwer Academic Publishers, 1988:144–148.
137. Antman K, Ryan L, Borden E, et al. Pooled results from three randomized adjuvant studies of doxorubicin versus observation in soft tissue sarcoma: 10 year results and review of the literature. In: Salmon SE, ed. Adjuvant therapy of cancer VI. Philadelphia, PA: WB Saunders, 1990:529–543.
138. Baker LH: Adjuvant therapy for soft tissue sarcomas. In: Ryan JR, Baker LO, eds. Recent concepts in sarcoma treatment. Dordrecht, the Netherlands: Kluwer Academic Publishers, 1988:130–135.
139. Petrioli R, Coratti A, Correale P, et al. Adjuvant epirubicin with or without ifosfamide for adult soft-tissue sarcoma. Am J Clin Oncol 2002;25:468–473.
140. Brodowicz T, Schwameis E, Widder J, et al. Intensified adjuvant IFADIC chemotherapy for adult soft tissue sarcoma: a prospective randomized feasibility trial. Sarcoma 2000;4:151–160.
141. Frustaci S, Gherlinzoni F, De Paoli A, et al. Adjuvant chemotherapy for adult soft tissue sarcomas of the extremities and girdles: results of the Italian randomized cooperative trial. J Clin Oncol 2001;19:1238–1247.
142. Adjuvant chemotherapy for localised resectable soft-tissue sarcoma of adults: meta-analysis of individual data. Sarcoma Meta-analysis Collaboration. Lancet 1997;350:1647–1654.
143. Bramwell VH. Adjuvant chemotherapy for adult soft tissue sarcoma: is there a standard of care? J Clin Oncol 2001;19:1235–1237.
144. Pervaiz N, Colterjohn N, Farrokhyar F, et al. A systematic meta-analysis of randomized controlled trials of adjuvant chemotherapy for localized resectable soft-tissue sarcoma. Cancer 2008;113:573–581.
145. Rosen G, Forscher C, Lowenbraun S, et al. Synovial sarcoma. Uniform response of metastases to high dose ifosfamide. Cancer 1994;73:2506–2511.
146. Karavasilis V, Seddon BM, Ashley S, et al. Significant clinical benefit of first-line palliative chemotherapy in advanced soft-tissue sarcoma: retrospective analysis and identification of prognostic factors in 488 patients. Cancer 2008;112:1585–1591.
147. O'Bryan RM, Luce JK, Talley RW, et al. Phase II evaluation of Adriamycin in human neoplasia. Cancer 1973;32:1–8.
148. Mouridsen HT, Bastholt L, Somers R, et al. Adriamycin versus epirubicin in advanced soft tissue sarcomas. A randomized phase II/phase III study of the EORTC Soft Tissue and Bone Sarcoma Group. Eur J Cancer Clin Oncol 1987;23:1477–1483.
149. Santoro A, Tursz T, Mouridsen H, et al. Doxorubicin versus CYVADIC versus doxorubicin plus ifosfamide in first-line treatment of advanced soft tissue sarcomas: a randomized study of the European Organization for Research and Treatment of Cancer Soft Tissue and Bone Sarcoma Group. J Clin Oncol 1995;13:1537–1545.
150. Le Cesne A, Judson I, Crowther D, et al. Randomized phase III study comparing conventional-dose doxorubicin plus ifosfamide versus high-dose doxorubicin plus ifosfamide plus recombinant human granulocyte-macrophage colony-stimulating factor in advanced soft tissue sarcomas: a trial of the European Organization for Research and Treatment of Cancer/Soft Tissue and Bone Sarcoma Group. J Clin Oncol 2000;18:2676–2684.
151. Gottlieb JA, Benjamin RS, Baker LH, et al. Role of DTIC (NSC-45388) in the chemotherapy of sarcomas. Cancer Treat Rep 1976;60:199–203.
152. Garcia del Muro X, Lopez-Pousa A, Martin J, et al. A phase II trial of temozolomide as a 6-week, continuous, oral schedule in patients with advanced soft tissue sarcoma: a study by the Spanish Group for Research on Sarcomas. Cancer 2005;104:1706–1712.
153. Trent JC, Beach J, Burgess MA, et al. A two-arm phase II study of temozolomide in patients with advanced gastrointestinal stromal tumors and other soft tissue sarcomas. Cancer 2003;98:2693–2699.
154. Woll PJ, Judson I, Lee SM, et al. Temozolomide in adult patients with advanced soft tissue sarcoma: a phase II study of the EORTC Soft Tissue and Bone Sarcoma Group. Eur J Cancer 1999;35:410–412.
155. Stuart-Harris RC, Harper PG, Parsons CA, et al. High-dose alkylation therapy using ifosfamide infusion with mesna in the treatment of adult advanced soft-tissue sarcoma. Cancer Chemother Pharmacol 1983;11:69–72.
156. Patel SR, Vadhan-Raj S, Papadopolous N, et al. High-dose ifosfamide in bone and soft tissue sarcomas: results of phase II and pilot studies—dose-response and schedule dependence. J Clin Oncol 1997;15:2378–2384.
157. van Oosterom AT, Mouridsen HT, Nielsen OS, et al. Results of randomised studies of the EORTC Soft Tissue and Bone Sarcoma Group (STBSG) with two different ifosfamide regimens in first- and second-line chemotherapy in advanced soft tissue sarcoma patients. Eur J Cancer 2002;38:2397–2406.
158. Worden FP, Taylor JM, Biermann JS, et al. Randomized phase II evaluation of 6 g/m^2 of ifosfamide plus doxorubicin and granulocyte colony-stimulating factor (G-CSF) compared with 12 g/m^2 of ifosfamide plus doxorubicin and G-CSF in the treatment of poor-prognosis soft tissue sarcoma. J Clin Oncol 2005;23:105–112.
159. Lorigan P, Verweij J, Papai Z, et al. Phase III trial of two investigational schedules of ifosfamide compared with standard-dose doxorubicin in advanced or metastatic soft tissue sarcoma: a European Organisation for Research and Treatment of Cancer Soft Tissue and Bone Sarcoma Group Study. J Clin Oncol 2007;25:3144–3150.
160. Svancarova L, Blay JY, Judson IR, et al. Gemcitabine in advanced adult soft-tissue sarcomas. A phase II study of the EORTC Soft Tissue and Bone Sarcoma Group. Eur J Cancer 2002;38:556–559.
161. Von Burton G, Rankin C, Zalupski MM, et al. Phase II trial of gemcitabine as first line chemotherapy in patients with metastatic or unresectable soft tissue sarcoma. Am J Clin Oncol 2006;29:59–61.
162. Patel SR, Gandhi V, Jenkins J, et al. Phase II clinical investigation of gemcitabine in advanced soft tissue sarcomas and window evaluation of dose rate on gemcitabine triphosphate accumulation. J Clin Oncol 2001;19:3483–3489.
163. Borden EC, Amato DA, Rosenbaum C, et al. Randomized comparison of three Adriamycin regimens for metastatic soft tissue sarcomas. J Clin Oncol 1987;5:840–850.
164. Gottlieb JA, Baker LH, Quagliana JM, et al. Chemotherapy of sarcomas with a combination of Adriamycin and dimethyl triazeno imidazole carboxamide. Cancer 1972;30:1632–1638.
165. Yap BS, Baker LH, Sinkovics JG, et al. Cyclophosphamide, vincristine, Adriamycin, and DTIC (CYVADIC) combination chemotherapy for the treatment of advanced sarcomas. Cancer Treat Rep 1980;64:93–98.
166. Elias A, Ryan L, Sulkes A, et al. Response to mesna, doxorubicin, ifosfamide, and dacarbazine in 108 patients with metastatic or unresectable sarcoma and no prior chemotherapy. J Clin Oncol 1989;7:1208–1216.
167. Patel SR, Vadhan-Raj S, Burgess MA, et al. Results of two consecutive trials of dose-intensive chemotherapy with doxorubicin and ifosfamide in patients with sarcomas. Am J Clin Oncol 1998;21:317–321.
168. Maki RG, Wathen JK, Patel SR, et al. Randomized phase II study of gemcitabine and docetaxel compared with gemcitabine alone in patients with metastatic soft tissue sarcomas: results of Sarcoma Alliance for Research Through Collaboration Study 002 [corrected]. J Clin Oncol 2007;25:2755–2763.
169. Zou CY, Smith KD, Zhu QS, et al. Dual targeting of AKT and mammalian target of rapamycin: a potential therapeutic approach for malignant peripheral nerve sheath tumor. Mol Cancer Ther 2009;8:1157–1168.
170. Forni C, Minuzzo M, Virdis E, et al. Trabectedin (ET-743) promotes differentiation in myxoid liposarcoma tumors. Mol Cancer Ther 2009;8:449–457.
171. Grosso F, Jones RL, Demetri GD, et al. Efficacy of trabectedin (ecteinascidin-743) in advanced pretreated myxoid liposarcomas: a retrospective study. Lancet Oncol 2007;8:595–602.
172. Stacchiotti S, Tamborini E, Marrari A, et al. Response to sunitinib malate in advanced alveolar soft part sarcoma. Clin Cancer Res 2009;15:1096–1104.
173. George S, Merriam P, Maki RG, et al. Multicenter phase II trial of sunitinib in the treatment of nongastrointestinal stromal tumor sarcomas. J Clin Oncol 2009;27:154–160.
174. Maki RG, D'Adamo DR, Keohan ML, et al. Phase II study of sorafenib in patients with metastatic or recurrent sarcomas. J Clin Oncol 2009;27:3133–3140.
175. McArthur GA, Demetri GD, van Oosterom A, et al. Molecular and clinical analysis of locally advanced dermatofibrosarcoma protuberans treated with imatinib: Imatinib Target Exploration Consortium Study B2225. J Clin Oncol 2005;23:866–873.
176. Tsuda M, Davis IJ, Argani P, et al. TFE3 fusions activate MET signaling by transcriptional up-regulation, defining another class of tumors as candidates for therapeutic MET inhibition. Cancer Res 2007;67:919–929.
177. Bu X, Bernstein L. A proposed explanation for female predominance in alveolar soft part sarcoma. Noninactivation of X; autosome translocation fusion gene? Cancer 2005;103:1245–1253.
178. Casanova M, Ferrari A, Bisogno G, et al. Alveolar soft part sarcoma in children and adolescents: a report from the Soft-Tissue Sarcoma Italian Cooperative Group. Ann Oncol 2000;11:1445–1449.
179. Kayton ML, Meyers P, Wexler LH, et al. Clinical presentation, treatment, and outcome of alveolar soft part sarcoma in children, adolescents, and young adults. J Pediatr Surg 2006;41:187–193.
180. Pappo AS, Parham DM, Cain A, et al. Alveolar soft part sarcoma in children and adolescents: clinical features and outcome of 11 patients. Med Pediatr Oncol 1996;26:81–84.
181. Ladanyi M, Lui MY, Antonescu CR, et al. The der(17)t(X;17)(p11;q25) of human alveolar soft part sarcoma fuses the TFE3 transcription factor gene to ASPL, a novel gene at 17q25. Oncogene 2001;20:48–57.
182. Argani P, Antonescu CR, Illei PB, et al. Primary renal neoplasms with the ASPL-TFE3 gene fusion of alveolar soft part sarcoma: a distinctive tumor entity previously included among renal cell carcinomas of children and adolescents. Am J Pathol 2001;159:179–192.
183. Clark J, Lu YJ, Sidhar SK, et al. Fusion of splicing factor genes PSF and NonO (p54nrb) to the TFE3 gene in papillary renal cell carcinoma. Oncogene 1997;15:2233–2239.
184. Yagihashi S. Alveolar soft part sarcoma. Are we approaching the goal of determining its histogenesis? Acta Pathol Jpn 1992;42:466–468.
185. Portera CA Jr, Ho V, Patel SR, et al. Alveolar soft part sarcoma: clinical course and patterns of metastasis in 70 patients treated at a single institution. Cancer 2001;91:585–591.

186. Lieberman PH, Brennan MF, Kimmel M, et al. Alveolar soft-part sarcoma. A clinicopathologic study of half a century. Cancer 1989;63:1–13.
187. Reichardt P, Lindner T, Pink D, et al. Chemotherapy in alveolar soft part sarcomas. What do we know? Eur J Cancer 2003;39:1511–1516.
188. Gardner K LM, Alvarez-Gutierrez M, Judson I, et al. Activity of the VEGFR/KIT tyrosine kinase inhibitor cediranib (AZD2171) in alveolar soft part sarcoma. London, UK: Connective Tissue Onoclogic Society, 2008.
189. Clark MA, Johnson MB, Thway K, et al. Clear cell sarcoma (melanoma of soft parts): The Royal Marsden Hospital experience. Eur J Surg Oncol 2008;34:800–804.
190. Kawai A, Hosono A, Nakayama R, et al. Clear cell sarcoma of tendons and aponeuroses: a study of 75 patients. Cancer 2007;109:109–116.
191. Ferrari A, Casanova M, Bisogno G, et al. Clear cell sarcoma of tendons and aponeuroses in pediatric patients: a report from the Italian and German Soft Tissue Sarcoma Cooperative Group. Cancer 2002;94:3269–3276.
192. Variend S, Bax NM, van Gorp J. Are infantile myofibromatosis, congenital fibrosarcoma and congenital haemangiopericytoma histogenetically related? Histopathology 1995;26:57–62.
193. Lucas DR, Nascimento AG, Sim FH. Clear cell sarcoma of soft tissues. Mayo Clinic experience with 35 cases. Am J Surg Pathol 1992;16:1197–1204.
194. Fletcher CD, Unni KK, Mertens F. World Health Organization Classification of Soft Tissue Tumours. Pathology and genetics tumours of soft tissue and bone. Lyon, France: IARC Press, 2002.
195. Reitamo JJ, Hayry P, Nykyri E, et al. The desmoid tumor, part I: incidence, sex-, age- and anatomical distribution in the Finnish population. Am J Clin Pathol 1982;77:665–673.
196. Ballo MT, Zagars GK, Pollack A, et al. Desmoid tumor: prognostic factors and outcome after surgery, radiation therapy, or combined surgery and radiation therapy. J Clin Oncol 1999;17:158–167.
197. Lev D, Kotilingam D, Wei C, et al. Optimizing treatment of desmoid tumors. J Clin Oncol 2007;25:1785–1791.
198. Spear MA, Jennings LC, Mankin HJ, et al. Individualizing management of aggressive fibromatoses. Int J Radiat Oncol Biol Phys 1998;40:637–645.
199. Faulkner LB, Hajdu SI, Kher U, et al. Pediatric desmoid tumor: retrospective analysis of 63 cases. J Clin Oncol 1995;13:2813–2818.
200. Gurbuz AK, Giardiello FM, Petersen GM, et al. Desmoid tumours in familial adenomatous polyposis. Gut 1994;35:377–381.
201. Nieuwenhuis MH, De Vos Tot Nederveen Cappel W, Botma A, et al. Desmoid tumors in a Dutch cohort of patients with familial adenomatous polyposis. Clin Gastroenterol Hepatol 2008;6:215–219.
202. Lazar AJ, Tuvin D, Hajibashi S, et al. Specific mutations in the beta-catenin gene (CTNNB1) correlate with local recurrence in sporadic desmoid tumors. Am J Pathol 2008;173:1518–1527.
203. Gronchi A, Casali PG, Mariani L, et al. Quality of surgery and outcome in extra-abdominal aggressive fibromatosis: a series of patients surgically treated at a single institution. J Clin Oncol 2003;21:1390–1397.
204. Guadagnolo BA, Zagars GK, Ballo MT. Long-term outcomes for desmoid tumors treated with radiation therapy. Int J Radiat Oncol Biol Phys 2008;71:441–447.
205. Merchant TE, Nguyen D, Walter AW, et al. Long-term results with radiation therapy for pediatric desmoid tumors. Int J Radiat Oncol Biol Phys 2000;47:1267–1271.
206. Azzarelli A, Gronchi A, Bertulli R, et al. Low-dose chemotherapy with methotrexate and vinblastine for patients with advanced aggressive fibromatosis. Cancer 2001;92:1259–1264.
207. Skapek SX, Ferguson WS, Granowetter L, et al. Vinblastine and methotrexate for desmoid fibromatosis in children: results of a Pediatric Oncology Group Phase II Trial. J Clin Oncol 2007;25:501–506.
208. Heinrich MC, McArthur GA, Demetri GD, et al. Clinical and molecular studies of the effect of imatinib on advanced aggressive fibromatosis (desmoid tumor). J Clin Oncol 2006;24:1195–1203.
209. Gega M, Yanagi H, Yoshikawa R, et al. Successful chemotherapeutic modality of doxorubicin plus dacarbazine for the treatment of desmoid tumors in association with familial adenomatous polyposis. J Clin Oncol 2006;24:102–105.
210. Gerald WL, Ladanyi M, de Alava E, et al. Clinical, pathologic, and molecular spectrum of tumors associated with t(11;22)(p13;q12): desmoplastic small round-cell tumor and its variants. J Clin Oncol 1998;16:3028–3036.
211. Lae ME, Roche PC, Jin L, et al. Desmoplastic small round cell tumor: a clinicopathologic, immunohistochemical, and molecular study of 32 tumors. Am J Surg Pathol 2002;26:823–835.
212. Saab R, Khoury JD, Krasin M, et al. Desmoplastic small round cell tumor in childhood: the St. Jude Children's Research Hospital experience. Pediatr Blood Cancer 2007;49:274–279.
213. Ordonez NG: Desmoplastic small round cell tumor, part I: a histopathologic study of 39 cases with emphasis on unusual histological patterns. Am J Surg Pathol 1998;22:1303–1313.
214. Wang LL, Perlman EJ, Vujanic GM, et al. Desmoplastic small round cell tumor of the kidney in childhood. Am J Surg Pathol 2007;31:576–584.
215. Kushner BH, LaQuaglia MP, Wollner N, et al. Desmoplastic small round-cell tumor: prolonged progression-free survival with aggressive multimodality therapy. J Clin Oncol 1996;14:1526–1531.
216. Lal DR, Su WT, Wolden SL, et al. Results of multimodal treatment for desmoplastic small round cell tumors. J Pediatr Surg 2005;40:251–255.
217. Ross HM, Lewis JJ, Woodruff JM, et al. Epithelioid sarcoma: clinical behavior and prognostic factors of survival. Ann Surg Oncol 1997;4:491–495.
218. Casanova M, Ferrari A, Collini P, et al. Epithelioid sarcoma in children and adolescents: a report from the Italian Soft Tissue Sarcoma Committee. Cancer 2006;106:708–717.
219. Chase DR, Enzinger FM: Epithelioid sarcoma. Diagnosis, prognostic indicators, and treatment. Am J Surg Pathol 1985;9:241–263.
220. Gross E, Rao BN, Pappo A, et al. Epithelioid sarcoma in children. J Pediatr Surg 1996;31:1663–1665.
221. Halling AC, Wollan PC, Pritchard DJ, et al. Epithelioid sarcoma: a clinicopathologic review of 55 cases. Mayo Clin Proc 1996;71:636–642.
222. Lualdi E, Modena P, Debiec-Rychter M, et al. Molecular cytogenetic characterization of proximal-type epithelioid sarcoma. Genes Chromosomes Cancer 2004;41:283–290.
223. Modena P, Lualdi E, Facchinetti F, et al. SMARCB1/INI1 tumor suppressor gene is frequently inactivated in epithelioid sarcomas. Cancer Res 2005;65:4012–4019.
224. Kuhnen C, Tolnay E, Steinau HU, et al. Expression of c-Met receptor and hepatocyte growth factor/scatter factor in synovial sarcoma and epithelioid sarcoma. Virchows Arch 1998;432:337–342.
225. Chbani L, Guillou L, Terrier P, et al. Epithelioid sarcoma: a clinicopathologic and immunohistochemical analysis of 106 cases from the French sarcoma group. Am J Clin Pathol 2009;131:222–227.
226. Miettinen M, Fanburg-Smith JC, Virolainen M, et al. Epithelioid sarcoma: an immunohistochemical analysis of 112 classical and variant cases and a discussion of the differential diagnosis. Hum Pathol 1999;30:934–942.
227. Hornick JL, Dal Cin P, Fletcher CD. Loss of INI1 expression is characteristic of both conventional and proximal-type epithelioid sarcoma. Am J Surg Pathol 2009;33:542–550.
228. Kohashi K, Izumi T, Oda Y, et al. Infrequent SMARCB1/INI1 gene alteration in epithelioid sarcoma: a useful tool in distinguishing epithelioid sarcoma from malignant rhabdoid tumor. Hum Pathol 2009;40:349–355.
229. de Visscher SA, van Ginkel RJ, Wobbes T, et al. Epithelioid sarcoma: still an only surgically curable disease. Cancer 2006;107:606–612.
230. Gupta H, Davidoff AM, Rao BN, et al. Neonatal epithelioid sarcoma: a distinct clinical entity? J Pediatr Surg 2006;41:e9–e11.
231. Callister MD, Ballo MT, Pisters PW, et al. Epithelioid sarcoma: results of conservative surgery and radiotherapy. Int J Radiat Oncol Biol Phys 2001;51:384–391.
232. Koscielniak E, Harms D, Schmidt D, et al. Soft tissue sarcomas in infants younger than 1 year of age: a report of the German Soft Tissue Sarcoma Study Group (CWS-81). Med Pediatr Oncol 1989;17:105–110.
233. Coffin CM, Dehner LP. Soft tissue tumors in first year of life: a report of 190 cases. Pediatr Pathol 1990;10:509–526.
234. Schofield DE, Fletcher JA, Grier HE, et al. Fibrosarcoma in infants and children. Application of new techniques. Am J Surg Pathol 1994;18:14–24.
235. Soule EH, Pritchard DJ. Fibrosarcoma in infants and children: a review of 110 cases. Cancer 1977;40:1711–1721.
236. Coffin CM, Jaszcz W, O'Shea PA, et al. So-called congenital-infantile fibrosarcoma: does it exist and what is it? Pediatr Pathol 1994;14:133–150.
237. Wilson MB, Stanley W, Sens D, et al. Infantile fibrosarcoma—a misnomer? Pediatr Pathol 1990;10:901–907.
238. Toguchida J, Yamaguchi T, Ritchie B, et al. Mutation spectrum of the p53 gene in bone and soft tissue sarcomas. Cancer Res 1992;52:6194–6199.
239. Ledet SC, Brown RW, Cagle PT. p53 immunostaining in the differentiation of inflammatory pseudotumor from sarcoma involving the lung. Mod Pathol 1995;8:282–286.
240. Alaggio R, Ninfo V, Rosolen A, et al. Primitive myxoid mesenchymal tumor of infancy: a clinicopathologic report of 6 cases. Am J Surg Pathol 2006;30:388–394.
241. Hays DM, Mirabal VQ, Karlan MS, et al. Fibrosarcomas in infants and children. J Pediatr Surg 1970;5:176–183.
242. Dobson L, Dickey LB. Spontaneous regression of malignant tumors; report of a twelve-year spontaneous complete regression of an extensive fibrosarcoma, with speculations about regression and dormancy. Am J Surg 1956;92:162–173.
243. Madden NP, Spicer RD, Allibone EB, et al. Spontaneous regression of neonatal fibrosarcoma. Br J Cancer Suppl 1992;18:S72–S75.
244. Kurkchubasche AG, Halvorson EG, Forman EN, et al. The role of preoperative chemotherapy in the treatment of infantile fibrosarcoma. J Pediatr Surg 2000;35:880–883.
245. Coffin CM, Dehner LP. Fibroblastic-myofibroblastic tumors in children and adolescents: a clinicopathologic study of 108 examples in 103 patients. Pediatr Pathol 1991;11:569–588.
246. Chung EB, Enzinger FM. Infantile myofibromatosis. Cancer 1981;48:1807–1818.
247. Zand DJ, Huff D, Everman D, et al. Autosomal dominant inheritance of infantile myofibromatosis. Am J Med Genet 2004;126A:261–266.
248. Narchi H. Four half-siblings with infantile myofibromatosis: a case for autosomal-recessive inheritance. Clin Genet 2001;59:134–135.
249. Alaggio R, Barisani D, Ninfo V, et al. Morphologic overlap between infantile myofibromatosis and infantile fibrosarcoma: a pitfall in diagnosis. Pediatr Dev Pathol 2008;11:355–362.
250. Gandhi MM, Nathan PC, Weitzman S, et al. Successful treatment of life-threatening generalized infantile myofibromatosis using low-dose chemotherapy. J Pediatr Hematol Oncol 2003;25:750–754.
251. Baerg J, Murphy JJ, Magee JF. Fibromatoses: clinical and pathological features suggestive of recurrence. J Pediatr Surg 1999;34:1112–1114.
252. Azzam R, Abboud M, Muwakkit S, et al. First-line therapy of generalized infantile myofibromatosis with low-dose vinblastine and methotrexate. Pediatr Blood Cancer 2009;52:308.
253. de Saint Aubain Somerhausen N, Fletcher CD. Leiomyosarcoma of soft tissue in children: clinicopathologic analysis of 20 cases. Am J Surg Pathol 1999;23:755–763.
254. Ferrari A, Bisogno G, Casanova M, et al. Childhood leiomyosarcoma: a report from the soft tissue sarcoma Italian Cooperative Group. Ann Oncol 2001;12:1163–1168.
255. Hwang ES, Gerald W, Wollner N, et al. Leiomyosarcoma in childhood and adolescence. Ann Surg Oncol 1997;4:223–227.
256. Cypriano MS, Jenkins JJ, Pappo AS, et al. Pediatric gastrointestinal stromal tumors and leiomyosarcoma. Cancer 2004;101:39–50.
257. Biggar RJ, Frisch M, Goedert JJ. Risk of cancer in children with AIDS. AIDS-Cancer Match Registry Study Group. JAMA 2000;284:205–209.
258. Timmons CF, Dawson DB, Richards CS, et al. Epstein-Barr virus-associated leiomyosarcomas in liver transplantation recipients. Origin from either donor or recipient tissue. Cancer 1995;76:1481–1489.
259. Hill MA, Araya JC, Eckert MW, et al. Tumor specific Epstein-Barr virus infection is not associated with leiomyosarcoma in human immunodeficiency virus negative individuals. Cancer 1997;80:204–210.
260. Bisogno G, Sotti G, Nowicki Y, et al. Soft tissue sarcoma as a second malignant neoplasm in the pediatric age group. Cancer 2004;100:1758–1765.
261. Chadwick EG, Connor EJ, Hanson IC, et al. Tumors of smooth-muscle origin in HIV-infected children. JAMA 1990;263:3182–3184.
262. Shen SC, Yunis EJ. Leiomyosarcoma developing in a child during remission of leukemia. J Pediatr 1976;89:780–782.
263. Swanson PE, Dehner LP, Maurer HM, et al. Pathology of soft tissue sarcomas in children and adolescents. In: Rhabdomyosarcoma and related tumors in children and adolescents. Boca Raton, FL: CRC Press, 1991:385–420.
264. Kaneko Y. Cytogenetics in pediatric solid tumors. Jpn Clin Pathol 1990;38:1047–1052.
265. Nibert M, Heim S. Uterine leiomyoma cytogenetics. Genes Chromosomes Cancer 1990;2:3–13.
266. Boghosian L, Dal Cin P, Turc-Carel C, et al. Three possible cytogenetic subgroups of leiomyosarcoma. Cancer Genet Cytogenet 1989;43:39–49.

267. Clary BM, DeMatteo RP, Lewis JJ, et al. Gastrointestinal stromal tumors and leiomyosarcoma of the abdomen and retroperitoneum: a clinical comparison. Ann Surg Oncol 2001;8:290–299.

268. Miyajima K, Oda Y, Oshiro Y, et al. Clinicopathological prognostic factors in soft tissue leiomyosarcoma: a multivariate analysis. Histopathology 2002;40:353–359.

269. Hensley ML, Blessing JA, Degeest K, et al. Fixed-dose rate gemcitabine plus docetaxel as second-line therapy for metastatic uterine leiomyosarcoma: a Gynecologic Oncology Group phase II study. Gynecol Oncol 2008;109:323–328.

270. Le Cesne A, Blay JY, Judson I, et al. Phase II study of ET-743 in advanced soft tissue sarcomas: a European Organisation for the Research and Treatment of Cancer (EORTC) Soft Tissue and Bone Sarcoma Group Trial. J Clin Oncol 2005;23:576–584.

271. Alaggio R, Coffin CM, Weiss SW, et al. Liposarcomas in young patients: a study of 82 cases occurring in patients younger than 22 years of age. Am J Surg Pathol 2009;33:645–658.

272. Knight JC, Renwick PJ, Cin PD, et al. Translocation t(12;16)(q13;p11) in myxoid liposarcoma and round cell liposarcoma: molecular and cytogenetic analysis. Cancer Res 1995;55:24–27.

273. Rabbitts TH, Forster A, Larson R, et al. Fusion of the dominant negative transcription regulator CHOP with a novel gene FUS by translocation t(12;16) in malignant liposarcoma. Nat Genet 1993;4:175–180.

274. Eneroth M, Mandahl N, Heim S, et al. Localization of the chromosomal breakpoints of the t(12;16) in liposarcoma to subbands 12q13.3 and 16p11.2. Cancer Genet Cytogenet 1990;48:101–107.

275. Weiss SW, Goldblum JR, Enzinger FM. Enzinger and Weiss' soft tissue tumors. 5th ed. Philadelphia, PA: Mosby Elsevier, 2008.

276. Ferrari A, Casanova M, Spreafico F, et al. Childhood liposarcoma: a single-institutional twenty-year experience. Pediatr Hematol Oncol 1999;16:415–421.

277. La Quaglia MP, Spiro SA, Ghavimi F, et al. Liposarcoma in patients younger than or equal to 22 years of age. Cancer 1993;72:3114–3119.

278. Cheng EY, Springfield DS, Mankin HJ. Frequent incidence of extrapulmonary sites of initial metastasis in patients with liposarcoma. Cancer 1995;75:1120–1127.

279. Issakov J, Soyfer V, Kollender Y, et al. Liposarcoma in adult limbs treated by limb-sparing surgery and adjuvant radiotherapy. J Bone Joint Surg Br 2006;88:1647–1651.

280. Engstrom K, Bergh P, Gustafson P, et al. Liposarcoma: outcome based on the Scandinavian Sarcoma Group Register. Cancer 2008;113:1649–1656.

281. Taamma A, Misset JL, Riofrio M, et al. Phase I and pharmacokinetic study of ecteinascidin-743, a new marine compound, administered as a 24-hour continuous infusion in patients with solid tumors. J Clin Oncol 2001;19:1256–1265.

282. Carli M, Ferrari A, Mattke A, et al. Pediatric malignant peripheral nerve sheath tumor: the Italian and German Soft Tissue Sarcoma Cooperative Group. J Clin Oncol 2005;23:8422–8430.

283. Ducatman BS, Scheithauer BW, Piepgras DG, et al. Malignant peripheral nerve sheath tumors. A clinicopathologic study of 120 cases. Cancer 1986;57:2006–2021.

284. Riccardi VM, Elder DW. Multiple cytogenetic aberrations in neurofibrosarcomas complicating neurofibromatosis. Cancer Genet Cytogenet 1986;23:199–209.

285. Decker HJ, Cannizzaro LA, Mendez MJ, et al. Chromosomes 17 and 22 involved in marker formation in neurofibrosarcoma in von Recklinghausen disease. A cytogenetic and in situ hybridization study. Hum Genet 1990;85:337–342.

286. Johannessen CM, Johnson BW, Williams SM, et al. TORC1 is essential for NF1-associated malignancies. Curr Biol 2008;18:56–62.

287. Johnson MR, Look AT, DeClue JE, et al. Inactivation of the NF1 gene in human melanoma and neuroblastoma cell lines without impaired regulation of GTP.Ras. Proc Natl Acad Sci U S A 1993;90:5539–5543.

288. Fletcher CD. Peripheral nerve sheath tumors. A clinicopathologic update. Pathol Annu 1990;25(Pt 1):53–74.

289. Meis JM, Enzinger FM, Martz KL, et al. Malignant peripheral nerve sheath tumors (malignant schwannomas) in children. Am J Surg Pathol 1992;16:694–707.

290. Enzinger FM, Weiss SW, Enzinger FM WSW. Malignant schwannomas, soft tissue tumors. St. Louis: CV Mosby, 1995:889–928.

291. Weiss SW, Langloss JM, Enzinger FM. Value of S-100 protein in the diagnosis of soft tissue tumors with particular reference to benign and malignant Schwann cell tumors. Lab Invest 1983;49:299–308.

292. Canter RJ, Qin LX, Maki RG, et al. A synovial sarcoma-specific preoperative nomogram supports a survival benefit to ifosfamide-based chemotherapy and improves risk stratification for patients. Clin Cancer Res 2008;14:8191–8197.

293. Ladanyi M, Antonescu CR, Leung DH, et al. Impact of SYT-SSX fusion type on the clinical behavior of synovial sarcoma: a multi-institutional retrospective study of 243 patients. Cancer Res 2002;62:135–140.

294. Guillou L, Benhattar J, Bonichon F, et al. Histologic grade, but not SYT-SSX fusion type, is an important prognostic factor in patients with synovial sarcoma: a multicenter, retrospective analysis. J Clin Oncol 2004;22:4040–4050.

295. Okcu MF, Munsell M, Treuner J, et al. Synovial sarcoma of childhood and adolescence: a multicenter, multivariate analysis of outcome. J Clin Oncol 2003;21:1602–1611.

296. de Leeuw B, Balemans M, Weghuis DO, et al. Molecular cloning of the synovial sarcoma-specific translocation (X;18)(p11.2;q11.2) breakpoint. Hum Mol Genet 1994;3:745–749.

297. Enzinger FM. Epithelioid sarcoma. A sarcoma simulating a granuloma or a carcinoma. Cancer 1970;26:1029–1041.

298. Terry J, Saito T, Subramanian S, et al. TLE1 as a diagnostic immunohistochemical marker for synovial sarcoma emerging from gene expression profiling studies. Am J Surg Pathol 2007;31:240–246.

299. Ferrari A, Gronchi A, Casanova M, et al. Synovial sarcoma: a retrospective analysis of 271 patients of all ages treated at a single institution. Cancer 2004;101:627–634.

300. Trassard M, Le Doussal V, Hacene K, et al. Prognostic factors in localized primary synovial sarcoma: a multicenter study of 128 adult patients. J Clin Oncol 2001;19:525–534.

301. Guadagnolo BA, Zagars GK, Ballo MT, et al. Long-term outcomes for synovial sarcoma treated with conservation surgery and radiotherapy. Int J Radiat Oncol Biol Phys 2007;69:1173–1180.

302. Lewis JJ, Antonescu CR, Leung DH, et al. Synovial sarcoma: a multivariate analysis of prognostic factors in 112 patients with primary localized tumors of the extremity. J Clin Oncol 2000;18:2087–2094.

303. Eilber FC, Brennan MF, Eilber FR, et al. Chemotherapy is associated with improved survival in adult patients with primary extremity synovial sarcoma. Ann Surg 2007;246:105–113.

304. Schultz KA, Ness KK, Whitton J, et al. Behavioral and social outcomes in adolescent survivors of childhood cancer: a report from the childhood cancer survivor study. J Clin Oncol 2007;25:3649–3656.

305. Hobbie WL, Stuber M, Meeske K, et al. Symptoms of posttraumatic stress in young adult survivors of childhood cancer. J Clin Oncol 2000;18:4060–4066.

306. Chapman CR, Gavrin J. Suffering: the contributions of persistent pain. Lancet 1999;353:2233–2237.

307. Hudson MM, Mertens AC, Yasui Y, et al. Health status of adult long-term survivors of childhood cancer: a report from the Childhood Cancer Survivor Study. JAMA 2003;290:1583–1592.

308. Park ER, Li FP, Liu Y, et al. Health insurance coverage in survivors of childhood cancer: the Childhood Cancer Survivor Study. J Clin Oncol 2005;23:9187–9197.

309. Crom DB, Lensing SY, Rai SN, et al. Marriage, employment, and health insurance in adult survivors of childhood cancer. J Cancer Surviv 2007;1:237–245.

310. Davis AM, Sennik S, Griffin AM, et al. Predictors of functional outcomes following limb salvage surgery for lower-extremity soft tissue sarcoma. J Surg Oncol 2000;73:206–211.

311. Ness KK, Hudson MM, Ginsberg JP, et al. Physical performance limitations in the Childhood Cancer Survivor Study Cohort. J Clin Oncol 2009;27:2382–2389.

312. Paulino AC. Late effects of radiotherapy for pediatric extremity sarcomas. Int J Radiat Oncol Biol Phys 2004;60:265–274.

313. Le Deley MC, Leblanc T, Shamsaldin A, et al. Risk of secondary leukemia after a solid tumor in childhood according to the dose of epipodophyllotoxins and anthracyclines: a case-control study by the Societe Francaise d'Oncologie Pediatrique. J Clin Oncol 2003;21:1074–1081.

314. Meadows AT, Friedman DL, Neglia JP, et al. Second neoplasms in survivors of childhood cancer: findings from the Childhood Cancer Survivor Study Cohort. J Clin Oncol 2009;27:2356–2362.

315. Carver JR, Shapiro CL, Ng A, et al. American Society of Clinical Oncology clinical evidence review on the ongoing care of adult cancer survivors: cardiac and pulmonary late effects. J Clin Oncol 2007;25:3991–4008.

316. Paulides M, Kremers A, Stohr W, et al. Prospective longitudinal evaluation of doxorubicin-induced cardiomyopathy in sarcoma patients: a report of the Late Effects Surveillance System (LESS). Pediatr Blood Cancer 2006;46:489–495.

317. Sorensen K, Levitt GA, Bull C, et al. Late anthracycline cardiotoxicity after childhood cancer: a prospective longitudinal study. Cancer 2003;97:1991–1998.

318. van Dalen EC, van der Pal HJ, Kok WE, et al. Clinical heart failure in a cohort of children treated with anthracyclines: a long-term follow-up study. Eur J Cancer 2006;42:3191–3198.

319. Green DM, Kawashima T, Stovall M, et al. Fertility of female survivors of childhood cancer: a report from the Childhood Cancer Survivor Study. J Clin Oncol 2009;27:2677–2685.

320. Green DM, Sklar CA, Boice JD Jr, et al. Ovarian failure and reproductive outcomes after childhood cancer treatment: results from the Childhood Cancer Survivor Study. J Clin Oncol 2009;27:2374–2381.

321. Sklar CA, Mertens AC, Mitby P, et al. Premature menopause in survivors of childhood cancer: a report from the childhood cancer survivor study. J Natl Cancer Inst 2006;98:890–896.

322. Greenfield DM, Walters SJ, Coleman RE, et al. Prevalence and consequences of androgen deficiency in young male cancer survivors in a controlled cross-sectional study. J Clin Endocrinol Metab 2007;92:3476–3482.

323. Kenney LB, Laufer MR, Grant FD, et al. High risk of infertility and long term gonadal damage in males treated with high dose cyclophosphamide for sarcoma during childhood. Cancer 2001;91:613–621.

324. Williams D, Crofton PM, Levitt G. Does ifosfamide affect gonadal function? Pediatr Blood Cancer 2008;50:347–351.

325. Sarosy G. Ifosfamide—pharmacologic overview. Semin Oncol 1989;16:2–8.

326. Stillwell TJ, Benson RC Jr. Cyclophosphamide-induced hemorrhagic cystitis. A review of 100 patients. Cancer 1988;61:451–457.

327. Burk CD, Restaino I, Kaplan BS, et al. Ifosfamide-induced renal tubular dysfunction and rickets in children with Wilms tumor. J Pediatr 1990;117:331–335.

328. Skinner R, Cotterill SJ, Stevens MC. Risk factors for nephrotoxicity after ifosfamide treatment in children: a UKCCSG Late Effects Group Study. United Kingdom Children's Cancer Study Group. Br J Cancer 2000;82:1636–1645.

329. Stohr W, Paulides M, Bielack S, et al. Ifosfamide-induced nephrotoxicity in 593 sarcoma patients: a report from the Late Effects Surveillance System. Pediatr Blood Cancer 2007;48:447–452.

CHAPTER 33 ■ EWING SARCOMA

DOUGLAS S. HAWKINS, TOBIAS BÖLLING, STEVEN DUBOIS, PANCRAS C.W. HOGENDOORN, HERIBERT JÜRGENS, MICHAEL PAULUSSEN, R. LOR RANDALL, AND STEPHEN L. LESSNICK

INTRODUCTION AND EPIDEMIOLOGY

Ewing sarcoma (ES) is the second most common primary malignant bone cancer in children and young adults, following osteosarcoma. The annual incidence of ES in the population younger than 20 years is approximately 2.9 per million.[1] It is slightly more common in males (1.2:1 male:female). Cases continue to be diagnosed through the third decade and later, with a decreasing incidence compared with the second decade. The oldest patient reported to date was 86 years old.[2] The most unusual feature of the epidemiology of ES is its predilection for Caucasians, in whom it is more frequent than among Asians, and six times more frequent than among Africans. This epidemiology is reproduced in sub-Saharan Africa, where rates of osteosarcoma and ES are similar to those seen in North American people of African ancestry. A partial explanation has been proposed: intron 6, near the translocation breakpoint region of *EWSR1* (see also "Biology"), is at least 50% smaller, because there are fewer Alu elements (interspersed repeat sequences) in approximately 8% of alleles in the African population.[3] Alu elements may be preferential sites of gene recombination in cancer.[4] The presence of a shorter sequence of such elements at the breakpoint region could account for a small fraction of the difference in incidence and suggests that further investigation of the details of the genetic structure of the breakpoint region and its associated polymorphisms may yield further clues. Epidemiologic studies have found associations between a history of hernia and paternal occupation and risk of developing ES.[5,6]

NOMENCLATURE

Classical ES of bone, extraskeletal ES, Askin tumor of the thoracic wall, and peripheral primitive neuroectodermal tumor (pPNET), also known as *peripheral neuroepithelioma*, are highly aggressive, poorly differentiated neoplasms with unknown histogenesis. For this group, the unifying terms *Ewing family of tumors* (EFT), *Ewing tumors* (ET), and *Ewing's sarcoma family of tumors* (ESFT) have been coined after molecular evidence was obtained for shared immunologic and genetic traits (see later).[7] The World Health Organization classification uses Ewing's sarcoma/primitive neuroectodermal tumor (ES/PNET) as an inclusive term.[8] For simplicity and reflecting the most common use currently, ES will be used throughout this chapter. The nomenclature referring to the translocation product (see "Biology" section, later) can be confusing at times, with a variety of similar, but nonidentical, terms used. Based on standard human gene nomenclature guidelines provided by the Human Genome Organization Gene Nomenclature Committee (HGNC), human gene symbols are capitalized and italicized, while protein names are capitalized in standard fonts. The officially recognized gene

name for the chromosome 22 translocation partner is *EWSR1*, indicating the ES Breakpoint Region 1.[9,10] The *EWSR1* gene encodes the EWSR1 protein, although most investigators refer to the protein product by its alias EWS. The officially recognized gene name for the chromosome 11 partner is *FLI1*, so named because of its homology to the murine Friend Leukemia Virus integration site 3.[11] The *FLI1* gene encodes the FLI1 protein (sometimes simply called FLI). It is incorrect to refer to the human proteins as Ews or Fli, as such a combination of capital and lowercase letters is reserved for murine proteins. This chapter refers to the gene fusion as *EWSR1-FLI1*, following the HGNC guidelines. However, given the most common usage in the literature, this chapter refers to the protein fusion as EWS-FLI1, recognizing that the literature contains many similar alternates, such as EWSR1-FLI1, EWS-FLI, EWSR1/FLI1, EWS/FLI, etc.

BIOLOGY

Genetic Definition

In comparison with osteosarcoma, ES is characterized by a relatively simple karyotype with only a few numerical and structural aberrations. Most consistently, a reciprocal chromosomal translocation between chromosomes 11 and 22, the t(11;22)(q24;q12), is present in about 85% of these tumors[12,13] and is therefore considered pathognomonic for the disease. Additional structural changes affect chromosomes 1 and 16 in about 20% of tumors, most frequently leading to a gain of 1q and a loss of 16q or the formation of a derivative chromosome der(1;16).[14,15] Among numerical chromosome changes, trisomy 8 and/or 12 is observed in half and one-third of cases, respectively.[15,16] These secondary abnormalities are present in primary tumors and a substantial number of widely used cell lines.[17] Deletion of the chromosomal region 9p21 housing the *ink4A* gene, which has been shown to be homozygously lost in about 25% of ES, remains cytogenetically cryptic in most patients.[18-20] Microarray-based approaches are beginning to define other cytogenetically cryptic abnormalities, but the consequences of these have yet to be defined.[21]

The best studied of the cytogenetic aberrations in ES is the t(11;22)(q24;q12).[9,10] The rearrangement results in the translocation of the 3′ portion of the *FLI1* (Friend leukemia virus integration site 1) gene from chromosome 11 to the 5′ portion of the ES breakpoint region gene *EWSR1* (encoding the EWS protein) on chromosome 22 (Fig. 33.1). As a result, a chimeric EWS-FLI1 RNA is expressed from the promoter of the rearranged *EWSR1* gene encoding for a novel fusion protein. The reciprocal translocation product *FLI1-EWSR1* is not expressed and is occasionally lost from ES cells. Using reverse transcriptase-polymerase chain reaction (RT-PCR) and fluorescence *in situ* hybridization (FISH), the presence of the t(11;22)(q24;q12) is confirmed in 85% of ES and correlates

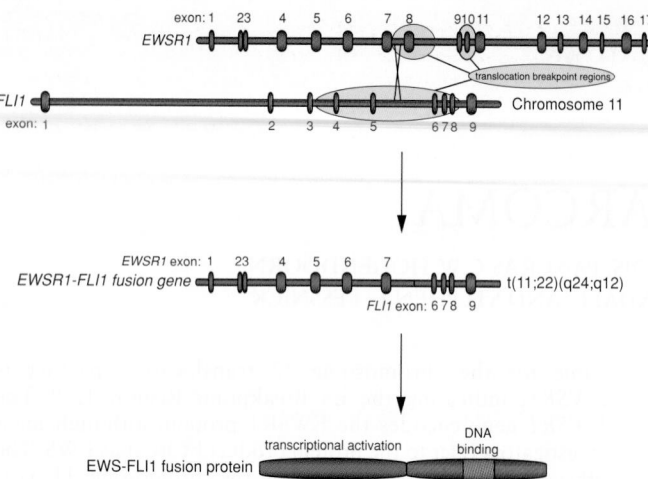

FIGURE 33.1 The reciprocal translocation between chromosomes 11 and 22 results in the formation of an *EWSR1-FLI1* fusion gene on the abnormal chromosome 22 that codes for a chimeric transcription factor with the N-terminal transcriptional regulatory domain deriving from EWS and the ETS specific DNA-binding domain derived from FLI1.

with high expression of the cell surface sialoglycoprotein CD99.[22–25] Experimental studies in model systems suggested that CD99 may be directly regulated by EWS-FLI1.[26,27]

About 15% of histopathologically defined CD99-positive ES lack the classical ES specific translocation. However, in the majority of these cases, evidence for *EWSR1* gene rearrangements can be obtained using probes flanking the ES breakpoint region on chromosome 22 in FISH analyses.[28] Molecular cloning identified the *FLI1*-related genes *ERG* on chromosome 21q22 in 10% of ES,[29,30] and *ETV1* on chromo-

some 7p22,[31] *E1AF* (*PEA3/ETV4*) on chromosome 17q12,[32] and *FEV*[33] on chromosome 2q33 in less than 1% of cases each as alternative *EWSR1* fusion partners in ES (Table 33.1). Common to all *EWSR1* fusion partners in ES is that they encode for members of the ETS transcription factor family that share a common DNA-binding domain structure, whereas rearrangements of the *EWSR1* gene with unrelated transcription factor genes are associated with other neoplasms[34] (Table 33.1). Although the *EWSR1* and the *FLI1* genes are oriented in the same direction on the long arms of

TABLE 33.1

CHROMOSOMAL TRANSLOCATIONS INVOLVING THE *EWSR1* GENE, OR THE RELATED *FUS* OR *TAF15* GENES

Tumor type	Translocation	Fusion gene
Ewing sarcoma	t(11;22)(q24;q12)	*EWSR1/FLI1*
	t(21;22)(q22;q12)	*EWSR1/ERG*
	t(7;22)(p22;q12)	*EWSR1/ETV1*
	t(17;22)(q12;q12)	*EWSR1/ETV4*
	t(2;22)(q35;q12)	*EWSR1/FEV*
	t(16;21)(p11;q22)	*FUS/ERG*
	t(2;16)(q35;p11)	*FUS/FEV*
Clear cell sarcoma	t(12;22)(q13;q12)	*EWSR1/ATF1*
Desmoplastic small round cell tumor	t(11;22)(p13;q12)	*EWSR1/WT1*
Extraskeletal myxoid chondrosarcoma	t(9;22)(q22;q12)	*EWSR1/NR4A3*
	t(9;17)(q22;q11)	*TAF15/NR4A3*
	t(9;15)(q22;q21)	*TCF12/NR4A3*
Myxoid liposarcoma	t(12;16)(q13;p11)	*FUS/DDIT3*
	t(12;22)(q13;q12)	*EWSR1/DDIT3*
Small round cell or undifferentiated sarcomas	t(1;22)(p36.1;q12)	*EWSR1/ZNF278*
	t(6;22)(p21;q12)	*EWSR1/POU5F1*
	t(2;22)(q31;q12)	*EWSR1/SP3*
	Ring chromosome containing portions of chromosomes 20 and 22	*EWSR1/NFATc2*
Angiomatoid fibrous histiocytoma	t(12;16)(q13;p11)	*FUS/ATF1*
Low grade fibromyxoid sarcoma	t(7;16)(q33;p11)	*FUS/CREB3L2*
Acute myelogenous leukemia	t(16;21)(p11;q22)	*FUS/ERG*
Acute myelogenous, lymphoblastic, or undifferentiated leukemia	t(12;22)(p13;q12)	*EWSR1/ZNF384*
	t(12;17)(p13;q11)	*TAF15/ZNF384*

chromosomes 22 and 11 allowing for simple translocation, *ERG* is oriented in the opposite direction on chromosome 21q. Thus, the cytogenetic equivalent of the *EWSR1-ERG* gene fusion is not always easily discernible and frequently involves interstitial translocations or complex rearrangements including more than two chromosomes.[35] Altogether, rearrangements of *EWSR1* with *FLI1*- or a *FLI1*-related gene characterize 98% of all ES. Additional reports have described fusions between *FUS (TLS)* and either *ERG* or *FEV* in ES as well.[36,37] FUS is highly related to EWS, and, along with TAF15 (TAF$_{II}$68/RPB56/TAF2N), encompasses the TET (FUS, EWS, TAF15) family of proteins that are involved in a variety of chromosomal rearrangements in malignancies (Table 33.1).

Taken together, "TET-ETS" fusions are present in nearly all cases of ES. Recent reports have described non-ETS fusions in small round cell tumors with histologic similarities to ES, such as EWS-ZNF278, EWS-POU5F1, EWS-SP3, and EWS-NFATc2.[38–42] It is unclear whether these tumors should be considered ES, based on morphology, or simply "small round cell" or "undifferentiated" sarcomas because of the lack of a TET-ETS fusion. The identification of such rare variants confounds the interpretation of a negative molecular genetic test for ES. Whether tumors harboring non–TET-ETS fusions respond adequately to standard ES therapies is also not known.

ES is currently defined by the presence of TET-ETS gene rearrangements and, as a surrogate marker, by high CD99 expression levels. Individual members of this tumor family are defined along a gradient of limited neuroglial differentiation with the poorly differentiated ES at one end and the more mature peripheral PNETs at the other. With the availability of molecular tools to unambiguously confirm the presence of TET-ETS gene rearrangements, the spectrum of ES-related neoplasms has recently been expanded to include rare CD99-positive extraskeletal tumors in various anatomic sites including kidney,[43–46] breast,[44] lung,[47] gastrointestinal tract,[48–51] prostate,[52] endometrium,[53] adrenal gland,[54] and meninges.[55]

Molecular Pathogenesis

Gene rearrangements of *EWSR1-ETS* and, rarely, *FUS-ETS* are thus pathognomonic of ES. The chimeric gene product is, therefore, likely crucial to malignant transformation in ES. The mechanisms of chromosomal translocation involving illegitimate recombination and genomic breakpoint structures do not explain the etiology of gene rearrangement.[55] Although the majority of *EWSR1-FLI1* gene rearrangements result in the production of chimeric proteins with the EWS amino terminus fused to the carboxy terminal protein portion of FLI1, about one-third of gene rearrangements in ES involve breakpoints in *EWSR1* exon 8 or intron 8 leading to out-of-frame fusions with *FLI1*. In these cases, the reading frame is always restored, primarily by splicing out of exon 8, resulting in consistent expression of a functional full-length fusion protein in the tumors.[30,56] This finding represents, perhaps, the best evidence for an essential role of EWS-ETS fusion proteins not only in the generation but also in the maintenance of the tumor. It is supported by two lines of experimental data: (a) EWS-FLI1 and related fusion proteins transform NIH3T3 (an immortalized murine fibroblast cell line) *in vitro* rendering it tumorigenic in nude mice[57–59] and (b) EWS-FLI1 antagonists (antisense RNA, antisense oligonucleotides, dominant negative constructs, small inhibitory RNA) block ES cell growth *in vitro* and tumor formation in mice.[34,60–67]

The phenotype of tumors obtained in immunodeficient mice after transplantation of EWS-ETS transformed NIH3T3 cells clearly differed from that obtained after transformation with other EWS transcription factor fusions, and resembled that of human ES with partial neural differentiation.[68,69] In this model, EWS and its close relatives FUS and TAF15 were functionally interchangeable, and the transcription factor moiety determined the tumor phenotype. This finding is also reflected by the structure of fusion genes observed in human tumors with both *EWSR1-CHOP* and *FUS-CHOP* characterizing myxoid liposarcoma, and with *EWSR1-TEC/CHN* and *TAF15-TEC/CHN* found in extraskeletal myxoid chondrosarcoma. In this respect, *FUS-ERG* appears to be somehow promiscuous, being present in both a small number of acute myeloid leukemias and a small number of ES.

The minimal transforming protein portion involves at least the first 82 amino acids of EWS (encoded by the first four exons) and the DNA-binding domain of the ETS partner (in *FLI1* encoded by the last exon, exon 9). For full transformation potential, however, *EWSR1* exons 1 to 7 and, in *EWSR1-FLI1* fusions, inclusion of the very C-terminal domain of FLI1 are required.[57,58,70] In fact, despite significant variation in the architecture of chimeric EWS-ETS RNAs in ES, *EWSR1* exons 1 to 7 and the DNA-binding domain encoding exons of the *ETS* fusion partner are always present in the translocation products of ES.[9,30] In *EWS-FLI1* fusions, *FLI1* exon 8, encoding for a highly conserved protein domain of unknown function, is also included in tumor-derived chimeric RNA. The most frequent gene fusions in ES join *EWSR1* exon 7 to *FLI1* exon 6 (type 1) or exon 5 (type 2) in 51% and 27% of cases, respectively.[71]

The region encoded by the EWS portion of the fusion proteins is composed of 31 repeats of a degenerate hexapeptide motif containing a critical tyrosine residue which, when combined with a DNA-binding domain, act as a potent transcriptional activation domain.[57,72,73] Transcriptional activation may be related to the normal function of germline EWS that, like its close relatives FUS and TAF15, has been found associated with the RNA polymerase II complex and to interact with several RNA processing proteins, possibly building a bridge between RNA transcription and maturation.[74–80] EWS- and FUS-transcription factor fusion proteins not only retain some of these interactions but also gain the ability to communicate with additional components of the RNA processing machinery and to interfere with normal RNA splicing at least in *in vitro* assays.[76,79–82] Thus, tumor-derived fusion proteins between EWS (or FUS) and the DNA-binding domain of a transcription factor are considered to exert much of their oncogenic activity via inappropriate activation of target genes. However, gene expression profiling studies in model systems revealed an almost equal number of genes suppressed as activated in response to ectopic EWS-FLI1 expression.[26,27,67,70,83–85] The first gene confirmed as a direct target of EWS-ETS fusions in ES, *TGFBR2*, is suppressed by these oncoproteins[86,87] although the mechanism of repression remains elusive. Data in NIH3T3 murine cells suggested that DNA binding is not absolutely required for EWS-FLIs oncogenic function, suggesting that transcription-independent functions may also contribute to the oncogenic properties of the chimeric fusion proteins, but this has not been validated in human-based systems.[88,89] The oncogenic function of EWS-ETS fusion proteins is not dependent on the presence of germline EWS, which is usually coexpressed from the second non–rearranged allele in ES.[90]

By whichever mechanism, expression of TET-ETS fusion genes leads to profound context specific changes of the transcriptome and eventually to distinct cell-type–dependent physiologic outcomes. For example, EWS-FLI1 induces cell death in primary mouse fibroblasts, which may either be rescued by loss of *p53* or *ink4A* gene function or a p53-dependent cell cycle arrest in immortalized human fibroblasts.[26,91] Pluripotent mesenchymal stromal cells are blocked from further differentiation by ectopic EWS-FLI1 expression,[92,93] whereas transdifferentiation is observed in human neuroblastoma and rhabdomyosarcoma cell lines.[27,84] In contrast, established fibroblast cell lines are either transformed or remain unchanged in response to EWS-FLI1.[57,58,91,94] More recently, model systems based on patient-derived ES cell lines have been used to investigate EWS-FLI1 function in its native cellular context.[66] The gross changes in gene expression profiles induced by ectopic expression of EWS-ETS proteins in model systems and by EWS-ETS antagonists in ES cells suggest that malignant conversion of the ES precursor cell is the result of changes in the activity of a multitude of EWS-ETS downstream genes rather than of single genes. Some of the best-validated candidates include the upregulated genes *NKX2.2* and *NR0B1*, and the repressed genes *IGFBP3* and *TGF-BRII*.[66,67,85,86] In some cases, linkages to known molecular pathways important for oncogenesis are apparent (such as modulation of insulin-like growth factor and transforming growth factor signaling), but in other cases, novel oncogenic pathways appear to be involved.

The difference in fate of primary and immortalized cells ectopically expressing EWS-FLI1, cell death or survival with an altered or blocked differentiation program and transformation, suggests the presence of a second mutational event in ES. Although in experimental systems abrogation of the p53 pathway by either *p53* mutation or *INK4A* deletion cooperates with EWS-FLI1 in transformation by stabilizing EWS-FLI1 expression,[91] these aberrations are relatively rare in ES, occurring with a frequency of less than 10% and about 25%, respectively.[18,19,95,96] The p53-dependent DNA damage response pathway has been shown to be largely intact in ES.[97,98] The p53 protein also plays a role as a guardian against oncogenic stress, and induction of cell death by ectopic EWS-FLI1 expression in primary fibroblasts may reflect this function. It therefore remains to be demonstrated why most ES tolerate EWS-ETS oncogene expression in the presence of wild-type p53. Inhibition of NOTCH signaling may be involved[99] or alternately autocrine growth factor loops may be involved, such as the insulin-like growth factor receptor 1 (IGF1R) circuit. Transformation of rodent fibroblasts by EWS-FLI1 has been demonstrated to require IGF1R expression[100]; EWS-FLI1 inhibits expression of IGFBP3,[66] which increases IGF1R signaling; and inhibition of IGF1R interferes with ES growth in nude mice.[101-103] An additional candidate that may affect the EWS-FLI1 pathway is the basic fibroblast growth factor circuit.[104] The possible roles of other autocrine and paracrine growth factor pathways that have been found to be active in ES, including platelet-derived growth factor beta, gastrin releasing peptide, and stem cell factor,[105-107] remain unknown.

Histogenesis

The histogenesis of ES has been a matter of controversy ever since the first description of ES as a diffuse endothelioma of bone by James Ewing in 1921[108] and has subsequently been ascribed to endothelial, mesenchymal, and hematopoietic stem cells based on ultrastructural features.[105-113] Further immunocytochemical and molecular studies and *in vitro* differentiation of ES cell lines using agents such as retinoic acid and dibutyryl adenosine cyclic monophosphate provided evidence for the neural differentiation potential of ES. This was interpreted as an argument for a descent from neural crest tissue.[100,107,112-120] Comparative gene expression profiling studies support this view and reveal a unique signature that clearly distinguishes ES from other small round cell tumors.[121] Because of the ability to synthesize choline acetyltransferase and the lack of appreciable synthesis of adrenergic pathway precursors, ES could be derive

from postganglionic parasympathetic primordial cells located throughout the parasympathetic autonomic nervous system. However, the observation that EWS-FLI1 expression in murine fibroblasts imposes a partial neural phenotype on the transformed cells and that introduction of the fusion protein into human neuroblastoma cells switches the adrenergic phenotype of ES to the cholinergic pattern of ES suggest a role for the chromosomal translocation in determining the pattern of differentiation marker expression in this disease.[27,68] EWS-ETS fusion proteins are transcription factors that probably bind to the same sequence motifs in the human genome as those recognized by their normal ETS counterparts. It is therefore possible that ES at least partially recapitulates the phenotype of tissues that express either FLI1 or ERG during normal development, such as hematopoietic tissues, endothelial cells, and neural crest cells.[122-125]

A recent hypothesis regarding the histogenesis of ES is that it might arise from mesenchymal stem cells.[126] Mesenchymal stem cells can be found in the bone-marrow–derived stromal cell compartment and have the ability to differentiate into multiple distinct lineages, including bone, cartilage, and fat cells. Initial studies demonstrated that expression of EWS-FLI1 in either murine bone-marrow–derived stromal cells, or in myoblasts, blocked those cells' ability to differentiate in tissue culture.[92,93] Subsequent studies found that inhibition of EWS-FLI1 expression in patient-derived ES cell lines caused those cells to adopt a mesenchymal stem cell phenotype.[127] This phenotype included a gene expression pattern that was similar to normal mesenchymal stem cells, the expression of characteristic mesenchymal stem cell surface markers, and the ability to differentiate into adipogenic, chondrogenic, and osteogenic lineages. Attempts to model ES through the introduction of EWS-FLI1 into human fibroblasts or mesenchymal stem cells have recapitulated the gene expression pattern of bona fide ES but have not resulted in oncogenic transformation, suggesting that additional events are required for this process.[26,128] Ultimately, the final proof of the long sought after ES cell of origin may have to await the development of animal models to test these hypotheses explicitly.

Biologic Determinants of Prognosis

At diagnosis, patients with ES either present with localized disease or clinically overt metastases. In the prechemotherapy era when local measures (surgery or radiation) were the only modes of therapy, more than 90% of patients died from tumor dissemination regardless of their stage at presentation.[129] With current multimodal treatment regimens, however, more than two-thirds of patients with localized disease can be cured. Survival rates of patients with metastatic disease remain very poor despite modern multi-modal therapy.

The availability of a unique and highly specific tumor marker, the *EWSR1-ETS* gene rearrangement, allows for high sensitivity tumor cell detection in tissues and body fluids by molecular techniques. The most widely used method is RT-PCR that uses short nucleotide sequences from the minimal regions present in all EWS-ETS chimeric products flanking the fusion point and a thermo-resistant DNA polymerase to specifically amplify the chimeric product from RNA, which has been reverse-transcribed into complementary DNA. The method allows for the detection of one tumor cell in a million normal cells and has therefore been used to screen peripheral blood and bone marrow of ES patients at diagnosis. Retrospective studies suggest that RT-PCR positivity of bone marrow may in fact be of prognostic relevance not only in patients with overt metastases but also in those with localized disease.[130-132] However, this finding has not yet been confirmed prospectively. In addition, the RT-PCR studies performed to date have revealed a number of critical technical issues and potential pitfalls. These include, most prominently, the mobilization of tumor cells into the blood during surgery; false positivity due to contamination problems; and false negativity due to inappropriate sampling, shipment, or storage of the tissue.[133] State-of-the-art prospective RT-PCR studies to uncover minimal disseminated disease in ES therefore have to consider the time of sampling (before biopsy); the site of sampling (to exclude false-positive bone-marrow results in patients with pelvic tumors due to sampling close to the involved site); and include controls for RNA and complementary DNA quality and sensitivity, specificity, and quality of the PCR reaction.

Among cytogenetic aberrations frequently accompanying the tumor-specific translocation of chromosome 22, controversial results have been obtained in terms of the potential prognostic impact of the gain of chromosomes 8 and 12.[14,15,47] Gain of 1q and loss of 16q have recently been described as associated with adverse outcome.[15] Patients with more complex karyotypes or with hyperdiploidy exceeding 50 chromosomes may have a worse outcome.[21,134] This may also be true for loss of 1p, which is associated with poor prognosis in neuroblastoma, in which it occurs at a much higher rate than in ES.[15] Among aberrations commonly associated with many cancers, aneuploidy, TP53 mutation (encoding p53 protein), INK4A gene deletion (encoding the p16 and ARF proteins), and telomerase expression have been described as unfavorable prognostic markers in ES, whereas P-glycoprotein expression has been found to be of no significance for the course of the disease.[19,135–139] All of these factors were evaluated in relatively low numbers of patients and none of these putative markers of prognosis has so far been evaluated prospectively. The same is true for a suggested impact of EWS-ETS RNA fusion type (exon composition) on outcome in patients with localized disease.[71,140]

Each of the cited studies assumed that single genetic or molecular markers may be sufficient to discriminate between different courses of disease. Genome-wide screening approaches allowing for hypothesis-free assessment of gene expression profiles are under way and are likely to result in the identification of characteristic patterns associated with distinct tumor biology.[141,142] From these studies, it can be expected that a small number of genes will be identified, whose expression correlates with the clinical course of the disease and which will eventually lead to a biology and risk-adopted stratification of patients for therapy.

Additional clinical variables have also been evaluated for possible prognostic impact. Histologic evaluation of response to neoadjuvant chemotherapy is a prognostic factor in ES, although applicable only to patients who undergo surgical resection after neoadjuvant chemotherapy.[143–147] Response to chemotherapy can also be assessed by magnetic resonance imaging (MRI).[148–150] Recent evidence suggests that fluorine-18 fluorodeoxyglucose positron emission tomography (FDG-PET) may provide a useful tool for monitoring response to therapy and outcome.[151]

Targeted Therapy

ES usually respond very well to chemotherapy and radiotherapy (RT). In addition, the bulky localized primary tumor mass is often surgically resectable. However, it was the introduction of systemic therapy that improved the survival rate of patients from less than 10% to approximately 60%, indicating that, to be potentially successful, tumor therapy has to target disseminated tumor cells. For high-risk patients, further intensification of therapy, including high-dose myeloablative chemotherapy

regimens with stem cell rescue, has not clearly improved outcome. Investigation of its role, particularly in patients with initially isolated pulmonary metastatic disease, continues. In addition, high-dose therapy is toxic and carries with it a high likelihood of life-threatening complications. Great hope and increasing efforts are consequently laid on the identification of tumor-specific therapeutic targets.

The ideal tumor-specific target would be the EWS-ETS fusion protein or critical gene products regulated by the fusion protein. Experimentally, proof of principle has been obtained by both antisense and RNA interference studies that demonstrated that modulation of EWS-FLI1 expression results in growth inhibition of ES in vitro and in vivo.[34,60–65] The clinical use of antisense RNA oligonucleotides or small inhibitory RNAs is impeded by the difficulty of efficiently delivering nucleic acids into disseminated tumor cells. One possible method to achieve this goal may be the inclusion of oligonucleotides (stabilized as phosphorothioates) into nanocapsules or nanospheres. This approach has been successfully applied to stop ES growth in xenotransplanted nude mice.[61,152,153] Another approach has been to identify available drugs, which may directly or indirectly modulate the expression of EWS-FLI1. One group performed a high-throughput screen and demonstrated that cytarabine downregulates the expression of EWS-FLI1.[153] This preclinical finding did not result in meaningful clinical activity in a phase II study of cytarabine in patients with refractory ES.[154]

CD99 may represent another promising candidate for targeted therapy in ES. Although neither a ligand for CD99 nor the mechanisms by which this antigen is involved in ES are known, in vitro studies on cell lines demonstrated that CD99 binding and silencing by specific antibodies induces rapid tumor cell death, enhanced by combination with conventional chemotherapeutic drugs. In vivo studies have been restricted to athymic mice subcutaneously xenografted with an ES cell line and indicated reduced ES growth on anti-CD99 treatment.[155] However, there is no direct homolog of CD99 in mice and thus toxicity of anti-CD99 treatment cannot be assessed in this model. Because of high-level expression of CD99 in hematopoietic stem cells, endothelial cells, and several cell types in the gonads and the pancreas in humans, clinical trials using anti-CD99 antibodies remain untested.

Tumor necrosis factor (TNF)–related apoptosis inducing ligand (TRAIL/Apo-2L) is a typical member of the TNF ligand family that induces apoptosis through activating death receptors. In recent years, considerable attention has been focused on the potential benefits of TRAIL in cancer therapy, because the majority of cancer cells are sensitive to TRAIL-induced apoptosis and most normal cells are TRAIL resistant.[156,157] This is particularly true for ES. Several in vitro studies suggest that ES may represent an ideal target for TRAIL therapy.[158–160] Furthermore, the use of TRAIL in combination with chemotherapeutic agents or irradiation strengthens its apoptotic effects.[156,157] Because apoptotic responsiveness to TRAIL is dependent on caspase-8 expression, which is frequently modulated in cancer by gene silencing, interferon gamma and demethylating agents may further improve ES sensitivity to TRAIL.[161,162]

BCL-2 is an important component of the mitochondrial pathway leading to apoptosis, the programmed cell death that is often disrupted in malignant disease.[163] BCL-2 may be overexpressed in ES cells, furthering the malignant process and engendering resistance to chemotherapy. Immunoperoxidase staining of tumor specimens from patients with localized ES showed a high percentage (>60%) of positive cells in 28 out of 41 tumors (68%). Interestingly, a trend to higher overall ($p = 0.16$) and event-free ($p = 0.09$) survival of ES patients with low levels of BCL-2 expression was observed, although the differences were not statistically significance.[164]

Angiogenesis, the formation of new blood vessels, is crucial to the progression of malignant disease, because otherwise the tumor would rapidly outgrow its nutrient supply.[165] A striking feature of ES is the presence of large blood lakes which are lined by tumour cells. It has been hypothesized that the tumor cell plasticity under hypoxic conditions contributes to this striking phenomenon.[166] The vascular endothelial growth factor (VEGF) pathway may be particularly important in cancer.[167] The EWS-ETS oncoprotein has been shown in an *in vitro* construct to activate the VEGF promoter, both directly and through an interaction with the transcription factor Sp1.[168] Seventeen of 31 ES tissue samples were immunostain positive for VEGF, and the 17 patients whose tumors expressed VEGF had an inferior outcome when compared with the 14 whose tumors were negative ($p = 0.0047$).[168] Similarly, serum VEGF was elevated in a small series of patients with ES at the time of initial diagnosis.[169] The endogenous antiangiogenic peptide, thrombospondin, is downregulated in ES.[170] Antiangiogenic therapies may be of interest as a targeted therapy of ES.

Recent attention has focused on the IGF1R pathway as a therapeutic target in ES since agents targeting this pathway have recently become available (see later). Several lines of evidence indicate that targeting IGF1R will be an effective strategy in the treatment of this disease. All but one ES cell line evaluated in two early studies demonstrated expression of both IGF1 and IGF1R.[101,171] Several studies have demonstrated that neutralizing antibodies against the IGF1R inhibit the growth of multiple ES cell lines.[101,103,171,172] These findings have also been observed in ES mouse xenografts.[102,103] Other *in vitro* studies have also demonstrated that treatment with an IGF1R monoclonal antibody markedly increases the sensitivity of ES cells to chemotherapy.[173]

CLINICAL PRESENTATION AND STAGING

Signs and Symptoms

ES can arise in almost every age group, but more than half of the patients are adolescents, the median age being 15 years (Fig. 33.2). Locoregional pain is the most common presenting symptom in patients with ES. Pain can be intermittent and may be less severe at night. However, pain often does not completely disappear during the night.[174] Because the majority of ES patients are in their second decade of life and physically active, pain is often mistaken for "bone growth" or injuries resulting from sports or everyday activities. Pain may be accompanied by paresthesia in some cases. Pain as the initial symptom may be followed by a palpable mass. The duration of symptoms prior to the definitive diagnosis can be weeks to months, or rarely even years, with a median of 3 to 9 months.[174–176] The delay between the first medical visit and the establishment of the definitive diagnosis in a Swedish cancer registry study was significantly longer for patients with ES than for those with osteosarcoma.[174] In more than two-thirds of patients, thorough physical examination will reveal reproducible pathologic findings, such as tenderness at the tumor location or a palpable mass, which should prompt further investigations. Tendinitis, hip inflammation, and osteomyelitis are common initial diagnoses. Pain without defined trauma adequate to explain the symptoms, pain lasting longer than a month, continuing at night, or with any other unusual features therefore should prompt early imaging studies. Slight or moderate fever and other nonspecific symptoms are more common in more advanced and/or metastatic stages, affecting about one-third of patients.[174–177]

Tumor growth will eventually lead to a visible or palpable swelling of the affected site. The tumor bulk, however, may be indiscernible for a long time in patients with pelvic, chest wall, or femoral tumors. As ES may arise in virtually any bone and from soft tissue, additional symptoms depending on the affected site may vary considerably. Spinal cord compression by tumors of the vertebral compartment requires emergency laminectomy, whereas patients with chest wall or pelvic primaries may experience significant complaints with locally advanced disease.

Laboratory Findings

No blood, serum, or urine test can specifically identify ES. Nonspecific signs of tumor or inflammation may be noted, such as an elevated erythrocyte sedimentation rate, moderate anemia, or leukocytosis. Elevated levels of serum lactate dehydrogenase correlate with tumor burden and for this reason with inferior outcome. In contrast to neuroblastoma, serum and urine catecholamine levels are always normal.

Tumor Sites

Most ES occur in bones. In contrast to osteosarcoma, flat bones of the axial skeleton are more commonly affected, and in long bones, ES (unlike osteosarcoma) tends to arise from the diaphyseal rather than the metaphyseal portion. The most

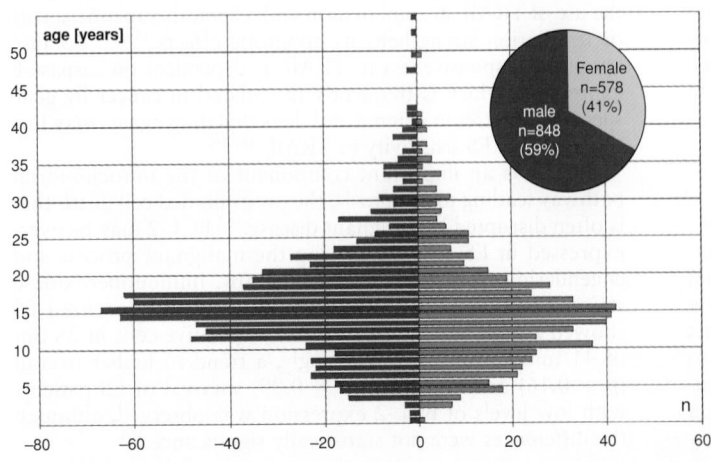

FIGURE 33.2 Age and gender of Ewing sarcoma patients. Data based on 1,426 patients from the European Intergroup Cooperative Ewing Sarcoma Studies (EI-CESS).

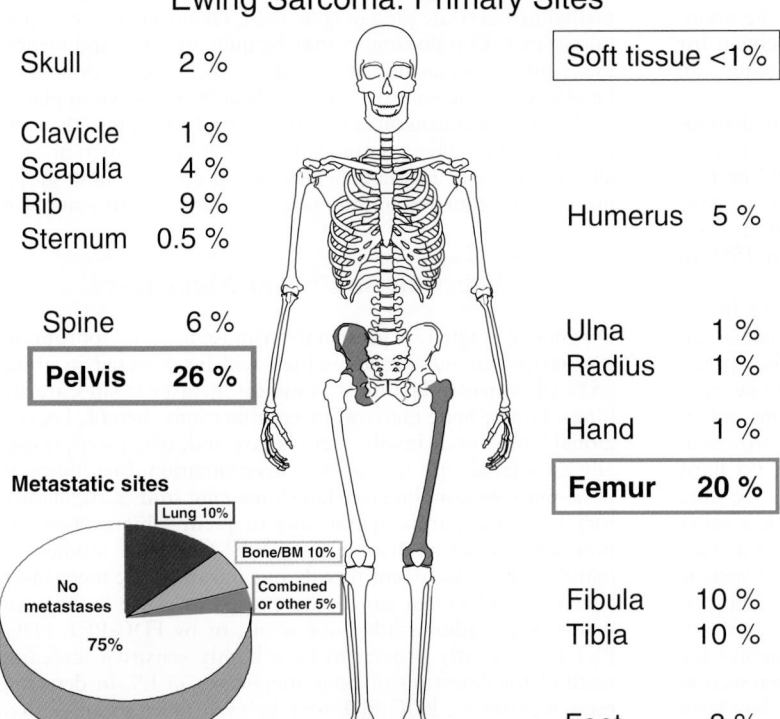

Ewing Sarcoma: Primary Sites

Skull	2 %
Clavicle	1 %
Scapula	4 %
Rib	9 %
Sternum	0.5 %
Spine	6 %
Pelvis	**26 %**

Soft tissue <1%

Humerus	5 %
Ulna	1 %
Radius	1 %
Hand	1 %
Femur	**20 %**
Fibula	10 %
Tibia	10 %
Foot	3 %

Metastatic sites

Lung 10%
Bone/BM 10%
Combined or other 5%
No metastases 75%

FIGURE 33.3 Primary tumor and metastatic sites in Ewing sarcoma. Data based on 1,426 patients from European Intergroup Cooperative Ewing Sarcoma Studies (EI-CESS) trials.

common sites of primary ES are the pelvic bones, the long bones of the lower extremities, and the bones of the chest wall (Fig. 33.3). Metastases in lungs, bone, bone marrow, or combinations thereof are detectable in about 25% of patients, with lung the most common site. Metastases to lymph nodes, liver, or central nervous system are rare.

Imaging Studies

The initial imaging investigation when an osseous lesion is suspected is usually a radiograph in two planes. Tumor-related osteolysis, detachment of the periosteum from the bone (Codman triangle), and spicula of calcification in soft tissue tumor masses may suggest the diagnosis of a malignant bone tumor. Diaphyseal location suggests an ES. The exact locoregional extent of the primary tumor requires assessment with MRI or computed tomography (CT). Although CT scans are of value to define cortical bone lesions, MRI investigations are superior to CT in revealing the relation to adjacent structures such as nerves or vessels and in more precisely delineating the intramedullary extension of bone lesions.[174,178–181] Precise documentation of the site and size of the primary tumor and its relation to relevant adjacent structures is of paramount importance to monitor response to initial treatment, as well as to plan local therapy.[182,183]

Biopsy Approaches

The initial surgical procedure for any bone tumor is the biopsy. Two types of biopsies are possible: incisional and excisional. Incisional biopsies include needle (closed) and open biopsies. Needle biopsies can be either fine needle or core. The type of biopsy must be carefully chosen after evaluating the size and location of the tumor, the differential diagnosis, and the age of the patient. The placement of the biopsy site relative to the location of the tumor and the anatomic structures of the patient is also of critical importance.

In general, if a malignant bone tumor such as ES is suspected, an excisional biopsy is rarely, if ever, utilized. Malignant tumors are often large at presentation, and neoadjuvant therapy is usually appropriate prior to definitive resection. Most bone tumors of uncertain biologic potential, where there is a significant suspicion for malignancy, are biopsied via an incisional approach. The location of the biopsy site is determined by a thorough prebiopsy assessment of the extent of local disease and its relationship to critical structures such as the neurovascular bundle. This must be determined on a case-by-case basis. It is strongly recommended that the biopsy be performed by the surgeon who will be performing the definitive resection so that the biopsy tract can be ellipsed within the planned surgical incision.[184] At the time of biopsy, the surgeon must be familiar with orthopedic oncologic principles, such as flap development and coverage when limb salvage is the proposed plan for definitive tumor resection. Needle (closed) biopsies can potentially expedite the diagnostic process when performed on an outpatient basis in an ambulatory setting. This can often be conducted using a local anesthetic. Most malignant bone tumors have a soft tissue component on their periphery. Conveniently, this is also the most representative tissue. Accordingly, deep deployment of the needle within the tumor is unnecessary and likely to lead to problems such as deep contamination and bleeding. Again, the needle biopsy site should be carefully planned so that it may be excised at time of resection. With a well-trained cytopathologist, fine needle biopsy is an option. A 0.7-mm diameter needle is generally used. Up to 90% diagnostic accuracy has been reported in general,[185] with the accuracy in cases of bone sarcoma exceeding 80%.[186] The drawback is that insufficient material may be obtained to perform cytogenetics, FISH, flow cytometry, gene profiling, and other tests that may help to establish the diagnosis.

Core biopsies are minimally invasive, can be performed under local anesthesia when appropriate, maintain the architecture of the tissue, and can obtain adequate specimen for advanced studies. Diagnostic accuracy for this technique can surpass 95%.[187]

Although needle biopsies are intended to facilitate diagnosis, they can also lead to a delay due to indeterminate results. Because no specific diagnosis of a malignancy should be rendered on a frozen analysis, the patient must wait several days until the results are finalized, particularly if special studies are necessary. An indeterminate needle biopsy occurs in 25% to 33% of cases even at experienced centers.[188]

An open incisional biopsy can potentially be done in the outpatient setting. However, for suspected bone malignancies, it is usually recommended that they be performed in the operating room and is the preferred method in children. In general, longitudinal incisions are the rule. Transverse incisions potentially contaminate flap planes and can compromise neurovascular structures. During the approach to the tumor, no flaps should be developed, to minimize contamination. The area where the tumor is most superficial is preferable unless other factors, such as an overlying vessel or nerve, preclude it. Furthermore, the preoperative imaging may suggest that a specific area within the tumor may be more diagnostic than another. Areas of extensive necrosis and/or hemorrhage can be misleading. Once the tumor is reached, the biopsy should involve the periphery only. Deep sampling is not necessary. A frozen section must be obtained to determine if diagnostic tissue has been retrieved but not to establish the definitive diagnosis. Careful communication with the pathologist should be done preoperatively to clarify the amount of tissue that may be necessary for special studies and any special processing of the tissue once it is explanted. Formaldehyde fixes the tissue, preventing the application of conventional cytogenetics and some molecular tests. Furthermore, RNA quality and cell viability rapidly diminishes once outside the body, which also compromises certain molecular and cellular tests optimized by fresh tissue, such as expression analyses, flow cytometry, and cytogenetic analysis; so expeditious handling of the specimen is very important.[189,190]

For those ES tumors that have not violated the cortex, controlled fenestration of the bone will be necessary. A trephine is usually adequate but if a larger window is required, it is imperative that it be round or oval, to minimize stress on the bone. A pituitary rongeur may then be used to retrieve tissue from within the medullary canal. The bone window may then be replaced and sealed with bone wax. Alternatively, a polymethylmethacrylate plug may be used. Hemostasis is of utmost importance. Certain tumors may be quite vascular and meticulous hemostasis may not be possible. In such cases, a drain must be placed, in line with the incision distally, and sewn in place.

The use of tourniquets is controversial. Although their use provides a bloodless approach, they must be let down prior to closure to ensure adequate hemostasis. If used, the limb should not be exsanguinated to minimize the risk of tumor embolism.

Detection of Distant Metastases

Diagnostic staging at presentation must include appropriate evaluation for metastases, which will be detected in about 25% of patients. The most common metastatic sites are the lungs, bones, bone marrow, or combinations thereof. Locoregional lymph node involvement is rare and, when seen, is usually associated with multi-organ dissemination. In addition to bone-marrow sampling (see later), imaging studies are mandatory to reveal parenchymal lung or pleural metastases and bone metastases at distant sites.[182,183] Chest CT studies are mandatory to document or rule out intrathoracic metastases. Skeletal involvement can be diagnosed by 99-m technetium whole-body radionuclide bone scans, or by FDG-PET. FDG-PET has recently proven to be a highly sensitive screening method for detection of bone metastases in ES. In detecting bone metastases, FDG-PET may be even more sensitive than whole-body MRI scans.[191] Table 33.2 lists appropriate staging investigations at diagnosis.

Microscopically detectable bone-marrow metastases occur in less than 10% of patients and are associated with a poor prognosis.[192] Because tumor cells may be focally distributed in bone marrow, bone-marrow samples should be harvested from multiple sites, conventionally both posterior iliac crests. Aspirates or trephine biopsies are analyzed by light microscopy. If the tumor is of pelvic origin, an aspirate or trephine may contain tumor from the primary site and not reflect metastatic disease.

Differential Diagnosis

On initial physical examination, tendinitis is a common suspected diagnosis in adolescent or adult patients, whereas synovitis and osteomyelitis are often suspected in younger

---

TABLE 33.2

STAGING INVESTIGATIONS AT DIAGNOSIS

Investigation	Primary tumor site	Staging for metastases
Radiograph in two planes, whole bone with adjacent joints	+ +	At suspicious sites
MRI and/or CT, affected bone(s) and adjacent joints	+ +	At suspicious sites
Biopsy: material for histology and molecular biology	+ +	At suspicious sites
Thoracic CT (lung window)		+ +
Bone-marrow biopsy and aspirates: microscopy (molecular biology still investigational)		+ +
Whole body 99 m-technetium bone scan	+ +	+ +
FDG-PET	±	±

CT, computed tomography; FDG-PET, fluorine-18 fluorodeoxyglucose positron emission tomography; MRI, magnetic resonance imaging; + +, mandatory; ±, indicated, if available.

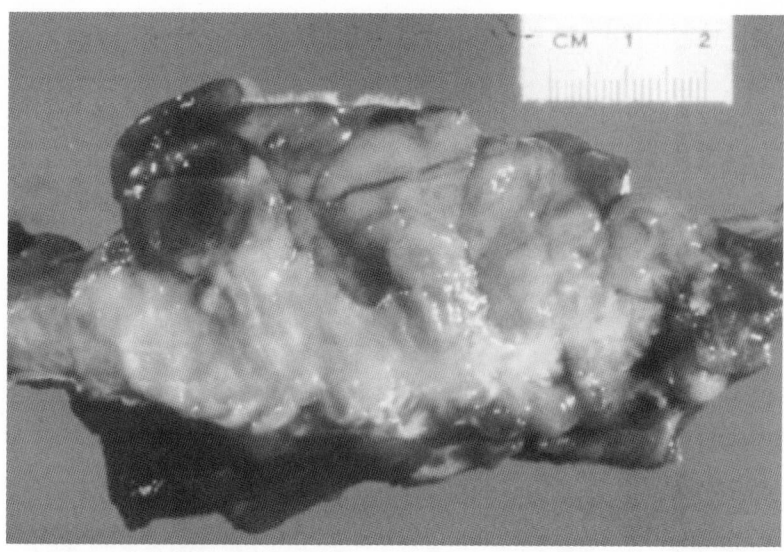

FIGURE 33.4 Typical gross appearance of Ewing sarcoma.

children.[159] Osteomyelitis may present a radiographic pattern similar to ES. In patients with metastatic disease, nonspecific symptoms such as malaise, fever, anorexia, and weight loss may resemble symptoms of infection. Osteosarcoma and lymphoma can have similar symptoms and radiographic findings. Children younger than the age of 5 years may thus present a constellation of symptoms similar to those of disseminated neuroblastoma. However, ES is extremely rare in children younger than 5 years.[193]

PATHOLOGY

Triaging and Processing Specimens

The primary purpose of the initial biopsy is to obtain adequate tissue for accurate diagnosis. Appropriate handling and triaging of specimens are critical, particularly when dealing with limited tissue from a core needle biopsy or fine needle aspirate. Ideally, tissue from a biopsy should be sent to the pathologist in the fresh state immediately after it is obtained. Assessment of viability is accomplished by visual inspection, complemented by touch preparations for rapid microscopic evaluation as deemed necessary. The tissue should be divided by the pathologist as follows: (a) imprints for FISH; (b) a portion in 10% neutral buffered formalin for routine histologic evaluation, immunohistochemical stains, and possibly for evaluation of chromosomal translocations by FISH; (c) a sample frozen at −70°C for molecular, RT-PCR, and specialized immunohistochemical studies; (d) a portion in glutaraldehyde for ultrastructural studies; and (e) a portion in tissue culture media for cytogenetics and flow-cytometric analysis of DNA ploidy and proliferation fraction. Ultrastructural and flow cytometry studies are rarely necessary for the diagnosis of ES and are not part of the routine pathologic evaluation in most institutions. After the specimen is appropriately triaged to ensure diagnosis, it is recommended that any residual fresh tissue be frozen at −70°C for possible future studies or for approved biologic studies to which the patient consents. Material obtained by fine needle aspiration should be triaged in a similar manner.[194,195]

Pathologic evaluation of the surgical resection specimen following neoadjuvant therapy is aimed at assessment of the bony and soft tissue resection margins for evidence of gross and/or microscopic involvement by tumor and of the histologic response to treatment. For the latter purpose, an entire section from the specimen representing the largest dimension of the tumor must be submitted in multiple blocks for histologic evaluation.

Gross Appearance

ES of bone has a permeative, destructive pattern of growth. Cortical infiltration and destruction, periosteal reaction with new bone formation, and soft tissue extension are often present at the time of presentation. On sectioning, these tumors have a fleshy, tan-white to gray-white, glistening appearance (Fig. 33.4). Tumor necrosis, cystic degeneration, hemorrhage, and fibrosis are variably present, depending on response to neoadjuvant therapy. Extraosseous ES has a similar appearance.

Histology and Ancillary Studies

ES encompasses tumors with a spectrum of histologic appearances and ultrastructural and immunohistochemical features. Classic ES, as first described by James Ewing in 1921,[108] is composed of a monotonous population of small round cells with high nuclear to cytoplasmic ratios arrayed in sheets (Fig. 33.5A). The cells have scant, faintly eosinophilic to amphophilic cytoplasm; indistinct cytoplasmic borders; and round nuclei with evenly distributed, finely granular chromatin, and inconspicuous nucleoli (Fig. 33.5B).[196–198] Mitotic activity is usually low. Cytoplasmic glycogen, which appears as periodic acid–Schiff (PAS)-positive diastase-digestible granules, is usually present. In contradistinction to lymphoma, which is included in the histologic differential diagnosis, ES lacks reticulin scaffolding. Foci of necrosis and hemorrhage are often present. Ultrastructural studies confirm the uniform, relatively undifferentiated nature of the constituent cells.[116,199] Cytoplasmic glycogen is usually abundant and may form pools; however, cytoplasmic organelles are scanty and consist predominantly of scattered mitochondria and polyribosomes. Only scattered rudimentary intercellular attachments are present. Variable numbers of Homer-Wright pseudorosettes may be present (Fig. 33.5C). The nuclei are round to oval with uneven, coarsely clumped chromatin and small to prominent nucleoli (Fig. 33.5D).[196–198] Increased mitotic activity is usually

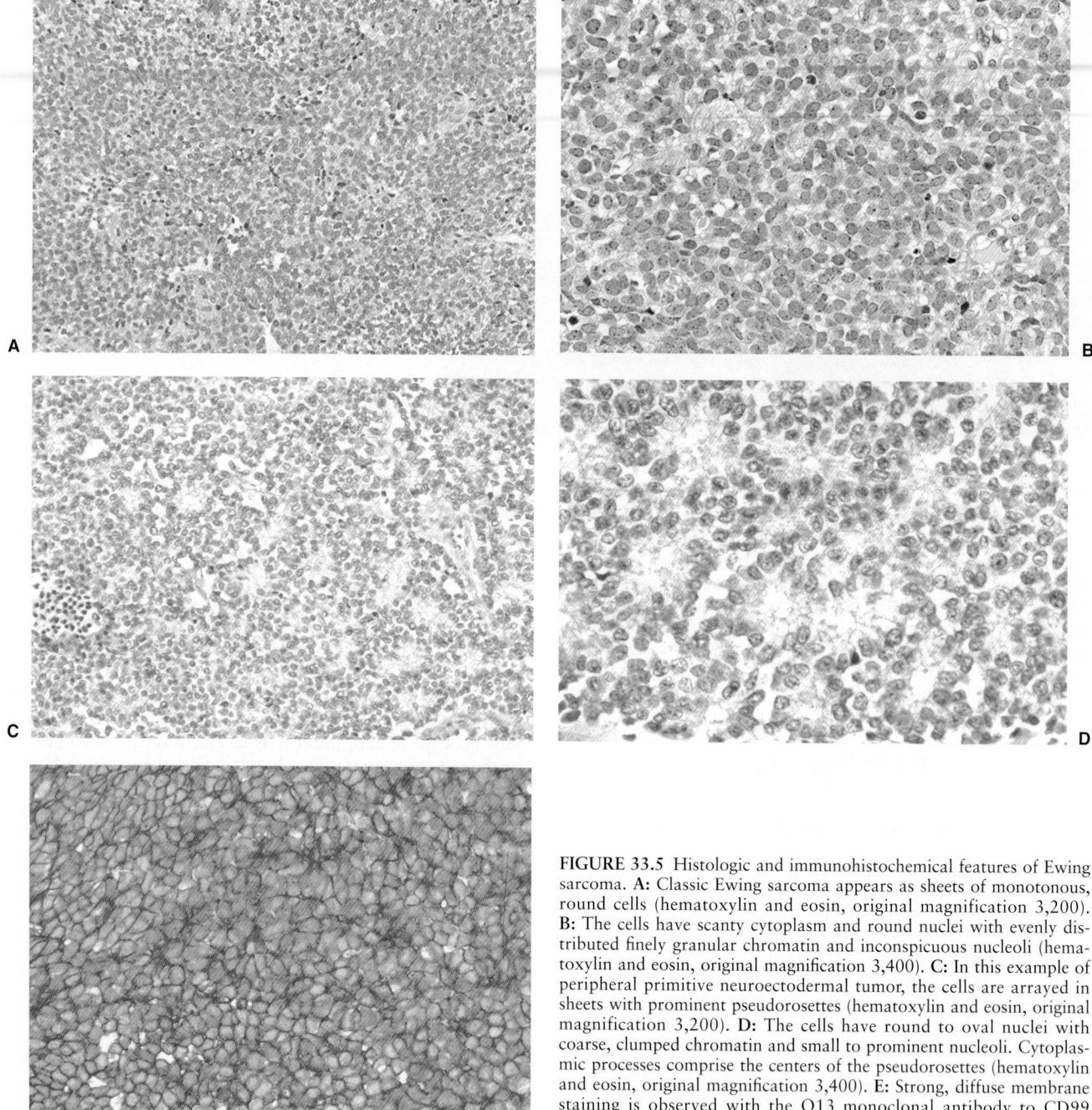

FIGURE 33.5 Histologic and immunohistochemical features of Ewing sarcoma. **A:** Classic Ewing sarcoma appears as sheets of monotonous, round cells (hematoxylin and eosin, original magnification 3,200). **B:** The cells have scanty cytoplasm and round nuclei with evenly distributed finely granular chromatin and inconspicuous nucleoli (hematoxylin and eosin, original magnification 3,400). **C:** In this example of peripheral primitive neuroectodermal tumor, the cells are arrayed in sheets with prominent pseudorosettes (hematoxylin and eosin, original magnification 3,200). **D:** The cells have round to oval nuclei with coarse, clumped chromatin and small to prominent nucleoli. Cytoplasmic processes comprise the centers of the pseudorosettes (hematoxylin and eosin, original magnification 3,400). **E:** Strong, diffuse membrane staining is observed with the O13 monoclonal antibody to CD99 (immunoperoxidase, original magnification 3,400).

evident. Foci of necrosis and hemorrhage are often present. Ultrastructural studies demonstrate neural differentiation, including neurite-like processes, irregular dense core granules, and, occasionally, neurofilaments and microtubules.[116,199] Intercellular attachments are relatively well developed.

Strong expression of the cell-surface glycoprotein CD99 is characteristic of ES, and strong, diffuse membrane staining is present in 95% to 100% of ES with one or more of the monoclonal antibodies to this antigen, including O13, 12E7, and HBA71 (Fig. 33.5E).[200–202] In addition, ES is immunoreactive for vimentin.[117,203,204] Immunohistochemical evidence of neural

differentiation in pPNET includes staining for neuron-specific enolase, S-100 protein, Leu-7, and/or PgP 9.5.[205] Infrequently, ES is focally immunoreactive for cytokeratins.

Because the histologic and immunophenotypic features of ES overlap to varying degrees with the other small round cell tumors of childhood, an expanded panel of immunohistochemical studies may be necessary to exclude other entities. Like ES, neuroblastoma is immunoreactive for neuron-specific enolase, S-100, and Leu-7, but in contrast to the PNET variant of ES, it is negative for vimentin and immunoreactive for neurofilament protein. Like ES, lymphoblastic lymphoma is strongly immunoreactive for CD99 in a membrane pattern, but unlike the former, lymphoblastic lymphoma is also immunoreactive for leukocyte common antigen (CD45) and other lymphoid markers. Rhabdomyosarcoma may also be immunoreactive with antibodies to CD99 (however, staining is usually focal, weak, and cytoplasmic) and in contradistinction to ES, rhabdomyosarcoma is immunoreactive for myogenin, myoD1, desmin, and actin. Rarely, focal desmin stain can be seen in ES.[206] The distinction between poorly differentiated small cell synovial sarcoma and poorly differentiated ES may be difficult in some cases. Although synovial sarcoma is immunoreactive for cytokeratin and/or epithelial membrane antigen, poorly differentiated small cell variants may be immunoreactive for CD99 in a membrane pattern and show only focal, weak staining for cytokeratin, thus mimicking poorly differentiated ES.

Molecular genetic studies, using FISH and/or RT-PCR, are valuable adjuncts for the evaluation of undifferentiated small round cell tumors of childhood, particularly in cases with indeterminate histologic and/or immunohistochemical features. Detection of characteristic translocations by these methods may allow for definitive diagnosis of ES, rhabdomyosarcoma, and synovial sarcoma.[207,208] Distinction between these tumors is critical, because their treatments are significantly different.

Atypical ES a term now abandoned but used in the past by some authors to denote a group of tumors with histologic features and evidence of neural differentiation intermediate between classic ES and PNET. Because a histologic continuum exists between classic ES and PNET, this distinction is no longer in use. There is currently no convincing evidence that atypical ES or other tumors in the ES/PNET spectrum with neural differentiation behave significantly differently from tumors with features of classic ES.[209]

INITIAL TREATMENT

Before the era of chemotherapy when patients with ES were treated with RT alone, fewer than 10% survived, despite the well-known radiosensitivity of this tumor.[210,211] Patients commonly died of metastases within 2 years, indicating the need for systemic treatment.[210] With application of modern multimodal therapeutic regimens including combination chemotherapy, surgery, and RT, cure rates of 60% and more can be achieved.[212-226] The treatment of ES patients worldwide is organized in cooperative trials, aiming to further improve treatment outcome.

Local Therapy

Cure from ES can only be achieved with both chemotherapy and local control. Current treatment schedules favor primary induction chemotherapy, followed by local therapy and adjuvant chemotherapy. For many years, RT was regarded as the standard local treatment modality. More recently, improvements in orthopedic surgery have allowed preservation of function without compromising survival rates.[226-230] In planning the optimal local therapy, an interdisciplinary approach involving experts experienced in this field is essential. The efficacy of this approach has been shown in two consecutive European trials by the reduction of local recurrences following the institution of centralized counseling regarding local therapy, including RT.[231]

There has been no randomized trial comparing local therapy modalities. Therefore, the question as to which modality, RT or surgery, is preferred for local therapy in ES remains controversial. From retrospective analyses of several groups, the impression has been that local control is improved when surgery is possible.[230,232-237] These data are usually confounded by the fact that there is a selection bias favoring patients in whom surgery is possible.[235] Currently, local treatment should be individually adapted depending on the site and size of the tumor, the adjacent anatomic structures, the patient's age, and individual preference.

Surgical Treatment of Ewing Sarcoma

The surgical management of malignant bone tumors has evolved and surgical approaches are now a function of the tumor type, location, and extent of disease. In general, patients with an isolated, resectable tumor after induction chemotherapy should have their tumor treated with surgery alone.[238-240] The use of postoperative RT due to poor histologic response (>10% viable tumor cells) is controversial, with some European clinical trials using it more widely,[230] whereas Children's Oncology Group (COG) trials reserve postoperative RT only for inadequate surgical margins regardless of histologic response.[241] After an unanticipated intralesional or marginal resections, postoperative RT may improve local control.[230,242] If postoperative RT is to be given, local control can be facilitated by treating within 60 days of surgery[243] (see also the section on "Radiotherapy").

The goal of any operation on a malignant tumor is to perform a complete, *en bloc* removal of the lesion with adequate margins. Limb-sparing surgery has become the norm with advances in imaging techniques, such as MRI. This, in combination with improved neoadjuvant therapy, has enabled the oncologic surgeon to obtain local control rates equivalent to amputation. However, in selected cases in which limb salvage may compromise the overall outcome and irradiation would lead to unacceptable morbidity, amputation is warranted.

Types of Reconstruction

Due to the complexity of the musculoskeletal system, different reconstructive operations are performed depending on the site of involvement. The main reconstructive options include autologous bone grafts, structural bone allografts (intercalary or osteoarticular), and metallic endoprosthetics. Allografts and endoprosthetics may also be used as part of a composite reconstruction. Autologous bone grafts may be vascularized (e.g., fibula). All three have inherent advantages and disadvantages. Which technique is employed is a function of the location of the tumor, age of the patient, and types of adjuvant therapies that will be employed (i.e., chemotherapy and/or radiation). Large structural allografts and endoprosthetics should generally be reserved for children older than 8 years. Nonvascularized autografts from the pelvis or other sites may be used in a limited fashion for relatively small defects and work well in children.[244] The advantage is a high incorporation rate, but there is also a potential for donor-site morbidity. Vascularized autografts, such as the fibula, are attractive because, when successful, the graft incorporates and may even hypertrophy and remodel because of the forces exerted across it.[245] Again, donor-site complications can occur. Because of the risk of severe vascular complications, vascularized autografts should be avoided if postoperative RT is anticipated.

Structural allografts have no donor-site morbidity. They provide a biologic solution that may be used in the reconstruction of the proximal humerus, distal femur, and proximal tibia and may last the lifetime of the patient.[246,247] Osteoarticular allografts may be used in the reconstruction of the

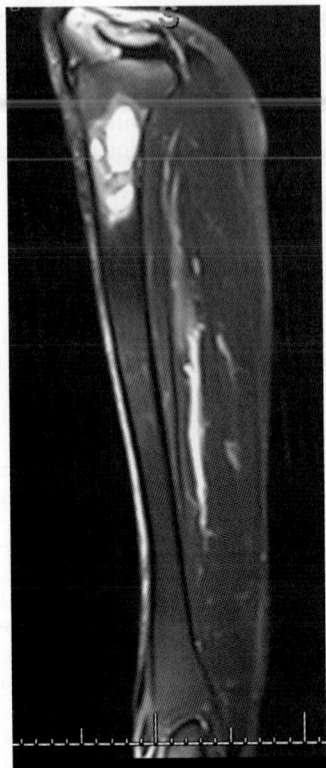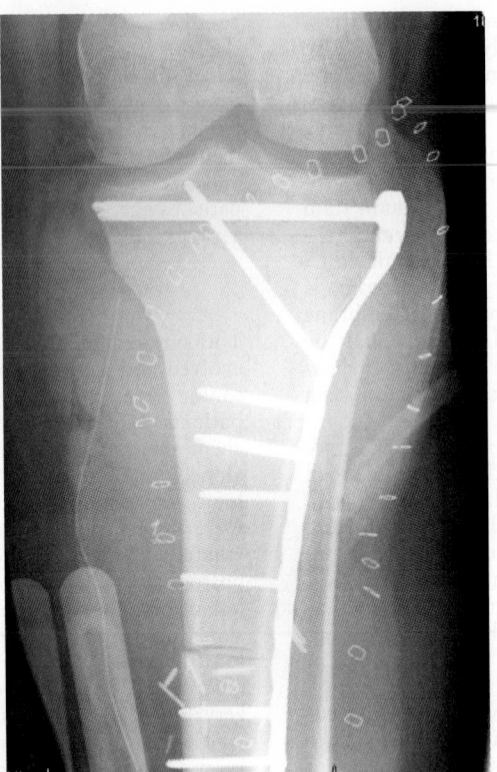

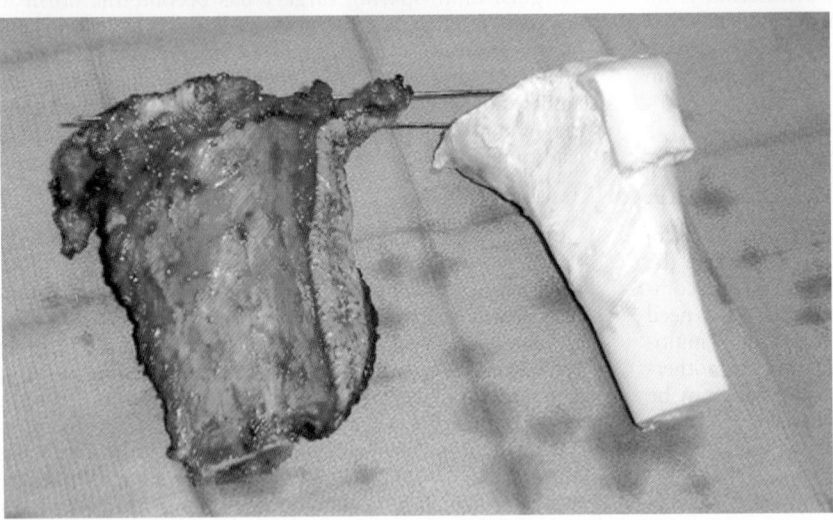

FIGURE 33.6 Allograft reconstruction of Ewing sarcoma involving the tibia. **A:** Preoperative sagittal MRI. Extent of anatomic involvement warrants intercalary allograft reconstruction to preserve the native knee joint. **B:** Postoperative radiograph. **C:** Resected tumor specimen and corresponding allograft prior to implantation.

proximal humerus, distal femur, and proximal tibia as well as potentially any joint.[248,249] Diaphyseal tumors can be reconstructed with intercalary allografts (Fig. 33.6), with good function.[248,250,251] The physis may sometimes serve as an adequate tumor barrier allowing preservation of the epiphysis and thus the joint surface. This must be carefully assessed preoperatively with MRI. The joint itself may be replaced with an allograft, but functional results are less satisfactory.[248,249] The major drawbacks of allografts are difficulty incorporating with the host bone (nonunion) and fracture.[252]

For osteoarticular allografts, satisfactory functional results can be anticipated in 60% to 70% of cases in which a high-grade sarcoma was removed and chemotherapy was utilized.[248,250] Function is generally better for intercalary reconstruction.[248,250] Impact activities are discouraged but compliance is not always common in younger patients. Fractures occur in

approximately 20% of cases.[253] Fractures can be managed by standard techniques but may necessitate a graft and/or implant removal and replacement. Vascularized fibular augmentation can be utilized as well.[254]

Metallic endoprosthetics (Fig. 33.7) provide an immediate stable reconstruction but suffer from eventual failure due to loosening and wearing of components.[255] Usually, the stem of the prosthesis is cemented in place with polymethylmethacrylate, but press fit stems and alternate fixation devices are used discretionarily as well.[256] They are generally cast from cobalt, chrome, or steel or machined from titanium. Infections are a significant risk with endoprosthetics as well.

Durability of endoprostheses varies, but the anticipated 5-year implant survival for proximal femoral reconstruction approaches 90%, whereas the rate for distal femoral reconstruction is about 60% and for the proximal tibia just over

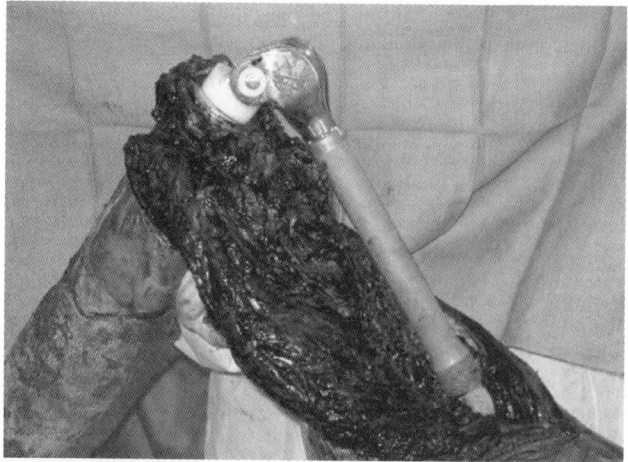

FIGURE 33.7 Typical distal femur/knee tumor endoprothesis used in limb salvage surgery. The patient's remaining native femur is on the right.

50%. Prosthetic reconstructions of the proximal humerus tend to be more durable because they are subject to lesser forces. Failure can result from loosening at the prosthesis-host interface or infection, which in up to a third of patients.[257] Improved metallurgy has resulted in a significant reduction in metal fatigue failure of the implants. In addition, newer cementless, porous ingrowth systems have been developed but have not yet replaced cement in most centers. A novel prestress compliant fixation device obviates the need for long intramedullary stems, thus minimizing the concentration of physical forces at focal points that may otherwise lead to fracture of the bone.[258] These devices facilitate osseous integration at the bone-implant interface.[259]

Allograft-prosthetic composites are another alternative for limb salvage surgery.[260] The advantage of this system is the hybridization of a more conventional arthroplasty with potential incorporation of the allograft for future bone stock. The construct may also prevent delayed allograft fracture.[261,262,263]

Arthrodesis remains an option in limb preservation surgery, but it is utilized with diminishing frequency as endoprostheses and allografts have improved.[264] The advantage to fusion is that once healed, the construct is very durable and may endure heavy activity. Because of the lack of motion, however, many patients are dissatisfied with the fusion process. It is better tolerated for the shoulder than the lower extremity,[265] with perhaps the exception of the ankle in select cases.[266,267]

Complications are far more frequent in limb salvage patients than in those who undergo amputation. However, as techniques evolve, the complication rate is steadily decreasing. Furthermore, patients who present with a pathologic fracture, or fracture during induction chemotherapy, may be poor candidates for limb salvage surgery, although this is not an absolute contraindication.[268–271]

Reconstruction as a Function of Location

For tumors of the shoulder and proximal humerus, limb salvage is generally possible with preservation of the neurovascular structures. Preservation of the hand is preferable, because the goal of the limb salvage is the ability to place the hand in front, and thus to enable self-feeding and grooming. However, activity that requires movement above the head is frequently not recovered in even the best-attempted reconstructions. In the lower extremity, the distal femur is the most common site. Again, the previously mentioned techniques may be used with good outcomes.

For certain sites, resection without reconstruction retains good function. These sites include the proximal fibula, clavicle, scapular body, and most areas of the ileum, ischium, and pubis of the pelvis. Approximately 10% of patients with ES have rib primary tumors. Neoadjuvant chemotherapy allows definitive surgical resection in three-fourths of such patients, avoiding the need for irradiation.[272]

Periacetabular pelvic lesions can be particularly troublesome in terms of resection and reconstruction, and irradiation may be a preferable alternative in severe cases. External hemipelvectomy (hind quarter amputation) historically was the only surgical option. Now internal hemipelvectomy (removal of the bony pelvis leaving a neurovascularly intact limb in place) can frequently be performed.[273] Reconstruction of the defect can be a challenge, however. It may be difficult to preserve adequate function and still ensure a complete oncologic resection. Even if internal hemipelvectomy is to be attempted, the goal must remain an adequate resection of the tumor, which can prove to be quite difficult. ES involving the axial musculoskeletal system is more commonly treated with definitive RT as the only mode of local control, although in cases with resectable lesions, strong consideration should be given to surgical management.

Special Considerations for the Skeletally Immature Child

The skeletally immature patient presents a particular challenge in that the reconstruction must be dynamic so as to accommodate future growth when a physis is sacrificed. In girls, the growth spurt occurs in pre- and early adolescence, whereas in boys it occurs later. Skeletal maturity is reached by age 14 to 15 years in girls and 16 to 17 years in boys. Most of the growth in the lower extremity is provided for by the physes about the knee (distal femur approximately 40%, proximal tibia approximately 30%), whereas the proximal femur and distal tibia have modest contributions of about 15% each. Because the physis does not survive in structural allografts, other options must be considered in the skeletally immature patient.

For expandable prostheses, the 5-year revision-free survival has been reported as low as 15%.[274] As with any reconstruction in the skeletally immature patient, the construct must be dynamic so as to facilitate skeletal growth. Expandable prosthetics are available with multiple, varying mechanisms for expansion.[275-277] Although some of these mechanisms may be easy to expand, the longevity of prosthetic implants is particularly poor in young children. Stress shielding and mechanical loosening are compounded by the continued diametrical growth of the host bone. Although revision surgery is possible, the resultant bone stock for refixation can be quite tenuous. Modular components are now available for both pediatric and adult patients making delay for customization the exception.

Limb lengthening via distraction osteogenesis is also an option,[278-280] but there remains concern in utilizing this complex technique concurrently with adjuvant multiagent chemotherapy.[281] Thus, this technique has only been embraced in a limited fashion, for very specialized cases. Alternatively, epiphysiodesis to arrest the growth of the contralateral leg results in near normal limb length when properly timed.

Intrinsic reconstructions such as rotationplasty and tibial turnup plasties are particularly attractive in the skeletally immature patient, especially in children younger than 8 years who will experience a significant amount of growth. Conceptually, rotationplasty is a resection of the hip or knee with

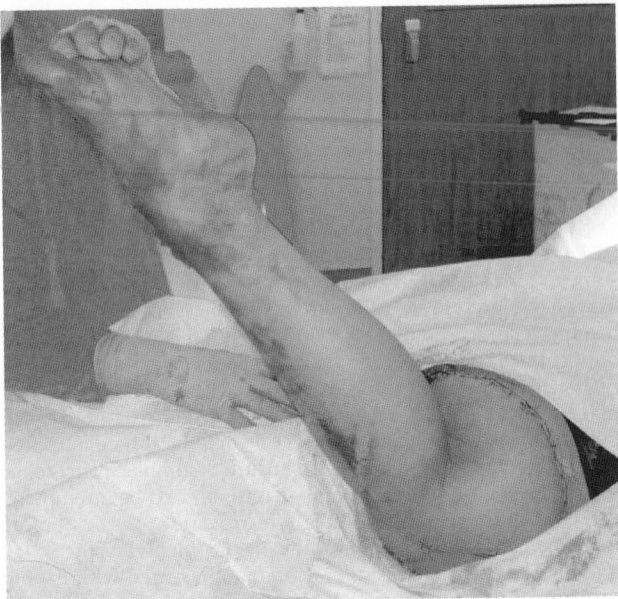

FIGURE 33.8 Double rotationplasty. The patient is lying supine with the distal femur having been rotated 180° and fixed to the supra-acetabular pelvis enabling the knee to function as a hip and the ankle to function as a knee with a modified below knee prosthesis.

subsequent reconstruction of the lost joint with the next joint below by rotating it 180° (Fig. 33.8). Most commonly, this is done for resection of the knee, where the ankle subsequently functions as a knee joint. A below knee prosthesis is then placed on the foot. Rotationplasty is a preferred method for skeletally immature patients with a large lesion about the knee, patients with large lesions that are not candidates for limb salvage, as an alternative to above-knee amputation, and as a salvage procedure for chronically infected prosthetic implants.[282–284] Interestingly, patients with rotationplasty were shown to be able to control their gait with their ankle, participate in hobbies to a significantly greater extent, and have less restriction in daily activities due to pain than patients who were treated with endoprosthetic replacements for similar conditions.[253,285–287] In addition, it is far more durable than other forms of reconstruction and retains the distal tibial physis for additional growth. The drawbacks relate to body image and cosmetic appearance.[253] Appropriate preoperative counseling should be performed, including images of patients that have undergone the procedure before and even meeting other such patients that have undergone the procedure.

Accordingly, many children and their families adjust very well to their new appearance and function.[288]

Radiotherapy

Definitive Radiotherapy

Patients who are selected to receive RT as the only local therapy modality usually represent an unfavorably selected group of patients. They frequently present with large tumors, tumors in unfavorable locations (e.g., vertebral tumors), or both, making RT difficult and surgery impossible. In an analysis of 1,058 patients with localized ES treated in the European Intergroup Cooperative Ewing Sarcoma Studies (EI-CESS) trials, 266 patients had RT alone. Local or combined local and systemic failures in this subgroup occurred in 26% of patients,[230,232] which was worse than the recurrence rate following surgery with or without RT (4% to 10%). It was not possible to define a subgroup of patients in whom the use of RT alone achieved the same local control rate as surgery. Even for the favorable subgroup of patients with small extremity tumors, local control with surgery was better than with definitive RT. In contrast, an analysis of patients with pelvic tumors from INT-001 demonstrated that radiation performed as well as surgery for attaining local control.[235] Given the risks of second malignancy with RT, current practice favors surgery when a wide resection is possible.

Definitive RT is indicated when only an intralesional resection is possible. In the experience of the European Cooperative Ewing Sarcoma Studies (CESS) and EI-CESS trials, patients who had an intralesional resection followed by RT had the same local control rate as patients who had RT alone.[230,232] Definitive RT may also be an alternative in selected subgroups of patients with small tumors that would require relatively morbid surgical procedures due to location, such as the sacrum. Using new RT modalities, including intensity-modulated radiotherapy (IMRT) or proton therapy, these patients are candidates for treatment without surgery.

Postoperative Radiotherapy

Postoperative RT is always indicated following intralesional resections. Debulking procedures do not improve local control and are associated with both additional unnecessary morbidity and delays in the administration of systemic therapy. In the analysis of the EI-CESS trials, local control with surgery alone was excellent in all patients who had a wide resection according to the Enneking classification[289] (Table 33.3) and with a good histologic response following initial chemotherapy (good histologic response: ≤10% viable tumor cells in the

TABLE 33.3

ENNEKING CLASSIFICATION OF SURGICAL INTERVENTION

Intralesional resection	Tumor opened during surgery, or surgical field contaminated, or microscopic or macroscopic residual disease
Marginal resection	Tumor removed *en bloc*; however, resection through the pseudocapsule of the tumor; microscopic residual disease likely
Wide resection	Tumor and its pseudocapsule removed *en bloc*, surrounded by healthy tissue, within the tumor-bearing compartment
Radical resection	The whole tumor-bearing compartment is removed *en bloc*, for example, above-knee amputation in lower leg tumor

From Enneking WF, Spanier SS, Goodman MA. A system for the surgical staging of musculoskeletal sarcoma. Clin Orthop 1980;153:106–120.

resected specimen).[290] Only one local failure in 101 patients occurred in this subgroup. Patients with wide resection and poor histologic response were at higher risk of local failure (12%). The local failure rate was lower in patients who received postoperative RT (6%).[230,232] This result has not yet been reproduced in other studies. Postoperative RT for patients with wide resection but poor histologic response has become standard in EI-CESS studies but not in COG studies. There was also a trend to benefit with the use of postoperative irradiation in patients who had a marginal resection.[291]

Preoperative Radiotherapy

The systematic use of preoperative RT was incorporated into the EI-CESS 92 trial. The governing objective was to sterilize the tumor compartment before surgery and thus to potentially reduce the rate of dissemination during surgery. With growing experience with the use of preoperative RT, it was used in this trial when narrow resection margins were expected. More than 40% of the EI-CESS patients were treated with preoperative RT. However, in an analysis of the data of these 246 patients, a reduction in systemic failure could not be demonstrated.[230] Although the local control rate following preoperative RT was excellent, there was not an improvement in local control among patients with wide resections.[230] In addition, preoperative RT may confound the response assessment to neoadjuvant chemotherapy.

Radiation Dose and Fractionation

To control ES, a radiation dose above 40 Gy is necessary. In the St. Jude's Children's Research Hospital experience with the use of lower radiation doses, a high rate of local recurrence was observed.[233] A clear dose response correlation at doses above 40 Gy has not yet been established. For definitive RT, doses between 55 and 60 Gy are usually given. When surgery precedes or follows RT, the doses range between 45 and 55 Gy, depending on the individual risk factors (i.e., resection margins and response). Usually, conventional fractionation with daily fractions of 1.8 to 2 Gy is given. In the CESS 86 and EI-CESS 92 trials, hyperfractionated RT with twice daily 1.6 Gy was also applied; after 22.4 Gy, a 10-day break was scheduled to permit the administration of chemotherapy. There has been no detectable difference in local control between the two different fractionation groups.[292] Hyperfractionated RT, however, is associated with higher acute toxicity in pediatric rhabdomyosarcoma patients.[293]

Target Volume Definition and Treatment Planning

In a randomized trial, the treatment of the whole tumor bearing compartment showed no better results than radiation to the tumor and an additional safety margin.[234] Therefore, the planning target volume is defined as the initial tumor extent on MRI with an additional longitudinal margin of at least 2 to 3 cm and lateral margins of 2 cm in long bones. If doses of more than 45 Gy are used, a shrinking field technique is applied. In patients with an axial tumor site, a minimum of a 2-cm margin around the initial tumor extent is necessary. In tumors protruding into body cavities (i.e., thorax, pelvis) without infiltration, the residual intracavitary tumor volume following chemotherapy is used for treatment planning. Surgically contaminated areas, scars, and drainage sites must be included in the radiation fields. Circumferential irradiation of extremities should be avoided to reduce the risk of lymphedema, with sparing of one-third of the extremity preferred. In growing children, growth plates must be considered. They should either be fully included in the radiation field or they should not be included at all. A dose gradient through the

epiphysis results in asymmetric growth and may lead to functional deficits. Similarly, vertebral bodies should either be fully included or spared from the radiation field to avoid scoliosis. For optimal dosimetry, three-dimensional conformal RT should be given in patients with ES. In selected cases, such as vertebral or pelvic tumors, newer techniques including IMRT or proton therapy may be beneficial. Figures 33.9, and 33.10 show examples of treatment planning.

Radiation of Metastatic Disease Sites

Lung Radiation. The efficacy of lung irradiation in ES was shown in the IESS I trial.[218] Patients with localized disease received one of three regimens: vincristine, dactinomycin, and cyclophosphamide (VAC); VACA (additional doxorubicin); and VAC plus lung irradiation. Although the best results were obtained with VACA, VAC plus lung irradiation was significantly better than VAC alone. It is uncertain whether the addition of prophylactic pulmonary irradiation would improve outcome beyond that achieved with modern chemotherapy. Prophylactic pulmonary irradiation is therefore not recommended for patients with initially localized disease as part of current standard management.

These results from IESS I have been applied to patients with documented lung metastases at initial presentation. Several studies have reported improved outcomes with the use of whole-lung irradiation in these patients.[192,294-296] Patients typically receive 12 to 20 Gy. Both acute and chronic complications appear to be limited with these regimens.[294,295] Based on this experience, the use of whole lung radiation has become common practice in patients with lung metastases at initial presentation. In the ongoing EURO-E.W.I.N.G. 99 trial, a regimen including standard chemotherapy and whole-lung irradiation is randomized against one incorporating high-dose chemotherapy followed by stem cell reinfusion for patients with lung metastases at initial diagnosis.

Bone Metastases. RT may be indicated in patients presenting with bone metastases. RT can be given to all initially involved sites if limited in number. Care must be taken to not irradiate overlapping fields from closely contiguous lesions, as this can then exceed normal tissue tolerance. In addition, normal structures such as the heart and kidneys may be unavoidably in the radiation field for some lesions. Irradiating those structures can augment the toxicity of chemotherapy. Similarly, irradiation of more than 50% of the estimated bone-marrow volume can result in significant myelosuppression and accentuate the toxicity of chemotherapy. In patients presenting with multiple bone metastases for whom irradiation to all initial sites of disease is not feasible, RT can be given to sites of residual tumor based on imaging studies. RT is also effective in relieving pain or to avoid neurologic complications even when used with palliative intent.

Toxicity

Because of the predominance of tumors in long bones and the pelvis, the primary late effects in the treatment of ES are changes in bones and soft tissue. RT results in growth deficits owing to damage to chondroblasts, with doses 10 to 20 Gy potentially leading to growth inhibition and doses above 20 Gy arresting further growth. The extent of the growth deficit depends on the age of the patient at the time of treatment and the contribution of a specific epiphysis in the radiation field to the total growth of the body or the limb. Hypoplasia of the soft tissues can occur after doses of at least 20 Gy. In addition to a reduction in the volume of the muscles and subcutaneous tissue, fibrosis can occur after higher doses and result in a limitation of movement.

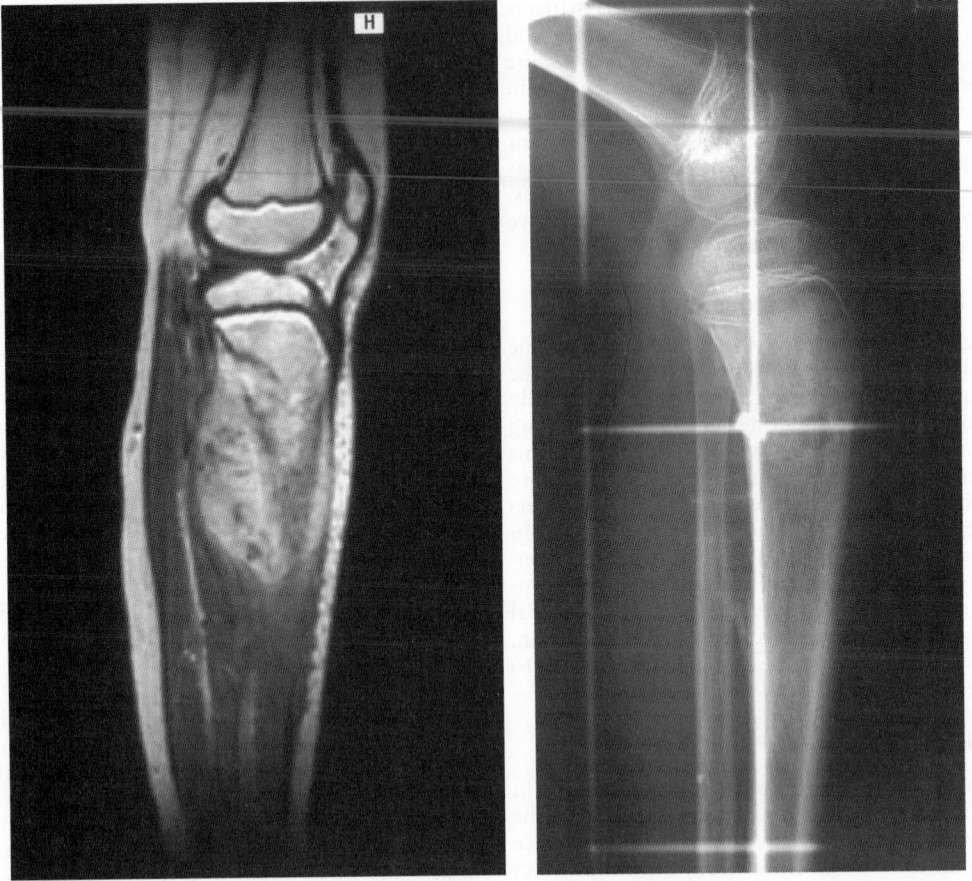

A   B

FIGURE 33.9 A: Magnetic resonance image of a Ewing sarcoma of the tibia. **B:** Radiation fields resulting from computed tomography–based three-dimensional treatment planning. The radiation portal covers the initial tumor extent with additional margins of at least 3 cm. Because it was not possible to avoid treating the epiphyses of the distal femur and proximal tibia, these are included in the fields to avoid asymmetric growth. Furthermore, lymphatic drainage is facilitated by avoiding radiotherapy of a dorsal longitudinal strip of tissue.

Surgical wound complications are more common when preoperative RT is utilized.[297,298] Although postoperative RT has not been shown to significantly increase the incidence of allograft nonunion and fracture alone,[299,300] the number of cases employing large structural allografts and concomitant RT is limited and there is some evidence that radiation may adversely affect structural allograft incorporation.[301] Radiation may also induce tissue fibrosis and interfere with joint mobility.

When RT is administered to the pelvis, care must be taken to limit doses delivered to the gonad, with testicular shielding and ovarian transposition used when possible. High dose irradiation of large volumes of the bowel should be avoided due

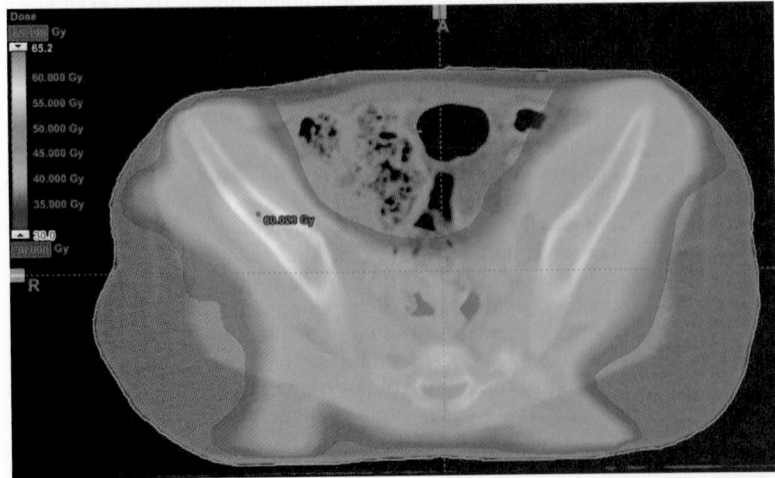

FIGURE 33.10 Intensity-modulated radiotherapy in patient with multifocal pelvic Ewing sarcoma. Using this technique, the volume of the bowel exposed to radiation doses exceeding 30 Gy can be limited. The figure shows the dose range from 30 Gy to the maximum dose of 65 Gy in primary tumor lesions.

to the risk of bowel obstruction and perforation. In ES of the chest wall, particular attention must be paid to limit doses to the lung and the heart, especially in the context of doxorubicin-containing chemotherapy. During RT, doxorubicin and dactinomycin should be withheld due to known radiosensitization. Patients who previously received busulfan-containing high-dose chemotherapy require special attention to minimize the additive toxicity with radiation on lungs, spinal cord, and intestine, which can be life-threatening.

Chemotherapy

The first reports of drug treatment of ES stem from the 1960s. These studies identified a series of active agents, including cyclophosphamide (CYC), dactinomycin (ACT), doxorubicin (DOX), ifosfamide (IFO), and vincristine (VCR).[211,302–314] The modern era of multimodality treatment of ES began with the report of sustained responses in five patients treated with the combination of CYC, VCR, and RT.[213] In 1976, Jaffe et al.[315] reported superior survival with VAC as compared with single-agent therapy. In 1974, Rosen from the Memorial Sloan Kettering Cancer Center (MSKCC) published the first results of a trial of RT given with a four-drug regimen consisting of VCR, ACT, CYC, and DOX used in combination rather than sequentially (VACD), leading to long-term survival in 12 patients with ES.[215] The first Intergroup Ewing Sarcoma Study, IESS-I, showed the superiority of the VACD four-drug regimen over a three-drug VAC regimen (without DOX), in terms of effectiveness of local control (96% vs. 86%) and EFS (60% vs. 24%).[218] The VACD regimen thus became a standard therapy for evaluation in numerous subsequent clinical trials (Table 33.4).

The importance of DOX, and especially of a high initial treatment intensity of DOX, was highlighted by a systematic meta-analysis of clinical trials in ES by Smith et al.,[316] concluding that of all drugs administered in ES, DOX is probably the most active, followed by alkylating agents. The authors clearly demonstrate that schedules with initial high dose intensity of DOX show the best survival rates, even when compared with schedules with identical cumulative doses of DOX and other drugs. This conclusion is also supported by an international study of patients with extraosseous ES which demonstrated improved outcomes with the use of DOX.[317]

In IESS-II, two schedules of the four-drug combination VACD were compared. The authors of the original report claim that a "high-dose intermittent" regimen with 3-weekly, higher doses of CYC was superior to a "low-dose continuous" schedule, in which lower doses of CYC were administered weekly, but with identical cumulative drug doses in both arms. There was, however, another significant difference between those two treatment schedules, with patients randomized to the high-dose intermittent regimen receiving higher initial DOX dose intensity, than those on the low-dose continuous schedule.[219] Smith et al. speculated that at least part of the superior outcome of the patients on the high-dose intermittent schedule may have been due to the higher initial DOX dose intensity.[316]

Because the total dose of DOX is limited by the risk of cardiomyopathy, cumulative dose intensification of alkylating agents has been studied, both using CYC as the main alkylator and using IFO as an alternative alkylating agent replacing or supplementing CYC. In parallel to these efforts, etoposide (ETO), a topoisomerase-II inhibitor, was also introduced into several studies. In St. Jude Children's Hospital EW-92 study, introduction of IFO and ETO increased patients' survival as compared with a previous VACD-based regimen, especially in larger localized tumors.[318] The Bologna group reported encouraging results with the combination of VCR, DOX,

CYC, ACT, IFO, and ETO, achieving 71% 5-year EFS.[319] The United Kingdom Children's Cancer Study Group (UKCCSG) performed two consecutive trials (ET-1 and ET-2), with VACD in ET-1, and VCR, ACT, IFO, and DOX (VAID) in ET-2, the latter achieving 5-year EFS of 62% as compared with 41% in ET-1.[176,221] Similarly, the German/Austrian/Dutch Pediatric Oncology/Hematology Group (GPOH) used VACD in CESS 81 high-risk patients (tumor volume >100 mL), resulting in 31% 3-year EFS. In CESS 86, in which IFO was given as part of a VAID schema, 51% 10-year EFS was observed in a comparable high-risk patient group.[217,223] MSKCC reported on a CYC dose intensified VDC schedule alternating with IFO and ETO (IE) (protocol P6), escalating CYC doses per course from conventional 1 to 1.5 g/m^2 to 4.2 g/m^2, resulting in a 2-year EFS of 77% for all patients and an 82% 4-year EFS for patients with localized disease.[224,320] Although most early studies suggested a benefit from the addition of IFO and/or ETO, the second French cooperative ES study did not demonstrate an improvement in outcome with substitution of IFO for CYC.[321]

The first Pediatric Oncology Group-Children's Cancer Group (POG-CCG) study INT-0091 randomized between VACD and VACD with IE. The VACD arm achieved 54% 5-year EFS in patients with localized disease, as compared with 69% EFS in the experimental arm with addition of IE.[225] It should be noted that the dose intensity of DOX was less in patients in the experimental arm as compared with that in the standard arm, suggesting that alternating therapy with other active agents can improve outcome, despite the reduction in DOX dose intensity. The combination of VACD alternating with IE then became standard for patients with localized ES in North America.

Another question related to the IE regimen is the importance of the individual components, IFO and ETO. In the European Intergroup Ewing Sarcoma Study, EI-CESS-92, researchers from the UKCCSG and the GPOH joined in an attempt to evaluate the efficacy of both drugs IFO and ETO in randomized studies. In a study for standard-risk ES patients, that is, those with localized disease and a tumor volume of less than 100 mL, patients were randomized to VACD versus VAID. In a study for high-risk patients (larger localized tumors, or metastatic disease), the addition of ETO to a VAID scheme was randomized.[322] In the standard-risk study, no significant difference was seen in 5-year EFS between the VACD (67%) and the VAID (68%) arms. A trend toward improved outcome was seen in the high-risk study, with 5-year EFS of 44% in the VAID arm, 52% in the EVAID arm, $p = 0.12$ (Table 33.4). Subgroup analysis of the high-risk patients suggested a trend toward a benefit for the addition of ETO to VAID for patients with large localized tumors.

Cytokines that ameliorate hematologic toxicity, in particular, granulocyte colony-stimulating factor (filgrastim), have allowed various dose-intensification strategies. The number of drugs may be increased in each cycle or the individual drug doses may be increased, as outlined previously.[224,320] A regimen combining VCR-IFO-DOX-ETO (VIDE) was tolerable in a pilot study and now forms the backbone for the ongoing Euro-Ewing 99 study.[323] The second POG-CCG Intergroup study included an investigational arm of alkylating agent dose intensification. The overall cumulative doses of the five medications (VDC, IE) were nearly identical, but, because of the increased alkylating agent dose fractions in the investigational arm, therapy was completed by 30 weeks as compared with 48 weeks in the standard arm. Despite dose intensification, no difference between treatment arms was seen.[241] COG study, AEWS 0031 used the strategy of interval compression, with therapy administered every 2 weeks in the experimental arm.[324] Time-dose intensity of all drugs is thus increased, perhaps interacting in a favorable way with cell cycle kinetics of

TABLE 33.4

TREATMENT RESULTS IN SELECTED CLINICAL STUDIES OF LOCALIZED ES

Study	References	Schedule	Patients	5-yr EFS	p^a	Comments
IESS Studies						
IESS-I (1973–1978)	218	VAC	342	24%	VAC/VAC + WLI: 0.001	Value of D
		VAC + WLI		44%	VAC/VACD: 0.001	Benefit of WLI?
		VACD		60%	VAC + WLI/ VACD: 0.05	
IESS-II (1978–1982)	219	VACD-HD	214	68%	0.03	Value of aggressive cytoreduction
		VACD-MD		48%		
First POG–CCG (INT-0091) (1988–1993)	225	VACD	200	54%	0.005	Value of combination IE in localized disease, no benefit in metastatic disease
		VACD + IE	198	69%		
Second POG–CCG (INT-0154) (1995–1998)	241	VCD + IE standard alkylating agent dose	231	72% (5 yr)	0.57	No benefit of alkylating agent dose intensification
		VCD + IE intensified alkylating agent dose	247	70% (5 yr)		
First COG (AEWS0031) (2001–2005)	324	VCD + IE every 3-week interval	284	65% (4 yr)	0.029	Dose compression improves outcome
		VCD + IE every 2-week interval	284	76% (4 yr)		
Memorial Sloan Kettering Cancer Center Studies						
T2 (1970–1978)	402	VACD (adjuvant)	20	75%		After local therapy only, cumulative dose of D up to 600 mg/m²
P6 (1990–1995)	320	HD-CVD + IE	36	77% (2 yr)		C dose escalation 4.2 g/m²/course
P6 (1991–2001)	224	HD-CVD + IE	68	Localized: 81% (4 yr); Metastatic: 12% (4 yr)		Good results in localized disease, poor outcome in metastatic patients
St. Jude Studies						
ES-79 (1978–1986)	403	VACD	52	82% <8 cm (3 yr) 64% ≥8 cm (3 yr)		Tumor size as prognostic factor
ES-87 (1987–1991)	404	Therapeutic window with IE	26	Clinical responses in 96%		Combination IE effective
EW-92 (1992–1996)	318	VCDIE × 3 VCD/IE Intensification	34	78% (3 yr)		Tumor size (</≥8 cm) loses prognostic relevance with more intensive treatment
ROI Bologna/Italy						
REN-3 (1991–1997)	319	VDC + VIA + IE	157	71%		Surgery in 78% of patients
SFOP/France						
EW-84 (1984–1987)	321	VIA-VID	49	50%		No improvement I over C with historic controls
EW-88 (1988–1991)	222	VD + VD/VA	141	58%		Histologic response better predictor of outcome compare with tumor volume

(continued)

TABLE 33.4

CONTINUED

Study	References	Schedule	Patients	5-yr EFS	p^a	Comments
SSG/Scandinavia						
SSG IX (1990–1999)	405	VID + PID	88	58% (metastases-free sur.)		70% overall survival after 5 yr
UKCCSG/MRC Studies						
ET-1 (1978–1986)	176	VACD	120	41% Extr. 52% Axial 38% Pelvic 13%		Tumor site as the most important prognostic factor
ET-2 (1987–1993)	221	VAID	201	62% Extr. 73% Axial 55% Pelvic 41%		Importance of the administration of high-dose alkylating agents (I)
CESS Studies						
CESS-81 (1981–1985)	217	VACD	93	<100 mL 80% ≥100 mL 31% (both 3 yr) Viable tumor <10%: 79% >10%: 31% (both 3 yr)		Tumor volume (</≥100 mL) and histologic response are prognostic factors
CESS-86 (1986–1991)	223	<100 mL (SR): VACD ≥100 mL (HR): VAID	301	52% (10 yr) 51% (10 yr)		Intensive treatment with I for high-risk patients Tumor volume (</≥200 mL) and histologic response as prognostic factors
EI-CESS Studies (CESS + UKCCSG)						
EI-CESS-92 (1992–1999)	322	SR: VAID/VACD	155	68%/67%	0.72	Stage, histologic response, type of local therapy as prognostic factors; randomized comparisons n.s.; randomized comparisons n.s.
		HR: VAID/EVAID	492	44%/52%	0.12	Included metastatic disease

EFS, event-free survival; A, actinomycin D; C, cyclophosphamide; D, doxorubicin; E, etoposide; I, ifosfamide; P, *cis*-platinum; V, vincristine; WLI, whole-lung irradiation; HD, high dose; MD, moderate dose; SR, standard risk; HR, high risk; n.s. not significant.
$^a p$ Values are given only for trials comparing randomized treatment arms.

the malignant cell population. Not only was interval compression feasible in a cooperative study, this trial demonstrated a significant improvement in 4-year EFS favoring the interval compressed arm, 76% versus 65%, $p = 0.029$. Toxicity was similar between the two treatment arms. With these results, interval compressed chemotherapy with cycles of VDC alternating every 2 weeks with IE has become the new standard regimen for North American patients with localized ES.

Another treatment intensification strategy in ES is high-dose chemotherapy with autologous hematopoietic stem cell rescue (HDT).[325] Because of the considerable toxicity of this approach, most studies investigate HDT for very high risk patients, most commonly those with metastatic disease at diagnosis or following recurrence (see later).[326–329] A controlled, randomized study of HDT in ES is one of the primary study questions of the Euro-E.W.I.N.G. 99 trial for patients with

large primary tumors locally treated with both surgery and irradiation, or small primary tumors (<200 mL) and an unfavorable histologic or radiologic response to induction chemotherapy (arm R2 loc). Accrual is ongoing.[323] Because of its intrinsic risk, high-dose therapy should be restricted to controlled clinical trials.[330,331]

Metastatic Disease

At initial diagnosis, approximately 25% of ES patients present with clinically detectable metastases in the lungs, bones, and/or bone marrow. The presence of metastatic disease is the most important adverse prognostic factor.[192,220,225,332] Patients with isolated lung metastases have been shown to have a better prognosis than those with extrapulmonary metastases;

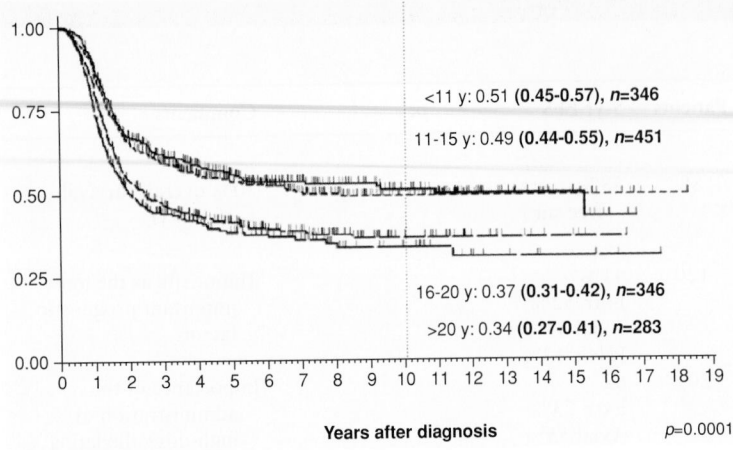

FIGURE 33.11 Event-free survival in Ewing sarcoma patients related to age at diagnosis (European Cooperative Ewing Sarcoma Studies [CESS]/European Intergroup Cooperative Ewing Sarcoma Studies [EI-CESS]) data, $n = 1,426$].

however, survival is still disappointing.[192,333,334] Whole lung irradiation appears to improve the outcome for these patients (see above). The COG joined the Euro-E.W.I.N.G. 99 randomized study comparing pulmonary irradiation with high-dose therapy for patients with initially isolated pulmonary metastatic disease (R2 pulm).[323] Patients with multiple bony metastases at initial diagnosis have an expected survival estimate below 20%.[192,224,332] Solitary or circumscribed bony metastases are typically irradiated at doses of 40 to 50 Gy, in addition to local therapy at the primary site and ES-directed chemotherapy. The discouraging results of treatment of metastatic disease has led to more aggressive approaches including intensified chemotherapy regimens, myeloablative high-dose therapy with stem cell rescue, and the use of novel biologic therapies.

Augmentation of chemotherapy regimens has not improved outcomes for patients with metastatic disease. In INT-0091, these patients did not benefit from the addition of IE to VACA chemotherapy.[225,334] Similarly, in EI-CESS-92, there was a trend to suggest that patients with high-risk localized disease benefited from the addition of ETO while patients with metastatic disease did not.[322] Two COG studies evaluating intensified chemotherapy doses have also not yielded improved outcomes for this population.[335,336] Notably, the use of interval compression as a means of increasing dose intensity has not yet been evaluated in patients with metastatic ES.

Multiple studies have evaluated further dose intensification as part of high-dose treatment regimens with autologous stem cell rescue.[327–329,337] Although some studies have suggested a possible improvement in outcome with this strategy, most prospective studies have had discouraging results.[328,329,331]

These results suggest that patients with metastatic disease are resistant to standard therapies. Recent studies have begun to evaluate biologically targeted therapies for these patients. In COG protocol AEWS02P1, patients received metronomic antiangiogenic therapy together with standard chemotherapy. The results of this study are not yet available. Planned studies are focusing on the use of IGF1R monoclonal antibodies combined with interval-compressed chemotherapy.

EWING SARCOMA IN ADOLESCENTS AND YOUNG ADULTS

ES typically arise in the second decade of life, the median age being 15 years (see "Clinical Presentation and Staging";

Fig. 33.2). Of the 1,426 patients in the database of the EI-CESS, 56% of patients were diagnosed between ages 10 and 20 years. Forty-four percent of patients were older than 15 years; 20% of patients were older than 20 years.

The prognosis for adolescents or young adults with ES has repeatedly been reported to be inferior to the outcome in the pediatric population.[1,220,221,225,226,338–342] Figure 33.11 shows the age-related outcome of ES patients from the EI-CESS registry. Although there seems to be no major difference in outcome between patients aged 16 and 20 years as compared with those older than 20 years, the outcome of the adolescent and adult population is significantly inferior to that of the pediatric age group.

Several reasons for the inferior outcome of adolescents have been proposed.[223,343–351]

- Different biologic behavior of ES in children and older patients (e.g., more central axis lesions, larger tumors, or increased resistance to chemotherapy)
- Patient-related covariables: such as comorbidities, decreased treatment tolerance (e.g., decreased drug metabolism—altered pharmacokinetics; increased toxicity from similar drug exposure—altered pharmacodynamics), poor treatment compliance
- Treatment-related or iatrogenic factors: differences in drug prescription, lower enrollment in clinical trials, differences between "pediatric" and "adult" treatment regimens.

Older ES patients present more commonly with larger tumors, or with metastatic disease, as compared with children (Table 33.5).[220,345–347] Unpublished data from the EI-CESS registry so far have not revealed significant differences in the pattern of chromosomal changes between both age groups (see Table 33.5). Adolescents and young adults with ES represent a typical example of cancer patients whose needs may not routinely be met by either pediatric or adult oncology institutions. The first adolescent cancer units have been launched in the United States and the United Kingdom to properly address this age group's specific needs, both in terms of medical and psychosocial care[344,349] (see also Chapter 15).

In a report from the United Kingdom, all ES patients aged 16 to 48 years were equally treated with an intensive "pediatric-type" regimen. Age was not found to influence survival.[347] Similarly, in a study on Italian patients aged 40 years or more, treated with a dose-intensive, pediatric-like regimen, Bacci et al.[350] described an outcome comparable with pediatric patients. Data from the CESS 86 study likewise did not show an impact of age on survival.[223] However, other reports of

TABLE 33.5

DISTRIBUTION OF UNFAVORABLE PROGNOSTIC FACTORS IN CHILDREN AND OLDER EWING SARCOMA PATIENTS

Variable	Age group n/n (%)		
	≤15 yr	>15 yr	$\chi^2 p$
Non–type 1 transcript	25/51 (49)	19/50 (38)	0.264
Metastatic stage	205/880 (23)	195/654 (30)	0.004
Tumor volume >200 mL	249/706 (35)	220/463 (48)	0.001
Poor histologic response	123/526 (23)	109/368 (30)	0.036

Data from the European Intergroup Cooperative Ewing Sarcoma Studies (EI-CESS) registry. Patient numbers vary between different variables due to data availability.

adolescents and/or adults on "pediatric" trials continue to describe an inferior outcome for older patients.[220,221,225] In a recent publication reporting the results of the POG-CCG study INT-0091, no differences in dose intensity between age groups were found to explain the inferior outcome of older patients.

In conclusion, the outcome of ES patients may be different between children and older patients. Factors such as tumor biology and drug tolerance may affect age-specific outcome.

RECURRENT DISEASE: NOVEL TREATMENT STRATEGIES

Improved multimodal therapeutic regimens that combine more intensive systemic treatment with chemotherapy, improved surgical approaches, and advanced RT planning have led to a reduced frequency of recurrent disease, in particular, of local recurrence.[217,352] Nevertheless, approximately 30% of patients still experience recurrent disease. The majority of relapses are either isolated distant relapse or combined distant and local relapse.[353–355] Patients with primary metastatic disease have a higher risk of relapse than those with localized disease.[220,352] The likelihood of long-term survival after recurrence is typically less than 20% to 25%.[353–358]

The timing and type of recurrence are important prognostic factors.[353–358] Patients with early relapse, within the first 2 years following initial diagnosis, have a poorer prognosis with 4% to 12% 5-year survival. Those with later recurrence experience a 23% to 48% 5-year survival.[353–358] Recurrence may be very late, as compared with most other pediatric and adolescent cancers. A report from the Dana-Farber Cancer Institute described late recurrences between 5.7 and 17.1 years after diagnosis.[359] Simultaneous local and distant recurrences have been observed to be associated with more aggressive disease with earlier recurrence and poorer outcome.[221,355,356,358,360]

Patients with suspected recurrence should be evaluated appropriately to assess the extent of relapse at local and distant sites. The majority of patients with local treatment failure have concomitant distant gross or microscopic disease. Recommended restaging studies at the time of relapse are similar to those recommended at the time of initial diagnosis. Imaging of the primary tumor site at the time of relapse may be difficult to interpret due to prior therapy.

There is no established treatment regimen for these patients with relapsed ES. Treatment of these patients requires careful understanding of the goals of therapy between patients, families, and the medical team. Options for second-line therapy include multiagent chemotherapy (particularly cooperative group phase II trials), local control measures with RT and surgery, novel therapies, or a combination of these as appropriate.

Patients with local recurrence are usually treated with surgery and further chemotherapy.[358] Recurrent distant disease involving the lungs or bones occurs in more than 50% of patients presenting with local recurrence and mandates further chemotherapy.[192,217,219,296,319,356,361] Whole-lung irradiation may improve the outcome for patients with lung metastases at relapse.[358]

Chemotherapy options are limited and dependent on the patient's prior treatment and possible impaired function of vital organs (e.g., heart and kidneys) at the time of relapse. IE had a particularly high response rate in patients with recurrent ES who had not previously received either agent.[362,363] Patients may respond to agents previously used as part of an initial treatment attempt.[364] A 34% response rate was seen in patients treated with higher dose IFO (15 grams/m^2/course) despite prior therapy with standard dose IFO.[365] Two camptothecin-based chemotherapy combinations have gained favor as salvage regimens for these patients. Although single-agent topotecan has a low response rate in ES,[366,367] the combination of topotecan and CYC has a 35% response rate in this setting.[368–370] More recent studies have suggested that the combination of irinotecan and temozolomide may have a similar response rate.[371,372] Given the tolerability of these regimens, they may provide a backbone on which to add biologically targeted therapies, including bevacizumab and IGF1R monoclonal antibodies.

Several studies have evaluated high-dose therapy with autologous hematopoietic stem cell reinfusion for patients with relapsed ES. The interpretation of these studies is hampered by the heterogeneity of treated patients, the heterogeneity of conditioning regimens, and the lack of randomized studies.[373] High-dose consolidation therapy with melphalan and ETO with hyperfractionated total body irradiation ± carboplatin, followed by autologous stem cell reinfusion, despite initial response, has failed to result in long-term remission in the treatment of early relapse.[329,374,375] Results from a hematopoietic stem cell transplantation regimen using combinations of active alkylating agents including busulfan and melphalan seem more encouraging and may improve the prognosis for patients at relapse.[325,337,353,375,376] However, the role of stem cell transplantation in the treatment of patients with recurrent disease remains unclear and further studies to define the best approach for these patients are needed.[325,329,374,377]

The presence of a specific molecular transcript, thought to play an active role in the ES tumorigenesis, suggests that specific molecular targets may provide future therapeutic approaches. Efforts are focused on directly inhibiting chimeric proteins (or their downstream targets) and on immunotherapy directed at tumor cell specific epitopes derived from chimeric products.[378] A variety of targeted therapies have been evaluated in patients with relapsed ES, with some agents showing more promise than other agents. Despite c-KIT expression on ES and *in vitro* evidence of efficacy, imatinib has not shown clinically relevant activity in patients with relapsed ES.[379] Likewise, the preclinical data supporting cytarabine as an agent targeting EWS/FLI did not translate into effective therapy for patients with relapsed ES.[153,154] In contrast, the use of bevacizumab in this patient population has shown early indications of activity, with prolonged stabilization of disease noted.[380] The COG is evaluating bevacizumab in combination with camptothecin-based chemotherapy for patients with relapsed ES.

Agents targeting the IGF1R and mTOR pathways have stimulated intense interest in recent years, based on preclinical evidence of efficacy in ES.[103,381] Several monoclonal antibodies against the IGF1R are undergoing evaluation in patients with relapsed ES. Preliminary reports suggest that these agents have activity in this setting and additional studies are ongoing.[382,383] One rapamycin analogue, deforolimus, has also been evaluated in patients with relapsed ES, with early evidence of clinical activity.[384,385] Studies of these compounds together with chemotherapy are planned for patients with relapsed and high-risk ES.

In an attempt to immunologically target the breakpoint region of tumor-specific fusion proteins expressed in ES, peptide pulsed vaccination has been investigated. To date, however, immune-directed therapies have failed to reach clinical applicability.[386,387] Further progress in developing high-density DNA microarrays as tools for the identification of tumor-specific gene expression profiles with obvious diagnostic value may lead to new therapeutic targets and additional new treatment strategies in patients with ES.

LATE EFFECTS

Survivors of ES face a number of potential late effects. These late effects include orthopedic issues, other organ toxicity, and risk of second malignancies (see also Chapter 49). As noted in the surgery section, preservation of the hand in patients with upper extremity primaries is associated with an improved functional outcome and better self-image. Orthopedic outcome for patients with lower extremity lesions can be quite satisfactory even if distal amputation is required.[388] Limb salvage procedures using massive internal prostheses or bone allografts can be complicated by late prosthetic failure or infection, requiring reoperation and, sometimes, delayed amputation.[388] At least two reports have indicated that overall function and quality of life do not differ based on use of amputation or limb salvage procedure for local control. Radiation therapy as a component of local control can be complicated by growth disturbances of both bone and soft tissue.

Organ-specific late effects are agent dependent,[389] and are reviewed in detail in Chapter 49. Briefly, anthracyclines, including DOX, induce a dose-related cardiomyopathy. Protocol doses are therefore usually limited to less than a lifetime total of 450 mg/m^2. In addition, administration is often either prolonged over a 48-hour period or, if given as a short intravenous bolus, preceded by the cardioprotectant dexrazoxane. Thoracic irradiation that includes the heart can augment the cardiotoxicity of anthracyclines. DOX is sometimes stopped at the lower cumulative dose of 300 mg/m^2 if thoracic irradiation is to be given. The alkylating agents CYC and IFO are

associated with infertility, especially male infertility. Sperm cryopreservation should be offered to postpubertal boys prior to the institution of chemotherapy. With improvements in technology, ovarian cryopreservation could similarly be offered to females. Gonadal irradiation is typically sterilizing. Shielding of the testes and transposition of the ovaries should be considered, particularly with pelvic primary sites. In addition, IFO can cause a persistent renal tubular electrolyte loss and, less commonly, a decrease in glomerular function, also in a dose-dependent fashion.[390]

ES survivors have two major risk factors for second malignancies: RT and intensive chemotherapy. The most common radiation-associated second malignant solid tumor is osteosarcoma. This is dose related, with a significant increase in rate at administered doses above 40 Gy, although an increased rate of osteosarcoma has been reported after as little as 10 Gy. Moreover, the onset may be late.[391,392] The cumulative incidence of second malignant solid tumors among ES patients treated with RT has been estimated as 1.4% to 5.5% at 10 years.[391–397]

Chemotherapy has been associated with secondary leukemia in ES survivors. There has been a 1% to 3% rate of secondary leukemia following treatment for ES, usually within 3 years of initial diagnosis. This risk has been associated with both alkylator and ETO exposure.[395,396,398] In INT-0091, there was no apparent difference in second malignancies between therapeutic arms with and without ETO, suggesting that, in the dose and schedule employed, the addition of ETO did not independently increase the risk of second malignancy.[225] A single-institution study suggested that more intensive protocols that included higher-doses of alkylators and ETO had a higher risk of secondary leukemia.[395] In addition, arm C of INT 0091 utilized very high cumulative doses of IFO (140 g/m^2) and CYC (17.6 g/m^2) and noted a cumulative incidence of therapy-related leukemia of approximately 11%.[398] In INT-0154, which compared a dose-intensified chemotherapy regimen to a standard regimen with similar cumulative alkylator and ETO doses, the rate of second leukemia was similar between treatment groups.[241] There may therefore be a threshold or stepwise effect, with a low rate of secondary leukemia with conventional dose treatment but a much higher rate at high cumulative doses.

Despite these concerns, the overall functioning of survivors of ES is reasonably good.[399] There is frequent need for medical services among survivors, even beyond 5 years from initial diagnosis. In one report, 7.6% of 5-year survivors had later adverse events, including relapse, second malignancies, and cardiac.[400] These findings underscore the need to ensure adequate follow-up and the provision of adequate resources is necessary.[401]

SUMMARY AND CONCLUSIONS

ES is the second most frequent primary bone cancer in children and young adults. Patients presenting with localized disease have an approximately two-thirds chance of being cured. Those whose disease is initially metastatic have a much worse outcome. Those with isolated pulmonary metastases experience an approximately 30% EFS, whereas those with more widespread disease, usually involving bone or bone marrow, have a less than 15% chance of cure with currently available therapy. Patients whose disease has recurred share this grim outlook. Advances in the biology of ES have led to increased knowledge concerning the underlying molecular basis of disease, as yet insufficient to have led to the new therapeutic approaches required to cure those with currently refractory disease and to cure all with fewer short- and long-term toxicities.

References

1. Gurney JG, Swensen AR, Bulterys M. Malignant bone tumors. In: Ries LAG, Smith MA, Gurney JG, et al., eds. Cancer incidence and survival among children and adolescents: United States SEER Program 1975–1995. Bethesda, MD: National Institutes of Health, 1999:99–110.
2. Kayhan B, Ozer D, Ozaslan E, et al. Ewing sarcoma in a geriatric patient. Aging Clin Exp Res 2005;17:347–349.
3. Zucman-Rossi J, Batzer MA, Stoneking M, et al. Interethnic polymorphism of EWS intron 6: genome plasticity mediated by Alu retroposition and recombination. Hum Genet 1997;99:357–363.
4. Kolomietz E, Meyn MS, Pandita A, et al. The role of Alu repeat clusters as mediators of recurrent chromosomal aberrations in tumors. Genes Chromosomes Cancer 2002;35: 97–112.
5. Winn DM, Li FP, Robison LL, et al. A case-control study of the etiology of Ewing's sarcoma. Cancer Epidemiol Biomarkers Prev 1992;1:525–532.
6. Holly EA, Aston DA, Ahn DK, et al. Ewing's bone sarcoma, paternal occupational exposure, and other factors. Am J Epidemiol 1992;135:122–129.
7. Delattre O, Zucman J, Melot T, et al. The Ewing family of tumors—a subgroup of small-round-cell tumors defined by specific chimeric transcripts. N Engl J Med 1994; 331:294–299.
8. Ushigome S, Machinami R, Sorensen PH. Ewing sarcoma/primitive neuroectodermal tumour (PNET). In: Fletcher CDM, Unni KK, Mertens F, eds. World Health Organization classification of tumours. Pathology and genetics. Tumours of soft tissue and bone. Lyon, France: IARC Press, 2002:297–300, Chapter 14.
9. Delattre O, Zucman J, Plougastel B, et al. Gene fusion with an ETS DNA-binding domain caused by chromosome translocation in human tumours. Nature 1992;359: 162–165.
10. Zucman J, Delattre O, Desmaze C, et al. Cloning and characterization of the Ewing's sarcoma and peripheral neuroepithelioma t(11;22) translocation breakpoints. Genes Chromosomes Cancer 1992;5:271–277.
11. Ben-David Y, Giddens EB, Bernstein A. Identification and mapping of a common proviral integration site Fli-1 in erythroleukemia cells induced by Friend murine leukemia virus. Proc Natl Acad Sci 1990;87:1332–1336.
12. Aurias A, Rimbaut C, Buffe D, et al. Translocation of chromosome 22 in Ewing's sarcoma. C R Seances Acad Sci III 1983;296:1105–1107.
13. Turc-Carel C, Aurias A, Mugneret F, et al. Chromosomes in Ewing's sarcoma. I. An evaluation of 85 cases of remarkable consistency of t(11;22)(q24;q12). Cancer Genet Cytogenet 1988;32:229–238.
14. Hattinger CM, Rumpler S, Strehl S, et al. Prognostic impact of deletions at 1p36 and numerical aberrations in Ewing tumors. Genes Chromosomes Cancer 1999;24: 243–254.
15. Hattinger CM, Potschger U, Tarkkanen M, et al. Prognostic impact of chromosomal aberrations in Ewing tumours. Br J Cancer 2002;86:1763–1769.
16. Maurici D, Perez-Atayde A, Grier HE, et al. Frequency and implications of chromosome 8 and 12 gains in Ewing sarcoma. Cancer Genet Cytogenet 1998;100:106–110.
17. Szuhai K, Ijszenga M, Tanke HJ, et al. Molecular cytogenetic characterization of four previously established and two newly established Ewing sarcoma cell lines. Cancer Genet Cytogenet 2006;166:173–179.
18. Kovar H, Jug G, Aryee DN, et al. Among genes involved in the RB dependent cell cycle regulatory cascade, the p16 tumor suppressor gene is frequently lost in the Ewing family of tumors. Oncogene 1997;15:2225–2232.
19. Wei G, Antonescu CR, de Alava E, et al. Prognostic impact of INK4 A deletion in Ewing sarcoma. Cancer 2000;89:793–799.
20. Savola S, Nardi F, Scotlandi K, et al. Microdeletions in 9p21.3 induce false negative results in CDKN2A FISH analysis of Ewing sarcoma. Cytogenet Genome Res 2007; 119:21–26.
21. Savola S, Klami A, Tripathi A, et al. Combined use of expression and CGH arrays pinpoints novel candidate genes in Ewing sarcoma family of tumors. BMC Cancer 2009; 9:17.
22. Ambros IM, Ambros PF, Strehl S, et al. MIC2 is a specific marker for Ewing's sarcoma and peripheral primitive neuroectodermal tumors. Evidence for a common histogenesis of Ewing's sarcoma and peripheral primitive neuroectodermal tumors from MIC2 expression and specific chromosome aberration. Cancer 1991;67:1886–1893.
23. Ladanyi M, Lewis R, Garin-Chesa P, et al. EWS rearrangement in Ewing's sarcoma and peripheral neuroectodermal tumor. Molecular detection and correlation with cytogenetic analysis and MIC2 expression. Diagn Mol Pathol 1993;2:141–146.
24. Hamilton G, Fellinger EJ, Schratter I, et al. Characterization of a human endocrine tissue and tumor-associated Ewing's sarcoma antigen. Cancer Res 1988;48:6127–6131.
25. Kovar H, Dworzak M, Strehl S, et al. Overexpression of the pseudoautosomal gene MIC2 in Ewing's sarcoma and peripheral primitive neuroectodermal tumor. Oncogene 1990;5:1067–1070.
26. Lessnick SL, Dacwag CS, Golub TR. The Ewing's sarcoma oncoprotein EWS/FLI induces a p53-dependent growth arrest in primary human fibroblasts. Cancer Cell 2002;1:393–401.
27. Rorie CJ, Thomas VD, Chen P, et al. The EWS/Fli-1 fusion gene switches the differentiation program of neuroblastomas to Ewing sarcoma/peripheral primitive neuroectodermal tumors. Cancer Res 2004;64:1266–1277.
28. Desmaze C, Zucman J, Delattre O, et al. Interphase molecular cytogenetics of Ewing's sarcoma and peripheral neuroepithelioma t(11;22) with flanking and overlapping cosmid probes. Cancer Genet Cytogenet 1994;74:13–18.
29. Sorensen PH, Lessnick SL, Lopez-Terrada D, et al. A second Ewing's sarcoma translocation, t(21;22), fuses the EWS gene to another ETS-family transcription factor, ERG. Nat Genet 1994;6:146–151.
30. Zucman J, Melot T, Desmaze C, et al. Combinatorial generation of variable fusion proteins in the Ewing family of tumours. Embo J 1993;12:4481–4487.
31. Jeon IS, Davis JN, Braun BS, et al. A variant Ewing's sarcoma translocation (7;22) fuses the EWS gene to the ETS gene ETV1. Oncogene 1995;10:1229–1234.
32. Urano F, Umezawa A, Yabe H, et al. Molecular analysis of Ewing's sarcoma: another fusion gene, EWS-E1AF, available for diagnosis. Jpn J Cancer Res 1998;89:703–711.
33. Peter M, Couturier J, Pacquement H, et al. A new member of the ETS family fused to EWS in Ewing tumors. Oncogene 1997;14:1159–1164.
34. Kovar H, Ban J, Pospisilova S. Potentials for RNAi in sarcoma research and therapy: Ewing's sarcoma as a model. Semin Cancer Biol 2003;13:275–281.
35. Desmaze C, Brizard F, Turc-Carel C, et al. Multiple chromosomal mechanisms generate an EWS/FLI1 or an EWS/ERG fusion gene in Ewing tumors. Cancer Genet Cytogenet 1997;97:12–19.
36. Shing DC, McMullan DJ, Roberts P, et al. FUS/ERG gene fusions in Ewing's tumors. Cancer Res 2003;63:4568–4576.
37. Ng TL, O'Sullivan MJ, Pallen CJ, et al. Ewing sarcoma with novel translocation t(2;16) producing an in-frame fusion of FUS and FEV. J Mol Diagn 2007;9:459–463.
38. Wang L, Bhargava R, Zheng T, et al. Undifferentiated small round cell sarcomas with rare EWS gene fusions: identification of a novel EWS-SP3 fusion and of additional cases with the EWS-ETV1 and EWS-FEV fusions. J Mol Diagn. 2007;9:498–509.
39. Yamaguchi S, Yamazaki Y, Ishikawa Y, et al. EWSR1 is fused to POU5F1 in a bone tumor with translocation t(6;22)(p21;q12). Genes Chromosomes Cancer. 2005;43: 217–22.
40. Mastrangelo T, Modena P, Tornielli S, et al. A novel zinc finger gene is fused to EWS in small round cell tumor. Oncogene 2000;19:3799–3804.
41. Szuhai K, Ijszenga M, de Jong D, et al. The NFATc2 gene is involved in a novel cloned translocation in a Ewing sarcoma variant that couples its function in immunology to oncology. Clin Cancer Res 2009;15:2259–2268.
42. Szuhai K, Ijszenga M, Tanke HJ, et al. Detection and molecular cytogenetic characterization of a novel ring chromosome in a histological variant of Ewing sarcoma. Cancer Genet Cytogenet 2007;172:12–22.
43. Marley EF, Liapis H, Humphrey PA, et al. Primitive neuroectodermal tumor of the kidney—another enigma: a pathologic, immunohistochemical, and molecular diagnostic study. Am J Surg Pathol 1997;21:354–359.
44. Sezer O, Jugovic D, Blohmer JU, et al. CD99 positivity and EWS-FLI1 gene rearrangement identify a breast tumor in a 60-year-old patient with attributes of the Ewing family of neoplasms. Diagn Mol Pathol 1999;8:120–124.
45. Sheaff M, McManus A, Scheimberg I, et al. Primitive neuroectodermal tumor of the kidney confirmed by fluorescence in situ hybridization. Am J Surg Pathol 1997;21: 461–468.
46. Kuroda M, Urano M, Abe M, et al. Primary primitive neuroectodermal tumor of the kidney. Pathol Int 2000;50:967–972.
47. Mikami Y, Nakajima M, Hashimoto H, et al. Primary pulmonary primitive neuroectodermal tumor (PNET). A case report. Pathol Res Pract 2001;197:113–119; discussion 121–122.
48. Kie JH, Lee MK, Kim CJ, et al. Primary Ewing's sarcoma of the duodenum: a case report. Int J Surg Pathol 2003;11:331–337.
49. Tokudome N, Tanaka K, Kai MH, et al. Primitive neuroectodermal tumor of the transverse colonic mesentery defined by the presence of EWS-FLI1 chimeric mRNA in a Japanese woman. J Gastroenterol 2002;37:543–549.
50. Shek TW, Chan GC, Khong PL, et al. Ewing sarcoma of the small intestine. J Pediatr Hematol Oncol 2001;23:530–532.
51. Maesawa C, Iijima S, Sato N, et al. Esophageal extraskeletal Ewing's sarcoma. Hum Pathol 2002;33:130–132.
52. Colecchia M, Dagrada G, Poliani PL, et al. Primary primitive peripheral neuroectodermal tumor of the prostate. Immunophenotypic and molecular study of a case. Arch Pathol Lab Med 2003;127:e190–e193.
53. Sinkre P, Albores-Saavedra J, Miller DS, et al. Endometrial endometrioid carcinomas associated with Ewing sarcoma/peripheral primitive neuroectodermal tumor. Int J Gynecol Pathol 2000;19:127–132.
54. Kato K, Kato Y, Ijiri R, et al. Ewing's sarcoma family of tumor arising in the adrenal gland—possible diagnostic pitfall in pediatric pathology: histologic, immunohistochemical, ultrastructural, and molecular study. Hum Pathol 2001;32:1012–1016.
55. Dedeurwaerdere F, Giannini C, Sciot R, et al. Primary peripheral PNET/Ewing's sarcoma of the dura: a clinicopathologic entity distinct from central PNET. Mod Patho 2002;15:673–678.
56. Zucman-Rossi J, Legoix P, Victor JM, et al. Chromosome translocation based on illegitimate recombination in human tumors. Proc Natl Acad Sci U S A 1998;95:11786–11791.
57. Lessnick SL, Braun BS, Denny CT, et al. Multiple domains mediate transformation by the Ewing's sarcoma EWS/FLI-1 fusion gene. Oncogene 1995;10:423–431.
58. May WA, Gishizky ML, Lessnick SL, et al. Ewing sarcoma 11;22 translocation produces a chimeric transcription factor that requires the DNA-binding domain encoded by FLI1 for transformation. Proc Natl Acad Sci U S A 1993;90:5752–5756.
59. Braunreiter CL, Hancock JD, Coffin CM, et al. Expression of EWS-ETS fusions in NIH3T3 cells reveals significant differences to Ewing's sarcoma. Cell Cycle 2006;5: 2753–2759.
60. Kovar H, Aryee DN, Jug G, et al. EWS/FLI-1 antagonists induce growth inhibition of Ewing tumor cells in vitro. Cell Growth Differ 1996;7:429–437.
61. Lambert G, Bertrand JR, Fattal E, et al. EWS fli-1 antisense nanocapsules inhibits Ewing sarcoma-related tumor in mice. Biochem Biophys Res Commun 2000;279:401–406.
62. Ouchida M, Ohno T, Fujimura Y, et al. Loss of tumorigenicity of Ewing's sarcoma cells expressing antisense RNA to EWS-fusion transcripts. Oncogene 1995;11:1049–1054.
63. Tanaka K, Iwakuma T, Harimaya K, et al. EWS-Fli1 antisense oligodeoxynucleotide inhibits proliferation of human Ewing's sarcoma and primitive neuroectodermal tumor cells. J Clin Invest 1997;99:239–247.
64. Toretsky JA, Connell Y, Neckers L, et al. Inhibition of EWS-FLI-1 fusion protein with antisense oligodeoxynucleotides. J Neurooncol 1997;31:9–16.
65. Dohjima T, Lee NS, Li H, et al. Small interfering RNAs expressed from a Pol III promoter suppress the EWS/Fli-1 transcript in an Ewing sarcoma cell line. Mol Ther 2003;7:811–816.
66. Prieur A, Tirode F, Cohen P, et al. EWS/FLI-1 silencing and gene profiling of Ewing cells reveal downstream oncogenic pathways and a crucial role for repression of insulin-like growth factor binding protein 3. Mol Cell Biol 2004;24:7275–7283.
67. Smith R, Owen LA, Trem DJ, et al. Expression profiling of EWS/FLI identifies NKX2.2 as a critical target gene in Ewing's sarcoma. Cancer Cell 2006;9:405–416.
68. Teitell MA, Thompson AD, Sorensen PH, et al. EWS/ETS fusion genes induce epithelial and neuroectodermal differentiation in NIH 3T3 fibroblasts. Lab Invest 1999;79:1535–1543.
69. Thompson AD, Teitell MA, Arvand A, et al. Divergent Ewing's sarcoma EWS/ETS fusions confer a common tumorigenic phenotype on NIH3T3 cells. Oncogene 1999;18: 5506–5513.

70. Arvand A, Welford SM, Teitell MA, et al. The COOH-terminal domain of FLI-1 is necessary for full tumorigenesis and transcriptional modulation by EWS/FLI-1. Cancer Res 2001;61:5311–5317.
71. Zoubek A, Dockhorn-Dworniczak B, Delattre O, et al. Does expression of different EWS chimeric transcripts define clinically distinct risk groups of Ewing tumor patients? J Clin Oncol 1996;14:1245–1251.
72. Bailly RA, Bosselut R, Zucman J, et al. DNA-binding and transcriptional activation properties of the EWS-FLI-1 fusion protein resulting from the t(11;22) translocation in Ewing sarcoma. Mol Cell Biol 1994;14:3230–3241.
73. Feng L, Lee KA. A repetitive element containing a critical tyrosine residue is required for transcriptional activation by the EWS/ATF1 oncogene. Oncogene 2001;20:4161–4168.
74. Bertolotti A, Lutz Y, Heard DJ, et al. hTAF(II)68, a novel RNA/ssDNA-binding protein with homology to the pro-oncoproteins TLS/FUS and EWS is associated with both TFIID and RNA polymerase II. Embo J 1996;15:5022–5031.
75. Bertolotti A, Melot T, Acker J, et al. EWS, but not EWS-FLI-1, is associated with both TFIID and RNA polymerase II: interactions between two members of the TET family, EWS and hTAFII68, and subunits of TFIID and RNA polymerase II complexes. Mol Cell Biol 1998;18:1489–1497.
76. Chansky HA, Hu M, Hickstein DD, et al. Oncogenic TLS/ERG and EWS/Fli-1 fusion proteins inhibit RNA splicing mediated by YB-1 protein. Cancer Res 2001;61:3586–3590.
77. Knoop LL, Baker SJ. The splicing factor U1 C represses EWS/FLI-mediated transactivation. J Biol Chem 2000;275:24865–24871.
78. Spahn L, Petermann R, Siligan C, et al. Interaction of the EWS NH2 terminus with BARD1 links the Ewing's sarcoma gene to a common tumor suppressor pathway. Cancer Res 2002;62:4583–4587.
79. Yang L, Chansky HA, Hickstein DD. EWS.Fli-1 fusion protein interacts with hyperphosphorylated RNA polymerase II and interferes with serine-arginine protein-mediated RNA splicing. J Biol Chem 2000;275:37612–37618.
80. Yang L, Embree LJ, Hickstein DD. TLS-ERG leukemia fusion protein inhibits RNA splicing mediated by serine-arginine proteins. Mol Cell Biol 2000;20:3345–3354.
81. Petermann R, Mossier BM, Aryee DN, et al. Oncogenic EWS-Fli1 interacts with hsRPB7, a subunit of human RNA polymerase II. Oncogene 1998;17:603–610.
82. Knoop LL, Baker SJ. EWS/FLI alters 5′-splice site selection. J Biol Chem 2001;276:22317–22322.
83. Braun BS, Frieden R, Lessnick SL, et al. Identification of target genes for the Ewing's sarcoma EWS/FLI fusion protein by representational difference analysis. Mol Cell Biol 1995;15:4623–4630.
84. Dauphinot L, de Oliveira C, Melot T, et al. Analysis of the expression of cell cycle regulators in Ewing cell lines: EWS-FLI-1 modulates p57KIP2 and c-Myc expression. Oncogene 2001;20:3258–3265.
85. Kinsey M, Smith R, Lessnick SL. NR0B1 is required for the oncogenic phenotype mediated by EWS/FLI in Ewing's sarcoma. Mol Cancer Res 2006;4:851–859.
86. Hahm KB, Cho K, Lee C, et al. Repression of the gene encoding the TGF-beta type II receptor is a major target of the EWS-FLI1 oncoprotein. Nat Genet 1999;23:222–227.
87. Im YH, Kim HT, Lee C, et al. EWS-FLI1, EWS-ERG, and EWS-ETV1 oncoproteins of Ewing tumor family all suppress transcription of transforming growth factor beta type II receptor gene. Cancer Res 2000;60:1536–1540.
88. Jaishankar S, Zhang J, Roussel MF, et al. Transforming activity of EWS/FLI is not strictly dependent upon DNA-binding activity. Oncogene 1999;18:5592–5597.
89. Welford SM, Hebert SP, Deneen B, et al. DNA binding domain-independent pathways are involved in EWS/FLI1-mediated oncogenesis. J Biol Chem 2001;276:41977–41984.
90. Kovar H, Jug G, Hattinger C, et al. The EWS protein is dispensable for Ewing tumor growth. Cancer Res 2001;61:5992–5997.
91. Deneen B, Denny CT. Loss of p16 pathways stabilizes EWS/FLI1 expression and complements EWS/FLI1 mediated transformation. Oncogene 2001;20:6731–6741.
92. Eliazer S, Spencer J, Ye D, et al. Alteration of mesodermal cell differentiation by EWS/FLI-1, the oncogene implicated in Ewing's sarcoma. Mol Cell Biol 2003;23:482–492.
93. Torchia EC, Jaishankar S, Baker SJ. Ewing tumor fusion proteins block the differentiation of pluripotent marrow stromal cells. Cancer Res 2003;63:3464–3468.
94. Zwerner JP, Guimbellot J, May WA. EWS/FLI function varies in different cellular backgrounds. Exp Cell Res 2003;290:414–419.
95. Hamelin R, Zucman J, Melot T, et al. p53 mutations in human tumors with chimeric EWS/FLI-1 genes. Int J Cancer 1994;57:336–340.
96. Kovar H, Auinger A, Jug G, et al. Narrow spectrum of infrequent p53 mutations and absence of MDM2 amplification in Ewing tumours. Oncogene 1993;8:2683–2690.
97. Kovar H, Jug G, Printz D, et al. Characterization of distinct consecutive phases in non-genotoxic p53-induced apoptosis of Ewing tumor cells and the rate-limiting role of caspase 8. Oncogene 2000;19:4096–4107.
98. Kovar H, Pospisilova S, Jug G, et al. Response of Ewing tumor cells to forced and activated p53 expression. Oncogene 2003;22:3193–3204.
99. Ban Kauer M, Schaefer KL, Poremba C, et al. EWS-FLI1 suppresses NOTCH-activated p53 in Ewing's sarcoma. Cancer Res 2008;68:7100–7109.
100. Toretsky JA, Kalebic T, Blakesley V, et al. The insulin-like growth factor-I receptor is required for EWS/FLI-1 transformation of fibroblasts. J Biol Chem 1997;272:30822–30827.
101. Scotlandi K, Benini S, Sarti M, et al. Insulin-like growth factor I receptor-mediated circuit in Ewing's sarcoma/peripheral neuroectodermal tumor: a possible therapeutic target. Cancer Res 1996;56:4570–4574.
102. Scotlandi K, Benini S, Nanni P, et al. Blockage of insulin-like growth factor-I receptor inhibits the growth of Ewing's sarcoma in athymic mice. Cancer Res 1998;58:4127–4131.
103. Kolb EA, Gorlick R, Houghton PJ, et al. Initial testing (stage 1) of a monoclonal antibody (SCH 717454) against the IGF-1 receptor by the pediatric preclinical testing program. Pediatr Blood Cancer 2008;50:1190–1197.
104. Girnita L, Girnita A, Wang M, et al. A link between basic fibroblast growth factor (bFGF) and EWS/FLI-1 in Ewing's sarcoma cells. Oncogene 2000;19:4298–4301.
105. Lawlor ER, Lim JF, Tao W, et al. The Ewing tumor family of peripheral primitive neuroectodermal tumors expresses human gastrin-releasing peptide. Cancer Res 1998;58:2469–2476.
106. Uren A, Merchant MS, Sun CJ, et al. Beta-platelet-derived growth factor receptor mediates motility and growth of Ewing's sarcoma cells. Oncogene 2003;22:2334–2342.
107. Ricotti E, Fagioli F, Garelli E, et al. c-kit is expressed in soft tissue sarcoma of neuroectodermic origin and its ligand prevents apoptosis of neoplastic cells. Blood 1998;91:2397–2405.
108. Ewing J. Diffuse endothelioma of bone. Proc N Y Pathol Soc 1921;21:17–24.
109. Mahoney JP, Alexander RW. Ewing's sarcoma. A light- and electron-microscopic study of 21 cases. Am J Surg Pathol 1978;2:283–298.
110. Bednar B. Solid dendritic cell angiosarcoma: re-interpretation of extraskeletal sarcoma resembling Ewing's sarcoma. J Pathol 1980;130:217–222.
111. Llombart-Bosch A, Peydro-Olaya A, Gomar F. Ultrastructure of one Ewing's sarcoma of bone with endothelial character and a comparative review of the vessels in 27 cases of typical Ewing's sarcoma. Pathol Res Pract 1980;167:71–87.
112. Mierau GW. Extraskeletal Ewing's sarcoma (peripheral neuroepithelioma). Ultrastruct Pathol 1985;9:91–98.
113. Shimada H, Newton WA Jr, Soule EH, et al. Pathologic features of extraosseous Ewing's sarcoma: a report from the Intergroup Rhabdomyosarcoma Study. Hum Pathol 1988;19:442–453.
114. Cavazzana AO, Miser JS, Jefferson J, et al. Experimental evidence for a neural origin of Ewing's sarcoma of bone. Am J Pathol 1987;127:507–518.
115. Noguera R, Triche TJ, Navarro S, et al. Dynamic model of differentiation in Ewing's sarcoma cells. Comparative analysis of morphologic, immunocytochemical, and oncogene expression parameters. Lab Invest 1992;66:143–151.
116. Navarro S, Cavazzana AO, Llombart-Bosch A, et al. Comparison of Ewing's sarcoma of bone and peripheral neuroepithelioma. An immunocytochemical and ultrastructural analysis of two primitive neuroectodermal neoplasms. Arch Pathol Lab Med 1994;118:608–615.
117. Navarro S, Gonzalez-Devesa M, Ferrandez-Izquierdo A, et al. Scanning electron microscopic evidence for neural differentiation in Ewing's sarcoma cell lines. Virchows Arch A Pathol Anat Histopathol 1990;416:383–391.
118. Lizard-Nacol S, Volk C, Lizard G, et al. Abnormal expression of neurofilament proteins in Ewing's sarcoma cell cultures. Tumour Biol 1992;13:36–43.
119. O'Regan S, Diebler MF, Meunier FM, et al. A Ewing's sarcoma cell line showing some, but not all, of the traits of a cholinergic neuron. J Neurochem 1995;64:69–76.
120. Hara S, Adachi Y, Kaneko Y, et al. Evidence for heterogeneous groups of neuronal differentiation of Ewing's sarcoma. Br J Cancer 1991;64:1025–1030.
121. Khan J, Wei JS, Ringner M, et al. Classification and diagnostic prediction of cancers using gene expression profiling and artificial neural networks. Nat Med 2001;7:673–679.
122. Truong AH, Ben-David Y. The role of Fli-1 in normal cell function and malignant transformation. Oncogene 2000;19:6482–6489.
123. Meyer D, Wolff CM, Stiegler P, et al. Xl-fli, the Xenopus homologue of the fli-1 gene, is expressed during embryogenesis in a restricted pattern evocative of neural crest cell distribution. Mech Dev 1993;44:109–121.
124. Meyer D, Stiegler P, Hindelang C, et al. Whole-mount in situ hybridization reveals the expression of the Xl-Fli gene in several lineages of migrating cells in Xenopus embryos. Int J Dev Biol 1995;39:909–919.
125. Vlaeminck-Guillem V, Carrere S, Dewitte F, et al. The Ets family member Erg gene is expressed in mesodermal tissues and neural crests at fundamental steps during mouse embryogenesis. Mech Dev 2000;91:331–335.
126. Sulva M-L, Riggi N, Stehle J-C, et al. Identification of cancer stem cells in Ewing's sarcoma. Cancer Res 2009;69:1776–1781.
127. Tirode F, Laud-Duval K, Prieur A, et al. Mesenchymal stem cell features of Ewing tumors. Cancer Cell 2007;11:421–429.
128. Riggi N, Suva ML, Suva D, et al. EWS-FLI-1 expression triggers a Ewing's sarcoma initiation program in primary human mesenchymal stem cells. Cancer Res 2008;68:2176–2185.
129. Falk S, Alpert M. Five-year survival of patients with Ewing's sarcoma. Surg Gynecol Obstet 1967;124:319–324.
130. Fagnou C, Michon J, Peter M, et al. Presence of tumor cells in bone marrow but not in blood is associated with adverse prognosis in patients with Ewing's tumor. Societe Francaise d'Oncologie Pediatrique. J Clin Oncol 1998;16:1707–1711.
131. Schleiermacher G, Peter M, Oberlin O, et al. Increased risk of systemic relapses associated with bone marrow micrometastasis and circulating tumor cells in localized Ewing tumor. J Clin Oncol 2003;21:85–91.
132. Zoubek A, Ladenstein R, Windhager R, et al. Predictive potential of testing for bone marrow involvement in Ewing tumor patients by RT-PCR: a preliminary evaluation. Int J Cancer 1998;79:56–60.
133. Zoubek A, Kovar H, Kronberger M, et al. Mobilization of tumour cells during biopsy in an infant with Ewing sarcoma. Eur J Pediatr 1996;155:373–376.
134. Roberts P, Burchill SA, Brownhill S, et al. Ploidy and karyotype complexity are powerful prognostic indicators in the Ewing's sarcoma family of tumors: a study by the United Kingdom Cancer Cytogenetics and the Children's Cancer and Leukaemia Group. Genes Chrom Cancer 2007;47:207–220.
135. Perotti D, Corletto V, Giardini R, et al. Retrospective analysis of ploidy in primary osseous and extraosseous Ewing family tumors in children. Tumori 1998;84:493–498.
136. de Alava E, Antonescu CR, Panizo A, et al. Prognostic impact of P53 status in Ewing sarcoma. Cancer 2000;89:783–792.
137. Ohali A, Avigad S, Cohen IJ, et al. Association between telomerase activity and outcome in patients with nonmetastatic Ewing family of tumors. J Clin Oncol 2003;21:3836–3843.
138. Perri T, Fogel M, Mor S, et al. Effect of P-glycoprotein expression on outcome in the Ewing family of tumors. Pediatr Hematol Oncol 2001;18:325–334.
139. Honoki K, Stojanovski E, McEvoy M, et al. Prognostic significance of p16INK4a alteration for Ewing sarcoma. Cancer 2007;110:1351–1360.
140. de Alava E, Kawai A, Healey JH, et al. EWS-FLI1 fusion transcript structure is an independent determinant of prognosis in Ewing's sarcoma. J Clin Oncol 1998;16:1248–1255.
141. Ohali A, Avigad S, Zaizov R, et al. Prediction of high risk Ewing's sarcoma by gene expression profiling. Oncogene 2004;23:8997–9006.
142. Scotlandi K, Remondini D, Castellani G, et al. Overcoming resistance to conventional drugs in Ewing sarcoma and identification of molecular predictors of outcome. J Clin Oncol 2009;27:2209–2216.
143. Delepine N, Delepine G, Cornille H, et al. Prognostic factors in patients with localized Ewing's sarcoma: the effect on survival of actual received drug dose intensity and of histologic response to induction therapy. J Chemother 1997;9:352–363.
144. Oberlin O, Patte C, Demeocq F, et al. The response to initial chemotherapy as a prognostic factor in localized Ewing's sarcoma. Eur J Cancer Clin Oncol 1985;21:463–467.
145. Picci P, Rougraff BT, Bacci G, et al. Prognostic significance of histopathologic response to chemotherapy in nonmetastatic Ewing's sarcoma of the extremities. J Clin Oncol 1993;11:1763–1769.

146. Wunder JS, Paulian G, Huvos AG, et al. The histological response to chemotherapy as a predictor of the oncological outcome of operative treatment of Ewing sarcoma. J Bone Joint Surg Am 1998;80:1020–1033.
147. Van der Woude HJ, Bloem JL, Taminiau AHM, et al. Classification of histopathologic changes following chemotherapy in Ewing's sarcoma of bone. Skeletal Radiol 1994;23: 501–507.
148. Van der Woude HJ, Bloem JL, Holscher HC, et al. Monitoring the effect of chemotherapy in Ewing's sarcoma of bone with MR imaging. Skeletal Radiol 1994;23:493–500.
149. Egmont-Petersen M, Hogendoorn PCW, Van der Geest R, et al. Detection of areas with viable remnant tumor in postchemotherapy patients with Ewing's sarcoma by dynamic contrast-enhanced MRI using pharmacokinetic modeling. Magn Reson Imaging 2000;18:525–535.
150. Van der Woude HJ, Bloem JL, Hogendoorn PCW. Preoperative evaluation and monitoring chemotherapy in patients with high-grade osteogenic and Ewing's sarcoma: review of current imaging modalities. Skeletal Radiol 1998;27:57–71.
151. Hawkins DS, Schuetze SM, Butrynski JE, et al. [18F]-fluorodeoxy-D-glucose positron emission tomography predicts outcome for Ewing sarcoma family of tumors. J Clin Oncol 2005;23:8828–8834.
152. Maksimenko A, Malvy C, Lambert G, et al. Oligonucleotides targeted against a junction oncogene are made efficient by nanotechnologies. Pharm Res 2003;20:1565–1567.
153. Stegmaier K, Wong JS, Ross KN, et al. Signature-based small molecule screening identifies cytosine arabinoside as an EWS/FLI modulator in Ewing sarcoma. PLoS Med 2007;4:e122.
154. DuBois SG, Krailo MD, Lessnick SL, et al. Phase II study of intermediate-dose cytarabine in patients with relapsed or refractory Ewing sarcoma: a report from the Children's Oncology Group. Ped Blood Cancer 2009;52:324–327.
155. Scotlandi K, Baldini N, Cerisano V, et al. CD99 engagement: an effective therapeutic strategy for Ewing tumors. Cancer Res 2000;60:5134–5142.
156. Wang S, El-Deiry WS. TRAIL and apoptosis induction by TNF-family death receptors. Oncogene 2003;22:8628–8633.
157. Shi J, Zheng D, Man K, et al. TRAIL: a potential agent for cancer therapy. Curr Mol Med 2003;3:727–736.
158. Kontny HU, Hammerle K, Klein R, et al. Sensitivity of Ewing's sarcoma to TRAIL-induced apoptosis. Cell Death Differ 2001;8:506–514.
159. Van Valen F, Fulda S, Truckenbrod B, et al. Apoptotic responsiveness of the Ewing's sarcoma family of tumours to tumour necrosis factor-related apoptosis-inducing ligand (TRAIL). Int J Cancer 2000;88:252–259.
160. Van Valen F, Fulda S, Schafer KL, et al. Selective and nonselective toxicity of TRAIL/Apo2L combined with chemotherapy in human bone tumour cells vs. normal human cells. Int J Cancer 2003;107:929–940.
161. Fulda S, Kufer MU, Meyer E, et al. Sensitization for death receptor- or drug-induced apoptosis by re-expression of caspase-8 through demethylation or gene transfer. Oncogene 2001;20:5865–5877.
162. Fulda S, Debatin KM. IFNgamma sensitizes for apoptosis by upregulating caspase-8 expression through the Stat1 pathway. Oncogene 2002;21:2295–2308.
163. Reed JC. Bcl-2: prevention of apoptosis as a mechanism of drug resistance. Hematol Oncol Clin North Am 1995;9:451–473.
164. Tsokos M, Steinberg SM, Stocker DM, et al. Bcl2 may be predictive of survival in patients with peripheral primitive neuroectodermal tumors (PNET). Lab Invest 1995; 72:145A (849).
165. Kaban K, Herbst RS. Angiogenesis as a target for cancer therapy. Hematol Oncol Clin North Am 2002;16:1125–1171.
166. van der Schaft DW, Hillen F, Pauwels P, et al. Tumor cell plasticity in Ewing sarcoma, an alternative circulatory system stimulated by hypoxia. Cancer Res 2005;65:11520–11528.
167. Rosen LS. Inhibitors of the vascular endothelial growth factor receptor. Hematol Oncol Clin North Am 2002;16:1173–1187.
168. Fuchs B, Inwards CY, Janknecht R. Vascular endothelial growth factor expression is up-regulated by EWS-ETS oncoproteins and Sp1 and may represent an independent predictor of survival in Ewing's sarcoma. Clin Cancer Res 2004;10:1344–1353.
169. Pavlakovic H, Von Schutz V, Rossler J, et al. Quantification of angiogenesis stimulators in children with solid malignancies. Int J Cancer 2001;92:756–760.
170. Potikyan G, Savene ROV, Gaulden JM, et al. EWS/FLI1 regulates tumor angiogenesis in Ewing's sarcoma via suppression of thrombospondins. Cancer Res 2007;67:6675–6684.
171. Yee D, Favoni RE, Lebovic GS, et al. Insulin-like growth factor I expression by tumors of neuroectodermal origin with the t(11;22) chromosomal translocation. A potential autocrine growth factor. J Clin Invest 1990;86:1806–1814.
172. van Valen F, Winkelmann W, Jürgens H. Type I and type II insulin-like growth factor receptors and their function in human Ewing's sarcoma cells. J Cancer Res Clin Oncol 1992;118:269–275.
173. Benini S, Manara MC, Baldini N, et al. Inhibition of insulin-like growth factor i receptor increases the antitumor activity of doxorubicin and vincristine against Ewing's sarcoma cells. Clin Cancer Res 2001;7:1790–1797.
174. Widhe B, Widhe T. Initial symptoms and clinical features in osteosarcoma and Ewing sarcoma. J Bone Joint Surg Am 2000;82:667–674.
175. Sneppen O, Hansen LM. Presenting symptoms and treatment delay in osteosarcoma and Ewing's sarcoma. Acta Radiol Oncol 1984;23:159–162.
176. Craft AW, Cotterill SJ, Bullimore JA, et al. Long-term results from the first UKCCSG Ewing's Tumour Study (ET-1). United Kingdom Children's Cancer Study Group (UKCCSG) and the Medical Research Council Bone Sarcoma Working Party. Eur J Cancer 1997;33:1061–1069.
177. Ferrari S, Bertoni F, Mercuri M, et al. Ewing's sarcoma of bone: relation between clinical characteristics and staging. Oncol Rep 2001;8:553–556.
178. Henk CB, Grampp S, Wiesbauer P, et al. Ewing sarcoma. Diagnostic imaging. Radiologe 1998;38:509–522.
179. Tateishi U, Gladish GW, Kusumoto M, et al. Chest wall tumors: radiologic findings and pathologic correlation: part 2. Malignant tumors. Radiographics 2003;23:1491–1508.
180. Frouge C, Vanel D, Coffre C, et al. The role of magnetic resonance imaging in the evaluation of Ewing sarcoma. A report of 27 cases. Skeletal Radiol 1988;17:387–392.
181. Cohen MD, Weetman RM, Provisor AJ, et al. Efficacy of magnetic resonance imaging in 139 children with tumors. Arch Surg 1986;121:522–529.
182. Meyer JS, Nadel HR, Marina N, et al. Imaging guidelines for children with Ewing sarcoma and osteosarcoma: a report from the Children's Oncology Group Bone Tumor Committee. Pediatr Blood Cancer 2008;51:163–170.
183. Paulussen M, Bielack S, Jürgens H, et al. ESMO Guidelines Working Group. Ewing's sarcoma of the bone: ESMO clinical recommendations for diagnosis, treatment and follow-up. Ann Oncol 2008;19:(suppl 2):ii97–ii98.
184. Mankin HJ, Mankin CJ, Simon MA. The hazards of the biopsy, revisited. Members of the Musculoskeletal Tumor Society. J Bone Joint Surg Am 1996;78:656–663.
185. Stewart CJ, Coldewey J, Stewart IS. Comparison of fine needle aspiration cytology and needle core biopsy in the diagnosis of radiologically detected abdominal lesions. J Clin Pathol 2002;55:93–97.
186. Nicol KK, Ward WG, Savage PD, et al. Fine-needle aspiration biopsy of skeletal versus extraskeletal osteosarcoma. Cancer 1998;84:176–185.
187. Pramesh CS, Deshpande MS, Pardiwala DN, et al. Core needle biopsy for bone tumours. Eur J Surg Oncol 2001;27:668–671.
188. Simon MA. Biopsy. In: Simon MA, Springfield DS, eds. Surgery for bone and soft-tissue tumors. Philadelphia, PA: Lippincott-Raven, 1998:55–65.
189. Hewitt SM, Lewis FA, Cao Y, et al. Tissue handling and specimen preparation in surgical pathology: issues concerning the recovery of nucleic acids from formalin-fixed, paraffin-embedded tissue. Arch Path Lab Med 2008;132:1929–1935.
190. Randall RL, Wade M, Albritton K, et al. Retrieval yield of total and messenger RNA in mesenchymal tissue ex vivo. Clin Orthop Relat Res 2003;415:59–63.
191. Daldrup-Link HE, Franzius C, Link TM, et al. Whole-body MR imaging for detection of bone metastases in children and young adults: comparison with skeletal scintigraphy and FDG PET. Am J Roentgenol 2001;177:229–236.
192. Paulussen M, Ahrens S, Burdach S, et al. Primary metastatic (stage IV) Ewing tumor: survival analysis of 171 patients from the EICESS studies. European Intergroup Cooperative Ewing Sarcoma Studies. Ann Oncol 1998;9:275–281.
193. van den Berg H, Dirksen U, Ranft A, et al. Ewing tumors in infants. Pediatr Blood Cancer 2008;50:761–764.
194. Guiter GE, Gamboni MM, Zakowski MF. The cytology of extraskeletal Ewing sarcoma. Cancer 1999;87:141–148.
195. Kumar RV, Rao CR, Hazarika D, et al. Aspiration biopsy cytology of primary bone lesions. Acta Cytol 1993;37:83–89.
196. Horowitz ME, Tsokos MG, DeLaney TF. Ewing's sarcoma. CA Cancer J Clin 1992; 42:300–320.
197. Tsokos M. Peripheral primitive neuroectodermal tumors. Diagnosis, classification, and prognosis. Perspect Pediatr Pathol 1992;16:27–98.
198. Dehner LP. Primitive neuroectodermal tumor and Ewing's sarcoma. Am J Surg Pathol 1993;17:1–13.
199. Mawad JK, Mackay B, Raymond AK, et al. Electron microscopy in the diagnosis of small round cell tumors of bone. Ultrastruct Pathol 1994;18:263–268.
200. Fellinger EJ, Garin-Chesa P, Su SL, et al. Biochemical and genetic characterization of the HBA71 Ewing's sarcoma cell surface antigen. Cancer Res 1991;51:336–340.
201. Ramani P, Rampling D, Link M. Immunocytochemical study of 12E7 in small round-cell tumours of childhood: an assessment of its sensitivity and specificity. Histopathology 1993;23:557–561.
202. Weidner N, Tjoe J. Immunohistochemical profile of monoclonal antibody O13: antibody that recognizes glycoprotein p30/32MIC2 and is useful in diagnosing Ewing's sarcoma and peripheral neuroepithelioma. Am J Surg Pathol 1994;18:486–494.
203. Lizard-Nacol S, Lizard G, Justrabo E, et al. Immunologic characterization of Ewing's sarcoma using mesenchymal and neural markers. Am J Pathol 1989;135:847–855.
204. Dierick AM, Roels H, Langlois M. The immunophenotype of Ewing's sarcoma. An immunohistochemical analysis. Pathol Res Pract 1993;189:26–32.
205. Shanfield RI. Immunohistochemical analysis of neural markers in peripheral primitive neuroectodermal tumor (pPNET) without light microscopic evidence of neural differentiation. Appl Immunohistochem Mol Morphol 1997;5:78–86.
206. Folpe AL, Goldblum JR, Rubin BP, et al. Morphologic and immunophenotypic diversity in Ewing family tumors: a study of 66 genetically confirmed cases. Am J Surg Pathol 2005;29:1025–1033.
207. Ladanyi M, Bridge JA. Contribution of molecular genetic data to the classification of sarcomas. Hum Pathol 2000;31:532–538.
208. Hill DA, O'Sullivan MJ, Zhu X, et al. Practical application of molecular genetic testing as an aid to the surgical pathologic diagnosis of sarcomas: a prospective study. Am J Surg Pathol 2002;26:965–977.
209. Parham DM, Hijazi Y, Steinberg SM, et al. Neuroectodermal differentiation in Ewing's sarcoma family of tumors does not predict tumor behavior. Hum Pathol 1999;30: 911–918.
210. Ewing J. Further report of endothelial myeloma of bone. Proc N Y Pathol Soc 1924;24: 93–100.
211. Jenkin RD. Ewing's sarcoma a study of treatment methods. Clin Radiol 1966;17: 97–106.
212. Phillips RF, Higinbotham NL. The curability of Ewing's endothelioma of bone in children. J Pediatr 1967;70:391–397.
213. Hustu HO, Holton C, James D Jr, et al. Treatment of Ewing's sarcoma with concurrent radiotherapy and chemotherapy. J Pediatr 1968;73:249–251.
214. Sutow WW, Vietti TJ, Fernbach DJ, et al. Evaluation of chemotherapy in children with metastatic Ewing's sarcoma and osteogenic sarcoma. Cancer Chemother Rep 1971;55: 67–78.
215. Rosen G, Wollner N, Tan C, et al. Proceedings: disease-free survival in children with Ewing's sarcoma treated with radiation therapy and adjuvant four-drug sequential chemotherapy. Cancer 1974;33:384–393.
216. Gasparini M, Barni S, Lattuada A, et al. Ten years experience with Ewing's sarcoma. Tumori 1977;63:77–90.
217. Jurgens H, Exner U, Gadner H, et al. Multidisciplinary treatment of primary Ewing's sarcoma of bone. A 6-year experience of a European Cooperative Trial. Cancer 1988;61:23–32.
218. Nesbit ME Jr, Gehan EA, Burgert EO Jr, et al. Multimodal therapy for the management of primary, nonmetastatic Ewing's sarcoma of bone: a long-term follow-up of the First Intergroup study. J Clin Oncol 1990;8:1664–1674.
219. Burgert EO Jr, Nesbit ME, Garnsey LA, et al. Multimodal therapy for the management of nonpelvic, localized Ewing's sarcoma of bone: intergroup study IESS-II. J Clin Oncol 1990;8:1514–1524.
220. Cotterill SJ, Ahrens S, Paulussen M, et al. Prognostic factors in Ewing's tumor of bone: analysis of 975 patients from the European Intergroup Cooperative Ewing's Sarcoma Study Group. J Clin Oncol 2000;18:3108–3114.
221. Craft A, Cotterill S, Malcolm A, et al. Ifosfamide-containing chemotherapy in Ewing's sarcoma: The Second United Kingdom Children's Cancer Study Group and the Medical Research Council Ewing's Tumor Study. J Clin Oncol 1998;16:3628–3633.
222. Oberlin O, Deley MC, Bui BN, et al. Prognostic factors in localized Ewing's tumours and peripheral neuroectodermal tumours: the third study of the French Society of Paediatric Oncology (EW88 study). Br J Cancer 2001;85:1646–1654.

223. Paulussen M, Ahrens S, Dunst J, et al. Localized Ewing tumor of bone: final results of the cooperative Ewing's Sarcoma Study CESS 86. J Clin Oncol 2001;19:1818–1829.

224. Kolb EA, Kushner BH, Gorlick R, et al. Long-term event-free survival after intensive chemotherapy for Ewing's family of tumors in children and young adults. J Clin Oncol 2003;21:3423–3430.

225. Grier HE, Krailo MD, Tarbell NJ, et al. Addition of ifosfamide and etoposide to standard chemotherapy for Ewing's sarcoma and primitive neuroectodermal tumor of bone. N Engl J Med 2003;348:694–701.

226. Bacci G, Forni C, Longhi A, et al. Long-term outcome for patients with non-metastatic Ewing's sarcoma treated with adjuvant and neoadjuvant chemotherapies. 402 patients treated at Rizzoli between 1972 and 1992. Eur J Cancer 2004;40:73–83.

227. Aparicio J, Munarriz B, Pastor M, et al. Long-term follow-up and prognostic factors in Ewing's sarcoma. A multivariate analysis of 116 patients from a single institution. Oncology 1998;55:20–26.

228. Carrie C, Mascard E, Gomez F, et al. Nonmetastatic pelvic Ewing sarcoma: report of the French Society of pediatric oncology. Med Pediatr Oncol 1999;33:444–449.

229. Bacci G, Ferrari S, Bertoni F, et al. Prognostic factors in nonmetastatic Ewing's sarcoma of bone treated with adjuvant chemotherapy: analysis of 359 patients at the Istituto Ortopedico Rizzoli. J Clin Oncol 2000;18:4–11.

230. Schuck A, Ahrens S, Paulussen M, et al. Local therapy in localized Ewing tumors: results of 1058 patients treated in the CESS 81, CESS 86, and EICESS 92 trials. Int J Radiat Oncol Biol Phys 2003;55:168–177.

231. Dunst J, Sauer R, Burgers JM, et al. Radiation therapy as local treatment in Ewing's sarcoma. Results of the Cooperative Ewing's Sarcoma Studies CESS 81 and CESS 86. Cancer 1991;67:2818–2825.

232. Schuck A, Hofmann J, Rube C, et al. Radiotherapy in Ewing's sarcoma and PNET of the chest wall: results of the trials CESS 81, CESS 86 and EICESS 92. Int J Radiat Oncol Biol Phys 1998;42:1001–1006.

233. Arai Y, Kun LE, Brooks MT, et al. Ewing's sarcoma: local tumor control and patterns of failure following limited-volume radiation therapy. Int J Radiat Oncol Biol Phys 1991;21:1501–1508.

234. Donaldson SS, Torrey M, Link MP, et al. A multidisciplinary study investigating radiotherapy in Ewing's sarcoma: end results of POG #8346. Pediatric Oncology Group. Int J Radiat Oncol Biol Phys 1998;42:125–135.

235. DuBois SG, Krailo MD, Cook EF, et al. Evaluation of local control in patients with non-metastatic Ewing sarcoma of the bone: a report from the Children's Oncology Group [abstract 10013]. J Clin Oncol 2007;25.

236. Bacci G, Longhi A, Briccoli A, et al. The role of surgical margins in treatment of Ewing's sarcoma family tumors: experience of a single institution with 512 patients treated with adjuvant and neoadjuvant chemotherapy. Int J Rad Onc Biol Phys 2006;65:766–772.

237. Rodríguez-Galindo C, Navid F, Liu T, et al. Prognostic factors for local and distant control in Ewing sarcoma family of tumors. Ann Oncol 2008;19:814–820.

238. Bernstein M, Kovar H, Paulussen M, et al. Ewing's sarcoma family of tumors: current management. Oncologist 2006;11:503–519.

239. Donati D, Yin J, Di Bella C, et al. Local and distant control in non-metastatic pelvic Ewing's sarcoma patients. J Surg Oncol 2007;96:19–25.

240. Indelicato DJ, Keole SR, Shahlaee AH, et al. Long-term clinical and functional outcomes after treatment for localized Ewing's tumor of the lower extremity. Int J Radiat Oncol Biol Phys 2008;70:501–509.

241. Granowetter L, Womer R, Devidas M, et al. Dose-intensified compared with standard chemotherapy for nonmetastatic Ewing sarcoma family of tumors: A Children's Oncology Group Study. J Clin Oncol 2009;27:2536–2541.

242. Laskar S, Mallick I, Gupta T, et al. Post-operative radiotherapy for Ewing sarcoma: when, how and how much? Pediatr Blood Cancer 2008;51:575–580.

243. Schuck A, Rube C, Konemann S, et al. Postoperative radiotherapy in the treatment of Ewing tumors: influence of the interval between surgery and radiotherapy. Strahlenther Onkol 2002;178:25–31.

244. Randall RL, Nork SE, James PJ. Aggressive aneurysmal bone cyst of the proximal humerus. A case report. Clin Orthop 2000;370:212–218.

245. Bae DS, Waters PM, Gebhardt MC. Results of free vascularized fibula grafting for allograft nonunion after limb salvage surgery for malignant bone tumors. J Pediatr Orthop. 2006;26:809–814.

246. Muscolo DL, Ayerza MA, Aponte-Tinao L, et al. Allograft reconstruction after sarcoma resection in children younger than 10 years old. Clin Orthop Relat Res. 2008;466:1856–1862.

247. Ramseier LE, Malinin TI, Temple HT, et al. Allograft reconstruction for bone sarcoma of the tibia in the growing child. J Bone Joint Surg Br. 2006;88:95–99.

248. Alman BA, de Bari A, Krajbich JI. Massive allografts in the treatment of osteosarcoma and Ewing sarcoma in children and adolescents. J Bone Joint Surg Am 1995;77:54–64.

249. Getty PJ, Peabody TD. Complications and functional outcomes of reconstruction with an osteoarticular allograft after intra-articular resection of the proximal aspect of the humerus. J Bone Joint Surg Am 1999;81:1138–1146.

250. Gebhardt MC, Flugstad DI, Springfield DS, et al. The use of bone allografts for limb salvage in high-grade extremity osteosarcoma. Clin Orthop 1991;270:181–196.

251. Deijkers RL, Bloem RM, Kroon HM, et al. Epidiaphyseal versus other intercalary allografts for tumors of the lower limb. Clin Orthop Relat Res 2005;439:151–160.

252. Potter BK, Adams SC, Pitcher JD Jr, et al. Proximal humerus reconstructions for tumors. Clin Orthop Relat Res 2009;467:1035–1041.

253. Finn HA, Simon MA. Limb-salvage surgery in the treatment of osteosarcoma in skeletally immature individuals. Clin Orthop 1991;262:108–118.

254. Ceruso M, Taddei F, Bigazzi P, et al. Vascularised fibula graft inlaid in a massive bone allograft: considerations on the bio-mechanical behaviour of the combined graft in segmental bone reconstructions after sarcoma resection. Injury 2008;39(suppl 3):S68–S74.

255. Jeys LM, Kulkarni A, Grimer RJ, et al. Endoprosthetic reconstruction for the treatment of musculoskeletal tumors of the appendicular skeleton and pelvis. J Bone Joint Surg Am 2008;90:1265–1271.

256. Gosheger G, Gebert C, Ahrens H, et al. Endoprosthetic reconstruction in 250 patients with sarcoma. Clin Orthop Relat Res 2006;450:164–171.

257. Horowitz SM, Glasser DB, Lane JM, et al. Prosthetic and extremity survivorship after limb salvage for sarcoma. How long do the reconstructions last? Clin Orthop 1993;293:280–286.

258. Bhangu AA, Kramer MJ, Grimer RJ, et al. Early distal femoral endoprosthetic survival: cemented stems versus the Compress implant. Int Orthop 2006;30:465–472.

259. O'Donnell RJ. Compressive osseointegration of modular endoprostheses. Current Opin Orthopedics 2007;18:590–603.

260. Donati D, Colangeli M, Colangeli S, et al. Allograft-prosthetic composite in the proximal tibia after bone tumor resection. Clin Orthop Relat Res 2008;466:459–465.

261. Gitelis S, Piasecki P. Allograft prosthetic composite arthroplasty for osteosarcoma and other aggressive bone tumors. Clin Orthop 1991;270:197–201.

262. Brien EW, Terek RM, Healey JH, et al. Allograft reconstruction after proximal tibial resection for bone tumors. An analysis of function and outcome comparing allograft and prosthetic reconstructions. Clin Orthop 1994;303:116–127.

263. Hejna MJ, Gitelis S. Allograft prosthetic composite replacement for bone tumors. Semin Surg Oncol 1997;13:18–24.

264. Donati D, Capanna R, Casadei R, et al. Arthrodesis of the knee after tumor resection: a comparison between autografts and allografts. Chir Organi Mov 1995;80:29–37.

265. Probyn LJ, Wunder JS, Bell RS, et al. A comparison of outcome of osteoarticular allograft reconstruction and shoulder arthrodesis following resection of primary tumours of the proximal humerus. Sarcoma 1998;2:163–170.

266. Niimi R, Matsumine A, Kusuzaki K, et al. Usefulness of limb salvage surgery for bone and soft tissue sarcomas of the distal lower leg. J Cancer Res Clin Oncol 2008;134:1087–1095.

267. Campanacci DA, Scoccianti G, Beltrami G, et al. Ankle arthrodesis with bone graft after distal tibia resection for bone tumors. Foot Ankle Int 2008;29:1031–1037.

268. Scully SP, Ghert MA, Zurakowski D, et al. Pathologic fracture in osteosarcoma: prognostic importance and treatment implications. J Bone Joint Surg Am 2002;84-A:49–57.

269. Scully SP, Temple HT, O'Keefe RJ, et al. The surgical treatment of patients with osteosarcoma who sustain a pathologic fracture. Clin Orthop 1996;324:227–232.

270. Jaffe N, Spears R, Eftekhari F, et al. Pathologic fracture in osteosarcoma. Impact of chemotherapy on primary tumor and survival. Cancer 1987;59:701–709.

271. Papagelopoulos PJ, Mavrogenis AF, Savvidou OD, et al. Pathological fractures in primary bone sarcomas. Injury 2008;39:395–403.

272. Shamberger RC, LaQuaglia MP, Gebhardt MC, et al. Ewing sarcoma/primitive neuroectodermal tumor of the chest wall: impact of initial versus delayed resection on tumor margins, survival, and use of radiation therapy. Ann Surg 2003;238:563–567; discussion 567–568.

273. Eilber FR, Grant TT, Sakai D, et al. Internal hemipelvectomy—excision of the hemipelvis with limb preservation. An alternative to hemipelvectomy. Cancer 1979;43:806–809.

274. Ward WG, Yang RS, Eckardt JJ. Endoprosthetic bone reconstruction following malignant tumor resection in skeletally immature patients. Orthop Clin North Am 1996;27:493–502.

275. Baumgart R, Hinterwimmer S, Krammer M, et al. The bioexpandable prosthesis: a new perspective after resection of malignant bone tumors in children. J Pediatr Hematol Oncol 2005;27:452–455.

276. Gupta A, Meswania J, Pollock R, et al. Non-invasive distal femoral expandable endoprosthesis for limb-salvage surgery in paediatric tumours. J Bone Joint Surg Br 2006;88:649–654.

277. Neel MD, Wilkins RM, Rao BN, et al. Early multicenter experience with a noninvasive expandable prosthesis. Clin Orthop Relat Res 2003;415:72–81.

278. Kapukaya A, Subasi M, Arslan H, et al. Technique and complications of callus distraction in the treatment of bone tumors. Arch Orthop Trauma Surg 2006;126:157–163.

279. Tsuchiya H, Abdel-Wanis ME, Sakurakichi K, et al. Osteosarcoma around the knee. Intraepiphyseal excision and biological reconstruction with distraction osteogenesis. J Bone Joint Surg Br 2002;84:1162–1166.

280. Tsuchiya H, Shirai T, Morsy AF, et al. Safety of external fixation during postoperative chemotherapy. J Bone Joint Surg Br 2008;90:924–928.

281. Dormans JP, Ofluoglu O, Erol B, et al. Case report: reconstruction of an intercalary defect with bone transport after resection of Ewing's sarcoma. Clin Orthop Relat Res. 2005;434:258–264.

282. Fuchs B, Kotajarvi BR, Kaufman KR, et al. Functional outcome of patients with rotationplasty about the knee. Clin Orthop Relat Res 2003;415:52–58.

283. Fuchs B, Sim FH. Rotationplasty about the knee: surgical technique and anatomical considerations. Clin Anat. 2004;17:345–353.

284. Sawamura C, Hornicek FJ, Gebhardt MC. Complications and risk factors for failure of rotationplasty: review of 25 patients. Clin Orthop Relat Res 2008;466:1302–1308.

285. McClenaghan BA, Krajbich JI, Pirone AM, et al. Comparative assessment of gait after limb-salvage procedures. J Bone Joint Surg Am 1989;71:1178–1182.

286. Winkelmann WW. Type-B-IIIa hip rotationplasty: an alternative operation for the treatment of malignant tumors of the femur in early childhood. J Bone Joint Surg Am 2000;82:814–828.

287. Hillmann A, Hoffmann C, Gosheger G, et al. Malignant tumor of the distal part of the femur or the proximal part of the tibia: endoprosthetic replacement or rotationplasty. J Bone Joint Surg 1999;81A:462–468.

288. Akahane T, Shimizu T, Isobe K, et al. Evaluation of postoperative general quality of life for patients with osteosarcoma around the knee joint. J Pediatr Orthop B 2007;164:269–272.

289. Enneking WF, Spanier SS, Goodman MA. A system for the surgical staging of musculoskeletal sarcoma. Clin Orthop 1980;153:106–120.

290. Salzer-Kuntschik M, Delling G, Beron G, et al. Morphological grades of regression in osteosarcoma after polychemotherapy—study COSS 80. J Cancer Res Clin Oncol 1983;106(Suppl):21–24.

291. Ozaki T, Hillmann A, Hoffmann C, et al. Significance of surgical margin on the prognosis of patients with Ewing's sarcoma. A report from the Cooperative Ewing's Sarcoma Study. Cancer 1996;78:892–900.

292. Dunst J, Jurgens H, Sauer R, et al. Radiation therapy in Ewing's sarcoma: an update of the CESS 86 trial. Int J Radiat Oncol Biol Phys 1995;32:919–930.

293. Donaldson SS, Meza J, Breneman JC, et al. Results from the IRS-IV randomized trial of hyperfractionated radiotherapy in children with rhabdomyosarcoma—a report from the IRSG. Int J Radiat Oncol Biol Phys 2001;51:718–728.

294. Bölling T, Schuck A, Paulussen M, et al. Whole lung irradiation in patients with solitary pulmonary metastases of Ewing tumors: toxicity analysis and treatment results of the EICESS 92 trial. Strahlenther Onkol 2008;184:193–197.

295. Spunt SL, McCarville MB, Kun L, et al. Selective use of whole-lung irradiation for patients with Ewing sarcoma family tumors and pulmonary metastases at the time of diagnosis. J Ped Hem Oncol 2001;23:93–98.

296. Paulussen M, Ahrens S, Craft AW, et al. Ewing's tumors with primary lung metastases: survival analysis of 114 (European Intergroup) Cooperative Ewing's Sarcoma Studies patients. J Clin Oncol 1998;16:3044–3052.

297. Peat BG, Bell RS, Davis A, et al. Wound-healing complications after soft-tissue sarcoma surgery. Plast Reconstr Surg 1994;93:980–987.

298. Cheng EY, Dusenbery KE, Winters MR, et al. Soft tissue sarcomas: preoperative versus postoperative radiotherapy. J Surg Oncol 1996;61:90–99.

299. Sorger JI, Hornicek FJ, Zavatta M, et al. Allograft fractures revisited. Clin Orthop 2001;382:66–74.

300. Hornicek FJ, Gebhardt MC, Tomford WW, et al. Factors affecting nonunion of the allograft-host junction. Clin Orthop 2001;382:87–98.
301. Ehrhart NP, Eurell JA, Constable PD, et al. The effect of host tissue irradiation on large-segment allograft incorporation. Clin Orthop Relat Res 2005;435:43–51.
302. Sutow WW, Sullivan MP. Cyclophosphamide therapy in children with Ewing's sarcoma. Cancer Chemother Rep 1962;23:55–60.
303. Pinkel D. Cyclophosphamide in children with cancer. Cancer 1962;15:42–49.
304. Haggard ME. Cyclophosphamide (NSC-26271) in the treatment of children with malignant neoplasms. Cancer Chemother Rep 1967;51:403–405.
305. Samuels ML, Howe CD. Cyclophosphamide in the management of Ewing's sarcoma. Cancer 1967;20:961–966.
306. Sutow WW. Vincristine (NSC-67574) therapy for malignant solid tumors in children (except Wilms' tumor). Cancer Chemother Rep 1968;52:485–487.
307. James DH Jr, George P. Vincristine in children with malignant solid tumors. J Pediatr 1964;64:534–541.
308. Oldham RK, Pomeroy TC. Treatment of Ewing's sarcoma with adriamycin (NSC-123127). Cancer Chemother Rep 1972;56:635–639.
309. Evans AE, Baehner RL, Chard RL Jr, et al. Comparison of daunorubicin (NSC-83142) with adriamycin (NSC-123127) in the treatment of late-stage childhood solid tumors. Cancer Chemother Rep 1974;58:671–676.
310. Gottlieb JA, Baker LH, Quagliana JM, et al. Chemotherapy of sarcomas with a combination of adriamycin and dimethyl triazeno imidazole carboxamide. Cancer 1972;30:1632–1638.
311. Tan C, Etcubanas E, Wollner N, et al. Adriamycin—an antitumor antibiotic in the treatment of neoplastic diseases. Cancer 1973;32:9–17.
312. Pomeroy TC, Johnson RE. Combined modality therapy of Ewing's sarcoma. Cancer 1975;35:36–47.
313. Cangir A, Morgan SK, Land VJ, et al. Combination chemotherapy with Adriamycin (NSC-123127) and dimethyl triazeno imidazole carboxamide (DTIC) (NSC-45388) in children with metastatic sold tumors. Med Pediatr Oncol 1976;2:183–190.
314. Van Dyk JJ, Falkson HC, Van der Merwe AM, et al. Unexpected toxicity in patients treated with iphosphamide. Cancer Res 1972;32:921–924.
315. Jaffe N, Paed D, Traggis D, et al. Improved outlook for Ewing's sarcoma with combination chemotherapy (vincristine, actinomycin D and cyclophosphamide) and radiation therapy. Cancer 1976;38:1925–1930.
316. Smith MA, Ungerleider RS, Horowitz ME, et al. Influence of doxorubicin dose intensity on response and outcome for patients with osteogenic sarcoma and Ewing's sarcoma. J Natl Cancer Inst 1991;83:1460–1470.
317. Castex M-P, Rubie H, Stevens MCG, et al. Extraosseous localized Ewing tumors: improved outcome with anthracyclines—The French Society of Pediatric Oncology and International Society of Pediatric Oncology. J Clin Oncol 2007;25:1176–1182.
318. Marina NM, Pappo AS, Parham DM, et al. Chemotherapy dose-intensification for pediatric patients with Ewing's family of tumors and desmoplastic small round-cell tumors: a feasibility study at St. Jude Children's Research Hospital. J Clin Oncol 1999;17:180–190.
319. Bacci G, Mercuri M, Longhi A, et al. Neoadjuvant chemotherapy for Ewing's tumour of bone: recent experience at the Rizzoli Orthopaedic Institute. Eur J Cancer 2002;38:2243–2251.
320. Kushner BH, Meyers PA, Gerald WL, et al. Very-high-dose short-term chemotherapy for poor-risk peripheral primitive neuroectodermal tumors, including Ewing's sarcoma, in children and young adults. J Clin Oncol 1995;13:2796–2804.
321. Oberlin O, Habrand JL, Zucker JM, et al. No benefit of ifosfamide in Ewing's sarcoma: a nonrandomized study of the French Society of Pediatric Oncology. J Clin Oncol 1992;10:1407–1412.
322. Paulussen M, Craft AW, Lewis I, et al. Results of the EICESS-92 Study: two randomized trials of Ewing's sarcoma treatment-cyclophosphamide compared with ifosfamide in standard-risk patients and assessment of benefit of etoposide added to standard treatment in high-risk patients. J Clin Oncol 2008;26:4385–4393.
323. Juergens C, Weston C, Lewis I, et al. Safety assessment of intensive induction with vincristine, ifosfamide, doxorubicin, and etoposide (VIDE) in the treatment of Ewing tumors in the EURO-E. W.I.N.G. 99 clinical trial. Pediatr Blood Cancer 2006;47:22–29.
324. Womer RB, West DC, Krailo MD, et al. Randomized comparison of every-two-week v. every-three-week chemotherapy in Ewing sarcoma family tumors (ESFT) [abstract 10504]. J Clin Oncol 2008;26.
325. Ladenstein R, Lasset C, Pinkerton R, et al. Impact of megatherapy in children with high-risk Ewing's tumours in complete remission: a report from the EBMT Solid Tumour Registry. Bone Marrow Transplant 1995;15:697–705.
326. Kinsella TJ, Glaubiger D, Diesseroth A, et al. Intensive combined modality therapy including low-dose TBI in high-risk Ewing's Sarcoma Patients. Int J Radiat Oncol Biol Phys 1983;9:1955–1960.
327. Burdach S, Jurgens H, Peters C, et al. Myeloablative radiochemotherapy and hematopoietic stem-cell rescue in poor-prognosis Ewing's sarcoma. J Clin Oncol 1993; 11:1482–1488.
328. Kushner BH, Meyers PA. How effective is dose-intensive/myeloablative therapy against Ewing's sarcoma/primitive neuroectodermal tumor metastatic to bone or bone marrow? The Memorial Sloan-Kettering experience and a literature review. J Clin Oncol 2001; 19:870–880.
329. Meyers PA, Krailo MD, Ladanyi M, et al. High-dose melphalan, etoposide, total-body irradiation, and autologous stem-cell reconstitution as consolidation therapy for high-risk Ewing's sarcoma does not improve prognosis. J Clin Oncol 2001;19:2812–2820.
330. Pinkerton CR. Intensive chemotherapy with stem cell support—experience in pediatric solid tumours. Bull Cancer 1995;82(suppl 1):61s–65s.
331. Meyers PA. High-dose therapy with autologous stem cell rescue for pediatric sarcomas. Curr Opin Oncol 2004;16:120–125.
332. Cangir A, Vietti TJ, Gehan EA, et al. Ewing's sarcoma metastatic at diagnosis. Results and comparisons of two intergroup Ewing's sarcoma studies. Cancer 1990;66:887–893.
333. Sandoval C, Meyer WH, Parham DM, et al. Outcome in 43 children presenting with metastatic Ewing sarcoma: the St. Jude Children's Research Hospital experience, 1962 to 1992. Med Pediatr Oncol 1996;26:180–185.
334. Miser JS, Krailo MD, Tarbell NJ, et al. Treatment of metastatic Ewing's sarcoma or primitive neuroectodermal tumor of bone: evaluation of combination ifosfamide and etoposide—a Children's Cancer Group and Pediatric Oncology Group Study. J Clin Oncol 2004:22:2873–2876.
335. Bernstein ML, Devidas M, Lafreniere D, et al. Intensive therapy with growth factor support for patients with Ewing tumors metastatic at diagnosis: Pediatric Oncology Group/Children's Cancer Group phase II study 9457—a report from the Children's Oncology Group. J Clin Oncol 2006;24:152–159.
336. Miser JS, Goldsby RE, Chen Z, et al Treatment of metastatic Ewing sarcoma/primitive neuroectodermal tumor of bone: Evaluation of increasing the dose intensity of chemotherapy—a report from the Children's Oncology Group. Pediatr Blood Cancer 2007;49:894–900.
337. Oberlin O, Rey A, Desfachelles AS, et al. Impact of high-dose busulfan plus melphalan as consolidation in metastatic Ewing tumors: a study by the Societe Francaise des Cancers de l'Enfant. J Clin Oncol 2006;24:3997–4002.
338. Sinkovics JG, Plager C, Ayala AG, et al. Ewing sarcoma: its course and treatment in 50 adult patients. Oncology 1980;37:114–119.
339. Klaassen R, Sastre-Garau X, Aurias A, et al. Ewing's sarcoma of bone in adults: an anatomic-clinical study of 30 cases. Bull Cancer 1992;79:161–167.
340. Moody AM, Norman AR, Tait D. Paediatric tumours in the adult population: the experience of the Royal Marsden Hospital 1974–1990. Med Pediatr Oncol 1996;26:153–159.
341. Baldini EH, Demetri GD, Fletcher CD, et al. Adults with Ewing's sarcoma/primitive neuroectodermal tumor: adverse effect of older age and primary extraosseous disease on outcome. Ann Surg 1999;230:79–86.
342. Eralp Y, Bavbek S, Basaran M, et al. Prognostic factors and survival in late adolescent and adult patients with small round cell tumors. Am J Clin Oncol 2002;25:418–424.
343. Albritton K, Bleyer WA. The management of cancer in the older adolescent. Eur J Cancer 2003;39:2584–2599.
344. Albritton K, Stock W, Paulussen M. Cancer at the interface between medical and pediatric oncology. Educational Book 2004, ed. Alexandria, VA: American Society of Clinical Oncology, 2004.
345. Fizazi K, Dohollou N, Blay JY, et al. Ewing's family of tumors in adults: multivariate analysis of survival and long-term results of multimodality therapy in 182 patients. J Clin Oncol 1998;16:3736–3743.
346. Verrill MW, Judson IR, Harmer CL, et al. Ewing's sarcoma and primitive neuroectodermal tumor in adults: are they different from Ewing's sarcoma and primitive neuroectodermal tumor in children? J Clin Oncol 1997;15:2611–2621.
347. Verrill MW, Judson IR, Wiltshaw E, et al. The use of paediatric chemotherapy protocols at full dose is both a rational and feasible treatment strategy in adults with Ewing's family tumours. Ann Oncol 1997;8:1099–1105.
348. Michelagnoli MP, Pritchard J, Phillips MB. Adolescent oncology—a homeland for the "lost tribe". Eur J Cancer 2003;39:2571–2572.
349. Whelan J. Where should teenagers with cancer be treated? Eur J Cancer 2003;39:2573–2578.
350. Bacci G, Ferrari S, Comandone A, et al. Neoadjuvant chemotherapy for Ewing's sarcoma of bone in patients older than thirty-nine years. Acta Oncol 2000;39:111–116.
351. Schiffer CA. Differences in outcome in adolescents with acute lymphoblastic leukemia: a consequence of better regimens? Better doctors? Both? J Clin Oncol 2003;21:760–761.
352. Ahrens S, Hoffmann C, Jabar S, et al. Evaluation of prognostic factors in a tumor volume-adapted treatment strategy for localized Ewing sarcoma of bone: the CESS 86 experience. Cooperative Ewing Sarcoma Study. Med Pediatr Oncol 1999;32:186–195.
353. Barker LM, Pendergrass TW, Sanders JE, et al. Survival after recurrence of Ewing's sarcoma family of tumors. J Clin Oncol 2005;23:4354–4362.
354. Shankar AG, Ashley S, Craft AW, et al. Outcome after relapse in an unselected cohort of children and adolescents with Ewing sarcoma. Med Pediatr Oncol 2003;40:141–147.
355. Leavey PJ, Mascarenhas L, Marina N, et al. Prognostic factors for patients with Ewing sarcoma (EWS) at first recurrence following multi-modality therapy: a report from the Children's Oncology Group. Pediatr Blood Cancer 2008;51:334–338.
356. Bacci G, Picci P, Ferrari S, et al. Neoadjuvant chemotherapy for Ewing's sarcoma of bone: no benefit observed after adding ifosfamide and etoposide to vincristine, actinomycin, cyclophosphamide, and doxorubicin in the maintenance phase—results of two sequential studies. Cancer 1998;82:1174–1183.
357. Klingebiel T, Pertl U, Hess CF, et al. Treatment of children with relapsed soft tissue sarcoma: report of the German CESS/CWS REZ 91 trial. Med Pediatr Oncol 1998;30:269–275.
358. Rodriguez-Galindo C, Billups CA, Kun LE, et al. Survival after recurrence of Ewing tumors: the St Jude Children's Research Hospital experience, 1979–1999. Cancer 2002; 94:561–569.
359. McLean TW, Hertel C, Young ML, et al. Late events in pediatric patients with Ewing sarcoma/primitive neuroectodermal tumor of bone: the Dana-Farber Cancer Institute/Children's Hospital experience. J Pediatr Hematol Oncol 1999;21:486–493.
360. Shankar AG, Pinkerton CR, Atra A, et al. Local therapy and other factors influencing site of relapse in patients with localised Ewing's sarcoma. United Kingdom Children's Cancer Study Group (UKCCSG). Eur J Cancer 1999;35:1698–1704.
361. Nesbit ME Jr, Perez CA, Tefft M, et al. Multimodal therapy for the management of primary, nonmetastatic Ewing's sarcoma of bone: an Intergroup Study. Natl Cancer Inst Monogr 1981;(56):255–262.
362. Kung FH, Pratt CB, Vega RA, et al. Ifosfamide/etoposide combination in the treatment of recurrent malignant solid tumors of childhood. A Pediatric Oncology Group Phase II study. Cancer 1993;71:1898–1903.
363. Miser JS, Kinsella TJ, Triche TJ, et al. Ifosfamide with mesna uroprotection and etoposide: an effective regimen in the treatment of recurrent sarcomas and other tumors of children and young adults. J Clin Oncol 1987;5:1191–1198.
364. Hayes FA, Thompson EI, Kumar M, et al. Long-term survival in patients with Ewing's sarcoma relapsing after completing therapy. Med Pediatr Oncol 1987;15:254–256.
365. Ferrari S, Brach del Prever A, Palmerini E, et al. Response to high-dose ifosfamide in patients with advanced/recurrent Ewing's tumours. Pediatr Blood Cancer 2009;52:581–584.
366. Hawkins DS, Bradfield S, Whitlock J, et al. Topotecan by 21-day continuous infusion in children with relapsed or refractory solid tumors: a Children's Oncology Group Study. Pediatr Blood Cancer 2006;47:790–794.
367. Nitschke R, Parkhurst J, Sullivan J, et al. Topotecan in pediatric patients with recurrent and progressive solid tumors: a Pediatric Oncology Group phase II study. J Pediatr Hem Oncol 1998:20:315–318.
368. Hunold A, Weddeling N, Paulussen M, et al. Topotecan and cyclophosphamide in patients with refractory or relapsed Ewing tumors. Pediatr Blood Cancer 2006;47:795–800.
369. Kushner BH, Kramer K, Meyers PA, et al. Pilot study of topotecan and high-dose cyclophosphamide for resistant pediatric solid tumors. Med Pediatr Oncol 2000;35:468–474.

370. Saylors RL III, Stine KC, Sullivan J, et al. Cyclophosphamide plus topotecan in children with recurrent or refractory solid tumors: a Pediatric Oncology Group phase II study. J Clin Oncol 2001;19:3463–3469.

371. Wagner LM, CrEWS KR, Iacono LC, et al. Phase I trial temozolomide and protracted irinotecan in pediatric patients with refractory solid tumors. Clin Cancer Res 2004;10: 840–848.

372. Wagner LM, McAllister N, Goldsby RE, et al. Temozolomide and intravenous irinotecan for treatment of advanced Ewing sarcoma. Pediatr Blood Cancer 2007;48:132–139.

373. Kalambakas SA, Moore TB, Feig SA. Megatherapy and stem cell transplantation for Ewing's family of tumors: a critical review of current literature. Pediatric Transplantation 2004;8(suppl 5):83–88.

374. Burdach S, Meyer-Bahlburg A, Laws HJ, et al. High-dose therapy for patients with primary multifocal and early relapsed Ewing's tumors: results of two consecutive regimens assessing the role of total-body irradiation. J Clin Oncol 2003;21:3072–3078.

375. Frohlich B, Ahrens S, Burdach S, et al. High-dosage chemotherapy in primary metastasized and relapsed Ewing's sarcoma (EI)CESS. Klin Padiatr 1999;211:284–290.

376. Hawkins D, Barnett T, Bensinger W, et al. Busulfan, melphalan, and thiotepa with or without total marrow irradiation with hematopoietic stem cell rescue for poor-risk Ewing-Sarcoma-Family tumors. Med Pediatr Oncol 2000;34:328–337.

377. Burdach S. Treatment of advanced Ewing tumors by combined radiochemotherapy and engineered cellular transplants. Pediatr Transplant 2004;8(suppl 5):67–82.

378. Kovar H. Ewing tumor biology: perspectives for innovative treatment approaches. Adv Exp Med Biol 2003;532:27–37.

379. Bond M, Bernstein ML, Pappo A, et al. A phase II study of imatinib mesylate in children with refractory or relapsed Ewing's tumors: results of a Children's Oncology Group study. Ped Blood Cancer 2008;50:254–258.

380. Glade Bender JL, Adamson PC, Reid JM, et al. Phase I trial and pharmacokinetic study of bevacizumab in pediatric patients with refractory solid tumors: a Children's Oncology Group Study. J Clin Oncol 2008;26:399–405.

381. Houghton PJ, Morton CL, Kolb EA, et al. Initial testing (stage 1) of the mTOR inhibitor rapamycin by the pediatric preclinical testing program. Pediatr Blood Cancer 2008;50:799–805.

382. Olmos D, Okuno S, Schuetze SM, et al. Safety, pharmacokinetics and preliminary activity of the anti-IGF-IR antibody CP-751,871 in patients with sarcoma [abstract 10501]. J Clin Oncol 2008;26.

383. Tolcher AW, Rothenberg ML, Rodon J, et al. A phase I pharmacokinetic and pharmacodynamic study of AMG 479, a fully human monoclonal antibody against insulin-like growth factor type 1 receptor (IGF-1R), in advanced solid tumors [abstract 3002]. J Clin Oncol 2007;25.

384. Chawla SP, Tolcher AW, Staddon AP, et al. Survival results with AP23573, a novel mTOR inhibitor, in patients (pts) with advanced soft tissue or bone sarcomas: Update of phase II trial [abstract 10076]. J Clin Oncol 2007;25.

385. Mita MM, Mita AC, Chu QS, et al. Phase I trial of the novel mammalian target of rapamycin inhibitor deforolimus (AP23573; MK-8669) administered intravenously daily for 5 days every 2 weeks to patients with advanced malignancies. J Clin Oncol 2008;26:361–367.

386. Dagher R, Long LM, Read EJ, et al. Pilot trial of tumor-specific peptide vaccination and continuous infusion interleukin-2 in patients with recurrent Ewing sarcoma and alveolar rhabdomyosarcoma: an inter-institute NIH study. Med Pediatr Oncol 2002;38: 158–164.

387. Mackall C, Berzofsky J, Helman LJ. Targeting tumor specific translocations in sarcomas in pediatric patients for immunotherapy. Clin Orthop 2000;373:25–31.

388. Nagarajan R, Clohisy DR, Neglia JP, et al. Function and quality-of-life of survivors of pelvic and lower extremity osteosarcoma and Ewing's sarcoma: the Childhood Cancer Survivor Study. Br J Cancer 2004;91:1858–1865.

389. Friedman DL, Meadows AT. Late effects of childhood cancer therapy. Pediatr Clin North Am 2002;49:1083–1106.

390. Stöhr W, Paulides M, Bielack S, et al. Ifosfamide-induced nephrotoxicity in 593 sarcoma patients: a report from the Late Effects Surveillance System. Pediatr Blood Cancer 2006;48:447–452.

391. Kuttesch JF Jr, Wexler LH, Marcus RB, et al. Second malignancies after Ewing's sarcoma: radiation dose-dependency of secondary sarcomas. J Clin Oncol 1996;14:2818–2825.

392. Dunst J, Ahrens S, Paulussen M, et al. Second malignancies after treatment for Ewing's sarcoma: a report of the CESS-studies. Int J Radiat Oncol Biol Phys 1998;42:379–384.

393. Le Vu B, de Vathaire F, Shamsaldin A, et al. Radiation dose, chemotherapy and risk of osteosarcoma after solid tumours during childhood. Int J Cancer 1998;77:370–377.

394. Bacci G, Longhi A, Barbieri E, et al. Second malignancy in 597 patients with Ewing sarcoma of bone treated at a single institution with adjuvant and neoadjuvant chemotherapy between 1972 and 1999. J Ped Hem/Onc 2005;27:517–520.

395. Navid F, Billups C, Liu T, et al. Second cancers in patients with the Ewing sarcoma family of tumours. Eur J Cancer 2008;44:983–991.

396. Paulussen M, Ahrens S, Lehnert M, et al. Second malignancies after Ewing tumor treatment in 690 patients from a cooperative German/Austrian/Dutch study. Ann Oncol 2001;12:1619–1630.

397. Goldsby R, Burke C, Nagarajan R, et al. Second solid malignancies among children, adolescents, and young adults diagnosed with malignant bone tumors after 1976: follow-up of a Children's Oncology Group cohort. Cancer 2008;113:2597–2604.

398. Bhatia S, Krailo MD, Chen Z, et al. Therapy-related myelodysplasia and acute myeloid leukemia after Ewing sarcoma and primitive neuroectodermal tumor of bone: a report from the Children's Oncology Group. Blood 2007;109:46–51.

399. Nagarajan R, Neglia JP, Clohisy DR, et al. Education, employment, insurance, and marital status among 694 survivors of pediatric lower extremity bone tumors: a report from the childhood cancer survivor study. Cancer 2003;97:2554–2564.

400. Bacci G, Balladelli A, Forni C, et al. Adjuvant and neo-adjuvant chemotherapy for Ewing's sarcoma family tumors and osteosarcoma of the extremity: further outcome for patients event-free survivors 5 years from the beginning of treatment. Ann Oncol 2007; 18:2037–2040.

401. Fuchs B, Valenzuela RG, Inwards C, et al. Complications in long-term survivors of Ewing sarcoma. Cancer 2003;98:2687–2692.

402. Rosen G, Caparros B, Mosende C, et al. Curability of Ewing's sarcoma and considerations for future therapeutic trials. Cancer 1978;41:888–899.

403. Hayes FA, Thompson EI, Meyer WH, et al. Therapy for localized Ewing's sarcoma of bone. J Clin Oncol 1989;7:208–213.

404. Meyer WH, Kun L, Marina N, et al. Ifosfamide plus etoposide in newly diagnosed Ewing's sarcoma of bone. J Clin Oncol 1992;10:1737–1742.

405. Elomaa I, Blomqvist CP, Saeter G, et al. Five-year results in Ewing's sarcoma. The Scandinavian Sarcoma Group experience with the SSG IX protocol. Eur J Cancer 2000; 36:875–880.

CHAPTER 34 ■ OSTEOSARCOMA: BIOLOGY, DIAGNOSIS, TREATMENT, AND REMAINING CHALLENGES

RICHARD GORLICK, STEFAN BIELACK, LISA TEOT, JAMES MEYER, R. LOR RANDALL, AND NEYSSA MARINA

INTRODUCTION

Historically, the outcome for patients with osteosarcoma treated with surgery and/or radiotherapy was poor with 2-year survivals of 15% to 20%.[1-4] The introduction of systemic chemotherapy dramatically improved outcome,[5,6] and most current series report 3-year event-free survivals of 60% to 70% for patients with localized, extremity osteosarcoma.[7-9] Our goal in this chapter is to discuss the epidemiology, biology, pathology, and therapeutic advances in the treatment of osteosarcoma. We will also discuss the remaining therapeutic challenges and therapy-related complications associated with treatment.

EPIDEMIOLOGY AND BIOLOGY

Epidemiology/Etiology

Several features about the epidemiology of osteosarcoma have provided some clues as to its pathogenesis. Osteosarcoma has a bimodal age distribution with the first peak in the second decade of life corresponding to the period of most rapid longitudinal bone growth. The second peak occurs among older adults in many cases associated with established risk factors such as the presence of Paget's disease.[10,11] There is some variability in annual incidence rates. The incidence by age is 4.4 per million in individuals under 24 years of age, 1.7 per million between 25 and 59 years, and 4.2 per million over the age of 60 years.[10,11] There are approximately 400 new cases of osteosarcoma each year in the United States in individuals younger than 20 years,[12] with similar incidence rates internationally.[13] Primary bone tumors account for approximately 5% to 10% of all new pediatric cancer diagnoses in the United States and osteosarcoma represents the most common pediatric bone cancer.[11] The male to female ratio is approximately 1.3:1 in the pediatric age range. The incidence in males is 5.2 per million as compared with 4.5 per million in females. Osteosarcoma is slightly more common in black children than in white children with an incidence of 5.2 per million in black individuals younger than 20 years compared with 4.6 per million in whites.[11] From the Surveillance Epidemiology and End Results (SEER) data, rates were higher in Hispanics and Asian-Pacific Islanders as well.[10]

The peak age for patients with osteosarcoma coincides with a period of rapid bone growth in young people, suggesting a correlation between rapid bone growth and the pathogenesis of osteosarcoma.[12,14] Other evidence supporting this relationship includes the higher incidence of osteosarcoma in large dog breeds as compared with small breeds,[15,16] the metaphyseal location of many of the tumors and the earlier peak age in girls as compared with boys, corresponding to their earlier growth spurt.[17] Greater height has been associated with a higher risk of osteosarcoma in some studies but has been refuted in other analyses and, therefore, remains somewhat controversial. A large study from the Children's Cancer Group suggested that relationship with height did not exist,[18] but many recent studies continue to suggest that taller individuals and those with earlier pubertal growth spurts are at higher risk for osteosarcoma.[19-21] It has been hypothesized that this may be related to polymorphisms in growth-related genes, with an association with a vitamin D receptor polymorphism found in a reported study.[22] The occurrence of osteosarcoma in the axial skeleton including the flat bones that undergo appositional bone growth rather than growth at the growth plate suggests that bone turnover or other etiologic factors may be important as well.

Radiation exposure is a well-documented risk factor for the development of osteosarcoma, but since the interval between irradiation and osteosarcoma is typically long this is not relevant to most pediatric patients.[12,23-29] The excess risk of osteosarcoma associated with radiation exposure has largely been calculated on the basis of both those treated with therapeutic radiation as well as atomic bomb survivors.[30,31] The excess risk has been found to be relatively linear and is approximately 1.8 for each gray of radiation exposure.[32] The lack of a clear threshold for this malignancy as well as others has been part of the concern with regard to avoiding diagnostic radiation exposure, particularly computed tomography scanning among normal children.[33,34] The incidence of osteosarcoma is dramatically increased among survivors of retinoblastoma particularly those with the hereditary form who harbor germline mutations of the retinoblastoma gene.[35,36] Patients with the hereditary form of retinoblastoma have a 19.8-fold excess risk of osteosarcoma, which makes osteosarcoma the most common secondary malignancy in this patient population.[37] The rate of osteosarcoma in patients with unilateral sporadic retinoblastoma, generally lacking germline mutations, is markedly lower.[38,39] They are reported to have a risk of osteosarcoma no higher than the general population. Germline mutations in the p53 gene (the basis of the Li-Fraumeni syndrome) can lead to a high risk of developing malignancies including osteosarcoma.[40,41] Rothmund-Thomson syndrome patients, particularly those with a RecQL4 mutation, are also at high risk of developing osteosarcoma.[17,42] Patients with Werner and Bloom syndrome are at a high risk of developing osteosarcoma among many other cancer predispositions.[43-45] Other predisposing factors include a history of disorders of bone metabolism (i.e., Paget's disease of the bone and fibrous dysplasia)[46-48] (see Table 34.1).

GENETIC CONDITIONS ASSOCIATED WITH OSTEOSARCOMA DEVELOPMENT

Hereditary cancer syndrome	Chromosome location	Gene	Function	Percentage of malignancies that are OS
Retinoblastoma	13q14.2	RB1	Cell cycle regulation	50%
Li-Fraumeni	17p13.1	P53	DNA damage response	10%
Paget's disease	18q21-q22 5q31 5q35	LOH18CR1 SQSTM1 MAPK8	IL-1/TNF signaling RANK signaling	Not applicable
Rothmund-Thomson syndrome	18q24.3	RTS (ReQL4)	DNA helicase	30%
Werner syndrome	8p12-p11.2	WRN (RecQL2)	DNA helicase Exonuclease activity	<10%
Bloom syndrome	15q26.1	15q26.1	DNA helicase	<10%

A viral etiology for osteosarcoma had been suggested on the basis of several lines of evidence. It had been suggested that contamination of poliovirus by SV40 was an etiologic factor in osteosarcoma.[49,50] It has subsequently been proven that SV40 is not a major epidemiologic factor in the development of osteosarcoma. Trauma is also often reported as part of the presenting history for patients with osteosarcoma, but little evidence exists to support a causal relationship.[12]

Biology

Osteosarcoma is genetically an extremely complex tumor.[51–54] Although many of the alterations present in the tumors have been elucidated, the molecular complexity precludes placing the tumor's pathogenesis into a simple conceptual framework.[17,23] Osteosarcoma is defined as a clinical entity by its production of disorganized osteoid.[55–57] However, the production of bony matrix is a cellular behavior or a phenotype, not a genetic marker. Considerable variability exists in the predominant matrix produced by osteosarcomas, usually described as a histologic subtype, but the presence of even a small area of osteoid in association with a malignant spindle cell is generally viewed by pathologists as sufficient to make a diagnosis. Cytogenetics, molecular markers, and immunohistochemistry are not typically used to aid in making a diagnosis.[56] Despite this phenotypic definition, the clinical behavior of high-grade osteosarcoma is homogeneous. Although once controversial, histologic subtype does not influence the chemotherapy utilized or the tendency to metastasize early in its natural history or to a great extent chemotherapy response or prognosis.[12,55,56] Given this phenotypic definition, it is perhaps not surprising that at the molecular level considerable variability exists, making understanding the fundamental biology of this tumor somewhat elusive.

Unlike the majority of tumors arising in adults, osteosarcoma does not have an obvious multistep progression. Although most adult malignancies are epithelial in origin, some sarcomas (common in adults) such as chondrosarcoma also have a stepwise progression from benign enchondromas through grade 3 high-grade sarcomas. Low-grade osteosarcomas cannot be identified as a precursor lesion in the majority of children, adolescents, or even adults that develop high-grade osteosarcoma.[58,59] The equivalent of a premalignant dysplastic lesion or a carcinoma in situ is not known to exist for osteosarcoma as is the case for most pediatric malignancies. When defining the molecular pathogenesis of osteosarcoma, the first lesion that can typically be analyzed is already a fully malignant tumor. This fact coupled with the tumor's molecular complexity makes it extremely difficult to define the molecular features essential to its pathogenesis. Despite these difficulties, a considerable amount is known about specific molecular features associated with the development of osteosarcoma.

Osteosarcoma Pathogenesis

Despite its genetic complexity, numerous clues exist as to which genetic pathway alterations may be associated with the pathogenesis of osteosarcoma. These clues are derived from mouse models of osteosarcoma, human predisposition syndromes, etiologic-environmental factors, and studies of genetic alterations in tumors.[17,23] In contrast to most cancers, a large number of models (rather than too few) produce osteosarcoma. Many of the same genetic alterations give rise to malignancies in adults, which arise at much higher frequencies. This suggests, given the relative rarity of osteosarcoma, that many of these genetic events are not clinically relevant or alternatively the development of osteosarcoma is restricted by other constraints. These constraints have not been identified but could be related to the target tissue/cell, temporal restrictions, or immune surveillance as several of many potential examples.[43] Models and analyses providing clues to the pathogenesis of osteosarcoma will be discussed subsequently.

Perhaps the most compelling data potentially defining the pathogenesis of osteosarcoma are humans with germline genetic alterations associated with an increased risk of developing osteosarcoma, which has been covered previously. Additional support for the importance of the Rb and p53 genes in osteosarcoma development derives from the frequent derangements of these pathways in tumor specimens.[36,60–62] It is important to note that in patients with sporadic osteosarcoma the incidence of unsuspected germline alterations in Rb and p53 is rare. The vast majority of Rb gene abnormalities are inherited in an autosomal-dominant manner and have high penetrance.[63] Hence, the lack of a history of prior retinoblastoma in virtually all patients who are diagnosed with sporadic osteosarcoma suggests that germline alterations of Rb in this patient population are not common. In large studies of sporadic osteosarcoma, only 3% of patients were found to harbor unsuspected alterations in germline p53.[64,65] Therefore, somatic alterations in either p53 or Rb do not explain the majority of sporadic osteosarcoma cases but suggest that these pathways may be involved in its pathogenesis (discussed subsequently). The data supporting RECQ DNA helicases involvement in the pathogenesis of sporadic osteosarcoma is even more limited. RECQ DNA helicases are conserved proteins that separate the complementary strands of DNA duplexes. The three RECQ DNA helicases involved in cancer predisposition syndromes are RECQL4 in Rothmund-Thomson syndrome, RECQL2 in Werner syndrome, and RECQL3 in Bloom syndrome. In sporadic osteosarcomas, RecQL4 is rarely altered suggesting that it does not play a role in the pathogenesis of these tumors even though it is associated with osteosarcoma in the context of Rothmund-Thomson syndrome.[66] Patients with Rothmund-Thomson syndrome have a 30% incidence of osteosarcoma, but less than 10% of patients with either Werner syndrome or Bloom syndrome develop osteosarcoma.[44,45]

Although genetic alterations in humans, which are associated with an increased risk of osteosarcoma, have directly established relevance, murine models offer additional evidence as to the genetic alterations and exposures that can predispose to osteosarcoma. A large number of murine models develop osteosarcoma. This, in part, may reflect lower barriers to developing malignancy in general in mice and their cells as compared to humans. Transgenic mice engineered to overexpress SV40 develop osteosarcoma, with the clinical pattern dependent upon the promoter driving expression.[67] This is supportive of the hypothesis that the p53 and Rb tumor suppressor genes have a role in osteosarcoma development as the SV40 large T antigen abrogates the function of both of these pathways.[67] Knockout mice with mutant or absent p53 develop osteosarcoma along with a variety of other tumors. Depending upon the particular p53 alteration, osteosarcoma develops in between 5% and 50% of the mice.[68–71] Knocking out the Rb gene is lethal at embryonic stages in mice; thus, it has not been possible to assess whether or not these mice are prone to developing osteosarcoma.[72] More recent studies have used conditional knockouts of p53 and Rb selectively in pre-osteoblasts to demonstrate that these models do indeed develop osteosarcoma.[43,73] Transgenic overexpression of several oncogenes, including myc and fos, can also produce osteosarcoma.[74,75] Almost 100% of transgenic mice that ubiquitously overexpress fos develop osteosarcoma.[74] Transgenic mice that conditionally overexpress myc in fibroblasts/osteoblasts also develop osteosarcoma.[75] Radiating mice leads to the development of osteosarcoma as does chronic exposure to parathyroid hormone.[76,77] A number of epidemiologic factors including growth are associated with the development of osteosarcoma. This has provided some support to the notion that the growth hormone–insulin-like growth factor (IGF) axis may be involved in osteosarcoma pathogenesis. Multiple studies have suggested that the incidence of this disease peaking during the second decade of life is related to the rapid longitudinal bone growth occurring during this period of time. Osteosarcoma has a predilection for rapidly growing long bones in the extremities, arising in the metaphysis, which is the site of new bone formation by the growth plates.[12,17,23,78] Other factors suggesting an association with growth include the association with height mentioned previously as well as its earlier peak incidence in females concordant with their earlier growth spurt.[18,20,21,48,79] Perhaps, among the more frequently cited data linking osteosarcoma to growth are its high incidence among large breed dogs and its almost complete absence among smaller breed dogs.[80–82] Recent studies, however, suggest that the incidence of osteosarcoma does not vary within canine breeds and that, perhaps, the determining factor may be their underlying genetics rather than height as a phenotype.[16,83] More recent explanations of canine breed height variability based on a finite number of polymorphisms in the IGF axis may give further support to that view.[84] Independent of growth, accelerated bone turnover may play a role in the etiology of osteosarcoma, given its association with disorders of bone metabolism (i.e., Paget's disease of the bone and fibrous dysplasia).[46,47,85] Other clear predisposing factors include exposure to nonspecific DNA-damaging agents such as ionizing radiation.[38,86–90] The mechanism by which these etiologic factors predispose to this specific malignancy remains unclear.

Multiple and variable molecular alterations resulting in inactivation of tumor suppressor genes and overexpression of oncogenes are observed in every osteosarcoma. With the multitude of genetic lesions, it is difficult to discern which of these events is fundamental to tumorigenesis.[17] The most consistent feature across human predisposition syndromes, murine predisposition syndromes, and analyses of human tumors is alterations of the Rb and p53 tumor suppressor pathways. The inactivation of these pathways is accomplished through a variety of genetic alterations, which occur in a nonoverlapping manner so that only one mechanism of Rb inactivation and one mechanism of p53 inactivation are present in each tumor. Genetic lesions in the Rb gene itself, mapped to 13q14, have been shown to be present in approximately 70% of primary osteosarcoma tumor samples.[36,60–62] In addition, approximately 60% of osteosarcoma tumors have loss of heterozygosity at 13q, the site of Rb. Gross structural rearrangements of the Rb gene are present in approximately 30% of osteosarcoma tumors.[36,60–62,91,92] Cyclin-dependent kinase-4 (CDK4) in complex with cyclin D1 (CCND1) is responsible for the phosphorylation of Rb, and therefore, amplification or overexpression of these genes results in functional inactivation of the Rb signaling pathway. Amplification of the 12q13–15 chromosomal region, which contains CDK4 or the gene itself, is observed in approximately 5% to 10% of osteosarcomas.[93] The INK4 A gene, localized to 9p21, encodes p16INK4 A; a tumor suppressor that inhibits the CDK4-CCND1 complex, thereby halting cell cycle transition. Alterations of INK4 A result in an Rb pathway disruption. Deletions in the INK4 A region are observed in approximately 5% to 10% of osteosarcomas.[93] Deletion of INK4 A, by virtue of an alternative reading frame that encodes another tumor suppressor p19INK4 A or p14ARF, functionally inactivates p53 as well.[94] Analogous to Rb, a significant proportion of sporadic osteosarcoma samples have some molecular modification abrogating normal p53 function. In osteosarcoma tumor samples, alterations in p53 consist of point mutations (occurs in 20% to 30%), gross gene rearrangements (occurs in 10% to 20%), and loss of one 17q allele (occurs in 75% to 80%).[64,95–98] Alterations in other genes encoding proteins that regulate p53 have also been implicated in the pathogenesis of osteosarcoma. MDM2, mapped to chromosome 12q13–14, which negatively modulates p53 function by binding the protein, concealing its activation site and facilitating its proteasomal degradation, is amplified in about 10% of osteosarcomas.[98] Another negative regulator of p53 is COPS3 (constitutive photomorphogenic homolog subunit 3), which is amplified in about 25% of cases of osteosarcoma.[99] COPS3 amplification, INK4 A deletion, MDM2 amplification, and TP53 mutations seem to be mutually exclusive; again suggesting that any of these alterations in the TP53 tumor suppressor pathway is sufficient in regard to the contribution of this pathway to tumorigenesis in osteosarcoma.[99] These molecular alterations provide a loss of cell cycle checkpoint function and normal DNA damage response, which are essential steps in malignant transformation.[100–102] The Rb gene plays an essential role in cell cycle regulation and the p53 gene product plays a major role in the cellular response to DNA damage a more full description of which is beyond the scope of this chapter.[103–106] While the invariable presence of alterations of Rb and p53 suggests that inactivation of these pathways may be essential for osteosarcoma development, this does not necessarily establish these events as early steps in tumor pathogenesis since other events may drive the development of these abnormalities and serve as the initiating genetic event.

Tumors may be defined by both the cells they originate from as well as the genetic events that lead to tumor formation. Osteosarcoma has traditionally been believed to arise from an osteoblast, but the data supporting this are limited.[55,56] Evidence may suggest that osteosarcoma has a more pluripotent potential and may, in fact, arise from a more primitive precursor.[43,73,107] Normal osteoblasts derive from a pluripotent mesenchymal stem cell that can differentiate into cartilage, muscle, stroma, fat, and fibrous tissue in accordance with well-defined differentiation pathways not unlike hematopoiesis. The presence of osteoid has led to the viewpoint that osteosarcoma is derived from osteoblasts. It is well known that great variability exists in the histological patterns seen in this tumor and in the degree of osteoid production. It is also known that these tumors are capable of differentiating toward fibrous tissue, cartilage, or bone with resulting chondroblastic, fibroblastic, and osteoblastic components. This suggests that the cell of origin has a more pluripotent potential than an osteoblast but may not reflect a more primitive origin as the pluripotent potential may be acquired as a result of transformation. Tumors with various patterns of differentiation are traditionally referred to as histologic subtypes. It is well established that many tumors have mixed patterns.[55,56] It is also known that the histologic subtype does not impact chemotherapy response or outcome and patients receive the same treatment regardless of histologic subtype, suggesting that these various patterns of differentiation are reflective of a single clinical entity. At present the factors that control histologic appearance in osteosarcoma are poorly understood.[55,56] Osteosarcoma could arise from a mesenchymal stem cell, which acquires patterns of osteoblastic differentiation during transformation. Similarly, osteosarcoma may arise from an osteoblast and the pluripotent capacity be acquired through dedifferentiation during the transformation process. The acquisition and loss of differentiation properties can be observed in the potentially analogous development of hematopoietic malignancies.[43,73] Some murine findings have implicated mesenchymal stem cells as a possible progenitor.[108] Two recent manuscripts reporting conditional p53 and Rb knockouts speculate on the cell of origin of osteosarcoma. One manuscript suggests that the preosteoblast is the cell of origin based on the conditional targeting of preosteoblasts resulting in an osteosarcoma-like tumor, while the other implicates a rare cell type that simultaneously expresses a more primitive differentiation marker and a preosteoblastic marker based on flow cytometric studies.[43,73] Even if one accepts mesenchymal stem cells, preosteoblasts, or osteoblasts as the cell of origin of osteosarcoma, these cells exist in various pools and anatomic locations. These pools include the bone marrow, growth plates, and the periosteum, and it is unclear which pool serves as the usual cell of origin.

Numerous studies have described the genetic abnormalities present in osteosarcoma tumor samples. Many of these will be discussed in the subsequent sections where they are considered in the context of functional roles as has been performed previously for the Rb and p53 pathways. In addition to the defined alterations, osteosarcomas have tremendous chromosomal complexity with numerous whole chromosome alterations as well as a large number of regions with consistent genetic gains and losses.[51,52,54,109] These sites have been characterized to a variable extent and many of the genes altered in osteosarcoma have not been fully identified or characterized.[85,110,111] Before reviewing some of these alterations, it may be worthwhile to mention that investigators have demonstrated that only a few genetic elements are necessary

to transform a normal cell into a cancerous one as only a few fundamental processes need to be deranged.[112] To become malignant, a normal cell needs to be able to progress through the cell cycle with loss of checkpoint control, telomere length stabilization, and loss of contact inhibition/dependence.[112] Osteosarcoma clearly does not need all of the alterations it possesses to achieve these tasks, and many genetic events are likely to be bystander effects related, perhaps, to genetic instability. The genetic instability can be attributed to alterations in specific genes resulting in loss of checkpoint control or to global issues in maintaining chromosomal integrity. This issue of redundant genetic alterations, which may be attributed to genetic instability, is perhaps most evident in the expression of growth factor receptors in osteosarcoma. Osteosarcoma has been reported to express IGF-1R (Insulin-like growth factor receptor-1), VEGF (vascular endothelial growth factor), EGF (endothelial growth factor), human epidermal growth factor receptor 2 (HER2), human epidermal growth factor 4 (ErbB-4), parathyroid hormone receptor (PTHR), and HGF (hepatocyte growth factor), among others.[113-131] Many, if not all, of these pathways are redundant. Additionally, there are numerous genetic abnormalities in osteosarcoma, a small subset of which could lead to the development of a malignancy. This redundancy makes it difficult to determine the relative timing and importance of each of these events.

Growth factor receptors and autocrine or paracrine stimulation pathways may contribute to abnormal cell proliferation in the pathogenesis of osteosarcoma. These feedback loops can lead to loss of external regulation of cell proliferation, motility, and angiogenesis. Insulin-like growth factor-1 (IGF-1), a major regulator of skeletal growth, has been found to be mitogenic in in vitro models of osteosarcoma.[123,132-135] Survival of osteosarcoma cell lines in vitro has been shown to be dependent on exogenous IGF-1, and proliferation of these cell lines can be inhibited by blocking signaling through the IGF-1 receptor via monoclonal antibodies or antisense oligonucleotides.[113,133,134] IGF-1R has been found to be abundantly expressed in osteosarcoma cells.[113] IGF-1R signaling may contribute not only to cellular proliferation but also, perhaps more importantly, to malignant transformation, and protection from apoptosis.[136] Overexpression of IGF-1 and its receptor may, therefore, play a role in the pathogenesis of osteosarcoma by contributing to oncogenic transformation and providing a proliferative and survival advantage.[136] Of the growth factor circuits involved in the pathogenesis of osteosarcoma, IGF-1/IGF-1R is currently believed to be of major importance.[137]

Overexpression of the c-met proto-oncogene tyrosine kinase receptor (Met) and its ligand, HGF or scatter factor, in osteosarcoma cell lines suggests a role for Met in the metastatic phenotype of osteosarcoma. Binding of the HGF or scatter factor to the Met/HGF receptor stimulates both cell proliferation and motility, which are associated with the malignant potential of tumor cells.[138,139] The predominant expression of the Met/HGF receptor on epithelial cells, along with its ligand being produced primarily by cells of mesenchymal origin, suggests a paracrine or autocrine signaling system in regulating stromal-epithelial interactions.[139-141] When primary and metastatic osteosarcomas from the same patient are compared, metastatic tumors have higher Met expression than the primary tumors, again suggesting its role in defining the metastatic phenotype.[137,140,141]

Platelet-derived growth factor (PDGF) is another potent mitogen for cells of mesenchymal origin. Coexpression of PDGF and its receptors has been observed in various human solid tumors and correlates with inferior prognosis and metastasis in some, suggesting an autocrine or paracrine mechanism driving cellular proliferation and differentiation, chemotaxis, and survival in these tumors.[142-150] The role of

PDGF/PDGF-R in osteosarcoma has been explored with studies reporting expression in at least a subset of tumors.[151] The relevance of this pathway to osteosarcoma's pathogenesis and clinical behavior is not completely defined.

Other tyrosine kinase receptors have been implicated in the pathogenesis of osteosarcoma. The c-erbB-2 proto-oncogene (also called HER2/neu), located on 17q12, encodes a protein structurally homologous to the epidermal growth factor receptor, although its actual ligand has not yet been identified. The importance of expression of ErbB family of tyrosine kinase receptors for tumor growth or clinical outcome has been demonstrated in a variety of human cancers, most notably in invasive breast cancers and non–small cell lung cancer. The data in osteosarcoma is controversial, with some investigators reporting overexpression (associated with either favorable or unfavorable prognosis) and other investigators reporting lack of overexpression of erb-B2.[116,120,125,128,152–162] Various explanations may account for the discrepancies between studies, including methodology and interpretation of immunohistochemical staining, antibody clones utilized, and cross-reactivity with other membrane antigens, along with inherent biologic variability among osteosarcoma samples tested in various institutions representing different geographical areas.

Identification of growth factor expression in osteosarcoma leads one to consider the downstream signal transduction pathways resulting from activation of their receptors. The majority of signaling by the aforementioned receptors is transduced by three interrelated parallel pathways: Ras/Raf/mitogen-activated protein kinases (MAPK), phosphatidylinositol 3'-kinase/Akt (PI3 K/Akt), and mammalian target of rapamycin (mTOR).[163–166] Each of these pathways is comprised of a series of kinases where signal is transmitted through phosphorylation of amino acids, tyrosine, serine, or threonine. Transmission of signal in this manner permits it to occur rapidly as no RNA or protein synthesis is required and it also permits marked signal amplification. The MAPK pathways play pivotal roles in cell proliferation, differentiation, and survival. Some data suggest that this pathway may mediate differentiation in osteoblasts.[167,168] To date, little information is available regarding the role of this pathway in osteosarcoma. Several sources of data suggest that this pathway may be constitutively active in osteosarcoma.[151]

The PI3 K/Akt and mTOR signal transduction pathways play an important role in transducing a variety of receptor signals. mTOR is believed to serve as the intracellular pathway through which IGF signaling is transduced.[166,169] In the context of osteosarcoma, little is known about these pathways although several publications demonstrate activation of these pathways with a variety of ligands and with associated biological effects. Analogous to the MAPK pathway both PI3 K/akt and mTOR have been suggested to be involved in the differentiation of mesenchymal stem cells toward the adipogenic lineage.[170] PI3 K/akt has been implicated in osteosarcoma's metastatic process as well as chemotherapy sensitivity.[171,172]

Many other cellular proto-oncogenes are altered in osteosarcoma and have been suggested as contributing to its molecular pathogenesis. The MYC proto-oncogene, localized to 8q24, functions in the regulation of cell proliferation, cell growth, inhibition of differentiation, and apoptosis. It has been found to be overexpressed in a subset of osteosarcoma tumor samples.[173–176] c-Myc expression has been suggested to be related with metastasis.[173] As mentioned previously, certain myc overexpressing transgenic mice have an osteosarcoma predisposition.[75] Fos was initially identified as being related to osteosarcoma through recognition that mice inoculated with FBJ murine virus developed these tumors.[177,178] The viral protein–inducing osteosarcoma is v-fos, which led to the identification of the structurally related c-fos protein as an oncogene.[178–180] Fos heterodimerizes with Jun to regulate the AP1 transcription factor. The AP1 transcription factor is known to be regulated by vitamin D, transforming growth factor beta and parathyroid hormone—all known to be involved in the regulation of bone growth, indicating a possible basis for its association with osteosarcoma development. Overexpression of Fos oncoprotein is found in the majority of osteosarcomas, and potentially associated with metastasis or recurrence.[173,181,182]

In addition to the known loss of tumor suppressor genes and gain of oncogenes, osteosarcoma has tremendous chromosomal complexity with numerous other genes affected by gross genetic changes. As one example of the genetic complexity, spectral karyotyping reveals an average of 39 chromosomal rearrangements per tumor.[183] Some of the genetic alterations appear to be random but recurrent regions of chromosomal gain and loss are present.[53,184,185] In many of these cases, the target of the genetic amplification or loss is known and in many cases it is not.[85,111] The most common genetic losses and regions with losses of heterozygosity involve chromosomes 2, 3, 6, 9, 10, 13, 17, and 18 with the Rb gene located on chromosome 13 and p53 located on chromosome 17.[53] Loss of heterozygosity on chromosome 18 is also seen in Paget's disease and chromosome 3 in Brachmann-de Lange syndrome, a bone dysmorphology syndrome.[46,110,111] The most common regions of amplification include regions within chromosomes 1, 5, 6, 8, 12, 16, and 17 with MYC located on chromosome 8 and MDM2 on chromosome 12. Candidate genes for some of the amplified regions include PRDM16, CDC5 L, NFKBIE, IFNG, MGRN1, PMP22, MYCD, TOP3 A, MAPK7, and COPS3.[53]

Immortalization heralded by telomere length stabilization has been explored as contributing to the pathogenesis of osteosarcoma. Telomeres cap chromosome ends and serve to potentiate the replicative process in cells by compensating for the loss of genetic material secondary to inability to replicate end DNA.[186,187] Maintaining telomere length is regarded as a fundamental necessity for overcoming cellular senescence in tumor cells. Maintaining telomere length is accomplished by most cancers via activation of an enzyme, telomerase (TERT).[112] TERT activity is only present in a minority of osteosarcomas and does not seem to be essential to tumorigenesis. The clinicopathological correlation of telomerase has varied: an inverse relationship was reported between TERT activity and pulmonary metastases, whereas another study found decreased survival associated with TERT expression in primary osteosarcoma tumor samples. Alternative mechanisms of telomere lengthening (ALT), a recombination-based method, is the mechanism of maintaining telomere length seen more often in osteosarcoma. About 60% of osteosarcoma tumor samples utilize ALT. The aggressiveness of osteosarcoma has been associated with telomere integrity: a subset of osteosarcoma patients that lacked both TERT activity and evidence of ALT demonstrated a more favorable prognosis.[188–190]

The complex molecular alterations in osteosarcoma may not only involve dysregulation of cellular pathways involved in proliferation and immortalization but also disruptions in differentiation. Osteosarcoma can be regarded as potentially evolving from a primitive pluripotent progenitor cell that retains its proliferative capacity while undergoing partial differentiation, or alternatively, a more differentiated precursor cell that dedifferentiates and regains an ability to proliferate. The differentiation status of osteosarcomas is variable. Transforming growth factor-β (TGF-β) isoforms play an important role in regulating bone formation.[191–193] Bone morphogenetic proteins (BMPs), part of the TGF-β superfamily, are multifunctional cytokines that regulate bone and skeletal development. BMPs are involved in the differentiation of mesenchymal cells to cells of osteoblastic lineage, and in the differentiation of immature osteoblasts into mature osteoblasts.[194,195] *In vitro* data suggest that BMPs stimulate growth of osteosarcoma cells.[195] Numerous BMPs and/or their receptors are highly expressed in osteosarcoma tumors, implicating their potential importance in autocrine or paracrine growth stimulation of osteosarcoma.[194] Overexpression of BMP Receptor II has been associated with poor prognosis and the metastatic potential of osteosarcoma.[194]

The process of osteoblast differentiation is driven by wingless (Wnt) signaling within the mesenchymal stem cell. In this signaling, pathway Wnt binds to the cell surface receptor frizzled (Frz) and the coreceptor lipoprotein related proteins 5 and 6 (LRP-5/6), leading to the stabilization and accumulation of β-catenin that in turn elicits a variety of cellular effects.[196–198] Aberrant activation of Wnt signaling is associated with many human cancers.[199] Cytoplasmic or nuclear accumulation of β-catenin has been found in a majority of osteosarcomas and has correlated with its metastatic potential.[200] PTH plays a central role in the regulation of bone and mineral metabolism and has been implicated in the pathogenesis of osteosarcoma.[129] In response to PTHrP, osteoclastic resorption of bone is stimulated, and as a result, growth factors such as transforming growth factor-β (TGF-β) and IGF-1 are released from the surrounding extracellular matrix, further stimulating PTHrP secretion and additional tumor growth.[129] This positive-feedback loop is believed to be involved in bone metastasis.[201]

Osteosarcoma's Biological Behavior

Metastasis is a complicated process that involves motility, migration, degradation of extracellular matrix, extravasation, survival during transit through vasculature, invasion, and growth.[202] Given the complicated nature of the process, many factors are likely to play a role in metastases. Chemokine stromal cell-derived factor 1 (SDF-1) is a cytokine-like protein expressed on the surface of vascular endothelial cells. Through binding to its chemokine receptor, CXCR4, it plays a role in cytoskeleton rearrangement, adhesion to endothelial cells, and chemotaxis.[203] CXCR4 mRNA has been reported to be expressed in osteosarcoma and associated with the presence of metastases at the time of diagnosis. These results have not been consistently supported.[124,204–208] Studies have demonstrated prevention of pulmonary metastasis in a murine model by the administration of a CXCR4 inhibitor, suggesting molecular strategies inhibiting this axis as a therapeutic target.[209]

Ezrin is a membrane-cytoskeleton linker protein that allows direct cellular interactions with the microenvironment, facilitating signal transduction through growth factor receptors and adhesion molecules, thereby regulating cell migration and metastasis among other processes. In an orthotopic model of murine osteosarcoma, ezrin expression was threefold higher in the more aggressive K7 M2 cell line, which correlated with its metastatic potential when compared with the less aggressive K12 cell line.[210] In follow-up experiments, ezrin expression was found to provide an early survival advantage for osteosarcoma metastatic to the lungs, which is in part mediated by AKT.[211] A significant correlation between high ezrin expression and poor outcome in osteosarcoma has been shown, supporting the animal model data.[210]

Other factors that may play a role in osteosarcoma metastases are expression of matrix metalloproteinases and other degradative enzymes. The expression of these enzymes is necessary to degrade the extracellular matrix, permitting extravasation into the vasculature.[212–215] Loss of expression of Fas appears to be necessary for survival of metastatic osteosarcoma cells in the lungs, since lung tissue highly expresses Fas ligand, and binding of Fas to Fas ligand activates apoptotic pathways in the malignant cell.[216–219]

In addition to cell proliferation and motility, another feature contributing to the behavior of tumors is the ability to induce the proliferation and migration of endothelial cells to allow the formation of new capillaries. VEGF is a peptide that acts as a mitogen for endothelial cells, directing new vessel formation.[114,118,121,124,220] The role of angiogenesis in the pathogenesis of osteosarcoma has been explored via expression analysis of VEGF, in tumor samples. VEGF expression has been assessed by immunostaining and correlated with poor prognosis and a higher metastatic rate.[220]

The efficacy of chemotherapy for the treatment of osteosarcoma can potentially be hindered by the presence of drug resistance. Mechanisms of drug resistance in osteosarcoma include alterations in a variety of proteins related to drug transport, drug efflux, drug metabolism, target interaction, and downstream response.[17] Of the potential mechanisms of resistance, P-glycoprotein expression has been the most extensively studied in osteosarcoma. P-glycoprotein is a transmembrane ATP-dependent efflux pump protein encoded by the multidrug resistance (MDR1) gene, which is responsible for the efflux of numerous chemotherapeutic agents, including doxorubicin.[116,221–232] Immunohistochemistry and/or RT-PCR quantification studies have explored P-glycoprotein expression in osteosarcoma, and demonstrated overexpression of P-glycoprotein in 23% to 45%, with decreased survival reported for patients with P-GP-positive tumors.[116,221–232] A meta-analysis also proposes that P-glycoprotein is associated with an increased risk of disease progression.[226] Though the literature suggests that P-glycoprotein may be a marker of drug resistance and aggressiveness in osteosarcoma, numerous studies contradict this finding and a prospective clinicopathological national intergroup study concluded that there was no correlation between P-glycoprotein expression and percentage of osteosarcoma tumor necrosis after induction chemotherapy or event-free survival in localized osteosarcoma.[232] Overexpression of MDR1, the gene encoding P-glycoprotein, has also been explored in regard to its role in the progression of osteosarcoma and its prognostic relevance.[230,231,233] Though a pilot study demonstrated a trend toward a worse outcome in patients exhibiting high levels of MDR1 expression, the larger, prospective investigation did not delineate any correlation between MDR1 expression and disease progression in patients with osteosarcoma, with patients with either very low or very high levels of MDR1 having a worse outcome.[231] The value of P-glycoprotein and MDR1 expression as predictors of prognosis remains extremely controversial.[222,229,232,234]

High-dose methotrexate (HD-MTX) with leucovorin rescue is a major component of current protocols for the treatment of osteosarcoma. HDMTX is much more effective than conventional dose methotrexate in the treatment of osteosarcoma—a finding that is not observed in other malignancies, implying a mechanism of intrinsic methotrexate resistance within osteosarcoma tumor cells.[235–239] Methotrexate is a potent inhibitor of dihydrofolate reductase, a key enzyme for intracellular folate metabolism. In experimental systems, resistance to methotrexate can occur through a variety of mechanisms, including impaired transmembrane transport of the drug via the reduced folate carrier, upregulation of dihydrofolate reductase, and diminished intracellular retention secondary to polyglutamylation.[240,241] Studies have demonstrated that impairment of methotrexate influx and upregulation of dihydrofolate reductase occur in osteosarcoma.[235–239,242,243] The alterations in influx are mediated by changes in reduced folate carrier expression and sequence.[235–239] Some studies have linked alterations conferring methotrexate resistance to clinical parameters.[235–239]

These studies have not been large enough to permit making definitive conclusions.

PATHOLOGY

Osteosarcoma is a malignant tumor characterized by production of osteoid by the neoplastic cells. In the current World Health Organization (WHO) Classification (see Table 34.2), osteosarcoma of bone is divided into conventional, telangiectatic, small cell, low-grade central, secondary, parosteal, periosteal, and high-grade surface variants.[244] The diagnosis and classification of osteosarcoma is based on correlation of the histologic findings with imaging studies.

The histologic diagnosis of conventional osteosarcoma,[245] which comprises the vast majority of tumors, is usually straightforward, although considerable variability exists between different tumors and, not uncommonly, within a single tumor. Conventional osteosarcoma is composed of pleomorphic, obviously malignant, cells that demonstrate at least focal evidence of osteoid production (Fig. 34.1). Pleomorphism is best seen in areas away from prominent osteoid formation, reflecting the tendency of the sarcomatous cells to become smaller and less pleomorphic as they become entrapped in the osteoid (so-called normalization). Matrix production varies from scant and inconspicuous to prominent, and ranges from a filigree pattern with thin, delicate, branching wisps of osteoid to a sclerotic pattern with densely packed, broad, irregular trabeculae of osteoid and woven bone. The osteoid and woven bone lack osteoblastic rimming. The constituent malignant cells of conventional osteosarcoma include round, ovoid, epithelioid, spindled, and bizarre mononuclear or multinucleated giant cells in varying numbers with interspersed benign-appearing osteoclastic giant cells. Mitotic figures, including abnormal forms, are readily identified.

In the current WHO Classification, conventional osteosarcoma is subdivided into osteoblastic, chondroblastic, and fibroblastic subtypes, on the basis of the predominant type of matrix.[245] In chondroblastic osteosarcoma, the defining chondroid matrix is usually hypercellular hyaline cartilage populated by pleomorphic to anaplastic chondrocytes. Fibroblastic osteosarcoma is composed of high-grade, malignant spindle cells with only scant osteoid. Giant-cell–rich and malignant fibrous histiocytoma-like osteosarcomas are also included under the fibroblastic subtype. The extreme paucity of matrix in fibroblastic osteosarcoma may result in a purely lytic appearance on imaging studies, which, combined with the absence of recognizable osteoid in a biopsy, may result in a misdiagnosis of fibrosarcoma. Similarly, histologic distinction between chondroblastic osteosarcoma and chondrosarcoma

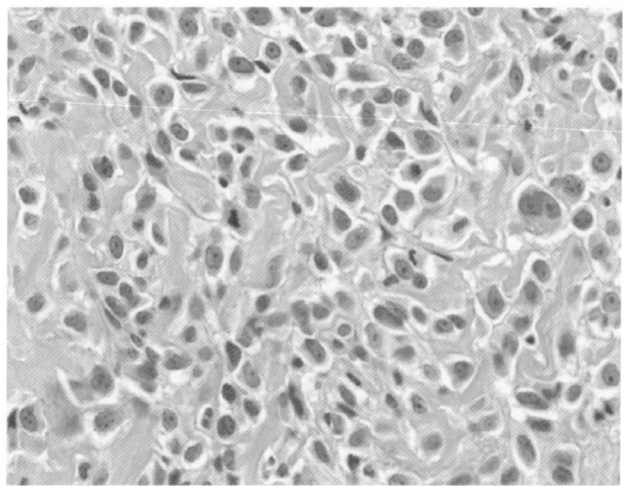

FIGURE 34.1 Conventional osteosarcoma demonstrating malignant cells associated with lace-like osteoid. Nuclear pleomorphism and mitotic figures are evident. (Hematoxylin and eosin, 400×)

may be difficult or impossible in biopsies with sparse or absent osteoid, respectively. Because treatment differs significantly between conventional osteosarcoma and chondrosarcoma, this distinction is essential and may justify further sampling in an effort to reach a definitive diagnosis. The value of subtyping conventional osteosarcoma is unclear given the heterogeneity within a single tumor and potential for sampling bias, particularly in a small diagnostic biopsy, as the prognosis appears to be similar.

Immunohistochemical stains are of little value in the diagnosis of osteosarcoma. Osteosarcoma is uniformly positive for vimentin. Osteocalcin and osteonectin, while usually positive, are of little value due to the broad range of staining observed with these antibodies. Osteosarcoma may also show staining for CD99, usually in a diffuse cytoplasmic pattern, smooth muscle actin, desmin, S100, cytokeratin, and epithelial membrane antigen.

Although detailed discussion of the rarer variants of osteosarcoma is beyond the scope of this chapter, these entities are noteworthy, primarily because they may be confused with other tumors, and are discussed briefly. Telangiectatic osteosarcoma[246] comprises approximately 4% of all osteosarcomas and on imaging studies typically appears as a purely lytic, destructive tumor without peripheral sclerosis. Cysts with fluid-fluid levels, reminiscent of aneurysmal bone cyst, are present. Histologically, telangiectatic osteosarcoma is characterized by large blood-filled spaces separated by variably thick septa. The septa are composed of anaplastic tumor cells admixed with benign-appearing multinucleated giant cells, bland mononuclear cells, and scant osteoid. When anaplastic cells and osteoid are inconspicuous, telangiectatic osteosarcomas may be confused with aneurysmal bone cysts. With current therapeutic regimens, the prognosis is similar to that of conventional osteosarcoma.[247]

Small cell osteosarcoma[248] comprises approximately 1.5% of all osteosarcomas and, as the name implies, it is composed of small round cells with scant cytoplasm. All have osteoid, although this is often scant, and a few have foci of cartilaginous matrix. These tumors may show strong, diffuse membrane staining for CD99, and like other osteosarcomas may be positive for smooth muscle actin and cytokeratin. In biopsies with inconspicuous osteoid, small cell osteosarcoma may be mistaken for other small round cell tumors including Ewing sarcoma, mesenchymal chondrosarcoma, lymphoma, and metastatic neuroblastoma. Small cell osteosarcoma lacks the t(11:22) chromosomal translocations associated with Ewing sarcoma. This variant has a slightly worse prognosis than conventional osteosarcoma.[249]

Low-grade central osteosarcoma[250] comprises 1% to 2% of all osteosarcomas. Aggressive features may be subtle or absent on diagnostic imaging studies. Low-grade central osteosarcoma is composed of relatively bland spindle cells within fibrous stroma. The cellularity is low or moderate, and cytologic atypia is usually subtle. Mitotic figures are present but not numerous. Woven or lamellar bone is present in variable patterns. Histologically, these tumors may be confused with fibrous dysplasia. This variant typically progresses more slowly and has a better prognosis than conventional osteosarcoma.[251,252] However, some recurrent tumors show a higher histologic grade or dedifferentiation with the potential for metastasis and death.

Parosteal, periosteal, and high-grade surface osteosarcomas are exophytic tumors arising from the periosteal surface of the bone and eroding the underlying cortical bone with minimal or no involvement of the subjacent medullary bone. High-grade surface osteosarcoma[253] comprises <1% of osteosarcomas and is histologically indistinguishable from conventional osteosarcoma. Treatment and prognosis are the same as for conventional osteosarcoma. Parosteal osteosarcoma[254] comprises 4% of osteosarcomas and is rare before the third decade of life. Histologically, the tumor is composed of well-formed bony trabeculae in parallel arrays with or without osteoblastic rimming separated by hypocellular, fibrous stroma. The spindle cells within the stroma show minimal or, occasionally, moderate cytologic atypia. Cartilaginous differentiation is present in about 50% of tumors, sometimes appearing as a cartilaginous cap. Foci of high-grade spindle cell sarcoma may be present at the time of original diagnosis or, more often, at the time of recurrence. Treatment is complete surgical resection and prognosis is excellent. However, in tumors with areas of high-grade spindle cell sarcoma, the prognosis is similar to that of conventional osteosarcoma. Periosteal osteosarcoma[255] comprises <2% of osteosarcomas, has a predilection for the diaphyseal or metadiaphyseal regions of long bones, and initially presents as a painless mass. Histologically, this tumor has features of an intermediate grade chondroblastic osteosarcoma. Treatment is complete surgical resection with or without chemotherapy. Marginal resection is associated with a recurrence rate of up to 70% and is not recommended. Prognosis is better than that of conventional osteosarcoma. Medullary involvement may be associated with a poorer prognosis.

Clinical Presentation

Osteosarcoma produces nonspecific symptoms and requires a high index of suspicion to detect the disease early and avoid potentially harmful diagnostic delays and misguided treatment attempts. Pain is the most common and first symptom in the majority of cases.[8,256–259] It may be intermittent at first, but later becomes continuous. In the typical physically active adolescent, pain caused by osteosarcoma is at first erroneously attributed to recent trauma, commonly related to a sports injury. Tumor-related swelling and loss of function of adjacent joints generally develop several weeks after the onset of pain (Fig. 34.2).[8] A small number of patients present with a pathological fracture. Pain at an osseous site other than the primary tumor may represent metastatic involvement. However, the most common metastatic site is the lungs,[260–266] and respiratory symptoms occur very late and only with the presence of exten-

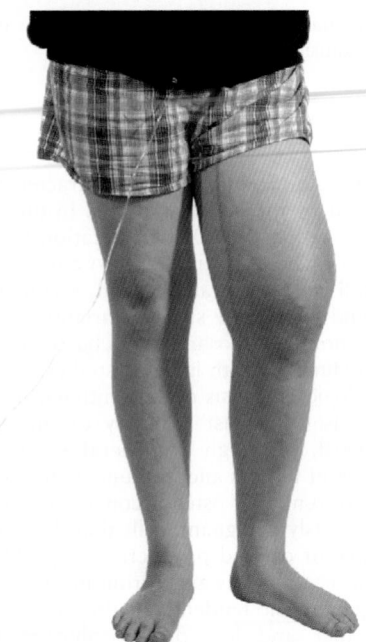

FIGURE 34.2 Massive swelling caused by a large osteosarcoma of the left distal femur in a 15-year-old male.

sive lung involvement. Systemic symptoms, such as fever, weight loss, and malaise are rare in the absence of far advanced disease. Therefore, the vast majority of osteosarcoma patients will not feel ill when the disease is first diagnosed.

The lag time between onset of symptoms and diagnosis ranges between 2 to 4 months for patients with localized extremity osteosarcoma in several North American and European studies,[8,256–258] but considerably longer in other parts of the world.[259] There is no correlation between the lag time between first symptoms and diagnosis and the likelihood of primary metastases,[8,256,258] but patients with axial primaries are usually diagnosed later than those with tumors located in the limbs.[8,257,258]

The differential diagnosis of osteosarcoma includes traumatic lesions, osteomyelitis, benign bone tumors such as osteochondroma, fibroma, osteoid-osteoma, chondroma, giant-cell tumor of bone, bone cysts, and others, as well as other primary malignancies of bone and bone metastases.

Only approximately 10% to 20% of patients present with radiologically apparent metastatic disease.[8,263,267] Nevertheless, 80% to 90% of seemingly unaffected patients will develop metastatic lung disease and die within 1 to 2 years from diagnosis if treatment efforts are limited to measures directed against the primary tumor.[2,4,5,268,269] Synchronous[260,261,263,265] and metachronous metastases[262,264] most commonly involve the lungs. In the two largest reported series of 202 primary metastatic osteosarcomas[270] and 532 metastatic recurrences[264] pulmonary involvement was observed in 81% and 88%, respectively; the lungs were the only metastatic site in 61% and 70%, respectively. Distant bones are the second most frequent site of metastatic deposits, combined with lung metastases in at least half of all metastatic cases.[263,264,266] Skip metastases, isolated tumor foci within the same bone as the primary tumor, represent another form of osseous dissemination.[271,272] While they occur only in a minority of patients, they must always be sought for by appropriate imaging of the total tumor bearing bone. Metastases to organs other than lungs or bones are rare in the absence of widespread disease and are associated with pulmonary or osseous involvement.[263,264] Death from progressive osteosarcoma is usually due to respiratory failure caused by extensive pulmonary metastases.

EVALUATION

Clinical Evaluation

The evaluation of a patient with suspected osteosarcoma begins with a full history, physical examination, laboratory evaluation, and plain radiographs. The focus of the clinical history is determining the extent and duration of physical symptoms as well as the associated physical limitations (if any). Most patients present with pain and swelling of the affected area lasting from 2 to 6 months. Physical examination is generally only remarkable for the presence of a soft tissue mass at the site of the primary tumor. There might also be redness and warmth on physical examination. The presence of regional and/or distant lymph node spread is rare.[273] The evaluation of a patient with osteosarcoma includes the use of imaging studies performed to determine the extent of disease. The most important prognostic factor is the presence of metastatic disease most commonly to the lungs,[23] which drastically worsens outcome.[265]

Laboratory Evaluation

There are no known laboratory parameters specific for osteosarcoma. Serum levels of alkaline phosphatase (ALP) and less frequently lactic dehydrogenase (LDH)[7,274] are elevated in a considerable number of patients. Elevated ALP levels do not necessarily correlate with disease extent but have been observed to correlate with an increased likelihood for recurrence.[7,274–277]

Several further laboratory tests must be performed before chemotherapy is started. These should aim to assess organ function and general health. Recommended baseline tests include a complete blood count and differential, tests for serum electrolytes including magnesium and phosphate, renal function evaluation including creatinine and (estimated) creatinine clearance, liver function studies, blood group typing, a coagulation profile, as well as tests for hepatitis and HIV infection.

Radiologic Evaluation

Diagnostic imaging plays a major role in the management of children with osteosarcoma. In most cases, it is findings on conventional radiographs that indicate the presence of a malignant bone tumor. Further imaging, usually with magnetic resonance imaging (MRI) or computed tomography (CT) of the involved area is then performed to determine the extent of local disease. Bone scintigraphy and chest CT are also performed to determine the presence and extent of metastatic disease. Additional imaging by F-18-fluoro-2-deoxy-D-glucose (FDG) positron emission tomography (PET), often combined with CT (PET/CT), thallium scintigraphy, or dynamic contrast-enhanced MRI (DCE-MRI), may also be performed to further assess the local tumor and in some cases to evaluate response to treatment.

On conventional radiography (Fig. 34.3), the classic high-grade intramedullary osteosarcoma presents as a large (>6 cm), mixed sclerotic and lucent metaphyseal lesion with fluffy, cloud-like calcific opacities characteristic of osteoid

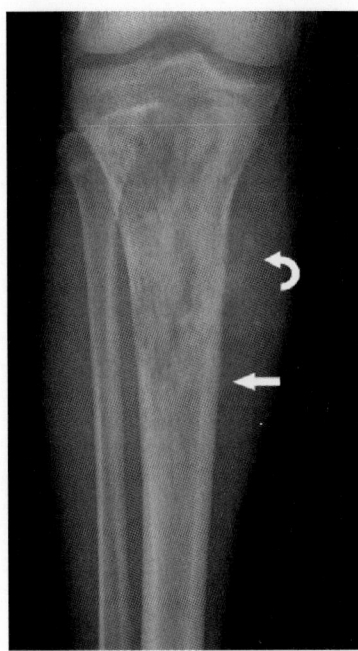

FIGURE 34.3 Conventional radiograph shows mixed lytic and sclerotic lesion with osteoid matrix (*curved arrow*) and Codman triangle (*straight arrow*) involving the proximal tibia.

matrix production.[278] There is usually a soft tissue mass with aggressive-appearing periosteal reaction often with a Codman triangle, which results from the soft tissue mass breaking through the overlying ossified periosteal new bone. The periosteal new bone may be spiculated or laminated and tumors that occur in the diaphyses may have onion-skin periosteal reaction that simulates Ewing sarcoma.[279]

Occasionally a classic high-grade intramedullary osteosarcoma is completely sclerotic or lucent. However, the telangiectatic subtype of osteosarcoma typically presents as a cystic, lucent lesion with subtle matrix mineralization and a geographic margin with a wide zone of transition.[280] Oblique parallel striations in the diaphysis thought to be secondary to intraosseous veins are an early radiographic sign.[281] On radiographs, these tumors may be confused with benign aneurysmal bone cysts. CT can be helpful in determining the correct diagnosis by showing subtle matrix mineralization, and either CT or MRI may show thick, solid, nodular-enhancing tissue surrounding the cystic spaces and the soft tissue mass that are present in a telangiectatic osteosarcoma.[280]

Juxtacortical osteosarcomas involve the bone surface and include intracortical, parosteal, periosteal, and high-grade surface lesions.[278] Parosteal osteosarcomas are the most common of these and typically involve the metaphysis of the long bones. On radiographs, these tumors appear as lobulated masses that attach to the cortex and are ossified centrally. Occasionally, parosteal osteosarcomas must be differentiated from myositis ossificans, which is ossified in the periphery and usually not attached to the cortex.[278] CT is particularly helpful for making this distinction.

Once a malignant bone tumor is suspected, advanced imaging by CT or MRI (Fig. 34.4) should be performed to determine the extent of the tumor within the bone and assess the relationship of the tumor to the nearby neurovascular bundle, muscles, and joints. MRI provides superb contrast resolution and multiplanar capabilities resulting in images that define the intraosseous and soft tissue components of the tumor and their relationship to adjacent structures. CT is also able to

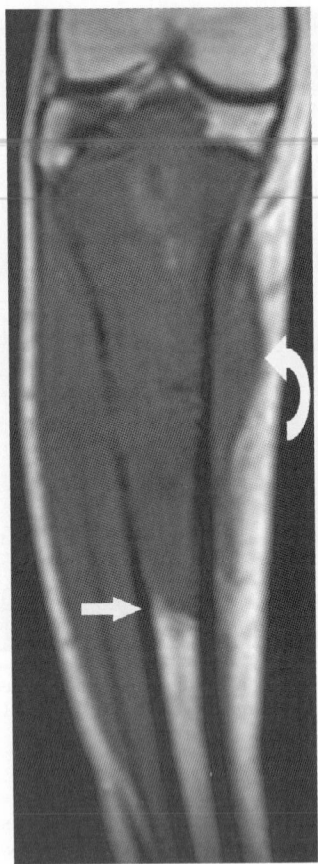

FIGURE 34.4 Coronal T1-weighted magnetic resonance imaging shows soft tissue mass (*curved arrow*) and demarcation (*arrow*) between low signal tumor and normal marrow.

that are equal in quality to direct CT acquisition in these orientations. Nonetheless, due to its superior contrast resolution and the absence of ionizing radiation, MRI is generally considered the imaging study of choice for the evaluation of the primary tumor in patients with osteosarcoma.[283]

Whether CT or MRI is performed for the assessment of the primary tumor, it is recommended that imaging be carried out prior to biopsy. The imaging findings can help in the selection of the optimal site for biopsy and this course of action will avoid distortion of the imaging findings by postbiopsy changes.[284] Imaging of the primary tumor should include coverage of the entire bone to look for the presence of skip lesions. For CT, the examination should be performed with intravenous (IV) contrast to improve the soft tissue contrast resolution. MRI should include long axis T1-weighted and/or short tau inversion recovery (STIR) sequences of the entire bone and axial imaging (Fig. 34.5) with T2-weighted and flow sensitive sequences to define the relationship of the tumor to the neurovascular bundle. High-resolution, relatively small field of view MRI in two planes is helpful when it is necessary to assess joint involvement and postgadolinium imaging is useful to assess the presence of tumor hemorrhage and necrosis.

On CT, the extent of intramedullary involvement is determined by the presence of mineralization or soft tissue attenuation material replacing the low attenuation of normal fatty marrow.[278] IV contrast is critical to opacify and help establish the location of the blood vessels. On MRI, tumors are low signal on T1-weighted images and heterogeneous high signal on T2-weighted and STIR images.[285] T1-weighted images are more accurate than STIR images to estimate the extent of an intraosseous tumor.[286] STIR sequences are very sensitive to fluid and as a result high-signal peritumoral edema or other benign tissue may simulate a tumor.

Additional imaging is performed to detect metastatic disease, the majority of which is in the lungs.[12] CT is superior to conventional radiography and is the imaging study of choice to detect lung metastases.[287-289] In cooperative patients, the CT scan should be performed using the spiral technique during a single breathhold with 5-mm or less slice collimation. Unless there is chest wall, hilar or mediastinal involvement, the CT should be performed without IV contrast. In addition, when possible the CT should be done prior to biopsy to avoid postsedation atelectasis or other postoperative processes that could simulate or obscure lung metastases.

Lung metastases (Fig. 34.6) are typically round or ovoid, sharply marginated, and located in the lung periphery.[289] The

define the intraosseous and soft tissue components of the tumor and is superior to MRI for the detection of small areas of mineralized matrix.[278] A multi-institutional study[282] found that CT and MRI were equally accurate for local staging without a statistically significant difference between the two imaging modalities for determining local tumor extent. In addition, newer CT scanners can acquire data in the axial plane and provide reconstructed images in long axis or oblique planes

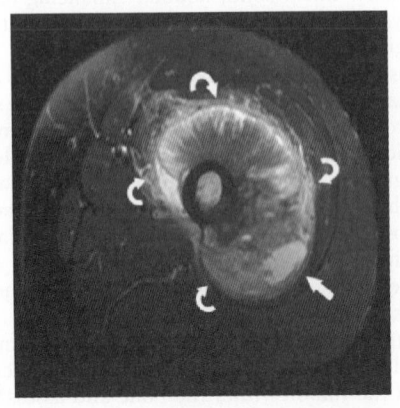
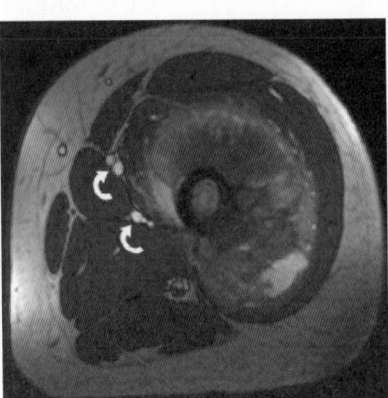
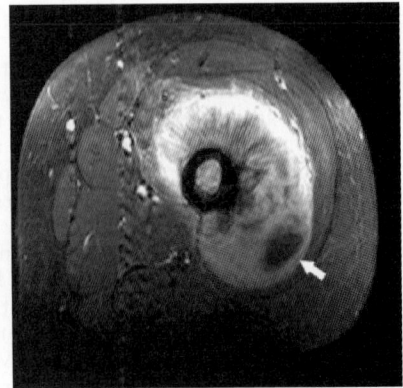

A,B   C

FIGURE 34.5 Axial magnetic resonance imaging images. **A:** T2-weighted fat-saturated image shows the tumor (*curved arrows*) involving and surrounding the femur and focal high signal area (*straight arrow*). **B:** Flow-sensitive image shows high signal intensity flow in blood vessels (*curved areas*) to help identify the neurovascular bundle. **C:** T1-weighted, fat-saturated image showing predominantly enhancing tumor with nonenhancing focus confirming that the high signal area in **A** is fluid (*straight arrow*).

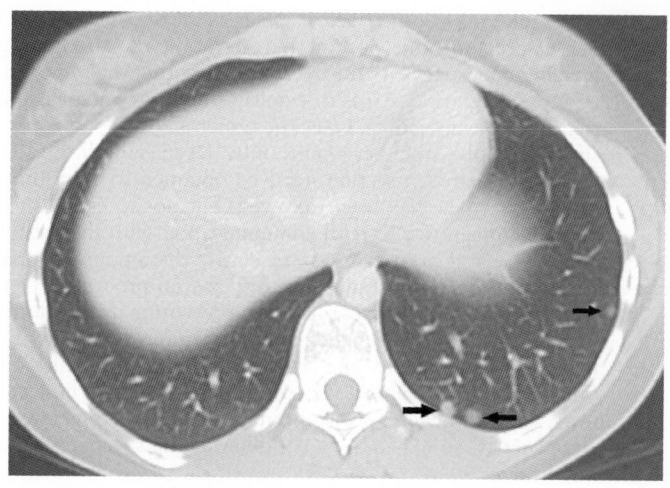
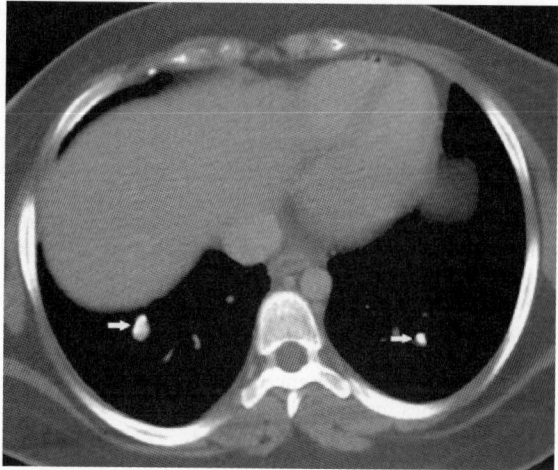

FIGURE 34.6 Lung metastases on CT. **A:** Axial image reviewed at lung windows shows multiple, small, well-defined peripheral nodules (*arrows*). **B:** Axial image reviewed at soft tissue windows shows high attenuation regions (*arrows*) corresponding to calcification within the lung metastases in a different patient.

metastases may or may not be calcified and differentiating benign from metastatic nodules can be difficult. This is particularly true for children who live in areas with endemic fungal disease, especially histoplasmosis, and have pulmonary nodules on chest CT. The size, number, and margins of the nodules can assist in making this distinction. Sharply marginated lesions larger than 5 mm in diameter, especially when multiple, are likely to be metastases,[290] while solitary nodules less than 5 mm with unsharp margins are likely to be benign.[290] Though there is no minimum number of nodules that excludes metastases, one study found that all patients with seven or more nodules at surgery had metastases.[291] Following nodules postchemotherapy can be helpful. Benign lesions are likely to remain unchanged in size, while lesions that increase or decrease in size are more likely to be metastases.[291] Criteria utilizing the nodule size and number have been established (Table 34.3) to guide the decision. However, in those uncertain cases wherein the diagnosis is crucial, nodule resection and biopsy are indicated.

Bone scintigraphy, typically with technetium-99m-methylene-diphosphonate (MDP) is performed for the assessment of bone metastases and skip lesions. Conventional radiographs are helpful to assess foci of increased uptake that are suspicious for bone metastases and occasionally MRI is needed to further evaluate these areas. Single photon emission tomography (SPECT) may be performed in conjunction with planar bone scintigraphy to characterize uptake at the primary tumor site and when there is suspicion for lung metastases.[292]

Numerous other imaging techniques and modalities are being used or developed for use in the assessment of osteosarcoma. Thallium-201 has shown value in evaluating tumor response to chemotherapy, but has not gained widespread application.[293,294] Similarly, DCE-MRI, which provides information on tissue vascularization and perfusion, capillary permeability, and the interstitial spaces has shown promise for the assessment of tumor response and disease prognosis.[295–297] DCE-MRI can be performed in conjunction with the contrast injection portion of a standard MRI and has been used successfully in a number of institutions. Diffusion-weighted MRI sequences, which also can be performed in conjunction with standard MRI, are also being investigated for the assessment of tumor response.[298] In addition, whole-body MRI has shown potential as a replacement for bone scintigraphy for the evaluation of bone metastases.[299]

Presently, however, FDG-PET and PET/CT seem to have the most potential for widespread application. FDG-PET is equal to or worse than MDP-bone scintigraphy for the detection of bone metastases[300,301] and worse than CT for the detection of lung metastases.[300] FDG-PET, however, has shown promise in the assessment of tumor response[302,303] and detection of recurrent disease.[304]

As imaging techniques evolve and new techniques are developed, the basic imaging assessment for children with osteosarcoma will continue to rely on conventional radiography, MRI, CT, and bone scintigraphy. There is general agreement on the need for MRI of the primary tumor at presentation and prior to local control and the use of bone scintigraphy and chest CT for the assessment of metastatic disease at presentation.[283,305] There are differing opinions regarding the timing and types of imaging that should be performed later in the patients' treatment course and during surveillance posttherapy.[283,305–307] These differences will likely continue until there is objective evidence on the value of a standard protocol of imaging studies to improve the outcome of children with osteosarcoma.

Biopsy

The initial surgical procedure for any bone tumor is a biopsy. Two types of biopsies are possible: incisional and excisional. Incisional biopsies include needle (closed) and open biopsies. Needle biopsies can be either fine needle or core. The type of

TABLE 34.3

CRITERIA FOR PULMONARY METASTATIC DISEASE FROM EURAMOS I TRIAL[16]

CT chest finding	Interpretation
One or more pulmonary/pleural lesion(s) ≥1 cm OR three or more lesions ≥0.5 cm maximum diameter	"Certain" pulmonary metastases
Fewer or smaller lesions	"Possible" metastatic disease

biopsy chosen must be carefully determined after evaluating the size and location of the tumor, the differential diagnosis as well as the age of the patient. The placement of the biopsy site relative to the location of the tumor and the anatomic structures of the patient is also of critical importance.

Small, superficial lesions are amenable to excisional biopsy. Generally, if a malignant bone tumor is suspected, an excisional biopsy is rarely, if ever, utilized. This is due to the fact that the tumor is often large at presentation and that neoadjuvant therapy is usually appropriate prior to definitive resection. If the lesion is most likely benign based upon the preoperative history, physical examination, and imaging studies, then at the time of excision a frozen section should be obtained. Primary excision of an expendable bone should only be considered by an experienced musculoskeletal oncologist. Expendable bones may include a rib, clavicle, sternum, ilium, scapular body, and perhaps, distal ulna.

Most bone tumors of uncertain biologic potential, where there is a significant suspicion for malignancy, are biopsied via an incisional approach. The location of the biopsy site is determined by a thorough prebiopsy assessment of the extent of local disease and its relationship to critical structures such as the neurovascular bundle. This must be determined on a case-by-case basis. It is strongly recommended that the biopsy be performed by the surgeon who will perform the definitive resection so that the biopsy tract can be ellipsed within the planned surgical incision.[308] At the time of biopsy, the surgeon must be familiar with orthopaedic oncologic principles of flap development, coverage, and even amputation, when definitive limb salvage is the proposed plan for a given bone tumor.

Needle (closed) biopsies can potentially expedite the diagnostic process when performed on an outpatient basis in the doctor's office. This can be conducted using a local anesthetic, which reduces the cost of the procedure. However, such techniques are generally not recommended for children. Most malignant bone tumors have a soft tissue component on its periphery. Conveniently, this is also the most representative tissue. Accordingly, deep deployment of the needle within the tumor is unnecessary and likely to lead to problems such as deep contamination and bleeding. Again the needle biopsy site must be carefully planned so that it may be excised at the time of definite resection. With a well-trained cytopathologist, fine needle biopsy is an option. A 0.7 mm diameter needle is generally used with reports of up to 90% diagnostic accuracy,[309] including higher than 80% accuracy in bone sarcomas.[310] The drawback of this approach is that insufficient material may be obtained to perform cytogenetics, fluorescent *in situ* hybridization, flow cytometry, gene expression profiling, and other tests that may help establish the diagnosis. Core biopsies are minimally invasive, can be performed under local anesthesia, maintain the architecture of the tissue, and can obtain adequate specimen for advanced studies. Diagnostic accuracy for this technique can surpass 95%.[311]

While needle biopsies are intended to facilitate diagnosis, they can also lead to a delay. Since the final diagnosis should not be based on the frozen section, the patient must wait until the results are finalized, which may take several days if special studies are necessary. If the specimen is indeterminate, which can occur in 25% to 33% of cases, even at experienced centers,[312] then a delay will most definitely occur.

An open incisional biopsy can potentially be done in the office. However for suspected bone malignancies, it is usually recommended that they be performed in the operating room. Generally speaking, longitudinal incisions are the rule since transverse incisions potentially contaminate flap planes and can compromise neurovascular structures. During the approach to the tumor, no flaps should be developed to minimize contamination. The area where the tumor is most superficial is

preferable unless other factors, such as an overlying vessel or nerve, preclude this option. Furthermore, the preoperative imaging may suggest that a specific area within the tumor may be more diagnostic. Areas of extensive necrosis and/or hemorrhage can be misleading. Once the tumor is reached, the biopsy should involve the periphery only. Deep sampling is not necessary. A frozen section must be obtained to determine if diagnostic tissue has been retrieved, but not to establish the definitive diagnosis. Careful communication with the pathologist is essential preoperatively to clarify the amount of tissue necessary for special studies and any special processing of the tissue. Formaldehyde fixes the tissue, preventing the application of conventional cytogenetics and some molecular tests. Furthermore, RNA quality and cell viability rapidly diminish once outside the body, which also compromises certain molecular tests, such as gene expression analyses, flow cytometry, and cytogenetics, so expeditious handling of the specimen is very important.[313,314]

For those bone tumors that have not violated the cortex, controlled fenestration will be necessary. A trephine is usually adequate but if a larger window is required it is imperative that it be round or oval to minimize stress risers. A pituitary rongeur may then be used to retrieve tissue from within the medullary canal. The bone window may then be impacted back in place and sealed with bone wax. Alternatively, a polymethylmethacrylate plug may be used instead. Hemostasis is of utmost importance. Certain tumors may be quite vascular and meticulous hemostasis may not be possible. In such cases, a drain must be placed, in line with the incision distally, and sewn in place.

The use of tourniquets is controversial. While their use provides for a bloodless approach, they must be let down prior to closure to assure adequate hemostasis. If used, the limb should not be exsanguinated to minimize the risk of tumor embolus.

Classification and Staging

Tumor extent (local and systemic) as well as malignant potential must be taken into account when classifying and staging bone tumors. For many years, clinicians, particularly orthopedic surgeons, have relied upon a staging system developed by the Musculoskeletal Tumor Society (MSTS), which recognizes these requirements. In the MSTS system, tumors are classified as either intra- (T1) or extracompartmental (T2) and as either low-grade (A) or high-grade (B) malignancies. Metastatic tumors are classified as T3.[315] Since extension through the cortex to the periosteum (present in virtually all osteosarcomas) defines extracompartmental involvement, the MSTS staging system classifies the majority of localized pediatric and adolescent osteosarcomas as stage IIB (Table 34.4).

TABLE 34.4

MUSCULOSKELETAL TUMOR SOCIETY (MSTS) CLASSIFICATION AND STAGING

Stage	T	N	M	Grade
Stage IA	T1	N0	M0	Low grade
Stage IB	T2	N0	M0	Low grade
Stage IIA	T1	N0	M0	High grade
Stage IIB	T2	N0	M0	High grade
Stage III	T3	N0	M0	Any grade
Stage IVA	Any T	N0	M1a	Any grade
Stage IVB	Any T	N1	Any M	Any grade
	Any T	Any N	Any M	Any grade

TABLE 34.5

SIXTH EDITION OF UICC TNM CLASSIFICATION OF MALIGNANT TUMORS

T, N, M	Definition
Tx	Primary tumor cannot be assessed
T0	No evidence of primary tumor
T1	Tumor ≤8 cm
T2	Tumor >8 cm
T3	Discontinuous tumors in the primary bone
Nx	Regional lymph nodes cannot be assessed
N0	No regional lymph node metastases
N1	Regional lymph node metastases
Mx	Distant metastases cannot be assessed
M0	No distant metastases
M1	Distant metastases
M1a	Lung
M1b	Other distant sites

The T-stages of the current 6th edition of the UICC TNM classification of malignant tumors,[316] an advancement over the MSTS staging system, distinguishes between smaller and larger primary tumors, with a cutoff at 8 cm in greatest dimension, and also allows for the description of skip metastases as T3 (see Table 34.5). The 6th edition of the UICC TNM classification also allows us to distinguish between pulmonary (M1a) and extrapulmonary (M1b) distant metastases. The resulting staging system is reminiscent of that of the original MSTS classification in that both grade of malignancy and local tumor extent are used for definitions.[244,316]

TREATMENT

Surgical Management

The surgical management of osteosarcoma has evolved into a complex field. Surgical approaches are a function of the osteosarcoma subtype, as well as the location and extent of disease at the time of initial diagnosis. The successful management of osteosarcoma has evolved into a multimodality approach. Advances in chemotherapy have significantly improved survival, and surgical extirpation generally occurs after a course of neoadjuvant chemotherapy. Surgery is then followed by further chemotherapy. It is of paramount importance that resumption of chemotherapy not be delayed postoperatively as a delay beyond 2 to 3 weeks has been associated with an increased risk of death.[317]

The goal of resection for any malignant tumor is to perform a complete, *en bloc* removal of the lesion with adequate margins. Limb-sparing surgery has become the standard approach with advances in imaging techniques, such as MRI. This, in combination with improved neoadjuvant therapy, has enabled the oncologic surgeon to obtain local control rates equivalent to amputation. However, in severe cases, where limb salvage may compromise the oncologic outcome, amputation is mandated.

Because of the complexity of the musculoskeletal system, different reconstructive options are performed depending upon the site of involvement. Generally, bone tumors arise in the distal femur, proximal tibia, proximal humerus, proximal femur, and the diaphyses of long bones. The spine, hand, and foot can also be involved, albeit less frequently.

Types of Reconstruction

Conceptually, reconstruction involves rebuilding the skeletal and soft tissue defect to enable optimal function for the patient. The main reconstructive options include autogenous bone grafts, structural bone allografts (intercalary or osteoarticular), and metallic endoprosthetics. Allografts and endoprosthetics may be used in conjunction as a composite reconstruction. Autogenous bone grafts may be vascularized (e.g., fibula). All three have inherent advantages and disadvantages. Which technique is employed remains a function of the location of the tumor, age of the patient, and types of adjuvant therapies employed (i.e., chemotherapy and/or radiation). Large structural allografts and endoprosthetics should generally be reserved for children older than 8 years. Nonvascularized autografts from the pelvis or other sites may be used in a limited fashion for relatively small defects and work well in children.[318] The advantage is a high incorporation rate but with potential donor site morbidity, such as pain and a second site infection. Vascularized autografts such as the fibula are attractive because, when successful, the graft incorporates and even may remodel itself secondary to the forces exerted across it.[319] Again, similar donor site complications can occur.

Structural allografts have no donor site morbidity. The major drawback to allografts is difficulty incorporating with the host bone (nonunion) and fracture.[320] Their advantage is that they are a biologic solution and if they heal and do not fracture they may last the lifetime of the patient.[321,322] Osteoarticular allografts may be used in the reconstruction of the proximal humerus, distal femur, and proximal tibia as well as potentially any joint (Fig. 34.7).[321,323–329] Diaphyseal tumors can be reconstructed with intercalary allografts (Fig. 34.8).[323,324,330–333] The physis may sometimes serve as an adequate tumor barrier allowing preservation of the epiphysis and thus the joint surface, but must be carefully assessed preoperatively with MRI. When this is possible, the durability and functional outcome will be superior to cases where the joint proper must be sacrificed (Fig. 34.9).

Infections can occur in 10% to 15% of allografts[323,325,329,334–336] and nonunion at the osteosynthesis site in 10% to 25% of cases.[324,329] Infection is a major complication requiring graft removal whereas nonunions can usually be managed by revision fixation and autogenous bone grafting. Both of these complications are more likely in patients receiving chemotherapy. Augmentation of the allograft with a vascularized fibula, while adding its own set of potential complications may facilitate osseous integration of the structural graft thereby preventing the inherent problems associated with allografts.[337,338]

For osteoarticular allografts, satisfactory functional results can be anticipated in 60% to 70% of cases in which a high-grade sarcoma was removed and chemotherapy was utilized.[324,325,328,336,339,340] Function is generally better for intercalary reconstructions.[323,326,332] In general, high impact activities are discouraged, but younger patients are not always compliant. Fractures occur in approximately 20% of cases.[341] Fractures can be managed by standard techniques but may necessitate graft and/or implant removal and replacement. In select cases, a combination of vascularized auto- and allografting techniques may be optimal.[337,338,342]

Metallic endoprosthetics provide an immediate stable reconstruction but suffer from the fact that they eventually fail because of loosening and failure of components, which is a substantive issue in pediatric and young adult patients surviving their disease.[343] Usually, the stem of the prosthesis is cemented in place with polymethylmethacrylate, but press fit stems and alternate fixation devices are used discretionarily as well.[344]

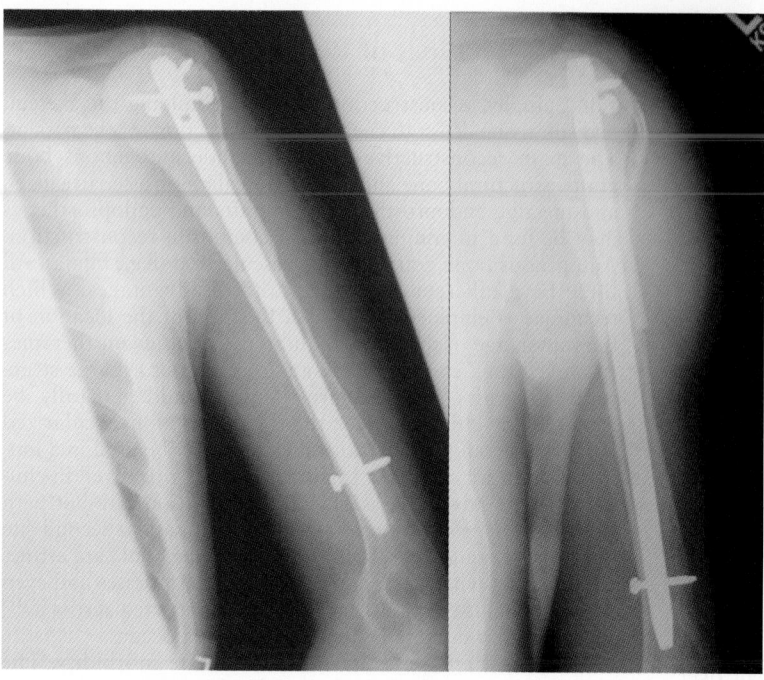

FIGURE 34.7 Reconstruction of the proximal humerus.

They are generally cast from cobalt, chrome, steel or machined from titanium. Infections are a significant risk with endoprosthetics as well, with rates ranging from 0% to 35%.[345–350]

The durability of any endoprosthesis is subject to a variety of influences but the anticipated event-free 5-year survival for proximal femur reconstructions approaches 90%, while for the distal femur is about 60% and the proximal tibia just over 50%.[351] Prosthetic reconstructions of the proximal humerus tend to be more durable as they are subject to less forces. Failure can result from loosening at the prosthesis-host interface or infection. Improved metallurgy has resulted in a significant

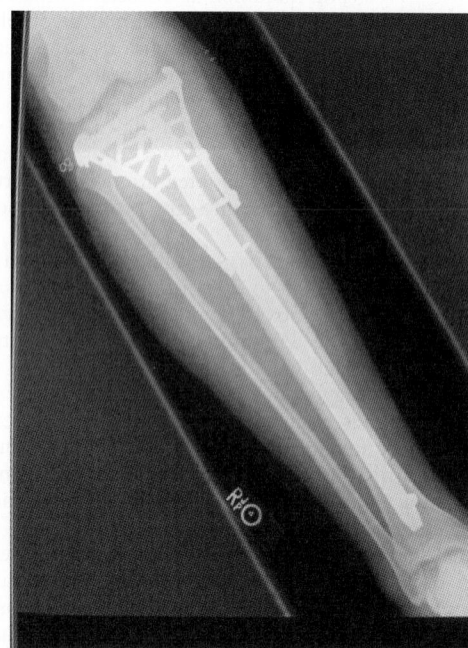

FIGURE 34.8 Intercalary allograft.

reduction in metal fatigue and failure of the implants. Articulating, moving components need revision at a rate in direct relation to the cyclical loading of the prosthesis. The more use, the more likely it is that a revision will be necessary. Sometimes failure can be catastrophic, as can be seen with late infections, necessitating a delayed amputation.

For expandable prostheses (Fig. 34.10), the 5-year revision-free survival has been reported as low as 15%.[352] As with any reconstruction in the skeletally immature patient, the construct must be dynamic so as to facilitate skeletal growth. Expandable prosthetics are available with multiple, varying mechanism for expansion.[339,345,352–362] While some of these mechanisms may be easy to expand, the longevity of prosthetic implants is poor in young children. Stress shielding and mechanical loosening are compounded by the continued diametrical growth of the host bone. While revision surgery is possible, the resultant bone stock for refixation can be quite tenuous. Modular components are now available for both pediatric and adult patients making the delay for customization the exception. The use of expandable prosthesis is a contentious topic and is influenced by cultural factors. More biologic reconstructive options, as discussed subsequently, are preferred by some surgeons, in the best interest of their patients, and yet the cosmetic considerations, which can be so heavy influential in some societies, is a counterargument endorsed by others.

For metallic prosthesis, newer cementless, porous ingrowth systems have been developed[346,363,364] but have not yet replaced cement in most centers. A novel prestress compliant fixation device, with encouraging early results, is also currently available that obviates the need for long intramedullary stems, thereby avoiding stress shielding.[365,366] This system is designed to facilitate osseous integration at the bone-implant interface; however, concern over the use of chemotherapy in the postoperative period interfering with bone-implant integration has been raised.[367]

Allograft-prosthetic composites are another alternative for limb salvage surgery.[324,329,331,339,368–375] The advantage of this system is the hybridization of a more conventional arthroplasty with potential incorporation of the allograft for future

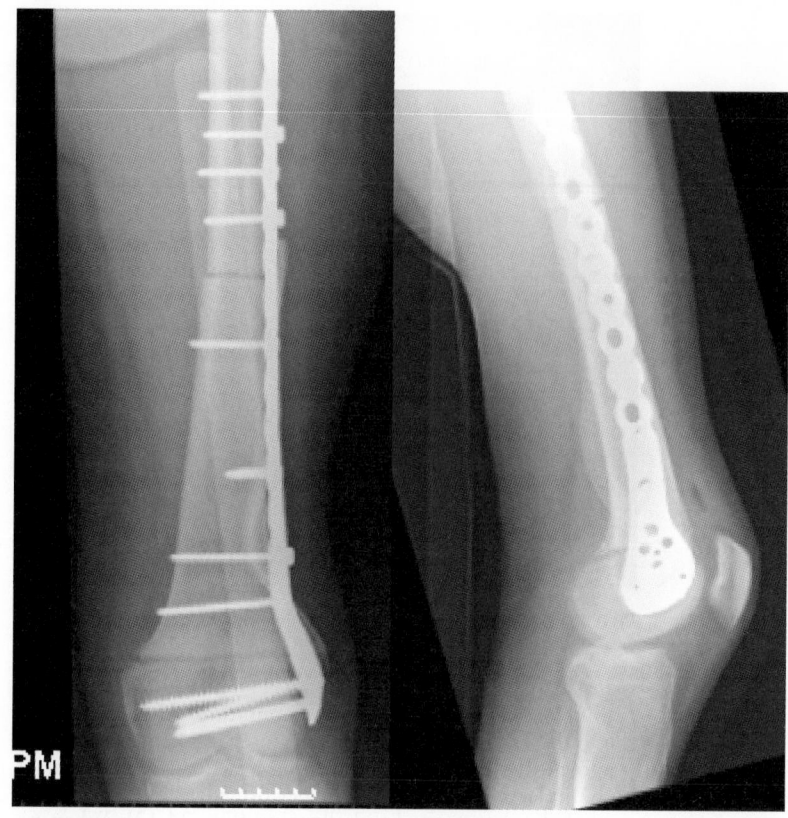

FIGURE 34.9 Epiphyseal preservation.

bone stock. The construct may also prevent delayed allograft fracture (Fig. 34.11).

Arthrodesis remains an option in limb preservation surgery, but it is utilized with diminishing frequency as endoprostheses and allografts have improved. The advantage to fusion is that once healed the construct is very durable and may endure heavy labor.[323,376–379] However, because of the lack of motion, many patients are dissatisfied. The procedure may be better tolerated in the upper rather than the lower extremity,[380] with perhaps the exception of the ankle in select cases.[381,382]

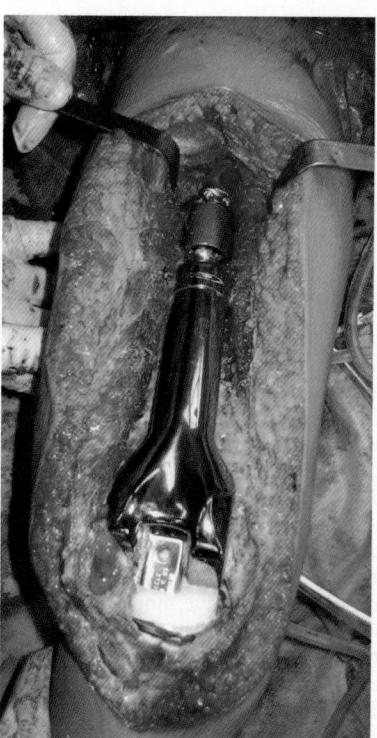

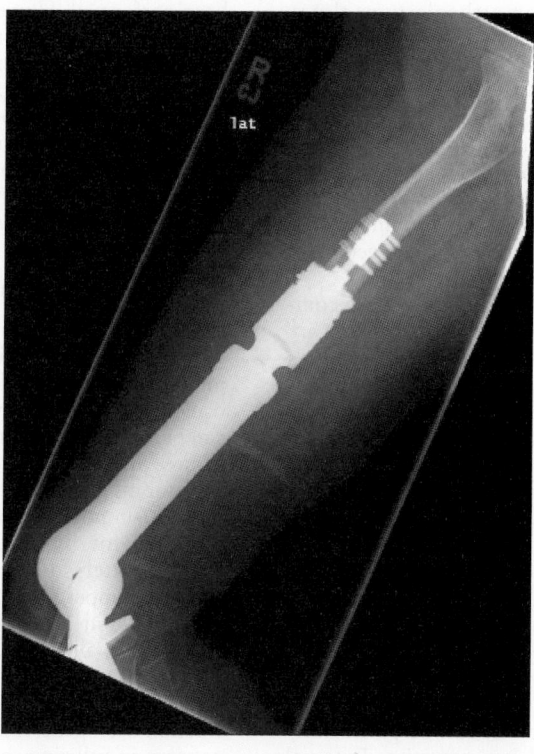

FIGURE 34.10 Expandable prosthesis.

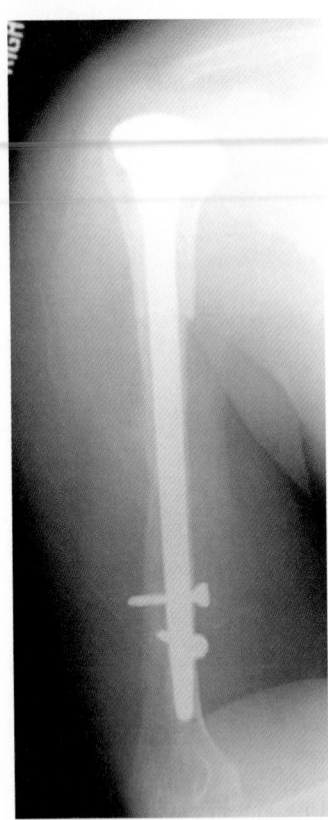

FIGURE 34.11 Allograft prosthetic composites.

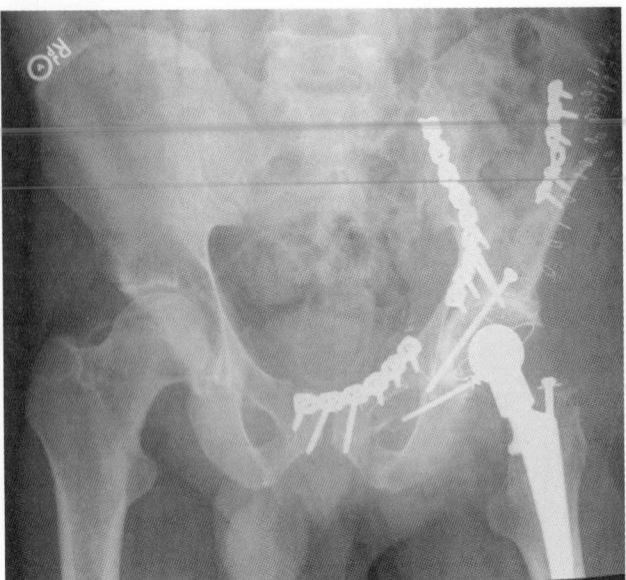

FIGURE 34.12 Internal hemipelvectomy with reconstruction.

Reconstruction as a Function of Location

For tumors of the shoulder and proximal humerus, limb salvage is generally possible with preservation of the neurovascular structures. Reconstruction options include those mentioned above. Arthrodesis rather than arthoplasty is also a viable alternative. One unique reconstructive option for the proximal humerus is the clavicula pro humero whereby the clavicle is disarticulated from the manubrium and rotated on its vascular pedicle and fused to the remaining distal humerus providing a very stable and durable reconstruction.[383,384] With or without reconstruction, preservation of the hand is preferable allowing placement of the hand in space in front of the patient as well as the ability to feed and clean/groom oneself. Even in the best reconstruction, overhead activity is generally not recovered.

In the lower extremity, the distal femur is the most common site. Again, the above techniques may be used. There are advantages and disadvantages to each modality and surgeon's experience and preference usually dictate which technique is used. The middle and proximal fibula, rib, clavicle, scapular body, and iliac wing can forgo reconstruction with good functional results.

In the pelvis, for iliac wing resections involving the sacroiliac joint and/or posterior column (Zone I), autografts, either non- or vascularized, can be employed to reconnect the supra-acetabular pelvis to the sacrum although reconstruction is not always necessary.[385] For more extensive sacral resections, lumbo-pelvic instrumentation and fusion may be indicated at the discretion of the surgeon.[386] Resection involving the pubis and ischium without acetabular involvement (Zone III) are generally not reconstructed.[387]

Periacetabular pelvic lesions (Zone II) can be particularly troublesome in terms of resection and reconstruction. External

hemipelvectomy (hind quarter amputation) historically was the only surgical option. Now internal hemipelvectomy (removal of the bony pelvis leaving a neurovascularly intact limb in place) can frequently be performed,[388] but reconstruction of the defect can be challenging (Fig. 34.12). When no reconstruction is performed, the space between the hip and residual pelvis/sacrum results in significant limb shortening (up to 4 inches) and poor function, albeit better than external hemipelvectomy. An attempt at creating a sling from synthetic material to prevent proximal migration, which is subsequently augmented by scarring, may assist in minimizing limb length inequality. Saddle endoprosthetic, allograft-hip arthroplasty composites, and complete endoprosthetic replacement have all been performed. However, each of these has significant disadvantages and complications.[389–396] Hip transposition has also been espoused as a viable reconstructive option where the proximal femur is utilized to rebuild the ring of the pelvis with proximal femur endoprosthetic replacement.[397,398] The type of reconstruction used is usually based on the preference and discretion of the surgeon. If internal hemipelvectomy is to be attempted, the goal must be an adequate resection of the tumor, which can prove to be quite difficult.[399–404]

Special Considerations for the Skeletally Immature

The skeletally immature patient presents a particular challenge in that the reconstruction must be dynamic in order to accommodate future growth when a physis is sacrificed. Because osteosarcoma generally arises in the child and adolescent, this can become a significant issue. In girls, the growth spurts occur in pre- and early adolescence, while in boys it happens later. Skeletal maturity is reached by age 14 to 15 years in girls and 16 to 17 in boys. Most of the growth in the lower extremity is provided for by the physes about the knee (distal femur approximately 40%, proximal tibia approximately 30%) while the upper femur and lower tibia have modest contributions of about 15% each. Because the physis does not survive in structural allografts, other options must be considered in the skeletally immature patient. A variety of expandable prostheses are available as described above. Limb lengthening via distraction osteogenesis is also an option,[405–407] but there remains concern in utilizing this complex technique concurrently with

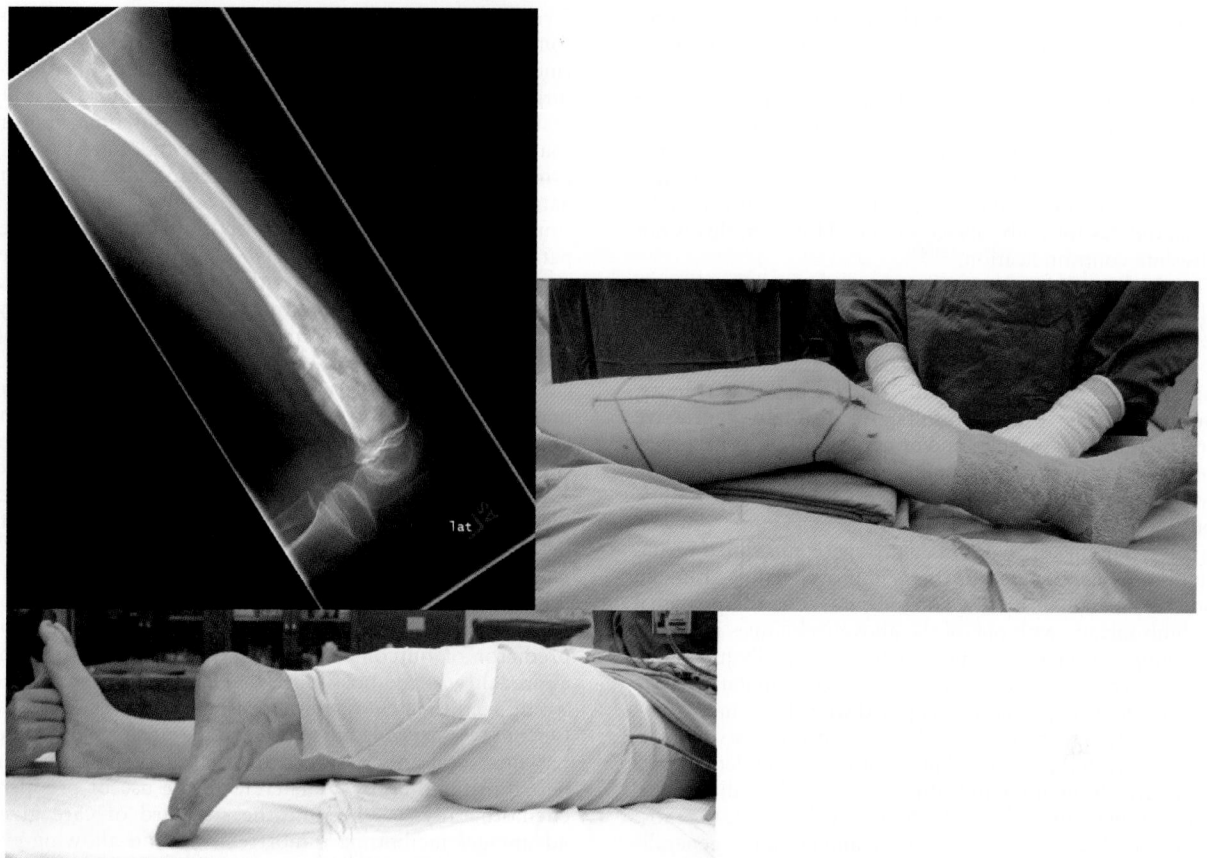

FIGURE 34.13 Rotationplasty of a distal femoral tumor.

adjuvant multiagent chemotherapy.[408] Thus, this technique has only been embraced in a limited fashion, at centers with a strong preference for this technique.

Intrinsic reconstructions such as rotationplasty and tibial turn up-plasties are particularly attractive in the skeletally immature patient, especially in children younger than 8 years, who will experience a significant amount of growth. Conceptually, rotationplasty is a resection of the hip or knee with subsequent reconstruction of the lost joint with the next joint below by rotating it 180° (Fig. 34.13). Most commonly, this is done for resection of the knee, where the ankle subsequently functions as a knee joint. A below knee prosthesis is then placed on the foot. Rotationplasty is a preferred method for skeletally immature patients with a large lesion about the knee, patients with large lesions that are not candidates for limb salvage, as an alternative to above-knee amputation, and as a salvage procedure for chronically infected prosthetic implants.[409–411] Interestingly, patients with rotationplasty were shown to be able to control their gait with their ankle, participate in hobbies to a significantly greater extent, and have less restriction in daily activities (because of pain) than patients who were treated with endoprosthetic replacements for similar conditions.[339,412,413] Additionally, it is far more durable than other forms of reconstruction and retains the distal tibial physis for additional growth. The drawbacks relate to body image and cosmetic appearance.[339] Appropriate, preoperative counseling should be performed, including images of patients that have undergone the procedure before and even meeting other such patients that have undergone the procedure. Accordingly, many children and their families adjust very well to their new appearance and function.[414]

Indications for Limb Salvage versus Amputation Surgery

In general, contemporary limb-sparing surgery results in a local recurrence rate of 5% to 10%, which is only slightly higher, and of questionable significance, when compared to amputation.[415] Amputation itself does not guarantee absolute local control. Noncontiguous disease ("skip lesions") proximal to the main tumor, if not detected, can result in recurrence within the stump in up to 20% of cases.[416] Historically, this leads surgeons to recommend radical resection of the entire bone that resulted in poor functional and esthetic outcomes and no improvement in overall survival.[415] Currently, with the availability of MRI, the entire involved bone must be imaged to detect any noncontiguous disease. Furthermore, the involvement of neurovascular structures, as meticulously assessed on MRI, may also preclude limb salvage. With the careful screening preformed by an experienced orthopaedic oncologist, contemporary limb salvage surgery does not appear to impart a survival disadvantage.[312,415,417,418] However, if there is a question about inadequate margins, amputation should be considered.[419]

After induction (neoadjuvant) chemotherapy, a preoperative follow-up assessment of the tumor must be performed.[283] The response to chemotherapy can be assessed by dynamic MRI[297] and quantitative contrast-enhanced ultrasonography,[420] although positron emission tomography (PET)[302,303,421] and perhaps thallium may also provide useful information.[294,422,423] In certain cases, an individual that was a questionable candidate for limb salvage may be eligible after induction chemotherapy. Nevertheless, if the margins are precarious at the preoperative staging evaluation, then amputation is necessary.

Complications are far more frequent in limb salvage patients than in those who undergo amputation. However, as techniques evolve, the complication rate is steadily decreasing. Furthermore, patients that either present with a pathologic fracture, or fracture during induction chemotherapy, may be poor candidates for limb salvage surgery. However, this is not an absolute contraindication.[424-427]

The decision to amputate is a complex one and must involve the entire team of health care providers. The age of the patient, location of the tumor, presence or absence of pathologic fracture, and the desires of the patient and family must be considered carefully. Functionally, in the upper extremity, amputation leads to poor results. Accordingly, aggressive reconstruction with vascular and/or nerve grafting as necessary should be done to save even limited hand and wrist function. However, if an adequate margin cannot be obtained, then amputation is necessary. In the lower extremity, external hemipelvectomy leads to a particularly poor functional result. A hip disarticulation at least permits improved sitting although prosthetic use remains poor. For tumors above the proximal tibia, limb salvage with one of the above techniques is preferable to amputation and can potentially give equally functional results. Patients undergoing above the knee amputation have increased energy expenditure compared with those undergoing endoprosthetic reconstruction.[428] A knee arthrodesis is intermediate between these two[429] but is not very well tolerated and has a relatively high complication rate.[430] Tibial diaphyseal lesions are often amenable to limb salvage; however, for those about the ankle and distal, below knee amputation is generally preferable to limb salvage.[381,382] Psychosocial adjustment and physical complaints have been reported more often in patients undergoing limb salvage, yet amputees tended to have lower self-esteem and experience more social isolation.[431] When specifically comparing education, employment, health insurance, and marriage, amputees and nonamputees appeared quite similar. However, gender and education often play a prominent role. When compared with siblings, amputees may benefit from additional support.[432]

Adjuvant Treatment

The outcome for patients with osteosarcoma treated with surgery and/or radiotherapy was poor with 2-year survivals of 15% to 20% in spite of adequate local control of the primary tumor.[1-4] Following local control measures, 80% to 90% of patients developed metastatic lung disease suggesting that most patients with apparently localized disease have microscopic lung metastases.[1-4] These findings led to the investigation of systemic chemotherapy to prevent metastatic spread following surgical resection.[433-437] Early trials identified cisplatin (DDP),[438-440] doxorubicin (DOX),[441,442] and high-dose methotrexate (HD-MTX)[443] as the most active agents. Ifosfamide (I) with[444] or without[261,445] etoposide (E) have shown promising activity, although their role in improving outcome has not been adequately evaluated.

Although early nonrandomized trials suggested that the addition of chemotherapy improved the outcome for patients with osteosarcoma,[433-437] some investigators were concerned that the reported improved outcome was related to patient selection, stage migration (related to the introduction of computed tomography), or improved surgical techniques.[446,447] On the basis of these concerns, investigators at the Mayo clinic conducted the first randomized controlled trial for patients with osteosarcoma.[448] The investigators reported an estimated

5-year relapse-free survival of 42% with no differences in outcome for patients treated with adjuvant chemotherapy with vincristine and HD-MTX compared with those treated with surgery followed by observation. The results of that trial suggested that the natural history of osteosarcoma had indeed changed. Two subsequent controlled randomized trials confirmed the importance of chemotherapy administration for patients with osteosarcoma.[5,6] The results of both trials were similar reporting a significantly improved outcome for patients receiving adjuvant chemotherapy (2-year relapse-free survival >50%) compared with observation (2-year relapse-free survival <20%)[5,6] confirming that the natural history had not changed and additionally establishing the importance of adjuvant chemotherapy.

In an effort to increase the number of patients able to undergo limb-sparing procedures, investigators at Memorial Sloan Kettering Cancer Center started using preoperative chemotherapy. The administration of chemotherapy allowed extra time for construction of prosthetic devices and also had the theoretical advantage of treating presumed micrometastatic disease.[449] This concept first introduced by Rosen,[450] not only facilitated surgical resection but also allowed for histological evaluation of response to treatment. Histological response to preoperative chemotherapy became an important predictor of outcome.[451-453] A potential concern with this approach was the possibility that delayed surgical resection would lead to chemotherapy resistance. However, a Pediatric Oncology Group study revealed equivalent outcome for patients randomly assigned to treatment with adjuvant or neoadjuvant therapy.[454] Therefore, the use of preoperative chemotherapy has become the standard of care given its advantages facilitating tumor removal and allowing evaluation of response to therapy.

The concept of altering therapy based on histological response in an effort to improve outcome was originally proposed by Rosen, who reported that altering therapy following surgical resection for patients with a poor histological response resulted in outcome similar to that of patients with a good histological response.[455] However, longer follow-up of that group of patients failed to confirm this improvement[456] and other investigators have been unable to reproduce the results reported by Rosen.[452,457] Memorial investigators have also evaluated the intensification of preoperative therapy to increase the number of patients with a good histological response. Although this strategy increases the number of good responders, in this setting histological response loses its predictive value.[458] Therefore, although histological response remains an important prognostic factor, attempts to improve outcome by increasing the number of good responders or by adjusting postoperative therapy to improve the outcome of poor responders have been generally unsuccessful.

Current Treatment Results

North America. Since osteosarcoma is a rare malignancy representing only about 3% of childhood cancer,[10,459] very few single institutions care for enough patients to perform single institution controlled clinical trials. This has led to the development of controlled clinical trials by cooperative groups under the auspices of the National Cancer Institute. Three different cooperative groups in North America: Pediatric Oncology Group (POG), Children's Cancer Group (CCG) and most recently the Children's Oncology Group (COG) have developed controlled clinical trials in osteosarcoma.[261,444,452,454,460] The most recent trial (INT-0133) enrolling patients between November 1993 and November 1997 included evaluation in a 2×2 factorial design of whether the addition of ifosfamide and/or muramyl tripeptide (MTP) improved the outcome for patients with osteosarcoma.[7] Muramyl tripeptide is a component of the *bacillus Calmette-Guerin* (BCG) cell wall. It is conjugated to phosphatidyl ethanolamine and encapsulated in liposomes to improve delivery to the reticuloendothelial system.[461,462] The primary rationale supporting the use of this relatively nonspecific immune adjuvant was the encouraging results obtained in a prospective randomized trial of this compound in canines,[463] and a couple of early phase trials in patients with recurrent osteosarcoma.[464–466] Results of INT-0133 have been difficult to interpret since the original publication[7] suggested an interaction between the experimental strategies precluding statistical analysis. However, further follow-up suggested no evidence of an interaction and a significant improvement in overall survival but not event-free survival for patients receiving MTP regardless of the chemotherapy regimen.[467] This has created significant controversy,[468–470] and although MTP has been approved in Europe, the destiny of MTP remains unclear partially because of the difficulties in interpreting the results of this trial.

Following completion of INT-0133, COG investigators conducted a series of pilot studies evaluating the feasibility of incorporation of high-dose IE with or without DOX dose-intensification.[471] The purpose of these pilots was to evaluate the tolerability of the regimens with the goal of identifying the best regimen to be studied in the next randomized controlled trial. The pilot studies evaluated the feasibility of administering methotrexate, cisplatin, and doxorubicin (MAP) with or without ifosfamide administering doxorubicin doses up to 600 mg/m² with the use of dexrazoxane. The third pilot evaluated the feasibility of combining MAP with high-dose ifosfamide and etoposide. The latter pilot provided the basis for the experimental regimen in poor responders in the EURAMOS trial.

Although systemic chemotherapy has dramatically improved the outcome of osteosarcoma patients,[7–9] we appeared to have reached a plateau in outcome. Detection of further improvements will likely require an understanding of the pathogenesis of osteosarcoma in order to develop treatment strategies that target these pathways. Alternatively, randomized controlled trials will need to involve accrual of a large number of patients. This will provide for the requisite number of *events* that will allow us to detect clinically relevant differences in survival among treatment arms. One of the strategies to enroll large numbers of patients relatively quickly is via international collaboration. With this goal in mind, investigators from four cooperative groups [COG, Cooperative Osteosarcoma Study Group (COSS), European Osteosarcoma Intergroup (EOI) and Scandinavia Sarcoma Group (SSG)] met in 2001 and agreed on the merits of collaboration. Recognizing the importance of histological response and the controversies surrounding improved outcome by altering postoperative therapy based on that response,[452,455–457] investigators agreed on a common three-drug control arm (HD-MTX, DOX, DDP) as well as agreed to ask two different questions. For patients with a poor histological response, investigators have chosen to evaluate whether the addition of high-dose IE to the three-drug therapy backbone improves outcome. While for patients with a good histological response, they have agreed to evaluate the role of maintenance therapy with pegylated interferon in outcome. This study is anticipated to complete accrual by June 2010.

In an effort to better understand the biological mechanisms of osteosarcoma development, the COG has developed a central repository of tumor specimens collected from patients diagnosed with osteosarcoma at member institutions. The goal of this tumor bank is to make samples available to investigators interested in evaluating the mechanisms of osteosarcoma development. This effort has resulted in the development of the largest osteosarcoma tumor bank, an available resource to interested investigators.

Worldwide

Soon after reports of positive effects of HD-MTX[472] and DOX[442] against osteosarcoma were published and parallel to the introduction of adjuvant multidrug regimens in North America,[436] European researchers from Italy[473] and the German speaking countries[474,475] initiated prospective, adjuvant, and in the latter case, multicenter trials for osteosarcoma. These trials included combination chemotherapy with DOX and HD-MTX as well as surgery. Since then, worldwide, chemotherapy for osteosarcoma consists of regimens combining several cytostatic agents. Most published protocols are still based upon DOX and/or HD-MTX, combined with DDP and/or I and sometimes other drugs.[476] (see Table 34.6).

Over the past decades, on the basis of the work of Rosen and coinvestigators,[450,455,486] most protocols from Europe and elsewhere have included preoperative (neoadjuvant) chemotherapy, followed by surgery of the primary tumor and postoperative (adjuvant) chemotherapy[476] (see Table 34.6). Most groups have confirmed the relationship between histological response to preoperative chemotherapy and the risk of recurrent, metastatic disease[8,451,457,477,480–482,487] using various grading methods.[488] In addition, researchers from Italy and Germany were also able to demonstrate that a poor histological response correlates with an increased risk of local recurrence after surgery.[489,490] While clinicians characterize osteosarcoma responses as good or poor, response must not be interpreted as an all-or-nothing phenomenon, but should be understood as a gradual effect. For instance, the German-Austrian-Swiss Cooperative Osteosarcoma Study Group (COSS) was able to demonstrate in 1,276 evaluable patients that increasing levels of tumor cell destruction conferred an ever-improving prognosis without a clear cutoff point. Even patients with more than 50% viable tumor cells seemed to have a better prognosis than patients without any response.[8]

European study groups have also demonstrated that the extent of histological response cannot be seen independently from the combination of drugs and the duration of preoperative treatment. The Rizzoli Institute from Bologna reported that adding a fourth drug, ifosfamide, to DDP, DOX, and HD-MTX preoperatively improved the response rate compared with their previous, three-drug regimen, but did not improve survival expectancies.[478] In their most recent randomized trial BO06/80931, the European Osteosarcoma Intergroup EOI gave either two or three of a total of six DDP/DOX cycles preoperatively, thereby increasing the response rate from 36% to 50%, but this did not translate into different progression-free or overall survival rates.[491] Therefore, increasing the response rate by using particularly intensive induction chemotherapy or by administering it over an extended time period may lead to increasing numbers of good responders, but will not necessarily improve survival rates.

As evidenced by the studies detailed in Table 34.4, DDP and DOX are almost universally accepted components of international osteosarcoma regimens.[476] However, there are concerns regarding the potential long-term toxicities of both drugs. In an Italian series of 755 patients with localized extremity osteosarcoma who had been treated with regimens including DOX, 13 (1.7%) developed clinically symptomatic cardiac toxicity. Six of those died, and three others needed a heart transplant.[492]

In an effort to increase the local efficacy of DDP, several investigators have advocated intra-arterial administration of this agent. Comparative analyses between cohorts treated with intensive preoperative chemotherapy including either intravenous or intra-arterial DDP argue against a substantial role of the intra-arterial route. In a prospective, nonrandomized comparison of the COSS group between 50 patients

TABLE 34.6

RESULTS WORLDWIDE

Study	N	Preoperative therapy	Response	Postoperative therapy	EFS (%)	Follow-up (yr)	Reference
IOR/OS-1	127	HD-MTX, DOX, DDP, BCD	All	HD-MTX, DOX, DDP, BCD	58	5	Bacci[477]
		ID-MTX, DOX, DDP, BCD	All	ID-MTX, DOX, DDP, BCD	42		
IOR/OS-2	164	HD-MTX, DOX, DDP	Good	HD-MTX, DOX, DDP	59	10	Bacci[260]
			Poor	HD-MTX, DOX, DDP, IE			
IOR/OS-4	133	HD-MTX, DOX, DDP, I	All	HD-MTX, DOX, DDP, I	56	5	Bacci[478]
IOR/SSG-pilot	68	HD-MTX, DOX, DDP, High I	All	HD-MTX, DOX, DDP, High I	73	5	Bacci[256]
SSG T10	97	HD-MTX	Good	HD-MTX, BCD	54	5	Sæter 1991[479]
			Poor	HD-MTX, DOX, DDP, BCD			
SSGVIII	113	HD-MTX, DOX, DDP	Good	HD-MTX, DOX, DDP	63	5	Smeland[274]
ISG.SSGI	182	HD-MTX, DOX, DDP, High I	All	HD-MTX, DOX, DDP, High I	64	5	Ferrari[9]
COSS-77	68	None	NA	HD-MTX, DOX, C	52	5	Winkler[474]
COSS-80	116	HD-MTX, DOX, DDP	All	HD-MTX, DOX, DDP	68	2.5	Winkler[451]
		HD-MTX, DOX, BCD	All	HD-MTX, DOX, BCD			
COSS-82	59	HD-MTX, DOX, DDP	Good	HD-MTX, DOX, DDP	68	5	Winkler[457]
			Poor	DDP, I, C, Act D			
	60	HD-MTX, BCD	Good	HD-MTX, BCD	45	5	
			Poor	DOX, DDP			
COSS-86	171	HD-MTX, DOX, DDP ± I	All	HD-MTX, DOX, DDP ± I	66	10	Fuchs[480]
EOI BO02.80831	99	DOX, DDP	All	DOX, DDP	57	5	Bramwell[481]
	99	HD-MTX, DOX, DDP	All	HD-MTX, DOX, DDP	41		
EOI BO05/80861	199	DOX, DDP	All	DOX, DDP	44	5	Souhami[482]
	192	HD-MTX, DOX, DDP, I, BCD, VCR	All	HD-MTX, DOX, DDP, I, BCD, VCR	44		
EOI BO06/80931	250	DOX, DDP	All	DOX, DDP	41	3	Lewis[483]
	254	DOX, DDP + GCSF	All	DOX, DDP + GCSF	46		
BOTG III/IV	168	I, Carbo, EPI	All	I, Carbo, EPI	46	5	Petrilli[484]
			All	HD-MTX, I, Carbo, EPI			
		DOX, DDP, Carbo	All	DOX, DDP, I, Carbo			
SFOP94	116	HD-MTX, DOX	Good	HD-MTX, DOX	58	5	LeDelay[485]
			Poor	IE			Fuchs[480]
	118	HD-MTX, IE	Good	HD-MTX, IE	66	5	
			Poor	DOX, DDP			Bramwell[481]

receiving intra-arterial and 59 receiving intravenous DDP together with HD-MTX, DOX and I, the fraction of histological good responders did not differ between both cohorts (34/50 [68%] vs. 41/59 [69%]).[493] Similarly, at the Rizzoli Institute, Bologna, Italy, while there was some evidence for enhanced local activity of intra-arterial DDP given as part of a three-drug regimen, the percentage of good histological responders was essentially the same for patients treated with intra-arterial or intravenous DDP (78% vs. 84%) in the two sequential studies where four drugs were used.[494] Therefore, choosing the intra-arterial route to administer DDP does not seem to improve local tumor response if DDP is given as just one component of an intensive multidrug regimen.

Currently, most European groups continue to incorporate HD-MTX into their osteosarcoma protocols because of its relative lack of myelotoxicity and late effects. HD-MTX may, however, be associated with severe acute toxicity. The incidence of nephrotoxicity above grade 2 was 1.8% in a transatlantic intergroup survey of 3,887 patients, and the mortality rate among affected patients was 4.4%.[495] The toxicity associated with reduced HD-MTX clearance can, however, be ameliorated by glucarpidase (carboxypeptidase G2), an enzyme that cleaves methotrexate.[495]

The role of HD-MTX in general and the potential importance of scheduled or received MTX-dose intensity or individual MTX pharmacokinetics have long been topics of intense debate.[496–499] The randomized IOR/OS-1 trial from Italy demonstrated that an otherwise identical combination regimen was more effective if it contained high-dose rather than moderate-dose methotrexate.[477] Some authors who used protocols devoid of HD-MTX, including those of a recent report on 53 patients from former East Germany, where 10-year survival was 67%[500] and those of the Brazilian Osteosarcoma Treatment Group (BTOG)[484] (see Table 34.6), have reported outcomes similar to those obtained with methotrexate. The EOI has performed two trials in which methotrexate-containing regimens were compared with a combination consisting of only two drugs, DOX and DDP. Their first trial (EOI BO02/80831) compared DOX 75 mg/m[2] and CDDP 100 mg/m[2] to be given every 3 weeks for 6 cycles with essentially the same schedule of DOX/CDDP but preceded 10 days earlier by 8 g/m[2] of HD-MTX.[481] Their second trial (EOI BO03/80861)[482] compared DOX/CDDP with a multidrug schedule based on the T10 regimen originally reported by Rosen.[455] In neither trial could an advantage for the methotrexate-containing regimen be demonstrated. However, it must be noted that the first EOI trial may not have truly evaluated whether adding methotrexate was beneficial, as the cumulative doses of DOX and DDP were reduced by one-third and the intervals between cycles extended by 50% in the HD-MTX arm.[481] Also, the HD-MTX dose prescribed in that trial, 8 g/m[2], may have been suboptimal. While no advantage of a more complex, HD-MTX-containing multidrug regimen over the DOX/DDP combination was detected in the second EOI trial, the achieved outcomes, 5-year overall and progression-free survival rates of 55% and 44%,[482] compared unfavorably with those obtained by others with similar multidrug regimens (see Table 34.4).[455,476] Therefore, it is difficult to draw definitive conclusions regarding the potential role of HD-MTX from the EOI trials.

The Société Francaise d'Oncologie Pédiatrique (SFOP) has investigated whether DOX and potentially also DDP could be avoided in a randomized comparison of preoperative chemotherapy with DOX plus HD-MTX with HD-MTX plus high-dose IE.[485] In that particular trial, a total of 234 eligible patients accrued over a period of 7 years. The response rate obtained with the three-drug combination was superior to that of the two-drug arm, 56% versus 39%. While there was a trend for improved event-free survival with the IE arm, the difference was not significant and overall survival for the entire population was similar in both arms at 76%. As poor responders to preoperative chemotherapy were scheduled to receive postoperative chemotherapy with other drugs (see Table 34.6), only 43% of the patients in the IE arm were actually event-free at 3 years without ever having received DOX or DDP. Therefore, the results of the SFOP-94 trial do not clarify the exact role of DOX and DDP in osteosarcoma but demonstrate that approaches other than the common HD-MTX, DOX, DDP induction may be feasible.[485]

Several European studies have addressed the question of salvage chemotherapy for osteosarcomas with a poor response to preoperative induction chemotherapy.[457,476] The failure of such a salvage approach was particularly apparent in a trial from the COSS group, where the effective but toxic agents DOX and DDP were deliberately omitted from preoperative chemotherapy in a randomized comparison with a more conventional preoperative regimen containing both drugs. In the experimental arm, DOX and DDP were then added postoperatively in the case of poor response. As expected, the response rate obtained in the experimental arm was lower than in the conventional arm, but the expectation that the outlook for poor responders would be improved by the postoperative addition of two very active agents was met with failure.[457] Similarly, salvage chemotherapy failed to improve the outlook for poor responders in several other, nonrandomized studies on both sides of the Atlantic.[476] Therefore, as of now, there is no proof that poor responders will benefit from postoperative

treatment modifications. One possible exception to the failure of salvage therapy is the high-dose IE combination, for which some efficacy was claimed on the basis of the results from an uncontrolled Italian study, where poor responders received these drugs combined with other drugs postoperatively and response was no longer an independent prognostic factor upon multivariate analysis.[501] In the Scandinavian Sarcoma Group's study SSG VIII, 113 patients received preoperative chemotherapy with HD-MTX, DDP and DOX. Poor responders were switched to salvage therapy consisting exclusively of IE, but this complete change of postoperative treatment did not improve the outcome. The authors concluded that the data obtained from their nonrandomized study did not support discontinuation and exchange of all drugs used preoperatively in the case of poor histological response.[274]

The dose intensity of treatment has been the focus of several reports from European study groups. Taken together, their results argue against an effect of increasing dose intensity above that normally encountered in modern protocols. The EOI performed a retrospective analysis of received dose intensity in 287 patients who had been randomized to receive a chemotherapy regimen of six DOX/DDP cycles in their trials BO02/80831 and BO05/80861.[502] On average, only 80% of the intended dose of chemotherapy was actually given, yet the mean time to completion of chemotherapy was 1.27 times longer than specified by the protocols. While progression-free survival was lower for patients who received less than all six scheduled cycles, there was no statistically significant correlation between either preoperative dose intensity and histological response or overall received dose intensity and overall or progression-free survival.[502] Furthermore, a retrospective analysis of 917 patients from neoadjuvant, multidrug COSS trials did not detect a correlation of either higher overall treatment intensity or of higher dose intensity of any of four individual agents (DOX, DDP, HD-MTX, I) with either overall or event-free survival.[503]

The EOI has also addressed the question of dose intensity in a prospective, randomized trial, BO06/80931. Using their two-drug regimen of three weekly DOX/DDP cycles as backbone, they asked whether it was feasible to shorten the interval between cycles to 2 weeks by adding the granulocyte colony stimulating factor, G-CSF, and whether this would improve outcomes. Patients in both arms were to receive a total of six chemotherapy cycles, and surgery was scheduled at week 6 in both arms, that is, after two cycles in the arm without and after three cycles in the arm with G-CSF. Thus, adding one cycle preoperatively, the response rate was indeed increased and the delivered dose intensity was higher in the experimental arm. There was, however, no evidence of a difference in overall or progression-free survival.[491] A recent Italian/Scandinavian study evaluating 182 patients treated with very intensive chemotherapy including high-dose I also failed to result in improved outcomes compared with less intense regimens.[9] Therefore, further increasing the doses or dose intensities of conventional chemotherapeutic agents may not be advantageous. In this context, it should be noted that attempts to improve the prognosis of patients with recurrent osteosarcoma by high-dose chemotherapy with blood stem cell rescue were met with failure.[504–506]

European groups and single institutions have evaluated adjuvant approaches other than chemotherapy with cytostatic agents. The European Organization for Research on Treatment of Cancer (EORTC) trial 20781, performed between 1978 and 1983, randomized 205 patients into either 9 months of adjuvant chemotherapy or bilateral lung irradiation with a total dose of 20 Gy, or 3 months of chemotherapy followed by lung irradiation. Four-year disease-free and overall survival were 24% and 43%, respectively, well below what would currently be considered standard, and there was no difference by treatment arm. Therefore, elective lung irradiation provided the same prognosis as the adjuvant chemotherapy given in that trial, but the combination of both did not lead to improved results.[507] Investigators from the Karolinska Hospital in Stockholm used adjuvant interferon-α without chemotherapy in a pilot series.[508,509] With a median follow-up of 12 years, 70 patients achieved 10-year metastasis-free and sarcoma-specific survival rates of 39% and 43%, respectively,[508] making this agent an attractive target for phase III trials. The European and American Osteosarcoma Study (EURAMOS1) evaluate-currently evaluates the efficacy of pegylated interferon-α maintenance treatment following standard chemotherapy in a prospective, randomized trial.

Around the world, prospective studies have generally focused on young patients with localized extremity osteosarcomas, and their results must be interpreted keeping this in mind, as other patients often have much poorer outcomes. For instance, patients with primary metastases had event-free survival expectancies of no more than 30% in series from Italy,[510] France,[511] and the German-speaking countries.[263] The number of metastatic lesions and the surgical remission status were uniformly identified as prognostic factors.

In summary, using the same general approaches worldwide, survival expectancies achieved in Europe[476,512] and for instance by selected South American[484,513] and Asian[487,514] groups are basically identical to those reported from North America. However, treatment outside of established infrastructures in economically advanced countries poses great challenges. Many patients worldwide still have a very limited chance to survive their disease, as evidenced by a 5-year survival rate of 7.5% for a series of 66 patients from a teaching hospital in southern Africa, most of whom presented with well-advanced local and distant spread.[515] Twinning programs may help to assure that patients in less affluent countries can benefit from the advantages of modern treatment. Within such a program, similar results were obtained for 22 patients treated in a single center in Santiago, Chile, and 48 patients treated at St. Jude Children's Research Hospital trials.[513] Results from Brazil demonstrate that multiinstitutional trials can also be conducted in countries with limited financial resources and that treatment within the infrastructure of such a trial can result in acceptable cure rates.[484]

Finally, it must be noted that the survival rates for osteosarcoma have not improved substantially over the past decades in the regions of the world with the most advanced health care systems. A study pooling the data from 59 population-based European cancer registries, thereby being able to evaluate 1,485 affected children and adolescents, demonstrated an improvement in 5-year survival rates between the time periods 1978–1982 and 1983–1987, 37% to 58%, but little change over the two following 5-year time spans, with 59% and 61% 5-year survival[512] Similar results were reported from the North American SEER Program, where survival increased significantly between 1973 and 1983 and between 1984 and 1993, but there was little change subsequently and survival rates reached a plateau just above 60%.[10] Innovative approaches are clearly required before the cure rate for osteosarcoma will once again increase substantially.

Treatment of Relapse

The treatment of patients with recurrent osteosarcoma remains challenging. The most common site of disease recurrence remains the lung and about 20% to 30% of patients are reported to be cured by exploration and complete surgical resection of all lung metastases.[516,517] Some recent series suggest that the outcome of patients with recurrent disease is poor and that as therapy has become more aggressive, cure with resection alone is not a realistic goal,[518] but this is not supported in all series.[264] Furthermore, a German series evaluating outcome for osteosarcoma patients following recurrence suggested that the most important factor predicting outcome was complete surgical resection. The series also suggested that for patients unable to undergo resection the use of chemotherapy might have a marginal effect, but that its role in the treatment of recurrence remained to be defined.[264] Furthermore, patients who develop subsequent recurrences have a slight chance of cure with aggressive resections.[519] Therefore, the management of patients with recurrent osteosarcoma remains controversial since the only proven curative strategy is complete surgical resection. The number of patients with recurrent disease available for evaluation precludes the performance of controlled randomized trials, which would be the only way to evaluate the role of postsurgical therapy in outcome. Many clinical trials have added promising agents to postsurgical therapy for patients with recurrent disease. Obviously, under those circumstances the interpretation of those trials is difficult.

Treatment of Osteosarcoma as a Second Malignancy

Several European groups have investigated treatment outcomes of patients in whom osteosarcoma arose as secondary malignancy. As evidenced by the results in 30 patients with secondary osteosarcoma from the COSS group, including 24 radiation-associated tumors,[520] 23 radiation-related osteosarcomas after treatment of childhood and adolescent cancer from France,[521] and 20 radioinduced osteosarcomas of the extremity from the Rizzoli Institute,[522] the prognosis of affected patients may approach that of otherwise comparable patients with primary osteosarcoma if treated by an appropriate multimodality approach.

Long-Term Outcome

The use of multiagent chemotherapy and surgical resection has drastically improved the outcome of osteosarcoma patients, and with modern therapy patients with localized, resectable osteosarcoma have a 3-year disease-free survival of 60% to 70%.[7,89,467] The survival improvement has raised concerns regarding the risk of posttherapy complications and their impact on the quality of life of survivors. Therapy-related complications include anthracycline-induced cardiomyopathy,[523–525] hearing loss,[526] kidney dysfunction,[527] second malignancies,[528] and sterility especially in patients receiving alkylating agents.[529] In addition, patients treated for osteosarcoma can have physical limitations resulting from the need for surgical resection. Review of the available literature would suggest that survivors adapt well to their resection.[530] Additionally, review of the available data suggests that mortality for cancer survivors is mostly related to recurrent disease,[531,532] suggesting that further efforts to improve survival are warranted.

FUTURE DIRECTIONS

With modern treatment, approximately 60% to 70% of newly diagnosed, resectable osteosarcoma patients can expect to be disease-free 3 years from diagnosis.[7,9,491] The outcome for patients with initially metastatic disease[260,261,263,444,460,533] and for those who develop recurrent disease[264] remains much worse with reported 2-year survivals of 10% to 30%. Likewise, despite intensive multimodal treatment, patients with osteosarcoma of the axial skeleton, particularly the pelvis[403,534–536] or the spine,[537] only obtained disease-free survival rates in a similar, unsatisfactory range. Local failure was a major problem in all reported series. Patients with osteosarcoma of the axial skeleton who achieve and maintain local tumor control may enjoy survival expectancies similar to those of patients with extremity primaries.[538]

North American efforts to improve the outcome of patients with osteosarcoma are focused on the evaluation of new chemotherapy[261,444] and/or biological agents.[539] These agents are incorporated into the treatment of patients with recurrent or metastatic disease to evaluate not only feasibility but also potential efficacy.[540] This strategy is based on the poor prognosis associated with the presence of initially metastatic disease[263,266] or the presence of recurrent disease[519] and the potential that new strategies may be beneficial to this subset of patients. New biologic agents under investigation include trastuzumab based on the fact that expression of HER2 in osteosarcoma appears to carry a worse prognosis,[155] inhaled granulocyte macrophage colony stimulating factor based on preliminary evidence suggesting that it might stimulate macrophages to become tumoricidal,[539] and zoledronic acid based on its preclinical activity against osteosarcoma.[541,542]

The IGF pathway is part of the endocrine system, stimulating linear body growth and bone formation, as well as promoting neuronal survival, myelination, and postnatal mammary development and lactation. The IGF system has two principal ligands: IGF-I and Insulin-like growth factor II (IGF-II). These ligands mediate their stimulatory effects via the IGF-IR, a transmembrane receptor tyrosine kinase.[543] The IGF-IR is structurally similar to the insulin receptor (IR), and with it forms active heterodimers. Upon ligand binding, autophosphorylation of the IGF-IR tyrosine kinase initiates activation of the MAPK and PI3 K/Akt pathways leading to proliferation, survival, and enhanced angiogenesis via downstream induction of VEGF.[544,545] The IGF-IR is expressed at high levels in a wide variety of cancers,[546,547] and appears to play a key role in the regulation of cellular activities including cell proliferation, differentiation, and apoptosis.[548]

The IGF signaling pathway appears to have a role in osteosarcoma development and IGF-I has been shown to drive proliferation, survival, and the metastatic phenotype in osteosarcoma.[123,133,135] In addition to the preclinical evidence suggesting a role for this pathway in osteosarcoma, the Pediatric Preclinical Testing Program (PPTP) has tested antibodies against osteosarcoma xenografts and demonstrated activity.[549] A number of drug companies are developing antibodies against this pathway on the basis of the preliminary evidence of *in vitro* efficacy and the limited toxicity of these agents. These agents are presently undergoing evaluation in the relapsed setting. It is likely that over the next few years, we will see a large number of trials evaluating these agents and likely incorporating them into frontline therapy.

References

1. Dahlin DC, Coventry MB. Osteogenic sarcoma. A study of six hundred cases. J Bone Joint Surg Am 1967;49:101–110.
2. Marcove RC, Mike V, Hajek JV, et al. Osteogenic sarcoma under the age of twenty-one. A review of one hundred and forty-five operative cases. J Bone Joint Surg Am 1970;52:411–423.
3. Weinfeld MS, Dudley HR. Osteogenic sarcoma: a follow-up study of the ninety-four cases observed at the Massachusetts General Hospital from 1920 to 1960. J Bone Joint Surg Am 1962;44A:269–276.
4. Friedman MA, Carter SK. The therapy of osteogenic sarcoma: current status and thoughts for the future. J Surg Oncol 1972;4:482–510.
5. Link MP, Goorin AM, Miser AW, et al. The effect of adjuvant chemotherapy on relapse-free survival in patients with osteosarcoma of the extremity. N Engl J Med 1986;314:1600–1606.
6. Eilber F, Giuliano A, Eckardt J, et al. Adjuvant chemotherapy for osteosarcoma: a randomized prospective trial. J Clin Oncol 1987;5:21–26.
7. Meyers PA, Schwartz CL, Krailo M, et al. Osteosarcoma: a randomized, prospective trial of the addition of ifosfamide and/or muramyl tripeptide to cisplatin, doxorubicin, and high-dose methotrexate. J Clin Oncol 2005;23:2004–2011.
8. Bielack SS, Kempf-Bielack B, Delling G, et al. Prognostic factors in high-grade osteosarcoma of the extremities or trunk: an analysis of 1,702 patients treated on neoadjuvant cooperative osteosarcoma study group protocols. J Clin Oncol 2002;20:776–790.
9. Ferrari S, Smeland S, Mercuri M, et al. Neoadjuvant chemotherapy with high-dose ifosfamide, high-dose methotrexate, cisplatin, and doxorubicin for patients with localized osteosarcoma of the extremity: a joint study by the Italian and Scandinavian Sarcoma Groups. J Clin Oncol 2005;23:8845–8852.
10. Mirabello L, Troisi RJ, Savage SA. Osteosarcoma incidence and survival rates from 1973 to 2004: data from the Surveillance, Epidemiology, and End Results Program. Cancer 2009;115:1531–1543.
11. Ries LAG. SEER Program (National Cancer Institute (U.S.)). Cancer incidence and survival among children and adolescents: United States SEER program 1975–1995 [edited by Lynn A. Gloecker Ries . . . et al.]. Bethesda, MD: National Cancer Institute, SEER Program, 1999.
12. Meyers PA, Gorlick R. Osteosarcoma. Pediatr Clin North Am 1997;44:973–989.
13. Mirabello L, Troisi RJ, Savage SA. International osteosarcoma incidence patterns in children and adolescents, middle ages and elderly persons. Int J Cancer 2009;125:229–234.
14. Arndt CA, Crist WM. Common musculoskeletal tumors of childhood and adolescence. N Engl J Med 1999;341:342–352.
15. Phillips JC, Stephenson B, Hauck M, et al. Heritability and segregation analysis of osteosarcoma in the Scottish deerhound. Genomics 2007;90:354–363.
16. Ru G, Terracini B, Glickman LT. Host related risk factors for canine osteosarcoma. Vet J 1998;156:31–39.
17. Gorlick R, Anderson P, Andrulis I, et al. Biology of childhood osteogenic sarcoma and potential targets for therapeutic development: meeting summary. Clin Cancer Res 2003; 9:5442–5453.
18. Buckley JD, Pendergrass TW, Buckley CM, et al. Epidemiology of osteosarcoma and Ewing's sarcoma in childhood: a study of 305 cases by the Children's Cancer Group. Cancer 1998;83:1440–1448.
19. Troisi R, Masters MN, Joshipura K, et al. Perinatal factors, growth and development, and osteosarcoma risk. Br J Cancer 2006;95:1603–1607.
20. Longhi A, Pasini A, Cicognani A, et al. Height as a risk factor for osteosarcoma. J Pediatr Hematol Oncol 2005;27:314–318.
21. Cotterill SJ, Wright CM, Pearce MS, et al. Stature of young people with malignant bone tumors. Pediatr Blood Cancer 2004;42:59–63.
22. Ruza E, Sotillo E, Sierrasesumaga L, et al. Analysis of polymorphisms of the vitamin D receptor, estrogen receptor, and collagen Ialpha1 genes and their relationship with height in children with bone cancer. J Pediatr Hematol Oncol 2003;25:780–786.
23. Marina N, Gebhardt M, Teot L, et al. Biology and therapeutic advances for pediatric osteosarcoma. Oncologist 2004;9:422–441.
24. Alpert LI, Abaci IF, Werthamer S. Radiation-induced extraskeletal osteosarcoma. Cancer 1973;31:1359–1363.
25. Chan LL, Czerniak BA, Ginsberg LE. Radiation-induced osteosarcoma after bilateral childhood retinoblastoma. AJR Am J Roentgenol 2000;174:1288.
26. Freeman CR, Gledhill R, Chevalier LM, et al. Osteogenic sarcoma following treatment with megavoltage radiation and chemotherapy for bone tumors in children. Med Pediatr Oncol 1980;8:375–382.
27. Haselow RE, Nesbit M, Dehner LP, et al. Second neoplasms following megavoltage radiation in a pediatric population. Cancer 1978;42:1185–1191.
28. Sim FH, Cupps RE, Dahlin DC, et al. Postradiation sarcoma of bone. J Bone Joint Surg Am 1972;54:1479–1489.
29. Varela-Duran J, Dehner LP. Postirradiation osteosarcoma in childhood. A clinicopathologic study of three cases and review of the literature. Am J Pediatr Hematol Oncol 1980;2:263–271.
30. Preston DL, Cullings H, Suyama A, et al. Solid cancer incidence in atomic bomb survivors exposed in utero or as young children. J Natl Cancer Inst 2008;100:428–436.
31. Preston DL, Ron E, Tokuoka S, et al. Solid cancer incidence in atomic bomb survivors: 1958–1998. Radiat Res 2007;168:1–64.
32. Le Vu B, de Vathaire F, Shamsaldin A, et al. Radiation dose, chemotherapy and risk of osteosarcoma after solid tumours during childhood. Int J Cancer 1998;77:370–377.
33. Brenner DJ, Elliston CD, Hall EJ, et al. Estimates of the cancer risks from pediatric CT radiation are not merely theoretical: comment on "point/counterpoint: in x-ray computed tomography, technique factors should be selected appropriate to patient size. against the proposition". Med Phys 2001;28:2387–2388.
34. Frush DP, Donnelly LF, Rosen NS. Computed tomography and radiation risks: what pediatric health care providers should know. Pediatrics 2003;112:951–957.
35. Hansen MF, Cavenee WK. Retinoblastoma and osteosarcoma: the prototypic cancer family. Acta Paediatr Jpn 1987;29:526–533.
36. Hansen MF, Koufos A, Gallie BL, et al. Osteosarcoma and retinoblastoma: a shared chromosomal mechanism revealing recessive predisposition. Proc Natl Acad Sci U S A 1985;82:6216–6220.
37. Yu CL, Tucker MA, Abramson DH, et al. Cause-specific mortality in long-term survivors of retinoblastoma. J Natl Cancer Inst 2009;101:581–591.
38. Abramson DH, Ellsworth RM, Kitchin FD, et al. Second nonocular tumors in retinoblastoma survivors. Are they radiation-induced? Ophthalmology 1984;91:1351–1355.
39. Dunkel IJ, Gerald WL, Rosenfield NS, et al. Outcome of patients with a history of bilateral retinoblastoma treated for a second malignancy: the Memorial Sloan-Kettering experience. Med Pediatr Oncol 1998;30:59–62.
40. Malkin D, Friend SH, Li FP, et al. Germ-line mutations of the p53 tumor-suppressor gene in children and young adults with second malignant neoplasms. N Engl J Med 1997;336:734.
41. Malkin D, Jolly KW, Barbier N, et al. Germline mutations of the p53 tumor-suppressor gene in children and young adults with second malignant neoplasms. N Engl J Med 1992;326:1309–1315.

42. Wang LL, Gannavarapu A, Kozinetz CA, et al. Association between osteosarcoma and deleterious mutations in the RECQL4 gene in Rothmund-Thomson syndrome. J Natl Cancer Inst 2003;95:669–674.

43. Berman SD, Calo E, Landman AS, et al. Metastatic osteosarcoma induced by inactivation of Rb and p53 in the osteoblast lineage. Proc Natl Acad Sci U S A 2008;105:11851–11856.

44. Ellis NA, Groden J, Ye TZ, et al. The Bloom's syndrome gene product is homologous to RecQ helicases. Cell 1995;83:655–666.

45. Goto M, Miller RW, Ishikawa Y, et al. Excess of rare cancers in Werner syndrome (adult progeria). Cancer Epidemiol Biomarkers Prev 1996;5:239–246.

46. Hansen MF, Nellissery MJ, Bhatia P. Common mechanisms of osteosarcoma and Paget's disease. J Bone Miner Res 1999;14(suppl 2):39–44.

47. Hansen MF, Seton M, Merchant A. Osteosarcoma in Paget's disease of bone. J Bone Miner Res 2006;21(suppl 2):P58–P63.

48. Gelberg KH, Fitzgerald EF, Hwang S, et al. Growth and development and other risk factors for osteosarcoma in children and young adults. Int J Epidemiol 1997;26:272–278.

49. Garcea RL, Imperiale MJ. Simian virus 40 infection of humans. J Virol 2003;77:5039–5045.

50. Mendoza SM, Konishi T, Miller CW. Integration of SV40 in human osteosarcoma DNA. Oncogene 1998;17:2457–2462.

51. Bridge JA, Nelson M, McComb E, et al. Cytogenetic findings in 73 osteosarcoma specimens and a review of the literature. Cancer Genet Cytogenet 1997;95:74–87.

52. Lau CC, Harris CP, Lu XY, et al. Frequent amplification and rearrangement of chromosomal bands 6p12-p21 and 17p11.2 in osteosarcoma. Genes Chromosomes Cancer 2004;39:11–21.

53. Man TK, Lu XY, Jaeweon K, et al. Genome-wide array comparative genomic hybridization analysis reveals distinct amplifications in osteosarcoma. BMC Cancer 2004;4:45.

54. Zielenska M, Bayani J, Pandita A, et al. Comparative genomic hybridization analysis identifies gains of 1p35 approximately p36 and chromosome 19 in osteosarcoma. Cancer Genet Cytogenet 2001;130:14–21.

55. Dorfman HD, Czerniak B. Bone tumors. St. Louis: Mosby, 1998.

56. Huvos AG. Bone tumors: diagnosis, treatment, and prognosis. 2nd ed. Philadelphia, PA: Saunders, 1991.

57. Dahlin DC, Unni KK. Bone tumors: general aspects and data on 8,542 cases. 4th ed. Springfield, IL: Thomas, 1986.

58. Borden EC, Baker LH, Bell RS, et al. Soft tissue sarcomas of adults: state of the translational science. Clin Cancer Res 2003;9:1941–1956.

59. Ladanyi M. The emerging molecular genetics of sarcoma translocations. Diagn Mol Pathol 1995;4:162–173.

60. Benassi MS, Molendini L, Gamberi G, et al. Alteration of pRb/p16/cdk4 regulation in human osteosarcoma. Int J Cancer 1999;84:489–493.

61. Wadayama B, Toguchida J, Shimizu T, et al. Mutation spectrum of the retinoblastoma gene in osteosarcomas. Cancer Res 1994;54:3042–3048.

62. Toguchida J, Ishizaki K, Sasaki MS, et al. Preferential mutation of paternally derived RB gene as the initial event in sporadic osteosarcoma. Nature 1989;338:156–158.

63. Harbour JW. Molecular basis of low-penetrance retinoblastoma. Arch Ophthalmol 2001;119:1699–1704.

64. McIntyre JF, Smith-Sorensen B, Friend SH, et al. Germline mutations of the p53 tumor suppressor gene in children with osteosarcoma. J Clin Oncol 1994;12:925–930.

65. Toguchida J, Yamaguchi T, Dayton SH, et al. Prevalence and spectrum of germline mutations of the p53 gene among patients with sarcoma. N Engl J Med 1992;326:1301–1308.

66. Nishijo K, Nakayama T, Aoyama T, et al. Mutation analysis of the RECQL4 gene in sporadic osteosarcomas. Int J Cancer 2004;111:367–372.

67. Knowles BB, McCarrick J, Fox N, et al. Osteosarcomas in transgenic mice expressing an alpha-amylase-SV40 T-antigen hybrid gene. Am J Pathol 1990;137:259–262.

68. Donehower LA, Harvey M, Slagle BL, et al. Mice deficient for p53 are developmentally normal but susceptible to spontaneous tumours. Nature 1992;356:215–221.

69. Jacks T, Remington L, Williams BO, et al. Tumor spectrum analysis in p53-mutant mice. Curr Biol 1994;4:1–7.

70. Liu G, McDonnell TJ, Montes de Oca Luna R, et al. High metastatic potential in mice inheriting a targeted p53 missense mutation. Proc Natl Acad Sci U S A 2000;97:4174–4179.

71. Olive KP, Tuveson DA, Ruhe ZC, et al. Mutant p53 gain of function in two mouse models of Li-Fraumeni syndrome. Cell 2004;119:847–860.

72. Khidr L, Chen PL. RB, the conductor that orchestrates life, death and differentiation. Oncogene 2006;25:5210–5219.

73. Walkley CR, Qudsi R, Sankaran VG, et al. Conditional mouse osteosarcoma, dependent on p53 loss and potentiated by loss of Rb, mimics the human disease. Genes Dev 2008;22:1662–1676.

74. Grigoriadis AE, Schellander K, Wang ZQ, et al. Osteoblasts are target cells for transformation in c-fos transgenic mice. J Cell Biol 1993;122:685–701.

75. Jain M, Arvanitis C, Chu K, et al. Sustained loss of a neoplastic phenotype by brief inactivation of MYC. Science 2002;297:102–104.

76. Erfle V, Schmidt J, Strauss GP, et al. Activation and biological properties of endogenous retroviruses in radiation osteosarcomagenesis. Leuk Res 1986;10:905–913.

77. Vahle JL, Sato M, Long GG, et al. Skeletal changes in rats given daily subcutaneous injections of recombinant human parathyroid hormone (1-34) for 2 years and relevance to human safety. Toxicol Pathol 2002;30:312–321.

78. Kufe DW, Holland JF, Frei E, American Cancer Society. Holland Frei cancer medicine 7. 7th ed. Lewiston, NY: BC Decker, 2006.

79. Fraumeni JF Jr. Stature and malignant tumors of bone in childhood and adolescence. Cancer 1967;20:967–973.

80. Withrow SJ. Osteosarcoma. Vet Q 1998;20(suppl 1):S19–S21.

81. Withrow SJ, Powers BE, Straw RC, et al. Comparative aspects of osteosarcoma. Dog versus man. Clin Orthop Relat Res 1991;270:159–168.

82. Tjalma RA. Canine bone sarcoma: estimation of relative risk as a function of body size. J Natl Cancer Inst 1966;36:1137–1150.

83. Cooley DM, Beranek BC, Schlittler DL, et al. Endogenous gonadal hormone exposure and bone sarcoma risk. Cancer Epidemiol Biomarkers Prev 2002;11:1434–1440.

84. Sutter NB, Bustamante CD, Chase K, et al. A single IGF1 allele is a major determinant of small size in dogs. Science 2007;316:112–115.

85. Nellissery MJ, Padalecki SS, Brkanac Z, et al. Evidence for a novel osteosarcoma tumor-suppressor gene in the chromosome 18 region genetically linked with Paget disease of bone. Am J Hum Genet 1998;63:817–824.

86. Hansen MR, Moffat JC. Osteosarcoma of the skull base after radiation therapy in a patient with McCune-Albright syndrome: case report. Skull Base 2003;13:79–83.

87. Koshy M, Paulino AC, Mai WY, et al. Radiation-induced osteosarcomas in the pediatric population. Int J Radiat Oncol Biol Phys 2005;63:1169–1174.

88. Kuttesch JF Jr, Wexler LH, Marcus RB, et al. Second malignancies after Ewing's sarcoma: radiation dose-dependency of secondary sarcomas. J Clin Oncol 1996;14:2818–2825.

89. Shaheen M, Deheshi BM, Riad S, et al. Prognosis of radiation-induced bone sarcoma is similar to primary osteosarcoma. Clin Orthop Relat Res 2006;450:76–81.

90. Wong FL, Boice JD Jr, Abramson DH, et al. Cancer incidence after retinoblastoma. Radiation dose and sarcoma risk. JAMA 1997;278:1262–1267.

91. Feugeas O, Guriec N, Babin-Boilletot A, et al. Loss of heterozygosity of the RB gene is a poor prognostic factor in patients with osteosarcoma. J Clin Oncol 1996;14:467–472.

92. Toguchida J, Ishizaki K, Sasaki MS, et al. Chromosomal reorganization for the expression of recessive mutation of retinoblastoma susceptibility gene in the development of osteosarcoma. Cancer Res 1988;48:3939–3943.

93. Wei G, Lonardo F, Ueda T, et al. CDK4 gene amplification in osteosarcoma: reciprocal relationship with INK4A gene alterations and mapping of 12q13 amplicons. Int J Cancer 1999;80:199–204.

94. Quelle DE, Zindy F, Ashmun RA, et al. Alternative reading frames of the INK4a tumor suppressor gene encode two unrelated proteins capable of inducing cell cycle arrest. Cell 1995;83:993–1000.

95. Miller CW, Aslo A, Tsay C, et al. Frequency and structure of p53 rearrangements in human osteosarcoma. Cancer Res 1990;50:7950–7954.

96. Overholtzer M, Rao PH, Favis R, et al. The presence of p53 mutations in human osteosarcomas correlates with high levels of genomic instability. Proc Natl Acad Sci U S A 2003;100:11547–11552.

97. Wunder JS, Gokgoz N, Parkes R, et al. TP53 mutations and outcome in osteosarcoma: a prospective, multicenter study. J Clin Oncol 2005;23:1483–1490.

98. Lonardo F, Ueda T, Huvos AG, et al. p53 and MDM2 alterations in osteosarcomas: correlation with clinicopathologic features and proliferative rate. Cancer 1997;79:1541–1547.

99. Yan T, Wunder JS, Gokgoz N, et al. COPS3 amplification and clinical outcome in osteosarcoma. Cancer 2007;109:1870–1876.

100. Nevins JR. The Rb/E2 F pathway and cancer. Hum Mol Genet 2001;10:699–703.

101. Nevins JR, Leone G, DeGregori J, et al. Role of the Rb/E2 F pathway in cell growth control. J Cell Physiol 1997;173:233–236.

102. Lane DP. Cancer. p53, guardian of the genome. Nature 1992;358:15–16.

103. Classon M, Harlow E. The retinoblastoma tumour suppressor in development and cancer. Nat Rev Cancer 2002;2:910–917.

104. Schmitt CA, Fridman JS, Yang M, et al. A senescence program controlled by p53 and p16INK4a contributes to the outcome of cancer therapy. Cell 2002;109:335–346.

105. Lowe SW. Cancer therapy and p53. Curr Opin Oncol 1995;7:547–553.

106. Lowe SW, Bodis S, Bardeesy N, et al. Apoptosis and the prognostic significance of p53 mutation. Cold Spring Harb Symp Quant Biol 1994;59:419–426.

107. Gibbs CP, Kukekov VG, Reith JD, et al. Stem-like cells in bone sarcomas: implications for tumorigenesis. Neoplasia 2005;7:967–976.

108. Tolar J, Nauta AJ, Osborn MJ, et al. Sarcoma derived from cultured mesenchymal stem cells. Stem Cells 2007;25:371–379.

109. Al-Romaih K, Bayani J, Vorobyova J, et al. Chromosomal instability in osteosarcoma and its association with centrosome abnormalities. Cancer Genet Cytogenet 2003;144:91–99.

110. Johnson-Pais TL, Nellissery MJ, Ammerman DG, et al. Determination of a minimal region of loss of heterozygosity on chromosome 18q21.33 in osteosarcoma. Int J Cancer 2003;105:285–288.

111. Kruzelock RP, Murphy EC, Strong LC, et al. Localization of a novel tumor suppressor locus on human chromosome 3q important in osteosarcoma tumorigenesis. Cancer Res 1997;57:106–109.

112. Hahn WC, Counter CM, Lundberg AS, et al. Creation of human tumour cells with defined genetic elements. Nature 1999;400:464–468.

113. Burrow S, Andrulis IL, Pollak M, et al. Expression of insulin-like growth factor receptor, IGF-1, and IGF-2 in primary and metastatic osteosarcoma. J Surg Oncol 1998;69:21–27.

114. Ek ET, Ojaimi J, Kitagawa Y, et al. Does the degree of intratumoural microvessel density and VEGF expression have prognostic significance in osteosarcoma? Oncol Rep 2006;16:17–23.

115. Fellenberg J, Krauthoff A, Pollandt K, et al. Evaluation of the predictive value of Her-2/neu gene expression on osteosarcoma therapy in laser-microdissected paraffin-embedded tissue. Lab Invest 2004;84:113–121.

116. Ferrari S, Bertoni F, Zanella L, et al. Evaluation of P-glycoprotein, HER-2/ErbB-2, p53, and Bcl-2 in primary tumor and metachronous lung metastases in patients with high-grade osteosarcoma. Cancer 2004;100:1936–1942.

117. Gorlick R, Cole P, Banerjee D, et al. Mechanisms of methotrexate resistance in acute leukemia. Decreased transport and polyglutamylation. Adv Exp Med Biol 1999;457:543–550.

118. Hoang BH, Dyke JP, Koutcher JA, et al. VEGF expression in osteosarcoma correlates with vascular permeability by dynamic MRI. Clin Orthop Relat Res 2004;426:32–38.

119. Hughes DP, Thomas DG, Giordano TJ, et al. Cell surface expression of epidermal growth factor receptor and Her-2 with nuclear expression of Her-4 in primary osteosarcoma. Cancer Res 2004;64:2047–2053.

120. Hughes DP, Thomas DG, Giordano TJ, et al. Essential erbB family phosphorylation in osteosarcoma as a target for CI-1033 inhibition. Pediatr Blood Cancer 2006;46:614–623.

121. Jung ST, Moon ES, Seo HY, et al. Expression and significance of TGF-beta isoform and VEGF in osteosarcoma. Orthopedics 2005;28:755–760.

122. Kilpatrick SE, Geisinger KR, King TS, et al. Clinicopathologic analysis of HER-2/neu immunoexpression among various histologic subtypes and grades of osteosarcoma. Mod Pathol 2001;14:1277–1283.

123. MacEwen EG, Pastor J, Kutzke J, et al. IGF-1 receptor contributes to the malignant phenotype in human and canine osteosarcoma. J Cell Biochem 2004;92:77–91.

124. Oda Y, Yamamoto H, Tamiya S, et al. CXCR4 and VEGF expression in the primary site and the metastatic site of human osteosarcoma: analysis within a group of patients, all of whom developed lung metastasis. Mod Pathol 2006;19:738–745.

125. Onda M, Matsuda S, Higaki S, et al. ErbB-2 expression is correlated with poor prognosis for patients with osteosarcoma. Cancer 1996;77:71–78.

126. Tsai JY, Aviv H, Benevenia J, et al. HER-2/neu and p53 in osteosarcoma: an immunohistochemical and fluorescence in situ hybridization analysis. Cancer Invest 2004;22:16–24.

127. Willmore-Payne C, Holden JA, Zhou H, et al. Evaluation of Her-2/neu gene status in osteosarcoma by fluorescence in situ hybridization and multiplex and monoplex polymerase chain reactions. Arch Pathol Lab Med 2006;130:691–698.
128. Yalcin B, Gedikoglu G, Kutluk T, et al. C-erbB-2 expression and prognostic significance in osteosarcoma. Pediatr Blood Cancer 2008;51(2):222–227.
129. Yang R, Hoang BH, Kubo T, et al. Over-expression of parathyroid hormone Type 1 receptor confers an aggressive phenotype in osteosarcoma. Int J Cancer 2007;121: 943–954.
130. Zhou H, Randall RL, Brothman AR, et al. Her-2/neu expression in osteosarcoma increases risk of lung metastasis and can be associated with gene amplification. J Pediatr Hematol Oncol 2003;25:27–32.
131. Coltella N, Manara MC, Cerisano V, et al. Role of the MET/HGF receptor in proliferation and invasive behavior of osteosarcoma. FASEB J 2003;17:1162–1164.
132. Bostedt KT, Schmid C, Ghirlanda-Keller C, et al. Insulin-like growth factor (IGF) I down-regulates type 1 IGF receptor (IGF 1R) and reduces the IGF I response in A549 non-small-cell lung cancer and Saos-2/B-10 osteoblastic osteosarcoma cells. Exp Cell Res 2001;271:368–377.
133. Kappel CC, Velez-Yanguas MC, Hirschfeld S, et al. Human osteosarcoma cell lines are dependent on insulin-like growth factor I for in vitro growth. Cancer Res 1994;54: 2803–2807.
134. Pollak M, Sem AW, Richard M, et al. Inhibition of metastatic behavior of murine osteosarcoma by hypophysectomy. J Natl Cancer Inst 1992;84:966–971.
135. Pollak MN, Polychronakos C, Richard M. Insulinlike growth factor I: a potent mitogen for human osteogenic sarcoma. J Natl Cancer Inst 1990;82:301–305.
136. Baserga R, Peruzzi F, Reiss K. The IGF-1 receptor in cancer biology. Int J Cancer 2003;107:873–877.
137. Scotlandi K, Manara MC, Nicoletti G, et al. Antitumor activity of the insulin-like growth factor-I receptor kinase inhibitor NVP-AEW541 in musculoskeletal tumors. Cancer Res 2005;65:3868–3876.
138. Rong S, Oskarsson M, Faletto D, et al. Tumorigenesis induced by coexpression of human hepatocyte growth factor and the human met protooncogene leads to high levels of expression of the ligand and receptor. Cell Growth Differ 1993;4:563–569.
139. Scotlandi K, Baldini N, Oliviero M, et al. Expression of Met/hepatocyte growth factor receptor gene and malignant behavior of musculoskeletal tumors. Am J Pathol 1996;149:1209–1219.
140. Ferracini R, Di Renzo MF, Scotlandi K, et al. The Met/HGF receptor is over-expressed in human osteosarcomas and is activated by either a paracrine or an autocrine circuit. Oncogene 1995;10:739–749.
141. Oda Y, Naka T, Takeshita M, et al. Comparison of histological changes and changes in nm23 and c-MET expression between primary and metastatic sites in osteosarcoma: a clinicopathologic and immunohistochemical study. Hum Pathol 2000;31:709–716.
142. McGary EC, Weber K, Mills L, et al. Inhibition of platelet-derived growth factor-mediated proliferation of osteosarcoma cells by the novel tyrosine kinase inhibitor STI571. Clin Cancer Res 2002;8:3584–3591.
143. Kawai T, Hiroi S, Torikata C. Expression in lung carcinomas of platelet-derived growth factor and its receptors. Lab Invest 1997;77:431–436.
144. Nakanishi K, Hiroi S, Kawai T, et al. Expression of platelet-derived growth-factor B-chain mRNA and tumor angiogenesis in invasive transitional cell carcinoma of the upper urinary tract. Mod Pathol 1997;10:341–347.
145. Sulzbacher I, Birner P, Trieb K, et al. Platelet-derived growth factor-alpha receptor expression supports the growth of conventional chondrosarcoma and is associated with adverse outcome. Am J Surg Pathol 2001;25:1520–1527.
146. Sulzbacher I, Traxler M, Mosberger I, et al. Platelet-derived growth factor-AA and -alpha receptor expression suggests an autocrine and/or paracrine loop in osteosarcoma. Mod Pathol 2000;13:632–637.
147. Mathew P, Thall PF, Bucana CD, et al. Platelet-derived growth factor receptor inhibition and chemotherapy for castration-resistant prostate cancer with bone metastases. Clin Cancer Res 2007;13:5816–5824.
148. Singh PK, Wen Y, Swanson BJ, et al. Platelet-derived growth factor receptor beta-mediated phosphorylation of MUC1 enhances invasiveness in pancreatic adenocarcinoma cells. Cancer Res 2007;67:5201–5210.
149. Li T, Wen H, Brayton C, et al. Epidermal growth factor receptor and notch pathways participate in the tumor suppressor function of gamma-secretase. J Biol Chem 2007; 282:32264–32273.
150. Wen YH, Koeppen H, Garcia R, et al. Epidermal growth factor receptor in osteosarcoma: expression and mutational analysis. Hum Pathol 2007;38:1184–1191.
151. Kubo T, Piperdi S, Rosenblum J, et al. Platelet-derived growth factor receptor as a prognostic marker and a therapeutic target for imatinib mesylate therapy in osteosarcoma. Cancer 2008;112:2119–2129.
152. Akatsuka T, Wada T, Kokai Y, et al. ErbB2 expression is correlated with increased survival of patients with osteosarcoma. Cancer 2002;94:1397–1404.
153. Akatsuka T, Wada T, Kokai Y, et al. Loss of ErbB2 expression in pulmonary metastatic lesions in osteosarcoma. Oncology 2001;60:361–366.
154. Flint AF, U'Ren L, Legare ME, et al. Overexpression of the erbB-2 proto-oncogene in canine osteosarcoma cell lines and tumors. Vet Pathol 2004;41:291–296.
155. Gorlick R, Huvos AG, Heller G, et al. Expression of HER2/erbB-2 correlates with survival in osteosarcoma. J Clin Oncol 1999;17:2781–2788.
156. Merimsky O, Kollender Y, Issakov J, et al. Induction chemotherapy for bone sarcoma in adults: correlation of results with erbB-4 expression. Oncol Rep 2003;10:1593–1599.
157. Rakesh Kumar V, Gupta N, Kakkar N, et al. Prognostic and predictive value of c-erbB2 overexpression in osteogenic sarcoma. J Cancer Res Ther 2006;2:20–23.
158. Valabrega G, Fagioli F, Corso S, et al. ErbB2 and bone sialoprotein as markers for metastatic osteosarcoma cells. Br J Cancer 2003;88:396–400.
159. Lee WI, Bacchni P, Bertoni F, et al. Quantitative assessment of HER2/neu expression by real-time PCR and fluorescent in situ hybridization analysis in low-grade osteosarcoma. Oncol Rep 2004;12:125–128.
160. Scotlandi K, Manara MC, Hattinger CM, et al. Prognostic and therapeutic relevance of HER2 expression in osteosarcoma and Ewing's sarcoma. Eur J Cancer 2005;41: 1349–1361.
161. Somers GR, Ho M, Zielenska M, et al. HER2 amplification and overexpression is not present in pediatric osteosarcoma: a tissue microarray study. Pediatr Dev Pathol 2005; 8:525–532.
162. Thomas DG, Giordano TJ, Sanders D, et al. Absence of HER2/neu gene expression in osteosarcoma and skeletal Ewing's sarcoma. Clin Cancer Res 2002;8:788–793.
163. Houghton PJ, Huang S. mTOR as a target for cancer therapy. Curr Top Microbiol Immunol 2004;279:339–359.
164. Huang S, Houghton PJ. Targeting mTOR signaling for cancer therapy. Curr Opin Pharmacol 2003;3:371–377.
165. Kurmasheva RT, Huang S, Houghton PJ. Predicted mechanisms of resistance to mTOR inhibitors. Br J Cancer 2006;95:955–960.
166. Kurmasheva RT, Houghton PJ. IGF-I mediated survival pathways in normal and malignant cells. Biochim Biophys Acta 2006;1766:1–22.
167. Cowley S, Paterson H, Kemp P, et al. Activation of MAP kinase kinase is necessary and sufficient for PC12 differentiation and for transformation of NIH 3T3 cells. Cell 1994;77:841–852.
168. Salasznyk RM, Klees RF, Hughlock MK, et al. ERK signaling pathways regulate the osteogenic differentiation of human mesenchymal stem cells on collagen I and vitronectin. Cell Commun Adhes 2004;11:137–153.
169. Thimmaiah KN, Easton J, Huang S, et al. Insulin-like growth factor I-mediated protection from rapamycin-induced apoptosis is independent of Ras-Erk1-Erk2 and phosphatidylinositol 3′-kinase-Akt signaling pathways. Cancer Res 2003;63:364–374.
170. Yu W, Chen Z, Zhang J, et al. Critical role of phosphoinositide 3-kinase cascade in adipogenesis of human mesenchymal stem cells. Mol Cell Biochem 2008;310:11–18.
171. Bjornsti MA, Houghton PJ. The TOR pathway: a target for cancer therapy. Nat Rev Cancer 2004;4:335–348.
172. Easton JB, Houghton PJ. mTOR and cancer therapy. Oncogene 2006;25:6436–6446.
173. Gamberi G, Benassi MS, Bohling T, et al. C-myc and c-fos in human osteosarcoma: prognostic value of mRNA and protein expression. Oncology 1998;55:556–563.
174. Ikeda S, Sumii H, Akiyama K, et al. Amplification of both c-myc and c-raf-1 oncogenes in a human osteosarcoma. Jpn J Cancer Res 1989;80:6–9.
175. Kochevar DT, Kochevar J, Garrett L. Low level amplification of c-sis and c-myc in a spontaneous osteosarcoma model. Cancer Lett 1990;53:213–222.
176. Ladanyi M, Park CK, Lewis R, et al. Sporadic amplification of the MYC gene in human osteosarcomas. Diagn Mol Pathol 1993;2:163–167.
177. Finkel MP, Biskis BO, Jinkins PB. Virus induction of osteosarcomas in mice. Science 1966;151:698–701.
178. Miller AD, Curran T, Verma IM. c-fos protein can induce cellular transformation: a novel mechanism of activation of a cellular oncogene. Cell 1984;36:51–60.
179. Curran T, MacConnell WP, van Straaten F, et al. Structure of the FBJ murine osteosarcoma virus genome: molecular cloning of its associated helper virus and the cellular homolog of the v-fos gene from mouse and human cells. Mol Cell Biol 1983;3:914–921.
180. Curran T, Verma IM. FBR murine osteosarcoma virus. I. Molecular analysis and characterization of a 75,000-Da gag-fos fusion product. Virology 1984;135:218–228.
181. Franchi A, Calzolari A, Zampi G. Immunohistochemical detection of c-fos and c-jun expression in osseous and cartilaginous tumours of the skeleton. Virchows Arch 1998;432:515–519.
182. Kakar S, Mihalov M, Chachlani NA, et al. Correlation of c-fos, p53, and PCNA expression with treatment outcome in osteosarcoma. J Surg Oncol 2000;73:125–126.
183. Bayani J, Zielenska M, Pandita A, et al. Spectral karyotyping identifies recurrent complex rearrangements of chromosomes 8, 17, and 20 in osteosarcomas. Genes Chromosomes Cancer 2003;36:7–16.
184. Squire JA, Pei J, Marrano P, et al. High-resolution mapping of amplifications and deletions in pediatric osteosarcoma by use of CGH analysis of cDNA microarrays. Genes Chromosomes Cancer 2003;38:215–225.
185. Zielenska M, Marrano P, Thorner P, et al. High-resolution cDNA microarray CGH mapping of genomic imbalances in osteosarcoma using formalin-fixed paraffin-embedded tissue. Cytogenet Genome Res 2004;107:77–82.
186. Holt SE, Shay JW, Wright WE. Refining the telomere-telomerase hypothesis of aging and cancer. Nat Biotechnol 1996;14:836–839.
187. Shay JW, Wright WE. Telomerase therapeutics for cancer: challenges and new directions. Nat Rev Drug Discov 2006;5:577–584.
188. Nakashima H, Nishida Y, Sugiura H, et al. Telomerase, p53 and PCNA activity in osteosarcoma. Eur J Surg Oncol 2003;29:564–567.
189. Sanders RP, Drissi R, Billups CA, et al. Telomerase expression predicts unfavorable outcome in osteosarcoma. J Clin Oncol 2004;22:3790–3797.
190. Ulaner GA, Huang HY, Otero J, et al. Absence of a telomere maintenance mechanism as a favorable prognostic factor in patients with osteosarcoma. Cancer Res 2003;63: 1759–1763.
191. Deshpande A, Hinds PW. The retinoblastoma protein in osteoblast differentiation and osteosarcoma. Curr Mol Med 2006;6:809–817.
192. Haydon RC, Luu HH, He TC. Osteosarcoma and osteoblastic differentiation: a new perspective on oncogenesis. Clin Orthop Relat Res 2007;454:237–246.
193. Tang N, Song WX, Luo J, et al. Osteosarcoma development and stem cell differentiation. Clin Orthop Relat Res 2008;466:2114–2130.
194. Guo W, Gorlick R, Ladanyi M, et al. Expression of bone morphogenetic proteins and receptors in sarcomas. Clin Orthop Relat Res 1999;365:175–183.
195. Ohta S, Hiraki Y, Shigeno C, et al. Bone morphogenetic proteins (BMP-2 and BMP-3) induce the late phase expression of the proto-oncogene c-fos in murine osteoblastic MC3T3-E1 cells. FEBS Lett 1992;314:356–360.
196. Hoang BH, Kubo T, Healey JH, et al. Dickkopf 3 inhibits invasion and motility of Saos-2 osteosarcoma cells by modulating the Wnt-beta-catenin pathway. Cancer Res 2004;64:2734–2739.
197. Hoang BH, Kubo T, Healey JH, et al. Expression of LDL receptor-related protein 5 (LRP5) as a novel marker for disease progression in high-grade osteosarcoma. Int J Cancer 2004;109:106–111.
198. Boland GM, Perkins G, Hall DJ, et al. Wnt 3 a promotes proliferation and suppresses osteogenic differentiation of adult human mesenchymal stem cells. J Cell Biochem 2004;93:1210–1230.
199. Polakis P. Wnt signaling and cancer. Genes Dev 2000;14:1837–1851.
200. Chen K, Fallen S, Abaan HO, et al. Wnt10b induces chemotaxis of osteosarcoma and correlates with reduced survival. Pediatr Blood Cancer 2008;51:349–355.
201. O'Keefe RJ, Guise TA. Molecular mechanisms of bone metastasis and therapeutic implications. Clin Orthop Relat Res 2003;415:S100–S104.
202. Fidler IJ, Yano S, Zhang RD, et al. The seed and soil hypothesis: vascularisation and brain metastases. Lancet Oncol 2002;3:53–57.
203. Bleul CC, Fuhlbrigge RC, Casasnovas JM, et al. A highly efficacious lymphocyte chemoattractant, stromal cell-derived factor 1 (SDF-1). J Exp Med 1996;184:1101–1109.
204. Laverdiere C, Hoang BH, Yang R, et al. Messenger RNA expression levels of CXCR4 correlate with metastatic behavior and outcome in patients with osteosarcoma. Clin Cancer Res 2005;11:2561–2567.

205. Miura K, Uniyal S, Leabu M, et al. Chemokine receptor CXCR4-beta1 integrin axis mediates tumorigenesis of osteosarcoma HOS cells. Biochem Cell Biol 2005;83:36–48.
206. Perissinotto E, Cavalloni G, Leone F, et al. Involvement of chemokine receptor 4/stromal cell-derived factor 1 system during osteosarcoma tumor progression. Clin Cancer Res 2005;11:490–497.
207. von Luettichau I, Nathrath M, Burdach S, et al. Mononuclear infiltrates in osteosarcoma and chemokine receptor expression. Clin Cancer Res 2006;12:5253–5254; author reply 4.
208. von Luettichau I, Segerer S, Wechselberger A, et al. A complex pattern of chemokine receptor expression is seen in osteosarcoma. BMC Cancer 2008;8:23.
209. Kim SY, Lee CH, Midura BV, et al. Inhibition of the CXCR4/CXCL12 chemokine pathway reduces the development of murine pulmonary metastases. Clin Exp Metastasis 2008;25:201–211.
210. Khanna C, Wan X, Bose S, et al. The membrane-cytoskeleton linker ezrin is necessary for osteosarcoma metastasis. Nat Med 2004;10:182–186.
211. Krishnan K, Bruce B, Hewitt S, et al. Ezrin mediates growth and survival in Ewing's sarcoma through the AKT/mTOR, but not the MAPK, signaling pathway. Clin Exp Metastasis 2006;23:227–236.
212. Uchibori M, Nishida Y, Nagasaka T, et al. Increased expression of membrane-type matrix metalloproteinase-1 is correlated with poor prognosis in patients with osteosarcoma. Int J Oncol 2006;28:33–42.
213. Heikkila P, Teronen O, Hirn MY, et al. Inhibition of matrix metalloproteinase-14 in osteosarcoma cells by clodronate. J Surg Res 2003;111:45–52.
214. Kido A, Tsutsumi M, Iki K, et al. Inhibition of spontaneous rat osteosarcoma lung metastasis by 3 S-[4-(N-hydroxyamino)-2R-isobutylsuccinyl]amino-1-methoxy-3,4-dihydrocarbostyril, a novel matrix metalloproteinase inhibitor. Jpn J Cancer Res 1999;90:333–341.
215. Himelstein BP, Asada N, Carlton MR, et al. Matrix metalloproteinase-9 (MMP-9) expression in childhood osseous osteosarcoma. Med Pediatr Oncol 1998;31:471–474.
216. Koshkina NV, Khanna C, Mendoza A, et al. Fas-negative osteosarcoma tumor cells are selected during metastasis to the lungs: the role of the Fas pathway in the metastatic process of osteosarcoma. Mol Cancer Res 2007;5:991–999.
217. Koshkina NV, Kleinerman ES, Li G, et al. Exploratory analysis of Fas gene polymorphisms in pediatric osteosarcoma patients. J Pediatr Hematol Oncol 2007;29:815–821.
218. Gordon N, Arndt CA, Hawkins DS, et al. Fas expression in lung metastasis from osteosarcoma patients. J Pediatr Hematol Oncol 2005;27:611–615.
219. Worth LL, Lafleur EA, Jia SF, et al. Fas expression inversely correlates with metastatic potential in osteosarcoma cells. Oncol Rep 2002;9:823–827.
220. Mizobuchi H, Garcia-Castellano JM, Philip S, et al. Hypoxia markers in human osteosarcoma: an exploratory study. Clin Orthop Relat Res 2008;466:2052–2059.
221. Baldini N, Scotlandi K, Barbanti-Brodano G, et al. Expression of P-glycoprotein in high-grade osteosarcomas in relation to clinical outcome. N Engl J Med 1995;333:1380–1385.
222. Baldini N, Scotlandi K, Serra M, et al. P-glycoprotein expression in osteosarcoma: a basis for risk-adapted adjuvant chemotherapy. J Orthop Res 1999;17:629–632.
223. Chan HS, Grogan TM, Haddad G, et al. P-glycoprotein expression: critical determinant in the response to osteosarcoma chemotherapy. J Natl Cancer Inst 1997;89:1706–1715.
224. Hornicek FJ, Gebhardt MC, Wolfe MW, et al. P-glycoprotein levels predict poor outcome in patients with osteosarcoma. Clin Orthop Relat Res 2000;373:11–17.
225. Kumta SM, Zhu QS, Lee KM, et al. Clinical significance of P-glycoprotein immunohistochemistry and doxorubicin binding assay in patients with osteosarcoma. Int Orthop 2001;25:279–282.
226. Pakos EE, Ioannidis JP. The association of P-glycoprotein with response to chemotherapy and clinical outcome in patients with osteosarcoma. A meta-analysis. Cancer 2003; 98:581–589.
227. Posl M, Amling M, Grahl K, et al. P-glycoprotein expression in high grade central osteosarcoma and normal bone cells. An immunohistochemical study. Gen Diagn Pathol 1997;142:317–325.
228. Serra M, Maurici D, Scotlandi K, et al. Relationship between P-glycoprotein expression and p53 status in high-grade osteosarcoma. Int J Oncol 1999;14:301–307.
229. Serra M, Picci P, Ferrari S, et al. Prognostic value of P-glycoprotein in high-grade osteosarcoma. J Clin Oncol 2007;25:4858–4860; author reply 60–61.
230. Wunder JS, Bell RS, Wold L, et al. Expression of the multidrug resistance gene in osteosarcoma: a pilot study. J Orthop Res 1993;11:396–403.
231. Wunder JS, Bull SB, Aneliunas V, et al. MDR1 gene expression and outcome in osteosarcoma: a prospective, multicenter study. J Clin Oncol 2000;18:2685–2694.
232. Schwartz CL, Gorlick R, Teot L, et al. Multiple drug resistance in osteogenic sarcoma: INT0133 from the Children's Oncology Group. J Clin Oncol 2007;25:2057–2062.
233. Trammell RA, Johnson CB, Barker JR, et al. Multidrug resistance-1 gene expression does not increase during tumor progression in the MGH-OGS murine osteosarcoma tumor model. J Orthop Res 2000;18:449–455.
234. Serra M, Pasello M, Manara MC, et al. May P-glycoprotein status be used to stratify high-grade osteosarcoma patients? Results from the Italian/Scandinavian Sarcoma Group 1 treatment protocol. Int J Oncol 2006;29:1459–1468.
235. Guo W, Healey JH, Meyers PA, et al. Mechanisms of methotrexate resistance in osteosarcoma. Clin Cancer Res 1999;5:621–627.
236. Yang R, Kolb EA, Qin J, et al. The folate receptor alpha is frequently overexpressed in osteosarcoma samples and plays a role in the uptake of the physiologic substrate 5-methyltetrahydrofolate. Clin Cancer Res 2007;13:2557–2567.
237. Yang R, Li WW, Hoang BH, et al. Quantitative correlation between promoter methylation and messenger RNA levels of the reduced folate carrier. BMC Cancer 2008;8:124.
238. Yang R, Qin J, Hoang BH, et al. Polymorphisms and methylation of the reduced folate carrier in osteosarcoma. Clin Orthop Relat Res 2008;466:2046–2051.
239. Yang R, Sowers R, Mazza B, et al. Sequence alterations in the reduced folate carrier are observed in osteosarcoma tumor samples. Clin Cancer Res 2003;9:837–844.
240. Bertino JR, Goker E, Gorlick R, et al. Resistance mechanisms to methotrexate in tumors. Oncologist 1996;1:223–226.
241. Gorlick R, Goker E, Trippett T, et al. Intrinsic and acquired resistance to methotrexate in acute leukemia. N Engl J Med 1996;335:1041–1048.
242. Scionti I, Michelacci F, Pasello M, et al. Clinical impact of the methotrexate resistance-associated genes C-MYC and dihydrofolate reductase (DHFR) in high-grade osteosarcoma. Ann Oncol 2008;19:1500–1508.
243. Serra M, Reverter-Branchat G, Maurici D, et al. Analysis of dihydrofolate reductase and reduced folate carrier gene status in relation to methotrexate resistance in osteosarcoma cells. Ann Oncol 2004;15:151–160.
244. World Health Organization Classification of Tumours: Pathology and Genetics: Tumours of Soft Tissue and Bone. Washington, DC: IARC Press, 2002.
245. Raymond AK, Ayala AG, Knuutila S. Conventional osteosarcoma. In: Kleihues P, Sobin L, Fletcher C, et al., eds. WHO classification of tumours: pathology and genetics of tumours of soft tissue and bone. Lyon, France: IARC Press, 2002:267–269.
246. Matsuno T, Okada K, Knuutila S. Telangiectatic osteosarcoma. In: Fletcher CDM, Unni KK, Mertens F, eds. WHO classification of tumours: pathology and genetics of tumours of soft tissue and bone. Lyon, France: IARC Press, 2002:271–272.
247. Weiss A, Khoury JD, Hoffer FA, et al. Telangiectatic osteosarcoma: the St. Jude Children's Research Hospital's experience. Cancer 2007;109:1627–1637.
248. Kalil R, Bridge JA. Small cell osteosarcoma. In: Fletcher CDM, Unni KK, Mertens F, eds. WHO classification of tumours: pathology and genetics of tumours of soft tissue and bone. Lyon, France: IARC Press, 2002:273–274.
249. Nakajima H, Sim FH, Bond JR, et al. Small cell osteosarcoma of bone. Review of 72 cases. Cancer 1997;79:2095–2106.
250. Inwards C, Knuutila S. Low grade central osteosarcoma. In: Fletcher CDM, Unni KK, Mertens F, eds. Health organization classification of tumours: pathology and genetics: tumours of soft tissue and bone. Lyons/Washington, DC: IARC Press, 2002:275–276.
251. Choong PF, Pritchard DJ, Rock MG, et al. Low grade central osteogenic sarcoma. A long-term followup of 20 patients. Clin Orthop Relat Res 1996;322:198–206.
252. Schwab JH, Antonescu CR, Athanasian EA, et al. A comparison of intramedullary and juxtacortical low-grade osteogenic sarcoma. Clin Orthop Relat Res 2008;466:1318–1322.
253. Wold L, McCarthy E, Knuutila S. High grade surface osteosarcoma. In: Fletcher CDM, Unni KK, Mertens F, eds. World health organization classification of tumours: pathology and genetics: tumours of soft tissue and bone. Lyons/Washington, DC: IARC Press, 2002:284–285.
254. Unni KK, Knuutila S. Parosteal osteosarcoma. In: Fletcher CDM, Unni KK, Mertens F, eds. World health organization classification of tumours: pathology and genetics: tumours of soft tissue and bone. Lyons/Washington, DC: IARC Press, 2002:279–281.
255. Ayala AG, Czerniak B, Raymond AK, et al. Periosteal osteosarcoma. In: Fletcher CDM, Unni KK, Mertens F, eds. World health organization classification of tumours: pathology and genetics: tumours of soft tissue and bone. Lyons/Washington, DC: IARC Press, 2002:282–283.
256. Bacci G, Ferrari S, Longhi A. High-grade osteosarcoma of the extremity: differences between localized and metastatic tumors at presentation. J Pediatr Hematol Oncol 2002;24:27–30.
257. Goyal S, Roscoe J, Ryder WDJ, et al. Symptom interval in young people with bone cancer. Eur J Cancer 2004;40:2280–2286.
258. Martin S, Ulrich C, Munsell M, et al. Delays in cancer diagnosis in underinsured young adults and older adolescents. Oncologist 2007;12:816–824.
259. Guerra RB, Tostes MD, Miranda LdC. Comparative analysis between osteosarcoma and Ewing's sarcoma: evaluation of the time from onset of signs and symptoms until diagnosis. Clinics 2006;61:99–106.
260. Bacci G, Briccoli A, Ferrari S, et al. Neoadjuvant chemotherapy for osteosarcoma of the extremities with synchronous lung metastases: treatment with cisplatin, adriamycin and high dose of methotrexate and ifosfamide. Oncol Rep 2000;7:339–346.
261. Harris MB, Gieser P, Goorin AM, et al. Treatment of metastatic osteosarcoma at diagnosis: a Pediatric Oncology Group Study. J Clin Oncol 1998;16:3641–3648.
262. Ferrari S, Briccoli A, Mercuri M, et al. Postrelapse survival in osteosarcoma of the extremities: prognostic factors for long-term survival. J Clin Oncol 2003;21:710–715.
263. Kager L, Zoubek A, Potschger U, et al. Primary metastatic osteosarcoma: presentation and outcome of patients treated on neoadjuvant Cooperative Osteosarcoma Study Group protocols. J Clin Oncol 2003;21:2011–2018.
264. Kempf-Bielack B, Bielack SS, Jurgens H, et al. Osteosarcoma relapse after combined modality therapy: an analysis of unselected patients in the Cooperative Osteosarcoma Study Group (COSS). J Clin Oncol 2005;23:559–568.
265. Marina NM, Pratt CB, Rao BN, et al. Improved prognosis of children with osteosarcoma metastatic to the lung(s) at the time of diagnosis [published erratum appears in Cancer 1993;71(9):2879]. Cancer 1992;70:2722–2727.
266. Meyers PA, Heller G, Healey JH, et al. Osteogenic sarcoma with clinically detectable metastasis at initial presentation. J Clin Oncol 1993;11:449–453.
267. Kaste SC, Pratt CB, Cain AM, et al. Metastases detected at the time of diagnosis of primary pediatric extremity osteosarcoma at diagnosis: imaging features. Cancer 1999; 86:1602–1608.
268. Foster L, Dall GF, Reid R, et al. Twentieth-century survival from osteosarcoma in childhood. Trends from 1933 to 2004. J Bone Joint Surg Br 2007;89:1234–1238.
269. Jaffe N, Frei IE. Osteogenic sarcoma: advances in treatment. CA Cancer J Clin 1976; 26:351–359.
270. Kager L, Zoubek A, Pötschger U, et al. Evaluating prognostic factors for outcomes in 186 patients presenting with high-grade metastatic osteosarcoma treated on neoadjuvant COSS protocols. Proc Am Soc Clin Oncol 2002;2002:1567a.
271. Kager L, Zoubek A, Kastner U, et al. Skip metastases in osteosarcoma: experience of the cooperative osteosarcoma study group. J Clin Oncol 2006;24:1535–1541.
272. Wuisman P, Enneking WF. Prognosis of patients who have osteosarcoma with skip metastasis. J Bone Joint Surg Am 1990;72:60–68.
273. Caceres E, Zaharia M, Calderon R. Incidence of regional lymph node metastasis in operable osteogenic sarcoma. Semin Surg Oncol 1990;6:231–233.
274. Smeland S, Muller C, Alvegard TA, et al. Scandinavian Sarcoma Group Osteosarcoma Study SSG VIII: prognostic factors for outcome and the role of replacement salvage chemotherapy for poor histological responders. Eur J Cancer 2003;39:488–494.
275. Bacci G, Longhi A, Ferrari S, et al. Prognostic significance of serum alkaline phosphatase in osteosarcoma of the extremity treated with neoadjuvant chemotherapy: recent experience at Rizzoli Institute. Oncol Rep 2002;9:171–175.
276. Bacci G, Picci P, Ferrari S, et al. Prognostic significance of serum alkaline phosphatase measurements in patients with osteosarcoma treated with adjuvant or neoadjuvant chemotherapy. Cancer 1993;71:1224–1230.
277. Ferrari S, Bertoni F, Mercuri M, et al. Predictive factors of disease-free survival for non-metastatic osteosarcoma of the extremity: an analysis of 300 patients treated at the Rizzoli Institute. Ann Oncol 2001;12:1145–1150.
278. Murphey MD, Robbin MR, McRae GA, et al. The many faces of osteosarcoma. Radiographics 1997;17:1205–1231.
279. Mirra JM, Gold RH, Piero P. Osseous tumors of intramedullary origin. In: Mirra JM, ed. Bone tumors: clinical, radiologic, and pathologic correlations. Philadelphia, PA: Lea & Febiger, 1989.
280. Murphey MD, wan Jaovisidha S, Temple HT, et al. Telangiectatic osteosarcoma: radiologic-pathologic comparison. Radiology 2003;229:545–553.
281. Suresh S, Saifuddin A. Radiological appearances of appendicular osteosarcoma: a comprehensive pictorial review. Clin Radiol 2007;62:314–323.

282. Panicek DM, Gatsonis C, Rosenthal DI, et al. CT and MR imaging in the local staging of primary malignant musculoskeletal neoplasms: report of the Radiology Diagnostic Oncology Group. Radiology 1997;202:237–246.
283. Meyer JS, Nadel HR, Marina N, et al. Imaging guidelines for children with Ewing sarcoma and osteosarcoma: a report from the Children's Oncology Group Bone Tumor Committee. Pediatr Blood Cancer 2008;51:163–170.
284. Brisse H, Ollivier L, Edeline V, et al. Imaging of malignant tumours of the long bones in children: monitoring response to neoadjuvant chemotherapy and preoperative assessment. Pediatr Radiol 2004;34:595–605.
285. Meyer JS, Dormans JP. Differential diagnosis of pediatric musculoskeletal masses. Magn Reson Imaging Clin N Am 1998;6:561–577.
286. Onikul E, Fletcher BD, Parham DM, et al. Accuracy of MR imaging for estimating intraosseous extent of osteosarcoma. AJR Am J Roentgenol 1996;167:1211–1215.
287. Cohen M, Grosfeld J, Baehner R, et al. Lung CT for detection of metastases: solid tissue neoplasms in children. AJR Am J Roentgenol 1982;139:895–898.
288. Vanel D, Henry-Amar M, Lumbroso J, et al. Pulmonary evaluation of patients with osteosarcoma: roles of standard radiography, tomography, CT, scintigraphy, and tomoscintigraphy. AJR Am J Roentgenol 1984;143:519–523.
289. Herold CJ, Bankier AA, Fleischmann D. Lung metastases. Eur Radiol 1996;6:596–606.
290. Grampp S, Bankier AA, Zoubek A, et al. Spiral CT of the lung in children with malignant extra-thoracic tumors: distribution of benign vs malignant pulmonary nodules. Eur Radiol 2000;10:1318–1322.
291. Picci P, Vanel D, Briccoli A, et al. Computed tomography of pulmonary metastases from osteosarcoma: the less poor technique. A study of 51 patients with histological correlation. Ann Oncol 2001;12:1601–1604.
292. Nadel HR. Nuclear oncology in children. In: Freeman LM, ed. Nuclear medicine annual. New York: Raven Press, 1996:143–194.
293. Sumiya H, Taki J, Tsuchiya H, et al. Midcourse thallium-201 scintigraphy to predict tumor response in bone and soft-tissue tumors. J Nucl Med 1998;39:1600–1604.
294. Imbriaco M, Yeh SD, Yeung H, et al. Thallium-201 scintigraphy for the evaluation of tumor response to preoperative chemotherapy in patients with osteosarcoma. Cancer 1997;80:1507–1512.
295. Verstraete KL, Van der Woude HJ, Hogendoorn PC, et al. Dynamic contrast-enhanced MR imaging of musculoskeletal tumors: basic principles and clinical applications. J Magn Reson Imaging 1996;6:311–321.
296. Dyke JP, Panicek DM, Healey JH, et al. Osteogenic and Ewing sarcomas: estimation of necrotic fraction during induction chemotherapy with dynamic contrast-enhanced MR imaging. Radiology 2003;228:271–278.
297. Reddick WE, Wang S, Xiong X, et al. Dynamic magnetic resonance imaging of regional contrast access as an additional prognostic factor in pediatric osteosarcoma. Cancer 2001;91:2230–2237.
298. Uhl M, Saueressig U, Koehler G, et al. Evaluation of tumour necrosis during chemotherapy with diffusion-weighted MR imaging: preliminary results in osteosarcomas. Pediatr Radiol 2006;36:1306–1311.
299. Goo HW, Choi SH, Ghim T, et al. Whole-body MRI of paediatric malignant tumours: comparison with conventional oncological imaging methods. Pediatr Radiol 2005;35: 766–773.
300. Volker T, Denecke T, Steffen I, et al. Positron emission tomography for staging of pediatric sarcoma patients: results of a prospective multicenter trial. J Clin Oncol 2007; 25:5435–5441.
301. Franzius C, Sciuk J, Daldrup-Link HE, et al. FDG-PET for detection of osseous metastases from malignant primary bone tumours: comparison with bone scintigraphy. Eur J Nucl Med 2000;27:1305–1311.
302. Hamada K, Tomita Y, Inoue A, et al. Evaluation of chemotherapy response in osteosarcoma with FDG-PET. Ann Nucl Med 2009;23:89–95.
303. Ye Z, Zhu J, Tian M, et al. Response of osteogenic sarcoma to neoadjuvant therapy: evaluated by 18 F-FDG-PET. Ann Nucl Med 2008;22:475–480.
304. Arush MW, Israel O, Postovsky S, et al. Positron emission tomography/computed tomography with 18fluoro-deoxyglucose in the detection of local recurrence and distant metastases of pediatric sarcoma. Pediatr Blood Cancer 2007;49:901–905.
305. Bielack S, Carrle D, Jost L. Osteosarcoma: ESMO clinical recommendations for diagnosis, treatment and follow-up. Ann Oncol 2008;19(suppl 2):ii94–ii96.
306. Dauer LT, St Germain J, Meyers PA. Let's image gently: reducing excessive reliance on CT scans. Pediatr Blood Cancer 2008;51:838; author reply 9–40.
307. Meyer JS, Nadel HR, Marina N, et al. Response to imaging guidelines for children with Ewing sarcoma and osteosarcoma: a report from the Children's Oncology Group Bone Tumor Committee. Pediatr Blood Cancer 2008;51:839–840.
308. Mankin HJ, Mankin CJ, Simon MA. The hazards of the biopsy, revisited. Members of the Musculoskeletal Tumor Society. J Bone Joint Surg Am 1996;78:656–663.
309. Stewart CJ, Coldewey J, Stewart IS. Comparison of fine needle aspiration cytology and needle core biopsy in the diagnosis of radiologically detected abdominal lesions. J Clin Pathol 2002;55:93–97.
310. Nicol KK, Ward WG, Savage PD, et al. Fine-needle aspiration biopsy of skeletal versus extraskeletal osteosarcoma. Cancer 1998;84:176–185.
311. Pramesh CS, Deshpande MS, Pardiwala DN, et al. Core needle biopsy for bone tumours. Eur J Surg Oncol 2001;27:668–671.
312. Simon MA. Limb salvage for osteosarcoma. J Bone Joint Surg Am 1988;70:307–310.
313. Hewitt SM, Lewis FA, Cao Y, et al. Tissue handling and specimen preparation in surgical pathology: issues concerning the recovery of nucleic acids from formalin-fixed, paraffin-embedded tissue. Arch Pathol Lab Med 2008;132:1929–1935.
314. Randall RL, Wade M, Albritton K, et al. Retrieval yield of total and messenger RNA in mesenchymal tissue ex vivo. Clin Orthop Relat Res 2003;415:59–63.
315. Enneking WF, Spanier SS, Goodman MA. A system for the surgical staging of musculoskeletal sarcoma. Clin Orthop 1980;153:106–120.
316. Sobin LH, Wittekind C. UICC TNM classification of malignant tumors. 6th ed. New York, NY: Wiley, 2002.
317. Imran H, Enders F, Krailo M, et al. Effect of time to resumption of chemotherapy after definitive surgery on prognosis for non-metastatic osteosarcoma. J Bone Joint Surg Am 2009;91:604–612.
318. Randall RL, Nork SE, James PJ. Aggressive aneurysmal bone cyst of the proximal humerus. A case report. Clin Orthop Relat Res 2000;370:212–218.
319. Bae DS, Waters PM, Gebhardt MC. Results of free vascularized fibula grafting for allograft nonunion after limb salvage surgery for malignant bone tumors. J Pediatr Orthop 2006;26:809–814.
320. Potter BK, Adams SC, Pitcher JD Jr, et al. Proximal humerus reconstructions for tumors. Clin Orthop Relat Res 2009;467:1035–1041.
321. Muscolo DL, Ayerza MA, Aponte-Tinao LA. Survivorship and radiographic analysis of knee osteoarticular allografts. Clin Orthop Relat Res 2000;373:73–79.
322. Ramseier LE, Malinin TI, Temple HT, et al. Allograft reconstruction for bone sarcoma of the tibia in the growing child. J Bone Joint Surg Br 2006;88:95–99.
323. Alman BA, De Bari A, Krajbich JI. Massive allografts in the treatment of osteosarcoma and Ewing sarcoma in children and adolescents. J Bone Joint Surg Am 1995;77:54–64.
324. Gebhardt MC, Flugstad DI, Springfield DS, et al. The use of bone allografts for limb salvage in high-grade extremity osteosarcoma. Clin Orthop Relat Res 1991;270:181–196.
325. Hornicek FJ Jr, Mnaymneh W, Lackman RD, et al. Limb salvage with osteoarticular allografts after resection of proximal tibia bone tumors. Clin Orthop Relat Res 1998;352:179–186.
326. Muscolo DL, Ayerza MA, Aponte-Tinao LA, et al. Use of distal femoral osteoarticular allografts in limb salvage surgery. J Bone Joint Surg Am 2005;87:2449–2455.
327. Clohisy DR, Mankin HJ. Osteoarticular allografts for reconstruction after resection of a musculoskeletal tumor in the proximal end of the tibia. J Bone Joint Surg Am 1994; 76:549–554.
328. Gebhardt MC, Roth YF, Mankin HJ. Osteoarticular allografts for reconstruction in the proximal part of the humerus after excision of a musculoskeletal tumor. J Bone Joint Surg Am 1990;72:334–345.
329. Mankin HJ, Gebhardt MC, Jennings LC, et al. Long-term results of allograft replacement in the management of bone tumors. Clin Orthop Relat Res 1996;324:86–97.
330. Deijkers RL, Bloem RM, Kroon HM, et al. Epidiaphyseal versus other intercalary allografts for tumors of the lower limb. Clin Orthop Relat Res 2005;439:151–160.
331. O'Connor MI, Sim FH, Chao EY. Limb salvage for neoplasms of the shoulder girdle. Intermediate reconstructive and functional results. J Bone Joint Surg Am 1996;78: 1872–1888.
332. Ortiz-Cruz E, Gebhardt MC, Jennings LC, et al. The results of transplantation of intercalary allografts after resection of tumors. A long-term follow-up study. J Bone Joint Surg Am 1997;79:97–106.
333. Weiner SD, Scarborough M, Vander Griend RA. Resection arthrodesis of the knee with an intercalary allograft. J Bone Joint Surg Am 1996;78:185–192.
334. Lord CF, Gebhardt MC, Tomford WW, et al. Infection in bone allografts. Incidence, nature, and treatment. J Bone Joint Surg Am 1988;70:369–376.
335. Dick HM, Strauch RJ. Infection of massive bone allografts. Clin Orthop Relat Res 1994;306:46–53.
336. Getty PJ, Peabody TD. Complications and functional outcomes of reconstruction with an osteoarticular allograft after intra-articular resection of the proximal aspect of the humerus. J Bone Joint Surg Am 1999;81:1138–1146.
337. Shapiro MS, Endrizzi DP, Cannon RM, et al. Treatment of tibial defects and nonunions using ipsilateral vascularized fibular transposition. Clin Orthop Relat Res 1993;296: 207–212.
338. Ozaki T, Hillmann A, Wuisman P, et al. Reconstruction of tibia by ipsilateral vascularized fibula and allograft. 12 cases with malignant bone tumors. Acta Orthop Scand 1997;68:298–301.
339. Finn HA, Simon MA. Limb-salvage surgery in the treatment of osteosarcoma in skeletally immature individuals. Clin Orthop Relat Res 1991;262:108–118.
340. Mnaymneh W, Malinin TI, Makley JT, et al. Massive osteoarticular allografts in the reconstruction of extremities following resection of tumors not requiring chemotherapy and radiation. Clin Orthop Relat Res 1985;197:76–87.
341. Gebhardt MC, Jaffe K, Mankin HJ. Bone allografts for tumors and other reconstructions in children. In: Langlais F, Tomeno, eds. Limb salvage-major reconstructions in oncologic and non-tumoral conditions. Berlin, Germany: Springer-Verlag, 1991: 561–572.
342. Ceruso M, Taddei F, Bigazzi P, et al. Vascularised fibula graft inlaid in a massive bone allograft: considerations on the bio-mechanical behaviour of the combined graft in segmental bone reconstructions after sarcoma resection. Injury 2008;39(suppl 3): S68–S74.
343. Jeys LM, Kulkarni A, Grimer RJ, et al. Endoprosthetic reconstruction for the treatment of musculoskeletal tumors of the appendicular skeleton and pelvis. J Bone Joint Surg Am 2008;90:1265–1271.
344. Gosheger G, Gebert C, Ahrens H, et al. Endoprosthetic reconstruction in 250 patients with sarcoma. Clin Orthop Relat Res 2006;450:164–171.
345. Grimer RJ, Belthur M, Carter SR, et al. Extendible replacements of the proximal tibia for bone tumours. J Bone Joint Surg Br 2000;82:255–260.
346. McDonald DJ, Capanna R, Gherlinzoni F, et al. Influence of chemotherapy on perioperative complications in limb salvage surgery for bone tumors. Cancer 1990;65: 1509–1516.
347. Wirganowicz PZ, Eckardt JJ, Dorey FJ, et al. Etiology and results of tumor endoprosthesis revision surgery in 64 patients. Clin Orthop Relat Res 1999;358:64–74.
348. Malawer MM, Chou LB. Prosthetic survival and clinical results with use of large-segment replacements in the treatment of high-grade bone sarcomas. J Bone Joint Surg Am 1995;77:1154–1165.
349. Ritschl P, Capanna R, Helwig U, et al. KMFTR (Kotz Modular Femur Tibia Reconstruction System) modular tumor endoprosthesis system for the lower extremity. Z Orthop Ihre Grenzgeb 1992;130:290–293.
350. Ward WG, Johnston-Jones K, Lowenbraun S, et al. Antibiotic prophylaxis and infection resistance of massive tumor endoprostheses during chemotherapy. J South Orthop Assoc 1997;6:180–185.
351. Horowitz SM, Glasser DB, Lane JM, et al. Prosthetic and extremity survivorship after limb salvage for sarcoma. How long do the reconstructions last? Clin Orthop Relat Res 1993;293:280–286.
352. Ward WG, Yang RS, Eckardt JJ. Endoprosthetic bone reconstruction following malignant tumor resection in skeletally immature patients. Orthop Clin North Am 1996;27:493–502.
353. Baumgart R, Hinterwimmer S, Krammer M, et al. The bioexpandable prosthesis: a new perspective after resection of malignant bone tumors in children. J Pediatr Hematol Oncol 2005;27:452–455.
354. Eckardt JJ, Safran MR, Eilber FR, et al. Expandable endoprosthetic reconstruction of the skeletally immature after malignant bone tumor resection. Clin Orthop Relat Res 1993;297:188–202.
355. Schiller C, Windhager R, Fellinger EJ, et al. Extendable tumour endoprostheses for the leg in children. J Bone Joint Surg Br 1995;77:608–614.
356. Gupta A, Meswania J, Pollock R, et al. Non-invasive distal femoral expandable endoprosthesis for limb-salvage surgery in paediatric tumours. J Bone Joint Surg Br 2006; 88:649–654.
357. Eckardt JJ, Kabo JM, Kelley CM, et al. Expandable endoprosthesis reconstruction in skeletally immature patients with tumors. Clin Orthop Relat Res 2000;373:51–61.

358. Schindler OS, Cannon SR, Briggs TW, et al. Stanmore custom-made extendible distal femoral replacements. Clinical experience in children with primary malignant bone tumours. J Bone Joint Surg Br 1997;79:927–937.
359. Schindler OS, Cannon SR, Briggs TW, et al. Use of extendable total femoral replacements in children with malignant bone tumors. Clin Orthop Relat Res 1998:157–170.
360. Kenan S, Bloom N, Lewis MM. Limb-sparing surgery in skeletally immature patients with osteosarcoma. The use of an expandable prosthesis. Clin Orthop Relat Res 1991;270:223–230.
361. Lewis MM, Bloom N, Esquieres EM, et al. The expandable prosthesis. An alternative to amputation for children with malignant bone tumors. AORN J 1987;46:457–470.
362. Neel MD, Wilkins RM, Rao BN, et al. Early multicenter experience with a noninvasive expandable prosthesis. Clin Orthop Relat Res 2003;415:72–81.
363. Ward WG, Johnston KS, Dorey FJ, et al. Extramedullary porous coating to prevent diaphyseal osteolysis and radiolucent lines around proximal tibial replacements. A preliminary report. J Bone Joint Surg Am 1993;75:976–987.
364. Kaste SC, Neel MD, Meyer WH, et al. Extracortical bridging callus after limb salvage surgery about the knee. Clin Orthop Relat Res 1999;363:180–185.
365. Bini SA, Johnston JO, Martin DL. Compliant prestress fixation in tumor prostheses: interface retrieval data. Orthopedics 2000;23:707–711; discussion 11–12.
366. Bhangu AA, Kramer MJ, Grimer RJ, et al. Early distal femoral endoprosthetic survival: cemented stems versus the Compress implant. Int Orthop 2006;30:465–472.
367. Avedian RS, Goldsby RE, Kramer MJ, et al. Effect of chemotherapy on initial compressive osseointegration of tumor endoprostheses. Clin Orthop Relat Res 2007;459:48–53.
368. Donati D, Colangeli M, Colangeli S, et al. Allograft-prosthetic composite in the proximal tibia after bone tumor resection. Clin Orthop Relat Res 2008;466:459–465.
369. Jensen KL, Johnston JO. Proximal humeral reconstruction after excision of a primary sarcoma. Clin Orthop Relat Res 1995;311:164–175.
370. Dick HM, Malinin TI, Mnaymneh WA. Massive allograft implantation following radical resection of high-grade tumors requiring adjuvant chemotherapy treatment. Clin Orthop Relat Res 1985;197:88–95.
371. Gitelis S, Piasecki P. Allograft prosthetic composite arthroplasty for osteosarcoma and other aggressive bone tumors. Clin Orthop Relat Res 1991;270:197–201.
372. Jofe MH, Gebhardt MC, Tomford WW, et al. Reconstruction for defects of the proximal part of the femur using allograft arthroplasty. J Bone Joint Surg Am 1988;70:507–516.
373. Brien EW, Terek RM, Healey JH, et al. Allograft reconstruction after proximal tibial resection for bone tumors. An analysis of function and outcome comparing allograft and prosthetic reconstructions. Clin Orthop Relat Res 1994;303:116–127.
374. McGoveran BM, Davis AM, Gross AE, et al. Evaluation of the allograft-prosthesis composite technique for proximal femoral reconstruction after resection of a primary bone tumour. Can J Surg 1999;42:37–45.
375. Hejna MJ, Gitelis S. Allograft prosthetic composite replacement for bone tumors. Semin Surg Oncol 1997;13:18–24.
376. Cheng EY, Dusenbery KE, Winters MR, et al. Soft tissue sarcomas: preoperative versus postoperative radiotherapy. J Surg Oncol 1996;61:90–99.
377. Kneisl JS. Function after amputation, arthrodesis, or arthroplasty for tumors about the shoulder. J South Orthop Assoc 1995;4:228–236.
378. Donati D, Capanna R, Casadei R, et al. Arthrodesis of the knee after tumor resection: a comparison between autografts and allografts. Chir Organi Mov 1995;80:29–37.
379. Enneking WF, Shirley PD. Resection-arthrodesis for malignant and potentially malignant lesions about the knee using an intramedullary rod and local bone grafts. J Bone Joint Surg Am 1977;59:223–236.
380. Probyn LJ, Wunder JS, Bell RS, et al. A comparison of outcome of osteoarticular allograft reconstruction and shoulder arthrodesis following resection of primary tumours of the proximal humerus. Sarcoma 1998;2:163–170.
381. Campanacci DA, Scoccianti G, Beltrami G, et al. Ankle arthrodesis with bone graft after distal tibia resection for bone tumors. Foot Ankle Int 2008;29:1031–1037.
382. Niimi R, Matsumine A, Kusuzaki K, et al. Usefulness of limb salvage surgery for bone and soft tissue sarcomas of the distal lower leg. J Cancer Res Clin Oncol 2008;134:1087–1095.
383. Nishida Y, Tsukushi S, Yamada Y, et al. Reconstruction of the proximal humerus after extensive extraarticular resection for osteosarcoma: a report of two cases with clavicula pro humero reconstruction. Oncol Rep 2008;20:1105–1109.
384. Tsukushi S, Nishida Y, Takahashi M, et al. Clavicula pro humero reconstruction after wide resection of the proximal humerus. Clin Orthop Relat Res 2006;447:132–137.
385. Beadel GP, McLaughlin CE, Aljassir F, et al. Iliosacral resection for primary bone tumors: is pelvic reconstruction necessary? Clin Orthop Relat Res 2005;438:22–29.
386. Court C, Bosca L, Le Cesne A, et al. Surgical excision of bone sarcomas involving the sacroiliac joint. Clin Orthop Relat Res 2006;451:189–194.
387. Dominkus M, Darwish E, Funovics P. Reconstruction of the pelvis after resection of malignant bone tumours in children and adolescents. Recent Results Cancer Res 2009;179:85–111.
388. Eilber FR, Grant TT, Sakai D, et al. Internal hemipelvectomy–excision of the hemipelvis with limb preservation. An alternative to hemipelvectomy. Cancer 1979;43:806–809.
389. Aboulafia AJ, Buch R, Mathews J, et al. Reconstruction using the saddle prosthesis following excision of primary and metastatic periacetabular tumors. Clin Orthop Relat Res 1995;314:203–213.
390. Bell RS, Davis AM, Wunder JS, et al. Allograft reconstruction of the acetabulum after resection of stage-IIB sarcoma. Intermediate-term results. J Bone Joint Surg Am 1997;79:1663–1674.
391. Delloye C, Banse X, Brichard B, et al. Pelvic reconstruction with a structural pelvic allograft after resection of a malignant bone tumor. J Bone Joint Surg Am 2007;89:579–587.
392. Falkinstein Y, Ahlmann ER, Menendez LR. Reconstruction of type II pelvic resection with a new peri-acetabular reconstruction endoprosthesis. J Bone Joint Surg Br 2008;90:371–376.
393. Gradinger R, Rechl H, Hipp E. Pelvic osteosarcoma. Resection, reconstruction, local control, and survival statistics. Clin Orthop Relat Res 1991;270:149–158.
394. Guo W, Li D, Tang X, et al. Reconstruction with modular hemipelvic prostheses for periacetabular tumor. Clin Orthop Relat Res 2007;461:180–188.
395. Harrington KD. The use of hemipelvic allografts or autoclaved grafts for reconstruction after wide resections of malignant tumors of the pelvis. J Bone Joint Surg Am 1992;74:331–341.
396. Ozaki T, Hillmann A, Winkelmann W. Treatment outcome of pelvic sarcomas in young children: orthopaedic and oncologic analysis. J Pediatr Orthop 1998;18:350–355.
397. Hoffmann C, Gosheger G, Gebert C, et al. Functional results and quality of life after treatment of pelvic sarcomas involving the acetabulum. J Bone Joint Surg Am 2006;88:575–582.
398. Gebert C, Gosheger G, Winkelmann W. Hip transposition as a universal surgical procedure for periacetabular tumors of the pelvis. J Surg Oncol 2009;99:169–172.
399. Kozlowski K, Campbell J, Beluffi G, et al. Primary bone tumours of the pelvis in childhood—Ewing's sarcoma of the ilium, pubis and ischium (report of 30 cases). (Part I). Australas Radiol 1989;33:354–360.
400. O'Connor MI, Sim FH. Salvage of the limb in the treatment of malignant pelvic tumors. J Bone Joint Surg Am 1989;71:481–494.
401. Estrada-Aguilar J, Greenberg H, Walling A, et al. Primary treatment of pelvic osteosarcoma. Report of five cases. Cancer 1992;69:1137–1145.
402. Fahey M, Spanier SS, Vander Griend RA. Osteosarcoma of the pelvis. A clinical and histopathological study of twenty-five patients. J Bone Joint Surg Am 1992;74:321–330.
403. Grimer RJ, Carter SR, Tillman RM, et al. Osteosarcoma of the pelvis. J Bone Joint Surg Br 1999;81:796–802.
404. Ham SJ, Kroon HM, Koops HS, et al. Osteosarcoma of the pelvis—oncological results of 40 patients registered by The Netherlands Committee on Bone Tumours. Eur J Surg Oncol 2000;26:53–60.
405. Kapukaya A, Subasi M, Arslan H, et al. Technique and complications of callus distraction in the treatment of bone tumors. Arch Orthop Trauma Surg 2006;126:157–163.
406. Tsuchiya H, Abdel-Wanis ME, Sakurakichi K, et al. Osteosarcoma around the knee. Intraepiphyseal excision and biological reconstruction with distraction osteogenesis. J Bone Joint Surg Br 2002;84:1162–1166.
407. Tsuchiya H, Shirai T, Morsy AF, et al. Safety of external fixation during postoperative chemotherapy. J Bone Joint Surg Br 2008;90:924–928.
408. Dormans JP, Ofluoglu O, Erol B, et al. Case report: reconstruction of an intercalary defect with bone transport after resection of Ewing's sarcoma. Clin Orthop Relat Res 2005;434:258–264.
409. Fuchs B, Kotajarvi BR, Kaufman KR, et al. Functional outcome of patients with rotationplasty about the knee. Clin Orthop Relat Res 2003;415:52–58.
410. Fuchs B, Sim FH. Rotationplasty about the knee: surgical technique and anatomical considerations. Clin Anat 2004;17:345–353.
411. Sawamura C, Hornicek FJ, Gebhardt MC. Complications and risk factors for failure of rotationplasty: review of 25 patients. Clin Orthop Relat Res 2008;466:1302–1308.
412. Hillmann A, Hoffmann C, Gosheger G, et al. Malignant tumor of the distal part of the femur or the proximal part of the tibia: endoprosthetic replacement or rotationplasty. Functional outcome and quality-of-life measurements. J Bone Joint Surg Am 1999;81:462–468.
413. McClenaghan BA, Krajbich JI, Pirone AM, et al. Comparative assessment of gait after limb-salvage procedures. J Bone Joint Surg Am 1989;71:1178–1182.
414. Akahane T, Shimizu T, Isobe K, et al. Evaluation of postoperative general quality of life for patients with osteosarcoma around the knee joint. J Pediatr Orthop B 2007;16:269–272.
415. Rougraff BT, Simon MA, Kneisl JS, et al. Limb salvage compared with amputation for osteosarcoma of the distal end of the femur. A long-term oncological, functional, and quality-of-life study. J Bone Joint Surg Am 1994;76:649–656.
416. Enneking WF, Kagan A. "Skip" metastases in osteosarcoma. Cancer 1975;36:2192–2205.
417. Lindner NJ, Ramm O, Hillmann A, et al. Limb salvage and outcome of osteosarcoma. The University of Muenster experience. Clin Orthop Relat Res 1999;358:83–89.
418. Gherlinzoni F, Picci P, Bacci G, et al. Limb sparing versus amputation in osteosarcoma. Correlation between local control, surgical margins and tumor necrosis: Istituto Rizzoli experience. Ann Oncol 1992;3(suppl 2):S23–S27.
419. Bacci G, Forni C, Longhi A, et al. Local recurrence and local control of non-metastatic osteosarcoma of the extremities: a 27-year experience in a single institution. J Surg Oncol 2007;96:118–123.
420. McCarville MB. New frontiers in pediatric oncologic imaging. Cancer Imaging 2008;8:87–92.
421. Schulte M, Brecht-Krauss D, Werner M, et al. Evaluation of neoadjuvant therapy response of osteogenic sarcoma using FDG PET. J Nucl Med 1999;40:1637–1643.
422. Sato O, Kawai A, Ozaki T, et al. Value of thallium-201 scintigraphy in bone and soft tissue tumors. J Orthop Sci 1998;3:297–303.
423. van der Woude HJ, Bloem JL, Hogendoorn PC. Preoperative evaluation and monitoring chemotherapy in patients with high-grade osteogenic and Ewing's sarcoma: review of current imaging modalities. Skeletal Radiol 1998;27:57–71.
424. Jaffe N, Spears R, Eftekhari F, et al. Pathologic fracture in osteosarcoma. Impact of chemotherapy on primary tumor and survival. Cancer 1987;59:701–709.
425. Papagelopoulos PJ, Mavrogenis AF, Savvidou OD, et al. Pathological fractures in primary bone sarcomas. Injury 2008;39:395–403.
426. Scully SP, Ghert MA, Zurakowski D, et al. Pathologic fracture in osteosarcoma: prognostic importance and treatment implications. J Bone Joint Surg Am 2002;84-A:49–57.
427. Scully SP, Temple HT, O'Keefe RJ, et al. The surgical treatment of patients with osteosarcoma who sustain a pathologic fracture. Clin Orthop Relat Res 1996;324:227–232.
428. Otis JC, Lane JM, Kroll MA. Energy cost during gait in osteosarcoma patients after resection and knee replacement and after above-the-knee amputation. J Bone Joint Surg Am 1985;67:606–611.
429. Harris IE, Leff AR, Gitelis S, et al. Function after amputation, arthrodesis, or arthroplasty for tumors about the knee. J Bone Joint Surg Am 1990;72:1477–1485.
430. Donati D, Giacomini S, Gozzi E, et al. Allograft arthrodesis treatment of bone tumors: a two-center study. Clin Orthop Relat Res 2002;400:217–224.
431. Postma A, Kingma A, De Ruiter JH, et al. Quality of life in bone tumor patients comparing limb salvage and amputation of the lower extremity. J Surg Oncol 1992;51:47–51.
432. Nagarajan R, Neglia JP, Clohisy DR, et al. Education, employment, insurance, and marital status among 694 survivors of pediatric lower extremity bone tumors: a report from the childhood cancer survivor study. Cancer 2003;97:2554–2564.
433. Pratt C, Shanks E, Hustu O, et al. Adjuvant multiple drug chemotherapy for osteosarcoma of the extremity. Cancer 1977;39:51–57.
434. Pratt CB, Rivera G, Shanks E, et al. Combination chemotherapy for osteosarcoma. Cancer Treat Rep 1978;62:251–257.
435. Sutow WW, Gehan EA, Dyment PG, et al. Multidrug adjuvant chemotherapy for osteosarcoma: interim report of the Southwest Oncology Group Studies. Cancer Treat Rep 1978;62:265–269.

436. Sutow WW, Sullivan MP, Fernbach DJ, et al. Adjuvant chemotherapy in primary treatment of osteogenic sarcoma. A Southwest Oncology Group study. Cancer 1975;36:1598–1602.
437. Goorin AM, Frei E III, Abelson HT. Adjuvant chemotherapy for osteosarcoma: a decade of experience. Surg Clin North Am 1981;61:1379–1389.
438. Ochs JJ, Freeman AI, Douglass HO, et al. cis-Dichlorodiammineplatinum (II) in advanced osteogenic sarcoma. Cancer Treat Rep 1978;62:239–245.
439. Gasparini M, Rouesse J, van Oosterom A, et al. Phase II study of cisplatin in advanced osteogenic sarcoma. European Organization for Research on Treatment of Cancer Soft Tissue and Bone Sarcoma Group. Cancer Treat Rep 1985;69:211–213.
440. Baum ES, Gaynon P, Greenberg L, et al. Phase II trail cisplatin in refractory childhood cancer: Children's Cancer Study Group Report. Cancer Treat Rep 1981;65:815–822.
441. Pratt CB, Shanks EC. Doxorubicin in treatment of malignant solid tumors in children. Am J Dis Child 1974;127:534–536.
442. Cortes EP, Holland JF, Wang JJ, et al. Amputation and adriamycin in primary osteosarcoma. N Engl J Med 1974;291:998–1000.
443. Jaffe N, Prudich J, Knapp J, et al. Treatment of primary osteosarcoma with intra-arterial and intravenous high-dose methotrexate. J Clin Oncol 1983;1:428–431.
444. Goorin AM, Harris MB, Bernstein M, et al. Phase II/III trial of etoposide and high-dose ifosfamide in newly diagnosed metastatic osteosarcoma: a pediatric oncology group trial. J Clin Oncol 2002;20:426–433.
445. Harris MB, Cantor AB, Goorin AM, et al. Treatment of osteosarcoma with ifosfamide: comparison of response in pediatric patients with recurrent disease versus patients previously untreated: a Pediatric Oncology Group study. Med Pediatr Oncol 1995;24: 87–92.
446. Taylor WF, Ivins JC, Pritchard DJ, et al. Trends and variability in survival among patients with osteosarcoma: a 7-year update. Mayo Clin Proc 1985;60:91–104.
447. Carter SK. Adjuvant chemotherapy in osteogenic sarcoma: the triumph that isn't? J Clin Oncol 1984;2:147–148.
448. Edmonson JH, Green SJ, Ivins JC, et al. A controlled pilot study of high-dose methotrexate as postsurgical adjuvant treatment for primary osteosarcoma. J Clin Oncol 1984;2:152–156.
449. Rosen G, Murphy ML, Huvos AG, et al. Chemotherapy, en bloc resection, and prosthetic bone replacement in the treatment of osteogenic sarcoma. Cancer 1976;37:1–11.
450. Rosen G, Marcove RC, Caparros B, et al. Primary osteogenic sarcoma: the rationale for preoperative chemotherapy and delayed surgery. Cancer 1979;43:2163–2177.
451. Winkler K, Beron G, Kotz R, et al. Neoadjuvant chemotherapy for osteogenic sarcoma: results of a Cooperative German/Austrian study. J Clin Oncol 1984;2:617–624.
452. Provisor AJ, Ettinger LJ, Nachman JB, et al. Treatment of nonmetastatic osteosarcoma of the extremity with preoperative and postoperative chemotherapy: a report from the Children's Cancer Group. J Clin Oncol 1997;15:76–84.
453. Bacci G, Avella M, Brach Del Prevert A, et al. Neoadjuvant chemotherapy for osteosarcoma of the extremities. Good response of the primary tumor after preoperative chemotherapy with high-dose methotrexate followed by cisplatinum and adriamycin. Preliminary results. Chemioterapia 1988;7:138–142.
454. Goorin AM, Schwartzentruber DJ, Devidas M, et al. Presurgical chemotherapy compared with immediate surgery and adjuvant chemotherapy for nonmetastatic osteosarcoma: Pediatric Oncology Group Study POG-8651. J Clin Oncol 2003;21:1574–1580.
455. Rosen G, Caparros B, Huvos AG, et al. Preoperative chemotherapy for osteogenic sarcoma: selection of postoperative adjuvant chemotherapy based on the response of the primary tumor to preoperative chemotherapy. Cancer 1982;49:1221–1230.
456. Meyers PA, Heller G, Healey J, et al. Chemotherapy for nonmetastatic osteogenic sarcoma: the Memorial Sloan- Kettering experience [see comments]. J Clin Oncol 1992; 10:5–15.
457. Winkler K, Beron G, Delling G, et al. Neoadjuvant chemotherapy of osteosarcoma: results of a randomized cooperative trial (COSS-82) with salvage chemotherapy based on histological tumor response. J Clin Oncol 1988;6:329–337.
458. Meyers PA, Gorlick R, Heller G, et al. Intensification of preoperative chemotherapy for osteogenic sarcoma: results of the Memorial Sloan-Kettering (T12) protocol. J Clin Oncol 1998;16:2452–2458.
459. Gurney JG, Swensen AR, Bulterys M. Malignant bone tumors. In: Ries LAG, Smith MA, Gurney JG, et al. eds. Cancer incidence and survival among children and adolescents: united states SEER program 1975–1995. Bethesda, MD: National Cancer Institute, SEER Program, 1999:99–110.
460. Ferguson WS, Harris MB, Goorin AM, et al. Presurgical window of carboplatin and surgery and multidrug chemotherapy for the treatment of newly diagnosed metastatic or unresectable osteosarcoma: Pediatric Oncology Group Trial. J Pediatr Hematol Oncol 2001;23:340–348.
461. Kleinerman ES, Raymond AK, Bucana CD, et al. Unique histological changes in lung metastases of osteosarcoma patients following therapy with liposomal muramyl tripeptide (CGP 19835A lipid). Cancer Immunol Immunother 1992;34:211–220.
462. Kleinerman ES, Snyder JS, Jaffe N. Influence of chemotherapy administration on monocyte activation by liposomal muramyl tripeptide phosphatidylethanolamine in children with osteosarcoma. J Clin Oncol 1991;9:259–267.
463. MacEwen EG, Kurzman ID, Rosenthal RC, et al. Therapy for osteosarcoma in dogs with intravenous injection of liposome-encapsulated muramyl tripeptide. J Natl Cancer Inst 1989;81:935–938.
464. Kleinerman ES, Gano JB, Johnston DA, et al. Efficacy of liposomal muramyl tripeptide (CGP 19835A) in the treatment of relapsed osteosarcoma. Am J Clin Oncol 1995;18: 93–99.
465. Kleinerman ES, Jia SF, Griffin J, et al. Phase II study of liposomal muramyl tripeptide in osteosarcoma: the cytokine cascade and monocyte activation following administration. J Clin Oncol 1992;10:1310–1316.
466. Kleinerman ES, Maeda M, Jaffe N. Liposome-encapsulated muramyl tripeptide: a new biologic response modifier for the treatment of osteosarcoma. Cancer Treat Res 1993;62:101–107.
467. Meyers PA, Schwartz CL, Krailo MD, et al. Osteosarcoma: the addition of muramyl tripeptide to chemotherapy improves overall survival—a report from the Children's Oncology Group. J Clin Oncol 2008;26:633–638.
468. Hunsberger S, Freidlin B, Smith MA. Complexities in interpretation of Osteosarcoma Clinical Trial results. J Clin Oncol 2008;26:3103–3104.
469. Bielack SS, Marina N, Ferrari S, et al. Osteosarcoma: the same old drugs or more? J Clin Oncol 2008;26:3102–3103; author reply 4–5.
470. Meyers PA, Schwartz CL, Krailo MD, et al. In reply. J Clin Oncol 2008;26:3104–3105.
471. Schwartz CL, Wexler LH, Devidas M, et al. P9754 therapeutic intensification in nonmetastatic osteosarcoma: a COG trial. In: American Society of Clinical Oncology; 2004. J Clin Oncol 2004;22:14S, ABSTRACT 8514.
472. Jaffe N. Recent advances in the chemotherapy of metastatic osteogenic sarcoma. Cancer 1972;30:1627–1631.
473. Pagani PA, Bacci G, Figus E, et al. Association of radical surgery and cyclic polychemotherapy (with vincristine, methotrexate and adriamycin) in the treatment of some forms of osteosarcoma. Preliminary results. Chir Organi Mov 1975;62:81–92.
474. Winkler K, Beron G, Schellong G, et al. Kooperative Osteosarkomstudie COSS-77: Ergebnisse nach über 4 Jahren. Klin Pädiatr 1982;194:251–256.
475. Winkler K, Gaedicke G, Grosch-Wörner I, et al. Chemotherapy of osteosarcoma. Dtsch Med Wochenschr 1977;102:1831–1835.
476. Bielack SS, Machatschek JN, Flege S, et al. Delaying surgery with chemotherapy for osteosarcoma of the extremities. Expert Opin Pharmacother 2004;5:1243–1256.
477. Bacci G, Picci P, Ruggieri P, et al. Primary chemotherapy and delayed surgery (neoadjuvant chemotherapy) for osteosarcoma of the extremities. The Istituto Rizzoli Experience in 127 patients treated preoperatively with intravenous methotrexate (high versus moderate doses) and intraarterial cisplatin. Cancer 1990;65:2539–2553.
478. Bacci G, Briccoli A, Ferrari S, et al. Neoadjuvant chemotherapy for osteosarcoma of the extremity: long-term results of the Rizzoli's 4th protocol. Eur J Cancer 2001;37: 2030–2039.
479. Seter G. Treatment of osteosarcoma of the extremities with the T-10 protocol, with emphasis on the effects of preoperative chemotherapy with single-agent high-dose methotrexate: a Scandinavian Sarcoma Group study. J Clin Oncol 1991;9:1766–1775.
480. Fuchs N, Bielack SS, Epler D, et al. Long-term results of the co-operative German-Austrian-Swiss osteosarcoma study group's protocol COSS-86 of intensive multidrug chemotherapy and surgery for osteosarcoma of the limbs. Ann Oncol 1998;9:893–899.
481. Bramwell VH, Burgers M, Sneath R, et al. A comparison of two short intensive adjuvant chemotherapy regimens in operable osteosarcoma of limbs in children and young adults: the first study of the European Osteosarcoma Intergroup. J Clin Oncol 1992;10: 1579–1591.
482. Souhami RL, Craft AW, Van der Eijken JW, et al. Randomised trial of two regimens of chemotherapy in operable osteosarcoma: a study of the European Osteosarcoma Intergroup. Lancet 1997;350:911–917.
483. Lewis IJ, Nooij MA, Whelan J, et al. Improvement in histologic response but not survival in osteosarcoma patients treated with intensified chemotherapy: a randomized phase III trial of the European Osteosarcoma Intergroup. J Natl Cancer Inst 2007;99: 112–128.
484. Petrilli AS, de Camargo B, Filho VO, et al. Results of the Brazilian Osteosarcoma Treatment Group Studies III and IV: Prognostic Factors and Impact on Survival. J Clin Oncol 2006;24:1161–1168.
485. Le Deley MC, Guinebretiere JM, Gentet JC, et al. SFOP OS94: a randomised trial comparing preoperative high-dose methotrexate plus doxorubicin to high-dose methotrexate plus etoposide and ifosfamide in osteosarcoma patients. Eur J Cancer 2007;4: 752–761.
486. Rosen G, Nirenberg A, Caparros B, et al. Osteogenic sarcoma: eight-percent, three-year, disease-free survival with combination chemotherapy (T-7). Natl Cancer Inst Monogr 1981;56:213–220.
487. Lee JA, Kim MS, Kim DH, et al. Risk Stratification based on the clinical factors at diagnosis is closely related to the survival of localized osteosarcoma. Pediatr Blood Cancer 2009;52:340–435.
488. Salzer-Kuntschik M, Brand G, Delling G. Determination of the degree of morphological regression following chemotherapy in malignant bone tumors. Pathologe 1983;4: 135–141.
489. Bielack S, Kempf-Bielack B, Winkler K. Osteosarcoma: relationship of response to preoperative chemotherapy and type of surgery to local recurrence. J Clin Oncol 1996; 14:683–684.
490. Picci P, Sangiorgi L, Rougraff BT, et al. Relationship of chemotherapy-induced necrosis and surgical margins to local recurrence in osteosarcoma. J Clin Oncol 1994;12: 2699–2705.
491. Lewis IJ, Nooij MA, Whelan J, et al. Improvement in histologic response but not survival in osteosarcoma patients treated with intensified chemotherapy: a randomized phase III trial of the European Osteosarcoma Intergroup. J Natl Cancer Inst 2007;99: 112–128.
492. Longhi A, Ferrari S, Bacci G, et al. Long-term follow-up of patients with doxorubicin-induced cardiac toxicity after chemotherapy for osteosarcoma. Anticancer Drugs 2007;18:737–744.
493. Winkler K, Bielack S, Delling G, et al. Effect of intraarterial versus intravenous cisplatin in addition to systemic doxorubicin, high-dose methotrexate, and ifosfamide on histologic tumor response in osteosarcoma (study COSS-86). Cancer 1990;66:1703–1710.
494. Bacci G, Ferrari S, Forni C, et al. The effect of intra-arterial versus intravenous cisplatinum in the neoadjuvant treatment of osteosarcoma of the limbs: the experience at the Rizzoli Institute. Chir Organi Mov 1996;81:369–382.
495. Widemann BC, Balis FM, Kempf-Bielack B, et al. High-dose methotrexate-induced nephrotoxicity in patients with osteosarcoma. Cancer 2004;100:2222–2232.
496. Aquerreta I, Aldaz A, Giráldez J, et al. Methotrexate pharmacokinetics and survival in osteosarcoma. Pediatr Blood Cancer 2004;42:52–58.
497. Delepine N, Delepine G, Bacci G, et al. Influence of methotrexate dose intensity on outcome of patients with high grade osteogenic osteosarcoma. Analysis of the literature. Cancer 1996;78:2127–2135.
498. Bielack S, Beron G, Winkler K. Influence of methotrexate dose intensity on outcome of patients with high grade osteogenic osteosarcoma: analysis of the literature. Cancer 1997;80:516–518.
499. Graf N, Winkler K, Betlemovic M, et al. Methotrexate pharmacokinetics and prognosis in osteosarcoma. J Clin Oncol 1994;12:1443–1451.
500. Tunn PU, Reichardt P. Chemotherapy for osteosarcoma without high-dose methotrexate: a 12-year follow-up on 53 patients. Onkologie 2007;30:228–232.
501. Bacci G, Ferrari S, Bertoni F, et al. Long-term outcome for patients with nonmetastatic osteosarcoma of the extremity treated at the Istituto Ortopedico Rizzoli according to the Istituto Ortopedico Rizzoli/Osteosarcoma-2 Protocol: an updated report. J Clin Oncol 2000;18:4016–4027.
502. Lewis IJ, Weeden S, Machin D, et al. Received dose and dose-intensity of chemotherapy and outcome in nonmetastatic extremity osteosarcoma. J Clin Oncol 2000;18:4028–4037.
503. Eselgrim M, Grunert H, Kuhne T, et al. Dose intensity of chemotherapy for osteosarcoma and outcome in the Cooperative Osteosarcoma Study Group (COSS) trials. Pediatr Blood Cancer 2006;47:42–50.

504. Colombat P, Biron P, Coze C, et al. Failure of high-dose alkylating agents in osteosarcoma. Solid Tumors Working Party. Bone Marrow Transplant 1994;14:665–666.

505. Fagioli F, Aglietta M, Tienghi A, et al. High-dose chemotherapy in the treatment of relapsed osteosarcoma: an Italian sarcoma group study. J Clin Oncol 2002;20:2150–2156.

506. Sauerbrey A, Bielack S, Kempf-Bielack B, et al. High-dose chemotherapy (HDC) and autologous hematopoietic stem cell transplantation (ASCT) as salvage therapy for relapsed osteosarcoma. Bone Marrow Transplant 2001;27:933–937.

507. Burgers JM, van Glabbeke M, Busson A, et al. Osteosarcoma of the limbs. Report of the EORTC-SIOP 03 trial 20781 investigating the value of adjuvant treatment with chemotherapy and/or prophylactic lung irradiation. Cancer 1988;61:1024–1031.

508. Muller CR, Smeland S, Bauer HC, et al. Interferon-alpha as the only adjuvant treatment in high-grade osteosarcoma: long term results of the Karolinska Hospital series. Acta Oncol 2005;44:475–480.

509. Strander H, Bauer HC, Brosjo O, et al. Long-term adjuvant interferon treatment of human osteosarcoma. A pilot study. Acta Oncol 1995;34:877–880.

510. Bacci G, Briccoli A, Rocca M, et al. Neoadjuvant chemotherapy for osteosarcoma of the extremities with metastases at presentation: recent experience at the Rizzoli Institute in 57 patients treated with cisplatin, doxorubicin, and a high dose of methotrexate and ifosfamide. Ann Oncol 2003;14:1126–1134.

511. Mialou V, Philip T, Kalifa C, et al. Metastatic osteosarcoma at diagnosis: prognostic factors and long-term outcome—the French pediatric experience. Cancer 2005;104:1100–1109.

512. Stiller CA, Bielack SS, Jundt G, et al. Bone tumours in European children and adolescents, 1978–1997. Report from the Automated Childhood Cancer Information System project. Eur J Cancer 2006;42:2124–2135.

513. Rivera GK, Quintana J, Villarroel M, et al. Transfer of complex frontline anticancer therapy to a developing country: the St. Jude osteosarcoma experience in Chile. Pediatr Blood Cancer 2008;50:1143–1146.

514. Abe S, Nishimoto Y, Isu K, et al. Preoperative cisplatin for initial treatment of limb osteosarcoma: its local effect and impact on prognosis. Cancer Chemother Pharmacol 2002;50:320–324.

515. Muthuphei MN, Mariba MT. Osteosarcoma in Ga-Rankuwa Hospital: a 10 year experience in an African population. Cent Afr J Med 2000;46:41–43.

516. Goorin AM, Delorey MJ, Lack EE. Prognostic significance of complete surgical resection of pulmonary metastases in patients with osteogenic sarcoma: analysis of 32 patients. J Clin Oncol 1984;2:425–431.

517. Meyer WH, Schell MJ, Kumar AP, et al. Thoracotomy for pulmonary metastatic osteosarcoma. An analysis of prognostic indicators of survival. Cancer 1987;59:374–379.

518. Hawkins DS, Arndt CA. Pattern of disease recurrence and prognostic factors in patients with osteosarcoma treated with contemporary chemotherapy. Cancer 2003;98:2447–2456.

519. Bielack SS, Kempf-Bielack B, Branscheid D, et al. Second and subsequent recurrences of osteosarcoma: presentation, treatment, and outcomes of 249 consecutive cooperative osteosarcoma study group patients. J Clin Oncol 2009;27:557–565.

520. Bielack SS, Kempf-Bielack B, Heise U, et al. Combined modality treatment for osteosarcoma occurring as a second malignant disease. Cooperative German-Austrian-Swiss Osteosarcoma Study Group. J Clin Oncol 1999;17:1164.

521. Tabone MD, Terrier P, Pacquement H, et al. Outcome of radiation-related osteosarcoma after treatment of childhood and adolescent cancer: a study of 23 cases. J Clin Oncol 1999;17:2789–2795.

522. Bacci G, Longhi A, Forni C, et al. Neoadjuvant chemotherapy for radioinduced osteosarcoma of the extremity: the Rizzoli experience in 20 cases. Int J Radiat Oncol Biol Phys 2007;67:505–511.

523. Goorin AM, Chauvenet AR, Perez-Atayde AR, et al. Initial congestive heart failure, six to ten years after doxorubicin chemotherapy for childhood cancer. J Pediatr 1990;116:144–147.

524. Lipshultz SE, Lipsitz SR, Mone SM, et al. Female sex and higher drug dose as risk factors for late cardiotoxic effects of doxorubicin therapy for childhood cancer. N Engl J Med 1995;332:1738–1743.

525. Scully RE, Lipshultz SE. Anthracycline cardiotoxicity in long-term survivors of childhood cancer. Cardiovasc Toxicol 2007;7:122–128.

526. Lewis MJ, DuBois SG, Fligor B, et al. Ototoxicity in children treated for osteosarcoma. Pediatr Blood Cancer 2009;52:387–391.

527. Marina NM, Poquette CA, Cain AM, et al. Comparative renal tubular toxicity of chemotherapy regimens including ifosfamide in patients with newly diagnosed sarcomas. J Pediatr Hematol Oncol 2000;22:112–118.

528. Goldsby R, Burke C, Nagarajan R, et al. Second solid malignancies among children, adolescents, and young adults diagnosed with malignant bone tumors after 1976: follow-up of a Children's Oncology Group cohort. Cancer 2008;113:2597–2604.

529. Meistrich ML, Chawla SP, da Cunha MF, et al. Recovery of sperm production after chemotherapy for osteosarcoma. Cancer 1989;63:2115–2123.

530. Nagarajan R, Clohisy DR, Neglia JP, et al. Function and quality-of-life of survivors of pelvic and lower extremity osteosarcoma and Ewing's sarcoma: the Childhood Cancer Survivor Study. Br J Cancer 2004;91:1858–1865.

531. Mertens AC, Liu Q, Neglia JP, et al. Cause-specific late mortality among 5-year survivors of childhood cancer: the Childhood Cancer Survivor Study. J Natl Cancer Inst 2008;100:1368–1379.

532. Mertens AC, Yasui Y, Neglia JP, et al. Late mortality experience in five-year survivors of childhood and adolescent cancer: the Childhood Cancer Survivor Study. J Clin Oncol 2001;19:3163–3172.

533. Seibel NL, Krailo M, Chen Z, et al. Upfront window trial of topotecan in previously untreated children and adolescents with poor prognosis metastatic osteosarcoma: Children's Cancer Group (CCG) 7943. Cancer 2007;109:1646–1653.

534. Donati D, Giacomini S, Gozzi E, et al. Osteosarcoma of the pelvis. Eur J Surg Oncol 2004;30:332–340.

535. Ozaki T, Flege S, Kevric M, et al. Osteosarcoma of the pelvis: experience of the Cooperative Osteosarcoma Study Group. J Clin Oncol 2003;21:334–341.

536. Matsuo T, Sugita T, Sato K, et al. Clinical outcomes of 54 pelvic osteosarcomas registered by Japanese musculoskeletal oncology group. Oncology 2005;68:375–381.

537. Ozaki T, Flege S, Liljenqvist U, et al. Osteosarcoma of the spine. Cancer 2002;94:1069–1077.

538. Bielack SS, Wulff B, Delling G, et al. Osteosarcoma of the trunk treated by multimodal therapy: experience of the Cooperative Osteosarcoma study group (COSS). Med Pediatr Oncol 1995;24:6–12.

539. Rao RD, Anderson PM, Arndt CA, et al. Aerosolized granulocyte macrophage colony-stimulating factor (GM-CSF) therapy in metastatic cancer. Am J Clin Oncol 2003;26:493–498.

540. Anderson PM, Wiseman GA, Dispenzieri A, et al. High-dose samarium-153 ethylene diamine tetramethylene phosphonate: low toxicity of skeletal irradiation in patients with osteosarcoma and bone metastases. J Clin Oncol 2002;20:189–196.

541. Evdokiou A, Labrinidis A, Bouralexis S, et al. Induction of cell death of human osteogenic sarcoma cells by zoledronic acid resembles anoikis. Bone 2003;33:216–228.

542. Heymann D, Ory B, Blanchard F, et al. Enhanced tumor regression and tissue repair when zoledronic acid is combined with ifosfamide in rat osteosarcoma. Bone 2005;37:74–86.

543. LeRoith D, Roberts CT Jr. The insulin-like growth factor system and cancer. Cancer Lett 2003;195:127–137.

544. Reinmuth N, Fan F, Liu W, et al. Impact of insulin-like growth factor receptor-I function on angiogenesis, growth, and metastasis of colon cancer. Lab Invest 2002;82:1377–1389.

545. Giorgetti S, Ballotti R, Kowalski-Chauvel A, et al. The insulin and insulin-like growth factor-I receptor substrate IRS-1 associates with and activates phosphatidylinositol 3-kinase in vitro. J Biol Chem 1993;268:7358–7364.

546. Ouban A, Muraca P, Yeatman T, et al. Expression and distribution of insulin-like growth factor-1 receptor in human carcinomas. Hum Pathol 2003;34:803–808.

547. Werner H, Shalita-Chesner M, Abramovitch S, et al. Regulation of the insulin-like growth factor-I receptor gene by oncogenes and antioncogenes: implications in human cancer. Mol Genet Metab 2000;71:315–320.

548. Pollak MN, Schernhammer ES, Hankinson SE. Insulin-like growth factors and neoplasia. Nat Rev Cancer 2004;4:505–518.

549. Kolb EA, Gorlick R, Houghton PJ, et al. Initial testing (stage 1) of a monoclonal antibody (SCH 717454) against the IGF-1 receptor by the pediatric preclinical testing program. Pediatr Blood Cancer 2008;50:1190–1197.

CHAPTER 35 ■ GERM CELL TUMORS

THOMAS A. OLSON, DOMINIK T. SCHNEIDER, AND ELIZABETH J. PERLMAN

Gonadal and extragonadal germ cell tumors are infrequent in childhood, occurring at a rate of 2.4 cases per million children and representing approximately 2% to 3% of cancers diagnosed in children and adolescents younger than 15 years.[1,2] Extracranial germ cell tumors account for 14% of all cancers in the 15 to 19 age group. A large population based analysis of pediatric germ cell tumors in German MAKEI trials from 1981 to 2000 showed a bimodal age distribution.[3] A small peak occurs during infancy and a larger peak after puberty. These separate groups were marked by distinct clinical and molecular features. Building on effective treatments developed for adults with testicular germ cell tumors, pediatric clinical trials have led to significant improvement in survival. Recently, trials have been developed to reduce therapy to minimize late effects, while maintaining excellent survival. This goal can only be achieved through ongoing cooperative studies. Advances in molecular understanding of these rare pediatric tumors may aid in the development of risk adaptive strategies.

EMBRYOGENESIS AND HISTOGENESIS OF GONADAL TUMORS

Germ cell tumors are presumed to share a common cell of origin, the primordial germ cell, yet they remain a heterogeneous group of tumors. Variations regarding age, sites of presentation, histopathology, and malignant potential stem from differences in the stage of germ cell development at tumorigenesis, differences in the tumor environment secondary to the gender of the patient and location of the clone, and specific genetic aberrations. Therefore, understanding the development of embryonic germ cells is critical to an appreciation of these issues.

There has been considerable debate whether heterogenous germ cell tumors, in particular extragonadal teratomas, may originate from midline somatic stem cells. This debate has been based on the experimental observation that teratoma-like tumors may develop at the injection site of cultured embryonal stem cells.[4] Moreover, the development of isochromosome 12p, the pathognomic marker of germ cell tumors in young men, has been described in long-term cultures of embryonal stem cells.[5] However, there is molecular evidence that both gonadal and extragonadal germ cell tumors originate from primordial germ cells at different stages of development. The examination of the epigenetic control of genomic imprinting reveals a methylation pattern that is characteristic of primordial germ cells during and after their migration during early embryonal development.[6,7] In addition, this methylation pattern distinguishes germ cell tumors from other embryonal tumors with presumed stem cell origins, such as nephroblastoma.[8]

The primordial germ cells first become evident in the extraembryonic yolk sac by the fourth week of gestation. By the fifth week (Fig. 35.1), the germ cells migrate through the mesentery to the gonadal ridge.[9] This migration appears to be mediated by the c-kit receptor and its ligand, stem-cell factor, or steel factor. Primordial germ cells express c-kit. The stem-cell factor is expressed with an increasing gradient from yolk sac to the gonadal ridge, guiding germ cells to the gonadal ridge.[10] In animal models, primordial germ cell tumors not expressing c-kit are unable to migrate to the gonad and proliferate during migration. The association of c-kit mutations with bilateral or familial germ cell tumors underlies the importance of this gene during germ cell development.[11] Germ cell migration is additionally directed by the chemotaxine/ligand pair soluble derived factor 1 (SDF-1) and its receptor CXCR-4.[12] Germ cells express CXCR-4 and migration is directed by the expression and secretion of SDF-1 in the mesenchyme of the gonadal ridge. In the absence of these factors, germ cells do not populate mouse gonads but may survive in the extragonadal environment.[13] However, no defects of SDF-1 or CXCR-4 have yet been reported in germ cell tumors. Extragonadal germ cell tumors are presumed to arise from germ cells that have migrated aberrantly.[14]

The fate of the germ cells, after their arrival at the gonadal ridge, depends on the sex of the individual. During a narrow window of opportunity in the sixth to seventh week, a gene on the Y chromosome (the SRY gene) initiates male sex determination. Ovarian differentiation commences either in the absence of a Y chromosome or if the window of opportunity is missed.[15] Testicular differentiation manifests by the abrupt development of cellular cords (sex cords) in the seventh week. Primordial germ cells populate these sex cords and then undergo mitotic arrest and remain in that state until puberty. The ovary does not demonstrate the defined sex cords seen in the testis. Instead, primordial germ cells populate the primitive gonad while continuing to divide and proliferate. At approximately 16 to 18 weeks' gestation, the germ cells gradually enter into meiosis I and are then arrested in the prophase of meiosis I. The follicular cells surround the oocytes. Primordial germ cells are not associated with follicular cells prior to entry into meiosis. The entry into meiosis of primordial germ cells is a gradual process that continues until birth; proliferation continues prior to entry into meiosis.

The gonads contain three cell types having neoplastic potential (Fig. 35.2). Germ cells give rise to germ cell tumors. The cells of the sex cords may rarely develop into stromal tumors, such as testicular Sertoli or Leydig cell tumors, ovarian granulosa cell tumors, or mixtures of these components. These tumors may sometimes display morphologic features that are discrepant from the sex of the patient, thus illustrating the bisexual differential potential of the gonadal stroma. Last, coelomic epithelium covering the ovary may evolve into epithelial neoplasms, found most often in adults.[16] Although exposure to female hormones during pregnancy has been suggested to play a role in germ cell tumor development, a case control study comparing children with germ cell tumors and normal controls failed to identify an association.[17] However, the paucity of pediatric germ cell tumors makes conclusions difficult.

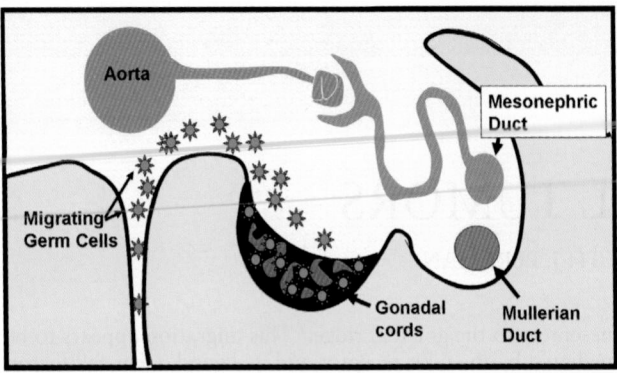

FIGURE 35.1 Migration of primordial germ cells through mesentery to gonadal ridge. Testicular development is manifested by abrupt development of sex cords. Ovaries do not demonstrate defined sex cords.

GENETICS AND MOLECULAR BIOLOGY

Genetic contributions to the pathogenesis of pediatric germ cell tumors include constitutional genetic changes leading to increased susceptibility and tumor-specific genetic changes. Little is known regarding the former, particularly with regard to infantile germ cell tumors. However, familial tumors appear to account for 1.5% to 2% of all adult germ cell tumors.[18] Therefore, the same contribution is likely for adolescent germ cell tumors. The association between sex-chromosomal abnormalities and the development of germ cell tumors is well established. In particular, individuals with 46,XY and 45,X/46,XY gonadal dysgenesis have a 10% to 50% risk of developing a gonadal germ cell tumor.[19] Patients with Klinefelter syndrome (47,XXY) have an increased risk of developing extragonadal germ cell tumors, in particular mediastinal germ cell tumors, although this risk level within this population is difficult to establish.[20] In general, the age of presentation at diagnosis of mediastinal germ cell tumors is 10 years younger in Klinefelter patients than in those with a normal constitutional karyotype. Approximately 50% of adolescents with mediastinal germ cell tumors have cytogenetic changes consistent with Klinefelter syndrome.[21]

In ovarian germ cell tumors, there is an association with Turner syndrome, in particular in patients with microscopic residues of Y-chromosomal sequences, and Swyer syndrome, a disorder characterized by a female appearance but with hypoplastic streak gonads in a cytogenetically male.

As we investigate molecular differences in germ cell tumors in children and adolescents, it must be emphasized that few pediatric germ cell tumors have been analyzed to date and differences may not be absolute.[22] When addressing tumor-specific genetic changes, the heterogeneity of the pediatric germ cell tumors is also evident in studies investigating their genetic and molecular properties. Four biologically distinct subcategories are distinguished in the pediatric population: tumors of the adolescent testis, tumors of the adolescent ovary, extragonadal tumors of adolescents, and tumors of infancy.

Genetic Characteristics of Testicular Tumors in Adolescents and Adults

Adolescent testicular germ cell tumors most commonly become clinically evident several years after puberty, suggesting that a critical genetic event occurs with, or is unmasked at, puberty. However, because these tumors have been shown to arise in premeiotic germ cells with erased genomic imprinting, some observers believe that the critical event occurs in the embryonic gonad.[23] Despite their histologic heterogeneity, tumors of the adolescent and adult testis are relatively homogeneous genetically, demonstrating an aneuploid DNA content and the isochromosome 12p or i(12p).[24] Postpubertal testicular teratomas may also present as clinically malignant tumors with metastatic spread and cytogenetic evidence of an i(12p).[25]

The i(12p) is composed of two copies of the short arm of chromosome 12, fused in the centromere, and can be demonstrated in more than 80% of postpubertal germ cell tumors (Fig. 35.3). Isochromosome negative adolescent germ cell tumors almost invariably show gain of chromosomal material of 12p, sometimes presenting as high level amplification at 12p11–12 (from the same parental origin).[26] Testicular tumors lacking i(12p) often show gain of 12p material within marker chromosomes.[27] The i(12p) has been documented by fluorescent *in situ* hybridization in intratubular germ cell neoplasia, a precursor lesion of testicular germ cell tumors. This finding provides further evidence that this genetic alteration occurs early in germ cell tumor pathogenesis.[28] Whether the critical genetic event is gain of 12p, loss of 12q, or both, is not fully understood. Murty et al.[29] noted loss of heterozygosity at the 12q13 and 12q22 regions in 41% and 47% of tumors, respectively. Genes implicated in the pathogenesis of other solid tumors that map to the 12q13 region, including INT1, GLI, and MDM2, are not altered in testicular germ cell tumors.

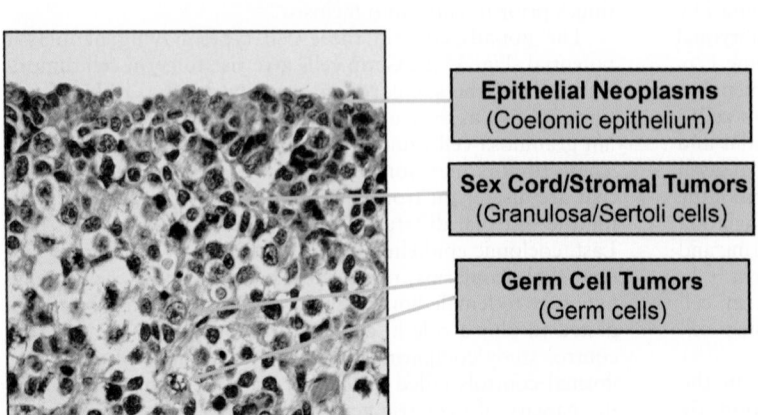

FIGURE 35.2 Fetal ovary at 18 weeks gestation. Coelomic epithelium is responsible for epithelial malignancies. This layer is lost in testicular development, thus low frequency of epithelial tumors in testes. Gonadal stromal tumors arise in a specialized stromal layer. Germ cell tumors arise within the primordial germ cells that migrate from yolk sac to gonad early in development.

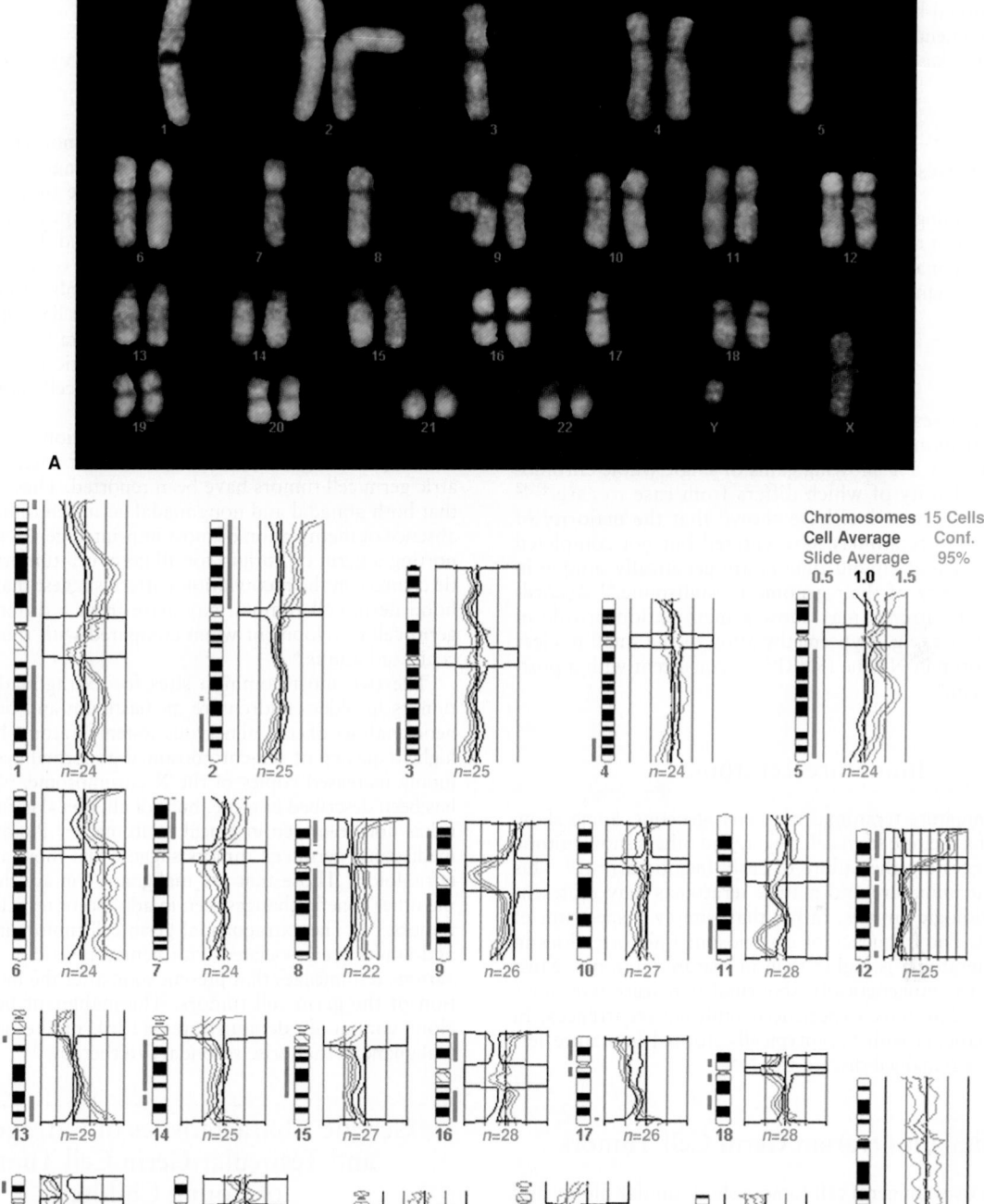

FIGURE 35.3 Comparative genomic hybridization of a male patient with a testicular mixed malignant germ cell tumor. **A:** Representative karyotype of DAPI-stained normal male chromosomes after co-hybridization against FITC stained (green) tumor DNA and Spectrum-Red stained reference DNA. Chromosomal regions with balanced hybridization signal are yellow, regions with amplification of tumor DNA green (e.g., 12p) and regions with chromosomal loss red. **B:** Corresponding calculated hybridization ratio. Balanced chromosomal regions lay within the reference interval, and regions with chromosomal gains or losses are shown as deviation to the right or left, respectively.

Testicular germ cell tumors have also exhibited loss of chromosome 13 (38%), gain of chromosome 21 (45%), gain of chromosome 8 (45%), gain of chromosome 1q (36%), and high-level gain of 12p11.2–12.1, suggesting amplification.[30] Other less frequent genetic changes include the following: loss of 1p,[31] K-ras, and N-ras mutations,[32] high N-myc expression without amplification,[33] absence of p53 mutation,[34] loss of heterozygosity for 11p13 and 11p15 with preferential loss of the paternal allele,[35] loss of 3p[36] and deletion of DCC.[37,38] Adolescent testicular germ cell tumors, like normal embryonic germ cells, demonstrate biallelic expression of multiple imprinted genes including H19 and insulin-like growth factor-2.[39] More functional-based technologies will be needed to determine environmental and genetic factors that lead to development of testicular germ cell tumors.[40]

Genetic Characteristics of Ovarian Tumors in Adolescents and Adults

The genetic biology of ovarian germ cell tumors is more complex than that of testicular germ cell tumors and is considered separately for mature teratomas, immature teratomas, and malignant ovarian germ cell tumors.

Teratomas

Cytogenetic assessment of more than 325 ovarian mature teratomas demonstrates that 95% are karyotypically balanced, with only 5% showing gains of single whole chromosomes, the identity of which differs from case to case.[41,42] Studies of molecular loci have shown that the majority of mature ovarian teratomas have entered but not completed meiosis.[41,43] These diploid tumors are genetically unique in that the majority of their genome is isodisomic.[44] Accordingly, these teratomas may show a methylation profile of imprinted genes (e.g., hypermethylation of the small nuclear ribonucleoprotein N gene (SNRPN)), consistent with a postmeiotic origin.[6]

Immature Teratomas

Ovarian immature teratomas are heterogeneous. Some show evidence of a meiotic stem-cell origin, and others show mitotic origins, suggesting the failure of early meiotic arrest.[45] This implies that immature and mature teratomas may represent different biologic entities, rather than simply a spectrum of maturation. The frequency of chromosomal abnormalities in immature teratoma is higher than in mature teratoma. Most patients with cytogenetically abnormal immature teratomas reported to date have experienced multiple recurrences. In contrast, patients with karyotypically normal immature teratomas have remained disease free.[45,46]

Malignant Ovarian Germ Cell Tumors

Malignant ovarian germ cell tumors show similar ploidy and genetic features when compared with their testicular counterparts. They are aneuploid: approximately 75% contain i(12p); 42% and 32% have gains of chromosomes 21 and 1q, respectively; 25% and 42% have loss of chromosomes 13 and 8, respectively.[47-49] DNA fingerprinting of four patients with dysgerminoma suggests an origin from premeiotic germ cells or germ cells at the beginning of the first meiotic division.[50] Also described was the development of a malignant endodermal sinus tumor with i(12p) and aneuploidy within an immature teratoma that had no i(12p) and was diploid. Such an event supports a genetic clonal evolution in this process.[47,48,50]

In summary, although malignant ovarian germ cell tumors appear to be equivalent to their adolescent testicular counterparts, immature and mature ovarian teratoma remain unique subcategories of germ cell tumors likely to have a different mechanism of origin. Immature teratomas may develop

genetic changes that are accompanied by histologic malignant transformations.

Genetic Characteristics of Extragonadal Germ Cell Tumors of Older Children

Aberrant or incomplete migration of primordial germ cells is one explanation for the origin of extragonadal germ cell tumors. Another hypothesis is that these tumors arise from totipotent embryonal cells that have escaped the influence of embryonic organizers controlling normal differentiation. This latter proposal is supported by a number of observations; the foremost being that ectopic germ cells only rarely have been reported to exist in human embryos, most having disappeared by 18 weeks' gestation.[9,51,52] Although data from animal models predict these tumors to be postmeiotic in origin,[53] other studies have shown extragonadal germ cell tumors in older children to be postmitotic in origin.[54,55]

More recently, studies of the methylation status of important imprinted genes within the different categories of pediatric germ cell tumors have been reported. These demonstrate that both gonadal and nongonadal germ cell tumors show the absence of methylation of most imprinted genes, strongly supporting a germ cell origin for all germ cell tumors. More subtle changes in the methylation pattern suggest that early childhood germ cell tumors may arise from a different stage of germ cell development when compared with those in adolescents and adults.[6]

The two most common sites for extragonadal germ cell tumors in older children are mediastinum and brain. Cytogenetic analyses of central nervous system teratoma have shown a high frequency of sex-chromosomal abnormalities, most commonly increased copies of the X chromosome.[56,57] The i(12p) has been described in some, but not all, pineal germinomas, but it has not been seen in pineal teratoma.[57,58] Ploidy analyses of mediastinal germ cell tumors suggest that most are diploid or tetraploid.[59] Those that are malignant contain the i(12p) and the other genetic changes seen in adolescent testicular germ cell tumors.[21,60] The extragonadal germ cell tumors in adolescents and adults are associated with hematopoietic malignancies of various cell lineages that present soon after the initial presentation of the germ cell tumors. The malignant hematopoietic clone commonly demonstrates i(12p), unlike hematopoietic malignancies that arise secondary to therapy.[61,62]

Genetic Characteristics of Extragonadal and Testicular Germ Cell Tumors of Young Children

In children younger than 4 years, germ cell tumors arising in gonadal and extragonadal sites are histologically, clinically, and genetically similar. Most teratomas in this age group are diploid, have normal karyotypes and, if completely resected, behave in a benign fashion regardless of degree of immaturity and site of origin.[25,55,63] Malignant germ cell tumors in these young children are almost exclusively yolk sac tumors, arising from a preexisting teratoma, and most often are diploid or tetraploid.[47,64] Recurrent cytogenetic abnormalities involve chromosomes 1, 3, and 6, among others, but only rarely the 12p (Fig. 35.1B).[47,63-65] In situ hybridization and loss of heterozygosity studies have demonstrated deletion of 1p36 in 80% to 100% of infantile malignant germ cell tumors arising from testicular and extragonadal sites.[66,67] Genetic surveys of regions of gain or loss in these infantile yolk sac tumors document recurrent loss of 6q24-qter, gain of 20q and 1q, and loss of 1p. A small number of tumors show evidence for c-myc or n-myc amplification.[68] The clinical significance for these markers is entirely unknown. Patterns of genetic expression have not been reported in these tumors.[69] Global gene expression was used to segregate germ cell tumors. Pediatric yolk sac tumors were enriched for genes associated with differentiation and seminomas with genes for proliferation.

PATHOLOGY

Germ cell tumors show numerous histologic subtypes. The histologic features of each subtype are independent of presenting clinical characteristics; tumor biology and clinical behavior vary with site of origin, stage, and age of the patient.[70,71] For example, mature teratoma in infants and in the ovary almost invariably are diploid and benign, whereas those in the adult testis, with the same histologic features, are aneuploid and potentially malignant.[72] The histologic classification of these tumors is shown in Table 35.1.

TABLE 35.1

HISTOLOGIC CLASSIFICATION OF PEDIATRIC GONADAL AND EXTRAGONADAL TUMORS

Ovarian
Germ cell
  Teratoma
    Mature (solid, cystic)
    Immature
    0. Mature tissue only
    1. Immature tissue, less than 1 low-power field per slide
    2. Immature tissue, 1–3 low-power fields per slide
    3. Abundant immature tissue
    Teratoma with associated malignant germ cell tumor component
    Teratoma with associated malignant somatic component (squamous carcinoma, glioblastoma, peripheral neuroectodermal tumor, etc.)
  Germinoma
  Yolk sac tumor (endodermal sinus tumor)
  Embryonal carcinoma
  Mixed malignant germ cell tumor
  Choriocarcinoma
  Gonadoblastoma
  Polyembryoma
Non–germ cell
  Epithelial (serous, mucinous)
  Sex cord–stromal (granulosa, Sertoli-Leydig, mixed, sclerosing, thecoma, SCT with annular tubules

Testicular
Germ cell
  Yolk sac tumor (endodermal sinus tumor)
  Embryonal carcinoma
  Teratoma
  Teratocarcinoma
  Gonadoblastoma
  Others (seminoma, choriocarcinoma, mixed germ cell)
Non–germ cell
  Sex cord–stromal (Leydig cell, Sertoli cell, etc.)

Extragonadal germ cell
Teratoma (sacral, mediastinal, retroperitoneal, pineal, other)
± Yolk sac tumor (endodermal sinus tumor).
± Embryonal carcinoma

Teratoma

Teratomas are the most common histologic subtype of childhood germ cell tumor arising in ovary and extragonadal locations. Mature teratomas of the gonads are encapsulated, multicystic, or solid tumors.[73–75] Extragonadal teratomas differ from those arising from the gonads only in the absence of a clearly defined external capsule. Teratomas can also be classified according to their histologic composition: mature, containing well-differentiated tissues; immature, containing varying degrees of immature fetal tissue, most often neuroectodermal; or malignant, containing at least one of the malignant germ cell elements.

The mature teratoma is composed of mature representative tissues from all three germ cell layers: ectoderm, mesoderm, and endoderm. Although any tissue type may be seen, the most common are skin and skin appendages, adipose tissue, mature brain, intestinal epithelium, and cystic structures lined by squamous, cuboidal, or flattened epithelium. Hematopoietic, pancreatic, or pituitary tissue frequently is found in mediastinal tumors and rarely in teratoma at other sites.[76]

Pediatric immature teratomas primarily occur in extragonadal sites in children and in the ovaries of girls near puberty.[77] Immature teratomas have a gross appearance similar to mature teratoma and are composed of representative tissues from all three germ layers. Unique to these tumors is the presence of various immature tissues, usually neuroepithelium, although immature ectodermal, mesodermal, and endodermal elements may also be observed. A number of grading systems have been established for immature teratoma, all of which are variations of the system originally devised by Thurlbeck and Scully.[78] All quantify the degree of immaturity in the lesion (Table 35.1). The grading of immature elements in childhood immature teratoma has not demonstrated prognostic significance. However, the risk of local recurrence is higher in immature teratomas, especially in the sacrococcygeal region, mostly due to a higher proportion of incomplete resections.[79] Immature teratomas in children behave in a malignant fashion, only if foci of malignant germ cell elements (usually yolk sac tumor) and specific clinical characteristics (usually advanced stage) are present. However, if resected completely, the presence of malignant yolk sac tumor foci does not impact on prognosis. Clusters of yolk sac tumors can be easily overlooked because they may be very small, associated intimately with the immature neural tissue, and they frequently do not stain positively for α-fetoprotein (AFP). Tumors containing such foci are likely responsible for the reports that immature teratoma may metastasize.

Yolk Sac Tumor

Yolk sac tumors are the most common pure malignant germ cell tumors in young children and are the most common germ cell tumors, benign or malignant, in the testes of infants and young boys.[72] Yolk sac tumor is the only malignant germ cell tumor type occurring in the sacrococcygeal region of infants.[70,75,80] Yolk sac tumors rarely occur in pure form in extragonadal sites of adolescents but more frequently are a component of the mixed malignant germ cell tumors occurring in these locations.[76,81] These tumors consist of friable, pale gray, mucoid tissue in which variable amounts of hemorrhage and necrosis are present. The microscopic features are varied and have been characterized fully only in the last two decades.[73,82,83] Individual cells may be small and pale, with scant cytoplasm, round to oval nuclei, and unapparent nucleoli, or they may be medium sized to large with clear vesicular nuclei and prominent nucleoli, resembling cells of an embryonal carcinoma or germinoma.

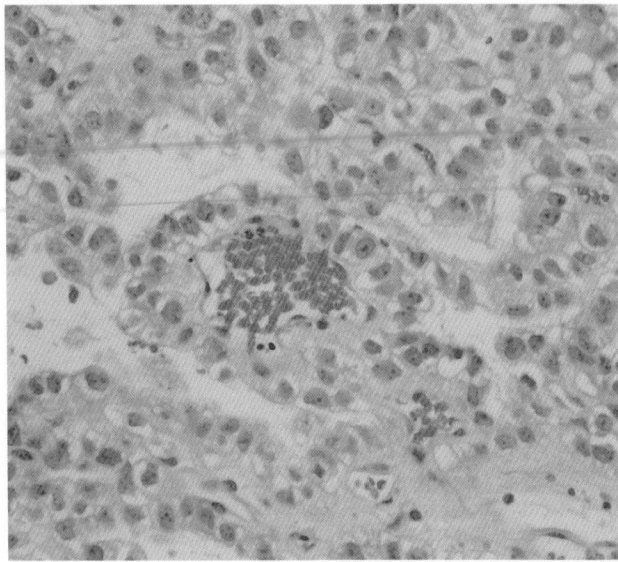

FIGURE 35.4 Yolk sac tumor. Schiller-Duval body is characterized by central blood vessel closely invested by a layer of tumor cells and separated from a second layer of tumor cells by a space, likened by some, to Bowman's space in glomerulus.

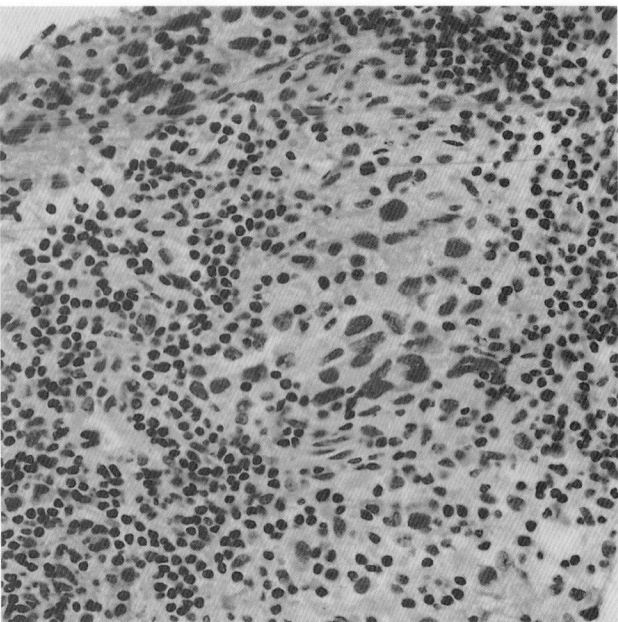

FIGURE 35.5 Germinoma (seminoma). Nests of monomorphic cells with abundant clear cytoplasm and round to oval vesicular nuclei with prominent nucleoli are separated by bands of connective tissue.

Mitoses range from few to many. Four general patterns and a number of variations have been recognized. These patterns are useful in the recognition of yolk sac tumors but have no other known clinical relevance.

The pseudopapillary or festoon pattern and the microcystic or reticular pattern are the most common and widely recognized. Both contain Schiller-Duval bodies, structures formed by a central small blood vessel closely invested by two layers of tumor cells (Fig. 35.4). The microcystic or reticular pattern is associated most often with eosinophilic globules and strands that only occasionally stain positively for AFP or α_1-antitrypsin. The pseudopapillary and parietal patterns are often observed after chemotherapy.[84] The solid pattern is usually found only focally and may resemble embryonal carcinoma, but the cells are smaller and less pleomorphic than those of embryonal carcinoma and tend to have nucleoli that are less prominent than those of either embryonal carcinoma or germinoma. A variant of the solid pattern is the hepatoid pattern, which closely resembles fetal liver.[85] A fourth pattern is the polyvesicular vitelline pattern, characterized by small, empty cystic structures lined by a single layer of malignant cells that merge from cuboidal to flat. The cells often are embedded in a loose, frequently myxoid stroma. Two other patterns have been described. The enteric pattern resembles the fetal human gastrointestinal tract and typically stains positively for AFP and chorionic embryonic antigen.[83,86,87] The mesenchyme-like pattern stains positively for cytokeratin and vimentin but not for AFP and has been implicated as the source of the sarcomas that occasionally occur in patients who have had a yolk sac tumor.[85] A proportion of yolk sac tumors may stain positive for the stem-cell marker CD34. In addition, the presence of immature hematopoietic foci in mediastinal yolk sac tumors of adults is associated with malignant transformation into acute myelogenous leukemia.

Germinoma

Germinomas, also termed dysgerminomas (ovary) or seminomas (testis), are the most common pure malignant germ cell tumors that occur in the ovary and central nervous system in children.[81,88] Pure seminomas represent the most common malignant germ cell tumor in men older than 20 years. However, pure seminomas are unusual in men younger than 20 years.[72] The exception is in patients with sex-chromosomal abnormalities or cryptorchidism, where tumors often present at an earlier age. Grossly, germinomas are encapsulated, solid, gray-pink tumors with a rubbery consistency and occasional small foci of hemorrhage and necrosis. Microscopically, the tumor cells are arranged in nests separated by bands of fibrous tissue in which variable numbers of lymphocytes are identified (Fig. 35.5). The cells are large, with clear cytoplasm, distinct cell membranes, and large round nuclei having one or two prominent nucleoli. Granulomas with giant cells frequently are present. Syncytiotrophoblasts may also be present, but they do not alter the prognosis of the tumor unless they are associated with cytotrophoblasts in foci of choriocarcinoma. Immunohistochemically, the germinoma cells have strong staining for placental alkaline phosphatase (PLAP) and c-kit, whereas the syncytiotrophoblasts stain for human chorionic gonadotropin beta-subunit (β-HCG). In addition, the stem-cell marker OCT-4, which stains positive in germinomas and embryonal carcinomas, has proven useful in the immunohistochemical assessment of germinomatous lesions, in particular in the differential distinction of testicular intratubular neoplasia.[11]

Embryonal Carcinoma

Embryonal carcinoma rarely occurs in a pure form in children and is more often a component of a mixed malignant germ cell tumor.[70,72] This component is seen in adolescent testicular germ cell tumors. They are characterized by large cells with large, overlapping nuclei and very large, round nucleoli (Fig. 35.6). The major pattern is epithelial and consists of large nests of cells with varying amounts of central necrosis. Pseudotubular and papillary patterns that may be confused with those of yolk sac tumors are frequent, but the cells are

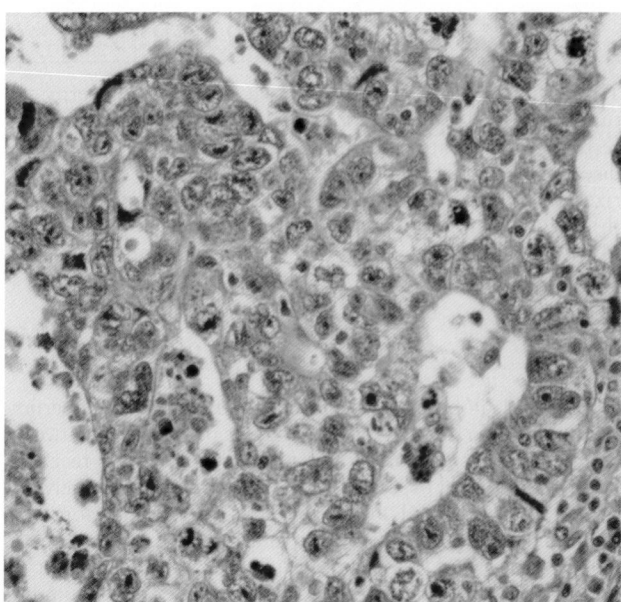

FIGURE 35.6 Embryonal carcinoma. Large, vesicular, overlapping nuclei with large prominent nucleoli and moderate amounts of eosinophilic cytoplasm are seen. Necrotic cells, typical of this histology, are present.

AFP-negative, and the tumors typically lack the eosinophilic hyaline globules characteristic of yolk sac tumors. They stain positive for OCT-4, and unlike other germ cell tumors, embryonal carcinoma is positive for CD30 by immunohistochemical staining.

Choriocarcinoma

Like embryonal carcinoma, choriocarcinoma rarely occurs outside the context of malignant mixed cell tumors in adolescents.[70,72] The rare case of pure choriocarcinoma detected in infants almost always represents metastasis from maternal or placental gestational trophoblastic primary tumor.[89] These tumors characteristically are very hemorrhagic and friable. Microscopically, two types of cells must be present to confirm the diagnosis: cytotrophoblasts, which classically appear as closely packed nests of relatively uniform, medium-sized cells having clear cytoplasm, distinct cell margins, and vesicular nuclei, and syncytiotrophoblasts, which represent multinucleate syncytial trophoblastic cells (Fig. 35.7). The syncytiotrophoblastic elements stain positively for β-HCG, accounting for the associated high concentrations of serum β-HCG in these patients.

Gonadoblastoma

Gonadoblastoma is a benign tumor found in dysgenetic gonads of phenotypic female subjects who have at least a portion of the Y chromosome. The tumors usually are small (1 to 3 cm in diameter), soft to firm, gray-tan to brown, and slightly lobulated. They are often gritty on cut sections because of the presence of multifocal calcification. Microscopic features include the proliferation of both germ cells and gonadal sex cord cells. The germ cells show positivity for PLAP and OCT-4.[70] Germinoma frequently develops with gonadoblastoma.[90] In addition, because gonadal dysgenesis may not come to clinical attention until adolescence, the presence of calcifications

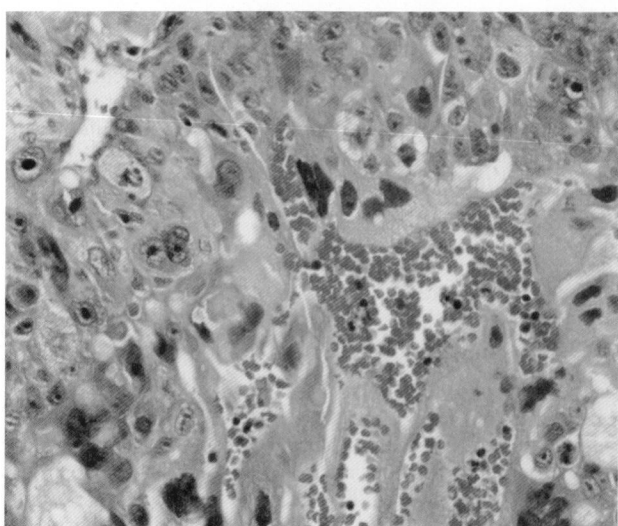

FIGURE 35.7 Choriocarcinoma. Nests of small cells with clear cytoplasm, round vesicular nuclei, and prominent nucleoli (cytotrophoblasts) are intimately associated with large, giant syncytiotrophoblasts.

within a dysgerminoma of an otherwise normal female patient suggests the prior presence of gonadoblastoma and, hence, merits evaluation of the patient for gonadal dysgenesis.

Sex Cord Stromal Tumors

Ovarian and testicular sex cord stromal tumors are a heterogeneous group of tumors developing from the gonadal nongerminative component of the ovary (granulosa, Sertoli, or Leydig cells).[91,92] According to the bisexual potential, tumors may display cellular differentiation divergent from the patient's sex or mixed histology. This phenomenon is illustrated by the term "gynandroblastoma" describing tumors with granulosa cell and Sertoli-Leydig cell differentiation. Juvenile granulosa cell tumors represent the most frequent subtype in children. Specific subtypes of sex cord stromal tumors (e.g., sex cord tumors with annular tubules) are associated with cancer predisposition syndromes such as Peutz-Jeghers syndrome.

Histologically, the diagnosis and categorization of sex cord stromal tumors may be challenging. The immunohistochemical profile shows coexpression of vimentin and cytokeratin, and most importantly, at least focal staining for inhibin. Inhibin staining may assist in differentiating juvenile granulose cell tumors from the rare small cell ovarian carcinoma of the hypercalcemic type. Histologic assessment must also include differentiation between the (rare) adult and (during childhood more frequent) juvenile granulosa cell tumor. A single somatic mutation of FOXL2 has been reported in most adult-type ovarian granulose cell tumors.[93] In addition, the description of Sertoli-Leydig cell tumors must include the grade of differentiation and an evaluation for the presence of heterologous elements such as cartilaginous or sarcomatous differentiation. The evaluation of the proliferative activity (most commonly assessed by the mitotic count) may serve as a prognostic marker.

Ovarian Small Cell Carcinoma of the Hypercalcemic Type

Due to the morphologic similarities between juvenile granulose cell tumors and ovarian small cell carcinomas of the hypercalcemic type, this differential diagnosis between these two types may be challenging. Both tumors show sheets of sometimes poorly differentiated and atypical cells with high proliferative activity and intermixed pseudofollicular structures. Differential diagnosis is aided by immunohistochemical staining, showing positive inhibin staining in juvenile granulosa cell tumors but negativity in ovarian small cell carcinoma. The clinical finding of hypercalcemia may additionally assist in the differential diagnosis.

Associated Pathologic Findings

Intratubular Germ Cell Neoplasia

Seminiferous tubules adjacent to testicular malignant germ cell tumors in adolescents and adults may show increased numbers of enlarged, atypical germ cells with abundant clear cytoplasm and prominent nucleoli. These cells show positivity for PLAP, c-kit, and OCT-4, similar to the cells of seminomas.[23,94] Such foci have been termed intratubular germ cell neoplasias and are thought to represent neoplasia *in situ*. The germ cells in the seminiferous tubules adjacent to infantile testicular malignant germ cell tumors may also be somewhat increased in number and slightly enlarged, with abundant, clear cytoplasm.[95] These cells are negative for the markers of intratubular neoplasia, OCT-4, PLAP, and c-kit, and therefore do not qualify as neoplastic precursor lesions.[23,70]

Gliomatosis Peritonei

A significant number of ovarian teratomas are associated with nodules of mature glial tissue implanted throughout the peritoneum or in lymph nodes.[96] Mature glial nodules have also been described in cervical lymph nodes in association with teratomas of the head and neck.[97] If these tissues are mature and composed only of glial tissue, this process is termed gliomatosis peritonei, and neither tumor stage nor prognosis is affected. It is not known if immature neural or other mature or immature nonneural tissues are associated with the same benign prognosis. Gliomatosis peritonei may rarely be detected in the absence of malignancy.[25] Accordingly, there is evidence that the glial tissue is reactive rather than neoplastic and does not belong to the same clonal origin as the teratoma.

CLINICAL MARKERS

The role of clinical markers in the diagnosis of germ cell tumors is well established. Their usefulness in predicting response or indicating the presence of residual or progressive disease is being examined. These markers have been categorized as follows: (a) oncofetoproteins (AFP and β-HCG); (b) cellular enzymes (lactate dehydrogenase [LDH] and PLAP); and (c) cytogenetic and molecular markers (see section "Genetics and Molecular Biology").

α-Fetoprotein (AFP)

AFP, an α-1-globulin, is the earliest and predominant serum-binding protein in the fetus, reaching its peak concentration at 12 to 14 weeks' gestation and gradually falling to reach an adult normal level of less than 10 ng/dL at approximately age 1 year.[98] As AFP levels begin to decline in fetal development, albumin becomes the principal serum-binding protein. In early embryogenesis, AFP is produced in the yolk sac and later by hepatocytes and the gastrointestinal tract. Elevated serum levels or positive immunohistochemical staining of germ cell tumors for AFP indicates the presence of malignant components, specifically yolk sac or embryonal carcinoma. The serum half-life ($t_{1/2}$) of AFP is 5 to 7 days.[99] Because of the wide variation in levels at birth, especially with infants of less than 40 weeks gestational age, and the wide variability in $t_{1/2}$ at different ages within the first year of life, difficulties arise in interpreting decay of serum AFP as an indication of residual or recurrent germ cell tumor in infants younger than 8 months. Normal ranges have been established to address these problems (Table 35.2).[100,101]

Increasing levels of serum AFP, however, are not necessarily indicative of tumor progression. Abrupt escalation in serum AFP can occur after chemotherapy-induced tumor lysis.[102] Spurious persistence of elevated serum AFP may reflect an alteration in hepatic function from such conditions as viral hepatitis (hepatitis B, hepatitis C, and human immunodeficiency virus–associated hepatitis), cholestasis secondary to anesthesia, or exposure to phenytoin or methotrexate.[102,103] Other conditions associated with elevated serum AFP include hepatoblastoma, pancreatic and gastrointestinal malignancies,

---

TABLE 35.2

NORMAL RANGES OF SERUM α-FETOPROTEIN IN INFANTS

	Wu et al.			Blohm et al.
Age	No. of patients	Mean ± SD (ng/mL)	Age	Mean (95% confidence interval)
Premature	11	134,734 ± 41,444	Premature	158,125 (31,261–799,834)
Newborn	55	48,406 ± 34,718	Newborn	41,687 (9,120–190,546)
Newborn–2 wk	16	33,113 ± 32,503	Day 8–14	9,333 (1,480–58,887)
2 wk–1 mo	12	9,452 ± 12,610	Day 15–28	1,396 (316–6,310)
2 mo	40	323 ± 278	Day 46–60	178 (16–1,995)
3 mo	5	88 ± 87	Day 61–90	80 (6–1,045)
4 mo	31	74 ± 56	Day 91–120	36 (3–417)
5 mo	6	46.5 ± 19.0	Day 120–150	20 (2–216)
6 mo	9	12.5 ± 9.8	Day 151–180	13 (1.25–129)
7 mo	5	9.7 ± 7.1		
8 mo	3	8.5 ± 5.5	Day 181–720	8 (0.8–87)

From Wu JT, Sudar K. Serum AFP levels in normal infants. Pediatr Res 1981;15:50, with permission; and Blohm MEG, Vesterling-Horner D, Calaminus G, et al. Alpha 1-fetoprotein (AFP) reference values in infants up to 2 years of age. Pediatr Hematol Oncol 1998;15(2):135–142.

lung cancers, and benign liver conditions, including hepatic dysfunction and cirrhosis.[104]

In adult germ cell tumors, AFP levels higher than 1000 µg/l are considered a poor prognostic factor[105] and the rate of decline of AFP during preoperative chemotherapy has been shown to correlate with outcome. These observations have not been confirmed in pediatric patients.

β-Subunit of Human Chorionic Gonadotropin

Human chorionic gonadotropin is a glycoprotein comprised of α- and β-peptide subunits and is normally synthesized during pregnancy by syncytiotrophoblasts of the placenta to maintain viability of the corpus luteum. The α-subunit is similar to α-peptides of other hormones, such as luteinizing hormone, follicle-stimulating hormone, and thyroid-stimulating hormone; the β-subunit is antigenically distinct, serving as the basis for the method of serum assay.[106] Minute amounts, less than 5 mIU/mL, are detected in serum of healthy adults; serum $t_{1/2}$ of β-HCG is 24 to 36 hours.

Elevation of serum β-HCG in patients with germ cell tumors implies the presence of clones of syncytiotrophoblasts, such as choriocarcinoma, or of syncytiotrophoblastic giant cells, found frequently in germinomas (pure seminomas or dysgerminomas) and occasionally in adult embryonal carcinoma. Immunoperoxidase staining of tumors for β-HCG detects these hormone-containing elements.[107]

Like serum AFP, sudden elevation of serum β-HCG occurs after cell lysis secondary to chemotherapy.[102] In adults, β-HCG levels higher than 10,000 IU/l are also associated with poor outcome, mostly related to metastatic choriocarcinoma. Iatrogenic hypogonadism secondary to bilateral orchiectomy, oophorectomy, or chemotherapy may also be associated with rising levels of serum β-HCG because of an increase in luteinizing hormone that results in immunologic cross-reactivity.[103] Other conditions in which modest elevations of serum β-HCG have been reported include multiple myeloma and other malignancies of liver, pancreas, gastrointestinal tract, breast, lung, and bladder.

Other Markers

Because some germ cell tumors with identifiable malignant elements do not produce measurable amounts of serum AFP or β-HCG, other markers with potential prognostic value have been investigated. Serum LDH, a glycolytic enzyme that appears to correlate with growth and regression of various solid neoplasms, has not shown specificity for a specific histologic subtype of germ cell tumors. In patients with dysgerminoma, serum levels of the LDH isoenzyme 1, the gene for which resides on 12p, correlate with the tumor burden and aid in the planning and assessment of surgical management.[108] However, in childhood GCTs (germ cell tumors) LDH is rarely elevated, and prognostic significance of LDH levels has not yet been demonstrated in prepubertal tumors. PLAP is a fetal isoenzyme of alkaline phosphatase that is elevated in the sera of up to 30% of patients with stage I disease and of almost 100% of cases with advanced seminoma.[109] As with AFP and β-HCG, immunohistochemical staining for PLAP sometimes is useful in determining the origin of histologically undifferentiated tumor.

Although elevated serum levels of carcinoembryonic antigen are reported in patients with ovarian tumors, the usefulness of this antigen has been hampered by lack of tumor specificity and correlation to disease natural history.[110] The carbohydrate antigen CA-125, which is related to the tissues of the coelomic epithelium and müllerian ducts, has been assessed in ovarian cancers of germ cell and epithelial origin. CA-125 has been reported to have some correlation with other tumor markers and to be of value in monitoring patients with ovarian tumors of germ cell, epithelial, and stromal origin.[111] The role of CA-19–9 is even less clear than that of CA-125.[110]

Ovarian sex cord stromal tumors may be associated with elevated levels of inhibin, a marker of steroid hormone production.

CLINICAL PRESENTATION

Ovarian Tumors

Ovarian tumors are rare, accounting for only about 1% of childhood malignancies.[112,113] The incidence increases after 8 years and peaks at 19 years. For children younger than 15 years, these tumors occur most commonly between the ages of 10 and 14.[114,115] The frequency of ovarian germ cell tumors parallels gonadotropin release, implicating hormonal factors in their etiology.[114,116] In contrast to adult ovarian tumors, two-thirds of pediatric ovarian tumors are of germ cell origin with tumors of epithelial and stromal origin occurring less frequently.[112,115,117,118]

Abdominal pain is the presenting symptom in up to 80% of patients.[114,115,119] The pain can be chronic, but may mimic an acute abdomen. Most latter cases have associated ovarian torsion and often undergo exploratory surgery for presumed acute appendicitis.[114,115] Other presenting signs and symptoms include a palpable abdominal mass, fever, constipation, amenorrhea, vaginal bleeding, and rarely frequency and dysuria.[115,120] Precocious puberty, more often associated with ovarian sex cord stromal tumors, has also been described in yolk sac tumor, choriocarcinoma, and mixed teratoma with sarcomatous and non–germ cell carcinomatous elements.[120]

Ultrasound is most often used for the initial evaluation of patients with abdominal or pelvic masses and will differentiate cystic from solid masses.[121] Although the presence of a solid ovarian mass raises the suspicion of malignancy, the majority of these will be benign teratoma.[114] Computed tomography (CT) of the abdomen and pelvis is helpful in identifying the site of origin, the extent of tumor, the presence of calcifications or fat, and metastatic disease. In a pediatric study evaluating CT for patients with ovarian masses, only 55% of children with teratomas had radiologic evidence of fat as compared with 94% of adult patients.[122] CT also appears useful in monitoring tumor response.[123] Tumor maturation, characterized radiographically by increased density, more circumscribed margins, and the presence of internal calcification with fatty areas and cystic changes, was observed and followed in seven patients with immature teratomas. At second-look surgery, all seven patients had mature teratoma without malignant elements and remained well from 1 to 6 years following treatment.

Because patients can develop metastatic disease to the thoracic lymph nodes, lung, and rarely to bone,[124,125] staging evaluation should include a chest CT, and 99mTc-pertechnetate–enhanced scintigraphy. Central nervous system metastases are rare.

Serum tumor markers AFP and β-HCG are essential because the majority of pediatric patients with ovarian germ cell tumors have a yolk sac tumor component, and mixed malignant germ cell tumors may also include significant choriocarcinoma components.[126,127]

TABLE 35.3

CHILDREN'S ONCOLOGY GROUP STAGING OF OVARIAN GERM CELL TUMORS

Stage	Extent of disease
I	Limited to ovary or ovaries; peritoneal washings negative for malignant cells No clinical, radiographic, or histologic evidence of disease beyond the ovaries Tumor markers normal after appropriate postsurgical half-life decline The presence of gliomatosis peritonei[a] does not upstage patient
II	Microscopic residual or positive lymph nodes (≤2 cm as measured by pathologist) Peritoneal washings negative for malignant cells Tumor markers positive or negative The presence of gliomatosis peritonei[a] does upstage patient
III	Lymph node with malignant metastatic nodule (>2 cm as measured by pathologist) Gross residual or biopsy only Contiguous visceral involvement (omentum, intestine, bladder) Peritoneal washings positive for malignant cells Tumor markers positive or negative
IV	Distant metastases, including liver

[a]Peritoneal nodules composed entirely of mature glial tissue and having no malignant elements.

The staging system designed by FIGO creates a framework for staging pediatric tumors.[128] Based on clinical, surgical, and pathologic findings, this system includes cytologic examination of any thoracic or peritoneal fluid. Stage I tumors are further characterized as stage Ib for bilateral tumors and stage Ic for tumors with malignant cells in peritoneal fluid or that have ruptured. A modification of this staging system (Table 35.3) was devised by the Pediatric Oncology Group (POG) and Children's Cancer Group (CCG) for intergroup studies. This surgicopathologic system refines the FIGO system by accounting for (a) the higher risk of tumor recurrence in patients with positive peritoneal washing who are therefore upstaged, (b) the utility of tumor markers for prediction of outcome, and (c) the lack of negative prognostic impact of gliomatosis peritonei if only mature glial tissue is present. In all ovarian tumors, cytologic evaluation of ascitic fluid or a peritoneal washing is mandatory. Clinical features to various ovarian tumors are summarized below.

Teratoma and Immature Teratoma

The mature cystic teratoma is the most common type of germ cell tumor and like all ovarian tumors is most common during the second decade of life. Approximately 10% of patients with teratomas have bilateral tumors[129] and, in this instance, every effort should be made to preserve fertility.[129,130] Although rare, between 1% and 3% of mature cystic teratomas present with ovarian torsion and an additional 1% to 3% can spontaneously rupture; a complication that can be fatal.[129,131] Rupture of the teratoma may be associated with two clinical pictures: acute peritonitis (sudden rupture of contents) or a granulomatous peritonitis, resulting from a chronically leaking tumor, which typically presents with multiple small peritoneal implants and adhesions. The solid teratoma is most frequently benign, although it can be associated with peritoneal implants and lymphatic spread.

An intergroup pediatric study of completely resected ovarian immature teratomas reported a median age of 10 years.[132] Thus, up to 50% of pediatric patients with ovarian immature teratoma might be premenarcheal. The most frequent complaint is abdominal pain occurring in 75% to 95% of patients and a palpable abdominal mass in 44% to 88%.[133,134] At laparotomy, the majority of tumors are unilateral, but spread beyond the ovary is documented in from 31% to 50%. Common metastatic sites include lymph nodes, liver, peritoneal surfaces, and rarely the lung.

Dysgerminoma

Dysgerminoma is the most common ovarian germ cell tumor of childhood and adolescence.[135,136] Although it can occur at any age during childhood, it is most frequent during adolescence, with a peak age at 19 years. The most common presenting signs and symptoms are similar to other ovarian tumors.[137,138] The majority of patients present with stage I disease, but the tumor can spread via the lymphatic system to the kidney and para-aortic region, and disseminate to the liver, lung, or supradiaphragmatic lymph nodes. Dysgerminoma can be bilateral in up to 20% of cases.[136]

Yolk Sac Tumor

Yolk sac tumor is the most common ovarian malignant germ cell tumor in pediatric patients and most patients have elevated levels of AFP.[126,127,139,140] The tumor can quickly spread to lymphatics and peritoneal structures, accounting for the acute onset of symptoms. Abdominal pain occurs in up to 80% of patients; 75% have abdominal masses. Distant metastases are seen in liver, lungs, lymph nodes, and rarely bone.[141]

Embryonal Carcinoma

In contrast to adult testicular tumors, embryonal carcinoma is a rare component of ovarian germ cell tumors and is most commonly seen as a component of mixed malignant germ cell tumors.[142] The median age at diagnosis is 14 years, and the most common presentation is an abdominal mass (80%) and/or abdominal pain (53%).[125] Because the tumor has multinucleated giant cells, similar to syncytiotrophoblasts (which can produce HCG), patients often present with precocious puberty, amenorrhea, or hirsutism.[141]

Choriocarcinoma

Pure ovarian choriocarcinomas are rare and most commonly a component of a mixed ovarian germ cell tumor.[142,143] The tumor typically produces β-HCG that can produce false-positive pregnancy tests and, in prepubertal patients, precocious puberty.[143] Choriocarcinomas can be either gestational or nongestational, but the diagnosis of nongestational choriocarcinoma is difficult in women of childbearing age and can only be confirmed in prepubertal patients.[143]

Choriocarcinoma is an aggressive subtype of germ cell tumor with a propensity for early metastases to lung, liver, and brain.

Malignant Mixed Germ Cell Tumor

Mixed malignant germ cell tumors comprise a subset of germ cell tumors containing more than one malignant component. Various reports suggest that 10% to 40% of patients with ovarian malignant germ cell tumors have mixed histology.[126,139] The median age at diagnosis is 16 years[124] and 40% of patients are prepubertal. Most patients present with abdominal pain, an abdominal mass, or both.[124] Approximately 30% of prepubertal patients have precocious puberty.[124]

Gonadoblastoma

Gonadoblastomas are tumors composed of germ cells intermixed with stromal cells (usually Sertoli or granulosa cells, with or without Leydig cells).[144,145] Most gonadoblastomas are small to medium sized and behave in a benign fashion unless there is overgrowth of a malignant germ cell element. Although most tumors are unilateral, up to 36% are bilateral. These neoplasms develop during the teenage years, most frequently in patients with XY gonadal dysgenesis, although a small number might occur in patients with 45, XO/46, XY mosaicism.[145,146] Patients are usually seen for evaluation of amenorrhea,[145] leading to chromosomal analysis. Patients may have a eunuchoid body habitus, elevated gonadotropin levels, the presence of streak gonads, and usually lack of secondary sexual characteristics.[145,147]

Sex Cord Stromal Tumors

Adult ovarian granulosa cell tumors are usually encountered in peri- and postmenopausal women and only about 5% occur in prepubertal girls or women younger than 30 years.[148,149] These tumors show a tendency to late relapses. Clinical presentation includes abdominal enlargement and a palpable mass. Additionally, up to 80% of prepubertal patients can have isosexual precocious puberty related to estrogen secretion.[148,149] Patients may present with bilateral tumors (5%) or disease beyond the ovary (10%). At diagnosis, hematogenous metastases to the lungs have not been reported in a total series of currently more than 100 children.

Sertoli-Leydig cell tumors are sex cord-stromal tumors exhibiting testicular direction of differentiation.[150] Approximately 75% of patients with these tumors are younger than 30 years and clinical features include evidence of androgen secretion and virilization.[151] they may present with precocious puberty and may be associated with Peutz-Jeghers syndrome.[152]

Testicular Tumors

Pediatric testicular tumors are rare, accounting for 2% of solid malignant neoplasms in boys.[153] Most present as a nontender scrotal mass but can be painful when the diagnosis is suspected torsion of the testis. The major risk factor for development of testicular tumors during childhood is the presence of an undescended testicle.[154] Considering that 10% of patients with testicular cancers are found to have undescended testicles and that the prevalence of undescended testicle is estimated at 0.23%, the theoretic risk for testicular cancer has been estimated to be 10- to 50-fold higher in boys and men with undescended testicles.[154,155]

Histologic abnormalities of germinal, tubular, or Sertoli tissue occur in 85% of undescended testicles, although only a few (<1%) are truly dysgenetic.[155] Because surgical relocation of the testes decreases the incidence of histologic anomalies, extrascrotal location appears more important than pathologic factors regarding malignant potential. The specific locale of the cryptorchid testicle does influence the risk of malignancy: The 8% to 22% of undescended testicles situated in the abdomen [156] account for approximately 45% of malignancies.[156] Typically, the histologic tumor types related to the cryptorchid testicle are seminoma and embryonal carcinoma, and presentation is typically in the fourth decade of life.[154,157]

Orchidopexy is advised on the undescended testicle after 6 months and before 18 months.[155] This earlier intervention, however, may not prevent the subsequent development of testicular germ cell tumors.[155,158]

Approximately 75% of childhood testicular tumors are of germ cell origin, as compared with more than 90% of those found in the adult population.[159] Two-thirds of the germ cell tumors are yolk sac tumors, and a smaller portion are teratomas. Rarely, a mixture of germ cell and stromal components (gonadoblastoma) is noted in a phenotypic female patient with dysgenetic gonads and male karyotype.

Almost all testicular tumors are identified as irregular, nontender scrotal masses. The paucity of associated signs or symptoms may lead to delays in evaluation for up to 6 months for germ cell tumors and 24 months for non–germ cell tumors. Although testicular tumors do not transilluminate, 20% may be associated with reactive hydroceles at the time of diagnosis.[160] Li and Fraumeni[161] reported a 21% incidence of concomitant inguinal hernias. Metastatic disease typically spreads to the lymph nodes of the retroperitoneum and chest.

Preoperative assessment of serum markers (AFP, β-HCG) is essential because it serves as the basis for staging and patient monitoring. Ultrasonography is instrumental in localizing the scrotal mass with respect to the testicle and for distinguishing a simple hydrocele from a reactive hydrocele associated with testicular tumor. Metastatic evaluation should include CT of the abdomen and pelvis to evaluate retroperitoneal lymph nodes, chest CT and bone scintigraphy with 99mTc-pertechnetate.

POG and CCG investigators developed staging criteria (Table 35.4) that account for tumor marker status and transscrotal surgical violation. Other pediatric groups, such as the German MAKEI, use the Lugano staging system for testicular tumors. Of note, the designation (stage I to IV) is not compatible between these different staging systems. Clinical features unique to the various histologic subtypes of testicular tumors are summarized below.

Teratoma and Immature Teratoma

Teratomas represent 10% of testicular neoplasms in children and occur most frequently before the age of 4 years.

TABLE 35.4

CHILDREN'S ONCOLOGY GROUP STAGING OF TESTICULAR TUMORS

Stage	Extent of disease
I	Limited to testes Completely resected by high inguinal orchiectomy or trans-scrotal orchiectomy with no spill No clinical, radiographic, or histologic evidence of disease beyond the testes Tumor markers normal after appropriate postsurgical half-life decline; patients with normal or unknown markers at diagnosis must have a negative ipsilateral retroperitoneal node dissection to confirm stage I
II	Trans-scrotal orchiectomy with gross spill of tumor Microscopic disease in scrotum or high in spermatic cord (<5 cm from proximal end) Retroperitoneal lymph node involvement (≤2 cm) Increased tumor marker after appropriate half-life
III	Retroperitoneal lymph node involvement (>2 cm) No visceral or extra-abdominal involvement
IV	Distant metastases, including liver

Approximately 15% of these tumors have poorly differentiated elements or immature neuroectodermal components. In prepubescent patients, these features do not impart an adverse prognosis, and essentially all such patients follow a benign clinical course after radical inguinal orchiectomy.[162] In contrast, postpubescent testicular teratomas are considered malignant even if these histologic features are not seen.

Yolk Sac Tumor

Yolk sac tumor is the malignant testicular tumor that occurs most frequently in children.[72–75] Synonyms include the following: endodermal sinus tumor, infantile embryonal carcinoma, orchidoblastoma, Teilum's tumor, and clear-cell adenoma.

From the perspectives of histopathology and natural history, yolk sac tumor of childhood is distinct from its adult counterpart.[72] In children, yolk sac tumor is characteristically pure or may occasionally be associated with teratoma, whereas yolk sac tumors in adults are usually components of mixed malignant components. Pediatric testicular yolk sac tumor is localized (stage I) in up to 85% of cases.

Embryonal Carcinoma

The adult-type embryonal carcinoma occurs rarely in young male individuals, usually in late adolescence or early adulthood.[73,75] Reports from POG[140] and the Pediatric Tumor Registry of Germany[75] documented a 7% incidence among 42 pediatric testicular malignant germ cell tumors. No embryonal carcinomas were noted among 61 cases of testicular cancer in the United Kingdom Children's Cancer Study Group study.[126] Symptoms include an enlarging scrotal mass, metastatic abdominal or mediastinal disease, or localized peripheral lymphadenopathy. Serum AFP and/or β-HCG may be elevated, and measurements should be obtained preoperatively.

Seminoma

The adult-type seminoma is rare in pediatric patients and is restricted to postpubertal males.

Sex Cord Stromal Tumors

Testicular sex cord stromal tumors are extraordinarily rare and develop mostly before puberty. Stromal tumors account for 10% to 30% of prepubertal testicular tumors.[163,164] Testicular sex cord stromal tumors may present with endocrinologic symptoms such as precocious puberty or gynecomastie. However, the most common presenting symptom is the detection of a painless testicular mass.

Extragonadal Tumors

Extragonadal germ cell tumors usually occur in midline sites as evidence of in vivo alteration in the complex migratory patterns of the embryonal gonads. In order of frequency, the most common locations are sacrococcygeal (Fig. 35.8), mediastinal, including pericardium, heart, and lung (Fig. 35.9), intracranial, retroperitoneal (Fig. 35.8), and uterine. Symptoms relate to the site and histology of the tumor, whether mature or immature teratoma or malignant germ cell tumor.

Sacrococcygeal Teratoma

Sacrococcygeal teratomas are the most common germ cell tumors of childhood, accounting for 40% of all, and up to 78% of extragonadal germ cell tumors.[71,74] They are also the most frequently recognized neoplasm of fetuses and neonates.[165,166] Approximately 75% of patients are female.[71,167,168] Congenital anomalies are observed in up to 18% of patients, with musculoskeletal and central nervous system defects being the most common (24% and 26%, respectively).[168] Altman et al.[71] reviewed the natural history data from 398 cases of sacrococcygeal teratoma and developed a descriptive classification that summarizes different patterns of clinical presentation due to different anatomical growth patterns. The Altman classification is not prognostic, given current multimodal treatment. The description does provide useful information for surgical planning.

Most teratomas in neonates and infants are exophytic and visible to external examination. Approximately 80% are

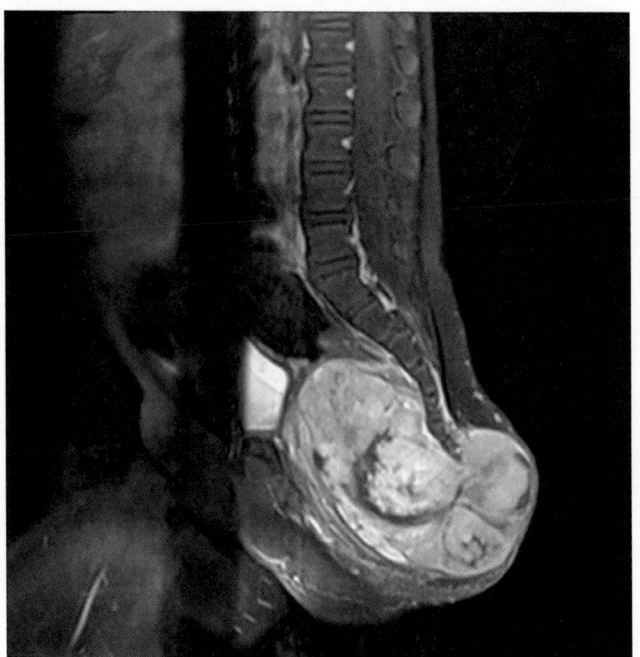

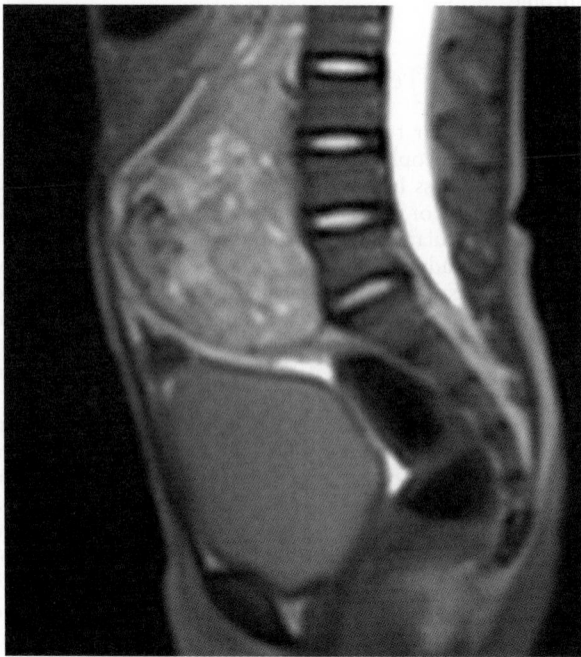

A

B

FIGURE 35.8 A: Abdominal MRI showing large sacrococcygeal teratoma with predominant yolk sac tumor histology. **B:** Abdominal MRI of retroperitoneal yolk sac tumor that is contained within pelvis.

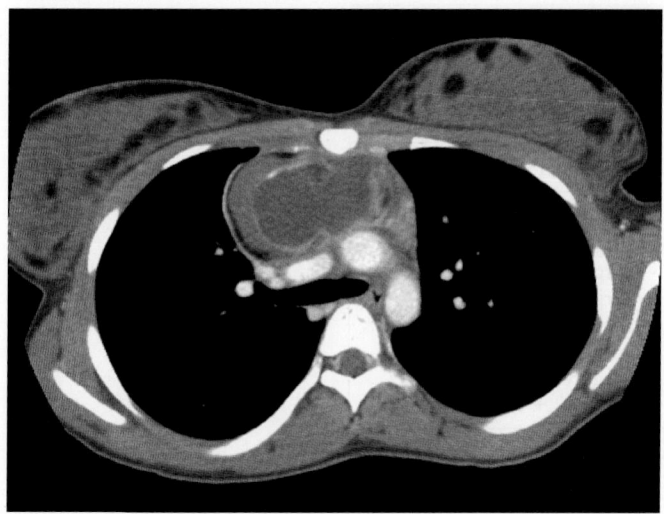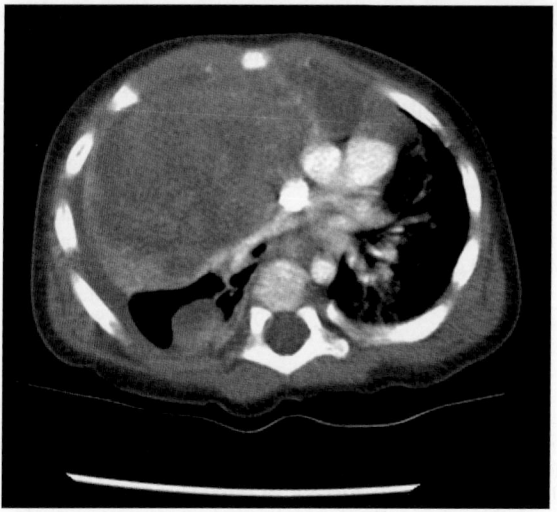

FIGURE 35.9 A: Chest CT scan with anterior mediastinal benign teratoma in a 15-year-old girl. Cystic lesions are noted. **B:** Chest CT showing a malignant mediastinal yolk sac tumor in a 4-year-old boy.

diagnosed within the first month of life. These exophytic tumors are less likely to be associated with malignant components. However, immunohistochemical analysis may detect microscopic foci of yolk sac tumor. If the tumors are resected completely, these microfoci do not affect prognosis.[79] Approximately 17% of sacrococcygeal teratomas exhibit malignant features.[71,167] The incidence of malignant components is related to surgical type (38% in type IV vs. 8% in type I), age at diagnosis, and gender but not to the size of the tumor.[71,140] A histologic grading system similar to that used for immature teratomas has been attempted in extragonadal tumors.[169,170] The German MAKEI group has applied the grading system according to Gonzalez-Crussi, and the prognostic significance of increasing immaturity has been demonstrated, in incompletely resected teratomas.[79,171] Nevertheless, it should be considered that even mature teratomas may recur, either with teratomatous or malignant yolk sac tumor histology.

Sacrococcygeal Yolk Sac Tumor

Sacrococcygeal yolk sac tumors may present as purely malignant tumors or with intermixed teratoma components. Compared with teratomas, the incidence distribution of yolk sac tumors is later, peaking at the age of 6 to 12 months. Some yolk sac tumor may present after removal of neonatal sacrococcygeal teratoma, and retrospectively, yolk sac tumor microfoci can be detected immunohistochemically in these tumors. These clinical observations illustrate the biologic relationship between sacrococcygeal teratomas and yolk sac tumors.

Mediastinal Tumors

Thoracic germ cell tumors usually (although not exclusively) are located in the anterior mediastinum,[172] and after puberty are more common in males.[173,174] Mediastinal germ cell tumors in adolescents and adults are frequently associated with Klinefelter syndrome, which tend to occur at a younger age.[20] In contrast, there is a slight female predominance in mediastinal germ cell tumors during infancy and childhood. Adolescents may be relatively asymptomatic, whereas infants and toddlers more often exhibit severe respiratory symptoms, including hemoptysis or upper airway obstruction.[175–177] During infancy and young childhood, the histologic subtypes are restricted to teratoma and yolk sac tumor. After the onset of puberty, histologic subtypes include most commonly yolk sac tumor,

germinoma, choriocarcinoma, teratoma, and immature teratoma either alone or as mixed elements.[178–182] Mediastinal teratomas occasionally have sarcomatous foci.[76] These foci are extremely aggressive, tend to overgrow the remaining teratoma, metastasize, and make treatment very difficult. Malignant germ cell tumors may also be associated with hematopoietic malignancies.[183,184] The source of these malignancies is controversial, but studies have shown that the cells in the hematopoietic malignancy have cytogenetic and molecular genetic identity and are immunohistochemically similar to pluripotential cells within the germ cell tumor rather than the host's own bone marrow cells. This evidence supports the contention that the germ cell tumor cells—and not the patient's host marrow—are the source of the second malignancy.[183,185,186] Rarely, such malignancies have been associated with gonadal tumors[70]; in most such cases, affected patients have been shown to have some form of XY gonadal dysgenesis.

Intracranial Tumors

Primary intracranial germ cell tumors may be located in the pineal gland (62%) or suprasellar region (31%), or they may span both areas (7%).[187,188] Symptomatology depends on the growth pattern and histology of the tumor and may include visual disturbances, diabetes insipidus, hypopituitarism, Parinaud syndrome (convergence nystagmus), anorexia, and precocious puberty.[189,190] Histologically, two-thirds of the tumors are germinomas, and the rest are nongerminomatous, some mixed with yolk sac tumor, choriocarcinoma, or teratocarcinoma.[188,190] Drop metastases to the spine and extracranial spread to lung and bone have been reported.[187,191]

TREATMENT OVERVIEW

An individualized, multimodality treatment plan is necessary due to the heterogeneity of pediatric germ cell tumors relative to the site of origin, age, histologic type, and stage.[3] In recent years, the timing and aggressiveness of surgery have been refined with the development of a variety of effective chemotherapeutic agents. The role of radiotherapy is established in pure germinomas, but not well studied in the treatment of other pediatric germ cell tumors. Currently, radiotherapy is not applied to extracranial GCTs in children

STANDARD TREATMENT APPROACHES FOR INFANTS AND CHILDREN YOUNGER THAN 15 YEARS WITH GERM CELL TUMORS BY HISTOLOGY, STAGE, AND PRIMARY SITE

Histology	Primary site	Stage	Treatment
Mature teratoma	All sites	Localized	Surgery + observation
Immature teratoma	All sites	Localized	Surgery + observation
Malignant germ cell tumors	Testicular	Stage I	Surgery + observation
		Stage II–IV[a]	Surgery + PEB
	Ovarian	Stage I	Surgery + observation/PEB?
		Stage II–IV	Surgery + PEB
	Extragonadal	Stage I–II	Surgery[b] + PEB
		Stage III–IV	Surgery[b] + PEB

[a]Patients ≥15 years with stage IV testicular tumors should be treated according to adult guidelines (IGCCC).
[b]The role for surgery at diagnosis for extragonadal tumors is age and site dependent and must be individualized. Depending on the clinical setting, the appropriate surgical approach may range from no surgery (e.g., mediastinal primary tumor in a patient with a compromised airway and elevated tumor markers), to biopsy, to primary resection. In some cases, an appropriate strategy is biopsy at diagnosis followed by subsequent surgery in selected patients who have residual masses following chemotherapy. All patients with stages III and IV extragonadal tumors treated with PEB have suboptimal outcome and should be considered for more intensive therapy on a clinical trial.

during first-line treatment. An outline of treatment strategies specific for site of tumor origin and histology is shown in Table 35.5. Details for specific sites and histology are described below. The establishment of clear treatment recommendations for pediatric germ cell tumors is difficult due to the inability to define widely accepted risk groups. Most pediatric trials do not contain sufficient numbers to achieve statistical power. A consensus meta-analysis has helped clarify the treatment strategy of adult patients with metastatic testicular germ cell tumors.[105] After completion of US pediatric intergroup trial, risk stratification was defined by response to therapy.[192,193] Low risk was defined by overall survival >95% with surgery, observation and salvage chemotherapy. Intermediate-risk patients had overall survival >92% and high-risk patients >84% with PEB (cisplatin, etoposide, and bleomycin).

Principles of Surgery

Surgical resection is the therapy of choice in benign tumors, such as teratomas. With malignant lesions, removal of the tumor including the organ of origin is indicated, if possible. However, given the availability of effective chemotherapy, resection should not be undertaken to the point of sacrificing vital structures. In this situation, biopsy may be appropriate and neoadjuvant chemotherapy should be administered. After initial chemotherapy, second-look surgery may help achieve complete response in selected patients. It must be emphasized that surgical recommendations may differ significantly for children and adolescents. In the United States, surgical staging of pediatric germ cell tumors has followed staging of other pediatric tumors.

Principles of Chemotherapy for Germ Cell Tumors

Substantial improvements in the cure rates for pediatric germ cell tumors have occurred. As single agents, actinomycin-D, vinblastine, bleomycin, doxorubicin, cisplatin, ifosfamide,

paclitaxel and etoposide have proved efficacious in treating germ cell tumors. Combinations of these agents demonstrating synergistic activity have served as the basis for numerous multidrug regimens. Most initial studies were conducted in adult patients. Before platinum, disease-free survival (DFS) ranged from 22% to 74%.[194] The advent of cisplatin and its incorporation into combination regimens resulted in a substantial increase in DFS, to between 68% and 92%.[195–197] Bosl et al.[196] compared a regimen of vinblastine, bleomycin, cyclophosphamide, cisplatin, and actinomycin-D to cisplatin and etoposide and reported similar rates of complete response (96% vs. 93%, respectively) and DFS (80% in both groups). Moreover, the two-drug regimen was associated with less toxicity. The improved clinical outcome in these patients suggested that the goal of future trials should be to reduce toxicity. In a randomized study of 184 patients with favorable-prognosis testicular tumors comparing outcome after three versus four courses of PEB, the rates of complete response and survival were identical, and less toxicity was observed in the short-course arm.[195] Bleomycin has played an important role in the treatment of adult testicular germ cell tumors. Pediatric studies have mirrored the adult experience. Combination chemotherapy is superior to single or dual agents, and the addition of cisplatin increased the efficacy of these regimens.[126,139,192,198–202] In the intergroup study conducted by the POG and the CCG, standard PEB was compared with a combination of high-dose cisplatin (200 mg/m^2) plus etoposide and bleomycin.[192] This regimen did differ from adult PEB treatments, because bleomycin was not administered weekly. Patients with localized gonadal germ cell tumors were treated with standard PEB.[193] All nonlocalized gonadal and all extragonadal germ cell tumors were randomized to standard PEB or a regimen with high-dose cisplatin. Although tumor control was better in high-risk patients who received high-dose cisplatin, significant toxicity appeared to limit its use. Studies conducted by the United Kingdom Children's Cancer Study Group suggest the superiority of carboplatin over standard-dose cisplatin in reducing permanent toxicity. Comparison was not made, however, to high-dose cisplatin.[199,203,204] Other groups (Germany, France, Brazil) have omitted bleomycin from first-line treatment to avoid

TABLE 35.6

CHEMOTHERAPEUTIC REGIMENS FOR PEDIATRIC GERM CELL TUMORS

Regimen	Components	Administration	Study
PVB	Cisplatin	20 mg/m^2 i.v. days 1–5	194
	Vinblastine	0.2 mg/kg i.v. days 1 and 2	
	Bleomycin	15 mg/m^2 i.v. days 2, 9, 16	
PEB	Cisplatin	20 mg/m^2 i.v. days 1–5	192
	Etoposide	100 mg/m^2 i.v. days 1–5	
	Bleomycin	15 mg/m^2 i.v. day 1	
JEB	Carboplatin	600 mg/m^2 i.v. day 1	203
	Etoposide	120 mg/m^2 i.v. days 1–3	
	Bleomycin	15 mg/m^2 i.v. day 2	
PE	Cisplatin	20 mg/m^2 i.v. days 1–5	205
	Etoposide	100 mg/m^2 i.v. days 1–5	
	Vinblastine	3 mg/m^2 i.v. day 1	
	Ifosfamide	1.5 g/m^2 i.v. days 1–5	
	Bleomycin	15 mg/m^2 i.v. day 1	
PEI	Cisplatin	20 mg/m^2 i.v. days 1–5	219
	Etoposide	100 mg/m^2 i.v. days 1–5	
	Ifosfamide	1.5 g/m^2 i.v. days 1–5	

B, bleomycin; E, etoposide; I, ifosfamide; J, carboplatin; P, cisplatin; V, vinblastine.

pulmonary toxicity. Cisplatin and etoposide (PE) were given to favorable-risk patients (Germany, Brazil) and ifosfamide was added (PEI; cisplatin, etoposide, and ifosfamide) for intermediate- or high-risk patients (Germany, France, Brazil).

The Brazilian pediatric germ cell tumor group applied a response-based strategy. Bleomycin was omitted for both intermediate- and high-risk patients. After three cycles, patients from both risk categories, who did not achieve complete response, were switched to ifosfamide, vinblastine, and bleomycin. Though the study was limited by small sample size, some patients were treated successfully without bleomycin.[205]

Specific recommendations for incorporating chemotherapy into the management of pediatric germ cell tumors are discussed separately for each tumor. The dosages and methods of administration of current regimens employed in pediatric germ cell tumors [cisplatin, vinblastine, and bleomycin (PVB); cisplatin, etoposide, and bleomycin (PEB); cisplatin, etoposide, and ifosfamide (PEI); and carboplatin, etoposide, and bleomycin (JEB)] are shown in Table 35.6.

OVARIAN TUMORS

Teratoma and Immature Teratoma

The standard treatment for mature teratomas is surgical resection. In a series of 81 ovarian teratomas (45 mature and 36 immature teratomas), three relapses of immature teratomas were observed, and one patient died after relapse. After surgery for ovarian mature teratomas, no recurrences were seen.[79] In a UK pediatric study of mature and immature teratomas, the 5-year event-free survival for ovarian mature teratomas was 97.1%.[206] Four girls with bilateral tumors were identified. Two mature and two immature teratomas were treated with bilateral oophorectomy.

Much controversy surrounds the management of immature teratoma in children. Norris et al.[133] described 58 women with ovarian immature teratoma and reported that 70% with grade 3 histology relapsed. This served as the basis of treatment recommendations that chemotherapy should be given to patients with incompletely resected grade 2 to 3 tumors.[134,207] A similar relationship of histologic grade to outcome has not been reported in pediatric patients with testicular and extragonadal immature teratomas.[162,208] In a prospective pediatric study, 44 patients with ovarian immature teratomas were treated with complete surgical resection followed by observation.[132] The 4-year event-free survival of this subset was 98% with only one patient developing recurrent tumor. On central pathologic review, 30% of these patients had microscopic foci of malignant elements, which did not appear to adversely impact outcome. It has been further demonstrated that in the case of complete resection of teratoma, the grade of immaturity and the presence of malignant microfoci do not impact on prognosis.[79] Therefore, the general recommendation is that completely resected teratomas and immature teratomas should be followed by close observation with serum tumor markers and diagnostic imaging.[77,132]

The prognostic significance of mature peritoneal implants (gliomatosis peritonei)[209] in patients with immature teratoma is uncertain. Although having peritoneal implants does not upstage the patient's disease, reports have cited malignant transformation of these elements[210] and growth during and after chemotherapy.[123,211,212] In the German MAKEI series, 12 of 36 immature teratomas were associated with gliomatosis peritonei, but only three showed progression of gliomatosis. Gliomatosis was not associated with unfavorable outcome.[79] Therefore, surgical resection of the biologically nonneoplastic lesions should be performed on an individual basis, if these lesions become clinically symptomatic.

Although there are adult reports that chemotherapy has a place in the treatment of immature teratomas,[134,207] the pediatric experience is limited. A German pediatric trial showed a recurrence rate of 18% that appeared related to the degree of resection.[79] Patients who are unable to undergo complete resection might be offered chemotherapy similar to that used for other germ cell tumors (i.e., PEB). Mann et al. reported that pediatric patients with residual or recurrent immature teratomas were treated with JEB without significant response.[206]

Dysgerminoma

Unlike other ovarian germ cell tumors, dysgerminomas were curable before the advent of effective chemotherapy, with survival rates ranging from 86% to 94% after surgery and radiotherapy.[136] Although radiotherapy produces very high cure rates, it has significant late sequelae that can be particularly severe in children who have not achieved their final adult height.[138,213] Increasing emphasis has been placed on attempts to treat patients with chemotherapy because the majority of patients with dysgerminoma present during their reproductive years and radiotherapy has the potential to cause infertility. The adult experience with this strategy confirms the chemosensitivity of this tumor.[214,215] On the basis of these data, the present recommendations are that patients with stage I dysgerminomas be observed after surgical resection. However, patients must be informed of the approximately 20% to 25% risk of recurrence, mostly in the para-aortic lymph nodes, which will require more intensive chemotherapy with generally four cycles of three-agent chemotherapy. Therefore, some authors would recommend the use of cisplatin-based therapy even in stage I patients, to reduce the risk of recurrent disease.[214] Patients with more advanced disease require four to six cycles of cisplatin-based therapy for cure.[214,215] Following this approach, sustained remissions are anticipated in 90% of patients[215,216] and up to 70% have normal menstrual function.[135]

Yolk Sac Tumor

The advent of cisplatin-based therapy for the treatment of yolk sac tumors has improved disease DFS for all stages to greater than 80%.[192,195,217] Excellent results in prepubertal girls with ovarian germ cell tumors have been reported by several groups.[218] In the US pediatric intergroup study, the surgical approach was conservative and did not include lymph node sampling. All patients were treated with PEB chemotherapy and the 6-year survival rates were: stage I 95.1%; stage II 93.8%; stage III 98.3%; and stage IV 93.3%.[192,193] However, surgical guidelines were followed in only 3/131 patients.[219] Outcomes were excellent because chemotherapy was given to all patients. In several European pediatric studies, stage I ovarian tumors were observed "watch and wait" and salvaged with chemotherapy.[220,221] Strict adherence to comprehensive staging may allow stage I patients to be treated with observation.[222]

EMBRYONAL CARCINOMA

Half the patients present with stage I embryonal carcinoma of the ovary undergo unilateral salpingo-oophorectomy only. However, the tumor may extend into peritoneal surfaces or metastasize to lymph nodes, lung, and liver.[141] After surgical resection, the survival is only 50%, suggesting the presence of micrometastases. As this tumor is rare, the data regarding the impact of chemotherapy on natural history are scant. However, based on the adult experience with testicular tumors,[223] the recommended treatment course is cisplatin-based therapy.[127]

Choriocarcinoma

Gestational choriocarcinomas are exquisitely sensitive to methotrexate[224] and are highly curable even in the presence of widespread metastases[225] In contrast, the small number of patients with nongestational choriocarcinomas may have a less favorable prognosis.[226] Such patients are usually managed as other patients with ovarian germ cell tumors.

Malignant Mixed Germ Cell Tumor

The most common histologic component is dysgerminoma, but immature teratoma, yolk sac tumor, choriocarcinoma, and embryonal carcinoma can also be detected. As with the other germ cell tumors, evaluation of tumor markers, at diagnosis, is essential, as patients with mixed germ cell tumors containing yolk sac tumor, embryonal carcinoma, choriocarcinoma, or dysgerminoma may have elevated tumor markers that are useful for diagnosis and follow-up. These patients are managed with cisplatin-based chemotherapy.

Polyembryoma

Polyembryomas are rare tumors of the ovary, often reported in combination with other neoplastic components.[227] Polyembryomas are very malignant tumors and, although not radiosensitive, have been reported to respond to chemotherapy similar to that used for other malignant germ cell tumors of the ovary.[228]

Gonadoblastoma

The management of patients with this gonadoblastoma may include prophylactic removal of their streak gonads (if present), because of the 30% risk for malignancy in patients with gonadal dysgenesis.[145] Although data are limited, chemotherapy used for other malignant germ cell tumors should be considered, depending on the malignant germ cell tumor element present and the stage of the disease.[229]

Despite the biologically benign nature of gonadoblastoma, the most challenging difficulty will be the counseling and psychosocial support of patients with female phenotype and male karyotype. These adolescent patients not only face infertility but may also develop problems with gender identity. Therefore, hormone replacement and long-term psychological support are recommended.

Sex Cord Stromal Tumors

Approximately 90% of patients with juvenile granulosa cell tumors of the ovary present with localized disease, stage I (FIGO classification), and complete resection is feasible. However, half of stage I patients may have microscopic tumor spread (stage Ic), either due to preoperative tumor rupture or malignant ascites or due to intraoperative rupture. The recurrence rate of patients with stage II and III tumors is high and, currently, cisplatin-based three-agent chemotherapy (PEI or PEB) is recommended.[148,149,230] The response to chemotherapy is associated with the mitotic activity. Tumors with more than 20 mitoses per 10 high power fields have a poorer response than those with lower mitotic index.[91,92]

The role of adjuvant chemotherapy in stage Ic tumors is controversial. According to the German series, rare relapses have been observed in stage Ic tumors with only intraoperative tumor violation, and therefore, observation is recommended.[92] In contrast, chemotherapy may be needed in stage Ic tumors with spontaneous preoperative tumor rupture or malignant ascites, the relapse rate exceeds 50%.[92] Therefore, cytologic evaluation of ascitic fluid or a peritoneal washing is mandatory in every ovarian tumor.

In the largest series of patients with Sertoli-Leydig tumors, the prognosis appears related to stage, mitotic index, and degree of differentiation.[150] Patients with well-differentiated tumors had 100% DFS compared with 41% DFS for patients with poorly differentiated tumors and 11% DFS for tumors with heterologous elements (i.e., carcinomas, sarcomas). Because these tumors are rare, controlled clinical trials are lacking and the role of adjuvant therapy has not been well studied. A recent German study suggested that chemotherapy might be beneficial for patients with advanced stage disease and high mitotic rate in the tumor.[91,92,150]

TESTICULAR TUMORS

The classic surgical approach for both diagnosis and treatment of testicular tumors is radical inguinal orchiectomy, with *en bloc* excision of spermatic cord structures and testicle. In adults, Giguere et al.[231] reported recurrence of tumor in inguinal and retroperitoneal sites in association with surgical procedures that violate the scrotum, tunica vaginalis, and tunica albuginea. Retroperitoneal lymph node dissection (RPLND) is often performed for staging of adult testicular germ cell tumors. Sufficient controversies on the management of stage I adult testicular germ cell studies still exist.[232] RPLND has not been used in pediatric trials for prepubertal boys, and the reports from the different prospective studies indicate that RPLND is not required in prepubertal germ cell tumors.[233]

Postpubertal boys with testicular germ cell tumors should be treated according to adult germ cell tumor guidelines. An adult International Germ Cell Classification System (IGCCC) has been recognized as standard risk assignment strategy for metastatic adult testicular germ cell tumor therapy and trials.[105] International pediatric groups have developed individual risk assignment strategies for pediatric patients, but no current standard exists. Data from the US intergroup trials were analyzed using the Children's Oncology Group and IGCCC criteria. Both segregated patients into nonconcordant risk groups, but neither was superior.[234]

Teratoma and Immature Teratoma

The treatment of testicular teratoma is orchiectomy. Mann et al. reported a 5-year event-free survival of 100% for both mature teratomas and immature teratomas in prepubertal boys.[206] In postpubertal boys, retroperitoneal metastatic recurrence from mature or immature teratoma has occurred, suggesting the presence of undetected microscopic malignant foci.[170] Postchemotherapy retroperitoneal lymph node resection of residual teratoma in adolescents may be necessary, given malignant transformation of testicular teratomas over 10 years.[235]

Yolk Sac Tumor

The overall survival rate for stage I YST in boys approaches 100%.[127,163,236,237] Patients are treated with orchiectomy and observation with salvage chemotherapy for recurrence. Considering that retroperitoneal lymphadenectomy identifies disease in few cases, with a significant risk of postoperative ejaculatory dysfunction, that serum AFP is elevated in 90% of patients,[238] and that three-fourths of patients are cured by orchiectomy alone,[236] the routine use of retroperitoneal lymphadenectomy in stage I prepubertal boys has been replaced with a more conservative approach.

After radical orchiectomy, patients are monitored by measurement of serum AFP and periodic evaluation of the chest and abdomen, permitting early identification of relapses and timely initiation of effective chemotherapy. Tumor recurrence after surgically managed stage I disease, is reported in retroperitoneal lymph nodes (69%) and in distant metastatic sites (15%).[193] Stage II tumor includes patients with surgical violations such as scrotal orchiectomy or biopsy, or relapse from surgically managed stage I tumor. Overall survival following chemotherapy retrieval has been excellent.[203,233] Because chemotherapy has proven effective, the need for subsequent retroperitoneal lymphadenectomy has also been challenged in prepubertal boys with stage III to IV disease and is currently limited to patients with persistent nodes after chemotherapy.[160,237,239] Children with higher stage disease require postoperative chemotherapy. Regimens containing cisplatin, vinblastine, and bleomycin have improved survival dramatically, even in patients with disseminated disease.[192,200,233] The treatment of adolescent males on pediatric trials has been limited. In the POG/CCG intergroup study, 25 males, ages 15 to 18, with stage IV testicular germ cell tumor had overall survival of 84% when treated with pediatric PEB (less bleomycin).[192] However, the small size of this cohort, the predominance of yolk sac histology, and infrequent embryonal carcinoma histology, limit conclusions in this age group.

Embryonal Carcinoma

Initial treatment consists of radical inguinal orchiectomy. On the basis of stage, various combinations of retroperitoneal lymphadenectomy, irradiation, and platinum-containing chemotherapy have been employed.

Seminoma

In the US pediatric intergroup trial, patients up to 18 years with testicular germ cell tumors were treated.[192,193] A few patients had seminoma as part of mixed tumors, but no treatment recommendations should be inferred from these scant data. Treatment of seminoma should be based on the current recommendations in adult testicular germ cell tumors.[105]

Mixed Germ Cell Tumors

Although pure yolk sac tumors are more common in males younger than 15 years, mixed malignant germ cell tumors predominate in males older than 15 years. This older group with stage IV tumors exhibits higher risk characteristics for recurrence and may benefit by more aggressive therapy.[192] In one study in adults, surveillance of stage I tumors, without initial chemotherapy, resulted in 74% with long-term disease control; this approached 90% when patients with predominant embryonal carcinoma or vascular invasion were excluded. Recurrent disease was controlled in 102 of 105 patients.[240] Reports of late recurrences indicate that 61% of metachronous tumors occur more than 5 years after the initial tumor, tending to be lower (1.4%) in patients with nonseminomatous histology.[241]

Testicular Sex Cord Stromal Tumors

The data from the US Prepubertal Testis Tumor Registry[163] and the German Childhood Tumor Registry[75] show that apart from a few Sertoli cell tumors in adolescents, virtually all testicular sex cord stromal tumors behave in a benign fashion. Most testicular sex cord stromal tumors are diagnosed as stage I tumors. Lymphatic or hematogenous metastases are usually not detected. Surgical therapy follows a high inguinal approach with early ligation of the spermatic vessels. The surgical approach has not been well studied in children.[242,243] Testis sparing surgery in specific tumors with suspected benign biology, i.e., in marker-negative tumors, is recommended. However, testis sparing surgery is only meaningful in the case of considerable remaining testicular tissue. This technique needs to be validated within prospective studies with regard to oncologic safety and testicular function, and should, therefore, certainly be restricted to specialized surgeons.

In the rare case of metastatic presentation of a testicular sex cord stromal tumor, therapy must follow an individual approach, because there are no prospectively validated data available. In general, high inguinal orchidectomy followed by chemotherapy analogous to malignant germ cell tumors is recommended. The approach is comparable to that in metastatic ovarian sex cord stromal tumors.

EXTRAGONADAL TUMORS

The POG/CCG Intergroup Study reported 80% event-free survival and 100% survival with complete resection alone in immature teratomas, all extracranial in presentation, even when microscopic foci of yolk sac tumor were present.[77] A conservative approach for extracranial teratomas, similar to that for low-stage gonadal germ cell tumors, has also been reported by the German cooperative study.[244] Marina et al. reported that multivariate Cox proportional hazards regression analysis identified age >12 years as a prognostic factor.[245] Using multivariate Cox regression analysis for survival, patients with a thoracic primary >12 years had a sixfold higher risk of death. The influence of site has also been reported by other groups.[246] Data from the German series show that mediastinal malignant nonseminomatous germ cell tumor patients >10 years of age have a worse prognosis compared with younger patients. However, the statistical significance was borderline due to small numbers.[21] A larger analysis of nongonadal germ cell tumors reported in the German studies showed a high-risk group defined by metastatic extragonadal germ cell tumors in adolescents >10 years. Of note, this difference correlates with differences in tumor biology. Prepubertal malignant germ cell tumors were yolk sac tumors, whereas other histotypes such as embryonal carcinomas and choriocarcinomas were limited to adolescent patients.

Sacrococcygeal Tumors

Sacrococcygeal Teratomas

In the case of detection of a teratoma with prenatal ultrasound, the growth velocity must be observed in regular intervals. If intrauterine tumor progression threatens fetal survival, premature delivery should be considered on an individual decision. Alternatively, intrauterine debulking may be performed (experimental), deferring definite surgery to the postnatal period.[247]

Early and complete excision of the presacral germ cell tumor has been the mainstay of successful management.[71] Preoperative establishment of the anatomic boundaries of the tumors, which are often nonencapsulated, evaluation for evidence of metastatic spread, and assessment of markers for malignancy (AFP) help adapt treatment planning for these individual risk factors. Operative principles that lead to the most successful outcome include the following: (a) sacral incision with removal of the entire coccyx; (b) early ligation of middle sacral arteries and veins; and (c) circumferential preparation of the torso and lower extremities should intraoperative changes be necessary. The sacrifice of vital organs is not indicated for benign neoplasms, and exenteration of untreated malignant lesions has not proven beneficial.

The German MAKEI series includes 132 patients with sacrococcygeal teratomas, among which 30 recurred and 4 patients died after relapse.[79] Half the recurrences presented with malignant yolk sac tumor histology. The most important risk factor for recurrence was incomplete resection. The UK pediatric study group reported 5-year event-free survival of 75% for both mature and immature sacrococcygeal teratomas.[206]

Cautious monitoring of patients with sacrococcygeal teratomas is required, because malignant germ cell tumors are well recognized to recur either from unnoticed malignant elements in the original tumor or from malignant transformation in residual tissue.[248-250] Until recently, only a 10% salvage rate for malignant lesions was expected. With the recognition that excision of primary malignant lesions alone has cured few

patients, the addition of chemotherapy, particularly platinum-containing regimens addressing the specific malignant element, has improved survival.[251,252] However, two long-term longitudinal national studies report significant problem with bowel and urinary incontinence and quality of life issues after surgery for sacrococcygeal teratoma as a child.[253,254]

Sacrococcygeal Yolk Sac Tumors

The therapy of sacrococcygeal yolk sac tumors is hampered by the close anatomical relation to the spinal canal, the sacral plexus, and the small pelvis. Therefore, attempt at complete resection at diagnosis may often fail, in particular in tumors with significant intrapelvic extension. The completeness of resection constitutes the most important prognostic factor.[255] Local control is essential, even in metastatic tumors. Neoadjuvant chemotherapy is an option in large sacrococcygeal tumors considered unsuitable for complete resection, based on initial imaging with MRI. In these patients, diagnosis may be established based on imaging and tumor markers.[256] Ideally, a biopsy should be obtained prior to chemotherapy, to support the diagnosis and facilitate biologic research.

In a study of 66 patients with sacrococcygeal yolk sac tumors including 30 metastatic tumors from the German MAKEI series treated between 1983 and 1995, event-free survival and overall survival were 76% and 81%, respectively.[255] Patients with locally advanced and metastatic disease had significantly better outcomes after neoadjuvant chemotherapy compared with initial surgery and adjuvant chemotherapy (83% vs. 45%). This difference can be explained by the higher rate of complete resections after neoadjuvant chemotherapy. The UK study supports these high cure rates, showing an event-free survival of 86% in 37 patients treated with JEB, including 24 malignant teratomas and 14 yolk sac tumors.[203] The recent analysis of the US Intergroup trial showed that dose intensification of cisplatin may further increase 6-year overall survival (81%) in stage III/IV extragonadal germ cell tumors.[192] However, an unacceptably high rate of ototoxicity was found.

Mediastinal Tumors

Data from pediatric studies suggest that, although this site is considered less favorable, treatment with platinum-based regimens improved event-free survival (57% to 88%).[199,201,202] Resection of the tumor, either at onset or as postinduction surgery, improved overall survival.[202,257] Despite encouraging data for mediastinal germ cell tumors in prepubertal children, mediastinal malignant germ cell tumors in adolescents and adults constitute the most prognostically unfavorable subgroup of germ cell tumors, with an overall survival less than 50%. A more intensive approach (even investigational) may be required in these patients to overcome the intrinsic treatment resistance in these tumors.

Intracranial Tumors

In the different national and international study groups, there are divergent diagnostic and therapeutic approaches to CNS germ cell tumors, described in detail in the section on CNS tumors. Diagnosis may be established on the basis of characteristic imaging and elevated tumor markers AFP and β-HCG in the serum and cerebrospinal fluid. In marker-negative tumors, initial management should include attempts to obtain a biopsy or to resect the primary tumor if this is possible without sequelae. Germinomas traditionally have been treated with radiotherapy. There are data that some of these tumors can be managed with a carboplatin-based chemotherapeutic regimen and restricted irradiation.[258] In contrast, all secreting tumors (yolk sac tumor, choriocarcinomas, and embryonal carcinomas) are treated with three-agent cisplatin-based chemotherapy (e.g., PEI in the SIOP CNS GCT study) followed by resection and radiation. Radiation is restricted to local in nonmetastatic tumors and craniospinal irradiation in the case of micro- or macroscopic metastasis.[259] The treatment of CNS teratomas is still controversial and is mainly based on surgical resection, potentially supported by chemotherapy and irradiation at high doses.

Tumors at Other Sites

Recent reports from the Intergroup study detail clinical presentation, surgical approach, and outcome in the retroperitoneal/abdominal[260] and genital[261] primary sites. Young and Scully[262] have previously studied tumors arising in the vaginal site; these germ cell tumors are exclusively yolk sac tumors, mostly without associated teratoma. They are characterized by an exquisite responsiveness to cisplatin-based chemotherapy. Therefore, the most important initial step is to establish diagnosis without performing extensive surgery, either based on radiographic imaging and tumor markers (AFP) or biopsy. With neoadjuvant chemotherapy, mutilating surgery may be avoided in many patients, with excellent survival rates approaching 100%.[205,263]

The orbit is another rare site of origin.[264,265] Although metastatic bone disease is infrequent, it has been reported in 3% of adult patients with newly diagnosed disease and in 9% of those with relapses. Other tumors, mostly teratomas in neonates and infants, present at the head-and-neck region. Clinically and radiographically, these may be misinterpreted as lymphangiomas. Although tumors at this site may present with dramatic extension, sometimes resulting in life-threatening upper airway obstruction at birth, the overall prognosis is favorable, both with regard to cure rates and to long-term quality of life.[266]

SALVAGE STRATEGIES

Most salvage data for patients with recurrent or persistent malignant germ cell tumors come from trials in adult patients. Motzer et al. reported a complete response rate of 77% with a 70% durable response with paclitaxel, ifosfamide, and cisplatin in patients who relapsed after cisplatin therapy.[267] The role of autologous marrow transplantation for relapsed or refractory malignant germ cell tumors has been studied in adult patients. In a retrospective review, relapsed patients treated with tandem high-dose chemotherapy and stem-cell rescue had approximately a 60% durable survival.[268] Other studies support a dose-intensified regimen with dose escalation of ifosfamide and etoposide or high-dose carboplatin, etoposide followed by autologous stem-cell transplantation.[269] The importance of retroperitoneal lymph node dissection postchemotherapy has been reported.[235,270] The prospective assessment of salvage therapies in recurrent or refractory pediatric germ cell tumors is limited by the small numbers of patients. In contrast to adult patients, who frequently present with disseminated relapse, the majority of children with recurrent tumors will have local relapses. Therefore, intensive local therapy, preferably a complete surgical resection, constitutes the mainstay of salvage therapy.[256] Neoadjuvant chemotherapy may facilitate complete resection, which should be attempted in specialized pediatric surgical centers. If local

control is insufficient, local irradiation with at least 45 Gy may be considered postoperatively.[256] The German MAKEI study has reported favorable response to PEI chemotherapy supported with locoregional hyperthermia in localized relapses, in particular in sacrococcygeal germ cell tumors. This combination has resulted in excellent local control facilitating complete resection on delayed surgery of the recurrence and good long-term outcome.[256,271]

Tumor recurrence must be distinguished from metachronous germ cell tumors, which may develop in the contralateral gonad.[272] The risk of syn- or metachronous bilateral gonadal tumors is approximately 5%, and the prognosis of metachronous tumors is comparable to that of the first tumor.

TOXICITY AND LATE EFFECTS

The use of cisplatin therapy has led to excellent improvement in survival but at the cost of significant toxicity and late effects. In the POG/CCG intergroup germ cell tumor trial, severe hearing loss was more pronounced in patients treated with high-dose cisplatin.[192] This study also highlighted the problem of standard ototoxicity reporting. When individual audiograms were examined by an independent skilled investigator, higher toxicity was seen with both standard and high-dose cisplatin.[273] Amifostine, which had been reported to protect patients from cisplatin toxicity, was studied with high-dose cisplatin. Patients with stage III/IV extragonadal germ cell tumors had event-free survival and overall survival of approximately 85%, but amifostine did not reduce grade 3 to 4 ototoxicity of 75%.[274] It is known that young children are particularly sensitive to toxic effects of cisplatin. It is clear that ototoxicity in younger children is under reported. Ototoxicity in a young child may lead to impaired academic and social development.[275] Data from an adult study suggest that cisplatin ototoxicity may be associated with specific glutathione S-transferase genotypes.[276] In addition, cisplatin ototoxicity is associated with genetic polymorphism of the megalin gene,[277] providing a diagnostic tool of assessing the risk of ototoxicity prospectively. This has not been studied in children, but perhaps, in the future we can identify those children who are at greatest risk for ototoxicity and adapt our treatment strategy.

In addition, cisplatin may be associated with nephrotoxicity that may be further enhanced by concurrent ifosfamide. The risk of pulmonary toxicity of bleomycin in toddlers and infants is controversial. In adult germ cell tumors, there are reports on an increased risk of cardiovascular disease, including atherosclerosis and coronary disease. However, there are no comparable long-term follow-up data available for patients treated for a germ cell tumor during childhood.

The risk of secondary neoplasms such as therapy-related acute myelogenous leukemias has been debated intensively, both for adult and pediatric patients treated with etoposide. According to the MAKEI series, the 10-year cumulative risk of secondary leukemia can be estimated to be approximately 1% in patients treated with chemotherapy alone and 4.2% in patients treated with both radio- and chemotherapy.[185] In the US pediatric intergroup study, there were four cases of acute myelocytic leukemia. None were associated with 11q23 abnormality.[192,193]

FUTURE CONSIDERATIONS

During the last decade, progress in understanding the biology and behavior of germ cell tumors of children has been substantial. The Intergroup studies (POG/CCG) in the United States and the ongoing trials in Europe, the United Kingdom, and Brazil demonstrate clearly that the next challenge will be to tailor specific therapy for these diverse tumors through the use of risk groupings. Although improving the numbers of children who become long-term survivors, higher doses of cisplatin cause ototoxicity, especially in young children.[192] Future emphasis needs to be directed at developing less toxic chemotherapy, specific chemoprotective agents, and retrieval therapies.

References

1. Ries LAG SM, Gurney JG, Linet M, et al., eds. Cancer Incidence and Survival among Children and Adolescents: United States SEER Program 1975–1995, National Cancer Institute, SEER Program. NIH Publication No. 99–4649. Bethesda, MD: National Cancer Institute, 1999.
2. Kaatsch P. German Childhood Cancer Registry and its favorable setting. Bundesgesundheitsblatt Gesundheitsforschung Gesundheitsschutz 2004;47(5):437–443.
3. Schneider DT, Calaminus G, Koch S, et al. Epidemiologic analysis of 1,442 children and adolescents registered in the German germ cell tumor protocols. Pediatr Blood Cancer. 2004;42(2):169–175.
4. Thomson JA, Itskovitz-Eldor J, Shapiro SS, et al. Embryonic stem cell lines derived from human blastocysts. Science 1998;282(5391):1145–1147.
5. Draper JS, Smith K, Gokhale P, et al. Recurrent gain of chromosomes 17q and 12 in cultured human embryonic stem cells. Nat Biotechnol 2004;22(1):53–54.
6. Schneider DT, Schuster AE, Fritsch MK, et al. Multipoint imprinting analysis indicates a common precursor cell for gonadal and nongonadal pediatric germ cell tumors. Cancer Res 2001;61(19):7268–7276.
7. Bussey KJ, Lawce HJ, Himoe E, et al. SNRPN methylation patterns in germ cell tumors as a reflection of primordial germ cell development. Genes Chromosomes Cancer 2001;32(4):342–352.
8. Sievers S, Alemazkour K, Zahn S, et al. IGF2/H19 imprinting analysis of human germ cell tumors (GCTs) using the methylation-sensitive single-nucleotide primer extension method reflects the origin of GCTs in different stages of primordial germ cell development. Genes Chromosomes Cancer 2005;44(3):256–264.
9. Jirasek JE. Morphogenesis of the genital system in the human. Birth Defects Orig Artic Ser 1977;13(2):13–39.
10. Strohmeyer T, Reese D, Press M, et al. Expression of the c-kit proto-oncogene and its ligand stem cell factor (SCF) in normal and malignant human testicular tissue. J Urol 1995;153(2):511–515.
11. Looijenga LH, Stoop H, de Leeuw HP, et al. POU5F1 (OCT3/4) identifies cells with pluripotent potential in human germ cell tumors. Cancer Res 2003;63(9):2244–2250.
12. Doitsidou M, Reichman-Fried M, Stebler J, et al. Guidance of primordial germ cell migration by the chemokine SDF-1. Cell 2002;111(5):647–659.
13. Molyneaux KA, Zinszner H, Kunwar PS, et al. The chemokine SDF1/CXCL12 and its receptor CXCR4 regulate mouse germ cell migration and survival. Development 2003;130(18):4279–4286.
14. Gonzalez-Crussi F. Extragonadal teratomas. Atlas of tumor pathology, 2nd series, fascicle 18. Washington, DC: Armed Forces Institute of Pathology, 1982.
15. O'Rahilly R. The timing and sequence of events in the development of the human reproductive system during the embryonic period proper. Anat Embryol (Berl) 1983; 166(2):247–261.
16. Stevens LC. The biology of teratomas including evidence indicating their origin form primordial germ cells. Annee Biol 1962;1:585–610.
17. Shankar S, Davies S, Giller R, et al. In utero exposure to female hormones and germ cell tumors in children. Cancer 2006;106(5):1169–1177.
18. Czene K, Lichtenstein P, Hemminki K. Environmental and heritable causes of cancer among 9.6 million individuals in the Swedish Family-Cancer Database. Int J Cancer 2002;99(2):260–266.
19. Rutgers JL, Scully RE. Pathology of the testis in intersex syndromes. Semin Diagn Pathol 1987;4(4):275–291.
20. Nichols CR, Heerema NA, Palmer C, et al. Klinefelter's syndrome associated with mediastinal germ cell neoplasms. J Clin Oncol 1987;5(8):1290–1294.
21. Schneider DT, Schuster AE, Fritsch MK, et al. Genetic analysis of mediastinal nonseminomatous germ cell tumors in children and adolescents. Genes Chromosomes Cancer 2002;34(1):115–125.
22. Palmer RD, Foster NA, Vowler SL, et al. Malignant germ cell tumours of childhood: new associations of genomic imbalance. Br J Cancer. 2007;96(4):667–676.
23. Jorgensen N, Rajpert-De Meyts E, Graem N, et al. Expression of immunohistochemical markers for testicular carcinoma in situ by normal human fetal germ cells. Lab Invest 1995;72(2):223–231.
24. Oosterhuis JW, Castedo SM, de Jong B, et al. Ploidy of primary germ cell tumors of the testis. Pathogenetic and clinical relevance. Lab Invest. 1989;60(1):14–21.
25. Harms D, Zahn S, Gobel U, et al. Pathology and molecular biology of teratomas in childhood and adolescence. Klin Padiatr 2006;218(6):296–302.
26. de Jong B, Oosterhuis JW, Castedo SM, et al. Pathogenesis of adult testicular germ cell tumors. A cytogenetic model. Cancer Genet Cytogenet 1990;48(2):143–167.
27. Rodriguez E, Houldsworth J, Reuter VE, et al. Molecular cytogenetic analysis of i(12p)-negative human male germ cell tumors. Genes Chromosomes Cancer 1993;8(4): 230–236.
28. Looijenga LH, Gillis AJ, Van Putten WL, et al. In situ numeric analysis of centromeric regions of chromosomes 1, 12, and 15 of seminomas, nonseminomatous germ cell tumors, and carcinoma in situ of human testis. Lab Invest 1993;68(2):211–219.
29. Murty VV, Houldsworth J, Baldwin S, et al. Allelic deletions in the long arm of chromosome 12 identify sites of candidate tumor suppressor genes in male germ cell tumors. Proc Natl Acad Sci U S A 1992;89(22):11006–11010.
30. Mostert MM, van de Pol M, Olde Weghuis D, et al. Comparative genomic hybridization of germ cell tumors of the adult testis: confirmation of karyotypic findings and identification of a 12p-amplicon. Cancer Genet Cytogenet 1996;89(2):146–152.
31. Mathew S, Murty VV, Bosl GJ, et al. Loss of heterozygosity identifies multiple sites of allelic deletions on chromosome 1 in human male germ cell tumors. Cancer Res 1994;54(23):6265–6269.
32. Ganguly S, Murty VV, Samaniego F, et al. Detection of preferential NRAS mutations in human male germ cell tumors by the polymerase chain reaction. Genes Chromosomes Cancer 1990;1(3):228–232.
33. Shuin T, Misaki H, Kubota Y, et al. Differential expression of protooncogenes in human germ cell tumors of the testis. Cancer 1994;73(6):1721–1727.
34. Heimdal K, Lothe RA, Lystad S, et al. No germline TP53 mutations detected in familial and bilateral testicular cancer. Genes Chromosomes Cancer 1993;6(2):92–97.
35. Lothe RA, Hastie N, Heimdal K, et al. Frequent loss of 11p13 and 11p15 loci in male germ cell tumours. Genes Chromosomes Cancer 1993;7(2):96–101.
36. Lothe RA, Fossa SD, Stenwig AE, et al. Loss of 3p or 11p alleles is associated with testicular cancer tumors. Genomics 1989;5(1):134–138.
37. Murty VV, Li RG, Houldsworth J, et al. Frequent allelic deletions and loss of expression characterize the DCC gene in male germ cell tumors. Oncogene 1994;9(11): 3227–3231.
38. Murty VV, Bosl GJ, Houldsworth J, et al. Allelic loss and somatic differentiation in human male germ cell tumors. Oncogene 1994;9(8):2245–2251.
39. van Gurp RJ, Oosterhuis JW, Kalscheuer V, et al. Biallelic expression of the H19 and IGF2 genes in human testicular germ cell tumors. J Natl Cancer Inst 1994;86(14): 1070–1075.
40. McIntyre A, Gilbert D, Goddard N, et al. Genes, chromosomes and the development of testicular germ cell tumors of adolescents and adults. Genes Chromosomes Cancer 2008;47(7):547–557.
41. Surti U, Hoffner L, Chakravarti A, et al. Genetics and biology of human ovarian teratomas. I. Cytogenetic analysis and mechanism of origin. Am J Hum Genet 1990;47(4): 635–643.
42. Linder D, McCaw BK, Hecht F. Parthenogenic origin of benign ovarian teratomas. N Engl J Med 1975;292(2):63–66.
43. Miura K, Obama M, Yun K, et al. Methylation imprinting of H19 and SNRPN genes in human benign ovarian teratomas. Am J Hum Genet 1999;65(5):1359–1367.
44. Mutter GL. Teratoma genetics and stem cells: a review. Obstet Gynecol Surv 1987; 42(11):661–670.
45. Ohama K, Nomura K, Okamoto E, et al. Origin of immature teratoma of the ovary. Am J Obstet Gynecol 1985;152(7, pt 1):896–900.
46. Gibas Z, Talerman A, Faruqi S, et al. Cytogenetic analysis of an immature teratoma of the ovary and its metastasis after chemotherapy-induced maturation. Int J Gynecol Pathol 1993;12(3):276–280.
47. Speleman F, De Potter C, Dal Cin P, et al. i(12p) in a malignant ovarian tumor. Cancer Genet Cytogenet 1990;45(1):49–53.
48. Hoffner L, Deka R, Chakravarti A, et al. Cytogenetics and origins of pediatric germ cell tumors. Cancer Genet Cytogenet 1994;74(1):54–58.
49. Riopel MA, Spellerberg A, Griffin CA, et al. Genetic analysis of ovarian germ cell tumors by comparative genomic hybridization. Cancer Res 1998;58(14):3105–3110.
50. Inoue M, Fujita M, Azuma C, et al. Histogenetic analysis of ovarian germ cell tumors by DNA fingerprinting. Cancer Res 1992;52(24):6823–6826.
51. Falin LI. The development of genital glands and the origin of germ cells in human embryogenesis. Acta Anat (Basel) 1969;72(2):195–232.
52. Upadhyay S, Zamboni L. Ectopic germ cells: natural model for the study of germ cell sexual differentiation. Proc Natl Acad Sci U S A 1982;79(21):6584–6588.
53. Zamboni L, Upadhyay S. Germ cell differentiation in mouse adrenal glands. J Exp Zool 1983;228(2):173–193.
54. Kaplan CG, Askin FB, Benirschke K. Cytogenetics of extragonadal tumors. Teratology 1979;19(2):261–266.
55. Mann BD, Sparkes RS, Kern DH, et al. Chromosomal abnormalities of a mediastinal embryonal cell carcinoma in a patient with 47,XXY Klinefelter syndrome: evidence for the premeiotic origin of a germ cell tumor. Cancer Genet Cytogenet 1983;8(3): 191–196.
56. Casalone R, Righi R, Granata P, et al. Cerebral germ cell tumor and XXY karyotype. Cancer Genet Cytogenet 1994;74(1):25–29.
57. Yu IT, Griffin CA, Phillips PC, et al. Numerical sex chromosomal abnormalities in pineal teratomas by cytogenetic analysis and fluorescence in situ hybridization. Lab Invest 1995;72(4):419–423.
58. de Bruin TW, Slater RM, Defferrari R, et al. Isochromosome 12p-positive pineal germ cell tumor. Cancer Res 1994;54(6):1542–1544.
59. Oosterhuis JW, Rammeloo RH, Cornelisse CJ, et al. Ploidy of malignant mediastinal germ-cell tumors. Hum Pathol 1990;21(7):729–732.
60. Dal Cin P, Drochmans A, Moerman P, et al. Isochromosome 12p in mediastinal germ cell tumor. Cancer Genet Cytogenet 1989;42(2):243–251.
61. Oosterhuis JW, van den Berg E, de Jong B, et al. Mediastinal germ cell tumor with secondary nongerm cell malignancy, and extensive hematopoietic activity. Pathology, DNA-ploidy, and karyotyping. Cancer Genet Cytogenet 1991;54(2):183–195.
62. Ladanyi M, Samaniego F, Reuter VE, et al. Cytogenetic and immunohistochemical evidence for the germ cell origin of a subset of acute leukemias associated with mediastinal germ cell tumors. J Natl Cancer Inst 1990;82(3):221–227.
63. Bussey KJ, Lawce HJ, Olson SB, et al. Chromosome abnormalities of eighty-one pediatric germ cell tumors: sex-, age-, site-, and histopathology-related differences–a Children's Cancer Group study. Genes Chromosomes Cancer 1999;25(2):134–146.
64. Perlman EJ, Cushing B, Hawkins E, et al. Cytogenetic analysis of childhood endodermal sinus tumors: a Pediatric Oncology Group study. Pediatr Pathol 1994;14(4): 695–708.
65. Oosterhuis JW, Castedo SM, de Jong B, et al. Karyotyping and DNA flow cytometry of an orchidoblastoma. Cancer Genet Cytogenet 1988;36(1):7–11.
66. Stock C, Ambros IM, Lion T, et al. Detection of numerical and structural chromosome abnormalities in pediatric germ cell tumors by means of interphase cytogenetics. Genes Chromosomes Cancer 1994;11(1):40–50.
67. Zahn S, Sievers S, Alemazkour K, et al. Imbalances of chromosome arm 1p in pediatric and adult germ cell tumors are caused by true allelic loss: a combined comparative genomic hybridization and microsatellite analysis. Genes Chromosomes Cancer 2006; 45(11):995–1006.

68. Perlman EJ, Hu J, Ho D, et al. Genetic analysis of childhood endodermal sinus tumors by comparative genomic hybridization. J Pediatr Hematol Oncol 2000;22(2):100–105.
69. Palmer RD, Barbosa-Morais NL, Gooding EL, et al. Pediatric malignant germ cell tumors show characteristic transcriptome profiles. Cancer Res 2008;68(11):4239–4247.
70. Hawkins E, Perlman EJ. Germ cell tumors in childhood: morphology and biology. In: Parham DM, ed. Pediatric neoplasia: morphology and biology. New York: Raven Press, 1996:297.
71. Altman RP, Randolph JG, Lilly JR. Sacrococcygeal teratoma: American Academy of Pediatrics Surgical Section Survey-1973. J Pediatr Surg 1974;9(3):389–398.
72. Young R, Scully R. Germ cell tumors: nonseminomatous tumors, occult tumors, effects of chemotherapy in testicular tumors. Chicago: ASCP Press, 1990.
73. Hawkins EP. Pathology of germ cell tumors in children. Crit Rev Oncol Hematol 1990; 10(2):165–179.
74. Dehner LP. Gonadal and extragonadal germ cell neoplasms: teratomas in childhood. In: Finegold MJ, Bennington J, ed. Pathology of neoplasia in children and adolescents. Philadelphia, PA: WB Saunders, 1986:282.
75. Harms D, Janig U. Germ cell tumours of childhood. Report of 170 cases including 59 pure and partial yolk-sac tumours. Virchows Arch A Pathol Anat Histopathol 1986; 409(2):223–239.
76. Dehner LP. Germ cell tumors of the mediastinum. Semin Diagn Pathol 1990;7(4): 266–284.
77. Marina NM, Cushing B, Giller R, et al. Complete surgical excision is effective treatment for children with immature teratomas with or without malignant elements: A Pediatric Oncology Group/Children's Cancer Group Intergroup Study. J Clin Oncol 1999;17(7):2137–2143.
78. Thurlbeck WM, Scully RE. Solid teratoma of the ovary. A clinicopathological analysis of 9 cases. Cancer 1960;13:804–811.
79. Gobel U, Calaminus G, Engert J, et al. Teratomas in infancy and childhood. Med Pediatr Oncol 1998;31(1):8–15.
80. Schropp KP, Lobe TE, Rao B, et al. Sacrococcygeal teratoma: the experience of four decades. J Pediatr Surg 1992;27(8):1075–1078; discussion 1078–1079.
81. Ho DM, Liu HC. Primary intracranial germ cell tumor. Pathologic study of 51 patients. Cancer 1992;70(6):1577–1584.
82. Ulbright TM, Roth LM, Brodhecker CA. Yolk sac differentiation in germ cell tumors. A morphologic study of 50 cases with emphasis on hepatic, enteric, and parietal yolk sac features. Am J Surg Pathol 1986;10(3):151–164.
83. Ulbright TM, Roth LM. Recent developments in the pathology of germ cell tumors. Semin Diagn Pathol 1987;4(4):304–319.
84. Ulbright TM, Michael H, Loehrer PJ, et al. Spindle cell tumors resected from male patients with germ cell tumors. A clinicopathologic study of 14 cases. Cancer 1990; 65(1):148–156.
85. Nakashima N, Fukatsu T, Nagasaka T, et al. The frequency and histology of hepatic tissue in germ cell tumors. Am J Surg Pathol 1987;11(9):682–692.
86. Clement PB, Young RH, Scully RE. Endometrioid-like variant of ovarian yolk sac tumor. A clinicopathological analysis of eight cases. Am J Surg Pathol 1987;11(10): 767–778.
87. Cohen MB, Friend DS, Molnar JJ, et al. Gonadal endodermal sinus (yolk sac) tumor with pure intestinal differentiation: a new histologic type. Pathol Res Pract 1987; 182(5):609–616.
88. Talerman A. Germ cell tumors of the ovary. In: Kurman RJ, ed. Blaustein's pathology of female genital tract. 3rd ed. New York: Springer-Verlag, 1987:659.
89. Belchis DA, Mowry J, Davis JH. Infantile choriocarcinoma. Re-examination of a potentially curable entity. Cancer 1993;72(6):2028–2032.
90. Scully RE. Gonadoblastoma. A review of 74 cases. Cancer 1970;25(6):1340–1356.
91. Schneider DT, Calaminus G, Wessalowski R, et al. Ovarian sex cord-stromal tumors in children and adolescents. J Clin Oncol 2003;21(12):2357–2363.
92. Schneider DT, Calaminus G, Harms D, et al. Ovarian sex cord-stromal tumors in children and adolescents. J Reprod Med 2005;50(6):439–446.
93. Shah SP, Kobel M, Senz J, et al. Mutation of FOXL2 in granulosa-cell tumors of the ovary. N Engl J Med 2009;360(26):2719–2729.
94. Burke AP, Mostofi FK. Placental alkaline phosphatase immunohistochemistry of intratubular malignant germ cells and associated testicular germ cell tumors. Hum Pathol 1988;19(6):663–670.
95. Manivel JC, Reinberg Y, Niehans GA, et al. Intratubular germ cell neoplasia in testicular teratomas and epidermoid cysts. Correlation with prognosis and possible biologic significance. Cancer 1989;64(3):715–720.
96. Harms D, Janig U, Gobel U. Gliomatosis peritonei in childhood and adolescence. Clinicopathological study of 13 cases including immunohistochemical findings. Pathol Res Pract 1989;184(4):422–430.
97. Dehner LP, Mills A, Talerman A, et al. Germ cell neoplasms of head and neck soft tissues: a pathologic spectrum of teratomatous and endodermal sinus tumors. Hum Pathol 1990;21(3):309–318.
98. Gitlin D, Perricelli A, Gitlin GM. Synthesis of fetoprotein by liver, yolk sac, and gastrointestinal tract of the human conceptus. Cancer Res 1972;32(5):979–982.
99. Lange PH, Vogelzang NJ, Goldman A, et al. Marker half-life analysis as a prognostic tool in testicular cancer. J Urol 1982;128(4):708–711.
100. Wu JT, Book L, Sudar K. Serum alpha fetoprotein (AFP) levels in normal infants. Pediatr Res 1981;15(1):50–52.
101. Blohm ME, Vesterling-Horner D, Calaminus G, et al. Alpha 1-fetoprotein (AFP) reference values in infants up to 2 years of age. Pediatr Hematol Oncol 1998;15(2): 135–142.
102. Vogelzang NJ, Lange PH, Goldman A, et al. Acute changes of alpha-fetoprotein and human chorionic gonadotropin during induction chemotherapy of germ cell tumors. Cancer Res 1982;42(11):4855–4861.
103. Germa JR, Llanos M, Tabernero JM, et al. False elevations of alpha-fetoprotein associated with liver dysfunction in germ cell tumors. Cancer 1993;72(8):2491–2494.
104. Bloomer JR, Waldmann TA, McIntire KR, et al. Serum alpha-fetoprotein in patients with massive hepatic necrosis. Gastroenterology 1977;72(3):479–492.
105. Group IGCCC. International germ cell consensus classification: a prognostic factor-based staging system for metastatic germ cell cancers. J Clin Oncol 1997;15(2): 594–603.
106. Vaitukaitis JL, Braunstein GD, Ross GT. A radioimmunoassay which specifically measures human chorionic gonadotropin in the presence of human luteinizing hormone. Am J Obstet Gynecol 1972;113(6):751–758.
107. Morinaga S, Ojima M, Sasano N. Human chorionic gonadotropin and alpha-fetoprotein in testicular germ cell tumors. An immunohistochemical study in comparison with tissue concentrations. Cancer 1983;52(7):1281–1289.
108. Schwartz PE, Morris JM. Serum lactic dehydrogenase: a tumor marker for dysgerminoma. Obstet Gynecol 1988;72(3, pt 2):511–515.
109. Koshida K, Nishino A, Yamamoto H, et al. The role of alkaline phosphatase isoenzymes as tumor markers for testicular germ cell tumors. J Urol 1991;146(1):57–60.
110. Hempling RE. Tumor markers in epithelial ovarian cancer. Clinical applications. Obstet Gynecol Clin North Am 1994;21(1):41–61.
111. Altaras MM, Goldberg GL, Levin W, et al. The value of cancer antigen-125 as a tumor marker in malignant germ cell tumors of the ovary. Gynecol Oncol 1986;25(2):150–159.
112. Bernstein L, Smith MA, Liu L, et al. Germ cell, trophoblastic and other gonadal neoplasms. In: Ries LAG SM, Gurney JG, Linet M, et al., eds. Cancer incidence and survival among children and adolescents: United States SEER Program 1975–1995, National Cancer Institute, SEER Program. Vol NIH Pub. No. 99–4649. Bethesda, MD: Cancer Statistics Branch, Cancer Surveillance Research Program, Division of Cancer Control and Population Sciences, National Cancer Institute, 1999:125–138.
113. Miller RW, Young JL Jr, Novakovic B. Childhood cancer. Cancer 1995;75(suppl 1): 395–405.
114. Cronen PW, Nagaraj HS. Ovarian tumors in children. South Med J 1988;81(4): 464–468.
115. Lovvorn HN III, Tucci LA, Stafford PW. Ovarian masses in the pediatric patient. AORN J 1998;67(3):568–576; quiz 577, 580–584.
116. Walker AH, Ross RK, Haile RW, et al. Hormonal factors and risk of ovarian germ cell cancer in young women. Br J Cancer 1988;57(4):418–422.
117. Brown MF, Hebra A, McGeehin K, et al. Ovarian masses in children: a review of 91 cases of malignant and benign masses. J Pediatr Surg 1993;28(7):930–933.
118. Raney RB Jr, Sinclair L, Uri A, et al. Malignant ovarian tumors in children and adolescents. Cancer 1987;59(6):1214–1220.
119. Gribbon M, Ein SH, Mancer K. Pediatric malignant ovarian tumors: a 43-year review. J Pediatr Surg 1992;27(4):480–484.
120. Harris BH, Boles ET Jr. Rational surgery for tumors of the ovary in children. J Pediatr Surg 1974;9(3):289–293.
121. Surratt JT, Siegel MJ. Imaging of pediatric ovarian masses. Radiographics 1991;11(4): 533–548.
122. Jabra AA, Fishman EK, Taylor GA. Primary ovarian tumors in the pediatric patient: CT evaluation. Clin Imaging 1993;17(3):199–203.
123. Moskovic E, Jobling T, Fisher C, et al. Retroconversion of immature teratoma of the ovary: CT appearances. Clin Radiol 1991;43(6):402–408.
124. Kurman RJ, Norris HJ. Malignant mixed germ cell tumors of the ovary. A clinical and pathologic analysis of 30 cases. Obstet Gynecol 1976;48(5):579–589.
125. Kurman RJ, Norris HJ. Embryonal carcinoma of the ovary: a clinicopathologic entity distinct from endodermal sinus tumor resembling embryonal carcinoma of the adult testis. Cancer 1976;38(6):2420–2433.
126. Mann JR, Pearson D, Barrett A, et al. Results of the United Kingdom Children's Cancer Study Group's malignant germ cell tumor studies. Cancer 1989;63(9):1657–1667.
127. Marina N, Fontanesi J, Kun L, et al. Treatment of childhood germ cell tumors. Review of the St. Jude experience from 1979 to 1988. Cancer 1992;70(10):2568–2575.
128. Cannistra SA. Cancer of the ovary. N Engl J Med 1993;329:1550.
129. Comerci JT Jr, Licciardi F, Bergh PA, et al. Mature cystic teratoma: a clinicopathologic evaluation of 517 cases and review of the literature. Obstet Gynecol 1994;84(1):22–28.
130. Jona JZ, Burchby K, Vitamvas G. Castration-sparing management of an adolescent with huge bilateral cystic teratomas of the ovaries. J Pediatr Surg 1988;23(10): 973–974.
131. Stern JL, Buscema J, Rosenshein NB, et al. Spontaneous rupture of benign cystic teratomas. Obstet Gynecol 1981;57(3):363–366.
132. Cushing B, Giller R, Ablin A, et al. Surgical resection alone is effective treatment for ovarian immature teratoma in children and adolescents: a report of the pediatric oncology group and the children's cancer group. Am J Obstet Gynecol 1999;181(2): 353–358.
133. Norris HJ, Zirkin HJ, Benson WL. Immature (malignant) teratoma of the ovary: a clinical and pathologic study of 58 cases. Cancer 1976;37(5):2359–2372.
134. Gershenson DM, del Junco G, Silva EG, et al. Immature teratoma of the ovary. Obstet Gynecol 1986;68(5):624–629.
135. Brewer M, Gershenson DM, Herzog CE, et al. Outcome and reproductive function after chemotherapy for ovarian dysgerminoma. J Clin Oncol 1999;17(9):2670–2675.
136. De Palo G, Lattuada A, Kenda R, et al. Germ cell tumors of the ovary: the experience of the National Cancer Institute of Milan. I. Dysgerminoma. Int J Radiat Oncol Biol Phys 1987;13(6):853–860.
137. Asadourian LA, Taylor HB. Dysgerminoma. An analysis of 105 cases. Obstet Gynecol 1969;33(3):370–379.
138. Teinturier C, Gelez J, Flamant F, et al. Pure dysgerminoma of the ovary in childhood: treatment results and sequelae. Med Pediatr Oncol 1994;23(1):1–7.
139. Ablin AR, Krailo MD, Ramsay NK, et al. Results of treatment of malignant germ cell tumors in 93 children: a report from the Childrens Cancer Study Group. J Clin Oncol 1991;9(10):1782–1792.
140. Hawkins EP, Finegold MJ, Hawkins HK, et al. Nongerminomatous malignant germ cell tumors in children. A review of 89 cases from the Pediatric Oncology Group, 1971–1984. Cancer 1986;58(12):2579–2584.
141. Kurman RJ, Norris HJ. Endodermal sinus tumor of the ovary: a clinical and pathologic analysis of 71 cases. Cancer 1976;38(6):2404–2419.
142. Dehner LP. Gonadal and extragonadal germ cell neoplasia of childhood. Hum Pathol 1983;14(6):493–511.
143. Wheeler CA, Davis S, Degefu S, et al. Ovarian choriocarcinoma: a difficult diagnosis of an unusual tumor and a review of the hook effect. Obstet Gynecol 1990;75(3, pt 2): 547–549.
144. Vilain E, Jaubert F, Fellous M, et al. Pathology of 46,XY pure gonadal dysgenesis: absence of testis differentiation associated with mutations in the testis-determining factor. Differentiation 1993;52(2):151–159.
145. Olsen MM, Caldamone AA, Jackson CL, et al. Gonadoblastoma in infancy: indications for early gonadectomy in 46XY gonadal dysgenesis. J Pediatr Surg 1988;23(3): 270–271.
146. Gadducci A, Madrigali A, Simeone T, et al. The association of ovarian dysgerminoma and gonadoblastoma in a phenotypic female with 46 XY karyotype. Eur J Gynaecol Oncol 1994;15(2):125–131.
147. Fisher RA, Salm R, Spencer RW. Bilateral gonadoblastoma/dysgerminoma in a 46 XY individual: case report with hormonal studies. J Clin Pathol 1982;35(4):420–424.
148. Calaminus G, Wessalowski R, Harms D, et al. Juvenile granulosa cell tumors of the ovary in children and adolescents: results from 33 patients registered in a prospective cooperative study. Gynecol Oncol 1997;65(3):447–452.

149. Young RH, Dickersin GR, Scully RE. Juvenile granulosa cell tumor of the ovary. A clinicopathological analysis of 125 cases. Am J Surg Pathol 1984;8(8):575–596.
150. Young RH, Scully RE. Ovarian Sertoli-Leydig cell tumors. A clinicopathological analysis of 207 cases. Am J Surg Pathol 1985;9(8):543–569.
151. Arhan E, Cetinkaya E, Aycan Z, et al. A very rare cause of virilization in childhood: ovarian Leydig cell tumor. J Pediatr Endocrinol Metab 2008;21(2):181–183.
152. Zung A, Shoham Z, Open M, et al. Sertoli cell tumor causing precocious puberty in a girl with Peutz–Jeghers syndrome. Gynecol Oncol 1998;70(3):421–424.
153. Pritchard J, Mitchell CD. Testicular tumors in children. In: Broecker BH, Klein FA, eds. Pediatric tumors of the genitourinary tract. New York: Alan R. Liss, 1988:187.
154. Giwercman A, Grindsted J, Hansen B, et al. Testicular cancer risk in boys with maldescended testis: a cohort study. J Urol 1987;138(5):1214–1216.
155. Palmer JM. The undescended testicle. Endocrinol Metab Clin North Am 1991;20(1): 231–240.
156. Krabbe S, Skakkebaek NE, Berthelsen JG, et al. High incidence of undetected neoplasia in maldescended testes. Lancet 1979;1(8124):999–1000.
157. Muller J, Skakkebaek NE, Nielsen OH, et al. Cryptorchidism and testis cancer. Atypical infantile germ cells followed by carcinoma in situ and invasive carcinoma in adulthood. Cancer 1984;54(4):629–634.
158. Pottern LM, Brown LM, Hoover RN, et al. Testicular cancer risk among young men: role of cryptorchidism and inguinal hernia. J Natl Cancer Inst 1985;74(2):377–381.
159. Weissbach L, Altwein JE, Stiens R. Germinal testicular tumors in childhood. Report of observations and literature review. Eur Urol 1984;10(2):73–85.
160. Exelby PR. Testicular cancer in children. Cancer 1980;45(suppl 7):1803–1809.
161. Li FP, Fraumeni JF. Testicular cancers in children: epidemiologic characteristics. J Natl Cancer Inst 1972;48(6):1575–1581.
162. Carney JA, Thompson DP, Johnson CL, et al. Teratomas in children: clinical and pathologic aspects. J Pediatr Surg 1972;7(3):271–282.
163. Ross JH, Rybicki L, Kay R. Clinical behavior and a contemporary management algorithm for prepubertal testis tumors: a summary of the Prepubertal Testis Tumor Registry. J Urol 2002;168(4, pt 2):1675–1678; discussion 1678–1679.
164. Pohl HG, Shukla AR, Metcalf PD, et al. Prepubertal testis tumors: actual prevalence rate of histological types. J Urol 2004;172(6, pt 1):2370–2372.
165. Havranek P, Rubenson A, Guth D, et al. Sacrococcygeal teratoma in Sweden: a 10-year national retrospective study. J Pediatr Surg 1992;27(11):1447–1450.
166. Flake AW. Fetal sacrococcygeal teratoma. Semin Pediatr Surg 1993;2(2):113–120.
167. Berry CL, Keeling J, Hilton C. Teratomata in infancy and childhood: a review of 91 cases. J Pathol 1969;98(4):241–252.
168. Conklin J, Abell MR. Germ cell neoplasms of sacrococcygeal region. Cancer 1967; 20(12):2105–2117.
169. Gonzalez-Crussi F, Winkler RF, Mirkin DL. Sacrococcygeal teratomas in infants and children: relationship of histology and prognosis in 40 cases. Arch Pathol Lab Med 1978;102(8):420–425.
170. Heifetz SA, Cushing B, Giller R, et al. Immature teratomas in children: pathologic considerations: a report from the combined Pediatric Oncology Group/Children's Cancer Group. Am J Surg Pathol 1998;22(9):1115–1124.
171. Gobel U, Calaminus G, Blohm M, et al. Extracranial non-testicular teratoma in childhood and adolescence: introduction of a risk score for stratification of therapy. Klin Padiatr 1997;209(4):228–234.
172. Noronha PA, Noronha R, Rao DS. Primary anterior mediastinal endodermal sinus tumors in childhood. Am J Pediatr Hematol Oncol 1985;7(3):312–316.
173. Lack EE, Weinstein HJ, Welch KJ. Mediastinal germ cell tumors in childhood. A clinical and pathological study of 21 cases. J Thorac Cardiovasc Surg 1985;89(6):826–835.
174. Sham JS, Fu KH, Chiu CS, et al. Experience with the management of primary endodermal sinus tumor of the mediastinum. Cancer 1989;64(3):756–761.
175. Lakhoo K, Boyle M, Drake DP. Mediastinal teratomas: review of 15 pediatric cases. J Pediatr Surg 1993;28(9):1161–1164.
176. Mogilner JG, Fonseca J, Davies MR. Life-threatening respiratory distress caused by a mediastinal teratoma in a newborn. J Pediatr Surg 1992;27(12):1519–1520.
177. Robertson JM, Fee HJ, Mulder DG. Mediastinal teratoma causing life-threatening hemoptysis. Its occurrence in an infant. Am J Dis Child 1981;135(2):148–150.
178. Arai K, Ohta S, Suzuki M, et al. Primary immature mediastinal teratoma in adulthood. Eur J Surg Oncol 1997;23(1):64–67.
179. Moran CA, Suster S. Primary germ cell tumors of the mediastinum: I. Analysis of 322 cases with special emphasis on teratomatous lesions and a proposal for histopathologic classification and clinical staging. Cancer 1997;80(4):681–690.
180. Moran CA, Suster S, Przygodzki RM, et al. Primary germ cell tumors of the mediastinum: II. Mediastinal seminomas—a clinicopathologic and immunohistochemical study of 120 cases. Cancer 1997;80(4):691–698.
181. Moran CA, Suster S. Primary mediastinal choriocarcinomas: a clinicopathologic and immunohistochemical study of eight cases. Am J Surg Pathol 1997;21(9):1007–1012.
182. Moran CA, Suster S, Koss MN. Primary germ cell tumors of the mediastinum: III. Yolk sac tumor, embryonal carcinoma, choriocarcinoma, and combined nonteratomatous germ cell tumors of the mediastinum—a clinicopathologic and immunohistochemical study of 64 cases. Cancer 1997;80(4):699–707.
183. Nichols CR, Roth BJ, Heerema N, et al. Hematologic neoplasia associated with primary mediastinal germ-cell tumors. N Engl J Med 1990;322(20):1425–1429.
184. Domingo A, Romagosa V, Callis M, et al. Mediastinal germ cell tumor and acute megakaryoblastic leukemia. Ann Intern Med 1989;111(6):539.
185. Schneider DT, Hilgenfeld E, Schwabe D, et al. Acute myelogenous leukemia after treatment for malignant germ cell tumors in children. J Clin Oncol 1999;17(10):3226–3233.
186. Hartmann JT, Nichols CR, Droz JP, et al. Hematologic disorders associated with primary mediastinal nonseminomatous germ cell tumors. J Natl Cancer Inst 2000;92(1): 54–61.
187. Jennings CD, Powell DE, Walsh JW, et al. Suprasellar germ cell tumor with extracranial metastases. Neurosurgery 1985;16(1):9–12.
188. Hoffman HJ, Otsubo H, Hendrick EB, et al. Intracranial germ-cell tumors in children. J Neurosurg 1991;74(4):545–551.
189. Dariano JA, Furlanetto TW, Costa SS, et al. Suprasellar germinoma: an unusual clinical presentation. Surg Neurol 1981;15(4):294–297.
190. Wara WM, Jenkin RD, Evans A, et al. Tumors of the pineal and suprasellar region: Childrens Cancer Study Group treatment results 1960–1975: a report from Childrens Cancer Study Group. Cancer 1979;43(2):698–701.
191. Gay JC, Janco RL, Lukens JN. Systemic metastases in primary intracranial germinoma. Case report and literature review. Cancer 1985;55(11):2688–2690.
192. Cushing B, Giller R, Cullen JW, et al. Randomized comparison of combination chemotherapy with etoposide, bleomycin, and either high-dose or standard-dose cisplatin in children and adolescents with high-risk malignant germ cell tumors: a Pediatric Intergroup Study—Pediatric Oncology Group 9049 and Children's Cancer Group 8882. J Clin Oncol 2004;22(13):2691–2700.
193. Rogers PC, Olson TA, Cullen JW, et al. Treatment of children and adolescents with stage II testicular and stages I and II ovarian malignant germ cell tumors: a Pediatric Intergroup Study—Pediatric Oncology Group 9048 and Children's Cancer Group 8891. J Clin Oncol 2004;22(17):3563–3569.
194. Einhorn LH, Williams SD, Troner M, et al. The role of maintenance therapy in disseminated testicular cancer. N Engl J Med 1981;305(13):727–731.
195. Einhorn LH, Williams SD, Loehrer PJ, et al. Evaluation of optimal duration of chemotherapy in favorable-prognosis disseminated germ cell tumors: a Southeastern Cancer Study Group protocol. J Clin Oncol 1989;7(3):387–391.
196. Bosl GJ, Geller NL, Bajorin D, et al. A randomized trial of etoposide + cisplatin versus vinblastine + bleomycin + cisplatin + cyclophosphamide + dactinomycin in patients with good-prognosis germ cell tumors. J Clin Oncol 1988;6(8):1231–1238.
197. Ozols RF, Ihde DC, Linehan WM, et al. A randomized trial of standard chemotherapy v a high-dose chemotherapy regimen in the treatment of poor prognosis nonseminomatous germ-cell tumors. J Clin Oncol 1988;6(6):1031–1040.
198. Haas RJ, Schmidt P, Gobel U, et al. Treatment of malignant testicular tumors in childhood: results of the German National Study 1982–1992. Med Pediatr Oncol 1994; 23(5):400–405.
199. Mann JR, Raafat F, Robinson K, et al. UKCCSG's germ cell tumour (GCT) studies: improving outcome for children with malignant extracranial non-gonadal tumours—carboplatin, etoposide, and bleomycin are effective and less toxic than previous regimens. United Kingdom Children's Cancer Study Group. Med Pediatr Oncol 1998; 30(4):217–227.
200. Pinkerton CR, Pritchard J, Spitz L. High complete response rate in children with advanced germ cell tumors using cisplatin-containing combination chemotherapy. J Clin Oncol 1986;4(2):194–199.
201. Baranzelli MC, Kramar A, Bouffet E, et al. Prognostic factors in children with localized malignant nonseminomatous germ cell tumors. J Clin Oncol 1999;17(4):1212.
202. Schneider DT, Calaminus G, Reinhard H, et al. Primary mediastinal germ cell tumors in children and adolescents: results of the German cooperative protocols MAKEI 83/86, 89, and 96. J Clin Oncol 2000;18(4):832–839.
203. Mann JR, Raafat F, Robinson K, et al. The United Kingdom Children's Cancer Study Group's second germ cell tumor study: carboplatin, etoposide, and bleomycin are effective treatment for children with malignant extracranial germ cell tumors, with acceptable toxicity. J Clin Oncol 2000;18(22):3809–3818.
204. Pinkerton CR, Broadbent V, Horwich A, et al. 'JEB'—a carboplatin based regimen for malignant germ cell tumours in children. Br J Cancer 1990;62(2):257–262.
205. Lopes LF, Macedo CR, Pontes EM, et al. Cisplatin and etoposide in childhood germ cell tumor: Brazilian Pediatric Oncology Society Protocol GCT-91. J Clin Oncol 2009; 27(8):1297–1303.
206. Mann JR, Gray ES, Thornton C, et al. Mature and immature extracranial teratomas in children: the UK Children's Cancer Study Group Experience. J Clin Oncol 2008;26(21): 3590–3597.
207. Bonazzi C, Peccatori F, Colombo N, et al. Pure ovarian immature teratoma, a unique and curable disease: 10 years' experience of 32 prospectively treated patients. Obstet Gynecol 1994;84(4):598–604.
208. Carter D, Bibro MC, Touloukian RJ. Benign clinical behavior of immature mediastinal teratoma in infancy and childhood: report of two cases and review of the literature. Cancer 1982;49(2):398–402.
209. Bahari CM, Lurie M, Schoenfeld A, et al. Ovarian teratoma with peritoneal gliomatosis and elevated serum alpha-fetoprotein. Am J Clin Pathol 1980;73(4):603–607.
210. Shefren G, Collin J, Soriero O. Gliomatosis peritonei with malignant transformation: a case report and review of the literature. Am J Obstet Gynecol 1991;164(6, pt 1): 1617–1620; discussion 1620–1611.
211. Logothetis CJ, Samuels ML, Trindade A, et al. The growing teratoma syndrome. Cancer 1982;50(8):1629–1635.
212. Tonkin KS, Rustin GJ, Wignall B, et al. Successful treatment of patients in whom germ cell tumour masses enlarged on chemotherapy while their serum tumour markers decreased. Eur J Cancer Clin Oncol 1989;25(12):1739–1743.
213. Mitchell MF, Gershenson DM, Soeters RP, et al. The long-term effects of radiation therapy on patients with ovarian dysgerminoma. Cancer 1991;67(4):1084–1090.
214. Gershenson DM, Morris M, Cangir A, et al. Treatment of malignant germ cell tumors of the ovary with bleomycin, etoposide, and cisplatin. J Clin Oncol 1990;8(4):715–720.
215. Williams SD, Blessing JA, Hatch KD, et al. Chemotherapy of advanced dysgerminoma: trials of the Gynecologic Oncology Group. J Clin Oncol 1991;9(11):1950–1955.
216. Gershenson DM, Wharton JT, Kline RC, et al. Chemotherapeutic complete remission in patients with metastatic ovarian dysgerminoma. Potential for cure and preservation of reproductive capacity. Cancer 1986;58(12):2594–2599.
217. Williams S, Blessing JA, Liao SY, et al. Adjuvant therapy of ovarian germ cell tumors with cisplatin, etoposide, and bleomycin: a trial of the Gynecologic Oncology Group. J Clin Oncol 1994;12(4):701–706.
218. De Backer A, Madern GC, Oosterhuis JW, et al. Ovarian germ cell tumors in children: a clinical study of 66 patients. Pediatr Blood Cancer 2006;46(4):459–464.
219. Billmire D, Vincour C, Rescorla F, et al. Outcome and staging evaluation in malignant germ cell tumors of the ovary in children and adolescents: an intergroup study. J Pediatr Surg 2004;39(3):424–429.
220. Gobel U, Schneider DT, Calaminus G, et al. Germ-cell tumors in childhood and adolescence. GPOH MAKEI and the MAHO study groups. Ann Oncol 2000;11(3):263–271.
221. Baranzelli MC, Bouffet E, Quintana E, et al. Non-seminomatous ovarian germ cell tumours in children. Eur J Cancer 2000;36(3):376–383.
222. Palenzuela G, Martin E, Meunier A, et al. Comprehensive staging allows for excellent outcome in patients with localized malignant germ cell tumor of the ovary. Ann Surg 2008;248(5):836–841.
223. Bosl GJ, Motzer RJ. Testicular germ-cell cancer. N Engl J Med 1997;337(4):242–253.
224. Lurain JR, Elfstrand EP. Single-agent methotrexate chemotherapy for the treatment of nonmetastatic gestational trophoblastic tumors. Am J Obstet Gynecol 1995;172(2, pt 1): 574–579.
225. Lurain JR. Management of high-risk gestational trophoblastic disease. J Reprod Med 1998;43(1):44–52.
226. Goldstein DP, Piro AJ. Combination chemotherapy in the treatment of germ cell tumors containing choriocarcinoma in males and females. Surg Gynecol Obstet 1972;134(1): 61–66.
227. King ME, Hubbell MJ, Talerman A. Mixed germ cell tumor of the ovary with a prominent polyembryoma component. Int J Gynecol Pathol 1991;10(1):88–95.

228. Takeda A, Ishizuka T, Goto T, et al. Polyembryoma of ovary producing alpha-fetoprotein and HCG: immunoperoxidase and electron microscopic study. Cancer 1982;49(9):1878–1889.

229. LaPolla JP, Fiorica JV, Turnquist D, et al. Successful therapy of metastatic embryonal carcinoma coexisting with gonadoblastoma in a patient with 46,XY pure gonadal dysgenesis (Swyer's syndrome). Gynecol Oncol 1990;37(3):417–421.

230. Schneider DT, Calaminus G, Wessalowski R, et al. Therapy of advanced ovarian juvenile granulosa cell tumors. Klin Padiatr 2002;214(4):173–178.

231. Giguere JK, Stablein DM, Spaulding JT, et al. The clinical significance of unconventional orchiectomy approaches in testicular cancer: a report from the Testicular Cancer Intergroup Study. J Urol 1988;139(6):1225–1228.

232. de Wit R, Fizazi K. Controversies in the management of clinical stage I testis cancer. J Clin Oncol 2006;24(35):5482–5492.

233. Haas RJ, Schmidt P, Gobel U, et al. Testicular germ cell tumors, an update. Results of the German cooperative studies 1982–1997. Klin Padiatr 1999;211(4):300–304.

234. Frazier AL, Rumcheva P, Olson T, et al. Application of the adult International Germ Cell Classification System to pediatric malignant non-seminomatous germ cell tumors: a report from the Children's Oncology Group. Pediatr Blood Cancer 2007;50(4):746–751.

235. Carver BS, Shayegan B, Serio A, et al. Long-term clinical outcome after postchemotherapy retroperitoneal lymph node dissection in men with residual teratoma. J Clin Oncol 2007;25(9):1033–1037.

236. Schlatter M, Rescorla F, Giller R, et al. Excellent outcome in patients with stage I germ cell tumors of the testes: a study of the Children's Cancer Group/Pediatric Oncology Group. J Pediatr Surg 2003;38(3):319–324; discussion 319–324.

237. Schmidt P, Haas RJ, Gobel U, et al. Results of the German Studies (MAHO) for treatment of Testicular Germ Cell Tumors in Children—an Update. Klin Padiatr 2002;214(4):167–172.

238. Flamant F, Nihoul-Fekete C, Patte C, et al. Optimal treatment of clinical stage I yolk sac tumor of the testis in children. J Pediatr Surg 1986;21(2):108–111.

239. Jewett MA, Kong YS, Goldberg SD, et al. Retroperitoneal lymphadenectomy for testis tumor with nerve sparing for ejaculation. J Urol 1988;139(6):1220–1224.

240. Sogani PC, Perrotti M, Herr HW, et al. Clinical stage I testis cancer: long-term outcome of patients on surveillance. J Urol 1998;159(3):855–858.

241. Theodore C, Terrier-Lacombe MJ, Laplanche A, et al. Bilateral germ-cell tumours: 22-year experience at the Institut Gustave Roussy. Br J Cancer 2004;90(1):55–59.

242. Agarwal PK, Palmer JS. Testicular and paratesticular neoplasms in prepubertal males. J Urol 2006;176(3):875–881.

243. Thomas JC, Ross JH, Kay R. Stromal testis tumors in children: a report from the prepubertal testis tumor registry. J Urol 2001;166(6):2338–2340.

244. Gobel U, Calaminus G, Teske C, et al. BEP/VIP in children and adolescents with malignant non-testicular germ cell tumors. A comparison of the results of treatment of therapy studies MAKEI 83/86 and 89P/89. Klin Padiatr 1993;205(4):231–240.

245. Marina N, London WB, Frazier AL, et al. Prognostic factors in children with extragonadal malignant germ cell tumors: a pediatric intergroup study. J Clin Oncol 2006;24(16):2544–2548.

246. De Backer A, Madern GC, Pieters R, et al. Influence of tumor site and histology on long-term survival in 193 children with extracranial germ cell tumors. Eur J Pediatr Surg 2008;18(1):1–6.

247. Graf JL, Housely HT, Albanese CT, et al. A surprising histological evolution of preterm sacrococcygeal teratoma. J Pediatr Surg 1998;33(2):177–179.

248. Hawkins E, Issacs H, Cushing B, et al. Occult malignancy in neonatal sacrococcygeal teratomas. A report from a Combined Pediatric Oncology Group and Children's Cancer Group study. Am J Pediatr Hematol Oncol 1993;15(4):406–409.

249. Rescorla FJ, Sawin RS, Coran AG, et al. Long-term outcome for infants and children with sacrococcygeal teratoma: a report from the Childrens Cancer Group. J Pediatr Surg 1998;33(2):171–176.

250. Huddart SN, Mann JR, Robinson K, et al. Sacrococcygeal teratomas: the UK Children's Cancer Study Group's experience. I. Neonatal. Pediatr Surg Int 2003;19(1–2):47–51.

251. Dewan PA, Davidson PM, Campbell PE, et al. Sacrococcygeal teratoma: has chemotherapy improved survival? J Pediatr Surg 1987;22(3):274–277.

252. Diez B, Richard L. Malignant germ cell sacrococcygeal tumors in children. Improved prognosis after introduction of cisplatin-containing multiple drug treatment. Acta Oncol 1989;28(2):249–251.

253. Cozzi F, Schiavetti A, Zani A, et al. The functional sequelae of sacrococcygeal teratoma: a longitudinal and cross-sectional follow-up study. J Pediatr Surg 2008;43(4):658–661.

254. Derikx JP, De Backer A, van de Schoot L, et al. Long-term functional sequelae of sacrococcygeal teratoma: a national study in The Netherlands. J Pediatr Surg 2007;42(6):1122–1126.

255. Gobel U, Schneider DT, Calaminus G, et al. Multimodal treatment of malignant sacrococcygeal germ cell tumors: a prospective analysis of 66 patients of the German cooperative protocols MAKEI 83/86 and 89. J Clin Oncol 2001;19(7):1943–1950.

256. Schneider DT, Wessalowski R, Calaminus G, et al. Treatment of recurrent malignant sacrococcygeal germ cell tumors: analysis of 22 patients registered in the German protocols MAKEI 83/86, 89, and 96. J Clin Oncol 2001;19(7):1951–1960.

257. Billmire D, Vinocur C, Rescorla F, et al. Malignant mediastinal germ cell tumors: an intergroup study. J Pediatr Surg 2001;36(1):18–24.

258. Balmaceda C, Heller G, Rosenblum M, et al. Chemotherapy without irradiation—a novel approach for newly diagnosed CNS germ cell tumors: results of an international cooperative trial. The First International Central Nervous System Germ Cell Tumor Study. J Clin Oncol 1996;14(11):2908–2915.

259. Nicholson JC, Punt J, Hale J, et al. Neurosurgical management of paediatric germ cell tumours of the central nervous system—a multi-disciplinary team approach for the new millennium. Br J Neurosurg 2002;16(2):93–95.

260. Billmire D, Vinocur C, Rescorla F, et al. Malignant retroperitoneal and abdominal germ cell tumors: an intergroup study. J Pediatr Surg 2003;38(3):315–318; discussion 315–318.

261. Rescorla F, Billmire D, Vinocur C, et al. The effect of neoadjuvant chemotherapy and surgery in children with malignant germ cell tumors of the genital region: a pediatric intergroup trial. J Pediatr Surg 2003;38(6):910–912.

262. Young RH, Scully RE. Endodermal sinus tumor of the vagina: a report of nine cases and review of the literature. Gynecol Oncol 1984;18(3):380–392.

263. Mauz-Korholz C, Harms D, Calaminus G, et al. Primary chemotherapy and conservative surgery for vaginal yolk-sac tumour. Maligne Keimzelltumoren Study Group. Lancet 2000;355(9204):625.

264. Berlin AJ, Rich LS, Hahn JF. Congenital orbital teratoma. Childs Brain 1983;10(3):208–216.

265. Chang DF, Dallow RL, Walton DS. Congenital orbital teratoma: report of a case with visual preservation. J Pediatr Ophthalmol Strabismus 1980;17(2):88–95.

266. Bernbeck B, Schneider DT, Koch S, et al. Germ cell tumors of the head and neck: report from the MAKEI Study Group. Pediatr Blood Cancer 2009;52(2):223–226.

267. Motzer RJ, Sheinfeld J, Mazumdar M, et al. Paclitaxel, ifosfamide, and cisplatin second-line therapy for patients with relapsed testicular germ cell cancer. J Clin Oncol 2000;18(12):2413–2418.

268. Einhorn LH, Williams SD, Chamness A, et al. High-dose chemotherapy and stem-cell rescue for metastatic germ-cell tumors. N Engl J Med 2007;357(4):340–348.

269. Schmoll HJ, Kollmannsberger C, Metzner B, et al. Long-term results of first-line sequential high-dose etoposide, ifosfamide, and cisplatin chemotherapy plus autologous stem cell support for patients with advanced metastatic germ cell cancer: an extended phase I/II study of the German Testicular Cancer Study Group. J Clin Oncol 2003;21(22):4083–4091.

270. Carver BS, Serio AM, Bajorin D, et al. Improved clinical outcome in recent years for men with metastatic nonseminomatous germ cell tumors. J Clin Oncol 2007;25(35):5603–5608.

271. Wessalowski R, Schneider DT, Mils O, et al. An approach for cure: PEI-chemotherapy and regional deep hyperthermia in children and adolescents with unresectable malignant tumors. Klin Padiatr 2003;215(6):303–309.

272. Hartmann JT, Fossa SD, Nichols CR, et al. Incidence of metachronous testicular cancer in patients with extragonadal germ cell tumors. J Natl Cancer Inst 2001;93(22):1733–1738.

273. Li Y, Womer RB, Silber JH. Predicting cisplatin ototoxicity in children: the influence of age and the cumulative dose. Eur J Cancer 2004;40(16):2445–2451.

274. Marina N, Chang KW, Malogolowkin M, et al. Amifostine does not protect against the ototoxicity of high-dose cisplatin combined with etoposide and bleomycin in pediatric germ-cell tumors: a Children's Oncology Group study. Cancer 2005;104(4):841–847.

275. Knight KR, Kraemer DF, Neuwelt EA. Ototoxicity in children receiving platinum chemotherapy: underestimating a commonly occurring toxicity that may influence academic and social development. J Clin Oncol 2005;23(34):8588–8596.

276. Oldenburg J, Kraggerud SM, Cvancarova M, et al. Cisplatin-induced long-term hearing impairment is associated with specific glutathione s-transferase genotypes in testicular cancer survivors. J Clin Oncol 2007;25(6):708–714.

277. Riedemann L, Lanvers C, Deuster D, et al. Megalin genetic polymorphisms and individual sensitivity to the ototoxic effect of cisplatin. Pharmacogenomics J 2008;8(1):23–28.

STEVEN G. WAGUESPACK, ANDREW J. BAUER, WINSTON HUH, AND ANITA K. YING

Endocrine tumors comprise a variety of benign and malignant neoplasms that arise from the endocrine glands or neuroendocrine tissues. Functioning tumors are associated with typical clinical syndromes related to the specific hormone(s) being secreted, whereas nonfunctioning tumors present incidentally or secondary to symptoms related to mass effect. Although most childhood endocrine tumors are sporadic without an identifiable mutation in germline DNA, others are familial, such as those that occur as part of the multiple endocrine neoplasia (MEN) syndromes. Endocrine tumors represent a minority of all neoplasms observed in the pediatric population and are generally clinically benign or low-grade cancers, although a small percentage of these tumors are high-grade malignancies requiring multimodality therapies. As with any rare childhood disease, treatment is best provided at tertiary care centers with multidisciplinary expertise in the management of such tumors.

PITUITARY TUMORS

Pituitary Adenomas

Epidemiology and Pathophysiology

A pituitary adenoma (PA) is generally a benign monoclonal neoplasm that arises from the anterior pituitary gland (adenohypophysis). PAs represent approximately 1.6% to 2.7% of all supratentorial tumors diagnosed during childhood, and 2% to 6% of all pituitary tumors treated surgically are in children.[1–3] Pubertal children represent the largest group, with more than 75% of PAs occurring in children older than 12 years, and females are more commonly affected than males.[1,2,4] The differential diagnosis for a sellar/suprasellar mass is broad and covered in recent reviews.[5,6] During adolescence and in patients with profound primary endocrine gland dysfunction (e.g., severe primary hypothyroidism), the pituitary may undergo significant hyperplasia and falsely resemble a neoplasm.[7] Pituitary hyperplasia and clinical syndromes of hormone excess can also rarely occur secondary to ectopic secretion of the hypothalamic hormones corticotropin releasing hormone (CRH) and growth hormone releasing hormone (GHRH). Tumors that metastasize to the pituitary gland are exceedingly rare in the pediatric population.

The development of a PA depends on genetic abnormalities, environmental factors, and/or physiological alterations at the hypothalamic, pituitary, and peripheral levels.[8,9] Genetic syndromes associated with PAs include multiple endocrine neoplasia type 1 (MEN1), familial isolated PAs, Carney complex (CNC), the tuberous sclerosis complex (TSC), and the McCune-Albright syndrome (MAS)[8–14] (Table 36.1). Furthermore, germline mutations in the human cyclin-dependent kinase inhibitor 1B gene (CDKN1B, which encodes p27^{Kip1}) have recently been identified in patients with PAs and MENX/MEN4.[15]

Clinical Presentation and Diagnosis

Pituitary tumors are usually diagnosed secondary to symptoms of hormone excess or mass effect, such as visual disturbance (classically a bitemporal hemianopsia), headache, or ophthalmoplegia. Patients may also present with delayed growth and pubertal development because of pituitary hormone hypersecretion, as seen with hyperprolactinemia, or hyposecretion, as seen with large PAs that compress the normal adenohypophyseal tissue.[1,4,8] Incidental identification of PAs is becoming more commonplace.[16] Pituitary apoplexy (infarction and/or hemorrhage into a pre-existing tumor) can also be the presenting feature of a PA, but central diabetes insipidus is not typical in the clinical presentation of a benign sellar mass.[2,8]

Pituitary tumors can be plurihormonal, secreting more than one hormone, most commonly a combination of growth hormone (GH) and prolactin (PRL).[1,2,5] Although the clinical and biochemical phenotype of a functioning PA generally correlates with immunohistochemical findings, this is not always the case, and immunohistochemistry alone does not make a diagnosis of a functional tumor.[2,5]

In a child with a PA, the initial workup includes imaging of the sella turcica, a comprehensive hormonal evaluation to assess for hyper- and hypopituitarism, and visual field testing for children with large tumors that involve the optic chiasm.[5] The best imaging modality for the diagnosis of PAs is T1-weighted spin-echo magnetic resonance imaging (MRI) of the pituitary in both coronal and sagittal planes (obtained at 3-mm intervals) before and after the intravenous administration of gadolinium[8] (Fig. 36.1). High-resolution computerized tomography can be useful in the identification of calcifications (pathognomonic for craniopharyngioma) and in those patients who otherwise cannot get an MRI. Microadenomas are defined as PAs ≤ 1 cm in greatest dimension whereas macroadenomas are > 1 cm (Fig. 36.1); the rare tumor that exceeds 4 cm is termed a giant adenoma.[8,17] Pituitary microadenomas are not always visible on MRI, which makes the diagnosis of certain diseases such as Cushing disease (CD) more complex. Newer MRI protocols such as dynamic contrast-enhanced MRI and spoiled gradient-recalled acquisition in the steady-state MRI may facilitate identifying these microadenomas.[18,19]

Staging and Prognosis

PAs are classified by the World Health Organization (WHO) into typical PAs, atypical PAs, and pituitary carcinomas. Atypical PAs are nonmetastatic tumors with morphologic features suggestive of aggressive behavior, including extensive nuclear staining for p53, an elevated mitotic index, and Ki-67 labeling index greater than 3%.[8] PAs may be locally invasive, but invasive growth into surrounding bone and dura does not necessarily portend a more dire clinical course. In pediatric patients with non–adrenocorticotropin (ACTH)-secreting PAs, disease-free survival is lower for macroadenomas, and these children typically require more aggressive multimodality therapy and have higher rates of hypopituitarism.[2] Although the mortality

TABLE 36.1

MAJOR GENETIC SYNDROMES ASSOCIATED WITH ENDOCRINE NEOPLASIA

	Gene (chromosome)	Type(s) of endocrine neoplasia	Other
Beckwith-Wiedemann syndrome	*CDKN1C* and other genes on 11p15.5 that undergo abnormal transcription and regulation	• ACT	• Macrosomia/organomegaly/macroglossia • Hemihypertrophy • Embryonal tumors (Wilms tumor, hepatoblastoma, neuroblastoma, rhabdomyosarcoma) • Omphalocele • Neonatal hypoglycemia • Anterior linear ear lobe creases/posterior helical ear pits • Renal abnormalities

Carney complex	*PRKAR1A* (17q23-q24) and unknown gene at chromosomal locus 2p16	• Mammosomatotroph hyperplasia/GH-secreting PA (10% of adults)
		• Primary pigmented nodular adrenocortical disease (25–60%)
		• Thyroid tumors (10–25%)
		  • Follicular adenomas
		  • Thyroid carcinoma (PTC & FTC)
		• Large-cell calcifying sertoli cell tumors (33–56% of males)
			• GH excess and hyperprolactinemia
			• Spotty skin pigmentation
			• Blue nevus
			• Cardiac, cutaneous, or breast myxomas
			• Psammomatous melanotic schwannoma

Cowden syndrome (*PTEN* hamartoma tumor syndrome)	*PTEN* (10q23.3)	• Thyroid adenomas and multinodular goiter (75%)
		• FTC (10%)
			• Mucocutaneous lesions
			  • Papillomatous lesions
			  • Trichilemmomas
			  • Acral keratoses
			• Breast cancer
			• Macrocephaly
			• Endometrial carcinoma/uterine fibroids
			• Genitourinary tumors

Familial adenomatous polyposis (Gardner syndrome)	*APC* (5q21-q22)	• ACT (~10%) • PTC (1–2%) • Cribriform variant	• Colorectal polyps/colorectal carcinoma • Osteomas • Desmoid tumors • Pancreas adenocarcinomas • Medulloblastoma • Hepatoblastoma
Familial isolated pituitary adenomas	*AIP* (11q13.3)	• GH-secreting adenomas (30%) • Prolactin-secreting adenomas (41%) • Nonfunctioning adenomas (17%)	• Aryl hydrocarbon receptor-Interacting Protein (AIP) mutations identified in only 15% of cases
CDC73-related hyper-parathyroidism (hyperparathyroidism-jaw tumor syndrome)	CDC73 [*HRPT2*] (1q25-q31)	• Parathyroid adenoma • Often cystic with atypical histology • Parathyroid carcinoma (10–15% of cases) • Possible thyroid neoplasia	• Ossifying fibroma(s) of the maxilla and/or mandible • Renal cystic disease/renal hamartomas • Wilms tumor • Benign and malignant uterine tumors
Li-Fraumeni syndrome	*TP53* (17p13.1)	• ACT (~10%)	• Sarcoma • Breast cancer • Leukemia • Melanoma • GI malignancies • Brain tumors • Gonadal germ cell tumors
McCune-Albright syndrome	*GNAS* (20q13)	• Mammosomatotroph hyperplasia/GH-secreting PA (20%) • Functioning thyroid nodules • Ovarian cysts • Macronodular ACT	• Peripheral precocious puberty • Polyostotic fibrous dysplasia • Café-au-lait macules with irregular margins • Cushing syndrome due to ACTs • GH excess and hyperprolactinemia

(continued)

TABLE 36.1

CONTINUED

	Gene (chromosome)	Type(s) of endocrine neoplasia	Other

MEN1	*MEN1* (11q13)	• Parathyroid adenomas/hyperplasia (100% by age 50 yr)
		• PA (up to 40%)
		• NETs
		  • PETs (40–50%)
		  • Thymic, bronchial, and gastric carcinoid tumors (10%)
		• ACT (~20–40%)
		• PHEO (<1%)
			• Lipomas/angiofibromas/collagenomas
			• Meningiomas
			• Ependymomas
			• Leiomyomas
			• Gastrinoma most common NET
			• Prolactinoma most common PA
			• NETs can over secrete ACTH (ectopic ACTH-dependent CS) and GHRH (GH excess)
			• ACTs usually nonfunctional

MEN2A (including familial MTC)	*RET* (10q11.2)	• MTC (almost 100%)
		• PHEO (50%)
		  • Sympathetic/adrenergic[a,b]
		  • Malignancy very rare
		• Parathyroid adenoma/hyperplasia (30%)
			• Codon-specific risk of MTC
			• Variants with cutaneous lichen amyloidosis and Hirschsprung disease
			• Ganglioneuroma identified in rare cases

MEN2B	*RET* (10q11.2)	• MTC (100%)
		• PHEO (50%)
		  • Sympathetic/adrenergic[a,b]
		  • Malignancy very rare
			• Very high risk for early onset and metastasis of MTC
			• Mucosal neuromas of the lips, tongue and eyelids
			• Medullated corneal nerve fibers
			• Distinctive facies with enlarged lips
			• Megacolon/ganglioneuromatosis of the GI tract
			• "Marfanoid" body habitus
			• Absent tears in infancy
			• Feeding difficulties and constipation in infancy
			• Ganglioneuroma identified in rare cases

MENX/MEN4	*CDKN1B*, which encodes p27[Kip1] (12p13)	• PA • Parathyroid adenoma/hyperplasia • Neuroendocrine cervical carcinoma	• Acromegaly and CD in two patients to date • Renal angiomyolipoma

NF1	*NF1* (17q11.2)	• PHEO
		  • Sympathetic/adrenergic[a,b]
		  • Malignancy rare
		• NETs
		  • Insulinoma (rare)
		  • Carcinoid (1%)
		    • + for somatostatin
			• Café-au-lait macules with smooth borders
			• Axillary and inguinal freckling
			• Dermal and plexiform neurofibromas
			• Lisch nodules of the iris
			• Learning disabilities
			• Scoliosis, vertebral dysplasia, pseudarthrosis, and bony overgrowth
			• Optic and other central nervous system gliomas
			• Malignant peripheral nerve sheath tumors
			• Vasculopathy
			• Macrocephaly

PGL1	*SDHD* (11q23)	• PGL (primarily head and neck)/PHEO
		  • Parasympathetic[a]
		  • Occasionally sympathetic/noradrenergic[b]
		  • Malignancy rare
		• PTC
			• 86% penetrance by age 50
			• Maternal imprinting, with disease caused only when inherited from the father
			• Rare cases of sympathetic PGL
			• Can be associated with GIST

PGL3	*SDHC* (1q21)	• PGL (head and neck)
		  • Parasympathetic[a]
		  • Malignancy rare
			• Rare cases of sympathetic PGL and PHEO
			• Can be associated with GIST

PGL4	*SDHB* (1p36.1-p35)	• PGL (primarily abdominal) and PHEO
		  • Sympathetic/noradrenergic[a,b]
		  • Malignancy common (50%)
		• ?PTC
			• 77% penetrance by age 50
			• Can be associated with GIST
			• RCC

(continued)

TABLE 36.1

CONTINUED

	Gene (chromosome)	Type(s) of endocrine neoplasia	Other

Tuberous sclerosis complex	*TSC1* (9q34)
	TSC2 (16p13.3)
		• PA
		• Parathyroid adenoma/hyperplasia
		• NETs
		  • PETs (chiefly insulinoma)
		  • Bronchial carcinoid (one case)
		• PHEO (one case)
			• Cutaneous findings associated with TSC include
			  • Hypomelanotic macules ("ash-leaf" spots)
			  • Facial angiofibromata (adenoma sebaceum)
			  • Ungual or periungual fibromas
			  • Shagreen patch
			• Neurologic disorders
			  • Epilepsy
			  • Mental retardation
			  • Autism
			• CNS lesions
			  • Cortical tuber
			  • Subependymal nodule
			  • Subependymal giant cell astrocytoma
			• Multiple retinal nodular hamartomas
			• Cardiac rhabdomyoma
			• Lymphangiomyomatosis
			• Renal angiomyolipoma

VHL	*VHL* (3p26-p25)	• PHEO (20% of cases)/PGL (5%)
		  • Sympathetic/noradrenergic[a,b]
		  • Malignancy rare (5%) and more likely with PGL
		• Nonfunctioning PETs (5–10%)
			• Hemangioblastomas of the CNS and retina
			• Renal cysts and clear cell RCC
			• Pancreatic cysts and cystadenomas
			• Endolymphatic sac tumors
			• Papillary cystadenomas of the epididymis (males) and round ligament (females)
			• Further subdivided into VHL types I and II based on phenotype (PHEO only in VHL type II and usually due to missense mutations in the VHL gene)

Werner syndrome	*WRN [RECQL]* (8p12-p11.2)	• PTC	• Premature aging
			• Cancer predisposition
			  • Sarcomas
			  • Acral lentiginous melanomas

ACT, adrenocortical tumor; ACTH, adrenocorticotropin; CD, Cushing disease; CNS, central nervous system; CS, Cushing syndrome; FTC, follicular thyroid carcinoma; GH, growth hormone; GHRH, growth hormone releasing hormone; GIST, gastrointestinal stromal tumor; MEN, multiple endocrine neoplasia; MTC, medullary thyroid carcinoma; NET, neuroendocrine tumor; NF, neurofibromatosis; PA, pituitary adenoma; PET, pancreatic endocrine tumor; PGL, familial paraganglioma syndrome or paraganglioma; PHEO, pheochromocytoma; PTC, papillary thyroid carcinoma; RCC, renal cell carcinoma; VHL, von Hippel-Lindau disease.

[a]*Sympathetic* tumors are functional and secrete catecholamines; *parasympathetic* tumors are nonfunctional. In general, head and neck PGL are parasympathetic while PHEO and abdominal PGL are sympathetic.

[b]*Noradrenergic* tumors almost exclusively secrete norepinephrine and normetanephrine, whereas *adrenergic* tumors primarily secrete epinephrine and metanephrine.

for children with PAs is low, there may be significant morbidity due to surgical complications and/or hypopituitarism.

Treatment and Follow-Up

In general, transsphenoidal resection is the treatment of choice for hormonally active tumors, with the notable exception of prolactinomas (see later). Surgery is also considered in macroadenomas causing mass effect or contributing to hypopituitarism; pituitary apoplexy; ineffectiveness or intolerance of medical therapy; and for smaller sellar masses associated with chronic severe headaches.[8,17,20] In the right hands, transsphenoidal resection is a safe and effective procedure, and it is imperative to identify a high-volume pituitary neurosurgeon.[21]

Microadenomas have a high surgical cure rate whereas complete resection of pituitary macroadenomas is often not possible, particularly with tumors greater than 2 cm and when cavernous sinus invasion and/or significant suprasellar extension is present.[17] Radiation therapy (either using conventional or radiosurgical techniques) has a limited role in the management of children with PAs, but can be considered in uncontrolled functional tumors or unresectable nonfunctioning tumors that are rapidly progressive.[22] Long-term follow-up should include periodic MRI and hormonal assessment based on the functional status of the PA and previous treatments required.

Late Effects/Complications of Treatment

Complications from surgery can include hypopituitarism, cavernous sinus hemorrhage, transient or permanent diabetes insipidus, the syndrome of inappropriate antidiuretic hormone secretion, cerebrospinal fluid leak, and meningitis.

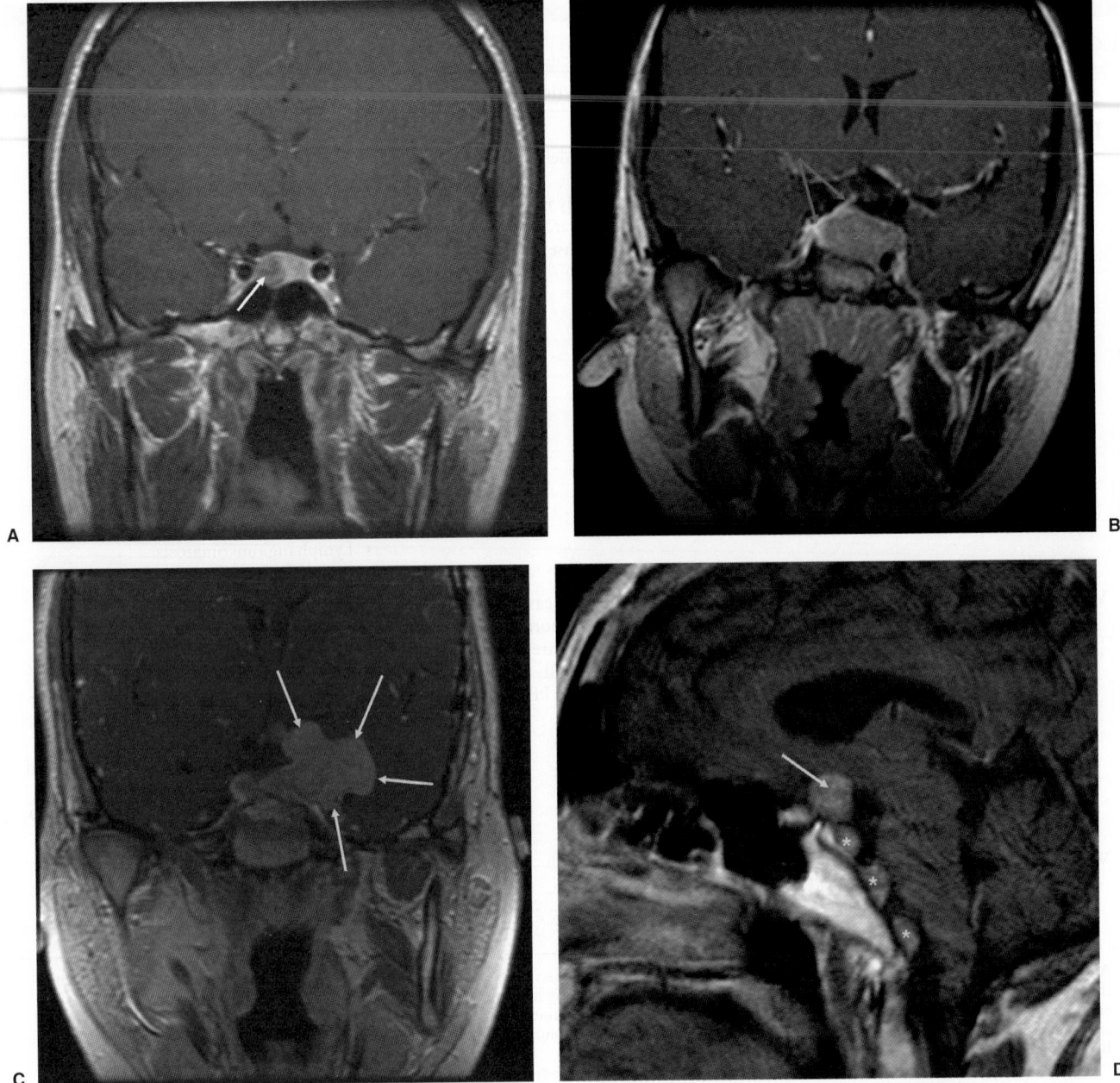

FIGURE 36.1 Various presentations of pituitary adenomas on T1-weighted MRI status post gadolinium contrast. **A:** Pituitary microadenoma (*white arrow*). **B:** Pituitary macroadenoma (*red asterisk*), note the normal pituitary gland and pituitary stalk (*red arrows*) deviated to the right. **C:** Invasive pituitary macroadenoma (*white arrows*). **D:** Pituitary carcinoma with primary residual tumor (*yellow arrow*) and drop metastases (*yellow asterisks*).

Hypopituitarism arising from surgery is immediate whereas hypopituitarism arising from radiation therapy is gradual and often insidious in its presentation, underscoring the need for long-term endocrine follow-up. Other late effects from radiation therapy can include visual deficits because of optic neuropathy, necrosis of normal brain tissue, second neoplasms (chiefly meningiomas and gliomas), cognitive impairment, and cerebrovascular accidents.[22]

Pituitary Adenoma Subtypes

Prolactin-Secreting Adenomas (Lactotroph Adenomas). Prolactinomas are the most common PA in childhood, representing approximately 50% of cases.[2,4] These tumors are diagnosed more commonly in girls and are rarely identified in the prepubertal child.[3,23,24] Prepubertal children present with symptoms of mass effect and/or delayed puberty whereas pubertal children present with amenorrhea (girls), galactorrhea (both genders), and rarely gynecomastia (boys).[23,24] Males are more likely to have macroadenomas and therefore tend to present with symptoms related to tumor size.[2,24]

The degree of hyperprolactinemia usually correlates with tumor size,[25] and the diagnosis of a prolactinoma is most likely when the PRL level is more than 100 to 200 ng/mL.[5,16,26] In order to establish the correct diagnosis, the possibilities of hyperprolactinemia because of stalk compression, macroprolactinemia, and the high-dose hook effect that occurs with large tumors and extremely elevated PRL levels should be considered.[5,16,25,27] Patients with elevated PRL levels and no tumor on MRI should have an evaluation for secondary hyperprolactinemia.[25,28] Primary hypothyroidism should always be ruled out as a cause of hyperprolactinemia and sellar mass. Due to the possibility of GH cosecretion, an insulin-like growth factor 1 (IGF-1) level should also be included in the evaluation.

Prolactinomas can effectively be treated with one of the available dopamine agonists (DAs), either bromocriptine or cabergoline, even in the presence of visual changes. Cabergoline is preferred due to less-frequent administration, fewer side effects, and greater efficacy.[23,25,29] Oral contraceptive pills are a reasonable alternative in adolescent girls with microadenomas and nonbothersome galactorrhea.[28,30] Sex steroids can exacerbate PRL hypersecretion and promote tumor growth[31,32], so caution should be undertaken when prescribing testosterone or estrogen replacement to adolescents with macroprolactinomas. The addition of an aromatase inhibitor may facilitate the use of testosterone replacement in males.[32]

Clinical improvement is usually seen before radiological tumor reduction. In most patients, treatment is continued until the PRL level normalizes (or at least stabilizes) and the tumor demonstrates significant shrinkage. Some patients will never achieve normal PRL levels, but many patients may ultimately be able to stop DA therapy.[25,30,33]

ACTH-Secreting Adenomas (Corticotroph Adenoma; Cushing Disease). ACTH-secreting adenomas causing CD are the second most common PA in children, occurring in approximately one third of children operated on for a pituitary tumor.[2,4] The median age of presentation is 14.1 years.[34] Corticotroph tumors are the most likely PA to be diagnosed in prepubertal children, and there have been several cases of

ACTH-secreting tumors presenting prior to the age of one year.[1,4] In general, there is a female to male predominance, except in prepubertal children.[1,35,36]

The onset of symptoms is usually insidious, and most children have a typical cushingoid phenotype (Fig. 36.2) with generalized weight gain, obesity, impairment of growth (namely in prepubertal patients), violaceous striae (chiefly in older children), hirsutism/premature pubarche, acne, and hypertension.[35,37–39] Clinical presentation can also include rounding of the face (moon facies), plethora, abnormal fat distribution with increased fat deposition in the supraclavicular fossae and upper back (Buffalo hump), acanthosis nigricans, easy bruising, hyperpigmentation (with significant ACTH elevation), muscle weakness, edema, impaired glucose tolerance/diabetes mellitus, pubertal delay, emotional lability, fatigue, headache, menstrual disturbance, low bone mass for age and fractures [3,35,37–43] (Fig. 36.2). Not every case of Cushing syndrome (CS) is classic, and the diagnosis can be hard to differentiate from exogenous obesity based on phenotype alone, as not all children with CS are short or have delayed bone ages as would be expected.[35,37] One of the most sensitive indicators of possible CS in a growing child is weight gain associated with a low growth velocity.[43]

These tumors are almost always microadenomas and are often not visualized on routine MRI.[34,35,38,44] Because of that, the diagnosis of CD is not always straightforward and care must be taken to differentiate an ACTH-secreting PA from ectopic ACTH secretion, such as from a thymic or bronchial carcinoid tumor. Fortunately, the latter situation is rare in children.

The diagnostic studies for CS have not been extensively validated in children. Screening studies to make the diagnosis include measurement of 24-hour urine-free cortisol, the overnight 1 mg (low dose) dexamethasone (DEX) suppression

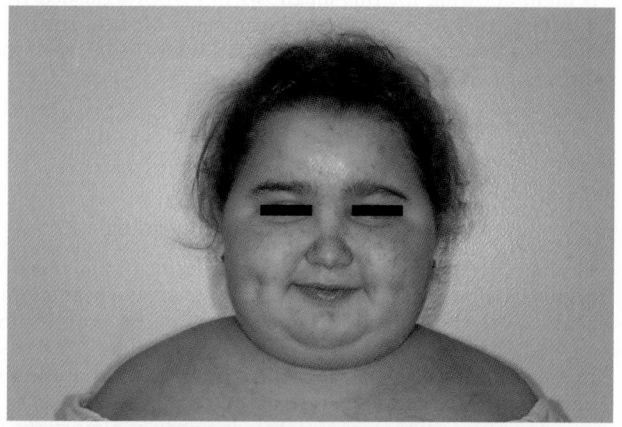

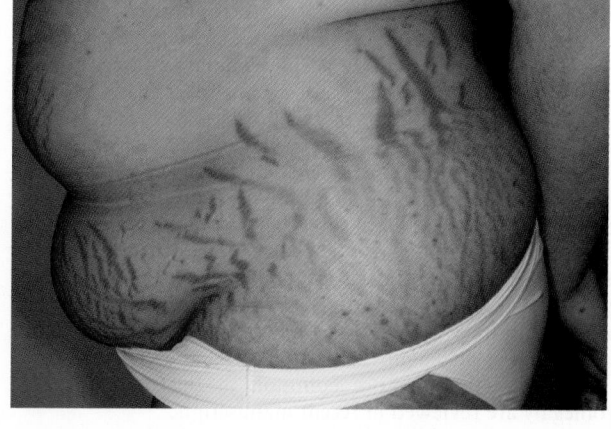

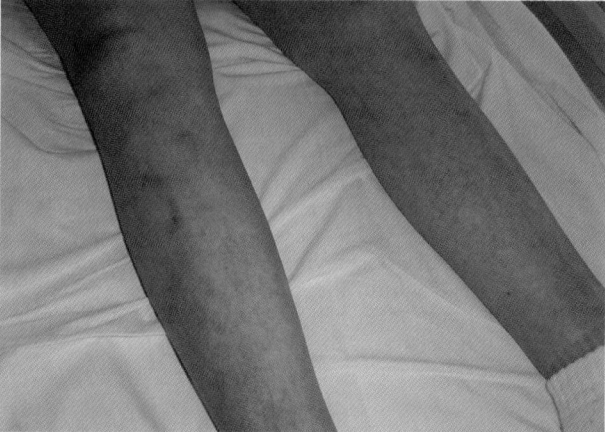

FIGURE 36.2 Signs of Cushing syndrome in three different patients. A: Typical appearance of Cushing syndrome with moon facies, acne, and abnormal fat distribution in the supraclavicular fossae. B: Central adiposity with classic violaceous wide striae. C: Thin extremities with easy bruising and thinning of the skin. (Photo courtesy of Dr. Rachel Edelen.)

test, the 2-day low dose DEX suppression test, and assessment of impaired circadian rhythm through the measurement of late evening salivary or serum cortisol levels.[34,35,39,42,43,45,46] The DEX/CRH test is utilized to distinguish CS from pseudo-CS states, although this test may not be as reliable in very obese children.[47] Once the diagnosis of ACTH-dependent CS (i.e., ACTH levels not less than 20 pg/mL[39]) has been made, the source of ACTH can generally be attributed to the pituitary if a clear adenoma is identified. If MRI findings are negative or equivocal, it is necessary to undertake additional testing to differentiate a pituitary from a peripheral source of ACTH production. These tests can include an overnight 8 mg (high dose) DEX suppression test, 2 day high-dose DEX suppression test, CRH test, CRH/desmopressin test, and CRH-stimulated inferior petrosal sinus sampling (IPSS).[35,39,42,43,45,48,49] IPSS obtained at the time of hypercortisolism appears to be the most definitive diagnostic test in the work up of ACTH-dependent CS and is safe and useful in children at experienced centers. Although IPSS can confirm a central source of ACTH production, its use solely for tumor lateralization is questionable.[34,50]

The management of CD includes the use of one or more inhibitors of cortisol synthesis, and currently available treatment options include metyrapone, ketoconazole, mitotane (o,p'-DDD; rarely used in nonmalignant conditions), etomidate, and mifepristone (RU-486).[39,44,51] In the patient who is not cured with surgery or radiotherapy and who continues to suffer from CS despite optimization of medical therapy, bilateral adrenalectomy is considered.[44,45] Although patients are committed to lifelong glucocorticoid and mineralocorticoid replacement, removal of all adrenocortical tissue is the best way to cure CS in the treatment-refractory patient. The development of Nelson syndrome (the association of an expanding pituitary tumor and a high ACTH concentration after adrenalectomy in patients with CD) is a concern in such children.[52]

Growth Hormone-Secreting Adenomas (Somatotroph Adenomas; Gigantism/Acromegaly). Somatotroph adenomas are the third most common PA in childhood, have a higher prevalence in males, are usually macroadenomas, and represent approximately 8% of all cases and 0.63% of surgically treated pituitary tumors in children.[4,53] Gigantism is the term used to describe the overgrowth that occurs because of GH excess in children with open epiphyses, whereas acromegaly describes GH excess occurring after epiphyseal closure. The clinical presentation is usually one of accelerating linear growth. Other common features include coarse facial features, frontal bossing, prognathism, and disproportionately large hands and feet with thick fingers and toes.[54] Symptoms related to tumor mass effect, pubertal delay, and menstrual irregularities can also be present at diagnosis.[53] Other signs and symptoms of GH excess that are more common in the patient with acromegaly are reviewed in recent manuscripts.[55,56]

During early childhood, gigantism is typically caused by mammosomatotroph tumors, secreting both GH and PRL, underscoring the genetic basis of these tumors[8] (Table 36.1). Sporadic adenomas can harbor somatic mutations in the GNAS complex locus, which encodes the stimulatory G-protein alpha subunit, in up to 40% of adult patients, but this is not generally seen in sporadic tumors identified in childhood.[13,57]

The best initial diagnostic test is measurement of an IGF-1 level, comparing it with age-matched normative ranges.[54,56] Confirmatory testing is accomplished through a 1.75 gm/kg (max 75 gm) oral glucose tolerance test, during which GH levels should fall to <1 ng/mL during the 2-hour testing period.[56,58] The sensitivity of the 1 ng/mL cutoff has recently been debated; using more sensitive GH assays and in milder cases of GH hypersecretion, GH should suppress to less than 0.2 to 0.4 ng/mL in normal individuals.[56,59–61] The clinician

must also consider the gender and pubertal status of the adolescent patient undergoing testing, as the nadir of GH after oral glucose ingestion may be higher than adults, especially in midpubertal girls.[62]

When surgery is not curative, pharmacologic inhibition of GH secretion and suppression of tumor growth are accomplished through the use of the somatostatin (SST) analogs (octreotide and lanreotide) and/or the DA cabergoline.[55,60,63,64] Pegvisomant is a competitive GH receptor antagonist that lowers IGF-1 levels but has no direct impact on tumor size.[55,65] Primary medical therapy can also be considered in patients who have surgically incurable tumors.

Clinically Nonfunctioning Adenomas (Null Cell Adenomas; Gonadotropin-Secreting Adenomas). Clinically nonfunctioning tumors include those neoplasms that silently produce hormones (e.g., ACTH) without clinical signs or symptoms, in addition to those PAs that produce no pituitary hormones (null cell adenomas), bioinactive hormones, or hormones such as the gonadotropins (luteinizing and/or follicle stimulating hormone) and α-subunit of the glycoprotein hormones that do not always cause clinical manifestations.[8,16] In contradistinction to adults, these tumors represent <5% of pediatric PAs.[2,4] Surgery is the mainstay of treatment, particularly in macroadenomas, which have a predisposition for enlargement and/or apoplexy over time.[16,66] Medical management with a DA or SST analog can also be considered in the appropriate clinical setting.

TSH-Secreting Adenomas (Thyrotroph Adenomas). PAs secreting thyroid stimulating hormone (TSH) are diagnosed due to elevated thyroxine and triiodothyronine levels and a nonsuppressed (and often elevated) TSH in the presence of a pituitary tumor on MRI. These tumors usually secrete excessive quantities of α-subunit, and the ratio of α-subunit to TSH is high, allowing for this diagnosis to be distinguished from pituitary resistance to thyroid hormone.[67] Medical treatment includes SST analogs and DAs, in addition to interventions directed at controlling the hyperthyroidism.

Pituitary Carcinoma

Epidemiology and Pathophysiology

Pituitary carcinomas are primary neoplasms of the adenohypophysis that arise from pre-existing invasive adenomas after a variable latency period and undergo craniospinal and/or systemic spread.[68–70] With less than 200 cases reported in the medical literature, primary pituitary malignancies are exceedingly rare, representing only 0.2% of resected pituitary tumors.[68,71] The diagnosis is almost always made in adulthood, but isolated pediatric case reports have been published.

Clinical Presentation and Diagnosis

The majority of pituitary carcinomas are functional tumors[68,69] and they present similarly to their benign counterparts; initial presentation with metastatic disease is rare. Sites of metastasis can include the brain, leptomeninges, liver, bones, lung, and lymph nodes. ACTH-secreting tumors are more likely to have systemic metastases, whereas prolactin-secreting tumors tend to spread within the craniospinal axis.[68] There is no single combination of histological features in the primary tumor that is diagnostic for pituitary carcinoma,[69,72] but early recurrence after initial surgery would suggest a possible malignancy.

Staging and Prognosis

The prognosis of pituitary carcinoma is poor, and most patients with systemic disease succumb to the disease within one year.[68,70] Mean survival is two years, although cases of prolonged survival have been documented.[73] There is no formal staging system for this rare cancer.

Treatment

Treatment is palliative in nature and should include a multidisciplinary approach utilizing surgery (sometimes with local instillation of chemotherapy-infused wafers), radiation therapy, medical therapy targeting hormonal hypersecretion, and systemic antineoplastic treatments.[69,72,74,75] Cytotoxic agents studied with variable success include lomustine and 5-fluorouracil (5-FU), carboplatin either as a single agent or combined with 5-FU or interferon α, cisplatin and etoposide, temozolomide, and cyclophosphamide with doxorubicin in combination with either 5-FU or dacarbazine.[69,71,72,76–78]

PARATHYROID TUMORS

Parathyroid Adenomas/Hyperplasia

Epidemiology and Pathophysiology

Primary hyperparathyroidism (HPT) results from benign parathyroid adenomas and multigland hyperplasia in approximately 93% and 6% of cases, respectively.[79] The incidence of primary HPT in children is 2 to 5 per 100,000/yr in children, and HPT is more common in older adolescents.[80–82] Studies are conflicting regarding gender predisposition.[80,81] The only identified environmental risk factor is exposure of the head and neck to ionizing radiation.[83] Familial syndromes (Table 36.1), chiefly MEN1, constitute as much as 30% to 50% of pediatric patients with primary HPT, compared with only 5% in adults.[80,81] In children presenting with PTH-mediated hypercalcemia, mutations in the calcium sensing receptor (*CaSR*) should also be considered.[84] Familial hypocalciuric hypercalcemia, also called familial benign hypercalcemia, is secondary to loss-of-function mutations in the *CaSR*. These patients have biochemical characteristics similar to neoplastic causes of HPT and are distinguished by their relative hypocalciuria.[85] As these patients do not have pathologic HPT, they do not require further treatment. Homozygotes or compound heterozygotes for mutations in the *CaSR* gene present at birth with severe neonatal HPT.[86]

Clinical Presentation and Diagnosis

Symptoms of HPT in children can be nonspecific, including polyuria, fatigue, headache, poor appetite, weight loss, abdominal pain, nausea, and emesis. Children with primary HPT are likely to have more severe symptoms compared with adults.[81,82] Because of delays in diagnosis, presenting features can also include nephrocalcinosis, nephrolithiasis, acute pancreatitis, band keratopathy, or bone involvement (brown tumors/osteitis fibrosa cystica in the most severe cases).[81,82]

The diagnosis of HPT is confirmed by demonstrating hypercalcemia and inappropriately normal or high serum concentrations of intact parathyroid hormone (PTH) in the absence of vitamin D deficiency. Phosphorus levels are often low and alkaline phosphatase levels can be elevated, with higher levels noted in HPT-induced bone disease.[81] Twenty-four hour or random urine measurement of calcium and creatinine for calculation of calcium clearance is necessary to rule out familial hypocalciuric

hypercalcemia. Bone radiographs may reveal characteristic lesions of osteitis fibrosa cystica and findings compatible with rickets. Assessment of bone density may demonstrate low bone mass for age. Imaging modalities used to localize parathyroid tumors include ultrasound (US), ^{99m}Tc-sestamibi scan with single photon emission computed tomography (SPECT) imaging, MRI, and high-resolution four-dimensional CT[87,88] (Fig. 36.3). The sensitivity of ^{99m}Tc-sestamibi is reduced in the presence of multigland disease, a finding more common to patients with familial syndromes such as MEN1.

Treatment and Follow-Up

Treatment of HPT consists of surgical removal of the affected parathyroid gland(s). For all pediatric patients with primary HPT, but especially in situations where multigland disease is suspected, imaging is negative, or a second surgical exploration is needed, locating an experienced endocrine surgeon is of paramount importance.[89] If preoperative localization studies identify a solitary adenoma, minimally invasive parathyroidectomy with the use of a rapid intraoperative PTH assay is generally the procedure of choice.[87] In patients with genetic syndromes predisposing to multigland involvement, cervical exploration of all parathyroid glands is recommended.[90] Possible surgical approaches in these patients include subtotal parathyroidectomy with viable remnant left in situ with a clip or total parathyroidectomy with forearm autograft.[91,92] The appropriate timing and indications for surgery in children with hereditary HPT has not been defined.[93] The medical management of hypercalcemia focuses on maintaining hydration, increasing urine calcium excretion, and diminishing bone resorption. Bisphosphonates or the calcimimetic, cinacalcet, can also be used in the acute management of severe HPT until surgery is undertaken.[94]

Vitamin D (25-hydroxy vitamin D) levels should be checked preoperatively and supplemented to reduce the risk of postoperative hypocalcemia. More severe postoperative hypocalcemia can occur in patients with pre-existing bone disease or vitamin D deficiency, a condition known as the "hungry bone syndrome" and manifested by hypocalcemia, hypophosphatemia, and hypomagnesemia.[95]

PTH levels drop immediately after successful surgical resection, and calcium levels follow in the next 24 to 48 hours.[96] Therefore, cure can be determined shortly after surgery. Despite normal calcium levels, PTH levels may remain elevated in a secondary fashion and should not be misinterpreted as recurrent or residual disease.[97] In pediatric patients with primary HPT, there is up to a 6% rate of recurrence.[81,82] This is more likely in patients with genetic syndromes of HPT, but recurrent adenomas can occur in sporadic cases. Thus, annual screening with calcium and PTH levels should be considered.

Parathyroid Carcinoma

Epidemiology and Pathophysiology

Parathyroid carcinoma (PTCa) is extremely rare, accounting for <1% of all cases of primary HPT.[98] The incidence in children is unknown, but PTCa occurs in all ages and has been reported as early as 8 years of age.[99] Gender distribution is about equal. Predisposing factors for the development of PTCa include a history of neck irradiation, prolonged secondary HPT, and end-stage renal disease on hemodialysis.[98] Malignant transformation from a pre-existing adenoma or hyperplasia does not appear to occur.[100] Somatic and germline mutations in *CDC73* (*HRPT2*) are a risk factor for PTCa.[101]

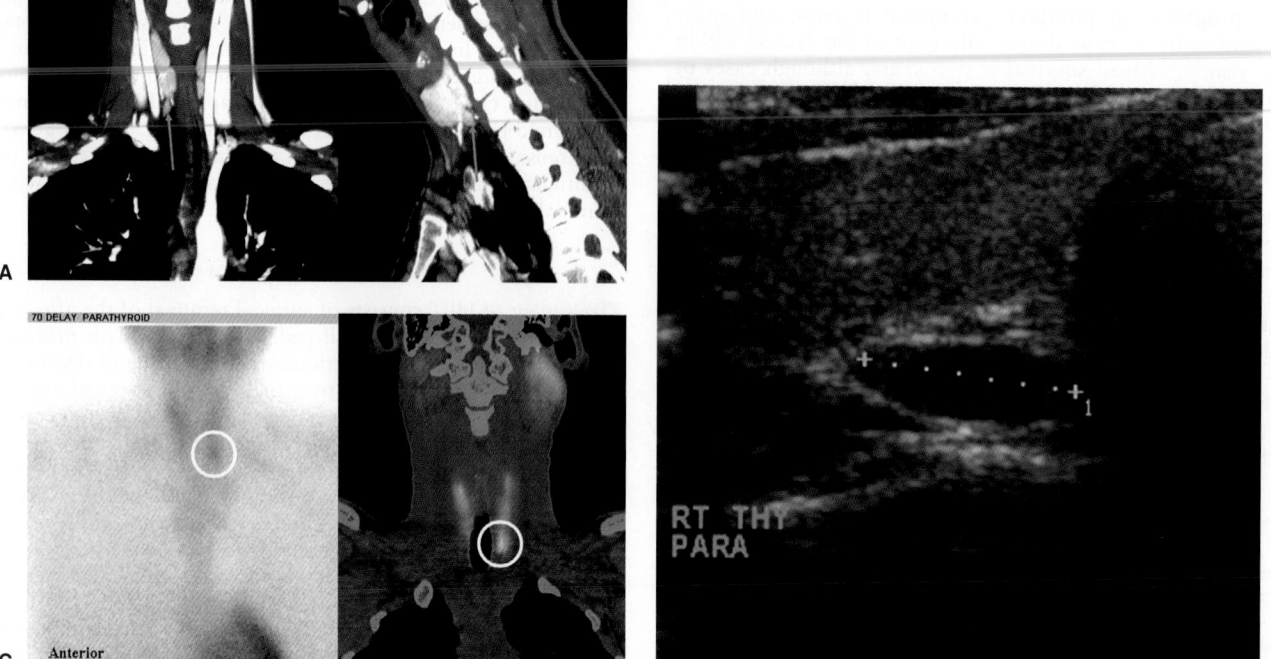

FIGURE 36.3 Imaging of parathyroid tumors. **A:** Coronal (*left*) and sagittal (*right*) four-dimensional computed tomography (CT) of a parathyroid adenoma (*green arrows*) with sporadic presentation. **B:** Ultrasound imaging of the same tumor (*green line*) presented in (**A**). **C:** ^{99m}Tc-Sestamibi scan (*left*) with fused single photon emission computed tomography (SPECT) coronal images (*right*) identifying a profoundly hyperplastic parathyroid gland (*white circle*) in a patient with primary hyperparathyroidism and MEN1.

Clinical Presentation and Diagnosis

The clinical features of PTCa are due to severe hypercalcemia and tumor mass infiltrating vital organs. Malignancy is suggested with a severe clinical presentation, palpable neck mass, serum calcium levels >14 mg/dL, significantly elevated PTH levels, and elevated alkaline phosphatase.[98,102,103] Pathologically, PTCa is difficult to distinguish from benign tumors. The diagnosis can be unequivocally made only in those tumors with documented metastases or in tumors that invade adjacent soft tissues, thyroid gland, blood vessels, and/or perineural spaces.[104] Given the possibility of *CDC73* mutations in PTCa, immunohistochemistry for parafibromin (the protein encoded by *CDC73*) may also assist in the pathologic diagnosis.[104] Fine needle aspiration is not recommended because of potential seeding of malignant cells and the inability to make an accurate histologic diagnosis.

Treatment

The recommended treatment for PTCa is an *en bloc* resection of the primary lesion together with the ipsilateral thyroid lobe and isthmus, central lymph nodes, thymic tongue, and any adherent tissue to the tumor, including the recurrent laryngeal nerve if needed. Extensive lateral neck dissection is not recommended unless there are grossly enlarged lymph nodes, and great care must be taken to avoid rupture of the capsule of the gland.[98,105] If the diagnosis is made postoperatively, re-exploration of the neck and more comprehensive resection may be indicated if the pathology appears aggressive or the patient remains hypercalcemic.

In appropriate cases, distant metastatic disease can be treated with surgical metastasectomy.[105] Systemic chemotherapy for PTCa is not well studied and has limited efficacy.

Agents that have been used include combinations of dacarbazine, cyclophosphamide, 5-FU, vincristine, and doxorubicin.[98,102,106] Radiation therapy may be helpful in terms of locoregional control.[102] The medical management of refractory symptomatic hypercalcemia includes intravenous bisphosphonates, parenteral salmon calcitonin, plicamycin (mithramycin), gallium nitrate, and/or cinacalcet.[98,107]

Prognosis

PTCa is a slow growing yet progressive tumor that tends to recur locally or spread to contiguous structures in the neck. Metastases occur later in the course of the disease via lymphatic or hematogenous spread. Cervical lymph nodes (30%), lung (40%), and liver (10%) are the most common metastatic sites.[98] Recurrence rates are high and the average time between surgery and first recurrence is approximately 3 years, noting that prolonged disease-free intervals have been reported. Disease-specific mortality usually results from uncontrolled hypercalcemia. Five-year survival has been reported between 40% and 85%.[102,108]

THYROID TUMORS

Benign Thyroid Neoplasms

Epidemiology and Pathophysiology

Palpable thyroid nodules are found in 2% of the pediatric population and represent approximately 5% of all nonfunctioning thyroid nodules.[109,110] The most common neoplasm identified in this age group is the follicular adenoma.[111,112] The likelihood

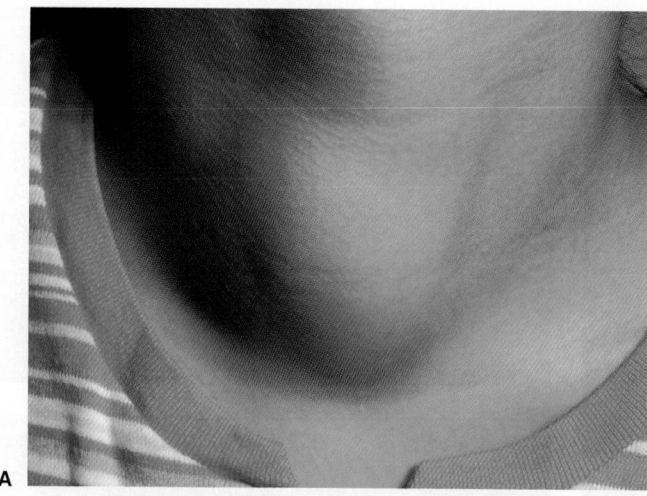
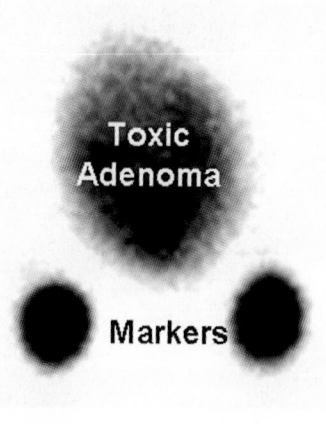

FIGURE 36.4 Functioning or "hot" nodule. **A:** A large thyroid nodule involving most of the right thyroid lobe is clearly visible on physical examination. **B:** On ^{123}I thyroid uptake and scan, only the toxic nodule is identified; the remainder of the normal thyroid tissue is appropriately suppressed.

of malignancy is higher in the pediatric age group, with approximately 25% of childhood thyroid nodules found to be malignant compared with 5% to 10% in adults.[109,111–113] Functioning nodules (Fig. 36.4) associated with subclinical or overt hyperthyroidism also occur, and these "hot" or toxic thyroid neoplasms have been associated with somatic mutations in the TSH receptor (*TSHR*) and *GNAS* genes.[13] Risk factors associated with developing thyroid nodules include iodine insufficiency, exposure to ionizing radiation, a family history of thyroid disease, and a personal history of autoimmune thyroid disease.[114] In addition, there is an increased prevalence of benign and malignant thyroid nodules in certain genetic syndromes (Table 36.1).

Clinical Presentation and Diagnosis

Thyroid nodules are usually asymptomatic, although those children with toxic nodules may have the classic signs and symptoms of hyperthyroidism. Many nodules are identified during routine physical exam, but an increasing number are incidentally discovered during an unrelated radiologic exam. Pediatric thyroid nodules should be evaluated with thyroid function testing, thyroid and neck US, and fine needle aspiration biopsy (FNAB). Although the routine measurement of calcitonin (CTN) is controversial, measuring thyroglobulin (TG) is not routinely recommended because elevated TG levels are identified in a variety of benign thyroid processes, thereby lowering the specificity of this diagnostic test.[115,116]

Thyroid US can provide information on size, location, echogenicity, blood flow, multiplicity, and potential involvement of regional lymph nodes by cancer (Fig. 36.5). US facilitates the accuracy of FNAB of both the primary thyroid lesion(s) and suspicious lymphadenopathy in the central and lateral neck, which greatly assists in surgical planning.[117] Benign US characteristics include a hyperechoic, homogenous internal architecture of the nodule; complete cystic composition; the presence of a translucent halo; eggshell calcifications; and/or a smooth, well-defined margin. In contrast, findings suggestive of malignancy include a hypoechoic pattern, subcapsular localization, increased peri- and intranodular vascularization, the presence of microcalcifications, and/or irregular/jagged margins.[109,115,118]

Nuclear scintigraphy using radioactive iodine (RAI) or ^{99m}Tc-pertechnetate[119] is not very useful in the initial evaluation of a thyroid nodule, except in patients with a low TSH (Fig. 36.4) or in those with an FNAB diagnosis of follicular lesion or neoplasm, in whom nodule functionality may help to determine management.[116,120]

FNAB is the most efficient and accurate method of evaluating the etiology of a thyroid nodule in pediatric patients.[109,116,121,122] Cytologic examination of the FNAB sample should be performed at the bedside in order to establish adequacy of the sample and determine if additional samples are needed for accurate diagnosis. Although surgery is not an unreasonable approach to the diagnosis of a thyroid nodule in a young child,[123] it is our feeling that FNAB allows for better operative planning and may minimize the need for a additional surgeries in children with cancer. In patients with multinodular disease, the selection of nodules to undergo FNAB should be based on US characteristics, not necessarily nodule size.[116]

Treatment and Follow-Up

In children with functional thyroid nodules, surgery is the preferred treatment, although RAI therapy can also be considered. For nonfunctional thyroid neoplasms, treatment and follow-up are determined by cytopathologic diagnosis. For patients with malignant/suspicious cytology or a diagnosis of follicular neoplasm, surgery is recommended (Table 36.2). In patients with nondiagnostic or indeterminate results, such as follicular lesion of undetermined significance, repeat FNAB or surgery is the most appropriate next step.[116,120,124] Given the lack of established cellular or biochemical markers to more accurately identify benign from malignant disease, the decision to proceed to surgery is based on clinical criteria such as age of the patient, family history, nodule size, US criteria, history of radiation exposure, and others.[109,115,120] In patients with benign cytology, annual physical exam and ultrasonography are appropriate, with repeat FNAB if the nodule grows significantly.[124] TSH suppression with exogenous levothyroxine is no longer recommended in the euthyroid patient.[109,115,116]

Malignant Thyroid Neoplasms

Thyroid carcinoma is the most common endocrine malignancy, with an estimated 37,200 new cases diagnosed in the

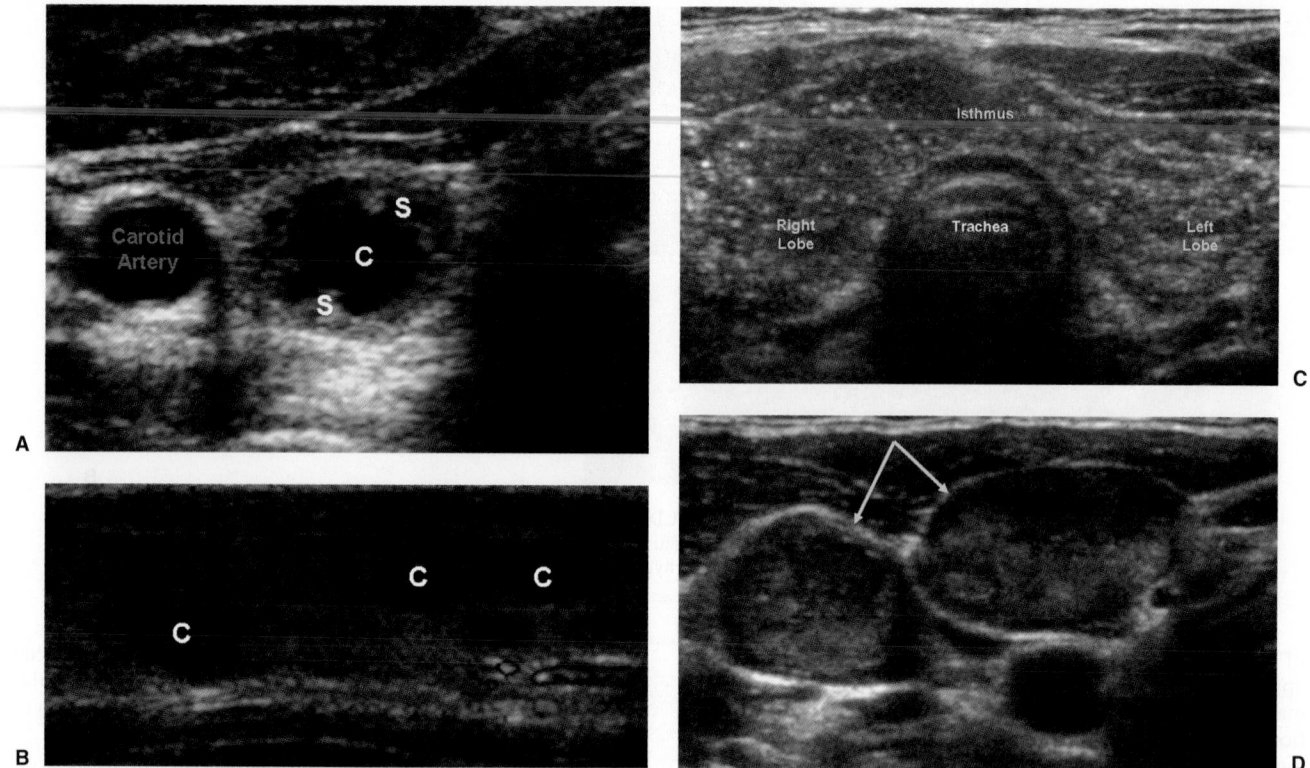

FIGURE 36.5 Ultrasound findings of benign and malignant thyroid neoplasms. **A:** Benign colloid nodule with mixed solid [S] and cystic [C] components. **B:** Multiple benign thyroid cysts [C] in a different patient. **C:** Papillary thyroid carcinoma diffusely involving the thyroid gland with characteristic scattered microcalcifications. **D:** Metastatic lymphadenopathy (*yellow arrows*) identified in the same patient as in (C).

United States during 2009, of which only 1.8% occur in individuals younger than 20 years.[125,126] The incidence is ≤1 case/million/yr in children younger than 10 years to 18 cases/million/yr in adolescents aged 15 to 19, the most commonly affected pediatric age group.[126–128]

Thyroid malignancies arise from the thyroid follicular epithelium (differentiated thyroid carcinoma [DTC]: papillary thyroid carcinoma [PTC], follicular thyroid carcinoma [FTC], and their variants) or the neural crest-derived parafollicular C cell (medullary thyroid carcinoma; MTC).[8] Anaplastic (undifferentiated) thyroid carcinomas and poorly DTCs are exceedingly rare in childhood, as are primary thyroid lymphomas and metastases to the thyroid gland. Several multidisciplinary guidelines[93,116,120,123,129–131] have been created to assist in clinical decision-making in the care of these patients, recognizing that there remains a dearth of evidence-based recommendations for the treatment of pediatric thyroid carcinoma.

Differentiated Thyroid Carcinoma

Epidemiology and Pathophysiology

DTC is the most common thyroid malignancy, with PTC representing 90% or more of cases.[128,132,133] PTC is typically a disease of young women, and the female:male incidence is greater than 5:1 in adolescents.[123,127] This gender difference is not pronounced in children younger than 10 years.[123] Subtypes of DTC include: follicular cell, tall cell, columnar cell, diffuse sclerosing, and encapsulated variants in PTC; and Hürthle-cell (oncocytic), clear cell, and insular (poorly differentiated) carcinoma in FTC.[8] In contrast to the classical type

found in older individuals, childhood PTC, particularly in patients younger than 10 years, may be unencapsulated, widely invasive throughout the gland, and have a follicular and solid architecture with unique nuclear features and abundant psammoma bodies.[134,135]

The major established environmental risk factor for the development of PTC is therapeutic radiation exposure to the head and neck.[136,137] Children, particularly those younger than 5 years, are much more sensitive to the tumorigenic effects of irradiation, which may be in part due to the higher rate of thyroid cell replication in children as compared with adults.[113,138,139] In the youngest children, radiation therapy not including the thyroid region can also increase the risk of PTC.[137] The risk of malignancy paradoxically appears to decline once the thyroid dose exceeds 200 cGy,[140] and radiation-induced PTC does not appear significantly different in clinical behavior compared with sporadic nonradiation-induced tumors.[141] Interestingly, thyroid cancer in childhood cancer survivors is increased even in those children who did not receive therapeutic radiation therapy.[142] Internal ionizing radiation, as seen with the large environmental exposure to RAI from the Chernobyl nuclear accident, is also associated with the development of PTC, particularly in children younger than 10 years when exposed.[128,143,144] The small doses of RAI used in diagnostic studies and in the treatment of hyperthyroidism appear to be below the threshold needed for tumorigenesis.[136] Iodine insufficiency is associated with an increased incidence of FTC[128,145] and, as with many other cancers, obesity may be an additional risk factor.[125]

Recent advances in the molecular and genetic basis of DTC have improved understanding of disease pathogenesis and provided new targets for therapeutic intervention. Activation

TABLE 36.2

SURGICAL MANAGEMENT OF THYROID CARCINOMA

Tumor	Surgical management of the neck	Surgical management of parathyroid glands that are devascularized/removed
Papillary thyroid carcinoma	• TT, consider prophylactic ipsilateral level VI ND in higher risk patients (tumor >1 cm, age > 45) • If clinical or radiographic evidence of level VI LN mets or large tumor size, perform level VI ND • If clinical or radiographic evidence of lateral LN mets, perform lateral neck dissection on that side	• Autograft in neck
Follicular thyroid carcinoma	• If known preoperatively (i.e., distant mets), TT • If Hürthle cell carcinoma or poorly differentiated cancer, extent of ND as per PTC recommendations • If not known preoperatively (i.e., follicular neoplasm), lobectomy followed by TT if tumor more than minimally invasive	• Autograft in neck
Medullary thyroid carcinoma		
Prophylactic thyroidectomy in MEN2/FMTC	• TT if normal US and normal or minimally elevated calcitonin (<40–50 pg/mL) • Performance of level VI ND based on *RET* mutation, age of the patient, serum calcitonin level, and cervical US findings	• Autograft in neck if *RET* mutation consistent with FMTC or MEN2B • Autograft in forearm for *RET* mutations consistent with MEN2A
Clinical MTC in MEN2/FMTC	• TT plus level VI ND • Lateral neck dissection if clinical or radiographic evidence of lateral LN mets (consider bilateral prophylactic lateral neck dissections in MEN2B)	• Autograft in neck if *RET* mutation consistent with FMTC or MEN2B • Cryopreserve/autograft in forearm for *RET* mutations consistent with MEN2A
Sporadic MTC (no germline *RET* mutation)	• TT plus level VI ND • Lateral neck dissection if clinical or radiographic evidence of lateral LN mets	• Autograft in neck

MEN, multiple endocrine neoplasia; FMTC, familial medullary thyroid cancer (MTC); TT, total thyroidectomy; ND, neck dissection; LN, lymph node; US, ultrasound.
From Ying AK, Huh W, Bottomley S, et al. Thyroid cancer in young adults. Semin Oncol 2009;36(3):258–274, with permission.

of the RAS-RAF-MEK-ERK (mitogen-activated protein kinase) signaling pathway is critical in tumorigenesis, and greater than 70% of adult PTCs are due to nonoverlapping genetic events in the genes *RAS*, *BRAF*, or *RET/PTC*.[146–148] One of the major early somatic events associated with the development of PTC is a chromosomal rearrangement linking the promotor region of an unrelated gene(s) ("*PTC*") to the carboxyl terminus of the *RET* (REarranged during Transfection) proto-oncogene.[113,138,143,148] The *RET/PTC* rearrangement produces a chimeric oncogene, resulting in a constitutively activated form of the *RET* receptor tyrosine kinase, which is normally not expressed in thyroid follicular cells.

Mutations in *BRAF* are the most common cause of PTC in adults, occurring in 36% to 83% of cases.[146] PTCs that are positive for a *BRAF* mutation are often interpreted as tall cell variants and are more clinically aggressive.[149] Children and young adults are less likely to harbor somatic *BRAF* mutations, and *RET/PTC* rearrangements are more common in this population.[128,148,150] Other genes and gene products involved in tumorigenesis include *RAS* (PTC and FTC); the *TRK* proto-oncogene (rearranged akin to *RET*, but found in a minority of PTCs); *Pax8-PPARγ1* translocations (follicular adenomas and FTCs only); *MET* overexpression (mostly in PTCs); the *p53* tumor suppressor gene (specifically involved in anaplastic thyroid cancer); *PIK3CA* (mostly FTC); and the *AKAP9–BRAF* gene fusion (radiation-induced PTC carcinomas developing after a short latency period).[113,138,146,148,151]

Up to 5% of patients with PTC have a family history of the disease.[113,152] Having familial nonmedullary thyroid carcinoma (FNMTC) may portend a worse prognosis and require more aggressive treatment.[153] Genetic anticipation has also been identified in such cases.[154] Although the genetic basis for familial nonmedullary thyroid carcinoma has not yet been elucidated, somatic mutations in *RAS* and *BRAF* have been identified in 52% of cases.[155] Other familial tumor syndromes in which there is an increased risk of DTC include familial adenomatous polyposis, Cowden syndrome, Werner syndrome, and CNC[8,113,156–159] (Table 36.1).

Clinical Presentation and Diagnosis

DTC usually presents as an asymptomatic neck mass, although occasionally the diagnosis may be made only after the discovery of distant metastases[160–162] (Fig. 36.6). DTC can uncommonly arise ectopically in a thyroglossal duct remnant or cyst or be identified incidentally after surgery for benign thyroid disease, such as Graves disease. Locally metastatic disease is present at diagnosis in the vast majority of pediatric PTC cases.[132,133,135,161,162] In addition, children more often have disseminated disease at diagnosis, with lung metastases identified in up to 20% of cases.[132,133,135,162–164] Metastases to other sites, such as bone and brain, are rare (Fig. 36.6).

PTC and FTC have key differences in clinical behavior,[165] likely due to different underlying mutational events. PTC is

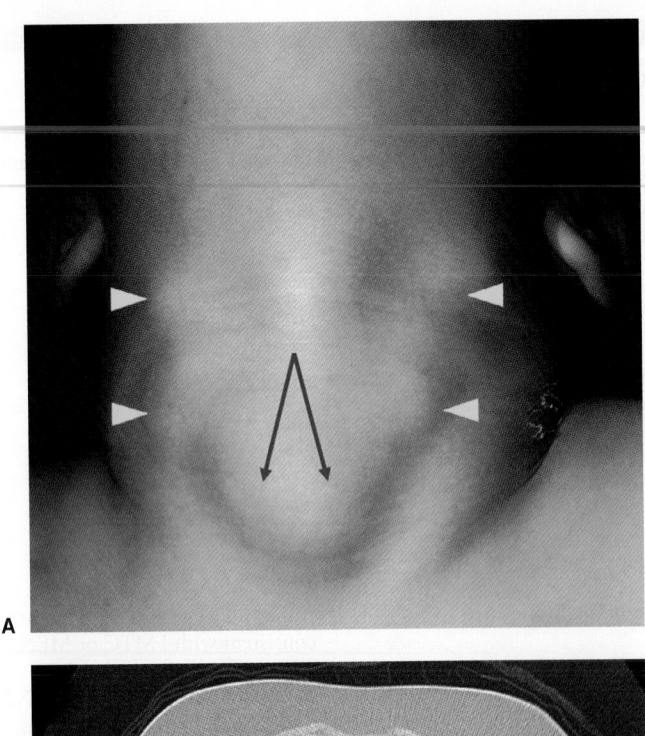

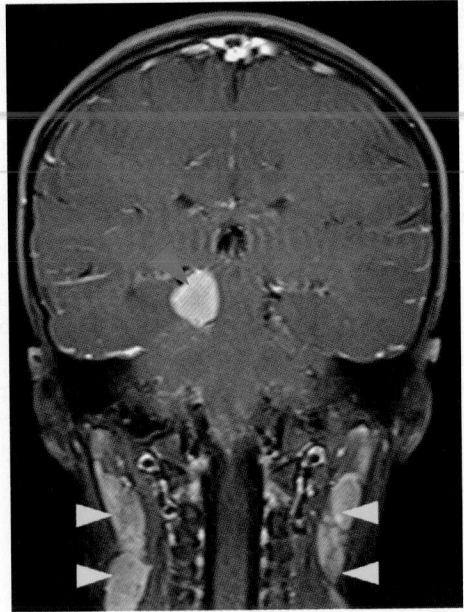

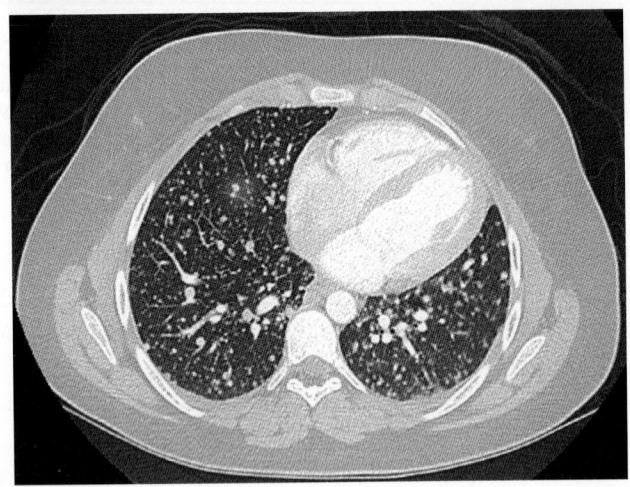

FIGURE 36.6 Clinical presentations of pediatric PTC. **A:** Large infiltrating thyroid mass (*blue arrows*) with bilateral palpable metastatic lymphadenopathy (*yellow arrowheads*). **B:** MRI of the same patient as in (**A**) demonstrating bulky metastatic lymphadenopathy (*yellow arrowheads*) and an incidental brain metastasis (*red arrowhead*). **C:** Lung metastases typically appear as multiple well-defined pulmonary nodules that are more prominent in the lung bases.

more likely to metastasize via lymphatic channels to regional neck lymph nodes, with hematogenous metastases, primarily to the lung, occurring less often and typically only when significant locoregional lymph node metastases are present.[133] FTC, on the other hand, is more prone initially to hematogenous metastases (affecting predominantly the lungs and bones). Metastasis to regional lymph nodes is uncommon, but can be seen with some of the less-differentiated FTC subtypes. Furthermore, PTC is more likely to be multifocal and bilateral; FTC, in contrast, is usually a unifocal tumor.

A high-quality neck US and FNAB of suspicious lymph nodes are critical in the initial evaluation of DTC (Fig. 36.5). Nuclear imaging studies are not helpful in the initial evaluation of thyroid cancer patients, and thyroid function studies are anticipated to be normal in most cases. DTC cells retain the ability to produce the thyroid-specific glycoprotein, TG. Once the diagnosis of DTC is established, a baseline TG will be useful for follow-up and for the potential identification of a large metastatic disease burden. TG autoantibodies should always be measured concomitantly, as these occur in up to 25% of thyroid cancer patients and render the TG level uninterpretable.[166] A chest x-ray or chest CT *without* contrast to assess for pulmonary metastases can also be considered at diagnosis, espe-

cially in those patients with significant locoregional disease, noting that many individuals with lung metastases may not have abnormalities visualized on plain radiographs.[162,164,167] Finally, cross sectional imaging of the neck (CT with contrast or MRI, depending on local expertise) is recommended for patients with significant metastatic neck lymphadenopathy, as the superior mediastinum and central compartment are not well visualized via US. Although the use of iodinated contrast will delay subsequent RAI therapy, the information gained should allow for better surgical planning and oncologic outcomes.

Staging and Prognosis

Although several prognostic staging systems have been described for thyroid cancer, specifically PTC,[116,168,169] a thorough discussion of these is beyond the scope of the current chapter. The pathological TNM (tumor-node-metastasis) classification was adopted by the American Joint Committee on Cancer and the International Union Against Cancer Committee as the international reference staging system for thyroid cancer.[170] By definition, however, the highest TNM stage that anyone younger than age 45 can achieve is stage II, distinguished from stage I only by the presence of distant metastases. Another frequently used staging system, the MACIS (distant Metastasis, patient Age, Completeness of resection, local Invasion, and tumor Size) score, may also be useful in children and adolescents but requires further validation.[171]

Most children with DTC have an excellent prognosis and survival over decades is generally the norm for these patients, even in the presence of distant metastases at diagnosis.[132,133,135,172–174] Cure rates are high, and 10-year survival is almost universally 100% in this age group.[123,133,135,163,172,173,175,176] For patients with stage II disease, micronodular lung metastases and iodine-avid disease (i.e., those cells that retain good expression of the sodium-iodide symporter) confer the best prognosis.[164,176,177] Some children with DTC will ultimately succumb to their disease or die from treatment-related complications.[172,178] Children diagnosed prior to age 10 appear to have a higher risk of recurrence and ultimately death from their disease.[134,174,179] It remains unknown why children with a similar extent of disease presentation have a much better prognosis compared with adults, but it is suspected that underlying mutational differences play a role, in addition to the knowledge that pediatric thyroid cancer tends to be more iodine-avid and responsive to TSH suppressive therapy.

Treatment and Follow-Up

Surgery. Surgery is the cornerstone of therapy for DTC (Table 36.2) and total thyroidectomy is the initial procedure of choice, since it has been associated with lower recurrence rates and better survival compared with lobectomy alone, particularly for tumors greater than 1 cm in size.[116,123,133,165,173,174,180–184] In addition, total thyroidectomy facilitates ^{131}I therapy. Lobectomy and isthmusectomy alone may suffice in the low-risk adolescent patient with a small unifocal PTC (without US evidence of lymphadenopathy or contralateral thyroid nodules).[116,120,123,182,183] The extent of lymph node dissection is based on the type of DTC and the clinical presentation[169] (Table 36.2). All lymph node dissections should be comprehensive and compartment focused because the rates of recurrence are higher when "berry picking" alone is undertaken.[185] Although total thyroidectomy and central compartment lymph node dissections are associated with higher risks, such as hypoparathyroidism and recurrent laryngeal nerve injury,[133,180,186] these risks should be minimized when the surgery is performed by a high-volume surgeon.[89,183]

The diagnosis of FTC is established only after the pathologic identification of capsular and/or vascular invasion of a resected "follicular lesion" or "follicular neoplasm." Although the prognosis of FTC may not be as dependent on the extent of the initial surgery, a total thyroidectomy facilitates the use of RAI to ablate the normal thyroid remnant, which permits an increased sensitivity to detect disease recurrence, thus improving outcomes for patients with FTC.[187] The lymph nodes should be managed similarly to PTC in poorly differentiated tumors and more aggressive variants such as Hürthle cell carcinoma (Table 36.2).

Radioactive Iodine/External Beam Radiation Therapy. The rationale for RAI treatment is to ablate normal remnant thyroid tissue, thus improving the sensitivity to identify residual or recurrent disease, and to treat iodine-avid metastatic disease.[165,184] RAI appears to lower recurrence rates and cancer-related mortality in patients whose tumors concentrate iodine.[176,181,188] However, recent studies in adults have demonstrated that low-risk patients may not clearly benefit from adjuvant RAI.[189,190] This issue has not been well-addressed in pediatric DTC, and the possible benefits of RAI must always be weighed against the potential side effects of therapy.

Following thyroidectomy, the child with DTC is usually rendered hypothyroid with plans to administer RAI when the TSH is above 30 μU/mL.[116,123,184,191] Recombinant human TSH (rhTSH; Thyrogen®) can also be used for RAI ablation of remnant thyroid tissue in low-risk patients,[192,193] and its use may result in a lower absorbed dose to the blood compared with RAI treatment after withdrawal.[194] However, prospective studies in children using rhTSH are lacking. A low iodine diet is followed for 2 weeks to facilitate RAI uptake by any remaining thyroid tissues. Most centers routinely obtain a pretherapy (or diagnostic) whole body scan using ^{131}I or ^{123}I to identify distant metastases and to determine the appropriate treatment dose.[116,191,195] In addition to the diagnostic scan, the administered dose of RAI also depends on histopathological features and the stimulated TG. There are no standardized recommendations for the use of therapeutic RAI in children, and the ^{131}I dose is based on a weight (or body surface area) adjustment of the typical adult dose used in that situation.[123,165,191] Dosimetric studies to limit whole body retention at 48 hours to less than 80 mCi and blood/bone marrow exposure to less than 200 cGy should be considered in those children anticipated to have significant diffuse lung uptake with RAI therapy and those children with more widespread distant metastases.[116,196] A posttreatment thyroid scan, sometimes coupled with SPECT imaging (Fig. 36.7), obtained 5 to 8 days after the therapeutic dose of ^{131}I is given, should be obtained to identify other sites of disease that were not apparent on the diagnostic study[116,164].

External beam radiation therapy to treat residual microscopic disease in the neck is not routinely offered to pediatric patients, except in the very rare case of a pathologically unfavorable thyroid carcinoma with known residual neck disease. As with any solid malignancy, radiation does play a role in palliation of distant metastases.

Thyroid-Stimulating Hormone Suppression. Most pediatric DTC remains well differentiated and because DTC can grow in response to the trophic effects of TSH, patients are treated with pharmacologic suppression of TSH, which decreases the risk of disease recurrence, progression, and mortality.[174,188,189,197] Consensus guidelines have recommended keeping the TSH suppressed below 0.1 mU/L in patients at high risk for morbidity and mortality and to keep the TSH minimally suppressed (between 0.1 and 0.5 mU/L) in low-risk patients (the vast majority of children).[116,120] The TSH can generally be kept in the low normal range in low-risk patients who have no evidence of disease after initial therapies.[197] Although unstudied, potential risks of long-term TSH suppression (such as negative effects on childhood growth, bone mineralization, and the heart) are expected to be minimal in the otherwise healthy pediatric population.

Chemotherapy and Targeted Therapy. In patients with progressive life-threatening disease that is not amenable to surgery and no longer responds to RAI, systemic therapy is warranted. Clinical trials are preferred in adults[116,120] but are not available for children with DTC, outside of phase I studies. Traditional cytotoxic chemotherapy has had limited success, and the most commonly used agent has been doxorubicin, either as a single agent or in combination with another drug such as cisplatin or interferon-α.[116,147,198,199] Carboplatin and paclitaxel are sometimes given to adult patients with advanced thyroid cancer requiring systemic therapy, but this regimen has not been studied formally. The advent of targeted therapies has revolutionized the management of DTC, with multiple different antiangiogenic agents showing promise in the treatment of this orphan disease[106,147,200] (Table 36.3). Sorafenib is the best studied and has shown benefit in treatment-refractory thyroid cancer.[207–209] Other oral tyrosine

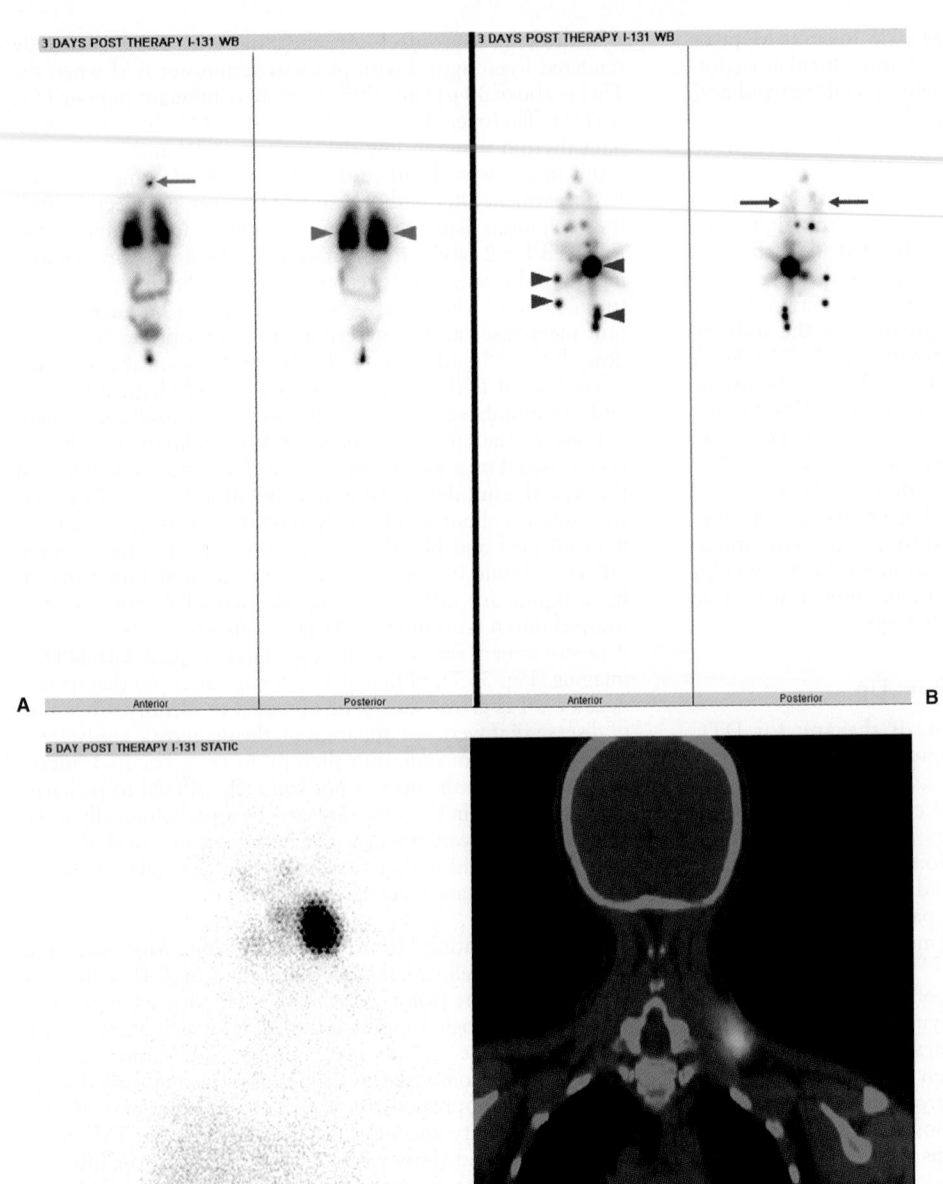

FIGURE 36.7 ^{131}I posttreatment scans in pediatric PTC. **A:** Neck uptake (red arrow) and diffuse pulmonary uptake (*red arrowheads*) in micronodular pulmonary metastases. **B:** Nodular pulmonary uptake (*blue arrows*) and bony metastases (*blue arrowheads*) in the patient from Figure 36.6 (**A**) and (**B**). **C:** RAI uptake in a metastatic left supraclavicular lymph node (*left*), well localized with concomitant SPECT imaging coronal images (*right*).

kinase inhibitors (TKIs) that have shown promise in the treatment of DTC include axitinib, motesanib, and sunitinib.[201–203,211]

Follow-Up. Children with DTC require lifelong surveillance, both to identify delayed recurrences and to assess for any late treatment effects. Given its indolent nature, DTC frequently becomes a chronic condition. In addition to TSH suppression, the long-term management of DTC includes periodic assessment of TG and TG antibody levels, routine neck US, and diagnostic RAI scans and cross sectional imaging as indicated, with the intensity of follow-up and treatment depending on initial and ongoing risk stratification for disease recurrence and progression.[116,120,165,184,191,213,214] If TG levels remain detectable while on levothyroxine therapy, the possibility of residual disease must be entertained and appropriate diagnostic studies ordered. In patients with detectable TG antibodies, the antibody titer itself should be followed.[215] A TSH-stimulated TG level and diagnostic thyroid scan after thyroid hormone withdrawal or rhTSH is typically obtained 12 months (earlier in the highest-risk patients) after initial

RAI therapy. Most patients with a rhTSH stimulated TG value of >2 ng/mL will have disease identified within 5 years, although some patients with a positive test may ultimately have resolution of their minimally elevated stimulated TG.[216] Therefore, there is some utility in repeating a stimulated TG in patients whose TG is negative on suppressive therapy but previously positive after THW or rhTSH, but it does not apply to patients in whom the stimulated and suppressed TG are undetectable, since these patients are likely cured.[216,217] Multiple repeated diagnostic thyroid scans are not necessary in the low-risk patient without evidence of disease after 1 year of follow-up.

In adult patients with elevated serum TG levels and negative imaging studies, or with a level of TG that appears out of proportion to the amount of disease identified, ^{18}F-Fluorodeoxyglucose (FDG)-positron emission tomography (PET) imaging can be helpful.[218,219] There is an inverse relationship between RAI and FDG avidity, and FDG-PET scans may also predict cancer-associated mortality in adults.[220]

In the patient identified to have a neck recurrence, surgery is the treatment of choice. If the recurrence is not amenable to

TABLE 36.3

PUBLISHED CLINICAL TRIALS/REPORTS USING ORAL TKIs FOR THYROID CARCINOMA

Drug and reference(s)	Clinical phase	Number of patients	Patient histology	Initial dose	Comments
Axitinib					
(201)	II	60	All subtypes	5 mg twice daily	PR in 30%; 38% SD ≥ 16 wk
Motesanib					
(202)	I	7	All subtypes	Various	PR in 43%; 43% SD ≥ 16 wk
(203)	II	93	DTC (57 PTC)	125 mg daily	14% PR; 35% SD ≥ 24 wk
Gefitinib					
(204)	II	27	All subtypes	250 mg daily	No PR; 12% SD at 12 mo
Imatinib					
(205)	II	9	MTC	600 mg daily	No PR; 55% SD ≤ 6 mo
(206)	II	15	MTC	600 mg daily	No PR; 26% SD at 24 mo
Sorafenib					
(207)	II	30	All subtypes	400 mg twice daily	23% PR; 53% SD ≥ 14 wk
(208)	II	41	PTC	400 mg twice daily	15% PR; 56% SD ≥ 6 mo
(209)	Report	1	PTC	200 mg twice daily	PR
Sorafenib and Tipifarnib					
(210)	Report; I	1	MTC	Sorafenib 400 mg/200 mg daily Tipifarnib 200 mg twice daily (21 d)	PR
Sunitinib					
(211)	Report; I	2	PTC and FTC	50 mg daily for 4/6 wk	PR/SD based on FDG-PET
(212)	Report	1	MTC	50 mg daily for 4/6 wk	PR

FTC, follicular thyroid carcinoma; MTC, medullary thyroid carcinoma; PR, partial response; PTC, papillary thyroid carcinoma; SD, stable disease; TKI, tyrosine kinase inhibitor.
Adapted from Ying AK, Huh W, Bottomley S, et al. Thyroid cancer in young adults. Semin Oncol 2009;36(3):258–274, with permission.

surgical therapy or if distant metastases are identified, assessment and treatment with RAI is appropriate, assuming that the disease readily concentrates the isotope on diagnostic imaging. RAI therapy should be used sparingly in indolent disease and only in those children in whom it will be beneficial.[221] Therefore, empiric dosing with RAI is not recommended with RAI-scan negative disease, unless the patient has evidence of disease progression and surgery is not an option. It should also be noted that TG levels may slowly continue to decline in children previously treated with RAI and that undetectable TG levels in children with pulmonary metastases may not be a feasible goal in all cases.[128,167,175,222]

Late Effects/Complications of Treatment. Treatment of pediatric DTC is generally well tolerated with limited side effects. However, with the prospect of decades of survivorship, it is important to maintain an awareness of the potential early and late adverse events that may impact the patient's quality of life.[186,189] Surgical resection can be associated with lifelong voice difficulties and hypoparathyroidism. The long-term consequences of ^{131}I therapy in children remain largely unstudied. Early and usually transient side effects of ^{131}I therapy may include nausea, vomiting, sialoadenitis, xerostomia, loss of taste, thyroiditis (if a sizable thyroid remnant remains after surgery), and bone marrow suppression (leukopenia and thrombocytopenia).[223,224] Other sequelae of RAI therapy can include gonadal dysfunction (particularly in men), permanent damage to the salivary glands resulting in chronic xerostomia or salivary duct stones, nasolacrimal duct obstruction, excessive dental caries, pulmonary fibrosis (in those with diffuse

pulmonary metastases), and the development of other cancers (chiefly leukemia but also stomach, bladder, colon, salivary gland, and breast carcinomas) after very high cumulative doses of [131]I.[222–228]

Medullary Thyroid Carcinoma

Epidemiology and Pathophysiology

MTC comprises a minority of childhood thyroid malignancies, with an incidence of 0.5 cases/million/yr.[127] Although sporadic MTC can rarely be diagnosed in adolescence, it is most appropriate to think of MTC in the pediatric population as a genetic disease arising secondary to dominantly inherited or *de novo* activating mutations of the *RET* (*RE*arranged during *T*ransfection) proto-oncogene.[131,229,230] Therefore, almost all children with MTC are afflicted with one of three hereditary cancer syndromes (Table 36.1): MEN type 2A or type 2B (Fig. 36.8) and familial MTC, noting that the latter is now considered a phenotypic variant of MEN2A.[131,231] In MEN2A, mutations are located mostly in the extracellular cysteine-rich domain of the *RET* proto-oncogene, usually in exon 10 (codons 609, 611, 618, or 620) or exon 11 (codon 634, the most common mutation). In patients with MEN2B, the mutation is almost exclusively in exon 16 (a change from methionine to threonine at codon 918), located in the intracellular tyrosine kinase domain of the gene. There is a well-established genotype-phenotype correlation in hereditary MTC, and the specific mutation predicts disease aggressiveness and the

Epidemiology and Pathophysiology

The specific incidence of NETs in children is unknown, but in all age groups, it is 5.25/100,000/yr.[246] The incidence of NETs has increased in recent years, which may be due to more sensitive diagnostic imaging and to more active surveillance for genetic syndromes associated with neuroendocrine tumors.[8]

NETs can be functional or nonfunctional, and the overproduction of gastrin, serotonin, glucagon, SST, and ectopic hormones such as ACTH, GHRH, PTH-related peptide, and CTN can occur in both carcinoids and PETs. Overproduction of insulin or vasoactive intestinal peptide (VIP) is generally from PETs.[245,247] Nonfunctional tumors, which represent almost 40% of PETs, can overproduce clinically silent hormones such as pancreatic polypeptide (PP).[8,247-249] Little is known about the oncogenesis of sporadic NETs, but several heritable tumor syndromes are clearly associated with the development of GEP-NETs, including MEN1, von Hippel-Lindau (VHL) disease, neurofibromatosis type 1 (NF1), and TSC[8,14] (Table 36.1).

Carcinoids are the most common gastrointestinal tumors in pediatric patients, and bronchial carcinoid tumors are the most common primary lung tumor of childhood. The mean age of diagnosis is in adolescence in most series, but cases have been reported in children younger than 10 years.[250,251] There is a female predominance in children, while there is no difference among gender in adults.[251] In children with PETs, insulinomas are the most frequent, with 10% of patients diagnosed younger than the 20 years.[8]

Clinical Presentation and Diagnosis

The signs and symptoms of GEP-NETs, which are often nonspecific and confused with irritable bowel syndrome, depend on the specific hormone hypersecreted or the location and size of a nonfunctioning tumor. Several neuroendocrine markers—chromogranin A (CgA), PP, and neuron-specific enolase—are elevated in NETs and can be especially useful in clinical follow-up. CgA is the most sensitive marker, with reports of 70% to 100% sensitivity.[252] False-positive elevations can occur in patients with renal insufficiency, liver failure, atrophic gastritis, inflammatory bowel disease, exercise, and proton pump inhibitor use.[253] PP is primarily produced by the pancreas and its function is not well-defined; for NETs, it has a sensitivity of 50% to 60% and specificity of 65% to 80%.[254] Neuron-specific enolase is a glycolytic isoenzyme located in central and peripheral neurons and neuroendocrine cells that can be a helpful tumor marker for poorly differentiated neuroendocrine tumors.[247]

Since GEP-NETs are often small and grow slowly, localization can be challenging and often multiple techniques are employed. NETs generally possess SST receptors, which can be exploited with SST receptor scintigraphy using ^{111}In-DTPA (diethylene triamine pentaacetic acid)-octreotide (octreotide scan). This is usually the initial imaging modality used to localize tumors and recommended as part of the screening studies in MEN1 patients.[93] Octreotide scanning is also helpful in determining which patients are more likely to respond to SST analog therapy. NETs are highly vascular tumors that are best appreciated on triple phase contrast-enhanced studies, and for PETs, MRI appears more sensitive than CT.[255] Endoscopic US is also useful in localizing smaller PETs.[8,248] FDG-PET is not routinely useful, except in poorly differentiated NETs.[248,256] Although not widely available, other PET tracers being studied that appear more diagnostically sensitive include ^{18}F-DOPA (dihydroxyphenylalanine), ^{11}C-labeled 5-HTP (hydroxytryptophan), and radiolabeled SST analogs (^{111}In-

DOTA-TOC, ^{68}Ga-DOTA-TOC, and ^{68}Ga-DOTA-NOC, among others).[256,257]

For all PETs, the criteria for malignancy are angioinvasion, gross invasion, lymph node or liver metastases, or a high mitotic rate with Ki-67 staining >2%.[258] Malignant potential is thought to be greatest when lesions are greater than 2 cm, but this may not be the case for MEN1-associated NETs.[245,259,260]

Treatment/Follow-Up

Surgical resection is the optimal treatment for GEP-NETs. Depending on the size, location and type of tumor, excision of the tumor and peripancreatic lymph nodes, pancreaticoduodenectomy (i.e., Whipple procedure), or distal pancreatectomy with or without splenectomy is recommended.[248] Even in the presence of liver metastases, surgical resection of the primary tumor in midgut carcinoids can provide significant palliation of symptoms and should be considered.[261] The indolent nature of many NETs means that a period of watchful waiting is appropriate for certain patients. Timing and extent of surgery is controversial in MEN1 patients.[93,260]

Resection of liver metastases is considered if the involvement is focal and if palliation of clinical symptoms is needed. In addition to surgery, other liver-directed therapies include hepatic arterial embolization or chemoembolization, laser-induced thermal ablation, and transplantation.[248,262-264]

Systemic therapy for GEP-NETs may be separated into therapy that provides supportive care therapy and that which is directed against the cancerous cells. Supportive care for GEP-NETs primarily involves the long-acting SST analogs, octreotide, and lanreotide.[265] Radiolabelled receptor-binding SST analogs are also showing promise in the treatment of malignant GEP-NETs.[266] Interferon-α has been used as a single agent and in combination with other systemic agents.[265,267] Traditional cytotoxic chemotherapy has generally been reserved for poorly differentiated neuroendocrine carcinomas, with malignant PETs responding better than metastatic carcinoid tumors.[267] Most studies have incorporated the alkylating agents streptozocin or temozolomide.[265,267-271] Due to the overall poor response to chemotherapy, there has been increased interest in utilizing targeted therapies, including bevacizumab, imatanib, sorafenib, sunitinib, and inhibitors of the mammalian target of rapamycin.[265,267,272-275]

GEP-NET Subtypes

Gastrinoma. Gastrin-secreting tumors are usually malignant and cause gastric acid hypersecretion and the Zollinger-Ellison syndrome. Typical manifestations of gastrinoma include peptic ulcer disease and its complications, such as abdominal pain, bleeding, perforation, and strictures. Some patients present with diarrhea because of passage of large amounts of acid into the duodenum. Metastasis to the lymph nodes and liver is present in 75% to 80% of patients at diagnosis, and bone metastasis is present in approximately 12%.[249] Most gastrinomas are located in the proximal duodenum.[249,276] Duodenal gastrinomas can metastasize to lymph nodes when they are very small; the more aggressive tumors with liver metastases are mostly seen in pancreatic primaries.[245,259] Surgery for metastatic gastrinoma is not generally curative. Therefore, the mainstay of therapy is acid reduction with proton pump inhibitors and H2 antagonists.[248]

Hypergastrinemia in the presence of acid hypersecretion (gastric pH <2.5) is diagnostic of gastrinoma. In selective patients, the secretin stimulation test can be utilized to confirm the diagnosis.[277] False elevations of gastrin can occur due to use of proton pump inhibitors or antacids (patients should be off such therapies for at least 1 week prior to testing); conditions of autoimmune chronic atrophic gastritis with achlorhydria; or chronic renal insufficiency.[278]

Insulinoma. The majority of insulinomas are benign. Patients present with symptoms of subacute glycopenia, primarily recurrent central nervous system dysfunction at times of physical exertion or fasting, and autonomic nervous system responses. Acute hypoglycemia episodes start with neuroglycopenic symptoms of confusion, amnesia, diplopia, or blurred vision, followed by the catecholamine response of sweating, weakness, hunger, tremor, and palpitations. Seizures and loss of consciousness can occur. Frequently, the patients are obese due to the lipogenic and antilipolytic effects of insulin.[8] The Whipple triad is necessary for the diagnosis of pathologic hypoglycemia and includes (1) symptoms of hypoglycemia, (2) plasma glucose < 55 mg/dL, and (3) complete relief of symptoms with glucose administration.

Endogenous hyperinsulinism is documented by hypoglycemia with a concomitant insulin of at least 3.0 μU/mL, C-peptide of at least 0.6 ng/mL, and proinsulin of at least 5.0 pmol/L.[279] Low ketone levels (β-hydroxybutyrate ≤ 2.7 mmol/L) and an increase in plasma glucose of at least 25 mg/dL after intravenous glucagon administration lend supporting evidence to insulin[280]-mediated hypoglycemia. A formal 72-hour fast may be required for definitive diagnosis. Measurement of insulin antibodies and screening for oral hypoglycemic agents should also be undertaken.[279] In addition to the imaging modalities discussed earlier, selective pancreatic arterial calcium injections with measurements of hepatic venous insulin levels can also be utilized in the diagnosis of insulinoma.[281]

Hypoglycemia should be managed with frequent carbohydrate intake. Medications that can be utilized to maintain euglycemia in the patient with metastatic or nonlocalized insulinoma include diazoxide, SST analogs, glucagon, and/or glucocorticoids.

Glucagonoma. Glucagon-secreting NETs are typically large tumors at presentation with a high rate of malignancy.[8,248,249] The characteristic glucagonoma syndrome is characterized by skin rash (necrolytic migratory erythema), diabetes mellitus, weight loss, stomatitis, and anemia.[249]

VIPoma. Hypersecretion of VIP is associated with the Verner-Morrison syndrome of watery diarrhea, hypokalemia, and achlorhydria (also known as the WDHA syndrome).[249,282] Less frequent signs include glucose intolerance, hypercalcemia with normal PTH levels, and episodes of cutaneous flushing. The latter two are because of cosecretion of VIP with CTN, serotonin, substance P, and some of the prostaglandins.[8] Fasting plasma VIP levels > 60 pmol/L is diagnostic of VIPoma. VIPomas are primarily large tumors that are located in the pancreas; malignancy rate is high.[8]

Somatostatinoma. Somatostatinomas are located in the pancreas or duodenum.[249] Pancreatic somatostatinomas are often malignant with hepatic metastases and produce a clinical syndrome characterized by hyperglycemia, cholelithiasis, diarrhea, and malabsorption. Diagnosis is confirmed by elevated SST levels in the presence of symptoms.[8] Duodenal somatostatinomas, as seen in NF1, do not produce the clinical syndrome above but present with obstructive jaundice, intestinal obstruction, or gastrointestinal bleeding due to being located in the ampullary region.

Nonfunctioning Pancreatic Endocrine Tumors. Nonfunctioning PETs are identified during routine screening for predispos-

ing genetic syndromes or when patients present with symptoms because of mass effect or metastases. There have been a few case reports of diarrhea and gastroduodenal ulcers with elevated PP levels.[248,283] The majority of nonfunctioning PETs are associated with malignant behavior and have a high rate of recurrence.[8,247]

Carcinoid. Carcinoid tumors can secrete various hormones, including serotonin, histamine, tachykinins, ACTH, gastrin, GHRH, human chorionic gonadotropin, and prostaglandins.[248] They originate throughout the GI tract and occur in extraintestinal locations, such as the thymus, bronchus, or ovary. In children, the appendix is the most common location and may be identified after surgery for acute appendicitis.[251] Carcinoid syndrome occurs in less than 10% of patients and only manifests when liver metastases from a midgut carcinoid are present. The typical syndrome consists of flushing, diarrhea, right-sided cardiac disease, wheezing, dyspnea, and pellagra.[249] Diagnosis of the carcinoid syndrome is made by measuring 24-hour urinary excretion of 5-hydroxyindoleacetic acid, a metabolite of serotonin.

ADRENAL TUMORS

Adrenocortical Tumors

Epidemiology and Pathophysiology

In children, tumors arising from the adrenal cortex are typically discussed as one group under the heading of adrenocortical tumors (ACTs) (Fig. 36.10) because the pathologic categorization of ACTs as benign or malignant does not always correlate to clinical behavior.[284] In the United States, less than 25 new cases of ACT are diagnosed annually (0.1–0.4 cases/million/yr, depending on age) and malignant ACTs comprise approximately 1% of all carcinomas diagnosed prior to 20 years of age.[285] ACT tend to present at an age <5 years (median age, 3–4 years), and may arise from the fetal zone in this age group.[123,286–289] Female predominance has been shown in the majority of studies, ranging from 1.6:1 to 3:1.[288,290–292] In Brazil, childhood ACT is 10 times more common than in the United States, secondary to the high population prevalence of germline mutations in the TP53 tumor suppressor gene.[288,293]

Pediatric ACTs can occur sporadically, but the early age of onset, distinct biologic activity, and association with several tumor syndromes strongly suggests a role for constitutional genetic abnormalities, underscoring the importance of genetic counseling and testing in such patients. Tumor syndromes that show an increased incidence of pediatric ACT include the Li-Fraumeni syndrome (LFS), Beckwith-Wiedemann syndrome, CNC, MAS, and MEN1.[8,294–297](Table 36.1) Alterations in TP53 are the most common cause of ACTs in childhood.[298] In the United States, this is most often seen in the context of LFS, but in southern Brazil, ACTs typically occur as an isolated neoplasm due to the R337H mutation in TP53.[289] CNC is associated with a specific form of ACT, called primary pigmented nodular adrenocortical disease.[299] Rarely, ACT may be associated with isolated hemihypertrophy and congenital adrenal hyperplasia.[123,300]

Somatic mutations are also common in pediatric ACT suggesting broader, and as of yet unidentified, pathways involved in the development and progression of these tumors. The most consistent finding is a gain in 9q34, a finding unrelated to the patients country of origin, tumor size or neoplastic characteristics.[301] Overexpression of the IGF-1 receptor and IGF-II may also play a role in malignant ACTs.[302]

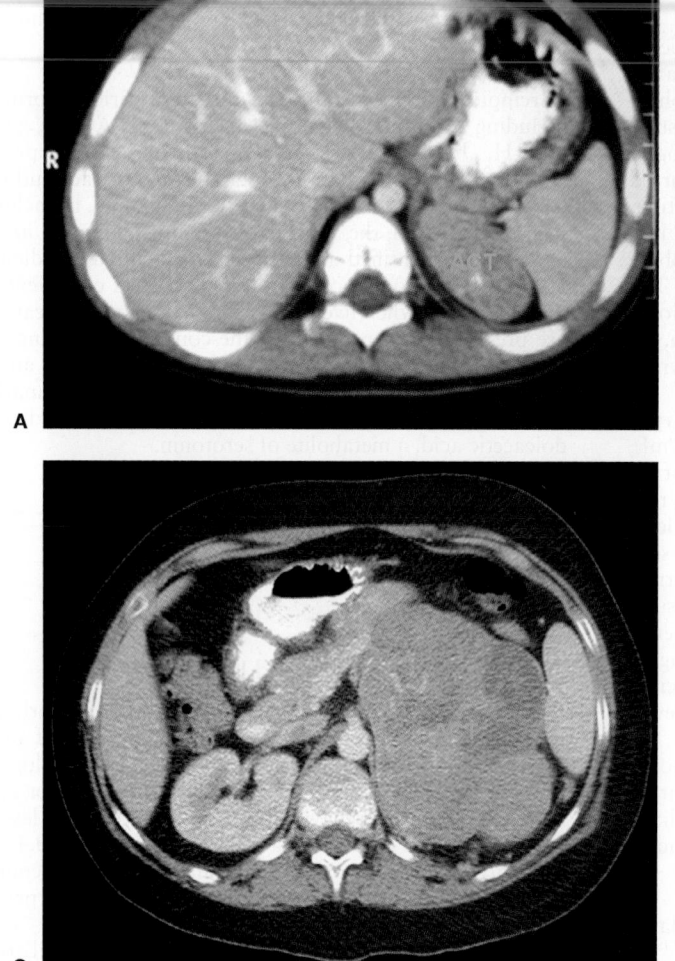
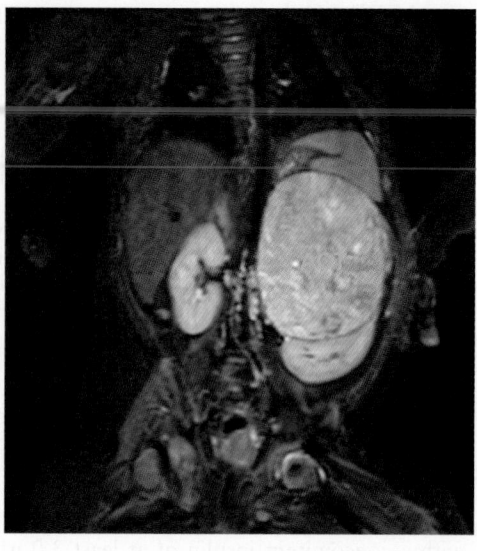

FIGURE 36.10 Adrenocortical tumors (ACT). **A:** Abdominal CT of a clinically benign virilizing ACT in a boy with Li-Fraumeni syndrome. **B:** Coronal MRI of a large malignant ACT arising from the left adrenal gland in an infant. **C:** CT of a malignant ACT presenting with Cushing syndrome in an adolescent; note the areas of necrosis and inhomogeneous nature of the tumor.

Clinical Presentation and Diagnosis

Similar to adults, the diagnosis of an ACT is usually delayed. It may present as an abdominal mass or pain, but frequently is identified earlier due to the high rate of concomitant endocrinopathy.[290] Most children (80–90%) present secondary to hormonal excess, with isolated virilization or a combination of hypercortisolism (CS) and virilization.[123,288,292,303] Less commonly, pediatric patients may present with isolated CS (Fig. 36.2), primary hyperaldosteronism, feminization or without any evidence of endocrine overactivity.

The hormonal evaluation of patients with suspected ACT should be comprehensive to aid in diagnosis and allow for assessment of tumor markers that may be useful to detect persistent or recurrent disease. Dehydroepiandrosterone sulfate levels are abnormal in the majority of cases and serve as a useful marker of ACTs.[304] In the absence of metastases, radiographic studies do not typically aid in establishing the diagnosis but are essential for staging and appropriate surgical planning. Cross sectional imaging with MRI or CT is generally preferred. Tumor size and Hounsfield units on CT may help to distinguish between benign and malignant ACTs.[287,305,306] Classic radiologic features of malignant ACTs include a large inhomogeneously enhancing mass that can contain areas of hemorrhage, necrosis, and calcification[8,287,306] (Fig. 36.10).

Radiographic evaluation must also include evaluation of the abdomen, chest, and bone to assess the common sites of metastasis as well as to evaluate the inferior vena cava and right atrium, common areas of vascular invasion, and thrombus formation[289,303,307,308] (Fig. 36.11). Although potentially useful, the clinical utility of FDG-PET in the evaluation and follow-up of pediatric ACT has not been clearly established.[306]

With the increased use of imaging studies in pediatrics, the discovery of an incidental adrenal lesion has become more commonplace. In adults, the majority of adrenal incidentalomas are benign adrenocortical adenomas, and consensus guidelines exist as to how to approach these patients.[309,310] In children, the differential diagnosis of an adrenal mass more commonly includes malignant lesions such as neuroblastoma, ganglioneuroblastoma, teratoma, and ACT. Therefore, after an appropriate hormonal evaluation, surgical resection may be preferred in all children with an incidental adrenal mass.[311]

Staging and Prognosis

The clinical behavior of ACT in childhood is different from that in adults, with the overall event free and disease survival being significantly better in the younger children and those with purely virilizing tumors.[288] Studies have also shown that prognosis is also dictated by tumor size, major blood vessel

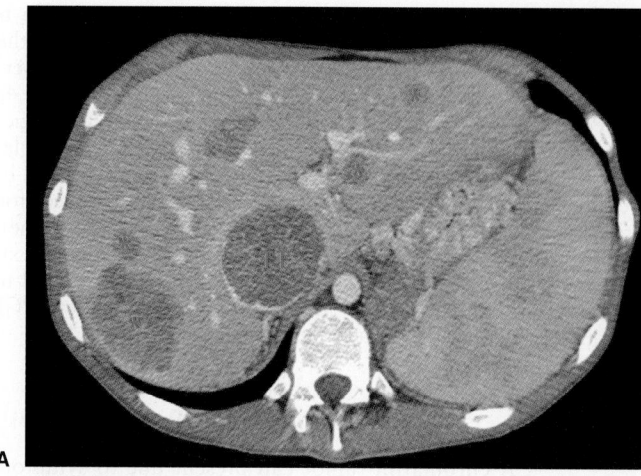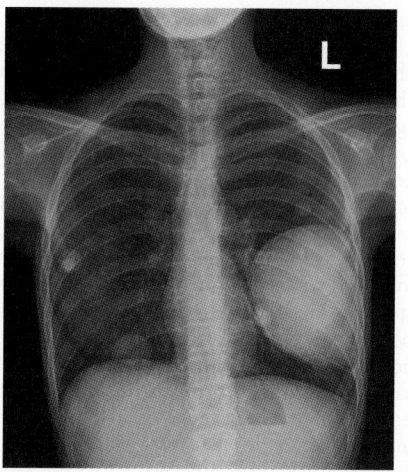

FIGURE 36.11 Patterns of metastases in malignant ACTs. **A:** CT demonstrating liver metastases (*red asterisks*) and tumor thrombus (TT) in the inferior vena cava in a teenage boy. **B:** Chest x-ray of macronodular pulmonary metastases in a girl with a metastatic virilizing ACT.

invasion, completeness of resection, tumor spillage during surgery, histologic features, and presence of distant metastases.

Several staging systems have been proposed for ACTs, and the most widely used is that based on TNM criteria and formulated in 2004 by the International Union Against Cancer Committee and the WHO.[303,306,312] Stage I and II patients can expect prolonged survival, but 5-year survival is usually 0% in children with stage IV disease.[290,303] However, prolonged survival in children with stage IV disease has also been described.[288]

Treatment and Follow-Up

Surgical resection is the mainstay of treatment of pediatric ACT. Preoperative FNAB is unhelpful and generally contraindicated.[123,313] For large tumors, a transabdominal approach with radical *en bloc* resection of the tumor and involved structures is recommended.[288,289,291,303,314] Because of tumor friability, capsule rupture with subsequent tumor spillage is not uncommon.[292] Laparoscopic resection should be avoided because of concerns of tumor spillage and diffuse peritoneal carcinomatosis.[315] All postsurgical patients with presurgical evidence of CS should be presumed to have adrenal insufficiency and placed on glucocorticoid replacement.

Given the rarity of the disease, the use of chemotherapy in the management of childhood ACT has not clearly been established. Systemic therapy (Table 36.4) is recommended for patients with unresectable or metastatic disease. Mitotane (o,p'-DDD) is a nonclassical antineoplastic derived from an insecticide that is the only adrenal-specific agent available for the treatment of malignant ACT. Mitotane can be effective in controlling endocrine hyperfunctioning and promoting tumor regression. It is used as monotherapy or in combination with cisplatin, etoposide, and doxorubicin.[316–318] The role of routine adjuvant mitotane therapy in completely resected disease remains unclear. Another commonly used chemotherapeutic regimen is streptozocin and mitotane.[319]

The therapeutic level for the adrenolytic effect of mitotane is 14 to 20 mg/L,[320] but the daily dose to achieve this level is variable and often limited by significant gastrointestinal and neurologic side effects.[321] All patients started on mitotane should be assumed to be adrenally insufficient and placed on replacement glucocorticoid and rarely mineralocorticoid therapy. Because of mitotane's effects on steroid metabolism and protein binding,[316] supraphysiologic dosing of steroids is usually required to prevent significant elevations of ACTH, which in turn could theoretically stimulate tumor growth. Monthly monitoring of mitotane levels should be initiated 6 weeks after starting therapy.[321]

Multiple other regimens have been utilized in malignant ACTs in adults without any one regimen proving superior.[322,323] As with other endocrine malignancies, there is significant interest in the use of targeted therapies. However, early results have been disappointing with minimal or no objective response seen in published studies using imatinib or erlotinib with gemcitabine.[324,325] Other novel therapies for malignant ACTs are the focus of recent excellent reviews.[106,314,323]

Although malignant ACTs are historically believed to be radioresistant, adjuvant radiation of the surgical bed has

---

TABLE 36.4

FIRST-LINE THERAPIES FOR MALIGNANT ADRENOCORTICAL TUMORS

Drug regimen	Dose and Comments
Mitotane[316,321]	• Start 1.5 gm/m²/d in divided doses and titrate to 4 gm/m²/d • Adjust dose based on tolerance and mitotane levels • Mean dose generally needed to achieve therapeutic levels between 14 and 20 mg/L is ~3 gm/m²/d[321] • Start concomitant glucocorticoid therapy (e.g., dexamethasone 0.5 mg/m²/d) and titrate based on adrenocorticotropin (ACTH) levels
EDP + mitotane[318,321]	• Etoposide 100 mg/m² on days 5–7 • Doxorubicin 20 mg/m² on days 1 and 8 • Cisplatin 40 mg/m² on days 1 and 9 • Mitotane as above
Streptozocin + mitotane[319]	• Streptozocin 1 gm/dᵃ for 5 days as induction, then 2 gmᵃ every 3 weeks • Mitotane as above

ᵃThis is the adult dose.

recently been associated with improved outcomes in adults.[326] In children, the efficacy of radiotherapy has not been established and therefore should be used with caution, particularly in view of the genetic susceptibility to tumor formation.[123]

The long-term follow-up of children considered cured includes routine radiographic and hormonal evaluations.[123,317] Those children on mitotane therapy should have levels monitored regularly to prevent toxicity and ensure a therapeutic concentration. In addition, ACTH and plasma renin activity levels, thyroid function studies, and routine biochemistries should be followed to assess for toxicities of therapy and hormonal replacement needs.[316] Recovery of the normal adrenal gland can be expected after stopping mitotane, noting that it may take months for mitotane levels to decline and for glucocorticoid production to return to normal.[316] Routine clinical surveillance for other malignancies is also required in those children identified to have a *TP53* germline mutation, and ongoing genetic counseling is advised.

Pheochromocytoma and Paraganglioma

Epidemiology and Pathophysiology

PHEOs (Fig. 36.12) and paragangliomas (PGL) (Fig. 36.13) occur in up to 1.7% of hypertensive children and have an incidence rate of 0.3 cases/million/yr or less.[123,327,328] Approximately 10% to 20% of cases are identified in childhood, and these tumors are diagnosed at an average age of 11 years, with a slight predominance in boys, particularly younger than 10 years.[123,329–332]

Catecholamine-secreting tumors arise from neural crest-derived endocrine cells or organs, known as paraganglia, and can occur in all locations where chromaffin tissue is found. PHEO is the term used to describe a PGL arising from the adrenal medulla (Fig. 36.12) whereas PGLs are extra-adrenal tumors.[8] PGLs are located anywhere from the base of the skull to the pelvis. They most commonly arise in the head and neck or in the abdomen near the renal vessels or the organ of Zuckerkandl (Fig. 36.13). Some authors use the term PHEO interchangeably with PGL, but it is best to maintain the distinction between the two tumor types due to underlying differences in genetics and malignant potential.

PHEOs represent the vast majority of these tumors in childhood and they synthesize and secrete catecholamines (dopamine, norepinephrine, and epinephrine) and their metabolites (homovanillic acid, normetanephrine, and metanephrine, respectively).[333,334] PGLs can be secretory (sympathetic) or non-secretory (parasympathetic), depending on the site of origin and underlying genetic events (Table 36.1). The vast majority of head and neck PGLs are nonfunctional whereas most intra-abdominal chromaffin tumors are functional. Areas of ganglioneuroblastoma, ganglioneuroma, or neuroendocrine carcinoma are sometimes admixed with PHEO or PGL, in which case the term composite PHEO or PGL is used.[8,334,335]

PHEOs often occur as sporadic tumors but can also develop, particularly in young children, as part of a hereditary syndrome, including VHL disease, MEN2A, MEN2B, NF1, the familial PGL syndromes because of mutations in subunits of the mitochondrial enzyme succinate dehydrogenase (SDH) gene, and rarely the TSC[8,14,123,336–338] (Table 36.1). VHL is responsible for the majority of cases in childhood.[329,330,336] Hereditary PHEOs and PGLs often occur multifocally and bilaterally, in the case of PHEO. Furthermore, a background of medullary hyperplasia is associated only with MEN2, and VHL-associated tumors have a distinct histologic phenotype that can distinguish such tumors from those arising in the setting of MEN2.[334,339]

Approximately 12% of pediatric chromaffin tumors are malignant, and based on a British tumor registry, the incidence of malignant PHEO is 0.02 per million children per year.[123,329] Some centers report a malignancy rate as high as 46%,[340] but this may reflect a referral bias. No single histologic feature or immunohistochemical profile is independently able to predict metastatic potential.[334] Malignancy is established by the presence of distant metastases in a site not typical for paraganglionic tissue (e.g., lymph nodes, liver, and/or bone).[334,335] The risk of malignant transformation is greater for extra-adrenal sympathetic PGLs than for PHEOs or head and neck PGLs; the highest risk is in SDHB-related sympathetic PGLs, with at least 50% of such tumors being malignant.[341]

Clinical Presentation and Diagnosis

A chromaffin tumor can present due to symptomatic catecholamine secretion or, less often, as an incidental radiographic finding, because of tumor mass effects, or because of family screening for one of the hereditary syndromes discussed earlier.[123,340] Symptoms include hypertension, usually sustained in the majority of cases; paroxysmal symptoms (e.g., the classic PHEO triad of headaches, palpitations, and diaphoresis); pallor; orthostatic hypotension and syncope; tremor; and anxiety.[329,333,336,340,342] Symptoms can also be nonspecific: blurred vision; abdominal pain, diarrhea, and other gastrointestinal symptoms; weight loss; hyperglycemia, with polyuria and polydipsia; low grade fever; and behavioral problems/decline in school performance.[333,336,342–344] Complications of catecholamine excess can include hypertensive crisis, cardiomyopathy, stroke, seizures, and even multiorgan failure and death.[336,342,344] Symptoms of parasympathetic tumors include hearing loss, tinnitus, and other symptoms of mass effect such as voice hoarseness, pharyngeal fullness, dysphagia, cough, and pain. Chromaffin tumors can very rarely cosecrete other hormones resulting in clinical syndromes of ectopic hormone excess or, in the case of bladder PGLs, present with hematuria and paroxysmal symptoms during micturition.[333] PHEOs and PGLs identified during the course of prospective screening within the context of a familial disorder are often asymptomatic.[345] There is no consensus as to how to approach such patients with small asymptomatic tumors, particularly in those settings with a low malignancy risk.

The best initial biochemical diagnostic test is assessment of fractionated plasma and/or urine metanephrines (metanephrines and normetanephrines), as these are highly sensitive tests with very few false-negative results.[346–348] An elevation of these analytes greater than fourfold above the reference interval is associated with almost 100% probability of the presence of a catecholamine-secreting tumor.[349] Very rarely do tumors secrete dopamine preferentially, and there is no pathognomonic constellation of symptoms that can lead to this diagnosis. Any drugs known to interfere with these assays (e.g., acetaminophen and decongestants) should be discontinued prior to testing,[346] and plasma analytes are best measured in the supine position 30 minutes after an indwelling needle or catheter is inserted into the vein, in order to avoid a false-positive result from procedure-induced stress.

CgA, a major secretory protein present in the soluble matrix of chromaffin granules, is an effective tumor marker that may correlate with tumor size and malignant potential and improve the sensitivity of diagnostic testing and long-term follow-up.[350–352] In patients with paroxysmal symptoms, confirmation of the diagnosis may be more easily achieved by biochemical screening just after an event. Clonidine suppression and glucagon stimulation tests[353] are not validated in the diagnosis of childhood PHEO or PGL.

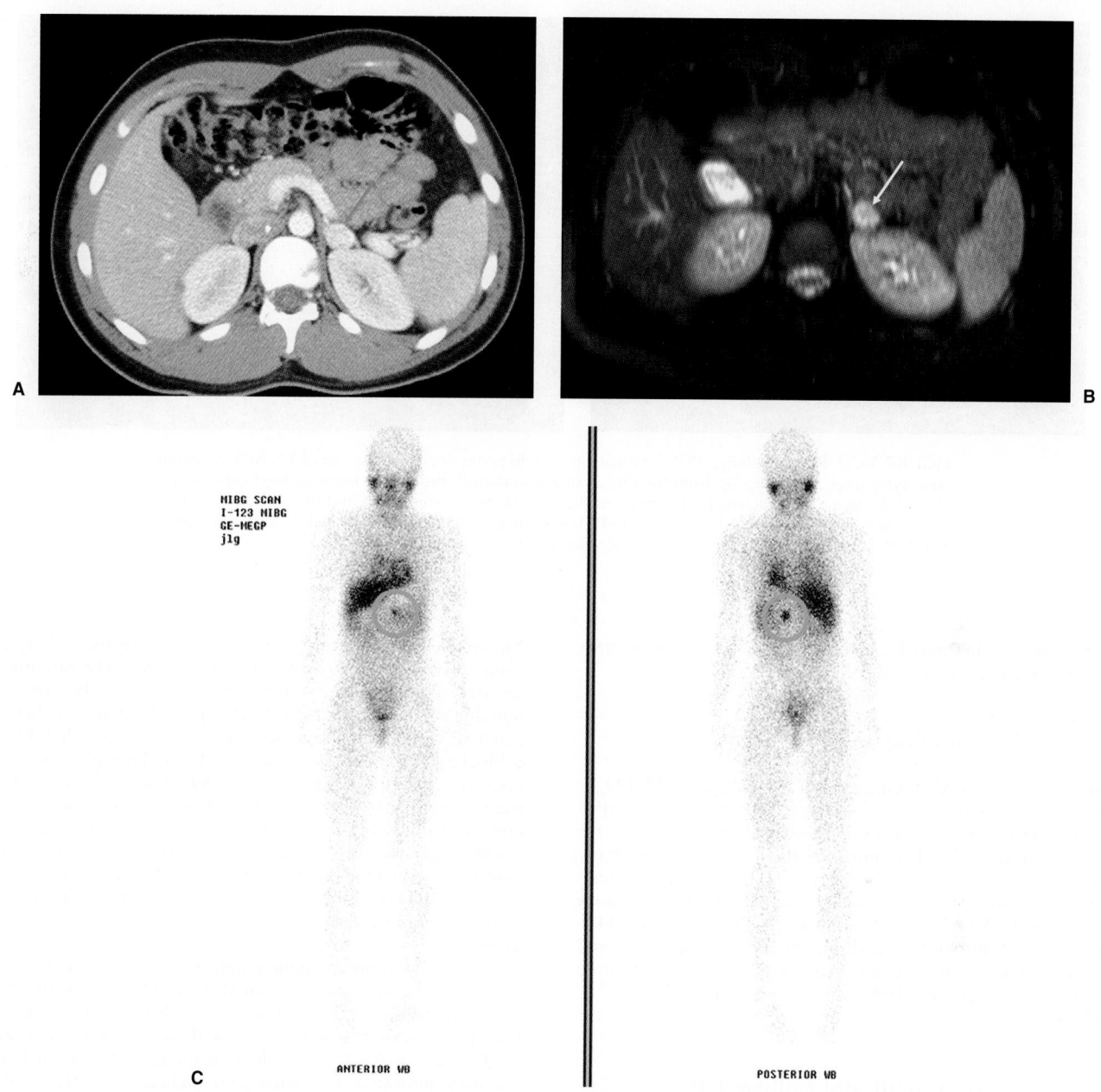

FIGURE 36.12 Imaging of pheochromocytoma in a teenager with von Hippel-Lindau (VHL) disease. **A:** Postcontrast CT reveals an enhancing left adrenal mass (*green arrow*). **B:** On MRI, the lesion (*white arrow*) appears bright on T2-weighted images. **C:** Nuclear scintigraphy with ^{123}I-MIBG (metaiodobenzylguanidine) (*orange circle*) documents the catecholamine-secreting nature of the tumor.

Once the biochemical diagnosis is established, radiographic studies are undertaken to identify the location of the tumor(s).[336] Cross sectional imaging (CT or MRI) of the abdomen and pelvis should be done initially and, if unrevealing, testing should expand to include imaging of the neck and chest.[346,348] If local expertise permits, abdominal US may also be considered in children. PHEOs and PGLs are vascular tumors that commonly contain cystic, necrotic, or hemorrhagic areas (Figs. 36.12 and 36.13). On MRI, they classically have a hyperintense appearance on T2-weighted images (Fig. 36.12). Functional testing with nuclear scintigraphy utilizing [123]I- (preferred) or ^{131}I-labeled metaiodobenzylguanidine (MIBG) is a highly specific test

that can confirm the catecholamine-secreting nature of a tumor, detect tumors not seen with cross sectional imaging, and identify other sites of disease[348,354,355] (Fig. 36.12). Prior to MIBG scanning, care should be taken to ensure that the patient is not taking medications, such as labetalol or over-the-counter decongestants, that are known to decrease MIBG uptake.[356] Other nuclear imaging modalities to be considered include: SST receptor scintigraphy using ^{111}In-DTPA-octreotide (octreotide scan) or ^{123}I-labeled Tyr3-DTPA-octreotide; 6-[^{18}F]F-DOPA (fluorodopamine) PET; [^{18}F]FDA (fluorodopa) PET; FDG-PET (Fig. 36.13); [^{18}F]-dihydroxyphenylalanine PET; [11C]-epinephrine PET; and [^{11}C]hydroxyephedrine PET.[348,357] Although some of these

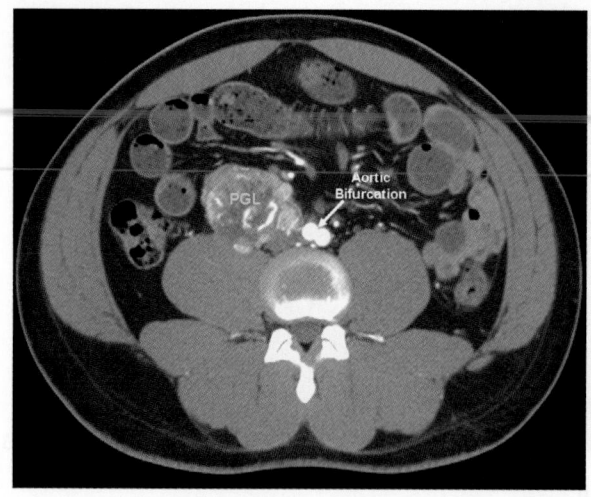 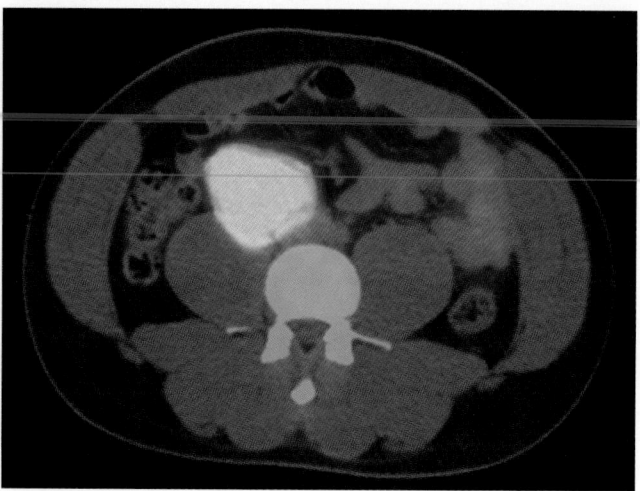

FIGURE 36.13 Paraganglioma (PGL) in a patient with hypertension since the age of 14. **A:** A noradrenergic sympathetic PGL arising from the Organ of Zuckerkandl, the largest extra-adrenal collection of chromaffin tissue located around the origin of the inferior mesenteric artery and the aortic bifurcation; note tumor hypervascularity. **B:** Fused FDG-PET scan images of the same tumor demonstrating significant FDG uptake with a standardized uptake value of 41.

functional studies may be superior to MIBG, not all of them are available at every medical center.

Staging and Prognosis

There is no clinical staging system for malignant PHEO or PGL. The prognosis for a completely resected chromaffin tumor, particularly a PHEO, is excellent. Life expectancy for malignant disease is determined by the location of metastatic disease, with survival younger than 5 years with liver and lung metastases and longer survival in those with metastatic lesions in bones.[348] Overall 5-year survival rate varies between 34% and 60%.[348] In children with malignant tumors, the 5- and 10-year disease-specific survival rates are estimated to be 78% and 31%, respectively, with a mean survival of 157 ± 32 months.[340]

Treatment and Follow-Up

Surgery is the mainstay in the treatment of chromaffin tumors, and the procedure of choice for PHEO is laparoscopic adrenalectomy.[358,359] In the setting of bilateral tumors, cortical-sparing procedures should be considered,[359,360] particularly in young children and children at risk for noncompliance with the lifelong glucocorticoid and mineralocorticoid replacement required after bilateral adrenalectomy. The surgical approach to PGLs depends on the location of the tumor(s).

Medical therapy should be initiated in preparation for surgery in order to minimize the complications that may arise from acute surges of catecholamines during induction of anesthesia and manipulation of the tumor.[332,336,361] No universal algorithm exists for the medical treatment of children. α_1-adrenergic blockade is usually the therapy of choice and the primary agent used in children is phenoxybenzamine (starting 0.2–1 mg/kg per day in divided doses[123,336,346,361]), but selective **α-blockers such as prazosin and doxazosin, and calcium channel blockers such as nifedipine and nicardipine can also be utilized.[332,353,362,363] The long action of phenoxybenzamine may increase the risk of postoperative hypotension.[332,353]

Metyrosine (starting dose 125–250 mg once or twice daily), a competitive inhibitor of tyrosine hydroxylase (the rate-limiting step of catecholamine biosynthesis) can also be given,[364] but due to its significant side effects and unclear utility in pediatric tumors, its use is not routinely recommended. Once α-blockade has been established, a β-blocking agent can be added to control reflex tachycardia; a β-blocker should not be used alone due to the possibility of worsening hypertension and symptoms due to unopposed catecholamine effects at α-adrenergic receptors. A few days before surgery, oral salt loading is recommended to expand blood volume and to try to prevent severe postoperative hypotension, and some centers routinely admit patients for intravenous fluids prior to surgery.[365]

Patients with unresectable malignant tumors or metastases can have excellent palliation of their symptoms through the use of the medications discussed earlier. Radiation therapy or radiofrequency ablation can help with symptomatic metastatic disease. Currently available systemic treatment modalities are only palliative in nature and include ^{131}I-MIBG, SST analogs, and chemotherapy.[106,341,366–370] The major chemotherapeutic regimen used in the treatment of malignant disease has been CVD (cyclophosphamide, vincristine, and dacarbazine), and this regimen can provide tumor regression and symptom relief in up to 50% of patients, but it does not prolong overall survival.[348,371] Recent reports of successful treatment using the oral TKI, sunitinib, suggest that these newer targeted therapies may hold promise for the treatment of this disease.[372]

Because PHEOs and PGLs can have unpredictable behavior and because children are at risk for the development of metachronous tumors, long-term follow-up with biochemical screening and intermittent imaging studies is required.[123,334,336] Since recurrence may be as high as 16%, diligent follow-up must also be taken in children who have had gland-sparing procedures for multicentric adrenal lesions.[331,340]

Genetic testing under the guidance of a qualified genetic counselor is available and recommended for all children who present with a PGL or PHEO, whether or not there is a positive family history.[123,336–338] Recommendations have been made to help the clinician prioritize genetic testing, with *VHL* being the gene of interest in children with PHEO and *SDHB* being the suspected gene in children with PGL and/or malignant disease. Testing for mutations in *RET* and *NF1* in the context of an apparently sporadic tumor will typically be of low yield, because MTC usually presents before PHEO in MEN2 and because NF1 is already diagnosed clinically in most patients.

References

1. Partington MD, Davis DH, Laws ER Jr, et al. Pituitary adenomas in childhood and adolescence. Results of transsphenoidal surgery. J Neurosurg 1994;80(2):209–216.
2. Kane LA, Leinung MC, Scheithauer BW, et al. Pituitary adenomas in childhood and adolescence. J Clin Endocrinol Metab 1994;79(4):1135–1140.
3. Lafferty AR, Chrousos GP. Pituitary tumors in children and adolescents. J Clin Endocrinol Metab 1999;84(12):4317–4323.
4. Kunwar S, Wilson CB. Pediatric pituitary adenomas. J Clin Endocrinol Metab 1999; 84(12):4385–4389.
5. Jagannathan J, Dumont AS, Jane JA Jr. Diagnosis and management of pediatric sellar lesions. Front Horm Res 2006;34:83–104.
6. Glezer A, Paraiba DB, Bronstein MD. Rare sellar lesions. Endocrinol Metab Clin North Am 2008;37(1):195–211, x.
7. Ehirim PU, Kerr DS, Cohen AR. Primary hypothyroidism mimicking a pituitary macroadenoma. Pediatr Neurosurg 1998;28(4):195–197.
8. DeLellis RA, Lloyd RV, Heitz PU, et al., eds. World Health Organization classification of tumours. Pathology and genetics of tumours of endocrine organs. Vol 8. Lyon, France: IARC Press, 2004.
9. Keil MF, Stratakis CA. Pituitary tumors in childhood: update of diagnosis, treatment and molecular genetics. Expert Rev Neurother 2008;8(4):563–574.
10. Asa SL, Ezzat S. The pathogenesis of pituitary tumors. Annu Rev Pathol 2009;4: 97–126.
11. Daly AF, Tichomirow MA, Beckers A. Update on familial pituitary tumors: from multiple endocrine neoplasia type 1 to familial isolated pituitary adenoma. Horm Res 2009;71(Suppl 1):105–111.
12. Verges B, Boureille F, Goudet P, et al. Pituitary disease in MEN type 1 (MEN1): data from the France-Belgium MEN1 multicenter study. J Clin Endocrinol Metab 2002; 87(2):457–465.
13. Lania AG, Mantovani G, Spada A. Mechanisms of disease: mutations of G proteins and G-protein-coupled receptors in endocrine diseases. Nat Clin Pract Endocrinol Metab 2006;2(12):681–693.
14. Dworakowska D, Grossman AB. Are neuroendocrine tumours a feature of tuberous sclerosis? A systematic review. Endocr Relat Cancer 2009;16(1):45–58.
15. Pellegata NS, Quintanilla-Martinez L, Siggelkow H, et al. Germ-line mutations in p27Kip1 cause a multiple endocrine neoplasia syndrome in rats and humans. Proc Natl Acad Sci U S A 2006;103(42):15558–15563.
16. Molitch ME. Nonfunctioning pituitary tumors and pituitary incidentalomas. Endocrinol Metab Clin North Am 2008;37(1):151–171, xi.
17. Chandler WF, Barkan AL. Treatment of pituitary tumors: a surgical perspective. Endocrinol Metab Clin North Am 2008;37(1):51–66, viii.
18. Batista D, Courkoutsakis NA, Oldfield EH, et al. Detection of adrenocorticotropin-secreting pituitary adenomas by magnetic resonance imaging in children and adolescents with Cushing disease. J Clin Endocrinol Metab 2005;90(9):5134–5140.
19. Friedman TC, Zuckerbraun E, Lee ML, et al. Dynamic pituitary MRI has high sensitivity and specificity for the diagnosis of mild Cushing's syndrome and should be part of the initial workup. Horm Metab Res 2007;39(6):451–456.
20. Fleseriu M, Yedinak C, Campbell C, et al. Significant headache improvement after transsphenoidal surgery in patients with small sellar lesions. J Neurosurg 2009;110(2): 354–358.
21. Barker FG II, Klibanski A, Swearingen B. Transsphenoidal surgery for pituitary tumors in the United States, 1996–2000: mortality, morbidity, and the effects of hospital and surgeon volume. J Clin Endocrinol Metab 2003;88(10):4709–4719.
22. Minniti G, Gilbert DC, Brada M. Modern techniques for pituitary radiotherapy. Rev Endocr Metab Disord 2009;10(2):135–144.
23. Colao A, Loche S, Cappa M, et al. Prolactinomas in children and adolescents. Clinical presentation and long-term follow-up. J Clin Endocrinol Metab 1998;83(8):2777–2780.
24. Fideleff HL, Boquete HR, Sequera A, et al. Peripubertal prolactinomas: clinical presentation and long-term outcome with different therapeutic approaches. J Pediatr Endocrinol Metab 2000;13(3):261–267.
25. Casanueva FF, Molitch ME, Schlechte JA, et al. Guidelines of the Pituitary Society for the diagnosis and management of prolactinomas. Clin Endocrinol (Oxf) 2006;65(2): 265–273.
26. Karavitaki N, Thanabalasingham G, Shore HC, et al. Do the limits of serum prolactin in disconnection hyperprolactinaemia need re-definition? A study of 226 patients with histologically verified non-functioning pituitary macroadenoma. Clin Endocrinol (Oxf) 2006;65(4):524–529.
27. Arafah BM, Nekl KE, Gold RS, et al. Dynamics of prolactin secretion in patients with hypopituitarism and pituitary macroadenomas. J Clin Endocrinol Metab 1995;80(12): 3507–3512.
28. Mancini T, Casanueva FF, Giustina A. Hyperprolactinemia and prolactinomas. Endocrinol Metab Clin North Am 2008;37(1):67–99, viii.
29. Webster J, Piscitelli G, Polli A, et al. A comparison of cabergoline and bromocriptine in the treatment of hyperprolactinemic amenorrhea. Cabergoline Comparative Study Group. N Engl J Med 1994;331(14):904–909.
30. Schlechte JA. Long-term management of prolactinomas. J Clin Endocrinol Metab 2007;92(8):2861–2865.
31. Garcia MM, Kapcala LP. Growth of a microprolactinoma to a macroprolactinoma during estrogen therapy. J Endocrinol Invest 1995;18(6):450–455.
32. Gillam MP, Middler S, Freed DJ, et al. The novel use of very high doses of cabergoline and a combination of testosterone and an aromatase inhibitor in the treatment of a giant prolactinoma. J Clin Endocrinol Metab 2002;87(10):4447–4451.
33. Colao A, Di Sarno A, Cappabianca P, et al. Withdrawal of long-term cabergoline therapy for tumoral and nontumoral hyperprolactinemia. N Engl J Med 2003;349(21): 2023–2033.
34. Savage MO, Chan LF, Afshar F, et al. Advances in the management of paediatric Cushing's disease. Horm Res 2008;69(6):327–333.

35. Magiakou MA, Mastorakos G, Oldfield EH, et al. Cushing's syndrome in children and adolescents. Presentation, diagnosis, and therapy. N Engl J Med 1994;331(10): 629–636.
36. Storr HL, Isidori AM, Monson JP, et al. Prepubertal Cushing's disease is more common in males, but there is no increase in severity at diagnosis. J Clin Endocrinol Metab 2004; 89(8):3818–3820.
37. Savage MO, Lienhardt A, Lebrethon MC, et al. Cushing's disease in childhood: presentation, investigation, treatment and long-term outcome. Horm Res 2001;55(Suppl 1): 24–30.
38. Kanter AS, Diallo AO, Jane JA Jr, et al. Single-center experience with pediatric Cushing's disease. J Neurosurg 2005;103(Suppl 5):413–420.
39. Pivonello R, De Martino MC, De Leo M, et al. Cushing's syndrome. Endocrinol Metab Clin North Am 2008;37(1):135–149, ix.
40. Savage MO, Besser GM. Cushing's disease in childhood. Trends Endocrinol Metab 1996;7(6):213–216.
41. Magiakou MA, Chrousos GP. Cushing's syndrome in children and adolescents: current diagnostic and therapeutic strategies. J Endocrinol Invest 2002;25(2):181–194.
42. Newell-Price J, Bertagna X, Grossman AB, et al. Cushing's syndrome. Lancet 2006; 367(9522):1605–1617.
43. Nieman LK, Biller BM, Findling JW, et al. The diagnosis of Cushing's syndrome: an Endocrine Society Clinical Practice Guideline. J Clin Endocrinol Metab 2008;93(5): 1526–1540.
44. Biller BM, Grossman AB, Stewart PM, et al. Treatment of adrenocorticotropin-dependent Cushing's syndrome: a consensus statement. J Clin Endocrinol Metab 2008;93(7): 2454–2462.
45. Findling JW, Raff H. Cushing's syndrome: important issues in diagnosis and management. J Clin Endocrinol Metab 2006;91(10):3746–3753.
46. Batista DL, Riar J, Keil M, et al. Diagnostic tests for children who are referred for the investigation of Cushing syndrome. Pediatrics 2007;120(3):e575–e586.
47. Batista DL, Courcoutsakis N, Riar J, et al. Severe obesity confounds the interpretation of low-dose dexamethasone test combined with the administration of ovine corticotrophin-releasing hormone in childhood Cushing syndrome. J Clin Endocrinol Metab 2008;93(11):4323–4330.
48. Chrousos GP, Schulte HM, Oldfield EH, et al. The corticotropin-releasing factor stimulation test. An aid in the evaluation of patients with Cushing's syndrome. N Engl J Med 1984;310(10):622–626.
49. Oldfield EH, Doppman JL, Nieman LK, et al. Petrosal sinus sampling with and without corticotropin-releasing hormone for the differential diagnosis of Cushing's syndrome. N Engl J Med 1991;325(13):897–905.
50. Batista D, Gennari M, Riar J, et al. An assessment of petrosal sinus sampling for localization of pituitary microadenomas in children with Cushing disease. J Clin Endocrinol Metab 2006;91(1):221–224.
51. Frank GR, Speiser PW, Griffin KJ, et al. Safety of medications and hormones used in pediatric endocrinology: adrenal. Pediatr Endocrinol Rev 2004;2(Suppl 1):134–145.
52. Assie G, Bahurel H, Coste J, et al. Corticotroph tumor progression after adrenalectomy in Cushing's Disease: a reappraisal of Nelson's Syndrome. J Clin Endocrinol Metab 2007;92(1):172–179.
53. Abe T, Tara LA, Ludecke DK. Growth hormone-secreting pituitary adenomas in childhood and adolescence: features and results of transnasal surgery. Neurosurgery 1999; 45(1):1–10.
54. Eugster EA, Pescovitz OH. Gigantism. J Clin Endocrinol Metab 1999;84(12): 4379–4384.
55. Chanson P, Salenave S. Acromegaly. Orphanet J Rare Dis 2008;3:17.
56. Cordero RA, Barkan AL. Current diagnosis of acromegaly. Rev Endocr Metab Disord 2008;9(1):13–19.
57. Metzler M, Luedecke DK, Saeger W, et al. Low prevalence of Gs alpha mutations in somatotroph adenomas of children and adolescents. Cancer Genet Cytogenet 2006; 166(2):146–151.
58. Giustina A, Barkan A, Casanueva FF, et al. Criteria for cure of acromegaly: a consensus statement. J Clin Endocrinol Metab 2000;85(2):526–529.
59. Pokrajac-Simeunovic A, Trainer PJ. Pitfalls in the diagnosis of acromegaly. Horm Res 2004;62(Suppl 3):74–78.
60. Melmed S, Colao A, Barkan A, et al. Guidelines for acromegaly management: an update. J Clin Endocrinol Metab 2009;94(5):1509–1517.
61. Freda PU, Reyes CM, Nuruzzaman AT, et al. Basal and glucose-suppressed GH levels less than 1 microg/L in newly diagnosed acromegaly. Pituitary 2003;6(4):175–180.
62. Misra M, Cord J, Prabhakaran R, et al. Growth hormone suppression after an oral glucose load in children. J Clin Endocrinol Metab 2007;92(12):4623–4629.
63. Kumar SS, Ayuk J, Murray RD. Current therapy and drug pipeline for the treatment of patients with acromegaly. Adv Ther 2009;26(4):383–403.
64. Moyes VJ, Metcalfe KA, Drake WM. Clinical use of cabergoline as primary and adjunctive treatment for acromegaly. Eur J Endocrinol 2008;159(5):541–545.
65. Goldenberg N, Racine MS, Thomas P, et al. Treatment of pituitary gigantism with the growth hormone receptor antagonist pegvisomant. J Clin Endocrinol Metab 2008; 93(8):2953–2956.
66. Dekkers OM, Pereira AM, Romijn JA. Treatment and follow-up of clinically nonfunctioning pituitary macroadenomas. J Clin Endocrinol Metab 2008;93(10):3717–3726.
67. Beck-Peccoz P, Persani L. Thyrotropinomas. Endocrinol Metab Clin North Am 2008;37(1):123–134, viii–ix.
68. Pernicone PJ, Scheithauer BW, Sebo TJ, et al. Pituitary carcinoma: a clinicopathologic study of 15 cases. Cancer 1997;79(4):804–812.
69. Scheithauer BW, Kurtkaya-Yapicier O, Kovacs KT, et al. Pituitary carcinoma: a clinicopathological review. Neurosurgery 2005;56(5):1066–1074; discussion 1066–1074.
70. Kaltsas GA, Nomikos P, Kontogeorgos G, et al. Clinical review: diagnosis and management of pituitary carcinomas. J Clin Endocrinol Metab 2005;90(5):3089–3099.

71. Kaltsas GA, Mukherjee JJ, Plowman PN, et al. The role of cytotoxic chemotherapy in the management of aggressive and malignant pituitary tumors. J Clin Endocrinol Metab 1998;83(12):4233–4238.

72. Lopes MB, Scheithauer BW, Schiff D. Pituitary carcinoma: diagnosis and treatment. Endocrine 2005;28(1):115–121.

73. Landman RE, Horwith M, Peterson RE, et al. Long-term survival with ACTH-secreting carcinoma of the pituitary: a case report and review of the literature. J Clin Endocrinol Metab 2002;87(7):3084–3089.

74. Kaltsas GA, Grossman AB. Malignant pituitary tumours. Pituitary 1998;1(1):69–81.

75. Laws ER Jr, Morris AM, Maartens N. Gliadel for pituitary adenomas and craniopharyngiomas. Neurosurgery 2003;53(2):255–269; discussion 259–260.

76. McCutcheon IE, Pieper DR, Fuller GN, et al. Pituitary carcinoma containing gonadotropins: treatment by radical excision and cytotoxic chemotherapy: case report. Neurosurgery 2000;46(5):1233–1239; discussion 1239–1240.

77. Fadul CE, Kominsky AL, Meyer LP, et al. Long-term response of pituitary carcinoma to temozolomide. Report of two cases. J Neurosurg 2006;105(4):621–626.

78. Lim S, Shahinian H, Maya MM, et al. Temozolomide: a novel treatment for pituitary carcinoma. Lancet Oncol 2006;7(6):518–520.

79. Ruda JM, Hollenbeak CS, Stack BC Jr. A systematic review of the diagnosis and treatment of primary hyperparathyroidism from 1995 to 2003. Otolaryngol Head Neck Surg 2005;132(3):359–372.

80. Allo M, Thompson NW, Harness JK, et al. Primary hyperparathyroidism in children, adolescents, and young adults. World J Surg 1982;6(6):771–776.

81. Kollars J, Zarroug AE, van Heerden J, et al. Primary hyperparathyroidism in pediatric patients. Pediatrics 2005;115(4):974–980.

82. Lawson ML, Miller SF, Ellis G, et al. Primary hyperparathyroidism in a paediatric hospital. QJM 1996;89(12):921–932.

83. Schneider AB, Gierlowski TC, Shore-Freedman E, et al. Dose-response relationships for radiation-induced hyperparathyroidism. J Clin Endocrinol Metab 1995;80(1):254–257.

84. Fuleihan Gel H. Familial benign hypocalciuric hypercalcemia. J Bone Miner Res 2002;17(Suppl 2):N51–N56.

85. Brown EM. Clinical lessons from the calcium-sensing receptor. Nat Clin Pract Endocrinol Metab 2007;3(2):122–133.

86. Pollak MR, Chou YH, Marx SJ, et al. Familial hypocalciuric hypercalcemia and neonatal severe hyperparathyroidism. Effects of mutant gene dosage on phenotype. J Clin Invest 1994;93(3):1108–1112.

87. Udelsman R, Pasieka JL, Sturgeon C, et al. Surgery for asymptomatic primary hyperparathyroidism: proceedings of the third international workshop. J Clin Endocrinol Metab 2009;94(2):366–372.

88. Mortenson MM, Evans DB, Lee JE, et al. Parathyroid exploration in the reoperative neck: improved preoperative localization with 4D-computed tomography. J Am Coll Surg 2008;206(5):888–895; discussion 895–886.

89. Sosa JA, Tuggle CT, Wang TS, et al. Clinical and economic outcomes of thyroid and parathyroid surgery in children. J Clin Endocrinol Metab 2008;93(8):3058–3065.

90. O'Riordain DS, O'Brien T, Grant CS, et al. Surgical management of primary hyperparathyroidism in multiple endocrine neoplasia types 1 and 2. Surgery 1993;114(6):1031–1037; discussion 1037–1039.

91. Stalberg P, Carling T. Familial parathyroid tumors: diagnosis and management. World J Surg 2009;33(11):2234–2243.

92. Lambert LA, Shapiro SE, Lee JE, et al. Surgical treatment of hyperparathyroidism in patients with multiple endocrine neoplasia type 1. Arch Surg 2005;140(4):374–382.

93. Brandi ML, Gagel RF, Angeli A, et al. Guidelines for diagnosis and therapy of MEN type 1 and type 2. J Clin Endocrinol Metab 2001;86(12):5658–5671.

94. Khan A, Grey A, Shoback D. Medical management of asymptomatic primary hyperparathyroidism: proceedings of the third international workshop. J Clin Endocrinol Metab 2009;94(2):373–381.

95. Eastell R, Arnold A, Brandi ML, et al. Diagnosis of asymptomatic primary hyperparathyroidism: proceedings of the third international workshop. J Clin Endocrinol Metab 2009;94(2):340–350.

96. Debruyne F, Delaere P, Vander Poorten V. Postoperative course of serum parathyroid hormone and calcium after surgery for primary hyperparathyroidism. Acta Otorhinolaryngol Belg 2001;55(2):153–157.

97. Dhillon KS, Cohan P, Darwin C, et al. Elevated serum parathyroid hormone concentration in eucalcemic patients after parathyroidectomy for primary hyperparathyroidism and its relationship to vitamin D profile. Metabolism 2004;53(9):1101–1106.

98. Shane E. Clinical review 122: parathyroid carcinoma. J Clin Endocrinol Metab 2001;86(2):485–493.

99. Hamill J, Maoate K, Beasley SW, et al. Familial parathyroid carcinoma in a child. J Paediatr Child Health 2002;38(3):314–317.

100. Schantz A, Castleman B. Parathyroid carcinoma. A study of 70 cases. Cancer 1973;31(3):600–605.

101. Shattuck TM, Valimaki S, Obara T, et al. Somatic and germ-line mutations of the HRPT2 gene in sporadic parathyroid carcinoma. N Engl J Med 2003;349(18):1722–1729.

102. Busaidy NL, Jimenez C, Habra MA, et al. Parathyroid carcinoma: a 22-year experience. Head Neck 2004;26(8):716–726.

103. Sandelin K, Auer G, Bondeson L, et al. Prognostic factors in parathyroid cancer: a review of 95 cases. World J Surg 1992;16(4):724–731.

104. Delellis RA. Challenging lesions in the differential diagnosis of endocrine tumors: parathyroid carcinoma. Endocr Pathol 2008;19(4):221–225.

105. Obara T, Okamoto T, Kanbe M, et al. Functioning parathyroid carcinoma: clinicopathologic features and rational treatment. Semin Surg Oncol 1997;13(2):134–141.

106. Fassnacht M, Kreissl MC, Weismann D, et al. New targets and therapeutic approaches for endocrine malignancies. Pharmacol Ther 2009;123(1):117–141.

107. Silverberg SJ, Rubin MR, Faiman C, et al. Cinacalcet hydrochloride reduces the serum calcium concentration in inoperable parathyroid carcinoma. J Clin Endocrinol Metab 2007;92(10):3803–3808.

108. Hundahl SA, Fleming ID, Fremgen AM, et al. Two hundred eighty-six cases of parathyroid carcinoma treated in the U.S. between 1985–1995: a National Cancer Data Base Report. The American College of Surgeons Commission on Cancer and the American Cancer Society. Cancer 1999;86(3):538–544.

109. Niedziela M. Pathogenesis, diagnosis and management of thyroid nodules in children. Endocr Relat Cancer 2006;13(2):427–453.

110. Belfiore A, Giuffrida D, La Rosa GL, et al. High frequency of cancer in cold thyroid nodules occurring at young age. Acta Endocrinol (Copenh) 1989;121(2):197–202.

111. Lafferty AR, Batch JA. Thyroid nodules in childhood and adolescence—thirty years of experience. J Pediatr Endocrinol Metab 1997;10(5):479–486.

112. Hung W. Solitary thyroid nodules in 93 children and adolescents. A 35-years experience. Horm Res 1999;52(1):15–18.

113. Schlumberger M, Pacini F. Thyroid tumors. Paris: Nucleon, 2003.

114. Wiersinga WM. Management of thyroid nodules in children and adolescents. Hormones (Athens) 2007;6(3):194–199.

115. Hegedus L, Bonnema SJ, Bennedbaek FN. Management of simple nodular goiter: current status and future perspectives. Endocr Rev 2003;24(1):102–132.

116. Cooper DS, Doherty GM, Haugen BR, et al. Management guidelines for patients with thyroid nodules and differentiated thyroid cancer. Thyroid 2006;16(2):109–142.

117. Kouvaraki MA, Shapiro SE, Fornage BD, et al. Role of preoperative ultrasonography in the surgical management of patients with thyroid cancer. Surgery 2003;134(6):946–954; discussion 954–955.

118. Lyshchik A, Drozd V, Demidchik Y, et al. Diagnosis of thyroid cancer in children: value of gray-scale and power doppler US. Radiology 2005;235(2):604–613.

119. Sarkar SD. Benign thyroid disease: what is the role of nuclear medicine? Semin Nucl Med 2006;36(3):185–193.

120. The NCCN Clinical Practice Guidelines in Oncology, Thyroid Carcinoma (Version 1.2009). http://www.NCCN.org. Accessed June 9, 2009.

121. Baloch ZW, LiVolsi VA, Asa SL, et al. Diagnostic terminology and morphologic criteria for cytologic diagnosis of thyroid lesions: a synopsis of the National Cancer Institute Thyroid Fine-Needle Aspiration State of the Science Conference. Diagn Cytopathol 2008;36(6):425–437.

122. Izquierdo R, Shankar R, Kort K, et al. Ultrasound-guided fine-needle aspiration in the management of thyroid nodules in children and adolescents. Thyroid 2009;19(7):703–705.

123. Spoudeas HA, ed. Paediatric endocrine tumours: a multi-disciplinary consensus statement of best practice from a working group convened under the auspices of the British Society of Paediatric Endocrinology and Diabetes and the United Kingdom Children's Cancer Study Group. West Sussex, UK: Novo Nordisk Ltd, 2005.

124. Layfield LJ, Abrams J, Cochand-Priollet B, et al. Post-thyroid FNA testing and treatment options: a synopsis of the National Cancer Institute Thyroid Fine Needle Aspiration State of the Science Conference. Diagn Cytopathol 2008;36(6):442–448.

125. American Cancer Society. Cancer facts & figures 2009. Atlanta: American Cancer Society, 2009.

126. Horner MJ, Ries LAG, Krapcho M, et al. SEER Cancer Statistics Review, 1975–2006. http://seer.cancer.gov/csr/1975_2006/. Accessed March 12, 2009.

127. Waguespack S, Wells S, Ross J, et al. Thyroid cancer. In: Bleyer A, O'Leary M, Barr R, et al., eds. Cancer epidemiology in older adolescents and young adults 15 to 29 years of age, including SEER incidence and survival 1975–2000. Vol NIH Pub. No. 06-5767. Bethesda, MD: National Cancer Institute, 2006:143–154.

128. Demidchik YE, Saenko VA, Yamashita S. Childhood thyroid cancer in Belarus, Russia, and Ukraine after Chernobyl and at present. Arq Bras Endocrinol Metabol 2007;51(5):748–762.

129. Cobin RH, Gharib H, Bergman DA, et al. AACE/AAES medical/surgical guidelines for clinical practice: management of thyroid carcinoma. American Association of Clinical Endocrinologists. American College of Endocrinology. Endocr Pract 2001;7(3):202–220.

130. British Thyroid Association, Royal College of Physicians. Guidelines for the management of thyroid cancer (Perros P, ed) 2nd edition. Report of the Thyroid Cancer Guidelines Update Group. London: Royal College of Physicians, 2007.

131. Kloos RT, Eng C, Evans DB, et al. Medullary thyroid cancer: management guidelines of the American Thyroid Association. Thyroid 2009;19(6):565–612.

132. Harness JK, Thompson NW, McLeod MK, et al. Differentiated thyroid carcinoma in children and adolescents. World J Surg 1992;16(4):547–553; discussion 553–554.

133. Demidchik YE, Demidchik EP, Reiners C, et al. Comprehensive clinical assessment of 740 cases of surgically treated thyroid cancer in children of Belarus. Ann Surg 2006;243(4):525–532.

134. Harach HR, Williams ED. Childhood thyroid cancer in England and Wales. Br J Cancer 1995;72(3):777–783.

135. Zimmerman D, Hay ID, Gough IR, et al. Papillary thyroid carcinoma in children and adults: long-term follow-up of 1039 patients conservatively treated at one institution during three decades. Surgery 1988;104(6):1157–1166.

136. Schneider AB. Radiation-induced thyroid cancer. UpToDate Online 17.1. www.uptodate.com. Accessed June 23, 2009.

137. Tucker MA, Jones PH, Boice JD Jr, et al. Therapeutic radiation at a young age is linked to secondary thyroid cancer. The Late Effects Study Group. Cancer Res 1991;51(11):2885–2888.

138. Alberti L, Carniti C, Miranda C, et al. RET and NTRK1 proto-oncogenes in human diseases. J Cell Physiol 2003;195(2):168–186.

139. Faggiano A, Coulot J, Bellon N, et al. Age-dependent variation of follicular size and expression of iodine transporters in human thyroid tissue. J Nucl Med 2004;45(2):232–237.

140. Ronckers CM, Sigurdson AJ, Stovall M, et al. Thyroid cancer in childhood cancer survivors: a detailed evaluation of radiation dose response and its modifiers. Radiat Res 2006;166(4):618–628.

141. Naing S, Collins BJ, Schneider AB. Clinical behavior of radiation-induced thyroid cancer: factors related to recurrence. Thyroid 2009;19(5):479–485.

142. Inskip PD, Curtis RE. New malignancies following childhood cancer in the United States, 1973–2002. Int J Cancer 2007;121(10):2233–2240.

143. Williams D. Cancer after nuclear fallout: lessons from the Chernobyl accident. Nat Rev Cancer 2002;2(7):543–549.

144. Farahati J, Demidchik EP, Biko J, et al. Inverse association between age at the time of radiation exposure and extent of disease in cases of radiation-induced childhood thyroid carcinoma in Belarus. Cancer 2000;88(6):1470–1476.

145. Sherman SI. Thyroid carcinoma. Lancet 2003;361(9356):501–511.

146. Sobrinho-Simoes M, Maximo V, Rocha AS, et al. Intragenic mutations in thyroid cancer. Endocrinol Metab Clin North Am 2008;37(2):333–362, viii.

147. Woyach J, Shah M. New therapeutic advances in the management of progressive thyroid cancer. Endocr Relat Cancer 2009;16(3):715–731.

148. Yamashita S, Saenko V. Mechanisms of disease: molecular genetics of childhood thyroid cancers. Nat Clin Pract Endocrinol Metab 2007;3(5):422–429.

149. Xing M, Westra WH, Tufano RP, et al. BRAF mutation predicts a poorer clinical prognosis for papillary thyroid cancer. J Clin Endocrinol Metab 2005;90(12):6373–6379.

150. Penko K, Livezey J, Fenton C, et al. BRAF mutations are uncommon in papillary thyroid cancer of young patients. Thyroid 2005;15(4):320–325.

151. Nikiforova MN, Tseng GC, Steward D, et al. MicroRNA expression profiling of thyroid tumors: biological significance and diagnostic utility. J Clin Endocrinol Metab 2008;93(5):1600–1608.
152. Kebebew E. Hereditary non-medullary thyroid cancer. World J Surg 2008;32(5): 678–682.
153. Alsanea O, Wada N, Ain K, et al. Is familial non-medullary thyroid carcinoma more aggressive than sporadic thyroid cancer? A multicenter series. Surgery 2000;128(6): 1043–1051.
154. Capezzone M, Marchisotta S, Cantara S, et al. Familial non-medullary thyroid carcinoma displays the features of clinical anticipation suggestive of a distinct biological entity. Endocr Relat Cancer 2008;15(4):1075–1081.
155. Cavaco BM, Batista PF, Martins C, et al. Familial non-medullary thyroid carcinoma (FNMTC): analysis of fPTC/PRN, NMTC1, MNG1 and TCO susceptibility loci and identification of somatic BRAF and RAS mutations. Endocr Relat Cancer 2008;15(1): 207–215.
156. Perrier ND, van Heerden JA, Goellner JR, et al. Thyroid cancer in patients with familial adenomatous polyposis. World J Surg 1998;22(7):738–742; discussion 743.
157. Liaw D, Marsh DJ, Li J, et al. Germline mutations of the PTEN gene in Cowden disease, an inherited breast and thyroid cancer syndrome. Nat Genet 1997;16(1): 64–67.
158. Goto M, Miller RW, Ishikawa Y, et al. Excess of rare cancers in Werner syndrome (adult progeria). Cancer Epidemiol Biomarkers Prev 1996;5(4):239–246.
159. Stratakis CA, Kirschner LS, Carney JA. Clinical and molecular features of the Carney complex: diagnostic criteria and recommendations for patient evaluation. J Clin Endocrinol Metab 2001;86(9):4041–4046.
160. Feinmesser R, Lubin E, Segal K, et al. Carcinoma of the thyroid in children—a review. J Pediatr Endocrinol Metab 1997;10(6):561–568.
161. Frankenthaler RA, Sellin RV, Cangir A, et al. Lymph node metastasis from papillary-follicular thyroid carcinoma in young patients. Am J Surg 1990;160(4):341–343.
162. Vassilopoulou-Sellin R, Klein MJ, Smith TH, et al. Pulmonary metastases in children and young adults with differentiated thyroid cancer. Cancer 1993;71(4): 1348–1352.
163. Schlumberger M, De Vathaire F, Travagli JP, et al. Differentiated thyroid carcinoma in childhood: long term follow-up of 72 patients. J Clin Endocrinol Metab 1987;65(6): 1088–1094.
164. Bal CS, Kumar A, Chandra P, et al. Is chest x-ray or high-resolution computed tomography scan of the chest sufficient investigation to detect pulmonary metastasis in pediatric differentiated thyroid cancer? Thyroid 2004;14(3):217–225.
165. Hung W, Sarlis NJ. Current controversies in the management of pediatric patients with well-differentiated nonmedullary thyroid cancer: a review. Thyroid 2002;12(8): 683–702.
166. Spencer CA, Takeuchi M, Kazarosyan M, et al. Serum thyroglobulin autoantibodies: prevalence, influence on serum thyroglobulin measurement, and prognostic significance in patients with differentiated thyroid carcinoma. J Clin Endocrinol Metab 1998;83(4): 1121–1127.
167. Samuel AM, Rajashekharrao B, Shah DH. Pulmonary metastases in children and adolescents with well-differentiated thyroid cancer. J Nucl Med 1998;39(9):1531–1536.
168. Lang BH, Lo CY, Chan WF, et al. Staging systems for papillary thyroid carcinoma: a review and comparison. Ann Surg 2007;245(3):366–378.
169. Grubbs EG, Rich TA, Li G, et al. Recent advances in thyroid cancer. Curr Probl Surg 2008;45(3):156–250.
170. Shaha AR. TNM classification of thyroid carcinoma. World J Surg 2007;31(5): 879–887.
171. Powers PA, Dinauer CA, Tuttle RM, et al. The MACIS score predicts the clinical course of papillary thyroid carcinoma in children and adolescents. J Pediatr Endocrinol Metab 2004;17(3):339–343.
172. Vassilopoulou-Sellin R, Goepfert H, Raney B, et al. Differentiated thyroid cancer in children and adolescents: clinical outcome and mortality after long-term follow-up. Head Neck 1998;20(6):549–555.
173. La Quaglia MP, Black T, Holcomb GW III, et al. Differentiated thyroid cancer: clinical characteristics, treatment, and outcome in patients under 21 years of age who present with distant metastases. A report from the Surgical Discipline Committee of the Children's Cancer Group. J Pediatr Surg 2000;35(6):955–959; discussion 960.
174. Landau D, Vini L, A'Hern R, et al. Thyroid cancer in children: the Royal Marsden Hospital experience. Eur J Cancer 2000;36(2):214–220.
175. Brink JS, van Heerden JA, McIver B, et al. Papillary thyroid cancer with pulmonary metastases in children: long-term prognosis. Surgery 2000;128(6):881–886; discussion 886–887.
176. Durante C, Haddy N, Baudin E, et al. Long-term outcome of 444 patients with distant metastases from papillary and follicular thyroid carcinoma: benefits and limits of radioiodine therapy. J Clin Endocrinol Metab 2006;91(8):2892–2899.
177. Patel A, Jhiang S, Dogra S, et al. Differentiated thyroid carcinoma that express sodium-iodide symporter have a lower risk of recurrence for children and adolescents. Pediatr Res 2002;52(5):737–744.
178. Lee YM, Lo CY, Lam KY, et al. Well-differentiated thyroid carcinoma in Hong Kong Chinese patients under 21 years of age: a 35-year experience. J Am Coll Surg 2002; 194(6):711–716.
179. Bal CS, Padhy AK, Kumar A. Clinical features of differentiated thyroid carcinoma in children and adolescents from a sub-Himalayan iodine-deficient endemic zone. Nucl Med Commun 2001;22(8):881–887.
180. Welch Dinauer CA, Tuttle RM, Robie DK, et al. Extensive surgery improves recurrence-free survival for children and young patients with class I papillary thyroid carcinoma. J Pediatr Surg 1999;34(12):1799–1804.
181. Jarzab B, Handkiewicz Junak D, Wloch J, et al. Multivariate analysis of prognostic factors for differentiated thyroid carcinoma in children. Eur J Nucl Med 2000;27(7): 833–841.
182. Bilimoria KY, Bentrem DJ, Ko CY, et al. Extent of surgery affects survival for papillary thyroid cancer. Ann Surg 2007;246(3):375–381; discussion 381–384.
183. Thompson GB, Hay ID. Current strategies for surgical management and adjuvant treatment of childhood papillary thyroid carcinoma. World J Surg 2004;28(12): 1187–1198.
184. Rachmiel M, Charron M, Gupta A, et al. Evidence-based review of treatment and follow up of pediatric patients with differentiated thyroid carcinoma. J Pediatr Endocrinol Metab 2006;19(12):1377–1393.
185. Musacchio MJ, Kim AW, Vijungco JD, et al. Greater local recurrence occurs with "berry picking" than neck dissection in thyroid cancer. Am Surg 2003;69(3):191–196; discussion 196–197.
186. van Santen HM, Aronson DC, Vulsma T, et al. Frequent adverse events after treatment for childhood-onset differentiated thyroid carcinoma: a single institute experience. Eur J Cancer 2004;40(11):1743–1751.
187. Taylor T, Specker B, Robbins J, et al. Outcome after treatment of high-risk papillary and non-Hurthle-cell follicular thyroid carcinoma. Ann Intern Med 1998;129(8): 622–627.
188. Mazzaferri EL, Jhiang SM. Long-term impact of initial surgical and medical therapy on papillary and follicular thyroid cancer. Am J Med 1994;97(5):418–428.
189. Jonklaas J, Sarlis NJ, Litofsky D, et al. Outcomes of patients with differentiated thyroid carcinoma following initial therapy. Thyroid 2006;16(12):1229–1242.
190. Sawka AM, Brierley JD, Tsang RW, et al. An updated systematic review and commentary examining the effectiveness of radioactive iodine remnant ablation in well-differentiated thyroid cancer. Endocrinol Metab Clin North Am 2008;37(2): 457–480, x.
191. Dinauer C, Francis GL. Thyroid cancer in children. Endocrinol Metab Clin North Am 2007;36(3):779–806, vii.
192. Pacini F, Ladenson PW, Schlumberger M, et al. Radioiodine ablation of thyroid remnants after preparation with recombinant human thyrotropin in differentiated thyroid carcinoma: results of an international, randomized, controlled study. J Clin Endocrinol Metab 2006;91(3):926–932.
193. Tuttle RM, Brokhin M, Omry G, et al. Recombinant human TSH-assisted radioactive iodine remnant ablation achieves short-term clinical recurrence rates similar to those of traditional thyroid hormone withdrawal. J Nucl Med 2008;49(5):764–770.
194. Hanscheid H, Lassmann M, Luster M, et al. Iodine biokinetics and dosimetry in radioiodine therapy of thyroid cancer: procedures and results of a prospective international controlled study of ablation after rhTSH or hormone withdrawal. J Nucl Med 2006;47(4):648–654.
195. Yaakob W, Gordon L, Spicer KM, et al. The usefulness of iodine-123 whole-body scans in evaluating thyroid carcinoma and metastases. J Nucl Med Technol 1999;27(4): 279–281.
196. Tuttle RM, Leboeuf R, Robbins RJ, et al. Empiric radioactive iodine dosing regimens frequently exceed maximum tolerated activity levels in elderly patients with thyroid cancer. J Nucl Med 2006;47(10):1587–1591.
197. Hovens GC, Stokkel MP, Kievit J, et al. Associations of serum thyrotropin concentrations with recurrence and death in differentiated thyroid cancer. J Clin Endocrinol Metab 2007;92(7):2610–2615.
198. Argiris A, Agarwala SS, Karamouzis MV, et al. A phase II trial of doxorubicin and interferon alpha 2b in advanced, non-medullary thyroid cancer. Invest New Drugs 2008;26(2):183–188.
199. Sherman SI. Advances in chemotherapy of differentiated epithelial and medullary thyroid cancers. J Clin Endocrinol Metab 2009;94(5):1493–1499.
200. Sherman SI. Early clinical studies of novel therapies for thyroid cancers. Endocrinol Metab Clin North Am 2008;37(2):511–524, xi.
201. Cohen EE, Rosen LS, Vokes EE, et al. Axitinib is an active treatment for all histologic subtypes of advanced thyroid cancer: results from a phase II study. J Clin Oncol 2008;26(29):4708–4713.
202. Rosen LS, Kurzrock R, Mulay M, et al. Safety, pharmacokinetics, and efficacy of AMG 706, an oral multikinase inhibitor, in patients with advanced solid tumors. J Clin Oncol 2007;25(17):2369–2376.
203. Sherman SI, Wirth LJ, Droz JP, et al. Motesanib diphosphate in progressive differentiated thyroid cancer. N Engl J Med 2008;359(1):31–42.
204. Pennell NA, Daniels GH, Haddad RI, et al. A phase II study of gefitinib in patients with advanced thyroid cancer. Thyroid 2008;18(3):317–323.
205. Frank-Raue K, Fabel M, Delorme S, et al. Efficacy of imatinib mesylate in advanced medullary thyroid carcinoma. Eur J Endocrinol 2007;157(2):215–220.
206. de Groot JW, Zonnenberg BA, van Ufford-Mannesse PQ, et al. A phase II trial of imatinib therapy for metastatic medullary thyroid carcinoma. J Clin Endocrinol Metab 2007;92(9):3466–3469.
207. Gupta-Abramson V, Troxel AB, Nellore A, et al. Phase II trial of sorafenib in advanced thyroid cancer. J Clin Oncol 2008;26(29):4714–4719.
208. Kloos RT, Ringel MD, Knopp MV, et al. Phase II trial of sorafenib in metastatic thyroid cancer. J Clin Oncol 2009;27(10):1675–1684.
209. Waguespack SG, Sherman SI, Williams MD, et al. The successful use of sorafenib to treat pediatric papillary thyroid carcinoma. Thyroid 2009;19(4):407–412.
210. Hong D, Ye L, Gagel R, et al. Medullary thyroid cancer: targeting the RET kinase pathway with sorafenib/tipifarnib. Mol Cancer Ther 2008;7(5):1001–1006.
211. Dawson SJ, Conus NM, Toner GC, et al. Sustained clinical responses to tyrosine kinase inhibitor sunitinib in thyroid carcinoma. Anticancer Drugs 2008;19(5):547–552.
212. Kelleher FC, McDermott R. Response to sunitinib in medullary thyroid cancer. Ann Intern Med 1 2008;148(7):567.
213. Tuttle RM, Leboeuf R. Follow up approaches in thyroid cancer: a risk adapted paradigm. Endocrinol Metab Clin North Am 2008;37(2):419–435, ix–x.
214. Mazzaferri EL, Robbins RJ, Spencer CA, et al. A consensus report of the role of serum thyroglobulin as a monitoring method for low-risk patients with papillary thyroid carcinoma. J Clin Endocrinol Metab 2003;88(4):1433–1441.
215. Chiovato L, Latrofa F, Braverman LE, et al. Disappearance of humoral thyroid autoimmunity after complete removal of thyroid antigens. Ann Intern Med 2003;139(5 Pt 1): 346–351.
216. Kloos RT, Mazzaferri EL. A single recombinant human thyrotropin-stimulated serum thyroglobulin measurement predicts differentiated thyroid carcinoma metastases three to five years later. J Clin Endocrinol Metab 2005;90(9):5047–5057.
217. Castagna MG, Brilli L, Pilli T, et al. Limited value of repeat recombinant human thyrotropin (rhTSH)-stimulated thyroglobulin testing in differentiated thyroid carcinoma patients with previous negative rhTSH-stimulated thyroglobulin and undetectable basal serum thyroglobulin levels. J Clin Endocrinol Metab 2008;93(1):76–81.
218. Kloos RT. Approach to the patient with a positive serum thyroglobulin and a negative radioiodine scan after initial therapy for differentiated thyroid cancer. J Clin Endocrinol Metab 2008;93(5):1519–1525.
219. Leboulleux S, Schroeder PR, Schlumberger M, et al. The role of PET in follow-up of patients treated for differentiated epithelial thyroid cancers. Nat Clin Pract Endocrinol Metab 2007;3(2):112–121.
220. Robbins RJ, Wan Q, Grewal RK, et al. Real-time prognosis for metastatic thyroid carcinoma based on 2-[18F]fluoro-2-deoxy-D-glucose-positron emission tomography scanning. J Clin Endocrinol Metab 2006;91(2):498–505.
221. Leboulleux S, Baudin E, Hartl DW, et al. Follicular cell-derived thyroid cancer in children. Horm Res 2005;63(3):145–151.
222. Dottorini ME, Vignati A, Mazzucchelli L, et al. Differentiated thyroid carcinoma in children and adolescents: a 37-year experience in 85 patients. J Nucl Med 1997;38(5): 669–675.

223. Meier DA, Brill DR, Becker DV, et al. Procedure guideline for therapy of thyroid disease with (131)iodine. J Nucl Med 2002;43(6):856–861.
224. Mandel SJ, Mandel L. Radioactive iodine and the salivary glands. Thyroid 2003;13(3): 265–271.
225. Sawka AM, Lakra DC, Lea J, et al. A systematic review examining the effects of therapeutic radioactive iodine on ovarian function and future pregnancy in female thyroid cancer survivors. Clin Endocrinol (Oxf) 2008;69:479–490.
226. Sawka AM, Lea J, Alshehri B, et al. A systematic review of the gonadal effects of therapeutic radioactive iodine in male thyroid cancer survivors. Clin Endocrinol (Oxf) 2008; 68(4):610–617.
227. Brown AP, Chen J, Hitchcock YJ, et al. The risk of second primary malignancies up to three decades after the treatment of differentiated thyroid cancer. J Clin Endocrinol Metab 2008;93(2):504–515.
228. Sawka AM, Thabane L, Parlea L, et al. Second primary malignancy risk after radioactive iodine treatment for thyroid cancer: a systematic review and meta-analysis. Thyroid 2009;19(5):451–457.
229. Mulligan LM, Kwok JB, Healey CS, et al. Germ-line mutations of the RET proto-oncogene in multiple endocrine neoplasia type 2A. Nature 1993;363(6428):458–460.
230. Carlson KM, Dou S, Chi D, et al. Single missense mutation in the tyrosine kinase catalytic domain of the RET protooncogene is associated with multiple endocrine neoplasia type 2B. Proc Natl Acad Sci U S A 1994;91(4):1579–1583.
231. Jimenez C, Hu MI, Gagel RF. Management of medullary thyroid carcinoma. Endocrinol Metab Clin North Am 2008;37(2):481–496, x–xi.
232. Elisei R, Cosci B, Romei C, et al. Prognostic significance of somatic RET oncogene mutations in sporadic medullary thyroid cancer: a 10-year follow-up study. J Clin Endocrinol Metab 2008;93(3):682–687.
233. Wolfe HJ, Melvin KE, Cervi-Skinner SJ, et al. C-cell hyperplasia preceding medullary thyroid carcinoma. N Engl J Med 1973;289(9):437–441.
234. Machens A. Early malignant progression of hereditary medullary thyroid cancer. N Engl J Med 2004;350(9):943.
235. Moley JF, DeBenedetti MK. Patterns of nodal metastases in palpable medullary thyroid carcinoma: recommendations for extent of node dissection. Ann Surg 1999;229(6): 880–887; discussion 887–888.
236. Wells SA Jr, Chi DD, Toshima K, et al. Predictive DNA testing and prophylactic thyroidectomy in patients at risk for multiple endocrine neoplasia type 2A. Ann Surg 1994;220(3):237–247; discussion 247–250.
237. Wray CJ, Rich TA, Waguespack SG, et al. Failure to recognize multiple endocrine neoplasia 2B: more common than we think? Ann Surg Oncol 2008;15(1):293–301.
238. Brauckhoff M, Machens A, Hess S, et al. Premonitory symptoms preceding metastatic medullary thyroid cancer in MEN 2B: an exploratory analysis. Surgery 2008;144(6): 1044–1050; discussion 1050–1053.
239. Waguespack SG. A perspective from pediatric endocrinology on the hereditary medullary thyroid carcinoma syndromes. Thyroid 2009;19(6):543–546.
240. Skinner MA, Moley JA, Dilley WG, et al. Prophylactic thyroidectomy in multiple endocrine neoplasia type 2A. N Engl J Med 2005;353(11):1105–1113.
241. Laure Giraudet A, Al Ghulzan A, Auperin A, et al. Progression of medullary thyroid carcinoma: assessment with calcitonin and carcinoembryonic antigen doubling times. Eur J Endocrinol 2008;158(2):239–246.
242. Yen TW, Shapiro SE, Gagel RF, et al. Medullary thyroid carcinoma: results of a standardized surgical approach in a contemporary series of 80 consecutive patients. Surgery 2003;134(6):890–899; discussion 899–901.
243. Fox E, Widemann BC, Whitcomb PO, et al. Phase I/II trial of vandetanib in children and adolescents with hereditary medullary thyroid carcinoma. J Clin Oncol 2009;27 (15s):10014.
244. Giraudet AL, Vanel D, Leboulleux S, et al. Imaging medullary thyroid carcinoma with persistent elevated calcitonin levels. J Clin Endocrinol Metab 2007;92(11):4185–4190.
245. Kloppel G, Perren A, Heitz PU. The gastroenteropancreatic neuroendocrine cell system and its tumors: the WHO classification. Ann N Y Acad Sci 2004;1014:13–27.
246. Yao JC, Hassan M, Phan A, et al. One hundred years after "carcinoid": epidemiology of and prognostic factors for neuroendocrine tumors in 35,825 cases in the United States. J Clin Oncol 2008;26(18):3063–3072.
247. Ehehalt F, Saeger HD, Schmidt CM, et al. Neuroendocrine tumors of the pancreas. Oncologist 2009;14(5):456–467.
248. The NCCN Clinical Practice Guidelines in Oncology, Neuroendocrine Tumors (Version 1.2009), 5/1/2009. http://www.nccn.org. Accessed June 9, 2009.
249. Tomassetti P, Migliori M, Lalli S, et al. Epidemiology, clinical features and diagnosis of gastroenteropancreatic endocrine tumours. Ann Oncol 2001;12(Suppl 2):S95–S99.
250. Broaddus RR, Herzog CE, Hicks MJ. Neuroendocrine tumors (carcinoid and neuroendocrine carcinoma) presenting at extra-appendiceal sites in childhood and adolescence. Arch Pathol Lab Med 2003;127(9):1200–1203.
251. Spunt SL, Pratt CB, Rao BN, et al. Childhood carcinoid tumors: the St Jude Children's Research Hospital experience. J Pediatr Surg 2000;35(9):1282–1286.
252. Eriksson B, Oberg K, Stridsberg M. Tumor markers in neuroendocrine tumors. Digestion 2000;62(Suppl 1):33–38.
253. Eriksson B, Arnberg H, Lindgren PG, et al. Neuroendocrine pancreatic tumours: clinical presentation, biochemical and histopathological findings in 84 patients. J Intern Med 1990;228(2):103–113.
254. Ardill JE. Circulating markers for endocrine tumours of the gastroenteropancreatic tract. Ann Clin Biochem 2008;45(Pt 6):539–559.
255. Sundin A, Vullierme MP, Kaltsas G, et al. ENETS Consensus Guidelines for the Standards of Care in Neuroendocrine Tumors: radiological examinations. Neuroendocrinology. 2009;90(2):167–183.
256. Rufini V, Calcagni ML, Baum RP. Imaging of neuroendocrine tumors. Semin Nucl Med 2006;36(3):228–247.
257. Eriksson B, Orlefors H, Oberg K, et al. Developments in PET for the detection of endocrine tumours. Best Pract Res Clin Endocrinol Metab 2005;19(2):311–324.
258. Solcia E, Kloppel G, Sobin LH, et al. Histological typing of endocrine tumours. WHO International histological classification of tumours. 2nd ed. Berlin: Springer, 2000.
259. Weber HC, Venzon DJ, Lin JT, et al. Determinants of metastatic rate and survival in patients with Zollinger-Ellison syndrome: a prospective long-term study. Gastroenterology 1995;108(6):1637–1649.
260. Kouvaraki MA, Shapiro SE, Cote GJ, et al. Management of pancreatic endocrine tumors in multiple endocrine neoplasia type 1. World J Surg 2006;30(5):643–653.
261. Makridis C, Oberg K, Juhlin C, et al. Surgical treatment of mid-gut carcinoid tumors. World J Surg 1990;14(3):377–383; discussion 384–385.
262. Phan AT, Yao JC, Evans DB. Treatment options for metastatic neuroendocrine tumors. Surgery. 2008;144(6):895–898.
263. Siperstein AE, Rogers SJ, Hansen PD, et al. Laparoscopic thermal ablation of hepatic neuroendocrine tumor metastases. Surgery 1997;122(6):1147–1154; discussion 1154–1155.
264. Olausson M, Friman S, Cahlin C, et al. Indications and results of liver transplantation in patients with neuroendocrine tumors. World J Surg 2002;26(8):998–1004.
265. Phan AT, Yao JC. Neuroendocrine tumors: novel approaches in the age of targeted therapy. Oncology (Williston Park) 2008;22(14):1617–1623; discussion 1623–1624, 1629.
266. Kaltsas GA, Papadogias D, Makras P, et al. Treatment of advanced neuroendocrine tumours with radiolabelled somatostatin analogues. Endocr Relat Cancer 2005;12(4): 683–699.
267. Chan JA, Kulke MH. Progress in the treatment of neuroendocrine tumors. Curr Oncol Rep 2009;11(3):193–199.
268. Kouvaraki MA, Ajani JA, Hoff P, et al. Fluorouracil, doxorubicin, and streptozocin in the treatment of patients with locally advanced and metastatic pancreatic endocrine carcinomas. J Clin Oncol 2004;22(23):4762–4771.
269. Ramage JK, Davies AH, Ardill J, et al. Guidelines for the management of gastroenteropancreatic neuroendocrine (including carcinoid) tumours. Gut 2005;54(Suppl 4): iv1–iv16.
270. Rivera E, Ajani JA. Doxorubicin, streptozocin, and 5-fluorouracil chemotherapy for patients with metastatic islet-cell carcinoma. Am J Clin Oncol 1998;21(1):36–38.
271. Ekeblad S, Sundin A, Janson ET, et al. Temozolomide as monotherapy is effective in treatment of advanced malignant neuroendocrine tumors. Clin Cancer Res 2007; 13(10):2986–2991.
272. Yao JC, Phan A, Hoff PM, et al. Targeting vascular endothelial growth factor in advanced carcinoid tumor: a random assignment phase II study of depot octreotide with bevacizumab and pegylated interferon alpha-2b. J Clin Oncol 2008;26(8): 1316–1323.
273. Kulke MH, Lenz HJ, Meropol NJ, et al. Activity of sunitinib in patients with advanced neuroendocrine tumors. J Clin Oncol 2008;26(20):3403–3410.
274. Duran I, Kortmansky J, Singh D, et al. A phase II clinical and pharmacodynamic study of temsirolimus in advanced neuroendocrine carcinomas. Br J Cancer 2006;95(9): 1148–1154.
275. Yao JC, Phan AT, Chang DZ, et al. Efficacy of RAD001 (everolimus) and octreotide LAR in advanced low- to intermediate-grade neuroendocrine tumors: results of a phase II study. J Clin Oncol 2008;26(26):4311–4318.
276. Norton JA, Fraker DL, Alexander HR, et al. Surgery to cure the Zollinger-Ellison syndrome. N Engl J Med 1999;341(9):635–644.
277. Berna MJ, Hoffmann KM, Long SH, et al. Serum gastrin in Zollinger-Ellison syndrome: II. Prospective study of gastrin provocative testing in 293 patients from the National Institutes of Health and comparison with 537 cases from the literature. Evaluation of diagnostic criteria, proposal of new criteria, and correlations with clinical and tumoral features. Medicine (Baltimore) 2006;85(6):331–364.
278. Arnold R. Diagnosis and differential diagnosis of hypergastrinemia. Wien Klin Wochenschr 2007;119(19–20):564–569.
279. Cryer PE, Axelrod L, Grossman AB, et al. Evaluation and management of adult hypoglycemic disorders: an Endocrine Society Clinical Practice Guideline. J Clin Endocrinol Metab 2009;94(3):709–728.
280. Goldman JA, Blanton WP, Hay DW, et al. False-positive secretin stimulation test for gastrinoma associated with the use of proton pump inhibitor therapy. Clin Gastroenterol Hepatol 2009;7(5):600–602.
281. Wiesli P, Brandle M, Schmid C, et al. Selective arterial calcium stimulation and hepatic venous sampling in the evaluation of hyperinsulinemic hypoglycemia: potential and limitations. J Vasc Interv Radiol 2004;15(11):1251–1256.
282. Perry RR, Vinik AI. Clinical review 72: diagnosis and management of functioning islet cell tumors. J Clin Endocrinol Metab 1995;80(8):2273–2278.
283. Mortenson M, Bold RJ. Symptomatic pancreatic polypeptide-secreting tumor of the distal pancreas (PPoma). Int J Gastrointest Cancer 2002;32(2–3):153–156.
284. Wieneke JA, Thompson LD, Heffess CS. Adrenal cortical neoplasms in the pediatric population: a clinicopathologic and immunophenotypic analysis of 83 patients. Am J Surg Pathol 2003;27(7):867–881.
285. Bernstein L GJ, ed. Carcinomas and other malignant epithelial neoplasms. In: Ries LAG, Smith MA, Gurney JG, et al., eds. Cancer and survival among children and adolescents: United States SEER program 1975–1995. Bethesda, MD: National Cancer Institute, SEER Program, 1999.
286. Mayer SK, Oligny LL, Deal C, et al. Childhood adrenocortical tumors: case series and reevaluation of prognosis—a 24-year experience. J Pediatr Surg 1997;32(6):911–915.
287. Agrons GA, Lonergan GJ, Dickey GE, et al. Adrenocortical neoplasms in children: radiologic-pathologic correlation. Radiographics 1999;19(4):989–1008.
288. Michalkiewicz E, Sandrini R, Figueiredo B, et al. Clinical and outcome characteristics of children with adrenocortical tumors: a report from the International Pediatric Adrenocortical Tumor Registry. J Clin Oncol 2004;22(5):838–845.
289. Rodriguez-Galindo C, Figueiredo BC, Zambetti GP, et al. Biology, clinical characteristics, and management of adrenocortical tumors in children. Pediatr Blood Cancer 2005;45(3):265–273.
290. Hanna AM, Pham TH, Askegard-Giesmann JR, et al. Outcome of adrenocortical tumors in children. J Pediatr Surg 2008;43(5):843–849.
291. Lack EE, Mulvihill JJ, Travis WD, et al. Adrenal cortical neoplasms in the pediatric and adolescent age group. Clinicopathologic study of 30 cases with emphasis on epidemiological and prognostic factors. Pathol Annu 1992;27(Pt 1):1–53.
292. Sandrini R, Ribeiro RC, DeLacerda L. Childhood adrenocortical tumors. J Clin Endocrinol Metab 1997;82(7):2027–2031.
293. Figueiredo BC, Sandrini R, Zambetti GP, et al. Penetrance of adrenocortical tumours associated with the germline TP53 R337 H mutation. J Med Genet 2006;43(1):91–96.
294. Malkin D, Li FP, Strong LC, et al. Germ line p53 mutations in a familial syndrome of breast cancer, sarcomas, and other neoplasms. Science 1990;250(4985):1233–1238.
295. Cohen MM Jr. Beckwith-Wiedemann syndrome: historical, clinicopathological, and etiopathogenetic perspectives. Pediatr Dev Pathol 2005;8(3):287–304.
296. Bertherat J, Horvath A, Groussin L, et al. Mutations in regulatory subunit type 1A of cyclic adenosine 5′-monophosphate-dependent protein kinase (PRKAR1A): phenotype analysis in 353 patients and 80 different genotypes. J Clin Endocrinol Metab 2009; 94(6):2085–2091.
297. Barlaskar FM, Hammer GD. The molecular genetics of adrenocortical carcinoma. Rev Endocr Metab Disord 2007;8(4):343–348.
298. Wagner J, Portwine C, Rabin K, et al. High frequency of germline p53 mutations in childhood adrenocortical cancer. J Natl Cancer Inst 1994;86(22):1707–1710.
299. Groussin L, Kirschner LS, Vincent-Dejean C, et al. Molecular analysis of the cyclic AMP-dependent protein kinase A (PKA) regulatory subunit 1A (PRKAR1A) gene in

patients with Carney complex and primary pigmented nodular adrenocortical disease (PPNAD) reveals novel mutations and clues for pathophysiology: augmented PKA signaling is associated with adrenal tumorigenesis in PPNAD. Am J Hum Genet 2002; 71(6):1433–1442.

300. Bauman A, Bauman CG. Virilizing adrenocortical carcinoma. Development in a patient with salt-losing congenital adrenal hyperplasia. JAMA 1982;248(23):3140–3141.

301. Figueiredo BC, Stratakis CA, Sandrini R, et al. Comparative genomic hybridization analysis of adrenocortical tumors of childhood. J Clin Endocrinol Metab 1999;84(3):1116–1121.

302. Almeida MQ, Fragoso MC, Lotfi CF, et al. Expression of insulin-like growth factor-II and its receptor in pediatric and adult adrenocortical tumors. J Clin Endocrinol Metab 2008;93(9):3524–3531.

303. Tucci S Jr, Martins AC, Suaid HJ, et al. The impact of tumor stage on prognosis in children with adrenocortical carcinoma. J Urol 2005;174(6):2338–2342, discussion 2342.

304. Ribeiro RC, Michalkiewicz EL, Figueiredo BC, et al. Adrenocortical tumors in children. Braz J Med Biol Res 2000;33(10):1225–1234.

305. Sturgeon C, Shen WT, Clark OH, et al. Risk assessment in 457 adrenal cortical carcinomas: how much does tumor size predict the likelihood of malignancy? J Am Coll Surg 2006;202(3):423–430.

306. Patalano A, Brancato V, Mantero F. Adrenocortical cancer treatment. Horm Res 2009;71(Suppl 1):99–104.

307. Godine LB, Berdon WE, Brasch RC, et al. Adrenocortical carcinoma with extension into inferior vena cava and right atrium: report of 3 cases in children. Pediatr Radiol 1990;20(3):166–168; discussion 169.

308. Ribeiro J, Ribeiro RC, Fletcher BD. Imaging findings in pediatric adrenocortical carcinoma. Pediatr Radiol 2000;30(1):45–51.

309. NIH state-of-the-science statement on management of the clinically inapparent adrenal mass ("incidentaloma"). NIH Consens State Sci Statements. 2002;19(2):1–23.

310. Young WF Jr. Clinical practice. The incidentally discovered adrenal mass. N Engl J Med 2007;356(6):601–610.

311. Masiakos PT, Gerstle JT, Cheang T, et al. Is surgery necessary for incidentally discovered adrenal masses in children? J Pediatr Surg 2004;39(5):754–758.

312. Fassnacht M, Johanssen S, Quinkler M, et al. Limited prognostic value of the 2004 International Union Against Cancer staging classification for adrenocortical carcinoma: proposal for a Revised TNM Classification. Cancer 2009;115(2):243–250.

313. Mazzaglia PJ, Monchik JM. Limited value of adrenal biopsy in the evaluation of adrenal neoplasm: a decade of experience. Arch Surg 2009;144(5):465–470.

314. Fassnacht M, Allolio B. Clinical management of adrenocortical carcinoma. Best Pract Res Clin Endocrinol Metab 2009;23(2):273–289.

315. Gonzalez RJ, Shapiro S, Sarlis N, et al. Laparoscopic resection of adrenal cortical carcinoma: a cautionary note. Surgery 2005;138(6):1078–1085; discussion 1085–1086.

316. Hahner S, Fassnacht M. Mitotane for adrenocortical carcinoma treatment. Curr Opin Investig Drugs 2005;6(4):386–394.

317. Allolio B, Fassnacht M. Clinical review: adrenocortical carcinoma: clinical update. J Clin Endocrinol Metab 2006;91(6):2027–2037.

318. Berruti A, Terzolo M, Sperone P, et al. Etoposide, doxorubicin and cisplatin plus mitotane in the treatment of advanced adrenocortical carcinoma: a large prospective phase II trial. Endocr Relat Cancer 2005;12(3):657–666.

319. Khan TS, Imam H, Juhlin C, et al. Streptozocin and o,p'DDD in the treatment of adrenocortical cancer patients: long-term survival in its adjuvant use. Ann Oncol 2000;11(10):1281–1287.

320. Baudin E, Pellegriti G, Bonnay M, et al. Impact of monitoring plasma 1,1-dichlorodiphenildichloroethane (o,p'DDD) levels on the treatment of patients with adrenocortical carcinoma. Cancer 2001;92(6):1385–1392.

321. Zancanella P, Pianovski MA, Oliveira BH, et al. Mitotane associated with cisplatin, etoposide, and doxorubicin in advanced childhood adrenocortical carcinoma: mitotane monitoring and tumor regression. J Pediatr Hematol Oncol 2006;28(8):513–524.

322. Fareau GG, Lopez A, Stava C, et al. Systemic chemotherapy for adrenocortical carcinoma: comparative responses to conventional first-line therapies. Anticancer Drugs 2008;19(6):637–644.

323. Berruti A, Ferrero A, Sperone P, et al. Emerging drugs for adrenocortical carcinoma. Expert Opin Emerg Drugs 2008;13(3):497–509.

324. Gross DJ, Munter G, Bitan M, et al. The role of imatinib mesylate (Glivec) for treatment of patients with malignant endocrine tumors positive for c-kit or PDGF-R. Endocr Relat Cancer 2006;13(2):535–540.

325. Quinkler M, Hahner S, Wortmann S, et al. Treatment of advanced adrenocortical carcinoma with erlotinib plus gemcitabine. J Clin Endocrinol Metab 2008;93(6):2057–2062.

326. Polat B, Fassnacht M, Pfreundner L, et al. Radiotherapy in adrenocortical carcinoma. Cancer 2009;115(13):2816–2823.

327. Wyszynska T, Cichocka E, Wieteska-Klimczak A, et al. A single pediatric center experience with 1025 children with hypertension. Acta Paediatr 1992;81(3):244–246.

328. Goodman MT, Gurney JG, Smith MA, et al. Sympathetic nervous system tumors. In: Ries LAG, Smith MA, Gurney JG, et al., eds. Cancer incidence and survival among children and adolescents: United States SEER Program 1975–1995. Bethesda, MD: National Cancer Institute, SEER Program, 1999:65–72. NIH Pub. No. 99-4649.

329. Barontini M, Levin G, Sanso G. Characteristics of pheochromocytoma in a 4- to 20-year-old population. Ann N Y Acad Sci 2006;1073:30–37.

330. Neumann HP, Bausch B, McWhinney SR, et al. Germ-line mutations in nonsyndromic pheochromocytoma. N Engl J Med 2002;346(19):1459–1466.

331. Beltsevich DG, Kuznetsov NS, Kazaryan AM, et al. Pheochromocytoma surgery: epidemiologic peculiarities in children. World J Surg 2004;28(6):592–596.

332. Ross JH. Pheochromocytoma. Special considerations in children. Urol Clin North Am Aug 2000;27(3):393–402.

333. Young WF Jr. Endocrine hypertension. In: Kronenberg HM, Melmed S, Polonsky KS, Larsen PR, eds. Williams Textbook of Endocrinology. 11 ed. Philadelphia, PA: Saunders Elsevier; 2008:505–537.

334. Tischler AS. Pheochromocytoma and extra-adrenal paraganglioma: updates. Arch Pathol Lab Med 2008;132(8):1272–1284.

335. Linnoila RI, Keiser HR, Steinberg SM, et al. Histopathology of benign versus malignant sympathoadrenal paragangliomas: clinicopathologic study of 120 cases including unusual histologic features. Hum Pathol 1990;21(11):1168–1180.

336. Armstrong R, Sridhar M, Greenhalgh KL, et al. Phaeochromocytoma in children. Arch Dis Child 2008;93(10):899–904.

337. Mannelli M, Castellano M, Schiavi F, et al. Clinically guided genetic screening in a large cohort of Italian patients with pheochromocytomas and/or functional or non-functional paragangliomas. J Clin Endocrinol Metab 2009;94(5):1541–1547.

338. Jimenez C, Cote G, Arnold A, et al. Review: should patients with apparently sporadic pheochromocytomas or paragangliomas be screened for hereditary syndromes? J Clin Endocrinol Metab 2006;91(8):2851–2858.

339. Koch CA, Mauro D, Walther MM, et al. Pheochromocytoma in von hippel-lindau disease: distinct histopathologic phenotype compared to pheochromocytoma in multiple endocrine neoplasia type 2. Endocr Pathol 2002;13(1):17–27.

340. Pham TH, Moir C, Thompson GB, et al. Pheochromocytoma and paraganglioma in children: a review of medical and surgical management at a tertiary care center. Pediatrics 2006;118(3):1109–1117.

341. Eisenhofer G, Bornstein SR, Brouwers FM, et al. Malignant pheochromocytoma: current status and initiatives for future progress. Endocr Relat Cancer 2004;11(3):423–436.

342. Januszewicz P, Wieteska-Klimczak A, et al. Pheochromocytoma in children: difficulties in diagnosis and localization. Clin Exp Hypertens A 1990;12(4):571–579.

343. Ein SH, Pullerits J, Creighton R, et al. Pediatric pheochromocytoma. A 36-year review. Pediatr Surg Int 1997;12(8):595–598.

344. Sullivan J, Groshong T, Tobias JD. Presenting signs and symptoms of pheochromocytoma in pediatric-aged patients. Clin Pediatr (Phila) 2005;44(8):715–719.

345. Walther MM, Reiter R, Keiser HR, et al. Clinical and genetic characterization of pheochromocytoma in von Hippel-Lindau families: comparison with sporadic pheochromocytoma gives insight into natural history of pheochromocytoma. J Urol 1999;162 (3 Pt 1):659–664.

346. Young WF Jr. Pheochromocytoma in Children. In: UpToDate, Basow DS (Ed), UpToDate, Waltham, MA, 2009.

347. Weise M, Merke DP, Pacak K, et al. Utility of plasma free metanephrines for detecting childhood pheochromocytoma. J Clin Endocrinol Metab 2002;87(5):1955–1960.

348. Pacak K, Eisenhofer G, Ahlman H, et al. Pheochromocytoma: recommendations for clinical practice from the First International Symposium. October 2005. Nat Clin Pract Endocrinol Metab 2007;3(2):92–102.

349. Eisenhofer G, Goldstein DS, Walther MM, et al. Biochemical diagnosis of pheochromocytoma: how to distinguish true- from false-positive test results. J Clin Endocrinol Metab 2003;88(6):2656–2666.

350. Bilek R, Safarik L, Ciprova V, et al. Chromogranin A, a member of neuroendocrine secretory proteins as a selective marker for laboratory diagnosis of pheochromocytoma. Physiol Res 2008;57(Suppl 1):S171–S179.

351. Algeciras-Schimnich A, Preissner CM, Young WF Jr, et al. Plasma chromogranin A or urine fractionated metanephrines follow-up testing improves the diagnostic accuracy of plasma fractionated metanephrines for pheochromocytoma. J Clin Endocrinol Metab 2008;93(1):91–95.

352. Grossrubatscher E, Dalino P, Vignati F, et al. The role of chromogranin A in the management of patients with phaeochromocytoma. Clin Endocrinol (Oxf) 2006;65(3):287–293.

353. Bravo EL, Tagle R. Pheochromocytoma: state-of-the-art and future prospects. Endocr Rev 2003;24(4):539–553.

354. Greenblatt DY, Shenker Y, Chen H. The utility of metaiodobenzylguanidine (MIBG) scintigraphy in patients with pheochromocytoma. Ann Surg Oncol 2008;15(3):900–905.

355. Lumachi F, Tregnaghi A, Zucchetta P, et al. Sensitivity and positive predictive value of CT, MRI and 123I-MIBG scintigraphy in localizing pheochromocytomas: a prospective study. Nucl Med Commun 2006;27(7):583–587.

356. Shulkin BL, Shapiro B. Current concepts on the diagnostic use of MIBG in children. J Nucl Med 1998;39(4):679–688.

357. Ilias I, Shulkin B, Pacak K. New functional imaging modalities for chromaffin tumors, neuroblastomas and ganglioneuromas. Trends Endocrinol Metab 2005;16 (2):66–72.

358. Walz MK, Alesina PF, Wenger FA, et al. Posterior retroperitoneoscopic adrenalectomy—results of 560 procedures in 520 patients. Surgery 2006;140(6):943–948; discussion 948–950.

359. Ludwig AD, Feig DI, Brandt ML, et al. Recent advances in the diagnosis and treatment of pheochromocytoma in children. Am J Surg 2007;194(6):792–796; discussion 796–797.

360. Yip L, Lee JE, Shapiro SE, et al. Surgical management of hereditary pheochromocytoma. J Am Coll Surg 2004;198(4):525–534; discussion 534–535.

361. Hack HA. The perioperative management of children with phaeochromocytoma. Paediatr Anaesth 2000;10(5):463–476.

362. Kocak S, Aydintug S, Canakci N. Alpha blockade in preoperative preparation of patients with pheochromocytomas. Int Surg 2002;87(3):191–194.

363. Lebuffe G, Dosseh ED, Tek G, et al. The effect of calcium channel blockers on outcome following the surgical treatment of phaeochromocytomas and paragangliomas. Anaesthesia 2005;60(5):439–444.

364. Perry RR, Keiser HR, Norton JA, et al. Surgical management of pheochromocytoma with the use of metyrosine. Ann Surg 1990;212(5):621–628.

365. Pacak K. Preoperative management of the pheochromocytoma patient. J Clin Endocrinol Metab 2007;92(11):4069–4079.

366. Scholz T, Eisenhofer G, Pacak K, et al. Clinical review: current treatment of malignant pheochromocytoma. J Clin Endocrinol Metab 2007;92(4):1217–1225.

367. Mukherjee JJ, Kaltsas GA, Islam N, et al. Treatment of metastatic carcinoid tumours, phaeochromocytoma, paraganglioma and medullary carcinoma of the thyroid with (131)I-meta-iodobenzylguanidine [(131)I-mIBG]. Clin Endocrinol (Oxf) 2001;55(1):47–60.

368. Loh KC, Fitzgerald PA, Matthay KK, et al. The treatment of malignant pheochromocytoma with iodine-131 metaiodobenzylguanidine (131I-MIBG): a comprehensive review of 116 reported patients. J Endocrinol Invest 1997;20(11):648–658.

369. Duet M, Guichard JP, Rizzo N, et al. Are somatostatin analogs therapeutic alternatives in the management of head and neck paragangliomas? Laryngoscope 2005;115(8):1381–1384.

370. Chrisoulidou A, Kaltsas G, Ilias I, et al. The diagnosis and management of malignant phaeochromocytoma and paraganglioma. Endocr Relat Cancer 2007;14(3):569–585.

371. Huang H, Abraham J, Hung E, et al. Treatment of malignant pheochromocytoma/paraganglioma with cyclophosphamide, vincristine, and dacarbazine: recommendation from a 22-year follow-up of 18 patients. Cancer 2008;113(8):2020–2028.

372. Jimenez C, Cabanillas ME, Santarpia L, et al. Use of the tyrosine kinase inhibitor sunitinib in a patient with von Hippel-Lindau disease: targeting angiogenic factors in pheochromocytoma and other von Hippel-Lindau disease-related tumors. J Clin Endocrinol Metab 2009;94(2):386–391.

CHAPTER 37 ■ MANAGEMENT OF INFREQUENT CANCERS OF CHILDHOOD

ALBERTO S. PAPPO, CARLOS RODRIGUEZ-GALINDO, AND WAYNE L. FURMAN

The preceding chapters have described in detail the diagnosis and management of the more common tumors of childhood. This chapter summarizes the clinical features and treatment of some of the less frequently encountered tumors in the pediatric population. A rare or infrequent childhood cancer is difficult to define given that pediatric cancer is a rare disease. Some authors have defined rare tumors as those that have an incidence of 2 or less per million and are not considered in other clinical trials.[1] However, the use of this definition would exclude some rare cancers such as melanoma and thyroid carcinoma that numerically exceed the numbers proposed by this definition (http://apps.nccd.cdc.gov/uscs/Table.aspx?Group= TableICCC&Year=2005&Display=n). Thus, in this chapter, we have opted to categorize rare tumors as those that are mostly of nonembryonal histology, which more commonly occur in adults but may be seen preferentially in the adolescent age group, and tumors for whom there has been no organized effort to study them within the context of a national cooperative group setting.

Some information about the staging of these tumors is required by the pediatric oncologist, who should confer with surgeons and pathologists to obtain information for patients, parents, and radiation oncologists. Reference to the sixth edition of the *American Joint Committee on Cancer (AJCC) Staging Handbook*[2] is required for tumors such as gastric, colon, renal cell, pancreatic, and nasopharyngeal carcinomas, as well as for melanoma. To facilitate access to information on pediatric rare tumors, the Children's Oncology Group is developing a Web-based rare tumor protocol and registry. This protocol will serve as an invaluable resource for clinical investigators involved in the care of pediatric patients with rare cancers. In this trial, biological samples and limited clinical information on selected rare cancers will be collected prospectively and, in addition, investigators will be able to access on line comprehensive literature reviews of selected rare cancers. A similar initiative called the Italian Study on Rare Tumors in Pediatric Age (TREP) project[1] has also been developed in Italy for rare tumors in the pediatric age group.

This chapter summarizes the infrequent cancers of childhood in descending anatomic order, from the nasopharynx through the trunk and skin.

OROPHARYNGEAL CANCER

The majority of oral lesions in children and adolescents are benign.[3–6] Oropharyngeal cancer is extremely rare in the pediatric age group; of the 35,000 cases diagnosed annually in the United States, only 0.6% affect children younger than 20 years (http://www.seer.cancer.gov/statfacts/html/oralcav. html). These tumors are extremely challenging to pediatric oncologists, surgeons, and radiotherapists. The most common of these cancers is nasopharyngeal carcinoma, which is discussed separately.

The risk factors for the development of oral and pharyngeal cancer include the use of any tobacco products, heavy alcohol use, certain viral infections such as human papillomavirus (HPV), low consumption of fruits and vegetables, marijuana use, older age, black race, and male sex.[7] It has been well documented that the use of smokeless tobacco and cigarette smoking increase the risk of oropharyngeal cancer as well as that of potentially malignant oral lesions such as leukoplakia, erythroplakia, palatal lesion of reverse cigar smoking, oral lichen planus, and submucosal fibrosis.[8] The Global Youth Tobacco Survey[9] estimates that about 17% of students aged between 13 and 15 years use tobacco products. The highest use was documented in America (22%) and the lowest in the Western Pacific and Southeast Asian regions. Boys were more likely than girls to use tobacco products in the Mediterranean, Southeast Asia, and Western Pacific regions. In this survey, about 9% of the population surveyed were current smokers and the highest rates were seen in the American and European regions. About 11% of the population surveyed used tobacco products other than cigarettes, with the highest rates being in Southeast Asia and Eastern Mediterranean areas. Among nonsmokers, 18% stated that they were susceptible to smoking within the coming year and over half of them had been exposed to second-hand smoke within the week preceding the survey. The consequences of using tobacco products in childhood are enormous and efforts to ameliorate the projected harm that will be caused by tobacco use needs to be urgently and aggressively addressed by developing comprehensive tobacco prevention and control programs.[9] Although tobacco cigarette use among high school students has decreased from the period of 1997 to 2003, the rates have remained stable from 2003 to 2007(http://www.cdc. gov/mmwr/preview/mmwrhtml/mm5725a3.htm).

Oral HPV infection is strongly associated with the number of recent oral sex partners or open-mouthed kissing partners,[10] and oral HPV infection is unequivocally associated with oropharyngeal cancer regardless of the use of tobacco or alcohol. The incidence of HPV-associated oropharyngeal cancer has significantly increased since 1973 particularly among white males aged 40 to 59 years.[11] Approximately 20% to 25% cases of head and neck cancer contain oncogenic HPV, mostly types 16, 31, and 33. In a study of 1,235 children, the prevalence of HPV in the oral cavity was 1.9% and the highest rates were seen in patients younger than 1 year and in those aged between 16 and 20 years.[12] HPV-associated oral cancers tend to occur in younger patients of high socioeconomic status, are associated with sexual behavior, more often involve the lingual and palatine tonsils, frequently have poorly differentiated basaloid features, express p16, and have a better prognosis and response to radiotherapy than other head and neck carcinomas.[11,13,14] Current preventive strategies using vaccine programs targeting the adolescent population may prove beneficial in decreasing the incidence of cervical and head and neck HPV-associated cancers.[15]

Other important predisposing conditions that should be considered when facing the diagnosis of oropharyngeal cancer in a pediatric patient include the following:

1. Recessive dystrophic epidermolysis bullosae[16]
2. Xeroderma pigmentosum[17]
3. Fanconi's anemia[18]
4. Mutations in the connexin 26 gene [Keratitis-ichthyosis-deafness (KID) syndrome][19]
5. Dyskeratosis congenita[20]

These tumors are treated using a multidisciplinary approach that often incorporate surgery, radiotherapy, and chemotherapy. In a recent randomized trial, the addition of docetaxel to cisplatin and 5-fluorouracil (5-FU) improved the survival and progression-free survival of adults with advanced stage head and neck squamous cell carcinoma.[21]

AERODIGESTIVE-TRACT CARCINOMAS ASSOCIATED WITH THE TRANSLOCATION (15;19) (MIDLINE CARCINOMAS WITH NUT REARRANGEMENTS)

These rare, highly aggressive, and lethal carcinomas account for 7% of poorly differentiated carcinomas of the aerodigestive tract in patients younger than 40 years.[22] These tumors are presumed to arise from the neural crest and are characterized by rearrangements of the NUT gene. About two-third of the cases have a t(15;19) that fuses the BRD4 gene in chromosome 19 with nearly the entire transcript of the NUT gene at chromosome band 15q13.[23] The BRD4-NUT transcript associates with chromatin and interferes with epithelial differentiation. It is estimated that up to 20% of undifferentiated carcinomas of the upper aerodigestive tract that are not caused by Epstein-Barr virus (EBV) will have NUT rearrangements.[24] About half of these tumors occur in patients younger than 20 years, and most arise in the midline of the aerodigestive tract or mediastinum and often involve the nasal cavity, sinuses, nasopharynx, mediastinum, orbit, lung, larynx, and occasionally the bladder.[24] Definitive diagnosis is made by demonstration of NUT rearrangements; however, this entity should be considered in the differential diagnosis of patients with EBV-negative poorly differentiated monomorphic midline neoplasms.[22] All but one of 22 reported cases have died at an average of 9 months from diagnosis.[24] Some authors have used a Ewing's-type regimen for the treatment of selected patients but results have been poor.[22]

NASOPHARYNGEAL CARCINOMA

Nasopharyngeal carcinoma, or lymphoepithelioma, is extremely rare in pediatric patients; only about 3% of all nasopharyngeal carcinomas occur in patients younger than 19 years.[25] This tumor accounts for less than 1% of all pediatric cancers but is responsible for 20% to 50% of all nasopharyngeal malignancies in children.[26,27]

Epidemiology

The incidence of nasopharyngeal carcinoma is highest in the south of China, southeast Asia, the Mediterranean basin, and Alaska, where the annual incidence is as high as 80 per 100,000 individuals.[25] In contrast, in the United States, the incidence is only approximately 1 case per 100,000 individuals per year. The tumor is more prevalent in the southern United States and in African American children.[25] The geographical and ethnic variation in the incidence of the disease strongly suggest that genetic and environmental factors play a role in its pathogenesis. In the Western hemisphere, the tumor is most commonly histologic type I (see later), occurs in a sporadic fashion, and is associated with behavioral risk factors such as alcohol and tobacco use.[25] The endemic form of the disease is associated with histologic types II and III (see later), is more common in southeast Asia and the Mediterranean basin, and is usually associated with environmental and genetic factors.[25] Consumption of salted cured fish and meat, which release volatile nitrosamines when cooked, has been associated with nasopharyngeal carcinoma in some ethnic groups.[25] An increased incidence of nasopharyngeal carcinoma has also been documented in patients with specific human leukocyte antigen (HLA) alleles such as HLA2 and HLABsin2, and AW19, BW46, and B17 haplotypes.[25,28] EBV infection has long been known to play an etiologic role, because high immunoglobulin G (IgG) and immunoglobulin G (IgA) titers against EBV early antigen or viral capsid antigens were observed in patients with nasopharyngeal carcinoma.[29] The full-length EBV genome is contained in all of the malignant epithelial cells but not in most infiltrating lymphocytes and the presence of the EBV DNA in the form of episomes suggests that the virus is present in the cell at the time of oncogenic transformation.[25,28,30] Nasopharyngeal carcinoma cells consistently express various EBV genes, including the EBV nuclear antigen 1 (EBNA1), the latent membrane protein I (LMP1), and EBV-encoded RNA 1 and 2 (EBERs 1 and 2).[25,31-33]

Pathology

The World Health Organization recognizes three types of nasopharyngeal carcinoma: Type I is the keratinizing squamous cell carcinoma that is usually associated with alcohol and tobacco use but can be associated with EBV infection in endemic areas. Type II is the nonkeratinizing epidermoid type, and type III, also referred to as lymphoepithelioma, is an undifferentiated carcinoma. Virtually all cases of pediatric nasopharyngeal carcinoma are of the histologic type III.[28]

Clinical Presentation

The median age at diagnosis is 13 years, and males and African Americans are more commonly affected.[28] In most cases, nasopharyngeal carcinoma arises from the fossa of Rosenmuller and presents as a painless mass in the upper neck. Palpable cervical lymphadenopathy is often found. Local tumor infiltration (Fig. 37.1) can cause hearing difficulties, serous otitis, tinnitus, nasal obstruction, epistaxis, and dysphasia. Involvement of cranial nerve XII can cause dysphonia, and involvement of cranial nerve VI can cause diplopia. Other symptoms may include loss of vision, dysphagia, taste disorders, and shoulder looseness. The median duration of symptoms is approximately 5 months. Metastases may be present in lung, bone, mediastinum, bone marrow, and visceral organs. Paraneoplastic syndromes such as hypertrophic osteoarthropathy, dermatomyositis, and syndrome of inappropriate antidiuretic hormone have all been described with widespread disease or relapse.[28,34,35]

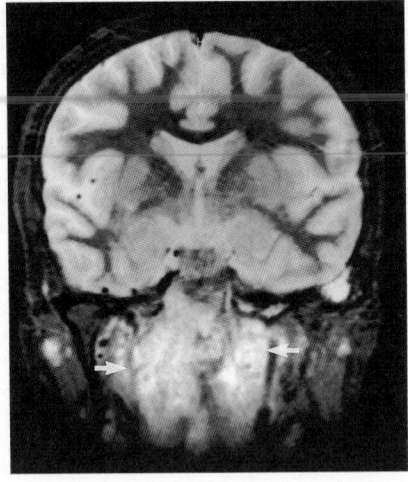
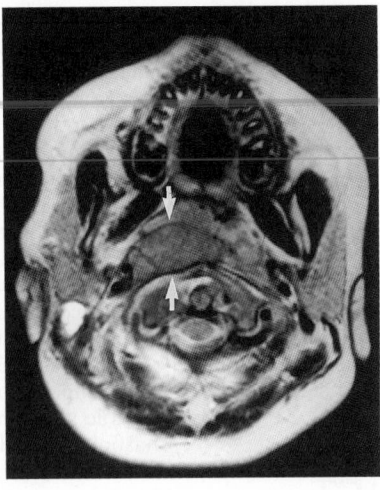

FIGURE 37.1 Coronal short inversion time inversion recovery (STIR) (**A**) and transverse T2-weighted (**B**) magnetic resonance images of nasopharyngeal carcinoma in a 12-year-old boy. The images demonstrate a large nasopharyngeal tumor (*arrows*) but do not show tumor extension to the dura, which was found on other views.

Differential Diagnosis

Differential diagnosis includes other malignancies that may present with primary or secondary tumors in the nasopharynx. Rhabdomyosarcoma and non-Hodgkin lymphoma are the most frequent malignant tumors, whereas angiofibroma is the most common benign tumor.[36] Less common malignancies that should be considered in the differential diagnosis include esthesioneuroblastoma and midline carcinoma with *NUT* rearrangements (see earlier). Thyroid carcinoma can also present with significant cervical adenopathy.

Staging and Prognosis

The extent of the tumor at diagnosis is described by the Tumor, Node, Metastasis (TNM) classification of the AJCC.[2] The majority of children with nasopharyngeal carcinoma present with advanced-stage disease (stage III or IV).[28] Serologic evidence of EBV infection is seen in most cases, usually revealing increases in both IgG and IgA antibodies against viral capsid antigen and early antigen. Anti-ZEBRA (replication activator protein) antibodies have also been detected in as many as 75% of patients with antibodies to EBV capsid antigen. Polymerase chain reaction can detect the viral DNA *in situ*. Circulating EBV DNA levels have been successfully used to screen, assess response, and predict disease recurrence in patients with nasopharyngeal carcinoma.[37] The presence of cell-free circulating hypermethylated gene promoter DNA has recently been described as a useful tool to screen for the disease and monitor for relapse.[38] Imaging is essential for accurate determination of the extent of disease. Magnetic resonance imaging (MRI) is most commonly used to determine this. Other recommended studies in the workup of patients with nasopharyngeal carcinoma include computed tomography (CT) of the chest, bone scan, and liver ultrasonography. Cytologic analysis of the spinal fluid is appropriate for patients who present with advanced stage disease or who have erosion of the skull base.

In children, just as in adults, the TNM stage at the time of diagnosis correlate with clinical outcome.[28,39] However, with more advanced diagnostic and staging techniques and improved treatments, while the presence of distant metastases continues to be associated with adverse outcome, T and N staging have lost prognostic significance.[40–43]

Treatment

Radiotherapy remains the mainstay of therapy for nasopharyngeal carcinoma. Patients with T1 and T2 lesions (tumors confined to nasopharynx or extension into the parapharyngeal spaces) can be adequately treated with radiation alone (doses of 65 to 70 Gy administered as 1.8- to 2.0-Gy daily fractions 5 days a week). Involved areas are rarely accessible for resection, and therefore the volume of radiation should include the nares, pharynx, posterior nasal cavity, posterior maxillary sinus, posterior ethmoid sinus, sphenoid sinus, base of skull, cervical lymphatics, and supraclavicular nodes.[28,44–47] Conformal intensity-modulated radiotherapy has recently gained popularity and may improve local control in children while limiting the side effects.[44–47]

Nasopharyngeal carcinoma is a very chemosensitive neoplasm. In order to improve outcome for children with advanced-stage disease, studies have investigated the use of neoadjuvant chemotherapy followed by local radiotherapy in small numbers of children with nasopharyngeal carcinoma. The most commonly used agents include cisplatin, methotrexate, leucovorin, and 5-FU. In a study at St. Jude Children's Research Hospital, 20 of 21 patients with advanced-stage disease were long-term survivors after receiving four preirradiation courses of these agents followed by radiotherapy. A subsequent study by the Pediatric Oncology Group used the same regimen to treat 17 patients and obtained a 4-year event-free survival estimate of 77%.[41] A multicenter German trial used a similar preradiation regimen of cisplatin, methotrexate, and 5-FU followed by radiation therapy and interferon beta for 6 months in a group of 59 children with nasopharyngeal carcinoma; 58 patients achieved a complete response, and the 4-year disease-free survival was 91%.[42] The role of chemotherapy in nasopharyngeal carcinoma continues to evolve, particularly with the use of concomitant chemoradiotherapy. Randomized studies performed in adults have demonstrated a benefit for the use of concomitant chemoradiation, and this approach is currently considered the standard of care. In a meta-analysis of 10 studies including 2,450 patients, and which randomized patients to conventional radiation therapy versus concomitant, neoadjuvant, or adjuvant chemotherapy, a significant survival advantage to the use of concomitant chemotherapy was found.[48] This advantage was the result of better locoregional and systemic control. The administration of neoadjuvant chemotherapy was also associated with better locoregional and systemic control, although its impact on outcome was less relevant. The use of neoadjuvant chemotherapy may be particularly relevant in children, as it may allow for the use of lower doses of radiation for patients with good responses. Using this tailored approach, radiation doses of 55 to 60 Gy to the primary tumor and 40 to 45 Gy to the neck may provide excellent disease control rates.[42,43] With the incorporation of concomitant chemoradiation, it is possible that lower radiation doses may be required. This is the approach currently followed by the Children's Oncology Group in the ARAR0331 protocol, where patients receive induction chemotherapy with cisplatin and 5-FU, followed by concurrent chemoradiation with cisplatin alone and three-dimensional conformal or intensity-modulated radiotherapy. Studies in adults have suggested that the incorporation of taxanes into the standard platinum-based regimens may result in improved outcome[49]; studies in pediatrics are currently ongoing. Finally, EBV-targeted cell therapy with autologous virus-specific cytotoxic T lymphocytes offers a very promising treatment for patients with recurrent disease.[50,51]

Side Effects of Treatment

Treatment of nasopharyngeal carcinoma can be associated with significant acute and long-term toxicity. The most common acute side effects of radiotherapy are mucositis, dermatitis, and xerostomia.[28,52] Studies in adults have shown that the administration of amifostine may reduce the incidence of radiation-induced xerostomia.[52] Late toxic effects related to radiation therapy to the head and neck area are relatively frequent and include hyposialosis, trismus, and dental complications. Late endocrine effects such as hypopituitarism and primary hypothyroidism are also very frequent among long-term survivors. Hearing loss, secondary malignancies, neck fibrosis, and encephalopathy have also been reported.[25]

AMELOBLASTOMA AND AMELOBLASTIC CARCINOMA

Ameloblastoma is an unusual locally aggressive odontogenic tumor that accounts for about 10% of all mandibular and maxillary neoplasms.[53] Ameloblastomas arise from the primitive dental lamina or from odontogenic cysts. About 10% to 20% of ameloblastomas occur in patients younger than 20 years, and the median age at presentation is 14 years.[54] The disease appears to be more prevalent in African and Asian children.[54] Ameloblastomas may be centrally or peripherally located. Central ameloblastomas arise in the jaw and can be further classified as multicystic/solid and unicystic. Multicystic/solid variants have a higher rate of recurrence. Peripheral ameloblastomas arise in the gingival area and do not involve bone.[53] In African children, there is a predominance of males, the disease often involves the mandible, and there is a higher incidence of the solid/multicystic subtype. In contrast, in children of Western origin, female sex predominates, and the disease is more often unicystic and involves the angle of the mandible.[54] Clinical symptoms at presentation include facial swelling, the presence of a submucosal mass, malocclusion, paresthesias, pain, and evidence of unerupted teeth in the affected area.[6,53] Analysis of small numbers of tumors suggest that p53, MDM2, and p14 may be responsible for tissue structuring and cytodifferentiation in ameloblastoma.[55] In addition, recent reports have documented the existence of a complex interaction that favors tumor formation and is mediated by the secretion of frizzled-related peptide (sFRP2), which impairs bone formation, as well as IL-6 and RANKL, which promote bone resorption.[56,57] Solid and multicystic ameloblastomas should be treated by surgical resection that includes a 1-cm margin of normal bone and soft tissue.[53,58] Unicystic ameloblastomas can be treated with simple enucleation followed by curettage and physicochemical therapy with either liquid nitrogen or Carnoy's solution.[58] Radiotherapy may be considered for patients with positive margins.[53] Local excision is sufficient for peripheral ameloblastomas. Malignant ameloblastomas have been reported. They often affect the mandible and can metastasize to lung and lymph nodes.[53] One case of metastatic disease has been reported to respond to chemotherapy with carboplatin and paclitaxel.[59]

Ameloblastic carcinoma is a rare odontogenic malignancy with features of ameloblastoma and cytologic atypia. In a series of 66 patients, only 9 were younger than 20 years. The tumor most often affects the mandible and can metastasize to bone, lung, and brain.[60] Recommended therapy includes surgical excision with a 2- to 3-cm bony margin. Lymph node dissection should be performed in the presence of palpable adenopathy. Chemotherapy with cisplatin, doxorubicin, and cyclophosphamide has been used in the presence of pulmonary metastatic disease. About 30% of patients are expected to die from their disease within 5 years from initial diagnosis.[60]

SALIVARY GLAND TUMORS

The diagnosis and management of salivary gland tumors is complicated by their diverse nature and relative infrequency.[61,62] Less than 5% of all salivary gland tumors occur in children, and most occur during the second decade of life.[63] Most of these neoplasms originate in the parotid gland, with 10% to 15% arising from submandibular, sublingual, or minor salivary glands.[64-67] These lesions may be primary or may be secondary to previous radiation therapy.[68-70] Approximately 75% of primary salivary gland tumors are benign, most commonly pleomorphic adenoma.[64,66,67] Among the cancerous lesions in children, mucoepidermoid carcinoma is the most common, followed in frequency by adenoid-cystic carcinoma, acinic cell carcinoma, undifferentiated carcinoma, and adenocarcinoma.[65,71,72] Most cases of mucoepidermoid carcinoma in children are low-grade and the differential diagnosis must include such tumors as hemangioma, mixed tumor, sarcomas, and other benign lesions.[66,67] The AJCC[2] system is used to assess the extent of disease and although distant metastases are very rare, nodal disease may occur in up to 50% of patients with high-grade tumors and advanced disease.[69] Surgical removal is the treatment of choice when feasible.[67,73,74] For pleomorphic adenomas, a lateral parotidectomy with en-bloc excision of the tumor within the surrounding tissues, preserving facial nerve integrity, is usually indicated; local recurrences in such cases are rare. For malignant tumors, more aggressive surgical approaches are required.[64] Adenoid-cystic carcinomas have a tendency for perivascular and perineural infiltration and are thus associated with a worse prognosis. Radiation therapy should be considered for lesions that may not be completely resected.[75] Cisplatin-based chemotherapy is usually reserved for palliation of disease not amenable to either surgery or irradiation or for distant metastatic disease.[73] Karyotypic abnormalities in mucoepidermoid carcinoma,[76] as well as association with EBV in other salivary gland tumors, have been reported.[77] In mucoepidermoid carcinoma, the translocation (11;19) fuses the MECT1 and MERML 1 genes and this fusion transcript appears to disrupt *notch* signaling.[78] The prognosis of patients with these tumors depends on the extent of disease and the success of surgical resection.

Salivary gland tumors in neonates, often called *sialoblastoma*, are even rarer.[63,79] These are distinct histologic entities with primitive embryonic histologic features of salivary gland tissue. Other names for these tumors include embryomas and adenoid cystic carcinomas. These tumors have a propensity for local recurrence if incompletely excised, but they do not metastasize.

LARYNGEAL CANCER

Carcinoma of the larynx is usually associated with high-risk behaviors such as smoking. This cancer is extremely rare in children, with fewer than 80 cases reported in the literature.[80,81] Approximately one-third of children with recurrent respiratory papillomatosis develop laryngeal cancer.[80,82-84] More than half of these patients had previously received radiation therapy. Recurrent respiratory papillomatosis, which is caused by HPV types 6 and 11, is the most common benign neoplasm of the larynx among children and the second most frequent cause of childhood hoarseness. After changes in voice, stridor is the second most common symptom, first inspiratory and then biphasic.[85] Infection in children has been associated with vertical transmission during vaginal delivery from an infected mother. Younger age at diagnosis is associated with more aggressive disease and the need for more frequent surgical procedures to decrease the airway burden. The disease can spread to the tracheobronchial tree in as many as 17% of cases.[86] Laser excision is the most commonly used treatment for papillomas. Other therapies have included interferon, acyclovir, retinoic acid, and cidofivir.[85-88]

Children with laryngeal cancer often present with dysphagia, dysphonia, stridor, and upper airway obstruction. Guidelines established for the treatment of laryngeal carcinoma in adults should be used for children or adolescents. T1 and T2 tumors (limited to one subsite of supraglottis with normal cord mobility or invasion of mucosa with one adjacent subsite) can usually be controlled with surgery or radiation therapy. Locally advanced disease can be treated with concurrent cisplatin and irradiation with excellent locoregional control and rates of laryngeal preservation.[89] Rehabilitative efforts should begin with preoperative counseling. An electronic speech device may be used immediately after surgery; approximately 10% of patients develop satisfactory esophageal speech. The electrolarynx transmits sounds from the neck or mouth, with speech from the neck being more easily understood than oral speech. The American Cancer Society offers rehabilitation services for pediatric patients, including information, support, and social outlets, patterned after those used for adults. Long-term attention should be directed toward thyroid size and function for survivors who have received radiation therapy.

LUNG CANCER

Primary lung cancers are extremely rare in childhood[90-92] and almost never (0.07%) diagnosed before the age of 30, according to a report from the Surveillance, Epidemiology, and End Results (SEER) database.[93] Among these rare tumors, most pediatric cases of bronchogenic carcinoma are undifferentiated or adenocarcinoma[91,94,95]; squamous cell carcinomas also have been reported.[96] Primary lung cancers may occur in children of any age, but they are more usually found during adolescence. These tumors may be associated with papillomato-

sis,[97] and patients with recurrent respiratory papillomatosis are at risk of developing lung involvement with lung cancer.[98] Most cases are symptomatic, with cough, recurrent pneumonia, or hemoptysis and frequently present with mediastinal and distant metastases.[94,95] Childhood bronchogenic carcinoma should be managed according to reasonable adult guidelines, with resection of operable tumors.[99] Radiation therapy and chemotherapy may be of some benefit to patients with unresectable tumors.[100]

PLEUROPULMONARY BLASTOMA

Pleuropulmonary blastoma is a rare dysontogenetic tumor of childhood that can present as a pleural or pulmonary mass.[101] Histologically, pleuropulmonary blastoma of childhood differs from adult pulmonary blastoma because of its primitive and embryonic stroma, absence of a carcinomatous component, and potential for sarcomatous differentiation.[102] Dehner and colleagues have defined three subtypes of pleuropulmonary blastoma of childhood: type I is exclusively cystic, type II exhibits both cystic and solid components (Fig. 37.2), and type III is a solid tumor without cystic spaces lined by epithelium.[101] Patients with type I tumors appear to have a better probability of survival; however, transition from type I to type III is possible.[103] The early form of the disease, cystic type I, can be clinically and pathologically deceptive because of its resemblance to some developmental lung cysts. Type I pleuropulmonary blastoma is a delicate multilocular cyst with variable numbers of primitive mesenchymal cells beneath a benign epithelial surface. Rhabdomyoblasts and cartilage nodules are seen in 40% to 50% of cases. Tumors in the youngest subset of patients, from birth to 2 months of age, are more uniform in composition and cellularity compared with those in older groups and have a subtle transition between normal developing lung and tumor.[104] The histologic origin of this malignancy is uncertain, but it is thought to be an expression of the somatopleural mesoderm or the thoracic splanchnopleura. Recurrent chromosomal abnormalities, including trisomy of chromosomes 8 and 2, have been reported in a few cases and have been confirmed by comparative genomic hybridisation (CGH), suggesting that a relevant gene may be located in these regions.[105,106] Mutations of *p53* and *MYCN* amplification have also been reported in a few cases.[107] Patients with the former alteration appear to have a poor prognosis, raising the possibility that inactivation of *p53*

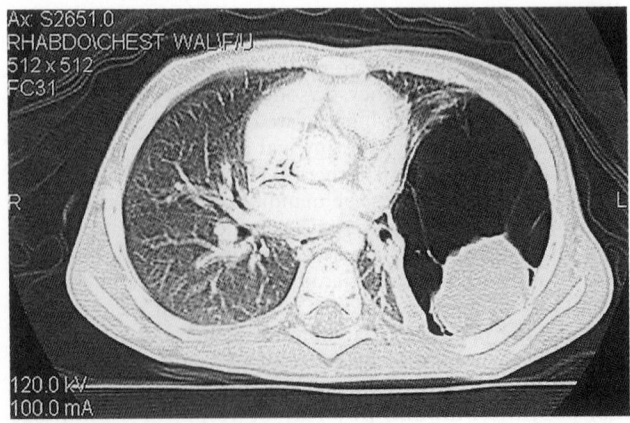

FIGURE 37.2 Axial computed tomography image of the chest of a 3-year-old child with a type II pleuropulmonary blastoma showing a round hyperdense tumor arising within a septate cystic lesion that involves the upper and lower lobes of the left lung.

could be a valuable predictor of outcome in these patients.[107] Nineteen of 82 patients registered in the pleuropulmonary blastoma registry (23%) have a constitutional or familial association with other neoplasias or dysplasias.[108] The most relevant is the association with cystic nephroma and other renal tumors; up to 9% of pleuropulmonary blastoma cases have been reported to develop cystic nephroma or Wilms' tumor, malignancies that are also more prevalent among family members.[109] Other neoplastic conditions reported in family members of patients with pleuropulmonary blastoma include germ cell and brain tumors, lymphoma, leukemia, sarcomas, histiocytosis, thyroid tumors, neuroblastoma, and Sertoli-Leydig tumor.[108] Recently, Hill and collaborators have identified heterozygous germ-line mutations of the gene DICER1, an endonuclease that participates in the generation of small RNAs, in familial cases of pleuropulmonary blastoma.[110] The median age at presentation of pleuropulmonary blastoma is 34 months, but those with type I tumors present at a younger age (10 months).[101] Presenting symptoms are not specific and commonly include respiratory distress, fever, chest or abdominal pain, pulmonary infections, pneumothorax, cough, anorexia, and malaise; 60% of the lesions are right-sided. Therapy includes surgical resection with lobectomy or pneumonectomy and chemotherapy and radiotherapy.[111] While a complete surgical resection is the most important prognostic factor, surgery alone even for type I lesions results in high relapse rates, usually as a type II or III tumor, suggesting that even patients with type I lesions should receive adjuvant chemotherapy.[105] Chemotherapy with sarcoma-targeted agents such as vincristine, dactinomycin, cyclophosphamide, ifosfamide, doxorubicin, and cisplatin has been used in the preoperative and adjuvant settings with mixed results.[111] The use of radiotherapy is controversial. Patients with type II and III pleuropulmonary blastomas have an increased risk for the development of brain metastasis, with a 5-year cumulative probability of 11% and 54%, respectively,[112] emphasizing the need for regular screening of this site in these patients. Detailed suggested guidelines for diagnosis and treatment can be found at www.ppbregistry.org. The overall prognosis is poor: half of all patients treated die within 2 years after diagnosis.[111,113] Patients with mediastinal or pleural involvement have a significantly poorer clinical outcome. Recurrence is usually local or involves the brain and the skeletal system.[113]

THYMOMA

Forty-three percent of mediastinal tumors in pediatric patients and 54% of mediastinal tumors in adult patients occur in the anterior mediastinum. Primary malignant lesions involving the anterior mediastinum include lymphomas, germ cell tumors, carcinoid tumors, carcinomas, thymolipomas, cysts, metastatic tumors, and thymoma, most of which are similar in their gross and microscopic appearance. Nearly half of all primary anterior mediastinal tumors in adults are thymoma, an epithelial malignancy arising from the thymus gland.[114] the epithelial cell is the cell of origin of thymomas and thymic carcinomas, whereas the lymphocytic component is considered benign.[115]

EPIDEMIOLOGY AND SYMPTOMATOLOGY

Less than 10% of thymomas occur in patients younger than 20 years, and less than 15% of the anterior mediastinal masses in this age group are thymomas; only about 30 cases

have been described in the medical literature.[116,117] Thymomas usually present in the fourth and fifth decades of life and have no clear sex predominance. At the time of initial diagnosis, the tumor is asymptomatic in nearly half of all adult patients and is discovered incidentally during imaging studies of the chest.[118] One-third of adult patients present with various symptoms, including cough, chest pain, hoarseness, superior vena cava syndrome, and dysphagia. Most patients with thymoma have one or more paraneoplastic disorders during their lifetime.[119,120] The most common associated disorder is myasthenia gravis, which occurs in approximately 30% of patients with thymoma.[118] This disorder has also been reported in children and is important to recognize prior to thoracotomy.[121] Ten percent to 15% of adult patients with myasthenia gravis have an underlying thymoma.[120] Various other paraneoplastic syndromes have been found to be associated with thymoma. These include pure red cell aplasia, hypogammaglobulinemia, nephrotic syndrome,[122] and autoimmune or immune disorders such as scleroderma, dermatomyositis, systemic lupus erythematosus, rheumatoid arthritis, and thyroiditis.[118] Endocrine disorders associated with thymoma include hyperthyroidism, Addison's disease, and panhypopituitarism.[119,123,124] Associated disorders are so common in patients with thymoma that lifelong surveillance for these disorders has been suggested in patients who have undergone therapy for thymoma.[119]

Pathology and Staging

Thymomas are generally located anterior to the great vessels of the mediastinum, which may be displaced posteriorly by the tumor. The masses are usually round with smooth or lobulated margins and may protrude to one or both sides of the mediastinum. Calcifications may be seen. The nomenclature for use in the pathologic classification of thymic neoplasms is still evolving. Thymomas can be subdivided into three main histologic categories: predominantly lymphocytic, mixed lymphoepithelial, and predominantly epithelial. The epithelial cell is well established as the malignant component of thymomas, and a predominance of these cells is associated with a greater risk of invasion and a poor clinical outcome.[120] A prominent organoid histologic pattern has been reported in pediatric thymomas.[125] However, the invasiveness of the tumor rather than the histologic architecture predicts clinical outcome.

Thymomas generally are slow-growing tumors and metastases at diagnosis are uncommon, with the pleura being the most frequent metastatic site.[126] Although almost all are potentially invasive, metastasis to distant organs or regional lymph nodes is rare. Involved organs have reportedly included bone, liver, kidney, brain, spleen, adrenal, thyroid and colon. Appropriate evaluation of patients with suspected thymoma or suspected other mediastinal tumors includes radiographic and CT examination of the chest. MRI can distinguish vascular structures from tumor but does not offer a clear advantage over CT. The differential diagnosis of other anterior mediastinal masses includes Hodgkin disease and non-Hodgkin lymphoma, thymolipoma, carcinoid tumors, germ cell tumors (e.g., primary germinoma, nonseminomatous and mixed germ cell tumors), and thymic carcinomas. In the Mississippi Valley, histoplasmosis should be included in the differential diagnosis of mediastinal tumors.

The staging system devised by Masaoka and colleagues[127] has been widely adopted.[126] This postsurgical staging system classifies thymomas as either noninvasive (stage I) or invasive (stages II to IV). Invasive thymomas can be further subclassified as minimally invasive (stage II), extensively invasive (III), or metastatic (IV). Prognosis is highly dependent on clinical stage. Five-year survival rates for patients with stage I tumors range from 83% to 100%, whereas only 46% to 70% of patients with stage III or IV tumors survive 5 years.[118,126]

Treatment

Surgery is the preferred modality for staging and treatment of thymoma. The surgical incision of choice is a median sternotomy.[126] This approach allows adequate visual assessment of the mediastinal structures and minimizes pain. An attempt should be made to resect all disease. Thymomas are usually staged at the time of initial surgical exploration, because invasive disease is found at this time in 30% of patients.[128,129] The intrathoracic failure rate is less than 5% after complete surgical excision of encapsulated tumors[118]; thus, adjuvant radiotherapy does not appear to offer a therapeutic advantage for these patients. Because thymomas are relatively radiosensitive, radiation therapy is recommended for patients with invasive disease regardless of the extent of surgical resection.[130] Among 21 patients with completely resected invasive disease who were treated with surgery alone, 38% had local tumor recurrence[131] compared with 0% to 5% when radiation therapy is added. Radiation dosage recommendations are based on the age of the child and the extent of tumor invasion. Total doses of 35 to 45 Gy delivered over 3 to 6 weeks are recommended for control of incompletely resected thymomas, although doses greater than 60 Gy have been advocated for patients with bulky residual disease.[118,130]

Chemotherapy is generally reserved for patients with advanced-stage disease that has not responded to irradiation or corticosteroid therapy. Doxorubicin and cisplatin are recognized as effective agents for the treatment of this tumor, although responses have been reported with alkylating agents as well.[126] The combination of cisplatin and etoposide has also proved active against metastatic or recurrent disease.[132] The addition of ifosfamide to this regimen has produced similar results (50% response rate). Taxol and carboplatin have been successful in selected cases of recurrent disease.[133] Preliminary results of a combined-modality therapy trial using cisplatin, doxorubicin, cyclophosphamide, vincristine, and radiotherapy have shown a 77% response rate in patients with advanced-stage disease.[129]

Because thymomas show high uptake of indium-labeled octreotide, trials using this somatostatin analogue have been recently conducted in patients with refractory disease. A durable complete remission has been obtained with high-dose octreotide and prednisone in a patient with pure red cell aplasia and heavily pretreated thymoma.[134] This combination was evaluated in an Eastern Cooperative Oncology Group Phase II trial in 42 patients; four patients had partial responses to octreotide alone and an additional eight patients responded with the addition of prednisone.[135]

Thymoma can recur decades after initial treatment, and therefore patients should receive lifelong monitoring. The long-term prognosis has been shown to depend on stage, tumor size, and the completeness of resection (which is the most important factor). The presence of symptoms at the time of diagnosis may portend a worse outcome.[125,136,137]

BRONCHIAL GLAND TUMORS

Historically, the term *bronchial adenoma* has been used to designate a diverse group of tumors including mucoepidermoid carcinoma, bronchial carcinoid, adenoid cystic carcinoma, and others. This misnomer implies a benign disease process and is no longer recommended.[138,139] Mucoepidermoid carcinoma accounts for approximately 10% of malignant lung tumors in children.[139,140] These tumors are histologically identical to the more common lesions involving the salivary glands. The tumors typically arise from mucous cells located within the respiratory tree and usually remain localized for prolonged periods of time.[141] The primary treatment is surgical resection alone, and with aggressive surgery the prognosis is excellent.[142] A review of all 31 children with mucoepidermoid carcinoma reported in the English language literature as of 1998 and treated with surgery alone identified no disease recurrence, with a mean follow-up of more than 5 years.[139] Another bronchial gland tumor, adenoid cystic carcinoma (cylindroma), is exceedingly rare. For example, a review of 151 cases of childhood primary pulmonary neoplasms included only four cases.[91] Because adenoid cystic carcinoma in adults tends toward extensive submucosal spread and late local recurrence, en bloc resection with hilar lymphadenectomy and careful examination of resection margins has been recommended. Bronchial carcinoid tumors are the most frequent primary pulmonary neoplasm of children and adolescents[143] and is discussed later in this chapter. Other lung tumors that may enter into a differential diagnosis include leiomyosarcoma, primary or secondary rhabdomyosarcoma, myofibroblastic tumors, and hemangioendotheliomas. Significant morbidity may be avoided if a neoplastic process is considered in the differential diagnosis of persistent cough, recurrent pneumonia, wheezing, hemoptysis, or a persistent radiographic abnormality in a child.[92,95,139,141]

MESOTHELIOMA

Malignant mesothelioma can arise in the mesothelial lining of the pleura, pericardium, peritoneum, and tunica vaginalis.[144–146] Thoracic mesotheliomas account for more than 90% of the cases, followed by abdominal primaries.[147] These tumors may occur as primary or secondary malignant neoplasms and may have epithelial, sarcomatous, and mixed histologic patterns.[148–150] In one report, secondary mesotheliomas were reported to occur after malignant ovarian teratoma, Hodgkin disease of the neck, and non-Hodgkin (Burkitt type) lymphoma of the abdomen in three patients who had previously undergone radiation and chemotherapy.[150] Asbestos and simian virus 40 have been implicated as causative agents of adult mesothelioma.[151] Mesotheliomas are primarily a tumor of the adult; more than 90% of the cases are diagnosed after the 5th decade.[147] Young household members of asbestos-exposed workers are also at risk of developing mesothelioma; however, the median latency is more than 40 years since initial exposure.[152] A widely accepted staging system is available only for pleural mesothelioma. The median survival estimate for patients with mesothelioma is 12 months. Adverse prognostic factors include nonepithelial tumor histology, poor performance status, male sex, older age, and advanced disease stage.[151] The benefit of surgery and chemotherapy in this disease is difficult to assess given the poor prognosis of the disease. The results of aggressive surgery (extrapleural pneumonectomy) alone have been disappointing, and pleurectomy with decortication appears to provide an attractive surgical alternative to these patients.[153] Radiation therapy is of limited effectiveness but intensity-modulated radiotherapy has been increasingly used in recent years.[153] Combination chemotherapy with pemetrexed and cisplatin appears very promising.[154] Overall survival at 5 years is less than 25%; however, when a multimodal treatment approach is used, nearly 50% of selected patients with stage I disease can be expected to survive 5 years.[147,155]

TUMORS OF THE HEART

Cardiac tumors are rare with a prevalence of 0.0017 to 0.28 in autopsy series.[156] However, the incidence of cardiac tumors during fetal life has been reported to be 0.14%.[156] The majority of cardiac tumors in children are benign, and the most common in order of decreasing frequency are rhabdomyomas, teratomas, fibromas, hemangiomas, and myxomas.[156] Malignant cardiac tumors in children are rare, and the majority are sarcoma including angiosarcoma, rhabdomyosarcoma, and fibrosarcoma. About 5% of malignant cardiac tumors in children are lymphomas. Metastatic tumors to the heart include neuroblastoma, leukemia, lymphoma, and melanoma. Presenting symptoms usually include dyspnea, orthopnea, irregular heart rhythm, embolic events, and cardiomegaly.[156,157] Systemic symptoms might include fever, fatigue, confusion, weight loss, embolic phenomena, and congestive heart failure.[156] When faced with a cardiac tumor in a pediatric patient, the practicing oncologist should be aware of important associations with certain genetic syndromes, in particular tuberous sclerosis and Carney complex (an autosomal dominant disorder characterized by endocrinopathy, cardiac myxomas, spotty skin pigmentation, and germ-line mutations of the PRKAR1 A gene).[158] It is estimated that 60% to 80% of patients with cardiac rhabdomyomas have tuberous sclerosis and that up to 7% of cardiac myxomas may occur within the setting of Carney complex.[158] The diagnosis of a cardiac tumor can be established with the use of transthoracic or transesophageal echocardiography, MRI imaging, and CT of the chest. Successful treatment requires surgery, which may include heart transplantation, and appropriate chemotherapy for the type of cancer being treated.[156,157]

CANCER OF THE ESOPHAGUS

An estimated 16,470 new cases of cancer of the esophagus were diagnosed in the United States in 2008,[159] but fewer than 10 cases of esophageal adenocarcinoma have been reported in patients younger than 25 years.[160] This tumor is much more frequent in boys, with an approximate 3:1 male predominance.[161] More than 90% of esophageal cancers are either adenocarcinoma or squamous cell carcinoma and both histologic types have been reported in children.[162-164] Adenocarcinomas of the esophagus in adults are usually associated with Barrett's esophagus and are thought to be the result of chronic gastrointestinal reflux. Although this effect is thought to develop over decades (the mean age at diagnosis is 67 years), this association has been reported in an 8-year-old child.[164] Other unusual tumors of the esophagus in children include lipomas and undifferentiated mesenchymal neoplasms.[165,166]

Adult and pediatric patients with this cancer present with dysphasia, difficulty swallowing, and weight loss. There may be associated vomiting, cough, hemoptysis, hematemesis, and regurgitation, and metastases may cause bone pain. The diagnosis must be made by histologic examination. Generally, barium-contrast radiography is followed by endoscopy and biopsy. A tissue biopsy should be obtained through endoscopy. Early-stage carcinomas of the esophagus are generally asymptomatic and may be detected incidentally. The standard of care has been surgery, although with this approach, 90% of patients eventually succumb to their disease.[161,167] Preoperative chemotherapy and radiation may result in superior survival, although the treatment for this difficult cancer is still evolving.

CANCER OF THE STOMACH

It is estimated that there were 21,500 new cases of cancer of the stomach in adults in the United States in 2008.[159] The incidence differs geographically, with Japan having the highest incidence rate and the United States one of the lowest.[168] On the other hand, this cancer is exceptionally rare in children and adolescents, with no appreciable variation in the rate of occurrence worldwide; only 1% to 3% of gastric carcinomas occur in patients younger than 30 years, and only about 0.05% occur in children or adolescents.[169]

Epidemiology

In 1936, gastric cancer was the leading cause of cancer-related death of men in the United States. The death rate and frequency of this disease have however declined worldwide since that time. There are no recognized genetic syndromes associated with gastric cancer, and familial occurrence is rare.

Pathology

The majority of malignancies of the stomach in children are gastrointestinal stromal tumors (GISTs) (see section on GIST in this chapter), lymphomas, or soft tissue sarcomas; fewer than 5% are carcinomas.[170-174] In contrast, approximately 95% of tumors of the stomach in all age groups are adenocarcinomas. Primary gastric adenocarcinoma in children accounts for less than 1% of all GI malignancies.[175] Gastric adenocarcinomas are classified according to the degree of histologic differentiation. Approximately half of all stomach neoplasms are located in the distal stomach[168,176]; nodal and omental involvement may be encountered. Other less frequent tumors include squamous cell carcinoma, carcinoid tumor, leiomyosarcoma, teratoma, and liposarcoma.[177-179] The differential diagnosis of gastric carcinoma in a child should include Peutz-Jeghers–type polyps in the stomach[180] and inflammatory myofibroblastic tumors,[181] among others. Gastric carcinomas spread via the lymphatic and blood vessels, by direct extension, and through seeding of the peritoneal surfaces. These lesions may infiltrate the submucosa, extend directly, and involve the duodenum or esophagus, liver, pancreas, or colon. Blood-borne metastases may involve the lungs, liver, and skin.

Clinical Presentation

The findings of most studies suggest that symptoms of gastric carcinoma in younger patients do not differ from those in older patients. Cancers of the stomach produce vague epigastric discomfort, which may or may not be associated with weight loss and anorexia.[176,182,183] Iron deficiency anemia may be present with occult blood in the stool. These cancers may not produce symptoms until they are metastatic. Therefore, individuals who experience weight loss and abdominal pain, nausea and vomiting, change in bowel habits, anorexia, dysphagia, weakness, hematemesis, or other vague abdominal symptoms should be investigated. The overall rarity of this diagnosis in children and the nonspecificity of the symptoms usually result in a delay in diagnosis.

Diagnosis

A gastroscopically obtained biopsy is the most accurate method of identifying gastric carcinoma. Fiberoptic endoscopy may be complemented with an upper gastrointestinal radiographic series. Chest radiographs, CT scans, and appropriate laboratory studies, including blood chemistries and a complete blood cell count, should be performed.

Staging

The tumor extent, lymph node status, and presence of metastases (TNM) classification of the AJCC is used for staging.[2] This information is obtained from surgical exploration and from clinical data when resection is not carried out.

Prognostic Considerations

A number of factors that increase the risk of gastric cancer have been identified in adults. These include *Helicobacter pylori* infection,[184] familial adenomatous polyposis (FAP), Barrett's esophagus, chronic atrophic gastritis, ethanol or nicotine use, limited consumption of fresh fruits or vegetables, and low socioeconomic status, among others. It is unknown whether any of these factors apply to children,[185] although an 8-year-old girl diagnosed with a signet cell adenocarcinoma of the gastric wall also had active chronic *Helicobacter pylori* gastritis.[175] The prognosis of carcinoma of the stomach depends on the extent of disease. There is little information about the outcomes of patients younger than 21 years at the time of diagnosis. However, in most reports, the survival rate, according to extent of disease at presentation, appears to be similar.[168,170]

Treatment and Complications

As with most rare tumors in children, treatment approaches are largely based on principles used in adults with similar histologies.[186] Complete surgical excision, with appropriate margins, is the procedure of choice for treatment of this cancer. Surgery should include subtotal gastrectomy with resection of associated lymph nodes. In a randomized trial of 711 patients (380 randomized to a limited [D1] lymph node dissection and 331 to an extended [D2] resection), more complications (43% vs. 25%; $p < 0.001$), and more postoperative deaths (10% vs. 4%; $p = 0.004$), were seen with D2 resections compared with D1 resections.[187] Although this tumor has been regarded as somewhat unresponsive to radiation because radiation therapy with curative intent is associated with tumor doses greater than the tolerance of surrounding tissues, it has recently been established as an integral part of treatment for patients with completely resected tumors.[188] As expected, there are no data available on radiation therapy for children.

Adjuvant chemotherapy with an oral fluoropyrimidine, S-1, has recently been shown to improve overall survival in stage II-III gastric cancer patients.[189] In a randomized trial of patients with metastatic or locally recurrent disease, the addition of docetaxel to cisplatin and fluorouracil (DCF) increased the time to progression, survival, and rate of response.[190] Adjuvant chemotherapy continues to be investigated. Other agents being used are epirubicin, mitomycin, irinotecan, oxaliplatin, and paclitaxel.[186] There are no available contemporary data on the results of therapy in children.

PANCREATIC CANCERS

In adults, pancreatic cancer is the fourth most frequent fatal malignancy, exceeded only by colon, lung, and breast cancers. In the United States, approximately 38,000 new cases of pancreatic cancer were diagnosed in 2008 and more than 30,000 patients died of this disease.[159] In a review of the SEER registry from 1973 to 2004, malignant pancreatic neoplasms were identified in 58 patients younger than 20 years. Of these, 31 were classified as exocrine, 19 as endocrine, and 5 were sarcomas. Exocrine tumors included 10 solid-cystic tumors, 4 acinar cell carcinomas, 7 ductal adenocarcinomas, and 10 pancreatoblastomas.[191] These data are consistent with previous reports, suggesting that the most common pancreatic tumor in childhood and adolescence is pancreatoblastoma.[192] There are some reports of the usual adult type of ductal adenocarcinoma in children, although these are exceptionally rare.[188,193,194] Other primary pancreatic tumors described in children and adolescents include pancreatic endocrine neoplasms such as insulinomas[195] and vasoactive intestinal polypeptide-secreting tumors (VIPomas), solid pseudopapillary tumors, acinar cell carcinomas, lymphomas, rhabdomyosarcoma, teratomas, and primitive neuroectodermal tumors.[196,197]

Multiple genetic abnormalities have been identified in adults with pancreatic cancer, and a number of hereditary syndromes are associated with an increased risk of pancreatic adenocarcinoma.[198,199] For example, there is evidence to suggest that melanoma-prone families with mutations that impair p16 (INK4a) function are at high risk of pancreatic cancer,[200] and it is believed that as many as one-third of young patients with adult-type pancreatic adenocarcinoma may have an underlying hereditary tumor syndrome.[188,201] Pancreatoblastoma, the most common type of pediatric pancreatic malignancy, has been associated with the Beckwith-Wiedemann syndrome.[202]

Pathogenesis, Natural History, and Patterns of Spread

The causes of pancreatic cancers in children are unknown. These tumors may arise in the head, body, or tail of the pancreas. In most instances, the tumors are nonfunctioning, and symptoms differ according to the site of origin. Functioning tumors may produce various symptoms. Islet cell carcinomas produce an overabundance of insulin, leading to hypoglycemia that may be associated with fatigue, restlessness, and malaise, followed by clouding of the sensorium, staggering gait, hyperthermia, and coma; these may appear as intermittent attacks, most frequently in the early morning hours. Nonfunctioning islet cell tumors are usually associated with peptic ulcers and the elaboration of gastrin by the tumor; some patients develop watery diarrhea, hypokalemia, and achlorhydria.

Most children present with vague gastrointestinal complaints, wasting, and pain. Other signs and symptoms include weight loss and a palpable abdominal mass.[196,201,203,204] Tumors at the head of the pancreas may cause mechanical obstruction of the duodenum and gastric outlet associated with jaundice and intestinal hemorrhage. Venous obstruction may lead to varices, hemorrhage, and ascites. Tumors of the body or tail of the pancreas may erode into the stomach and cause hemorrhage. Ascites associated with involvement of the liver and peritoneum may result in hepatic failure, and patients may die because of progressive weight loss and anorexia. Metastases commonly occur in the liver, lymph nodes, and lung; tumor may spread locoregionally to the stomach, spleen, gallbladder, and omentum.[203,205,206]

Diagnosis

The usual diagnostic imaging studies should be used, along with evaluation of the chest by CT, to establish the diagnosis and the extent of disease. The differential diagnosis includes benign neoplasms such as papillary cystic tumor and hemangiomas. Radiographic studies should include contrast studies of the gastrointestinal tract, abdominal ultrasonography, and CT or MRI scans of the abdomen. Primary tumors of the head of the pancreas may cause deformity of the duodenal C loop, or gastric antrum, and may be associated with mucosal abnormalities detected by gastroscopy. Retrograde endoscopic cholangiopancreatography may be helpful, as may be arteriography, when resection is being considered.

Serum markers including carcinoembryonic antigen, alphafetoprotein, cancer antigen (CA) 125, CA19-9, and pancreatic oncofetal antigen may be of value in the diagnosis and follow-up.[207,208] Serum alpha-fetoprotein levels are often elevated in children with pancreatoblastoma. Other markers such as amylase, lipase, alkaline phosphatase, lactic dehydrogenase, transaminases, leucine aminopeptidase, and pancreatic ribonuclease may aid in diagnosis and in evaluation of the success of treatment.

Pathology

Pediatric malignant tumors of the pancreas include malignant papillary cystic carcinoma and pancreatoblastoma as well as tumors of islet cell origin such as insulinoma and gastrinoma. Other cancers of duct cell origin are adenocarcinoma and squamous cell carcinoma; acinar cell carcinoma, peripheral neuroepithelioma, and lymphoma may involve the pancreas.[209–212] Surgical staging of this tumor uses the grading system of the AJCC; the reader is referred to the most recent edition of that handbook.[2]

Prognostic Considerations

Less than 10% of adult patients with carcinoma of the pancreas survive, but better results have been sporadically reported in children. Most tumors of the pancreas are not radiosensitive or chemosensitive; thus, cure is possible only when the diagnosis is made at an early stage and when the tumor is confined to the body of the pancreas. In such cases, surgical resection provides the only chance of long-term disease-free survival. Pancreatoblastoma may have a more favorable clinical course.[213]

Treatment

The principles of treatment for pediatric pancreatic tumors are derived from the experience in adults.[214–216] Various surgical resection methods developed since 1935 include pancreatoduodenectomy, total pancreatectomy, regional pancreatectomy, and distal pancreatectomy. The standard resection approach is pancreaticoduodenectomy, referred to as the *Whipple procedure*. Too few pediatric patients have been treated with radiation therapy for pancreatic carcinoma or pancreatoblastoma to allow meaningful conclusions. For adults, a radiation dose of 45 to 54 Gy is given over 4 to 6 weeks, usually with concurrent 5-FU. Concurrent gemcitabine and radiation may be equally as effective.[216] Complications may include bowel obstruction, biliary obstruction, and biliary fistula. Studies to evaluate the use of adjunctive conventional or intraoperative radiation therapy are under way in adults.

Localized Tumors

Chemotherapy for pancreatic carcinoma differs from that given for pancreatoblastoma and is usually ineffective. The agents used to treat metastatic pancreatic carcinoma include 5-FU, capecitabine, streptozotocin, mitomycin C, gemcitabine, doxorubicin, irinotecan, docetaxel, erlotinib, and oxaliplatin. The reported rates of response to these agents range from 7% to 36%,[215–217] although gemcitabine is the only cytotoxic agent that has even a modest impact on survival or disease-related symptoms.[217] For pediatric patients with pancreatoblastoma, the usual agents include vincristine, cyclophosphamide, doxorubicin, cisplatin or carboplatin, dactinomycin, and bleomycin.[192,213] Unresectable lesions at presentation must undergo surgical excision and radiation therapy after a response to chemotherapy to prevent regrowth of tumors.[218,219]

GASTROINTESTINAL STROMAL TUMORS

GISTs are the most common mesenchymal tumor of the gastrointestinal tract in adults with an estimated annual incidence of 6.8 to 14.5 per million.[220,221] In the past, GISTs were classified as leiomyomas, cellular leiomyomas, leiomyoblastomas, and leiomyosarcomas. The recognition of GISTs as a distinct clinicopathologic entity has resulted in a 25-fold increase in the age-adjusted incidence of GISTs from 1992 to 2002 in the SEER database.[221] GISTs are thought to arise from a primitive precursor mesenchymal cell related to the interstitial cells of Cajal, which regulates motility and autonomic nerve function of the intestinal tract.[222] In 1998, Hirota and colleagues demonstrated that GISTs have gain-of-function mutations in the c-KIT protooncogene,[223] and on immunocytochemical analysis, more than 95% of GISTs express KIT (CD117). Recent studies with large numbers of patients have confirmed that 85% to 90% of adult GISTs harbor KIT or PDGR mutations.[224–226]

GISTs can arise within the context of four tumor predisposition syndromes:

1. Familial GISTs: GISTs develop late, at a median age of 46 years, and patients often have other associated symptoms and findings including abnormalities in skin pigmentation and dysphagia.[227]
2. Neurofibromatosis type 1: GISTs develop late, at a median age of 49 years; usually involves the small intestine and lack KIT or PDGFR mutations.[228]
3. Carney triad[229]: GISTs develop early at a median age of 20 years and is associated with pulmonary chondromas and paragangliomas.[230]
4. Carney-Stratakis dyad: GISTs develop early at a median age of 19 years. Associated with paragangliomas. Caused by germ-line mutations or deletions of the succinate hydrogenase (SDH) B, C, or D genes.[231]

GISTs commonly affect middle-aged individuals with a median age at the time of presentation of 60 years. They most commonly arise in the stomach (50% to 60%) (Fig. 37.3), followed by the small intestine (20% to 30%), the large bowel (10%), and other sites including the esophagus (10%).[232] Presenting symptoms depend on the size and site of the tumor. Small tumors may go unrecognized until incidentally detected

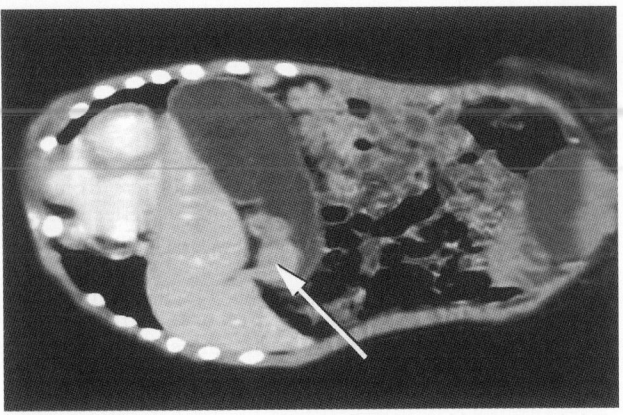

FIGURE 37.3 Reformatted coronal computed tomography image of a 6-year-old child with a gastrointestinal stromal tumor. A lobulated hyperdense mass (*arrow*) is seen arising from the superior aspect of the gastric antrum.

during laparotomy. Symptomatic tumors can present with abdominal pain, ulceration, gastrointestinal hemorrhage, bleeding, perforation, or an externally palpable abdominal mass. Evaluation should include endoscopic visualization of the mass and CT of the abdomen. PET imaging may also be used. Standard therapy for sarcoma is ineffective against these tumors.[233–236] The risk of recurrence is determined by the size and site of the tumor and mitotic count[234] (Table 37.1). Imatinib mesylate, a small molecule tyrosine kinase inhibitor of KIT, PDGFR, and ABL, has proven to be highly effective in the treatment of these tumors, with a documented clinical benefit (partial responses and stable disease) of about 80%[237,238] The median survival period in adults treated with imatinib is 57 months.[239] The likelihood of response to imatinib is higher (83%) in patients who have an exon 11 mutation.[240] Sunitinib has proved to be efficacious in patients with imatinib-resistant tumors.[241]

The incidence and prevalence of pediatric GISTs is unknown, but isolated institutional reports estimate that pediatric GISTs account for about 2% of all nonrhabdomyosarcomatous soft-tissue sarcomas or for 2% of all GISTs.[242,243] In a review of 121 reported patients with GISTs, the median age at presentation was approximately 14 years and 74% of affected patients were female.[229] The most common presenting symptoms were gastrointestinal bleeding and a palpable mass; obstructive symptoms were more commonly reported in very young patients. About 85% of tumors arose in the stomach, and the most common histologic subtype was epithelioid or a mix of spindle and epithelioid cells. Pediatric GISTs have a higher incidence of nodal involvement and are often slow growing and multifocal.[229] Ten percent of reported cases had evidence of Carney triad or dyad and two patients had a history of malignancy (neuroblastoma and osteosarcoma).[229] Analysis of tumor cells of patients with pediatric GISTs demonstrate few large scale chromosome changes[244] and infrequent KIT or PDGFR mutations; only 7 of 64 (11%) tumors analyzed had mutations and these were evenly distributed in exons 11 and 9 of the KIT protooncogene and the PDGFR gene.[229] Recent studies also demonstrate that IGF1R is amplified and overexpressed in pediatric and adult wild-type GISTs, suggesting that clinical benefit might be derived from targeting this pathway in these patients who traditionally do not respond well to imatinib.[245,246].

Suggested management guidelines for pediatric patients with GISTs have been recently published but have not been prospectively validated.[229] Surgery, when feasible, remains the mainstay of therapy, and tissue samples should be sent for mutational analysis. At the time of surgery, abnormal lymph nodes should be sampled since pediatric GISTs have a propensity for nodal dissemination.[246] For patients who have KIT or PDGFR mutations, physicians should follow the guidelines published for adult GISTs.[247] In the absence of KIT or PDGFR mutations, the tumor should be resected when feasible (avoiding extensive morbid procedures such as total gastrectomy), and the patient be closely followed at 3- to 6-month intervals. Although adjuvant imatinib has been shown to improve recurrence-free survival in adult patients with high-risk resected GISTs, this strategy has not been prospectively studied in pediatric patients and therefore cannot be recommended.[248] For patients with unresectable or metastatic disease who are asymptomatic, close follow-up is recommended. In the presence of symptoms or progression, surgical resection should be performed when feasible. Although pediatric GISTs have a lower rate of response to kinase inhibitors when compared with adult GISTs, a trial of imatinib is indicated in the presence of worsening clinical symptoms and limited surgical options.[229] For patients who experience progression or recurrence after imatinib therapy, the administration of sunitinib has shown promising activity.[249]

TABLE 37.1

FEATURES PREDICTIVE OF RECURRENCE IN GASTROINTESTINAL STROMAL TUMORS[222]

Tumor parameters			Patients with progressive disease and malignant potential (%)	
Group	Size (cm)	Mitotic rate per 50 high power field (HPF)	Gastric	Small intestine
1	≤2	≤5	0 Very low	0 Very low
2	>2, ≤5	≤5	1.9 Low	4.3 Low
3a	>5, ≤10	≤5	3.6 Low	24 Intermediate
3b	>10	≤5	12 Intermediate	53 High
4	≤2	>5	0 Low	50 High
5	>2, ≤5	>5	16 Intermediate	73 High
6a	>5, ≤10	>5	55 High	85 High
6b	>10	>5	86 High	90 High

COLORECTAL CARCINOMA

Although colorectal carcinoma (CRC) is one of the most frequent tumors of adults, it rarely occurs before the age of 20 years.

Epidemiology

CRC is more common in developed countries. Thus, it is seen more frequently in Europe and North America than in Africa or Asia, with the exception of Japan, where the incidence approaches that in other developed countries.[250] The reasons for this disparity are poorly understood. However, dietary differences have been suggested as one explanation. In general, an increased intake of red meats and fats and decreased intake of vegetables and fruits is characteristic of diets in more developed countries. Red meat, especially when cooked at high temperatures, has an increased content of carcinogens such as heterocyclic amines,[251,252] and a relatively low-fiber diet is thought to prolong the transit time of fecal material containing these carcinogens. However, the geographic variation is likely to reflect a complex interaction of lifestyle, environmental and dietary factors, and genetic factors.[253]

There are approximately 150,000 new cases of CRC in adults in the United States annually.[159] However, it accounts for only about 2% of all cancers in adolescents and young adults between the ages of 15 and 29 years and for less than 1% of all cases in children younger than 20 years.[254,255] Thus, the incidence is approximately one case per million in this age group. In children and adolescents, these tumors may occur at any site in the large bowel and are not usually associated with a family history of large-bowel cancer.[256-264] However, an increased incidence of uterine/cervical cancer in the families of younger patients with CRC has been suggested.[265] CRC shows no gender predilection, and among patients younger than 20 years, there is a peak incidence around age 15 years.[262,266] Most of the case reports have come from the central Mississippi Valley, where some patients had been exposed to pesticides and herbicides.[266] Patients with long-standing ulcerative colitis are at increased risk; the risk increases with the duration and severity of colitis, increasing to approximately 20% after age 40 years.[267] Over the past several decades the predominant sites of primary lesions have shifted from the left to the right colon and African Americans have a higher occurrence of CRC than do white Americans.[268]

Genetics

Several recognized conditions may be associated with the development of CRC in young patients (Table 37.2).[255,269] Studies of familial clustering show that 20% to 30% of all cases of CRC have a potentially definable inherited cause. However, the specific genes remain to be characterized in most such cases.[270] Well-defined CRC predisposition syndromes account for only about 3% to 5% of all cases of colon cancer; these include Peutz-Jeghers syndrome, familial juvenile polyposis, hereditary mixed polyposis syndrome, hereditary nonpolyposis colon cancer, and FAP. The most common genetic polyposis syndrome is FAP, inherited as a dominant trait with 90% penetrance, which may be associated with the appearance of multiple cancers by the age of 37 years. Early diagnosis and total colectomy eliminates the risk of CRC for these patients. Other syndromes associated with CRC in young people include Turcot syndrome,[271] in which the adenomatous polyposis coli gene is frequently mutated,[272] Oldfield syndrome[273]; and Gardner syndrome.[274] There may be an association between neurofibromatosis and polyposis coli,[275] and one reported individual with multiple adenomatous polyps, multiple colon carcinomas, and neurofibromatosis had a constitutional deletion of *p53*.[275]

A stepwise model for the development of CRC was proposed by Fearon and Vogelstein.[276] They proceeded from the observation that most CRCs arise from adenomas that have undergone mutational activation of an oncogene in addition to the loss of several tumor suppressor genes. They surmised that mutations in the adenomatous polyposis coli tumor suppressor gene occur early in the development of polyps, followed by Ki-ras mutations during the adenomatous stage. Finally, loss of sequences on several chromosomes, such as

TABLE 37.2

POLYPOSIS SYNDROMES ASSOCIATED WITH COLORECTAL CARCINOMA

Name	Description	Reference
Familial adenomatous polyposis (FAP)	>100 polyps in teens, colon adenomas, small bowel adenomas, gastric polyposis, congenital hypertrophy of retinal pigment epithelium, odontomas, osteomas, fibromas, lipomas, epidermoid cysts, desmoid tumors	180, 443
Variant FAP syndromes		
Gardner syndrome	Osteomas, polyposis, multiple sebaceous cysts	269, 274
Turcot syndrome	FAP associated with central nervous system tumors	271
Attenuated FAP	Average of 30 polyps, predominantly right-sided colonic adenomas	180, 443
Hereditary flat adenoma syndrome	<100 small flat polyps, predominantly in right colon	269
Muir-Torre syndrome	Multiple skin lesions with <100 adenomatous polyps	444
Hamartomatous polyposis syndromes		
Peutz-Jeghers	Numerous hamartomatous polyps in the gastrointestinal tract, mucocutaneous pigmentation of lips, perioral region, buccal mucosa	269
Juvenile polyposis	10 juvenile polyps, skin lesions, intestinal hamartomas, congenital abnormalities (malrotation of midgut; cardiac and genitourinary abnormalities)	445
Cowden syndrome	Hamartomas in intestine and other tissues, trichilemmoma, central nervous system abnormalities; possible increased risk of colorectal carcinoma	446

17p and 18q (the DCC gene, deleted in colon cancer),[277] coincide with malignant transformation of the polyp. This model has been confirmed by other investigators, and the specific cellular pathways perturbed by these changes are increasingly being elucidated.[278] The scant molecular data available for childhood CRC indicate that a different molecular pathway(s) may be involved.[279,280]

There is no evidence that a family history of bowel cancer increases the risk of bowel cancer before age 20 years. The risk for persons younger than 20 years who belong to families with hereditary CRC, familial cancer syndromes, or familial juvenile polyposis is unclear. Most affected family members do not develop CRC until after the third decade of life. For example, the mean age of diagnosis of CRC in patients with FAP is 39 years.[281] Therefore, prophylactic colectomy is usually not recommended until late adolescence or early adulthood. However, there is one report of a 5-year-old child with FAP who presented with rectal bleeding and found to have hundreds of sessile polyps. At colectomy, many adenomatous polyps were identified. However, none had extended beyond the muscularis mucosae[282] (Fig. 37.4). Individuals with the Peutz-Jeghers syndrome may develop cancers in the stomach, duodenum, or small bowel as well as the large bowel, because the hamartomatous polyps characteristic of this syndrome may occur anywhere in the gastrointestinal tract.[180]

Clinical Presentation

Signs and symptoms may be absent. A change in bowel habits, such as constipation or diarrhea, and a change in the caliber of stools may be observed before the development of tarry stools, rectal bleeding, or other changes. There may be decreased appetite and weight loss. Abdominal pain is usually the most common presenting symptom and is frequently severe enough to suggest an acute abdomen.[261,263,264,283] The signs and symptoms of CRC are related to its primary site within the large bowel. Tumors involving the cecum and descending colon, which may be associated with familial colon carcinoma, may become bulky before symptoms appear. Tumors of the rectum and sigmoid colon may be associated

with changes in the caliber of the stool, dyschezia, hematochezia, and anemia.

The diagnosis of CRC in young patients is often delayed because it is seldom suspected. Acute bowel symptoms necessitate immediate abdominal exploration, at which time perforation of the large bowel with multiple metastatic deposits may be observed.[264,284]

The natural history of CRC in young individuals differs from that in adults, in that tumors of the young are more advanced at diagnosis.[263,264,283,285] These tumors, therefore, may not be resectable. They may spread throughout the peritoneal cavity to involve the omentum, peritoneum, mesenteric lymph nodes, liver, and ovaries, and they may spread through the bloodstream to the lungs and eventually the brain, bones, or both. Peritoneal seeding in female patients frequently involves the ovaries, which may become extremely enlarged. More than half of the reported neoplasms of the colon in younger patients, but only approximately 15% of those in adults, are mucinous adenocarcinomas.[264,286]

Ancillary Clinical Tests

Examination of the stool for occult blood may produce positive test results when no gross blood or bloody discoloration can be seen in the stool. Test results of hepatic and renal function are rarely abnormal initially, although metastatic involvement of the liver may cause abnormal liver function test results. Anemia may be related to blood loss or malnutrition. There is very little information about the value of various tumor markers in children with CRC.[287] Carcinoembryonic antigen should be assayed preoperatively. A concentration greater than 5 ng per mL in adults has been associated with advanced stage and poorer prognosis. Unfortunately, only a minority of children with CRC may produce this protein, possibly because poorly differentiated adenocarcinomas produce less carcinoembryonic antigen.[288] Other markers that are being evaluated include CA 19-9, interleukin-6, tumor expression of the DCC and p27^{Kip1} genes, p53, Ras, thymidine synthase, 18q loss of heterozygosity, dihydropyrimidine dehydrogenase, and microsatellite instability (MSI). However, none are recommended for use outside the research setting.[289]

Imaging Studies

Any patient with suspected CRC should undergo fiberoptic examination of the entire colon, because the occurrence of synchronous tumors may change the surgical approach.[270] Conventional radiographic studies include barium enema with air contrast to define the tumor and the remainder of the colon. These radiographs, performed together with CT scans of the abdomen, pelvis, and chest, may define areas of spread to the liver, lungs, or lymph nodes and metastases involving the pelvis and cul de sac, especially the ovaries. More recently, (18 F)-fluorodeoxy-D-glucose positron emission tomography (FDG-PET) has appeared to be more useful than standard radiologic techniques in detecting hepatic or peritoneal disease.[290,291] In a retrospective review of 71 adults with presumably resectable liver metastases, FDG-PET identified additional metastatic disease not appreciated by conventional CT scans in 23 patients and resulted in a change in management in 17 cases. Eleven patients (15%) had false-negative FDG-PET scans; two of these had mucinous tumors.[292] Others have reported that only about 60% of mucinous carcinomas (16 of 25) are FDG-PET–avid.[293] Because mucinous adenocarcinoma is the most common histologic type of CRC in children, this imaging modality may have limited usefulness for

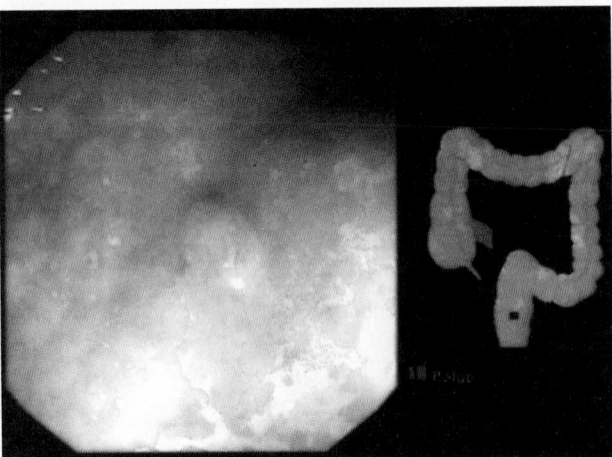

FIGURE 37.4 Endoscopic photograph of an adenomatous polyp in the rectum of a 20-year-old man. At age 10 years, after he had experienced bloody stools and pain, a stage III mucinous adenocarcinoma of the cecum was diagnosed. Additional polyps were removed the following year, and a colon resection to the peritoneal reflection was performed during the succeeding year. The figure demonstrates a polyp seen 8 years after resection.

the evaluation of many children with CRC. More experience is needed in the use of FDG-PET scans to evaluate patients with CRC, especially children.

Pathology

Most colorectal cancers in adults are moderately differentiated or well-differentiated adenocarcinomas; in contrast, more than half of reported cases of childhood CRC are poorly differentiated mucinous adenocarcinoma, and many are of the signet-ring cell type.[264,294,295]

CRC arises from the mucosal surface of the bowel, usually at the site of an adenomatous polyp overgrowth. Tumor may extend into the muscularis area to the serosa, perforate the serosa, and penetrate the omental fat, lymph nodes, liver, ovaries, and other loops of bowel. Some lesions may obstruct the bowel lumen. There also may be implants along the abdominal scar, at the anastomotic site, or throughout the peritoneum. Rarely are multiple tumors present simultaneously.[270] Multiple lesions may show the same or different histology and the same or different stages of development.

The gross appearance of colonic lesions depends on the extent of involvement of the lumen and the extent of the disease outside the bowel wall. Because these tumors are derived from endoderm, all of their cytologic characteristics will be those of carcinoma, yet they may be well differentiated or poorly differentiated and contain pools of mucin. These tumors may grow to remarkable sizes, and in females, ovarian involvement may be massive and may complicate the differential diagnosis of bowel cancer versus ovarian cancer.

The differential diagnosis includes malignant carcinoid tumor, leiomyosarcoma, malignant fibrous histiocytoma, and metastatic tumor from other sites. All may have similar presentations; metastases may be identified only by histology or metastatic site. When patients present with an acute abdomen, associated pain, and possible perforation, the diagnosis of acute appendicitis is most often considered.

Staging

Several staging systems have been proposed for this tumor over the past 50 years, including the Dukes classification, the Astler-Coller modification, the Gastrointestinal Tumor Study Group (GITSG) classification, and the TNM classification. The TNM classification of the AJCC has been used most frequently to define the reporting requirements of tumor registries.[2]

Treatment

Biopsy is required for the diagnosis of CRC. A biopsy may be obtained during colonoscopy or laparotomy, at which time definitive surgery may or may not be feasible. The treatment of choice is surgical resection. In fact, if patients cannot be rendered surgically free of disease, they are rarely cured. Radical surgery with curative intent is the mainstay of treatment. The basic surgical principles are removal of the major vascular pedicle supplying the tumor and its lymphatics and en bloc resection of any organs or structures attached to the tumor. A margin of at least 5 cm of normal bowel should be removed on either side of the tumor to minimize the possibility of anastomotic recurrence. Adequate lymph node resection is imperative, because some patients with stage III tumors can be cured by surgery alone. A minimum of 12 negative lymph nodes should be examined to define node-negative disease.[296]

Unfortunately, many children's initial surgery is not planned as a cancer operation. In these cases, reexploration of the abdomen, with the goals of radical resection of tumor with adequate margins and adequate lymph node sampling, should be done at a center experienced in this type of surgery. Other surgical staging procedures include biopsy of the ovaries in female patients, resection of the omentum, and examination and possible biopsy of the liver. Complete excision is the goal of surgery, whereas secondary aims are related to palliation by resection of bulky tumors or metastases. Debulking provides little benefit for the patient with extensive metastatic disease. However, removal of single or multiple hepatic metastases may be a life-saving procedure for patients whose other sites of disease have been successfully resected.

Chemotherapy and Radiation Therapy

Tumor involvement of the rectosigmoid area or anus that is considered unresectable at the time of diagnosis is treated initially with a combination of 5-FU–based chemotherapy and radiation therapy before resection is attempted. Localized, completely resected tumors (T_{is}, T_1, T_2, N0, M0 lesions) are usually cured by surgery alone. For patients with more advanced disease, chemotherapy options are expanding beyond the use of 5-FU with leucovorin.[297] Other approved agents include irinotecan,[298] oxaliplatin,[299] two monoclonal antibodies against the epidermal growth factor receptor (cetuximab; Erbitux and panitumumab),[300,301] and a monoclonal antibody against the vascular endothelial growth factor receptor (bevacizumab; Avastin).[302] Standard chemotherapy recommendations for stage III disease (T_{1-4}, N1–2, M0) currently include either FOLFOX4 or mFOLFOX6.[303,304] Therapy options for patients with metastatic disease are under active investigation and changing rapidly.

Complications of Therapy

Complications of therapy and disease are sometimes difficult to distinguish; they may be nutritional or obstructive or may be related to the effects of metastatic disease on other organ systems. Patients who have survived colon carcinoma experience a relatively high quality of life although some have reported ongoing problems with diarrhea and depression.[305]

Therapeutic Trends

Current therapies are unsatisfactory for patients with stage III and IV tumors, and the failure to consider CRC when a teenager has diffuse abdominal discomfort or mass adds to the problem. Surgery is the only modality known to be curative, although adjuvant chemotherapy extends life. Few patients with extensive metastatic disease are cured, although options for their treatment have improved with the approval of several new agents, including irinotecan, oxaliplatin, and the monoclonal antibodies cetuximab and bevacizumab. Other, more specific targeted agents, such as erlotinib, PTK785, gefitinib, and panitumumab, may soon follow.[306,307]

Annual colonoscopy has been recommended for individuals at high risk of primary or recurrent CRC. For children, this procedure should probably be performed once every 2 years. Screening of pediatric patients for fecal occult blood has not proved to be of significant value.

MSI is a distinct pattern of genetic alteration in tumor DNA characterized by general instability of short, tandem repeats of DNA sequences known as *microsatellites*.[308] This pattern is found in most hereditary nonpolyposis colorectal cancers.[309] In a study of 607 adults with CRC, 17% had MSI. These patients were more likely than others to be in a young age group at diagnosis, have poorly differentiated or right-sided tumors, have a higher risk of metachronous tumors, and have a favorable prognosis. The survival advantage was independent of all standard prognostic factors, including tumor stage, and patients with MSI had less likelihood of metastasis to regional lymph nodes.[309] In contrast, Datta et al. of Memorial Sloan-Kettering Cancer Center reported MSI in 6 of 13 children younger than 21 years at diagnosis. They found neither an improved prognosis nor any distinct histologic or clinical features associated with MSI.[280] These results may indicate that other molecular events account for the development of CRC in children. More study is needed. It is conceivable that continued research will allow the molecular characterization of tumors and the customized tailoring of therapy in the near future.[310,311] Observations that nonsteroidal antiinflammatory drugs (NSAIDs) inhibit the growth of colon tumors in various animal models encourage the hope that one day CRC will be preventable. Inhibition of the cyclooxygenase enzyme pathway is thought to be responsible for these effects, although the exact mechanism is still the subject of intense research.[312,313] The chemopreventive effects of NSAIDs on CRC have been investigated in a number of trials in humans. Most of the randomized studies have been investigations of FAP. For example, in a randomized, double-blind, placebo-controlled study in 22 patients with FAP, the NSAID sulindac, a nonselective cyclooxygenase inhibitor, reduced both the number and the size of colorectal adenomas.[314] However, the long-term gastrointestinal effects of sulindac argue against its widespread use. Another trial with celecoxib, a more specific cyclooxygenase-2 (COX-2) inhibitor with a more favorable toxicity profile, was shown to have the same effect.[315] Other epidemiologic studies are consistent with these findings. For example, in a prospective mortality study of 662,424 adults, death rate from colon cancer decreased as the frequency of aspirin use increased in both men and women.[316] In an extension of these results in another trial, 1,561 subjects who had adenomas removed within 3 months of enrollment were randomly assigned to celecoxib ($n = 933$) or placebo ($n = 638$). Celecoxib reduced the rate of advanced adenomas detected through 3 years compared with those who received placebo (5.3% vs. 10.4%; relative risk, 0.49; 95% confidence interval, 0.33 to 0.73; $p < 0.001$).[317] Unfortunately, patients in the celecoxib group also experienced an increase in serious cardiovascular events. These results led to the approval of celecoxib as a preventative agent for CRC in high-risk patients with FAP. Although these trials confirm an association between the COX-2 enzyme and development of precancerous lesions of the colon, they cannot be routinely recommended for CRC prevention because of the associated increase in risk of serious cardiovascular events. Other agents being evaluated include polyamine inhibitors, bile salts, statins, complex dietary interventions, and micronutrients such as organoselenium, calcium, and vitamins E, C, and D.[318,319]

PAPILLARY SEROUS CARCINOMA OF THE PERITONEUM

Papillary serous carcinoma of the peritoneum is an unusual tumor that may arise on the surface of the ovaries and spread to the omentum and the abdominal and pelvic peritoneum.[320–322] This tumor has also been called *multifocal extraovarian serous carcinoma, serous borderline tumor of the peritoneum,* and *serous surface carcinoma of the peritoneum.*

The tumor rarely affects adolescents and resembles papillary carcinoma of the ovaries in adults.[323,324] The presenting signs are abdominal distension and pain. Serum CA125 may be elevated at presentation in some patients.[325] Treatment usually consists of debulking and cisplatin-based therapy,[320] with or without paclitaxel.[323] Heated intraoperative and early postoperative intraperitoneal chemotherapy has also been used in selected patients.[326] The prognosis for long-term survival is poor, yet individuals may have an indolent course with recurrences over many years. The differential diagnosis includes mesothelioma of the peritoneum and surface carcinoma of the ovary.

CARCINOMA OF THE BLADDER

Bladder cancer is an occupationally acquired industrial disease and cigarette smoking is associated with two- or threefold excess risk. Thus, primary carcinomas of the bladder are extremely rare in childhood.[327,328] The most frequent bladder cancer in children is rhabdomyosarcoma (see Chapter 31). A review of literature revealed fewer than 30 cases of bladder carcinoma in children younger than 10 years. As in adults, there is a male predominance with ratios ranging from 3:1 to 9:1 and exposure to paternal cigarette smoking may be associated with increased risk of developing this cancer.[329–331] The most common carcinoma is transitional cell carcinoma, which may be encountered as a second malignant neoplasm after extensive treatment with cyclophosphamide.[332–334] A case of transitional cell carcinoma has been described in association with the Costello syndrome.[335] Transitional cell carcinoma of the bladder in children must be distinguished from a separate entity called papillary urothelial neoplasm of low malignant potential (PUNLMP), which, using the 2004 WHO Bladder Consensus Classification, may account for up to 40% of pediatric bladder neoplasms previously diagnosed as carcinomas.[330] The main presenting symptom or urothelial neoplasms is usually gross, painless hematuria. The tumors appear as pedunculated lesions; most patients have PUNLMP or grade I transitional cell carcinoma, and surgical resection via cystoscopy is usually possible. The general principles of staging and treatment are the same for children and adolescents and for adults. Finally, although rare, inflammatory pseudotumor of the bladder must be included in the differential diagnosis of bladder neoplasms.[336]

CERVICAL, VAGINAL, AND VULVAR TUMORS

Tumors of the cervix, vagina, and vulva are extremely rare in children and adolescents.[337–339] Rhabdomyosarcoma is the most common tumor in these sites, yet squamous cell tumors may also occur. Cervical squamous cell carcinoma is observed more frequently with increasing age, through adolescence.[340] Infection with HPV oncogenic types 16 and 18 is the most significant risk/causative factor in cervical cancer etiology. In 2006, Merck's quadrivalent vaccine was approved by the Food and Drug Administration. It targets four HPV types (6, 11, 16, and 18) that are involved in cervical cancer, high- and low-grade squamous intraepithelial lesions, and anogenital warts. Results from combined Phase II/III studies show an efficacy rate of 95% to 100% against low- and high-grade squamous intraepithelial lesions caused by HPV 16 and 18 and that the vaccine use led to a 99% reduction in the incidence of genital warts (related to HPV 6 and 11).[341] The Advisory Committee on Immunization Practices recommends HPV immunization to all girls aged 11 to 12 years, and this practice is expected to decrease the burden of HPV-related disease.[342] Cervical carcinoma has also been described in association with the use of radiation therapy in survivors of pediatric pelvic tumors.[343]

Adenocarcinomas accounts for less than 10% of all primary vaginal malignancies. However, in female patients younger than 20 years, adenocarcinomas account for almost all vaginal carcinomas. Approximately 70% of adenocarcinomas of the cervix and vagina in young patients are clear cell adenocarcinomas, an entity that in the 1970s was linked with intrauterine exposure to diethylstilbestrol. Mesonephric adenocarcinomas account for the remaining 30% of the cases.[344] A review of 38 reported pediatric cases of clear cell carcinoma and mesonephric adenocarcinoma of the cervix or vagina revealed that the most common presenting symptom was vaginal bleeding and that the median age at diagnosis was 15 years. Most patients were white (89%), and 62% reported a history of exposure to diethylstilbestrol. The vagina was the most common primary site, and 20% of the patients had metastatic disease (most commonly pelvic and para-aortic nodes). Surgical resection with nodal exploration is the treatment of choice and yields a long-term survival rate above 70%.[344] The role of radiation is not clearly defined. Other tumors of these sites include carcinomas, papillomas, nodular fasciitis, and sweat gland tumors. Their appropriate treatment depends on the site, stage, and pathologic features.

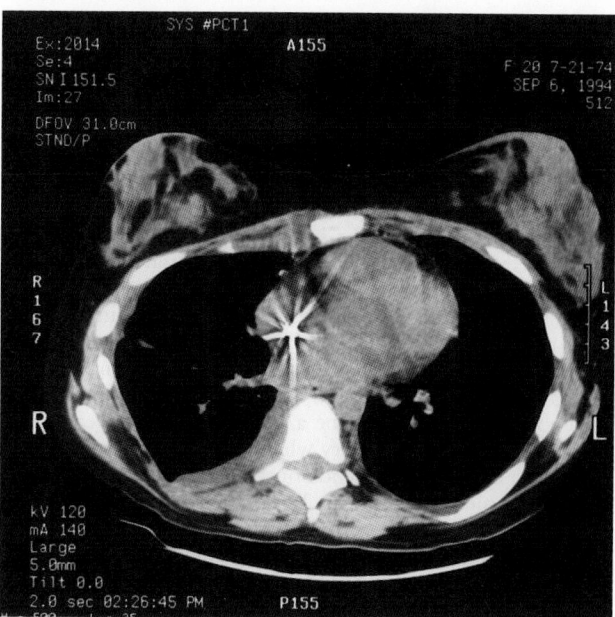

FIGURE 37.5 Axial noncontrast computed tomographic scans of the thorax demonstrating multiple bilateral breast metastases of a paraspinal alveolar rhabdomyosarcoma in a 20-year-old woman. A right pleural effusion and erosion of a right posterior rib are also seen.

CANCER OF THE BREAST

Breast tumors of children and adolescents are usually benign; only about 0.2% of primary breast carcinomas occur before age 20 years.[345] A review of the SEER registry data from 1973 to 2004 revealed only 75 cases of breast cancer occurring in females 19 years of age or younger, for an annual age-adjusted incidence of 0.08 cases per 100,000.[346] Only 15% of the cases were considered to be in-situ malignancies, whereas the remaining were invasive. Carcinomas (mostly of the ductal type) accounted for 55% of the cases, whereas sarcomas accounted for the remaining cases. Most sarcomas (85%) were phyllodes tumors, with the remaining cases being fibrosarcoma, leiomyosarcoma, rhabdomyosarcoma, and hemangiosarcoma. Carcinomas were regionally advanced in 26% of the cases, and 7% of the patients had distant metastases. In contrast, all sarcomatous lesions were localized. The 5-year survival estimates were 89% for sarcomas and 63% for carcinomas.[346]

A breast mass in a young boy or girl may arise from normal and abnormal breast development. Other causes of masses include infection, trauma, and cyst formation. After onset of puberty, most cases of breast enlargement arise from benign fibroadenoma in girls and gynecomastia in boys.[347,348] Other cancers such as rhabdomyosarcoma, neuroblastoma, leukemia, or lymphoma may originate in the breast (Fig. 37.5).[349-351] Breast carcinomas can affect either males or females. Secondary neoplasms, which include carcinomas, can also affect the breasts. These tumors generally follow radiation therapy delivered to the chest to treat lymphoma (usually Hodgkin disease); survivors of Hodgkin disease have significantly increased risk of breast cancer that is more than 20 times that of age- and race-matched controls.[352,353] Another rare tumor of the breast is cystosarcoma phyllodes, which can mimic a giant fibroadenoma. Phyllodes tumors are rare and unique in their suspected stromal and epithelial origin and their propensity to recur despite surgical resection. Current surgical treatment of this sarcoma does not include sampling of regional lymph nodes as it infrequently spreads to the

lymph nodes.[354,355] This tumor has been reported to metastasize in as many as 9% of adults; additional therapy is usually reserved for multiple recurrences or very large tumors, giant fibroadenomas, which may occur after puberty. These tumors may be disfiguring or may cause pressure necrosis of the skin and should be resected to rule out malignancy and preserve breast architecture.

It is difficult to make general recommendations about surgery, radiation therapy, and chemotherapy for breast carcinoma in children and adolescents.[356] However, invasive breast cancer that occurs in young women is often more aggressive than in other patients and has a worse prognosis.[357] In addition, young women who undergo breast-conserving surgery are at higher risk of local recurrence than others.[358] For this reason, aggressive surgery and adjuvant therapy that includes doxorubicin and docetaxel should be strongly considered, regardless of lymph node status.[359] Breast cancer in children is even more unusual than in older adolescents and may have a less aggressive course.

Epidemiologic studies of breast cancer aggregation in families with Li-Fraumeni syndrome have been discussed in Chapter 2.[360] The most important risk factor for the development of breast cancer is a family history of breast cancer. Germline mutations in the breast cancer–associated genes 1 and 2 (*BRCA1* and *BRCA2*) account for many of these hereditary cases.[361]

CARCINOID TUMORS

Carcinoid tumors occur in 1 to 1.42 children per million younger than 15 years,[362] are more common in females, and occur commonly in the appendix in most pediatric series.[362-364] In larger adult series, most occur in the small intestine (45%), but they can occur in the bronchi or elsewhere in the bowel.[365] These tumors are of epithelial origin and may be benign or malignant.[366,367] A carcinoid tumor is found in approximately 1 in 200 appendices removed because of acute appendicitis. Generally, these tumors require no treatment unless there is evidence of metastatic spread to lymph nodes or omentum or a tumor size greater than 2 cm.[368] These tumors are derived from chromaffin cells and are able to secrete vasoactive peptides such as serotonin. Elevated blood concentration of these vasoactive peptides may produce symptoms referred to as the *carcinoid syndrome*.[363,369] Affected patients have periodic flushing, diarrhea, bronchial constriction, peripheral vasomotor symptoms, and cyanosis. These symptoms and signs are attributed to circulating 5-hydroxytryptamine (serotonin) and histamine. These tumors secrete various tachykinins and other hormones, including insulin, serotonin, gastrin, vasoactive intestinal peptide, and corticotropin.[370] The urine concentration of 5-hydroxyindoleacetic acid, a serotonin metabolite, is often elevated. Plasma levels of chromogranin A may also be a useful tumor marker.[371] The treatment of choice is surgery when possible. The appropriate diagnostic evaluation depends on the tumor site. Octreotide scans and measurement of 24-hour urinary excretion of 5-hydroxyindoleacetic acid or other hormones or tumor markers such as chromogranin A may confirm the diagnosis.

If the tumor is malignant and has spread in a manner similar to CRC, chemotherapy (usually doxorubicin-based) may be beneficial to some patients.[372] However, combination chemotherapy has not improved overall survival. Treatment is usually focused on control of symptoms by use of somatostatin analogues, such as octreotide and ondansetron.[373] Regional ileocolectomy has been advocated for carcinoid tumor that extends to the mesoappendix and serosal fat, when adequate surgical resection margins are uncertain or unfeasible.

Although malignant carcinoid is rare, it may present with massive hepatic enlargement, metastases, and the carcinoid syndrome. Carcinoid tumor is rarely suspected at the time of initial presentation, and therefore the diagnosis may be delayed. Patients who have metastatic disease at diagnosis fare poorly. Complete surgical resection remains the only chance for cure. Other options include laser treatment, radiofrequency ablation, and chemoembolization.[374] Octreotide and its analogs may palliate the symptoms, and in some patients they result in significant clinical responses.[375]

Bronchial carcinoids are neuroendocrine tumors that arise from Kulchitsky cells in the bronchial mucosa. The carcinoid syndrome is rarely seen in these patients. They often present with evidence of obstructive bronchial disease or pneumonia. These tumors should be considered in the differential diagnosis of persistent cough, pneumonitis, wheezing, or hemoptysis.[370] Although most bronchial carcinoid tumors are not malignant, lobectomy may be necessary for tumor resection.

CHORDOMA

This rare primary bone tumor has an annual incidence rate of less than 0.1 per 100,000 per year in adults, afflicting about 25 persons in the United States annually.[376] About 5% of chordomas occur in children.[377] This neoplasm arises from notochordal remnants in the midline of the neuraxis and involves adjacent bone. In children, chordomas most often involve the skull base, but other sites such as coccyx and sacrum can be involved.[377-379] The most common complaints of patients with sacrococcygeal tumors are pain, constipation, and sensory loss. Patients with cranial chordomas present with symptoms of increased intracranial pressure, long tract signs, and cranial nerve palsies.[378] The conventional and chondroid variants of chordoma predominate in older children, whereas patients younger than 5 years have a higher incidence of atypical or poorly differentiated histology, a feature that is associated with a very poor prognosis.[378,380] Chordomas have frequent loss of 1p36, evidence of microsatellite instability, and PDGFRβ overexpression and activation.[376,381] Surgical removal and postoperative radiotherapy are the main treatment modalities for this disease. Newer radiation therapy techniques, such as proton-beam and intensity-modulated radiotherapy, have produced encouraging results in several adult and pediatric series.[382,383] Chordomas are not sensitive to chemotherapy, but the use of the tyrosine kinase inhibitor imatinib mesylate has produced encouraging responses in 44 adults with chordoma.[384] The effects of imatinib might be explained by inhibition of an autocrine/paracrine loop that involves PDGFRβ, PDGFRα, and KIT.[381] Long-term survival for pediatric patients with chordoma ranges from 65% to 80%, but patients younger than 5 years fare worse. The most common sites of metastases are lung, liver, bones, and lymph nodes.[377,378]

CANCER OF UNKNOWN PRIMARY SITE

This group of malignancies is characterized by the presence of metastatic disease in the absence of clinical evidence of a primary tumor despite a standardized diagnostic evaluation.[385] The SEER data estimates that 31,500 such cases (about 2% of all malignancies) were diagnosed in the United States in 2008.[159] In adults, the most frequent cancer of unknown primary site (CUP) tumors are adenocarcinoma (50%), undifferentiated or poorly differentiated carcinoma (30%), squamous cell carcinoma (15%), and undifferentiated neoplasm (5%). The latter group has been better characterized in recent years and includes neuroendocrine tumors, lymphomas, germ cell tumors, sarcomas, and embryonal malignancies.[386] In children, the most common CUP tumors are melanoma and embryonal malignancies such as rhabdomyosarcoma, neuroblastoma, and Ewing's sarcoma.[387] Immunocytochemistry, electron microscopy, and serum markers can aid in the diagnosis. A primary site can be detected with the use of CT in as many as 35% of adult patients with CUP, and PET scanning is particularly useful in identifying occult primary tumors in the head and neck area.[385] However, despite the availability of these diagnostic tools, a primary site is identified antemortem in less than 20% of patients.[385] More recently, molecular profiling of CUP has been successfully conducted in 87% of 120 biopsy specimens of adults with CUP and identified a putative origin, most commonly lung, pancreas, and colon cancer.[386] Treatment should be based on the results of the diagnostic imaging and pathology studies, regardless of knowledge of the primary site. Prompt initiation of treatment may lead to clinical response and occasional cures.[387]

CANCERS OF THE SKIN

In 2008, more than 1 million new cases of basal cell and squamous cell carcinoma and more than 62,000 cases of melanoma were diagnosed in the United States.[159] Basal cell carcinoma is the most common skin cancer in adults and accounts for 80% of the cases and for about one-fourth of all cancers diagnosed in the United States.[388] The mortality rate for basal and squamous cell carcinoma is low, but for melanoma is high, with more than 8,000 deaths from the disease in 2008.[159]

The most common risk factors associated with basal cell and squamous cell carcinomas is ultraviolet radiation.[16] These cancers are usually curable with surgery and radiation therapy and are not discussed at length in this chapter. The small molecule inhibitor GDC-09449, which targets the hedgehog pathway, has recently shown promising clinical activity in a trial of 33 adult patients with metastatic or locally advanced basal cell carcinoma.[389]

Epidemiology of Melanoma

Childhood melanoma is rare, accounting for less than 3% of all pediatric malignancies and for 0.9% of all cases of melanoma.[390] Despite this, the incidence of melanoma in the pediatric population has increased by 2.9% per year from the period 1973–2001.[391] Melanoma is extremely rare during the prepubertal years, but it accounts for 7.1% of all cancers in patients 15 to 19 years of age.[392] Melanoma in children is more common during the second decade of life, more commonly affects whites and females, often arises in the extremities or torso, is predominantly of the superficial spreading subtype, and is localized in 80% of the cases.[391] Patients younger than 10 years are more commonly nonwhite, have a predominance of head and neck primaries, nodular histology, advanced stage disease, and a history of cancer in the family.[391] The following contributing factors, or conditions, are associated with the development of pediatric melanoma:

1. Congenital and infantile melanoma: The majority develop before birth or during the first year of life and arise from medium-sized or giant congenital nevi.[393] Melanoma is the most common transplacentally acquired malignancy in newborns (six documented cases), and the affected infants have a very poor outcome.[394] Unaffected infants of mothers who have placental metastases should be closely evaluated during routine well-child visits and should have a chest radiograph, liver function tests, and lactate dehydrogenase assay at 6-month intervals during the first 2 years postpartum.

2. Giant congenital melanocytic nevi affect fewer than 1 in 20,000 newborns and are precursor lesions of melanoma (Fig. 37.6).[395] The lifetime risk of melanoma in these patients is estimated to be 4.1% to 8.5%.[395–397] The melanomas may arise in noncutaneous sites, including the central nervous system and retroperitoneum.[395] The vast majority of melanomas in these patients develop during the first decade of life, and the risk of melanoma appears to be increased in patients with larger size nevi and an increased number of satellite nevi.[398]

3. Xeroderma pigmentosum is a rare (annual incidence, 1 in 500,000), inherited excisional DNA repair disorder characterized by photosensitivity, neurologic abnormalities, and a greater than 1,000-fold increase in the risk of skin cancer including melanoma.[399] Melanomas in these patients occur at a median age of 19 years and most commonly involve the face, the head, and the neck.[17,400]

4. Werner syndrome: An autosomal recessive disorder characterized by premature aging and caused by mutations of the WRN gene, which belongs to the REcQ family of helicases. Melanomas in these patients occur in unusual locations such as feet, nasal cavity, and esophagus.[401,402]

5. Immunosuppression and history of malignancy: Children with immunodeficiencies have a risk of melanoma three to six times that of others, and those with Hodgkin disease have an eightfold risk.[397] Melanoma has also been described after renal transplantation, after administration of immunosuppressive therapy, and after solid organ and bone marrow transplantation.[403,404] Survivors of hereditary retinoblastoma are also at increased risk of developing melanoma.[405]

6. Neurocutaneous melanosis is a rare syndrome characterized by large or multiple congenital nevi associated with

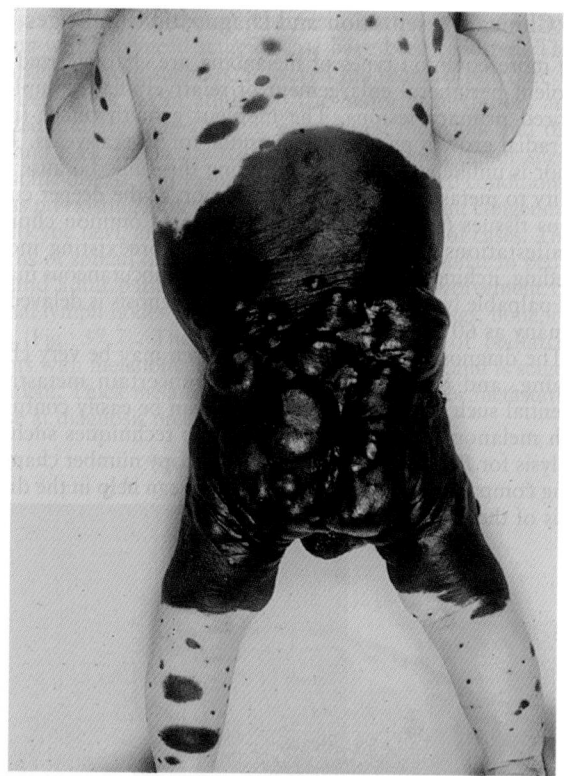

FIGURE 37.6 Giant pigmented nevus in a 2-year-old child. Notice the "bathing trunk" pattern of the nevus, the verrucous appearance of the nevus, and the presence of numerous satellites.

meningeal melanosis or melanoma.[395,406] Most patients have giant pigmented lesions along the posterior midline or in the head and neck region. In symptomatic cases, neurologic manifestations including hydrocephalus, seizures, papilledema, headaches, and mental retardation are evident by age 2 years. Prognosis is poor; leptomeningeal melanoma develops in 64% of patients, and only 18% are long-term survivors.[407] An asymptomatic form of neurocutaneous melanosis characterized by brain abnormalities evident on MRI (T1 shortening in the amygdala, cerebellum, or pons) has recently been described and affects 23% of patients with large nevi of the dorsal spine or scalp. Only 1 of 46 patients evaluated developed neurologic symptoms.[408]

7. Environmental and genetic factors: An estimated 44% of melanomas in people younger than 30 years arise in a small nevus that was present at birth or during early childhood.[409] Environmental and genetic factors associated with the development of melanoma in children and adolescents include skin pigmentation, number of melanocytic nevi, tanning ability, freckling, race, and sex.[410,411]

8. Dysplastic nevi or clinically atypical moles affect as much as 5% of the U. S. population and are potential precursors of melanoma, thus defining a population at high risk of early onset melanoma.[412] Inactivating germ-line mutations of the *CDKN2 A* gene, which encodes the tumor suppressor p16 and P14ARF, have been described in as many as 40% of families in which three or more first-degree relatives have melanoma and in 15% of patients with multiple primary melanomas.[413] However, the incidence of *CDKN2 A* mutations in sporadic early onset melanoma is very low (1.6%).[414] Individuals with germ-line *CDKN2 A* mutations are also at increased risk of pancreatic cancer.[200]

Treatment of Primary Disease

Surgical Resection. As in adults, early detection and early surgical removal of primary melanoma are the most effective treatment for children. Suspect skin lesions (i.e., those with irregular borders, pigmentation, or texture) should be surgically removed and examined histopathologically. If melanoma is documented, the invasiveness and depth of the lesion should be determined. Lesions 1 mm or less in thickness should be resected with a 1-cm margin; those 1 to 4 mm thick are excised with a 2-cm margin. To minimize the risk of local recurrence, margins of at least 2 cm are recommended for lesions greater than 4 mm in thickness.[426]

Adjuvant Therapy. The role of adjuvant therapy in pediatric melanoma has not been prospectively studied. Two single-institution trials have confirmed that the administration of high-dose interferon is feasible in pediatric patients.[427,428] Four consecutive multicenter randomized trials in adults conducted by the Eastern Cooperative Oncology Group have documented a statistically significant improvement in relapse-free survival among patients with high-risk resected melanoma who were treated with high-dose adjuvant interferon alpha 2b.[429] Because of the unavailability of clinical trials of adjuvant therapy for children with melanoma, the Children's Oncology Group is participating in one Intergroup Southwest Oncology Group (SWOG) trial of adjuvant therapy for adults with high-risk melanoma.

Treatment of Disseminated Disease

Chemotherapy. Few chemotherapy trials for pediatric melanoma have been conducted. Dacarbazine has been used before surgery with encouraging results in four children with melanoma.[430] Hayes and Green reported responses to vincristine, dactinomycin, and cyclophosphamide in seven of nine children with advanced-stage melanoma.[431] In adults, dacarbazine and temozolomide produce objective response rates in less than 15% of patients.[432] In a randomized adult trial, the combination of taxol and carboplatin with or without sorafenib produced responses in less than 15% of patients.[433]

Interleukin 2 and Biochemotherapy. Interleukin 2 (IL-2) has modest activity against adult melanoma,[434] and two pediatric trials that used IL-2 for refractory disease failed to show any significant activity against melanoma.[435,436] The use of biochemotherapy that combines cisplatin, vinblastine, dacarbazine, interferon, and IL-2 has not been prospectively studied in pediatric melanoma; however, in adults with metastatic disease, this therapy has failed to show a survival benefit when compared with chemotherapy alone.[437]

Newer Therapies. In adults, the molecular classification of melanoma is becoming a reality and therapies that target the *KIT* and *BRAF* oncogenes will increasingly play a role in the treatment of this disease.[438,439]

Adoptive immunotherapy using autologous tumor-infiltrating lymphocytes has shown promise in selected adults patients with metastatic melanoma,[440] and cytotoxic T lymphocyte-associated antigen 4 (CTLA4) blockade with tremelimumab has produced responses in 10% of adults with metastatic melanoma.[441]

Nevoid Basal Cell Carcinoma Syndrome (Gorlin Syndrome)

Gorlin syndrome is an autosomal dominant disorder characterized by developmental abnormalities, including rib and craniofacial anomalies, odontogenic keratocysts of jaws, epidermal skin cysts, and palmar or plantar pits (Fig. 37.8). In addition, these patients are prone to the development of various tumors, including fibromas of the ovaries and heart. Medulloblastoma is also diagnosed in approximately 5% of patients with Gorlin syndrome, and as many as 10% of patients with medulloblastoma are estimated to have Gorlin syndrome. The *patched* gene at chromosome band 9q22, which is mutated in Gorlin syndrome, influences development by regulating transcription of several genes, including *gli*, members of the tumor growth factor b family, and the Wnt family of transcription factors.[442]

References

1. Ferrari A, Bisogno G, De Salvo GL, et al. The challenge of very rare tumours in childhood: the Italian TREP project. Eur J Cancer 2007;43:654–659.
2. Edge SB, Byrd DR, Compton CC, et al. AJCC cancer staging manual. New York, Springer, 2010.
3. Trobs RB, Mader E, Friedrich T, et al. Oral tumors and tumor-like lesions in infants and children. Pediatr Surg Int 2003;19:639–645.
4. Ulmansky M, Lustmann J, Balkin N. Tumors and tumor-like lesions of the oral cavity and related structures in Israeli children. Int J Oral Maxillofac Surg 1999;28:291–294.
5. Das S, Das AK. A review of pediatric oral biopsies from a surgical pathology service in a dental school. Pediatr Dent 1993;15:208–211.
6. Tanaka N, Murata A, Yamaguchi A, et al. Clinical features and management of oral and maxillofacial tumors in children. Oral Surg Oral Med Oral Pathol Oral Radiol Endod 1999;88:11–15.
7. Silverman S Jr. Demographics and occurrence of oral and pharyngeal cancers. The outcomes, the trends, the challenge. J Am Dent Assoc 2001;132(suppl):7S–11S.
8. Napier SS, Speight PM. Natural history of potentially malignant oral lesions and conditions: an overview of the literature. J Oral Pathol Med 2008;37:1–10.
9. Warren CW, Jones NR, Eriksen MP, et al. Patterns of global tobacco use in young people and implications for future chronic disease burden in adults. Lancet 2006;367: 749–753.
10. D'Souza G, Agrawal Y, Halpern J, et al. Oral sexual behaviors associated with prevalent oral human papillomavirus infection. J Infect Dis 2009;199:1263–1269.
11. Vidal L, Gillison ML. Human papillomavirus in HNSCC: recognition of a distinct disease type. Hematol Oncol Clin North Am 2008;22:1125–1142, vii.
12. Smith EM, Swarnavel S, Ritchie JM, et al. Prevalence of human papillomavirus in the oral cavity/oropharynx in a large population of children and adolescents. Pediatr Infect Dis J 2007;26:836–840.
13. Lassen P, Eriksen JG, Hamilton-Dutoit S, et al. Effect of HPV-associated p16INK4 A expression on response to radiotherapy and survival in squamous cell carcinoma of the head and neck. J Clin Oncol 2009;27:1992–1998.
14. Fakhry C, Westra WH, Li S, et al. Improved survival of patients with human papillomavirus-positive head and neck squamous cell carcinoma in a prospective clinical trial. J Natl Cancer Inst 2008;100:261–269.

15. Ragin CC, Modugno F, Gollin SM. The epidemiology and risk factors of head and neck cancer: a focus on human papillomavirus. J Dent Res 2007;86:104–114.
16. Fine JD, Johnson LB, Weiner M, et al. Epidermolysis bullosa and the risk of life-threatening cancers: the National EB Registry experience, 1986–2006. J Am Acad Dermatol 2009;60:203–211.
17. Kraemer KH, Lee MM, Scotto J. Xeroderma pigmentosum: cutaneous, ocular, and neurologic abnormalities in 830 published cases. Arch Dermatol 1987;123:241–250.
18. Blanche PA. Cancer in Fanconi anemia, 1927–2001. Cancer 2003;97:425–440.
19. Mazereeuw-Hautier J, Bitoun E, Chevrant-Breton J, et al. Keratitis-ichthyosis-deafness syndrome: disease expression and spectrum of connexin 26 (GJB2) mutations in 14 patients. Br J Dermatol 2007;156:1015–1019.
20. Alter BP, Giri N, Savage SA, et al. Cancer in dyskeratosis congenita. Blood 2009; 113(26):6549–6557.
21. Vermorken JB, Remenar E, van Herpen C, et al. Cisplatin, fluorouracil, and docetaxel in unresectable head and neck cancer. N Engl J Med 2007;357:1695–1704.
22. French CA. Molecular pathology of NUT midline carcinomas. J Clin Pathol 2010;63: 492–496.
23. French CA, Kutok JL, Faquin WC, et al. Midline carcinoma of children and young adults with NUT rearrangement. J Clin Oncol 2004;22:4135–4139.
24. Stelow EB, Bellizzi AM, Taneja K, et al. NUT rearrangement in undifferentiated carcinomas of the upper aerodigestive tract. Am J Surg Pathol 2008;32:828–834.
25. Spano JP, Busson P, Atlan D, et al. Nasopharyngeal carcinomas: an update. Eur J Cancer 2003;39:2121–2135.
26. Richey LM, Olshan AF, George J, et al. Incidence and survival rates for young blacks with nasopharyngeal carcinoma in the United States. Arch Otolaryngol Head Neck Surg 2006;132:1035–1040.
27. Greene MH, Fraumeni JF, Hoover R. Nasopharyngeal cancer among young people in the United States: racial variations by cell type. J Natl Cancer Inst 1977;58:1267–1270.
28. Ayan I, Kaytan E, Ayan N. Childhood nasopharyngeal carcinoma: from biology to treatment. Lancet Oncol 2003;4:13–21.
29. Neel HB III, Pearson GR, Taylor WF. Antibodies to Epstein-Barr virus in patients with nasopharyngeal carcinoma and in comparison groups. Ann Otol Rhinol Laryngol 1984;93:477–482.

30. Niedobitek G, Agathanggelou A, Nicholls JM. Epstein-Barr virus infection and the pathogenesis of nasopharyngeal carcinoma: viral gene expression, tumour cell phenotype, and the role of the lymphoid stroma. Semin Cancer Biol 1996;7:165–174.
31. Huang DP, Ho HC, Henle W, et al. Presence of EBNA in nasopharyngeal carcinoma and control patient tissues related to EBV serology. Int J Cancer 1978;22:266–274.
32. Vasef MA, Ferlito A, Weiss LM. Nasopharyngeal carcinoma, with emphasis on its relationship to Epstein-Barr virus. Ann Otol Rhinol Laryngol 1997;106:348–356.
33. Pagano JS. Epstein-Barr virus: the first human tumor virus and its role in cancer. Proc Assoc Am Physicians 1999;111:573–580.
34. Roebuck DJ. Skeletal complications in pediatric oncology patients. Radiographics 1999;19:873–885.
35. Bass IS, Haller JO, Berdon WE, et al. Nasopharyngeal carcinoma: clinical and radiographic findings in children. Radiology 1985;156:651–654.
36. Witt TR, Shah JP, Sternberg SS. Juvenile nasopharyngeal angiofibroma. A 30 year clinical review. Am J Surg 1983;146:521–525.
37. Lo YM, Chan AT, Chan LY, et al. Molecular prognostication of nasopharyngeal carcinoma by quantitative analysis of circulating Epstein-Barr virus DNA. Cancer Res 2000; 60:6878–6881.
38. Wong TS, Kwong DL, Sham JS, et al. Quantitative plasma hypermethylated DNA markers of undifferentiated nasopharyngeal carcinoma. Clin Cancer Res 2004;10: 2401–2406.
39. Perez CA, Devineni VR, Marcial-Vega V, et al. Carcinoma of the nasopharynx: factors affecting prognosis. Int J Radiat Oncol Biol Phys 1992;23:271–280.
40. Ozyar E, Selek U, Laskar S, et al. Treatment results of 165 pediatric patients with nonmetastatic nasopharyngeal carcinoma: a rare cancer network study. Radiother Oncol 2006;81:39–46.
41. Rodriguez-Galindo C, Wofford M, Castleberry RP, et al. Preradiation chemotherapy with methotrexate, cisplatin, 5-fluorouracil, and leucovorin for pediatric nasopharyngeal carcinoma. Cancer 2005;103:850–857.
42. Mertens R, Granzen B, Lassay L, et al. Nasopharyngeal carcinoma in childhood and adolescence: concept and preliminary results of the cooperative GPOH study NPC-91. Gesellschaft fur Padiatrische Onkologie und Hamatologie. Cancer 1997;80:951–959.
43. Orbach D, Brisse H, Helfre S, et al. Radiation and chemotherapy combination for nasopharyngeal carcinoma in children: radiotherapy dose adaptation after chemotherapy response to minimize late effects. Pediatr Blood Cancer 2008;50:849–853.
44. Leibel SA, Fuks Z, Zelefsky MJ, et al. Intensity-modulated radiotherapy. Cancer J 2002;8:164–176.
45. Wolden SL, Zelefsky MJ, Hunt MA, et al. Failure of a 3D conformal boost to improve radiotherapy for nasopharyngeal carcinoma. Int J Radiat Oncol Biol Phys 2001;49: 1229–1234.
46. Lee N, Xia P, Quivey JM, et al. Intensity-modulated radiotherapy in the treatment of nasopharyngeal carcinoma: an update of the UCSF experience. Int J Radiat Oncol Biol Phys 2002;53:12–22.
47. Hsiung CY, Yorke ED, Chui CS, et al. Intensity-modulated radiotherapy versus conventional three-dimensional conformal radiotherapy for boost or salvage treatment of nasopharyngeal carcinoma. Int J Radiat Oncol Biol Phys 2002;53:638–647.
48. Langendijk JA, Leemans CR, Buter J, et al. The additional value of chemotherapy to radiotherapy in locally advanced nasopharyngeal carcinoma: a meta-analysis of the published literature. J Clin Oncol 2004;22:4604–4612.
49. Chan AT, Ma BB, Lo YM, et al. Phase II study of neoadjuvant carboplatin and paclitaxel followed by radiotherapy and concurrent cisplatin in patients with locoregionally advanced nasopharyngeal carcinoma: therapeutic monitoring with plasma Epstein-Barr virus DNA. J Clin Oncol 2004;22:3053–3060.
50. Straathof KC, Bollard CM, Popat U, et al. Treatment of nasopharyngeal carcinoma with Epstein-Barr virus–specific T lymphocytes. Blood 2005;105:1898–1904.
51. Comoli P, Pedrazzoli P, Maccario R, et al. Cell therapy of stage IV nasopharyngeal carcinoma with autologous Epstein-Barr virus-targeted cytotoxic T lymphocytes. J Clin Oncol 2005;23:8942–8949.
52. Bourhis J, Rosine D. Radioprotective effect of amifostine in patients with head and neck squamous cell carcinoma. Semin Oncol 2002;29:61–62.
53. Mendenhall WM, Werning JW, Fernandes R, et al. Ameloblastoma. Am J Clin Oncol 2007;30:645–648.
54. Ord RA, Blanchaert RH Jr, Nikitakis NG, et al. Ameloblastoma in children. J Oral Maxillofac Surg 2002;60:762–770; discussion 770–771.
55. Kumamoto H, Izutsu T, Ohki K, et al. p53 gene status and expression of p53, MDM2, and p14 proteins in ameloblastomas. J Oral Pathol Med 2004;33:292–299.
56. Sathi GA, Inoue M, Harada H, et al. Secreted frizzled related protein (sFRP)-2 inhibits bone formation and promotes cell proliferation in ameloblastoma. Oral Oncol 2009;45:856–860.
57. Sathi GS, Nagatsuka H, Tamamura R, et al. Stromal cells promote bone invasion by suppressing bone formation in ameloblastoma. Histopathology 2008;53:458–467.
58. Pogrel MA, Montes DM. Is there a role for enucleation in the management of ameloblastoma? Int J Oral Maxillofac Surg 2009;38:807–812.
59. Grunwald V, Le Blanc S, Karstens JH, et al. Metastatic malignant ameloblastoma responding to chemotherapy with paclitaxel and carboplatin. Ann Oncol 2001;12: 1489–1491.
60. Benlyazid A, Lacroix-Triki M, Aziza R, et al. Ameloblastic carcinoma of the maxilla: case report and review of the literature. Oral Surg Oral Med Oral Pathol Oral Radiol Endod 2007;104:e17–e24.
61. Johns ME, Goldsmith MM. Incidence, diagnosis, and classification of salivary gland tumors. Part 1. Oncology (Huntingt) 1989;3:47–56; discussion 56, 58, 62.
62. Neely MM, Rohrer MD, Young SK. Tumors of minor salivary glands and the analysis of 106 cases. J Okla Dent Assoc 1996;86:50–52.
63. Garrido A, Humphrey G, Squire RS, et al. Sialoblastoma. Br J Plast Surg 2000;53: 697–699.
64. Ellies M, Schaffranietz F, Arglebe C, et al. Tumors of the salivary glands in childhood and adolescence. J Oral Maxillofac Surg 2006;64:1049–1058.
65. Shapiro NL, Bhattacharyya N. Clinical characteristics and survival for major salivary gland malignancies in children. Otolaryngol Head Neck Surg 2006;134:631–634.
66. Laikui L, Hongwei L, Hongbing J, et al. Epithelial salivary gland tumors of children and adolescents in west China population: a clinicopathologic study of 79 cases. J Oral Pathol Med 2008;37:201–205.
67. Guzzo M, Ferrari A, marcon I, et al. Salivary gland neoplasms in children: the experience of the Istituto Nazionale Tumori of Milan. Pediatr Blood Cancer 2006;47:806–810.
68. Ron E, Saftlas AF. Head and neck radiation carcinogenesis: epidemiologic evidence. Otolaryngol Head Neck Surg 1996;115:403–408.
69. Vedrine PO, Coffinet L, Temam S, et al. Mucoepidermoid carcinoma of salivary glands in the pediatric age group: 18 clinical cases, including 11 second malignant neoplasms. Head Neck 2006;28:827–833.
70. Kaste SC, Hedlund G, Pratt CB. Malignant parotid tumors in patients previously treated for childhood cancer: clinical and imaging findings in eight cases. AJR Am J Roentgenol 1994;162:655–659.
71. Krolls SO, Trodahl JN, Boyers RC. Salivary gland lesions in children. A survey of 430 cases. Cancer 1972;30:459–469.
72. Luna MA, Batsakis JG, el-Naggar AK. Salivary gland tumors in children. Ann Otol Rhinol Laryngol 1991;100:869–871.
73. Johns ME, Goldsmith MM. Current management of salivary gland tumors. Part 2. Oncology (Huntingt) 1989;3:85–91; discussion 94, 99.
74. Vaughan ED. Management of malignant salivary gland tumours. Hosp Med 2001;62:400–405.
75. Kamal SA, Othman EO. Diagnosis and treatment of parotid tumours. J Laryngol Otol 1997;111:316–321.
76. El-Naggar AK, Lovell M, Killary AM, et al. A mucoepidermoid carcinoma of minor salivary gland with t(11;19)(q21;p13.1) as the only karyotypic abnormality. Cancer Genet Cytogenet 1996;87:29–33.
77. Kuo T, Hsueh C. Lymphoepithelioma-like salivary gland carcinoma in Taiwan: a clinicopathological study of nine cases demonstrating a strong association with Epstein-Barr virus. Histopathology 1997;31:75–82.
78. Tonon G, Modi S, Wu L, et al. t(11;19)(q21;p13) translocation in mucoepidermoid carcinoma creates a novel fusion product that disrupts a Notch signaling pathway. Nat Genet 2003;33:208–213.
79. Brandwein M, Al-Naeif NS, Manwani D, et al. Sialoblastoma: clinicopathological/ immunohistochemical study. Am J Surg Pathol 1999;23:342–348.
80. Siddiqui F, Sarin R, Agarwal JP, et al. Squamous carcinoma of the larynx and hypopharynx in children: a distinct clinical entity? Med Pediatr Oncol 2003;40:322–324.
81. Chow CW, Tabrizi SN, Tiedemann K, et al. Squamous cell carcinomas in children and young adults: a new wave of a very rare tumor? J Pediatr Surg 2007;42:2035–2039.
82. McGuirt WF Jr, Little JP. Laryngeal cancer in children and adolescents. Otolaryngol Clin North Am 1997;30:207–214.
83. Gabbott M, Cossart YE, Kan A, et al. Human papillomavirus and host variables as predictors of clinical course in patients with juvenile-onset recurrent respiratory papillomatosis. J Clin Microbiol 1997;35:3098–3103.
84. Chaput M, Ninane J, Gosseye S, et al. Juvenile laryngeal papillomatosis and epidermoid carcinoma. J Pediatr 1989;114:269–272.
85. Derkay CS, Wiatrak B. Recurrent respiratory papillomatosis: a review. Laryngoscope 2008;118:1236–1247.
86. Kendall KA. Current treatment for laryngeal papillomatosis. Curr Opin Otolaryngol Head Neck Surg 2004;12:157–159.
87. Fischer RA, Wharam MD, Kashima HK. Nasopharyngeal carcinoma in siblings. Ear Nose Throat J 1979;58:93–97.
88. Kashima H, Leventhal B, Clark K, et al. Interferon alfa-n1 (Wellferon) in juvenile onset recurrent respiratory papillomatosis: results of a randomized study in twelve collaborative institutions. Laryngoscope 1988;98:334–340.
89. Forastiere AA, Goepfert H, Maor M, et al. Concurrent chemotherapy and radiotherapy for organ preservation in advanced laryngeal cancer. N Engl J Med 2003;349:2091–2098.
90. Kantar M, Cetingul N, Veral A, et al. Rare tumors of the lung in children. Pediatr Hematol Oncol 2002;19:421–428.
91. Hartman GE, Shochat SJ. Primary pulmonary neoplasms of childhood: a review. Ann Thorac Surg 1983;36:108–119.
92. Dishop MK, Kuruvilla S. Primary and metastatic lung tumors in the pediatric population: a review and 25-year experience at a large children's hospital. Arch Pathol Lab Med 2008;132:1079–1103.
93. Ramalingam S, Pawlish K, Gadgeel S, et al. Lung cancer in young patients: analysis of a surveillance, epidemiology, and end results database. J Clin Oncol 1998;16:651–657.
94. Epstein DM, Aronchick JM. Lung cancer in childhood. Med Pediatr Oncol 1989;17: 510–513.
95. Lal DR, Clark I, Shalkow J, et al. Primary epithelial lung malignancies in the pediatric population. Pediatr Blood Cancer 2005;45:683–686.
96. Niitu Y, Kubota H, Hasegawa S, et al. Lung cancer (squamous cell carcinoma) in adolescence. Am J Dis Child 1974;127:108–111.
97. Dallimore NS. Squamous bronchial carcinoma arising in a case of multiple juvenile papillomatosis. Thorax 1985;40:797–798.
98. Gelinas JF, Manoukian J, Cote A. Lung involvement in juvenile onset recurrent respiratory papillomatosis: a systematic review of the literature. Int J Pediatr Otorhinolaryngol 2008;72:433–452.
99. Onn A, Vaporciyan A, Chang JY, et al. Cancer of the lung. In: Kufe DW Bast RC, Haiut WN, et al. eds. Cancer medicine. 7th ed. Hamilton, ON: Decker Inc., 2006:1179–1224.
100. Tajiri T, Suita S, Shono K, et al. Lung cancer in a child with a substantial family history of cancer. Eur J Pediatr Surg 1999;9:409–412.
101. Priest JR, McDermott MB, Bhatia S, et al. Pleuropulmonary blastoma: a clinicopathologic study of 50 cases. Cancer 1997;80:147–161.
102. Manivel JC, Priest JR, Watterson J, et al. Pleuropulmonary blastoma. The so-called pulmonary blastoma of childhood. Cancer 1988;62:1516–1526.
103. Priest JR, Hill DA, Williams GM, et al. Type I pleuropulmonary blastoma: a report from the International Pleuropulmonary Blastoma Registry. J Clin Oncol 2006;24: 4492–4498.
104. Hill DA, Jarzembowski JA, Priest JR, et al. Type I pleuropulmonary blastoma: pathology and biology study of 51 cases from the international pleuropulmonary blastoma registry. Am J Surg Pathol 2008;32:282–295.
105. Yang P, Hasegawa T, Hirose T, et al. Pleuropulmonary blastoma: fluorescence in situ hybridization analysis indicating trisomy 2. Am J Surg Pathol 1997;21:854–859.
106. Roque L, Rodrigues R, Martins C, et al. Comparative genomic hybridization analysis of a pleuropulmonary blastoma. Cancer Genet Cytogenet 2004;149:58–62.
107. Kusafuka T, Kuroda S, Inoue M, et al. P53 gene mutations in pleuropulmonary blastomas. Pediatr Hematol Oncol 2002;19:117–128.
108. Priest JR, Watterson J, Strong L, et al. Pleuropulmonary blastoma: a marker for familial disease. J Pediatr 1996;128:220–224.
109. Boman F, Hill DA, Williams GM, et al. Familial association of pleuropulmonary blastoma with cystic nephroma and other renal tumors: a report from the International Pleuropulmonary Blastoma Registry. J Pediatr 2006;149:850–854.
110. Hill DA, Ivanovich J, Priest JR, et al. DICER1 mutations in familial pleuropulmonary blastoma. Science 325:965, 2009.

111. Romeo C, Impellizzeri P, Grosso M, et al. Pleuropulmonary blastoma: long-term survival and literature review. Med Pediatr Oncol 1999;33:372–376.
112. Priest JR, Magnuson J, Williams GM, et al. Cerebral metastasis and other central nervous system complications of pleuropulmonary blastoma. Pediatr Blood Cancer 2007; 49:266–273.
113. Indolfi P, Bisogno G, Casale F, et al. Prognostic factors in pleuro-pulmonary blastoma. Pediatr Blood Cancer 2007;48:318–323.
114. Morgenthaler TI, Brown LR, Colby TV, et al. Thymoma. Mayo Clin Proc 1993;68: 1110–1123.
115. Loehrer PJ Sr, Wick MR. Thymic malignancies. Cancer Treat Res 2001;105:277–302.
116. Spigland N, Di Lorenzo M, Youssef S, et al. Malignant thymoma in children: a 20-year review. J Pediatr Surg 1990;25:1143–1146.
117. Rose JS, McCarthy J, Mutchler RW, et al. Thymoma in childhood. N Y State J Med 1978;78:82–84.
118. Thomas CR, Wright CD, Loehrer PJ. Thymoma: state of the art. J Clin Oncol 1999; 17:2280–2289.
119. Souadjian JV, Enriquez P, Silverstein MN, et al. The spectrum of diseases associated with thymoma. Coincidence or syndrome? Arch Intern Med 1974;134:374–379.
120. Tormoehlen LM, Pascuzzi RM. Thymoma, myasthenia gravis, and other paraneoplastic syndromes. Hematol Oncol Clin North Am 2008;22:509–526.
121. Furman WL, Buckley PJ, Green AA, et al. Thymoma and myasthenia gravis in a 4-year-old child. Case report and review of the literature. Cancer 1985;56:2703–2706.
122. Kilis-Pstrusinska K, Medynska A, Zwolinska D, et al. Lymphoepithelioma-like thymic carcinoma in a 16-year-old boy with nephrotic syndrome—a case report. Pediatr Nephrol 2008;23:1001–1003.
123. Drachman DB. Myasthenia gravis (first of two parts). N Engl J Med 1978;298:136–142.
124. Drachman DB. Myasthenia gravis (second of two parts). N Engl J Med 1978;298: 186–193.
125. Pescarmona E, Giardini R, Brisigotti M, et al. Thymoma in childhood: a clinicopathological study of five cases. Histopathology 1992;21:65–68.
126. Casey EM, Kiel PJ, Loehrer PJ Sr. Clinical management of thymoma patients. Hematol Oncol Clin North Am 2008;22:457–473.
127. Masaoka A, Monden Y, Nakahara K, et al. Follow-up study of thymomas with special reference to their clinical stages. Cancer 1981;48:2485–2492.
128. Maggi G, Giaccone G, Donadio M, et al. Thymomas. A review of 169 cases, with particular reference to results of surgical treatment. Cancer 1986;58:765–776.
129. Lara PN Jr. Malignant thymoma: current status and future directions. Cancer Treat Rev 2000;26:127–131.
130. Ariaratnam LS, Kalnicki S, Mincer F, et al. The management of malignant thymoma with radiation therapy. Int J Radiat Oncol Biol Phys 1979;5:77–80.
131. Curran WJ Jr, Kornstein MJ, Brooks JJ, et al. Invasive thymoma: the role of mediastinal irradiation following complete or incomplete surgical resection. J Clin Oncol 1988;6: 1722–1727.
132. Giaccone G, Ardizzoni A, Kirkpatrick A et al. Cisplatin and etoposide combination chemotherapy for locally advanced or metastatic thymoma. A phase II study of the European Organization for Research and Treatment of Cancer Lung Cancer Cooperative Group. J Clin Oncol 1996;14:814–820.
133. Jan N, Villani GM, Trambert J, et al. A novel second line chemotherapy treatment of recurrent thymoma. Med Oncol 1997;14:163–168.
134. Palmieri G, Lastoria S, Colao A, et al. Successful treatment of a patient with a thymoma and pure red-cell aplasia with octreotide and prednisone. N Engl J Med 1997;336: 263–265.
135. Loehrer PJ Sr, Wang W, Johnson DH, et al. Octreotide alone or with prednisone in patients with advanced thymoma and thymic carcinoma: an Eastern Cooperative Oncology Group Phase II Trial. J Clin Oncol 2004;22:293–299.
136. Johnson SB, Eng TY, Giaccone G, et al. Thymoma: update for the new millennium. Oncologist 2001;6:239–246.
137. Blumberg D, Port JL, Weksler B, et al. Thymoma: a multivariate analysis of factors predicting survival. Ann Thorac Surg 1995;60:908–913; discussion 914.
138. Gaissert HA, Mark EJ. Tracheobronchial gland tumors. Cancer Control 2006;13: 286–294.
139. Welsh JH, Maxson T, Jaksic T, et al. Tracheobronchial mucoepidermoid carcinoma in childhood and adolescence: case report and review of the literature. Int J Pediatr Otorhinolaryngol 1998;45:265–273.
140. Mullins JD, Barnes RP. Childhood bronchial mucoepidermoid tumors: a case report and review of the literature. Cancer 1979;44:315–322.
141. Torres AM, Ryckman FC. Childhood tracheobronchial mucoepidermoid carcinoma: a case report and review of the literature. J Pediatr Surg 1988;23:367–370.
142. Fauroux B, Aynie V, Larroquet M, et al. Carcinoid and mucoepidermoid bronchial tumours in children. Eur J Pediatr 2005;164:748–752.
143. Wang LT, Wilkins EW Jr, Bode HH. Bronchial carcinoid tumors in pediatric patients. Chest 1993;103:1426–1428.
144. Kelsey A. Mesothelioma in childhood. Pediatr Hematol Oncol 1994;11:461–462.
145. Stein N, Henkes D. Mesothelioma of the testicle in a child. J Urol 1986;135:794.
146. Wunsch L, Flemming P, Reiter A. Long-term follow-up of a well-differentiated mesothelioma of the peritoneum in a 2-year-old girl. Med Pediatr Oncol 1998;31:123–124.
147. Rodriguez D, Cheung MC, Housri N, et al. Malignant abdominal mesothelioma: defining the role of surgery. J Surg Oncol 2009;99:51–57.
148. Weissmann LB, Corson JM, Neugut AI, et al. Malignant mesothelioma following treatment for Hodgkin's disease. J Clin Oncol 1996;14:2098–2100.
149. Hofmann J, Mintzer D, Warhol MJ. Malignant mesothelioma following radiation therapy. Am J Med 1994;97:379–382.
150. Pappo AS, Santana VM, Furman WL, et al. Post-irradiation malignant mesothelioma. Cancer 1997;79:192–193.
151. Robinson BW, Lake RA. Advances in malignant mesothelioma. N Engl J Med 2005; 353:1591–1603.
152. Miller A. Mesothelioma in household members of asbestos-exposed workers: 32 United States cases since 1990. Am J Ind Med 2005;47:458–462.
153. Tsao AS, Wistuba I, Roth JA, et al. Malignant pleural mesothelioma. J Clin Oncol 2009;27:2081–2090.
154. Milano E, Pourroy B, Rome A, et al. Efficacy of a combination of pemetrexed and multiple redo-surgery in an 11-year-old girl with a recurrent multifocal abdominal mesothelioma. Anticancer Drugs 2006;17:1231–1234.
155. Sugarbaker DJ, Flores RM, Jaklitsch MT, et al. Resection margins, extrapleural nodal status, and cell type determine postoperative long-term survival in trimodality therapy of malignant pleural mesothelioma: results in 183 patients. J Thorac Cardiovasc Surg 1999;117:54–63; discussion 63–65.
156. Uzun O, Wilson DG, Vujanic GM, et al. Cardiac tumours in children. Orphanet J Rare Dis 2007;2:11.
157. Butany J, Nair V, Naseemuddin A, et al. Cardiac tumours: diagnosis and management. Lancet Oncol 2005;6:219–228.
158. Wilkes D, Charitakis K, Basson CT. Inherited disposition to cardiac myxoma development. Nat Rev Cancer 2006;6:157–165.
159. Jemal A, Siegel R, Ward E, et al. Cancer Statistics, 2008. CA Cancer J Clin 2008;58: 71–96.
160. Pultrum BB, Bijleveld CM, de Langen ZJ, et al. Development of an adenocarcinoma of the esophagus 22 years after primary repair of a congenital atresia. J Pediatr Surg 2005; 40:e1–e4.
161. Koshy M, Esiashvilli N, Landry JC, et al. Multiple management modalities in esophageal cancer: combined modality management approaches. Oncologist 2004;9: 147–159.
162. Hoeffel JC, Nihoul-Fekete C, Schmitt M. Esophageal adenocarcinoma after gastroesophageal reflux in children. J Pediatr 1989;115:259–261.
163. Hassall E, Dimmick JE, Magee JF. Adenocarcinoma in childhood Barrett's esophagus: case documentation and the need for surveillance in children. Am J Gastroenterol 1993;88:282–288.
164. Gangopadhyay AN, Mohanty PK, Gopal SC, et al. Adenocarcinoma of the esophagus in an 8-year-old boy. J Pediatr Surg 1997;32:1259–1260.
165. Hasan N, Mandhan P. Respiratory obstruction caused by lipoma of the esophagus. J Pediatr Surg 1994;29:1565–1566.
166. Jollimore JV, Zamakhshary M, Giacomantonio M, et al. Undifferentiated mesenchymal neoplasm of the esophagus in a child: case report and comparison with gastrointestinal stromal tumor. Pediatr Dev Pathol 2003;6:257–260.
167. Enzinger PC, Mayer RJ. Esophageal cancer. N Engl J Med 2003;349:2241–2252.
168. Schwartz MG, Sgaglione NA. Gastric carcinoma in the young: overview of the literature. Mt Sinai J Med 1984;51:720–723.
169. McGill TW, Downey EC, Westbrook J, et al. Gastric carcinoma in children. J Pediatr Surg 1993;28:1620–1621.
170. Curtis JL, Burns RC, Wang L, et al. Primary gastric tumors of infancy and childhood: 54-year experience at a single institution. J Pediatr Surg 2008;43:1487–1493.
171. Moschovi M, Menegas D, Stefanaki K, et al. Primary gastric Burkitt lymphoma in childhood: associated with Helicobacter pylori? Med Pediatr Oncol 2003;41:444–447.
172. Mahour GH, Isaacs H Jr, Chang L, Primary malignant tumors of the stomach in children. J Pediatr Surg 1980;15:603–608.
173. Jacquemart C, Guidi O, Etienne I, et al. Pediatric gastric lymphoma: a rare entity. J Pediatr Hematol Oncol 2008;30:984–986.
174. Skinner MA, Plumley DA, Grosfeld JL, et al. Gastrointestinal tumors in children: an analysis of 39 cases. Ann Surg Oncol 1994;1:283–289.
175. Harting MT, Blakely ML, Herzog CE, et al. Treatment issues in pediatric gastric adenocarcinoma. J Pediatr Surg 2004;39:e8–e10.
176. Goto S, Ikeda K, Ishii E, et al. Carcinoma of the stomach in a 7-year-old boy—a case report and a review of the literature on children under 10 years of age. Z Kinderchir 1984;39:137–140.
177. Lack EE. Leiomyosarcomas in childhood: a clinical and pathologic study of 10 cases. Pediatr Pathol 1986;6:181–197.
178. Ogami H, Ikeda K, Koga Y, et al. Gastric teratoma in infancy and childhood: report of three cases and review of literature. Jpn J Surg 1973;3:218–228.
179. Ferrari A, Casanova M, Spreafico F, et al. Childhood liposarcoma: a single-institutional twenty-year experience. Pediatr Hematol Oncol 1999;16:415–421.
180. Corredor J, Wambach J, Barnard J. Gastrointestinal polyps in children: advances in molecular genetics, diagnosis, and management. J Pediatr 2001;138:621–628.
181. Karnak I, Senocak ME, Ciftci AO, et al. Inflammatory myofibroblastic tumor in children: diagnosis and treatment. J Pediatr Surg 2001;36:908–912.
182. Black RE. Linitis plastica in a child. J Pediatr Surg 1985;20:86–87.
183. Pisters P, Kelsen D, Tepper J. Cancer of the stomach. In: DeVita V, Lawrence T, Rosenberg A, eds. Cancer principles and practice of oncology. 8th ed. Philadelphia, PA: Lippincott Williams & Wilkins, 2008:1043–1078.
184. Correa P. Helicobacter pylori and gastric carcinogenesis. Am J Surg Pathol 1995; 19:(suppl 1):S37–S43.
185. Siegel SE, Hays DM, Romansky S, et al. Carcinoma of the stomach in childhood. Cancer 1976;38:1781–1784.
186. Catalano V, Labianca R, Beretta GD, et al. Gastric cancer. Crit Rev Oncol Hematol, 2009.
187. Bonenkamp JJ, Hermans J, Sasako M, et al. Extended lymph-node dissection for gastric cancer. N Engl J Med 1999;340:908–914.
188. Macdonald JS, Smalley SR, Benedetti J, et al., Chemoradiotherapy after surgery compared with surgery alone for adenocarcinoma of the stomach or gastroesophageal junction. N Engl J Med. 2001;345(10):725–730.
189. Sakuramoto S, Sasako M, Yamaguchi T, et al. Adjuvant chemotherapy for gastric cancer with S-1, an oral fluoropyrimidine. N Engl J Med 2007;357:1810–1820.
190. Van Cutsem E, Moiseyenko VM, Tjulandin S, et al. Phase III study of docetaxel and cisplatin plus fluorouracil compared with cisplatin and fluorouracil as first-line therapy for advanced gastric cancer: a report of the V325 Study Group. J Clin Oncol 2006;24: 4991–4997.
191. Perez EA, Gutierrez JC, Koniaris LG, et al. Malignant pancreatic tumors: incidence and outcome in 58 pediatric patients. J Pediatr Surg 2009;44:197–203.
192. Defachelles AS, Martin De Lassalle E, Boutard P, et al. Pancreatoblastoma in childhood: clinical course and therapeutic management of seven patients. Med Pediatr Oncol 2001;37:47–52.
193. Tsukimoto I, Watanabe K, Lin JB, et al. Pancreatic carcinoma in children in Japan. Cancer 1973;31:1203–1207.
194. Taxy JB. Adenocarcinoma of the pancreas in childhood. Report of a case and a review of the English language literature. Cancer 1976;37:1508–1518.
195. Panamonta O, Areemit S, Srinakarin J, et al. Insulinoma in childhood. J Med Assoc Thai 2001;84:136–142.
196. Shorter NA, Glick RD, Klimstra DS, et al. Malignant pancreatic tumors in childhood and adolescence: The Memorial Sloan-Kettering experience, 1967 to present. J Pediatr Surg 2002;37:887–892.
197. Eisenhuber E, Schoefl R, Wiesbauer P, et al. Primary pancreatic lymphoma presenting as acute pancreatitis in a child. Med Pediatr Oncol 2001;37:53–54.
198. Lynch HT, Brand RE, Deters CA, et al. Hereditary pancreatic cancer. Pancreatology 2001;1:466–471.
199. Cowgill SM, Muscarella P. The genetics of pancreatic cancer. Am J Surg 2003;186: 279–286.

200. Goldstein AM, Fraser MC, Struewing JP, et al. Increased risk of pancreatic cancer in melanoma-prone kindreds with p16INK4 mutations. N Engl J Med 1995;333: 970–974.
201. Bowlby LS. Pancreatic adenocarcinoma in an adolescent male with Peutz-Jeghers syndrome. Hum Pathol 1986;17:97–99.
202. Drut R, Jones MC. Congenital pancreatoblastoma in Beckwith-Wiedemann syndrome: an emerging association. Pediatr Pathol 1988;8:331–339.
203. Tersigni R, Arena L, Alessandroni L, et al. Pancreatic carcinoma in childhood: case report of long survival and review of the literature. Surgery 1984;96:560–566.
204. Moynan RW, Neerhout RC, Johnson TS. Pancreatic carcinoma in childhood: case report and review. J Pediatr 1964;65:711–720.
205. Lack EE, Cassady JR, Levey R, et al. Tumors of the exocrine pancreas in children and adolescents. A clinical and pathologic study of eight cases. Am J Surg Pathol 1983;7: 319–327.
206. Grosfeld JL, Vane DW, Rescorla FJ, et al. Pancreatic tumors in childhood: analysis of 13 cases. J Pediatr Surg 1990;25:1057–1062.
207. Iseki M, Suzuki T, Koizumi Y, et al. Alpha-fetoprotein-producing pancreatoblastoma. A case report. Cancer 1986;57:1833–1835.
208. Sharma MP, Gregg JA, Loewenstein MS, et al. Carcinoembryonic antigen (CEA) activity in pancreatic juice of patients with pancreatic carcinoma and pancreatitis. Cancer 1976;38:2457–2461.
209. Reed DN Jr, Turcotte JG. Papillary epithelial neoplasm of the pancreas in the pediatric population. J Surg Oncol 1986;32:182–183.
210. Vannier JP, Flamant F, Hemet J, et al. Pancreatoblastoma: response to chemotherapy. Med Pediatr Oncol 1991;19:187–191.
211. Lewis MA, Lilleyman JS, Variend S. Benign metastatic islet cell tumour of the pancreas. Med Pediatr Oncol 1985;13:97–100.
212. Mah PT, Loo DC, Tock EP. Pancreatic acinar cell carcinoma in childhood. Am J Dis Child 1974;128:101–104.
213. Klimstra DS, Wenig BM, Adair CF, et al. Pancreatoblastoma. A clinicopathologic study and review of the literature. Am J Surg Pathol 1995;19:1371–1389.
214. Yeo TP, Hruban RH, Leach SD, et al. Pancreatic cancer. Curr Probl Cancer 2002; 26:176–275.
215. Haller DG. Future directions in the treatment of pancreatic cancer. Semin Oncol 2002;29:31–39.
216. NCCN clinical practice guidelines in oncology. Pancreatic adenocarcinoma. National Comprehensive Cancer Network, 2009. Available at www.hccn.org.
217. Moore M. Activity of gemcitabine in patients with advanced pancreatic carcinoma. A review. Cancer 1996;78:633–638.
218. Chun Y, Kim W, Park K, et al. Pancreatoblastoma. J Pediatr Surg 1997;32:1612–1615.
219. Vossen S, Goretzki PE, Goebel U, et al. Therapeutic management of rare malignant pancreatic tumors in children. World J Surg 1998;22:879–882.
220. Nilsson B, Bumming P, Meis-Kindblom JM, et al. Gastrointestinal stromal tumors: the incidence, prevalence, clinical course, and prognostication in the preimatinib mesylate era—a population-based study in western Sweden. Cancer 2005;103:821–829.
221. Perez EA, Livingstone AS, Franceschi D, et al. Current incidence and outcomes of gastrointestinal mesenchymal tumors including gastrointestinal stromal tumors. J Am Coll Surg 2006;202:623–629.
222. Miettinen M, Lasota J. Gastrointestinal stromal tumors: review on morphology, molecular pathology, prognosis, and differential diagnosis. Arch Pathol Lab Med 2006; 130:1466–1478.
223. Hirota S, Isozaki K, Moriyama Y, et al. Gain-of-function mutations of c-kit in human gastrointestinal stromal tumors. Science 1998;279:577–580.
224. Corless CL, Fletcher JA, Heinrich MC. Biology of gastrointestinal stromal tumors. J Clin Oncol 2004;22:3813–3825.
225. Corless CL, Schroeder A, Griffith D, et al. PDGFRA mutations in gastrointestinal stromal tumors: frequency, spectrum and in vitro sensitivity to imatinib. J Clin Oncol 2005; 23:5357–5364.
226. Debiec-Rychter M, Dumez H, Judson I, et al. Use of c-KIT/PDGFRA mutational analysis to predict the clinical response to imatinib in patients with advanced gastrointestinal stromal tumours entered on phase I and II studies of the EORTC Soft Tissue and Bone Sarcoma Group. Eur J Cancer 2004;40:689–695.
227. Li FP, Fletcher JA, Heinrich MC, et al. Familial gastrointestinal stromal tumor syndrome: phenotypic and molecular features in a kindred. J Clin Oncol 2005;23:2735–2743.
228. Miettinen M, Fetsch JF, Sobin LH, et al. Gastrointestinal stromal tumors in patients with neurofibromatosis 1: a clinicopathologic and molecular genetic study of 45 cases. Am J Surg Pathol 2006;30:90–96.
229. Pappo AS, Janeway KA. Pediatric gastrointestinal stromal tumors. Hematol Oncol Clin North Am 2009;23:15–34, vii.
230. Carney JA. Gastric stromal sarcoma, pulmonary chondroma, and extra-adrenal paraganglioma (Carney Triad): natural history, adrenocortical component, and possible familial occurrence. Mayo Clin Proc 1999;74:543–552.
231. Pasini B, McWhinney SR, Bei T, et al. Clinical and molecular genetics of patients with the Carney-Stratakis syndrome and germline mutations of the genes coding for the succinate dehydrogenase subunits SDHB, SDHC, and SDHD. Eur J Hum Genet 2008;16: 79–88.
232. Quek R, George S. Gastrointestinal stromal tumor: a clinical overview. Hematol Oncol Clin North Am 2009;23:69–78, viii.
233. Plaat BE, Hollema H, Molenaar WM, et al. Soft tissue leiomyosarcomas and malignant gastrointestinal stromal tumors: differences in clinical outcome and expression of multidrug resistance proteins. J Clin Oncol 2000;18:3211–3220.
234. Dematteo RP, Gold JS, Saran L, et al. Tumor mitotic rate, size, and location independently predict recurrence after resection of primary gastrointestinal stromal tumor (GIST). Cancer 2008;112:608–615.
235. Dematteo RP, Heinrich MC, El-Rifai WM, et al. Clinical management of gastrointestinal stromal tumors: before and after STI-571. Hum Pathol 2002;33:466–477.
236. DeMatteo RP, Lewis JJ, Leung D, et al. Two hundred gastrointestinal stromal tumors: recurrence patterns and prognostic factors for survival. Ann Surg 2000;231:51–58.
237. Verweij J, van Oosterom A, Blay JY, et al. Imatinib mesylate (STI-571 Glivec, Gleevec) is an active agent for gastrointestinal stromal tumours, but does not yield responses in other soft-tissue sarcomas that are unselected for a molecular target. Results from an EORTC Soft Tissue and Bone Sarcoma Group phase II study. Eur J Cancer 2003;39: 2006–2011.
238. Demetri GD, von Mehren M, Blanke CD, et al. Efficacy and safety of imatinib mesylate in advanced gastrointestinal stromal tumors. N Engl J Med 2002;347:472–480.
239. Blanke CD, Demetri GD, von Mehren M, et al. Long-term results from a randomized phase II trial of standard versus higher-dose imatinib mesylate for patients with unresectable or metastatic gastrointestinal stromal tumors expressing KIT. J Clin Oncol 2008;26:620–625.
240. Heinrich MC, Corless CL, Demetri GD, et al. Kinase mutations and imatinib response in patients with metastatic gastrointestinal stromal tumor. J Clin Oncol 2003;21: 4342–4329.
241. Demetri GD, van Oosterom AT, Garrett CR, et al. Efficacy and safety of sunitinib in patients with advanced gastrointestinal stromal tumour after failure of imatinib: a randomised controlled trial. Lancet 2006;368:1329–1338.
242. Cypriano MS, Jenkins JJ, Pappo AS, et al. Pediatric gastrointestinal stromal tumors and leiomyosarcoma. Cancer 2004;101:39–50.
243. Prakash S, Sarran L, Socci N, et al. Gastrointestinal stromal tumors in children and young adults: a clinicopathologic, molecular, and genomic study of 15 cases and review of the literature. J Pediatr Hematol Oncol 2005;27:179–187.
244. Janeway KA, Liegl B, Harlow A, et al. Pediatric KIT wild-type and platelet-derived growth factor receptor alpha-wild-type gastrointestinal stromal tumors share KIT activation but not mechanisms of genetic progression with adult gastrointestinal stromal tumors. Cancer Res 2007;67:9084–9088.
245. Tarn C, Rink L, Merkel E, et al. Insulin-like growth factor 1 receptor is a potential therapeutic target for gastrointestinal stromal tumors. Proc Natl Acad Sci USA 2008; 105:8387–8392.
246. Agaram NP, Laquaglia MP, Ustun B, et al. Molecular characterization of pediatric gastrointestinal tumors. Clin Cancer Res 2008;14:3204–3215.
247. Demetri GD, Benjamin RS, Blanke CD, et al. NCCN Task Force report: management of patients with gastrointestinal stromal tumor (GIST)—update of the NCCN clinical practice guidelines. J Natl Compr Canc Netw 2007;(suppl 2):S1–S29; quiz S30.
248. Dematteo RP, Ballman KV, Antonescu CR, et al. Adjuvant imatinib mesylate after resection of localised, primary gastrointestinal stromal tumour: a randomised, double-blind, placebo-controlled trial. Lancet 2009;373:1097–1104.
249. Janeway KA, Albritton KH, Van Den Abbeele AD, et al. Sunitinib treatment in pediatric patients with advanced GIST following failure of imatinib. Pediatr Blood Cancer 2009; 52:767–771.
250. Libutti SK, Saltz LB, Tepper JE. Colon cancer. In: DeVita VT, Lawrence TS, Rosenberg S, eds. Cancer principles and practice of oncology. 8th ed. Philadelphia, PA: Lippincott Williams & Wilkins, 2008:1232–1285.
251. Berlau J, Glei M, Pool-Zobel BL. Colon cancer risk factors from nutrition. Anal Bioanal Chem 2004;378:737–743.
252. Corpet DE, Stamp D, Medline A, et al. Promotion of colonic microadenoma growth in mice and rats fed cooked sugar or cooked casein and fat. Cancer Res 1990;50: 6955–6958.
253. Potter JD. Colorectal cancer: molecules and populations. J Natl Cancer Inst 1999;91: 916–932.
254. Ries LA, Wingo PA, Miller DS, et al. The annual report to the nation on the status of cancer, 1973–1997, with a special section on colorectal cancer. Cancer 2000;88: 2398–2424.
255. Saab R, Furman WL. Epidemiology and management options for colorectal cancer in children. Paediatr Drugs 2008;10:177–192.
256. Kern WH, White WC. Adenocarcinoma of the colon in a 9-month-old infant; report of a case. Cancer 1958;11:855–857.
257. Andersson A, Bergdahl L. Carcinoma of the colon in children: a report of six new cases and a review of the literature. J Pediatr Surg 1976;11:967–971.
258. Hoerner MT. Carcinoma of the colon and rectum in persons under twenty years of age. Am J Surg 1958;96:47–53.
259. Middelkamp JN, Haffner H. Carcinoma of the colon in children. Pediatrics 1963; 32:558–571.
260. Lewis CT, Riley WE, Georgeson K, et al. Carcinoma of the colon and rectum in patients less than 20 years of age. South Med J 1990;83:383–385.
261. Rao BN, Pratt CB, Fleming ID, et al. Colon carcinoma in children and adolescents. A review of 30 cases. Cancer 1985;55:1322–1326.
262. Pratt CB, Rao BN, Merchant TE, et al. Treatment of colorectal carcinoma in adolescents and young adults with surgery, 5-fluorouracil/leucovorin/interferon-alpha 2a and radiation therapy. Med Pediatr Oncol 1999;32:459–460.
263. LaQuaglia MP, Heller G, Filippa DA, et al. Prognostic factors and outcome in patients 21 years and under with colorectal carcinoma. J Pediatr Surg 1992;27:1085–1089; discussion 1089–1090.
264. Hill DA, Furman WL, Billups CA, et al. Colorectal carcinoma in childhood and adolescence: a clinicopathologic review. J Clin Oncol 2007;25:5808–5814.
265. Bhatia S, Pratt CB, Sharp GB, et al. Family history of cancer in children and young adults with colorectal cancer. Med Pediatr Oncol 1999;33:470–475.
266. Caldwell GG, Cannon SB, Pratt CB, et al. Serum pesticide levels in patients with childhood colorectal carcinoma. Cancer 1981;48:774–778.
267. Lashner BA. Colorectal cancer in ulcerative colitis patients: survival curves and surveillance. Cleve Clin J Med 1994;61:272–275.
268. Obrand DI, Gordon PH. Continued change in the distribution of colorectal carcinoma. Br J Surg 1998;85:246–248.
269. Dean PA. Hereditary intestinal polyposis syndromes. Rev Gastroenterol Mex 1996; 61:100–111.
270. Arenas RB, Fichera A, Mhoon D, et al. Incidence and therapeutic implications of synchronous colonic pathology in colorectal adenocarcinoma. Surgery 1997;122:706–709; discussion 709–710.
271. Turcot J, Despres JP, St Pierre F. Malignant tumors of the central nervous system associated with familial polyposis of the colon: report of two cases. Dis Colon Rectum 1959;2:465–468.
272. Hamilton SR, Liu B, Parsons RE, et al. The molecular basis of Turcot's syndrome. N Engl J Med 1995;332:839–847.
273. Oldfield MC. The association of familial polyposis of the colon with multiple sebaceous cysts. Br J Surg 1954;41:534–541.
274. Gardner EJ. Follow-up study of a family group exhibiting dominant inheritance for a syndrome including intestinal polyps, osteomas, fibromas and epidermal cysts. Am J Hum Genet 1962;14:376–390.
275. Pratt CB, Jane JA. Multiple colorectal carcinomas, polyposis coli, and neurofibromatosis, followed by multiple glioblastoma multiforme. J Natl Cancer Inst 1991;83:880–881.
276. Vogelstein B, Fearon ER, Hamilton SR, et al. Genetic alterations during colorectal-tumor development. N Engl J Med 1988;319:525–532.
277. Fearon ER, Cho KR, Nigro JM, et al. Identification of a chromosome 18q gene that is altered in colorectal cancers. Science 1990;247:49–56.

278. Lynch JP, Hoops TC. The genetic pathogenesis of colorectal cancer. Hematol Oncol Clin North Am 2002;16:775–810.
279. Liu B, Farrington SM, Petersen GM, et al. Genetic instability occurs in the majority of young patients with colorectal cancer. Nat Med 1995;1:348–352.
280. Datta RV, LaQuaglia MP, Paty PB. Genetic and phenotypic correlates of colorectal cancer in young patients. N Engl J Med 2000;342:137–138.
281. Burt RW. Colon cancer screening. Gastroenterology 2000;119:837–853.
282. Distante S, Nasioulas S, Somers GR, et al. Familial adenomatous polyposis in a 5 year old child: a clinical, pathological, and molecular genetic study. J Med Genet 1996;33:157–160.
283. Radhakrishnan CN, Bruce J. Colorectal cancers in children without any predisposing factors. A report of eight cases and review of the literature. Eur J Pediatr Surg 2003; 13:66–68.
284. Enker WE, Palovan E, Kirsner JB. Carcinoma of the colon in the adolescent: a report of survival and an analysis of the literature. Am J Surg 1977;133:737–741.
285. Sharma AK, Gupta CR. Colorectal cancer in children: case report and review of literature. Trop Gastroenterol 2001;22:36–39.
286. Symonds DA, Vickery AL. Mucinous carcinoma of the colon and rectum. Cancer 1976;37:1891–1900.
287. Angel CA, Pratt CB, Rao BN, et al. Carcinoembryonic antigen and carbohydrate 19–19 antigen as markers for colorectal carcinoma in children and adolescents. Cancer 1992;69:1487–1491.
288. Bhatnagar J, Tewari HB, Bhatnagar M, et al. Comparison of carcinoembryonic antigen in tissue and serum with grade and stage of colon cancer. Anticancer Res 1999;19: 2181–2187.
289. Locker GY, Hamilton S, Harris J, et al. ASCO 2006 update of recommendations for the use of tumor markers in gastrointestinal cancer. J Clin Oncol 2006;24:5313–5327.
290. Ruers TJ, Langenhoff BS, Neeleman N, et al. Value of positron emission tomography with [F-18]fluorodeoxyglucose in patients with colorectal liver metastases: a prospective study. J Clin Oncol 2002;20:388–395.
291. Tanaka T, Kawai Y, Kanai M, et al. Usefulness of FDG-positron emission tomography in diagnosing peritoneal recurrence of colorectal cancer. Am J Surg 2002;184:433–436.
292. Joyce DL, Wahl RL, Patel PV, et al. Preoperative positron emission tomography to evaluate potentially resectable hepatic colorectal metastases. Arch Surg 2006;141:1220–1226; discussion 1227.
293. Whiteford MH, Whiteford HM, Yee LF, et al. Usefulness of FDG-PET scan in the assessment of suspected metastatic or recurrent adenocarcinoma of the colon and rectum. Dis Colon Rectum 2000;43:759–767; discussion 767–770.
294. Taguchi T, Suita S, Hirata Y, et al. Carcinoma of the colon in children: a case report and review of 41 Japanese cases. J Pediatr Gastroenterol Nutr 1991;12:394–399.
295. Heys SD, O'Hanrahan TJ, Brittenden J, et al. Colorectal cancer in young patients: a review of the literature. Eur J Surg Oncol 1994;20:225–231.
296. Wright FC, Law CH, Berry S, et al. Clinically important aspects of lymph node assessment in colon cancer. J Surg Oncol 2009;99:248–255.
297. Pratt CB, Meyer WH, Howlett N, et al. Phase II study of 5-fluorouracil/leucovorin for pediatric patients with malignant solid tumors. Cancer 1994;74:2593–2598.
298. Saltz L. Irinotecan-based combinations for the adjuvant treatment of stage III colon cancer. Oncology (Williston Park) 2000;14:47–50.
299. Andre T, Boni C, Mounedji-Boudiaf L, et al. Oxaliplatin, fluorouracil, and leucovorin as adjuvant treatment for colon cancer. N Engl J Med 2004;350:2343–2351.
300. Cunningham D, Humblet Y, Siena S, et al. Cetuximab monotherapy and cetuximab plus irinotecan in irinotecan-refractory metastatic colorectal cancer. N Engl J Med 2004;351:337–345.
301. Van Cutsem E, Peeters M, Siena S, et al. Open-label phase III trial of panitumumab plus best supportive care compared with best supportive care alone in patients with chemotherapy-refractory metastatic colorectal cancer. J Clin Oncol 2007;25:1658–1664.
302. Hurwitz H, Fehrenbacher L, Novotny W, et al. Bevacizumab plus irinotecan, fluorouracil, and leucovorin for metastatic colorectal cancer. N Engl J Med 2004;350: 2335–2342.
303. Rothenberg ML, Oza AM, Bigelow RH, et al. Superiority of oxaliplatin and fluorouracil-leucovorin compared with either therapy alone in patients with progressive colorectal cancer after irinotecan and fluorouracil-leucovorin: interim results of a phase III trial. J Clin Oncol 2003;21:2059–2069.
304. NCCN clinical practice guidelines in oncology. Colon cancer. National Comprehensive Cancer Network, 2009.
305. Ramsey SD, Berry K, Moinpour C, et al. Quality of life in long term survivors of colorectal cancer. Am J Gastroenterol 2002;97:1228–1234.
306. Smith RE, Renaud RC, Hoffman E. Colorectal cancer market. Nat Rev Drug Discov 2004;3:471–472.
307. Kohne CH, Lenz HJ. Chemotherapy with targeted agents for the treatment of metastatic colorectal cancer. Oncologist 2009;14:478–488.
308. Thibodeau SN, Bren G, Schaid D. Microsatellite instability in cancer of the proximal colon. Science 1993;260:816–819.
309. Gryfe R, Kim H, Hsieh ET, et al. Tumor microsatellite instability and clinical outcome in young patients with colorectal cancer. N Engl J Med 2000;342:69–77.
310. Watanabe T, Wu TT, Catalano PJ, et al. Molecular predictors of survival after adjuvant chemotherapy for colon cancer. N Engl J Med 2001;344:1196–1206.
311. Iqbal S, Lenz HJ. Molecular predictors of treatment and outcome in colorectal cancer. Curr Gastroenterol Rep 2003;5:399–405.
312. Chan TA. Nonsteroidal anti-inflammatory drugs, apoptosis, and colon-cancer chemoprevention. Lancet Oncol 2002;3:166–174.
313. Rayyan Y, Williams J, Rigas B. The role of NSAIDs in the prevention of colon cancer. Cancer Invest 2002;20:1002–1011.
314. Giardiello FM, Hamilton SR, Krush AJ, et al. Treatment of colonic and rectal adenomas with sulindac in familial adenomatous polyposis. N Engl J Med 1993;328:1313–1316.
315. Steinbach G, Lynch PM, Phillips RK, et al. The effect of celecoxib, a cyclooxygenase-2 inhibitor, in familial adenomatous polyposis. N Engl J Med 2000;342:1946–1952.
316. Thun MJ, Namboodiri MM, Heath CW Jr. Aspirin use and reduced risk of fatal colon cancer. N Engl J Med 1991;325:1593–1596.
317. Arber N, Eagle CJ, Spicak J, et al. Celecoxib for the prevention of colorectal adenomatous polyps. N Engl J Med 2006;355:885–895.
318. Half E, Arber N. Colon cancer: preventive agents and the present status of chemoprevention. Expert Opin Pharmacother 2009;10:211–219.
319. Gustin DM, Brenner DE. Chemoprevention of colon cancer: current status and future prospects. Cancer Metastasis Rev 2002;21:323–348.
320. Ransom DT, Patel SR, Keeney GL, et al. Papillary serous carcinoma of the peritoneum. A review of 33 cases treated with platin-based chemotherapy. Cancer 1990;66:1091–1094.
321. Truong LD, Maccato ML, Awalt H, et al. Serous surface carcinoma of the peritoneum: a clinicopathologic study of 22 cases. Hum Pathol 1990;21:99–110.
322. Fromm GL, Gershenson DM, Silva EG. Papillary serous carcinoma of the peritoneum. Obstet Gynecol 1990;75:89–95.
323. Wall JE, Mandrell BN, Jenkins JJ III, et al. Effectiveness of paclitaxel in treating papillary serous carcinoma of the peritoneum in an adolescent. Am J Obstet Gynecol 1995;172:1049–1052.
324. Ulbright TM, Morley DJ, Roth LM, et al. Papillary serous carcinoma of the retroperitoneum. Am J Clin Pathol 1983;79:633–637.
325. Koutselini HA, Lazaris AC, Thomopoulou G, et al. Papillary serous carcinoma of peritoneum: case study and review of the literature on the differential diagnosis of malignant peritoneal tumors. Adv Clin Path 2001;5:99–104.
326. Look M, Chang D, Sugarbaker PH. Long-term results of cytoreductive surgery for advanced and recurrent epithelial ovarian cancers and papillary serous carcinoma of the peritoneum. Int J Gynecol Cancer 2004;14:35–41.
327. Fitch LB, Rubenstone AI. Carcinoma of the bladder in childhood. J Urol 1962;87: 549–552.
328. Castellanos RD, Wakefield PB, Evans AT. Carcinoma of the bladder in children. J Urol 1975;113:261–263.
329. Patel R, Tery T, Ninan GK. Transitional cell carcinoma of the bladder in first decade of life. Pediatr Surg Int 2008;24:1265–1268.
330. Fine SW, Humphrey PA, Dehner LP, et al. Urothelial neoplasms in patients 20 years or younger: a clinicopathological analysis using the world health organization 2004 bladder consensus classification. J Urol 2005;174:1976–1980.
331. Hemminki K, Chen B. Parental lung cancer as predictor of cancer risks in offspring: clues about multiple routes of harmful influence? Int J Cancer 2006;118:744–748.
332. Keetch DW, Manley CB, Catalona WJ. Transitional cell carcinoma of bladder in children and adolescents. Urology 1993;42:447–449.
333. Agarwala S, Hemal AK, Seth A, et al. Transitional cell carcinoma of the urinary bladder following exposure to cyclophosphamide in childhood. Eur J Pediatr Surg 2001;11: 207–210.
334. Worth PH. Cyclophosphamide and the bladder. Br Med J 1971;3:182.
335. Urakami S, Igawa M, Shiina H, et al. Recurrent transitional cell carcinoma in a child with the Costello syndrome. J Urol 2002;168:1133–1134.
336. Montgomery EA, Shuster DD, Burkart AL, et al. Inflammatory myofibroblastic tumors of the urinary tract: a clinicopathologic study of 46 cases, including a malignant example inflammatory fibrosarcoma and a subset associated with high-grade urothelial carcinoma. Am J Surg Pathol 2006;30:1502–1512.
337. Tscherne G. Female genital tract malignancies during puberty. Uterine and cervical malignancies. Ann N Y Acad Sci 1997;816:331–337.
338. Fivozinsky KB, Laufer MR. Vulvar disorders in adolescents. Adolesc Med 1999;10: 305–319, vii.
339. Dillon MB, Rosenshein NB, Parmley TH, et al. The diagnosis and management of cervical intraepithelial neoplasia in the patient under the age of twenty-one. Int J Gynaecol Obstet 1981;19:97–102.
340. Hannemann M, Weeks J, Evans A, et al. Incidence, pathology and outcome of gynaecological cancer in patients under the age of 21 years in South-west England 1995–2004: comparison of data from regional, national and international registries. J Obstet Gynaecol 2008;28:722–727.
341. Ghazal-Aswad S. Cervical cancer prevention in the human papilloma virus vaccine era. Ann N Y Acad Sci 2008;1138:253–256.
342. Fisher R, Darrow DH, Tranter M, et al. Human papillomavirus vaccine: recommendations, issues and controversies. Curr Opin Pediatr 2008;20:441–445.
343. Navid F, Billups C, Liu T, et al. Second cancers in patients with the Ewing sarcoma family of tumours. Eur J Cancer 2008;44:983–991.
344. McNall RY, Nowicki PD, Miller B, et al. Adenocarcinoma of the cervix and vagina in pediatric patients. Pediatr Blood Cancer 2004;43:289–294.
345. Simmons PS. Breast disorders in adolescent females. Curr Opin Obstet Gynecol 2001; 13:459–461.
346. Gutierrez JC, Housri N, Koniaris LG, et al. Malignant breast cancer in children: a review of 75 patients. J Surg Res 2008;147:182–188.
347. Chung EM, Cube R, Hall GJ, et al. From the archives of the AFIP: breast masses in children and adolescents: radiologic-pathologic correlation. Radiographics 2009;29:907–931.
348. Tea MK, Asseryanis E, Kroiss R, et al. Surgical breast lesions in adolescent females. Pediatr Surg Int 2009;25:73–75.
349. Rogers DA, Lobe TE, Rao BN, et al. Breast malignancy in children. J Pediatr Surg 1994; 29:48–51.
350. Hays DM, Donaldson SS, Shimada H, et al. Primary and metastatic rhabdomyosarcoma in the breast: neoplasms of adolescent females, a report from the Intergroup Rhabdomyosarcoma Study. Med Pediatr Oncol 1997;29:181–189.
351. Simmons PS. Diagnostic considerations in breast disorders of children and adolescents. Obstet Gynecol Clin North Am 1992;19:91–102.
352. Constine LS, Tarbell N, Hudson MM, et al. Subsequent malignancies in children treated for Hodgkin's disease: associations with gender and radiation dose. Int J Radiat Oncol Biol Phys 2008;72:24–33.
353. Alm El-Din MA, Hughes KS, Finkelstein DM, et al. Breast cancer after treatment of Hodgkin's lymphoma: risk factors that really matter. Int J Radiat Oncol Biol Phys 2009;73:69–74.
354. Belkacemi Y, Bousquet G, Marsiglia H, et al. Phyllodes tumor of the breast. Int J Radiat Oncol Biol Phys 2008;70:492–500.
355. Gullett NP, Rizzo M, Johnstone PA. National surgical patterns of care for primary surgery and axillary staging of phyllodes tumors. Breast J 2009;15:41–44.
356. Shannon C, Smith IE. Breast cancer in adolescents and young women. Eur J Cancer 2003;39:2632–2642.
357. Mintzer D, Glassburn J, Mason BA, et al. Breast cancer in the very young patient: a multidisciplinary case presentation. Oncologist 2002;7:547–554.
358. Kurtz JM, Jacquemier J, Amalric R, et al. Why are local recurrences after breast-conserving therapy more frequent in younger patients? J Clin Oncol 1990;8:591–598.
359. Goldhirsch A, Glick JH, Gelber RD, et al. Meeting highlights: International Consensus Panel on the Treatment of Primary Breast Cancer. Seventh International Conference on Adjuvant Therapy of Primary Breast Cancer. J Clin Oncol 2001;19:3817–3827.
360. Gonzalez KD, Noltner KA, Buzin CH, et al. Beyond Li Fraumeni syndrome: clinical characteristics of families with p53 germline mutations. J Clin Oncol 2009;27:1250–1256.
361. Eby N, Chang-Claude J, Bishop DT. Familial risk and genetic susceptibility for breast cancer. Cancer Causes Control 1994;5:458–470.
362. Parkes SE, Muir KR, al Sheyyab M, et al. Carcinoid tumours of the appendix in children 1957–1986: incidence, treatment and outcome. Br J Surg 1993;80:502–504.

363. Spunt SL, Pratt CB, Rao BN, et al. Childhood carcinoid tumors: the St Jude Children's Research Hospital experience. J Pediatr Surg 2000;35:1282–1286.
364. Moertel CL, Weiland LH, Telander RL. Carcinoid tumor of the appendix in the first two decades of life. J Pediatr Surg 1990;25:1073–1075.
365. Pinchot SN, Holen K, Sippel RS, et al. Carcinoid tumors. Oncologist 2008;13:1255–1269.
366. Godwin JD II. Carcinoid tumors. An analysis of 2,837 cases. Cancer 1975;36:560–569.
367. Soga J. Statistical evaluation of 2001 carcinoid cases with metastases, collected from literature: a comparative study between ordinary carcinoids and atypical varieties. J Exp Clin Cancer Res 1998;17:3–12.
368. Assadi M, Kubiak R, Kaiser G. Appendiceal carcinoid tumors in children: does size matter? Med Pediatr Oncol 2002;38:65–66.
369. King MD, Young DG, Hann IM, et al. Carcinoid syndrome: an unusual cause of diarrhoea. Arch Dis Child 1985;60:269–271.
370. Moraes TJ, Langer JC, Forte V, et al. Pediatric pulmonary carcinoid: a case report and review of the literature. Pediatr Pulmonol 2003;35:318–322.
371. Campana D, Nori F, Piscitelli L, et al. Chromogranin A: is it a useful marker of neuroendocrine tumors? J Clin Oncol 2007;25:1967–1973.
372. Moertel CG, Hanley JA. Combination chemotherapy trials in metastatic carcinoid tumor and the malignant carcinoid syndrome. Cancer Clin Trials 1979;2:327–334.
373. O'Toole D, Ducreux M, Bommelaer G, et al. Treatment of carcinoid syndrome: a prospective crossover evaluation of lanreotide versus octreotide in terms of efficacy, patient acceptability, and tolerance. Cancer 2000;88:770–776.
374. Oberg K. Diagnosis and treatment of carcinoid tumors. Expert Rev Anticancer Ther 2003;3:863–877.
375. Leong WL, Pasieka JL. Regression of metastatic carcinoid tumors with octreotide therapy: two case reports and a review of the literature. J Surg Oncol 2002;79:180–187.
376. Chugh R, Tawbi H, Lucas DR, et al. Chordoma: the nonsarcoma primary bone tumor. Oncologist 2007;12:1344–1350.
377. Hoch BL, Nielsen GP, Liebsch NJ, et al. Base of skull chordomas in children and adolescents: a clinicopathologic study of 73 cases. Am J Surg Pathol 2006;30:811–818.
378. Borba LA, Al-Mefty O, Mrak RE, et al. Cranial chordomas in children and adolescents. J Neurosurg 1996;84:584–591.
379. Tekkok IH, Acikgoz B. Pediatric intracranial chordomas. J Neurosurg 85:990, 1996.
380. Coffin CM, Swanson PE, Wick MR, et al. Chordoma in childhood and adolescence. A clinicopathologic analysis of 12 cases. Arch Pathol Lab Med 1993;117:927–933.
381. Tamborini E, Miselli F, Negri T, et al. Molecular and biochemical analyses of platelet-derived growth factor receptor (PDGFR) B, PDGFRA, and KIT receptors in chordomas. Clin Cancer Res 2006;12:6920–6928.
382. Hug EB, Sweeney RA, Nurre PM, et al. Proton radiotherapy in management of pediatric base of skull tumors. Int J Radiat Oncol Biol Phys 2002;52:1017–1024.
383. Nguyen QN, Chang EL. Emerging role of proton beam radiation therapy for chordoma and chondrosarcoma of the skull base. Curr Oncol Rep 2008;10:338–343.
384. Casali PG, Stacchiotti S, Sangalli C, et al. Chordoma. Curr Opin Oncol 2007;19:367–370.
385. Pavlidis N, Briasoulis E, Hainsworth J, et al. Diagnostic and therapeutic management of cancer of an unknown primary. Eur J Cancer 2003;39:1990–2005.
386. Varadhachary GR, Talantov D, Raber MN, et al. Molecular profiling of carcinoma of unknown primary and correlation with clinical evaluation. J Clin Oncol 2008;26: 4442–4448.
387. Kuttesch JF Jr, Parham DM, Kaste SC, et al. Embryonal malignancies of unknown primary origin in children. Cancer 1995;75:115–121.
388. Rubin AI, Chen EH, Ratner D. Basal-cell carcinoma. N Engl J Med 2005;353:2262–2269.
389. Von Hoff DD, LoRusso PM, Rudin CM, et al. Inhibition of the hedgehog pathway in advanced basal-cell carcinoma. N Engl J Med 2009;361:1164–1172.
390. Ries L SM, Gurney J, Tamra T, et al. Cancer incidence and survival among children and adolescents: United States SEER Program 1975–1995. National cancer Institute SEER Program NIH Pub 99–4649. Bethesda, MD, 1999.
391. Strouse JJ, Fears TR, Tucker MA, et al. Pediatric melanoma: risk factor and survival analysis of the surveillance, epidemiology and end results database. J Clin Oncol 2005;23:4735–4741.
392. Bleyer A, O'leary M, Barr R, Ries LAG. Cancer epidemiology in older adolescents and young adults 15 to 29 years of age, including SEER incidence and survival: 1975–2000. NIH Pub No 06–5767. Bethesda, MD, 2006.
393. Richardson SK, Tannous ZS, Mihm MC Jr. Congenital and infantile melanoma: review of the literature and report of an uncommon variant, pigment-synthesizing melanoma. J Am Acad Dermatol 2002;47:77–90.
394. Alexander A, Samlowski WE, Grossman D, et al. Metastatic melanoma in pregnancy: risk of transplacental metastases in the infant. J Clin Oncol 2003;21:2179–2186.
395. Bittencourt FV, Marghoob AA, Kopf AW, et al. Large congenital melanocytic nevi and the risk for development of malignant melanoma and neurocutaneous melanocytosis. Pediatrics 2000;106:736–741.
396. Ruiz-Maldonado R, Tamayo L, Laterza AM, et al. Giant pigmented nevi: clinical, histopathologic, and therapeutic considerations. J Pediatr 1992;120:906–911.
397. Ceballos PI, Ruiz-Maldonado R, Mihm MC Jr. Melanoma in children. N Engl J Med 1995;332:656–662.
398. Hale EK, Stein J, Ben-Porat L, et al. Association of melanoma and neurocutaneous melanocytosis with large congenital melanocytic naevi—results from the NYU-LCMN registry. Br J Dermatol 2005;152:512–517.
399. Lambert WC, Kuo HR, Lambert MW. Xeroderma pigmentosum. Dermatol Clin 1995; 13:169–209.
400. Cleaver JE. Cancer in xeroderma pigmentosum and related disorders of DNA repair. Nat Rev Cancer 2005;5:564–573.
401. Shibuya H, Kato A, Kai N, et al. A case of Werner syndrome with three primary lesions of malignant melanoma. J Dermatol 2005;32:737–744.
402. Goto M, Miller RW, Ishikawa Y, et al. Excess of rare cancers in Werner syndrome (adult progeria). Cancer Epidemiol Biomarkers Prev 1996;5:239–246.
403. Curtis RE, Rowlings PA, Deeg HJ, et al. Solid cancers after bone marrow transplantation. N Engl J Med 1997;336:897–904.
404. Euvrard S, Kanitakis J, Claudy A. Skin cancers after organ transplantation. N Engl J Med 2003;348:1681–1691.
405. Kleinerman RA, Tucker MA, Abramson DH, et al. Risk of soft tissue sarcomas by individual subtype in survivors of hereditary retinoblastoma. J Natl Cancer Inst 2007;99: 24–31.
406. DeDavid M, Orlow SJ, Provost N, et al. Neurocutaneous melanosis: clinical features of large congenital melanocytic nevi in patients with manifest central nervous system melanosis. J Am Acad Dermatol 1996;35:529–538.
407. Kadonaga JN, Frieden IJ. Neurocutaneous melanosis: definition and review of the literature. J Am Acad Dermatol 1991;24:747–755.
408. Foster RD, Williams ML, Barkovich AJ, et al. Giant congenital melanocytic nevi: the significance of neurocutaneous melanosis in neurologically asymptomatic children. Plast Reconstr Surg 2001;107:933–941.
409. Mackie RM, Watt D, Doherty V, et al. Malignant melanoma occurring in those aged under 30 in the west of Scotland 1979–1986: a study of incidence, clinical features, pathological features and survival. Br J Dermatol 1991;124:560–564.
410. Youl P, Aitken J, Hayward N, et al. Melanoma in adolescents: a case-control study of risk factors in Queensland, Australia. Int J Cancer 2002;98:92–98.
411. Whiteman DC, Valery P, McWhirter W, et al. Risk factors for childhood melanoma in Queensland, Australia. Int J Cancer 1997;70:26–31.
412. Goldstein AM, Fraser MC, Clark WH Jr, et al. Age at diagnosis and transmission of invasive melanoma in 23 families with cutaneous malignant melanoma/dysplastic nevi. J Natl Cancer Inst 1994;86:1385–1390.
413. Goldstein AM, Tucker MA. Genetic epidemiology of cutaneous melanoma: a global perspective. Arch Dermatol 2001;137:1493–1496.
414. Pappo AS. Melanoma in children and adolescents. Eur J Cancer 2003;39:2651–2661.
415. Saenz NC, Saenz-Badillos J, Busam K, et al. Childhood melanoma survival. Cancer 1999;85:750–754.
416. Ludgate MW, Fullen DR, Lee J, et al. The atypical Spitz tumor of uncertain biologic potential: a series of 67 patients from a single institution. Cancer 2009;115:631–641.
417. Mones JM, Ackerman AB. "Atypical" Spitz's nevus, "malignant" Spitz's nevus, and "metastasizing" Spitz's nevus: a critique in historical perspective of three concepts flawed fatally. Am J Dermatopathol 2004;26:310–333.
418. Bastian BC, Olshen AB, LeBoit PE, et al. Classifying melanocytic tumors based on DNA copy number changes. Am J Pathol 2003;163:1765–1770.
419. Gill M, Renwick N, Silvers DN, et al. Lack of BRAF mutations in Spitz nevi. J Invest Dermatol 2004;122:1325–1326.
420. Gerami P, Jewell SS, Morrison LE, et al. Fluorescence in situ hybridization (FISH) as an ancillary diagnostic tool in the diagnosis of melanoma. Am J Surg Pathol 2009;33: 1146–1156.
421. Balch CM, Gershenwald JE, Soong SJ, et al. Final version of 2009 AJCC melanoma staging and classification. J Clin Oncol 2009;27(36):6199–6206.
422. Kaste SC, Pappo AS, Jenkins JJ III, et al. Malignant melanoma in children: imaging spectrum. Pediatr Radiol 1996;26:800–805.
423. Acland KM, Healy C, Calonje E, et al. Comparison of positron emission tomography scanning and sentinel node biopsy in the detection of micrometastases of primary cutaneous malignant melanoma. J Clin Oncol 2001;19:2674–2678.
424. Morton DL, Thompson JF, Cochran AJ, et al. Sentinel-node biopsy or nodal observation in melanoma. N Engl J Med 2006;355:1307–1317.
425. Rao BN, Hayes FA, Pratt CB, et al. Malignant melanoma in children: its management and prognosis. J Pediatr Surg 1990;25:198–203.
426. Harris MN, Shapiro RL, Roses DF. Malignant melanoma. Primary surgical management (excision and node dissection) based on pathology and staging. Cancer 1995;75: 715–725.
427. Navid F, Furman WL, Fleming M, et al. The feasibility of adjuvant interferon alpha-2b in children with high-risk melanoma. Cancer 2005;103:780–787.
428. Chao MM, Schwartz JL, Wechsler DS, et al. High-risk surgically resected pediatric melanoma and adjuvant interferon therapy. Pediatr Blood Cancer 2004.
429. Kirkwood JM, Manola J, Ibrahim J, et al. A pooled analysis of eastern cooperative oncology group and intergroup trials of adjuvant high-dose interferon for melanoma. Clin Cancer Res 2004;10:1670–1677.
430. Boddie AW Jr, Cangir A. Adjuvant and neoadjuvant chemotherapy with dacarbazine in high-risk childhood melanoma. Cancer 1987;60:1720–1723.
431. Hayes FA, Green AA. Malignant melanoma in childhood: clinical course and response to chemotherapy. J Clin Oncol 1984;2:1229–1234.
432. Middleton MR, Grob JJ, Aaronson N, et al. Randomized phase III study of temozolomide versus dacarbazine in the treatment of patients with advanced metastatic malignant melanoma. J Clin Oncol 2000;18:158.
433. Hauschild A, Agarwala SS, Trefzer U, et al. Results of a phase III, randomized, placebo-controlled study of sorafenib in combination with carboplatin and paclitaxel as second-line treatment in patients with unresectable stage III or stage IV melanoma. J Clin Oncol 2009;27:2823–2830.
434. Smith FO, Downey SG, Klapper JA, et al. Treatment of metastatic melanoma using interleukin-2 alone or in conjunction with vaccines. Clin Cancer Res 2008;14: 5610–5618.
435. Ribeiro RC, Rill D, Roberson PK, et al. Continuous infusion of interleukin-2 in children with refractory malignancies. Cancer 1993;72:623–628.
436. Bauer M, Reaman GH, Hank JA, et al. A phase II trial of human recombinant interleukin-2 administered as a 4-day continuous infusion for children with refractory neuroblastoma, non-Hodgkin's lymphoma, sarcoma, renal cell carcinoma, and malignant melanoma. A Childrens Cancer Group study. Cancer 1995;75:2959–2965.
437. Atkins MB, Hsu J, Lee S, et al. Phase III trial comparing concurrent biochemotherapy with cisplatin, vinblastine, dacarbazine, interleukin-2, and interferon alfa-2b with cisplatin, vinblastine, and dacarbazine alone in patients with metastatic malignant melanoma (E3695): a trial coordinated by the Eastern Cooperative Oncology Group. J Clin Oncol 2008;26:5748–5754.
438. Curtin JA, Fridlyand J, Kageshita T, et al. Distinct sets of genetic alterations in melanoma. N Engl J Med 2005;353:2135–2147.
439. Hodi FS, Friedlander P, Corless CL, et al. Major response to imatinib mesylate in KIT-mutated melanoma. J Clin Oncol 2008;26:2046–2051.
440. Rosenberg SA, Dudley ME. Adoptive cell therapy for the treatment of patients with metastatic melanoma. Curr Opin Immunol 2009;21:233–240.
441. Camacho LH, Antonia S, Sosman J, et al. Phase I/II trial of tremelimumab in patients with metastatic melanoma. J Clin Oncol 2009;27:1075–1081.
442. Gorlin RJ. Nevoid basal cell carcinoma (Gorlin) syndrome. Genet Med 2004;6: 530–539.
443. Grady WM. Genetic testing for high-risk colon cancer patients. Gastroenterology 2003; 124:1574–1594.
444. Cohen PR, Kohn SR, Davis DA, et al. Muir-Torre syndrome. Dermatol Clin 1995;13: 79–89.
445. Veale AM, McColl I, Bussey HJ, et al. Juvenile polyposis coli. J Med Genet 1966;3: 5–16.
446. Mallory SB. Cowden syndrome (multiple hamartoma syndrome). Dermatol Clin 1995; 13:27–31.

SECTION 5 ■ SUPPORTIVE CARE OF CHILDREN WITH CANCER

CHAPTER 38 ■ ONCOLOGIC EMERGENCIES

MICHAEL J. FISHER AND SUSAN R. RHEINGOLD

Emergencies can occur at any time during a child's course of care for cancer. Some emergencies are the initial manifestation of cancer or develop as the diagnosis is being made; others arise as a consequence of therapy, and some develop at the time of cancer progression or recurrence. All physicians who care for children with cancer must be able to recognize life-threatening emergencies and triage or treat them quickly and appropriately.

This chapter addresses pediatric oncologic emergencies by system—cardiothoracic, gastrointestinal (GI), genitourinary, neurologic, and metabolic; as well, it summarizes the etiology and differential of cardiovascular collapse and shock, the end result of uncompensated emergent situations. Chapter 39 reviews management of emergencies associated with cytopenias and abnormal hemostasis and use of blood component therapy; Chapter 40 covers infectious complications; and Chapter 42 covers the principles of pain management.

CARDIOTHORACIC EMERGENCIES

Respiratory distress is a common presenting symptom of intrathoracic malignancies and is often the sole symptom of a cardiothoracic emergency occurring at any time. Respiratory distress can be caused by mediastinal lesions compressing the airway and vasculature (superior vena cava syndrome [SVCS] and superior mediastinal syndrome [SMS]); intrapulmonic processes such as infiltrates, pneumothoraces, masses, and fibrosis; intrapleural processes such as masses and effusions; and cardiac processes such as masses, effusions, fibrosis, and failure.

Superior Vena Cava Syndrome and Superior Mediastinal Syndrome

SVCS refers to the signs and symptoms resulting from compression, obstruction, or thrombosis of the superior vena cava. The term *SMS* is used when tracheal compression also occurs. In children with mediastinal masses, tracheal compression and respiratory embarrassment usually coexist with SVCS; therefore, SVCS and SMS are often used synonymously.

Etiology and Pathogenesis

The most common primary cause of SVCS in children is compression by malignant mediastinal masses, with thrombotic complications of cardiovascular surgery being the most common secondary cause.[1] Mediastinal granulomas, infections such as histoplasmosis, or venous thrombosis from central venous lines (CVL) may cause SVCS and SMS symptomatically indistinguishable from other etiologies.[1–3] Table 38.1 lists the frequency of SVCS among 3,721 children with cancer treated at St. Jude Children's Research Hospital.[2] Almost 70%

of patients with non-Hodgkin lymphomas (NHL) and 30% with Hodgkin disease (HD) presented with mediastinal masses. Patients with neuroblastoma, germ cell tumors, sarcomas, thymic tumors, and acute lymphoblastic leukemia (ALL) also were found to have mediastinal masses at diagnosis.

The SVC is a thin-walled vessel with low intraluminal pressure. It is surrounded by lymph nodes and the thymus. Tumor or infection in the mediastinal nodes or thymus can compress the SVC, causing venous stasis. The adjacent pericardium and coronary or collateral vessels fill with tumor or clot. Compression, clotting, and edema combine to minimize tracheal airflow and reduce venous return from the head, neck, and upper thorax, causing the signs and symptoms of both SVCS and SMS. The trachea and right mainstem bronchus in young children are more compliant and compressible than in the adult. Symptoms of compression are especially pronounced in infants and toddlers, as their tracheas and bronchi have small intraluminal diameters.

Evaluation

The most common symptoms of SVCS and SMS in children are dyspnea, cough, orthopnea, dysphagia, and hoarseness (Table 38.2).[1,2,4,5] Anxiety, confusion, lethargy, headache, distorted vision, and syncope indicate carbon dioxide retention and central venous stasis. Symptoms are typically aggravated when the patient is supine, such as for a computed tomographic (CT) scan, bone marrow, or lumbar puncture (LP). Characteristic physical findings include head and neck edema, plethora, and cyanosis of the face, neck, and upper extremities; cervical and thoracic venous distention; conjunctival suffusion and edema; and wheezing or stridor.[1,2,4,5] Signs of pleural and pericardial effusions may coexist. In adults, onset of SVCS caused by a malignant tumor, usually lung cancer, is insidious. In children and adolescents, the symptoms often progress rapidly over days.

Management of children with mediastinal malignancies can be challenging, as respiratory distress and cardiovascular compromise are often the presenting symptoms in a previously well child. A child with a single or many of these signs and symptoms needs both a posterior-anterior and lateral chest radiograph (CXR). Most children with SVCS will have a mass in the anterior superior mediastinum. Pleural and pericardial effusions are more common in NHL than in HD or other malignancies.[4] A CXR may show tracheal deviation. Patients with tumors that are greater than 45% of the transthoracic diameter are more likely to be symptomatic than smaller tumors with ratios less than 30%.[4,6] CT scans can delineate the distortions of normal anatomy and more accurately assess the extent of tracheal compression. Figure 38.1 shows compression of the trachea and superior vena cava by an anterior mediastinal lymphoma. The CT scan can be obtained in the prone position if the supine position aggravates the respiratory distress. If there is concern that the symptoms are being caused by a thromboembolism or pericardial

TABLE 38.1

INCIDENCE OF MEDIASTINAL MASS AND SUPERIOR VENA CAVA SYNDROME (SVCS) AT ST. JUDE CHILDREN'S RESEARCH HOSPITAL BETWEEN 1973 AND 1988

Diagnosis	No. of patients	Mediastinal mass (%)	SVCS with mediastinal mass (%)
Acute lymphoblastic leukemia	1,464	130 (8.4)	6 (4.6)
Acute nonlymphocytic leukemia	392	9 (2.3)	0
Hodgkin disease	333	102 (30.6)	2 (2.0)
Non-Hodgkin lymphoma	330	230 (69.7)	8 (3.4)
Neuroblastoma	332	69 (20.8)	3 (4.3)
Germ cell tumors	114	10 (8.8)	2 (20.0)
Sarcomas	696	26 (3.7)	3 (11.0)

From Ingram L, River G, Shapiro DDN. Superior vena cava syndrome associated with childhood malignancy. Analysis of 24 cases. Med Pediatr Oncol 1990;18:476, with permission.

effusion, an echocardiogram should be obtained. Pulmonary function tests and volume flow loop assess pulmonary reserve and resilience.

When cancer is the probable cause of SVCS or SMS, it is desirable to obtain a tissue specimen for diagnosis. It is imperative that the diagnosis be made by the least invasive procedure possible, as respiratory and cardiovascular failure may occur with sedation or general anesthesia.[4,5,7] During general anesthesia, respiratory muscle tone decreases, abdominal muscle tone increases, the caudal movement of the diaphragm disappears, bronchial smooth muscle relaxes, and lung volume diminishes.[4] These changes aggravate the effects of extrinsic compression of the vena cava. Tracheal intubation may be extremely difficult, even impossible, and some patients will not tolerate extubation until the tumor bulk has been reduced. Conscious sedation or anti-anxiolytics may also be contraindicated as they decrease respiratory drive and dilate peripheral vessels, thereby reducing venous return. Studies have evaluated anesthetic risk according to tracheal cross section on CT, mediastinal mass width on CT, and, more recently, peak expiratory flow rate by pulmonary function testing.[4,8] Both tracheal area greater than 50% of predicted and peak expiratory flow rate greater than 50% of predicted value are associated with low anesthetic risk.[4,8] Great vessel and tracheal compression noted on CT and increasing number of

respiratory signs and symptoms have been predictive of anesthetic complications.[5,7] Although no single measure is predictive of anesthetic outcome, they can all provide important information in regard to risk.

Diagnosis should be made in the least invasive manner possible. Several reports suggest a stepwise approach to diagnosis.[4,8] An algorithm appropriate for pediatric patients is shown in Figure 38.2. A complete blood cell count (CBC) or a bone marrow aspirate performed with local anesthesia only with the patient upright may reveal leukemic blasts. Pleurocentesis or pericardiocentesis may offer immediate relief and provide diagnostic material by cytology or cytogenetics. If there is an enlarged peripheral lymph node, node biopsy is faster and less invasive than a mediastinal biopsy. Anterior mediastinal biopsies can be performed under local anesthesia via anterior mediastinoscopy or mediastinotomy using ultrasound or CT guidance in older children.[9,10]

Therapy

In a child who presents with SVCS or SMS as an initial symptom of malignancy, establishing a tissue diagnosis may be impossible; it may be medically necessary to start empiric therapy. Historically, emergency therapy was irradiation, because

TABLE 38.2

SYMPTOMS AND PHYSICAL FINDINGS IN PATIENTS WITH SUPERIOR VENA CAVA SYNDROME AT INITIAL PRESENTATION

Finding	No. (%)
Cough/dyspnea	11 (68)
Dysphagia/orthopnea	10 (63)
Wheezing	5 (31)
Hoarseness	3 (19)
Facial edema	2 (12)
Chest pain	1 (6)
Pleural effusion	8 (50)
Pericardial effusion	3 (19)

From Ingram L, River G, Shapiro DDN. Superior vena cava syndrome associated with childhood malignancy. Analysis of 24 cases. Med Pediatr Oncol 1990;18:476, with permission.

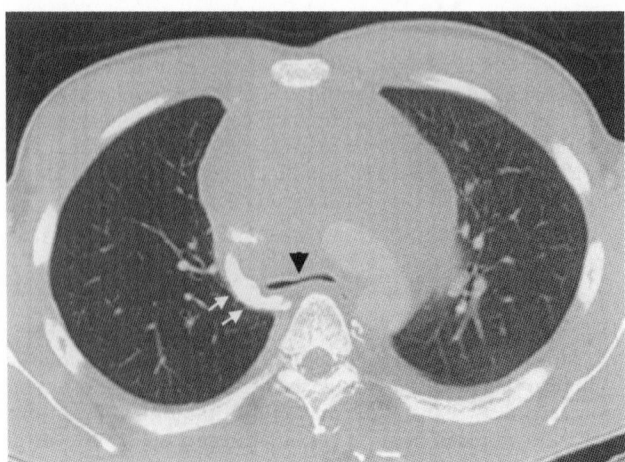

FIGURE 38.1 CT (computed tomographic) scan of the chest revealing compression of the trachea (*black arrow*) and superior vena cava (*white arrows*) by a mediastinal lymphoma.

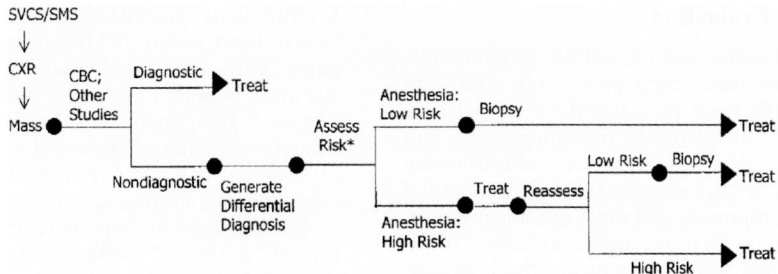

FIGURE 38.2 Assessment and management of a child with respiratory distress, superior mediastinal syndrome (SMS), or superior vena cava syndrome (SVCS) and an anterior mediastinal mass. Initial assessment for anesthetic risk may include computed tomography of the chest, echocardiography, pulmonary function tests, and flow volume loop. If the patient cannot tolerate these studies, or if the studies indicate severely compromised cardiopulmonary reserve, the patient is a high anesthetic risk. CBC, complete blood cell count; CXR, chest radiograph.

most leukemias and lymphomas are exquisitely radiosensitive. Between 1988 and 1994, 10% of pediatric oncology patients at the Children's Hospital of Philadelphia referred for emergent radiation therapy had respiratory difficulties associated with SMS; 83% responded to the radiation therapy.[11] In NHL, radiotherapy is effective, and improvement can occur within 12 hours.[11] However, some lymphomas are so radioresponsive that doses as low as 200 cGy to a circumscribed area of the tumor can cause rapid dissolution of the mass and regional lymph nodes, making subsequent tissue diagnosis impossible. Loeffler and associates reported that out of 19 patients with mediastinal masses, emergency prebiopsy irradiation rendered the histologic specimen uninterpretable in 8 patients.[12] Seven of the eight patients were treated empirically for HD or NHL. Four had no tumor recurrence; three had recurrence with the disease they were assumed to have had; and recurrent seminoma developed in the one untreated patient. The authors point out that patient management was not altered by prebiopsy therapy or by continued empiric therapy.

Respiratory deterioration, presumably from tracheal swelling, can follow hours after irradiation. The phenomenon of postirradiation deterioration seems limited to children and adolescents, perhaps because of the greater compressibility of their respiratory structures and the inability of their more narrow lumina to accommodate postirradiation edema. If the patient's symptoms worsen because of airway edema during empiric irradiation, a dose of IV methylprednisolone (1 mg/kg) every 6 hours may be unavoidable. Radiation oncologists now use highly focused radiation portals, such as a small field centered on the trachea only to circumvent the problem of swelling of small airways.[11,13] Another option consists of using small bilateral opposing fields encompassing the trachea, superior vena cava, and proximal right auricle. The daily dose is governed by the presumed radiosensitivity of the tumor with 100 to 200 cGy given twice daily for radioresponsive tumors such as lymphoblastic lymphoma or leukemia. Less responsive neoplasms such as teratoma, neuroblastoma, germ cell tumor, or benign tumors may not respond quickly to radiation therapy, making surgical resection inevitable.

Use of emergent systemic steroids and chemotherapy in suspected leukemic and lymphomatous masses is now the standard of care. Chemotherapy, including steroids, cyclophosphamide (CPM), vincristine, and/or an anthracycline, is a reasonable alternative to irradiation and is readily available in any hospital. Administration of urate oxidase can prevent the metabolic and renal complications of rapid tumor dissolution (see subsequent discussion on "Tumor Lysis Syndrome"). Unfortunately, chemotherapy can also confound the diagnosis, as it may render the histologic picture uninterpretable within 48 hours.[6] Borenstein et al. reviewed the diagnostic outcome of 23 children with mediastinal lymphoma treated with IV steroids prior to biopsy due to respiratory compromise.[14] Of the 23 children, steroids had an adverse effect on diagnosis in 5 (22%). Two had a delay in diagnosis, two had no definitive diagnosis and were treated presumptively, and one had a failure of staging.[14] Failure to persist with treatment for a presumed leukemia or lymphoma, even if a histologic diagnosis is not made, may allow the disease to progress to a more advanced stage.[12]

In emergency situations or with vascular compromise, arterial extracorporeal membrane oxygenation has been used successfully to support a patient through diagnosis and early treatment with chemotherapy.[15] Tracheal stents have also been placed in emergent situations or for end-stage palliation.[16]

If signs or symptoms of SVCS develop in a child with a CVL and no mediastinal mass, one must evaluate for a venous thromboembolism (VTE). Although often asymptomatic, CVL-associated VTEs should be treated with anticoagulation in children with cancer.[17,18] In children who are symptomatic, infusional thrombolytic therapy may be indicated. Fibrinogen, fibrin split products, platelet count, prothrombin time (PT), and activated partial thromboplastin time (aPTT) should be monitored closely during thrombolysis. Systemic or low-molecular-weight heparin (LMWH) therapy begins either during or immediately following thrombolytic therapy. LMWH is rapidly becoming the antithrombotic of choice in children with cancer due to its better safety profile and lack of drug interaction. Extrapolating from adult dosing, LMWH should be started at 1 mg/kg BID in children older than 2 years with higher doses for younger children.[18] Goal antifactor Xa levels are 0.5 to 1 U/mL.[18] Anticoagulation should continue for a minimum of 3 months with subcutaneous LMWH or oral coumadin.[17,18] Placement of a CVL into the SVC should be delayed until SVCS resolves.

Pleural and Pericardial Effusions

Etiology and Pathogenesis

An effusion represents the escape of fluid into a potential space and can be exudative or transudative. Exudates are generally caused by malignancy or infection and result from inflammation.[19] In contrast, transudates result from a sympathetic response to tumor in the chest or abdomen, fluid overload, heart failure, or hypoproteinemia. Exudates have protein concentrations greater than 2.5 g/dL, a specific gravity greater than 1.015, and a high cell count. Protein concentration, specific gravity, and cell counts are low in transudates.

Evaluation

Symptoms of both pericardial and pleural effusions include dyspnea, tachypnea, orthopnea, chest pain, retractions, and cough.[19-21] Small, clinically silent pleural and pericardial effusions are often detected incidentally on radiographs and echocardiograms. Although an asymptomatic effusion may not require intervention, a large accumulation of pericardial fluid can cause cardiac tamponade and rapid decompensation. Emergent thoracentesis or pericardiocentesis can relieve respiratory or cardiac distress, obtain diagnostic fluid, or can eliminate a potential reservoir for drugs such as methotrexate. Laboratory evaluation of the fluid should include cell count, protein content, cytology, gram stain, culture, cytogenetics, and assays of appropriate immunologic and biologic markers.

Therapy

In a child with untreated cancer and respiratory distress, removal of the fluid one time often suffices, as the fluid usually does not reaccumulate once therapy is under way. In contrast, children with advanced malignant disease may develop recurrent effusions that compromise their duration and quality of life. Palliative measures include repeated centesis, placement of a percutaneous catheter, or thorascopic instillation of a sclerosing agent into pleural or pericardial cavities to cause irritation and adhesion of the potential space.[19] Historically, talc and tetracycline were commonly used sclerosing agents for both pleural and pericardial effusions but are now difficult to obtain. A review of 1,168 patients showed a 93% success rate with talc.[20] Talc itself is inexpensive, but its instillation requires thoracoscopy and usually general anesthesia. Bleomycin and cisplatin have both been used successfully and safely in the treatment of malignant pleural effusions.[22,23] In 8 of 11 children with malignant solid tumors, intracavitary cisplatin at 100 to 200 mg/m² with 16 to 52 g/m² of thiosulfate (300 mL/m² in infant) in 2 L of warmed normal saline or 50 to 210 mg/m² cisplatin without thiosulfate rescue eliminated the intracavitary disease.[23] Intracavitary therapy achieved drug concentrations 40-fold higher than systemic therapy.[23] If sclerosing agents fail, pleural abrasion, surgical pleurectomy, or pericardiectomy may be necessary, but surgery risks substantial morbidity and potential mortality for patients with resistant metastatic disease.

Cardiac Tamponade

Etiology and Pathogenesis

Cardiac tamponade occurs when the left ventricle fails to maintain output because of compression by pericardial fluid or leukemic infiltration, inflammation or infection of the pericardium, constrictive fibrosis from previous radiation, or occlusion from tumors of the cardiac muscle or endocardium.[21,24,25] Infectious pericarditis or myocarditis is probably the most common cause of tamponade in immunocompromised children with cancer. Intracardiac masses such as marantic vegetations or clots can also cause cardiac tamponade. A Wilms' tumor thrombus can extend from the renal vein through the tricuspid valve to fill the right cardiac chambers. Although leukemia may cause pericardial effusions at diagnosis,[21] cardiac tamponade is rarely the presenting symptom of an undiagnosed malignancy.

Evaluation

Gradual accumulation of fluid allows the pericardium to accommodate a large volume, but rapid accumulation of several hundred milliliters can cause sudden decompensation.

Symptoms of impending tamponade resemble those of congestive heart failure (CHF): cough, chest pain, dyspnea, hiccups, and abdominal pain. Signs include tachycardia, cyanosis, hypotension, and a pulsus paradoxus of more than 10 mm.[26] Tamponade must be differentiated from CHF, infectious pericarditis or myocarditis, and therapy-induced cardiomyopathy. Constrictive pericarditis may cause friction rubs, diastolic murmurs, and atrial arrhythmias.

Radiographs of large pericardial effusions often show a typical "waterbag" cardiac shadow on anterior/posterior view and an abnormal space between the pericardial fat and pericardium on the lateral view. Pleural effusions may also be noted. The echocardiogram may show low-voltage QRS complexes, flattened or inverted T-waves and electrical atrial and ventricular alternans.[26] Echocardiography of the posterior wall shows two echoes, one from the cardiac muscle and one from the pericardium. An echocardiogram may also reveal a thickening of the pericardium consistent with pericarditis or pericardial tumor.

Therapy

Supportive care for malignant pericardial effusion and constrictive pericarditis consists of hydration, oxygen, and positioning the patient to maximize cardiac output. Diuretics are contraindicated as hypovolemia decreases stroke volume.[26] Definitive treatment of tamponade caused by an effusion is immediate removal of fluid under echocardiographic guidance. Of nine pediatric patients treated by percutaneous catheter drainage at Memorial Sloan-Kettering, all experienced symptomatic relief, and eight showed complete echocardiographic resolution.[24] Alternative, but more invasive, procedures such as subxiphoid pericardiotomy or pericardial window have high diagnostic accuracy, low morbidity and mortality, and a high rate of success.[25] These procedures are the treatment of choice for persistent symptomatic effusion unresponsive to medical management and tamponade from constrictive pericarditis. Pericardial fluid should be sent for protein, cell count, gram stain, culture, cytogenetics, and cytology. Instillation of sclerosing agents should be reserved for palliation in patients with recurrent or refractory tumor. In patients with a Wilms' tumor thrombus extending into the right side of the heart, if the mass does not occlude the chambers, therapy with dactinomycin and vincristine may reduce the size of thrombus within a week (see Chapter 29).

Massive Hemoptysis

Etiology and Evaluation

Massive blood loss into the respiratory tree can cause thrombus formation within the bronchial tree, leading to asphyxiation or, less likely, exsanguination. In general, pediatric tumors do not cause massive hemoptysis. The most common etiology of mild hemoptysis in an oncology patient is aspiration of blood from epistaxis. The most common cause of massive hemoptysis is invasive pulmonary aspergillosis (IPA). The underlying lesion may consist of a mycetoma cavity surrounded by many collateral vessels from the bronchial, axillary, or subclavian arteries. The majority of patients with IPA leading to massive hemoptysis are patients with acute leukemia recovering from a period of prolonged neutropenia.[27,28] The increasing white blood cell (WBC) count accelerates the process of necrosis and increases the risk of hemorrhage by arterial perforation. A CXR often reveals a nodular or cavitary lesion or a peripheral wedge-shaped infiltrate. Thoracic CT may reveal a halo sign, a localized infiltrate with a halo of ground glass appearance, and an air-crescent sign,

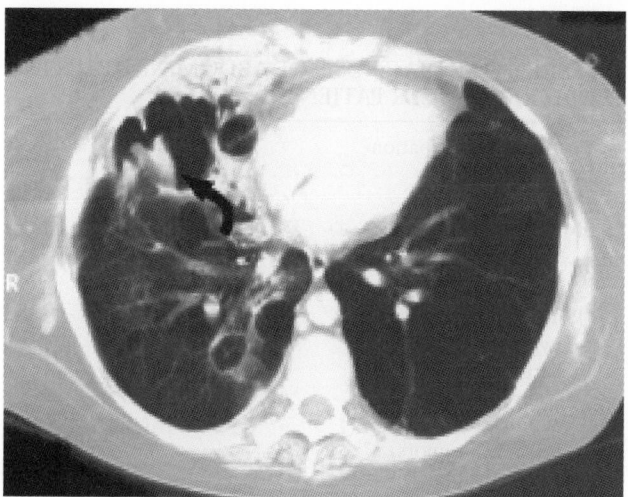

FIGURE 38.3 Computed tomographic image of the chest viewed at lung windows shows a fungus ball (*curved arrow*) within an air cyst in a 20-year-old woman with Langerhans' cell histiocytosis. Note extensive cystic disease and parenchymal destruction in both lungs. (Courtesy of James S. Meyer, MD, Children's Hospital of Philadelphia.)

representing late cavitation.[27,28] Figure 38.3 shows pulmonary aspergillosis in a patient with hemoptysis. The differential diagnosis includes all invasive fungi and, less frequently, bacterial pneumonias and consolidations with invasive organisms such as *Staphylococcus aureus*, *Klebsiella*, and *Pseudomonas*. A CBC, along with a PT, aPTT, fibrinogen, and fibrin split products, should be obtained immediately to look for coagulation abnormalities.

Therapy

Therapeutic objectives are to prevent asphyxiation, localize the site of the bleeding, and arrest hemorrhage. Thrombocytopenia and coagulopathy should be corrected and erythrocytes transfused as needed. For epistaxis, start with direct pressure by external compression of the nares with the patient in an upright position. Unreconstituted topical thrombin powder can be rubbed directly into the bleeding nare for local hemostasis. It should not be given intravenously. For repetitive or persistent epistaxis, an otolaryngologist should be consulted for proper packing or cautery.

If the site of pulmonary bleeding is known, the patient should lie on the side of the hemorrhage to prevent collection of blood into the normal lung. Preventing asphyxiation may require intubation. Oropharyngeal tubes should be big enough to allow passage of a bronchoscope.[26] Nasotracheal intubation may cause epistaxis, making localization of the bleed difficult.[26] Systemic antifungal therapy should be initiated. When the patient has been stabilized, a chest CT should be obtained to localize the lesion. Bronchial artery embolization using selective intrabronchial coagulation with embolic agents such as polyvinyl alcohol particles or spherical embolic agents, or occlusion of the hemorrhaging vessel with a balloon catheter have met with success in patients with massive pulmonary hemorrhage from causes other than *Aspergillus*.[27,29] Unfortunately, these procedures are rarely successful in abating hemoptysis from *Aspergillus* with its extensive collateral vessel network. Caillot and colleagues report very good outcomes with prophylactic resection of large aspergillomas near pulmonary vessels prior to bone marrow recovery.[28] In most cases of hemoptysis, the bleeding eventually stops. In a patient with known fungal disease experiencing recurrent episodes of

hemoptysis, the lesion should be excised. It is becoming more common to medically treat mild hemoptysis from pulmonary aspergillosis because many of the cavities seal off and form linear scars. If an undiagnosed malignancy is found to be the cause of the hemoptysis, surgical resection is indicated when possible. Initiating chemotherapy or emergent radiation therapy can also improve symptoms rapidly.

Pneumothorax or Pneumomediastinum

Etiology and Evaluation

A pneumothorax is air in the pleural space; pneumomediastinum is air in the mediastinum, often with subcutaneous emphysema. A tension pneumothorax arises when inspired air accumulates in the pleural space and is not expelled due to a one-way valve effect. A tension pneumothorax will eventually cause mediastinal shift and circulatory collapse.

Pneumothorax or pneumomediastinum is a rare presenting symptom of an undiagnosed malignancy. They are more likely due to infection, chemotherapy-induced emesis, esophageal perforation, recurrent or metastatic disease, pulmonary fibrosis from radiation or bleomycin, pulmonary histiocytosis, or idiopathic causes.[30–32]

Patients present with cough, dyspnea, or pleuritic chest pain, but often a pneumothorax is found incidentally on CXR. Examination may reveal decreased breath sounds on the affected side, tachycardia, tachypnea, shifting of the trachea, hyperresonance to percussion, or subcutaneous emphysema.[30] A CXR may show a collapsed lung. In pneumomediastinum, air can be seen tracking through the soft tissue and under the skin.[31] Shifting of the cardiac shadow and trachea indicates a tension pneumothorax that must be relieved immediately. Pulse oximetry or an arterial blood gas can be used to assess oxygenation. CT with contrast esophagography can rule out esophageal perforation as a cause of pneumomediastinum.[31]

Therapy

The patient should be placed on 100% oxygen immediately. If the lesion is small, oxygen may suffice. If the lesion is large or a tension pneumothorax or pneumomediastinum is present, the excess pleural or mediastinal air must be evacuated.[33] Needle thoracentesis can be performed acutely, but a chest tube should be placed for long-term evacuation.[32,33] Tension pneumomediastinum can be relieved using a subxiphoid incision and placement of a chest tube retrosternally.[31] In the case of recurrent pneumothoraces, pleurodesis with mechanical abrasion or a chemical agent (see "Pleural and Pericardial Effusions") can prevent recurrence. Treatment of the underlying problem, such as antibiotics for infection or steroids for pulmonary fibrosis, should be started as soon as the patient is stabilized.[31]

Acute Promyelocytic Leukemia Differentiation Syndrome

Etiology and Evaluation

Differentiation syndrome (DS), formerly known as retinoic acid syndrome, is a life-threatening complication during induction in patients treated for acute promyelocytic leukemia (APL) with all-*trans*-retinoic acid (ATRA) or arsenic trioxide. Diagnosis of the syndrome should be suspected clinically in the presence of one or several of the following signs or symptoms: respiratory distress, infiltrates on CXR, unexplained fever, edema, weight gain, pleural and pericardial effusions, hypotension, and renal failure.[34] Symptoms have been noted as early as 2 days to several weeks after starting ATRA.[34] Incidence of moderate to severe DS ranges from 2% to 27%, but overall mortality rate has fallen from 13% to less than 1% due to prophylactic treatment with steroids, and earlier recognition and treatment of the syndrome.[34] A recent multivariate analysis found that a WBC $> 5 \times 10^9$/L and an abnormal serum creatinine at diagnosis put patients at increased risk of developing DS.[34] Use of concurrent cytotoxic chemotherapy appears to mitigate the risk of DS.[34,35] The pathogenesis is unknown, but several mediators have been identified that enhance capillary permeability and cell adhesion, and upregulate endothelial cell expression; and the development of DS often coincides with the ATRA-induced proliferation and differentiation of leukemic promyelocytes.[36] DS should be considered in any patient in whom respiratory distress develops while receiving ATRA. A CXR may reveal pulmonary edema or infiltrates and a pleural or pericardial effusion. The differential diagnosis includes pneumonia or sepsis with bacteria or fungi, CHF, acute respiratory distress syndrome, or any other causes of interstitial pneumonitis.

Therapy

At the earliest clinical suspicion of DS, dexamethasone, 10 mg IV every 12 hours in adults and 0.5 to 1 mg/kg every 12 hours in children, should be initiated.[36] ATRA, arsenic, and other chemotherapy should be held only if the symptoms are life-threatening. When the symptoms resolve, dexamethasone can be stopped and ATRA or arsenic resumed.[36] Prophylactic use of steroids in patients with elevated WBC counts has shown decreased morbidity in uncontrolled studies; randomized, controlled trials have yet to be performed.

GASTROINTESTINAL EMERGENCIES

In the 1970s and early 1980s, gastrointestinal (GI) emergencies in cancer patients had poor outcomes. Today advances in diagnostic imaging, interventional radiology, endoscopy, and surgical laparoscopy allow earlier diagnosis with less invasive management.[37–39]

Etiology and Pathogenesis

Although a child with cancer can develop an acute abdomen for the same reasons as any other child, an acute abdomen unrelated to the underlying malignancy or its treatment is unusual.[37] Many uncommon abdominal emergencies occur commonly in the immunocompromised host: esophagitis, gastric hemorrhage, typhlitis, perirectal abscess, hemorrhagic pancreatitis, and massive acute hepatic enlargement from tumor and venoocclusive disease.[37,40,41]

GI emergencies in the child with cancer arise because of hemorrhage, mechanical obstruction, perforation, and inflammation (Table 38.3).[37,40] Hemorrhage may result from thrombocytopenia, coagulopathy, mucosal ulceration, or abnormal tumor vessels. Obstruction results from compression of a GI lumen by a tumor or abscess or from medication-induced ileus. Perforation can result from unresolved obstruction, localized ulceration, and segmental necrosis. Abdominal processes that are localized in healthy children may be generalized in the neutropenic or immunosuppressed child. Moreover, the inflammatory response may be blunted by a lack of WBCs. Wound healing may be slow because of the effects of

TABLE 38.3

DIFFERENTIAL DIAGNOSIS OF ABDOMINAL PAIN IN PEDIATRIC CANCER PATIENTS

Constipation/obstipation
Vincristine
Narcotics
Amitriptyline
Distention
Ascites
Primary tumor
Lymphoma
Sarcoma
Neuroblastoma
Wilms' tumor
Germ cell tumors
Hepatosplenomegaly
Nerve compression
Retroperitoneal nodes
Inflammation
Appendicitis
Colitis/typhlitis
Ulceration
Referred pain
Pneumonitis
Pleural effusion
Pleural or pulmonary tumor
Retroperitoneal tumor

malnutrition and chemotherapy, notably corticosteroids, on fibroblast proliferation and collagen production.

Evaluation

Pain is the principal symptom of an acute abdominal process, no matter how compromised the patient. It is important to determine the location, quality, and timing of pain in relation to status of the cancer, recent medications, and surgical history. GI hemorrhage is a sign of a serious intra-abdominal process. Changes in vital signs, including fever, hypertension or hypotension, and tachycardia; the presence of blood in vomitus or stool; abdominal distention; and absence of flatus or stool are less specific indications of an acute abdomen.

The examiner should perform the examination causing as little discomfort as possible. On observation, one should note whether the child lies still, is willing to move, or winces with cough, movement, or motion of the bed. Observation may also reveal distension, asymmetry, and surgical scars. Auscultation can help differentiate ileus from obstruction. Compressing the head of the stethoscope gently into the abdomen during auscultation can reveal guarding or tenderness. Inspection of the oropharyngeal mucosa may provide insight into the state of the esophageal or gastric mucosa. Inspection of the perineum and anus is important in the febrile neutropenic patient. Pain detected on perineal examination may be the result of generalized serositis, mucositis, or abscess.

Laboratory and Diagnostic Studies

Selective use of laboratory and radiographic studies may differentiate the child who requires immediate surgical intervention from one who will respond to medical management. Serial CBCs can help monitor hemorrhage and reveal neutropenia that interferes with pus and abscess formation. Persistently positive blood cultures despite treatment with appropriate antibiotics may indicate the presence of an abscess or necrotic bowel. Electrolyte changes may reveal metabolic deficits from fluid shifts before they are clinically apparent. Traditionally, abdominal paracentesis and diagnostic lavage were performed to provide information about extraluminal bleeding, intestinal perforation, or infection. These techniques are being replaced by better imaging and laparoscopy, which permits therapeutic intervention as well as diagnostic potential.[38]

Diagnostic radiologic studies begin with supine, erect, and left lateral decubitus abdominal radiographs.[39] Obstruction, especially high small bowel obstruction, pneumatosis intestinalis, and intra-abdominal free air, can be diagnosed by these studies. In a large retrospective study, the presence of peritoneal signs on examination and pneumatosis intestinalis on radiograph were highly associated with the presence of an acute surgical process in children receiving chemotherapy.[37] A CXR may reveal pneumonia as the etiology of upper quadrant abdominal pain. Barium studies may help diagnose esophagitis or colitis, but direct examination with endoscopy or colonoscopy has replaced contrast studies in the evaluation of the GI tract in both compromised and healthy children.[39] Abdominal ultrasound (US), CT, magnetic resonance imaging (MRI), and angiography may all be used to locate and characterize mass lesions, peritoneal fluid, and abnormal bowel mucosa.

Gastrointestinal Hemorrhage

Esophageal Varices

Esophageal varices can develop as a consequence of fibrosis, cholangitis, and cirrhosis. They occur in patients with Langerhans cell histiocytosis, refractory abdominal tumors compressing the portal vein, portal hypertension, or chronic viral hepatitis. Variceal bleeding is brisk and patients may have associated hematemesis and melena. A CBC, PT, aPTT, and blood type and cross match should be obtained immediately. Initial management includes elevation of the head of the bed to 30 to 45 degrees, judicious volume expansion with normal saline or Ringer's lactate, and correction of anemia. Overzealous volume expansion may contribute to continued bleeding, thrombocytopenia, and coagulation abnormalities.[42] Febrile patients should receive broad-spectrum antibiotics because bleeding varices may be a sign of sepsis in a patient with cirrhosis. Passage of a nasogastric tube and gastric lavage may be initiated as follows: 50 mL volumes of normal saline at room temperature through a 12 French tube in infants; 100 to 200 mL through a 14-16 French tube in older children.[42] Lavage should continue for 5 to 10 minutes with recording of volumes in and out.[42]

Emergent management is indicated for persistence of bright red blood in the lavage fluid. Systemic infusion of vasopressin through a large bore intravenous line or CVL decreases blood flow through the portal circulation.[42] Infusion should continue for 12 to 24 hours with cardiac monitoring for evidence of myocardial ischemia or arrhythmias and frequent observation for signs and symptoms of limb ischemia. If bleeding persists, endoscopy with endoscopic variceal ligation or sclerotherapy is indicated, preferably performed within hours of the onset of bleeding.[42] Balloon tamponade under direct observation with a Sengstaken-Blakemore tube or Linton tube may control refractory bleeding but is associated with considerable morbidity and mortality.[42]

Upper Gastrointestinal Hemorrhage

Hematemesis and melena may consist of blood swallowed from epistaxis or oropharyngeal mucositis or may signify upper GI hemorrhage. Children with cancer taking high-dose corticosteroids, those with increased intracranial pressure (ICP), and those who underwent high-dose irradiation are prone to develop multiple, punctate, shallow gastric, and duodenal ulcers (i.e., stress ulcers, Cushing's ulcers).[43,44] Chemotherapy-induced emesis can cause Mallory-Weiss tears, which are mucosal lacerations at the gastroesophageal junction resulting from large gradients between the intragastric and intrathoracic pressure during emesis.

Children with ICP receiving steroids for central nervous system (CNS) tumors and those receiving long-term steroids should receive prophylactic antacids, H_2 blockers, or proton-pump inhibitors.[42] Medical management of bleeding consists of initiating H_2 blockers, proton-pump inhibitors, antacids, lavage, and correction of thrombocytopenia and coagulation abnormalities as described for esophageal varices.[44] Self-limited hematemesis or coffee-ground emesis can be treated expectantly, whereas brisk bleeding may require lavage as described above. Endoscopy is indicated for uncontrolled or recurrent bleeding and hemostasis may be achieved with a heater probe or multipolar electrocoagulation.[42] Sclerotherapy is not indicated. Surgery for persistent bleeding must be individualized but most often entails vagotomy, pyloroplasty, and oversewing of the ulcer.

Lower Gastrointestinal Hemorrhage

Infections with *Clostridium difficile*, cryptosporidium, fungi, and typhlitis are associated with bloody stools. Neutropenic enterocolitis is the most common cause of lower GI bleeds in adults with acute leukemia and is discussed in more detail below.[45] Intussusception due to tumor, surgery, or an abscess can cause pain, intermittent bleeding, or currant jelly stools.[46] Most major lower GI hemorrhage in the pediatric cancer patient is multifactorial, for example, *C. difficile* enterocolitis in a child with thrombocytopenia and coagulopathy. Melena is usually a sign of an upper GI bleed.[45] Hemorrhoids and anal fissures occasionally cause bleeding in children with cancer. Rarely does this cause significant bleeding and is often reported as blood in the toilet bowl or on the toilet paper. Management is directed at each of the underlying causes.

Gastrointestinal Obstruction

Although bowel obstruction from primary cancer is rare in children, it may be the presenting symptom of Burkitt's lymphoma of the abdomen. Small bowel intussusception is the presenting symptom in 17% to 25% of abdominal Burkitts (Fig. 38.4).[46] The differential diagnosis of bowel obstruction in the child who has had adjuvant therapy or previous abdominal surgery includes obstipation or paralytic ileus induced by vinca alkaloids or narcotics, adhesions or strictures, and intussusception.[47] Abdominal compartment syndrome, defined as elevated intra-abdominal pressure (≥ 20 mm Hg) associated with respiratory compromise and renal insufficiency, can be seen in patients with bulky abdominal tumors at diagnosis or as a postoperative complication.[48] GI obstruction may also complicate palliative care in patients with refractory sarcomas, particularly desmoplastic small cell sarcoma, or with typical adult colon or ovarian stromal cell cancer. Presacral teratomas and pelvic sarcomas may occlude the rectum.

History, physical examination, and plain radiographs that document obstipation can help differentiate narcotic or vincristine-related ileus from a surgical abdomen. Small bowel

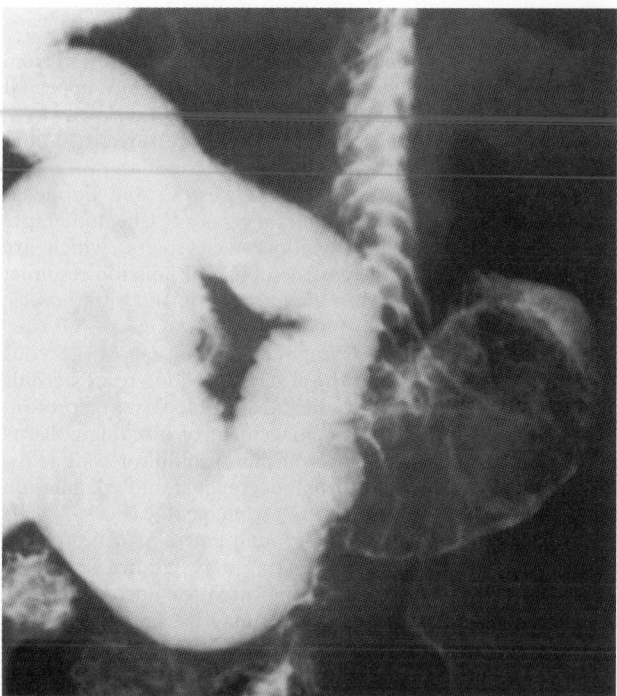

FIGURE 38.4 Contrast study of a 3-year-old girl 6 days after removal of a Wilms' tumor shows evidence of complete small-bowel obstruction. The study illustrates a filling defect from small-bowel intussusception.

obstruction is initially managed by making a patient NPO and placing a nasogastric tube for decompression. Evaluation for the underlying etiology should proceed as described in laboratory and diagnostic studies. Intussusception is often diagnosed and temporarily reduced by air-contrast or barium enema, but surgical reduction is generally necessary for intussusception caused by leading edge tumors.[46]

Gastrointestinal Perforation

Perforation may be the outcome of unresolved obstruction, ulcers or gastritis unresponsive to medical therapy, infections such as typhlitis, or erosion by the primary tumor.[40,42] In the case of abdominal Burkitt's lymphoma, perforation may occur at presentation, during steroid therapy, or after clinical improvement in association with necrosis of the underlying tumor.[49] Upright abdominal radiographs may reveal air under the diaphragm, tracking into the liver, or along the flank on a decubitus view. Perforations are a surgical emergency and are managed either by resection of the affected area and secondary closure or by primary reanastomosis.[49] In massively disseminated, abdominal Burkitt's tumor, cytotoxic therapy may be necessary to reduce the tumor burden before surgical access is possible.

Gastrointestinal Infection and Inflammation

Typhlitis, also referred to as neutropenic enterocolitis, is a necrotizing colitis typically localized to the terminal ileum and cecum. Traditionally, it was defined as the triad of neutropenia, abdominal pain, and fever, primarily seen in patients with acute leukemia. Improved imaging, revealing bowel wall thickening and pneumatosis, has enabled diagnosis of typhli-

tis in both neutropenic and non–neutropenic patients, and in children with solid tumors. Symptoms in order of frequency include abdominal pain (90%), fever (84%), diarrhea (72%), and, less frequently, nausea and emesis. The incidence of typhlitis in children with cancer is reported at 2% to 6%.[50-52] Although typhlitis usually follows cytotoxic chemotherapy, it has been documented in children with ALL at presentation.[53]

Bacterial or fungal invasion of cecal mucosa may progress from inflammation to full-thickness infarction, necrosis, and perforation. Gram-negative bacteria, such as *Pseudomonas* species, *Escherichia coli*, and Clostridium species are the most common bacterial pathogens, but *Staphylococcus*, *Streptococcus, and Enterococcus* species have been identified.[51,54-57] In a recent meta-analysis, fungal pathogens were identified in 6% of typhlitis cases, of which 94% were *Candida* species.[58] Fungus, including *Candida* and *Aspergillus* species, was found at postmortem examination in 24% of patients with leukemia and typhlitis.[55]

Radiographic studies may demonstrate thickening of the bowel wall (>0.3 mm), free air or pneumatosis intestinalis.[51] In a retrospective review of 24 children with typhlitis, Sloas et al. found that CT scan and ultrasound were more sensitive than plain radiographs: false-negative rates were 15% for CT, 23% for ultrasound, and 48% for plain radiographs.[54] Figure 38.5 exhibits the appearance of typhlitis on CT scan. Cartoni et al. have shown that symptomatic patients with acute leukemia and sonographically detected thickening of the bowel wall of greater than 10 mm are more likely to have a worse outcome.[52]

In the past, the mortality rate from typhlitis ranged from 20% to almost 100% with either surgical or medical treatment, but now stands at 2.5%, primarily with medical treatment alone.[50,51,54,55] Shamberger and associates have proposed four criteria for surgical intervention in typhlitis: (a) persistent GI bleeding despite resolution of thrombocytopenia and correction of clotting abnormalities; (b) evidence of free air; (c) need for vasopressor support or large volumes of fluid, suggesting uncontrolled sepsis from intestinal infarction; and (d) development of symptoms of an intra-abdominal process that would normally require an operation.[59] Pneumatosis and localized peritoneal signs are not sufficient to warrant surgical exploration in the absence of one or more of the above

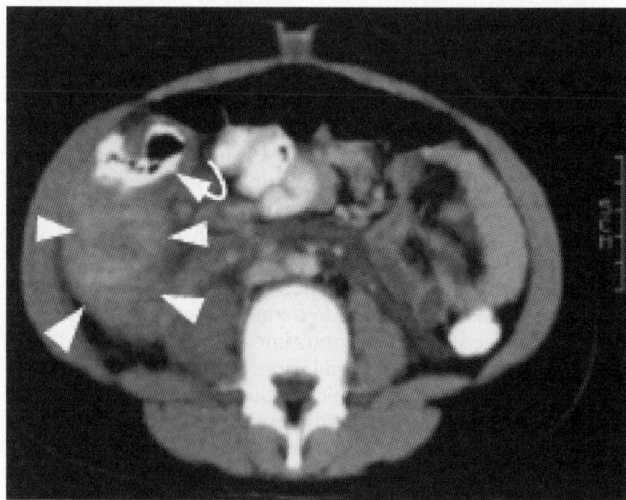

FIGURE 38.5 Computed tomographic scan showing a poorly defined soft tissue mass and indicating a phlegmon (*arrowheads*) and thickened cecal wall (*curved arrow*) in a patient with typhlitis. (Courtesy of James S. Meyer, MD, Children's Hospital of Philadelphia.)

indications. Using these criteria, most patients can be managed medically with broad-spectrum antibiotics to cover gram-negative pathogens, clindamycin or metronidazole for GI anaerobes, and fungal coverage.[54] In two recent reports, only 4% to 8% of patients with typhilitis ultimately required a surgical intervention.[50,51]

Typhilitis and appendicitis have very similar presentations in children with cancer. Appendicitis also presents with abdominal pain, but typhilitis is more frequently associated with fever, diarrhea, and prolonged neutropenia.[60] Incidence rates of appendicitis range from 0.5% to 1.5% and is primarily seen in children with leukemia or lymphoma.[60,61] Despite the sensitive imaging modalities of US and CT, one-third of oncology patients with appendicitis have a delay in diagnosis due to blunted inflammatory response and a broad differential of abdominal pain.[39,60,61] Case reports exist of appendicitis being treated successfully with conservative medical management alone.[62]

Patients who do not have typhilitis but have signs and symptoms of enterocolitis may have transverse colitis, intussusception, or antibiotic-related pseudomembranous or clostridial enterocolitis.[56] *C. difficile* colitis is now the major cause of nosocomial diarrhea in the United States and Western Europe.[57] Although use of second- and third-generation cephalosporins, clindamycin, ampicillin, and amoxicillin is associated with the highest risk of *C. difficile* colitis, even a single dose of almost any antibiotic can predispose a patient to *C. difficile* colitis.[57] The specific therapy for *C. difficile* colitis is oral metronidazole or oral vancomycin.[57]

Perirectal Abscess

Anorectal pain, tenderness, and discomfort with bowel movements may indicate a perirectal abscess or fistula. Perirectal abscesses occur in patients with neutropenia, especially those with acute myelogenous leukemia (AML).[63,64] Superficial lesions are obvious; deeper lesions require cautious rectal examination. In a neutropenic patient, the only physical finding may be tender, brawny, woody edema with a dense cellulitic reaction. Most abscesses are caused by a mixture of aerobes including staphylococci, *E. coli*, pseudomonas, and streptococci and fecal anaerobes.[63] Initial therapy includes antibiotics to cover aerobic and anaerobic gram-negative and gram-positive bacteria. Sitz baths may relieve pain. If the abscess or induration is well circumscribed or progresses, the lesion may need to be incised and drained.[64] Early aggressive medical management often eliminates the need for incision and drainage, particularly while the patient is neutropenic.

Cholecystitis and Biliary Obstruction

Inflammation of the liver and biliary tract can present as localized right upper quadrant pain or jaundice. The most common cause of hyperbilirubinemia, often asymptomatic, is temporary hepatic toxicity from chemotherapy. Acute cholecystitis and particularly acute acalculous cholecystitis occur in children who are septic, stressed, and volume depleted. Biliary obstruction as a result of primary tumor is rare: lymphoma and neuroblastoma occasionally block biliary flow and rhabdomyosarcoma of the common duct occurs.[65]

Ultrasonography or CT scan can differentiate calculus from acalculous cholecystitis.[66] Hydration, broad-spectrum antibiotics, and nasogastric decompression usually treat the acute cholecystitis. Antibiotics should cover gram-negative bacilli and, in the neutropenic patient, fungi. Endoscopic or combined endoscopic-cutaneous decompression is successful

in most patients, and stent placement may provide effective palliation for up to 6 months.[67,68]

Veno-occlusive Disease

Veno-occlusive disease (VOD), also referred to as hepatic sinusoidal obstruction syndrome, consists of rapid and often massive hepatic enlargement with resultant right upper quadrant pain, liver tenderness, jaundice, weight gain, and ascites. VOD is most frequently a complication of cytoreductive therapy for bone marrow transplantation and can range from mild to severe.[41] Mild-to-moderate reversible VOD has also occurred following vincristine and actinomycin D with or without CPM therapy for rhabdomyosarcoma and Wilms' tumor.[69,70] Those younger than 36 months was found to be the primary risk factor for the development of hepatopathy after treatment with vincristine, actinomycin-D, and CPM for rhabdomyosarcoma, with an incidence of 5%.[69] Gemtuzumab therapy for AML is associated with a 15% to 24% incidence of VOD, primarily developing days to weeks into bone marrow transplant (BMT).[71] In both Children's Cancer Group and United Kingdom pediatric ALL trials that randomized 6-mercaptopurine with thioguanine in maintenance, thioguanine was associated with a significantly increased incidence of VOD during treatment.[72,73]

Treatment of VOD is primarily supportive in the nontransplant setting. Withholding vincristine or actinomycin-D generally leads to symptomatic improvement.[69,70] Despite discontinuation of thioguanine, more than 10% of affected patients have persistent splenomegaly and thrombocytopenia, as well as evidence of varices, abnormal liver biopsies, and portal hypertension requiring close follow-up by a gastroenterologist.[74]

Historically, children who developed irreversible VOD post-BMT had a mortality rate approaching 100%.[41,75] Systemic anticoagulation and antithrombotic therapies salvaged a small percentage of children.[76] More recently, the use of defibrotide (a fibrinolytic, antithrombotic, and antiischemic agent) has been associated with complete response rates between 35% and 60% and a 35% to 50% survival at 100 days post-BMT.[41,75,76]

Acute Massive Hepatomegaly in Neuroblastoma

Massive hepatomegaly may complicate stage IV-S neuroblastoma in the neonate and may be fatal.[77] Unless life-threatening respiratory embarrassment is present, supportive care and observation are sufficient until the disease resolves spontaneously. If hepatomegaly compromises respiratory function, the therapeutic options include standard neuroblastoma chemotherapy and emergent radiation.[77] Radiation therapy involves lateral portals with the child supine and fields encompassing most of the liver, but sparing the ovaries and kidneys, and extending from the dome to the posterior portion of the right hepatic lobe. A midplane dose of 150 cGy given on 3 successive days has been sufficient to ameliorate life-threatening hepatomegaly resistant to chemotherapy.[77]

Pancreatitis

When vomiting and abdominal pain occur in a child receiving L-asparaginase or corticosteroids or in a child with ICP, pancreatitis should be included in the differential diagnosis.[78–80] The reported incidence of asparaginase associated pancreatitis ranges from 1% to 18%, tending to occur early in ALL/NHL therapy.[79,80] Studies have shown that pancreatitis is associated with concomitant steroid use and older age.[79,80] An elevated pancreatic amylase and lipase often make the diagnosis, and a US or CT scan of the pancreas should be obtained. A CT scan with contrast may show a phlegmon as a diffuse homogenous area and an abscess may appear as loculations of various densities within the pancreas.[39]

The majority of patients with clinically symptomatic pancreatitis require inpatient admission, complete bowel rest, and intravenous narcotics for pain management. Parenteral nutrition may be necessary.[81] Placement of a nasogastric tube is indicated for intractable emesis or an ileus. Antibiotics should be started for evidence of pancreatic necrosis, abscess, or phlegmon and should include gram-negative and anaerobic coverage. Octreotide, a synthetic somatostatin analog, may ameliorate the clinical course of pancreatitis in children.[82,83] Most cases of pancreatitis are self-limited and can be treated medically. Indications for surgical drainage of a pancreatic abscess or pseudocyst depends on the child's condition and the evolution of the process on sequential US or CT examinations.[39,84] Necrotizing pancreatitis often requires emergent surgical drainage. Percutaneous CT-guided drainage by an interventional radiologist may also be effective.[84]

GENITOURINARY EMERGENCIES

Renal complications in children with malignancies can be divided into primary complications caused by the tumor itself, such as obstruction of the urinary tract and renal vein thrombosis,[85] and those that are secondary to the therapy, such as hemorrhagic cystitis, acute renal failure, or hypertension.[86]

Oliguria or Anuria

When a child has reduced or absent urine output, it is necessary to determine whether the cause is pre-renal, renal, or postrenal. In children receiving cancer treatment, septic shock is the most common pre-renal cause of reduced urine output. Chemotherapy-induced emesis, profuse infectious diarrhea, negligible oral intake, and metabolic abnormalities all can cause intravascular depletion and oliguria.[85] Bulky abdominal or pelvic tumors, including retroperitoneal sarcomas and lymphomas, germ cell tumors, ovarian tumors, and adrenal or celiac axis neuroblastomas, may compress or obstruct the ureters or bladder, causing postrenal failure as illustrated in Figure 38.6.[85,87] Abdominal compartment syndrome from bulky tumors can also result in renal insufficiency and oliguria.[48] Intravesicular blood clots from hemorrhagic cystitis can lead to ureteral or bladder outlet obstruction.[39] Chemotherapy (methotrexate, cisplatin, CPM, ifosfamide [IFOS]), antibiotics, and antifungals can cause renal insufficiency.[85] Narcotics, vincristine, phenothiazines, and herpes zoster can affect the sacral nerves and cause urinary retention.

In a child presenting with a new abdominal or pelvic mass, one should inquire about urinary or bowel dysfunction and obtain a blood urea nitrogen (BUN) and creatinine (Cr). CT or US of the abdomen and pelvis can reveal both a large mass and renomegaly.[39,88] If there is no evidence of impending renal failure, contrast may be used. Delayed filling of the bladder may be noted. Postrenal oliguria from compression or obstruction must be differentiated from tumor lysis syndrome (TLS) as both can present with elevated uric acid, potassium, and phosphorus, although a very elevated BUN and Cr are more consistent with postrenal obstruction.

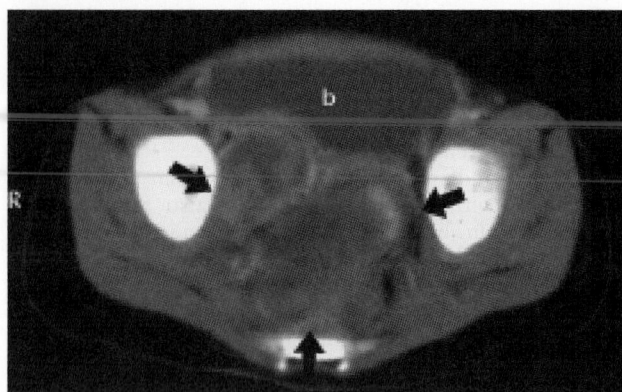

FIGURE 38.6 Computed tomographic image of the pelvis viewed at soft tissue windows shows lobulated presacral mass (*arrows*), displacing the bladder (b) anteriorly in a 2-year-old girl with a sacrococcygeal teratoma. Masses in these locations often compress the ureters and cause upper urinary tract obstruction. (Courtesy of James S. Meyer, MD, Children's Hospital of Philadelphia.)

Therapy

Vigorous hydration quickly corrects oliguria in patients with pre-renal failure but should be avoided in postrenal failure. In most cases of obstructive uropathy with resultant hydronephrosis, decompression of the obstructed kidney by emergent placement of a urinary catheter, percutaneous nephrostomy tube, or ureteral stents will lead to rapid improvement.[87] Treatment of the underlying tumor with surgery, radiation, or chemotherapy will ultimately relieve the obstruction. Nephrotoxic drugs may have to be stopped and replaced with less toxic agents.

Hypertension

Etiology and Pathogenesis

Hypertension is defined as systolic or diastolic blood pressure above the 95th percentile for age and gender.[89,90] Symptoms include headache, irritability, lethargy, confusion, and, if untreated, seizures and coma. The most common cause of hypertension in children with cancer is pain or anxiety and is typically associated with tachycardia. Hypertension can also be a secondary effect of medications such as corticosteroids, cyclosporine A, and amphotericin, or due to fluid overload. Hypertension can be due to renal artery or renal parenchymal compression by tumor, leading to increased renin production.[91] This most commonly occurs in nephroblastoma, neuroblastoma, ganglioneuroblastoma, abdominal lymphomas, and pheochromocytomas. Wilms' tumors, pheochromocytomas, teratomas, and neuroblastomas have also been documented to produce renin ectopically and cause a secondary hyperaldosteronism.[91,92] Renal vein thrombosis can cause arterial systolic hypertension and hematuria.[93] Cushing's triad, consisting of hypertension, bradycardia, and respiratory depression, indicate ICP in a child with a brain tumor, CNS leukemia, or a CNS infection.

Evaluation

Vital signs with frequent blood pressures, using an appropriate sized blood pressure cuff, should be followed. Crying, fever, or pain may temporarily elevate the blood pressure. The abdomen should be examined for the presence of a mass, and radiologic evaluation should include a CT scan of the abdomen to rule out an underlying malignancy and a Doppler US to evaluate renal blood flow. Signs of ICP warrant an emergent CT scan of the brain. Urine and plasma catecholamine levels and plasma renin levels may be elevated in paraneoplastic hypertension.[92,93]

Therapy

Treatment of hypertension typically results in rapid improvement of neurologic sequelae. A modest reduction in blood pressure can prevent stroke, encephalopathy, and CHF. Excessively rapid reduction in blood pressure reduces perfusion of end organs. Recommended emergent IV therapy for patients with normal renal function includes nitroprusside (0.5 to 8 mg/kg/min infusion), diazoxide (2 to 5 mg/kg/dose IV), and hydralazine (0.2 to 0.4 mg/kg/dose IV).[89,90] If a patient is fluid overloaded, furosemide (0.5 to 1 mg/kg) is indicated. Sublingual nifedipine (5 to 10 mg/dose for children weighing >10 kg) acts rapidly and is especially useful to treat asymptomatic hypertension. A long-acting angiotensin-converting enzyme inhibitor or calcium channel blocker dosed once or twice a day provides long-term control.[89,90] For hypertension caused by ICP, dexamethasone or mannitol can decrease cerebral edema, in turn decreasing the blood pressure (see "Neurologic Emergencies"). Definitive treatment of hypertension caused by a tumor is surgical resection of the tumor (pheochromocytoma) or shrinkage of the tumor using cytotoxic or radiation therapy (neuroblastoma, nephroblastoma, and lymphoma).

Hemorrhagic Cystitis

Etiology and Evaluation

Signs and symptoms of hemorrhagic cystitis are hematuria or clots in the urine caused by bleeding and inflammation of the bladder, leading to dysuria, urgency, and frequency. Substantial blood loss and urinary obstruction can result. Therapy with CPM and IFOS are the most common causes of hemorrhagic cystitis.[86] Acrolein, their principal metabolite, is toxic when it precipitates in the bladder. The early phases of hemorrhagic cystitis are mucosal edema, ulceration, epithelial necrosis, and submucosal fibrosis.[86,94] Hemorrhagic cystitis may occur hours to months after CPM or IFOS administration. Long-term complications include bladder fibrosis and contraction, urinary reflux, renal failure, and transitional cell bladder tumors.[86,94] In the immunosuppressed patient, adenovirus, cytomegalovirus, JC virus, and polyomavirus BK can also cause hemorrhagic cystitis.[86,95] In patients who have received CPM or IFOS with prolonged hematuria, viral studies should be sent.

The diagnosis is made by history and urinalysis. Patients usually present with gross hematuria and the passing of painful clots. Ultrasonography may demonstrate a boggy, edematous, hemorrhagic bladder or possibly a fibrotic bladder with hemorrhage. Direct examination may be necessary to locate large areas of bleeding.

Therapy

Chemotherapy-induced cystitis is best prevented by vigorous hydration and brisk diuresis to reduce accumulation of acrolein in the bladder during CPM or IFOS infusion.[94,96] Concurrent use of the uroprotective agent sodium-2-mercaptoethanesulfonate (MESNA), which binds acrolein, has decreased the need for prophylactic bladder irrigation and hyperhydration.[94]

If prevention fails, immediate treatment consists of hydration, correction of thrombocytopenia and coagulation abnormalities, transfusion of packed red blood cells, and placement

of a double-lumen Foley catheter for continuous bladder irrigation. Bladder spasms may be controlled with oral oxybutynin chloride (Ditropan), baclofen, or opioids. Concurrent bladder irradiation and chemotherapy with radiomimetic agents should be stopped. Patients who continue to bleed may need endoscopy and electrocoagulation. If electrocoagulation fails, instillation of formalin, alum, or prostaglandin E$_2$ may be helpful.[96,97] Traditionally, treatment consisted of instillation of a 0.25% solution of formalin into the bladder through a Foley catheter while the patient was under anesthesia.[86,98] The risks of formalin includes obstruction, extravasation, and bladder constriction. In patients with reflux, formalin is contraindicated and alum instillation is preferred. A newer, less toxic therapy is prostaglandin E$_2$. In one study, the instillation of prostaglandin E$_2$ resulted in resolution of hematuria in all 10 patients within 5 days of infusion without any systemic side effects.[97] Antivirals can be used to treat viral-induced hemorrhagic cystitis.[95]

NEUROLOGIC EMERGENCIES

Neurologic emergencies in children with cancer can result from the direct effects of the malignancy, such as spinal cord compression from a paraspinal neuroblastoma or ICP from a CNS tumor. More often, they result from secondary tumor-associated abnormalities of metabolism, hemostasis, or organ system dysfunction or from the neurologic toxicities of cancer therapy or supportive care agents.

A thorough neurologic examination is essential in evaluating a child with cancer and acute neurologic deterioration. A formal neurologic evaluation should not be omitted because the child is considered too weak, too uncooperative, or in too much pain. The reason for the child's misery frequently lies in the CNS impairment itself. Without neurologic localization of the deficit, unnecessary, potentially harmful investigations may be undertaken, further delaying diagnosis and possibly increasing morbidity and mortality.

Increased Intracranial Pressure

Increased intracranial pressure (ICP) occurs when a mass lesion blocks the flow of cerebrospinal fluid, usually at the level of the third or fourth ventricle (obstructive hydrocephalus), or compresses the cerebellum and brainstem, forcing it through the foramen magnum (Fig. 38.7).

Etiology and Pathogenesis

CNS infections were formerly the most common cause of increased ICP. Today brain tumors and blocked shunts in patients with brain tumors are a relatively common cause of elevated ICP. Pseudotumor cerebri can cause elevated ICP in patients treated with glucocorticoids, those with APL treated with ATRA, and those with disseminated subarachnoid tumor in its early stages when it is not yet visible on MRI scans. Abscesses, massive cerebrovascular accidents (CVAs), CNS hemorrhage, and extensive meningeal tumor can also cause increased ICP.

Signs and symptoms of elevated ICP vary with age. In infants and toddlers, history may reveal changes in personality, irritability and lethargy, head holding or banging, vomiting, developmental delay or loss of previously acquired motor skills, failure to thrive, and seizures. Physical examination can show accelerated increase in head circumference, bulging fontanelle, prominent scalp veins, and strabismus. In children and adolescents, headache is the most common symptom. The

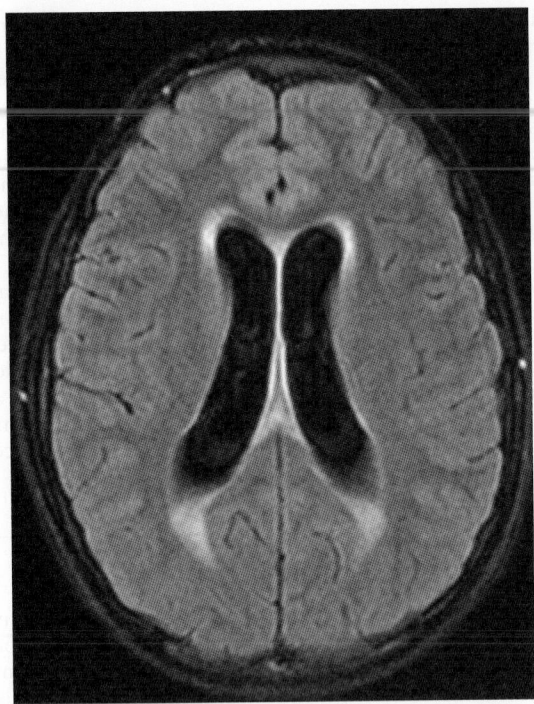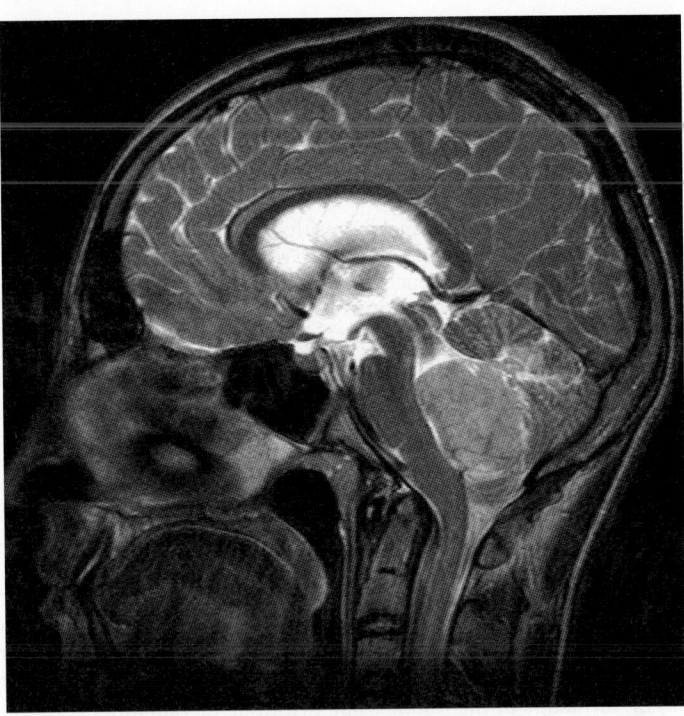

FIGURE 38.7 Magnetic resonance imaging (MRI) of the brain revealing obstructive hydrocephalus. **A:** Axial FLAIR sequence reveals enlarged lateral ventricles with transependymal edema. **B:** Sagittal T2-weighted sequence reveals enlarged 3rd and lateral ventricles caused by obstruction of the fourth ventricle by a brain tumor.

headaches are often vague and intermittent initially but rapidly progress to severe headaches every day. Classic headaches from elevated ICP are occipital in location, and are present when the patient awakens. They are generally followed by vomiting, which may relieve the pain. Repetitive morning vomiting, with or without nausea, is also a common presenting symptom. The patient may also complain of double vision. Poor upgaze and unilateral or bilateral VI nerve palsy with inability to bury sclera is an early finding on physical examination. Strabismus, esotropia, and sometimes nystagmus may be seen. Papilledema is a late finding. Ataxia, hemiparesis, speech disturbance, stiff neck, dizziness, lethargy, and coma are also late manifestations of increased ICP.

Herniation is the end result of progressive increase in ICP or of sudden shifts in pressure as can occur when a LP is performed in a patient with a mass lesion. Transtentorial herniation occurs when supratentorial brain structures are displaced downward through the tentorium, compressing the upper brainstem. Uncal herniation occurs when a unilateral mass pushes the ipsilateral uncus and temporal lobe; ipsilateral pupillary dilatation from compression of the third nerve is the first sign, followed in rapid succession by signs of acute herniation: third nerve palsy (with ptosis and medial gaze paresis), ipsilateral hemiplegia, Cushing's triad (bradycardia, hypertension, and irregular breathing), decerebrate posturing, quadriparesis, fixed and dilated pupils, Cheyne-Stokes respiration, and respiratory arrest. Foramen magnum herniation occurs when the cerebellar tonsils are forced through the foramen magnum compressing the medulla and upper cervical cord. Symptoms include neck pain, bradycardia, hypertension, and altered consciousness. Upward herniation can occur when ventricular pressure is released by a ventriculostomy or ventricular shunt in the presence of an expanding mass in the posterior fossa.[99]

Evaluation and Treatment

Emergent CT scan is the radiologic study of choice; CT is superior to MRI to rule out a hemorrhagic CVA. It can also demonstrate ventriculomegaly and herniation. MRI with diffusion-weighted imaging is used to define the area of ischemia in a thrombotic CVA, and MR angiography can determine the vessel of origin of a hemorrhagic CVA. In cases of presumed herniation, treatment is necessary before the diagnostic procedure. Patients with signs and symptoms of increased ICP should receive dexamethasone (first dose, 1 to 2 mg/kg, then 0.25 to 0.5 mg/kg every 6 hours) and those with acute manifestations of herniation (altered consciousness and respiratory or circulatory collapse) from increased ICP require mannitol (0.5 to 1 g/kg IV over 30 to 60 minutes), endotracheal intubation to achieve mild hyperventilation (pCO_2 of 30 to 35 mm Hg), and placement of a ventriculostomy.[99] Removal of the mass lesion, when possible, is the definitive therapy for increased ICP.

Acute Alterations in Consciousness

Etiology and Pathogenesis

Acute alterations in consciousness (AAC) range from lethargy, where the patient has difficulty maintaining an aroused state, to coma, where the patient is unresponsive to all pain and stimuli. A state of full awareness depends on the integrity of the cerebral hemispheres and the ascending reticular activating system (ARAS), a polysynaptic neuronal network lying in the central core of the brainstem, thalamus, and hypothalamus.[100] The ARAS receives input from and projects to all portions of the CNS. Coma or other forms of alteration in consciousness result from diffuse derangement of cerebral function or damage to the ARAS. Drugs usually cause alterations in consciousness by derangements of diffuse bilateral cerebral function. Increased ICP from a localized mass may cause herniation or compression of the brainstem and disruption of the ARAS (see previous discussion on "Increased Intracranial Pressure").[100]

The causes of AAC can be focal or diffuse (Table 38.4). Focal intracranial mass lesions that cause AAC with or without localizing signs include primary CNS tumors, infarctions, hemorrhages, metastases, and abscesses. Acute thrombotic or, rarely, embolic CVAs can cause neurologic deterioration (see subsequent discussion on "Cerebrovascular Accidents").[101] Spontaneous hemorrhage into intracranial tumors, especially

---

TABLE 38.4

ETIOLOGY OF ACUTE ALTERATIONS IN CONSCIOUSNESS IN CHILDREN WITH CANCER

Tumor
  Primary central nervous system tumor
  Metastatic tumor
  Leukemic meningitis
  Hyperleukocytosis

Infection
  Meningitis: bacterial, fungal
  Viral encephalitis
  Brain abscess
  Septic shock

Cerebrovascular accident

Seizure/postictal state

Disseminated intravascular coagulation

Treatment
  Cytotoxic chemotherapy
    Methotrexate
    Cytosine arabinoside
    Corticosteroids
    Ifosfamide
    5-Fluorouracil
    Arabinofuranosyl guanine (Ara-G)
  Supportive care
    Narcotics
    Benzodiazepines
    Antihistamines
    Anticonvulsants
    Tricyclic antidepressants

Leukoencephalopathy

Metabolic abnormality
  Hyponatremia/hypernatremia
  Hypoglycemia/hyperglycemia
  Hypomagnesemia/hypocalcemia/hypercalcemia
  Uremia

Postradiotherapy somnolence syndrome

Hypotension/hypertension

Dehydration

Hypoxia

Anemia

Liver failure

Depression

---

medulloblastomas and high-grade gliomas, or into metastatic tumors, may occur with normal platelet counts and normal coagulation. Metastatic spread of tumor to the CNS occurs late in the disease in children with sarcomas, lymphomas, and primary renal tumors. Children with cancer who are immunosuppressed, especially those who have recently undergone neurosurgery, are prone to fungal or bacterial brain abscesses and meningitis (see Chapter 40).[102]

Diffuse disorders causing up to one-fourth of encephalopathy and mental status changes in children with cancer include metabolic derangements, drug toxicity, infectious encephalitis, meningeal leukemia or carcinomatosis, and rare neurologic paraneoplastic syndromes.[103] Metabolic derangements that alter consciousness include anoxia, ischemia, uremia, hyperammonemia, hypernatremia, hyponatremia, and hypercalcemia. Metabolic disturbances infrequently lead to increased pressure and central herniation. Viral encephalitis, most commonly from varicella or herpes simplex, may result in acute coma. Seizures cause more than 50% of acute mental status changes in young patients; therefore, the postictal state must be differentiated from other changes in consciousness.

Drugs are the most common cause of AAC in both adults and children with cancer, and opiates are the most frequently identified drugs.[104,105] Table 38.4 lists the commonly used chemotherapeutic and supportive care agents that acutely alter level of consciousness. Neurotoxic agents prime the CNS for neurologic compromise. In this setting, relatively mild metabolic derangements or sedative drugs may suppress consciousness seemingly out of proportion to the insult. High-dose narcotics can sedate profoundly and their rapid termination can lead to withdrawal symptoms. Benzodiazepines, widely used for conscious sedation, may cause acute dysphoria. Poor excretion of narcotics due to hepatic dysfunction or overdoses due to malfunction of patient-controlled analgesia devices can lead to toxic drug levels. Transdermal fentanyl or scopolamine patches can cause sedation and when placed behind the ear, ipsilateral pupillary constriction.

Many forms of chemotherapy cause AAC. Corticosteroids may cause personality changes and occasionally hallucinations and psychosis. The putative mechanisms involve hippocampal damage and changes in excitatory amino acids, glucose metabolism and neurotrophic factors.[106,107] Repetitive high doses of cytosine arabinoside may cause symptoms of cerebellar dysfunction, seizures, coma, or death during an infusion or days later.[108,109] Both high-dose parenteral methotrexate and intrathecal (IT) methotrexate can cause transient encephalopathy or seizures, believed to be secondary to a direct toxic effect on the brain.[110,111] High-dose methotrexate can also cause focal neurologic deficits presumably due to acute intracellular metabolic derangements.[110,112] Ara-G (nelarabine), a T-cell–specific deoxyguanosine derivative, has been associated with weakness, ataxia, confusion, seizures, and coma at high doses.[113] It has also been associated with Guillain-Barré syndrome.[113] IFOS is associated with acute somnolence, neurologic deterioration, and coma, especially after prior cisplatin exposure or in patients with renal insufficiency.[114,115] The introduction of new drugs, higher doses of standard drugs, and the wider use of means to overcome the blood-brain barrier such as intra-arterial infusion are introducing more acute neurotoxicity. Intra-arterial infusions of BCNU and cisplatin have been related to acute neurologic deterioration, seizures, strokes, and encephalopathy.[116,117] AAC may occur in patients with a familial deficiency of dihydropyrimidine deaminase receiving 5-fluorouracil.[118] Thiotepa and BCNU, given in high doses in BMT regimens, can result in severe, life-threatening encephalopathy.[116,117] Retinoids such as ATRA and fenretinide may lead to pseudotumor cerebri, a complication especially common in children.[34,119]

Biologic response modifiers can also cause AAC. Up to half of adult patients receiving high-dose interleukin-2 (IL-2) experience disorientation and confusion; less common are paranoia and combativeness; somnolence and coma are rare.[120] These have not been noted in children given IL-2 as 24-hour infusion for 4 to 10 days.[121] The interferons can cause subacute somnolence, altered cognition, psychiatric symptoms, conceptual disorganization, focal neurologic deficits, cortical blindness, coma, and death.[120] Antiangiogenic agents may be associated with an increased risk of hemorrhage, particularly tumor-related bleeding.[122]

Evaluation and Differential Diagnosis

The evaluation of a child with AAC begins with a rapid assessment of the airway, breathing, and circulation and emergent stabilization as indicated. It then proceeds with a history and formal neurologic examination. A focused history includes the patient's affect and behavior leading up to the acute change, history of similar episodes, seizure activity, recent illness, fever or other infectious symptoms, recent medications, chemotherapy and radiation therapy, and status of the malignancy.

The differential diagnosis includes all the entities listed in Table 38.4. History and physical examination can help classify the process as diffuse or focal. Altered breathing pattern, unequal or abnormal pupillary size and reactivity, abnormal extraocular movements, lack of spontaneous motor function, and reduced response to verbal or physical stimuli may indicate cerebral herniation. When the diagnosis is unclear, a screening laboratory evaluation includes a CBC with differential, PT and aPTT, serum electrolytes, BUN, Cr, hepatic enzymes, serum ammonia, pH, blood cultures in febrile patients, and urine or serum toxin screen. If there are signs and symptoms of increased ICP, LP should be deferred. Patients with presumed mass lesions, unexplained coma, or focal neurological deficits should undergo emergent CT scanning or MRI once they are medically stable. Osmotic contrast agents are contraindicated in the presence of hyperviscosity or hyperosmolality. Diffusion-weighted MRI may help in the diagnosis of CVA or methotrexate neurotoxicity.[123]

Therapy

First, life-threatening respiratory and circulatory disturbances must be corrected. Symptoms or signs of increased ICP should be managed as described in the previous section. In patients with signs or symptoms of elevated ICP in whom sepsis or meningitis is suspected, broad-spectrum antibiotics should be given prior to imaging. Neurosurgical intervention may be indicated for mass lesions or hydrocephalus unresponsive to medical management. LP should not be performed until a mass lesion has been ruled out. Thrombocytopenia and/or a coagulopathy should be corrected as the patient evaluation is ongoing, and before LP or surgery.

For chemotherapy-related neurologic alterations that threaten life or function, the medication should be discontinued or the dose reduced. The specific antidote for IFOS encephalopathy is methylene blue.[124] In the situation of high-dose Ara-C and Ara-G–induced neurologic dysfunction, the drug should be discontinued. Steroids may ameliorate the neurologic effects of IL-2 but may interfere with efficacy. Acute CNS deterioration from methotrexate at any dose or due to elevated methotrexate levels stemming from either altered clearance or overdose can be treated with dextromethorphan (1 to 2 mg/kg/dose),[125] leucovorin, or carboxypeptidase (see chemotherapy complications). Acute methotrexate encephalopathy is usually reversible, and many patients tolerate subsequent use of methotrexate. Management of radiation-induced vascular change is primarily supportive.

When large areas of focal necrosis are present, surgical debulking may be helpful.[126] Although hyperbaric oxygenation and anticoagulation have been recommended for the treatment of radiation-induced necrosis, their efficacy is unproven.[127,128] In children receiving narcotics with AAC, naloxone (1 to 2 mg) can be given IV, IM, or sublingually to rapidly reverse the sedation. The antidote for midazolam is flumezapine 0.01 mg/kg initially, then 0.005 mg/kg every minute to a maximum dose of 1 mg.

Cerebrovascular Accidents

Etiology

Although all children with cancer are at risk for CVAs, children with acute leukemia are at greatest risk. In children with cancer, CVAs are most frequently due to cerebral arterial or venous thrombosis, intracerebral hemorrhage, local or metastatic spread of tumor, antineoplastic agents, hematologic abnormalities, or primary CNS infections; embolic causes are exceptional.[101] When a CVA occurs at the presentation of cancer, it is usually caused by disease-related coagulation abnormalities. During treatment, most CVAs are related to a specific chemotherapeutic agent (such as IT or high-dose methotrexate) or infection. At the end stages of disease, sepsis, disseminated intravascular coagulation (DIC), CNS infection, and progressive tumor are common causes of CVA. Strokes occurring months to years after children have completed therapy are sometimes the result of radiation-induced vascular damage.[129] Bulky medulloblastomas, high-grade gliomas, ependymomas, and choroid plexus tumors are prone to intratumoral hemorrhage even in the absence of coagulopathy.

Pathogenesis

Patients with AML, especially APL, myelodysplasia, or any form of leukemia with hyperleukocytosis (see "Hyperleukocytosis"), are at especially high risk for stroke at diagnosis or early in treatment.[36,130–132] Leukemic promyelocytes enhance thrombin activation, and their high levels of expression of annexin II increase production of plasmin, a fibrinolytic protein, causing DIC and CVA.[36,133] The CVA usually occurs early in treatment of APL and may even be the presenting symptom.

L-Asparaginase, as a single agent or in combination with vincristine and prednisone, is associated with increased risk of venous thrombosis, especially near the end of induction therapy for ALL.[134] A prospective screening study of children with ALL and CVL treated with L-asparaginase found a thromboembolism prevalence of 36%, primarily in the upper central venous system.[135] The majority of symptomatic thromboses occur in the CNS.[136] Children receiving L-asparaginase acquire a deficiency of antithrombin-III (AT-III) and of proteins S and C, thereby having an enhanced thrombin formation, creating a prothrombotic state.[134] A study of antithrombin replacement is ongoing in this high risk population; preliminary data suggest benefits to replacement.[137] IT methotrexate occasionally causes CVA.[138]

During induction treatment for ALL or NHL, visual hallucinations progressing to confusion and stroke-like episodes may occur. They are associated with bilateral cortical or subcortical white matter lesions. The etiology of these spells is believed to be vascular, possibly associated with hypertension or vincristine.[139] Transient ischemic events, similar to complicated migraine, may occur after cranial irradiation and chemotherapy.[140]

Radiation therapy may cause delayed large and small vessel occlusions.[129,141] Total doses of radiation therapy in excess of 3,000 to 5,000 cGy have been associated with an increase risk of stroke.[129,142] The peak incidence of large vessel occlusions is 6 months to 3 years after treatment, but occlusions may take place up to 2 decades later.[141] Rarely, patients develop a CVA after lower dose radiation. More commonly, radiation therapy causes small, focal vascular occlusions. Mineralizing microangiopathy with dystrophic calcification is seen histopathologically in many children who have died of cancer but is rarely reported in children who have received less than 2,000 cGy. IT or parenteral methotrexate and cytosine arabinoside potentiate the risk of radiation-induced damage.[143]

Hemorrhagic CVA can occur preterminally, especially in children with neuroblastoma metastatic to the dura or torcula and in those with platelet-resistant thrombocytopenia.[103] Neuroblastoma may also cause lateral and transverse sinus thrombosis by compression from metastases to the calvarium adjacent to the venous channels.[103]

Evaluation and Differential Diagnosis

In evaluating a child with cancer and a presumed CVA, it is important to consider the type, extent, and status of the cancer, the antineoplastic treatment, and any associated medical conditions. In a critically ill child with uncontrollable cancer, no specific evaluation may be indicated. CVAs usually present as acute impairments in motor function or speech and are often associated with severe or unremitting headache, altered mental status, and seizures. A major CVA, such as a sagittal sinus thrombosis or a brain stem stroke, can cause obtundation, which must be differentiated from lethargy or coma due to other causes.

Any new-onset focal deficit should prompt appropriate imaging to rule out a structural CNS lesion. When the child is medically stable, emergent CT should be performed to evaluate for hemorrhage or a mass lesion. Evidence of ischemic stroke may be lacking in the first 24 hours on CT scan. MRI with diffusion-weighted imaging is more sensitive and may reveal evidence of ischemia within minutes of onset of symptoms.[144] MR angiography can help confirm a specific diagnosis, such as postradiation vessel occlusive vasculopathy[129] but is rarely needed at the onset of symptoms. MR venogram should be performed if sinus thrombosis is suspected. Follow-up imaging studies may be necessary to document infarction and demonstrate the full extent of damage.[145] Care should be taken to evaluate the torcular region of the calvarium and dura in children with neuroblastoma, to rule out the possibility of a sinus thrombosis.[103] If the CT or MRI does not show a focal mass lesion, LP can be performed for analysis of opening pressure, protein, glucose, cell count, cytology, and bacterial, viral, and fungal cultures.

Therapy

Traditionally, the management of a child with a CVA has been primarily supportive, with platelets and plasma to correct deficiencies. The platelet count in children with hemorrhagic strokes should be kept above 75,000/mL to prevent further bleeding. Although surgery may be lifesaving in the child with an intracerebral hemorrhage, operative intervention may be unwarranted in patients with uncontrolled coagulopathy or at the end stage of their disease. For arterial ischemic strokes, patients should remain supine for at least 48 hours after the CVA to maximize perfusion to the compromised area. They should be rendered normothermic, normoglycemic (i.e., blood glucose concentration between 80 and 120 g/L), and normotensive or minimally hypertensive, never hypotensive. Intravenous fluids should be isotonic without dextrose unless serum glucose is below normal. If CVA is a presenting or early symptom of malignancy, treating the underlying disease with cytotoxic therapy may prevent

additional CVAs. Antibiotics or antifungals should be started if there is concern of infection.

The use of heparin in stroke management is controversial. It is contraindicated in the presence of an intracranial hemorrhage or in patients undergoing neurosurgery. Heparin may be useful in patients whose CVA is thromboembolic in nature. In a cohort study that included 30 children with sinovenous thrombosis, deVeber and associates found no evidence of intracranial bleeding in the 12 children who received LMWH and one silent hemorrhage in the 10 children who received standard heparin.[146] Johnson and associates reported on 15 children with sinovenous thrombosis who received a variety of agents, and none had recurrence or hemorrhage.[147] Stam et al. reviewed two randomized trials of anticoagulation that involved 79 patients and concluded that relative risk of death with anticoagulation is 0.33 (95% CI, 0.08 to 1.21) and of dependency is 0.46 (95% CI, 0.16 to 1.31).[148] The PAARKA randomized controlled trial of AT-III therapy in preventing thrombosis in children receiving L-asparaginase showed a trend to safety and efficacy, but the study included all thromboses, not just sinovenous thrombosis.[137] The aggregated evidence suggest that anticoagulation for cerebral sinus thrombosis is generally not harmful and may be of benefit, but there are too few pediatric cancer patients in these studies to know if these results should be generalized. Aspirin is often recommended for those with arterial ischemic stroke but is usually avoided in patients actively being treated with myelosuppressive therapy. Thrombolytic therapy is recommended for adults with ischemic stroke diagnosed within the first 3 hours,[149] and recent evidence suggests its utility for up to 4.5 hours[150]; however, the safety and efficacy of thrombolytic use in children is unproven.

The use of ATRA to treat APL often resolves the coagulopathy in 5 to 7 days[36,133]; however, many CVAs occur at presentation. Supportive care with transfusion of platelets, fresh-frozen plasma, fibrinogen, and/or cryoprecipitate should be instituted immediately in patients with suspected APL and coagulopathy.[34] In patients with L-asparaginase–related CVA or coagulation abnormalities, prophylactic treatment with fresh-frozen plasma (10 mL/kg) has been investigated, but it does not affect the AT-III deficiency.[134] The use of AT-III concentrates is controversial. In children with neuroblastoma metastatic to the torcular region, emergency radiation to the sinus area can resolve the symptoms rapidly.[103]

Seizures

Etiology and Pathogenesis

Seizures are transient involuntary alterations of consciousness, behavior, motor function, sensation, or autonomic function due to excessive rate and hypersynchrony of neuronal discharges. Table 38.5 lists common causes of seizures in children with cancer. Seizures account for up to 60% of neurologic consults on pediatric oncology services.[103,151] They are primarily due to the underlying malignancy, especially primary CNS tumors, tumors metastatic to the CNS, and meningeal leukemia, and to antineoplastic therapy. IT cytarabine and IT and high-dose IV methotrexate can cause seizures, especially in children who have received cranial irradiation.[103,111] It is unclear whether vincristine directly causes seizures; however, vincristine can cause hyponatremia due to syndrome of inappropriate antidiuretic hormone secretion (SIADH) with resultant seizures. Radiation-induced small vessel disease, cerebral necrosis, and leukoencephalopathy also provoke seizures.[126] CVAs, CNS infections, and metabolic derangements also cause seizures.[103]

TABLE 38.5

ETIOLOGY OF SEIZURES IN CHILDREN WITH CANCER

Tumor
  Primary central nervous system tumor
  Metastatic tumor
  Leukemic meningitis
  Hyperleukocytosis

Central nervous system infection
  Viral
  Bacterial
  Fungal
  Protozoal

Cerebrovascular accident
  Treatment
  Intrathecal methotrexate
  Intrathecal cytosine arabinoside
  L-Asparaginase

Metabolic abnormality

Hypoxia

Evaluation and Differential Diagnosis

A seizure is a symptom of an underlying pathologic process. The investigation of the seizure is similar to that previously discussed for AAC and CVA and should take place as soon as the seizure is controlled. A history of any previous seizures, family history of seizures, a list of medications, and cancer chemotherapy or radiation therapy should be obtained. A CBC, serum electrolytes (including magnesium, calcium, phosphorus), renal and hepatic function, and coagulation studies should be checked. Emergent CT or MRI with and without contrast is indicated to look for hemorrhage or a mass lesion. On T2-weighted images, methotrexate-induced encephalopathy and seizures may appear as diffuse hyperintensities in the white matter and cerebral subcortical calcifications.[111] Diffusion-weighted imaging may allow for early detection of methotrexate toxicity.[152] Cerebral spinal fluid (CSF) analysis, after CT or MRI reveals no mass lesion, should include cell count, glucose, protein, cytology, bacterial culture, and viral titers, as clinically indicated. Electroencephalogram (EEG) can localize abnormal electrical activity in the brain.

Therapy

Most seizures are self-limited; a prolonged seizure requires emergent management.[153] Adequate ventilation and circulation must be secured and metabolic abnormalities corrected, followed by the initiation of anticonvulsants. Table 38.6 lists recommended anticonvulsants and their doses. For status epilepticus unresponsive to therapies directed at the cause, diazepam or lorazepam are the usual initial therapy because of their rapid onset of action.[153,154] For treatment of prolonged or multiple seizures, phenytoin can be used. Carbamazepine should be avoided due to its potential marrow suppression.

Most children with cancer and seizures receive antiepileptic medication while evaluation is underway. Those without markedly abnormal EEGs and normal neuroimaging can usually discontinue therapy without a recurrence. Many seizures associated with chemotherapeutic agents do not recur, even when the drugs are given again, unless an associated metabolic abnormality also recurs. Children whose first seizure is prolonged or who have repetitive seizures experience an increased incidence of seizure recurrence and generally require prolonged therapy with anticonvulsants.[103]

Antibiotics are indicated in febrile neutropenic patients, those with meningeal signs or symptoms, and those in whom infection is a concern. In the case of CNS infection, metabolic abnormalities, and most therapy-related seizures, antiepileptics can be withdrawn after correction of the underlying abnormality, if the follow-up EEG shows no epileptiform activity and there is no residual focal CNS defect.

Intrathecal Chemotherapy Overdoses or Errors

IT chemotherapy is used frequently in the treatment of ALL, AML, and NHL and unfortunately overdoses and errors in administration occur. The symptoms noted with IT methotrexate overdoses range from none to headache for doses less than

TABLE 38.6

ANTICONVULSANTS FOR STATUS EPILEPTICUS IN CHILDREN WITH CANCER

Drug	Dose (mg/kg)	Duration of action	Advantages	Disadvantages
Diazepam	i.v.: 0.2–0.5 (max. 10 mg) p.r.: 0.2–0.5 (max. 30 mg)	i.v.: 20–30 min p.r.: up to 4 hr	Rapid onset, rectal formulation	Short duration, respiratory depression, hypotension
Lorazepam	i.v.: 0.05–0.1 mg/kg/dose	12–24 hr	Rapid onset, longer duration of action	Respiratory depression hypotension, drowsiness
Phenytoin	i.v.: 10–20 mg/kg bolus at 1–2 mg/kg/min	Up to 12 hr	Rapid onset, minimal sedation	Arrhythmia, wide QT interval
Phenobarbital	i.v.: 10–20 mg/kg bolus at 1 mg/kg/min (max. 30 mg/kg)	Up to 24 hr	Long half-life	Sedation, respiratory depression, bradycardia
Fosphenytoin sodium	i.m.: 10–20 mg PE/kg, 3 mg PE/kg/min (max. 150 mg/min)	Up to 12 hr	Intramuscular formulation	Emesis, ataxia, cost, pruritus

PE, phenytoin equivalent.
Adapted from Bebin M. The acute management of seizures. Pediatr Ann 1999;28(4):225–229, with permission.

100 mg to seizure, coma, and cardiopulmonary compromise within 1 hour for doses greater than 500 mg.[155,156] The only reported overdose of IT cytarabine (200 mg) was associated with dilated pupils for an hour.[157] Two inadvertent instillations of IT anthracyclines were notable for their delayed onset (16 and 17 days) of neurologic symptomatology; one ended in death.[158] Infusion of IT vincristine, a CNS neurotoxin, causes a rapid ascending paralysis and coma,[159] and is usually fatal at any dose.[158]

Treatment

Immediate action is necessary for any chance of complete recovery after an IT overdose or error. If the interval between the overdose and recognition of the problem is less than 2 hours, as much CSF as possible should be drained.[155,156] Thirty percent to 50% of the initial drug dose can be recovered by simple CSF drainage within 1 to 2 hours of infusion.[158,160,161] If more time has elapsed, CSF can be exchanged with saline or lactated Ringer's. Ventricular catheter placement for ventriculo-lumbar perfusion should be considered if the patient's clinical condition continues to deteriorate or if the overdose is severe.

Overdoses of less than 100 mg methotrexate need minimal intervention; higher doses require prompt, aggressive intervention to minimize neurologic sequelae. With the advent of IT carboxypeptidase G_2 (CPDG$_2$), survival without sequelae has occurred following IT methotrexate doses of greater than 500 mg, even when noted several hours after the initial instillation.[156] CPDG$_2$ rapidly hydrolyzes methotrexate to nontoxic metabolites *in vitro* and in patients with or without CSF exchange decreased CSF methotrexate concentrations by more than 98%.[156] Present recommendations for the treatment of IT methotrexate overdoses of more than 100 mg include immediate drainage of CSF by gravity, followed by ventriculo-lumbar CSF exchange (when feasible), and IT administration of 2,000 units of CPDG$_2$. High-dose systemic leucovorin (100 mg every 6 hours for 4 doses) and IV dexamethasone (0.5 mg/kg) every 6 hours for 24 to 72 hours should be administered concomitantly to decrease systemic toxicity and chemical meningitis.[156] CNS drainage and systemic leucovorin usually suffice for IT methotrexate doses of less than 100 mg.[162] Leucovorin should not be administered IT.[161]

Only 3 of 10 children reported in the medical literature survived accidental administration of IT VCR.[158,159,163] The surviving children had CSF drained within 5 minutes of administration, followed by three CSF exchanges with lactated Ringer's and fresh-frozen plasma and prolonged ventriculo-lumbar perfusion with the same. All children received glutamic acid (IV 10 g over 24 hours, then 250 mg orally every 8 hours), two received leucovorin and pyroxidine, and one received caffeine in addition.[158,159,163]

Spinal Cord Compression

Etiology and Pathogenesis

A mass compromising the integrity of the spinal cord, conus medullaris, or cauda equina requires urgent attention to minimize long-term neurologic dysfunction. Epidural compression may occur with a known malignancy or may be the presenting symptom of an undiagnosed malignancy. Acute compression of the spinal cord occurs in 3% to 5% of children with cancer, often at diagnosis.[164,165] Another 5% to 10% of patients develop back pain that must be differentiated from spinal cord compression. Table 38.7 shows the frequency of epidural metastases among 2,259 children with

TABLE 38.7

INCIDENCE OF SPINAL CORD COMPRESSION IN CHILDREN WITH SOLID MALIGNANT TUMORS

Pathology	No. of cases of SCC (%)	Total cases
Ewing's sarcoma	30 (17.9)	168
Neuroblastoma	32 (7.9)	402
Osteogenic sarcoma	16 (6.5)	243
Rhabdomyosarcoma	14 (4.9)	287
Hodgkin disease	8 (2.0)	404
Soft tissue sarcoma	4 (3.9)	102
Germ cell tumor	5 (3.8)	130
Wilms' tumor	2 (0.7)	290
Hepatoma	1 (1.4)	69
Other[a]	—	164
Total	113 (5.0)	2,259

SCC, spinal cord compression due to epidural metastatic disease.
[a]Patients with other tumors who did not develop epidural spinal metastases.
Reproduced from Klein SL, Sanford RA, Muhlbauer MS. Pediatric spinal epidural metastases. J Neurosurg 1991;74:70, with permission.

malignant solid tumors at St. Jude Children's Research Hospital from 1962 to 1987.[165] Sarcomas account for most spinal cord metastases, with neuroblastoma, germ cell tumors, lymphoma, and dropped metastases from primary CNS tumors accounting for most of the remainder.[165] Spinal cord compression has occurred with almost any tumor type, including Wilms' tumor[166] and leukemia.[167]

The spinal cord and cauda equina may be compressed by tumor in the epidural or subarachnoid space, or, less commonly, by metastatic spread to the cord parenchyma. Epidural compression occurs by extension of a paravertebral tumor through the intervertebral foramina. Compression of the vertebral venous plexus by the tumor causes vasogenic cord edema, venous hemorrhage, and ischemia.[10] Metastatic involvement of the vertebral bodies and secondary compression of the spinal cord, common in adults with cancer, is rare in childhood.[168] Treatment-related myelitis may mimic cord compression.[168,169]

Evaluation and Differential Diagnosis

Children with cancer and back pain should be considered to have spinal cord compression until proven otherwise. Local or radicular back pain occurs in 80% of children with cord compression and is often worse at night and when the patient lies flat.[164] Pain can start weeks to months before diagnosis. Other symptoms of cord compression include weakness, sensory abnormalities, and sphincter disturbances (urinary and fecal incontinence or retention).[169] The latter is a poor prognostic sign of neurological outcomes and is a late symptom of cord involvement but may occur earlier with compression of the conus medullaris.[170] Once neurologic abnormalities are apparent, paraplegia and quadriplegia can occur rapidly and may be irreversible.[169]

Detailed neurologic examination with attention to extremity strength, reflexes, and determination of a sensory level is essential. A rectal examination assesses sphincter tone. Localized tenderness to vertebral percussion occurs in many patients, and the level of maximal spinal tenderness is a reliable localizing sign. Most patients have objective loss of motor strength in the extremities at the time of diagnosis. On the basis of clinical findings, the level of spinal cord involvement can usually be determined (Table 38.8), but the absence

TABLE 38.8

CLINICAL LOCALIZATION OF EPIDURAL CORD COMPRESSION

Sign	Location		
	Spinal cord	Conus medullaris	Cauda equina
Weakness	Symmetric; profound	Symmetric; variable	Asymmetric; may be mild
Tendon reflexes	Increased or absent	Increased knee; decreased ankle	Decreased; asymmetric
Babinski	Extensor	Extensor	Plantar
Sensory	Symmetric; sensory level	Symmetric; saddle	Asymmetric; radicular
Sphincter abnormality	Spared until late	Early involvement	May be spared
Progression	Rapid	Variable; may be rapid	Variable; may be rapid

of weakness or sensory abnormalities does not exclude spinal cord compression. History and physical examination can usually rule out vincristine neuropathy as the etiology of back pain.

MRI (T1- and T2-weighted and postgadolinium sequences) is the gold standard for diagnosis.[145] MRI demonstrates epidural disease, intraparenchymal spread of tumor, and small lesions compressing nerve roots in the cauda equina.[145,169,171] Any child who is not ambulatory at the time of clinical presentation, independent of the duration of dysfunction before evaluation, should undergo imaging immediately. In those children with localizing back pain and no focal findings on neurologic examination, MRI can be arranged within 24 hours. If MRI is not available or is contraindicated, CT myelography should be performed.[10] Spine radiographs and radionuclide bone scanning are not as sensitive as MRI and provide less information.[171]

Therapy

Dexamethasone is the initial treatment for cord compression and improves long-term ambulatory rates[172]; however, the appropriate dosing of dexamethasone is unclear. High-dose dexamethasone (100 mg loading dose followed by 96 mg/day) is recommended for use in adults with rapidly declining motor function or who are nonambulatory, while moderate dosing (10 mg loading dose followed by 16 mg/day) is more appropriate for patients with minimal neurologic findings.[170] Others have suggested that dexamethasone may be deferred in a select group of patients with minimal cord compression and good neurological function.[173] For children, loading doses of 1.0 to 2.0 mg/kg followed by 0.25 to 0.5 mg/kg every 6 hours has been suggested.[168,169]

If an epidural mass is compressing the spinal cord, the cord must be decompressed immediately. Although dexamethasone reduces vasogenic cord edema and often results in neurologic improvement, it is not an alternative to definitive spinal decompression. Local radiation therapy, surgical decompression, and chemotherapy all have their advocates. There are no randomized controlled studies or prospective studies to compare short- and long-term outcomes. A clear indication for surgery is the unknown primary. For the child with epidural disease without known dissemination, surgery offers the dual benefit of decompression plus identification of the tumor type. Because pediatric tumors frequently enter the spinal canal by way of the intervertebral foramina, surgery involves laminectomy and posterior decompression.[169] Resection of multiple vertebral lamina in an infant or young child causes problems of growth and spinal stability. Surgery should be considered in patients with radiation and chemotherapy-resistant tumors,[174] and in those whose symptoms progress despite these other treatments.[175] For the rare child or adolescent with spinal cord compression from vertebral body metastases, vertebral body resection may be needed.

If the diagnosis is known and the tumor is radioresponsive, radiation therapy is often the treatment of choice. The portal should include the full volume implicated on radiographic study plus a margin, depending on disease and patient-related factors. The optimum fractionation schedule is controversial, although one large adult series reported similar functional outcomes with doses of 200 to 800 cGy, but lower recurrence rates for lower doses used in protracted schedules.[176] In children, daily doses between 180 and 400 cGy are given with concomitant dexamethasone. Total dose depends on tumor histology and response to initial therapy. In an infant or young child, high-dose wide-field XRT will impair growth of the spine, spinal cord, and surrounding tissues. The functional outcomes for patients with radiosensitive tumors are similar for radiation alone versus surgery plus radiation.[177]

A third alternative, chemotherapy, may be appropriate for patients with spinal cord compression due to lymphoma, leukemia, and neuroblastoma.[167,178,179] High-dose dexamethasone and systemic chemotherapy often result in prompt symptomatic improvement and reduction in mass size.[167] However, surgery should be considered for patients with further neurological decline during chemotherapy[180] and those without noticeable tumor regression or functional improvement. For children with less chemosensitive tumors, such as sarcomas, surgery is indicated.[171,180] Ultimately, the optimal treatment often involves a combination of XRT, surgery, and chemotherapy planned by a multidisciplinary team.

The prognosis for patients with spinal cord compression depends on the neurologic findings and presentation. Patients who are ambulatory when treatment is started usually remain ambulatory.[169] In adults, patients who are paraplegic at the time of treatment rarely regain function.[175] In contrast, up to half of children who were not ambulatory at the beginning of treatment regained the ability to walk after emergency treatment.[164] Others have shown that the rate of motor deficit development is inversely related to functional outcome.[176]

Hyperleukocytosis

Etiology

Hyperleukocytosis is defined as a peripheral leukocyte count exceeding 100,000/mL, but clinically significant hyperleukocytosis occurs with WBC counts of greater than 200,000/mL in AML, and greater than 300,000/mL in ALL and chronic myelogenous leukemia (CML). Hyperleukocytosis occurs in 8% to 13% of children with ALL, 5% to 25% of children with AML,

TABLE 38.9

EARLY COMPLICATIONS IN PATIENTS WITH HYPERLEUKOCYTOSIS

Complications	ALL (N = 161)	ANLL (N = 73)	p Value[a]
Metabolic[b]	22	4	0.08
Hyperkalemia	16	2	
Decreased calcium, increased phosphorus	15	3	
Acute renal failure	5	4	
Respiratory	0	6	<0.001
Hemorrhagic	4	14	<0.001
Central nervous system	2	9	
Gastrointestinal	0	2	
Pulmonary	2	3	
Pericardial	0	1	
Death	8	17	<0.001

[a]For comparison of frequencies of the indicated complication in patients with ALL versus those with ANLL.
[b]Some patients experienced more than one complication.
ALL, acute lymphocytic leukemia; ANLL, acute nonlymphocytic leukemia.
From Bunin NJ, Piu CH. Differing complications of hyperleukocytosis in children with acute lymphoblastic or acute nonlymphoblastic leukemia. J Clin Oncol 1985;3:1590, with permission. Copyright 1985, Grune & Stratton, Inc.

and almost all children with CML.[130–132,181,182] Hyperleukocytosis is more common in infant with ALL and AML, blast phase of CML, T-cell ALL with a mediastinal mass, and leukemia with translocations involving 11q23.[130,181,182]

Hyperleukocytosis can cause death by CNS hemorrhage or thrombosis, pulmonary leukostasis, and the metabolic derangements that accompany tumor lysis. Table 38.9 classifies complications of 234 children with acute leukemia and hyperleukocytosis. Of the 73 patients with AML, 23% died during early induction from pulmonary leukostasis or intracerebral hemorrhage. In contrast, 5% of 161 patients with ALL died of complications of TLS.[131] With improved modern management, early mortality attributable to hyperleukocytosis has declined sharply to less than 5% for ALL and AML, although incidence of symptomatic leukostasis has not changed.[130,181]

Pathogenesis

Traditionally, hyperleukocytosis was thought to directly increase blood viscosity by increasing the packed leukocyte volume and indirectly increase blood viscosity by the formation of leukemic cell aggregates and thrombi.[182,183] Myeloblasts are almost twice the size of lymphoblasts and are felt to be "stickier."[181–183] Increasing evidence points not to increased blood viscosity but to the adhesive interactions between damaged endothelium and the leukemic blasts causing leukostasis.[182,184] The leukemic blasts respond to cytokines and toxins released by the damaged endothelium, explaining why symptoms of leukostasis occasionally develop in patients with WBC counts less than 100,000/mL.[184] Cerebral and pulmonary hemorrhage exacerbate the symptoms of leukostasis.

Evaluation and Differential Diagnosis

Frequently, a CBC revealing the significantly elevated WBC is obtained prior to arrival at a tertiary care center. The child

with a WBC greater than 100,000/mL should be evaluated for signs and symptoms of hyperleukocytosis. Many will be asymptomatic, but others will present with mental status changes, headaches, blurred vision, seizures, coma, symptoms of stroke, papilledema, and retinal artery or vein distention, all attributable to leukostasis in the cerebral vessels.[130,181,183]

Pulmonary leukostasis and secondary pulmonary hemorrhage causes tachypnea, dyspnea, hypoxia, cyanosis, and pulmonary infiltrates on CXR.[130,181] Priapism, clitoral engorgement, and dactylitis have also been described with hyperleukocytosis.[130,185] Additional laboratory studies include serum electrolytes, uric acid, renal function tests, and a coagulation profile. A CXR may reveal a mediastinal mass and/or diffuse interstitial infiltrates.

Therapy

There are no controlled studies of the management of hyperleukocytosis. As outlined in Table 38.10, IV hydration at two to four times maintenance, allopurinol with alkalinization, or urate oxidase should be started immediately.[181,184] Patients with platelet counts of less than 20,000/mL should receive platelet transfusions to prevent cerebral hemorrhage as platelets do not add substantially to blood viscosity. In a study of adult patients, the risk of death prior to therapy initiation is higher during periods of concomitant thrombocytopenia.[186] In contrast, packed red cells increase viscosity.[182,184] If a child is hemodynamically stable, packed red blood cell transfusion should be avoided until therapy for the hyperleukocytosis is initiated.[130] Coagulation abnormalities should be corrected. Exchange transfusion and/or leukapheresis can rapidly lower the WBC and may improve coagulopathy but is contraindicated in APL.[182,185] Pediatric studies found a 52% to 66% mean reduction in WBC with exchange transfusion and 48% to 62% reduction with leukapheresis.[130,181] Maurer and associates noted a significantly lower incidence of severe TLS in patients with ALL and WBC greater than 200,000/mL who underwent leukapheresis compared with those who did not.[187] Neurologic abnormalities, respiratory distress, and priapism have improved after leukapheresis in patients with AML, ALL, and CML.[185] Whether leukophoresis reduces the risk of CNS hemorrhage in AML is unknown and prophylactic cranial irradiation is no longer an accepted practice.[185] Problems associated with leukapheresis are the need for anticoagulation, difficulty with access in small children, and limited availability in many hospitals. Exchange transfusion and leukapheresis are only temporizing. Systemic antileukemic therapy must be initiated as soon as problems such as SVCS or SMS and compromised renal function have been addressed.

METABOLIC EMERGENCIES

Tumor Lysis Syndrome

Tumor lysis syndrome (TLS) consists of the metabolic abnormalities that result from the death of tumor cells and release of their contents into the circulation. The classic triad of TLS includes hyperuricemia, hyperphosphatemia, and hyperkalemia. Symptomatic hypocalcemia can develop secondary to formation of calcium phosphate from the hyperphosphatemia. Although TLS can occur prior to any cytotoxic therapy, its manifestations usually appear 12 to 72 hours from the initiation of therapy.

Etiology and Pathogenesis

TLS laboratory abnormalities are reported in 25% to 50% of children with high-risk malignancies, but clinical TLS is much

TABLE 38.10

MANAGEMENT OF PATIENTS AT RISK FOR TUMOR LYSIS SYNDROME

Hydration	D_5¼ NS with 40 mEq/L $NaHCO_3$—no K^+, Ca^+, PO_4 2–4 times maintenance fluid rate Maintain urine output at >100 mL/m²/hr, urine specific gravity <1.010
Alkalinization	Maintain urine pH at 7.0–7.5; increase $NaHCO_3$ as needed. Not required if urate oxidase is used Stop $NaHCO_3$ when cytotoxic therapy is initiated or the urine pH >7.5
Diuresis	Avoid if hypovolemia present Furosemide (0.5–1.0 mg/kg) Mannitol (0.5 g/kg over 15 min)
Uric acid reduction	Start allopurinol (300 mg/m²/day or 10 mg/kg/day) or urate oxidase (0.2 mg/kg/day for 1 or 2 days)
Metabolic abnormalities	Monitor electrolytes, Ca, Mg, PO_4 q4–8 hr
Hyperkalemia	Kayexalate (1 g/kg with 50% sorbitol) Calcium gluconate (100–200 mg/kg) Insulin (0.1 U/kg) and 25% glucose (2 mL/kg)
Hyperphosphatemia	Aluminum hydroxide (15 mL q4–8 hr), sevelamer (adult dosing of 800–1,600 mg t.i.d.)
Hypocalcemia	Calcium gluconate slow i.v. infusion *only* if symptomatic
Dialysis indications	Volume overload: pleural, pericardial effusions Renal failure Hyperkalemia Hyperphosphatemia Hyperuricemia Symptomatic hypocalcemia

D_5 ¼ NS, 5% dextrose with 0.25% normal saline; $NaHCO_3$, sodium bicarbonate; K^+, potassium; Mg, magnesium; Ca+, calcium; PO_4, phosphorus. t.i.d., three times a day; i.v., intravenously.

less frequent, occurring in 4% to 8% of patients.[188] TLS occurs in patients with tumors that have a high growth fraction, large volume, or wide dissemination and that are sensitive to cytotoxic therapy. It occurs most commonly in Burkitt's lymphoma, lymphoblastic lymphoma, and acute leukemias, particularly T-lineage ALL with hyperleukocytosis and extensive extramedullary disease. TLS has also been noted in HD, large-cell lymphoma, CML, and rarely in pediatric solid tumors.[188] The literature contains descriptions of children who present with hyperuricemia and acute renal failure as the initial manifestation of occult lymphoproliferative malignancy.[189] Other risk factors found to be associated with the development of TLS include bulky abdominal Burkitt's lymphoma, hepatosplenomegaly, hyperleukocytosis, mediastinal mass, elevated pretreatment serum uric acid and lactic dehydrogenase, and poor urine output or low glomerular filtration rate (GFR).[188,190,191] Andreoli and coworkers found that older age (10.4 ± 5.4 years), but not high WBC, correlated with development of renal failure in children with ALL.[191] This may, in part, be due to the progressive decline in the fractional excretion and clearance of uric acid that accompanies advancing age.

TLS is a direct result of the release into the circulation of the nuclear and cytoplasmic degradation products of malignant cells. Potassium, the principal intracellular cation, increases in the serum and its excretion is exacerbated by renal insufficiency. A rapid rise in potassium can cause cardiac arrest in minutes or hours. Elevated uric acid comes from the breakdown of the released nucleic acids. In the presence of hyperuricemia, renal excretion of uric acid initially increases, but then decreases as uric acid crystals precipitate in the collecting ducts of the renal tubules due to the acid environment of the kidney.[188] Lymphoblasts are especially rich in phosphate, having four times the content of normal lymphocytes.[188,192] Elevated levels of serum phosphate are also exacerbated by a metabolic acidosis, which induces a shift of intracellular phosphate into the extracellular space. When the solubility product factor (Ca X P) reaches 60, calcium phosphate precipitates in the microvasculature, causing a secondary hypocalcemia.[192] Precipitation of uric acid crystals and calcium phosphate within the renal tubules and microvasculature leads to acute renal failure.

Evaluation and Differential Diagnosis

In a patient at risk for TLS, pertinent historical information includes the time of onset of symptoms referable to the malignancy, abdominal pain or fullness, back pain, vomiting, diarrhea, signs and symptoms of dehydration, and anorexia, vomiting, cramps, spasms, tetany, seizure, and alterations in consciousness suggestive of hypocalcemia. On examination, special attention should be given to blood pressure, cardiac rate and rhythm, abdominal masses, presence of pleural effusions or ascites, signs of SVCS or SMS, and signs of cerebral anoxia.

Initial studies include a CBC, serum sodium, potassium, chloride, bicarbonate, calcium, phosphorus, uric acid, BUN, and Cr levels. If the serum calcium is low, an ionized calcium and serum albumin should be obtained as well. An electrocardiogram

(ECG) is essential if the serum potassium level is greater than 6.0 mEq/L. It may show QRS widening and peaked T waves. Patients with electrocardiographic abnormalities should be placed on a cardiac monitor. Hypocalcemia can cause a prolonged QT_C interval on electrocardiography.

Because acute renal insufficiency due to obstruction can have manifestations similar to those of TLS, a US or CT should be performed in any child with an abdominal or pelvic mass to rule out obstructive renal failure. Obstructive renal failure can be improved rapidly with catheterization and is exacerbated by hydration.[88]

Therapy

Attempts have been made to stratify risk of TLS based upon diagnosis, extent of disease, and baseline uric acid.[188] Monitoring only, for patients at low risk of developing TLS, is controversial.[193] Early and aggressive intervention effectively reduces the morbidity associated with TLS. Patients with newly diagnosed leukemia or NHL should receive hydration, and either alkalinization and allopurinol or urate oxidase (Table 38.10). For most patients, this regimen suffices to prevent clinically significant tumor lysis and renal failure. When severe metabolic abnormalities have improved, cytotoxic therapy can commence.

Hydration is probably the most critical factor in preventing TLS. Increased hydration translates to increased urinary outflow and improved GFR. Patients should receive two to four times maintenance fluid volume as 5% dextrose in 0.25% normal saline with 40 to 80 mEq of sodium bicarbonate per liter to produce a urine pH of 7.0 to 7.5. Urine output should be maintained at greater than 100 mL/m^2/hr with a specific gravity of no more than 1.010. Potassium, calcium, and phosphorus should not be added to hydration fluids unless a patient has symptomatic deficiencies. Although diuretics and mannitol are contraindicated in the patient with volume depletion, they may be indicated in patients with poor urine output because of accumulation of the infused fluid in the third space.[188]

Allopurinol (250 to 500 mg/m^2/day, maximum 800 mg) directly inhibits the formation of uric acid by blocking the enzyme xanthine oxidase that converts uric acid to hypoxanthine and xanthine. A new alternative, recombinant urate oxidase, is now available for the treatment of children at high risk of developing TLS. Urate oxidase converts uric acid to allantoin, a much more urine-soluble product than uric acid, and does not require alkalinization.[188,194,195] Recent studies demonstrated a fivefold reduction in plasma uric acid levels within hours of a single dose of urate oxidase (0.2 mg/kg/day).[188,194,195] In one study, serum creatinine decreased significantly in 24 hours, and no patient developed renal insufficiency or required dialysis.[189,195] The drug is contraindicated in patients with G6PD deficiency.

Alkalinization of the urine aids in solubilizing uric acid. Sodium bicarbonate should be discontinued when plasma levels of uric acid normalize and cytotoxic therapy begins.[196] Overzealous alkalinization (urine pH, >7.5) can lead to worsening nephropathy. At a pH above 7.5, xanthine and hypoxanthine stones (from allopurinol therapy) may form and at a pH of 8 or above, calcium phosphate may crystallize in the kidneys.[196] Alkalinization is not needed if urate oxidase is used to treat hyperuricemia.

Serum electrolytes should be monitored closely. In a child with pre–B-cell ALL, a low WBC, and minimal hepatosplenomegaly, tumor lysis labs can be monitored every 8 to 12 hours. In a patient with disseminated Burkitt's lymphoma who presents with evidence of TLS, metabolic studies should be repeated 4 hours after initiation of therapy and monitored

six times a day. Additional interventions should be started when metabolic abnormalities are worsening, in an attempt to avoid dialysis. Aluminum hydroxide, a phosphate binder (15 mL every 8 hours escalated to a continuous nasogastric infusion as needed), will increase excretion of phosphate. Case reports exist of successfully using sevelamer hydrochloride, a non–calcium-containing phosphate binder in capsule form, in lieu of aluminum hydroxide, for TLS-associated hyperphosphatemia.[197]

Kayexalate (1 g/kg orally with 50% sorbitol), a potassium-binding resin, may help lower rising potassium. Calcium gluconate (100 to 200 mg/kg/dose, administered via slow infusion with ECG monitoring) can shift potassium intracellularly and stabilize myocardial conduction. Insulin (0.1 U/kg of rapid-acting insulin with 2 mL/kg of 25% glucose in water) as an intravenous bolus also promotes intracellular influx of potassium.[188] When hyperphosphatemia is present, treatment of hypocalcemia with IV infusions of calcium gluconate (100 to 200 mg/kg/dose) should be reserved only for those individuals with signs and symptoms of hypocalcemia (such as tetany, arrhythmias, or seizures), as increasing the serum calcium will also increase the calcium/phosphorus solubility factor product favoring calcium phosphate deposition and renal failure. When medical interventions fail to correct electrolyte disturbances or oliguria persists, dialysis may be necessary. Table 38.10 outlines the indications for starting dialysis. Hemodialysis is preferable to peritoneal dialysis because it corrects electrolyte abnormalities more rapidly. Peritoneal dialysis is contraindicated with an abdominal or pelvic tumor. Continuous venovenous hemofiltration has been used prophylactically in patients with Burkitt's lymphoma to prevent renal failure,[198] but the benefits are unclear. Although no controlled studies have been performed, some have advocated leukapheresis or exchange transfusion to reduce the tumor load and prevent TLS in the setting of hyperleukocytosis.

Hypercalcemia

Although common in adults with cancer, severe hypercalcemia (serum calcium, >12 mg/dL) complicating childhood malignancy is rare, with an incidence of only 0.4% to 1.3%.[199,200] In about half of cases, hypercalcemia is present at diagnosis, the rest occurring during therapy or at relapse. Hypercalcemia of malignancy has been documented in almost every type of childhood cancer but is most commonly seen in hematologic malignancies, rhabdomyosarcoma, and neuroblastoma.[199,200]

Etiology and Pathogenesis

In children, malignant hypercalcemia can be caused by a paraneoplastic syndrome, bone or bone marrow invasion, a defect in renal excretion and immobilization. Hypervitaminosis A or D, granulomatous disease, adrenal insufficiency, and fractures may also contribute. The most common etiology is paraneoplastic syndrome, in which the tumor itself produces an ectopic hormone that causes parathyroid hormone (PTH)–like effects: increased osteoclastic bone resorption, increased renal resorption of calcium, and increased renal phosphate loss. PTH itself is rarely elevated in these patients, but a parathyroid hormone-related peptide (PTHrP) or other cytokines such as IL-6 or tumor necrosis factor are elevated.[200,201] In osteolytic hypercalcemia, osteoclasts activated at the site of bone metastases or in the bone marrow resorb bone with the participation of various cytokines. Osteoclast-activating factor has been associated with hypercalcemia in patients with multiple myeloma and Burkitt's lymphoma.[199,201] Renal insufficiency with water and electrolyte imbalances often exacerbates poor calcium excretion.

Hypercalcemia has been reported in children in remission with prolonged immobilization and no other abnormalities.[200]

Evaluation and Differential Diagnosis

The likelihood of symptoms correlates with the calcium level at presentation. Early nonspecific symptoms are often gastrointestinal: nausea/vomiting, anorexia, and constipation (Table 38.11).[199,200] Asthenia, polyuria/polydipsia, irritability, and bone pain are also seen. Increasing serum calcium levels lead to profound muscle weakness, renal insufficiency, bradyarrhythmias, and coma. Anorexia, vomiting, and polyuria initiate a self-sustaining spiral of dehydration that leads to a decreased GFR and reduced renal calcium excretion. The early symptoms can mimic TLS in the newly diagnosed patient with leukemia, and the two disorders can overlap. Pediatric patients with malignant hypercalcemia tend to have elevated BUN and uric acid levels, normal or increased phosphorus concentration, and a metabolic alkalosis.[199,200] Serum calcium, phosphate, BUN, Cr, uric acid, and ionized calcium should be obtained. Serum levels of PTH, PTHrP, as well as 25-(OH) vitamin D and 1,25-(OH)$_2$ may help define the origin of the hypercalcemia. An electrocardiograph may reveal a prolonged PR interval with broad T waves. A bone scan or skeletal survey may show bony metastases.

Therapy

Calcium levels above 12.0 mg/dL require immediate correction. Treatment has four components: hydration, increasing the renal calcium excretion, decreasing the calcium mobilization from bone, and treatment of the underlying malignancy. First-line therapy for hypercalcemia is hyperhydration with furosemide diuresis.[191,200,202] Furosemide blocks calcium resorption by the kidney and can decrease serum calcium by 3 mg/dL in 48 hours. Forced diuresis requires monitoring of intravascular

volume and serum and urine electrolytes; profound fluid shifts and potassium and magnesium losses may accompany sodium, calcium, and fluid excretion. Medications that exacerbate hypercalcemia of malignancy; such as thiazide diuretics, oral contraceptives, tamoxifen, vitamin D, retinoic acid, antacids with calcium carbonate, and lithium, should be avoided. In children with calcium levels of less than 14 mg/dL, this may suffice.

Glucocorticoids slowly reduce serum calcium if hypercalcemia is mediated by osteoclast-activating factor, prostaglandin E$_2$, and/or calcitriol. Calcitonin, mithramycin, and gallium nitrate, traditional therapies for hypercalcemia, have fallen out of favor with the development of the bisphosphonates. Bisphosphonates inhibit osteoclast-mediated resorption of bone and reduce osteoclast viability. Side effects include transient lymphopenia, fever, myalgia, GI upset, and, most seriously, prolonged hypocalcemia, hypophosphatemia, and hypomagnesemia. Although most data exist in adults, the literature on their use in the pediatric population is growing. The bisphosphonate most studied in pediatrics to date is IV pamidronate.[200,203] Clinical response occurs in 24 to 48 hours, and serum calcium levels usually normalize within 2 to 4 days. A recommended starting dose for children is 0.5 to 1 mg/kg infused over 4 to 6 hours with close monitoring of serum calcium, phosphate, and magnesium for 2 weeks.[200,203] A subsequent dose of 1 mg/kg can be given if necessary. Oral bisphosphonates are also now available, but pediatric experience with them is limited.

Syndrome of Inappropriate Secretion of Antidiuretic Hormone/Hyponatremia

Excessive secretion of antidiuretic hormone (ADH) accompanying a normal or low plasma osmolality or serum sodium concentration is termed "inappropriate" because it further depresses the sodium level. Symptoms of excessive ADH secretion are not usually apparent until the plasma sodium falls below 125 mmol/L. A rapid fall in the serum sodium level to below 125 mmol/L within 24 hours or a gradual decrease in serum sodium to less than 115 mmol/L can be life-threatening.

Etiology and Pathogenesis

SIADH is characterized, in most cases, by the release of ADH without any relation to plasma osmolality. Excessive secretion of ADH increases water resorption by the kidneys with a resultant dilutional hyponatremia.[162,204] Hyponatremia due to SIADH is associated with the use of vincristine, vinblastine, cyclophosphamide, IFOS, cisplatin, and melphalan.[205,206]

SIADH can also occur with CNS injury or CNS disease; with stress, pain, surgery, or positive-pressure ventilation; with pulmonary infection and inflammation; and with tumors, such as small-cell lung carcinoma, lymphoma, or GI carcinoma.[207] CNS disease stimulates release of ADH from the posterior pituitary gland.

Evaluation and Differential Diagnosis

Most hyponatremia is asymptomatic and is usually diagnosed by routine laboratory evaluation. Early symptoms include fatigue, headache, nausea, and myalgias; later manifestations are lethargy, confusion, hallucinations, seizures, and coma.[204,207] Although severe hyponatremia in children with cancer is often related to SIADH, the most common cause of mild hyponatremia is iatrogenic: simple overhydration with a hypotonic solution such as 5% dextrose in 0.25% normal saline. Hyponatremia can also be caused by failure to

---

TABLE 38.11

SIGNS AND SYMPTOMS OF HYPERCALCEMIA OF MALIGNANCY

Gastrointestinal
  Anorexia
  Nausea
  Vomiting
  Constipation
  Ileus

Neuromuscular
  Asthenia
  Lethargy
  Depression
  Fatigue
  Hypotonia
  Obtundation
  Stupor
  Coma
  Bone pain

Cardiovascular
  Bradycardia
  Arrhythmia

Renal
  Polyuria/polydipsia
  Nocturia

administer stress doses of glucocorticoids in a patient who has recently discontinued systemic steroids. Hypothyroidism, heart failure, acute renal failure, pancreatitis, and use of diuretics may exacerbate hyponatremia. Diabetes insipidus occurs in children with Langerhans cell histiocytosis or with suprasellar tumors, either from the tumors or after tumor resection. Diabetes insipidus usually presents with polydipsia, polyuria, and hypernatremic volume depletion; however, if the patient has been replacing losses with water or other hypotonic solutions, hyponatremia may develop. In patients with CNS tumors and renal damage, SIADH may need to be differentiated from cerebral salt wasting (CSW).[208,209]

The following studies should be obtained in the evaluation of hyponatremia: renal and liver function tests; serum osmolality; urinalysis, including a specific gravity; and urine sodium, Cr, and osmolality. Like SIADH, CSW is associated with a low serum and inappropriately high urine osmolality (urine to serum osmolality ratio often >1) and an elevated urine sodium concentration (>20 mEq/L), although CSW tends to have higher urine sodium losses. The main distinguishing feature of SIADH and CSW is plasma volume, which is decreased in CSW and generally normal in SIADH. Other helpful differences include urine output (generally high in CSW and decreased to normal in SIADH) and serum uric acid concentration (low in SIADH, normal in CSW).[208,209]

Therapy

Fluid restriction is the mainstay of therapy for mild hyponatremia (Na > 125 mmol/L) due to water intoxication, chronic SIADH, or acute SIADH if the patient is asymptomatic.[204,207] If fluid restriction is contraindicated (e.g., hydration needed to prevent hemorrhagic cystitis), consider furosemide and sodium replacement with hypertonic saline as described later. In cases of acute, severe symptomatic hyponatremia, 3% hypertonic saline should be infused to replace sodium losses, and some advocate addition of furosemide to diurese free water. The rate of sodium correction should not exceed 1 to 2 mmol/L/hr, as too rapid a correction of sodium can cause pontine myelinolysis with further neurologic deterioration. Once symptoms improve, the rate of sodium correction should be decreased, so as not to exceed 8 to 12 mmol/L correction in the first 24 hours. For patients with severe hyponatremia and moderate symptoms, slow correction (0.5 to 2 mmol/L/hr) may be achieved with 0.9% saline.

In CSW, replacement of urine sodium losses and volume is needed.[210] High-dose fludrocortisone (0.2 to 0.4 mg/day), a mineral corticoid, may be useful in some resistant cases. As with SIADH, too rapid a correction of sodium should be avoided. No matter what the cause of hyponatremia, urine output should be monitored closely along with frequent serum electrolytes.

SHOCK

Shock occurs when cardiovascular dysfunction results in inadequate perfusion of vital organs. The body attempts to compensate first by increasing heart rate and then by reducing perfusion to vital end organs.[211] Only when these mechanisms fail to compensate, does hypotension ensue. Hypovolemic distributive shock is due to vasodilation, and cardiogenic shock is caused by cardiac dysfunction.

Etiology and Pathogenesis

In pediatric cancer patients, the most common cause of shock is sepsis. Bacterial endotoxins and proteins trigger vasodila-

tion and capillary leak, leading to hypotension and, if untreated, multiorgan system failure. Other causes of distributive shock in oncology patients include drug-related anaphylaxis, severe pancreatitis, and CNS injury (Table 38.12). Hypovolemic shock is caused by decreased circulating blood perfusion. Oncology patients are often anemic and thus more

---

TABLE 38.12

COMMON CAUSES OF SHOCK IN THE CHILD WITH CANCER

Hypovolemic shock
- Sepsis
- Hemorrhage
- Bladder (drug; adenovirus)
- Intestine
- Typhlitis
- *Clostridium difficile*
- Massive hemoptysis
- *Aspergillus*
- Tumor invasion
- Intractable emesis
- Pancreatitis
- L-Asparaginase
- Glucocorticoid
- Central nervous system lesion
- Addisonian crisis, after glucocorticoid
- Diabetes mellitus
- After glucocorticoid
- After pancreatitis
- Malignant hypercalcemia

Distributive shock
- Anaphylaxis
- Etoposide
- Carboplatin
- L-Asparaginase
- Cytosine arabinoside
- Amphotericin-B
- Blood products
- Gamma globulin
- Vitamin K
- Interleukin-2
- Tumor necrosis factor
- Sepsis
- Veno-occlusive disease

Cardiogenic shock
- Treatment related
- Anthracycline
- Cyclophosphamide (bone marrow transplantation)
- Radiotherapy
- Cardiac tamponade
- Intracardiac tumor
- Intracardiac thrombus
- Pericardial effusion
- Constrictive pericarditis
- Fungus ball
- Myocarditis
- Viral
- Fungal
- Bacterial
- Metabolic
- Hyperkalemia
- Hypokalemia
- Hypocalcemia

sensitive to blood loss via hemorrhage, plasma loss from hypoproteinemia, or free water loss from vomiting, diarrhea, diuresis, or fever. Hypovolemic shock may also occur with an addisonian crisis in patients who have received high doses of glucocorticoids and recently discontinued them.

Cardiogenic shock occurs in patients who have received moderate or high doses of anthracyclines with or without cardiac irradiation. It can occur following high-dose cyclophosphamide use during BMT cytoreduction. A mass within the cardiac chambers or constrictive or effusive pericarditis can lead to cardiogenic shock.

Evaluation and Differential Diagnosis

The respiratory and cardiovascular systems must be assessed rapidly. Increased heart and respiratory rates; signs of respiratory distress (air hunger, nasal flaring, retractions, stridor, grunting, use of accessory muscles); weak peripheral pulses; pale, gray, or mottled skin; and cold extremities may be indications of impending cardiovascular collapse. Repeated blood pressure measurements with the appropriate sized cuff should be obtained to monitor for decompensation. Capillary refill time should be used to assess peripheral perfusion. The status of the brain is best assessed by the level of consciousness, the patient's ability to respond to normal stimuli and to pain, the patient's generalized muscle tone and pupil size, and the presence of posturing or seizures.

Therapy

For detailed management of shock, the reader is referred to the *Textbook of Pediatric Emergency Medicine*.[211] Thera-

pies include establishing an airway and providing 100% oxygen by the least traumatic means possible. Initial fluid resuscitation should be 20 mL/kg of 0.9% normal saline or Ringer's lactate given as a rapid bolus over 10 to 20 minutes. A large bore peripheral IV may need to be placed as limited fluid resuscitation may be performed through a central line alone. If there is no response, a second fluid bolus or packed red blood cell infusion (if anemic) may be needed.[211] Concomitantly, the underlying etiology should be sought and treated. If the cause is presumed to be sepsis, cultures should be obtained and appropriate antibiotics started without delay. A CXR is needed if the patient has respiratory symptoms. A CBC, electrolytes, and tests of renal and hepatic function are necessary to determine proper replacement of fluids and end-organ damage. If there is evidence of hemorrhage, the patient should receive packed red cells (see Chapter 39), platelets, coagulation factors, and a surgical evaluation if a surgically correctable cause of hemorrhage is present.

In anaphylactic shock, the suspected drug should be discontinued immediately. Epinephrine should be given subcutaneously. Antihistamines, both H1 (diphenhydramine or hydroxyzine) and H2 antagonists (ranitidine), should be given. The use of steroids in anaphylaxis may prevent late-phase reactions. Steroids are often used for blood product reactions.

In cardiogenic shock, an ECG and an echocardiogram should be obtained immediately. An abnormal rhythm must be appropriately corrected. Use of adrenergic agents should be planned with the consultation of cardiologists and intensivists.

References

1. Issa PY, Brinhi ER, Janin Y, et al. Superior vena cava syndrome in childhood. Pediatrics 1983;71:337.
2. Ingram L, Rivera GK, Shapiro DN. Superior vena cava syndrome associated with childhood malignancy: analysis of 24 cases. Med Pediatr Oncol 1990;18(6):476–481.
3. Gaebler JW, Kleiman MB, Cohen M, et al. Differentiation of lymphoma from histoplasmosis in children with mediastinal masses. J Pediatr 1984;104:706.
4. Perger L, Lee EY, Shamberger RC. Management of children and adolescents with a critical airway due to compression by an anterior mediastinal mass. J Pediatr Surg 2008; 43(11):1990–1997.
5. Anghelescu DL, Burgoyne LL, Liu T, et al. Clinical and diagnostic imaging findings predict anesthetic complications in children presenting with malignant mediastinal masses. Paediatr Anaesth 2007;17(11):1090–1098.
6. Maity A, Goldwein JW, Lange BJ, et al. Mediastinal masses in children with Hodgkin's disease. Cancer 1992;69:2755–2760.
7. Ng A, Bennett J, Bromley P, et al. Anaesthetic outcome and predictive risk factors in children with mediastinal tumours. Pediatr Blood Cancer 2007;48(2):160–164.
8. Ricketts RR. Clinical management of anterior mediastinal tumors in children. Semin Pediatr Surg 2001;10(3):161–168.
9. Dosios T, Theakos N, Chatziantoniou C. Cervical mediastinoscopy and anterior mediastinotomy in superior vena cava obstruction. Chest 2005;128(3):1551–1556.
10. Rendina EA, Venuta F, De Giacomo T, et al. Biopsy of anterior mediastinal masses under local anesthesia. Ann Thorac Surg 2002;74(5):1720–2; discussion 1722–1723.
11. Bertsch H, Rudoler S, Needle MN, et al. Emergent/urgent therapeutic irradiation in pediatric oncology: patterns of presentation, treatment, and outcome. Med Pediatr Oncol 1998;30:101–105.
12. Loeffler JS, Leopold KA, Recht A, et al. Emergency prebiopsy radiation for mediastinal masses. Impact on subsequent pathologic diagnosis and outcome. J Clin Oncol 1986; 4:716.
13. Armstrong BA, Perez CA, Simpson JR, et al. Role of irradiation in the management of superior vena cava syndrome. Int J Radiat Oncol Biol Phys 1987;13(4):531–539.
14. Borenstein SH, Gerstle T, Malkin D, et al. The effects of prebiopsy corticosteroid treatment on the diagnosis of mediastinal lymphoma. J Pediatr Surg 2000;35(6): 973–976.
15. Frey TK, Chopra A, Lin, RJ, et al. A child with anterior mediastinal mass supported with veno-arterial extracorporeal membrane oxygenation. Pediatr Crit Care Med 2006;7(5):479–481.
16. Lee J, Won JH, Kim HC, et al. Emergency dilation by self-expandable tracheal stent for upper airway obstruction in a patient with a giant primary thyroid lymphoma. Thyroid 2009;19(2):193–195.
17. Bajzar L, Chan AK, Massicotte MP, et al. Thrombosis in children with malignancy. Curr Opin Pediatr 2006;18(1):1–9.
18. Monagle P, Chalmers E, Chan A, et al. Antithrombotic therapy in neonates and children: American College of Chest Physicians Evidence-Based Clinical Practice Guidelines (8th Edition). Chest 2008;133(suppl 6):887S–968S.
19. Beers SL, Abramo TJ. Pleural effusions. Pediatr Emerg Care 2007;23(5):330–334; quiz 335–338.
20. Vaitkus PT, Herrmann HC, LeWinter MM, Treatment of malignant pericardial effusion. JAMA 1994;272:59.
21. Arya LS, Narain S, Thavaraj V, et al. Leukemic pericardial effusion causing cardiac tamponade. Med Pediatr Oncol 2002;38:282–284.
22. Ostrowski MJ. Intracavitary therapy with bleomycin for the treatment of malignant pleural effusions. J Surg Oncol Suppl 1989;1:7–13.
23. Boyer MW, Moertel CL, Priest JR, et al. Use of intracavitary cisplatin for the treatment of childhood solid tumors in the chest or abdominal cavity. J Clin Oncol 1995;13:631.
24. Medary I, Steinherz LJ, Aronson DC, et al. Cardiac tamponade in the pediatric oncology population: treatment by percutaneous catheter drainage. J Pediatr Surg 1996; 31(1):197–200.
25. da Costa CML, de Camargo BY, Lamelas RG, et al. Cardiac tamponade complicating hyperleukocytosis in a child with leukemia. Med Pediatr Oncol 1999;32:120–123.
26. Maguire WM. Mechanical complications of cancer. Emerg Med Clin North Am 1993; 11(2):421–430.
27. Gorelik O, Cohen N, Shpirer I, et al. Fatal haemoptysis induced by invasive pulmonary aspergillosis in patients with acute leukaemia during bone marrow and clinical remission: report of two cases and review of the literature. J Infect 2000;41(3):277–282.
28. Caillot D, Mannone L, Cuisenier B, et al. Role of early diagnosis and aggressive surgery in the management of invasive pulmonary aspergillosis in neutropenic patients. Clin Microbiol Infect 2001;7(2):54–61.
29. Roebuck DJ, Barnacle AM. Haemoptysis and bronchial artery embolization in children. Paediatr Respir Rev 2008;9(2):95–104.
30. Stein ME, Shklar Z, Drumea K, et al, Chemotherapy-induced spontaneous pneumothorax in a patient with bulky mediastinal lymphoma: a rare oncologic emergency. Oncology 1997;54:15–18.
31. Briassoulis G, Hatzis, T, Paphitis C, et al. Acute spontaneous pneumomediastinum in a child with Hodgkin's disease and pulmonary fibrosis. Pediatr Hem and Oncol 1999; 16:175–180.
32. Chalumeau M, Amigo ME, Delgado R, et al, Pneumomediastinum: a rare, impressive but benign complication of chemotherapy-induced emesis in children. Med Pediatr Oncol 1998;31:182–184.
33. Langenburg SE, Lelli JL. Minimally invasive surgery of the lung: lung biopsy, treatment of spontaneous pneumothorax, and pulmonary resection. Semin Pediatr Surg 2008; 17(1):30–33.
34. Montesinos P, Bergua JM, Vellenga E, et al. Differentiation syndrome in patients with acute promyelocytic leukemia treated with all-trans retinoic acid and anthracycline chemotherapy: characteristics, outcome, and prognostic factors. Blood 2009;113(4): 775–783.
35. DeBotton S, Chevret S, Coiteux V, et al. Early onset of chemotherapy can reduce the incidence of ATRA syndrome in newly diagnosed acute promyelocytic leukemia (APL) with low white blood cell counts: results from APL 93 trial. Leukemia 2003;18(2):339–342.

36. Sanz MA, Grimwade D, Tallman MS, et al. Management of acute promyelocytic leukemia: recommendations from an expert panel on behalf of the European Leukemi-aNet. Blood 2009;113(9):1875–1891.

37. Silliman CC, Haase GM, Strain JD, et al. Indictions for surgical intervention for gastrointestinal emergencies in children receiving chemotherapy. Cancer 1994;74:203.

38. Easter DW, Cuschieri A, Nathanson LK, et al. The utility of diagnostic laparoscopy for abdominal disorders. Arch Surg 1992;127:379.

39. Kaste SC, Rodriguez-Galindo C, Furman WL. Imaging pediatric oncologic emergencies of the abdomen. AJR Am J Roentgenol 1999;173(3):729–736.

40. Wiener ES. Pediatric surgical oncology. Curr Opin Pediatr 1993;5:110–116.

41. Reiss U, Cowan M, McMillan A, et al. Hepatic venoocclusive disease in blood and bone marrow transplantation in children and young adults: incidence, risk factors and outcome in a cohort of 241 patients. J Pediatr Hem/Onc 2002;24(9):746–750.

42. Durbin D, Liacouras C. Gastrointestinal emergencies. In: Fleisher GR, Ludwig S, Henretig FM. eds. Textbook of pediatric emergency medicine. 5th ed. 2006:1087–1111.

43. Ross AJ III, Siegel KR, Bell W, et al. Massive gastrointestinal hemorrhage in children with posterior fossa tumors. J Pediatr Surg 1987;22:633.

44. Athale UH, Chan AK. Hemorrhagic complications in pediatric hematologic malignancies. Semin Thromb Hemost 2007;33(4):408–415.

45. Soylu AR, Buyukasik Y, Cetiner D, et al. Overt gastrointestinal bleeding in haematologic neoplasms. Dig Liver Dis 2005;37(12):917–922.

46. Gupta H, Davidoff AM, Pui CH, et al. Clinical implications and surgical management of intussusception in pediatric patients with Burkitt lymphoma. J Pediatr Surg 2007;42(6):998–1001; discussion 1001.

47. Kaste SC, Williams J, Rao BN. Postoperative small-bowel intussusception in children with cancer. Pediatr Radiol 1995;25(1):21–23.

48. Hendrick JM, Kaste SC, Tamburro RF, et al. Abdominal compartment syndrome in a newly diagnosed patient with Burkitt lymphoma. Pediatr Radiol 2006;36(3):254–257.

49. Goldberg SR, Godder K, Lanning DA. Successful treatment of a bowel perforation after chemotherapy for Burkitt lymphoma. J Pediatr Surg 2007;42(3):E1–E3.

50. Mullassery D, Bader A, Battersby AJ, et al. Diagnosis, incidence, and outcomes of suspected typhlitis in oncology patients—experience in a tertiary pediatric surgical center in the United Kingdom. J Pediatr Surg 2009;44(2):381–385.

51. McCarville MB, Adelman CS, Li C, Xiong X, et al. Typhlitis in childhood cancer. Cancer 2005;104(2):380–387.

52. Cartoni C, Dragoni F, Micozzi A, et al. Neutropenic enterocolitis in patients with acute leukemia: prognostic significance of bowel wall thickening detected by ultrasonography. J Clin Oncol 2001;19(3):756–761.

53. Wilson DB, Rao A, Hulbert M, et al. Neutropenic enterocolitis as a presenting complication of acute lymphoblastic leukemia: an unusual case marked by delayed perforation of the descending colon. J Pediatr Surg 2004;39(7):e18–e20.

54. Sloas MM, Flynn PM, Caste SC, et al. Typhlitis in children with cancer. A thirty-year experience. J Clin Infect Dis 1993;17:484.

55. Katz JA, Wagner ML, Gresik MV, et al. Typhlitis: an 18-year experience and post-mortem review. Cancer 1990;65:1041–1047.

56. Kelly CP, Pothoulakis C, Lamont JT. *Clostridium difficile* colitis. N Engl J Med 1994; 330:251.

57. Gorbach SL. Antibiotics and clostridium difficile. N Engl J Med 1999;341(22): 1690–1691.

58. Gorschluter M, Mey U, Strehl J, et al. Invasive fungal infections in neutropenic enterocolitis: a systematic analysis of pathogens, incidence, treatment and mortality in adult patients. BMC Infect Dis 2006;6:35.

59. Shamberger RC, Weinstein HJ, Delorey MJ, et al. The medical and surgical management of typhlitis in children with acute nonlymphocytic (myelogenous) leukemia. Cancer 1986;57(3):603–609.

60. Hobson MJ, Carney DE, Molik KA, et al. Appendicitis in childhood hematologic malignancies: analysis and comparison with typhilitis. J Pediatr Surg 2005;40(1):214–219; discussion 219–220.

61. Angel CA, Rao BN, Wrenn Jr, et al. Acute appendicitis in children with leukemia and other malignancies: still a diagnostic dilemma. J Pediatr Surg 1992;27(4):476–479.

62. Wiegering VA, Kellenberger CJ, Bodmer N, et al. Conservative management of acute appendicitis in children with hematologic malignancies during chemotherapy-induced neutropenia. J Pediatr Hematol Oncol 2008;30(6):464–467.

63. Brook I, Frazier EH. The aerobic and anaerobic bacteriology of perirectal abscesses. J Clin Microbiol 1997;35(11):2974–2976.

64. North JH Jr, Weber TK, Rodriguez-Bigas MA, et al. The management of infectious and noninfectious anorectal complications in patients with leukemia. J Am CollSurg 1996; 183(4):322–328.

65. Ruymann FB, Raney RB Jr, Crist WM, et al. Rhabdomyosarcoma of the biliary tree in childhood. A report from the Intergroup Rhabdomyosarcoma Study. Cancer 1984; 56(3):575–581.

66. Coughlin JR, Mann DA. Detection of acute cholecystitis in children. Can Assoc Radiol J 1990;41(4):213–216.

67. Marsh WH, Cunningham JT. Endoscopic stent placement for obstructive jaundice secondary to metastatic malignancy. Am J Gastroenterol 1992;87(8):985–990.

68. van den Bosch RP, van der Schelling GP, Klinkenbihl JHG, et al. Guidelines for the application of surgery and endoprostheses in the palliation of obstructive jaundice in advanced cancer of the pancreas. Ann Surg 1994;219:18.

69. Arndt C, Hawkins D, Anderson JR, et al. Age is a risk factor for chemotherapy-induced hepatopathy with vincristine, dactinomycin, and cyclophosphamide. J Clin Oncol 2004;22(10):1894–1901.

70. Ortega JA, Donaldson SS, Ivy SP, et al. Venoocclusive disease of the liver and chemotherapy with vincristine, actinomycin D and cyclophosphamide for the treatment of rhabdomyosarcoma: a report of the Intergroup Rhabdomyosarcoma Study Group. Cancer 1997;79(12):2435–2439.

71. Arceci RJ, Sande J, Lange B, et al. Safety and efficacy of gemtuzumab ozogamicin in pediatric patients with advanced CD33+ acute myeloid leukemia. Blood 2005; 106(4):1183–1188.

72. Stork LC, Sather H, Hutchinson RJ, et al. Comparison of mercaptopurine (MP) with thioguanine (TG) and IT methotrexate (ITM) with IT "triples" (ITT) in children with SR-ALL: results of CCG-1952. Blood 2002;100(11):156a.

73. Stoneham S, Lennard L, Coen P, et al. Veno-occlusive disease in patients receiving thiopurines during maintenance therapy for childhood acute lymphoblastic leukaemia. Br J Haematol 2003;123:100–102.

74. Ravikumara M, Hill FG, Wilson, et al. 6-Thioguanine-related chronic hepatotoxicity and variceal haemorrhage in children treated for acute lymphoblastic leukaemia—a dual-centre experience. J Pediatr Gastroenterol Nutr 2006;42(5):535–538.

75. Richardson PG, Murakami C, Zhezhen J, et al. Multi-institutional use of defibrotide in 88 patients after stem cell transplantation with severe veno-occlusive disease and multi-system organ failure: response without significant toxicity in a high-risk population and factors predictive of outcome. Blood 2002;100(13):4337–4343.

76. Ho VT, Linden E, Revta C, et al. Hepatic veno-occlusive disease after hematopoietic stem cell transplantation: review and update on the use of defibrotide. Semin Thromb Hemost 2007;33(4):373–388.

77. Hsu LL, Evans AE, D'Angio GJ. Hepatomegaly in neuroblastoma stage 4s: criteria for treatment of vulnerable neonate. Med Ped Oncol 1996;27(6):521–528.

78. Eichelberger MR, Chatten J, Bruce DA, et al. Acute pancreatitis and increased intracranial pressure. J Pediatr Surg 1981;16:562.

79. Knoderer HM, Robarge J, Flockhart DA. Predicting asparaginase-associated pancreatitis. Pediatr Blood Cancer 2007;49(5):634–639.

80. Kearney SL, Dahlberg SE, Levy DE, et al. Clinical course and outcome in children with acute lymphoblastic leukemia and asparaginase-associated pancreatitis. Pediatr Blood Cancer 2009;53(2):162–167.

81. Latifi R, McIntosh JK, Dudrick SJ. Nutritional management of acute and chronic pancreatitis. Surg Clin North Am 1991;71:579.

82. Wu SF, Chen AC, Peng CT, et al. Octreotide therapy in asparaginase-associated pancreatitis in childhood acute lymphoblastic leukemia. Pediatr Blood Cancer 2008; 51(6):824–825.

83. Paran H, Neufeld D, Mayo A, et al. Preliminary report of a prospective randomized study of octreotide in the treatment of severe acute pancreatitis. J Am Coll Surg 1995; 181(2):121–124.

84. Top PC, Tissing WJ, Kuiper JW, et al. L-asparaginase-induced severe necrotizing pancreatitis successfully treated with percutaneous drainage. Pediatr Blood Cancer 2005;44(1):95–97.

85. Rossi R, Kleta R, Ehrich JHH. Renal involvement in children with malignancies. Pediatr Nephrol 1999;13:153–162.

86. deVries CR, Freiha FS. Hemorrhagic cystitis: a review. J Urol 1990;143:1–9.

87. Leslie JA, Cain MP. Pediatric urologic emergencies and urgencies. Pediatr Clin North Am 2006;53(3):513–527, viii.

88. Mantadakis E, Aquino WM, Strand WR, et al. Acute renal failure due to obstruction in Burkitt lymphoma. Pediatr Nephrol 1999;13:237–240.

89. Sinaiko AR. Treatment of hypertension in children. Pediatr Nephrol 1994;8(5): 603–609.

90. National Heart, Lung, and Blood Institute. The fourth report on the diagnosis, evaluation, and treatment of high blood pressure in children and adolescents. Pediatrics 2004;114(2):555–576.

91. de Graaf JH, Tamminga RYJ, Kamps WA. Paraneoplastic manifestations in children. Eur J Pediatr 1994;153:784–791.

92. Pursell RN, Quinlan PM. Secondary hypertension due to a renin-producing teratoma. Am J Hypertens 2003;16:592–595.

93. Murray JC, Dorfman SR, Brandt ML, et al. Renal venous thrombosis complicating acute myeloid leukemia with hyperleukocytosis. J Pediatr Hematol Oncol 1996;18(3): 327–330.

94. Haselberger MB, Schwinghammer TL. Efficacy of mesna for prevention of hemorrhagic cystitis after high-dose cyclophosphamide therapy. Ann Pharmacother 1995;29:918–921.

95. Cheerva AC, Raj A, Bertolone SJ, et al. BK virus-associated hemorrhagic cystitis in pediatric cancer patients receiving high-dose cyclophosphamide. J Pediatr Hematol Oncol 2007;29(9):617–621.

96. Russo P. Urologic emergencies in the cancer patient. Semin Oncol 2000;27(3):284–298.

97. Laszlo D, Bosi A, Guidi S, et al. Prostaglandin E2 bladder instillation for the treatment of hemorrhagic cystitis after allogeneic bone marrow transplantation. Haematologica 1995;80(5):421–425.

98. Shrom SH, Donaldson MH, Duckett JW, et al. Formalin treatment for intractable hemorrhagic cystitis. A review of the literature with 16 additional cases. Cancer 1976; 38:1785.

99. Greenes DS. Neurotrauma. In: Fleisher CR, Ludwig S, Henretig FM, eds. Textbook of pediatric emergency medicine. 5th ed. 2006:1361–1388.

100. Nelson D. Coma and altered level of consciousness. In: Fleisher CR, Ludwig S, Henretig FM, eds. Textbook of pediatric emergency medicine. 5th ed. 2006:201–212.

101. Packer RJ, Rorke LB, Lange BJ, et al. Cerebrovascular accidents in children with cancer. Pediatrics 1985;76(2):194–201.

102. Sommers LM, Hawkins DS. Meningitis in pediatric cancer patients: a review of forty cases from a single institution. Pediatr Infect Dis J 1999;18(10):902–907.

103. DiMario FJ Jr, Packer RJ. Acute mental status changes in children with systemic cancer. Pediatrics 1990;85(3):353–360.

104. Tuma R, DeAngelis LM. Altered mental status in patients with cancer. Arch Neurol 2000;57(12):1727–1731.

105. Antunes NL. Mental status changes in children with systemic cancer. Pediatr Neurol 2002;27(1):39–42.

106. Alderson AL, Novack TA. Neurophysiological and clinical aspects of glucocorticoids and memory: a review. J Clin Exp Neuropsychol 2002;24(3):335–355.

107. Uno H, Eisele S, Sakai A, et al. Neurotoxicity of glucocorticoids in the primate brain. Horm Behav 1994;28(4):336–348.

108. Herzig RH, Hines JD, Herzig GP, et al. Cerebellar toxicity with high-dose cytosine arabinoside. J Clin Oncol 1987;5(6):927–932.

109. Rubin EH, Andersen JW, Bert DT, et al. Risk factors for high-dose cytarabine neurotoxicity: an analysis of a cancer and leukemia group B trial in patients with acute myeloid leukemia. J Clin Oncol 1992;10(6):948–953.

110. Jaffe N, Tkaue Y, Anzae T, et al. Transient neurologic disturbances induced by high-dose methotrexate treatment. Cancer 1985;56:1356.

111. Lovblad KO, Kelkar P, Ozdoba C, et al. Pure methotrexate encephalopathy presenting with seizures: CT and MRI features. Pediatr Radiol 1998;28:86–91.

112. Walker RJ, Allen JC, Rosen G, et al. Transient cerebral dysfunction secondary to high-dose methotrexate. J Clin Oncol 1986;4:1845.

113. Kisor DF, Plunkett W, Kurtzberg J, et al. Pharmacokinetics of nelarabine and 9-beta-D-arabinofuranosyl guanine in pediatric and adult patients during a phase I study of nelarabine for the treatment of refractory hematologic malignancies. J Clin Oncol 2000;18:995–1003.

114. Gieron MA, Barak LS, Estrada J. Severe encephalopathy associated with ifosfamide administration in two children with metastatic disease. J Neurooncol 1988;6:29.

115. Pratt CB, Horowitz ME, Meyer WH, et al. Phase II trial of ifosfamide in children with malignant solid tumors. Cancer Treat Rep 1987;71:131.

116. Mahaley MS, Whaley RA, Blue M, et al. Central neurotoxicity following intracarotid BCNU chemotherapy for malignant glioma. J Neurooncol 1986;3:297.

117. Schold SC, Fay JW. Central nervous system toxicity from high-dose BCNU treatment of systemic cancer. Neurology 1980;30:429.
118. Harris BE, Carpenter JT, Diasio RB. Severe 5-fluorouracil toxicity secondary to dihydropyrimidine dehydrogenase deficiency. A potentially more common pharmacogenetic syndrome. Cancer 1991;68(3):499–501.
119. Schroeter T, Lanvers C, Herding H, et al. Pseudotumor cerebri induced by all-trans-retinoic acid in a child treated for acute promyelocytic leukemia. Med Pediatr Oncol 2000;34:284–286.
120. Forman AD. Neurologic complications of cytokine therapy. Oncology 1994;8:105.
121. Seivers E, Lange BJ, Sondel P, et al. Phase II study of interleukin-2 after consolidation chemotherapy for acute myelogenous leukemia: a report from the Children's Cancer Group. J Clin Oncol 1998;16:914–919.
122. Cabebe E, Wakelee H. Role of anti-angiogenesis agents in treating NSCLC: focus on bevacizumab and VEGFR tyrosine kinase inhibitors. Curr Treat Options Oncol 2007; 8(1):15–27.
123. Davis DP, Robertson T, Imbesi SG. Diffusion-weighted magnetic resonance imaging versus computed tomography in the diagnosis of acute ischemic stroke. J Emerg Med 2006;31(3):269–277.
124. Patel PN. Methylene blue for management of Ifosfamide-induced encephalopathy. Ann Pharmacother 2006;40(2):299–303.
125. Drachtman RA, Cole PD, Golden CB, et al. Dextromethorphan is effective in the treatment of subacute methotrexate neurotoxicity. Pediatr Hematol Oncol 2002;19(5): 319–327.
126. Edwards MS, Wilson CB. Treatment of radiation necrosis. In: gilbert HA, Kagan AR, eds. Radiation damage to the nervous system. A delayed therapeutic hazard. New York: Raven Press, 1980:129.
127. Chuba PJ, Aronin P, Bhambhani K, et al. Hyperbaric oxygen therapy for radiation-induced brain injury in children. Cancer 1997;80(10):2005–2012.
128. Glantz MJ, Burger PC, Friedman AH, et al. Treatment of radiation-induced nervous system injury with heparin and warfarin. Neurology 1994;44(11):2020–2027.
129. Omura M, Aida N, Sekido K, et al. Large intracranial vessel occlusive vasculopathy with radiation therapy in children: clinical features and usefulness of magnetic resonance imaging. Int J Radiat Oncol 1997;38(2):241–249.
130. Lowe EJ, Pui CH, Hancock ML, et al. Early complications in children with acute lymphoblastic leukemia presenting with hyperleukocytosis. Pediatr Blood Cancer 2005; 45(1):10–15.
131. Bunin NJ, Piu CH. Differing complications of hyperleukocytosis in children with acute lymphoblastic or acute nonlymphoblastic leukemia. J Clin Oncol 1985;3:1590.
132. Rowe JM, Lichtman MA. Hyperleukocytosis and leukostasis. Common features of childhood chronic myelogenous leukemia. Blood 1984;63:1230.
133. Menell JS, Cesarman GM, Jacovina AT, et al. Annexin II and bleeding in acute promyelocytic leukemia. N Engl J Med 1999;340(13):994–1004.
134. Mitchell L, Hoogendoorn H, Giles AR, et al. Increased endogenous thrombin generation in children with acute lymphoblastic leukemia: risk of thrombotic complications in L-asparaginase-induced antithrombin III deficiency. Blood 1994;83(2):386–391.
135. Mitchell LG, PARKAA Group. A prospective cohort study determining the prevalence of thrombotic events in children with acute lymphoblastic leukemia and a central venous line who are treated with L-asparaginase. Results of the prophylactic antithrombin replacement in kids with acute lymphoblastic leukemia treated with asparaginase (PARKAA) study. Cancer 2003;97(2):508–516.
136. Nowak-Gottl U, Wermes C, Junker R, et al. Prospective evaluation of the thrombotic risk in children with acute lymphoblastic leukemia carrying the MTHFR TT 677 genotype, the prothrombin G20210 A variant, and further prothrombotic risk factors. Blood 1999;93(5):1595–1599.
137. Mitchell L, Andrew M, Hanna K, et al. Trend to efficacy and safety using antithrombin concentrate in prevention of thrombosis in children receiving L-asparaginase for acute lymphoblastic leukemia. Results of the PAARKA study. Thromb Haemost 2003; 90(2):235–244.
138. Yim YS, Mahoney DH, Oshman DG. Hemiparesis and ischemic changes of the white matter after intrathecal therapy for children with acute lymphocytic leukemia. Cancer 1991;67:2058.
139. Pihko M, Tyni T, Virkola K, et al. Transient ischemic cerebral lesions during induction chemotherapy for acute lymphoblastic leukemia. J Pediatr 1993;123:718.
140. Shuper A, Packer RJ, Vezina LG, et al. Complicated migraine-like episodes in children following cranial irradiation and chemotherapy. Neurology 1995;45:1837.
141. Grenier Y, Tomita T, Marymont MH, et al. Late postirradiation occlusive vasculopathy in childhood medulloblastoma. Report of two cases. J Neurosurg 1998;89(3):460–464.
142. Bowers DC, Liu Y, Leisenring W, et al. Late-occurring stroke among long-term survivors of childhood leukemia and brain tumors: a report from the Childhood Cancer Survivor Study. J Clin Oncol 2006;24(33):5277–5282.
143. Bleyer WA. Central nervous system leukemia. Pediatr Clin North Am 1988;35(4): 789–814.
144. Moustafa RR, Baron JC. Clinical review: Imaging in ischaemic stroke—implications for acute management. Crit Care 2007;11(5):227.
145. Packer RJ, Zimmerman RA, Sutton LN, et al. Magnetic resonance imaging (MRI) of spinal cord disease of childhood. Pediatrics 1986;78:251.
146. deVeber G, Chan A, Monagle P, et al. Anticoagulation therapy in pediatric patients with sinovenous thrombosis: a cohort study. Arch Neurol 1998;55(12):1533–1537.
147. Johnson MC, Parkerson N, Ward S, et al. Pediatric sinovenous thrombosis. J Pediatr Hematol Oncol 2003;25(4):312–315.
148. Stam J, de Bruijn S, deVeber G. Anticoagulation for cerebral sinus thrombosis. Stroke 2003;34:1054–1055.
149. Adams HP Jr, del Zoppo G, Alberts MJ, et al. Guidelines for the early management of adults with ischemic stroke: a guideline from the American Heart Association/American Stroke Association Stroke Council, Clinical Cardiology Council, Cardiovascular Radiology and Intervention Council, and the Atherosclerotic Peripheral Vascular Disease and Quality of Care Outcomes in Research Interdisciplinary Working Groups: the American Academy of Neurology affirms the value of this guideline as an educational tool for neurologists. Stroke 2007;38(5):1655–1711.
150. Lansberg MG, Bluhmki E, Thijs VN. Efficacy and safety of tissue plasminogen activator 3 to 4.5 hours after acute ischemic stroke: a metaanalysis. Stroke 2009;40(7):2438–2441.
151. Antunes NL, DeAngelis LM. Neurologic consultations in children with systemic cancer. Pediatr Neurology 1999;20(2):121–124.
152. Fisher MJ, Khadernian ZP, Simon EM, et al. Diffusion-weighted MR imaging of early methotrexate-related neurotoxicity in children. AJNR Am J Neuroradiol 2005;26(7): 1686–1689.
153. Bebin M. The acute management of seizures. Pediatr Ann 1999;28(4):225–229.
154. Shnecker BF, Fountain NB. Epilepsy. Dis Mon 2003;49:426–478.
155. Jardine LF, Ingram LC, Bleyer WA. Intrathecal leucovorin after intrathecal methotrexate overdose. J Pediatr Hematol Oncol 1996;18(3):302–304.
156. Widemann BC, Balis FM, Shalabi A, et al. Treatment of accidental intrathecal methotrexate overdose with intrathecal carboxypeptidase G2. J Natl Cancer Inst 2004;96(20):1557–1559.
157. Lafolie P, Liliemark J, Bjork O, et al. Exchange of cerebrospinal fluid in accidental intrathecal overdose of cytarabine. Med Toxicol Adverse Drug Exp 1988;3(3): 248–252.
158. Trinkle R, Wu JK. Errors involving pediatric patients receiving chemotherapy: a literature review. Med Pediatr Oncol 1996;26(5):344–351.
159. Zaragoza MR, Ritchey ML, Walter A. Neurourologic consequences of accidental intrathecal vincristine: a case report. Med Pediatr Oncol 1995;24:61–62.
160. Kosmidis HV, Bouhoutsou DO, Varvoutsi MC, et al. Vincristine overdose: experience with 3 patients. Pediatr Hematol Oncol 1991;8(2):171–178.
161. O'Marcaigh AS, Johnson CM, Smithson WA, et al. Successful treatment of intrathecal methotrexate overdose in using ventriculolumbar perfusion and intrathecal instillation of carboxypeptidase G2. Mayo Clin Proc 1996;71:161–165.
162. Pimentel L. Medical complications of oncologic disease. Emerg Med Clin North Am 1993;11(2):407–419.
163. Michelagnoli MP, Bailey CC, Wilson I, et al. Potential salvage therapy for inadvertent intrathecal administration of vincristine. Br J Haematol 1997;99(2):364–367.
164. Lewis DW, Packer RJ, Raney B, et al. Incidence, presentation and outcome of spinal cord diseases in child with systemic cancer. Pediatrics 1986;78:438.
165. Klein SL, Stanford RA, Muhlbauer MS. Pediatric spinal epidural metastases. J Neurosurg 1991;74:70.
166. Ebb DM, Karasidis M, Vezina G, et al. Spinal cord compression in widely metastatic Wilms' tumor. Paraplegia in two children with anaplastic Wilms' tumor. Cancer 1992;69:2726.
167. Geetha N, Hussain BM, Ratheesan K, et al. Intraspinal leukemia with cord compression. Med Pediatr Oncol 1999;33:132–133.
168. Boogerd W, van der Sande JJ. Diagnosis and treatment of spinal cord compression in malignant disease. Cancer Treatment Rev 1993;19:129.
169. Byrne TN. Spinal cord compression from epidural metastases. N Engl J Med 1992; 327:614.
170. Cole JS, Patchell RA. Metastatic epidural spinal cord compression. Lancet Neurol 2008;7(5):459–466.
171. Mut M, Schiff D, Shaffrey ME. Metastasis to nervous system: spinal epidural and intramedullary metastases. J Neurooncol 2005;75(1):43–56.
172. Sorensen S, Helweg-Larsen S, Mouridsen H, et al. Effect of high-dose dexamethasone in carcinomatous metastatic spinal cord compression treated with radiotherapy: a randomised trial. Eur J Cancer 1994;30A(1):22–27.
173. Maranzano E, Latini P, Beneventi S, et al. Radiotherapy without steroids in selected metastatic spinal cord compression patients. A phase II trial. Am J Clin Oncol 1996;19(2):179–183.
174. Patchell RA, Tibbs PA, Regine WF, et al. Direct decompressive surgical resection in the treatment of spinal cord compression caused by metastatic cancer: a randomised trial. Lancet 2005;366(9486):643–648.
175. Loblaw DA, Laperriere NJ. Emergency treatment of malignant extradural spinal cord compression: an evidence-based guideline. J Clin Oncol 1998;16(4):1613–1624.
176. Rades D, Heidenreich F, Karstens JH. Final results of a prospective study of the prognostic value of the time to develop motor deficits before irradiation in metastatic spinal cord compression. Int J Radiat Oncol Biol Phys 2002;53(4):975–979.
177. Young RF, Post EM, King GA. Treatment of spinal epidural metastases. Randomized prospective comparison of laminectomy and radiotherapy. J Neurosurg 1980;53(6): 741–748.
178. De Bernardi B, Balwierz W, Bejent J, et al. Epidural compression in neuroblastoma: Diagnostic and therapeutic aspects. Cancer Lett 2005;228(1–2):283–299.
179. Sanderson IR, Pritchard J, Marsh HT. Chemotherapy as initial treatment of spinal cord compression due to disseminated neuroblastoma. J Neurosurg 1989;70:685.
180. Spinazze S, Caraceni A, Schrijvers D. Epidural spinal cord compression. Crit Rev Oncol Hematol 2005;56(3):397–406.
181. Inaba H, Fan Y, Pounds S, et al. Clinical and biologic features and treatment outcome of children with newly diagnosed acute myeloid leukemia and hyperleukocytosis. Cancer 2008;113(3):522–529.
182. Porcu P, Farag S, Marcucci G, et al. Leukocytoreduction for acute leukemia. Ther Apher 2002;6(1):15–23.
183. Lichtman MA, Rowe JM. Hyperleukocytic leukemias. Rheological, clinical, and therapeutic considerations. Blood 1982;60:279.
184. Porcu P, Cripe LD, Ng EW, et al. Hyperleukocytic leukemias and leukostasis: a review of pathophysiology, clinical presentation and management. Leuk Lymphoma 2000; 39(1–2):1–18.
185. Bunin NJ, Kunkel K, Callihan TR. Cytoreductive procedures in the early management in cases of leukemia and hyperleukocytosis in children. Med Pediatr Oncol 1987;15: 232–235.
186. Nowacki P, Zdziarska B, Fryze C, et al. Co-existence of thrombocytopenia and hyperleukocytosis ('critical period') as a risk factor of haemorrhage into the central nervous system in patients with acute leukaemias. Haematologia 2002;31(4): 347–355.
187. Maurer HS, Steinherz PG, Gaynon PS, et al. Management of hyperleukocytosis (HL) in childhood with acute lymphoblastic leukemia. J Clin Oncol 1988;6:1425.
188. Coiffier B, Altman A, Pui CH, et al. Guidelines for the management of pediatric and adult tumor lysis syndrome: an evidence-based review. J Clin Oncol 2008;26(16): 2767–2778.
189. Larsen G, Loghman-Adham M. Acute renal failure with hyperuricemia as initial presentation of leukemia in children. J Pediatr Hematol Oncol 1996;18(2):191–194.
190. Truong TH, Beyene J, Hitzler J, et al. Features at presentation predict children with acute lymphoblastic leukemia at low risk for tumor lysis syndrome. Cancer 2007; 110(8):1832–1839.
191. Andreoli SP, Clark JH, McGuire WA, et al. Purine excretion during tumor lysis in children with acute lymphocytic leukemia receiving allopurinol. Relationship to acute renal failure. J Pediatr 1986;109:292.
192. Vachvanichsanong P, Maipang M, Dissaneewate P, et al. Severe hyperphosphatemia following acute tumor lysis syndrome. Med Pediatr Oncol 1995;24:63–66.
193. Feusner JH, Ritchey AK, Cohn SL, et al. Management of tumor lysis syndrome: need for evidence-based guidelines. J Clin Oncol 2008;26(34):5657–5658; author reply 5658–5689.

194. Goldman SC, Holcenberg JS, Finklestein JZ, et al. A randomized comparison between rasburicase and allopurinol in children with lymphoma or leukemia at high risk for tumor lysis. Blood 2001;97(10):2998–3003.

195. Pui CH, Mahmoud HH, Wiley JM, et al. Recombinant urate oxidase for the prophylaxis or treatment of hyperuricemia in patients with leukemia or lymphoma. J Clin Oncol 2001;19(3):697–704.

196. Ten Harkel ADJ, Kist-Van Holthe JE, Van Weel M, et al. Alkalinization and the tumor lysis syndrome. Med Pediatr Oncol 1998;31:27–28.

197. Abdullah S, Diezi M, Sung L, et al. Sevelamer hydrochloride: a novel treatment of hyperphosphatemia associated with tumor lysis syndrome in children. Pediatr Blood Cancer 2008;51(1):59–61.

198. Saccente SL, Kohaut EC, Berkow RL. Prevention of tumor lysis syndrome using continuous veno-venous hemofiltration. Pediatr Nephrol 1995;9:569–573.

199. McKay C, Furman WL. Hypercalcemia complicating childhood malignancies. Cancer 1993;72:256–260.

200. Kerdudo C, Aerts I, Fattet S, et al. Hypercalcemia and childhood cancer: a 7-year experience. J Pediatr Hematol Oncol 2005;27(1):23–27.

201. Seymour JF, Gagel RF. The major humoral mediator of hypercalcemia in Hodgkin's disease and non-Hodgkin lymphoma. Blood 1993;82:1383.

202. Bilezikan JP. Management of acute hypercalcemia. N Engl J Med 1992;326:1196.

203. Young G, Shende A. Use of pamidronate in the management of acute cancer-related hypercalcemia in children. Med Pediatr Oncol 1998;30:117–121.

204. Adrogue HJ, Madias NE. Primary care: hyponatremia. NEJM 2000;342(21):1581–1589.

205. Sorensen JB, Andersen MK, Hansen HH. Syndrome of inappropriate secretion of antidiuretic hormone (SIADH) in malignant disease. J Int Med 1995;238:97–110.

206. Kirch C, Gachot B, Germann N, et al. Recurrent ifosfamide-induced hyponatraemia. Eur J Cancer 1997;33(14):2438–2439.

207. Ellison DH, Berl T. Clinical practice. The syndrome of inappropriate antidiuresis. N Engl J Med 2007;356(20):2064–2072.

208. Kappy MS, Ganong CA. Cerebral salt wasting in children: the role of atrial natriuretic hormone. Adv Pediatr 1996;43:271–308.

209. Cerda-Esteve M, Cuadrado-Godia E, Chillaron JJ, et al. Cerebral salt wasting syndrome: review. Eur J Int Med 2008;19(4):249–254.

210. Albanese A, Hindmarsh P, Stanhope R. Management of hyponatraemia in patients with acute cerebral insults. Arch Dis Child 2001;85(3):246–251.

211. Bell LM. Shock. In: Fleisher CR, Ludwig S, Henretig FM, eds. Textbook of pediatric emergency medicine. 5th ed. Philadelphia, PA: Lippincott, Williams & Wilkins, 2000:47.

CHAPTER 39 ■ HEMATOLOGIC SUPPORTIVE CARE FOR CHILDREN WITH CANCER

ANURAG K. AGRAWAL, CAROLINE A. HASTINGS, AND JAMES FEUSNER

Transfusion therapy has been the key to successful management of children with cancer or hematologic diseases and recipients of hematopoietic stem cell transplants. In this chapter, we provide a comprehensive review of the indications for transfusion, along with a discussion of the pathophysiology, risks, and benefits of transfusion therapy. Where possible, we furnish guidelines for management; in addition, we review the current status of cytokine therapy for children with malignancies.

ANEMIA

Definition and Prevalence

Anemia is classically defined as a deficiency of red blood cells (RBCs) or hemoglobin leading to a reduction in the oxygen-carrying capacity of blood. No consistent definition of what constitutes anemia in pediatric oncology has been adopted. The incidence of anemia in children with solid tumors or Hodgkin disease at the time of diagnosis has been reported to be 51% to 74%.[1] Several other pediatric studies report a high incidence of anemia (>50%) requiring intervention with transfusion in children with Wilms' tumor, acute lymphoblastic leukemia, and osteosarcoma.[2–4] Although baseline hemoglobin values differ by age, type of cancer, and intensity of therapy, a recent European pediatric survey reported that >80% of children receiving chemotherapy were anemic.[5] Regardless of the specific definition of anemia, it is clearly common during the course of treatment of childhood cancer. In one large pediatric study, the incidence of anemia in children with leukemia was reported to be 97%. Treatment of anemia in these children was almost exclusively blood transfusion (typically given when hemoglobin levels dropped below 5.5 to 8.0 g per dL).[5]

Pathophysiology and Etiology

Anemia occurs as a result of blood loss and impaired production. Cancer-related anemia is multifactorial and often has both acute and chronic components.[1,6,7] Blood loss may be due to hemorrhage (facilitated by concomitant thrombocytopenia), repetitive blood sampling, infection, and hemolysis. Impaired production results from infiltration of the marrow by malignant cells, suppression of erythropoiesis related to chemotherapy, radiation treatment or infection, shortened RBC survival secondary to treatment, iron deficiency and impaired use of iron stores, and low endogenous erythropoietin (EPO) levels suggestive of impaired production secondary to underlying chronic disease.[8,9] Direct infiltration of the marrow by malignant cells produces a slow decrement in the hemoglobin level. Both serum iron and transferrin saturation may be low; however, the ferritin may be moderately elevated because it is an acute phase reactant.

Infections may have a significant impact on blood counts and suppress marrow production of RBCs. Infection with parvovirus B19, the cause of erythema infectiosum, has been reported in children with acute leukemia and following bone marrow transplantation.[10–17] Manifestations of this infection are varied and include fever, rash, neutropenia, reticulocytopenia, and prolonged severe anemia. Parvovirus immunoglobulin G (IgG) and immunoglobulin M (IgM) levels may not be diagnostic, and if highly suspected, an assessment for parvovirus B19 in the DNA should be performed. Acute and chronic parvovirus B19 infections have been treated successfully with immune globulin infusions.[11,12,17] Infection secondary to other viruses, such as cytomegalovirus (CMV) and Epstein-Barr virus (EBV), has also been implicated in chronic anemia or pancytopenia in children with cancer.[18–22]

Signs and Symptoms of Anemia

At the presentation of leukemia or a malignancy with significant marrow involvement, the child often is anemic. The anemia is usually normochromic and normocytic with a low reticulocyte count. A slow decline in erythrocyte production typically results in an insidious onset with pallor and gradual onset of fatigue. These signs and symptoms are related to the degree of reduction in oxygen-carrying capacity of the blood, change in blood volume, rate at which these changes occur, and the ability of the cardiovascular and hematopoietic systems to compensate. One study found that anemic pediatric patients are in a state of relative oxygen deficit and are able to adapt physiologically to function in this state.[23] How this finding may be extrapolated to pediatric cancer patients is not known.

The clinical signs of anemia are often related to its severity, rapidity of onset, and underlying malignancy. General symptoms can include poor feeding, loss of appetite, headaches, dizziness, fatigue, vertigo, tinnitus, dyspnea, irritability, faintness, inactivity, loss of concentration, change in behavior, and poor school performance.[24,25] Cardiac enlargement and evidence of congestive heart failure may be present with either blood loss or chronic severe anemia. Tachycardia, prominent arterial pulses, bruits, tachypnea, dyspnea, and postural hypotension can be detected in patients with modest to severe anemia. Hemic murmurs reflect an increase in cardiac output, stroke volume, and heart rate associated with decreased peripheral resistance and decreased blood viscosity. Gallop rhythm may be present in a hemodynamically compromised state. These signs and symptoms respond rapidly to treatment with transfusion.

It is uncertain what risk anemia poses to the child or adolescent with cancer; the level of hemoglobin at which it is best to intervene is also unknown. Children are potentially at risk for acute and long-term effects of severe or moderate anemia. The acute effects are usually evident in the history and physical examination of the patient. Physical signs such as pallor, hypoxia, or a change in vital signs (increased heart rate and decreased blood pressure) may be present. Patients may experience transient cognitive dysfunction, including decreased mental alertness, poor concentration, and memory problems. The long-term effects of chronic anemia in young patients with cancer are poorly understood but may include neurocognitive sequelae.[26] Children receiving immune suppressive therapies for extended periods may experience chronic anemia with little opportunity between cycles of chemotherapy or radiation to recover fully. Chronic anemia in young children may have an adverse impact on growth and development.

Fatigue is a frequently unrecognized and undertreated complication of anemia and is a relatively universal symptom among oncology patients.[8,24,27,28] Vogelzang et al. interviewed 419 adult oncology patients, and they reported fatigue being a more important factor than pain (61% vs. 19%), although in a comparable survey of oncologists, the oncologists felt that pain adversely affected their patients more than fatigue (61% vs. 37%).[29] The recognition of fatigue and its possible implications for quality of life (QOL) in cancer patients are now being studied in children and adolescents.[26,30,31] Fatigue is often present at diagnosis. Both disease and treatment-associated factors contribute to its development.[7] Fatigue affected the ability to participate in social activities, maintain interpersonal relationships, and carry out simple cognitive tasks. It also had a remarkably negative impact on employment and financial status. Cancer patients are often tired at rest and may have a decreased capability to carry out activities of daily living, with slow physical recovery from tasks. Concentration may be impaired and patients may have reduced efficiency in responding to stimuli. Chronic pathologic fatigue may result in asthenia. Chronic fatigue is often not alleviated by rest and can become a stressful condition.[9]

Maintaining a higher hemoglobin concentration during chemotherapy results in a better QOL and may possibly affect survival.[24,26,32–36] QOL measures typically take into consideration the effect of fatigue on physical, functional, emotional, and social well-being of the patient.[37] In these studies, general scores for QOL, fatigue, and sensations of physical and functional well-being are significantly higher among patients with hemoglobin levels above 12 g per dL. Other interventions for the treatment of fatigue include exercise; optimal nutrition; and psychosocial interventions including stress management, energy conservation, sleep therapy, and restorative therapy in addition to adjunctive pharmacologic treatment.[24,38–40] Factors contributing to fatigue in children and adolescents with cancer include loss of muscle mass, medications, immobility, altered sleep patterns, anxiety, and depression.[26,41] Maintaining a higher hemoglobin level (i.e., 9 to 11 g per dL) in these children and adolescents for an extended time may have a positive effect on health-related QOL, especially neurocognitive function, although this must be assessed on an individual basis.[9,26,32] The clinical manifestations of anemia compound the consequences of the malignancy and its treatment, adding to the serious deterioration in QOL for young patients, as well as complicating effective therapy. Therefore, assessment of the impact of fatigue on QOL should be considered when deciding on a transfusion threshold for an individual patient.[42] In addition, global interventions to address the physical, developmental, and psychosocial impact of anemia should be addressed by the health care team.

Red Cell Transfusion Guidelines

The traditional therapy for chemotherapy-induced anemia has been the use of RBC transfusions, despite their short-lived effects and inherent risks. Transfusion therapy is simple, fast, effective, available, and relatively safe, and it provides a measurable, direct benefit. In deciding when to transfuse a child, it is important to have evidence-based guidelines. Because these are not currently available, it is reasonable to abandon a quest for a specific hemoglobin level at which to transfuse, and rather tailor transfusion to the patient's needs.[43,44] Considerations include the clinical condition of the patient, anticipated procedures, presence of comorbidities, especially pulmonary or cardiac disease, concomitant thrombocytopenia, and attendant risk of prolonged bleeding. The patient should be assessed with attention to physical signs and symptoms. Transfusion need not be given if the child is clinically stable and recovery from chemotherapy-induced aplasia is imminent. Consideration should also be given to individual variation in tolerance of fatigue, QOL, and patient preference.[45] Restrictive strategies may safely reduce the need for frequent transfusions with their resultant potential complications and cost.[46,47]

Severe anemia (<7 g per dL) requiring RBC transfusion is a frequent manageable complication of pediatric cancer therapy.[48,49] The need for immediate RBC transfusion is determined by the etiology and expected duration of the anemia, in addition to the patient's ability to compensate for the decreased blood volume and resultant decreased oxygen-carrying capacity. The use of blood transfusions typically increases as the intensity of therapy increases.[48,50] A hemoglobin level of less than 6 to 7 g per dL with symptoms of lassitude, malaise, decreased activity, or irritability often warrant intervention with transfusion support.[51,52] Management of moderate anemia (>7 g per dL) may only require close monitoring.[51] Again, the decision to transfuse or not in cases of moderate anemia must be based on a constellation of physical findings and potential detriment to the patient's physical, mental, and developmental status.

The goal of prophylactic transfusion therapy is to improve or maintain the overall well-being of the patient, or to ensure safety for the patient anticipating a surgical procedure or blood loss. Therefore, considerations for prophylactic transfusion should include multiple factors, in addition to signs or symptoms of anemia (Table 39.1). In general, children tolerate lower hemoglobin levels than do adults because of their greater ability to compensate for the anemia, and the fact that the normal baseline hemoglobin level in children is lower than that in adults.[49,53,54] Adolescents as well as younger children often do not tolerate the symptoms of anemia. Consideration should be given to maintaining a hemoglobin level of 8 g per dL or higher in symptomatic adolescent patients or younger children with chronic anemia to prevent impairment of growth or development. The timing of prophylactic transfusions should take into account recovery from the effects of chemotherapy or radiation-induced aplasia.

A child with a past history of severe anemia due to hemorrhage should be maintained at a higher hemoglobin level. A suggested level is 8 to 10 g per dL in severely thrombocytopenic patients at risk for hemorrhage or with a history of prior hemorrhage. Prophylaxis with platelet transfusions should also be considered, and is discussed later.[55,56] RBC transfusion may improve outcomes of medical or surgical treatment by providing temporary support and increased oxygen delivery in patients undergoing anesthesia. In patients having an invasive or surgical procedure, maintenance of a moderate hemoglobin level of 8 to 10 g per dL is suggested to minimize the degree of anemia when perioperative blood loss is anticipated. A relationship between hematocrit and platelet function has been suggested.[43,57] A higher hematocrit appears to improve platelet function in uremic patients.[58–60]

Red Cell Component Therapy

The risks and benefits of blood transfusion must be carefully considered, and the patient and family need to be well

TABLE 39.1

PROPHYLACTIC RED BLOOD CELL TRANSFUSION GUIDELINES FOR CHILDREN
AND ADOLESCENTS WITH CANCER

Clinical scenario		Hemoglobin level to transfuse (g/dL)
Stable	Asymptomatic child, imminent hemoglobin and platelet recovery	<7
Vital sign changes	Tachycardia, tachypnea, hypotension	<8
Oxygen requirement	Pulmonary or cardiac comorbidities	8–10
Thrombocytopenia	History of prior hemorrhage and PRBC requirement	8–10
Procedure	Anticipation of blood loss	8–10
Fatigue	Negative effect on quality of life, especially in adolescents	8–10
Chronic anemia	Impact on development	8–10
Infants	Impact on growth or development	8–10
Radiation (controversial; see text for details)		8–10

PRBC, packed red blood cells.

informed about both. Major risks of transfusion include receiving blood products of the wrong type, transmission of infections, and transfusion reactions. Informed consent is a vital part of the transfusion process and is required by local, state, and national health and safety codes (such as the Paul Gann Blood Safety Code in the state of California).[61] The physician is obliged to explain to the patient and family the indications, potential benefits, risks, and alternatives to transfusion therapy and to provide appropriate documentation of this discussion in the medical record. After consent is obtained, the patient who is to be transfused should have a type and screen performed and kept on file in the blood bank. Viral serologies to CMV, and hepatitis A, B, and C are recommended before transfusion. If the patient is seronegative, titers should be obtained again at the completion of therapy or, if clinical infection is suspected, to determine potential transfusion-associated transmission. Knowledge of the CMV status is particularly important in high-risk populations, such as potential bone marrow transplant recipients, to allow for proper screening of blood products.

RBC products may be collected and prepared in either citrate phosphate dextrose adenine (CPDA) or adsol (AS). CPDA RBCs typically contain 200 mL of RBCs and 50 mL of plasma. AS RBCs are more commonly used because of their longer storage life (42 days vs. 35 days). The hematocrit is lower in AS units (55% to 60%) than in CPDA units (70% to 80%) because of the addition of 100 mL of adenine saline solution. Therefore, the expected increase in hemoglobin or hematocrit level is lower when receiving an AS unit.[62] These factors must be considered when calculating the amount of blood required to correct anemia.[63]

Leukoreduction

Leukofiltration, ultraviolet irradiation, and washing of RBCs are special preparative methods to prevent specific complications of transfusion associated with white blood cells (WBCs). WBCs primarily distribute themselves within the cellular components of the blood product during processing. These "passenger" leukocytes are implicated as important contributors to the majority of transfusion-associated reactions.[64,65] It is well established that leukoreduction reduces the frequency of

platelet alloimmunization; febrile nonhemolytic transfusion reactions (FNHTR); infections with viral, bacterial, and protozoal pathogens; prion transmission; and the likelihood of CMV transmission with subsequent infection or reactivation.[66–76] Recent reports quantifying a decrease in sepsis secondary to indwelling catheters as well as infections after elective cardiac and orthopedic surgery in adult patients have been conflicting, but a majority of data reflects a decrease in significant infection that can be related to leukoreduction.[77–79] Transfusion-related immunomodulation (TRIM), thought to be secondary to the accumulation of immunosuppressive cytokines in nonleukoreduced blood, may play a role in this decreased rate of infection with leukoreduction although the actual effects of TRIM have not been well quantified or studied.[80] Rates of allergic reactions as well as transfusion-associated graft-versus-host disease (TA-GVHD) and transfusion-related acute lung injury (TRALI) are likely not affected by leukoreduction, although Yazer et al. did show a decrease in TRALI in patients receiving leukoreduced platelets and RBCs.[74,76,81–83]

Leukoreduction is achieved by filtration either at the time of collection or at the bedside. The current standards from the American Association of Blood Banks (AABB) and guidelines from the U.S. Food and Drug Administration (FDA) stipulate that RBC and apheresis platelets contain less than 5×10^6 leukocytes per unit while retaining greater than 85% of the therapeutic component.[84,85] Current estimates suggest that approximately 80% of the nation's blood supply is leukoreduced.[80] Although universal leukoreduction performed at the time of collection and blood component preparation currently is in place in Canada and much of Europe, it remains a controversial topic in the United States.[66,68,80,86,87] It continues to be speculated that universal leukoreduction will soon become standard of practice in the United States. Given the high percentage of centers that already practice universal leukoreduction, it seemingly has already become the standard.[80,87]

Leukoreduction of blood products should, in theory, reduce the incidence of transmission of leukotropic viruses, such as CMV and less importantly EBV.[88] Leukoreduction achieves a four-log decrease in EBV genomic copy number and renders EBV infectivity extremely minimal.[89] Similarly, studies have shown a two to three-log decrease in CMV genomic number although CMV is not completely removed from blood components.[90] The degree of WBC removal to prevent CMV infection is unknown.[71,91] Latently infected mononuclear cells appear to be the vector for transfusion-associated CMV infection in susceptible hosts and primary CMV infection or reactivation of latent CMV infection can cause morbidity and death in immunocompromised patients.[22,92,93] Transmission of CMV usually occurs following close contact with an infected person shedding the CMV into body fluids. The virus may be community acquired, transplacentally transmitted, passed through breast milk, or transmitted via transfusion. In the setting of pediatric transfusion, the two main strategies to prevent the transmission of CMV are leukoreduction and transfusion of CMV-seronegative blood products. Both strategies have been shown to reduce the incidence of transfusion-transmitted CMV although several studies support a higher degree of safety in at-risk patients with seronegative units.[88,91,94–97] Although it remains somewhat controversial in the literature, consensus guidelines recommend CMV-seronegative, leukoreduced products in patients at high risk such as hematopoietic stem cell transplant recipients, premature infants of CMV-negative mothers, and patients with immune deficiencies.[52,98] Leukoreduction only is possibly sufficient for apheresis platelet transfusions.[96]

Irradiation

Irradiation of platelets and RBCs is recommended for immunocompromised patients and is effective in preventing TA-GVHD by halting donor T-cell replication and engraftment in the host.[99–101] This often-fatal immunologic complication was first reported over 20 years ago in individuals with hematologic malignancies and in infants with immune deficiencies who received a blood transfusion.[102] Recently, investigators have demonstrated transfusion-associated microchimerism in the circulation of otherwise healthy transfusion recipients 3 to 5 days later, although it appears to occur most frequently in trauma patients who receive a significant amount of relatively fresh blood products and amongst those who receive blood transfusion and live in a more homogeneous population secondary to the increased incidence of one-way histocompatibility between the donor and the recipient, leading to increased survival of donor leukocytes.[103–106] Persistence of microchimerism can be detected at the 0.01% level. Its biological consequences in the adult and pediatric population are yet to be determined.[105,107] The development of TA-GVHD occurs in the setting of one-way histocompatibility between the donor and recipient and is affected by the presence of immunocompetent cells in the graft (blood) and the recipient's inability to reject the immunocompetent cells. Clinical manifestations of TA-GVHD present like hematopoietic stem cell transplant GVHD and include fever, anorexia, vomiting and diarrhea, and skin rash of variable severity. Pancytopenia and hepatic dysfunction with hyperbilirubinemia can also be present and may be severe and life threatening. Clinical suspicion may warrant a skin biopsy, liver biopsy, and/or bone marrow aspirate. Irradiation of blood products can effectively prevent TA-GVHD in patients at risk from immune compromise (i.e., premature infants, patients with immune deficiency or malignancy, recipients of a hematopoietic stem cell transplant) or those receiving blood from a likely histocompatible donor (transfusion from a blood relative).[71,105,108] Ionizing radiation results in the inactivation of T lymphocytes by damaging nuclear DNA or indirectly by generating ions and free radicals. A dose of 2,500 cGy is recommended to optimize inactivation of T-lymphocyte proliferation.[105,109,110]

Newer methods of prevention of TA-GVHD as well as infections such as CMV are in development and include photochemical treatment using psoralens and long-wavelength ultraviolet irradiation (pathogen-inactivation technologies).[71,99,105,111] Washing RBCs is an uncommon practice and usually indicated in the event of severe allergic or anaphylactic transfusion reactions, selective immunoglobulin A (IgA) deficiency, hyperkalemia, or large-volume transfusions, such as during extracorporeal membrane oxygenation procedures.[108]

Directed Donation

A directed blood donation is one in which a donor gives blood to be used by a specific recipient. Concerns about the safety of the blood pool have influenced some individuals to believe directed donor blood may be safer than that obtained from the general inventory. No definitive data supports this hypothesis.[112] Conventional blood donors are educated about blood safety and are screened by history and laboratory assessments. Donors are anonymous and are not paid for their donation. In contrast, it is thought that family or friends who are asked to become designated donors may not be as forthcoming in sharing their medical or personal history. While safety is the key concern, volunteer donors have not been found to impose increased risk over designated donors. Moreover, several potential dangers are raised when biological parents wish to serve as blood donors for their infants or for children who may become recipients of hematopoietic stem cell transplants from a family member. These complications include microchimerism, TA-GVHD, TRALI, and development of significant RBC antibodies.[113,114] The pros and cons of directed donation should be addressed with every family and include a discussion of cost, safety, immediate availability and time for laboratory screening, and health concerns for the recipient.

Dosage of Packed Red Blood Cell

Before ordering a packed RBC transfusion, the desired hemoglobin level should be determined to estimate the required transfusion volume. This level is dependent on the patient's diagnosis, clinical status, anticipated blood loss associated with procedures, and expected recovery of hematopoietic precursors. Care should be taken to minimize exposure to multiple units and maximize the use of each unit of RBCs. Children and adolescents who are anemic typically receive 10 to 20 mL per kg of RBCs, rounded off to the nearest RBC unit, if possible, to avoid wastage. Each 10 to 15 mL per kg of RBC volume is routinely given over 4 hours, although this paradigm has not been well studied in hemodynamically stable infants and children. The expected increase in the hemoglobin level is dependent on the hematocrit concentration of the blood and should increase by approximately 2 g per dL for each 10 mL per kg transfused of blood contained in AS (hematocrit concentration of approximately 55% to 60%).[63] Of note, anecdotal teaching that one must wait 4 hours after RBC transfusion is complete to get an accurate measurement of hemoglobin concentration is poorly studied and likely unnecessary.[63,115]

Special Considerations for Transfusion of Red Blood Cells

Severe Anemia

The rate of infusion of RBCs is determined by assessment of the absolute hemoglobin level, severity and acuteness of blood loss, ongoing blood loss such as with bleeding or hemolysis, and the patient's cardiovascular status. Patients with evidence of cardiac failure or a gallop rhythm warrant a slow transfusion. Children with severe anemia of gradual onset may safely tolerate a transfusion rate of 2 mL per kg per hour.[116] Historic teaching has recommended a slow transfusion (i.e., 5 mL per kg over 4 hours) for children with a hemoglobin level less than 5 g per dL, based on the assumption that total blood volume will be increased too quickly with rapid transfusion and lead to hemodynamic decompensation or collapse (transfusion-associated circulatory overload [TACO]). Children and adults with a chronic severe anemia have a compensatory increase in their plasma blood volume to near normal levels prior to transfusion; therefore, rapid transfusion or large volume transfusion is at risk for creating cardiogenic pulmonary edema and cardiac decompensation. In infants and children who are hemodynamically stable with normal underlying cardiopulmonary function, TACO secondary to rapid transfusion with underlying severe chronic anemia has not been examined. With the judicious use of diuretics during and after the transfusion, is it likely unnecessary to limit the rate of transfusion in this population. Since rate of transfusion in patients with hemoglobin levels of less than 5 g per dL has not been well studied in pediatrics, we can only recommend continuing with the current conservative practice until evidence-based guidelines emerge. If the desired posttransfusion hemoglobin level will likely not be met following 4 hours of slow transfusion, the RBCs should be divided into smaller bags in the blood bank to allow for proper storage until needed and to reduce exposure to additional donors.

Hyperleukocytosis

Hyperleukocytosis, defined as a WBC of 100,000 per mm^3 or greater, can be seen in acute lymphocytic leukemia (ALL), acute myeloid leukemia (AML), and chronic myelogenous leukemia. The patient with hyperleukocytosis is at risk for clinical complications because of the rapid proliferation of leukemic blasts, increased blood viscosity, and tumor lysis syndrome. Leukostasis in the pulmonary and central nervous system microvasculature may cause respiratory compromise leading to hypoxia and dyspnea and neurologic effects ranging from confusion or somnolence to seizures and coma. Rapid proliferation and breakdown of leukemic blasts may release procoagulants and induce a coagulopathy, predisposing patients to hemorrhage or thrombosis.[117,118] Every effort should be made to perform diagnostic studies rapidly and safely and initiate therapy. Special consideration must be given for transfusion safety in these patients.

Blood viscosity is a function of the plasma viscosity and the deformability of the cellular components of the blood in the capillaries. In patients with hyperleukocytosis, the bulk viscosity of blood is often not elevated because of a compensatory decrease in the erythrocrit.[117,119] Leukocytes, lymphoblasts, and myeloblasts are larger and less deformable than RBCs, thus the viscosity increases more dramatically as the fractional volume of leukocytes (leukocrit) increases.[119] A leukocrit of more than 10% to 15% is required to be significantly more viscous than the equivalent volume of RBCs. Therefore, an increased number of circulating blasts may result in decreased flow and decreased oxygen transport to the tissues. In addition, leukemic blast cells have an elevated oxygen consumption rate.[119,120] As a result of these rheologic properties, patients with elevated blast counts typically experience symptoms of cerebral or pulmonary leukostasis with hypoxia, tachypnea, dyspnea, disorientation, agitation, seizures, or coma.

Hyperleukocytosis requires emergent intervention with dilution of the leukemic blast cells (e.g., exchange, leukapheresis) and treatment of the underlying disease. An exception to this rule may be acute promyelocytic leukemia (APL) where leukapheresis may worsen the underlying coagulopathy although data are extremely limited and have not been

reported in a randomized controlled study.[121,122] Care must be taken not to transfuse large quantities of RBCs before the leukocyte count is reduced, because this may result in hyperviscosity and deleterious consequences.[123,124] A hemoglobin level above 10 g per dL is an adverse risk factor when the blast cell count exceeds 100 per mm^3 and care should be taken to not transfuse a patient above this level.[123,124] Many of these patients are hemodynamically stable at low hemoglobin levels and often will not require RBC support. A partial exchange may be performed to obtain an isovolemic increase in the hemoglobin level.[117] Transfusion with platelets is generally deemed safe and does not affect blood viscosity.

Jehovah's Witnesses

The religious beliefs and practices of Jehovah's Witnesses forbid the ingestion of blood according to the literal interpretation of the Bible. Accepting blood and blood products in any form or by any method, such as intravenously, are traditionally prohibited. This prohibition can prove challenging when a child may receive lifesaving therapies that lead to severe anemia. This situation can compromise the child's QOL or put the child at risk for preventable morbidity or mortality. Jehovah's Witnesses believe that the prohibition applies at all times, even in emergencies, and that accepting blood transfusion therapy could potentially jeopardize one's position in the congregation.

Medical ethics teaches physicians and medical caregivers to assume the important responsibility of balancing beneficence and nonmaleficence, while respecting autonomy and justice for our patients.[125] We have an equally important role to explore the values and religious beliefs of our patients and consider their wishes. When a patient's beliefs clash with those of his or her caregivers, it challenges our personal and professional boundaries of what is ethical, compassionate, and appropriate therapy.

When meeting with family members who have stated their preference not to receive blood products, it is critical to discuss all potential options of therapy and adverse effects of refusing some parts of treatment. Conflicts emerge when communication is not clear and consistent. Families need to fully understand the risks of treating the primary malignancy, including the risks of developing anemia or thrombocytopenia, and the risk of nontransfusion. Stimulation of erythropoiesis with agents such as EPO should be considered and instituted if medically applicable albeit knowing that these agents may come with potential risks and are currently not recommended in the general pediatric oncology population. Also, consideration should be given to establishing a lower transfusion threshold and minimizing blood draws, dependent, of course, on the clinical status.[126] Physicians should not consider suboptimal therapy with increased risk of recurrence or refractoriness to avoid the possibility of transfusion. Although treating any patient with a malignancy involves a balance between treating the disease and avoiding treatment toxicities, this balance becomes much more tenuous for patients who refuse blood products.[127–129]

The issues physicians and medical caregivers face in these circumstances can challenge personal beliefs in the science of medicine, the legal system, and personal religious beliefs, including the right to choose. Pediatricians are taught to first do best for the child, while always considering and respecting the rights of the parents and their personal values. The courts have upheld the rights of adult Jehovah's Witnesses to refuse lifesaving blood transfusions. However, the right of parents to refuse this therapy for their child has been challenged by the legal system. When the medical caregivers feel that the child's life is in danger, a court order has frequently been issued to administer the lifesaving therapy.[130] Many families have found this acceptable.

Infants

Guidelines for transfusion of neonates and infants are controversial and have a wide variety of recommendations. In general, RBC transfusions are given to maintain a hemoglobin level most desirable for the existing clinical condition.[131] Consideration should be given to prematurity and the physiologic nadir expected at 10 to 12 weeks of age in the healthy infant (which occurs earlier in the sick or premature infant). In addition, blood loss secondary to phlebotomy may play a key role in the anemia of infancy when serial laboratory studies are needed to monitor therapy. Infants requiring high volumes of oxygen or with severe cardiac disease may need more RBC support to maintain a higher hemoglobin level (i.e., 11 to 15 g per dL) than an infant with mild to moderate respiratory disease or perioperative care (i.e., 10 g per dL).[52,132,133] Stable infants who become symptomatic from anemia (i.e., tachycardia, tachypnea, poor feeding) may need transfusion to maintain a hemoglobin level of 7 g per dL or greater.[52,133] Premature infants and low-birth-weight infants are at higher risk for TA-GVHD and should receive irradiated blood.[52,134] Premature infants from CMV-seronegative mothers should receive CMV-seronegative blood products, while term infants from CMV-seronegative mothers may benefit from CMV-seronegative blood products although some suggest that leukoreduced blood is sufficient.[52,98]

Radiation Therapy

Tumor hypoxia likely has a role in the effectiveness of radiation therapy in causing tumor cell death.[135,136] Yet, determining what role underlying anemia has in tissue hypoxia is as yet to be fully understood. Brizel et al. importantly showed that even in nonanemic patients, 50% of tumors were still poorly oxygenated.[137] Studies in patients with solid tumors, head and neck cancers, and cervical cancers undergoing radiation therapy have shown that patient outcomes are worse with underlying anemia.[45,136–140] Yet, it is not well understood whether anemia causes poor outcomes secondary to the ineffectiveness of therapy or, plausibly, is a marker of tumor aggressiveness and the severity of the underlying disease.[138,139] Most important, there is no evidence to date which suggests that correction of anemia improves prognosis.[138] Further research is required before any recommendations can be made regarding transfusion as a method to enhance radiation therapy.

End-of-Life Management of Anemia

Patients receiving palliative care may develop anemia related to chronic disease, marrow invasion, blood loss, or toxicity of therapy. Anemia is quite prevalent in the palliative care setting in adults.[141] A recent report on end-of-life issues in children found that patients and families reported fatigue as the most common symptom contributing to suffering.[142] The etiology of fatigue is multifactorial and includes natural progression of the disease, depression, poor nutritional status, and anemia. Certainly no effective treatment is available for some of these factors, but anemia can be alleviated by transfusion or possibly erythropoiesis-stimulating agents. Although ample data are available to demonstrate the benefits of transfusion in actively treated oncology patients, little is known about the benefits of transfusion in the palliative setting, especially in pediatrics. Studies in adults have shown that up to 50% of patients do not gain a symptomatic benefit from blood transfusion, likely because anemia is only one of many factors

contributing to the patient's symptoms.[143,144] Patients with a longer prognosis are likely to gain more from transfusion than do patients who are end-stage.[145] In addition, anemia is not thought to be painful in the dying child and the decision to transfuse may conflict with the family's goal to minimize interventions.[146] Transfusion will likely not improve or prolong life in the end-stage patient.[145] Symptom management with pain medication may prove useful for headaches secondary to anemia. Caregivers must balance the needs of the patient and the desires of the family members in making the decision as how best to manage anemia in this setting.

THROMBOCYTOPENIA

Intensive therapies currently used to treat leukemia and solid tumors in children often lead to severe and sustained thrombocytopenia or platelet dysfunction, or both. Thrombocytopenia may be a direct result of marrow replacement by tumor cells. In addition, factors contributing to thrombocytopenia include bleeding (spontaneous and iatrogenic), consumption secondary to infection, disseminated intravascular coagulation (DIC), organ sequestration (splenomegaly), and RBC transfusion (dilutional effect).[147] Platelet dysfunction may occur secondary to uremia or a medication effect.[60,148,149] Immune-mediated thrombocytopenia rarely occurs in pediatric cancer.

Platelet transfusions are indicated for the prevention and treatment of hemorrhage in patients with thrombocytopenia or platelet dysfunction. The decision to transfuse must be based on an assessment of risk versus benefit. Platelet transfusion has become routine in the supportive care of pediatric malignancy, because thrombocytopenia is a major, if not the principal, cause of bleeding in these patients.[51,150–154] Prophylactic platelet transfusions represent a large percentage of the total number of platelet products consumed.[155–158]

Practice Guidelines for Prophylactic Platelet Transfusions

Severe spontaneous or life-threatening hemorrhage is currently an unusual complication, despite the large number of oncology patients being treated.[55,159–164] Although this may be due to the use of prophylactic platelet infusions, recent efforts have addressed the concern that patients may be receiving too many platelet transfusions and, in fact, may be safe at levels lower than previously realized.[160,161,165–167] Platelet transfusions are expensive and are associated with several adverse effects including fever, allergic reaction, transmission of viral and bacterial infections, circulatory congestion, TRALI, and alloimmunization.[159,168–174] Important reasons to minimize transfusion include decreasing alloimmunization and alleviating the demand on already strained resources. In addition, in some clinical situations, the practice of frequent transfusion and resultant sensitization may affect the success of future therapies, as evidenced by the inferior outcome of bone marrow transplantation in multiply transfused children with aplastic anemia.[175]

Platelet transfusion in the patient with bone marrow failure, such as that caused by malignancy or chemotherapy, may be considered either prophylactic or therapeutic, depending on whether the goal is to prevent bleeding or stop it. Contemporary clinical practice has adopted the prophylactic approach as standard of care.[55,56,147,155–166,171,176,177] The use of prophylactic transfusion is based on a threshold platelet count below which there is a significantly increased risk of serious bleeding. The literature has been reviewed with respect to the threshold for platelet transfusion for various clinical scenarios, and the guidelines presented here are a synopsis of this evidence-based approach. An effort has been made to balance the clinical benefits, optimize safety, and reduce costs associated with transfusion or added complications of therapy. In addition, the improvement in QOL with fewer hospital stays, decreased infection transmission, and decreased alloimmunization are important considerations.

Practice guidelines for platelet transfusion have been developed by an expert panel commissioned by the American Society of Clinical Oncology (ASCO) to improve care, minimize inappropriate clinical practice, and decrease cost and overutilization of a product that is difficult to procure.[159] Although no pediatric oncology representative was on this panel, several clinical trials involving children with malignancy were reviewed. The data have been incorporated into the following discussion and recommendations.

A therapeutic platelet transfusion is typically given based on the presence of clinical factors predisposing to bleeding, or before a surgical procedure (Table 39.2). They are given to individuals with thrombocytopenia or functional platelet impairment, or both, who have significant bleeding. Primary hemostasis is impaired when the platelet count drops below the normal range (150,000 to 400,000 per mm³). The bleeding time is prolonged when the platelet count is below 100,000 per mm³.[178] Easy bruisability, excessive menstrual blood loss, and epistaxis are reported more frequently when the platelet count drops below 75,000 per mm³. These symptoms become even more clinically significant when the platelet count drops below 20,000 per mm³. Petechiae, spontaneous hemorrhage, and mucosal bleeding are exacerbated at platelet counts of 10,000 to 20,000 per mm³. Mild mucosal hemorrhage, petechiae, trace guaiac-positive stool, or trace blood in the urine do not necessarily indicate a higher risk of bleeding. It is unusual for a life-threatening hemorrhage to occur at this platelet level unless aggravating clinical factors are present.[59,147,151,161,179,180] Unfortunately, it is impossible to predict bleeding sites, and the first hemorrhage may be into a vital organ, resulting in severe morbidity or mortality.

The decision to transfuse platelets depends on many clinical factors including the platelet count; cause of thrombocytopenia;

time of expected resolution; rapidity of platelet count drop; the functional ability of the platelets; and the clinical condition of the patient including the presence of fever, infection, coagulopathy, or bleeding. As the platelet count decreases, an increasing number of available (transfused) platelets are required to meet the need for hemostasis.[181] A minimal number of platelets may be required to maintain the integrity of the microvasculature.[181,182] This may explain why patients with chronic severe thrombocytopenia are more susceptible to spontaneous bleeding.

In one of the earliest publications on platelet transfusion in thrombocytopenic children and adults with leukemia, Gaydos et al. found that a quantitative relationship existed between platelet counts and risk of bleeding (Table 39.3).[151] Because this study was conducted during a time when aspirin was the drug of choice for treatment of fever, it is not possible to extrapolate their findings of platelet thresholds and bleeding manifestations to modern times and therapies. No threshold platelet level could be determined. An association between onset of gross hemorrhage and falling platelet counts (a low platelet turnover state) was noted. Others have found that a drop in the platelet count in the prior 24 hours preceded significant hemorrhagic episodes.[59,185] Avoidance of a low hemoglobin/hematocrit level in patients with thrombocytopenia has been reported to reduce the risk of hemorrhage.[55,186,187] The degree of thrombocytopenia that should trigger the use of prophylactic platelet transfusion continues to be debated in the literature, as evidenced by a wide spectrum of clinical practice.[55,56,177,188]

Studies performed over the past 20 years suggest that the platelet transfusion point can safely be set below 20,000 per mm³ in the clinically stable child (Table 39.3).[56,147,179,184,189] Murphy et al. performed a randomized trial in 56 children with leukemia, comparing prophylactic and therapeutic platelet transfusions.[189] The children in the prophylactic group received transfusion when the platelet count dropped to 20,000 per mm³. There was no difference in survival. Patients in the prophylactic group had fewer days with hemorrhage. However, patients in the prophylactic group had more significant hemorrhage in the last month of life, possibly due to frequent platelet support and development of alloimmunization. The authors concluded that the philosophy of platelet transfusion, whether therapeutic or prophylactic, had but a minor influence on survival.

Gmür et al. reported their 10-year experience of prophylactic platelet transfusion in 102 adolescents and adults with acute leukemia followed in a prospective nonrandomized study.[160] They developed and tested an algorithm for routine administration of platelets for three different platelet ranges and considered the clinical condition of the patient on the basis of a perception of bleeding risk. When the count dropped below 5,000 per mm³ (confirmed by a manual count), platelets were transfused in all cases. If fever (temperature >38.0°C) or minor hemorrhage was present, the threshold for transfusion was 10,000 per mm³. Platelets were administered at levels of 10,000 to 20,000 per mm³ in patients with a coagulation disorder and/or heparin therapy, or before a lumbar puncture or bone marrow biopsy. In the presence of major bleeding, or in anticipation of minor surgical procedures, platelets were transfused to ensure a platelet count of more than 20,000 per mm³. Most of the patients in this study received fresh platelets, given within 6 hours of collection. When extended storage methods became available, platelets were given within 72 hours of collection. Platelet counts were done manually if the automated counter determined the count to be below 50,000 per mm³. Three fatal hemorrhages occurred (3% incidence); two patients had coexisting coagulopathies, and one was refractory to platelet transfusion. Of note, serious episodes of bleeding

---

TABLE 39.2

CLINICAL FACTORS AFFECTING THE RISK OF BLEEDING IN THROMBOCYTOPENIC CHILDREN

- Precipitous drop in platelet count
- History of brisk or life-threatening hemorrhage (requiring resuscitative efforts or immediate PRBC transfusion)
- Solid tumors: location (GI, bladder, pelvis); necrosis, radiation, recent biopsy
- Comorbidities: fever, sepsis/infection, DIC, liver disease
- Medications: amphotericin (addressed in text, data on vancomycin, and cotrimoxazole not as clear as amphotericin)
- Phase of therapy: induction therapy in acute leukemia
- Coagulopathy, disease-related (APL, NBL, tumor lysis, hyperleukocytosis) or acquired (liver disease, DIC)
- Splenomegaly
- Alloimmunization

APL, acute promyelocytic leukemia; DIC, disseminated intravascular coagulation; GI, gastrointestinal; NBL, neuroblastoma; PRBC, packed red blood cells.

TABLE 39.3

CLINICAL STUDIES EXAMINING PLATELET TRANSFUSION THRESHOLDS

Author (year)	Number of patients, age, and diagnosis	Type of study, transfusion strategy	Prophylaxis benefit	Comments
Gaydos et al. (1962)[151]	40 adults 52 children 34 AML 57 ALL	None (retrospective)	N/A	Era of aspirin use. Defined relationship between incidence of bleeding and platelet level. Eight patients with ICH (all with platelet counts <5,000/mm³). Questioned accuracy of determining low platelet counts (especially <5,000/mm³). No "threshold" level.
Higby et al. (1974)[155]	18 (15–76 yr) AML	Randomized to receive platelet transfusion or plasma when <30,000/mm³	N/A	Fever preceded hemorrhage in 10 out of 13 patients. Infection thought to initiate bleeding (no associated coagulopathies.) Increase in clinically significant bleeding in plasma transfusion arm.
Solomon et al. (1978)[165]	31 (16–71 yr) ANLL, induction (no APL)	Randomized: Prophylactic group (n = 17): Transfuse for <20,000/mm³ and clinically significant bleeding Therapeutic group (n = 12): Transfuse for clinically significant bleeding *or* platelet count <20,000/mm³ with >50% decline over prior 24 h	N/A	Two patients in prophylactic group died of ICH. Recommend platelet transfusion for specific indications (bleeding or rapid decline with platelet count <20,000 mm³).
Murphy et al. (1982)[183]	56 children ALL, ANLL	Prophylactic group: Transfuse for <20,000/mm³ Therapeutic group: Transfuse for clinically significant bleeding and thrombocytopenia	Yes	Similar survival curves. Prophylactic transfusion delays first episode of bleeding and number of bleeding days, except for terminal month of life.
Gmür et al. (1991)[160]	102 (15–71 yr) ANLL n = 87 (APL n = 7) ALL n = 15	Prospective study: Transfusion threshold stratified on the basis of platelet count and clinical condition (four groups)	Yes	Increased bleeding noted when platelets <10,000/mm³ and more notable when <5,000/mm³. One case of ICH in a patient with platelets <1,000/mm³ and alloimmunization. Two fatal hemorrhages in association with coagulopathies (one APL) both with platelet counts >35,000/mm³. No prophylaxis failures. 32% serious bleeds seen in association with fevers.
Heckman et al. (1997)[184]	78, acute leukemia, induction (no APL)	Randomized: Transfuse for >10,000/mm³ versus 10–20,000 mm³	Yes, safe at >10,000 mm³	No difference noted between arms with respect to PRBC requirements, hospital days, fever, number of thrombocytopenic days, remission, or death. Patients with >20,000/mm³ received more platelet transfusions for prophylaxis with greater total number of transfusions despite more transfusions being given for bleeding in >10,000/mm³ group. No fatal hemorrhage.
Rebulla et al. (1997)[179]	255 (16–70 yr) AML (no APL)	Randomized: Transfuse for >10,000/mm³, 10–20,000/mm³ and fever or bleeding or surgery, >20,000/mm³	Safe at >10,000/ mm³	Similar risk of bleeding between groups. One fatal ICH (at platelet 32,000/mm³, in >10,000/mm³ group). Increased incidence of GI bleeding in >10,000/mm³ group. No difference in PRBC transfusion requirements. Reduced use of platelet transfusion in >10,000/mm³ group. Recommend level of 20,000/mm³ if fever present.

(continued)

TABLE 39.3

CONTINUED

Author (year)	Number of patients, age, and diagnosis	Type of study, transfusion strategy	Prophylaxis benefit	Comments
Wandt et al. (1998)[56]	105 (17–73 yr) AML (no APL)	Multicenter study (n = 17) Each choose to participate as: Group A (transfuse at >10,000/mm³), n = 58 Or Group B (transfuse at >20,000/mm³), n = 47 Both groups: Transfuse >15,000/mm³ with fever >38.5°C, rapid decline in platelet count, coagulopathy, or hyperleukocytosis Transfuse >20,000/mm³ for bleeding or procedures	Safe at >10,000/mm³	Similar outcome. Decreased platelet transfusion requirements in group A. Based on results, the authors posed a strategy of platelet transfusion for active bleeding only.

AML, acute myeloid leukemia; ANLL, acute nonlymphocytic leukemia; APL, acute promyelocytic leukemia; ICH, intracranial hemorrhage; PRBC, packed red blood cells.

occurred in this study in patients with relatively high platelet counts, making it clear that none could have been prevented by simply using a 20,000 per mm³ threshold. The data emphasize the importance of clinical factors in the etiology of bleeding. This restrictive transfusion policy proved to be safe for the 102 patients receiving induction therapy.

Heckman et al. performed a prospective randomized trial in 78 adults undergoing induction therapy for acute leukemia.[184] The investigators demonstrated a reduction in the utilization of platelet transfusions for patients using a lower threshold of 10,000 per mm³ versus 20,000 per mm³ and found no statistical difference between the two groups regarding remission rate, hospital days, death during induction, RBC transfusion requirements, febrile days, or platelet refractoriness. No patient in either group died from hemorrhage. Patients with APL, a known bleeding diathesis, coagulopathy, or platelet refractoriness, were excluded from the study. The authors looked at febrile patients in a separate analysis to determine if prolonged fever increased the risk of bleeding. In both groups, febrile patients received more platelet transfusions; however, there was no difference in incidence of severe hemorrhage. They suggested the threshold of 10,000 per mm³ was safe for febrile patients as long as therapeutic platelets were administered as needed for high-risk situations such as fever or presence of a coagulopathy.

In a large Italian multicenter randomized trial, Rebulla et al. evaluated 255 adults undergoing remission induction for AML, excluding those with French-American-British M3 subtype (APL).[179] Patients were randomized to a threshold of 20,000 or 10,000 per mm³ when in stable condition and a threshold of less than 20,000 per mm³ in the presence of fresh hemorrhage, fever of more than 38°C, or anticipation of invasive procedures. The threshold of 10,000 per mm³ was associated with a significant reduction in platelet requirements, and there were no significant differences in the number of patients experiencing severe hemorrhage, number of RBC products transfused, or induction deaths. The authors note that they selected a manual platelet count of 10,000 per mm³, because they could not rely upon the accuracy of the platelet count at

this level with automated blood analyzers. Unfortunately, this can be a difficult dilemma in clinical practice as manual platelet counts may be time intensive or unavailable.[190]

Wandt et al. also confirmed the effectiveness and safety of a stringent policy using a threshold of 10,000 per mm³ as a prophylactic trigger for platelet transfusion.[56] They compared prospectively the risk of bleeding complications in 105 patients (age range 17 to 73 years) with acute leukemia, excluding APL, undergoing induction and consolidation therapy. At the start of the study, each of the 17 participating institutions chose a prophylactic platelet trigger of either 10,000 per mm³ (group A, eight centers) or 20,000 per mm³ (group B, nine centers). Patients in group A had a significantly longer period of thrombocytopenia; however, this did not result in a higher bleeding risk. Minor bleeding complications occurred in both groups with approximately equal frequency. Group A patients received fewer platelet transfusions. There was no difference in the number of RBC transfusions administered. This comparison held when type of platelet product was compared (single donor apheresis vs. random donor pooled concentrates). Two patients died as a result of hemorrhage, with platelet counts of 36,000 and 50,000 per mm³. Provisions for transfusion were made in both groups in the presence of fever, rapid decrease in the platelet count, plasma coagulation factor deficiencies due to sepsis or leukemia, hyperleukocytosis, before surgical procedures (bone marrow biopsy excluded) or in the case of major bleeding. Patients with APL were excluded, because this type of leukemia is associated with a well-known high risk for bleeding during induction therapy due to significant anomalies in plasma coagulation factors. The authors feel, however, that a similar stringent platelet transfusion policy could be applied to this group of patients after they have achieved remission. This study emphasizes again the importance of assessing clinical conditions known to be associated with increased risk of bleeding when deciding on a transfusion threshold for platelets.

The above studies demonstrate that a stringent platelet transfusion policy is feasible, safe, and cost effective. The data support the use of a prophylactic platelet threshold of less

TABLE 39.4

PLATELET TRANSFUSION GUIDELINES

Clinical scenario	Transfuse when platelet count falls below (thousand per mm³)[a]	
Well, stable		10
Procedures	Lumbar puncture (use lower number for clinically stable, sedated patients and experienced practitioner)	10–20
	For diagnostic LP and to avoid introduction of blasts	100[b]
	Bone marrow aspirate	Not indicated
	Surgery: minor (central venous catheter)	50
	Surgery: major (CNS, ophthalmologic, solid tumor biopsy/resection with anticipated blood loss)	100
Signs/symptoms	Bleeding: minor (mucosal, epistaxis)	20
	Bleeding: major (hemoptysis, hemorrhagic cystitis, GI, CNS, tumor necrosis)	100
	Fever	20
	Organomegaly, hypersplenism	Per clinical indication
	Medication-induced dysfunction	Per clinical indication
	Newborns (BT reduced when transfused to 30/mm³)	30
	Radiation (dependent on extent of marrow radiation or solid tumor necrosis)	Per clinical indication
	APL (induction)	50
	CNS metastases (e.g., choriocarcinoma, melanoma, testicular carcinoma)	50
Coexisting laboratory abnormalities	Hyperleukocytosis	20
	Rapid fall of platelet count (pattern of recent platelet counts)	50
	Coagulation abnormalities	50
	DIC, elevated FDP	50

[a]Consideration for prophylaxis must take into account the presence of individual risk factors and overall clinical condition of the patient.
[b]Refer to text.
APL, acute promyelocytic leukemia; BT, bleeding time; CNS, central nervous system; DIC, disseminated intravascular coagulation; FDP, fibrin degradation product; GI, gastrointestinal.

than 10,000 per mm³ in patients without risk factors for hemorrhage (Table 39.4).[56,147,157,160,179,183,184] Although some authors have suggested that a pretransfusion threshold of 5 per mm³ may be sufficient for many stable patients,[157,188] the lack of accuracy of platelet quantitation by automated counters argues against this approach.[160,179,190]

With improved supportive care and better understanding of the clinical situations predisposing to life-threatening hemorrhage, a logical next step may be to evaluate whether platelet transfusions should be administered only in the actively bleeding patient or in those with antecedent risk factors. In deciding when to transfuse, it is important to consider not only the absolute platelet count, but also the number of functional platelets. Posttransfusion platelet increments may not accurately predict function, and use of the platelet function analysis (PFA) may prove to be useful in the uncontrolled bleeding patient not adequately treated with platelet transfusion (Table 39.5).

Clinical factors such as history of prior bleeding, site, presence of fever or infection, degree of anemia, coexisting coagulopathy, rate of platelet count decrement, platelet consumptive states or medications, or hyperleukocytosis may predispose to bleeding at lesser degrees of thrombocytopenia than in the clinically stable patient.[55,155,160,165,176,184,185,191] An additional factor to consider is access to emergent medical care. Hospitalized patients tend to be closely observed, have frequent laboratory studies, and have access to rapid intervention, and they are less likely to be involved in trauma.[59] Outpatients, especially those living at a great distance from health care providers, may be more at risk due to less frequent monitoring, and transfusion support may be less readily accessible.[192]

No randomized trials exist to answer the questions of what is the risk of bleeding in patients with severe, chronic, stable thrombocytopenia, and what is the ideal clinical treatment of such patients. Patients with myelodysplasia, aplastic anemia, and platelet refractoriness often have sustained and severe thrombocytopenia. Clinical experience suggests these patients may have no or minimal bleeding for long periods despite the low platelet counts.[159,188] Gmür et al. reported an increased

TABLE 39.5

FACTORS AFFECTING THE POSTTRANSFUSION PLATELET INCREMENT

Blood bank factors	• Compatibility of platelet concentrate: ABO, HLA, platelet-specific antigens • Dose • Duration of storage (age of product) • Collection method • Platelet activation, cytokine release
Patient factors	• Anticipated nadir and time to recovery of thrombocytopenia • Consumptive states: active bleeding, sepsis, fever, splenomegaly, DIC • Immune-mediated states: alloimmunization, medications

DIC, disseminated intravascular coagulation; HLA, human leukocyte antigen.

incidence of severe hemorrhage (one lethal) in four patients with platelet alloimmunization who experienced delays in transfusion due to difficulty obtaining human leukocyte antigen (HLA)-matched products.[160] Some patients may indeed be at risk for a severe or fatal hemorrhage, but it is not clear whether transfusing platelets when there is no incremental change will provide any benefit.

Children with solid tumors often experience prolonged aplasia as an adverse effect of chemotherapy or radiation. Five retrospective observational studies support the clinical benefit of prophylactic platelet transfusion at a threshold of 10,000 per mm^3.[185,193–196] As in patients with leukemia, clinical factors must be considered when deciding on an individual platelet threshold. Tumor location and intratumor bleeding and necrosis predispose to life-threatening hemorrhage.[194,196] Radiation may also increase tissue friability, and consideration should be given to transfusion at a higher threshold, perhaps 20,000 per mm^3. Tumors located in the gastrointestinal tract or bladder may have an increased tendency to hemorrhage and also be considered for the higher threshold. Prior severe hemorrhage from the tumor or tumor necrosis should prompt the clinician to use individual judgment in setting an appropriate hemoglobin and platelet threshold to avoid a life-threatening situation.[193,197]

Although a therapeutic platelet transfusion policy has been proposed, its efficacy is unproven given the small numbers of patients and possible other confounding factors.[155,165,183] It is now reasonable to assess the safety and feasibility of this therapeutic algorithm in the current generation of young cancer patients. Giving platelets to patients for specific indications is likely to reduce the use of platelet transfusions. Given the lack of clinical studies elucidating a clear platelet transfusion policy, it is not surprising that tremendous variability exists in platelet transfusion and dosing strategies amongst pediatric oncologists.[44] Clear criteria for both prophylactic and therapeutic indications remains an area of tremendous interest and need.[198]

Recommendations Regarding Surgical or Invasive Procedures in Thrombocytopenic Patients

Cancer patients frequently require invasive diagnostic or therapeutic procedures. These procedures include placement of central venous access devices, tumor biopsy or resection, bone marrow aspirates and biopsies, and lumbar punctures. Occasionally, the ill patient will also require bronchial-alveolar lavage (BAL), paranasal sinus aspirations, or endoscopic biopsies. No randomized studies have been performed to determine accurate, safe platelet thresholds for major or minor procedures in children with malignancy. In fact, only a modest amount of literature is available on this subject. On the basis of an accumulated clinical experience, consensus panels have concluded that a platelet count of 50,000 per mm^3 is sufficient for major surgery and 20,000 per mm^3 is safe for the performance of minor procedures.[55,147,159,199] This consensus assumes the absence of associated coagulation abnormalities. Bone marrow aspiration and biopsy can be performed in patients with severe thrombocytopenia without platelet support, providing that adequate surface pressure is applied.[199]

Bishop et al. reported on 95 patients (age range 16 to 73 years) with acute leukemia who had 167 operations, 70% of which were major procedures (laparotomy, craniotomy, thoracotomy) and 30% were minor procedures (central venous catheter insertion, tracheotomy, and tooth extractions).[200] Patients were transfused preoperatively to

achieve platelet counts higher than 50,000 per mm^3 (to a median of 56,000 per mm^3) and maintained postoperatively for 3 days at platelet counts higher than 40,000 per mm^3 for major surgery and higher than 30,000 per mm^3 for minor surgery. There were no deaths from bleeding attributable to surgery within 1 month of the procedure. Patients with preoperative fever or coagulation abnormalities required more RBC transfusion support. This significant retrospective study found that the risk for perioperative bleeding was most influenced by type of surgery (major), preoperative fever, and perioperative coagulation abnormalities. The investigators conclude that cytopenic patients with acute leukemia can safely undergo surgical procedures with transfusion supportive care.

Several investigators have evaluated performance of procedures in thrombocytopenic patients and have emphasized that factors other than platelet count must be considered when determining risk of hemorrhage. Weiss et al. performed 66 fiberoptic bronchoscopy and BAL in bone marrow transplant recipients.[201] Complications of minor bleeding occurred at a median platelet count of 37,000 per mm^3 and were reported in 12% of patients. Sixty-seven percent of patients had platelet counts lower than 50,000 per mm^3 and 20% had platelet counts less than 20,000 per mm^3. The level of platelet count did not correlate with the rate of complications. The factor most predictive of bleeding was prior life-threatening hemorrhage, rather than baseline platelet count.[202]

Conventional wisdom among oncologists has been that the most experienced practitioner available should perform the procedure. Supervision by an experienced practitioner is advisable for those in training. Bleeding complications from procedures are often related to procedural problems and lack of experience rather than patient factors, such as the platelet count.[203–208] This has been most effectively demonstrated in a study by Howard et al. investigating potential risk factors for traumatic lumbar punctures in children with acute lymphoblastic leukemia.[204] Practitioner experience was evaluated, and experience level was determined to be a more important predictor of outcome than practitioner education. As procedural technique is often linked to complications, it may be reasonable to recommend that all procedures on thrombocytopenic children be performed by experienced practitioners.

Lumbar Puncture

Lumbar puncture is perhaps the most common procedure performed on children with leukemia, for diagnostic purposes and to instill intrathecal chemotherapy. Most pediatric oncologists administer prophylactic platelet transfusions to thrombocytopenic patients before lumbar puncture. However, this practice is controversial because a safe platelet count has not been determined for this procedure. Thrombocytopenia is not a proven risk factor for permanent neurologic injury.[209]

A retrospective review of children with newly diagnosed leukemia who underwent a diagnostic lumbar puncture did not report serious complications, regardless of platelet count.[209] The reviewers evaluated 5,223 procedures performed during remission induction or consolidation for ALL; 941 had platelet counts less than 50,000 per mm^3 and 199 had platelet counts of 20,000 per mm^3 or less. They concluded that prophylactic platelet transfusion is not necessary in children with platelet counts higher than 10,000 per mm^3. Only 29 spinal taps were performed in children with a platelet count less than 10,000 per mm^3, precluding a statistically significant conclusion on its safety. Interestingly, they noted a 10.5% rate of traumatic lumbar punctures (defined as 500 or more RBCs per high-powered microscopic field). A smaller study in 24 children with ALL who underwent lumbar punctures with platelet counts less than 50,000 per mm^3, (5 of which were less than 20,000 per mm^3), observed no hemorrhagic complications.[210] Thus, owing to small numbers, the safety of lumbar puncture when performed at a platelet level of 10,000 per mm^3 or less cannot be proven. Again, these authors note a rather high incidence of traumatic taps (7 out of 24) and one patient with prolonged oozing. There are no randomized studies to determine if the incidence of traumatic taps would be lessened with a higher platelet threshold or if a traumatic spinal tap is detrimental to patient care.

A large retrospective study (by the same investigators as above) evaluated 5,609 lumbar punctures and looked at several modifiable and unmodifiable risk factors of traumatic (10 RBCs per μL) or bloody (500 RBCs per μL) spinal taps.[204] They found that African American race, young age (<1 year), prior traumatic tap within 2 weeks, or prior lumbar puncture performed while the platelet count was 50,000 per mm^3 or less, were factors that increased risk for a traumatic tap. Modifiable risk factors included lack of general anesthesia, platelet count of 100,000 per mm^3 or less, an interval of 15 days or less between lumbar punctures, or a less experienced practitioner. Although the authors had previously determined that 10,000 per mm^3 was a safe platelet level for routine lumbar puncture with instillation of chemotherapy, they now recommend, on the basis of this study, that the initial diagnostic lumbar puncture be performed with a platelet count of 100,000 per mm^3.[204,209] This is to ensure that the interpretation of the cerebrospinal fluid is not obscured by excessive RBCs. In addition, the authors reviewed data suggesting that bloody spinal taps may be of prognostic significance with respect to possible introduction of circulating leukemic blasts into the cerebrospinal fluid.[204,211] However, a recent report demonstrates that the presence of a low number of leukemic blasts in the cerebrospinal fluid does not affect outcome in childhood leukemia.[212]

Placement of a Central Venous Access Device

A number of studies support the safe practice of central venous catheter insertion in a stable patient with a platelet count of 50,000 per mm^3.[207,208,213,214] Several investigators have performed such procedures, including implantable infusion ports and tunneled Silastic catheters, at platelet levels of 30,000 to 50,000 per mm^3 with acceptable side effects.[215–217] No pediatric experience has been reported in thrombocytopenic patients with Broviac catheter insertion. Central venous catheters should be placed by skilled physicians in patients with severe thrombocytopenia.[208] If coexisting coagulopathy is present, corrective measures should be taken to optimize safety and decrease risk of bleeding. The patient should be evaluated for possible confounding factors, such as plasma coagulation factor deficiencies or infection. This can be done with simple screening studies including prothrombin time (PT) and activated partial thromboplastin time (aPTT), in addition to a complete physical examination and assessment of vital signs. Platelet counts can be determined quickly and accurately immediately after transfusion and not cause delay in performing the procedure.[218]

Platelet Component Preparation

Platelets for transfusion can be prepared by apheresis from single donors or by separation of platelet concentrates (PC) from whole blood. In routine circumstances, either product can be used because they offer the same potential benefit of posttransfusion increment, platelet survival, and hemostatic effect.[219–222] However, pooled PCs are less costly. Single-donor platelets are often preferred for individuals requiring frequent or large quantities of platelets due to the lessened exposure to numerous blood donors and the theoretical benefit of decreased risk of disease transmission or alloimmunization. Other potential advantages of single-donor units are decreased risk of bacterial contamination and ease of handling, because the need to pool platelets is eliminated.

Apheresis (single donor) platelets are collected from donors in 90-minute procedures and yield 3 to 8 × 10^{11} platelets in 200 to 300 mL of plasma and anticoagulant.[223] The resultant apheresis product contains the number of platelets equivalent to 6 to 10 PC units. Apheresis platelet units may be split into two products to accommodate smaller recipient size. Current platelet pheresis procedures produce a leukodepleted platelet product.[224,225] PCs are not usually leukoreduced at the time of collection and must be subsequently filtered to remove leukocytes.[222] These differences in platelet product acquisition and preparation result in a differential cost, with the single-donor product remaining more expensive, even when considering possible additional steps of pooling products and filtration.[226–228]

Platelet preparations can be stored (with good maintenance of platelet viability) for up to 5 days after collection at 20°C to 24°C using continuous gentle horizontal agitation.[229] Longer storage periods increase the risk of bacterial proliferation and cytokine-related reactions.[171,230] Current storage bags have been designed to permit the exchange of O$_2$ and CO$_2$ to optimize platelet quality.[231–236]

Dosage for Platelet Transfusion

The dose of platelets given to children is determined on the basis of weight or body surface area. PCs typically containing 0.7 × 10^{11} platelets should result in a platelet count increment of 5,000 to 10,000 per mm^3 in an average-sized adult. When calculating the dose of platelets for a child, 10 mL per kg of either a random or apheresis unit should result in an increase of 50 to 100,000 per mm^3.[133,237] For children weighing more than 10 kg, a dose of 1 unit per 10 kg should result in an increase in the platelet count of 50,000 to 100,000 per mm^3.[133,237–240] Apheresis units are ordered by single units for children weighing 30 kg or more, or have a total body surface area more than 0.5 m^2. One-half of a pheresed unit is appropriate for a child weighing between 10 and 30 kg, or with a total body surface area of less than 0.5 m^2. Subsequent transfusion doses and frequency should be determined by the child's weight, starting platelet count, prior platelet increment in response to transfusion, and clinical condition. In addition, when given therapeutically to treat active bleeding, a larger dose of platelets may be indicated.

An optimal platelet dose of 0.07 × 10^{11} per kg is suggested for stable thrombocytopenic patients and 0.15 × 10^{11} per kg for patients with clinical factors known to result in platelet consumption.[179] These doses are similar to those proposed in recent Platelet Transfusion Therapy Consensus guidelines (1 PC per 10 kg of body weight).[162] Although these doses may produce optimal increments and intertransfusion intervals, they have not been shown to be superior to smaller, more frequent transfusions in the prevention of bleeding. In addition, improvement in platelet count following transfusion may not necessarily indicate improvement in platelet function.[241] A PFA assay may be a more sensitive measure of primary hemostatic capacity in situations in which other confounding factors interfere with optimal platelet function.

The 1-hour corrected count increment (CCI) is a very accurate determination of the response to platelet transfusion.[159,222,237,242–245] The CCI used is as follows:

$$CCI = \text{absolute increment} \times \text{body surface area (m}^2\text{)}/ \text{number of platelets transfused} \times 10^{11}$$

The expected CCI is about 15,000 per m² of body surface per unit of platelets. If the CCI is less than 5,000 per m² per unit after two successive platelet transfusions, the patient is considered to be refractory.[159]

Alternatively, an ASCO expert panel suggests using a rough estimate of 2,000 per unit of PC to be equivalent to a CCI of 5,000 per m² per unit. This is based on an average size adult with a body surface area of 1.76 m² and an average unit of PC containing 0.7×10^{11} platelets. For children, an approximate equivalent calculation for the absolute increment is 3,500 per m² per unit.

There is a direct correlation between posttransfusion platelet increment and level of thrombocytopenia, which becomes more significant when the platelet count falls below 100,000 per mm³. It is logical, then, to assume that a higher platelet increment obtained by a high volume of platelets may result in a more sustained platelet count, therefore decreasing the frequency of transfusion. Roy et al. compared a moderately low dose with a high dose of platelets given prophylactically to children, and compared this to a historical group of children who had not received prophylactic transfusions.[156] The two groups receiving transfusion prophylactically fared better with respect to bleeding than the historical controls. They concluded that a moderate dose of platelets would suffice to prevent bleeding.

Norol et al. compared the effects of four different platelet dosages and found that they could increase the interval between transfusions at the higher levels.[246,247] The investigators performed a dose-response study with platelet transfusions in a group of 82 patients, 13 children and 69 adults. Patients received fresh (<24 hours old) ABO-identical platelets. They evaluated four dose levels and found that the higher platelet doses resulted in greater posttransfusion increments and significant lengthening of the intertransfusion interval (2.6 to 4.1 days). The positive effect of the higher dose was observed regardless of the pretransfusion clinical status but was more marked in patients without clinical factors known to impair platelet recovery. Although transfusion events decreased with the larger doses of platelets, there was no difference in hemorrhagic events.

Infusion Volumes and Rates

Platelets should be infused through a dedicated line. Platelets may be infused safely over 30 to 60 minutes, depending on the volume. During the transfusion, and especially within the initial 15 minutes, the patient should be monitored for signs of infection from product contamination, allergy, or anaphylaxis. Mild reactions may be treated by discontinuing or slowing the infusion and administering diphenhydramine. Severe reactions (hypotension, tachycardia, tachypnea) require immediate cessation of the transfusion and administration of supportive or resuscitative care.

The potential benefits of rapid infusions include a more rapid correction of thrombocytopenia, decreased patient time if given in the outpatient setting, increased time available for other parenteral agents if given in the inpatient setting, and decrease in costs of nursing care and associated facility costs.[242] Rapid infusion rates (10 mL per kg per hour) have not been shown to adversely affect the quality of transfused platelets and may provide direct benefit to the patient.[242]

Posttransfusion Platelet Count

Because of rapid equilibration of transfused platelets, platelet counts can be monitored 10 minutes after transfusion.[218]

Platelet counts may decrease between 10 and 60 minutes in patients with clinical conditions associated with platelet consumption. However, an immediate posttransfusion count is suitable for decisions regarding surgical procedures and refractoriness.

Leukoreduction of Platelet Products

In general, it is preferable to use leukoreduced blood for all patients with hematologic malignancies and those receiving chemotherapy. Leukocyte reduction is accomplished by passing the PC through a polyester-based filter or by apheresis technology. Filtration removes 99.9% of the leukocytes, resulting in 1 to 5×10^6 residual leukocytes per concentrated platelet pool.[66,84,85,223,248,249] The purpose of leukocyte depletion is to reduce the potential complications associated with the leukocytes in the PC, such as FNHTRs, transmission of infectious organisms, immune modulation, and alloimmunization. Transfusion reactions are rare in the infant and neonate; however, prevention of infections, such as CMV infection, warrants leukodepleted blood products in this age group.

Leukocyte reduction may also be accomplished by ultraviolet B (UVB) irradiation of the blood product. WBCs are inactivated by UVB, without a survival effect on RBCs or platelets.[250,251] Ultraviolet irradiation appears to intervene with cell activation, including calcium mobilization and transmembrane signaling, and by modulation of cell surface antigens. This abrogation of the antigen-presenting capability likely is the reason UVB irradiation is associated with decreased alloimmunization and platelet refractoriness.

The relationship between the number of platelet units received and development of refractoriness has been debated and may not be as relevant now given contemporary screening and testing techniques.[159,222,244,252] Platelet components given to severely immunocompromised patients should be irradiated to reduce the risk of TA-GVHD.[105,109] Some patients with malignancies who are CMV seronegative may be appropriate candidates for CMV-screened blood products, especially if they are potential or actual candidates for allogeneic bone marrow or stem cell transplantation, although leukoreduction only is possibly sufficient for apheresis platelet transfusions.[96] Platelets should be infused as soon as they are released from the blood bank.

Platelet Refractoriness and Alloimmunization

Platelet refractoriness is the condition in which patients cease to respond to repeated platelet transfusion with appropriate and sustained increments in the platelet count, regardless of the etiology. Refractoriness has been specifically defined as a poor increment in the posttransfusion platelet count in the multiply transfused patient, obtained at 1 hour and 8 to 24 hours after transfusion, on at least two occasions. Alloimmunization refers to an immune response and is defined as a specific alloantibody-mediated clearance of vulnerable transfused platelets. It is the most important long-term complication of platelet transfusion.[253]

Patients can become refractory to platelet transfusion for a variety of independent and coincident reasons. The two major categories of platelet refractoriness are nonimmune and immune (destruction by antibodies to HLA class I antigens).[254,255] Nonimmune causes may be more prevalent than immune causes of platelet refractoriness.[256] These include DIC, fever, sepsis, massive hemorrhage, splenomegaly, bone marrow transplantation, graft-versus-host disease, veno-occlusive disease, viral and bacterial infections, concurrent amphotericin B, and the number of concurrent antibiotics.[155,180,190,256–264] Immune causes such as platelet-specific antibodies or ABO-incompatible platelets less commonly lead to refractoriness.[252,265–271] A recent study evaluating the efficacy of ABO-major mismatched platelet transfusion in children with oncologic or hematologic diagnoses clearly demonstrated inferior platelet recovery posttransfusion.[272] In addition, using flow cytometric and fluorescent microscopy techniques, the study was able to identify increased clearance of subgroups of platelets expressing A antigens on the cell surface. However, there is no evidence that D-incompatible platelet transfusion results in D-alloimmunization since Rh antigens are not expressed on platelet membranes.[237,273] The most common immune cause of refractoriness is HLA antibody mediated. Alloimmunization occurs in recipients of multiple random-donor platelet transfusions with an estimated frequency of 25% to 50% in newly diagnosed AML and less commonly in ALL.[59,222,244,245,252,255,257]

Certain antibiotics and medications may inhibit platelet function and render the transfusion ineffective. Drugs known to interfere directly with platelet function include aspirin and nonsteroidal anti-inflammatory drugs. Other medications may cause direct marrow suppression or induce immune-mediated platelet destruction. Vancomycin has been reported to induce IgG antibodies to platelet glycoproteins IIb and IIIa.[274] Cotrimoxazole is a potent antimicrobial agent advocated for prophylaxis for *Pneumocystis jiroveci* pneumonia and other serious bacterial infections in children undergoing immune suppressive therapy for cancer.[275] Diminished platelet survival due to the production of antibodies directed against the trimethoprim component has been reported.[191] Intravenous amphotericin B has also been associated with thrombocytopenia and transfusion platelet refractoriness.[257,276,277] The precise mechanism of this effect is unknown, although it is thought amphotericin B may cause direct membrane damage by binding to sterols. Indications for the above medications should be clearly defined in patients with platelet support problems.

Leukocytes contaminating platelet preparations are the primary stimulus for alloimmunization.[278,279] Primary HLA alloimmunization requires the recognition of class I (A, B, C) and class II (DR, DQ, DP) HLA antigens by the recipient. Platelets do not express class II antigens and there is much evidence that passenger leukocytes in blood products are the primary cause of HLA alloimmunization.[280,281] Filtration of platelets to remove the offending leukocytes may theoretically help reduce HLA sensitization. Leukofiltration can be performed during collection or at the time of infusion. Filtration does increase the cost of transfusion and there may be an appreciable loss in the quantity of transfused platelets with the potential for an increased requirement in transfusion products.[85]

A number of clinical trials have focused on leukocyte removal from platelet and RBC products to reduce development of alloimmunization and shown a positive outcome.[72,282–285] A large, blinded, randomized, multicenter trial (Trial to Reduce Alloimmunization to Platelets [TRAP]), assessed whether platelet transfusion leukoreduced by filtration or UVB irradiation would prevent the formation of antiplatelet alloantibodies and refractoriness to platelet transfusions.[222] Six hundred three adult patients with newly diagnosed AML were randomized to receive PCs (control group), filtered PC (leukoreduced), leukofiltered apheresis platelets, or UVB-irradiated PC. Filtration was performed at the blood bank and not at the bedside. There was a statistically significant reduction in the development of anti-HLA antibody in all three groups receiving leukofiltration or UVB manipulation of the platelets. There was no advantage noted between the filtered, pooled PCs and the filtered apheresis, single-donor

platelet product. Reduction of leukocytes by filtration or UVB irradiation proved to be equally effective in the prevention of alloimmunization and refractoriness to platelet transfusion during therapy for AML.

Leukocyte-reduced platelet products are now the standard of practice for patients with cancer and those likely to require frequent transfusion support. This approach is cost effective and may also provide additional benefits of decreasing infections associated with transfusion.[159,286,287] Leukocyte filtration done at the blood bank before storage may be more efficient and offer better cost saving, given recent evidence that cytokines released from the leukocytes during storage may contribute to the development of febrile transfusion reactions.[170]

Before determining a diagnosis of platelet refractoriness, at least two transfusions with ABO-compatible, fresh platelets (stored <72 hours) should be given.[268] In addition, nonimmune causes of platelet consumption should be addressed medically before pursuing an evaluation for immune-mediated platelet destruction.

The management of platelet alloimmunization requires a dual approach: donor selection and platelet product preparation to reduce immunogenicity (Table 39.6).[169,288,289] Patients who require long-term platelet support should receive leukodepleted, ABO-identical platelets to delay the development of platelet alloimmunization. In a prospective study, Heal et al. demonstrated that transfusion of ABO-identical platelets is associated with a significantly higher CCI and reduced number of platelet transfusions in the first 30 days of therapy.[265,266] Transfusion of ABO-mismatched platelets may accelerate the development of platelet refractoriness.[269] Transfusion of "Rh-positive" platelets to Rh-negative individuals should be discouraged because it could affect future transfusions and pregnancies secondary to the small number of Rh-positive RBCs in the transfusion.[237] Antibodies against platelet-specific antigens are an infrequent cause of alloimmunization.[231,253]

Crossmatching platelets at the blood bank may help identify suitable donors.[289–291] The patient's serum can be screened

TABLE 39.6

STRATEGIES TO TREAT AND PREVENT PLATELET REFRACTORINESS

1. Ensure ABO-compatible units on at least two occasions. ABO incompatibility between donor and recipient may contribute to reduced intravascular recovery and survival of transfused platelets
2. Give at least one transfusion of platelets 1 to 3 days old
3. Identify and treat any correctable clinical factor that may cause platelet refractoriness
4. Ensure that the patient is receiving the correct dose of platelets
5. Determine whether or not the patient has HLA- or platelet-specific antibodies
6. Give transfusions of either crossmatched or HLA-matched platelets, whichever is available sooner
7. Monitor response with 1-hour and 8- to 24-hour platelet counts
8. Consider a family donor
9. Transfuse judiciously, only for clinical bleeding. There is no role for prophylaxis above 10,000 mm³ without bleeding or an anticipated procedure

HLA, human leukocyte antigen.

for the presence of alloantibodies against platelet components. One study confirmed the effectiveness of such a strategy with a significantly improved posttransfusion platelet count in more than 50% of refractory patients.[292] If HLA typing cannot be performed, the patient does not respond to HLA-matched platelets, or has a rare HLA type, then platelet crossmatching techniques may substitute for HLA matching.[288,291,293]

Patients with suspected alloimmune refractory thrombocytopenia should have antibody testing performed to confirm the diagnosis. HLA-matched platelets may have to be reserved for refractory patients. Platelet products partially mismatched, at one or two HLA antigens, may be just as effective in increasing circulating platelet levels as perfectly matched platelets.[294] This strategy may increase the potential donor pool, especially for rare HLA types. Approximately 50% to 60% of patients receiving HLA-matched platelets demonstrate adequate increments in the posttransfusion platelet count.[159,258]

There is currently no evidence to support the prophylactic transfusion of unmatched platelets to patients who are refractory and have no demonstrable increment in the platelet count. Such patients should receive transfusion only in the event of hemorrhage. However, transfusion of massive quantities of PCs may benefit patients who are actively bleeding, either as a result of a transient decrease in the antibody titer or a fortuitous compatible unit.[55,293,295] Therapies such as those used in idiopathic thrombocytopenia purpura have been tried in the setting of platelet alloimmunization with little success. Randomized studies have not shown a beneficial effect of intravenous immune globulin.[296-298] Of note, antibody levels and specificity may decrease with time, so patients with known alloimmunization may be rechallenged again in the future with a successful outcome.[236,299,300]

Pharmacologic Adjuncts to Platelet Transfusion

The role of pharmacologic adjuncts to reduce bleeding in thrombocytopenic patients is uncertain (Table 39.7). The antifibrinolytic agent, epsilon aminocaproic acid, has been shown to be safe and effective in the control of minor and severe bleeding in patients with immune (e.g., immune thrombocytopenia purpura) and nonimmune (e.g., amegakaryocytic thrombocytopenia, bone marrow transplant) causes of chronic thrombocytopenia.[263,301,302] Patients tolerated a long-term low-dose regimen (up to 7 months). However, there are no data at this time to suggest its use in the bleeding thrombocytopenic oncology patient, other than as an adjunct after other known methods have failed. Desmopressin (DDAVP) is well known to improve platelet function in patients with von Willebrand's disease and may possibly improve platelet function in cardiac surgery patients pretreated with aspirin or other antiplatelet medications.[303,304] Whether DDAVP will improve hemostasis in thrombocytopenic cancer patients with normally functioning platelets has not been determined.

In addition to therapeutic measures to prevent or control bleeding, simple physical measures can be taught and quickly implemented to prevent excessive blood loss. Development of an epistaxis protocol (Table 39.8) has proven to be a simple but successful measure at our institution.[305]

Granulocyte Transfusion

Patients with an anticipated long period of profound neutropenia secondary to myelosuppressive therapy are at very high risk for a serious bacterial or fungal infection.[306-310] In the

TABLE 39.7

THERAPEUTIC APPROACHES TO BLEEDING IN THE THROMBOCYTOPENIC PATIENT

Clinical assessment	Obtain vital signs
	Identify source and rate of bleeding
	Determine current platelet count and hemoglobin level
	Assess for concurrent coagulopathy
Transfusion intervention	Transfuse platelets; transfuse red blood cells as needed for anemia or rapid blood loss; transfuse plasma for correction of coagulopathy
Medications to treat or prevent bleeding	Antifibrinolytic agents such as Amicar (epsilon aminocaproic acid) may help maintain a clot in a mucosal hemorrhage
	Desmopressin (DDAVP) enhances platelet adhesion to vascular endothelium and shortens bleeding time (of unclear value when platelet count is below 50,000/mm^3)
	Oral contraceptives to prevent/ decrease menstrual blood losses in postmenarchal girls
	Avoidance of antiplatelet agents; ibuprofen, naproxen, aspirin
Procedures	Apply pressure after intramuscular injection, venipuncture, bone marrow aspirates for 5–15 min
Develop institutional protocols/staff education	Epistaxis protocol (see example in Table 39.8)

severely neutropenic patient (absolute neutrophil count [ANC] <500 cells per mm^3), combinations of antimicrobial agents may not be effective in eradicating a life-threatening infection. Recent approaches in the supportive care of these patients have led to earlier detection of serious infection, improved antibacterial and antifungal therapies, and the acceleration of neutrophil recovery by cytokine stimulation or granulocyte transfusions.[311] It is generally agreed that the prognosis of systemic fungal disease in the immunocompromised patient is dependent upon the recovery of the neutrophil count.[312,313] Unfortunately, beneficial effects of granulocyte transfusions in profoundly neutropenic patients remains controversial due to the paucity of randomized controlled trials (RCTs).[314-319] A phase III RCT is currently underway in adult patients to help answer this important question.[320]

Many observational studies are available in the pediatric population as best documented most recently by van de Wetering et al.[315] Overall these studies show a high rate of survival with limited side effects, but without any randomized controlled data it is impossible to report a potential benefit to this therapy. Renewed enthusiasm for the use of granulocyte transfusions in the profoundly neutropenic and septic patient is largely due to the increased yield of granulocytes obtained after donor mobilization with granulocyte colony-stimulating factor (G-CSF), with or without the use of dexamethasone.[321-326] Further trials have also shown that G-CSF-derived neutrophils maintain their ability to appropriately migrate to sites of infection.[327] The dose of granulocytes is the most important factor

TABLE 39.8

EPISTAXIS: A STEP-BY-STEP MANAGEMENT OF ANTERIOR EPISTAXIS IN THE ONCOLOGY PATIENT

Purpose: To restore nasal hemostasis in hematology/oncology patients

Supportive data:
- Objectives: To arrest nasal bleeding in a standardized fashion
- Indications: Hematology/oncology division patients experiencing nasal bleeding
- Contraindications: Known allergy to polyvinyl alcohol, thrombin topical

Equipment list:
- Merocel Standard Nasal Packing 4.5 cm (product no. 400400) or 8 cm (product no. 400403) depending on age/size of patient
- Polyvinyl alcohol foam, an open-cell foam capable of compression when dry and expansion when wet. The expansion produces both active and passive absorption, and places gentle pressure on the mucosa, thus stopping the bleeding. The advantages of foam pack are its ease of insertion and decreased trauma during removal. The nasal sponge/tampon should fit snugly through the nare and be placed along the floor of the nasal cavity
- Neosporin
- Topical Thrombin Powder 10,000 units (1 for each nostril)
- Scissors
- Cotton-tipped swabs
- 1-inch cloth tape
- Normal saline bolus
- Tincture of Benzoin
- 2 × 2 gauze
- Face mask or face shield

Content:
1. Assess patient for initiation of bleeding episode, any events to halt bleeding, events before initiation of bleeding
2. Wash hands and gather supplies. Be mindful of Standard Precautions
3. Apply pressure to nares for 20 min with following technique. **If manual pressure is stopped momentarily to change dressings or to examine, the patient may need to start the 20-min process all over again if bleeding resumes**
   (a) Place patient in a sitting position to decrease venous pressure and to prevent blood from draining into the nasopharynx
      - Keep the head higher than the level of the heart. Do not have the patient lie flat
      - Flex neck anteriorly, with the chin touching the chest
      - If the patient is recumbent in bed, turn the head slightly laterally to the side
   (b) With the thumb and index finger, have the patient pinch all the soft parts of the nose. The correct location is below the nasal bones, on the ala nasi (i.e., hold pressure on the lower half of the nose)
      - Press firmly toward the face, compressing the pinched parts of the nose against the bones of the face. Applying pressure in this area will compress arteries in the anterior portion of the nose in the region of Kiesselbach's plexus, also called Little's area. The upper half of the nose (near the bridge of the nose) has the nasal bones, and applying pressure there will not compress the inner portions of the nose
      - If bleeding continues while pressure is applied, assume that the nose is being held in the wrong spot and pressure should be applied in the correct spot for the full 20 min
   (c) Evaluate presence/amount of bleeding after 20 min of pressure
      - If bleeding stops and recurs, repeat but pinch nose **firmly** on both sides for at least 20 minutes. Holding the nose tightly closed allows the blood to clot and seal the damaged blood vessels
      - If actively bleeding and clot(s) can be visualized, pull the clot(s) out from the patient's nose, then reapply digital pressure for at least 20 min
      - It is still unknown if ice placed on the posterior neck area, ice placed over the middle of the face, or if pressure on the upper lip will promote vasoconstriction, but most will agree that these maneuvers do not cause the bleeding to worsen
   (d) Instruct patient not to blow his/her nose, but rather to allow the blood to ooze on its own. If blood is in the patient's mouth, have the patient expectorate into an emesis basin
   (e) Advise the patient not to blow his/her nose for 12 h after bleeding stops to avoid dislodging the blood clot
4. **Pack the nasal cavity with compressed sponge** (polyvinyl alcohol) when bleeding persists for more than 20 min with continuous digital pressure. Anterior packing can be done by a trained RN or a resident
   (a) Place Neosporin at the end of the PVA packing to act as an antimicrobial agent as well as lubrication for ease of insertion
   (b) Place Topical Thrombin Powder (hemostatic agent) or NeoSynephrine (vasoconstrictor) to the nasal packing to help with the bleeding
   (c) Insert the packing into the patient's nare along the nasal floor of the nasal cavity
   (d) Tape the strings to the cheek of the patient to facilitate removal; do not cut the strings at the end of the packing
   (e) Tape the packing down toward the nostrils to prevent accidental removal
   (f) Leave anterior packs in place for at least 24 h and up to 5 days. However, 24 h *maximum* in immunocompromised patients
   (g) Other supportive care:
      - Consider offering humidification by mouth to prevent drying and crusting of oral mucous membranes as nasal packing necessitates mouth breathing
      - Consider nasal saline spray after 24–48 h to hasten dissolution
      - Initiate/administer antibiotics per orders (covers staph and sinus flora)
      - Consider stool softeners to prevent Valsalva's maneuver during bowel movement

(continued)

TABLE 39.8

CONTINUED

(h) Removal of anterior packing should be done by an RN or resident only when appropriate staff is present. Appropriate staffing is defined as at least one physician on unit and two RNs nearby in the event of a sudden severe onset of bleeding once packing is removed
- It is recommended to use saline (saline bullets) or sterile water to dampen packing before removal to prevent tissue injury before removal

(i) Provide additional care to monitor patient per orders:
- Evaluate laboratory values per orders: complete blood cell count, prothrombin time, partial thromboplastin time, type and crossmatch
- Consider transfusion of platelets and packed red blood cells per parameters

Documentation:
1. Describe the following on the nursing progress report:
- Site of bleeding
- Amount of blood loss (estimate if possible)
- Duration of bleeding
- Action(s) taken to restore hemostasis
- Record patient's vital signs and mental status
2. Describe patient's response to any/all interventions
3. Document notification of physician support and any/all actions taken subsequent to that notification
4. Document any/all patient education per unit standard

RN, registered nurse.

---

in determining the success of the transfusion.[314,316,322,328,329] The dose of granulocytes, however, does not correlate with the incremental change in the peripheral WBC count in the recipient.[322] Factors that may modify the absolute posttransfusion WBC count include dose and age of the transfused granulocytes, consumption of granulocytes in areas of infection, fever, and prior mobilization with cytokines.[307,329]

Preparation of Granulocyte Concentrates

Donor mobilization is recommended with G-CSF (5 mg per kg or 300 mg IV or subcutaneously) and dexamethasone (8 mg orally) administered 12 hours before collection. This increases the yield of granulocytes by five- to tenfold.[321,322,326,327,329,330] The range of neutrophil yield in mobilized concentrates varies from 3 to 10×10^{10} cells.[328] These medications are well tolerated by healthy donors. Mild side effects may be expected from G-CSF and include mild bone pain, myalgias, arthralgias, and headache. Donors should be in good health without a history of hypertension, diabetes, or peptic ulcers. These conditions may be aggravated by the use of steroids.[321,329] Mobilization does not appear to hinder granulocyte function.[327,331] In fact, cytokine stimulation may augment the microbicidal activity of polymorphonuclear cells.[332,333] It remains to be seen if higher doses of mobilized granulocytes increase survival in septic neutropenic children. Limited randomized controlled data in neonates with sepsis to date have failed to show a significant benefit from granulocyte transfusion.[334]

Granulocytes are collected by apheresis for a specific patient and must be transfused within 24 hours of collection. Ideally, granulocytes should be transfused within 8 to 12 hours of collection; however, storage at 20°C to 24°C is safe with good survival and functional activity.[311] Hubel et al. recently reported that storage at 10°C might be superior to storage at 22°C.[335] The collection process takes approximately 2 to 3 hours. The final concentrate is commonly 200 to 300 mL and contains a rich supply of granulocytes in addition to RBCs, platelets, and citrated plasma. The RBC contamination requires the product to be ABO compatible and crossmatched before transfusion. Collections are typically

obtained daily for 4 to 7 days since granulocytes have a half-life of only 7 hours, dependent on the needs of the recipient and availability of donors.[317] Granulocyte concentrates contain T-lymphocytes capable of causing TA-GVHD; therefore, 2,500 cGy of irradiation before use is recommended.[329] In addition, CMV-seronegative recipients should receive CMV-negative products.[317]

Adverse Effects of Granulocyte Transfusions

Granulocyte transfusions are generally well tolerated in the pediatric population but come with many of the same risks as other transfusion modalities.[315,336] Immediate transfusion reactions include fever, chills, and acute pulmonary symptoms including dyspnea, chest tightness, hypoxia, and pulmonary infiltrates.[329,337] Alloimmunization and platelet refractoriness may occur. Premedication with acetaminophen and diphenhydramine is recommended before administration of a granulocyte transfusion. Corticosteroids may be helpful in ameliorating a severe transfusion reaction. A high incidence of CMV infection has been demonstrated in CMV-seronegative patients who received granulocyte transfusions from CMV-seropositive donors compared with CMV-seropositive recipients.[93] Because transmission of CMV infection in severely immunocompromised patients can result in a severe and fatal outcome, CMV-seronegative donors should be utilized for these patients.

Concurrent administration of amphotericin B and granulocyte transfusion in neutropenic patients is potentially associated with severe pulmonary reactions.[338] This initial data though have not been subsequently confirmed.[339,340] The most significant reactions have been reported to occur if amphotericin B is administered within 4 hours of granulocyte transfusion or if the granulocyte transfusion is given before amphotericin B. Under these circumstances, amphotericin B can potentially induce granulocyte aggregates, enhance pulmonary leukostasis, and damage granulocytes, leading to lysis and release of neutrophil proteases.[307,329] The observation of an interaction between these two therapies is confounded by other potential causes of pulmonary problems in critically ill patients. A practical approach is to separate the infusion of amphotericin B and transfusion of granulocytes by at least 4 to 6 hours, in lieu of confirmatory evidence.[307,317] Newer lipid formulations of amphotericin are associated with a lower incidence of side effects and less *in vitro* aggregation of neutrophils.[341]

Clinical Recommendations for Granulocyte Transfusion

The decision to transfuse granulocytes must take into consideration the clinical factors and potential benefits and risks, especially in light of a lack of prospective controlled clinical trials. There is currently no role for prophylactic granulocyte transfusions in neutropenic patients although one recent RCT in patients after allogeneic hematopoietic stem cell transplant posed some potential benefits that require further study.[342,343] Based on current available literature, it is reasonable to consider therapeutic granulocyte transfusions in severely neutropenic patients in whom bacterial or fungal infection has been refractory or progressive on appropriate, aggressive antibacterial and/or antifungal therapy, and neutropenia is expected to continue for at least one or more weeks further.[317] Allogeneic granulocyte donors should be mobilized with G-CSF and dexamethasone 12 hours before collection by pheresis and transfused as soon as possible. A dose of at least 1×10^{10} or 1×10^{10} per m^2 should be infused daily at a rate of 1 to 2×10^{10} cells per hour for a minimum of 4 to 7 days.[311,314] In children, a minimum dose of 1×10^9 cells per kg per day should be given.[307] Granulocyte transfusions should be obtained from ABO-compatible, crossmatched donors. HLA matching is indicated for alloimmunized patients. The increment in WBC count should not be used as a measurement of successful transfusion. Clearance of the infection and/or recovery of the recipient's own neutrophil count obviate the need for further transfusions.

Plasma

The transfusion of fresh frozen plasma (FFP) is indicated for bleeding or before an invasive procedure when a patient has a documented coagulation factor deficiency, or a significantly prolonged PT or aPTT. FFP is obtained from single donors, with each unit removed from a unit of whole blood, frozen within 6 to 8 hours of collection and stored at $-18°C$ or colder. FFP is administered in doses of 10 to 20 mL per kg given over 1 to 2 hours, or as tolerated. This is expected to increase the concentration of coagulation factors by 25% to 50%.[51,237] Isohemagglutinins are present in FFP and can be responsible for severe hemolytic transfusion reactions (HTRs) or result in a positive direct antiglobulin (Coombs) test (DAT). Therefore, FFP should be ABO compatible. The majority of WBCs are killed or made nonfunctional during the freezing process, therefore leukoreduction and irradiation of FFP are unnecessary.[237]

Cryoprecipitate

Cryoprecipitate, a supernatant of FFP, contains concentrated FVIII, FXIII, fibrinogen, and von Willebrand factor, allowing for a more rapid correction of these factors at a reduced volume and is used mainly for bleeding secondary to dysfibrinogenemia, hypofibrinogenemia, or afibrinogenemia. Cryoprecipitate is given as a dose of 1 unit (10 to 15 mL) per 5 kg of body weight. One unit bag per 5 kg of cryoprecipitate should increase fibrinogen by approximately 100 mg per dL.[237] This product does not contain RBCs, and

therefore ABO compatibility is not necessary. Similar to FFP, leukoreduction and irradiation are unnecessary.

Recombinant Activated Factor VII

Recombinant activated factor VII (rFVIIa) is specifically licensed by the FDA for use in hemophilia A and B patients who are refractory to treatment secondary to the development of inhibitors.[344] Unlicensed use of rFVIIa has become more widespread over the last several years.[345] No RCTs in pediatrics outside of its licensed usage have been reported in the literature. Although the side effect profile of rFVIIa appears significantly low, the risk of thromboembolism still remains and "off-label" use of this expensive medication should be considered with caution.[346] Case reports have shown potential benefits for pediatric patients with brain tumors to control intraoperative bleeding.[347,348] Potential benefit for hemorrhagic cystitis may exist but is tempered by the short half-life of the medication and results of the only RCT in adolescents and adults showed no benefit.[349–351] In addition, as rFVIIa relies on tissue factor and activation of platelets to form a more stable thrombin plug, oncology patients with severe thrombocytopenia are less likely to benefit.[344]

Complications of Transfusion

Improvement in the quality of blood components has resulted in impressive incremental increased blood safety. Optimal blood safety measures require the accurate collection and labeling of samples, proper storage, appropriate transfusion indications, and accurate blood administration at the bedside.[352] In the past, the major cause of transfusion-related death was clerical error in the proper identification of the intended transfusion recipient, either at the time of phlebotomy for pretransfusion testing, or before administration of blood.[353–355] Now with the improvement in quality control measures, TRALI, in its increased recognition, especially in adults, has become the most likely cause of death and major morbidity.[356,357] Measurable and dramatic reductions in the risk of transfusion-related human immunodeficiency virus (HIV), hepatitis B virus (HBV), and hepatitis C virus (HCV) have occurred as a result of efforts of the national blood banks to improve product testing and safety. Now, acute, noninfectious risks are much more common than infection transmission.[357]

Adverse reactions to blood component therapy may range from brief episodes of fever to life-threatening reactions such as acute hemolysis and shock. Short-term complications are common. The challenge for the clinician is the prompt recognition of potentially serious reactions that may present with seemingly mild and common symptoms, such as fever. Acute reactions are defined as those occurring within the initial 24 hours following administration of a blood component. Delayed reactions occur after at least 24 hours. Transfusion recipients may experience immune-mediated hemolytic reactions, FNHTRs, allergic reactions, TRALI, TACO, and TA-GVHD in addition to infectious complications (Table 39.9). Iron overload and alloimmunization are potential problems experienced by those patients who are chronically transfused.

Hemolytic Transfusion Reactions

HTRs can be either acute or delayed. Acute HTRs (AHTRs) classically present with fever, chills, nausea, and vomiting. Young children may exhibit signs of generalized discomfort or anxiety. Low back pain, dyspnea, hypotension or shock, oliguria, hemoglobinuria, hemoglobinemia, and DIC are

TABLE 39.9

ADVERSE REACTIONS TO TRANSFUSION: RECOGNITION AND MANAGEMENT

Type	Time of onset	Clinical presentation	Laboratory features	Treatment	Prevention
AHTR (acute hemolytic transfusion reaction)	Immediate, during red cell transfusion	Fever, apprehension, back pain, hypotension, DIC, renal failure	• Hemoglobinemia • Hemoglobinuria • Positive direct antiglobin test	Stop transfusion • Supportive, hydration IV (e.g., normal saline 10–20 mL/kg) • Furosemide (1–2 mg/kg/dose) IV to maintain urine flow (1 mL/kg/h) • Dopamine (1–5 mg/kg/min) for hypotension • FFP, platelets, cryoprecipitate for bleeding/DIC	Strict adherence to proper donor and recipient identification procedures at time of collection, testing, and prior to transfusion
FNHTR (febrile nonhemolytic transfusion reaction)	During transfusion or within 4 h (more common following platelet transfusion)	Fever (rise of temperature >1°C), chills, rigors, nausea/vomiting, headache	None	Stop transfusion • Acetaminophen (10–15 mg/kg/dose orally) • Transfusion may be restarted following clinical assessment (rule out AHTR or bacterial contamination) and defervescence of fever	For history of FNHTR, consider premedication with acetaminophen 30–60 min prior to subsequent transfusions, use prestorage leukocyte reduced blood components, consider washed blood components for recurrent FNHTRs despite premedication
Allergic transfusion reaction	Immediate, during transfusion (mild allergic reaction may become apparent several hours following the transfusion, whereas severe allergic reactions [anaphylaxis] tend to occur within minutes)	Cutaneous manifestations: urticaria, pruritus, flushing, facial edema, angioedema Respiratory manifestations: wheezing, stridor, dyspnea, cough, shortness of breath, retractions Cardiovascular manifestations: hypotension, weak pulse, LOC Gastrointestinal manifestations: abdominal cramps, nausea, vomiting	None	Stop transfusion Mild allergic reaction: • Diphenhydramine, orally or IV (1 mg/kg/dose) • Inhaled beta-2 agonists for bronchospasm: nebulized albuterol 0.05 mL/kg of 0.5% solution (max dose 1 mL diluted in 1–2 mL normal saline) Severe allergic reaction: • Resuscitation team and equipment accessed due to medical emergency • Epinephrine (1:1000) subcutaneously 0.01 mg/kg/dose (0.01 mL/kg) (max dose 0.4 mg = 0.4 mL) • Diphenhydramine IV 1 mg/kg/dose (max dose 50 mg)	Mild allergic reaction: consider premedication with antihistamine 1 h prior to transfusion. Moderate to severe reactions: avoid transfusion if possible, autologous blood donation for elective procedures, consider oral prednisone 1–2 mg/kg/dose Q6 h beginning 24 h prior to transfusion in addition to antihistamine

(continued)

TABLE 39.9

CONTINUED

Type	Time of onset	Clinical presentation	Laboratory features	Treatment	Prevention
				• Methylpred-nisolone IV 1–2 mg/kg/dose (max dose 125 mg) • Albuterol nebulizer 0.01–0.05 mL/kg of 0.5% solution (max dose 1 mL)	
DHTR (delayed hemolytic transfusion reaction)	>24 h after red cell transfusion (usually first 2 weeks)	Fever, chills, jaundice, malaise, back pain; rarely renal failure	• Anemia; less than expected increment posttransfusion • Evidence of extra-vascular hemolysis: spherocytes and reticulocytes on peripheral smear, increase in total and unconjugated bilirubins, increased LDH • Diagnosis supported by positive DAT (may be negative if all transfused cells have lysed) • Serial testing to detect red cell alloantibodies	• Usually mild and no treatment necessary, may require repeat transfusion, screen for antigen of corresponding newly discovered antibody • Adequate hydration for ongoing hemolysis and monitoring of renal function	Prompt identification and accurate record keeping of clinically significant red cell alloantibodies with repeat pretransfusion testing for specific antibody detection and compatibility tests
TRALI (transfusion-related acute lung injury)	1–2 h after initiation of transfusion, becoming severe within 6 h. All plasma-containing blood components have been implicated	Dyspnea, hypoxemia, fever, noncardio-genic pulmonary edema, hypotension not responsive to fluid resuscitation or diuretics	• No typical findings • HLA- or granulo-cyte-specific antibodies in donor or recipient plasma strongly suggestive of diagnosis	• Oxygen; supportive care including mechanical ventilation may be necessary • Pressor support may be helpful • Corticosteroids may be of benefit	Minimization of transfusion, especially in those with underlying cardiopulmonary dysfunction, consider plasma-containing blood components from male donors

DAT, direct antiglobin (Coombs) test; DIC, disseminated intravascular coagulation; FFP, fresh frozen plasma; HLA, human leukocyte antigen; IV, intravenous; LDH, lactate dehydrogenase; LOC, loss of consciousness.

potential serious complications of AHTRs and should alert the clinician to intervene immediately. The mechanism of action of AHTRs is thought to be acute intravascular hemolysis, usually due to IgM antibodies to anti-A and anti-B isohemagglutinins, but can also be caused by other IgG and IgM antibodies, which induce complement fixation on transfused RBCs with resultant lysis. In addition, bystander hemolysis can lead to lysis of the transfusion recipient's own RBCs. The severity of the reaction is extremely variable and usually is reflective of the volume and rate of transfused blood although severe symptoms have been reported after the transfusion of only 10 to 15 mL of blood.[358] Inadvertent ABO incompatibility is the most common cause of AHTRs. Pediatric oncology patients who receive large volumes of plasma incompatible platelets may receive a high bolus of ABO antibodies; therefore, only plasma compatible platelets

should be administered to prevent hemolytic reactions and decrease alloimmunization.[359,360] Volume-reduced, plasma-incompatible platelets may be necessary on occasion when compatible units are not available.[361] Acute intravascular hemolysis may be caused by other immune and nonimmune mechanisms such as physical damage to RBCs by blood warmers, incompatible intravenous fluids, incorrect preparation of frozen RBCs, and bacterial contamination in the unit. Clinical conditions associated with intravascular hemolysis include autoimmune and drug-induced hemolytic anemia.

Delayed HTRs (DHTRs) classically present with milder symptoms such as low-grade fever, jaundice, and a posttransfusion hemoglobin increment lower than expected. These symptoms typically are evident 2 to 14 days after transfusion. DHTRs are thought to occur primarily in previously sensitized patients with no detectable circulating antibody at the time of crossmatching. The result is complement fixation by IgG-mediated antibodies, clinically manifested by extravascular hemolysis.[362,363]

Evaluation of a Suspected Hemolytic Transfusion Reaction. In the event of a transfusion reaction, all blood components are suspect. If a child has received multiple products or units, each unit must be evaluated. A bedside check of each unit's labeling should be conducted and the unit should be sent to the blood bank for further investigation. The laboratory evaluation of an AHTR should include a thorough assessment by the blood bank for clerical error with repeat typing and crossmatching, visual inspection of the patient's plasma after transfusion compared with a pretransfusion specimen, and performance of a DAT. Visual inspection is a sensitive method of detecting intravascular hemolysis that results in hemoglobinemia. Icteric plasma suggests a hemolytic process that has been ongoing for several hours. The DAT detects antibody or complement binding to circulating RBCs. A negative DAT may reflect complete destruction and clearance of transfused, incompatible cells and may be accompanied by hemoglobinemia and/or hemoglobinuria. Additional laboratory studies consistent with intravascular hemolysis include an elevated plasma-free hemoglobin and decreased haptoglobin. DHTRs have a more insidious onset and lead to extravascular hemolysis. Laboratory findings include a decreased hemoglobin level, increased reticulocytes, increased unconjugated (indirect) bilirubin, positive DAT, and increased lactate dehydrogenase.

Management of a Hemolytic Transfusion Reaction. In the event of an acute transfusion reaction, the transfusion should be discontinued immediately and supportive care initiated with intravenous fluids. Adequacy of renal perfusion is critical and should be monitored by careful measurement of urine output for at least 18 to 24 hours. The urine flow rate should be maintained above 1 mL per kg per hour with intravenous normal saline and diuretics as needed. Dopamine may be needed to treat hypotension and increase cardiac output and renal blood flow. Patients with DIC and active bleeding may require administration of platelets, FFP, and cryoprecipitate. Administration of further units of RBCs should be avoided if possible secondary to continued bystander hemolysis, but may be necessary in patients with active bleeding. If patient identification issues remain unresolved, the safest blood product is uncrossmatched, group O-negative RBCs.

Febrile Nonhemolytic Transfusion Reactions

An FNHTR is defined as a temperature increase of >1°C (1.8°F) associated with a transfusion, not attributed to any other cause. Prior to near universal leukoreduction, FNHTRs were far more frequent, occurring in as much as 30% of transfusions.[364,365] The major cause of FNHTRs from PCs and RBCs is likely due to the presence of pyrogenic cytokines that are released from leukocytes during storage.[170,237] Several studies have shown a significant decrease in FNHTRs with prestorage WBC reduction in both PCs and RBCs.[74–76] A recent review of 2,509 transfusions in a pediatric intensive care unit setting resulted in an overall 0.9% rate of FNHTRs.[366]

Assessment and Management of Febrile Nonhemolytic Transfusion Reactions. The diagnosis of an FNHTR is one of exclusion. Bacterial contamination, AHTR, and TRALI must be considered and ruled out. Fever may occur during the transfusion or within 4 hours of completion and may be associated with chills, rigors, and general discomfort, making it initially difficult to determine the causative etiology. The transfusion

should be discontinued until an AHTR can be ruled out. The laboratory evaluation should proceed as with an AHTR, and blood cultures should be drawn to rule out infectious causes. Fever associated with an FNHTR is often self-limited and usually resolves within 1 to 2 hours after the transfusion has been stopped. Antipyretics can be administered to provide comfort and lessen the duration of the fever although they likely provide little benefit for the associated chills, rigors, and general discomfort.[365] The decision to complete the transfusion should be guided by the patient's clinical status, urgency of the transfusion, and results of the AHTR investigation.

Prevention of Febrile Nonhemolytic Transfusion Reactions. Premedication with acetaminophen remains controversial. Recent RCTs show little benefit, even in patients with a history of multiple previous FNHTRs.[367–370] This is partly due to FNHTRs being rare for patients receiving leukoreduced blood products. Therefore, the routine use of premedications for transfusion is unnecessary. Similarly, antihistamines are not indicated for prophylaxis of FNHTRs. Antipyretic premedication can be considered for patients who have experienced two or more febrile reactions to transfusion knowing that it may not be effectual and will not treat the associated symptoms of an FNHTR. For the patient who continues to experience FNHTRs despite premedication with antipyretics and transfusion with leukoreduced units, a trial of washed blood components could be considered. A major disadvantage of this procedure is the loss of a substantial portion of the RBCs or platelets in the unit.[364]

Allergic Transfusion Reactions

Allergic transfusion reactions typically present with signs and symptoms of histamine release, most likely secondary to a type I hypersensitivity reaction secondary to antigens in the plasma of blood components. Allergic reactions are the most common acute transfusion reaction, complicating 1% to 5% of all transfusions and more likely occurring with platelets or plasma derivatives than RBCs.[364,371] Allergic reactions to blood components have variable severity and onset, with the majority being mild and beginning within an hour of starting the transfusion. Anaphylaxis, however, tends to occur within minutes. Cutaneous manifestations may be limited to urticaria, flushing, itching, or swelling. Systemic symptoms dominate in more serious reactions and may or may not be preceded by urticarial lesions. Severe respiratory, gastrointestinal, or cardiac symptoms may occur. Absence of fever and the specificity of urticaria help distinguish allergic reactions from other types of transfusion reactions.

Management of an Allergic Transfusion Reaction. Treatment of an allergic reaction is generally symptomatic. The transfusion should be discontinued and medications given as necessary to treat the symptoms. An antihistamine (diphenhydramine 1 to 1.5 mg per kg per dose orally or intravenously) is indicated to alleviate mild cutaneous symptoms. If the patient has a good response to antihistamines, the transfusion may be completed within the 4-hour requisite time. If systemic symptoms are present, resuming the transfusion is not advisable. Medical treatment is primarily supportive, and generally antihistamines are sufficient. Wheezing, cough, chest tightness, or pain may require intervention with nebulized albuterol or other beta-2 agonists. Oxygen, rapid volume expansion, epinephrine, or steroids may be required for the treatment of severe systemic or anaphylactic reactions.

Patients who experience a systemic allergic reaction or anaphylaxis should be tested for IgA deficiency and the presence of anti-IgA antibodies. Although IgA deficiency is relatively common, anaphylaxis is a rare event, and a majority of allergic reactions are not related to IgA deficiency. Allergic reactions to food, drugs, or latex can occur coincidentally with a transfusion. All exposures to known allergens within 4 hours of transfusion should be investigated.

Prevention of an Allergic Transfusion Reaction. Leukoreduction has not been shown to decrease allergic transfusion reactions.[76] As with antipyretics, premedication with antihistamines remains controversial, even in patients with a history of allergic transfusion reactions. The results of the majority of RCTs show no benefit to premedication.[367–370] No RCTs exist for the use of prophylactic corticosteroids. Antihistamines (e.g., diphenhydramine) can be considered for the patient who has had multiple allergic reactions. In such a patient if antihistamine prophylaxis is ineffectual, the addition of corticosteroids to the premedication regimen can be considered although evidence-based guidelines are lacking. Dexamethasone, prednisone, or methylprednisolone can all be considered for single or multiple pretransfusion doses. If the patient continues to have severe allergic reactions or has a history of anaphylaxis or IgA deficiency, washed blood products should be utilized.

Transfusion-Related Acute Lung Injury

TRALI is a life-threatening complication following transfusion of plasma-containing blood products.[372] TRALI remains an uncommon complication of blood product transfusion but is an increasingly recognized cause of major morbidity and death.[356,357] A 2004 consensus conference defined TRALI as a new episode of acute lung injury (ALI) presenting within 6 hours after completion of transfusion without any competing cause of ALI being present during that time frame.[373,374] Signs of ALI include hypoxemia and bilateral infiltrates on chest radiograph without evidence of circulatory overload. Clinical symptoms that have been noted to be present for patients with TRALI include dyspnea, fever, hypotension, tachypnea, tachycardia, inability to oxygenate without mechanical ventilation, and frothy endotracheal aspirates.[373]

Some authors argue that TRALI can present beyond the 6-hour period in patients with other risk factors for the development of acute respiratory distress syndrome.[375] True incidence of TRALI is not well understood secondary to the varying definitions that have been used in the past, and even less information is available regarding pediatric patients. Silliman et al. reported the largest number of pediatric patients, with TRALI occurring in 46 patients, 15 of which were younger than 17 years. A majority of the patients had a hematologic malignancy, many of which were receiving induction or consolidation chemotherapy, and only two had an underlying cardiopulmonary process. Of note, TRALI was more common as platelet age at time of transfusion increased.[168] Other pediatric reviews highlight the paucity of data in pediatric patients although in these few patients it does appear that the pathogenesis and course of TRALI are similar to those of adults, with a majority of them recovering within a 48- to 96-hour period, although three fatalities have been reported.[376,377] Pathogenesis of TRALI continues to be somewhat controversial though it appears that the most likely etiology is a "two-hit" model. Kelher et al. recently showed in a mouse model that only mice first injected with lipopolysaccharide to mimic active infection were subject to ALI secondary to antibodies directed against major histocompatibility complex class I antigens from plasma in stored RBCs.[82] This implies that those patients with underlying risk factors are more likely subject to TRALI, possibly explaining its extremely low incidence in the pediatric population and making the data of

pediatric incidence from Silliman et al. more difficult to explain.[168] Low incidence in the pediatric population could be secondary to a lack of proper diagnosis and reporting and is currently hard to corroborate. Some authors argue for other models for the development of TRALI. Some believe that the presence of donor antibodies in plasma is sufficient to cause TRALI without any underlying risk factors, although most patients who receive plasma with donor antibodies are asymptomatic.[378] As antibody detection is not universal in donors or recipients of suspected TRALI cases, other possible mechanisms have been considered as inciting agents including neutrophil priming agents such as lipids or cytokines.[373,378]

Passive transfer of antibody and/or neutrophil priming agent from donor plasma to the recipient appears to set off a chain of reactions involving complement fixation and neutrophil influx into the lung. The neutrophils release their proteases and oxygen radicals, causing damage to the pulmonary microvasculature and subsequent extravasation of protein-laden fluid into the adjacent interstitium.[372,379–381] This process is likely heightened in patients with a predisposing clinical condition, which induces pulmonary vascular endothelium activation.[378] Neutrophil activation is corroborated by the finding of transient leukopenia in recipients of neutrophil-specific antibodies from donor plasma, with a range of severity in pulmonary dysfunction.[374,382] One could assume that neutropenic patients are less likely to experience TRALI, but this has not been specifically addressed in the literature.[383]

TRALI is a clinical spectrum and fortunately a majority of patients recover quickly and completely. There is no pathognomonic sign or test for TRALI; the diagnosis is often one of exclusion. Those with milder symptoms are most likely to go unrecognized. Approximately 10% to 15% of patients die from complications related to the pulmonary insult.[237] All patients will require oxygen support and many may need short-term mechanical ventilation. The hypotension is frequently unresponsive to fluid resuscitation because these patients typically have a normal central venous pressure.[374] Pressor agents may be useful in cases of sustained hypotension. Diuretics are not helpful because the injury involves microvascular damage rather than fluid overload. Corticosteroids may be of value but have unproven utility.[384] Recognition of the syndrome is vital to provide optimal medical management and also to potentially demonstrate the presence of neutrophil-specific antibodies.

Although TRALI is rare, the recognition that it is an important cause of major morbidity and death has led to increased work to determine the best prevention strategies. Review of fatalities secondary to TRALI by the American Red Cross has implicated FFP as the most likely contributing blood product. Equally important, a female antibody-positive donor was identified in a disproportionate number of these cases.[385] Multiparous females obviously pose the highest risk. Directed maternal donation is a potential cause of TRALI secondary to sensitization to paternally derived antigens.[377] Increased risk of TRALI in a homogeneous population as is seen with TA-GVHD has not been reported to date. To address this issue, more than 90% of FFP obtained in England now comes from male donors.[378] Although Yazer et al. showed decreased incidence of TRALI after leukoreduction, both nonleukoreduced and leukoreduced blood products have been implicated as causing TRALI.[82,84,378] Washing of blood products with a known donor antibody can be considered.[237]

Transfusion-Associated Circulatory Overload

TACO, like TRALI, is a poorly understood transfusion complication that is becoming more widely recognized. TACO is cardiogenic pulmonary edema that likely is due to too rapid transfusion or too large a volume of transfusion and is more likely to occur in the patient with underlying poor cardiac function.[385] Clinical signs are similar to TRALI and include dyspnea, tachypnea, hypoxemia, and tachycardia. Hypertension is more likely than hypotension secondary to systemic and pulmonary overcirculation. Fluid balance should be positive and B-type (brain) natriuretic peptide (BNP), a measure of congestive heart failure, should be elevated.[374] TACO appears more likely in the very young and very old although the true incidence is poorly quantified.[385] TACO may occur with smaller transfusion volumes or slower rates of transfusion for not well-understood reasons. Unlike TRALI, TACO should be managed with aggressive diuresis. Risks and incidence of TACO in the pediatric population has not been well quantified but is likely quite small.

Transfusion-Associated Graft-Versus-Host Disease

Nonirradiated platelet and RBC transfusions are at risk for causing TA-GVHD, especially in immunocompromised patients or in those receiving blood from a likely histocompatible donor. The development of TA-GVHD occurs secondary to one-way histocompatibility between donor T-lymphocytes and the recipient's inability to reject these cells. Clinical manifestations of TA-GVHD present like hematopoietic stem cell transplant GVHD and include fever, anorexia, vomiting and diarrhea, and skin rash of variable severity. Pancytopenia and hepatic dysfunction with hyperbilirubinemia can also be present and may be severe and life threatening. Clinical suspicion may warrant a skin biopsy, liver biopsy, and/or bone marrow aspirate.

Infectious Complications of Transfusion

Improved donor screening and the development of more sensitive serologic tests have lead to continuing downward trends for transfusion-transmitted infection. This may in part also be due to a decreased prevalence and incidence in the donor population and overall population in general.[386] Continued risk of infection from donor blood products is due in large part to the window period in which serologic tests are negative but the donor has active infection. Most recent estimates of infection risk include HIV-1, 1 in 2.3 million, HCV, 1 in 1.8 million, and HBV, 1 in 350,000 donations.[386,387]

Hepatitis

Posttransfusion hepatitis is caused almost exclusively by viruses, including hepatitis A virus (HAV), HBV, HCV, hepatitis E virus (HEV), CMV, and EBV. HAV and HEV are enterically transmitted viruses with no carrier state. The viremic individual is usually clinically ill and not a candidate to donate blood. Blood donors with HBV or HCV may be asymptomatic carriers. Many patients with transfusion-associated hepatitis (TAH) develop transaminitis not attributable to underlying disease, medications, or other forms of viral hepatitis.[388] Hepatitis secondary to CMV and EBV is usually clinically insignificant in the absence of severe immunosuppression. However, TAH, which may cause only a mildly persistent elevation in the alanine aminotransferase level, can lead to significant hepatic disease.

There has been a marked reduction in the incidence of transfusion-transmitted HCV infection since the introduction of an effective anti-HCV antibody-screening test. Oncology patients today are at little risk for acquiring HCV via transfusion. However, cancer survivors from the 1980s represent a population at risk; they should be screened for hepatitis C by polymerase chain reaction analysis at least once on a routine evaluation.[389] Acute HCV infection is commonly asymptomatic but often results in chronic disease. The spectrum of disease ranges from elevation of liver transaminases to cirrhosis, hepatocellular carcinoma, and end-stage liver disease. Chronic liver disease may not appear for decades.[390,391] A recent study in children who underwent cardiac surgery before the implementation of blood-donor screening found a higher rate of spontaneous recovery and a milder clinical course, unlike adults with transfusion-associated HCV.[392] Spontaneous clearance of the virus has also been reported in children treated for malignancy.[393,394] However, care must be taken to repeat testing in individuals with a history of HCV, because RNA levels can fluctuate and periodically dip below levels of detection. In patients with elevated transaminases and an initial negative result, repeat analyses over several years should be performed, to rule out persistent infection.[395]

Cytomegalovirus Infection

CMV can be transmitted via transfusion and presents with a wide spectrum of clinical symptoms. Transfusion recipients may develop a mononucleosis-type infection with fever, adenopathy, lymphocytosis, pharyngitis, and hepatitis. Immunocompromised individuals may experience more severe manifestations such as retinitis, nephritis, colitis, interstitial pneumonitis, or cytopenias.[396] Primary infection occurs in the setting of a seronegative recipient receiving blood or a transplant from a donor with active or latent CMV infection. Secondary infection is defined as reactivation or coinfection. A CMV-seropositive recipient who receives blood from a seronegative or seropositive donor may experience reactivation of CMV, with a significant rise in the CMV IgG titer.[397] Reactivation of latent CMV is most often subclinical, with the exception of immunocompromised recipients. Coinfection occurs when a seropositive recipient is exposed to a different strain of CMV from that which caused the original infection.

Transfused RBCs, platelets, and granulocyte concentrates have all been implicated in the transmission of CMV.[94,398] Monocytes are thought to be the major cell reservoir harboring the CMV virion.[399] Measures taken to reduce or eliminate leukocytes from blood products have been successful in decreasing the risk of transmission of CMV although the degree of WBC removal to prevent CMV infection is unknown.[70,71,91,94,95,400] All patients receiving immunosuppressive therapies should receive leukocyte-filtered blood products to reduce the risk of primary or secondary transfusion-transmitted CMV. Although leukodepletion is effective in reducing transmission of CMV, patients at very high risk of infection may be safer with CMV-seronegative blood products.[88,91,94-97] Although it remains somewhat controversial in the literature, patients undergoing hematopoietic stem cell transplantation should receive CMV-seronegative blood products, unless the recipient is known to be CMV seropositive. Similarly, premature infants of CMV-negative mothers and patients with immune deficiencies should receive CMV-seronegative blood products.[52,98] Leukoreduction alone is possibly sufficient for apheresis platelet transfusions.[96]

Human Immunodeficiency Virus Infection

Transmission of the HIV virus via transfusion has dramatically declined due to modifications of donor screening and development of sensitive serologic assays.[390] The great majority of HIV transmission occurred before the discovery of the virus and institution of blood donor screening. The first reported cases of transfusion-associated acquired immunodeficiency syndrome (AIDS) were in hemophiliacs and recipients of blood components in 1982. Epidemiologic studies were able to target high-risk populations, in particular homosexual or bisexual men and intravenous drug users. Donors have since been screened with respect to high-risk behaviors. The discovery of HIV in 1984 as the etiologic agent for AIDS facilitated the development of serologic assays used by blood banks as part of routine donor screening. HIV-2 is a second retrovirus that can cause immune deficiency.[401] At present, antibody testing for HIV-1 and HIV-2 is required for screening of all blood donors. Additional laboratory steps to reduce HIV infection have been implemented with the specific aim of shortening the 25-day seronegative window period.[402] Nucleic acid testing for HIV was implemented in 1999 to reduce this window period, which is now 16 days.[403,404] These interventions have successfully reduced the transmission of HIV by transfusion to a rare event.

Bacterial Infections

Bacterial infection is the most common microbiological cause of transfusion-associated morbidity and mortality. These infections are associated with a rapid onset of symptoms with high morbidity and mortality. In the past, bacterial contamination of blood components was the most frequently reported cause of transfusion-related fatalities after incorrectly matched blood products, although this has changed with the increasing recognition of TA-GVHD and TRALI as important causes of major morbidity and death and with improved methods to screen blood products for contamination.[357,386,405] Blood components are often contaminated at the time of collection through introduction of skin flora, or during processing.[406] Careful skin preparation may reduce transfusion-transmitted infection with Gram-positive organisms but is unlikely to prevent the majority of deaths, which are mainly associated with Gram-negative organisms. The incidence of bacterial-related reactions from contaminated units of RBCs and platelets is significantly associated with prolonged storage time.[407] Interestingly, however, fatal infection following a platelet transfusion is more common in units stored for 3 days or less and may be due to endotoxin production by Gram-negative organisms.[408] Infection with Gram-positive organisms is more often associated with platelet units stored from 3 to 5 days. Overall, bacterial infections are much more common following platelet transfusions than RBC transfusions since platelets are stored at or near room temperature. Single-donor platelet transfusions are associated with a decreased incidence of septic transfusion reactions due to decreased donor exposure as well as the collection process and method for white cell reduction.[409]

Clinical signs and symptoms of infection due to a unit of contaminated RBCs are usually more severe than those due to contaminated platelets. The most common organism responsible for RBC contamination is *Yersinia enterocolitica*, occurring primarily in units stored for more than 25 days.[408] Most infections related to platelet transfusion are skin flora, such as *Staphylococcus epidermidis*. Factors that affect the severity of infection include bacterial virulence, concentration of transfused bacteria, immune status of the patient, and the rapidity with which the complication is recognized and treated.

If bacterial contamination is suspected, the transfusion should be stopped immediately. Treatment of the recipient should not be delayed for confirmation by either Gram stain or bacterial culture from the suspected unit. Treatment consists of administration of intravenous fluids; initiation of broad-spectrum antibiotics; antipyretics; and therapy for DIC, shock, or renal failure, if indicated.

Prevention of Transfusion-Related Bacterial Infection. A variety of strategies have been devised to reduce the risk of transfusion-associated sepsis. Platelet transfusions are most often implicated, likely due to the storage of PCs in a growth media as well as at a temperature, which facilitates bacterial growth.[410] Improved strategies to prevent and detect bacterial growth in blood components include bacterial detection by automated detection systems; improved technique in collection, processing, and storage; reducing recipient exposure by judicious use of blood components; and the introduction of pathogen inactivation methodology.[410–413] Other approaches to reduce the risk of bacterial contamination include filtration to remove leukocytes and bacteria, improved donor skin cleansing, and diversion of an initial aliquot of blood during donation.

Other Potential Transfusion-Related Pathogens

Blood product transmission of human T-lymphotropic retrovirus is extremely low (one in several million).[386] Risk for human herpesvirus-8 through blood transfusion has been demonstrated but true incidence and consequences of such transmission are unknown.[386] Parvovirus B19 causes transient viremia in potential blood donors and is not routinely screened for secondary to the rarity of blood product transmission and the mild illness it usually causes.[414] This can be a potential issue for patients with hematologic malignancies in which such infection could lead to prolonged reticulocytopenia and anemia. The recent emergence of bovine spongiform encephalopathy raised concerns about the ability to transmit variant Creutzfeldt-Jakob disease (vCJD) through blood transfusion. Although classic Creutzfeldt-Jakob disease does not appear to be transmissible through blood products, reports have confirmed transmission of vCJD in England.[386] After the emergence of West Nile virus (WNV), the virus was soon thereafter found to be transmissible through blood transfusion. Screening was implemented quite quickly but raises the concern for transmission of other similar viruses or of influenza during a pandemic situation.[386]

Iron Overload from Chronic Transfusion

Transfusion-related iron overload in children with cancer is an iatrogenic complication of supportive care. With the intensive therapies given to children, especially with AML, solid tumors, and hematopoietic stem cell transplant, we may expect to see this complication more often in survivors of childhood cancer. Total body iron stores are approximately 3 g, of which 1 g is in the liver and 2 g is in the blood. Each milliliter of packed RBCs contains 1 mg of iron. Therefore, multiple transfusions of RBCs, over weeks to months, can add up to large amounts of transfused iron. Ferritin levels are an inexpensive and noninvasive measure of hepatic iron but values can be confounded by chronic inflammation.[415] Accurate quantification of total body iron can be accomplished by liver biopsy, measurement with a superconducting quantum interference device (SQUID), or proton magnetic resonance imaging (R2 MRI).[416–420] SQUID is a very sensitive magnetometer used to measure small magnetic fields, such as those created by iron in the human body but has extremely limited availability. Liver iron concentration (LIC) by liver biopsy remains the gold standard; however, noninvasive methods are becoming more widely utilized. Although Angelucci et al. showed that LIC accurately reflects total body iron stores, T2* MRI is emerging as the new standard for cardiac iron assessment.[417,421]

Iron overload has been implicated as a risk factor for severe infection and invasive aspergillosis after stem cell transplantation.[422,423] Other clinical manifestations are typically not evident for many years in patients receiving chronic transfusion therapy. Children who have received intensive short-term transfusion may be at risk for late adverse effects of iron overload. The organ systems most profoundly affected are the liver, heart, and endocrine glands. When confounded by potential late effects of other therapies, including chemotherapy and radiation, the organ toxicity may be dramatic.

Iron overload has been shown to occur in children after treatment of acute lymphoblastic leukemia.[424] Therefore, *all* childhood cancer survivors should be screened for transfusional iron overload. Screening should include an assessment of quantity of transfused cells (and an approximation of transfused iron), a serum ferritin level, and transferrin saturation.[424] If these studies indicate iron overload, the patient should also be screened for hereditary hemachromatosis. Should the screening indicate substantial iron overload, determination of total iron body stores with liver biopsy, SQUID assessment, or R2 MRI may be indicated.

Halonen et al. have shown that a majority of young children have reversible iron overload during growth without further treatment.[424] Other approaches to iron overload include phlebotomy and chelation. No published guidelines exist, but patients who no longer require transfusion support and have recovered from the marrow-suppressive effects of therapy are most likely to benefit from phlebotomy, especially adolescent males. We recommend that those children with persistently elevated serum ferritin of more than 1,000 μg per L have measurement of total body iron stores by liver biopsy or a noninvasive method and then institute monthly phlebotomy therapy. Depending on clinical response to treatment, 1 to 2 years of phlebotomy may be required and efficacy as measured by decreasing ferritin levels and total body iron stores should be monitored at 6- to 12-month intervals. Therapy can be stopped once serum ferritin levels and LIC have reached the normal range (LIC < 1.6 mg per g dry weight liver).

Alloimmunization

As previously outlined, alloimmunization directed against class I HLA or platelet-specific antigens is a common problem with frequent platelet transfusion. Primary alloimmunization can be reduced by avoiding unnecessary transfusions. Patients who develop platelet refractoriness secondary to platelet antibodies may potentially benefit from crossmatched or HLA-matched platelet transfusions. In addition, patients who are undergoing intensive chemotherapy for AML, solid tumors, and those receiving hematopoietic stem cell transplants are likely to require multiple RBC transfusions and are at greater risk for the development of RBC alloimmunization as well. Any patient with a delayed HTR should have a work-up to determine the underlying RBC alloantibody to avoid repeat transfusion with these implicated RBC antigens.[425]

HEMATOPOIETIC COLONY-STIMULATING FACTORS

This section discusses the use of hematopoietic growth factors as supportive care for children with cancer. There are a multitude of publications on cytokine use in oncology, especially in adults. The focus here is on the highest quality data: final

reports of prospective RCTs or meta-analyses of such trials. Reference to adult data will be made only when data are lacking in children.

Several excellent general reviews are recommended.[426–429] The reader should also be aware of the extensive guidelines provided by ASCO and the American Society of Hematology (ASH), although these are directed primarily at the adult patient.[430,431]

Erythropoietins

EPO is a 14- to 39-kDa sialoglycoprotein whose gene is located on chromosome 7 and is primarily produced in the cortical region of the kidney. Its production is intimately linked to hypoxia, and its receptors are found primarily on erythroblasts and erythrocyte colony-forming unit cells. The main effect of EPO is the induction of proliferation and terminal differentiation of RBC progenitors. Recombinant human EPO alfa (rHuEPO) and darbepoetin alfa, which contains two additional carbohydrate chains leading to a two to threefold longer circulating half-life, are the current FDA-approved products (EPO-stimulating agents, herein ESAs).[432] Although darbepoetin has undergone a phase I trial in pediatric patients with chemotherapy-induced anemia, which showed adequate pharmacokinetics and no toxicity, it is currently not approved in the pediatric population.[433]

Multiple RCT studies in adults have demonstrated the ability of ESAs to increase hemoglobin in patients being treated with chemotherapy or radiotherapy, reduce the need for RBC transfusions, and improve QOL, especially anemia-associated fatigue.[434,435] The majority of the data in the literature regard adults and there are only six RCTs in the pediatric population published as peer-reviewed full manuscripts, most recently reviewed by Shankar.[436–442] These reports have included a mixture of patients with solid tumors, lymphomas, and ALL and utilized differing rHuEPO doses including 150 U per kg three times per week, 200 U per kg daily, and 450 to 900 U per kg weekly administered subcutaneously or intravenously. Like the adult studies, most of these pediatric studies report an increase in hemoglobin levels and decrease in RBC transfusions in the rHuEPO group. Specifically, three out of the five studies, which reported hemoglobin data, report a statistically significant increase in hemoglobin level, averaging 1.5 g per dL higher than that at randomization. Five out of the six studies reported RBC transfusion data and of these five, three report a significant reduction in transfusions amongst the rHuEPO group. Of note, one of these studies additionally showed a statistically significant decrease in the number of necessary platelet transfusions as well.[436] QOL data were collected by three studies, the largest of which showed no difference overall, although there was a significant improvement in the subset of patients aged from 5 to 7 years.[440] Two smaller studies, which contained only 30 and 15 patients, respectively, did show a trend toward improved performance status with the tools they used.[437,441]

Two recent trials of rHuEPO in adults were concerning for poor response rates and higher death rates in the rHuEPO treatment arm as compared with placebo control. One trial in women with metastatic breast cancer was stopped early due to an increased mortality rate in the patients receiving rHuEPO; the second trial in head and neck cancer patients reported an increase in disease recurrence in the rHuEPO treatment group as compared with controls.[443,444] Concern has also arisen as to the increased risk of venous thromboembolism with ESAs. A recent comprehensive meta-analyses by Bohlius et al., which included relevant studies from 1985 to 2005 including 57 trials involving 9,353 adult cancer patients reported: (a) a significantly reduced risk of blood transfusion (relative risk [RR] = 0.64, 95% confidence interval [CI] = 0.60 to 0.68), (b) significantly increased risk of thromboembolic events (RR = 1.67, 95% CI = 1.35 to 2.06), and (c) survival not improved and possibly even decreased in those treated with ESAs (hazard ratio [HR] = 1.08, 95% CI = 0.99 to 1.18).[434] Bohlius et al. hypothesize that the more recent trials aimed at a higher hemoglobin range (i.e., 12 to 14 g per dL for women and 13 to 15 g per dL for men) and this may have attributed to a higher relative risk for thromboembolism and subsequent decreased survival, although per their study this could not be concretely ascertained. Bennett et al. conducted a meta-analysis of the risk of venous thromboembolism and mortality and analyzed 51 trials with 13,611 patients with mortality data and 38 trials with 8,172 patients with venous thromboembolism data and reported (a) significantly increased risk of venous thromboembolism (RR = 1.57, 95% CI = 1.31 to 1.87) and (b) significantly increased mortality (HR = 1.10, 95% CI = 1.01 to 1.20) in the ESA-treated group as compared with controls.[445] Only one pediatric study has analyzed survival as an endpoint and reported no significant difference in progression-free survival and overall survival.[439] None of the pediatric studies have reported any cases of venous thromboembolism. Concern has also been raised in the past regarding recombinant EPO-induced pure RBC aplasia, but reports are rare and seem to be confined to patients with chronic renal failure and those mainly who have used EPO beta (Eprex, Johnson & Johnson), which is not licensed by the FDA for use in the United States.[446]

Concern has also been raised that decrease in survival may be secondary to the ubiquitous expression of EPO receptor (EPO-R) in cancer cells, and it has been hypothesized that the exogenous use of ESAs may have a direct effect on tumor cells by stimulation of tumor growth, inhibition of apoptosis, stimulation of angiogenesis within the tumor bed, or modulation of the effectiveness of chemoradiation. Batra et al. reported the expression of EPO and EPO-Rs in various pediatric tumors including neuroblastoma, Ewing's sarcoma, pediatric brain tumors (medulloblastoma, ependymoma, astrocytoma), Wilms' tumor, rhabdomyosarcoma, and hepatoblastoma.[447] In vitro exogenous EPO was shown to increase expression of antiapoptotic genes and increase production and secretion of angiogenic growth factors. Yasuda et al. reported similar results and postulated on the deprivation of EPO signaling as a potential oncologic therapy with a similar mechanism to the currently studied vascular endothelial growth factor inhibitors and angiogenesis inhibitors.[448] Similarly, Sartelet et al. reported an increased expression of EPO-R in neuroblastoma cell lines.[449] In their in vitro study, exogenous EPO did not contribute to tumor cell proliferation. No studies have been published which show an in vivo effect of ESAs on tumor growth or modulation of the effectiveness of chemoradiation.

Although multiple guidelines exist for adults, little is available in terms of pediatric guidelines. The updated ASH and ASCO guidelines by Rizzo et al. recommend rHuEPO or darbepoetin as a treatment option in adults with chemotherapy-induced anemia with a hemoglobin at or near 10 g per dL and cautioned against the use of ESAs in patients not receiving chemotherapy and in those at increased risk of thromboembolism.[431] The French National Cancer Institute is the first to publish pediatric guidelines and they conclude (a) systematic administration of ESAs is not recommended in pediatric cancer patients with anemia, (b) ESAs can be considered on a case-by-case basis in those patients with a contraindication to RBC transfusion, and (c) intravenous ESA use is the preferred method of administration.[450] The published literature implies an equipotency of ESAs whether given intravenously or

subcutaneously, but recent studies in the adult hemodialysis literature conclude that subcutaneous injection is approximately 30% more effective.[451–453] If ESAs are to be best utilized, serum iron and total iron-binding capacity should be monitored to detect relative iron deficiency that may limit the efficacy of the cytokine.[431,454] ESAs have not been evaluated in AML due to concerns about possible stimulation of leukemic cells.[455] In his editorial response to the French guidelines, Feusner agrees that currently there is not enough information to support the use of ESAs in pediatric patients with chemotherapy-induced anemia, and further studies are needed to delineate the true cost-effectiveness, true change in QOL, effect on tumor progression and survival as well as risks of side effects, especially venous thromboembolism, in the pediatric population prior to recommending their potential usage.[456]

Granulocyte Colony-Stimulating Factors

Improved survival in pediatric oncology is due in large part to increasingly more intense chemoradiotherapeutic treatments. Children receiving such treatment are at risk of serious infectious complications during periods of pronounced and especially prolonged neutropenia. Attempts to prevent this severe neutropenia have included delay or reduction of chemotherapy dosing, and prophylactic antibiotics. The former method is generally not compatible with increased survival, and the latter has often led to emergence of resistant microbes and is generally discouraged by infectious disease experts. During the last 20 years neutrophilic CSFs (i.e., G-CSF, granulocyte-macrophage CSF [GM-CSF], PEG-GCSF) have been studied intensively in adult oncology patients, and have been shown to be beneficial in certain situations. The data in children are fewer and will be discussed below.

Homeostasis of Neutrophil Production

The CSFs are proteins that are produced in response to a reduction in numbers of the peripheral blood elements. They can be generally thought of as those acting on early hematopoietic progenitors (interleukin-3 [IL-3], IL-6, IL-11, stem-cell factor, and flt3 ligand) and those acting later with effects primarily restricted to a single lineage (G-CSF, GM-CSF, and erythropoietin). Under normal conditions, serum levels of the CSFs are low, but they can increase in response to specific stimuli, such as infection or reduction in the number of terminally differentiated cells.[457] The actual level of G-CSF appears to be controlled by changes in both its rate of production and its clearance. High neutrophil levels increase the clearance of CSF.[458] Normal levels are approximately 25 pg per mL, whereas levels of 1,000 pg per mL or more can be seen in response to severe infection.[459]

GM-CSF is a 127-amino acid, 14- to 35-kDa glycosylated protein whose gene is located on chromosome 5q21–32. It has activity on multiple cell lineages, including monocytes as well as neutrophils. It was the first FDA-approved cytokine used to stimulate myelopoiesis in the posttransplant setting.

G-CSF (filgrastim) is a 207-amino acid, 18- to 22-kDa protein whose gene is located on chromosome 17q11–22. It is lineage specific to the neutrophil. The newest form of therapeutic CSF in this category is pegfilgrastim, a pegylated form of G-CSF. It has been evaluated in several adult trials and is claimed to provide similar granulocyte protection as the native G-CSF but with reduced frequency of administration.[460] It has received FDA approval for use in adults with nonmyeloid malignancies being treated with myelosuppressive chemotherapy.

To date, there have only been four published reports of pegfilgrastim use in children.[461–464] None of these reports are RCTs comparing this agent to the standard filgrastim. They were each single institutional reports of pegfilgrastim use in mainly older children (10 to 18 years of age) with various solid tumors. There were a total of 68 children treated with 219 injections of the agent at the usual dose of 100 µg per kg (no single dose > 6 mg). The reported side effects were quite minimal: only a 7.7% incidence, with most being mild bone pain. Before the role of this new agent can be properly assessed, there needs to be RCTs to determine its effectiveness, best dosage, and cost benefit compared with standard filgrastim.

Clinical Use of Neutrophilic Growth Factors

The use of myeloid CSFs has been described in four scenarios: (a) an attempt to ameliorate myelosuppression after chemotherapy (primary prophylaxis); (b) an attempt to prevent a recurrence of febrile neutropenia or a delay in subsequent chemotherapy administration (secondary prophylaxis); (c) treatment of established neutropenia to prevent an infection; and (d) treatment of an established episode of febrile neutropenia.

ASCO has developed guidelines for use of these agents (G-CSF and GM-CSF) based on rigorous review of the best available published data (generally RCTs). These were first published in 1994 and have been updated thrice since then: in 1996, 2000, and most recently in 2006.[430] The clearly indicated situations for the use of these CSFs in adults in nontransplant settings include: (a) prophylactic use in patients in whom the expected incidence of chemotherapy-induced neutropenia is at least 20%: and (b) in patients who have already suffered from an episode of chemotherapy-induced febrile neutropenia. The panel has concluded that the pediatric data are not conclusive, but in general suggest the guidelines for adult patients are applicable to children as well. The available prospective randomized trials in children are discussed later. The interested reader is referred to several excellent comprehensive reviews of the data in children.[427,465,466]

Primary Prophylaxis. Until very recently, the prevailing opinion was that the pediatric data did not clearly support a practice of primary prophylactic use of neutrophilic growth factors in children. There were some reports suggesting a benefit, but patient numbers were small and study designs were problematic. However, two recently published meta-analyses strongly suggest the available data does in fact support such a practice.[465,466]

Sung et al. have carefully analyzed the best data, sifting through 971 titles and abstracts, to find 53 full articles to review.[465] They identified 16 such reports that met their strict criteria of study populations consisting of patients younger than 18 years, randomizations occurring between CSF and placebo or no treatment, CSFs given after chemotherapy and before onset of neutropenia, and identical chemotherapy used immediately before the CSF or placebo/no treatment. These reports included use of G-CSF (11 studies) as well as GM-CSF (5 studies). They found a significant reduction in febrile neutropenia (rate ratio, 0.80; 95% CI, 0.67 to 0.95; $p = 0.01$), in hospitalization length (−1.9 days; 95% CI, −2.7 to −1.1 days; $p < 0.00001$), a reduction in documented infections (rate ratio, 0.78; 95% CI, 0.62 to 0.97; $p = 0.02$), and a reduction in amphotericin use (rate ratio, 0.50; 95% CI, 0.28 to 0.87; $p = 0.02$). There was, however, no significant reduction in infection-related mortality (rate ratio, 1.02; 95% CI, 0.34 to 3.06; $p = 0.97$). Of importance, the mean rate of febrile neutropenia in the control arms in this analysis was 57% (range, 39% to 100%). More recently, Wittman et al. conducted another meta-analysis of the pediatric data and arrived at essentially the same conclusions as did Sung et al.[466]

This suggests, at the least, that CSF use in this setting could reduce morbidity, and perhaps cost, in children being treated with moderate to severe myelosuppressive chemotherapy.

Secondary Prophylaxis. There are no randomized trials of G-CSF or GM-CSF in children who have sustained episodes of febrile neutropenia with prior cycles of chemotherapy. In adults, the data are very limited and not sufficient to warrant a recommendation by ASCO. A more recent review of hematopoietic growth factors in pediatric oncology does not discuss this issue.[427] Overall, it would appear that use of these growth factors for this purpose cannot be justified by the available data.

Treatment of Febrile Neutropenia. Published recommendations from expert panels are discrepant on the issue of treatment of febrile neutropenia. European experts (pediatric oncology and bone marrow transplant specialists) concluded in a 1998 report that CSF support was indicated for children with chemotherapy-induced febrile neutropenia if they are at increased risk.[426] This included patients with any of the following: proven pseudomonal or fungal infection, multiorgan dysfunction, pneumonia, prolonged neutropenia (>28 days), uncontrolled sepsis, or age less than 12 months. In a later review of this topic, Lehrnbecher and Welte came to similar but not as inclusive conclusions.[427] They conclude that use of growth factors in patients with factors "predictive of clinical deterioration" might be reasonable. These factors included pneumonia, hypotension, multiorgan dysfunction, or fungal infection. The latest update by ASCO concludes that CSFs should not be routinely used in patients with "uncomplicated" fever and neutropenia.[430] Their definition of "uncomplicated" was quite broad: fever of less than 11 days' duration; no evidence of pneumonia, cellulitis, abscess, sinusitis, hypotension, multiorgan dysfunction, or invasive fungal infection; and no uncontrolled malignancy. This recommendation goes on to suggest (similar to the two other reviews cited earlier) that patients with certain features suggestive of increased risk might benefit from CSF use: profound neutropenia (ANC <100), uncontrolled primary disease, pneumonia, hypotension, multiorgan dysfunction, and invasive fungal infection.

In pediatrics, there have been three randomized prospective trials of CSF use in the setting of febrile neutropenia.[467–469] Mitchell et al. found in 112 patients that G-CSF (5 mg per kg per day) shortened median hospital stay (5 vs. 7 days; $p = 0.04$), days of antibiotic use (5 vs. 6 days; $p = 0.02$), and reduced the cost of treatment of the febrile neutropenic episode by 29%.[467] Riikonen et al. used GM-CSF in 58 episodes of febrile neutropenia in 40 children, at a dose of 5 mg per kg per day.[468] They also found benefit: a reduction in days receiving antibiotics (7.0 vs. 8.5 days; $p < 0.05$), a nonsignificant reduction in time to resolution of febrile neutropenia, and, most significant, a reduction in total hospital days (9.0 vs. 10.0 days; $p < 0.05$). Most recently, a study of 66 patients in the Children's Oncology Group (COG) was stopped early owing to a significant reduction in duration of febrile neutropenia (4 vs. 9 days; $p < 0.0001$) and in hospital days (4 vs. 5 days; $p < 0.04$) between the treatment group (G-CSF at 5 mg per kg per day) and the matched control group.[469]

Although none of the above pediatric studies demonstrated a difference in overall survival, they did show significant reductions of other endpoints, which should improve the QOL and reduce overall expense (especially regarding reduction in length of hospitalization). Taken in aggregate, these data support the use of growth factors, especially in the higher-risk patients with febrile neutropenia. This conclusion also appears to be supported by the very recent exhaustive review by the Cochrane group of the published literature through 2002 on this topic.[470]

Use of Colony-Stimulating Factors to Enhance Chemotherapy Dose Intensity

Several laboratory studies and retrospective analyses in adult patients have correlated chemotherapeutic efficacy with the dose intensity of the chemotherapy delivered.[471,472] Early phase I and II trials of both G-CSF and GM-CSF achieved reductions in delays of scheduled full-dose chemotherapy.[473,474] These data suggest that CSF prophylaxis may permit increases in dose intensity of chemotherapy, with the possibility of consequent improvement in antineoplastic efficacy. Several pediatric studies have evaluated chemotherapeutic regimens in which the doses of agents were escalated beyond the usual maximal doses by using CSF support. These studies demonstrated the relative safety of this practice, but whether this translated into better eventual disease control and patient survival was not evaluated.[475–477]

Of the published trials in pediatrics of CSF-supported intensive chemotherapy with controls, only two were prospective, randomized, and concurrently controlled.[478–483] Michel et al. evaluated G-CSF in 67 children with high-risk ALL.[480] They found that the dose intensity of chemotherapy was increased in the G-CSF group, while the days febrile, days of intravenous antibiotic use, and days in hospital were all significantly reduced. There was, however, absolutely no improvement in the 3-year disease-free survival. Michon et al., in a similarly designed trial in metastatic neuroblastoma (59 patients), found that G-CSF reduced the duration of severe neutropenia and intravenous antibiotic use after the first cycle of chemotherapy, but did not reduce the duration of hospital stay or the incidence of febrile neutropenia.[481] They found a trend for prolongation in event-free survival (2.4 years median for G-CSF group vs. 1.3 years for the controls; $p = 0.072$). Thus, the best-quality data published in pediatric patients have not shown a clear survival benefit for CSF use in this manner.

Another method for increasing dose intensity is to compress the interval between chemotherapy courses, with CSF support. A prospective randomized trial of this approach in pediatric AML was performed and did show enhanced antineoplastic effect and eventual improvement in long-term survival for children treated with more intensified chemotherapy.[484] The role of G-CSF in this improvement, however, was determined to be negligible and G-CSF is not routinely used in current AML trials in the COG.[485]

In conclusion, randomized trials to date have not convincingly shown a benefit in overall survival or disease-free survival for most tumors when the dose of chemotherapy was maintained and secondary prophylaxis with myeloid CSFs was used. Some, but not all, have shown a decrease in intravenous antibiotic usage or in hospital stay. The 2006 ASCO guidelines recommend that except for curable tumors or tumors for which data exist to maintain dose intensity, chemotherapy dose reduction should be considered, rather than CSF use, after neutropenic fever or prolonged neutropenia following prior cycles of chemotherapy.[430] The use of CSFs to maintain dose intensity should be limited to clinical research protocols. The excellent and very thorough recent review of this topic by Lehrnbecher and Welte comes to the same conclusion.[427]

Comparison of Granulocyte Colony-Stimulating Factor to Granulocyte-Macrophage Colony-Stimulating Factor

There have been very few published trials of G-CSF versus GM-CSF and only one focusing on children.[486] The Lydaki trial involved 39 children with malignant disease randomized to G-CSF or GM-CSF following chemotherapy.[486] All patients received the cytokine during two cycles of chemotherapy at the same dose of 5 mg per kg per day, given subcutaneously, starting 1 day following the end of chemotherapy and continuing until either the ANC exceeded 1,500 per mm³ or for a maximum of 14 days. There was a significant delay in ANC recovery for the patients treated with GM-CSF (2 to 4 days to reach ANC of 1,000), but no differences in IV antibiotic use, or in mean length of hospital stays. There also was no significant difference in toxicity observed: 2 out of 25 children receiving G-CSF had mild bone pain; 1 out of 14 children getting GM-CSF had mild pruritus.

A much larger study in adults compared the relative effectiveness of these two cytokines (at the same dose of 5 mg per kg per day), compared with placebo, when added to antibiotics for adults with chemotherapy-induced febrile neutropenia.[487] There were no statistically significant differences in ANC recovery, days with fever, hospital days, infection-related deaths, or estimated costs between these cytokines. Toxicity was mild and consisted of CSF-related fever in one patient receiving G-CSF compared with four patients receiving GM-CSF.

An even larger study of adults with solid tumors who became neutropenic after moderately intense chemotherapy had similar findings.[488] One hundred seventy patients were randomized between G-CSF and GM-CSF at doses of 5 mg per kg per day and 250 mg per m² per day, respectively. The cytokines were initiated from study enrollment (ANC < 500 per mm³) until the ANC rose to 1,500 per mm³. The time to reach ANC of greater than 500 per mm³ was no different, although the time to reach ANCs of 1,000 and 1,500 per mm³ was significantly shorter in the G-CSF patients, but of doubtful clinical significance (<1 full day difference). There was no difference in hospital admissions for neutropenic fever, mean length of hospitalization, or adverse events due to the cytokine administered.

The available data would suggest no clinically significant difference in efficacy between G-CSF and GM-CSF when used at doses of approximately 5 mg per kg and 250 mg per m², respectively. There appears to be a slightly higher incidence of fever and local reactions with GM-CSF.

Optimal Dose of Colony-Stimulating Factors

There has been one published full manuscript RCT and one randomized sequential crossover trial regarding the optimal dose of CSFs in pediatric patients.[489,490]

The earliest reported trial was a short one describing the effects of 100 versus 200 mg per m² per day of G-CSF (given IV over 1 hour) in 29 children with a mixture of leukemia and solid tumor diagnoses.[490] The trial design was a randomization of the two doses of G-CSF with crossover to the alternate dose following the next (identical) chemotherapy course. Effects were analyzed after just the two cycles of chemotherapy. The duration of severe neutropenia (ANC < 500 per mm³) and median time from neutrophil nadir to recovery (ANC > 500 per mm³) were significantly shorter following the higher G-CSF dose. However, the median duration of febrile neutropenia was not shortened significantly. Other clinically significant endpoints such as hospital days, use of antibiotics, relapse-free or overall survival, or costs were not evaluated. It should also be noted that the details of diagnoses, prior therapy, or chemotherapy used in this CSF trial were not reported.

The RCT evaluated G-CSF at doses of 5 versus 10 mg per kg per day starting 24 hours after ICE chemotherapy (ifosfamide, carboplatin, etoposide) in 123 children with relapsed or refractory solid tumors.[490] The analysis was limited to effects seen following the first two cycles of this chemotherapy. There were no significant differences found in either the hematologic parameters (time to ANC 1,000 per mm^3, time to platelet count > 100,000 per mm^3, or incidence of ANC < 500 per mm^3) or clinical endpoints evaluated (incidence of bacterial or fungal infections, days febrile, incidence of hospitalization for parenteral antibiotics, tumor response, or overall survival). The only positive finding in support of the higher dose was a lower rate of grade IV thrombocytopenia (58% vs. 78%, $p = 0.022$). This finding was unexplained.

Based on these two studies, there is no published data to support an initial dose of greater than approximately 3 to 5 mg per kg of G-CSF or 250 mg per m^2 GM-CSF in pediatric patients for the purpose of ameliorating marrow toxicity following nonmyeloablative chemotherapy. The Europeans have come to the same conclusion.[334]

Optimal Timing of Colony-Stimulating Factor Use

When to Start

There has been only one RCT of the optimal starting time for CSFs following myelosuppressive chemotherapy in children.[491] In this trial, 18 children with mainly solid tumors (one with ALL) were randomized to start G-CSF (5 mg per kg per day subcutaneously) at 1 day (d +1) or 5 days (d +5) after completion of chemotherapy. Each group received the same chemotherapy for two successive cycles with a start time of d +1 for one course, and d +5 for the other. The mean duration of neutropenia (ANC < 500 per mm^3) was 6.8 versus 7.4 days; there were seven febrile neutropenic episodes versus five; and the mean number of hospital days on parenteral antibiotics was 2.3 versus 3.3 days in the d +1 group versus the d +5 group, respectively. None of these were statistically significant differences.

In adults, this question has been evaluated in several RCTs, all of which show that delay in starting the CSF is safe. These include patients with ALL during remission induction and patients in the transplant setting.[492-496]

When to Stop

The standard recommendation, to continue G-CSF until the ANC has reached 10,000 per mm^3 beyond the expected neutrophil nadir, has no good evidence-based support.[497] In the study by Beveridge et al. comparing G-CSF to GM-CSF, the CSF was continued until the ANC reached 1,500 per mm^3.[488] They found, in 181 adults, there were no readmissions to the hospital for fever with neutropenia using ANC of 1,500 per mm^3 as the stopping point for CSF administration. The exact duration of CSF use past the chemotherapy nadir that should be adopted is still not clear, but it would appear there has been sufficient study of this issue to conclude that the traditional ANC level to be attained (10,000 per mm^3) is excessive.

Route of Administration

CSFs can be given either intravenously or subcutaneously. Although the official company recommendation for G-CSF is to use the same dose for either route of administration, there are data from adults to suggest they are not equivalent (D. Woo, Amgen, personal communication, 2002). Kaneko et al. found that in adults with lymphoma, the optimal dose for primary prophylaxis was 50 mg per m^2 for subcutaneous administration versus 100 to 200 mg per m^2 for intravenous administration of G-CSF.[498] Similarly, Eguchi et al. found the dose of G-CSF to alleviate neutropenia in patients with advanced lung cancer undergoing chemotherapy to be 50%

less when given subcutaneously as compared to intravenously.[499] There are similar reports regarding GM-CSF.[500,501] There are no published prospectively collected data in pediatric oncology patients comparing intravenous versus subcutaneous administration of CSFs. The current practice appears to be to use the same dose, but it is not clearly supported by the literature.

Platelet Growth Factors

Platelet transfusions are currently the only effective acute treatment for severe thrombocytopenia. Although generally well tolerated in the early phases of treatment, problems can develop (e.g., transmission of infection, transfusion reactions, alloimmunization), and there is a relatively limited supply of this product.[502-504] This has been a stimulus for the ongoing search for specific and effective platelet growth factors.

Multiple growth factors are known to have stimulatory effects on platelet production *in vitro* including thrombopoietin (TPO), stem cell factor (SCF), stromal cell-derived factor-1 (SDF-1), fibroblast growth factor, IL-1, IL-3, IL-6, IL-11, GM-CSF, leukemia inhibitory factor, and EPO.[505-507] *In vivo* activity has been limited to TPO and SCF although IL-11 has also shown benefit in some patients.[508,509] Only IL-11 is currently licensed in the United States for use in thrombocytopenia due to myelosuppressive chemotherapy. TPO receptor agonists have recently been approved for the treatment of adult immune thrombocytopenic purpura (ITP) and are being studied for other purposes. IL-1, IL-3, IL-6, and GM-CSF have shown *in vitro* activity and some benefit in clinical studies but have been discontinued from clinical trials secondary to unacceptable toxicities or an insignificant increase in platelet counts.[510] PIXY 321, an IL-3/GM-CSF chimeric molecule has been withdrawn after disappointing results in adults and the development of neutralizing antibodies.[511-513] Similarly, promegapoietin, a TPO/IL-3 chimeric molecule, which showed promising primate results, has been discontinued from clinical trials secondary to the development of antibody formation.[514,515]

Thrombopoietin Receptor Agonists

TPO is the ligand for the c-Mpl receptor and is the primary physiologic regulator of megakaryocyte and platelet development. It has been shown *in vitro* and *in vivo* to stimulate megakaryocyte number and ploidy, as well as to increase the platelet count in 5 to 14 days in a normal marrow.[516-518] Two different TPO products were originally developed: a glycosylated recombinant human TPO (rHuTPO) that is identical to the native molecule, and a recombinant nonglycosylated and truncated molecule called megakaryocyte growth and development factor (rHuMGDF). In preclinical trials these products were shown to increase platelet counts in 5 to 14 days. Both products were discontinued after clinical trials reported the development of late-appearing platelet-neutralizing antibodies in volunteers and patients to rHuMGDF.[519,520]

RHuMGDF and rHuTPO had demonstrated some effect on platelet transfusions secondary to chemotherapy-induced thrombocytopenia in adults and children after solid tumors and lymphoma.[521-528] Of the seven noted adult studies, five utilized PEG-rHuMGDF and two used rHuTPO. All deemed exogenous TPO useful with overall results showing a trend toward avoidance of platelet transfusions and improvement in the platelet nadir. Only three adult studies reported as to whether delays in chemotherapy were avoided and this occurred in two of the three studies. Survival was not a reported end result in any of the studies and important side effects included an increased risk of thromboembolism and a dose-dependent risk of thrombocytosis. The sole pediatric study was limited to only 12 patients and although it did show an improvement in hematologic time to recovery and number of platelet transfusions, it was not an RCT, using historical controls instead. In addition, there were no reportable side effects although this was limited by the small sample size.[528] Similar trials in patients with AML failed to demonstrate any clinically meaningful benefit, with no avoidance of platelet transfusion or improvement in platelet nadir.[529–532] The timing and therefore optimization of rHuTPO administration relative to the chemotherapy given and the myelosuppressive intensity of the chemotherapy was an area that was noted to need further investigation.[526,533]

Considering the early promising results with rHuMDGF and rHuTPO, second-generation TPO-receptor agonists are currently being studied. These drugs include TPO peptide mimetics: AMG-531 (Romiplostim), Fab 59 and PEG-TPOmp, TPO nonpeptide mimetics: Eltrombopag and AKR-501 as well as TPO agonist antibodies: TPO minibodies [VB22B sc(Fv)2] and domain subclass-converted TPO agonist antibodies (MA01G4G344).[429] Indications currently under investigation in adults include autoimmune thrombocytopenia, thrombocytopenia associated with chronic liver disease, thrombocytopenia associated with the treatment of HCV infection, thrombocytopenia induced by chemotherapy for malignancy, thrombocytopenia associated with intrinsic marrow abnormalities, thrombocytopenia associated with the treatment of hematologic malignancy, and potentially for improvement of stem cell mobilization.[534] Phase I/II clinical trials for Romiplostim and Eltrombopag have shown dose-dependent increases in platelet counts without the development of neutralizing antibodies.[534–537] Eltrombopag and Romiplostim have both been recently FDA approved for adults with ITP after Phase III studies showed a durable platelet response in this patient population with a tolerable side effect profile.[538] Further study on potential side effects including thrombocytosis, thrombosis, tumor/leukemia cell growth, interaction with other cytokines, formation of neutralizing antibodies crossreactive with native TPO, stem cell depletion, platelet activation and vascular aggregation (seen in baboons with recombinant TPO), increased bone marrow reticulin or collagen deposition (secondary to TGFβ), and rebound thrombocytopenia below baseline upon sudden cessation of therapy are warranted.[429,539] No studies to date using the TPO-R agonists have been published in chemotherapy-induced thrombocytopenia.[537] No pediatric data are available to date. TPO-R agonists may play a role in mobilization of stem cells for hematopoietic stem cell transplantation but further studies are warranted.[540,541]

Interleukin-11

IL-11 stimulates the maturation of megakaryocytes through increasing the ploidy of the cells.[542–544] In preclinical trials, it stimulated platelet production in mice, resulting in a maximum increase in platelet count at 14 to 21 days.[543,545] IL-11 exerts pleiotropic effects on bone remodeling, chondrocytes, neurons, adipocytes, gastrointestinal and bronchial epithelium in addition to its effects on hematopoiesis.[546] Eight notable studies were found in the literature: two in adult patients with breast cancer, one in adult patients with a variety of solid tumors and lymphoma, three in adult patients with AML, one after autologous transplant in adults with breast cancer, and one study in children with solid tumors or lymphoma.[547–554] In the adult studies in solid tumors and lymphoma, including the study after autologous transplant, the data were promising for an increase in platelet counts with IL-11. Gordon et al. showed a dose-dependent increase in platelet count with a mean 19% decrease in hematocrit with 75 μg per kg as the maximally tolerated dose.[547] Antibody formation was confirmed in one patient and possible in a second with five patients being removed from study due to adverse effects possibly secondary to recombinant IL-11 therapy. Isaacs et al. and Tepler et al. showed a significant decrease in platelet transfusion in their placebo-controlled randomized studies whereas Vredenburgh et al. reported a trend toward decreased transfusions.[548,549,553] Side effects were concerning for fluid retention leading to palpitations, dyspnea, edema, headache, and symptomatic atrial arrhythmias. On the other hand, IL-11 had no effect in the three studies in patients with AML.[550–552] None of the studies in adults showed any benefit in overall survival.[547–553] Finally, in the one phase I/II study in pediatrics, Cairo et al. looked at 47 patients with a mean age of 10.5 years with a maximal tolerated dose of 50 μg per kg per day.[554] Although there appeared to be a decrease in median time to platelet recovery and median number of platelet transfusions after ICE chemotherapy, this was compared with historic controls as the study was not a randomized placebo-controlled trial. One patient was noted to develop anti-IL-11 antibodies. In addition, the study was concerning for clinically important adverse side effects (percent affected) including papilledema (15.9%), periosteal bone changes (11.4%), cardiomegaly (20.5%), edema (29.5%), and tachycardia (45.5%). This limited data strongly suggest that IL-11 use in pediatric oncology currently be restricted to clinical trials in order to better define its proper role in therapy.

References

1. Hockenberry MJ, Hinds PS, Barrera P, et al. Incidence of anemia in children with solid tumors or Hodgkin disease. J Pediatr Hematol Oncol 2002;24:35–37.
2. Green DM, Breslow NE, Beckwith JB, et al. Comparison between single-dose and divided-dose administration of dactinomycin and doxorubicin for patients with Wilms' tumor: a report from the National Wilms' Tumor Study Group. J Clin Oncol 1998;16:237–245.
3. Nachman J, Sather HN, Cherlow JM, et al. Response of children with high-risk acute lymphoblastic leukemia treated with and without cranial irradiation: a report from the Children's Cancer Group. J Clin Oncol 1998;16:920–930.
4. Borsi JD, Ferencz T, Csaki C, et al. Transfusion requirements of children with cancer and the use of recombinant erythropoietin for the prevention and treatment of cytostatics induced anemia in children [abstract]. Can J Infect Dis 1995;6(suppl C):235C.
5. Michon J. Incidence of anemia in pediatric cancer patients in Europe: results of a large, international survey. Med Pediatr Oncol 2002;39:448–450.
6. Groopman JE, Itri LM. Chemotherapy-induced anemia in adults: incidence and treatment. J Natl Cancer Inst 1999;91:1616–1634.
7. Sobrero A, Puglisi F, Guglielmi A, et al. Fatigue: a main component of anemia symptomatology. Semin Oncol 2001;28(2, suppl 8):15–18.
8. Cazzola M. Mechanisms of anaemia in patients with malignancy: implications for the clinical use of recombinant human erythropoietin. Med Oncol 2000;17(suppl 1):S11–S16.
9. Stasi R, Abriani L, Beccaglia P, et al. Cancer-related fatigue: evolving concepts in evaluation and treatment. Cancer 2003;98:1786–1801.
10. Cohen BJ, Beard S, Knowles WA, et al. Chronic anemia due to parvovirus B19 infection in a bone marrow transplant patient after platelet transfusion. Transfusion 1997;37:947–952.
11. Corbett TJ, Saw H, Popat U, et al. Successful treatment of parvovirus B19 infection and red cell aplasia occurring after an allogeneic bone marrow transplant. Bone Marrow Transplant 1995;16:711–713.
12. Koch WC, Massey G, Russell CE, et al. Manifestations and treatment of human parvovirus B19 infection in immunocompromised patients. J Pediatr 1990;116:355–359.

13. Rao SP, Miller ST, Cohen BJ. Severe anemia due to B19 parvovirus infection in children with acute leukemia in remission. Am J Pediatr Hematol Oncol 1990;12:194–197.

14. El-Mahallawy HA, Mansour T, El-Din SE, et al. Parvovirus B19 infection as a cause of anemia in pediatric acute lymphoblastic leukemia patients during maintenance chemotherapy. J Pediatr Hematol Oncol 2004;26:403–406.

15. Parsyan A, Candotti D. Human erythrovirus B19 and blood transfusion—an update. Transfusion Med 2007;17:263–278.

16. Eid AJ, Brown RA, Patel R, et al. Parvovirus B19 infection after transplantation: a review of 98 cases. Clin Infect Dis 2006;43:40–48.

17. Tang JW, Lau JS, Wong SY, et al. Dose-by-dose virological and hematological responses to intravenous immunoglobulin in an immunocompromised patient with persistent parvovirus B19 infection. J Med Virol 2007;79:1401–1405.

18. Hagihara M, Tsuchiya T, Hyodo O, et al. Clinical effects of infusing anti-Epstein-Barr virus (EBV)-specific cytotoxic T-lymphocytes into patients with severe chronic active EBV infection. Int J Hematol 2003;78:62–68.

19. Kaptan K, Beyan C, Ural AU, et al. Successful treatment of severe aplastic anemia associated with human parvovirus B19 and Epstein-Barr virus in a healthy subject with allo-BMT. Am J Hematol 2001;67:252–255.

20. Alpert G, Fleisher GR. Complications of infection with Epstein-Barr virus during childhood: a study of children admitted to the hospital. Pediatr Infect Dis 1984;3:304–307.

21. Almeida-Porada GD, Ascensao JL. Cytomegalovirus as a cause of pancytopenia. Leuk Lymphoma 1996;21:217–223.

22. Adachi N, Kiwaki K, Tsuchiya H, et al. Fatal cytomegalovirus myocarditis in a seronegative ALL patient. Acta Paediatr Jpn 1995;37:211–216.

23. Grant MJ, Huether SE, Witte MK. Effect of red blood cell transfusion on oxygen consumption in the anemic pediatric patient. Pediatr Crit Care Med 2003;4:459–464.

24. Mock V, Olsen M. Current management of fatigue and anemia in patients with cancer. Semin Oncol Nurs 2003;19(4, suppl 2):36–41.

25. Cunningham RS. Anemia in the oncology patient: cognitive function and cancer. Cancer Nurs 2003;26(6 suppl):38S–42S.

26. Hockenberry-Eaton M, Hinds PS. Fatigue in children and adolescents with cancer: evolution of a program of study. Semin Oncol Nurs 2000;16:261–272, discussion 272–278.

27. Hofman M, Ryan JL, Figueroa-Moseley CD, et al. Cancer-related fatigue: the scale of the problem. Oncologist 2007;12(S1):4–10.

28. Wagner LI, Cella D. Fatigue and cancer: causes, prevalence and treatment approaches. Brit J Cancer 2004;91:822–828.

29. Vogelzang NJ, Breitbart W, Cella D, et al. Patient, caregiver, and oncologist perceptions of cancer-related fatigue: results of a tripart assessment survey. The fatigue coalition. Semin Hematol 1997;34(3, suppl 2):4–12.

30. Hockenberry MJ, Hinds PS, Barrera P, et al. Three instruments to assess fatigue in children with cancer: the child, parent and staff perspectives. J Pain Symptom Manage 2003;25:319–328.

31. Hinds PS, Hockenberry M, Tong X, et al. Validity and reliability of a new instrument to measure cancer-related fatigue in adolescents. J Pain Symptom Manage 2007;34:607–618.

32. Knight K, Wade S, Balducci L. Prevalence and outcomes of anemia in cancer: a systematic review of the literature. Am J Med 2004;116(suppl 7A):11S–26S.

33. Van-Steenkiste J. Pharmacotherapy of chemotherapy-induced anaemia. Expert Opin Pharmacother 2003;4:2221–2227.

34. Estrin JT, Schocket L, Kregenow R, et al. A retrospective review of blood transfusions in cancer patients with anemia. Oncologist 1999;4:318–324.

35. Caro JJ, Salas M, Ward A, et al. Anemia as an independent prognostic factor for survival in patients with cancer: a systemic, quantitative review. Cancer 2001;91:2214–2221.

36. Glaspy J. The impact of epoetin alfa on quality of life during cancer chemotherapy: a fresh look at an old problem. Semin Hematol 1997;34(3, suppl 2):20–26.

37. Cella D. The Functional Assessment of Cancer Therapy-Anemia (FACT-An) Scale: a new tool for the assessment of outcomes in cancer anemia and fatigue. Semin Hematol 1997;34(3, suppl 2):13–19.

38. Mustian KM, Morrow GR, Carroll JK, et al. Integrative nonpharmacologic behavioral interventions for the management of cancer-related fatigue. Oncologist 2007;12(S1):52–67.

39. Carroll JK, Kohli S, Mustian KM, et al. Pharmacologic treatment of cancer-related fatigue. Oncologist 2007;12(S1):43–51.

40. Minton O, Richardson A, Sharpe M, et al. A systematic review and meta-analysis of the pharmacological treatment of cancer-related fatigue. J Natl Cancer Inst 2008;100:1155–1166.

41. Hinds PS, Hockenberry M, Rai SN, et al. Nocturnal awakenings, sleep environment interruptions, and fatigue in hospitalized children with cancer. Oncol Nurs Forum 2007;34:393–402.

42. Bosanquet N, Tolley K. Treatment of anaemia in cancer patients: implications for supportive care in the National Health Service Cancer Plan. Curr Med Res Opin 2003;19:643–650.

43. Buchanan GR. Blood transfusions in children with cancer and hematologic disorders: why, when, and how? (Commentary). Pediatr Blood Cancer 2005;44:114–116.

44. Wong EC, Perez-Albuerne E, Moscow JA, et al. Transfusion management strategies: a survey of practicing pediatric hematology/oncology specialists. Pediatr Blood Cancer 2005;44:119–127.

45. Rossetto CL, McMahon JE. Current and future trends in transfusion therapy. J Pediatr Oncol Nurs 2000;17:160–173.

46. Hardy JF. Should we reconsider triggers for red blood cell transfusion? Acta Anaesthesiol Belg 2003;54:287–295.

47. Lacroix J, Hébert PC, Hutchinson JS, et al. Transfusion strategies for patients in paediatric intensive care units. N Engl J Med 2007;365:1609–1619.

48. Marec-Berard P, Blay JY, Schell M, et al. Risk model predictive of severe anemia requiring RBC transfusion after chemotherapy in pediatric solid tumor patients. J Clin Oncol 2003;21:4235–4238.

49. Ruggiero A, Riccardi R. Interventions for anemia in pediatric cancer patients. Med Pediatr Oncol 2002;39:451–454.

50. Tas F, Eralp Y, Basaran M, et al. Anemia in oncology practice: relation to diseases and their therapies. Am J Clin Oncol 2002;25:371–379.

51. Barnard D, Rogers ZR. Blood component therapy. In: Altman A, ed. Supportive care of children with cancer: current therapy and guidelines from the Children's Oncology Group. Baltimore and London: The Johns Hopkins University Press, 2004:39–57.

52. Gibson BE, Todd A, Roberts I, et al. Transfusion guidelines for neonates and older children. Br J Haematol 2004;124:433–453.

53. Wu WC, Rathore SS, Wang Y, et al. Blood transfusion in elderly patients with acute myocardial infarction. N Engl J Med 2001;345:1230–1236.

54. Davies SC, Kinsey SE. Clinical aspects of paediatric blood transfusion: cellular components. Vox Sang 1994;67(suppl 5):50–53.

55. Norfolk DR, Ancliffe PJ, Contreras M, et al. Consensus Conference on Platelet Transfusion, Royal College of Physicians of Edinburgh, 27–28 November 1997. Synopsis of background papers. Br J Haematol 1998;101:609–617.

56. Wandt H, Frank M, Ehninger G, et al. Safety and cost effectiveness of a $10 \times 10(9)/L$ trigger for prophylactic platelet transfusions compared with the traditional $20 \times 10(9)/L$ trigger: a prospective comparative trial in 105 patients with acute myeloid leukemia. Blood 1998;91:3601–3606.

57. Ho CH. The hemostatic effect of packed red cell transfusion. Transfusion 1998;38:1011–1014.

58. Livio M, Gotti E, Marchesi D, et al. Uraemic bleeding: role of anaemia and beneficial effect of red cell transfusions. Lancet 1982;2:1013–1015.

59. Rintels PB, Kenney RM, Crowley JP. Therapeutic support of the patient with thrombocytopenia. Hematol Oncol Clin North Am 1994;8:1131–1157.

60. Fernandez F, Goudable C, Sie P, et al. Low haematocrit and prolonged bleeding time in uraemic patients: effect of red cell transfusions. Br J Haematol 1985;59:139–148.

61. Paul Gann Blood Safety Act. In: California Codes, Health and Safety Code Section 1645, 1991.

62. Josephson CD, Hillyer CD. Blood components. In: Hillyer C, Strauss R, Luban NL, eds. Handbook of pediatric transfusion medicine. San Diego, CA: Academic Press, 2004:27–44.

63. Davies P, Robertson S, Hedge S, et al. Calculating the required transfusion volume in children. Transfusion 2007;47:212–216.

64. Walker RH. Special report: transfusion risks. Am J Clin Pathol 1987;88:374–378.

65. Raife TJ. Adverse effects of transfusions caused by leukocytes. J Intraven Nurs 1997;20:238–244.

66. Logdberg LE. Leukoreduced products: prevention of leukocyte-related transfusion associated adverse effects. In: Hillyer C, Strauss R, Luban NL, eds. Handbook of pediatric transfusion medicine. San Diego, CA: Academic Press, 2004:85–92.

67. Corwin HL, AuBuchon JP. Is leukoreduction of blood components for everyone? JAMA 2003;289:1993–1995.

68. Goodnough LT. Universal leukoreduction of cellular blood components in 2001? No. Am J Clin Pathol 2001;115:674–677.

69. Vamvakas EC, Blajchman MA. Universal WBC reduction: the case for and against. Transfusion 2001;41:691–712.

70. Chu RW. Leukocytes in blood transfusion: adverse effects and their prevention. Hong Kong Med J 1999;5:280–284.

71. Dzik WH. Leukoreduction of blood components. Curr Opin Hematol 2002;9:521–526.

72. van Marwijk Kooy M, van Prooijen HC, Moes M, et al. Use of leukocyte-depleted platelet concentrates for the prevention of refractoriness and primary HLA alloimmunization: a prospective, randomized trial. Blood 1991;77:201–205.

73. Heddle NM. Universal leukoreduction and acute transfusion reactions: putting the puzzle together. Transfusion 2004;44:1–4.

74. Yazer MH, Podlosky L, Clarke G, et al. The effect of prestorage WBC reduction on the rates of febrile nonhemolytic transfusion reactions to platelet concentrates and RBC. Transfusion 2004;44:10–15.

75. King KE, Shirey RS, Thoman SK, et al. Universal leukoreduction decreases the incidence of febrile nonhemolytic transfusion reactions to RBCs. Transfusion 2004;44:25–29.

76. Paglino JC, Pomper GJ, Fisch GS, et al. Reduction of febrile but not allergic reactions to RBCs and platelets after conversion to universal prestorage leukoreduction. Transfusion 2004;44:16–24.

77. Blumberg N, Zhao H, Wang H, et al. The intention-to-treat principle in clinical trials and meta-analyses of leukoreduced blood transfusions in surgical patients. Transfusion 2007;47:573–581.

78. Blumberg N, Fine L, Gettings KF, et al. Decreased sepsis related to indwelling venous access devices coincident with implementation of universal leukoreduction of blood transfusions. Transfusion 2005;45:1632–1639.

79. Llewelyn CA, Taylor RS, Todd AA, et al. The effect of universal leukoreduction on postoperative infections and length of hospital stay in elective orthopedic and cardiac surgery. Transfusion 2004;44:489–500.

80. Cervia JS, Wenz B, Ortolano GA. Leukocyte reduction's role in the attenuation of infection risks among transfusion recipients. Clin Infect Dis 2007;45:1008–1013.

81. Utter GH, Nathens AB, Lee TH, et al. Leukoreduction of blood transfusions does not diminish transfusion-associated microchimerism in trauma patients. Transfusion 2006;46:1863–1869.

82. Kelher MR, Masuno T, Moore EE, et al. Plasma from stored packed red blood cells and MHC class I antibodies causes acute lung injury in a 2-event in vivo rat model. Blood 2009;113:2079–2087.

83. Vamvakas EC, Blajchman MA. Transfusion-related mortality: the ongoing risks of allogeneic blood transfusion and the available strategies for their prevention. Blood 2009;113:3406–3417.

84. Gregory KR. Leukocyte reduction guidance. December 13, 2001. Statement of the American Association of Blood Banks before the Blood Products Advisory Committee.

85. Kao KJ, Mickel M, Braine HG, et al. White cell reduction in platelet concentrates and packed red cells by filtration: a multicenter clinical trial. The Trap Study Group. Transfusion 1995;35:13–19.

86. Seftel MD, Growe GH, Petraszko T, et al. Universal prestorage leukoreduction in Canada decreases platelet alloimmunization and refractoriness. Blood 2004;103:333–339.

87. Shapiro MJ. To filter blood or universal leukoreduction: what is the answer? Crit Care 2004;8(S2):S27–S30.

88. Roback JD. Preparation of blood components to reduce cytomegalovirus and other infectious risks. In: Hillyer C, Strauss R, Luban NL, eds. Handbook of pediatric transfusion medicine. San Diego, CA: Academic Press, 2004:93–100.

89. Qu L, Xu S, Rowe D, et al. Efficacy of Epstein-Barr virus removal by leukoreduction of red blood cells. Transfusion 2005;45:591–595.

90. Visconti MR, Pennington J, Garner SF, et al. Assessment of removal of human cytomegalovirus from blood components by leukocyte depletion filters using real-time quantitative PCR. Blood 2004;103:1137–1139.

91. Vamvakas EC. Is white blood cell reduction equivalent to antibody screening in preventing transmission of cytomegalovirus by transfusion? A review of the literature and meta-analysis. Transfusion Med Rev 2005;19:181–199.

92. Roback JD, Drew WL, Laycock ME, et al. CMV DNA is rarely detected in healthy blood donors using validated PCR assays. Transfusion 2003;43:314–321.
93. Winston DJ, Ho WG, Howell CL, et al. Cytomegalovirus infections associated with leukocyte transfusions. Ann Intern Med 1980;93:671–675.
94. Bowden RA, Slichter SJ, Sayers M, et al. A comparison of filtered leukocyte-reduced and cytomegalovirus (CMV) seronegative blood products for the prevention of transfusion-associated CMV infection after marrow transplant. Blood 1995;86:3598–3603.
95. Hillyer CD, Emmens RK, Zago-Novaretti M, et al. Methods for the reduction of transfusion-transmitted cytomegalovirus infection: filtration versus the use of seronegative donor units. Transfusion 1994;34:929–934.
96. Nichols WG, Price TH, Gooley T, et al. Transfusion-transmitted cytomegalovirus infection after receipt of leukoreduced blood products. Blood 2003;101:4195–4200.
97. Ljungman P. Risk of cytomegalovirus transmission by blood products to immunocompromised patients and means for reduction. Br J Haematol 2004;125:107–116.
98. Blajchman MA, Goldman M, Freedman JJ, et al. Proceedings of a consensus conference: prevention of post-transfusion CMV in the era of universal leukoreduction. Transfus Med Rev 2001;15:1–20.
99. Wong EC. Irradiated products. In: Hillyer C, Strauss R, Luban NLC, eds. Handbook of pediatric transfusion medicine. San Diego, CA: Academic Press, 2004:101–112.
100. Anderson KC, Goodnough LT, Sayers M, et al. Variation in blood component irradiation practice: implications for prevention of transfusion-associated graft-versus-host disease. Blood 1991;77:2096–2102.
101. Moroff G, Luban NL. Prevention of transfusion-associated graft-versus-host disease. Transfusion 1992;32:102–103.
102. von Fliedner V, Higby DJ, Kim U. Graft-versus-host reaction following blood product transfusion. Am J Med 1982;72:951–961.
103. Lee TH, Donegan E, Slichter S, et al. Transient increase in circulating donor leukocytes after allogeneic transfusions in immunocompetent recipients compatible with donor cell proliferation. Blood 1995;85:1207–1214.
104. Lee TH, Paglieroni T, Ohto H, et al. Survival of donor leukocyte subpopulations in immunocompetent transfusion recipients: frequent long-term microchimerism in severe trauma patients. Blood 1999;93:3127–3139.
105. Dwyre DM, Holland PV. Transfusion-associated graft-versus-host disease. Vox Sang 2008;95:85–93.
106. Utter GH, Reed WF, Lee TH, et al. Transfusion-associated microchimerism. Vox Sang 2007;93:188–195.
107. Reed WF, Lee TL, Trachtenberg E, et al. Detection of microchimerism by PCR is a function of amplification strategy. Transfusion 2001;41:39–44.
108. Klein HG, Spahn DR, Carson JL. Red blood cell transfusion in clinical practice. Lancet 2007;370:415–426.
109. Luban NL, Drothler D, Moroff G, et al. Irradiation of platelet components: inhibition of lymphocyte proliferation assessed by limiting-dilution analysis. Transfusion 2000;40: 348–352.
110. Pelszynski MM, Moroff G, Luban NL, et al. Effect of gamma irradiation of red blood cell units on T-cell inactivation as assessed by limiting dilution analysis: implications for preventing transfusion-associated graft-versus-host disease. Blood 1994;83:1683–1689.
111. Grass JA, Wafa T, Reames A, et al. Prevention of transfusion-associated graft-versus-host disease by photochemical treatment. Blood 1999;93:3140–3147.
112. Strauss RG, Barnes A Jr, Blanchette VS, et al. Directed and limited-exposure blood donations for infants and children. Transfusion 1990;30:68–72.
113. Thaler M, Shamiss A, Orgad S, et al. The role of blood from HLA-homozygous donors in fatal transfusion-associated graft-versus-host disease after open-heart surgery. N Engl J Med 1989;321:25–28.
114. Kruskall MS, Eynon EE, Awdeh Z, et al. Identification of HLA-B44 subtypes associated with extended MHC haplotypes. Immunogenetics 1987;26:216–219.
115. Glatstein M, Oron T, Barak M, et al. Posttransfusion equilibration of hematocrit in hemodynamically stable neonates. Pediatr Crit Care Med 2005;6:707–708.
116. Jayabose S, Tugal O, Ruddy R, et al. Transfusion therapy for severe anemia. Am J Pediatr Hematol Oncol 1993;15:324–327.
117. Rowe JM, Lichtman MA. Hyperleukocytosis and leukostasis: common features of childhood chronic myelogenous leukemia. Blood 1984;63:1230–1234.
118. Lowe EJ, Pui CH, Hancock ML, et al. Early complications in children with acute lymphoblastic leukemia presenting with hyperleukocytosis. Pediatr Blood Cancer 2005;45: 10–15.
119. Lichtman MA, Rowe JM. Hyperleukocytic leukemias: rheological, clinical, and therapeutic considerations. Blood 1982;60:279–283.
120. Lichtman MA, Kearney EA. The filterability of human normal and leukemic leukocytes. Blood Cells 1976;2:491–506.
121. Vahdat L, Maslak P, Miller WH Jr, et al. Early mortality and the retinoic acid syndrome in acute promyelocytic leukemia: impact of leukocytosis, low-dose chemotherapy, PMN/RAR-alpha isoform, and CD13 expression in patients treated with all-trans retinoic acid. Blood 1994;84:3843–3849.
122. Blum W, Porcu P. Therapeutic apheresis in hyperleukocytosis and hyperviscosity syndrome. Semin Thromb Hemost 2007;33:350–354.
123. Thompson DS, Goldstone AH, Parry HF, et al. Leukostasis in chronic myeloid leukaemia. BMJ 1978;2:202.
124. Harris AL. Leukostasis associated with blood transfusion in acute myeloid leukaemia. BMJ 1978;1:1169–1171.
125. Sazama K. The ethics of blood management. Vox Sang 2007;92:95–102.
126. Tenenbaum T, Hasan C, Kramm CM, et al. Oncological management of pediatric cancer patients belonging to Jehovah's Witnesses: a two-institutional experience report. Onkologie 2004;27:131–137.
127. Penson RT, Amrein PC. Faith and freedom: leukemia in Jehovah Witness minors. Onkologie 2004;27:126–128.
128. Cothren C, Moore EE, Offner PJ, et al. Blood substitute and erythropoietin therapy in a severely injured Jehovah's Witness. N Engl J Med 2002;346:1097–1098.
129. Aguilera P. Blood transfusions in Jehovah's Witnesses. Rev Med Chil 1993;121: 447–451.
130. Ridgway D. Court-mediated disputes between physicians and families over the medical care of children. Arch Pediatr Adolesc Med 2004;158:891–896.
131. Strauss RG. Red blood cell transfusion practices in the neonate. Clin Perinatol 1995;22: 641–655.
132. Strauss RG. Red blood cell transfusions in the neonate, infant, child, and adolescent. In: Hillyer C, Strauss R, Luban NL, eds. Handbook of pediatric transfusion medicine. San Diego, CA: Academic Press, 2004:131–136.
133. Roseff SD, Luban NL, Manno CS. Guidelines for assessing appropriateness of pediatric transfusion. Transfusion 2002;42:1398–1413.
134. Galel SA, Fontaine MJ. Hazards of neonatal blood transfusion. NeoReviews 2008;7: e69–e74.
135. Stuben G, Thews O, Pöttgen C, et al. Impact of anemia prevention by recombinant human erythropoietin on the sensitivity of xenografted glioblastomas to fractionated irradiation. Strahlenther Onkol 2003;179:620–625.
136. Vaupel P, Thews O, Hoeckel M. Treatment resistance of solid tumors: role of hypoxia and anemia. Med Oncol 2001:18:243–259.
137. Brizel DM, Dodge RK, Clough RW, et al. Oxygenation of head and neck cancer: changes during radiotherapy and impact on treatment outcome. Radiother Oncol 1999;53:113–117.
138. Prosnitz RG, Yao B, Farrell CL, et al. Pretreatment anemia is correlated with the reduced effectiveness of radiation and concurrent chemotherapy in advanced head and neck cancer. Int J Radiat Oncol Biol Phys 2005;61:1087–1095.
139. Harrison L, Blackwell K. Hypoxia and anemia: factors in decreased sensitivity to radiation therapy and chemotherapy? Oncologist 2004;9(S5):31–40.
140. Dische S, Anderson PJ, Sealy R, et al. Carcinoma of the cervix–anaemia, radiotherapy and hyperbaric oxygen. Br J Radiol 1983;56:251–255.
141. Dunn A, Carter J, Carter H. Anemia at the end of life: prevalence, significance, and causes in patients receiving palliative care. J Pain Symptom Manage 2003;26:1132–1139.
142. Wolfe J, Grier HE, Klar N, et al. Symptoms and suffering at the end of life in children with cancer. N Engl J Med 2000;342:326–333.
143. Gleeson C, Spencer D. Blood transfusion and its benefits in palliative care. Palliat Med 1995;9:307–313.
144. Monti M, Castellani L, Berlusconi A, et al. Use of red blood cell transfusions in terminally ill cancer patients admitted to a palliative care unit. J Pain Symptom Manage 1996;12:18–22.
145. Brown E, Bennett M. Survey of blood transfusion practice for palliative care patients in Yorkshire: implications for clinical care. J Palliat Med 2007;10:919–922.
146. Friebert S, Hilden JM. Palliative care. In: Altman AJ, ed. Supportive care of children with cancer: current therapy and guidelines from the Children's Oncology Group. Baltimore and London: The Johns Hopkins University Press, 2004:379–396.
147. Rebulla P. Platelet transfusion trigger in difficult patients. Transfus Clin Biol 2001;8: 249–254.
148. Eberst ME, Berkowitz LR. Hemostasis in renal disease: pathophysiology and management. Am J Med 1994;96:168–179.
149. Noris M, Remuzzi G. Uremic bleeding: closing the circle after 30 years of controversies? Blood 1999;94:2569–2574.
150. Freireich EJ, Kliman A, Gaydos LA, et al. Response to repeated platelet transfusion from the same donor. Ann Intern Med 1963;59:277–287.
151. Gaydos L, Freireich EJ, Mantel N. The quantitative relation between platelet count and hemorrhage in patients with acute leukemia. N Engl J Med 1962;266:905–909.
152. Hersh EM, Bodey GP, Nies BA, et al. Causes of death in acute leukemia: a ten-year study of 414 patients from 1954–1963. JAMA 1965;193:105–109.
153. Bierman HR, Cohen P, McClelland JN, et al. The effect of transfusions and antibiotics upon the duration of life in children with lymphogenous leukemia. J Pediatr 1950;37: 455–462.
154. Freireich EJ, Gehan EA, Sulman D, et al. The effect of chemotherapy on acute leukemia in the human. J Chronic Dis 1961;14:593–608.
155. Higby DJ, Cohen E, Holland JF, et al. The prophylactic treatment of thrombocytopenic leukemic patients with platelets: a double blind study. Transfusion 1974;14:440–446.
156. Roy AJ, Jaffe N, Djerassi I. Prophylactic platelet transfusions in children with acute leukemia: a dose response study. Transfusion 1973;13:283–290.
157. Murphy WG. Prophylactic platelet transfusion in acute leukaemia. Lancet 1992;339: 120, author reply 120–121.
158. McCullough J, Steeper TA, Connelly DP, et al. Platelet utilization in a university hospital. JAMA 1988;259:2414–2418.
159. Schiffer CA, Anderson KC, Bennett CL, et al. Platelet transfusion for patients with cancer: clinical practice guidelines of the American Society of Clinical Oncology. J Clin Oncol 2001;19:1519–1538.
160. Gmür J, Burger J, Schanz U, et al. Safety of stringent prophylactic platelet transfusion policy for patients with acute leukaemia. Lancet 1991;338:1223–1226.
161. Slichter SJ, Harker LA. Thrombocytopenia: mechanisms and management of defects in platelet production. Clin Haematol 1978;7:523–539.
162. Consensus conference. Platelet transfusion therapy. JAMA 1987;257:1777–1780.
163. Contreras M. The appropriate use of platelets: an update from the Edinburgh Consensus Conference. Br J Haematol 1998;101(suppl 1):10–12.
164. Athale UH, Chan AK. Hemorrhagic complications in pediatric hematologic malignancies. Semin Thromb Hemost 2007;33:408–415.
165. Solomon J, Bofenkamp T, Fahey JL, et al. Platelet prophylaxis in acute non-lymphoblastic leukaemia. Lancet 1978;1:267.
166. Beutler E. Platelet transfusions: the 20,000/microL trigger. Blood 1993;81:1411–1413.
167. Beutler E. An iconoclastic view of conventional wisdoms in hematology. Arch Intern Med 1979;139:221–223.
168. Silliman CC, Boshkov LK, Mehdizadehkashi Z, et al. Transfusion-related acute lung injury: epidemiology and a prospective analysis of etiologic factors. Blood 2003;101: 454–462.
169. Slichter SJ. Optimizing platelet transfusions in chronically thrombocytopenic patients. Semin Hematol 1998;35:269–278.
170. Heddle NM, Klama L, Singer J, et al. The role of the plasma from platelet concentrates in transfusion reactions. N Engl J Med 1994;331:625–628.
171. Saxonhouse M. Platelet transfusions in the infant and child. In: Hillyer C, Strauss R, Luban NL, eds. Handbook of pediatric transfusions medicine. San Diego, CA: Academic Press, 2004:253–270.
172. Brecher ME, Holland PV, Pineda AA, et al. Growth of bacteria in inoculated platelets: implications for bacteria detection and the extension of platelet storage. Transfusion 2000;40:1308–1312.
173. Dodd RY. Viral contamination of blood components and approaches for reduction of infectivity. Immunol Invest 1995;24:25–48.
174. Rao PL, Strausbaugh LJ, Liedtke LA, et al. Bacterial infections associated with blood transfusion: experience and perspective of infectious disease consultants. Transfusion 2007;47:1206–1211.
175. Champlin RE, Horowitz MM, van Bekkum DW, et al. Graft failure following bone marrow transplantation for severe aplastic anemia: risk factors and treatment results. Blood 1989;73:606–613.
176. Aderka D, Praff G, Santo M, et al. Bleeding due to thrombocytopenia in acute leukemias and reevaluation of the prophylactic platelet transfusion policy. Am J Med Sci 1986;291:147–151.

177. Pisciotto PT, Benson K, Hume H, et al. Prophylactic versus therapeutic platelet transfusion practices in hematology and/or oncology patients. Transfusion 1995;35:498–502.
178. Harker LA, Slichter SJ. The bleeding time as a screening test for evaluation of platelet function. N Engl J Med 1972;287:155–159.
179. Rebulla P, Finazzi G, Marangoni F, et al. The threshold for prophylactic platelet transfusions in adults with acute myeloid leukemia. Gruppo Italiano Malattie Ematologiche Maligne dell'Adulto. N Engl J Med 1997;337:1870–1875.
180. Bishop JF, Matthews JP, McGrath K, et al. Factors influencing 20-hour increments after platelet transfusion. Transfusion 1991;31:392–396.
181. Hanson SR, Slichter SJ. Platelet kinetics in patients with bone marrow hypoplasia: evidence for a fixed platelet requirement. Blood 1985;66:1105–1109.
182. Kitchens CS, Pendergast JF. Human thrombocytopenia is associated with structural abnormalities of the endothelium that are ameliorated by glucocorticosteroid administration. Blood 1986;67:203–206.
183. Murphy S, Litwin S, Herring LM, et al. Indications for platelet transfusion in children with acute leukemia. Am J Hematol 1982;12:347–356.
184. Heckman KD, Weiner GJ, Davis CS, et al. Randomized study of prophylactic platelet transfusion threshold during induction therapy for adult acute leukemia: 10,000/microL versus 20,000/microL. J Clin Oncol 1997;15:1143–1149.
185. Belt RJ, Leite C, Haas CD, et al. Incidence of hemorrhagic complications in patients with cancer. JAMA 1978;239:2571–2574.
186. Hellem AJ, Borchgrevink CF, Ames SB. The role of red cells in haemostasis: the relation between haematocrit, bleeding time and platelet adhesiveness. Br J Haematol 1961;7:42–50.
187. Blajchman MA, Bordin JO, Bardossy L, et al. The contribution of the haematocrit to thrombocytopenic bleeding in experimental animals. Br J Haematol 1994;86:347–350.
188. Sagmeister M, Oec L, Gmür J. A restrictive platelet transfusion policy allowing long-term support of outpatients with severe aplastic anemia. Blood 1999;93:3124–3126.
189. Gil-Fernández JJ, Alegre A, Fernández-Villalta MJ, et al. Clinical results of a stringent policy on prophylactic platelet transfusion: nonrandomized comparative analysis in 190 bone marrow transplant patients from a single institution. Bone Marrow Transplant 1996;18:931–935.
190. Hanseler E, Fehr J, Keller H. Estimation of the lower limits of manual and automated platelet counting. Am J Clin Pathol 1996;105:782–787.
191. Claas FH, van der Meer JW, Langerak J. Immunological effect of co-trimoxazole on platelets. BMJ 1979;2:898–899.
192. Benjamin RJ, Anderson KC. What is the proper threshold for platelet transfusion in patients with chemotherapy-induced thrombocytopenia? Crit Rev Oncol Hematol 2002;42:163–171.
193. Goldberg GL, Gibbon DG, Smith HO, et al. Clinical impact of chemotherapy-induced thrombocytopenia in patients with gynecologic cancer. J Clin Oncol 1994;12:2317–2320.
194. Dutcher JP, Schiffer CA, Aisner J, et al. Incidence of thrombocytopenia and serious hemorrhage among patients with solid tumors. Cancer 1984;53:557–562.
195. Fanning J, Hilgers RD, Murray KP, et al. Conservative management of chemotherapeutic-induced thrombocytopenia in women with gynecologic cancers. Gynecol Oncol 1995;59:191–193.
196. Elting L, Rubenstein EB, Martin CG, et al. Risk and outcomes of chemotherapy (chemo)-induced thrombocytopenia (TCP) in solid tumor patients [abstract]. Proc Am Soc Clin Oncol 1997;16:412a.
197. Avvisati G, Tirindelli MC, Annibali O. Thrombocytopenia and hemorrhagic risk in cancer patients. Crit Rev Oncol Hematol 2003;48(suppl):S13–S16.
198. Cameron B, Rock G, Olberg B, et al. Evaluation of platelet transfusion triggers in a tertiary-care hospital. Transfusion 2007;47:206–211.
199. British Committee for Standards in Hematology (BCSH). Guidelines of the use of platelet transfusions. Br J Haematol 2003;122:10–23.
200. Bishop JF, Schiffer CA, Aisner J, et al. Surgery in acute leukemia: a review of 167 operations in thrombocytopenic patients. Am J Hematol 1987;26:147–155.
201. Weiss SM, Hert RC, Gianola FJ, et al. Complications of fiberoptic bronchoscopy in thrombocytopenic patients. Chest 1993;104:1025–1028.
202. Friedmann AM, Sengul H, Lehmann H, et al. Do basic laboratory tests or clinical observations predict bleeding in thrombocytopenic oncology patients? A reevaluation of prophylactic platelet transfusions. Transfus Med Rev 2002;16:34–45.
203. Wolcott GJ, Grunnet ML, Lahey ME. Spinal subdural hematoma in a leukemic child. J Pediatr 1970;77:1060–1062.
204. Howard SC, Gajjar AC, Cheng C, et al. Risk factors for traumatic and bloody lumbar puncture in children with acute lymphoblastic leukemia. JAMA 2002;288:2001–2007.
205. Masdeu JC, Breuer AC, Schoene WC. Spinal subarachnoid hematomas: clue to a source of bleeding in traumatic lumbar puncture. Neurology 1979;29:872–876.
206. Breuer AC, Tyler HR, Marzewski DJ, et al. Radicular vessels are the most probable source of needle-induced blood in lumbar puncture: significance for the thrombocytopenic cancer patient. Cancer 1982;49:2168–2172.
207. Stellato TA, Gauderer MW, Lazarus HM, et al. Percutaneous silastic catheter insertion in patients with thrombocytopenia. Cancer 1985;56:2691–2693.
208. Doerfler ME, Kaufman B, Goldenberg AS. Central venous catheter placement in patients with disorders of hemostasis. Chest 1996;110:185–188.
209. Howard SC, Gajjar AC, Ribeiro RC, et al. Safety of lumbar puncture for children with acute lymphoblastic leukemia and thrombocytopenia. JAMA 2000;284:2222–2224.
210. Mainwaring C, Natarajan A, Peckham C, et al. Untreated thrombocytopenia and lumbar puncture-related bleeding risk at diagnosis of childhood acute-lymphoblastic leukemia (ALL) [abstract]. Br J Hematol 1998;101(suppl 1):73.
211. Gajjar A, Harrison PL, Sandlund JT, et al. Traumatic lumbar puncture at diagnosis adversely affects outcome in childhood acute lymphoblastic leukemia. Blood 2000;96:3381–3384.
212. te Loo DM, Kamps WA, van der Does-van den Berg A, et al. Dutch Childhood Oncology Group. Prognostic significance of blasts in the cerebrospinal fluid without pleocytosis or a traumatic lumbar puncture in children with acute lymphoblastic leukemia: experience of the Dutch Pediatric Oncology Group. J Clin Oncol 2006;24:2332–2336.
213. Ray CE Jr, Shenoy SS. Patients with thrombocytopenia: outcome of radiologic placement of central venous access devices. Radiology 1997;204:97–99.
214. Barrera R, Mina B, Huang Y, et al. Acute complications of central line placement in profoundly thrombocytopenic cancer patients. Cancer 1996;78:2025–2030.
215. Lowell JA, Bothe A Jr. Venous access. Preoperative, operative, and postoperative dilemmas. Surg Clin North Am 1991;71:1231–1246.
216. Coit DG, Turnbull AD. A safe technique for the placement of implantable vascular access devices in patients with thrombocytopenia. Surg Gynecol Obstet 1988;167:429–431.
217. Loh AH, Chui CH. Port-A-Cath insertions in acute leukemia: does thrombocytopenia affect morbidity? J Pediatr Surg 2007;42:1180–1184.
218. O'Connell B, Lee EJ, Schiffer CA. The value of 10-minute posttransfusion platelet counts. Transfusion 1988;28:66–67.
219. Patel IP, Ambinder E, Holland JF, et al. In vitro and in vivo comparison of single-donor platelets and multiple-donor pooled platelets transfusions in leukemic patients. Transfusion 1978;18:116–119.
220. Turner VS, Hawker RJ, Mitchell SG, et al. Paired in vivo and in vitro comparison of apheresis and "recovered" platelet concentrates stored for 5 days. J Clin Apheresis 1994;9:189–194.
221. Daly PA, Schiffer CA, Aisner J, et al. A comparison of platelets prepared by the Haemonetics Model 30 and multiunit bag plateletpheresis. Transfusion 1979;19:778–781.
222. Leukocyte reduction and ultraviolet B irradiation of platelets to prevent alloimmunization and refractoriness to platelet transfusions. The Trial to Reduce Alloimmunization to Platelets Study Group. N Engl J Med 1997;337:1861–1869.
223. Burghardt DC. Component preparation and storage. In: Hillyer C, Strauss R, Luban NL, eds. Handbook of pediatric transfusion medicine. San Diego, CA: Academic Press, 2004:11–26.
224. Kuriyan M, Opalka A. Leukoreduced platelet apheresis production with a modified COBE spectra collection protocol. J Clin Apheresis 1995;10:85–86.
225. Fournel JJ, Zingsem J, Riggert J, et al. A multicenter evaluation of the routine use of a new white cell-reduction apheresis system for collection of platelets. Transfusion 1997;37:487–492.
226. Lopez-Plaza I, Weissfeld J, Triulzi DJ. The cost-effectiveness of reducing donor exposures with single-donor versus pooled random-donor platelets. Transfusion 1999;39:925–932.
227. Sweeney JD, Petrucci J, Yankee R. Pooled platelet concentrates: maybe not fancy, but fiscally sound and effective. Transfus Sci 1997;18:575–583.
228. Sloand EM, Yu M, Klein HG. Comparison of random-donor platelet concentrates prepared from whole blood units and platelets prepared from single-donor apheresis collections. Transfusion 1996;36:955–959.
229. Schiffer CA, Lee EJ, Ness PM, et al. Clinical evaluation of platelet concentrates stored for one to five days. Blood 1986;67:1591–1594.
230. Klein HG, Dodd RY, Ness PM, et al. Current status of microbial contamination of blood components: summary of a conference. Transfusion 1997;37:95–101.
231. Kunicki TJ, Tuccelli M, Becker GA, et al. A study of variables affecting the quality of platelets stored at "room temperature." Transfusion 1975;15:414–421.
232. Handin RI, Valeri CR. Hemostatic effectiveness of platelets stored at 22 degrees C. N Engl J Med 1971;285:538–543.
233. Becker GA, Tuccelli M, Kunicki T, et al. Studies of platelet concentrates stored at 22°C and 4°C. Transfusion 1973;13:61–68.
234. Scott EP, Slichter SJ. Viability and function of platelet concentrates stored in CPD-adenine (CPDA-1). Transfusion 1980;20:489–497.
235. Holme S, Vaidja K, Murphy S. Platelet storage at 22 degrees C: effect of type of agitation on morphology, viability, and function in vitro. Blood 1978;52:425–435.
236. Filip DJ, Aster RH. Relative hemostatic effectiveness of human platelets stored at 4 degrees and 22 degrees C. J Lab Clin Med 1978;91:618–624.
237. Fasano R, Luban NL. Blood component therapy. Pediatr Clin N Am 2008;55:421–455.
238. Platelet transfusion therapy. National Institutes of Health Consensus Conference. Transfus Med Rev 1987;1:195–200.
239. Strauss RG. Clinical perspectives of platelet transfusions: defining the optimal dose. J Clin Apheresis 1995;10:124–127.
240. Herman JH, Kamel HT. Platelet transfusion. Current techniques, remaining problems, and future prospects. Am J Pediatr Hematol Oncol 1987;9:272–286.
241. Salama ME, Raman S, Drew MJ, et al. Platelet function testing to assess effectiveness of platelet transfusion therapy. Transfus Apheresis Sci 2004;30:93–100.
242. Norville R, Hinds P, Wilimas J, et al. The effects of infusion rate on platelet outcomes and patient responses in children with cancer: an in vitro and in vivo study. Oncol Nurs Forum 1997;24:1789–1793.
243. Hutchinson RE, Kunkel KD, Schell MJ, et al. Beneficial effect of brief pretransfusion incubation of platelets at 37 degrees C. Lancet 1989;1:986–988.
244. Dutcher JP, Schiffer CA, Aisner J, et al. Alloimmunization following platelet transfusion: the absence of a dose-response relationship. Blood 1981;57:395–398.
245. Dutcher JP, Schiffer CA, Aisner J, et al. Long-term follow-up patients with leukemia receiving platelet transfusions: identification of a large group of patients who do not become alloimmunized. Blood 1981;58:1007–1011.
246. Norol F, Ducdari N, Kuentz M, et al. Comparison of different doses of platelet transfusion. Blood 1995;86(suppl 1):353a.
247. Norol F, Bierling P, Roudot-Thoraval F, et al. Platelet transfusion: a dose-response study. Blood 1998;92:1448–1453.
248. Heddle NM. The efficacy of leukodepletion to improve platelet transfusion response: a critical appraisal of clinical studies. Transfus Med Rev 1994;8:15–28.
249. Confer D. The prevention of HLA alloimmunization. In Kurtz SR, ed. Clinical decisions in platelet therapy. Arlington, VA: American Association of Blood Banks, 1992.
250. Deeg HJ. Transfusions with a tan. Prevention of allosensitization by ultraviolet irradiation. Transfusion 1989;29:450–455.
251. Pamphilon DH, Potter M, Cutts M, et al. Platelet concentrates irradiated with ultraviolet light retain satisfactory in vitro storage characteristics and in vivo survival. Br J Haematol 1990;75:240–244.
252. Howard JE, Perkins HA. The natural history of alloimmunization to platelets. Transfusion 1978;18:496–503.
253. Schiffer CA. Prevention of alloimmunization against platelets. Blood 1991;77:1–4.
254. Murphy MF, Waters AH. Platelet transfusions: the problem of refractoriness. Blood Rev 1990;4:16–24.
255. DeCoteau J, Haddad S, Blanchette V, et al. Refractoriness to platelet transfusions in children with acute leukemia. J Pediatr Hematol Oncol 1995;17:306–310.
256. Doughty HA, Murphy MF, Metcalfe P, et al. Relative importance of immune and non-immune causes of platelet refractoriness. Vox Sang 1994;66:200–205.
257. Bishop JF, McGrath K, Wolf MM, et al. Clinical factors influencing the efficacy of pooled platelet transfusions. Blood 1988;71:383–387.
258. Engelfriet CP, Reesink HW, Aster RH, et al. Management of alloimmunized, refractory patients in need of platelet transfusions. Vox Sang 1997;73:191–198.
259. Alcorta I, Pereira A, Ordinas A. Clinical and laboratory factors associated with platelet transfusion refractoriness: a case-control study. Br J Haematol 1996;93:220–224.
260. Rio B, Andreu G, Nicod A, et al. Thrombocytopenia in venoocclusive disease after bone marrow transplantation or chemotherapy. Blood 1986;67:1773–1776.

261. Hussein MA, Lee EJ, Schiffer CA. Platelet transfusions administered to patients with splenomegaly. Transfusion 1990;30:508–510.
262. Norol F, Kuentz M, Cordonnier C, et al. Influence of clinical status on the efficiency of stored platelet transfusion. Br J Haematol 1994;86:125–129.
263. Benson K, Fields K, Hiemenz J, et al. The platelet-refractory bone marrow transplant patient: prophylaxis and treatment of bleeding. Semin Oncol 1993;20(5, suppl 6): 102–109.
264. McFarland JG, Anderson AJ, Slichter SJ. Factors influencing the transfusion response to HLA-selected apheresis donor platelets in patients refractory to random platelet concentrates. Br J Haematol 1989;73:380–386.
265. Heal JM, Rowe JM, McMican A, et al. The role of ABO matching in platelet transfusion. Eur J Haematol. 1993;50:110–117.
266. Heal JM, Rowe JM, Blumberg N. ABO and platelet transfusion revisited. Ann Hematol 1993;66:309–314.
267. Heal JM, Kenmotsu N, Rowe JM, et al. A possible survival advantage in adults with acute leukemia receiving ABO-identical platelet transfusions. Am J Hematol 1994;45: 189–190.
268. Lee EJ, Schiffer CA. ABO compatibility can influence the results of platelet transfusion. Results of a randomized trial. Transfusion 1989;29:384–389.
269. Carr R, Hutton JL, Jenkins JA, et al. Transfusion of ABO-mismatched platelets leads to early platelet refractoriness. Br J Haematol 1990;75:408–413.
270. Kickler T, Kennedy SD, Braine HG. Alloimmunization to platelet-specific antigens on glycoproteins IIb-IIIa and Ib/IX in multiply transfused thrombocytopenic patients. Transfusion 1990;30:622–625.
271. Evans CM. Alloimmunization and refractoriness to platelet transfusion. Lab Med 1992;23:528–532.
272. Julmy F, Ammann RA, Taleghani BM, et al. Transfusion efficacy of ABO major-mismatched platelets (PLTs) in children is inferior to that of ABO-identical PLTs. Transfusion 2009;49:21–33.
273. Molnar R, Johnson R, Sweat LT, et al. Absence of D alloimmunization in D- pediatric oncology patients receiving D-incompatible single-donor platelets. Transfusion 2002;42:177–182.
274. Christie DJ, van Buren N, Lennon SS, et al. Vancomycin-dependent antibodies associated with thrombocytopenia and refractoriness to platelet transfusion in patients with leukemia. Blood 1990;75:518–523.
275. Altman AJ, Wolff LJ. The prevention of infection. In: Altman A, ed. Supportive care of children with cancer: current therapy and guidelines from the Children's Oncology Group. Baltimore and London: The Johns Hopkins University Press, 2004:1–12.
276. Kulpa J, Zaroulis CG, Good RA, et al. Altered platelet function and circulation induced by amphotericin B in leukemic patients after platelet transfusion. Transfusion 1981;21: 74–76.
277. Brajtburg J, Elberg S, Schwartz DR, et al. Involvement of oxidative damage in erythrocyte lysis induced by amphotericin B. Antimicrob Agents Chemother 1985;27:172–176.
278. Claas FH, Smeenk RJ, Schmidt R, et al. Alloimmunization against the MHC antigens after platelet transfusions is due to contaminating leukocytes in the platelet suspension. Exp Hematol 1981;9:84–89.
279. Slichter SJ, Weiden PL, Kane PJ, et al. Approaches to preventing or reversing platelet alloimmunization using animal models. Transfusion 1988;28:103–108.
280. Eriksson L, Shanwell A, Gulliksson H, et al. Platelet concentrates in an additive solution prepared from pooled buffy coats. In vivo studies. Vox Sang 1993;64:133–138.
281. Heaton WA, Rebulla P, Pappalettera M, et al. A comparative analysis of different methods for routine blood component preparation. Transfus Med Rev 1997;11:116–129.
282. Simon TL, Sierra ER. Concentration of platelet units into small volumes. Transfusion 1984;24:173–175.
283. Schiffer CA, Dutcher JP, Aisner J, et al. A randomized trial of leukocyte-depleted platelet transfusion to modify alloimmunization in patients with leukemia. Blood 1983; 62:815–820.
284. Murphy MF, Metcalfe P, Thomas H, et al. Use of leucocyte-poor blood components and HLA-matched-platelet donors to prevent HLA alloimmunization. Br J Haematol 1986; 62:529–534.
285. Saarinen UM, Koskimies S, Myllyla G. Systematic use of leukocyte-free blood components to prevent alloimmunization and platelet refractoriness in multitransfused children with cancer. Vox Sang 1993;65:286–292.
286. Heal JM, Blumberg N. Optimizing platelet transfusion therapy. Blood Rev 2004;18: 149–165.
287. Blumberg N, Heal JM, Kirkley SA, et al. Leukodepleted-ABO-identical blood components in the treatment of hematologic malignancies: a cost analysis. Am J Hematol 1995;48:108–115.
288. Friedberg RC, Donnelly SF, Mintz PD. Independent roles for platelet crossmatching and HLA in the selection of platelets for alloimmunized patients. Transfusion 1994;34: 215–220.
289. Friedberg RC, Donnelly SF, Boyd JC, et al. Clinical and blood bank factors in the management of platelet refractoriness and alloimmunization. Blood 1993;81:3428–3434.
290. Welch HG, Larson EB, Slichter SJ. Providing platelets for refractory patients. Prudent strategies. Transfusion 1989;29:193–195.
291. Kickler TS, Ness PM, Braine HG. Platelet crossmatching. A direct approach to the selection of platelet transfusions for the alloimmunized thrombocytopenic patient. Am J Clin Pathol 1988;90:69–72.
292. Gelb AB, Leavitt AD. Crossmatch-compatible platelets improve corrected count increments in patients who are refractory to randomly selected platelets. Transfusion 1997; 37:624–630.
293. O'Connell BA, Lee EJ, Rothko K, et al. Selection of histocompatible apheresis platelet donors by cross-matching random donor platelet concentrates. Blood 1992;79: 527–531.
294. Duquesnoy RJ, Filip DJ, Rodey GE, et al. Successful transfusion of platelets "mismatched" for HLA antigens to alloimmunized thrombocytopenic patients. Am J Hematol 1977;2:219–226.
295. Nagasawa T, Kim BK, Baldini MG. Temporary suppression of circulating antiplatelet alloantibodies by the massive infusion of fresh, stored, or lyophilized platelets. Transfusion 1978;18:429–435.
296. Lee EJ, Norris D, Schiffer CA. Intravenous immune globulin for patients alloimmunized to random donor platelet transfusion. Transfusion 1987;27:245–247.
297. Schiffer CA, Hogge DE, Aisner J, et al. High-dose intravenous gammaglobulin in alloimmunized platelet transfusion recipients. Blood 1984;64:937–940.
298. Kickler T, Braine HG, Piantadosi S, et al. A randomized, placebo-controlled trial of intravenous gammaglobulin in alloimmunized thrombocytopenic patients. Blood 1990;75:313–316.
299. Murphy MF, Metcalfe P, Ord J, et al. Disappearance of HLA and platelet-specific antibodies in acute leukaemia patients alloimmunized by multiple transfusions. Br J Haematol 1987;67:255–260.
300. Lee EJ, Schiffer CA. Serial measurement of lymphocytotoxic antibody and response to nonmatched platelet transfusions in alloimmunized patients. Blood 1987;70:1727–1729.
301. Gardner FH, Helmer RE III. Aminocaproic acid. Use in control of hemorrhage in patients with a megakaryocytic thrombocytopenia. JAMA 1980;243:35–37.
302. Bartholomew JR, Salgia R, Bell WR. Control of bleeding in patients with immune and nonimmune thrombocytopenia with aminocaproic acid. Arch Intern Med 1989;149: 1959–1961.
303. Salzman EW, Weinstein MJ, Reilly D, et al. Adventures in hemostasis. Desmopressin in cardiac surgery. Arch Surg 1993;128:212–217.
304. Mannucci PM. Desmopressin: a nontransfusional form of treatment for congenital and acquired bleeding disorders. Blood 1988;72:1449–1455.
305. Khunhausen S, Nichols DJ, Noonan N, et al. Epistaxis Procedure, Children's Hospital Oakland Department of Nursing. Poster presented at: Association of Pediatric Oncology Nurses Conference Philadelphia, 2003; Philadelphia.
306. Pizzo PA. Management of fever in patients with cancer and treatment-induced neutropenia. N Engl J Med 1993;328:1323–1332.
307. Chanock SJ, Gorlin JB. Granulocyte transfusions. Time for a second look. Infect Dis Clin North Am 1996;10:327–343.
308. Chanock S. Evolving risk factors for infectious complications of cancer therapy. Hematol Oncol Clin North Am 1993;7:771–793.
309. Donowitz GR, Maki DG, Crnich CJ, et al. Infections in the neutropenic patient—new views of an old problem. Hematology Am Soc Hematol Educ Program 2001;113–139.
310. Hughes WT, Armstrong D, Bodey GP, et al. 2002 Guidelines for the use of antimicrobial agents in neutropenic patients with cancer. Clin Infect Dis 2002;34:730–751.
311. Klein HG, Strauss RG, Schiffer CA. Granulocyte transfusion therapy. Semin Hematol 1996;33:359–368.
312. Bodey G, Buckley M, Sathe YS, et al. Quantitative relationship between circulating leukocytes and infections in patients with acute leukemia. Ann Intern Med 1966;64: 328–340.
313. Boutati EI, Anaissie EJ. Fusarium, a significant emerging pathogen in patients with hematologic malignancy: ten years' experience at a cancer center and implications for management. Blood 1997;90:999–1008.
314. Massey E, Paulus U, Doree C, et al. Granulocyte transfusions for preventing infections in patients with neutropenia or neutrophil dysfunction. Cochrane Database Syst Rev 2009;(1):CD005341.
315. van de Wetering MD, Weggelaar N, Offinga M, et al. Granulocyte transfusions in neutropaenic children: a systematic review of the literature. Eur J Cancer 2007;43: 2082–2092.
316. Peters C. Granulocyte transfusions in neutropenic patients: beneficial effects proven? Vox Sang 2009;96:275–283.
317. Bishton M, Chopra R. The role of granulocyte transfusions in neutropenic patients. Br J Haematol 2004;127:501–508.
318. Robinson SP, Marks DI. Granulocyte transfusion in the G-CSF era. Where do we stand? Bone Marrow Transplant 2004;34:839–846.
319. Seidel MG, Peters C, Wacker A, et al. Randomized phase III study of granulocyte transfusions in neutropenic patients. Bone Marrow Transplant 2008;42:679–684.
320. Dale DC, Price TH. Granulocyte transfusion therapy: a new era? Curr Opin Hematol 2009;16:1–2.
321. Dale DC, Liles WC. Return of granulocyte transfusions. Curr Opin Pediatr 2000;12: 18–22.
322. Price TH, Bowden RA, Boeckh M, et al. Phase I/II trial of neutrophil transfusions from donors stimulated with G-CSF and dexamethasone for treatment of patients with infections in hematopoietic stem cell transplantation. Blood 2000;95:3302–3309.
323. Strauss RG. Rebirth of granulocyte transfusions: should it involve pediatric oncology and transplant patients? J Pediatr Hematol Oncol 1999;21:475–478.
324. Liles WC, Huang JE, Llewellyn C, et al. A comparative trial of granulocyte-colony-stimulating factor (G-CSF) and dexamethasone, separately and in combination, for the mobilization of neutrophils in the peripheral blood of normal human volunteers. Transfusion 1997;37:182–187.
325. Price TH, Gurkamal S, Chatta GS, et al. The effect of recombinant granulocyte colony-stimulating factor on neutrophil kinetics in normal young and elderly humans. Blood 1996;88:335–340.
326. Bensinger WI, Price TH, Dale DC, et al. The effects of daily recombinant human granulocyte colony-stimulating factor administration on normal granulocyte donors undergoing leukapheresis. Blood 1993;81:1883–1888.
327. Dale DC, Liles WC, Llewellyn C, et al. Neutrophil transfusions: kinetics and functions of neutrophils mobilized with granulocyte colony-stimulating factor and dexamethasone. Transfusion 1998;38:713–721.
328. Strauss RG. Therapeutic granulocyte transfusions in 1993. Blood 1993;81:1675–1678.
329. Sulis ML, Harrison L, Cairo MS. Granulocyte transfusions in the neonate and child. In: Hillyer C, Strauss R, Luban NL, eds. Handbook of pediatric transfusion medicine. San Diego: Academic Press, 2004;167–180.
330. Liles WC, Rodger E, Dale DC. Combined administration of G-CSF and dexamethasone for the mobilization of granulocytes in normal donors: optimization of dosing. Transfusion 2000;40:642–644.
331. Caspar CB, Seger RA, Burger J, et al. Effective stimulation of donors for granulocyte transfusions with recombinant methionyl granulocyte colony-stimulating factor. Blood 1993;81:2866–2871.
332. Roilides E, Pizzo PA. Modulation of host defenses by cytokines: evolving adjuncts in prevention and treatment of serious infections in immunocompromised hosts. Clin Infect Dis 1992;15:508–524.
333. Roilides E, Walsh TJ, Pizzo PA, et al. Granulocyte colony-stimulating factor enhances the phagocytic and bactericidal activity of normal and defective human neutrophils. J Infect Dis 1991;163:579–583.
334. Mohan P, Brocklehurst P. Granulocyte transfusions for neonates with confirmed or suspected sepsis and neutropaenia. Cochrane Database Syst Rev 2003;4:CD003956.
335. Hubel K, Rodger E, Gaviria JM, et al. Effective storage of granulocytes collected by centrifugation leukapheresis from donors stimulated with granulocyte-colony stimulating factor. Transfusion 2005;45:1876–1889.
336. Sachs UJ, Reiter A, Walter T, et al. Safety and efficacy of therapeutic early onset granulocyte transfusions in pediatric patients with neutropenia and severe infections. Transfusion 2006;46:1909–1914.
337. Adkins DR, Goodnough LT, Shenoy S, et al. Effect of leukocyte compatibility on neutrophil increment after transfusion of granulocyte colony-stimulating factor-mobilized

prophylactic granulocyte transfusions and on clinical outcomes after stem cell transplantation. Blood 2000;95:3605–3612.

338. Wright DG, Robichaud KJ, Pizzo PA, et al. Lethal pulmonary reactions associated with the combined use of amphotericin B and leukocyte transfusions. N Engl J Med 1981; 304:1185–1189.

339. Dutcher JP, Kendall J, Norris D, et al. Granulocyte transfusion therapy and amphotericin B: adverse reactions? Am J Hematol 1989;31:102–108.

340. Dana BW, Durie BG, White RF, et al. Concomitant administration of granulocyte transfusions and amphotericin B in neutropenic patients: absence of significant pulmonary toxicity. Blood 1981;57:90–94.

341. Sulis ML, Van de Ven C, Henderson T, et al. Liposomal amphotericin B (AmBisome) compared with amphotericin B +/− FMLP induces significantly less in vitro neutrophil aggregation with granulocyte-colony-stimulating factor/dexamethasone-mobilized allogeneic donor neutrophils. Blood 2002;99:384–386.

342. Vamvakas EC, Pineda AA. Determinants of the efficacy of prophylactic granulocyte transfusions: a meta-analysis. J Clin Apheresis 1997;12:74–81.

343. Oza A, Hallemeier C, Goodnough L, et al. Granulocyte-colony-stimulating factor-mobilized prophylactic granulocyte transfusions given after allogeneic peripheral blood progenitor cell transplantation result in a modest reduction of febrile days and intravenous antibiotic usage. Transfusion 2006;46:14–23.

344. Roberts HR, Monroe DM, White GC. The use of recombinant factor VIIa in the treatment of bleeding disorders. Blood 2004;104:3858–3864.

345. Heller M, Lau W, Pazmino-Canizares J, et al. A comprehensive review of rFVIIa use in a tertiary care pediatric center. Pediatr Blood Cancer 2008;50:1013–1017.

346. Abshire T, Kenet G. Recombinant factor VIIa: review of efficacy, dosing regimens and safety in patients with congenital and acquired factor VIII and IX inhibitors. J Thromb Haemost 2004;2:899–909.

347. Heisel M, Nagib M, Madsen L, et al. Use of recombinant factor VIIa (fVIIa) to control intraoperative bleeding in pediatric brain tumor patients. Pediatr Blood Cancer 2004; 43:703–705.

348. Hartmann M, Sucker C, Messing M. Recombinant activated factor VII in the treatment of near-fatal bleeding during pediatric brain tumor surgery. J Neurosurg 2006;104: 55–58.

349. Ritchey M, Ferrer F, Shearer P, et al. Late effects on the urinary bladder in patients treated for cancer in childhood: a report from the Children's Oncology Group. Pediatr Blood Cancer 2009;52:439–446.

350. Franchini M, Veneri D, Lippi G. The potential role of recombinant activated FVII in the management of critical hemato-oncological bleeding: a systematic review. Bone Marrow Transplant 2007;39:729–735.

351. Pihusch M, Bacigalupo A, Szer J, et al. Recombinant activated factor VII in treatment of bleeding complications following hematopoietic stem cell transplantation. J Thromb Haemost 2005;3:1935–1944.

352. Dzik WH. Emily Cooley Lecture 2002: transfusion safety in the hospital. Transfusion 2003;43:1190–1199.

353. Myhre BA, McRuer D. Human error—a significant cause of transfusion mortality. Transfusion 2000;40:879–885.

354. Linden JV, Wagner K, Voytovich AE, et al. Transfusion errors in New York State: an analysis of 10 years' experience. Transfusion 2000;40:1207–1213.

355. Williamson LM, Lowe S, Love EM, et al. Serious hazards of transfusion (SHOT) initiative: analysis of the first two annual reports. BMJ 1999;319:16–19.

356. Bolton-Maggs PH, Murphy MF. Blood transfusion. Arch Dis Child 2004;89:4–7.

357. Stainsby D, Jones H, Asher D, et al. Serious hazards of transfusion: a decade of hemovigilance in the UK. Transfus Med Rev 2006;20:273–282.

358. Sazama K. Reports of 355 transfusion-associated deaths: 1976 through 1985. Transfusion 1990;30:583–590.

359. Larsson LG, Welsh VJ, Ladd DJ. Acute intravascular hemolysis secondary to out-of-group platelet transfusion. Transfusion 2000;40:902–906.

360. Duguid JK, Minards J, Bolton-Maggs PH. Lesson of the week: incompatible plasma transfusions and haemolysis in children. BMJ 1999;318:176–177.

361. Moroff G, Friedman A, Robkin-Kline L, et al. Reduction of the volume of stored platelet concentrates for use in neonatal patients. Transfusion 1984;24:144–146.

362. Friedberg RC. Issues in transfusion therapy in the patient with malignancy. Hematol Oncol Clin North Am 1994;8:1223–1253.

363. Eder AF. Transfusion reactions. In: Hillyer C, Strauss R, Luban NL, eds. Handbook of pediatric transfusion medicine. San Diego, CA: Academic Press, 2004:301–316.

364. Brecher ME. Technical manual. 13th ed. Arlington, VA: American Association of Blood Banks, 2002.

365. Heddle NM, Klama LN, Griffith L, et al. A prospective study to identify the risk factors associated with acute reactions to platelet and red cell transfusions. Transfusion 1993;33:794–797.

366. Gauvin F, Lacroix J, Robillard P, et al. Acute transfusion reactions in the pediatric intensive care unit. Transfusion 2006;46:1899–1908.

367. Wang SE, Lara PN, Lee-OW A, et al. Acetaminophen and diphenhydramine as premedication for platelet transfusions: a prospective randomized double-blind placebo-controlled trial. Am J Hematol 2002;70:191–194.

368. Sanders RP, Maddirala SD, Geiger TL, et al. Premedication with acetaminophen or diphenhydramine for transfusion with leucoreduced blood products in children. Br J Haematol 2005;130:781–787.

369. Geiger TL, Howard SC. Acetaminophen and diphenhydramine premedication for allergic and febrile nonhemolytic transfusion reactions: good prophylaxis or bad practice? Transfus Med Rev 2007;21:1–12.

370. Kennedy LD, Case LD, Hurd DD, et al. A prospective, randomized, double-blind controlled trial of acetaminophen and diphenhydramine pretransfusion medication versus placebo for the prevention of transfusion reactions. Transfusion 2008;48:2285–2291.

371. Couban S, Carruthers J, Andreou P, et al. Platelet transfusions in children: results of a randomized, prospective, crossover trial of plasma removal and a prospective audit of WBC reduction. Transfusion 2002;42:753–758.

372. Popovsky MA. Transfusion-related acute lung injury. Curr Opin Hematol 2000;7: 402–407.

373. Kleinman S, Caulfield T, Chan P, et al. Towards an understanding of transfusion-related acute lung injury: statement of a consensus panel. Transfusion 2004;44:1774–1789.

374. Andreu G. Transfusion-associated circulatory overload and transfusion-related acute lung injury: diagnosis, pathophysiology, management and prevention. ISBT Science Series 2009;4:63–71.

375. Marik PE, Corwin HL. Acute lung injury following blood transfusion: expanding the definition. Crit Care Med 2008;36:3080–3084.

376. Sanchez R, Toy P. Transfusion related acute lung injury: a pediatric perspective. Pediatr Blood Cancer 2005;45:248–255.

377. Church GD, Price C, Sanchez R, et al. Transfusion-related acute lung injury in the paediatric patient: two case reports and a review of the literature. Transfus Med 2006;16: 343–348.

378. Goldman M, Webert KE, Arnold DM, et al. Proceedings of a consensus conference: towards an understanding of TRALI. Transfus Med Rev 2005;19:2–31.

379. Jacob HS, Craddock PR, Hammerschmidt DE, et al. Complement-induced granulocyte aggregation: an unsuspected mechanism of disease. N Engl J Med 1980;302:789–794.

380. Hammerschmidt DE, Jacob HS. Adverse pulmonary reactions to transfusion. Adv Intern Med 1982;27:511–530.

381. Craddock PR, Hammerschmidt DE, Moldow CF, et al. Granulocyte aggregation as a manifestation of membrane interactions with complement: possible role in leukocyte margination, microvascular occlusion, and endothelial damage. Semin Hematol 1979; 16:140–147.

382. Fadeyi EA, Muniz MD, Wayne AS, et al. The transfusion of neutrophil-specific antibodies causes leucopenia and a broad spectrum of pulmonary reactions. Transfusion 2007;47:545–550.

383. Sheppard CA, Lögdberg LE, Zimring JC, et al. Transfusion-related acute lung injury. Hematol Oncol Clin North Am 2007;21:163–176.

384. Barrett NA, Kam PC. Transfusion-related acute lung injury: a literature review. Anaesthesia 2006;61:777–785.

385. Eder AF, Herron R, Strupp A, et al. Transfusion-related acute lung injury surveillance (2003–2005) and the potential impact of the selective use of plasma from male donors in the American Red Cross. Transfusion 2007;47:599–607.

386. Dodd RY. Current risk for transfusion transmitted infections. Curr Opin Hematol 2007;14:671–676.

387. Busch MP, Glynn SA, Stramer SL. A new strategy for estimating risks of transfusion-transmitted viral infections based on rates of detection of recently infected donors. Transfusion 2005;45:254–264.

388. Dienstag JL, Purcell HR, Alter HJ, et al. Non-A, non-B posttransfusion hepatitis. Lancet 1977;1:560–562.

389. Randall RJ. Hepatitis C virus infection and long-term survivors of childhood cancer: issues for the pediatric oncology nurse. J Pediatr Oncol Nurs 2001;18:4–15.

390. Jamali F, Ness P. Infectious complications. In: Hillyer C, Strauss R, Luban NLC, eds. Handbook of pediatric transfusion medicine. San Diego, CA: Academic Press, 2004: 329–342.

391. Alter M, Mast EE, Moyer LA, et al. Hepatitis C. Infect Dis Clin North Am 1998;12: 13–26.

392. Vogt M, Lang T, Frösner G, et al. Prevalence and clinical outcome of hepatitis C infection in children who underwent cardiac surgery before the implementation of blood-donor screening. N Engl J Med 1999;341:866–870.

393. Cesaro S, Petris MG, Rossetti F, et al. Chronic hepatitis C virus infection after treatment for pediatric malignancy. Blood 1997;90:1315–1320.

394. Locasciulli A, Testa M, Pontisso P, et al. Prevalence and natural history of hepatitis C infection in patients cured of childhood leukemia. Blood 1997;90:4628–4633.

395. Fujisawa T, Komatsu H, Inui A, et al. Spontaneous remission of chronic hepatitis C in children. Eur J Pediatr 1997;156:773–776.

396. Rubin RH, Tolkoff-Rubin NE, Oliver D, et al. Multicenter seroepidemiologic study of the impact of cytomegalovirus infection on renal transplantation. Transplantation 1985;40:243–249.

397. Söderberg-Nauclér C, Fish KN, Nelson JA. Reactivation of latent human cytomegalovirus by allogeneic stimulation of blood cells from healthy donors. Cell 1997; 91:119–126.

398. Bowden R, Sayers M. The risk of transmitting cytomegalovirus infection by fresh frozen plasma. Transfusion 1990;30:762–763.

399. Larsson S, Söderberg-Nauclér C, Wang FZ, et al. Cytomegalovirus DNA can be detected in peripheral blood mononuclear cells from all seropositive and most seronegative healthy blood donors over time. Transfusion 1998;38:271–278.

400. Sayers MH, Anderson KC, Goodnough LT, et al. Reducing the risk for transfusion-transmitted cytomegalovirus infection. Ann Intern Med 1992;116:55–62.

401. O'Brien TR, George JR, Holmberg SD. Human immunodeficiency virus type 2 infection in the United States. Epidemiology, diagnosis, and public health implications. JAMA 1992;267:2775–2779.

402. Busch MP, Lee LL, Sateen GA, et al. Time course of detection of viral and serologic markers preceding human immunodeficiency virus type 1 seroconversion: implications for screening of blood and tissue donors. Transfusion 1995;35:91–97.

403. Busch MP, Stramer SL, Kleinman SH. Evolving applications of nucleic acid amplification assays for prevention of virus transmission by blood components and derivatives. In: Garratty G, ed. Applications of molecular biology to blood transfusion medicine. Bethesda, MD: American Association of Blood Banks, 1997:123–176.

404. Dodd RY, Notari EPT, Stramer SL. Current prevalence and incidence of infectious disease markers and estimated window-period risk in the American Red Cross blood donor population. Transfusion 2002;42:975–979.

405. Kuehnert MJ, Roth VR, Haley NR, et al. Transfusion-transmitted bacterial infection in the United States, 1998 through 2000. Transfusion 2001;41:1493–1499.

406. Wagner S. Transfusion-related bacterial sepsis. Curr Opin Hematol 1997;4:464–469.

407. Morrow JF, Braine HG, Kickler TS, et al. Septic reactions to platelet transfusions. A persistent problem. JAMA 1991;266:555–558.

408. Arduino MJ, Bland LA, Tipple MA, et al. Growth and endotoxin production of Yersinia enterocolitica and Enterobacter agglomerans in packed erythrocytes. J Clin Microbiol 1989;27:1483–1485.

409. Ness P, Braine H, King K, et al. Single-donor platelets reduce the risk of septic platelet transfusion reactions. Transfusion 2001;41:857–861.

410. Blajchman MA, Goldman M, Baeza F. Improving the bacteriological safety of platelet transfusions. Transfus Med Rev 2004;18:11–24.

411. Grass JA, Hei DJ, Metchette K, et al. Inactivation of leukocytes in platelet concentrates by photochemical treatment with psoralen plus UVA. Blood 1998;91:2180–2188.

412. Munksgaard L, Albjerg L, Lillivang ST, et al. Detection of bacterial contamination of platelet components: six years' experience with the BacT/ALERT system. Transfusion 2004;44:1166–1173.

413. Fang CT, Chambers LA, Kennedy J, et al. Detection of bacterial contamination in apheresis platelet products: American Red Cross experience, 2004. Transfusion 2005; 45:1845–1852.

414. Kaur P, Basu S. Transfusion-transmitted infections: existing and emerging pathogens. J Postgrad Med 2005;51:146–151.

415. Brittenham GM, Cohen AR, McLaren CE, et al. Hepatic iron stores and plasma ferritin concentration in patients with sickle cell anemia and thalassemia major. Am J Hematol 1993;42:81–85.
416. Brittenham GM, Sheth S, Allen CJ, et al. Noninvasive methods for quantitative assessment of transfusional iron overload in sickle cell disease. Semin Hematol 2001;38(1, suppl 1):37–56.
417. Angelucci E, Brittenham GM, McLaren CE, et al. Hepatic iron concentration and total body iron stores in thalassemia major. N Engl J Med 2000;343:327–331.
418. Fischer R, Tiemann CD, Engelhardt R, et al. Assessment of iron stores in children with transfusion siderosis by biomagnetic liver susceptometry. Am J Hematol 1999;60: 289–299.
419. St. Pierre TG, Clark PR, Chau-anusorn W, et al. Noninvasive measurement and imaging of liver iron concentrations using proton magnetic resonance. Blood 2005;105: 855–861.
420. Wood JC, Enriquez C, Ghugre N, et al. MRI R2 and R2* mapping accurately estimates hepatic iron concentration in transfusion-dependent thalassemia and sickle cell disease patients. Blood 2005;106:1460–1465.
421. Anderson LJ, Holden S, Davis B, et al. Cardiovascular T2-star (T2*) magnetic resonance for the early diagnosis of myocardial iron overload. Eur Heart J 2001;22: 2171–2179.
422. Altes A, Remacha AF, Sarda P, et al. Frequent severe liver iron overload after stem cell transplantation and its possible association with invasive aspergillosis. Bone Marrow Transplant 2004;34:505–509.
423. Miceli MH, Dong L, Grazziutti ML, et al. Iron overload is a major risk factor for severe infection after autologous stem cell transplantation: a study of 367 myeloma patients. Bone Marrow Transplant 2006;37:857–864.
424. Halonen P, Mattila J, Suominen P, et al. Iron overload in children who are treated for acute lymphoblastic leukemia estimated by liver siderosis and serum iron parameters. Pediatrics 2003;111:91–96.
425. Eder AF, Chambers LA. Noninfectious complications of blood transfusion. Arch Pathol Lab Med 2007;131:708–718.
426. Schaison G, Eden OB, Henze G, et al. Recommendations on the use of colony-stimulating factors in children: conclusions of a European panel. Eur J Pediatr 1998; 157:955–966.
427. Lehrnbecher T, Welte K. Haematopoietic growth factors in children with neutropenia. Br J Haematol 2002;116:28–56.
428. Feusner J, Hastings C. Recombinant human erythropoietin in pediatric oncology: a review. Med Pediatr Oncol 2002;39:463–468.
429. Kuter DJ. New thrombopoietic growth factors. Blood 2007;109:4607–4616.
430. Smith T, Khatcheressian J, Lyman G, et al. 2006 Update of Recommendations for the use of white blood cell growth factors: an evidence-based clinical practice guideline. J Clin Oncol 2006;24:3187–3205.
431. Rizzo JD, Somerfield MR, Hagerty KL, et al. Use of epoetin and darbopoietin in patients with cancer: 2007 American Society of Hematology/American Society of Clinical Oncology clinical practice guideline update. Blood 2008;111:25–41.
432. Zamboni WC, Stewart CE. An overview of the pharmacokinetic disposition of darbepoetin alfa. Pharmacotherapy 2002;22:133S-140S.
433. Blumer J, Berg S, Adamson PC, et al. Pharmacokinetic evaluation of darbepoetin alfa for the treatment of pediatric patients with chemotherapy-induced anemia. Pediatr Blood Cancer 2007;49:687–693.
434. Bohlius J, Wilson J, Seidenfeld J, et al. Recombinant human erythropoietins and cancer patients: updated meta-analysis of 57 studies including 9353 patients. J Natl Cancer Inst 2006;98:708–714.
435. Bokemeyer C. EORTC guidelines for the use of erythropoietic proteins in anaemic patients with cancer. Eur J Cancer 2004;40:2201–2216.
436. Porter JC, Leahey A, Polise K, et al. Recombinant human erythropoietin reduces the need for erythrocyte and platelet transfusions in pediatric patients with sarcoma: a randomized, double-blind, placebo-controlled trial. J Pediatr 1996;129:656–660.
437. Csáki C, Ferencz T, Schuler D, et al. Recombinant human erythropoietin in the prevention of chemotherapy-induced anaemia in children with malignant solid tumors. Eur J Cancer 1998;34:364–367.
438. Büyükpamukçu M, Varan A, Kutluk T, et al. Is epoetin alfa a treatment option for chemotherapy-related anemia in children? Med Pediatr Oncol 2002;39:455–458.
439. Wagner L, Billups CA, Furman WL, et al. Combined use of erythropoietin and granulocyte colony-stimulating factor does not decrease blood transfusion requirements during induction therapy for high-risk neuroblastoma: a randomized controlled trial. J Clin Oncol 2004;22:1886–1893.
440. Razzouk BI, Hord JD, Hockenberry M, et al. Double-blind, placebo-controlled study of quality of life, hematologic end points, and safety of weekly epoetin alfa in children with cancer receiving myelosuppressive chemotherapy. J Clin Oncol 2006;24: 3583–3589.
441. Abdelrazik N, Fouda M. Once weekly recombinant human erythropoietin treatment for cancer-induced anemia in children with acute lymphoblastic leukemia receiving maintenance chemotherapy: a randomized case-controlled study. Hematology 2007;12: 533–541.
442. Shankar AG. The role of recombinant erythropoietin in childhood cancer. Oncologist 2008;13:157–166.
443. Leyland-Jones B. Breast cancer trial with erythropoietin terminated unexpectedly. Lancet Oncol 2003;4:459–460.
444. Henke M, Laszig R, Rübe C, et al. Erythropoietin to treat head and neck cancer patients with anaemia undergoing radiotherapy: randomised, double-blind, placebo-controlled trial. Lancet 2003;362:1255–1260.
445. Bennett CL, Silver SM, Djulbegovic B, et al. Venous thromboembolism and mortality associated with recombinant erythropoietin and darbopoietin administration for the treatment of cancer-associated anemia. JAMA 2008;299:914–924.
446. McKoy JM, Stonecash RE, Cournoyer D, et al. Epoeitin-associated pure red cell aplasia: past, present, and future considerations. Transfusion 2008;48:1754–1762.
447. Batra S, Perelman N, Luck LR, et al. Pediatric tumor cells express erythropoietin and a functional erythropoietin receptor that promotes angiogenesis and tumor cell survival. Lab Invest 2003;83:1477–1487.
448. Yasuda Y, Fujita Y, Matsuo T, et al. Erythropoietin regulates tumour growth of human malignancies. Carcinogenesis 2003;24:1021–1029.
449. Sartelet H, Fabre M, Castaing M, et al. Expression of erythropoietin and its receptor in neuroblastomas. Cancer 2007;110:1096–1105.
450. Marec-Berard P, Chastagner P, Kassab-Chahmi D, et al. 2007 Standards, Options, and Recommendations: use of erythropoiesis-stimulating agents (ESA: epoetin alfa, epoetin beta, and darbopoietin) for the management of anemia in children with cancer. Pediatr Blood Cancer 2009;53:7–12.
451. Kaufman JS. Subcutaneous compared with intravenous epoetin in patients receiving hemodialysis. N Engl J Med 1998;339:578–583.
452. Galliford JW, Malasana R, Farrington K. Switching from subcutaneous to intravenous erythropoietin α in haemodialysis patients requires a major dose increase. Nephrol Dial Transplant 2005;20:1956–1962.
453. Vercaigne LM, Collins DM, Penner SB. Conversion from subcutaneous to intravenous erythropoietin in a hemodialysis population. J Clin Pharmacol 2005;45:895–900.
454. Glaspy J, Cavill I. Role of iron in optimizing responses of anemic cancer patients to erythropoietin. Oncology 1999;13:461–473, discussion 477–478, 483–488.
455. Takeshita A, Shinjo K, Higuchi M, et al. Quantitative expression of erythropoietin receptor (EPO-R) on acute leukaemia cells: relationships between the amount of EPO-R and CD phenotypes, in vitro proliferative response, the amount of other cytokine receptors and clinical prognosis. Japan Adult Leukaemia Study Group. Br J Haematol 2000;108:55–63.
456. Feusner J. Guidelines for Epo use in children with cancer. Pediatr Blood Cancer 2009; 53:7–12.
457. Lieschke GJ, Burgess AW. Granulocyte colony-stimulating factor and granulocyte-macrophage colony-stimulating factor (1). N Engl J Med 1992;327:28–35.
458. Layton JE, Hockman H, Sheridan WP, et al. Evidence for a novel in vivo control mechanism of granulopoiesis: mature cell-related control of a regulatory growth factor. Blood 1989;74:1303–1307.
459. Kawakami M, Tsutsumi M, Kumakawa T, et al. Levels of serum granulocyte colony-stimulating factor in patients with infections. Blood 1990;76:1962–1964.
460. Holmes FA, O'Shaughnessy JA, Vukelja S, et al. Blinded, randomized, multicenter study to evaluate single administration pegfilgrastim once per cycle versus daily filgrastim as an adjunct to chemotherapy in patients with high-risk stage II or stage III/IV breast cancer. J Clin Oncol 2002;20:727–731.
461. Wendelin G, Lackner H, Schwinger W, et al. Once-per-cycle pegfilgrastim versus daily filgrastim in pediatric patients with Ewing sarcoma. J Pediatr Hematol Oncol 2005;27: 449–451.
462. te Poele EM, Kamps WA, Tamminga RY, et al. Pegfilgrastim in pediatric cancer patients. J Pediatr Hematol Oncol 2005;27:627–629.
463. André N, Kababri ME, Bertrand P, et al. Safety and efficacy of pegfilgrastim in children with cancer receiving myelosuppressive chemotherapy. Anticancer Drugs 2007;18: 277–281.
464. Dallorso S, Berger M, Caviglia I, et al. Prospective single-arm study of pegfilgrastim activity and safety in children with poor-risk malignant tumours receiving chemotherapy. Bone Marrow Transplant 2008;42:507–513.
465. Sung L, Nathan PC, Lange B, et al. Prophylactic granulocyte colony-stimulating factor and granulocyte-macrophage colony-stimulating factor decrease febrile neutropenia after chemotherapy in children with cancer: a meta-analysis of randomized controlled trials. J Clin Oncol 2004;22:3350–3356.
466. Wittman B, Horan J, Lyman G. Prophylactic colony-stimulating factors in children receiving myelosuppressive chemotherapy: a meta-analysis of randomized controlled trials. Cancer Treat Rev 2006;32:289–303.
467. Mitchell PL, Morland B, Stevens MC, et al. Granulocyte colony-stimulating factor in established febrile neutropenia: a randomized study of pediatric patients. J Clin Oncol 1997;15:1163–1170.
468. Riikonen P, Saarinen UM, Mäkipernaa A, et al. Recombinant human granulocyte-macrophage colony-stimulating factor in the treatment of febrile neutropenia: a double blind placebo-controlled study in children. Pediatr Infect Dis J 1994;13:197–202.
469. Ozkaynak MF, Krailo M, Chen Z, et al. Randomized comparison of antibiotics with and without granulocyte colony-stimulating factor in children with chemotherapy-induced febrile neutropenia: a report from the Children's Oncology Group. Pediatr Blood Cancer 2005;45:274–280.
470. Clark OA, Lyman G, Castro AA, et al. Colony stimulating factors for chemotherapy induced febrile neutropenia. Cochrane Database Syst Rev 2003;(3):CD003039.
471. Kwak LW, Halpern J, Olshen RA, et al. Prognostic significance of actual dose intensity in diffuse large-cell lymphoma: results of a tree-structured survival analysis. J Clin Oncol 1990;8:963–977.
472. Bonadonna G, Valagussa P. Dose-response effect of adjuvant chemotherapy in breast cancer. N Engl J Med 1981;304:10–15.
473. Antman KS, Griffin JD, Elias A, et al. Effect of recombinant human granulocyte-macrophage colony-stimulating factor on chemotherapy-induced myelosuppression. N Engl J Med 1988; 319:593–598.
474. Bronchud MH, Howell A, Crowther D, et al. The use of granulocyte colony-stimulating factor to increase the intensity of treatment with doxorubicin in patients with advanced breast and ovarian cancer. Br J Cancer 1989;60:121–125.
475. Kushner BH, LaQuaglia MP, Bonilla MA, et al. Highly effective induction therapy for stage 4 neuroblastoma in children over 1 year of age. J Clin Oncol 1994;12:2607–2613.
476. Kushner BH, Meyers PA, Gerald WL, et al. Very-high-dose short-term chemotherapy for poor-risk peripheral primitive neuroectodermal tumors, including Ewing's sarcoma, in children and young adults. J Clin Oncol 1995;13:2796–2804.
477. White L, McCowage G, Kannourakis G, et al. Dose-intensive cyclophosphamide with etoposide and vincristine for pediatric solid tumors: a phase I/II pilot study by the Australia and New Zealand Childhood Cancer Study Group. J Clin Oncol 1994;12: 522–531.
478. Saarinen-Pihkala UM, Lanning M, Perkkiö M, et al. Granulocyte-macrophage colony-stimulating factor support in therapy of high-risk acute lymphoblastic leukemia in children. Med Pediatr Oncol 2000;34:319–327.
479. Jones CA, Shaw PJ, Stevens MM. Use of granulocyte colony stimulating factor to reduce the toxicity of super-VAC chemotherapy in advanced solid tumours in childhood. Med Pediatr Oncol 1995;25:84–89.
480. Michel G, Landman-Parker J, Auclerc MF, et al. Use of recombinant human granulocyte colony-stimulating factor to increase chemotherapy dose-intensity: a randomized trial in very high-risk childhood acute lymphoblastic leukemia. J Clin Oncol 2000;18: 1517–1524.
481. Michon JM, Hartmann O, Bouffet E, et al. An open-label, multicentre, randomised phase 2 study of recombinant human granulocyte colony-stimulating factor (filgrastim) as an adjunct to combination chemotherapy in paediatric patients with metastatic neuroblastoma. Eur J Cancer 1998;34:1063–1069.
482. Kushner BH, Heller G, Kramer K, et al. Granulocyte-colony stimulating factor and multiple cycles of strongly myelosuppressive alkylator-based combination chemotherapy in children with neuroblastoma. Cancer 2000;89:2122–2130.

483. Fernandez MC, Krailo MD, Gerbing RR, et al. A phase I dose escalation of combination chemotherapy with granulocyte-macrophage-colony stimulating factor in patients with neuroblastoma. Cancer 2000;88:2838–2844.
484. Woods WG, Kobrinsky N, Buckley J, et al. Intensively timed induction therapy followed by autologous or allogeneic bone marrow transplantation for children with acute myeloid leukemia or myelodysplastic syndrome: a Children's Cancer Group pilot study. J Clin Oncol 1993;11:1448–1457.
485. Alonzo TA, Kobrinsky NL, Aledo A, et al. Impact of granulocyte colony-stimulating factor use during induction for acute myelogenous leukemia in children: a report from the Children's Cancer Group. J Pediatr Hematol Oncol 2002;24:627–635.
486. Lydaki E, Bolonaki E, Stiakaki E, et al. Efficacy of recombinant human granulocyte colony-stimulating factor and recombinant human granulocyte-macrophage colony-stimulating factor in neutropenic children with malignancies. Pediatr Hematol Oncol 1995;12:551–558.
487. Mayordomo JI, Rivera F, Díaz-Puente MT, et al. Improving treatment of chemotherapy-induced neutropenic fever by administration of colony-stimulating factors. J Natl Cancer Inst 1995;87:803–808.
488. Beveridge RA, Miller JA, Kales AN, et al. A comparison of efficacy of sargramostim (yeast-derived RhuGM-CSF) and filgrastim (bacteria-derived RhuG-CSF) in the therapeutic setting of chemotherapy-induced myelosuppression. Cancer Invest 1998;16: 366–373.
489. Kubota M, Akiyama Y, Mikawa H, et al. Comparative effect of 100 versus 250 micrograms/m²/day of G-CSF in pediatric patients with neutropenia induced by chemotherapy. Pediatr Hematol Oncol 1995;12:393–397.
490. Cairo MS, Shen V, Krailo MD, et al. Prospective randomized trial between two doses of granulocyte colony-stimulating factor after ifosfamide, carboplatin, and etoposide in children with recurrent or refractory solid tumors: a children's cancer group report. J Pediatr Hematol Oncol 2001;23:30–38.
491. Rahiala J, Perkkio M, Riikonen P. Prospective and randomized comparison of early versus delayed prophylactic administration of granulocyte colony-stimulating factor (filgrastim) in children with cancer. Med Pediatr Oncol 1999;32:326–330.
492. Elonen E, Jantunen E, Koistinen P, et al. G-CSF (lenograstim) following chemotherapy in the induction treatment of acute lymphoblastic leukemia (ALL) in adults [abstract]. Blood 1996;88(10):213a.
493. Hofmann WK, Seipelt G, Langenhan S, et al. Prospective randomized trial to evaluate two delayed granulocyte colony stimulating factor administration schedules after high-dose cytarabine therapy in adult patients with acute lymphoblastic leukemia. Ann Hematol 2002;81:570–574.
494. Hägglund H, Ringdén O, Oman S, et al. A prospective randomized trial of Filgrastim (r-metHuG-CSF) given at different times after unrelated bone marrow transplantation. Bone Marrow Transplant 1999;24:831–836.
495. Lee KH, Lee JH, Choi SJ, et al. Randomized comparison of two different schedules of granulocyte colony-stimulating factor administration after allogeneic bone marrow transplantation. Bone Marrow Transplant 1999;24:591–599.
496. Ciernik IF, Schanz U, Gmür J. Delaying treatment with granulocyte colony-stimulating factor after allogeneic bone marrow transplantation for hematological malignancies: a prospective randomized trial. Bone Marrow Transplant 1999;24:147–151.
497. Physician's Desk Reference. 58th ed. Montvale, NJ: Thomson PDR, 2004:53.
498. Kaneko T, Takaku F, Ogawa M. Outline of clinical studies on recombinant human granulocyte colony stimulating factor (KRN 8601) in Japan. Tokai J Exp Clin Med 1991;16:51–61.
499. Eguchi K, Shinkai T, Sasaki Y, et al. Subcutaneous administration of recombinant human granulocyte colony- stimulating factor (KRN8601) in intensive chemotherapy in patients with advanced lung cancer. Jpn J Cancer Res 1990;81:1168–1174.
500. Honkoop AH, Hoekman K, Wagstaff J, et al. Continuous infusion or subcutaneous injection of granulocyte-macrophage colony-stimulating factor: increased efficacy and reduced toxicity when given subcutaneously. Br J Cancer 1996;74:1132–1136.
501. Stute N, Furman WL, Schell M, et al. Pharmacokinetics of recombinant human granulocyte-macrophage colony-stimulating factor in children after intravenous and subcutaneous administration. J Pharm Sci 1995;84:824–828.
502. Novotny VM. Prevention and management of platelet transfusion refractoriness. Vox Sang 1999;76:1–13.
503. Chiu EK, Yuen KY, Lie AK, et al. A prospective study of symptomatic bacteremia following platelet transfusion and of its management. Transfusion 1994;34:950–954.
504. Chambers LA, Kruskall MS, Pacini DG, et al. Febrile reactions after platelet transfusion: the effect of single versus multiple donors. Transfusion 1990;30:219–221.
505. Broudy VC, Lin NL, Kaushansky K. Thrombopoietin (c-mpl ligand) acts synergistically with erythropoietin, stem cell factor, and interleukin-11 to enhance murine megakaryocyte colony growth and increases megakaryocyte ploidy in vitro. Blood 1995;85: 1719–1726.
506. Kuter DJ, Cebon J, Harker LA, et al. Platelet growth factors: potential impact on transfusion medicine. Transfusion 1999;39:321–332.
507. Kaushansky K. The molecular mechanisms that control thrombopoiesis. J Clin Invest 2005;115:3339–3347.
508. Zeuner A, Signore M, Martinetti D, et al. Chemotherapy-induced thrombocytopenia derives from the selective death of megakaryocyte progenitors and can be rescued by stem cell factor. Cancer Res 2007;67:4767–4773.
509. Bhatia M, Davenport V, Cairo MS. The role of interleukin-11 to prevent chemotherapy-induced thrombocytopenia in patients with solid tumors, lymphoma, acute myeloid leukemia and bone marrow failure syndromes. Leuk Lymphoma 2007;48:9–15.
510. Demetri GD. Targeted approaches for the treatment of thrombocytopenia. Oncologist 2001;6(S5):15–23.
511. O'Shaughnessy JA, Tolcher A, Riseberg D, et al. Prospective, randomized trial of 5-fluorouracil, leucovorin, doxorubicin, and cyclophosphamide chemotherapy in combination with the interleukin-3/granulocyte-macrophage colony-stimulating factor (GM-CSF) fusion protein (PIXY321) versus GM-CSF in patients with advanced breast cancer. Blood 1996;87:2205–2211.
512. Jones SE, Khandelwal P, McIntyre K, et al. Randomized, double-blind, placebo-controlled trial to evaluate the hematopoietic growth factor PIXY321 after moderate-dose fluorouracil, doxorubicin, and cyclophosphamide in stage II and III breast cancer. J Clin Oncol 1999;17:3025–3032.
513. Miller LL, Korn EL, Stevens DS, et al. Abrogation of the hematological and biological activities of the interleukin-3/granulocyte-macrophage colony-stimulating factor fusion protein PIXY321 by neutralizing anti-PIXY321 antibodies in cancer patients receiving high-dose carboplatin. Blood 1999;93:3250–3258.
514. Farese AM, Smith WG, Giri JG, et al. Promegapoietin-1 a, an engineered chimeric IL-3 and Mpl-L receptor agonist, stimulates hematopoietic recovery in conventional and abbreviated schedules following radiation-induced myelosuppression in nonhuman primates. Stem Cells 2001;19:329–338.
515. Vadhan-Raj S, Cohen V, Bueso-Ramos C. Thrombopoietic growth factors and cytokines. Curr Hematol Rep 2005;4:137–144.
516. Kuter DJ, Beeler DL, Rosenberg RD. The purification of megapoietin: a physiological regulator of megakaryocyte growth and platelet production. Proc Natl Acad Sci U S A 1994;91:11104–11108.
517. Kaushansky K, Lok S, Holly RD, et al. Promotion of megakaryocyte progenitor expansion and differentiation by the c-Mpl ligand thrombopoietin. Nature 1994;369: 568–571.
518. Kaushansky K. Thrombopoietin. N Engl J Med 1998;339:746–754.
519. Li J, Yang C, Xia Y, et al. Thrombocytopenia caused by the development of antibodies to thrombopoietin. Blood 2001;98:3241–3248.
520. Basser RL, O'Flaherty E, Green M, et al. Development of pancytopenia with neutralizing antibodies to thrombopoietin after multicycle chemotherapy supported by megakaryocyte growth and development factor. Blood 2002;99:2599–2602.
521. Basser RL, Rasko JE, Clarke K, et al. Randomized, blinded, placebo-controlled phase I trial of pegylated recombinant human megakaryocyte growth and development factor with filgrastim after dose-intensive chemotherapy in patients with advanced cancer. Blood 1997;89:3118–3128.
522. Fanucchi M, Glapsy J, Crawford J, et al. Effects of polyethylene glycol-conjugated recombinant human megakaryocyte growth and development factor on platelet counts after chemotherapy for lung cancer. N Engl J Med 1997;336:404–409.
523. Crawford J, Glapsy J, Belani C, et al. A randomized, placebo-controlled, blinded, dose scheduling trial of pegylated recombinant human megakaryocyte growth and development factor in non small cell lung cancer patients treated with paclitaxel and carboplatin during multiple cycles of chemotherapy [abstract]. Proc Am Soc Clin Oncol 1998;17:73a.
524. Basser RL, Underhill, Davis I, et al. Enhancement on platelet recovery after myelosuppressive chemotherapy by recombinant human megakaryocyte growth and development factor in patients with advanced cancer. J Clin Oncol 2000;18:2852–2861.
525. Vadhan-Raj S, Verschraegen CF, Bueso-Ramos C, et al. Recombinant human thrombopoietin attenuates carboplatin-induced severe thrombocytopenia and the need for platelet transfusions in patients with gynecologic cancer. Ann Intern Med 2000;132: 364–368.
526. Vadhan-Raj S, Patel S, Bueso-Ramos C, et al. Importance of predosing of recombinant human thrombopoietin to reduce chemotherapy-induced early thrombocytopenia. J Clin Oncol 2003;21:3158–3167.
527. Moskowitz CH, Hamlin PA, Gabrilove J, et al. Maintaining the dose intensity of ICE chemotherapy with a thrombopoietic agent, PEG-rHuMGDF, may confer a survival advantage in relapsed and refractory aggressive non-Hodgkin lymphoma. Ann Oncol 2007;18:1842–1850.
528. Angiolillo AL, Davenport V, Bonilla MA, et al. A phase I clinical, pharmacologic, and biologic study of thrombopoietin and granulocyte colony-stimulating factor in children receiving ifosfamide, carboplatin, and etoposide chemotherapy for recurrent or refractory solid tumors: a Children's Oncology Group experience. Clin Cancer Res 2005;11: 2644–2650.
529. Cripe L, Neuberg D, Tallman M, et al. A pilot study of recombinant human thrombopoietin and GM-CSF following induction therapy in patients older than 55 years with acute myelogenous leukemia [abstract]. Blood 2000;96:616a.
530. Archimbaud E, Ottmann OG, Yin JA, et al. A randomized, double-blind, placebo-controlled study with pegylated recombinant human megakaryocyte growth and development factor (PEG-rHuMGDF) as an adjunct to chemotherapy for adults with de novo acute myeloid leukemia. Blood 1999;94:3694–3701.
531. Geissler K, Yin JA, Ganser A, et al. Prior and concurrent administration of recombinant human megakaryocyte growth and development factor in patients receiving consolidation chemotherapy for de novo acute myeloid leukemia-a randomized, placebo-controlled, double-blind safety and efficacy study. Ann Hematol 2003;82:677–683.
532. Schiffer CA, Miller K, Larson RA, et al. A double-blind, placebo-controlled trial of pegylated recombinant human megakaryocyte growth and development factor as an adjunct to induction and consolidation therapy for patients with acute myeloid leukemia. Blood 2000;95:2530–2535.
533. Vadhan-Raj S, Murray LJ, Bueso-Ramos C, et al. Stimulation of megakaryocyte and platelet production by a single dose of recombinant human thrombopoietin in patients with cancer. Ann Intern Med 1997;126:673–681.
534. Bussel JB, Kuter DJ, George JN, et al. AMG 531, a thrombopoiesis-stimulating protein, for chronic ITP. N Engl J Med 2006;355:1672–1681.
535. Jenkins JM, Williams D, Deng Y, et al. Phase 1 clinical study of eltrombopag, an oral, nonpeptide thrombopoietin receptor agonist. Blood 2007;109:4739–4741.
536. Bussel JB, Cheng G, Saleh MN, et al. Eltrombopag for the treatment of chronic idiopathic thrombocytopenic purpura. N Engl J Med 2007;357:2237–2247.
537. Andemariam B, Psaila B, Bussel JB. Novel thrombopoietic agents. Hematol Am Soc Hematol Educ Program 2007;(1):106–113.
538. Kuter DJ, Bussel JB, Lyons RM, et al. Efficacy of romiplostim in patients with chronic immune thrombocytopenia purpura: a double-blind randomized controlled trial. Lancet 2008;371:395–403.
539. Gernsheimer T. The pathophysiology of ITP revisited: ineffective thrombopoiesis and the emerging role of thrombopoietin receptor agonists in the management of chronic immune thrombocytopenic purpura. Hematol Am Soc Hematol Educ Program 2008:219–226.
540. Somlo G, Sniecinski I, ter Veer A, et al. Recombinant human thrombopoietin in combination with granulocyte colony-stimulating factor enhances mobilization of peripheral blood progenitor cells, increases peripheral blood platelet concentration, and accelerates hematopoietic recovery following high-dose chemotherapy. Blood 1999;93: 2798–2806.
541. Gajewski JL, Rondon G, Donato ML, et al. Use of thrombopoietin in combination with chemotherapy and granulocyte colony-stimulating factor for peripheral blood progenitor cell mobilization. Biol Blood Marrow Transplant 2002;8:550–556.
542. Orazi A, Copper RJ, Tong J, et al. Effects of recombinant human interleukin-11 (Neumega rhIL-11 growth factor) on megakaryocytopoiesis in human bone marrow. Exp Hematol 1996;24:1289–1297.
543. Musashi M, Yang YC, Paul SR, et al. Direct and synergistic effects of interleukin 11 on murine hemopoiesis in culture. Proc Natl Acad Sci U S A 1991;88:765–769.
544. Teramura M, Kobayashi S, Hoshino S, et al. Interleukin-11 enhances human megakaryocytopoiesis in vitro. Blood 1992;79:327–331.
545. Du X, Neben T, Goldman S, et al. Effects of recombinant human interleukin-11 on hematopoietic reconstitution in transplant mice: acceleration of recovery of peripheral blood neutrophils and platelets. Blood 1993;81:27–34.

546. Du X, Williams DA. Interleukin-11: review of molecular, cell biology, and clinical use. Blood 1997;89:3897–3908.

547. Gordon MS, McCaskill-Stevens WJ, Battiato LA, et al. A phase I trial of recombinant human interleukin-11 (neumega rhIL-11 growth factor) in women with breast cancer receiving chemotherapy. Blood 1996;87:3615–3624.

548. Tepler I, Elias L, Smith JW II, et al. A randomized placebo-controlled trial of recombinant human interleukin-11 in cancer patients with severe thrombocytopenia due to chemotherapy. Blood 1996;87:3607–3614.

549. Isaacs C, Robert NJ, Bailey FA, et al. Randomized placebo-controlled study of recombinant human interleukin-11 to prevent chemotherapy-induced thrombocytopenia in patients with breast cancer receiving dose-intensive cyclophosphamide and doxorubicin. J Clin Oncol 1997;15:3368–3377.

550. Giles FJ, Kantarjian HM, Cortes JE, et al. Adaptive randomized study of idarubicin and cytarabine alone or with interleukin-11 as induction therapy in patients aged 50 or above with acute myeloid leukemia or high-risk myelodysplastic syndromes. Leuk Res 2005;29:649–652.

551. Cripe LD, Rader K, Tallman MS, et al. Phase II trial of subcutaneous recombinant human interleukin 11 with subcutaneous recombinant human granulocyte-macrophage colony stimulating factor in patients with acute myeloid leukemia (AML) receiving high-dose cytarabine during induction: ECOG 3997. Leuk Res 2006;30: 823–827.

552. Usuki K, Urabe A, Ikeda Y, et al. A multicenter randomized, double-blind, placebo-controlled late-phase II/III study of recombinant human interleukin 11 in acute myelogenous leukemia. Int J Hematol 2007;85:59–69.

553. Vredenburgh JJ, Hussein A, Fisher D, et al. A randomized trial of recombinant human interleukin-11 following autologous bone marrow transplantation with peripheral blood progenitor cell support in patients with breast cancer. Biol Blood Marrow Transplant 1998;4:134–141.

554. Cairo MS, Davenport V, Bessmertny O, et al. Phase I/II dose escalation study of recombinant human interleukin-11 following ifosfamide, carboplatin and etoposide in children, adolescents and young adults with solid tumors or lymphoma: a clinical, haematological and biological study. Br J Haematol 2004;128:49–58.

CHAPTER 40 ■ INFECTIOUS COMPLICATIONS IN PEDIATRIC CANCER PATIENTS

ANDREW Y. KOH AND PHILIP A. PIZZO

Infectious diseases are major causes of morbidity and mortality in pediatric patients with cancer. The advances in supportive care during the past *several* decades have permitted patients to successfully recover from the impact of cytotoxic cancer chemotherapy, hematopoietic stem cell transplantation (HSCT), radiation therapy, surgical intervention, and profound immunosuppression. The advances of pediatric infectious diseases supportive care have contributed substantially to the improved survival and outcome from infectious complications.

This chapter reviews the epidemiology, clinical manifestations, and strategies for managing infectious diseases in pediatric oncology patients. Formidable challenges, however, continue to threaten and undermine these successes, including the inexorable rise of multidrug-resistant bacteria, emergence of invasive fungal infections, and development of refractory viral infections. Moreover, for a number of these infections (especially the invasive mycoses), there are limited or no effective therapies. Further compounding these challenges are the increasing uncertainties of the impact of new immunosuppressive therapies on host defenses (Fig. 40.1).

HOST DEFENSES: INNATE AND ADAPTIVE IMMUNITY

Host defenses against bacterial, fungal, viral, and parasitic pathogens are often classified as innate or adaptive. Innate host defenses include mucocutaneous barriers, phagocytic cells, cytokine regulatory networks, the toll-like receptor system, natural killer cells, and nonclonal T and B cells. Adaptive immunity encompasses the production of pathogen-specific antibodies and T-lymphocyte cell-mediated immunity.

Mucocutaneous Barriers: The First Line of Innate Host Defense

The skin and mucosal surfaces constitute the primary innate host defense against invasion by endogenous and exogenous microorganisms. In addition to providing a physical barrier, mucocutaneous cells express unique biochemical, mechanical, and immunologic defenses against microbial invasion. For example, ciliated and mucus-producing cells of the pseudostratified columnar epithelium of the lower respiratory tract provide a mucociliary "escalator" that propels organisms out of the lungs. Pulmonary surfactant molecules belong to the collection class of molecules and serve to opsonize bacterial and fungal pathogens.[1–3] Pentraxin, a secreted pattern-recognition receptor that has a nonredundant role in resistance to selected microbial agents, in particular to the opportunistic fungal pathogen *Aspergillus fumigatus*, is another key molecule that has been found to be critical to pulmonary host defenses.[4] Other classes

of antimicrobial peptides also play key roles in mucosal host defenses.[5–7] For example, defensins are cysteine-rich antimicrobial peptides that contribute to host defense against bacterial, fungal, and viral infections. The alpha-defensins are present in neutrophils polymorphonuclear lymphocytes (PMNs) and Paneth cells of the small intestine, and beta-defensins protect the skin and the mucosal surfaces of the respiratory, gastrointestinal (GI), and urinary tracts. Among the specialized cells of the GI tract, parietal cells elaborate gastric acid that serves as a potent barrier against potential enteric pathogens. Paneth cells of the intestinal tract synthesize and release antimicrobial molecules that protect the luminal surface of the epithelial cells.

Pediatric oncology patients sustain disruptions of the mucocutaneous integrity because of their underlying cancer and its treatment, resulting in increased susceptibility to infection. For example, mucocutaneous integrity may be disrupted by local tumor invasion or as a result of surgery, irradiation, or cytotoxic chemotherapy. The disruption of mucocutaneous barriers provides a key portal of entry for bacterial and fungal pathogens.

The use of vascular catheters provides a striking example of the impact of cutaneous disruptions. Vascular catheters, whether temporary or chronically indwelling, disrupt cutaneous barriers and provide a direct access of microorganisms through the catheter lumen and into the bloodstream in oncology patients.[8–10] One study reported an estimated four-fold increase in the incidence of bacteremia in neutropenic cancer patients who had catheters compared with those who did not.[11] Foreign devices other than vascular catheters have been implicated in the risk of infectious complications in cancer patients (e.g., Omaya intraventricular reservoirs and prosthetic bone-joint hardware).[12] Increasing recognition of the role of biofilms underscores mechanisms by which these organisms may perpetuate seeding of the bloodstream and promote emergence of resistance.[13,14]

Several antineoplastic compounds administered in patients with hematologic malignancies may induce severe mucosal disruption. These include high-dose methotrexate, cytosine arabinoside (Ara-C), anthracyclines (daunorubicin, doxorubicin), and etoposide. Radiation therapy to the abdomen or thorax may result in similar disruption of the GI epithelium in the esophagus or in the small and large intestines, respectively. GI barriers may also be disrupted by mucosal disruption due to herpes simplex virus (HSV) or cytomegalovirus (CMV). Graft-versus-host disease (GVHD) may also compromise GI mucosal integrity and permit bacteria and/or fungi to translocate from the mesenteric capillary bed and portal venous system.

Other disruptions of mucocutaneous barriers in pediatric oncology patients include ventricular drains, ventriculostomies, nasogastric tubes, endotracheal tubes, chest tubes, surgical drains, dialysis catheters, nephrostomy tubes, urinary catheters, finger sticks, venipunctures, and bone marrow aspirations. These disruptions alter the epidermal integument and provide a

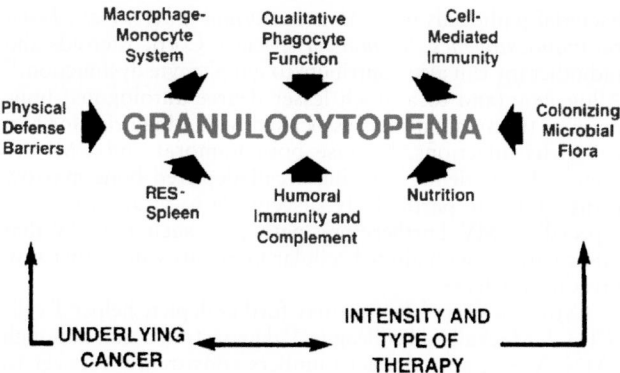

FIGURE 40.1 Interactions of the defense matrix that delineates the compromised host.

potential nidus for colonization, local infection, and hematogenous dissemination of bacterial and fungal pathogens.

Microbial Colonization: Normal Microflora Serving as an Extension of Mucocutaneous Barriers

Most bacterial and fungal infectious episodes in immunocompromised patients are preceded by colonization with the infecting organism. Colonization by normal bacterial flora provides a competitive microbiologic barrier to colonization by extrinsically acquired bacterial and fungal organisms. This normal bacterial flora may be abrogated by antibiotics or by the onset of illness. The mechanisms by which this bacterial barrier is maintained are not well understood. In healthy persons, integumentary and mucosal attachment sites are populated with a quantitative predominance of aerobic gram-positive bacteria and various anaerobic bacteria with relatively low virulence.[15] However, within 24 hours of hospitalization, seriously ill patients undergo a change in their indigenous microflora toward one of aerobic gram-negative organisms.[16,17] The mechanisms of this microbiologic shift are unclear; however, underlying disease and exposure to broad-spectrum antibiotics likely contribute to these changes in bacterial adherence and colonization.

Schimpff et al.[17] demonstrated that approximately one-half of the responsible pathogens causing infections are acquired by oncology patients after initial admission to the hospital. They further found that more than 80% of the microbiologically documented infections that occur in adult patients with acute myelogenous leukemia (AML) are caused by organisms that were a component of the endogenous mucosal organisms, usually at sites at or near the source of infection.

Phagocytic Cells: The Second Line of Innate Host Defense

The innate host defense system includes the repertoire of phagocytic cells consisting of PMNs, circulating monocytes (MNCs), and tissue macrophages. These cells assert their antimicrobial effects of phagocytosis, oxidative and nonoxidative mediators, and the release of cytokines. PMNs possess the greatest degree of oxidative capacity and response to a microbial stimulus followed by MNCs and then by macrophages. Pulmonary alveolar macrophages, splenic macrophages, and

Küpfer cells constitute an important residual phagocytic barrier during neutropenia, when PMNs and MNCs may be depleted. Both MNCs and macrophages serve as important immunoregulatory cells by expressing cytokines and chemokines to activate and regulate host response.

Phagocytic cells may be quantitatively or qualitatively impaired. Patients with quantitative or qualitative defects of their PMNs are subject primarily to infections due to bacteria (*Escherichia coli, Klebsiella pneumoniae, Pseudomonas aeruginosa*, and more recently an expanding range of resistant gram-negative organisms) and fungi (particularly *Candida* species, *Aspergillus* species, *Fusarium* species, and Zygomycetes), and does not, *per se*, appear to increase the incidence or severity of viral and parasitic infections.[18]

The most important determinants of risk of infection associated with neutropenia are (1) the absolute neutrophil count (ANC), (2) the rate of decline of the ANC, and (3) the duration of neutropenia. The ANC is a critical determinant of susceptibility to most bacterial and fungal pathogens in patients receiving cytotoxic chemotherapy. Cytotoxic chemotherapy, total body irradiation, aplastic anemia, and bone marrow infiltration by leukemic cells may all cause neutropenia. The seminal work of Bodey and colleagues[19] demonstrated that a decline in ANC to less than 500 cells/mL significantly increased the risk of infection and that profound neutropenia (<100 cells/mL) precipitously increased the risk of bacterial and fungal infections.

The rate of decline of circulating PMNs is also critical. For example, patients with rapidly declining ANCs following therapy for acute leukemia appear to be at greater risk for infectious complications than patients with chronic neutropenia (e.g., aplastic anemia).[20]

Finally, neutropenia that persists for more than 7 to 10 days is associated with increasing risk for severe, recurrent, or new bacterial and fungal infections.[20] On the other hand, those in whom no infection has been documented, who defervesce rapidly on empirical antimicrobial therapy, and recover from neutropenia within 1 week of the febrile episode are more likely to pursue an uncomplicated course. As discussed later, the duration of neutropenia is an important variable in assessment of patients for oral administration of empirical antibacterial therapy and for preventive strategies for management of invasive fungal infections.

In addition to quantitative declines of PMNs and MNCs, functional changes may occur in pediatric oncology patients. Qualitative abnormalities of PMN function may occur as a consequence of the underlying malignancy (especially acute leukemia) or secondary to antineoplastic therapy. For example, the PMNs from patients with leukemia or lymphoma exhibit suboptimal chemoattractant responsiveness, bactericidal activity, and superoxide production.[21,22] Antineoplastic chemotherapy and radiotherapy also cause qualitative abnormalities of PMN function.[23] Deficiencies of PMN function iatrogenically induced by the administration of various medications (e.g., opiates, corticosteroids, antibiotics) may have a detrimental effect.[24] For example, corticosteroids suppress oxidative metabolism in superoxide production, impair phagocytosis, and reduce the microbicidal activity of PMNs against bacteria and fungi.[25–27]

The advent of corticosteroid-sparing immunosuppressive agents may also indirectly impair PMN and MNC function because of their suppressive effects on activating cytokines. For example, infliximab, which is used in the management of corticosteroid-refractory GVHD through inhibition of tumor necrosis factor alpha (TNF-α), may result in an increased risk for reactivation of tuberculosis and for development of invasive aspergillosis.

Cytokines and Toll-Like Receptors

The innate host defense mechanisms include an elaborate network of immunoregulatory cytokines and chemokines.[28] TNF-α, interleukin-1 (IL-1), interferon-gamma (INF-γ), interleukin 2 (IL-2), interleukin 6 (IL-6), and interleukin 12 (IL-12) are proinflammatory cytokines that upregulate phagocytic response against bacteria, mycobacteria, fungi, and viruses. IL-1, TNF-α, INF-γ, and IL-12 promote increased microbicidal activity against most bacteria, mycobacteria, and fungi mediated by a T-helper 1–type response. By comparison, the molecules interleukin 4 (IL-4) and interleukin 10 (IL-10) promote a downregulation of host response against these pathogens; these molecules are characteristic of a T-helper 2–type response.

Toll-like receptors (TLRs) are key components of innate host response that are responsible for recognition of pathogens and cytokine response to surface molecules.[29,30] The family of TLRs recognizes pathogen-associated molecular patterns. Different pathogens interact with certain TLRs through distinct patterns of molecules on their cell surface in the form of carbohydrates, proteins, and glycoproteins. Binding of pathogen-associated molecular patterns to TLRs activates signal transduction pathways that lead to cytokines, interferons, and chemokines that, in turn, may activate host response to the infecting pathogen. As this process occurs independent of adaptive immunity, the TLR system may be especially relevant to immunocompromised patients when adaptive immunity is significantly suppressed. For instance, a recent study suggests an association between a donor TLR4 haplotype and the risk of invasive aspergillosis among recipients of hematopoietic stem cell transplants from unrelated donors.[31] Similarly, other TLR4 single-nucleotide polymorphisms have been associated with susceptibility to infections caused by gram-negative bacteria,[32] C. albicans,[33] and respiratory syncytial virus.[34]

Adaptive Immunity

Adaptive immunity is composed of B-cell and T-cell populations that mediate humoral and cell-mediated immunity (CMI), respectively. The B cell–plasma cell axis of humoral immunity provides a host with antibody and response to bacterial, viral, and some fungal pathogens. However, during the course of chemotherapy or during hypogammaglobulinemia, there may be substantial qualitative and quantitative defects in antibody response. Defective immunoglobulin synthesis or hypogammaglobulinemia leads to an increase in the susceptibility to encapsulated bacteria, particularly Streptococcus pneumoniae, Haemophilus influenzae type B (HIB), and Neisseria meningitidis.[35] Despite effective vaccination against HIB, a recent study estimated that HIB caused about 8.13 million serious illnesses worldwide in 2000, with an estimated 371,000 deaths in children aged 1 to 59 months (8,100 human immunodeficiency virus (HIV)-positive; 363,000 HIV-negative).[36] Similarly, about 14.5 million cases of serious pneumococcal disease were estimated to occur worldwide in 2000, with 826,000 deaths in children aged 1 to 59 months (91,000 HIV-positive; 735,000 HIV-negative); of the deaths in HIV-negative children, more than 61% occurred in 10 African and Asian countries where the pneumococcal vaccine is not readily available.[37]

Patients with Hodgkin disease or non-Hodgkin lymphoma have an impaired CMI that can persist even when the cancer is in remission.[38,39] Patients with deficiencies of cellular immunity are prone to fungal, viral, and intracellularly replicating bacterial pathogens (e.g., Mycobacterium tuberculosis, Listeria monocytogenes, Salmonella species). Corticosteroids and radiotherapy can also contribute to lymphocyte dysfunction.[40] Allogeneic (and to a much lesser degree autologous) bone marrow transplantation is associated with a high risk for herpes virus infections, because both humoral and CMI are impaired.[41] Patients receiving T-cell–depleted bone marrow transplants are particularly susceptible to viral pathogens, especially CMV. Furthermore, pathogens such as CMV that infect patients with altered cellular immunity can further suppress host defenses.[42]

Cytotoxic chemotherapy may further deplete helper T cells (CD4+). Mackall and colleagues[43] demonstrated that although PMN, MNC, and platelet numbers consistently recover to greater than 50% of pretreatment values after sequential cycles of therapy, lymphocyte numbers do not recover promptly, and lymphopenia may persist for many months after the completion of a chemotherapy regimen. The capacity for CD4+ T-cell regeneration after chemotherapy seems to diminish with age, such that younger children have significantly greater recovery of T cells 6 months after chemotherapy than do young adults, who have persistent, severe T-cell depletion. Prolonged T-cell depletion probably contributes to the development of opportunistic infections such as herpes zoster or Pneumocystis carinii pneumonia during the months after chemotherapy.

Spleen and Reticuloendothelial System

The spleen is a key organ of both innate and adaptive immunity. The spleen acts as a mechanical filter and as an immune effector organ. At the same time, the spleen also is the principal organ involved in the production of antibodies to polysaccharide antigens, filtering damaged cells and opsonized organisms from the circulation.[44] Splenectomized patients are deficient in antibody production when challenged with particulate antigens and have decreased levels of immunoglobulin M (IgM) and properdin (a component of the alternate complement pathway). Asplenic patients are at increased risk for fulminant and rapidly fatal septicemia caused by encapsulated bacterial pathogens, especially S. pneumoniae, H. influenzae, and N. meningitidis.[45] S. pneumoniae, which is the most common cause of sepsis in the asplenic patient, may be penicillin-resistant, particularly in patients on chronic penicillin prophylaxis. Several other pathogens also are associated with a fulminant course in asplenic patients: Capnocytophaga canimorsus dysgonic fermenter (formerly known as DF-2), Salmonella species, Babesia microti, and Plasmodium falciparum. Fulminant sepsis due to C. canimorsus is typically associated with dog bites. B. microti, which is transmitted by the bite of Ixodes tick, occurs in the same regions as Lyme disease. Patients with severe combined immunodeficiency (SCID) are predisposed to developing bacteremia, or even splenic abscesses, secondary to functional asplenia.[46]

Neurologic, Mechanical, and Nutritional Factors Contributing to Immune Impairment

Alterations in central nervous system (CNS) function or decreased levels of awareness due to tumor or opioids increase the risk of aspiration pneumonia. Aspirated pharyngeal organisms, most commonly aerobic gram-negative bacilli, can colonize, invade, and disseminate from a pulmonary source. The risk of an aspiration pneumonia and subsequent disseminated infection is heightened by decreased mucosal clearance mechanisms and damage mediated by antineoplastic therapy.

Mechanical obstruction of hollow viscus by a primary or metastatic tumor mass can promote an infection by the organisms colonizing the site of obstruction. For example, obstruction of the bronchus by osteogenic sarcoma may lead to postobstructive pneumonia, obstruction of the GI tract by a pelvic rhabdomyosarcoma may cause perforation and peritonitis, and obstruction of the ureter may lead to hydronephrosis and pyelonephritis.

The compromising effect of a malnourished state on immune function is well documented.[47] Nutritional deficiencies affect B and T lymphocytes, PMNs, mononuclear phagocytes, complement system function, and cytokine immunoregulation. Increasing data indicate that proteosome activation may severely deplete total body protein[48] with profound implications for mechanical and cellular host defenses.

CARE OF FEBRILE CANCER PATIENTS

General Principles

Fever in the neutropenic patient is a common manifestation of infection in pediatric oncology.[49] Left untreated, febrile neutropenic patients may sustain devastating complications of bacterial sepsis. Hence, fever in a neutropenic patient should be managed as a potential medical emergency. The localizing signs initially may be muted owing to the paucity of inflammatory cells.[50] A careful history and physical examination directed toward identifying possible foci of infection is important as a guide to selection of antimicrobial therapy and any adjunctive supportive measures, such as surgical intervention. Less commonly but importantly, neutropenic patients can have serious and life-threatening infection in the absence of fever (e.g., nonfebrile, neutropenic patients with *Clostridium septicum* can present with severe abdominal pain and can ultimately develop septic shock and rapidly progressive necrotizing fasciitis with myonecrosis). Accordingly, if a neutropenic patient develops signs or symptoms suggestive of a localizing infection, he or she should be managed according to the same principles as the neutropenic patient who presents with fever. Supportive culture data and diagnostic imaging procedures will further define the microbiologic etiology and location of the infection. Ultimately, continued reevaluation of these patients is critical to their successful outcome.

Mechanisms of Fever

Fever (defined as an oral temperature >38.3°C) is a common clinical manifestation among children with cancer.[49] The production of fever in humans is mediated by the actions of several proinflammatory cytokines, primarily IL-1, TNF-α, and IL-6. Although MNCs and macrophages are the major cellular source for these cytokines, multiple other cell types produce these proinflammatory cytokines. These cytokines share a number of proinflammatory properties that inhibit bacterial replication, including the induction of fever; hepatic synthesis of acute-phase reactants (e.g., C-reactive protein and fibrinogen); activation of T and B cells; and metabolic changes such as mobilization of amino acids, decreases in serum iron and zinc, and an increase in serum copper. By inducing the synthesis of other cytokines and chemokines, IL-1 and TNF-α also stimulate PMN, lymphocyte, and MNC migration and activate mature PMN functions such as chemotaxis, phagocytosis, and killing of bacteria and fungi. IL-1 and TNF-α also

appear to mediate the development of septic shock in humans. The elaboration of these cytokines results in a coordinated proinflammatory and immunoregulatory host response against an infectious pathogen.[51]

Initial Manifestations of Infection in Neutropenic Patients

Although fever in cancer patients is frequently caused by infection, noninfectious causes must also be considered in the differential diagnosis. The initial manifestations of acute lymphoblastic leukemia (ALL) commonly include fever due to the primary neoplastic process; by comparison, fever in patients with AML is seldom due to the leukemic process and is more likely to be due to a concomitant infection. In addition to the malignant process, pyrogenic medications (e.g., bleomycin and Ara-C), blood product transfusions, and allergic reactions are potential sources of a febrile response. Nonetheless, in a neutropenic patient, fever may be the first and only sign of infection.[52] Other clinical signs and symptoms frequently indicative of an infectious process (i.e., pain, erythema, swelling) may be blunted or lacking. Alternatively, localized pain and signs of inflammation may occur in the absence of fever in a neutropenic patient. For example, neutropenic patients with intraabdominal sepsis may complain only of localizing pain despite a perforated bowel. Thus, in an afebrile, neutropenic patient with localizing pain, hemodynamic instability, or altered mental status, prompt initiation of empirical antibacterial therapy is indicated.

Patients with an ANC, including PMNs plus band forms, of 500 cells/mL or less are considered to be neutropenic and at increased risk for infection. However, patients who have recently received chemotherapy may present with an ANC greater than 500 but less than 1,000 cells/mL. Because these patients likely have rapidly declining counts, they are managed in a manner similar to those whose counts are already declining.

Pediatric Versus Adult Patients

Pediatric cancer patients are different from their adult counterparts in numerous ways. These include the spectrum of oncologic diagnoses, the intensity of chemotherapeutic regimens (with a larger percentage of children with cancer who are treated very intensely with a curative goal), and the incidence and severity of comorbid medical conditions preceding the diagnosis of cancer. In addition, the use of prophylactic antimicrobials, the percentage of patients with indwelling central venous catheters, the community exposures to infectious pathogens, and maturation of the immune system may be different based on age.

These differences between adult and pediatric patients affect the frequency and nature of episodes of fever and neutropenia. A review of results from four European Organization for Research and Treatment of Cancer (EORTC) studies reported that the sites of infection and spectrum of infecting organisms are different in children and adults.[52] Children more often do not have a clinically apparent site of infection and consequently have a higher rate of fever without a source. When a defined site is present, children were more likely than their adult counterparts to have upper respiratory tract findings. The overall incidence of bacteremia is similar; however, the rate of death during fever and neutropenia was 1% in children compared with 4% in adults.

Evaluation of Patients with Fever and Neutropenia

A careful history and meticulous physical examination is essential to the initial assessment of patients with fever and neutropenia. Neutropenic hosts have a decreased ability to manifest an inflammatory response and thus even subtle signs and symptoms should be considered significant. The history and physical examination should focus on areas at special risk in patients receiving cytotoxic therapy, including the oropharynx, respiratory tract, perianal area, central venous line sites, any site of recent invasive procedures, and the skin and soft tissues.

Blood cultures should be obtained from all lumens of central venous lines, when present. Volume of blood cultures is the most important factor for detection of circulating bacteria and fungi. Given the additional time, discomfort, and increased risk of contamination, peripheral blood cultures are not necessary in patients with a vascular access device when two or more sets of blood cultures have been obtained through the catheter. A meta-analysis showed little benefit in two-site culturing in patients with cancer with vascular access devices.[53] Most catheter-related bacteremias can be managed on a pathogen-based approach rather than on a quantitative culture or time-based approach. Urine cultures should be obtained routinely. Other cultures (e.g., stool, cerebrospinal fluid [CSF]) should be obtained based on clinical suspicion.

A chest radiograph should be considered for all patients. Although the yield of routine chest radiographs in asymptomatic neutropenic patients is small,[54] the study can serve as an important baseline for comparison with later films. The presence of a pulmonary infiltrate should also prompt consideration for subsequent evaluation by computed tomography (CT) or even bronchoscopy for a more definitive microbiologic diagnosis.

Following the completion of history, physical examination, and cultures, broad-spectrum antibiotics should be started promptly in all febrile neutropenic patients. Should the chest radiograph prove to be positive, additional coverage for community-acquired pneumonia or invasive fungal infections should also be considered.

Evaluation of Afebrile Neutropenic Patients with Localizing Signs

Fever may be absent in some cases of subsequently documented infection in neutropenic patients, particularly those with profound neutropenia and those receiving corticosteroids. The presence of infection in this setting may be detected only by attention to seemingly minor complaints from the patient or by subtle physical findings. It is critical that the physician acknowledge these complaints or findings seriously and pursue them vigorously. Abdominal pain, for example, may signify an evolving intraabdominal infection (e.g., typhlitis), whereas erythema and tenderness along a subcutaneous catheter tunnel track usually indicates the presence of a deep soft-tissue infection, even if the patient is afebrile.[55] In these situations, it is most prudent to obtain cultures of blood and any other pertinent sites, and then to immediately begin antibiotics directed against probable pathogens. Although colonization with microorganisms often precedes development of significant infection, routine surveillance cultures are rarely helpful in a neutropenic patient. Any delay in antibiotic therapy while awaiting the results of cultures may permit the unchecked progression of infection in the neutropenic host.

Risk Assessment in Cancer Patients with Fever and Neutropenia

Traditionally, empirical antibacterial therapy for oncology patients with fever and neutropenia has involved admission to the hospital and administration of broad-spectrum intravenous (IV) antibiotics. More recently, it has become clear that not all patients with fever and neutropenia are at equal risk for significant morbidity or mortality from infection.[56,57] The identification of a low-risk subset may allow for modifications of therapy in this group with a goal of reduced therapy-related toxicity, an improved quality of life, and decreased cost of treatment.

A retrospective study performed by Talcott et al.[56] evaluated risk factors for serious medical complications and death during episodes of fever and neutropenia in adult oncology patients. A "high-risk" group was defined as those patients who were inpatients at the time of diagnosis with fever and neutropenia and those presenting as outpatients with either concurrent comorbidity or uncontrolled cancer. The "low-risk" group was, by exclusion, those patients presenting with fever and neutropenia as outpatients without comorbidity or progressive cancer. Importantly, the information required to stratify a patient as either high or low risk was available to the clinician at the time of the patient's presentation with fever and neutropenia. The medical course in the two groups was found to be significantly different. The rates of serious complications ranged from 31% to 55% in the high-risk group compared with 2% in the low-risk group. Similarly, rates of death ranged from 14% to 23% in the high-risk group compared with no deaths in the low-risk group.

Although no definitive consensus exists regarding the criteria used to distinguish high-risk from low-risk patient, several key factors that may increase the risk of infectious complications have been surmised for numerous studies that have been conducted: anticipated duration of neutropenia[58]; significant medical comorbidity[56,58]; cancer status and cancer type; documented infection on presentation (i.e., pneumonia, IV cathersite infection); evidence of bone marrow recovery (e.g, absolute monocyte count)[59,60]; and magnitude of fever.[52,59]

Numerous studies have investigated the use of oral antibiotic therapy (pefloxacin,[61] ofloxacin,[62–64] ciprofloxacin,[65,66] cefixime,[67,68] and moxifloxacin[69]) for empiric coverage in low-risk febrile cancer patients with neutropenia). Although the results of these studies are promising, many of these trials were statistically underpowered and limited by methodologic issues. In contrast, two large, prospective randomized clinical trials of low-risk febrile and neutropenic cancer patients being treated with oral ciprofloxacin plus oral amoxicillin-clavulanate compared with parenteral antibiotic therapies administered in the inpatient setting showed that the efficacy of the oral and IV regimens was comparable.[70,71] But the authors of both of these trials were quick to warn that their findings should not be used to justify the widespread implementation of the use of empirical oral antibiotic therapy to treat low-risk febrile and neutropenic patients. Before adapting an institutional policy for transferring care of febrile neutropenic children to an outpatient setting of oral therapy, careful consideration of infrastructural support is needed. The challenge in administering oral antibacterial empirical therapy is to identify and validate criteria for the truly low-risk patients within one's own institution. Practitioners must have a validated system to accurately prognosticate a pediatric cancer patient's risk of serious complications or death from infection. The length of time of inpatient observation, if any, and design of outpatient follow-up need to be determined to ensure the efficacy and safety of such regimens. In addition, the potential burden on patients and families, satisfaction with care in the inpatient versus outpatient settings, and cost, including level of reimbursement for services and out-of-pocket expenses for patients and their families, need to be assessed. Other factors that need to be addressed are the availability of reliable telecommunications, proximity to a hospital for emergency transfer, a reliable caregiver to ensure compliance with oral therapy, and the availability of transportation to a medical facility.

Evaluation of Febrile Nonneutropenic Patients

Evaluation of a febrile nonneutropenic cancer patient begins with a careful history and physical examination. Blood cultures are generally obtained on febrile nonneutropenic pediatric oncology patients—especially those with indwelling catheters. Patients with localized symptoms or signs should undergo the appropriate diagnostic procedures (e.g., stool cultures in patients with diarrhea, lumbar puncture for patients with meningeal irritation). Patients with focal findings should receive appropriate therapy based on the site involved (e.g., amoxicillin for otitis, cephalexin or dicloxacillin for cellulitis of the catheter exit site). If blood cultures are negative in such patients, then the empirical antibacterial therapy may be discontinued. Patients who are nonneutropenic, clinically well, without any identifiable focus of infection and without an indwelling central venous catheter may be observed without empirical antibacterial therapy. By comparison, patients who are febrile and nonneutropenic, clinically well, without any identifiable focus of infection but who have an indwelling central venous catheter should receive empirical antibacterial therapy (e.g., ceftriaxone), pending results of blood cultures.

Patients with an indwelling venous access catheter (i.e., Hickman, Broviac) who become febrile present a special problem. The frequency of infectious complications in patients with intravascular devices can be high with central line–associated bacterial bloodstream infections being of greatest concern. Blood cultures should be obtained from each port of a multilumen catheter. The catheter exit site should be examined carefully for signs of erythema, tenderness, or discharge, and any discharge material should be cultured. If signs of infection or clinical instability are observed, an antibiotic regimen designed to cover the most commonly encountered line-related pathogens (i.e., *Staphylococcus aureus, Staphylococcus epidermidis*, and gram-negative aerobes) should be initiated. A broad-spectrum third-generation cephalosporin (e.g., ceftriaxone) offers adequate initial coverage in the absence of an obvious tunnel infection. Vancomycin is recommended for empirical therapy in health care settings with an elevated prevalence of methicillin-resistant *Staphylococcus aureus* (MRSA); daptomycin can be used as an alternative but linezolid is not recommended.[72] Antibiotics should be continued for a 48- to 72-hour trial. If the preantibiotic blood and catheter culture results are negative and no site of infection is determined, the antibiotics may be withdrawn, whether or not fever persists. This allows for a thorough evaluation of the cause of fever, without the confounding influence of antibiotics. If the cultures are positive, a full therapeutic course is warranted (Fig. 40.2). For further details, please refer to the 2009 guidelines of the Infectious Diseases Society of America (IDSA) for the diagnosis and management of intravascular catheter-related infection.[72]

EMPIRICAL ANTIBACTERIAL TREATMENT OF FEBRILE NEUTROPENIC PATIENTS

General Considerations

Perhaps the single most important advance in infectious diseases oncology supportive care leading to improved survival has been the prompt initiation of empirical antibacterial antibiotics when the neutropenic cancer patient becomes febrile. Before this approach was instituted in the early 1970s, the mortality rate from gram-negative infections, especially that of *P. aeruginosa, E. coli*, and *K. pneumoniae*, approached 80%.[73,74] With the widespread use of effective empirical antibiotics, the overall mortality has declined to approximately 10% to 40% for infections caused by gram-negative bacteria.

An ideal empirical antibacterial regimen should provide a broad spectrum of activity against a wide variety of pathogenic organisms, including but not limited to *Pseudomonas*; be bactericidal in the absence of neutrophils; and have low potential for adverse effects. The choice of a specific agent or combination should also be predicated on the specific patterns of bacterial infection in one's own institution, as well as antibiotic susceptibility profiles, cost, toxicity, and standards used at one's center.

Approximately 85% to 90% of pathogens that are documented to be associated with new fevers in neutropenia patients are gram-positive and gram-negative bacteria (Table 40.1). Hence, an empirical antibiotic regimen must cover a broad spectrum of bacteria, provide high serum bactericidal drug levels, be stable against the emergence of resistant bacteria, and be as nontoxic and as simple to administer as possible. These conditions have traditionally required the combination of two or more antibiotics.[75] Several regimens, usually consisting of a cephalosporin, an aminoglycoside, and extended-spectrum penicillin, have been employed.[73,74]

Combination Therapy

Combination antibacterial therapy was especially important in earlier days of antibiotic development. The objective was to provide expanded antibacterial spectrum, enhance potential synergistic interaction, and prevent the emergence of resistance. Antimicrobial synergy was particularly relevant to gram-negative bacteria. A synergistic combination would enhance the efficacy and lower the effective minimum inhibitory concentration (MIC) of each compound when used in combination. However, with the advent of third- and fourth-generation cephalosporins and carbapenems, which have significantly lower MICs than earlier β-lactams, the combining of two agents to achieve enhanced synergistic activity was no longer important. Moreover, third- and fourth-generation cephalosporins and carbapenems possess the broader spectrum of the combination of conventional β-lactam/aminoglycoside combinations. Finally, third- and fourth-generation cephalosporins and carbapenems are more resistant to the β-lactamases that emerged in organisms resistant to the earlier carboxypenicillins and acylureidopenicillins.

Antibiotic Monotherapy

The development of third- and fourth-generation cephalosporins (e.g., ceftazidime and cefepime, respectively) and carbapenems

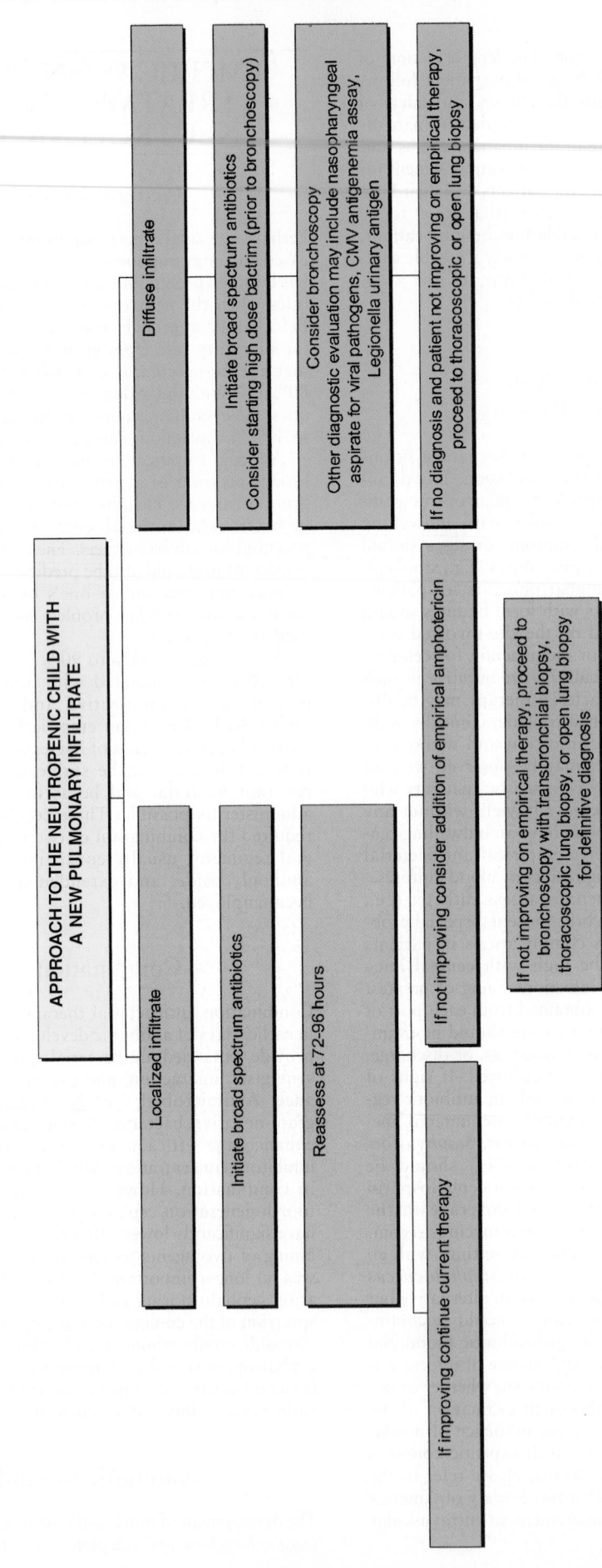

FIGURE 40.2 Algorithm for the management of the child with neutropenia and a pulmonary infiltrate.

TABLE 40.1

PREDOMINANT PATHOGENS IN PEDIATRIC CANCER PATIENTS

Gram-positive bacteria
Staphylococcus species (e.g., *S. epidermidis* and *S. aureus*)
Streptococcus species (α-hemolytic; e.g., *S. mitis*)
Enterococcus species (e.g., *E. faecium, E. faecalis*)
Corynebacterium species (e.g., *C. jeikeium*)
Listeria monocytogenes
Bacillus species (*B. cereus, B. circulans, B. licheniformis*)
Clostridium species (*C. difficile, C. septicum, C. tertium*)

Gram-negative bacteria
Enterobacteriaceae (*Escherichia coli, Klebsiella* species,
    Enterobacter species, *Serratia* species)
Pseudomonas aeruginosa (similar oxidase-positive
    multiresistant gram-negative organisms) *Stenotrophomonas
    maltophilia*
Anaerobes (e.g., *Bacteroides* species and *Prevotella* species)

Fungi
Candida species (e.g., *C. albicans, C. glabrata, C. tropicalis,*
    C. krusei)
Aspergillus species (e.g., *A. fumigatus, A. flavus,* and
    A. terreus)
Zygomycetes (e.g., *Rhizopus oryzae*)
Fusarium species (e.g., *F. solani* and *F. oxysporum*)
Scedosporium species (*S. apiospermum* and *S. inflatum*)
Cryptococcus neoformans
Pneumocystis jiroveci (formerly, *P. carinii*)

Viruses
Herpes simplex virus
Varicella-zoster virus
Cytomegalovirus
Epstein-Barr virus
Respiratory syncytial virus
Adenovirus
Influenza virus
Parainfluenza virus
Human herpes virus 6
Polyoma viruses (e.g., BK virus, JC virus)

Protozoa and helminths
Toxoplasma gondii
Cryptosporidium species
Strongyloides stercoralis

TABLE 40.2

MANAGEMENT OF CENTRAL VENOUS CATHETERS IN PATIENTS WITH BACTEREMIA

Criteria for central venous line removal
1. Evidence of a local tunnel infection
2. Persistently positive blood cultures
3. Recurrently positive blood cultures with the same
   pathogen
4. Positive blood cultures for:
   - *Candida* species
   - Polymicrobial infections
   - Vancomycin-resistant enterococci
   - Atypical mycobacteria (e.g., *M. fortuitum, M. chelonae,
     M. abscessus*)
   - *Bacillus* species

Criteria for probable central venous line removal
1. Exit site or pocket space infection with *Pseudomonas
   aeruginosa, Stenotrophomonas maltophilia,* or atypical
   mycobacteria
2. Clinical deterioration with known positive blood cultures
3. Positive blood cultures for:
   - *S. aureus*
   - Viridans group streptococci

patients based on large randomized controlled trials: ceftazidime, cefepime, imipenem, and meropenem.

Ceftazidime

The proof of concept of monotherapy as an initial strategy for empirical antimicrobial therapy was first demonstrated by the results of a prospective randomized trial at the National Cancer Institute (NCI) in which ceftazidime was compared with the combination of cephalothin, carbenicillin, and gentamicin for the initial empirical management of 550 episodes of fever and neutropenia.[76] For ceftazidime and the combination regimen, the study demonstrated equivalent rates of success, as measured by patient survival through neutropenia, with or without antibiotic modifications of the initial regimen. However, significantly more modifications were required among patients randomized to ceftazidime, reflecting the need for anaerobic coverage in patients who developed necrotizing gingivitis or perianal cellulitis, as well as the greater need for vancomycin for patients with documented gram-positive infections. Patients with documented infections more frequently required changes in antimicrobial therapy than those with unexplained fever; however, the need was the same (59%) for those receiving monotherapy or combination therapy.

A large multicenter, randomized European study by dePauw et al.[77] subsequently evaluated ceftazidime versus piperacillin plus tobramycin in 876 episodes of fever and neutropenia. The majority of patients had acute leukemia or were HSCT recipients. The mean duration of neutropenia was 18 days. The two regimens were similar in rates of defervescence, control, and eradication of infections and infection-related mortality; however, fewer adverse reactions occurred in patients enrolled into the ceftazidime arm. This study confirmed that ceftazidime monotherapy is a viable empirical regimen in high-risk febrile neutropenic patients.

Many centers have adopted ceftazidime monotherapy as a standard of care for the initial management of the febrile neutropenic patient. Nonetheless, several concerns have been raised

(e.g., imipenem and meropenem) provides alternatives to the more traditional aminoglycoside-containing combination regimens (Table 40.2).[76–78] Several of these compounds are able to provide breadth of antimicrobial spectrum and high bactericidal levels when used as single agents. The use of antibiotic monotherapy for the empirical management of the febrile neutropenic patient is attractive because of the ease of administration, lower cost, and lesser toxicity of a single drug, particularly without the use of an aminoglycoside.

As oncology centers have different patterns of microbial isolates and antibiotic resistance, the clinical decisions about appropriate antibacterial empirical regimens must ultimately be individualized for each institution. The 2002 guidelines of the IDSA) for the use of antimicrobial agents in neutropenic patients with cancer underscore the need to adjust empirical therapy to local patterns of infection and to individual patient characteristics.[79] This document identified the following four antibiotics to be appropriate as empirical monotherapy in febrile neutropenic

regarding the use of ceftazidime monotherapy. First, the relative lack of *in vitro* activity of third-generation cephalosporins against gram-positive cocci, particularly *S. aureus* and some strains of alpha-hemolytic streptococci, prompted some investigators to advocate inclusion of vancomycin in the primary regimen.[80,81] However, the concerns of *S. aureus* are overstated, because ceftazidime maintains adequate time spent above the MIC (the key pharmacodynamic variable of β-lactam antibiotics) of most strains of oxacillin-susceptible *S. aureus*. Second, some have advocated the inclusion of an aminoglycoside in the initial regimen to maximize the activity against gram-negative pathogens and to decrease the emergence of resistant organisms.[78] However, the need for an aminoglycoside is probably not tenable in most centers unless there is a high frequency of relative resistance to ceftazidime by gram-negative bacilli. The problem of ceftazidime resistance due to gram-negative pathogens with extended spectrum β-lactamases and chromosomally mediated inducible β-lactamases has clearly become a threat to the utility of ceftazidime as initial monotherapy in some centers.

Cefepime

Cefepime is a potent broad-spectrum fourth-generation cephalosporin with enhanced activity against gram-positive and gram-negative aerobes, including some pathogens resistant to other cephalosporins. Its *in vitro* spectrum includes viridans streptococci (e.g., *Streptococcus mitis* and gram-negative bacilli expressing Amp-C type 1 β-lactamases). The toxicity profile of cefepime is similar to that of ceftazidime. Cefepime has been compared to ceftazidime, imipenem, and piperacillin/tazobactam in a series of clinical trials evaluating monotherapy for fever and neutropenia. In each of these studies, the regimens were similar in terms of efficacy or toxicity.[82,83] Cefepime is the only cephalosporin that is Food and Drug Administration (FDA) approved for empirical antibacterial therapy in febrile neutropenic patients. A recent meta-analysis investigating the efficacy and safety of cefepime came to the conclusion that all-cause mortality was higher with cefepime than with other β-lactams.[84] In November 2007, the FDA posted an alert regarding the use of cefepime and the announcement of an investigation to review the safety of administering cefipime. In June 2009, the FDA released a meta-analysis based on additional data beyond those included in the Yahav et al. publication.[84] In the FDA analysis, no statistically significant increase in mortality was seen in cefepime-treated patients compared with comparator-treated patients.[85]

Carbapenems: Imipenem and Meropenem

Imipenem and meropenem are members of the class of β-lactam antibiotics called *carbapenems*. Although their mechanism of bactericidal activity involves interference with bacterial cell wall synthesis, imipenem and meropenem uniquely possesses the broadest antimicrobial spectrum of any currently available β-lactam antibiotic. In addition to activity against gram-negative aerobes, including *P. aeruginosa* and the Enterobacteriaceae, imipenem and meropenem act against many gram-positive organisms (e.g., *S. aureus*, *Enterococcus* species, and some coagulase-negative staphylococci) and most anaerobic organisms.

Imipenem is impervious to destruction by Amp-C chromosomally mediated β-lactamases that are commonly produced by *Enterobacter*, *Citrobacter*, and *Serratia* species.[86] Treatment of infections caused by these pathogens by ceftazidime (or another β-lactam agent) may induce β-lactamase production

and, accordingly, lead to therapeutic failures. Because imipenem offers the advantage of β-lactamase stability as well as efficacy against most of these organisms, it is an appropriate treatment for serious infections caused by *Enterobacter* species and related species or as empirical therapy in ill patients previously treated with multiple antibiotics, in whom the likelihood of resistant organisms is increased.

Imipenem was found to be comparable to ceftazidime for empirical coverage in febrile neutropenic adults and children in a randomized trial at the NCI.[87] However, despite the broader spectrum of imipenem, modifications were required as frequently by those receiving that drug as by those receiving ceftazidime with the exception of fewer modifications for anaerobic coverage with imipenem.

Several adverse effects of imipenem therapy have been identified that may limit its use. Nausea and vomiting are well-documented adverse effects of imipenem. There is also an increased frequency of *Clostridium difficile* colitis observed among imipenem recipients, presumably related to alterations in normal anaerobic bowel flora. Imipenem also is known to decrease the seizure threshold in seriously ill patients and in those with CNS pathology, and it should be avoided in these patients.[88] Imipenem-associated seizures also occur in the setting of renal impairment and increased plasma concentrations.

Meropenem is another carbapenem that shares similar *in vitro* antimicrobial properties of imipenem.[79] A large trial, evaluating more than 1,000 episodes of fever and neutropenia, that compared monotherapy with meropenem versus combination therapy with ceftazidime and amikacin showed the two regimens to be similarly effective and both well tolerated.[89,90] Meropenem has the potential advantage over imipenem of less GI toxicity and does appear to alter the seizure threshold. There also have been several smaller studies comparing meropenem to ceftazidime alone or to imipenem with results suggesting equivalency.[90,91]

As *Stenotrophomonas maltophilia* is usually resistant to imipenem and meropenem, this organism should be considered as among the most likely pathogens emerging as a cause of infection in immunocompromised patients receiving one of these carbapenems.[92] Hence, an oxidase-negative gram-negative bacillus causing bacteremia in a febrile neutropenic patient who is already receiving imipenem is likely to be *S. maltophilia*. Trimethoprim-sulfamethoxazole (TMP-SMX) is the preferred antibiotic against *S. maltophilia*. Some strains of *S. maltophilia* initially may appear susceptible to other antibiotics, such as fluoroquinolones; however, resistance may emerge during the course of therapy.[93] Multidrug-resistant *P. aeruginosa* may also emerge during the course of carbapenem therapy.

Ertapenem is a new carbapenem with the advantage of once daily IV administration in comparison with the three times daily IV administration of imipenem and meropenem.[94] Although similar to those of meropenem and imipenem, the *in vitro* antimicrobial spectrum of ertapenem does not include *P. aeruginosa*, which ultimately may exclude its use in febrile, neutropenic cancer patients.

Vancomycin

Vancomycin is a glycopeptide antibiotic with microbicidal activity against a broad range of gram-positive bacteria. Its widespread use has been associated in the last decade with the emergence of vancomycin-resistant enterococcus (VRE) species (*Enterococcus faecium* and *Enterococcus faecalis*), as well as vancomycin-intermediate *S. aureus* and vancomycin-resistant *S. aureus*. Other gram-positive bacteria that are resistant to vancomycin include *Enterococcus gallinarum*, *Enterococcus casseliflavus, Leuconostoc mesenteroides, Pediococcocus* species, *Lactobacillus* species, and *Erysipelothrix rushiopathiae*.

Empirical administration of vancomycin is not recommended for routine use in patients with fever and neutropenia.[79] However, certain neutropenic populations at risk for *S. mitis* infections and MRSA are appropriate candidates for vancomycin.[95] *The 2002 Guidelines for the Use of Antimicrobial Agents in Neutropenic Patients with Cancer* from IDSA recommend that vancomycin should "probably" be used as initial empirical therapy in institutions with high rates of gram-positive organisms leading to fulminant infections (i.e., *Streptococcus viridans*, MRSA). Empirical vancomycin is also recommended for certain patient groups, including those with obvious serious central line infections (e.g., catheter entrance and exit site infections and tunnel infections), those receiving intensive chemotherapy leading to severe mucositis (particularly high-dose Ara-C for AML), those who have received fluoroquinolone prophylaxis prior to their febrile episode, patients with known colonization with organisms treatable only with vancomycin, and patients presenting with hypotension. If vancomycin is initiated empirically and a gram-positive infection is not subsequently microbiologically documented, it may be discontinued. If a gram-positive organism is identified that is oxacillin-susceptible, then a penicillinase-resistant β-lactam or alternative agent is recommended.

Daptomycin, Linezolid, and Quinupristin-Dalfopristin

As the challenges of infections caused by VRE, MRSA, and other resistant gram-positive cocci continue to mount worldwide, daptomycin, linezolid, and quinupristin-dalfopristin have become increasingly important resources in management of immunocompromised patients.

Daptomycin is a lipopeptide antimicrobial agent with bactericidal activity against MRSA and *Enterococcus* species, including VRE.[96] Administered parenterally once daily, daptomycin may be particularly useful in modification of initial therapy in neutropenic patients after VRE is documented as a cause of serious infection. Although combination therapy is necessary to achieve microbicidal activity for treatment of enterococcal sepsis in neutropenic patients (e.g., ampicillin plus aminoglycoside), daptomycin achieves bactericidal activity as a single agent against *Enterococcus* species. As multidrug-resistant VRE may preclude such combination therapy, daptomycin may be particularly effective in neutropenic hosts as a single agent for treatment of this emerging pathogen. The use of daptomycin for pulmonary infections (e.g., MRSA pneumonia), however, is not recommended since pulmonary surfactant inactivates daptomycin.[97] Dosage and pharmacokinetics of daptomycin in children remain to be studied.

Linezolid is the first of a new class of synthetic antimicrobial agents, the oxazolidinones, which exert a unique mechanism of action through inhibition of protein synthesis via interference of formation of the initiation complex.[96] Because of its unique mode of action, linezolid does not exhibit cross-resistance with other antimicrobial agents. It is active against gram-positive bacteria, including MRSA, VRE (including *E. faecium* and *E. faecalis*), as well as β-lactam-resistant strains of *S. pneumoniae*.[98] Linezolid is administered parenterally and orally with excellent oral bioavailability. In a randomized clinical trial of patients with MRSA infections, linezolid demonstrated efficacy similar to that of vancomycin, as well as in treatment of patients with nosocomial pneumonia in which linezolid and vancomycin were each paired with aztreonam.[99,100] In an open-label salvage therapy study for treatment of resistant gram-positive infections, linezolid was effective and well-tolerated in treating resistant gram-positive infections in neutropenic patients with neoplastic diseases.[101] The toxicity profile of linezolid is favorable; however, reversible thrombocytopenia, anemia, and neutropenia may occur in patients receiving prolonged therapy, especially exceeding 2 weeks. Peripheral neuropathy and optic neuropathy also may develop during prolonged administration. As linezolid also is a weakly active but reversible monoamine oxidase inhibitor, it may interact with adrenergic or serotonergic agents.

Quinupristin-dalfopristin is a 30:70 mixture of quinupristin and dalfopristin, which are semisynthetic streptogramin antibiotics.[96] The antibacterial spectrum of quinupristin-dalfopristin is similar to that of linezolid; however, quinupristin-dalfopristin is active against isolates of *E. faecium* but not of *E. faecalis*. Quinupristin-dalfopristin is effective in treatment of serious infections caused by vancomycin-resistant *E. faecium*, nosocomial pneumonia, as well as in complicated soft-tissue infections due to resistant gram-positive cocci.[102,103] The toxicity profile of quinupristin-dalfopristin includes myalgias and arthralgias in approximately 10% of patients, as well as conjugated hyperbilirubinemia and cholestatic jaundice. Because quinupristin-dalfopristin causes local pain, inflammation, and thrombophlebitis during peripheral venous infusion, it should be administered through a central venous catheter. Because of its inhibition of metabolism of agents cleared through cytochrome P-450 3A4, adverse drug interactions may occur.

Piperacillin/Tazobactam

Tazobactam is an irreversible inhibitor of TEM-1 (Bush-Medeiros type 2) β-lactamases that has been paired with the extended-spectrum antipseudomonal piperacillin to yield a broad-spectrum agent that is relatively stable and active in the presence of many of the clinically important gram-positive and gram-negative aerobes and anaerobes. Piperacillin/tazobactam in combination with aminoglycosides and as monotherapy has been evaluated in a series of small trials.[80,104,105]

Piperacillin/tazobactam was recently compared with cefepime in an open-label, randomized study of empirical therapy in febrile neutropenic patients with hematologic malignancies.[106] The analyses demonstrated noninferiority for piperacillin-tazobactam at all time points. Adverse events were similar. This large clinical trial supports the use of piperacillin/tazobactam as an acceptable agent of monotherapy for empirical antibacterial therapy in febrile neutropenic patients.

As piperacillin/tazobactam has become more widely used as empirical antibacterial therapy in febrile neutropenic patients, an antigenic cross-reactivity in the galactomannan enzyme immunoassay (GM-EIA) system for detection of invasive aspergillosis has been observed.[107,108] Neutropenic patients who are at high risk for invasive aspergillosis may be prospectively monitored by serial serum GM-EIA levels. If such patients are also receiving piperacillin-tazobactam, their serum may have positive reactions to a GM-like antigen in the antibiotic formulation and convey a false-positive interpretation for the presence of invasive aspergillosis.

Fluoroquinolones

The fluoroquinolones constitute a group of synthetic antibiotics that possess a broad spectrum of microbicidal activity against most medically important aerobic gram-positive and gram-negative bacteria but are virtually devoid of activity against the clinically important anaerobic bacteria. Ciprofloxacin, nor-floxacin, and ofloxacin comprise the first generation of fluoro-quinolones that were developed. The second generation of fluoroquinolones includes levofloxacin, gatifloxacin, and moxi-floxacin. This newer generation of fluoroquinolones has reliable activity against most isolates of penicillin-resistant pneumo-cocci; however, quinolone-resistant pneumococcal isolates have become more frequent in association with the increased use of these agents.[109] Levofloxacin and moxifloxacin provide excel-lent bioavailability, once daily dosing, tolerability, and im-proved gram-positive spectrum, including most strains of penicillin-resistant *S. pneumoniae.*

Fluoroquinolones exert bactericidal activity through a unique mechanism of action via inhibition of the DNA gyrase responsible for supercoiling and packaging of bacterial DNA. Because they are structurally unrelated to the β-lactams or to any other antibiotic class, cross-resistance through a common mechanism between the fluoroquinolones and other antibi-otics is uncommon. Fluoroquinolones are usually active against multiresistant organisms; ciprofloxacin, for example, exhibits activity against many of the resistant gram-negative rods, including *P. aeruginosa, Serratia, Enterobacter,* and *Klebsiella* species that are responsible for serious infections in neutropenic and otherwise immunocompromised patients. Ciprofloxacin activity against streptococcal species, particu-larly alpha-hemolytic streptococci (e.g., *Streptococcus mitis, Streptococcus sanguis*) is often inadequate.[110]

As the result of the paucity of reliable activity against strep-tococcal and staphylococcal pathogens, ciprofloxacin is not useful as a single agent for empirical therapy in febrile neu-tropenic patients. However, the addition of vancomycin or a penicillinase-protected penicillin to IV ciprofloxacin yields a regimen that compares favorably with more traditional com-binations of a β-lactam plus an aminoglycoside.[111,112]

The combination of an antipseudomonal β-lactam with a quinolone empirical therapy for febrile neutropenic patients provides broad-spectrum activity against gram-negative bacilli and avoids aminoglycoside-related nephrotoxicity. In a large randomized study consisting of 471 evaluable febrile episodes, ciprofloxacin plus piperacillin was as effective as tobramycin plus piperacillin as empirical therapy for febrile neutropenic patients.[113] However, the combination of ciprofloxacin plus piperacillin-tazobactam confers substantially greater gram-positive activity to this fluoroquinolone-based regimen.

Laboratory findings of chondrotoxicity in beagle puppies treated with fluoroquinolones have limited use of this class of antibiotics in pediatric patients. Nonetheless, ciprofloxacin is being given with increasing frequency to children with cystic fibrosis who are colonized with *P. aeruginosa* and to children with other refractory gram-negative infections. A report on more than 1,700 young patients who received ciprofloxacin therapy had only a few cases of transient arthralgias that resolved promptly after discontinuation of the drug.[114,115] Sim-ilarly, Schaad et al.[115] conducted extensive serial physical and radiographic examinations, including magnetic resonance imaging (MRI), of children taking ciprofloxacin for 3 months; this study revealed no evidence of joint toxicity. These encour-aging findings, however, do not preclude a low frequency of clinically delayed development of arthropathy in pediatric patients treated with fluoroquinolone. Thus, for children with cancer who are at risk for severe infections and in whom a very potent oral antibiotic would facilitate the possibility of outpa-tient therapy, the benefits of fluoroquinolone therapy in selected cases may be found to outweigh the risk of chondro-toxicity. Such patients should also be monitored for Achilles tendon rupture, which may also ensue in patients of any age and could be potentiated in patients receiving glucocorticoid therapy.

Aztreonam

Aztreonam is a monobactam antimicrobial agent with activity that is exclusively against aerobic gram-negative bacteria.[116] The *in vitro* antimicrobial spectrum of aztreonam includes the Enterobacteriaceae (e.g., most isolates of *E. coli, Klebsiella, Serratia, Enterobacter*) and *P. aeruginosa.* Because there is no gram-positive or anaerobic coverage, aztreonam is not used as a single agent for empirical antibacterial therapy in febrile neutropenic patients. Aztreonam has been used successfully in combination with vancomycin for empirical treatment of febrile neutropenic patients with cancer.[117,118]

The absence of the thiazolidine component in the monobac-tam molecule substantially reduces the antigenic cross-reactiv-ity between aztreonam and β-lactam antibiotics.[119] Thus, aztreonam is most useful for patients with significant allergy to penicillin or other β-lactams in whom an antipseudomonal agent is desirable or required. The gram-negative spectrum and absence of renal toxicity allow the use of aztreonam as an alternative to aminoglycosides in certain instances.

ANTIFUNGAL AGENTS

During the past 30 years, the armamentarium of systemically administered antifungal compounds has expanded from amphotericin B as the only available compound for treatment of life-threatening invasive fungal infections to the new classes of lipid formulations of amphotericin B (LFABs), antifungal triazoles, and echinocandins. The antifungal and pharmaco-logic properties of these compounds are summarized in the following section.

Amphotericin B

Amphotericin B is a polyene antifungal agent with a broad spec-trum against yeast-like and filamentous fungi. Deoxycholate amphotericin B (D-AmB) has been the cornerstone of antifungal therapy in most critically ill pediatric patients with deeply invasive fungal infections for the past 50 years. However, newer agents, including the LFABs, antifungal triazoles, and echino-candins, with an improved therapeutic index are providing safer alternatives with similar or superior efficacy. The principal mechanism of action of amphotericin B, as of other polyenes, is the binding to ergosterol, which is found in fungal cell mem-branes but not in mammalian cell membranes. Amphotericin B forms pore-like ionic channels, which result in altered mem-brane permeability and leakage of monovalent and divalent cations from the fungal cell. Amphotericin B also binds to a lesser extent to other sterols, such as cholesterol, which accounts for much of the toxicity associated with its usage. Yet another mechanism of action of amphotericin B is the induction of lipoperoxidation of the fungal cell membrane. Amphotericin B also modulates host response by cytokine and oxidation-dependent enhancement of the effector functions of macro-phages, MNCs, and PMNs.[120,121]

The pharmacokinetic profile of amphotericin B in children differs from that in adults. Children older than 3 months have a smaller volume of distribution and a faster clearance than what is usually found in adults. There is a strong inverse correlation between patient age and total clearance of ampho-tericin B, suggesting that higher dosages may be better toler-ated in patients between 3 months and 9 years of age.

Acute or infusion-related toxicity of D-AmB is character-ized by fever, chills, rigor, nausea, vomiting, and headache. Fever, chills, and rigors may be mediated by TNF and IL-1, cytokines that are released from human peripheral MNCs or tissue macrophages in response to D-AmB. These acute reactions may possibly be blunted by corticosteroids, acetaminophen, aspirin, other nonsteroidal antiinflammatory drugs, or meperidine. Corticosteroids should be used only in relatively low dosages (e.g., 0.5 to 1.0 mg/kg of hydrocortisone). Meperidine in low doses (0.2 to 0.5 mg/kg) interdicts development of rigors; it is not usually effective for prevention of rigors. Acetaminophen may decrease fever but appears to have little effect on rigors. Aspirin should be avoided in thrombocytopenic patients. Although diphenhydramine is used in many centers for prevention of acute infusion reactions, the rationale for this anti-H_1-receptor inhibitor is not pharmacologically clear, as most acute reactions due to D-AmB are not histamine-mediated. Any perceived benefits of diphenhydramine for D-AmB–associated acute infusion reactions are more likely related to its sedating effects.

Nephrotoxicity (glomerular or tubular) is the most significant dose-limiting adverse effect of D-AmB. The clinical and laboratory manifestations of glomerular toxicity include a decrease in glomerular filtration rate and renal blood flow, as evidenced by azotemia. Tubular toxicity is manifested as the presence of urinary casts, hypokalemia, hypomagnesemia, renal tubular acidosis, and nephrocalcinosis. Hypomagnesemia may be more profound in patients with cancer who develop a divalent cation-losing nephropathy associated with cisplatin or ifosfamide. Although azotemia in most pediatric patients is usually reversible, renal function may not return to normal levels after cessation of D-AmB in children who have received previous repeated or prolonged courses of this polyene. Moreover, return to pretreatment levels may require several months in some cases.

Foremost among the important drug interactions with amphotericin B is the nephrotoxicity caused by concomitant aminoglycosides, cyclosporine, and foscarnet; where possible, D-AmB should not be used in conjunction with these nephrotoxic agents. Acute pulmonary reactions (hypoxemia, acute dyspnea, and radiographic evidence of pulmonary infiltrates) have been associated with simultaneous transfusion of granulocytes and infusion of amphotericin B.[122] Although some investigators have disputed the causality of amphotericin B in such reactions, a rational approach is to separate the infusions of amphotericin B and granulocytes by the longest possible time period.

Lipid Formulations of Amphotericin B

Three engineered LFABs have been approved in North America and Europe: a small unilamellar vesicle formulation of liposomal amphotericin B (L-AmB or AmBisome), amphotericin B lipid complex (ABLC or Abelcet), and amphotericin B colloidal dispersion (Amphotec or Amphocil). The introduction of LFABs has been an important therapeutic advance in improving the therapeutic index of amphotericin B. Because toxicity is the major dose-limiting factor of this drug, lipid formulations have been developed to reduce toxicity and permit larger doses to be administered. Although classically considered as liposomal formulations of amphotericin B, the investigational and clinically approved formulations of amphotericin B have a wider diversity of lipid structure. Liposomes (defined as phospholipid bilayers of one or more closed concentric structures) and other lipid formulations have been used as vehicles for amphotericin B with encouraging results. The lipid formulation may provide a selective diffusion gradient toward the fungal cell membrane and away from mammalian cell membrane.

ABLC was the first lipid formulation approved in the United States by the FDA in November 1995 for both children

and adults. ABLC, 5 mg/kg/day IV, under an emergency compassionate release protocol, was found to be active in treatment of immunocompromised pediatric patients with refractory mycoses and those with intolerance to conventional amphotericin B.[123] This study found little dose-limiting nephrotoxicity of ABLC. These findings were subsequently confirmed in a large open-label prospective study of pediatric patients receiving ABLC.[124] A phase I-II study of ABLC in children with hepatosplenic (chronic disseminated) candidiasis found that the compound administered at 2.5 mg/kg for 6 weeks was effective, had no dose-limiting nephrotoxicity, and appeared to reach steady-state plasma pharmacokinetics by 7 days.[125]

Two phase I-II studies of the safety, tolerability, and activity of L-AmB in oncology patients demonstrated that dosages of as much as 15 mg/kg/day were not dose limiting and were effective in empirical antifungal therapy as well as in treatment of invasive filamentous fungal infections. Although the optimal dosage for treatment of invasive fungal infections is controversial,[126,127] we recommend that treatment of invasive candidiasis should begin with 3 mg/kg/day and of invasive aspergillosis and other filamentous fungal infections at 5 mg/kg/day.

Although LFABs are associated with less nephrotoxicity, they may confer their own patterns of toxicity. For example, the multilamellar LFAB induced reversible hypoxemia, pulmonary hypertension, and depression of cardiac output during infusion.[128] ABLC is more commonly associated with the infusion-related reactions of the well-known fever, chills, and rigors typical of D-AmB.[129] Although historically associated with less infusion-related toxicity than that of D-AmB and ABLC, L-AmB may cause a syndrome of severe acute infusion-related reactions characterized by substernal chest pain, hypoxia, flank and abdominal pain, and urticarial eruptions.[130] Infusion-related toxicity with amphotericin B colloidal dispersion was found to be more severe than that of D-AmB.[131]

Despite the relatively greater expense of the LFABs, an expanding body of data underscores the risk of D-AmB–induced irreversible nephrotoxicity and the expense of renal impairment in management of seriously ill patients.[132] An LFAB is appropriate as initial empirical therapy or as definitive therapy for proven mycoses in high-risk patients receiving concomitant nephrotoxic agents ([e.g., cyclosporine, aminoglycosides] in diabetes mellitus, preexisting renal impairment), in those with preexisting renal impairment, and in those with an anticipated course of protracted neutropenia during which dose-limiting nephrotoxicity may ensue.

Flucytosine

Historically, 5-fluorocytosine (5FC) has been most frequently used as an adjunct to amphotericin B therapy in the treatment of cryptococcal meningitis. This combination was originally proposed because of the observation that amphotericin B potentiates the uptake of 5FC by increasing fungal cell membrane permeability. Because of rapid emergence of resistant strains, 5FC is used only in combination with another antifungal agent, most commonly amphotericin B. The strongest clinical data support the use of D-AmB plus 5FC in treatment of CNS cryptococcosis. Although experimental data support the use of 5FC in combination with D-AmB in treatment of experimental disseminated candidiasis, there are no controlled clinical trials to test this hypothesis.

Dose-dependent myelosuppression is the most serious toxicity associated with administration of 5FC. GI side effects, such as diarrhea, nausea, and vomiting, are the most common symptomatic side effects and are dose dependent. Abnormal elevation of hepatic transaminases also has been reported in approximately 5% of patients receiving the drug. Other than its use in treatment of cryptococcal meningoencephalitis, 5FC is seldom used owing in part to its narrow therapeutic index.

Antifungal Imidazoles and Triazoles

The antifungal azoles include imidazoles (clotrimazole, miconazole, and ketoconazole) and triazoles (itraconazole, fluconazole, and voriconazole). Clotrimazole and miconazole are available in topical applications. Ketoconazole has been generally supplanted in its use by itraconazole and fluconazole in the pediatric oncology setting. Accordingly, only fluconazole and itraconazole are discussed in this section.

The antifungal azoles are synthetic compounds that demonstrate less toxicity than D-AmB, have flexibility for oral administration, and have comparable or superior efficacy against certain infections. The antifungal azole agents function principally by inhibition of the fungal cytochrome P-450 enzyme lanosterol 14a-demethylase, which is involved in the synthesis of ergosterol.

Fluconazole

Fluconazole, available in both oral and parenteral formulations, has been shown to be effective against infections caused by *Candida* species, *Cryptococcus neoformans*, and other fungi in patients with neoplastic diseases, HIV infection, and other immunocompromised states. Fluconazole is a relatively small molecule with rapid absorption and excellent bioavailability. The concentration-time curves of orally and parenterally administered fluconazole are almost superimposable. Fluconazole exhibits linear plasma kinetics and is only slightly metabolized. In the setting of renal impairment, the dosage of fluconazole is adjusted to reflect glomerular filtration. A 50% reduction of dosage is recommended in patients with a creatinine clearance of 21 to 50 mL/min and a 75% reduction in those with a clearance of less than 21 mL/min. Oral absorption of fluconazole does not depend on a low intragastric pH, feeding, fasting, or mucosal integrity.

The plasma half-life of fluconazole in children aged 5 to 15 years was substantially reduced in comparison with the half-life in adults (17 hours in children vs. reports of 27 and 37 hours in adults).[133] In light of this more rapid clearance of fluconazole, life-threatening fungal infections in children are treated with 12 mg/kg/day in two divided doses (assuming normal renal function) to approximate the dosage equivalency in adults of 400 mg once daily (approximately 6 mg/kg in a 70-kg adult).

Fluconazole penetrates well into the CSF.[134] It has been well tolerated with few dose-limiting side effects in different pediatric populations. Nausea, other GI symptoms, and elevated hepatic transaminases occur infrequently and are usually reversible.

The drug interactions of fluconazole are noteworthy and are similar to those of other azoles. For example, fluconazole has been reported to precipitate phenytoin toxicity because of inhibition of metabolism, thus warranting monitoring of phenytoin concentrations during coadministration of fluconazole. Concentrations of cyclosporin may be increased, and the effects of warfarin may be potentiated.

Itraconazole

Itraconazole, although structurally similar to ketoconazole, has a broader spectrum of antifungal activity, less toxicity, a longer plasma half-life, and the capacity to penetrate into brain tissue. The spectrum of itraconazole includes *Candida* species, *C. neoformans*, *Trichosporon* species, *Aspergillus* species, dematiaceous molds, and the endemic dimorphic fungi, including *Histoplasma capsulatum*, *Blastomyces dermatitidis*, *Coccidioides immitis*, and *Paracoccidioides brasiliensis*. Despite this extended spectrum and greater safety profile, itraconazole has limited bioavailability. Itraconazole is soluble only at low pH, as in the normal gastric milieu.

Plasma levels of itraconazole are substantially decreased by antacids and by histamine H_2-receptor blocking agents (e.g., ranitidine) or proton pump inhibitors because of elevated gastric pH, which impairs absorption of the drug. This erratic bioavailability compromises the role of itraconazole in neutropenic patients, particularly those with chemotherapy- or radiotherapy-induced mucosal disruption.

Attainment of adequate plasma concentrations is critical for optimal antifungal effect of itraconazole.[135] Because itraconazole is highly protein bound with only 0.2% available as free drug, concentrations in body fluids equivalent to body water, such as saliva and CSF, are negligible. However, tissue concentrations, including those of the CNS, are two to five times higher than those in plasma, and they persist for longer, explaining the efficacy of the drug despite low plasma concentrations. Because the primary route of excretion is the biliary tract, no adjustment of dosage is necessary in patients with renal impairment.

Itraconazole has properties of drug interaction with cyclosporin, rifampin, phenytoin, phenobarbital, antihistamines, Coumadin, and oral hypoglycemic agents. Important drug interactions between itraconazole and other agents can prolong the plasma half-life of cyclosporin, which may lead to cyclosporin-induced nephrotoxicity or neurotoxicity. Consequently, serum cyclosporin levels should be closely monitored, and dosages of cyclosporin should be adjusted in patients receiving itraconazole. Itraconazole's inhibition of the metabolism of some concomitant antihistamines may lead to widening QT intervals and cardiac ventricular arrhythmias, including torsades de pointes: pimozide, dofetilide, quinidine, and cisapride. The serum concentrations of itraconazole may be markedly decreased with concomitant administration of drugs that induce hepatic microsomal enzymes, such as rifampin, phenobarbital, and phenytoin. Caution should also be exerted in the co-administration of itraconazole with vinca alkaloids, Coumadin, and oral hypoglycemic agents, because the increased concentrations of these drugs may cause increased neuropathy, bleeding, and hypoglycemia, respectively.

Itraconazole is well-tolerated with long-term use and has a relatively low incidence of hepatic toxicity. Most of the reported adverse reactions are transient: GI disturbances, dizziness, and headache, and no adverse effect on steroidogenesis.

A parenteral formulation of itraconazole has become available, but because of the potential nephrotoxicity of the vehicle, use of the compound is not approved beyond 2 weeks. Although studies of the safety, pharmacokinetics, and tolerability of the oral formulations of itraconazole have been completed in immunocompromised pediatric patients,[136] the parenteral formulation of itraconazole has not been studied in children.

Voriconazole

Voriconazole was developed from fluconazole by substituting a fluoropyrimidine ring for one of the azole groups to enhance the spectrum, and adding an alpha-methyl group to provide fungicidal activity against *Aspergillus* and other filamentous fungi. Voriconazole has broad *in vitro*, *in vivo*, and clinical antifungal activity against most medically important yeasts (*Candida* species, *C. neoformans*, *Trichosporon* species, and endemic dimorphic fungi) as well as *Aspergillus* species, *Fusarium* species, *Scedosporium apiospermum*, and other filamentous fungi. Voriconazole, however, has no activity against Zygomycetes (the agents of zygomycosis or mucormycosis).

Voriconazole is administered orally and parenterally. Oral voriconazole is rapidly and nearly completely absorbed in the fasted state. High-fat meals result in reduced plasma concentrations. Voriconazole penetrates well into multiple tissues, including those of the CNS. Metabolism and elimination of voriconazole is primarily via hepatic cytochrome P-450 enzymes. CYP 2C19 plays a major role in voriconazole metabolism and demonstrates allelic polymorphism, with individuals of Asian descent having a greater likelihood of being poor metabolizers and requiring higher levels. As voriconazole is a substrate for CYP 2C19, 2C9, and 3A4, drug interactions are also probable. The dosing regimen most widely studied for IV voriconazole is a standard loading dose of 6 mg/kg IV every 12 hours for two doses followed by 4 mg/kg IV every 12 hours. However, voriconazole pharmacokinetics are nonlinear in adults but are linear in children at the maintenance dosage of 4 mg/kg, resulting in lower drug exposure in pediatric patients.[137] Although this dosage has been found to be effective in treatment of invasive aspergillosis, scedosporiosis, and other life-threatening mycoses in pediatric patients,[138] higher dosages of 7 mg/kg may be necessary in order to achieve comparable adult drug exposure.

Based on a large international, randomized, open-label trial against D-AmB that resulted in a significant 22% survival advantage, voriconazole is considered the drug of choice for primary treatment of invasive aspergillosis.[139] Further supporting the role of voriconazole in the primary treatment of invasive aspergillosis is the observation that some species, such as *A. terreus*, are resistant to amphotericin B but susceptible to antifungal triazoles.[140,141]

Although voriconazole is generally well tolerated, there are four specific concerns of safety with its use: hepatotoxicity, visual adverse events, cutaneous reactions, and visual hallucinations. Hepatic enzyme abnormalities (elevated aspartate transaminase and alanine transaminase) are dose-limiting adverse events for voriconazole. Transient altered perception of light, photopsia, or photophobia may occur following oral or IV dosing; these visual effects tend to appear and resolve early in the course of therapy over several days. Erythematous macular and desquamative rashes, most of which are mild, may occur in as many as 15% to 20% of patients receiving voriconazole. However, severe cutaneous reactions, including Stevens-Johnson, toxic epidermal necrolysis, and intense photosensitivity reactions, may occur.[142] Visual hallucinations occur significantly more often in patients receiving voriconazole versus L-AmB[143]; these hallucinations are distinct from the infusion-related visual side effects and may be dose related.

Posaconazole

In 2006, the FDA approved the use of posaconazole for prophylaxis against the development of invasive Aspergillus and Candida infections in immunocompromised patients 13 years of age and older. Posaconazole, available only in an oral formulation and requiring frequent dosing, is structurally similar to itraconazole and has broad *in vitro*, *in vivo*, and clinical efficacy against most yeasts and filamentous fungi. This triazole is distinct in having been successfully used in salvage treatment of infections due to Zygomycetes. It is not indicated in the primary treatment of zygomycosis. Furthermore, posaconazole's efficacy as an empiric antifungal agent in febrile and neutropenic patients has not been investigated.

Echinocandins

Echinocandins are semisynthetic cyclic hexapeptide antifungal compounds that interrupt cell biosynthesis by noncompetitive inhibition of 1,3 B-D-glucan synthase. The polymer, 1,3 B-D-glucan, is a key component of the fungal cell wall of *Candida* species and *Aspergillus* species Echinocandins have N-acyl aliphatic or aryl side chains that expand the antifungal spectrum to include *Candida* species, *Aspergillus* species, and *P. carinii* but not *C. neoformans*, *Trichosporon* species, and *Rhodotorula* species. Three echinocandins have been studied in recent clinical trials: caspofungin, micafungin, and anidulafungin. These three echinocandins, which are currently available only in parenteral formulation, have been generally well tolerated and associated with few drug interactions.

Caspofungin

Caspofungin has documented *in vitro*, *in vivo*, and clinical activity against *Candida* species (including azole-resistant non-*albicans Candida* species) and *Aspergillus* species.[144,145] Caspofungin was found to be effective with an overall success rate of 45% (similar to success rates using LFABs in salvage treatment) in the treatment of 90 patients with invasive aspergillosis refractory to or intolerant of standard therapy.[144]

An international randomized, double-blind study demonstrated that caspofungin was similar in efficacy to D-AmB for treatment of invasive candidiasis.[145] Approximately 50% of patients in this trial also had non-*albicans Candida* species infection; most had a successful outcome. However, caution is warranted in the treatment of candidemia due to *C. parapsilosis*. Approximately 20% in each group had *C. parapsilosis* isolated at baseline, and five caspofungin versus no D-AmB patients had persistently positive blood cultures for *C. parapsilosis*. There are few studies of treatment of pediatric patients. One report of caspofungin in pediatric oncology patients found this echinocandin to be well tolerated.[146] Another recent report documents the successful treatment with caspofungin of 10 newborn infants with refractory candidemia, endocarditis, and meningoencephalitis.[147]

Caspofungin undergoes hepatic metabolism and is not removed with hemodialysis. No dosage adjustments are recommended for renal insufficiency or during hemodialysis. The plasma pharmacokinetics of caspofungin in children is different from that in adults. To achieve comparable drug exposure, 50 mg/m^2 is recommended for pediatric patients who are 2 to 17 years of age.[148]

Micafungin and Anidulafungin

These two echinocandins also demonstrate *in vitro*, *in vivo*, and clinical activity against *Candida* species and *Aspergillus* species Both compounds have been found to be effective in treatment of esophageal candidiasis. Micafungin was found to be effective in prevention of invasive fungal infections in neutropenic HSCT recipients in a randomized controlled trial against fluconazole.[149] Anidulafungin was highly active for treatment of candidemia, achieving an approximately 80% response rate, in an open label study,[150] and recently shown to be synergistic with voriconazole (at a dose of 5 mg/kg/day) and antagonistic at higher doses (10 mg/kg/day) in an experimental invasive pulmonary aspergillosis model in rabbits.[151] Current studies indicate that both echinocandins are well tolerated in pediatric oncology patients.[152,153]

Combination Antifungal Therapy

Not all antifungal combinations are beneficial; indeed, some combinations may be antagonistic and potentially deleterious to improved patient outcome. With the exception of D-AmB plus 5FC for cryptococcal meningoencephalitis, combination antifungal therapy is clinically unproved and expensive; as such, it should be considered as an investigational modality. Different organisms respond differently to antifungal combinations. For example, the combination of fluconazole plus 5FC appears experimentally to be synergistic against cryptococcal meningitis, whereas the same combination has no benefit above single agent against disseminated candidiasis. The combination of amphotericin B and antifungal triazoles should be considered potentially antagonistic against *Aspergillus* species and is thus not recommended. The combination of an echinocandin with a triazole or with a formulation of amphotericin may be additive or synergistic *in vitro* and *in vivo* against experimental invasive aspergillosis[154,155]; however, these combinations have not been shown or studied in prospective randomized clinical trials to be superior to standard monotherapy.

ANTIVIRAL AGENTS

Immunocompromised pediatric oncology patients are at risk for a wide range of viral infections : those due to the herpesviruses group (HSV, CMV, varicella zoster virus [VZV], human herpesvirus 6 [HHV-6], and Epstein-Barr virus [EBV]), community-acquired respiratory viruses (influenza, parainfluenza, and respiratory syncytial virus [RSV]), adenoviruses, and polyoma viruses (JC virus and BK virus [BKV]). Members of the herpesviruses group cause acute infections and are subsequently maintained in a state of latency, specifically within dorsal root ganglia in the case of HSV and VZV and probably within MNCs in the case of CMV. Latent herpesviruses are apparently held in abeyance and prevented from reactivation by the presence of effective cellular immune function. Immunosuppression, as a consequence of either cancer chemotherapy or the underlying malignancy itself, has a permissive effect in inducing reactivation of herpesvirus from latency. Reactivation of viral replication may be detected as asymptomatic shedding of virus, circulating antigenemia or elevated polymerase chain reaction (PCR) signal without disease (e.g., CMV), or clinically overt end-organ disease. The common disease manifestations of the herpesvirus group in immunocompromised pediatric oncology patients are HSV stomatitis and esophagitis, localized or disseminated zoster, CMV-related interstitial pneumonitis and GI hemorrhage, HHV-6–associated encephalitis, and EBV-related lymphoproliferative disorders. Influenza, parainfluenza, and RSV can cause lethal pneumonic processes. In addition to causing respiratory tract infections, adenoviruses may cause diarrhea and hepatitis in immunocompromised children. JC virus and BKV are etiologic agents, respectively, in progressive multifocal leukoencephalopathy and hemorrhagic cystitis, particularly in HSCT recipients. Antiviral agents have been developed for some but certainly not all of these viral infections. These agents are discussed in the following sections.

Acyclovir

Acyclovir was the first widely available antiviral agent effective against HSV and VZV and has become an essential element in the supportive care of children and adults with cancer.

Acyclovir is a guanine nucleoside analog that, when triphosphorylated, is selectively recognized by viral DNA polymerase as a nucleotide. Acyclovir triphosphate acts as an inhibitor of herpesvirus DNA polymerase and stops viral DNA synthesis. The selective antiviral action of acyclovir and other similar compounds is caused by preferential phosphorylation (i.e., activation of the drug) by the virus-encoded thymidine kinase (TK) enzyme. This virus-specific TK-dependent activation of acyclovir also carries important implications for resistance, as a common mechanism of HSV resistance to acyclovir is low expression of TK activity.

Acyclovir is effective for prophylaxis and treatment of both primary infections and reactivations of HSV types 1 and 2 in immunocompromised patients.[156–158] It is used prophylactically in seropositive persons who are undergoing intensive therapy or bone marrow transplantation. Although acyclovir itself has no therapeutic efficacy against established CMV disease, it also may prevent reactivations of CMV in HSCT recipients who receive it prophylactically.[159–161] When valacyclovir (the valine esterified analog of acyclovir with high oral bioavailability) was compared with acyclovir as prophylaxis in a randomized study of allogeneic HSCT recipients, it was more effective than acyclovir in preventing CMV reactivation (28% vs. 40%, respectively).[159] However, as neither acyclovir nor valacyclovir are completely adequate agents for CMV prophylaxis, prospective surveillance and preemptive therapy with ganciclovir or foscarnet are still indicated.

Balfour et al.[162] demonstrated that IV acyclovir treatment of localized zoster in immunocompromised patients also prevented dissemination and reduced mortality from visceral VZV infection. In immunocompetent children with chickenpox, oral acyclovir marginally reduces the duration of symptoms, whereas IV acyclovir remains the standard of care in immunocompromised patients. Because VZV is relatively less susceptible to acyclovir, the IV dosages of acyclovir required to treat VZV disease (500 mg/m² every 8 hours or 10 mg/kg every 8 hours) are double those used for HSV therapy (250 mg/m² every 8 hours or 5 mg/kg every 8 hours). Acyclovir is associated with few adverse effects; however, high IV doses should be given with adequate hydration to avoid nephrotoxicity, particularly involving the renal tubules. Seizures and ataxia may ensue if acyclovir dosage is not adjusted for renal impairment.

Ganciclovir

Ganciclovir is a deoxyguanosine nucleoside analog that is active against HSV, VZV, and CMV but that is also more potent than acyclovir against CMV. The significant myelotoxic effects of ganciclovir preclude its routine use to treat HSV or VZV. It is used almost exclusively for treatment and prevention of disease caused by CMV.[163,164] For invasive CMV disease (i.e., colitis, pneumonitis, hepatitis, retinitis), ganciclovir induction therapy at 5 mg/kg twice daily for 2 to 4 weeks is often followed by a prolonged maintenance therapy period until resolution of signs, symptoms, and CMV antigenemia or PCR signal. For preemptive therapy, ganciclovir is initiated in allogeneic HSCT recipients based on the presence of CMV antigenemia in a nonneutropenic host or in the presence of a positive PCR signal in a neutropenic host.[159] Because of its dose-dependent effects of myelosuppression, the use of ganciclovir for routine prophylaxis in allogeneic HSCT recipients is not recommended. Instead, the use of antigen or PCR-guided preemptive therapy provides a more balanced approach between myelosuppression and prevention of CMV disease.[165,166] The oral formulation of valganciclovir provides a more effective means of managing patients on maintenance therapy on an ambulatory basis.[167]

Foscarnet

Foscarnet directly inhibits the DNA polymerases of the herpesviruses. Unlike acyclovir and ganciclovir, foscarnet does not require TK and phosphorylation for activation. The unique function of foscarnet has made it particularly useful for the treatment of infections caused by HSV, VZV, and CMV that have become resistant to the standard nucleoside analogs. Typically, these resistant herpesviruses have, by mutation, lost the viral TK activity that normally activates acyclovir and ganciclovir.

Although electrolyte disturbances, hypocalcemia, and azotemia are the major toxicities associated with foscarnet, a more recent study suggests that these toxicities may be manageable in a preemptive setting. Reusser et al.[168] report in a randomized clinical trial of foscarnet versus ganciclovir for preemptive CMV therapy in allogeneic HSCT recipients that ganciclovir was more frequently discontinued prematurely for either neutropenia or thrombocytopenia. Notably, renal impairment was observed only in 5% of foscarnet recipients.

For many allogeneic HSCT recipients requiring IV therapy for CMV patients receiving concomitant nephrotoxic agents, including cyclosporine, amphotericin B, and aminoglycosides, there appears to be increased risk of foscarnet-associated nephrotoxicity and they may better tolerate ganciclovir. Alternatively, foscarnet may be preferred in patients with limited marrow reserve and preexisting neutropenia or thrombocytopenia.

Valacyclovir and Famciclovir

Valacyclovir and famciclovir are prodrugs designed to enhance the bioavailability of their parent antiviral compounds. Valacyclovir and famciclovir have pharmacokinetic profiles that permit less frequent oral dosing for treatment of herpes zoster in immunocompetent patients. Twice-daily dosing of famciclovir and thrice-daily dosing of valacyclovir provide clear advantages for the patient when compared with the five times daily oral acyclovir dose that is recommended for immunocompetent adults. Both agents appear to be as effective as orally administered acyclovir for treatment of HSV infection in these patients.

The plasma pharmacokinetics of valacyclovir administered as tablets have been studied in immunocompromised pediatric patients.[169,170] Eksborg et al.[169] found that the bioavailability of acyclovir after oral administration of valacyclovir was 45% in neutropenic children with mucositis. However, it should be noted that a pediatric formulation of valacyclovir is unavailable and that crushed tablets (used for children) have a very unpleasant taste. There are also few data on the pharmacokinetics and use of famciclovir in children.

Cidofovir

Cidofovir is a nucleotide analog of deoxycytidine monophosphate with demonstrable activity against all of the human herpesviruses and other DNA viruses, including adenoviruses. Cidofovir's activity does not depend upon virus-specific phosphorylation and hence it is active against TK-deficient and TK-mutated strains of HSV, as well as ganciclovir-resistant CMV due to mutations in the UL-97 gene encoding the viral phosphotransferase. It acts as a competitive inhibitor of dCTP

and viral DNA polymerase. Cidofovir's long intracellular half-life of as much as 60 hours (plasma half-life of approximately 2.5 hours) permits a once weekly dosing of 5 mg/kg. For induction therapy, the dosage is 5 mg/kg once weekly with maintenance dose of 5 mg/kg once every 2 weeks. Cidofovir is cleared by glomerular filtration and tubular secretion. Cidofovir-induced nephrotoxicity is characterized by azotemia, proteinuria, and proximal tubular toxicity manifested by glycosuria and metabolic acidosis. Hydration and probenecid (which reduces tubular secretion, increases plasma concentrations, and diminishes nephrotoxicity) are used to reduce the nephrotoxic effects of cidofovir. An alternative dosage of 1 mg/kg three times weekly has been attempted in some patients as a strategy for reduction of nephrotoxicity without an apparent loss of efficacy.[171]

Cidofovir is used in the treatment of CMV disease after failure or intolerance to ganciclovir or foscarnet.[172] Encouraging data have emerged in the use of cidofovir for treatment of adenovirus infections in pediatric and adult allogeneic HSCT recipients.[171,173]

Ribavirin

Ribavirin is a synthetic virostatic nucleoside with antiviral properties *in vitro* against various RNA and DNA viruses. It is a small-particle aerosol usually given in a dose of 20 mg/mL in 300 mL of distilled water nebulized in an oxygen hood, tent, or mask over 12 to 18 hours for every 24-hour period. Shorter-duration therapy with high-dose aerosolized ribavirin appears to be efficacious and is more convenient. Ribavirin is associated with few side effects; nausea, headache, and bronchospasm occur at low frequency. Data have suggested that health care workers are not at significant risk for adverse effects with the minimal exposure that occurs during care of a child receiving aerosolized ribavirin, although pregnant women are advised to avoid areas where ribavirin therapy is administered because of concerns about the uncertain teratogenic potential of the drug in humans.[174]

The use of ribavirin for treatment of RSV pneumonia was originally studied in infants with severe disease. The efficacy of this drug has shown mixed results, with some studies showing improvement in overall severity of illness[175] and others showing no difference[176,177] in the ribavirin-treated group. The ambiguity of the data prompted the American Academy of Pediatrics to change its recommendation from ribavirin "should be used" to "may be considered" for selected infants and young children at high risk for serious disease.[178] These include children with chronic lung disease, congenital heart disease, prematurity, or those who are immunosuppressed. The mortality rate from RSV pneumonia in adults undergoing therapy for AML and in bone marrow transplant patients is high.[179,180] The data regarding the efficacy of ribavirin therapy in these patients are somewhat limited and are based primarily on reports of case series compared with historical controls. There is a suggestion from pilot studies that the early initiation of ribavirin therapy, often given in conjunction with immune globulin, may have some beneficial effect.[181]

IV ribavirin in conjunction with interferon-a2b is now the standard of care for patients with chronic hepatitis C infection.[182] This combination has been shown to increase sustained response rates to 40% in those individuals who are treatment naïve and to 50% in those who have relapsed after initially responding to interferon alone. Response is dependent to some degree on viral genotype, with 60% of those individuals with non-1 genotype having sustained responses compared with 30% in those individuals with genotype 1.[183] This therapy is unfortunately associated with significant side effects, most notably flulike symptoms from the interferon and dose-related hemolytic anemia from ribavirin, making it not tolerable for a subset of patients.

Palivizumab (Synergis) and Respiratory Syncytial Virus Immune Globulin (Respigam)

Palivizumab is a monoclonal antibody directed at the F glycoprotein of RSV, a surface protein highly conserved among RSV isolates, and was licensed by the FDA in 1998 for the prevention of RSV in premature infants and in those with chronic lung disease. It is given monthly during the RSV season at a dose of 15 mg/kg, administered intramuscularly (IM). With this regimen it was shown in a randomized placebo-controlled trial involving 1,502 patients with chronic lung disease who were younger than 24 months or in patients with a gestational age less than 35 weeks and were less than 6 months old that prophylaxis during the RSV season decreased hospitalization, intensive care unit days, and severity of disease.[184] RSV can be a serious pathogen in oncology patients, especially in those with acute leukemia and those undergoing bone marrow transplantation. Although palivizumab appears to be well tolerated in cancer patients,[185] there is, however, no data substantiating the utility of this agent for prophylaxis in these patient groups.

RSV immune globulin (RSV-IG) is a blood product prepared from donors selected for high titers of RSV neutralizing antibodies.[186] The range of RSV antibody titer is 1:2,400 to 1:8,000, whereas unselected immune globulin usually has anti-RSV antibody titers of less than 1:1,000. Licensed by the FDA in 1996 also for the prevention of RSV pneumonia in premature infants and for those with chronic lung disease, RSV-IG is given intravenously once a month at a dose of 750 mg/kg. Again, however, there are no data evaluating this agent for prophylaxis in oncology patients.

The American Academy of Pediatrics recommends palivizumab for infants and young children with hemodynamically significant congenital heart disease and further stated that palivizumab is preferred for most high-risk infants and children because of ease of IM administration.[187] Monthly administration of palivizumab during the RSV season resulted in a 45% to 55% decrease in the rate of hospitalization attributable to RSV.

There are a number of small case series in adult oncology and bone marrow transplant patients using RSV Ig or palivizumab[185,188] in combination with ribavirin for the treatment of severe lower tract disease with a suggestion of improved outcomes over historical controls. However, as palivizumab and RSV-IG are expensive and difficult to obtain, a more practical approach in immunocompromised pediatric oncology patients may be to detect RSV infection early and promptly initiate intravenous immune globulin (IVIG) (in which anti-RSV titers approach those of RSV-IG) and aerosolized ribavirin.[181]

Amantadine and Rimantadine

Influenza is a potentially life-threatening infection in immunocompromised patients.[189] Amantadine and rimantadine were the first agents available for treatment of influenza.[190] They inhibit uncoating of the viral RNA within host cells, ultimately blocking viral replication. Both compounds have activity against influenza A but not against influenza B, are well-absorbed orally, and are usually well tolerated, with no

serious organ toxicities. The most common side effects of amantadine and rimantadine are mild GI discomfort, including loss of appetite and nausea. Amantadine, however, is associated with CNS effects such as nervousness, lightheadedness, difficulty in concentrating, and insomnia, particularly in older adults. Rimantadine causes fewer CNS effects.

Both drugs have proved to be effective for prophylaxis and treatment of influenza A infections in immunocompetent patients, and there are reported successes of amantadine in immunocompromised patients with influenza A pneumonia. Although the improvements in symptoms and in viral shedding that are seen in patients treated with amantadine or rimantadine are better than those seen with aspirin or placebo treatment, they are modest, and there have been no trials in immunocompromised patients or in patients with life-threatening influenza A.[190] Wild-type viruses are usually susceptible to both drugs, but resistance (and cross-resistance) emerge rapidly. Resistant influenza A virus has been isolated from children receiving rimantadine treatment and in family members receiving postexposure prophylaxis.[191] This finding is of concern, and for this reason it is suggested that simultaneous therapy and prophylaxis in the same household be avoided. Amantadine doses of 2.2 to 4.4 mg/kg twice per day up to 150 mg/day are suggested for young children (1 to 10 years old), and older children may receive 100 mg twice daily for prophylaxis or treatment of influenza A. Amantadine, however, has essentially been supplanted by the neuraminidase inhibitors for prevention and treatment of influenza.

Oseltamivir and Zanamivir

Oseltamivir and zanamivir are potent and specific neuraminidase inhibitors of influenza A and B. Oseltamivir is administered orally, whereas zanamivir is administered intranasally. When administered early in the course of infection with influenza A or B, both agents have been shown to decrease the duration of illness and the severity of symptoms of infection.[192,193] Given the data in immunocompromised individuals, use of these agents for prophylaxis of high-risk patients with significant exposures is warranted. Zanamivir also has been studied in immunocompetent children older than the age of 5 years with similar results in terms of efficacy and tolerability as were found in adult studies.[194]

Nichols and colleagues reported that among patients who suffered influenza while undergoing HSCT, influenza pneumonia tended to develop more frequently among those infected earlier after transplantation.[195] Pneumonia developed in 6 (18%) of 34 untreated patients, whereas pneumonia developed in 1 (13%) of 8 patients treated with rimantadine and 0 of 9 treated with oseltamivir.

In addressing the concern about the emergence of resistance to neuraminidase inhibitors, Kiso et al.[196] documented the emergence of resistant influenza A viruses in 50 children treated with oseltamivir for documented infection. Mutations in the neuraminidase gene and *in vitro* phenotypic resistance were documented in nine patients (18%); however, the clinical significance of this emergence of resistance was not reflected in clinical outcome. Children continued to shed nonresistant virus after as much as 5 days of therapy. On the other hand, a study from Australia demonstrated that there has been no emergence of resistance in influenza isolates since the introduction of the neuraminidase inhibitors.[197] At this juncture, emergence of strains resistant to neuraminidase inhibitors does not appear to be a direct clinical problem. However, the genetic studies of Kiso et al. indicate that the potential exists for high-level resistance to neuraminidase inhibitors in influenza A.

ANTI-*PNEUMOCYSTIS* PNEUMONIA AGENTS

A number of agents are in common usage for the prophylaxis and treatment of *Pneumocystis* pneumonia (PCP) due to *Pneumocystis jiroveci* (formerly *carinii*). Although the data describing their efficacy originated from patients with AIDS, there are also substantial data in oncology patients and HSCT recipients.

Trimethoprim-Sulfamethoxazole

Hughes and colleagues demonstrated in 1977 that prophylaxis with TMP-SMX was highly effective in preventing PCP in high-risk pediatric oncology patients.[198] The use of PCP prophylaxis has since become a routine part of the management of childhood leukemia. The recommended prophylactic regimen is TMP-SMX with 150 mg TMP/m²/day and 750 mg/m²/day of SMX given orally in divided doses twice a day during three consecutive days per week. Most oncology patients are able to tolerate TMP-SMX; however, adverse events, including myelosuppression and rash, sometimes make alternative therapy necessary. TMP-SMX is also used for proven PCP at a dosage of 20 mg/kg in four divided doses.

Dapsone

Dapsone, a synthetic sulfone, is effective in the treatment and prevention of PCP and acts through the inhibition of folic acid synthesis in susceptible organisms.[199] For prophylaxis, it is administered at a dose of 2 mg/kg/day. Adverse effects include rash, anemia, methemoglobinemia, agranulocytosis, and hepatic dysfunction.

Pentamidine

Pentamidine in its aerosolized form is another agent that has been studied extensively in both children and adults with HIV as a prophylactic agent for PCP. It has been shown to be an effective regimen when administered at a dose of 300 mg via Respirgard inhaler monthly. In small children, it is often considered difficult to administer this drug because of the mechanics of the inhaler therapy. IV pentamidine has undergone only limited evaluation as a preventive regimen but is associated with potentially debilitating adverse drug reactions, including pancreatitis, hypoglycemia, diabetes mellitus, and renal impairment.[200]

Atovaquone

Atovaquone has broad antiprotozoal activity, as well as proven efficacy against PCP. Atovaquone was shown to be as effective as dapsone for PCP prophylaxis in patients with AIDS who were intolerant of TMP-SMX.[201] The most common adverse effects are mild upper GI symptoms and diarrhea. The drug is significantly more bioavailable in suspension form and therefore is routinely given in that form. Pharmacokinetic studies in children[202] indicate once daily dosing of children from 0 to 3 months; for those greater than 24 months at 30 mg/kg/day and for those 3 to 24 months at 45 mg/kg/day. That the cost of atovaquone is substantially greater than that of other oral agents used for PCP warrants consideration in selecting an agent.

MANAGEMENT OF UNEXPLAINED FEVER IN THE NEUTROPENIC PATIENT

Duration of Antibiotic Therapy

Once antibiotics have been initiated empirically, duration of therapy should be defined if a site of infection is not documented. Low-risk patients do well when antibiotics are continued until recovery from neutropenia (>500 cells/mm³). Alternatively, there is evidence that antibiotics may be discontinued in these low-risk patients if their PMN counts are rising before reaching more than 500 cells/mm³. In a prospective study of 131 children with fever and neutropenia hospitalized for IV antibiotic treatment, 70 had their antibiotics discontinued and were discharged after they met the following criteria: afebrile for 24 hours, appeared clinically well, had negative cultures for at least 48 hours, exhibited control of local infection, and had evidence of bone marrow recovery for at least 1 day, as measured by rising ANC or PMN count or platelet count. Only 1 of the 70 children required readmission for recurrent fever, whereas 6 of 8 patients inadvertently discharged without signs of marrow recovery required readmission. Substantial savings in hospital costs were estimated for early discharge patients, and this approach is a reasonable option for those patients who fit specific low-risk criteria.[57,203] However, these guidelines do not apply to high-risk patients who remain neutropenic for more than 1 week and who do not demonstrate evidence of bone marrow recovery. Stopping antibiotic therapy too early can lead to clinical deterioration in patients who remain granulocytopenic, particularly if they are persistently febrile.

The management of high-risk patients with prolonged neutropenia is addressed in a series of prospective clinical studies that stratified according to those who defervesced after the initiation of broad-spectrum antibiotics or who remained persistently febrile (Fig. 40.3).[204] Among patients with prolonged neutropenia who defervesced on therapy, 41% again became febrile within 3 days of stopping antibiotics on day 7; new bacterial isolates from those with documented infections were susceptible to the antibiotics that had been withdrawn. On the other hand, no subsequent infections were observed among patients who continued antibiotics.

Empirical Antifungal Therapy

The situation is more complicated for patients who remain persistently granulocytopenic and febrile despite antibiotic therapy. In a randomized clinical trial, 56% of patients with unexplained fever who remained febrile after receiving empirical antibiotics developed complications within 3 days of stopping therapy.[205] Of these, 38% became hypotensive. Strikingly, 31% of these patients eventually developed invasive fungal infections. These fungal infections were probably related to continued antibiotic therapy and protracted granulocytopenia.

The rationale for the empirical use of an antifungal compound are based on several lines of reasoning. First, antemortem diagnosis of invasive fungal disease is difficult in an immunocompromised host. Second, withholding antifungal therapy pending a definitive diagnosis may allow local progression or dissemination to occur. Third, the outcome of an invasive fungal infection in an immunocompromised patient is improved by early institution of therapy. Fourth, it is possible to identify patients who are at greatest risk for invasive mycoses. Neutropenic patients who remain febrile despite a

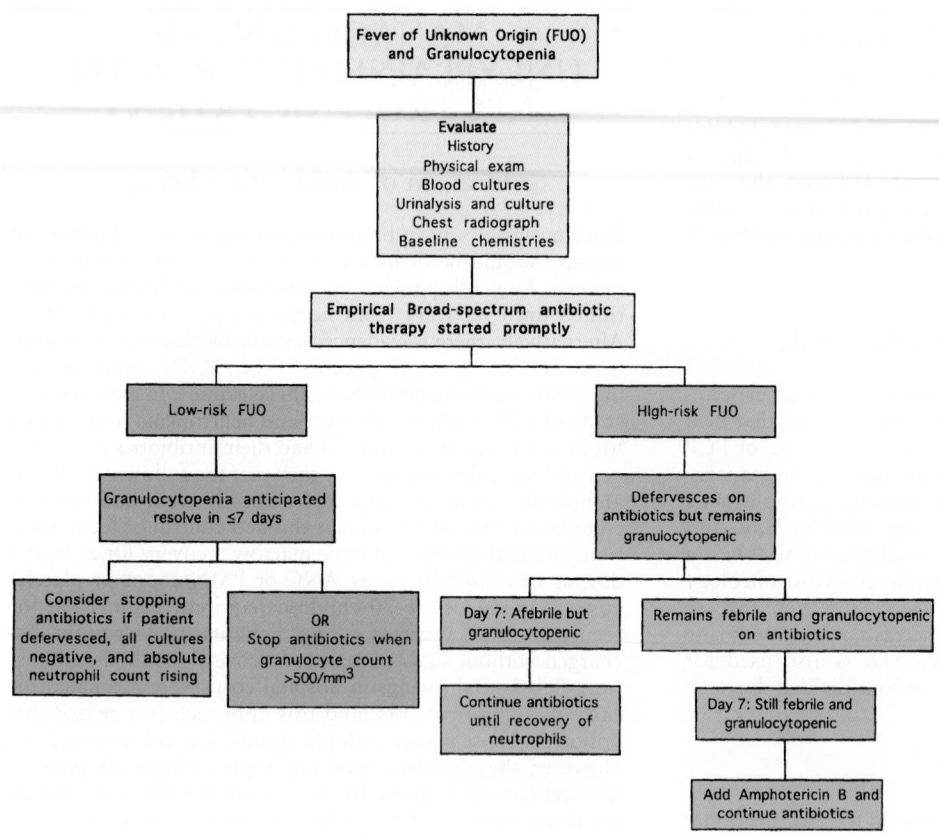

FIGURE 40.3 Algorithm for the initial management of the child who has unexplained fever and neutropenia (see text for details).

4- to 7-day trial of broad-spectrum antimicrobial therapy are particularly prone to fungal disease.[205] The use of empirical antifungal therapy would be expected to provide a dual benefit: the suppression of the fungal overgrowth that accompanies broad-spectrum antimicrobial therapy and the early treatment of subclinical, localized mycotic disease.

A prospective, randomized trial performed by the EORTC corroborated the benefit of empirical amphotericin B therapy with D-AmB for persistently febrile neutropenic patients. In that study, there were six documented fungal infections, four of which were fatal, among 64 patients who did not receive antifungal therapy, compared with only one fungemia and no deaths among 68 patients treated empirically with amphotericin (0.6 mg/kg/day or 1.2 mg/kg every other day) on or after day 4 of broad-spectrum antibiotic therapy.[206]

The point at which antifungal therapy was initiated varied in these studies. The arbitrary designation of day 7, used in the NCI trials, avoids the overuse of antifungal agents in patients who are slow to defervesce with empirical antibiotics and those who recover their granulocyte counts before day 7. Despite theoretical and clinical evidence substantiating the efficacy of empirical antifungal therapy, the dose-limiting nephrotoxicity of D-AmB limits the utility of this compound for empirical use. Thus, less toxic alternatives were sought for this indication.

A multicenter study therefore investigated whether L-AmB may be used instead of conventional D-AmB for empirical antifungal therapy in a randomized, double-blind trial design of L-AmB versus D-AmB in neutropenic children and adults with persistent fever despite broad-spectrum antibiotics.[207] Among 687 randomized patients, the composite success rate was equivalent and independent of administration of antifungal prophylaxis or use of colony- stimulating factors. There were fewer proven breakthrough fungal infections in patients

treated with L-AmB versus D-AmB and also were fewer infusion-related fevers, chills/rigors, and cardiorespiratory events (dyspnea, hypotension, tachycardia, hypertension, and hypoxia) for L-AmB versus D-AmB, respectively. Moreover, there was reduced nephrotoxicity in patients treated with L-AmB (19%) versus D-AmB (34%). Thus, this study concluded that L-AmB was equivalent to D-AmB in therapeutic success for empirical antifungal therapy in neutropenic patients but superior in reducing proven treatment-emergent fungal infections, infusion-related toxicity, and nephrotoxicity. These findings are consistent with those of Prentice et al. who found similar results of L-AmB for empirical antifungal therapy.[208]

With the advent of second-generation triazoles, a multicenter international study tested the hypothesis that voriconazole would be comparable to L-AmB as empirical antifungal therapy in persistently febrile neutropenic patients.[143] Although voriconazole did not meet the prespecified statistical end point for noninferiority, it was associated with significantly fewer breakthrough invasive fungal infections, particularly those due to invasive aspergillosis. Moreover, a prespecified secondary efficacy analysis in the category of high-risk neutropenic patients (relapsed leukemia and allogeneic HSCT) found that voriconazole was comparable to L-AmB and resulted in a significant reduction of invasive fungal infections. Voriconazole was associated with more infusion-related visual side effects, as well as visual hallucinations, whereas L-AmB was associated with more nephrotoxicity.

A subsequent multicenter double-blind international study investigated the hypothesis that the safety and efficacy of an echinocandin would be comparable to that of L-AmB for empirical antifungal therapy in persistently febrile neutropenic patients.[209] Patients receiving caspofungin and L-AmB had similar overall success rates, fulfilling statistical criteria for noninferiority. Among patients with baseline invasive fungal infections, a higher proportion treated with caspofungin had a successful outcome. The proportion of patients who survived at least 7 days posttherapy also was greater in the caspofungin group. Premature study discontinuation occurred more often in the L-AmB group. Breakthrough fungal infections and resolution of fever during neutropenia were similar in both groups. Fewer patients who received caspofungin sustained nephrotoxicity, an infusion-related toxicity, one or more drug-related adverse events, or discontinued therapy because of drug-related adverse events. This study concluded that caspofungin was at least as effective as L-AmB and was generally better tolerated as empirical antifungal therapy in persistently febrile neutropenic patients.

Itraconazole and fluconazole also have been studied for this indication in comparison with D-AmB.[210,211] Itraconazole was studied in adult patients with acute leukemia, and fluconazole was studied in patients with relatively short durations of neutropenia for empirical antifungal therapy.

Thus, D-AmB, L-AmB, voriconazole, caspofungin, and itraconazole have been well characterized for empirical antifungal therapy for persistent fever in high-risk neutropenic patients. Selection of an agent for empirical antifungal therapy will depend on the patterns of infection in one's institution; use, if any, of prophylactic agents; drug acquisition cost; and the presence of or risk for end-organ toxicity (e.g., renal or hepatic dysfunction).

For patients who remain neutropenic, antifungal therapy should be continued until the resolution of neutropenia. Persistence or recrudescence of fever should prompt a meticulous investigation for nonfungal infectious causes (e.g., bacterial or viral superinfections) or for a fungus that is resistant to initial empirical antifungal coverage (e.g., *Aspergillus* species, *Trichosporon*, *Fusarium* species, *Pseudallescheria boydii*, *Scedosporium* species, and Zygomycetes). Patients who develop a documented fungal infection should be treated with the appropriate antifungal agent.

As LFABs and other more recently introduced antifungal agents are more costly than conventional D-AmB, targeting the highest risk patients who may optimally benefit from empirical antifungal therapy is important. Such patients include those with preexisting renal insufficiency, concomitant nephrotoxic agents, and anticipated protracted neutropenia. The use of D-AmB may be associated with severe nephrotoxicity and excess mortality.[212] As exemplified in a pharmacoeconomics analysis that analyzed the impact of nephrotoxicity on total cost of hospitalization and the cost/benefit ratios of D-AmB and L-AmB, drug-acquisition cost alone is not sufficient in assessing the potential cost-to-benefit and risk-to-benefit ratios of antifungal therapy beyond D-AmB.[213]

EVALUATION AND MANAGEMENT OF DOCUMENTED INFECTIONS

Bacteremia

Approximately 10% to 30% of all febrile neutropenic cancer patients are bacteremic at presentation.[76] In low-risk patients, the rate of bacteremia is consistently less than 10%. Until the late 1970s, aerobic gram-negative bacilli (especially *E. coli*, *K. pneumoniae*, and *P. aeruginosa*) were the most frequently isolated pathogens. Subsequently, the pattern of infections has shifted toward gram-positive bacteria. Among the factors possibly contributing to this shift in gram-positive isolates are increased use of indwelling central venous catheters, fluoroquinolone prophylaxis, and high-dose chemotherapy-induced oral mucositis.

The gram-positive pathogens most commonly isolated include *S. aureus*, *S. epidermidis*, *Streptococcus* species (particularly *S. viridans*), and *Enterococcus* species. Species of *Corynebacterium* (e.g., *Corynebacterium jeikeium*) and *Bacillus* species are less frequently isolated and tend to occur in patients with long episodes of granulocytopenia or those with indwelling vascular access devices, respectively.[214] Metallo-β-lactamase–producing *S. maltophilia*, Amp-C stably derepressed β-lactamase–producing *Enterobacter* species, and extended-spectrum β-lactamase–producing *E. coli* and *K. pneumoniae* are now increasingly emerging as the most frequently isolated aerobic gram-negative bacilli with high-level resistance to many of the front-line empirical regimens. These isolates also may carry resistance genes encoding quinolone resistance.

Resistance patterns in gram-positive pathogens isolated from febrile neutropenic patients also have emerged as an increasing challenge. *Enterococcus* species that are resistant to vancomycin, ampicillin, and/or aminoglycosides, have been increasingly reported and are associated with high mortality in immunocompromised patients.[215,216] Some isolates of viridans streptococci are resistant to penicillin and cephalosporins and therefore require vancomycin for therapy. Isolates of *S. pneumoniae* with either intermediate or high-level penicillin resistance are now relatively common in many parts of the United States which has clinical implications for asplenic patients and patients post-HSCT with chronic GVHD who are at particularly high risk for pneumococcal sepsis.

The attributable morbidity and mortality rates associated with infections due to coagulase-negative staphylococci and enterococci are lower than those caused by gram-negative bacilli. However, bacteremia caused by α-hemolytic streptococci may cause sudden onset of hypotension, with progression in approximately one-fourth of cases to a syndrome that can include shock, respiratory failure due to adult respiratory distress syndrome, acute renal failure, and neurologic manifestations. Palmar erythema and subsequent desquamation may also be a feature of this syndrome. Although there is considerable variability between centers of mortality related to viridans streptococcal sepsis, the median death rate is approximately 10%.[217] The antecedent administration of high-dose Ara-C is a strongly correlative risk factor for the development of α-hemolytic streptococcal sepsis.[218] A number of other distinct risk factors have been associated with this syndrome, including the presence of mucositis, the administration of antacids or H₂-blockers, and prophylactic treatment with TMP-SMX or fluoroquinolone antibiotics, both of which allow for breakthrough growth of α-hemolytic streptococci.[219]

The most important therapeutic intervention for patients ultimately shown to be bacteremic is the prompt initiation of empirical antibiotic treatment at the time of the patient's presentation with fever and neutropenia. A reasonable antibiotic regimen could include a β-lactam and aminoglycoside or monotherapy with a β-lactam (e.g., ceftazidime, cefipime, or meropenem). Necessary modifications of the initial regimen should be based on the antimicrobial susceptibility pattern of the bloodstream isolate (Table 40.3) while maintaining broad empirical coverage.

Catheter-Associated Bacteremia

With the increased use of indwelling venous access devices, catheter-associated bacteremic episodes have become more frequent.[9] The strict diagnosis of a catheter-related versus noncatheter-related bacteremia is often difficult. Positive

TABLE 40.3

COMMONLY USED ANTIMICROBIAL AGENTS FOR PEDIATRIC CANCER PATIENTS

Class	Agent	Spectrum[a]	Daily dose (maximum)	Comments
Antibacterial agents				
Third-generation cephalosporin	Ceftazidime	Enteric bacteria, some gram-positive aerobes, no anaerobic coverage	100 mg/kg divided every 8 h (max 6 g/d)	Only ceftazidime covers *Pseudomonas aeruginosa*
Fourth-generation cephalosporin	Cefepime	Enteric bacteria, gram-positive aerobes	100 mg/kg divided every 8 h (6 g/d)	Active against some *P. aeruginosa*, *Enterobacter* species, and *Serratia* species resistant to ceftazidime; broader gram-positive spectrum
Carbapenems	Imipenem	Most gram-negative and gram-positive aerobes, including *P. aeruginosa*, enterococci; excellent anaerobic coverage	50 mg/kg divided every 6 h (4 g/d)	*Stenotrophomonas maltophilia* and *Burkholderia cepacia* not covered
	Meropenem	Similar to imipenem	60–120 mg/kg divided every 8 h (3 g/d)	Less likely than imipenem to cause seizures
Extended-spectrum penicillins	Piperacillin, azlocillin, mezlocillin	Enteric aerobes, including some *P. aeruginosa*, *Enterobacter* species, *Serratia* species; anaerobes	300 mg/kg divided every 4 h (21 g/d)	Must be paired with an aminoglycoside for coverage of *P. aeruginosa*
	Piperacillin-tazobactam	Similar to piperacillin, increased activity versus some β-lactamase producing gram-positive cocci, gram-negative bacilli, and anaerobes	300 mg/kg divided every 4 h (12 g/d)	Not adequate as monotherapy for *P. aeruginosa*; aminoglycoside should be added
Monobactams	Aztreonam	Exclusively aerobic gram-negative aerobes including *P. aeruginosa*	100–150 mg/kg divided every 6 h (4 g/d)	Limited spectrum requires pairing with gram-positive agent, not cross-reactive with β-lactams so can be used in penicillin or cephalosporin allergic patients
Glycopeptide	Vancomycin	Exclusively gram-positive	25–40 mg/kg divided every 6–12 h (3 g/d) IV	No need to add vancomycin routinely for empirical coverage for fever and neutropenia
Lipopeptide	Daptomycin	Exclusively gram-positive, including ORSA and susceptible strains of VRE	4 mg/kg/d IV	Data in pediatrics are limited at this time
Oxazolidinone	Linezolid	Exclusively gram-positive, including ORSA, susceptible strains of VRE, and penicillin and cephalosporin-resistant *S. pneumoniae*	10 mg /kg q12h	Excellent oral bioavailability
Streptogramin	Quinupristin/dalfopristin	Exclusively gram-positive, similar to linezolid but spectrum does not include *E. faecalis*	7.5 mg/kg q8h	Venous irritation, should be given via central venous catheter

Antifungal agents

Agent	Spectrum	Dosage	Comments
Amphotericin B			
Deoxycholate amphotericin B	Very broad antifungal activity including *Candida* species, *Aspergillus* species, Zygomycetes, *Cryptococcus neoformans*, *Histoplasma capsulatum*	0.5 mg/kg once daily for empirical therapy, higher doses (1.0–1.5 mg/kg) are necessary for documented infections due to *Aspergillus* species and other filamentous fungi	Significant nephrotoxicity may be reduced by saline hydration before daily infusion
Lipid formulations (amphotericin B lipid complex, amphotericin B colloidal dispersion, and liposomal amphotericin B)	Same spectrum as deoxycholate formulation	3 mg/kg/d for empirical therapy, 5 mg/kg/d (or greater) for documented infections due to *Aspergillus* species and other filamentous fungi	Significantly less nephrotoxicity with efficacy at least equal to that of deoxycholate amphotericin B
Triazole			
Fluconazole	*Candida* species (not *C. krusei* and not some strains of *C. glabrata*); *C. neoformans*, *Trichosporon* species, and *Coccidioides immitis*	3–12 mg/kg/d Dosage of 12 mg/kg/d is required for life-threatening infections to achieve comparable plasma drug exposure attained in adults with 400 mg/d (see text)	Excellent bioavailability, independent of gastric acidity
Itraconazole	*Aspergillus* species, *Candida* species, *H. capsulatum*, *Blastomyces dermatitidis*, and *C. immitis*	3–5 mg/kg/d PO[b]	Absorption erratic but increased with taking drug with meals or by using cyclodextrin formulation
Voriconazole	*Candida* species, *Aspergillus* species, *Trichosporon* species and some strains of *Scedosporium* species, and *Fusarium* species	3 mg/kg q12h for empirical therapy and 4 mg/kg q12h IV for documented infections; higher dosages in pediatric patients may be necessary in order to achieve comparable adult drug exposures (see text)	Pediatric suspension is available; bioavailability is reliable and is enhanced with empty stomach
Posaconazole	*Candida* species, *Aspergillus* species, Zygomycetes	For patients ≥ 13 y.o., prophylactic dosing of 200 mg PO three times a day.	
Echinocandin			
Caspofungin	*Candida* species and *Aspergillus* species	50 mg/m^2/d IV to achieve comparable plasma concentrations in adults receiving 50 mg/d IV	

(continued)

1211

TABLE 40.3

CONTINUED

Class	Agent	Spectrum[a]	Daily dose (maximum)	Comments
Antiviral agents Antiherpetic	Acyclovir	HSV, VZV	HSV: 750 mg/m² divided q8h or 5 mg/kg q8h VZV: 1,500 mg/m² divided q8h or 10 mg/kg q8h	IV dose for VZV is twice that for HSV. Hydration should be ensured when administering high doses
	Ganciclovir	CMV, HSV, VZV, HHV-6	For CMV: 5 mg/kg q12h for 14 d induction, then 5 mg/kg/d for maintenance	Granulocytopenia is the major dose-limiting toxicity; not routinely used for HSV, VZV but dose used for CMV is effective for the other herpesviruses
	Foscarnet	HSV, VZV, CMV (including most acyclovir- and ganciclovir-resistant strains)	CMV: 60 mg/kg/d q8h for 14 d then 90–120 mg/kg/d for maintenance VZV, HSV: 40 mg/kg q8h	Nephrotoxicity is dose-limiting effect, renal function and electrolytes require close monitoring
	Trimethoprim-sulfamethoxazole	*Pneumocystis jiroveci* (formerly, *P. carinii*), also is active against many gram-positive and gram-negative bacteria, including *S. maltophilia* and *B. cepacia*	20 mg/kg/d IV in two divided doses for PCP treatment	May cause bone marrow suppression in high doses
Anti-PCP agents	Pentamidine	*P. jiroveci*	4 mg/kg/d IV for treatment	Adverse effects include pancreatitis, hypoglycemia, hypocalcemia, infusional hypotension
	Dapsone	*P. jiroveci*	2 mg/kg/d (for prophylaxis)	High incidence of hemolytic reactions, can also cause methemoglobinemia
	Atovaquone	*P. jiroveci*	30 mg/kg/d, max 1,500 mg/d	Suspension formulation has better bioavailability

VRE, vancomycin-resistant enterococci; ORSA, oxacillin-resistant *Staphylococcus aureus*; HSV, herpessimplex virus; VZV, varicella zoster virus; CMV, cytomegalovirus; HHV-6, human herpes virus 6; PCP, *Pneumocystis* pneumonia.
[a]Spectrum depicted here is for summary purposes and is not a complete list.
[b]IV formulation for itraconazole is available but dosage and pharmacokinetics have not been defined inpediatric patients.

blood cultures drawn through an indwelling venous catheter can be considered to have arisen from one of three possible sources: infection of the line from external sources (skin and catheter hub); hematogenous seeding of the catheter from internal sources; and, rarely, contaminated infusate (e.g., platelets with bacterial contamination). For suspected catheter-related bloodstream infections, paired blood samples, drawn from the catheter and a peripheral vein, should be cultured prior to the initiation of antimicrobial therapy.[72] However, because peripheral blood cultures in pediatric patients are painful and are associated with increased contamination from cutaneous flora, they are infrequently performed when an indwelling device is in place. The volume of blood drawn is the critical determinant for recovery of bacteria from bloodstream infections. Thus, 2 or more blood cultures through the central venous catheter (one set through each lumen) will provide a yield similar to that of central cultures plus peripheral cultures but without the patient discomfort and the potential for increased contamination from cutaneous flora.

Removal of chronic indwelling central venous catheters is best determined by the type of organism recovered, the hemodynamic stability of the patient, and the presence of persistent bacteremia. Removal and replacement of chronic indwelling catheters carries the risk of general anesthesia, pneumothorax, and hemorrhage, particularly in thrombocytopenic patients. The majority of patients with fever and neutropenia and a central line–associated bacteremia do not need to have their chronic indwelling central silastic catheters removed.[220] However, there are certain clinical situations and infectious pathogens that require line removal for cure of infection. Among the organisms causing catheter-related bloodstream infections that warrant removal of a chronic indwelling central silastic venous catheter are *S. aureus*, *Bacillus* species, atypical mycobacteria, *Candida* species, and polymicrobial infections. Catheter-related bacteremia due to *S. maltophilia* also may cause refractory bacteremia and warrants catheter removal.

Although catheter-related bacteremia due to *S. aureus* can be treated without line removal, relapses after completion of therapy in those patients whose line was not removed can sometimes occur.[221] Although *Bacillus* species may appear to be susceptible to standard antibiotics, their propensity for forming tenacious biofilms usually requires catheter removal to cure the infection.[214] Patients with polymicrobial catheter-related bacteremia and those with candidemia should have their catheters removed.

Most catheter-associated infections caused by coagulase-negative staphylococci can be controlled without removal of the catheter.[221] In addition, many catheter-related bacteremias due to gram-negative bacilli can be treated with intravenously delivered antibiotics and without removal of the catheter. In patients with double- or triple-lumen catheters, the antibiotic infusions should be infused simultaneously in split doses among the lumens or rotated among each of the catheter lumens. If, despite these measures, blood cultures remain persistently positive more than 72 hours later, the catheter should be removed. Nevertheless, removal of the catheter should be considered when there is recurrent bacteremia with the same organism after an appropriate course of therapy. Additional medical indications for removal of catheters in patients with catheter-associated infections include severe sepsis, suppurative thrombophlebitis, and endocarditis.[72]

Catheter-Associated Candidemia

Candida species are the fourth most common bloodstream isolates following coagulase-negative *Staphylococcus* species,

S. aureus, and *Enterococcus* species[222] Historically, *Candida albicans* has been the most common species isolated, constituting approximately 50% of isolates, and non-*albicans Candida* species (predominantly *Candida glabrata*, *Candida tropicalis*, *Candida parapsilosis*, and *Candida krusei*) account for the remaining half of bloodstream isolates.[223,224] A recent study analyzing the epidemiology and outcomes of candidemia in 2,019 patients from 2004 to 2008, however, revealed that the incidence of candidemia caused by non-*Candida albicans Candida* species (54.4%) was higher than the incidence of candidemia caused by *C. albicans* (45.6%). Crude 12-week mortality was 35.2%. Interestingly, *C. parapsilosis* had the lowest mortality (27.9%) and was less likely to be associated with patients who were neutropenic, receiving steroids, or receiving other immunosuppressive mediations. In contrast, *C. krusei* candidemia was most commonly associated with prior use of antifungal agents (and is virtually always resistant to fluconazole[225]), hematologic malignancy, stem cell transplantation, neutropenia, and corticosteroid treatment. Patients with *C. krusei* candidemia had the highest mortality in this series (52.9%).[226] Therefore, the identification of *Candida* species carries important clinical implications. *C. glabrata* has variable levels of resistance, shows an unpredictable susceptibility to antifungal triazoles and to amphotericin B, and results in poorer outcomes than in patients with *C. albicans* candidemia.[224,227] *C. tropicalis* has a more severe clinical course than does *C. albicans* in neutropenic patients: associated disproportionately with a syndrome of cutaneous dissemination, arthralgias, and myalgias, and renal failure appears to be more common.[228] Some isolates of *Candida lusitaniae* and *Candida guilliermondii* are resistant to amphotericin B.[229,230]

The recommended management of catheter-related candidemia includes antifungal therapy (echinocandins or, in selected patients, fluconazole[72]) and removal of the vascular catheter; however, the practice of catheter removal for candidemia in oncology and HSCT patients is controversial.[231–233] Nucci and Anaissie maintain that because the GI tract is the principal portal of entry for *Candida* species in oncology-HSCT patients, catheter removal may not improve outcome.[232,233] On the other hand, vascular catheters also may become the target for seeding by organisms hematogenously disseminated from the GI tract. A reasonable approach to this question in catheter-related candidemia would be to remove vascular catheters, where feasible, unless there are extenuating circumstances such as limited vascular access or transfusion-refractory thrombocytopenia.[234]

Local Infections of Vascular Catheters

Local infections of chronic indwelling vascular catheters include exit site infections, pocket space abscesses, pocket space cellulitis, and tunnel infections.[235] Warmth, erythema, and tenderness at the exit site are highly suggestive of an infectious etiology; and purulence or cellulitis at the catheter exit site, without associated bacteremia, is evidence of a local exit site infection. Exit site infections can often be managed without catheter removal; however, if *P. aeruginosa* is cultured from the exit site, catheter removal may be required, particularly for resistant organisms.

In contrast to exit site infections, pocket-space infections present with fluctuance around the subcutaneous catheter hub with signs of inflammation or cellulitis of the overlying skin, and tunnel infections are characterized by spreading cellulitis in the subcutaneous tissues along the tunnel tract of long-term IV catheters. Unlike exit site infections, these infections are often associated with serious local morbidity and bacteremias.

Removal of the vascular device is often warranted in these circumstances. The pathogens involved in tunnel infections are most commonly gram-positive cocci; however, gram-negative bacilli, including *Pseudomonas* species, and *Mycobacterium* species (*Mycobacterium fortuitum, Mycobacterium chelonae, and Mycobacterium abscessus*), are also reported.[236] These infections are best managed by rapid removal of the catheter and treatment with IV antibiotics. The infected tunnel tract may require surgical debridement in advanced infections.

Ear Infections

Children with cancer may develop the same infectious problems as immunocompetent patients but may do so with recurrent and persistent infections. Children with anatomic alterations (e.g., radiation damage) of the external or middle ear or eustachian tube are particularly susceptible to recurrent infectious episodes. Clinical findings suggesting an ear infection range from the classic complaints (e.g., ear pain, drainage, fever, irritability) to minimal findings (e.g., slight tympanic erythema) in profoundly neutropenic children. Although the most likely pathogens may be the same as those isolated from immunocompetent hosts (e.g., *S. pneumoniae*, non-typable *H. influenzae*), other gram-positive or gram-negative bacteria that may have colonized the oropharynx and nasopharynx may cause infection in neutropenic patients. Therefore, broad-spectrum antibiotic therapy is necessary in pediatric oncology and HSCT patients unless a specific pathogen has been identified. Patients should receive 10 to 14 days of therapy.

Although mastoiditis has become an uncommon complication of otitis media, immunosuppressed patients, particularly those with an anatomic abnormality of the middle ear, are at increased risk for the development of mastoiditis. In addition to the usual bacterial pathogens associated with this disorder, individuals with prolonged neutropenia or other forms of chronic immunosuppression are at risk for fungal mastoiditis, which requires surgical management for cure.[237] Patients should undergo appropriate evaluation, including CT scans of the involved area, particularly if they have symptoms or signs (e.g., localized erythema, swelling, tenderness) referable to the mastoid. Surgical drainage of the infected mastoid sinus in immunocompromised patients is often necessary. Lack of an aggressive management of mastoiditis may lead to chronic osteomyelitis, subdural empyema, cortical vein thrombosis, septic thrombosis of the transverse venous sinus, and cerebral abscess.

Malignant otitis externa, an invasive and potentially life-threatening infection of the external ear and skull base, requires urgent diagnosis and treatment. It occurs primarily in immunocompromised individuals, particularly those with diabetes mellitus, and the most common pathogen is *Pseudomonas aeruginosa*. Patients complain of severe otalgia that worsens at night and otorrhea. Definitive diagnosis requires culturing of ear secretions, pathologic examination of granulation tissue from the infection site, and imaging studies, such as CT. Treatment includes modification of immunosuppression, when possible, local treatment of the auditory canal, long-term systemic antibiotic therapy, and, in selected patients, surgery.[238]

Bacterial and Fungal Sinusitis

Acute bacterial sinusitis in the immunocompetent child is most commonly caused by *S. pneumoniae, H. influenzae, and Moraxella catarrhalis*.[239] Chronic sinusitis is most commonly caused by *S. aureus*, gram-negative bacilli (including *P. aeruginosa*), and anaerobic bacterial species. Patients with obstruction of the sinuses by tumor (e.g., nasopharyngeal carcinoma, Burkitt's lymphoma, rhabdomyosarcoma) are especially at risk for acute or chronic sinusitis. However, because the true bacterial etiology of an acute sinusitis is difficult to discern, a pediatric otolaryngologist should be consulted to help identify the microbial pathogen. Until such microbiologic results are available, broad-spectrum empirical antibacterial therapy is instituted. Also essential to establishing a definitive treatment plan is the importance of distinguishing between bacterial and fungal etiologies.

Fungal sinusitis in neutropenic patients and HSCT recipients is most commonly due to *Aspergillus* species, Zygomycetes, and *Fusarium* species[240,241] Patients with acute leukemia, aplastic anemia, and HSCT are especially susceptible to fungal sinusitis. The diagnosis of acute sinusitis is usually suggested by complaints of facial pain, local tenderness, and (assuming a patent outlet and an adequate granulocyte count) purulent nasal drainage. With involvement of the ethmoid sinus, edema of the eyelids and excessive tearing may also be observed. In young children, a nonproductive cough and fetid breath may indicate a sinus infection. However, these findings are often muted, delayed, or absent in immunocompromised patients with fungal sinusitis. Hence, a high index of suspicion must be maintained, particularly in persistently febrile, neutropenic patients receiving broad-spectrum antibiotics. Any sinus tenderness or even minimal complaints of nasal congestion in a neutropenic child should be pursued with a CT scan and a detailed nasopharyngeal examination. Subtle findings on otolaryngologic examination (e.g., crusting ulcers on the nasal turbinates) may be indicative of an invasive fungal infection. Such lesions should be sampled and submitted for microbiologic identification.

Radiologic examination of the sinuses is useful for diagnosis of sinusitis in children older than 1 year. The findings of sinus opacity, an air-fluid interface, or mucosal thickening in immunocompromised children correlate with acute infection. Radiologic evidence of erosion of bone is an insensitive radiologic marker and its absence should not be used to exclude invasive fungal sinusitis. In patients with chronic sinusitis, radiographic findings are less helpful because of the persistence of abnormalities related to the chronic infection. Serial CT or MRI scans may prove helpful in immunosuppressed patients with chronic sinus disease, because they are more sensitive to subtle changes and more specific than plain radiographs.[242]

The presence of ethmoidal fungal sinusitis requires urgent otolaryngologic and medical intervention in neutropenic patients. Invasion by fungi through the lamina papyracea causes postseptal periorbital infection, threatens the ocular globe, entraps extraocular muscles, and may result in the orbital apex syndrome with infarction of the optic nerve and central retinal artery. As the cavernous sinuses receive the venous drainage of the ethmoid sinus, fungal ethmoidal sinusitis may result in cavernous sinus thrombosis and invasion of the cranial nerves II, IV, V-1, V-2, and VI, as well as the internal carotid artery.

Antimicrobial therapy for bacterial sinusitis is tailored to the organisms and clinical situation. The new onset of acute bacterial sinusitis in a nonneutropenic patient may be managed with amoxicillin plus clavulanic acid or TMP-SMX.[243] For neutropenic patients, broad-spectrum antimicrobial therapy is necessary. Decongestants are an essential adjunct to antimicrobial therapy, to provide drainage of the sinuses. If a neutropenic patient with presumptive bacterial sinusitis does not improve after 72 hours of treatment, aspiration or biopsy of the sinus should be performed. For patients with chronic or recurrent sinusitis, particularly those with a local tumor mass or damage secondary to radiotherapy, an antral window may be necessary to allow adequate drainage.

The diagnosis and treatment of fungal sinusitis in neutropenic and other immunocompromised patients remain difficult. A microbiologic diagnosis is important, particularly to distinguish aspergillosis from zygomycosis. Voriconazole is used for primary treatment of *Aspergillus* sinusitis, whereas amphotericin B is used for zygomycosis. Given the heightened probability of zygomycosis as a cause of sinusitis in immunocompromised patients,[244] the broader spectrum amphotericin B formulation is used initially pending a definitive microbiologic diagnosis.

A high level of clinical suspicion is essential to establishing a definitive diagnosis. Plain radiographs often appear normal although CT or MRI scans reveal the presence of extensive disease. Patients with prolonged neutropenia in whom fever and mild symptoms of nasal congestion or bleeding develop should undergo such scanning to identify invasive fungal disease. Fungal sinusitis caused by *Aspergillus* species or Zygomycetes (e.g., *Rhizopus* species or *Mucor* species) can progress to the rhinocerebral syndrome through invasion from the ethmoid sinuses, frontal sinuses, sphenoid sinuses, or cribriform plate and into the CNS. Early institution of antifungal therapy is imperative for successful interdiction of this progression. Surgical debridement of involved tissue is often required in an effort to remove necrotic and inflammatory material. Even with these aggressive therapeutic maneuvers, a successful outcome depends on the recovery from neutropenia and reversal of other forms of immunosuppression.

Infections of the Lower Respiratory Tract

The respiratory tract is a site for infectious complications in immunosuppressed cancer patients. Colonization of the upper airway provides a ready source of pathogenic organisms in direct proximity to the lower respiratory tract. Altered mucosal and humoral immune mechanisms (e.g., subnormal mucociliary function, decreased secretory immunoglobulins) provide for less effective clearance of aspirated organisms, and the absence or suboptimal functioning of the phagocytic effector cells (e.g., PMNs, pulmonary macrophages) permits establishment of a local infection and frequently hematogenous dissemination of respiratory pathogens.

The relatively large number of infectious and noninfectious causes of pulmonary infiltrates that must be considered in the differential diagnosis, including progression of the underlying malignancy, drug reactions, emboli, and hemorrhage secondary to vascular erosion or severe thrombocytopenia, are among the principal problems in management of pulmonary infiltrates in immunocompromised hosts. The most practical approach for the evaluation of an immunocompromised patient with a pulmonary infiltrate is to categorize the patient according to the anatomic distribution of the infiltrative lesion (i.e., localized or diffuse) and the PMN count (i.e., neutropenic or not). This classification permits rapid evaluation, identification of likely pathogens, and prompt institution of appropriate therapy to optimize the probability for a successful therapeutic intervention (Fig. 40.4).

Diagnosis of Pneumonia in Immunocompromised Patients

Because pulmonary infections in immunocompromised patients can progress rapidly to respiratory failure, initial evaluation needs to be performed expeditiously. Evaluation of the neutropenic or immunocompromised child with suspected pneumonia includes a chest radiograph, CT scan when possible, blood cultures, hematologic indices, pulse oximeter reading (or arterial blood gases in more critical situations), and

collection and examination of available culture material. Nasopharyngeal washes for viral pathogens, including respiratory RSV, parainfluenza, influenza, and adenovirus, are important in patients with concomitant upper respiratory tract symptoms.

Radiographic evaluation with a CT scan is more sensitive than conventional chest radiography and may provide information regarding the pattern and extent of disease that may not be evident on plain film alone.[245] Specific findings of a "halo" sign, crescent sign, nodular infiltrate, or wedge-shape infiltrate are indicative of a possible angioinvasive filamentous fungus, including, but not limited to, *Aspergillus* species.[246,247] Pulmonary infiltrates due to aspergillosis and other filamentous fungi in neutropenic patients are due to angioinvasion, thrombosis, infarction, and hemorrhage, representing a direct effect of organism-mediated pulmonary injury, which may evolve rapidly.[248] Hence, localized pulmonary infiltrates in neutropenic patients should prompt an urgent assessment of the etiology. Chest CT scans facilitate detection of pulmonary aspergillosis in patients with persistent neutropenic fever leading to earlier initiation of therapy, which, in turn, may be associated with an improved outcome.[249] It is important to remember, however, that the radiographic presentation may be highly variable for any given etiology and that the differential diagnosis of most radiographic findings remains broad, thus necessitating a more definitive diagnosis where feasible.

Flexible fiberoptic bronchoscopy can provide evidence for a specific diagnosis in immunocompromised patients with pneumonia. The yield of bronchoscopy depends on the clinical situation and the extent of prior therapy. Bronchoalveolar lavage (BAL) can yield a specific diagnosis in approximately 80% of cases of PCP, whereas it is significantly less sensitive for detection of invasive fungal infections or bacterial infections in patients who have received prior antibiotic therapy. In a series of 89 bone marrow transplant patients with pulmonary complications of unclear etiology, approximately 50% had a diagnosis made by BAL, including findings of infectious (PCP, bacterial, CMV, RSV) and noninfectious (diffuse alveolar hemorrhage) causes.[250] Although transbronchial biopsy may increase the diagnostic yield in some situations, this procedure is limited in very small children by size of the equipment required and may be fraught with hemorrhagic complications.

Transthoracic needle biopsy can be useful for the assessment of disease that is focal and in the periphery of the lung parenchyma. Video-assisted thorascopically (VAT) guided lung biopsy can provide excellent pathologic samples as well as an ability to visualize superficial lesions; however, this procedure is limited in small children by the size of the instruments required. Open lung biopsy remains the time-honored "gold standard" for the diagnosis of pulmonary pathology. Open biopsy allows for sampling of an affected area and can obtain more tissue for pathologic analysis. In patients not responding to appropriate empirical antimicrobial therapy with a nondiagnostic workup, an open lung biopsy is often indicated. Open lung biopsy may also provide definitive therapy by permitting resection of solitary infectious lesions, such as a focus of invasive fungal infection.

Localized Pulmonary Infiltrates in Nonneutropenic Patients

The common causes of localized pulmonary infiltrates in non-neutropenic cancer patients are similar to those of an immunocompetent child. Common bacterial, viral, and mycoplasmal organisms are most frequently isolated (Table 40.4), and therapeutic considerations are similar to those for an immunocompetent child.

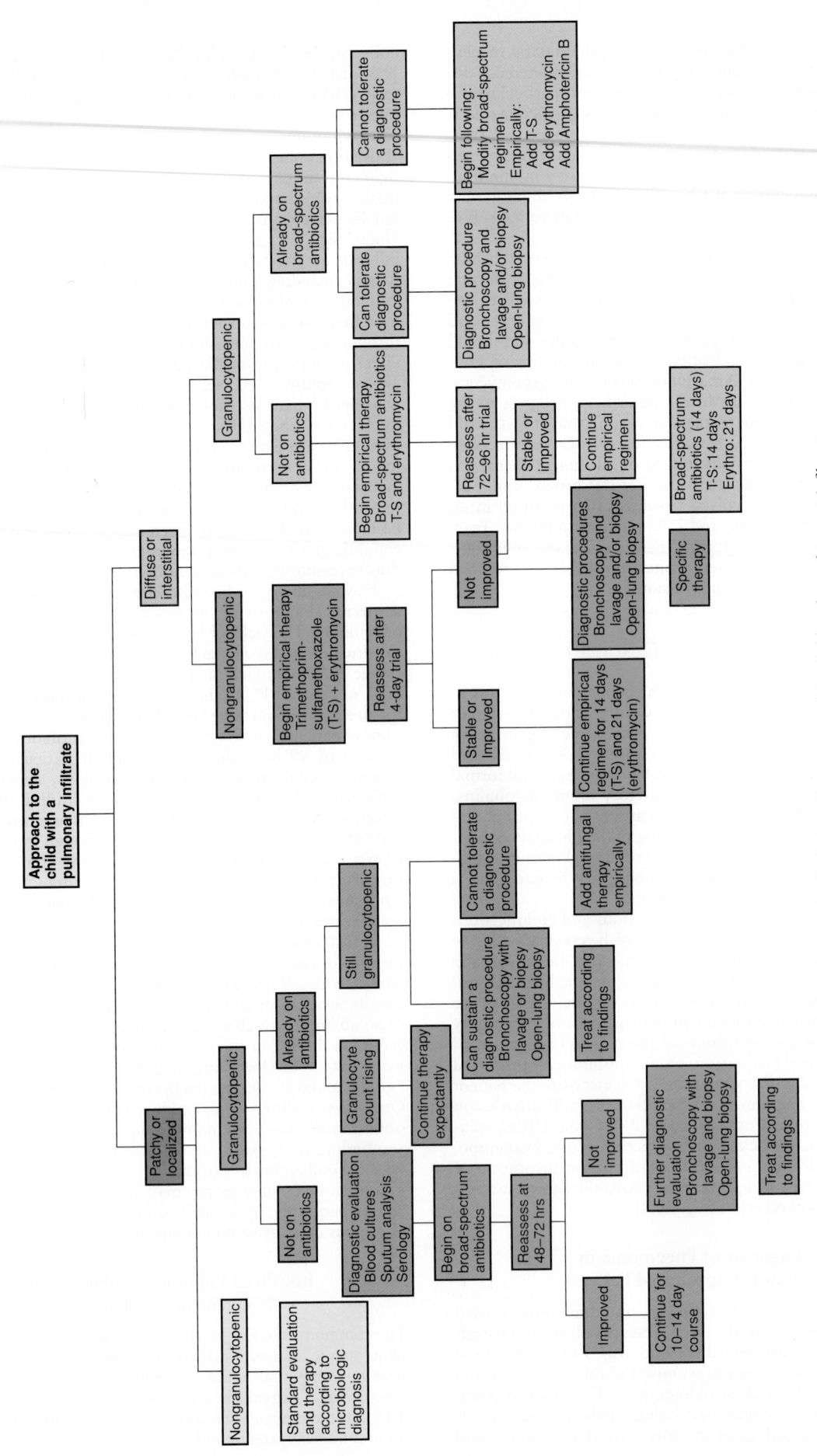

FIGURE 40.4 Algorithm for the management of the child with a pulmonary infiltrate.

TABLE 40.4

MODIFICATIONS OF INITIAL ANTIMICROBIAL REGIMENS FOR FEBRILE NEUTROPENIC CANCER PATIENTS

Status or symptoms	Modifications of primary regimen
Fever	
Persistent for >5 d	Add empirical antifungal therapy
Recurrence after 5 d or later in patient with persistent neutropenia	Add empirical antifungal therapy
Persistent or recurrent fever at time of recovery from neutropenia	Evaluate liver and spleen by CT, ultrasonography, or MRI, for hepatosplenic candidiasis, and evaluate need for antifungal therapy. If evaluation is negative, consider chest CT for evaluation of untreated or partially treated pneumonia
Bloodstream	
Cultures drawn before initiation of initial antibiotic therapy	
Gram-positive organism	Add vancomycin pending further identification
Gram-negative organism	Maintain regimen if patient is hemodynamically stable and if isolate is susceptible. If *Pseudomonas aeruginosa, Enterobacter* species, *Serratia* species, or *Citrobacter* species are isolated or if found to be resistant to cephalosporin, add a carbapenem
Organism isolated during initial antibiotic therapy	
Gram-positive organism	Add vancomycin
Gram-negative organism	Change to new combination regimen (e.g., imipenem or meropenem plus aminoglycoside)
Head, eyes, ears, nose, throat	
Necrotizing or marginal gingivitis	Add specific antianaerobic agent (clindamycin or metronidazole) to empirical therapy
Vesicular or ulcerative lesions	Suspect HSV infection. Culture and begin acyclovir therapy
Sinus congestion, tenderness or nasal ulcerative lesions	Suspect invasive fungal infection with *Aspergillus* or Zygomycetes; obtain imaging studies and ENT consultation. Adjust antifungal therapy according to organism recovered
Gastrointestinal tract	
Retrosternal burning pain	Suspect candida or herpetic esophagitis, or both. Add antifungal therapy and, if no response, acyclovir. Bacterial esophagitis also is a possibility. For patients not responding within 48 h, endoscopy should be considered
Acute abdominal pain	Suspect typhlitis, as well as appendicitis, if pain in right lower quadrant, even in the absence of fever. Add specific antianaerobic coverage (e.g., metronidazole to ceftazidime; or substitution of imipenem or meropenem for ceftazidime) to empirical regimen and monitor closely for need for surgical intervention
Perianal tenderness	Evaluate for anal fissures, perianal cellulitis, perianal fistulas, or perirectal abscesses (see text). Add specific antianaerobic drug to empirical regimen, as indicated, and monitor need for surgical intervention, especially when patient is recovering from neutropenia
Respiratory tract	
New focal lesion(s) in patient recovering from neutropenia	Observe carefully, as such lesions may be a consequence of inflammatory response to previously occult pneumonic process detected in concert with neutrophil recovery
New focal lesion(s) in patient with continuing neutropenia	Invasive pulmonary aspergillosis is the chief concern. Rule out other causes of fungal pneumonia. Perform BAL or transthoracic needle aspirate with appropriate direct examinations and cultures. Add voriconazole or lipid formulation of amphotericin B, depending on findings (do not administer voriconazole and amphotericin B simultaneously)
New interstitial pneumonitis	Attempt diagnosis by examination of induced sputum or BAL. If patient is symptomatic, begin empirical treatment with trimethoprim-sulfamethoxazole, pending procedure. Consider noninfectious causes and need for open lung biopsy if diagnosis is not established

BAL, bronchoalveolar lavage; CT, computed tomography; ENT, ear, nose, and throat; MRI, magnetic resonance imaging.

Immunocompromised patients who are not neutropenic, such as HSCT recipients receiving immunosuppressive therapy, are also at risk for less common pathogens, including *M. tuberculosis*, atypical mycobacteria, *Nocardia* species, *Legionella* species, *Chlamydia* species, and fungi, such as *Aspergillus* species, *C. neoformans*, and certain endemic mycoses such as *C. immitis* and *H. capsulatum*. Pulmonary histoplasmosis may present as a solitary focal lesion, multiple small focal lesions, or a diffuse reticular nodular infiltrate in HSCT recipients. A rapid definitive diagnosis of pulmonary histoplasmosis can be established with lysis centrifugation of blood cultures, bone marrow aspirate, clot section, and biopsy, and *Histoplasma* urinary antigen.[251]

Specific mycobacterial identification is especially important to distinguish atypical isolates (particularly *Mycobacterium avium-intracellulare*) from *M. tuberculosis*. Children with documented drug-sensitive *M. tuberculosis* should receive 9 to 12 months of therapy with at least two effective antituberculosis agents (e.g., isoniazid and rifampin). However, it is critical to consider the possibility of multidrug-resistant strains of tuberculosis, particularly in patients who live in areas where those strains are endemic.[252]

Legionella species are also important pathogens to consider as possible causes of localized pneumonia in an immunosuppressed child. Patients with impaired cellular immunity are at particularly increased risk for legionellosis. Within the pediatric oncology population, patients at high risk include those receiving high-dose corticosteroids, fludarabine, and allogeneic HSCT recipients. *Legionella* species are commonly found in water sources and may be found in the hospital environment, leading to nosocomial acquisition. *Legionella* pneumonia in immunosuppressed pediatric patients is heralded by abrupt onset of nonspecific symptoms such as fever, malaise, anorexia, lethargy, and headache. A nonproductive cough develops in most patients; chest pain, dyspnea, diarrhea, and neurologic symptoms may be prominent features.[253] A lobar, patchy alveolar infiltrate is most common, although diffuse infiltrates also may occur.[254]

A definitive diagnosis of *Legionella* pneumonia is made by culture of the organism from respiratory secretions. Because this organism grows optimally on buffered charcoal yeast agar, the clinical microbiology laboratory should be alerted when *Legionella* pneumonia is suspected. The combination of culture of respiratory secretions or BAL fluid and urinary antigen assay optimizes diagnostic sensitivity for detection of *Legionella* pneumonia.[255] The urinary antigen test is specific only for *Legionella pneumophila* type 1, which causes approximately 80% of cases.[256] Other rapid tests for diagnosis of *Legionella* infection (direct fluorescent antibody stain, DNA probe) lack the sensitivity and specificity of culture. Erythromycin or azithromycin given for 3 weeks is the treatment of choice in pediatric patients. Rifampin may be added for seriously ill patients. Fluoroquinolones, such as ciprofloxacin and levofloxacin, are also effective in the treatment of legionellosis but should be employed only in pediatric patients who are refractory to or intolerant of the macrolide antibiotics.

Nocardia species, particularly *Nocardia asteroides,* also present most frequently as a localized or nodular pulmonary infiltrate,[257] although miliary and microcavitary patterns have been reported but are distinctly less common.[258] Approximately 30% of patients with a pulmonary infection caused by *N. asteroides* also have cutaneous infection and CNS involvement (usually brain abscesses). *Nocardia* infections are most frequent in patients with impaired T-cell immunity. Diagnosis depends on positive cultures or histopathologic demonstration of tissue invasion by the organisms. TMP-SMX (15 mg/kg/day trimethoprim component) for 6 months is the most widely employed therapy. A carbapenem with an aminoglycoside is an alternative for patients who are intolerant of or refractory to TMP-SMX for treatment of nocardiosis.

Pulmonary aspergillosis is increasingly recognized as a cause of localized or nodular pulmonary infiltrates in nonneutropenic HSCT recipients in the postengraftment phase of transplantation.[259,260] With an increasing burden of immunosuppression in HSCT applied to management of GVHD, pulmonary aspergillosis has emerged as the most common cause of infectious pneumonic mortality in HSCT recipients and a common cause of community-acquired pneumonia after patients are discharged.

Among the noninfectious causes of localized pulmonary infiltrates in a nonneutropenic patient to be considered in the differential diagnosis are progression of the underlying malignancy, an atelectatic segment of lung (potentially caused by narrowing of the airway by adjacent or endobronchial tumor), intraalveolar hemorrhage, radiation injury, and pulmonary embolus.

Localized Pulmonary Infiltrates in Neutropenic Patients

Among the opportunistic pathogens that cause localized infiltrates in neutropenic patients are gram-positive or gram-negative bacteria, fungi, and viruses, as well as those pathogens listed in the section on localized infiltrates in nonneutropenic patients (Table 40.4). Bacterial pathogens predominate in patients with neutropenia lasting less than 10 to 14 days. Patients with longer periods of neutropenia and those in certain clinical settings (e.g., allogeneic HSCT) are more prone to develop a fungal (e.g., *Aspergillus*) or viral (e.g., CMV) infection. Unless the clinical presentation suggests otherwise, it is appropriate to initiate a 48- to 72-hour trial of broad-spectrum antibiotics before proceeding to an invasive diagnostic procedure. If the patient has stabilized or improved by 72 hours, a 10- to 14-day course of treatment is necessary. If the patient has not stabilized or improved, a BAL, percutaneous needle aspirate, VAT biopsy, or open lung biopsy should be performed.

Invasive aspergillosis is the most frequently encountered cause of a localized pulmonary infiltrate in patients with protracted neutropenia, particularly if the patient already is receiving broad-spectrum antibiotics.[261,262] Although *Aspergillus* species are most often responsible for localized pulmonary infiltrates in patients with protracted neutropenia, *Scedosporium* species, *Fusarium* species, *Trichosporon beigelii*, and the Zygomycetes (e.g., *Rhizopus* species) may also play a role.[263] Occasionally, *Candida* species (especially *C. albicans* and *C. tropicalis*) may cause primary pulmonary candidiasis.[264] Other fungi, including *H. capsulatum*, *C. immitis*, and *C. neoformans*, can also cause focal pneumonia in neutropenic patients receiving corticosteroids; however, infections with these organisms are more commonly manifested as a diffuse or nodular pulmonary pattern.[265,266] Although some radiographic features, including the halo sign, in neutropenic patients may distinguish angioinvasive fungi from other pathogens, these findings are subjective and not specific for aspergillosis. A definitive diagnosis depends on microbiologic or histopathologic confirmation in specimens obtained from BAL or other procedure. The recent development and introduction of the double-sandwich enzyme-linked immunosorbent assay (ELISA) system for detection of galactomannan antigenemia is an important advance in the nonculture diagnosis of invasive aspergillosis in neutropenic patients and HSCT recipients. Depending on the patient population, several studies have demonstrated a sensitivity ranging from 50% to 95% and specificity ranging from 87% to 99% for diagnosis of invasive aspergillosis.[267–269] Additional studies in animal models and patients indicate that serial serum galactomannan antigen levels permit therapeutic monitoring and have prognostic implications.[270,271] Coupled with a CT scan that is radiographically compatible with invasive pulmonary aspergillosis in the appropriate host population, a positive serum galactomannan assay may suggest a diagnosis of probable invasive aspergillosis in neutropenic patients and HSCT recipients,[272] although a positive culture remains the gold standard.

A common scenario for development of invasive aspergillosis in pediatric oncology is that of a profoundly and persistently neutropenic patient who develops localized, progressive pulmonary infiltrates while receiving broad-spectrum antibiotics. The incidence of pulmonary infections caused by *Aspergillus* species has increased and has been observed in clusters in various hospitals.[273] Infections caused by *Aspergillus fumigatus* are the most common; however, an increasing spectrum of non-*fumigatus Aspergillus* species are being recognized as emerging pathogens.[273] Because of the tendency for *Aspergillus* species to invade blood vessels, a necrotizing bronchopneumonia is characteristic, with the possibility of life-threatening hemoptysis.[274] Disseminated aspergillosis occurs in approximately 30% of cases, with involvement of the CNS, liver, kidneys, skin, and spleen. Despite this propensity for widespread disease, blood cultures are virtually never positive.

Successful management of invasive pulmonary aspergillosis requires an early diagnosis and prompt intervention. Based on the compelling findings of the international randomized trial demonstrating that voriconazole conferred a significant benefit of survival and overall therapeutic response, primary therapy of invasive pulmonary aspergillosis should be initiated with voriconazole.[140] However, several points of caution should be noted. Recent plasma pharmacokinetic studies demonstrate that plasma clearance of voriconazole in pediatric patients is significantly greater than that observed in adults,[137] prompting a recommendation for higher dosages, preferably at 7 mg/kg every 12 hours. For patients with pre-existing hepatic transaminase elevation, consideration should be given to avoiding triazoles and initiating an LFAB at 5 mg/kg/day.[275] LFABs offer the potential of treating sinopulmonary aspergillosis with higher dosages and less nephrotoxicity. These compounds may be particularly important in patients receiving concomitant nephrotoxic agents, such as aminoglycosides, cyclosporin, and foscarnet. Even with potent pharmacologic intervention, the most important prognosticator of a successful outcome is recovery from neutropenia. Subsequent cycles of chemotherapy-induced neutropenia may result in recurrence of *Aspergillus* pneumonia unless antifungal therapy is continued during these periods of immunosuppression.[276]

Surgical resection of pulmonary lesions in invasive pulmonary aspergillosis and other mycoses due to these filamentous fungi may provide definitive and potentially life-saving therapy.[277,278] Patients who undergo subsequent myelosuppressive procedures may benefit from surgical resection of isolated lesions. Surgical resection should be considered in the following situations: hemoptysis from a single cavitary lesion; progression of a solitary lesion despite antifungal therapy; and infiltration into contiguous structures, including pericardium, great vessels, esophagus, or chest wall while receiving antifungal therapy.

Other filamentous fungi, such as *Scedosporium* species, *Fusarium* species, dematiaceous molds, and the Zygomycetes, especially *Rhizopus* species, can cause pulmonary infiltrates that are similar to those associated with *Aspergillus*. These organisms may also cause sinus infections and the rhinocerebral syndrome. Diagnosis requires documentation of tissue invasion, particularly to distinguish zygomycosis from other infections. Treatment of zygomycosis consists of amphotericin B (1 mg/kg/day) or an LFAB (5 mg/kg/day) and, where appropriate, aggressive surgical debridement.[279] Nevertheless, treatment results remain poor unless PMN recovery ensues.[280] Treatment of scedosporiosis, fusariosis, and infections due to dematiaceous molds also is challenging. However, successful outcomes have been achieved in oncology patients with either voriconazole for scedosporiosis and fusariosis or with amphotericin B against fusariosis.[281]

Diffuse Pulmonary Infiltrates in Patients with Cancer

Diffuse pulmonary infiltrates in pediatric oncology patients can be caused by bacterial, viral, and fungal pathogens, as well as noninfectious causes. Among the noninfectious causes of diffuse pulmonary infiltrates in patients with cancer are antineoplastic agents (e.g., bleomycin, cyclophosphamide, and methotrexate) and neoplastic processes (e.g., lymphoid malignancies).

Pneumocystis jiroveci (carinii) is an important treatable cause of diffuse pulmonary infiltrates in pediatric oncology patients. For purposes of taxonomic accuracy, *P. jiroveci* is considered in this chapter as a fungus and not a protozoan.[282] The probability of having a specific bacterial or fungal pathogen is influenced by whether the patient is neutropenic

(Table 40.4). However, a febrile nonneutropenic patient with a diffuse pulmonary infiltrate is more likely to have a viral infection or PCP than a bacterial process.[283] This observation is particularly apparent in an immunosuppressed child who may be recovering from neutropenia following chemotherapy. However, both neutropenic and nonneutropenic patients are at risk for severe infection from *P. jiroveci (carinii)* and various viral pathogens. In assessing a priori risk, the probability of developing PCP is increased in relation to impaired T-cell immunity.

Because virtually all normal children possess detectable antibody to *P. jiroveci (carinii)*, development of PCP is thought to result from a reactivation of latent cysts. However, patient-to-patient transmission has been suggested by reports of nosocomial clusters of cases.[284] Patients with PCP most commonly present with fever, a nonproductive cough, tachypnea, dyspnea, and hypoxemia. The time course of the symptoms ranges from a chronic, indolent course (characteristic of AIDS patients) to an acute, fulminant presentation, more commonly observed in pediatric oncology patients.[285] Although adventitious lung sounds are not usually detectable on auscultation in most cases of PCP, patients receiving corticosteroids may have evidence of rales. Radiographic examination usually reveals bilateral diffuse alveolar-interstitial infiltrates, often originating at the hilum and extending peripherally. Rarely, the chest radiograph is atypical, ranging from normal to a lobar or nodular infiltrate. Pleural effusions are rare.

Diagnosis of PCP requires demonstration of cysts or trophozoites in pulmonary material from patients with a clinically compatible course. In patients with AIDS, positive specimens may readily be obtained from induced sputum samples stained with toluidine blue O, a modified Giemsa stain, or with monoclonal antibodies to human *Pneumocystis* organisms.[20] The sensitivity of sputum examination in an HIV-infected patient population has increased from initial reports of 55% with the routine stains to as high as 92% with monoclonal antibody stains detected by indirect immunofluorescence.[286] A specificity of almost 100% has been reported from experienced laboratories. In cancer patients, *Pneumocystis* organisms may not be as abundant as in patients with AIDS. Thus, the diagnosis of PCP in an immunosuppressed cancer patient may sometimes be made by monoclonal staining techniques on induced sputum, and this should be the first diagnostic approach whenever possible. However, the demonstration of *Pneumocystis* cysts or trophozoites in oncology patients often requires BAL or, in some cases, a VAT or open lung biopsy.

In evaluation of a patient with diffuse pulmonary infiltrates for the risk of PCP, the importance of impaired T-cell immunity should be underscored. For example, Sepkowitz et al. reported that corticosteroid use was associated with 204 of 227 (90%) cases of PCP in patients without AIDS at Memorial Sloan-Kettering Cancer Center between 1963 and 1992.[287] Yet another setting for the development of PCP is during the tapering phase of a course of corticosteroid-induced immunosuppression in oncology patients. When such patients manifest dyspnea, tachypnea, hypoxia, and diffuse alveolar interstitial infiltrates, the suspicion for PCP should be high in the differential diagnosis.[288]

In clinical situations in which the likelihood of PCP is great, examination of induced sputum is a reasonable first step in high-risk older children. If the specimen is not attainable or if there is a negative result, a BAL is performed while initiating an empirical course of TMP-SMX. A response to TMP-SMX may not be apparent for 4 to 5 days; however, stabilization or slight improvement in alveolar air exchange usually occurs within 72 to 96 hours. Acutely ill patients who do not respond to TMP-SMX should receive an alternative regimen, such as clindamycin plus primaquine, dapsone plus pyrimethamine, or IV pentamidine.[289,290] However, pentamidine has been associated with myriad toxicities, including metabolic and hematologic abnormalities, pancreatitis, hypotension, and nausea and vomiting. Orally administered atovaquone is another option for patients who are not acutely ill.[291]

Adjunctive administration of corticosteroids has a role in the management of pediatric oncology-HSCT patients with moderate to severe PCP. For adult patients with AIDS who have moderate or severe PCP, as defined by a room air arterial partial pressure of oxygen of 70 mm Hg or an alveolar-arterial gradient greater than 35 mm Hg on presentation, the early use of adjunctive corticosteroids has been shown to improve outcome. Decreases in respiratory failure and death rates were observed among patients who received corticosteroids with standard anti-PCP therapies, compared with those who did not receive corticosteroids.[292,293] Based on this information, the practice of initiating a short course of corticosteroids in children with moderate or severe PCP has been adopted by many pediatric oncology centers; however, the optimal dosage and duration of corticosteroid therapy in children have not been defined. The recommendation for adults is for 40-mg prednisone (or the equivalent corticosteroid) twice daily for the first 5 days of treatment, 40 mg once daily for the next 5 days, and then 20 mg once daily for 11 days, for a total treatment course of 21 days. An estimated equivalent for children is 1 mg/kg twice daily for the first 5 days, 1 mg/kg daily for the next 5 days, and 0.5 mg/kg daily for the remainder of a 14- to 21-day course of therapy.

Mycoplasma pneumoniae and *Chlamydia pneumoniae* can cause diffuse pulmonary infiltrates and severe disease in immunocompromised children.[294,295] Often underestimated as causes of community-acquired pneumonias in pediatric oncology patients, *M. pneumoniae* and *C. pneumoniae* have been historically difficult to accurately diagnose as causes of lower respiratory tract infections. However, considerable advances have been achieved in evaluation of BAL fluid by PCR for detection of *Mycoplasma* and *Chlamydia* DNA, enabling more specific pathogen-directed therapy.[296] If reliable diagnostic assays are not available, an empirical course of azithromycin is warranted in immunocompromised children with diffuse pulmonary infiltrates.

Among the important viral causes of diffuse interstitial infiltrates in nonneutropenic patients are CMV and RSV. Prior to routine prophylaxis and strategies for preemptive therapy (see later), CMV pneumonitis was a common cause of viral pneumonia, after HSCT.[297] Seropositive recipients are at the greatest risk of developing CMV disease.[298] Among CMV-seronegative recipients of HSCT from seropositive donors, there is a high risk of death caused by bacterial infections and mycoses due likely to the indirect immunosuppressive effects of CMV.[299] CMV pneumonitis also has been seen in a very small percentage of patients with acute leukemia and after autologous bone marrow transplantation.[179] The most frequent causes of CMV infection and subsequent disease are reactivation of latent virus in seropositive patients and acquisition of CMV from donor marrow in seronegative patients. CMV pneumonitis most often occurs between day 30 and day 100 after allogeneic bone marrow transplantation, coinciding with the period of highest risk for the development of acute GVHD. CMV pneumonitis is characterized radiographically by diffuse bilateral linear or nodular infiltrates. However, CMV pneumonitis occasionally may present as a lobar or segmental consolidation or as a solitary nodule.

The use of CMV antigenemia assays as well as CMV PCR has allowed for the rapid diagnosis of CMV infection. CMV antigenemia can be utilized only in nonneutropenic patients, while PCR does not require the presence of leukocytes.

Routine screening during the period of highest risk, for example with twice weekly CMV antigen assays, has proven to be a highly effective strategy to prevent invasive disease. Detection of CMV virus or antigen in blood buffy coat post–bone marrow transplantation is a sign of CMV reactivation that is highly predictive of impending invasive disease.[300] Such findings should prompt the institution of a treatment course with ganciclovir. However, because ganciclovir therapy has significant myelotoxicity, primarily causing granulocytopenia, patients should be monitored carefully. Foscarnet is an appropriate alternative to ganciclovir, particularly in those at risk for myelotoxicity or who are intolerant of or refractory to ganciclovir.[168]

The diagnosis of CMV pneumonia can be made by isolation of CMV from BAL fluid, demonstration of either CMV antigen or nucleic acid in pulmonary alveolar macrophages, or characteristic histopathology. Until recently, CMV pneumonitis has been associated with an extremely high mortality. Combined therapy with ganciclovir and IVIG (pooled or CMV hyperimmune) has improved survival to more than 50% in allogeneic HSCT recipients with CMV pneumonitis.[301,302] Despite the limited enrollment and uncontrolled nature of these trials, the dramatic results have led to an acceptance of the ganciclovir and immune globulin combination as a standard of care for patients with CMV pneumonitis. Whether IVIG is a useful adjunct to ganciclovir for CMV colitis or in non-HSCT patients is not well understood.

Other herpesviruses, particularly VZV and HSV, can also cause diffuse pneumonitis in immunocompromised patients. VZV may reactivate late in the course of HSCT, particularly in those not receiving acyclovir suppressive therapy.[303] These viruses, however, rarely cause isolated pulmonary disease but instead are associated with cutaneous disease and visceral dissemination.

RSV can cause severe lower respiratory tract disease with a high mortality rate especially in patients undergoing therapy for AML or HSCT.[179,180] RSV usually can be diagnosed rapidly, using a direct immunofluorescent antibody stain performed on a nasopharyngeal wash specimen. Although no randomized controlled studies have addressed the utility of ribavirin in immunocompromised cancer patients, it may be appropriate to extrapolate from existing data in other pediatric populations that suggest that there may be a benefit of this therapy.[175,177,181] There is anecdotal evidence from several small case series reports that adult bone marrow transplantation and acute leukemia patients with lower tract RSV respond favorably to ribavirin aerosol in addition to therapy with IVIG or RSV immune globulin.[181] Survival appears to be improved particularly if ribavirin is administered early in the course of infection.

Parainfluenza, influenza, adenovirus, and HHV-6 have been described as causes of interstitial pneumonitis in pediatric cancer patients.[304,305] However, these respiratory RNA viruses more commonly cause tracheobronchitis and bronchopneumonia rather than a diffuse interstitial process. Therapeutic options for pneumonia due to these viruses are limited and are associated with a high rate of morbidity and mortality. With increasing globalization of medicine and referrals, clinicians also must remain vigilant for infections caused by coronavirus-induced severe acute respiratory syndrome (SARS).

In March 2009, an outbreak of a respiratory illness later proved to be caused by novel swine-origin influenza A (H1N1) virus (S-OIV) was identified in Mexico.[306] S-OIV infection can cause severe illness, the acute respiratory distress syndrome, and death in previously healthy persons, particularly children and young adults. Very few individuals younger than 30 years have protective levels of cross-reactive neutralizing antibodies against the H1N1 virus.[307] In the United

States, among persons with H1N1 infection hospital admission was more common for pregnant women (32.4%) than for the general population (4.2%), and pregnant women accounted for only 0.62% of all confirmed and probably H1N1 cases from April to May 2009 but 13% of deaths.[308] A monovalent, inactivated vaccine (hemagglutinin antigen injected intramuscularly) and an attenuated H1N1 virus administered intranasally were manufactured and made available. In July 2009, the CDC's Advisory Committee on Immunization Practices (ACIP) made recommendations on who should be given priority in receiving the H1N1 vaccine: pregnant women, persons who live with or provide care for infants younger than 6 months, health care and emergency medical services personnel, children and young adults aged 6 months to 24 years, and persons aged 25 to 64 years who have medical conditions that put them at higher risk for influenza-related complications.[309] In terms of antiviral therapy against H1N1, as of April 2009, the CDC reported that all tested viruses from confirmed S-OIV cases in the United States were resistant to amantadine and rimantadine but were susceptible to oseltamivir and zanamivir.[310]

Infections of the Cardiovascular System

Cardiovascular infections are relatively uncommon among cancer patients. Viridans streptococcal infections in neutropenic patients are more likely to cause a fulminant septic event in comparison with nonneutropenic patients who are more likely to have endocarditis.[311] Nevertheless, cancer patients who have predisposing factors for a cardiovascular infection, such as dental abscess, a history of illicit IV drug use, or a congenital cardiac anomaly, are at risk for this complication. Right-sided endovascular infections are more likely with the increased use of indwelling venous access catheters.[312] Although gram-positive bacterial species (e.g., *Enterococcus*, viridans streptococci, and *S. aureus*) most commonly cause endovascular infections, aerobic gram-negative bacilli and fungi may also cause disease. These latter pathogens are particularly difficult to eradicate, and morbidity and mortality remain discouragingly high.

The clinical manifestations of endocarditis in immunosuppressed patients are similar to those in immunocompetent patients. Nonspecific complaints of fever, chills, malaise, fatigue, night sweats, and weight loss are common, but these complaints are nondescript, and the degree of diagnostic specificity that may be ascribed to them is slight. In most instances, the diagnosis must be made on the basis of the physical and laboratory evaluations. The numerous physical stigmata of endocarditis (e.g., heart murmurs, splinter hemorrhages, Roth's spots, splenomegaly) should be sought, but other than splenomegaly the other physical findings are quite rare. Ultimately, the diagnosis is confirmed by the isolation of an organism from multiple blood cultures.

The complications of endovascular infection in immunocompromised patients are similar to those described for patients without cancer. Valvular insufficiency resulting in congestive heart failure, emboli, and renal failure are the most serious. Fungal endocarditis is particularly likely to cause large-vessel embolization.[313,314] Patients with *Candida* or *Aspergillus* endocarditis are treated with valve replacement and antifungal chemotherapy (amphotericin B or echinocandin). Fungal infection of a prosthetic valve may require lifelong suppressive therapy.[315]

Therapy of endocarditis is directed at the specific pathogen. The isolation of *S. aureus* or *S. epidermidis* from multiple blood samples, even if the patient has an indwelling catheter, is not a sufficient criterion for prolonged antibiotic therapy unless a valvular infection can be confirmed. A standard 10- to 14-day course of therapy suffices for these patients.

Pericarditis is another cardiovascular complication in oncology patients. The differential diagnosis of pericarditis includes radiation therapy, neoplastic infiltration, and several major infectious etiologies (bacterial, viral, and fungal). Aspergillosis pericarditis is a particularly devastating complication in immunosuppressed oncology patients.[316] Arising often from an endomyocardial focus or a contiguous pulmonary lesion, pericardial aspergillosis may evolve rapidly with pericardial effusion and tamponade. Initial management requires percutaneous pericardial drainage and systemic antifungal therapy. Pericardial resection is usually required for definitive eradication of infection.[317]

Infections of the Gastrointestinal Tract

The GI tract is frequently a portal of entry of enteric blood-borne pathogens, as well as a primary focus of infections in neutropenic patients and HSCT recipients. The GI mucosa is in direct contact with the external environment. Normally, it acts as a mechanical barrier, but it can be disrupted by tumor invasion or by damage from chemotherapy or radiotherapy. The mucosal ulceration induced by these treatments offers a potential site for bacterial, fungal, viral, and parasitic infection. The normal microbial balance of the GI tract is also altered by serious illness, mechanical factors (e.g., surgery, altered motility), hospital exposures, and antimicrobial therapy.

Infections of the Oral Cavity

Oropharyngeal candidiasis ("thrush") is the most common oral mucosal infection encountered in the immunosuppressed oncology patient. Oropharyngeal candidiasis is a superficial infection caused most commonly by *C. albicans*. The lesions of oropharyngeal candidiasis usually appear as whitish plaques with slightly raised indurated borders. This infection is easily controlled in most cases by topical antifungal agents, such as clotrimazole troches or nystatin suspension. If there is no response to topical therapy, fluconazole at doses of 2 to 3 mg/kg/day is highly effective for the treatment and prevention of oropharyngeal candidiasis.[318]

HSV is the most common viral pathogen isolated from mucosal lesions in pediatric oncology patients. Perioral and intraoral HSV lesions usually appear as clear vesicular eruptions, frequently in clusters or "crops" on an erythematous base. However, intraoral lesions may be nondescript, often ulcerative, and can be confused with the stomatotoxicity usually attributed to chemotherapy. Diagnosis may be confirmed by rapid shell vial culture (requiring 24 to 48 hours) by a positive fluorescent-antibody reaction. Herpetic stomatitis may be a serious complication in an immunosuppressed patient. The severity of the local tissue involvement, inflammation, and eschar formation has deleterious consequences, causing discomfort and also serving as a nidus for bacterial and fungal superinfections. Acyclovir (750 mg/m^2/day divided every 8 hours or 5 mg/kg every 8 hours) is the preferred treatment because of its infrequent toxicity, ease of administration, and documented efficacy in reducing the duration of viral shedding and shortening the time to healing.[156] HSV-seropositive patients undergoing bone marrow transplantation or induction regimens for acute leukemia should receive prophylactic acyclovir, orally or parenterally, to prevent HSV reactivations.

The initial management of painful chemotherapy or radiation-related mucosal ulcerations should be directed toward establishing an infectious etiology by obtaining appropriate cultures for HSV. Pending HSV cultures, acyclovir may be initiated in conjunction with topical and systemic analgesic therapy for pain. If cultures are negative for HSV, acyclovir may be discontinued. If cultures are positive, specific therapy will have been initiated early and facilitate management of the patient's oral mucositis.

Periodontal disease (including gingivitis and periodontitis) is especially problematic among adults, and the incidence of periodontal disease in the general population increases with age. However, periodontal disease may be found among pediatric cancer patients and is related to the adverse effects of the antineoplastic therapy on the host defense mechanisms normally operative in the oral mucosa. The periodontium is the most common site, and cultures of infected sites reveal mixed aerobic and anaerobic flora.[319] *Capnocytophaga ochracea* (formerly DF-1) may cause necrotizing gingivitis and gram-negative sepsis in patients receiving cytotoxic chemotherapy.[320] The presence of marginal or necrotizing gingivitis, characterized by an erythematous periapical gingiva, is caused by anaerobes and should be treated with antianaerobic agents such as clindamycin, metronidazole, or carbapenem.

Esophageal Infections

Clinically overt esophageal infection may result from infectious or noninfectious causes. A syndrome clinically identical to infectious esophagitis occurs in patients who have received extensive chest wall or mediastinal irradiation, or it may result from the severe mucosal toxicity that is associated with certain chemotherapeutic regimens. Infectious esophagitis most commonly occurs among neutropenic patients. Patients most often present with subacute onset of retrosternal burning chest pain, dysphagia, and odynophagia. Fungal, viral, and bacterial organisms can all cause an infectious esophagitis in the immunocompromised host.

The occurrence of infectious esophagitis in a nonneutropenic patient is uncommon. In nonneutropenic patients, esophagitis is most commonly caused by chemical irritation of the distal esophagus by refluxed gastric contents, as may be associated with chemotherapy-induced emesis. These patients are best managed with judicious use of antacids, histamine antagonists, or omeprazole. If the nonneutropenic patient has a persistent esophageal discomfort, esophagoscopy with brushings for culture and biopsy should be performed.

Chemotherapy-induced mucositis, neutropenia, mediastinal radiation, and gastroesophageal reflux are important risk factors for esophageal candidiasis. Concomitant infections caused by HSV, CMV, and bacteria may coincide with or precede esophageal candidiasis. The absence of oral lesions cannot be used to discount the presence of esophageal candidiasis in neutropenic patients. Unlike the experience in patients with AIDS, the absence of oropharyngeal candidiasis is not sufficiently reliable to exclude a diagnosis of esophageal candidiasis in a patient with compatible symptoms. Although esophagoscopy with mucosal biopsy is the most definitive method for establishing a diagnosis, this may not be feasible, practical, or safe in many children. Accordingly, an empirical approach is often warranted in children with suspected esophageal candidiasis. Initial therapy with fluconazole is often effective; however, failure to symptomatically respond promptly is an indication for empirical amphotericin B or an echinocandin for treatment of possible azole-resistant *Candida* species. Echinocandins have been extensively studied experimentally and clinically in treatment of esophageal candidiasis due to fluconazole-susceptible and fluconazole-resistant *Candida* species.[321,322] Furthermore, the resolution of symptoms does not necessarily signify the eradication of esophageal candidiasis in granulocytopenic patients and therapy should continue until the resolution of the neutropenia.

Persistent symptoms may indicate the presence of another infectious process, such as HSV, CMV, or bacterial esophagitis. If the patient has persistent symptoms after 48 hours of IV amphotericin B, an empirical course of acyclovir (750 mg/m²/day, given at 8-hour intervals) is reasonable, because the second most likely pathogen (or copathogen) is HSV. If the patient symptomatically responds to acyclovir, antiviral therapy should be given for 7 days.

Intraabdominal Infections: Typhlitis (Neutropenic Colitis) and *C. difficile* Colitis

The clinical presentation of common intraabdominal processes such as appendicitis or infectious diarrheal syndromes can be altered by granulocytopenia and compounded by complications of cancer or its treatment. For example, obstructive lesions may be caused by primary or metastatic cancer, cholangitis or a conjugated hyperbilirubinemia may be caused by extrahepatic biliary obstruction by tumor, and chronic abdominal pain or diarrheal syndromes may be secondary to bowel wall infiltration by malignant disease or infection.

Intraabdominal pain must be expeditiously evaluated with a thorough physical examination. Repetitive rectal examinations must not be performed in the neutropenic patient, because bacteremia and local infection may result. Appropriate studies include routine hematologic and serum chemistry values, amylase, total and direct bilirubin, and flat and upright abdominal radiographs. Abdominal or pelvic ultrasound or CT or MRI scan should be pursued in the appropriate settings. Invasive diagnostic or radiographic procedures such as barium enema and endoscopy should be avoided in the neutropenic patient.

Typhlitis or neutropenic colitis is a necrotizing infection of the cecum restricted almost entirely to cancer patients.[323] Typhlitis most commonly occurs in association with prolonged granulocytopenia in patients with acute leukemia although any granulocytopenic patient is at risk. Patients most often present with subacute or acute onset of right lower quadrant abdominal pain and tenderness, which frequently becomes generalized over several hours, with fever, diarrhea, and prostration. As fever may be absent early in the course of neutropenic colitis, the presence of abdominal pain in a neutropenic patient should prompt the administration of empirical antibacterial therapy for aerobic and anaerobic pathogens.

The etiologic agents responsible for typhlitis include anaerobes and gram-negative bacilli, especially *P. aeruginosa*. *C. difficile* is recognized increasingly as an important cause of typhlitis. Optimal management initially involves supportive care, including nasogastric suction, adequate fluid replacement, and adjustment of antimicrobial therapy to cover resistant gram-negative and anaerobic species. A carbapenem is a reasonable choice for a single antibacterial agent. However, if typhlitis develops in a patient who has diarrhea and has received previous antibacterial therapy, then ceftazidime or cefepime plus metronidazole is the logical choice. Metronidazole should be administered parenterally for successful treatment of *C. difficile* colitis and concomitant typhlitis. CT scan, which is the most sensitive diagnostic imaging technique for assessment of suspected neutropenic colitis, should be performed in all neutropenic patients with right lower quadrant pain for prompt diagnosis. CT imaging may reveal localized thickening of the bowel wall, mucosal edema, right lower quadrant inflammatory mass, and pericecal fluid. Although the cecum is the most common site of infection, abnormalities may extend beyond this region. Typhlitis was the most common disease in a review of neutropenic patients with GI abnormalities identified by CT scan; other abnormalities in descending order included *C. difficile* colitis, GVHD of the bowel, CMV colitis, and bowel ischemia.[324]

Most patients with typhlitis can be medically managed without surgical resection of the involved segment of colon. Aggressive surgical intervention to resect necrotic bowel may be beneficial for a subset of patients, and the timing of such intervention is critical. Criteria that have been proposed for sending a patient to surgery are persistent GI bleeding after resolution of neutropenia; thrombocytopenia and clotting abnormalities; evidence of free intraperitoneal perforation; clinical deterioration requiring support with vasopressors or large volumes of fluid, suggesting uncontrolled sepsis; and development of symptoms of an intraabdominal process, in the absence of neutropenia, which would normally require surgery.[325]

There may be considerable overlap in the clinical presentation between typhlitis and antibiotic-associated *C. difficile* colitis in neutropenic patients. *C. difficile* colitis has long been associated with the administration of clindamycin, ampicillin, and broad-spectrum β-lactam antibiotics.[326] Symptomatic disease is related to *C. difficile* colonization of the gut after some perturbation of the normal gut flora, followed by overgrowth and toxin production by the organism.[327] Hospitalized patients commonly become colonized with *C. difficile* and may acquire the organism from nosocomial transmission.[328] Antineoplastic agents and antibiotics contribute to the alteration of intestinal flora and increase the risk of *C. difficile* colitis in pediatric oncology patients. *C. difficile* colitis classically presents with acute generalized abdominal pain, fever, leukocytosis, and watery or mucoid, foul-smelling diarrhea. A high index of suspicion is necessary because of the occurrence of similar abdominal symptoms in oncology patients receiving chemotherapy or periabdominal radiation. Fever and abdominal pain may be muted in neutropenic patients. Oncology patients with diarrhea with or without fever and abdominal pain should be evaluated with routine stool cultures and a *C. difficile* toxin assay. The commercial enzyme immunoassays detect *C. difficile* toxins A or B with sensitivities of approximately 80% and specificities of nearly 100%.[329] Toxin production, not just a culture positive for *C. difficile*, is necessary for diagnosis, because hospitalized patients receiving antibiotics may be culture positive but not toxin positive. Blood cultures should also be monitored during the course of therapy of *C. difficile* colitis in light of the increased risk of bacteremia by enteric pathogens, including VRE.[330]

Primary treatment of documented *C. difficile*-associated colitis is accomplished with metronidazole. Oral vancomycin is reserved for patients intolerant of or refractory to metronidazole. The use of vancomycin as first-line therapy is discouraged because of concern about emergence of resistant gram-positive organisms. Although there is a 10% to 20% rate of relapse to either metronidazole or vancomycin, most patients respond to a second course with the same or alternative therapy. For patients who cannot ingest oral agents, IV metronidazole should be given, as exudation from the inflamed colon and biliary excretion of the drug can deliver effective intraluminal concentrations of the drug against *C. difficile*.[331]

For patients who have repetitive episodes of *C. difficile* diarrhea with each cycle of chemotherapy, documentation with *C. difficile* toxin assay and early initiation of antimicrobial therapy is important. Long-term prophylaxis with either vancomycin or metronidazole in such patients is not recommended. Because *C. difficile* may be nosocomially transmitted, patients who are diagnosed as having documented *C. difficile*–associated colitis should be placed on enteric precautions.

Other Abdominal Infections

Clostridium species arise from the GI tract to cause fulminant intraabdominal, musculoskeletal, and disseminated infections.[332] Infections caused by *Clostridium perfringens* and *Clostridium septicum* are the most common clostridial bloodstream infections in patients with cancer. *Clostridium tertium* is a less common but highly virulent cause of clostridial bacteremia.[333] Patients with clostridial peritonitis classically have a fulminant clinical course with fever, tachycardia, abdominal wall ecchymoses and crepitance, and significant hemolysis. Bacteremia due to *C. perfringens* may cause severe intravascular hemolysis. *C. septicum* may arise from the GI tract to hematogenously seed skeletal muscle to cause an extensive and rapidly evolving myonecrosis. Serious infections with *Clostridium* (especially *C. septicum*) can occur in the absence of fever and should be considered in the afebrile neutropenic patient with abdominal pain. Nonneutropenic patients with GI tumors also may suffer bacteremia and myonecrosis due to *C. septicum*. Most *Clostridium* species are susceptible *in vitro* to the penicillins, metronidazole, clindamycin, and vancomycin. *C. tertium*, however, is resistant to penicillins and clindamycin and hence requires vancomycin or metronidazole therapy.

The hyperinfection syndrome caused by the intestinal nematode *Strongyloides stercoralis* is an infrequently encountered but potentially lethal clinical problem.[334] Endemic in tropical and subtropical regions, *S. stercoralis* is also observed in Europe and rural areas in the southeastern United States. *S. stercoralis* initially establishes an asymptomatic chronic GI infection through internal autoinfection. The hyperinfection syndrome then occurs in chronically infected patients who become immunosuppressed. The clinical syndrome of fever, nausea, vomiting, diarrhea, and abdominal pain is caused by invasion and ulceration of the GI mucosa by the filariform larvae. Chemotherapy is thought to promote the maturation of these larvae from a quiescent rhabditiform stage. Polymicrobial bacteremia may accompany this intestinal invasion. Overwhelming pulmonary and meningeal involvement may occur in immunocompromised patients.

Successful management of hyperinfection syndrome requires early detection and initiation of therapy. Diagnosis requires demonstration of the rhabditiform larvae in feces or duodenal fluid and should be sought in patients who have resided in subtropical climates or endemic regions. The clinical microbiology laboratory should be alerted to the clinical suspicion of strongyloidiasis. Treatment of asymptomatic infestation is accomplished with ivermectin, 200 mg/kg, with thiabendazole (25 mg/kg twice daily for 2 days) as an alternative. Ivermectin has evolved as the preferred drug with efficacy comparable to that of thiabendazole but with less toxicity. Immunocompromised patients with the hyperinfection syndrome should be treated for 2 to 3 weeks; however, the mortality rate remains high despite such long-term treatment.[335] Because of its long half-life, ivermectin may be used on days 1, 2, 13, and 14 of a 2-week treatment cycle.

Morbidity and mortality due to strongyloidiasis in immunocompromised oncology patients can be ultimately reduced by screening patients from high-risk areas and treating asymptomatic chronic infection. However, because laboratory detection methods for *S. stercoralis* have limited sensitivity, some have advocated that a more cost-effective approach is to preventively treat all patients from high-risk geographic areas with ivermectin before the initiation of immunosuppressive therapy.[336]

Hepatic Infections

Hepatitis may be caused by various infectious agents, including those that infect the liver primarily (e.g., hepatitis A, B, C, and the delta agent) and those that infect secondarily (e.g., HSV, CMV, EBV, VZV, Coxsackie B virus, adenovirus, *Toxoplasma gondii*, and *Candida* species). In addition, many chemotherapeutic agents and other medications that immunocompromised cancer patients may be receiving are associated with noninfectious hepatitis. In addition to the morbidity (e.g., fever, nausea, emesis, arthritis, and arthralgia) and deaths directly attributable to hepatitis, significant alteration in hepatic function can affect the pharmacokinetics of antineoplastic agents and other medications and should be taken into consideration when dosing drugs.

Hepatitis C virus (HCV) is now well-recognized as the predominant cause of classic transfusion- associated non-A, non-B hepatitis.[337] More recently, HCV has been recognized as an important factor in long-term survivors of childhood cancer. In one study of pediatric oncology patients who had been transfused between 1961 and 1992, 6.6% were found to be infected with HCV.[338] At the time of HCV infection, most cases are subclinical but can be characterized by fatigue and hepatomegaly with elevated or fluctuating levels of transaminases. Incubation is about 8 weeks, with the onset of symptoms, if any, typically occurring 5 to 12 weeks after exposure. Approximately 85% of patients infected with HCV will develop chronic infection.[339] Among those patients with chronic hepatitis, 20% to 25% will develop cirrhosis, and 2% to 9% will die owing to complications of cirrhosis or hepatocellular carcinoma.

Persistent anti-hepatitis C antibody is usually, but not always, found in patients with chronic disease, whereas those with the acute, self-limited illness may have only a transient rise in antibody titers. The development of antibody after hepatitis C exposure is usually delayed, with a mean interval of approximately 20 weeks and occasionally much longer. Late serologic testing is therefore essential for the diagnosis of chronic hepatitis C.[339] All patients positive for HCV antibodies by EIA and/or by recombinant immunoblot assay should be tested for HCV RNA by PCR. In addition, the viral genotype should be determined as this information may impact therapy.[182]

Some patients with chronic HCV infection can be effectively treated with a combination of interferon (both subtypes alpha-2a and alpha-2b were recently shown to be equally effective)[340] and ribavirin. The decision of who and when to treat is based on a number of factors, including severity of disease, concurrent comorbidity, and preexisting contraindications to ribavirin or interferon-a2b. There have been two large randomized controlled trials of combination therapy in patients with documented HCV infection and persistently elevated transaminases and without significant coexisting medical conditions or decompensated hepatic cirrhosis. In both of these studies, patients had improved outcomes with combined therapy as compared with monotherapy.[341,342] In these studies, the overall rate of sustained response for the combination regimen was 64% to 69% in patients with genotype 2 and 3 and 28% for those with genotype 1. The combination regimen had significant side effects that required discontinuation of study drugs in 8% to 19%. A recent study showed that the addition of telaprevir, a specific inhibitor of the HCV serine protease, to standard treatment regimens including interferon and/or ribavirin lead to a significantly higher rate of sustained virologic response as compared with standard therapy alone.[343]

Hepatitis B virus (HBV) may result in acute or chronic infections, including chronic active hepatitis, chronic persistent hepatitis, and asymptomatic carrier states. The prevalence of hepatitis B was previously as high as 10% to 20% among cancer patients, but with the introduction of effective prophylactic measures, particularly widespread use of the hepatitis B vaccine and efficient screening methods to detect infected blood donors, the number of patients affected has fallen dramatically. Immunosuppressive therapy may increase the likelihood of development of a chronic carrier state among patients infected with HBV, making it important to know the patient's hepatitis status before initiating antineoplastic therapy.

Although the presence of circulating hepatitis B surface antigen (HBsAg) is not a contraindication to chemotherapy, an acute hepatic failure syndrome may result from acute HBV infection in an immunosuppressed patient.[344] Among HBsAg-positive autologous HSCT recipients, the pretransplant HBV DNA viral load was found to be the most important risk factor for posttransplant HBV reactivation. Thus, lowering the HBV DNA viral load before chemotherapy or HSCT with lamivudine (3TC) may improve outcome.[345] Consistent with this premise, lamivudine (3TC) starting 1 week before and continuing until 52 weeks after allogeneic HSCT significantly reduced HBV exacerbation in a small randomized clinical trial.[346]

A note of caution is necessary for the pediatric oncologist in interpreting the serology of HBV. First, chronic hepatitis due to HBV may occur in patients with negative serology.[347] For example, among 23 cases of histologically proven HBV infection in children with leukemia and hepatitis, none had detectable HBsAg or hepatitis B surface antibody (HBsAb).[348] Second, seroconversion in HBV-infected patients may occur after remission of leukemia and discontinuation of immunosuppressive therapy. For example, 8 (35%) of the 23 of the previously HBV seronegative children subsequently were seropositive within 15 months of discontinuing chemotherapy.[348] Third, HBV reactivation may occur in patients, despite previously established HBV immunity (HBsAb-positive and hepatitis B core antibody [HBcAb]-positive) resulting in a form of reverse seroconversion to HBsAg-positive status, particularly in allogeneic HSCT recipients.[349]

Several viruses may involve the liver secondarily as part of a more widespread systemic infection: EBV, CMV, HSV, VZV, rubella, rubeola, mumps, adenovirus, and Coxsackie B virus. All have been associated with hepatic transaminase elevations. The hepatic dysfunction attending these secondary infections is usually self-limited and less severe than that associated with primary viral hepatitis. However, fulminant hepatic necrosis, coma, and death have been described with several of these viral pathogens, especially HSV, CMV, and VZV, in immunocompromised oncology patients. Immunocompromised patients with acute hepatitis caused by HSV or VZV should receive acyclovir, and those with CMV hepatitis are candidates for ganciclovir or foscarnet.

All cancer patients with clinical or biochemical evidence of hepatitis should undergo a serologic evaluation to attempt to characterize the etiologic agent. Serum tests for HBsAg and for HBsAb, as well as antibodies to hepatitis A (IgM and IgG), and hepatitis B core antibodies (HBcAb IgM and HBcAb IgG) can identify patients with hepatitis A or B. Repeated testing for the development of antibody to hepatitis C over a period of weeks to months may be required to diagnose this infection in addition to evaluation by PCR for HCV RNA. Patients with a negative antibody screen for all of these viruses can have hepatitis caused by an agent other than the classic hepatitis viruses or a noninfectious cause. In addition to viral infection, hepatic enzyme elevation or hyperbilirubinemia can occur with bacterial sepsis, toxoplasmosis, or hepatic candidiasis.

Hepatic Candidiasis. A syndrome referred to as *hepatic candidiasis* (also known as *hepatosplenic candidiasis* or *chronic disseminated candidiasis*) occurs in patients following recovery from a relatively long period (usually >7 days) of neutropenia during which time they have sustained hematogenous seeding of *Candida* species to the liver and other tissue sites.[350,351] The infection may have been manifest only as an earlier episode of candidemia but may have had no evidence of antecedent candidemia until recovery from neutropenia. Patients have persistent fever after recovery from an episode of neutropenia, frequently with right upper quadrant discomfort, nausea, weight loss, and increased serum alkaline

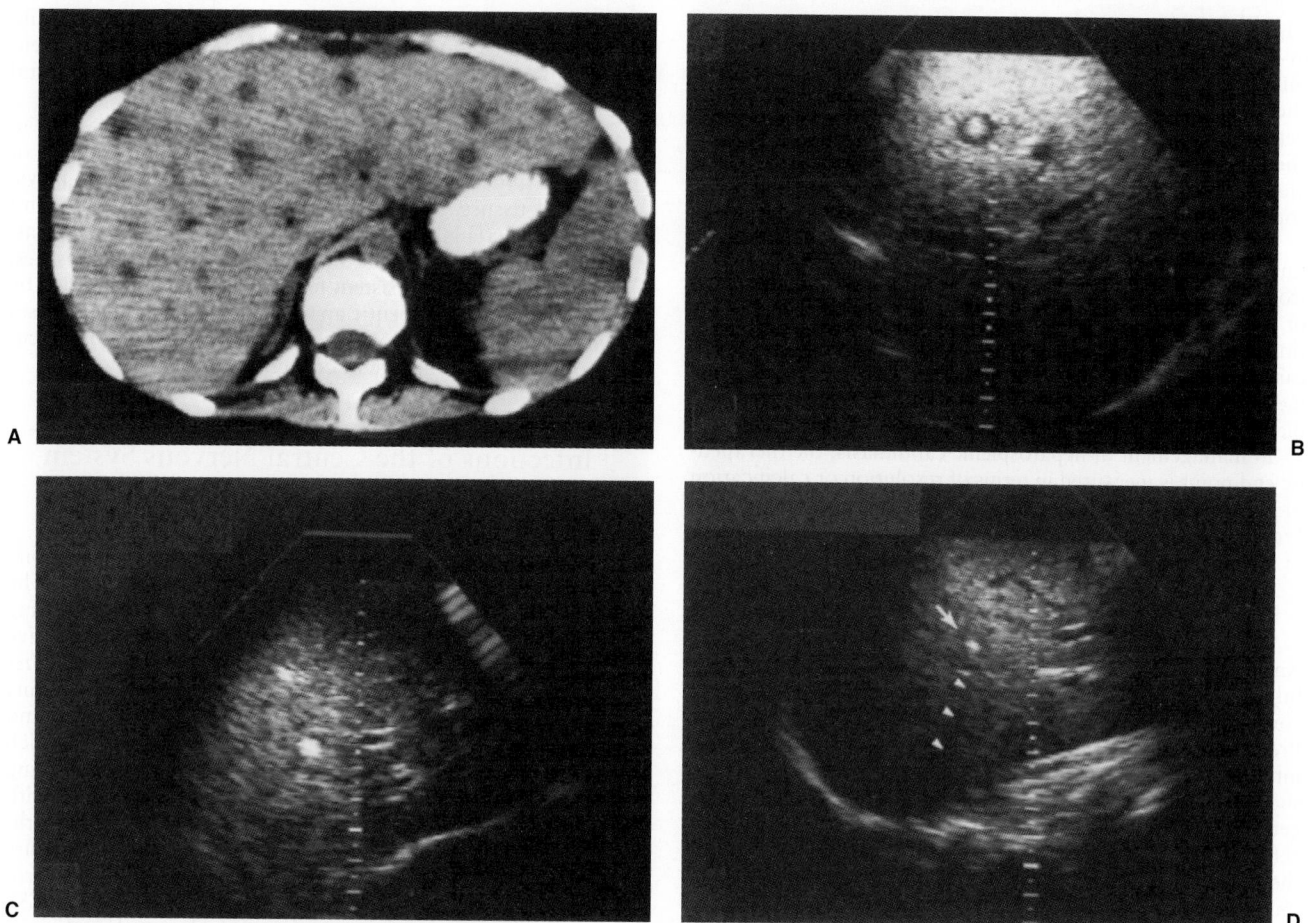

FIGURE 40.5 A: Computed tomography scan of the liver shows numerous rounded areas of decreased attenuation compatible with the diagnosis of hepatic candidiasis. This is a nonspecific finding. **B:** Ultrasound examination in the same patient shows the typical bull's-eye lesion of candidiasis characterized by a central echogenic nidus surrounded by a radiolucent halo. This is seen early in the natural history of the disease. **C:** The radiolucent halo is now less obvious than in B. This illustrates the variable appearances of candida abscesses on ultrasound studies at different times in the same patient. **D:** Later in the course of the disease, the microabscesses become denser (*arrow*). Note the acoustical shadow posterior to the lesion, caused by attenuation of the sound beam (*arrowheads*). (From Thaler M, Bader O'Leary T, Pizzo PA. Hepatic candidiasis in immunocompromised patients. Ann Intern Med 1988;108:88–100, with permission.)

phosphatase. It is characterized by the presence of multiple "bull's eye" lesions in the liver on ultrasound or CT scan (Fig. 40.5). These lesions are not apparent in patients who are neutropenic but rather become recognizable at the time of PMN recovery. The lesions are granulomas and consist of an inner core of necrosis (where the yeast and pseudohyphae can be found) surrounded by a ring of inflammatory cells and an outer ring of fibrosis. These imaged lesions change over time and with treatment and resolution may become calcified (an important end point of therapy).

The pathogenesis of hepatic candidiasis is one of chronic disseminated candidiasis; that is, the liver, as well as the spleen, kidneys, lungs, brain, eyes, and other tissues, may be infected by antecedent candidemia. Blood cultures may be negative prior to the diagnosis of hepatic candidiasis and are almost invariably negative upon recovery from neutropenia. Marcus et al.[352] found that multiple hepatic abscesses may be due to *Candida* species or bacteria, whereas solitary hepatic abscesses were caused by bacterial infections but not by candidiasis.

The diagnosis of hepatic candidiasis is based on a high index of suspicion and ideally should be confirmed with liver biopsy. Other conditions that may radiologically resemble

hepatic candidiasis include the underlying or new neoplastic disease (e.g., lymphoma, neuroblastoma), atypical mycobacterial infections, disseminated nocardiosis, and non-*Candida* fungal infections (e.g., aspergillosis). Hepatic tissue may be obtained by a small midline open incision in children and by laparoscopy in adolescents and adults. Splenic lesions may be the only apparent abscesses on CT scan. However, on laparoscopy or biopsy, the liver in these cases is usually found to be infected by small lesions below the threshold of detection of CT scan. MRI scans with gadolinium contrast may reveal lesions that are not otherwise visible on CT scans. The detection of the *Candida* enolase antigen and D-arabinitol in blood has been employed as an adjunctive tool for diagnosing invasive candidiasis, including hepatic candidiasis.[353,354]

Hepatic candidiasis poses a therapeutic challenge. Historically, long courses of treatment are necessary, with the average duration of D-AmB administered approximately 6 to 12 months. Experimental data and several encouraging reports indicate that fluconazole also has favorable efficacy in the treatment of hepatosplenic candidiasis in patients in whom amphotericin B has failed to control the infection or who have had serious amphotericin B–related toxicities.[355] Fluconazole has been increasingly used as initial therapy in stable patients in an outpatient setting. However, failures of fluconazole in this setting have also been described, suggesting that caution should be exercised in closely monitoring patients with hepatosplenic candidiasis. A reasonable approach is to treat children initially with amphotericin B and after the patient is afebrile or has response of lesions to change therapy to fluconazole at 6 mg/kg/day.[231]

Whether patients with hepatosplenic candidiasis should continue to receive antineoplastic therapy, which may cause neutropenia with the risk for progressive hepatosplenic involvement or breakthrough fungemia, can be a major dilemma. This infection in patients with cancer can be treated successfully under careful observation through repeated courses of chemotherapy-induced neutropenia without progression of hepatosplenic candidiasis or breakthrough fungemia.[356]

In management of hepatosplenic candidiasis, the therapeutic end point is measured in terms of resolution or calcification of lesions. Children tend to calcify lesions more so than adults. Premature discontinuation of therapy may lead to recurrence of symptoms and progression of lesions.

Anorectal Infections

Anorectal infections present as perianal fissures, perianal cellulitis, and perirectal infections. Anal fissures are the most common cause of anorectal infections in neutropenic patients. Presenting as painful linear tears in the mucocutaneous integrity of the anal orifice, uncomplicated anal fissures can be successfully treated with an initial antibacterial regimen targeting aerobic gram-negative bacilli, such as ceftazidime or cefepime. Broadening coverage to antianaerobic activity for these superficial but painful fissures usually is not necessary unless there is evidence of concomitant perianal cellulitis. If symptoms of perianal fissure do not improve within 48 hours, broadening of initial antibacterial empirical therapy to include anaerobes is warranted.

Perianal cellulitis presents as pain, tenderness, and erythema extending beyond the anal orifice. Extension of tenderness and erythema into the surrounding soft tissue may involve anaerobic flora. Hence, the presence of perianal cellulitis warrants the addition of antianaerobic coverage, such as metronidazole, to ceftazidime or cefepime, or the substitution of the initial empirical antimicrobial by a carbapenem or piperacillin-tazobactam. The overall incidence of perianal cellulitis has decreased in recent years, presumably because of the early use of empirical antibiotics when granulocytopenic patients become febrile. Nonetheless, the risk for perianal cellulitis remains, especially for patients in the high-risk category, those with chronic (>7 days) and profound (<100 cells/mm³) granulocytopenia. Predisposing factors include perianal mucositis caused by chemotherapy or localized radiotherapy, hemorrhoids, anal fissures, and any type of rectal manipulation (e.g., barium enema, anoscopy, sigmoidoscopy). Accordingly, constipation should be avoided, because passage of hard stool promotes the formation of anal fissures and increases the risk of perianal infection.

The most common pathogens in perianal cellulitis are aerobic gram-negative bacilli (e.g., *P. aeruginosa, K. pneumoniae, E. coli*), enterococci, and bowel anaerobes. Because of the potential involvement of anaerobic organisms, antibiotic coverage must include a specific antianaerobic agent such as metronidazole or clindamycin in addition to broad-spectrum aerobic coverage. A diagnosis of perianal fissure and perianal cellulitis should be pursued at the first complaints of tenderness. Additional supportive measures include sitz baths three or four times daily, stool softeners, a low-bulk diet, and avoidance of unnecessary rectal manipulation, especially

repetitive digital examinations. Surgical intervention should be restricted to those cases that demonstrate the development of an abscess or progressive involvement of the ischiorectal fossa despite optimal antimicrobial therapy.[357]

True perirectal infections are uncommon complications in neutropenic patients. Developing as the result of disruption of the rectal mucosa and extension of infection into the pelvic perirectal tissues, the diagnosis is suspected in patients with intractable perianal cellulitis; development of perianal fistulas, suggesting a tract between the skin and deeper pelvic tissues; and the presence of persistent fever. Diagnosis is confirmed by pelvic CT scan. Therapeutic approaches to perirectal abscesses include antianaerobic coverage and timely surgical or percutaneous catheter drainage of collections.

Infections of the Central Nervous System

Shunt and Reservoir Infections

Children with intraventricular shunts and Ommaya reservoirs are at high risk for development of CNS infection. The responsible pathogens are most commonly those colonizing the adjacent skin: coagulase-positive and coagulase-negative staphylococci, *Corynebacterium* species, and *Propionibacterium acnes*; rarely, they are gram-negative bacilli.[358] Patients may have fever, headache, increased intracranial pressure, and meningismus. Patients also may be asymptomatic, in which case the diagnosis may be made by noting CSF cultures being repetitively positive for the same organism. Most patients with Ommaya reservoir infections can be treated successfully without the need to remove the device; however, this may require a combination of intraventricular and IV therapy. Antimicrobial therapy is directed at the organism recovered from CSF and usually consists of vancomycin, which may be administered parenterally and intraventricularly.

Meningitis

Infectious meningitis in cancer patients is uncommon but associated with significant morbidity and mortality.[359] Meningitis in cancer patients can be subtle in presentation. Children with cancer presenting with fever and signs or symptoms of CNS dysfunction should be promptly evaluated. Radiographic evaluation, a head CT scan with contrast or an MRI scan with gadolinium, should be preformed if there is concern for a potential focal process. Evaluation of CSF should include aerobic culture and Gram stain, cryptococcal antigen, fungal culture, and cytologic analysis in addition to cell count and differential, protein, and glucose.

In a retrospective series of 40 pediatric cancer patients with meningitis, recent neurosurgical manipulation was found to be the most common risk factor in 65% of cases.[360] Among those patients who were neutropenic, most presented with fever and altered mental status but without meningismus. The pathogens causing infection were similar to those that are commonly associated with bacteremia in this patient population, including gram-positive organisms (*S. epidermidis, S. aureus*, alpha-hemolytic *streptococci, and Enterococcus* species), gram-negative organisms (*E. coli, K. pneumoniae, P. aeruginosa*), and fungi (*C. albicans and Aspergillus* species). Neutropenia at presentation was the primary risk factor for death related to meningitis in this series.

Encephalitis

Various viral, bacterial, parasitic, fungal, and rickettsial agents can be associated with encephalitis or encephalomyelitis. The relative prevalence of the various etiologic agents is altered in different populations of immunodeficient patients. For example, patients with humoral immune abnormalities, especially hypogammaglobulinemia, may have a chronic encephalitis caused by poliovirus or echovirus.[361] Encephalitis may be caused by other viral pathogens, such as EBV, CMV, VZV, and HHV-6. Increasing data indicate that HHV-6 is an increasingly common cause of infectious encephalitis in allogeneic HSCT recipients.[362] Detected by PCR in the CSF, HHV-6 may cause a fatal encephalopathy.[363]

West Nile virus (WNV) is the most recently recognized cause of mosquito-borne encephalitis in North America that clearly poses a threat particularly to ambulatory pediatric oncology patients. Although most human cases of WNV infection are acquired via bites from an infected mosquito, blood products and transplanted cells and tissues are other potential vehicles of transmission. Allogeneic HSCT increases the risk for severe WNV infection due to prolonged immune impairment.[364]

Patients with encephalitis or encephalomyelitis commonly present with signs of meningeal irritation (e.g., fever, headache, nuchal rigidity) and evidence of altered mentation. Confusion may progress to stupor and finally to coma. Focal neurologic signs and seizures are relatively common. Patients with WNV infection may present with flaccid paralysis of the lower extremities. CSF examination may demonstrate a pleocytosis (10 to 2,000 cells/mm^3), with a predominance of mononuclear cells. An increased number of erythrocytes have been reported with HSV encephalitis. Protein levels are usually elevated, and the glucose level characteristically remains within the normal range except for a decreased level in mumps infection.

For the cancer patient with focal neurologic deficits or altered mentation, it is important to separate infectious, metabolic, toxic, and neoplastic causes. CT scan or MRI of the brain may help in some instances, especially if a focal lesion is visualized, but specific diagnosis of encephalitis in an immunocompromised patient is often difficult.

The use of PCR to detect viral DNA in CSF is supplanting some of the older and less precise immunodiagnostic procedures. The impact of PCR on diagnosis of HSV encephalitis is especially apparent. Previously requiring a brain biopsy, PCR of CSF now allows for prompt, sensitive, and highly specific diagnostic accuracy for HSV encephalitis with excellent correlation with brain biopsy results. Nevertheless, when PCR is not available, acute and convalescent serum antibody titers against herpesviruses, echoviruses, and the less common arboviruses should be measured. Specific CSF antibody may be detected in cases of mumps, HSV, or VZV.

Toxoplasmosis of the CNS is a treatable infection that can present as encephalitis in an immunosuppressed oncology patient or HSCT recipient.[365,366] Caused by the obligate intracellular protozoan, *T. gondii*, toxoplasmosis may represent newly acquired or reactivated infection and is rarely limited to the CNS, usually occurring in concert with fever, lymphadenopathy, hepatitis, pneumonia, myocarditis, and pericarditis. The CSF typically manifests a mononuclear pleocytosis, elevated protein, and a normal glucose concentration. Definitive diagnosis requires demonstration of the parasite within tissue sections.[367] Recent advances in PCR of CSF may detect CNS toxoplasmosis noninvasively.

Pyrimethamine combined with sulfadiazine, with the addition of folinic acid to reduce pyrimethamine-induced myelotoxicity, is considered standard treatment of active toxoplasmosis. For immunodeficient patients, therapy should be continued for 4 to 6 weeks after the resolution of all clinical symptoms and signs. The combination of high-dose IV clindamycin with the usual doses of pyrimethamine appears to be

a useful alternative for treatment of toxoplasmosis in patients who are unable to tolerate sulfonamide-based drugs. Other agents combined with pyrimethamine, such as atovaquone, dapsone, or the newer macrolides, may also be effective in treatment of toxoplasmosis in immunocompromised hosts.

Brain Abscesses

The important differential diagnosis in a cancer patient with evidence of a focal lesion within the CNS is between metastatic or primary malignancy and a brain abscess. Predisposing factors for brain abscess include a contiguous infected site (e.g., otitis, sinusitis, dental abscess), a history of recent neurosurgery, congenital cardiac disease, bacterial endocarditis, and pulmonary infection. The organisms most often causing brain abscesses in immunocompetent and immunosuppressed patients are typically aerobic and anaerobic bacteria derived from the oral cavity. However, because pediatric oncology patients are immunosuppressed, nocardiosis and invasive fungal infections also rank high in the differential diagnosis for brain abscess in this population.[368,369] Consequently, a definitive microbiologic diagnosis of the cause of brain abscess in pediatric oncology patients is necessary.

Early evaluation and specific diagnosis are crucial in the management of brain abscess, because effective antimicrobial or neurosurgical therapy is available. Diagnosis is commonly made by radiographic demonstration of a localized mass and followed by an open or closed procedure to aspirate or resect the localized lesion. Because CNS nocardiosis and invasive fungal infections are usually associated with preceding pulmonary infiltrates, a less invasive diagnostic approach is to establish a microbiologic cause of the lung infection.

Underscoring the importance of CNS fungal infections as a cause of brain abscesses in immunocompromised oncology patients, a review of brain abscesses complicating HSCT found that 53 (92%) of 58 cases were caused by fungi.[369] *Aspergillus* species were the most common pathogen, followed by *Candida* species. Only four (7%) had a bacterial brain abscess, and one patient had cerebral toxoplasmosis. *Aspergillus* species accounted for ~60% of isolates and one-third were caused by *Candida* species. Mortality associated with these treatable infections was 97%.

Manifestations of CNS aspergillosis include focal seizures, hemiparesis, cranial nerve palsies, and hemorrhagic infarcts due to vascular invasion.[370] CSF cultures are usually negative. Interestingly, the presence of pulmonary infiltrates and focal neurologic deficits in an immunocompromised patient were significantly more predictive of CNS aspergillosis than for CNS candidiasis or cryptococcosis in a multivariate discriminant analysis of autopsy-proven CNS mycoses.[371] Although a specific diagnosis of CNS aspergillosis historically has been difficult to establish, recent case reports illustrate that galactomannan detected by EIA in CSF may permit a noninvasive means of detecting this frequently lethal infection,[372] although as noted before positive culture continues to be the gold standard.

Infections of the Genitourinary Tract

Although infections of the GI tract are infrequent in immunocompromised children, local obstruction resulting from tumor, neurologic dysfunction mediated by spinal cord compression or medications (e.g., vincristine, narcotics), and local therapeutic maneuvers (e.g., radiotherapy, surgery, bladder catheterization) can predispose cancer patients to genitourinary infections. Gram-negative aerobic bacilli (e.g., *E. coli*, *Klebsiella* species, *Proteus* species, *P. aeruginosa*) or enterococci are the most common causative agents. In a neutropenic patient, urine culture of a single organism should prompt antibiotic intervention whether or not the patient is symptomatic. The presence or absence of leukocytes in the urine should not be used as a diagnostic criterion in neutropenic hosts.

Differentiation between colonization and tissue invasion is particularly difficult for fungal pathogens. Fungal colonization is especially prevalent among patients with indwelling urinary catheters and those receiving broad-spectrum antimicrobial therapy. Unlike the typical situation with bacterial pathogens, in which clinical signs and symptoms are apparent, fungal invasion of the genitourinary tract may be insidious. The repetitive isolation of a particular fungal species (usually *C. albicans*, *C. tropicalis*, or *C. glabrata*) in association with fever, deteriorating renal function, or, rarely, flank pain should prompt the institution of systemic antifungal therapy. Heavily colonized bladders or superficial bladder infections manifested by persistence of positive urine cultures despite removal of predisposing factors may be effectively treated by fluconazole, which is highly concentrated in the urine. If the patient is not receiving azole prophylaxis or empirical therapy, fluconazole should be used as initial therapy in neutropenic patients. If the infection represents an emergence through azole therapy, amphotericin B, which can achieve fungicidal concentrations in the urine, should be used.

Hemorrhagic cystitis may occur as the result of mucosal injury due to cyclophosphamide or ifosfamide-based cytotoxic regimens during or soon after completion of a cycle of chemotherapy or an HSCT preparative regimen. Later in the course of HSCT, adenovirus, particularly type 11, and BKV also may cause hemorrhagic cystitis. Bladder pain and gross hematuria may occur suddenly and can be very difficult to control. Urinary tract infections may be localized, but in some cases they precede a disseminated adenovirus infection. Detection of adenovirus as well as defining serotype is possible by PCR.[373] Case reports of successful control of adenoviral and BKV-associated hemorrhagic cystitis with IV ribavirin, vidarabine, ganciclovir, and cidofovir have yet to be confirmed by larger studies.[373]

Infections of the Skin and Soft Tissues

The skin can be infected primarily or in association with bacteremia (e.g., *P. aeruginosa*, *S. maltophilia*, *Aeromonas hydrophila*, and *Bacillus* species), fungemia (*Aspergillus* species, *Candida* species, *Trichosporon* species, *Fusarium* species, and *C. neoformans*), or viremia (e.g., HSV, VZV, and CMV).[374-378] Skin lesions may lead to the early diagnosis of an infection, and new lesions should be aspirated or biopsied and the material stained (e.g., Gram stain, wet mount, and methylene blue) and cultured. If the lesions are vesicular, the base should be scraped, smeared on a glass slide, and submitted for a direct fluorescent antibody test to detect HSV or VZV.

Several bacterial and fungal skin and soft-tissue infections have distinctive clinical features. Ecthyma gangrenosum is a classic cutaneous lesion of *P. aeruginosa*. The lesions of ecthyma gangrenosum range from the more typical necrotic ulcerative lesion and black eschars to vesiculobullous or diffuse macular lesions that may progress to the more classical lesions. Other aerobic gram-negative bacilli that may cause lesions of ecthyma gangrenosum include *Aeromonas* species and *S. maltophilia*.[377] For patients with a history of swimming or wading in brackish waters, *Aeromonas hydrophila* and *Vibrio vulnificus* may cause rapidly bullous and ulcerative cutaneous lesions. Toxin-producing group A streptococci tend to cause localized foci of serpiginous erythema. By comparison, viridans streptococci, such as *S. mitis*, commonly cause a

truncal macular rash followed by a desquamative eruption on the palms and soles in the wake of its acute septic syndrome.[379] Clostridial infections of skin and soft tissue may develop as the result of direct traumatic inoculation or hematogenous dissemination.[332] When inoculated directly, these infections progress rapidly from small necrotic cutaneous foci to extensive infection of the skin, fascia, and muscle. With primary muscle infection by *Clostridium* species, fever, pain, tenderness, and edema of an extremity develop initially and are followed later by dusky cutaneous lesions. Notably, examination of the extent of these clostridial cutaneous lesions may markedly underestimate the degree of primary deep fascial and muscle infections until the time of surgery.

Aspergillus species and Zygomycetes are angioinvasive and also may cause cutaneous lesions of ecthyma gangrenosum as the result of direct inoculation; hematogenously disseminated lesions of aspergillosis tend to cause deep dermal nonulcerative nodular lesions.[378] The ulcerative cutaneous lesions of Zygomycetes are usually the result of direct inoculation. *Candida* species, particularly *C. tropicalis*, cause a syndrome of candidemia, cutaneous lesions, myalgias, arthralgias, and multiorgan dysfunction; the cutaneous lesions initially may appear as macular lesions with a small central vesicular or necrotic focus.[380] *Trichosporon* species cause a syndrome of fungemia, multiple macular or nodular lesions, chorioretinitis, renal impairment, and pulmonary infiltrates often emerging while receiving amphotericin B.[381] The cutaneous lesions of hematogenously disseminated *Fusarium* species begin typically as dermal nodules that may expand to involve the epidermis with a central ring of ischemia surrounded by a peripheral ring of erythema, suggesting a peripheral toxin production.[382] Another characteristic feature of fusariosis is a painful paronychia of the great toe due to fusarial invasion of the periungual tissues. Although staphylococcal paronychia is part of the differential diagnosis, fusarial paronychia is reported to occur in neutropenic patients who are already receiving broad-spectrum antibiotics. Hospital water and water distribution systems, such as showers, may be the source of nosocomial fusarial paronychial infections.[383] By comparison, the cutaneous lesions of disseminated cryptococcosis typically appear as umbilicated nodules resembling molluscum contagiosum.

Primary varicella is an important concern for the child with cancer, because the mortality in untreated patients ranges from 7% to 20%, usually owing to visceral dissemination to the liver, lung, and CNS.[384] Severe abdominal pain, back pain, or evidence of inappropriate antidiuretic hormone secretion may herald multisystem involvement, indicating the need for prompt use of acyclovir.[385] High doses of IV acyclovir (500 mg/m² every 8 hours or 10 mg/kg every 8 hours) are indicated for the treatment of primary varicella or herpes zoster in immunosuppressed patients.

Scabies infestation may present as papules, excoriations, or vesicles located particularly in the interdigital spaces and on the palms and soles, face, neck, and scalp. A severe clinical variant of scabies, called *Norwegian* or *crusted scabies*, occurs in immunodeficient patients and is characterized by widespread, hyperkeratotic, and crusted lesions. As these lesions contain heavy burdens of mites and their eggs, Norwegian scabies is highly contagious. Lindane 1% lotion has been the standard treatment for scabies, although it is not recommended for young children because it is percutaneously absorbed and may cause neurologic side effects. Permethrin 5% cream is recommended for children as it is poorly absorbed and may be more effective than lindane. The antiparasitic agent, ivermectin, has been shown to be highly effective in curing both routine cases and Norwegian scabies

TABLE 40.5

CAUSES OF PNEUMONIA IN PEDIATRIC ONCOLOGY PATIENTS

Localized infiltrates	Diffuse infiltrates
Nonneutropenic patients Bacteria: *Streptococcus pneumoniae, Moraxella* species, *Legionella* species, mycobacteria, *Nocardia* species Fungi: *Cryptococcus neoformans, Histoplasma capsulatum, Coccidioides immitis*; and *Aspergillus* species (the latter especially HSCT recipients postengraftment) Viruses: RSV, adenovirus, influenza, CMV	**Nonneutropenic patients** Fungi: *Pneumocystis jiroveci, Cryptococcus neoformans, Histoplasma capsulatum* Bacteria: mycobacteria, *Mycoplasma pneumoniae, Chlamydia pneumoniae,* and less commonly *Legionella* species *and Nocardia* species Viruses: RSV, adenovirus, HSV, VZV, CMV, influenza, swine-origin influenza Protozoa: *Toxoplasma gondii* Drugs: bleomycin, busulfan, cyclophosphamide, methotrexate, cytosine arabinoside Radiation pneumonitis
Neutropenic patients Bacteria: any gram-positive or gram-negative; mycobacteria, *Legionella* species, *Nocardia* species Fungi: *Pneumocystis jiroveci, Cryptococcus neoformans, Histoplasma capsulatum* Viruses: RSV, adenovirus, influenza	**Neutropenic patients** Bacteria: any gram-positive or gram-negative; mycobacteria, *Mycoplasma pneumoniae, Chlamydia pneumoniae,* and less commonly *Legionella* species *and Nocardia* species Fungi: *Aspergillus* species, Zygomycetes, *Fusarium* species, *Scedosporium* species, and other filamentous fungi (see text) Viruses: RSV, adenovirus, HSV, VZV, CMV, influenza Protozoa: *T. gondii* Radiation pneumonitis

CMV, cytomegalovirus; HSCT, hematopoietic stem cell transplantation; HSV, herpes simplex virus; RSV, respiratory syncytial virus; VZV, varicella zoster virus.

after a single oral dose; the simplicity and efficacy of this therapy may preclude use of the topical agents.[386]

Noninfectious causes of cutaneous lesions in oncology patients and HSCT recipients are prevalent and may simulate infectious processes. Unless recognized, these conditions may lead to the inappropriate use of antibiotics. Maculopapular eruptions due to drugs are commonly encountered particularly in relation to β-lactam antibiotics. Erythema multiforme and Stevens-Johnson syndrome may also occur, especially as a reaction to sulfonamides. Cutaneous lesions in oncology patients may be paraneoplastic manifestations of the primary neoplastic process but simulate infectious processes. For example, Sweet syndrome is associated with hematologic malignancies and is characterized by fever and nodular or ulcerative skin lesions. Biopsy of the lesions of Sweet syndrome may be deceptive as they histologically may demonstrate a dense neutrophilic infiltrate of the papillary and reticular dermis.

Occasionally, tumor infiltration of the skin by a chloroma, lymphoid malignancy, melanoma, or metastatic tumor may ulcerate and become superinfected usually by *Staphylococcus* species or by water-borne organisms, such as *P. aeruginosa* or *S. maltophilia*. Cutaneous GVHD in HSCT recipients may appear as a bacterial cellulitis, a toxin-mediated infection (e.g., group A streptococci), or furuncle. In the absence of concomitant GVHD of the liver or GI tract, biopsy of suspicious isolated cutaneous lesions usually establishes a diagnosis.

PREVENTION OF INFECTION IN CHILDREN WITH CANCER

In a multitude of clinical trials investigating the efficacy of various measures to prevent or reduce infection, the most important antiinfective measure identified has been the simplest: careful handwashing practices.[387] Several approaches have

been taken to decrease the acquisition of new organisms or to suppress those already colonizing cancer patients (Table 40.5). However, no method has stood out as singularly effective and each has both promise and problems.

Preventing the Acquisition of New Organisms

Because most of the organisms responsible for infections in patients with cancer are derived from the endogenous flora, and almost half of this flora is acquired from the hospital environment, much attention has been directed toward preventing the acquisition of potential pathogens. Inanimate objects within the hospital environment (e.g., faucet aerators, showerheads, respirators, plants, and floors) are reservoirs of pathogenic organisms. Although epidemiologic studies have, for the most part, investigated nonimmunocompromised patients, they also suggest that transmission from inanimate sources often requires a human vector. Therefore, the most efficacious and practical intervention that can be performed is adherence to strict handwashing precautions. The easiest way to enforce such a policy is to educate the child and parents to disallow contact with anyone who has neglected to wash his or her hands.

A second maneuver to decrease the acquisition of new organisms is to maintain a cooked diet during periods of granulocytopenia, with avoidance of fresh fruits and vegetables and nonprocessed diary products, because these foods are naturally contaminated with gram-negative bacteria, especially *E. coli, K. pneumoniae,* and *P. aeruginosa*.[388]

Environmental sources can contribute to fungal (especially *Aspergillus* species, *Fusarium* species, and Zygomycetes) and bacterial (*Legionella* species, *Pseudomonas* species, *Acinetobacter* species) colonization and infection. In medical centers where *Aspergillus* species and *Fusarium* species are a significant problem, special air filtration systems, such as high-efficiency particulate air (HEPA) filters, and close attention to cleaning bathroom facilities may be helpful.[389]

Although the technique of reverse isolation has often been used, it does not significantly reduce the acquisition of new organisms in an environment in which handwashing techniques are strictly followed. Hence, there is no compelling reason to enforce this policy, particularly because the extra expense, time consumption, and inconvenience are not balanced by a beneficial effect.[390]

Total protective isolation is a comprehensive regimen designed to reduce patients' endogenous microbial burden while preventing the acquisition of new organisms (Table 40.5). A sterile environment is created in a clean-air room with constant positive-pressure airflow. It is maintained by an aggressive program of surface decontamination and sterilization of all objects that enter the room and by an intensive regimen to disinfect the patient, including oral nonabsorbable antibiotics, skin antiseptics, antibiotic sprays and ointments, and a low-microbial diet. The total protective environment reduces the number of infections in profoundly granulocytopenic patients. However, a total protective environment is expensive, and because of the improvement in treating established infections, it does not offer a survival advantage to patients. Total protective isolation is not necessary for the routine care of cancer patients. Modifications of the approach are used, on occasion, for patients undergoing allogeneic bone marrow transplantation and for patients who are likely to experience periods of 30 or more days of profound neutropenia.

PROPHYLACTIC ANTIBIOTICS

Antibacterial Prophylaxis

Because the GI tract is the source of many of the pathogens causing microbiologically defined infections in oncology patients, investigators initially evaluated the efficacy of reducing the endogenous GI flora with oral nonabsorbable antibiotics (e.g., vancomycin, gentamicin, polymyxin B, nystatin, framycetin, colistin). This technique has not been especially valuable because the agents used are unpalatable and poorly tolerated, making compliance a significant problem, especially among patients receiving emetogenic chemotherapy. Equally disturbing has been the emergence of resistant bacterial strains among patients receiving aminoglycoside-containing regimens. Therefore, prophylactic regimens aimed solely at reducing the total endogenous GI flora cannot be recommended.

A modified technique is selective decontamination of the GI tract with antibiotics that preserve the anaerobic flora while reducing the aerobic bacteria. This approach is based on experimental data showing that preservation of the anaerobic flora of the GI tract provides colonization resistance against aerobic and fungal organisms.[391,392] The most commonly investigated agent for selective decontamination has been TMP-SMX. Early trials of this drug in children and adults demonstrated a reduction in all infections and in bacteremic episodes. However, many follow-up clinical trials have yielded conflicting results, perhaps because of variability in study design, nonuniform patient populations, and failure to properly monitor compliance. The potential for reduction in infectious morbidity and mortality must be balanced against two important adverse effects observed with the prophylactic use of TMP-SMX: the prolongation of granulocytopenia and emergence of resistant organisms. Successful selective decontamination of the GI tract requires excellent patient compliance and close microbiologic monitoring to

adjust the antimicrobial regimen properly for resistant or newly emerging species. However, strict compliance with the oral regimens is often difficult, and surveillance cultures are costly in time and money.[393–396]

The fluoroquinolone antibiotics (norfloxacin, ciprofloxacin, and levofloxacin) have been used as oral prophylaxis in neutropenic patients. A meta-analysis of published randomized trials of quinolone prophylaxis found that total infections, microbiologically documented infections (particularly gram-negative bacteria), and fevers were significantly reduced. The incidence of gram-positive infections and more importantly infection-related deaths, however, was not reduced.[397] Two independent recent studies investigating the use of prophylactic oral levofloxacin in patients receiving chemotherapy for either solid tumors or lymphomas[398] or hematologic malignancies[399] both documented a reduction in infections. Finally, a comprehensive meta-analysis of all types of antibiotic prophylaxis in neutropenic cancer patients (a total of 95 trials conducted between 1973 and 2004) concluded that antibiotic prophylaxis significantly decreased the risk for death when compared with placebo or with no treatment at all.[400] When further analyzing only trials that tested quinolones, a significant reduction in the risk for all-cause mortality, infection-related mortality, and microbiologically documented infections was reported. However, the strongest argument against the use of prophylactic fluoroquinolones is the increasing rates of antimicrobial resistance to quinolones reported in many of these same studies.[399–401] Ultimately, the use of prophylactic antibiotics in pediatric cancer patients is best guided by clinical guidelines and protocols.

Antifungal Prophylaxis

Because of the increasing incidence of invasive mycoses in immunocompromised hosts, antifungal prophylaxis also has been extensively studied. Orally administered and topically applied nystatin, amphotericin B, miconazole, and clotrimazole; orally administered and systemically absorbed ketoconazole, fluconazole, itraconazole, and posaconazole; and parenterally administered amphotericin B and micafungin have all been evaluated as prophylactic antifungal agents in neutropenic patients. Most prophylactic regimens have been aimed at reducing invasive infections caused by *Candida* species and, by virtue of the antifungal activity of the agents employed, would not be expected to have a significant impact against *Aspergillus* or filamentous fungal pathogens.

Two randomized, placebo-controlled studies demonstrated that the prophylactic administration of fluconazole to recipients of allogeneic bone marrow transplant reduced the incidence of both disseminated and mucosal candidiasis.[402,403] These and other studies employing prophylactic antifungal regimens observed a shift in the colonization pattern of fungal organisms, usually toward more resistant fungi. Prophylactic regimens may eradicate susceptible fungi, while permitting overgrowth and ultimate invasion by more resistant species, including *C. glabrata, Candida krusei, Candida parapsilosis, Aspergillus,* and other filamentous fungi. Fluconazole is most beneficial in prevention of disseminated candidiasis in neutropenic allogeneic bone marrow transplant recipients. Fluconazole is the only compound that is FDA-approved for prevention of deeply invasive fungal infections in neutropenic patients and HSCT recipients. The decision to use fluconazole or other prophylactic antifungal agents in other patient populations depends on the institution, the cytotoxic regimen employed, and the patient. More recent studies involving pediatric patients demonstrate that micafungin was superior to fluconazole in prevention of proven and suspected invasive fungal infections in neutropenic HSCT patients.[149] Finally, in a recent randomized multicenter study, those patients with AML or myelodysplastic syndrome who were treated with prophylactic posaconazole had a lower incidence of proven or probable fungal disease (particularly invasive aspergillosis) compared with those patients treated with fluconazole or itraconazole.[404]

Antiviral Prophylaxis

Several antiviral agents can be used for selective prophylaxis. Amantadine has proven prophylactic activity against influenza A (although not against influenza B) in school children treated with 100 mg/day, and it is likely to be similarly efficacious in the immunocompromised host.[405] Rimantadine has equivalent protective efficacy but is associated with fewer CNS effects than amantadine. Postexposure prophylaxis of family members is also effective with both drugs, although it is recommended that simultaneous prophylaxis and treatment of influenza A be avoided within a household, so that resistant virus strains do not become a significant problem.[406] The use of the newer neuraminidase inhibitors in immunocompromised patients as prophylactic agents has been studied recently in pediatric and adult populations.[407,408]

Acyclovir, given orally or intravenously, is effective prophylaxis against reactivations of HSV in seropositive HSCT recipients and in those undergoing intensive chemotherapy for acute leukemia.[157,158] IV doses ranging from 250 mg/m² every 8 hours to 5 mg/kg every 12 hours, and oral doses of 400 mg given three times daily, are effective in preventing reactivation of HSV in seropositive individuals. Although acyclovir is therapeutically less active against VZV or CMV, prophylactic acyclovir given to HSCT recipients may nonetheless decrease the occurrence of zoster and invasive CMV disease during the posttransplant period.[160,409]

Acyclovir-resistant strains of HSV have been recognized with increasing frequency, particularly in patients with HIV infection. In HSCT recipients and in those with HIV infection, resistant HSV is associated with indolent disease, characterized by the persistence of low-grade, chronic mucocutaneous lesions that may be painful and refractory to routine or even high-dose acyclovir therapy. The clinical presentation of resistant HSV infection is preceded by a prolonged continuous or intermittent course of acyclovir, such as a prophylactic regimen. Discontinuation of acyclovir often allows the reemergence of a sensitive virus strain from the mixed pool of latent virus. Refractory lesions may be responsive to foscarnet.[410]

Ganciclovir prophylaxis can reduce the frequency of invasive CMV disease in HSCT recipients. However, the marked myelosuppressive effects of ganciclovir are problematic for most patients, making it an unattractive routine prophylactic agent. Targeting of those who are at highest risk for severe CMV disease has yielded the practice of "preemptive" ganciclovir therapy, that is, treatment of patients who have evidence of CMV reactivation in surveillance assays (CMV antigenemia, CMV PCR). This approach has been shown to effectively suppress CMV culture positivity in most patients and, accordingly, it is associated with dramatically fewer cases of invasive CMV disease.[163,411]

Pneumocystis Prophylaxis

Successful prophylaxis for PCP was originally described using TMP-SMX in high-risk oncology patients.[198,283] In the 1980s, PCP emerged as the most common opportunistic infection in individuals with AIDS. Most large studies of prophylactic regimens with newer agents since that time have been undertaken in the HIV population, with results then abstracted for the use in other immunocompromised groups.

The decision to administer antimicrobial prophylaxis to oncology patients should be based on underlying disease and the type and intensity of immunosuppressive therapy. The reported frequency of PCP in patients before the routine use of prophylaxis was 22% to 43% in children with ALL, 25% in patients being treated for rhabdomyosarcoma,[283] 16% in those having undergone a bone marrow transplant,[412] and 27% in those children with severe combined immunodeficiency syndrome. In some centers almost half of the cases of PCP occur in patients with solid tumors.[287] In addition, patients with brain tumors receiving significant doses of corticosteroids are also at risk.[288,413]

There are several effective regimens for PCP prophylaxis. The choice among them often depends on the patient's tolerance of their various side effects. TMP-SMX, given twice a day for 3 days a week, is considered the first-line regimen.[414] For patients who can tolerate this regimen, protection against PCP is virtually complete.[415] The use of TMP-SMX is limited, however, in a significant number of individuals by rash, neutropenia, and GI symptoms.

Alternative compounds for prevention of PCP in patients who are intolerant of or refractory to TMP-SMX include dapsone, atovaquone, and aerosolized pentamidine. Dapsone administered at a dose of 2 mg/kg/day (with a maximum dose of 100 mg/day) is also effective for PCP prophylaxis. The rate of reported failure of prophylactic dapsone ranges from 0% to 21%.[199] The side effects of dapsone include rash, anemia, methemoglobinemia, agranulocytosis, and hepatitis. The frequency of treatment-limiting adverse reactions is estimated to be similar to that of TMP-SMX.

Atovaquone has been shown to be as effective as dapsone in a single large trial of adult HIV patients who were intolerant of TMP-SMX.[416] Atovaquone also was better tolerated in patients who were not already receiving dapsone at the time of randomization. The most common adverse events of atovaquone include upper GI symptoms and diarrhea. Pharmacokinetic studies have been performed in children with HIV, giving rise to dosing recommendations of 30 mg/kg/day in children aged 1 to 3 months and 45 mg/kg/day for those between 3 and 24 months. These dosages were chosen to attain a serum level of 15 mg/mL, which in adult patients is associated with a therapeutic success of greater than 95%.[202] Aerosolized pentamidine administered monthly is also effective in prevention of PCP in HIV-infected pediatric patients.[417] Bronchospasm at the time of administration is the primary side effect of aerosolized pentamidine. The use of aerosolized pentamidine is often limited in very young children because of technical difficulties in inhalational administration and compliance. IV pentamidine has been associated with breakthrough infections in HIV-infected children and should not be used for prophylaxis.

IMMUNIZATION

Immunizations are an important part of the care of healthy children. The routine vaccination schedule will often be disrupted for younger children undergoing therapy for cancer. There are no universally accepted recommendations for immunizing children undergoing therapy for cancer, but some general guidelines can be applied. The American Academy of Pediatrics and the CDC regularly publish updated guidelines regarding immunization practices in healthy and immunocompromised pediatric patients.[418,419] Guidelines for vaccination of HSCT recipients and household members also have been published by the CDC.[420] In considering reasonable vaccine strategies in pediatric oncology patients, information about the host's risks for infection need to be balanced with the safety and efficacy of each vaccine in this population. Two main concerns must be considered: (a) Will the patient be able to mount (or maintain) an antibody response? and (b) Could the vaccine itself (in the case of attenuated live organisms) cause disease?

Live Attenuated Viruses

Measles-mumps-rubella (MMR) is a live attenuated virus vaccine that is contraindicated in patients undergoing active chemotherapy. If immunocompromised patients with cancer are exposed to measles, immunoglobulin should be administered regardless of previous vaccination status.[421,422] In the early development of the vaccine, one of eight children vaccinated with the Edmonton b strain measles vaccine died of the disease. Immunization has been shown to be safe and is recommended for patients with ALL after completion of therapy, generally waiting for 3 to 6 months following the completion of chemotherapy to allow for T-cell reconstitution. However, Ambrosino et al.[421] recommended that patients having completed therapy for Hodgkin disease not be vaccinated because of their prolonged T-cell deficits. Household contacts can be safely vaccinated because transmission of the vaccine virus does not occur. Children with severe immunosuppression (for definition see Table 40.6) due to HIV infection should not receive the MMR vaccine either; however, HIV-infected children with mild or moderate immune suppression can follow the normal immunization schedules.[421] The risk associated with wild-type measles is considered to be higher than the risk for vaccine-related complications.[423] For HSCT recipients, administration of MMR vaccine is recommended at 24 months or later after transplantation if the HSCT patient is not receiving immunosuppressive therapy and is considered immunocompetent.[420]

Oral polio vaccine is a live virus vaccine that is also contraindicated in immunocompromised patients and their household contacts. Inactivated polio vaccine (IPV) can be used safely during treatment for nonimmunized patients. Reimmunization with inactivated polio vaccine after the completion of chemotherapy or HSCT is generally recommended.[420]

The current varicella vaccine uses the live attenuated Oka strain and has been extensively studied in immunocompromised children. Varicella vaccine is now universally recommended for healthy individuals in early childhood and for susceptible older children and adolescents. It is not contraindicated in household contacts of immunosuppressed individuals.[418,419] Household contacts and health care workers who have no history of varicella and who are sero-negative for VZV should receive the vaccine to prevent infection by and prevent transmission of wild-type varicella. Contact with immunocompromised patients should be avoided if a varicella-like rash developed following vaccination.

The vaccine is safe in children with ALL, with the most common toxicity being a mild rash occurring in 50% of those treated.[424,425] The efficacy of the vaccine is apparent in the degree of protection from acquiring the disease from household contacts, with 14% developing mild disease and complete protection from severe varicella. There has been concern about varicella zoster in immunocompromised vaccinees; however, leukemic vaccinees are less likely to develop zoster than comparable children with leukemia who had wild-type infection. Although Gershon and colleagues found that the varicella vaccine is safe and effective in children with leukemia, it is still considered investigational in the United

TABLE 40.6

IMMUNIZATIONS IN PEDIATRIC CANCER PATIENTS[a]

Patients receiving chemotherapy for cancer	
DtaP	For children younger than 7 yr, given 3–6 mo after completion of therapy
HIB	Given 3–6 mo after completion of therapy
IPV	OPV should not be given to patients or their household contacts, IPV given 3–6 mo postcompletion of therapy
MMR	Given 3–6 mo postcompletion of therapy
VZV	Should be considered in ALL patients after remission for 1 yr, otherwise at 3–6 mo postcompletion of therapy
Influenza	Should be given each autumn, household contacts should also be immunized
Pediatric hematopoietic stem cell transplant patients[420]	
Td	Given at 12, 14, and 24 mo posttransplant for those ≥7 yr of age
DTaP	Given at 12, 14, and 24 mo posttransplant for those <7 yr of age
HIB	Given at 12, 14, and 24 mo posttransplant
Pneumovax	Given at 12 and 24 mo posttransplant
MMR	Given at 24 mo posttransplant in those patients without significant GVHD
VZV	Contraindicated for HSCT patients
IPV	Given at 12, 14, and 24 mo posttransplant, OPV should not be given
Influenza	Given each autumn (>6 mo posttransplant), household contacts should also be immunized
Hep B	Given at 12, 14, and 24 mo posttransplant

dT, diphtheria-tetanus; DTaP, diphtheria-tetanus-acellular pertussis; GVHD, graft-versus-host disease; HIB, *Haemophilus influenzae* type B; IPV, inactivated polio vaccine; MMR, measles-mumps-rubella; OPV, oral polio vaccine; VZV, varicella zoster virus.
[a]Recommendations are based on limited data. Immunization schedules may need to be individualized based on the patient's underlying disease and degree of immunosuppression.

States in immunocompromised patients.[424,425] Given the lack of access of immunocompromised patients to the live attenuated varicella vaccine, passive immunoprophylaxis either with varicella zoster immune globulin within 96 hours of exposure or regular infusions of gamma-globulin are indicated in the high-risk children with no reliable history of varicella. If inadvertent contact occurs between an immunocompromised child and a recent varicella vaccine recipient, administration of varicella zoster immune globulin is not recommended as the transmission rate is low and varicella from the Oka strain, albeit unlikely, would be mild and self-limiting. Finally, one should be aware that the varicella vaccine might not be fully protective against varicella, particularly in an outbreak setting.[426]

Live Attenuated Bacteria

Bacillus Calmette-Guérin (BCG) vaccine is the only common live bacterium that potentially could be used in a childhood immunization. Although not used in the United States, BCG is still recommended in more than 100 countries worldwide.[427] Because disseminated BCG infection can occur in immunocompromised children, it is generally contraindicated in that population.[428]

Inactivated Bacteria, Inactivated Viruses, Polysaccharide-Protein Conjugates, and Toxoids

The diphtheria-pertussis-tetanus (DPT) vaccine is immunogenic and protective in young infants with neuroblastoma and in children receiving maintenance therapy for various malignancies.[429] The vaccine containing the acellular form of the pertussis component (diphtheria-tetanus-acellular pertussis [DTaP]) decreases the risk of seizures and is currently recommended for all children. Although some experts suggest that children should receive DTaP at scheduled times even while undergoing active chemotherapy, an alternative approach to ensure greater immunogenicity is to immunize at the end of antineoplastic therapy. For HSCT recipients, the current guidelines recommend administration of three doses of DTaP, as well as inactivated polio, HIB, and HBV vaccines at 12, 14, and 24 months post-HSCT.

Patients with ALL, as well as those with Hodgkin disease who were treated with splenectomy, are at a higher risk for invasive pneumococcal and HIB disease.[430,431] Where possible, immunization against encapsulated bacteria should be performed at least 2 weeks before splenectomy. Otherwise immunization after splenectomy is still advisable with a possible reimmunization every 5 years thereafter.[432,433]

The pneumococcal polysaccharide vaccine covering 23 serotypes is only moderately immunogenic in oncology and transplantation populations. The newer heptavalent conjugated pneumococcal polysaccharide vaccine is well tolerated and immunogenic in immunocompetent children. Studies in immunocompetent patients thus far demonstrate a significant reduction in pneumococcal-related otitis media and a trend toward reduction in severe pneumococcal disease.[434,435] A shift toward colonizing serotypes not recognized by the vaccine has been seen in nasopharyngeal cultures in vaccinated patients. However, there are few data at this point describing the safety and immunogenicity in immunosuppressed children. The most practical approach would be to administer the heptavalent conjugated pneumococcal polysaccharide vaccine after immunosuppressive chemotherapy to pediatric oncology patients.

The HIB conjugate vaccines have been tested in children who were receiving cancer chemotherapy or who had completed treatment for ALL. Although the responses were not normal, those patients who did respond had protective antibodies that were measurable for 12 months.[436] Current guidelines recommend the vaccination of all immunosuppressed individuals with pneumococcal, HIB, and, where appropriate, meningococcal vaccines.[418-420]

Impacting particularly on the young, elderly, and immunocompromised, influenza is the most common cause of seasonal excess mortality in the United States. In a small retrospective study of pediatric patients with ALL, immunization decreased the frequency of influenza infection compared with unimmunized controls.[437] Most authorities recommend annual influenza vaccination of all immunocompromised children and their household contacts before the onset of influenza season.[418,419] For HSCT recipients, lifelong seasonal administration of influenza vaccine is recommended before HSCT and resuming 6 months post-HSCT.[420]

GRANULOCYTE TRANSFUSIONS

Although the principle of granulocyte transfusions in neutropenic patients with refractory infections is physiologically sound, the data supporting this clinical practice have been the subject of considerable controversy. Some early randomized studies demonstrated a clinical benefit for the PMN transfusion group compared with controls,[438,439] whereas others showed no overall benefit although demonstrating efficacy in certain subgroups of patients,[440] and still others reported no benefit at all.[441] Foremost among the confounding variables contributing to the lack of consistency across studies is the variable amount of cells transfused. Those studies transfusing larger amounts of cells per transfusion demonstrated improved efficacy compared with those with lower doses of infused cells.[442]

Recent technical advances in the ability to collect substantially larger numbers of PMNs per pheresis have opened new potential for the therapeutic benefit of this adjunctive modality. The use of granulocyte colony-stimulating factor (G-CSF) to mobilize granulocytes in normal healthy donors has been shown to be safe and effective, allowing for the collection of significantly more PMNs per cycle of pheresis.[443,444]

In addition to total number of cells transfused, human leukocyte antigen (HLA)-match is also thought to be an important factor in the efficacy of granulocyte transfusions.[445] Alloimmunization to HLA antigens decreases cell recovery in the recipient and may also correlate with the frequency of transfusion reactions.[446] Given the technical advances in G-CSF mobilization, WBC collection, and donor matching, a randomized trial is warranted to investigate the use of granulocyte transfusions in neutropenic patients with refractory infections. However, standardization of collection methods, HLA matching, dose of granulocytes, and type of patients enrolled present daunting challenges to a multicenter trial. Until such studies are available, selection of candidate patients to receive granulocyte transfusions must be made by an individual assessment of risk and benefit.

Administration of granulocyte transfusions carries risks of alloimmunization and respiratory distress. Not all profoundly neutropenic patients with refractory infections are appropriate candidates for granulocyte transfusions. Because of alloimmunization, patients who receive granulocyte transfusions during aplastic anemia may have a worsened prognosis following HSCT. Patients with underlying chronic lung disease or limited pulmonary reserve may not be able to tolerate the respiratory toxicity associated with granulocyte transfusions. CMV-seronegative allogeneic HSCT recipients should receive transfusions from CMV-seronegative granulocyte donors, where feasible. Given the adverse reactions and expense, granulocyte transfusions are not indicated for prophylaxis of infections or in treatment of infections that may be managed with antimicrobial therapy alone. Instead, they may be indicated for the treatment of infections that are refractory to conventional antimicrobial therapy in patients with persistent but potentially reversible neutropenia.

RECOMBINANT HUMAN CYTOKINES

The development of recombinant human (rh) cytokines and colony-stimulating factors (CSFs) for adjunctive therapy in oncology patients has been an important advance in helping to attenuate the myelotoxic effects of cancer chemotherapy, radiotherapy, and HSCT. Recombinant human CSFs have acquired an important role in the care of pediatric oncology patients but should be used judiciously to maximize medical benefit, limit potential toxicity, and be cost effective. G-CSF (filgrastim) and granulocyte-macrophage-CSF (GM-CSF, sargramostim) have undergone the most intense study for their potential to decrease infectious morbidity of chemotherapy.

G-CSF increases the proliferation and maturation of committed PMN precursors, as well as the function of mature PMNs. GM-CSF additionally enhances the number and function of cells of the MNC-macrophage lineage.[447] The indications for G-CSF and GM-CSF in oncology patients have been delineated in guidelines from the American Society of Clinical Oncology (ASCO).[448]

The standard dosages of G-CSF and GM-CSF, respectively, are 5 µg/kg/day and 250 µg/m²/day. These dosages of G-CSF have been associated with reduced durations of neutropenia and decreased frequency of infectious complications.[449–451] The use of higher doses has not been associated with improved clinical outcome.[450] The exception to this dosage recommendation is in the setting of donor stimulation for peripheral blood stem cell pheresis, where there may be an advantage to the use of 10 µg/kg/day of G-CSF. In either setting, rounding the dose to the closest vial size is likely to save costs without detriment to the patient. The CSFs should be administered subcutaneously but may also be given intravenously.

Primary Prophylaxis: Use of Granulocyte Colony-Stimulating Factors or Granulocyte-Macrophage Colony-Stimulating Factors in the Prevention of Fever and Neutropenia

The use of CSFs for primary prevention involves their administration immediately following a course of myelotoxic chemotherapy in an attempt to decrease the depth and duration of neutropenia, reduce the risk of infection, and shorten the duration of hospitalization.[452–454] However, there are a paucity of data to demonstrate any significant effect of rhCSFs on disease-free or overall survival. Moreover, the use of G-CSF as primary prophylaxis for patients undergoing less aggressive chemotherapeutic regimens, with a low frequency of fever and neutropenia, is of unclear medical or economic benefit. If the number of patients receiving the cytokine injections far exceeds those who would potentially experience any beneficial effects, the expense of the growth factor and the discomfort of daily injections in all patients could offset the advantage to a few patients.

The original ASCO guidelines recommend the use of G-CSF and GM-CSF for primary prophylaxis if the anticipated rate of fever and neutropenia for a given chemotherapeutic regimen is greater than 40%.[448] In addition to those groups of patients with anticipated high rate of fever and neutropenia, there may be individuals who may benefit from primary prophylaxis, such as patients who have received extensive prior chemotherapy or radiation therapy to their pelvis or spine and are therefore expected to have more significant myelotoxicity from any given regimen.

Secondary Prophylaxis: Use of Granulocyte Colony-Stimulating Factors or Granulocyte-Macrophage Colony-Stimulating Factors in Patients with a Previous Episode of Fever and Neutropenia

The restriction of CSF administration to patients with a history of a prior episode of fever and neutropenia may provide a more select patient population that may benefit from CSFs. In addition, this strategy may avoid their use, and associated toxicities and costs, in a group of patients for which they would provide limited or no benefit. The original ASCO

recommendations encourage dose adjustment of chemotherapy for subsequent treatment cycles for patients who have developed fever and neutropenia on a prior cycle unless there is evidence that maintaining dose intensity is beneficial to patient outcome. If maintaining dose intensity is important, then CSFs should be considered for secondary prophylaxis. Notably, in a survey of practicing pediatric oncologists, dosage modification was seldom selected as a mode of secondary prophylaxis and conversely, CSF use was common.[455] This observation is consistent with a difference in pediatric malignancies in which curative intent is sought in chemotherapy-responsive malignancies.

Tertiary Prophylaxis: Use of Granulocyte Colony-Stimulating Factors or Granulocyte-Macrophage Colony-Stimulating Factors in Patients with Known Neutropenia but Without Fever

There have been several clinical trials that have investigated the efficacy of initiation of CSFs at the time of the patient's diagnosis with neutropenia.[450,456] Although the number of days of neutropenia was shortened, there was no measurable clinical benefit in terms of days in the hospital, days of antibiotic therapy, or documented infections. Given these data, CSFs should not be routinely initiated for patients presenting with neutropenia alone.

Use of Granulocyte Colony-Stimulating Factors or Granulocyte-Macrophage Colony-Stimulating Factors for the Adjunctive Treatment of Fever and Neutropenia

There have been a series of prospective, randomized controlled trials addressing the question of whether administration of G-CSF or GM-CSF as adjunctive therapy to antibiotics, beginning at the time of diagnosis of fever and neutropenia, has beneficial effects on patient outcome.[457–459] Similar to other randomized trials, these studies in general have shown that G-CSF or GM-CSF decrease the duration of neutropenia, days of fever, days of antibiotic administration, and days of hospitalization. However, none have found a discernible impact on infection-related mortality. Thus, the ASCO guidelines on use of CSFs recommend that G-CSF and GM-CSF not routinely be initiated as adjunctive therapy for the patient presenting with fever and neutropenia.[448]

Use of Granulocyte Colony-Stimulating Factors or Granulocyte-Macrophage Colony-Stimulating Factors in Documented Infections in Immunocompromised Hosts

G-CSF and GM-CSF enhance the antimicrobial activity of granulocytes and MNCs *in vitro* and *in vivo*. Accordingly, they may augment microbicidal activity of these effector cells in the immunocompromised patient and may therefore be useful as adjuncts to antimicrobial agents in the treatment of ongoing infections. Although there are some data from animal models to suggest a survival benefit of CSFs given during bacterial sepsis,[459] one small clinical study in leukemic children showed no apparent benefit to the delayed addition of G-CSF at the time of documented sepsis.[460] However, there are experimental data and clinical observations supporting the use of G-CSF or GM-CSF in the adjunctive treatment of invasive fungal infections in immunocompromised hosts.[461,462] Multicenter randomized controlled trials are needed in proven invasive fungal infections in order to further define the roles of G-CSF, GM-CSF, and other recombinant cytokines.

Use of Colony-Stimulating Factors in Stem Cell Transplantation

The effects of G-CSF and GM-CSF in prevention of infections in neutropenic patients are perhaps best illustrated in the impact of these agents on stem cell mobilization in HSCT donors. Transfusion of peripheral mobilized stem cells has led to a substantial reduction in depth and duration of neutropenia.[463–465] G-CSF and GM-CSF also are used in HSCT recipients as part of most immediate posttransplant regimens for their impact on shortening the duration of neutropenia. The effects on the incidence of fever or documented infections, antibiotic usage, or duration of hospitalization have been more variable and dependent on clinical trial design. Notably, as these cytokines do not augment platelet recovery, thrombocytopenia remains a challenging problem for HSCT recipients. G-CSF or GM-CSF is continued until engraftment is documented and an adequate circulating PMN count has been observed on successive days. In selected circumstances, G-CSF or GM-CSF may be indicated in HSCT recipients who demonstrate delayed engraftment or PMN recovery.

Interferon-γ

Human recombinant IFN-γ augments cell-mediated and innate host defenses against intracellular as well as extracellular bacteria, fungi, viruses, and parasites. IFN-γ enhances chemotaxis, phagocytosis, oxidative metabolism, and microbicidal activity of PMNs and MNCs, as well as increases phagocytosis and antimicrobial activity of tissue macrophages. Despite these properties, IFN-γ data supporting its clinical usage are limited.

IFN-γ is licensed for prevention of serious infections in patients with chronic granulomatous disease.[466] It has been used in combination with antimycobacterial agents for treatment of refractory atypical mycobacterial infections in patients with defective IFN-γ production.[467] IFN-γ also was found to be active in the treatment of AIDS-associated cryptococcal meningitis in a pilot dose-response study.[468] Several individual case reports also point to the potential utility of

IFN-γ as adjunctive immunotherapy. It has been reported as adjunctive therapy in combination with GM-CSF or G-CSF and antifungal therapy in two children with scedosporiosis and zygomycosis, as well as in the management of hepatosplenic candidiasis complicating AML, hepatosplenic *Blastoschizomyces capitatus* infection in ALL, and aspergillosis and scedosporiosis in chronic granulomatous disease and normal hosts.[469–471]

Clearly, there is a need for controlled clinical trials to further evaluate the potential adjunctive antimicrobial activity of IFN-γ. If IFN-γ is used in the management of a refractory infection, several caveats bear note. First, IFN-γ may induce fever, thus abrogating a useful marker of therapeutic response, and, second, it should be avoided in allogeneic HSCT recipients unless studied in a clinical trial, as there is a theoretical risk of acceleration of GVHD.

FUTURE DIRECTIONS

Infectious diseases have remained an important cause of morbidity and mortality in children with cancer. Infections may ensue as the result of the primary neoplastic process or the result of antineoplastic therapy. Advances in infectious diseases supportive care have been paramount to improving survival and reducing the suffering of children with cancer over the past 30 years. Despite these advances, new infectious diseases, including those due to multidrug-resistant bacteria, emerging fungal pathogens, and an expanding array of viruses, pose ongoing threats to these achievements and to the lives of our patients.

New antimicrobial agents will need to be developed for safety and efficacy in light of these emerging microbial threats. It is critical that as new drugs are developed, knowledge about their appropriate use in children is obtained. Further understanding of the components and function of the immune system in the "normal" host and how it is affected by cancer and its therapy will continue to inform the best clinical care. Understanding risk factors for infection, spectrum of clinical presentations of infectious disease in different hosts, and the appropriate use of diagnostic tests and therapeutic agents will continue to be challenges in the care of the child with cancer.

With the evolution of new cancer therapies there will continue to be new challenges in the assessment and management of infections in children with cancer. The use of novel chemotherapeutic agents, monoclonal antibodies, and immunomodulators will provide new challenges in the assessment of their impact on the child's immune function and the associated infectious complications. Continued laboratory and clinical investigation through robust translational research are critical to ensuring new advances in infectious diseases supportive care for future pediatric oncology patients.

References

1. Beachey EH. Bacterial adherence: adhesin-receptor interactions mediating the attachment of bacteria to mucosal surface. J Infect Dis 1981;143:325–345.
2. Hawgood S, Brown C, Edmondson J, et al. Pulmonary collectins modulate strain-specific influenza a virus infection and host responses. J Virol 2004;78:8565–8572.
3. Hussain S. Role of surfactant protein A in the innate host defense and autoimmunity. Autoimmunity 2004;37:125–130.
4. Garlanda C, Hirsch E, Bozza S, et al. Non-redundant role of the long pentraxin PTX3 in anti-fungal innate immune response. Nature 2002;420:182–186.
5. Ayabe T, Ashida T, Kohgo Y, et al. The role of Paneth cells and their antimicrobial peptides in innate host defense. Trends Microbiol 2004;12:394–398.
6. De Lucca AJ, Walsh TJ. Antifungal peptides: novel therapeutic compounds against emerging pathogens. Antimicrob Agents Chemother 1999;43:1–11.
7. Lehrer RI. Primate defensins. Nat Rev Microbiol 2004;2:727–738.
8. Lecciones JA, Lee JW, Navarro EE, et al. Vascular catheter-associated fungemia in patients with cancer: analysis of 155 episodes. Clin Infect Dis 1992;14:875–883.
9. Raad II, Hanna HA. Intravascular catheter-related infections: new horizons and recent advances. Arch Intern Med 2002;162:871–878.
10. Salzman MB, Rubin LG. Intravenous catheter-related infections. Adv Pediatr Infect Dis 1995;10:337–368.
11. Hiemenz J, Skelton J, Pizzo PA. Perspective on the management of catheter-related infections in cancer patients. Pediatr Infect Dis 1986;5:6–11.
12. Gaur AH, Liu T, Knapp KM, et al. Infections in children and young adults with bone malignancies undergoing limb-sparing surgery. Cancer 2005;104:602–610.
13. Fux CA, Stoodley P, Hall-Stoodley L, et al. Bacterial biofilms: a diagnostic and therapeutic challenge. Expert Rev Anti Infect Ther 2003;1:667–683.

14. Kuhn DM, Ghannoum MA. Candida biofilms: antifungal resistance and emerging therapeutic options. Curr Opin Investig Drugs 2004;5:186–197.
15. Johanson WG, Pierce AK, Sanford JP. Changing pharyngeal bacterial flora of hospitalized patients. Emergence of gram-negative bacilli. N Engl J Med 1969;281:1137–1140.
16. Johanson WG Jr., Woods DE, Chaudhuri T. Association of respiratory tract colonization with adherence of gram-negative bacilli to epithelial cells. J Infect Dis 1979;139: 667–673.
17. Schimpff SC, Young VM, Greene WH, et al. Origin of infection in acute nonlymphocytic leukemia. Significance of hospital acquisition of potential pathogens. Ann Intern Med 1972;77:707–714.
18. Pizzo PA, Rubin M, Freifeld A, et al. The child with cancer and infection. II. Nonbacterial infections. J Pediatr 1991;119:845–857.
19. Bodey GP, Buckley M, Sathe YS, et al. Quantitative relationships between circulating leukocytes and infection in patients with acute leukemia. Ann Intern Med 1966;64: 328–340.
20. Pizzo PA. After empiric therapy: what to do until the granulocyte comes back. Rev Infect Dis 1987;9:214–219.
21. McCormack RT, Nelson RD, Bloomfield CD, et al. Neutrophil function in lymphoreticular malignancy. Cancer 1979;44:920–926.
22. Pickering LK, Anderson DC, Choi S, et al. Leukocyte function in children with malignancies. Cancer 1975;35:1365–1371.
23. Baehner RL, Neiburger RG, Johnson DE, et al. Transient bactericidal defect of peripheral blood phagocytes from children with acute lymphoblastic leukemia receiving craniospinal irradiation. N Engl J Med 1973;289:1209–1213.
24. Hersh EV, Gutterman JU, Mavligit GM. Effect of haematological malignancies and their treatment on host defence factors. Clin Haematol 1976;5:425–448.
25. Berenguer J, Allende MC, Lee JW, et al. Pathogenesis of pulmonary aspergillosis. Granulocytopenia versus cyclosporine and methylprednisolone-induced immunosuppression. Am J Respir Crit Care Med 1995;152:1079–1086.
26. Lionakis MS, Kontoyiannis DP. Glucocorticoids and invasive fungal infections. Lancet 2003;362:1828–1838.
27. Roilides E, Uhlig K, Venzon D, et al. Prevention of corticosteroid-induced suppression of human polymorphonuclear leukocyte-induced damage of Aspergillus fumigatus hyphae by granulocyte colony-stimulating factor and gamma interferon. Infect Immun 1993;61:4870–4877.
28. Walsh TJ, Roilides E, Cortez K, et al. Control, immunoregulation, and expression of innate pulmonary host defenses against Aspergillus fumigatus. Med Mycol 2005; 43(suppl 1):S165–S172.
29. Akira S, Takeda K. Toll-like receptor signalling. Nat Rev Immunol 2004;4:499–511.
30. Beutler B. Inferences, questions and possibilities in toll-like receptor signalling. Nature 2004;430:257–263.
31. Bochud PY, Chien JW, Marr KA, et al. Toll-like receptor 4 polymorphisms and aspergillosis in stem-cell transplantation. N Engl J Med 2008;359:1766–1777.
32. Agnese DM, Calvano JE, Hahm SJ, et al. Human toll-like receptor 4 mutations but not CD14 polymorphisms are associated with an increased risk of gram-negative infections. J Infect Dis 2002;186:1522–1525.
33. Van der Graaf CA, Netea MG, Morre SA, et al. Toll-like receptor 4 Asp299Gly/ Thr399Ile polymorphisms are a risk factor for Candida bloodstream infection. Eur Cytokine Netw 2006;17:29–34.
34. Tal G, Mandelberg A, Dalal I, et al. Association between common Toll-like receptor 4 mutations and severe respiratory syncytial virus disease. J Infect Dis 2004;189: 2057–2063.
35. Fahey JL, Scoggins R, Utz JP, et al. Infection, antibody response and gamma globulin components in multiple myeloma and macroglobulinemia. Am J Med 1963;35: 698–707.
36. Watt JP, Wolfson LJ, O'Brien KL, et al. Burden of disease caused by *Haemophilus influenzae* type b in children younger than 5 years: global estimates. Lancet 2009;374: 903–911.
37. O'Brien KL, Wolfson LJ, Watt JP, et al. Burden of disease caused by *Streptococcus pneumoniae* in children younger than 5 years: global estimates. Lancet 2009;374:893–902.
38. Fisher RI, DeVita VT Jr, Bostick F, et al. Persistent immunologic abnormalities in long-term survivors of advanced Hodgkin's disease. Ann Intern Med 1980;92:595–599.
39. Slivnick DJ, Nawrocki JF, Fisher RI. Immunology and cellular biology of Hodgkin's disease. Hematol Oncol Clin North Am 1989;3:205–220.
40. Donaldson SS, Glatstein E, Vosti KL. Bacterial infections in pediatric Hodgkin's disease: relationship to radiotherapy, chemotherapy and splenectomy. Cancer 1978;41: 1949–1958.
41. Hiemenz JW, Greene JN. Special considerations for the patient undergoing allogeneic or autologous bone marrow transplantation. Hematol Oncol Clin North Am 1993;7: 961–1002.
42. Rouse BT, Horohov DW. Immunosuppression in viral infections. Rev Infect Dis 1986;8: 850–873.
43. Mackall CL, Fleisher TA, Brown MR, et al. Age, thymopoiesis, and CD4+ T-lymphocyte regeneration after intensive chemotherapy. N Engl J Med 1995;332:143–149.
44. Rosse WF. The spleen as a filter. N Engl J Med 1987;317:704–706.
45. Eraklis AJ, Kevy SV, Diamond LK, et al. Hazard of overwhelming infection after splenectomy in childhood. N Engl J Med 1967;276:1225–1229.
46. Cavenagh JD, Joseph AE, Dilly S, et al. Splenic sepsis in sickle cell disease. Br J Haematol 1994;86:187–189.
47. Santos JI. Nutrition, infection, and immunocompetence. Infect Dis Clin North Am 1994;8:243–267.
48. Chamberlain JS. Cachexia in cancer—zeroing in on myosin. N Engl J Med 2004;351: 2124–2125.
49. Pizzo PA, Robichaud KJ, Wesley R, et al. Fever in the pediatric and young adult patient with cancer. A prospective study of 1001 episodes. Medicine (Baltimore) 1982;61: 153–165.
50. Sickles EA, Greene WH, Wiernik PH. Clinical presentation of infection in granulocytopenic patients. Arch Intern Med 1975;135:715–719.
51. Dinarello CA. The proinflammatory cytokines interleukin-1 and tumor necrosis factor and treatment of the septic shock syndrome. J Infect Dis 1991;163:1177–1184.
52. Hann I, Viscoli C, Paesmans M, et al. A comparison of outcome from febrile neutropenic episodes in children compared with adults: results from four EORTC studies. International Antimicrobial Therapy Cooperative Group (IATCG) of the European Organization for Research and Treatment of Cancer (EORTC). Br J Haematol 1997;99: 580–588.
53. Safdar N, Fine JP, Maki DG. Meta-analysis: methods for diagnosing intravascular device-related bloodstream infection. Ann Intern Med 2005;142:451–466.
54. Korones DN, Hussong MR, Gullace MA. Routine chest radiography of children with cancer hospitalized for fever and neutropenia: is it really necessary? Cancer 1997;80: 1160–1164.
55. Siegman-Igra Y, Anglim AM, Shapiro DE, et al. Diagnosis of vascular catheter-related bloodstream infection: a meta-analysis. J Clin Microbiol 1997;35:928–936.
56. Talcott JA, Finberg R, Mayer RJ, et al. The medical course of cancer patients with fever and neutropenia. Clinical identification of a low-risk subgroup at presentation. Arch Intern Med 1988;148:2561–2568.
57. Buchanan GR. Approach to treatment of the febrile cancer patient with low-risk neutropenia. Hematol Oncol Clin North Am 1993;7:919–935.
58. Talcott JA, Siegel RD, Finberg R, et al. Risk assessment in cancer patients with fever and neutropenia: a prospective, two-center validation of a prediction rule. J Clin Oncol 1992;10:316–322.
59. Rackoff WR, Gonin R, Robinson C, et al. Predicting the risk of bacteremia in children with fever and neutropenia. J Clin Oncol 1996;14:919–924.
60. Klaassen RJ, Goodman TR, Pham B, et al. "Low-risk" prediction rule for pediatric oncology patients presenting with fever and neutropenia. J Clin Oncol 2000;18: 1012–1019.
61. Gardembas-Pain M, Desablens B, Sensebe L, et al. Home treatment of febrile neutropenia: an empirical oral antibiotic regimen. Ann Oncol 1991;2:485–487.
62. Malik IA, Abbas Z, Karim M. Randomised comparison of oral ofloxacin alone with combination of parenteral antibiotics in neutropenic febrile patients. Lancet 1992;339: 1092–1096.
63. Malik IA, Khan WA, Aziz Z, et al. Self-administered antibiotic therapy for chemotherapy-induced, low-risk febrile neutropenia in patients with nonhematologic neoplasms. Clin Infect Dis 1994;19:522–527.
64. Malik IA, Khan WA, Karim M, et al. Feasibility of outpatient management of fever in cancer patients with low-risk neutropenia: results of a prospective randomized trial. Am J Med 1995;98:224–231.
65. Rubenstein EB, Rolston K, Benjamin RS, et al. Outpatient treatment of febrile episodes in low-risk neutropenic patients with cancer. Cancer 1993;71:3640–3646.
66. Aquino VM, Herrera L, Sandler ES, et al. Feasibility of oral ciprofloxacin for the outpatient management of febrile neutropenia in selected children with cancer. Cancer 2000;88:1710–1714.
67. Paganini HR, Sarkis CM, De Martino MG, et al. Oral administration of cefixime to lower risk febrile neutropenic children with cancer. Cancer 2000;88:2848–2852.
68. Shenep JL, Flynn PM, Baker DK, et al. Oral cefixime is similar to continued intravenous antibiotics in the empirical treatment of febrile neutropenic children with cancer. Clin Infect Dis 2001;32:36–43.
69. Chamilos G, Bamias A, Efstathiou E, et al. Outpatient treatment of low-risk neutropenic fever in cancer patients using oral moxifloxacin. Cancer 2005;103:2629–2635.
70. Freifeld A, Marchigiani D, Walsh T, et al. A double-blind comparison of empirical oral and intravenous antibiotic therapy for low-risk febrile patients with neutropenia during cancer chemotherapy. N Engl J Med 1999;341:305–311.
71. Kern WV, Cometta A, De Bock R, et al. Oral versus intravenous empirical antimicrobial therapy for fever in patients with granulocytopenia who are receiving cancer chemotherapy. International Antimicrobial Therapy Cooperative Group of the European Organization for Research and Treatment of Cancer. N Engl J Med 1999;341: 312–318.
72. Mermel LA, Allon M, Bouza E, et al. Clinical practice guidelines for the diagnosis and management of intravascular catheter-related infection: 2009 Update by the Infectious Diseases Society of America. Clin Infect Dis 2009;49:1–45.
73. Schimpff S, Satterlee W, Young VM, et al. Empiric therapy with carbenicillin and gentamicin for febrile patients with cancer and granulocytopenia. N Engl J Med 1971;284: 1061–1065.
74. Schimpff SC, Gaya H, Klastersky J, et al. Three antibiotic regimens in the treatment of infection in febrile granulocytopenic patients with cancer. The EORTC International Antimicrobial Therapy Project Group. J Infect Dis 1978;137:14–29.
75. Walsh TJ, Schimpff SC. Antibiotic combinations for the empiric treatment of the febrile neutropenic patient. Schweiz Med Wochenschr Suppl 1983;14:58–63.
76. Pizzo PA, Hathorn JW, Hiemenz J, et al. A randomized trial comparing ceftazidime alone with combination antibiotic therapy in cancer patients with fever and neutropenia. N Engl J Med 1986;315:552–558.
77. De Pauw BE, Deresinski SC, Feld R, et al. Ceftazidime compared with piperacillin and tobramycin for the empiric treatment of fever in neutropenic patients with cancer. A multicenter randomized trial. The Intercontinental Antimicrobial Study Group. Ann Intern Med 1994;120:834–844.
78. Ceftazidime combined with a short or long course of amikacin for empirical therapy of gram-negative bacteremia in cancer patients with granulocytopenia. The EORTC International Antimicrobial Therapy Cooperative Group. N Engl J Med 1987;317: 1692–1698.
79. Chen HY, Livermore DM. In-vitro activity of biapenem, compared with imipenem and meropenem, against *Pseudomonas aeruginosa* strains and mutants with known resistance mechanisms. J Antimicrob Chemother 1994;33:949–958.
80. Rubin M, Hathorn JW, Marshall D, et al. Gram-positive infections and the use of vancomycin in 550 episodes of fever and neutropenia. Ann Intern Med 1988;108:30–35.
81. Cometta A, Kern WV, De Bock R, et al. Vancomycin versus placebo for treating persistent fever in patients with neutropenic cancer receiving piperacillin-tazobactam monotherapy. Clin Infect Dis 2003;37:382–389.
82. Biron P, Fuhrmann C, Cure H, et al. Cefepime versus imipenem-cilastatin as empirical monotherapy in 400 febrile patients with short duration neutropenia. CEMIC (Study Group of Infectious Diseases in Cancer). J Antimicrob Chemother 1998;42:511–518.
83. Cherif H, Bjorkholm M, Engervall P, et al. A prospective, randomized study comparing cefepime and imipenem-cilastatin in the empirical treatment of febrile neutropenia in patients treated for haematological malignancies. Scand J Infect Dis 2004;36:593–600.
84. Yahav D, Paul M, Fraser A, et al. Efficacy and safety of cefepime: a systematic review and meta-analysis. Lancet Infect Dis 2007;7:338–348.
85. Information for Healthcare Professionals: Cefepime (marketed as Maxipime). 2009. Available at: http://www.fda.gov/Drugs/DrugSafety/PostmarketDrugSafetyInformationforPatientsandProviders/DrugSafetyInformationforHeathcareProfessionals/ucm167254.htm. Accessed September 2009.
86. Chow JW, Fine MJ, Shlaes DM, et al. Enterobacter bacteremia: clinical features and emergence of antibiotic resistance during therapy. Ann Intern Med 1991;115:585–590.
87. Freifeld AG, Walsh T, Marshall D, et al. Monotherapy for fever and neutropenia in cancer patients: a randomized comparison of ceftazidime versus imipenem. J Clin Oncol 1995;13:165–176.

88. Salata RA, Gebhart RL, Palmer DL, et al. Pneumonia treated with imipenem/cilastatin. Am J Med 1985;78:104–109.
89. Cometta A, Calandra T, Gaya H, et al. Monotherapy with meropenem versus combination therapy with ceftazidime plus amikacin as empiric therapy for fever in granulocytopenic patients with cancer. The International Antimicrobial Therapy Cooperative Group of the European Organization for Research and Treatment of Cancer and the Gruppo Italiano Malattie Ematologiche Maligne dell'Adulto Infection Program. Antimicrob Agents Chemother 1996;40:1108–1115.
90. Lindblad R, Rodjer S, Adriansson M, et al. Empiric monotherapy for febrile neutropenia—a randomized study comparing meropenem with ceftazidime. Scand J Infect Dis 1998;30:237–243.
91. Equivalent efficacies of meropenem and ceftazidime as empirical monotherapy of febrile neutropenic patients. The Meropenem Study Group of Leuven, London and Nijmegen. J Antimicrob Chemother 1995;36:185–200.
92. Denton M, Kerr KG. Microbiological and clinical aspects of infection associated with Stenotrophomonas maltophilia. Clin Microbiol Rev 1998;11:57–80.
93. Trigo Daporta M, Munoz Bellido JL, Garcia-Rodriguez JA. Topoisomerases mutations and fluoroquinolone resistance in Stenotrophomonas maltophilia. Int J Antimicrob Agents 2004;24:520–521.
94. Curran M, Simpson D, Perry C. Ertapenem: a review of its use in the management of bacterial infections. Drugs 2003;63:1855–1878.
95. Hughes WT, Armstrong D, Bodey GP, et al. 2002 guidelines for the use of antimicrobial agents in neutropenic patients with cancer. Clin Infect Dis 2002;34:730–751.
96. Lundstrom TS, Sobel JD. Antibiotics for gram-positive bacterial infections: vancomycin, quinupristin-dalfopristin, linezolid, and daptomycin. Infect Dis Clin North Am 2004;18:651–668, x.
97. Silverman JA, Mortin LI, Vanpraagh AD, et al. Inhibition of daptomycin by pulmonary surfactant: in vitro modeling and clinical impact. J Infect Dis 2005;191:2149–2152.
98. Chien JW, Kucia ML, Salata RA. Use of linezolid, an oxazolidinone, in the treatment of multidrug-resistant gram-positive bacterial infections. Clin Infect Dis 2000;30: 146–151.
99. Rubinstein E, Cammarata S, Oliphant T, et al. Linezolid (PNU-100766) versus vancomycin in the treatment of hospitalized patients with nosocomial pneumonia: a randomized, double-blind, multicenter study. Clin Infect Dis 2001;32:402–412.
100. Stevens DL, Herr D, Lampiris H, et al. Linezolid versus vancomycin for the treatment of methicillin-resistant *Staphylococcus aureus* infections. Clin Infect Dis 2002;34: 1481–1490.
101. Smith PF, Birmingham MC, Noskin GA, et al. Safety, efficacy and pharmacokinetics of linezolid for treatment of resistant Gram-positive infections in cancer patients with neutropenia. Ann Oncol 2003;14:795–801.
102. Eliopoulos GM. Quinupristin-dalfopristin and linezolid: evidence and opinion. Clin Infect Dis 2003;36:473–481.
103. Linden PK, Moellering RC Jr, Wood CA, et al. Treatment of vancomycin-resistant *Enterococcus faecium* infections with quinupristin/dalfopristin. Clin Infect Dis 2001;33: 1816–1823.
104. Hess U, Bohme C, Rey K, et al. Monotherapy with piperacillin/tazobactam versus combination therapy with ceftazidime plus amikacin as an empiric therapy for fever in neutropenic cancer patients. Support Care Cancer 1998;6:402–409.
105. Bohme A, Shah PM, Stille W, et al. Piperacillin/tazobactam versus cefepime as initial empirical antimicrobial therapy in febrile neutropenic patients: a prospective randomized pilot study. Eur J Med Res 1998;3:324–330.
106. Bow EJ, Rotstein C, Noskin GA, et al. A randomized, open-label, multicenter comparative study of the efficacy and safety of piperacillin-tazobactam and cefepime for the empirical treatment of febrile neutropenic episodes in patients with hematologic malignancies. Clin Infect Dis 2006;43:447–459.
107. Adam O, Auperin A, Wilquin F, et al. Treatment with piperacillin-tazobactam and false-positive Aspergillus galactomannan antigen test results for patients with hematological malignancies. Clin Infect Dis 2004;38:917–920.
108. Sulahian A, Touratier S, Ribaud P. False positive test for aspergillus antigenemia related to concomitant administration of piperacillin and tazobactam. N Engl J Med 2003;349: 2366–2367.
109. Chen DK, McGeer A, de Azavedo JC, et al. Decreased susceptibility of *Streptococcus pneumoniae* to fluoroquinolones in Canada. Canadian Bacterial Surveillance Network. N Engl J Med 1999;341:233–239.
110. McWhinney PH, Patel S, Whiley RA, et al. Activities of potential therapeutic and prophylactic antibiotics against blood culture isolates of viridans group streptococci from neutropenic patients receiving ciprofloxacin. Antimicrob Agents Chemother 1993;37: 2493–2495.
111. Kelsey SM, Wood ME, Shaw E, et al. A comparative study of intravenous ciprofloxacin and benzylpenicillin versus netilmicin and piperacillin for the empirical treatment of fever in neutropenic patients. J Antimicrob Chemother 1990;25:149–157.
112. Smith GM, Leyland MJ, Farrell ID, et al. A clinical, microbiological and pharmacokinetic study of ciprofloxacin plus vancomycin as initial therapy of febrile episodes in neutropenic patients. J Antimicrob Chemother 1988;21:647–655.
113. Peacock JE, Herrington DA, Wade JC, et al. Ciprofloxacin plus piperacillin compared with tobramycin plus piperacillin as empirical therapy in febrile neutropenic patients. A randomized, double-blind trial. Ann Intern Med 2002;137:77–87.
114. Hampel B, Hullmann R, Schmidt H. Ciprofloxacin in pediatrics: worldwide clinical experience based on compassionate use—safety report. Pediatr Infect Dis J 1997;16: 127–129; discussion 160–162.
115. Schaad UB, abdus Salam M, Aujard Y, et al. Use of fluoroquinolones in pediatrics: consensus report of an International Society of Chemotherapy commission. Pediatr Infect Dis J 1995;14:1–9.
116. Sobel JD. Imipenem and aztreonam. Infect Dis Clin North Am 1989;3:613–624.
117. Jones PG, Rolston KV, Fainstein V, et al. Aztreonam therapy in neutropenic patients with cancer. Am J Med 1986;81:243–248.
118. Raad II, Whimbey EE, Rolston KV, et al. A comparison of aztreonam plus vancomycin and imipenem plus vancomycin as initial therapy for febrile neutropenic cancer patients. Cancer 1996;77:1386–1394.
119. Adkinson NF Jr, Saxon A, Spence MR, et al. Cross-allergenicity and immunogenicity of aztreonam. Rev Infect Dis 1985;7(suppl 4):S613–S621.
120. Roilides E, Lyman CA, Filioti J, et al. Amphotericin B formulations exert additive antifungal activity in combination with pulmonary alveolar macrophages and polymorphonuclear leukocytes against Aspergillus fumigatus. Antimicrob Agents Chemother 2002;46:1974–1976.
121. Simitsopoulou M, Roilides E, Dotis J, et al. Differential expression of cytokines and chemokines in human monocytes induced by lipid formulations of amphotericin B. Antimicrob Agents Chemother 2005;49:1397–1403.
122. Wright DG, Robichaud KJ, Pizzo PA, et al. Lethal pulmonary reactions associated with the combined use of amphotericin B and leukocyte transfusions. N Engl J Med 1981; 304:1185–1189.
123. Walsh TJ, Seibel NL, Arndt C, et al. Amphotericin B lipid complex in pediatric patients with invasive fungal infections. Pediatr Infect Dis J 1999;18:702–708.
124. Wiley JM, Seibel NL, Walsh TJ. Efficacy and safety of amphotericin B lipid complex in 548 children and adolescents with invasive fungal infections. Pediatr Infect Dis J 2005; 24:167–174.
125. Walsh TJ, Whitcomb P, Piscitelli S, et al. Safety, tolerance, and pharmacokinetics of amphotericin B lipid complex in children with hepatosplenic candidiasis. Antimicrob Agents Chemother 1997;41:1944–1948.
126. Ellis M, Spence D, de Pauw B, et al. An EORTC international multicenter randomized trial (EORTC number 19923) comparing two dosages of liposomal amphotericin B for treatment of invasive aspergillosis. Clin Infect Dis 1998;27:1406–1412.
127. Karp JE, Merz WG. Randomized trial of lipid-based amphotericin B for invasive aspergillosis in neutropenic hosts is an important step forward. Clin Infect Dis 1998;27: 1413–1414.
128. Levine SJ, Walsh TJ, Martinez A, et al. Cardiopulmonary toxicity after liposomal amphotericin B infusion. Ann Intern Med 1991;114:664–666.
129. Walsh TJ, Yeldandi V, McEvoy M, et al. Safety, tolerance, and pharmacokinetics of a small unilamellar liposomal formulation of amphotericin B (AmBisome) in neutropenic patients. Antimicrob Agents Chemother 1998;42:2391–2398.
130. Roden MM, Nelson LD, Knudsen TA, et al. Triad of acute infusion-related reactions associated with liposomal amphotericin B: analysis of clinical and epidemiological characteristics. Clin Infect Dis 2003;36:1213–1220.
131. White MH, Anaissie EJ, Kusne S, et al. Amphotericin B colloidal dispersion vs. amphotericin B as therapy for invasive aspergillosis. Clin Infect Dis 1997;24:635–642.
132. Rex JH, Walsh TJ. Estimating the true cost of amphotericin B. Clin Infect Dis 1999;29: 1408–1410.
133. Lee JW, Seibel NL, Amantea M, et al. Safety and pharmacokinetics of fluconazole in children with neoplastic diseases. J Pediatr 1992;120:987–993.
134. Arndt CA, Walsh TJ, McCully CL, et al. Fluconazole penetration into cerebrospinal fluid: implications for treating fungal infections of the central nervous system. J Infect Dis 1988;157:178–180.
135. Berenguer J, Ali NM, Allende MC, et al. Itraconazole for experimental pulmonary aspergillosis: comparison with amphotericin B, interaction with cyclosporin A, and correlation between therapeutic response and itraconazole concentrations in plasma. Antimicrob Agents Chemother 1994;38:1303–1308.
136. Groll AH, Wood L, Roden M, et al. Safety, pharmacokinetics, and pharmacodynamics of cyclodextrin itraconazole in pediatric patients with oropharyngeal candidiasis. Antimicrob Agents Chemother 2002;46:2554–2563.
137. Walsh TJ, Karlsson MO, Driscoll T, et al. Pharmacokinetics and safety of intravenous voriconazole in children after single- or multiple-dose administration. Antimicrob Agents Chemother 2004;48:2166–2172.
138. Walsh TJ, Lutsar I, Driscoll T, et al. Voriconazole in the treatment of aspergillosis, scedosporiosis and other invasive fungal infections in children. Pediatr Infect Dis J 2002; 21:240–248.
139. Walsh TJ, Petraitis V, Petraitiene R, et al. Experimental pulmonary aspergillosis due to Aspergillus terreus: pathogenesis and treatment of an emerging fungal pathogen resistant to amphotericin B. J Infect Dis 2003;188:305–319.
140. Herbrecht R, Denning DW, Patterson TF, et al. Voriconazole versus amphotericin B for primary therapy of invasive aspergillosis. N Engl J Med 2002;347:408–415.
141. Steinbach WJ, Benjamin DK Jr, Kontoyiannis DP, et al. Infections due to Aspergillus terreus: a multicenter retrospective analysis of 83 cases. Clin Infect Dis 2004;39:192–198.
142. Denning DW, Ribaud P, Milpied N, et al. Efficacy and safety of voriconazole in the treatment of acute invasive aspergillosis. Clin Infect Dis 2002;34:563–571.
143. Walsh TJ, Pappas P, Winston DJ, et al. Voriconazole compared with liposomal amphotericin B for empirical antifungal therapy in patients with neutropenia and persistent fever. N Engl J Med 2002;346:225–234.
144. Maertens J, Raad I, Petrikkos G, et al. Efficacy and safety of caspofungin for treatment of invasive aspergillosis in patients refractory to or intolerant of conventional antifungal therapy. Clin Infect Dis 2004;39:1563–1571.
145. Mora-Duarte J, Betts R, Rotstein C, et al. Comparison of caspofungin and amphotericin B for invasive candidiasis. N Engl J Med 2002;347:2020–2029.
146. Franklin JA, McCormick J, Flynn PM. Retrospective study of the safety of caspofungin in immunocompromised pediatric patients. Pediatr Infect Dis J 2003;22:747–749.
147. Walsh TJ, Adamson PC, Seibel NL, et al. Pharmacokinetics, safety, and tolerability of caspofungin in children and adolescents. Antimicrob Agents Chemother 2005;49: 4536–4545.
148. Odio CM, Araya R, Pinto LE, et al. Caspofungin therapy of neonates with invasive candidiasis. Pediatr Infect Dis J 2004;23:1093–1097.
149. van Burik JA, Ratanatharathorn V, Stepan DE, et al. Micafungin versus fluconazole for prophylaxis against invasive fungal infections during neutropenia in patients undergoing hematopoietic stem cell transplantation. Clin Infect Dis 2004;39:1407–1416.
150. Krause DS, Reinhardt J, Vazquez JA, et al. Phase 2, randomized, dose-ranging study evaluating the safety and efficacy of anidulafungin in invasive candidiasis and candidemia. Antimicrob Agents Chemother 2004;48:2021–2024.
151. Petraitis V, Petraitiene R, Hope WW, et al. Combination therapy in treatment of experimental pulmonary aspergillosis: in vitro and in vivo correlations of the concentration- and dose-dependent interactions between anidulafungin and voriconazole by Bliss independence drug interaction analysis. Antimicrob Agents Chemother 2009;53: 2382–2391.
152. Seibel NL, Schwartz C, Arrieta A, et al. Safety, tolerability, and pharmacokinetics of Micafungin (FK463) in febrile neutropenic pediatric patients. Antimicrob Agents Chemother 2005;49:3317–3324.
153. Benjamin DK Jr, Driscoll T, Seibel NL, et al. Safety and pharmacokinetics of intravenous anidulafungin in children with neutropenia at high risk for invasive fungal infections. Antimicrob Agents Chemother 2006;50:632–638.
154. Petraitis V, Petraitiene R, Sarafandi AA, et al. Combination therapy in treatment of experimental pulmonary aspergillosis: synergistic interaction between an antifungal triazole and an echinocandin. J Infect Dis 2003;187:1834–1843.
155. Kirkpatrick WR, Perea S, Coco BJ, et al. Efficacy of caspofungin alone and in combination with voriconazole in a Guinea pig model of invasive aspergillosis. Antimicrob Agents Chemother 2002;46:2564–2568.
156. Meyers JD, Wade JC, Mitchell CD, et al. Multicenter collaborative trial of intravenous acyclovir for treatment of mucocutaneous herpes simplex virus infection in the immunocompromised host. Am J Med 1982;73:229–235.

157. Saral R, Burns WH, Laskin OL, et al. Acyclovir prophylaxis of herpes-simplex-virus infections. N Engl J Med 1981;305:63–67.
158. Wade JC, Newton B, Flournoy N, et al. Oral acyclovir for prevention of herpes simplex virus reactivation after marrow transplantation. Ann Intern Med 1984;100:823–828.
159. Ljungman P, de La Camara R, Milpied N, et al. Randomized study of valacyclovir as prophylaxis against cytomegalovirus reactivation in recipients of allogeneic bone marrow transplants. Blood 2002;99:3050–3056.
160. Meyers JD, Reed EC, Shepp DH, et al. Acyclovir for prevention of cytomegalovirus infection and disease after allogeneic marrow transplantation. N Engl J Med 1988;318:70–75.
161. Prentice HG, Gluckman E, Powles RL, et al. Impact of long-term acyclovir on cytomegalovirus infection and survival after allogeneic bone marrow transplantation. European Acyclovir for CMV Prophylaxis Study Group. Lancet 1994;343:749–753.
162. Balfour HH Jr, Bean B, Laskin OL, et al. Acyclovir halts progression of herpes zoster in immunocompromised patients. N Engl J Med 1983;308:1448–1453.
163. Goodrich JM, Bowden RA, Fisher L, et al. Ganciclovir prophylaxis to prevent cytomegalovirus disease after allogeneic marrow transplant. Ann Intern Med 1993;118:173–178.
164. Winston DJ, Ho WG, Bartoni K, et al. Ganciclovir prophylaxis of cytomegalovirus infection and disease in allogeneic bone marrow transplant recipients. Results of a placebo-controlled, double-blind trial. Ann Intern Med 1993;118:179–184.
165. Boeckh M, Gooley TA, Myerson D, et al. Cytomegalovirus pp65 antigenemia-guided early treatment with ganciclovir versus ganciclovir at engraftment after allogeneic marrow transplantation: a randomized double-blind study. Blood 1996;88:4063–4071.
166. Einsele H, Ehninger G, Hebart H, et al. Polymerase chain reaction monitoring reduces the incidence of cytomegalovirus disease and the duration and side effects of antiviral therapy after bone marrow transplantation. Blood 1995;86:2815–2820.
167. Freeman RB. Valganciclovir: oral prevention and treatment of cytomegalovirus in the immunocompromised host. Expert Opin Pharmacother 2004;5:2007–2016.
168. Reusser P, Einsele H, Lee J, et al. Randomized multicenter trial of foscarnet versus ganciclovir for preemptive therapy of cytomegalovirus infection after allogeneic stem cell transplantation. Blood 2002;99:1159–1164.
169. Eksborg S, Pal N, Kalin M, et al. Pharmacokinetics of acyclovir in immunocompromised children with leukopenia and mucositis after chemotherapy: can intravenous acyclovir be substituted by oral valacyclovir? Med Pediatr Oncol 2002;38:240–246.
170. Nadal D, Leverger G, Sokal EM, et al. An investigation of the steady-state pharmacokinetics of oral valacyclovir in immunocompromised children. J Infect Dis 2002;186(suppl 1):S123–S130.
171. Hoffman JA, Shah AJ, Ross LA, et al. Adenoviral infections and a prospective trial of cidofovir in pediatric hematopoietic stem cell transplantation. Biol Blood Marrow Transplant 2001;7:388–394.
172. Ljungman P, Deliliers GL, Platzbecker U, et al. Cidofovir for cytomegalovirus infection and disease in allogeneic stem cell transplant recipients. The Infectious Diseases Working Party of the European Group for Blood and Marrow Transplantation. Blood 2001;97:388–392.
173. Ljungman P, Ribaud P, Eyrich M, et al. Cidofovir for adenovirus infections after allogeneic hematopoietic stem cell transplantation: a survey by the Infectious Diseases Working Party of the European Group for Blood and Marrow Transplantation. Bone Marrow Transplant 2003;31:481–486.
174. Krilov LR. Safety issues related to the administration of ribavirin. Pediatr Infect Dis J 2002;21:479–481.
175. Hall CB, McBride JT, Walsh EE, et al. Aerosolized ribavirin treatment of infants with respiratory syncytial viral infection. A randomized double-blind study. N Engl J Med 1983;308:1443–1447.
176. Meert KL, Sarnaik AP, Gelmini MJ, et al. Aerosolized ribavirin in mechanically ventilated children with respiratory syncytial virus lower respiratory tract disease: a prospective, double-blind, randomized trial. Crit Care Med 1994;22:566–572.
177. Wheeler JG, Wofford J, Turner RB. Historical cohort evaluation of ribavirin efficacy in respiratory syncytial virus infection. Pediatr Infect Dis J 1993;12:209–213.
178. Reassessment of the indications for ribavirin therapy in respiratory syncytial virus infections. American Academy of Pediatrics Committee on Infectious Diseases. Pediatrics 1996;97:137–140.
179. Harrington RD, Hooton TM, Hackman RC, et al. An outbreak of respiratory syncytial virus in a bone marrow transplant center. J Infect Dis 1992;165:987–993.
180. Khushalani NI, Bakri FG, Wentling D, et al. Respiratory syncytial virus infection in the late bone marrow transplant period: report of three cases and review. Bone Marrow Transplant 2001;27:1071–1073.
181. Whimbey E, Champlin RE, Englund JA, et al. Combination therapy with aerosolized ribavirin and intravenous immunoglobulin for respiratory syncytial virus disease in adult bone marrow transplant recipients. Bone Marrow Transplant 1995;16:393–399.
182. Gutfreund KS, Bain VG. Chronic viral hepatitis C: management update. CMAJ 2000;162:827–833.
183. Boyer N, Marcellin P. Pathogenesis, diagnosis and management of hepatitis C. J Hepatol 2000;32:98–112.
184. Palivizumab, a humanized respiratory syncytial virus monoclonal antibody, reduces hospitalization from respiratory syncytial virus infection in high-risk infants. The IMpact-RSV Study Group. Pediatrics 1998;102:531–537.
185. Boeckh M, Berrey MM, Bowden RA, et al. Phase 1 evaluation of the respiratory syncytial virus-specific monoclonal antibody palivizumab in recipients of hematopoietic stem cell transplants. J Infect Dis 2001;184:350–354.
186. Rodriguez WJ, Gruber WC, Groothuis JR, et al. Respiratory syncytial virus immune globulin treatment of RSV lower respiratory tract infection in previously healthy children. Pediatrics 1997;100:937–942.
187. American Academy of Pediatrics Subcommittee on Diagnosis and Management of Bronchiolitis. Diagnosis and management of bronchiolitis. Pediatrics 2006;118:1774–1793.
188. Chavez-Bueno S, Mejias A, Merryman RA, et al. Intravenous palivizumab and ribavirin combination for respiratory syncytial virus disease in high-risk pediatric patients. Pediatr Infect Dis J 2007;26:1089–1093.
189. Whimbey E, Englund JA, Couch RB. Community respiratory virus infections in immunocompromised patients with cancer. Am J Med 1997;102:10–18; discussion 25–26.
190. Douglas RG Jr. Prophylaxis and treatment of influenza. N Engl J Med 1990;322:443–450.
191. Hayden FG, Belshe RB, Clover RD, et al. Emergence and apparent transmission of rimantadine-resistant influenza A virus in families. N Engl J Med 1989;321:1696–1702.
192. Hayden FG, Osterhaus AD, Treanor JJ, et al. Efficacy and safety of the neuraminidase inhibitor zanamivir in the treatment of influenzavirus infections. GG167 Influenza Study Group. N Engl J Med 1997;337:874–880.
193. Treanor JJ, Hayden FG, Vrooman PS, et al. Efficacy and safety of the oral neuraminidase inhibitor oseltamivir in treating acute influenza: a randomized controlled trial. US Oral Neuraminidase Study Group. JAMA 2000;283:1016–1024.
194. Hedrick JA, Barzilai A, Behre U, et al. Zanamivir for treatment of symptomatic influenza A and B infection in children five to twelve years of age: a randomized controlled trial. Pediatr Infect Dis J 2000;19:410–417.
195. Nichols WG, Guthrie KA, Corey L, et al. Influenza infections after hematopoietic stem cell transplantation: risk factors, mortality, and the effect of antiviral therapy. Clin Infect Dis 2004;39:1300–1306.
196. Kiso M, Mitamura K, Sakai-Tagawa Y, et al. Resistant influenza A viruses in children treated with oseltamivir: descriptive study. Lancet 2004;364:759–765.
197. Hurt AC, Barr IG, Durrant CJ, et al. Surveillance for neuraminidase inhibitor resistance in human influenza viruses from Australia. Commun Dis Intell 2003;27:542–547.
198. Hughes WT. Five-year absence of *Pneumocystis carinii* pneumonitis in a pediatric oncology center. J Infect Dis 1984;150:305–306.
199. Hughes WT. Use of dapsone in the prevention and treatment of *Pneumocystis carinii* pneumonia: a review. Clin Infect Dis 1998;27:191–204.
200. Gupta M, Stephenson K, Gauar S, et al. Intravenous pentamidine as an alternate for *Pneumocystis carinii* pneumonia prophylaxis in children with HIV infection. Pediatr Pulmonol Suppl 1997;16:199–200.
201. Hughes W, Leoung G, Kramer F, et al. Comparison of atovaquone (566C80) with trimethoprim-sulfamethoxazole to treat *Pneumocystis carinii* pneumonia in patients with AIDS. N Engl J Med 1993;328:1521–1527.
202. Hughes W, Dorenbaum A, Yogev R, et al. Phase I safety and pharmacokinetics study of micronized atovaquone in human immunodeficiency virus-infected infants and children. Pediatric AIDS Clinical Trials Group. Antimicrob Agents Chemother 1998;42:1315–1318.
203. Mullen CA, Petropoulos D, Roberts WM, et al. Outpatient treatment of fever and neutropenia for low risk pediatric cancer patients. Cancer 1999;86:126–134.
204. Pizzo PA, Robichaud KJ, Gill FA, et al. Duration of empiric antibiotic therapy in granulocytopenic patients with cancer. Am J Med 1979;67:194–200.
205. Pizzo PA, Robichaud KJ, Gill FA, et al. Empiric antibiotic and antifungal therapy for cancer patients with prolonged fever and granulocytopenia. Am J Med 1982;72:101–11.
206. Empiric antifungal therapy in febrile granulocytopenic patients. EORTC International Antimicrobial Therapy Cooperative Group. Am J Med 1989;86:668–672.
207. Walsh TJ, Finberg RW, Arndt C, et al. Liposomal amphotericin B for empirical therapy in patients with persistent fever and neutropenia. National Institute of Allergy and Infectious Diseases Mycoses Study Group. N Engl J Med 1999;340:764–771.
208. Prentice HG, Hann IM, Herbrecht R, et al. A randomized comparison of liposomal versus conventional amphotericin B for the treatment of pyrexia of unknown origin in neutropenic patients. Br J Haematol 1997;98:711–718.
209. Walsh TJ, Teppler H, Donowitz GR, et al. Caspofungin versus liposomal amphotericin B for empirical antifungal therapy in patients with persistent fever and neutropenia. N Engl J Med 2004;351:1391–1402.
210. Boogaerts M, Winston DJ, Bow EJ, et al. Intravenous and oral itraconazole versus intravenous amphotericin B deoxycholate as empirical antifungal therapy for persistent fever in neutropenic patients with cancer who are receiving broad-spectrum antibacterial therapy. A randomized, controlled trial. Ann Intern Med 2001;135:412–422.
211. Winston DJ, Hathorn JW, Schuster MG, et al. A multicenter, randomized trial of fluconazole versus amphotericin B for empiric antifungal therapy of febrile neutropenic patients with cancer. Am J Med 2000;108:282–289.
212. Bates DW, Su L, Yu DT, et al. Mortality and costs of acute renal failure associated with amphotericin B therapy. Clin Infect Dis 2001;32:686–693.
213. Cagnoni PJ, Walsh TJ, Prendergast MM, et al. Pharmacoeconomic analysis of liposomal amphotericin B versus conventional amphotericin B in the empirical treatment of persistently febrile neutropenic patients. J Clin Oncol 2000;18:2476–2483.
214. Cotton DJ, Gill VJ, Marshall DJ, et al. Clinical features and therapeutic interventions in 17 cases of Bacillus bacteremia in an immunosuppressed patient population. J Clin Microbiol 1987;25:672–674.
215. Kapur D, Dorsky D, Feingold JM, et al. Incidence and outcome of vancomycin-resistant enterococcal bacteremia following autologous peripheral blood stem cell transplantation. Bone Marrow Transplant 2000;25:147–152.
216. Montecalvo MA, Horowitz H, Gedris C, et al. Outbreak of vancomycin-, ampicillin-, and aminoglycoside-resistant *Enterococcus faecium* bacteremia in an adult oncology unit. Antimicrob Agents Chemother 1994;38:1363–1367.
217. Shenep JL. Viridans-group streptococcal infections in immunocompromised hosts. Int J Antimicrob Agents 2000;14:129–135.
218. Gamis AS, Howells WB, DeSwarte-Wallace J, et al. Alpha hemolytic streptococcal infection during intensive treatment for acute myeloid leukemia: a report from the Children's cancer group study CCG-2891. J Clin Oncol 2000;18:1845–1855.
219. Bochud PY, Calandra T, Francioli P. Bacteremia due to viridans streptococci in neutropenic patients: a review. Am J Med 1994;97:256–264.
220. Riikonen P, Saarinen UM, Lahteenoja KM, et al. Management of indwelling central venous catheters in pediatric cancer patients with fever and neutropenia. Scand J Infect Dis 1993;25:357–364.
221. Raad I, Narro J, Khan A, et al. Serious complications of vascular catheter-related *Staphylococcus aureus* bacteremia in cancer patients. Eur J Clin Microbiol Infect Dis 1992;11:675–682.
222. Edmond MB, Wallace SE, McClish DK, et al. Nosocomial bloodstream infections in United States hospitals: a three-year analysis. Clin Infect Dis 1999;29:239–244.
223. Pfaller MA, Diekema DJ, Jones RN, et al. Trends in antifungal susceptibility of *Candida* spp. isolated from pediatric and adult patients with bloodstream infections: SENTRY Antimicrobial Surveillance Program, 1997 to 2000. J Clin Microbiol 2002;40:852–856.
224. Viscoli C, Girmenia C, Marinus A, et al. Candidemia in cancer patients: a prospective, multicenter surveillance study by the Invasive Fungal Infection Group (IFIG) of the European Organization for Research and Treatment of Cancer (EORTC). Clin Infect Dis 1999;28:1071–1079.
225. Wingard JR, Merz WG, Rinaldi MG, et al. Increase in *Candida krusei* infection among patients with bone marrow transplantation and neutropenia treated prophylactically with fluconazole. N Engl J Med 1991;325:1274–1277.
226. Horn DL, Neofytos D, Anaissie EJ, et al. Epidemiology and outcomes of candidemia in 2019 patients: data from the prospective antifungal therapy alliance registry. Clin Infect Dis 2009;48:1695–1703.

227. Bodey GP, Mardani M, Hanna HA, et al. The epidemiology of *Candida glabrata* and *Candida albicans* fungemia in immunocompromised patients with cancer. Am J Med 2002;112:380–385.
228. Kontoyiannis DP, Vaziri I, Hanna HA, et al. Risk factors for *Candida tropicalis* fungemia in patients with cancer. Clin Infect Dis 2001;33:1676–1681.
229. Dick JD, Rosengard BR, Merz WG, et al. Fatal disseminated candidiasis due to amphotericin-B-resistant *Candida guilliermondii*. Ann Intern Med 1985;102:67–68.
230. Merz WG. *Candida lusitaniae*: frequency of recovery, colonization, infection, and amphotericin B resistance. J Clin Microbiol 1984;20:1194–1195.
231. Pappas PG, Rex JH, Sobel JD, et al. Guidelines for treatment of candidiasis. Clin Infect Dis 2004;38:161–189.
232. Nucci M, Anaissie E. Revisiting the source of candidemia: skin or gut? Clin Infect Dis 2001;33:1959–1967.
233. Nucci M, Anaissie E. Should vascular catheters be removed from all patients with candidemia? An evidence-based review. Clin Infect Dis 2002;34:591–599.
234. Walsh TJ, Rex JH. All catheter-related candidemia is not the same: assessment of the balance between the risks and benefits of removal of vascular catheters. Clin Infect Dis 2002;34:600–602.
235. Greene JN. Catheter-related complications of cancer therapy. Infect Dis Clin North Am 1996;10:255–295.
236. Raad II, Vartivarian S, Khan A, et al. Catheter-related infections caused by the Mycobacterium fortuitum complex: 15 cases and review. Rev Infect Dis 1991;13: 1120–1125.
237. Slack CL, Watson DW, Abzug MJ, et al. Fungal mastoiditis in immunocompromised children. Arch Otolaryngol Head Neck Surg 1999;125:73–75.
238. Carfrae MJ, Kesser BW. Malignant otitis externa. Otolaryngol Clin North Am 2008;41: 537–549, viii–ix.
239. Wald ER, Milmoe GJ, Bowen A, et al. Acute maxillary sinusitis in children. N Engl J Med 1981;304:749–754.
240. Robinson MR, Fine HF, Ross ML, et al. Sino-orbital-cerebral aspergillosis in immunocompromised pediatric patients. Pediatr Infect Dis J 2000;19:1197–1203.
241. Berkow RL, Weisman SJ, Provisor AJ, et al. Invasive aspergillosis of paranasal tissues in children with malignancies. J Pediatr 1983;103:49–53.
242. Diament MJ. The diagnosis of sinusitis in infants and children: x-ray, computed tomography, and magnetic resonance imaging. Diagnostic imaging of pediatric sinusitis. J Allergy Clin Immunol 1992;90:442–444.
243. Wald ER. Antimicrobial therapy of pediatric patients with sinusitis. J Allergy Clin Immunol 1992;90:469–473.
244. Kontoyiannis DP, Lionakis MS, Lewis RE, et al. Zygomycosis in a tertiary-care cancer center in the era of Aspergillus-active antifungal therapy: a case-control observational study of 27 recent cases. J Infect Dis 2005;191:1350–1360.
245. Heussel CP, Kauczor HU, Heussel GE, et al. Pneumonia in febrile neutropenic patients and in bone marrow and blood stem-cell transplant recipients: use of high-resolution computed tomography. J Clin Oncol 1999;17:796–805.
246. Kim MJ, Lee KS, Kim J, et al. Crescent sign in invasive pulmonary aspergillosis: frequency and related CT and clinical factors. J Comput Assist Tomogr 2001;25:305–310.
247. Kuhlman JE, Fishman EK, Siegelman SS. Invasive pulmonary aspergillosis in acute leukemia: characteristic findings on CT, the CT halo sign, and the role of CT in early diagnosis. Radiology 1985;157:611–614.
248. Walsh TJ, Garrett K, Feurerstein E, et al. Therapeutic monitoring of experimental invasive pulmonary aspergillosis by ultrafast computerized tomography, a novel, noninvasive method for measuring responses to antifungal therapy. Antimicrob Agents Chemother 1995;39:1065–1069.
249. Forrest GN, Walsh TJ. Approaches to management of invasive fungal infections in patients with hematologic malignancies. Support Cancer Ther 2004;2:21–30.
250. Huaringa AJ, Leyva FJ, Signes-Costa J, et al. Bronchoalveolar lavage in the diagnosis of pulmonary complications of bone marrow transplant patients. Bone Marrow Transplant 2000;25:975–979.
251. Wheat LJ, Garringer T, Brizendine E, et al. Diagnosis of histoplasmosis by antigen detection based upon experience at the histoplasmosis reference laboratory. Diagn Microbiol Infect Dis 2002;43:29–37.
252. American Thoracic Society, CDC, and Infectious Diseases Society of America. Treatment of tuberculosis. MMWR Recomm Rep 2003;52:1–77.
253. Andersen RD, Lauer BA, Fraser DW, et al. Infections with *Legionella pneumophila* in children. J Infect Dis 1981;143:386–390.
254. Kirby BD, Peck H, Meyer RD. Radiographic features of Legionnaires' disease. Chest 1979;76:562–565.
255. Murdoch DR. Diagnosis of Legionella infection. Clin Infect Dis 2003;36:64–69.
256. Birtles RJ, Harrison TG, Samuel D, et al. Evaluation of urinary antigen ELISA for diagnosing *Legionella pneumophila* serogroup 1 infection. J Clin Pathol 1990;43:685–690.
257. Torres HA, Reddy BT, Raad II, et al. Nocardiosis in cancer patients. Medicine (Baltimore) 2002;81:388–397.
258. Smego RA Jr, Gallis HA. The clinical spectrum of Nocardia brasiliensis infection in the United States. Rev Infect Dis 1984;6:164–180.
259. Alangaden GJ, Wahiduzzaman M, Chandrasekar PH. Aspergillosis: the most common community-acquired pneumonia with gram-negative Bacilli as copathogens in stem cell transplant recipients with graft-versus-host disease. Clin Infect Dis 2002;35:659–664.
260. Marr KA, Carter RA, Boeckh M, et al. Invasive aspergillosis in allogeneic stem cell transplant recipients: changes in epidemiology and risk factors. Blood 2002;100: 4358–4366.
261. Commers JR, Robichaud KJ, Pizzo PA. New pulmonary infiltrates in granulocytopenic cancer patients being treated with antibiotics. Pediatr Infect Dis 1984;3:423–428.
262. Young RC, Bennett JE, Vogel CL, et al. Aspergillosis. The spectrum of the disease in 98 patients. Medicine (Baltimore) 1970;49:147–173.
263. Walsh TJ, Groll A, Hiemenz J, et al. Infections due to emerging and uncommon medically important fungal pathogens. Clin Microbiol Infect 2004;10(suppl 1):48–66.
264. Haron E, Vartivarian S, Anaissie E, et al. Primary Candida pneumonia. Experience at a large cancer center and review of the literature. Medicine (Baltimore) 1993;72: 137–142.
265. Allende M, Pizzo PA, Horowitz M, et al. Pulmonary cryptococcosis presenting as metastases in children with sarcomas. Pediatr Infect Dis J 1993;12:240–243.
266. Kauffman CA, Israel KS, Smith JW, et al. Histoplasmosis in immunosuppressed patients. Am J Med 1978;64:923–932.
267. Herbrecht R, Letscher-Bru V, Oprea C, et al. Aspergillus galactomannan detection in the diagnosis of invasive aspergillosis in cancer patients. J Clin Oncol 2002;20: 1898–1906.
268. Maertens J, Van Eldere J, Verhaegen J, et al. Use of circulating galactomannan screening for early diagnosis of invasive aspergillosis in allogeneic stem cell transplant recipients. J Infect Dis 2002;186:1297–1306.
269. Marr KA, Balajee SA, McLaughlin L, et al. Detection of galactomannan antigenemia by enzyme immunoassay for the diagnosis of invasive aspergillosis: variables that affect performance. J Infect Dis 2004;190:641–649.
270. Boutboul F, Alberti C, Leblanc T, et al. Invasive aspergillosis in allogeneic stem cell transplant recipients: increasing antigenemia is associated with progressive disease. Clin Infect Dis 2002;34:939–943.
271. Petraitiene R, Petraitis V, Groll AH, et al. Antifungal activity and pharmacokinetics of posaconazole (SCH 56592) in treatment and prevention of experimental invasive pulmonary aspergillosis: correlation with galactomannan antigenemia. Antimicrob Agents Chemother 2001;45:857–869.
272. Ascioglu S, Rex JH, de Pauw B, et al. Defining opportunistic invasive fungal infections in immunocompromised patients with cancer and hematopoietic stem cell transplants: an international consensus. Clin Infect Dis 2002;34:7–14.
273. Walsh TJ, Groll AH. Overview: non-fumigatus species of Aspergillus: perspectives on emerging pathogens in immunocompromised hosts. Curr Opin Investig Drugs 2001;2: 1366–1367.
274. Panos RJ, Barr LF, Walsh TJ, et al. Factors associated with fatal hemoptysis in cancer patients. Chest 1988;94:1008–1013.
275. Walsh TJ, Goodman JL, Pappas P, et al. Safety, tolerance, and pharmacokinetics of high-dose liposomal amphotericin B (AmBisome) in patients infected with Aspergillus species and other filamentous fungi: maximum tolerated dose study. Antimicrob Agents Chemother 2001;45:3487–3496.
276. Karp JE, Burch PA, Merz WG. An approach to intensive antileukemia therapy in patients with previous invasive aspergillosis. Am J Med 1988;85:203–206.
277. Caillot D, Mannone L, Cuisenier B, et al. Role of early diagnosis and aggressive surgery in the management of invasive pulmonary aspergillosis in neutropenic patients. Clin Microbiol Infect 2001;7(suppl 2):54–61.
278. Salerno CT, Ouyang DW, Pederson TS, et al. Surgical therapy for pulmonary aspergillosis in immunocompromised patients. Ann Thorac Surg 1998;65:1415–1419.
279. Gonzalez CE, Rinaldi MG, Sugar AM. Zygomycosis. Infect Dis Clin North Am 2002; 16:895–914, vi.
280. Gonzalez CE, Couriel DR, Walsh TJ. Disseminated zygomycosis in a neutropenic patient: successful treatment with amphotericin B lipid complex and granulocyte colony-stimulating factor. Clin Infect Dis 1997;24:192–196.
281. Nucci M, Anaissie EJ, Queiroz-Telles F, et al. Outcome predictors of 84 patients with hematologic malignancies and Fusarium infection. Cancer 2003;98:315–319.
282. Edman JC, Kovacs JA, Masur H, et al. Ribosomal RNA sequence shows *Pneumocystis carinii* to be a member of the fungi. Nature 1988;334:519–522.
283. Hughes WT, Kuhn S, Chaudhary S, et al. Successful chemoprophylaxis for *Pneumocystis carinii* pneumonitis. N Engl J Med 1977;297:1419–1426.
284. Gerberding JL. Nosocomial transmission of opportunistic infections. Infect Control Hosp Epidemiol 1998;19:574–577.
285. Kovacs JA, Hiemenz JW, Macher AM, et al. *Pneumocystis carinii* pneumonia: a comparison between patients with the acquired immunodeficiency syndrome and patients with other immunodeficiencies. Ann Intern Med 1984;100:663–671.
286. Kovacs JA, Ng VL, Masur H, et al. Diagnosis of *Pneumocystis carinii* pneumonia: improved detection in sputum with use of monoclonal antibodies. N Engl J Med 1988; 318:589–593.
287. Sepkowitz KA, Brown AE, Telzak EE, et al. *Pneumocystis carinii* pneumonia among patients without AIDS at a cancer hospital. JAMA 1992;267:832–837.
288. Slivka A, Wen PY, Shea WM, et al. *Pneumocystis carinii* pneumonia during steroid taper in patients with primary brain tumors. Am J Med 1993;94:216–219.
289. Leoung GS, Mills J, Hopewell PC, et al. Dapsone-trimethoprim for *Pneumocystis carinii* pneumonia in the acquired immunodeficiency syndrome. Ann Intern Med 1986; 105:45–48.
290. Toma E, Thorne A, Singer J, et al. Clindamycin with primaquine vs. trimethoprim-sulfamethoxazole therapy for mild and moderately severe *Pneumocystis carinii* pneumonia in patients with AIDS: a multicenter, double-blind, randomized trial (CTN 004). CTN-PCP Study Group. Clin Infect Dis 1998;27:524–530.
291. Dohn MN, Weinberg WG, Torres RA, et al. Oral atovaquone compared with intravenous pentamidine for *Pneumocystis carinii* pneumonia in patients with AIDS. Atovaquone Study Group. Ann Intern Med 1994;121:174–180.
292. Bozzette SA, Sattler FR, Chiu J, et al. A controlled trial of early adjunctive treatment with corticosteroids for *Pneumocystis carinii* pneumonia in the acquired immunodeficiency syndrome. California Collaborative Treatment Group. N Engl J Med 1990;323: 1451–1457.
293. Gagnon S, Boota AM, Fischl MA, et al. Corticosteroids as adjunctive therapy for severe *Pneumocystis carinii* pneumonia in the acquired immunodeficiency syndrome. A double-blind, placebo-controlled trial. N Engl J Med 1990;323:1444–1450.
294. Hammerschlag MR. *Chlamydia trachomatis* and *Chlamydia pneumoniae* infections in children and adolescents. Pediatr Rev 2004;25:43–51.
295. Waites KB, Talkington DF. *Mycoplasma pneumoniae* and its role as a human pathogen. Clin Microbiol Rev 2004;17:697–728, table of contents.
296. Miyashita N, Saito A, Kohno S, et al. Multiplex PCR for the simultaneous detection of *Chlamydia pneumoniae*, *Mycoplasma pneumoniae* and *Legionella pneumophila* in community-acquired pneumonia. Respir Med 2004;98:542–550.
297. Wingard JR, Piantadosi S, Burns WH, et al. Cytomegalovirus infections in bone marrow transplant recipients given intensive cytoreductive therapy. Rev Infect Dis 1990; 12(suppl 7):S793–S804.
298. Ljungman P, Brand R, Einsele H, et al. Donor CMV serologic status and outcome of CMV-seropositive recipients after unrelated donor stem cell transplantation: an EBMT megafile analysis. Blood 2003;102:4255–4260.
299. Nichols WG, Corey L, Gooley T, et al. High risk of death due to bacterial and fungal infection among cytomegalovirus (CMV)-seronegative recipients of stem cell transplants from seropositive donors: evidence for indirect effects of primary CMV infection. J Infect Dis 2002;185:273–282.
300. Nichols WG, Corey L, Gooley T, et al. Rising pp65 antigenemia during preemptive anticytomegalovirus therapy after allogeneic hematopoietic stem cell transplantation: risk factors, correlation with DNA load, and outcomes. Blood 2001;97:867–874.
301. Emanuel D, Cunningham I, Jules-Elysee K, et al. Cytomegalovirus pneumonia after bone marrow transplantation successfully treated with the combination of ganciclovir and high-dose intravenous immune globulin. Ann Intern Med 1988;109:777–782.
302. Reed EC, Bowden RA, Dandliker PS, et al. Treatment of cytomegalovirus pneumonia with ganciclovir and intravenous cytomegalovirus immunoglobulin in patients with bone marrow transplants. Ann Intern Med 1988;109:783–788.
303. Locksley RM, Flournoy N, Sullivan KM, et al. Infection with varicella-zoster virus after marrow transplantation. J Infect Dis 1985;152:1172–1181.

304. Hale GA, Heslop HE, Krance RA, et al. Adenovirus infection after pediatric bone marrow transplantation. Bone Marrow Transplant 1999;23:277–282.
305. Wendt CH, Weisdorf DJ, Jordan MC, et al. Parainfluenza virus respiratory infection after bone marrow transplantation. N Engl J Med 1992;326:921–926.
306. Perez-Padilla R, de la Rosa-Zamboni D, Ponce de Leon S, et al. Pneumonia and respiratory failure from swine-origin influenza A (H1N1) in Mexico. N Engl J Med 2009;361(7):680–689.
307. Hancock K, Veguilla V, Lu X, et al. Cross-reactive antibody responses to the 2009 pandemic H1N1 influenza virus. N Engl J Med 2009;361(20):1945–1952.
308. Jamieson DJ, Honein MA, Rasmussen SA, et al. H1N1 2009 influenza virus infection during pregnancy in the USA. Lancet 2009;374:451–458.
309. Centers for Disease Control and Prevention (CDC). Update on influenza A (H1N1) 2009 monovalent vaccines. MMWR Morb Mortal Wkly Rep 2009;58:1100–1111.
310. Centers for Disease Control and Prevention (CDC). Update: drug susceptibility of swine-origin influenza A (H1N1) viruses, April 2009. MMWR Morb Mortal Wkly Rep 2009;58:433–435.
311. Westling K, Ljungman P, Thalme A, et al. *Streptococcus viridans* septicaemia: a comparison study in patients admitted to the departments of infectious diseases and haematology in a university hospital. Scand J Infect Dis 2002;34:316–319.
312. Martino P, Micozzi A, Venditti M, et al. Catheter-related right-sided endocarditis in bone marrow transplant recipients. Rev Infect Dis 1990;12:250–257.
313. Mullen P, Jude C, Borkon M, et al. Aspergillus mural endocarditis. Clinical and echocardiographic diagnosis. Chest 1986;90:451–452.
314. Rubinstein E, Noriega ER, Simberkoff MS, et al. Fungal endocarditis: analysis of 24 cases and review of the literature. Medicine (Baltimore) 1975;54:331–334.
315. Johnston PG, Lee J, Domanski M, et al. Late recurrent Candida endocarditis. Chest 1991;99:1531–1533.
316. Walsh TJ, Bulkley BH. Aspergillus pericarditis: clinical and pathologic features in the immunocompromised patient. Cancer 1982;49:48–54.
317. Le Moing V, Lortholary O, Timsit JF, et al. Aspergillus pericarditis with tamponade: report of a successfully treated case and review. Clin Infect Dis 1998;26:451–460.
318. Groll AH, Just-Nuebling G, Kurz M, et al. Fluconazole versus nystatin in the prevention of candida infections in children and adolescents undergoing remission induction or consolidation chemotherapy for cancer. J Antimicrob Chemother 1997;40:855–862.
319. Peterson DE, Minah GE, Overholser CD, et al. Microbiology of acute periodontal infection in myelosuppressed cancer patients. J Clin Oncol 1987;5:1461–1468.
320. Parenti DM, Snydman DR. Capnocytophaga species: infections in nonimmunocompromised and immunocompromised hosts. J Infect Dis 1985;151:140–147.
321. Krause DS, Simjee AE, van Rensburg C, et al. A randomized, double-blind trial of anidulafungin versus fluconazole for the treatment of esophageal candidiasis. Clin Infect Dis 2004;39:770–775.
322. Petraitis V, Petraitiene R, Groll AH, et al. Dosage-dependent antifungal efficacy of V-echinocandin (LY303366) against experimental fluconazole-resistant oropharyngeal and esophageal candidiasis. Antimicrob Agents Chemother 2001;45:471–479.
323. Sloas MM, Flynn PM, Kaste SC, et al. Typhlitis in children with cancer: a 30-year experience. Clin Infect Dis 1993;17:484–490.
324. Kirkpatrick ID, Greenberg HM. Gastrointestinal complications in the neutropenic patient: characterization and differentiation with abdominal CT. Radiology 2003;226: 668–674.
325. Shamberger RC, Weinstein HJ, Delorey MJ, et al. The medical and surgical management of typhlitis in children with acute nonlymphocytic (myelogenous) leukemia. Cancer 1986;57:603–609.
326. Larson HE, Price AB, Honour P, et al. *Clostridium difficile* and the aetiology of pseudomembranous colitis. Lancet 1978;1:1063–1066.
327. Bartlett JG, Chang TW, Gurwith M, et al. Antibiotic-associated pseudomembranous colitis due to toxin-producing clostridia. N Engl J Med 1978;298:531–534.
328. McFarland LV, Mulligan ME, Kwok RY, et al. Nosocomial acquisition of *Clostridium difficile* infection. N Engl J Med 1989;320:204–210.
329. Doern GV, Coughlin RT, Wu L. Laboratory diagnosis of *Clostridium difficile*-associated gastrointestinal disease: comparison of a monoclonal antibody enzyme immunoassay for toxins A and B with a monoclonal antibody enzyme immunoassay for toxin A only and two cytotoxicity assays. J Clin Microbiol 1992;30:2042–2046.
330. Roghmann MC, McCarter RJ Jr, Brewrink J, et al. *Clostridium difficile* infection is a risk factor for bacteremia due to vancomycin-resistant enterococci (VRE) in VRE-colonized patients with acute leukemia. Clin Infect Dis 1997;25:1056–1059.
331. Bolton RP, Culshaw MA. Faecal metronidazole concentrations during oral and intravenous therapy for antibiotic associated colitis due to *Clostridium difficile*. Gut 1986; 27:1169–1172.
332. Bodey GP, Rodriguez S, Fainstein V, et al. Clostridial bacteremia in cancer patients. A 12-year experience. Cancer 1991;67:1928–1942.
333. Thaler M, Gill V, Pizzo PA. Emergence of *Clostridium tertium* as a pathogen in neutropenic patients. Am J Med 1986;81:596–600.
334. Igra-Siegman Y, Kapila R, Sen P, et al. Syndrome of hyperinfection with *Strongyloides stercoralis*. Rev Infect Dis 1981;3:397–407.
335. Liu LX, Weller PF. Strongyloidiasis and other intestinal nematode infections. Infect Dis Clin North Am 1993;7:655–682.
336. Keiser PB, Nutman TB. *Strongyloides stercoralis* in the immunocompromised population. Clin Microbiol Rev 2004;17:208–217.
337. American Academy of Pediatrics. Committee on Infectious Diseases. Red book: report of the Committee on Infectious Diseases. Elk Grove Village, IL: American Academy of Pediatrics, 2000:v.
338. Strickland DK, Riely CA, Patrick CC, et al. Hepatitis C infection among survivors of childhood cancer. Blood 2000;95:3065–3070.
339. Tong MJ, el-Farra NS, Reikes AR, Co RL. Clinical outcomes after transfusion-associated hepatitis C. N Engl J Med 1995;332:1463–1466.
340. McHutchison JG, Lawitz EJ, Shiffman ML, et al. Peginterferon alfa-2b or alfa-2a with ribavirin for treatment of hepatitis C infection. N Engl J Med 2009;361:580–1593.
341. McHutchison JG, Gordon SC, Schiff ER, et al. Interferon alfa-2b alone or in combination with ribavirin as initial treatment for chronic hepatitis C. Hepatitis Interventional Therapy Group. N Engl J Med 1998;339:1485–1492.
342. Poynard T, Marcellin P, Lee SS, et al. Randomised trial of interferon alpha2b plus ribavirin for 48 weeks or for 24 weeks versus interferon alpha2b plus placebo for 48 weeks for treatment of chronic infection with hepatitis C virus. International Hepatitis Interventional Therapy Group (IHIT). Lancet 1998;352:1426–1432.
343. Hezode C, Forestier N, Dusheiko G, et al. Telaprevir and peginterferon with or without ribavirin for chronic HCV infection. N Engl J Med 2009;360:1839–1850.
344. Chen PM, Chiou TJ, Fan FS, et al. Fulminant hepatitis is significantly increased in hepatitis B carriers after allogeneic bone marrow transplantation. Transplantation 1999; 67:1425–1433.
345. Lau GK, Leung YH, Fong DY, et al. High hepatitis B virus (HBV) DNA viral load as the most important risk factor for HBV reactivation in patients positive for HBV surface antigen undergoing autologous hematopoietic cell transplantation. Blood 2002;99: 2324–2330.
346. Lau GK, He ML, Fong DY, et al. Preemptive use of lamivudine reduces hepatitis B exacerbation after allogeneic hematopoietic cell transplantation. Hepatology 2002;36:702–709.
347. Brechot C, Degos F, Lugassy C, et al. Hepatitis B virus DNA in patients with chronic liver disease and negative tests for hepatitis B surface antigen. N Engl J Med 1985;312: 270–276.
348. Vergani D, Locasciulli A, Masera G, et al. Histological evidence of hepatitis-B-virus infection with negative serology in children with acute leukaemia who develop chronic liver disease. Lancet 1982;1:361–364.
349. Dhedin N, Douvin C, Kuentz M, et al. Reverse seroconversion of hepatitis B after allogeneic bone marrow transplantation: a retrospective study of 37 patients with pretransplant anti-HBs and anti-HBc. Transplantation 1998;66:616–619.
350. Kontoyiannis DP, Luna MA, Samuels BI, et al. Hepatosplenic candidiasis. A manifestation of chronic disseminated candidiasis. Infect Dis Clin North Am 2000;14:721–739.
351. Thaler M, Pastakia B, Shawker TH, et al. Hepatic candidiasis in cancer patients: the evolving picture of the syndrome. Ann Intern Med 1988;108:88–100.
352. Marcus SG, Walsh TJ, Pizzo PA, et al. Hepatic abscess in cancer patients. Characterization and management. Arch Surg 1993;128:1358–1364; discussion 1364.
353. Walsh TJ, Hathorn JW, Sobel JD, et al. Detection of circulating candida enolase by immunoassay in patients with cancer and invasive candidiasis. N Engl J Med 1991;324: 1026–1031.
354. Walsh TJ, Merz WG, Lee JW, et al. Diagnosis and therapeutic monitoring of invasive candidiasis by rapid enzymatic detection of serum D-arabinitol. Am J Med 1995;99: 164–172.
355. Kauffman CA, Bradley SF, Ross SC, et al. Hepatosplenic candidiasis: successful treatment with fluconazole. Am J Med 1991;91:137–141.
356. Walsh TJ, Whitcomb PO, Revankar SG, et al. Successful treatment of hepatosplenic candidiasis through repeated cycles of chemotherapy and neutropenia. Cancer 1995;76: 2357–2362.
357. Glenn J, Cotton D, Wesley R, et al. Anorectal infections in patients with malignant diseases. Rev Infect Dis 1988;10:42–52.
358. Browne MJ, Dinndorf PA, Perek D, et al. Infectious complications of intraventricular reservoirs in cancer patients. Pediatr Infect Dis J 1987;6:182–189.
359. Lukes SA, Posner JB, Nielsen S, et al. Bacterial infections of the CNS in neutropenic patients. Neurology 1984;34:269–275.
360. Sommers LM, Hawkins DS. Meningitis in pediatric cancer patients: a review of forty cases from a single institution. Pediatr Infect Dis J 1999;18:902–907.
361. Wilfert CM, Buckley RH, Mohanakumar T, et al. Persistent and fatal central-nervous-system ECHOvirus infections in patients with agammaglobulinemia. N Engl J Med 1977;296:1485–1489.
362. Drobyski WR, Dunne WM, Burd EM, et al. Human herpesvirus-6 (HHV-6) infection in allogeneic bone marrow transplant recipients: evidence of a marrow-suppressive role for HHV-6 in vivo. J Infect Dis 1993;167:735–739.
363. Wilborn F, Brinkmann V, Schmidt CA, et al. Herpesvirus type 6 in patients undergoing bone marrow transplantation: serologic features and detection by polymerase chain reaction. Blood 1994;83:3052–3058.
364. Hong DS, Jacobson KL, Raad II, et al. West Nile encephalitis in 2 hematopoietic stem cell transplant recipients: case series and literature review. Clin Infect Dis 2003;37: 1044–1049.
365. Israelski DM, Remington JS. Toxoplasmosis in patients with cancer. Clin Infect Dis 1993;17(suppl 2):S423–S435.
366. Slavin MA, Meyers JD, Remington JS, et al. *Toxoplasma gondii* infection in marrow transplant recipients: a 20 year experience. Bone Marrow Transplant 1994;13:549–557.
367. Conley FK, Jenkins KA, Remington JS. *Toxoplasma gondii* infection of the central nervous system. Use of the peroxidase-antiperoxidase method to demonstrate toxoplasma in formalin fixed, paraffin embedded tissue sections. Hum Pathol 1981;12:690–698.
368. Choucino C, Goodman SA, Greer JP, et al. Nocardial infections in bone marrow transplant recipients. Clin Infect Dis 1996;23:1012–1019.
369. Hagensee ME, Bauwens JE, Kjos B, et al. Brain abscess following marrow transplantation: experience at the Fred Hutchinson Cancer Research Center, 1984–1992. Clin Infect Dis 1994;19:402–408.
370. Walsh TJ, Hier DB, Caplan LR. Aspergillosis of the central nervous system: clinicopathological analysis of 17 patients. Ann Neurol 1985;18:574–582.
371. Walsh TJ, Hier DB, Caplan LR. Fungal infections of the central nervous system: comparative analysis of risk factors and clinical signs in 57 patients. Neurology 1985;35: 1654–1657.
372. Viscoli C, Machetti M, Gazzola P, et al. Aspergillus galactomannan antigen in the cerebrospinal fluid of bone marrow transplant recipients with probable cerebral aspergillosis. J Clin Microbiol 2002;40:1496–1499.
373. Echavarria MS, Ray SC, Ambinder R, et al. PCR detection of adenovirus in a bone marrow transplant recipient: hemorrhagic cystitis as a presenting manifestation of disseminated disease. J Clin Microbiol 1999;37:686–689.
374. Bodey GP. Dermatologic manifestations of infections in neutropenic patients. Infect Dis Clin North Am 1994;8:655–675.
375. Boutati EI, Anaissie EJ. Fusarium, a significant emerging pathogen in patients with hematologic malignancy: ten years' experience at a cancer center and implications for management. Blood 1997;90:999–1008.
376. Henrickson KJ, Shenep JL, Flynn PM, et al. Primary cutaneous bacillus cereus infection in neutropenic children. Lancet 1989;1:601–603.
377. Vartivarian SE, Papadakis KA, Palacios JA, et al. Mucocutaneous and soft tissue infections caused by Xanthomonas maltophilia. A new spectrum. Ann Intern Med 1994; 121:969–973.
378. Walsh TJ. Primary cutaneous aspergillosis—an emerging infection among immunocompromised patients. Clin Infect Dis 1998;27:453–457.
379. Elting LS, Bodey GP, Keefe BH. Septicemia and shock syndrome due to viridans streptococci: a case-control study of predisposing factors. Clin Infect Dis 1992;14:1201–1207.
380. Wingard JR, Merz WG, Saral R. *Candida tropicalis*: a major pathogen in immunocompromised patients. Ann Intern Med 1979;91:539–543.
381. Walsh TJ, Orth DH, Shapiro CM, et al. Metastatic fungal chorioretinitis developing during Trichosporon sepsis. Ophthalmology 1982;89:152–156.

382. Nucci M, Anaissie E. Cutaneous infection by Fusarium species in healthy and immuno-compromised hosts: implications for diagnosis and management. Clin Infect Dis 2002; 35:909–920.

383. Anaissie EJ, Kuchar RT, Rex JH, et al. Fusariosis associated with pathogenic fusarium species colonization of a hospital water system: a new paradigm for the epidemiology of opportunistic mold infections. Clin Infect Dis 2001;33:1871–1878.

384. Feldman S, Lott L. Varicella in children with cancer: impact of antiviral therapy and prophylaxis. Pediatrics 1987;80:465–472.

385. Shepp DH, Dandliker PS, Meyers JD. Treatment of varicella-zoster virus infection in severely immunocompromised patients. A randomized comparison of acyclovir and vidarabine. N Engl J Med 1986;314:208–212.

386. Meinking TL, Taplin D, Hermida JL, et al. The treatment of scabies with ivermectin. N Engl J Med 1995;333:26–30.

387. Doebbeling BN, Stanley GL, Sheetz CT, et al. Comparative efficacy of alternative hand-washing agents in reducing nosocomial infections in intensive care units. N Engl J Med 1992;327:88–93.

388. Pizzo PA, Purvis DS, Waters C. Microbiological evaluation of food items. For patients undergoing gastrointestinal decontamination and protected isolation. J Am Diet Assoc 1982;81:272–279.

389. Anaissie EJ, Stratton SL, Dignani MC, et al. Cleaning patient shower facilities: a novel approach to reducing patient exposure to aerosolized Aspergillus species and other opportunistic molds. Clin Infect Dis 2002;35:E86–E88.

390. Nauseef WM, Maki DG. A study of the value of simple protective isolation in patients with granulocytopenia. N Engl J Med 1981;304:448–453.

391. van der Waaij D, Berghuis-de Vries JM. Selective elimination of Enterobacteriaceae species from the digestive tract in mice and monkeys. J Hyg (Lond) 1974;72:205–211.

392. van der Waaij D, Berghuis-de Vries JM, Lekkerkerk L-v. Colonization resistance of the digestive tract in conventional and antibiotic-treated mice. J Hyg (Lond) 1971;69:405–411.

393. Gurwith MJ, Brunton JL, Lank BA, et al. A prospective controlled investigation of pro-phylactic trimethoprim/sulfamethoxazole in hospitalized granulocytopenic patients. Am J Med 1979;66:248–256.

394. Gualtieri RJ, Donowitz GR, Kaiser DL, et al. Double-blind randomized study of pro-phylactic trimethoprim/sulfamethoxazole in granulocytopenic patients with hemato-logic malignancies. Am J Med 1983;74:934–940.

395. Kauffman CA, Liepman MK, Bergman AG, et al. Trimethoprim/sulfamethoxazole pro-phylaxis in neutropenic patients. Reduction of infections and effect on bacterial and fungal flora. Am J Med 1983;74:599–607.

396. Wilson JM, Guiney DG. Failure of oral trimethoprim-sulfamethoxazole prophylaxis in acute leukemia: isolation of resistant plasmids from strains of Enterobacteriaceae caus-ing bacteremia. N Engl J Med 1982;306:16–20.

397. Engels EA, Lau J, Barza M. Efficacy of quinolone prophylaxis in neutropenic cancer patients: a meta-analysis. J Clin Oncol 1998;16:1179–1187.

398. Cullen M, Steven N, Billingham L, et al. Antibacterial prophylaxis after chemotherapy for solid tumors and lymphomas. N Engl J Med 2005;353:988–998.

399. Reuter S, Kern WV, Sigge A, et al. Impact of fluoroquinolone prophylaxis on reduced infection-related mortality among patients with neutropenia and hematologic malig-nancies. Clin Infect Dis 2005;40:1087–1093.

400. Gafter-Gvili A, Fraser A, Paul M, et al. Meta-analysis: antibiotic prophylaxis reduces mortality in neutropenic patients. Ann Intern Med 2005;142:979–995.

401. Bucaneve G, Micozzi A, Menichetti F, et al. Levofloxacin to prevent bacterial infection in patients with cancer and neutropenia. N Engl J Med 2005;353:977–987.

402. Goodman JL, Winston DJ, Greenfield RA, et al. A controlled trial of fluconazole to pre-vent fungal infections in patients undergoing bone marrow transplantation. N Engl J Med 1992;326:845–851.

403. Slavin MA, Osborne B, Adams R, et al. Efficacy and safety of fluconazole prophylaxis for fungal infections after marrow transplantation—a prospective, randomized, double-blind study. J Infect Dis 1995;171:1545–1552.

404. Cornely OA, Maertens J, Winston DJ, et al. Posaconazole vs. fluconazole or itracona-zole prophylaxis in patients with neutropenia. N Engl J Med 2007;356:348–359.

405. Crawford SA, Clover RD, Abell TD, et al. Rimantadine prophylaxis in children: a follow-up study. Pediatr Infect Dis J 1988;7:379–383.

406. Monto AS, Arden NH. Implications of viral resistance to amantadine in control of influenza A. Clin Infect Dis 1992;15:362–367; discussion 368–369.

407. Chik KW, Li CK, Chan PK, et al. Oseltamivir prophylaxis during the influenza season in a paediatric cancer centre: prospective observational study. Hong Kong Med J 2004; 10:103–106.

408. Hayden FG, Belshe R, Villanueva C, et al. Management of influenza in households: a prospective, randomized comparison of oseltamivir treatment with or without postex-posure prophylaxis. J Infect Dis 2004;189:440–449.

409. Perren TJ, Powles RL, Easton D, et al. Prevention of herpes zoster in patients by long-term oral acyclovir after allogeneic bone marrow transplantation. Am J Med 1988;85:99–101.

410. Erlich KS, Jacobson MA, Koehler JE, et al. Foscarnet therapy for severe acyclovir-resistant herpes simplex virus type-2 infections in patients with the acquired immunod-eficiency syndrome (AIDS). An uncontrolled trial. Ann Intern Med 1989;110:710–713.

411. Schmidt GM, Horak DA, Niland JC, et al. A randomized, controlled trial of prophylac-tic ganciclovir for cytomegalovirus pulmonary infection in recipients of allogeneic bone marrow transplants: The City of Hope-Stanford-Syntex CMV Study Group. N Engl J Med 1991;324:1005–1011.

412. Meyers JD, Pifer LL, Sale GE, et al. The value of Pneumocystis carinii antibody and antigen detection for diagnosis of Pneumocystis carinii pneumonia after marrow trans-plantation. Am Rev Respir Dis 1979;120:1283–1287.

413. Henson JW, Jalaj JK, Walker RW, et al. Pneumocystis carinii pneumonia in patients with primary brain tumors. Arch Neurol 1991;48:406–409.

414. Hughes WT, Rivera GK, Schell MJ, et al. Successful intermittent chemoprophylaxis for Pneumocystis carinii pneumonitis. N Engl J Med 1987;316:1627–1632.

415. Ioannidis JP, Cappelleri JC, Skolnik PR, et al. A meta-analysis of the relative efficacy and toxicity of Pneumocystis carinii prophylactic regimens. Arch Intern Med 1996;156:177–188.

416. El-Sadr WM, Murphy RL, Yurik TM, et al. Atovaquone compared with dapsone for the prevention of Pneumocystis carinii pneumonia in patients with HIV infection who cannot tolerate trimethoprim, sulfonamides, or both. Community Program for Clinical Research on AIDS and the AIDS Clinical Trials Group. N Engl J Med 1998;339:1889–1895.

417. Principi N, Marchisio P, Onorato J, et al. Long-term administration of aerosolized pen-tamidine as primary prophylaxis against Pneumocystis carinii pneumonia in infants and

children with symptomatic human immunodeficiency virus infection. The Italian Pedi-atric Collaborative Study Group on Pentamidine. J Acquir Immune Defic Syndr Hum Retrovirol 1996;12:158–163.

418. Centers for Disease Control Advisory Committee on Immunization Practices; American Academy of Pediatrics; American Academy of Family Physicians. Recommended immu-nization schedule for persons aged 7–18 years—United States 2008. S D Med 2008; 61:223.

419. Centers for Disease Control Advisory Committee on Immunization Practices; American Academy of Pediatrics; American Academy of Family Physicians. Recommended immu-nization schedule for persons aged 0–6 years—United States 2008. S D Med 2008; 61:222.

420. Centers for Disease Control and Prevention; Infectious Disease Society of America; American Society of Blood and Marrow Transplantation. Guidelines for preventing opportunistic infections among hematopoietic stem cell transplant recipients. MMWR Recomm Rep 2000;49:1–125, CE1–CE7.

421. Ambrosino DM, Molrine DC. Critical appraisal of immunization strategies for preven-tion of infection in the compromised host. Hematol Oncol Clin North Am 1993;7:1027–1050.

422. Palumbo P, Hoyt L, Demasio K, et al. Population-based study of measles and measles immunization in human immunodeficiency virus-infected children. Pediatr Infect Dis J 1992;11:1008–1014.

423. Kaplan LJ, Daum RS, Smaron M, et al. Severe measles in immunocompromised patients. JAMA 1992;267:1237–1241.

424. Gershon AA, Steinberg SP. Persistence of immunity to varicella in children with leukemia immunized with live attenuated varicella vaccine. N Engl J Med 1989;320:892–897.

425. Hardy I, Gershon AA, Steinberg SP, et al. The incidence of zoster after immunization with live attenuated varicella vaccine. A study in children with leukemia. Varicella Vac-cine Collaborative Study Group. N Engl J Med 1991;325:1545–1550.

426. Galil K, Lee B, Strine T, et al. Outbreak of varicella at a day-care center despite vacci-nation. N Engl J Med 2002;347:1909–1915.

427. Skinner R, Appleton AL, Sprott MS, et al. Disseminated BCG infection in severe com-bined immunodeficiency presenting with severe anaemia and associated with gross hypersplenism after bone marrow transplantation. Bone Marrow Transplant 1996;17:877–880.

428. Talbot EA, Perkins MD, Silva SF, et al. Disseminated bacille Calmette-Guerin disease after vaccination: case report and review. Clin Infect Dis 1997;24:1139–1146.

429. Kung FH, Orgel HA, Wallace WW, et al. Antibody production following immunization with diphtheria and tetanus toxoids in children receiving chemotherapy during remis-sion of malignant disease. Pediatrics 1984;74:86–89.

430. Chilcote RR, Baehner RL, Hammond D. Septicemia and meningitis in children splenec-tomized for Hodgkin's disease. N Engl J Med 1976;295:798–800.

431. Feldman S, Gigliotti F, Shenep JL, et al. Risk of Haemophilus influenzae type b disease in children with cancer and response of immunocompromised leukemic children to a conjugate vaccine. J Infect Dis 1990;161:926–931.

432. Kobel DE, Friedl A, Cerny T, et al. Pneumococcal vaccine in patients with absent or dysfunctional spleen. Mayo Clin Proc 2000;75:749–753.

433. Molrine DC, Siber GR, Samra Y, et al. Normal IgG and impaired IgM responses to polysaccharide vaccines in asplenic patients. J Infect Dis 1999;179:513–517.

434. Lucero MG, Dulalia VE, Parreno RN, et al. Pneumococcal conjugate vaccines for pre-venting vaccine-type invasive pneumococcal disease and pneumonia with consolidation on x-ray in children under two years of age. Cochrane Database Syst Rev 2004: CD004977.

435. Pelton SI, Loughlin AM, Marchant CD. Seven valent pneumococcal conjugate vaccine immunization in two Boston communities: changes in serotypes and antimicrobial sus-ceptibility among Streptococcus pneumoniae isolates. Pediatr Infect Dis J 2004;23:1015–1022.

436. Shenep JL, Feldman S, Gigliotti F, et al. Response of immunocompromised children with solid tumors to a conjugate vaccine for Haemophilus influenzae type b. J Pediatr 1994;125:581–584.

437. Brydak LB, Rokicka-Milewska R, Machala M, et al. Immunogenicity of subunit triva-lent influenza vaccine in children with acute lymphoblastic leukemia. Pediatr Infect Dis J 1998;17:125–129.

438. Herzig RH, Herzig GP, Graw RG Jr, et al. Successful granulocyte transfusion therapy for gram-negative septicemia. A prospectively randomized controlled study. N Engl J Med 1977;296:701–705.

439. Vogler WR, Winton EF. A controlled study of the efficacy of granulocyte transfusions in patients with neutropenia. Am J Med 1977;63:548–555.

440. Alavi JB, Root RK, Djerassi I, et al. A randomized clinical trial of granulocyte transfu-sions for infection in acute leukemia. N Engl J Med 1977;296:706–711.

441. Winston DJ, Ho WG, Gale RP. Therapeutic granulocyte transfusions for documented infections. A controlled trial in ninety-five infectious granulocytopenic episodes. Ann Intern Med 1982;97:509–515.

442. Price TH. The current prospects for neutrophil transfusions for the treatment of granu-locytopenic infected patients. Transfus Med Rev 2000;14:2–11.

443. Anderlini P, Przepiorka D, Seong D, et al. Clinical toxicity and laboratory effects of granulocyte-colony-stimulating factor (filgrastim) mobilization and blood stem cell apheresis from normal donors, and analysis of charges for the procedures. Transfusion 1996;36:590–595.

444. Bensinger WI, Price TH, Dale DC, et al. The effects of daily recombinant human gran-ulocyte colony-stimulating factor administration on normal granulocyte donors under-going leukapheresis. Blood 1993;81:1883–1888.

445. McCullough J, Clay M, Hurd D, et al. Effect of leukocyte antibodies and HLA match-ing on the intravascular recovery, survival, and tissue localization of 111-indium gran-ulocytes. Blood 1986;67:522–528.

446. Stroncek DF, Leonard K, Eiber G, et al. Alloimmunization after granulocyte transfu-sions. Transfusion 1996;36:1009–1015.

447. Gerhartz HH, Engelhard M, Meusers P, et al. Randomized, double-blind, placebo-controlled, phase III study of recombinant human granulocyte-macrophage colony-stimulating factor as adjunct to induction treatment of high-grade malignant non-Hodgkin's lymphomas. Blood 1993;82:2329–2339.

448. Smith TJ, Khatcheressian J, Lyman GH, et al. 2006 update of recommendations for the use of white blood cell growth factors: an evidence-based clinical practice guideline. J Clin Oncol 2006;24:3187–3205.

449. Crawford J, Ozer H, Stoller R, et al. Reduction by granulocyte colony-stimulating fac-tor of fever and neutropenia induced by chemotherapy in patients with small-cell lung cancer. N Engl J Med 1991;325:164–170.

450. Mitchell PL, Morland B, Stevens MC, et al. Granulocyte colony-stimulating factor in established febrile neutropenia: a randomized study of pediatric patients. J Clin Oncol 1997;15:1163–1170.

451. Ohno R, Tomonaga M, Kobayashi T, et al. Effect of granulocyte colony-stimulating factor after intensive induction therapy in relapsed or refractory acute leukemia. N Engl J Med 1990;323:871–877.

452. Fossa SD, Kaye SB, Mead GM, et al. Filgrastim during combination chemotherapy of patients with poor-prognosis metastatic germ cell malignancy. European Organization for Research and Treatment of Cancer, Genito-Urinary Group, and the Medical Research Council Testicular Cancer Working Party, Cambridge, United Kingdom. J Clin Oncol 1998;16:716–724.

453. Phillips KA, Tannock IF. Design and interpretation of clinical trials that evaluate agents that may offer protection from the toxic effects of cancer chemotherapy. J Clin Oncol 1998;16:3179–3190.

454. Savarese DM, Hsieh C, Stewart FM. Clinical impact of chemotherapy dose escalation in patients with hematologic malignancies and solid tumors. J Clin Oncol 1997;15:2981–2995.

455. Parsons SK, Mayer DK, Alexander SW, et al. Growth factor practice patterns among pediatric oncologists: results of a 1998 Pediatric Oncology Group Survey. Economic Evaluation Working Group the Pediatric Oncology Group. J Pediatr Hematol Oncol 2000;22:227–241.

456. Maher DW, Lieschke GJ, Green M, et al. Filgrastim in patients with chemotherapy-induced febrile neutropenia. A double-blind, placebo-controlled trial. Ann Intern Med 1994;121:492–501.

457. Ravaud A, Chevreau C, Cany L, et al. Granulocyte-macrophage colony-stimulating factor in patients with neutropenic fever is potent after low-risk but not after high-risk neutropenic chemotherapy regimens: results of a randomized phase III trial. J Clin Oncol 1998;16:2930–2936.

458. Riikonen P, Saarinen UM, Makipernaa A, et al. Recombinant human granulocyte-macrophage colony-stimulating factor in the treatment of febrile neutropenia: a double blind placebo-controlled study in children. Pediatr Infect Dis J 1994;13:197–202.

459. Wakiyama H, Tsuru S, Hata N, et al. Therapeutic effect of granulocyte colony-stimulating factor and cephem antibiotics against experimental infections in neutropenic mice induced by cyclophosphamide. Clin Exp Immunol 1993;92:218–224.

460. Liang DC, Chen SH, Lean SF. Role of granulocyte colony-stimulating factor as adjunct therapy for septicemia in children with acute leukemia. Am J Hematol 1995;48:76–81.

461. Abzug MJ, Walsh TJ. Interferon-gamma and colony-stimulating factors as adjuvant therapy for refractory fungal infections in children. Pediatr Infect Dis J 2004;23:769–773.

462. Roilides E, Walsh T. Recombinant cytokines in augmentation and immunomodulation of host defenses against Candida spp. Med Mycol 2004;42:1–13.

463. Beyer J, Schwella N, Zingsem J, et al. Hematopoietic rescue after high-dose chemotherapy using autologous peripheral-blood progenitor cells or bone marrow: a randomized comparison. J Clin Oncol 1995;13:1328–1335.

464. Korbling M, Przepiorka D, Huh YO, et al. Allogeneic blood stem cell transplantation for refractory leukemia and lymphoma: potential advantage of blood over marrow allografts. Blood 1995;85:1659–1665.

465. Schmitz N, Linch DC, Dreger P, et al. Randomised trial of filgrastim-mobilised peripheral blood progenitor cell transplantation versus autologous bone-marrow transplantation in lymphoma patients. Lancet 1996;347:353–357.

466. A controlled trial of interferon gamma to prevent infection in chronic granulomatous disease. The International Chronic Granulomatous Disease Cooperative Study Group. N Engl J Med 1991;324:509–516.

467. Holland SM, Eisenstein EM, Kuhns DB, et al. Treatment of refractory disseminated nontuberculous mycobacterial infection with interferon gamma. A preliminary report. N Engl J Med 1994;330:1348–1355.

468. Pappas PG, Bustamante B, Ticona E, et al. Recombinant interferon-gamma 1b as adjunctive therapy for AIDS-related acute cryptococcal meningitis. J Infect Dis 2004;189:2185–2191.

469. DeMaio J, Colman L. The use of adjuvant interferon-gamma therapy for hepatosplenic Blastoschizomyces capitatus infection in a patient with leukemia. Clin Infect Dis 2000;31:822–824.

470. Poynton CH, Barnes RA, Rees J. Interferon gamma and granulocyte-macrophage colony-stimulating factor for the treatment of hepatosplenic candidosis in patients with acute leukemia. Clin Infect Dis 1998;26:239–240.

471. Rodriguez-Adrian LJ, Grazziutti ML, Rex JH, et al. The potential role of cytokine therapy for fungal infections in patients with cancer: is recovery from neutropenia all that is needed? Clin Infect Dis 1998;26:1270–1278.

CHAPTER 41 ■ NUTRITIONAL SUPPORTIVE CARE

SONIA ARORA BALLAL, LORI J. BECHARD, TOM JAKSIC, AND CHRISTOPHER DUGGAN

INTRODUCTION

The high prevalence of malnutrition in pediatric[1] patients with cancer has been appreciated for decades and continues to be documented.[2–5] Although the prognostic significance of nutritional status among patients with cancer remains controversial,[6–8] it is generally accepted that nutritional support is an important component of medical therapy (Table 41.1). An increasing prevalence of obesity in the healthy pediatric population, combined with additional risks associated with cancer treatment,[19,20] has prompted care providers to appropriately confront the potential for obesity-related chronic diseases among childhood cancer survivors. Hence, tailored nutritional intervention is essential from diagnosis, through treatment, and beyond to long-term survival. Each newly diagnosed child with cancer warrants a systematic, comprehensive survey of his/her nutrition status, with periodic reassessments. Parents of children with cancer are often quite concerned about issues of appetite and other gastrointestinal symptoms, even when death is imminent.[21] The frequent use of complementary and alternative dietary supplements among patients with cancer also underlines the importance that families attach to nutritional therapy.[22,23] We review the definitions, epidemiology, etiology, and practical therapy of nutritional problems of the pediatric patient with cancer.

DEFINITION OF CANCER CACHEXIA

Cachexia has been defined as a severe state of malnutrition characterized by anorexia, weight loss, muscle wasting, and anemia.[9,24] Roubenoff et al.[25] have proposed that the terms wasting, cachexia, and sarcopenia be considered as three distinctly defined entities (Table 41.2). Wasting is defined as involuntary weight loss, and is found in patients with anorexia nervosa, cancer, advanced HIV infection, and marasmus. Cachexia, in contrast, is defined as involuntary loss of fat-free mass in the setting of minimal or no overall weight loss. This type of malnutrition can be seen in some patients with cancer, as well as those with critical illness and early HIV infection. In this scenario, patients of normal weight can still be malnourished due to reduced lean body mass. A decline in lean body mass has important functional and prognostic significance, even in the setting of stable or increasing weight. Sarcopenia refers to the involuntary loss of muscle mass that occurs with aging.

The pattern of weight loss and changes in body composition in patients with illness are important to be considered because differential loss of body fat versus fat-free mass implies a different etiology and prognosis of malnutrition. For example, prolonged fasting in the absence of metabolic perturbation (as can be seen in adolescents with anorexia nervosa) leads to a predictable decrement first in body fat, then in body protein stores.[26] In these cases, energy repletion is usually successful with the provision of adequate energy, protein, and micronutrients.

In contrast, weight loss in the setting of cancer, infection, or other metabolic stress is composed of both fat and fat-free mass.[27] Because the energy density of fat-free mass is lower than that of fat, the body's use of lean body mass as an energy and amino acid source can lead to weight loss that can be quite profound and rapid. It is this loss of fat-free mass that is of significance, because loss of lean body mass is associated with important functional changes such as loss of strength, decreased immune function, decreased pulmonary function, increased disability, and death.[28,29]

More importantly, the provision of nutritional support to these patients may not be adequate to reverse the catabolic effects of the underlying condition. In the early days of parenteral nutrition use, it was hypothesized that aggressive parenteral nutrition could overcome the catabolism of cancer and other critical illnesses[30]; however, this has not proven to be the case. Instead, a more realistic appreciation for the limitations of nutritional support has emerged.[18] Methodologies and nutritional prescriptions for children with cancer are explored in the following sections.

OBESITY AND THE PEDIATRIC PATIENT WITH CANCER

Over the last few decades, the prevalence of obesity in children has increased substantially, with currently 15% of children and adolescents falling into that category.[31] In certain populations, this number is even higher. Such numbers demand that pediatric oncologists feel comfortable in approaching the overweight/obese patient who is also diagnosed with cancer. One major concern is the effect of therapeutics and toxicities in the obese patient. One study of 621 acute lymphoblastic leukemia (ALL) patients that examined the influence of body mass index (BMI) on the pharmacokinetics, toxicity, and outcome of chemotherapy found that overall survival and toxicity did not vary across groups with different BMIs.[32] Another study noted increased mortality because of treatment-related events, namely infection, in both underweight and overweight patients with acute myelogenous leukemia, although the increased mortality seen in the overweight population did not appear to be secondary to higher doses of chemotherapy, or reduced clearance of toxic substances.[33] In contrast, children with greater than 30% body fat were found to have decreased clearance of doxorubicinol, compared with children with less body fat, as measured by dual-energy x-ray absorptiometry (DXA).[34]

Obesity is an increasingly noted health problem among cancer survivors. Multiple theories exist regarding the alarming number of obese cancer survivors. A reduction in physical activity and thus a change in body composition of leukemia survivors may explain the subsequent onset of obesity.[35] The frequent use of glucocorticoids in cancer treatment may also

TABLE 41.1

RATIONALE FOR NUTRITION SCREENING AND INTERVENTION IN PEDIATRIC PATIENTS WITH CANCER

The rationale for identifying, treating, and preventing malnutrition among pediatric patients with cancer may be summarized as follows:

1. **Malnutrition is common among patients with cancer.** Both upon presentation and with subsequent anti-tumor therapy, weight loss, deficits in weight for height (wasting), and deficits in height for age (stunting) are observed. Even in the absence of these gross anthropometric deficits, more subtle changes in body composition and metabolic handling of nutritional substrates occur.[9,10] Catabolic patients with cancer who are outwardly well nourished still benefit from specialized nutritional intervention.[11]

2. **There are no known disease processes wherein malnutrition is advantageous to the host.** There is an extensive literature documenting increased morbidity from malnutrition in hospitalized patients, including delayed wound healing, increased infectious complications, decreased immune competence, reduced respiratory and other muscle strength, and increased length of stay.[12] The nutrition literature in pediatrics confirms wasting as an important risk factor for early death; mid-upper arm circumference is highly predictive of mortality and is used as a triage instrument in the setting of famine. Moreover, acute malnutrition is marked by depression and apathy, and chronic malnutrition by delayed neurodevelopment.[13] All of the morbidities named earlier are common in pediatric patients with cancer.

3. **Malnutrition in pediatric and adult[14] patients with cancer has been associated with intolerance to chemotherapy[15] and increased mortality rates.**[7] The possible contribution of malnutrition to infectious and immunologic morbidities has been less well studied,[16] but is conceivably additive to the insults from chemo- and radiotherapy. The role of malnutrition in cancer and neuropsychiatric well-being has not been well addressed in the literature.

4. **Early recognition of the patient at risk for malnutrition can obviate the need for more aggressive nutritional support subsequently in the patient's course.** The efficacy of parenteral nutrition (PN) has been proven in those undergoing bone marrow transplantation.[17] PN is also commonly used for patients with malnutrition and/or poor oral intake who are undergoing standard chemotherapy, although concerns about increased infectious morbidity have been raised. Moreover, PN is an expensive therapy that carries the risk of multiple metabolic complications. Successful nutritional support with oral or enteral supplements may reduce the need to use PN.[18] Because malnutrition is associated with a variety of complications of cancer and its therapy, it is generally believed that nutritional support may enhance therapy, decrease complications, improve immunologic status, and perhaps improve survival.

help explain a high prevalence of obesity. One study observed increased fat mass in children with ALL.[36] Glucocorticoids may be associated not only with this rise in fat mass, but also decreased adult height. As many as half of childhood leukemia survivors in one study became obese young adults.[37] This incidence may be related to the impact of therapy on final adult height. A cohort of bone marrow transplant survivors, engrafted before or at the onset of puberty, had a significant

decrease in final height, compared with pretransplant height standard deviation scores. However, most of the patients achieved a height considered to be normal.[38] A study of 33 childhood leukemia survivors followed for a median of 16.2 years found that 36% were obese. All patients had reduced height standard deviation scores during treatment; however, only patients who received cranial radiation with chemotherapy (versus chemotherapy alone) had reductions in

TABLE 41.2

PARADIGMS OF WEIGHT LOSS/BODY COMPOSITION CHANGES IN ILLNESS

	Cachexia	Wasting	Sarcopenia
Decreased BCM	Yes	Yes	Yes, skeletal muscle cells
Weight loss	None or little compared to loss of BCM	Yes	Not necessarily
Elevated REE	Often	Not necessarily	Not necessarily
Decreased functional status	Yes	Yes	Yes
Increased cytokine production	Yes	No	?
Increased mortality	Yes	Yes	?
Treatment	?Anti-cytokine agents, ?anabolic hormones	Increased intake (adequate to increase BCM)	Progressive resistance training
Clinical examples	Critical illness with adequate nutritional support, liver disease, early renal failure, rheumatoid arthritis, HIV infection without opportunistic infection, kwashiorkor	Critical illness without adequate nutritional support, advanced AIDS, end stage renal or liver disease, marasmus	Aging

BCM, body cell mass; REE, resting energy expenditure; AIDS, acquired immunodeficiency syndrome.
Adapted from Roubenoff R, Heymsfield SB, Kehayias JJ, et al. Standardization of nomenclature of body composition in weight loss. Am J Clin Nutr 1997;66:192–196.

final adult height.[39] Cranial irradiation has also been linked with the development of metabolic syndrome and growth hormone deficiency, laying the foundation for adult development of diabetes and heart disease.[40] In children, cranial irradiation may alter the leptin receptor in the hypothalamus, causing decreased sensitivity posttreatment. An examination of a polymorphism of the leptin receptor could lead to targeted attempts to identify individuals more susceptible to obesity after radiation therapy.[41] Some investigations suggest a gender divide, with a predilection for the development of obesity among female patients with cancer, while other studies find no difference between males and females.

EPIDEMIOLOGY

The occurrence of wasting among patients with cancer is determined by host susceptibility, tumor type and location, and anti-cancer regimen. Since during infancy and adolescence there are increased energy needs for growth, children in these age groups are at increased risk of malnutrition. Other patients at higher risk of malnutrition are those with advanced disease, metastatic solid tumors, and those needing protracted chemotherapy (Table 41.3). A striking example of malnutrition is the diencephalic syndrome in which a hypothalamic tumor presents with severe weight loss in the setting of a normal appetite.[42,43]

In contrast, most patients with low-risk ALL, those with nonmetastatic solid tumors, and patients in remission are generally able to maintain a normal weight. Weight loss, however, may be the final step in a long process of nutritional

TABLE 41.3

RISK FACTORS FOR MALNUTRITION IN PEDIATRIC PATIENTS WITH CANCER

High nutritional risk
Advanced diseases during initial intense treatment
Unfavorable histology Wilms tumor
Stages III and IV neuroblastoma, especially unfavorable biology
Advanced stage rhabdomyosarcoma
Advanced stage Ewing sarcoma
Some non-Hodgkin lymphoma
Tumors of the head and neck (e.g., nasopharyngeal carcinomas)
Acute myelogenous leukemia
Some poor prognosis acute lymphoblastic leukemias
Acute lymphoblastic leukemias during induction
Multiple relapse leukemia
Medulloblastoma and other high grade brain tumors
Stem cell transplantation, especially with graft-versus-host disease
Low nutritional risk
Good prognosis acute lymphoblastic leukemia
Nonmetastatic solid tumors
Advanced diseases in remission during maintenance treatment

Adapted from Mauer AM, Burgess JB, Donaldson SS, et al. Special nutritional needs of children with malignancies: a review. JPEN J Parenter Enteral Nutr 1990;14:315–324; Rickard K, Grosfeld J, Coates T, et al. Advances in nutrition care of children with neoplastic diseases: a review of treatment, research, and application. J Am Diet Assoc 1986;86:1666–1676.

perturbation in patients with cancer, and as such may not be a sufficiently sensitive marker for malnutrition. For example, one study of prepubertal children with low risk ALL followed body weight and lean body mass over time (as measured by sum of four skinfold measurements and bioelectrical impedance). Although body weight in the patients with cancer was no different than age- and sex-matched controls, lean body mass declined substantially with the use of chemotherapy.[44] Another study of ALL survivors compared BMI values and whole body percent fat as measured by DXA with controls. ALL survivors had significantly higher percent body fat, while their BMI remained similar to controls.[45] Thus, mere reliance on body weight to document normal nutritional status may lead to an underestimate of lean body mass depletion or fat accumulation.

ETIOLOGY AND PATHOPHYSIOLOGY

It is axiomatic that patients with weight loss exhibit reduced dietary intake, malabsorption or maldigestion of foods, or altered energy and nutrient needs. The challenge of nutritional care of pediatric patients with cancer is that all three mechanisms may be at play, so that the clinician's diagnostic and therapeutic tools must be broadly considered.

In brief, weight loss or gain is due to energy imbalance, which ensues when energy intake differs from total energy expenditure (TEE). TEE in turn is considered to be the sum of several components of the energy equation. That is, in a steady state,

$$\text{Energy intake} = \text{TEE} = \text{REE} + E_{activity} + E_{growth} + E_{losses} + \text{SDA}$$

where REE = resting energy expenditure (an estimate of basal metabolic rate)

$E_{activity}$ = energy needs for activity
E_{growth} = energy needs for normal growth
E_{losses} = energy needs for obligatory losses in urine and stool
SDA = specific dynamic action of food, the energy needs for digestion and absorption.

Weight loss will occur when any of the components of TEE are higher than expected and are not matched by a compensatory increase in energy intake. Weight gain occurs when energy intake exceeds TEE. Although an increase in energy intake is the most common reason for overweight, reduction in energy of activity has also been implicated in the development of obesity.[46]

Decreased Nutrient Intake

There are multiple reasons for decreased nutrient intake in the child receiving chemo- or radiotherapy.[47] One is the well-known occurrence of circulating cytokines, including tumor necrosis factor alpha that induces anorexia.[24] The effects of proinflammatory cytokines have been studied as the etiology of multiple metabolic phenomena of cancer and its treatment and are more fully considered later.

Another important reason for decreased nutrient intake is anorexia and other gastrointestinal side effects of chemo- and radio-therapy. Mucosal damage is generally dose-related, with increased risk of mucosal toxicity with high-dose induction therapy and combination chemotherapy treatments. High-dose chemotherapy and total body irradiation as conditioning for hematopoietic stem cell transplantation (HSCT) often produce painful oral mucositis that can reduce nutritional intake for days to weeks. Other gastrointestinal side effects of cancer treatment include esophagitis, enteritis with malabsorption, and diarrhea; these are more fully described in Chapter 10. Taste perception has also been shown to be altered in patients with cancer receiving chemotherapy, with an increasing sensitivity to bitter tastes; this phenomenon may lead to reduced food intake, and may make the use of oral supplements difficult.

Psychological factors are also important to consider in evaluating the reasons behind inadequate dietary intake. Depression-related anorexia is probably underappreciated as a cause. Appetite and feeding behaviors are inherently complicated activities of all children, and this behavior can obviously be affected by the onset of illness, its treatment, as well as the psychosocial impact that cancer has on the child and family. The nature of cancer medical care is such that parents often feel that they are relinquishing much of their usual care-giving behavior to the medical and nursing staff. Some parents understandably cling to the provision of food and nutrients as a critical part of parenting; indeed, the terms nutrition, nursing, and nurture all share the same Latin root.

Changes in Energy Expenditure: REE

Although decreased nutrient intake is common in cancer, anorexia alone cannot wholly explain the common development of malnutrition since some patients maintain an excellent intake but still suffer progressive weight loss. Much research has focused on the possible role of increased energy expenditure of patients with cancer in trying to explain cancer cachexia;[48–50] however, the issue has not been consistently resolved.

Early studies suggested that the energy needs of rapidly dividing cells of the tumor increased basal metabolic demands of the host from 20% to 90% over predicted needs. More recent data have confirmed that hypermetabolism can occur but not in all patients at all times. Knox et al.[51] studied 200 adult patients with cancer using the technique of indirect calorimetry, a noninvasive bedside measure of REE, the clinical estimate of basal metabolic rate. They found that one-third of patients were hypometabolic (REE was < 90% of predicted levels), one-fourth were hypermetabolic (REE > 110% predicted), and the remaining 40% had normal REE (between 90% and 110% predicted).

In children, changes in REE have been observed in a variety of clinical scenarios. Stallings et al. measured REE in nine patients with ALL and found that patients with a higher tumor burden (elevated WBC count, organomegaly) had an increased REE.[52] A study of 26 patients with ALL or solid tumors in remission showed no evidence of an increased resting energy expenditure, when compared with age- and sex-matched healthy controls.[53] Changes in REE measured by indirect calorimetry have been demonstrated by two studies of children undergoing HSCT. Ringwald-Smith et al. compared weekly measured REE in 34 children undergoing autologous or allogeneic HSCT with standardized equations and found that REE was significantly less than predicted except at 14 days posttransplant.[54] Another prospective study of 37 children undergoing allogeneic transplantation described a significant decline in REE from baseline to week 3 after HSCT, as well as significant decline in mid-arm muscle area, suggesting that REE changes may be related to reductions in lean body mass incurred during transplant.[55] Further explorations of REE changes in pediatric cancer warranted.

Changes in Energy Expenditure: Energy of Activity

As noted earlier, total energy requirements include energy needed for physical activity. Reilly et al.[56] studied 20 preadolescent children with ALL with doubly labeled water, a technique that reliably measures TEE in free-living individuals.[57] Compared with healthy controls matched for age, sex, and body composition, children with ALL had significantly lower TEE than controls, mostly due to reduced physical activity. A similar study, using a combination of indirect calorimetry and ambulatory heart rate monitoring to measure REE and TEE, also concluded that ALL patients have lower levels of energy expenditure for activity.[35] The implications of these findings for obesity prevention in ALL survivors, as well as children at large, may be significant.

Alterations in Macronutrient Metabolism

Children with cancer manifest changes in macronutrient utilization markedly different than that evident with starvation. The tumor itself seems to impose a pattern of perturbations that lead to catabolism; however, the extent of this response is variable. This may be due to the heterogeneity of tumor types and sizes, treatment protocols, and baseline nutritional status. A general understanding of these alterations is useful in anticipating potential metabolic complications and planning nutritional therapy.

Carbohydrate

The changes seen in carbohydrate metabolism associated with malignancy generally include glucose intolerance, increased gluconeogenesis (the conversion of amino acid carbon skeletons to glucose),[58] and increased Cori cycling (the hepatic conversion of lactate to glucose).[59] Glucose intolerance in patients with cancer is at least partially due to the presence of insulin resistance.[60] This has been demonstrated with various tumors by documenting decreased glucose uptake under steady states of hyperinsulinemia induced during glucose clamp studies. The augmented conversion of lactate to glucose may be secondary to increased lactate production by selected tumors. Overall the enhanced production of glucose provides the tumor with a substrate that is readily metabolized under both aerobic and anaerobic conditions.

Lipid

Lipid metabolism is also affected by cancer. Alterations include increased free fatty acid turnover, free fatty acid oxidation, glycerol turnover, and lipolysis. Lipogenesis is reduced. A lipid-mobilizing factor has been isolated from the urine of cachectic patients with cancer and shows bioactivity with isolated murine adipocytes.[61] As may be expected these changes are accompanied by a marked loss of body fat that can occur early in the evolution of the malignancy. Children with ALL and widespread solid tumors tend to have elevated triglycerides as do children in remission treated with L-asparaginase.[62] The provision of glucose does not seem to resolve the high rates of fatty acid and glycerol turnover evident in weight losing patients with cancer.[63] Treatment with chemotherapy is associated with decreased fat utilization in children newly diagnosed with ALL.[52]

Protein

Another salient derangement of macronutrient metabolism accompanying cancer is the presence of protein catabolism. Hypoalbuminemia is common while the synthesis of acute-phase proteins remains high.[64] Some tumors such as hepatocellular cancer manifest very high rates of protein turnover and increased protein degradation.[65] An increase in the muscle protein breakdown mobilizes amino acids that may afford tumor growth as well as fuel gluconeogenesis. This increased protein breakdown in pediatric patients with cancer may be related to falling levels of insulin-like growth factor 1 and insulin-like growth factor-binding proteins.[66] In other patients, decreased skeletal muscle protein synthesis seems to be of primary importance.[67] Although the mechanism remains uncertain, a net loss of skeletal muscle protein is a common finding with malignancy and is particularly problematic in the growing child.

Cytokines

Proinflammatory cytokines commonly associated with cancer cachexia include tumor necrosis factor alpha (TNF-α), interleukin-6 (IL-6), interleukin-1, and interferon-γ. These cytokines are secreted by macrophages and lymphocytes and may represent the host response to cancer. TNF-α was first identified as a mediator of cachexia in an animal model of infection.[68] In humans, the acute administration of TNF-α produces effects associated with cancer cachexia including: increased fatty acid turnover, elevated glycerol turnover, and increased whole body protein turnover.[69] Not all patients with cancer cachexia have detectable levels of TNF-α, hence a paracrine or autocrine mechanism of action may be responsible. Other factors also seem to be involved with the catabolic response to cancer. Circulating IL-6 levels are generally elevated in patients with cancer and transfection of the IL-6 gene into nude mice does engender cachexia.[70] As with TNF-α, the precise mechanism of action of IL-6 is unknown. The metabolic roles of interleukin-1 and interferon-γ are less well characterized in tumor models; however, as with TNF-α and IL-6 they appear to inhibit lipoprotein lipase and hence facilitate lipolysis. Various medications with cytokine inhibitory properties such as pentoxyfylline and megestrol acetate are being evaluated as possible therapies for cancer cachexia,[71] although a report of severe, symptomatic adrenal suppression associated with the use of megestrol acetate suggests caution and monitoring when utilizing this drug.[72]

CLINICAL ASSESSMENT OF NUTRITIONAL STATUS

The assessment of a child with cancer includes standard elements of a nutritional evaluation: history of past and present illness, review of dietary intake, physical examination, and anthropometric measurements. Attention should also be directed to the significance of body composition changes as well as a review of pertinent laboratory measures.

History

A detailed medical history is essential to the nutritional evaluation of a patient, including the type and stage of the tumor, the intensity of the planned anti-tumor therapy, and the presence or absence of remission. As noted earlier, there are important risk factors for the development of malnutrition in patients with cancer[73] (Table 41.3).

Nutritional history should include (1) elicitation of current symptoms of cancer and its therapy and their effect on nutrient intake, absorption, and retention; (2) past history, including past growth data; previous anti-tumor therapy and its effects on nutritional status; (3) developmental status, with special attention to milestones of feeding skills and swallowing function; (4) known or perceived food allergies or intolerances;

(5) medications, with special attention to those with gastrointestinal side effects; (6) family history, parental heights, and sibling growth patterns; and (7) social history, food preferences/beliefs, and food availability.

The ability of children to eat at their appropriate developmental level may affect the nutritional adequacy of their diet. Anorexia, mucositis, and other effects of cancer treatment may interrupt the normal progression of feeding skills in infants and young children. Once arrested, the development of these skills may be difficult to restore. Poor swallowing and chewing abilities will lengthen the time required to complete a meal and thus may lead to inadequate consumption of many required nutrients. Children may refuse to eat their preferred foods due to adverse associations or other impairments and thus may self-restrict their intake.

A thorough diet history obtained from the patient and/or caregivers may be analyzed to detail the nutritional intake of the child with cancer. A 24-hour dietary recall, which is the most rapid dietary intake method, can be easily incorporated into the general history and physical examination. A prospective food diary, in which a subject measures and records all intake for 3 to 7 days, may be the most reliable and valid clinical tool for evaluating usual nutritional intake. Proper interpretation of these diet records requires consultation with a qualified dietitian. Prospective diet records should generally be performed while the patient is feeling well, free of the effects of acute illness, and should include at least one weekend day in school-age children.

Formal nutrition screening tools have been examined among adults with cancer. These screens aid the practitioner in quickly determining those individuals at nutrition risk, and therefore requiring further nutrition intervention. The Malnutrition Screening Tool is a short, three-item set of questions that probes the patient about weight, percentage weight loss, and appetite.[74] The Patient-Generated Subjective Global Assessment (PGSGA)[75] was designed specifically for the oncology population and consists of four questions for the patient around weight history, symptoms, food intake, and activity level. The second portion of the PGSGA is directed toward the health care professional and includes an evaluation of metabolic demand, diagnosis, and comorbidities in relation to nutrition requirements and elements of the physical examination. Both the Malnutrition Screening Tool and the PGSGA have been validated in specific adult oncology populations, though their applicability in the pediatric population is unknown.

Physical Examination

The physical characteristics of a child with cancer may suggest the presence of nutritional problems. Indeed, the predisposition of chemotherapy to affect tissues of rapid turnover (e.g., hair and gastrointestinal mucosa) mirrors the symptoms of deficiency of a wide range of nutrients (e.g., stomatitis with some B vitamins, alopecia with biotin deficiency). Careful inspection and palpation of subcutaneous fat and muscle stores are particularly important in the physical examination, because deficits of these two components of body stores are common in malnutrition.

The general physical examination may show edema as a result of low concentrations of circulating albumin. This can be a subtle finding with only mild hypoalbuminemia. Edema may actually mask progressive muscle wasting and loss of lean body mass. Edema on physical examination may reflect edema of the bowel, which can contribute to malabsorption. Hypoalbuminemia may be due to poor liver function related to tumor or treatment, inadequate protein intake, or nutrient losses in excess of intake.[76] Painful mouth or esophageal sores caused by mucositis can negatively impact a child's oral intake and thus be an impetus to consider nutritional support.[77] Alopecia and stomatitis, commonly associated with chemotherapy, can also be caused by vitamin or mineral deficiencies. Recognition of significant changes in the physical examination is a valuable clue to the overall nutritional assessment of a child with cancer.

Anthropometrics

Weight and height measured over time are the mainstays of nutritional monitoring and evaluation. When compared with age and sex-appropriate standards, these data can provide objective measures of nutritional status and provide the most information for the least inconvenience and cost. Weight should be measured daily in the hospital setting and at each office visit for outpatients. Accurate technique is critical to the validity of the measures; detailed methodologies are outlined elsewhere.[78,79] Length should be measured every 1 to 3 months in infants, and at least yearly for older patients. Measurements should be plotted on the National Center for Health Statistics (NCHS) growth curve and compared with established norms for age and sex and the corresponding percentiles determined. Reference curves are published by the NCHS of the Centers for Disease Control and Prevention (CDC) at http://www.cdc.gov/growthcharts/.

The most widely used anthropometric screening criteria for malnutrition in children are those of Waterlow.[80] These criteria recognize that children who are underweight may be either short and well proportioned (so-called "stunted") or truly underweight for their height (so-called "wasted"). Wasted children have an acute deficit of body mass and suffer a variety of functional deficits (e.g., decreased muscle strength, impaired immune function, and decreased organ mass among others). The incidence of weight and height deficits in children with cancer has been reported to be quite high, depending on the severity and type of cancer and its treatment.[73,81]

Due to the increased incidence of obesity in children and the predisposition of some pediatric patients with cancer to become obese, it is equally important to screen for overweight. For children younger than 3 years, this can be done by calculating the weight-for-height percentage standard using the NCHS growth curves. For older children, BMI[82] is a more reasonable measure of body fatness. Children with BMIs greater than the 85th percentile for age and sex are termed overweight, whereas those with BMIs greater than the 95th percentile are obese. Reference values for BMIs are available[83] and are also included with the NCHS growth curves.

Arm Anthropometrics

Arm anthropometrics are an inexpensive, noninvasive and widely accepted technique for estimating body composition against established normal values. Mid-arm circumference is measured with a nonstretchable flexible tape at the midpoint between the acromion and the olecranon. Triceps skinfold is measured on the back of the arm at this same point with a caliper exerting a constant pressure of 10 g/mm[2]. With these two measurements, the mid-arm muscle area (MAMA) can be calculated:

$$MAMA = \frac{(MUAC - \pi TSF)^2}{4\pi}$$

where MAMA is the mid-arm muscle area (cm[2]), MUAC is mid-upper arm circumference (cm), TSF is triceps skinfold (cm), and $\pi = 3.1416$.

Percentiles and standards for comparisons for triceps skinfolds and MAMA are available[84] and may indicate the presence of malnutrition when weight or height is unavailable or invalid.

A study of 16 boys with newly diagnosed cancer revealed no significant deviation from normal with respect to weight, height, and weight for height. However, when comparing the mid-arm circumference, triceps skinfold, and subscapular skinfold to normal values, significant reductions were found in the patients with cancer.[85] Another study compared weight for height values with MUAC and TSF of children with solid tumors and controls. Although all children presented with normal weights and heights compared with national standards, children with solid tumors, particularly those with intra-abdominal tumors, had significantly lower values of MUAC and TSF.[86] These studies suggest that arm anthropometrics may be more sensitive indicators of undernutrition than are weight and height, especially when significant tumor weight is expected. A study of 23 children with various oncologic conditions examined the validity of different anthropometric measurements in assessing nutritional status. Researchers confirmed that measurements of triceps skinfolds and percentage of ideal body weight were accurately reflective of percentage of body fat, and should be incorporated into the routine assessment of the pediatric patients with cancer.[87]

Measures of Body Composition

Anthropometric measurements may be confounded by technique, inaccuracy of equipment, lack of patient cooperation, and discrepancies between weight and protein energy reserves. Lean body mass is the metabolically active component of the body. It would be ideal, therefore, to characterize weight by some measure of lean body mass in order to accurately assess the need for and/or response to nutritional intervention.[85] Patients with solid tumors prior to reduction or excision are particularly susceptible to inaccurate weight measurements. In a study of 19 children with malignant solid tumors, regional ultrasonography of the femoral quadriceps muscle was more sensitive than anthropometrics and measurements of visceral proteins in detecting reduced muscle protein reserves compared with age and sex matched controls,[88] suggesting the need for further analysis of body composition in assessing nutritional status.

Bioelectrical impedance (BIA) is an inexpensive and increasingly available method of assessing body composition. The technique relies on the principle that fat-free mass, being composed of water and ions, conducts an electrical charge faster than fat mass.[89] Lean body mass therefore has a lower resistance to current. Reactance, a measure of cell membrane capacitance, is also measured by BIA, and together with resistance can be used to estimate total body water, both intra- and extracellular. Using assumptions about its water content, fat-free mass is calculated. When compared with other techniques, BIA appears to be a reliable measure of body composition.[90]

DXA is becoming increasingly available for clinical use. DXA measures lean body mass, fat mass, and bone mass, thereby accounting for any abnormalities in bone mineral density.[91] Specifically, DXA scanning determines bone mineral content, bone mineral density, and total body bone mineral content. Some instruments assess total body bone mineral content, nonbone lean tissue, and fat, thereby providing body composition information using a three compartment model.

A number of studies have compared measurements of fat mass with DXA versus results obtained from under water weighing (hydrodensitometry),[92] and the correlations between the methods have generally been high. Unlike hydrodensitometry, DXA also measures the composition of particular body parts, thus allowing one to compare visceral and subcutaneous adiposity. Studies regarding the validity of DXA as an appropriate measure of body composition are conflicting. One group examined patients aged 4 to 20 years and found that percentage of body fat, fat mass, lean tissue mass, and bone mineral content correlated significantly between DXA and BMI.[93] Other studies suggest that the fat mass component, which can lead to overweight/obesity according to BMI, may vary greatly in growing children, especially females.[94] Although the ultimate applicability of DXA scanning to nutritional assessment is still evolving,[95] it is now widely used as a reasonable method of assessing body composition.[96]

Laboratory Evaluation

Although laboratory evaluation of the pediatric patient with cancer is commonly performed to assess the hematologic and metabolic response to cancer and its treatment, the clinician should also monitor nutritional status with select biochemical parameters. A specific metabolic emergency termed "tumor lysis syndrome" occurs when the tumor mass is suddenly reduced with initial chemotherapy. The massive cell lysis can lead to life-threatening electrolyte abnormalities, as discussed in detail in Chapter 38 "Oncologic Emergencies."

Proteins synthesized by the liver are often used to assess nutritional status, because decreased levels presumably reflect a reduced supply of amino acid precursors and/or decreased hepatic and other visceral protein mass. Blood concentrations of these proteins, however, are dependent on their rates of synthesis, degradation, and escape from the circulatory system. Serum proteins are also affected by infectious or catabolic processes. The concentrations of positive acute-phase proteins (e.g., C-reactive protein, ferritin, and ceruloplasmin) are increased in infectious or other catabolic illnesses, whereas negative acute-phase proteins (e.g., albumin, prealbumin, transferrin, and retinol-binding protein) are decreased in these circumstances.

Albumin is the most abundant serum protein, making up nearly 5 of the 10 g/dL of total protein in the serum. Because more than half of the body albumin is extravascular (primarily in skin and muscle), maintenance of normal serum levels can occur from mobilization of these stores despite prolonged energy or protein inadequacy. Combined with its long half-life of 20 days, these factors make serum albumin a relatively insensitive marker of nutritional status. Hypoalbuminemia is not necessarily diagnostic of malnutrition; it can occur in situations of decreased synthesis (e.g., liver disease, age over 70 years, malignancy), increased losses (e.g., nephrosis, protein-losing enteropathy, burn injuries), or increased losses to extravascular spaces (e.g., acute catabolic stress with capillary leak syndrome). Fluid overload can also dilute albumin concentrations, and bed rest can decrease levels by 0.5 g/dL.

Prealbumin is another visceral protein, named because of its proximity to albumin on an electrophoretic strip. Prealbumin circulates in plasma in a 1:1 ratio with retinol-binding protein. Its short half-life (2 days) and high ratio of essential to nonessential amino acids make it a good measure of visceral protein status, more sensitive than albumin as a measure of nutritional recovery. Studies have shown prealbumin to correlate well with nitrogen balance,[97,98] and it may be the best available serum marker of nutritional status. Like albumin, concentrations fall with an acute-phase protein response or liver disease. Levels increase with renal failure.

It may also be helpful to assess vitamin and mineral nutritional status, particularly in the patient on total enteral or parenteral nutritional support. At the time of diagnosis, the effect of tumor burden on metabolic processes may be profound, as demonstrated by laboratory analysis. In a study of 40 children with ALL, >70% of children had low plasma 1,25-dihydroxy vitamin D levels, 73% had low osteocalcin levels, and 64% had hypercalciuria at the time of diagnosis. This is an indication of the effect of leukemia on vitamin D metabolism and bone turnover. The use of steroids and nephrotoxic agents may worsen hypercalciuria, putting patients at a greater risk for osteopenia and fractures. Excessive renal losses of magnesium during treatment with these medications were also demonstrated, with only 50% of patients able to maintain normal serum magnesium levels despite parenteral supplementation.[99]

Antioxidant nutrients, including vitamins A and E, β-carotene, zinc, and selenium have also been studied. Children with a variety of cancers had lower concentrations of retinol, β-carotene, vitamin E, and zinc prior to treatment compared with controls, but were not significantly different than controls following treatment. When separated by diagnosis, however, zinc concentrations in patients with central nervous system tumors and malignant bone tumors were persistently lower following 6 months of treatment.[100] Zinc deficiency was also found to be common in children following stem cell transplantation. Nineteen of 28 children developed biochemical zinc deficiency at a median of 7 days posttransplant.[101] Selenium deficiency has been reported in adult and pediatric oncology patients.[102–104] Additional research is needed to further elucidate the relationship of these nutrients with clinical outcomes.

NUTRITION INTERVENTION TECHNIQUES

The method of nutrition support chosen is based on the clinical assessment and the child's nutrient requirements.[105] Some children may require minor alterations to their oral diet; others may require specialized enteral or parenteral support. There is substantial evidence that enteral support is a less expensive, safer, and effective way of nourishing the child with cancer than parenteral nutrition.[106] Patients and their family members should of course be included in the discussion of nutrition options, with accurate depiction of the risks and benefits of the possible methods of nutrition support given the patient's current situation.

When treating the malnourished child, it is imperative to consider the manifestations of refeeding the body in a starved state. A profound hypophosphatemia, in particular, can characterize the rapid cellular influx of nutrients during the anabolic phase following starvation. Severe metabolic complications may be avoided by the slow advancement of macronutrients over a period of days to weeks as well as close laboratory monitoring of electrolytes, glucose, and minerals.

Oral Feeding

Modifications to the oral diet for pediatric oncology patients include reduced bacteria,[107] texture changes, adjustments to electrolyte or mineral content, and calorie supplementation. Although the efficacy of low bacteria diets to reduce infections has not been proven, some centers continue to use them

TABLE 41.4

SANITARY FOOD PRACTICES FOR IMMUNOCOMPROMISED PATIENTS

- Good hand washing before and after preparing and eating meals
- Do not share food with others
- Avoid foods from street vendors, salad bars, shared bins of foods in grocery stores
- Wash raw foods well prior to eating
- Cook meat until well done
- Avoid raw eggs
- Avoid soft French style cheeses, pates, uncooked hot dogs, and sliced deli meats
- Avoid alfalfa sprouts and unpasteurized juices
- Keep foods at <40° F or >140° F to minimize growth of bacteria
- Clean all preparation items thoroughly before and after use to avoid cross-contamination
- Keep refrigerated leftovers for no more than 3 d

Adapted from Bechard L. Oncology and bone marrow transplantation. In: Hendricks K, Duggan C, Walker W, eds. Manual of pediatric nutrition. 3rd ed. Hamilton, Ontario: B.C. Decker, 2000.

TABLE 41.5

STRATEGIES FOR IMPROVING ORAL INTAKE DURING CANCER TREATMENT

Loss of appetite
- Small frequent feedings (6–8 meals/snacks per day)
- Encourage nutrient-dense beverages between meals
- Offer favorite nutritious foods during treatment-free periods to prevent learned food aversions

Nausea and vomiting
- Feed 3–4 h before therapy that typically causes nausea and vomiting
- Offer small amounts of cool foods and encourage slow eating; avoid strong odors
- Offer clear liquids between meals; using a straw in a covered cup may facilitate sipping

Mouth sores
- Serve soft or pureed bland food or liquids
- Add butter, gravy, sauce or salad dressing to moisten foods
- Avoid highly seasoned or hard, rough foods

Altered taste perception
- Use stronger seasonings; avoid excessively sweet foods
- Offer salty foods, e.g., hot dogs, pizza, canned pasta
- Try new flavors of foods

Adapted from Bechard L. Oncology and bone marrow transplantation. In: Hendricks K, Duggan C, Walker W, eds. Manual of pediatric nutrition. 3rd ed. Hamilton, Ontario: B.C. Decker, 2000.

routinely, particularly in the stem cell transplant setting. General principles of cautious food safety should be followed for any immunocompromised child (Table 41.4).

Children with mucositis often better tolerate a soft diet. A diet high in magnesium or potassium may be useful for the child with excessive urinary losses of minerals because of chemotherapies or antibiotics. Calorie supplementation may be required to assist with weight gain or weight maintenance during cancer treatment. This can be accomplished with usual foods, or in combination with commercial supplemental drinks or calorie additives. Techniques for increasing oral energy intake are listed in Table 41.5.

Some children, particularly long-term survivors of cancer with activity limitations, may be aided by the instruction of moderate calorie and low-fat diet principles when obesity is a concern (Table 41.6).

Enteral Feeding

If children are unable to meet their nutrient needs orally, tube feedings should be considered as a means of preserving or obtaining optimal nutritional status. In children newly diagnosed with cancer, nasogastric tube feedings have been given in addition to volitional oral intake with successful weight gain.[108] Several studies have reported the use of nasogastric feedings in children after HSCT with varying results. One group demonstrated improved weight gain in 21 patients, compared with 8 children receiving dietary counseling alone. There was a positive correlation between increases in weight and mid-arm circumference and the duration of enteral feedings. However, 8 of the 21 patients stopped feedings after 10 days because of vomiting or diarrhea. Six of these patients were then switched to parenteral nutrition support.[109] Langdana et al. retrospectively analyzed their intensive enteral feeding protocol for children undergoing HSCT, which included routine insertion of nasogastric tubes during conditioning or when oral intake had decreased. Of their 49 evaluable patients, 86% were maintained on enteral nutrition alone, including 8% who took adequate oral intake.[110] A

more recent study compared tube feeding with parenteral nutrition in a group of children undergoing allogeneic HSCT, with just 3 of 34 patients supported exclusively by tube feeding; the remainder required partial or total parenteral nutrition. Cholestasis occurred significantly less often in children who received at least some tube feeding compared with children who were exclusively parenterally fed; nutritional costs were also less in children receiving tube feeding.[111] These studies suggest the feasibility of nasogastric feeding as a method of nutrition support for pediatric cancer and HSCT patients, although clearly some patients will be unable to tolerate the

TABLE 41.6

HEALTHY EATING GUIDELINES FOR CHILDHOOD CANCER SURVIVORS

Aim for fitness
- Aspire to a healthy weight
- Be active each day within personal limitations

Build a healthy base
- Eat a variety of whole grains, fruits, and vegetables each day
- Consume 3–4 servings of high calcium foods daily

Choose sensibly
- Select a diet low in saturated fat and cholesterol
- Limit sugary foods and beverages
- Choose and prepare foods with less salt.

Adapted from Excerpt of the Report of the Dietary Guidelines Advisory Committee on Dietary Guidelines for Americans, 2000, United States Department of Agriculture. http://www.health.gov/dietary guidelines/dga2000/document/frontcover.htm

required volumes to support their nutritional requirements. Gastrostomy tube feedings are generally considered to be more cosmetically acceptable and more comfortable than nasogastric feedings, while still providing the same advantages over parenteral nutrition. The use of surgically placed or percutaneous endoscopic gastrostomy feedings in pediatric patients with cancer has been examined by several groups. Almost all the groups documented that the majority of patients maintained or gained weight with percutaneous endoscopic gastrostomy feeds. Severe complications, such as systemic infections, were a rarity and not observed in all studies. Minor complications were noted, and included leakage of gastric juice leading to site irritation, bleeding at the site, and superficial infections.[112–114]

Nutritionally complete formulas for oral supplementation or tube feeding are available for a variety of ages and conditions (Table 41.7). Most pediatric patients with cancer will tolerate intact protein, 1 kcal/mL formulas either orally or via tube feeding. On rare occasions, a specialized formula for tube feeding may be indicated. Formulas with elemental (free amino acids) or semielemental (small peptides) protein are available, primarily for the purpose of allergy or intolerance. Medium chain triglycerides are also used in many formulas intended for patients with fat malabsorption. An abundance of defined formula diets are available for varying conditions and ages.

Parenteral Feeding

When the gastrointestinal tract is nonfunctional or unavailable, nutrients may be infused via central venous catheters. Parenteral nutrition (PN) has been widely used in the oncology population due to the cytotoxic effects of many treatment regimens. Many chemotherapy agents commonly cause some degree of nausea and vomiting. Radiation therapy, when directed to gastrointestinal organs, also causes cell damage that may impair digestive or absorptive function. High-dose chemotherapeutic regimens and total body irradiation, used in preparation for stem cell transplantation, may cause a severe mucositis and enteritis, making significant oral or enteral intake difficult for many patients to achieve for several weeks. Gastrointestinal graft-versus-host disease, a complication of allogeneic stem cell transplantation, typically causes impaired absorption of nutrients, either because of anorexia and diminished oral intake in its mildest cases, or as profuse, bloody diarrhea in its more severe cases.

The value of PN in patients with cancer has been questioned; in fact, its routine use in adults undergoing chemotherapy has been discouraged due to the risks of infectious complications.[115] HSCT, however, is one of the few clinical situations where PN has demonstrated benefit. Studies in the 1980s suggested sooner engraftment,[116] better survival, lengthier time to relapse, and improved disease-free survival grouping patients receiving PN.[17] These studies were instrumental in making PN an integral part of supportive care to HSCT patients.

When indicated, PN goals should be based on estimated requirements for age and nutritional assessment. Fluid requirements and venous access must also be considered in formulating the PN prescription. Electrolytes, pediatric multivitamin, and trace element preparations should be added according to usual requirements.

The risks of PN can be significant, and include infections, hepatotoxicity, suppression of oral intake, and metabolic abnormalities. Most children undergoing aggressive cancer treatment will require indwelling central venous catheters for chemotherapy, but the use of PN has been associated with a 2.4-fold increase in the risk of infection in children receiving chemotherapy who have central access devices in place.[117] The

---

TABLE 41.7

COMMON FORMULAS FOR ORAL OR TUBE FEEDING IN PEDIATRIC ONCOLOGY

Formula	Caloric density (kcal/mL)	Nutrient sources			Indications
		Carbohydrate	Protein	Fat	
Boost[a]	1.01	Sucrose, corn syrup solids	Milk protein concentrate	Canola, high oleic sunflower, and corn oils	Complete oral/enteral supplement
Ensure[b]	1.06	Sucrose, corn syrup, corn maltodextrin	Milk protein concentrate, soy protein concentrate	Soy, canola, and corn oils	Complete oral/enteral supplement
Pediasure[b]	1.0	Sucrose, corn maltodextrin	Milk protein concentrate, whey protein concentrate, soy protein isolate	High oleic safflower, soy, and medium chain triglyceride oils	Complete feeding for 1–13 yr
Nutren junior[a]	1.0	Maltodextrin, sugar	Milk protein concentrate, whey protein concentrate	Soy, canola, and medium chain triglyceride oils	Enteral feeding for 1–10 yr
Peptamen junior[a]	1.0	Maltodextrin, corn starch	Enzymatically hydrolyzed whey protein	Medium chain triglyceride, soy, and canola oils	Peptide based feeding for 1–10 yr
Neocate junior[c]	1.0 (standard dilution)	Corn syrup solids	100% free amino acids	Fractionated coconut, canola, and high oleic safflower oils	Hypoallergenic feeding for 1–10 yr

[a]Nestle Nutrition. www.nestle-nutrition.com, www.boost.com.
[b]Abbott Nutrition. www.ensure.com, www.pediasure.com.
[c]Nutricia North America. www.shsna.com.
From product information.

TABLE 41.8

NUTRITIONAL MONITORING SCHEDULE OF CHILDREN WITH CANCER

Parameter	Hospitalized patients on parenteral nutrition	Hospitalized patients on oral/tube feedings	Outpatients on parenteral nutrition	Outpatients on oral/tube feedings
Weight	Daily	Daily	Weekly	Monthly
Height	Monthly	Monthly	Monthly	Monthly
Head circumference (<36 mo)	Weekly	Weekly	Monthly	Monthly
Arm anthropometrics	Monthly	As indicated	Monthly	As indicated
Intake/output	Daily	Daily	Daily to weekly	Weekly to monthly
Electrolytes, glucose	Daily	Weekly	Weekly	Monthly
Blood urea nitrogen, creatinine	Weekly	Weekly	Weekly	Monthly
Calcium, phosphorus, magnesium	Daily to weekly	Weekly	Weekly	Monthly
Triglyceride	Weekly	Monthly	Weekly	As indicated
Liver function tests	Weekly	Weekly	Monthly	Monthly
Trace elements	Monthly	As indicated	Biannually	As indicated
Carnitine	Monthly	As indicated	Biannually	As indicated
Vitamin levels	Monthly	As indicated	Biannually	As indicated

Adapted from Davis AM. Initiation, monitoring, and complications of pediatric parenteral nutrition. In: Baker RD Jr, Baker SS, Davis AM, eds. Pediatric parenteral nutrition. New York: Chapman & Hall, 1997:212–237.

specific role of intravenous fats in increasing infectious complications was evaluated in a randomized trial of more than 500 children and adults undergoing HSCT. There was no increased risk of bacteremia or fungal infections in those receiving standard amounts of intravenous lipids (25–30% of energy) versus those receiving only 6% to 8% of energy as fat.[118]

Many of the medicines used in oncologic treatment can cause liver injury. The use of PN, singly or in combination with these medicines, may cause biliary dysfunction or steatosis.[119] The use of intravenous omega-3 fatty acids in the treatment of PN-associated liver disease has been described in infants with short bowel syndrome; its role in pediatric patients with cancer should be evaluated. Another potential risk of PN administration is the generation of peroxide compounds, which may have harmful effects in neonates and others with immune dysfunction and/or reduced antioxidant defenses.[120] Covering PN bags and intravenous tubing with opaque plastic coloring may reduce this effect.[121]

PN may also cause early satiety and decreased oral intake. In a randomized controlled trial of children and young adults following marrow transplantation, outpatient PN delayed resumption of oral intake by 6 days as compared with 5% dextrose hydration. The clinical outcome of both groups was not significantly different.[122] Nausea and vomiting have been linked with children receiving PN at home.[123] Metabolic derangements are also associated with PN. Over- or underhydration, electrolyte imbalance, hyperglycemia, and hypoglycemia are among the most common concerns.[124]

Although the weight of evidence still seems to support a role for PN in selected pediatric patients with cancer, close monitoring of laboratory values and clinical condition in addition to the specifics of the PN prescription are necessary to prevent complications (Table 41.8).

VITAMINS IN TREATING THE PEDIATRIC PATIENT WITH CANCER

Surveys suggest that 24% to 90% of pediatric patients with cancer have used some form of complementary or alternative

therapy.[125] Chapter 52 discusses "Complementary and Alternative Medical Therapies in Pediatric Oncology", though it is worth mentioning that certain nutrition supplements fall into this category, including antioxidants, homeopathic treatment for mucositis, and glutamine as a nutraceutical, or nutrition therapy.

Antioxidants, those chemicals or nutrients that help prevent the accumulation of highly reactive oxygen species, are thought to stave off the adverse effects of cancer treatment, aid the anti-cancer effects of conventional therapy, and prevent second malignancies.[126] Some data support these postulates in pediatric patients with cancer. A study of 103 children with ALL associated higher plasma concentrations of vitamin A, E, total carotenoids, total antioxidant capacity, and 8-oxo-2'-deoxyguanosine with fewer dose reductions, fewer infections, improved quality of life, less delay in chemotherapy treatment schedule, reduced toxicity, and fewer days spent in the hospital.[127] Although such research supports an antioxidant-rich diet, further studies are needed to validate these observations before routine supplementation of antioxidants can be recommended to the pediatric patient with cancer.

Clearly vitamins have a critical role in both enteral and parenteral nutritional intervention. More recently, though, research suggests that vitamins may be linked to the prevention of certain childhood cancers and the decrease of certain adverse effects of chemotherapy.[128] Prenatal maternal multivitamin use has been connected to a reduction in the risk of neuroblastoma in a sample size of 500 cases and 500 controls. Mothers who took a daily multivitamin 1 month prior and during each trimester of the pregnancy had a 30% to 40% reduction in the risk of neuroblastoma.[129] Details regarding the protective element in the multivitamin are yet to be elucidated. Another study of 80 children with ALL and 166 control families links a protective effect between iron or folate during pregnancy and ALL.[130] Increased vitamin E intake at 3 months post chemotherapy offers a protective effect against infection, while β-carotene intake at 6 months decreases toxicity.[131] In a cohort of children with Down syndrome, a decreased risk of leukemia was observed with maternal use of periconceptional vitamins.[132] These studies all hint at the potential benefits of vitamins in treating the pediatric patient with cancer, and will undoubtedly lead to further investigation.

NUTRITIONAL CONCERNS OF LONG-TERM SURVIVORS OF CHILDHOOD CANCER

Most nutritional issues during cancer treatment are associated with weight loss or poor growth. Although it is true that many cancer survivors become underweight adults,[133] there is also a notable risk of obesity. This risk of obesity can be connected to the development of insulin resistance and metabolic syndrome in pediatric cancer survivors, with severe implications for adult health. Conflicting reports of a greater prevalence of osteopenia in childhood cancer survivors have been published.[134,135] One recent study of 74 long-term ALL survivors used population normative data to conclude that osteopenia was more prevalent than expected.[136] As the number of pediatric cancer survivors continues to increase, understanding the long-term nutritional concerns will be critical in managing their health as adults.

CONCLUSION

The nutritional care of children with cancer is a challenge that lasts from diagnosis to many years after treatment. Because children must be expected to show acceptable growth during extended treatment courses as well as following therapy, serial nutritional assessments should be performed with appropriate follow-up. Malnutrition should not be accepted as an unavoidable consequence of cancer and/or its therapy. Similarly, every effort should be made to prevent obesity and other chronic diseases of adulthood in long-term cancer survivors. Children should be taught healthy diet principles and acceptable activity options for weight maintenance and control (Table 41.6). A multidisciplinary approach of extensive nutritional intervention and counseling can assist with the supportive care of the pediatric patient with cancer to improve health outcomes and quality of life.

References

1. Donaldson S, Wesley M, DeWys W, et al. A study of the nutritional status of pediatric cancer patients. Am J Dis Child 1981;135:1107.
2. Costelli P, Baccino F. Cancer cachexia: from experimental models to patient management. Curr Opin Clin Nutr Metab Care 2000;3:177–181.
3. Reilly JJ, Weir J, McColl JH, et al. Prevalence of protein-energy malnutrition at diagnosis in children with acute lymphoblastic leukemia. J Pediatr Gastroenterol Nutr 1999;29:194–197.
4. Elhasid R, Laor A, Lischinsky S, et al. Nutritional status of children with solid tumors. Cancer 1999;86:119–125.
5. Kumar R, Marwaha RK, Bhalla AK, et al. Protein energey malnutrition and skeletal muscle wasting in childhood acute lymphoblastic lukemia. Indian Pediatr 2000;37:720–726.
6. Weir J, Reilly J, McColl J, et al. No evidence for an effect of nutritional status at diagnosis on prognosis in children wtih acute lymphoblastic leukemia. J Pediatr Hematol Oncol 1998;20:534–538.
7. Viana M, Murao M, Ramos G, et al. Malnutrition as a prognostic factor in lymphoblastic leukaemia: a multivariate analysis. Arch Dis Child 1994;71:304–310.
8. Lobato-Mendizabal E, Lopez-Martinez B, Ruiz-Arguelles GJ. A critical review of the prognostic value of the nutritional status in the outcome of therapy of children with acute lymphoblastic leukemia. Rev Invest Clin 2003;55:31–35.
9. Kern K, Norton J. Cancer cachexia. JPEN J Parenter Enteral Nutr 1988;12:286–298.
10. Burt M, Stein T, Schwade J, et al. Whole-body protein metabolism in cancer-bearing patients: effect of total parenteral nutrition and associated serum insulin response. Cancer 1984;53:1246–1252.
11. Ziegler TR, Young LS, Benfell K, et al. Clinical and metabolic efficacy of glutamine-supplemented parenteral nutrition after bone marrow transplantation. A randomized, double-blind, controlled study. Ann Int Med 1992;116:821–828.
12. Martyn CN, Winter PD, Coles SJ, et al. Effect of nutritional status on use of health care resources by patients with chronic disease living in the community. Clin Nutr 1998;17:119–123.
13. Galler J, Ramsey F, Soliman G, et al. The influence of early malnutrition on subsequent behavioral development: 1. Degree of impairment in intellectual performance. J Am Acad Child Adolesc Psychiatry 1983;22:8.
14. Andreyev HJ, Norman AR, Oates J, et al. Why do patients with weight loss have a worse outcome when undergoing chemotherapy for gastrointestinal malignancies? Eur J Cancer 1998;34:503–509.
15. Rickard K, Loghmani E, Gorsfeld J, et al. Short- and long-term effectiveness of enteral and parenteral nutrition in reversing or preventing protein energy malnutrition in advanced neuroblastoma: a prospective randomized study. Cancer 1985;56:2881–2897.
16. Taj M, Pearson A, Mumford D, et al. Effect of nutritional status on the incidence of infection in childhood cancer. Pediatr Hematol Oncol 1993;10:283–287.
17. Weisdorf S, Lysne J, Wind D, et al. Positive effect of prophylactic total parenteral nutrition on long-term outcome of bone marrow transplantation. Transplantation 1987;43:833–838.
18. Souba W. Nutritional support. N Engl J Med 1997;336:41–48.
19. Oeffinger KC, Mertens AC, Sklar CA, et al. Obesity in adult survivors of childhood acute lymphoblastic leukemia: a report from the Childhood Cancer Survivor Study. J Clin Oncol 2003;21:1359–1365.
20. Lustig RH, Post SR, Srivannaboon K, et al. Risk factors for the development of obesity in children surviving brain tumors. J Clin Endocrinol Metab 2003;88:611–616.
21. Wolfe J, Grier HE, Klar N, et al. Symptoms and suffering at the end of life in children with cancer. N Engl J Med 2000;342:326–333.
22. Fernandez CV, Stutzer CA, MacWilliam L, et al. Alternative and complementary therapy use in pediatric oncology patients in British Columbia: prevalence and reasons for use and nonuse. J Clin Oncol 1998;16:1279–1286.
23. Kemper KJ, Wornham WL. Consultations for holistic pediatric services for inpatients and outpatient oncology patients at a children's hospital. Arch Pediatr Adolesc Med 2001;155:449–454.
24. Tisdale MJ. Cancer cachexia: metabolic alterations and clinical manifestations. Nutrition 1997;13:1–7.
25. Roubenoff R, Heymsfield SB, Kehayias JJ, et al. Standardization of nomenclature of body composition in weight loss. Am J Clin Nutr 1997;66:192–196.
26. Moley JF, Aamodt R, Rumble W, et al. Body cell mass in cancer-bearing and anorexic patients. JPEN J Parenter Enteral Nutr 1987;11:219–222.
27. Tisdale M. Wasting in cancer. J Nutr 1999;129:243S–246S.
28. Cunningham JJ. Body composition and nutrition support in pediatrics: what to defend and how soon to begin. Nutr Clin Pract 1995;10:177–182.
29. Castaneda C, Charnley JM, Evans WJ, et al. Elderly women accommodate to a low-protein diet with losses of body cell mass, muscle function, and immune response. Am J Clin Nutr 1995;62:30–39.
30. Brennan M. Total parenteral nutrition in the cancer patient. N Engl J Med 1981;305:375–382.
31. Dietz WH, Robinson TN. Overweight children and adolescents. N Engl J Med 2005;352:2100–2109.
32. Hijiya N, Panetta JC, Zhou Y, et al. Body mass index does not influence pharmacokinetics or outcome of treatment in children with acute lymphoblastic leukemia. Blood 2006;108:3997–4002.
33. Lange BJ, Gerbing RB, Feusner J, et al. Mortality in overweight and underweight children with acute myeloid leukemia. JAMA 2005;293:203–211.
34. Thompson PA, Rosner GL, Matthay KK, et al. Impact of body composition on pharmacokinetics of doxorubicin in children: a Glaser Pediatric Research Network study. Cancer Chemother Pharmacol 2009;64(2):243–251.
35. Warner JT, Bell W, Webb DK, et al. Daily energy expenditure and physical activity in survivors of childhood malignancy. Pediatr Res 1998;43:607–613.
36. Murphy AJ, Wells JCK, Williams JE, et al. Body composition in children in remission from acute lymphoblastic leukemia. Am J Clin Nutr 2006;83:70–74.
37. Didi M, Didcock E, Davies HA, et al. High incidence of obesity in young adults after treatment of acute lymphoblastic leukemia in childhood. J Pediatr 1995;127:63–67.
38. Cohen A, Rovelli A, Van-Lint M, et al. Final height of patients who underwent bone marrow transplantation during childhood. Arch Dis Child 1996;74:437–440.
39. Birkebaek N, Clausen N. Height and weight pattern up to 20 years after treatment for acute lymphoblastic leukemia. Arch Dis Child 1998;79:161–164.
40. Gurney JG, Ness KK, Sibley SD, et al. Metabolic syndrome and growth hormone deficiency in adult survivors of childhood acute lymphoblastic leukemia. Cancer 2006;107:1303–1312.
41. Ross JA, Oeffinger KC, Davies SM, et al. Genetic variation in the leptin receptor gene and obesity in survivors of childhood acute lymphoblastic leukemia: a report from the Childhood Cancer Survivor Study. J Clin Oncol 2004;22:3558–3562.
42. Ertem D, Acar Y, Alper G, et al. An uncommon and often overlooked cause of failure to thrive: diencephalic syndrome. J Pediatr Gastroenterol Nutr 2000;30:453–457.
43. Greenes D, Woods M. Case report: a 4-month old boy with severe emaciation, normal linear growth, and a happ affect. Curr Opin Pediatr 1996;8:50–57.
44. Delbecque-Boussard L, Gottrand F, Ategbo S, et al. Nutritional status of children with acute lymphoblastic leukemia: a longitudinal study. Am J Clin Nutr 1997;65:95–100.
45. Nysom K, Holm K, Michaelsen KF, et al. Degree of fatness after treatment for acute lymphoblastic leukemia in childhood. [erratum appears in J Clin Endocrinol Metab 2001;86(4):1758]. J Clin Endocrinol Metab 1999;84:4591–4596.
46. Strauss R. Childhood obesity. Curr Problems Pediatr 1999;29:1–36.
47. van Eys J. Nutrition and cancer: physiological interrelationships. Ann Rev Nutr 1985;5:435–461.
48. Silver S, Poroto P, Crohn E. Hypermetabolic states without hyperthyroidism (nonthyrogenous hypermetabolism). Arch Int Med 1950;85:479–482.
49. Waterhouse C, Fenninger L, Keutmann E. Nitrogen exchange and caloric expenditure in patients with malignant neoplasm. Cancer 1951;4:500–514.
50. Young VR. Energy metabolism and requirements in the cancer patient. Cancer Res 1977;37:2336–2347.
51. Knox LS, Crosby LO, Feurer ID, et al. Energy expenditure in malnourished cancer patients. Ann Surg 1983;197:152–162.

52. Stallings VA, Vaisman N, Chan HS, et al. Energy metabolism in children with newly diagnosed acute lymphoblastic leukemia. Pediatr Res 1989;26:154–157.
53. Bond SA, Han AM, Wootton SA, et al. Energy intake and basal metabolic rate during maintenance chemotherapy. Arch Dis Child 1992;67:229–232.
54. Ringwald-Smith KA, Heslop HE, Krance RA, et al. Energy expenditure in children undergoing hematopoietic stem cell transplantation. Bone Marrow Transplant 2002; 30:125–130.
55. Duggan C, Bechard L, Donovan K, et al. Changes in resting energy expenditure among children undergoing allogeneic stem cell transplantation. Am J Clin Nutr 2003;78: 104–109.
56. Reilly JJ, Ventham JC, Ralston JM, et al. Reduced energy expenditure in preobese children treated for acute lymphoblastic leukemia. Pediatr Res 1998;44:557–562.
57. Schoeller DA, Ravussin E, Schutz Y, et al. Energy expenditure by doubly labeled water: validation in humans and proposed calculation. Am J Physiol 1986;250:R823–R830.
58. Lundholm K, Holm G, Schersten T. Insulin resistance in patients with cancer. Cancer Res 1978;38:4665–4670.
59. Holroyde CP, Gabuzda TG, Putnam RC, et al. Altered glucose metabolism in metastatic carcinoma. Cancer Res 1975;35:3710–3714.
60. Yoshikawa T, Noguchi Y, Doi C, et al. Insulin resistance was connected with the alterations of substrate utilization in patients with cancer. Cancer Lett 1999;141: 93–98.
61. Todorov PT, McDevitt TM, Meyer DJ, et al. Purification and characterization of a tumor lipid-mobilizing factor. Cancer Res 1998;58:2353–2358.
62. Halton JM, Nazir DJ, McQueen MJ, et al. Blood lipid profiles in children with acute lymphoblastic leukemia. Cancer 1998;83:379–384.
63. Shaw JH, Wolfe RR. Fatty acid and glycerol kinetics in septic patients and in patients with gastrointestinal cancer. The response to glucose infusion and parenteral feeding. Ann Surg 1987;205:368–376.
64. Fearon KC, McMillan DC, Preston T, et al. Elevated circulating interleukin-6 is associated with an acute-phase response but reduced fixed hepatic protein synthesis in patients with cancer. Ann Surg 1991;213:26–31.
65. O'Keefe SJ, Ogden J, Ramjee G, et al. Contribution of elevated protein turnover and anorexia to cachexia in patients with hepatocellular carcinoma. Cancer Res 1990;50: 1226–1230.
66. Attard-Montalto SP, Camacho-Hubner C, Cotterill AM, et al. Changes in protein turnover, IGF-I and IGF binding proteins in children with cancer. Acta Paediatr 1998;87:54–60.
67. Dworzak F, Ferrari P, Gavazzi C, et al. Effects of cachexia due to cancer on whole body and skeletal muscle protein turnover. Cancer 1998;82:42–48.
68. Beutler B, Greenwald D, Hulmes JD, et al. Identity of tumour necrosis factor and the macrophage-secreted factor cachectin. Nature 1985;316:552–554.
69. Starnes HF Jr, Warren RS, Jeevanandam M, et al. Tumor necrosis factor and the acute metabolic response to tissue injury in man. J Clin Invest 1988;82:1321–1325.
70. Black K, Garrett IR, Mundy GR. Chinese hamster ovarian cells transfected with the murine interleukin-6 gene cause hypercalcemia as well as cachexia, leukocytosis and thrombocytosis in tumor-bearing nude mice. Endocrinology 1991;128:2657–2659.
71. Haslett PA. Anticytokine approaches to the treatment of anorexia and cachexia. Semin Oncol 1998;25:53–57.
72. Orme LM, Bond JD, Humphrey MS, et al. Megestrol acetate in pediatric oncology patients may lead to severe, symptomatic adrenal suppression. Cancer 2003;98:397–405.
73. Mauer AM, Burgess JB, Donaldson SS, et al. Special nutritional needs of children with malignancies: a review. JPEN J Parenter Enteral Nutr 1990;14:315–324.
74. Huhmann MB, August DA. Review of American Society for Parenteral and Enteral Nutrition (A.S.P.E.N.) Clinical Guidelines for Nutrition Support in Cancer Patients: Nutrition Screening and Assessment. Nutr Clin Pract 2008;23:182–188.
75. Bauer JCS, Ferguson M. Use of the scored Patient-Generated Subjective Global Assessment (PG-SGA) as a nutrition assessment tool in patients with cancer. Eur J Clin Nutr 2002;56:779–785.
76. Papadopoulou A, Nathavitharana K, Williams M, et al. Diarrhea and weight loss after bone marrow transplantation in children. Pediatr Hematol Oncol 1994;11: 601–611.
77. Tyc V, Vallelunga L, Mahoney S, et al. Nutritional and treatment-related characteristics of pediatric oncology patients referred or not referred for nutritional support. Med Pediatr Oncol 1995;25:379–388.
78. Anonymous. Guide to the growth assessment of infants in clinical studies. Columbus, OH: Ross Laboratories, 1992.
79. Rombeau J, Caldwell M, Forlaw L, et al. Atlas of nutritional support techniques. Boston: Little, Brown and Company, 1989.
80. Waterlow J. Classification and definition of protein-calorie malnutrition. Br Med J 1972;3:566–569.
81. Bakish J, Hargrave D, Tariq N, et al. Evaluation of dietetic intervention in children with medulloblastoma or supratentorial primitive neuroectodermal tumors. Cancer 2003; 98:1014–1020.
82. Dietz WH, Bellizzi MC. Introduction: the use of body mass index to assess obesity in children. Am J Clin Nutr 1999;70:123S–125S.
83. Must A, Dallal G, Dietz W. Reference data for obesity: 85th and 95th percentiles of body mass index (wt/ht2) and triceps skinfold thickness. Am J Clin Nutr 1991;53: 839–846.
84. Frisancho A. New norms of upper limb fat and muscle areas for assessment of nutritional status. Am J Clin Nutr 1981;34:2540.
85. Brennan BMD. Sensitive measures of the nutritional status of children with cancer in hospital and in the field. Int J Cancer 1998;11:10–13.
86. Oguz A, Karadeniz C, Pelit M, et al. Arm anthropometry in evaluation of malnutrition in children with cancer. Pediatr Hematol Oncol 1999;16:35–41.
87. White M, Davies P, Murphy A. Validation of percent body fat indicators in pediatric oncology nutrition assessment. J Pediatr Hematol Oncol 2008;30:124–129.
88. Taskinen M, Saarinen-Pihkala UM. Evaluation of muscle protein mass in children with solid tumors by muscle thickness measurement with ultrasonography, as compared with anthropometric methods and visceral protein concentrations. Eur J Clin Nutr 1998;52: 402–406.
89. Yanovski S, Hubbard V, Heymsfield S, et al. Bioelectrical impedance analysis in body composition measurement. Am J Clin Nutr 1994;64:387S–532S.
90. Lewy VD DK, Arslanian S. Determination of body composition in African-American children: validation of bioelectrical impedence with dual energy X-ray absorptiometry. J Pediatr Endocrinol Metab 1999;12:443–448.
91. Zemel BS, Riley EM, Stallings VA. Evaluation of methodology for nutritional assessment in children: anthropometry, body composition, and energy expenditure. Ann Rev Nutr 1997;17:211–235.
92. Kohrt W. Dual-energy x-ray absorptiometry: research issues and equipment. In: Carlson-Newberry S, Costello R, eds. Emerging technologies for nutrition research. Washington, DC: National Academy Press, 1997:151–167.
93. Boot AM, Bouquet J, de Ridder MA, et al. Determinants of body composition measured by dual-energy X-ray absorptiometry in Dutch children and adolescents. Am J Clin Nutr 1997;66:232–238.
94. Taylor RW, Jones IE, Williams SM, et al. Body fat percentages measured by dual-energy X-ray absorptiometry corresponding to recently recommended body mass index cutoffs for overweight and obesity in children and adolescents aged 3–18 y. Am J Clin Nutr 2002;76:1416–1421.
95. Roubenoff R, Kehayias J, Dawson-Hughes B, et al. Use of dual-energy x-ray absorptiometry in body-composition studies: not yet a "gold standard". Am J Clin Nutr 1993; 58:589–591.
96. Warner JT, Evans WD, Webb DK, et al. Body composition of long-term survivors of acute lymphoblastic leukaemia. Med Pediatr Oncol 2002;38:165–172.
97. Fletcher J, Little J, Guest P. A comparison of serum transferrin and serum prealbumin as nutritional parameters. JPEN J Parenter Enteral Nutr 1987;11:144–147.
98. Hawker FH, Stewart PM, Baxter RC, et al. Relationship of somatomedin-C/insulin-like growth factor I levels to conventional nutritional indices in critically ill patients. Crit Care Med 1987;15:732–736.
99. Atkinson SA, Halton JM, Bradley C, et al. Bone and mineral abnormalities in childhood acute lymphoblastic leukemia: influence of disease, drugs and nutrition. Int J Cancer Suppl 1998;11:35–39.
100. Malvy DJM, Arnaud J, Burtschy B, et al. Antioxidant micronutrients and childhood malignancy during oncological treatment. Med Pediatr Oncol 1997;29:213–217.
101. Papadopoulou A, Nathavitharana K, Williams MD, et al. Diagnosis and clinical associations of zinc depletion following bone marrow transplantation. Arch Dis Child 1996; 74:328–331.
102. Postovsky S, Arush MWB, Diamond E, et al. The prevalence of low selenium levels in newly diagnosed pediatric cancer patients. Pediatr Hematol Oncol 2003;20:273–280.
103. Pazirandeh A, Assadi Nejad M, et al. Determination of selenium in blood serum of children with acute leukemia and effects of chemotherapy on serum selenium level. J Trace Elements Med Biol 1999:242–246.
104. Ozgen IT, Dagdemir A, Elli M, et al. Hair selenium status in children with leukemia and lymphoma. J Pediatr Hematol Oncol 2007;29:519–522.
105. Bowman LC, Williams R, Sanders M, et al. Algorithm for nutritional support: experience of the Metabolic and Infusion Support Service of St. Jude Children's Research Hospital. Int J Cancer Suppl 1998;11:76–80.
106. Deswarte-Wallace J, Firouzbakhsh S, Finklestein JZ. Using research to change practice: enteral feedings for pediatric oncology patients. J Pediatr Oncol Nurs 2001;18: 217–223.
107. Aker SN, Cheney CL. The use of sterile and low microbial diets in ultraisolation environments. J Parenter Enteral Nutr 1983;7:390–397.
108. denBroeder E, Lippens R, van'tHof M, et al. Effects of naso-gastric tube feeding on the nutritional status of children with cancer. Eur J Clin Nutr 1998;52:494–500.
109. Papadopoulou A, MacDonald A, Williams MD, et al. Enteral nutrition after bone marrow transplantation. Arch Dis Child 1997;77:131–136.
110. Langdana A, Tully N, Molloy E, et al. Intensive enteral nutrition support in paediatric bone marrow transplantation. Bone Marrow Transplant 2001;27:741–746.
111. Hopman GD, Pena EG, Le Cessie S, et al. Tube feeding and bone marrow transplantation. Med Pediatr Oncol 2003;40:375–379.
112. Skolin I, Hernell O, Larsson MV, et al. Percutaneous endoscopic gastrostomy in children with malignant disease. J Pediatr Oncol Nurs 2002;19:154–163.
113. Pedersen AM, Kok K, Petersen G, et al. Percutaneous endoscopic gastrostomy in children with cancer. Acta Paediatr 1999;88:849–852.
114. Mathew P, Bowman L, Williams R, et al. Complications and effectiveness of gastrostomy feedings in pediatric cancer patients. J Pediatr Hematol Oncol 1996;18: 81–85.
115. American College of Physicians. Parenteral nutrition in patients receiving cancer chemotherapy. Ann Intern Med 1989;110:734–736.
116. Weisdorf S, Hofland C, Sharp H, et al. Total parenteral nutrition in bone marrow transplantation: a clinical evaluation. J Pediatr Gastroenterol Nutr 1984;3:95–100.
117. Christensen ML, Hancock ML, Gattuso J, et al. Parenteral nutrition associated with increased infection rate in children with cancer. Cancer 1993;72:2732–2738.
118. Lenssen P, Bruemmer BA, Bowden RA, et al. Intravenous lipid dose and incidence of bacteremia and fungemia in patients undergoing bone marrow transplantation. Am J Clin Nutr 1998;67:927–933.
119. Copeman MC. Use of total parenteral nutrition in children with cancer: a review and some recommendations. Pediatr Hematol Oncol 1994;11:463–470.
120. Laborie S, Lavoie JC, Chessex P. Paradoxical role of ascorbic acid and riboflavin in solutions of total parenteral nutrition: implication in photoinduced peroxide generation. Pediatr Res 1998;43:601–606.
121. Laborie S, Lavoie JC, Pineault M, et al. Protecting solutions of parenteral nutrition from peroxidation. JPEN J Parenter Enteral Nutr 1999;23:104–108.
122. Charuhas P, Fosberg K, Bruemmer B, et al. A double-blind randomized trial comparing outpatient parenteral nutrition with intravenous hydration: effect on resumption of oral intake after marrow transplantation. J Parenter Enteral Nutr 1997;21: 157–161.
123. Nicol J, Hoagland R, Heitlinger L. The prevalence of nausea and vomiting in pediatric patients receiving home parenteral nutrition. Nutr Clin Pract 1995;10:189–192.
124. Davis AM. Initiation, monitoring, and complications of pediatric parenteral nutrition. In: Baker RD Jr, Baker SS, Davis AM, eds. Pediatric parenteral nutrition. New York: Chapman & Hall, 1997:212–237.
125. Kelly K. Complementary and alternative medicines for use in supportive care in pediatric cancer. Support Care Cancer 2007;15:457–460.
126. Kelly KM. Bringing evidence to complementary and alternative medicine in children with cancer: focus on nutrition-related therapies. Pediatr Blood Cancer 2008;50: 490–493.

127. Kennedy DD, Ladas E, Rheingold SR, et al. Antioxidant status decreases in children with acute lymphoblastic leukemia during the first six months of chemotherapy treatment. Pediatr Blood Cancer 2005;44:378–385.

128. Stallings VA. Childhood cancer and vitamins: prevention and treatment. Pediatr Blood Cancer 2008;50:442–444.

129. Olshan AF, Smith JC, Bondy ML, et al. Maternal vitamin use and reduced risk of neuroblastoma. Epidemiology 2002;13:575–580.

130. Thompson FR, Gerald P, Willoughby ML, et al. Maternal folate supplementation in pregnancy and protection against acute lymphoblastic leukemia in childhood: a case control study. Lancet 2001;358:1935–1940.

131. Kennedy DD, Tucker KL, Ladas ED, et al. Low antioxidant vitamin intakes are associated with increases in adverse effects of chemotherapy in children with acute lymphoblastic leukemia. Am J Clin Nutr 2004;79:1029–1036.

132. Ross JA, Blair C, Olshan AF, et al. Periconceptional vitamin use and leukemia risk in children with Down syndrome. Cancer 2005;104:405–410.

133. Meacham LR, Gurney JG, Mertens AC, et al. Body mass index in long-term adult survivors of childhood cancer. Cancer 2005;103:1730–1739.

134. Kadan-Lottick N, Marshall JA, Baron AE, et al. Normal bone mineral density after treatment for childhood acute lymphoblastic leukemia diagnosed between 1991 and 1998. J Pediatr 2001;138:898–904.

135. Arikoski P, Komulainen J, Riikonen P, et al. Reduced bone density at completion of chemotherapy for a malignancy. Arch Dis Child 1999;80:143–148.

136. Thomas IH, Donohue J, Ness KK, et al. Bone mineral density in young adult survivors of acute lymphoblastic leukemia. Cancer 2008;113:3248–3256.

CHAPTER 42 ■ PAIN AND SYMPTOM MANAGEMENT

ELLIOT J. KRANE, JACQUELINE CASILLAS, AND LONNIE K. ZELTZER

OVERVIEW OF CHILDHOOD CANCER

There are approximately 12,400 children diagnosed with cancer each year in the United States. As recently as the 1970s, a diagnosis of childhood cancer was considered uniformly fatal. Today, there is an overall 80% survival rate across the major 12 diagnostic categories of childhood cancer, and many malignancies have survival rates equivalent to or better than those of common pediatric diseases.

Despite the low incidence rates of pediatric malignancies and because of the increasing survivability of childhood cancer, there is a growing population of children in active treatment, as well as increasing numbers of childhood cancer survivors. These growing populations result from better supportive care and use of aggressive, multimodal treatment strategies of chemotherapy, radiation, and surgery. As a result, there are periods of discomfort, side effects, and anxiety resulting in greater pain for pediatric cancer patients during their cancer treatment continuum. However, with careful planning, an effective pain management regimen can be developed and implemented.

The result of the aggressive treatment regimens for pediatric cancer patients is a success story. However, despite these advances for 5-year survival rates, there continues to be a high risk for the development of late effects (chronic health impairment) months and years after cancer treatment is completed. Complications of treatment include risk for second malignant neoplasms, cardiac and/or pulmonary dysfunction, skeletal disease, and neurocognitive deficits.[1] Indeed, there is nearly a 75% risk of childhood cancer patients having a chronic health problem by 30 years postdiagnosis.[2] Another important childhood cancer statistic that has implications for the field of pain management is the current estimated prevalence rate of childhood cancer survivors, now more than 300,000 in the United States.[3] Given this rapidly growing population of childhood cancer survivors, it is important to be familiar with the unique challenges faced both during and after completion of treatment of cancer during childhood because the increasing population of survivors has unique pain management issues, as this chapter will describe.

WHAT IS PAIN?

The International Association for the Study of Pain (IASP) defines *pain* as an unpleasant sensory and emotional experience associated with actual or potential tissue damage or described in terms of such damage. The IASP definition of pain begs the question of whether infants and small children, or indeed nonverbal adults, can feel pain, as they do not have the ability to report or describe such an unpleasant sensory and emotional experience. Therefore, it is useful to break pain down into its components, nociception, the physiological response to nociception, and the psychological/emotional response to nociception, that is, suffering, to deflect the debate from whether infants can feel pain, to the more useful discussion of whether the phenomenon of pain is one that deserves treatment without self-report or memory of pain.

Nociception is the unconscious sensation of noxious stimuli, tissue injury, or inflammation, and is an important biologic function that alerts an individual to potential or ongoing injury and prompts the avoidance or limitation of further injury. This definition is not to be confused with pain, *per se*, which is a conscious experience. Lack of protective sensation can lead to a variety of medical complications, including limb injury or decubitus ulcers. Conversely, some nociception (e.g., metastatic cancer, migraine) carries no protective significance.

Nociceptors in deep and superficial tissues can be activated by chemical, thermal, or mechanical stimuli to send afferent impulses through myelinated Aδ fibers or unmyelinated C fibers.

Between the initiation of tissue damage in the periphery and the perception of pain that follows in the brain, there occurs a complex series of physiologic events. Nociception can thus be divided into four processes:

> transduction;
> transmission;
> modulation;
> perception.[4]

Transduction refers to the process in which noxious stimuli are translated into electrical signals at the sensory nerve endings and transmitted to the spinal cord via Aδ and C fibers (Fig. 42.1).

Aδ fibers are myelinated, rapidly conducting fibers (10 to 40 m/s), ending in specialized nerve endings (high-threshold mechanoreceptors). These fibers are primarily responsible for sensations of well-localized, sharp, stabbing pain, otherwise known as *first pain*. Aδ fibers have a high threshold for firing in response to mechanical-thermal stimuli, but once activated, they dramatically increase their firing rate as the stimulus intensity increases.

C-polymodal fibers are unmyelinated fibers with free nerve endings. They respond to noxious mechanical, thermal, and chemical stimuli at a much slower rate (<2 m/s), leading to pain characterized as dull, aching, burning, and poorly localized. This pain is known as *second pain* because it is usually perceived after the first pain sensation. Substances that mediate and intensify the stimulation of these nerve endings include bradykinin, prostaglandins, leukotrienes, substance P, acetylcholine, histamine, hydrogen ions, and potassium.

Sensitization is the process by which activation of neural impulses occurs at a lower than normal threshold of activation. Both Aδ and C-polymodal nociceptors are capable of

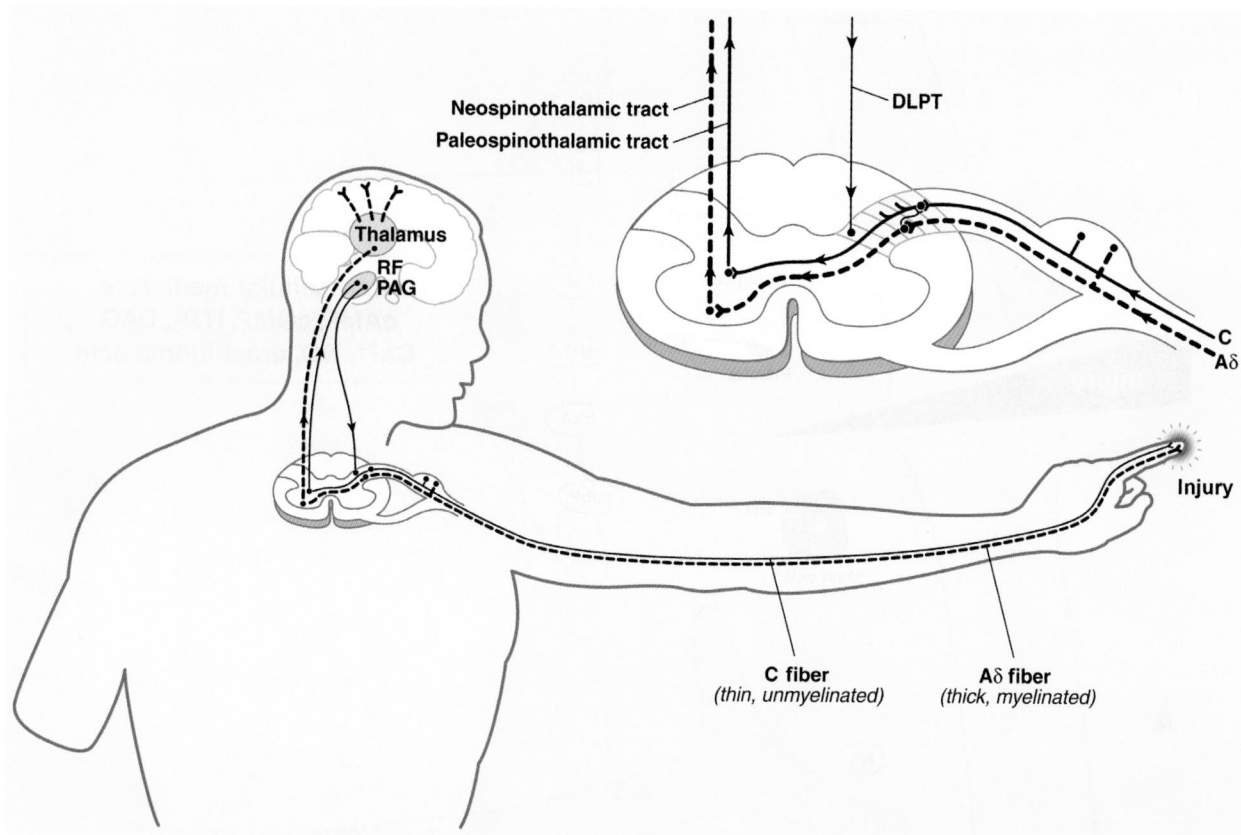

FIGURE 42.1 Transduction of mechanical or chemical tissue injury to electrical activity in the nociceptive pathway, and conduction of impulses in the Aδ and C fibers to the central nervous system. DLPT, Dorsolateral Pontine Tegmentum; PAG, Periaqueductal Gray; RF, Reticular Formation.

sensitization. C-polymodal nociceptors may also widen their receptive fields and are capable of prolonged discharge relative to the stimulus duration.

In addition to the above-mentioned mediators, the sympathetic system may itself be sensitized and may activate primary afferent neurons (Fig. 42.2). This may involve norepinephrine (noradrenaline) and other substances acting at α_2-adrenoreceptors on the afferent neurons. This phenomenon is certainly present in the early stages of the neuropathic pain syndromes but may also play a role in acute tissue trauma in the absence of nerve injury.[5]

Transmission refers to propagation of the impulse through the sensory nervous system via primary afferent fibers, which synapse in the dorsal horn of the spinal cord, second-order neurons in the lamina of the dorsal horn, and ascending neurons projecting to brainstem, thalamus, and thalamocortical projections (Fig. 42.1).

Modulation denotes the alteration of nociceptive information by endogenous mechanisms. This modulation may result in either attenuation or amplification of the initial signal. Perhaps, the most important of these sites is the dorsal horn of the spinal cord. Modulation occurs between neurons, as well as via pathways of descending inhibition originating in the thalamus and brainstem. Neurons within these pathways release inhibitory neurotransmitters, including norepinephrine, serotonin, γ-aminobutyric acid, glycine, enkephalin, and other endogenous opioids that block the release of substance P, glutamate, and other excitatory neurotransmitters (Fig. 42.3).

Finally, *perception* reflects the impact of the nociceptive information upon the existing cognitive-psychological framework. Perception is the emotional and cognitive experience of physical pain. That experience then changes the framework itself and thereby affects subsequent painful experiences. The term *unpleasant*, within the context of the IASP definition of pain, commonly means painful or painfulness in a broad sense. In contrast to the sensory dimension, it generally refers to the affective dimension of pain. This aspect of pain produces *suffering*, which is described as an individual's affective experience of unpleasantness, and *aversion* associated with harm, real or perceived, or the threat of harm. It is this dimension, suffering, that mandates the effective treatment of pain from the humanitarian perspective.

Nociception also produces a physiological and endocrine response separate from its conscious perception and subsequent cognitive and emotional behavioral responses. These biological responses are measurable, are sometimes useful for quantifying pain in pre- or nonverbal patients (particularly in the research setting), and are generally medically adverse in their physiological consequences. These adverse effects include tachycardia and hypertension, activation of glucose counterregulatory hormones, muscle spasms, and an overall increase in metabolic demands as a consequence of these effects. This dimension of pain mandates effective treatment from the medical and medicoeconomic perspectives. While pain is generally associated with a process of tissue injury, or potential injury, clinicians and researchers have long observed a lack of correlation between the extent of tissue injury and the intensity of pain or suffering. The experience of pain is therefore and obviously quite subjective and, as such, is modulated by developmental, familial, situational, emotional, and other factors. Assessment of the extent to which one or more of these

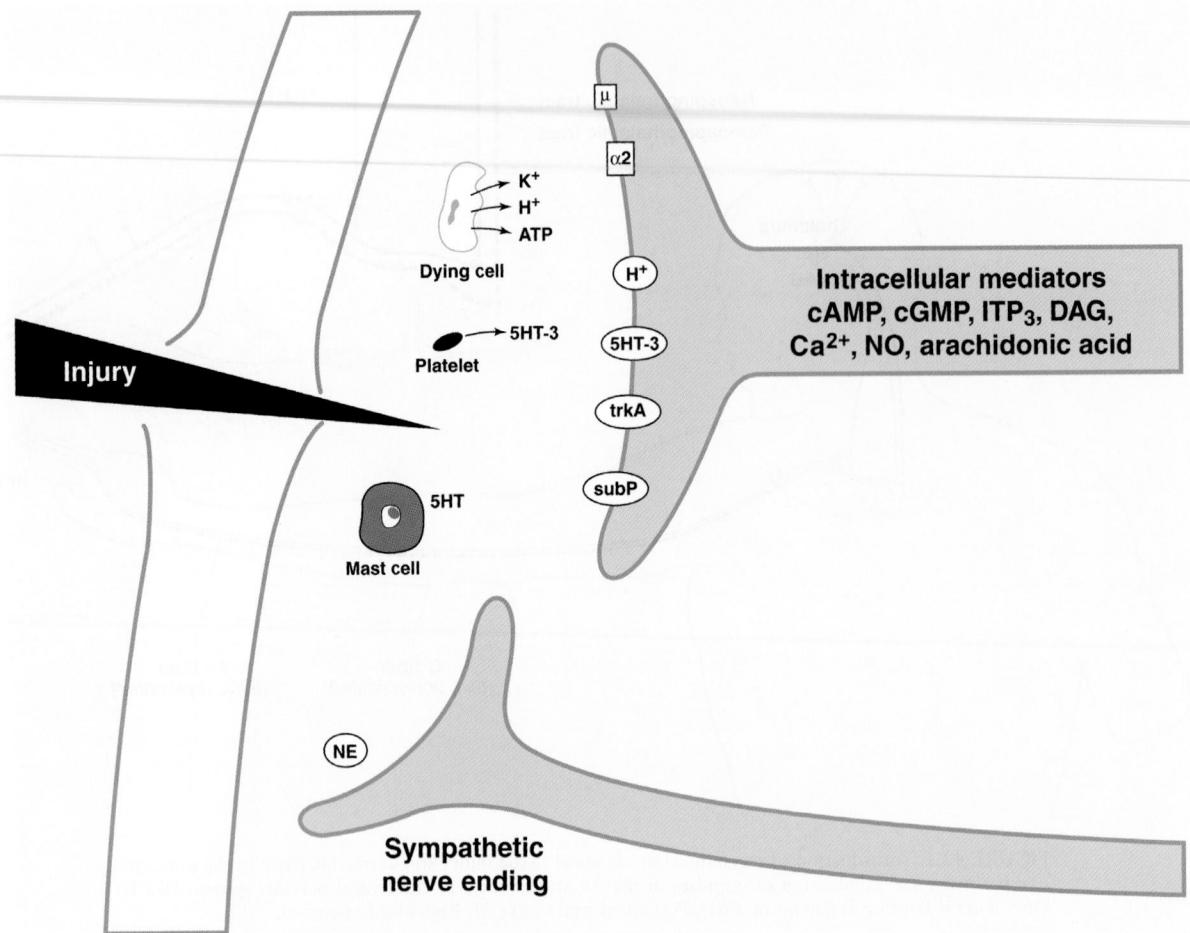

FIGURE 42.2 Intracellular mediators involved in the transduction of tissue injury into painful nerve impulses; note that the sympathetic nervous system is closely involved in the modulation and amplification of this process.

modulating factors require specific intervention is critical to the effective treatment of pain.

PAIN IN CHILDREN: HOW DOES IT DIFFER FROM THAT IN ADULTS?

Before a discussion can exist about the differences of pain in adults and children, it is useful to define pain within the context of childhood. The Cartesian model for conceptualizing medical conditions in general, and pain specifically, the mind-body duality has long been abandoned in favor of the current thinking of pain as a comprehensive phenomenon consisting not only of a physical domain but also of intimately intertwined psychological and social domains; this construct is termed the *biopsychosocial model*. As is well known to the pediatric oncologist, childhood is a period in which there are complex and rapid neurodevelopmental changes occurring from birth to young adulthood. In children, the biopsychosocial model of pain is yet more complex than in the adult because the developmental level of the child needs is integrated. Children grow and develop through five stages of development: (1) infancy; (2) toddlerhood; (3) a preschool period; (4) a school-age period; and (5) adolescence; the relevance of these periods is projected not only to psychological effects of pain and its treatment but also to the pharmacokinetics and pharmacodynamics of pain therapy and to anatomical and physiological considerations in performing nerve blocks or other interventions to manage pain. These levels of development are also important because they directly effect the assessment of pain in children.

Newborns–Infants

It was previously believed that newborns and infants could not experience pain because they possessed immature neurological systems and that only as a child developed could pain be experienced. However, ongoing basic research has dispelled this myth and proven that newborns and infants possess all the anatomical and neurological structures needed for nociception to occur from the time of birth, do indeed respond to nociceptive stimuli, and mount a hormonal stress response to noxious stimuli that may even exceed that seen in adults. In fact, the partial development of the immature nervous system preserves nociception but may paradoxically amplify pain because the descending pain inhibitory system is the one neu-

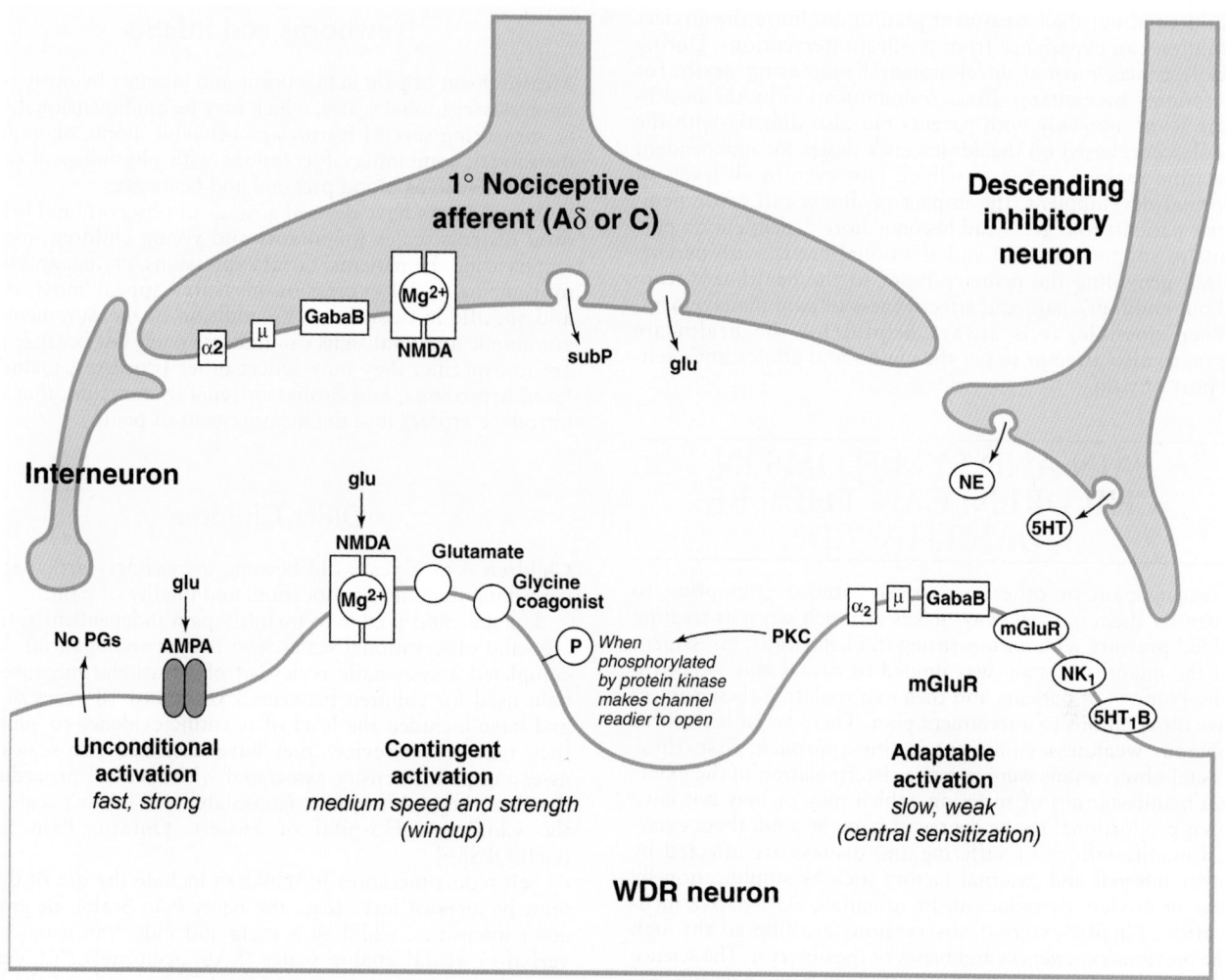

FIGURE 42.3 The transmission of nociception from the peripheral nervous system to the central nervous system and the propagation of nerve impulses to higher centers is modulated and amplified by a wide variety of neurotransmitters and receptor blockers, all of which present pharmacologic targets for therapeutic agents. Abbreviation: NMDA, N-methyl-D-aspartate; WDR, Wide Dynamic Range; GabaB, gamma-aminobutyric acid type B; subP, substance P; glu, glutamate; NE, norepinephrine; 5HT, 5-hydroxytryptamine; NK1, neurokinin 1; PGs, prostaglandins; AMPA, α-amino-3-hydroxyl-5-methyl-4-isoxazole-propionate.

roanatomical feature of pain physiology that is not fully mature at birth; therefore, a painful stimulus transmitted through the neural afferent system to the newborn brain may prove to be *more* painful to the newborn than it would be to the older child or adult![6]

Infants–Preschool

From birth through early childhood, there is complete maturation of the neuroanatomy and physiology of nociception; the principle differentiating factor that distinguishes a child at this age from older peers is in the domain of intellect, psychology, and personality. A normal developmental assessment evaluates five main areas: gross motor skills, fine motor skills, language skills, personal/social skills, and cognitive skills. Changes occurring in these areas, in turn, affect the pain assessment and emotional response of the child to the painful stimuli. For example, the language skills of a 2-year-old include a 50-word vocabulary and the ability to construct two-word sentences. During this period, the child is not able to effectively describe the pain sensation and is unable to quantify it, and if inadequate pain treatment occurs as a consequence, there can be more fear and anxiety with each subsequent painful procedure. One year later, at 3 years of age, there is an expected 250-word vocabulary, 3-word sentences, and speech is intelligible to strangers 75% of the time. These children may be more able to effectively communicate with parents and doctors and have treatment of the pain anticipated and initiated more promptly, a factor related to these enhanced communication skills that can serve to decrease anxiety for future procedures.

School-age–Adolescence

School-aged children will have a progressively increasing ability to communicate effectively with the healthcare team. In turn, the providers must clearly communicate with these children about their treatment plan to minimize the anxiety children can experience from medical interventions. During adolescence, normal developmental increasing desire for autonomy necessitates direct communication by the healthcare team, not only with parents but also directly with the adolescent, based on the adolescent's desire for independent decision making (when possible). However, in all levels of normal development, the impact of illness can cause pediatric patients to regress and become more dependent on parents to support physical and emotional needs, with parents often providing the primary input to the healthcare team about children's pain and effectiveness of pain management. When possible, it is always helpful for the healthcare team to also attempt to get the child's and adolescent's self-report of pain.

PAIN AND SYMPTOMS IN CHILDREN: CAN THEY BE QUANTITATED?

Treating pain or other symptoms without attempting to quantify them in some way makes as much sense as treating blood pressure without measuring it. Historically, assessment of the quantity of pain was limited to casual and subjective observations of patients and then extrapolating these subjective observations to a treatment plan. There are at least three obvious weaknesses inherent in this approach; first, these casual observations were in fact a determination of the external manifestations of suffering, which may or may not have been proportional to the degree of pain. Second, these external manifestations of suffering and distress are affected by other internal and external factors such as amplification by fear or anxiety or reduction by nonanalgesic sedative medication. Finally, external observations are filtered through the previous experiences and biases of the observer. The science of pain measurement is imperfect and evolving; nevertheless, it is important to attempt to quantify pain in all circumstances.

In the final analysis, pain is a subjective experience known only to the patient, whereas to the clinician it is a secondhand experience. Therefore, the most reliable measure of pain is self-report, but because children vary widely in their developmental and intellectual capabilities to express pain in a quantifiable manner, several tools have been developed that are age and development specific. Although many symptom assessment instruments have been developed and validated for adults in a variety of clinical settings, there are few symptom assessment tools for children with cancer. The validated symptom assessment tools in pediatrics have focused on three common symptoms: pain, nausea, and fatigue. In contrast to instruments measuring nausea and vomiting, instruments measuring pain in children have largely been validated in predominantly the noncancer setting. These are summarized in Table 42.1.

In addition to making an attempt in order to quantify pain, determining its qualitative characteristics will provide the clinician important clinical clues regarding both its etiology and appropriate treatment. For example, abdominal pain that is central and colicky in nature suggests a bowel obstruction or dysmotility, whereas abdominal pain that is constant, localized to a quadrant, and radiates to the back is more suggestive of solid organ pathology. Similarly, limb pain that is burning, lancinating, shooting, and associated with skin sensitivity suggests a neuropathic process. This will be discussed in further detail in sections of this chapter to follow.

Newborns and Infants

Measurement of pain in newborns and infants obviously relies upon observational scales, which may be unidimensional, that is, measuring several features of behavior alone, or multidimensional, combining observations with physiological measurements such as blood pressure and heart rate.

Investigators have devised a range of observational behavioral distress scales for infants and young children, mostly emphasizing the patients' facial expressions, crying, and body movement. Facial expression measures appear most useful and specific in neonates. The addition of measurements of autonomic and vital signs can indicate pain, but because they are nonspecific, they may reflect other processes, including fever, hypoxemia, and cardiac or renal dysfunction, that may introduce artifact into the measurement of pain.

Older Children

Children 3 to 7 years old become increasingly articulate in describing the intensity, location, and quality of pain.

For the child unable to quantify pain independently, there are valid observational scales. von Baeyer and Spagrud[7] have completed a systematic review of observational measures of pain used for children between 3 years and 18 years of age and have included the level of scientific evidence to support their use. In this review, they have identified two scales for assessing pain intensity associated with medical procedures, the Face, Legs, Arms, Cry, Consolability (FLACC) scale and the Children's Hospital of Eastern Ontario Pain Scale (CHEOPS).[8,9]

Self-report measures for children include the use of drawings, pictures of faces (e.g., the Faces Pain Scale), or graded color intensities. Children 8 years and older can usually use verbal or visual analog scales (VAS) accurately.[10,11] Verbal numerical ratings are now preferred and considered the gold standard; studies show valid and reliable ratings from children 8 years and older.[12] The Numerical Rating Scale (NRS), or Likert scale, consists of numbers from 0 to 10, where 0 represents *no pain* and 10 represents *very severe pain*. (There is debate about the label for the anchor expression for the highest pain rating, but the current agreement is *not* to use the worst pain possible since children can always imagine a greater pain.)

Cognitively Impaired Children

Measuring pain in cognitively impaired children remains a challenge; investigators are studying methods of assessing pain in this group.[13,14] Understanding pain expression and experience in this population is important because behaviors may be misinterpreted as indicating that cognitively impaired children are more insensitive to pain than cognitively competent children. Children with trisomy 21 may express pain less precisely and more slowly than the general population. Pain in children with autism spectrum disorders may be difficult to assess because they may be both hyposensitive and hypersensitive to many different types of sensory stimuli and they may have limited communication abilities. While self-reports of pain can be elicited from some children who are cognitively impaired, observational measures have better research validation across children. The Noncommunicating Child's Pain Checklist—Postoperative Version is recommended for

TABLE 42.1

PAIN MEASUREMENT TOOLS

Name	Features	Age range	Advantages	Validation and uses	Limitations
Visual analog scale (VAS)	Horizontal 10-cm line; subject marks a spot on the line between anchors of "no pain" (or neutral face) and "most pain imaginable" (or sad face)	6–8 yr and older	Good psychometric properties; validated for research purposes	Acute pain Surgical pain Chronic pain	Cannot be used in younger children or in those with cognitive limitations. Requires language skills and numerical processing; upper anchor of "most pain" Requires an experiential reference point lacking in many children
Likert scale	Integers from 0 to 10, inclusive, corresponding to no pain to most pain	6–8 yr and older	Good psychometric properties; validated for research purposes	Acute pain Surgical pain Chronic pain	Same as VAS
Faces Scales (e.g., FACES-R, Wong-Baker, Oucher, Bieri, McGrath scales)	Subjects rate their pain by identifying with line drawings of faces, or photos of children	4 yr and older	Can be used at younger ages than the VAS or Likert scale	Acute pain Surgical pain	Choice of "no pain" face affects responses (neutral vs. smiling); not culturally universal
Behavioral or combined behavioral-physiologic scales (e.g., FLACC, N-PASS, CHEOPS, OPS, FACS, NIPS)	Scoring of observed behaviors (e.g., facial expression, limb movement) ± heart rate and blood pressure	Some work for any ages; some work for specific age groups, including preterm infants	May be used in both infants and nonverbal children	FLACC, N-PASS: Acute pain Surgical pain	Nonspecific; overrates pain in toddlers and preschool children; underrates persistent pain; some measures are convenient; others require videotaping and complex processing; vital sign changes unrelated to pain can occur and affect total score
Autonomic measures (e.g., heart rate, blood pressure, heart rate spectral analyses)	Scores changes in heart rate, blood pressure, or measures of heart rate variability (e.g., "vagal tone")	All ages	Can be used at all ages; useful for patients receiving mechanical ventilation		Nonspecific; vital sign changes unrelated to pain may occur and may artifactually increase or decrease score
Hormonal-metabolic measures	Plasma or salivary sampling of "stress" hormones (e.g., cortisol, epinephrine)	All ages	Can be used at all ages		Nonspecific; changes unrelated to pain can occur; inconvenient; cannot provide "real-time" information; standard normal values not available for every age bracket

children aged up to 18 years. In addition, maladaptive behavior and reduction in functions may also indicate pain. Studies have shown that children with severe cognitive impairments experience pain frequently, mostly not because of accidental injury. Children with the fewest abilities experience the most pain.

Measurement of Pain in Research and Drug Development

Although many pain assessment scales exist for use in infants and children, relatively few have been rigorously, statistically validated to be used in research and therapeutic drug development. When selecting a tool for pain measurement, confirm that (1) the tool has been validated in the relevant age group and (2) the tool has validity for the model of pain (e.g., chronic pain, acute surgical pain, neuropathic pain) under investigation. It is common to see a pain scale validated in one clinical circumstance applied to a different pain model without justification or statistical validity. Table 42.1 lists the statistically validated pain scales and the clinical circumstances in which they have been validated.[15]

Instruments for the Assessment of Nausea in Children With Cancer

A rating scale for nausea and vomiting utilizing verbal descriptors was used in a series of assessment studies in children with cancer aged 5 to 18 years.[16–19] Children younger than 10 years had faces included above numbers on the scale. There was 80% agreement between parent and child ratings when they were assessed independently.

A comparison of child and parental ratings of children's nausea and emesis symptoms was assessed among 33 children (aged 1.7 to 17.5 years, median 4.7 years) with acute lymphoblastic leukemia (ALL) receiving identical chemotherapy.[20] The measures used nausea and vomiting vignettes designed to assess the frequency and severity of nausea and emesis symptoms as reported by children and their parents on the basis of previous chemotherapy experience of these children. The vignettes, based on the work of Zeltzer et al.,[21] consisted of 12 questions separately assessing nausea and emesis at three time intervals: prior to, during, and after chemotherapy. A 5-point Likert-type rating scale, ranging from *not at all* to *all the time* for the frequency items and from *not bad* to *real bad* on the severity items, was employed. A composite nausea/vomiting score was determined by calculating the mean of the 12 frequency and severity items. Children younger than 5 years were not asked to complete this measure because of their difficulty understanding the instructions. This study demonstrated a significant correlation between child and parent ratings of nausea. Significant interrater correlations for nausea frequency and severity but not for emesis frequency or severity were found.

Instruments for the Assessment of Fatigue in Children With Cancer

Hockenberry-Eaton, Hinds, and their colleagues[22–24] have developed and validated rating scales for fatigue in children and adolescents with cancer. Versions are available for child and adolescent self-report and for observational rating by parents. Ratings assess both the frequency and intensity of fatigue-related symptoms.

The Memorial Symptom Assessment Scales for Children[25,26]

The measurement of symptoms is one aspect of quality-of-life (QOL) assessment. All recently developed validated measures of cancer-specific QOL for adults assess a selected group of prevalent symptoms within a broader assessment of physical, social, and psychological functioning.[27–30] Understanding symptom prevalence and characteristics in children with cancer has been hampered by the lack of symptom assessment tools validated in this population. Neither of the two QOL measures developed for children with cancer, the single-item observer-rated Play Performance Scale for Children[31] and the 21-item, parent-rated Pediatric Quality of Life Scale,[32] measures symptoms. Symptom-specific scales available for children with cancer either evaluate pain, using either self-report or observer rating, or assess chemotherapy-related nausea and vomiting, using self-report.

The Memorial Symptom Assessment Scale (MSAS) 10–18 is a 30-item patient-rated instrument adapted from a previously validated adult version to provide multidimensional information about the symptoms experienced by children with cancer. This instrument was administered to 160 children with cancer aged 10 to 18 years (45 inpatients, 115 outpatients). To confirm the instrument's reliability and validity, additional data about symptoms were collected from both the parents and the medical charts and retesting was performed on a subgroup of inpatients.

The scale was easily completed by patients in a mean time of 11 minutes. The analyses supported the reliability and validity of the MSAS 10–18 subscale scores as measures of physical, psychological, and global symptom distress, respectively. Symptom prevalence ranged from 49.7% for lack of energy to 6.3% for problems with urination. The mean ± SD number of symptoms per inpatient was 12.7 ± 4.9 (range, 4 to 26), significantly more than the mean 6.5 ± 5.7 (range, 0 to 28) symptoms per outpatient. Patients who had recently received chemotherapy had significantly more symptoms than patients who had not received chemotherapy for more than 4 months (11.6 ± 6.0 vs. 5.2 ± 5.1), and those patients with solid tumors had significantly more symptoms than patients with either hematologic or central nervous system (CNS) malignancies. The most common symptoms (prevalence 35%) were lack of energy, pain, drowsiness, nausea, cough, and lack of appetite and psychological symptoms (feeling sad, feeling nervous, worrying, feeling irritable). Of the symptoms with prevalence rates greater than 35%, those that caused high distress in more than one-third of patients were feeling sad, pain, nausea, lack of appetite, and irritable. Subscale scores demonstrated large variability in symptom distress and could identify subgroups with high distress.

The prevalence, characteristics, and distress associated with physical and psychological symptoms could be quantified using the MSAS 10–18, a reliable and valid multidimensional instrument for symptom assessment, in older children with cancer. The data confirm a high prevalence of symptoms overall and the existence of subgroups with high distress associated with one or multiple symptoms. Symptom distress is relatively higher among inpatients, children with solid tumors, and children who are undergoing antineoplastic treatment.

A revised MSAS was created as an instrument for the assessment of symptoms in children with cancer aged 7 to 12 years. Validity was evaluated by comparison with the medical record, parental report, and concurrent assessment on the VAS for selected symptoms. The data provide evidence of the reliability and validity of MSAS 7–12 and demonstrated that children with cancer as young as 7 years could report clinically relevant and consistent information about their symptom experience. The completion rate for MSAS 7–12 was high, and the majority of children completed the instrument in a short period of time and with little difficulty. The instrument appeared to be age appropriate and may be helpful to older children unable to independently complete MSAS 10–18.

CANCER PAIN IN CHILDREN

The vast majority of pediatric cancer patients do not have a chronic medical condition at the time of diagnosis and therefore have not experienced chronic or recurrent pain. Instead, their pain experience typically has been limited to acute, intermittent self-limiting episodes associated with immunizations, infections, or minor injuries. It is thus not surprising that the diagnosis and rapid initiation of treatment of cancer can overwhelm a child with fear and anxiety because of the number of invasive, painful medical and surgical procedures that are required for which the child is psychologically unprepared. In addition, acute pain associated with the first medical procedure at the time of diagnosis can set the expectations of pain to be experienced by the child for all future procedures. Studies have demonstrated that even posttraumatic stress symptoms can be experienced by childhood cancer survivors because of memory recall of invasive procedures during treatment, and these painful memories continue well beyond the treatment into the survivorship period.[33]

Pain Evaluation and Treatment Plans for Children With Cancer

The importance of eliciting and listening to all details of the pain narrative of pediatric cancer patients is critical. Again, what is asked of children and expected of the children is dependent on their developmental level. For school-aged children or adolescents, the pain assessment should occur early on, where there is the support of family, and in a nonthreatening environment. In tertiary care centers that care for large numbers of pediatric cancer patients, there are child life services available and serve as another resource to help elucidate a clear description of the pain narrative. For infants or toddlers, the healthcare provider is dependent on the parents' narratives of the painful experience since they are the source for safety and communication for their young children. Across the entire developmental continuum of pediatrics, the physical examination is critical to provide additional information about physical factors that contribute to the experience of pain. During the physical examination, it is also critical for the healthcare provider to recognize and identify psychosocial factors, such as parental fear or anxiety, that can also increase the suffering associated with pain for pediatric cancer patients. After a careful history and physical examination, a targeted treatment plan can then be developed. Further details of treatment plans for the various etiologies of pain in the pediatric cancer population are discussed in the following sections.

TREATMENT OF PAIN IN PEDIATRIC CANCER PATIENTS

There are seven main categories of pain in children with cancer: (1) pain associated with medical procedures used for cancer diagnosis and treatment; (2) pain associated with bone marrow infiltration by malignant disease; (3) neuropathic pain and pain due to CNS tumors; (4) bone pain and amputation pain; (5) visceral pain; (6) pain associated with the complications of bone marrow transplantation (BMT), such as oral mucositis; and (7) stress, anxiety, and other symptoms.

Pain Related to Medical Procedures

Invasive, painful procedures for the childhood cancer patient include diagnostic tests such as bone marrow biopsies, lumbar punctures (LPs), surgery for tissue biopsy, venipuncture for diagnosis and/or treatment administration, access of subcutaneous central venous catheter ports, and removal of central venous access catheters. Not only do pediatric cancer patients face many painful stimuli repeatedly but also these pain-evoking procedures can occur in a relatively short time (within a few days, weeks, to months). Besides the physical pain that invasive procedures cause related to tissue damage by insertion of a needle or device through the skin and/or bone, the procedures themselves produce a great deal of psychological distress including fear and anxiety.[34] This anxiety can, in turn, result in a quick recall of the procedure that, in turn, will influence future pain management for all future painful procedures. Children with ALL on current treatment protocols, for example, receive LPs on a regular basis ranging from once weekly to once every 3 months. The initial LPs that are done at time of diagnosis and for the initial induction treatment therefore set the stage for the pain anticipated and experienced for children during their 2 to 3 years of ongoing chemotherapy. Studies in ALL cancer patients have demonstrated that children do indeed have accurate memories of their painful procedures. The more negative a memory a child had about a previous procedure, the higher the likelihood of increasing distress related to future procedures.[35]

There may also be specific groups of pediatric cancer patients who are at higher risk for distress due to painful, invasive procedures. Early studies have suggested that differences in reactions to painful stimuli can be attributed, at least in part, to a child's temperament, including the dimensions of distractibility and conversely persistence.[36–39] Chen et al.[40] have shown that having a higher level of pain sensitivity (i.e., *pain perception*) is associated with greater anxiety and pain both prior to and during an LP procedure. In addition, the psychological stress and corresponding coping experienced by the parent, in turn, affect the child's coping responses to the painful stressor. For example, mothers of childhood cancer survivors experience posttraumatic stress symptoms well into the survivorship period, years after their children were treated for cancer.[41] Thus, given that children are dependent on their parents for both physical and emotional support throughout the cancer care continuum, they can be at increased risk for distress due to pain if their caretaker is not able to soothe or provide a safe, consistent environment because of caretaker's own maladaptive coping.

Treatment plans for first-time invasive procedures for a pediatric cancer patient should be made preemptively and include the use of pharmacologic treatment of the pain. A child's first LP, for example, ideally includes the integration of a pediatric pain service and/or pediatric anesthesia team so that effective systemic anesthesia (in addition to local anesthesia) can be administered by qualified personnel with appropriate physiologic monitoring to minimize risk associated with the pharmacologic intervention. Anesthesia or deep sedation with propofol, an intravenous general anesthetic agent with rapid onset and short offset, has become the standard of care in many cancer centers for patients who have intravenous access. Anesthetic depth and can be easily titrated to produce a deep level of sedation or general anesthesia to eliminate awareness, painful stimulation, and the formation of memory the child would experience during the procedure.[11] Local anesthetics, such as lidocaine, should be administered even when the patient is receiving light or moderate sedation or propofol anesthesia so that the total dose of sedatives and hypnotics required is minimized while pain control is maximized. There are data to suggest that bolus dosing of propofol results in a more rapid recovery after completion of the invasive procedure because it results in a smaller cumulative dose of the anesthetic.[42]

Equally important, there are several cognitive-behavioral interventions that can be employed to minimize the anxiety associated with painful procedures. These can include an emphasis on the family-centered care model, which includes the parent being present with the patient while undergoing induction anesthesia and at the time the pediatric cancer patient regains consciousness. Child life services can assist with preparing the patient to understand the various mechanical procedures that will occur, from the trivial matters of povidone-iodine (Betadine) skin cleansing to palpation of landmarks to the more painful injection of local anesthetic agents. Relaxation therapies that can be used for painful procedures include focused attention such as mindfulness meditation and hypnosis/guided imagery,[43,44] which has been shown to lower postoperative pain ratings, decrease hospitalization stays, and decrease anxiety in pediatric patient populations.[45–51]

Distraction methods are also another category of cognitive-behavioral therapies employed to decrease the pain experience during invasive medical therapies. They include use of bubbles, music therapy, mutual storytelling, pop-up books, videos, and simple conversation so that the attention is taken away from the procedure and focused onto another target. For example, by offering music therapy to the adolescent who may feel a lack of control due to the required invasive procedure, the opportunity to exert some autonomy over the painful experience (such as through singing) can occur through the freedom of expression of his or her feelings about the procedure as well as the change in focus of attention.[52–55]

Pain Due to Bone Marrow Infiltration

Acute leukemias, ALL and acute myelogenous leukemia, are the most common form of pediatric cancer.[56] The rapid growth of leukemic blasts within the bone marrow commonly results in the experience of diffuse bone pain. The clinical presentation of the bone pain, however, is variable depending on the age of the patient. Very young children, such as toddlers, who are most commonly affected by ALL, may present with a limp or inability to walk. A school-aged child who is able to provide a pain narrative may report diffuse total body pain that is poorly localized. An adolescent patient may have back pain that he or she associates with a sports injury and may localize the pain to a specific area in a long bone. There are also solid tumors, such as neuroblastoma, which most commonly present during the toddler years and which can metastasize to either bone marrow or bone and also present as a limp or as localized pain to a specific boney area.

The most effective method of eradication of pain due to bone marrow infiltration begins with treatment of the primary disease. For ALL, induction chemotherapy regimens generally place children into remission within a 1-month treatment course.[57] For most standard risks ALL patients, by day 7 of treatment, there is a significant reduction in the leukemic burden to less than 25% of the bone marrow being affected. This decrease in leukemic burden, in turn, results in marked improvement in the bone pain. Adolescents with acute leukemias, however, often have more resistant disease and may have longer periods of acute pain due to the persistence of blasts within the bone marrow and may require analgesics throughout the induction chemotherapy regimen.[58] For patients with bone metastases from solid tumors, such as neuroblastoma, effective treatment may also include local radiation therapy to the affected site.

Pharmacologic regimens for the treatment of pain from bone marrow infiltration for both children and adolescents include the use of parenteral opioids, such as morphine or hydromorphone. Opioid analgesics may be administered through bolus dosing regimens if the pain is not constant. However, for patients experiencing continuous pain, the delivery of the opioid should include the use of a patient-controlled analgesia (PCA) component.

Often, healthcare providers use adjuvant pain medications, such as acetaminophen (APAP) or nonsteroidal anti-inflammatory drugs (NSAIDs), together with opioid analgesics, to optimize pain control and minimize the side effects of opioids such as respiratory depression at high doses.[59] However, in the patient with bone marrow infiltration, there is frequently thrombocytopenia. As a result, the use of NSAIDs is not recommended for these patients because of the antiplatelet effects of this class of analgesics that may place the pediatric cancer patient at increased risk for hemorrhage secondary to both the quantitative and qualitative platelet defects. Analgesia with an oral coxib, celecoxib, is an excellent alternative in this circumstance (see the following text).

Neuropathic Pain

Pediatric cancer patients can experience neuropathic pain for a variety of reasons including nerve invasion and inflammation of a nerve root due to the malignancy or infectious process, or from cancer treatment side effects. These etiologies include (1) chemotherapy-related peripheral neuropathies, such as with vincristine or vinblastine neurotoxicity[60]; (2) neural compression or invasion by tumors, such as pelvic sarcomas; and (3) infectious etiologies, such as postherpetic neuralgia and neuropathies secondary to herpes zoster reactivation associated with immunosuppression. In addition, direct injury to or compression of nerve or spinal cord can occur with soft tissue sarcomas arising in the pelvis, such as Ewing's sarcoma or rhabdomyosarcoma; such a patient can present with complaints of abdominal pain, lower extremity weakness, and/or bladder and bowel dysfunction from involvement of the sacral nerves.

The medications that are most effective for the management of neuropathic pain are not the opioids but rather the tricyclic antidepressants (TCAs), such as amitriptyline, the newer selective serotonin norepinephrine reuptake inhibitors (SSNRIs), such as duloxetine, the antiepileptic drugs (AEDs), such as, gabapentin and pregabalin, and local anesthetics including the local topical application of the 5% lidocaine patch or intravenous administration of lidocaine.[61–63] In addition, a recent Cochrane review of the adult pain literature recommended that future research on the treatment of neuropathic pain include the assessment of effectiveness for other naturally occurring antidepressants such as St Johns wort and L-tryptophan since there are currently insufficient data to support their use or disuse.[64]

Opioids, including the long-acting opioid methadone, can also be used for severe neuropathic pain that has not been effectively treated with TCAs or anticonvulsant medications, although neuropathic pain is notoriously resistant to opioid analgesia.[65] However, opioids are associated with a risk profile that has not been widely studied in children. Thus, when considering the use of opioids for neuropathic pain, one should first maximize the total recommended daily dose of TCAs and AEDs, given their relatively low toxicity profile, before initiating a long-term opioid regimen.

Mechanical approaches are also important to consider in the treatment regimen for neuropathic pain. These include the use of physical therapy and acupuncture. Physical therapy should be considered for those patients who have neuropathic pain particularly due to vinca alkaloids, since these agents also cause motor weakness. Although physical therapy can be an effective therapeutic modality itself, there are several barriers to its utilization in cancer patients,[66] including financial and/or insurance barriers. A pediatric cancer patient may be too fatigued to engage in physical conditioning and exercises. With persistence, and pairing of the child to a single therapist with whom he or she can form a relationship of trust and who can then motivate the patient to participate regularly in the recommended exercise regimen, physical therapy is an effective, nonpharmacologic modality to supplement pharmacologic regimens that are insufficient *per se* at relieving the neuropathic pain.

Pain Associated With Central Nervous System Tumors

Central nervous system tumors are the most common solid tumors diagnosed during childhood. Because of the mass effect of the brain tumor or mechanical obstruction of cerebrospinal fluid (CSF) flow and secondary hydrocephalus, children usually present with symptoms of headaches due to increased intracranial pressure. To decrease the intracranial pressure and thereby treat the pain/headache of children, different therapeutic approaches can be used. For some brain tumors that are locally invasive but without metastatic potential, such as low-grade gliomas (astrocytomas), complete surgical removal is the treatment of choice.

Dexamethasone is usually used in the preoperative period to relieve the cytotoxic cerebral edema that surrounds malignancies, and this is often remarkably effective in relieving the head pain associated with brain tumors even before surgical excision.

If the child with a brain tumor continues to report headaches postoperatively, NSAIDs, such as ibuprofen, can be considered 24 hours after surgery if there is no plan for bone marrow–inhibiting chemotherapy and/or radiation therapy. Celecoxib may safely be used in these circumstances. If an NSAID is used in the pain treatment regimen, a histamine H2-receptor antagonist to inhibit stomach acid production is thought to provide protection against gastritis or ulceration, particularly in the patient treated with dexamethasone.

For malignant brain tumors with metastatic potential, such as medulloblastomas, chemotherapy and radiation therapy follow the surgical treatment regimen. Not all primary resections of malignant brain tumors result in complete surgical removal of the tumor; therefore, pain may persist because of residual disease. Opioids, such as morphine sulfate, administered intravenously are the preferred pharmacologic medication of choice. When using high dose or prolonged courses of opioids for the treatment of CNS pain from brain tumors, the treatment plan must also include a bowel regimen to reduce the likelihood of constipation. This is discussed in more detail later in this chapter.

Benzodiazepines, such as midazolam and lorazepam, may be used as an adjunct for the treatment of pain due to CNS tumors, even though this class of medications has no direct analgesic effect. Its utility includes decreasing anxiety, decreasing muscle spasm that may occur postoperatively, and facilitating sleep.[67] Postoperatively after the resection of a CNS tumor, children typically remain within the intensive care unit (ICU) for intracranial pressure monitoring or external CSF drainage; here, benzodiazepines are commonly used by continuous infusion or bolus dosing to minimize anxiety and agitation.[68] Benzodiazepines are often used concomitantly with opioid analgesics outside the ICU when significant postoperative pain is reported, observed, or expected, or to alleviate painful cervical muscle spasm and pain following posterior fossa craniotomies.

Pain Associated With Primary Malignant Bone Tumors

Primary malignant bone tumors, osteosarcoma, and Ewing's sarcoma result in significant pain, pain resulting from both destruction of normal trabecular bone from direct tumor invasion and intense tissue inflammation surrounding the malignancy. Thus, the pain can often be very severe and requires the use of opioid analgesic medications or interventional pain techniques.

Because bone tumors have such an inflammatory component, the pain is remarkably responsive to NSAIDs, which should be considered with caution given the risk for bleeding in the patient receiving chemotherapy. Coxibs are alternatives that are not associated with platelet inhibition. Because most common primary malignant bone tumors usually occur during adolescence, PCA is the preferred method for the delivery of parenteral opioids. For continuous, long-term pain associated with bone tumors for outpatient management, long-acting oral opioids such as methadone or controlled release oxycodone is the best alternative for long pharmacologic half-life and duration of effect.

Phantom Limb Pain

Amputation as well as limb-salvage procedures may be used to achieve local control of a bone tumor, and each in turn can result in chronic pain perceived to originate in the amputated limb. There are several etiologies for the occurrence of phantom limb pain, including spontaneous electrical activity of amputated nerve trunks and abnormal regrowth of nerve trunks (neuromas), each resulting in painful electrical discharges to the spinal cord and the brain. There may also be abnormalities in the CNS in response to the loss of limb, in which there may be loss of inhibitory sensory input from the amputated limb. Phantom limb pain is often severe and very challenging to treat.

Systematic analyses of studies to effectively treat chronic postoperative phantom limb pain have not clearly demonstrated an effective treatment option.[69,70] Central strategies, such as hypnotherapy, aimed at altering metabolic activity in pain perception areas of the brain, such as the anterior cingulate cortical area, show promise over peripheral strategies or opioids.

Because the incidence of phantom limb pain may be correlated with the incidence of presurgical pain in the diseased limb,[71] the first important principle in the treatment of phantom limb pain is to effectively treat the bone pain preoperatively before the amputation. This can include the use of regional anesthetic techniques, such as continuous epidural analgesia, with the use of opioids and local anesthetic to reduce dorsal horn sensitization prior to surgical resection.[72]

Preemptive use of nonconventional analgesics that slow the rate of spontaneous neuronal discharge, the AEDs, may also have a role in preventing phantom pain.

Following the surgical amputation, treatment of the acute postoperative pain must be initiated promptly in attempt to minimize the development of a chronic pain syndrome. Strategies for the acute postoperative pain for amputees include continuous peripheral nerve blocks, continuous plexus blocks, or epidural blocks. Given that long-term opioid use is not usually effective for the phantom limb pain syndrome, AEDs and/or TCAs may be empirically initiated or continued from the preoperative period, though there is no literature support for this recommendation.[73,74]

Complementary and alternative medicine (CAM) options for the treatment of chronic pain due to phantom limb pain include the use of hypnotherapy, massage, and acupuncture.[75-77] While no randomized clinical studies provide support for using nonpharmacologic strategies to treat phantom limb pain, neuroimaging research demonstrates that specific areas of the brain show decreased arousal associated with these practices, interpreted as a reinterpretation of the chronic pain experience.[78]

Visceral Pain

The four major etiologies of visceral pain include (1) organ invasion with capsular wall stretching; (2) organ compression; (3) hollow organ obstruction (e.g., ureter or bowel); and (4) or peritoneal cavity bleeding. For all etiologies of visceral abdominal pain, it is important to initiate the treatment of the pain early in an attempt to prevent visceral hyperalgesia and subsequent centralization of pain. Visceral hyperalgesia results from an insult, such as tumor invasion or surgical manipulation, to the celiac plexus (consisting of the hepatic plexus, splenic plexus, gastric plexuses, pancreatic plexus, supra/renal plexuses, testicular plexus, superior mesenteric plexus, and the inferior mesenteric plexus). If treatment of the visceral pain is not initiated promptly or effectively, ongoing nociception ultimately may result in a central pain syndrome, which can be very difficult to treat.

For visceral pain due to organ invasion with capsular wall stretching or tumor regrowth, the primary treatment to decrease the pain is to decrease the tumor size by surgery, chemotherapy, and/or radiation therapy. Of course, surgical resection of an abdominal tumor will result in significant postoperative pain; therefore, a treatment plan should be in place to manage the surgical pain to expedite postoperative recovery. The management of surgical pain with parenteral opioids, regional anesthetic infusions, adjunctive agents, and other techniques is discussed elsewhere.[79-81]

Regional nerve blocks and abdominal plexus blocks are also a consideration for the treatment of visceral pain due to tumor invasion of a solid organ or abdominal nerve plexus. They can be used in the pediatric population by experienced pediatric anesthesia or pain management consultants for the management of pain in unresponsive abdominopelvic tumors, such as bladder rhabdomyosarcoma or neuroblastoma.

Visceral abdominal pain can also be due to intestinal obstruction either from the tumor mass or from intestinal adhesions that are the consequence of prior abdominal surgical procedures. The treatment of the pain of a bowel obstruction is, of course, mechanical relief of the bowel distention first by nasogastric suction and then, ultimately, by surgical resection of the obstruction. Opioids are an effective measure to temporize while awaiting definitive surgical treatment and act by their analgesic properties as well as by decreasing the peristaltic activity of the gut.

Pain Associated With Bone Marrow Transplantation

Pediatric cancer patients requiring BMT as part of their treatment regimen are considered a high-risk group of patients for the development of acute and chronic pain, given the intensity of this treatment regimen. Mechanisms of acute pain associated with BMT include mucositis, graft-versus-host disease (GVHD), and infectious complications. Thus, pain management is critical in the care of the BMT patient, and if pain is not treated adequately, it can result in decreased QOL.

Mucositis

Although mucositis occurs when chemotherapy alone is given, mucositis is often more prolonged and severe in BMT patients.[82] The grading scale for describing the severity of oral mucositis established by the World Health Organization (WHO) begins with mild, or grade I mucositis, in which the oral mucosa is red and tender, to severe, grade IV mucositis, in which the pediatric cancer patient is unable to eat and maintain his or her own nutrition.[83] The severity of the mucositis often corresponds to the description of the severity of the pain by the patient. Grade I mucositis may only require intermittent bolus dosing of an opioid analgesic. In the BMT setting, however, mucositis pain usually requires use of an opioid, ideally administered by both continuous intravenous administration and PCA, given the duration of pain over a period that may last for 2 or more weeks and the extensive tissue injury involving the entire gastrointestinal tract.[84] When marrow engraftment occurs and counts recover, the PCA is usually weaned relatively quickly and discontinued.

Graft-Versus-Host Disease

Acute GVHD manifested by skin rash, right upper quadrant pain, and/or diarrhea is a source of peripheral somatic and abdominal pain. The skin rash ranges from mild erythema of the palms and soles of the feet to painful bullous desquamation in the severe form. Chronic GVHD occurs 100 days beyond the hematopoietic stem cell infusion and is thought to be an autoimmune process. Chronic GVHD primarily has skin manifestations that include scleroderma-type changes often accompanied by joint stiffness and immobility.

Treatment of Pain Due to GVHD

Treatment of pain due to acute gastrointestinal GVHD, often presenting as crampy abdominal pain due to the diffuse enteritis, requires the use of an opioid analgesic in the form of a PCA both for analgesia and to reduce hypermotility. Chronic GVHD is usually an outpatient disease requiring a long-term pain management plan since the autoimmune process can cause muscle and organ invasion resulting in chronic neuropathic pain. In the setting of chronic pain, oral opioid use may be required until the neuropathic pain is adequately treated with alternative agents, including AEDs such as gabapentin or TCAs such as amitriptyline. Nonpharmacologic therapies, including the use of acupuncture, massage therapy, and other relaxation strategies, may also be considered. No randomized controlled analgesic trials have been published to guide the management of pain in chronic GVHD.

Other Factors Important to Pain Assessment and Development of the Treatment Plan for BMT Pediatric Patients

There often is significant anxiety experienced by the pediatric patients who have undergone BMT, due to prolonged hospitalization, frequent procedures and episodes of pain, and fear of impending death. Thus, both pharmacologic and psychological services to decrease anxiety of the children are useful. Facilitation of night sleep is also valuable and may be enhanced by the pharmacologic use of psychotropic drugs, such as amitriptyline or trazodone, with sedative side effects.

TREATMENT OF SIDE EFFECTS AND SYMPTOMS IN PEDIATRIC CANCER PATIENTS

Nausea and Vomiting

The intensification of both chemotherapeutic and radiotherapeutic programs has resulted in both increased efficacy in and increased toxicity to cancer patients. Nausea and vomiting, which are experienced by almost all cancer patients, are among the most troublesome side effects. Without effective prophylaxis and treatment, these symptoms become debilitating, and patients are physically incapable of receiving further chemotherapy or are so psychologically distressed that they or their parents may refuse subsequent treatments.

During the last two decades, major advances have led to better control of nausea and emesis. These advances stem from improved understanding of the physiology of nausea and vomiting, the development of the 5-hydroxytryptamine subtype 3 (5-HT3) receptor antagonist class of antiemetics, and improved differentiation of anticipatory, acute, and delayed symptoms. Despite these advances, nausea and vomiting remain the first and third most distressing side effects of chemotherapy in adults and continue to occur in most adult and pediatric patients.[85,86]

Chemotherapy-Induced Vomiting

Chemotherapeutic agents may induce vomiting either by stimulation of the vomiting center itself (located in the medullary lateral reticular formation) or via direct or indirect stimulation of the chemoreceptor trigger zone (CTZ). The CTZ, a distinct medullary center located in the floor of the fourth ventricle in the vicinity of the area postrema, activates the vomiting center to produce nausea and vomiting.

Serotonin (5-HT) receptors, particularly subtype 3 receptors (5-HT3), play a role in the mediation of chemotherapy-induced nausea and vomiting. Selective antagonists of 5-HT3 receptors are potent antiemetics. Enterochromaffin cells in the gastrointestinal tract are major producers of serotonin, and studies in ferrets have demonstrated that cisplatin-induced emesis can be prevented with depletion of body serotonin stores.[87] Human studies have shown a rise in serotonin metabolites in the urine after administration of cisplatin.[88] This rise correlates with the onset and intensity of emesis. 5-HT3 receptors are located throughout the human brain, including a high concentration in the area postrema, where the CTZ is located.[89] In addition, metoclopramide, which previously was known to act on dopaminergic receptors, now has been shown to act on serotonin receptors as well.[90] Whether the predominant clinical effect of 5-HT3 receptor antagonists is central, on receptors in the area postrema, or peripheral, on receptors in the gastrointestinal tract wall or vagal afferents, remains unclear.

Radiation-Induced Vomiting

Radiation-induced nausea and vomiting appear to be mediated through both CTZ and peripheral mechanisms.[91] Total-body, cranial, and abdominal radiation are all emetogenic, particularly the latter.[92] The role of serotonin in emesis induction is suggested by the findings that higher urine serotonin metabolite levels have been correlated with more emetogenic radiation and that 5-HT3 receptor antagonists are effective in controlling radiation-induced emesis.[93]

Disease-Induced Vomiting

Nausea and vomiting result from various sequelae of cancer. Metastatic disease may produce tumor exudate or sloughing of tissue, which, in turn, produces toxic central effects. Abnormally high or low intracranial pressure, stretching of the capsule of an organ, inflammation of the gastrointestinal tract (gastritis or gastroenteritis), or gastrointestinal obstruction may also initiate nausea and vomiting. The exact mechanisms of symptoms are not clearly defined for these states. However, some of these states can respond to both surgical and pharmacologic intervention. Opioid-induced vomiting and opioid-induced ileus leading to vomiting are common among patients at all stages of illness. Opioids produce nausea and vomiting by both brainstem and direct enteral afferent mechanisms.

Clinical Presentation

Great variability occurs in symptom presentation, intensity, time to onset, and duration. Some of this variability can be predicted from the specific treatment modalities used, but great variability among patients in response to identical regimens also exists. Symptoms include nausea, retching, and vomiting and tend to occur in a cyclic fashion if not properly treated early in therapy. Retching is identical to vomiting in that the same physiologic mechanisms are occurring, but gastric contents are not expelled. Clinically, retching often is perceived by the patient to be more debilitating than vomiting, because the abdominal musculature can be significantly strained and no relief is achieved. *Acute* symptoms occur during the first 24 hours after the administration of chemotherapy. *Delayed* nausea and vomiting occur 24 to 120 hours after emetogenic treatment. Almost all patients experience delayed symptoms after cisplatin administration; nearly half do so after moderately emetogenic treatment.[94] *Anticipatory (psychogenic) vomiting*, the onset of nausea and vomiting before the administration of chemotherapy, is difficult to treat because it is a conditioned response and may be related to anxiety. Despite major improvements in the management of acute and delayed symptoms, more than one-half of pediatric patients experience anticipatory symptoms.[95–97] Patient factors that increase the probability of severe clinical symptoms in adults include a prior chemotherapeutic experience, a predisposition to nausea and vomiting (e.g., motion sickness), anxiety, and female gender.[98] A multivariate analysis found that prechemotherapy nausea, low social functioning, and female gender were extremely predictive of an increased incidence of symptoms.[99] Better control of acute nausea and vomiting is associated with a lower incidence of delayed nausea and vomiting.[100,101] Pediatric studies addressing risk factors are very limited.

Treatment of Nausea and Vomiting

The origin of vomiting must be identified before any therapy is initiated. In addition to chemotherapy, other causes of vomiting common to pediatric cancer patients include stretching of the capsule of an organ, vestibular reflexes (motion sickness), inflammation of the gastrointestinal tract (gastritis, gastroenteritis), gastrointestinal obstruction, increased intracranial pressure, opioid administration, and ileus. The latter may be induced by chemotherapeutic agents that affect the peripheral nervous system (e.g., vincristine), by opioids or by direct gastrointestinal tract damage from disease or treatment. The etiology of vomiting may change with the patient's condition. For example, the same chemotherapy that directly caused acute and delayed symptoms may then cause gastrointestinal inflammation, leading to continued vomiting. Although treatment-induced symptoms generally are predictable, unusual severity, timing, or duration should prompt development of a differential diagnosis and not just a reflexive modification of the antiemetic regimen. Such symptoms could be the manifestation of a completely different process, such as intestinal obstruction or increased intracranial pressure.

To prevent treatment-induced nausea and vomiting, the receptors for the emetic stimulus must be blocked before the stimulus occurs and the blockade must be continued as long as symptoms are likely to occur. If the emetic stimuli are not drug induced (e.g., infection or metabolic derangement), therapy cannot be initiated before symptoms become established. Because nausea and vomiting in patients receiving chemotherapy or radiotherapy are predictable, a planned approach to prophylactic antiemetic therapy is indicated. Scheduled doses must be administered in a timely fashion, regardless of whether symptoms appear. The duration of follow-up therapy is determined by both the patient's previous patterns of nausea and vomiting and the expected duration of emetic activity of the stimulus. Intravenous therapy was once the standard of care for all patients. Newly available oral agents offer good bioavailability and marked efficacy in adults but have not been well studied in children.[102-104]

Knowledge of the emetogenic potential and patterns of vomiting associated with the various chemotherapeutic agents helps to predict the severity and duration of the anticipated symptoms. The severity and duration of vomiting also differ among patients, as does the time of onset. Acute symptoms may appear immediately (mechlorethamine) or 6 to 12 hours after administration (cyclophosphamide or actinomycin-D). Delayed symptoms do not appear until at least 24 hours after administration. When these agents are used in combination, antiemetic prophylaxis should be based on the most emetic component of the regimen. When combinations of moderately emetogenic agents are used, prophylaxis for severely emetogenic treatment should be considered. The severity of nausea and vomiting usually is increased with increasing dose and decreased with increasing infusion time.[105] Increasing use of multiday chemotherapeutic regimens, recognition of delayed vomiting, and availability of effective antiemetics with few side effects have led to longer administration of antiemetics. Nausea and vomiting associated with radiotherapy are less well understood. Abdominal radiation almost always causes nausea and vomiting, whereas the occurrence and severity of nausea and vomiting from cranial radiation are more variable. The pharmacologic management of nausea and vomiting is discussed in further detail in the following sections.

Somnolence, Fatigue, and Insomnia

Sleep disorders, daytime sedation, fatigue, and lack of mental clarity are common problems among children undergoing cancer treatment, in the setting of advanced cancer, and in some long-term cancer survivors. Fatigue or lack of energy is extremely common among children with cancer.[24,106] These symptoms can occur during treatment with chemotherapy or radiation, after surgery, in the setting of advanced disease, or even in long term in disease-free survivors. The causes of fatigue often are multifactorial and may reflect a combination of medical and psychosocial factors. Sleep disturbance, depression, and anxiety often are associated with daytime fatigue. Depressed mood and anxiety are common in patients with cancer; in most cases, these subjects had no history of mood disorders prior to the onset of the cancer.

One's approach to the child with fatigue should include identification of remediable medical factors (e.g., anemia, cachexia, and endocrine or electrolyte disturbances). When depression or anxiety is present, consideration should be given to psychotherapy and pharmacologic treatment. Fatigue often coexists with sleep disturbance. Lifestyle change, including improved sleep hygiene and avoidance of caffeine in the evening, may be helpful to improve sleep. Low doses of an antidepressant are our preferred pharmacologic treatment of persistent sleep disturbance. Fatigue and somnolence, especially in patients taking opioids, may improve with the administration of methylphenidate or other stimulants.[107] Graded aerobic exercise programs have shown promise;[108] they may also improve sleep and ameliorate depressed mood.

Constipation

Constipation is common among patients with cancer. Often, but not exclusively, it is due to opioids.[109] Some studies suggest differences among opioids in the severity of constipation. For example, in some studies, transdermal fentanyl was found to produce less constipation than oral morphine.[110]

When using high dose or prolonged courses of opioids for the treatment of pain, the treatment plan should also include a bowel regimen to reduce the likelihood of constipation, certainly the most troubling opioid side effect to patients. Constipation may already be a significant problem in children prior to the use of opioids since certain types of chemotherapeutic agents, such as the vinca alkaloids, used to treat solid tumors of childhood can cause severe impairment of normal peristalsis.

Pruritus

Pruritus is common among children with cancer, due to a variety of causes, including opioid therapy. Although antihistamines are most commonly prescribed, it should be emphasized that histamine release is only one among several mechanisms that produce the sensation of itch.[111-113] Antihistamines can produce sedation and other mental status changes, particularly when excessive doses are used or when combined with other medications that produce central anticholinergic effects, including scopolamine and TCAs.[114,115] Other classes of medications that have been used to treat pruritus include very low-dose opioid antagonists, κ-opioid agonists, 5-HT3 receptor antagonists, and antidepressants.[116,117]

DRUGS FOR PAIN AND SYMPTOM MANAGEMENT

Medication management of pain in children requires awareness of the developmental differences in drug metabolism and effect and consideration of the use of several classes of analgesic medications.

Developmental Pharmacology

Drug dosing in infants and younger children is often extrapolated, using weight-based scaling, from studies in adults and older children because of the paucity of pharmacokinetic (PK) and pharmacodynamic (PD) studies in children. Yet, the PK/PD of analgesics vary with age; drug responses in infants and young children differ from those in older children and adults. The elimination half-life of most analgesics is prolonged in neonates and young infants because of their immature hepatic enzyme systems. Clearance of analgesics may also be variable in young infants and children. Renal blood flow, glomerular filtration, and tubular secretion increase dramatically in the first few weeks, approaching adult values by 3 to 5 months of age. Renal clearance of analgesics is often greater in toddlers and preschool-aged children than in adults, whereas in premature infants clearance is reduced. Age-related differences in body composition and protein binding also exist. Total body water as a fraction of body weight is greater in neonates than in children or adults. Tissues with high perfusion, such as the brain and heart, account for a larger proportion of body mass in neonates than do other tissues, such as muscle and fat. Because of decreased serum concentrations of albumin and α_1-acid glycoprotein, neonates have reduced protein binding of some drugs, resulting in higher amounts of free, unbound, pharmacologically active drug.

Acetaminophen, Aspirin, and Nonsteroidal Anti-inflammatory Drugs

Acetaminophen and NSAIDs have replaced aspirin as the most commonly used antipyretics and oral, nonopioid analgesics (Table 42.2). Acetaminophen, a generally safe, nonopioid analgesic and antipyretic that has the advantage of rectal and oral routes of administration, is expected soon to be available as an intravenous preparation in the United States as it is now in Europe. In addition, APAP is not associated with the gastrointestinal or antiplatelet effects of aspirin and NSAIDs, making it a particularly useful drug in patients with cancer. Unlike NSAIDs and aspirin, APAP has only mild anti-inflammatory action. Acetaminophen toxicity can result from either large, single doses or cumulative, excessive dosing over days or weeks. A single, massive overdose overwhelms the normal glucuronidation and sulfation metabolic pathways in the liver, whereas chronic overdosing exhausts supplies of the sulfhydryl donor glutathione, leading to alternative cytochrome P450–catalyzed oxidative metabolism and the production of the hepatotoxic metabolite N-acetyl-p-benzoquinone imine (NAPQI). Toxicity manifests as fulminant hepatic necrosis and failure in infants, children, and adults. In general, drug biotransformation processes are immature in neonates, very active in young children, and somewhat less active in adults. Acetaminophen metabolism follows this pattern, with small differences between age groups. Infants are actually more resistant to APAP-induced hepatotoxicity than adults as a result of metabolism differences: sulfation predominates over glucuronidation, leading to a reduction in NAPQI production.

The NSAIDs are used widely to treat pain and fever in children. In children with juvenile rheumatoid arthritis, ibuprofen and aspirin are equally effective, but ibuprofen is associated with fewer side effects and better compliance. NSAIDs used adjunctively in surgical patients reduce opioid requirements (and therefore opioid side effects) by as much as 35% to 40%. NSAIDs are particularly useful in the management of bone pain due to metastatic processes in cancer patients and for the management of orofacial pain for which it is more efficacious than opioids.

Ketorolac, an intravenous NSAID, is useful in treating moderate to severe acute pain when patients are unable or unwilling to swallow oral NSAIDs. In addition, intravenous ibuprofen was recently approved in the United States for the management of pain and fever for 5 days or less, although there is no pediatric indication in the package labeling. Although we lack clinical experience with intravenous ibuprofen in the United States, we expect it will be widely used in the future. In Europe, intravenous ibuprofen is already used to treat pediatric pain; it is also used to induce closure of newborn patent ductus arteriosus.

The antiplatelet effects frequently limit the usefulness of this class of medications in children with cancer who are or will become thrombocytopenic. Other adverse effects of NSAIDs are uncommon, but they may be serious when they occur. They include gastritis with pain and bleeding; decreased renal blood flow that may reduce glomerular filtration, in some cases, leading to tubular necrosis; and hepatic dysfunction and liver failure. Renal injury from short-term use of NSAIDs in euvolemic children is quite rare; the risk is increased by hypovolemia or cardiac dysfunction. The safety of both NSAIDs and APAP for short-term use is well established.

NSAIDs and aspirin act by nonspecific inhibition of both isotypes of cyclo-oxygenase (COX-1 and COX-2), the enzyme that catalyzes the production of prostanoids to form arachidonic acid. However, COX has two predominant isoenzymes: a constitutively synthesized form (COX-1) found in platelets, the gastric mucosa, liver, and kidneys and an inducible form (COX-2) found in monocytes, peripheral nerves, kidney, and spinal cord and induced by injury and inflammation. Inhibition of COX-1 produces most unwanted NSAID side effects, and inhibition of COX-2 produces analgesia. A relatively new class of drugs, the coxibs, are COX-2–specific inhibitors. COX-2 inhibitors (coxibs) are generally safer NSAIDs because they are not associated with platelet inhibition, and the rate of gastric bleeding is dramatically reduced. Although these agents are indeed associated with fewer gastric side effects, initial sponsored studies of their efficacy in elderly adults with cardiovascular disease showed an increased rate of stroke and myocardial infarction, the mechanism of which was undefined, resulting in the withdrawal from the market or from the U.S. Food and Drug Administration (FDA) regulatory pathway, leaving only celecoxib (Celebrex) available in the United States.

Interestingly, subsequent studies have demonstrated similar increased risk of cardiovascular complications in at-risk patients associated with the preoperative use of the conventional mixed COX-1 and COX-2 NSAIDs ibuprofen and naproxen. Celecoxib, therefore, may be a particularly useful agent in the setting of childhood cancer because of its potent analgesia and absence of platelet inhibition and gastrointestinal side effects. Generally, children with cancer are not considered at increased risk of thrombotic stroke or myocardial infarction.

Opioid Analgesics

Opioid analgesia in children include the use of typical μ-opioid agonists (e.g., morphine sulfate and methadone), atypical opioid analgesics (e.g., tramadol), μ-opioid antagonists (e.g.,

TABLE 42.2

COMMONLY USED NONOPIOID MEDICATIONS

Acetaminophen	10–15 mg/kg PO q4 h 20–30 mg/kg/PR q4 h 40 mg/kg/PR q6–8 h Maximum daily dosing: 90 mg/kg/24 h (children) 60 mg/kg/24 h (infants) 30–45 mg/kg/24 h (neonates)	Little anti-inflammatory action; no antiplatelet or adverse gastric effects; overdosing can produce fulminant hepatic failure
Aspirin	10–15 mg/kg PO q4 h Maximum daily dosing: 120 mg/kg/24 h (children)	Anti-inflammatory; prolonged antiplatelet effects; may cause gastritis; associated with Reye syndrome
Ibuprofen	8–10 mg/kg PO q6 h	Anti-inflammatory; transient antiplatelet effects; may cause gastritis; extensive pediatric safety experience
Naprosyn	5–7 mg/kg PO q8–12 h	Anti-inflammatory; transient antiplatelet effects; may cause gastritis; more prolonged duration than that of ibuprofen
Ketorolac	Loading dose 0.5 mg/kg and then 0.25–0.3 mg/kg IV q6 h to a maximum of 5 days; maximum dose 30 mg loading with maximum dosing of 15 mg q6 h	Anti-inflammatory; reversible antiplatelet effects; may cause gastritis; useful for short-term situations when oral dosing is not feasible
Celecoxib	3–6 mg/kg PO q12–24 h	Anti-inflammatory; no antiplatelet or gastric effects; cross-reactivity with sulfa allergies
Choline magnesium salicylate	10–20 mg/kg PO q8–12 h	Weak anti-inflammatory; lower risk of bleeding and gastritis than with conventional NSAIDs
Nortriptyline, amitriptyline, desipraminebe	0.1–0.5 mg/kg PO qhs	For neuropathic pain; facilitates sleep; may enhance opioid effect; may useful in sickle-cell pain; risk of dysrhythmia in prolonged QTc syndrome; may cause fatal dysrhythmia in overdose; the U.S. Food and Drug Administration states that it may enhance suicidal ideation
Gabapentin	100 mg bid or tid titrated to up to 3600 mg/24 h	For neuropathic pain; associated with sedation, dizziness, ataxia, headache, and behavioral changes
Quetiapine, risperidone, Thorazine, haloperidol	Quetiapine: 6.25 or 12.5 mg PO qd (hs); may use q6 h prn acute agitation with pain. Escalate dose to 25 mg/dose, if needed Risperidone: useful for PDD, spectrum disorder, or tic disorder and chronic pain; 0.25–1 mg (in 0.25-mg increments) qd or bid; see PDR for other dosing	Useful when arousal is amplifying pain; often used when first starting SSRI and then weaned after at least 2 wk; check for normal QTc before initiating; side effects include extrapyramidal reactions (diphenhydramine may be used to treat) and sedation; in high doses, can lower the seizure threshold
Fluoxetine	10–20 mg PO qd (usually in morning)	SSRI for children with anxiety disorders in which arousal amplifies sensory signaling; useful in PDD and spectrum disorders in very low doses; best to use in conjunction with psychiatric evaluation
Sucrose solution via pacifier or gloved finger	Preterm infants (gestational age): 28 wk: 0.2 mL swabbed into mouth; 28–32 wk: 0.2–2 mL, depending on suck/swallow; >32 wk: 2 mL Term infants: 1.5–2 mL PO over 2 min	Allow 2 min before starting procedure; analgesia may last up to 8 min; the dose may be repeated once

NSAIDs, nonsteroidal anti-inflammatory drugs; PDD, pervasive developmental disorder; PDR, Physicians' Desk Reference; QTc, corrected QT interval on an electrocardiogram; SSRI, selective serotonin reuptake inhibitor.

naloxone, naltrexone, or methylnaltrexone) in low doses to ameliorate unwanted side effects of opioids, and the *N*-methyl-D-aspartate (NMDA) antagonist ketamine in some cases, which may reverse or retard the development of opioid tolerance. While opioid monotherapy is a highly effective method for treating moderate to severe pain,[118] its effectiveness may be limited by the development opioid tolerance and opioid-induced hyperalgesia.[119] Furthermore, the analgesic response to any given opioid depends on the primary endogenous tolerance of the patient as well as induced secondary tolerance. Adverse effects of opioid analgesics, for both opioid-naive patients and opioid-tolerant patients, include somnolence, constipation, pruritus, nausea, vomiting, urinary retention, and diaphoresis. Long-term opioid therapy has also been associated with alterations in immune function and hormone levels, the clinical significance of which is speculative.[120]

Patient controlled analgesia is the most effective method for intravenous administration of opioids in appropriate patients because with it there is no lag time between the need and demand for and the delivery of the analgesic; there can be both continuous and demand delivery; and there are lock-out mechanisms for total doses given per period of time, thereby increasing the safety profile. Hospitals have different protocols in place for the use of PCAs in young children, such that some do not allow for their use, because it requires a parent or nurse to administer the boluses, and is no longer patient controlled. Alternatively, other hospitals, such as those with well-integrated pain management services within their pediatric oncology division, do allow for the use of PCA by proxy; in other words, parent-controlled or nurse-controlled analgesia for the child too young to understand the concept or for the cognitively impaired child.[121–123]

The choice of opioid for intravenous or enteral administration is guided by personal experience of the clinician, preference of the patient, and drug availability for each route of administration. Virtually no clinical investigations show superiority of one μ-opioid over another in efficacy, patient satisfaction, or risk of adverse events. Coda et al.[124] compared intravenous PCA with morphine, sufentanil (a very infrequently used potent synthetic opioid), and hydromorphone in adolescents following BMA. The primary utility of their publication was the precise pharmacologic calculation of potency ratios for morphine and hydromorphone (1:5) in this population. Their double-blind, crossover model demonstrated a very slight patient preference for morphine, as evidenced by slightly fewer patient-initiated crossover models, to the other study medications in those teenagers receiving morphine PCA.

Besides the usual parenteral intravenous route of administration and the oral-enteral route of administration of opioids, there are three delivery systems of opioids that are useful in the pediatric cancer population. The oral transmucosal delivery of fentanyl citrate (including Actiq [a fentanyl-containing raspberry-flavored lozenge on a handle] and Fentora [an effervescent orally dissolvable transmucosally absorbed tablet]) are formulations that are commercially available with approved indications for the treatment of breakthrough pain in opioid-tolerant adult patients.[125] They result in the rapid absorption of fentanyl. A transdermal PCA device, which delivers fentanyl transdermally on demand, developed by Alza Pharmaceuticals, was recently FDA approved but has not achieved clinical acceptance. Under clinical investigation are transnasal and inhaled delivery devices for potent synthetic opioids.

The fentanyl transdermal therapeutic systems (Duragesic) has been approved for use in both adults and children for the management of pain *in opioid-tolerant patients*. (The pharmaceutical industry's definition of opioid tolerant is generally a patient receiving the equivalent of 1 mg/kg per day of oral morphine for 1 week or more.) The transdermal drug delivery method allows for an alternative route to oral administration in patients unable or unwilling to swallow medications. Several investigations have defined the pharmacokinetics of the fentanyl transdermal therapeutic system in children and are discussed in a recent review by Zernikow et al.,[126] who defined the approximate conversion factor of 45 mg per day of morphine (or morphine equivalents; see Table 42.3) to fentanyl transdermal therapeutic system equal to 12.5 μg/h for initial therapy for both children and adolescents who require long-term opioid therapy. The data supporting the use of the trans-

dermal route over traditional routes of administration are scant, but there are data that demonstrate child and parent satisfaction with the transdermal therapeutic delivery system of fentanyl in both pain relief and QOL in the pediatric palliative care setting.[127]

Tramadol hydrochloride is an atypical opioid that has a weak affinity for μ-opioid receptors, as well as being a weak inhibitor of serotonin and noradrenaline reuptake. The advantage of tramadol is that it has negligible respiratory depression.[128] It is hepatically metabolized and renally excreted, factors that must be taken into consideration when using this medication in pediatric cancer patients since chemotherapy can result in hepatotoxicity. The active metabolite is O-desmethyltramadol (M1), and recent pharmacokinetic studies in children have demonstrated that it is possible to produce enough of the active metabolite to achieve adequate pain relief.[129] Safe dosing regimens for children older than 12 months include 1 to 2 mg/kg by mouth every 4 to 6 hours, with a maximum dose of 8 mg/kg per day.[130]

Dependence and Addiction

There may be barriers to the use of opioid analgesia in children due to parents' and healthcare providers' concerns regarding the risk of dependence or addiction.[131] While fear of addiction is common in our society, addiction is, in fact, a complex psychopathology, the tendency to which is largely genetically determined; it is characterized by the compulsive use of a drug, psychological craving, and use in spite of harm and is commonly associated with sociopathic behaviors. Addiction is not and cannot be induced by the mere pharmacologic use of opioids for pain management in a patient not genetically at risk for its development, nor is it commonly seen in the pediatric population. Addiction may be observed in older adolescents who have complex psychosocial issues resulting in maladaptive coping to pain. Generally, the incidence of opioid addiction and misuse in the pain population mirrors that of the general society and is estimated to be about 0.5%; in other words, were opioid therapy capable of inducing opioid addiction, then the incidence would be much higher than that of our general society.

Pseudoaddiction, however, is commonly seen in the cancer population and refers to the phenomenon of the exhibition of addiction-like behaviors (clock-watching, drug seeking, and symptom amplification) that is the result of undertreatment of pain by well-meaning clinicians prescribing inadequate doses of opioids at excessive dose intervals.[132–134]

Tolerance to Opioids

The presence of tolerance, dependence, and risk of withdrawal are not indicative of or synonymous with addiction, but of course are the pharmacologic consequences of the appropriate use of opioids for more than several days or a week and are no different from the development of tolerance and withdrawal to a large number of pharmacologic substances (note that society does not refer to insulin-tolerant patients as addicted; society reserves that pejorative descriptor to patients managed with opioids).

Tolerance, dependence, and therefore the predilection to exhibit opioid withdrawal (also termed opioid abstinence syndrome) usually go hand in hand; that is to say that it is safe to assume that patients exhibiting tolerance to opioids are opioid dependent and at risk of developing abstinence syndrome if the opioids were to be discontinued or weaned too rapidly. The more common symptoms of withdrawal in children with

TABLE 42.3

PEDIATRIC DOSAGE GUIDELINES FOR OPIOID ANALGESICS

Drug	Equianalgesic doses		Parenteral dosing		IV: Po dose ratio	Oral dosing		Comments
	IV	Oral	<50 kg	>50 kg		<50 kg	>50 kg	
Codeine	N/A	20 mg	N/A	N/A	1:2	0.5–1 mg/kg q3–4 h	30–60 mg q3–4 h	Weak opioid; typically given with acetaminophen; not for severe pain; 33% of patients are not codeine responders
Fentanyl	10 µg	100 µg	0.5–1 µg/kg q1–2 h 0.5–1.5 µg/kg/h	0.5–1 µg/kg q1–2 h 0.5–1.5 µg/kg/h	Oral Transmucosal 1:10 Transdermal 1:1	Oral transmucosal: 10 µg/kg Transdermal: 12.5–50 µg/kg	Transdermal patches available; patch reaches steady state at 24 h and should be changed q72 h	70–100 times as potent as morphine with rapid onset and shorter duration. With high doses and rapid administration, can cause chest wall rigidity. Useful for short procedures; transdermal form should be used only in opioid-tolerant patients with chronic pain
Hydrocodone	N/A	1.5 mg	N/A	N/A	N/A	0.15 mg/kg	10 mg	Weak opioid; preferable to codeine; typically prescribed in form with acetaminophen
Hydromorphone	0.2 mg	0.6 mg	0.01 mg q2–4 h 0.002 mg/kg/h	0.01 mg q2–4 h 0.002 mg/kg/h	1:3	0.04–0.08 mg/kg q3–4 h	2–4 mg q3–4 h	5× potency of morphine; no histamine release and fewer adverse events than morphine
Meperidine	10 mg	30 mg	0.5 mg/kg q2–4 h	0.5 mg/kg q2–4 h	1:4	2–3 mg/kg q3–4 h	100–150 mg q3–4 h	Primary use in low doses is for treatment of rigors and shivering after anesthesia or with amphotericin or blood products. Not appropriate for repeated dosing

Methadone	1 mg	2 mg	0.1 mg/kg q8–24 h	0.1 mg/kg q8–24 h	1:2	0.2 mg/kg q8–12 h PO; available in liquid or tablet	5–10 mg q6–8 h	12- to 24-h duration; useful in certain types of chronic pain; requires additional vigilance, because it will accumulate over 72 h and produce delayed sedation. When patients who are tolerant to opioids switch to methadone, they show incomplete cross-tolerance and improved efficacy
Morphine	1 mg	3 mg	0.05 mg/kg q2–4 h 0.01–0.03 mg/kg/h	Bolus: 5–8 mg q2–4 h	1:3	Immediate release: 0.3 mg/kg q3–4 h Sustained release: 20–35 kg: 10–15 mg q8–12 h 35–50 kg: 15–30 mg q8–12 h	Immediate release: 15–20 mg q3–4 h Sustained release: 30–90 mg q8–12 h	Potent opioid for moderate/ severe pain; may cause histamine release Sustained-release form must be swallowed whole; cannot be crushed or it becomes immediate acting leading to acute overdose
Oxycodone	N/A	3 mg	N/A	N/A	N/A	0.1–0.2 mg q3–4 h; available in liquid (1 mg/mL)	Immediate release: 5–10 mg q4 h; Sustained release: 10–120 mg q8–12 h	Strong opioid; potent and preferable to hydrocodone Sustained-release form must be swallowed whole; cannot be crushed or it becomes immediate-acting leading to acute overdose

N/A, not available.

tolerance and dependence include severe dysphoria, diarrhea, abdominal cramps, and nasal congestion and the behavioral symptoms of anxiety and restlessness. The symptoms observed in young children may vary from those observed in adults. For example, an infant can have a high-pitched cry and inability to be soothed with a pacifier, bottle, or swaddling. A toddler's signs of withdrawal may include only diarrhea and temperature instability.

Given that tolerance to opioid analgesics can limit their clinical effectiveness and dependence to opioids creates the risk of abstinence syndrome, various approaches have been used in an attempt to prevent or reverse tolerance in children who require prolonged exposure to high-dose opioids. One proposed approach to prevent tolerance includes the use of a NMDA antagonist concomitantly with the opioid. Ketamine has been studied and shown to have a role in mitigating opioid-induced tolerance in children and adolescents who experience cancer pain. Finkel and colleagues[135] used ketamine at low doses, 0.1 to 1.0 mg/kg/h, in patients who had signs of opioid tolerance or severe side effects such as profound sedation. With this regimen, they found that adjuvant ketamine infusions used in combination with opioid analgesics (including morphine, methadone, and hydromorphone) resulted in improved pain control. Under investigation is the combined use of μ-opioid agonists and antagonists, the latter in ultralow dose. There is no pediatric experience with this combination, but it holds some promise for the future.[136,137]

When using high-dose or prolonged courses of opioids for the treatment of pain, the treatment plan must also include a bowel regimen to reduce the likelihood of constipation, certainly the most troubling opioid side effect in patients. Constipation may already be a significant problem for children prior to the use of opioids since certain types of chemotherapeutic agents used to treat solid tumors of childhood, such as the vinca alkaloids, can cause severe impairment of normal peristalsis. There are several alternatives that can be used to treat or prevent constipation including polyethylene glycol (Miralax, often preferable since it is a tasteless and odorless powder that can be mixed with any liquid), senna (Senakot, a stimulant laxative), docusate (Dulcolax, a lubricating laxative), milk of magnesia (magnesium hydroxide, an osmotic laxative), and mineral oil (a lubricant).

Local Anesthetics

Local anesthetics are widely used in children for topical application, cutaneous infiltration, peripheral nerve block, epidural neuraxial blocks, intrathecal infusions, and intravenous administration. Local anesthetics can be used with excellent safety and effectiveness. However, excessive systemic concentrations can cause seizures, CNS depression, arrhythmia, or cardiac depression. Unlike opioids, local anesthetics require a strict maximum dosing schedule. Pediatricians should be aware of the need to calculate these doses and adhere to guidelines. Topical local anesthetic preparations can reduce pain in diverse circumstances: suturing lacerations, placing peripheral intravenous catheters, performing LPs, and accessing indwelling central venous ports. Intravenous administration of lidocaine is useful in the management of neuropathic pain and refractory pain from mucositis.

EMLA, a topical eutectic mixture of lidocaine and prilocaine used to anesthetize intact skin, is commonly applied for venipuncture, lumbar puncture, and other needle procedures. It is generally safe for use, but in neonates, it has been associated with prilocaine-induced methemoglobinemia. Lidocaine cream (5% Elemax) has replaced EMLA in many pediatric centers.

Lidocaine is the most commonly used local anesthetic for cutaneous infiltration. Maximum safe dose of lidocaine is 5 mg/kg without epinephrine and 7 mg/kg with epinephrine. Although concentrated solutions (2%) are commonly available from hospital pharmacies, more dilute solutions such as 0.25% to 0.5% are as equally effective as 1% to 2% solutions for subcutaneous infiltration. The diluted solutions cause less burning discomfort on injection and permit use of larger volumes without achieving toxic doses.

In the surgical setting, cutaneous wound infiltration and regional nerve blocks are more often performed with bupivacaine 0.25% or ropivacaine 0.2% because of the much longer duration of effect. The maximum dose of these long-acting amide anesthetics is 2 to 4 mg/kg, or 0.5 to 0.6 mg/kg/h if administered as a continuous epidural or nerve block infusate.

Neuropathic pain may respond to the local application of a lidocaine topical patch (Lidoderm) for 12 hours per day. Neuropathic pain may also respond well to intravenous lidocaine administration, which may be used in hospital settings for refractory pain associated with neuropathic pain syndromes and pain associated with mucositis following BMT. In these instance, 1 to 2 mg/kg/h may be administered and the infusion titrated to achieve a blood lidocaine level in the 2- to 5-μg/mL range, using twice-daily therapeutic blood monitoring.

Unconventional Analgesics

The term *unconventional analgesic medication* refers to a wide variety of drugs developed for other indications but that have been found to have analgesic properties. These drugs include some antidepressants, antiepileptics, and neurotropic drugs.

The unconventional analgesics are generally used to manage neuropathic pain conditions in cancer patients, but they are generally not used to manage routine surgical, somatic, or musculoskeletal pain. Figure 42.4 presents a decision-making tree that will help the physician select the appropriate analgesic category for various types of pain.

Most of the currently used off-label pharmacologic strategies are extrapolated from adult trials, without evidence of their efficacy in children and adolescents. Although several unconventional analgesics have been approved by the FDA for analgesic uses, few have been specifically approved for use in youth with pain. Thus, they should be used with caution, with a focus on mitigating pain to allow children to participate effectively in therapies and return to normal activity as soon as possible. The use of psychotropic medications should be guided by the same principles that are applied to pharmacologic treatment of any symptom or disease. Target symptoms should be identified and medication side effects monitored. To determine dosing regimens, consider the child's weight and the effects of medical condition and other medications, such as psychotropic drugs, may have on the child's metabolism. When available, therapeutic blood-level monitoring should be performed. Side effects should be addressed in detail with both parents and children and specific instructions given for responding to possible adverse events. It may be necessary to directly address concerns about addiction, dependence, and tolerance to decrease treatment-related anxiety and increase compliance.

Antidepressant Medications

Antidepressant medications have been demonstrated as useful in adults with chronic pain, including neuropathic pain, headaches, and rheumatoid arthritis, independent of their effects on depressive disorders. Animal models of pain clearly demonstrate that analgesic properties of antidepressants

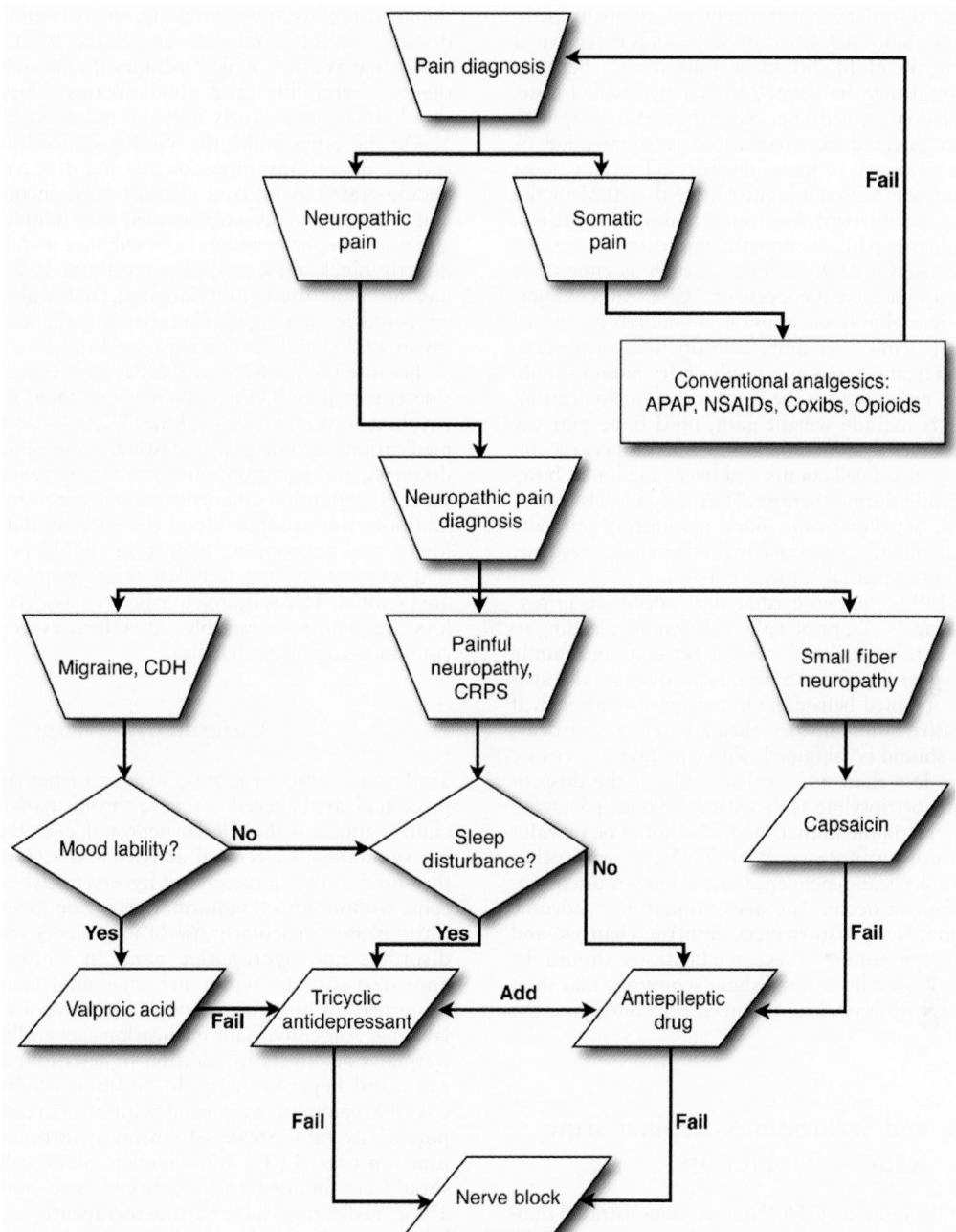

FIGURE 42.4 A decision tree for the management of cancer pain, showing the use of conventional and nonconventional analgesics and interventional nerve blocks. Abbreviations: CDH, chronic daily headache; CRPS, complex regional pain syndrome; APAP, acetaminophen; NSAIDs, nonsteroidal anti-inflammatory drugs.

inhibit norepinephrine reuptake in the CNS. In children, because clinical trials have been limited, practitioners should use antidepressants cautiously to treat chronic pain or associated depressive or anxiety symptoms. The FDA issued a Black Box Warning, its strongest warning, to inform the public of a small but significant increase in suicidal thoughts and attempts. A meta-analysis of studies involving children and adolescents receiving antidepressants indicated that no suicides had been attempted.[138] Pediatricians should address this fact with parents of patients treated with antidepressants and develop monitoring plans consistent with current FDA recommendations.

Tricyclic Antidepressants

Tricyclic antidepressants, which have been most studied in children with chronic pain, have been found effective in pain relief for symptoms including neuropathic pain, functional abdominal pain, and migraine. The efficacy of TCAs may be based on inhibition of the neurochemical pathways involved in norepinephrine and serotonin reuptake and their interference with other neurochemicals involved in the perception or neural conduction of pain. Because sedation is their most common side effect, these medications are also effective in treating the sleep disorders that frequently accompany pediatric pain. Because biotransformation of TCAs is extensive in healthy children, the child should be started on a bedtime dose, which should then be titrated to a daily divided dose, giving the larger dose at bedtime. Note that pain symptoms usually remit at lower doses than those recommended or required for the treatment of mood disorders. Typically, most children and adolescents do not require more than 0.25 mg/kg of amitriptyline or nortriptyline once a day at bedtime. Attention should be paid to hepatic microsomal enzyme metabolism because CYP2D6 inhibitors, such as cimetidine and quinidine, can increase the levels of TCAs. Anticholinergic side effects, remarkably uncommon in children compared with adults, often remit over time. Constipation, orthostatic hypotension, and dental caries as a result of dry mouth should be addressed by emphasizing the importance of hydration. Other side effects include weight gain, mild bone marrow suppression, and liver dysfunction. Some practitioners recommend monitoring blood cell counts and liver function at baseline and periodically during therapy. TCA blood levels can be obtained as well, but therapeutic blood monitoring generally should occur individually, particularly if adherence, overdose, or sudden changes in mental status are issues.

In the early 1990s, sudden cardiac death occurred in several children taking TCAs, principally desipramine, leading to concerns about cardiotoxicity. A careful personal and family history regarding cardiac arrhythmias, heart disease, and syncope should be obtained before the initiation of treatment. If there is any positive family history, then a baseline electrocardiogram (ECG) should be obtained, with care taken to ensure that the QTc is less than 445 milliseconds. If the dose of amitriptyline or nortriptyline is increased beyond 0.5 mg/kg per day, then we recommend that the ECG should be reevaluated with each dosing increase. With TCAs, as with other antidepressants, physical dependence and a known discontinuation syndrome can occur. The discontinuation syndrome includes agitation, sleep disturbances, appetite changes, and gastrointestinal symptoms. These medications should be tapered slowly to assist in distinguishing symptoms that indicate rebound or withdrawal or the need for continuing the medication.

Serotonin and Serotonin Norepinephrine Reuptake Inhibitors

Serotonin reuptake inhibitors (SSRIs) have demonstrated minimal efficacy in the treatment of a variety of pain syndromes in adults, leading to a supposition that noradrenergic pathways are more significant than serotonergic pathways in the treatment of pain. However, SSRIs are very useful when symptoms of depressive or anxiety disorders are present and cannot be addressed adequately by nonpharmacologic means such as psychotherapy. Although many SSRIs are used in practice with children, only fluoxetine has been approved by the FDA for use in children and adolescents. SSRIs have a significantly milder side effect profile than TCAs (most side effects are transient), and they cause no anticholinergic side effects. Chief side effects include gastrointestinal symptoms, headaches, agitation, insomnia, sexual dysfunction, and anxiety. Rarely, hyponatremia, or the syndrome of inappropriate antidiuretic hormone, may occur. Interactions with other medications with serotonergic effects (tramadol, trazodone, tryptophan, and triptan migraine medication) may also occur. When these medications are used in combination, there is increased likelihood that a life-threatening serotonergic syndrome may occur, with associated symptoms of myoclonus, hyperreflexia, autonomic instability, muscle rigidity, and delirium. There is also a discontinuation syndrome associated with shorter acting SSRIs (paroxetine), which includes dizziness, lethargy, paresthesias, irritability, and vivid dreams. These medications should be tapered slowly over several weeks.

On the other hand, the SSNRIs duloxetine and the non-specific neurotransmitter-potentiating drug venlafaxine have demonstrated significant efficacy with chronic neuropathic and other pain syndromes because they inhibit both serotonin and norepinephrine reuptake or enhance its release. They may directly block associated pain receptors as well. Venlaxafine has no pain indication labeling, but duloxetine is FDA approved for managing neuropathic pain (diabetic neuropathy in adults) and fibromyalgia syndrome.

Because both SSRIs and SSNRIs have fewer anticholinergic side effects than TCAs, adherence to them is better than in psychiatric populations taking TCAs. Side effects of both medications include gastrointestinal symptoms, hyperhidrosis, dizziness, and agitation, but these effects generally wane over time. Hypertension and orthostatic hypotension may occur; in addition, the patient's blood pressure should be closely followed and appropriate hydration should be stressed. Note that whereas appetite stimulation and weight gain are associated with all TCAs, duloxetine is often associated with weight loss, frequently a desirable side effect, especially in weight-conscious adolescent females.

Antiepileptic Drugs

Traditional anticonvulsants, such as carbamazepine and valproic acid, are believed to relieve chronic pain by blocking calcium channels at the cellular neuronal level, thereby suppressing spontaneous electrical activity and restoring the normal threshold to depolarization of hypersensitive nociceptive neurons, without affecting normal nerve conduction. These medications are particularly useful in patients with labile mood disorders and neuropathic pain. In adults, the FDA has approved carbamazepine for trigeminal neuralgia and valproic acid for migraine prophylaxis, which are their only pain labeling. Anticonvulsant medications generally have gastrointestinal side effects in addition to sedation, anemia, ataxia, rash, and hepatotoxicity. In addition, carbamazepine and oxcarbazepine are associated with an increased incidence of potentially fatal Stevens-Johnson syndrome. Baseline liver function tests (LFTs) and complete blood cell (CBC) counts should be obtained and monitored with both these agents. These medications have narrow therapeutic windows and may have extreme variability in therapeutic blood medication levels as well as multiple drug-drug interactions. They may produce liver disease and renal impairment. These concerns are particularly cogent in the cancer population; therefore, less toxic drugs should always be tried first. Drug levels should be obtained with each dose increase and periodically thereafter. Carbamazepine, in particular, autoinduces hepatic microsomal enzymes, which can further complicate obtaining a therapeutic medication level. Frequent pregnancy tests are useful with menstruating female adolescents taking valproic acid, because severe neural tube defects are associated with this medication.

In the last decade, newer, far less toxic AEDs have arrived, almost entirely supplanting the use of valproate an carbamazepine in the pain population. While these newer agents have their own, and sometimes troubling, side effect profiles, they are far less toxic than their predecessors. They do not require monitoring of liver function, bone marrow function, or therapeutic blood levels. They are also far less lethal in accidental or deliberate overdose.

The first of these new AEDs is gabapentin, the most widely prescribed AED for the management of pain disorders, with demonstrated efficacy in treating children with chronic pain, particularly neuropathic pain. Studies using gabapentin to treat chronic headaches, reflex sympathetic dystrophy, and chronic regional pain syndrome have shown great promise. The mechanism of action of this medication is unclear. It is theorized that it increases gabaminergic transmission and decreases glutaminergic transmission while binding to the voltage-dependent calcium channels, producing antineuralgic effects, and inhibiting spontaneous and inappropriate discharge of nociceptive fibers. Gabapentin has a relatively benign side effect profile and few drug interactions. Side effects include somnolence, dizziness, and ataxia. Interestingly, children demonstrate side effects not reported in adults—severe impulsive or oppositional behavior, agitation, and occasionally depression. These side effects do not seem to be a dose related.

A second newer AED is pregabalin, which works by similar mechanisms to gabapentin but appears to have a better side effect profile. Because it undergoes virtually no hepatic metabolism, it has no significant drug interactions, a concern in patients with chronic pain who frequently take multiple medications, which are for both pain and the underlying medical or surgical condition causing the pain. Because it is eliminated by the kidneys, dosing adjustment must be made for patients with renal impairment.

A third newer AED is topiramate, which has demonstrated greater success than traditional anticonvulsants in treating trigeminal neuralgia in adults and in preventing migraines. Its increased efficacy is likely related to its multiple mechanisms of action. However, topiramate very frequently results in cognitive dysfunction and short-term memory loss, particularly problematic with school-aged children. Pediatricians who dose this medication should consider its effects on school performance. The pediatrician should also be aware that in female adolescents topiramate is associated with anorexia and weight loss—frequently a desirable side effect except in the cancer patient—whereas other anticonvulsants are typically associated with appetite stimulation and weight gain.

Benzodiazepines

Children and adolescents with chronic pain have significantly more psychiatric disorders than healthy children: depressive, sleep, and anxiety disorders, including generalized anxiety disorder, separation anxiety, posttraumatic stress disorder, and panic attacks. Pervasive developmental disorders are also common among this population. The increase in comorbid psychiatric disorders may be explained by the disruption of the serotonergic and noradrenergic systems that are the common pathways in both pain disorders and psychiatric disorders. Even without diagnosable psychiatric comorbidity, psychologic factors can negatively affect a youth's ability to cope with a pain disorder—a conditioned response to pain may be to feel out of control, leading to increased anxiety, and increased pain. Conversely, the feeling of helplessness can prime the pain, leading children to perseverate on the pain, think catastrophically, and feel hopeless, resulting in increased pain experience and development of a depressive disorder.

Benzodiazepines are anxiolytic medications that also have muscle-relaxant effects. They are particularly appropriate in acute pain as valuable adjuncts to the management of pain in the hospital setting, both because they inhibit painful muscle spasms in surgical patients and, more important, because they suppress the anxiety that virtually every hospitalized child experiences—anxiety that interferes with restorative sleep and amplifies the child's perception of pain. Studies have demonstrated that benzodiazepines are useful to calm children with anxiety and anticipatory anxiety about planned, painful procedures.

Because dependence, tolerance, and withdrawal may occur with prolonged use, benzodiazepines are generally not recommended for the routine management of chronic pain. However, in concert with psychotherapy, they help control anxiety disorders that amplify the symptoms of perception of pain. Infrequently, benzodiazepines may cause behavioral disinhibition and psychosis-like behaviors or, in large doses, respiratory depression, but fortunately these effects are uncommon. When dosing these medications, pediatricians should consider that many benzodiazepines are metabolized by the P450 microsomal enzyme system before conjugation, decreasing their duration of action. This effect may be less significant in benzodiazepines such as lorazepam and oxazepam, which undergo first-pass hepatic conjugation. Side effects common to benzodiazepines include sedation, ataxia, anemia, increased bronchial secretions, and depressed mood. If administered for several and consecutive days, benzodiazepines should be slowly tapered over 2 or more weeks; if abruptly discontinued, symptoms may include autonomic instability, delirium, seizures, and profound insomnia.

Antipsychotics and Major Sedatives

Low doses of antipsychotic medications are often used to address more severe anxiety and agitation sometimes associated with pain in youth. The use of these medications is controversial because the associated adverse events may be severe. Typical antipsychotics, including thioridazine (Mellaril), haloperidol, and chlorpromazine, are associated with a decrease in seizure threshold, agranulocytosis, weight gain, cardiac conduction disturbances, tardive dyskinesia, orthostatic hypotension, hepatic dysfunction, and life-threatening laryngeal dystonia. These side effects are generally less severe with newer atypical antipsychotics. However, because they may still occur, the pediatrician should obtain baseline ECG, LFTs, and CBC counts and act accordingly. If the pediatrician is using typical antipsychotics, an inventory of movement disturbances, such as the Abnormal Voluntary Movement Scale (AIMS) test, should be performed at baseline and at every follow-up visit, because movement disorders can worsen with abrupt withdrawal of medications or become irreversible.

Atypical antipsychotics are generally associated with less severe side effect profiles, particularly with regard to dyskinesias and dystonias. Use of olanzapine, which is particularly helpful with insomnia, requires assessing and monitoring levels of blood glucose, cholesterol, and triglycerides, and its side effects may include diabetes, hypercholesterolemia, or significant weight gain. The anticholinergic side effects associated with quetiapine warrant frequent monitoring of blood pressure. Risperidone at doses of more than 6 mg may cause side effects similar to those of typical antipsychotics. Clozapine, which causes increased incidence of life-threatening agranulocytosis, should generally be avoided as a treatment of children and adolescents with chronic pain. All antipsychotics are associated with the rare but potentially lethal neuroleptic malignant syndrome, which includes severe autonomic instability, muscular rigidity, hyperthermia, catatonia, and altered mental status.

The utility of unconventional analgesic medications in the treatment of children with chronic pain is apparent. These medications, when used judiciously, have proven successful, even when common psychiatric comorbidities, such as depression and anxiety, are not apparent. Gabapentin, pregabalin, topiramate, and duloxetine are among the most promising of these medications, because of their efficacy, mild, side effect profiles, and limited medication interactions; however, further testing in children should be pursued. Low-dose quetiapine also appears similarly useful for children with symptoms of agitation or severe anxiety. Most important when working with these medications is the team approach. A relationship with a consulting child and adolescent psychiatrist is extremely useful, in light of the complexities of working with antipsychotic medications. A psychiatrist or a team psychologist should also be consulted to define common psychiatric comorbidities or isolated symptoms, such as feelings of helplessness and hopelessness, which may complicate the medical picture and decrease the patient's level of functioning.

Pharmacologic Treatment of Nausea and Vomiting

Drugs used in the prevention of nausea and vomiting include both true antiemetics and ancillary agents. The latter are not always true antiemetics but are used to potentiate the effects of true antiemetics, to treat anxiety, or to induce sleep. True antiemetics can be classified on the basis of their therapeutic index, which accounts for both efficacy and side effects. Side effects include not only such obvious problems as extrapyramidal symptoms and hallucinations but also more subtle symptoms such as dysphoria or soporific effects. Because the vast majority of the antiemetic literature, including most randomized, controlled antiemetic studies, have included only adult patients, we are forced to extrapolate from the adult literature approaches to antiemetic management in children. These studies do not account for potential differences between adults and children with regard to antiemetic half-life or side effects or in terms of the emetogenic potential of various drugs.

In pediatric patients, route of administration and available dose forms can greatly affect the efficacy of an agent. Developmental or psychological reasons may prevent administration of oral tablets or capsules in some children. For other children, the only available oral or transdermal dose forms may be inappropriately high. Thus, clinical practice guidelines developed in the adult setting may not be fully applicable to children.

5-HT3 Receptor Antagonists

The 5-HT3 receptor antagonists are potent antiemetics with a wide therapeutic margin. Their development in the 1980s and widespread use in the 1990s have revolutionized the prevention of nausea and vomiting in cancer patients. Prior to the availability of these agents, the efficacy of the most widely used antiemetics, metoclopramide and the phenothiazines, was severely limited because of their extrapyramidal side effects. Initial research on different 5-HT3 receptor antagonists focused on each individual agent to determine appropriate dosing, efficacy as compared with metoclopramide and phenothiazines, and optimal use of concomitant agents. More recent research has shown a threshold effect but no dose response, relative equivalence of oral and parenteral routes, and remarkable therapeutic and toxic equivalence between the different 5-HT3 receptor antagonists. Their role in the control of delayed symptoms is unclear at best.

On the basis of the published literature, finding an efficacy or toxicity rationale to support the use of one 5-HT3 receptor antagonist as opposed to another is difficult. In general, all the 5-HT3 receptor antagonists share a number of characteristics, including a wide therapeutic margin, a threshold effect with little or no dose response, minimal toxicity, and high cost. Although the pediatric literature is very limited, major differences from the adult literature have not been identified. Some studies have demonstrated decreased efficacy for tropisetron or dolasetron as compared with ondansetron and granisetron, but final conclusions about differences cannot be determined. One randomized, double-blind pediatric study found no differences between ondansetron and granisetron in the bone marrow transplant setting.[139]

Ondansetron was the first 5-HT3 receptor antagonist commercially available in the United States. For the control of acute symptoms in adults, ondansetron is highly effective[140] and superior to metoclopramide. Its efficacy is enhanced by the addition of dexamethasone. The majority of the early studies in adults used a three-dose intravenous regimen of 0.15 mg/kg per dose or 8 mg per dose, with or without subsequent oral maintenance. Subsequent adult studies have shown that single-dose regimens of 16 to 32 mg are at least as effective as divided-dose regimens and benefit from the addition of dexamethasone. Oral regimens offer good bioavailability. They have been shown to be effective for moderately and highly emetogenic chemotherapy but have not been studied as extensively as intravenous therapy. Toxicity in most studies has been minimal and consists primarily of headache (10% to 15%), transient elevation of hepatic transaminases (6% to 8%), and constipation (5%).

Nonrandomized pediatric studies have shown ondansetron to be effective in children receiving a variety of chemotherapeutic agents and radiation. Randomized pediatric studies with ondansetron have shown better efficacy compared to metoclopramide, that doses greater than 5 mg/m² do not add to efficacy, and that the addition of dexamethasone improves efficacy. Some pediatric studies show a lower incidence of headache Although pharmacokinetic studies in adults have shown trends toward correlations between antiemetic efficacy and the area under the blood concentration-time curve, the clinical effect of the shorter half-life of ondansetron in children as compared with adults is unknown.

Few data regarding ondansetron dosing in children are available. Most published studies have used divided-dose regimens with three daily doses of 0.15 mg/kg per dose or 5 mg/m² per dose. Oral ondansetron twice daily has been given after the initial intravenous administration of drug in many studies. A two-dose regimen of 0.15 mg/kg has been effective in mildly and moderately emetogenic chemotherapy. When ondansetron first became available in the United States, our clinical practice was to administer 0.15 mg/kg per dose before and 8 and 16 hours after chemotherapy.

Granisetron, the next 5-HT3 receptor antagonist to become commercially available in the United States, is usually administered as a single intravenous or oral dose prior to the administration of emetogenic chemotherapy. Conflicting data appeared in earlier studies regarding the optimal dose, schedule, and route of administration. Current adult consensus guidelines and recent studies use a dose of 2 mg by mouth daily. For the control of acute symptoms, the combination of dexamethasone and granisetron is more effective than granisetron alone. Limited pediatric granisetron data are consistent with adult data in terms of efficacy.[139] The appropriate pediatric dosage of granisetron is unclear at present. Despite the manufacturer's recommended dose of 10 µg/kg, at least one study has shown lack of efficacy at that dose. Data regarding the relative efficacy of 20 and 40 µg/kg are conflicting. Data regarding the use of oral granisetron in children are not found in the literature.

Dolasetron, the 5-HT3 receptor antagonist most recently available in the United States, is usually administered as a single intravenous or oral dose of 100 or 1.8 mg/kg. Pediatric studies with small numbers of patients suggested the possibility of increased efficacy with a single dose of 1.8 mg/kg given either intravenously or orally.

Steroids

Although their mechanism of action is not understood, steroids have been used as antiemetic agents. Dexamethasone is the most extensively evaluated steroid, with doses ranging from 5 to 48 mg in single and multiple doses. Recent studies focus on doses of 10 to 20 mg per day, but administration of five daily doses totaling 120 mg per day have been reported. Dexamethasone and metoclopramide have been shown to have similar efficacy in adults receiving moderately and highly emetogenic chemotherapy. For adults receiving moderately emetogenic chemotherapy, ondansetron was somewhat more effective than dexamethasone. Although only moderately effective when used alone, dexamethasone is highly effective when used to potentiate the efficacy of other antiemetics. The addition of dexamethasone significantly improves emesis control in patients receiving metoclopramide and all the 5-HT3 receptor antagonists. Overall, dexamethasone appears to be a safe, effective adjunct to antiemetic regimens.

No clear dexamethasone dose guidelines are available for children. Starting dosage is typically 10 mg/m^2 to a maximum dose of 10 mg, given once daily. In the most symptomatic patients, the total daily dosage is doubled and divided into a twice-daily regimen, with a maximum of 10 mg given twice daily.

Phenothiazines

Prior to the availability of 5-HT3 receptor antagonists, phenothiazines and metoclopramide were the mainstay of therapy for children. At the usual therapeutic doses, many phenothiazines appear to depress CTZ activity and also may directly depress the vomiting center. Two distinct chemical classes of phenothiazines exist, each with its own therapeutic and toxic characteristics. The aliphatic class, of which chlorpromazine (Thorazine) is the prototype, has limited antiemetic activity and is associated with a high incidence of orthostatic hypotension, sedation, prolongation of the sedative effects of narcotics and barbiturates, and blood dyscrasias. The piperazine class, which includes prochlorperazine (Compazine), thiethylperazine (Torecan), and perphenazine (Trilafon), has pronounced antiemetic activity but is associated with an increased incidence of extrapyramidal effects. The major disadvantages of these agents—the development of extrapyramidal reactions or agitation—can be decreased by very slow (45 to 60 minutes) intravenous administration with coadministration of an antihistamine such as diphenhydramine (Benadryl). Although generally immediate, the extrapyramidal side effects can appear as much as 48 hours after drug administration. Thus, repeated dosing of diphenhydramine for an additional 24 hours is recommended for patients who receive prolonged courses of phenothiazines.

The doses and routes of administration vary among the phenothiazines. Thiethylperazine, available for intravenous, intramuscular, oral, and rectal administration, should be given in 10- mg doses every 6 to 8 hours for children 12 years or older and in 5-mg doses for younger children. Use of thiethylperazine is not recommended for children younger than

2 years. The recommended loading dose of perphenazine is 2 to 5 mg intravenously over 60 minutes, depending on the age of the child. The loading dose can be followed by either a continuous infusion of 0.25 to 0.5 mg/h or an oral dose of 2 to 4 mg every 4 hours. Prochlorperazine is considered to be the safest phenothiazine in children younger than 5 years but has only minimal antiemetic efficacy. The development and widespread use of the serotonin receptor antagonists led to the near abandonment of the phenothiazines.

Metoclopramide

Metoclopramide (Reglan), a procainamide derivative, has both central and peripheral antiemetic actions. It inhibits chemotherapy-induced vomiting and accelerates gastric emptying. Because of its short half-life, it must be administered frequently. The standard regimen in adults has been 2 mg/kg every 30 minutes before chemotherapy and again at 1.5, 3.5, 5.5, and (sometimes) 8.5 hours after chemotherapy. Anecdotal evidence suggest a that a dose of 1 mg/kg intravenously over 60 minutes repeated every 2 to 4 hours for a total of five doses is effective. Children are at higher risk for extrapyramidal symptoms than are adults and so prophylaxis with diphenhydramine is recommended. The incidence of akathisia and extrapyramidal reactions increases greatly at doses in excess of 1.5 mg/kg. Note that much lower doses of metoclopramide (e.g., 0.2 mg/kg every 6 hours) are effective for postoperative nausea or for acceleration of gastric emptying.

Miscellaneous Agents

Although not a true antiemetic, lorazepam has proved particularly useful in combination. Lorazepam is useful for its amnestic and anxiolytic effects. It produces anterograde amnesia and therefore is useful in allaying anticipatory nausea and vomiting by causing patients to forget their previous experiences with chemotherapy. Lorazepam should always be used in combination with a true antiemetic. The initial dosage of lorazepam is 0.025 mg/kg intravenously or orally, administered 30 minutes before chemotherapy and repeated every 6 hours, as needed. To avoid perception disturbances associated with higher doses, it is prudent to start with a lowest appropriate dose and avoid exceeding 1 mg.

Scopolamine (hyoscine) is a potent anticholinergic agent available in a transdermal patch for the treatment of motion sickness. It has been reported to be effective as a single agent in preventing emesis due to methotrexate and in combination to prevent cisplatin-induced emesis. Its major side effects are sedation and dry mouth. The transdermal patch should be applied the evening before or the morning of intended chemotherapy. Because of the fixed dosing, it cannot be used in small children.

Cannabinoids, which are the active ingredients of marijuana, have proven antiemetic properties. Delta-9-tetrahydrocannabinol (THC) has been shown to be more effective than both placebo and prochlorperazine in preventing vomiting in patients receiving antineoplastic drugs. Although the exact mechanism of action is unknown, recent work suggests that THC acts as a ligand for a newly described class of specific cannabinoid receptors, both in the peripheral nervous system and in the CNS. Many patients report relief of nausea while reporting no sedation. Interest in the cannabinoids has led to the development of synthetic analogues of THC, one of which is commercially available as dronabinol (Marinol). Although cannabinoids are not considered first-line therapy, they have been effective in children, in dosages ranging from 2.5 to 7.5 mg/m². Side effects range from drowsiness to dysphoria, the most common side effect being the development of a high.

Droperidol (Inapsine), a butyrophenone, is a potent inhibitor of the CTZ. In numerous studies using doses ranging from 0.5 to 2.5 mg as single or multiple doses or by continuous infusion, droperidol has been found to be somewhat effective. Reported toxicities include hypotension, tachycardia, somnolence, agitation, arrhythmias, and extrapyramidal effects. Experience with droperidol in young children is very limited. In older children, a loading dose of 2.5 mg intravenously over 60 minutes followed by a continuous infusion of 1 mg/h is recommended. As with other neuroleptics, coadministration of diphenhydramine is recommended to reduce the risk of extrapyramidal reactions. Recent reports of serious arrhythmias in adults at risk for prolongation of the Q-T interval have led to the recommendation to limit the use of droperidol and to monitor the electrocardiogram routinely during administration.

Many antihistamines have mild antiemetic properties, but no correlation can be drawn between antihistaminic potency and antiemetic activity. Dimenhydrinate (Dramamine), hydroxyzine (Atarax, Vistaril), and diphenhydramine are effective antiemetics for motion sickness and may be used in combination with other antiemetic therapy either to potentiate effectiveness or to decrease toxicity.

Treatment of Constipation

There are several alternatives that can be used to treat or prevent constipation including polyethylene glycol (Miralax, often preferable since it is a tasteless and odorless powder that can be mixed with any liquid), senna (Senakot, a stimulant laxative), docusate (Dulcolax, a lubricating laxative), milk of magnesia (magnesium hydroxide, an osmotic laxative), and mineral oil (a lubricant).

Recently, a μ-opioid antagonist, methylnaltrexone (Relistor), has been approved for use in the United States for the management of chronic opioid-induced constipation. Methylnaltrexone does not cross the blood-brain barrier and enter the CNS, and therefore does not reverse opioid analgesia; rather, its site of action is peripheral. Administration of a single dose of methylnaltrexone by subcutaneous injection usually results in evacuation of the colon within a few hours; the recommended dosing in adults is 12 mg by subcutaneous injection 2 or 3 times per week.[141] The drug has not been evaluated in children.

INTERVENTIONAL PROCEDURES FOR PAIN MANAGEMENT

In the last 25 years, the use of regional nerve blocks in children has increased because of several factors: (1) better knowledge of the pharmacology of local anesthetic agents in the child, (2) the availability of equipment adapted for children's anatomy, (3) recognition of the remarkable hemodynamic stability of young children following a neuraxial block, (4) the advent of ultrasonography, computed tomography (CT), and magnetic resonance imaging of nerves and block needles, and (5) the recognition of the need to treat pain aggressively not only in the operative period but also in other disease states such as cancer.[142] Interventional neuraxial and peripheral nerve blocks provide not only intraoperative anesthesia but also postoperative analgesia, the treatment of acute pain complicating malignancies or chemotherapy (e.g., pathologic long-bone fracture and the pain of acute pancreatitis), and the management of chronic cancer pain.

Performing these blocks usually requires special training and supervision. Described are individual blocks' actions, benefits, and risks; several regional anesthesia textbooks detail techniques and discuss pitfalls and complications for the reader who wishes further detail.[143,144] They are described in the following text so that cancer specialists may recognize their utility and propose their use for their patient to a consulting anesthesiologist or understand their use if initiated by an anesthesiologist providing surgical care to their patient.

Regional anesthesia provides several benefits: (1) it is an alternative to or augmentation of opioid-based pain control and is well recognized to be ovoid sparing, thereby minimizing opioid-induced side effects of nausea, vomiting, somnolence, respiratory depression, pruritus, and constipation; (2) it generally provides better quality pain relief because it interrupts nociceptive pathways and more profoundly inhibits the endocrine stress responses; (3) it results in earlier ambulation and functional restoration in recovering surgical patients; and (4) it helps prevent atelectasis in the setting of severe chest pain by permitting deep breathing and coughing.

Regional anesthesia is considered safe and effective, if performed by trained staff with the proper equipment. Most nerve blocks are performed by an anesthesiologist or pain management physician; a few may be easily performed by a nonanesthesiologist with appropriate training. Giaufre et al.[145] prospectively reviewed pediatric regional anesthesia and demonstrated both the utility and safety of regional anesthesia in children.

Head and Neck Blocks

Primary pain syndromes of the head, such as trigeminal neuralgia, are distinctly unusual in the pediatric population, and few malignancies or surgeries of the head and neck are amenable to regional anesthesia.

Upper Extremity Blocks

The brachial plexus block controls pain during surgical procedures or malignant lesions of the upper extremities. This block also protects the extremity from movement, reduces arterial spasm, and blocks sympathetic outflow to the upper extremity. The brachial plexus, responsible for cutaneous and motor innervation of the upper extremity, is an arrangement of nerve fibers originating from spinal nerves C5, C6, C7, C8, and T1 extending from the neck into the axilla, arm, and hand. The brachial plexus innervates the entire upper limb, except for the trapezius muscle and an area of skin near the axilla. If pain is located proximal to the elbow, the brachial plexus may be blocked above the clavicle (roots and trunks); if the pain is located distal to the elbow, the brachial may be blocked below it (cords). The block may be given as a single injection with a long-acting anesthetic (bupivacaine or ropivacaine) to provide up to 20 hours of analgesia or given via a catheter (to infuse local anesthetic) attached to a pump that can provide continuous analgesia over days or even weeks.[146]

Trunk and Abdominal Visceral Blocks

Trunk blocks provide somatic and visceral analgesia and anesthesia for pain or surgery of the thorax and abdominal areas. Sympathetic, motor, and sensory blockade may be obtained. These blocks are often used in combination to provide optimal relief. Intercostal and paravertebral blocks may be beneficial in those patients for whom an epidural injection or catheter is contraindicated, for example, in the presence of a coagulopathy. Respiratory function is usually well maintained, and the side effects of opioid therapy are reduced or eliminated.

The paravertebral, rectus sheath, and transverse abdominal plane blocks are the most useful trunk blocks for pediatric unilateral chest and abdominal wall pain. When pain is bilateral, an epidural block and catheter is more appropriate (see the following text).

The celiac plexus block is useful for visceral hepatic pain caused by cancer- or chemotherapy-induced pancreatitis. These blocks are best performed by an experienced anesthesiologist or pain physician.

The paravertebral block, an alternative to intercostal nerve block or epidural analgesia, is useful for pain associated with thoracotomy, breast surgery, or unilateral abdominal surgery such as nephrectomy or splenectomy. The thoracic paravertebral space, lateral to the vertebral column, contains the sympathetic chain, rami communicantes, and dorsal and ventral roots of the spinal nerves. Since it is a continuous space, local anesthetic injection will provide sensory, motor, and sympathetic blockade to several dermatomes. As for many blocks, the paravertebral block may be performed as a single injection or, for a very prolonged effect, as a continuous infusion over several days or weeks via a catheter inserted in the paravertebral space.

The celiac plexus block is indicated for surgery or pain of the pancreas and upper abdominal viscera. The celiac plexus receives sympathetic fibers from the greater, lesser, and least splanchnic nerves, as well as from parasympathetic fibers from the vagus nerve. Autonomic and nociceptive nerve fibers from the liver, gallbladder, pancreas, stomach, spleen, kidneys, intestines, and adrenal glands originate from the celiac plexus. This block requires CT guidance or fluoroscopy to provide direct visualization of the appropriate landmarks and to confirm correct needle placement. The close proximity of neighboring structures such as the aorta and the vena cava make this a technical procedure best performed by an anesthesiologist, an interventional pain physician, or a radiologist. There have been recent reports of newer radiographic techniques, including three-dimensional rotational angiography, to facilitate the correct placement of celiac plexus blocks in children.[147]

Lower Extremity Blocks

Lumbar plexus and sciatic nerve blocks provide pain control for painful malignancies or surgical procedures of the lower extremities, with the benefit of providing analgesia to only one extremity while preserving the motor and sensory functions of the opposite leg. In contrast to dense lumbar epidural blocks, the patient may still bear weight. The lumbar plexus arises from L2 to L4 and divides into three nerves, the lateral femoral cutaneous, femoral, and obturator nerves, that supply the muscles and sensation of the anterior and medial thigh, with a sensory branch of the femoral nerve extending below the knee to innervate the medial aspect of the foreleg, ankle and foot (the saphenous nerve). The sacral plexus arises from L4 to S3 and divides into the sciatic, tibial, and common peroneal nerves, which, in turn, provide sensation to the muscles of the pelvis, posterior thigh, and entire lower leg and foot except for medial sensation. The lumbar plexus can be blocked in the back, resulting in analgesia of the femoral, lateral femoral cutaneous, and obturator nerves. Or, any of these three nerves can be individually anesthetized more distally, depending on the location of the pain. Similarly, the sciatic nerve can be anesthetized proximally as it emerges from the

pelvis deep into the gluteus muscles, more distally in the posterior thigh, or along its major branches yet more distally.

Epidural Anesthesia (Thoracic, Lumbar, and Caudal)

Epidural anesthesia and analgesia are indicated for surgical pain below the clavicles, management of cancer pain unresponsive to systemic opioids, and pain limited by opioid side effects.

The three layers of the spinal meninges—the dura mater (outermost), the arachnoid mater (middle), and the pia mater (innermost)—envelop the spinal neural tissue. The subarachnoid space contains CSF between the arachnoid mater and the pia mater. The epidural space extends from the foramen magnum to the sacral hiatus. The epidural space, which contains fat, lymphatics, blood vessels, and the spinal nerves as they leave the spinal cord, separates the dura mater from the periosteum of the surrounding vertebral bodies.

Epidural local anesthetics block both sensory and sympathetic fibers, and, if the local anesthetic is of sufficient concentration, also motor fibers. Hypotension may occur because of the sympathetic nerve block, although unusual in children younger than 8 years. In addition to using local anesthetics, it is routine to use opioids and/or α-agonists in the epidural space. These agents have their primary site of action in the spinal cord, where they diffuse from their epidural depot. Side effects associated with epidural opioid administration include delayed respiratory depression, particularly when hydrophilic opioids such as morphine are used. This risk indicates that children receiving epidural opioids by intermittent injection or continuous infusion be monitored by continuous pulse oximetry and nursing observation, particularly during the first 24 hours of therapy or after significant dose escalations. Respiratory depression occurring after the first 24 hours of epidural opioid administration is distinctly unusual and is unheard of in opioid tolerant patients.

Epidural clonidine, an α$_2$-agonist with distinct analgesic properties, is associated with minimal risk and side effects. Although product labeling indicates its use only in children with severe cancer pain, it is commonly used for milder postsurgical pain. Mild sedation is the most common side effect of epidural clonidine, and it is not associated with respiratory depression beyond the newborn period.

Intrathecal Analgesia

Implanted intrathecal catheters infused with opioids, clonidine, the novel calcium-channel blocking analgesic ziconotide, and/or local anesthetics are highly effective and useful for pediatric patients with intractable pain from cancer that cannot be managed by conventional means. Typically, intrathecal catheters inserted are attached with an implanted electronic pump containing a drug reservoir sufficient for several weeks or months of dosing. Because the pump is bulky, roughly the size of a hockey puck, it is not suitable for smaller children or very thin older children; in these cases, the catheter may be attached to a subcutaneous port that may be accessed percutaneously and infused via an external pump. Once popular, chronically implanted epidural catheters have been all but replaced by the implanted intrathecal catheter because of the 10-fold reduction in drug dose and volume and because epidural catheters frequently become occluded by scar tissue over time. In children, the technique is generally reserved for terminally ill children, largely because the long-term effects of intrathecal drug infusion on the developing nervous system have not been defined. The technique is technical and best performed by an experienced pain management physician.

Nerve Ablation and Destruction

Infrequently, pediatric cancer pain may remain refractory in spite of maximal reliance upon oral and intravenous medications and nerve blockade. In these instances, temporary (ablation) or permanent (chemolytic or surgical) destruction of one or more nerves may be performed. These situations are rather extraordinary in children, and these techniques should be carefully weighed against the consideration of inducing permanent nerve injury with its attendant functional effects in a growing child with decades of life ahead. On the other hand, when pain is severe in life-limiting disease processes, then the long-term considerations are less concerning and these techniques should be discussed with a pain management specialist skilled in their performance.

PALLIATIVE CARE FOR PEDIATRIC CANCER PATIENTS

A chapter on pain management for children with cancer is not complete without highlighting the important topic of palliative care, given that 20% of children will not be cured of their disease. Chapter 49 treats this topic in greater detail.

The WHO's definition of palliative care is the active total care of patients whose disease is not responsive to curative treatment. Control of pain, of other symptoms, and of psychological, social, and spiritual problems is paramount. The goal of palliative care is achievement of the best possible QOL for patients and their families.[148] The other symptoms in addition to pain that can be experienced by children without the option of curative therapy include fatigue, dyspnea, poor appetite, nausea, vomiting, constipation and/or diarrhea.[149] Thus, symptom control for children facing end of life is imperative. When the multidisciplinary approach of palliative care is employed, families and patients report improved satisfaction with their care, improved informed decision making, and a decrease in the number of emergency room visits and inpatient admissions.[150]

The American Academy of Pediatrics has put forth a policy statement promoting the use of palliative care at the end of life for children with life-limiting disease. Their statement highlights that palliative care can improve the QOL for terminally ill patients and their families through the treatment of symptoms and by addressing the psychological, social, or spiritual aspects of facing a noncurable disease.[151] Despite this policy statement on the importance of the provision of palliative care services for children with life-threatening disease, there are barriers that currently exist and thereby impede its implementation across our healthcare system. First, there can be differences in parents' understanding of prognosis of their children's illness and their healthcare providers' knowledge, a discrepancy that, in turn, can affect parental informed decision making for end-of-life care, including pain management.[152] Second, for parents whose children have an incurable cancer diagnosis, they rate doctor-patient communication as the principal determinant of high-quality physician care. Conversely, physicians' care ratings depend on biomedical rather than doctor-patient relationship aspects of care.[153] It is, therefore, critical for physicians caring for dying children to listen to the concerns of these patients and their parents, particularly for those related to descriptions of pain. By listening to a patient's description of

pain and thereby classifying the etiology of the pain, one can determine the best therapeutic approach (as discussed above). By aggressively exercising symptom management, the pain and suffering at the end of life for a terminally ill pediatric cancer patient can be minimized.[154]

Pediatric palliative care requires frequent evaluation and reevaluation of symptoms. In addition to the assessment of pain, the provider needs to assess symptoms of fatigue, dyspnea, anxiety, nausea, and sleep patterns. There should also be determination of caretaker function and support since fatigue or anxiety in the primary caretaker can, in turn, affect the symptoms associated with pain manifested by the child. Treatment of other end-of-life symptoms, such as dyspnea, can require the use of morphine to decrease air hunger. If the child is heavily sedated and the family or caretaker has minimal awake time with the child, psychostimulants (e.g., methylphenidate, modafinil) can be used in the morning to counteract the sedative side effects of high-dose opioids needed for pain. In addition, nonpharmacologic therapies, such as music therapy or hypnotherapy, can be used concurrently with pain medications. The pediatric palliative care model as described above can be delivered both in the inpatient setting and in the home if pediatric hospice services are available. In either setting, the goal of maximizing QOL for the quantity of time that remains for a child without curative therapy should be emphasized. It should be noted that many clinicians now consider palliative care to begin with a serious diagnosis, such as cancer, even if the likelihood for cure is high, since some children even with low-risk cancers, such as ALL in young children, will die in spite of all expectations. Thus, a focus on maximizing QOL and reducing distressing symptoms should be as important a focus on the child with cancer as is the aim for cure.

COMPLEMENTARY AND ALTERNATIVE MEDICINE FOR PEDIATRIC CANCER PATIENTS

There are multiple nonpharmacologic therapies that can be employed for pain management in pediatric cancer patients (Table 42.4). These include massage, yoga, hypnotherapy, meditation, biofeedback, relaxation, spirituality, acupuncture, botanicals, physical therapy, and energy therapies, including the use of magnets, some of which will be described in detail in the following text.

The definition of CAM are those interventions that are not generally provided by U.S. hospital clinics, nor widely taught in medical school.[155] Thus, although these CAM techniques may not be familiar territory for physicians trained within the

TABLE 42.4

COMPLEMENTARY AND ALTERNATIVE MEDICINE THERAPIES TO BE CONSIDERED IN THE TREATMENT OF PEDIATRIC CANCER PAIN

Acupuncture
Hypnotherapy
Massage
Biofeedback
Botanicals
Magnets
Spirituality/religiosity
Therapeutic yoga

United States, there is an emerging body of literature discussing the state-of-the-science CAM use in both adult and pediatric populations.[156] In addition, the latest literature in medical education has documented a clear trend of higher usage rates of CAM by anesthesia training programs across the United States.[157] Thus, CAM interventions should be considered as adjuvant therapy for the treatment of pediatric cancer pain.

Acupuncture

Acupuncture consists of inserting fine needles into the skin's surface, or using heat, pressure, or other stimulation in areas that correspond to specific points along meridians (i.e., hypothesized energy channels within the body). These meridians, or channels, in which the body's life forces (spiritual, emotional, mental, and physical) are said to flow are thought by acupuncture practitioners to be out of balance and cause the physical sensation of pain, imbalance, and sickness. Insertion of the needles into specific points along meridians restores the balance of forces within the body and thereby eliminate the pain by achieving a flow of energy or Qi (pronounced chi) in this way of thinking. Although the practice of acupuncture is more widely accepted within Eastern societies, the use of acupuncture for the treatment of pain has been increasing across the United States.[158,159]

There is a growing body of literature evaluating its effectiveness for alleviating pain.[160,161] The available literature on the use and effectiveness of acupuncture in the treatment of pain in the pediatric population suggests it being an acceptable treatment modality for adolescents with certain types of chronic pain, as well as being an effective modality for other common symptoms experienced by the childhood cancer patient, including headache, nausea, and vomiting and opioid withdrawal symptoms.[162–164] Nonetheless, acupuncture has not been widely disseminated into pain treatment regimens for the pediatric population. One reason is the preexisting beliefs by healthcare practitioners in the United States that children are afraid of needles and thus they do not make referrals for acupuncture.[156,165] On the contrary, it has been shown that for those children who have been referred to acupuncture for various chronic pain syndromes, more than two-thirds report that it was a positive experience and was an effective modality for treatment of their pain.[157] Acupuncture, therefore, can be considered as a possible adjuvant treatment modality for neuropathic pain and symptom management in pediatric cancer patients.

Hypnotherapy

Hypnosis is a cognitive strategy that helps children achieve a narrowed focus of attention, relax, and learn how to dissociate from the current sensory environment. Liossi and others[49,166,167] in randomized controlled studies of children with cancer undergoing medical procedures have shown hypnotherapy to be effective in reducing procedure-related pain and anxiety. In addition, a recent review article by Wood and Bioy[168] provides a succinct review on the effectiveness of this technique, an understanding of the physiologic effect of hypnosis and the practical application of its use to treat pain in children. For example, Rainville and colleagues[169] have demonstrated increased blood flow to the occipital cortical areas through the use of positive emission tomographic changes in regional cerebral blood flow when hypnosis is used. This increase in blood flow to the occipital region is though to result in a reduction of inhibitory processes that occur normally during high levels of attention.[78] Thus,

hypnosis results in an acceptance of specific altered sensations, thereby mediating changes in perception of the painful experience.

Several studies on the effect of hypnosis for symptom management in children, including the effect on pain perception, anxiety, and nausea/vomiting have been completed. Early studies have demonstrated the feasibility of being able to hypnotize children.[170] Subsequent studies by Zeltzer et al.[171] have demonstrated the effectiveness of hypnosis in decreasing other symptoms, including nausea, experienced by pediatric cancer patients. More recent studies have demonstrated the effectiveness of hypnosis in decreasing pain and anxiety in children undergoing the invasive painful procedures of lumbar punctures and bone marrow biopsies.[172] Thus, there continues to be increasing evidence of both the feasibility of administration and the effectiveness of hypnosis in the pediatric population and should be considered when a pediatric cancer patient is undergoing invasive, painful procedures. As the review paper by Wood and Bioy[168] discusses, practical considerations of using hypnosis include the child's age (as younger children are more responsive to the hypnosis than adolescents), the cognitive development and therapeutic relationship with his or her provider.

Massage

Massage is the practice of light body stroking or deep tissues stroking that is thought to work by increasing serotonin levels and reducing cortisol levels. The basic principle of massage is that when muscles are overworked, there is a release of chemical waste products that accumulate in the area that can be relieved using the hands of the therapist to manipulate muscles and surrounding tissues. Massage therapy has been used as an adjuvant therapy in pain management, with a number of studies demonstrating its effectiveness. For example, it has been shown that when massage therapy was used in addition to a standard pharmacologic regimen for postoperative pain management, the experimental group demonstrated decreased pain intensity, pain unpleasantness, and anxiety when compared with the control group.[173] Massage therapy is also a CAM modality that can be easily instituted at the bedside of cancer patients.[174] There are few studies to date completed in the pediatric population on the use and effectiveness of massage therapy. Nonetheless, the studies that have been completed demonstrate decreased pain in the group receiving a standardized massage protocol.[175] In a study of children with ALL, a daily massage over a 1-month period was found to have an effect on the immune system as demonstrated by an increase in white blood cell count, as well as an improvement in children's negative affect.[176] Given the promising application of massage therapy to decrease pain in children, future research is warranted to evaluate the effectiveness of the healing powers of touch (i.e., massage) in a randomized controlled trial for pediatric cancer patients.

Biofeedback

Biofeedback involves measuring physiologic parameters, including blood pressure, heart rate, skin temperature, sweating, and muscle tension, and conveying these changes that occur while the child is learning breathing and imagery strategies to alter these bodily processes. This bodily feedback information can be provided through the use of computer-generated, audio-generated, or other form of visual-generated systems, with skin temperature or muscle contraction being the most commonly measured parameter. The basic concept of biofeedback is that by providing physiological information to a patient who is usually unaware of these bodily processes, while also teaching the child cognitive and breathing strategies that alter these processes, the child can learn to reduce muscle tension and autonomic arousal, thereby reducing pain. For children, it provides proof that the mind can affect the body by being able to gain physiologic control of the part of the nervous system that is activated by pain or stress.

Studies on the use of biofeedback have primarily been focused on adult patients, particularly for those with headaches. Meta-analysis of this mind-body approach for the treatment of headache pain indicates that it is effective when used alone or in combination with other CAM modalities.[138] Studies completed in pediatric patients again are limited in number, but those that have been completed also have focused on the treatment of pediatric migraine headache. Similar to the adult literature, meta-analysis on the use of biofeedback as well as other behavioral methodologies to treat headache in children demonstrate that it can be considered as an important adjunct to the pain treatment regimen.[177] Given that there are minimal side effects and there are data suggesting its effectiveness, biofeedback can also be considered as another adjunctive therapy to pain management in pediatric cancer patients. There is no license to practice biofeedback, although the majority of practitioners have other medical licensures, such as registered nursing, physical therapy, or marriage and family therapy. Hospitals and clinics with pediatric pain programs can often provide referral lists of biofeedback therapists.

Botanicals

The use of herbal or alternative medicines requires at least brief mention in the treatment of cancer pain, given the increasing frequency of use within the U.S. population with or without data suggesting its effectiveness.[178] The studies that have evaluated the use of herbal medicine in pediatric patients have been for the treatment of otalgia and have been completed outside the United States.[179] One such study evaluating the use of the naturopathic ear drop, Otikon, concluded that it was as effective as anesthetic ear drops for acute otitis media associated with ear pain.[180] Thus, given the paucity of studies documenting effectiveness of botanicals, this CAM option cannot be recommended in the treatment of pediatric cancer pain. The lesson that must be taken away, however, is that it is important for practitioners to ask whether botanicals (including megavitamins and herbs) are being used by parents to help treat their children's pain because there may be drug interactions that may interfere with the cancer treatment regimen.

Remembering the significant placebo response rate in analgesic trials, that is as high as 40% to 50%, there may be a placebo effect for patients who use various forms of CAM, including magnet therapy, botanicals, and herbal remedies.[181]

Spirituality/Religiosity

Spirituality (i.e., religiosity) is an important domain that must be considered when conceptualizing the model of palliative care for children with pain.[182] It must be discussed as another CAM modality since it is commonly used by cancer patients to cope with their diagnosis, aggressive treatment plans, and the associated painful experiences. Spirituality has been shown to be an important coping mechanism for adult cancer patients. For example, it has been shown that breast cancer patients who rate their spirituality as high have lower rates of depression, although no effect on pain ratings.[139] Similarly, when mothers of childhood cancer patients were asked to rate their religiosity concomitantly with the measurement of depression using the Beck Depression Inventory—II, it was shown that those mothers who reported lower levels of religious beliefs and behaviors had higher rates of depressive symptoms.[183] It has therefore been recommended that healthcare providers consider—when they have patients practicing prayer or prayer-like behaviors—to include a discussion on the benefit of this behavior on improving health through the mind-body connection that was discussed earlier in this chapter.[184] In addition, given that most major medical centers caring for children with cancer have access to a chaplain/spiritual support, this service should be considered (where appropriate) for consultation when developing a pain management plan for pediatric cancer patients.

SUMMARY

Although pediatric cancer statistics are currently at an all time high with an overall survival rate of 80%, cancer-related morbidity including the risk for the development of significant acute and chronic pain persists.[185] Thus, a comprehensive approach to pain and symptom management in pediatric cancer patients, especially through empowerment of these children through a mind-body therapeutic approach to their pain management, is critical. There are several pharmacologic treatments that can be used to treat the various types of pediatric cancer pain including μ-opioid analgesics, NMDA antagonist agents, nonsteroidal anti-inflammatory medications, atypical opioid medications, TCAs, and anticonvulsants. Integration of CAM modalities as an adjuvant or alternative to pharmacologic interventions is also important since there can be limitations in the traditional pharmacologic approach to pain, particularly for chronic pain syndromes. Although not all CAM therapies have a long track record in the scientific literature regarding their effectiveness, it does not mean that these options should be excluded from pain management consideration but rather a discussion with families of the strengths and limitations of such approaches is warranted.

In summary, the foundation to the pain evaluation and treatment plans for children with cancer is a focus on the whole child. The importance of eliciting and listening to all details of the pain narrative of pediatric cancer patients is critical. Child self-report will be dependent on the developmental level of the child and child pain evaluation encompasses the parental role in the pain experience, a proxy reporter of the pain narrative. For both children and the parents, the pain assessment should occur early on, in a nonthreatening environment, where the strong triad relationship between the pediatric cancer patient, the parent, and the healthcare provider can be an effective one. In this family-centered care approach, the common goal of alleviating children's pain can be achieved through education, empowerment, and the provision of mind-body therapeutics.

References

1. Hudson MM, Mertens AC, Yasui Y, et al. Health status of adult long-term survivors of childhood cancer: a report from the Childhood Cancer Survivor Study. JAMA 2003;290:1583–1592.
2. Oeffinger KC, Mertens AC, Sklar CA, et al. Childhood Cancer Survivor Study. Chronic health conditions in adult survivors of childhood cancer. N Engl J Med 2006;355:1572–1582.
3. Reis LAG, Eisner MP, Kosary CL, et al. SEER cancer statistics review, 1973–1998. Bethesda, MD: National Cancer Institute, 2001.
4. Fields HL. Pain. New York, NY: McGraw-Hill, 1987:1–78.
5. Janig W, Levine JD, Michaelis M. Interactions of sympathetic and primary afferent neurons following nerve injury and tissue trauma. Progr Brain Res 1996;113:161–184.
6. Anand, KJ. Clinical importance of pain and stress in preterm neonates. Biol Neonate 1998;73:1–9.
7. von Baeyer CL, Spagrud LJ. Systematic review of observational (behavioral measures of pain for children and adolescents aged 3 to 18 years. Pain 2007;127:40–150.
8. McGrath PJ, Hohnson G, Goodman JT, et al. CHEOPS: a behavioral scale for rating post-operative pain in children. In: Fields HL, Dubner R, Cervero F, eds. Advances in pain research and therapy. Vol 9. New York, NY: Raven Press, 1985:395–402.
9. Merkel SI, Voepel-Lewis T, Shayevitz JR, et al. The FLACC: A behavioral scale for scoring postoperative pain in young children. Pediatr Nurs 1997;23:293–297.
10. Van Hulle VC. Nurses' knowledge, attitudes, and practices regarding children's pain. MCN Am J Matern Child Nurs 2005;30:177–183.
11. Vetter T, Heiner E. Disconcordance between patient self-reported visual analog scale pain scores and observed pain-related behavior in older children after surgery. J Clin Anesth 1996;8:371–375.
12. LeBaron S, Zeltzer L. Assessment of acute pain and anxiety in children and adolescents by self-reports, observer reports, and a behavior checklist. J Consult Clin Psychol 1984;52:729–738.
13. Breau LM, Burkitt C. Assessing pain in children with intellectual disabilities. Pain Res Manag 2009;14:116–120.
14. Voepel-Lewis T, Malviya S, Tait AR, et al. A comparison of the clinical utility of pain assessment tools for children with cognitive impairment. Anesth Analg 2008;106:72–78.
15. Cohen LL, Lemanek K, Blount RL, et al. Evidence-based assessment of pediatric pain. J Pediatr Psychol 2008;33:939–955; discussion 956–957.
16. Zeltzer L, Kellerman J, Ellenberg L, et al. Hypnosis for reduction of vomiting associated with chemotherapy and disease in adolescents with cancer. J Adolesc Health Care 1983;4:77–84.
17. Zeltzer LK, LeBaron S, Zeltzer PM. A prospective assessment of chemotherapy-related nausea and vomiting in children with cancer. Am J Pediatr Hematol Oncol 1984;6:5–16.
18. Lebaron S, Zeltzer L. Behavioral intervention for reducing chemotherapy-related nausea and vomiting in adolescents with cancer. J Adolesc Health Care 1984;5:178–182.
19. Zeltzer L, LeBaron S. Effects of the mechanics of administration on doxorubicin-induced side effects: a case report. Am J Pediatr Hematol Oncol 1984;6:212–215.
20. Tyc VL, Mulhern RK, Fairclough D, et al. Chemotherapy induced nausea and emesis in pediatric cancer patients: external validity of child and parent emesis ratings. J Dev Behav Pediatr 1993;14:236–241.
21. Zeltzer LK, LeBaron S, Richie DM, et al. Can children understand and use a rating scale to quantify somatic symptoms: Assessment of nausea and vomiting as a model. J Consult Clin Psychol 1988;56:567–572.
22. Hinds PS, Hockenberry-Eaton M, Quargnenti A, et al. Fatigue in 7- to 12-year-old patients with cancer from the staff perspective: an exploratory study. Oncol Nurs Forum 1999;26:37–45.
23. Hinds PS, Hockenberry-Eaton M, Gilger E, et al. Comparing patient, parent, and staff descriptions of fatigue in pediatric oncology patients. Cancer Nurs 1999;22:277–288.
24. Hockenberry-Eaton M, Hinds PS, Alcoser P, et al. Fatigue in children and adolescents with cancer. J Pediatr Oncol Nurs 1998;15:172–182.
25. Collins JJ, Byrnes ME, Dunkel I, et al. The memorial symptom assessment scale (MSAS): validation study in children aged 10–18. J Pain Symptom Manage 2000;19:363–367.
26. Collins JJ, Devine TD, Dick GS, et al. The measurement of symptoms in young children with cancer: the validation of the Memorial Symptom Assessment Scale in children aged 7–12. J Pain Symptom Manage 2002;23:10–16.
27. Cella DF, Tulsky DS, Gray G, et al. The Functional Assessment of Cancer Therapy scale: development and validation of the general measure. J Clin Oncol 1993;11:570–579.
28. Aaronson NK, Ahmedzai S, Bergman B, et al. The European Organization for Research and Treatment of Cancer QLQ-C30: a quality-of-life instrument for use in international clinical trials in oncology. J Natl Cancer Inst 1993;85:365–376.
29. Schipper H, Clinch J, McMurray A, et al. Measuring the quality of life in cancer patients: the functional living index-cancer. Development and validation. Qual Life Res 1992;1:19–29.
30. Ganz PA, Schag CA, Lee JJ, et al. The CARES: a generic measure of health-related quality of life for patients with cancer. Qual Life Res 1992;1:19–29.
31. Lansky SB, List MA, Lansky LL, et al. The measurement of performance in childhood cancer patients. Cancer 1987;60:1651–1656.
32. Goodwin DAJ, Boggs SR, Graham-Pole J. Development and validation of the Pediatric Oncology Quality of Life Scale. Psychol Assess 1994;6:321–328.
33. Stuber Ml, Kazak AE, Meeske K, et al. Predictors of post-traumatic stress symptoms in childhood cancer survivors. Pediatrics 1997;100:958–964.
34. Jay SM, Elliot CH, Ozolins M, et al. Behavioral management of children's distress during painful procedures. Behav Res Ther 1985;23:513–520.
35. Chen E, Zeltzer LK, Craske MG, et al. Children's memories for painful cancer treatment procedures: implications for distress. Child Dev 2000;71:933–947.
36. Schecter NL, Bernstein BA, Beck A, et al. Individual differences in children's response to pain: role of temperament and parental characteristics. Pediatrics 1991;87:171–177.
37. Goldsmith HH, Buss AH, Plomin R, et al. Roundtable: what is temperament? Four approaches. Child Dev 1987;58:505–529.
38. Broom ME, Rehwaldt M, Fogg L. Relationships between cognitive behavioral techniques, temperament, observed distress, and pain reports in children and adolescents during lumbar puncture. J Pediatr Nurs 1998;13:48–54.
39. Helgadottir HL, Wilson ME. Temperament and pain in 3 to 7-year-old children undergoing tonsillectomy. J Pediatr Nurs 2004;19:204–213.
40. Chen E, Craske MG, Katz ER, et al. Pain-sensitive temperament: does it predict procedural distress and response to psychological treatment among children with cancer? J Pediatr Psychol 2000;25:269–278.
41. Stuber ML, Kazak AE, Meeske K, et al. Is posttraumatic stress a viable model for understanding responses to childhood cancer? Child Adolesc Psychiatr Clin N Am 1998;7:169–182.
42. Klein SM, Hauser GJ, Anderson BD, et al. Comparison of intermittent versus continuous infusion of propofol for elective procedures in children. Pediatr Crit Care Med 2003;4:78–82.
43. Ott MJ. Mindfulness meditation in pediatric clinical practice. Pediatr Nurs 2002;28:487–490.
44. Yuan-Chi L, Lee ACC, Kemper KJ, et al. Use of complimentary and alternative medicine in pediatric pain management service: a survey. Pain Med 2005;6:452–458.
45. Lambert SA. The effects of hypnosis/guided imagery on the postoperative course of children. J Dev Behav Pediatr 1996;17:307–310.
46. Liossi C, White P, Hatira P. A randomized clinical trial of a brief hypnosis intervention to control venipuncture-related pain of paediatric cancer patients. Pain 2009;142:255–263.
47. Power N, Liossi C, Franck L. Helping parents to help their child with procedural and everyday pain: practical, evidence-based advice. J Spec Pediatr Nurs 2007;12:203–209.
48. Liossi C, White P, Franck L, et al. Parental pain expectancy as a mediator between child expected and experienced procedure-related pain intensity during painful medical procedures. Clin J Pain 2007;23:392–399.
49. Liossi C, White P, Hatira P. Randomized clinical trial of local anesthetic versus a combination of local anesthetic with self-hypnosis in the management of pediatric procedure-related pain. Health Psychol 2006;25:307–315.
50. Liossi C, Hatira P. Clinical hypnosis in the alleviation of procedure-related pain in pediatric oncology patients. Int J Clin Exp Hypn 2003;51:4–28.
51. Liossi C, Hatira P. Clinical hypnosis versus cognitive behavioral training for pain management with pediatric cancer patients undergoing bone marrow aspirations. Int J Clin Exp Hypn 1999;47:104–116.
52. Chetta HD. The effect of music and desensitization on preoperative anxiety in children. J Music Ther 1981;18:74–87.
53. Avers L, Mathur A, Kamat D. Music therapy in pediatrics. Clin Pediatr 2007;46:575–579.
54. Cohen LL. Behavioral approaches to anxiety and pain management for pediatric venous access. Pediatrics 2008;122:S134–S139.
55. MacLaren JE, Cohen LL, Larkin KT, et al. Training nursing students in evidence- based techniques for cognitive-behavioral pediatric pain management. J Nurs Educ 2008;47:351–358.
56. Jemal A, Thomas A, Murray T, et al. Cancer statistics, 2002. CA Cancer J Clin 2002;52:23–47.
57. Reaman GH. Pediatric cancer research from past successes through collaboration to future transdisciplinary research. J Pediatr Oncol Nurs 2004;21:123–127.
58. Albritton K, Bleyer WA. The management of cancer in the older adolescent. Eur J Cancer 2003;39:2584–2599.
59. Guindon J, Walczak JS, Beaulieu P. Recent advances in the pharmacological management of pain. Drugs 2007;67:2121–2133.
60. Ozyurek H, Turker H, Akbalik M, et al. Pyridoxine and pyridostigmine treatment in vincristine-induced neuropathy. Pediatr Hematol Oncol 2007;24:447–452.
61. Finnerup NB, Otto M, Jensen TS, et al. An evidence-based algorithm for the treatment of neuropathic pain. MedGenMed 2007;9:36.
62. Collins JJ, Kerner J, Sentivany S, et al. Intravenous amitriptyline in pediatrics. J Pain Symptom Manage 1995;10:471–475.
63. Krane EJ, Leong MS, Golianu B, et al. Treatment of pediatric pain with nonconventional analgesics. In: Schechter NL, Berde CS, Yaster M, eds. Pain in infants, children, adolescents. 2nd ed. New York, NY: Lippincott Williams & Wilkins, 2002:225–240.
64. Saarto T, Wiffen PJ. Antidepressants for neuropathic pain. Cochrane Database Syst Rev. 2007 Oct 17;(4):CD005454.
65. Altier N, Dion D, Boulanger A, et al. Management of chronic neuropathic pain with methadone: a review of 13 cases. Clin J Pain 2005;21:364–369.
66. Silver J, Mayer RS. Barriers to pain management in the rehabilitation of the surgical oncology patient. J Surg Oncol 2007;95:427–435.
67. Richtsmeier AJ, Barkin RL, Alexander M. Benzodiazepines for acute pain in children. J Pain Symptom Manage 1992;7:492–495.
68. Tobias JD, Rasmussen GE. Pain management and sedation in the pediatric intensive care unit. Pediatr Clin North Am 1994;41:1269–1292.
69. Halbert J, Crotty M, Cameron ID. Evidence for the optimal management of acute and chronic phantom pain: a systematic review. Clin J Pain 2002;18:84–92.
70. Mishra S, Bhatnagar S, Singhal AK. High-dose morphine for intractable phantom limb pain. Clin J Pain 2007;23:99–101.
71. Krane EJ, Heller LB. The prevalence of phantom sensation and pain in pediatric amputees. J Pain Symptom Manage 1995;10:21–29.
72. Baron R, Maier C. Phantom limb pain: are cutaneous nociceptors and spinothalamic neurons involved in the signaling and maintenance of spontaneous and touch-evoked pain? A case report. Pain 1995;60:223–228.
73. Nikolajsen L, Finnerup NB, Kramp S, et al. A randomized study of the effects of gabapentin on postamputation pain. Anesthesiology 2006;105:1008–1015.
74. Robinson LR, Czerniecki JM, Ehde DM, et al. Trial of amitriptyline for relief of pain in amputees: results of a randomized controlled study. Arch Phys Med Rehabil 2004;85:1–6.
75. Douglas DB. Hypnosis: useful, neglected, available. Am J Hosp Palliat Care 1999;16:665–670.
76. Leskowitz ED. Phantom limb pain treated with therapeutic touch: a case report. Arch Phys Med Rehabil 2000;81:522–524.

77. Bradbrook D. Acupuncture treatment of phantom limb pain and phantom limb sensation in amputees. Acupunct Med 2004;22:93–97.
78. Rainville P, Hofbauer RK, Bushnell MC, et al. Hypnosis modulates activity in brain structures involved in the regulation of consciousness. J Cogn Neurosci 2002;1: 139–150.
79. Schechter NL, Berde CB, Yaster M. Pain in infants, children, and adolescents. 2nd ed. Philadelphia, PA: Lippincott Williams & Wilkins, 2003.
80. Motoyama EK, Davis P. Smith's anesthesia for infants and children. 7th ed. Philadelphia, PA: Mosby, 2006.
81. Golianu B, Krane EJ. Treatment of Pain in Children. In: Healy TEJ, Knight PR, eds. Wylie and Churchill-Davidson's a practice of anaesthesia. 7th ed. London: Arnold, 2003:1267–1290.
82. Silverman S Jr. Diagnosis and management of oral mucositis. J Support Oncol 2007; 5:13–21.
83. http://www.cdc.gov/nchs/ppt/icd9/att_mucositis_sep05.ppt. Accessed January 11, 2008.
84. Friedrichsdorf SJ, Finney D, Bergin M, et al. Breakthrough pain in children with cancer. J Pain Symptom Manage 2007;34:209–216.
85. Osoba D, Zee B, Pater J, et al. Determinants of postchemotherapy nausea and vomiting in patients with cancer. Quality of Life and Symptom Control Committees of the National Cancer Institute of Canada Clinical Trials Group. J Clin Oncol 1997;15: 116–123.
86. Orchard PJ, Rogosheske J, Burns L, et al. A prospective randomized trial of the anti-emetic efficacy of ondansetron and granisetron during bone marrow transplantation. Biol Blood Marrow Transplant 1999;5:386–393.
87. Barnes NM, Barry JM, Costall B. Antagonism by parachlorophenylalanine of cisplatin-induced emesis. Br J Pharmacol 1987;92(Suppl):469.
88. Cubeddu LX, Hoffman IS, Fuenmayor NT, et al. Antagonism of serotonin S3 receptors with ondansetron prevents nausea and emesis induced by cyclophosphamide-containing chemotherapy regimens. J Clin Oncol 1990;8:1721–1727.
89. Barnes JM, Barnes NM, Costall B, et al. Identification and distribution of 5-HT3 recognition sites within the human brainstem. Neurosci Lett 1990;111:80–86.
90. Barnes NM, Ge J, Jones WG, et al. Cisplatin induced emesis: preliminary results indicative of changes in plasma levels of 5-hydroxytryptamine. Br J Cancer 1990;62: 862–864.
91. Wang SC, Renzi AA, Chinn SL. Mechanisms of emesis following x-irradiation. Am J Physiol 1958;198:335–339.
92. Scarantino CW, Ornitz RD, Hoffman LG, et al. On the mechanism of radiation-induced emesis: the role of serotonin. Int J Radiat Oncol Biol Phys 1994;30:825–830.
93. Hunter AE, Prentice HG, Pothecary K, et al. Granisetron, a selective 5-HT3 receptor antagonist, for the prevention of radiation induced emesis during total body irradiation. Bone Marrow Transplant 1991;71:439–441.
94. Morrow GR, Hickok JT, Burish TG, et al. Frequency and clinical implications of delayed nausea and delayed emesis. Am J Clin Oncol 1996;19:199–203.
95. Tyc VL, Mulhern RK, Bieberich AA. Anticipatory nausea and vomiting in pediatric cancer patients: an analysis of conditioning and coping variables. J Dev Behav Pediatr 1997;118:27–33.
96. Morrow GR, Asbury R, Hammon S, et al. Comparing the effectiveness of behavioral treatment for chemotherapy-induced nausea and vomiting when administered by oncologists, oncology nurses, and clinical psychologists. Health Psychol 1992;11:250–256.
97. Dolgin MJ, Katz ER, McGinty K, et al. Anticipatory nausea and vomiting in pediatric cancer patients. Pediatrics 1985;75:547–552.
98. Morrow GR. The effect of a susceptibility to motion sickness on the side effects of cancer chemotherapy. Cancer 1985;55:2766–2770.
99. Osoba D, Zee B, Warr D, et al. Effect of postchemotherapy nausea and vomiting on health-related quality of life. The Quality of Life and Symptom Control Committees of the National Cancer Institute of Canada Clinical Trials Group. Support Care Cancer 1997;5:307–313.
100. Kris mg, Gralla RJ, Tyson LB, et al. Controlling delayed vomiting: double-blind, randomized trial comparing placebo, dexamethasone alone, and metoclopramide plus dexamethasone in patients receiving cisplatin. J Clin Oncol 1989;7:108–114.
101. Sorbe B, Hogberg T, Himmelmann A, et al. Efficacy and tolerability of tropisetron in comparison with a combination of tropisetron and dexamethasone in the control of nausea and vomiting induced by cisplatin-containing chemotherapy. Eur J Cancer 1994:5:629–634.
102. Hsyu PH, Pritchard JF, Bozigian HP, et al. Oral ondansetron pharmacokinetics: the effect of chemotherapy. J Clin Pharmacol 1994;34:767–773.
103. Ettinger DS, Eisenberg PD, Fitts D, et al. A double-blind comparison of the efficacy of two dose regimens of oral granisetron in preventing acute emesis in patients receiving moderately emetogenic chemotherapy. Cancer 1996;78:144–151.
104. Rubenstein EB, Gralla RJ, Hainsworth JD, et al. Randomized, double blind, dose-response trial across four oral doses of dolasetron for the prevention of acute emesis after moderately emetogenic chemotherapy. Oral Dolasetron Dose-Response Study Group. Cancer 1997;79:1216–1224.
105. Hesketh PJ, Kris MG, Grunberg SM, et al. Proposal for classifying the acute emetogenicity of cancer chemotherapy. J Clin Oncol 1997;15:103–109.
106. Collins JJ, Byrnes ME, Dunkel IJ, et al. The measurement of symptoms in children with cancer. J Pain Symptom Manage 2000;19:363–377.
107. Yee JD, Berde CB. Dextroamphetamine or methylphenidate as adjuvants to opioid analgesia for adolescents with cancer. J Pain Symptom Manage 1994;9:122–125.
108. Dimeo F, Rumberger BG, Keul J. Aerobic exercise as therapy for cancer fatigue. Med Sci Sports Exerc 1998;30:475–478.
109. Sykes NP. The relationship between opioid use and laxative use in terminally ill cancer patients. Palliat Med 1998;12:375–382.
110. Radbruch L, Sabatowski R, Loick G, et al. Constipation and the use of laxatives: a comparison between transdermal fentanyl and oral morphine. Palliat Med 2000; 14:111–119.
111. Greaves MW, Khalifa N. Itch: more than skin deep. Int Arch Allergy Immunol 2004; 135:166–172.
112. Ikoma A, Rukwied R, Stander S, et al. Neurophysiology of pruritus: interaction of itch and pain. Arch Dermatol 2003;139:1475–1478.
113. Stander S, Steinhoff M, Schmelz M, et al. Neurophysiology of pruritus: cutaneous elicitation of itch. Arch Dermatol 2003;139:1463–1470.
114. Antunes NL. Mental status changes in children with systemic cancer. Pediatr Neurol 2002;27:39–42.
115. DiMario FJ Jr, Packer RJ. Acute mental status changes in children with systemic cancer. Pediatrics 1990;85:353–360.
116. Porzio G, Aielli F, Narducci F, et al. Pruritus in a patient with advanced cancer successfully treated with continuous infusion of granisetron. Support Care Cancer 2004; 12:208–209.
117. Zylicz Z, Krajnik M, Sorge AA, et al. Paroxetine in the treatment of severe non- dermatological pruritus: a randomized, controlled trial. J Pain Symptom Manage 2003; 26:1105–1112.
118. Zernikow B, Smale H, Michel E, et al. Paediatric cancer pain management using the WHO analgesic ladder—results of a prospective analysis from 2265 treatment days during a quality improvement study. Eur J Pain 2006;10:587–595.
119. Angst MS, Clark JD. Opioid-induced hyperalgesia: a qualitative systematic review. Anesthesiology 2006;104:570–587.
120. Borner C, Warnick B, Smida M, et al. Mechanisms of opioid-mediated inhibition of human t cell receptor signaling. J Immunol 2009;183:882–889.
121. Anghelescu DL, Burgoyne LL, Oakes LL, et al. The safety of patient-controlled analgesia by proxy in pediatric oncology patients. Anesth Analg 2005;101:1623–1627.
122. Voepel-Lewis T, Marinkovic A, Kostrzewa A, et al. The prevalence of and risk factors for adverse events in children receiving patient-controlled analgesia by proxy or patient-controlled analgesia after surgery. Anesth Analg 2008;107:70–75.
123. Krane EJ. Patient-controlled analgesia: proxy-controlled analgesia? Anesth Analg 2008;107:15–17.
124. Coda BA, O'Sullivan B, Donaldson G, et al. Comparative efficacy of patient-controlled administration of morphine, hydromorphone, or sufentanil for the treatment of oral mucositis pain following bone marrow transplantation. Pain 1997;72:333–346.
125. Mystakidou K, Tsilika E, Tsiatas M, et al. Oral transmucosal fentanyl citrate in cancer pain management: a practical application of nanotechnology. Int J Nanomed 2007; 2:49–54.
126. Zernikow B, Michel E, Anderson B. Transdermal fentanyl in childhood and adolescence: a comprehensive literature review. J Pain 2007;8:187–207.
127. Noyes M, Irving H. The use of transdermal fentanyl in pediatric oncology palliative care. Am J Hosp Palliat Care 2001;18:411–416.
128. Payne KA, Roelofse JA. Tramadol drops in children: analgesic efficacy, lack of respiratory effects, and normal recovery times. Anesth Prog 1999;46:91–96.
129. Garrido MJ, Habre W, Rombout F, et al. Population pharmacokinetic/pharmacodynamic modelling of the analgesic effects of tramadol in pediatrics. Pharm Res 2006; 23:2014–2023.
130. Payne KA, Roelofse JA, Shipton EA. Pharmacokinetics of oral tramadol drops for post-operative pain relief in children aged 4 to 7 years—a pilot study. Anesth Prog 2002; 49:109–112.
131. Von Roenn JH, Cleeland CS, Gonin R, et al. Physician attitudes and practice in cancer pain management. A survey from the Eastern Cooperative Oncology Group. Ann Intern Med 1993;119:121–126.
132. Porter-Williamson K, Heffernan E, Von Gunten CF. Pseudoaddiction. J Palliat Med 2003;6:937–939.
133. Lusher J, Elander J, Bevan D, et al. Analgesic addiction and pseudoaddiction in painful chronic illness. Clin J Pain 2006;22:316–324.
134. Bell K, Salmon A. Pain, physical dependence and pseudoaddiction: redefining addiction for "nice" people? Int J Drug Policy 2009;20:170–178.
135. Finkel JC, Pestieau SR, Quezado Z. Ketamine as an adjuvant for treatment of cancer pain in children and adolescents. J Pain 2007:8:515–521.
136. Cruciani RA, Lussier D, Miller-Saultz D, et al. Ultra-low dose oral naltrexone decreases side effects and potentiates the effect of methadone. J Pain Symptom Manage 2003;25:491–494.
137. Largent-Milnes TM, Guo W, Wang HY, et al. Oxycodone plus ultra-low-dose naltrexone attenuates neuropathic pain and associated mu-opioid receptor-GS coupling. J Pain 2008;9:700–713.
138. Vitiello B, Silva SG, Rohde P, et al. Suicidal events in the Treatment for Adolescents with Depression Study (TADS). J Clin Psychiatry 2009;70:741–747.
139. Sierpina V, Astin J, Giordano J, et al. Mind-body therapies for headache. Am Fam Physician 2007;76:1518–1522.
140. Aukst-Margetić B, Jakovljević M, Margetić B, et al. Religiosity, depression and pain in patients with breast cancer. Gen Hosp Psychiatry 2005;27:250–255.
141. Yuan CS, Foss JF. Oral methylnaltrexone for opioid-induced constipation. JAMA 2000;284:1383–1384.
142. Collins JJ, Grier HE, Sethna NF, et al. Regional anesthesia for pain associated with terminal pediatric malignancy. Pain 1996;65:63–69.
143. Hadzic A. New York School of Regional Anesthesia. Textbook of regional anesthesia and acute pain management. New York, NY: McGraw-Hill, Medical Pub. Division, 2007.
144. Cousins MJ, Bridenbaugh PO. Cousins and Bridenbaugh's neural blockade in clinical anesthesia and pain medicine. 4th ed. Philadelphia, PA: Lippincott Williams & Wilkins, 2009.
145. Giaufre E, Dalens B, Gombert A. Epidemiology and morbidity of regional anesthesia in children: a one-year prospective survey of the French-language Society of Pediatric Anesthesiologists. Anesth Analg 1996;83:904–912.
146. Cooper MG, Keneally JP, Kinchington D. Continuous brachial plexus neural blockade in a child with intractable cancer pain. J Pain Symptom Manage 1994;9:277–281.
147. Goldschneider KR, Racadio JM, Weidner NJ. Celiac plexus blockade in children using a three-dimensional fluoroscopic reconstruction technique: case reports. Reg Anesth Pain Med 2007;32:510–515.
148. http://www.who.int/cancer/palliative/definition/en/. Accessed June 19, 2007.
149. Wolfe J, Grier HE, Klar N, et al. Symptoms and suffering at the end of life in children with cancer. N Engl J Med 2000;342:326–433.
150. Jennings PD. Providing pediatric palliative care through a pediatric supportive care team. Pediatr Nurs 2005;31:195–200.
151. American Academy of Pediatrics. Committee on Bioethics and Committee on Hospital Care. Palliative Care for Children. Pediatrics 2000;106:351–357.
152. Wolfe J, Klar N, Grier HE, et al. Understanding of prognosis among parents of children who died of cancer: impact on treatment goals and integration of palliative care. JAMA 2000;284:2469–2475.
153. Mack JW, Hilden JM, Watterson J, et al. Parent and physician perspectives on quality of care at the end of life in children with cancer. J Clin Oncol 2005;23:9155–9161.
154. Calabrese CL. ACT—for pediatric palliative care. Pediatr Nurs 2007;33:532–534.
155. Eisenberg DM, Kessler RC, Foster C, et al. Unconventional medicine in the United States: prevalence, costs, and patterns of use. N Engl J Med 1993;328:246–252.
156. Tsao JCI, and Zeltzer LK. Complementary and alternative medicine approaches for pediatric pain: a review of the state-of-the-science. eCAM. Evid Based Complement Altern Med 2005;2149–159.

157. Lin YC, Lee AC, Kemper KJ, et al. Use of complementary and alternative medicine in pediatric pain management service: a survey. Pain Med 2005;6:452–458.

158. Itoh K, Kitakoji H. Acupuncture for chronic pain in Japan: a review. Evid Based Complement Altern Med 2007;4:431–438.

159. Kundu A, Berman B. Acupuncture for pediatric pain and symptom management. Pediatr Clin N Am 2007;54:885–889.

160. Furlan AD, van Tulder M, Cherkin D, et al. Acupuncture and dry-needling for low back pain: an updated systematic review within the framework of the Cochrane Collaboration. Spine 2005;30:944–963.

161. Wang SM, Kain ZN, White PF. Acupuncture analgesia, part II: clinical considerations. Anesth Analg 2008;106:611–621.

162. Tsao JC, Meldrum M, Kim SC, et al. Treatment preferences for CAM in children with chronic pain. Evid Based Complement Altern Med 2007;4:367–374.

163. Gottschling S, Meyer S, Gribova I, et al. Laser acupuncture in children with headache: a double-blind, randomized, bicenter, placebo-controlled trial. Pain 2008;137:405–412.

164. Reindl TK, Geilen W, Hartmann R, et al. Acupuncture against chemotherapy-induced nausea and vomiting in pediatric oncology. Interim results of a multicenter crossover study. Support Care Cancer. 2006;14:172–176.

165. Kemper KJ, Sarah R, Silver-Highfield E, et al. On pins and needles? Pediatric pain patients' experience with acupuncture. Pediatrics 2000;105:941–994.

166. Liossi C, Hatira P. Clinical hypnosis versus cognitive behavioral training for pain management with pediatric cancer patients undergoing bone marrow aspirations. Int J Clin Exp Hypn 1999;47:104–116.

167. Liossi C, Hatira P. Clinical hypnosis in the alleviation of procedure-related pain in pediatric oncology patients. Int J Clin Exp Hypn 2003;51:4–28.

168. Wood C, Bioy A. Hypnosis and pain in children. J Pain Symptom Manage 2008;35:437–446.

169. Rainville P, Hofbauer RK, Paus T, et al. Cerebral mechanisms of hypnotic induction and suggestion. J Cogn Neurosci 1999;11:110–125.

170. LeBaron S, Zeltzer LK, Fanurik D. Imaginative involvement and hypnotizability in childhood. Int J Clin Exp Hypn 1988;36:284–295.

171. Zeltzer LK, Dolgin MJ, LeBaron S, et al. A randomized, controlled study of behavioral intervention for chemotherapy distress in children with cancer. Pediatrics 1991;88:34–42.

172. Butler LD, Symons BK, Henderson SL, et al. Hypnosis reduces distress and duration of an invasive medical procedure for children. Pediatrics 2005;115:e77–e85.

173. Mitchinson AR, Kim HM, Rosenberg JM, et al. Acute postoperative pain management using massage as an adjuvant therapy: a randomized trial. Arch Surg 2007;142:1158–1167.

174. Gatlin CG, Schulmeister L. When medication is not enough: nonpharmacologic management of pain. Clin J Oncol Nurs 2007;11:699–704.

175. Field T, Hernandez-Reif M, Seligman S, et al. Juvenile rheumatoid arthritis: benefits from massage therapy. J Pediatr Psychol 1997;22:607–617.

176. Field T, Cullen C, Diego M, et al. Leukemia immune changes following massage therapy. J Bodyw Mov Ther 2001;5:271–274.

177. Andrasik F. Behavioral treatment of migraine: current status and future directions. Expert Rev Neurother 2004;4:403–413.

178. Eisenberg DM, Davis RB, Ettner SL, et al. Trends in alternative medicine use in the United States, 1990–1997: results of a follow-up national survey. JAMA 1998;280:1569–1575.

179. Sarrell EM, Cohen HA, Kahan E. Naturopathic treatment for ear pain in children. Pediatrics 2003;111:e574–e579.

180. Sarrell EM, Mandelberg A, Cohen HA. Efficacy of naturopathic extracts in the management of ear pain associated with acute otitis media. Arch Pediatr Adolesc Med 2001;155:796–799.

181. Carter R, Hall T, Aspy CB, et al. The effectiveness of magnet therapy for treatment of wrist pain attributed to carpal tunnel syndrome. J Fam Pract 2002;51:38–40.

182. Donnelly JP, Huff SM, Lindsey ML, et al. The needs of children with life-limiting conditions: a healthcare-provider-based model. Am J Hosp Palliat Care 2005;22:259–267.

183. Elkin TD, Jensen SA, McNeil L, et al. Religiosity and coping in mothers of children diagnosed with cancer: an exploratory analysis. J Pediatr Oncol Nurs 2007;24:274–278.

184. Krebs K. The spiritual aspect of caring–an integral part of health and healing. Nurs Adm Q 2001;25:55–60.

185. Centers for Disease Control and Prevention. Trends in childhood cancer mortality–United States, 1990–2004. MMWR Morb Mortal Wkly Rep 2007;56:1257–1261.

CHAPTER 43 ■ NURSING SUPPORT OF THE CHILD WITH CANCER

MARILYN J. HOCKENBERRY AND NANCY E. KLINE

Pediatric oncology nurses are essential contributors to the successful diagnosis, treatment, and cure of children with cancer. As a member of the multidisciplinary care team, the nurse works with physicians, social workers, child life specialists, schoolteachers, psychologists, chaplains, and other specialists to provide comprehensive care for the child and family. Innovative technologies require that nurses caring for children with cancer become experts in critical care management as well as in the provision of psychological support to the child and family. The expert oncology nurse often functions as the coordinator of patient care, facilitating communication among team members.

Pediatric oncology nursing roles are diverse and allow for opportunities in direct patient care, education, management, and research (Table 43.1). Advanced practice nurses (nurse practitioners and clinical nurse specialists) have made significant contributions toward providing continuity of care for children with cancer. Children are followed by advanced practice nurses in various patient care settings including the hospital, outpatient setting, and home environment.

DIRECT PATIENT CARE NURSING ROLES

Nurses caring for the child with cancer in the hospital setting must keep pace with the complex advances in treatment as well as with advanced technology. The trend in pediatric oncology continues with more therapies being administered in clinic setting with inpatient settings used for the management of acute life-threatening complications and administration of chemotherapy regimens that cannot be given in the ambulatory setting. Nurses with highly specialized skills staff the pediatric oncology inpatient care settings.[1]

The nurse working with children in the tertiary care setting recognizes acute as well as long-term side effects caused by the disease and the treatment. Expert nursing care requires the ability to assess the child's condition on the basis of extensive knowledge of childhood cancer, to develop a plan of care in collaboration with other health care professionals, to provide direct nursing care for the child, and to evaluate the child's condition on the basis of specific nursing outcomes.[2] Nurses caring for children with cancer must competently manage symptoms of common side effects of treatment such as nausea and vomiting, pain, mucositis, fatigue, and anorexia. Pediatric oncology nurses are essential for providing education and support to families with a child newly diagnosed with cancer. Crisis intervention and the ability to provide emotional support are important aspects of the role. The nurse serves as a child advocate, ensuring proper preparation prior to invasive procedures and treatment. Because many patients receive frequent admissions for treatment, nurses develop long-term relationships providing continuity of care for these families.

The nurse working in the outpatient clinic setting is often the direct link between the community and the cancer treatment center. Pediatricians who follow cases of children with cancer in community settings may communicate directly with the nursing staff regarding specific side effects or laboratory findings. Outpatient clinic nurses frequently provide education regarding administration of chemotherapy in the pediatrician's office. Extensive knowledge of the side effects of treatment allows the nurse to provide families with an understanding of what may occur at home. Information regarding specific restrictions and changes in activities for the child is communicated with the family.

Children are now receiving in the outpatient clinic setting chemotherapy that could previously be administered only in a hospital. The use of moderate sedation before invasive procedures is a common practice in childhood cancer centers. Outpatient clinic nurses have extensive knowledge regarding assessment and management of children receiving complicated chemotherapy regimens and sedation. As a consequence of intensive chemotherapy regimens, blood product support is also frequently necessary and is administered in the outpatient setting by nurses who are knowledgeable regarding possible reactions and who expertly manage side effects related to blood product transfusion.

Families who have children with cancer return to the outpatient setting frequently for treatment and follow-up. The nurse becomes a major support to the child and family throughout treatment. Once therapy is completed, families continue to use the nurse as a major resource for their questions and concerns. A parent described the pediatric oncology nurse as a source of information, reassurance, and comfort. The nurse was quoted as being a "lifeline" for parents of a child with cancer that continues long after treatment is completed.[3]

ADVANCED PRACTICE ROLES

One of the most significant contributions of nursing has been the development of advanced practice roles. Advanced clinical practice in pediatric oncology nursing requires preparation at the master's degree level. Graduate programs are designed to prepare advanced practice nurses to think independently, to function autonomously, and to participate actively within an interdisciplinary team.[4] An extensive knowledge base in physiology, pharmacology, child health assessment, growth and development, health promotion, disease prevention, and management of common problems of childhood is essential. Once a foundation of knowledge regarding well-child care is established, graduate-nursing programs should provide opportunities for experiences in the care of the child with cancer. Didactic content in the pathophysiology, diagnosis, and management of the various types of childhood cancer is essential; yet, general pediatric graduate programs often do not include these

NURSING ROLES IN PEDIATRIC ONCOLOGY

Nursing role	Education	Registration	Certification
Nurses in tertiary care and outpatient clinic settings	Nursing Diploma Associate Degree in Nursing Baccalaureate Degree in Nursing	Registered Nurse (RN)	Certified Pediatric Oncology Hematology Nurse (CPHON)
Advanced practice nursing	Master's Degree	RN	CPHON, Pediatric Nurse Practitioner, or Clinical Nurse Specialist
Research	Master's Degree and/or PhD	RN	None specific to research role

topics in the curriculum.[4] Nurses seeking to specialize in pediatric oncology should pursue opportunities to care for children with cancer during graduate nursing study.

Many advanced practice nurses who join comprehensive childhood cancer centers have limited knowledge of the diagnosis, treatment, and management of cancer. Cancer centers must consider developing innovative educational opportunities that provide the knowledge necessary to pursue advanced practice roles. Short-term fellowship programs that allow for clinical participation under the supervision of experienced nurses may become an important investment as nurses' functions become more independent in the future.

Nurse Practitioners

Since the conception of the advanced practice role, nurse practitioners have demonstrated ability to provide appropriate, cost-effective care for a range of health services, including primary care, management of chronic illness, and treatment of episodic health problems. Positions for nurse practitioners have been created in critical care areas and bone marrow transplant units, as physicians and health care administrators have recognized the quality and cost-effectiveness of the role.

Nurse practitioners serve as the coordinators of care among hospital, clinic, and community settings. The nurse practitioner must understand the assessment and management of children with cancer. Proficient in performing physical assessments and diagnostic procedures such as bone marrow aspiration and lumbar punctures and in diagnosing common pediatric illnesses, the nurse practitioner role has evolved as a vital role in the pediatric oncology specialty.

Clinical Nurse Specialists

The clinical nurse specialist complements the role of the nurse practitioner by providing continuity between the clinic and the hospital. Whereas the nurse practitioner directly cares for a selected population of patients, the clinical nurse specialist often serves as a coordinator of care for all children who are hospitalized. Clinical nurse specialists use their expertise by helping other team members to coordinate care, usually during the patient's hospitalization. Communication between staff nurses and the clinical nurse specialist is key in providing information from the health care team managing the child's care. The clinical nurse specialist is instrumental in implementing organized teaching programs for parents and children. Both the clinical nurse specialist and the nurse practitioner serve as resources for other nurses.

Administrators

Nurses in administrative roles face the challenge of implementing cost-effective, high-quality care to increasingly ill patients who have complex health care needs. These nurses must have an extensive background in nursing as well as in business. Managed care is changing health care, and nurses in administration will be instrumental in coordinating care in accordance with specific health care plans in the future. Administrative nurses must support the specialization of oncology nursing while meeting the demands of changing health care systems. A major concern is to direct efforts toward recruitment and retention of professional, that is the skilled pediatric oncology nurses who will deliver high-quality care to these children and their families.

RESEARCH ROLES

Nurses with diverse educational backgrounds and experience are involved in research roles. Educational preparation influences the type of research role nurses pursue. Baccalaureate level nurses typically participate in research by evaluating its applicability for nursing practice. They assist in the identification of research problems and are involved in research implementation by serving as data collectors and by obtaining subjects for study.

Numerous cancer centers also use baccalaureate-prepared research nurses as coordinators of clinical trials. The research nurse ensures that the study is implemented according to protocol and that data collection is accurate. Phase I clinical trials are excellent examples of studies coordinated by research nurses; the research nurse implements labor-intensive regimens according to protocol and closely monitors side effects and toxicity data.

The National Institute of Nursing Research convened a working group to evaluate the state of the science of pediatric oncology nursing.[5] This conference reviewed the knowledge gained from biobehavioral and sociocultural research findings and identified gaps that are important for future research endeavors. Examples of important research areas for nursing include symptom assessment and management, quality of life, long-term survivors, and end of life care.

The pediatric oncology nurse with a master's degree has the expertise to identify practical problems for clinical relevance and to facilitate using evidence to improve nursing care. Pediatric oncology nurses have paved the way in demonstrating the importance of using evidence to improve the care they provide. Examples of the impact nurses have had on patient care include implementing symptom management interventions, promoting professional collaboration in care, establishing support groups for children and adolescents, understanding the impact of having a child with cancer on the parent, and developing strategies for educating children and families on the type of cancer and treatment.[6–13]

The nurse in advanced practice enhances the value of research among other nurses by participating in collaborative research endeavors. Doctoral prepared nurses are increasing in number and serve as nursing research directors at numerous institutions. They promote interest in research and are instrumental in implementing funded nursing research projects.

NURSING STANDARDS OF CARE

The image of pediatric oncology nursing is reflected in the standards of care practiced daily by nurses. The outcome standards of pediatric oncology nursing practice, established by the Association of Pediatric Oncology Nurses, reflect the comprehensive involvement of nursing in the care of children with cancer.[14] These standards assist in identifying the future focus of pediatric oncology nursing care and include providing expert clinical care though assessment, diagnosis, outcomes identification, planning, and implementation. The pediatric oncology nurse serves as a coordinator of patient care and an educator for health care teaching and health promotion. Patient and family education, psychosocial support, and growth and development assessment also are major aspects of the clinical nursing role.

PROVIDING EXPERT CLINICAL NURSING CARE

Expert nurses are able to assess the child's condition using extensive knowledge of childhood cancer, to develop a plan of care in collaboration with other health care professionals, to provide direct nursing care, and to evaluate the child's condition based on specific nursing outcomes.[2] Pediatric oncology nurses play a major role in managing disease-related and treatment-related side effects, coordinating care for central venous lines, administering chemotherapy, and preparing the child for invasive procedures. As more children are treated in the outpatient or home environment, nurses have become the coordinators of care in these settings.

Managing Side Effects

Children with cancer frequently experience side effects and often live with unrelieved symptoms. These distressing symptoms occur frequently owing to aggressive therapy regimens designed to cure the disease.[15–19] Multiple symptoms frequently occur as reported by 509 pediatric oncology nurses participating in a national survey evaluating nurses' management of patient symptoms.[20] The average number of symptoms experienced was six, with pain being the most commonly report symptom. Pain was also identified by these nurses as the most effectively treated symptom compared to fatigue, which was perceived as the symptom least effectively managed by nurses.[20] Woodgate and Degner[15] described the presence of cancer symptoms as a series of transition periods reflecting the dynamic nature of the childhood cancer experience. Hedstrom et al.[16] discovered that the most common causes of distress in a group of 121 children with cancer were treatment-related pain, nausea, and fatigue. Collins[18] described the most common physical symptoms (prevalence 35%) in a group of 160 children with cancer as lack of energy, pain, drowsiness, nausea, cough, and lack of appetite. Woodgate and Degner[17] evaluated expectations and beliefs about childhood cancer symptoms in children and their family members and found that these individuals expected to experience suffering as part of the cancer treatment. The families felt that unrelieved or uncontrolled symptoms were necessary for cure. Docherty[19] completed a review of the published research literature on symptom experiences of children and adolescents with cancer. The most frequent symptoms found in the literature include infection, bleeding, anemia, nutritional concerns, nausea and vomiting, mucositis, fatigue, and pain.[15–20] Common flaws in symptom management nursing research studies include no longitudinal symptom management study designs, limited use of conceptual models or theories, frequent adaptation of adult instruments as symptom measures, and no attention to the impact of these symptoms on the children's lives.

Myelosuppression and Consequent Infection

Chemotherapy agents and radiation therapy cause myelosuppression. In addition, certain malignancies that metastasize to the bone marrow (e.g., leukemia, lymphoma, neuroblastoma, sarcomas) cause a decrease in the number of normal blood cell precursors. When the myelosuppressive effect is severe enough, the child becomes predisposed to infection, anemia, or bleeding, depending on which blood cell line is affected.

Infection resulting from neutropenia may be life threatening (see Chapter 40). The bone marrow cannot produce an adequate number of neutrophils to protect against infection after cytotoxic chemotherapy is administered, or during long courses of radiotherapy. A patient with an absolute neutrophil count of less than 500 mm^3 is considered neutropenic. Children who have prolonged periods of neutropenia (i.e., >7 days) are at high risk for developing infection. The neutropenic child will not demonstrate the normal signs and symptoms of infection, and fever may be the only indication that infection is present.

The nurse plays an important role in minimizing the risk of infection in these children. Most infections in the neutropenic child are caused by endogenous flora (e.g., *Staphylococcus*, *Escherichia coli*, *Candida*) and adequate protection from infection is the best defense. Handwashing before and after contact with each patient minimizes the risk of microbial transmission, and is the single most important method of preventing nosocomial infection.[21,22] Administration of biologic response modifiers (e.g., granulocyte colony stimulating factor [G-CSF], granulocyte-macrophage colony stimulating factor [GM-CSF]) has decreased the duration of neutropenia after cytotoxic chemotherapy. The use of these agents for patients with a short period of neutropenia is generally not indicated (see Chapters 39 and 40).[23]

When a neutropenic child develops fever, blood cultures from both central (e.g., implanted central venous access device [CVAD]) and peripheral sources are obtained, as well as cultures of other appropriate body fluids or sites (e.g., urine, stool, throat, wound, lesions, catheter exit site). Broad-spectrum intravenous (IV) antibiotics are initiated. Antibiotic therapy is modified based on the culture and sensitivity of the organisms isolated.

Nursing care of the child hospitalized with fever and neutropenia is directed toward monitoring for signs of septic shock. Vital signs must be monitored frequently to identify temperature fluctuations (very low or very high), heart rate, respiratory rate, and blood pressure. Because hypotension is usually a late sign of shock in children, peripheral perfusion should be checked frequently. Delayed capillary refill and tachycardia are early signs of impending shock. Strict intake and output must be measured to monitor renal function. The child's level of consciousness must be assessed continually for irritability, lethargy, or unresponsiveness. Temperature measurement by the rectal route and the use of suppositories and enemas must be avoided. Mouth care and perianal hygiene must be done on a regular schedule. If the child is febrile (temperature 38.3°C), blood cultures are obtained, and acetaminophen is administered. The parents should be given an opportunity to ask questions during the period of acute serious illness (e.g., fever and neutropenia, septic shock) because this time is often confusing and stressful for the family.

Parents and children must be educated regarding the prevention of infection. All members of the family must practice strict handwashing to decrease the spread of pathogens among each other. The parents must know when the period of neutropenia is likely to occur following chemotherapy. If fever is suspected, they should take the child's temperature by the oral or axillary route, but never rectally. If the child's temperature is 38.0°C on two or more occasions in a 24-hour period, or 38.3°C or higher on one occasion, the parents should notify the nurse or physician immediately and should not administer acetaminophen unless instructed to do so.

Adequate nutrition is an important component in the prevention of infection. Cancer treatments often cause anorexia, nausea, and vomiting, which make adequate dietary intake difficult to achieve. Food should never be forced on the child, and should alternate feeding plans be required (e.g., gastric tube feedings, total parenteral nutrition), care must be taken to use the appropriate sterile technique to prevent infection.

Primary varicella-zoster virus infection can present a potentially life-threatening danger to the immunosuppressed child (see Chapter 40.) Therefore, if the child has never had chickenpox, the parents must educate school nurses, teachers, neighbors, and parents of playmates regarding this danger so that they can be notified if any contacts develop chickenpox. Infected persons are contagious for 1 to 2 days before the appearance of the vesicular rash and throughout the duration of eruption until all lesions have crusted. If the immunocompromised child is directly exposed to an infected person, varicella-zoster immune globulin (VZIG) (125 units/10 kg, maximum dose, 625 units) should be administered intramuscularly within 96 hours.[23,24] Direct exposure is defined as having an infected household contact, 1 hour or more of indoor play with an infected person, or hospital exposure through prolonged face-to-face contact with an infected health care worker or patient. The exact duration of effectiveness of VZIG is unknown. If another exposure occurs longer than 3 weeks after the injection, the dose is administered again. Hospitalized children with varicella-zoster virus must be placed in strict isolation for up to 28 days after exposure. Immunocompromised children who develop varicella infection may be treated with IV acyclovir alone,[25] although some children with mild or uncomplicated cases may receive IV acyclovir followed by oral acyclovir and reduce the duration of IV treatment and hospitalization.[25] Health care workers who have not had chickenpox should be advised to receive the varicella vaccine and should follow their institution's guidelines regarding any special precautions following immunization.[26]

After an individual has had chickenpox, varicella-zoster virus persists in the dorsal root ganglia in a latent form. Immunosuppression from chemotherapy or radiation can reactivate the virus resulting in herpes zoster ("shingles"). Vesicular lesions appear in the distribution of one to three sensory dermatomes. The eruption of lesions is often preceded by a prodrome of pain or tingling. Some immunosuppressed patients may not manifest the typical vesicular cutaneous changes and may only describe sensations of pain or tingling, which may or may not lie within a dermatome. Treatment of

patients who have zoster is similar to that of patients with primary varicella infection.[25]

Nursing care of the child with varicella infection requires strict attention to good hygiene and hydration, fever control, and management of pruritus or pain. These children must be continually assessed for evidence of disseminated infection or secondary bacterial infection. Hemorrhagic varicella is more commonly seen in immunocompromised patients. Ocular involvement, pneumonia, hepatitis, meningitis, and encephalitis (i.e., progressive disseminated varicella) may occur.[27]

Pneumocystis carinii generally is not pathogenic in a healthy host, but it can cause a life-threatening pneumonia (*Pneumocystis carinii* pneumonia [PCP]) in persons who are immunosuppressed.[28] Fortunately, this condition is almost entirely preventable. Trimethoprim-sulfamethoxazole (TMP-SMZ), 150 mg/m^2 of the trimethoprim component, by mouth divided into two doses, given three consecutive days each week, is adequate prophylaxis.[29] For patients who are unable to take TMP-SMZ because of hypersensitivity reaction or bone marrow suppression, dapsone, 2 mg/kg (maximum 100 mg/day) by mouth, given once daily, is also effective.[29] Aerosolized pentamidine 300 mg/dose is another option for PCP prophylaxis and is administered once monthly.[30] The patients must be old enough (usually 5 years of age or older) to cooperate with aerosolized drug administration via the Respirgard II inhaler and must come into the clinic to receive the medication. Pentamidine may also be given intravenously, but it is expensive and is associated with side effects (e.g., hypotension, hypoglycemia). Although pentamidine has been shown to prevent PCP, its administration is labor intensive, and it is certainly more costly than the medications that can be administered at home.

Respiratory syncytial virus (RSV) and cytomegalovirus (CMV) are other potentially problematic infections for children with cancer, especially those undergoing bone marrow transplantation. Other respiratory viruses, including adenovirus and influenza, generally do not cause more severe disease in children with cancer than in more immunocompetent patients.

Administration of Immunizations

Live virus vaccines are contraindicated in children receiving immunosuppressive therapy because of potentially serious adverse effects.[24] Vaccine-strain poliomyelitis, measles virus, and vaccinia have been reported in immunocompromised children after administration of live virus vaccines. Immunologically normal household contacts of immunocompromised children should receive inactivated poliovirus (IPV) vaccine, because live poliovirus is transmissible following immunization with oral poliovirus vaccine (OPV).[24] Live measles, mumps, and rubella (MMR) vaccine can be administered to the siblings and household contacts of immunosuppressed children because these viruses are not transmissible after vaccination. Varicella vaccine has been given to nonimmune household contacts of children with cancer without transmission of the virus to the immune suppressed child. Therefore, this vaccine is recommended for susceptible contacts of these children.[24] Children who have received chemotherapy or radiation therapy should not be given live virus vaccines until at least 3 months after immunosuppressive treatments have ceased. The degree of immunosuppression and its duration may vary among patients, however.[24] Other routine childhood immunizations, such as diphtheria-tetanus-pertussis, *Haemophilus influenzae* type-b conjugate, and hepatitis B, can be administered safely on a standard schedule, although immunogenicity may be reduced. Children who have Hodgkin disease and are 24 months old or older should receive pneumococcal and meningococcal vaccines because these children are at increased risk of infection from these organisms.[24]

Bleeding and Anemia

Children with cancer are at risk of developing bleeding related to thrombocytopenia or coagulopathy.[31] Anemia may occur because of blood loss or a decrease in the production of red blood cells related to bone marrow suppression from cancer treatment or malignancy (see Chapter 39). Children who are at risk for bleeding (platelet count below 100,000 per mm^3) should be placed on precautions, so the potential for bleeding can be decreased. Spontaneous internal hemorrhage does not occur until the platelet count is 20,000 per mm^3. Nurses should educate the family and child to avoid ibuprofen, aspirin, and aspirin-containing products. Minor pain and fever without neutropenia are treated with acetaminophen. The child's body temperature should not be taken rectally. Venipunctures and other invasive procedures (e.g., lumbar puncture and bone marrow aspiration) should be performed with caution when platelet counts are low.

The use of razors should be avoided, and a soft toothbrush should be used for dental care. Children should avoid using dental floss and not eat or chew sharp foods (e.g., tortilla chips, ice) to prevent gingival bleeding. Adolescent female patients may be given oral contraceptives or hormone therapy to suppress menses to decrease the risk of excessive bleeding. Contact sports or activities that may cause injury or bleeding (e.g., football, soccer, bicycle riding, skateboards, tree climbing) should not be permitted during periods of thrombocytopenia.

If the child experiences epistaxis, the parents should be instructed to pinch the child's nostrils together with a gauze pad held between the thumb and index finger for at least 10 minutes. If there is persistent epistaxis, or if the patient experiences hematuria or hematochezia, the child should be evaluated at the hospital. If the child is admitted to the hospital with thrombocytopenia, nursing interventions include measures to prevent injury, inspection of body fluids for evidence of blood, monitoring of vital signs and peripheral perfusion for evidence of blood loss, and administration of platelet transfusions.

Children may become anemic from blood loss or as a consequence of chemotherapy-induced myelosuppression. Children are amazingly resilient and tolerate low hemoglobin concentrations well. Signs and symptoms of anemia include pallor, headache, dizziness, shortness of breath, fatigue, tachycardia, and heart murmur. Packed red blood cell transfusion is generally required when the hemoglobin falls below 7 g/dL.

When red blood cell transfusions are required, leukocyte-depleted or irradiated blood products are often administered. Lymphocyte reduction of packed red blood cells and platelets is used to prevent HLA-alloimmunization and refractoriness to allogeneic platelet transfusion, nonhemolytic transfusion febrile reactions, and graft-versus-host disease (GVHD).[32,33] Irradiation of cellular blood components is used to prevent posttransfusion GVHD.[34] The decision to administer lymphocyte-depleted or irradiated blood products depends on the child's immunologic status and on the intensity of the chemotherapy regimen. All children who are bone marrow transplant recipients should receive leukocyte-depleted, irradiated blood products.

Transfusion of blood products may cause transfusion reactions, manifested by fever, chills, body aches, urticaria, pruritus, and, in severe cases, wheezing and respiratory compromise. If a transfusion reaction occurs, the transfusion should be discontinued and IV normal saline should be infused. Antihistamines, steroids, or acetaminophen may be administered.[35,36] Parents may prefer to limit blood and platelet transfusions to

designated donor products if the situation is not an emergency or if the child is not a potential bone marrow transplant recipient. The use of designated donor blood products may reduce the incidence of transfusion reaction if a parent or sibling's blood products are compatible. The institutional blood bank can provide information and instructions regarding specific designated donor programs.

Nutritional Changes

Adequate nutrition continues to be a major concern during childhood cancer treatment. Altered nutrition has been reported in between 8% to 32% of all children treated for cancer.[37] Alterations in nutritional status in the child undergoing cancer treatment are common (see Chapter 41). The disease itself and the side effects of therapy (e.g., nausea, vomiting, anorexia, stomatitis, dysphagia, changes in taste) often interfere with adequate caloric intake. Conversely, the use of glucocorticoids (i.e., prednisone, dexamethasone) causes an increased appetite and an intense craving for salty foods. When these drugs are given, weight gain may be excessive. In either case, the patient's weight should be checked at each visit and plotted at regular intervals on a growth curve.

When metabolic needs exceed caloric intake, the child may benefit from a nutritional supplement given between meals. Methods to increase caloric intake include providing high-protein snacks or high-calorie ingredients in recipes. Small, frequent meals may be more appetizing if the child is suffering from nausea. If the child continues to lose weight, or drops off the growth curve, a dietitian should be consulted. The child may require total parenteral nutrition or placement of a feeding tube to prevent malnourishment[38-40] (see Chapter 41).

Nutrition in pediatric bone marrow transplant patients has become a focus for nursing research in recent years.[38-43] Bone marrow transplant patients are a high-risk population who frequently experience gastrointestinal side effects that can result in poor nutrition.[43] Nurse researchers are exploring risk factors that can lead the way to earlier nutritional interventions and nutrient support. Other nursing research focus areas evaluated enteral feedings in pediatric oncology patients[39,40] and parental perception of their child's food intake during chemotherapy.[43]

Nausea and Vomiting

Cancer chemotherapy agents are emetogenic, and nausea and vomiting can severely alter fluid balance in the pediatric patient (see Chapter 42). Even when chemotherapy administration is preceded by antiemetic therapy, nausea and vomiting may still occur. Some patients receiving cisplatin or carboplatin experience delayed nausea and vomiting several days after the drugs are administered. While chemotherapy agents or IV hydration is infusing, the nurse must monitor intake and output closely and note any discrepancy that would indicate dehydration or overhydration. Patients receiving radiation therapy to the chest, abdomen, pelvis, or craniospinal axis may experience nausea, vomiting, anorexia, and diarrhea. Antiemetic or antispasmodic therapy may be indicated for these patients to provide symptomatic relief (see Chapter 42). Certain patients who suffer from anticipatory or treatment-associated nausea and vomiting may benefit from relaxation techniques or guided imagery.

Patient assessment prior to chemotherapy administration can provide insight into strategies that can decrease nausea and vomiting. A pre-chemotherapy assessment is found in Table 43.2. Nurses can educate the patient and family regarding these nonpharmacologic methods. Standards for care of a child with nausea and vomiting include screening at each clinic visit, prophylaxis for acute and delayed emesis in

TABLE 43.2

NAUSEA AND VOMITING ASSESSMENT

Assessment time	History
Prior to first chemotherapy course	• Prior experiences with motion sickness • Previous bad experience with nausea and vomiting • Fatigue • Anxiety during treatment • Sensitivity to odors
With each chemotherapy course	• Chemotherapy being administered • Previous history of nausea and vomiting • If patient has received the treatment before, determine how the treatment was tolerated: what worked and what contributed to the symptoms • Preferred antiemetic regimen • Supporting interventions that help decrease the symptoms; does the patient use relaxation techniques, distraction, biofeedback, etc. • Document the patient's treatment preferences to control nausea and vomiting

children receiving moderately to highly emetic chemotherapy and follow-up after treatment for nausea and vomiting symptoms.[44] Strategies for decreasing nausea and vomiting and preventing anorexia are found in Table 43.3.

Mucositis

Gastrointestinal cell damage from chemotherapy or radiation can cause ulcerations in the mucosal surface of the alimentary canal.[45] Ulcers occurring in the oral cavity are referred to as *stomatitis* and appear as edematous, erythematous, eroded lesions. These lesions may extend down into the esophagus. Anorexia commonly occurs, because eating and drinking cause extreme pain.

Meticulous oral hygiene assists in preventing or lessening the deleterious effects of mucositis. In infants and small children, gingival care is achieved by wrapping a gauze pad around a finger, soaking the gauze pad in saline solution, and swabbing the patient's gums, palate, and buccal mucosa. This should be done after eating or drinking, or as often as every 2 hours. Older children can cleanse their own teeth and gums with a soft toothbrush and use a saline-based oral solution to rinse the mouth. Because orthodontic appliances may harbor debris and cause infection, these appliances may need to be removed during chemotherapy. Nursing management of the child with mucositis involves implementing an oral hygiene regimen, monitoring hydration, and encouraging the child to choose foods that are best tolerated.

Prevention of infection and treatment of pain are the main objectives in treating oral mucositis.[46] Various oral care measures, including pharmacologic management of mucositis, are summarized in Table 43.4. Daily oral care, antiseptics, topical anesthetics, coating agents, lubricants, mechanical debridement, and miscellaneous agents are used. Fluid intake can be facilitated by the use of a straw to bypass tender oral mucosa. Anorexia is expected in these children, and as the ulcerations heal, they will start to eat and drink normally. Subsequent chemotherapy regimens may require dose modification to prevent similar episodes.

TABLE 43.3

STRATEGIES FOR NAUSEA AND VOMITING AND ANOREXIA

Nausea and vomiting	Anorexia

• Eat foods served cold or at room temperature
• Drink sips of clear liquids when nausea is severe
• Eat light meals throughout the day; try easy-to-digest food such as gelatin, toast, rice, dry cereals, and crackers
• Avoid foods that are fried, greasy, very sweet, spicy, hot, or strong-flavored
• Maintain good oral hygiene, rinse mouth with lemon water
• Avoid eating or drinking 1 to 2 hours before and after chemotherapy
• Use distraction such as music, television, games and reading before, during and after chemotherapy
• Listen to relaxation tapes or use visual imagery before, during and after chemotherapy
 	
Exercise when possible
	• Evaluate extent of appetite loss, vomiting, diarrhea, and drug side effects
	• Recognize risk factors associated with malnutrition in children with cancer[4]
	  • Advanced cancer (unfavorable histology Wilms' tumor, neuroblastoma, rhabdomyosarcoma, Ewing's sarcoma)
	  • Tumors of the head and neck
	  • Poor prognosis leukemia, multiple relapse leukemia
	  • High-grade brain tumors
	  • Stem cell transplantation
	• Realize that some children gain weight during cancer treatment. Certain chemotherapy regimens containing steroids, inactivity, electrolyte imbalances, and fluid retention are common causes of weight gain
	• Monitor weight closely; if <10th percentile or <1 kg/year prepubertal or <1 kg/6 months pubertal, consult dietician and or nutritionist

Advice for parents
• Don't push the child to eat
• Try to get the foods they ask for
• Explain reasons behind the need for good nutrition
• Offer food six times a day: three meals and three snacks
• Encourage the child to finish what he or she started eating
• "Power pack" the food so that each bite counts by adding extra margarine, cheese, gravy, or sauce to foods.
• Offer the high-fat version of a food such as fried chicken instead of baked

TABLE 43.4

GUIDELINES FOR ORAL CARE[a]

Category	Agents	Action	Comments
Rinses	Saline rinse (salt in warm water to taste) Sodium bicarbonate rinse (1 teaspoon baking soda to 1 pint water)	Removes particulate matter from teeth, tongue, and gingival tissue	Safe, effective, economical
Antiseptics	Chlorhexidine gluconate 12% (Peridex) Hexylresorcinol 0.1%, glycerin 28.2%, sodium bisulfate (ST-37)	Antibacterial activity	Chlorhexidine may stain teeth Generally well tolerated
Topical anesthetics	Maalox plus diphenhydramine Viscous lidocaine (Xylocaine) 2%	Antacids reduce acidity, diphenhydramine has a mild anesthetic effect Anesthetic effect	Give 15 to 20 min before meals; effect brief Limit use if swallowing to prevent systemic toxicity. Numbness may increase danger of oral trauma or aspiration
Coating agents	Orabase (with or without benzocaine) Sucralfate suspension	Provides protective barrier Cryoprotectant	Odorless and tasteless Soothes inflamed tissue
Lubricants	Xero-Lube (artificial salve)	Provides moisture	Tasteless; thick consistency
Other topical agents	Vitamin E Tretinoin (vitamin A derivative)	Antioxidant Stimulates wound healing	Tasteless; sticky consistency Mild odor; tasteless
Mechanical debridement	Soft-bristle toothbrush Foam swabs (toothettes)	Removes debris	Use gently if neutropenic or thrombocytopenic Also useful for application of topical medications

[a]See text for details.

Nurses play a key role in assessment of the oral cavity during childhood cancer treatment. Challenges to accurate oral assessment are numerous when caring for children who are often uncooperative. The need for assessment tools that are simple, quick to complete, and easy to use to assess most children is evidence in the literature. The lack of validated oral assessment instruments for infants, for children with cancer stresses the need for future research studies.[9,47,48]

Fatigue in Children with Cancer

Fatigue is described as one of the most distressing symptoms experienced during childhood cancer treatment.[49] Since 1998, numerous research publications evaluating fatigue in children with cancer have been published, the majority of which have been published in nursing journals.[50] This symptom has been evaluated from both qualitative and quantitative research perspectives. There are numerous causes of fatigue, and examples are given in Table 43.5. The qualitative findings indicate that fatigue is defined differently by children, adolescents, and their parents[49–51] and that different types of fatigue exist in pediatric oncology patients.[52] Fatigue changes throughout the courses of treatment for childhood cancer, increases during the first few days; medical procedures and the hospital environment are major causative factors of fatigue.[49–51,53] Newly developed fatigue measurement instruments have been tested during the past 5 years.[50,54] Further research is needed regarding fatigue as a single symptom and also in relation to other symptoms. Adolescents with the cluster of increased fatigue and sleep disturbances experienced more depressive symptoms and behavior changes.[55] The prevalence of this symptom confirms the need to explore the interrelationships between fatigue and other symptoms commonly experienced by children with cancer, as treating one symptom may diminish the presence or intensity of other related symptoms.

One mechanism contributing to cancer-related fatigue involves abnormalities in adenosine triphosphate synthesis

TABLE 43.5

FACTORS RELATED TO FATIGUE IN CHILDREN WITH CANCER

Factors	Causes
Treatment related	Chemotherapy, radiation therapy, surgery, biologic response modifiers, myelosuppression
Environmental	Long waits in the clinic and hospital, altered schedules or routines, hospital noise, sleep/rest interruptions in the hospital
Personal/Behavioral	Cognitive/developmental stage, emotions, moods, worry, boredom
Cultural/Family	Parent cues, expectations of others (e.g., family, relatives or friends), being pushed too hard, lacking a schedule

caused by carnitine deficiency.[56] Carnitine, a nutrient, has an important role in how muscles metabolize energy.[56] Studies indicate that several anti-cancer drugs interfere with the carnitine network, resulting in a less efficient aerobic muscle metabolism.[57,58] In a recent study of 67 children and adolescents who had received prior chemotherapy consisting of ifosfamide, cisplatin, or doxorubicin experienced increased fatigue in the presence of decreased carnitine levels.[59]

Certain types of interventions are now being tested to decrease fatigue during treatment. These include pharmacologic measures, sleep hygiene education, schedules for regular physical activity, and distraction techniques. More research into matching the type of fatigue and intervention is needed.

Pain Management

One of the most important roles of the nurse is the assessment and management of pain in children with cancer (see also Chapter 42). Supportive care for children in pain starts with a developmentally appropriate assessment to establish effective pain interventions. Interventions designed to decrease pain in children should include nonpharmacologic strategies as well as medications, when possible.

Common Myths About Children in Pain. Myths and misconceptions about the child's ability to perceive pain interfere with accurate assessment and treatment of pain. Some of these are as follows[60]: (a) a child's ability to feel pain is inhibited because children have an immature nervous system; (b) a child cannot communicate the location and intensity of pain; (c) children do not remember painful events; (d) it is always possible to determine whether a child is faking pain or is truly suffering from pain; (e) pain must have an evident stimulus, and if one is not noted, then the child cannot be feeling pain; (f) a child reports pain to the nurse or doctor; and (g) if the child does not complain of pain, then the child is not suffering from pain.

If any member of the health care team believes any of the foregoing myths regarding a child's ability to perceive pain, pain management will be inadequate, as the entire assessment and intervention process will be impaired.[61,62] Pain management in children has always been suboptimal, and if this situation is to be remedied, each health care professional needs to be aware of and dispel these myths.

Developmental Considerations. Children's perceptions of pain are influenced by the child's stage of cognitive development, cultural environment, and parent-child relationships.[60] These influences are important to consider when assessing the child's pain as well as when developing appropriate management strategies. Another important consideration is that the child with a chronic illness such as cancer may be more medically sophisticated than other children of the same age. Children with cancer are often advanced in their knowledge of medical treatment and are acutely aware of its effects. However, they may not be cognitively able to comprehend the meaning of the treatment and its importance to survival. This discrepancy can create confusion for the health provider caring for the 4-year-old patient who can explain the technical details of bone marrow aspiration, yet is combative and uncontrollable during the procedure.

Children develop their understanding of pain similar to Piaget's[63] conceptualization of cognitive development, recognizing the considerable overlap in these categories (Table 43.3). Younger children who are generally in the preoperational stage of development communicate their perceptions of pain much differently from older children who are capable of abstract thought. The toddler or preschool child often perceives that he or she has done something wrong to cause the pain and does not understand why treatment or a procedure is necessary. Children of this age cannot comprehend that painful treatment is sometimes necessary to prevent the disease from recurring. For this reason, the young toddler, unable to understand the purpose of a bone marrow aspiration, should have the procedure completed as quickly and painlessly as possible. In very young children, or children with developmental delay, the use of pharmacologic interventions is more appropriate and effective than trying to explain the importance of the procedure.[64]

Children between the ages of 7 and 11 years begin to develop concrete thinking skills and are able to understand situations that infants, toddlers, and preschool children are generally unable to comprehend. During this stage, however, children have vivid imaginations and often fear that pain may lead to death. Preparation of the school-aged child before the procedure is essential to assist in alleviating unfounded fears and anxiety. Past experiences often play a major role in how the 6- to 12-year-old child perceives pain caused by cancer or required treatment. For example, a difficult procedure performed by an unskilled health care professional can cause the child to fear the procedure and to become uncooperative during future attempts. Every effort should be made to prevent experiences that unnecessarily increase the child's pain and discomfort.

Children older than 12 years generally begin to develop the capabilities for formal operational thought.[63] They are able to understand the differences between disease-related pain and the side effects of treatment. During this stage of development, adolescents may express their reaction to pain by withdrawing from others or by becoming depressed. Open, honest discussions between the health care provider and the adolescent regarding the disease and its treatment may assist the patient in coping with the associated discomfort. These dialogues allow for the development of effective coping skills.

The influence of the child's cultural environment should not be overlooked. Cultural beliefs can play a major role in the family and child's perception of cancer and the associated treatment. Pain expression by children and interpretation by caregivers may be affected by the culture of the patient or the caregiver.[65] Cultural beliefs regarding pain and suffering in children should be considered when implementing intervention strategies for the child. Family assessment should include specific questions regarding the meaning of the illness and perceptions of treatment. Accurate family assessment can provide helpful information when establishing interventions for the child in pain.

Parent-child relationships directly influence the child's perception of pain, regardless of the age of the child. Parents who are distraught and are unable to control their fears and concerns often are a detriment to the child's ability to cope with the painful effects of the disease and treatment. Early intervention with parents is essential in developing effective coping skills. Parental support positively influences the child's ability to adjust to painful experiences.

Assessment of Pain in Children. To achieve effective pain management, pain intensity and relief obtained from interventions must be assessed at regular intervals. Because children cannot, or do not, report pain consistently to health care providers, the nurse must carry a high index of suspicion regarding the presence of pain. Pain assessment in infants and children is not necessarily straightforward. Chronologic and developmental ages influence the accurate assessment of pain. In infants, properties of their cry, facial movements, and body posturing all give clues to the presence of pain. Whereas a shrill, uncontrollable cry, contortion of facial features, restlessness, and arching of the back are indicators of pain, a silent, lethargic, submissive infant or child may also be in pain. The goal is to prevent pain from becoming severe by initiating early intervention, rather than facing the difficult task of treating established pain.

Early intervention is possible only if a thorough patient assessment is obtained. As mentioned previously, signs of pain may not be readily apparent. The nurse must use age-appropriate assessment techniques or instruments. Physiologic responses to pain are manifested by tachycardia, tachypnea, hyperventilation, hypertension, diaphoresis, and nausea and vomiting. These responses are all measurable. Self-report instruments are appropriate for use in children 4 years of age and older. These tools are in the form of graphic rating scales, visual analog scales, numeric scales, and color scales.[1] To assess pain in children less than 4 years of age, an instrument such as the FLACC may be used. The FLACC uses physiologic and behavioral cues (Face, Legs, Activity, Cry, Consolability) for the nurse to quantify the rating of the infant or child's pain.[66] The use of instruments is necessary for obtaining a baseline and for periodic reassessment of pain intensity. It is important to use pain-rating instruments that have been tested for reliability and validity. If the child is unable to report pain, the parent should be asked to assist in determining the presence or severity of pain by evaluating changes in behavior (e.g., eating less, playing less, crying more, sleeping more). Once a plan of pain assessment has been established, the same methods should be used consistently. Physiologic indicators, behavioral responses, and self-report instruments should be used for reassessment at least every 2 hours after instituting interventions for pain management.[1]

Procedure-Related Pain. Invasive procedures are the most painful and traumatic events experienced by children receiving treatment for cancer.[67] Aggressive treatments such as high-dose chemotherapy for cancer are also major sources of pain and discomfort for children. Although procedure-related pain represents an acute, brief experience, it is accompanied by fear and anxiety. Bone marrow aspirations and lumbar punctures are perceived as extremely painful by children with cancer. Previous studies have shown that children do not adapt to the discomfort associated with invasive procedures, and they experience greater levels of anxiety with repeated painful experiences.[68] Children often experience symptoms such as depression, insomnia, and anorexia before the clinic or hospital visit when such procedures are scheduled.

Researchers continue to build on the knowledge of how best to prepare children for invasive procedures. Specifically, preparation before the procedure includes providing children with sensory and procedural information in an age-appropriate manner and providing training in coping skills.[67] Teaching parents and children cognitive behavioral interventions (i.e., distraction, relaxation, guided imagery) for support during invasive procedures continue to be effective in decreasing pain and distress. Consensus among professionals caring for children with cancer supports a developmental approach to manage the pain associated with invasive procedures.[69]

1. The child and parents must be prepared, with specific methods indicated for the parent to help the child relax.
2. The child must be evaluated to assess effectiveness of treatment in reducing pain and anxiety.
3. As pleasant an environment as possible should be created in the treatment room.
4. The treatment approach should be multimodal and should meet the child's needs.
5. Treatment of pain and anxiety should be maximal for the initial procedure, to reduce the development of subsequent anticipatory anxiety symptoms.
6. Local anesthetics should be considered even for simple procedures.
7. Staff responsible for procedures must be knowledgeable about behavioral and pharmacologic treatment of acute pain and anxiety.
8. Appropriate monitoring and resuscitative equipment must be readily available.
9. Staff must demonstrate competence in performing invasive procedures.

Pharmacologic management of procedural pain should include analgesic and sedative agents. Procedural sedation is used at many institutions and is defined as a minimally depressed level of consciousness that retains the patient's ability to maintain a patent airway independently and continuously, and respond appropriately to physical stimulation and/or verbal command. Various pharmacologic approaches are used, most of which combine an opioid analgesic with a benzodiazepine for anxiolysis and sedation. General anesthesia (i.e., propofol) is a safe, effective anesthetic intervention. Table 43.6 describes specific nursing responsibilities related to sedation of patients for invasive procedures.

Topical anesthetics are used extensively in the management of procedure-related pain. EMLA cream and LMX4 cream are topical anesthetic preparations that penetrate intact skin. The depth of anesthesia obtained from using the topical anesthetic is approximately 5 mm, and the duration of action is 4 hours. A thick layer of the topical anesthetic (about 2 mm) is significantly more effective than thinner layers. The anesthetic effects of the cream depend on thorough hydration of the skin; the skin should be covered with an occlusive dressing after application. A 30-minute application of LMX4 is as effective as a 60-minute application of EMLA cream.[70] For more invasive procedures such as bone marrow aspiration or lumbar puncture, the most complete anesthesia occurs 90 to 120 minutes after application of the EMLA cream. Patients who are seen in the outpatient setting can have their cream applied at home to prevent delays in the clinic.

A traumatic experience during a child's first invasive procedure may affect the child's ability to cope with future procedures.[68,69] Parental participation is helpful to the child, particularly for toddlers and preschool children, in whom separation issues are paramount. Parents who are present during invasive procedures should receive specific information beforehand as to what will take place and suggestions as to what they can do to help their child during the procedure. Involving the parents during a procedure provides a source of support for the child. During minor procedures, such as venipuncture or IV access, the parent can hold and hug the child while assisting in isolating and restraining a limb or body part. During more extensive procedures (e.g., bone marrow aspiration, lumbar puncture) the parent can be positioned close to the child, within the child's view, to talk with and soothe the child. Parents who are uncomfortable in this role and who prefer not to accompany the child into the procedure room should be reassured that the child will be treated well. Another adult can assume the role of the parent in this situation.

Tactile stimulation and relaxation techniques are behavioral methods that can be used to diminish procedure-related pain as well as acute pain.[64,67] An infant can be provided with a pacifier or sucrose nipple to suck during episodes of pain.[71] Relaxation techniques reduce muscle tension, which often accompanies pain. Infants can be swaddled in a warm blanket, held securely, and rocked. Toddlers and preschool children may also benefit from being held and rocked. Older children can be instructed in relaxation techniques such as closing their eyes and deep breathing. Practicing these methods along with them reinforces these techniques.[67]

TABLE 43.6

NURSING RESPONSIBILITIES RELATED TO SEDATION OF PEDIATRIC PATIENTS FOR INVASIVE PROCEDURES

Before procedure	During procedure	After procedure until recovery
Ensure that appropriate monitoring and resuscitation equipment is available and functioning in both procedure and recovery room.	Maintain physical and verbal contact with the child. Continuously assess for airway patency and monitor pulse oximeter.	Position child to maintain airway patency and prevent aspiration. Continuously monitor child's status with pulse oximeter. Assess skin color, nail beds, and mucosa at 2- to 3-min intervals.
Ensure that emergency cart is in close proximity.	Assess child's color (skin, nail beds, lips, mucosa) at 1- to 2-min intervals.	Asses heart rate, respiratory rate, responsiveness at 5-min intervals until child is alert and cardiovascular, respiratory rate, and responsiveness have returned to pre-sedation status.
Obtain and document child's vital signs (including height and weight).	Assess heart rate, respiratory rate, and responsiveness at 2- to 3-min intervals.	Evaluate efficacy of treatment plan for pain, anxiety in conjunction with child, parent, and other caregivers; plan individualized treatment approach for future procedures.
Obtain child's current health history (including allergies and current medications).	Initiate appropriate behavioral interventions for child and parent.	Instruct child and parent concerning follow-up care and future treatment plan.
Assess child's current health status (including responsiveness, skin and nail bed color).	Document child's tolerance of procedure, vital signs, and pulse oximeter reading.	Document vital signs, color, responsiveness, general health status, efficacy of treatment plan, future treatment plan, and plan for follow-up care in medical record.
Review sedation order (including drug, dosage, route, in relation to child's current health status).		
Assess child's and parent's psychological preparation, knowledge, and coping skills related to procedure.		
Initiate behavior interventions appropriate to age and health status.		
Apply pulse oximeter.		
Administer sedation as ordered.		
Document medication administration, including child's tolerance.		

Medical play is an innovative method used to instruct and educate the child regarding diagnostic tests and procedures. As the procedure is explained, the child has the opportunity to ask questions and to examine equipment. The child is encouraged to perform the procedure on a doll. Anxiety related to the procedure is relieved as the child gains understanding of the procedure and the sensations they will experience.

Distraction and guided imagery are two cognitive methods of nonpharmacologic pain management.[72] Distraction involves concentrating on an event or object other than the pain. Infants and toddlers are easily distracted because of their short attention span. Older children can be distracted with activities such as video games, television, and music. Guided imagery works well with school-aged and older children who can visualize an enjoyable experience or pleasant memory. The child describes the event in detail as he or she visualizes it. The effectiveness of this method may be enhanced by the use of a coach. The coach may be a parent or other adult who discusses the event with the child and who keeps the image alive. Physical tactics may also be employed as nonpharmacologic methods of pain management. Many times, these are useful in older children who do not require pharmacologic management for minor procedures or discomfort. These methods include application of heat or cold, immobilization of the affected limb or body part, or massage therapy. A recent study describing a self-hypnosis intervention in children with cancer undergoing venipuncture suggested that patients in the local anesthetic plus hypnosis group reported less anticipatory anxiety, less procedure-related pain and anxiety, and were rated as demonstrating less behavioral distress during the procedure. The parents of these children also experienced less anxiety during their child's procedure.[73]

Disease-Related and Treatment-Related Pain. Nurses must be knowledgeable about the basic pathophysiology of cancer pain and treatment-related side effects. The World Health Organization's three-step analgesic pain ladder should be incorporated into the approach to pain management for every child with cancer.[74] Nurses must acquire extensive knowledge of common analgesics and narcotics used in pediatric pain management. Interdisciplinary pain management teams are used in numerous pediatric cancer centers. These teams serve as consultants and provide expertise in the assessment and management of pain. The nurse often serves as the coordinator of care, playing a key role in cancer pain management.

Pharmacologic management of disease-related pain involves various methods, discussed in detail in Chapter 43. More than a trial of one type of medication may be necessary to find the appropriate agent to manage the child's pain. The route of administration must be considered as well. Providing pain relief by administering deep intramuscular injections, as an alternative to the IV, is not appropriate therapy, because many oral and transdermal preparations are now available with comparable efficacy. Nonsteroidal antiinflammatory drugs (NSAIDs), acetaminophen with codeine, morphine, and fentanyl are commonly used in the management of disease-related pain. Appropriate dosing is imperative. Doses should be titrated to increase the amount of analgesia and to minimize side effects.

Pain management at end-of-life may be particularly challenging. Unfortunately, analgesia is often insufficient due to a lack of knowledge concerning the prescribing and adjustment of opioid doses. Morphine continues to be the first line opioid of choice in pediatric palliative care, and extended-release oral morphine remains the dominant formulation for long-term use with hydromorphone slow-release preparations being used when there are severe adverse effects from morphine. The fentanyl transdermal patch is also being used in children with cancer-related pain.[75] Ketamine, an IV anesthetic with analgesic properties, when used in low doses, may be useful in managing pediatric cancer pain at the end of life. A recent case report documented how ketamine was used in two children with cancer at the end of life, providing adequate pain control in the home without sedation or other difficult opioid-associated side effects.[76]

Central Line Care

Patients on prolonged or intensive treatment regimens will require a vascular access device (VAD). These devices are used for administration of blood products and IV fluids, chemotherapy, parenteral nutrition, peripheral blood stem cell (PBSC) harvest and PBSC or bone marrow reinfusion, antibiotics, repeated blood specimens, and for pain and symptom management at the end of life.[77] Nontunneled catheters include short peripheral cannulas, midlines, and PICC (peripherally inserted central catheter) lines. Tunneled catheters include Hickman, Broviac and Groshong catheters, and ports (e.g., Infusaport, Portacath, Mediport). Chapter 12 discusses these catheters in detail. Groshong catheters do not require the instillation of heparin to maintain patency.

Nurses caring for children with venous access devices must be aware of the complications related to indwelling catheters. These include infection, bleeding, thrombus formation, and catheter damage.[78] Patient and parent education regarding the care of external catheters should be based on institutional guidelines. Instruction must include a detailed discussion of sterile technique, flushing with saline and heparin when appropriate, and dressing changes. Meticulous hand hygiene is imperative in preventing infection in patients with central lines.[79]

Standard guidelines to determine when removal of the catheter is necessary include positive blood cultures beyond 72 hours of antimicrobial therapy based on susceptibility testing or evidence of a tunnel infection, catheter occlusion unresponsive to thrombolytic or chemical treatments, and a suspected or documented catheter-related infection causing septic shock. When antibiotics are administered to patients with double-lumen or triple-lumen catheters, the doses must be rotated to each of the ports and lumina, to avoid persistent bacterial colonization of an untreated lumen. When infections are treated and the CVAD is not removed, the length of therapy depends on the duration of infection and the immunologic status of the patient.

Chemotherapy Administration

An understanding of the actions and side effects of chemotherapeutic agents is essential for nurses caring for children with cancer (see Chapter 10). Most institutions require nurses to complete a chemotherapy certification course before administering these drugs. Chemotherapy courses for nurses should include an overview of the principles of chemotherapy, classification and actions of specific agents, side effects, special considerations (e.g., interactions with other drugs), proper administration and handling, disposal of materials, and precautions to be taken with vesicants (Table 43.7). Nurses should be observed administering chemotherapy and should demonstrate competence before completion of the certification course. Specific guidelines for safe practice in the administration of chemotherapy have now been established and are described in Table 43.8.[80]

Chemotherapeutic agents must be given through a free-flowing IV line. The infusion should be stopped immediately if any sign of infiltration occurs (i.e., pain, stinging, erythema, swelling). Agents such as vincristine, vinblastine, mitomycin-C, and doxorubicin pose significant clinical problems when they become extravasated into subcutaneous tissue.[80]

If extravasation occurs, the chemotherapy infusion should be immediately discontinued, and aspiration of any residual drug and blood should be attempted from the tubing, needle, and site. If the nurse is not able to aspirate the drug in the tubing, the needle or catheter should be removed. Direct pressure to the extravasation site should be avoided. When an antidote

TABLE 43.7

OBJECTIVES FOR EDUCATIONAL PROGRAMS PREPARING NURSES TO ADMINISTER CHEMOTHERAPY OR BIOTHERAPY

Before administering chemotherapy or biotherapy, the nurse should be able to do the following:

Demonstrate familiarity with cancer chemotherapeutic or biotherapeutic agents (pharmacokinetics, dosage, interactions, stability, administration, side effects, toxicities, and latent effects).

Interpret laboratory values that determine need for delay in treatment administration or dose adjustment.

Plan for the management of treatment side effects.

Plan for potential extravasation (chemotherapy) or anaphylaxis (chemotherapy and biotherapy).

Initiate procedure for nursing interventions in emergency situations.

Verify the appropriateness of the drug dosage ordered by the physician by verifying the dosage with the protocol and confirming it with a second person.

Educate patients and families about the treatment.

When applying knowledge in a clinical setting, the nurse should be able to do the following:

Select an appropriate site for therapy; when administering vesicant chemotherapy peripherally, select an appropriate vein, perform the venipuncture, and anchor the needle safely.

Administer the chemotherapy and biotherapy safely according to the facility's procedure.

Document chemotherapy or biotherapy administration and patient's reaction to treatment.

Dispose of all materials and unused chemotherapeutic or biotherapeutic agents safely.

TABLE 43.8

GUIDELINES FOR SAFE HANDLING OF CHEMOTHERAPEUTIC AGENTS

Use care and strict aseptic technique in handling chemotherapeutic agents to prevent any physical contact with the substance.

Prepare drugs in a properly ventilated room or biologic safety cabinet (incorporates protective front panel and vertical laminar airflow to reduce potential for inhalation during preparation).

Wear disposable gloves and protective clothing and discard in special container after each use.

Use a sterile gauze pad when priming intravenous tubing, connecting and disconnecting tubing, inserting syringes into vials, breaking glass ampules, or any other procedure in which antineoplastic drugs may be inadvertently discharged.

Dispose of all contaminated needles, syringes, intravenous tubing, and other contaminated equipment in a leak-proof and puncture-resistant container; do not recap or break needles.

TABLE 43.9

ASSESSMENT OF HOME CARE SERVICES FOR A CHILD WITH CANCER

Does the agency employ nurses with pediatric experience? If so, how many nurses?

Do the nurses have experience with cancer patients?

Are the nurses certified or competent in chemotherapy administration?

Do the nurses have experience with long-term venous access devices (e.g., Broviac, Hickman)?

Can blood product transfusion be administered in the home?

Are the nurses familiar with side effects of cancer therapy?

Are appropriate precautions followed to minimize exposure to infectious organisms?

What kind of coverage is provided (i.e., 24 h)?

is available, it should be instilled through the catheter. If the catheter has been removed, the nurse should inject the antidote into the subcutaneous tissue at the location of the extravasation using a 25-gauge needle. Warm or cold compresses discussed for use in the extravasation of specific agents should be used for 20-minute intervals four times a day for 24 to 48 hours. The affected arm should be elevated if possible for 48 hours. The site should be observed for induration, pain, erythema, swelling, blistering, and necrosis.

Planning for Care at Home

Planning for discharge to home should begin when the child is admitted to the hospital. The nurse must be familiar with resources available to assist the patient's family members in meeting their needs after hospital discharge. Coordination of care between hospital and home is essential. Many families require home care services provided by public agencies, hospitals, or organized home care agencies. Home care nurses are generalists who provide advanced technical skills and supportive nursing care for many different pediatric problems. Children with cancer may require hyperalimentation, IV antibiotic therapy, chemotherapy, central line care, pain management, and psychosocial support. Coordination of care in the home requires that the pediatric oncology team and the home care agency work together to develop and implement a plan of care. The pediatric oncology nurse initiates the first contact with the home care nurse and provides a detailed overview of the child' diagnosis, treatment plan, and specific needs in the home setting. Answers to specific questions about the ability of the home care agency to care for children with cancer adequately should be obtained (Table 43.9).

As care delivery continues to shift from inpatient admission for chemotherapy administration, more complicated regimens are being given in the outpatient setting. At one center in New York, chemotherapy regimens such as high-dose methotrexate; 5-day high-dose ifosfamide and etoposide; cyclophosphamide, doxorubicin, and vincristine; ifosfamide, carboplatin, and etoposide; and cisplatin and doxorubicin are administered in the outpatient setting and IV hydration and supportive medications (e.g., Mesna, antiemetics) are administered in the home

at night. This level of care requires extensive coordination of care, but allows the child to return home at night and decreases hospital admission.[81]

Providing Information on the Disease and Treatment

The pediatric oncology nurse works with other members of the interdisciplinary team to provide education for the family and patient regarding the diagnosis, treatment, and psychosocial issues of childhood cancer. At the initial diagnostic talk, the nurse should be present. During subsequent discussions, the nurse reinforces and reviews information and answers the questions and concerns of the patients and family. Most pediatric cancer centers have structured education programs for families that include written materials, handbooks for parents, formal teaching sessions, videotapes, tours of the hospital and clinic, and structured play activities for the child to learn more about the illness and treatment. Parent and patient education is ongoing and continues throughout treatment and after completion of therapy.

Educational programs for families and patients should include discussion of the pathophysiology of the different types of cancer, various treatment options, general side effects of treatment, growth and development concerns, and family issues. Parents must become familiar with the special needs of their child. Psychomotor skills such as central line care and subcutaneous injections may need to be acquired by the parents and child and are taught by the nurse before hospital discharge. Assessment and evaluation of specific teaching given to families and patients should be documented in the patient's record. The nurse should be aware of the numerous educational resources that exist for children and families with cancer. Organizations that provide these materials are found in Chapter 55.

Nurses caring for children with cancer must understand that patient education must relate to the child's developmental stage. Knowledge of growth and development helps the nurse to communicate with the child before painful procedures or unfamiliar tests and to understand the child's uncertainty about hospitalization. For example, when dealing with a preschool child, it may be more appropriate to use medical play to demonstrate how a bone marrow aspiration is performed. In comparison, the adolescent needs a detailed discussion of the procedure, a description of the experience, and instructions about what to do. Programs targeting preparation for radiation therapy have been developed at some centers to familiarize the child with equipment and procedures in order to decrease anxiety.[82] Chapter 48 describes specific considerations when discussing the disease and treatment with children at various ages.

Facilitating Psychosocial Support

Nurses work with the interdisciplinary care team to provide psychosocial support for the patient and family. The nurse must understand family systems and the role each member plays in the family. The expert nurse considers cultural influences on the child and family and conducts a detailed assessment of the family's support system including their strengths and weaknesses. Evaluation of community resources is an integral part of the family assessment.

Diagnosis, treatment, discontinuation of therapy, relapse, and terminal illness are crisis points for families who have a child with cancer. At the time of diagnosis, anxiety, fear, anger, and depression are commonly felt by family members. Coping with the crisis of childhood cancer requires that the family develop new attitudes, behaviors, and coping techniques. Nurses provide support by helping family members work together. During the treatment period, nurses are resources for the family; they teach the family members about the disease and treatment and provide support during stressful situations. Nurses play a major role in preventing parental overprotec-

tion and isolation of the child. Families must be reassured that maintaining discipline during treatment is in the best interest of the child. Many children who are diagnosed with cancer are successfully treated and go on to lead normal adult lives. Maintaining discipline during childhood enables them to become well-adjusted adults. Essential coping tasks for the family during the diagnostic period and initiation of treatment are described in Table 43.10. Over time, the family ideally learns to adjust to the changes brought on by treatment of childhood cancer. Cessation of therapy can bring with it new fears for the child and family. Preparation for discontinuation of therapy is as essential as the education provided at the time of initial diagnosis. Nurses must encourage the parents to verbalize their fears. Table 43.11 identifies specific interventions for families at the time of discontinuation of therapy.

Recurrent disease brings with it a crisis for the entire family. Adequate time must be spent in counseling and providing support during the period when families must face the failure of treatment. Parents frequently feel guilty, and they may be angry. Parents may question why the disease has recurred despite all they have done. Nurses caring for children and families experiencing a relapse must be excellent listeners and must create a caring atmosphere amid the turmoil. Table 43.12 reviews specific nursing interventions for families during this time.

At the time of the initial cancer diagnosis, families with a child who has cancer are confronted with the possibility of death. Return of the disease brings with it the realization that

TABLE 43.10

FAMILY COPING TASKS AND INTERVENTIONS DURING DIAGNOSIS AND TREATMENT

Essential coping tasks	Interventions
Diagnosis	
Gaining control of emotions	Allow time for parents to be alone to grieve.
Alleviating acute anxiety	Maintain hope for the child no matter how serious the situation.
	Allow the family to express their feelings and fears.
Understanding the diagnosis	Spend time discussing the diagnosis and its meaning before presenting a plan for treatment.
Explaining cancer to the child	Use terms the child can understand; tell the child about cancer and the need for treatment.
Establishing the treatment regimen	Begin discussions with parents and the child about the treatment regimen and side effects.
Preventing anxiety regarding discharge and home care	Begin early to discuss care for the child at home.
	Identify key individuals who will assist the family at home.
Allowing for participation of family members	Discuss with siblings and other family members the child's diagnosis and treatment.
	Encourage siblings to visit the child.
Treatment	
Accepting the diagnosis	Allow for ongoing discussion of the diagnosis with parents and family members.
	Reinforce with parents that it is normal to have continued fears and doubts.
Understanding treatment and its side effects	Throughout the treatment, continue discussions of treatment and its side effects to increase family's understanding.
Identifying support systems	Assist the family in identifying individuals and groups who will support the family during times of crisis.
Establishing alternative routines, lifestyle	Provide opportunities for the family to begin reestablishing their lifestyle to meet each family member's needs.
	Encourage activities the family participated in before diagnosis.
	Stress importance of child's return to school.
Providing support for the child	Allow the child to express his or her own thoughts and feelings, separate from the parents.
	Provide opportunities for age-appropriate play therapy, especially for invasive procedures.
	Provide the child with explanations for body changes occurring from the disease or treatment.
	Allow the child to participate in care actively.
Encouraging siblings' participation	Stress importance of including siblings in conversations and care.
	Allow siblings to accompany the child to the hospital when possible.
	Stress that parents need to provide time alone with other siblings at home.

Adapted from Hockenberry MJ, Coody DK. Pediatric oncology and hematology: perspectives on care. St. Louis, MO: Mosby, 1986.

TABLE 43.11

FAMILY COPING TASKS AND INTERVENTIONS AT DISCONTINUATION OF THERAPY

Essential coping tasks	Interventions
Adapting to discontinuing treatment	Begin discussions several months before therapy is discontinued. Allow time for parents and child to ask questions and verbalize concerns.
Recognizing fear of relapse	Discuss openly the possibility of relapse. Review concerns for parents and child regarding what to expect if relapse should occur.
Realizing impact of parent's attitude	Discuss importance of parents' attitude and how it affects the child. Stress importance of verbalizing fears while recognizing the positive situation of discontinuing therapy.
Supporting child's needs and preventing fears	Reassure the child that therapy would not be discontinued unless he or she was doing well. Allow the child to express fears separately from parents (provide support and stress need for courage and trust).

Adapted from Hockenberry MJ, Coody DK. Pediatric oncology and hematology: perspectives on care. St. Louis, MO: Mosby, 1986.

TABLE 43.12

FAMILY COPING TASKS AND INTERVENTIONS WITH RELAPSE

Essential coping tasks	Interventions
Alleviating initial shock of relapse	Allow parents to express shock and disbelief. Provide time for grieving before initiating discussion of treatment plan.
Understanding the impact of relapse	Discuss the seriousness of relapse; yet, provide hope in the situation. Offer facts regarding possible outcome of the disease.
Discussing relapse with the child	Express importance of being truthful with the child. Discuss the relapse with the child and the need to begin therapy again (realize the child will perceive the seriousness of the situation by observing parents and staff).
Expressing appropriate feelings of grief	Encourage expression of feelings and need for family to maintain a realistic outlook toward the situation. Identify key support individuals to maintain close follow-up with all family members.

Adapted from Hockenberry MJ, Coody DK. Pediatric oncology and hematology: perspectives on care. St. Louis, MO: Mosby, 1986.

the child may not survive. Parents facing the loss of a child to cancer have been through numerous crises since diagnosis but none so difficult as the awareness that their child may die. Nurses can assist the family during this crisis by helping to identify strengths that will support them throughout this difficult time. Nursing interventions that promote effective coping tasks include helping the family accept the terminal status of their child's disease, allowing the family to participate in the child's care as much as possible, including hospice support (see Chapter 49), encouraging expression of emotions and guilt feelings, and planning for the future (Table 43.13).

Promoting Normal Growth and Development

Cancer therapy has the potential to cause significant developmental and growth delays.[83] The nurse must continually assess the child's growth and development during treatment and after cessation of therapy. Evaluation of the child's weight and height should be documented on standardized growth charts at regular intervals. Children younger than 3 years should have head circumferences documented. Changes in weight or lack of expected growth in height or weight should be followed closely. Any percentile change on the growth chart, or weight loss of 5% or more, should be evaluated. Specific nutritional interventions described in Chapter 41 should be started immediately once changes in weight occur.

Nurses can facilitate normal development by ensuring that the child is treated at an age-appropriate level when visiting the clinic or hospital. The importance of meeting basic needs and supporting developmental tasks should be emphasized at each visit. Family support should be given to encourage normal childhood development at home. Accurate assessment of any disruption in growth or development allows for early intervention.

Returning to school is an important milestone for children with cancer. Every attempt must be made to ensure that the child has the opportunity to return to the classroom, despite the disease and treatment. Chapter 50 discusses the importance of school reentry programs for children with cancer. Nurses are instrumental in assisting with the child's return to school.[84,85] Visits to the school by the nurse, to meet with teachers and to talk to the child's peers, are commonly offered by most comprehensive childhood cancer centers. At times, a child with cancer must refrain from returning to school, often because of the intensity of the treatment program. When a child must have homebound instruction before returning to the classroom, ongoing communication between the child and classmates should be encouraged. Successful school reentry is a goal for all children and must be perceived as such by all members of the patient's care team. The nurse must be vigilant in attempting to help the child return to school when at all possible.

Following up Long-Term Survivors

Nurses who provide care for survivors of childhood cancer must understand the late effects of therapy and should have an extensive knowledge of normal growth and development.

TABLE 43.13

FAMILY COPING TASKS AND INTERVENTIONS DURING END-STAGE DISEASE

Essential coping tasks	Interventions
Accepting the child's impending death	Allow the parents to verbalize their fears of the child's death. Discuss any questions they may have to decrease their worries and concerns. When possible, listen to the parent's wishes and demands.
Participating in the child's care	Encourage the family to remain involved with the child's care. (This involvement allows them to comfort the child while giving the parents a sense of belonging and need; it will also assist in preparing them for the inevitable loss.)
Expressing appropriate emotions	Stress the importance of expressing grief. Identify key individuals who will provide comfort and reassurance. Encourage relatives and significant others to be involved to give parents an opportunity to rest and maintain physical strength.
Resolving guilt feelings and sense of helplessness	Reassure parents that they could have done nothing to prevent the child's death. Assure them that they are doing everything possible by providing comfort and support. Stress that the most important role is their presence with the child.
Planning for the future	Stress the need for the family to look toward the future.

Adapted from Hockenberry MJ, Coody DK. Pediatric oncology and hematology: perspectives on care. St. Louis, MO: Mosby, 1986.

Current collaborative practice models designed to follow these patients include nurses as direct care providers. These models provide a more comprehensive approach to meet the complex needs of children and adolescents who have survived cancer. Nurses, usually in advanced practice roles, are able to perform physical assessment, to provide growth and development evaluation, and to conduct screening tests for specific late effects related to the type of cancer or its treatment.[83] A major aspect of the nursing role is patient and family education regarding possible late psychological or physical consequences of childhood cancer. Chapter 47 discusses specific late effects in detail.

Nurses must be knowledgeable regarding the long-term complications of specific chemotherapeutic agents.[80] Toxicity related to therapy can result in long-term disability. Anthracyclines, which include doxorubicin (Adriamycin) and daunomycin, can produce irreversible cardiac damage.[84] Cumulative doses of anthracyclines must be closely monitored by the nurse, and examination of left ventricular function should be ordered periodically as part of the overall medical management plan (see Chapter 47). Agents known to cause renal or bladder complications include cisplatin, ifosfamide, and cyclophosphamide.[83] Long-term kidney damage can occur

with other agents as well. Nurses must be aware of these complications and should monitor the patient for signs of bladder toxicity such as hemorrhagic cystitis after cyclophosphamide therapy. Renal function should be evaluated by obtaining serum chemistry determinations on each return visit. Children who have undergone bone marrow transplantation have the potential for developing long-term pulmonary toxicities and must be evaluated periodically for signs and symptoms or respiratory compromise.[83] These individuals should avoid tobacco products after transplantation and be treated aggressively for respiratory illnesses. The nurse should assess the patient for symptoms such as dyspnea, shortness of breath, cough, or fever. Chest radiographs and pulmonary function tests should be performed routinely in these individuals. Several agents, such as methotrexate, chlorambucil, 6-mercaptopurine, daunomycin, and doxorubicin, are associated with long-term liver toxicity.[86] Nurses must be aware of the potential for development of hepatitis, hepatic fibrosis, and cirrhosis in these patients. Gastrointestinal toxicities are most frequently caused by combined chemotherapy and radiation therapy. Signs and symptoms include abdominal pain, nausea, vomiting, diarrhea, constipation, and gastrointestinal bleeding. Bone growth is usually not affected by chemotherapy alone; however, prolonged use of methotrexate and corticosteroid may cause osteoporosis, bone pain, and increased susceptibility to fractures.[86] Nurses must be comprehensive in their assessment for musculoskeletal complications in children after treatment of cancer.

Nurses caring for survivors of cancer who received cranial irradiation and intrathecal methotrexate at a young age must be aware of the possible neurocognitive late effects associated with this treatment. Intellectual and motor function may be impaired because of interference with neural development before maturation of the brain is complete. Memory loss may occur in children receiving high doses of irradiation. Children younger than 3 years are at the highest risk of this complication.[85,87] Assessment of these children must include an extensive neurologic evaluation that includes cognitive function. Nurses should assess school attendance and performance because problems with mathematics and reading may occur.[87]

Radiation therapy can cause bone growth to cease and can decrease the function of reproductive glands responsible for manufacturing growth hormones.[88,89] Nurses must document growth by assessing height and weight at each visit. Changes in growth velocity should be referred for further evaluation. Further assessment must include measuring parental heights, obtaining a radiograph of the patient's left wrist to predict further growth potential, and assessing gonadal development and pituitary function. An endocrinologist should be consulted when abnormalities are found or are suspected.

Knowledge of the effects of radiation therapy and alkylating agents on hormonal function, fertility, and sterility is important for the nurse caring for the cancer survivor. The potential for gonadal dysfunction depends on the child's age at the time of diagnosis, the child's sex, the type of treatment, and the duration and total dose of treatment.[89,90] Nursing assessment must include careful documentation of sexual development using the Tanner staging scale and a detailed history.

Survivors who have undergone radiation therapy to developing bone or cartilage need close observation of the irradiated bone to detect abnormalities such as spinal kyphosis or scoliosis, leg-length discrepancy, and skull or facial disfigurement. Because irradiated bones are more fragile, the survivor is at risk for bone fractures, often has functional limitations, and heals more slowly in the presence of infection.[88] Osteoporosis may develop. Children who have received irradiation to the mandibular area are at risk for dental caries, arrested tooth development, and incomplete dental calcification.

A complete assessment of the oral cavity at every clinic visit is essential in children who have received irradiation to the mandible.

PROFESSIONAL DEVELOPMENT

Pediatric oncology nurses must continue to pursue ways to maintain their professional competence. Participation in professional organizations such as the Association of Pediatric Hematology Oncology Nurses (APHON) ensures ongoing involvement in continuing education, professional development, and research. Pediatric hematology oncology nursing certification is now available through Oncology Nursing Certification Corporation. Nurses who successfully pursue certification in pediatric oncology demonstrate a commitment to the specialty and obtain the credentials associated with specialization. Pediatric oncology nurses must continue to be committed to their colleagues as well as to the ongoing development of collaborative relationships. Through these relationships, the role of the nurse in pediatric oncology can be realized.

References

1. Hockenberry M, Wilson D, eds. Nursing care of infants and children. 8th ed. St. Louis, MO: Mosby, 2007.
2. Kline NE, Hobbie WL, Hooke MC, et al., eds. Essentials of pediatric hematology oncology nursing: a core curriculum. 3rd ed. Glenview, IL: AMC, 2007.
3. Buell L. The gift of nursing. Pediatr Nurs 2008;34:477–479.
4. Hamric A, Spross J, Hanson J. Advanced nursing practice: an integrative approach. 4th ed. Philadelphia, PA: Saunders, 2008.
5. Hare ML, Hinds PS. Moving the research agenda forward for children and adolescents with cancer. J Pediatr Oncol Nurs 2004;21:121–122.
6. Woodgate RL. Feeling states: a new approach to understanding how children and adolescent with cancer experience symptoms. Cancer Nurs 2008;3:229–238.
7. Bayat M, Erdem E, Gul Kuzucu E. Depression, anxiety, hopelessness, and social support levels of the parents of children with cancer. J Pediatr Oncol Nurs 2008;25:247–253.
8. Huang IC, Mu PF, Chiou TM. Parental experience of family resources in single-parent families having a child with cancer. J Clin Nurs 2008;17:2741–2749.
9. Tomlinson D, Gibson F, Treister N, et al. Challenges of mucositis assessment in children: expert opinion. Eur J Oncol Nurs 2008;12:469–475.
10. Horvath B, Norville R, Lee D, et al. Reducing central venous catheter-related bloodstream infections in children with cancer. Oncol Nurs Forum 2009;36:232–238.
11. Eilertsen ME, Reinfjell T, Vik T. Value of professional collaboration in the care of children with cancer and their families. Eur J Cancer Care 2004;12:349–355.
12. Eilertsen ME, Kristiansen K, Reinfjell T, et al. Professional collaboration-support for children with cancer and their families. J Interprof Care 2009;29:1–14.
13. Klassen AF, Klaasen R, Dix D, et al. Impact of caring for a child with cancer on parents' health-related quality of life. J Clin Oncol 2008;26:5884–5889.
14. Nelson MB, Forte K, Freiburg D, et al. Pediatric oncology nursing: scope and standards of practice. Glenview, IL: Association of Pediatric Hematology/Oncology Nurses, 2007.
15. Woodgate RL, Degner LF. Cancer symptom transition periods of children and families. J Adv Nurs 2004;46:358–368.
16. Hedstrom M, Haglund K, Skolin I, et al. Distressing events for children and adolescents with cancer: child, parent, and nurse perceptions. J Pediatr Oncol Nurs 2003;20:120–132.
17. Woodgate RL, Degner LF. Expectations and beliefs about children's cancer symptoms: perspective of children with and their families. Oncol Nurs Forum 2003;30:479–491.
18. Collins JJ, Byrnes MM, Dunkel IJ, et al. The measurement of symptoms in children with cancer. J Pain Symptom Manage 2000;19:363–373.
19. Docherty SL. Symptom experiences of children and adolescents with cancer. Annu Rev Nurs Res 2003;21:123–149.
20. Rheingans JI. Pediatric oncology nurses' management of patients' symptoms. J Pediatr Oncol Nurs 2008;25:303–311.
21. Barbacane JL. Back to the basics: handwashing. Geriat Nurs 2004;25:90–92.
22. Smith MJ. Catheter-related bloodstream infection in children. Am J Infect Control 2008;36:S173.e1–S173.e3.
23. Levine JE, Boxer LA. Clinical application of hematopoietic growth factors in pediatric oncology. Curr Opin Hematol 2002;9:222–227.
24. American Academy of Pediatrics. Red book: 2006 report of the Committee on Infectious Diseases. 27th ed. Elk Grove Village, IL: American Academy of Pediatrics, 2006.
25. Carcao MD, Lau RC, Gupta A, et al. Sequential use of intravenous and oral acyclovir in the therapy of varicella in immunocompromised children. Pediatr Infect Dis J 1998;17:626–631.
26. Schulster L, Chinn RY. Guidelines for environmental infection control in health-care facilities. Recommendations of CDC and Healthcare Infection Control Practices Advisory Committee (HICPAC). MMWR Recomm Rep 2003;52(RR-10):1–42.
27. Centers for Disease Control and Prevention. Outbreak of varicella among vaccinated children—Michigan 2003. MMWR Recomm Rep 2004;53(18):389–392.
28. Poulsen A, Demeny AK, Bang Plum C, et al. Pneumocystis carinii pneumonia during maintenance treatment of childhood acute lymphoblastic leukemia. Med Pediatr Oncol 2001;37:20–23.
29. Shankar SM, Nania JJ. Management of pneumocystis jiroveci pneumonia in children receiving chemotherapy. Paediatr Drugs 2007;9:301–309.
30. Kim SY, Dabb AA, Glenn DJ, et al. Intravenous pentamidine is effective as second line Pneumocystis pneumonia prophylaxis in pediatric oncology patients. Pediatr Blood Cancer 2008;50:779–783.
31. Wazny LD, Ariano RE. Evaluation and management of drug-induced thrombocytopenia in the acutely ill patient. Pharmacotherapy 2000;20:292–307.
32. Pruss A, Kalus U, Radtke H, et al. Universal leukodepletion of blood components results in a significant reduction of febrile non-hemolytic but not allergic transfusion reactions. Transfus Apheresis Sci 2004;30:41–46.
33. Enright H, Davis K, Gernsheimer T, et al. Factors influencing moderate to severe reactions to platelet transfusions: experience of the TRAP multicenter clinical trial. Transfusion 2003;43:1545–1552.
34. Grass JA, Wafa T, Reames A, et al. Prevention of transfusion-associated graft-versus-host disease by photochemical treatment. Blood 1999;93:3140–3147.
35. James V. Bloody easy: blood transfusions, blood alternatives and transfusion reactions—a guide to transfusion medicine. Transfus Med 2004;14:193–194.
36. Herberg A. Blood product administration. In: Bowden VR, Smith Greenberg C, eds. Pediatric nursing procedures. Philadelphia, PA: Lippincott Williams & Wilkins, 2003: 122–132.
37. Bryant R. Managing side effects of childhood cancer treatment. J Pediatr Nurs 2003;18:113–125.
38. Langdana A, Tully N, Molloy E, et al. Intensive enteral nutrition support in paediatric bone marrow transplantation. Bone Marrow Transplant 2001;27:741–746.
39. Pietsch JB, Ford C, Whitlock JA. Nasogastric tube feedings in children with high-risk cancer: a pilot study. J Pediatr Hematol Oncol 1999;21:111–114.
40. DeSwarte-Wallace J, Firouzbakhsh S, Finklestein JZ. Using research to change practice: enteral feedings for pediatric oncology patients. J Pediatr Oncol Nurs 2001;18:217–223.
41. Muscaritoli M, Grieco G, Capria S, et al. Nutritional and metabolic support in patients undergoing bone marrow transplantation. Am J Clin Nutr 2002;75:183–190.
42. Rodgers C, Walsh T. Nutritional issues in adolescents after bone marrow transplant: a literature review. J Pedatr Oncol Nurs 2008;25:254–264.
43. Skolin I, Ulla-Kaisa KH, Wahlin YB. Parents' perception of their child's food intake after the start of chemotherapy. J Pediatr Oncol Nurs 2001;18:124–136.
44. Naeim A, Dy SM, Lorenz KA, et al. Evidence-based recommendations for cancer nausea and vomiting. J Clin Oncol 2008;26:3903–3909.
45. Rubenstein EB, Peterson DE, Schubert M, et al. Mucositis Study Section of the Multinational Association for Supportive Care in Cancer; International Society for Oral Oncology. Clinical practice guidelines for the prevention and treatment of cancer therapy-induced oral and gastrointestinal mucositis. Cancer 2004;100(9 suppl):2026–2046.
46. El-Housseiny AA, Saleh SM, Ei-Masry AA, et al. Assessment or oral complications in children receiving chemotherapy. J Clin Pedatr Dent 2007;31:267–273.
47. Eilers J, Epstein JB. Assessment and measurement of oral mucositis. Semin Oncol Nurs 2004;20:22–29.
48. Tomlin D, Juddd P, Hendershot E, et al. Establishing literature-based items for an oral mucositis assessment tool in children. J Pediatr Oncol Nurs 2008;25:139–147.
49. Hockenberry-Eaton M, Hinds PS, Alcoser P, et al. Fatigue in children and adolescents with cancer. J Pediatr Oncol Nurs 1998;15:172–182.
50. Hinds PS, Hockenberry-Eaton M, Quargnenti A, et al. Fatigue in 7- to 12-year-old patients with cancer from the staff perspective: an exploratory study. Oncol Nurs Forum 1999;26:37–45.
51. Hockenberry MJ, Hinds PS, Barrera P, et al. Three instruments to assess fatigue in children with cancer: the child, parent and staff perspectives. J Pain Symptom Manage 2003;25:319–328.
52. Davies B, Whitsett SF, Bruce A, et al. A typology of fatigue in children with cancer. J Pediatr Oncol Nurs 2002;19:12–21.
53. Perdikaris P, Merkouris A, Patiraki E, et al. Changes in children's fatigue during the course of treatment for paediatric cancer. Int Nurs Rev 2008;55:412–419.
54. Varni JW, Burwinkle TM, Katz ER, et al. The PedsQL in pediatric cancer: reliability and validity of the Pediatric Quality of Life Inventory Generic Core Scales, Multidimensional Fatigue Scale, and Cancer Module. Cancer 2002;94:2090–2106.
55. Hockenberry MJ, Hooke MC, Gegurich MA, et al. Symptoms clusters in children/adolescents receiving cisplatin, doxorubicin, or ifosamide chemotherapy. Oncol Nurs Forum 2010;37(1):E16–27.
56. Peluso PJ, Nicolai R, Reda E, et al. Cancer and anticancer therapy-induced modifications on metabolism mediated by carnitine system. J Cell Physiol 2000;182:339–350.
57. Yaris N, Akyuz C, Coskun T, et al. Serums carnitine levels of pediatric cancer patients. Pediatr Hematol Oncol 2002;19(1):1–8.
58. Graziano F, Bisonni R, Catalano V, et al. Potential role of levocarnitine supplementation for the treatment of chemotherapy-induced fatigue in non-anaemic cancer patients. Br J Cancer 2002;86:1854–1857.
59. Hockenberry MJ, Hooke MC, Gegurich MA, et al. Carnitine plasma levels and fatigue in children/adolescents receiving cisplatin, ifosfamide or doxorubicin. J Pediatr Hematol Oncol 2009;31(9):664–669.
60. Christo PJ, Mazloomdoost D. Cancer pain and analgesia. Ann N Y Acad Sci 2008;1138:278.
61. Subhashini L, Vatsa M, Lodha R. Knowledge, attitude and practices among health care professionals regarding pain in children [published online ahead of print May 27, 2009]. Indian J Pediatr 2009;76(9):913–916.
62. Simons J, Moseley L. Influences on nurses' scoring of children's post-operative pain. J Child Health Care 2009;13(2):101.
63. Piaget J. The theory of stages in cognitive development. New York: McGraw-Hill, 1969.
64. Maclaren JE, Cohen LL. Interventions for paediatric procedure-related pain in primary care. Paediatr Child Health 2007;12(2):111.
65. Finley GA, Kristjánsdóttir O, Forgeron PA. Cultural influences on the assessment of children's pain. Pain Res Manag 2009;14(1):33.

66. Silva FCD, Thuler LCS. Cross-cultural adaptation and translation of two pain assessment tools in children and adolescents. JPediatr (Rio J). 2008;84(4):344.

67. Cohen LL. Behavioral approaches to anxiety and pain management for pediatric venous access. Pediatrics 2008;122(suppl 3):S134.

68. Kennedy RM, Luhmann J, Zempsky WT. Clinical implications of unmanaged needle-insertion pain and distress in children. Pediatrics 2008;122(suppl 3):S130.

69. American Pain Society. Guideline for the management of cancer pain in adults and children. Glenview: IL. AMC, 2005.

70. Zempsky WT. Pharmacologic approaches for reducing venous access pain in children. Pediatrics 2008;122(suppl 3):S140.

71. Sexton S, Natale R. Risks and benefits of pacifiers. Am Fam Physician 2009;79(8):681.

72. Murphy G. Distraction techniques for venepuncture: a review. Paediatr Nurs 2009;21 (3):18.

73. Liossi C, White P, Hatira P. A randomized clinical trial of a brief hypnosis intervention to control venepuncture-related pain of paediatric cancer patients. Pain 2009;142(3):255.

74. Ripamonti C, Bandieri E. Pain therapy. Crit Rev Oncol Hematol 2009;70(2):145.

75. Zernikow B, Michel E, Craig F, et al. Pediatric palliative care: use of opioids for the management of pain. Paediatr Drugs 2009;11(2):129.

76. Conway M, White N, Jean CS, et al. Use of continuous intravenous ketamine for end-stage cancer pain in children. J Pediatr Oncol Nurs 2009;26(2):100.

77. Gallieni M, Pittiruti M, Biffi R. Vascular access in oncology patients. CA Cancer J Clin 2008;58(6):323.

78. Pittiruti M, Hamilton H, Biffi R, et al; ESPEN. ESPEN guidelines on parenteral nutrition: central venous catheters (access, care, diagnosis and therapy of complications) [published online ahead of print May 21 2009]. Clin Nutr 2009;28(4):365–377.

79. Larson EL, Quiros D, Lin SX. Dissemination of the CDC's hand hygiene guideline and impact on infection rates. Am J Infect Control 2007;35(10):666.

80. Kline NE, Echtenkamp DS, Rae-Zahradnik ML, et al., eds. The pediatric chemotherapy and biotherapy curriculum. 2nd ed. Glenview, IL: AMC, 2007.

81. Lashlee M, O'hanlon Curry J. Pediatric home chemotherapy: infusing "quality of life". J Pediatr Oncol Nurs 2007;24(5):294.

82. Filin A, Treisman S, Peles Bortz A. Radiation therapy preparation by a multidisciplinary team for childhood cancer patients aged 31/2 to 6 years. J Pediatr Oncol Nurs 2009; 26(2):81.

83. Diller L, Chow EJ, Gurney JG, et al. Chronic disease in the childhood cancer survivor study cohort: a review of published findings. J Clin Oncol 2009;27(14):2339.

84. Kavey RW, Allada V, Daniels SR, et al. Cardiovascular risk reduction in high-risk pediatric patients: a scientific statement from the American Heart Association expert panel on population and prevention science the councils on cardiovascular disease in the young, epidemiology and prevention, nutrition, physical activity and metabolism, high blood pressure research, cardiovascular nursing, and the kidney in heart disease and the interdisciplinary working group on quality of care and outcomes research. J Cardiovasc Nurs 2007;22(3):218.

85. Mulhern RK, Palmer SL, Merchant TE, et al. Neurocognitive consequences of risk-adapted therapy for childhood medulloblastoma. J Clin Oncol 2005;23(24):5511.

86. Tonorezos ES, Oeffinger KC. Survivorship after childhood, adolescent, and young adult cancer. Cancer J 2008;14(6):388.

87. Nathan PC, Patel SK, Dilley K, et al. Guidelines for identification of, advocacy for, and intervention in neurocognitive problems in survivors of childhood cancer: a report from the children's oncology group. Arch Pediatr Adolesc Med 2007;161(8):798.

88. Lipman TH, Hench KD, Benyi T, et al. A multicentre randomised controlled trial of an intervention to improve the accuracy of linear growth measurement. Arch Dis Child 2004;89(4):342.

89. Cohen LE. Endocrine late effects of cancer treatment. Endocrinol Metab Clin North Am 2005;34(3):769.

90. Laughton SJ, Merchant TE, Sklar CA, et al. Endocrine outcomes for children with embryonal brain tumors after risk-adapted craniospinal and conformal primary-site irradiation and high-dose chemotherapy with stem-cell rescue on the SJMB-96 trial. J Clin Oncol 2008;26(7):1112.

91. Koh JL, Harrison D, Myers R, et al. A randomized, double-blind comparison study of EMLA and ELA-max for topical anesthesia in children undergoing intravenous insertion. Pediatr Anaesth 2004;14(12):977.

CHAPTER 44 ■ REHABILITATION OF THE CHILD WITH CANCER

DAVID W. PRUITT, MARY A. MCMAHON, STEPHANIE R. RIED,
SUSAN D. APKON, AND LINDA J. MICHAUD

The comprehensive rehabilitation of children with cancer requires an interdisciplinary team approach across the continuum of care. Extraordinary improvement in survival of children with a wide variety of cancer types is the result of advances in treatment previously discussed in this text. Accompanying this success are new challenges resulting from morbidity in the survivors, due to the cancer itself or its interventions. Physical, psychological, and social function may be affected. Minimizing the consequences of these sequelae on future quality of life is the overall goal of rehabilitation.

The process of general cancer rehabilitation can be grouped into one of four broad categories, often referred to as the Dietz classification.[1] *Preventative rehabilitation* emphasizes early intervention and education in order to prevent or delay the symptoms of tumor progression or treatment.[2] Interventions might include range of motion in order to maintain joint flexibility in a spastic extremity or prophylaxis for deep venous thrombosis in inpatient rehabilitation. *Restorative rehabilitation* attempts to assist patients return to their premorbid functional status without substantial residual disability. *Supportive rehabilitation* occurs in those patients who sustain permanent, residual impairments as a result of their cancer or its treatment and focuses on maximizing functional independence in an optimal environment. *Palliative rehabilitation* is utilized in those patients with a recurrent or progressive cancer and focuses primarily on comfort, caregiver education, minimizing burden of care, and appropriate equipment recommendations.[3]

The focus in rehabilitation is typically on disability management. Dimensions of disablement and functioning include *impairment, activity,* and *participation.*[4] *Impairment* refers to the loss or abnormality of psychological, physical, or anatomic structure or function, and it is at the *organ* system level of function. Specific impairments, in this case different types of cancer, may have an impact on the child's age-appropriate activity, affecting mobility, self-care, communication, cognition, and/or psychological and social function (Table 44.1). *Disability* is the *limitation in activity,* in the manner or within the range considered normal, due to impairment. The same impairment may or may not result in activity limitations in different children. *Handicap* exists when an impairment or disability *restricts participation* in a role that is normal for age and gender within the social and cultural milieu. Participation restrictions are external to the individual, such as those imposed by architectural or attitudinal barriers.

Goals of pediatric disability management include minimizing the impairment and maximizing activity and participation in age-appropriate life roles: school, play and recreation, and work. Major objectives include facilitating independent child function in each area of functioning, or domain, that is affected, and also minimizing the burden of disability for the parents and caregivers. Function is promoted in mobility, self-care, communication, cognition, and/or psychosocial domains. Efforts are directed toward achieving maximum independence despite the disorder, primarily through six categories of intervention strategies to help mitigate disability.[5] These include: preventing or correcting additional secondary disability; enhancing function in the affected system; enhancing function in systems unaffected; using adaptive equipment to promote function; modifying the social and vocational environment; and using psychological techniques to enhance patient performance and patient/family education. In pediatric rehabilitation, prescriptions for therapy programs, adaptive equipment, orthoses, and prostheses must be appropriate to the age and developmental level of the child and include considerations related to ongoing growth and development.[6,7]

The interdisciplinary pediatric rehabilitation team evaluating and addressing individualized goals for the child with disability can include one or more of the following specialists: pediatric physiatrist (specialist in physical medicine and rehabilitation), rehabilitation nurse, physical therapist, occupational therapist, speech-language pathologist, psychologist, social worker, therapeutic recreation specialist, prosthetist-orthotist, special educator, and vocational counselor. Care should be coordinated, comprehensive, and family-centered.

Significant functional gains follow rehabilitation of adult patients with cancer.[8–10] While similar evidence has not been directly evaluated for rehabilitation of children with cancer, extrapolation from adults with cancer and from children with other disabling conditions support provision of pediatric rehabilitative services to children with cancer.

In the first section of this chapter, the focus is on the common issues of limitations in activity and restrictions in participation that cross malignancies involving different organ systems. The second section focuses on specific functional limitations associated with the major specific types of pediatric cancer that result in a significant incidence of disability.

I. REHABILITATION PROBLEMS

Mobility

Deficits in functional mobility may occur with the generalized deconditioning associated with prolonged or chronic illness and immobility, which is discussed in further detail in the next section of this chapter, as it is such a significant issue in the population of children with cancer. Due either to the tumor or its treatments, central neurologic involvement of the motor strip, long tracts, basal ganglia, cerebellum, or spinal cord, or peripheral neurologic involvement can result in problems in motor function due to weakness or paralysis,

TABLE 44.1

IMPACT OF ANTICANCER THERAPIES ON FUNCTION

Treatment	Pathophysiology	Impairment	Disability	Qualifiers
Surgical resection	Unclear	Deficits dependent on location and extent of surgery, age, and tumor type	Functional limitations related to areas of deficit	
Posterior fossa surgery	Unclear	Cerebellar mutism; may see high-level linguistic and cognitive deficits	Limited verbal communication, may affect social skills and school performance	
Cranial irradiation	Neural/glial degeneration Gliosis Proliferative/sclerosing angiopathy Demyelination	Cognitive dysfunction learning disabilities ↓ memory attention problems Language deficits ↓ executive function ↓ verbal and performance IQ	↓ academic potential ↓ communication skills to language disorder/delay may impact behavior, social competence, and vocational potential	Impact related to dose and volume of CNS irradiated and inversely related to age of child at time of exposure. Effects potentiated by IT* or high-dose intravenous methotrexate
	Ischemic events related to cerebral vasculopathy		Functional deficits related to location and extent of ischemia	Rehabilitation managed as in stroke
	Progressive, necrotizing leukoencephalopathy		Potential for marked functional impairments in all affected areas, including dementia, dysarthria, ataxia and/or spasticity	Usually seen when treatment has included methotrexate
	Negative impact on GHRH* when posterior fossa involved	Short stature	May affect self-image, social competence	Cosmesis included in problem list for adolescents
Spinal irradiation	May cause radiation myelitis	Spastic quadriplegia or paraplegia	Functional impairments in mobility and ADLs dependent on level of injury	
		Neurogenic bowel and bladder	May require special program for evacuation of bladder and bowel	Management as in spinal cord injury
	Failure of vertebral growth	Short stature, ↑ risk of scoliosis or kyphosis	Potential altered self-image and ↓ social competence	Cosmesis of particular psychosocial impact for adolescents
Mediastinal irradiation	Vascular damage, fibrosis	Pulmonary fibrosis Pneumonitis	Disability dependent on degree of restrictive lung changes and can significantly limit ADLs, exercise tolerance when severe	Decrease in radiation-induced late pulmonary toxicity seen over last decade due to refinements in radiation therapy
	In very young, possible interference with both lung and chest wall growth	Decreases in lung volume, compliance, and CO_2 diffusing capacity		
	Fibrosis of the parietal pericardium (most common), intimal proliferation of myofibroblasts, collagen and lipid accumulation	Constrictive pericarditis, myocardial damage (rare), conduction system defects, coronary artery disease	Functional limitations related to degree of cardiac dysfunction	
Methotrexate	Neurotoxicity including acute, stroke-like encephalopathy, chronic leukoen-cephalopathy (progressive demyelinating encephalopathy)	Cognitive impairment, developmental delay, learning problems, potential motor impairment with deficits in coordination and high-level skills With intrathecal dosing, can see ascending radiculopathy, similar to GBS	May affect school performance, ↓ age-appropriate ADL independence, may limit participation in athletics, team sports, impact self-esteem and social competence Loss of motor function with consequent mobility and ADL deficits dependent on extent of weakness	Neurotoxicity potentiated by cranial irradiation Alert parents to monitor for school problems developing in upper grades when ↑ independence and efficiency required

(continued)

TABLE 44.1

CONTINUED

Treatment	Pathophysiology	Impairment	Disability	Qualifiers
Methotrexate (cont.)	Osteopathy	Osteoporosis/↑ risk of pathologic fractures, bone pain	Limitations in mobility and ADLs related to areas involved	Toxicity cumulative
Corticosteroids	Preferential atrophy of type II muscle fibers	Myopathy	Decreased mobility related to proximal muscle weakness	Reversible when drug withdrawn or dose reduced
		Osteoporosis	↑ risk of pathologic fracture	↑ risk for osteonecrosis of weight-bearing joints in children when ↑ doses used
		Avascular necrosis	Hip pain, gait abnormality	
		Growth failure	Impacts self-esteem and social competence	
Vincristine/ Vinblastine	Axonal sensorimotor polyneuropathy		Paresthesias, neuritic pain, distal weakness which may impair hand function, cause foot drop and walking difficulty	Neurotoxicity more prominent in presence of CMT
	Impairment of efferent and afferent pathways from the sacral spinal cord, autonomic neuropathy	Impaired rectal emptying	Constipation which may alter ADLs, comfort	Usually recovers with end of therapy or ↓ dose
				Neurotoxicity usually minimal with vinblastine
Anthracycline (doxorubicin, daunorubicin)		Can cause arrhythmias, conduction abnormalities, ↓ left ventricular function, chronic cardiomyopathy	Diminished capacity to perform age-appropriate ADLs, ↓ endurance, ↓ exercise tolerance, limited ability to participate in sports, may impact self esteem and social competence	Potentiates radiation reactions Increased toxicity with lower age
Cisplatin	Injury to hair cells of the organ of Corti	High-frequency sensorineural hearing loss Tinnitus	Affects communication skills and potentially speech/ language development in the young child; may impact social competence	Ototoxic and neurotoxic effects are cumulative
		Reversible sensory peripheral neuropathy	Paresthesias/neuritic pain may interfere with ADLs, comfort	Symptoms may progress after discontinuation
Carboplatin	Minor or absent loss of hair cells of the organ of Corti	High-frequency sensorineural hearing loss	Affects communication skills and potentially speech/ language development in the young child; may impact social competence	Effects are cumulative Ototoxicity & neurotoxicity milder than cisplatin
Cyclophosphamide/ Ifosfamide		Reversible neurotoxicity with somnolence, disorientation, lethargy, hallucinations	Negative impact on ability to perform age-appropriate ADLs	Risk of neurotoxicity ↑ with prior use of high dose cisplatin. Reversible or preventable with methylene blue.
		Avascular necrosis	Pain may limit ADLs, ambulation	
	Can cause hemorrhagic cystitis secondary to urotoxic metabolite acrolein	Potential loss of renal function		Occurrence decreased by use of MESNA

GHRH, growth hormone releasing hormone; IT, intrathecal; ADLs, activities of daily living; GBS, Guillain-Barrè Syndrome; CMT, Charcot-Marie-Tooth Disease; IQ, intelligence quotient; CNS, central nervous system; IT, intrathecal; ↑, increased; ↓, decreased.

spasticity, and/or deficits in balance and coordination, often associated with limited endurance. The physical and occupational therapists work with the child and family to ameliorate specific motor deficits, prevent secondary complications such as contractures, provide training in compensatory strategies, limit use of abnormal movement patterns, and recommend use of orthotic and assistive devices as appropriate.

Progression of ambulation retraining may involve use of gait aids, often beginning with those providing more support, such as a walker, and weaning to crutches and possibly to canes before independence is reestablished. Bracing, most typically with ankle-foot-orthoses (AFOs), may be indicated. Design of the AFO is determined by multiple factors, including ankle strength, range of motion, presence of spasticity, and medial-lateral ankle stability. Alternative means of mobility to ambulation may be indicated, temporarily or permanently, for some children with a variety of types of cancer. Some may require a manual wheelchair; however, others may benefit from power wheelchair use for independence in mobility.

As endurance improves, intensity of exercise regimens can be increased. Exercise programs for children in the acute phase of their management may initially focus on passive range of motion to maintain joint flexibility. As the child is able, active participation is progressively increased, with particular activities selected to focus on the child's specific individualized therapy goals, which are advanced as possible. Participation in sports and recreational activities should be encouraged, whenever possible. Aquatic therapy often allows movement, due to buoyancy and elimination of gravity, which is not possible out of the water. Again, progression can occur, as the child is able, often to the level of competitive sports participation in the longterm.

Immobility

Prolonged bed rest and immobility affect almost every organ system and can negatively impact a child's functional capacity. Muscle strength and endurance decrease due to the inactivity and reduced force of gravity associated with bed rest. With complete bed rest, a muscle loses 1.0% to 1.5% of its strength per day or 10% to 15% per week.[11] Immobilized muscles have also been shown to have a more rapid depletion of glycogen and an increased production of lactic acid during work.[12] Muscles immobilized in a shortened position are also at risk for contracture, associated with segmental necrosis, disorganization of myofibrils, and a reduction in the number of sarcomeres.[13] Connective tissue contracts and reorganizes within 1 week of a joint becoming immobile, further increasing the risk for contracture development. Inactivity also results in increased bone resorption that may result in osteoporosis and risk for pathological fractures.[14]

Immobilization also has significant effects on the cardiovascular system. Increased sympathetic activity leads to an increased heart rate.[15] Cardiac output, stroke volume, and left ventricular function decline and orthostatic hypotension increases.[16] A decrease in cardiac output combined with a peripheral oxygen utilization deficiency causes a decline in maximal oxygen consumption.[17] Blood volume decreases with prolonged bed rest. Plasma volume decreases more than red cell mass resulting in increased blood viscosity.[17] Increased blood viscosity combined with immobility places the patient at increased risk for deep venous thrombosis.

Respiratory complications of immobility can be life threatening. Potential changes include diminished diaphragmatic movement in the supine position, decreased chest excursion, and decreased range of motion of the costovertebral and costochondral joints. These changes can result in a decrease in the vital capacity and functional reserve capacity of 25% to 50%.[17] The ventilation-to-perfusion ratio may be altered in dependent areas of the lung, resulting in arteriovenous shunting and reduced oxygenation.[18] Impaired ability to clear secretions can lead to atelectasis and increased risk for pneumonia.

Immobility can also negatively affect metabolism and the endocrine system. A decrease in total body sodium is associated with diuresis during early bed rest. Potassium levels also decrease during the early stages of immobility.[17] Serious electrolyte abnormalities, however, rarely occur with the exception of hypercalcemia, most commonly seen in patients with high bone turnover, such as children and adolescents.[18] Glucose intolerance and nitrogen loss due to an increase in protein catabolism are also not uncommon in immobilized patients.[18]

Pressure ulcers are another complication of immobility that can occur when external pressure is greater than capillary pressure for prolonged periods. Poor nutrition, moisture, insensate skin, and shear forces are additional risk factors for skin breakdown. Supine patients are at risk for pressure ulcers over their occiput, sacrum, and heels. Patients lying on their sides are at risk for breakdown over their greater trochanters and patients who sit for prolonged periods are at risk for ulcers over their ischial tuberosities.

Activities of Daily Living

All members of the rehabilitation team, but specifically the occupational therapist, work with the child to increase independence in age-appropriate daily care activities such as eating, grooming, bathing, toileting, and play, with use of adaptive equipment as needed. Bladder and bowel dysfunction, in particular, pose common special management challenges and so are discussed in detail. Family education is provided and family members are encouraged to allow the child to function at the highest level of independence at which he or she is capable.

Bladder Dysfunction

Various combinations of urinary storage and voiding impairment may occur with tumors along the neural axis from the pons to the cauda equina, due to lower urinary tract dysfunction. Incontinence with lesions above the level of the pons is usually due to disinhibition. Neural pathways that modulate bladder function traverse the length of the spinal cord between the pons and the sacral spinal cord, with events coordinated in the pontine micturition center. Interruption of these pathways result in storage or voiding dysfunction or detrusor-sphincter dyssynergia (DSD), when there is loss of the coordinated function of the detrusor and the external striated urethral sphincter. Lesions at the level of the pons may also impair the coordinated functioning of the lower urinary tract. As seen in spinal cord lesions, manifestations are usually upper motor neuron in nature with involuntary detrusor contractions, non-relaxation of the external sphincter during detrusor contractions, and subsequent development of bladder wall thickening, trabeculations, and decreased compliance and storage capacity due to detrusor hyperactivity. Fluorourodynamics is the most informative study to evaluate children with neuropathic vesicourethral dysfunction. This study superimposes pressure measurements on the simultaneous fluoroscopic appearance of the bladder and urethra and provides valuable information on the function of the bladder and urethra during filling and voiding. Clean intermittent catheterization is an effective method of bladder emptying and may be used alone or in combination with anticholinergic or alpha-adrenergic medications to protect the upper tracts while achieving satisfactory continence. Fluid intake should be regulated so that only 4 to 5 catheterizations are necessary to not exceed the bladder capacity (age [years] + 2 = ounces).[19] If high volume of fluid is necessary due to the chemotherapy regimen, placement of an indwelling catheter may be necessary for short term. At 5 to 7 years of age, children with adequate hand function can begin self-catheterization.

Bowel Dysfunction

Constipation, defined as infrequent, excessively hard, and dry bowel movements, is a common problem for children with cancer. Decreased rectal filling or emptying may be due to poor intake, dehydration, decreased activity, narcotic analgesics, tumor-related neurologic injury, or neurotoxic chemotherapeutic agents. Vincristine and vinblastine are neurotoxic alkaloids, which commonly disrupt bowel function via their neuropathic effects, including peripheral neuropathy. Nonfunctional afferent and efferent pathways from the sacral cord result in impaired rectal emptying similar to that seen in neurogenic bowel due to spinal cord injury.

Management includes promoting mobility, providing appropriate positioning for the nonambulatory child, increasing dietary fiber and fluid intake, and minimizing use of medications that decrease gastrointestinal motility, if possible.

Fluid intake is critical, particularly when strategies to address the constipation include the addition of bulk to the diet. Bulk without adequate hydration increases risk of impaction. If activity is limited or ongoing administration of narcotic or neurotoxic agents is required, a stool softener or mild laxative may be given with adjustment of the dose and frequency to ensure good bowel evacuation at least every other day. The goal of a bowel program is to have the bowel empty regularly and adequately.

The child with a neurogenic bowel may require a formal bowel program with digital stimulation or a suppository, in addition, to stimulate evacuation from below. Use of digital stimulation and suppositories may have to be limited when a child is neutropenic. Alternative bowel programs may need to be utilized during those times. The presence of an anal wink indicates an upper motor neuron lesion and a better prognosis for continence, since sphincter tone is usually adequate to retain the stool. When this reflex is absent, as in lower motor neuron lesions, there may be a flaccid sphincter and inabilities to either expel or retain feces. Constant stool leakage can occur. Routine and consistency are critical to the successful bowel program, therefore a convenient, relaxed time should be selected to perform the bowel program each day and should vary as little as possible from day to day. Trying to evacuate the bowels 30 minutes after a meal will take advantage of the gastrocolic reflex.

Problems with bowel management may represent a significant source of emotional turmoil for both the child and his or her family, particularly in the older, previously continent child. Successful bowel management enhances the potential of the child to achieve age-appropriate independence and social acceptability.

Communication

Children with cancer may experience communication disorders as a consequence of their primary disease, particularly with primary brain tumors, central nervous system (CNS) metastasis, or as a late effect of cranial irradiation. Depending upon the area of the brain affected and the age of the child, communication may be impaired due to deficits in speech, language, cognition, memory, and/or personality. While speech and voice problems are related to motor dysfunction, either due to weakness of the involved structures or incoordination, language skills are more reflective of cognitive functioning (Table 44.2). For this reason, language processing may be further compromised by concomitant impairments in critical cognitive or information-processing skills, such as memory, perception, attention, or organization, as well as behavioral impairment, such as disinhibition, poor self-monitoring, limited frustration tolerance, or poor judgment.[20]

In older children with established language, the processing and use of language is usually abruptly disrupted. The pattern of speech and language deficits is dependent upon the area of

TABLE 44.2

ACQUIRED COMMUNICATION IMPAIRMENTS

Language	
Aphasia	Communication disorder caused by brain injury and characterized by complete or partial impairment of language comprehension, formulation, and use. It excludes disorders associated with primary sensory deficits, general mental retardation, or psychiatric disorders. May affect spoken or written skills. *Expressive aphasia*—primarily involves ability to produce language *Receptive aphasia*—primarily involves language comprehension skills
Pragmatics	Functional use of language in social context, e.g., use of language to interact socially, fulfill personal functions, or to regulate behavior of others
Motor speech disorders	
Apraxia	Loss of ability to carry out familiar, purposeful movements in the absence of paralysis or other motor or sensory impairment. May be limited to oral-motor movements (oral apraxia) or word production (verbal apraxia) or a combination of both. Due to difficulty with motor planning.
Aphonia	Absence or impairment of phonation due to vocal cord dysfunction
Spastic dysphonia	Difficulty controlling tone or inflection of speech due to velar or vocal cord spasticity
Dysarthria	Impaired articulation of speech due to disturbances of muscular control due to central or peripheral nervous system damage, bulbar dysfunction
Aprosodia	Lack of inflection of speech, which may be due to motor dysfunction, or related to affective dysfunction
Cerebellar mutism	A period of transient loss of speech following posterior fossa surgery due to motor speech dysfunction and evidence of concomitant high-level linguistic and cognitive deficits

the brain injury. These may be related to receptive and/or expressive language problems or motor dysfunction, including dysarthria with weakness of the oral musculature, apraxia due to motor incoordination, or phonation deficits due to velopharyngeal insufficiency or vocal cord paralysis. The child with severe expressive language deficits and good comprehension may benefit from and augmentative or alternative communication system. Pragmatics may be a problem when there is frontal or right hemisphere involvement. In the very young child, who has not yet fully developed language skills, the pattern of language dysfunction is less predictable than that seen in the older child with a similar lesion. The child may present with a developmental language disorder, secondary either to specific neurologic involvement or as a part of the global developmental delay often seen in children with serious and chronic illness early in life. There is little in the literature on the treatment-related effects or neuroplasticity in this setting and unfortunately, due to the limited former skill acquisition, these children have few compensatory strategies available to them. As language development parallels cognition, in general, factors that affect cognition will have a similar impact on language skills. Following evaluation, communication deficits may be addressed with individual and/or group within a developmental format.

Thorough speech and language assessment should be completed by the speech pathologist and a therapeutic program planned to address communication deficits in a manner appropriate to the child's age and medical condition. For the child who has lost the capacity for verbal communication, it is important to provide some form of functional communication as a means of self-expression and to indicate needs. Simple communication boards, electronic augmentative communication devices, keyboards, and sign language are among the available options.

Cognition

Cranial irradiation, as well as both intrathecal and high-dose intravenous methotrexate have long been associated with leukoencephalopathy and learning disability.[21] Also, studies have suggested that the administration of high-dose methotrexate potentiates the deleterious effects of cranial irradiation on cognition.[22] The impact on cognitive function is an often devastating late effect of cancer therapy, which significantly impacts quality of life, particularly in very young children. The age at the time of treatment is a major factor in the development of cognitive decline following cranial irradiation. Children with leukemia, lymphoma, or brain tumors treated before 4 or 5 years of age are at higher risk for cognitive impairment, in comparison to older children.[21] The deleterious effects can have major impact on intellectual and academic performance, social competence, behavior, and vocational potential. Cognitive dysfunction in children who survive brain tumors is covered later in this chapter.

Psychosocial

Issues related to psychological adjustment to chronic illness and disability, family adaptation, and sibling adjustment are critical to the long-term outcomes of children with cancer. It is crucial that comprehensive rehabilitation, in addition to directing efforts to maximize independent function in the domains discussed earlier, also addresses school reentry and eventual work entry, as well as inclusion with the family and peers in social and recreational activities. These issues are comprehensively covered elsewhere in this text.

II. SPECIFIC CHILDHOOD CANCERS: REHABILITATION ISSUES

Brain Tumors

Intracranial tumors represent the second most common type of childhood cancer, with peak incidence in early childhood.[23] Children with brain tumors experience significant functional deficits related to the primary disease process and also as a consequence of its treatment. As in adults, childhood brain tumors represent a heterogeneous group of tumors, which vary in pathologic characteristics, tumor biology, response to therapy, anatomic location, and age at diagnosis. With the advances in diagnostic strategies, neurosurgical techniques, and cooperative therapeutic trials over the past 30 years, more than 50% of children with these neoplasms are now surviving. With this improved survival has come increased recognition of the significance of the long-term sequelae of the tumor, its treatment, and the impact of consequent functional deficits on quality of life.

Each treatment modality may be associated with both transient and long-term effects, which may have an impact on duration of survival, functional outcome, and quality of life.[24] Despite the significantly decreased surgical morbidity due to improvements in surgery, anesthesia, and postoperative care, surgical resections may be associated with significant neurological morbidity related to the age and preoperative clinical status of the child, type of tumor, location, and extent of resection.[25]

Although the introduction of radiation therapy has significantly improved duration of survival in a number of CNS tumors, it is well recognized that cranial radiation has long-term effects that are progressive and potentially devastating. The extent of the radiation-induced injury is directly related to dose and volume of CNS irradiated, in addition to the age of the child. Histological changes in the brain following cranial irradiation may include neuronal dropout, gliosis, and proliferative and sclerosing angiopathy.[26] Long-term complications associated with these changes include cognitive deficits, endocrinopathies, vasculopathies, hearing loss, radiation necrosis and second primary neoplasms.[27,28] Radiation myelitis with spastic paraplegia or tetraplegia may result from spinal cord irradiation. Additionally, radiation to the vertebrae in the young child increases the risk of scoliosis and kyphosis.

The effects of chemotherapy on the developing nervous system are less well understood. Leukoencephalopathy is a late complication associated with both radiation and chemotherapy, particularly methotrexate given intrathecally or in high-dose intravenously. It is characterized clinically by dementia, ataxia, and focal motor deficits, and it can progress to coma and death. Other delayed toxic effects of chemotherapy that impact significantly on function include peripheral neuropathies, myopathies, and hearing loss.

Children with brain tumors may experience a wide range of functional deficits related to the effects of the primary lesion or treatment complications. These include motor and sensory deficits, speech and language dysfunction, cognitive impairment, and psycho-emotional disorders. The nature and extent of impairment depends upon the age and developmental level of the child at time of diagnosis, the location of the lesion, and the degree of neurologic compromise. With the exception of cognition, there is a paucity of information related to rehabilitation issues in the literature. The basic tenets of neurorehabilitation are heavily impairment-driven, with the goal to maximize function and minimize caregiver and societal burden for all etiologies of acquired brain injuries

(ABI).[29] Common impairments in persons with brain tumors undergoing rehabilitation include weakness (hemiparesis and general debility), cognitive and visual-perceptive deficits, ataxia, cranial nerve dysfunction, bowel and bladder problems, aphasia, dysphagia, and dysarthria.[30,31] Overlapping impairment profiles suggest that the rehabilitation team can approach brain tumor survivors much like more familiar etiologies of ABI.[29] Creating a rehabilitation program for optimization of functional independence necessitates identification of appropriate goals and phases of rehabilitation care as well as clear communication of realistic goals to the patient and family.

Children with brain tumors may require acute inpatient rehabilitation, outpatient rehabilitation, or home-based therapy. Often, children are admitted to the inpatient rehabilitation unit following craniotomy for gross total resection, surgical debulking or biopsy and they sustain impairments and disabilities as a result of the tumor or side effects of treatment. An inpatient pediatric rehabilitation environment assists in optimizing a therapeutic schedule and environment, typically including therapeutic services for 3 or more hours per day. A functional neurologic examination by the team at the time of admission assesses strength, coordination, reflexes, muscle tone, sensation and levels of independence with mobility, activities of daily living, communication, and cognition. The clinician should consider how impairments in multiple areas (musculoskeletal, neurologic, mood, cognitive, visual, and vestibular) collectively affect limitations in activity and participation.[29] Impairment-specific tests may assist in providing objective assessments in outlining and developing a plan of care. Currently, there are no objective measurements for functional assessments specific to pediatric brain tumors, so measurements for other ABI are utilized when needed (i.e., Romberg Test, Childhood Orientation and Amnesia Test). Once evaluations are completed, the team formulates and communicates the rehabilitation plan of care on the basis of the goals identified by the team, family, and patient. Integral to this formulation is identifying appropriate Dietz category and assuring that the goals are realistically well defined, consider the prognosis, and involve the caregiver.[29]

Rehabilitation strategies utilized in other ABI are also employed in the rehabilitation care of children with impairments and disabilities as a result of a brain tumor and its treatments. Constraint-induced motor therapy (CIMT); partial weight-supported ambulation; functional electrical stimulation; spasticity management; and cognitive, visual, and vestibular rehabilitation are all used in the appropriate clinical circumstance.[29] For example, a child with a cerebellar astrocytoma may present with vestibular dysfunction, ataxia, dysmetria, and nystagmus and may benefit from incorporating vestibular adaptation and habituation activities as the primary focus. A child with a frontoparietal juvenile pilocytic astrocytoma may present with a dense hemiparesis with evolving hypertonia and spasticity. A trial of a number of therapeutic interventions including CIMT of the unaffected upper extremity and partial weight-supported treadmill training may assist in cortical reintegration. Treatment of spastic muscles with antispasticity medication if generalized spasticity is observed or focal management with botulinum toxin injections to selected muscles may also assist in functional recovery. In some cases of restorative and more cases of supportive rehabilitation, evaluation of appropriate equipment or devices to obtain or maintain functional independence is necessary. Examples of such equipment might include a walker or wheelchair for mobility, adaptive utensils for activities of daily living or augmentative communication devices for communication. A thorough evaluation is necessary for identifying appropriate equipment, and knowledge of Dietz

category is helpful in identification of appropriate equipment needs of both the child and the caregivers. Reevaluation at follow-up visits is also integral in evaluating the current rehabilitation program and optimization of the child's functional independence.

For the child who is receiving rehabilitation services while undergoing radiation and/or chemotherapy, it is particularly critical to have good communication and cooperation between the rehabilitation and neuro-oncology teams. The rehabilitation team must be aware of the treatment planned and any potential complications. They must be sensitive to problems of pain, nausea, anorexia, constipation, and poor endurance, which may limit the child's ability to participate fully in the rehabilitation process. When pain is an issue, adequate pain management must be provided, including medication and adjunct strategies and services such as counseling, relaxation techniques, therapeutic modalities, and biofeedback when appropriate. Rehabilitation schedules should be modified appropriately to accommodate the antitumor treatments and allow rest periods. The occupational therapist can address energy conservation strategies and pacing with the family and child. Additionally, the team must be vigilant for subtle signs and symptoms of treatment complications or disease progression and address these with the neuro-oncologist.

Aside from the disease process itself, both radiation and chemotherapy can have a deleterious effect on appetite with dire nutritional consequences. Poor nutrition can impair wound healing, growth, that is, it can diminish overall well being and reduce the ability to participate in age-appropriate activities and in the overall rehabilitation process. Nutritional status should be closely monitored and deficits should be aggressively addressed. In some cases, hyperphagia may occur with potential for rapid weight gain. Nutrition issues are addressed in more detail elsewhere in this text.

Highlighted below are specific areas of dysfunction that present frequent challenges for the child with a brain tumor, with significant potential for impact on quality of life.

Physical Performance

Physical disability can have significant impact on educational, vocational, and economic potential. The Childhood Cancer Survivor Study (CCSS) recently reported on physical performance limitations and associated participation restrictions in young cancer survivors.

The highest prevalence of physical performance limitations in the CCSS cohort were among survivors of bone (36.9%) and brain tumors (26.6%).[32] Treatment with radiation and treatment with a combination of alkylating agents or anthracyclines were risk factors for physical performance limitations and consequent participation restrictions. Survivors treated with radiation were most likely to report limitations in physical performance and participation restrictions in self care activities, routine activities, school, or work.[33]

Sensory Deficits

Sensory deficits may occur due to direct involvement of the tumor or due to the antitumor therapy. Visual loss, visual field deficits, gaze palsies, and involuntary ocular movements may all impair vision and result in significant functional impairment. Visual disturbances are quite common in craniopharyngiomas due to compression of the optic chiasm. Thorough ophthalmologic assessment should be completed and visual function monitored as part of the rehabilitation plan. This is particularly important in young children with oculomotor abnormalities who may require treatment to prevent amblyopia. Of note, focal pathology does not always signify focal disease. For example, the abducens nerve has a long free intracranial course and passes in close proximity to bony structures. It may be compromised due to elevation of intracranial pressure, with resultant sixth nerve palsy and diplopia. The occupational therapist can address compensatory strategies for visual deficits, in addition to addressing visual-motor and visual-perceptual deficits. With severe vision impairment, a low-vision specialist should be part of the rehabilitation team. Adjunct service providers are usually available through the state agency for the blind, the school district, or special schools for the blind/visually impaired. If visual impairment is severe, referral should always be made to the state commission for the blind for adjunct services and equipment needs.

Hearing loss can result from tumor involvement or as a consequence of radiation or chemotherapy agents such as cisplatin and carboplatin. Cisplatin produces high-frequency sensorineural hearing loss and tinnitus, the latter of which usually subsides. The hearing loss is almost always permanent and is primarily due to injury to the hair cells of the organ of Corti, although damage to the stria vascularis has also been described. Factors associated with a higher risk of cisplatin toxicity include prior or concomitant cranial irradiation, preexisting hearing loss, decreased renal function, concomitant use of other ototoxic drugs, faster infusion rate, higher peak plasma concentration, very young age or older age, higher cumulative dose, in addition to individual susceptibility.[34] Recent research suggests that amifostine may ameliorate the risk of severe ototoxicity; however, further investigation is warranted.[35]

With carboplatin, studies have revealed high-frequency hearing loss, but minor or no loss of hair cells. Baseline audiologic evaluation should be provided for all children, with regular reevaluation determined by type of treatment provided. Hearing assessment should precede initiation of speech and language therapy services. Depending upon the deficits, amplification may be warranted in the form of a hearing aid or auditory trainer. For the young child with severe hearing loss, instruction in sign language may be appropriate, in addition to training in oral language skills. For the child who has been exposed to chemotherapeutic agents that are ototoxic, care must be taken to limit further exposure to ototoxic agents, even in the absence of hearing deficits, as the toxic effects may be cumulative.

Impairment of smell and taste are less recognized sensory deficits, but can be seen with tumors, which involve the region of the olfactory nerve. These deficits become significant when they affect appetite and therefore nutrition.

Cognitive Impairment

At diagnosis, cognitive impairment is most common with hemispheric and supratentorial midline tumors. Deficits in memory, language acquisition and comprehension, attention, and academic skills vary with age at diagnosis, gender, type and duration of presenting symptoms, tumor extent, and treatment. With improved survival, the impact of cranial irradiation on cognitive function and academic potential has gained increased significance. Radiation therapy is associated with a significant decline in cognitive function that is inversely related to age at diagnosis. A mean IQ (intelligence quotient) loss of 27 points has been demonstrated 2 years following cranial radiation in children younger than 7 years, while no significant difference was seen in the performance of older children at reevaluation.[36] Younger children, particularly those younger than 3 years, have been found to be more susceptible to the negative cognitive effects of radiation therapy, possibly due to decreased plasticity following global impact to a very young brain, with reported drops in IQ as much as 40 points. Treatment approaches may be adapted, for example, delaying radiation treatment, to ameliorate impact on cognitive function. It is unclear why

female gender has also been recognized a risk factor for neurocognitive deficits but may be related to gender differences in brain development. Deficits have included significant impairments in verbal and performance IQ.[37] Problems in attention/concentration, processing speed, working memory, and nondominant hemisphere function, such as visual-motor integration and visual-spatial functions are the most common cognitive deficits among brain tumor survivors.[37]

It is essential to identify and understand factors other than radiotherapy that may contribute to neuropsychological impairment in survivors of brain tumors. A more accurate assessment of the neuropsychological status of a child with a brain tumor may be obtained by considering the accumulation of pre- and post-diagnostic medical events resulting in brain injury, in addition to the treatment-related complications that affect cognition.[38]

When feasible, baseline neuropsychological assessment should be done prior to or shortly after initiating treatment. When deficits exist, therapeutic and educational services should be instituted, if appropriate, based on the child's status. A multicenter, randomized trial evaluating cognitive remediation programming to address deficits revealed significant improvement in academic achievement in the areas of language and math and improved attention and concentration on parental report for those children participating in the cognitive rehabilitation program (CRP). Despite the fact that these children consistently demonstrated improvement in academic performance after the CRP, there were no significant differences on individual neurocognitive variables. Strategies proposed to address cognitive deficits may include pharmacologic interventions to address attention as well as cognitive rehabilitation.[39] When no deficits are present, cognitive status should be monitored on a regular basis with neuropsychological reassessments. Children under the age of 3 years should be referred to an early childhood intervention program for monitoring and stimulation of developmental progress, appropriate therapies, and parent education. An advantage of this type of program is that services can be provided in the child's home, which decreases risks of exposures to the common communicable diseases for the child who is immunosuppressed.

For the school-age child, close communication between the treatment team and the child's educational program is critical to ensure appropriate bi-directional flow of information regarding the child's level of function, academic, therapeutic, and psycho-emotional status, and recommended services. Behavior and emotional problems are commonly reported in children returning to school following treatment for brain tumor.[40] The Children's Oncology Group has published "Guidelines for identification of, advocacy for, and intervention in neurocognitive problems in survivors of childhood cancer" which includes recommendations for screening and management of late effects of treatment as well as address advocacy and school issues.[41] The importance of providing an appropriate educational program is discussed subsequently in this text.

Communication Deficits

In addition to deficits in speech and language discussed earlier, cerebellar mutism syndrome may specifically occur following posterior fossa surgery. One of the remarkable features of this poorly understood syndrome is the delayed onset. In the immediate postoperative period and for as long as 5 days afterwards, there may be normal speech production. This is followed by a sudden cessation of speech, with preservation of symbolic functions and without evidence of impairment of cranial nerves or peripheral organs of speech. In most cases, resolution of the muteness is followed by an "ataxic dysarthria" speech is characterized by slurring, scanning, slow rhythm, and fluctuation of pitch.[42] Persistent impairment due to cerebellar mutism syndrome (CMS) has been demonstrated to be more common than previously recognized with long-term adverse neurological, cognitive, and psychological deficits. These include ataxia, speech and language dysfunction, and other cognitive deficits. In a prospective study, the Children's Oncology Group found that impairments in these areas were present 1 year post onset of the syndrome and were correlated with severity of CMS.[43] Children with cerebellar mutism have also demonstrated significant high-level linguistic and cognitive deficits on formal speech-language and neuropsychological testing. These deficits are consistent with those aspects of cognition associated with the cerebellum in recent literature, for example, processing speed, memory, and cognitive planning.[44] Although medulloblastoma and vermal location appear to be risk factors, pathophysiology of CMS remains open to debate.[42]

Oral Motor Dysfunction

With involvement of the lower cranial nerves and bulbar dysfunction that can occur with tumors of the posterior fossa, swallowing and deglutition dysfunction may occur. The speech and language pathologist is responsible for providing clinical evaluation of the swallowing mechanism, and he or she participates with the radiologist in videofluoroscopic evaluation when warranted to insure that the child can safely be fed orally. It is critical to recognize that silent aspiration is a common finding with bulbar dysfunction, especially in the presence of pharyngeal sensory deficits.

Lifespan Counseling

As childhood brain tumor survivors age, it has become apparent that consequences beyond school reentry and academic performance must be addressed. It is helpful to prepare families by presenting a lifespan perspective very early in management and providing the families and survivors with tools to mange their experience through the stages of development.[45] Career development and vocational counseling programs parallel survivorship clinics and psychosocial programs for adolescents and young adults.[37] Cognitive reserve, plasticity, and impact of aging will be future concerns. As childhood brain tumor survivors enter later adulthood, changes in patterns of health care needs and new vulnerabilities should be anticipated.[45] Long-term survivor studies point to deficits in social functioning and psychosocial domains, such as employment, ability to drive, dating history, and independent living that will need to be addressed if quality of life for these survivors is to be optimized.[46–48]

Spinal Cord Tumors

Spinal cord dysfunction occurs in up to 4% of children with systemic cancer.[49] Sarcomas account for the majority of epidural metastases, followed by neuroblastoma, lymphoma, and leukemia. Symptoms of metastatic cord compression include back pain, weakness, sphincter dysfunction, and sensory abnormalities.[49] Primary spinal cord tumors are a relatively rare diagnosis and account for 1% to 10% of all pediatric central nervous system tumors.[50] The most common spinal cord tumors are intramedullary with pathology consistent with astrocytoma and medulloblastoma.[50,51] The initial evaluation and medical management are covered elsewhere in this text.

The neurological examination of a child with a spinal cord tumor should be performed by a professional familiar with American Spinal Injury Association (ASIA) examination (Fig. 44.1). The ASIA examination classifies patients with spinal cord injuries based on their clinical examination rather than radiographic findings. The components of the examination include assessment of 10 index muscles (5 in the upper extremities and 5 in the lower extremities), 28 dermatomes, and a rectal examination assessing for sensation and voluntary contraction. Findings on this examination determine the neurological level as well as the ASIA Impairment Scale, which determines the completeness of the injury. These findings are very useful in predicting the functional outcome of the patient as well as for prognosticating functional or medical decline if tumor progresses. (Table 44.3)

A number of medical complications may affect the child's ability to participate in therapy following a spinal cord injury (SCI). Impairments in respiratory function can be observed in children with cervical or thoracic level spinal cord injuries. Normal pulmonary function requires the diaphragm (C3 to C5) and the intercostal muscles (T1 to T12). Paralysis of these muscles can lead to respiratory complications including an impaired cough, pneumonia, and the need for a temporary or permanent tracheostomy tube and ventilator dependency (high cervical injury above C4). Aggressive management is necessary to decrease complications. Treatments include positioning the child in an upright position and out of bed as much as possible, assisted cough either manually or with mechanical insufflation-exsufflation, and, when necessary, the use of non-invasive ventilation such as BiPAP. Evaluation of sleep-disordered breathing can be performed using polysomnography.

Sympathetic outflow is interrupted in lesions above thoracic level 6. Unopposed vagal tone may result in bradycardia, and decreased systemic vascular resistance may result in postural hypotension. Autonomic dysreflexia (AD) is a massive reflex sympathetic discharge following a noxious stimulation below the level of the spinal cord lesion in people with injuries above the T6 level. Common causes include a distended bladder or stool impaction; however, any noxious stimulus below the level of the lesion should be considered. Symptoms include headache, flushing, sweating, decreased or increased heart rate, and hypertension. AD is a medical emergency that can lead to cerebral hemorrhage, seizures, and even death. If AD is suspected, the patient should be placed in an upright position to lower the blood pressure, and a cause of the noxious stimuli should be sought. Typically, when the focus is removed, the blood pressure quickly returns to baseline.

Children with SCI are at risk for deep venous thrombosis (DVT). The exact incidence of DVT in pediatric spinal cord injuries is unknown; one study reported an incidence of 10% in children aged 15 to 18 years and 5% in children younger than 15 years.[52] There are no standard recommendations for pediatric DVT prophylaxis in children who are immobile as a result of spinal cord tumors.[53] The Consortium for Spinal Cord Medicine has published guidelines for prophylaxis in adults.[54] Recommendations include the use of compression hose or pneumatic devices for all patients with SCI during the first 2 weeks. Anticoagulant prophylaxis with either low-molecular-weight heparin or adjusted-dose unfractionated heparin should be started in those considered at high risk within 72 hours of injury, if there are no contraindications.

Decreased sensation is frequently observed in children with spinal cord involvement. It is critical for team members including the family, nursing, and therapists to understand the extent of the sensory loss and risk of developing pressure sores. If the child is not able to be out of bed, it is important to change their positions every couple of hours to prevent pressure sores. Careful attention to the sacrum and heels is needed, as these are frequently problematic in a child who

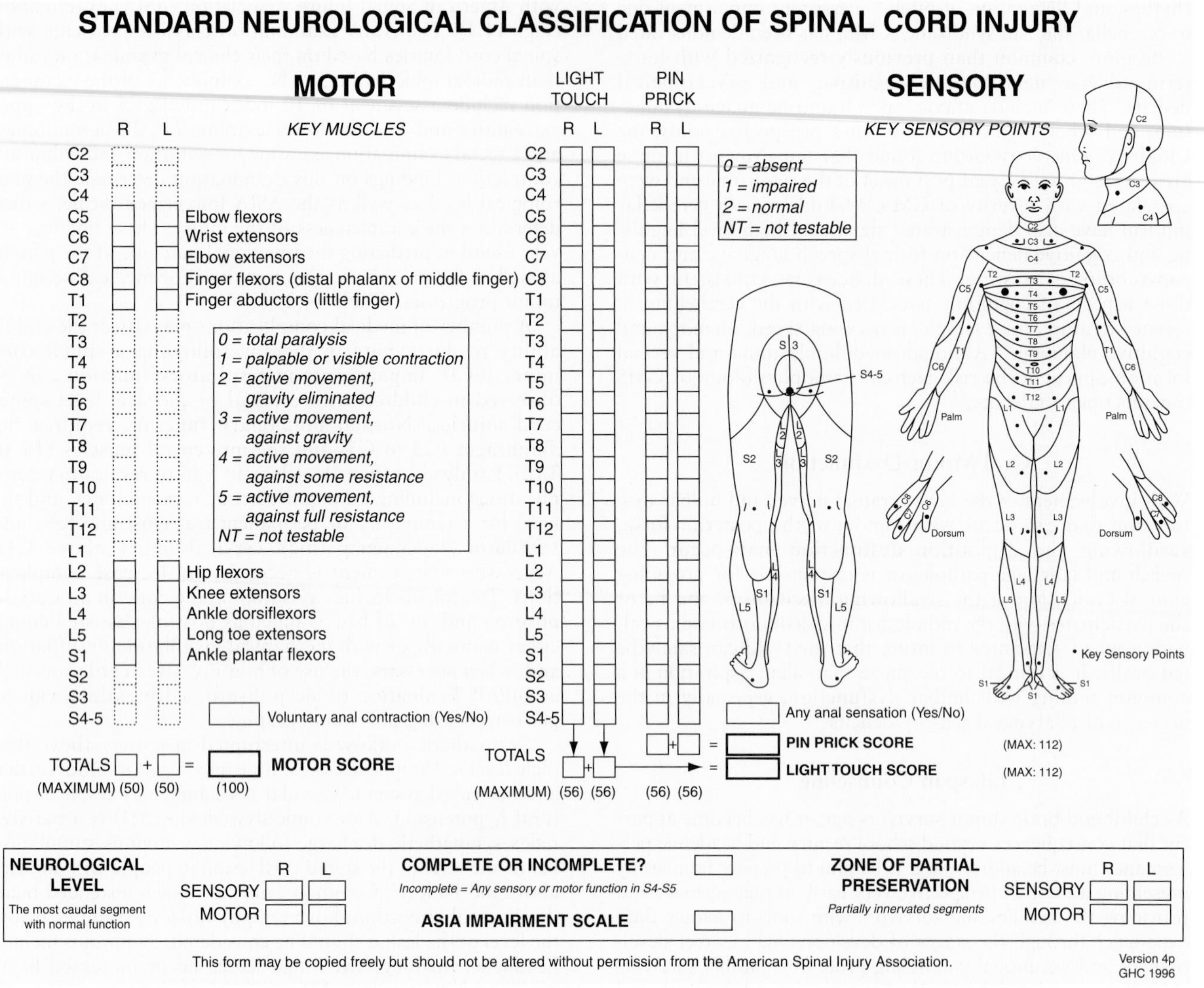

Figure 44.1 American Spinal Injury Association flow sheet. (From American Spinal Injury Association/ International Spinal Cord Society (ISCoS). International standards for neurological and functional classification of spinal cord injury patients. Chicago, IL: 2002, with permission.)

is supine. One should consider use of a pressure-relieving mattress for the child who is going to have prolonged bedrest. When the child is permitted to sit, the therapists should train the child and/or family in pressure-relieving techniques (wheelchair push-ups, shifting side-to-side, or use of a tilt-in-space wheelchair). Specialized wheelchair cushions can be obtained to decrease the risk of sacral or ischial pressure sores in the child who is wheelchair dependent.

Immobilization results in increased urinary excretion of calcium that may last many months, predisposing patients to uroliathisis.[55] Immobilization hypercalcemia presents typically in males 4 to 12 weeks after injury. Signs and symptoms such as lethargy, alteration of mood, nausea, anorexia, and polyuria are nonspecific, therefore serum calcium should be periodically monitored.[55]

Spasticity often occurs after upper motor neuron lesions including spinal cord or brain tumors. Spasticity can cause pain, decreased range of motion, and interference with mobility and self care activities. Similar to autonomic dysreflexia, spasticity can be caused by noxious stimuli. Treatment should begin with removal of any potential stimuli followed by positioning, stretching, and splinting. Oral medications such as use of a GABA

(gamma aminobutyric acid) agonist (baclofen or diazepam) should be considered when the spasticity is leading to joint contractures, causing pain, or interfering with function. Focal injections with botulinum toxin or phenol can be effective treatments of spasticity when specific muscle groups are targeted.

Rehabilitation efforts are aimed at maximizing muscle strength and range of motion and facilitating independence in activities of daily living and mobility. Greater independence can be expected with lower spinal cord levels of injury and with incomplete injuries (Table 44.3). Adults with neurological levels as high as C7 can live a completely independent life. As described above, the ASIA neurological level assists the rehabilitation team in identifying appropriate goals to work on during the course of an inpatient hospital stay. The age and developmental level of the patient will also dictate the skills that will be worked on in therapy.

During acute rehabilitation, children work with occupational therapists and nursing on self care skills such as dressing, hygiene, and feeding. Orthotic devices such as universal cuffs, balanced forearm orthoses and wrist-driven flexor hinge orthoses may increase a child's level of independence when they have a cervical level diagnosis and subsequent hand

TABLE 44.3

PROJECTED FUNCTIONAL OUTCOMES AT 1 YEAR POST-INJURY/DIAGNOSIS BY NEUROLOGIC LEVEL OF INJURY

	C1–C4	C5	C6	C7	C8–T1
Feeding	Dependent	Independent with adaptive equipment after setup	Independent with or w/o adaptive equipment	Independent	Independent
Grooming	Dependent	Minimal assistance with equipment after setup	Some assistance to independent with adaptive equipment	Independent with adaptive equipment	Independent
Upper extremity dressing	Dependent	Requires assistance	Independent	Independent	Independent
Lower extremity dressing	Dependent	Dependent	Requires assistance	Some assistance to independent with adaptive equipment	Usually independent
Bathing	Dependent	Dependent	Some assistance to independent with equipment	Some assistance to independent with equipment	Independent with equipment
Bed Mobility	Dependent	Assistance	Assistance	Independent to some assistance	Independent
Weight shifts	Independent in power; dependent in manual wheelchair	Assistance unless in power wheelchair	Independent	Independent	Independent
Transfers	Dependent	Maximum assistance	Some assistance to independence on level surfaces	Independence with or without board for level surfaces	Independent
Wheelchair propulsion	Independent with power Dependent with manual	Independent in power; independent to some assistance in manual with adaptations on level surfaces	Independent—manual with coated rims on level surfaces	Independent—except curbs and uneven terrain	Independent
Driving	Unable	Independent with adaptations	Independent with adaptations	Car with hand controls or adapted van	Car with hand controls or adapted van

	T2–T9	T10–L2	L3–L5
ADLs (Grooming, feeding, dressing, bathing)	Independent	Independent	Independent
Bowel/Bladder	Independent	Independent	Independent
Transfers	Independent	Independent	Independent
Ambulation	Standing in frame, tilt table, or standing wheelchair Exercise only	Household ambulation with orthosis	Community ambulation is possible

From Kirshblum SC, Ho C, Druin E, et al. Rehabilitation after spinal cord injury. In: Kirshblum SC, Campagnolo D, DeLisa JE, eds. Spinal cord medicine. Philadephia, PA: Lippincott Williams & Wilkins, 2002:275–298.

involvement. A number of factors influence a child's use of orthoses, including the size and weight of the orthosis, the child's understanding of the purpose of the orthosis, parental support, and independent ability to use it at school.[56] There are a wide variety of adaptive devices that may also be useful, such as built-up utensil handles, scoop dishes, sock loops, button hooks, adapted mirrors, and long-handled sponges. Children with tetraplegia are at risk for deformities of the upper extremities particularly elbow flexion, forearm supination, and metacarpophalangeal extension contractures. The occupational therapists will train the families to perform range of motion exercises to prevent these deformities.

There are many aspects of mobility that need to be addressed, even if ambulation is not a goal. Therapists should address turning in bed; assuming a sitting position; sitting balance; transfers between wheelchair, bed, toilet, and car; and wheelchair skills. Ambulation is possible for children with paraplegia. Children with levels T11–L2 can be functional indoor ambulators with long-leg braces and an assistive device. However, community ambulation requires a level of L3 or lower. Above T11, ambulation is quite slow and best viewed as exercise.[55] For those children who will remain wheelchair dependent, the physical therapist will assist with ordering a custom wheelchair which will provide appropriate positioning and independence in pushing. Power mobility is typically utilized by children with a higher- to mid-level cervical spinal cord injury.

The family and medical team should be familiar with the child's capabilities, in order to maximize the child's independence across settings including the community. Community reentry activities are essential for the child to become familiar with negotiating common architectural barriers such as curbs, heavy doors, and inaccessible areas so that they can learn to solve problems related to negotiating barriers or ask for assistance. Discharge planning should address independence in the child's home, school, and community, including recreational activities.

Bone Tumors

After the introduction of neo-adjuvant chemotherapy in the 1970s, survival after treatment for a bone sarcoma has improved dramatically and today the 5-year survival for non-metastatic osteosarcoma and Ewing's sarcoma is approximately 70%.[57–59] Historically, amputation was the prescribed treatment for these tumors of the extremities in children, but limb-sparing surgery has been increasingly used with a substantial decrease in the rate of amputation.[60,61] There are currently several surgical options to amputation, and rehabilitation involvement currently includes, but is no longer limited to, provision of external prostheses.[60] Prior planning of the rehabilitation is recommended for any of the surgical options in order to maximize functional independence during and following treatment.[62]

The variations of limb-sparing surgery include an endoprosthetic reconstruction, allograft reconstruction, a composite endoprosthetic allograft reconstruction, and arthrodesis.[63] Physical maturity is an important consideration in deciding the type of surgical procedure, especially if the sarcoma involves a growth plate. If there is significant growth potential, the surgical options include an expanding endoprostheses, rotationplasty reconstruction, or an amputation as discussed elsewhere in this text. Future growth, functional demands, individual preference, and life expectancy should all be considered.[62] Many variables contribute to the potential limb-length discrepancy, such as systemic chemotherapy, slowing of the preserved growth plate in the affected joint,

muscle atrophy, muscle loss, and overgrowth of the contralateral limb. Each of these must be considered when estimating the final growth of a patient and the final limb-length discrepancy.

Optimizing estimations of final height at skeletal maturity is important in the reconstruction of a segmental long bone defect in the skeletally immature patient and may be reliably completed with use of the Green-Anderson growth remaining charts, the Moseley straight-line graph, and the Menelaus chronological age-growth remaining method.[64] Utilizing these methods, the length of the unaffected limb and hence the projected leg-length discrepancy can be estimated. Leg-length discrepancies less than 2 cm tend to have minimal functional or clinical significance and can be typically managed with shoe lifts and are often purposeful in allowing for clearance of the foot in case of nerve palsy intraoperatively.[64] Discrepancies greater than 2 cm are typically associated with gait abnormalities and often require further surgical intervention with epiphysiodesis of the contralateral physis or distraction osteogenesis of the shortened limb.[65,66] Assessment of the optimal surgical and reconstructive procedure to reconstruct large skeletal defects and simultaneously address the ensuing leg-length discrepancy is necessary in order to optimize long-term functional outcomes in these children and adolescents.

The relative functional advantages of a rotationplasty over the endoprosthetic options are the relatively low rate of complications, excellent functional outcomes with the ability to participate in sports in many children at a level approaching the activity level of a child with a below-knee amputation, and accommodation for future growth of the extremities.[67] It is recommended as an alternative to endoprosthetic replacement for skeletally immature individuals, in particular for those who place function ahead of cosmesis.[67] Some surgeons advocating for strong consideration of age in the selection of procedure recommend rotationplasty for children who are less than 10 years of age.[68] Frequently mentioned disadvantages to the rotationplasty are cosmesis and potential adverse psychologic impact.[67] However, assessment at least 1 year after rotationplasty reveals levels of psychosocial functioning, general quality of life, and social support that are highly comparable to those of healthy peers in adults and older teenagers.[69] Based on their responses to quality-of-life questionnaires, patients who had undergone rotationplasties could participate in daily weight-bearing and sports activities to a significantly greater degree than did patients who had undergone limb salvage surgery.[64]

Occasionally, still, amputations are performed in the treatment of extremity sarcomas and these patients should also be offered the services of a pediatric rehabilitation team. Rehabilitation management following amputation includes initial skin management and eventual soft dressings for promotion of wound healing and edema control. Therapies initially focus on preprosthetic training with goals of maintenance of range of motion in joints proximal to the amputation, strengthening the gluteus medius and maximus, as well as mobility and transfer training using a mobility device if needed prior to prosthetic fit. Following prosthetic fitting, gait and balance training with the prosthesis on all surfaces and training on proper donning and doffing of prosthesis as well as skin care is important. Monitoring for complications of amputations including bony overgrowth, leg-length discrepancy, prosthetic device malfunction in addition to skin breakdown related to prosthetic wear is an important role of the rehabilitation team.

Limb salvage therapy, combining wide tumor resection with endoprosthetic replacement and adjuvant chemotherapy, has become a popular option to amputation or rotationplasty for primary bone sarcoma.[60,70] The consensus of the Committee of Pediatric Orthopaedics of the American Academy of

Orthopaedic Surgeons is that limb salvage surgery is preferable to amputation when survival is not compromised, with upper limb salvage more important than lower limb salvage.[62] Endoprosthetic reconstructions give satisfying cosmetic and functional results in most patients.[60,70] Patients with distal femoral endoprosthetic reconstruction achieve the highest functional outcomes, and patients with total or push-through femoral replacements achieve the lowest functional outcomes.[70] During the first 6 months postoperatively, 80% of patients in one study, two-thirds of whom had reconstruction with modular prosthetic arthroplasties, were unable to walk without support.[71] Function generally progressively improves throughout the second 6-month period and the first and second years after amputation, rotationplasty, or limb salvage procedures.[71]

Physical rehabilitation following limb-sparing procedures is more difficult than that following amputation.[72] Early and more aggressive rehabilitation programs result in better outcomes.[70] The patient and his or her family must be committed not only to the procedure but also to the long rehabilitation process. Failure to participate in rehabilitation can lead to fixed flexion contractures and poor functional results. Although excellent flexion may be achieved in the immediate postoperative period, flexion contractures of up to 20 to 30 degrees can develop in as short a time as 2 weeks, and correction of the flexion contractures often requires further operative intervention.[64] Specific regimens vary with the site, surgical procedure, and surgeon. Exercise regimens can often start 1 to 2 days postoperatively.[60,70] Range of motion exercise provided by a continuous passive motion machine can also be initiated after distal femoral reconstruction either in the recovery room[73] or 1 to 2 days postoperatively, with active range-of-motion exercise started subsequently.[70] After proximal tibial replacement, a less aggressive approach may be indicated; gentle range of motion exercises may not be indicated until after a 2- to 3-week period of casting in full extension.[70,73] Standing may be appropriate within a week after endoprosthetic replacement surgery, unless a muscle flap was performed.[60] Gradual weight bearing using two crutches may be possible 2 weeks after surgery, with progression to full weight bearing after a few months,[70] although ambulation with the use of a knee immobilizer is begun a few days after surgery following distal femoral reconstruction.[73] Bracing at the knee can augment stability following procedures involving the femur or tibia.[60] Continuous passive-motion machines can be used after discharge for another 1 to 2 months at home.[73] For patients with total or proximal femur replacements, bed rest with hip abduction for 2 to 4 weeks, followed by hip abduction bracing for 3 months, may be recommended.[73] Upper extremity endoprosthetic reconstruction can be followed by shoulder immobilization for 2 to 3 weeks before beginning physical therapy to maximize shoulder and elbow range of motion.[73] These regimens result in fewer difficulties establishing extremity function than earlier methods in which primary wound healing was achieved prior to initiating assisted active exercise.[70]

Almost half of children who have resection of primary bone tumors with expandable endoprosthetic replacement will not require use of an orthosis or gait aid.[60] Unassisted ambulation is more likely if the quadriceps mechanism is preserved, either following expandable endoprosthetic replacement[60] or after prosthetic knee replacement following distal femur bone tumor resection.[68] More extensive loss of the active quadriceps mechanism with endoprosthetic replacement at the level of the proximal tibia results in loss of active knee extension and knee instability and a worse functional outcome than for distal femur replacement.[60] Rehabilitative needs of children who undergo limb-sparing surgery include early mobilization, gait training, and continued follow-up to monitor activity restriction.[60] Shoe lifts can be utilized on the contralateral limb to address the leg-length discrepancy between lengthening procedures.[60]

Some functional limitations can be expected after endoprosthetic reconstruction. Patients may be advised following lower extremity endoprosthetic reconstruction to use a cane out-of-doors permanently and not to participate in sports other than swimming.[70] While children with endoprostheses are restricted from high-speed, high-impact sports and activities requiring a high degree of coordination, specifically football, tennis, soccer, and field hockey, using a stationary bicycle, walking, hiking with a cane, and participating in a modified program of physical education at school are permitted, in addition to swimming.[60]

Children with expandable endoprostheses may also face issues related to adjustment to the need for repeated hospitalizations for lengthening.[60] Several studies of children and adolescents with acquired limb loss show remarkably good psychosocial adjustment in this population, regardless of surgical approach.[72] There have not been significant differences in comparisons of quality of life or global physical and psychological functioning, assessed 1 to 3 years after surgery, between children and adolescents managed with limb-sparing procedures and adjuvant therapy and those managed with amputations and adjuvant chemotherapy.[72]

Several studies from the Childhood Cancer Survivor Study (CCSS) have looked at the long-term outcomes of childhood cancer survivors. One study from the CCSS assessed the health status of childhood cancer survivors including general health, mental health, functional impairment, activity limitations, pain, and anxiety. Bone sarcoma survivors were more likely to report adverse health outcomes in all domains, except mental health, when compared to leukemia survivors. Functional limitations, activity status, and pain as a result of cancer or its treatment were most affected.[74] A second study focused primarily on physical performance and daily activities and found that one-third of survivors of bone sarcomas reported physical limitations, and 11% reported that poor health restricted their ability to attend work or school. Overall, bone sarcoma survivors, again, were among the most likely to report performance limitations, having restricted ability to do routine activities, and having restricted ability to attend work or school.[32] A third study looked at self-reported quality of life and function of survivors of a lower extremity or pelvic bone sarcoma and had relatively good quality of life and function, but certain subgroups were at risk.[75] Although the bone sarcoma survivors were treated in an earlier era which may not reflect current management and surgical techniques, these studies are important in demonstrating the need for long-term assessments to assist with maximizing functional outcome.

Although it is currently more likely that a child or adolescent with a primary bone tumor will be offered a limb salvage operation and reconstruction instead of an amputation, it remains unclear which type of surgical intervention results in a superior functional result.[76] A single comparison study of patients treated for pediatric malignant bone tumors with either amputation or limb-sparing surgery showed no significant differences at a median of 14 years after surgery in functional limitations, educational or occupational status, pain, self-image, interpersonal interactions, or overall satisfaction with their surgical procedure.[77] In each group in this study, approximately 90% of patients reported limitations in running and lifting heavy objects, 75% to 90% reported limitations in contact or team sports, and 50% reported limitations in recreational activities and bending, kneeling, and stooping.

Acute Lymphoblastic Leukemia

The majority of children diagnosed with acute lymphoblastic leukemia (ALL) will survive into adulthood. The rehabilitation team needs to address not only the effects of the leukemia itself but also consider the long-term effects of treatment. A wide variety of neuromuscular and musculoskeletal complications are associated with ALL, such as pain, paresthesias, muscle cramps, muscle weakness, reduced ankle dorsiflexion, impaired gross and fine motor performance, decreased energy expenditure, avascular necrosis, osteopenia, osteoporosis and learning disabilities.[78] In addition, ALL also has the potential for remissions and exacerbations, and the emphasis of rehabilitation is likely to change over time.

Bone pain caused by proliferation of hemopoietic tissue within the medullary cavity is a frequent occurrence in ALL. The pain most commonly occurs in the lower extremities and is usually intermittent, well-localized, sharp, severe, and sudden in onset.[79] Radiographic skeletal changes may include osteopenia, radiolucent metaphyseal bands, lytic lesions, sclerotic lesions, or pathological fractures.[80] There is no widely accepted method for determining the risk of a pathological fracture in involved bone. The risk may be higher with painful lytic lesions where the ratio between the width of the metastasis and bone is greater than 0.6, or if there is cortical destruction of the circumference greater than or equal to 50%.[81] Attempts should be made to reduce weight bearing through areas at risk and resistive strengthening activities should be avoided. Isometric strengthening and aerobic exercise such as swimming or riding a stationary bike should be considered. With spinal compression fractures, flexion activities of the spine should be avoided and a corset or custom molded spinal orthosis may be helpful if significant pain is present.

Reduced bone mineral density (BMD) is common in ALL.[82,83] Potential causes for low BMD include leukemic infiltration of bone, side effects of chemotherapy agents, the influence of steroid therapy on bone metabolism, cranial radiation's effect on the hypothalamic or pituitary function, nutritional factors, or decreased physical activity. There is conflicting evidence as to whether long-term survivors of ALL have lower BMD compared to healthy age-matched controls. Some studies suggest that decreased BMD becomes more common with increasing time after diagnosis,[82] while other studies report normal BMD in the years following therapy.[84,85] Many of the studies that support a prolonged decrease in BMD had a high proportion of subjects with cranial radiation, but the current practice is to limit radiation therapy. This may account for the findings of improved BMD. Immobility related to prolonged hospitalizations is also less common and this may impact BMD positively. The risk for decreased BMD remains and all patients with ALL should be encouraged to optimize their calcium and vitamin D intake, as well as participate in weight-bearing exercise.

Osteonecrosis (ON), also known as aseptic or avascular necrosis of the bone, presents in up to 15% of patients with ALL.[86] The etiology of ON is not well understood, but it is believed to be secondary to an ischemic insult to the bone and bone marrow. Risk factors for ON include older age at diagnosis, glucocorticoid therapy, alkylator therapy, methotrexate, history of any radiation therapy, radiation to the hypothalamic-pituitary region, radiation to the gonads, and older treatment era.[87] The most common sites for ON are the hips, shoulders, and knees, and it is commonly multi-articular.[87] The clinical manifestations are variable; some patients may be asymptomatic, but the majority of patients will develop a variable degree of pain and decreased range of motion. The potential for articular collapse is also present. Treatment consists of analgesic medications, range of motion, and limited weight bearing of the affected joint. The use of bisphosphonates is also being studied. Orthopedic surgical intervention is occasionally necessary as well.

There is increasing evidence for a variety of motor impairments associated with ALL. A number of therapeutic agents can negatively impact motor performance, including vincristine, steroids, and cranial radiation. Physical activity may be limited by frequent hospitalizations, anthracycline-related cardiotoxicity, and over-protective parents. In addition, the motor impairments themselves may cause decreased self-confidence and desire to participate in activities, resulting in further inactivity and lack of opportunity to improve motor performance.

The actual prevalence of motor impairments in ALL is not known. A number of studies have demonstrated decreased strength,[88,89] balance,[90,91] and motor proficiency[92,93] in survivors when compared to age-matched controls. In addition, physical fitness, as assessed by peak oxygen uptake (VO_{2peak}), is reduced.[94,95] Impaired motor skills and physical fitness likely play a significant role in the increased incidence of obesity reported in survivors of ALL.[74] Recent evidence suggests that survivors have a reduced total daily energy expenditure, related to low participation in physical activity, which would also place them at additional risk for obesity.[96] Other factors that may contribute to increased weight gain include hypothalamic pituitary dysfunction following cranial radiation, weight gain associated with steroid therapy, and limitations in activity related to anthracycline-induced cardiomyopathy.

Peripheral neuropathy or myopathy may occur in ALL and should be considered in patients with progressive weakness. Myopathy is a common complication of corticosteroid therapy and a rare complication of vincristine therapy. It classically presents with the insidious onset of painless, symmetric, proximal muscle weakness that leads to difficulties in rising from a low chair, climbing stairs, and performing overhead activities. The electrodiagnostic exam may reveal few abnormalities, due to the preferential atrophy of type II fibers that are not evaluated by electromyography.[97] The myopathy is usually reversible if the drug is withdrawn, or the dose is reduced.[98] The rehabilitation program should include passive stretching and proper positioning of the hip, knee, and shoulder with particular focus on the hip flexors, hamstrings, iliotibial bands, and shoulder adductors and internal rotators. Strengthening and endurance exercise can lessen but cannot eliminate glucocorticoid-induced muscle atrophy and weakness.[99]

Vincristine therapy commonly causes an axonal, sensorimotor polyneuropathy. Loss of ankle reflexes and complaints of numbness and tingling in the feet and/or hands usually precedes the onset of distal weakness. The weakness may progress to involve the more proximal limbs but generally recovers rapidly if the drug is stopped, or the dose is reduced.[98] Therapy should focus on passive stretching of the wrist and finger flexors as well as the gastrocnemius-soleus complex. If the weakness is severe, a resting wrist-hand splint may be worn at night and periodically during the day to maintain range of motion. A splint may also be used at the ankle to maintain at least a neutral position (0 degrees) in dorsiflexion. If the weakness causes foot drop during ambulation, a custom molded ankle-foot-orthosis should be considered.

Anthracyclines and cardiac radiation have the potential to cause acute and long-term cardiotoxicity, including ventricular dysfunction, pericarditis, electrocardiographic abnormalities, and arrhythmias.[100,101] The risk for cardiac abnormalities is dose-dependent; however, a recent study of long-term survivors of ALL who received doses of less than 300 mg/m^2 demonstrated impaired cardiac function.[102] This adds to the growing evidence that even relatively low doses of anthracycline may lead to cardiac dysfunction over time. Survivors of ALL, treated with anthracycline, should therefore receive lifelong surveillance for late cardiac effects. Periodic evaluations should include an echocardiogram, a resting ECG, and a history of exercise intolerance.[103] A pediatric cardiologist should be consulted to provide safe exercise precautions in patients with cardiac abnormalities.

The increased risk for motor impairments, decreased physical fitness and obesity suggest that exercise may play an important role in minimizing potential side effects and improving quality of life in ALL. A small non-randomized study of younger children receiving maintenance therapy for ALL reported increased strength and functional mobility following an 8 week in hospital, supervised training program combining cardiorespiratory and resistance exercises.[94] Another small study, on a similar group of children, demonstrated greater physical activity and fitness in children who were randomized to a 12-month home-based exercise and nutrition program compared to age-matched controls.[104]

An evidenced-based guideline for safe and effective exercise for patients with ALL does not exist. Hematologic abnormalities may impact the patient's mobility and ability to perform exercise. Low platelet counts increase the risk for cerebral, intramuscular, and joint hemorrhage during exercise. In a study of patients with ALL, visible hemorrhage was rare with platelet counts greater than 20,000, and no intracranial hemorrhage occurred with platelet counts greater than 10,000.[105] In general, moderately vigorous exercise can be pursued when platelet counts are at least 30,000–50,000 and low-impact aerobic, but not resistive activities, can be considered with counts greater than 10,000 to 20,000.[106] Exercise is not recommended with platelet counts less than 10,000.[107] It has also been suggested that exercise be discontinued with a hemoglobin less than 7.5 grams and white blood cell count less than 3,000.[106] Exercise can produce favorable changes in the function of the cellular and humoral components of the immune systems in healthy children, but there is little data on the effects of exercise on the immune response in childhood ALL. A pilot study reported a similar increase in basal levels of circulating leukocytes following 30 minutes of vigorous exercise in subjects on maintenance therapy versus healthy controls and no significant negative neutrophil responses were noted.[108] This suggests that neutrophils in children with ALL may respond to acute exercise similarly to neutrophils in healthy children, lessening the concern for a negative effect of exercise on the immune system in ALL.

Some general guidelines have been suggested for physical activity in ALL,[109] but exercise recommendations should be individualized for each patient. In the induction and consolidation phase of therapy, very light levels of physical activity may help decrease late effects of treatment. In the maintenance phase of treatment, children should participate in light-to-moderate intensity lifestyle activities such as walking, riding a bike, helping with chores, or recreational swimming. Once a child is ready for more strenuous aerobic activity, they should start with short intervals (5 to 10 minutes) and progress slowly to longer periods. Muscular strength and endurance-building activities are very important. Traditional weight lifting is not recommended for any young child. The use of stability balls, resistance bands, and fun activities that require muscle strength, such as gymnastics or swimming, are preferred methods of strengthening.

Long-term cognitive deficits and academic difficulties in survivors of ALL are common following cranial radiation and intrathecal methotrexate therapy. Cranial radiation is believed to be largely responsible for these changes and therefore it is no longer used in most ALL treatment protocols. Unfortunately, CNS chemotherapy is potentially neurotoxic as well. A review of 21 controlled studies of cognitive function in children who received only CNS chemotherapy (no cranial radiation) revealed evidence of subtle long-term deficits.[110] In particular, deficits in attention and executive functioning were noted with relatively preserved global intellectual function. Young age at diagnosis and female sex appeared to be risk factors for poorer outcome. Deficits were also associated with poorer academic achievement and behavior disorders. Abnormalities in conventional imaging do not correlate with neurocognitive deficits; therefore, it is recommended that children with academic or behavioral deficits be screened with neuropsychological testing. Preliminary studies suggest that there may be some benefit to cognitive remediation or neuro stimulants in the treatment of the cognitive deficits associated with ALL.[110]

References

1. Dietz JH Jr. Rehabilitation of the cancer patient. Med Clin North Am 1969;53(3): 607–624.
2. Hill CI, Nixon CS, Ruehmeier JL, et al. Brain tumors. Phys Ther 2002;82(5):496–502.
3. Dietz JH Jr. Adaptive rehabilitation of the cancer patient. Curr Probl Cancer 1980; 5(5):1–56.
4. ICIDH-2: International Classification of Impairments, Activities, and Participation. A manual of dimensions of disablement and functioning. Beta-1 draft for field trials. Geneva: World Health Organization, 1997.
5. Delisa JA Currie DM, Martin GM. Rehabilitation medicine: past, present, and future. In: Delisa JA, Gans BM, eds. Rehabilitation medicine: principles and practice. Vol 3. Philadelphia, PA: Lippincott-Raven, 1998:3–32.
6. Michaud LJ. Childhood disability and rehabilitation. In: Rudolph CD, Rudolph AM, Hostetter MK, et al., eds. Rudolph's pediatrics. 21st ed. Philadelphia, PA: McGraw-Hill, 2003.
7. Hays RM, Michaud LJ. Principles of pediatric rehabilitation. In: Hays RM, Kraft GH, Stolov WC, eds. Chronic disease and disability: a contemporary rehabilitation approach to medical practice. New York: Demos Publications, 1994:215–229.
8. Marciniak CM, Sliwa JA, Spill G, et al. Functional outcome following rehabilitation of the cancer patient. Arch Phys Med Rehabil 1996;77(1):54–57.
9. O'Dell MW, Barr K, Spanier D, et al. Functional outcome of inpatient rehabilitation in persons with brain tumors. Arch Phys Med Rehabil 1998;79(12):1530–1534.
10. Philip PA, Ayyangar R, Vanderbilt J, et al. Rehabilitation outcome in children after treatment of primary brain tumor. Arch Phys Med Rehabil 1994;75(1):36–39.
11. Muller EA. Influence of training and of inactivity on muscle strength. Arch Phys Med Rehabil 1970;51(8):449–462.
12. Booth FW, Gollnick PD. Effects of disuse on the structure and function of skeletal muscle. Med Sci Sports Exerc 1983;15(5):415–420.
13. Baker JH, Matsumoto DE. Adaptation of skeletal muscle to immobilization in a shortened position. Muscle Nerve 1988;11(3):231–244.
14. Minaire P. Immobilization osteoporosis: a review. Clin Rheumatol 1989;8(suppl 2): 95–103.
15. Dittmer DK, Teasell R. Complications of immobilization and bed rest. Part 1: Musculoskeletal and cardiovascular complications. Can Fam Physician 1993;39:1428–1432, 1435–1427.
16. Chobanian AV, Lille RD, Tercyak A, et al. The metabolic and hemodynamic effects of prolonged bed rest in normal subjects. Circulation 1974;49(3):551–559.
17. Halar EM, Bell KR. Physiological and functional changes and effects of inactivity on body functions. In: JA DeLisa, Gans BM, eds. Rehabilitation medicine: principles and practice. Philadelphia, PA: Lippincott-Raven, 1998:1015–1034.
18. Teasell R, Dittmer DK. Complications of immobilization and bed rest. Part 2: Other complications. Can Fam Physician 1993;39:1440–1442, 1445–1446.
19. Koff SA. Estimating bladder capacity in children. Urology 1983;21(3):248.
20. Smith C, Hill J. Language development and disorders of communication and oral motor function. In: Molnar GE, Alexander MA, eds. Pediatric rehabilitation. Philadelphia, PA: Hanley & Belfus, Inc., 1999:57–80.
21. Duffner PK, Cohen ME. The long-term effects of central nervous system therapy on children with brain tumors. Neurol Clin 1991;9(2):479–495.

22. Waber DP, Tarbell NJ, Fairclough D, et al. Cognitive sequelae of treatment in childhood acute lymphoblastic leukemia: cranial radiation requires an accomplice. J Clin Oncol 1995;13(10):2490–2496.
23. Bleyer WA. The impact of childhood cancer on the United States and the world. CA Cancer J Clin 1990;40(6):355–367.
24. Siffert J, Greenleaf M, Mannis R, et al. Pediatric brain tumors. Child Adolesc Psychiatr Clin N Am 1999;8(4):879–903, x.
25. Packer RJ. Childhood medulloblastoma: progress and future challenges. Brain Dev 1999;21(2):75–81.
26. Poussaint TY, Siffert J, Barnes PD, et al. Hemorrhagic vasculopathy after treatment of central nervous system neoplasia in childhood: diagnosis and follow-up. AJNR Am J Neuroradiol 1995;16(4):693–699.
27. Mostow EN, Byrne J, Connelly RR, et al. Quality of life in long-term survivors of CNS tumors of childhood and adolescence. J Clin Oncol 1991;9(4):592–599.
28. Janss AJ, Grundy R, Cnaan A, et al. Optic pathway and hypothalamic/chiasmatic gliomas in children younger than age 5 years with a 6-year follow-up. Cancer 1995;75(4):1051–1059.
29. O'Dell MW, Lin CD, Schwabe E, et al. Rehabilitation of patients with brain tumors. In: Stubblefield MD, O'Dell MW, eds. Cancer rehabilitation: principles and practice. New York: Demos Medical Publishing, 2009:517–532.
30. Marciniak CM, Sliwa JA, Heinemann AW, et al. Functional outcomes of persons with brain tumors after inpatient rehabilitation. Arch Phys Med Rehabil 2001;82(4): 457–463.
31. Mukand JA, Blackinton DD, Crincoli MG, et al. Incidence of neurologic deficits and rehabilitation of patients with brain tumors. Am J Phys Med Rehabil 2001;80(5): 346–350.
32. Ness KK, Mertens AC, Hudson MM, et al. Limitations on physical performance and daily activities among long-term survivors of childhood cancer. [summary for patients in Ann Intern Med 2005143(9):I30; PMID: 16263881]. Ann Intern Med 2005;143(9): 639–647.
33. Ness KK, Hudson MM, Ginsberg JP, et al. Physical performance limitations in the Childhood Cancer Survivor Study cohort. J Clin Oncol 2009;27(14):2382–2389.
34. Freilich RJ, Kraus DH, Budnick AS, et al. Hearing loss in children with brain tumors treated with cisplatin and carboplatin-based high-dose chemotherapy with autologous bone marrow rescue. Med Pediatr Oncol 1996;26(2):95–100.
35. Fouladi M, Chintagumpala M, Ashley D, et al. Amifostine protects against cisplatin-induced ototoxicity in children with average-risk medulloblastoma. J Clin Oncol 2008;26(22):3749–3755.
36. Radcliffe J, Packer RJ, Atkins TE, et al. Three- and four-year cognitive outcome in children with noncortical brain tumors treated with whole-brain radiotherapy. Ann Neurol 1992;32(4):551–554.
37. Butler RW, Sahler OJ, Askins MA, et al. Interventions to improve neuropsychological functioning in childhood cancer survivors. Dev Disabil Res Rev 2008;14(3):251–258.
38. Ater JL, Moore BD III, Francis DJ, et al. Correlation of medical and neurosurgical events with neuropsychological status in children at diagnosis of astrocytoma: utilization of a neurological severity score. J Child Neurol 1996;11(6):462–469.
39. Butler RW, Copeland DR, Fairclough DL, et al. A multicenter, randomized clinical trial of a cognitive remediation program for childhood survivors of a pediatric malignancy. J Consult Clin Psychol 2008;76(3):367–378.
40. Upton P, Eiser C. School experiences after treatment for a brain tumour. Child Care Health Dev 2006;32(1):9–17.
41. Nathan PC, Patel SK, Dilley K, et al. Guidelines for identification of, advocacy for, and intervention in neurocognitive problems in survivors of childhood cancer: a report from the Children's Oncology Group. Arch Pediatr Adolesc Med 2007;161(8): 798–806.
42. Wells EM, Walsh KS, Khademian ZP, et al. The cerebellar mutism syndrome and its relation to cerebellar cognitive function and the cerebellar cognitive affective disorder. Dev Disabil Res Rev. 2008;14(3):221–228.
43. Robertson PL, Muraszko KM, Holmes EJ, et al. Incidence and severity of postoperative cerebellar mutism syndrome in children with medulloblastoma: a prospective study by the Children's Oncology Group. J Neurosurg 2006;105(suppl 6):444–451.
44. Vandeinse D, Hornyak JE. Linguistic and cognitive deficits associated with cerebellar mutism. Pediatr Rehabil 1997;1(1):41–44.
45. Rey-Casserly C, Meadows ME. Developmental perspectives on optimizing educational and vocational outcomes in child and adult survivors of cancer. Dev Disabil Res Rev 2008;14(3):243–250.
46. Ribi K, Relly C, Landolt MA, et al. Outcome of medulloblastoma in children: long-term complications and quality of life. Neuropediatrics 2005;36(6):357–365.
47. Maddrey AM, Bergeron JA, Lombardo ER, et al. Neuropsychological performance and quality of life of 10 year survivors of childhood medulloblastoma. J Neurooncol 2005;72(3):245–253.
48. Hjern A, Lindblad F, Boman KK. Disability in adult survivors of childhood cancer: a Swedish national cohort study. J Clin Oncol 2007;25(33):5262–5266.
49. Lewis DW, Packer RJ, Raney B, et al. Incidence, presentation, and outcome of spinal cord disease in children with systemic cancer. Pediatrics 1986;78(3):438–443.
50. Wilson PE, Oleszek JL, Clayton GH. Pediatric spinal cord tumors and masses. J Spinal Cord Med 2007;30(suppl 1):S15–S20.
51. Farwell JR, Dohrmann GJ, Flannery JT. Central nervous system tumors in children. Cancer 1977;40(6):3123–3132.
52. Radecki RT, Gaebler-Spira D. Deep vein thrombosis in the disabled pediatric population. Arch Phys Med Rehabil 1994;75(3):248–250.
53. Monagle P, Chan A, Massicotte P, et al. Antithrombotic therapy in children: the Seventh ACCP Conference on Antithrombotic and Thrombolytic Therapy. Chest 2004; 126(suppl 3):645S–687S.
54. Consortium for Spinal Cord Medicine. Prevention of thromboembolism in spinal cord injury. J Spinal Cord Med 1997;20:259–283.
55. Massagli TL, Jaffe KM. Pediatric spinal cord injury: treatment and outcome. Pediatrician 1990;17(4):244–254.
56. Mulcahey MJ. Unique management needs of pediatric spinal cord injury patients: rehabilitation. J Spinal Cord Med 1997;20(1):25–30.
57. Elomaa I, Blomqvist CP, Saeter G, et al. Five-year results in Ewing's sarcoma: the Scandinavian Sarcoma Group experience with the SSG IX protocol. Eur J Cancer 2000; 36:875–880.
58. Bacci G, Ferrari S, Bertoni F, et al. Long-term outcome for patients with nonmetastatic osteosarcoma of the extremity treated at the istituto ortopedico rizzoli according to the istituto ortopedico rizzoli/osteosarcoma-2 protocol: an updated report. J Clin Oncol 2000;18(24):4016–4027.
59. Fuchs B, Valenzuela RG, Inwards C, et al. Complications in long-term survivors of Ewing sarcoma. Cancer 2003;98(12):2687–2692.
60. Frieden RA, Ryniker D, Kenan S, et al. Assessment of patient function after limb-sparing surgery. Arch Phys Med Rehabil 1993;74(1):38–43.
61. Aksnes LH, Bauer HC, Jebsen NL, et al. Limb-sparing surgery preserves more function than amputation: a Scandinavian sarcoma group study of 118 patients. J Bone Joint Surg Br 2008;90(6):786–794.
62. Dormans JP. Limb-salvage surgery versus amputation for children with extremity sarcomas. In: Herring JA, Birch JG, eds. The child with a limb deficiency. Rosemont, IL: American Academy of Orthopedic Surgeons, 1998:289–303.
63. Link MP, Gebhardt MC, Meyers PA. Osteosarcoma. In: Pizzo PA, Poplack DG, eds. Principles and practice of pediatric oncology. 5th ed. Philadelphia, PA: Lippincott Williams & Wilkins, 2006:1074–1115.
64. Lewis VO. Limb salvage in the skeletally immature patient. Curr Oncol Rep 2005;7(4):285–292.
65. Dominkus M, Krepler P, Schwameis E, et al. Growth prediction in extendable tumor prostheses in children. Clin Orthop Relat Res 2001(390):212–220.
66. Horton GA, Olney BW. Epiphysiodesis of the lower extremity: results of the percutaneous technique. J Pediatr Orthop 1996;16(2):180–182.
67. Krajbich JI. Modified Van Nes rotationplasty in the treatment of malignant neoplasms in the lower extremities of children. Clin Orthop Relat Res 1991;262:74–77.
68. Kawai A, Muschler GF, Lane JM, et al. Prosthetic knee replacement after resection of a malignant tumor of the distal part of the femur: medium to long-term results. J Bone Joint Surg Am 1998;80(5):636–647.
69. Veenstra KM, Sprangers MA, van der Eyken JW, et al. Quality of life in survivors with a Van Ness-Borggreve rotationplasty after bone tumour resection. J Surg Oncol 2000;73(4):192–197.
70. Ham SJ, Schraffordt Koops H, Veth RP, et al. Limb salvage surgery for primary bone sarcoma of the lower extremities: long-term consequences of endoprosthetic reconstructions. Ann Surg Oncol 1998;5(5):423–436.
71. Zunino JH, Johnston JO. Early results of lower limb surgery for osteogenic sarcoma of bone. Orthopedics 1998;21(1):47–50.
72. Tyc VL. Psychosocial adaptation of children and adolescents with limb deficiencies: a review. Clin Psychol Rev 1992;12:275–291.
73. Eckardt JJ, Kabo JM, Kelley CM, et al. Expandable endoprosthesis reconstruction in skeletally immature patients with tumors. Clin Orthop Relat Res 2000;373:51–61.
74. Hudson MM, Mertens AC, Yasui Y, et al. Health status of adult long-term survivors of childhood cancer: a report from the Childhood Cancer Survivor Study [see comment]. JAMA 2003;290(12):1583–1592.
75. Nagarajan R, Clohisy DR, Neglia JP, et al. Function and quality-of-life of survivors of pelvic and lower extremity osteosarcoma and Ewing's sarcoma: the Childhood Cancer Survivor Study. Br J Cancer 2004;91(11):1858–1865.
76. Enneking WF, Dunham W, Gebhardt MC, et al. A system for the functional evaluation of reconstructive procedures after surgical treatment of tumors of the musculoskeletal system. Clin Orthop Relat Res 1993;286:241–246.
77. Hudson MM, Tyc VL, Cremer LK, et al. Patient satisfaction after limb-sparing surgery and amputation for pediatric malignant bone tumors. J Pediatr Oncol Nurs 1998;15(2): 60–69; discussion 70–61.
78. Marchese VG, Chiarello LA, Lange BJ. Effects of physical therapy intervention for children with acute lymphoblastic leukemia. Pediatr Blood Cancer 2004;42(2): 127–133.
79. Gallagher D, Heinrich SD, Craver R, et al. Skeletal manifestations of acute leukemia in childhood. Orthopedics 1991;14(4):485–492.
80. Rogalsky RJ, Black GB, Reed MH. Orthopaedic manifestations of leukemia in children. J Bone Joint Surg Am 1986;68(4):494–501.
81. Menck H, Schulze S, Larsen E. Metastasis size in pathologic femoral fractures. Acta Orthop Scand 1988;59(2):151–154.
82. Kaste SC, Rai SN, Fleming K, et al. Changes in bone mineral density in survivors of childhood acute lymphoblastic leukemia. Pediatr Blood Cancer 2006;46(1):77–87.
83. van der Sluis IM, van den Heuvel-Eibrink MM, Hahlen K, et al. Altered bone mineral density and body composition, and increased fracture risk in childhood acute lymphoblastic leukemia. J Pediatr 2002;141(2):204–210.
84. Kadan-Lottick N, Marshall JA, Baron AE, et al. Normal bone mineral density after treatment for childhood acute lymphoblastic leukemia diagnosed between 1991 and 1998. J Pediatr 2001;138(6):898–904.
85. Marinovic D, Dorgeret S, Lescoeur B, et al. Improvement in bone mineral density and body composition in survivors of childhood acute lymphoblastic leukemia: a 1-year prospective study. Pediatrics 2005;116(1):e102–e108.
86. Ribeiro RC, Fletcher BD, Kennedy W, et al. Magnetic resonance imaging detection of avascular necrosis of the bone in children receiving intensive prednisone therapy for acute lymphoblastic leukemia or non-Hodgkin lymphoma. Leukemia 2001;15(6): 891–897.
87. Kadan-Lottick NS, Dinu I, Wasilewski-Masker K, et al. Osteonecrosis in adult survivors of childhood cancer: a report from the childhood cancer survivor study. J Clin Oncol 2008;26(18):3038–3045.
88. Ness KK, Baker KS, Dengel DR, et al. Body composition, muscle strength deficits and mobility limitations in adult survivors of childhood acute lymphoblastic leukemia. Pediatr Blood Cancer 2007;49(7):975–981.
89. Hovi L, Era P, Rautonen J, et al. Impaired muscle strength in female adolescents and young adults surviving leukemia in childhood. Cancer 1993;72(1):276–281.
90. Wright MJ, Galea V, Barr RD. Proficiency of balance in children and youth who have had acute lymphoblastic leukemia. Phys Ther 2005;85(8):782–790.
91. Galea V, Wright MJ, Barr RD. Measurement of balance in survivors of acute lymphoblastic leukemia in childhood. Gait Posture 2004;19(1):1–10.
92. Reinders-Messelink HA, Schoemaker MM, Hofte M, et al. Fine motor and handwriting problems after treatment for childhood acute lymphoblastic leukemia. Med Pediatr Oncol 1996;27(6):551–555.
93. Wright MJ, Halton JM, Martin RF, et al. Long-term gross motor performance following treatment for acute lymphoblastic leukemia. Med Pediatr Oncol 1998;31(2):86–90.
94. San Juan AF, Chamorro-Vina C, Mate-Munoz JL, et al. Functional capacity of children with leukemia. Int J Sports Med 2008;29(2):163–167.
95. van Brussel M, Takken T, van der Net J, et al. Physical function and fitness in long-term survivors of childhood leukaemia. Pediatr Rehabil 2006;9(3):267–274.
96. Warner JT. Body composition, exercise and energy expenditure in survivors of acute lymphoblastic leukaemia. Pediatr Blood Cancer 2008;50(suppl 2):456–461; discussion 468.
97. Dumitru D. Electrodiagnostic medicine. Philadelphia, PA: Hanley & Belfus, 1995.

98. Stubgen JP. Neuromuscular disorders in systemic malignancy and its treatment. Muscle Nerve 1995;18(6):636–648.

99. Sliwa JA. Acute weakness syndromes in the critically ill patient. Arch Phys Med Rehabil 2000;81(3 suppl 1):S45–S52; quiz S53–S44.

100. Larsen RL, Jakacki RI, Vetter VL, et al. Electrocardiographic changes and arrhythmias after cancer therapy in children and young adults. Am J Cardiol 1992;70(1):73–77.

101. Lipshultz SE, Colan SD, Gelber RD, et al. Late cardiac effects of doxorubicin therapy for acute lymphoblastic leukemia in childhood. N Engl J Med 1991;324(12):808–815.

102. Rathe M, Carlsen NL, Oxhoj H. Late cardiac effects of anthracycline containing therapy for childhood acute lymphoblastic leukemia. Pediatr Blood Cancer 2007;48(7):663–667.

103. Jakacki RI, Larsen RL, Barber G, et al. Comparison of cardiac function tests after anthracycline therapy in childhood: implications for screening. Cancer 1993;72(9): 2739–2745.

104. Moyer-Mileur LJ, Ransdell L, Bruggers CS. Fitness of children with standard-risk acute lymphoblastic leukemia during maintenance therapy: response to a home-based exercise and nutrition program. J Pediatr Hematol Oncol 2009;31(4):259–266.

105. Gaydos LA, Freireich EJ, Mantel N. The quantitative relation between platelet count and hemorrhage in patients with acute leukemia. N Engl J Med 1962;266:905–909.

106. Gerber LH, Vargo M. Rehabilitation for patients with cancer diagnoses. In: Delisa JA, Gans BM, eds. Rehabilitation medicine: principles and practice. 3rd ed. Philadelphia, PA: Lippincott-Raven, 1998:1293–1317.

107. James MC. Physical therapy for patients after bone marrow transplantation. Phys Ther 1987;67(6):946–952.

108. Ladha AB, Courneya KS, Bell GJ, et al. Effects of acute exercise on neutrophils in pediatric acute lymphoblastic leukemia survivors: a pilot study. J Pediatr Hematol Oncol 2006;28(10):671–677.

109. White J, Flohr JA, Winter SS, et al. Potential benefits of physical activity for children with acute lymphoblastic leukaemia. Pediatr Rehabil 2005;8(1):53–58.

110. Buizer AI, de Sonneville LM, Veerman AJ. Effects of chemotherapy on neurocognitive function in children with acute lymphoblastic leukemia: a critical review of the literature. Pediatr Blood Cancer 2009;52(4):447–454.

CHAPTER 45 ■ PSYCHIATRIC AND PSYCHOSOCIAL SUPPORT FOR THE CHILD AND FAMILY

LORI S. WIENER, STEPHEN P. HERSH, AND MELISSA A. ALDERFER

Since the 1960s advances in treatment techniques, as well as supportive care, have created dramatic improvements in the survival of children with cancer. As a result, in this early part of the 21st century, pediatric oncology treatment goes beyond seeking cures to include a focus on the short and long-term quality of life of the child or adolescent patient, their siblings, and parents. Successful developmental and psychosocial outcomes for the patient and family hinge on thoughtful assessment, dedication to prevention of physical, neurocognitive and psychosocial late effects, and well-orchestrated collaboration by a multidisciplinary health care team.

This chapter addresses the multidimensional impact of childhood cancers on the child, family members, and the family system. We examine the phases of illness from diagnosis through the stages of treatment and posttreatment and discuss specific issues such as reentry into school and the community, relapse, and the transition to long-term survivorship. Vulnerabilities, stressors, and potential disruptions at each stage of the illness are reviewed and educational, psychological, and psychiatric supports to foster adjustment are presented. Interventions and strategies recommended within this chapter are aimed at building on child and family strengths, providing support, enhancing adaptive coping skills, accepting change, and mobilizing support systems.

PRINCIPLES AND ESSENTIAL KNOWLEDGE FOR HEALTH PROFESSIONALS

Childhood cancer has a powerful and lasting impact on the patient, the family, and their immediate community. Families must endure the transition from feeling safe and in control of their lives to living with vulnerability and uncertainty. Many families experience difficulties adjusting to dependence on the medical system for answers and cure and on extended family/ friends for emotional support. No family member—sibling, grandparent, or other relative—is unaffected.

With current state-of-the-art treatments, most children diagnosed with cancer can be cured; yet, they are likely to have long-term complications. When faced with a diagnosis of cancer, fears of death, disfigurement, pain and suffering, and loss of control are common. The emotionally charged nature of a cancer diagnosis, the demands of treatment (e.g., invasive procedures, hospitalizations, repeated outpatient appointments), and uncertainty associated with long-term outcome have a large impact on the family. Marriages, careers, and relationships are significantly affected.[1] Some families, particularly those with higher levels of adaptability become more cohesive, developing increased strengths and a positive redefi-

nition of values.[2–4] Others, often those with preexisting vulnerabilities and poor intrafamilial communication, suffer various degrees of chronic disequilibrium. When a child dies of his or her disease, the family faces a different challenge. The death of a child can be one of the most difficult losses to grieve.[5]

Given the complexity of the diagnosis and treatment, alongside the unique needs of each individual family, no single health professional can meet a family's needs completely. However, through collaborative, multidisciplinary efforts, a health care team can provide comprehensive care that supports the entire family through the disease course. Screening families on factors known to be predictive of ongoing psychological difficulties can help the team anticipate the psychologic adjustment of families and provide a means for quickly and efficiently providing psychosocial care to families, on the basis of their needs.

An essential component of this screening approach includes an assessment of the family's strengths and vulnerabilities (Table 45.1). This information can be gathered and synthesized during one to three intake meetings, each lasting 45 to 60 minutes. A team member with training in child development and mental health should conduct the intake. The setting should be as relaxed and unthreatening as possible. Intake is the optimal time for identification of families who are at high risk for the development of significant psychosocial problems over the course of the child's illness. Examples of preexisting psychosocial problems include (a) growth and development lags; (b) clinical psychiatric conditions (e.g., anxiety disorders, depression, patterns of impulsive behaviors, and poor judgment); (c) consistent impairment in school or work performance; and (d) family system dysfunction (e.g., abuse, lack of communication, isolation from the community, noncompliance or overt sabotage of medical care). One example of a screening instrument for families of children with cancer is the Psychosocial Assessment Tool (PAT)[6,7] that assesses family risk across eight areas: family structure and resources; social support; child's cognitive, emotional, and behavioral concerns; marital or family problems; sibling problems; family beliefs; and parent stress reactions. Based on findings in the intake, the team can initiate psychosocial interventions, which include crisis intervention, insight-oriented psychotherapy, the use of psychotropic medication or other treatments, such as behavioral techniques (which address specific problems), support groups, and family therapy for members of the family. Although evaluation of family functioning is best formulated at the time of diagnosis or on entry into a new medical environment, evaluation needs to be ongoing, to reassess the family throughout the stages of the child's disease course.

Intake is the best time to begin the ongoing process of assessing family strengths and educating the child and family

SUGGESTED AREAS OF INQUIRY FOR OUTLINING THE FAMILY'S STRENGTHS AND VULNERABILITIES

Illness and history
How the illness presented itself
Was the illness identified and diagnosed rapidly
Did parents feel a sense of competence in their handling of
    the situation
Stage of child's disease at diagnosis and prognosis
Previous child and family experiences with physical health
    problems and trauma, behavioral, and psychological problems,
    including substance abuse
Family's ways of coping, especially family's cohesiveness and
    communication style

Child patient as a person
How child responds to diagnosis
Pre-illness relationships with parents, siblings, peers,
    significant others
Parent in whom child confides when troubled
Energy level, moods, sleeping, and eating habits before and
    after illness
As seen by parents, the child's basic trust, sense of self, ability to
    deal with separation, level of self-care, ability to use fantasy
    and play, orientation toward and ability to deal with
    others, curiosity
Pre-illness functioning in school, plus any existing standardized
    test information (e.g., Wide Range Achievement Test, Wechsler
    Intelligence Scale for Children)
Previous psychological testing and/or psychiatric treatment

Parents
Family constellation and extended nuclear family
Length of marriage
Marital relationship before the diagnosis: level of collaboration in
    parenting, any prior actual or contemplated separations,
    differences in coping styles, communication patterns, trust,
    mutual respect
If separated/divorced, legal and custody arrangements
Physical health, previous losses, mental health, alcohol or drug
    abuse, self-esteem
Comfort with parent role, nurturing interests and capacities,
    abilities to set limits and allow independence, knowledge of
    child's nonverbal cues, awareness of importance of role-
    modeling, knowledge of growth and development, ability to be
    protective yet separate

Each family member's roles/responsibilities
Social (family, community, school) adjustment
Perceptions of parents' attitudes toward them
Quality of current and past relationship to ill child
Ability to express feelings
Understanding of illness
How informed about illness and by whom
Degree of involvement in the diagnosis, treatment, and care
Capacity to ask questions
Parent in whom child confides when he/she has a problem

Environment
Housing
If blended family, quality of relationships
Number of moves over child's lifetime
Sleeping arrangements within the home
Quality of neighborhood and community support
Financial status
Involvement within the community before illness
Distance in miles and travel time to treatment center

Grandparents
Number
Ages
Understanding of cancer
Physical and mental health
Residence
Social adjustment
Expectations and sense of the future
Relationship to own children and to grandchildren; trust in
    and respect for children's autonomy and functioning as
    parents

Siblings
Ages and sexes
Health
Coping support system
Special needs
Coping styles

about the illness, medical system, and treatment. Ideally, these sessions engage the child and parents as active members of the treatment team. Over the course of the intake sessions, the older child and the child's parents can be informed about skills they can learn (through biofeedback, hypnosis, relaxation training) to help deal with their experiences. They can also learn how to work with doctors and maintain social functioning, school attendance, appropriate limit setting, family chores, and work during treatment.

INITIAL DIAGNOSTIC PERIOD: A TIME OF CRISIS

Family's Reaction to Diagnosis

How the diagnosis of cancer is presented to parents and their child not only significantly influences initial responses to med-

ical interventions but also sets the attitudes that affect collaboration, compliance, and trust over the course of the illness.[8,9] Sophisticated oncologists develop an empathic but direct style of disclosing a cancer diagnosis, a style tailored to the characteristics (culture, education, language skills) and needs of each family, patient, and situation. The need to repeat information cannot be overemphasized.

Parents see themselves as providers for their children, whom they are supposed to outlive and protect from fear, hurt, and pain.[5] The diagnosis of cancer represents an assault on a parent's identity and their sense of adequacy as guardian.[2] Shock, confusion, disbelief, guilt, anger, numbness, and fear are the usual emotional reactions experienced by parents after their child's diagnosis. In response to these emotions, most parents struggle to understand the diagnosis and recommended treatments. Driven by a wish to reverse the implications of the diagnosis, families may seek second or more opinions as well as spend long hours talking to friends, visiting medical libraries, and accessing information on the

Internet. Parents may talk only to those friends or relatives who promote unrealistic hopes or who encourage disbelief in what the doctors have told them. Initial disbelief allows the reality to be approached and integrated at a pace that does not overwhelm defenses[10] and therefore, can be protective. It reduces what could otherwise be intolerable anxiety, guilt, and anger.

As the diagnosis is accepted, guilt and anger can become significant emotions, directed in many ways. Anger, in particular, may be aimed at physicians, other staff members, or the hospital at large. Those who were involved in the initial presentation of the diagnosis may, for a short time, be the focus of significant negative feelings. Guilt is expressed in ruminations as parents seek an explanation for their child's illness. Many parents pass through a period of self-blame during which they focus on transgressions they may have committed and for which they feel they are now being punished. They may begin searching for evidence that they failed to pay sufficient attention to early signs of less than optimal health in their child. Some parents may berate themselves for not taking complaints seriously enough, for having children when "cancer runs in the family," for smoking, or for living in polluted urban or industrial areas.

Careful listening (in the context of awareness of the family's cultural and linguistic background) and supportive attention by the oncology staff are important to families. Families need reassurance that they are not responsible for causing the disease,[11,12] so they can redirect their energies toward providing the extensive emotional support needed by their sick child and the child's siblings and mobilizing their own support systems.

An important task for parents is disclosing the cancer diagnosis to their child. Factors including when, how, and what to tell their child about the diagnosis are important to consider as children, as well as parents, later recall vividly what took place when the diagnosis was revealed. Ideally, the parents should be the ones to share this information with their child. Parents need much guidance in this task. Parents often use euphemisms and attempt to protect their child (and themselves) from the harsh realities of the diagnosis and the illness itself. Therefore, they need help in understanding why such information must be presented both honestly and calmly, how (including the timing issue of "when") to communicate information about the nature of the illness as well as the impending changes in activities, appearance, and energy.[13] Many parents benefit from repeated explanation that honest discussion, when properly timed and tailored to the age and developmental level of the child, is essential in order to establish trust with the medical team, decrease the child's anxiety, explain why unpleasant treatments and procedures are necessary, and increase the likelihood of cooperation from the child.[9] Such communication avoids the distortions of secrets held, promises not kept, and misinformation given.[14] Family stress can be better managed once the child understands and accepts the diagnosis. This paves the way for more open communication within the family.[15,16]

Establishing a strong collaborative relationship with the child's treatment team is key for the family. Families find themselves in the situation of needing to absorb a great deal of highly technical information at a time when they are feeling overwhelmed. In addition, they must hear this information from people who they do not yet know or necessarily trust. For these reasons, it is especially important for the medical team to make collaborative efforts in supporting the family while understanding that the child's age and developmental level significantly influence the experience of illness-related events (See Table 45.2).

Family's Reaction to Initiation of Treatment

A new adaptive equilibrium in the family occurs as treatment is initiated. This equilibrium incorporates the illness, as the family reaches for a new sense of normality. Along with a treatment plan comes a sense of hope for the future. As one mother stated, "After I found out what needed to be done, I felt like I had something to hold on to, a chance for a cure. Almost immediately, I felt as if I had some control back. Now we had something to fight with."

Along with feelings of relief, optimism, and improved mood, the initiation of treatment stimulates anxiety, particularly concerning side effects. Eliciting from families their understanding and expectations of the illness and diagnostic and treatment procedures, correcting these impressions as needed, and providing further education, all become essential activities. Misunderstandings commonly occur at this time because of the "selective" hearing of the parents—retaining information that reinforces their hopefulness and "forgetting" information with negative implications. Perceiving the physician as "too busy" gives the parent a comfortable reason to avoid confirmation of valid fears about the child's condition. Coping with the treatment process is often affected by the length of the prediagnostic period: a rapid diagnosis, without uncertainty, demands much less of the family's resources than a prolonged prediagnostic period of professional uncertainty. Equally important, the physician needs to clarify with the family the nature of his or her involvement throughout the treatment process: how much care the physician will administer directly, what will be done by others, and what will be the physician's supervisory role.

It is important to remember that throughout the first few weeks and months of cancer treatment, parental (particularly maternal) distress is very high and can take the form of depression, anxiety, and posttraumatic stress.[17–26] Rates of traumatic stress are particularly remarkable. In one study, 51% of mothers and 40% of fathers within 2 weeks of their child's cancer diagnosis met Diagnostic and Statistical Manual of Mental Disorders (DSM-IV) criteria for Acute Stress Disorder.[27] In a second report, 68% of mothers and 57% of fathers of children under treatment for at least 2 months reported posttraumatic stress symptoms in the moderate to severe range.[28]

Informed Consent

Informing parents and their child about treatments is similar to informing them about the diagnosis of cancer. The approach, the setting, the need for repetition, and the awareness of each family's unique strengths and limitations all remain important. Careful explanations of the disease and its treatment that are tailored to the understanding of each family can significantly improve compliance. It is a positive sign of coping and adaptation when the family asks questions, openly expresses concern, and actively seeks to increase understanding of the child's disease and treatment.[29] Parents should be encouraged to take notes; we suggest offering pads and pencils as this often assists parents in recalling and in formulating questions. For parents who are not literate or who speak another language, a team member assigned as a patient advocate or a translator should be present (see the section Cultural Considerations). Only the physicians involved in the child's treatment should be responsible for informed consent. Nine steps can assist families through this process.[29,30]

1. A full explanation of the treatment and associated procedures must be presented. The language should avoid

TABLE 45.2

CHILD'S REACTION TO DIAGNOSIS AND INITIATION OF TREATMENT: DEVELOPMENTAL CONSIDERATIONS

Developmental stage	Potential issues	Beneficial interventions
Infancy	• Burden of diagnosis weighs on caregivers • Delay in growth, development	• Facilitate parental bonding with infant • Provide support in caring for a medically ill infant

Toddlers/Preschoolers	• Heightened anxiety, depression related to:
	  • unfamiliar hospital setting and medical staff;
	  • separation from parents;
	  • changes in daily routine; and
	  • perceived illness, a punishment
	• Physical stressors
	• Possible regression in skills
		• Educate toddler in an age-appropriate manner.
		• Repetition is necessary to ensure understanding
		• Reassurance from parents addressing cause of illness and periods of separation
		• Staff should inform children in an age-appropriate and honest manner of all procedures and expectations. It is also helpful to familiarize child with medical equipment, staff, etc.
		• Implement positive incentives to award bravery and cooperation
		• Teach relaxation/distraction techniques
		• Do not punish regressive behaviors, rather help child build coping skills

School age	• Heightened anxiety, depression related to:
	  • unfamiliar hospital setting and medical staff;
	  • separation from parents; and
	  • changes in daily routine
	• Physical stressors
	• Psychosomatic complaints
	• Absence from school
		• Education regarding disease and treatment
		• Have child participate in discussions with doctors/staff
		• Facilitate development of self-regulatory skills
		• Teach relaxation/distraction techniques
		• Utilize hospital school services, facilitate reentry into academic setting, and assist with peer education

Adolescence	• Concerns related to independence, appearance, acceptance, sexuality • Difficulties losing control and managing forced dependence • School absence • Disruption of plans for the future	• Facilitate/encourage adolescent independence, especially in regard to self-care • Allow control where appropriate • Include adolescent in family meetings and treatment decision making • Provide a safe environment for adolescent to express concerns and ask questions • Provide counseling to facilitate coping • Facilitate academic assistance and school reentry

professional images and jargon. Professional terms that are unavoidable should be explained in lay images and words.

2. The purposes and expected benefits of the treatments need to be listed.
3. Common morbidities from procedures as well as common morbidities and side effects of treatments should be outlined. Overinforming verbally (e.g., presenting extensive lists of all possible side effects) generates confusion and anxiety and should be avoided.
4. Alternative (complementary) treatments need to be acknowledged and discussed.
5. At this point, the physician should stop and review both questions and emotional reactions with the parents. This recognition of the parents' feelings and thoughts invariably enhances their positive reaction to the physician. It also helps to quiet anxiety. This is the time to inquire about the known or expected reactions from grandparents, other relatives, and friends; these caring people may pressure the parents with their own disbelief about the diagnosis, their anxieties, and advice. Learning about such pressures helps the physician to understand the parents' questions and emotional responses more clearly.[29]
6. The voluntary nature of treatment must be made clear.

7. Parental awareness of the right to withdraw from treatment should be explained carefully, including the meaning of withdrawal "against medical advice." Describe, if necessary, those situations in which the physician will vigorously pursue treatment over parental objections, even to the point of obtaining a court order supporting treatment.
8. The foregoing steps are summarized in the patient's medical chart; at the very least, the date, time, and those present when informed consent was obtained are to be noted.
9. Written consent forms are signed when appropriate or required.

Consent forms almost always cause families considerable stress. Studies reveal that most consent forms "obfuscate, intimidate, and alienate."[8] The readability of these forms is often at a college or higher educational level. In clinical research settings, the realities of informed consent are compounded by requests to participate in randomized treatment trials. Such trials tend to provoke feelings of helplessness, anxiety, guilt, and anger.[31–33] Parents fear the complications of procedures and treatments. Their desire to postpone these interventions—especially in a child who seems well—coupled with being unsettled by not fully understanding information presented through consent forms threatens physician-family relationships.

Families often undergo periods of questioning their decisions to pursue treatment. Side effects such as infections, toxicity, hair loss, muscle weakness, and ataxia can arouse feelings of guilt in the parents. As one parent described it, "I can't stand watching the chemo being administered. I feel as if I'm permitting my son to be poisoned." Many parents struggle with the changes in their child's appearance: "I know she's the same person and I love her every bit as much as I always have. But she looks so different." In the case that an amputation may be the best or only treatment for the disease, health care professionals are cautioned not to overlook the effect that an amputation may have on parents.[29] The loss of a child's limb is experienced as a loss for the parents as well. Clarifying expectations, prognosis, and physical changes associated with treatment is important when obtaining consent, so families can appropriately prepare themselves. Receiving this information from someone they trust is most helpful.[34] Thus, *true informed consent is a process that extends beyond a few formal meetings and printed consent forms.*

Assent

Ideally, in addition to parents' permission, the child's assent to participate in the research should be obtained. The amount and specificity of information provided to the child should be appropriate for his or her stage of development and understanding. Generally, assent is unobtainable from children younger than 7 years.[35] Understanding of research participation is often related more to emotional factors than age or cognitive development. Providing medical environments that decrease anxiety and increase control may enhance children's and adolescents' understanding of the research process.[36]

Parental Adjustment during the Initial Treatment Period

Following the period after the child's diagnosis, parents face a number of new demands. They must maintain employment and/or home responsibilities despite considerable disruption to personal and family routines. In two-parent families, the mother is likely to assume the burden of care of the child with cancer, being more likely than fathers to stay overnight during hospitalizations and to be responsible for outpatient visits. The mother's career and social activities may fall to the wayside, and caregiving to well children and housekeeping may fall to the father and older siblings, taxing the marital relationship and family functioning.[37] Decisions regarding how roles shift related to financial support, management, and care of the home and family appear to be influenced by the location of treatment (out patient or in patient; close to or far from home), the burdens it causes, parental employment, the age of the affected child and siblings, the support available to the family, and the ability of the parents to communicate openly and to share tasks.[38] Open communication allows spouses to negotiate the reallocation of roles more effectively, resulting in a more cohesive, less conflictual family environment.[33]

A mutually supportive marital relationship is a significant variable in the family's ability to cope with the stress imposed by childhood cancer.[39,40] However, the diagnosis of cancer gives rise to a continuous state of uncertainty, anxiety, and stress, all of which have an affect on the parents' marital relationship. Some relationships are adversely affected while others may be strengthened by the experience.[41] Parents, who have supported each other through previous crises; who can share with each other expressions of sadness, anger, frustration, and hope; and who are able to make their child's illness a priority, often eventually find their relationship strengthened. For others, the stress of a child's cancer exacerbates previous marital problems. The child's parents may appear to be emotionally distant, coping with the situation in isolation from each other or using it to fight their unresolved battles. Such marital disharmony negatively affects the entire family's emotional adjustment and thus requires intervention.[42]

Several factors have been identified as creating additional strain on the marriage including the parents' need to "make the child as happy as possible," a sense of guilt regarding the child's disease, fear of leaving the child alone or in someone else's care (compounded by the fear of permanent separation and loss of one's child), disregard of their own needs or those of other family members, and the separation of family members from one another.[43] Some parents may be faced with the difficult task of making decisions independently about their child for the first time. When both partners are forced by their child's illness to assume different roles and responsibilities, problems can arise if the parents remain emotionally invested in their relinquished roles.[44] "Dyssynchrony" of coping styles may occur[45] and may reflect general gender differences.[46] This often leads to isolation of family members from one another and feelings of abandonment and lack of empathy.[47] When differences of coping styles are identified and addressed, tension within the marriage and family is often considerably alleviated. The longer the child is ill, the more resources are depleted, and the prolonged state of stress can lead to a state of marital exhaustion. Marital strengths are important resources to build upon when helping families under stress.[48]

Although the team is encouraged to support parents as a unit, they must also treat each parent as a unique person with his or her own experiences, needs, and roles within the family structure. One parent may require more information, whereas the other may want more support. One parent may want to be involved in every decision, whereas another may want to relinquish responsibility to the team. Such efforts at understanding enhance the family's ability and willingness to place trust in the hospital staff.

In general, the literature on families of children with cancer is based heavily on mothers because the patient's mother most often remains present at the treatment facility. Consequently, her strengths and vulnerabilities can be identified more readily than those of the child's father. Yet, the role of fathers is essential to understand the context in which the child lives.[49] Unfortunately, fathers tend to receive less support, have limited opportunity to share their concerns with others, and often feel guilty and excluded from the daily aspects of the child's life and care.[50–57] In fact, fathers have posttraumatic stress symptoms (PTSS) at a level similar to mothers, and many cases in which a parent has clinically significant PTSS would be missed if only mothers were assessed.[58,59] When given the opportunity, fathers describe the difficulty of having to perform at work and at home, constantly altering work schedules for family obligations, missing life "as it was," and feeling helpless. They value meeting face-to-face with health care professionals to receive information, to determine what and how much information to give their ill child and how to cope with stress.[60] Therefore, efforts should be made to involve both the parents in the child's care. This will facilitate parents (a) obtaining accurate information; (b) addressing questions/concerns; and, (c) developing an understanding of day-to-day responsibilities that are required in looking after their child.[32] Open communication and involvement of both parents is essential to the well-being of their child.

Additional resources are available and beneficial, including support groups in which families can learn from one another how to meet their own needs as well as those of their sick child. Individual or family therapy allows issues of communication, intimacy, or differences in coping styles to be addressed.[47,61] The Candlelighters Childhood Cancer Foundation and the American Cancer Society have local chapters which can be sources of support for families interested in self-help groups within their home community and for those who wish to obtain a bibliography of reading materials and/or films pertaining to their child's disease. Other resources exist as well and are readily available through the Internet (Table 45.3).

ADAPTATION PERIOD

Early Remission and Ongoing Treatment

After the induction of therapy, parents often describe "coming to terms" with the cancer diagnosis. Following initiation of treatment, the child often has a period of remission or tumor regression. The child is able to go home for extended periods, returning to the hospital on a scheduled basis to receive treatments. This process may continue for years.

Parental and Family Adaptation

Subsequent to the distress and disruptions associated with the diagnosis and initiation of cancer treatment, most families adjust to these changes with consistent improvements noted in overall psychological well-being over the first year after diagnosis. Although there is variability in these patterns and in psychological outcomes,[20] in general, there is stability in the overall course of adjustment. Surprisingly, the extent of psychological difficulties in response to diagnosis and treatment is not consistently related to more objective measures of the severity of the illness or intensity of the treatment.[62] Those families that cope and adjust most adaptively at diagnosis tend to continue to do so over the course of treatment and into survivorship.[63] Alternatively, those families that experience the greatest distress at diagnosis are likely to warrant greater attention to their psychosocial needs across time.

Given the improved survival rate in childhood cancer, health care professionals emphasize normalcy throughout the treatment. Recent data also suggests that families maintain a sense of normalcy in their lives during the early period of the cancer trajectory.[64–67] This is challenging as the family is faced with the task of reorganizing itself, changing previous priorities and expectations, and reassigning roles.[68] Optimally, both parents are physically and emotionally available to share the responsibility of the child's care. The themes discussed above regarding parental reactions to the initiation of treatment continue to be important during this adaptation phase, including unequal burden of care on mothers[38] and fathers struggling with the pressure to maintain employment and support their families emotionally when they are feeling overwhelmed themselves. Families who live in communities without local cancer treatment options face additional problems: the need to travel for treatment; separation from home and the family support system during a stressful time; and the additional financial strain associated with time away from work, transportation, child care, and meals and accommodations away from home.

Particularly when the initial hospitalization has been lengthy, families anxiously await the day their child is well enough to return home. Some parents, however, find the return to home particularly stressful as the hospital is often perceived as a safe environment, a place where the child's medical and psychosocial needs are continuously met. Parents may worry about the added responsibility and question their ability to care for their child's physical well-being at home. Despite their concerns, parents are typically successful in the transition to create as normal a life as possible within the confines of the diagnosis.[69] Over time, a new day-to-day routine is established, encompassing the needs of the marital relationship and the well siblings in addition to those of the sick child.

When it is time for the child to return for further treatment, some parents resent having to yield some of their parental responsibilities to the medical system again. Others look forward to being assured that their child is doing well or will be receiving treatments that can cure the disease. These responses are appropriate. Over time, families settle into the routine of the hospital visits while obtaining a comprehensive grasp of the medical treatments and procedures.

It is normative and understandable to see parental distress across treatment.[25,70] Parents fear for their child's life and struggle to make sense of the diagnosis. There are underlying processes of grief and mourning that also impact their behavior. All people have their own way of handling stress and coping with crises.[61] Emotions may change quickly and are influenced by the child's medical state and resources available. Specific factors associated with adaptive family functioning during treatment include open communication about the illness within the family, an attitude of living in the present, lack of other concurrent stresses (marital, financial, illness of other family members), positive family relationships, previous adaptive coping of all family members, and adequacy of the support system. Maladaptive coping may include excessive concern about relapse and death, reluctance to allow the child to return to everyday activities, interpersonal strife, emotional distress and persistent and/or escalating anxiety or depression, behavioral symptoms in the well siblings, difficulties making clinic visits or treatments, reluctance to interact with other patients or families, and ongoing pessimism. In more extreme situations, magical thinking, regressive forms of behavior, or withdrawal from reality may be evident.[63]

Understanding what parents believe and how they experience and interpret their child's illness and treatment may be important in helping families. Beliefs related to self-efficacy facilitate adjustment during difficult times and may guide psychosocial assessment.[71] These include beliefs about the life threat and potentially devastating impact on the family, beliefs about suffering from side effects of treatment, thoughts that reflect a sense of competence in handling difficult situations, feeling supported by family, friends and the health care team, and beliefs that show progress towards making meaning of the experience.[58]

In time, most families develop a "new normal" in their lives. They become hopeful that the disease will respond to treatment and start to make future plans. Still, an infection or unexpected side effect necessitating hospitalization will interfere with family adjustment.[72] When the physical health of the child is stabilized and time between hospital visits is lengthened, families may begin to worry that the details of their child's "case" have been forgotten. Such feelings may be more exaggerated in teaching hospitals in which physicians frequently rotate assignments. These feelings are surmountable when attention is given to the emotional needs of families in remission.

The need for psychosocial intervention during treatment cannot be overemphasized. Information gathered during the initial screening will help tailor and guide the nature and intensity of psychosocial support according to the specific

TABLE 45.3

INTERNET AND BOOK RESOURCES

Internet support organizations for children & teens living with cancer and siblings

Ability Online Support System: www.ablelink.org

Ashley Foundation: www.theashleyfoundation.org

2bMe: www.2bme.org

Blood counts information for children with cancer:
http://pedspain.nursing.uiowa.edu/BCounts/index.HTM

Cancer kids: http://www.cancerkids.org

Common thread: www.commonthread.org

Captain chemo: http://www.royalmarsden.org/captchemo

Fertile hope: http://www.fertilehope.org

Kidscope: http://www.kidscope.org

Kids' home at NCI: www.cancer.gov.cancerinformation

Melinda home page: www.monkey-boy.com/melinda

OncoLink for kids: www./oncolink.com

Group loup: teens talk center online: http://www.grouploop.org/

Outlook: life beyond childhood cancer: http://www.outlook-life.org

PatchWorx: www.patchworx.org

Peanut butter and spinach on wheat toast: www.oncolink.upenn.edu/
psychosocial/books/pbswt

Planet cancer: http://www.planetcancer.org

Starbright world: www.starbright.org

Supersibs.org: http://www.supersibs.org

Teens living with cancer: teenslivingwithcancer.org

Books for Children

Rita Berglund and Katy Tartakoff. An alphabet about kids with cancer. Denver: The Children's Legacy, 1991

Marilyn Hershey. Oncology, stupidology. I want to go home! Cochranville, PA: Butterfly Press, 1999

Jason Gaes. My book for kids with cancer: a child's autobiography of hope. Melius Pub. Corp., 1987

Nancy Keene and Trevor Romain. Chemo, craziness & comfort: my book about childhood cancer. Kensington, MD: Candlelighters

Amy Klett. The amazing Hannah: look at everything I can do! Candlelighters Childhood Cancer Foundation, 2002

Trudy Krisher. Kathy's hats: A story of hope. Morton Grove, IL: Albert Whitman and Company, 1992

Sarah Marston. Sarah: a six-year-old who is unafraid of cancer. Arcadia, CA: National Childhood Cancer Foundation

Sandra J. Philipson. Annie loses her leg but finds her way. Chagrin Falls, OH: Chagrin River, 1999

David Saltzman. The jester has lost his jingle. Jester Books, 1995

Alice Trillin. Dear Bruno. New York: The New Press, 1996

Lori Wiener. This is my world (workbook). Washington, DC: Child Welfare League of America, 1999

Books for Teens

Lance Armstrong. It's not about the bike: my journey back to life. Putnam, 2000.

Leslie Bowden and Brian Bowden. Magical story: a teenager's inspiring battle with Hodgkin's disease. Lucky Press, 2002

Elena Dorfman. The C-word: teenagers and their families living with cancer. Elena Dorfman, 1998

Karen Gravelle and Bertram John. Teenagers: face to face with cancer. Julian Messner, 1986

Miriam Kaufman. Easy for you to say: Q and As for teenagers living with chronic illness or disability. Firefly Books, 2005

Edith Pendleton, ed. Too old to cry, too young to die. Nashville: Thomas Nelson Publishers, 1980

Geraldo Rivera. A special kind of courage. New York: Simon and Schuster, 1976

Internet support organizations for parents

American Psychosocial Oncology Society helpline: www.apos-society.org/survivors/helpline

CancerCare, Inc.: http://www.cancercare.org

CancerNet: www.cancernet.nci.nih.gov

CarePages: www.carepages.com

Caring Bridge: http://www.caringbridge.org

Children's Brain Tumor Foundation: http://www.cbtf.org

The Childhood Brain Tumor Foundation: http://www.childhoodbraintumor.org

Candlelighters Childhood Cancer Foundation: http://www.candlelighters.org

Children's Hospice International: http://www.chionline.org

Children's Legacy: www.members.aol.com/Tclphoto

Families of Children with Cancer: www.fcco.org

Family Voices: http://www.familyvoices.org

Fertile Hope: http://www.fertilehope.org

Foundation for the Children's Oncology Group: www.ConquerKidsCancer.org

Gilda's Club Worldwide: http://www.gildasclub.org

Kids Cope: www.kidscope.org

Kids' Hospital Network: www.bearabletimes.org

Look Good . . . Feel Better: http://www.lookgoodfeelbetter.org

Make-A-Wish Foundation: http://www.wish.org

MUMS National Parent-to-Parent Network: http://www.netnet.net/mums

National Association for Home Care: http://www.nahc.org

National Bone Marrow Transplant Link: http://www.comnet.org/nbmtlink

National Coalition for Cancer Survivorship: http://www.canceradvocacy.org

National Family Caregivers Association: http://www.nfcacares.org/

National Hospice and Palliative Care Organization: http://www.nhpco.org

National Marrow Donor Program: http://www.marrow.org

National Childhood Cancer Foundation: http://www.nccf.org

National Children's Cancer Society: http://www.children-cancer.com

Neuroblastoma Children's Cancer Society: http://www.neuroblastomacancer.org

Outlook: Life Beyond Childhood Cancer: http://www.outlook-life.org

Padres Contra El Cáncer: www.iamhope.org

Patient Advocacy Foundation: www.patientadvocate.org

Pediatric Oncology Resource Center: www.acor.org/ped-onc

People Living with Cancer: www.plwc.org

(continued)

TABLE 45.3

INTERNET AND BOOK RESOURCES (CONTINUED)	
Books for Teens Kathy Ruccione, Nancy Keene, and Wendy Hobbie. Childhood cancer survivors: a practical guide to your future. 2nd Ed. O'Reilly Media, Inc., 2006. Mary A. Kjosness and Laura A. Rudolph. What happened to you happened to me. Seattle: Children's Orthopedic Hospital and Medical Center, 1980 **Books for Siblings** K. Ballard. When your brother or sister gets cancer. Birmingham Children's Hospital Sibling Group and UKCCSG Sibling Project Group Michael Dodd. Oliver's story: for 'sibs' of kids with cancer. Candlelighters Childhood Cancer Foundation, 2004 Jordan Sonnenblick. Drums, GIRLS AND DANGEROUS PIE. DayBue Publishing, 2004	**Internet support organizations for parents** The Children's Cause: http://www.childrenscause.org The National Children's Cancer Society: www.children-cancer.com The Never-Ending Squirrel Tale: www.squirreltales.com The Starlight Starbright Foundation, http://www.starlight.org The Wellness Community: www.thewellnesscommunity.org The Ulman Cancer Fund for Young Adults: http://www.ulmanfund.org

Although we tried to include all potentially useful resources, this list is not exhaustive; new and additional resources may be available.

needs of the family. Most families will benefit from individual or family supportive counseling to find ways in which the family can further unite and strengthen relationships. Education about the disease and its management are critical and should address psychosocial aspects as well as medical and/or nursing implications. Interventions offered at their cancer treatment center may also be helpful and are appreciated by families.[73] One example is "problem-solving therapy" for mothers of children with cancer, which has been found to reduce negative affectivity in mothers and enhance their ability to resolve problems related to the care of their child.[74] In many cases, the expertise of social workers and/or case managers is vitally important in assuring that families have the tangible resources necessary to travel to the hospital and pay bills. There are many helpful resources available to families (Table 45.3) and these organizations typically provide written materials for families and may sponsor support groups or other programs for children with cancer and their families. Increasingly, the Internet is also a source of information and support for families.

Many cancer treatment programs offer the services of social workers, child-life specialists, educators, psychologists, and psychiatrists to assist families. However, the provision of such care has generally lessened across centers in the past 10 to 15 years due to increased health care costs and the fiscal challenges inherent in sustaining these programs.

Parental Expectations and Discipline

As treatment continues, fears related to the disease become less prominent, and other concurrent stresses are perceived as more troublesome.[75] Parents often find themselves in a quandary in deciding how to "parent" their own child. Parenting the child or adolescent in a "normal" way requires parents to control their fears enough to return to modified pre-illness expectations of achievement, independence, and responsibility. Doing so allows the child to become a well-functioning and responsible adult.[76] Feelings of uneasiness, guilt, and anxiety about the disease and possible relapse may interfere with the parents' ability to act in the child's best interest.[77]

"I thought because his treatments were going well, he should be able to continue football practice and be as content and easygoing as before. It wasn't until I found him alone and

sobbing one day that I realized that my expectations were unrealistic. I just wanted him to be normal like before."

"I remember when I turned 15 and my mother took me to the Social Security office. We didn't need the money but she told me that it was better to apply for disability now so I could be assured of an income later on. I assumed this meant that I could never be well enough to work and that I would be permanently sick. She was wrong—there are plenty of things I can do. That wasn't fair."

Many parents experience a natural tendency to care for their children in a way that encourages dependency.[78] For example, they may overindulge or overprotect their child, and find it difficult to administer any discipline. This situation exacerbates the child's perception of himself or herself as different and "singled-out" and places the child in an uncomfortable position with peers and siblings, who resent unequal attention. This unequal attention may also be perceived by the child as meaning that the prognosis is worse than what he or she had been told. Children may encounter overprotectiveness in one parent and overindulgence in another, or both reactions in the same parent. These inconsistencies challenge the child's understanding and coping skills.[79]

Parents need to be informed by the medical team as to what the child can and cannot realistically do in comparison with abilities before the cancer diagnosis.[80] Parents need to be encouraged to allow the child to live as full and as normal a life as possible within the restrictions imposed by the disease. They need to find a balance between overindulging the child and setting too many limits.[81] Parents feel less guilty saying "no" to their child when the physician or other significant persons on the health care team have sanctioned limit-setting.

Social Reintegration of the Child

Cancer disrupts the typical avenues of social activity and forces the young patient to temporarily relinquish usual roles for that of a patient in an unfamiliar system of doctors and nurses.[82] The family is the immediate social setting in which the child copes with his or her cancer. Thus, the family has the opportunity to set the tone for the child's adjustment.[83] By structuring daily living for the child with cancer in accordance with normal expectations for a well child at a parallel developmental stage, a family can help to alleviate the child's feelings of being alone and different.[84] When medically able, the child should be encouraged to resume social activities and roles. Interaction within the community and with the peers is critical for social development. The roles of son or daughter, sibling, friend, student, and possibly athlete and boyfriend or girlfriend and corresponding arenas of social interaction provide necessary vehicles for development. When the child is not medically able to resume all previous activities, contact with friends can be encouraged by planning short visits and making telephone calls.[82] Today, more and more children use e-mail and Internet messaging services or social networking sites (e.g., Facebook) to stay in touch with one another. Children with primary central nervous system (CNS) involvement tend to be at greatest risk for peer problems[85] and particular attention should be given to their social relationships and functioning.

A top priority for the family should be to reestablish patterns and routines of daily life that were disrupted by initial treatment or hospitalization. For young children, familiar routines related to bedtime, toileting, feeding, naps, and play provide a sense of control and security. For older children and adolescents, attention should be paid to reestablishing the child's role in the family. Parents are encouraged to maintain consistent discipline. Those who become lax in their expectations of ill children, overprotective or overindulgent often establish a cycle, which results in significant behavioral problems and/or reduction in the child's sense of self-worth (i.e., feeling they cannot care for themselves or maintain their role). The absence of appropriate limits leads to a sense of lack of control and insecurity in all children, particularly those threatened by a serious illness. In addition, emotional and behavioral consequences can occur in siblings who recognize disparity between rules and expectations.

No consistent, comprehensive, and generalizable protocol is available for promoting the social adaptation of the child with cancer. At present, institutions differ in the number and type of social activities (e.g., playroom, volunteer programs, special camps) and interventions (e.g., child-life or support groups) available to the children they treat. A critical next step is to measure the social performance of these children systematically,[86] to follow their progress over time, and to develop interventions (e.g., social-skills training) to minimize developmental interruptions.

Return to School

A child's life is organized around school, and successful reentry demands rapid return to this environment. School provides for the development of academic abilities, peer contacts, and social activities. A child who misses as little as 4 weeks of school in a year may encounter problems in building the skills necessary for academic progress, as well as miss out on the shared experiences that make up friendships. In addition to possible academic and peer difficulties, school absence has been related to serious stress and adjustment problems.[87,88] Children and adolescents who are receiving treatment for cancer often identify fatigue as one of the most distressing treatment-related symptoms.[89,90] The illness and its treatment may also be associated with reduced concentration, memory deficits, slowed processing speed, and other executive functioning impairments[87,91] that further interfere with academic and social learning.

For the child with cancer, school plays a vital role as the most immediate and important part in normalizing the child's life and counteracting the anxiety, depression, and isolation that may accompany illness and treatment.[92–95] Successful rehabilitation must start with reentry into school. This is a challenge since children with cancer often have difficulty in returning to school and/or maintaining attendance.[96–98] They

show high rates of absenteeism and school refusal, missing an average of 21 to 45 days per year.[97,99] Long-term survivors have reported school absenteeism to be one of the most significant and disruptive consequences of having cancer. Reasons for absenteeism extend beyond necessary clinic visits, hospitalizations, and treatment side effects. Children must also cope with fears of death, the reactions of others, fatigue, and activity restriction, and changes in physical appearance caused by weight gain or loss, alopecia, or amputation. Resulting anxieties and embarrassment and possibly depression significantly contribute to the child's reluctance to attend school.[93] The development of a dependent-protective relationship between the parent and child may also reinforce school absences.[100]

Interventions facilitating school attendance and experiences are imperative.[101] Prevention of school problems is possible by establishing a system for early and ongoing communication among the family, school, and medical personnel. As suggested by Katz and Gonzalez-Morkos,[102] home instruction should begin in the hospital or as soon as a child returns home, if not medically ready to return to school. The home teacher should be oriented to the child's illness, treatment, and schedule as well as to special family and cultural issues. A plan for returning the child to school as soon as medically possible should be created. Special assistance plans (e.g., 504 plans) should be put in place to accommodate the physical and educational needs of the child related to their cancer treatment. Children who received Special Education services through an Individualized Education Plan before getting ill should have the plan revised as needed during the period of home instruction to ensure proper assistance is in place when they return.

At the same time, to minimize feelings of isolation, the patient and family can be encouraged to maintain contact with the child's school friends and teachers. It is extremely important that children receiving home or hospital instruction maintain friendships and connections with peers at school. This may be done through webcams to the classroom or classmate visits to the hospital or home. The patient, classmates, and school personnel all need to be prepared for the child's return to the classroom. For the patient, concerns about being unable to resume previous activities and the reactions, questions, or misunderstandings of classmates are the foremost. Opportunities to rehearse explanations often decrease anxiety. It is usually best to tell the child to respond to questions or comments briefly, directly, and honestly. The child's specific response depends on his or her comfort and developmental level. Some children have benefited greatly from watching videos about the reentry process prior to returning to school. Such videos include the "Back to School Video" in the *Videos with Attitude Series* of the Starbright Foundation (1999) (Table 45.3). Children who resist returning to school or interacting with healthy peers may benefit from professional guidance to remain connected to their friends. These videos and others similar to them can be used in schools and classrooms to help the other children understand their peers' experiences.

Classmates and peers often may benefit from preparation in order to dispel myths and misconceptions about what has happened to the ill child during their absence. Teachers can obtain permission from the family to prepare the class in advance for the child's return by describing events openly and answering questions honestly. Alternatively, some children with cancer are interested in talking to their class as a group. Presentations or projects, such as a show-and-tell for young children or science or health projects for older children, may be used to inform the class about the disease and its treatment.[103,104]

School personnel need information about childhood cancer and its implications in the academic setting. Specifically, teachers require a description of the child's medical status, treatment side effects, prognosis, and daily functioning. Detailed information about any physical changes or restrictions, potential absenteeism, and treatment schedules further alleviates the teacher's own anxieties and uncertainties.[93] Conferences, workshops, and telephone contacts all are useful ways to convey this information. Teachers have responded with reassurance and appreciation for such opportunities to ask questions and to clarify misconceptions.[105–109]

Play

Play occupies a central role in the mental and physical growth of all children. Serious illness and its accompanying stress and physical restriction interrupt natural play and socialization.[110,111] As such, specific developmental tasks, such as the toddler's exploratory behaviors or the adolescent's identification with peers, may be diverted. Parents may be fearful of injury or anxious about their child being with other children. An important task for the oncology team is to encourage the child to resume previous play as much as possible and to participate in available supervised experiences.

In many pediatric oncology centers, the child with cancer has access to established supportive activities ranging from hospital or clinic playrooms to structured groups to special summer camps. The child's participation in such play and recreational programs is important beginning at diagnosis and continuing through treatment and remission to long-term survival. Hospital and clinic playrooms provide the patient with a child-centered environment. They offer a safe place, a setting free of medical procedures in which the patient can restore, in part, normal aspects of living. Over the course of illness, these activities may assume varying functions, helping to prepare the child for medical procedures, forestalling major developmental disruptions, and facilitating the child's social development. Play activities provide a needed source of pleasure and a medium for self-exploration as well as offer the patient an opportunity for mastery and control as opposed to the passivity and dependence enforced by illness. Play may reduce anxiety by helping the child to overcome fears and to cope with frustrations.

Medication Adherence

Ongoing adherence with medical regimens is an important part of living with and adapting to cancer. This includes following prescribed drug protocols, enduring multiple medical procedures, and attending appointments. Noncompliance represents a significant, though often unrecognized issue for pediatric patients with cancer and their families as it can hinder or negate attempts to provide optimal treatment and can compromise the young patient's chances of survival.[112–115] Nonadherence can also lead to misjudging medications as ineffective, ordering unnecessary diagnostic tests, and initiating alternative treatments. Undetected nonadherence also precludes reliable assessment of new or experimental treatment regimens, resulting in erroneous conclusions. Finally, the extent to which nonadherence contributes to poorer outcomes in certain groups of patients (e.g., adolescents with leukemia) remains an unanswered question.

To date, few comprehensive studies of adherence issues in pediatric oncology populations have been conducted. Several factors including history of psychological or psychiatric problems, limited cognitive functioning in child or parent, high family conflict and poor communication, the aversiveness of procedures, the complexity and prolonged nature of drug protocols, mastery over and confidence in the treatment, sense of control, and the patient's age[114,116] likely contribute to poor adherence. In addition, patient anxiety surrounding diagnosis

and treatment, as well as feelings of discouragement and/or hopelessness can also contribute to nonadherence.

Compared with younger children, adolescents are less adherent with oral medication[117] and, in general, less cooperative with their medical care.[118–120] This pattern is consistent with developmental expectations—adolescents seek to exert and maintain control of their lives and develop their independence. Although the adolescent is beginning to assume some adult responsibilities and aspects of their cancer care, these are probably carried out inconsistently. Confusion about responsibility for certain functions increases the chances of missing appointments or medication doses. Adolescents also struggle with wanting to assimilate to their peers and become their own person. Complicated medical regimens and side effects often challenge these attempts. Alternatively, nonadherence may represent the adolescent's denial of illness and its life-threatening consequences.[121]

Routine assessments of adherence are indicated throughout the treatment course. When adherence difficulties are identified, interventions should be delivered immediately. Ongoing management of adherence includes several factors. First, the adolescent must be an active participant in treatment-related decision making. To the extent of the youth's capability, the adolescent should be given as much choice as is possible (e.g., scheduling treatments when they will least interfere with other activities). Second, the oncology team can help the family to set clear expectations and to clarify roles. Decisions about who will be responsible for administering medications or for remembering appointments should be made early, before problems arise. In this regard, if indicated, it can be helpful to both physicians and adolescents to set up a contract, a system of expected behavior and consequent reward. Family members or friends can be recruited to assume supportive or supervisory roles. Third, medical personnel should provide written directions and should make sure that patients understand the purpose and dosage of each medication as well as the timing frequency and method of administration. Visual or auditory signals may be helpful to remind adolescents when it is time to take their medication. For example, the patient can learn to identify a daily routine that can be linked to the taking of medication or utilize a watch or cell phone alarm as reminders. Adjusting medication schedules in order to minimize interference with normative adolescent activities, increased monitoring, treatment by a mental health specialist for behavioral intervention strategies, and in extreme cases, hospitalization for stabilization, education, or the involvement of child protective services may also be needed.[114]

Completion of Therapy

Completion of therapy and discharge to long-term follow-up is a significant milestone. Discontinuation of treatment encourages an increased sense of hope for extended survival. The family may be full of joy, pride, and a sense of accomplishment at the end of treatment. They may also experience a concomitant sense of anxiety, sadness, and fear, however, due to recalling other patients who had relapses or died and losing the routine of taking medication to maintain security and optimism. Separation from the treatment team, on whom the family has depended for so long, also generates fear and uneasiness in parents and the older adolescent who may believe that not actively fighting the disease may make relapse more likely.

Families require extra support and education at this junction. Physicians must outline reasons for discontinuation of therapy, the possibility of relapse with or without treatment, and the risks of continuing therapy longer than necessary.[122,123]

Physicians can be helpful to the family by explaining the meaning of the word "cure," by discussing the follow-up care provided, and by reviewing symptoms that should be reported without delay. Treatment options in the event of a relapse should be explained to the parents. Families can also be reassured by the knowledge that the child is still a patient and will be monitored closely. Changes and growth that have taken place in each family member should be discussed at this time, encouraging an awareness of achievement while preparing the family for the challenges of long-term cancer survival. Finally, patient, siblings, and parents should be instructed about and given written guidelines for self-care. Family members may, at this point, find it useful to increase their use of available communication resources, including chat rooms, through the Internet (Table 45.3). The anxiety felt when therapy is completed dissipates slowly as months pass and the child remains free of disease.[124]

RELAPSES AND RECURRENCES

A Second Crisis

Although an increasing number of children with cancer are able to achieve and maintain freedom from disease, some inevitably experience a relapse or recurrence. In certain ways, this second crisis can be more devastating than the initial stress of diagnosis.[125,126]

Parents often describe the first relapse or recurrence as the most difficult time emotionally, especially when treatment appeared to be going well and no obvious symptoms were present, or when the remission was of long duration. Denial of the illness and fantasies of cure become much more difficult to maintain. After confirmation of a relapse, feelings of shock, anxiety, disbelief, fear, guilt, anger, and sadness are common. Families faced with reinitiating treatment must start over again, but with a smaller chance for successful outcome. The crisis and stress of the diagnosis are reactivated, the threat to life is relived, and new adjustments are required.[81,127] Encouraging the family once again to adopt a positive attitude toward treatment is a challenge to the oncology team. Families can gain a sense of hope from the knowledge that further action will be taken against the disease. Optimal communication among the child, family, and oncology team is essential at this time. Yet, feelings of guilt and failure may hamper communication. Support must also be given to staff members who have worked most closely with the child and family. More than ever before, parents require the availability of team members.

Krulik[128] refers to the time between the first relapse (recurrence) and second remission as the midstage of illness. Hopes for another treatment response are rekindled when the family is encouraged to begin reinduction or another treatment regimen promptly.[126] Attempts to recreate equilibrium within the family are difficult. Intensive treatments once again limit the family's time for other activities. Work habits, social activities, friendship patterns, relationships within the family, and expression of feelings are again altered. Within the hospital environment itself, the family may experience a change of identity because they are no longer part of the "successful" remission group.[128] The family may also feel a change in the attitudes of health care team members toward the child and toward them. Team members may be struggling with their own feelings of disappointment, frustration, sadness, and possibly defeat.

When the disease recurs, relatives and friends may encourage families to seek other treatments or new second opinions or to try an unorthodox method of therapy. Newspapers, magazines, the Internet, fund-raising events, and television talk shows disseminate information about cancer research "breakthroughs" and unconventional treatment in such a dramatic way that it is difficult for the general public to evaluate these reports (see Chapter 51). At this time, the physician may refer the child to another treatment center for participation in a particular randomized clinical trial. The request to consider such a referral can challenge the trust between family and physician, particularly if the family interprets the referral to be a dismissal from care because their child's case is now "hopeless."[129] This misunderstanding can be eliminated and confidence in the professional relationship can be reestablished if a pattern of open, honest communication is encouraged and maintained. The physician needs to reassure the child and family that the relationship that he or she has with the family will not be severed.

In most instances, parents continue treatment with their current medical team and refuse to subject their child to unproved methods. Nonetheless, they may experience guilt and anxiety about rejecting a possible "miracle cure." The treatment team can help to minimize this stress by discussing with the family any treatment information they have received. A commitment to care for the emotional needs of the patient and family, to provide pain control, if necessary, and not to abandon the family if the disease progresses, is essential. Each family searches for ways to cope with the renewed threat to life and to emotional equilibrium. At relapse, increased psychosocial support, exploration of the family's strengths, and focusing on enhancing quality of life together help many to rediscover hope and courage.[81]

Most families manage to cope adequately through their second round of treatment. As was the case during the first treatment course, coping patterns are influenced by treatment side effects, length of hospitalization, and concurrent stresses (e.g., financial pressures, career obligations, family problems). The altered prognosis elicits feelings of sadness and fears of separation and loss; yet, an investment in "going on" persists. Maladaptive coping is manifested by an overly pessimistic attitude about the future that may immobilize parents in their day-to-day functioning. Emotional or physical withdrawal from the child, inability to normalize the child's life, and refusal to follow through with medical care are other signs indicating the need for intervention. Crisis intervention with individual or family sessions can help the family to alter maladaptive coping.

If another remission is achieved, the termination of active treatment often activates a crisis that requires additional education and support from the staff. Parents fear another relapse and the lack of future treatment options. The treatment team must remain in close contact with the family. Not only is frequent medical follow-up required, but the quality of the family's life also needs continual assessment as the family copes with fear and tremendous uncertainty.

Some parents do pursue complementary medicine and unproved methods of treatment or faith healing in addition to, or instead of, traditional or conventional care. Regardless of prognosis, the health care team should present to the family all the information regarding the success rate of conventional treatments. Should parents refuse to pursue conventional treatments, one should enlist the help of extended family members as well as clergy, if appropriate, as a way of convincing them not to turn their back on conventional care.[130] Use of the child abuse and neglect statutes is, on infrequent occasions, the only way to ensure that a child with a treatable disease receives appropriate therapy. Such measures should be taken only after all efforts to secure the parents' willing participation in the treatment regimen have been exhausted.

Parents should be reassured that the medical care team remains interested in them and the child's welfare and is willing to provide any care needed.

Treatment Refusal

When the child or adolescent refuses treatment, the underlying motivations may include hopelessness about the outcome, feelings of helplessness, loss of control, distress about the side effects of treatment, or a combination thereof. By refusing treatment, some adolescents are asserting their independence and are demonstrating that they are in charge of their own destiny. This is another situation in which preventive measures are far more effective than trying to intervene in a crisis. While the specific preventive measures should be tailored to the age of the adolescent, it is important to include the adolescent in the discussion and decision-making process from the beginning. Support groups for teenagers may be effective in this regard because the members confront one another when poor decisions are made, just as they share coping skills with one another and general support. In the event that staff and family must intervene during a crisis, the staff needs to calmly sort out which factors are influencing the decision and proceed in an orderly manner to discuss them. Sometimes the patient feels that the parent is making all the decisions. This situation can usually be handled directly by encouraging the parents to work collaboratively with the adolescent. For patients and parents who believe that treatment is hopeless, the risk-to-benefit ratio of further treatments must be presented clearly, particularly when the treatment is palliative. Quality of life must be discussed and examined. The distress and discomfort of side effects are the most common reasons for refusing further treatment. In such instances, a mental health professional not directly involved in the child's care can be of assistance.[131] It should be remembered that 18-year-olds, as long as they are not deemed incompetent to make treatment decisions, can refuse treatment.

When Treatments are No Longer Effective

Although survival of childhood cancer is more prevalent now than in the past, the course of cancer for some children is characterized by a series of treatment responses and relapses leading to a time when curative options are exhausted. There have been recent developments in how care is provided to children who may (or will) die that include consideration of psychosocial factors from earlier in the disease process than has typically been evidenced.[132,133]

Specifically, the practice of pediatric palliative care offers a model of treatment for children with life-threatening conditions and their families that combines aggressive symptom control with provision of timely, accurate information and support in decision making.[133] Such care provides a broad frame of reference, including consideration that some children who will not die would still benefit from attention to "comprehensive, compassionate and developmentally appropriate palliative care."[134] As outlined by Himelstein et al.,[134] there are five spheres of practice in pediatric palliative care, each of which has significant psychosocial impact: physical concerns (e.g., pain); psychosocial concerns (fears, coping, communication, resources); spiritual concerns (hopes, life meaning, religious beliefs, and behavior); advance care planning (goals and related care plans); and practical concerns (communication and coordination with treatment team, location of care,

school and functional issues, financial concerns). The goal is to provide consistent, competent care that meets not only the child's physical needs but his or her emotional, spiritual, and cultural ones as well.

The point at which curative treatments are unlikely to be successful is typically a crisis point for the family. Factors that influence the recognition by parents and professionals of this time include the specific form of cancer; the length and course of the illness and treatment; the child's physiology; the child's and family's threshold of tolerance for physical pain and loss of control; their levels of hope; and their beliefs.[135]

Most training programs provide little formal education for physicians, nurses, psychologists, or social workers regarding death and working with children and their families at the end of life. This gap has been increasingly recognized, as the discordance among patients, families, and staff can be an obstacle to care.[136] Differences between parents' reports of their child's symptoms and the documentation of the symptoms by the health care team can create barriers to effective communication about pain and suffering and its treatment.[137] A series of meetings with the family should be held to discuss the transition in care associated with palliation. The staff members who have been most intimately involved with the child and family during the course of the disease ideally should be present at these meetings. The leader of these meetings, generally the patient's oncologist, should elicit from parents their understanding of the situation, selectively sharing impressions with them and remaining open to a range of emotional reactions and unfolding questions. The child may or may not attend these meetings, depending on his or her age, developmental stage, and other circumstances. If the child is not present, relevant information should be communicated to the child in a developmentally appropriate manner. Staff members who are closest to the child and family should be present at these meetings if the parents wish them to be present. The patient and family should be informed of both physical and emotional expectations and possibilities.

Once they understand that treatment is no longer effective, parents begin the process of accepting that their child will die. They may experience preparatory (anticipatory) grief. Many of their thoughts focus on preparing for death (this may include rehearsing the funeral in their imaginations) while continuing to hope for cure or recovery.[138] Parents become increasingly vulnerable during this period to the promises of nontraditional or even fraudulent healers and healing rituals as well as to misguided advice from Internet sites. The opposing forces arising from experiencing moments of hopefulness while simultaneously thinking of the child's funeral generate guilt. Guilt can be diminished in parents by simply informing them of the normality of these responses.[139]

Hope can be redefined by redirecting energies toward enhancing the child's quality of life and planning for the child's comfort in death (absence of anxiety and pain combined with the presence of loved ones) as much as possible. Comprehensive care for the dying child involves maximizing physical and emotional comfort. Open communication, pain control, involvement with friends and family, distractions, and the maintenance of familiar routines all convey a sense of security that is important in reassuring the dying child. The family itself needs ongoing emotional support as well as specific information and assistance with difficult decisions and preparations. This is where the many excellent hospice staff can be extremely helpful (see Chapter 49). Painful decisions must be made regarding home versus hospital care for the dying child, autopsy, and funeral arrangements. The decision-making process is facilitated through open discussion ahead of time. This can be accomplished by linking medical care, supportive home care, hospice, and community services.[140]

Talking to the Dying Child

Struggling with their own anticipations and fears of separation and death, the family needs assistance in addressing their child's thoughts and concerns. Many parents are unable to discuss the imminence of death with their child.[136,141] Some believe that the child is unaware of the prognosis and approaching death. Two models of communication are currently described in the literature.[142] These are labeled as *the protective approach* in which the ill child is shielded from knowledge of the disease diagnosis and prognosis and *the open approach*, which encourages providing an environment in which the child feels free to express concerns and ask questions about his or her condition.[143]

In the past, it was frequently assumed that children did not understand death and that creating an atmosphere of cheerful normality would protect the child from the seriousness of the illness as well as from the awareness of death as a possibility. Nonetheless, research has shown that children who exhibited a higher level of adaptation to the illness were members of families in which open discussion was allowed and maintained. Waechter[144] conducted a study of hospitalized and fatally ill children and stated that giving a child the opportunity to discuss issues related to death does not heighten anxiety. These findings support the prediction that "understanding, acceptance, and conveyance of permission to discuss any aspect of the illness decreases feelings of isolation and alienation from parents and other meaningful adults and gives the child the sense that his or her illness is not too terrible to discuss."[144]

Children generally have two main questions. The first is, "Am I going to die?" When the answer is understood to be yes, the second questions is, "When?" It is helpful to point out to the child what can and cannot be done regarding the illness. Telling the child that cure is no longer a possibility is not only the most difficult but also the most important message to convey. It is easy for caregivers to camouflage difficult messages in professional jargon. Instead, one must relay prognosis in an open, straightforward manner without appearing uncaring. The child needs at this time a feeling of security and trust maintained through honest communication.

In telling dying children that a cure is no longer possible, one must also leave room for hope by redirecting the focus from cure to comfort. Comfort includes having people around who they love, being free of further diagnostic or treatment procedures, and having pain controlled. Although adolescents may need some time alone, one of the greatest fears of young patients is being abandoned by or separated from family and friends. If these children are in the hospital, a nonrestrictive visiting policy for family should be provided, and interaction with friends and other patients should be encouraged. Even children cared for at home need repeated reassurances that they will not be left alone. Providing comfort also involves acknowledgment and acceptance of the range of feelings that come and go. Children should be told that it is all right to feel confused, sad, or angry—and to talk about these feelings, or, at times, to remain silent. To the extent possible, children should be encouraged to participate in normal daily routines. Continued attendance at school (even if part-time) and involvement in family functions counteract boredom and boost quality of life. Each day can be organized so that even children confined to bed feel that they are important contributors to their world. Preserving familiar behaviors and schedules also serves to minimize feelings of being a burden.

Once discussion surrounding death is initiated, children often begin to ask specific questions such as (a) what will death be like; (b) what will happen to me after I die; (c) will the "bad things" I have done or thought cause me to be punished; (d) will my family be all right after my death; (e) will dying hurt. Parents benefit from being informed that they might be asked such questions. Parents also benefit from exploring their own spirituality. Such explorations, with or without the help of clergy, provide strength to parents as they provide support for both their dying and their healthy children.

Depending on the child's religious upbringing, spiritual concerns and questions may arise. For example, children experiencing considerable guilt and conflict or feelings of isolation may become frightened and preoccupied about whether "the devil is in their heart" or whether "God will stop watching over them." Consultation with a chaplain specializing in work with terminally ill children can allay the child's fears and bring in the child and family a sense of comfort and peace. Parents often need help understanding their child's questions and providing answers appropriate to their developmental stage and knowledge of the disease.[145] Some children may keep their thoughts about death to themselves due to fear of emotional abandonment by family members and significant others. They may feel that discussing their own death may compound the emotional burden on parents and siblings.[146] Through play, art, drama, and therapeutic conversation, mental health professionals can ascertain the child's private perceptions and concerns and can correct distortions, dispel fantasies, and promote self-esteem through mastery of fears.[147,148] Parents should be encouraged to participate in this process.

As death approaches, it is important to help families believe they have done all they could for their child. Parents trying to hold on to any semblance of control may seem less cooperative or easily frustrated and annoyed. Such responses are appropriate given the sequence of experiences leading to the terminal phase of illness. Living with a dying child is a significant additional stress for families.[149] One needs to respect each family's readiness, delicately balancing life issues with those related to palliative care, death, and loss. The medical team's participation and investment in caring for the dying child is extremely important to and is greatly appreciated by all families.

The terminal phase of illness is an especially crucial time to involve all significant family members. As separation anxiety is heightened, feelings of helplessness and despair may prevail. Family members often find it helpful to participate in the child's physical and emotional care. This care can take place in the hospital or at home and can include anything from having a sibling help the child eat to having a parent administer medications and oxygen. Family members vividly recollect these terminal events. They can either be plagued by them or find solace in their remembrance.[142] Parents, siblings, and others close to the child benefit greatly from having someone available with whom to share their thoughts, fears, and concerns. Sensitive assistance should be given to the family with difficult decisions and preparations. Parents need repeated reassurance about the importance of their vigil with the child and how this vigil reduces their child's feelings of isolation and abandonment through the moment of death. Home hospice staff usually can provide assistance and guidance to parents and other family members.

Pain Control

One of the child's most frequently posed questions is, "will it hurt?" Children ask this about medical procedures and surgical interventions and may raise this question in discussions about dying (see Chapters 42 and 49). The multidisciplinary health care team has the responsibility to provide the most effective pain management possible. The treatment team's goal is freedom from pain with as little sedation as possible. Pain is made worse by anxiety as well as by depression. Both often occur simultaneously. Anxiety, depression, posttraumatic stress, and disordered sleep must all be addressed for optimal pain control. Properly used combinations of non-pharmacologic methods (psychological interventions, complementary, and alternative medical practices) and pharmacological methods (drug therapy as well as interventional or invasive anesthesia techniques such as nerve blocks, epidural catheters, and electric stimulators) can significantly reduce pain and suffering. Comprehensive care that integrates symptom control, psychosocial support, and palliative care into the routine care of the seriously ill child is strongly advised.[150,151]

Hypnotic techniques may be helpful to the young child as they help focus attention and mobilize children's imaginations. Some older children and adolescents are very responsive to hypnotic focusing of attention and distraction while others respond best to guided imagery and fantasy under the direction of a trained professional with the help of a caregiver.[152] Proper pain control enhances the child's capacity to respond to all treatments, improve self-care, as well as to engage with caregivers, family members, and school.[146]

Advance Care Planning

"Helping a child on his way" and "ending the child's suffering" are sometimes whispered or become unspoken issues during the terminal stage of illness. More open and frank appraisal of these and other delicate issues by health professionals with patients and families is occurring more often now than in the past. The process of advance care planning may be thought of as a series of steps,[134] beginning with the identification of the decision makers and including the role of the child or adolescent in this process. In fact, developmentally appropriate advance-care planning may play an important role in the care of seriously ill adolescents and young adults. In a study designed to explore whether youth living with a potentially life-limiting disease find an advance care planning guide helpful, participants reported such a document would be appropriate and unlikely to elicit significant stress.[153] As we listen to the concerns and provide counsel to our adolescent and young adult patients throughout treatment, it is important that providers do the same about their thoughts about death and how they would like to be remembered in the years to come. Providing an avenue to share such intimate views and wishes promotes communication, fosters decision-making, and can augment dignity and respect of self-autonomy and determination in the face of death.[154] Discussions about treatments that may sustain life (e.g., resuscitation, feeding tubes, hydration, treatment of infection) and their use help in the formulation of a plan with the patient and family that is medically, legally, and ethically acceptable. The advance-care planning process can facilitate wishes to ease the pain of dying through more aggressive use of pain medications or through the removal of those treatments that slow the pace of the dying.

Although many health care professionals agree that children should not be allowed to die in agony, children do sometimes die that way.[155,156] The health care team ideally should be open to parents who inquire about helping their child die in comfort and to the children who prefer to leave these decisions in their parents' hands. The physician can serve as a special listener, selectively interpreting and responding to the parent's concerns about suffering. When a parent wishes to ease the pain of dying through more aggressive use of pain medications or through the removal of treatments that slow the pace of the dying, the physician must examine parental wishes in the context of physician's knowledge of the child's clinical status. If the physician finds his or her perceptions concordant with those of the parent, we believe it appropriate to stand by that parent, to be an advocate for the needs of the dying child while adhering to local laws and medical ethics. The intent to relieve suffering is ethical and legal, but intent to hasten death or end life is not.[157]

After the child's death, the involved professional needs to be available to the parents. The mourning process extends over several years and those making the decision of passive euthanasia need time to absorb that reality into their lives and values structure. Be aware that the echoes and emotional doubts over these actions linger for extended periods of time. As health professionals, we should be available to listen to the parents quietly and acceptingly.

Bereavement in the Family

The death of a child is one of life's great tragedies. It disrupts a family system in multiple ways. In our society, the bereavement process may have even greater consequences than in earlier times because of the absence of general familiarity with death and its rituals. Death in children accounts for less than 5% of mortality in the United States.[158] Cancer is the third leading case of death among children aged 1 to 4 years, and the second leading cause of death among children aged 5 to 14 years,[159] accounting for 8% of that pediatric mortality.[160,161] This means that families who lose a child to cancer are an isolated minority, with relatively few social supports for their grief.

The child's death marks the major milestone in a bereavement process initiated when the cancer diagnosis was first heard. Varying degrees of family disruption consequent to such a death have been identified.[149,162–165] Included are rates of marital separation and divorce ranging from 5% to 70%.[166,167] Bereavement after the death of a child has been found to be "more intense grief reactions of somatic types, greater depression, anger and guilt with accompanying feelings of despair" when compared to bereavement over a spouse or parent.[168] No parent ever "gets over" the death of his or her child.

The parents suffer from both the loss of the child and of what the child represented to them. In our culture, children represent continuity of their parents' lives into the future, beyond death.[169] Children also are vessels into which parents tend to pour hopes and dreams not only for the child but also for themselves through the child's growth. Mothers and fathers may differ from one another in their responses based on their own personalities, life experiences, and beliefs. A child's death may precipitate guilt in parents. This usually involves wishes that "it would all finally end."[170] When this kind of guilt is left unresolved, unexposed, and unexamined, it is a significant psychological risk factor for the parent. Other special vulnerabilities arise depending upon the deceased child's role in the family. For example, the more emotionally dependent the family was on the child and the more the child was viewed by one or both parents as an emotional extension of self, the more disruptive the child's death is to the family system.[149,169,171] The same is true for a child who served as the essential bond or the "communicator" between the parents.

Spinetta et al.[3] found that certain families' coping efforts during the course of illness can make a difference in their adaptation after the death. Better adjustment was seen in

(a) parents who had a viable and ongoing "significant other" to turn to for help during the course of illness; (b) those who had an open and responsive communication with the child during the illness and who gave their child the information and emotional support he or she needed; and (c) those who had a consistent philosophy of life that helped the family to accept the diagnosis and cope with its consequences. Participation in the care of the child during his or her life is associated with healthier bereavement responses. Similarly, attendance to the child during the dying process makes a significant difference, attenuating guilt feelings and anger.

Families generally do not seek professional help to deal with bereavement. If they were involved in hospice, follow-up counseling is supposed to be offered. Parents, siblings, and grandparents benefit from the opportunity to reflect on and review the illness-dying-death experience until acceptance occurs.[172] When the atmosphere of the treatment site is accepting, families may return over a period of many years for spontaneous visits to the oncology service where their child was treated. Ongoing availability and interest in the health of these families should not stop at the point of the child's death.[2,127,172,173]

SURVIVORSHIP

Despite the real possibility that a child with cancer will die, today, 78% of children under 20 years of age diagnosed with cancer are expected to survive for 5 years or more.[174] With the diminishing of concerns about disease recurrence, other worries have become relevant including fears about the long-term sequelae of the illness and treatment. According to a recent report of cancer survivorship, as many as two-thirds of childhood cancer survivors experience at least one late effect, with one-fourth of survivors reporting a late effect that is severe or life threatening.[175]

Among the earliest and most widely recognized late effects of childhood cancer are neuropsychological deficits, particularly deficits in memory, metacognition, visual-spatial/motor skills, and processing speed.[176–179] Interventions to remediate neurocognitive difficulties have focused on collaborative relationships between families and schools and advocacy for the educational needs and concerns of survivors. However, cognitive remediation or retraining and pharmacological interventions have also been explored.[180] A Cognitive Remediation Program has been evaluated in a multisite randomized clinical trial demonstrating improvements in academic achievement.[178,180,181] Pharmacologically, methylphenidate has also been investigated as a potential treatment for neurocognitive late effects, demonstrating some success.[182–184]

Other late effects can involve changes in appearance (e.g., obesity, physical disabilities left by surgery), defects in major organ systems (e.g., cardiac, liver, renal), fertility problems, and the risk of second malignant neoplasms.[185–205] Recent studies are revealing some delays in young adult developmental milestones for survivors of childhood cancer[206] and concerns about health behaviors.[207] Routine follow-up of the long-term cancer survivor should include screening for these potential late effects as well as age-appropriate education regarding special lifelong health risks and necessary health maintenance practices[208,209] (see Chapter 47).

The experience of childhood cancer may also have lasting psychological effects. Developmental disruptions experienced during treatment have undeniable implications for future psychosocial adjustment though the degree to which these disruptions affect the child's later adjustment varies.[210] Older children and adolescents are particularly sensitive to disruptions in their developing peer and intimate relationships, school and extracurricular activities, and future lifestyle and occupation plans.[203] Evidence has suggested that pediatric cancer survivors with CNS involvement may experience difficulties in social competence and peer interactions including social isolation, fewer best friends than same-age peers, and less participation in peer activities than other children.[85,211]

The risk of psychological/psychiatric illness remains unclear however,[212] as investigations designed to examine psychological outcomes in long-term survivors of childhood cancer have produced inconsistent findings.[213–215] A few studies suggest that survivors are at increased risk for maladaptive psychosocial sequelae and psychiatric symptoms[210,212] including depression,[216,217] behavioral adjustment problems,[217–219] and anxiety.[220–222] Most studies, however, report that childhood cancer survivors as a group have no higher prevalence rates of anxiety,[223,224] depression,[224–226] overall mood disorder,[227] adjustment problems,[187,201,212] or lowered self-concept[228] and are relatively well adjusted when compared to healthy controls, non-ill siblings, and standardized norms.[221,228–236] Similarly, adolescent and young adult survivors of cancer report normal psychological functioning.[221,226,228,237–239] Even though survivors in the large multi-site Childhood Cancer Survivors Study (CCSS) reported more depressive and somatic symptoms than their siblings, their rates of depressive and somatic symptoms were in the normal range.[220]

Several studies suggest that childhood cancer survivors are better adjusted compared to normative groups.[63,216,229,240–242] The apparent emotional health of childhood cancer survivors, however, has not been accepted without question and there are subgroups that are at risk for emotional difficulties. The absence of anxiety and depression in child and adolescents survivors of cancer has been explained in terms of a tendency to minimize distress, using a repressive coping style.[234,243] Furthermore, there is emerging evidence that childhood cancer survivors are vulnerable to psychosocial difficulties during the transition to early adulthood. Adult survivors of childhood cancer report more negative moods, tension, and depression than their siblings[244] and may report increased suicidal symptoms and global psychological distress.[244,245]

Posttraumatic stress has emerged as a helpful model for understanding the cancer-related distress of families of survivors. Low rates of posttraumatic stress disorder (PTSD) are typically found for young cancer survivors, in the range of 5% to 10%,[18,23,59,246–248] however, many survivors experience posttraumatic stress symptoms (PTSS) such as intrusive thoughts about cancer, arousal and a desire to avoid cancer-related reminders.[18,247,249–251] Studies typically find higher rates of PTSS and PTSD in young adults who survived childhood cancer compared to adolescents but not all find this pattern.[251–256]

Young-adult survivors also face additional concerns including the acute and long-term physical effects of their treatment, dating and fertility, employment, obtaining their own health and life insurance, as well as fear of recurrence or death. Research is emerging that demonstrates that young adult survivors of childhood cancer are achieving milestones of adulthood such as autonomy, independence, and psychosexual development, at a slower rate than healthy peers.[206,257] Investigation of health-related quality of life (HRQOL) in survivors of childhood cancer is growing. One's "quality of life" is a subjectively reported multidimensional construct that includes aspects of physical functioning, psychological adjustment, social functioning, and an overall sense of well-being.[258] HRQOL can be measured in school-age children as young as age 8[259] and a variety of measures exist.[260] Survivors of childhood cancer have been found to have poorer HRQOL compared to healthy peers.[259,261] Follow-up care should assess survivor HRQOL and interventions tailored to the needs of survivors at different developmental stages are needed.

In addition, the health behaviors of childhood cancer survivors are important to consider. Limiting risky health behaviors and engaging in health-protective behaviors are important for cancer survivors given their increased risk for secondary cancers and physical late effects. Adolescent and young adult cancer survivors engage in healthy habits (e.g., medical follow-up, exercise, healthy diet, sunscreen use) at low to moderate rates, similar to their peers.[207] They engage in unhealthy behaviors (e.g., tobacco and alcohol use) at similar or lower rates than their peers.[210,262] Health behavior interventions for childhood cancer survivors, such as the Survivors Health and Resilience Education (SHARE) program, are being developed and evaluated.[263]

The impact of childhood cancer on the close family members of the diagnosed child is significant and variable over time. In the longest-term study to date, investigating parents of survivors 10 years posttreatment, on average, psychiatric symptomatology and psychological adjustment of parents was within normal ranges.[63] Parents of children at least 5-years posttreatment are also within normal ranges on anxiety and depression with 10% falling in the clinical range for distress.[264] Similar results have also been reported for parents of children 1- to 5-years posttreatment[265] and parents of children who had undergone bone marrow transplant 1 to 10 years previously.[266] In this last study, 14% of parents indicated ongoing emotional distress. In sum, it seems that only about 10% to 14% of parents of children off treatment more than 1 year experience high levels of anxiety and depression. Nevertheless, a series of reports has documented PTSS and/or PTSD in parents of childhood cancer survivors.[18,24,59,229,267-271] The prevalence of these symptoms can be marked; for example, in a study of 150 families of adolescent survivors of childhood cancer, 20% of the families had at least one parent with current PTSD[59] and in an investigation of patterns of posttraumatic stress symptoms across parents, the majority of families had at least one parent with moderate to severe PTSS.[272] Not surprisingly, those parents with higher rates of distress during treatment were more likely to have persistent PTSS after treatment ended.[267,273] Looking at other members of the family, Alderfer et al.[274] found that 32% of adolescent siblings of cancer survivors had PTSS in the moderate to severe range.

PTSS have emerged as a target for intervention across family members. Surviving Cancer Competently Intervention Program (SCCIP)[275] takes such an approach and integrates cognitive-behavioral and family therapy in a four-session, one-day program involving groups of families of adolescent cancer survivors. The results of a randomized clinical trial of 150 families indicate that those randomized to SCCIP showed significant reductions in PTSS, particularly for survivors and fathers.[276] A two-session intervention based on SCCIP has also been developed and piloted with young adult survivors.[253]

Specific educational and occupational achievements and choices may be affected by cancer survival. The academic ability of the long-term survivor may potentially be affected by intellectual[277-281] and learning problems.[282,283] Potential learning problems, coupled with disruptions in school attendance, may limit the child's educational achievement and occupational attainment.[284] Early results of interventions using a psychologically based outpatient rehabilitation program in order to remediate treatment-related cognitive effects appear promising.[285] Even when they are successful in overcoming learning and educational barriers, long-term cancer survivors may encounter difficulties in the community and workplace as a result of their cancer history. Hiring discrimination, ineligibility for health and life insurance, and employers' attitudes about cancer may all complicate the cancer survivor's entry into the work force.[91,286,287]

Routine screening for psychological late effects should be standard care in follow-up clinics. Educational interventions during the follow-up visit are important, especially given the significant gaps that young adults have demonstrated regarding knowledge of their medical history and vulnerability.[288] Informal interventions include giving survivors information regarding their medical late effects while minimizing the anxiety that such education may provoke[289] and providing anticipatory guidance about normative psychosocial symptoms (e.g., anxiety and worry about medical late effects, distress when reminded of cancer and late effects). Formal educational interventions can include standardized methods of educating survivors about medical and psychosocial risks[290] or more targeted behavioral efforts to modify health risk behaviors.[291,292]

It is important to note that while childhood cancer is generally viewed as a traumatic event, positive outcomes may be identified as well. The experience of surviving cancer may be an opportunity and a catalyst for personal growth.[293,294] Relationships may be enhanced as people value their friends or family more. Greater strength or wisdom to face life challenges may evolve and each day be more fully appreciated after treatment for a disease, which was potentially life-limiting.[295] Thus, as part of the assessment of psychosocial stressors, identifying areas of growth is also warranted. Prospective studies should further refine the definition of post-trauma growth as well as determinants for both post-trauma stress and growth outcomes.

FAMILY CONSIDERATIONS

Siblings

The effects of childhood cancer on the healthy siblings within the family deserve special attention. While the effects of illness on families and individual family members is multifaceted and reciprocal,[64,65,296] only in recent years has it been recognized that the needs of siblings are met less sufficiently than for other members of the family.[297,298] Support for the healthy siblings should begin at the time of diagnosis and continue throughout the course of the illness, and as part of bereavement support if appropriate.

Identifying siblings at high risk of difficulty is essential as soon after the diagnosis of cancer as possible. The strengths and vulnerabilities of each well sibling should be included in the initial family assessment. If possible, well siblings old enough to understand who express an interest in gaining more information should attend early family conferences to obtain information and be more included in the process.[298] The siblings' early involvement minimizes feelings of isolation from the family and establishes an atmosphere of openness and understanding that sets the stage for communications among family members.[299]

Siblings experience a range of reactions after a diagnosis of cancer including shock, disbelief, helplessness, sadness, loneliness, rejection, anxiety, anger, jealousy, and guilt.[17,54,300-315] This emotional intensity is accompanied by feelings of insecurity, vulnerability[306,314,316] and worry.[307,313] There is tremendous change within the lives of siblings, including losses (e.g., parental attention, normal family roles, sense of self) and gains (e.g., family closeness, independence, maturity, empathy).[297] Particularly during the first year or two after the diagnosis, a siblings' quality of life is significantly affected.[317-322] A subset (about one-third) experience moderate to severe posttraumatic stress symptoms[23,308,321,323,324] and parents often report increases in behavioral problems.[325] Most siblings, however, do not experience clinical levels of behavioral problems, anxiety, or depression,[17,213,308,317,321,323,326-336] though within 2 years of the cancer diagnosis these youngsters worry about their own health[302,312,314,337,338] and school-age siblings may be at greater risk for somatic distress than their peers.[317-319,330] Some healthy children may wish they were the ones with the disease; others fear the day that they too will develop cancer. Whenever distress, traumatic stress or somatic symptoms, depression, anxiety, or behavioral problems start to interfere with daily functioning, referrals for psychosocial care should be made.

As the child proceeds throughout treatment, the healthy sibling often feels a sense of isolation and deprivation. Family separations and disruptions of daily routines can result in decreased social contact with important sources of emotional and social support.[17] Often, healthy siblings share less of the parents' time and may begin to question whether they still are loved. Lengthy hospitalizations or limited financial resources may cause siblings to be deprived of parental supervision and opportunities for social activities. They may experience an increased need for instrumental support (e.g., transportation) to maintain friendships and social pursuits.[298,313,314,337] When fewer opportunities are available to communicate cancer-related worries, beliefs, and feelings, behavioral, social, and emotional problems can ensue,[17] creating a family environment that is even more highly charged with emotion.[339] While envy and rivalry among children exist in every family, healthy siblings often feel resentment and jealousy because of the special care and parental attention given to the sick child, which sets the stage for experiencing guilt. Although siblings often feel neglected, most fear confronting their parents with such negative feelings.[340]

Healthy siblings can also experience difficulties in school. Disruptions in academic performance and behavior may occur due to changes in routine, fatigue, worry, and sibling-reported conflicts in loyalty (wanting to be with the child with cancer instead of at school).[305,307,308,311,337] Siblings have also been found to have problems with concentration, memory, and learning within the first 2 years after the cancer diagnosis.[321,322,329,330,341] The possibility of such difficulties should be explained to the family so that problems in the classroom are not perceived as mere cries for attention.

Considering the multitude of individual, family, and illness variables that may moderate the impact of childhood cancer, understanding sibling adjustment is a complex task.[329] Empathy[329] and high levels of social support[17] appear to play a protective role in the psychological adjustment of siblings and therefore possible opportunities for support, either formally through individual or group counseling[327] or through community agencies; school or camping programs could be greatly beneficial. Several other measures can be helpful in easing the emotional stress on siblings. The parents or treatment team need to discuss the ill child's diagnosis, treatment, and prognosis with siblings at a level they can easily understand.[342] Siblings need to be prepared for the physical changes that their brother or sister will undergo and for the possible role realignments in the family. Siblings must believe that their thoughts, concerns, and questions are important and acceptable. This includes feelings of anger toward their parents and jealousy or hostility toward the sick child. Siblings need to be reassured that they will be kept up-to-date on their brother's or sister's treatment progress and, whenever possible, will be included in their care and management. (The free Internet site, www.caringbridge.com, may make keeping up with progress and problems easier.) When treatment requires parental absence from home, a regularly scheduled time should be arranged for the parents and siblings and ill child to talk by telephone. This helps lessen separation anxiety and provides the sibling with a sense of belonging and contact while including them in the sick child's care.

Importantly, along with inherent challenges, many siblings report positive responses to the experiences associated with childhood cancer.[314,343] Many show increased maturity,

responsibility, and independence, as well as increased empathy, sensitivity, and compassion.[306,311,314,337,344,345] These positive outcomes may co-occur with and mask difficulties with adjustment.

Few investigations have reported children's reactions to the death of a sibling from cancer. Spinetta et al.[3] found that siblings' symptoms or unresolved feelings persisted in most families, including crying spells, health fears, feelings of remorse and guilt, and refusal to discuss the deceased child even 2 or 3 years after the child's death. In a study based on parental report, Lewis[173] reported that more than half of the siblings required some sort of medical consultation after the death of the affected child. In a study based on psychiatric patients, Cain et al.[346] found that the surviving children had a heightened awareness and fear of death, believing that it could strike someone close to them at any time or themselves when they reached the same age as the deceased sibling. All authors agree that the experience of a child's death has a profound effect on the siblings. The factors that determine a child's immediate and long-term reactions to the death of a sibling include (a) the level of communication with the sibling during his or her life; (b) the parents' explanation of the diagnosis, treatment, and prognosis to the surviving child; (c) the child's ability to express both positive and negative feelings about the sibling, and the disease; (d) the age, sex, and developmental level of the surviving sibling; (e) the child's preexisting relationship with the sibling and parents; and (f) the parents' reactions (expressed thoughts and behaviors) to the death and their subsequent attitude toward their remaining children.

There is no strong evidence regarding which siblings are most at-risk for problems adapting to childhood cancer. The reality is, unfortunately, that our evaluations do not sufficiently emphasize siblings. Unless a crisis occurs, problems with siblings are rarely brought to the attention of the oncology staff. Oncology staff and other health care professionals can assist families considerably by directing their attention to the needs of their well children and by encouraging open communication among all family members. While the siblings' problems may appear temporary and less burdensome than the difficulties their ill brothers or sisters are facing[171] or the worries their parents face, we now know they can be lifelong.

Family Structure

The traditional definition of family has changed for many members of society. Therefore, when considering the "family" with whom the child with cancer lives, it is important to be respectful of variations in the family structure.

Single Parents

The proportion of children in two-parent homes has decreased significantly in the last 30 years. A major problem for most single-parent families is task overload.[347] Struggling to work, provide childcare, maintain a home and finances, while caring for their sick child, and possibly dealing with visitation arrangements can be overwhelming. With often limited support to share the responsibility of the sick child's care or day-to-day decisions, single parents may feel especially isolated, alone, overwhelmed, sad, and without an adequate support system to meet the crisis. They may also experience considerable anger toward former mates, who may provide little if any emotional or financial assistance.

The health care team can assist single-parent families by identifying the financial, emotional, social, and support resources needed early in the child's treatment. Each family member's strengths and limitations as they relate to the child's care must be assessed. Parents need to be encouraged to turn to staff, extended families, or other supports for help in reassignment of home responsibilities and financial assistance (especially travel and child care costs) when needed. Individual and family counseling often helps single parents find the strength needed to cope with daily demands and the overwhelming stress with which they are confronted. With caring and sensitive intervention, these families may discover new resources within themselves, their families, and their extended or nonfamily supports that can be used again through the course of the child's illness.[153,348]

Separation and Divorce

If the child's parents are separated or divorced, special efforts need to be made by the health care team to keep both parents informed about the child's diagnosis, treatments, and progress. Parents maintaining a friendship after separation or divorce tend to handle the stresses associated with disease and treatment better than parents who have difficulty in communicating or being in the same place together. The latter situation often presents a dilemma for staff. In an attempt to gain a sense of control and feel included in the child's care, some parents vie for alignments with certain staff members. The staff must not become enmeshed in the family system by splitting their alliances between parents. In such cases, the child often is caught in the middle and is left feeling guilty, alone, and without support. The health care team also needs to be aware of custody decisions, parental visitation arrangements, and possible remarriage and stepfamily relationships.

Blended Families

"Blended families" is a relatively new term that refers to a situation in which a child from a previous relationship is included in a family created by a new marriage/union. There are an increasing number of children living in a blended home environment; therefore, it is important to inquire about who the child considers to be members of his or her family; how recently the child's parents have been separated, divorced, or remarried; who is involved in the child's daily medical care; how resources are mobilized; whether roles in the family are clearly defined; and whether the child's cancer diagnosis and treatment unifies the family or causes additional family stress. It is critical that the health care team assess decision-making and communication between biological parents, stepparents, grandparents, and significant nonfamily members early in treatment to assure that the family is supported and roles are clearly defined.[9]

Cultural Considerations

Our growing multicultural society presents health care providers with a difficult task of providing appropriate care for individuals who have diverse life experiences, beliefs, value systems, religions, languages, and notions of health care. As cultural practice and spiritual beliefs are the foundations on which many lives are based, providing quality care requires that providers be culturally sensitive and competent. Families need the opportunity to carry out important religious and/or cultural rituals during the child's life. This is especially vital when a child has a potentially life-limiting illness, such as cancer.[348,349] Clinicians must move beyond the limitations of traditional approaches, learning how to determine the impact of cultural differences, poverty, discrimination, and acculturation issues.[350] Such differences affect how each family perceives and responds to illness, treatment, and death.[351] For example, different cultures have different expectations of the medical system, different beliefs and attitudes about patient care and disease causation, and different attitudes about death and rituals around death. The effects of cultural barriers on communication have a major impact on both the family's reactions to their child's illness and their ability to place trust in the health care team.[352]

Misunderstanding, confusion, and alienation often result from the failure of the medical team to consider sociocultural factors in the child's care. Learning about the beliefs, attitudes, and behaviors of the family's ethnic group enhances the therapeutic alliance. Explore with the family their understanding of the illness, their expectations of the staff and of the treatment offered, and the role of religion in their daily lives. For instance, a common definition of disease from Chinese tradition is based on retribution for past sin or God's punishment.[116] The health care team ideally will identify whether (a) conflict exists between religious beliefs and treatment decisions; (b) the parents can meet their child's need for information; (c) problems exist because of language differences or difficulty in using the supports available within the medical environment or community; (d) parents are able to accept assistance from others whose lifestyles differ from their own; and (e) parents respond better to informal or formal interactions with staff. Families are often eager to share with staff information about the family structure, culture, roles within the family, and belief systems when an interest is expressed. But the health professional must create the interpersonal atmosphere that signals to them an interest, a caring about learning this information. Caution must be used to determine that words as well as images used have the same meaning to the family as they do to the professional. Once this information has been elicited, it may be possible to mobilize available sources of support that could further reduce the stresses of being in a different environment and assist in the family's adjustment. If the family does not speak English, regularly scheduled meetings with the family are essential. The meetings should include the child's physicians, nurse, and social worker, as well as a staff member or reliable volunteer who speaks the language, understands the culture, and is trusted by the family. Such meetings avoid miscommunications and enhance the quality of patient-family-staff relations.

Costs

Chapter 50 discusses financial issues in pediatric cancer care. No family undergoes the rigors of cancer treatment and follow-up without economic stress.[353] Early assessment of the family's financial situation is essential to lessen current and future economic stress on the family. Many families find it helpful to keep a record of all incurred expenses.

The cost of treatment can be divided into direct medical charges and nonmedical expenses. Nonmedical costs, including extra food and clothing, transportation, long-distance telephone calls to doctors and family members, meals, temporary housing near the hospital, care for siblings, time lost from work, and miscellaneous items, such as decreased efficiency and effectiveness because of emotional pain and suffering all have a great impact on the family's budget. Direct medical costs for cancer treatment vary with diagnosis, with a large spread between cancers requiring intensive treatment and those involving more routine follow-up. Studies have found that the diagnostic and terminal stages of illness account for more than 50% of these charges with outstanding debts to the cancer center as long as 3 years after the child's death.[354,355]

Economic impact adds significantly to the family's overall distress. Even when the financial hardship is less extreme, it has long-lasting deleterious effects on all family members because of both the depletion and redirection of resources over an extended period. Parents and siblings have fewer needs met because such a large proportion of the family budget goes toward the care of the sick child. There are no simple solutions for the financial plight of these families. Early assessment of socioeconomic vulnerability may include evaluation of insurance coverage, the availability of community resources, and job-related issues.[47] At best, such an assessment facilitates planning for the support needed.[356]

PSYCHOSOCIAL AND PSYCHIATRIC INTERVENTIONS

Psychological and developmental problems in the patient or any family member add significantly to the burden of dealing with a chronic, life-threatening condition. Preexisting conditions such as anxiety and phobic disorders, mood disorders, psychosis, severe personality disorders, substance abuse, severe learning disabilities, and attention deficit and hyperactivity disorders in the cancer patient or family members add complications to cancer treatment. Any one of these disorders can deplete a family's time, and exhaust its emotional and financial resources. Even dramatic psychiatric symptoms can be reactive, at least in part, to the stresses and disruptions of the cancer diagnosis and treatment course. Knowledge of these conditions can help the health care team anticipate problems and provide them with the time to engage additional resources, as needed.

Psychosocial Interventions

Throughout this chapter, various interventions have been discussed at key points of the cancer experience. Psychosocial support for the child with cancer and his or her family members is an important component of comprehensive cancer care[356,357] but often is not adequately provided.[358]

As discussed in the preceding sections, most families with a child with cancer adjust well and are able to meet the challenges of childhood cancer. This requires psychosocial interventions to adopt preventative, competence-based models of care (Table 45.4). Such models of care provide broad-based education about cancer and supportive care to all families to foster their resilience and promote the conduct of systematic screening of families to identify those with elevated or escalating distress and provide targeted interventions to reduce that distress.[359]

A recent meta-analysis of psychological interventions in pediatric oncology concluded that these interventions are effective in reducing distress and improving adaptation of parents of children with cancer; however, significant effects were not seen for decreasing the distress of the children themselves.[360] Examples of interventions include Maternal Problem Solving delivered during the first few months of treatment and SCCIP-Newly Diagnosed.[23,275,361,362]

Psychopharmacological Interventions

When psychiatric symptoms present, consultation from a psychiatrist is indicated, especially if the patient has or had an immediate family member with a psychiatric history, has been prescribed psychotropic medications, exhibits depressive symptoms associated with extreme guilt, anxiety, and/or suicidal thoughts, is confused, hallucinating, agitated, or violent.[135] All treatment teams should have an experienced clinical social worker, psychologist or psychiatrist available to them. Medications (see Table 45.5) to treat psychiatric disorders require great sophistication on the part of treating physicians and

TABLE 45.4
INTERVENTIONS THROUGHOUT TREATMENT

Education	*Psychological/Psychiatric Interventions*
Disease and its management	Family counseling, including:
Care activities for daily living	• Dealing with separation
Finances	• Dealing with regression
Nutrition	Joint counseling to address
Physical activity	preexisting conflicts,
Touching and holding	including
Stress-management training	• Marriage/couples
Common emotional reactions	counseling
	• Parent/child counseling
Mobilization of resources and environmental change	Individual psychotherapy, cognitive-behavioral therapy and/or hypnosis, for:
Transportation and travel	• Anxiety
Employment issues	• Depression
Childcare	• Phobias
	• Panic reactions
Self-help groups	• Sleep disorders
Education resource	• Enhancing strengths
information	• Promoting growth
Isolation v. legitimization	Group therapy, for:
Channeling feelings	• Enhancing feelings of
Encouraging advocacy	support
	• Decreasing isolation, helplessness, and separation
	• Promoting goal-setting
	Medication, for:
	• Anxiety
	• Depression
	• Panic reactions

nurses concerning drug-drug interactions since many of these agents can be powerful inhibitors or inducers of hepatic enzyme systems.[364] Up-to-date drug interaction resources can be found at several internet websites (e.g., http://medicine.iupui.edu/flockhart/).

Psychiatric Emergencies

Most psychiatric emergencies fall into the categories of (a) acute toxic, psychotic reactions; (b) chronic sleep cycle disruption; (c) anxiety reactions that have escalated to panic attacks; or (d) depression, with suicidal ideation and behaviors, or severe withdrawal. The existence of a competent professional team and early recognition is essential to address such emergencies.

Acute, toxic psychotic reactions show themselves through significant changes in the patient's ability to communicate nonverbally (eye contact, touch, etc.) and verbally, and through their behaviors (agitation, severe restlessness, etc.) These reactions are not usually from a primary psychiatric disorder, rather secondary to electrolyte imbalances, systemic infection, toxic reactions to medications (steroids, some antibiotics, some drug-drug interactions), and CNS metastases. Treatment of toxic reactions is urgent. The environment should be made as reassuring as possible for the patient, and temperature, hydration, and vital signs should be carefully

TABLE 45.5

MAJOR CATEGORIES OF PSYCHOTROPIC MEDICATIONS

Anti-anxiety agents
  Benzodiazepines[a] (lorazepam[b], clonazepam)
  Antihistamines (diphenhydramine, hydroxyzine, promethazine)
Mood stabilizing agents
  (lamotrigine, carbamazepine, lithium, valproic acid, topiramate)
Psycho-stimulants
  (Methylphenidate[a], mixed amphetamine salts[a], dextroamphetamine[a], modafinil)
Anti-psychotics
  Traditional (haloperidol[ab], chlorpromazine)
  Atypical (risperidone[b], quetiapine, ziprasidone, clozapine—as of 2009, all are "Black Boxed" by the FDA)
Anti-depressants
  Tricyclics (amitriptyline[a], desipramine, nortriptyline)
  Serotonin Reuptake Inhibitors (SSRI's) (fluoxetine[ab], sertraline[ab], paroxetine, citalopram[b], escitalopram, fluvoxamine[a])
  Monamine Oxidase Inhibitors (MAOI's) (phenelzine, tranylcypromine, orphenadrine)
  Novel antidepressants (bupropion, mirtazapine, nefazodone, venlafaxine, duloxetine, trazodone)

[a]FDA approval for use in children/adolescents.
[b]liquid formulation available.
Note: The effectiveness of these medications may be enhanced or diminished by simultaneous use of: SSRI's; diphenhydramine; anti-viral agents; some antibiotics (Biaxin, Clarithromycin, Ciprofloxacin, Erythromycin); anti-fungals (ketoconazole, triaconazole); nefazodone; valproic acid; phenytoin; oral contraceptives; alcohol; caffeine; grapefruit juice; St. John's Wort; smoking; watercress; broccoli; brussel sprouts; charbroiled food.[363] This is only a partial listing of medications available in each category.

monitored until the primary cause(s) of the acute psychotic reaction are identified. Safety may be assured through appropriate physical and chemical restraints. Expert oncologist-psychiatrist collaboration is essential with respect to chemical restraints, given the many complex side effects of neuroleptic medications, including possible effects on cardiac function.

Chronic sleep cycle disruption can arise from reactions to altered routines, altered nutrition, treatments and treatment settings, pain, drug side effects, and any combination of these factors. Sleep cycle disruption, when chronic, produces an irritable child, more vulnerable to anxiety reactions, depression, behavioral problems, and may impair immune system function. Intervention begins with recognition that the child or adolescent has an abnormal diurnal cycle. The team of parents, social workers, and psychologists should work collaboratively with the treating oncologists to identify the contributing factors. Attention should be paid to sleep hygiene and setting in the context of the chronological and developmental age of the child. Interventions may take time but must be directed toward

reestablishing a normal diurnal cycle. Always obtain the reference point of the child's pre-morbid sleep patterns.

Anxiety reactions escalating into panic attacks may evolve as a result of the anxieties and fears of the particular child. They are often amplified by a pre-cancer history of anxiety problems. These reactions should be carefully evaluated in order to determine the appropriate interventions. Ideally, anxiety and panic reactions are anticipated and dealt with through psychological means such as desensitization, relaxation training, guided imagery, cognitive-behavioral and play therapy.

Depression is often overlooked. Sadness is not the same as clinical depression. Depression is associated with loss of interest and motivation, increased negative thoughts, inability to receive pleasure from play or other activities that had been pleasurable, loss of interest in peers, poor sleep, and possibly increased irritability and non-goal-directed agitation. Suicidal thoughts often may not be voluntarily expressed. They also may be expressed indirectly through drawings, play, songs, and poems. Sometimes the themes presented are simply those of not waking up. An experienced professional must investigate suspicion of clinical depression. The treatment team (including the parents) should be made aware of the findings. Interventions include the appropriate uses of psychotherapy (cognitive-behavioral and supportive) combined with appropriate medications and environmental changes. Certain medications, including antibiotics, can themselves induce clinical depression. This must be considered part of the diagnostic and intervention puzzle. Finally, medications do not help instantly with depression beyond the placebo effect of hope. Thus, vigilance, with close clinical follow-up, must be maintained for a minimum of 3 weeks from the time of diagnosis.[365]

FINAL WORD

Despite the life-disrupting and life-threatening nature of childhood cancer, most families display remarkable resilience in adaptation.[366] Working to mobilize the strengths of families adds enormously to the effectiveness of the oncology treatment team. An attitude on the part of the physicians and nurses that child and parents be included as members of the treatment team is essential. An ongoing multidisciplinary approach to the psychosocial care of children and adolescents and their families is basic to responsible modern treatment. Ignoring at the outset signs of significant vulnerabilities can wreak havoc with the most brilliant treatment protocols. Because oncologic diseases are chronic processes, comprehensive psychosocial care begins with early assessment of family strengths and vulnerabilities. Interventions and strategies aimed at identifying the continuum of coping responses, building on family strengths, assisting families with special needs, and enhancing adaptive coping skills are essential to facilitating both family growth and survival through the crises generated by childhood cancer and should continue throughout and beyond the course of the disease. One hopes that the economics of "managed care" in the United States and countries around the globe will allow for incorporation of this concept into all oncology programs.

References

1. Brody A, Simmons L. Family resiliency during childhood cancer: the father's perspective. J Pediatr Oncol Nurs 2007;24:152–165.
2. Futterman E, Hoffman I. Crisis and adaptation in the families of fatally ill children. In: Anthony E, Koupernik E, eds. The child and his family. New York, NY: Wiley & Sons, 1973:127.
3. Spinetta JJ, Swarner JA, Sheposh JP. Effective parental coping following the death of a child from cancer. J Pediatr Psychol 1981;6:251–263.
4. Alderfer M, Kazak A. Family issues when a child is on treatment for cancer. In: Brown R, ed. Pediatric hematology/oncology: a biopsychosocial approach. New York, NY: Oxford University Press, 2006:53–74.

5. Worden W, Monahan J. Caring for bereaved parents. In: Armstrong-Dailey A, Zarbock S, eds. Hospice care for children. 2nd ed. New York, NY: Oxford University Press, 2001:137–156.
6. Pai AL, Patino-Fernandez AM, McSherry M, et al. The psychosocial assessment tool (PAT 2.0): psychometric properties of a screener for psychosocial distress in families of children newly diagnosed with cancer. J Pediatr Psychol 2008;33:50–62.
7. Kazak AE, Cant MC, Jensen MM, et al. Identifying psychosocial risk indicative of subsequent resource use in families of newly diagnosed pediatric oncology patients. J Clin Oncol 2003;21:3220–3225.
8. Hersh S. Psychological aspects of patients with cancer. In: DeVita VJ, Hellman S, Rosenberg S, eds. Principles and practice of oncology. 2nd ed. Philadelphia, PA: JB Lippincott, 1985:2051.
9. Breyer J. Talking to children and adolescents. In: Wiener L, Pao M, Kazak A, Kupst M, Patenaude A, eds. Quick reference for Pediatric Oncology Clinicians: the psychiatric and psychological dimensions of pediatric cancer symptom management. Charlottesville, VA: IPOS Press, 2009:4–22.
10. Kubler-Ross E. On death and dying. New York, NY: Macmillan Publishing Co, Inc., 1969.
11. Evans AE, Edin S. If a child must die. N Engl J Med 1968;278:138–142.
12. Stephens J, Lascari AD. Psychological follow-up of families with childhood leukemia. J Clin Psychol 1974;30:394.
13. Clarke S, Davies H, Jenney M, et al. Parental communication and children's behaviour. Psychooncology 2005;14(4):274–281.
14. Kaplan D. Interventions for acute stress experiences. In: Spinetta JJ, Deasy-Spinetta P, eds. Living with childhood cancer. St. Louis, MO: CV Mosby, 1981:41.
15. Kupst M, Bingen K. Stress and coping in the pediatric cancer experience. In: Brown RT, ed. Comprehensive handbook of childhood cancer and sickle cell disease: a biopsychosocial approach. New York, NY: Oxford University Press, 2006:35–52.
16. Patenaude AF, Kupst MJ. Psychosocial functioning in pediatric cancer. J Pediatr Psychol 2005;30:9–27.
17. Barrera M, Fleming CF, Khan FS. The role of emotional social support in the psychological adjustment of siblings of children with cancer. Child Care Health Dev 2004;30: 103–111.
18. Brown RT, Madan-Swain A, Lambert R. Posttraumatic stress symptoms in adolescent survivors of childhood cancer and their mothers. J Trauma Stress 2003;16:309–318.
19. Dahlquist LM, Czyzewski DI, Jones CL. Parents of children with cancer: a longitudinal study of emotional distress, coping style, and marital adjustment two and twenty months after diagnosis. J Pediatr Psychol 1996;21:541–554.
20. Dolgin MJ, Phipps S, Fairclough DL, et al. Trajectories of adjustment in mothers of children with newly diagnosed cancer: a natural history investigation. J Pediatr Psychol 2007;32:771–782.
21. Frank NC, Brown RT, Blount RL, et al. Predictors of affective responses of mothers and fathers of children with cancer. Psychooncology 2001;10:293–304.
22. Kazak AB L. Parenting stress and quality of life during treatment for childhood leukemia predicts child and parent adjustment after treatment ends. J Pediatr Psychol 1997;22:749–758.
23. Kazak AE, Alderfer M, Rourke MT, et al. Posttraumatic stress disorder (PTSD) and posttraumatic stress symptoms (PTSS) in families of adolescent childhood cancer survivors. J Pediatr Psychol 2004;29:211–219.
24. Manne S, DuHamel K, Ostroff J, et al. Anxiety, depressive, and posttraumatic stress disorders among mothers of pediatric hematopoietic stem cell transplantation. Pediatrics 2004;113(6):1700–1708.
25. Sloper P. Predictors of distress in parents of children with cancer: a prospective study. J Pediatr Psychol 2000;25:79–91.
26. Steele RG, Dreyer ML, Phipps S. Patterns of maternal distress among children with cancer and their association with child emotional and somatic distress. J Pediatr Psychol 2004;29:507–517.
27. Patiño-Fernández AM, Pai A, Alderfer M, et al. Acute stress in parents of children newly diagnosed with cancer. Pediatr Blood Cancer 2008;50:289–292.
28. Kazak AE, Boeving CA, Alderfer MA, et al. Posttraumatic stress symptoms during treatment in parents of children with cancer. J Clin Oncol 2005;23:7405–7410.
29. Prugh D. The psychosocial aspects of pediatrics. Philadelphia, PA: Lea & Febiger, 1983.
30. Carparulo F, Kempton W. Sexual health needs of the mentally retarded adolescent female. Issues Health Care Women 1981;3:35.
31. Pfefferbaum B. Mental health aspects of neoplasm in children. In: Grossman H, Stubblefield R, eds. The physician and the mental health of the child. Vol II: the psychosocial concomitants of illness. Monroe, WI: American Medical Association, 1980:113.
32. Johnson FL, Rudolph LA, Hartmann JR. Helping the family cope with childhood cancer. Psychosomatics 1979;20:241, 245–247, 251.
33. Vess J, Moreland JR, Schwebel AI. An empirical assessment of the effects of cancer on family role functioning. J Psychosoc Oncol 1985;3:1.
34. Howarth RV. The psychiatry of terminal illness in children. Proc R Soc Med 1972;65: 1039–1040.
35. Wiener L, Septimus A, Grady C. Psychological support and ethical issues for the child and family. In: Pizzo PA, Wilfert C, eds. Pediatric AIDS: the challenge of HIV infection in infants, children, and adolescents. 3rd ed. Philadelphia, PA: Lippincott, Williams and Wilkins, 1998:703–727.
36. Dorn LD, Susman EJ, Fletcher JC. Informed consent in children and adolescents: age, maturation and psychological state. J Adolesc Health 1995;16:185–190.
37. Williams P, Lorenzo F, Borja M. Pediatric chronic illness: effects on siblings and mothers. Matern Child Nurs J 1993;21:111–121.
38. Burr C. Impact on the family of a chronically ill child. In: Hobbs N, Perrin J, eds. Issues in the care of children with chronic illness. San Francisco, CA: Jossey-Bass, 1985:24.
39. Hamovitch M. The parent and the fatally ill child. Los Angeles, CA: Delmar, 1964.
40. Dahlquist LM, Czyzewski DI, Copeland KG, et al. Parents of children newly diagnosed with cancer: anxiety, coping, and marital distress. J Pediatr Psychol 1993;18:365–376.
41. Gaither R, Bingen K, Hopkins J. When the bough breaks: the relationship between chronic illness in children and couple functioning. In: Sher TB, Schmaling KB, eds. The psychology of couples and illness: theory, research, and practice. Washington, DC: American Psychological Association, 2000:337–365.
42. Murstein B. The effects of long-term illness of children on the emotional adjustment of parents. Child Dev 1960;31:157.
43. Taylor G. Helping families cope when a child has cancer. Med Times 1981;109: 24s–27s.
44. Freund BL, Siegel K. Problems in transition following bone marrow transplantation: psychosocial aspects. Am J Orthopsychiatry 1986;56:244–252.
45. Christ G. "Dis-synchrony" of coping among children with cancer, their families and the treating staff. In: Christ AE, Flomenhaft K, eds. Psychosocial family interventions in chronic pediatric illness. New York, NY: Plenum Press, 1982:85.
46. Lavee Y. Correlates of change in marital relationships under stress: the case of childhood cancer. Families in Society 2005;86:112–120.
47. Adams-Greenly M. Psychological staging of pediatric cancer patients and their families. Cancer 1986;58:449–453.
48. Lavee Y, Mey-Dan M. Patterns of change in marital relationships among parents of children with cancer. Health Soc Work 2003;28:255–263.
49. Seagull EA. Beyond mothers and children: finding the family in pediatric psychology. J Pediatr Psychol 2000;25:161–169.
50. McGrath P, Huff N. Including the fathers' perspective in holistic care. Part 1: findings on the fathers' experience with childhood acute lymphoblastic leukaemia. Aust J Holist Nurs 2003;10:4–12.
51. McKeever PT. Fathering the chronically ill child. Matern Child Nurs 1981;6:124–128.
52. Biller H. Father, child and sex role: paternal determinants in personality development. Lexington, MA: Heath and Co., 1971.
53. O'Connell D. Benefits for all when dads get involved. Hemalog 2002;13:11–14.
54. McGrath P. Identifying support issues of parents of children with leukemia. Cancer Practice 2001;9:198–205.
55. Mu P, Ma F, Hwang B, et al. Families of children with cancer: the impact on anxiety experienced by fathers. Cancer Nurs 2002;25:66–73.
56. Wiener LS, Vasquez MJ, Battles HB. Brief report: fathering a child living with HIV/AIDS: psychosocial adjustment and parenting stress. J Pediatr Psychol 2001;26: 353–358.
57. Laws T. Fathers struggling for relevance in the care of their terminally ill child. Contemp Nurse 2004;18:34–45.
58. Kazak A, McClure K, Alderfer M, et al. Cancer related parental beliefs: the Family Illness Beliefs Inventory (FIBI). J Pediatr Psychol 2004;29(7):531–542.
59. Kazak A, Alderfer M, Rourke M, et al. Posttraumatic stress symptoms (PTSS) and posttraumatic stress disorder in families of adolescent childhood cancer survivors. J Pediatr Psychol 2004;29:211–219.
60. Ljungman G, McGrath PJ, Cooper E, et al. Psychosocial needs of families with a child with cancer. J Pediatr Hematol Oncol 2003;25:223–231.
61. Ross JW. Social work intervention with families of children with cancer: the changing critical phases. Soc Work Health Care 1978;3:257–272.
62. Vannatta K, Gerhardt K. Pediatric oncology: psychosocial outcomes for children and families. In: Roberts M, ed. Handbook of pediatric psychology. 3rd ed. New York, NY: Guilford, 2003.
63. Kupst MJ, Natta MB, Richardson CC, et al. Family coping with pediatric leukemia: ten years after treatment. J Pediatr Psychol 1995;20:601–617.
64. Clarke-Steffen L. A model of the family transition to living with childhood cancer. Cancer Practice 1993;1:285–292.
65. Clarke-Steffen L. Reconstructing reality: family strategies for managing childhood cancer. J Pediatr Nurs 1997;12:278–287.
66. Tarr J, Pickler R. Becoming a cancer patient: a study of families with acute lymphocytic leukemia. J Pediatr Oncol Nur 1999;16:44–50.
67. Woodgate RL, Degner LF. A substantive theory of Keeping the Spirit Alive: the Spirit Within children with cancer and their families. J Pediatr Oncol Nurs 2003;20:103–119.
68. Alderfer MA. Use of family management styles in family intervention research. J Pediatr Oncol Nurs 2006;23:32–35.
69. McQuown L. The parents of children with cancer: a view from those who suffer most. In: Spinetta JJ, Deasy-Spinetta P, eds. Living with childhood cancer. St Louis, MO: CV Mosby, 1981:198.
70. Yeh CH. Gender differences of parental distress in children with cancer. J Adv Nurs 2002;38:598–606.
71. Lazarus RS. Stress and emotion: a new synthesis. New York, NY: Springer, 1999.
72. Ross J. The role of the social worker with long term survivors of childhood cancer and their families. Soc Work Health Care 1982;7:1–13.
73. Kazak AE. Evidence-based interventions for survivors of childhood cancer and their families. J Pediatr Psychol 2005;30(1):29–39.
74. Sahler OJ, Varni JW, Fairclough DL, et al. Problem-solving skills training for mothers of children with newly diagnosed cancer: a randomized trial. J Dev Behav Pediatr 2002; 23:77–86.
75. Kalnins I, Churchill MP, Terry GE. Concurrent stresses in families with a leukemic child. J Pediatr Psychol 1980;5:81–92.
76. Bluebond-Langner M. The private worlds of dying children. Princeton, NJ: Princeton University Press, 1990.
77. Steele R, Long A, Reddy K, et al. Changes in maternal distress and child-rearing strategies across treatment for childhood cancer. J Pediatr Psychol 2003:447–452.
78. Heffron W, Bommelaere K, Masters R. Group discussions with the parents of leukemic children. Pediatrics 1973;52:831–840.
79. Levine AS, Hersh SP. The psychosocial concomitants of cancer in young patients. In: Levine AS, ed. Cancer in the young. New York, NY: Masson Publishing, 1982:367.
80. Hymovich D. Child-rearing concerns of parents with cancer. Oncol Nurs Forum 1993; 20:1355–1360.
81. Adams D, Deveau EJ. Coping with childhood cancer: where do we go from here? Reston, VA: Reston Publishing Co., 1984.
82. Ellis JA. Coping with adolescent cancer: it's a matter of adaptation. J Pediatr Oncol Nurs 1991;8:10–17.
83. Spinetta JJ, Deasy-Spinetta P. The patient's socialization in the community and school during therapy. Cancer 1986;58:512–515.
84. Wong DL. Transition from hospital to home for children with complex medical care. J Pediatr Oncol Nurs 1991;8:3–9.
85. Vannatta K, Gartstein MA, Short A, et al. A controlled study of peer relationships of children surviving brain tumors: teacher, peer, and self ratings. J Pediatr Psychol 1998; 23:279–287.
86. Mulhern R, Ochs J, Armstrong FD, et al. Assessment of quality of life among pediatric patients with cancer. J Consult Clin Psychol 1989;2:130.
87. Katz E, Rubinstein CL, Hubert NC, et al. School and social reintegration of children with cancer. J Psychosoc Oncol 1988;6:123.
88. Cairns N, Lansky SB, Klopovich P. Meeting educational needs of children with cancer. In: Paper presented at the annual conference of the American Psychological Association; August, 1979; New York.
89. Hockenberry-Eaton M, Hinds PS. Fatigue in children and adolescents with cancer: evolution of a program of study. Semin Oncol Nurs 2000;16:261–272; discussion 272–268.

90. Clarke-Steffen L, Hockenberry-Eaton M, Hinds PS, et al. Consensus statements: analyzing a new model to evaluate fatigue in children with cancer. J Pediatr Oncol Nurs 2001;18:21–23.
91. Feldman F. Work and cancer health histories. Oakland, CA: California Division: American Cancer Society, 1980.
92. Zwarnes W, Education of the child with cancer. In: Paper presented at the National Conference on the Care of the Child with Cancer. Boston, MA: American Cancer Society, 1978:150.
93. Moore I, Triplett JL. Students with cancer: a school nursing perspective. Cancer Nurs 1980;3:265–270.
94. Henning J, Fritz GK. School re-entry in childhood cancer. Psychosomatics 1983;24: 261–269.
95. Sposto R, Hammond GD. Survival in childhood cancer. Clin Oncol 1985;4:195–204.
96. Stehbens J, Kisker CT, Wilson BK. School behavior and attendance during the first year of treatment for childhood cancer. Psychol Sch 1983;20:223.
97. Lansky S, Cairns N, Zwarnes W. School attendance among children with cancer: a report from two centers. J Psychosoc Oncol 1983;1:75.
98. Lansky S, Ritter-Sterr C, List M, et al. Rates and patterns of school attendance. In: Proceedings of the American Society of Clinical Oncology; May 1990; Washington, DC.
99. Cairns N, Klopovich P, Hearne E, et al. School attendance of children with cancer. J Sch Health 1982;52:152–155.
100. Lansky S, Gendel M. Symbiotic regressive behavior patterns in childhood malignancy. Clin Pediatr 1978;17:133.
101. Katz E, Kellerman J, Rigler D, et al. School intervention with pediatric cancer patients. J Pediatr Psychol 1977;2:72.
102. Katz E, Gonzalez-Morkos B. School and academic planning. In: Wiener L, Pao M, Kazak A, Kupst M, Patenaude A, eds. Quick reference for pediatric oncology clinicians: the psychiatric and psychological dimensions of pediatric cancer symptom management. Charlottesville, VA: IPOS Press, 2009:223–235.
103. Komp D, Crocket J. Educational needs of the child with cancer. In: Presented at the American Cancer Society Second National Conference on Human Values and Cancer; 1977; Chicago, IL.
104. Klopovich P, Rosen D, Cairns N, et al. Cancer in the classroom: how do you cope? (A teacher's guide to cancer in children). Kansas City, KS: Mid-American Cancer Center, University of Kansas Medical Center, 1980.
105. Wear E, Blessing P. Child with cancer: facilitating the return to school. In: Peterson BH, Kellogg CJ, eds. Current practice in oncologic nursing. St Louis, MO: CV Mosby, 1976:222.
106. Deasy-Spinetta P, Spinetta JJ. The child with cancer in school: teacher's appraisal. Am J Pediatr Hematol Oncol 1980;2:89.
107. Ross J, Scarvalone SA. Facilitating the pediatric cancer patient's return to school. Soc Work 1982;27:256–261.
108. Ross J. Resolving nonmedical obstacles to successful school re-entry for children with cancer. J Sch Health 1984;54:84–86.
109. McEvoy M, Duchon D, Schaefer DS. Therapeutic play group for patients and siblings in a pediatric oncology ambulatory care unit. Top Clin Nurs 1985;7:10–18.
110. Adams M. A hospital play program: helping children with serious illness. Am J Orthopsychiatry 1976;46:416–424.
111. Gibbons M, Boren H. Stress reduction: a spectrum of strategies in pediatric oncology nursing. Nurs Clin North Am 1985;20:83–103.
112. Kennard BD, Stewart SM, Olvera R, et al. Nonadherence in adolescent oncology patients: preliminary data on psychological risk factors and relationships to outcome. J Clin Psychol Med Settings 2004;11:30–39.
113. Spinetta JJ, Masera G, Eden T, et al. Refusal, non-compliance, and abandonment of treatment in children and adolescents with cancer: a report of the SIOP Working Committee on Phychosocial Issues in Pediatric Oncology. Med Pediatr Oncol 2002;38: 114–117.
114. Pai A, Drotar D. Medication adherence in pediatric oncology. In: Wiener L, Pao M, Kazak A, Kupst M, Patenaude A, eds. Quick reference for pediatric oncology clinicians: the psychiatric and psychological dimensions of pediatric cancer symptom management. Charlottesville, CA: IPOS Press, 2009:90–96.
115. Koren G, Ferrazini G, Sulh H, et al. Systemic exposure to mercaptopurine as a prognostic factor in acute lymphocytic leukemia in children. N Engl J Med 1990;323: 17–21.
116. Yeh CH. Dynamic coping behaviors and process of parental response to child's cancer. Appl Nurs Res 2003;16:245–255.
117. Smith SD, Rosen D, Trueworthy RC, et al. A reliable method for evaluating drug compliance in children with cancer. Cancer 1979;43:169–173.
118. Dolgin MJ, Katz ER, Zeltzer LK, et al. Behavioral distress in pediatric patients with cancer receiving chemotherapy. Pediatrics 1989;84:103–110.
119. Dolgin MJ, Phipps S, Harow E, et al. Parental management of fear in chronically ill and healthy children. J Pediatr Psychol 1990;15:733–744.
120. Jamison RN, Lewis S, Burish TG. Cooperation with treatment in adolescent cancer patients. J Adolesc Health Care 1986;7:162–167.
121. Zeltzer L. The adolescent with cancer. In: Kellerman J, ed. Psychological aspects of childhood cancer. Springfield, IL: Charles C Thomas, 1980:70.
122. Pfefferbaum B, Lucas RH. Management of acute psychologic problems in pediatric oncology. Gen Hosp Psychiatry 1979;1:214–219.
123. Duffey-Lind E, Holleran E., Healey M, et al. Transitioning to survivorship: a pilot study. J Pediatr Oncol Nurs 2006:335–343.
124. Peck B. Effects of childhood cancer on long-term survivors and their families. BMJ 1979;1:1327–1329.
125. Jones P. Malignant disease in childhood: the problems in general practice. Aust Fam Physician 1977;6:237–239.
126. Kupst MJ, Tylke L, Thomas L, et al. Strategies of intervention with families of pediatric leukemia patients: a longitudinal perspective. Soc Work Health Care 1982;8:31–47.
127. Holland JC. Psychological aspects of oncology. Med Clin North Am 1977;61:737–748.
128. Krulik T. Helping parents of children with cancer during the midstage of illness. Cancer Nurs 1982;5:441–445.
129. Levine R. Referral of patients with cancer for participation in randomized clinical trials: ethical considerations. Cancer 1986;36:95–99.
130. Lansky S, Vats T, Cairns NU. Refusal of treatment. Am J Pediatr Hematol Oncol 1979; 1:277–282.
131. Greer S, Moorey S, Baruch JD, et al. Adjuvant psychological therapy for patients with cancer: a prospective randomised trial. BMJ 1992;304:675–680.
132. American Academy of Paediatrics; Committee of Bioethics and Committee of Hospital Care. Palliative care for children. Pediatrics 2000;106:351–357.
133. Medicine IO. When Children Die: improving palliative and end of life care for children and their families. Washington, DC: National Academies Press, 2003.
134. Himelstein B, Hilden J, Boldt A, et al. Pediatric palliative care. N Eng J Med 2004;350: 1752–1762.
135. Rosenstein D, Cai J, Pao M. Psychopharmacologic management in the Oncology Setting in Bethesda. In: Abraham J, Allegra CJ, Gulley JL, eds. Handbook of clinical oncology. 2nd ed. Philadelphia, PA: Lippincott Williams and Wilkins.
136. Beale EA, Baile WF, Aaron J. Silence is not golden: communicating with children dying from cancer. J Clin Oncol 2005;23:3629–3631.
137. Wolfe J, Hammel JF, Edwards KE, et al. Easing of suffering in children with cancer at the end of life: is care changing? J Clin Oncol 2008;26:1717–1723.
138. Chapman JA, Goodall J. Helping a child to live whilst dying. Lancet 1980;1:753–756.
139. Hersh S. How can we help? In: KJ D, ed. Children mourning/mourning children. Washington, DC: Hospice Foundation of America, 1995:93.
140. Summer L. Lighting the way: improving the way children die in America. Caring 2003;12:143–148.
141. Frantz T. When your child has a life-threatening illness. Washington, DC: association for the Care of Children's Health and the Candlelighters Foundation. 1983.
142. Share L. Family communication in the crisis of a child's fatal illness: a literature review and analysis. Omega 1972;3:187.
143. Spinetta J, Maloney LT. The child with cancer: patterns of communication and denial. J Consult Clin Psychol 1978;46:1540–1541.
144. Waechter E. Children's awareness of fatal illness. Am J Nurs 1971;71:1168–1172.
145. Doka K. Children mourning/mourning children. Washington, DC: Hospice Foundation of America, 1995.
146. Greenham DE, Lohmann RA. Children facing death: recurring patterns of adaptation. Health Soc Work 1982;7:89–94.
147. Adams-Greenly M. Helping children communicate about serious illness and death. J Psychosoc Oncol 1984;2:61.
148. Stuber M, Houskamp B. Spirituality in children confronting death. Child Adolesc Psychiatr Clin N Am 2004;13:127–136.
149. Herz F. The impact of death and serious illness on the family life cycle. In: Carter E, McGoldrick M, eds. The family life cycle: a framework for family therapy. New York, NY: Gardner Press, 1980:223.
150. Hilden JM, Emanuel EJ, Fairclough DL, et al. Attitudes and practices among pediatric oncologists regarding end-of-life care: results of the 1998 American society of clinical oncology survey. J Clin Oncol 2001;19:205–212.
151. Zeltzer L, Krane E. Pain. In: Wiener L, Pao M, Kazak A, Kupst M, Patenaude A, eds. Quick reference for pediatric oncology clinicians: the psychiatric and psychological dimensions of pediatric cancer symptom management. Charlottesville, VA: IPOS Press, 2009:108–120.
152. Kuttner L, Bowman M, Teasdale M. Psychological treatment of distress, pain, and anxiety for young children with cancer. J Dev Behav Pediatr 1988;9:374–381.
153. Brown RT, Wiener L, Kupst MJ, et al. Single parents of children with chronic illness: an understudied phenomenon. J Pediatr Psychol 2008;33:408–421.
154. Wiener L, Ballard E, Brennan T, et al. How I wish to be remembered: the use of an advance care planning document in adolescent and young adult populations. J Palliat Med 2008;11:1309–1313.
155. Wolfe J, Grier HE, Klar N, et al. Symptoms and suffering at the end of life in children with cancer. N Engl J Med 2000;342:326–333.
156. McGivney WT, Crooks GM. The care of patients with severe chronic pain in terminal illness. JAMA 1984;251:1182–1188.
157. McIntyre A. The double life of double effect. Theor Med Bioeth 2004;25:61–74.
158. Howell DA. A child dies. Semin Hematol 1966;3:168–173.
159. Minino A, Smith BL. Deaths: preliminary data for 2000. Natl Vital Stat Rep 2001;49: 1–40.
160. Society AC. Cancer Facts and Figures, 2000. Atlanta, GA: American Cancer Society, 2000.
161. Board NCP, Hewitt M, Weiner S, et al., eds. Chidlhood cancer survivorship: improving care and quality of life. Washington, DC: The National Academies Press 2003.
162. Owen G, Fulton R, Marknsen E. Death at a distance: a study of family survivors. Omega 1982–1983;13:191.
163. Tietz W, McSherry L, Britt B. Family sequelae after a child's death due to cancer. Am J Psychother 1977;31:417–425.
164. Binger C. Childhood leukemia: emotional impact on siblings. In: Anthony E, Koupernik E, eds. The child and his family. New York, NY: John Wiley & Sons, 1973:195.
165. Morrow GR, Hoagland A, Carnrike CL Jr. Social support and parental adjustment to pediatric cancer. J Consult Clin Psychol 1981;49:763–765.
166. Kaplan DM, Grobstein R, Smith A. Predicting the impact of severe illness in families. Health Soc Work 1976;1:71–82.
167. Lansky SB, Cairns NU, Hassanein R, et al. Childhood cancer: parental discord and divorce. Pediatrics 1978;62:184–188.
168. Sanders C. A comparison of adult bereavement in the death of a spouse, child and parent. Omega 1979–1980;10:303.
169. Hersh S. Reactions to particular types of bereavement. In: Osterweis M Solomon F, Green M, eds. Bereavement reactions, consequences, and care. Washington, DC: National Academy Press, 1984:71.
170. Lewis M Lewis D. Death and dying in children and their families. In: Grossman H, Stubblefield R, eds. The physician and the mental health of the child. Vol II: the psychosocial concomitants of illness. Monroe, WI: American Medical Association, 1980:121.
171. Bowen M. Family reaction to death. In: Guerin P, ed. Family therapy: therapy and practice. New York, NY: Gardner Press, 1976:335.
172. Koch CR, Hermann J, Donaldson MH. Supportive care of the child with cancer and his family. Semin Oncol 1974;1:81–86.
173. Lewis I. Leukemia in childhood: its effects on the family. Aust Pediatr J 1967;3:244.
174. Reis L, Eisner MP, Kosary CL, et al., eds. SEER cancer statistics review, 1973–1999. Bethesda, MD: National Cancer Institute, 2002.
175. Hewitt M, Weiner S, Simone J, et al. Childhood cancer survivorship: improving care and quality of life. Washington, DC: National Academies Press, 2003.
176. Armstrong F, Briery B. Childhood cancer and the school. In: Brown R, ed. Handbook of pediatric psychology in the school setting. Mahwah, NJ: Lawrence Erlbaum, 2003: 263–282.
177. Armstrong FD, Mulhern R. Acute leukemia and brain tumors. In: Brown RT, ed. Cognitive aspects of chronic illness in children. NY: Guilford, 1999:47–77.
178. Butler RC, Copeland DR. Attentional processes and their remediation in children treated for cancer: a literature review and the development of a therapeutic approach. J Int Neuropsychol Soc 2002;8:115–124.

179. Butler RW, Haser JK. Neurocognitive effects of treatment for childhood cancer. Ment Retard Dev Disabil Res Rev 2006;12:184–191.
180. Butler RW, Sahler OJ, Askins MA, et al. Interventions to improve neuropsychological functioning in childhood cancer survivors. Dev Disabil Res Rev 2008;14:251–258.
181. Spencer J. The role of cognitive remediation in childhood cancer survivors experiencing neurocognitive late effects. J Pediatr Hematol/Oncol Nurs 2006;23:321–325.
182. Thompson S, Leigh L, Christensen R, et al. Immediate neurocognitive effects of methylphenidate on learning-impaired survivors of childhood cancer. J Clin Oncol 2001;19:1802–1808.
183. Conklin HM, Khan RB, Reddick WE, et al. Acute neurocognitive response to methylphenidate among survivors of childhood cancer: a randomized, double-blind, cross-over trial. J Pediatr Psychol 2007;32:1127–1139.
184. Daly BP, Brown RT. Scholarly literature review: management of neurocognitive late effects with stimulant medication. J Pediatr Psychol 2007;32:1111–1126.
185. Meadows A, Krejmas NL, Belasco JB. The medical cost of cure: sequelae in survivors of childhood cancer. In: van Eys J Sullivan MP, eds. Status of the curability of childhood cancers. New York, NY: Raven Press; 1980:263–276.
186. Li F, Cassady JR, Jaffe N. Risk of second tumors in survivors of childhood cancer. Cancer 1975;35:1230–1235.
187. Li F, Stone R. Survivors of cancer in childhood. Ann Intern Med 1976;84:551–553.
188. Li F. Follow-up survivors of childhood cancer. Cancer 1977;39:1776–1778.
189. Li F. Second malignant tumors after cancer in childhood. Cancer 1977;40:1899.
190. Li F, Myers MH, Heise HW, et al. The course of 5-year survivors of cancer in childhood. J Pediatr 1978;93:185–187.
191. Li FP, Fine W, Jaffe N, et al. Offspring of patients treated for cancer in childhood. J Natl Cancer Inst 1979;62:1193–1197.
192. DíAngio G. The child cured of cancer: a problem for the internist. Semin Oncol 1982;9: 143.
193. DíAngio G. Early and delayed complications of therapy. Cancer 1983;51:2515.
194. Jaffe N. Non-oncologic sequelae of cancer chemotherapy. Radiology 1975;114:167.
195. Biancaniello T, Meyer RA, Wong KY, et al. Doxorubicin cardiotoxicity in children. J Pediatr 1980;97:45–50.
196. Dawson W. Growth impairment following radiotherapy in childhood. Clin Radiol 1968;19:241–256.
197. Jaffe N, Toth BB, Hoar RE, et al. Dental and maxillofacial abnormalities in long-term survivors of childhood cancer: effects of treatment with chemotherapy and radiation to the head and neck. Pediatrics 1984;73:816–823.
198. Brown I, Lee TJ, Eden OB, et al. Growth and endocrine function after treatment for medulloblastoma. Arch Dis Child 1983;58:722.
199. Zee P, Chen CH. Obesity in children after therapy for acute lymphoblastic leukemia. Am J Pediatr Hematol Oncol 1986;814:294–299.
200. Novakovic B, Fears TR, Wexler LH, et al. Experiences of cancer in children and adolescents. Cancer Nurs 1996;19:54–59.
201. Holmes HA, Holmes FF. After ten years, what are the handicaps and life styles of children treated for cancer? An examination of the present status of 124 such survivors. Clin Pediatr (Phila) 1975;14:819–823.
202. Chang PN. Psychosocial needs of long-term childhood cancer survivors: a review of literature. Pediatrician 1991;18:20–24.
203. Kellerman J, Zeltzer L, Ellenberg L, et al. Psychological effects of illness in adolescence. I. Anxiety, self-esteem, and perception of control. J Pediatr 1980;97:126–131.
204. Zebrack BJ, Zeltzer LK. Living beyond the sword of Damocles: surviving childhood cancer. Expert Rev Anticancer Ther 2001;1:163–164.
205. Ness KK, Gurney JG. Adverse late effects of childhood cancer and its treatment on health and performance. Annu Rev Public Health 2007;28:279–302.
206. Van Dijk EM, Kaspers GJ, van Dulmen-den Broder E, et al. Psychosexual functioning of childhood cancer survivors. Psychooncology 2008;17:506–511.
207. Ford J, Ostroff J. Health behaviors of childhood cancer survivors: what we've learned. J Clin Psychol Med Settings 2006;13:151–167.
208. Geenen MM, Cardous-Ubbink MC, Kremer LC, et al. Medical assessment of adverse health outcomes in long-term survivors of childhood cancer. JAMA 2007;297:2705–2715.
209. Van den Berg H, Langeveld N. Parental knowledge of fertility in male childhood cancer survivors. Psychooncology 2008;17:287–291.
210. Koocher GP, O'Malley JE, Gogan JL, et al. Psychological adjustment among pediatric cancer survivors. J Child Psychol Psychiatry 1980;21:163–173.
211. Reiter-Purtill J, Noll R. Peer relationships of children with chronic illness. In: Roberts M, ed. Handbook of pediatric psychology. 3rd ed. New York, NY: Guilford, 2003.
212. Lansky SB, List MA, Ritter-Sterr C. Psychosocial consequences of cure. Cancer 1986; 58:529–533.
213. Zebrack BJ, Zeltzer LK, Whitton J, et al. Psychological outcomes in long-term survivors of childhood leukemia, Hodgkin's disease, and non-Hodgkin's lymphoma: a report from the Childhood Cancer Survivor Study. Pediatrics 2002;110:42–52.
214. Kokkonen J, Vainionpaa L, Winqvist S, et al. Physical and psychosocial outcome for young adults with treated malignancy. Pediatr Hematol Oncol 1997;14:223–232.
215. Teta MJ, Del Po MC, Kasl SV, et al. Psychosoical consequences of childhood and adolescent cancer survival. J Chronic Dis 1986;39:751–759.
216. Fritz GK, Williams JR, Amylon M. After treatment ends: Psychosocial sequelae in pediatric cancer survivors. Am J Orthopsychiatry 1988;58:552–561.
217. Mulhern RK, Wasserman AL, Friedman AG, et al. Social competence and behavioral adjustment of children who are long-term survivors of cancer. Pediatrics 1989;83: 18–25.
218. Fritz GK, Williams JR. Issues of adolescent development for survivors of childhood cancer. J Am Acad Child Adolesc Psychiatry 1988;27:712–715.
219. Madan-Swain A, Brown RT. Cognitive and psychosocial sequelae for children with acute lymphocytic leukemia survivors and their families. Clin Psychol Rev 1991;11: 267–294.
220. Zebrack BJ, Chesler MA. Quality of life in childhood cancer survivors. Psychooncology 2002;11:132–141.
221. Pendley JS, Dahlquist LM, Dreyer Z. Body image and psychological adjustment in adolescent cancer survivors. J Pediatr Psychol 1997;22:29–43.
222. Neff EJ, Beardslee CI. Body knowledge and concerns of children with cancer as compared with the knowledge and concerns of other children. J Pediatr Nurs 1990;5: 179–189.
223. Schmale AH, Morrow GR, Schmitt MH, et al. Well-being of cancer survivors. Psychosom Med 1983;45:163–169.
224. Greenberg H, Kazak A, Meadows A. Psycholoic functioning in 8- to 16 year old cancer survivors and their parents. J Pediatr 1989;114:488–493.
225. Greenberg HS, Kazak AE, Meadows AT. Psycholoic functioning in 8-to 16 year old cancer survivors and their parents. J Pediatr 1989;114:488–493.
226. Ross L, Johansen C, Oksbjerg Dalton S, et al. Psychiatric hospitalizations among survivors of cancer in childhood or adolescence. N Engl J Med 2003;349:650–657.
227. Gray R, Doan B, Shermer P, et al. Surviving childhood cancer: a descriptive approach to understanding the impact of life-threatening illness. Psychooncology 1992;1:235–245.
228. Anholt U, Fritz GK, Keener M. Self-concept in survivors of childhood and adolescent cancer. J Psychosocial Oncol 1993;11:1–16.
229. Barakat L, Kazak A, Meadows A, et al. Families surviving childhood cancer: a comparison of posttraumatic stress symptoms with families of healthy children. J Pediatr Psychol 1997;22:843–859.
230. Brown RT, Kaslow NJ, Hazzard AP, et al. Psychiatric and family functioning in children with leukemia and their parents. J Am Acad Child Adolesc Psychiatry 1992;31: 495–502.
231. Canning E, Canning R, Boyce W. Depressive symptoms and adaptive style in children with cancer. J Am Acad Child Adolesc Psychiatry 1992;31:1120–1124.
232. Kazak A. ed. Implications of survival: pediatric oncology patients and their families. New York, NY: Oxford University Press, 1994.
233. Martinson LM, Bossert E. The psychological status of children with cancer. J Child Adolesc Psychiatr Nurs 1994;7:16–23.
234. Phipps S, Steele RG, Hall K, et al. Repressive adaptation children with cancer: a replication and extension. Health Psychol 2001;20:445–451.
235. Radcliffe J, Bennett D, Kazak AE, et al. Adjustment in childhood brain tumor survival: child, mother, and teacher report. J Pediatr Psychol 1996;21:529–539.
236. Sloper T, Larcombe IJ, Charleston A. Psychosocial adjustment of five-year survivors of childhood cancer. J Cancer Educ 1994;9:163–169.
237. Elkin TD, Phipps S, Mulhern RK, et al. Psychological functioning of adolescent and young adult survivors of pediatric malignancy. Med Pediatr Oncol 1997;29:582–588.
238. Mackie E, Hill J, Kondryn H, et al. Adult psychosocial outcomes in long-term survivors of acute lymphoblastic leukaemia and Wilms' tumour: a controlled study. Lancet 2000; 355:1310–1314.
239. Magglioni A, Grassi R, Adamoli L, et al. Self-image of adolescent survivors of long-term childhood leukemia. J Pediatr Hematol/Oncol 2000;22:417–421.
240. Kazak A. Posttraumatic distress in childhood cancer survivors and their parents. Med Pediatr Oncol 1998;(suppl 1):60–68.
241. Cella DF, Tross S. Psychological adjustment to survival from Hodgkin's disease. J Consult Clin Psychol 1986;54:616–622.
242. Chesler M, Zebrack B. An updated report on our studies of long-term survivorship of childhood cancer and a brief review of the psychosocial literature. Ann Arbor, MI: Center for Research on Social Organization, University of Michigan, 1997.
243. Phipps S. Repressive adaptation in children with cancer. Health Psycholo 1997;16: 521–528.
244. Glover D, Byrne J, Mills J, et al. Impact of CNS treatment on mood in adult survivors of childhood leukemia: a report from the Children's Cancer Group. J Clin Oncol 2003; 21:4395–4401.
245. Recklitis C, O'Leary T, Diller L. Utility of routine psychological screening in the childhood cancer survivor clinic. J Clin Oncol 2003;21,:787–792.
246. Butler RW, Rizzi LP, Handwerger BA. Brief report: the assessment of Posttraumatic Stress Disorder in pediatric cancer patients and survivors. J Pediatr Psychol 1996;21: 499–504.
247. Erickson SJ, Steiner H. Trauma and personality correlates in long term pediatric cancer survivors. Child Psychiatry Hum Dev 2002;31:195–213.
248. Pelcovitz D, Libov B, Mandel F, et al. Posttraumatic stress disorder and family functioning in adolescent cancer. J Trauma Stress 1998;11:205–221.
249. Kazak A, Barakat L, Alderfer M, et al. Posttraumatic stress in survivors of childhood cancer and mothers: development and validation of the Impact of Traumatic Stressors Interview Schedule (ITSIS). J Clin Psychol Med Settings 2001;8:307–323.
250. Stuber M, Christakis D, Houskamp B, et al. Posttrauma symptoms in childhood leukemia survivors and their parents. Psychosomatics 1996;37:254–261.
251. Langeveld N, Grootenhuis M, Voute P, et al. Posttraumatic stress symptoms in adult survivors of childhood cancer. Pediatr Blood Cancer 2004;42:604–610.
252. Hobbie WL, Stuber M, Meeske K, et al. Symptoms of Posttraumatic Stress in Young Adult Survivors of Childhood Cancer. J Clin Oncol 2000;18:4060–4066.
253. Rourke M, Hobbie W, Kazak A. Posttraumatic stress in young adult survivors of childhood cancer (poster). In: 7th International Conference on Long-Term Complications of Treatment of Children and Adolescents for Cancer; June, 2002; Niagra-on-the-Lake, Ontario, Canada.
254. Lee Y, Santacroce S. Posttraumatic stress in long-term young adult survivors of childhood cancer: a questionnaire survey. J Nurs Stud 2007;44:1406–1417.
255. Meeske KA, Ruccione K, Globe DR, et al. Posttraumatic stress, quality of life, and psychological distress in young adult survivors of childhood cancer. Oncol Nurs Forum 2001;28:481–489.
256. Schwartz L, Drotar D. Posttraumatic stress and related impairment in survivors of childhood cancer in early adulthood compared to healthy peers. J Pediatr Psychol 2006; 31:356–366.
257. Stam H, Grootenhuis M, Last B. The course of life of survivors of childhood cancer. Psychooncology 2005;14:227–238.
258. Cantrell M. Health-related quality of life in childhood cancer: state of the science. Oncol Nurs Forum 2007;34:103–111.
259. Varni J, Limbers C, Burwinkle T. Literature review: health-related quality of life measurement in pediatric oncology. J Pediatr Psychol 2007;32:1151–1163.
260. Eiser C. Beyond survival: quality of life and follow-up after childhood cancer. J Pediatr Psychol 2007;32:1140–1150.
261. Stam H, Grootenhuis M, Caron H, et al. Quality of life and current coping in young adult survivors of childhood cancer: positive expectations about the further course of the disease were correlated with better quality of life. Psychooncology 2006;15:31–43.
262. Lown EA, Goldsby R, Mertens A, et al. Alcohol consumption patterns and risk factors among childhood cancer survivors compared to siblings and general population peers. Addiction 2008;103:1139–1148.
263. Donze J, Tercyak K. The Survivor Health and Resilience Education (SHARE) program: development and evaluation of a health behavior intervention for adolescent survivors of childhood cancer. J Clin Psychol Med Settings 2006;13:169–176.
264. Kazak A, Christakis D, Alderfer M, et al. Young adolescent cancer survivors and their parents: adjustment, learning problems, and gender. J Fam Psychol 1994;8:74–84.
265. Grootenhuis MA, Last BF. Adjustment and coping by parents of children with cancer: a review of the literature. Support Care Cancer 1997;5:466–484.

266. Sormanti M, Dungan S, Reiker PP. Pediatric bone marrow transplantation: psychosocial issues for parents after a child's hospitalization. Journal Psychosoc Oncol 1994;12: 23–42.
267. Kazak AE, Barakat LP. Brief report: parenting stress and quality of life during treatment for childhood leukemia predicts child and parent adjustment after treatment ends. J Pediatr Psychol 1997;22:749–758.
268. Kazak AE, Stuber ML, Barakat LP, et al. Predicting posttraumatic stress symptoms in mothers and fathers of survivors of childhood cancers. J Am Acad Child Adolesc Psychiatry 1998;37:823–831.
269. Manne SL, Du Hamel K, Gallelli K, et al. Posttraumatic stress disorder among mothers of pediatric cancer survivors: diagnosis, comorbidity, and utility of the PTSD checklist as a screening instrument. J Pediatr Psychol 1998;23:357–366.
270. Manne S, DuHamel K, Nereo N, et al. Predictors of PTSD in mothers of children undergoing bone marrow transplantation: the role of cognitive and social processes. J Pediatr Psychol 2002;27:607–617.
271. Fuemmeler B, Mullins L, Van Pelt J, et al. Posttraumatic stress symptoms and distress among parents of children with cancer. Children's Health Care 2005;34:289–303.
272. Alderfer MA, Cnaan A, Annunziato RA, et al. Patterns of posttraumatic stress symptoms in parents of childhood cancer survivors. J Fam Psychol 2005;19:430–440.
273. Best M, Streisand R, Catania L, et al. Parental distress during pediatric leukemia and parental posttraumatic stress symptoms after treatment ends. J Pediatr Psychol 2002; 26:299–307.
274. Alderfer MA, Labay LE, Kazak AE. Brief report: does posttraumatic stress apply to siblings of childhood cancer survivors? J Pediatr Psychol 2003;28:281–286.
275. Kazak A, Simms S, Barakat L, et al. Surviving Cancer Competently Intervention Program (SCCIP): a cognitive-behavioral and family therapy intervention for adolescent survivors of childhood cancer and their families. Family Process 1999;38:175–191.
276. Kazak AE, Alderfer MA, Streisand R, et al. Treatment of posttraumatic stress symptoms in adolescent survivors of childhood cancer and their families: a randomized clinical trial. J Fam Psychol 2004;18(3):493–504.
277. Meadows AT, Gordon J, Massari DJ, et al. Declines in IQ scores and cognitive dysfunctions in children with acute lymphocytic leukaemia treated with cranial irradiation. Lancet 1981;2:1015–1018.
278. Duffner PK, Cohen ME, Thomas P. Late effects of treatment on the intelligence of children with posterior fossa tumors. Cancer 1983;51:233–237.
279. Eiser C. Intellectual abilities among survivors of childhood leukaemia as a function of CNS irradiation. Arch Dis Child 1978;53:391–395.
280. Lansky SB, Cairns NU, Lansky LL, et al. Central nervous system prophylaxis: studies showing impairment in verbal skills and academic achievement. Am J Pediatr Hematol Oncol 1984;6:183–190.
281. Robison LL, Nesbit ME Jr, Sather HN, et al. Factors associated with IQ scores in long-term survivors of childhood acute lymphoblastic leukemia. Am J Pediatr Hematol Oncol 1984;6:115–121.
282. Haupt R, Fears TR, Robison LL, et al. Educational attainment in long-term survivors of childhood acute lymphoblastic leukemia. JAMA 1994;272:1427–1432.
283. Challinor J, Karl D. Educational attainment in survivors of ALL. JAMA 1995;274: 1134–1135.
284. Chang P, Nesbit ME, Youngren N, et al. Personality characteristics and psychosocial adjustment of long-term survivors of childhood cancer. J Psychosoc Oncol 1987;5:43.
285. Butler RW, Hill JM, Steinherz PG, et al. Neuropsychologic effects of cranial irradiation, intrathecal methotrexate, and systemic methotrexate in childhood cancer. J Clin Oncol 1994;12:2621–2629.
286. Faboir P, Hoppe RT, Bloom J, et al. Psychosocial problems among survivors of Hodgkin's disease. J Clin Oncol 1986;4:805–814.
287. Dietz J. How doctors can help solve cancer patients' employment problems. Legal Aspects Med Practice 1978;6:25–29.
288. Kadan-Lottick NS, Robison L, Gurney JG, et al. Childhood cancer survivors' knowledge about their past diagnosis and treatment: Childhood Cancer Survivor Study. JAMA 2002;287:1832–1839.
289. Hudson M, Mertens A, Yasui Y, et al. Health status of adult long-term survivors of childhood cancer. JAMA 2003;290:1583–1592.
290. Eiser C, Hill JJ, Blacklay A. Surviving cancer: what does it mean for you? An evaluation of a clinic based intervention for survivors of childhood cancer. Psychooncology 2000; 9(3):214–220.
291. Emmons KM, Butterfield RM, Puleo E., et al. Smoking among participants in the childhood cancer survivors cohort: the Partnership for Health Study. Journal of Clinical Oncology 2003;21:189–196.
292. Hudson M, Tyc V, Srivastava D, et al. Multi-component behavioral intervention to promote health protective behaviors in childhood cancer survivors: the protect study. Med Pediatr Oncol 2002;39:2–11.
293. Barakat L, Alderfer M, Kazak A. Posttraumatic growth in adolescent survivors of cancer and their mothers and fathers. J Pediatr Psychol 2006;31:413–419.
294. Parry C, Chesler MA. Thematic evidence of psychosocial thriving in childhood cancer survivors. Qual Health Res 2005;15:1055–1073.
295. Joseph SL, Linley PA. Growth following adversity: theoretical perspectives and implications for clinical practice. Clinical Psychol Rev 2006;26:1041–1053.
296. Wright LM, Leahey M. Nurses and families: a guide to family assessment and intervention. 3rd ed. Philadelphia, PA: F. A. Davis Co., 2000.
297. Wilkins KL, Woodgate R. A review of qualitative research on the childhood cancer experience from the perspective of siblings: a need to give them a voice. J Pediatr Oncol Nursing 2005;22:305–319.
298. Murray JS. A qualitative exploration of psychosocial support for siblings of children with cancer. J Pediatr Nurs 2002;17:327–337.
299. Perin G, Kramer RF. The child and family facing death. In: Waechter EH, Phillips J, Holaday B, eds. Nursing care. Philadelphia, PA: JB Lippincott, 1985:1333.
300. Bjork M, Wiebe T, Hallstrom I. Striving to survive: families' lived experiences when a child is diagnosed with cancer. J Pediatr Oncol Nurs 2005;22:265–275.
301. Freeman K, O'Dell C, Meola C. Childhood brain tumors: children's and siblings' concerns regarding the diagnosis and phase of illness. J Pediatr Oncol Nurs 2003;20: 133–140.
302. Grinyer A, Thomas C. Young adults with cancer: the effect of the illness on parents and families. Int J Palliat Nurs 2001;7:162–170.
303. Lehna C. A childhood cancer sibling's oral history. J Pediatr Oncol Nurs 1998;15: 163–171.
304. MacLeod K, Whitsett S, Mash E, et al. Pediatric sibling donors of successful and unsuccessful hematopoietic stem cell transplants. J Pediatr Psychol 2003;28:223–231.
305. McGrath P, Paton M, Huff N. Beginning treatment for pediatric acute myeloid leukemia: the family connection. Issues Compr Pediatr Nurs 2005;18:97–114.
306. Murray JS. The lived experience of childhood cancer: one sibling's perspective. Issues Compr Pediatr Nurs 1998;21:217–227.
307. Nolbris M, Enskar K, Hellstrom A. Experience of siblings of children treated for cancer. Eur J Oncol Nurs 2007;22:227–233.
308. Packman W, Crittenden M, Rieger FJ, et al. Sibling's perceptions of the bone marrow transplantation process. J Psychosoc Oncol 1997;15:81–105.
309. Packman W, Beck V, VanZutphen K, et al. The human figure drawing with donor and nondonor siblings of pediatric bone marrow transplant patients. Art Ther: J Amer Assoc 2003;20:83–91.
310. Patterson J, Holm K, Gurney J. The impact of childhood cancer on the family: a qualitative analysis of strains, resources, and coping behaviors. Psychooncology 2004;13: 390–407.
311. Phuphaibul R, Muensa W. Negative and positive adaptive behaviors of Thai school-aged children who have a sibling with cancer. J Pediatr Nurs 1999;14:342–348.
312. Scott-Findlay S, Chalmers K. Rural families' perspectives on having a child with cancer. J Pediatr Oncol Nurs 2001;18:205–216.
313. Sidhu R, Passmore A, Baker DA. An investigation into parent perceptions of the needs of siblings of children with cancer. J Pediatr Oncol Nurs 2005;22:276–287.
314. Sloper P. Experiences and support needs of siblings of children with cancer. Health Soc Care Community 2000;8:298–306.
315. Woodgate R. Siblings' experiences with childhood cancer. Cancer Nurs 2006;29: 404–414.
316. McGrath P. Treatment for childhood acute lymphoblastic leukaemia: the fathers' perspective. Aust Health Rev 2001;24:135–142.
317. Houtzager BA, Grootenhuis MA, Caron HN, et al. Quality of life and psychological adaptation in siblings of paediatric cancer patients, 2 years after diagnosis. Psychooncology 2004;13:499–511.
318. Houtzager BA, Grootenhuis MA, Caron HN, et al. Sibling self-report, parental proxies, and quality of life: the importance of multiple informants for siblings of a critically ill child. Pediatr Hematol Oncol 2005;22:25–40.
319. Houtzager BA, Grootenhuis MA, Hoekstra-Weebers JE, et al. Psychosocial functioning in siblings of paediatric cancer patients one to six months after diagnosis. Eur J Cancer 2003;39:1423–1432.
320. Houtzager BA, Oort FJ, Hoekstra-Weebers JE, et al. Coping and family functioning predict longitudinal psychological adaptation of siblings of childhood cancer patients. J Pediatr Psychol 2004;29:591–605.
321. Packman W, Gong K, vanZutphen K, et al. Psychosocial adjustment of adolescent siblings of hematopoietic stem cell transplant patients. J Pediatr Oncol Nurs 2004;21:233–248.
322. Packman W, Greenhalgh J, Chesterman B, et al. Siblings of pediatric cancer patients: the quantitative and qualitative nature of quality of life. J Psychosoc Oncol 2005;23: 87–108.
323. Alderfer M, Labay LE, Kazak AE. Brief report: does posttraumatic stress apply to siblings of childhood cancer survivors? J Adv Nurs 2003;28:281–286.
324. Kazak AE, Alderfer MA, Streisand R, et al. Treatment of posttraumatic stress symptoms in adolescent survivors of childhood cancer and their families: a randomized clinical trial. J Fam Psychol 2004;18:493–504.
325. Sahler OJ, Roghmann KJ, Mulhern RK, et al. Sibling Adaptation to Childhood Cancer Collaborative Study: the association of sibling adaptation with maternal well-being, physical health, and resource use. J Dev Behav Pediatr 1997;18:233–243.
326. Barrera M, Chung JYY, Greenberg M, et al. Preliminary investigation of a group intervention for siblings of pediatric cancer patients. Child Health Care 2002;31:131–142.
327. Barrera M, Chung JYY, Fleming CF. Group intervention for siblings of padiatric cancer patients. J Psychosoc Oncol, 2004;22(2):21–39.
328. Dolgin M, Blumensohn R, Mulhern R, et al. Sibling adaptation to childhood cancer collaborative study: cross cultural aspects. J Psychosoc Oncol 1997;15:1–14.
329. Labay LE, Walco GA. Brief report: empathy and psychological adjustment in siblings of children with cancer. J Pediatr Psychol 2004;29:309–314.
330. Lahteenmaki P, Sjoblom J, Korhonen T, et al. The siblings of childhood cancer patients need early support: a follow up study over the first year. Arch Dis Child 2004;89: 1008–1013.
331. Wellisch D, Crater B, Wiley F, et al. Psychosocial impacts of a camping experience for children with cancer and their siblings. Psychooncology 2006;15:56–65.
332. Zeltzer L, Chen E, Weiss K, et al. Comparison of psychological outcome in adult survivors of childhood acute lymphoblastic leukemia versus sibling controls a Cooperative Children's Cancer Group and National Institutes of Health Study. J Clinic Oncol 1997; 15:547–556.
333. Houtzager BA, Grootenhuis MA, Last BF. Supportive groups for siblings of pediatric oncology patients: impact on anxiety. Psychooncology 2001;10:315–324.
334. Lim JW, Zebrack B. Caring for family members with chronic physical illness: a critical review of caregiver literature. Health Qual Life Outcomes 2004;2:50.
335. Zebrack B, Zevon M, Turk N. Psychological distress in long-term survivors of solid tumors diagnoses in childhood. Pediatr Blood Cancer 2007;49:47–51.
336. Zeltzer L, Lu Q, Leisenring W, et al. Psychosocial outcomes and health-related quality of life in adult childhood cancer survivors. Cancer Epidemiol Biomarkers Prev 2008;17: 435–446.
337. Freeman K, O'Dell C, Meola C. Issues in families of children with brain tumor. Oncol Nurs Forum 2000;27:843–848.
338. Cuttini M, Da Fre M, Haupt R, et al. Survivors of childhood cancer: using siblings as a control group. Pediatrics 2003;112:1454–1455; author reply 1454–1455.
339. Adams M. Helping the parents of children with malignancy. J Pediatr 1978;93: 734–738.
340. Cairns NU, Clark GM, Smith SD, et al. Adaptation of siblings to childhood malignancy. J Pediatr 1979;95:484–487.
341. Houtzager BA, Grootenhuis MA, Hoekstra-Weebers JE, et al. One month after diagnosis: quality of life, coping and previous functioning in siblings of children with cancer. Child Care Health Dev 2005;31:75–87.
342. Blotcky A. Helping adolescents with cancer cope with their disease. Semin Oncol Nurs 1986;2:117–122.
343. Wiener L, Steffen-Smith E, Battles H, et al. Sibling stem cell donor experiences at a single institution. Psychooncology 2008;17:304–307.
344. Chao CC, Chen SH, Wang CY, et al. Psychosocial adjustment among pediatric cancer patients and their parents. Psychiatry Clin Neurosci 2003;57:75–81.
345. Heffernan S, Zanelli A. Behavior changes exhibited by siblings of pediatric oncology patients: a comparison between maternal and sibling description. J Pediatr Oncol Nurs 1997;14:3–14.

346. Cain A, Fast I, Erickson ME. Children's disturbed reactions to the death of a sibling. Am J Orthopsychiatry 1964;34:741.

347. Beal E. Separation, divorce, and single-parent families. In: Carter EA, McGoldrick M, eds. The family life cycle: a framework for family therapy. New York, NY: Gardner Press, 1980:241–264.

348. Koenig B, Davies E. Cultural dimensions of care at life's end for children and their families. In: Field M, Behrman R, eds. When children die: improving palliative and end-of-life care for children and their families. Washington, DC: National Academies Press, 2003.

349. Levetown M. Palliative care in the intensive care unit. New Horiz 1998;6:383–397.

350. Canino I, Spurlock J. Culturally diverse children and adolescents: assessment, diagnosis, and treatment. New York, NY: Guilford Press, 1994.

351. Thibodeaux AG, Deatrick J. Cultural influence on family management of children with cancer. J Pediatr Oncol Nurs 2007;24:227–233.

352. Thoma M. The effects of a cultural awareness program on the delivery of health care. Health Soc Work 1977;2:124–136.

353. Brown M, Yabroff K. Economic impact of cancer in the United States. In: Schottenfeld D, Fraumeni JF, eds. Cancer epidemiology and prevention. 3rd ed. New York: Oxford University, 2009.

354. Lansky SB, Black JL, Cairns NU. Childhood cancer. Medical costs. Cancer 1983;52:762–766.

355. Cairns N, Clark GM, Black J, et al. Childhood cancer: nonmedical costs of the illness. In: Spinetta JJ, Deasy-Spinetta P, eds. Living with childhood cancer. St Louis, MO: CV Mosby, 1981.

356. American Academy of Pediatrics. Guidelines for the pediatric cancer center and the role of such centers in diagnosis and treatment. Pediatrics 1997;99:139–140.

357. Noll R, Kazak A. Psychosocial care. In: Altman AJ, ed. Supportive care of children with cancer: current therapy and guidelines form the children's oncology group. 3rd ed. Baltimore, MD: Johns Hopkins Press, 2004:237–353.

358. Cantrell M. The art of pediatric oncology nursing practice. J Pediatr Oncol Nurs 2007;24:132–138.

359. Kazak AE, Rourke MT, Alderfer MA, et al. Evidence-based assessment, intervention and psychosocial care in pediatric oncology: a blueprint for comprehensive services across treatment. J Pediatr Psychol 2007;32:1099–1110.

360. Pai AL, Drotar D, Zebracki K, Moore M, et al. A meta-analysis of the effects of psychological interventions in pediatric oncology on outcomes of psychological distress and adjustment. J Pediatr Psychol 2006;31:978–988.

361. Kazak AE, Simms S, Alderfer MA, et al. Feasibility and preliminary outcomes from a pilot study of a brief psychological intervention for families of children newly diagnosed with cancer. J Pediatr Psychol 2005;30:644–655.

362. Lutz Stehl M, Kazak AE, Alderfer MA, et al. The feasibility of conducting a randomized clinical trial of an intervention for parent/caregivers of children newly diagnosed with cancer. J Pediatr Psychol. 2009;34(8):803–816.

363. Armstrong S, Cozza K, Benedek DM. Med-psych drug-drug interactions. New York: American Psychiatric Association, 2004.

364. DeVane CL, Nemeroff CB. Guide to Psychotropic drug interactions. Prim Psychiatry 2002;9:28–57.

365. Galanter C, Jensen P. DSM-IV-TR casebook and treatment guide for child mental. Arlington VA: American Psychiatric Publishing, 2009.

366. Hamburg DA. Coping behavior in life-threatening circumstances. Psychother Psychosom 1974;23:13–25.

CHAPTER 46 ■ ETHICAL CONSIDERATIONS IN PEDIATRIC ONCOLOGY

STEVEN JOFFE, JENNIFER KESSELHEIM, AND SUSAN B. SHURIN

The notion of an ethical dilemma is familiar to those who care for or conduct research with children with cancer. Indeed, few fields are as rich in ethical challenges as pediatric oncology. We want both to be truthful with the child who has cancer and to respect parents' roles in guiding their families. We want to honor families' religious beliefs while ensuring that a child does not die for lack of a blood transfusion. We want to avoid burdensome interventions at the end of life while keeping open any possibility that the child may recover.

Understanding of and commitment to ethical values and principles are central to professionalism in medical and research practice. The fundamental principles of professional practice include the primacy of patient welfare, autonomy, and social justice.[1] Specific obligations include commitments to honesty with patients, confidentiality, respect for appropriate boundaries, a just distribution of finite resources, and management of conflicts of interest. Importantly, increasing evidence suggests that professionalism can be taught and learned, and that it must be a core component at all stages of medical education.[2]

Medical ethics can be understood on at least two levels.[3] An analogy to mental health helps clarify the distinction between them. One can be psychologically healthy yet unfamiliar with Freud and Jung. Psychology is a 2nd-order discipline, one that studies human behavior and emotion. By analogy, many adults are models of moral integrity yet know little of Mill and Kant. Ethics is also a 2nd-order discipline, an attempt to understand moral behavior and to use this understanding to guide and justify the best course of action when confronted with ethical challenges. This chapter is an attempt to use systematic analysis to shed light on ethical questions that arise in pediatric oncology.

In what follows, we concentrate on selected areas relevant to clinicians and investigators caring for and conducting research with children with cancer. We begin with discussions of informed consent and of the ethics of human subjects research. This is followed by comments on confidentiality, genetic testing, and ethics in end-of-life care. Finally, we consider financial incentives and conflicts of interest. We contend that, in every area of pediatric oncology, professionalism requires attention to the ethical dimensions of clinical and research practice.

INFORMED CONSENT

Few areas of bioethics have evolved as dramatically over the past 50 years as has the discussion of the rights and responsibilities of patients and their physicians. For centuries, both physicians and patients assumed that the physician knew what was best, and therefore bore responsibility for medical decisions. The Hippocratic Oath directed physicians to "follow that system of regimen which, according to my ability and judgment, I consider for the benefit of my patients."[4] Physicians, not patients, were the ultimate decision makers about care.

Medicine has always been both art and science. As the scientific basis of medical practice has solidified, both physicians and patients have come to expect an evidence base for recommendations and decisions. As a result, the locus of authority for medical decisions has shifted decisively to the patient. In some instances, this means that patients are burdened with decisions when a modicum of paternalism or at least of wise guidance might be helpful. Respect for persons, or respect for autonomy, is operationalized in the practice of informed consent. It would not have occurred to Hippocrates' patients to ask, "Doctor, how do you know this is the best thing for me? What is the evidence, and what are my options?" As evidence and options have increased, the concept of consent—meaningful only when informed—has acquired a central place in bioethics.

The notion of informed consent has matured over time. Scattered legal cases from the 1700s to the early 1900s emphasized the need for consent—usually without considering how or whether the patient became informed—and viewed infractions of the consent requirement as tantamount to battery. Since the mid-1900s, legal cases have developed the requirement for *informed* consent, and consequently for sufficient disclosure by the physician about the relevant facts.[5–8] The mandate that consent be *informed* was not firmly established in U.S. case law until 1957.[8] The legal system has generally viewed violations of the disclosure requirement as professional negligence rather than as battery.

The historical origins of consent to treatment and to research differ. Consent to treatment evolved as a legal doctrine, as patients successfully brought malpractice actions for violations of consent. In contrast, the requirement for consent to research developed through a combination of ethical codes—beginning with the Nuremberg Code in response to the Nazis' abuses[9]—and prospective regulation of research.[10,11]

Several factors complicate discussions of informed consent in pediatric oncology. First, many conversations and decisions take place primarily between clinicians and parents, with increasing involvement of children as they mature. Second, the remarkable proportion of patients cared for within trials demands understanding of both clinical and research consent. Third, investigators enrolling subjects on clinical trials are usually also clinicians responsible for the patient's care. Fourth, the protracted nature of cancer treatment underscores the point that informed consent is a process—an ongoing conversation between the patient, responsible relatives or caregivers, and a team of physicians and nurses—rather than a discrete event.

We start with the simplest case—the competent adult deciding about nonresearch clinical care—before addressing consent in pediatrics. We discuss the special issues raised by consent to research in the section on "Human Subjects Research."

Informed Consent for Competent Adults

The doctrine of informed consent is most straightforward when applied to individuals "of adult years and sound mind."[12] Five criteria together constitute valid informed consent: (a) voluntariness, (b) capacity, (c) disclosure, (d) understanding, and (e) decision.[13]

Competence and Capacity

Competence and *capacity* are often used interchangeably. However, they have distinct if related meanings. Competence is a legal term that specifies if a person has authority to manage her own affairs in a particular domain of life. Capacity denotes the perceptual, cognitive, and communicative ability to perform a particular task. It reflects a clinical rather than a legal judgment, and therefore falls within the domain of physicians and others with appropriate clinical expertise. For example, although the average older teen may have capacity to make most medical decisions, she will generally be presumed legally incompetent in most jurisdictions.

Decision-making capacity can be judged in relation to four abilities: (a) the ability to make a choice; (b) the ability to understand relevant information; (c) the ability to appreciate the consequences of a decision for one's situation; and (d) the ability to manipulate information rationally.[14] Many clinicians take a "sliding scale" approach to capacity determinations, whereby standards become increasingly stringent as the consequences of a decision and the degree to which it deviates from what seems reasonable increase.[15] Patients with capacity should be included in the consent process, regardless of their competence in the legal sense.

Disclosure

Disclosure refers to the information that must be communicated to the patient, including: (a) the nature and purpose of the proposed treatment; (b) the foreseeable risks and discomforts; (c) the potential benefits; and (d) available alternatives. Although this requirement seems onerous, any reasonable interpretation recognizes the need for selectivity in the amount and type of information shared.[16] As a rule, common complications should be disclosed regardless of severity, and serious or irreversible risks should be disclosed regardless of frequency.

Three standards are available to guide physicians in deciding what information to present to patients. Two are used by courts to determine whether physicians have met their disclosure requirements. Under the professional standard, the physician must provide the information that a *reasonable physician* would disclose in similar circumstances. Under the reasonable-person standard, the physician must provide all the information that a *reasonable decision maker* would want to know (i.e., that is material to the decision). A third standard, the subjective standard, is an ethical ideal that has no specific correlate in the law. Under this standard, the clinician should provide the information that is material not just for a reasonable person, but for *this particular person*. For example, even if most patients would not wish to know of the rare risk of mild peripheral neuropathy from a chemotherapeutic, this information might be of crucial importance to a professional pianist. Meeting this standard requires that the physician know the patient well enough to anticipate that such information would be subjectively relevant.

Failures of disclosure undermine the validity of informed consent through willful or unintentional deception. Distortion or omission of key facts deprives patients of the information they need to make decisions. Some commentators and courts have carved out a "therapeutic privilege" exception to disclosure requirements. This exception may be invoked when the information disclosed is so threatening as potentially to impair a patient's ability to make rational decisions, or might be harmful to the patient's health. This exception opens the door wide open to inappropriate paternalism and therefore should be sparingly invoked.

Understanding

It is easier to determine what a clinician has disclosed than what a patient has understood. Furthermore, even when disclosure is exemplary, understanding can be difficult to achieve, particularly in settings such as pediatric oncology in which fear, desperation, and other emotions can so profoundly influence patients' and parents' decision-making processes. Courts have therefore generally looked to evidence of disclosure rather than of understanding to judge the adequacy of consent. Nevertheless, understanding remains an important ethical aspiration.

To achieve shared decision making, clinicians should regularly assess patients' understanding of the diagnostic and treatment alternatives. This can be particularly difficult around choices involving risk. Studies have shown, for example, that individuals will choose different treatments, depending on whether the risks are presented as the probability of success or of failure.[17] Such framing can have powerful consequences in pediatric oncology if, for example, a clinician optimistically presents her preferred option in terms of its chances for disease control while presenting the alternatives in terms of their probabilities of recurrence.

Voluntariness

To be valid, consent must be free as well as informed. Choices can be influenced by persuasion or coercion. Physicians may ethically employ persuasion.[18] When, for example, a patient refuses chemotherapy for a potentially curable malignancy because of concerns over side effects, the physician should not hesitate to challenge him. Indeed, not attempting to persuade in these circumstances would be ethically inappropriate.

Coercion differs from persuasion in that it involves the use of credible threats to influence decisions.[19] For example, a clinician may tell parents that, if they refuse chemotherapy, hospital attorneys will seek a court order to initiate treatment. Involving legitimate outside authorities may be justified when the situation requires examination for broader societal concerns, but such threats should only be used when efforts at persuasion have been made repeatedly and have failed. Punitive threats, such as refusing to treat pain unless parents agree to the physician's preferred cancer treatment regimen, are always unjustified. Finally, only situations in which a decision puts others at risk (e.g., harm to third parties from a contagious disease) justify the use of coercion to influence the decision of a competent adult patient.

Decision

Because of the legal view of informed consent, many clinicians see consent as signature on the bottom of a form. The transitive verb *to consent (him or her)* has emerged in hospital jargon to describe this activity as another procedure performed upon the patient. Consent should be viewed as a process rather than as an event.[13] Particularly in pediatric oncology, where patients and families generally are faced with multiple decisions that must be navigated over the course of the illness, obtaining a signature is only a way station in the process of informed consent.

Informed Consent, Surrogate Authorization, and Incompetent Adults

The model of autonomous consent is such a powerful paradigm for medical decision making that it has overwhelmed other possible models. The law has sought to define ways in which partially or fully incapacitated patients can exercise these rights indirectly via surrogates.

Two standards have evolved to guide decision making by surrogates. The *substituted-judgment standard* seeks decisions based on actual values and preferences that patients had before becoming incompetent. Substituted judgment is most readily implemented in situations in which the incompetent person's wishes are known or can be inferred, and fits poorly when making decisions for never-competent persons or for those whose wishes cannot be deduced.[20]

The desire to base decisions on patients' actual wishes has motivated efforts to have patients articulate these wishes before losing capacity through advance directives. One type of directive, the living will, allows patients to specify the extent to which they would like to have life-sustaining medical treatments provided should they develop specific medical problems while incompetent. Living wills have proved problematic, however; few people complete them, individuals have difficulty predicting their wishes in serious and unfamiliar circumstances, it is difficult to articulate those preferences, and clinicians and surrogates do not reliably act on them.[21] An alternate approach is the durable power of attorney for health care (or health care proxy), a document that assigns decision-making authority to a particular person in the event of incapacity. The Patient Self-Determination Act of 1990 requires hospitals in the United States to inquire whether adult patients currently have an advance directive, and to give them an opportunity to create one if they do not.[22,23]

The *best-interests standard* is generally used for patients who never have been competent or whose preferences about care are not known. Although this standard provides useful guidance for surrogates, it does not resolve situations in which views about how best to advance the interests of affected patients differ, and does not adequately clarify surrogates' range of discretion. To address these problems, Dresser has proposed "clear harm" as the criterion for determining which proxy decisions are unacceptable when a patient's wishes are unknown.[24]

Informed Consent and Children

Analyses of medical decision making for children often begin with the conceptual model of the noncompetent patient. Children, however, differ from noncompetent adults. Most of the sentinel legal cases involving noncompetent adults involved patients who never were expected to regain capacity (i.e., adults with chronic, usually progressive illness). In contrast, in most cases children's decision-making capacity is in a state of growth and evolution. The goal is to respect the *former* autonomy of adults; with children, the challenge is to protect their *future* autonomy.

Until the early 20th century, children were considered property of their parents, who were empowered to make decisions on children's behalf. The presumption of parental authority has several bases: (a) parents are motivated powerfully to make decisions in their children's best interests;

(b) children are expected to grow up to espouse many of their parents' values, so parental decisions are most likely to resemble the kinds of decisions that children will make when they become competent; (c) parents have to live with the consequences of the decisions they make for their children; and (d) parents make most nonmedical decisions involving their children (e.g., schooling), so they should have responsibility for medical decisions as well. In making difficult decisions for young children, the best interests standard provides the best available guidance about the appropriate treatment.

The American Academy of Pediatrics (AAP) has argued that "in most cases, physicians have an ethical (and legal) obligation to obtain *parental permission* to undertaken recommended medical interventions. In many circumstances, physicians should also solicit *patient assent* when developmentally appropriate. In cases involving emancipated or mature minors with adequate decision-making capacity, or when otherwise permitted by law, physicians should seek *informed consent* directly from patients.[25] According to the AAP, *consent* is appropriately given only by patients with "appropriate decisional capacity and legal empowerment."

The benefits of initial therapy for pediatric cancer are usually sufficiently clear that a child's objection will be overruled. However, it becomes increasingly important to solicit the child's agreement in circumstances, such as relapse with a poor prognosis, where the benefit-risk ratio of treatment is less clear. Also, as we discuss in the following text, the weight of the assent requirement in childhood cancer research is controversial.

Involvement of Children in Consenting to Treatment and to Research Participation

Few topics in pediatric bioethics are as challenging as the concept of "assent" by children to undergo medical procedures or participate in research. Assent for treatment has been incorporated into professional ethical guidelines. According to the AAP,[25] elements of assent include:

1. Helping the patient achieve a developmentally appropriate awareness of her condition;
2. Explaining what the child should expect with tests or treatment;
3. Assessing the child's understanding, as well as any pressure to accept treatment;
4. Soliciting an expression of the child's willingness to accept care. The AAP notes, however, that "in situations in which the patient will have to receive medical care despite his or her objection, the patient should be told that fact and should not be deceived."

Emancipated and Mature Minors

Two legal categories—emancipated minor and mature minor—give special decision-making status to patients under the age of majority.[26] State laws defining emancipation vary, but typically minors may be emancipated by virtue of either (a) their status as independent from their parents (living apart, financial self-sufficiency, marriage) or (b) the presence of a specified condition (sexually transmitted diseases, pregnancy, mental illness, substance use). Status-based emancipation is generally justified by the fact that the parents no longer have responsibility for or authority over the teen, whereas condition-based emancipation is thought to serve the public health by encouraging teens to seek treatment for sensitive conditions. Minors emancipated by virtue of status can generally give or withhold consent in any treatment setting, whereas those with a specified condition may only be granted the right to make independent decisions about the particular condition. An important corollary of emancipation is that the minor generally has the right to decide who (including her parents) may receive access to her medical record. It is important to recognize that emancipation does not necessarily imply mature decision-making facility (indeed, some reasons for emancipation, such as pregnancy, may suggest the converse). As a result, efforts to assist emancipated minors in making reasonable decisions are often ethically appropriate.

Many states have case law regarding treatment of mature minors. Mature minors are not emancipated, but nevertheless may have a legally enforceable decision making role based on their capacity to give informed consent. If a minor evidences such capacity in connection with a proposed treatment, including the ability to understand its nature and risks, he or she may have the legal right to consent to or refuse treatment.[26-28] Even when there is substantial risk, as in a case involving an older adolescent Jehovah's Witness who declines transfusion, it may be ethically appropriate and legally acceptable to respect the minor's decision.[29]

Ethical Dilemmas Regarding Informed Consent in Pediatric Oncology

When Parents Do Not Want Their Child to Know the Diagnosis

Communication of cancer diagnosis and prognosis with patients and families is heavily influenced by cultural norms, varying with national context and subculture expectations.[30] Early in the medical experience with chemotherapy for childhood cancer, it was felt to be unethical to inform children with leukemia of their diagnosis, as they needed to be protected from the psychological harms of knowing of their life-threatening illness.[31] By the late 1970s, however, cultural changes had led to a reversal of this view, with recommendations for full disclosure to adults and disclosure as appropriate to children.[31] It is also not easy to keep secrets when a child comes to a cancer clinic for therapy. Although variability among children and families precludes the identification of age-based rules, practical as well as ethical considerations favor disclosing the diagnosis to patients, while working with parents to inform children in a sensitive and individualized manner. It may be helpful to solicit parents' agreement that children's direct questions will be answered truthfully and that clinicians will never deliberately lie to the child.

When an Older Child Dissents from Medically Necessary Diagnostic or Therapeutic Procedures

Directly related to the issue of assent for treatment is the management of active dissent, primarily by adolescents, from unwanted treatment. Active dissent from research participation is more likely to be respected than dissent from standard therapy, unless participation in research is likely to bring the child substantial benefit that is not available otherwise.

Although teenagers lack adults' nearly unqualified right to refuse medical therapy, parents cannot easily mandate their treatment. There is no simple way to resolve the dilemmas that result when adolescents refuse recommended therapy. At a minimum, providers should explore the teen's decision-making capacity, the reasons behind the refusal, how it fits with deeply held values such as religious beliefs, where it falls on the spectrum of reasonableness, and the parents' views. Attempts at persuasion are appropriate. Factors that favor respecting a teen's refusal include older age, rational reasons for the refusal, parental concurrence, and an ambiguous

benefit-risk ratio. Assistance from consultants such as psychosocial clinicians, clergy, ethics committees, or legal counsel should be sought in difficult cases.

Parental Refusal of Therapy on Cultural or Other Grounds

Not all families subscribe to Western allopathic approaches to medicine. Furthermore, alternative approaches to healing are widely employed by patients and families either exclusively or in combination with allopathic treatments.[32,33] Some parents refuse treatment on cultural, religious, or other grounds. Both groups within Western cultures and individuals and groups who have immigrated may come in conflict with the broadly accepted values enunciated in this chapter. The resulting clashes of cultures tend to be more dramatic in cases involving children than adults. A striking example of such culture clash involving a Hmong family was described in 1998.[34] Should cultural differences be privileged over other reasons for treatment refusal? How can one know when to attribute parents' views to culture as opposed to idiosyncratic or even irrational opinion? One of the hallmarks of good ethical decision making is that similar cases should be decided similarly: if the clinicians would seek a court order to treat a U.S.-born child in similar circumstances, what arguments could justify not seeking a court order for a child from another country?

In many areas of pediatric practice, clinicians have a low threshold for overriding parents' refusals of prescribed therapy, even when those refusals derive from religious or cultural grounds. When clinicians believe that failure to transfuse will lead to permanent harm, they frequently obtain court orders for blood transfusion against the wishes of parents who are Jehovah's Witnesses. However, cancer is a chronic disease that is treated over a period of months or years, requiring a long-term therapeutic alliance and adherence to multiple complex medications and cooperation with procedures. This may require concessions to family demands that deviate from optimal medical management but are felt to carry acceptable incremental risk. These concessions may be necessary to maintain a family's cooperation with core cancer therapy. In many cases, the only alternative is to place the child in foster care for the duration of treatment, with all the family disruption and psychological trauma that this entails. It is more difficult to accede to parents' wishes that place the child at serious risk of preventable harm.

In cases of treatment refusal, it is important to distinguish among situations in which (a) parents lack decision-making capacity, (b) parents with capacity act on irrational beliefs, and (c) parents act rationally in the service of unusual but deeply held beliefs.[35] Because parents have a moral duty to act rationally in their children's best interests, it is easier to challenge or override their decisions in the first two circumstances than in the third. These situations transcend the relationship between the family and the medical teams, implicate societal values, and involve legal conflicts. The most contentious situations arise when the parties involved fail to understand the context of each others' positions and decisions. Clinicians tend to approach such situations from a perspective of compromise, whereas legal engagements are often adversarial. Often, by the time the courts are involved, the therapeutic alliance has been damaged or destroyed, and no satisfactory solution is possible.

HUMAN SUBJECTS RESEARCH

Pediatric oncologists are justifiably proud of the remarkable advances in the treatment of childhood cancer during the past five decades.[36] This success can largely be attributed to an extraordinary integration of research with care; at some point during their illness, perhaps 70% of patients take part in a trial.[37] Given the heterogeneity of childhood cancer and the small numbers of patients, progress would have been much slower without the cooperative clinical trials effort and infrastructure that made it possible.

Despite its achievements, the merging of research and routine care demands caution. As we discuss later, the aims of research and of treatment differ.[38] Although it is often possible to achieve both sets of objectives simultaneously, this happy outcome is not automatic. Thus pediatric oncology, perhaps more than any other field of medicine, requires attention to and clarity about the complex intersection between clinical research and clinical care.[39]

A Conceptual Model for Human Subjects Research

The notions of "therapeutic" and "nontherapeutic" research are widely invoked. They featured prominently in the first five versions of the World Medical Association's (WMA's) *Declaration of Helsinki*, which until recently stated that "a fundamental distinction must be recognized between medical research in which the aim is essentially diagnostic or therapeutic for a patient, and medical research, the essential object of which is purely scientific..."[40] Ethicists have challenged the idea of "research in which the aim is ... diagnostic or therapeutic for a patient" as incoherent.[41] The WMA abandoned the distinction in the *Declaration's* 5th (2000) revision.

The *Belmont Report* offers an alternative conceptual framework.[38] Though best known for its principles of respect for persons, beneficence, and justice, the *Report's* articulation of the boundary between practice (treatment) and research is equally important. The *Report* defines *practice* as "interventions ... designed solely to enhance the well being of an individual patient or client and that have a reasonable expectation of success." In contrast, *research* is "an activity designed to test an hypothesis, permit conclusions to be drawn, and thereby to develop or contribute to generalizable knowledge." The *Report* thus views research and treatment as conceptually distinct endeavors, albeit ones that may be conducted jointly within a trial.

The Role of the Clinical Researcher

When a patient enrolls in a trial, the physician-patient relationship changes.[42–44] The physician is now also an investigator and the patient also a subject. The investigator takes on obligations to science—fidelity to the protocol and its objectives—distinct from his or her fiduciary duties to the patient. This dual obligation requires a unique professionalism on the part of the clinician–investigator, one appropriate to his or her complex role.[42] Some have even argued that, in light of this dual role, enrolling in a study—particularly one that involves random assignment—amounts to a renunciation of "personal care," and is therefore ethically problematic.[45–47] In our view, this criticism is too strong; pediatric oncology has largely succeeded in aligning the investigator–subject and the physician-patient relationships inherent in trials. Nevertheless, there is a need for recognition of the unavoidable tension between these relationships,[43] and for rigorous justification when study design requires deviating from a strict conception of the participant's best interests (such as a study that involves extra research-specific bone marrows or lumbar punctures). Miller and Brody have decried the prevalent "therapeutic orientation to clinical trials," which leads to blurring of the boundaries between clinical and research roles.[48] Joffe and Miller have

called for reconceptualizing the clinical investigator as someone engaged in scientific experimentation, albeit within constraints imposed by the rights and interests of the human subject, rather than as a clinician who is also engaged in research.[49] This is especially true of the principal investigator, who assumes overall responsibility for the conduct of the study, but also extends to collaborating investigators by virtue of their responsibility to carry out the study with fidelity to protocol requirements.

The Therapeutic Misconception and Informed Consent to Research

If research is a conceptually different activity from care, then it is important that patients or their parents understand the implications of study enrollment. These include the constraints on individualized care necessitated by the research aims and the fact of participation in an endeavor whose primary purpose is to advance knowledge or improve treatment. Failure to understand this has been termed the "therapeutic misconception,"[50,51] defined by the National Bioethics Advisory Commission (NBAC) as "the belief that the purpose of a clinical trial is to benefit the individual patient rather than to gather data for the purpose of contributing to scientific knowledge."[52] (Importantly, NBAC also emphasized that "It is not a misconception to believe that participants probably will receive good clinical care during research. But it is a misconception to believe that the purpose of clinical trials is to administer treatment rather than to conduct research.") Though the evidence is imperfect, accumulating data suggest that therapeutic misconceptions are prevalent among research subjects and inhibit their ability to recognize salient distinctions between research participation and ordinary clinical care.[53–55] If so, then countering subjects' tendencies towards therapeutic misconceptions must be among the primary tasks of those who seek valid informed consent for research.

Kodish et al. recently articulated important guidance for investigators who discuss clinical trials with patients and parents. Their model emphasizes the need for a strategic, sequenced approach that focuses first on the understanding of a child's diagnosis and prognosis, followed by a discussion of current treatment for her disease. Only after these objectives have been accomplished should the investigator raise the option of clinical trial participation.[56] More generally, the available evidence suggests that extended contact with a knowledgeable clinician or member of the study team is the most effective means of enhancing research participant understanding.[57]

An Ethical Framework for Clinical Research

Various ethical codes, dating to the Nuremberg Code of 1947, have offered guidance for the appropriate conduct of human subjects research. Each provided important new insights, but none offered a comprehensive account. Emanuel et al. have attempted to articulate such a model.[10] Their framework invokes seven principles derived from previous codes that, applied sequentially, facilitate systematic judgments about which studies should be permitted to go forward (Table 46.1).

Special Requirements for Research with Children

In addition to the *Belmont Report*, the National Commission published a separate report on pediatric research that recommended several special considerations for studies involving children.[58] First, the Commission developed the concepts of assent (i.e., affirmative agreement) and parental permission. Because of the other-directed nature of clinical research, the obligation to solicit a child's agreement takes on greater

ETHICAL PRINCIPLES GUIDING THE DESIGN AND CONDUCT OF HUMAN SUBJECTS RESEARCH

Principle	Explanation
Social or scientific value	Research should address an important question, and should have the potential to improve health, well-being, or scientific understanding
Scientific validity	Research should involve methods that make it likely that the study question will be answered successfully
Fair subject selection	Eligibility criteria and recruitment strategies should be based on considerations of science and risk, not vulnerability
Favorable risk-benefit ratio	Risks should be minimized, consistent with the scientific objectives of the study Sum of benefits to subjects and society should justify risks to subjects
Independent review	Study design and procedures must be justified to individuals who are otherwise unaffiliated with the research; facilitates accountability
Informed consent	Salient information about the research must be disclosed to prospective subjects so that they can make reasoned decisions about study participation In pediatric research, model of surrogate permission, with or without the assent of the child, applies
Respect for enrolled subjects	Investigators should: • attend to the welfare of subjects • protect subjects' privacy • permit withdrawal from the research • provide new information about risks, benefits, or alternatives • inform subjects of study results

importance in the research context than it does in ordinary care. Under current United States federal regulations, the affirmative agreement of pediatric research subjects is required unless either: (a) they are incapable of providing meaningful agreement by virtue of age, maturity, or psychological state; or (b) the research offers the prospect of direct benefit that is unavailable outside the research context.[59] In addition, though not mentioned in the regulations, some children who are developmentally incapable of providing affirmative agreement may still express "deliberate objection." Such dissent should be respected unless there are compelling reasons to the contrary.

Despite the mandate to obtain the child's agreement, the notion remains challenging. First, it views the child's decision as radically separate from the parents', and therefore ignores the interconnected nature of decision making within families.[60,61] Second, it allows the child to veto the parents' decision, which some have criticized as failing to respect parents' appropriate role in guiding their children's moral development.[62] Third, the dichotomous nature of the decision to require or not require assent ignores the complex and nonlinear trajectory of children's cognitive and moral development,[60] and fails to recognize the practical complexities of engaging acutely ill children in these conversations.[63] Fourth, there are no agreed-upon standards for what constitutes "meaningful" assent. And finally, while several studies suggest that, under optimal circumstances, children aged 14 or older can achieve levels of comprehension approaching those of adults, the extent to which younger children can engage in these deliberations is controversial.[61,62,64–68] The Children's Oncology Group has offered guidance in an effort to fill in these gaps in the concept and practice of assent (Table 46.2).[69]

Although mature individuals can altruistically agree to take part in high-risk research studies without the prospect for compensating benefit, surrogate permission cannot justify enrolling children in such studies.[70,71] To deal with questions of maximum permissible risk, the National Commission

defined four categories of pediatric research. These combine judgments about risk (i.e., minimal risk, minor increment over minimal risk, or more than a minor increment above minimal risk) with determinations about whether the research holds the prospect of direct benefit (Table 46.3). U.S. regulations governing pediatric research incorporate this framework.[59] The regulations define minimal-risk research as research in which "the probability and magnitude of harm or discomfort . . . are not greater in and of themselves than those ordinarily encountered in daily life or during the performance of routine physical or psychological examinations or tests," but do not directly specify what constitutes a minor increment over minimal risk.[72]

Although this framework serves reasonably well, two important problems bear mention. First, the validity and consistency of judgments about the level of risk associated with a particular procedure are questionable.[73,74] Second, the framework presupposes that each study fits uniquely into one of the four categories. However, many protocols involve multiple research elements. For example, a trial might both administer an investigational agent that offers the prospect of direct benefit and require serial bone marrow aspirates performed for research purposes. Judging such a protocol as a whole, rather than in terms of its individual parts, succumbs to the "fallacy of the package deal."[75] It is preferable to evaluate each component individually,[76] and in particular to avoid using the benefits of one element (e.g., access to an investigational agent) to justify the burdens of another (e.g., protocol bone marrows).

The U.S. Institute of Medicine (IOM) recently undertook a comprehensive review of the ethical and regulatory issues related to children's participation in research.[61] The IOM's report included recommendations addressing definitions of risk thresholds and the relationship of risk to the condition and age of the patient; the need for institutional review board (IRB) review to focus attention to the details of the parental permission and assent processes, with a focus on the process

TABLE 46.2

CHILDREN'S ONCOLOGY GROUP RECOMMENDATIONS REGARDING CHILDREN'S PARTICIPATION IN RESEARCH DECISIONS[69]

1. *Provision of information to children*: All children should be given developmentally appropriate information about their diagnosis, treatment, and the proposed research study

2. *Inclusion of children in decisions*: Children's involvement in decisions about research should be viewed along a continuum, from no involvement when a child is very young or incapacitated to mature authority for many older adolescents

3. *Integration of family decision making*: In most cases, investigators should seek a unified family decision rather than separate decisions from the parents and the child

4. *Assent as a process*: Assent should be viewed as a process, with key decisions revisited at important milestones or as the child matures over time

5. *Waivers of assent requirements based on a prospect of direct benefit*: Waivers of the assent requirement based on a prospect of direct benefit should be limited to those cases in which there is good reason to believe that the child's outcome is likely to be better in research as compared with receipt of nonresearch therapy

6. *Waivers of assent requirements based on lack of decision-making capacity*: As a general rule, few children under the age of 9–10 are able to make informed decisions about participation in complex research, whereas most children aged 14 and above can make reasonably mature decisions. Especially in the gray zone between these ages, investigators and IRBs should permit considerable flexibility, rather than invoking age-based rules, in deciding which children have the capacity for assent. Appropriate consultation should be sought when capacity is in doubt

7. *Determining capacity to assent*: In addition to considering age, maturity, and psychological state, investigators and IRBs should consider capacity as it relates to the complexity of the decision task. In evaluating capacity, investigators should pay particular attention to the reasons a child gives for his preference regarding research participation

8. *Documentation of assent*: Documentation requirements should emphasize the investigator's responsibility to describe the child's role in the decision, and his or her preference, in the medical or research record. Requiring signatures from younger children may be inappropriate if children are unable to comprehend the symbolic or quasi-contractual nature of signing a document

9. *The role of older adolescents*: Older adolescents can play a mature role in research decisions, ethically co-equal with their parents. It may be appropriate, in order to recognize this role, to ask them to cosign the consent form with their parents

10. *Resolving disagreements*: Disagreements between children and parents about research participation are probably rare. Investigators and IRBs should establish fair processes for resolving such disagreements, such as appointing an advocate for the child, involving a consent monitor, or seeking ethics consultation

11. *Defining, understanding, and improving assent*: Pediatric oncology professionals should support research intended to enhance the quality and practice of assent

12. *Educating professionals*: Pediatric oncologists and others who participate in the consent and assent processes require education in the relevant regulations and best practices

---

rather than the signed documents; the essential role of improved parental education regarding the research process so that they can ask questions relevant to the implications of participation on their children and their families; and the training of clinical investigators. These recommendations have important implications for pediatric oncology practice.

Applications

Randomized Trials

The roles of clinician and investigator can conflict in studies that randomly assign patients to a control or an experimental arm. Some argue that it is only ethical for physicians to participate in such trials if they have no preference for one treatment over the other (i.e., are in "personal equipoise").[45] Others believe that this standard is unreasonably strict, and that it is ethical to assign patients at random as long as a subgroup within the expert medical community prefers each treatment.[77] According to this argument, when the treatment recommended depends primarily on which physician the patient happens to see, the medical community is in a state of "clinical equipoise," and random assignment does not violate a physician's fiduciary duties.

The concept of clinical equipoise fails, however, to resolve completely the conflict between the clinician and investigator roles. First, it assumes that because of uncertainty within the medical community regarding optimal treatment, patients will

be satisfied with having their therapy determined by a flip of the coin. Rather, patients generally expect physicians to integrate consensus views and available evidence with personal experience and "clinical judgment." Thus, even when equipoise obtains, trial participants may not receive some aspects of the personalized care that physicians typically render.

Second, just because equipoise may exist within the medical community, patients may not be indifferent about which treatment they receive.[78–81] Consider a trial evaluating chemotherapy with or without radiotherapy for low-stage Hodgkin disease. Even if oncologists are uncertain which treatment offers the best outcomes, patients or parents may have strong preferences based on such factors as short- and long-term sequelae.

Finally, clinical trials generally are designed to terminate when one treatment proves statistically superior to the other according to some predetermined threshold. Yet well before this threshold is reached, there will be a trend favoring the treatment that ultimately proves more successful. Neither patients nor physicians are permitted access to these data, in part because the information could affect willingness to enroll or continue in the trial and thereby jeopardize the chance that the study will reach a definitive conclusion. Withholding the data may be important for the successful conduct of research, but is difficult to justify from the perspective of the participant, who presumably would like all available information as part of the decision-making process.[82] Most randomized controlled trials (RCTs) have data monitoring committees and predefined stopping rules to address these tensions, but the

FOUR CATEGORIES OF PEDIATRIC RESEARCH, AS DEFINED IN U.S. FEDERAL REGULATIONS

Prospect for direct benefit	Maximum permissible risk	Criteria for approval by an IRB
No	Minimal risk	• Permission of parent or guardian • Assent of child, if capable

Yes	No maximum	• Risk justified by anticipated benefits to subjects
		• Relation of benefits to risks is at least as favorable as that presented by available alternatives
		• Permission of parent or guardian
		• Assent of child, unless
		  • child is incapable, *or*
		  • prospect for benefit is important to the health of the child and is available only in the context of the research

No	Minor increment over minimal risk	• Intervention or procedure presents experiences that are "reasonably commensurate with those inherent in [the subjects'] actual or expected medical, dental, psychological, social, or educational situations." • Study likely to yield knowledge that is of *vital importance about the subjects' condition* • Permission of *both* parents (if both are reasonably available) or of guardian • Assent of child, if capable
No	More than a minor increment over minimal risk	• Research presents a reasonable opportunity to further the understanding, prevention or alleviation of a serious problem affecting children • Research will be conducted in accordance with sound ethical principles • Permission of both parents (if both are reasonably available) or of guardian • Assent of child, if capable • Federal approval after consultation with an expert panel

Adapted from 45 CFR 46. Subpart D–Additional Protections for Children Involved as Subjects in Research. Federal Regist 1983 March 8; 48:9818.

optimum procedures and rules for early termination are ethically contested.[82-85] In sum, RCTs unavoidably highlight the tensions between rigorous science and the fiduciary duties of physicians to patients.

Some dissenters reject equipoise as the ethical basis for RCTs. Miller and Brody argue that equipoise mistakenly judges research according to criteria appropriate to individualized care.[44] In their view, equipoise need not obtain for a study to be ethical, so long as the trial is not exploitative when assessed according to criteria appropriate to research.[10]

Phase I Trials

Pediatric phase I trials seek to "define a safe and appropriate dose and schedule for new agents that can subsequently be used in phase II trials to test for activity against specific childhood malignancies."[86] They also provide preliminary information about toxicity and pharmacokinetics. They do not seek primarily to evaluate efficacy.

In a typical phase I trial, initial participants receive a low dose of a new agent that is unlikely to be either beneficial or toxic. Doses are increased in successive cohorts until an excessive number of participants experience dose-limiting toxicity (DLT). The dose level just below this threshold—the maximum tolerated dose (MTD)—is taken forward into phase II trials.

Phase I trials in pediatric oncology are necessary because MTDs for children and adults often differ.[87] Unless there are biological reasons to test an agent in a particular childhood cancer, pediatric trials typically begin only after the adult MTD is known. This policy reflects a desire to minimize the risks and maximize the benefits of phase I trials for children, but entails some delay in evaluating new agents for pediatric

cancer. The starting dose is generally just below the adult MTD, thereby minimizing the number of children who receive suboptimal doses.[86]

Phase I trials, especially in children, are ethically controversial.[54,88-99] Objections center on the low likelihood of direct benefit to participants in the face of what is perceived to be substantial risk, the fact that primary endpoints relate to safety rather than to efficacy, and the challenges of informed decision making for terminally ill patients or their parents. Agrawal and Emanuel recently reviewed the literature on phase I trials in an attempt to answer these objections.[88]

There is room for disagreement about how favorable or unfavorable the risk-benefit ratio of pediatric phase I trials is. Complete and partial response rates, which range from 6% to 8%,[100,101] are higher than those seen in adult trials.[102,103] However, responses are generally short lived, with a median duration in one study of 60 days.[100] Toxic deaths in pediatric trials are relatively uncommon, with 2.8% of participants dying from infection, hemorrhage or direct toxicity in one study and 1.4% dying from toxicity or aplasia in another.[100,101]

Given risks and benefits of these magnitudes, can IRBs approve pediatric oncology phase I trials under U.S. federal regulations? It seems clear that they involve more than a minor increment over minimal risk. Thus, to approve them, IRBs must determine that (a) they involve the prospect for direct benefit, (b) the risks are justified by the anticipated benefits to subjects, and (c) the relation of benefits to risks is at least as favorable as that presented by available alternatives (Table 46.3).[59] A crucial question is what the alternatives are for purposes of comparative risk-benefit assessment.[98] In our view, unless in a particular case an available alternative offers a more favorable balance of risks and benefits, well-designed phase I trials can meet federal criteria for approvable research.

Concerns about informed consent center on the potential desperation of patients or their parents, and on evidence suggesting that subjects overestimate benefits and misunderstand how design constraints intersect with therapeutic considerations.[54,94] Work by Daugherty and others suggests that participants generally enroll for reasons of personal benefit, and few understand that the primary objectives of phase I trials address toxicity and dose-finding rather than efficacy.[54,104] Even more concerning, many participants quantitatively overestimate the magnitude of expected benefit; in one adult study, respondents on average predicted a 65% likelihood that the phase I agent would "control their cancer."[96]

It is important to know whether misunderstandings among participants derive in part from inaccurate information provided by investigators. One study, involving audiotaping of consent conferences, suggested that most investigators clearly stated the novelty of the agent, the potential for risk, and the limited prospects for benefit.[105] A review of consent forms showed that most explained the research nature of the trial, the fact that it was designed to evaluate safety or appropriate dose, and the possibility of serious or life-threatening harms.[92] However, a minority clearly distinguished clinical from research procedures, and virtually all made unqualified references to the study agent as "therapy," thereby perhaps fostering therapeutic misconceptions.

Integrating these considerations, we conclude that phase I trials in pediatric oncology are ethically acceptable provided (a) no alternatives can be identified that offer a more favorable risk-benefit ratio, (b) there is scrupulous attention to the informed consent and permission process, and (c) children's wishes regarding enrollment are honored.[106] The latter requirement is particularly important in light of the difficulty that parents often have in "giving up the fight." Finally, the alternative of palliative care should be offered explicitly, and high-quality symptom care should be provided to all children who enroll.[95] Fortunately, despite the traditional belief that phase I trials and palliative care are mutually exclusive alternatives, there seems to be increasing recognition of the fact that they can peacefully coexist.

Laboratory Research Involving Biological Specimens

Historically, laboratory investigators who wished to conduct studies involving stored biological specimens faced few regulatory barriers. More recently, however, such research has generated substantial debate. This controversy, driven by worries about the power of genetic technologies and increased attention to privacy and confidentiality in health care, has raised concerns that the promise of such research will not fully be realized.[107–110]

Researchers who wish to conduct studies on *existing* specimens that were originally collected for clinical rather than research purposes must address two questions. First, is the study considered human subjects research, and therefore is it within IRBs' jurisdiction? And second, is it necessary to obtain participant's consent before including a specimen in a research project?

According to the Common Rule (the federal regulations governing clinical research), a living individual becomes a human subject when an investigator (a) obtains data through intervention or interaction with the person, or (b) obtains identifiable private information.[72] The regulations specifically exempt research involving existing data or specimens from IRB review "if the information is recorded by the investigator in such a manner that subjects cannot be identified, directly or through identifiers linked to the subjects."[72] Though the

Common Rule does not regulate research involving deceased persons, separate privacy regulations do apply.[111]

Given these definitions, investigators should engage their IRBs whenever they propose to conduct research involving human samples that are linked directly or through a code to the identity of the source. Even when the samples are currently identified but there are plans to de-identify them before proceeding with the research, investigators should discuss with their IRBs whether review is required. In many cases, studies will meet criteria for expedited review.[112]

Questions about consent are more complicated. There is a strong view that individuals should control what is done with their bodies and personal information, but inflexible consent requirements might unreasonably hinder research. Data on public attitudes vary.[113–115] For research that falls under IRB jurisdiction, the Common Rule permits consent waivers if four conditions are met: (a) the research involves no more than minimal risk; (b) the waiver will not adversely affect the rights and welfare of the subjects; (c) the research could not practicably be carried out without the waiver; and (d) whenever appropriate, subjects will be provided with additional pertinent information after participation.[72] Many research projects involving stored tissue will meet these criteria, particular if the study includes rigorous systems for protecting confidentiality.

Considerations differ when prospectively collecting research samples. There is an emerging consensus that patients or parents should be asked about their willingness to permit excess tissue to be saved.[107–110,116] From a practical point of view, this mandate requires systems for educating patients, obtaining their decision, and recording it in a way that can be linked to the specimen and data. Controversy surrounds the nature of the questions that should be asked.[107] At one extreme, patients might be asked simply whether or not they wish their samples to be available for research purposes in the future. At the other, they might be given a detailed list of options, including such questions as whether the tissue can be shared with commercial entities, whether it can be used for research on an unrestricted set of conditions or only for studies of particular diseases, whether germline genetic studies are permissible, and whether specimens must be anonymized.[107] A literature review suggested that most individuals are willing to provide one-time general consent for use of their tissue for future research studies.[117] Questions arise, however, as to whether such one-time general consent satisfies the Privacy Rule under the Health Insurance Portability and Accountability Act (HIPAA), because the Rule has been interpreted to require authorization for specified rather than open-ended research. Wendler has argued that such general consent is consistent with the Privacy Rule, so long as an IRB approves any subsequent research that was not covered by the original consent and, as part of that approval, grants the investigator who proposes the subsequent research a waiver of study-specific authorization for disclosure of Protected Health Information (PHI).[118]

Whole-genome Research

The last several years have seen an explosion of whole-genome research, especially genome-wide association studies (GWAS).[119] Even more powerful technologies, such as whole-genome sequencing, are on the horizon. Such approaches raise difficult policy questions.[120] For example, there is an increasing expectation that datasets, which often require substantial taxpayer funds, be made publicly available through archives such as the National Library of Medicine's database of Genotypes and Phenotypes (dbGaP, http://www.ncbi.nlm.nih.gov/sites/entrez?Db=gap), to maximize their value for discovery. The uniquely individual nature of DNA, however, suggests the risk that individuals may be reidentified from their DNA signatures, especially if a reference sample is available, and therefore that true de-identification of samples or data is impossible.[121,122] The issues of public release of whole-genome data and of re-identification suggest pressing challenges related to consent and confidentiality that the scientific community has yet to fully address. These questions are even more complicated in pediatrics, with some arguing against the release of children's specimens or genomic data from population-based banks until the children can legally give autonomous consent.[123] In addition, whole-genome research may identify genetic information of potential clinical significance to the research participant, raising the question of whether that information should be made available to participants. We address this subject in the following text.

Return of Aggregate and Individual Research Results

Research participants and families are increasingly recognized as partners who are owed an opportunity to learn the results of studies in which they took part. Participants, including parents of children with cancer and adolescent patients, desire access to research results.[124,125] Cancer clinicians and research ethics board chairs generally support the concept of returning study result to participants, and participants report high levels of satisfaction after receiving results.[126–128] However, some clinicians express concerns about adverse effects on participants, especially those who received inferior treatments or experienced poor outcomes.[129] In addition, questions about how best to implement this imperative, such as how to notify participants, how to maintain contact information, and how to cover the costs of notification, remain.[124,126]

In some studies involving genetics, the question of return of individual test results to participants arises.[130] Guidance regarding the return of individual test results varies, with some authors advocating a broad duty to offer results grounded in respect for the autonomy of participants.[131] The dominant view, however, endorses a duty to offer return of individual genetic test results only when certain criteria are met: (a) the test has established validity; (b) the excess risk for disease associated with a positive test is substantial; (c) the disease has important health implications; and (d) interventions to prevent or ameliorate the condition are available.[132,133] Although sparse, empirical data on participants' views support the practice of offering return of individual genetic test results when clinically informative.[125] When disclosure is planned, investigators should provide or refer for appropriate genetic counseling.[134]

Publication Ethics

Over 20 years ago, Simes demonstrated that positive trials are more likely to be published than negative trials; this "publication bias" makes new treatments appear more effective than they are.[135] A robust literature confirms the existence of this bias.[136–138] To counter this bias, Simes presciently called for prospective registration of clinical trials in a publicly accessible database. In the last five years, two important developments have turned this vision into a reality. First, the International Committee of Medical Journal Editors (ICMJE), which represents the editors of 11 major medical journals, has decided that its member journals will only publish clinical trials (with the exception of phase I and selected other trials, such as pharmacokinetic studies) that were registered in an approved public database prior to enrolling the first participant.[139] Second, the Food and Drug Amendments Act, enacted by Congress in 2007, requires that clinical trials (again, excepting phase I trials) be registered in the ClinicalTrials.gov database prior to inception, and also that selected trial results be made available

in the database.[140] As of January, 2009, more than 67,000 trials were registered on ClinicalTrials.gov.[140]

PRIVACY AND CONFIDENTIALITY

Confidentiality has always been central to medical care. The Hippocratic Oath has physicians pledge that "Whatsoever in the course of practice I see or hear . . . that ought never to be published abroad, I will not divulge, but consider such things to be holy secrets."[141] Concern about privacy and confidentiality is increasing, fueled by growth of electronic medical records and databases that allow easy exchange of patient information.[142] Another source of concern is the commercial sale of patient information. Similarly, suspicion of insurers and managed care companies has raised worries about how they use patient information. Finally, advances in genetics and the sense that genetic knowledge is a type of intimate personal knowledge with potential for discriminatory use have increased attention to privacy and confidentiality.

The traditional ethical standard of confidentiality is justified by many considerations. The first is intrinsic: respect for persons.[143] Confidentiality recognizes that privacy is essential to being a free, autonomous person; it is fundamental to human dignity and to the ability to form relationships.[144] A further instrumental reason applies: presumably, people will be less likely to seek medical attention and reveal important health-related information to health care providers unless information is kept confidential. The failure to reveal health-related information to clinicians can have significant consequences not just for an affected individual but, as with communicable diseases, for others.[144] Finally, confidentiality of health information is a widespread social expectation that defines norms of acceptable practice. Indeed, a "commitment to patient confidentiality" is essential to medical professionalism.[1]

Nevertheless, the right to confidentiality is not absolute.[144] There are a number of legitimate reasons why patients' expectations of confidentiality can or even must occasionally be breached.[143,145] Unfortunately, providing specific guidance about when confidentiality can be breached is difficult. Judgments depend upon the balancing of competing values that are subjectively defined and weighed by patients and clinicians. In general, confidentiality can be breached for three broad reasons: avoiding harm to others, benefiting the patient, and preserving public health for the benefit of others. For example, when Tatiana Tarasoff was murdered by Prosenjit Poddar, her parents took legal action against Poddar's psychiatrist. Poddar had disclosed his intention to commit the murder during counseling sessions, prompting the psychiatrist to alert police but not the victim herself. The courts determined that breaching patient confidentiality would have been appropriate because the patient presented a credible threat to the life of another person.[144,146] Further, some states mandate breaches of confidentiality by health providers in cases of child or elder abuse and neglect, justified by the belief that such disclosures ultimately will be for the patient's best interest. Public health laws also may require reporting a variety of information, ranging from communicable diseases to the provision of certain interventions.[143,145] Finally, it is important to recognize that the law may require disclosure of medical information for a variety of reasons unrelated to the actual provision of health care: as part of child custody cases, for reimbursement of health care services, as part of regulatory audits, and the like.[145]

In pediatrics, the question of the child's right to confidentiality from his or her parents arises. Withholding information from parents and guardians is justified mainly in those circumstances in which disclosures are thought to harm the child, when the child's agreement to treatment depends on an assurance of privacy, or when the child meets statutory criteria for emancipation (see the section on "Informed Consent"). Thus, many states permit the withholding of medical information from parents and guardians if the information is related to (a) sexual activity, pregnancy, or abortion; (b) treatment for alcohol or drug abuse; (c) psychiatric treatment; or (d) treatment for communicable diseases, especially sexually transmitted diseases. Obviously, these exceptions can apply only to adolescents and mature minors who are capable of making their own decisions. In such cases, physicians should assess the circumstances and, when appropriate, encourage adolescents to discuss these situations with their parents or guardians, providing support and counseling in the process.

In the United States, the most important recent change regarding confidentiality practices is related to the Privacy Rule under HIPAA.[111] HIPAA applies to protected health information (PHI), defined as "any information, whether oral or recorded in any form or medium, that . . . relates to the past, present, or future physical or mental health or condition of an individual, the provision of health care to an individual or the past, present, or future payment for the provision of health care to an individual" and that could reasonably be used to identify the individual.

The default position of HIPAA is that disclosure of PHI, including within the research setting, requires the patient's or guardian's written authorization.[143,147,148] This authorization must include a description of the information to be disclosed, to whom, for what purpose, and expiration date of use of the information. There are a few exceptions to this default, permitting release of information without the patient's authorization. First, HIPAA permits use of PHI without patient authorization for (a) provisions of care, such as obtaining a medical consultation; (b) billing; and (c) operations, such as quality monitoring or improvement. Second, data that have been de-identified, or stripped of the 18 individual identifiers specified in the Privacy Rule,[149] may be used without authorization. Third, data may be disclosed for legally authorized public health monitoring purposes.[150] There is also a role for professional judgment to inform physicians' decisions to disclose PHI for incidental disclosures, such as to family members who are closely involved with a patient's treatment, that are meant to optimize patient care.[151]

In the setting of clinical research, a Privacy Board or IRB can permit a waiver of patient authorization under some circumstances. Researchers can receive this waiver in order to do preparatory work for research or to work with data related to deceased patients. More important, a waiver can be requested when research with medical records cannot be conducted with de-identified information and yet it is impracticable to obtain each patient's authorization. In these cases, the researchers must have adequate plans to protect the patients' identifiers and destroy the identifiable information at the earliest possible time.[152] When applied to clinical research, HIPAA attempts to balance individual research subjects' autonomy and interest in privacy with society's interest in promoting ethical research.[153] However, a recent report from the Institute of Medicine[154] argues that the HIPAA Privacy Rule inadequately protects confidentiality of PHI in the research setting. Moreover, both the IOM report and empirical research surveying epidemiologists about their experiences with the Privacy Rule concluded that the Rule serves as a barrier to health research and likely inhibits medical advances.[155]

Critics, both those who think HIPAA too onerous and those who think it does not go far enough or has too many loopholes, agree that it is unnecessarily complex.[152,156,157] An

additional level of complexity arises because HIPAA provides minimum standards for confidentiality practices; states can exceed those standards when they see fit.[158] Thus, despite HIPAA, current legal standards of confidentiality still vary from state to state. Importantly, in the pediatric setting, state law controls parental access to minor children's medical information.

GENETIC TESTING

Increasingly, genetic tests are available to determine whether a person carries a mutation that might affect her developing cancer, response to therapy, or risk of toxicity with treatment. The availability of such tests has raised numerous questions: Who should be tested and under what circumstances? How should genetic information related to cancer predisposition or treatment be handled? How should further research on genetic causes of cancer be approached?

Genetic tests are perceived to differ from other diagnostic tests for several reasons.[159] First, they have implications for family members; a germline mutation in one member means that relatives could be affected. Second, because of incomplete penetrance, genetic tests usually entail information about risks and probabilities. This complicates deliberations about their implications for particular patients. Finally, although all genetic testing raises the issues of psychological risks, the effect may be particularly pronounced for children, because so many fundamental life choices—education, career, marriage, reproduction—have not yet been made.

Ethical considerations in performing a genetic test vary depending on whether the test will be performed in a clinical or research setting. In the clinical setting, genetic testing can be performed for several reasons: to screen a population for presence of genes that distinguish high-risk from average-risk individuals; to diagnose a cancer predisposition in an individual identified by personal or family history as potentially at increased risk; and to predict efficacy or side effects of therapeutic interventions. Currently, there are no situations in which population genetic screening for cancer risk is recommended.[160,161] More controversy surrounds the clinical use of genetic testing to determine an individual's cancer predisposition. The American Society of Clinical Oncology (ASCO) has recommended that predictive genetic testing should only occur if three criteria are fulfilled: (a) the individual's medical or family history suggests a genetic susceptibility to cancer; (b) the genetic test can be adequately interpreted; and (c) the results will aid in the medical or surgical management of the patient or family members.[162] Such management might include instituting a monitoring regimen for early detection, utilizing an effective prophylactic or treatment intervention, or influencing reproductive choices. For children, many commentators argue that genetic testing should occur only if cancer may develop during childhood or an effective preventive or treatment intervention (or occasionally reproductive choice) is available before the age of majority.[159,162] When testing would not result in clearly established medical benefits and the cancer will not develop during childhood, it is "advisable to defer testing until adulthood," at which time children can make their own decisions.[162,163]

Although indications for testing are satisfied for adults in some circumstances, such as BRCA1 and 2, there is disagreement about which cases fulfill them in childhood. Multiple endocrine neoplasia type IIb, which may be diagnosed by testing for a *RET* gene mutation and for which thyroidectomy is an effective prophylactic intervention, is perhaps the clearest example of a syndrome for which testing is indicated.[164] Conversely, a prototypically difficult case is the child whose family history is consistent with Li-Fraumeni syndrome.[165] This condition is associated with onset of malignancy during childhood, but whether or not screening improves outcomes is unclear. According to ASCO's guidelines, testing of such children may be permissible at the parents' insistence, but clinicians should first ensure that parents understand the strong reasons to consider deferring testing until the child reaches adulthood.[162]

In offering genetic testing in the clinical setting, great emphasis has been placed on ensuring informed consent.[159,160,166] Because genetic testing is rarely urgent, the consent process can occur over several meetings that include introduction of information, discussion of the implications of the test results, and appropriate pre-test counseling.

The ability to identify individuals' genetic predispositions to illness has generated great concern about the possibility of discrimination on the basis of genetic risk. The Genetic Information Nondiscrimination Act, which was recently signed into U.S. law, provides protection against genetic discrimination in health insurance and employment, but not in other areas of insurance such as life, disability and long-term care insurance.[167]

Issues related to genetic testing in the research setting, including informed consent and the challenge of return of individual-level genetic research results and incidental findings, are discussed in the section on "Human Subjects Research."

ETHICAL ISSUES AT THE END OF LIFE

Clarifying the Goals of Care

Developing an ethically sound approach to end-of-life care depends on achieving clarity on the goals of care. Clinicians, patients, and family members must communicate to become mutually aligned in their understanding of these goals. Decisions about such topics as life-sustaining therapies or the ethical use of sedatives and analgesia, all discussed in the following text are greatly complicated by disagreement or lack of clarity surrounding the overall goals of care.

All too often, clinicians, families, and children must face the realization that cure is no longer a realistic possibility, and that goals must shift toward providing the best care possible through the dying process. Such discussions demand the highest levels of honesty, integrity, and professionalism.[1,168] Studies exploring this transition have found that a more prompt recognition by parents that their child was dying or had no realistic chance for cure is associated with earlier introduction of elements of palliative care, including hospice or quality home care services, into the child's treatment.[169,170] Additionally, better communication between providers and families that cure is no longer a realistic possibility allows for comfort to become the primary treatment goal.[169]

Studies and guidelines have argued that palliative care can be integrated throughout the care of patients at the end of life.[171-175] Patients and families need not relinquish hope for cure in order to benefit from an emphasis on symptom management and prevention of suffering.[173,176,177] Recent data indicate that pediatric oncologists are increasing their incorporation of palliative care in the setting of pediatric cancer.

Decision Making About Life-Sustaining Treatments

Over the past several decades, medicine has seen dramatic advances in its ability to sustain life. As a consequence, there has been a corresponding increase in the need for active decisions about withholding or withdrawing life-sustaining treatment. Most adults and children who die in an ICU do so following the decision to withhold or withdraw life-sustaining treatments.[176,178,179]

Recommendations for ethical decision making regarding limitations of life-sustaining treatments, as well as the appropriate care of patients once a decision has been made, were put forth as early as 1983 by the President's Commission for the Study of Ethical Problems in Medicine and Biomedical and Behavioral Research.[180] Consensus guidelines and recommendations for clinicians on decision making for dying patients have also been put forth by the American Academy of Pediatrics and other organizations.[174,175,181-184]

When approaching decisions about life-sustaining therapies, parents of dying children prioritize quality of life, likelihood of improvement, and freedom from pain.[185] Physicians also consider patient preferences about life support and prognostic factors, such as the likelihood of survival and the likely functional outcome.[186] In addition, decisions about life-sustaining treatment are now commonly approached from a patient- and family-centered perspective with new emphasis on communication, surrogate satisfaction, and shared choices.[176,187,188] What are the ethical principles and historical precedents that should guide decisions about the withholding or withdrawal of life-sustaining treatments?

Paradigm Cases Regarding the Provision of Life-Sustaining Therapies

I. The "Baby Doe" Regulations

Perhaps the most controversial and misunderstood framework for decision making about life-sustaining treatments in pediatrics is the so-called "Baby Doe" regulations.[189,190] Baby Doe was an infant with Down syndrome and tracheoesophageal fistula born in Bloomington, Indiana in 1982. He died after his parents declined corrective surgery on the grounds that he would never achieve a "minimally acceptable quality of life." The case generated public controversy, and the federal Department of Health and Human Services subsequently promulgated regulations designed to prevent parents or health care providers from withholding care from handicapped infants. Following a number of appeals, the final Baby Doe regulation was passed by Congress as the 1984 Amendments to the Child Abuse Prevention and Treatment Act. This legislation required all states to create a regulatory system to investigate cases where medically indicated treatment is withheld from handicapped infants, or risk losing federal funding for children's services. According to stipulations in the final legislation:

> The term "withholding of medically indicated treatment" means the failure to respond to the infant's life threatening conditions by providing treatment (including appropriate nutrition, hydration, and medication) which, in the treating physician's reasonable medical judgment, will be most likely to be effective in ameliorating or correcting all such conditions, except that the term does not include the failure to provide treatment (other than appropriate nutrition, hydration, or medication) to an infant when, in the

treating physician's reasonable medical judgment any of the following circumstances apply:

A. The infant is chronically and irreversibly comatose;
B. The provision of such treatment would merely prolong dying, not be effective in ameliorating or correcting all of the infant's life-threatening conditions, or otherwise be futile in terms of survival of the infant; or
C. The provision of such treatment would be virtually futile in terms of survival of the infant and the treatment itself under such circumstances would be inhumane.

Many argue that the Baby Doe regulations are not helpful in decision making for infants because of ambiguity surrounding the term "appropriate." This framework is not recommended for ethical decision-making at the end of life in pediatrics.[191]

II. Medical Futility and Baby K

Another controversial concept encountered in end-of-life decision making is futility. Conflicts can arise between physicians, parents, and (sometimes) patients about whether life-sustaining therapies should be initiated or continued. Typically these disagreements can be resolved through ongoing discussions. In some situations, however, dialogue leads not to agreement but to intractable conflict over whether a life-sustaining treatment is "futile." The concept of futility has been debated in the medical literature for decades, as clinicians have struggled with requests from caregivers to provide treatments with uncertain benefits. Scholarly exploration of futility initially focused on defining the term.[192] This process involved identifying either severe clinical conditions or dire prognostic criteria that would indicate that further treatment should not be pursued.[193] One widely cited definition proposed that "when physicians conclude (either through personal experience, experiences shared with colleagues, or consideration of published empiric data) that in the last 100 cases a medical treatment has been useless, they should regard that treatment as futile."[194] However, these attempts to define futility in this way have been problematic as they typically hinged on arbitrary distinctions that lacked an empirical basis, expert consensus, or societal endorsement.[193,195] Medical experts and patients may differ over the value of a treatment. Although some may value preserving life at all costs, others may conclude that when the quality of life is poor, death is the preferred outcome. The definitional approach falsely casts futility in an objective light, whereas in reality, controversy around futility often centers on subjective values that will not be resolved by scientific means. For example, must an oncologist provide aggressive cancer-directed therapy to a patient without a realistic chance for cure because the patient's parents feel it to be justified? Similarly, must intensive life-sustaining interventions be continued for a critically ill child when there is agreement among clinicians that recovery is no longer possible? How low must the likelihood of benefit be to substantiate an oncologist's refusal to provide such therapy?

Consider, for example, one of the most publicized pediatric cases of intractable conflict between parents and physicians.[196] Baby K was an infant born with anencephaly in Virginia in the early 1990s. Her mother demanded that physicians provide mechanical ventilation during multiple hospitalizations for aspiration pneumonia. The clinicians refused, stating that mechanical ventilation could not reverse the anencephalic infant's malformation and therefore was not indicated. Her mother responded by saying that she understood the medical facts about anencephaly and the natural history of the malformation, "but the value of this kind of life is God's secret."

That is, there was no disagreement about the facts of the case, but these "medical facts" were valued differently. In such a situation, whose values predominate? Can patients or their surrogates demand care that clinicians believe violates their professional conscience? In the case of Baby K, a Federal Appeals Court sided with the child's mother, ruling that the hospital was legally required to provide care to any patient seeking emergency treatment.[197] The court did not, however, address the merits of the futility argument, thereby leaving open the question of how futility should be defined and whether and how personal values become relevant.

Despite the failure of efforts to define futility, medicine has an obligation to provide wise stewardship over scarce medical resources, to articulate situations where the use of such resources is inadvisable, to consider the interests of clinicians who are asked to administer treatments they believe are unreasonably burdensome in light of their limited benefits, and to develop an approach to disputes over futility. In 1999, the American Medical Association stated that, "since definitions of futile care are value laden, universal consensus on futile care is unlikely to be achieved. Rather, the American Medical Association Council on Ethical and Judicial Affairs recommends a process-based approach to futility determinations."[198]

Such statements led hospitals and professional groups to develop procedures for resolving disagreements about futility.[193,199] The Society of Critical Care Medicine (SCCM) stated:

> Policies to limit inadvisable treatment should have the following characteristics: (a) be disclosed in the public record; (b) reflect moral values acceptable to the community; (c) not be based exclusively on prognostic scoring systems; (d) articulate appellate mechanisms; and (e) be recognized by the courts.[200]

Over the past several years, a consensus has emerged around principles like these that emphasize a fair process for deciding about futile and otherwise inappropriate care. Several states, including Texas, have incorporated this approach into legislation. Legislation of this type gives the recommendations of the hospital ethics committee the force of law, thereby enforcing the view of clinicians who believe treatments to be futile.[193]

Guidelines for Decision Making

The framework put forward in 1983 by the President's Commission is frequently cited as a useful construct for decisions at the end of life.[180] The Commission proposed five considerations for determining a child's best interests in these situations: (a) the amount of suffering, and the potential for relief; (b) the severity of dysfunction and the potential for restoration of function; (c) the expected duration of life; (d) the potential for personal satisfaction and enjoyment of life; and (e) the possibility of developing the capacity for self-determination. The Commission then advocated applying these criteria to proposed treatments for children based on three assessments of the proposed treatment plan: clearly beneficial, ambiguous or uncertain, and clearly not beneficial. The Commission further stated that if the proposed treatment is either ambiguous/uncertain or clearly not beneficial, and the parents prefer to forgo treatment, then the clinicians should withdraw life-sustaining therapy.

Moral Accountability for End-of-Life Decisions and Actions

Although some clinicians believe that distinctions such as "ordinary versus extraordinary" or "withholding versus withdrawing" are helpful in guiding end-of-life decision making, most view these distinctions as confusing rather than clarifying actions. Consider the ordinary versus extraordinary distinction. One interpretation would be that ordinary treatments are obligatory, whereas extraordinary treatments are not. A simple appeal to what is customary, however, cannot suffice as a justification for what is morally required. Similarly misleading is the distinction between withholding and withdrawing treatments. Is there a moral difference between deciding not to intubate a patient because we think that the patient will not benefit from mechanical ventilation, and extubating a patient who has not improved despite a period of mechanical ventilation? In the landmark Cruzan case, the U.S. Supreme Court stated that there is no legal difference between the two actions.[201,202] In addition, there is a broad ethical consensus that such a distinction is not morally relevant. Although one understandably feels more responsible for the outcome when it results from the withdrawal rather than the withholding of a therapy, there is no fundamental logical difference between the two decisions.

Sedatives and Analgesics in the Care of the Dying

There is some evidence that symptom management for children at the end of life may be improving. In 2000, Wolfe et al. found that 89% of 103 parents whose children died of cancer in a hospital setting reported that their child experienced "a lot" or "a great deal" of suffering from at least one symptom in their last month of life.[203] Of children treated for specific symptoms, treatment was successful, by parents' assessments, in a minority of those with pain or dyspnea. More recently, the authors published a follow-up cohort study in which reports of "a great deal" or "a lot" of suffering decreased for many symptoms, including pain and dyspnea.[204]

The bioethics community as well as the U.S. Supreme Court have supported and protected physicians' abilities to treat the pain and suffering of terminally ill patients, even when such treatment may hasten the patient's death. The ethical principle relevant to this question is the Doctrine of Double Effect, originally developed by Catholic theologians but subsequently accepted broadly by other religious traditions, law, and philosophy.[205] The doctrine states that when an action has two effects, of which one is inherently good and the other inherently bad, it can be justified if certain conditions are met:

1. The action in itself is, be good or at least morally indifferent.
2. The clinician must intend only the good effect and not the evil effect. The evil effect is foreseen, not intended. For example, when administering morphine to a terminally ill patient, the physician must intend only the relief of the patient's suffering. The risk of an earlier death may be foreseeable, but it is not the clinician's objective.
3. The evil effect cannot be a means to the good effect. For example, the physician may not administer potassium chloride instead of morphine. By administering potassium chloride, the evil effect (death) becomes the means to the good effect (relief from suffering). In contrast, morphine does not depend on the side effect of death to relieve pain.
4. The good intended must outweigh the evil permitted. In the case of morphine administration to a suffering patient who is imminently dying, the benefit of pain relief clearly outweighs the risk of death. This would not be true if the patient were not imminently dying.

Whether double-effect reasoning is an appropriate guide to the use of sedation and analgesia in end-of-life care is controversial. For example, what is the difference between practice by the doctrine of double effect and the performance of euthanasia? The key difference lies in the intention of the physician. Although another's intentions and motives cannot be validated with certainty, if the physician's intention is to treat the patient's pain and suffering, the administration of analgesics and sedatives is ethically permitted under the doctrine of double effect. When the physician's intention is to kill the patient, then the line between accepted practice and euthanasia has been crossed. Critics of the doctrine argue that it relies on an overly simplistic notion of intent that is impossible to verify externally. These critics believe that the only morally relevant consideration is the patient's informed consent, not the clinician's intentions.[206]

Other critics claim that strict adherence to the doctrine of double effect may paradoxically constrain some clinicians from providing adequate relief of suffering because they fear violating the absolute prohibition against intentionally causing death. In addition, empirical evidence suggests that the use of opioids and sedatives to relieve symptoms at the end of life in no way shortens life, obviating the need for the doctrine of double-effect as an ethical justification.[207-209] In the final analysis, however, double-effect reasoning provides a defensible rationale for assuring the comfort of the patient among practitioners who support neither euthanasia at one extreme, nor the practice of allowing patients to die with untreated suffering on the other.

How much analgesia or sedation for a terminally ill child is too much? There is no arbitrary amount of narcotic that is necessarily excessive in any given case.[210] According to the American Academy of Pediatrics, "On occasion, the relief of severe, progressive symptoms such as pain or dyspnea may require rapid escalation in the doses of administered analgesics and sedatives."[172] Regardless of the doses required to effectively treat pain and suffering, it is essential to document thoroughly the signs and symptoms of suffering that patients report or clinicians observe, and the rationale behind the regimen chosen to treat these symptoms.

In rare circumstances, children must be sedated to unconsciousness in order to relieve suffering.[211-213] This practice has been termed "terminal" or—preferably—"palliative" sedation, and should be employed only as a last resort.[214] Typically barbiturates or benzodiazepines are used as sedatives, although propofol has also been employed. Once unconscious, patients typically die after several days from dehydration or another complication of treatment.

Some have argued that terminal sedation is a covert form of euthanasia. Once the patient is unconscious, no attempt is typically made to restore him to consciousness, and medical nutrition and hydration are terminated. Others have defended terminal sedation under the rule of double effect.[215] In addition, the U.S. Supreme Court implicitly endorsed the practice in two decisions concerning physician-assisted suicide (PAS), citing the technique as an alternative to PAS that could assure, at least theoretically, that no patient should die with "untreatable" pain.[216,217]

Withholding or Withdrawal of Medical Nutrition and Hydration

A consensus in bioethics holds that the withholding or withdrawal of medical nutrition and hydration should be justified by a burdens/benefits assessment of that therapy for that patient, just as it is for decisions to withhold or withdraw mechanical ventilation and other forms of life-sustaining treatment.[218,219] For many, however, withholding something so basic to human existence diminishes patients' dignity and caregivers' humanity, and is tantamount to abandonment. Despite these concerns, courts have ruled that medically administered nutrition and hydration are medical interventions that may be discontinued on the same grounds as any other treatment. This position holds that there is no logically valid distinction between the withholding or withdrawal of a tube from the trachea that provides life-sustaining treatment and the withholding or withdrawal of a tube from the intestine that provides life-sustaining treatment. In the Cruzan case, the U.S. Supreme Court ruled that artificial hydration and nutrition are considered medical therapies, which patients, or their surrogates speaking for them, have a constitutional right to refuse.[220] Concurring with the majority ruling, Justice Sandra Day O'Connor concluded, "Artificial feeding cannot readily be distinguished from other forms of medical treatment . . . Accordingly, the liberty guaranteed by the Due Process Clause must protect, if it protects anything, an individual's deeply personal decision to reject medical treatment, including the artificial delivery of food and water."

FINANCIAL INCENTIVES AND CONFLICT OF INTEREST

A conflict of interest (COI) exists when a professional judgment regarding a primary interest risks being unduly influenced by a secondary interest.[221] COIs can arise when individuals simultaneously play several roles, and therefore serve several interests. A physician's primary interest is the patient's health, welfare, and dignity. An investigator's primary interest includes contributing to new knowledge. Secondary interests, which might include advancing one's reputation or supporting one's family, are not intrinsically bad, but must not compromise primary interests.[42] Although there are many types of secondary interests, we focus on financial interests, including benefits that accrue to a physician or to a health care institution. We emphasize financial interests not because they are necessarily the most prevalent or problematic type of secondary interest, but because they are the most optional, the easiest to identify and regulate, and have the highest profile with the lay public and government.

Translating basic science insights into new therapies is the major goal of physician-investigators, academic health centers, and the taxpayer funds that support them. Bringing these benefits to patients requires private sector involvement.[222] Technology transfer fosters increasingly close relationships between industry and universities, health care systems, physicians and investigators; these fruitful relationships facilitate advances that no single partner can achieve alone. Although they have been likened to "dancing with the porcupine,"[223] relationships with industry are here to stay; the challenge is how to manage them in a way that preserves the priority of patients', research participants', and the public's interests.

Types of Financial Interests

Financial interests arise in both the clinical and the research setting. In clinical settings, physicians might benefit financially from referring patients to entities, such as radiology or physical therapy facilities, in which they have an interest.[224,225] Alternately, they might receive gifts from industry or derive income from service on speakers bureaus. Even more fundamentally, fee-for-service medicine creates incentives to provide more billable care, whereas in capitated systems, incentives favor reducing expensive care. In both instances, the best interests of the patient may be compromised. In the research context, investigators might have consulting income, royalties from the licensing of intellectual property, equity in a company that stands to benefit or lose from study results, or simply an interest in preserving funding for their research.

Although individual physicians' or investigators' financial relationships have received most notice, academic medical centers' and universities' institutional relationships are under increasing scrutiny. These relationships include philanthropic support, funding for research or continuing medical education, licensing of intellectual property, and equity interests. The Association of American Medical Colleges (AAMC) and a group of academic leaders have recently published recommendations for eliminating, minimizing, or managing these institutional relationships.[226,227] It is important to recognize that the financial ties of leaders such as hospital presidents, deans, and department chairs constitute institutional as well as individual COIs.[228]

Prevalence of Financial Ties

Limited data are available regarding the prevalence of financial ties among practicing physicians; none specifically address pediatric oncology. A survey of members of the American College of Physicians-American Society of Internal Medicine in Maryland found that 22% participated in industry-sponsored clinical trials and 27% gave industry-sponsored lectures.[229] Participation in industry-sponsored activities was positively associated with subspecialty practice, group or academic practice setting, and dissatisfaction with income.

Policy initiatives have encouraged academic-industry collaborations to bring better treatments to patients. The Bayh-Dole Act of 1980 affirmed that ownership and control of patents derived from federally funded research belonged to the performing institution, and insulated the process of commercial development from political interference.[230] Later amendments allowed nonprofit organizations to offer exclusive licenses, providing incentives for investment in university technology, and required institutions to share proceeds with inventors. As a result, investigators may be better able to bring new diagnostics and therapies to patients, but they also now have significant financial stakes in the commercialization of intellectual property.[231,232]

A number of studies have documented a high prevalence of financial ties to industry among investigators both generally and in cancer medicine. One systematic review suggested that, on average, about 25% of investigators across all fields of medicine have relationships with industry.[233] More recent studies in oncology confirm this general estimate, and indicate that consulting relationships, honoraria, and research funding are the most prevalent financial ties.[234-237] Little is known about academic-industry relationships in pediatric oncology specifically. Although the orphan status of childhood cancer has likely limited such relationships, policy initiatives that create incentives for manufacturers to study drugs and devices in children are likely to increase the number and intensity of these ties.[238]

Impact of Financial Interests and of Relationships with Industry

Evidence suggests that physicians' and trainees' relationships with industry influence patient care.[239] Ownership interests in free-standing radiology facilities or physical therapy practices are associated with increased referrals, higher costs, and indicators of inferior quality.[224,225] Such self-referral is now prohibited by the "Stark II" amendments to the Omnibus Budget Reconciliation Act of 1993.[234] Contact with industry representatives during residency affects physicians' attitudes and behaviors after completion of training.[235] Attendance at industry-sponsored symposia is associated with increased prescribing of the sponsor's product, and requests for formulary additions are associated with industry contacts.[236,237] More broadly, social science research compellingly demonstrates how even small gifts can bias individuals' attitudes and behaviors; there is no support for the argument that physicians are immune to such bias.[240]

In the research setting, data suggest that financial ties are associated with conclusions favorable to industry. A systematic review from 2003 found that industry sponsorship was associated with pro-industry conclusions, with a pooled odds ratio of 3.6 (95% CI, 2.6–4.9).[233] Meta-analyses limited to cancer trials generally confirm this finding.[241–243] The reasons for this association are not well understood, although several hypotheses stand out. First, industry-sponsored trials are more likely than other trials to use inactive (including placebo) controls rather than active comparators, which may predispose studies to favor the investigational agent.[242] Second, one study suggests a greater disjunction between quantitative results and authors' conclusions or recommendations in industry-funded trials than in other settings.[244] Less is known about the relationship between authors' personal financial ties and study outcomes, although one study in psychiatry suggests a positive association.[245]

Commercial support has also been associated with decreased openness in science. Studies reviewed by Bekelman demonstrated a consistent relationship between industry sponsorship or involvement in startups and restrictions on or delay of publication, withholding of data, and refusal to share research materials.[233]

Third, there is a great deal of concern about the possibility that financial ties may put research participants at risk. Despite anecdotal examples such as Jesse Gelsinger's death in a gene transfer trial in 1999,[246] however, we are unaware of systematic data that address whether source of funding or investigators' financial ties to industry are associated with increased risks to subjects.

Finally, poor handling of financial relationships with industry risks compromising public trust in physicians, investigators, and academic medical institutions. Legislative and regulatory initiatives in response to allegations of research misconduct or undisclosed financial relationships are likely to increase scrutiny and transparency of such ties in the coming years.[247,248]

Approaches to the Challenge of Conflicts of Interest

Recognition, disclosure, and appropriate management of COIs are essential to the maintenance of public trust and professional integrity. Factors that influence how a conflict is managed include: (a) the importance of the secondary interest to physicians or investigators; (b) the degree of the physician's or investigator's discretion and accountability in exercising judgment; (c) the risks to patients, research subjects, the medical profession, or scientific investigation if conflicts exert undue influence; and (d) the financial magnitude of the interests.

The AAMC provided a template for addressing financial COIs in research in a 2001 report.[249] The report identified several core components of an institutional mechanism for overseeing financial COIs, including naming a responsible official and standing committee, specifying a process for gathering information about COIs and making that information available to decision makers including the IRB, and putting in place a written policy on financial interests in research. Substantive elements of the policy should include: a rebuttable presumption that individuals with significant financial interests may not conduct human subjects research; a process for deciding when compelling circumstances justify rebutting this presumption; procedures for monitoring research involving financially interested individuals; a requirement for disclosure of significant financial interests to stakeholders; a prohibition of payments conditioned on results; a statement of investigator accountability for the integrity of any study publication or communication that bears his or her name; and affirmation of the investigator's right to receive, analyze, and interpret study data and to publish results.

Consistent with the AAMC report, most COI policies outline three principal strategies for responding to financial COIs. The first is *disclosure*. Investigators might be required to inform interested individuals of their financial ties. Such individuals might include journal editors and readers, meeting organizers and attendees, sponsors, and research participants. For example, the ICMJE states that "when authors submit a manuscript, whether an article or a letter, they are responsible for disclosing all financial and personal relationships that might bias their work."[250] Though essential to transparency, disclosure is problematic as the sole response to financial ties because it is not clear how recipients of disclosure should use that information. Evidence from randomized trials of disclosure suggests that, rightly or wrongly, journal readers are more skeptical of and less interested in articles that disclose financial ties than they are in the same articles without the financial disclosures.[251,252] Data on attitudes of research participants to disclosure of investigators' financial ties are more mixed. Although such disclosures are unlikely to affect many individuals' decisions about participation, a substantial minority of participants favor disclosure and at least some are troubled by knowledge of investigators' financial ties.[253–255]

In response to revelations of undisclosed COIs, several states have enacted laws requiring pharmaceutical companies to disclose payments to physicians.[256,257] Increasing Congressional interest has led to the introduction of a proposed federal law, the Physician Payments Sunshine Act of 2009.[247]

A second strategy for responding to financial COIs is *management*. For example, an independent reviewer may be appointed to oversee the physician or investigator as she fulfills her primary interest, thereby limiting the impact of a secondary interest without totally eliminating it. Such oversight invokes additional mechanisms of accountability to supplement those ordinarily in place for unconflicted relationships and activities. U.S. Public Health Service regulations require grantee institutions to identify and manage investigators' significant financial interests relevant to the research (defined as equity or income of over $10,000), but do not specify the precise manner in which they must be managed.[258]

The third strategy is *prohibition* or *divestiture*. For example, the American Society of Clinical Oncology's (ASCO's) COI policy states that "the role of the principal investigator [PI] . . . is so pivotal that further restrictions should apply in appropriate cases in order to promote public confidence in the clinical trial process."[259] As a result, during a trial, PIs of non-NIH sponsored studies may not hold a secondary financial interest that could affect the research. Prohibited interests including equity, royalties or licensing fees, patents, leadership positions, sponsor-paid travel unrelated to the trial, research payments substantially exceeding costs, or honoraria, or gifts from the sponsor. Absent special permission, trials whose PIs have prohibited interests may not be published in ASCO journals or presented at ASCO meetings. Rigorous elimination of conflicts has had a particularly powerful impact within the U.S. Department of Health and Human Services, including the National Institutes of Health and the Food and Drug Administration.[260]

CONCLUSION

COIs are a prevalent feature of medical practice and of clinical research. Failure of the profession to develop appropriate mechanisms for recognizing and managing these conflicts has materially injured the image of the medical profession and of biomedical science, with resultant legal and regulatory responses. COIs are likely to increase, given the overlap of patient care and research, the involvement of industry in providing patients with access to new technology, the powerful and conflicting pressures of the health care industry, and incentives related to the economic interests of third parties. Although such conflicts cannot be eliminated, they must be carefully managed to preserve patients', research participants', and the public's trust in health care and in the biomedical research enterprise.

References

1. ABIM Foundation; American Board of Internal Medicine; ACP-ASIM Foundation; American College of Physicians-American Society of Internal Medicine; European Federation of Internal Medicine. Medical professionalism in the new millennium: a physician charter. Ann Intern Med 2002;136:243–246.
2. Stern DT, Papadakis M. The developing physician–becoming a professional. N Engl J Med 2006;355:1794–1799.
3. Curran CE. Bioethics: an overview. In: Levin DL, Morriss FC, eds. Essentials of pediatric intensive care. New York, NY: Churchill Livingstone, 1997:1063–1068.
4. Hurwitz B, Richardson R. Swearing to care: the resurgence in medical oaths. BMJ 1997;315:1671–1674.
5. Berg JW, Appelbaum PS, Lidz CW, et al. Informed consent: legal theory and clinical Practice. 2nd ed. Oxford: Oxford University Press, 2001.
6. *Canterbury v. Spence.* 464 F.2d 772 (D.C. Cir. 1972).
7. *Natanson v. Kline.* 186 Kan. 393, 350 P.2d 1093, opinion on denial of motion for rehearing, 187 Kan. 186, 354 P.2d 670 (1960).
8. *Salgo v. Leland Stanford Jr. Board of Trustees.* 317 P.2d 170 (Cal Ct. App. 1957).
9. Seidelman WE. The path to Nuremberg in the pages of JAMA, 1933–1939. JAMA 1996;276:1693–1696.
10. Emanuel EJ, Wendler D, Grady C. What makes clinical research ethical? JAMA 2000;283:2701–2711.
11. Advisory Committee on Human Radiation Experiments. The Human Radiation Experiments. New York, NY: Oxford University Press, USA, 1996.
12. *Schloendorff v. Society* of New York Hospitals. 211 N.Y. 125 (1914).
13. Meisel A, Roth L, Lidz C. Toward a model of the legal doctrine of informed consent. Am J Psychiatry 1977;134:285–289.
14. Appelbaum P, Grisso T. Assessing patients' capacities to consent to treatment. N Engl J Med 1988;319:1635–1638.
15. Drane J. The many faces of competency. Hastings Cent Rep 1985;15:17–21.
16. Faden RR, Beauchamp TL. A history and theory of informed consent. New York, NY: Oxford University Press, 1986.
17. Tversky A, Kahneman D. The framing of decisions and the psychology of choice. Science 1981;211:453–458.
18. Emanuel EJ, Emanuel LL. Four models of the physician-patient relationship. JAMA 1992;267:2221–2226.
19. Wertheimer A. Coercion. Princeton, NJ: Princeton University Press, 1987.
20. Shalowitz DI, Garrett-Mayer E, Wendler D. The accuracy of surrogate decision makers – a systematic review. Arch Intern Med 2006;166:493–497.
21. Ditto PH, Danks JH, Smucker WD, et al. Advance Directives as Acts of Communication: a Randomized Controlled Trial. Arch Intern Med 2001;161:421–430.
22. La Puma J, Orentlicher D, Moss RJ. Advance directives on admission Clinical Implications and analysis of the Patient Self-Determination Act of 1990. JAMA 1991;266:402–405.
23. Omnibus Reconciliation Act 1990. In: Title IV Section 4206. USA; 1990:Congressional Record, October 26, 1990;12638.
24. Dresser R. Standards for family decisions: replacing best interests with harm prevention. Am J Bioeth 2003;3:54–55.
25. Committee on Bioethics of the American Academy of Pediatrics. Informed consent, parental permission, and assent in pediatric practice. Pediatrics 1995;95:314–317.
26. Holder AR. Minors' rights to consent to medical care. JAMA 1987;257:3400–3402.
27. Santelli J. Human subjects protection and parental permission in adolescent health research. J Adolesc Health 1997;21:384–387.
28. Sigman G, Silber TJ, English A, et al. Confidential health care for adolescents: position paper of the Society for Adolescent Medicine. J Adolesc Health 1997;21:408–415.
29. Ellement J. Ruling clarifies minors' rights; court gives weight to medical wishes. Boston Globe February 17, 1999:Sect. B1.
30. Oken D. What to tell cancer patients: a study of medical attitudes. JAMA 1961;175:1120–1128.
31. Evans AE, Edin S. If a child must die. N Engl J Med 1968;278:138–142.
32. Fernandez C, Stutzer C, MacWilliam L, et al. Alternative and complementary therapy use in pediatric oncology patients in British Columbia: prevalence and reasons for use and nonuse. J Clin Oncol 1998;16:1279–1286.
33. Eisenberg DM, Davis RB, Ettner SL, et al. Trends in alternative medicine use in the United States, 1990–1997: results of a follow-up national survey. JAMA 1998;280: 1569–1575.
34. Fadiman A. The spirit catches you and you fall down. New York, NY: Farrar, Straus and Giroux, 1998.
35. Brock DW, Wartman SA. When competent patients make irrational choices. N Engl J Med 1990;322:1595–1599.
36. Bleyer WA. The U.S. pediatric cancer clinical trials programmes: international implications and the way forward. Eur J Cancer 1997;33:1439–1447.
37. Tejeda HA, Green SB, Trimble EL, et al. Representation of African-Americans, Hispanics, and whites in National Cancer Institute cancer treatment trials. J Natl Cancer Inst 1996;88:812–816.
38. National Commission for the Protection of Human Subjects of Biomedical and Behavioral Research. The Belmont Report: Ethical principles and guidelines for the protection of human subjects of biomedical and behavioral research. Washington, DC: U.S. Government Printing Office, 1979.
39. Joffe S, Weeks JC. Views of American oncologists about the purposes of clinical trials. J Natl Cancer Inst 2002;94:1847–1853.
40. World Medical Association Declaration of Helsinki. Recommendations guiding physicians in biomedical research involving human subjects. JAMA 1997;277: 925–926.
41. Levine RJ. Ethics and regulation of clinical research. 2nd ed. New Haven: Yale University Press, 1986.
42. Miller FG, Rosenstein DL, DeRenzo EG. Professional integrity in clinical research. JAMA 1998;280:1449–1454.
43. Brody H, Miller FG. The clinician-investigator: unavoidable but manageable tension. Kennedy Inst Ethics J 2003;13:329–346.
44. Miller FG, Brody H. A critique of clinical equipoise. Therapeutic misconception in the ethics of clinical trials. Hastings Cent Rep 2003;33:19–28.
45. Fried C. Medical experimentation: personal integrity and social policy. New York, NY: American Elsevier Publishing Co., Inc., 1974.
46. Hellman S, Hellman DS. Of mice but not men. Problems of the randomized clinical trial. N Engl J Med 1991;324:1585–1589.
47. Marquis D. Leaving therapy to chance. Hastings Cent Rep 1983;13:40–47.
48. Miller FG, Rosenstein DL. The therapeutic orientation to clinical trials. N Engl J Med 2003;348:1383–1386.
49. Joffe S, Miller FG. Bench to bedside: mapping the moral terrain of clinical research. Hastings Cent Rep 2008;32:30–42.
50. Appelbaum PS, Roth LH, Lidz C. The therapeutic misconception: informed consent in psychiatric research. Int J Law Psychiatry 1982;5:319–329.
51. Appelbaum PS, Roth LH, Lidz CW, et al. False hopes and best data: consent to research and the therapeutic misconception. Hastings Cent Rep 1987;17:20–24.
52. National Bioethics Advisory Commission. Ethical and policy issues in International research: clinical trials in developing countries. Bethesda, MD: National Bioethics Advisory Commission, 2001.
53. Joffe S, Cook EF, Cleary PD, et al. Quality of informed consent in cancer clinical trials: a cross-sectional survey. Lancet 2001;358:1772–1777.
54. Daugherty C, Ratain MJ, Grochowski E, et al. Perceptions of cancer patients and their physicians involved in phase I trials. J Clin Oncol 1995;13:1062–1072.
55. Kodish E, Eder M, Noll RB, et al. Communication of randomization in childhood leukemia trials. JAMA 2004;291:470–475.
56. Eder ML, Yamokoski AD, Wittmann PW, et al. Improving informed consent: suggestions from parents of children with leukemia. Pediatrics 2007;119:e849–e859.
57. Flory J, Emanuel EJ. Interventions to improve research participants' understanding in informed consent for research: a systematic review. JAMA 2004;292:1593–1601.
58. National Commission for the Protection of Human Subjects of Biomedical and Behavioral Research. Research involving children: report and recommendations. Washington, DC: 1977. DHEW Publication No. (OS) 77-0004.
59. U.S. Department of Health and Human Services. 45 CFR 46. Subpart D–Additional Protections for Children Involved as Subjects in Research. Fed Regist 1983 March 8;48:9818.
60. Joffe S. Rethink "affirmative agreement," but abandon "assent". Am J Bioeth 2003;3: 9–11.
61. Institute of Medicine Committee on Clinical Research Involving Children. Ethical conduct of clinical research involving children. Washington, DC: National Academies Press, 2004.
62. Ackerman TF. Fooling ourselves with child autonomy and assent in nontherapeutic clinical research. Clin Res 1979;27:345–348.
63. Olechnowicz JQ, Eder M, Simon C, et al. Assent observed: children's involvement in leukemia treatment and research discussions. Pediatrics 2002;109:806–814.
64. Weithorn LA, Campbell SB. The competency of children and adolescents to make informed treatment decisions. Child Dev 1982;53:1589–1598.
65. Susman EJ, Dorn LD, Fletcher JC. Participation in biomedical research: the consent process as viewed by children, adolescents, young adults, and physicians. J Pediatr 1992;121:547–552.
66. Tait AR, Voepel-Lewis T, Malviya S. Do they understand? (part II): assent of children participating in clinical anesthesia and surgery research. Anesthesiology 2003;98:609–614.
67. Leikin S. Minors' assent, consent or dissent to medical research. IRB 1993;15:5.
68. Geller G, Tambor ES, Bernhardt BA, et al. Informed consent for enrolling minors in genetic susceptibility research: a qualitative study of at-risk children's and parents' views about children's role in decision-making. J Adolesc Health 2003;32:260–271.

69. Joffe S, Fernandez CV, Pentz RD, et al. Involving children with cancer in decision-making about research participation. J Pediatr 2006;149:862–868.

70. Brock DW. Ethical issues in exposing children to risks in research. In: Grodin MA, Glantz LH, eds. Children as research subjects: science, ethics, and law. New York, NY: Oxford University Press, 1994;81–101.

71. Ramsey P. The Patient as Person. New Haven: Yale University Press, 1970.

72. U.S. Department of Health and Human Services. 45 CFR 46. Fed Regist 1991 June 18;56:28012.

73. Shah S, Whittle A, Wilfond B, et al. How do institutional review boards apply the federal risk and benefit standards for pediatric research? JAMA 2004;291:476–482.

74. Janofsky J, Starfield B. Assessment of risk in research on children. J Pediatr 1981;98:842–846.

75. Levine RJ. The need to revise the Declaration of Helsinki. N Engl J Med 1999;341:531–534.

76. Weijer C. The ethical analysis of risk. J Law Med Ethics 2000;28:344–361.

77. Freedman B. Equipoise and the ethics of clinical research. N Engl J Med 1987;317:141–145.

78. Veatch RM. Indifference of subjects: an alternative to equipoise in randomized clinical trials. Soc Philos Policy 2002;19:295–323.

79. Angell M. Patients' preferences in randomized clinical trials. N Engl J Med 1984;310:1385–1387.

80. Ashcroft R. Giving medicine a fair trial. Trials should not second guess what patients want. BMJ 2000;320:1686.

81. Lilford RJ. Ethics of clinical trials from a bayesian and decision analytic perspective: whose equipoise is it anyway? BMJ 2003;326:980–981.

82. Lilford RJ, Braunholtz D, Edwards S, et al. Monitoring clinical trials–interim data should be publicly available. BMJ 2001;323:441–442.

83. National Breast Cancer Coalition. NBCC raises concerns about halting of letrozole clinical trial. 2003. http://www.stopbreastcancer.org//index.php?option=com_content&task=view&id=145&Itemid=170. Accessed January 30, 2008.

84. Cannistra SA. The ethics of early stopping rules: who is protecting whom? J Clin Oncol 2004;22:1542–1545.

85. Bryant J, Wolmark N. Letrozole after tamoxifen for breast cancer–what is the price of success? N Engl J Med 2003;349:1855–1857.

86. Smith M, Bernstein M, Bleyer WA, et al. Conduct of phase I trials in children with cancer. J Clin Oncol 1998;16:966–978.

87. Pratt CB. The conduct of phase I-II clinical trials in children with cancer. Med Pediatr Oncol 1991;19:304–309.

88. Agrawal M, Emanuel EJ. Ethics of phase 1 oncology studies: reexamining the arguments and data. JAMA 2003;290:1075–1082.

89. Annas GJ. The changing landscape of human experimentation: Nuremberg, Helsinki, and beyond. Health Matrix 1992;2:119–140.

90. Annas GJ. Questing for grails: duplicity, betrayal and self-deception in postmodern medical research. J Contemp Health Law Policy 1996;12:297–324.

91. Estlin EJ, Cotterill S, Pratt CB, et al. Phase I trials in pediatric oncology: perceptions of pediatricians from the United Kingdom Children's cancer study group and the pediatric oncology group. J Clin Oncol 2000;18:1900–1905.

92. Horng S, Emanuel EJ, Wilfond B, et al. Descriptions of benefits and risks in consent forms for phase 1 oncology trials. N Engl J Med 2002;347:2134–2140.

93. Kodish E, Stocking C, Ratain MJ, et al. Ethical issues in phase I oncology research: a comparison of investigators and institutional review board chairpersons. J Clin Oncol 1992;10:1810–1816.

94. Miller M. Phase I cancer trials. A collusion of misunderstanding. Hastings Cent Rep 2000;30:34–43.

95. Oberman M, Frader J. Dying children and medical research: access to clinical trials as benefit and burden. Am J Law Med 2003;29:301–317.

96. Weinfurt KP, Castel LD, Li Y, et al. The correlation between patient characteristics and expectations of benefit from Phase I clinical trials. Cancer 2003;98:166–175.

97. Ackerman TF. Phase I pediatric oncology trials. J Pediatr Oncol Nurs 1995;12:143–145.

98. Joffe S, Miller FG. Rethinking risk-benefit assessment for phase I cancer trials. J Clin Oncol 2006;24:2987–2990.

99. Miller FG, Joffe S. Benefit in phase 1 oncology trials: therapeutic misconception or reasonable treatment option? Clin Trials 2008;5:617–623.

100. Furman W, Pratt C, Rivera G. Mortality in pediatric phase I clinical trials. J Natl Cancer Inst 1989;81:1193–1194.

101. Shah S, Weitman S, Langevin AM, et al. Phase I therapy trials in children with cancer. J Pediatr Hematol Oncol 1998;20:431–438.

102. Estey E, Hoth D, Simon R, et al. Therapeutic response in phase I trials of antineoplastic agents. Cancer Treat Rep 1986;70:1105–1115.

103. Decoster G, Stein G, Holdener EE. Responses and toxic deaths in phase I clinical trials. Ann Oncol 1990;1:175–181.

104. Pentz RD, Flamm AL, Sugarman J, et al. Study of the media's potential influence on prospective research participants' understanding of and motivations for participation in a high-profile phase I trial. J Clin Oncol 2002;20:3785–3791.

105. Tomamichel M, Sessa C, Herzig S, et al. Informed consent for phase I studies: evaluation of quantity and quality of information provided to patients. Ann Oncol 1995;6:363–369.

106. Nitschke R, Humphrey GB, Sexauer CL, et al. Therapeutic choices made by patients with end-stage cancer. J Pediatr 1982;101:471–476.

107. National Bioethics Advisory Commission. Research Involving Human Biological Materials: Ethical Issues and Policy Guidance. Rockville, MD: National Bioethics Advisory Commission, 1999.

108. Clayton EW, Steinberg KK, Khoury MJ, et al. Informed consent for genetic research on stored tissue samples. JAMA 1995;274:1786–1792.

109. ASHG report. Statement on informed consent for genetic research. The American Society of Human Genetics. Am J Hum Genet 1996;59:471–474.

110. ACMG statement. Statement on storage and use of genetic materials. American College of Medical Genetics Storage of Genetics Materials Committee. Am J Hum Genet 1995; 57:1499–1500.

111. Office of Civil Rights of the Department of Health and Human Services. Standards for privacy of individually identifiable health information: final rule. Fed Regist 2002;67:53182–53272.

112. Office for Human Research Protections. Categories of Research That May Be Reviewed by the Institutional Review Board (IRB) through an Expedited Review Procedure. Fed Regist 1998;63:60364–60367. http://www.hhs.gov/ohrp/humansubjects/guidance/expedited98.htm. Accessed June 18, 2010.

113. Wendler D, Martinez RA, Fairclough D, et al. Views of potential subjects toward proposed regulations for clinical research with adults unable to consent. Am J Psychiatry 2002;159:585–591.

114. Jack AL, Womack C. Why surgical patients do not donate tissue for commercial research: review of records. BMJ 2003;327:262.

115. Stegmayr B, Asplund K. Informed consent for genetic research on blood stored for more than a decade: a population-based study. BMJ 2002;325:634–635.

116. Medical Research Council. Human tissue and biological samples for use in research: operational and ethical guidelines. London: Medical Research Council, 2001.

117. Wendler D. One-time general consent for research on biological samples. BMJ 2006;332:544–547.

118. Wendler D. One-time general consent for research on biological samples: is it compatible with the health insurance portability and accountability act? Arch Intern Med 2006;166:1449–1452.

119. Hardy J, Singleton A. Genomewide association studies and human disease. N Engl J Med 2009;360:1759–1768.

120. Caulfield T, McGuire AL, Cho M, et al. Research ethics recommendations for whole-genome research: consensus statement. PLoS Biol 2008;6:e73.

121. Lowrance WW, Collins FS. Ethics. Identifiability in genomic research. Science 2007; 317:600–602.

122. McGuire AL, Gibbs RA. Genetics. No longer de-identified. Science 2006;312:370–371.

123. Gurwitz D, Fortier I, Lunshof JE, et al. Research ethics. Children and population biobanks. Science 2009;325:818–819.

124. Fernandez C, Gao J, Strahlendorf C, et al. Providing research results to participants: attitudes and needs of adolescents and parents of children with cancer. J Clin Oncol 2009;27:878–883.

125. Shalowitz DI, Miller FG. Communicating the results of clinical research to participants: attitudes, practices, and future directions. PLoS Med 2008;5:e91.

126. Partridge AH, Hackett N, Blood E, et al. Oncology physician and nurse practices and attitudes regarding offering clinical trial results to study participants. J Natl Cancer Inst 2004;96:629–632.

127. MacNeil SD, Fernandez CV. Attitudes of research ethics board chairs towards disclosure of research results to participants: results of a national survey. J Med Ethics 2007; 33:549–553.

128. Partridge AH, Wolff AC, Marcom PK, et al. The impact of sharing results of a randomized breast cancer clinical trial with study participants. Breast Cancer Res Treat 2009; 115:123–129.

129. Partridge AH, Wong JS, Knudsen K, et al. Offering participants results of a clinical trial: sharing results of a negative study. Lancet 2005;365:963–964.

130. Wolf SM, Lawrenz FP, Nelson CA, et al. Managing incidental findings in human subjects research: analysis and recommendations. J Law Med Ethics 2008;36:219–248, 211.

131. Shalowitz DI, Miller FG. Disclosing individual results of clinical research: implications of respect for participants. JAMA 2005;294:737–740.

132. Knoppers BM, Joly Y, Simard J, et al. The emergence of an ethical duty to disclose genetic research results: international perspectives. Eur J Hum Genet 2006;14:1170–1178.

133. Bookman EB, Langehorne AA, Eckfeldt JH, et al. Reporting genetic results in research studies: summary and recommendations of an NHLBI working group. Am J Med Genet 2006;140:1033–1040.

134. Fuller BP, Kahn MJ, Barr PA, et al. Privacy in genetics research. Science 1999;285:1359–1361.

135. Simes RJ. Publication bias: the case for an international registry of clinical trials. J Clin Oncol 1986;4:1529–1541.

136. Melander H, Ahlqvist-Rastad J, Meijer G, et al. Evidence b(i)ased medicine–selective reporting from studies sponsored by pharmaceutical industry: review of studies in new drug applications. BMJ 2003;326:1171–1173.

137. Stern JM, Simes RJ. Publication bias: evidence of delayed publication in a cohort study of clinical research projects. BMJ 1997;315:640–645.

138. Krzyzanowska MK, Pintilie M, Tannock IF. Factors associated with failure to publish large randomized trials presented at an oncology meeting. JAMA 2003;290:495–501.

139. DeAngelis CD, Drazen JM, Frizelle FA, et al. Clinical trial registration: a statement from the International Committee of Medical Journal Editors. JAMA 2004;292: 1363–1364.

140. Wood AJ. Progress and deficiencies in the registration of clinical trials. N Engl J Med 2009;360:824–830.

141. The Hippocratic Oath. BMJ 1998;317:1110B.

142. Rothstein MA, Talbott MK. Compelled disclosure of health information: protecting against the greatest potential threat to privacy. JAMA 2006;295:2882–2885.

143. Moskop JC, Marco CA, Larkin GL, et al. From Hippocrates to HIPAA: privacy and confidentiality in emergency medicine–Part I: conceptual, moral, and legal foundations. Ann Emerg Med 2005;45:53–59.

144. Beauchamp TL, Childress JF. Principles of biomedical ethics. 4th ed. New York, NY: Oxford University Press, 1994.

145. van Eys J. Confidentiality of medical records in pediatric cancer care. Myths, perceptions, and reality. Am J Pediatr Hematol Oncol 1984;6:415–423.

146. Tarasoff v. Regents of the University of California. In: 17 Cal 3d. 425; 1976.

147. Gunn PP, Fremont AM, Bottrell M, et al. The Health Insurance Portability and Accountability Act Privacy Rule: a practical guide for researchers. Med Care 2004;42:321–327.

148. Annas GJ. HIPAA regulations – a new era of medical-record privacy? N Engl J Med 2003;348:1486–1490.

149. Office of Civil Rights of the Department of Health and Human Services. Standards for privacy of individually identifiable health information: final rule. Fed Register 2002; 67(157):53182–53272.

150. HIPAA privacy rule and public health. Guidance from CDC and the U.S. Department of Health and Human Services. MMWR Morb Mortal Wkly Rep 2003;52(Suppl):1–17, 9–20.

151. Lo B, Dornbrand L, Dubler NN. HIPAA and patient care: the role for professional judgment. JAMA 2005;293:1766–1771.

152. Kulynych J, Korn D. The effect of the new federal medical-privacy rule on research. N Engl J Med 2002;346:201–204.

153. Rothstein MA. Currents in contemporary ethics. Research privacy under HIPAA and the common rule. J Law Med Ethics 2005;33:154–159.

154. Beyond the HIPAA Privacy Rule: enhancing privacy, improving health through research. 2009. www.nap.edu. Accessed July 7, 2009.

155. Ness RB. Influence of the HIPAA Privacy Rule on health research. JAMA 2007;298:2164–2170.

156. Rothstein MA. Currents in contemporary ethics. Research privacy under HIPAA and the common rule. J Law Med Ethics 2005;33:154–159.

157. Feld AD. The Health Insurance Portability and Accountability Act (HIPAA): its broad effect on practice. Am J Gastroenterol 2005;100:1440–1443.

158. Brous EA. HIPAA vs. law enforcement. A nurses' guide to managing conflicting responsibilities. Am J Nurs 2007;107:60–63.

159. Geller G, Botkin JR, Green MJ, et al. Genetic testing for susceptibility to adult-onset cancer. The process and content of informed consent. JAMA 1997;277:1467–1474.

160. Kodish E, Wiesner GL, Mehlman M, et al. Genetic testing for cancer risk: how to reconcile the conflicts. JAMA 1998;279:179–181.

161. National Advisory Council for Human Genome Research. Statement on use of DNA testing for presymptomatic identification of cancer risk. JAMA 1994;271:785.

162. American Society of Clinical Oncology. American Society of Clinical Oncology policy statement update: genetic testing for cancer susceptibility. J Clin Oncol 2003;21: 2397–2406.

163. Wertz DC, Fanos JH, Reilly PR. Genetic testing for children and adolescents. Who decides? JAMA 1994;272:875–881.

164. Brandi ML, Gagel RF, Angeli A, et al. Guidelines for diagnosis and therapy of MEN type 1 and type 2. J Clin Endocrinol Metab 2001;86:5658–5671.

165. Li FP, Garber JE, Friend SH, et al. Recommendations on predictive testing for germ line p53 mutations among cancer-prone individuals. J Natl Cancer Inst 1992;84:1156–1160.

166. Reilly PR, Boshar MF, Holtzman SH. Ethical issues in genetic research: disclosure and informed consent. Nat Genet 1997;15:16–20.

167. Hudson KL, Holohan MK, Collins FS. Keeping pace with the times–the Genetic Information Nondiscrimination Act of 2008. N Engl J Med 2008;358:2661–2663.

168. Fallat ME, Glover J. Professionalism in pediatrics: statement of principles. Pediatrics 2007;120:895–897.

169. Wolfe J, Klar N, Grier HE, et al. Understanding of prognosis among parents of children who died of cancer: impact on treatment goals and integration of palliative care. JAMA 2000;284:2469–2475.

170. Hechler T, Blankenburg M, Friedrichsdorf SJ, et al. Parents' perspective on symptoms, quality of life, characteristics of death and end-of-life decisions for children dying from cancer. Klin Padiatr 2008;220:166–174.

171. Himelstein BP, Hilden JM, Boldt AM, et al. Pediatric palliative care. N Engl J Med 2004;350:1752–1762.

172. American Academy of Pediatrics. Committee on Bioethics and Committee on Hospital Care. Palliative care for children. Pediatrics 2000;106:351–357.

173. Mack JW, Wolfe J. Early integration of pediatric palliative care: for some children, palliative care starts at diagnosis. Curr Opin Pediatr 2006;18:10–14.

174. Institute of Medicine Committee on Care at the End of Life. Approaching death: improving care at the end of life. Washington, DC: National Academies Press, 1997.

175. Institute of Medicine: Committee on Palliative and End-of-Life Care for Children and their Families. When children die: improving palliative and end-of-life care for children and their families. Washington, DC: National Academies Press, 2003.

176. Gerstel E, Engelberg RA, Koepsell T, et al. Duration of withdrawal of life support in the intensive care unit and association with family satisfaction. Am J Respir Crit Care Med 2008;178:798–804.

177. Back AL, Arnold RM, Quill TE. Hope for the best, and prepare for the worst. Ann Intern Med 2003;138:439–443.

178. Varelas PN, Abdelhak T, Hacein-Bey L. Withdrawal of life-sustaining therapies and brain death in the intensive care unit. Semin Neurol 2008;28:726–735.

179. Inwald D. The best interests test at the end of life on PICU: a plea for a family-centred approach. Arch Dis Child 2008;93:248–250.

180. President's Commission for the Study of Ethical Problems in Medicine and Biomedical and Behavioral Research. Deciding to forego life-sustaining treatments. Washington, D.C: U.S. Government Printing Office, 1983.

181. Council on Ethical and Judicial Affairs of the American Medical Association. Decisions near the end of life. JAMA 1992;267:2229–2233.

182. American Academy of Pediatrics Committee on Bioethics. Guidelines on foregoing life-sustaining medical treatment. Pediatrics 1994;93:532–536.

183. Truog RD, Cist AF, Brackett SE, et al. Recommendations for end-of-life care in the intensive care unit: The Ethics Committee of the Society of Critical Care Medicine. Crit Care Med 2001;29:2332–2348.

184. Council on Ethical and Judicial Affairs of the American Medical Association. Good care of the dying patient. JAMA 1996;275:474–478.

185. Meyer EC, Burns JP, Griffith JL, et al. Parental perspectives on end-of-life care in the pediatric intensive care unit. Crit Care Med 2002;30:226–231.

186. Cook D, Rocker G, Marshall J, et al. Withdrawal of mechanical ventilation in anticipation of death in the intensive care unit. N Engl J Med 2003;349:1123–1132.

187. Giannini A, Messeri A, Aprile A, et al. End-of-life decisions in pediatric intensive care. Recommendations of the Italian Society of Neonatal and Pediatric Anesthesia and Intensive Care (SARNePI). Paediatr Anaesth 2008;18:1089–1095.

188. Munson D. Withdrawal of mechanical ventilation in pediatric and neonatal intensive care units. Pediatr Clin North Am 2007;54:773–785, xii.

189. Lantos J. Baby Doe five years later. Implications for child health. N Engl J Med 1987; 317:444–447.

190. Pless JE. The story of Baby Doe. N Engl J Med 1983;309:664.

191. Kopelman LM, Irons TG, Kopelman AE. Neonatologists judge the "Baby Doe" regulations. N Engl J Med 1988;318:677–683.

192. Lo B, Jonsen AR. Clinical decisions to limit treatment. Ann Intern Med 1980;93: 764–768.

193. Burns JP, Truog RD. Futility: a concept in evolution. Chest 2007;132:1987–1993.

194. Schneiderman LJ, Jecker NS, Jonsen AR. Medical futility: its meaning and ethical implications. Ann Intern Med 1990;112:949–954.

195. Bernat JL. Medical futility: definition, determination, and disputes in critical care. Neurocrit Care 2005;2:198–205.

196. Post SG. Baby K. Medical futility and the free exercise of religion. J Law Med Ethics 1995;23:20–26.

197. Annas GJ. Asking the courts to set the standard of emergency care–the case of Baby K. N Engl J Med 1994;330:1542–1545.

198. Plows C. Medical futility in end-of-life care–Report of the Council on Ethical and Judicial Affairs. JAMA 1999;281:937–941.

199. Singer PA, Barker G, Bowman KW, et al. Hospital policy on appropriate use of life-sustaining treatment. University of Toronto Joint Centre for Bioethics/Critical Care Medicine Program Task Force. Crit Care Med 2001;29:187–191.

200. Consensus statement of the Society of Critical Care Medicine's Ethics Committee regarding futile and other possibly inadvisable treatments. Crit Care Med 1997;25: 887–891.

201. Orentlicher D. From the Office of the General Counsel. The right to die after Cruzan. JAMA 1990;264:2444–2446.

202. Annas GJ. Nancy Cruzan and the right to die. N Engl J Med 1990;323:670–673.

203. Wolfe J, Grier HE, Klar N, et al. Symptoms and suffering at the end of life in children with cancer. N Engl J Med 2000;342:326–333.

204. Wolfe J, Hammel JF, Edwards KE, et al. Easing of suffering in children with cancer at the end of life: is care changing? J Clin Oncol 2008;26:1717–1723.

205. May WF. Double effect. In: Reich WT, ed. Encyclopedia of bioethics. New York, NY: Free Press, 1978;316–320.

206. Quill TE, Dresser R, Brock DW. The rule of double effect–a critique of its role in end-of-life decision making. N Engl J Med 1997;337:1768–1771.

207. Sykes N, Thorns A. The use of opioids and sedatives at the end of life. Lancet Oncol 2003;4:312–318.

208. Sykes N, Thorns A. Sedative use in the last week of life and the implications for end-of-life decision making. Arch Intern Med 2003;163:341–344.

209. Fohr SA. The double effect of pain medication: separating myth from reality. J Palliat Med 1998;1:315–328.

210. Brody H, Campbell ML, Faber-Langendoen K, et al. Withdrawing intensive life-sustaining treatment–recommendations for compassionate clinical management. N Engl J Med 1997;336:652–657.

211. Truog RD, Berde CB, Mitchell C, et al. Barbiturates in the care of the terminally ill. N Engl J Med 1992;327:1678–1682.

212. Postovsky S, Moaed B, Krivoy E, et al. Practice of palliative sedation in children with brain tumors and sarcomas at the end of life. Pediatr Hematol Oncol 2007;24: 409–415.

213. Cowan JD, Walsh D. Terminal sedation in palliative medicine–definition and review of the literature. Support Care Cancer 2001;9:403–407.

214. National Ethics Committee, Veteran's Health Administration. The ethics of palliative sedation as a therapy of last resort. Am J Hosp Palliat Care 2006;23:483–491.

215. Sulmasy DP, Pellegrino ED. The rule of double effect: clearing up the double talk. Arch Intern Med 1999;159:545–550.

216. McStay R. Terminal sedation: palliative care for intractable pain, post Glucksberg and Quill. Am J Law Med 2003;29:45–76.

217. Quill TE, Byock IR. Responding to intractable terminal suffering: the role of terminal sedation and voluntary refusal of food and fluids. ACP-ASIM End-of-Life Care Consensus Panel. American College of Physicians-American Society of Internal Medicine. Ann Intern Med 2000;132:408–414.

218. Nelson LJ, Rushton CH, Cranford RE, et al. Forgoing medically provided nutrition and hydration in pediatric patients. J Law Med Ethics 1995;23:33–46.

219. Levi BH. Withdrawing nutrition and hydration from children: legal, ethical, and professional issues. Clin Pediatr (Phila) 2003;42:139–145.

220. *Cruzan v. Director of Missouri Department of Health.* In: 110 S. Ct 2841; 1990.

221. Thompson DF. Understanding financial conflicts of interest. N Engl J Med 1993;329: 573–576.

222. Bodenheimer T. Uneasy Alliance–Clinical Investigators and the Pharmaceutical Industry. N Engl J Med 2000;342:1539–1544.

223. Lewis S, Baird P, Evans RG, et al. Dancing with the porcupine: rules for governing the university-industry relationship. CMAJ 2001;165:783–785.

224. Mitchell JM, Scott E. Physician ownership of physical therapy services. Effects on charges, utilization, profits, and service characteristics. JAMA 1992;268: 2055–2059.

225. Hillman BJ, Joseph CA, Mabry MR, et al. Frequency and costs of diagnostic imaging in office practice–a comparison of self-referring and radiologist-referring physicians. N Engl J Med 1990;323:1604–1608.

226. AAMC Task Force on Financial Conflicts of Interest in Clinical Research. Protecting subjects, preserving trust, promoting progress II: principles and recommendations for oversight of an institution's financial interests in human subjects research. Acad Med 2003;78:237–245.

227. Brennan TA, Rothman DJ, Blank L, et al. Health industry practices that create conflicts of interest: a policy proposal for academic medical centers. JAMA 2006;295:429–433.

228. Campbell EG, Weissman JS, Ehringhaus S, et al. Institutional academic industry relationships. JAMA 2007;298:1779–1786.

229. Ashar BH, Miller RG, Getz KJ, et al. Prevalence and determinants of physician participation in conducting pharmaceutical-sponsored clinical trials and lectures. J Gen Intern Med 2004;19:1140–1145.

230. University and Small Business Patent Procedures Act. In: 35 USC 200–212; 1980.

231. Eisenberg RS, Nelson RR. Public vs. proprietary science: a fruitful tension? Acad Med 2002;77:1392–1399.

232. Ledbetter DH. Gene patenting and licensing: the role of academic researchers and advocacy groups. Genet Med 2008;10:314–319.

233. Bekelman JE, Li Y, Gross CP. Scope and impact of financial conflicts of interest in biomedical research: a systematic review. JAMA 2003;289:454–465.

234. Stark RFP. H. Conf Rep. No. 213, 103d Cong., 1st Sess. 810. In; 1993.

235. McCormick BB, Tomlinson G, Brill-Edwards P, et al. Effect of restricting contact between pharmaceutical company representatives and internal medicine residents on posttraining attitudes and behavior. JAMA 2001;286:1994–1999.

236. Orlowski JP, Wateska L. The effects of pharmaceutical firm enticements on physician prescribing patterns. There's no such thing as a free lunch. Chest 1992;102:270–273.

237. Chren MM, Landefeld CS. Physicians' behavior and their interactions with drug companies. A controlled study of physicians who requested additions to a hospital drug formulary. JAMA 1994;271:684–689.

238. Steinbrook R. Testing medications in children. N Engl J Med 2002;347:1462–1470.

239. Wazana A. Physicians and the pharmaceutical industry: is a gift ever just a gift? JAMA 2000;283:373–380.

240. Dana J, Loewenstein G. A social science perspective on gifts to physicians from industry. JAMA 2003;290:252–255.

241. Peppercorn J, Blood E, Winer E, et al. Association between pharmaceutical involvement and outcomes in breast cancer clinical trials. Cancer 2007;109:1239–1246.

242. Djulbegovic B, Lacevic M, Cantor A, et al. The uncertainty principle and industry-sponsored research. Lancet 2000;356:635–638.

243. Jagsi R, Sheets N, Jankovic A, et al. Frequency, nature, effects, and correlates of conflicts of interest in published clinical cancer research. Cancer 2009;115:2783–2791.

244. Als-Nielsen B, Chen W, Gluud C, et al. Association of funding and conclusions in randomized drug trials: a reflection of treatment effect or adverse events? JAMA 2003;290:921–928.

245. Perlis RH, Perlis CS, Wu Y, et al. Industry sponsorship and financial conflict of interest in the reporting of clinical trials in psychiatry. Am J Psychiatry 2005;162:1957–1960.

246. Stolberg SG. The Biotech Death of Jesse Gelsinger. New York Times. November 28, 1999:136–140, 149–150.

247. Meier B. An rx for ethics. New York Times January 24, 2009.

248. Steinbrook R. Standards of ethics at the National Institutes of Health. N Engl J Med 2005;352:1290–1292.

249. AAMC Task Force on Financial Conflicts of Interest in Clinical Research. Protecting subjects, preserving trust, promoting progress I: policy and guidelines for the oversight of individual financial interests in human subjects research. Acad Med 2003;78:225–236.

250. Uniform Requirements for Manuscripts Submitted to Biomedical Journals: Ethical Considerations in the Conduct and Reporting of Research: Conflicts of Interest. 2009. http://www.icmje.org/ethical_4conflicts.html. Accessed September 27, 2009.

251. Chaudhry S, Schroter S, Smith R, et al. Does declaration of competing interests affect readers' perceptions? A randomised trial. BMJ 2002;325:1391–1392.

252. Schroter S. Does the type of competing interest statement affect readers' perceptions of the credibility of research? Randomised trial. BMJ 2004;328:742–743.

253. Hampson LA, Agrawal M, Joffe S, et al. Patients' views on financial conflicts of interest in cancer research trials. N Engl J Med 2006;355:2330–2337.

254. Weinfurt KP, Hall MA, Dinan MA, et al. Effects of disclosing financial interests on attitudes toward clinical research. J Gen Intern Med 2008;23:860–866.

255. Weinfurt KP, Hall MA, Friedman JY, et al. Effects of disclosing financial interests on participation in medical research: a randomized vignette trial. Am Heart J 2008;156:689–697.

256. Ross JS, Lackner JE, Lurie P, et al. Pharmaceutical company payments to physicians: early experiences with disclosure laws in Vermont and Minnesota. JAMA 2007;297:1216–1223.

257. Brennan TA, Mello MM. Sunshine laws and the pharmaceutical industry. JAMA 2007;297:1255–1257.

258. Office of Research Integrity of the U.S. Department of Health and Human Services. 42 CFR 50, Subpart F–Responsibility of Applicants for Promoting Objectivity in Research for Which PHS Funding Is Sought. Fed Register. July 11 and 31, 1995;60:35815 and 39076.

259. American Society of Clinical Oncology. Revised conflict of interest policy. J Clin Oncol 2006;24:519–521.

260. Office of Government Ethics. 5 CFR Pt. 5501 and 5502–Supplemental standards of ethical conduct and financial disclosure requirements for employees of the Department of Health and Human Services. 61 Federal Register 39763, July 30, 1996; 70 Federal Register 5543, February 3, 2005; and 70 Federal Register 51559, August 31, 2005.

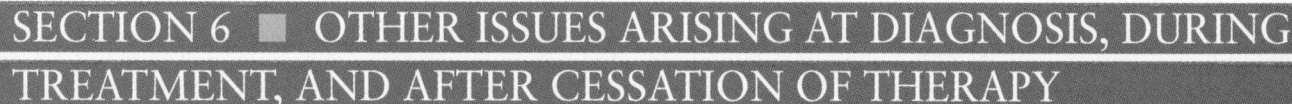

SECTION 6 ■ OTHER ISSUES ARISING AT DIAGNOSIS, DURING TREATMENT, AND AFTER CESSATION OF THERAPY

CHAPTER 47 ■ LATE EFFECTS OF CHILDHOOD CANCER AND ITS TREATMENT

SARO H. ARMENIAN, ANNA T. MEADOWS AND SMITA BHATIA

More than 12,000 children and adolescents are diagnosed with cancer each year in the United States.[1] With the use of risk-based therapies, the overall 5-year survival rate is approaching 80%.[1] This improvement in survival has resulted in a growing population of childhood cancer survivors. In 2005, there were an estimated 328,652 survivors of childhood cancer[2]; of these 24% had survived more than 30 years since diagnosis; and ~27% were 40 years of age or older. This translates into 1 in 1000 individuals being a childhood cancer survivor; constituting 3% of the total cancer survivor population in the United States.[1]

Unlike adults, the growing child tolerates the acute side effects of therapy relatively well. However, the use of cancer therapy at an early age can produce complications that may not become apparent until years later as the child matures—hence the term "late effect" for late-occurring or chronic outcome, either physical or psychological, that persists or develops beyond 5 years from the diagnosis of cancer.

Research leading to our current state of knowledge began more than three decades ago in the setting of single institutions and multi-institution consortia. With the recognition that large cohorts of survivors would be needed to evaluate the effects of multiple therapies on individuals treated for a variety of neoplasms at different ages, the Childhood Cancer Survivor Study (CCSS) was established with funding from the National Cancer Institute.[3]

BURDEN OF MORBIDITY

Several investigators have described the burden of morbidity by quantifying the chronic medical problems experienced by this population;[4,5] Table 47.1 summarizes these issues. These reports suggest that approximately two-thirds of the survivors experience at least one chronic medical problem and one-third experience a late effect that is severe or life-threatening. In a recent study, Oeffinger et al. confirmed these findings in a cohort of 10,397 adult survivors of childhood cancer.[6] Overall, the survivors were at an 8-fold higher risk of reporting a severe chronic health condition, when compared with age- and sex-matched siblings. Individuals identified to be at highest risk included those treated for Hodgkin lymphoma (HL) or brain tumors, and those exposed to chest radiation and anthracyclines. These studies demonstrate quite conclusively that the implications of cure are not trivial, and that the burden of morbidity carried by childhood cancer survivors is quite substantial. Furthermore, these data support a critical need for continuing follow-up of childhood cancer survivors into adult life. There exists an urgent need for survivors and their healthcare providers to be aware of "at risk" populations in order to develop appropriate surveillance strategies.

KNOWLEDGE ABOUT PAST DIAGNOSIS AND TREATMENT

An investigation of childhood cancer survivors' knowledge about past cancer diagnosis and treatment demonstrated that only 72% of the cancer survivors were able to accurately and precisely report their cancer diagnosis.[7] Furthermore, only 70% of the childhood cancer survivors exposed to radiation could accurately describe the site of radiation. Most importantly, only 35% of the survivors understood that serious health problems could result from past treatment.

STANDARDIZED RECOMMENDATIONS FOR FOLLOW-UP OF CHILDHOOD CANCER

The Institute of Medicine has recognized the need for a systematic plan for lifelong surveillance that incorporates risks based on therapeutic exposures, genetic predisposition, health-related behaviors, and comorbid health conditions.[8] In response to this, the Children's Oncology Group (COG) developed risk-based, exposure-related guidelines (Long-Term Follow-Up Guidelines for Survivors of Childhood, Adolescent, and Young Adult Cancers)[9] specifically designed for follow-up care of patients who have completed treatment for pediatric malignancies. Specially tailored patient education materials, known as "Health Links" accompany the guidelines, offering detailed information on guideline-specific topics in order to enhance health promotion in this population with specialized healthcare needs. The Guidelines and the Health Links can be downloaded from www.survivorshipguidelines.org. Plans are underway to develop an automated version of the COG *Long-Term Follow-Up Guidelines* to generate individualized follow-up recommendations in collaboration with the Texas Children's Cancer Center and the Baylor College of Medicine through an initiative called the Passport For Care[SM] (PFC). When fully operationalized, the PFC will be able to generate individualized guidelines for screening and evaluation and survivor education resources that are customized to the needs of each patient based on their disease and treatment. The eventual goal of this project is to develop a national resource that will serve as the model for meeting the needs of cancer survivors. Regardless of the setting for follow-up, the first step in any evaluation is to develop an outline of the patient's medical history, including a treatment summary, and other elements listed in Table 47.2. Once completed, the treatment summary allows the survivor or their healthcare provider to interface with the COG Long-Term Follow-Up Guidelines to determine recommended

TABLE 47.1

COMMONLY OCCURRING LATE EFFECTS IN CHILDHOOD CANCER SURVIVORS

Adverse outcome	Therapeutic exposures associated with increased risk	Factors associated with highest risk
Hearing loss	Cranial radiation, platinum-based chemotherapy	Younger age (<4 yr) at treatment, increasing radiation and chemotherapy dose
Cataracts	Cranial irradiation, steroids	Higher radiation dose, combination of steroids and radiation, single daily fraction
Dental abnormalities	Cranial irradiation	Younger age at treatment
Neurocognitive deficits	Cranial irradiation, intrathecal methotrexate, cytarabine	Female sex, younger age (<5 yr) at treatment, cranial irradiation, and intrathecal chemotherapy
Cardiomyopathy/congestive heart failure	Anthracyclines	High cumulative doses (>500 mg/m^2), females, younger than 5 yr at treatment, mediastinal radiation
Myocardial infarction	Radiation to chest	Underlying risk factors for coronary artery disease (smoking, hypertension, hyperlipidemia, obesity, etc.)
Pulmonary fibrosis/interstitial pneumonitis	Bleomycin, radiation to chest, carmustine	Younger age at treatment, bleomycin dose >400 U/m^2
Therapy-related myelodysplasia	Alkylating agents, topoisomerase II inhibitors, anthracyclines, platinum compounds	Increasing dose of chemotherapeutic agents, older age at therapeutic exposure
Thyroid cancer	Radiation to the thyroid gland (neck, mantle, etc.)	Increasing dose upto 29 Gy, female sex, younger age at radiation
Skin cancer (basal cell, squamous cell, melanoma)	Radiation therapy	Orthovoltage radiation (prior to 1970)—delivery of greater dose to skin, additional excessive exposure to sun, tanning booths
Secondary brain tumor	Cranial irradiation	Increasing dose, younger age at treatment
Hypothyroidism	Radiation to the thyroid gland (neck, mantle, etc.)	Increasing dose, female sex, age at treatment
Hypogonadism	Alkylating agents, craniospinal irradiation, abdomino-pelvic irradiation, gonadal irradiation	Males sex, treatment during peripubertal or post-pubertal period in girls, higher cumulative doses of alkylators
Precocious puberty	Cranial irradiation	Female sex, younger age at treatment, radiation dose >18 Gy
Renal insufficiency	Platinum-based therapy, ifosfamide, high-dose methotrexate, abdominal radiation, surgery	High-dose chemotherapy, younger age, abdominal radiation, and chemotherapy
Bladder complications	Alkylating agents, abdominal radiation, surgery	Use of high-dose alkylating agents without bladder uroprophylaxis, abdominal radiation
Chronic Hepatitis C Virus (HCV) infection and HCV-related sequelae	Transfusions before 1992	Living in hyperendemic area
Short stature	Cranial irradiation, corticosteroids, total body irradiation	Younger age at treatment, cranial radiation dose >18 Gy, unfractionated (10 Gy) total body irradiation
Obesity	Cranial irradiation	Younger age at treatment (<8 yr), female sex, cranial irradiation dose >20 Gy
Osteopenia/osteoporosis	Corticosteroids, craniospinal irradiation, gonadal irradiation, total body irradiation	Associated hypothyroidism, hypogonadism, growth hormone deficiency
Avascular necrosis	Corticosteroids, high-dose radiation to any bone	Dexamethasone, adolescence, female sex

follow-up care. Before the survivor graduates from a pediatric oncologist's care, this treatment record and possible long-term problems should be reviewed with the family and, in the case of adolescents or young adults, with the patient. Correspondence between the pediatric oncologist and subsequent caretakers should address these same issues.

In the sections below, we review some of the known and emerging late effects in survivors of childhood cancer, and the relationship between these late effects and specific therapeutic exposures, in order to suggest reasonable starting points for evaluation of specific long-term problems using the screening recommendations from the COG guidelines. Detailed exam-

ples of specific screening strategies outlined within the COG guidelines are summarized in Table 47.3.

AUDITORY, OCULAR, ORAL, AND DENTAL COMPLICATIONS

Auditory Impairment

Several potentially ototoxic agents are commonly used in the management of childhood cancer. These agents include

TABLE 47.2

KEY ELEMENTS OF A COMPREHENSIVE TREATMENT SUMMARY

Key elements	Details
Demographics	Name, date of birth, treating institution, treatment team
Diagnosis	Initial diagnosis type, date, stage, site(s) relapses(s) with date(s) and site(s), if applicable
	Subsequent malignant neoplasms with type and site(s), if applicable
Therapeutic exposures:	
Chemotherapy	List of all agents received including route of administration
	Include cumulative doses (per m^2) for alkylators, anthracyclines, and bleomycin
	If available, include cumulative doses for all agents
	If patient received IV methotrexate or IV cytarabine, indicate whether any doses were in the intermediate/high dose range (>1000 mg/m^2)
Radiation	Dates, type, fields (laterality), total dose, no. of fractions/dose per fraction
Surgical procedures	Type(s), date(s)
Hematopoietic cell transplant	Type(s), date(s), GVHD prophylaxis/treatment
Completion of therapy	Date

GVHD, graft-versus-host disease; IV, intravenous.

platinum-based chemotherapy, aminoglycoside antibiotics, loop diuretics, and radiation therapy; all these agents are capable of causing sensorineural hearing loss.[10] Risk factors for hearing loss include, treatment with platinum-based chemotherapy in combination with cranial irradiation; treatment involving multiple ototoxic agents; and young age (less than 4 years) at exposure to ototoxic agents.[10] Diagnoses commonly associated with hearing loss include brain and germ cell tumors, neuroblastoma, and osteosarcoma.

Platinum-containing chemotherapy, particularly cisplatin and myeloablative doses of carboplatin, has been well established as risk factors for therapy-related hearing loss. Platinum-related ototoxicity results from destruction of cochlear hair cells. Because these specialized hair cells are arranged tonotypically (in order of pitch), the initial hearing loss is generally in the high frequency ranges (> 2000 Hz). As cumulative doses of platinum chemotherapy increase, so does the progression of injury toward the cochlear apex where lower frequencies (500–2000 Hz) are affected.[11] Similar to platinum-related ototoxicity, radiation-induced injury is caused by dose-dependent injury to the cochlea, and specifically affects high frequency hearing. Hearing loss is infrequent ($< 3\%$) when cochlear radiation dose is limited to 35 Gy or less.[12] However, mild-to-moderate hearing loss occurs in as many as 37% of children exposed to doses exceeding 60 Gy.[12] Treatment with higher dose radiation has also been associated with tympanosclerosis, otosclerosis, and Eustachian tube dysfunction.[13] Concomitant use of platinum agents with radiation may have synergistic sensorineural ototoxicity.[14] Use of proton beam radiation has made it possible to limit cochlear radiation doses to nearly zero.[15]

Recommendations for Screening and Follow-up

Very young children who received ototoxic agents during their cancer treatment and whose speech has not yet developed fully, should undergo audiologic evaluations to determine whether they require intervention. Interventions to assist children experiencing hearing loss include the use of hearing aids and other assistive devices, along with preferential seating in the classroom. For more severely affected children, placement in special educational environments for the hearing impaired may be required. Affected patients should be counseled to avoid exposure to loud noise, to use ear protection in noisy environments, and to avoid further exposure to ototoxic agents (e.g., aminoglycosides, loop diuretics) in order to prevent additional hearing loss. All children with hearing loss should receive ongoing follow-up from a pediatric audiologist or otologist.

Ocular Complications

Ocular and visual complications can occur as a result of surgery, radiation, or treatment with corticosteroids. Common conditions observed in long-term survivors include cataracts, glaucoma, retinopathy, xerophthalmia (dry eyes), or orbital hypoplasia.[16] Children at risk for cataract formation include those who received treatment with busulfan, long-term corticosteroids, total body irradiation (TBI), or radiation to the brain, head, or orbit.[16–18] The risk of cataracts is greatest in those treated with radiation doses greater than 15 Gy, with combination of corticosteroids and radiation, or those exposed to single daily fraction of TBI.[16,17] TBI and cranial irradiation may result in xerophthalmia, and the prevalence is especially high in individuals who develop chronic graft versus host disease (GvHD) following allogeneic hematopoietic cell transplantation (HCT).[19] Orbital irradiation may place survivors at risk for dry eyes, corneal ulceration, optic nerve damage, retinitis, iritis, glaucoma, blepharitis, and orbital hypoplasia.[16,20] Retinopathy, a rare complication, can occur years after radiation, and is more likely in individuals who were young at exposure or who received high-dose (>45 Gy) therapy to their orbit.[20]

TABLE 47.3

SELECTED EXPOSURE-BASED SCREENING RECOMMENDATIONS

Category	Therapeutic exposure	Potential late effect	Recommended screening
Auditory	Platinum-based chemotherapy Radiation involving the ear	Hearing loss (sensorineural, conductive, mixed)	Baseline audiologic assessment; repeat every 5 yr if radiation dose >30 Gy
Ocular	Glucocorticoids Busulfan Radiation involving the eye	Cataracts Cataracts Other adverse effects related to eye irradiation	Yearly fundoscopic exam and assessment of visual acuity Yearly fundoscopic exam and assessment of visual acuity Full ophthalmologic evaluation for those who received radiation involving the eye (frequency based on radiation dose)
Dental	Any chemotherapy administered prior to achieving permanent dentition Radiation impacting the oral cavity (including neck, mantle, cranial)	Enamel and structural malformation of developing teeth Increased risk of dental caries	Dental evaluation and cleaning every 6 mo
Neurocognitive	Radiation involving the brain Intrathecal methotrexate Intermediate/high-dose IV methotrexate or cytarabine	Neurocognitive deficit	Baseline neuropsychological assessment Yearly assessment of vocational/educational progress
Cardiac	Anthracycline chemotherapy Chest irradiation	Cardiomyopathy Cardiomyopathy Early-onset atherosclerotic heart disease Valvular disease	Yearly history and physical exam Baseline electrocardiogram Periodic echocardiogram as indicated based on exposure dose, age, and mediastinal radiation Fasting glucose and lipid profile every 2 yr Cardiac consultation as indicated for symptomatic patients with subclinical abnormalities on screening evaluations, and for patients who are pregnant or considering pregnancy who have received cumulative anthracycline doses $\geq$300 mg/m^2 or <300 mg/m^2 if combined with radiation potentially impacting the heart
Pulmonary	Carmustine Lomustine Busulfan Bleomycin Radiation impacting the lungs	Pulmonary fibrosis Interstitial pneumonitis Acute respiratory distress syndrome Pulmonary fibrosis Delayed interstitial pneumonitis Restrictive/obstructive lung disease	Yearly history and physical exam Baseline measure of pulmonary function, including DLCO and spirometry Baseline chest radiograph Repeat evaluations prior to general anesthesia and as clinically indicated
Gastrointestinal/ hepatic	Methotrexate Thioguanine Radiation impacting the liver Exploratory laparotomy	Hepatic dysfunction Hepatic fibrosis Cirrhosis Adhesive/obstructive complications	Yearly history and physical exam Baseline ALT, AST, bilirubin If abnormal, obtain prothrombin time for evaluation of hepatic synthetic function History and physical exam if symptomatic

(continued)

information-processing deficits resulting in academic difficulties, and are prone to problems with receptive and expressive language, attention span, and visual and perceptual motor skills. Younger children and those treated for brain tumors may experience significant drops in intelligence quotient (IQ) scores, with irradiation- or chemotherapy-induced destruction in normal white matter over time, partially explaining intellectual and academic achievement deficits in these survivors.[27,29,31] Recent studies indicated that patients with medulloblastoma exposed to lower doses of whole-brain irradiation (23.5 Gy) are at reduced risk of neurocognitive dysfunction.[32,33] Additionally, there is preliminary evidence to suggest that survivors of medulloblastoma with glutathione S-transferase M1 and T1 gene polymorphisms may be at an increased risk of neurotoxicity and intellectual impairment.[34]

Treatment of ALL patients with cranial irradiation at a dose of 24 Gy is also associated with cognitive deficits; the deficits are not as profound as those seen among brain tumor patients treated with a similar dose of cranial irradiation.[26] This difference may be because of the impact of the intracranial tumor itself, neuronal injury due to intracranial pressure, or a result of surgery. Nevertheless, leukemia and brain tumor survivors have been shown to use special education services more than with age- and sex-matched siblings.[35] There is evidence of subtle long-term neurocognitive deficits in survivors of childhood ALL after treatment with chemotherapy alone. These deficits are restricted to attention, executive function, and complex fine-motor functioning; global intellectual function is relatively preserved. Younger patients and females are at higher risk for these deficits.[36]

Recommendations for Screening and Follow-up

A baseline neuropsychological evaluation is recommended for patients who received therapy that may impact neurocognitive function. This should be repeated as clinically indicated and at key transition points (transitioning from grade school to middle/junior high school); an annual assessment of their vocational or educational progress should also be monitored.

CARDIOVASCULAR FUNCTION

The anthracyclines doxorubicin and daunomycin are well-known causes of cardiomyopathy. Anthracyclines have a wide range of clinical activity against pediatric cancers, and it is estimated that as many as 60% of childhood cancer survivors have been treated with anthracyclines, making it one of the more common therapeutic exposures.[37] Anthracycline cardiotoxicity is thought to be related to direct myocardial injury due to formation of free radicals. Over time, the left ventricular wall thins, leading to increased myocardial stress and decreased contractility.[38] Progressive cardiomyopathy can occur early within the first year of treatment or can be delayed, being diagnosed years following completion of therapy; the risk of disease is dose-dependent.[37] The incidence of congestive heart failure (CHF) is less than 10% in patients exposed to cumulative dose of anthracycline of less than 500 mg/m^2, and approaches 36% for doses exceeding 600 mg/m^2.[39] With longer follow-up of childhood cancer survivors, it has become apparent that lower cumulative doses of anthracyclines may place children at risk for cardiac compromise, suggesting that there is no "safe" dose of anthracyclines.[40] Advances in noninvasive cardiac imaging have allowed investigators to identify a growing population of survivors with asymptomatic left ventricular dysfunction who may be at risk for late CHF,

setting the stage for potential interventions to prevent the progression to clinical CHF.[40,41] The risk of anthracycline-related cardiomyopathy is modified by younger age (< 5 years) at exposure, female gender, pre-existing heart disease, and concomitant mediastinal irradiation.[39,42] Clinical CHF is associated with poor prognosis; 5-year overall survival rates are reported to be less than 50%.[43]

It is increasingly evident that well-recognized clinical and therapeutic risk factors may not fully explain the wide inter-individual variability in susceptibility to therapy-related CHF. Significant cardiotoxicity has been reported at cumulative doses of less than 250 mg/m^2 in some patients,[44] whereas doses that exceed 1000 mg/m^2 have been tolerated without long-term sequelae by some.[45] Investigators have begun examining the role of genetic susceptibility in the development of therapy-related CHF. Using a candidate gene approach, studies have identified genetic polymorphisms involved in metabolism of anthracyclines, the myocardial response to the drug, as well as others thought to play a role in susceptibility to *de novo* disease, which could place survivors at increased risk for therapy-related CHF.[46,47] A recent report from the CCSS[47] a trend towards an association between a polymorphism in carboxyl reductase 3, *CBR3* V244M and risk of CHF (OR = 8.16, P = 0.056 for G/G vs. A/A; OR = 5.44, P = 0.09 for G/A vs. A/A), suggesting that functional *CBR3* V244M polymorphism may impact the risk of anthracycline-related CHF by modulating the intracardiac formation of cardiotoxic anthracycline alcohol metabolites.

Mediastinal radiotherapy has been implicated in the development of constrictive pericarditis, cardiomyopathy, valvular heart disease, coronary artery disease, and conduction abnormalities.[38] Exposure to mediastinal radiation is associated with valvular fibrosis or insufficiency in 40% to 60% of HL survivors, whereas conduction defects are present in as many as 75%.[48] Although clinically evident CHF is rare following mediastinal radiation alone; when present, it is primarily in the form of diastolic dysfunction, as opposed to systolic disease seen following anthracycline exposure.[38,48]

Coronary artery disease [26] has been reported following radiation to the mediastinum, with a cumulative risk of 21% at 20 years.[49] The morphologic changes in radiation-induced vascular disease are similar to those observed in spontaneous atherosclerosis. Coronary ostia and left anterior descending artery are frequently involved. The exact mechanism by which radiation produces atherosclerosis is not well understood, but it is likely that endothelial injury secondary to radiation initiates the process. However, significant radiation-associated CAD rarely occurs in the absence of other cardiovascular risk factors such as dyslipidemia, hypertension, and obesity.[50]

The pericardium is one of the most commonly affected structures of the heart after radiotherapy. Patients can present with chronic pericardial effusions, constrictive pericarditis, or sometimes with chronic effusions in association with pancarditis.[49] Although total-heart radiation at a dose of 40 Gy appears to be the usual threshold, pericarditis has been reported following doses as low as 15 Gy, even in the absence of radiomimetic chemotherapy.[49]

Prevention of cardiotoxicity is currently being intensively explored. Analogs of doxorubicin and daunomycin and liposomal anthracyclines, with a potential for decreased cardiotoxicity while retaining equivalent antitumor activity have been studied.[37] Dexrazoxane, a chelator of intracellular iron, has been shown to be the most promising cardioprotectant for use in conjunction with anthracyclines.[42] In a randomized trial of children diagnosed with ALL, those who received dexrazoxane prior to doxorubicin were significantly less likely to have cardiac injury during treatment, as measured by cardiac troponin levels.[51] Several trials have since shown that it is possible to use dexrazoxane to prevent cardiomyopathy without compromising disease-related outcome.[42] The role of pharmacologic intervention for prevention of CHF in asymptomatic survivors with left ventricular dysfunction is less well-studied. A randomized placebo-controlled study using angiotensin-converting enzyme (ACE) inhibitors demonstrated that while ACE-inhibitors did not prevent decline in ventricular function, they were able to provide some respite in the form of afterload reduction.[52]

Recommendations for Screening and Follow-up

Patients exposed to anthracyclines need ongoing monitoring for late-onset cardiomyopathy using serial noninvasive testing (echocardiogram) and physical examination.[41] The frequency of echocardiograms can range from yearly to every 5 years, depending on cumulative anthracycline dose, age at exposure, and treatment with mediastinal radiation. Aerobic exercise is generally safe and should be encouraged for most patients. However, intensive isometric activities (i.e.,: heavy weight lifting, wrestling) should be avoided. Pregnant women previously treated with anthracyclines should be closely monitored, as changes in volume during the third trimester could add significant stress to a potentially compromised myocardium. In addition to monitoring for cardiomyopathy, survivors who received radiation involving the heart field also need monitoring for potential early-onset atherosclerosis. Heart-healthy lifestyles should be encouraged for all survivors, including implementation of a regular exercise program, dietary recommendations, as well as screening for dyslipidemia. Additional specific recommendations for monitoring, based on age and therapeutic exposure, are delineated within the COG *Long-Term Follow-Up Guidelines* available at www.survivorshipguidelines.org.

PULMONARY FUNCTION

Lungs are particularly susceptible to radiation-induced injury. Radiation-related complications such as pulmonary fibrosis and pneumonitis are most often seen in patients with malignant diseases of the chest, notably HL and solid tumors with pulmonary metastases such as in Wilms tumor and Ewing sarcoma. Asymptomatic abnormal radiographic findings or restrictive changes in pulmonary function testing have been reported in greater than 30% of patients who received radiation to the lungs.[53,54] These changes can be detected months to years after completion of therapy, and are most prevalent in individuals with a history of pneumonitis as an acute complication of therapy. The incidence and severity of radiation-associated lung damage is related to the total dose, fractionation of that dose, type of radiation, total volume of lung irradiated, and age at exposure.[53,54]

Radiation-related pulmonary injury is likely mediated by cytokines, which stimulate septal fibroblasts, increasing collagen production, resulting in pulmonary fibrosis.[55] The basis for respiratory damage in young children appears to be different from that in the adult or adolescent, and is likely because of resulting chest wall hypoplasia and compromised lung parenchymal growth. As many as 30% of children with Wilms tumor treated with bilateral pulmonary irradiation for metastatic disease are reported to have dyspnea on exertion and radiographic evidence of interstitial and pleural thickening 7 to 14 years after completion of therapy.[19] In contrast to older children and adults, these findings in younger children are consistent with a proportionate interference with growth of the lungs and chest wall. The incidence of radiation-induced late pulmonary toxicity has dramatically decreased

in the past decade secondary to refined radiation therapy techniques.[56]

Certain chemotherapeutic agents can also compromise pulmonary function.[57] Bleomycin toxicity is the prototype for chemotherapy-related lung injury. Clinically apparent bleomycin pneumonopathy (interstitial pneumonitis and pulmonary fibrosis) is more frequent in older adolescents and adults.[58] The chronic lung toxicity usually follows persistence or progression of abnormalities which develop within 3 months of completion of therapy. Dose-dependent toxicity occurs at treatment doses greater than 400 units, and can be exacerbated by concurrent or previous radiation therapy to the mediastinum.[57] Above this dose, 10% of adult patients experience fibrosis;[57] data are limited for such high drug doses in children because few are exposed.

As with bleomycin, pulmonary toxicity associated with alkylating agents such as carmustine (BCNU) and lomustine (CCNU) is dose-related. Cumulative BCNU doses exceeding 1,500 mg/m^2 can result in symptomatic lung fibrosis and restrictive disease in more than 50% of patients.[57] Pulmonary fibrosis has also been observed in 16% to 40% of HCT recipients treated with cytotoxic conditioning agents including BCNU at doses of 500 to 600 mg/m^2; the incidence of fibrosis declines when doses are limited to less than 300 to 450 mg/m^2.[59]

Cyclophosphamide can cause delayed-onset pulmonary fibrosis with severe restrictive lung disease.[60] Melphalan and busulfan are also known to cause pulmonary fibrosis in a dose-related manner. Busulfan toxicity is most predictable in doses exceeding 500 mg and may be associated with a progressive, potentially fatal restrictive lung disease, characterized by diffuse interstitial fibrosis and bronchopulmonary dysplasia.[57,60]

Pulmonary complications are a leading cause of morbidity and mortality in long-term HCT survivors, where both restrictive and obstructive lung disease can significantly complicate the medical management of these survivors.[61,62] The intensity of therapy in patients undergoing HCT and the additive effects of previous therapies magnify the risk. Patients who received unfractionated, single dose, TBI as part of their conditioning regimen have the highest risk for late pulmonary complications. Fractionated TBI has reduced the risk for many of these complications.[62] Obliterative bronchiolitis (BO), a chronic, irreversible, obstructive lung disease can be diagnosed months to years after transplantation.[63] Chest radiographs show hyperinflation, and chest CT scans demonstrate parenchymal hypoattenuation and air trapping.[63,64] The treatment of BO remains a challenge; many patients with BO succumb to their pulmonary disease.[61]

Recommendations for Screening and Follow-up

Monitoring for pulmonary dysfunction in childhood cancer survivors includes assessment of symptoms such as chronic cough or dyspnea on annual follow-up. Risks of smoking and exposure to secondhand smoke should be discussed with all patients. The best approach to chronic pulmonary toxicity of anticancer therapy is preventive and includes respecting cumulative dosage restrictions of bleomycin and alkylators, limiting radiation dosage and port sizes, and avoidance of primary or secondhand smoke. Pulmonary function tests and chest x-ray are recommended as a baseline upon entry into long-term follow-up for patients at risk, repeated as clinically indicated in symptomatic patients and in those with subclinical abnormalities identified on screening evaluation. Repeat evaluation should also be considered for at-risk patients prior to general anesthesia. Influenza and pneumococcal vaccines are encouraged in survivors at risk for pulmonary compromise.

GENITOURINARY ABNORMALITIES

Renal

Long-term renal complications in childhood cancer survivors can occur as a result of chemotherapy (cisplatin, carboplatin, ifosfamide, and methotrexate), radiation or surgery. Chemotherapy-induced nephrotoxicity can manifest as acute irreversible renal failure, slow progressive chronic renal failure, or renal tubular dysfunction.[65] Clinical manifestations of renal injury include hypertension, proteinuria, and varying degrees of renal insufficiency.[65,66] Radiation nephropathy can present with many of the clinical symptoms seen in chemotherapy-related nephrotoxicity, whereas survivors who have undergone nephrectomy are at risk for additional complication such as hyperfiltration injury.[65]

Ifosfamide nephrotoxicity typically manifests as proximal tubular dysfunction, and, less often, as decreased glomerular filtration rate (GFR).[67,68] It is estimated that approximately 30% of ifosfamide-treated children develop a persistent nephropathy, and 5% have clinically significant Fanconi renal syndrome (hypokalemia, hypophosphatemia, glucosuria, proteinuria, renal tubular acidosis, and rickets).[69] Risk factors for chronic nephrotoxicity include higher cumulative dose ($\geq$ 60 gm/m^2), young age (< 5 years) at treatment, concurrent or previous platinum-based therapy, irradiation involving the kidneys at a dose exceeding 15 Gy, and unilateral nephrectomy.[69,70]

Cisplatin can damage the glomerulus and distal renal tubules, potentially causing diminished GFR and electrolyte wasting, most commonly involving magnesium, calcium, potassium, and sodium.[65] Hypomagnesemia may persist in some patients, and can be severe enough to require magnesium supplementation.[71] It is estimated that up to 50% of patients remain hypomagnesemic, and the risk is greatest for those exposed to other nephrotoxic agents such as ifosfamide.[65]

Irradiation to the kidney can result in radiation nephritis or nephropathy after a latent period of 3 to 12 months. Doses in excess of 20 Gy can result in significant nephropathy.[65] The prevalence of renal insufficiency, as defined by hypertension, approached 10% in one study of 5-year Wilms tumor survivors.[70]

Recommendations for Screening and Follow-up

Surveillance in at risk survivors should include monitoring of serum creatinine, blood urea nitrogen, and serum chemistries at baseline at entry into long-term follow-up; and should be repeated as clinically indicated. Urinalysis and measurement of blood pressure should be performed at baseline and annually thereafter. Ongoing management may include electrolyte replacement, treatment of hypertension, and avoidance of further nephrotoxic agents. In children with a history of radiation to the renal artery who develop hypertension, radiologic studies for stenosis of the renal artery should be ordered and, if stenosis is present, surgical correction should be undertaken. Patients with a history of nephrectomy should be counseled regarding the importance of protecting the remaining single kidney. These patients should be cautioned to avoid nephrotoxic agents (e.g., ibuprofen, aminoglycosides); to maintain normal weight; to seek early intervention for urinary tract infections; and to consult with their physician prior to participating in contact sports.

Bladder

Well-recognized complications involving the bladder include hemorrhagic cystitis, bladder fibrosis, and neurogenic bladder. Hemorrhagic cystitis is a condition in which irritation of the lining of the bladder leads to exposure of the submucosal blood vessels and bleeding.[72,73] Treatment with alkylating agents such as cyclophosphamide, ifosfamide, and radiation has been implicated in the development of HC.[72,73] Patients who receive both chemotherapy and radiation are at highest risk.[72] Patients may report urinary urgency, frequency, dysuria, and suprapubic pain. Although hemorrhagic cystitis typically occurs during therapy, it may become a chronic recurring problem after completion of therapy. The incidence of HC has been reported to be 15% in Ewing sarcoma patients treated with cyclophosphamide.[73] Uroprophylaxis with 2-mercaptoethane (mesna)[74] in conjunction with cyclophosphamide administration has decreased the incidence of HC; mesna administration is now the standard of care for protocols utilizing high-dose cyclophosphamide and ifosfamide.

Radiation to the pelvis or bladder can result in fibrosis and scarring, with resultant decreased bladder capacity and predisposition to urinary tract infections.[73] Changes in bladder function with diminished bladder compliance are noted within 6 to 9 months after irradiation and correlate with radiation dose.[75] Patients exposed to radiation dose greater than 45 Gy to the whole bladder are at highest risk for late fibrosis and contractures.[73]

Surgery involving the lower genitourinary tract has the potential to impair normal function of the bladder and normal voiding mechanisms. Myogenic and neurogenic impairment may occur as a result of bladder or peripheral nerve injury during surgery to remove portions of the bladder or adjacent pelvic tumors.[76,77] In addition, neural innervation to the bladder can be compromised if there is injury to the central nervous system or at the spinal cord level, resulting in inability to void and/or incontinence.[73] In patients with bladder rhabdomyosarcoma, partial cystectomy can affect bladder function by reducing bladder volume. The extent of resection generally predicts severity of bladder function compromise.[73,77]

Recommendations for Screening and Follow-up

Evaluation of bladder function in at-risk patients should begin with a careful history with an emphasis on voiding pattern, characterization of urinary stream, and degree of incontinence. Survivors treated with cyclophosphamide should undergo annual urinalysis screen for microscopic hematuria. Patients with culture-negative microscopic hematuria (defined as >5 red blood cells/high power field on at least 2 occasions) and abnormal ultrasound and/or abnormal calcium/creatinine ratio should be referred to a nephrologist for further evaluation. Those with culture-negative macroscopic hematuria or those with evidence of bladder dysfunction should receive urologic evaluation.

GASTROINTESTINAL FUNCTION

Enteritis and fibrosis are the most common abnormalities of the gastrointestinal tract observed in long-term survivors of cancer. These can arise as late complications of radiation to any site from the esophagus to the rectum and have been associated with adhesions or stricture formation, sometimes with obstruction, ulcers, fistulae, and chronic enterocolitis or incontinence.[78,79] The frequency depends on radiation dose. The stomach and small intestine appear to be more radiation sensitive than the colon or rectum.[80] Overall, the prevalence of fibrosis after 40 to 50 Gy is 5% and as high as 36% when radiation dose exceeds 60 Gy.[81] Intestinal fibrosis usually manifests itself within 5 years, but strictures have developed as late as 20 years after treatment.[70]

Chronic liver toxicity has been reported in survivors treated with now obsolete doses of radiation to the liver (>20 Gy).[82] In addition, chemotherapy even in the absence of radiation may be a late cause of chronic hepatopathy. With intermediate doses of intravenous methotrexate, the prevalence of fibrosis has been less than 5%.[83] In general, methotrexate-related hepatic fibrosis stabilizes or resolves after discontinuation of the drug.

Veno-occlusive disease, an often fatal, but sometimes reversible acute complication of conventional therapy, has been reported in patients treated with 6-thioguanine (6-TG) as part of maintenance therapy for ALL.[84] There is emerging evidence that patients treated with 6-TG remain at risk for chronic hepatotoxicity and portal hypertension months to years after completion of therapy, regardless of whether VOD occurred as an acute complication of therapy.[85]

Viral hepatitis, most often related to transfusion of blood products prior to 1992, may be another cause of chronic liver disease in long-term survivors. In a retrospective series of 658 survivors of childhood cancer treated prior to routine screening of blood products, 117 (17.8%) were seropositive for hepatitis C.[86] A third of the long-term survivors of pediatric leukemia, who received an HCT prior to 1991 are estimated to be seropositive for hepatitis B or C, and hepatitis C is a major risk factor for late onset of cirrhosis.[86]

Recommendations for Screening and Follow-up

Because the confirmatory diagnosis of cirrhosis requires an invasive procedure such as a liver biopsy, and cannot always be identified by abnormalities in liver function or in the physical examination, it has been difficult to suggest screening guidelines for early identification. Patients at risk for gastrointestinal complications should be monitored by history or physical examination for hepatomegaly, icterus, and malabsorption. For those with a history of acute hepatotoxicity during therapy or those treated with hepatectomy, 6-TG, or with hepatic radiation (or right-sided abdominal irradiation as sometimes used in Wilms tumor), potential consequences of excessive alcohol use and other high-risk behaviors should be emphasized. In such patients, a post-treatment baseline screen including transaminase and bilirubin levels should be considered. Prothrombin time and serum albumin for evaluation of liver synthetic function may be indicated. If persistent abnormalities are detected, further evaluation should be in collaboration with a gastroenterologist. The Centers for Disease Control (CDC) now recommend hepatitis C screening for patients transfused or transplanted before 1992, even when transaminase levels are normal.[87] Hepatitis A and B testing should be performed in nonimmunized patients with abnormal liver function tests. Routine liver scans or biopsies are not recommended.

THYROID ABNORMALITIES

Complications involving the thyroid gland include hypothyroidism (primary or central), hyperthyroidism, and thyroid tumors (benign or malignant). These complications are primarily seen in patients treated with radiation to fields involving the thyroid gland (e.g., cranial, naso- or oropharyngeal, cervical, supraclavicular, mantle, and total body).[88] Risk factors include female gender, young age at treatment, and radiation dose.[88,89] The risk for hypothyroidism or thyroid nodules is especially high for those treated with radiation doses in excess of 20 Gy.[89] The risk of thyroid malignancies demonstrates a linear relation with radiation dose up to 29 Gy, beyond which the risk declines.[90] Shielding of the thyroid gland during irradiation, elimination of radiation, or the use of lower doses and avoidance of the concurrent use of radiation and iodide-containing contrast materials should help decrease the incidence of thyroid abnormalities.

Hodgkin lymphoma (HL) survivors have been reported to be at a 17-fold increased risk of hypothyroidism when compared with a sibling comparison group.[89] Although the risk is highest in the first five years after radiation, incident cases have been observed for up to 20 years after radiation. The cumulative incidence of developing hypothyroidism is 30% at 20 years following a radiation dose of 35 to 45 Gy to the thyroid gland; increasing to 50% for doses exceeding 45 Gy. In comparison, for patients treated with chemotherapy alone, the cumulative incidence of hypothyroidism is reported to be 7.6%, and is comparable to the sibling comparison group.

Central hypothyroidism in the setting of cranial radiation is primarily a result of deficiency of thyrotropin-releasing hormone (hypothalamic) and thyroid stimulating hormone (pituitary) in children who have received greater than 40 Gy of radiation.[91] The risk of central hypothyroidism with lower doses of cranial radiation, as seen in patients with ALL is very low.[88]

Hyperthyroidism is observed in 5% of patients after radiation therapy for HL[89,92] or after TBI for HCT.[93,94] The symptoms are similar to those observed in Grave's disease, that is, diffusely enlarged thyroid gland, elevated thyroid hormone levels in conjunction with suppression of thyroid-stimulating hormone, increased uptake of radioactive iodine, and development of thyroid autoantibodies.[93]

Recommendations for Screening and Follow-up

The diagnostic evaluation of thyroid dysfunction relies on history and physical examination, as well as annual thyroid function tests (free thyroxine, thyroid stimulating hormone). Survivors with abnormalities on the history and physical examination or screening tests should be referred to an endocrinologist for hormone replacement therapy.

GONADAL FUNCTION

Male Patients

All therapeutic modalities (radiation, surgery, and chemotherapy) can cause both germ (Sertoli) cell depletion as well as abnormalities of gonadal endocrine function (Leydig cells) among male cancer survivors. Production of mature sperm cells starts at age 12 to 14 years (spermarche), after which new spermatozoa are produced through life. Leydig cells produce testosterone in response to luteinizing hormone (LH); testosterone along with follicle-stimulating hormone (FSH) stimulates Sertoli cells, which provide support for spermatogenesis. The germinal epithelium has a high mitotic rate and is more sensitive to radiation and cytotoxic effects of chemotherapy than the testosterone-producing Leydig cells. Thus, unlike in females, it is possible to have impaired germ cell function (azoospermia) without evidence of gonadal endocrine dysfunction in males.

Radiation to the testes is known to result in germinal loss with decrease in testicular volume and sperm production, and increase in FSH. Radiation-related effects are dose-dependent, and can typically be seen following fractionated exposures of 0.1 to 6 Gy.[95] At doses of 1 to 3 Gy, azoospermia may be reversible; at doses of 3 to 6 Gy, azoospermia may persist for at least 3 to 5 years and is much less likely to reverse; doses greater than 6 Gy cause irreversible injury.[88,96] Azoospermia following HCT occurs in large part as a result of chemotherapy. However, older transplantation strategies such as use of unfractionated TBI at a single dose of 10 Gy resulted in infertility in nearly all patients.[88] Data regarding germ cell function in pre-pubertal boys treated with radiation alone is limited, although there is evidence that pre-pubertal testicular germ cells may be more radiosensitive than those exposed to radiation following completion of spermarche.[97]

Chemotherapy-related germ cell injury primarily occurs following treatment with alkylating agents, heavy metals, and nonclassic alkylators such as procarbazine and dacarbazine. Alkylating agents such as busulfan, procarbazine, and mechlorethamine have been shown to be particularly gonadotoxic.[98] Many of these agents decrease spermatogenesis in a dose-dependent manner, regardless of pubertal status at the time of exposure. Gonadal injury has been reported to be reversible in up to 70% of patients after therapy-free intervals of several years following cumulative cyclophosphamide doses lower than 7.5 gm/m^2 (or 200 mg/kg, as used in HCT).[99] Doses exceeding 7.5 gm/m^2 result in prolonged (2 to 4 years), and in some cases, permanent azoospermia.[98,99] Among pubertal or adult males treated for HL, exposure to five or more cycles of mechlorethamine, vincristine, prednisone, and procarbazine (MOPP) has been associated with prolonged or permanent azoospermia in up to 80% to 100% of survivors.[100,101] Patients treated with doxorubicin, bleomycin, vinblastine, and dacarbazine (ABVD) have a lower prevalence of azoospermia (36% to 54%), and a higher likelihood of recovery (up to 100%) when compared to patients exposed to MOPP-based therapy.[102]

Gonadal endocrine dysfunction occurs less frequently in males than females. Preservation of Leydig function in the setting of abnormal germ cell function in long-term male survivors is not uncommon. Radiation doses required to damage Leydig cells are higher than those toxic to germ cells. As summarized by Sklar,[103] radiation-related Leydig cell damage is dose-dependent and inversely related to age at treatment. Boys treated prepubertally or peripubertally with radiation doses exceeding 20 Gy for testicular leukemia, in addition to having significant germ cell depletion, are at high risk of delayed sexual maturation associated with decreased testosterone levels, despite high LH levels.[103] Adolescent and young adult males are able to tolerate fractionated doses greater than 30 Gy to the testes, with only 50% developing Leydig cell failure. Administration of fractionated doses of less than 12 Gy to the prepubertal testis is compatible with normal pubertal maturation in most patients, although often at the expense of compensated Leydig cell failure (normal testosterone levels with elevated LH levels).[103,104]

The effects of surgery on the gonads include impotence or retrograde ejaculation after bilateral retroperitoneal lymph node dissection or partial or complete pelvic exenteration. In patients with brain tumors involving the hypothalamus or pituitary, surgical resection may cause secondary hypogonadism.[105] Hydroceles have been seen in survivors of Wilms tumor[106] and paratesticular rhabdomyosarcoma[78] after surgery or radiation therapy.

The gonadal toxicities listed in this section, although not life-threatening, are of serious concern to patients and their families, particularly in the case of young men who have not already had children at the time of diagnosis. This concern has popularized pre-treatment sperm banking. Cryopreserved semen from adults has produced normal children.[107] Despite the fact that patients with HL and primary testicular cancer may have lower-than-expected sperm counts and decreased sperm motility at the time of diagnosis,[108] discussion of sperm banking is strongly encouraged. The use of chemotherapeutic regimens such as ABVD that may be less toxic but as effective, as well as refinement of radiation techniques, has been advocated.

Recommendations for Screening and Follow-up

Screening for impairment in gonadal function with an age-appropriate history, Tanner staging, with specific attention to problems with libido, impotence, or fertility and examination for gynecomastia, should be part of the follow-up of all male survivors. Hormonal evaluation, including at least a single measurement of serum LH, FSH, and testosterone levels, has been recommended as a baseline at age 11 years and in boys whose puberty appears to be delayed. Male patients at risk of infertility may request semen analysis when honest and sensitive discussions of fertility are part of the follow-up visit. When abnormalities in testicular function are detected, close cooperation with an endocrinologist is essential in planning hormone replacement therapy or in monitoring patients for spontaneous recovery. When no abnormalities are noted on history and physical examination but sexual maturity has not been completed, these studies should be repeated every 1 to 2 years. Conversely, reminders about contraception should be given in light of the potential for recovery of spermatogenesis and inter-patient variations in gonadal toxicity.

Female Patients

In contrast to males, in females germ cell failure and loss of ovarian endocrine function are synchronous. Depending on the extent of damage to the ovaries, two forms of premature ovarian failure have been described. Survivors who lose ovarian function during cancer treatment or shortly thereafter are classified as having premature ovarian failure (POF). Some survivors are able to retain ovarian function after the completion of therapy yet will experience menopause before 40 years of age.[109,110] Older age at treatment, exposure to abdominal or pelvic radiation, and chemotherapy with alkylating agents have been associated with increased risk of ovarian failure in female cancer survivors.[103,109,110]

Prepubertal ovaries are relatively radioresistant, and despite higher doses of radiation (12 to 50 Gy), POF was reported in only 68% of patients treated at a mean age of 6.9 years.[111] In one series, only 23% of prepubertal and adolescent girls in whom at least one ovary was at the edge of the radiation field (and therefore had received a dose of 0.9 to 10 Gy) had ovarian failure.[109,112] Unfractionated TBI (10 Gy) has been associated with primary amenorrhea and absent secondary sexual characteristics in most patients.[93] Patient age at the time of TBI appears to be critical in determining outcome of ovarian function.[93] Approximately 50% of prepubertal girls given conventional fractionated TBI will enter puberty spontaneously and achieve menarche at a normal age. On the other hand, ovarian failure is seen in nearly all who are older than 10 years at TBI.[113]

Ovarian failure has also been associated with chemotherapy. Although the morbidity is less than in male survivors, single alkylating agents (cyclophosphamide, busulfan, nitrogen mustard) and MOPP are the best-described agents.[103,110] As with radiation therapy, chemotherapy results in dose- and age-dependent toxicity. Women older than 40 years may develop amenorrhea with as little as one to four cycles of MOPP.[114] In contrast, 30% of women less than 35 years of age require 3 to 12 cycles to become amenorrheic. Measurement of serum anti-Müllerian hormone and inhibin levels, and sonographic measure of ovarian size, suggest that subclinical abnormalities of ovarian function may occur despite normal menses and gonadotropin levels.[115] After myeloablative doses of alkylating agents, permanent ovarian failure can be expected at all ages.[116]

There is increasing evidence that many females who do not develop amenorrhea following exposure to radiation to the ovaries and/or alkylators therapy remain at risk for eventually developing POF, with cessation of hormone production and infertility.[109] Many females who develop these symptoms are at increased risk of developing a variety of adverse health-related outcomes, including osteoporosis, cardiovascular diseases, and psychosexual dysfunction. In the CCSS cohort, female survivors had a greater than 13-fold risk of developing nonsurgical premature menopause when compared to the female sibling comparison group.[109] Risk factors included older attained age, exposure to increasing doses of radiation to the ovaries, increasing alkylating agent score, and a diagnosis of HL. For patients treated with alkylating agents plus abdominal-pelvic radiation, cumulative incidence of nonsurgical premature menopause approached 30%.[117] Unilateral oophorectomy does not appear to compromise gonadal function,[118] although long-term follow-up data regarding onset of menopause have not been reported.

In an attempt to prevent gonadal failure, some investigators have explored suppression of ovulation with a lack of convincing results. Harvesting and freezing of ova prior to cancer treatment is currently under investigation.[107,119]

Recommendations for Screening and Follow-up

The diagnostic evaluation of ovarian dysfunction rests on history (primary or secondary amenorrhea, menstrual irregularity, and pregnancies or difficulties in becoming pregnant), Tanner staging, and serum gonadotropin and estradiol levels. In the absence of clinical evidence of puberty (menarche, development of secondary sexual characteristics), baseline studies should be obtained at the expected time of onset of puberty, to assess the need for hormone therapy to induce puberty. Furthermore, because young women may progress to POF, they should have ongoing follow-up. Survivors with concerns regarding fertility are urged to seek consultation with reproductive endocrinologists.

Pregnancy Outcomes

For survivors who are fertile after anticancer therapy, concerns remain about the ability to have normal pregnancies and healthy children. Abnormal outcomes appear to vary with the therapeutic regimen and, especially, with timing of the pregnancy with respect to drug exposure. Teratogenicity, by definition, is limited to exposure to therapeutic agents during the first trimester of the embryo and fetus. A detailed summary of the effects of anticancer agents administered during pregnancy is reported elsewhere.[120] Whether therapy completed before pregnancy is a risk to subsequent offspring, is a problem more relevant to the long-term survivor of childhood anticancer therapy. As previously reviewed,[120] numerous reports have suggested that intensive chemotherapy completed before pregnancy, including myeloablative chemotherapy prior to HCT, is compatible with normal offspring. A recent report of 4,029 pregnancies in 1,915 female survivors of childhood cancer, did not identify excess adverse pregnancy outcomes.[109] A companion study of 2,323 pregnancies in partners of 1,427 male survivors identified 69% live births, 1% stillbirths, 13% miscarriages, and 13% abortions (5% of outcomes were not accounted for).[121] The probability of a pregnancy ending in a live birth was significantly less than that for partners of male sibling comparison group.

Radiation involving the pelvis is more likely than chemotherapy to result in pregnancy-related complications. Reports document an increased risk of perinatal death, prematurity, and low birth weight in the offspring of female long-term survivors. Malposition of the fetus, early or threatened labor, birth weight less than 2500 g, and gestation of less than 36 weeks correlate with radiation in a dose-related manner.[122]

The possibility of mutagenic (as opposed to teratogenic) effects of anticancer therapy also has been raised. One cytogenetic study showed nonclonal chromosomal abnormalities in peripheral blood lymphocytes of long-term survivors of childhood ALL at a median of 7 years after therapy, a finding suggesting that genetic damage can be sustained.[123] However, accumulating studies of several thousands of offspring of long-term survivors who had been treated during childhood or adolescence with chemotherapy with or without radiation therapy have failed to demonstrate an increased overall risk of childhood cancer in offspring of childhood cancer survivors.[124,125]

Patients who desire to have children after completion of therapy may require care in high-risk obstetrical clinics, especially those who have received abdominal or pelvic irradiation. Because much remains unknown about the problems of children born to survivors of childhood cancer, long-term general follow-up should be emphasized.

GROWTH

Decreased linear growth is a common problem during therapy in children with cancer. Although catch-up growth may occur, such that the premorbid growth status is regained, in some instances short stature is permanent or even progressive. Severe growth retardation, defined as a standing height below the fifth percentile, has been observed in as many as 30% to 35% of survivors of childhood brain tumors[126] and in 10% to 15% of patients treated with some antileukemia regimens.[127,128]

One major risk factor for short stature is whole-brain irradiation. Severe growth retardation is seen in more than 50% of patients with brain tumors, when radiation doses exceed 30 Gy to the hypothalamus or pituitary gland.[126] Growth retardation after 18 or 24 Gy, as used in children with ALL, is less frequent,[127,129] although survivors of ALL treated with 24 Gy of cranial irradiation have a decrease in median height of about 5 to 10 cm.[130,131] The effects of cranial irradiation are age-related, and children younger than 5 years at therapy are particularly susceptible.

The precise mechanism by which cranial irradiation induces short stature is not clear. Doses as low as 24 Gy have caused growth hormone deficiency, as indicated by uniform although sometimes transient, blunting of spontaneous growth hormone pulses.[132] However, other biochemical evidence of growth hormone deficiency, including low plasma insulin-like growth factor 1 (IGF-1 [somatomedin C]) levels and blunted growth hormone responses to different provocative stimuli, has varied.[133] Early onset of puberty in girls with ALL, also reported as a consequence of cranial irradiation may contribute to loss of final height.

Direct inhibition of vertebral growth by spinal irradiation also contributes to short stature. This change is seen most commonly in patients with brain tumors whose entire spinal columns have received doses in excess of 35 Gy.[134–136] Nearly 30% of children with ALL who received 12 Gy of abdominal irradiation in addition to 18 to 24 Gy of craniospinal irradiation had standing heights less than the fifth percentile.[130] This result may have been due to irradiation of the gonads or thyroid, or to scatter radiation to the femoral heads. When lower doses (10 to 25 Gy) are given to part or all of the spine, patients, although not necessarily short, have reduced sitting heights (measured from crown to rump).[134,137] This problem has been seen particularly in children who are either younger than 6 years of age or who are undergoing their adolescent growth spurt at the time of radiation therapy.

The long-term effects on height of TBI are well described.[138] After 10 Gy given as a single fraction, long-term, severe decreases in growth rates appear in most children. Fractionation of TBI appears to decrease growth retardation. The pathogenesis of short stature in these children includes factors other than radiation, notably GvHD and its management.

In contrast to the effects of radiation, when chemotherapy is given alone, growth retardation is usually temporary and patients catch up with their peers. Some chemotherapeutic agents such as high-dose prednisone and methotrexate appear to mediate this effect by direct inhibition on bone growth. Nonetheless, growth hormone deficiency and short stature have been reported in some patients following chemotherapy alone.[127,139]

Current approaches to cancer therapy in children include attempts to spare adverse effects on growth. Leukemia protocols are attempting to use high-dose methotrexate, cytosine arabinoside, or both, or intrathecal chemotherapy alone in lieu of radiation for CNS prophylaxis (see Chapter 19). Hyperfractionation schedules for radiation therapy and chemotherapy-only regimens are being implemented for treatment of brain tumors and as conditioning regimens for HCT. Whether these changes will permit long-term survivors to have normal growth remains to be seen.

Recommendations for Screening and Follow-up

Monitoring long-term survivors for growth problems relies on the use of standardized curves available online at www.cdc.gov/growthcharts. Because single values for heights and weights are unreliable for children, serial measurements to establish each child's pattern of growth are recommended. Endocrine consultation may be indicated for children whose height crosses percentiles; is less than the third percentile; or whose growth velocity is less than 4 to 5 cm per year. Treatment with growth hormone prior to closure of epiphyses in patients with documented growth hormone deficiency usually results in near normalization of final height, unless the spinal axis has also been irradiated.

OBESITY

Obesity, as measured by weight or body mass index (BMI), is being increasingly recognized as a late sequela in children with ALL;[140,141] the reported prevalence of obesity in survivors ranges from 11% to 40%.[140,141] Obesity developing during adolescence or young adulthood is strongly associated with the subsequent development of health problems in adulthood, such as adult-onset diabetes mellitus, hypertension, dyslipidemia, cardiovascular disease, osteoarthritis, and possibly breast and colon cancer.[142] ALL survivors are at the highest

risk, largely as a consequence of cranial radiation. The contribution of specific chemotherapeutic agents, particularly corticosteroids to the development of obesity is unclear. Other risk factors include: higher radiation dosage (exceeding 20 Gy to the hypothalamus),[126,140] age less than 8 years at treatment, female gender,[140,142,143] higher BMI at diagnosis,[144] and medical conditions, including hypothyroidism and familial dyslipidemias.[142]

A possible mechanism of radiation-related obesity is leptin-insensitivity compounded by growth hormone deficiency that can result from radiation-mediated disruption of the hypothalamic-pituitary axis. Leptin is a hormone secreted almost exclusively by adipocytes, and it plays an important role in long-term regulation of body weight and metabolism.[145] Leptin is thought to act as a satiety signal in a feedback loop with hypothalamic centers that control feeding behavior and hunger, energy expenditure, and body temperature.

Ross and colleagues examined the potential association between the Gln223Arg polymorphism in the *LEPR* gene and risk of obesity in a large cohort of ALL survivors. Survivors with BMI $\geq$25 kg/m^2 were significantly more likely to be Arg homozygous compared with those with BMI less than 25 kg/m^2, an observation that was limited to females. The risk was especially great for Arg homozygous females who received $\geq$20 Gy CRT (OR, 6.1, 2.1–22.0). These preliminary findings support the role for the *LEPR* polymorphism in modifying risk of obesity. However, the limitation of this association to female survivors reinforces the complex nature of a likely polygenic trait.

There is emerging evidence that cancer survivors are at risk for metabolic syndrome.[146,147] Metabolic syndrome is a cluster of disorders related to insulin resistance that includes central obesity, elevated plasma glucose, dyslipidemia, hypertension, and a prothrombotic and proinflammatory state. Growth hormone deficiency has emerged as a contributor to central obesity and related metabolic disorders, including insulin resistance and dyslipidemia. Preliminary evidence indicates that long-term growth hormone deficiency may be associated with adverse cardiovascular disease and diabetes risk as a consequence of cranial irradiation.[148]

Recommendations for Screening and Follow-up

Monitoring for metabolic syndrome should encompass annual physical examination including BMI to check for obesity and associated comorbidities such as hypertension. Fasting blood glucose and lipid profile are recommended every 2 years, or more frequently if indicated, for patients who have received cranial radiation or TBI. A thorough nutritional evaluation should be conducted on all cancer survivors, and those identified to be at risk for being overweight or obese should work with a nutritionist to improve dietary choices and be encouraged to adopt a healthy lifestyle.

MUSCULOSKELETAL AND RELATED TISSUES

Functional and cosmetic disabilities involving bone, muscle, and other soft tissues are common and are reported in up to a third of survivors of various pediatric cancers, notably solid tumors. Most clinically significant problems involve bony abnormalities, such as scoliosis, atrophy or hypoplasia, avascular necrosis (AVN), and osteoporosis (bone density > 2.5 SD below mean)/ osteopenia (bone density 1 to 2.5 SD below

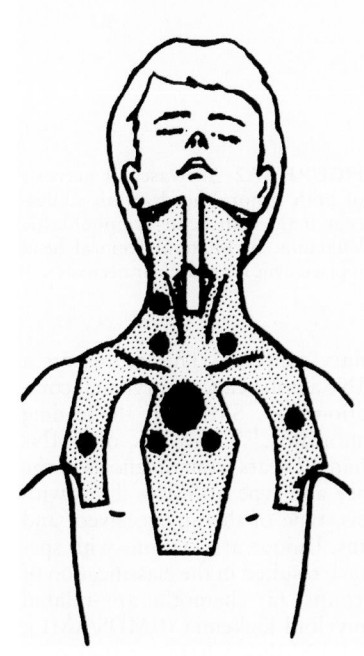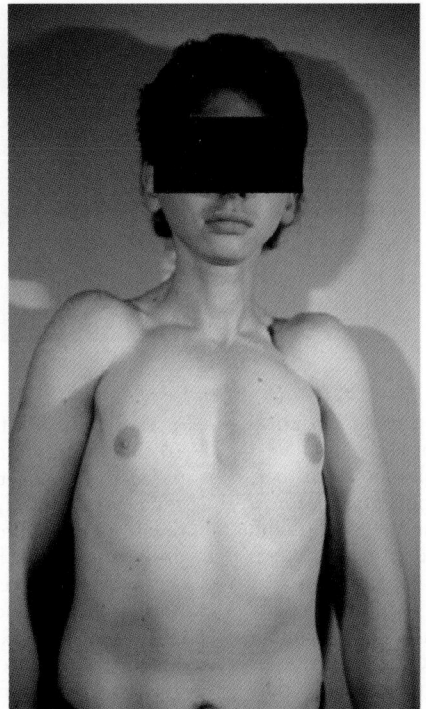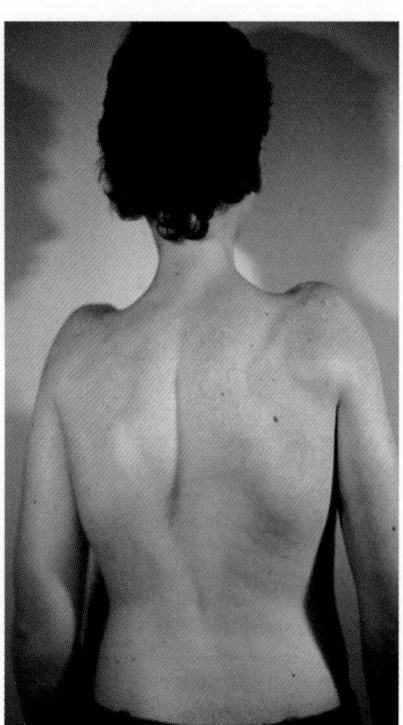

FIGURE 47.1 Growth impairment after radiation therapy.

mean). Scoliosis is a delayed consequence of radiation therapy to segments of the spinal column.[149,150] The concavity of the deformity is on the side of irradiation, and worsens during the adolescent growth spurt, irrespective of the age of the patient at radiation (Fig. 47.1). In addition, with current techniques including symmetric irradiation of the entire spine, sparing large volumes of the adjacent soft tissue, as in the treatment of medulloblastoma or as in total nodal irradiation for HL, the risk of scoliosis is low. Other factors that may contribute to the development of scoliosis include vertebral changes from metastatic tumor, laminectomy, and osteoporosis. In addition to causing scoliosis by direct effects on vertebral growth, abdominal irradiation for Wilms tumor may result in hypoplasia of the ileum and atrophy of muscle, soft tissue, and skin within the field.[70] These fibrosed tissues "act as a bow string across the vertebrae,"[151] increasing the degree of curvature. With better staging systems, the number of children requiring vertebral or paravertebral radiation therapy for Wilms tumor or rhabdomyosarcoma has decreased. Atrophy or hypoplasia has been reported to follow radiation of long bones in children with soft tissue sarcomas of an extremity and the facial skeleton.[152,153] Doses of radiation exceeding 20 Gy and involvement of epiphyses in the radiation field increase the risk. When patients have already achieved their maximum growth at the time of diagnosis, leg length discrepancy does not appear to be a significant problem even when the entire bone receives as much as 70 Gy.[154] However, soft tissue deformities and leg length discrepancy may occur following amputation or endoprostheses (discussed in Chapters 33 and 35).

Young adult survivors of childhood cancer may also have reduced bone density, as measured by DEXA scans. Although some studies have demonstrated decreased bone density at diagnosis in children with ALL, osteopenia and osteoporosis are well recognized to progress after steroid administration or radiation therapy in doses used in children with ALL, soft tissue sarcomas, or Ewing sarcoma.[155] Osteopenia in survivors

of childhood ALL, has been related to cranial irradiation.[156] Antimetabolites have been linked to decreased bone density in a dose-dependent manner, primarily during therapy with resolution once the drug has been discontinued.[155] Both genders are at equal risk for reduced bone mineral density;[155] whites are at greater risk than African-Americans.[155,157] Contributing factors include treatment-related gonadal and growth hormone failure, hypothyroidism, poor calcium intake, and increased body weight.[155]

AVN can develop during therapy, although latency periods as long as 13 years after treatment have been reported.[158] The diagnosis is made with plain radiographs, but magnetic resonance imaging (MRI) is more sensitive and can provide early detection. Estimates for the incidence of AVN vary, ranging from 1%[159] to 9%,[160] when based on clinical presentation, to nearly 15%, when based on MRI screening.[161] In the CCSS cohort,[159] cancer survivors were 6.2 times more likely than a sibling comparison to report AVN. The risk was greatest among leukemia survivors who had undergone allogeneic HCT (ALL, RR = 26.9; AML, RR = 66.5). Among individuals with nonhematologic malignancies, the greatest risk was for those with bone sarcoma (RR = 7.3).

The association between glucocorticoids and AVN is well established.[158] Dexamethasone appears to have more bone toxicity than equivalent doses of prednisone, and continuous cumulative exposure conveys higher risk.[158–160] The cumulative risk of AVN in ALL patients receiving two 21-day dexamethasone on a legacy COG trial was 23.1%.[160] Other risk factors have included older age at exposure, female gender, radiation exposure, and white race.[158] AVN most commonly involves the femoral heads (Fig. 47.2), where it may be accompanied by a slipped capital femoral epiphysis, but it has been described in virtually all locations and commonly is multifocal.

The mechanisms by which glucocorticoids cause AVN can be complex and may include suppression of osteoblasts, apoptosis of osteocytes, intra-medullary lipocyte proliferation (affecting

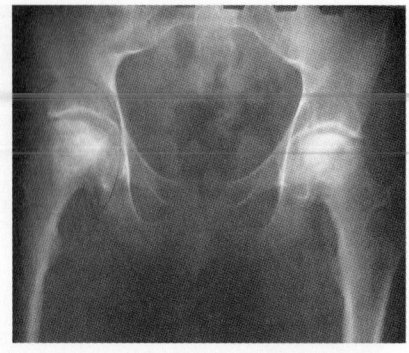
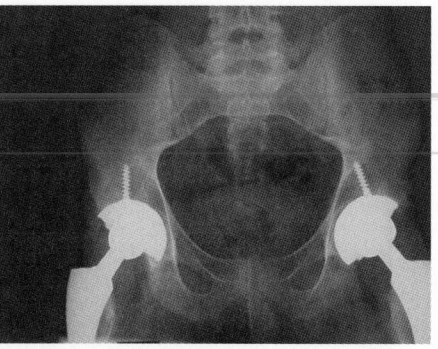

FIGURE 47.2 A: Avascular necrosis of both femoral heads in an adolescent male with acute lymphoblastic leukemia. **B:** Bilateral femoral head replacement for avascular necrosis.

sinusoidal circulation), and fat embolization to subchondral arteries.[162] This has prompted a unifying theory of "cumulative cell stress"[158] to explain the complex pathophysiology of therapy-related AVN that is based on three components: anatomic location (weight bearing), systemic illness, and glucocorticoid exposure. In this hypothesis, it is recognized that glucocorticoids play a "necessary but not sufficient" role, and that clear host-exposure differences exist that account for heterogeneity of clinical presentation. Relling[161] demonstrated that thymidylate synthase (*TYMS*) low activity 2/2 enhancer repeat genotype and vitamin D receptor Fok1 start site CC genotype were independent predictors of AVN (OR = 4.5 and 7.4, respectively). The *TYMS* 2/2 genotype is associated with low *TYMS* expression, rendering cells more susceptible to toxic effects of methotrexate. Subsequent associations with polymorphisms in the plasminogen activator inhibitor (PAI-1) gene[163] have further improved our understanding of the pathogenesis of AVN, and may be useful for the development of interventional strategies.

Recommendations for Screening and Follow-up

Detection and diagnosis of musculoskeletal and connective tissue sequelae depends largely on anticipating these issues in vulnerable hosts, on taking a careful history, and on performing a thorough physical examination. For patients at high risk for the development of scoliosis, follow-up visits may need to be scheduled every 6 months during the adolescent growth spurt. Although soft tissue or bony asymmetries may be obvious, pain or a history of fractures may be the only indication of AVN or osteoporosis. The need for diagnostic radiographs and appropriate referral in the case of clinically apparent disease is obvious. The relative benefit of surveillance radiographs of bones encompassed by radiation ports, and of bone densitometry, is less clear. However, because of progress with various interventions (including the use of calcium supplementation, calcitonin, bisphosphonates, and hormone replacement in patients with gonadal failure), a baseline DEXA or quantitative CT scan has been recommended when survivors reach 18 years of age, with repeat studies as clinically indicated.

SECOND MALIGNANT NEOPLASMS

Second malignant neoplasms (SMNs) are defined as histologically distinct malignancies developing at least 2 months after completion of the treatment for the primary malignancy. The cumulative incidence of SMNs approaches 15% at 20 years

after diagnosis of the primary cancer.[164] This represents a 10-fold increased risk of SMNs among cancer survivors, compared to the general population.[165–167] SMNs are the leading cause of nonrelapse late mortality.[168] The risk of SMNs remains elevated for more than 20 years from diagnosis of the primary cancer. The incidence and type of SMNs differ with the primary cancer diagnosis, type of therapy received, and presence of genetic conditions. Unique associations with specific therapeutic exposures have resulted in the classification of SMNs into two distinct groups: (a) chemotherapy-related myelodysplasia and acute myeloid leukemia (t-MDS/AML); and (b) radiation-related solid SMNs. Characteristics of t-MDS/AML include a short latency (< 3 years from primary cancer diagnosis) and association with alkylating agents and/or topoisomerase II inhibitors.[169] Solid SMNs have a strong and well-defined association with radiation, and are characterized by a latency that exceeds 10 years.[169] Figure 47.3 shows the risk of SMNs in a cohort of 1,380 patients diagnosed with HL and followed for a median of 17 years, depicting clearly that the risk of solid tumors continues to climb with increasing follow-up, whereas that of t-MDS/AML plateaus after 10 to 15 years.[170]

Therapy-Related Leukemia

t-MDS/AML has been reported after treatment of HL, NHL, ALL, and sarcomas, with the cumulative incidence approaching 2% at 15 years after therapy.[169,170] t-MDS/AML is a clonal disorder characterized by distinct chromosomal changes. Two types are recognized by the WHO classification: alkylating agent-related type and topoisomerase II inhibitor-related type.[171]

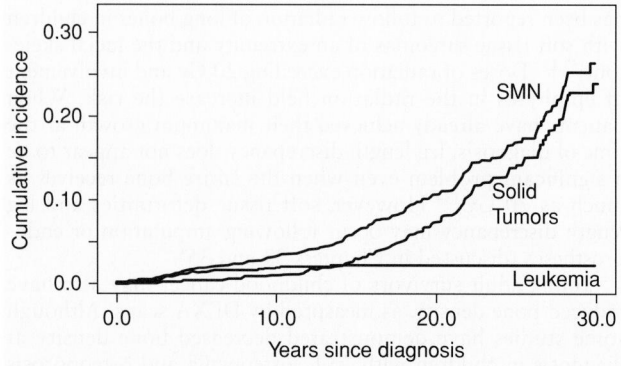

FIGURE 47.3 Cumulative incidence of subsequent malignant neoplasms after extended follow-up of childhood Hodgkin lymphoma.

Alkylating agent-related t-MDS/AML: Alkylating agents associated with t-MDS/AML include cyclophosphamide, ifosfamide, mechlorethamine, melphalan, busulfan, nitrosureas, chlorambucil, dacarbazine, and platinum compounds.[172] Mutagenicity is related to the ability of alkylating agents to form crosslinks and/or transfer alkyl groups to form DNA monoadducts. The risk of alkylating agent-related t-MDS/AML is dose-dependent, with a latency of 3 to 5 years after exposure;[172] it is associated with abnormalities involving chromosomes 5 (−5/del[5q]) and 7 (−7/del[7q]).[172]

Topoisomerase II inhibitor-related t-MDS/AML: Topoisomerase II catalyzes the relaxation of supercoiled DNA by covalently binding and transiently cleaving and re-ligating both strands of the DNA helix. DNA topoisomerase II inhibitors (epipodophyllotoxins and anthracyclines) stabilize the enzyme-DNA covalent intermediate, decrease the religation rate, and cause chromosomal breakage. These events initiate apoptosis, required for antineoplastic activity.[173,174] Occasionally, repair of chromosomal damage results in chromosomal translocations, leading to leukemogenesis.[173,175,176] Most of the translocations disrupt a breakpoint cluster region between exons 5 and 11 of the band 11q23 and fuse mixed lineage leukemia (MLL) with a partner gene.[172] Topoisomerase II inhibitor-related t-AML presents as overt leukemia after a latency of 6 months to 3 years and is associated with balanced translocations involving chromosome bands 11q23 or 21q22.[177]

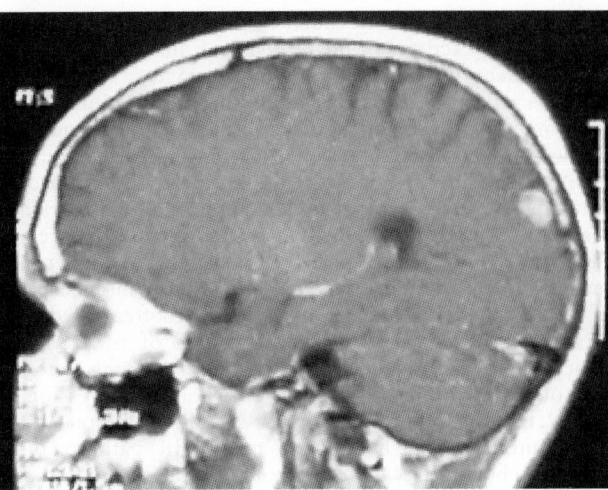

FIGURE 47.4 A dural-based enhancing lesion in the right parietooccipital region consistent with meningioma developing 22 years after 24 Gy of cranial irradiation for acute lymphoblastic leukemia.

Therapy-Related Solid SMNs

Therapy-related solid SMNs demonstrate a strong relation with ionizing radiation. The risk of solid SMNs is highest when the exposure occurs at a younger age, increases with the total dose of radiation, and with increasing follow-up after radiation.[165] Solid SMNs account for 80% of the largest burden of SMNs. Some of the well-established radiation-related solid SMNs include breast, lung, thyroid cancer, brain tumors, sarcomas, and basal cell carcinomas (BCC).[169]

Breast Cancer is the most common solid SMN after HL, largely due to high-dose chest radiation for treatment of HL (standardized incidence ratio [SIR] of second breast cancer = 25 to 55).[170,178] For female HL patients treated with chest radiation at less than 16 years of age, the cumulative incidence of breast cancer approaches 20% by age 45 years.[170] The latency after chest radiation ranges from 8 to 10 years, and the risk of second breast cancer increases in a linear fashion with radiation dose (*p* for trend <0.001).[179]

Thyroid cancer is observed after neck radiation for HL, ALL, brain tumors and after TBI for HCT.[165,169] The risk of thyroid cancer has been reported to be 18-fold that of the general population.[89] Radiation therapy at a young age is the major risk factor for the development of second thyroid cancers. A linear dose-response relationship between thyroid cancer and radiation is observed up to 29 Gy, with a decline in the odds ratio at higher doses, especially in children younger than 10 years of age at treatment, demonstrating evidence for a cell kill effect.[180]

Brain tumors develop after cranial radiation for histologically distinct brain tumors[181] or for management of disease among ALL or NHL patients (Fig. 47.4).[165,169,182] The risk for second brain tumors also demonstrates a linear relationship with radiation dose.[181]

Bone tumors: The risk of second bone tumors has been reported to be 133-fold that of the general population, with an estimated 20-year cumulative risk of 2.8%.[183] Survivors of hereditary retinoblastoma, Ewing sarcoma, and other malignant bone tumors are at a particularly increased risk.[184]

Radiation therapy is associated with a linear dose-response relation.[184,185] After adjustment for radiation therapy, treatment with alkylating agents has also been linked to bone cancer, with the risk increasing with cumulative drug exposure.[184]

Lung cancer has been reported after chest irradiation for HL. The risk rises with increasing follow-up. Smoking has been linked with the occurrence of lung cancer developing after radiation for HL. The increase in risk of lung cancer with increasing radiation dose is greater among the patients who smoke after exposure to radiation than among those who refrain from smoking (*p* = 0.04).[186]

SMNs and Genetic Susceptibility

Literature clearly supports the role of chemotherapy and radiation in the development of SMNs. However, interindividual variability exists, suggesting a role for genetic variation in susceptibility to genotoxic exposures, or because of genetic susceptibility syndrome conferring an increase risk of cancer such as the Li-Fraumeni syndrome. Previous studies have demonstrated that childhood cancer survivors with either a family history of cancer, but more so, presence of Li-Fraumeni syndrome, carry an increased risk of developing an SMN.[187,188] The risk of SMNs could potentially be modified by mutations in high-penetrance genes that lead to these serious genetic diseases, for example, Li-Fraumeni syndrome[189] However, the attributable risk is expected to be very small because of their extremely low prevalence. The interindividual variability in risk of SMNs is more likely related to common polymorphisms in low-penetrance genes that regulate the availability of active drug metabolite, or those responsible for DNA repair. Gene-environment interactions may magnify subtle functional differences resulting from genetic variations.

Drug-metabolizing enzymes: Metabolism of genotoxic agents occurs in two phases. Phase I involves activation of substrates into highly reactive electrophilic intermediates that can damage DNA—a reaction principally performed by the cytochrome p450 (CYP) family of enzymes. Phase II enzymes (conjugation) function to inactivate genotoxic substrates. The phase II proteins comprise the glutathione S-transferase (GST), NAD(P)H:quinone oxidoreductase-1 (NQO1), and others. The balance between the two sets of enzymes is critical to the cellular response to xenobiotics; for example, high activity of phase I enzyme and low activity of a phase II enzyme can result in DNA damage.

DNA repair: DNA repair mechanisms protect somatic cells from mutations in tumor suppressor genes and oncogenes that can lead to cancer initiation and progression. An individual's DNA repair capacity appears to be genetically determined.[190] A number of DNA repair genes contain polymorphic variants, resulting in large inter-individual variations in DNA repair capacity.[190] Mismatch repair (MMR) functions to correct mismatched DNA base pairs that arise as a result of misincorporation errors that have avoided polymerase proofreading during DNA replication.[191] Approximately 50% of t-MDS/AML patients have microsatellite instability, associated with methylation of the MMR family member MLH1, low expression of MSH2, or polymorphisms in MSH2.[192-194] RAD51 is one of the central proteins in the homologous repair (HR) pathway, functioning to bind to DNA and promote ATP-dependent homologous pairing and strand transfer reactions. RAD51-G-135 C polymorphism is significantly over-represented in patients with t-MDS/AML compared with controls (C allele: OR = 2.7).[192] XRCC3 also functions in the HR DSB repair pathway by directly interacting with and stabilizing RAD51.[195,196] XRCC3 is a paralog of RAD51, also essential for genetic stability.[197,198] Although XRCC3-Thr241Met was not associated with t-MDS/AML (OR = 1.4, 95% CI, 0.7–2.9), a synergistic effect resulting in an 8-fold increased risk of t-MDS/AML (OR = 8.1, 95% CI, 2.2–29.7) was observed in the presence of XRCC3–241Met and RAD51–135 C allele in patients with t-MDS/AML compared with controls.[192] Base Excision Repair (BER) pathway corrects individually damaged bases occurring as a result of ionizing radiation and exogenous xenobiotic exposure. The XRCC1 protein plays a central role in the BER pathway and also in the repair of single strand breaks, by acting as a scaffold and recruiting other DNA repair proteins.[199,200] The presence of XRCC1–399Gln has been shown to be protective for t-MDS/AML.[201]

Recommendations for Screening and Follow-up

Vigilant screening is important for those at risk. t-MDS/AML usually manifests within 10 years following exposure. Recommendations include monitoring with annual complete blood count for 10 years after exposure to alkylating agents or topoisomerase II inhibitors. Most other SMNs are associated with radiation exposure. Screening recommendations include careful annual physical examination of the skin and underlying tissues in the radiation field. Because outcome after breast cancer is closely linked to stage at diagnosis, close surveillance resulting in early diagnosis should confer survival advantage.[202] Mammography, the most widely accepted screening tool for breast cancer in the general population, may not be the ideal screening tool by itself, for radiation-related breast cancers occurring in relatively young women with dense breasts, hence the American Cancer Society recommends including adjunct screening with MRI.[203] Thus, the following are recommendations for females who received radiation with potential impact to the breast (i.e., radiation doses of 20 Gy or higher to the mantle, mediastinal, whole lung, and axillary fields): monthly breast self-examination beginning at puberty; annual clinical breast examinations beginning at puberty until age 25 years; and a clinical breast examination every 6 months, with annual mammograms and MRIs beginning 8 years after radiation or at age 25 (whichever occurs later). Screening of those at risk for early-onset colorectal cancer (i.e., radiation doses of 30 Gy or higher to the abdomen, pelvis, or spine) should include colonoscopy every 5 years beginning at age 35 years or 10 years following radiation (whichever occurs last).

LATE MORTALITY AMONG CHILDHOOD CANCER SURVIVORS

Childhood cancer survivors remain at risk for disease- and treatment-associated late mortality, and the excess mortality persists long after diagnosis.[168] Recurrent disease is the most common cause of premature death. Overall mortality among survivors has been described to be 8-fold that of the general population. Increases in cause-specific mortality are seen for deaths due to SMNs (SMR = 5.2, 95% CI = 13.9–16.6), cardiac (SMR = 7.0, 95% CI, 5.9–8.2), and pulmonary (SMR = 8.8, 95% CI = 6.8–11.2) causes.

CANCER SURVIVORSHIP— FUTURE RESEARCH OPPORTUNITIES

The growing childhood cancer survivor population provides numerous opportunities for research relating to the etiopathogenesis of cancer and other late effects, including evaluating interventions for early detection and prevention of adverse outcomes. The advantages of studying outcomes in cancer survivors, including detailed knowledge of the therapeutic exposures coupled with close follow-up after these exposures, enables researchers to study testable hypotheses and determine the effects of host and therapy-related factors in the development of adverse outcomes ranging from carcinogenesis and organ dysfunction to psychosocial consequences. Opportunities also exist to explore gene-environment interactions that may modify susceptibility to develop adverse outcomes, thus providing insights into the identification of high-risk populations.

The growing population of childhood cancer survivors carries a significant burden of morbidity, necessitating comprehensive long-term follow-up of these survivors. This follow-up should ideally begin at the completion of active therapy, with a documented summarization of therapeutic exposures and recommendations for follow-up, thus ensuring standardization of care received by the survivors. However, many barriers prevent effective follow-up—the most fundamental barrier being the lack of knowledge regarding survivorship issues demonstrated by both the long-term survivors and the primary care physicians caring for them. Shortcomings of the healthcare system also pose potential barriers, and include logistical issues such as a lack of capacity within centers, training and educational deficiencies, inadequate communication between pediatric oncologists, and primary care physicians that subsequently provide the large bulk of follow-up. Finally, a major obstacle faced by survivors of childhood cancer in the United States is the difficulty in obtaining affordable health insurance, especially for young adults, making it impossible for survivors to seek and obtain appropriate long-term care, even if they are aware and willing.[204]

Attention also needs to focus on development of interventional strategies, such as behavior modification, educational interventions, and chemoprevention. Execution of these intervention strategies in the setting of clinical trials would permit evaluation of interventions in early detection, leading to a reduction in morbidity and mortality and, ultimately, improvement in the overall quality of life of childhood cancer survivors.

Despite these unique opportunities, conduct of survivorship research faces several challenges. Cancer survivorship research can be expected to evolve during the next several years as better treatment options, new agents, and combinations of agents are developed for the more than 20% of pediatric cancer patients who do not now survive. Targeted therapies such as imatinib mesylate and other growth factor inhibitors likely will contribute to increased survivorship. Evaluation of their late effects will need to keep in step with their increased usage. Refinements in radiation therapy such as conformal radiation, and popularization of minimally invasive surgeries, are intended to minimize late effects. Evidence-based research will need to determine whether they will live up to this expectation. Advances in supportive care, including

transfusions and hematopoietic growth factors, also require ongoing surveillance for identification of late effects. Furthermore, the influence of genetic profiles on susceptibility to late effects, as well as their interaction with lifestyle exposures such as tobacco, alcohol, and diet, is of growing interest and has not been fully explored. However, the multifactorial etiology of the adverse effects, coupled with the heterogeneous nature of the patient population, necessitates large sample sizes within the context of well-characterized cohorts with complete long-term follow-up, and this remains the greatest challenge to sound survivorship research.

References

1. Ries LAG, Melbert D, Krapcho M, et al. SEER Cancer Statistics Review, 1975–2005. Bethesda, MD: National Cancer Institute, 2007.
2. Mariotto AB, Rowland JH, Yabroff KR, et al. Long-term survivors of childhood cancers in the United States. Cancer Epidemiol Biomarkers Prev 2009;18:1033–1040.
3. Robison LL, Armstrong GT, Boice JD, et al. The Childhood Cancer Survivor Study: a national cancer institute-supported resource for outcome and intervention research. J Clin Oncol 2009;27:2308–2318. http://www.stjude.org/ccss. Accessed November 30, 2009.
4. Diller L, Chow EJ, Gurney JG, et al. Chronic disease in the childhood cancer survivor study cohort: a review of published findings. J Clin Oncol 2009;27(14):2339–55.
5. Stevens MC, Mahler H, Parkes S. The health status of adult survivors of cancer in childhood. Eur J Cancer 1998;34:694–698.
6. Oeffinger KC, Mertens AC, Sklar CA, et al. Chronic health conditions in adult survivors of childhood cancer. N Engl J Med 2006;355:1572–1582.
7. Kadan-Lottick NS, Robison LL, Gurney JG, et al. Childhood cancer survivors' knowledge about their past diagnosis and treatment. Childhood Cancer Survivor Study. JAMA 2002;287:1832–1839.
8. Hewitt M WS, Simone JV (Eds.). Childhood cancer survivorship: improving care and quality of life. Washington, DC: National Academies Press, 2003.
9. Landier W, Bhatia S, Eshelman DA, et al. Development of risk-based guidelines for pediatric cancer survivors: the children's oncology group long-term follow-Up guidelines from the children's oncology group late effects committee and nursing discipline. J Clin Oncol 2004;22:4979–4990.
10. Schell MJ, McHaney VA, Green AA, et al. Hearing loss in children and young adults receiving cisplatin with or without prior cranial irradiation. J Clin Oncol 1989;7:754–760.
11. Roland JT, Cohen NL. Vestibular and auditory toxicity, In: Cummings CW, Fredrickson JM, Harker LA, et al (eds). Otolaryngology head and neck surgery. 3rd ed. St. Louis, MO: Mosby, 1998:3186–3197.
12. Hua C, Bass JK, Khan R, et al. Hearing loss after radiotherapy for pediatric brain tumors: effect of cochlear dose. Int J Radiat Oncol Biol Phys 2008;72:892–899.
13. Paulino AC, Simon JH, Zhen W, et al. Long-term effects in children treated with radiotherapy for head and neck rhabdomyosarcoma. Int J Radiat Oncol Biol Phys 2000;48:1489–1495.
14. Low WK, Toh ST, Wee J, et al. Sensorineural hearing loss after radiotherapy and chemoradiotherapy: a single, blinded, randomized study. J Clin Oncol 2006;24:1904–1909.
15. Merchant TE, Hua CH, Shukla H, et al. Proton versus photon radiotherapy for common pediatric brain tumors: comparison of models of dose characteristics and their relationship to cognitive function. Pediatr Blood Cancer 2008;51:110–117.
16. Abramson DH, Servodidio CA. Ocular complications due to cancer treatment, In: Schwarz CL, Hobbie WL, Constine LS, et al., eds. Survivors of childhood cancer: assessment and management. St. Louis: Mosby, 1994:111–131.
17. Gurney JG, Ness KK, Rosenthal J, et al. Visual, auditory, sensory, and motor impairments in long-term survivors of hematopoietic stem cell transplantation performed in childhood: results from the Bone Marrow Transplant Survivor Study. Cancer 2006;106:1402–1408.
18. Soysal T, Bavunoglu I, Baslar Z, et al. Cataract after prolonged busulphan therapy. Acta Haematol 1993;90:213.
19. Tichelli A, Duell T, Weiss M, et al. Late-onset keratoconjunctivitis sicca syndrome after bone marrow transplantation: incidence and risk factors. european droup or blood and marrow transplantation (EBMT) working party on late effects. Bone Marrow Transplant 1996;17:1105–1111.
20. Oberlin O, Rey A, Anderson J, et al. Treatment of orbital rhabdomyosarcoma: survival and late effects of treatment–results of an international workshop. J Clin Oncol 2001;19:197–204.
21. Kaste SC, Hopkins KP, Bowman LC, et al. Dental abnormalities in children treated for neuroblastoma. Med Pediatr Oncol 1998;30:22–27.
22. Kaste SC, Hopkins KP, Jones D, et al. Dental abnormalities in children treated for acute lymphoblastic leukemia. Leukemia 1997;11:792–796.
23. Kaste SC, Hopkins KP, Bowman LC. Dental abnormalities in long-term survivors of head and neck rhabdomyosarcoma. Med Pediatr Oncol 1995;25:96–101.
24. Guchelaar HJ, Vermes A, Meerwaldt JH. Radiation-induced xerostomia: pathophysiology, clinical course and supportive treatment. Support Care Cancer 1997;5:281–288.
25. Bras J, de Jonge HK, van Merkesteyn JP. Osteoradionecrosis of the mandible: pathogenesis. Am J Otolaryngol 1990;11:244–250.
26. Campbell LK, Scaduto M, Sharp W, et al. A meta-analysis of the neurocognitive sequelae of treatment for childhood acute lymphocytic leukemia. Pediatr Blood Cancer 2007;49:65–73.
27. Reimers TS, Ehrenfels S, Mortensen EL, et al. Cognitive deficits in long-term survivors of childhood brain tumors: identification of predictive factors. Med Pediatr Oncol 2003;40:26–34.
28. Walter AW, Mulhern RK, Gajjar A, et al. Survival and neurodevelopmental outcome of young children with medulloblastoma at St Jude Children's Research Hospital. J Clin Oncol 1999;17:3720–3728.
29. Palmer SL, Gajjar A, Reddick WE, et al. Predicting intellectual outcome among children treated with 35–40 Gy craniospinal irradiation for medulloblastoma. Neuropsychology 2003;17:548–555.
30. Silber JH, Radcliffe J, Peckham V, et al. Whole-brain irradiation and decline in intelligence: the influence of dose and age on IQ score. J Clin Oncol 1992;10:1390–1396.
31. Mulhern RK, Reddick WE, Palmer SL, et al. Neurocognitive deficits in medulloblastoma survivors and white matter loss. Ann Neurol 1999;46:834–841.
32. Ris MD, Packer RJ, Goldwein J, et al. Intellectual outcome after reduced-dose radiation therapy plus adjuvant chemotherapy for medulloblastom: a Children's Cancer Group study. J Clin Oncol 2001;19:3470–3476.
33. Mulhern RK, Kepner JL, Thomas PR. Neuropsychologic functioning of survivors of childhood medulloblastoma randomized to receive conventional or reduced-dose craniospinal irradiation: a Pediatric Oncology Group Study. J Clin Oncol 1998;16:1723–1728.
34. Barahmani N, Carpentieri S, Li XN, et al. Glutathione S-transferase M1 and T1 polymorphisms may predict adverse effects after therapy in children with medulloblastoma. Neuro Oncol 2009;11:292–300.
35. Haupt R, Fears TR, Robison LL, et al. Educational attainment in long-term survivors of childhood acute lymphoblastic leukemia: a report from the NIH and the CCG. JAMA 1994;272:1427–1432.
36. Buizer AI, de Sonneville LM, Veerman AJ. Effects of chemotherapy on neurocognitive function in children with acute lymphoblastic leukemia: a critical review of the literature. Pediatr Blood Cancer 2009;52(4):447–454.
37. Lipshultz SE, Alvarez JA, Scully RE. Anthracycline associated cardiotoxicity in survivors of childhood cancer. Heart 2008;94:525–533.
38. Adams MJ, Lipshultz SE. Pathophysiology of anthracycline- and radiation-associated cardiomyopathies: implications for screening and prevention. Pediatr Blood Cancer 2005;44:600–606.
39. Kremer LC, van Dalen EC, Offringa M, et al. Frequency and risk factors of anthracycline-induced clinical heart failure in children: a systematic review. Ann Oncol 2002;13:503–512.
40. Hudson MM, Rai SN, Nunez C, et al. Noninvasive evaluation of late anthracycline cardiac toxicity in childhood cancer survivors. J Clin Oncol 2007;25:3635–3643.
41. Shankar SM, Marina N, Hudson MM, et al. Monitoring for cardiovascular disease in survivors of childhood cancer: report from the Cardiovascular Disease Task Force of the Children's Oncology Group. Pediatrics 2008;121:e387–e396.
42. Giantris A, Abdurrahman L, Hinkle A, et al. Anthracycline-induced cardiotoxicity in children and young adults. Crit Rev Oncol Hematol 1998;27:53–68.
43. Felker GM, Thompson RE, Hare JM, et al. Underlying causes and long-term survival in patients with initially unexplained cardiomyopathy. N Engl J Med 2000;342:1077–1084.
44. van Dalen EC, van der Pal HJ, Kok WE, et al. Clinical heart failure in a cohort of children treated with anthracyclines: a long-term follow-up study. Eur J Cancer 2006;42:3191–3198.
45. Henderson IC, Allegra JC, Woodcock T, et al. Randomized clinical trial comparing mitoxantrone with doxorubicin in previously treated patients with metastatic breast cancer. J Clin Oncol 1989;7:560–571.
46. Deng S, Wojnowski L. Genotyping the risk of anthracycline-induced cardiotoxicity. Cardiovasc Toxicol 2007;7:129–134.
47. Blanco JG, Leisenring WM, Gonzalez-Covarrubias VM, et al. Genetic polymorphisms in the carbonyl reductase 3 gene CBR3 and the NAD(P)H:quinone oxidoreductase 1 gene NQO1 in patients who developed anthracycline-related congestive heart failure after childhood cancer. Cancer 2008;112:2789–2795.
48. Glanzmann C, Kaufmann P, Jenni R, et al. Cardiac risk after mediastinal irradiation for Hodgkin's disease. Radiother Oncol 1998;46:51–62.
49. Adams MJ, Hardenbergh PH, Constine LS, et al. Radiation-associated cardiovascular disease. Crit Rev Oncol Hematol 2003;45:55–75.
50. Jurado J, Thompson PD. Prevention of coronary artery disease in cancer patients. Pediatr Blood Cancer 2005;44:620–624.
51. Barry EV, Vrooman LM, Dahlberg SE, et al. Absence of secondary malignant neoplasms in children with high-risk acute lymphoblastic leukemia treated with dexrazoxane. J Clin Oncol 2008;26:1106–1111.
52. Silber JH, Cnaan A, Clark BJ, et al. Enalapril to prevent cardiac function decline in long-term survivors of pediatric cancer exposed to anthracyclines. J Clin Oncol 2004;22:820–828.
53. Abid SH, Malhotra V, Perry MC. Radiation-induced and chemotherapy-induced pulmonary injury. Curr Opin Oncol 2001;13:242–248.
54. Meyer S, Reinhard H, Gottschling S, et al. Pulmonary dysfunction in pediatric oncology patients. Pediatr Hematol Oncol 2004;21:175–195.

55. Rubin P, Finkelstein J, Shapiro D. Molecular biology mechanisms in the radiation induction of pulmonary injury syndromes: interrelationship between the alveolar macrophages and septal fibroblast. Int J Radiat Oncol Biol Phys 1992;24:93.
56. Villani F, Viviani S, Bonfante V, et al. Late pulmonary effects in favorable stage I and IIA Hodgkin's Disease treated with radiotherapy alone. Am J Clin Oncol 2000;23:18.
57. Liles A, Blatt J, Morris D, et al. Monitoring pulmonary complications in long-term childhood cancer survivors: guidelines for the primary care physician. Cleve Clin J Med 2008;75:531–539.
58. Eigen H, Wyszomierski D. Bleomycin lung injury in children: pathophysiology and guidelines for management. Am J Pediatr Hematol Oncol 1985;7:71
59. Wheeler C, Antin JH, Churchill WH, et al. Cyclophosphamide, carmustine, and etoposidewith autologous bone marrow transplantation in refractory Hodgkin's disease and non-Hodgkin's lymphoma: a dose-finding study. J Clin Oncol 1990;8:648–656.
60. Kreisman H, Wolkove N. Pulmonary toxicity of antineoplastic therapy. Semin Oncol 1992;19:508–520.
61. Collaco JM, Gower WA, Mogayzel PJ, Jr. Pulmonary dysfunction in pediatric hematopoietic stem cell transplant patients: overview, diagnostic considerations, and infectious complications. Pediatr Blood Cancer 2007;49:117–126.
62. Gower WA, Collaco JM, Mogayzel PJ, Jr. Pulmonary dysfunction in pediatric hematopoietic stem cell transplant patients: non-infectious and long-term complications. Pediatr Blood Cancer 2007;49:225–233.
63. Kurland G, Michelson P. Bronchiolitis obliterans in children. Pediatr Pulmonol 2005;39:193–208.
64. Siegel MJ, Bhalla S, Gutierrez FR, et al. Post-lung transplantation bronchiolitis obliterans syndrome: usefulness of expiratory thin-section CT for diagnosis. Radiology 2001; 220:455–462.
65. Jones DP, Spunt SL, Green D, et al. Renal late effects in patients treated for cancer in childhood: a report from the Children's Oncology Group. Pediatr Blood Cancer 2008; 51:724–731.
66. Keaney CM, Springate JE. Cancer and the kidney. Adolesc Med Clin 2005;16:121–148.
67. Berrak SG, Pearson M, Berberoglu S, et al. High-dose ifosfamide in relapsed pediatric osteosarcoma: therapeutic effects and renal toxicity. Pediatr Blood Cancer 2005; 44:215–219.
68. Stohr W, Paulides M, Bielack S, et al. Ifosfamide-induced nephrotoxicity in 593 sarcoma patients: a report from the Late Effects Surveillance System. Pediatr Blood Cancer 2007;48:447–452.
69. Skinner R. Chronic ifosfamide nephrotoxicity in children. Med Pediatr Oncol 2003; 41:190–197.
70. Paulino A, Wen BC, Brown CK, et al. Late effects in children treated with radiation therapy for Wilms tumor. Int J Radiat Oncol Biol Phys 2000;46:1239–1246.
71. Ariceta G, Rodriguez-Soriano J, Vallo A, et al. Acute and chronic effects of cisplatin therapy on renal magnesium homeostasis. Med Pediatr Oncol 1997;28:35–40.
72. Sklar CA, LaQuaglia MP. The long-term complications of chemotherapy in childhood genitourinary tumors. Urol Clin North Am 2000;27:563–568,x.
73. Ritchey M, Ferrer F, Shearer P, et al. Late effects on the urinary bladder in patients treated for cancer in childhood: a report from the Children's Oncology Group. Pediatr Blood Cancer 2009;52:439–446.
74. Brock N, Pohl J, Stekar J. Detoxification of urotoxic oxazaphosphorines by sulfhydryl compounds. J Cancer Res Clin Oncol 1981;100:311–320.
75. Dorr W, Beck-Bornholdt HP. Radiation-induced impairment of urinary bladder function in mice: fine structure of the acute response and consequences on late effects. Radiat Res 1999;151:461–467.
76. Mosiello G, Gatti C, De Gennaro M, et al. Neurovesical dysfunction in children after treating pelvic neoplasms. BJU Int 2003;92:289–292.
77. Raney B, Anderson J, Jenney M, et al. Late effects in 164 patients with rhabdomyosarcoma of the bladder/prostate region: a report from the international workshop. J Urol 2006;176:2190–2194; discussion 2194–2195.
78. Heyn R, Raney RB, Hayes DM, et al. Late effects of therapy in patients with paratesticular rhabdomyosarcoma. J Clin Oncol 1992;10:614–623.
79. Lal DR, Foroutan HR, Su WT, et al. The management of treatment-related esophageal complications in children and adolescents with cancer. J Pediatr Surg 2006;41:495–499.
80. Emami B, Lyman J, Brown A, et al. Tolerance of normal tissue to therapeutic irradiation. Int J Radiat Oncol Biol Phys 1991;21:109–122.
81. Mahboubi S, Silber JH. Radiation-induced esophageal strictures in children with cancer. Eur Radiol 1997;7:119–122.
82. Lawrence TS, Robertson JM, Anscher MS, et al. Hepatic toxicity resulting from cancer treatment. Int J Radiat Oncol Biol Phys 1995;31:1237–1248.
83. McIntosh S, Davidson DL, O'Brien RT, et al. Methotrexate hepatotoxicity in children with leukemia. J Pediatr 1977;90:1019.
84. Vora A, Mitchell CD, Lennard L, et al. Toxicity and efficacy of 6-thioguanine versus 6-mercaptopurine in childhood lymphoblastic leukaemia: a randomised trial. Lancet 2006;368:1339–1348.
85. De Bruyne R, Portmann B, Samyn M, et al. Chronic liver disease related to 6-thioguanine in children with acute lymphoblastic leukaemia. J Hepatol 2006;44:407–410.
86. Locasciulli A, Testa M, Pontisso P, et al. Prevalence and natural history of hepatitis C infection in patients cured of childhood leukemia. Blood 1997;90:4628.
87. Workowski KA, Berman SM. Sexually transmitted diseases treatment guidelines, 2006. MMWR Recomm Rep 2006;55:1–94.
88. Nandagopal R, Laverdiere C, Mulrooney D, et al. Endocrine late effects of childhood cancer therapy: a report from the Children's Oncology Group. Horm Res 2008;69: 65–74.
89. Sklar C, Whitton J, Mertens A, et al. Abnormalities of the thyroid in survivors of Hodgkin's disease: data from the Childhood Cancer Survivor Study. J Clin Endocrinol Metab 2000;85:3227–3232.
90. Ronckers CM, Sigurdson AJ, Stovall M, et al. Thyroid cancer in childhood cancer survivors: a detailed evaluation of radiation dose response and its modifiers. Radiat Res 2006;166:618–628.
91. Gurney JG, Kadan-Lottick NS, Packer RJ, et al. Endocrine and cardiovascular late effects among adult survivors of childhood brain tumors: Childhood Cancer Survivor Study. Cancer 2003;97:663–673.
92. Hancock SL, Cox RS, McDougall IR. Thyroid diseases after treatment of Hodgkin's disease. N Eng J Med 1991;325:599–605.
93. Chemaitilly W, Sklar CA. Endocrine complications of hematopoietic stem cell transplantation. Endocrinol Metab Clin North Am 2007;36:983–998,ix.
94. Cohen A, Bekassy AN, Gaiero A, et al. Endocrinological late complications after hematopoietic SCT in children. Bone Marrow Transplant 2008;41(Suppl 2):S43–S48.
95. Rowley MM, Leach DR, Warner GA, et al. Effect of graded doses of ionizing radiation on the human testes. Radiat Res 1974;59:665.
96. Clifton DK, Bremner WJ. The effect of testicular x-irradiation on spermatogenesis in man. J Androl 1983;4:387
97. Shalet SM, Beardwell CG, Jacobs HS, et al. Testicular function following irradiation of the human prepubertal testes. Clin Endocrinol 1978;9:483.
98. Meistrich ML. Male gonadal toxicity. Pediatr Blood Cancer 2009;53(2):261–266.
99. Rivkees SA, Crawford JD. The relationship of gonadal activity and chemotherapy-induced gonadal damage. JAMA 1988;259:2123–2125.
100. Whitehead E, Shalet SM, Morris-Jones PH, et al. Gonadal function after combination chemotherapy for Hodgkin's disease in childhood. Arch Dis Child 1982;57:287.
101. Sherins RJ, Olweny CLM, Ziegler JL. Gynecomastia and gonadal dysfunction in adolescent boys treated with combination chemotherapy for Hodgkin's disease. N Engl J Med 1978;299:12.
102. Viviani S, Santoro A, Ragni G, et al. Gonadal toxicity after combination chemotherapy for Hodgkin's disease. Comparative results of MOPP vs ABVD. Eur J Cancer Clin Oncol 1985;21:601–605.
103. Sklar C. Reproductive physiology and treatment-related loss of sex hormone production. Med Pediatr Oncol 1999;33:2.
104. Couto-Silva AC, Trivin C, Thibaud E, et al. Factors affecting gonadal function after bone marrow transplantation during childhood. Bone Marrow Transplant 2001;28:67–75.
105. Thomsett MJ, Conte FA, Kaplan SL, et al. Endocrine and neurologic outcome in childhood craniopharyngioma: review of effect of treatment on 42 patients. J Pediatr 1980; 97:728.
106. Ginsberg JP, Hobbie WL, Ogle SK, et al. Prevalence of and risk factors for hydrocele in survivors of Wilms' tumor. Pediatric Blood Cancer. 2004;42:361–363.
107. Wallace WH, Thomson AB. Preservation of fertility in children treated for cancer. Arch Dis Child 2003;88:493–496.
108. Chapman RM, Sutcliffe SB, Malpas JS. Male gonadal dysfunction in Hodgkin's disease: a prospective study. JAMA 1981;245:1323.
109. Green DM, Sklar CA, Boice JD Jr., et al. Ovarian failure and reproductive outcomes after childhood cancer treatment: results from the Childhood Cancer Survivor Study. J Clin Oncol 2009;27(14):2374–2381.
110. Chemaitilly W, Mertens AC, Mitby P, et al. Acute ovarian failure in the childhood cancer survivor study. J Clin Endocrinol Metab 2006;91:1723–1728.
111. Stillman RJ, Schinfeld JS, Schiff I, et al. Ovarian failure in long-term survivors of childhood malignancy. Am J Obstet Gynecol 1981;139:62.
112. Ortin TTS, Shostak CA, Donaldson SS. Gonadal status and reproductive function following treatment for Hodgkin's disease in childhood: the Stanford experience. Int J Radiat Oncol Biol Phys 1990;19:873.
113. Sarafoglou K, Boulad F, Gillio A, et al. Gonadal function after bone marrow transplantation for acute leukemia during childhood. J Pediatr 1997;130:210–216.
114. Nicosia SV, Matus-Ridley M, Meadows AT. Gonadal effects of cancer therapy in girls. Cancer 1985;55:2364.
115. Bath LE, Wallace WH, Shaw MP, et al. Depletion of ovarian reserve in young women after treatment for cancer in childhood: detection by anti-mullerian hormone, inhibin B and ovarian ultrasound. Hum Reprod. 2003;1811:2368–2374.
116. Afify Z, Shaw PJ, Clavano-Harding A, et al. Growth and endocrine function in children with acute myeloid leukaemia after bone marrow transplantation using busulfan/ cyclophosphamide. Bone Marrow Transplant 2000;25:1087–1092.
117. Sklar CA, Mertens AC, Mitby P, et al. Premature menopause in survivors of childhood cancer: a report from the childhood cancer survivor study. J Natl Cancer Inst 2006;98: 890–896.
118. Brewer M, Gershenson DM, Herzog CE, et al. Outcome and reproductive function after chemotherapy for ovarian dysgerminoma. J Clin Oncol 1999;17:2670–2675.
119. Wallace WH, Anderson R, Baird D. Preservation of fertility in young women treated for cancer. Lancet Oncol 2004;5:269–270.
120. Blatt J. Pregnancy outcome following anticancer therapy. In: Bern MM, Frigoletto FD, eds. Hematologic disorders in maternal-fetal medicine. New York, NY: Alan R. Liss, 1990:569.
121. Green DM, Whitton JA, Stovall M, et al. Pregnancy outcome of partners of male survivors of childhood cancer: a report from the Childhood Cancer Survivor Study. J Clin Oncol 2003;21:716–721.
122. Kalapurakal JA, Peterson S, Peabody EM, et al. Pregnancy outcomes after abdominal irradiation that included or excluded the pelvis in childhood Wilms tumor survivors: a report from the National Wilms Tumor Study. Int J Radiat Oncol Biol Phys 2004; l58:1364–1368.
123. Rubin CM, Robison LL, Nesbit ME, et al. Cytogenetic studies of long-term survivors of childhood acute lymphoblastic leukemia: a follow-up report. Med Pediatr Oncol 1986; 14:295.
124. Mulvihill JJ, Myers MH, Connelly RR, et al. Cancer in offspring of long-term survivors of childhood and adolescent cancer. Lancet 1987;2:813.
125. Hawkins MM, Draper GJ, Winter DL. Cancer in the offspring of survivors of childhood leukaemia and non-Hodgkins lymphomas. Br J Cancer 1995;71:1335.
126. Gurney JG, Ness KK, Stovall M, et al. Final height and body mass index among adult survivors of childhood brain cancer: Childhood Cancer Survivor Study. J Clin Endocrinol Metab 2003;88:4731–4739.
127. Chow EJ, Friedman DL, Yasui Y, et al. Decreased adult height in survivors of childhood acute lymphoblastic leukemia: a report from the Childhood Cancer Survivor Study. J Pediatr 2007;150:370–375, 375 e1.
128. Sklar C, Mertens A, Walter A, et al. Final height after treatment for childhood acute lymphoblastic leukemia: comparison of no cranial irradiation with 1800 and 2400 centigrays of cranial irradiation. J Pediatr 1993;123:59–64.
129. Dalton VK, Rue M, Silverman LB, et al. Height and weight in children treated for acute lymphoblastic leukemia: relationship to CNS treatment. J Clin Oncol 2003;21: 2953–2960.
130. Robison LL, Nesbit ME, Sather HN, et al. Height of children successfully treated for acute lymphoblastic leukemia: a report from the late effects study Committee of Children's Cancer Study Group. Med Pediatr Oncol 1985;13:14.
131. Schriock EA, Schell MJ, Carter M, et al. Longitudinal growth patterns and final height of long term survivors of childhood leukemia. J Clin Oncol 1991;9:400.
132. Livesay EA, Hindmarsh PC, Brook CG, et al. Endocrine disorders following treatment of childhood brain tumours. Br J Cancer 1990;61:622–625.
133. Darzy KH, Pezzoli SS, Thorner MO, et al. The dynamics of growth hormone (GH) secretion in adult cancer survivors with severe GH deficiency acquired after brain irradiation in childhood for nonpituitary brain tumors: evidence for preserved pulsatility and diurnal variation with increased secretory disorderliness. J Clin Endocrinol Metab 2005;90:2794–2803.

134. Oberfield SE, Allen JC, Pollack J, et al. Long-term endocrine sequelae after treatment of medulloblastoma: prospective study of growth and thyroid function. J Pediatr 1986;108:219.

135. Pasqualini T, Diez B, Domene H, et al. Long-term endocrine sequelae after surgery, radiotherapy, and chemotherapy in children with medulloblastoma. Cancer 1987;59:801–806.

136. Kiltie AE, Lashford LS, Gattamaneni HR. Survival and late effects in medulloblastoma patients treated with craniospinal irradiation under three years old. Med Pediatr Oncol 1997;28:348–54.

137. Schell MJ, Ochs JJ, Schriock EA, et al. A method of predicting adult height and obesity in long-term survivors of childhood acute lymphoblastic leukemia. J Clin Oncol 1992;10:128.

138. Sanders JE. Growth and development after hematopoietic cell transplant in children. Bone Marrow Transplant 2008;41:223–227.

139. Rose SR, Schreiber RE, Kearney NS, et al. Hypothalamic dysfunction after chemotherapy. J Pediatr Endocrinol Metab 2004;17:55–66.

140. Oeffinger KC, Mertens AC, Sklar CA, et al. Obesity in adult survivors of childhood acute lymphoblastic leukemia: a report from the Childhood Cancer Survivor Study. J Clin Oncol 2003;21:1359–1365.

141. Nathan PC, Jovcevska V, Ness KK, et al. The prevalence of overweight and obesity in pediatric survivors of cancer. J Pediatr 2006;149:518–525.

142. Rogers PC, Meacham LR, Oeffinger KC, et al. Obesity in pediatric oncology. Pediatr Blood Cancer 2005;45:881–891.

143. Ross JA, Oeffinger KC, Davies SM, et al. Genetic variation in the leptin receptor gene and obesity in survivors of childhood acute lymphoblastic leukemia: a report from the Childhood Cancer Survivor Study. J Clin Oncol 2004;22:3558–3562.

144. Razzouk BI, Rose SR, Hongeng S, et al. Obesity in survivors of childhood acute lymphoblastic leukemia and lymphoma. J Clin Oncol 2007;25:1183–1189.

145. Clement K, Ferre P. Genetics and the pathophysiology of obesity. Pediatr Res 2003;53:721–725.

146. Ness KK, Oakes JM, Punyko JA, et al. Prevalence of the metabolic syndrome in relation to self-reported cancer history. Ann Epidemiol 2005;15:202–206.

147. Link K, Moell C, Garwicz S, et al. Growth hormone deficiency predicts cardiovascular risk in young adults treated for acute lymphoblastic leukemia in childhood. J Clin Endocrinol Metab 2004;89:5003–5012.

148. Gurney JG, Ness KK, Sibley SD, et al. Metabolic syndrome and growth hormone deficiency in adult survivors of childhood acute lymphoblastic leukemia. Cancer 2006;107:1303–1312.

149. Paulino AC, Fowler BZ. Risk factors for scoliosis in children with neuroblastoma. Int J Radiat Oncol Biol Phys 2005;61:865–869.

150. de Jonge T, Slullitel H, Dubousset J, et al. Late-onset spinal deformities in children treated by laminectomy and radiation therapy for malignant tumours. Eur Spine J 2005;14:765–771.

151. Thomas PRM, Griffith KD, Fineberg BB, et al. Late effects of treatment for Wilms tumor. Int J Radiat Oncol Biol Phys 1983;9:651.

152. Larson DL, Kroll S, Jaffe N, et al. Long-term effects of radiotherapy in childhood and adolescence. Am J Surg 1990;160:348.

153. Fletcher BD. Effects of pediatric cancer therapy on the musculoskeletal system. Pediatr Radiol 1997;27:623–636.

154. Marcus RB Jr, Cantor A, Heare TC, et al. Local control and function after twice-a-day radiotherapy for Ewing's sarcoma of bone. Int J Radiat Oncol Biol Phys 1991;21:1509–1515.

155. Wasilewski-Masker K, Kaste SC, Hudson MM, et al. Bone mineral density deficits in survivors of childhood cancer: long-term follow-up guidelines and review of the literature. Pediatrics 2008;121:e705–e713.

156. Haddy TB, Mosher RB, Reaman GH. Osteoporosis in survivors of acute lymphoblastic leukemia. Oncologist 2001;6:278–285.

157. Kaste SC, Jones-Wallace D, Rose SR, et al. Bone mineral decrements in survivors of childhood acute lymphoblastic leukemia: frequency of occurrence and risk factors for their development. Leukemia 2001;15:728–734.

158. Sala A, Mattano LA Jr, Barr RD. Osteonecrosis in children and adolescents with cancer – an adverse effect of systemic therapy. Eur J Cancer 2007;43:683–689.

159. Kadan-Lottick NS, Dinu I, Wasilewski-Masker K, et al. Osteonecrosis in adult survivors of childhood cancer: a report from the childhood cancer survivor study. J Clin Oncol 2008;26:3038–3045.

160. Mattano LA, Sather HN, Trigg ME, et al. Osteonecrosis as a complication of treating acute lymphoblastic leukemia in children: a report from the Children's Cancer Group. J Clin Oncol 2000;18:3262–3272.

161. Relling MV, Yang W, Das S, et al. Pharmacogenetic risk factors for osteonecrosis of the hip among children with leukemia. J Clin Oncol 2004;22:3930–3936.

162. Assouline-Dayan Y, Chang C, Greenspan A, et al. Pathogenesis and natural history of osteonecrosis. Semin Arthritis Rheum 2002;32:94–124.

163. French D, Hamilton LH, Mattano LA Jr, et al. A PAI-1 (SERPINE1) polymorphism predicts osteonecrosis in children with acute lymphoblastic leukemia: a report from the Children's Oncology Group. Blood 2008;111:4496–4499.

164. Meadows AT, Friedman DL, Neglia JP, et al. Second neoplasms in survivors of childhood cancer: findings from the Childhood Cancer Survivor Study cohort. J Clin Oncol 2009;27:2356–2362.

165. Neglia JP, Friedman DL, Yutaka Y, et al. Second malignant neoplasms in five-year survivors of childhood cancer: childhood cancer survivor study. J Natl Cancer Inst 2001;93:618–629.

166. Mike V, Meadows AT, D'Agio GJ. Incidence of second malignant neoplasms in children: results of an international study. Lancet 1982;2(8311):1326–1331.

167. Olsen JH, Garwicz S, Hertz H, et al. Second malignant neoplasms after cancer in childhood or adolescence. Nordic Society of Paediatric Haematology and Oncology Association of the Nordic Cancer Registries. BMJ 1993;307:1030–1036.

168. Mertens AC, Liu Q, Neglia JP, et al. Cause-specific late mortality among 5-year survivors of childhood cancer: the Childhood Cancer Survivor Study. J Natl Cancer Inst 2008;100:1368–1379.

169. Bhatia S, Sklar C. Second cancers in survivors of childhood cancer. Nat Rev Cancer 2002;2:124–132.

170. Bhatia S, Yasui Y, Robison LL, et al. High risk of subsequent neoplasms continues with extended follow-up of childhood Hodgkin's disease: report from the Late Effects Study Group. J Clin Oncol 2003;21:4386–4394.

171. Vardiman JW, Harris NL, Brunning RD. The World Health Organization (WHO) classification of the myeloid neoplasms. Blood 2002;100:2292–2302.

172. Thirman MJ, Larson RA. Therapy-related myeloid leukemia. Hematol Oncol Clin North Am 1996;10:293–320.

173. Felix CA, Walker AH, Lange BJ, et al. Association of CYP3A4 genotype with treatment-related leukemia. Proc Natl Acad Sci U S A 1998;95:13176–13181.

174. Corbett AH, Osheroff N. When good enzymes go bad: conversion of topoisomerase II to a cellular toxin by antineoplastic drugs. Chem Res Toxicol 1993;6:585–597.

175. Lovett BD, Strumberg D, Blair IA, et al. Etoposide metabolites enhance DNA topoisomerase II cleavage near leukemia-associated MLL translocation breakpoints. Biochemistry 2001;40:1159–1170.

176. Megonigal MD, Cheung NK, Rappaport EF, et al. Detection of leukemia-associated MLL-GAS7 translocation early during chemotherapy with DNA topoisomerase II inhibitors. Proc Natl Acad Sci U S A 2000;97:2814–2819.

177. Pedersen-Bjergaard J, Philip P. Balanced translocations involving chromosome bands 11q23 and 21q22 are highly characteristic of myelodysplasia and leukemia following therapy with cytostatic agents targeting at DNA-topoisomerase II. Blood 1991;78:1147–1148.

178. Bhatia S, Robison LL, Oberlin O, et al. Breast cancer and other second neoplasms after childhood Hodgkin's disease. N Engl J Med 1996;334:745–751.

179. Travis LB, Hill D, Dores GM, et al. Cumulative absolute breast cancer risk for young women treated for Hodgkin lymphoma. J Natl Cancer Inst 2005;97:1428–1437.

180. Sigurdson AJ, Ronckers CM, Mertens AC, et al. Primary thyroid cancer after a first tumour in childhood (the Childhood Cancer Survivor Study): a nested case-control study. Lancet 2005;365:2014–2023.

181. Neglia JP, Robison LL, Stovall M, et al. New primary neoplasms of the central nervous system in survivors of childhood cancer: a report from the Childhood Cancer Survivor Study. J Natl Cancer Inst 2006;98:1528–1537.

182. Neglia JP, Meadows AT, Robison LL, et al. Second neoplasms after acute lymphoblastic leukemia in childhood. N Engl J Med 1991;325:1330–1336.

183. Tucker MA, D'Angio GL, Boice JD Jr, et al. Bone sarcomas linked to radiotherapy and chemotherapy in children. N Engl J Med 1987;317:588–593.

184. Hawkins MM, Wilson LM, Burton HS, et al. Radiotherapy, alkylating agents, and risk of bone cancer after childhood cancer. J Natl Cancer Inst 1996;88:270–278.

185. Le Vu B, de Vathaire F, Shamsaldin A, et al. Radiation dose, chemotherapy and risk of osteosarcoma after solid tumours during childhood. Int J Cancer 1998;77:370–377.

186. Van Leeuwen FE, Klokman WJ, Stovall M, et al. Roles of radiotherapy and smoking in lung cancer following Hodgkin's disease. J Natl Cancer Inst 1995;87:1530–1537.

187. Andersson A, Enblad G, Tavelin B, et al. Family history of cancer as a risk factor for second malignancies after Hodgkin's lymphoma. Br J Cancer 2008;98:1001–1005.

188. Hisada M, Garber JE, Fujng CY, et al. Multiple primary cancers in families with Li-Fraumeni syndrome. J Natl Cancer Inst 1998;90:606–611.

189. Alter BP. Cancer in Fanconi anemia, 1927–2001. Cancer 2003;97:425–440.

190. Collins A, Harrington V. Repair of oxidative DNA damage: assessing its contribution to cancer prevention. Mutagenesis 2002;17:489–493.

191. Karran P, Offman J, Bignami M. Human mismatch repair, drug-induced DNA damage, and secondary cancer. Biochimie 2003;85:1149–1160.

192. Seedhouse C, Faulkner R, Ashraf N, et al. Polymorphisms in genes involved in homologous recombination repair interact to increase the risk of developing acute myeloid leukemia. Clin Cancer Res 2004;10:2675–2680.

193. Worrillow LJ, Travis LB, Smith AG, et al. An intron splice acceptor polymorphism in hMSH2 and risk of leukemia after treatment with chemotherapeutic alkylating agents. Clin Cancer Res 2003;9:3012–3020.

194. Horiike S, Misawa S, Kaneko H, et al. Distinct genetic involvement of the TP53 gene in therapy-related leukemia and myelodysplasia with chromosomal losses of Nos 5 and/or 7 and its possible relationship to replication error phenotype. Leukemia 1999;13:1235–1242.

195. Bishop DK, Ear U, Bhattacharyya A, et al. Xrcc3 is required for assembly of Rad51 complexes in vivo. J Biol Chem 1998;273:21482–21488.

196. Liu N, Lamerdin JE, Tebbs RS, et al. XRCC2 and XRCC3, new human Rad51-family members, promote chromosome stability and protect against DNA cross-links and other damages. Mol Cell 1998;1:783–793.

197. Tebbs RS, Zhao Y, Tucker JD, et al. Correction of chromosomal instability and sensitivity to diverse mutagens by a cloned cDNA of the XRCC3 DNA repair gene. Proc Natl Acad Sci U S A 1995;92:6354–6358.

198. Pierce AJ, Johnson RD, Thompson LH, et al. XRCC3 promotes homology-directed repair of DNA damage in mammalian cells. Genes Dev 1999;13:2633–2638.

199. Caldecott KW, McKeown CK, Tucker JD, et al. An interaction between the mammalian DNA repair protein XRCC1 and DNA ligase III. Mol Cell Biol 1994;14:68–76.

200. Kubota Y, Nash RA, Klungland A, et al. Reconstitution of DNA base excision-repair with purified human proteins: interaction between DNA polymerase beta and the XRCC1 protein. EMBO J 1996;15:6662–6670.

201. Seedhouse C, Bainton R, Lewis M, et al. The genotype distribution of the XRCC1 gene indicates a role for base excision repair in the development of therapy-related acute myeloblastic leukemia. Blood 2002;100:3761–3766.

202. Diller L, Medeiros Nancarrow C, Shaffer K, et al. Breast cancer screening in women previously treated for Hodgkin's disease: a prospective cohort study. J Clin Oncol 2002;20:2085–2091.

203. Saslow D, Boetes C, Burke W, et al. American Cancer Society guidelines for breast screening with MRI as an adjunct to mammography. CA Cancer J Clin 2007;57:75–89.

204. Bhatia S, Meadows AT. Long-term follow-up of childhood cancer survivors: future directions for clinical care and research. Pediatr Blood Cancer 2006;46:143–148.

CHAPTER 48 ■ EDUCATIONAL ISSUES FOR CHILDREN WITH CANCER

LAURIE D. LEIGH AND HEATHER M. CONKLIN

Each year in the United States, approximately 10,000 new cases of cancer occur in children younger than 15 years.[1] With medical advances, childhood cancer has come to be viewed as a life-threatening chronic illness rather than a terminal illness. In the United States alone, there are almost 300,000 cancer survivors, including 1 in 640 adults between the ages of 20 and 39.[2] As the rate of survival increases, the quality of life of survivors takes on added importance. In his book, *The Truly Cured Child*, Van Eys[3] challenged professionals working with children with cancer to reconsider the definition of cure. He defined a cured child as one with "social, mental, and physical well-being" and a "child who becomes an adult able to live to the full extent of his talents."[3] Because education is crucial to the realization of a child's full potential, a partnership between health care professionals and school personnel is important to patients' and survivors' quality of life.[4] Communication among professionals who participate in children's care, including school personnel, is not a luxury but an essential element in the total care of children.

Children with cancer present a unique set of challenges to any school system. Some problems, such as absences and resulting poor performance, may be of short duration, whereas others may be long-term developmental problems that require ongoing assessment.[5] This chapter approaches school re-entry and intervention as the ongoing processes they must be. This process starts at diagnosis and requires a continuing commitment from health care professionals, school personnel, and the family of the child with cancer. Proactive, preventive assessment and intervention must be made an integral part of children's treatment and the long-term follow-up process.[6]

THE IMPORTANCE OF SCHOOL RE-ENTRY INTERVENTION

School is the work of childhood. It presents each child with a daily opportunity to feel productive, master the environment, learn social skills, and receive peer support. As Maul-Mellott and Adams[7] stated in *Childhood Cancer: A Nursing Overview*, "The regular achievement and long-range planning required in the school setting validate the future for children. The acquisition of skills and mastery of complex principles are aimed toward preparing the child for the larger arena of life. In this way, participation in school reinforces the fact of the future for all children. It affirms the probability of living to use the skills gained." Thus, children denied school participation are, in effect, denied an important opportunity to engage in age-appropriate, goal-oriented behavior.[8] Such children may acquire a sense of learned helplessness that reinforces feelings of hopelessness and despair, obstructing their ability to cope with their illness and the rehabilitation process.[8]

Many authors have advised that children and adolescents with cancer return to normal activities such as school as soon as medically possible.[9–13] Getting back to school and attending regularly has been linked to a better quality of life even many years after treatment.[14] Regular school attendance translates to children and adolescents who are involved in social activities and who do not miss as many learning opportunities in the school day.[15] In this manner, at least a part of their lives is returned to normalcy in the midst of their illness and medical treatment. Van Eys[3] wrote, "A child's development continues when he has cancer . . . But the environment must be conducive to normal development. That environment is not just the one created by the parents at home, but the sum total of all experiences that the child has during his illness. The child must be allowed normal development during abnormal circumstances." Thus, school re-entry becomes a part of the treatment process, and teachers and school system become a part of the treatment team.

Problems that sometimes create a barrier to school re-entry include a patient's anxiety about peer teasing because of the visible effects of treatment, continued school absences, parents' reticence to allow a child to return to school, a child's school phobia or separation anxiety, a teacher's overindulgence or unrealistic expectations about a child's abilities, a child's illness-related disabilities (e.g., fatigue, pain), and the need for special services or accommodations.[8,10,16–18] However, children and adolescents often find that most of the social and emotional support they need for the return to school comes from classmates who have received education about their illness and treatment.[19] They report that a continuing emphasis on education is extremely important and helps focus their attention on something familiar and productive.[20] Research conducted over the past 30 years on the problems of school re-entry for children with cancer and other chronic illnesses indicates that intervention increases the likelihood of successful re-entry. Prevatt and colleagues reviewed 14 journal articles describing school re-entry programs done between 1977 and 1998 and classified them into three categories: school personnel workshops, peer education programs, and comprehensive programs.[21] Below are examples of the three categories of programs:

School Personnel Workshops

Ross and Scarvalone[22] described an intervention program for school personnel using a seminar format. The seminar offered general information about childhood cancer, treatment, and side effects; information about the psychosocial aspects of cancer treatment and ways in which school personnel can be helpful; a tour of the hospital; and small group discussions. Evaluation of the program indicated that the school personnel who were given information about the child with cancer, and cancer as a disease, its treatment, and related psychosocial issues felt more confident, were able to answer the questions of patients and classmates, could deal more effectively with parents, and could treat patients more as normal students.

Peer Education Programs

Benner and Marlow[23] described an intervention for first-, second-, and third-graders who had a classmate with cancer. The 30-minute presentation provided general information about childhood cancer, treatment, side effects, and the emotional aspects of cancer. After the presentation, the classmates showed increased knowledge of childhood cancer and an increased desire to interact with the child with cancer.

Comprehensive Programs

Comprehensive programs include both school personnel and peer education components as well as other components to enhance collaboration between family, school, and hospital.[21] Rynard and colleagues[24] reported the results of year-end teacher and parent evaluations of a school support program. The basic components of the program were: (a) discussion with patient and parent and phone contact with school personnel to explain services; (b) provision of information to the school; (c) a meeting with school personnel, peers, and the child; (d) follow-up with the child and school personnel; and (e) an annual workshop for teachers, parents, and health professionals to provide additional information. Parents and teachers viewed the program as "highly useful."[24] The teachers found the school conference to be the most important component. Parents also rated provision of information to the school as very important. The results of this study strongly support the importance of links between school, hospital, and home.[24]

Katz and colleagues[9] studied the psychological and social functioning of children with cancer using a two-group design. The components of the intervention were (a) preparatory activities, including parent-child counseling and phone communication with school personnel, (b) face-to-face conferences with school personnel, (c) classroom presentation, and (d) follow-up. The parents of children in the intervention group reported fewer behavior problems than did the parents of children in the control group. Children in the intervention group were also less anxious, less depressed, and had greater social competence after returning to school. Patients, parents, and teachers perceived the intervention as successful.

Finally, Varni and colleagues[25] went beyond the usual school re-entry intervention. Their intervention was designed to improve the social competence of children with chronic illness, thereby facilitating positive social interaction with teacher and classmates. The results of this study suggested that social skills' training may add to the benefits offered by the standard school reintegration intervention through a significant reduction in behavior problems, a significant increase in classmate and teacher social support, and a significant increase in social competence after nine months.

Despite the demonstrated benefits of school re-entry programs, many hospitals that treat pediatric cancer patients do not offer these services. A recent telephone survey was conducted with each of the 37 National Cancer Institute-designated comprehensive cancer centers with a 100% response rate.[26] School re-entry programs for post-treatment pediatric cancer survivors were identified at only seven centers. There was little mention of efforts to address re-entry for college students or adults into the workforce.

Moore and colleagues[27] studied the perceptions of nurses, school personnel, and parents about school re-entry for children with cancer. Respondents indicated that school personnel and nurses did little to assist with school re-entry, but parents indicated that what they did was helpful. There was also agreement among the groups that school re-entry services were inadequate. Furthermore, there was evidence that part of the problem was confusion about health care provider and school personnel roles. These findings strongly suggest a need for a designated school liaison to coordinate school re-entry services.

PHASES OF SCHOOL RE-ENTRY

In previous editions of this chapter we used, as a framework for our discussion of school re-entry, a three-phase model first described by Madan-Swain and colleagues.[28] Here we use a modified version of this model that includes the following three phases: (a) initial diagnosis and hospitalization, (b) preparation for school re-entry and re-entry, and (c) follow-up. In addition to these phases, we include a stratification of student disabilities that can be used at re-entry and throughout affected children's scholastic careers. This chapter also addresses school intervention for children with cancer, including how to obtain special education services and special classroom accommodations based on federal legislation. Finally, the difficult case of terminal illness is discussed.

Phase 1: Initial Diagnosis and Hospitalization

The process of school re-entry should begin shortly after diagnosis. Principal considerations in this phase include identification of a hospital-school liaison, involvement of the treating physician, alternative arrangements for interim education, providing classmates with initial illness-related information, and assessing the patient's level of cognitive disability.[9,28]

Identification of a Hospital-School Liaison

As early as possible, the child's treatment team should obtain parental consent to assign a school liaison. The liaison should be a professional who can work with parents as an advocate for the child and serve as a bridge between the hospital and school personnel.[13,29] As mentioned previously, Moore describes one barrier to school re-entry as being confusion regarding professional roles.[27] Having a designated liaison should decrease this confusion and open the pathway for a smoother school re-entry process. The school liaison should contact the child's school to discuss the child's diagnosis and initial absence from school. The liaison also may use this opportunity to discuss any pertinent premorbid history, such as scholastic achievement, peer acceptance, and general social adjustment in the school environment as well as the parents' history of supporting the child's achievement in school, their cooperation, and their attitude toward school personnel.[6]

This information is helpful not only for anticipating school re-entry needs but for understanding a child's learning style or possible learning disabilities and foreseeing what assistance a child may need in understanding the diagnosis and treatment plan. Generally, children who have a history of premorbid learning or adjustment problems are at greater risk of difficult school re-entry.[8,10,1,18,30] As the re-entry process proceeds, the liaison will continue to act as a coordinator to bring appropriate personnel and information together. This is very important because one predictor of successful school re-entry is the ability of all *parties involved to have questions answered and information available*; in other words, a very open line of communication between. Other predictors include the child's participation in some form of alternative education while away from school and continued communication with peers/classmates while away from school.

Physician Emphasis on the Importance of Returning to School

Early in the treatment process, the child's physician should discuss the importance of returning to school and other normal activities and give parents a clear timeline, if possible, to think about re-entry. Parents who see the return to school as a normal expectation and part of the treatment plan are more likely to feel comfortable with the prospect of school re-entry and to comply with the plan.[13] Although many parents and patients are eager to discuss school re-entry, some parents are more reticent about sending their child back to school because of anxiety about infection or potential peer rejection. Some parents also become emotionally enmeshed with their child during illness, and both parent and child experience separation anxiety.[17] School phobia can begin at this time.

At least one study indicated predictors of school re-entry difficulties. These include avoidance of the topic of school and passive or active resistance to participation in alternative school services, such as hospital bound instruction.[17] These issues necessitate ongoing communication among parent, child, and physician about the continuation of education and school re-entry. This communication will provide physicians an opportunity to gauge children's and parents' adjustment and compliance; will provide information to reassure anxious parents; and will arrange for the participation of other professionals, such as a psychologist or social worker, whose help may be needed. It will also give the patient and parents an opportunity to ask questions about any concerns about school re-entry.

Alternative Arrangements for Instruction

It is very important that children have some type of alternative educational services while they are unable to attend school. Although important for every child, ongoing instruction and learning are most significant for children who are beginning their education and are building foundation skills in mathematics and reading, for children with a history of learning disability, and for older adolescents who are near graduation.[6,10,31,32] An emphasis on continuation of school even while in the hospital or at home for extended periods reassures children with cancer about an expectation for a future.[33] In her study of 51 survivors of childhood cancer, Bessell reported that the survivors felt that continuing with school was very important. It made them feel "worth educating because survival was in the picture," but it also created a focus on normal and productive activity. Also, appropriate homebound or hospital bound education serves to decrease anxiety and hesitation about school re-entry.[33] Sometimes, school system personnel tell parents not to worry about school but rather concentrate on the health of the child and worry about catching up later. This advice is not usually helpful and can cause a child to repeat a grade as retention is still one solution school systems use to deal with absenteeism due to cancer treatments.[20,34]

Several options are available for the continuation of children's education during hospitalization or confinement at home because of immunosuppression or other side effects of treatment. If children are at home or are hospitalized near their home, their school is responsible for providing a homebound teacher. If children are hospitalized at such a distance from the home community that such provision is not possible, the hospital will probably have teachers or can access teachers in the hospital community. The school liaison can assist the parents in finding the most appropriate option for the continuation of school.

For homebound services to be approved, the physician may need to document the need for services in a letter or by his signature on a form from the child's school system. The liaison can assist the parent with this process by contacting school personnel to get the form or letter signed by the physician and back to school personnel. Once school services begin, the hospital or homebound teacher should communicate with the home community teacher so that books and assignments can be sent.[7,35] Such an arrangement will help to keep children with cancer in touch with what their classmates are doing. School re-entry will be easier if children know they have been doing the same work from the same books as their classmates.

Teachers of hospital- or homebound students probably will meet with children for two to four sessions per week. Therefore, self-discipline on the part of these children and support from the parents is needed if children are to keep up with assignments. Parental assistance and additional instruction may be required to supplement the limited number of school provided hours. Basic skills development is of utmost importance for younger children and building foundation skills in mathematics and reading is vital.[7,10,35] During this time, students probably will not be able to complete every assignment for every class. This is especially true for adolescents who may have several difficult subjects. The assignments should be prioritized for the students so that the teachers only communicate what is essential to complete. Also, some classes, such as drama and art, cannot be taught in the home or hospital setting; adolescents must be excused or be given alternative assignments.[6]

Respondents in Bessell's study indicated much frustration in negotiating with the school system in getting homebound services started as well as with the quantity and quality of homebound services. They specifically reported problems with the homebound teacher communicating with the classroom teacher, knowing what was happening in the classroom and/or having appropriate materials from the classroom teacher. They also reported that the quality of instruction was poor and did not meet the needs of special education or advanced placement students.[20] Certainly, homebound instruction can vary widely from district to district. An adolescent who has more specialized subjects like algebra or chemistry may find that he has a homebound teacher with no experience in those subjects, so may not be able to receive appropriate instruction in those subjects.[36]

Parents can ask the homebound teacher to make sure the materials match what is happening in the classroom as much as possible. They can also keep track of communication by asking that any e-mail communication between the community school teacher and the homebound teacher be copied to them. If they need further assistance in getting the homebound teacher or school system to cooperate, they can ask for the school liaison to provide assistance with advocacy.[20]

Technology is changing how some students receive homebound school services. Some school systems now lend laptop computers to students so they can keep up through video teleconferencing and online courses. Many teachers also use e-mail to update students on assignments and have progress reports available online so parents and students can make sure the student is receiving appropriate credit for work completed. The video teleconferencing and online courses may work well to provide supplemental instruction for a student whose needs are not being addressed adequately by homebound instruction.

The school liaison should work with parents and their children's school system to find the most appropriate method for continuing their children's education and to design a plan whereby patients receive appropriate credit for work completed. In helping parents with decisions about continued instruction, health, social/emotional, and academic factors need to be considered.[36] In a small study done by Searle, Askins, and Bleyer, homebound, hospital bound, and community school services for adolescents during treatment were compared. Results revealed homebound services were the least favorable option of the three, but would work best for the adolescent who was an excellent student and taking part in many extracurricular activities prior to diagnosis. Students who had academic problems prior to diagnosis may benefit more from hospital bound school or as much school attendance as possible.[36] A combination of school attendance and hospital bound or homebound services when the child cannot attend school may work well.[20,36]

Providing Information to Classmates About a Child's Illness

The child or adolescent may not return to school for several weeks to several months so it may not be best to wait until the re-entry presentation to give information to classmates. When children are absent from school for a period, peers will have questions about where they are and what is happening to them. In the case of a child with cancer, the news can spread quickly, but inaccurate information also may spread.[37] Classmates may overhear inaccurate information from parents and teachers or may fabricate an explanation when their questions are not answered. Myths about cancer, such as its being contagious, also abound, even among older adolescents and adults, and can lead to the child's isolation from peers. Sometimes, for older adolescents, such misinformation can include the association between cancer and acquired immunodeficiency syndrome. Other children in the class may become worried about their own physical symptoms. They may become afraid that normal headaches and other body aches they experience mean they have cancer. They need to be reassured that cancer is a rare diagnosis and every child has illnesses not related to cancer.

The only experience many children and adolescents have had with cancer is that of an adult in the family. They need to know adult cancer is different from childhood cancer. They should be told that children, for the most part, respond very well to treatment. If the child with cancer's prognosis is unfavorable, those around him should be told of the possibility of death if they ask, with emphasis on "things are going well for now."[37]

With the parent's permission, the school liaison can work with the teacher, counselor, or both to provide appropriate information to a child's classmates about the diagnosis, treatment, and anticipated length of absence. The liaison also can provide written materials, such as *Helping Schools Cope with Childhood Cancer: Current Facts and Creative Solutions*, authored by Chambers and colleagues,[38] and *Cancervive Teacher's Guide for Kids with Cancer*, written by Nessim and Katz.[32] These booklets can provide the teacher with direction about how to talk with classmates and answer their questions if there is no one available from the hospital to make the presentation. It is also important to remember that siblings will be affected by their brother or sister's diagnosis and treatment and there are times when a classroom presentation for the sibling classroom is appropriate. This is especially true for siblings who are close in age and may attend the same school. Other resources for the school presentation will be presented later in the chapter.

At this point we should mention HIPPA issues with the communication of medical information to school personnel and classmates. Certainly, HIPPA rules apply in the release of medical information to teachers and classmates. This is never done without the parents' and patient's permission. School personnel will need to be reminded of HIPPA as there is some laxity in some schools in discussion of these issues in common areas such as the school office and other areas where students and other adults can hear.

Classmates should be encouraged to communicate with the child in the hospital or at home. Keeping in contact with classmates will give a child with cancer a sense that they remain a part of the classroom, and are not forgotten by peers. Classmates may not be sure how to accomplish this on their own, so the teacher should offer ideas such as using e-mail, cards, phone calls, audiotaped or videotaped messages, hand-drawn posters and, if possible, personal visits. Children undergoing treatment for cancer have noted that continuing support from their friends and school throughout their hospital stay greatly improved their confidence in re-entering school and reduced anxiety about peer rejection.[10]

Assessment of Level of Disability

In the section on stratification of disability levels, we present a schema based on premorbid disabilities and chronic illness- and treatment-related disabilities. The level of disability should be assessed many times over a child's scholastic career, and changes in level should be expected. In phase 1, information should be gathered about the child's premorbid functioning. Any premorbid history of learning or physical disability will be the first pieces of information to be considered in determining level of disability.

The next information to be considered is the presence of any chronic illness- or treatment-related disability. Such diagnoses as brain tumor or acute lymphocytic leukemia (ALL) for which central nervous system-directed therapies are used, are associated most often with chronic illness-related disabilities. With regard to brain tumors, disabilities may be caused by the tumor itself or by the effects of surgical resection.[39] In the case of slow-growing tumors, learning difficulties that appeared before the diagnosis of cancer may have been caused by the tumor. Hence, a learning disability, cognitive deficit, or delay that was in evidence before diagnosis may be disease related. In some cases, the children's cognitive or academic functioning may improve after tumor resection and recovery from surgery.

Children who receive central nervous system-directed therapies, including certain chemotherapeutic agents and radiation therapy, are at significant risk for delayed emergence of cognitive problems.[40,41] Although global declines on measures of intellectual functioning and academic achievement are most commonly reported,[41–43] more recent findings suggest that attention, working memory, and processing speed deficits may be underlying causes for these declines. Risk factors associated with cognitive declines include younger age at treatment, longer time since treatment, female gender, higher treatment intensity (e.g., radiation dose), and complicating medical factors (e.g., hydrocephalus or meningitis).[41,42] Health care providers are working to reduce treatment-related cognitive effects, while still maintaining a high survival rate, thorough use of risk-adapted therapies that save the most aggressive therapies for children with the poorest prognostic indicators (e.g., radiation therapy for relapsed versus initially presenting ALL)[43] and use of therapeutic approaches that reduce treatment intensity (e.g., conformal or proton beam radiation rather than cranial spinal radiation therapy for localized brain tumors).[44–46] Efforts to date suggest that these treatment advances have successfully reduced cognitive late effects; yet, for many of these children, there continue to be deficits that will require interventions and accommodations.[43,45,47] Children with other malignancies may have impairments such as limb amputation or visual impairment due to enucleation of one or both eyes. Chronic illness- or treatment-related disability will have the greatest effect on children's disability rating over time, as the long-term effects of treatment on learning emerge.

Also, during this initial phase, patients may begin serial assessment of their neuropsychological functioning. This monitoring is most important for children who receive central nervous system-directed therapies, such as those who have ALL or brain tumors.[39] Repeated assessment will be essential for the detection of emerging treatment-related disabilities that may not be seen for several years after treatment.[5] Close monitoring of cancer survivors is a necessity as they are moving targets with respect to cognitive abilities because of late emerging cognitive problems as well as changes in teacher expectations with increasing age that may reveal previously existing problems. Results from current neuropsychological assessments allow for the development of targeted, individualized, educational recommendations that can assist in optimizing academic performance.

Phase 2: Preparation for School Re-entry and Re-entry

In phase 2, work should be directed toward discussion with the child with cancer, the parent, the child's physician, and school personnel to get ready for the return to school. Children with cancer will go back to school, if possible, and a classroom presentation will assist with school re-entry. In planning for school re-entry, the different perspectives, expectations, and needs of all the participants must be considered. School re-entry should not be an all or none issue, and the child should be able to return to school on a part-time basis with the continued support of homebound services. Fatigue and frequent absences because of treatment may make full-time school attendance difficult or impossible. Considering the positive aspects of school attendance, it is important to accommodate these issues so that the child can return to school as soon as possible.[36] Specific accommodations will be discussed in greater detail later in the chapter.

Child and Adolescent

Planning for school re-entry always should begin with an interview with the child with cancer. Although common concerns usually are expressed by children and adolescents, all children should be given the opportunity to express their individual concerns.[12] The concerns most often expressed include peer rejection or ridicule because of hair loss or other changes in appearance, falling behind academically or having to repeat a grade, and relating to teachers and other school staff.[8,10,16–18,20,34]

These problems are intensified for adolescents. Academic pressures are greater as adolescents move closer to graduation, so that the fear of falling behind or not graduating on time is greater. Adolescents also must interact with several teachers, each with their own perspective on the student's illness and how best to accommodate returning students. Peer and social relationships are more complex at this age, as adolescents usually are more independent and spend more time with peers. Duffey-Lind and colleagues conducted focus group interviews with recently treated adolescent cancer patients to identify their greatest concerns.[48] Most of the adolescents revealed concerns regarding return to school and feeling different from their peers. They indicated that they often lost friends shortly after diagnosis and had difficulty building new friendships after school re-entry.

Children or adolescents also may be concerned about potentially stigmatizing situations, such as nausea, extreme fatigue, or frequent need to use the restroom during classes. Children and adolescents with physical impairments may be concerned about being knocked down while navigating a crowded hallway or stairway.

Before the interview with the child with cancer, it is important to gather as much information as possible about their current level of disability and their premorbid school adjustment and level of achievement. Children and adolescents who disliked school or were poor achievers before their illness may have more difficulty with school re-entry.[6] Any other problems children may have had in school in the past, such as discipline issues or peer relationship issues, will affect what fears and concerns they have now.

Parents

Parents have many concerns about their child's school re-entry. The attitudes of parents range from thankfulness that their child can return to the normalcy of school to feeling that they do not want them to suffer more by being forced back to school.[49] Parents may be overprotective and feel that their child is too vulnerable to go out into the world.[30] Parents and children also may develop a mutual separation anxiety that can lead to school phobia and can cause parents to refuse to allow school re-entry.[17] In a survey by Charlton and colleagues,[35] parents of children who had solid tumors and were returning to school listed the best and worst things about school re-entry. In the "best" category were: returning to normal, seeing their child happy and reuniting with friends, and ensuring that the child did not get too far behind in work. On the "worst" list were: worries about the child's inability to cope with school, possibility of physical injury, loss of hair, teasing by peers, and being behind in schoolwork. These parents also reported that they had received discouraging opinions about school re-entry from others in the family, such as grandparents, who may have had outmoded ideas about childhood cancer. Similarly, interviews by McCarthy and colleagues conducted with parents prior to school re-entry revealed primary concerns related to their child being teased, becoming physically injured, or becoming ill secondary to infection. Interestingly, mothers did not express concerns regarding their child's academic progress and responses indicated that they felt their child could catch up easily. Although mothers reported feeling knowledgeable about their children's cancer diagnosis and treatment, they did not feel confident presenting this information to the school.

Parents' level of anxiety or comfort about school re-entry and return to other normal activities definitely influences how children with cancer respond[8,16,35] and, in fact, can be crucial to school re-entry success.[30] Those parents who had little premorbid school participation may not believe that school re-entry is very important and may not have skills necessary to help their children.[8,34] On the opposite end of the spectrum are those parents who not only want the child back in school as soon as possible, but may have unrealistic expectations about the child's level of school attendance and level of achievement. This pressure can be just as detrimental and may set the child up for failure early in the re-entry process. Parents need education about appropriate expectations for their child and how to support their child's re-entry.

Information received by the school liaison about the parents' premorbid school involvement should be shared with other professionals. Everyone working with returning children should understand parents' attitudes toward school re-entry and scholastic achievement in general, and should work in a proactive manner to assist the parents in recognizing the positive aspects of school re-entry while providing reassurance and information to decrease anxiety about problems children may encounter. Any professional who detects a problem should alert other professionals working with the family to ensure the family receives the needed support, such as referral to a psychologist or social worker.

For parents of children who have illness- or treatment-related impairment, the prospect of school re-entry may be especially intimidating. Such parents worry about teasing and the possibility of injury to their children and also must navigate through the school system's bureaucracy to get special services (i.e., special education, classroom accommodations, or both) needed by returning children. It is essential that such parents—and all parents of children with cancer—have access to information about available services, how they are accessed, what federal laws mandate, and how to become an effective advocate for their child. Older adolescents also should have this knowledge. As adolescents transition to college or work settings, they will become their own advocate and will be required to communicate their needs for academic services or vocational assistance. The school liaison should provide this information to parents and young adult patients to help them to understand this process better. The school liaison also should attend, with the parents, any important school meetings about the child or adolescent. If the school liaison cannot attend such meetings because of distance, the possibility of a conference call during the meeting should be explored. Empowering parents and adolescents in this way can help them to regain a sense of control and a more positive outlook about school re-entry.

Teachers

The low prevalence of childhood cancer means that for most teachers, and other school personnel, having a child with cancer in the classroom is a new experience.[14,49,50] The teacher plays a crucial role in adjustment to school re-entry by influencing the tone of the classroom and helping classmates to understand returning children's physical changes and limitations.[51] Most respondents in Bessell's study of childhood cancer survivors saw the teacher as a "key individual in creating a successful school environment."[20] It is, therefore, vital that these teachers have a full understanding of the child's diagnosis and treatment and have access, through school liaisons or parents, to any other pertinent medical information.

Teachers experience anxiety about their lack of knowledge of childhood cancer, what their expectations of the child with cancer's performance should be, what medical problems might arise in the classroom, and how to deal with them.[4,11] Teachers want and need information but feel uncomfortable about asking parents for it directly for fear of exacerbating their sadness about their children's illnesses.[4,19,22,30,51] This lack of information may lead to teachers overprotecting children.[4] Under these circumstances, returning students are not challenged to live up to their potential.

Conversely, involved teachers may lack information about the true limitations of such children and may have unrealistic expectations that lead to frustration and discouragement.[30] If teachers were familiar with returning children before the advent of their illness, their expectations may not take into account changes that the children have undergone. When several teachers are involved, as in the case of adolescents, this problem is intensified. Teachers who are provided inadequate information may also try to fit cancer survivors into more familiar learning disability categories such as Attention Deficit Hyperactivity Disorder (ADHD) that could lead to an oversimplification of their needs.

Teachers may feel uncertain and unprepared to answer questions from classmates about returning children's illness and prognosis. Also, teachers may feel some conflict about the attention needed by children with cancer and may fear a conflict with the needs of the other children in the class. Teachers have reported being concerned about the entire class, the adjustment of the child with cancer, and the adjustment of the child's classmates to the knowledge that a peer had a life-threatening disease.[34] The one factor that can prevent or alleviate these problems and fears is *communication*. Several studies have shown that teachers feel the need for more communication with the child with cancer's medical team. Such teachers seek the provision of more medical information or information about the child's functional level and performance expectations.[10,11,16,19,22,35] A review by Vance and Eiser found that the teachers' reported information provided to them was often inadequate and should focus more on behavioral and psychological problems.[52] Following school re-entry intervention programs, teachers reported increased knowledge of childhood cancer and improved confidence in working with these children.[52] According to the previously mentioned study by Rynard and colleagues,[19] teachers rated the importance of a school conference very highly.

Once the date of school re-entry is known, the school liaison can meet with (or telephone) the teacher, other school personnel, and parents to make specific plans and to discuss expectations for performance, changes in level of ability and level of physical activity, and any accommodations or special services the returning child may need. The child's teachers should communicate with the homebound/hospital bound teacher about what skills have been learned and the level at which the child will be re-entering school. Teachers and school personnel also need to know what, if any, medical problems may arise at school, what to do or whom to call, and what medications the child may need to take. Also important is information about infectious diseases; teachers should inform involved parents as soon as possible about any possible cases of influenza or exposure to chickenpox.

Peers

Peer socialization is an essential part of children's lives and provides them with opportunities to learn how to interact socially and build skills in conflict resolution and leadership. School is the primary place where these skills are learned and practiced. As adolescents start to experience more independence from parents, their peer relationships take on even more importance.[18,33] For a child with cancer who must be absent a lot, maintenance of good peer relationships throughout treatment is essential. Varni and colleagues studied how children with newly diagnosed cancer were affected by perceived social support. The study revealed that perceived social support from classmates was identified as the most consistent predictor of adaptation. This further establishes the importance of the school as a social environment for the child or adolescent and the importance of maintaining peer support during treatment.[53] In fact, there is evidence that a program of social skills training as prescribed in an earlier study by Varni and colleagues may serve to increase perceived classmate and teacher social support.[25]

The importance of the school as a social environment in the eyes of children and adolescents also leads to fears of peer teasing and rejection at the time of school re-entry. Some teasing is a normal part of the school experience, but sometimes children with cancer are targeted because of their perceived vulnerability or because of the visible signs of their disease.[16] Vance and Eiser's review of the school re-entry literature revealed that children with cancer were more often nominated by their peers and teachers for sensitive-isolated roles than healthy children, even though the child with cancer may not view themselves as more eligible for these roles.[52] Several authors have also noted that most incidents of teasing come from students in other classes.[10,35,54] Although children can be cruel, some tease because they do not know how to act around children with cancer. They may wait for cues from the child with cancer and otherwise see how they behave before feeling comfortable with interacting with them.[16] On the other hand, peers can become overly nice or doting, and this behavior may be perceived just as negatively as teasing, especially by adolescent patients.[33] Most children and adolescents just want to be treated like normal.[16,20]

Peer education after diagnosis and before school re-entry can be a bridge toward making peers and the child with cancer more comfortable with each other. When presented with clear, accurate information at an age-appropriate level, peers can become the patient's main source of support and sometimes can act to protect them from teasing.[10]

Much misinformation can be spread through rumors and other student's overhearing teacher's and peer conversations. As mentioned earlier, HIPPA regulations apply in the school setting and teachers and students both need to be aware of the privacy protections, which are part of HIPPA. Peers need accurate information about the returning child's diagnosis; treatment; side effects of treatment, including any transient or chronic impairments (especially those that are visible); the course of treatment, including information about absences; and how they can assist in re-entry, with an emphasis on the need to treat them normally. They also need the opportunity to ask questions and should receive straightforward answers to their questions, including those about death. However, many adolescents do not want a presentation and prefer to share the information with a few close friends and have the school liaison talk with the teachers.

Services or Support Available to Assist Re-entry

After fears and concerns are discussed, information should be provided about services available to assist re-entry. Services may include a school re-entry presentation and/or assistance with getting needed accommodations or special education services. Evaluation of a child's learning needs and social/emotional functioning would also be helpful in making sure any deficits or weaknesses are documented. This is especially true for those children who are receiving CNS-directed therapy.[46,55,56]

After an evaluation is done, discussion should address any need for special education or classroom accommodations and the federal laws that mandate the provision of these services to children with disabilities (discussed in the section on federal laws). This information will assist in alleviating some fears and concerns of patients and parents.

Associating the need for special education services with the impact of the disease process and treatment, and identifying new deficits as "acquired," may help returning patients to avoid perceptions that the services or the difficulties reflect on them personally. Reframing the condition as a side effect, as something the disease or treatment has done to them, may help to protect children's sense of self-worth. Special education services can be viewed as a way to optimize a child's ability to succeed in school through leveling of the playing field with their peers by lessening the impact of new challenges.

Presentation About Illness and Treatment to Classmates or Teachers. Even if there has been a post-diagnosis presentation to the classmates, the child who is returning to school may want another presentation. In some cases, the child may be going to a different grade or even to a different school and will have classmates who were not involved in the first presentation. Elementary school children usually want someone from the hospital to go to their school. The case is less well defined with middle-school and high-school students, for whom the

need to not be different is paramount. Adolescents sometimes wish to tell only teachers and a close group of friends. It is important to respect such patients' wishes in this regard, but equally important is to ensure that they are fully aware of available services and support and how these services can benefit them. If patients have agreed to a classroom or teacher presentation, the exact content of the presentation should be reviewed. *Always* ensure that children are fully aware of, and agree to, everything that will be covered in the presentation. At this time, also, children should be assisted in anticipating some of the questions they are likely to encounter.

Being Present and Participating in the Discussion with Classmates and Teacher. Most children and adolescents want to be there during the presentation and may wish to participate as an "expert" on their illness. They may want to give part of the presentation or just be available for the question/answer session during or after the presentation. Discuss with the child how they wish to participate and if they need any help with formulating some "stock" answers to difficult questions. Providing children with examples of what can be said or how situations have been handled by other children may ease some of their uncertainty or concerns. On the other hand, some children and adolescents do not want to participate or even be present during the presentation. Their wishes should be respected as well.

If the child lives at a distance from the hospital, telephone consultation with school personnel and provision of appropriate written materials and/or videos can be done.

School Re-entry Plan

Materials for a school presentation are available through multiple sources such as Cancervive, which has a Back to School Kit, and the Leukemia/Lymphoma Society, which has the Trish Greene Back to School Program, Candlelighter's Childhood Cancer Foundation, American Cancer Society, and Starlight Children's Foundation. There are also individual journal articles outlining school re-entry programs such as Worchel-Prevatt and colleagues.[57] The programs from Cancervive and Leukemia/Lymphoma Society offer written materials and videos to put together a presentation for different age groups. The child may also make their own video of the hospital and a typical day at the hospital with the assistance of nurses or child life specialists. Table 48.1 is a template for a school presentation that was first presented in a chapter in the revision of the book *Educating the Child with Cancer* (Table 48.1).[58]

Whatever combination of peer education and teacher education is used in a school re-entry plan, one must keep in mind that every child is an *individual* with individual needs regarding school re-entry. Although certain information almost always should be presented, the needs of returning children should be foremost in rendering school re-entry a positive experience. Communication among the school, parent, and school liaison should be frequent in the days after school re-entry to ensure that any problems or questions can be handled quickly. School liaisons should clarify to school personnel that they can be contacted at any time in the future with questions or concerns regarding the child.

Federal Laws Protecting the Educational Rights of Children with Disabilities

Three federal laws protect the rights of children between the ages of 3 and 21 who have disabilities that impede their ability to benefit from their educational environment. These laws are the Individuals with Disability Education Act (IDEA); the Rehabilitation Act of 1973 (Section 504); the Americans with

TABLE 48.1

TEMPLATE FOR A SCHOOL PRESENTATION FOR RE-ENTRY OF CHILDREN WITH CANCER

Topics to be discussed with peers	General information about cancer	Specific information about the child's diagnosis and treatment	Effects of cancer and treatment	What classmates can do to assist the child
Discussion points	• Facts and myths about cancer • Cancer is not contagious • You do not get cancer because of bad behavior	• Type of cancer • Treatment • Venous access/line subcutaneous port • Other medical appliances such as shunts	• Changes in appearance • Energy level • Suppressed immune system • School absences	• Ask classmates for ideas and ask them to think about how they would like to be treated in the same situation.

Disabilities Act (ADA). These laws apply to every level of education, from infant and toddler to college and vocational education, and they guarantee every citizen the right to education regardless of physical, mental, or health impairment. Although these laws are federal, local and state governments interpret and implement them differently. It is important that parents contact their state's department of education for guidelines governing the ways in which these laws are implemented. Also, every state department of education has a Web site so parents can look at state guidelines themselves and find out whom to contact for further clarification.

Any services needed by children in school, such as special education or classroom accommodations, should be formalized with a written plan using the IDEA or section 504 of the Rehabilitation Act. The written, signed plan will protect the rights of the child with cancer and provide documentation needed by parents if the services are not provided appropriately. Parents working with cooperative educators may not feel the need to document services in writing but written documentation is crucial for sharing information among different teachers and across grades, as well was for documenting progress or failure to make progress that requires adjustments to the plan. Documentation of the services provided is necessary to obtain accommodations on tests such as ACT and SAT and to transfer accommodations to college. Additionally, documentation is especially important in times such as these when federal and state resources are constrained. School system personnel may say that certain services are not available because of lack of adequate funding. This is inappropriate because, by law, services are provided because of need, not funding. Having good documentation of the need for services and an advocate who can respond appropriately when any request for services is denied because of funding issues will be most helpful.

Individuals With Disabilities Education Act. The IDEA is a revision of an earlier law, PL 94–142 (Education of the Handicapped Act). The IDEA is a federal law that establishes a grant program to assist states in providing a free, appropriate public education, which includes special education and related services, to meet the unique needs of all disabled individuals between the ages of 3 and 21 [34 Code of Federal Regulations (CFR), Sec. 300.1(a)]. To receive special education under provisions of the IDEA, children must meet criteria for classification under one of 13 categories. In 2004, IDEA was reauthorized as the Individuals with Disabilities Education Improvement Act of 2004 with some amendments affecting the individual education plan (IEP) process, due process, and discipline provisions. The changes are too numerous to include in this

chapter; however, an explanation can be found in the Wrightslaw Web site at www.wrightslaw.com.

Most children diagnosed with cancer are eligible for services under the category *other health impairment*, defined as "a child who has limited strength, vitality, or alertness due to chronic or acute health problems, such as heart condition, tuberculosis, rheumatic fever, nephritis, asthma, sickle anemia, hemophilia, epilepsy, lead poisoning, leukemia, or diabetes which adversely affects educational performance" (34 CFR, Sec. 300.7).

Special education includes services ranging from simple classroom accommodations in a regular classroom to all-day placement in a resource room environment to instruction in the home, hospital, or other institution. Related services such as physical and occupational therapy can also be provided through special education. Classroom accommodations that children with cancer may receive include use of a scribe or tape recorder to take notes, shortened class or homework assignments, provision of information instead of copying from a board or book, preferential seating, more time for tests or written work, oral testing, books on tape, use of a word processor to complete assignments, multiple choice versus open-ended exam questions, one-on-one organizational assistance and permission to leave class early to avoid accidental injury caused by travel through crowded hallways.

To receive these services, qualifying children must be referred to the school's principal or to the special education coordinator for the school or school district. Anyone can make the referral including the parent and, it is best for the referral to be in writing. This assists all involved by making sure there is a record of the referral. Once the referral is made, the school system has a certain amount of time to evaluate such children or to review the evaluation performed by other agencies.

If a child with cancer has received neuropsychological, physical, or occupational therapy evaluations while in the hospital, the school liaison can provide these reports to the appropriate school personnel, with parental permission. Information about diagnosis, course of treatment, and any illness- or treatment-related impairments that impact education may be needed or the school system may have a form for physicians to sign verifying the medical diagnosis.

If the child is deemed eligible for special education services, a meeting will be scheduled to write the IEP. The meeting should include, at the least, the parents, any teacher involved, a school administrator, and others involved in the child's care. It is advisable to have someone from the hospital, probably the school liaison, at the meeting to ensure that the pertinent aspects of the children's medical care, illness, and any transient or chronic impairments are well understood by the IEP team. The IEP constructed at the meeting should consist of certain elements[6] such as present level of academic and cognitive functioning and a statement of needs as identified by assessments. The plan also should include a statement regarding accommodations needed for state- or district-wide achievement tests.

After the IEP is signed by all participants at the meeting, it becomes a legal document that, by law, the state is required to carry out as written. Parents should keep a file or binder of all appropriate documents, including the IEP, and a copy should go into the child's medical records. The goals and objectives of the IEP are reviewed annually, and the IEP is rewritten. Every 3 years, the child is reassessed. Children with cognitive late effects can have progressive changes that occur more rapidly than the 3-year window for reassessment as prescribed by IDEA. The need for a different reassessment schedule can be documented and written into the IEP or the parents can opt to have a private evaluation. Also, parents or any other member of the IEP team can call for another IEP meeting and it can be scheduled to reassess a child's placement and services. For a timeline for the development and review of the IEP, please go to www.wrightslaw.com or www.nichcy.org.

IDEA mandates early intervention services for infants and toddlers who are disabled or at risk of developmental delays. Services are provided either by school systems or the state health department. The law requires that services be provided to affected children and their families. Rather than an IEP, an individual family service plan (IFSP) is written.

Transition services—The purpose of transition services is to provide students with disabilities with the skills and knowledge that will facilitate a successful transition to adult life (34 CFR, Sec. 300.43) to facilitate the child's movement from school to post-school activities, including post-secondary education, vocational training, integrated employment (including supported employment), continuing and adult education, adult services, independent living, or community participation. The IEP should contain information about the actions that will be taken to prepare the child for the move from high school to adult life in their community. More specifically, there should be goals related to courses of study and any other support, training, or employment counseling the child will need. Also, other agencies will be identified that are likely to be responsible for providing or paying for transition services and will be invited to send a representative to the IEP meeting. The age requirements have also changed with transition planning now beginning at the first IEP to be in effect when the child is 16. Some states have retained 14 years as the age to begin transition planning such that anyone working with a patient who needs transition planning will need to check with specific state special education regulations.

Section 504 of the Rehabilitation Act of 1973. Section 504 of the Rehabilitation Act of 1973 (re-authorized in 1998) is not an education law or a federal grant program. It is an anti-discrimination law that requires that the educational needs of disabled students are met as adequately as the needs of students without disabilities. It also mandates the provision of a free appropriate public education to students who qualify under Section 504, but who do not meet criteria to qualify under IDEA.[59] This is generally used for those children who are in need of accommodations in the regular classroom, but do not need a different classroom placement. This law applies also to colleges, universities, and private schools that receive federal funds and is the avenue for college students to receive accommodations. In addition to stipulating conditions in academic settings, the Rehabilitation Act prohibits discrimination in employment practices; program accessibility; health, welfare, and other social services; nonacademic and extracurricular activities, including clubs; counseling services; transportation; and health services.[6]

In order to receive services under Section 504, some school districts will require documentation that the disability "substantially limits" one or more major life activity. As there are no definitions provided for this term in the law, school districts are instructed to define the term themselves.[60] This has led to variability across school districts in who is considered eligible. If a child with cancer is denied a 504 Plan, it would be helpful for the parents to get further assistance from the school liaison or an advocate. Children and adolescents with diagnosed cancer are usually eligible to receive services under Section 504 because learning, which is one of the "major life activities" defined in the law, is limited by absences or side effects of treatment.[61,62] Each school system should have a Section 504 coordinator who oversees compliance with this law and a referral to this person is the beginning of the process toward the development of a 504 Plan. Once eligibility is determined, a meeting similar to an IEP meeting is held to discuss specific accommodations and the 504 Plan is written. Review of the plan occurs periodically and the plan can be modified as needed at any time. Although Section 504 of the Rehabilitation Act of 1973 does not mandate transition planning, it can be part of the 504 Plan and the 1998 amendments to the Rehabilitation Act do facilitate access to resources for transition, such as the Council for Independent Living and vocational rehabilitation services.

American with Disabilities Act (ADA) of 1990 provides a wider range of protection for all persons with disabilities. All persons with diagnosed cancer, even long-term survivors, are eligible for protection under the provisions of the ADA.[63] It prohibits discrimination against persons with disabilities and applies to all state and local agencies (not just those receiving federal funds), including private businesses. The ADA not only prohibits discrimination against persons with disabilities but also requires that persons with disabilities receive "reasonable accommodation." Although it is not an education law, its provisions do apply to education, including nonsectarian private schools. It provides a second layer of protection, in addition to section 504, to ensure that schools provide reasonable accommodations for students with disabilities.[61]

On January 1, 2009, the American with Disabilities Amendments Act of 2008 became effective. This act officially rejected Supreme Court decisions that reduced protections for some people with disabilities under ADA of 1990. Because ADA and Section 504 define disability in a similar way, ADA case law applies to 504 cases. This law supports a broad definition of "disability" by: (a) expanding the definition of "major life activities" to include two non-exhaustive lists, one of general activities and one of bodily functions; (b) stipulating that mitigation of the disability by medication, assistive technology, or learned behavioral adaptations does not disqualify anyone from protection under ADA or 504; and (c) clarifying that an impairment that is episodic or in remission is still a disability if it would substantially limit a major life activity when active.[64,65]

Federal Laws and Public Versus Private School Placement. Because private schools do not take federal funds, they are not bound by IDEA or Section 504 to provide special education services. They are bound by ADA and should provide "reasonable" classroom accommodations to students with disabilities. There are even some private schools that are primarily for students with disabilities or students who have not done well in the public classroom environment.

One area of confusion with regard to federal laws is what obligation public school systems have to provide special education services to private school students. We are specifically addressing students with disabilities whose parents choose to place them in a private school. The law states that children with disabilities who are placed by their parents in private schools have no individual right to receive all or some of the special education and related services that the child would receive if enrolled in a public school (34 CFR 300.137). The Local Education Agency (LEA) will provide some special education services to some students with disabilities, but not the total range of possible special educations services to all students with disabilities in private schools.

Certainly, if there is a child with cancer who may have a disability enrolled in a private school, the parents should ask for an evaluation as per the child fund requirements. If the child is determined to be eligible for special education services, the parents should ask that these services be provided by the LEA; however, they need to understand the limitations of the federal law in provision of these services.

Please refer to any of the Web site resources cited here for further information about these laws.

Web site resources for educational services and advocacy:

> Individuals with Disabilities Education Act: http://.idea.ed.gov
> [Information on IDEA implementation regulations including a Q & A area]
> Special Education Resources on the Internet (SERI): www.seriweb.com
> [A collection of internet accessible information and resources related to special education]
> Council of Parent Attorneys and Advocates: www.copaa.net
> [Information and resources for securing special education advocacy]
> National Parent Information Network: www.npin.org
> [Education software and services for middle school, high school, and college students]
> Council for Exceptional Children: www.cec.sped.org
> [Professional organization dedicated to the educational success of children with disabilities and/or those who are gifted]
> Educational Register: www.vincentcurtis.com
> [Information and advice about private schools and summer programs]
> National Center on Secondary Education and Transition: www.ncset.org
> [Information and resources about secondary education and transitional services]
> National Dissemination Center for Children with Disabilities: www.nichcy.org
> [Information on disabilities, IDEA, NCLB, and effective education practices]
> National Center for Learning Disabilities: www.ncld.org
> [Information on learning disabilities from legislation to teaching strategies]
> Wrightslaw: www.wrightslaw.com
> [Information on special education law and advocacy for children with disabilities].

Stratification of Disability Levels. Cancer survivors will vary both with respect to their premorbid level of functioning, including the presence of any pre-existing disability, as well as the extent to which they experience chronic illness- or treatment-related impairment. Premorbid disabilities may include attention deficit-hyperactivity disorder; learning disability; hearing, vision, or speech impairment; mental retardation; behavioral problems; or affective disorders. Any premorbid learning or adjustment problems, along with the school absences related to the child with cancer's treatment, will render school re-entry more difficult.[8,10,16,18,30,38] In this chapter, we propose that a level of disability be identified at the time of school re-entry and throughout a child with cancer's scholastic career to identify the resources needed and discern which children are at risk of long-term learning problems. School re-entry needs are determined by the level of disability.

Children can be categorized into four levels—level 1: no premorbid disability and no chronic illness- or treatment-related impairment; level 2: premorbid disability and no chronic illness- or treatment-related impairment; level 3: no premorbid disability but chronic illness- or treatment-related impairment; and level 4: premorbid disability and chronic illness- or treatment-related impairment. These levels of disability will determine the need for temporary versus long-term educational services, parental familiarity with special education rights and procedures, the extent of required services, recommendations regarding monitoring and serial assessments, and the degree to which parents may need to adjust expectations regarding their child's future academic trajectory.

Children classified at level 1 or 2, who are not likely to experience chronic illness- or treatment-related impairment, may experience transient problems related to school absence, fatigue, and restrictions in physical activity. They may not be able to play on the playground or participate in physical education for a period. They also may need to make up work missed in their absence and will have future absences because of follow-up clinic visits. School re-entry may mean a modified schedule of only half-days or a 2- to 3-day week. Use of homebound services can continue to supplement educational services when they cannot attend school. Shortened or modified assignments also may be used to assist with staying abreast of schoolwork. These accommodations should be included in a section 504 Plan.

Parents of children who have no history of premorbid disability, level 1 or 3, will require information regarding special education procedures. Because such children are unlikely to have received previous special services, school re-entry planning should include discussion with parents about their rights and their children's rights under the provisions of the IDEA and section 504 of the Rehabilitation Act, so as to obtain any needed services or classroom accommodations. The school liaison should provide information about the referral process and assist them with meeting with school personnel.

Children with premorbid disabilities, level 2 or 4, may have had some level of special education services or classroom accommodations and may have an IEP or a section 504 plan. Possibly, previous services were, or may have become, inadequate or inappropriate. Children at level 4 may be the most impaired, because problems related to the premorbid condition may be exacerbated by the illness or treatment-related impairment.[56] School re-entry planning should include a review of the child's previous special education services or accommodations and discussion of any additional or more intensive services needed because of chronic illness- or treatment-related impairment. Professionals at the hospital, such as a psychologist or the school liaison, can review children's previous services and make recommendations for improvement, if necessary. Neuropsychological testing also may be helpful or necessary to assist with school re-entry. Professionals involved in the children's care should discuss specific school recommendations with the child's parents. Parents can call school personnel to arrange a meeting for revision of an IEP or 504 plan.

Chronic impairment usually is associated with central nervous system-directed therapy for ALL or brain tumors.[5,39,41-44,66] School re-entry planning, as one would expect, is more complex for chronically impaired children and may involve coordination with other professionals in a multidisciplinary format. For such impairments as hemiparesis or vision, hearing, or speech impairment, a qualified professional should perform an assessment to determine the level of therapy or support needed by children with cancer. A neuropsychological assessment should also be conducted to determine level of cognitive functioning and document any learning disabilities or deficits (e.g., slow processing speed, memory problems, or attention difficulties). Given the evolving nature of cognitive deficits in childhood cancer survivors due to late emerging treatment-related changes, the interaction of neurodevelopment with pre-existing lesions and the exacerbation of deficits due to changes in environmental support, children will likely need to be monitored closely and formally assessed more frequently. There are also predictable time points (e.g., the transition to junior high school with increased expectancies for independence) at which increased support may need to be provided. Evaluation reports can be sent to the school system after children have been referred for special services. Children with cancer may need occupational therapy, physical therapy, or speech therapy or a special teacher for the visually impaired or hearing impaired to assist in a regular classroom. Full-time placement in the regular classroom may not be possible; children may have to spend part or all of their days in a resource room environment where the student-teacher ratio is lower and each child can work at his or her level. All recommendations regarding therapy, alternative class placement, and alternative educational services should be outlined clearly in the IEP or section 504 plan. For the IEP or 504 Plan meeting at the school, it is advisable to have someone such as the school liaison at the meeting to discuss any pertinent medical issues, answer any questions, and act as a child-parent advocate. If a school liaison cannot attend the meeting, the liaison can be part of a conference call during the meeting. Parents may also contact the state advocacy agency if they need an advocate more than someone to answer medically related questions. There are listings of many different education agencies including advocacy agencies by state at www.nichcy.org.

One additional issue that must be raised with children with chronic illness- or treatment-related disability is the fact that changes in cognitive or physical abilities may necessitate changes in expectations for the future. Plans for college may change to plans for vocational training or for a 2-year degree, and plans for an athletic scholarship or career may have to be set aside. Concomitantly, both parents and children may need support to develop acceptance of their need to reset expectations. All parents want their children to live up to their potential, but when that potential is changed by a cognitive or physical impairment, parents may have difficulty in understanding and accepting what was once possible for their child is no longer within reach. They experience disappointment, even grief, for the loss of their premorbid children. Psychologists and physicians who evaluate and treat chronically impaired children must be aware of these possible problems and should carefully explain to both parents and children any illness- or treatment-related impairment, how the impairment changes affected children's ability to function cognitively or physically, and how these changes will affect plans for the future. The psychologist or physician should assess parents' and children's understanding and acceptance of this information and provide further information and counseling as necessary to assist with this process. In follow-up, they should maintain discussion with both parents and children and assist them as necessary in finding a new direction for their children's future.

Empirically-Supported Interventions. The efficacy of school-based interventions for pediatric cancer patients who return to school manifesting cognitive late effects continues to be under investigation. Preliminary studies suggested the potential effectiveness of stimulant medications in addressing the problems with attention and arousal experienced by children whose cancer had been treated with cranial irradiation or intrathecal chemotherapy.[67] Extension of this work has now revealed significant, sustained, benefits based on parent and teacher ratings of attention and social skills.[68,69] Further, as a group, childhood cancer survivors tolerate stimulant medication well with the frequency and severity of side effects similar to those reported for children diagnosed with ADHD.[70,71]

The most systematic approaches to cognitive remediation in survivors of childhood cancer have been developed by Butler and Copeland.[72] These researchers developed a tripartite model, the Cognitive Remediation Program (CRP), that uses techniques from brain injury rehabilitation (e.g., massed practice of sustained, selective, and divided attention tasks), special education (e.g., instruction in metacognitive strategies such as task preparedness, on-task performance, and post task evaluation), and clinical psychology (e.g., cognitive behavioral interventions such as reframing cognitive struggles in a positive light, monitoring negative internal dialogue, and stress inoculation).[73] A recently published multi-center, randomized controlled trial in 167 childhood cancer survivors revealed that CRP participants experienced a significant improvement in academic achievement, incorporated more metacognitive strategies in problem solving, and showed improvement on a parent-rated measure of attention.[74] Some of the strategies used in CRP can be implemented by a special educator and/or psychologist within the school setting.

Although group-based empirical studies continue to examine interventions for pediatric cancer patients experiencing cognitive late effects, the need may be for individually customized approaches with delineation of specific academic skill goals rather than for "pre-packaged" programs.[75] School personnel need to draw from research from other populations as well as from the general field of cognitive psychology in order to develop the nature of the individual student's deficits and to develop interventions tailored to the particular student with close monitoring of their effectiveness in a "single case study" model. Educators may need to attempt interventions that have proved effective with other populations showing similar deficits and closely monitor the outcomes for the individual student. For example, Armstrong and Briery have proposed that language-based cognitive abilities can serve as the basis for development of compensatory strategies and interventions for deficits arising in visual-motor learning and performance.[55] This is because language skills, appearing earlier in the course of brain development as the brain structures associated with these processes complete their maturation sooner, may be more resistant to disruption by chemotherapy or cranial radiation in pediatric cancer patients. In contrast, later developing processes controlled by later maturing brain structures, such as attention and behavioral regulation, memory organization and retrieval, and higher-order problem-solving may be more vulnerable to disruption by the same therapeutic agents.[55] Given this consideration, a logical case could be made for attempting to correct for attention and/or behavior regulation difficulties in a childhood cancer survivor through the use of self-coaching techniques, verbal mediation-based strategies or externalization of processing approaches such as those delineated by Kendal and Braswell, Meichenbaum and Goodman, and Douglas and colleagues.[59,76,77] Cognitive psychology also offers guidance regarding design of school interventions through careful definition of cognitive constructs and their component processes. Take memory as an example. Using knowledge of the component processes of memory allows neuropsychologists to move beyond treatment of memory as a unitary construct in recommending interventions to school personnel. Careful examination of a child's approach to a standardized memory test and their pattern of errors allows us to isolate the step(s) at which memory problems are encountered. For example, classic list learning tasks allow us to identify whether a child has specific difficulty with memory encoding, retention and/or retrieval, as well as whether they profit from repetition or categorical cueing. For a child with encoding difficulties, use of "depth of processing"[78] principles can guide psychologists and school personnel in designing interventions that incorporate linking new information to old or previously mastered information, use of "active" versus passive learning modalities, and use of multisensory instruction and information. In contrast, for the child who is demonstrating isolated difficulty with retrieval, teaching strategies might include instruction in the use of mnemonics that assist in organizing the way in which information is encoded to facilitate retrieval as well as the use of recognition testing formats (e.g., true/false and multiple choice) versus free recall formats (e.g., open-ended questions). A degree of logic should prevail in the planning of accommodations and interventions for pediatric cancer patients or survivors returning to school with new educational needs and cognitive deficits. For example, with a student now requiring significantly more time to process information or a student now more prone to physical and mental fatigue, elimination of timed testing and reduction in the workload or volume of assignments seem natural conclusions.

Phase 3: Follow-up Contact

Initial Follow-up

In the weeks and months after re-entry to school, school personnel and the school liaison should continue to communicate frequently to assess how children are adjusting to the school environment. Any further assistance should be given as necessary. If there is an IEP or section 504 plan, the school liaison can assist the parents in ensuring that their children are receiving the services according to the plan.

Long-Term Follow-up

In our model of school re-entry, follow-up for children with cancer continues for years, through high school and college or vocational training. Long-term follow-up is necessary because of long-term or late neuropsychological effects of therapy for cancer. As defined by Mulhern,[39] there are "pathological changes in the child's central nervous system (CNS) secondary to cancer or its treatment that are manifested by stable changes in the child's behavior." For our purposes, *behavior* includes cognitive and academic skills.

Not all children treated for cancer receive treatment that affects the central nervous system or its functioning.[79] Significant physical and psychosocial effects relate to diagnosis and treatment of any childhood cancer, but the transient impairments resolve with few or no long-term sequelae.[50] However, 50% of children treated for cancer, specifically those with ALL or brain tumors, receive cranial radiotherapy or systemic or intrathecal methotrexate. Several recent studies have shown that such children are at increased risk of neuropsychological late effects from their illness or from treatment

that significantly limits their attainment of educational and vocational goals.[41–43,78]

Testing of long-term survivors of ALL and brain tumors indicates that cognitive deficits usually do not begin to appear until 2 to 4 years after the start of treatment and the magnitude of the deficit increases with time after treatment.[39,79–81,82] Psychometric scores also decline progressively over 2 to 4 years.[5,39,79] Cognitive deficits seen on neuropsychological testing include deficits in sequential memory, arithmetic, processing speed, visuomotor integration, attention and concentration, and fine motor coordination.[5,39,81,83] The decline in standard scores usually is not representative of a progressive deterioration of abilities but of a significant slowing of the rate of development of abilities relative to the rate demonstrated by others in the patient's age cohort.[5] This information, combined with the facts that younger children have greater deficits and that specific abilities associated with prefrontal cortex function (e.g., attention and executive functions) are impaired, led Armstrong and Horn[5] to propose a model of developmental emergence of deficits. According to this model, treatment with central nervous system-directed therapies interferes with the normal development of the prefrontal cortex, thus interrupting or delaying functions that would have emerged as part of the normal development course.[5]

Multiple lines of research have revealed that the prefrontal cortex is protracted in neurodevelopment, with increases in white matter extending into the third decade of life.[84] White matter, or myelin, facilitates the speed and efficiency of communication among brain regions.[85] Given that children treated for cancer with central nervous system-direct therapies demonstrate a loss of white matter, in contrast to expected developmental maturation, functions supported by the prefrontal cortex that typically mature during adolescence are particularly vulnerable.[86] This model helps to explain why a child's performance on tests of neuropsychological function is within normal limits during a given year but becomes significantly impaired a few years later.

At the time of development that the specific cognitive ability would have been expected to become evident normally and thereby testable, it fails to be manifested by the child experiencing late cognitive effects secondary to cranial irradiation or intrathecal chemotherapy. At that time, the presence of the deficit becomes documented psychometrically. A final point regarding this phenomenon is that the nature of the child's inability to perform the specific cognitive task or process at the prescribed developmental time-point is generally unknown. There are four possible explanations: (a) the inability reflects a true deficit; that is, the loss of, or failure to develop, the capacity; (b) there is a delay such that the ability and process will eventually develop and be manifested at some later point in development; (c) it is a disruption such that the process is present but there is interference with its effective manifestation or application; or (d) there is a deviation such that the process or ability is developing but in an altered fashion.

The neuropsychologist, school, or clinical psychologist evaluating the child can be helpful in delineating the apparent nature of the deficit by providing qualitative information as well as quantitative data about the child's performance on testing. Most scores from a child's performance on the most frequently used norm-referenced psychometric measures merely represent the child's relative percentile ranking within the cohort of his age peers and are not measures of the quality of a cognitive, academic, or neuropsychological ability or process. Consequently, for school personnel to better target the selection of curriculum materials for the amelioration of identified deficits, it is paramount that the evaluator incorporate into the assessment report descriptions and qualitative analysis of the types and nature of errors the child made that contribute to the problematic testing score. It is insufficient for a psychologist to report, in the documentation of a child's testing results, only the child's standard score. For example, on one of the tests of story recall that are part of verbal memory test batteries, a child could attain that same score through a variety of means. The child could recall a certain number of details from only the beginning of the story, the same number of details from only the end of the story, or the same number of details that were scattered about within the whole story. Each performance suggests a different functional dynamic to the child's verbal memory functioning (e.g., primacy effect dominance, recency effect dominance, or poor memory organization), which would necessitate significantly different intervention and educational strategies for correction. Yet which dynamic is at play is unknown when merely the standard score is reported to school personnel. Similarly, it should be unacceptable for the psychologist to merely report that on academic achievement testing the child, for example, "performed within the Borderline range" "or at an early-2nd grade level equivalency" when doing written math calculations. Far more informative to school personnel in planning the child's IEP would be an additional statement such as, "While able to perform addition and subtraction when regrouping was not necessary, the child made numerous errors where the operations required carrying or borrowing as the child tended to extract quantities from or relocate values to the wrong column."

The fact that these neuropsychological deficits are not readily observable[5] suggests that even in the light of average academic performance, neuropsychological abilities should be assessed at regular intervals, according to a plan of surveillance.[39] Often, school and medical professionals do not have information about premorbid functioning of children and do not consider that some of such children were above average in function before the administration of central nervous system-directed therapies, and average performance in these children may represent a slowing of the acquisition of skills. Although they appear to be doing well, such students may need special accommodations or services to retain as much of their previous learning potential and scholastic performance as possible.

Provision of special educational services or classroom accommodations for children with cancer may be complicated, because their disabilities do not always conform to the concepts of specific learning disabilities (SLD) and ADHD that educators and others rely on when considering a child for special education services. The reauthorization of IDEA in 2004 changed how a determination of SLD is made such that the formula of a severe discrepancy between IQ and achievement used in the past can no longer be used and the law further states that the evaluation "cannot rely on any single procedure as the sole criterion for determining eligibility for special education and related services," but must use a variety of tools in the process of evaluation.[87] The new regulations, while improved over the discrepancy formula, still require the child be identified as "at risk" by having test scores fall below a certain cut-off before any academic interventions can begin. There are other problems with the process as well.[88] This is why it continues to be true that the best avenue for a child who is a survivor of cancer to receive accommodations or other special education services is to be identified as "Other Health Impaired" under IDEA or receive services under Section 504.

School personnel, including school psychologists, often have little or no experience with children with cancer and do not understand the potential impact of treatment for ALL or brain tumors. Problems with attention or memory may be interpreted by school personnel as laziness, lack of motivation, or other emotional difficulties.[89] School psychologists also may lack experience with the kinds of neuropsychological assessment needed to define the cognitive deficits experienced by childhood cancer survivors. Therefore, it is important that the child be assessed by a neuropsychologist through the auspices of the hospital.[5,39,80] Guidelines have been proposed for the assessment of school problems to assist professionals with this process.[54,79,80] These authors recommended that a re-evaluation should take place every 18 to 24 months and that both raw score and standard score changes be examined.[55] They also urge that, in addition to neuropsychological tests, curriculum-based measures be used to track the progress of individual children.

This prescribed frequency of formal assessment is greater than the reassessment rate traditionally undertaken by school systems and prescribed by special education legislation as the minimum (which is every 36 months). Therefore, more frequent serial neuropsychological and psychoeducational testing of the child may need to be delineated and scheduled within the formal goals of the child's IEP.

The foregoing findings corroborate the need for pediatric oncology professionals, parents, and school personnel to work together to evaluate the school performance and neuropsychological abilities of children at risk. To facilitate this vigilance, the long-term neuropsychological effects of disease and treatment must be explained carefully and explicitly to parents and older children who can participate in decision making.[39] In addition, they should be made aware of the need for the regular assessments as outlined previously. For school personnel to become full partners in this process, they also should have access to such information.

As stated, professionals also need to assess the parents' and children's understanding and acceptance of any changes in functioning and the need to reset expectations for children's future. Further information and counseling should be provided as necessary to help parents and children with this process.

College and Vocational Training

Not all high school graduates can or will attend college, but the presence of any learning disability related to disease or treatment should not keep young adults from considering the possibility of college attendance. As mentioned previously, a plan for transitional services should be included in an adolescent's IEP or Section 504 plan.

Colleges and universities must accommodate students with disabilities, according to provisions of the Rehabilitation Act of 1973 and the ADA. Having an IEP or section 504 Plan in high school will provide the documentation necessary to assist students in obtaining appropriate services in college. If students are attending college when disabilities are discovered or when they become severe enough to affect school performance, appropriate assessment will provide the documentation needed to obtain a 504 Plan.

Most colleges have a person designated to work specifically with students with disabilities through an official "office for students with disabilities." The college's Web site will have information about their programs for students with disabilities, the name of a person to contact for further information, forms that can be printed to fill out about the student's disabilities and needs, and information about the steps the student will need to take to receive services. Once the student has been approved to receive accommodations and is officially registered as a student with disabilities, self-advocacy will be essential. Every semester, it will be the role of the student to discuss accommodations with the individual instructors. Some accommodations, like having a note taker, will not need to come to the attention of the instructor, but instructors will need to know if extended time for projects or tests is needed.

Professionals from the office for students with disabilities can provide some assistance in the form of official written documentation of the 504 Plan if a professor does not cooperate with providing the accommodations, but much of the communication about needed accommodations will come from the student. To help students to determine which college may have the best program for a specific student, they may consult several books that list colleges and universities that provide specialized programs (e.g., Peterson's *Colleges for Students with Learning Disabilities or Attention Deficit Disorders*).[90] Those students who do not want to attend a 4-year college or who cannot because of their level of functioning have alternatives, including 2-year training programs through community colleges and vocational or technical training. The process of obtaining needed accommodations in these programs is similar. Sheltered workshop programs are available for those who are more severely impaired.

Terminally Ill Children

School re-entry and intervention programs emphasize the hopeful aspect of childhood cancer. However, sometimes children's cancer progresses and all curative treatment has been exhausted and children enter the terminal phase. When should school services end? Davis[91] chose to answer the question by looking at the range of school services available.

Terminally ill children probably have been in the chronic phase of treatment and have been attending school.[91] School participation can change from school attendance to homebound services or any combination of the two to accommodate terminally ill children's physical problems or minimize their discomfort. Continued school participation is very important to the emotional well-being of terminally ill children, and it may be one of the few normal activities in which such children can continue to participate.[31,92] Engaging in normal daily activities as much as possible is supportive for the child and family as a whole. In addition, adolescents may find hope in the goal of high school graduation.[56] The importance of school attendance in the face of impending death was also made clear by Lansky and colleagues[93] in a review of absenteeism in children with cancer. These authors found that children attended school one-half the time during the year they died. It is vitally important that teachers continue to see such children for as long as the children desire. If contact with these children is stopped suddenly against their wishes, they will feel "abandoned, lonely, and helpless."[91] At some time, academics no longer will be appropriate, and teachers may want to engage such children in other activities.

Another issue is support for teachers and classmates. Teachers will be trying to support a terminally ill child's classmates but will need support as well. This is an additional time during which the school liaison will be very important. As the child moves closer toward the end of life, the teacher may not feel comfortable communicating with the family and may need assistance from the liaison. Classmates may see the child decline physically over time and have questions about the child's condition. There may be a need to dispel any rumors or inaccurate information that circulate among classmates. They will need some preparation before the child dies and may even wish to say goodbye through personal visits, cards, or e-mails.[55] This will depend on how close the child was with the classmates and how much the child has been in class and in contact with classmates. A school psychologist or local mental health professional may also be of assistance in working with the classmates. Each situation is as unique as the child and must be handled with sensitivity to ensure that the needs of the child, family, and school are met.[56]

Grief Issues in the Classroom

Many times when a child dies, they may not have been in the classroom for a few weeks or months. Classmates may not be aware when death is imminent or that the child with cancer has died. If nothing is said about it in the classroom by the teacher or a counselor, classmates may feel awkward about their feelings of grief and not know how to cope with those feelings. Everyone deals with grief differently, and some classmates may not want to experience grief in a group setting, yet others may find the experience a validation of their feelings and find solace in talking with peers and teachers/counselors in this setting.

Dealing with grief in the classroom, the teacher must take into account developmental issues and the individuality of each student's reaction to the child or adolescent's death.[55] Consultation with a bereavement professional, school psychologist, or other school mental health professional would be appropriate before considering how best to discuss the death of a classmate.[28,55,56] Madan-Swain and colleagues present a very good overall discussion of grief issues in the classroom setting and provide some ideas for age-appropriate activities that can be carried out in the classroom.[94] There are also other resources to review:

1. American Hospice Association—www.americanhospice.org—has materials for a grief workshop for teacher, counselors, etc.
2. Centering Corporation—www.centering.org—provides books to assist with grief issues in the classroom.

CONCLUSION

It is important that the process of school re-entry and intervention begin at the time of diagnosis and continue through the transition to college or vocational training and into adulthood. Educational intervention continues to be one of the most exciting areas of research in pediatric oncology. It is also one of the most promising because, as survival rates increase, the quality of life of survivors becomes ever more important. Because education is necessary for successful entry into employment and adulthood, it is imperative that children and adolescents with cancer receive the services they need to realize their cognitive potential fully. Toward this end, it is imperative also that parents and professionals who work with children with cancer, including physicians, psychologists, and teachers, have a clear and thorough understanding of the educational issues involved. They must also be prepared and committed to work together as a team to provide the long-term continuing intervention and follow-up needed.

Parents of children with cancer need information and support to become effective advocates for their children. As children grow to adolescence and young adulthood, they also must have this information and become advocates for themselves. Through an integrated, developmental approach to school re-entry and continued school intervention, the survivor of childhood cancer can look more optimistically forward to successful adult life.

Although research investigating the benefits of school re-entry for cancer survivors has largely been positive, there is considerable need for ongoing research in this area. The role and responsibilities of the physician in early school planning should be examined. Homebound instructional programs should be carefully studied to investigate ways to improve teacher-to-teacher communication and maximize limited instruction time. With the range of re-entry services offered by different medical centers, a study that compares the relative costs, benefits, and efficacy of different interventions is required. There is a great need for empirical validation of specific school-based interventions and accommodations designed to address cognitive late effects. Such studies should include measures of pre- to post-intervention changes including parent and teacher knowledge, as well as student academic performance and adjustment. Potentially the most meaningful line of investigation would be assessing the ultimate impact of school re-entry programs on long-term career success, vocational satisfaction, and quality of life for cancer survivors.

ACKNOWLEDGMENTS

The authors wish to express appreciation to the American Lebanese Syrian Associated Charities for the support it has provided to the School Program of St. Jude Children's Hospital, at which many of the principles related in this chapter have been developed and applied. We also wish to acknowledge Mark Miles as he was a contributing author on this chapter in the two previous editions.

References

1. American Cancer Society. Cancer facts and figures. Atlanta, GA: American Cancer Society, 2007.
2. Hudson M. Survivors of childhood cancer: coming of age. Hematol Oncol Clin N Am 2008;22:211–231.
3. Van Eys J. What do we mean by the "truly cured child"? In: Van Eys J, ed. The truly cured child, the new challenge in pediatric cancer. Baltimore, MD: University Park Press, 1977:81–96.
4. Herman S. School re-entry following a diagnosis of cancer. In: Hockenberry MJ, Coody DK, eds. Pediatric oncology and hematology: perspectives on care. St Louis, MO: CV Mosby, 1986;463–468.
5. Armstrong FD, Horn M. Educational issues in childhood cancer. Sch Psychol Q 1995; 10:292–304.
6. Deasy-Spinetta P. Educational issues for children with cancer. In: Pizzo PA, Poplack DG, eds. Principles and practice of pediatric oncology. 4th ed. New York: Lippincott-Raven, 1997:1331–1341.
7. Maul-Mellot SK, Adams JN. Childhood cancer: a nursing overview. Boston/Monterey: Jones & Bartlett Publishers, 1987.
8. Katz ER. Illness impact and social integration. In: Kellerman J, ed. Psychological aspects of cancer in children. Springfield, IL: Charles C Thomas, 1980:14–46.
9. Katz ER, Rubenstein CL, Hubert NC, et al. School and social reintegration of children with cancer. J Psychosoc Oncol 1988;6:123–139.
10. Chekryn J, Deegan M, Reid J. Normalizing the return to school of the child with cancer. J Asssoc Pediatr Oncol Nurs 1986;3:20–24.
11. Eiser C. How leukaemia affects a child's schooling. Br J Soc Clin Psychol 1980;19: 365–368.
12. Kagen-Goodheart L. Re-entry: living with childhood cancer. Am J Orthopsychiatry 1977;47:651–658.
13. Deasy-Spinetta P. The school and the child with cancer. In: Spinetta J, Deasy-Spinetta P, eds. Living with childhood cancer. St. Louis, MO: Mosby, 1981:153–168.
14. Armstrong FD. Childhood cancer and education. In: Keene N, ed. Educating the child with cancer. Bethesda, MD: Candlelighter's Childhood Cancer Foundation, 2003:15–23.
15. Katz ER. Education in the hospital and home. In: Keene N, ed. Educating the child with cancer. Bethesda, MD: Candlelighter's Childhood Cancer Foundation, 2003:27–33.
16. Chesler M, Barbarin O. Childhood cancer and the family: meeting the challenge of stress and support. New York: Brunner/Mazel, 1974.
17. Lansky S, Lowman J, Vats T, et al. School phobia in children with malignant neoplasms. Am J Dis Child 1975;129:42–46.
18. Katz ER, Kellerman J, Rigler D, et al. School intervention with pediatric cancer patients. J Pediatr Psychol 1977;2:72–76.
19. Chekryn J, Deegan M, Reid J. Impact on teachers when a child with cancer returns to school. Child Health Care 1987;15:161–165.
20. Bessell AG. Children surviving cancer: psychosocial adjustment, quality of life and school experiences. Except Child 2001;67(3):345–359.
21. Prevatt FF, Heffer RW, Lowe PA. A review of school re-integration programs for children with cancer. J Sch Psychol 2000;38:447–467
22. Ross J, Scarvalone S. Facilitating the cancer patient's return to school. Social Work 1982;27:256–261.
23. Benner A, Marlow L. The effect of a workshop on childhood cancer on student's knowledge, concerns, desire to interact with a classmate with cancer. Child Health Care 1992;20:101–107.
24. Rynard D, Chambers A, Klinck AM, et al. School support programs for chronically ill children: evaluating the adjustment of children with cancer at school. Child Health Care 1998;27:31–46.
25. Varni J, Katz ER, Colegrove R, et al. The impact of social skills training on the adjustment of children with newly diagnosed cancer. J Pediatr Psychol 1993;18:751–767.
26. Tesauro GM, Rowland JH, Lustig C. Survivorship resources for post-treatment cancer survivors. Cancer Pract 2002;10:277–283.
27. Moore JB, Kaffenberger C, Goldberg P, et al. School re-entry for children with cancer: perception of nurses, school personnel and parents. J Pedatr Oncol Nurs 2009;26:86–99.
28. Madan-Swain A, Fredrick LD, Wallander JL. Returning to school after a serious illness or injury. In: Brown R, ed. Cognitive aspects of chronic illness in children. New York: Guilford Press, 1999:312–332.
29. Wissler KA. Advice to educators. In: Keene N, ed. Educating the child with cancer. Bethesda, MD: Candlelighter's Childhood Cancer Foundation, 2003:83–90.
30. Sexson S, Madan-Swain A. School re-entry for the child with chronic illness. J Learn Disabil 1993;26:115–125.
31. American Cancer Society. Back to school: a handbook for teachers of children with cancer. New York: American Cancer Society, 1988.
32. Nessim S, Katz ER. Cancervive Teacher's Guide for kids with cancer. California: Bristol-Myers Squibb, 1995.
33. Battista E. Educational needs of the adolescent with cancer and his family. Semin Oncol Nurs 1986;2:123–125.
34. McCarthy AM, Williams J, Plumer C. Evaluation of a school re-entry nursing intervention for children with cancer. J Pediatr Oncol Nurs 1998;15:143–152.
35. Charlton A, Pearson D, Morris-Jones PH. Children's return to school after treatment for solid tumors. Soc Sci Med 1986;22:1337–1346.
36. Searle NS, Askins M, Bleyer WA. Homebound schooling is the least favorable option for continued education of adolescent cancer patients, a preliminary study. Med Pediatr Oncol 2003;40:380–384.
37. Rolsky JT. Your child has cancer: a guide to coping. Philadelphia: Committee to Benefit the Children, St. Christopher's Hospital for Children, 1992.
38. Chambers A, Klinck A, Rynard D. Helping schools cope with childhood cancer: current facts and creative solutions. Ontario, Canada: Pediatric Division of Victoria Hospital, 1996.
39. Mulhern R. Neuropsychological late effects. In: Bearison DJ, Mulhern RK, eds. Pediatric Psychooncology. New York: Oxford University Press, 1994:99–121.
40. Moore BD. Neurocognitive outcomes in survivors of childhood cancer. J Pediatr Psych 2005;30:51–63.
41. Mulhern RK, Butler RW. Neurocognitive sequelae of childhood cancers and their treatment. Ped Rehab 2004;7:1–14.
42. Mulhern RK, Merchant TE, Gajjar A, et al. Late neurocognitive sequelae in survivors of brain tumours in childhood. Lancet 2004;5:399–408.
43. Moleski M. Neuropsychological, neuroanatomical, and neurophysiological consequences of CNS chemotherapy for acute lymphoblastic leukemia. Arch Clin Neuropsych 2000;15:603:630.
44. MacDonald SM, Safai S, Trofimov A, et al. Proton radiotherapy for childhood ependymoma: initial clinical outcomes and dose comparisons. Int J Radiat Oncol Biol Phys 2008;71:979–986.
45. Merchant TE, Mulhern RK, Krasin MJ, et al. Preliminary results from a phase II trial of conformal radiation therapy and evaluation of radiation-related CNS effects for pediatric patients with localized ependymoma. J Clin Oncol 2004;22:156–162.
46. Yock TI, Tarbell NJ. Technology insight: proton beam radiotherapy in pediatric brain tumors. Nat Clin Pract Oncol 2004;1:97–103.
47. Conklin HM, Li C, Xiong X, et al. Predicting change in academic abilities after conformal radiation therapy for localized ependymoma. J Clin Oncol 2008;26:3965–3970.
48. Duffey-Lind EC, O'Holleran E, Healey M, et al. Transitioning to survivorship: a pilot study. J Pediatr Oncol Nurs 2006;23:335–343.
49. Adams D, Deveau E. Coping with childhood cancer: where do we go from here? Ontario, Canada: Kinbridge Publications, 1998.
50. Larcombe IJ, Walker J, Charlton A, et al. Impact of childhood cancer on return to normal schooling. BMJ 1990;301:169–171.
51. Greene P. The child with leukemia in the classroom. Am J Nurs 1975;75:86–87.
52. Vance YH, Eiser C. The school experience of the child with cancer. Child Care Health Dev 2002;28:5–19.
53. Varni J, Katz E, Colegrove RJ, et al. Perceived social support and adjustment of children with newly diagnosed cancer. J Dev Behav Pediatr 1994;15:20–26.
54. Varni J, Setoguchi Y, Rappaport L, et al. Effects of stress, social support, and self-esteem on depression in children with limb deficiencies. Arch Phys Med Rehabil 1991;72: 1053–1058.
55. Armstrong FD, Briery BG. Childhood cancer and the school. In Brown RT, ed. Handbook of pediatric psychology in school settings. Mahwah, NJ: Lawrence Erlbaum Associates, 2003:263–281.
56. Katz ER, Madan-Swan A. Maximizing school, academic, and social outcomes in children and adolescents with cancer. In: Brown R, ed. Comprehensive handbook of childhood cancer and sickle cell disease a biopsychosocial approach. New York: Oxford University Press, 2006:313–338.
57. Worchel-Prevatt FF, Heffer RW, Prevatt BC, et al. A school reentry program for chronically ill children. J Sch Psychol 1998;36:261–279.
58. Leigh L. School re-entry. In: Keene N, ed. Educating the child with cancer. Bethesda, MD: Candlelighter's Childhood Cancer Foundation, 2003:41–48.
59. Meichenbaum DH, Goodman J. Training impulsive children to talk to themselves: a means of developing self-control. J Abnormal Psychol 1971;77:115–126.
60. Richards DM. (n.d.) Overview of section 504. http://www.504idea.org/504overview. html. Accessed April 12, 2009.
61. Council for Exceptional Children. The rights of children with disabilities under ADA and Section 504: a companion To IDEA. Reston, VA: Author, 1994.
62. National Center for Learning Disabilities. (n.d.) Section 504 and IDEA comparison chart [Fact sheet]. www.ncld.org/content/view/1127/456169/. Accessed May 15, 2009.
63. Monaco GP, Smith GP. Special education: the law. In: Keene N, ed. Educating the child with cancer. Bethesda, MD: Candlelighter's Childhood Cancer Foundation, 2003: 193–204.
64. Council of Parents, Attorneys, and Advocates, Inc. 2008. ADAAA becomes law strengthens 504 and ADA. www.wrightslaw.com/law/504/ADAAA.law.pdf. Accessed April 22, 2009.
65. North Dakota Protection and Advocacy Project. 2008. America with Disabilities Amendment Act of 2008. www.ndpanda.org/news/2008/. Accessed April 22, 2009.
66. Copeland D. Neuropsychological and psychosocial effects of childhood leukemia and its treatment. CA Cancer J Clin 1992;42:283–295.
67. Thompson SJ, Leigh L, Christensen R, et al. Immediate neurocognitive effects of methylphenidate on learning-impaired survivors of childhood cancer. J Clin Oncol 2001;19:1802–1808.

68. Mulhern RK, Khan RB, Kaplan S, et al. Short-term efficacy of methylphenidate: a randomized, double-blind, placebo-controlled trial among survivors of childhood cancer. J Clin Oncol 2004;22:4795–4803.

69. Conklin HM, Reddick WE, Ashford J, et al. Long term efficacy of methylphenidate in enhancing attention, regulation, social skills and academic abilities in childhood cancer survivors. J Clin Onc (in press).

70. Conklin HM, Lawford J, Jasper BW, et al. Side effects of methylphenidate in survivors of childhood cancer: a randomized, placebo-controlled trial. Pediatrics 2009;124:226–233.

71. Efron D, Jarman F, Barker M. Side effects of methylphenidate and dexamphetamine in children with attention deficit hyperactivity disorder: a double-blind, crossover trial. Pediatrics 1997;100:662–666.

72. Butler RW, Copeland DR. Attentional processes and their remediation in children treated for cancer: a literature review and the development of a therapeutic approach. J Inter Neuropsych Soc 2002;8:115–124.

73. Butler RW, Mulhern RK. Neurocognitive interventions for children and adolescents surviving cancer. J Ped Psychol 2005;30:65–78.

74. Butler RW, Copeland DR, Fairclough DL, et al. A multicenter, randomized clinical trial of a cognitive remediation program for childhood survivors of a pediatric malignancy. J Consult Clinic Psychol 2008;76:367–378.

75. Crowley JA, Miles MA. Cognitive remediation in pediatric head injury: a case study. J Pediatr Psychol 1991;16:611–627.

76. Kendall PC, Braswell L. Cognitive-behavioral therapy for impulsive children. 2nd ed. New York: Guilford Press, 1993.

77. Douglas VI, Parry P, Marton P, et al. Assessment of a cognitive training program for hyperactive children. J Abnormal Child Psychol 1976;4:389–410.

78. Eysenck MW, Keane MT. Cognitive psychology: A student's handbook. Hove, UK: Lawrence Erlbaum Associates, 1990.

79. Armstrong D, Mulhern R. Acute lymphoblastic leukemia and brain tumors. In: Brown R, ed. Cognitive aspects of chronic illness in children. New York: Guilford Press, 1999:47–77.

80. Mulhern R, Armstrong D, Thompson S. Function-specific neuropsychological assessment. Med Pediatr Oncol 1998;suppl 1:34–40.

81. Cousens P, Ungerer JA, Crawford JA, et al. Cognitive effects of childhood leukemia therapy: a case for four specific deficits. J Pediatr Psychol 1991;16:474–488.

82. Brown R, Madan-Swain A, Waco GA, et al. Cognitive and academic late effects among children previously treated for acute lymphocytic leukemia receiving chemotherapy as CNS prophylaxis. J Pediatr Psychol 1998;23:333–340.

83. Brouwers P, Poplack D. Memory and learning sequelae in long-term survivors of acute lymphoblastic leukemia: association with attention deficits. Am J Pediatr Hematol Oncol 1990;12:174–181.

84. Casey BJ, Giedd JN, Thomas KN. Structural and functional brain development and its relation to cognitive development. Bio Psychol 2000;54:241–257.

85. Giedd JN. The anatomy of mentalization: a view from developmental neuroimaging. Bull Menninger Clin 2003;67:132–142.

86. Reddick WE, Russell JM, Glass JO, et al. Subtle white matter volume differences in children treated for medulloblastoma with conventional or reduced dose craniospinal irradiation. Mag Res Imag 2000;18:787–793.

87. Hale JB. Response to intervention: guidelines for parents and practitioners. 2008. http://www.wrightslaw.com. Accessed April 22, 2010.

88. Strangeman N, Hitchcock C, Hall T, et al. Response to instruction and universal design for learning: how might they intersect in the general education classroom? 2006. http://www.ldonline.org/article/13002. Accessed April 22, 2010.

89. Kazak AE. Implications for survival: pediatric oncology patients and their families. In: Bearison DJ, Mulhern RK, eds. Pediatric Psychooncology. New York: Oxford University Press, 1994:99–121.

90. Seghers L, ed. Peterson's colleges for students with learning disabilities or attention deficit disorders. 8th ed. New Jersey: Peterson's, 2007.

91. Davis K. Educational needs of terminally ill children. Issues Compr Pediatr Nurs 1989;12:235–245.

92. Faulkner KW, Armstrong-Dailey A. Care of the dying child. In: Pizzo PA, Poplack DG, eds. Principles and practice of pediatric oncology. 3rd ed. New York: Lippincott–Raven, 1997:1343–1359.

93. Lansky S, Cairns N, Zwartjes W. School attendance among children with cancer: a report from two centers. J Psychosoc Oncol 1983;1:75–82.

94. Madan-Swain A, Austin H, Taylor-Cook P. Grief issues in the classroom. In: Keene N, ed. Educating the child with cancer. Bethesda, MD: Candlelighter's Childhood Cancer Foundation, 2003:287–308.

CHAPTER 49 ■ PALLIATIVE CARE FOR THE CHILD WITH CANCER

CHRISTINA ULLRICH, BARBARA SOURKES, AND JOANNE WOLFE

Life is so strange. Sometimes you feel it's like a book with chapters to fill, never ending.

Sometimes it's like a chess game where you have to make each move so carefully.

Other times it's like a mystery where each hidden chamber reveals its secrets.

It is even a war where to live it is to win it.

—Karen Beth Josephson, age 10.[1] (p. 23)

These profound and poignant opening words exemplify the experience of the child living with a life-threatening condition. Uncertainty, vigilance, determination, and hope mark the uncharted horizons that lie ahead for both the child and the family. From an emotional point of view, the child who is confronted with life and death issues longs for understanding and comfort. Through drawings and words, a teenager described the hardship of these extraordinary life circumstances (Figs. 49.1 and 49.2).

Although the healthy siblings live through the illness experience with the same intensity as the patient and parents, they often stand outside the spotlight of professional and family attention.[2,3] This is particularly ironic—and tragic—since these are children who go on to live their lives marked by the implications of premature loss (Fig. 49.3).

INTEGRATING PALLIATIVE CARE

Approximately 20% of children diagnosed with cancer eventually die of their disease (SEER 2008). This makes cancer the leading cause of nonaccidental death in childhood.[4] High-quality palliative care is now an expected standard.[5–8] The American Academy of Pediatrics set the following as a minimum standard for pediatric palliative care: "Excellence in pediatric palliative care is essential for hospitals and other facilities caring for children. Program development in pediatric palliative care, along with community outreach and public education, must be a priority of tertiary care centers serving children."[5] Furthermore, the Institute of Medicine published its comprehensive report on improving palliative and end-of-life care for children and their families in 2003 calling for improvements in all aspects of care including clinical models, education, finance restructuring, and research.[8]

According to the World Health Organization (WHO), palliative care for children with life-threatening conditions is the active total care of the child's body, mind, and spirit, and it also involves giving support to the family.[9] It begins when illness is diagnosed and continues regardless of whether or not a child receives treatment directed at the disease. Health providers must evaluate and alleviate a child's physical, psychological, and social distress. Effective palliative care requires a broad interdisciplinary approach that includes the family and makes use of available community resources; it can

be successfully implemented even if resources are limited. It can be provided in tertiary care facilities, in community health centers, and in children's homes.[10] Although palliative care services are increasingly available, they are not yet ubiquitous. For example, a palliative care team exists in only 58% of Children's Oncology Group centers.[11]

In children with cancer, it is not always possible to determine whether the disease will be responsive to cancer-directed therapy, nor is it possible to determine which type of trajectory the dying process will take (Fig. 49.4).[12] Some children may die suddenly and unexpectedly—for example, the child undergoing bone marrow transplant who experiences a treatment-related complication (Fig. 49.4A). Others may experience a steady and fairly predictable decline (Fig. 49.4B), such as the child with a progressive brainstem glioma after radiation therapy. Most children with progressive cancer will experience varying periods of chronic illness punctuated by crises, one of which may prove fatal (Fig. 49.4C). An example of this type of trajectory may involve a child with relapsed metastatic neuroblastoma who may be palliated long term, before experiencing a life-ending event.

In the context of such prognostic uncertainty, at times, palliative care may not be introduced until late in the illness trajectory. However, when the care team focuses solely on life-extending therapy, as opposed to concurrent integration of quality of life, patients and families may be deprived of optimal comfort care.[13] Thus, optimal care of the child with life-threatening illness requires recognition on the part of the care team that it may not be clear if or when a child is dying, but if death is a *potential* outcome, palliative care should be a priority.

Another challenge to the institution of palliative care is the viewpoint that palliative care can only be implemented to the exclusion of disease-directed therapy. This is one of the most common reasons for pediatricians to delay referral to a palliative care program.[14] In addition, this perspective promotes an abrupt transition from life-prolonging to symptom-oriented care (Fig. 49.5A).[13] If palliative care is conceptualized as always being a part of the care paradigm (Fig. 49.5B), the transition to predominantly comfort care can occur gradually and intuitively. This approach is supported by the views of parents of children with cancer, who favor concurrent pursuit of cancer-directed therapy and optimizing child's quality of life.[15,16] Understanding that palliative care is not synonymous with end-of-life care facilitates the timely introduction of palliative care, even as disease-directed or life-prolonging measures are pursued.

INTERDISCIPLINARY CARE

The care of a child with advanced cancer is best met through an interdisciplinary team, working to address the physical, emotional, and spiritual needs of the child, parents, siblings, and community. For example, Wolfe and colleagues showed

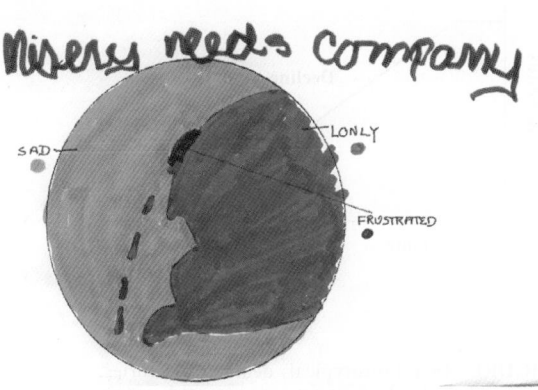

FIGURE 49.1 Misery Needs Company. I feel so lonely. I feel like the man in the moon who is crying. This moon will never be happy unless there's another moon, and of course, that is not likely. I feel *lonely (blue)* because I don't have anyone to be with. *Sad* is *orange*. I hate orange—it's a yucky color. And I hate being sad. And I hate the combination of blue and orange. I can't help being *frustrated (black)*. This is all too much.

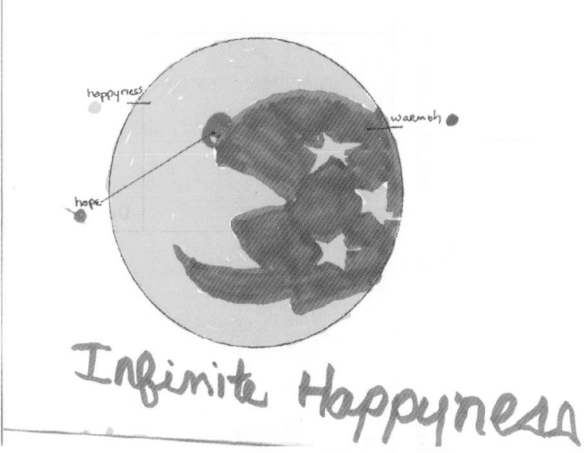

FIGURE 49.2 Infinite Happiness [sic]. Psychologist: "How would the man in the moon feel if another moon did appear?" The moon would feel infinite happiness. It would change from a color I hate (orange) to the *happiness* of *yellow*. *Warmth* is *purple*—a combination of home-like colors. *Hope* is *green*, for Irish. I am Irish and I am studying about the Irish coming to America with hope.

that communication about a child's poor prognosis was more effective if a psychologist or social worker was involved in the child's care.[15] Above all, families must be reassured that they are not alone, whether the child is cared for in the hospital or at home. The trained interdisciplinary team should recognize the long-term needs of families and ensure continuity of service through time. The team should facilitate a family-oriented approach that fosters open communication, intensive symptom management, psychosocial and spiritual support, and timely access to care, with the primary goal of enabling meaningful experiences. This support must include the care and counsel of siblings, friends, and school peers. Ideally, a

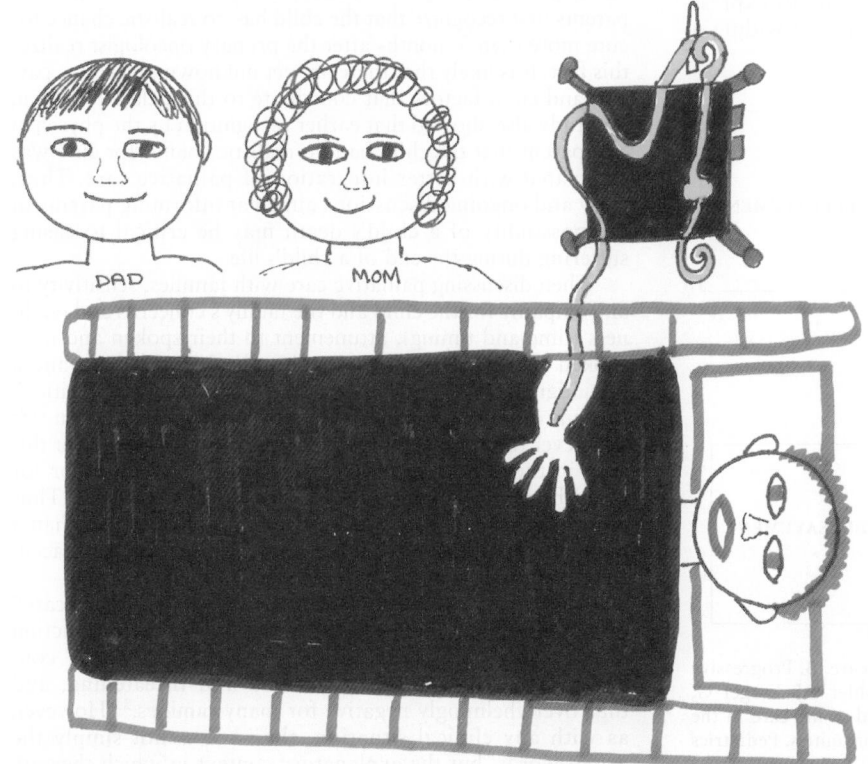

FIGURE 49.3 Don't brothers and sisters count too? Siblings who were participating in a support group designed a poster "to educate the public about the plight of healthy brothers and sisters with a seriously ill child in the family." The children drew a child in a hospital bed, hooked up to medical equipment, with parents at bedside. No siblings are present in the poster. The caption reads starkly: "Don't brothers and sisters count too?"

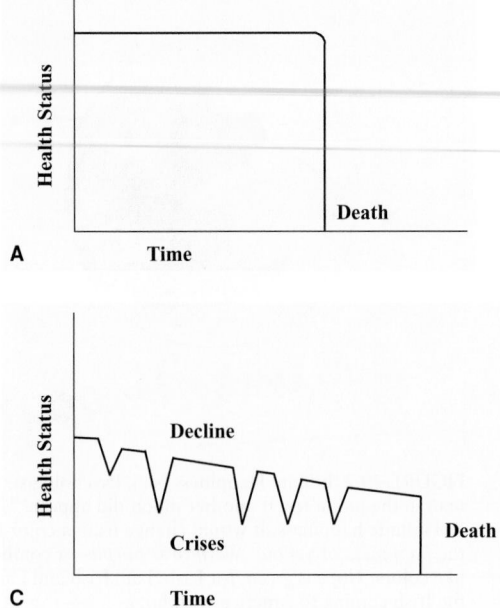

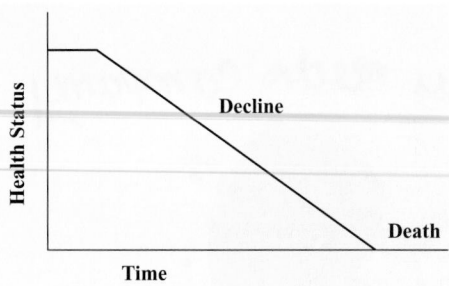

FIGURE 49.4 Prototypical death trajectories. A: Sudden death from an unexpected cause. B: Steady decline from a progressive disease with a "terminal" phase. C: Advanced illness marked by slow decline with periodic crises and "sudden" death. (Adapted from Field MJ, Cassel CK; Institute of Medicine (U.S.). Committee on Care at the End of Life. Approaching death: improving care at the end of life. Washington, DC: National Academy Press, 1997:29.)

well-established team should mobilize the community to ensure that the child, family, and friends receive appropriate support and counseling well before and long after the child dies.

BREAKING BAD NEWS

Much has been written about communication strategies for breaking bad news.[17–20] Recommendations have focused on ensuring privacy and adequate time; assessing the families' understanding of the condition; providing information simply and honestly; encouraging patients and parents to express their feelings and empathizing with them; and providing a

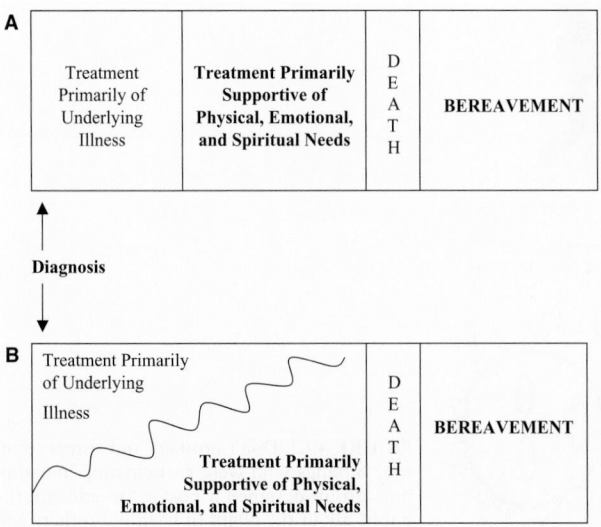

FIGURE 49.5 A: Abrupt transition to palliative care. B: Progressive transition to palliative care. (Adapted from Sahler OJ, Frager G, Levetown M, et al. Medical education about end-of-life care in the pediatric setting: principles, challenges, and opportunities. Pediatrics 2000;105:575–584.)

strategy for approaching the situation and a summary of what was discussed. It is critical to end such discussions by assuring the family that there will be follow-up opportunities for ongoing discussions that address continued concerns.

DISCUSSING PALLIATIVE CARE WITH FAMILIES

Optimal palliation requires the establishment of open and ongoing communication between all care team members, the child, and the family. Wolfe and colleagues[15] have shown that parents first recognize that the child has no realistic chance for cure more than 3 months after the primary oncologist realizes this fact. It is likely that there are yet unknown physician, parent, and child factors that contribute to this delay. However, the study also showed that earlier recognition by the physician and parent that the child had no realistic chance for cure was associated with better integration of palliative care. Thus, early and ongoing discussions aimed at informing parents of the possibility of a child's death may be critical to easing suffering during the end of a child's life.

When discussing palliative care with families, sensitivity to and empathy for the child and the family's concerns and readiness (time and timing), attunement to their spoken and nonspoken cues, respect for their cultural/spiritual beliefs, and a nonjudgmental attitude on the part of the team are critical. Hope is a universal underpinning of any communication.[21,22] Whatever the meaning of hope for the child and family at this time in the illness trajectory (e.g., hope for comfort or for going home), it is essential to convey a sense of hope. Thus presenting palliative care as an added resource, rather than a redirection of care, is often the most helpful, and most accurate, approach from this perspective.

Controversy exists as whether the words "palliative care" or "hospice" should be used with parents at the introduction of discussions. Some caregivers believe that the words' connotation is still too misunderstood and threatening, and thus overwhelmingly negative for many families.[23] However, as with any clinical situation, the issue is not simply the actual words, but the explanatory context in which they are embedded. An approach that one author (BMS) has found effective is to introduce the concept of palliative care very much in the context of "options," "planning for now or the future," and "decision-making for your child and family during this most difficult chapter of the illness." The words "option" and "decision-making" have a positive, proactive slant, and families appreciate understanding palliative care from this perspective.[24]

Lo and colleagues[25] have proposed starting with open-ended questions to begin to address some of these issues with patients and families. Such questions can be adapted to the needs of children as well,[26] for example, What concerns you most about your child's illness? How is treatment going for you/your child and your family? As you think about your/your child's illness, what are the best and worst that might happen? What are your/your child's hopes (expectations, fears) for the future? These open-ended questions provide a means to explore the possibility of a child's dying.

DISCUSSING PALLIATIVE CARE WITH CHILDREN

One side of my head says: "Think optimistic." The other side says: "What if this treatment doesn't work?" (Eleven-year-old child)[27] p. 156

While empirical research regarding communication about palliative care with children is in its earliest stages, clinical experience has shown that many children can face and negotiate discussions about their care to a remarkable degree. An important consideration is the extent to which children should be included in the decision-making process.

> Psychologist: Do you remember what we talked about last time?
>
> Child (aged 5 years): (without hesitation) About dying. . . .
> (A few minutes later)
>
> If I don't feel like talking about dying today, there will be other days.[27] (p. 121)

In the past, professionals relied on "normal" (i.e., not seriously ill) children's developmental understanding of death to judge their involvement. However, these "norms" do not reflect the sophistication of children who are living the living/dying process themselves. In general, children with advanced illness may have a precocious understanding of the concepts of death and their personal mortality.[28–31] A child's likely developmental understanding of death based on age is helpful when engaging them in conversations about death, recognizing that it is through such an exchange that an individual's conceptualization of death can be known.

Most children learn to recognize when something is "dead" before they reach the age of 3 years, but at this early age, death, separation, and sleep are almost synonymous in the child's mind. As children grow to preschool age, they come to recognize that a dead person cannot function, but they are likely to believe that death is temporary. Their egocentric reasoning makes them vulnerable to believing they can cause death with their thoughts or actions. However, most preschoolers do not understand why people die.

School-aged children are typically problem solvers, who have begun to develop logical thoughts. During these years, they normally acquire a much more complete understanding of death, including its irreversibility, universality (i.e., that everyone will die), and that people die from both internal and external causes. They are interested in the specific details of death, and in the latter part of this phase they are able to envision their own deaths.

As children become teenagers, their thinking about death is usually consistent with reality. They are ready to add to their complete definition of death the effect it has on other people and on society as a whole. Their future orientation makes it difficult for them to recognize their own deaths as a present possibility, although they can conceive this occurring at some point in the future.

The seriously ill child's awareness of the life-threatening implications of his or her condition can be conceptualized along a continuum and begins at the time of diagnosis.[27,32] At one end, the child acknowledges being "very sick" or having a "bad disease"; however, there is no prognostic statement referring to life or death. In the middle, the child expresses some awareness that his or her life might be in jeopardy—uncertainty about *living*—but without a focus on death. At the other end of the continuum, the child is explicitly conscious that he or she could die of the illness. Awareness is gleaned from many sources. Primary is the "wisdom of the body": the child's irrefutable recognition of how sick he or she is. Other cues include the child's knowledge of the illness, the urgency and intensity of treatment, the emotions of family and caregivers, and encounters with other patients. Awareness is a fluid, not a static state. During the terminal phase, the child's awareness of dying becomes more focused. No longer a distant and abstract threat, death takes on an identity of its own. Rather than being a possible outcome, death is *the* outcome, its time of occurrence the only unknown. References to its proximity can be quite direct and explicit. If an open climate has been established from the beginning of the illness, it will be reflected in how the child talks about death.

A 13-year-old girl with widespread disease recounted to the therapist: "I know how to read palms, and I read my own. I'll be famous. I'll be married once. I see a break in my life when I'm about seventeen. I wonder what that is. . . ."[33](p. 268)

An 11-year-old girl commented matter-of-factly: "Some of my friends have died. I wish I could talk to those kids' parents to see what their symptoms were, so that I would know what is happening to me."[27](p. 157)

It is important to emphasize that it is impossible to lie to a child and preserve a relationship that is built on trust and caring. According to Hilden and colleagues,[34] children will often know when they are dying and may feel tremendous isolation if they are not given permission to talk openly about their illness and impending death. Candor is just as crucial in communicating with the siblings, as evidenced in the following drawing and commentary by a 10-year-old child (Fig. 49.6).

During the last decade, there has been increased recognition of the child's participation in making treatment decisions.[35–38] In a survey of 50 children with cancer aged 8 to 17 years, 95% of patients wanted to be told if they were dying.[39] Although most of the children felt that treatment decisions were up to the physicians, 63% of the adolescents and 28% of the younger children wanted to make their own decisions about palliative therapy. Nitschke and colleagues[40] reported on their experience of including children aged between 6 and 20 years in a "final stage conference" in which progression of disease, minimal chance of cure, imminence of death, and therapeutic options were discussed. These children appeared capable of making rational decisions about further therapy.[40] Others have suggested that children younger than 11 years may not be able to grasp these concepts.[41,42] The approach should be tailored to the individual child and family. Crucial to this process is an assessment of the child's ability to appreciate the nature and consequences of a specific medical decision. This becomes particularly complex when the wishes of the child differ from those of the parents. Although by law, parental views supersede those of children, when the illness is in the

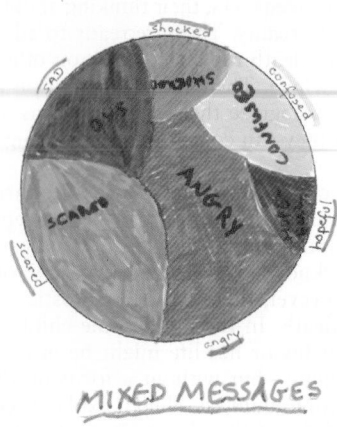

FIGURE 49.6 Mixed messages: I feel *scared (green)*—I feel as if I do not really know what is happening. *Sad* is *blue*—at first my parents just told me that my brother needed an operation. They didn't say it was cancer. *Confused* is *yellow*—just all mixed feelings–I don't know what to think. *Hopeful* is *purple*—bright—I don't really have a lot of hope, but maybe just a little. *Angry* is *red* because that is a mad color. Why him? What did it have to happen to him? My drawing is called "Mixed Messages" because I have all of these different feelings and everyone is telling me different things. Like they say mostly that he is going to be okay, but they—and I—don't really believe it. . . .

advanced stages, it is crucial to find the means to reconcile differing perspectives. This is often a juncture when input from members of the interdisciplinary team can be crucial: children often express their understanding, awareness, and thoughts about treatment options and living or dying to individuals other than their parents or primary physician. Frequently, their most candid disclosures evolve within the context of psychotherapy (Fig. 49.7).

An 11-year-old child who had been offered radiation therapy for palliative symptom control confided to her therapist: "I'm scared because I'm not so good at making decisions. My parents want me to have radiation, but a little voice in me tells me not to. . . . My mother always said that if I die, she wants me to die happy and at home. If I had radiation, I'd have to come into the hospital every day. And I don't know if radiation will really help, or if I would die anyway." This child had been through many remission-relapse cycles and had been informed and involved in all aspects of her illness and treatment from the beginning. Nonetheless, her statements highlight the "burden" of decision making that children may feel at critical junctures of their illness, particularly at end-stage. Furthermore, despite what had been her clear understanding of the reason for radiation therapy (exclusively for palliative symptom management), her intense emotion and hope have overridden the intellectual as she wonders whether the radiation will help her to live longer "or would I die anyway."[1] p. 156[37]

In communicating with children, the individual child's competence and vulnerability serve as the context for decisions regarding disclosure.[27,43] Considerations about what, or how much to tell, include the child's age, cognitive and emotional maturity, family structure and functioning, cultural background, and history of loss. In communication with the life-threatened child at any juncture, "the truth is not a principle nor a duty nor a rule. The truth is an atmosphere of exchange, of listening, and of respect for the child and his needs. The truth is a state."[43] (p. 473) The precedent for a climate that enables such honest interchange is created from the time of diagnosis. In this way, parents may avoid experiencing

regret about not having discussed death with their child, as seen in 27% of parents who felt regret in one recent survey.[44]

It is important to stay open and receptive when the child initiates a conversation. "Teachable moments" may be fleeting, and an immediate response is necessary to capitalize on them. Recognize that many children communicate best through nonverbal means such as artwork or music. They may also be more willing to "talk things over" through puppets or stuffed animals rather than with real people.[1,27]

RESUSCITATION STATUS

Discussion of appropriateness of initiating cardiopulmonary resuscitation for children with advanced cancer is a very emotional topic.[45] For this reason, medical caregivers often avoid these conversations until respiratory or cardiac collapse seems imminent.[46] Clearly, parents would be better able to consider this decision if they were not in the midst of a crisis. It is our experience that when broached in advance, in a thoughtful and sensitive manner, many parents appreciate the opportunity to think ahead, before a crisis arises. Thus, advanced discussions regarding resuscitation status are strongly recommended.

We have often approached this sensitive topic by framing it in the following manner "We are hoping for the best of all possible outcomes, however, it is also helpful to prepare for the worst, to ensure that no matter what happens we are taking the best possible care of your child. [pause, listen, allow for reflection] We would like to decide together whether your child should undergo cardiopulmonary resuscitation if we believe she or he has an irreversible problem." This approach along with reassurance that a life-threatening event is not imminent enables parents to maintain hope while facing this decision. It is also helpful to reassure parents that should the child's condition improve, the decision would be reconsidered. Even if a family is unable to make a decision about resuscitation status during the initial conversations, it is helpful for them to have heard that they may have to face this decision in the future.

Careful thought should be given to the exact words used during a discussion regarding resuscitation status. Parents often think that agreeing not to resuscitate is choosing death over life for their children. It is helpful to explain that it is the uncontrolled cancer that would cause the death. To some parents, the phrase "do not resuscitate" implies that if these interventions were performed, they would be successful. Experience tells us that among children with advanced cancer, the likelihood of a patient being extubated and leaving the hospital is very low. Thus, when approaching families about this issue, it is preferred to use the phrase "do not attempt resuscitation (DNAR)." Others advocate changing the term to a more affirmative statement, for example, several institutions now use, "allow natural death (AND)" orders, and some suggest that this phrase is softer, and more comforting and implies that the team will continue caring for the family member.[47] Although this phrase may be more family centered, some providers feel that it is also more ambiguous.[48] A change in semantics alone will not necessarily improve communication.[49] Furthermore, AND terminology may be received differently by parents of dying children. The state of Oregon has developed, Physician Orders for Life-Sustaining Treatment (POLST).[50] At Children's Hospital Boston, we are currently piloting "Intervention Orders for Persons with Advanced Illness," which try to encompass the spectrum of decisions that families face when a child's illness is advancing.

Importantly, it is not always possible to know for certain whether a change in clinical status that necessitates resuscitation efforts is an irreversible event. For example, apnea related

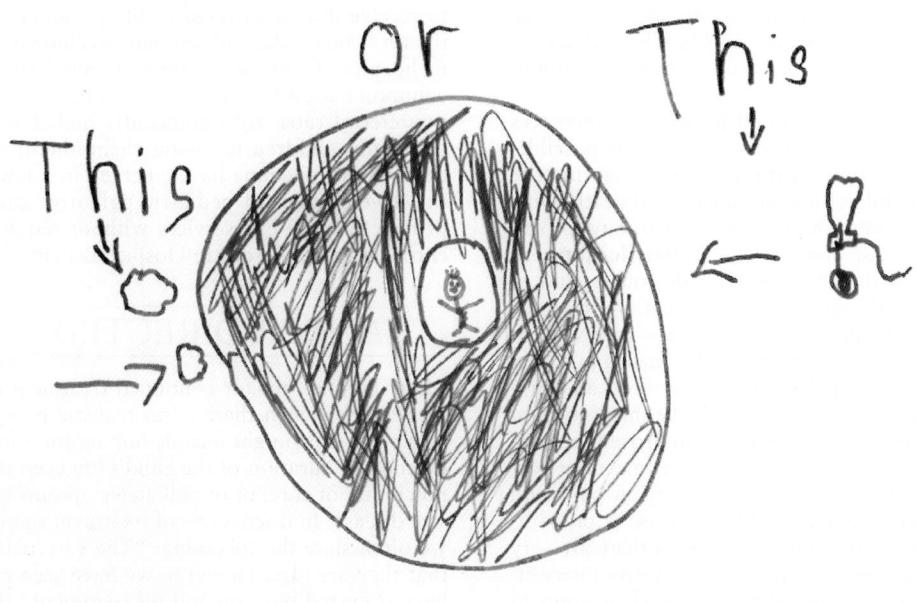

FIGURE 49.7 "This or This." Mikaela, a 10-year-old child who had just relapsed drew a picture entitled "This or This." On one side of a doughnut she depicted tumor cells, on the other side she drew a needle for spinal taps. In the middle of the doughnut is a little stick figure of a person. At the time of drawing the picture the child said: "I hate needles and spinal taps, but I also don't want my tumor to come back. If I don't have all the needles, then more tumor cells will grow. So if I don't want them to grow, I have to have all those awful needles. That's why I feel as if I am stuck in the middle of a doughnut." Reflecting back on the drawing months later, the child elaborated more explicitly: "What I mean by 'I was stuck in a dough-nut' is that I had two choices and I didn't want to take either of them. One of the choices was to get nee-dles and pokes and all that stuff and make the tumor go away. My other choice was letting my tumor get bigger and bigger and I would just go away up to heaven. . . . My mom wanted me to get needles and pokes. But I felt like I just had had too much—too much for my body—too much for me. . . . So I kind of wanted to go up to heaven that time. . . . But then I thought about how much my whole entire family would miss me and so just then I was kind of like stuck in a doughnut. . . ." (Reprinted from Sourkes BM. The psychological impact of life-limiting illness. In: Goldman A, Hain RD, Liben S, eds. The Oxford text-book of pediatric palliative care. 1st ed. Oxford, NY: Oxford University Press, 2006:98 with permission).

to administration of seizure medications may well be a reversible event. Thus, documentation should always specify under which circumstances a DNAR order is applicable. In the outpatient setting, it is helpful to provide the family with a letter to keep with the patient at all times, which briefly sum-marizes the patient's medical condition and documents the details of the resuscitation status discussion. In several states, there is also an official DNAR verification form, such as the Comfort Care Form in Massachusetts, which permits emer-gency medical teams to honor DNAR orders written in the hospital or clinic.

LOCATION OF CARE

Studies have found that slightly more than one-half of children with progressive cancer die at home.[51–53] Data on how pedi-atric families make the choice of hospital, hospice, or home—as well as follow-up outcome data—are preliminary and

scarce. Thus it is critical that the professional team's values do not pressure the parents, especially toward taking a child home. Future efforts need to be aimed at better understanding why some families choose to remain primarily at home, whereas other parents prefer their child to die in the hospital. Some have suggested that family adjustment after the death is better if the child dies in the home.[54,55] The beneficial effects of care in the home on parental functioning have been attributed to fewer feelings of helplessness and the broad opportunity for family intimacy offered by home care. Given the retrospective nature of these studies, however, cause-and-effect relationships cannot be established with certainty. Parents who choose home care may have premorbid differences with respect to personal-ity traits and coping. Others have found family relationships to be better when the child died in the hospital.[56] Although many have suggested that most children prefer to die at home, this, too, has not been systematically evaluated. Higginson and Thompson report that children from families who are impov-erished are less likely to die at home.[57,58] Thus, creating the opportunity for a home death may be dependent on availability of services. A serious omission in the decision making and implementation of the care plan is the fact that siblings are rarely included in the information and discussion process, either by parents or professionals (B.M.S. The impact on healthy children of a family member dying at home: a cautionary note. Submitted).

Regardless, it is critically important to discuss preferences regarding the primary location of care as early as possible. More important than *actual* location is giving parents the opportunity to *plan* a child's location of care and death. Dussel et al. found that parents who had the opportunity to plan were more likely to choose home as the primary location, to feel better prepared for the child's end-of-life course, and to experience less decisional regret about the location of care.[59] Location options include inpatient care or home care with or without the support of a home care team. Increasing numbers of hospitals are developing palliative care services, and preliminary data suggest that concurrent with the integration of a palliative care service, key outcomes are improved. Specifically, fewer children are dying in the intensive care unit; parents also report diminished child suffering from pain and other prevalent symptoms and an improved sense of preparation for the child's end-of-life course. Although there are very few inpatient pediatric hospice units, one innovative intervention is the development of hospital-based homelike suites to allow for inpatient care of the child in an environment that accommodates the entire family.[60]

Home care teams might include a visiting nurse association, bridge programs, or hospice. There are very few inpatient pediatric hospice units. A parental decision to care for their terminally ill child at home involves the consideration of medical, psychological, social, and cultural factors together with such practical considerations as the availability of respite care, physician access, and financial resources.[61] Furthermore, whatever the decision is regarding the primary location of care, families should be reassured that they can change from one option to another and that the primary team will remain closely involved.

There are special challenges that we face regarding home care for terminally ill children. Specifically, because death from chronic illness in childhood is uncommon, the low census makes it difficult to maintain a staff of caregivers experienced in pediatric issues. Pediatric programs often face financial difficulties and are hard to sustain in the long term. Furthermore, caregivers skilled in the care of dying adults lack the expertise to deal with the unique medical and psychological needs of children.[62] In addition, communication between the primary hospital- or clinic-based team and the home care team is often suboptimal because these medical caregivers are not familiar to one another. Finally, parents may be reluctant to accept hospice because they equate this with giving up.

When families are able to embrace hospice, however, assistance from these programs can be invaluable. Support by the hospice team may include not only the nurse, physician, and home health aide but also the social worker, chaplain, and volunteers.[63] Optimal hospice care for children incorporates physical care for the child, home care, pain and symptom management, psychosocial support for child and family, respite care, staff support for health care providers, and special services such as transportation. Importantly, hospice programs are required to provide bereavement follow-up for family members. It is helpful to understand, however, that to be eligible for the hospice benefit, the physician must consider the child's life span to be no longer than 6 months.[63] Furthermore, reimbursement mechanisms for hospice differ from typical home care. Specifically, the Medicare Hospice Benefit provides a *per diem* reimbursement for care.[64,65] Because philosophi-

cally hospice programs encourage a natural, simple, and cost-effective approach to end-of-life care, this reimbursement mechanism is not usually problematic. However, children tend to receive disease-directed or life-prolonging treatments until the very end of life, and this may preclude them from enrolling in hospice. Continued cancer-directed therapy is the most common reason for children to not be referred to hospice, and nonreferral rates are significantly higher when hospice does not admit children receiving chemotherapy.[66] Possible solutions to this dilemma have emerged in a few states, including the development of pediatric palliative care programs that provide hospice-like services without requiring a child to be enrolled on the Medicare Hospice Benefit.[67,68]

CANCER-DIRECTED THERAPY

Many families opt for continued treatment of the underlying cancer even when there is no realistic prospect for cure.[15,16] Their rationale might include hoping for a miracle, a desire to extend the duration of the child's life even though there is no possibility of cure, or to palliate symptoms related to progressive disease. In discussions of treatment options with families, we often state the following: "The very nature of miracles is that they are rare. However, we have seen miracles, and they have occurred both on and off treatment." In other words, a child does not have to continue on cancer-directed therapy to preserve hope, especially when the therapy significantly impacts the child's remaining quality of life. Generally, decisions regarding continued cancer-directed therapy need to be carefully considered, weighing the potential for life extension and the impact on quality of life.

CHEMOTHERAPY

An inherent conflict exists in advanced cancer care between life-extending measures and efforts to minimize global suffering. Palliative cancer therapy can prolong life and lessen suffering. Alternatively, administration of treatments may result in increased numbers of physician-patient interactions, visits to clinic, admissions to the hospital, and most important, treatment-related complications requiring augmentation of supportive care. Nevertheless, several studies show improved quality of life among adult patients receiving chemotherapy compared with those who were not.[69-73] Several possible reasons for this include placebo effect, provision of hope, or increased medical attention associated with being on treatment. The role of palliative chemotherapy in children has not been well studied. The benefits may depend on the developmental stage of the child and his or her awareness of disease state. For example, increased interactions with medical personnel may outweigh any improvements in quality of life for the child. Parents may also have differing views on the role of continued cancer-directed therapy. Wolfe and colleagues[15] found that only 13% of parents reported that the primary goal of cancer-directed therapy for their child during the end-of-life care period was to lessen suffering. Most parents maintained a primary goal of extending life. Communication about this issue must be very clear and tailored to the individual family.

Several agents have been shown to be well tolerated in children and to have some antitumor effect. For example, oral etoposide has antitumor effect with limited toxicity in children with refractory neuroblastoma, brain tumors, and other solid tumors.[74-76] Relapsed acute lymphoblastic leukemia may be temporarily controlled with regimens including vincristine, methotrexate, prednisone, and 6-mercaptopurine. The decision about whether to continue cancer-directed therapy must carefully balance considerations of efficacy, potential treatment-related complications, and psychological impact.

PHASE I TRIALS

The goal of phase I research is to determine the toxicities and maximum-tolerated doses of an investigational drug or drugs. Yet Daugherty et al.[77] found that only one-third of adults enrolled in a phase I trial were able to state the purpose of the trial. They also found that cancer patients who participate in phase I trials are strongly motivated by the hope of therapeutic benefit and this is also true of parents of children with advanced cancer.[78] Altruistic feelings appear to have a limited and inconsequential role in motivating patients to participate in these trials. Yet overall, the chance of tumor response in phase I trials is low, ranging from 4% to 6%.[77,79] In children, the response rate is similar.[80] It is important to note, however, that the chance of fatal toxicity is also low, at approximately 0.5%.[79,80] In general, physicians also tend to assume more positive potential benefit from experimental chemotherapy than statistics would warrant.[77] Although these biases are not presented to the family with any intention of doing harm, they may make the informed consent process exceedingly difficult and potentially raise serious ethical questions.[81]

Similar to discussions about palliative chemotherapy, it is critical to ensure effective communication when discussing phase I therapy for children with advanced cancer. Furthermore, it is strongly recommended that children give their assent to participation in clinical trials.[82] Finally, further consideration about linking palliative care support with enrollment in phase I trials is warranted.[83]

RADIATION THERAPY

Given with the intent of relieving symptoms, and without significant concern for late effects, palliative radiation is typically delivered in larger fraction sizes over shorter time frames.[84–86] This treatment approach explains the observation that while approximately 40% of adults with cancer receive palliative radiation, 25% of all radiation treatments are given with palliative intent.[87]

Such single-fraction regimens, when compared with multiple-fraction regimens, provide equal palliation with lower medical and societal costs.[88] However, reimbursement issues remain a barrier to patients enrolled on hospice.[89]

In the pediatric population, studies evaluating radiation for palliative purposes are sparse. Retrospective reviews of children with metastatic Ewing's sarcoma or advanced neuroblastoma indicate that 70% to 80% of children receive at least a partial reduction in pain.[90,91] In addition to pain, common indications for palliative radiation include the following:

Pain relief from bony or pulmonary metastases and tumors causing nerve root and soft tissue infiltration
Control of bleeding
Control of fungation and ulceration
Relief of impeding or actual obstruction—(e.g., upper airway obstruction)
Shrinkage of symptomatic tumor masses—(e.g., brain metastases, skin lesions, and other sites)
Oncological emergencies—(e.g., spinal cord compression, superior vena caval obstruction)

Although infrequently used in pediatrics, radiopharmaceuticals can effectively reduce bone pain and may be particularly attractive when numerous osseous metastases are present.

Bone-seeking radiopharmaceuticals, such as Samarium-153, form metal complexes that preferentially localize to bone in proportion to the osteoblastic activity present. Myelotoxicity may occur with extensive metastatic disease.

SYMPTOM MANAGEMENT

Wolfe and colleagues[52] demonstrated that according to their parents, children with terminal cancer experience a high prevalence of symptoms during the last month of life, with fatigue, pain, and dyspnea resulting in significant suffering (Fig. 49.8). Parents also reported limited success in treating symptoms. Increased availability of palliative care services, however, is associated with improvement in symptom control (Fig. 49.3).[53] Intensive symptom management is a priority in patients with advanced cancer. Symptoms that are out of control should be considered a medical emergency requiring direct evaluation of the patient and immediate implementation of interventions.

Fatigue

Fatigue is the most common symptom experienced by children with terminal cancer.[52,92] Cancer-related fatigue is unlike everyday fatigue in its impact on everyday activities and lack of responsiveness to rest. Children are apt to describe fatigue in physical terms, whereas adolescents may refer to both physical and mental aspects of this symptom.[93]

Despite its prevalence, little is known about the pathogenesis or treatment of fatigue in this population. In all likelihood, the etiology of cancer-related fatigue is multifaceted, including factors related to the underlying disease; treatment of the disease; factors associated with intercurrent illness including anemia, infection, respiratory compromise, malnutrition, and cardiac, renal, and hepatic compromise; sleep disturbances; uncontrolled symptoms; medication side effects; and psychosocial factors such as anxiety, and depression.[94–96]

Thus, treatment of fatigue requires careful evaluation of the child aimed at identifying treatable underlying causes. In

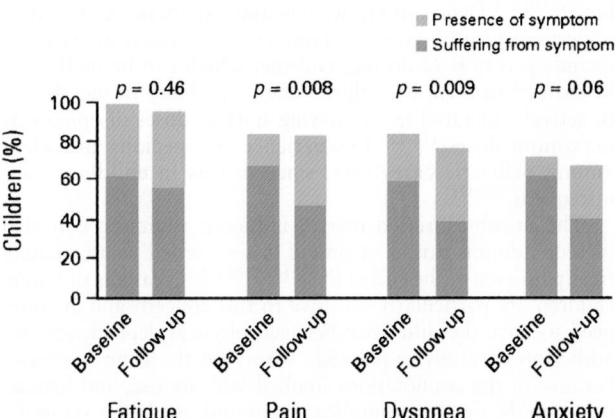

FIGURE 49.8 Prevalence and degree of suffering from common symptoms in the last month of life in baseline (before implementation of a palliative care service) and follow-up cohorts. Proportions of children who, according to parental report, had a specific symptom in the last month of life and who had "a great deal" or "a lot" of suffering as a result are illustrated. (Adapted from Wolfe J, Hammel J, Edwards K, et al. Easing of suffering in children with cancer at the end of life: is care changing? J Clin Oncol 2008;26(10):1717–1723.)

some situations, such as fatigue primarily related to advanced disease or organ failure, expectations for reversal of the symptom are limited. This should be explained to the patient and parents as a part of a plan to improve adaptation. However, some primary interventions pose relatively little burden for the patient. For example, the drug therapies administered to the patient should be reviewed whenever fatigue is prominent with specific attention to centrally acting drugs. Increasingly, methylphenidate or dextroamphetamine is recommended for symptomatic relief of fatigue, regardless of the suspected etiology.[97,98] The threshold for intervening to reduce insomnia,[95,99] some metabolic abnormalities, or depressed mood should be low. Exercise has been shown to be effective in relieving fatigue in adult cancer patients.[100,101] Moderate physical activity as tolerated may also be efficacious for children, even near the end of life. The sections that follow address treatment of other factors contributing to fatigue.

Pain

Incidence of Terminal Pain[102]

Most of the pain experienced by children with cancer occurs because of therapy rather than disease, particularly in the earlier stages of illness.[103,104] In the child with advanced cancer, however, the pain most likely is related to the disease. Studies of the incidence of terminal pain in pediatric patients have provided insights about when pain may be anticipated to be a problem. More than 80% of children with advanced cancer will experience pain, regardless of the underlying diagnosis.[52,105-107] However, patients with hematologic malignancy may experience pain for shorter duration in comparison to those with solid tumors.[105] If patients with solid tumors have impingement on the spine and major nerves, effective pain relief may require more invasive measures such as placement of an epidural catheter.[108,109]

Barriers to Effective Pain Management

To ensure effective pain management in children with advanced cancer, it is important to be familiar with common barriers leading to undertreatment of pain at the end of life.[102,110-114] Deficit in knowledge and experience can lead to undertreatment of pain.[115] Examples of ineffective approaches include *pro re nata* dosing, codeine, which can be ineffective in more than 30% of children due to inability to metabolize to active[116] metabolite, or viewing starting doses of opioids as maximum doses.[117-120] Inexperience is especially prevalent among pediatric caregivers, since deaths in childhood are infrequent.[121-126]

The unsubstantiated fear of inducing addiction can also impede administration of opioid doses needed to adequately treat pain even at the end of life.[121,124,125,127-130] Parents of young children are particularly sensitive to this concern and at times need to have the difference between physical dependence and addiction carefully explained. We avoid the term *narcotics* because of the connotations implied with its use, and instead use *opioids*. Further complicating opioid use is the symbolic meaning of opioids and the implication that beginning a "morphine drip" means giving up on the patient.[12,121,129] Again the emphasis here should be that maximizing comfort does not preclude continued hope and treatment of the underlying disease.

What appears to be the most significant barrier among health care providers to administering adequate pain medication is the fear of hastening death through respiratory depression, excess sedation, or both.[102,131] However, there are virtually

no empiric data that support the belief that appropriate use of opioids hastens death in patients dying from cancer or other causes.[132] In fact, it is possible that the proper treatment of pain may prolong rather than shorten life.[133,134] Nonetheless, caregivers continue to be concerned that the cardiopulmonary side effects of the medications used to relieve the pain and suffering of dying patients have the potential to hasten the patient's death. In these circumstances, an ethical justification for intensive efforts to relieve suffering, including rapid escalation of opioids or administration of sedation to reduce distress is the *principle of double effect*.[132,135,136] This principle stems from Roman Catholic moral theology and states that an action with both a good and a bad effect is ethically permissible if the following conditions are met:

The action itself must be morally good or at least indifferent.
Only the good effect must be intended (even though the bad or secondary effect is foreseen).
The good effect must not be achieved by way of the bad effect.
The good effect must outweigh the bad result.

Thus, the good effect (pain control) is intended, whereas the bad or secondary effect (hastening death) is foreseen but not intended. This doctrine has been used to justify an intensive approach to pain and comfort, even to the point of using barbiturates with the goal of inducing sedation, when appropriate.[137]

Open communication regarding these issues among medical caregivers and the family may be an important means of overcoming these barriers.

Assessing Pediatric Pain

The reliable assessment of children's pain is both a science and an art. It requires an understanding of child development so that the practitioner can choose an appropriate tool with which to undertake the assessment.[138] In addition to choosing the best assessment tool, it is most important for the caregiver to use that tool consistently. It has been shown repeatedly that there is poor correlation of pain perception between patients and caregivers in the absence of regular assessment.[139,140] Increasingly, pain assessment has been integrated as a fifth vital sign; that is, pain is assessed on a regular basis for all patients, independent of their clinical status.[141]

PAIN MANAGEMENT

A comprehensive discussion of pain control in the cancer patient is found in Chapter 42. The basic approach to the child in pain uses the WHO Analgesic Ladder Program.[9] This is a stepwise approach to escalating therapy from weak analgesics (e.g., acetaminophen or nonsteroidal anti-inflammatory drugs [NSAIDs]) to strong ones (e.g., morphine, fentanyl, or hydromorphone). However, there is little role for "weak" opioids in the treatment of cancer pain. In a randomized trial of 100 adult patients with cancer comparing the WHO guidelines to first-line treatment with "strong opioids" they found that patients started on strong opioids had significantly better pain relief, required fewer changes in therapy, and patients reported greater satisfaction with treatment as compared to the "WHO" guidelines group. Furthermore, there was no tolerance to opioids or serious adverse events. Importantly, however, a multimodal approach should be considered in which medications, cognitive interventions, local anesthetics, and other pain therapies are used from the onset to limit pain perception and the pathologic responses to pain.[142] Practitioners should also have access to pediatric pain or palliative care services to help relieve the symptoms of the small group of patients who do not benefit from the standard approach.[5]

Pain Management: Setting the Stage

Before the initiation of therapy for pain, it is worthwhile to clarify the meaning of pain with the patient and to establish mutual goals of therapy. There may be many factors that influence the child's perception of pain in addition to the physical damage initiating that pain.[143,144] The practitioner should assess whether the family's cultural, religious, or medical interpretation of the pain will affect the treatment plan.

In addition, the team should attempt to help the patient and family devise reasonable therapeutic goals. Although ideally pain can be eliminated using nonpharmacologic approaches, often these are more effectively used as adjuvant rather than primary therapy. If medication is used to control pain, there are frequently side effects in addition to pain relief.[145,146] The goal from the standpoint of both the medical team and the patient and family is to obtain pain relief with neither euphoria nor sedation, and with effective control of any other side effects. If this goal proves to be impossible in a given patient's situation, the family and patient need to know that their decision about what is an acceptable toxicity profile will be respected by the team.

Families need to be educated about pain management. They need to know that opioid administration titrated against pain does not hasten death, that it does not lose its effectiveness over time, and that the dose can be increased as needed without a fixed ceiling. They should be taught that pain medications work most effectively when given around the clock so that pain does not have to be experienced to be relieved, that opioid administration rarely causes addiction in the cancer patient with pain, and that side effects most often can be managed without an interruption in pain relief. Finally, patients and families need to know that they have access to medical personnel 24 hours a day for help with control of pain or other symptoms.

Pharmacologic Treatment of Pain

Some basic principles in treating pain in children with advanced cancer are as follows. The choice of a specific opioid agent should be directed primarily by the child's previous opioid experience.

Keep the approach to pain management simple and consistent. Medications should be administered enterally or transbuccally (i.e., absorbed through the buccal mucosa) whenever possible, with rectal, transdermal, subcutaneous, and intravenous (IV) routes reserved for situations in which the caregiver is unable to reliably administer oral medication or pain escalation is so rapid that the oral route is not providing quick enough relief. Note that the rectal route of administration should be reserved for patients who are not neutropenic, unless there are no other options.

Work with the patient and family to choose one drug on the basis of pain assessment, and opioid history. For the caregivers, this is easier than multiple medication shifts, it is the most cost-effective way of treating pain, and it allows the care team to become very familiar with the therapeutic effect and toxicity profiles of a limited number of drugs.

For mild pain, acetaminophen is the drug of choice (Table 49.1). If the pain originates from bony metastases, an NSAID should be considered.[147] Although ibuprofen has been found

---

TABLE 49.1

PAIN MANAGEMENT GUIDELINES

Intensity	Drug preference[a]	Starting oral dose	Maximum dosage
Mild	Acetaminophen (Tylenol, others)[b]	10 mg/kg q4h	15 mg/kg q4h
	Choline magnesium salicylate (Trilisate)[b]	25 mg/kg t.i.d.	25 mg/kg t.i.d.
	Ibuprofen (Motrin, others)[b]	10 mg/kg q8h	10 mg/kg q6h
Moderate	Oxycodone (Roxicodone)	0.05–0.15 mg/kg q4–6h	No ceiling
	Hydrocodone with acetaminophen (Vicodin, others)	0.2 mg/kg hydrocodone q4h	No ceiling for hydrocodone; 15 mg/kg acetaminophen q4h
	Oxycodone with acetaminophen (Percocet, others)	0.05–0.15 mg/kg oxycodone q4–6h	No ceiling for oxycodone; 15 mg/kg acetaminophen q4h
Severe	Immediate-release morphine sulfate (MSIR, Roxanol)[b]	0.3 mg/kg q4h 0.1 mg/kg for infants	Titrate by 50%–100% per dose without ceiling <1 yr q4h
	Immediate-release morphine sulfate (MSIR, Roxanol)[b]	25%–33% of long-acting morphine dose	Every 1–2 h prn
	Long-acting morphine sulfate (MS Contin, Oramorph)	15 mg q12h	No ceiling
	Long-acting oxycodone (OxyContin)	0.3 mg/kg q12h	No ceiling
	Hydromorphone (Dilaudid)	0.05–0.1 mg/kg per dose q4h	No ceiling
	Methadone (Dolophine, others)[b]	0.1–0.15 mg/kg q4h	No ceiling

[a]When a change is made to short half-life opioids in an opioid-tolerant patient, the new drug should be given at 50% of the equianalgesic dose (because of incomplete tolerance) and titrated to effect.
[b]Available in liquid form.

to be safe in normal children, many children with cancer have compromised platelet numbers, so their function becomes critical.[148] Choline magnesium trisalicylate and the selective COX II inhibitor, celecoxib, had been used with increasing frequency since many of the effects on platelet functioning, renal blood flow, and the gastrointestinal (GI) tract may be minimized.[149]

For moderate pain, morphine or oxycodone is the first-choice drug in treatment. Both are available in concentrated liquid form. Because there is no ceiling dose, these drugs could conceivably be used to carry a patient through the entire course of the illness.[148] However, dosing may be limited when it is administered in combination with nonopioid agents such as acetaminophen. Many practitioners discourage the use of codeine. The toxic effects of nausea, vomiting, and constipation with codeine seem higher than that with oxycodone or hydrocodone,[150] and it provides pain relief comparable to nonopioid analgesics. Furthermore, relatively common genetic polymorphisms in the *CYP2D6* gene lead to wide variation in codeine metabolism. "Poor metabolizers" cannot metabolize codeine into morphine, and therefore receive suboptimal analgesia, whereas others are "ultra metabolizers" who may develop respiratory depression from rapid metabolism of codeine into morphine.[116]

For control of chronic, severe pain in cancer patients, the use of immediate-release and long-acting morphine or oxycodone is advocated. In most situations, therapy begins with liquid or oral immediate-release opioid, allowing patient-controlled titration of the dosing for 24 to 48 hours. During this time, the caregiver should be in constant consultation with the family to monitor the need to increase or decrease the dose or timing interval. After the patient's analgesic needs are established, the dose is converted to long-acting opioid (if the opioid requirement is high enough to be able to use the lowest-concentration dose). Methadone is an alternative long-acting opioid medication that is available in a liquid formulation, and is an N-methyl-D-aspartic acid (NMDA) receptor antagonist. Because the NMDA receptor may mediate opioid tolerance, opioid hyperalgesia, and neuropathic pain, methadone may be the preferred opioid in these situations. Methadone can be used as a first-line opioid,[151] however, because of its extended terminal half-life, rapid titration guidelines for other opioids do not apply to methadone. It is recommended to increase methadone no more frequently than every 3 days. Notably, methadone may prolong the QTc interval, particularly when administered with other agents that cause QTc prolongation,[152] and this is associated with an increased incidence of sudden cardiac arrest in adults.[153] For this reason, it should be used with caution in children with underlying cardiac conditions or those at risk for prolonged QTc.

After the patient is receiving long-acting morphine, the initial titrating solution is used as a breakthrough medication. Concentrated morphine solution can be made as concentrated as is feasible for the individual patient (up to 20 mg/mL) so that it may be given buccally if the patient is unable to swallow pills in the last days of life. Generally a rescue dose should equal 50% to 200% of the hourly dose or approximately 5% to 10% of the daily opioid requirements.[154] With rapidly progressive disease in the terminal phase, opioids may reach surprisingly large and well-tolerated doses.[108] Opioid titration for these opioid-tolerant patients should be made in significant increments, such as increases of 30% to 50%. In addition, it is important not only to increase the continuous dose but also to increase proportionally the breakthrough or rescue dose.

Other options are available when oral administration is either unacceptable to the child or precluded by physical conditions. Fentanyl is available via transdermal delivery through a skin patch.[155] The patient must have relatively stable opioid needs, however, because this transdermal application takes 12 to 16 hours to reach effect once a change is made and therefore does not lend itself to frequent dose titration changes. Further, the lowest transdermal dose may be too high for a smaller pediatric patient.

Once pain management is initiated, it is critical *to monitor the patient closely for the development of treatment-related side effects*. Caregivers should aggressively treat, or prevent, the development of the more common side effects of drug therapy. There are three side effects that often occur in the first days after therapy is started. They are usually temporary (48 to 72 hours) but may persist and be problematic. The first of these is sedation and somnolence. This side effect can be exacerbated if the patient was experiencing sleep deprivation before the initiation of opioid therapy. There is often a period of "catch up" sleep once a patient is comfortable. No treatment for this condition is needed except education and reassurance. If the symptom is persistent, however, both dextroamphetamine and methylphenidate have been shown to be effective in pediatric cancer patients in relieving unacceptable levels of somnolence.[98] Opioid-induced pruritus has been shown to be effectively treated with opioid antagonists[156] or opioid rotation. Although opioids do cause histamine release from mast cells, this does not account for most of the pruritus due to opioids. Therefore, antihistamines do not reliably ameliorate pruritus due to opioids. Nausea and vomiting can be another troublesome immediate toxicity associated with institution of opioid therapy. This symptom should be treated aggressively but not prophylactically unless a patient is already experiencing GI symptomatology. In this case, antiemetics, should be initiated before the development of aversion to the opioid therapy.

Constipation is a chronic, persistent side effect of opioid therapy for most patients. It is one that is best treated prophylactically, usually with sodium docusate or senna therapy. These medications may need to be supplemented with other treatment regimens to ensure regular bowel movements. The dose should be increased concomitantly with increases in the opioid dose. Methylnaltrexone is an opioid receptor antagonist with a limited ability to cross the blood-brain barrier. Preliminary investigations in adults suggest that it can prevent opioid side effects, while not affecting opioid analgesic action. However, there are as yet no data in children.[157,158]

At high doses of opioid therapy, myoclonus can be a disturbing side effect.[159,160] This symptom should be treated vigorously by attempts to lower the opioid dose if possible or by use of agents such as baclofen, diazepam, or clonazepam drug therapy.[161] Persistent myoclonus or myoclonus progressing to seizures is the reason to change to another class of opioids for pain relief.

Although respiratory depression is extremely rare among patients receiving chronic opioid therapy for cancer pain, it is nonetheless a constant concern for the physicians and families as the patient approaches death.[131] If the physician or family is concerned that the opioid drug therapy could be contributing to the patient's decreased responsiveness or lowered respirations, attempts can made to lower the opioid dose. It should not be abruptly discontinued because of the possibility of precipitating physiologic withdrawal symptoms. This therapeutic trial usually shows that the pain returns rapidly and that it is the patient's overall condition that is deteriorating. Administration of an opioid antagonist, such as naloxone, can cause extreme distress and is almost never required.

For unremitting side effects, opioid rotation is the strategy of choice. Drake and colleagues retrospectively assessed the value of opioid rotation in a large pediatric oncology center.[162] Twenty-two children (14%) on opioid therapy underwent 30 opioid rotations. The favored rotations were from morphine to fentanyl (67%) and fentanyl to hydromorphone (20%). Adverse opioid effects were resolved in 90% of cases, all failures occurred when morphine was rotated to fentanyl. There was no significant loss of pain control or increase in mean morphine equivalent dose requirement.

ADJUVANT DRUG THERAPIES

A number of adjuvant therapies have been shown to be clinically effective for treatment of pain in children with advanced cancer, particularly in the following situations.

Bony Metastases

Bony metastases should prompt the initiation of an NSAID, such as ibuprofen. Bisphosphonates, such as pamidronate [163] and ibandronate,[164,165] have also been shown to decrease the experience of pain in adult patients with bony metastases, but their use for this purpose in children has not yet been investigated.[163]

Neuropathic Pain

Neuropathic pain is caused by compression or infiltration of neural tissue by tumor. This type of pain can be notoriously difficult to treat and is frequently resistant to opioids.[166,167] These patients require different classes of drugs, such as tricyclic antidepressants and anticonvulsants, to control pain.[168] Gabapentin (or a related sodium channel blocker, pregabalin) is often used as first-line treatment of neuropathic pain.[169,170] The principle side effect is sedation, which requires slow increase to therapeutic doses. Gabapentin is available as a liquid. Other anticonvulsants such as valproate, carbamazepine, and topiramate can be tried successfully in patients who have either not responded satisfactorily to, have contraindications to, or have experienced adverse effects to gabapentin.[171] A child with pain and insomnia would do well with a sedating agent, such as amitriptyline.[142] Children bothered by anticholinergic side effects, such as sedation and dry mouth, can be treated with desipramine (which is relatively stimulating) or nortriptyline (which is less activating).[168] Tramadol is a norepinephrine and serotonin-reuptake inhibitor with a major metabolite that is a μ-opioid agonist, and has been shown to be very effective for neuropathic pain.[172] Families should be informed that this medication interacts with many other medications. Although this medication is not available in liquid formulation, the tablet is scored. If neuropathic pain is refractory to these strategies, invasive techniques, such as epidural or intrathecal catheters and neurolytic nerve blocks, may be required and should be considered early rather than as a preterminal therapy.[173] Furthermore, nonopioid infusions such as lidocaine[174] or ketamine[175,176] may be beneficial.

Corticosteroids

Corticosteroids can have dramatically beneficial effects, but the adverse effects may be severe and occasionally devastating. Pain secondary to visceral distention, bony destruction, or cerebral edema can be mitigated with the use of steroids, either prednisone or dexamethasone.[177–179] Other positive effects can include appetite stimulation, combating nausea, and promoting euphoria.[142,178,179] Alternatively, these medications can lead to severe cushingoid appearance, hypertension, and glucose intolerance and neurobehavioral changes. Thus,

the use of corticosteroids must be carefully considered, and review of the child's past experience with these medications can be helpful in deciding whether they should be initiated. It is recommended that corticosteroids be stopped if no therapeutic effect becomes evident within 3 to 5 days.[178]

ADJUVANT NONDRUG THERAPIES

There are a multitude of nonpharmacologic strategies, including guided imagery, hypnosis, meditation, acupuncture, and acupressure.[180] For example, Zeltzer and colleagues demonstrated that a combined acupuncture/hypnosis intervention for children with chronic pain was both feasible and acceptable. Preliminary results also showed that the intervention led to significant improvements in pain.[181] Very often, the pediatric oncology patient has used one or more of these techniques effectively to cope with the side effects of therapy or procedure-associated pain. A survey of parents of children with cancer in the State of Washington showed that 73% children used at least one alternative treatment or therapy.[182] Most patients used alternative medicine to cope with disease symptoms or the side effects of the medical treatments. This mastery allows the child to apply these methods to help control symptoms associated with the terminal phase.

Involvement of a therapist skilled in nonverbal communication can also be very helpful. This person may be trained in child life therapy or in the use of music, art, or movement therapy.[183–186] Reiki and therapeutic touch are currently under investigation as adjuvant approaches to pain management in patients with advanced cancer.[187–189] This type of therapy can be taught to parents of terminally ill children. Involving the parent in administering therapeutic touch can be a very meaningful experience for the entire family.[190]

PSYCHOLOGICAL/ PSYCHIATRIC SYMPTOMS

A physician asked a 10-year-old child how she was feeling. She answered: "Medically I'm fine, but psychologically I'm not so fine, but I'll discuss that with my psychologist."[27] (p. 11)

Ideally, the psychological status of each child should be evaluated, in the same way as medical and nursing assessments are carried out (American Psychological Association. Task Force on Children and End-of-Life. In preparation).[27,37,191] Under optimal circumstances, psychological intervention can play a pivotal role in the integration of the child's comprehensive palliative care. The contribution of child psychology and psychiatry, as well as other mental health disciplines, provides specialized knowledge and skills. The specific and unique interventions include evaluation of the child's psychological status, diagnosis of psychological/psychiatric symptoms and disturbance, role of psychotherapy and psychotropic medication, consultation to families and the team.

Psychological symptoms in seriously ill children are often multiply determined and in flux.[27,191–192] Physical pain, metabolic imbalance, neurologic dysfunction, infection, and the impact of medications are closely linked, if not at times inseparable from psychological distress. Most common are diagnoses in the broad categories of anxiety and depression. Anxiety represents a widely diverse group of developmentally appropriate and pathological coping responses, ranging from preexistent anxieties exacerbated under the stress of illness, to cumulative generalized anxiety, and even posttraumatic stress disorder. Yet, sleep deprivation and delirium may present as anxiety and agitation. The psychological and somatic symptoms of depression can be hard to differentiate from effects of the illness and treatment. Furthermore, there is often confusion between sadness/anticipatory grief and clinical depression: what is a "normal" response to impending loss versus the "symptom" of depression that should be treated with psychotropic medication? Psychotic and organic brain syndromes often present with cognitive and perceptual disturbances. Delirium may also present as anxiety or oppositional or aggressive behavior; parents frequently report sensing something is "different" about their child but are unable to describe specifically the change. It is for reasons such as these that definitive psychiatric diagnosis can at times be elusive. Because of these diagnostic ambiguities, one often proceeds with psychological or psychotropic intervention on the basis of managing specific symptoms rather than treatment of a presumed underlying psychiatric disorder.[191]

Although many psychological problems of the child may be categorized as adjustment reactions, more severe psychopathology can emerge. This is especially true in the child with preexistent vulnerabilities, or when there is a prior psychiatric history in the child or a family member. Although it is important not to overemphasize pathology in the child, there is also a risk in minimizing or not recognizing it.

It is a fact that the availability of psychological consultation in pediatric palliative care is often limited. Although it is true that psychological treatment is not universally necessary, the ability to identify "high-risk" children and intervene in a timely fashion is often missed. The challenge, under these circumstances, is to provide thoughtful emotional support for the child in a carefully planned manner. This support ranges from an openness to listen and answer questions, to regular visits at expected times, to creative art and play activities that allow the child expression of feelings and concerns.

On a cautionary note, there are risks when untrained or inadequately skilled personnel attempt to undertake a more profound psychotherapeutic role.[192] These include opening up too much vulnerability in the child and then not knowing how to contain the emotion; interpreting—beyond simply clarifying—the child's disclosures; promising confidentiality that may set up competition, rather than collaboration, with the parents; and becoming over-involved with the child beyond appropriate boundaries. As a pediatric oncologist stated: "Psychological intervention is no less a professionally skilled phenomenon than giving chemotherapy."

Depression

Depression can contribute to psychological distress and suffering in terminally ill adults and their families and poses challenges in diagnosis and treatment.[193] Preliminary data suggest that depression may also be prevalent among children with cancer.[52] Diagnosing and treating depression in patients with advanced illness involve unique challenges. Evidence of hopelessness, helplessness, worthlessness, guilt, and suicidal ideation may be better indicators of depression in this context than are neurovegetative symptoms. Chochinov and colleagues[194] found that simply asking, Are you depressed? was the best screening tool among adult patients. However, it is uncertain whether this approach would be useful for children.

Caregivers should have a low threshold for treating depression in children with advanced cancer. Psychological interventions—including eliciting concerns and conveying the potential for connection, meaning and reconciliation, and closure in the dying process—can facilitate coping.[195] Although tricyclic antidepressants are helpful for neuropathic pain, there is little evidence to support the use of tricyclics for the treatment of depression in children.[196] Psychostimulants and selective serotonin reuptake inhibitors are the mainstay of treatment for depression in terminally ill patients. They are particularly useful for children who may be too compromised to engage meaningfully in psychotherapy at a given time, or for those children or parents who decline such intervention.[97,156,197–200] Psychostimulants, such as dextroamphetamine or methylphenidate, deserve special consideration in treating depression near the end of life, because they take effect quickly.[97,156,197,198] Unfortunately, the antidepressant activity of these drugs has not been studied in children with advanced cancer.

Anxiety

Many children have anxiety disorders, especially when trying to cope with advanced illnesses.[201] Cognitive behavioral therapy and selective serotonin reuptake inhibitors can help children and adolescents with anxiety.[195,202,203] Although empirical data concerning the efficacy of these treatments in children and adolescents who are coping with advanced cancer are lacking, psychological/psychiatric evaluation and a clear treatment plan are imperative for such children, particularly those receiving palliative care.[203]

Anxiety may also be a complicating factor in the pain management of children with cancer. In situations in which the anxiety is interfering with pain relief, lorazepam may be used as adjunctive therapy. Although there is a long-standing debate about whether the benzodiazepines possess analgesic property, they frequently have a positive effect on a patient's mood and level of anxiety.[204] Benzodiazepines are best limited to short-term or intermittent use; prolonged administration may lead to a decline in anxiolytic effect and cumulative psychomotor impairment.[205]

Sleep Disturbance

Sleep disturbance is a common and distressing problem in patients with advanced cancer, and this may also be true in children.[95,99,206–209] However, both patients and clinicians often consider insomnia as an inevitable part of an advanced cancer diagnosis. As a consequence, many patients receive hypnotic medication on a long-term basis often with unclear benefit, and little attention is paid to the underlying causes of patients' sleep disturbance.[210] In a retrospective review, Hugel and colleagues found that uncontrolled physical symptoms, most often pain, were the commonest cause of insomnia in patients admitted to hospice.[99] Thus, improved symptom control should be a priority in the management of insomnia in patients with advanced cancer.

Furthermore, a multidimensional treatment approach should be undertaken to improve sleep behavior, including directive parent education, behavior modification, chronotherapy, and short-term pharmacological treatment.[211,212]

Children's sleep disturbances—whether insomnia, restlessness, hypervigilance or nightmares—frequently reflect anxiety, much exacerbated by the dark and quiet of night. Frightening dreams are common in a healthy child, so it is not surprising that a seriously ill child may report them even more frequently. However, a child who has constant nightmares, such that sleep becomes a dreaded time, is clearly overwhelmed by the confluence of intrapsychic and external realities. When children can express their fears through words and drawings in psychotherapy, the intensity and frequency of frightening dreams often diminish dramatically, as do the episodes of wakefulness and agitation.

Although pediatricians commonly prescribe hypnotics and sedatives in children with sleep disturbances,[213] a recent review found little empiric data supporting their use.[211] Although benzodiazepines are the most commonly used pharmacological treatment for sleep disturbance in palliative care, there are no randomized controlled studies justifying their use.[214] Short-term use of benzodiazepines may be useful in treating insomnia related to anticipatory anxiety, but the potential for addiction and tolerance are ongoing concerns.[211,215] Trazodone is commonly prescribed to adults in clinical practice as a sleeping aid for insomnia associated with depression, or insomnia associated with selective serotonin reuptake inhibitor activation.[211,216,217] However, there are few data to support the use of trazodone in nondepressed subjects.[218] Low doses of tricyclic antidepressants may also be useful, especially when pain is a significant contributing component to the sleep disturbance.[216,219]

ANEMIA AND BLEEDING

In children with hematologic malignancies or solid tumors metastatic to bone marrow, anemia and thrombocytopenia often occur in the terminal phases. The medical team should have a candid discussion with the family about how to handle symptoms associated with underlying marrow failure.

Anemia

If aligned with family goals, it may be helpful to keep laboratory investigation to a minimum, with the team concentrating instead on evaluation of the symptoms and the response to intervention such as transfusion. If the patient demonstrates symptoms from anemia (e.g., decreased strength, dizziness, shortness of breath, tachycardia) or has signs of continued blood loss, periodic transfusion of red blood cells may be an appropriate palliative course of action.[220,221] There should be no assumption that transfusions need to be continued after they are started, because the clinical situation may change, and there may come a time when further transfusions are unlikely to benefit the patient.[222] The impact of erythropoietin on health-related quality of life in children receiving myelosuppressive chemotherapy is unclear[223,224] and has not been evaluated in children with advanced disease. Erythropoietin therapy may be of benefit in certain circumstances (e.g., erythropoietin deficiency secondary to renal disease).

Thrombocytopenia and Bleeding

In adults, 6% to 10% of patients with advanced cancer will experience hemorrhage.[225] When visible, it can be particularly distressing to patients and their caregivers.[226] Local interventions such as packing, dressings, and hemostatic agents such as thrombin should be considered.[227] Depending on the child's hepatic and/or nutritional status, vitamin K may also be helpful.[227] Octreotide, an analog of somatostatin, has been used to manage upper GI bleeding.[228]

If the child is anticipated to be thrombocytopenic and begins to manifest bleeding symptoms (e.g., nosebleeds, GI oozing), then the possibility of platelet transfusion support should be discussed with the family.[226] Generally, the child must travel to a medical center for this transfusion, and because platelets are more short lived, this is a more intrusive form of palliative support. Massive external bleeding is unusual in the terminal pediatric cancer patient, so the medical team should feel comfortable in supporting whatever approach is desired by the patient and family.

CENTRAL NERVOUS SYSTEM SYMPTOMS

Seizures

Seizures can be a very distressing symptom for patients and families when they occur during the terminal phase. Although most common in the presence of brain tumors or metastases of other cancers to the brain, they sometimes occur spontaneously with metabolic disturbances or central nervous system bleeding due to thrombocytopenia or hypocoagulability. For new onset of seizures, in whom discovery of an intracranial mass may result in a course of radiation therapy for palliation, it may be reasonable to investigate the cause through imaging.

Prophylactic anticonvulsants have not been proven to be effective in seizure prevention in patients with supratentorial primary or metastatic brain tumors.[229] However, in children who are at higher risk for seizures it is highly recommended to have a benzodiazepine readily available.[230] If seizures occur in a patient who is taking anticonvulsant therapy, they can often be controlled by increasing the dose of the medications already prescribed. If this is inappropriate because of problems with the route of administration or the long half-life of the drugs the patient is taking, a short-acting benzodiazepine can be used to suppress the seizures quickly. Some hospices use the IV solution of diazepam, which can be administered rectally with the use of a special bulb syringe. An alternative is to use lorazepam, which can be administered buccally to the seizing child.

Increased Intracranial Pressure

Increased intracranial pressure is sometimes problematic in children who have an advanced brain tumor. If maximum radiation doses have previously been administered, as is frequently the case, the main therapeutic option left is to increase the dose of dexamethasone. It is important to involve the patient and family in the decision to increase steroid doses to control symptoms of headache, nausea, vomiting, and increased somnolence. The side effects of long-term dexamethasone therapy, including weight gain and the development of a cushingoid appearance, can be so disturbing to some children that they place limits on the amount of drug that they are willing to take on a chronic basis. There are no data regarding the risks and benefits of shunt placement in the setting of increased intracranial pressure for children with advanced cancer. The tradeoffs between the morbidity of the procedure and possible later complications, and the potential benefit of relieving pressure need to be carefully considered. Fluid status should also be carefully considered. It is not uncommon to continue hydration in children with advanced cancer. However, in the setting of increased intracranial pressure this may exacerbate discomfort, and fluid restriction may be beneficial to the patient's overall well-being.

Spinal Cord Compression

Spinal cord compression resulting from epidural metastases, although uncommon, can result in significant morbidity in the child with advanced cancer. Thus, new onset back pain should be carefully evaluated. Normal findings on physical examination do not diminish the probability of cord compression, and magnetic resonance imaging is the preferred evaluation technique. If a patient is treated while he or she is still ambulatory, the probability of remaining ambulatory is 89% to 94%.[231] Even if the patient loses some function, earlier intervention can lead to improved outcomes. Corticosteroid therapy decreases cord edema and pain, helps preserve neurological function, and improves overall outcome after specific therapy.[232] Radiation therapy may be helpful for radiosensitive tumors.[233] In addition, for children able to undergo surgery, laminectomy may also relieve the effects of spinal cord compression.

Fever and Infections

When assessing the child with fever to determine whether a diagnostic workup should be attempted or antibiotic therapy begun (or both), it is most important to focus on the current goals of the patient and family. The approach can range from a complete workup with IV antibiotic administration to empiric treatment of infections contributing to the child's discomfort, such as dysuria with frequency due to a urinary tract infection. Similarly, if a child should develop a fever and cough, chest x-ray films may not be necessary for confirmation. After many months of constant vigilance against infection while the child was on chemotherapy, however, it may be difficult for families to watch the development of fever in the child and not take the typical approach. It is therefore critical to carefully explain the options to families and determine together what is best for the child. Factors to consider include how responsive the infection may be to antibiotics, whether they can be administered in the patient's setting of choice, whether there is significant toxicity from the antibiotics or their administration, and how uncomfortable the child may be were they to be withheld.[234]

Many hospices choose to treat relatively straightforward infections, such as pneumonia, urinary tract infections, and skin infections, with oral antibiotics in the home. More invasive infections such as sepsis or widespread fungal disease may be difficult to control without significant toxicity to the child. It is important to explain to families that death resulting from sepsis can be very peaceful, and in certain circumstances, intervening with IV. Antibiotics may only serve to prolong suffering.

The discomfort of fever can usually be controlled with acetaminophen alone or with acetaminophen combined with ibuprofen. Environmental manipulation will also help to keep the child comfortable.

GASTROINTESTINAL SYMPTOMS

Nutrition and Hydration

Nutrition and hydration in the child with advanced cancer are complex issues evoking intense emotional response in medical caregivers and families. The cancer anorexia-cachexia syndrome is extremely common in children with advanced cancer and is often associated with a patient's decline and death.[52,235] Its cause is multifactorial, and it is most often irreversible, even in the face of hyperalimentation or vigorous nutritional support.[236]

The use of supplemental hydration and nutrition in children with advanced cancer is controversial.[237] Some have argued that the naturally occurring decreased oral intake is not associated with symptoms of hunger and thirst in most patients.[238-240] Others contend that dehydration may contribute to patients suffering.[241] Family members often find these symptoms most distressing.[242] Clinical studies do suggest that terminally ill cancer patients may achieve adequate hydration with much lower volumes than recommended for the average patient.[243] For these reasons, it is important to educate families about the normalcy of decreased appetite and thirst in the dying child. The goal of nutrition and fluid management should be to alleviate any hunger and thirst, to reduce anxiety, and to preserve the social aspects of mealtimes.[244] Patients may find consumption of small, frequent meals more manageable than large meals.

Magestrol acetate can be used to stimulate appetite and promote weight gain in patients with advanced cancer.[245,246] However, this medication has recently been found to be associated with significant adrenal suppression in children with cancer.[247] Cyproheptadine and dronabinol have also been used for cancer-induced anorexia.[248,249] The use of more invasive strategies such as gastrostomy tubes or IV hydration or nutrition should be carefully considered in light of individual patient and family needs.[250]

Nausea and Vomiting

Nausea and vomiting, either because of tumor invasion or a consequence of medications, can be a problem in the child with advanced cancer. It is helpful to attempt to establish the cause of the nausea before treatment.[251] In addition to reviewing the medications of the patient and signs of abdominal tumor involvement, it is important to rule out impaction from chronic constipation. Nausea resulting from increased intracranial pressure may be alleviated with dexamethasone.

There are many empiric pharmacologic approaches to the treatment of nausea and vomiting in children, and the practitioner must make a decision based on the patient's previous experience with antiemetics and an evaluation of the current problem.[252] Metoclopramide and scopolamine are effective antiemetics commonly used in patients with advanced cancer.[253,254] Selective 5-hydroxytryptamine antagonists have been found to be effective for patients with advanced cancer, whether or not they are receiving chemotherapy.[255,256] Aprepitant is a substance P inhibitor that is particularly effective for delayed chemotherapy-induced nausea,[257] but is effective in other circumstances as well. In general, phenothiazines provide little benefit over other antiemetics, and should be used with caution because of concern for extrapyramidal side effects. For this reason, if used they should be administered with concomitant diphenhydramine. Case reports suggest that olanzapine may be superior to haloperidol in refractory nausea and vomiting in patients with advanced cancer, with lower risks of extrapyramidal side effects.[258] The addition of dexamethasone and lorazepam should be considered with refractory symptoms.

Constipation

Knowledge of the underlying cause of constipation helps in both prophylaxis and treatment. The most important of these are immobility, poor fluid and dietary intake, and drugs, particularly opioids (as previously discussed).[259] Less commonly GI obstruction or neurological compromise results in constipation. Effective management of constipation starts with a careful assessment of the patient, including history of the frequency and difficulty of defecation. When the diagnosis of obstruction is unclear, an abdominal x-ray may be helpful.[260]

The management of constipation extends well beyond the use of laxatives. Attention to other symptoms, especially pain, and advice on diet, fluid intake, mobility, and other activities of daily living contribute to an effective outcome. As soon as a patient is begun on opioids, a bowel regimen should be instituted. Specifically, a softener such as sodium docusate or lactulose should be used in combination with a stimulant such as senna. Although not favored by most children, rectal laxatives may be necessary to treat severe constipation or impaction.

Intestinal Obstruction

Surgery is the primary treatment of malignant intestinal obstruction. For patients with advanced cancer, medical strategies to relieve symptoms may be more consistent with their goals of care. Many of the symptoms of GI obstruction can be relieved with a combination of analgesic, antiemetic, and antisecretory drugs, such as scopolamine, and haloperidol.[261] and may obviate the need for a venting nasogastric tube. Corticosteroids have also been useful for patients with intestinal obstruction.[262] Octreotide is a somatostatin analog, which reduces GI secretions. When administered in combination with standard pharmacological treatment, it can be very effective in the symptomatic management of inoperable bowel obstruction.[263–265]

Dyspnea

Dyspnea has been defined as an "uncomfortable awareness of breathing." Dyspnea is a common symptom among children with advanced cancer and can result in substantial suffering.[52,206,266,267] It is important for the team to consider the cause of the respiratory distress and adopt the most efficacious treatment. For example, dyspnea resulting from pneumonia may be effectively treated with an oral antibiotic regimen. Congestive heart failure is, in general, unusual in pediatric cancer patients, but there are times when cardiomyopathy or chemotherapy cardiac toxicity is a significant problem.[268] Drug therapy including an angiotensin-converting enzyme inhibitor or diuretic may be beneficial. Drainage of even small quantities of fluid can greatly relieve dyspnea resulting from pleural effusion; however, rapid reaccumulation of fluid is common, and the relief from thoracentesis may be quite temporary. More invasive approaches to pleural fluid, including chest tube placement and instillation of sclerosant drugs, should be carefully considered.[269,270] In very weak patients with a short life expectancy, the discomforts resulting from this approach may outweigh any benefit in control of symptoms.[271]

The most common cause of respiratory distress in pediatric cancer patients is pulmonary metastases that interfere with oxygen exchange. Important to the success of managing this symptom is routine systematic assessment. The Dalhousie Dyspnea Scale assesses dyspnea in children aged 8 years or older can use it reliably. This instrument has been tested in children with asthma or cystic fibrosis but not in children with cancer.[272] Most studies have found that systemic opioids of different types are effective in treating dyspnea by relieving feelings of suffocation.[273,274] Supplemental administration of as little as 25% of the equivalent 4-hour dose can provide substantial relief.[275] Nebulized opioids have not proved to be beneficial thus far.[276,277] Studies comparing oxygen with air, in patients with and without hypoxemia have shown no clear benefit of oxygen over air.[97,278] Benzodiazepines have a place in managing dyspnea even in patients who do not have prominent anxiety.[279] Finally, nonpharmacological interventions such as self-hypnosis have been found to be useful in children who had normal pulmonary function,[280] and may be helpful for children with advanced cancer as well.

MEANINGFULNESS AND QUALITY OF LIFE AT THE END OF LIFE

Adequate pain and symptom management, strengthening relationships with loved ones, and avoiding inappropriate prolongation of dying are among a set of priorities elicited from adult patients with terminal illness.[281] Hinds and colleagues have shown that children also hold existential concerns.[282] Furthermore, families must have the opportunity to carry out important family, religious, or cultural rituals during the child's end-of-life care period.[8,283] The families' sense of spirituality or engagement in a religious community may provide a structure for positive coping strategies for both parent and child.[284] "The goal is to add life to the child's years, not simply years to the child's life."[5] Facilitating memory building during this period can be the greatest gift to the child and family.

School

For many children, the social context of school and friendship is most important (Fig. 49.9).

Bouffet and colleagues followed 30 French school children with incurable cancer and found that 60% of the children demonstrated a genuine desire to attend school until the advanced stages of their disease.[285] Reading, mathematics, and computer work were their favorite subjects, increasing physical disability and fatigue diminished their motivation over time. Refusal to attend school occurred in 40% of children, many of whom had poorly controlled pain. The care team should encourage the child's continued participation in a school setting, even if attendance is limited by the child's physical deterioration to "social" visits. Whether the child is based at home or in an institution, regular social contact with other children and adults should be strongly encouraged. School participation may be enhanced through health care team contact with the school staff provided there is parental permission and child assent.

Spirituality

Most Americans consider themselves either religious or spiritual, with 9 out of 10 believing in God or a higher power.[286] Among adult patients in the United States, many view spirituality as a vital aspect of the illness experience.[287–290] Research also indicates that among cancer patients, religion and spirituality are positively associated with better quality of life, psychological adjustment and well-being.[291,292] In a survey of pastoral care providers at children's hospitals throughout the United States, respondents reported that among the patients they visited, 34% were chronically ill and 21% were clearly dying.[293] Half or more of children were thought to have spiritual care needs regarding feeling fearful or anxious, coping with pain or other physical symptoms, and regarding their relationship to their parents or the relationship between their parents. Among parents, 68% to 80% were estimated to question why they and their child were going through the experience, asked about the meaning or purpose of suffering, and felt guilty. Three barriers to attending to spiritual distress were identified through this study, including inadequate staffing of the pastoral care office, inadequate training of health care

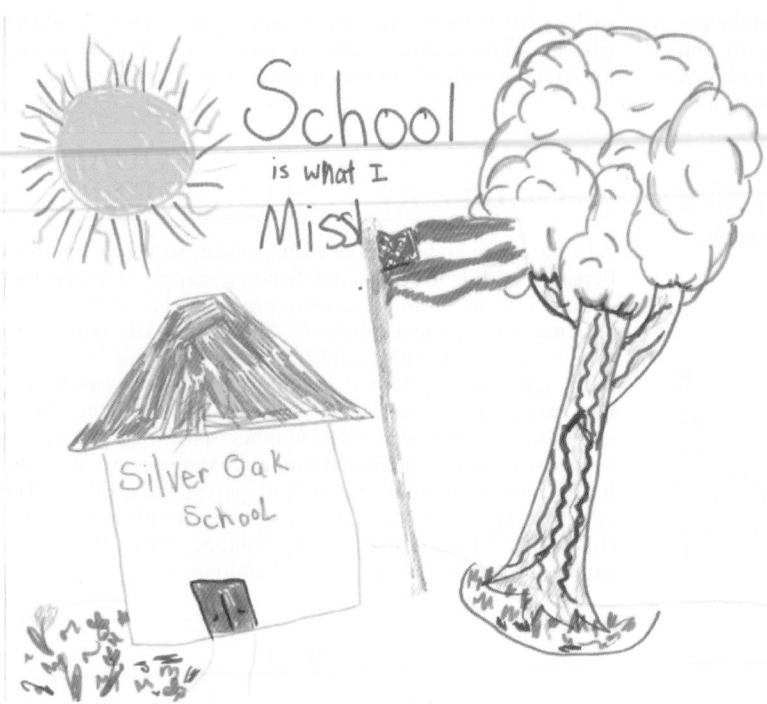

FIGURE 49.9 School is what I miss. Three weeks before her death, a 10-year-old child was asked what she had missed the most in her life during her protracted illness. Her response was immediate: "Being in school!"

providers to detect patients' spiritual needs, and being called to visit with patients and families too late to provide all the care that could have been provided. There is clearly a need to ensure that all children with advanced illness and their families receive the best spiritual care possible.

The seriously ill child can be quite pensive about the meaning of life and death. The child tries to make sense of what has happened to put his or her individual situation into a broader context. Issues of faith—and loss of faith—arise even in the very young child. Although some children's sense of trust may be shaken ("How could God let this happen to me?"), most find comfort in their beliefs. When the child has a question related to his or her own religion, it is prudent to encourage discussion of the issue with the parents, or a member of the clergy. Caregivers must take utmost care not to intrude on the family's belief system, either through ignorance or contradictory ideas.

When Death is Imminent

The endpoint of the terminal phase is often marked by a turning inward, away from the external world, on the part of the child. Cognitive and emotional horizons narrow, as all energy is needed simply for physical survival. A generalized irritability is not uncommon. The child may talk very little, and may even retreat from physical contact. Although such withdrawal is not universal, a certain degree of quietness is almost always evident. The child is pulling into him or herself, not away from others. It is critical to explain this behavior (as a normal and expectable precursor to death) to the parents, so that they do not interpret it as rejection.[1,27]

During the last few days of life, patients also experience increasing weakness and immobility, loss of interest in food and drink, difficulty swallowing, and drowsiness.[294] This phase usually can be anticipated, but sometimes a deterioration can be sudden and distressing. Control of symptoms and family support take priority, and the nature of the primary illness becomes less important. This is a time when levels of anxiety, stress, and emotion can be high for patients, families, and other caregivers.

There are several key principles in managing the child's final days. An analytical approach to symptom control continues but usually relies on clinical findings rather than investigation. Drugs should be reviewed regarding the need and route of administration. Some patients manage to take oral drugs until near to death, but many require an alternative route. Finally, it is essential that the care team maintains effective communication during this time and ensures that support is in place for the family. A daily visit for inpatients or a daily phone call at a planned time can be very reassuring for families. In our experience, physician home visits are greatly appreciated throughout the entire palliative care course, and data suggest that this is especially valued at the end of a patient's life.[295]

Importantly, even when the child may be comfortable and symptoms well controlled, simply being a presence during the final period can be very comforting to family members. Such a presence reinforces that the dying patient's welfare remains important, and it provides support and guidance to the family at a time of extreme stress. It is critical to inform the family that although death may be imminent, the time frame may be hours to days. It is essential to ensure that someone will be available to pronounce the child, especially when the child is not in the hospital.

Palliative Sedation

For symptoms refractory to intensive efforts, palliative sedation may relieve suffering by reducing a child's level of consciousness. Palliative sedation is most often used for intractable pain, dyspnea, or agitation, but is not necessarily limited to these indications. It is critical to be clear and honest in describing to the family and to the other caregivers the aims and endpoints of palliative sedation and how sedation will affect the child. Opportunities for such communication are important both before and during the provision of sedation. Although opioids should be continued to provide analgesia and prevent withdrawal, palliative sedation should never be attempted through administration of opioids alone. Instead, medications such as midazolam, pentobarbital, or propofol should be employed. Sedatives should be administered via continuous infusion with dose escalation by 50% as needed. Vigilance for breakthrough symptoms or adverse effects is warranted.

Death Rattle

Breathing can become particularly noisy when death is imminent, often described as the *death rattle*. This is more common in patients with primary lung disease or brain tumors.[296] It is critically important to prepare family members for this possibility. Because this symptom is often present when the child is already unconscious, the child may not experience this as uncomfortable. However, transdermal scopolamine, L-hyoscyamine drops for smaller patients and glycopyrrolate can be helpful in drying secretions and diminishing this symptom.[297–299] We believe that treatment of perceived suffering by family members should be a priority, even if there are differences of opinion within the care team.

Autopsy

When a child dies from progressive cancer, medical caregivers may feel that there is no reason to perform an autopsy.[300] However, postmortem examinations may provide a great deal of additional information. Sirkia and colleagues[301] found that in 40 children who died of progressive cancer autopsy examinations afforded totally new information in 20% of cases and important additional information in 55%. In a retrospective case series of 100 pediatric deaths in a large tertiary care hospital, Feudtner and colleagues found that information yielded by autopsy could further clarify the causes(s) of death in 53% of cases.[302] In addition, whether or not new information is uncovered, families report that knowing the findings at autopsy is helpful for them, and the vast majority who consent believe that autopsy of their child would at least be helpful to other patients. The autopsy also provides an opportunity for families to return for a follow-up discussion, often an important step in bereavement.[303]

Importantly, the decision to perform an autopsy should not be influenced by the place of death. In the experience of the Midwest Children's Cancer Center at Milwaukee Children's Hospital, home care did not reduce the incidence of postmortem examinations for research purposes. In their series, autopsies were performed on 57% of the children who died at home, compared with 47% of cancer-related hospital deaths.[304]

In order for this important decision to be fully considered, families should be given the opportunity to consider this request before the child dies. Given the sensitive nature of the request, it is best discussed with a member of the primary care team.[303]

Bereavement

My little brother thought that you were a checkup doctor! But I explained to him: "You know how our older sister died?. . . . Well, Dr Sourkes tries to get the sadness out of our hearts." (10 year old child)

Bereaved families face inordinate psychic challenges that test their resilience to the utmost.[305] Bereavement follow-up by the professional team is an intrinsic component of comprehensive pediatric palliative care. Families often express the sentiment of a double loss: loss of their child, and loss of their professional "family"—the treatment team whom they have known and trusted, often over months and years.[306,307] Contact from a team member after the child's death not only assuages the family's sense of abandonment; it can serve a crucial preventive role by identifying families at particular risk and identifying resources for them.

The death of a child has a profound and lasting impact on the family unit.[308] Most parents work through the grief associated with losing a child to cancer, and opportunities to share the emotional burden with others facilitates the grieving process.[309] However, parents who report not being able to work through their grief are at increased risk of long-term mental and physical morbidity, increased health service use, and increased sick leave.[310]

During this long period of mourning and reorganization, parents and siblings can be supported in several ways. At some interval after the child's death, review with the family the medical events surrounding the illness and terminal phase. If a postmortem examination has been performed, the results can be included in this discussion. Parents often have significant medical questions that need to be answered before the psychological work of mourning can take place. Ideally, a physician or nurse familiar with the case should initiate this contact so that the questions and concerns can be answered specifically. Siblings of a dying child often hold misconceptions and misunderstandings that cause confusion in the weeks and months after the death. Specific, concrete information about the deceased child's illness as well as the siblings' own health may do much to allay fears.[311]

Offer educational materials about the process of grief and mourning. Anticipate such challenging times at the first holiday season, the first birthday, and the first anniversary of the death. There are many resources written for adults about the grieving process.[311]

In addition, many children's books on dying, death, and bereavement are available for families to use in helping siblings mourn.[312,313]

Identify abnormal patterns of grief within the family. The bereavement practitioner should be cognizant of high-risk mourning situations in both parents and children so that pathologic grief may be recognized.

Invite Bereaved Parents and Siblings to Receive Support from Others

There are a variety of resources for the family of a deceased child. These include special interest groups, such as The Compassionate Friends,[314] as well as the bereavement groups of hospices and hospitals. The bereavement specialist should also be aware of therapists in the geographic area who can provide expert counseling to those who would prefer individual consideration. In addition to time-limited or ongoing children's bereavement groups, some hospices and hospitals also offer camps experience for bereaved children.

Consider attending the funeral, sending a sympathy card, sending a card on birthdays/anniversaries, or visiting the family at home. Such acts to demonstrate support for families and to commemorate their child are greatly appreciated by bereaved parents. And, families notice when staff do not engage in these activities.[315]

Establish memorial rituals for families of deceased children. These can take place either in the context of the tertiary medical center or in the community. They provide both a powerful reaffirmation of the importance of the deceased child and a time when parents and siblings can reunite with those who cared for their child.

Be prepared to follow bereaved families for a long time. The death of a child is so shockingly abnormal that the parents' bereavement period often extends for months, if not years, longer than is usual for other, more anticipated deaths.[316] In addition, as siblings grow through different developmental phases, they will probably find it helpful to reprocess the death in light of their newfound knowledge and emotional capabilities. For this reason, it is important for the bereavement counselor to remain available for long periods after a child has died.

Although it can be said that families never "get over" the death of a child, in most cases they are able to accomplish the tasks of mourning and find meaning and purpose in life once more. It is the task and commitment of the care team to stand with the family, ready to give support if needed throughout their work of grief and mourning.

Care of the Caregivers

Thank you for giving me aliveness. (six-year-old child)[3] (p. 167)

The care of terminally ill children and their families is extremely rewarding. Yet, professional caregivers often experience distress in a sort of parallel process to the families.[1,27,306,307,317,318] The professional often feels anguish and helplessness in witnessing a child endure pain and suffering—physical or psychic. He or she often identifies with the parents of the child; for the caregiver who does not yet have children, the specter of a fatally ill child may loom threateningly. In a recent survey,[306] staff cited the *personal pain* of losing a child as the most difficult experience in their work with dying children.

There is little doubt that repeated losses experienced by medical caregivers become a significant source of personal stress. In a large study on stress, 56% of 600 randomly surveyed oncologists reported experiencing burnout in their professional lives. The reasons given included feelings of frustration or failure (56%), depression (34%), loss of interest (20%), and boredom (18%).[319] Sources of distress for the medical provider include the frequent reminder that death is an existential fact, emphasizing our finite nature, the cumulative grief associated with frequent unresolved losses, and the pressure of a health care system fueled by the medical information explosion.[318]

Physicians are frequently unable to achieve the ideals embraced by holistic medical care, and when treatment fails and death is imminent, health care providers may question the meaning of their work. Yet despite the sadness involved in caring for children at the end of life, we believe that medical caregivers have a rare opportunity to uncover meaning and fulfillment in their work. Dying children seem to find a way to live in the "precious present." Much can be learned and discovered from both patient and family by acknowledging the significant burdens that they face, by communicating honestly and sensitively, and by simply listening.[318]

For all these reasons, the professionals who engage in this extraordinarily rich and demanding work articulate significant needs for support themselves.[306] Strategies useful in the prevention and management of stress include the encouragement of increased awareness of stress in self and colleagues, the clarification of appropriate goals and priorities, encouragement of appropriate limit setting, the clarification of team roles and organizational patterns, the establishment of team support meetings and favorable working conditions, exercise, and the clarification and working through of previously unresolved personal psychodynamic issues.[320] A cohesive team and/or the opportunity for consultation, psychotherapy, and support groups are crucial for those who are intimately engaged in repeated cycles of attachment and loss with dying children and their families.

Ongoing Challenges in the Care of the Child with Advanced Cancer

Optimal care of the dying child requires the unified effort of an interdisciplinary team. Although the principles of pediatric palliative care have been defined and refined over the last two decades, notable challenges remain.

The tertiary pediatric oncology center and the community agency must forge a respectful partnership in caring for children and their families. They should recognize and acknowledge one another's areas of expertise and allow the family to draw strength from both sources.

The medical professional should advocate for governmental and legal support for symptom-free living in an environment of the patient's choosing. Although pediatric palliative care services in the community are increasingly available, many legal and health care reimbursement policy impediments to administration of optimal hospice home care remain.[26,321,322]

The medical professionals should work toward assuring that all children with advanced illness and their families receive the support of a trained interdisciplinary team.[5] They must also recognize the long-term needs of families and ensure the continuity of service through time. This requires creating a supportive environment for staff so that they are able to maintain a high level of commitment to the field and enjoyment and satisfaction in their work. Pediatric palliative care is

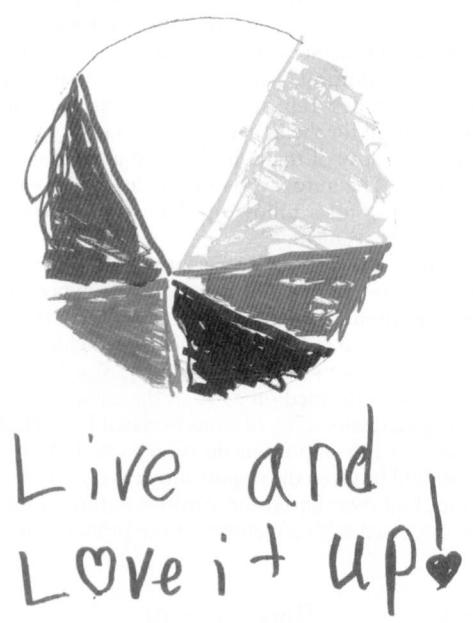

FIGURE 49.10 Live and Love it up! This drawing [shows how I felt last week when I heard that my friend had died. I was *happy (blue)* because I know he will have a happier life up in the sky. But I am *sad (purple)* for me and his family. I was really *shocked (yellow)* that he died, even though I knew he was not doing well. When my mother told me, my heart just freezed [sic]. Now I am starting to feel a little less shocked—a little tame. . . . Like you know when a tiger gets more tame, you feel less afraid. The *white* space is for love and sadness. . . . He was a really really really close friend, closer than close. . . . *Alone (pinkish)*—I feel really alone without him. He had the exact same thing as me.

emerging as a newly formed subspecialty developing clinical, educational, and investigational expertise focused on enhancing quality of life and comfort in children with advanced illness and their families. With time, models for blending this subspecialty with pediatric oncology will emerge with the goal of shared expertise leading to the best possible care.[323,324]

Formal education about palliative care is lacking across disciplines and at all levels of experience.[13,325–327] In a survey of American Society of Clinical Oncology members, pediatric oncologists reported a lack of formal courses in pediatric palliative care, a strikingly high reliance on trial and error in learning to care for dying children, and a need for strong role models in this area.[115] Increasingly, initiatives are under development to enhance learning about pediatric palliative care.[328–332] However, these programs need to be integrated into training on a routine basis and carefully evaluated. Finally, the field of pediatric palliative care is in need of rigorous research efforts aimed at developing ways to enhance communication, symptom management, and quality of life for children with advanced illness. Significant challenges exist to conducting the critically needed research on children with advanced cancer and their families, including small numbers of patients with diverse life-threatening illnesses, an insufficient number of clinical investigators with experience in conducting pediatric palliative care research, reluctance of institutional review boards to approve such research because of concerns related to the risk/benefit ratios, the need for targeted funding for testing of guidelines or care models, and a national mechanism (such as a consortium) to conduct pediatric palliative research that will yield representative findings related to the characteristics of pediatric deaths and effectiveness of interventions to prevent or diminish suffering of the child and of the bereaved survivors.[333,334] Just as the pediatric oncology community has made tremendous strides in curing cancer, so too can we join together as a community to win the battle on suffering. Outstanding care of children facing the end of life and their families is worthy of societies' attention and support.[335]

Live and love it up!
Live the best life you can.
Love everyone you love as long as you can.
"My Motto" (Mikaela, age 10)[335] (p. 28)

The resilient spirit, love, identification, and wisdom expressed by Mikaela highlight the depth of the pediatric palliative care experience for the children, their families, and the professional caregivers (Fig. 49.10).

References

1. Sourkes BM. The deepening shade : psychological aspects of life-threatening illness, contemporary community health series. Pittsburgh, PA: University of Pittsburgh Press, 1982:23.
2. Sourkes BM. Siblings of the child with a life-threatening illness. J Child Contemp Soc 1987;13:158–184.
3. DeVita-Raeburn E. The empty room : surviving the loss of a brother or sister at any age. New York, NY: Scribner, 2004.
4. Hamilton BE, Minino AM, Martin JA, et al. Annual summary of vital statistics: 2005. Pediatrics 2007;119:345–360.
5. American Academy of Pediatrics, Committee on Bioethics and Committee on Hospital Care. Palliative care for children. Pediatrics 2000;106:351–357.
6. Good care of the dying patient. Council on Scientific Affairs, American Medical Association. JAMA 1996;275:474–478.
7. Cancer care during the last phase of life. J Clin Oncol 1998;16:1986–1996.
8. Field MJ, Behrman RE; Institute of Medicine (U.S.). Committee on Palliative and End-of-Life Care for Children and Their Families: When children die: improving palliative and end-of-life care for children and their families. Washington, DC: National Academy Press, 2003.
9. World Health Organization. Cancer pain relief and palliative care in children. Geneva, Switzerland: World Health Organization, 1998.
10. World Health Organization. Cancer pain relief and palliative care. Report of a WHO Expert Committee. Geneva, Switzerland: World Health Organization, 1990.
11. Johnston DL, Nagel K, Friedman DL, et al. Availability and use of palliative care and end-of-life services for pediatric oncology patients. J Clin Oncol 2008;26:4646–4650.
12. Field MJ, Cassel CK; Institute of Medicine (U.S.). Committee on Care at the End of Life. Approaching death: improving care at the end of life. Washington, DC: National Academy Press, 1997.
13. Sahler OJ, Frager G, Levetown M, et al. Medical education about end-of-life care in the pediatric setting: principles, challenges, and opportunities. Pediatrics 2000;105: 575–584.
14. Thompson LA, Knapp C, Madden V, et al. Pediatricians' perceptions of and preferred timing for pediatric palliative care. Pediatrics 2009;123:e777–e782.
15. Wolfe J, Klar N, Grier HE, et al. Understanding of prognosis among parents of children who died of cancer: impact on treatment goals and integration of palliative care. JAMA 2000;284:2469–2475.
16. Bluebond-Langner M, Belasco JB, Goldman A, et al. Understanding parents' approaches to care and treatment of children with cancer when standard therapy has failed. J Clin Oncol 2007;25:2414–2419.
17. Buckman R. How to break bad news. Baltimore, MD: Johns Hopkins University Press, 1992.
18. Girgis A, Sanson-Fisher RW. Breaking bad news: consensus guidelines for medical practitioners. J Clin Oncol 1995;13:2449–2456.
19. Suchman AL, Markakis K, Beckman HB, et al. A model of empathic communication in the medical interview [see comments]. JAMA 1997;277:678–682.
20. Mack JW, Grier HE. The day one talk. J Clin Oncol 2004;22:563–566.
21. Back AL, Arnold RM, Quill TE. Hope for the best, and prepare for the worst. Ann Intern Med 2003;138:439–443.
22. Kirk P, Kirk I, Kristjanson LJ. What do patients receiving palliative care for cancer and their families want to be told? A Canadian and Australian qualitative study. BMJ 2004; 328:1343.
23. van Kleffens T, Van Baarsen B, Hoekman K, et al. Clarifying the term 'palliative' in clinical oncology. Eur J Cancer Care (Engl) 2004;13:263–271.
24. Billings JA. What is palliative care? J Palliat Med 1998;1:73–82.
25. Lo B, Quill T, Tulsky J. Discussing palliative care with patients. ACP-ASIM End-of-Life Care Consensus Panel. American College of Physicians-American Society of Internal Medicine. Ann Intern Med 1999;130:744–749.
26. Hurwitz CA, Duncan J, Wolfe J. Caring for the child with cancer at the close of life: "there are people who make it, and I'm hoping I'm one of them." JAMA 2004; 292: 2141–2149.
27. Sourkes BM. Armfuls of time: the psychological experience of the child with a life-threatening illness. Pittsburgh, PA: University of Pittsburgh Press, 1995.
28. Schonfeld DJ. Talking with children about death. J Pediatr Health Care 1993;7: 269–274.
29. Spinetta J, Rigler D, Karon M. Anxiety in the dying child. Pediatrics 1973;52:841–845.
30. Spinetta J. The dying child's awareness of death: a review. Psychol Bull 1974;81: 256–260.
31. Greenham DE, Lohmann RA. Children facing death: recurring patterns of adaptation. Health Soc Work 1982;7:89–94.
32. Blueblond-Langner M. The private worlds of dying children. Princeton, NJ: Princeton University Press, 1978.
33. Sourkes B. Psychotherapy with the dying child. In: Chochinov HM, Breitbart W, eds. Handbook of psychiatry in palliative medicine. Oxford, NY: Oxford University Press, 2000:xx, 435.
34. Hilden JM, Watterson J, Chrastek J. Tell the children [in process citation]. J Clin Oncol 2000;18:3193–3195.
35. Bartholome WG. Informed consent, parental permission, and assent in pediatric practice [letter; comment]. Pediatrics 1995;96:981–982.
36. National Hospice and Palliative Care Organization. ChiPPS workgroup on decision making. www.nhpco.org. Accessed June 14, 2010.
37. Abrahm JL, Soukes B. Palliative care. In: Hoffman R, ed. Hematology : basic principles and practice. 4th ed. Philadelphia, PA: Churchill Livingstone, 2005:1639–1645.
38. McConnell Y, Frager G. Decision-making in pediatric palliative care—Module 12. Ian Anderson Continuing Education Program in End-of-Life Care. University of Toronto Web site. www.cme.utoronto.ca/endoflife/. June 14, 2010.
39. Ellis R, Leventhal B. Information needs and decision-making preferences of children with cancer. Psychooncology 1993;2:277–284.
40. Nitschke R, Humphrey GB, Sexauer CL, et al. Therapeutic choices made by patients with end-stage cancer. J Pediatr 1982;101:471–476.
41. Leikin SL, Connell K. Therapeutic choices by children with cancer. Pediatrics 1983;103: 167.
42. Shumway CN, Grossman LS, Sarles RM. Therapeutic choices by children with cancer. Pediatrics 1983;103:168.
43. Charest M, Douesnard S. La verite sort de la bouche des enfants. Prisme 1992;2: 473.
44. Kreicbergs U, Valdimarsdottir U, Onelov E, et al. Talking about death with children who have severe malignant disease. N Engl J Med 2004;351:1175–1186.
45. Goold SD, Williams B, Arnold RM. Conflicts regarding decisions to limit treatment: a differential diagnosis [see comments]. JAMA 2000;283:909–914.
46. A controlled trial to improve care for seriously ill hospitalized patients. The study to understand prognoses and preferences for outcomes and risks of treatments (SUPPORT). The SUPPORT Principal Investigators [see comments] [published erratum appears in JAMA 1996;275(16):1232]. JAMA 1995;274:1591–1598.
47. Cohen RW. A tale of two conversations. Hastings Cent Rep 2004;34:49.
48. Jones BL, Parker-Raley J, Higgerson R, et al. Finding the right words: using the terms allow natural death (AND) and do not resuscitate (DNR) in pediatric palliative care. J Healthc Qual 2008;30:55–63.
49. Chessa F. "Allow natural death"—not so fast. Hastings Cent Rep 2004;34:4.
50. Hickman SE, Tolle SW, Brummel-Smith K, et al. Use of the Physician Orders for Life-Sustaining Treatment program in Oregon nursing facilities: beyond resuscitation status. J Am Geriatr Soc 2004;52:1424–1429.
51. Sirkia K, Saarinen UM, Ahlgren B, et al. Terminal care of the child with cancer at home [see comments]. Acta Paediatr 1997;86:1125–1130.

52. Wolfe J, Grier HE, Klar N, et al. Symptoms and suffering at the end of life in children with cancer [see comments]. N Engl J Med 2000;342:326–333.
53. Wolfe J, Hammel JF, Edwards KE, et al. Easing of suffering in children with cancer at the end of life: is care changing? J Clin Oncol 2008;26:1717–1723.
54. Lauer ME, Mulhern RK, Wallskog JM, et al. A comparison study of parental adaptation following a child's death at home or in the hospital. Pediatrics 1983;71:107–112.
55. Lauer ME, Mulhern RK, Schell MJ, et al. Long-term follow-up of parental adjustment following a child's death at home or hospital. Cancer 1989;63:988–994.
56. Birenbaum LK, Robinson MA. Family relationships in two types of terminal care. Soc Sci Med 1991;32:95–102.
57. Feudtner C, Silveira MJ, Christakis DA. Where do children with complex chronic conditions die? Patterns in Washington State, 1980–1998. Pediatrics 2002;109:656–660.
58. Higginson IJ, Thompson M. Children and young people who die from cancer: epidemiology and place of death in England (1995–9). BMJ 2003;327:478–479.
59. Dussel V, Kreicbergs U, Hilden JM, et al. Looking beyond where children die: determinants and effects of planning a child's location of death. J Pain Symptom Manage 2009;37:33–43.
60. Duncan J, Spengler E, Wolfe J. Providing pediatric palliative care: PACT in action. MCN Am J Matern Child Nurs 2007;32:279–287.
61. Liben S, Goldman A. Home care for children with life-threatening illness. J Palliat Care 1998;14:33–38.
62. Morgan ER, Murphy SB. Care of children who are dying of cancer [editorial; comment] [see comments]. N Engl J Med 2000;342:347–348.
63. Boling A, Lynn J. Hospice: current practice, future possibilities. Hosp J 1998;13:29–32.
64. Buntin MB, Huskamp H. What is known about the economics of end-of-life care for Medicare beneficiaries? Gerontologist 2002;42(3):40–48.
65. Huskamp HA, Buntin MB, Wang V, et al. Providing care at the end of life: do Medicare rules impede good care? Health Aff (Millwood) 2001;20:204–211.
66. Fowler K, Poehling K, Billheimer D, et al. Hospice referral practices for children with cancer: a survey of pediatric oncologists. J Clin Oncol 2006;24:1099–1104.
67. Massachusetts Pediatric Palliative Care Network. http://www.mass. gov/ppcn. Accessed June 14, 2010.
68. Knapp CA, Madden VL, Curtis CM, et al. Partners in care: together for kids: Florida's model of pediatric palliative care. J Palliat Med 2008;11:1212–1220.
69. Cassileth BR, Lusk EJ, Guerry D, et al. Survival and quality of life among patients receiving unproven as compared with conventional cancer therapy [see comments]. N Engl J Med 1991;324:1180–1185.
70. Ellis PA, Smith IE, Hardy JR, et al. Symptom relief with MVP (mitomycin C, vinblastine and cisplatin) chemotherapy in advanced non-small-cell lung cancer. Br J Cancer 1995; 71:366–370.
71. Geels P, Eisenhauer E, Bezjak A, et al. Palliative effect of chemotherapy: objective tumor response is associated with symptom improvement in patients with metastatic breast cancer. J Clin Oncol 2000;18:2395–2405.
72. Kiebert GM, Jonas DL, Middleton MR. Health-related quality of life in patients with advanced metastatic melanoma: results of a randomized phase III study comparing temozolomide with dacarbazine. Cancer Invest 2003;21:821–829.
73. Ernst DS, Tannock IF, Winquist EW, et al. Randomized, double-blind, controlled trial of mitoxantrone/prednisone and clodronate versus mitoxantrone/prednisone and placebo in patients with hormone-refractory prostate cancer and pain. J Clin Oncol 2003;21: 3335–3342.
74. Kushner BH, Kramer K, Cheung NK. Oral etoposide for refractory and relapsed neuroblastoma. J Clin Oncol 1999;17:3221–3225.
75. Chamberlain MC. Recurrent supratentorial malignant gliomas in children. Long-term salvage therapy with oral etoposide. Arch Neurol 1997;54:554–558.
76. Kebudi R, Gorgun O, Ayan I. Oral etoposide for recurrent/progressive sarcomas of childhood. Pediatr Blood Cancer 2004;42:320–324.
77. Daugherty C, Ratain MJ, Grochowski E, et al. Perceptions of cancer patients and their physicians involved in phase I trials [see comments] [published erratum appears in J Clin Oncol 1995;13(9):2476]. J Clin Oncol 1995;13:1062–1072.
78. Deatrick JA, Angst DB, Moore C. Parents' views of their children's participation in phase I oncology clinical trials. J Pediatr Oncol Nurs 2002;19:114–121.
79. Decoster G, Stein G, Holdener EE. Responses and toxic deaths in phase I clinical trials. Ann Oncol 1990;1:175–181.
80. Shah S, Weitman S, Langevin AM, et al. Phase I therapy trials in children with cancer. J Pediatr Hematol Oncol 1998;20:431–438.
81. Emanuel EJ. A phase I trial on the ethics of phase I trials [editorial; comment]. J Clin Oncol 1995;13:1049–1051.
82. Informed consent, parental permission, and assent in pediatric practice. Committee on Bioethics, American Academy of Pediatrics [see comments]. Pediatrics 1995;95: 314–317.
83. Ulrich CM, Grady C, Wendler D. Palliative care: a supportive adjunct to pediatric phase I clinical trials for anticancer agents? Pediatrics 2004;114:852–855.
84. Gaze MN, Kelly CG, Kerr GR, et al. Pain relief and quality of life following radiotherapy for bone metastases: a randomised trial of two fractionation schedules. Radiother Oncol 1997;45:109–116.
85. Chow E, Danjoux C, Wong R, et al. Palliation of bone metastases: a survey of patterns of practice among Canadian radiation oncologists. Radiother Oncol 2000;56: 305–314.
86. Wu JS, Wong R, Johnston M, et al. Meta-analysis of dose-fractionation radiotherapy trials for the palliation of painful bone metastases. Int J Radiat Oncol Biol Phys 2003; 55:594–605.
87. Janjan NA. An emerging respect for palliative care in radiation oncology. J Palliat Med 1998;1:83–88.
88. van den Hout WB, van der Linden YM, Steenland E, et al. Single- versus multiple-fraction radiotherapy in patients with painful bone metastases: cost-utility analysis based on a randomized trial. J Natl Cancer Inst 2003;95:222–229.
89. McCloskey SA, Tao ML, Rose CM, et al. National survey of perspectives of palliative radiation therapy: role, barriers, and needs. Cancer J 2007;13:130–137.
90. Koontz BF, Clough RW, Halperin EC. Palliative radiation therapy for metastatic Ewing sarcoma. Cancer 2006;106:1790–1793.
91. Paulino AC. Palliative radiotherapy in children with neuroblastoma. Pediatr Hematol Oncol 2003;20:111–117.
92. Drake R, Frost J, Collins JJ. The symptoms of dying children. J Pain Symptom Manage 2003;26:594–603.
93. Hinds PS, Hockenberry-Eaton M, Gilger E, et al. Comparing patient, parent, and staff descriptions of fatigue in pediatric oncology patients. Cancer Nurs 1999;22:277–288; quiz 288–289.
94. Miaskowski C, Portenoy RK. Update on the assessment and management of cancer-related fatigue. Support Oncol 1998;1:1–10.
95. Mercadante S, Girelli D, Casuccio A. Sleep disorders in advanced cancer patients: prevalence and factors associated. Support Care Cancer 2004;12:355–359.
96. Ullrich CVD, Hilden JM, Sheaffer JW, et al. Fatigue in children with cancer at the end of life. J Pain Symptom Manage 2009. In press.
97. Bruera E, Driver L, Barnes EA, et al. Patient-controlled methylphenidate for the management of fatigue in patients with advanced cancer: a preliminary report. J Clin Oncol 2003;21:4439–4443.
98. Yee JD, Berde CB. Dextroamphetamine or methylphenidate as adjuvants to opioid analgesia for adolescents with cancer. J Pain Symptom Manage 1994;9:122–125.
99. Hugel H, Ellershaw JE, Cook L, et al. The prevalence, key causes and management of insomnia in palliative care patients. J Pain Symptom Manage 2004;27:316–321.
100. Mock V, Dow KH, Meares CJ, et al. Effects of exercise on fatigue, physical functioning, and emotional distress during radiation therapy for breast cancer. Oncol Nurs Forum 1997;24:991–1000.
101. Dimeo FC, Stieglitz RD, Novelli-Fischer U, et al. Effects of physical activity on the fatigue and psychologic status of cancer patients during chemotherapy. Cancer 1999; 85:2273–2277.
102. Wolfe J. Suffering in children at the end of life: recognizing an ethical duty to palliate. J Clin Ethics 2000;11:157–163.
103. Miser AW, Dothage JA, Wesley RA, et al. The prevalence of pain in a pediatric and young adult cancer population. Pain 1987;29:73–83.
104. Ljungman G, Gordh T, Sorensen S, et al. Pain variations during cancer treatment in children: a descriptive survey. Pediatr Hematol Oncol 2000;17:211–221.
105. Sirkia K, Hovi L, Pouttu J, et al. Pain medication during terminal care of children with cancer. J Pain Symptom Manage 1998;15:220–226.
106. Kreicbergs U, Valdimarsdottir U, Onelov E, et al. Care-related distress: a nationwide study of parents who lost a child to cancer. J Clin Oncol 2005;23:9162–9171.
107. Jalmsell L, Kreicbergs U, Onelov E, et al. Symptoms affecting children with malignancies during the last month of life: a nationwide follow-up. Pediatrics 2006;117: 1314–1320.
108. Collins JJ, Grier HE, Kinney HC, et al. Control of severe pain in children with terminal malignancy. J Pediatr 1995;126:653–657.
109. Tobias JD. Applications of intrathecal catheters in children. Paediatr Anaesth 2000;10: 367–375.
110. Wanzer SH, Federman DD, Adelstein SJ, et al. The physician's responsibility toward hopelessly ill patients. A second look [see comments]. N Engl J Med 1989;320: 844–849.
111. Portenoy RK, Coyle N. Controversies in the long-term management of analgesic therapy in patients with advanced cancer. J Palliat Care 1991;7:13–24.
112. Ingham JM, Foley KM. Pain and the barriers to its relief at the end of life: a lesson for improving end of life health care. Hosp J 1998;13:89–100.
113. Buchan ML, Tolle SW. Pain relief for dying persons: dealing with physicians' fears and concerns. J Clin Ethics 1995;6:53–61.
114. Angell M. The quality of mercy [editorial]. N Engl J Med 1982;306:98–99.
115. Hilden JM, Emanuel EJ, Fairclough DL, et al. Attitudes and practices among pediatric oncologists regarding end-of-life care: results of the 1998 American Society of Clinical Oncology Survey. J Clin Oncol 2001;19:205–212.
116. Williams DG, Patel A, Howard RF. Pharmacogenetics of codeine metabolism in an urban population of children and its implications for analgesic reliability. Br J Anaesth 2002;89:839–845.
117. American Pain Society. Principles of analgesic use in the treatment of acute pain and cancer pain. 4th ed. Glenview, IL: American Pain Society, 1999.
118. Kaiko RF, Foley KM, Grabinski PY, et al. Central nervous system excitatory effects of meperidine in cancer patients. Ann Neurol 1983;13:180–185.
119. Marinella MA. Meperidine-induced generalized seizures with normal renal function. South Med J 1997;90:556–558.
120. Abrahm JL. A physician's guide to pain and symptom management in cancer patients. Baltimore, MD: The Johns Hopkins University Press, 2000.
121. Von Roenn JH, Cleeland CS, Gonin R, et al. Physician attitudes and practice in cancer pain management. A survey from the Eastern Cooperative Oncology Group. Ann Intern Med 1993;119:121–126.
122. Porter J, Jick H. Addiction rare in patients treated with narcotics [letter]. N Engl J Med 1980;302:123.
123. Levin DN, Cleeland CS, Dar R. Public attitudes toward cancer pain. Cancer 1985;56: 2337–2339.
124. Fife BL, Irick N, Painter JD. A comparative study of the attitudes of physicians and nurses toward the management of cancer pain. J Pain Symptom Manage 1993;8: 132–139.
125. Elliott TE, Murray DM, Elliott BA, et al. Physician knowledge and attitudes about cancer pain management: a survey from the Minnesota cancer pain project. J Pain Symptom Manage 1995;10:494–504.
126. Weinstein SM, Laux LF, Thornby JI, et al. Physicians' attitudes toward pain and the use of opioid analgesics: results of a survey from the Texas Cancer Pain Initiative. South Med J 2000;93:479–487.
127. Aranda S, Yates P, Edwards H, et al. Barriers to effective cancer pain management: a survey of Australian family caregivers. Eur J Cancer Care (Engl) 2004;13:336–343.
128. Anderson KO, Richman SP, Hurley J, et al. Cancer pain management among underserved minority outpatients: perceived needs and barriers to optimal control. Cancer 2002;94:2295–2304.
129. Potter VT, Wiseman CE, Dunn SM, et al. Patient barriers to optimal cancer pain control. Psychooncology 2003;12:153–160.
130. Letizia M, Creech S, Norton E, et al. Barriers to caregiver administration of pain medication in hospice care. J Pain Symptom Manage 2004;27:114–124.
131. Solomon MZ, O'Donnell L, Jennings B, et al. Decisions near the end of life: professional views on life-sustaining treatments [see comments]. Am J Public Health 1993;83: 14–23.
132. Fohr SA. The double effect of pain medication: separating myth from reality. J Palliate Med 1998;1:315–328.
133. Manfredi PL, Morrison RS, Meier DE. The rule of double effect [letter; comment]. N Engl J Med 1998;338:1390.
134. Morita T, Tsunoda J, Inoue S, et al. Improved accuracy of physicians' survival prediction for terminally ill cancer patients using the Palliative Prognostic Index. Palliat Med 2001;15:419–424.
135. Quill TE, Dresser R, Brock DW. The rule of double effect—a critique of its role in end-of-life decision making [see comments]. N Engl J Med 1997;337:1768–1771.

136. Sulmasy DP, Pellegrino ED. The rule of double effect: clearing up the double talk [see comments]. Arch Intern Med 1999;159:545–550.
137. Truog RD, Berde CB, Mitchell C, et al. Barbiturates in the care of the terminally ill [see comments]. N Engl J Med 1992;327:1678–1682.
138. Franck LS, Greenberg CS, Stevens B. Pain assessment in infants and children. Pediatr Clin North Am 2000;47:487–512.
139. Au E, Loprinzi CL, Dhodapkar M, et al. Regular use of a verbal pain scale improves the understanding of oncology inpatient pain intensity. J Clin Oncol 1994;12:2751–2755.
140. Treadwell MJ, Franck LS, Vichinsky E. Using quality improvement strategies to enhance pediatric pain assessment. Int J Qual Health Care 2002;14:39–47.
141. Merboth MK, Barnason S. Managing pain: the fifth vital sign. Nurs Clin North Am 2000; 35:375–383.
142. Galloway KS, Yaster M. Pain and symptom control in terminally ill children. Pediatr Clin North Am 2000;47:711–746.
143. Pfefferbaum B, Adams J, Aceves J. The influence of culture on pain in Anglo and Hispanic children with cancer. J Am Acad Child Adolesc Psychiatry 1990;29:642–647.
144. Garro LC. Culture, pain and cancer. J Palliat Care 1990;6:34–44.
145. Lyss AP, Portenoy RK. Strategies for limiting the side effects of cancer pain therapy. Semin Oncol 1997;24:S16–S28-34.
146. Collins JJ. Cancer pain management in children. Eur J Pain 2001;5(Suppl A):37–41.
147. Mercadante S, Casuccio A, Agnello A, et al. Analgesic effects of nonsteroidal anti-inflammatory drugs in cancer pain due to somatic or visceral mechanisms. J Pain Symptom Manage 1999;17:351–356.
148. Lesko SM, Mitchell AA. An assessment of the safety of pediatric ibuprofen. A practitioner-based randomized clinical trial [see comments]. JAMA 1995;273:929–933.
149. Tobias JD. Weak analgesics and nonsteroidal anti-inflammatory agents in the management of children with acute pain. Pediatr Clin North Am 2000;47:527–543.
150. Schecter NL, Weisman SJ. Management of pain in childhood cancer. In: Patt RD, ed. Cancer pain. Philadelphia, PA: J.B. Lippincott, 1993:509.
151. Bruera E, Palmer JL, Bosnjak S, et al. Methadone versus morphine as a first-line strong opioid for cancer pain: a randomized, double-blind study. J Clin Oncol 2004;22: 185–192.
152. Maremmani I, Pacini M, Cesaroni C, et al. QTc interval prolongation in patients on long-term methadone maintenance therapy. Eur Addict Res 2005;11:44–49.
153. Chugh SS, Socoteanu C, Reinier K, et al. A community-based evaluation of sudden death associated with therapeutic levels of methadone. Am J Med 2008;121:66–71.
154. Frager G. Palliative care and terminal care of children. Child Adolesc Psychiatr Clin N Am 1997;6:889–909.
155. Noyes M, Irving H. The use of transdermal fentanyl in pediatric oncology palliative care [see comment]. Am J Hosp Palliat Care 2001;18:411–416.
156. Rozans M, Dreisbach A, Lertora JJ, et al. Palliative uses of methylphenidate in patients with cancer: a review. J Clin Oncol 2002;20:335–339.
157. Chamberlain BH, Cross K, Winston JL, et al. Methylnaltrexone treatment of opioid-induced constipation in patients with advanced illness. J Pain Symptom Manage 2009; 38:683–690.
158. Slatkin N, Thomas J, Lipman AG, et al. Methylnaltrexone for treatment of opioid-induced constipation in advanced illness patients. J Support Oncol 2009;7:39–46.
159. Sjogren P, Jonsson T, Jensen NH, et al. Hyperalgesia and myoclonus in terminal cancer patients treated with continuous intravenous morphine. Pain 1993;55:93–97.
160. Tiseo PJ, Thaler HT, Lapin J, et al. Morphine-6-glucuronide concentrations and opioid-related side effects: a survey in cancer patients. Pain 1995;61:47–54.
161. Cherny N, Ripamonti C, Pereira J, et al. Strategies to manage the adverse effects of oral morphine: an evidence-based report. J Clin Oncol 2001;19:2542–2554.
162. Drake R, Longworth J, Collins JJ. Opioid rotation in children with cancer. J Palliat Med 2004;7:419–422.
163. Body JJ, Bartl R, Burckhardt P, et al. Current use of bisphosphonates in oncology. International Bone and Cancer Study Group [see comments]. J Clin Oncol 1998;16: 3890–3899.
164. Heidenreich A, Ohlmann C, Body JJ. Ibandronate in metastatic bone pain. Semin Oncol 2004;31:67–72.
165. Mancini I, Dumon JC, Body JJ. Efficacy and safety of ibandronate in the treatment of opioid-resistant bone pain associated with metastatic bone disease: a pilot study. J Clin Oncol 2004;22:3587–3592.
166. Collins JJ, Berde CB, Grier HE, et al. Massive opioid resistance in an infant with a localized metastasis to the midbrain periaqueductal gray. Pain 1995;63:271–275.
167. Dougherty M, DeBaun MR. Rapid increase of morphine and benzodiazepine usage in the last three days of life in children with cancer is related to neuropathic pain. J Pediatr 2003;142:373–376.
168. Dworkin RH, Backonja M, Rowbotham MC, et al. Advances in neuropathic pain: diagnosis, mechanisms, and treatment recommendations. Arch Neurol 2003;60: 1524–1534.
169. Caraceni A, Zecca E, Martini C, et al. Gabapentin as an adjuvant to opioid analgesia for neuropathic cancer pain. J Pain Symptom Manage 1999;17:441–445.
170. Caraceni A, Zecca E, Bonezzi C, et al. Gabapentin for neuropathic cancer pain: a randomized controlled trial from the Gabapentin Cancer Pain Study Group. J Clin Oncol 2004;22:2909–2917.
171. Lussier D, Huskey AG, Portenoy RK. Adjuvant analgesics in cancer pain management. Oncologist 2004;9:571–591.
172. Duhmke RM, Cornblath DD, Hollingshead JR. Tramadol for neuropathic pain. Cochrane Database Syst Rev 2004;3:CD003726.
173. Collins JJ, Grier HE, Sethna NF, et al. Regional anesthesia for pain associated with terminal pediatric malignancy. Pain 1996;65:63–69.
174. Massey GV, Pedigo S, Dunn NL, et al. Continuous lidocaine infusion for the relief of refractory malignant pain in a terminally ill pediatric cancer patient. J Pediatr Hematol Oncol 2002;24:566–568.
175. Subramaniam K, Subramaniam B, Steinbrook RA. Ketamine as adjuvant analgesic to opioids: a quantitative and qualitative systematic review. Anesth Analg 2004;99: 482–495, Table of contents.
176. Fine PG. Low-dose ketamine in the management of opioid nonresponsive terminal cancer pain. J Pain Symptom Manage 1999;17:296–300.
177. Watanabe S, Bruera E. Corticosteroids as adjuvant analgesics. J Pain Symptom Manage 1994;9:442–445.
178. Mercadante S, Fulfaro F, Casuccio A. The use of corticosteroids in home palliative care. Support Care Cancer 2001;9:386–389.
179. Gannon C, McNamara P. A retrospective observation of corticosteroid use at the end of life in a hospice. J Pain Symptom Manage 2002;24:328–334.
180. Rusy LM, Weisman SJ. Complementary therapies for acute pediatric pain management. Pediatr Clin North Am 2000;47:589–599.
181. Zeltzer LK, Tsao JC, Stelling C, et al. A phase I study on the feasibility and acceptability of an acupuncture/hypnosis intervention for chronic pediatric pain. J Pain Symptom Manage 2002;24:437–446.
182. Neuhouser ML, Patterson RE, Schwartz SM, et al. Use of alternative medicine by children with cancer in Washington state. Prev Med 2001;33:347–354.
183. Murrant GM, Rykov M, Amonite D, et al. Creativity and self-care for caregivers. J Palliat Care 2000;16:44–49.
184. Daveson BA, Kennelly J. Music therapy in palliative care for hospitalized children and adolescents. J Palliat Care 2000;16:35–38.
185. Tyler J. Nonverbal communication and the use of art in the care of the dying. Palliat Med 1998;12:123–126.
186. Barrera ME, Rykov MH, Doyle SL. The effects of interactive music therapy on hospitalized children with cancer: a pilot study. Psychooncology 2002;11:379–388.
187. Snyder JR. Therapeutic touch and the terminally ill: healing power through the hands. Am J Hosp Palliat Care 1997;14:83–87.
188. Giasson M, Bouchard L. Effect of therapeutic touch on the well-being of persons with terminal cancer. J Holist Nurs 1998;16:383–398.
189. Olson K, Hanson J, Michaud M. A phase II trial of Reiki for the management of pain in advanced cancer patients. J Pain Symptom Manage 2003;26:990–997.
190. Moore J. Compassionate endings. Am J Hosp Palliat Care 1997;14:75–80.
191. Spiegel L. Pediatric psychopharmacology. In: Holland JC, Breitbart W, eds. Psychooncology. Oxford, NY: Oxford University Press, 1998:954–961.
192. Sourkes BM. The psychological impact of life-limiting illness. In: Goldman A, Hain RD, Liben S, eds. The Oxford textbook of pediatric palliative care. 1st ed. Oxford, NY: Oxford University Press, 2006:95–107.
193. Block SD. Assessing and managing depression in the terminally ill patient. ACP-ASIM End-of-Life Care Consensus Panel. American College of Physicians—American Society of Internal Medicine. Ann Intern Med 2000;132:209–218.
194. Chochinov HM, Wilson KG, Enns M, et al. "Are you depressed?" Screening for depression in the terminally ill [see comments]. Am J Psychiatry 1997;154:674–676.
195. Compton SN, March JS, Brent D, et al. Cognitive-behavioral psychotherapy for anxiety and depressive disorders in children and adolescents: an evidence-based medicine review. J Am Acad Child Adolesc Psychiatry 2004;43:930–959.
196. Hazell P, O'Connell D, Heathcote D, et al. Tricyclic drugs for depression in children and adolescents. Cochrane Database Syst Rev 2000;(3):CD002317.
197. Homsi J, Walsh D, Nelson KA. Psychostimulants in supportive care. Support Care Cancer 2000;8:385–397.
198. Homsi J, Nelson KA, Sarhill N, et al. A phase II study of methylphenidate for depression in advanced cancer. Am J Hosp Palliat Care 2001;18:403–407.
199. Fisch MJ, Loehrer PJ, Kristeller J, et al. Fluoxetine versus placebo in advanced cancer outpatients: a double-blinded trial of the Hoosier Oncology Group. J Clin Oncol 2003; 21:1937–1943.
200. Wagner KD, Ambrosini P, Rynn M, et al. Efficacy of sertraline in the treatment of children and adolescents with major depressive disorder: two randomized controlled trials. JAMA 2003;290:1033–1041.
201. Lavigne JV, Faier-Routman J. Psychological adjustment to pediatric physical disorders: a meta-analytic review. J Pediatr Psychol 1992;17:133–157.
202. Fluvoxamine for the treatment of anxiety disorders in children and adolescents. The Research Unit on Pediatric Psychopharmacology Anxiety Study Group. N Engl J Med 2001;344:1279–1285.
203. Gothelf D, Cohen IJ. Pediatric palliative care. N Engl J Med 2004;351:301–302; author reply 301–302.
204. Reddy S, Patt RB. The benzodiazepines as adjuvant analgesics. J Pain Symptom Manage 1994;9:510–514.
205. Barraclough J. ABC of palliative care. Depression, anxiety, and confusion. BMJ 1997; 315:1365–1368.
206. Collins JJ, Byrnes ME, Dunkel IJ, et al. The measurement of symptoms in children with cancer. J Pain Symptom Manage 2000;19:363–377.
207. Rosen GM, Bendel AE, Neglia JP, et al. Sleep in children with neoplasms of the central nervous system: case review of 14 children. Pediatrics 2003;112:e46–e54.
208. Savard J, Morin CM. Insomnia in the context of cancer: a review of a neglected problem. J Clin Oncol 2001;19:895–908.
209. Collins JJ, Devine TD, Dick GS, et al. The measurement of symptoms in young children with cancer: the validation of the Memorial Symptom Assessment Scale in children aged 7–12. J Pain Symptom Manage 2002;23:10–16.
210. Bruera E, Fainsinger RL, Schoeller T, et al. Rapid discontinuation of hypnotics in terminal cancer patients: a prospective study. Ann Oncol 1996;7:855–856.
211. Younus M, Labellarte MJ. Insomnia in children: when are hypnotics indicated? Paediatr Drugs 2002;4:391–403.
212. Quesnel C, Savard J, Simard S, et al. Efficacy of cognitive-behavioral therapy for insomnia in women treated for nonmetastatic breast cancer. J Consult Clin Psychol 2003;71: 189–200.
213. Owens JA, Rosen CL, Mindell JA. Medication use in the treatment of pediatric insomnia: results of a survey of community-based pediatricians. Pediatrics 2003;111: e628–e635.
214. Hirst A, Sloan R. Benzodiazepines and related drugs for insomnia in palliative care. Cochrane Database Syst Rev 2002;(4):CD003346.
215. Morita T, Tei Y, Inoue S. Correlation of the dose of midazolam for symptom control with administration periods: the possibility of tolerance. J Pain Symptom Manage 2003; 25:369–375.
216. Gursky JT, Krahn LE. The effects of antidepressants on sleep: a review. Harv Rev Psychiatry 2000;8:298–306.
217. Kaynak H, Kaynak D, Gozukirmizi E, et al. The effects of trazodone on sleep in patients treated with stimulant antidepressants. Sleep Med 2004;5:15–20.
218. James SP, Mendelson WB. The use of trazodone as a hypnotic: a critical review. J Clin Psychiatry 2004;65:752–755.
219. Hajak G, Rodenbeck A, Voderholzer U, et al. Doxepin in the treatment of primary insomnia: a placebo-controlled, double-blind, polysomnographic study. J Clin Psychiatry 2001;62:453–463.
220. Monti M, Castellani L, Berlusconi A, et al. Use of red blood cell transfusions in terminally ill cancer patients admitted to a palliative care unit [see comments]. J Pain Symptom Manage 1996;12:18–22.
221. Gleeson C, Spencer D. Blood transfusion and its benefits in palliative care. Palliat Med 1995;9:307–313.

222. Thomas ML. Anemia and quality of life in cancer patients: impact of transfusion and erythropoietin. Med Oncol 1998;15(Suppl 1):S13–S18.

223. Razzouk BI, Hord JD, Hockenberry M, et al. Double-blind, placebo-controlled study of quality of life, hematologic end points, and safety of weekly epoetin alfa in children with cancer receiving myelosuppressive chemotherapy. J Clin Oncol 2006;24:3583–3589.

224. Hinds PS, Hockenberry M, Feusner J, et al. Hemoglobin response and improvements in quality of life in anemic children with cancer receiving myelosuppressive chemotherapy. J Support Oncol 2005;3:10–11.

225. Pereira J, Mancini I, Bruera E. The management of bleeding in patients with advanced cancer. In: Portenoy RK, Bruera E, eds. Topics in palliative care. Oxford, NY: Oxford University Press, 2000:163–183.

226. Gagnon B, Mancini I, Pereira J, et al. Palliative management of bleeding events in advanced cancer patients. J Palliat Care 1998;14:50–54.

227. Pereira J, Phan T. Management of bleeding in patients with advanced cancer. Oncologist 2004;9:561–570.

228. Lamberts SW, van der Lely AJ, de Herder WW, et al. Octreotide. N Engl J Med 1996;334:246–254.

229. Forsyth PA, Weaver S, Fulton D, et al. Prophylactic anticonvulsants in patients with brain tumour. Can J Neurol Sci 2003;30:106–112.

230. Wrede-Seaman LD. Management of emergent conditions in palliative care. Prim Care 2001;28:317–328.

231. Loblaw DA, Laperriere NJ. Emergency treatment of malignant extradural spinal cord compression: an evidence-based guideline. J Clin Oncol 1998;16:1613–1624.

232. Abrahm JL. Management of pain and spinal cord compression in patients with advanced cancer. ACP-ASIM End-of-life Care Consensus Panel. American College of Physicians-American Society of Internal Medicine [see comments]. Ann Intern Med 1999;131:37–46.

233. Abrahm JL. Assessment and treatment of patients with malignant spinal cord compression. J Support Oncol 2004;2:377–388, 391; discussion 391–393, 398, 401.

234. Pereira J, Watanabe S, Wolch G. A retrospective review of the frequency of infections and patterns of antibiotic utilization on a palliative care unit. J Pain Symptom Manage 1998;16:374–381.

235. Nelson KA. The cancer anorexia-cachexia syndrome. Semin Oncol 2000;27:64–68.

236. Torelli GF, Campos AC, Meguid MM. Use of TPN in terminally ill cancer patients. Nutrition 1999;15:665–667.

237. Burns JP, Truog RD. Ethical controversies in pediatric critical care. New Horiz 1997;5:72–84.

238. Meares CJ. Terminal dehydration: a review. Am J Hosp Palliat Care 1994;11:10–14.

239. McCann RM, Hall WJ, Groth-Juncker A. Comfort care for terminally ill patients. The appropriate use of nutrition and hydration [see comments]. JAMA 1994;272:1263–1266.

240. Vullo-Navich K, Smith S, Andrews M, et al. Comfort and incidence of abnormal serum sodium, BUN, creatinine and osmolality in dehydration of terminal illness [see comments]. Am J Hosp Palliat Care 1998;15:77–84.

241. Steiner N, Bruera E. Methods of hydration in palliative care patients. J Palliat Care 1998;14:6–13.

242. Morita T, Tsunoda J, Inoue S, et al. Perceptions and decision-making on rehydration of terminally ill cancer patients and family members. Am J Hosp Palliat Care 1999;16:509–516.

243. Bruera E, Belzile M, Watanabe S, et al. Volume of hydration in terminal cancer patients. Support Care Cancer 1996;4:147–150.

244. Watanabe S, Bruera E. Anorexia and cachexia, asthenia, and lethargy. Hematol Oncol Clin North Am 1996;10:189–206.

245. De Conno F, Martini C, Zecca E, et al. Megestrol acetate for anorexia in patients with far-advanced cancer: a double-blind controlled clinical trial. Eur J Cancer 1998;34:1705–1709.

246. Wood L, Palmer M, Hewitt J, et al. Results of a phase III, double-blind, placebo-controlled trial of megestrol acetate modulation of P-glycoprotein-mediated drug resistance in the first-line management of small-cell lung carcinoma. Br J Cancer 1998;77:627–631.

247. Orme LM, Bond JD, Humphrey MS, et al. Megestrol acetate in pediatric oncology patients may lead to severe, symptomatic adrenal suppression. Cancer 2003;98:397–405.

248. Bruera E. Is the pharmacological treatment of cancer cachexia possible? Support Care Cancer 1993;1:298–304.

249. Desport JC, Gory-Delabaere G, Blanc-Vincent MP, et al. Standards, options and recommendations for the use of appetite stimulants in oncology (2000). Br J Cancer 2003;89(Suppl 1):S98–S100.

250. Bachmann P, Marti-Massoud C, Blanc-Vincent MP, et al. Summary version of the standards, options and recommendations for palliative or terminal nutrition in adults with progressive cancer (2001). Br J Cancer 2003;89(Suppl 1):S107–S110.

251. Baines MJ. ABC of palliative care. Nausea, vomiting, and intestinal obstruction. BMJ 1997;315:1148–1150.

252. Roila F, Aapro M, Stewart A. Optimal selection of antiemetics in children receiving cancer chemotherapy. Support Care Cancer 1998;6:215–220.

253. Glare P, Pereira G, Kristjanson LJ, et al. Systematic review of the efficacy of antiemetics in the treatment of nausea in patients with far-advanced cancer. Support Care Cancer 2004;12:432–440.

254. Bruera E, Moyano JR, Sala R, et al. Dexamethasone in addition to metoclopramide for chronic nausea in patients with advanced cancer: a randomized controlled trial. J Pain Symptom Manage 2004;28:381–388.

255. Mystakidou K, Befon S, Liossi C, et al. Comparison of the efficacy and safety of tropisetron, metoclopramide, and chlorpromazine in the treatment of emesis associated with far advanced cancer. Cancer 1998;83:1214–1223.

256. Currow DC, Coughlan M, Fardell B, et al. Use of ondansetron in palliative medicine. J Pain Symptom Manage 1997;13:302–307.

257. Gore L, Chawla S, Petrilli A, et al. Aprepitant in adolescent patients for prevention of chemotherapy-induced nausea and vomiting: a randomized, double-blind, placebo-controlled study of efficacy and tolerability. Pediatr Blood Cancer 2009;52:242–247.

258. Srivastava M, Brito-Dellan N, Davis MP, et al. Olanzapine as an antiemetic in refractory nausea and vomiting in advanced cancer. J Pain Symptom Manage 2003;25:578–582.

259. Fallon M, O'Neill B. ABC of palliative care. Constipation and diarrhoea. BMJ 1997;315:1293–1296.

260. Mancini I, Bruera E. Constipation in advanced cancer patients [see comments]. Support Care Cancer 1998;6:356–364.

261. Ripamonti C, Mercadante S, Groff L, et al. Role of octreotide, scopolamine butylbromide, and hydration in symptom control of patients with inoperable bowel obstruction and nasogastric tubes: a prospective randomized trial. J Pain Symptom Manage 2000;19:23–34.

262. Laval G, Girardier J, Lassauniere JM, et al. The use of steroids in the management of inoperable intestinal obstruction in terminal cancer patients: do they remove the obstruction? Palliat Med 2000;14:3–10.

263. Choi YS, Billings JA. Opioid antagonists: a review of their role in palliative care, focusing on use in opioid-related constipation. J Pain Symptom Manage 2002;24:71–90.

264. Ripamonti C, Panzeri C, Groff L, et al. The role of somatostatin and octreotide in bowel obstruction: pre-clinical and clinical results. Tumori 2001;87:1–9.

265. Mystakidou K, Tsilika E, Kalaidopoulou O, et al. Comparison of octreotide administration vs conservative treatment in the management of inoperable bowel obstruction in patients with far advanced cancer: a randomized, double-blind, controlled clinical trial. Anticancer Res 2002;22:1187–1192.

266. Hain RD, Patel N, Crabtree S, et al. Respiratory symptoms in children dying from malignant disease. Palliat Med 1995;9:201–206.

267. Hongo T, Watanabe C, Okada S, et al. Analysis of the circumstances at the end of life in children with cancer: symptoms, suffering and acceptance. Pediatr Int 2003;45:60–64.

268. Giantris A, Abdurrahman L, Hinkle A, et al. Anthracycline-induced cardiotoxicity in children and young adults. Crit Rev Oncol Hematol 1998;27:53–68.

269. Chen YM, Shih JF, Yang KY, et al. Usefulness of pig-tail catheter for palliative drainage of malignant pleural effusions in cancer patients. Support Care Cancer 2000;8:423–426.

270. Sartori S, Tassinari D, Ceccotti P, et al. Prospective randomized trial of intrapleural bleomycin versus interferon alfa-2b via ultrasound-guided small-bore chest tube in the palliative treatment of malignant pleural effusions. J Clin Oncol 2004;22:1228–1233.

271. Ripamonti C. Management of dyspnea in advanced cancer patients [see comments]. Support Care Cancer 1999;7:233–243.

272. McGrath PJ, Pianosi PT, Unruh AM, et al. Dalhousie dyspnea scales: construct and content validity of pictorial scales for measuring dyspnea. BMC Pediatr 2005;5:33.

273. Bruera E, MacEachern T, Ripamonti C, et al. Subcutaneous morphine for dyspnea in cancer patients [see comments]. Ann Intern Med 1993;119:906–907.

274. Abernethy AP, Currow DC, Frith P, et al. Randomised, double blind, placebo controlled crossover trial of sustained release morphine for the management of refractory dyspnea. BMJ 2003;327:523–528.

275. Allard P, Lamontagne C, Bernard P, et al. How effective are supplementary doses of opioids for dyspnea in terminally ill cancer patients? A randomized continuous sequential clinical trial. J Pain Symptom Manage 1999;17:256–265.

276. Noseda A, Carpiaux JP, Markstein C, et al. Disabling dyspnea in patients with advanced disease: lack of effect of nebulized morphine. Eur Respir J 1997;10:1079–1083.

277. Joyce M, McSweeney M, Carrieri-Kohlman VL, et al. The use of nebulized opioids in the management of dyspnea: evidence synthesis. Oncol Nurs Forum 2004;31:551–561.

278. Booth S, Kelly MJ, Cox NP, et al. Does oxygen help dyspnea in patients with cancer? Am J Respir Crit Care Med 1996;153:1515–1518.

279. Davis CL. ABC of palliative care. Breathlessness, cough, and other respiratory problems. BMJ 1997;315:931–934.

280. Anbar RD. Self-hypnosis for management of chronic dyspnea in pediatric patients. Pediatrics 2001;107:E21.

281. Singer PA, Martin DK, Kelner M. Quality end-of-life care: patients' perspectives [see comments]. JAMA 1999;281:163–168.

282. Hinds PS, Drew D, Oakes LL, et al. End-of-life care preferences of pediatric patients with cancer. J Clin Oncol 2005;23:9146–9154.

283. Levetown M. Palliative care in the intensive care unit. New Horiz 1998;6:383–397.

284. Barnes LJ, Plotnikoff GA, Fox K, et al. Spirituality, religion, and pediatrics: intersecting worlds of healing. Pediatrics 2000;104:899–908.

285. Bouffet E, Zucchinelli V, Costanzo P, et al. Schooling as a part of palliative care in paediatric oncology. Palliat Med 1997;11:133–139.

286. Bishop G. Americans' belief in God. Public Opin Q 1999;63:421–434.

287. Ehman JW, Ott BB, Short TH, et al. Do patients want physicians to inquire about their spiritual or religious beliefs if they become gravely ill? Arch Intern Med 1999;159:1803–1806.

288. Maugans TA, Wadland WC. Religion and family medicine: a survey of physicians and patients. J Fam Pract 1991;32:210–213.

289. King DE, Bushwick B. Beliefs and attitudes of hospital inpatients about faith healing and prayer. J Fam Pract 1994;39:349–352.

290. King DE, Sobal J, Haggerty J III, et al. Experiences and attitudes about faith healing among family physicians. J Fam Pract 1992;35:158–162.

291. Daugherty CK, Fitchett G, Murphy PE, et al. Trusting God and medicine: spirituality in advanced cancer patients volunteering for clinical trials of experimental agents. Psychooncology 2005;14:135–146.

292. Brady MJ, Peterman AH, Fitchett G, et al. A case for including spirituality in quality of life measurement in oncology. Psychooncology 1999;8:417–428.

293. Feudtner C, Haney J, Dimmers MA. Spiritual care needs of hospitalized children and their families: a national survey of pastoral care providers' perceptions. Pediatrics 2003;111:e67–e72.

294. Adam J. ABC of palliative care. The last 48 hours. BMJ 1997;315:1600–1603.

295. Cherin DA, Enguidanos SM, Jamison P. Physicians as medical center "extenders" in end-of-life care: physician home visits as the lynch pin in creating an end-of-life care system. Home Health Care Serv Q 2004;23:41–53.

296. Morita T, Tsunoda J, Inoue S, et al. Risk factors for death rattle in terminally ill cancer patients: a prospective exploratory study. Palliat Med 2000;14:19–23.

297. Wildiers H, Menten J. Death rattle: prevalence, prevention and treatment. J Pain Symptom Manage 2002;23:310–317.

298. Bennett M, Lucas V, Brennan M, et al. Using anti-muscarinic drugs in the management of death rattle: evidence-based guidelines for palliative care. Palliat Med 2002;16:369–374.

299. Back IN, Jenkins K, Blower A, et al. A study comparing hyoscine hydrobromide and glycopyrrolate in the treatment of death rattle. Palliat Med 2001;15:329–336.

300. O'Grady G. Death of the teaching autopsy. BMJ 2003;327:802–803.

301. Sirkia K, Saarinen-Pihkala UM, Hovi L, et al. Autopsy in children with cancer who die while in terminal care. Med Pediatr Oncol 1998;30:284–289.

302. Feinstein JA, Ernst LM, Ganesh J, et al. What new information pediatric autopsies can provide: a retrospective evaluation of 100 consecutive autopsies using family-centered criteria. Arch Pediatr Adolesc Med 2007;161:1190–1196.

303. Bates C, Burgess H. A case for autopsy in palliative medicine? Palliat Med 2004;18: 652–653.

304. Lauer ME, Camitta BM. Home care for dying children: a nursing model. J Pediatr 1980; 97:1032–1035.

305. Les enfant en deuil: Portrait du chagrin [Bereaved Children: Portraits of Grief]. Paris, France: Frison-Roche, 1997.

306. Contro NA, Larson J, Scofield S, et al. Hospital staff and family perspectives regarding quality of pediatric palliative care. Pediatrics 2004;114:1248–1252.

307. Contro N, Larson J, Scofield S, et al. Family perspectives on the quality of pediatric palliative care. Arch Pediatr Adolesc Med 2002;156:14–19.

308. Martinson IM, McClowry SG, Davies B, et al. Changes over time: a study of family bereavement following childhood cancer. J Palliat Care 1994;10:19–25.

309. Kreicbergs UC, Lannen P, Onelov E, et al. Parental grief after losing a child to cancer: impact of professional and social support on long-term outcomes. J Clin Oncol 2007; 25:3307–3312.

310. Lannen PK, Wolfe J, Prigerson HG, et al. Unresolved grief in a national sample of bereaved parents: impaired mental and physical health 4 to 9 years later. J Clin Oncol 2008;26:5870–5876.

311. The pediatrician and childhood bereavement. American Academy of Pediatrics. Committee on Psychosocial Aspects of Child and Family Health. Pediatrics 2000;105: 445–447.

312. Corr C, ed. Special issue: death-related literature for children. Omega 2004;48:4.

313. The Dougy Center. http://www.dougy.org/. Accessed June 14, 2010.

314. The compassionate friends. www.compassionatefriends.org. Accessed June 14, 2010.

315. Macdonald ME, Liben S, Carnevale FA, et al. Parental perspectives on hospital staff members' acts of kindness and commemoration after a child's death. Pediatrics 2005; 116:884–890.

316. Saunders CM. A comparison of adult bereavement in the death of a spouse, child, and parent. Omega 1979–1980;10:302–322,.

317. Sourkes BM. The child with a life-threatening illness. In: Brandell JR, ed. Countertransference in psychotherapy with children and adolescents. Northvale, NJ: J. Aronson Inc., 1992:267–284.

318. Mount BM. Dealing with our losses. J Clin Oncol 1986;4:1127–1134.

319. Whippen DA, Canellos GP. Burnout syndrome in the practice of oncology: results of a random survey of 1,000 oncologists. J Clin Oncol 1991;9:1916–1920.

320. Rushton CH. Caregiver suffering is a dimension of end-of-life care. Am Nurse 2001;33: 9, 23.

321. Joranson DE, Berger JW. Regulatory issues in pain management [in process citation]. J Am Pharm Assoc (Wash) 2000;40:S60–S61.

322. Orentlicher D, Caplan A. The Pain Relief Promotion Act of 1999: a serious threat to palliative care [see comments]. JAMA 2000;283:255–258.

323. von Gunten CF, Lupu D. Development of a medical subspecialty in palliative medicine: progress report. J Palliat Med 2004;7:209–219.

324. von Gunten CF, Lupu D. Recognizing palliative medicine as a subspecialty: what does it mean for oncology? J Support Oncol 2004;2:166–174.

325. Hain R, Goldman A. Training in paediatric palliative medicine. Palliat Med 2003;17: 229–231.

326. Khaneja S, Milrod B. Educational needs among pediatricians regarding caring for terminally ill children [see comments]. Arch Pediatr Adolesc Med 1998;152: 909–914.

327. Arnold R. The challenges of integrating palliative care into postgraduate training. J Palliat Med 2003;6:801–807.

328. ELNEC Pediatric Palliative Care Training Program.www.aacn.nche.edu/elnec. Accessed June 14, 2010.

329. Initiative for Pediatric Palliative Care. www.ippcweb.org. Accessed June 14, 2010.

330. Bagatell R, Meyer R, Herron S, et al. When children die: a seminar series for pediatric residents. Pediatrics 2002;110:348–353.

331. Browning D. To show our humanness—relational and communicative competence in pediatric palliative care. Bioethics Forum 2002;18:23–28.

332. Serwint JR, Rutherford LE, Hutton N, et al. "I learned that no death is routine": description of a death and bereavement seminar for pediatrics residents. Acad Med 2002;77:278–284.

333. Hinds PS, Schum L, Baker J, et al. Key factors affecting dying children and their families. J Palliat Med 2005;8:S70–S78.

334. Graham R, Dussel V, Wolfe J. Research in palliative care. In: Hain R, Goldman A, Liben S, eds. Textbook of pediatric palliative care. 1st ed. Oxford, NY: Oxford University Press, 2006:615–647.

335. Sourkes BM. "Live the best life you can": Pediatric palliative care. Hospice Palliat Care Insights 2004;2:28–33.

CHAPTER 50 ■ ECONOMIC ISSUES IN PEDIATRIC CANCER

SUSAN K. PARSONS, JOSHUA T. COHEN, AND MELISSA L. LICHTE

The rapid rise in health care costs in the United States has become an increasingly dominant news story in both the popular press and in academic medical journals. In part, this trend reflects the unprecedented growth in the number of older Americans. By 2030, nearly one in five Americans will be at least 65 years old.[1] The disproportionate utilization of medical services by this group is expected to contribute substantially to further increases in health care spending, which is expected to balloon to more than 20% of GDP by 2018, from its already large share of approximately 16% in 2007.[2] The projected increase in the number of individuals diagnosed with cancer is a case in point. Because cancer diagnoses are more common in older adults, the total cancer incidence is expected to increase by 45% from 1.6 million in 2010 to 2.3 million by 2030.[3] The rapidly growing population of older Americans is not the only cause of increasing health care costs, however. New, more expensive technologies and medications are also a critical factor. This is where childhood cancer fits into the picture. Although the incidence of cancer in children aged 14 and younger has remained relatively steady at 15 per 100,000 over the past 5 years,[4] the cost of therapy continues to increase.

For adults and children, emerging therapies and diagnostics are extremely expensive, and these costs are borne by patients and families, the health care sector, and society. In a recent analysis, Bach[5] estimated that average monthly cancer drug costs exceed $5000 per patient. As illustrated in Figure 50.1, these costs have increased substantially in recent years. Bach attributed this increase primarily to "a unique legislative and regulatory framework that shields cancer drugs . . . from the strategies that health care payers such as Medicare typically use to hold down the price and utilization of drugs and other health care goods."

Resorting to the use of more and more expensive treatments to extend survival is consistent with what some observers have described as a uniquely American tendency to believe that the provision of care should not be influenced by cost considerations. This perspective is evident in the rejection in 1989 of a proposal that would have permitted Medicare to take into account care costs when making coverage decisions. Among the reasons for the failure of this proposal identified by Neumann[6] (p. 1516) are "Americans' affinity for new medical technology, a distaste for explicit limit setting, a sense of entitlement with regard to Medicare funds, [and] the perception that in a vast and wealthy country, health care resources are not really constrained. . . ." Efforts by the state of Oregon in the 1980s to prioritize its coverage of Medicaid services based on health benefits per dollar spent were likewise rejected[6] and no state since has attempted to introduce that kind of prioritization scheme.[7] A 2009 survey conducted by the Kaiser Family Foundation, National Public Radio, and the Harvard School of Public Health[8] revealed a similar sentiment among a majority of Americans older than 18 years. In that

survey, 56% of respondents stated that insurance companies should be required to cover expensive treatments even if those treatments have not been shown to be superior to less expensive options.

American oncologists also resist the idea that cost should be a factor in treatment decisions. In a survey of members of the American Society of Clinical Oncology,[9] 67% of respondents stated that patient access to effective cancer treatment should not be influenced by cost. Nonetheless, oncologists recognize the inevitable impact of costs, with 56% saying that drug costs influence their treatment recommendations, and even more (84%) saying that patient out-of-pocket expenses influence their decisions.

There can be little doubt that for cancer interventions in general, and in the case of pediatric oncology in particular, the role of cost in the provision of care will continue to be controversial. On one hand, cancer survival rates for both adults and children continue to improve as new, effective therapies emerge[4] and significant progress is made in early detection and treatment. On the other hand, as costs grow, trade-offs must be confronted even when new therapies improve outcomes. Hillner and Smith[10] pointed out that it is easy to support payment for so-called "home run" therapies that provide substantial health benefits. They add, however, that "The much stickier issue will be drugs that add a small benefit at a high cost . . . [A]s oncologists we have to discuss these issues with our patients." Recent publications suggest approaches for discussing monetary concerns with patients with cancer and mark an emerging interest among oncologists to understand the impact of economic issues on patient care.[11,12]

To fully address this situation, two issues must be confronted. First, how do we determine whether an intervention's health benefits are sufficiently large to justify its costs? The first part of this chapter reviews the tools developed by health economists to assess the value of an intervention. Second, if the benefits are sufficiently large, how do we finance the provision of care? The second part of this chapter describes the available financing mechanisms in the United States and explores their limitations.

METHODS OF ECONOMIC EVALUATION

The need to make health care more economically sustainable has stimulated demand for evaluations of intervention costs. This demand gave rise to *cost analysis*, which formally reviews what is being spent on the intervention being evaluated, where, and by whom. Cost analysis aids identification of gaps or the problems with current expenditures and helps delineate future trends. Analysis of costs is particularly salient in the context of cancer treatment due to the use of new and expensive technologies and the aging of the population.

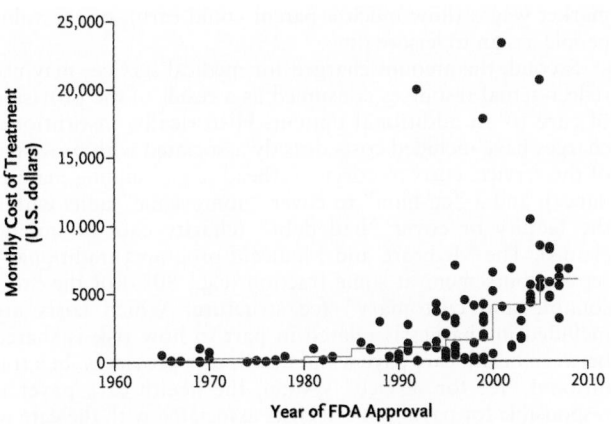

FIGURE 50.1 Monthly costs for cancer treatment medications.

The value of conducting economic evaluations of health care expenditures is based on the assumption that although demand for services is essentially infinite, resources for health care are scarce.[13] This assumption implies that decreasing expenditures on interventions that deliver limited value can be beneficial because the saved resources can be reallocated to more beneficial applications. In particular, the saved resources can be spent on health care interventions that deliver better value, thus improving overall population health. *Cost-effectiveness* and *cost-utility* analysis are methodologies that assess the extent to which reallocation of resources from one health care intervention to another can improve population health. Alternatively, resources appropriated from an inefficient health care intervention can be spent on goods and services people value outside the health care sector. *Cost-benefit* analysis addresses the question of whether such a reallocation is worthwhile.

The assumption of scarce health care resources is most evident in countries with a single-payer health care system because (excluding private purchases of health care outside the public system) the payer's budget represents the national cap on health care spending. In the context of the decentralized reimbursement system in the United States, where health care is covered by a mix of public programs (e.g., Medicare and Medicaid), a huge number of private employers, and individuals, the finite nature of the resources available for health care is less obvious. Economic analysis in health care results in the unusual wedding of principles of economics and clinical decision making—linking planning decisions on behalf of the community with clinical decisions made on behalf of the individual patient.

Components of Cost and Analysis Perspective

Before describing the different analysis methods just mentioned, it is useful to consider the different components of *costs* and why those components may be included or omitted from a particular economic analysis. "Costs" refer to impacts that deny resources for other uses.[14] Three common categories considered are those costs incurred by the patient and/or family, costs incurred by the health care system (health care delivery institutions and payers), and costs incurred by any sector in society.[15]

The perspective of an analysis—that is, the identity of the decision maker for whom the analysis is conducted—determines which cost categories are included. Consider a program that decreases inpatient care by having more of the care conducted at home. An insurer will be interested in the impact on health care sector costs, including inpatient hospital care costs, and the cost of professional in-home care providers, but

may not be concerned with patient/family costs, including the burden on the family of providing patient care. A societal perspective analysis would take account for all of these costs. It would also consider the cost of parent absenteeism from work incurred by employers. It can be useful to conduct an analysis from different perspectives. For example, the intervention in this example could have a favorable impact on costs from the health care perspective but an unfavorable impact from the patient/family perspective. Other cost categories (and perspectives) may be appropriate, depending on what question the analysis is addressing and for what audience. For example, an analysis could limit consideration to those incurred by the employer in order to help a company identify preventive measures that will best promote profitability.

Patient/Family Costs

These costs include copayments and expenditures on health care goods and services not covered by health insurance. Copayments can be substantial in the context of high-cost oncology medications. They also include time and out-of-pocket expenses associated with receiving treatment. Repeated visits to hospital facilities for chemotherapy treatments can require a substantial amount of parental time. Visits to distant institutions for treatments not available at a local facility can involve substantial travel expenses. Finally, patient/family costs include reduced salary associated with time lost at work, for example, due to the demands of caring for a child with cancer.

Health Care Sector

These costs include those expenses borne by public and private payers, including Medicare, Medicaid, and private health care insurance companies.

Society

The "societal perspective" accounts for costs incurred by the patient/family and the health care sector (earlier). It also accounts for costs incurred by other sectors (e.g., time spent by volunteers caring for a patient). Finally, it includes economic losses suffered by employers when employee productivity is adversely affected by health conditions (net of decreased wages). Productivity losses are sometimes considered a distinct, fourth cost category.[14]

Other Cost Categorization Schemes

Some writers classify costs into three major categories: direct, indirect, and intangibles. In recent years, however, use of these terms has fallen out of favor, in part because they have been used inconsistently and tend to lead to confusion (p. 24).[14] *Direct costs* refer to costs affecting the health care sector, but are sometimes also used to refer to costs incurred by patients/families and by other sectors for health care sector goods and services. The term *"Indirect costs"* has often been used to refer to time spent by patients and their families to receive treatments, and to productivity losses. The term has lead to confusion because accountants use it to refer to "overhead costs." Finally, the term *intangibles* has been used to refer to impacts whose monetary value is difficult to measure (e.g., changes in health status or pain and suffering associated with treatment). These impacts, however, are not costs as defined earlier because they do not deny the use of resources for another purpose.

Types of Analyses

Whereas the analysis perspective (and resulting determination of which costs are to be included) are driven by *who* is the decision maker, the options available drive what type of analysis is most appropriate (see Table 50.1).

Cost Analysis

A cost analysis is appropriate in cases where a decision maker is interested in understanding the resource consumption impacts of alternative interventions. Two examples from large cooperative group analyses illustrate the use of cost analysis and exemplify useful methodologies. First, Green et al.,[16] from the National Wilms Tumor Study Group, compared two treatment regimens for children with newly diagnosed Wilms tumor that varied by treatment duration (short, 6 months; long, 15 months). Because 4-year relapse-free survival did not significantly differ by treatment duration, the difference in costs for the two approaches became the most salient distinguishing factor. Annual total cost (medical costs, estimated from relative value units and Medicare charges) for the short duration was 50% of that of the long duration, with an estimated aggregate savings of $730,000 per annum. In a second example, Bennett et al.[17] reported a cost analysis of filgrastim in children with T-cell leukemia and advanced lymphoblastic leukemia. This study was conducted retrospectively, using data on resource use from participants enrolled in a Pediatric Oncology Group randomized clinical trial. The Bennett et al. study is exemplary because it estimated costs based on resource use as tabulated on study case report forms, an approach that minimized work from the cooperative group personnel. The study also identified cost drivers, a process that could be replicated in prospective analyses to focus efforts on collection of the most important cost information. Key limitations acknowledged by the authors included the lack of statistical power in the economic analysis due to the extent of variance in cost estimates.

As outlined by Drummond et al.,[14] cost estimation involves a number of considerations, some of which are particularly relevant to the evaluation of interventions to address pediatric cancer. First, because parents care of pediatric patient with cancer can consume a substantial amount of time, how the analysis assigns a value to parent time can influence the results. For example, time can be assigned a value based on market wages (how much a parent could earn), or the value people assign to leisure time.

Second, the amount charged for medical services may not reflect actual resources consumed as a result of the provision of care to an additional patient. Historically, institutional charges have included costs directly associated with provision of the service, costs to cover overhead (e.g., building maintenance), and a "cushion" to cover "nonrevenue" units within the facility or cover "bad debt" (charity care or unpaid claims). The Medicare and Medicaid programs traditionally set reimbursement at some fraction (e.g., 80%) of the "reasonable and customary" fee structure. Which costs are included in charges is related in part to how risk is shared between health care payers and health care providers. In a traditional "fee for service" system, the health care payer is responsible for paying for all costs associated with the care of a patient, even when costs rise dramatically due to unforeseen events. Under a "capitated" system (e.g., prepaid health care), charges are more closely tied to a prespecified level that depends on the condition being treated. Unforeseen costs are absorbed by the health care provider (although some plans have offered oncology services as a "carve out," based on negotiated discount). Importantly, in a capitated system, charges do not necessarily represent costs for a particular patient. Instead, charges represent average costs for a population of patients, assuming that it is possible to properly estimate the mix of patients, costs associated with typical "base case" patients, and costs associated with "outlier" patients.

Third, results depend on the analysis "time horizon," which determines how far into the future costs are tracked. Long-term costs depend on morbidity and the proportion of childhood cancer survivors who will enjoy extended survival. Long-term care costs relate not only to cancer-related morbidity but also to noncancer illnesses for which the survivor is at risk due to extended survival. The use of a shorter time horizon (e.g., 1-year, 5-year) for which outcomes are better elucidated, although methodologically easier, ignores the long-term survival cost impacts.

A related issue is the use of "discounting" to make costs occurring at very different points in time comparable. Health economists consider the use of discounting critical in order to properly account for the general preference of people to defer costs (and to consume goods and services as soon as possible). Generally, discounting decreases the importance of costs that occur at more distant points in the future. In practice,

TABLE 50.1

TYPES OF ECONOMIC ANALYSIS

Type	Features	Context
Cost analysis	Description of costs (typically health care sector costs)	Compare resource impact or budget impact of alternative programs
Cost-effectiveness	Comparison of intervention incremental costs and incremental benefits, expressed in any type of unit, such as cases prevented and life years saved	Compare interventions that affect similar health outcomes—e.g., two treatments for the same kind of cancer
Cost-utility	Comparison of interventions incremental costs and incremental benefits, expressed using the standardized quality adjusted life year (QALY) metric	Compare any pair of interventions whose main benefit is improved health
Cost-benefit	All intervention consequences quantified in monetary terms, and interventions compared based on net benefit	Compare value of health care interventions to other possible uses for resources outside the health sector

discounting converts "future costs" into "present costs" by scaling the future costs downward by a discount factor that grows exponentially with time. For example, if the annual discount rate is 3% (a common, recommended value),[18] a cost incurred 1 year in the future is scaled by $0.97 = \frac{1}{(1.03)^1}$, whereas a cost incurred 20 years in the future is scaled by $0.55 = \frac{1}{(1.03)^{20}}$. Use of modestly larger discount rates (e.g., 5% annually) can have a dramatic impact on cost estimates, and this impact is greater for costs that are further in the future. The use of discounting is particularly relevant for evaluations of pediatric cancer interventions due to the potential life expectancy of pediatric patients. For example, at even a 3% annual discount rate, the present value of costs incurred 70 years in the future is reduced by approximately a factor of 8.

Fourth, the cost of technology can change over time. The learning curve with new technologies or drugs may be steep, resulting in an exaggeration of cost early on.[19] Drug costs can change substantially when they come off patent. However, full accounting of start-up costs is not routinely examined. In a recent review of 181 articles of cost analysis, only 14 (14.4%) of studies including actual cost data (97 of 181) accounted for start-up costs.

Finally, analysis results can depend on the inclusion of *non*health costs influenced by health care interventions. For example, curing a child of fatal cancer can result in a lifetime of productivity gains. Whether nonhealth costs should be included in cost analyses (or other types of economic analysis) can depend in part on perspective (e.g., productivity impacts may be omitted from analyses conducted from the health care payer perspective, whereas they should be included for analyses conducted from a societal perspective).

A major limitation of cost analysis is that it does not consider an intervention's benefits. For example, a more costly intervention can still be desirable so long as its incremental benefits are sufficiently large to justify its incremental costs. Cost analysis has no way to address that possibility. The remaining types of analyses all consider benefits, as well as costs.

Cost-Effectiveness Analysis

Cost-effectiveness analysis compares an intervention to a "comparator" by computing the cost-effectiveness ratio, defined to be the incremental costs of the intervention divided by its incremental benefits. For example, Kievit et al.[20] evaluated a new strategy for identifying patients with a gene mutation placing them at elevated risk of colon cancer and reported that the new strategy cost 141 euros more per patient than contemporary practice. On the other hand, the new strategy boosted detection of carriers with the genetic mutation by 1.9%. The cost-effectiveness ratio for the new strategy amounted to an incremental cost of 7330 euros per additional mutation carrier detected.

Cost-effectiveness analysis can be used to compare programs whose benefits can all be measured using the same units. For that reason, it is most useful when considering alternatives for allocating a fixed budget to address a specific health care goal. For example, the analysis described by Kievit et al. could be used to compare alternative approaches for identifying individuals with important gene mutations. The intervention with the smallest cost-effectiveness ratio—that is, the lowest "price" per individual detected—is most efficient.

Comparing cost-effectiveness ratios to identify the most efficient option makes sense only if the ratios compare interventions with the same comparator. For example, it makes sense to compare the cost-effectiveness of targeted screening for cancer based on family history and the cost-effectiveness of targeted screening based on physical symptoms only if both strategies

are compared with the same thing (e.g., universal screening). For example, it would not make sense to compare cost-effectiveness ratios for these two targeted strategies if one cost-effectiveness ratio compared its strategy with universal screening and the other compared its strategy with no screening.

Cost-Utility Analysis

Because cost-effectiveness ratios can be compared only if the benefits are expressed in the same units, highly specialized measures (e.g., cost per identified individual with a specific gene mutation) can limit comparisons to a narrow collection of interventions. More general benefit measures, such as lives saved, make it possible to compare a broader set of interventions that all reduce fatalities. It may be desirable to account for other aspects of benefit, however. For example, quantifying benefits in terms of life years saved can help distinguish programs that prevent childhood fatalities from programs that prevent adult fatalities. Although the life years saved measure accounts for mortality impacts, it does not account for impacts on morbidity. For example, two medications that have the same impact on cancer survival may have very different side effect profiles.

The quality adjusted life year (QALY) is a common measure that accounts for the impact of interventions on both length and quality of life (e.g., freedom from pain and ability to take part in normal activities). A year in perfect health has a value of 1 QALY, whereas a year with an adverse condition generally has a value between 0 and 1 QALY. The more severe the condition, the less one year with that condition is worth. Being dead has a value of 0 QALYs. A program's incremental benefit is the amount by which it increases the number of QALYs an individual gains by increasing life expectancy, improving average quality of life, or some combination of the two.

Analyses quantifying intervention benefits in terms of QALYs are known as "cost-utility analyses" and are a special subset of cost-effectiveness analyses. (The term "utility" refers to the "utility weights" that scale life years to account for quality of life.) The cost-effectiveness ratio (CE) for these analyses is computed as follows:

$$CE = \frac{\Delta Cost}{\Delta QALY} = \frac{Cost_{Int} - Cost_{Comp}}{QALY_{Int} - QALY_{Comp}},$$

where the "Int" subscript refers to the intervention that is the focus of the analysis, and the "Comp" subscript refers to the comparator with which the intervention of interest is compared.

Cost-effectiveness ratios can be graphically illustrated in a Cartesian plane with ΔQALY on the horizontal axis and ΔCost on the vertical axis (Fig. 50.2). When both ΔQALY and ΔCost are positive (i.e., when the intervention not only increases costs but also improves health), the ratio is plotted in the "northeast" quadrant of this figure. The shallower the slope of the line from the origin to the point corresponding to this ratio, the more favorable it is—that is, the smaller ΔCost is relative to ΔQALY. Ratios plotted in the "northwest" quadrant of the cost-effectiveness plane represent interventions that make health worse (ΔQALY < 0) and increase costs. These interventions are sometimes referred to as "dominated." Interventions that make health better and decrease costs ("southeast" quadrant) are sometimes referred to as "dominant." Finally, interventions plotted in the "southwest" quadrant make health worse but save money. In theory, interventions in the southwest quadrant can be desirable if they achieve substantial savings (that can in theory be redeployed to other interventions) with minimal loss of health benefits. A review

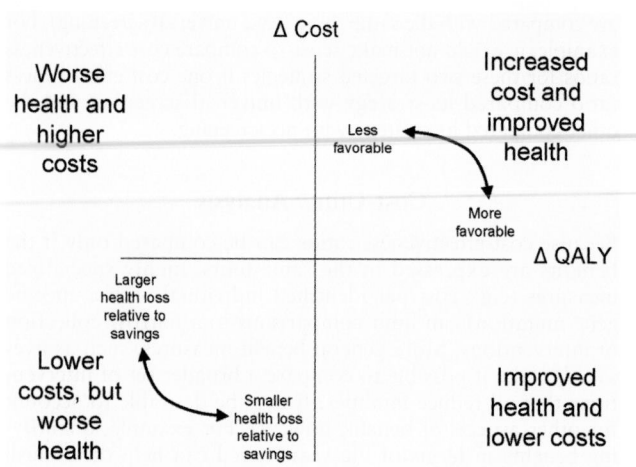

FIGURE 50.2 A graphical illustration of cost-effectiveness ratios.

TABLE 50.2

QALY WEIGHTS FOR SELECTED HEALTH CONDITIONS

Condition	Utility Weight	Reference
Untreated hyperactivity in a child—assumed to cause slight social disability and moderate emotional distress	0.88	25
Child with cystic fibrosis	0.7	26
Kidney dialysis	0.41–0.68	27
Below knee amputation	0.61–0.8	27
Liver cancer	0.1–0.49	27

of the cost-effectiveness literature revealed that very few reviewed interventions fall into this category.[21]

Interventions with ratios that are in the northeast quadrant can be divided into groups comprised of those that are favorably "cost-effective" (i.e., those with a sufficiently low ratio to indicate good value for money) and those that are not. A common dividing line for these two categories is an incremental cost of $50,000 to $100,000 for each QALY gained.[22] Critics claim that these cutoffs are too stringent, that is, that a QALY is worth more than $50,000 to $100,000. For example, based on information quantifying how much society (willingly) spent to improve health between 1950 and 2003, and data on the cost of unsubsidized health insurance (which people are generally reluctant to purchase), Braithwaite et al.[23] estimated that a QALY is worth approximately $110,000 to $300,000. In any case, the fact that there is no market for QALYs makes estimates of a QALY value uncertain.

Estimation of dollar-per-QALY cost-effectiveness ratios requires development of "utility weight" values between 0 and 1 quantifying the severity of the relevant health conditions. Utility weight values can be estimated using a "standard gamble" technique[14] that asks respondents to choose between two hypothetical options. One option is a treatment that will either cure the individual of the condition (without changing life expectancy), but might also result in death. The other option is to decline the treatment and live with the condition in question. The respondent is asked how low the probability of death must be to make the two options equally preferable. Presumably, the more severe the condition, the more willing a respondent will be to accept a treatment that has a higher chance of death and a lower risk of cure. The probability of cure (one minus the probability of death) that makes the patient indifferent between the two options is the utility weight for the condition.[24] Table 50.2 lists some examples of utility weights. Another common elicitation approach, the time trade-off method,[14] asks respondents what fraction of their life expectancy they would be willing to sacrifice in exchange for eliminating the health condition in question. The more severe the health condition, the larger the fraction respondents are willing to sacrifice. The utility score for the condition is one minus this fraction. Figure 50.3 illustrates both the standard gamble and time trade-off elicitation approaches.

Elicitation of new utility weight values for every health condition, however, can be burdensome. Pediatric conditions present additional complications because it is not clear that children can competently answer elicitation questions. That

problem raises questions about whether proxies (e.g., parents) must be used to develop utility weight estimates. Nonetheless, a 2007 survey of the cost-effectiveness analysis literature identified some three dozen studies that used utility weights for pediatric health conditions.[28]

Because elicitation of new utility weight values for every health condition can be burdensome, researchers have developed generic multiattribute utility scales. For example, the Health Utility Index (Mark 3) scale estimates utility weights based on a condition's impact on speech, ambulation, dexterity, emotion, cognition, and pain.[14] Although use of multiattribute utility scales facilitates estimation of utilities, these measures can be inaccurate if they omit a particularly salient attribute for a particular condition. Nonetheless, these tools can be useful for pediatric conditions because they sidestep the need to elicit utilities directly from children. Feeny et al.[29] compared utilities estimated using the Health Utilities Index (HUI) (Mark 2) and HUI (Mark 3) to utilities elicited directly from teenage survivors of extremely low birth weight using the standard gamble technique. They found that the there was reasonable agreement between the mean standard gamble weights and the mean HUI 2 and HUI 3 weights, but poor correlation across instruments at the individual level. From this result, the authors concluded that the HUI system is a reasonable substitute for the standard gamble for groupwise comparisons. They argued further that more meaningful comparisons between treatments would result if the same system of preferences were used (i.e., provided by a consistently used multiattribute classification system).[30]

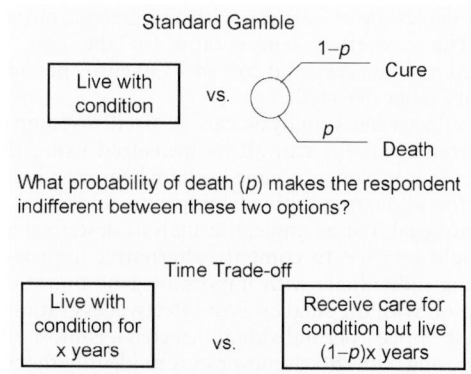

FIGURE 50.3 Methods for eliciting quality adjusted life year utility weights.

Although elicitation of utility weights can pose a challenge, especially in the context of pediatric conditions, their importance must be kept in perspective. In some cases, the values used will not have a strong impact on the result of the analysis, especially in cases where the major benefit of the treatment being evaluated is its impact on mortality, rather than quality of life. Chapman et al.[31] found that in many cases, use of unweighted life years in place of QALYs (equivalent to using a utility weight of 1 for all nondeath health states) did not substantially influence results for the vast majority of cost-effectiveness analyses they reviewed. On the other hand, for an evaluation of a new medication whose main advantage is its side effect profile, the utility weight estimates used will be much more critical.

Utility weight assignments are only one set of assumptions that must be developed to conduct a cost-utility analysis. Quantification of an intervention's impacts on QALYs gained requires estimation of its impact on both life expectancy and morbidity. Because such information is rarely available in a single empirical dataset, cost-utility analysis often demands the integration of multiple datasets, computer simulation of disease histories, and even the incorporation of subjective judgments to make the needed projections. For example, an evaluation of a pediatric cancer treatment might estimate its impact on survival by combining information from multiple sources, including: (1) the treatment's 5-year survival rate, (2) the impact of the treatment on the risk of cancer later in life, and (3) the morbidity and mortality associated with the sequalae cancers. Sensitivity analysis can quantify the resulting uncertainty associated with each assumption by systematically varying each over its plausible range while the other assumptions are held to their "base case" value, and recording the resulting range of cost-effectiveness ratios. "Probabilistic sensitivity analysis" can evaluate the simultaneous impact of uncertainty for multiple assumptions. By quantifying how uncertain the cost-effectiveness analysis ratio is, sensitivity analysis can help decision makers understand how robust the evidence base is for evaluating an intervention. By quantifying the contribution to uncertainty from each assumption, this type of analysis helps to identify research priorities.

During the last three decades, cost-utility analysis has become an increasingly popular approach for evaluating medical interventions but has yet to be used extensively in interventions targeting children. The Tufts Cost-Effectiveness Analysis Registry lists more than 1700 cost-utility analyses published in the peer-reviewed literature. A survey of this literature identified 200 analyses of interventions to address cancer.[32] This set of articles, however, includes only four analyses that specifically target pediatric interventions. Zbrozek et al.[33] evaluated the use of an anti-nausea medication (Ondansetron) in both adults and children undergoing chemotherapy; Lundkvist et al.[34] compared proton radiation therapy with conventional radiation therapy and surgery in children with medulloblastoma; Medina[35] evaluated the use of diagnostic imaging for children with headache and suspected brain tumor; finally, Goldie et al.[36] evaluated vaccination of 12 year-old girls to prevent infection from human papilloma virus (HPV) and hence reduce the risk of cervical cancer.

Cost-Benefit Analysis

Cost-benefit analysis characterizes the value of an intervention in terms of its nets benefits, that is, the difference between the monetized value of its benefits and costs. Quantifying benefits in monetary terms has the advantage of effectively comparing the benefits of a health care intervention to the benefits that can be achieved by spending resources on other goods and services. Classical economic theory implies that an intervention with positive net benefits (i.e., monetized benefits > costs) represents an opportunity to improve the overall "welfare" of the parties whose perspective the analysis takes.

On one hand, the monetization of health benefits is objectionable because it implies that health outcomes are "goods" that can be compared in value with any other good that money can buy. In fact, the strong tradition of using cost-effectiveness (and cost-utility) analysis to evaluate health interventions stems from the position "that the fulfillment of health needs should be exempt from direct competition with other claims on resources, and that health cannot be measured with the same currency as other goods or services" (p. 27).[37] Monetization of health benefits is further complicated by productivity impacts. The question is, how do we estimate production gains, based on future earnings in a way that is equitable? Basing future earnings on current earnings or other proxies of societal position or employability penalizes low-income groups, the elderly, and the handicapped.

On the other hand, monetization avoids some of the ethical pitfalls of QALYs. In particular, quantifying benefits in terms of QALYs puts a higher value on the lives of individuals with the greatest life expectancy.[37] Within this framework, the lives of children are worth more than the lives of adults. It also means, however, that the lives of children who are destined to suffer life-shortening sequalae are worth less than the lives of children who have a normal life expectancy. Monetization of benefits makes it possible to side step this dilemma by placing a value on lives, rather than on an outcome that depends on life expectancy.

Monetization of lives, life years, or QALYs, however, represents a key methodological challenge for cost-benefit analysis. Because health outcomes are not explicitly bought and sold, values must be estimated indirectly. Approaches fall into two categories. "Revealed preference" methods infer estimates from decisions to purchase products to improve their person safety (e.g., installation of smoke detectors), and wage premiums demanded for more risky jobs. This approach is limited by confounding (e.g., more risky jobs may also be less physically pleasant, making it necessary to statistically disentangle the contribution of these two factors). It is also based on the assumption that individuals have knowledge regarding the magnitude of the risks associated with their decisions. "Expressed preference" methods get around these limitations by asking people what value they place on reducing personal risks. Evidence indicates, however, that survey respondents overstate how much they would be willing to pay with real money.[38] A review of the literature revealed estimates for the "value of a statistical life" spanning more than a factor of 10.

Finally, the elicitation methods just described suffer from the ethical shortcoming that an individual's economic circumstances can influence both behavior (in the case of revealed preferences) and responses to valuation surveys (in the case of expressed preference elicitation). Estimates based on these methods assume perfect knowledge, unobstructed access, and voluntary choice. Rarely do we have access to these three requisites.[13,39]

FINANCING CARE

Public or private health insurance covers the majority of medical costs for most pediatric patients. Gaps in coverage, inadequate insurance, and the nonmedical costs of care often strain family finances, however. This section will review the most common types of health insurance for children with cancer, their limitations, and some of the prominent reforms that aim to improve health care access.

Types of Insurance Coverage

Studies have found that insurance status, meaning the type of insurance coverage an individual has, has a marked impact on cancer prevention, diagnosis, and survival. Insurance can reduce the financial burden of cancer care on families and help children maintain access to timely quality care. Lack of health insurance or underinsurance is associated with delayed diagnosis and treatment.[40] In a study that measured the relationship between insurance type and time to diagnosis in a cohort of 15 to 29 year olds at the University of Texas MD Anderson Cancer Center, Martin et al.[41] found that among patients with public insurance or no health insurance, the mean lag time between first symptoms and definitive diagnosis was 13.1 weeks longer than among patients with private health insurance. Similarly, a national retrospective analysis of patients registered in the US National Cancer Database found that uninsured and Medicaid-insured patients had an increased risk of presenting with advanced-stage cancer at diagnosis.[42] Another study of adult patients with cancer found that Medicare-insured patients were less likely to receive guideline therapy.[43] These studies had limitations, including a limited sample size, sample characteristics that limit the extent to which findings can be generalized to the U.S. population, and potential confounding between socioeconomic status and health outcomes.[44,45] Nonetheless, the findings lend credence to the idea that insurance coverage influences access to interventions to both detect and treat pediatric cancer.

Lack of insurance or underinsurance is particularly problematic for childhood cancer survivors with (or at risk for) chronic health care issues.[46] Specifically, lack of insurance reduces access to care for childhood cancer survivors who require ongoing surveillance and management of treatment sequelae for years after the conclusion of active treatment. Nathan et al. report that 29% of uninsured childhood cancer survivors had not received medical care within the past 2 years in comparison with 9% of insured survivors.[47]

Cancer survivors who sustained expensive treatments may reach a lifetime cap on insurance coverage and be limited to inadequate or expensive policies due to preexisting conditions.[48] Reports from the Childhood Cancer Survivor Study indicate that cancer survivors have more difficulty obtaining insurance compared with siblings. Park et al. found that 29% of survivors had difficulty obtaining coverage compared with 3% of siblings.[49]

Private Insurance

Approximately 60% of American children are covered under employer-sponsored health plans, though the percentage covered is declining.[50,51] This reduction coincides with increasing premiums, which averaged $4704 for individuals and $12,680 for families in 2008. The reduction in coverage has been offset to a limited extent by growth in public insurance coverage but has also been associated with larger increases in the uninsurance rate.[50,51] Even among those who have retained employer-provided insurance have experienced the impact of rising premiums. Monthly employee contributions for insurance have more than doubled since 1999. In 2008, average contributions for family insurance amounted to $3354 per year.[52] The financial burden of copayments and insurance premiums was particularly profound among the working poor. Rasell et al.[53] reported that low-income families spent five times as much of their income on premiums as did high-income families.

Private insurance plans often have cost-control measures that influence the type of care subscribers receive. According to 2008 figures from the Kaiser Family Foundation Employer Health Benefits Survey, most employers offer managed care options that encourage subscribers to get their care from a predesignated list of health care providers. In particular, 41% of employers offered health maintenance organization plans, 77% offering preferred provider organization plans, and 24% offer point of service plans. The survey also revealed that 25% of employers offer high-deductible health plans with savings options. Only 8% of employers offer conventional fee-for-service plans. Private insurance plans may also place limits on the type of care covered. For example, plans may exclude coverage of therapies by care site or route of administration. These factors can influence treatment. For example, anecdotal evidence suggests that individuals with high-deductible health plans linked to a health savings account have a particularly difficult time evaluating whether their coverage is adequate and forgo preventive and routine medical appointments to avoid having to pay initial out-of-pocket costs of care.[54]

Medicaid

Approximately 25% of children younger than 18 years diagnosed with cancer are covered by Medicaid and the State Children's Health Insurance Program (SCHIP) administered by the states and the US Department of Health and Human Services.[40] In 2007, Medicaid provided insurance coverage for 13.2% of the American population, including 29 million children.[55]

More children than adults are eligible for coverage. Forty-four states provide Medicaid or SCHIP coverage for children in families with incomes at or below 200% of the federal poverty line.[55] Eligibility limits for adults are much more stringent: 33 states provide Medicaid coverage to only those adults who are below the federal poverty line.[56] Because of differences in adult and child eligibility requirements for these programs, there has been a significant increase in the proportion of families with a mixture of both public and private insurance. Vistnes and Schone[57] reported that between 1997 and 2005, the proportion of families with adults covered by private insurance and children covered by public insurance grew from 5.1% to 15.5%.

The rise in the U.S. unemployment rate that accompanied the recession that started in 2007 increased the number of people eligible for Medicaid. Between December 2007 and February 2009, the unemployment rate climbed from 4.9% to 8.1% and the demand for public coverage was commensurate with this increase. In general, for every 1% point increase in the national unemployment rate, an additional 1 million Americans seek Medicaid coverage and 1.1 million more become uninsured.[56]

State Children's Health Insurance Program

In 1997, the General Accounting Office reported a 9.6% reduction in the number of children with private insurance in the period from 1989 to 1995, nearly twofold the rate of adults younger than 65 years.[58] The growing number of uninsured children and the steady erosion of free care served as the impetus for the 1997 Children's Health Insurance Provides Security (CHIPS) Act, creating the SCHIP. The program was flexible in allowing individual states to offer coverage by broadening Medicaid, creating a separate state insurance program, or offering a hybrid of both. The initiative targeted families that earned too much to be eligible for Medicaid but too little to afford private health insurance. The initial impact of these initiatives on uninsurance rates was disappointing, with an actual increase in the number of uninsured children.[59]

By 1999, data suggest that 20% of all children did not have health insurance.[60] This increase was explained in part by a continued drop in the number of children with private insurance, particularly for those families earning less than 200% of the federal poverty level. From 2001 to 2003, as many as 9 million people lost their employer coverage, with changes in employment status and the increased cost of insurance likely responsible. As a result of loss of employer coverage, approximately 5 million children, previously covered by private insurance, were added to government programs, including Medicaid and SCHIP.[61] These programs have served as an important safety net in curbing the rate of uninsurance, particularly among children. In 2007, 11% of children were uninsured, down from 13.9% in 1997.[51,62] Adolescents have also fared well with the expansion of public insurance programs. According to estimates from the Current Population Survey, an average of 12% of adolescents were uninsured between 1999 and 2007.[63] This is down from 14.1% measured by the National Health Interview Survey in 1995.[64]

In an effort to maintain these positive trends, CHIP was reauthorized under the Children's Health Insurance Program Reauthorization Act of 2009 (CHIPRA), and allocates an additional $33 billion dollars in federal funds to cover an additional 6.5 million children under CHIP and Medicaid by 2013. The legislation included performance targets and financial incentives for states in order to maximize enrollment of eligible children.[55] Amidst hopeful outlooks, there are continued concerns that due to greater pressure on state budgets, these programs will not be able to sustain their positive impact.

Social Security Disability Insurance and Medicare

The Social Security Administration oversees two federally funded programs for the disabled. Eligibility requirements for the two programs differ. The Supplemental Security Income (SSI) program, originally enacted in 1974, assists low-income children and adults with disabilities. As of December 2007, 1.1 million children received SSI benefits, with 61.8% receiving the maximum monthly payment of $623.[65] Applicants must meet criteria for financial eligibility (income and resources) and have a disabling condition that results in "marked and severe functional limitations." The Social Security Disability Insurance (SSDI) program provides coverage for adults who are unable to work due to an extended disability (one that lasts at least 12 months or is fatal). In general, SSDI coverage requires a history of employment with payment into the Social Security system through employment taxes, although adults who became disabled before the age of 22 can qualify for coverage if at least one parent is collecting social security due to retirement or disability, or if a parent has died and worked long enough to qualify for social security.

In addition to monthly cash benefits, each program also provides access to health coverage. The mechanism of that coverage may vary from state to state. SSDI recipients automatically become eligible for Medicare after 2 years of SSDI eligibility. Further, SSDI recipients can become eligible for Medicaid in most states by "spending down" personal savings and income to meet income requirements for Medicaid.[48]

SSI recipients are eligible for Medicaid in most states. Over the past decade, the number of children on SSI has increased fourfold. Kuhlthau et al. recently reported that in a four-state study of Medicaid expenditures, Medicaid paid 2.9 to 9.4 times more for SSI recipients than for non-SSI Medicaid recipients.[66] Moreover, expenditures exceeded $10,000 per year for approximately 10% (7.2–12.4%) of SSI recipients, accounting for 63.4% to 81% of all Medicaid expenditures. In contrast, expenditures exceeded $10,000 per year among only 0.8% to 1.7% of individuals not receiving SSI, accounting for 14.4% to 28.2% of total Medicaid expenditures. Children with SSI and high expenditures were more likely to have a chronic medical condition and developmental chronic conditions than children not receiving SSI. To curb the continued rapid growth of the SSI program, the 1996 Welfare Reform Act (Personal Responsibility and Work Opportunity Act) imposed a more restrictive definition of disability. In the years 1997 through 2000, SSI enrollment of children generally declined, although enrollment increased during the years 2001 through 2006.[67]

It is difficult to predict the impact of these changes on childhood patients with cancer or survivors. In addition to restricting enrollment, both SSI and SSDI have recently developed work incentive programs to encourage disabled persons to seek employment and ultimately gain financial independence.

Issues and Solutions

Efforts to ensure adequate care of children with cancer fall into two categories. The first category includes measures to maintain insurance coverage of families in the face of possible employment loss or job change. The Consolidated Omnibus Budget and Reconciliation Act (COBRA) and the Health Insurance Portability and Accountability Act (HIPPA) statutes are examples of such legislation. The second category includes steps to provide care at substantially reduced prices, or even for free. As described later, hospitals are reducing their provision of free care.

COBRA and HIPAA

Several recent legislative efforts address insurance issues germane to children with cancer and their families. Under the Consolidated Omnibus Budget and Reconciliation Act of 1987, parents who either lose or leave their job can continue coverage with their group insurance for up to 18 months (22 months if disabled). COBRA also allows for continued coverage for up to 36 months for dependents as old as 19 years of age (or 22 years of age if they are disabled). Eligible parents are responsible for the payment of insurance premiums. This eligibility applies either until the covered period expires or new coverage is obtained.[68]

The lack of occupational mobility continues to plague patients with cancer and survivors. In a 1995 survey of patients with cancer in treatment at the M.D. Anderson Cancer Center in Houston, Texas, 58% of respondents reported that they would not leave their current (employment) position due to the health insurance. The proportion that were "job locked" ranged from 40% of those employed by small firms to 88% of respondents employed by large firms.[69] Further, insurance coverage is becoming more difficult to maintain. In a recent analysis of Survey of Income and Program Participation data, Cutler et al. reported that children younger than 18 years had a higher probability of losing insurance coverage during a 12-month period between 2001 and 2004 than during a corresponding period between 1983 and 1986.[70] Three quarters of employees eligible for employee-based insurance face a waiting period before coverage is available.[52]

The Health Insurance Portability and Accountability Act of 1996 (HIPAA) was designed to decrease the impact of preexisting health conditions on health insurance coverage during changes in employment. The major features of HIPAA include (a) restriction of the waiting period for the previously uninsured to 12 months based on preexisting conditions and (b) elimination of the waiting period for those who had previously been insured (with paid-up premiums). These requirements minimize the impact of job changes and help to address the problem of job lock. It is important to note that the law does not prevent companies from raising the cost of premiums or leaving smaller markets completely.[58] Ongoing evaluation of the impact of this law is imperative.

Charity Care/Uncompensated Care

Historically, faced with an inability to pay for health care, the uninsured or underinsured patients have either postponed care, sought alternative venues to obtain care that often turn out to be more expensive (e.g., emergency departments),[71] or turned to charity (uncompensated) care. Resources expended on uncompensated care more than doubled between the mid-1980s and the mid-1990s.[72] However, with increased enrollment in public programs such as Medicaid and CHIP, the provision of uncompensated care has decreased. Reduced provision of these services leaves the medically indigent without access to care. Conversely, given other fiscal changes, the provision of uncompensated care has a dramatic impact on the institutions attempting to deliver it. Recent legislative efforts have sought to expand free care programs based on the premise that hospitals should "earn" their nonprofit status by providing such care. Hospital advocacy organizations contend that an expanded provision of free care is not warranted, however, because demand for free care is decreasing and hospitals provide benefits to their communities in other ways.[73]

Health Reform Initiatives

State and national health reform efforts offer further opportunities to increase insurance enrollment and improve access to care. In April 2006, Massachusetts enacted the Health Care Access and Affordability Act. The act created a quasi-government agency that provides low-cost alternatives to COBRA and includes a low-cost individual plan targeting young adults aged 19 to 26 who cannot obtain employer-based coverage.[74] The law also includes individual and employer mandates, obligating Massachusetts residents older than 18 years to have health insurance and requiring firms with 11 or more full-time employees to contribute to insurance premiums.[75] Though the program is still too new for systematic analysis, mixed review abound. Proponents highlight the results from the 2008 Massachusetts Health Insurance Survey indicating that the rate of being uninsured for all residents had dropped to 2.6% and the uninsurance rate for children dropped to 1.2%.[38] Critics of the reform question the sustainability of funding and fear that these new insurance products do not provide comprehensive coverage. Further, recent analysis suggests that rising health care costs in Massachusetts have made health care less affordable since the implementation of the 2006 legislation.[76] Notwithstanding these challenges, federal lawmakers are considering the feasibility of replicating elements of the Massachusetts program on a national scale.

FAMILY IMPACT

Even if families maintain their insurance coverage, they must still contend with numerous burdens not addressed by insurance. First, they must make out-of-pocket payments for both medical and nonmedical costs. Second, due to the burden of caring for a child with cancer, patient family members sometimes cut back on work hours or take other steps that result in lower take home pay. Third, family members end up devoting substantial time and effort to the care of the child diagnosed with cancer. Finally, over the long term, childhood survivors of cancer face more obstacles to securing and maintaining employment.

Out-of-Pocket Expenses

Adequate health insurance, although vitally important, does not offer patients and their families full protection from high health care costs. Families are subject to significant out-of-pocket expenses related to their medical care. These expenses are classified as medical or nonmedical costs. Out-of-pocket (OOP) medical costs are those associated with the provision of medical services (e.g., copayments for medication, procedures or diagnostic assessments, insurance premiums, and fees for professional services),[77] while costs associated with accommodations needed to seek care (e.g., transportation, alternate child care, changes in job) are referred to as nonmedical expenses.

A 2007 telephone survey of 18,000 Americans found that one in five had trouble paying medical bills and of those respondents who reported difficulty, more than 40% had OOP expenses exceeding $1000 in the past year.[78] Banthin et al. analyzed data from the Medical Expenditure Panel Survey (MEPS) between 2001 and 2004 and found that the increase in families' financial burden was being encountered entirely by people with private health insurance.[79]

It is difficult to precisely estimate the nonmedical financial burden of cancer on families. Some OOP expenditures individually may seem trivial, particularly compared with the burden of dealing with the disease itself. The full impact of such costs, however, can be substantial when aggregated, and in the extent to which they exceed usual household expenditures. Many families may not recognize that they have already made accommodations (job change, reduction of hours), highlighting the need to compare their work status and income with the premorbid state. For example, if one of the parents is already not working, there may be no additional childcare expenses because the accommodation has already occurred.

Several researchers have developed cost diaries to be completed by patients and their families regarding OOP (direct nonmedical costs) and lost wages. A 1979 landmark study of the pediatric oncology population by Lansky et al.,[80] collected cost information from 70 families of children with cancer. These data revealed that because of nonmedical expenses and a cut in take home income, more than half of the families effectively experienced a loss of more than 25% of their income.[80] Factors influencing cost included level of care, the patient's performance status, distance from the treatment center, and family size. In a follow-up study in 1983, Lansky et al.[81] demonstrated that costs varied by treatment phase with the diagnostic (early) and terminal phases of illness involving the greatest expenses. More recently, Barr et al.[82] used prospective cost diaries to demonstrate that family-borne costs represented at least one-third of the average family's after-tax income during the treatment of three pediatric malignancies—acute lymphoblastic leukemia, neuroblastoma, and Wilms tumor. These findings are noteworthy. First, families bear substantial costs despite first-dollar and universal coverage in the Canadian system. Second, the level of expenditure among study participants is nearly tenfold greater than the estimated 2% of after-tax income spent by the general population on health care, and approaches what is typically spent on food and transportation or shelter. Equally important is the likelihood that this result understates true costs because it does not account for relapses.[82] A 2006 survey of U.K. families caring for children undergoing outpatient cancer treatment found that 55% of the 145 families surveyed spent £50 to 100 more per week on health care than they did before their child became ill.[83]

In a study of adults receiving outpatient chemotherapy, Houts et al.,[84] reported that 28% of patients spent more than 25% of their weekly income on health care; 14% spent more than 50%. These data, based on a modification of the Birenbaum cost diary, also revealed the regressive nature of OOP expenses, as the lowest income groups incurred the same financial burdens as higher income patients.[84] The following year, Houts et al.[85]

identified three risk factors for financial burden related to cancer care: age less than 65 years, income below $20,000, and inpatient stay exceeding 2 days over the previous 6 months. Among patients with cancer with all the three risk factors, 20% of the sample spent more than half of their income on cancer and its treatment. This result compared with none of those without any of these risk factors spending more than 10% of income on health care. The regressive nature of OOP expenditures was also noted in the 1987 National Medical Expenditure Survey,[53,86] the Rand Health Insurance Experiment,[87] and the most recent results of the 2006 MEPS survey.[88]

The results of the 1987 National Medical Expenditure Survey indicated that among the nonelderly, OOP expenditures accounted for 21% of total health care expenditures. For low-income families, these OOP expenditures represented a 6.6-fold greater burden (as a share of income) than they did among higher income families.[53] Dicker and Sunshine[86] reported that 27% of older families and 20% of younger, lower income families had total OOP expenses for health of at least 10% of their income; for younger, better off families, the corresponding figure was 4%.[86] The 1999 and 2000 MEPS survey results for lower income families of children with disabilities showed that these families incurred a greater fiscal burden than higher income families of children with disabilities. In particular, lower income families were 19 times more likely than higher income families to have OOP expenditures exceeding 5% of the family's income.[89]

Increased OOP expenditures for health care have pernicious effects not only for these families but also for the larger society. First, health care expenditures at this level may leave families without sufficient resources to acquire other needed services. Second, inadequate use of health care may increase costs incurred when care is ultimately sought because delays can allow disease to progress and the comorbid conditions to develop.

Lost Income

Because of the time needed to care for a child with cancer, family members often experience a depletion of banked paid time off from work (e.g., sick time and vacation time) or reduced take home pay because they cut back their regular and overtime hours at work. For example, Barr et al.[82] found that 39% of families reported losing half a day per week of paid employment for the duration of the child's treatment. Mothers were more likely than fathers to lose time from work, refuse promotions, or agree to relocate. Houts et al.[84] estimated that lost wages accounted for 55% of the nonmedical costs of outpatient chemotherapy. In a survey of U.K. parents, Eiser[83] found that 34.7% of working mothers gave up all paid employment after their child was diagnosed with cancer. Only 1.7% of working fathers gave up all paid employment after diagnosis, but 37.3% had reduced their hours.

The Study to Understand Prognoses and Preferences for Outcomes and Risks of Treatments (SUPPORT) of seriously ill hospitalized adults reported that 31% of families lost most or all of their savings, particularly those with younger, poorer, or more functionally dependent patients.[90] In addition, 29% of the respondents (n 52,123) lost a major source of income.[91] Similarly, care in the terminal phases of illness has been shown to result in exodus from the labor force as well as more lost time from work among those who remain employed.[90] This appears to be especially true among lower income families that may not be able to afford alternative care arrangements.[92]

Efforts to reduce costs to the health care system by treating children with cancer in an outpatient setting have shifted some costs to families. In a study of children with cancer receiving terminal care at home, Birenbaum and Clarke-Steffen[93] demonstrated that although overall costs are lower when the child is cared for at home, direct nonmedical and indirect costs are higher. Moreover, this study estimated that 12% to 24% of the costs of care were borne by the family.[93] The authors caution that the ability to pay the additional costs may influence the site of terminal care. Most of the existing cost analyses focus on patients in the active phases of treatment. Less clear are the economic consequences of care over time—specifically, the services being delivered and in which settings over the disease trajectory and the duration of survival.

Cost of Informal Caregiving

Although the determination of OOP nonmedical expenses and lost wages poses methodologic challenges, it pales in comparison to the estimation of the cost or value of informal caregiving, generally provided by patients' families. This type of care is uncompensated (in monetary terms) and thus lies outside of the market economy.[94] In a 2007 AARP issue brief, Gibson and Houser estimated that the economic value of informal caregiving for adults approaches $350 billion per year.[95] Although estimation of informal care costs for pediatric conditions in general, or for pediatric oncology in particular is uncertain at best, it should be noted that parental caregiving for children with chronic diseases is extensive. In the 1997 National Caregiver Survey, 19% of the 817 survey respondents were parents providing care for children, 64% of whom were younger than 20 years. One in three of these caregivers indicated that providing care resulted in financial burdens for his or her family.[96] Parents caring for children were reported to provide the highest level of care based on hours of care per week and the type of care (related to activities of daily living). In the aggregate, more than 60% of caregivers provided more than 40 hours per week of caregiving. Although 47% of the total sample was employed, 71% of the employed reported working more than 30 hours per week in addition to their caregiving activity.[96] Recent updates to the national caregiver survey only include data for care recipients older than 18 years.

Several studies that have evaluated caregiver impacts have reported that this group experiences a decline in physical health and emotional well-being.[97-99] The implications of program initiatives shifting care away from institutional-based care to home-based care must include a careful analysis of the true cost—financial and human—of informal caregiving. In addition, the impact of federal cutbacks to paid home health care on informal caregiving must be carefully assessed. The Congressional Budget Office estimated that between 1998 and 2002, upward of $69 billion was taken away from home health care.[100] These cutbacks stemmed from concerns about corruption and excessive payment among home care providers. The economic downturn that started at the end of 2007 made it more difficult for family caregivers to balance care provision with their own financial needs.[101] Health reform proposals advocate for an expansion of home health care services as a cost saving measure.[102]

Special Considerations for Childhood Cancer Survivors

Several studies have demonstrated higher rates of unemployment among survivors of childhood cancer.[103,104] For example, a meta-analysis of 177,969 participants revealed that cancer survivors are 1.37 times more likely to be unemployed than control participants. Job discrimination was cited as a major factor for unemployment.[105] Without employment, cancer survivors lack access to employer-based insurance coverage. In addition, cancer survivors are less likely than gender-matched siblings to be accepted into the armed forces.[106,107] Younger survivors also report differential levels of educational attainment and employment opportunities than controls.[107,108]

Because younger survivors were not in the work force before their diagnosis, they may require specially tailored programs such as educational and vocational training in contrast to rehabilitation and retraining for older survivors. In-depth research is needed to characterize more fully the barriers to employment for childhood cancer survivors.

The Americans with Disabilities Act of 1990 helps to protect childhood cancer survivors against selected types of job discrimination, provided that the "essential functions" of the job can be performed. Employees requiring additional time to complete the job functions are also allowed "reasonable accommodation" under the law. In addition, employers cannot ask prospective applicants about their cancer history.[68] The law also prevents discrimination with respect to offered employee benefits.

Despite these safeguards, patients with cancer and survivors continue to face cancer-based discrimination, though recent analysis suggests progress is being made.[109] More contemporary and more complete information is needed to evaluate the impact of recent legislation, entitlement programs, and vocational programs on equalizing opportunities for patients with cancer and survivors.[110] This information is crucial, particularly within the context of the growing numbers of young adults who are uninsured.

CONCLUSION

Pediatric cancer confronts the health care system with a formidable challenge. Cancer is a particularly dreaded disease, and children are among the most vulnerable members of society. Moreover, preventing childhood cancer deaths can extend lives by many decades. Nonetheless, addressing cancer is expensive because it involves the use of sophisticated diagnostic tools and new medications. Rising health care costs associated with new technologies threaten the financial viability of a health care system already struggling to deal with the growing number of older Americans. The unreimbursed costs associated with care also place the families of childhood patients with cancer in financial peril.

The finite nature of the resources available to address pediatric cancer necessitates the use of economic evaluation tools to help us identify those that provide benefits sufficiently large to justify their costs. Which tool is most appropriate depends on the questions that are asked, and in particular on the contemplated alternative uses for the resources. A narrow question might ask which of two diagnostic technologies for a particular form of childhood cancer represents the best

opportunity to invest health care resources. In that case, cost-effectiveness analysis is a useful tool because it can characterize the value of each technology in terms of its cost per case correctly diagnosed. A somewhat broader question might ask whether a medication to treat a particular childhood cancer represents good value compared with other potential health care investments, such as investments to reduce the risk of diabetes. In that case, cost-utility analysis can be used to compare interventions in terms of cost per QALY, a common metric that accounts for both life expectancy and quality of life impacts. Finally, cost-benefit analysis can be used to compare a medical intervention to uses of resources outside the health care sector. For example, resources expended on health care cannot be devoted to other worthwhile priorities, like education and housing. Ultimately, the trade-offs between technologies to address pediatric cancer, or between treatment of different diseases, or between health care and other societal priorities cannot be avoided. The tools described in this chapter will not "make the decision" between competing priorities, but they can help us understand what we give up and what we gain by making one choice over another.

Once worthwhile interventions are identified, adequate means of financing must be secured. The means currently available have substantial limitations. Evidence suggests that public insurance coverage does not confer the same health benefits as private coverage. Even in cases where children have desirable private insurance coverage, families struggle with OOP expenses not reimbursed by their policies. The substantial time required to care for a child with cancer can substantially reduce a family's take home wages. On top of the lost income, families must contend with the burden associated with actually providing care not provided by paid professionals. Finally, survivors of childhood cancer must confront less optimistic prospects for employment, which in turn limits their access to health insurance critical to their being able to manage the sequelae of their original disease.

Beyond the clinical discoveries and expert care that is necessary to fight pediatric cancer, successfully negotiating its economic challenges depends on two requirements. First, our society must be willing to make the hard choices to identify those interventions that do provide good value and those for which the benefits do not warrant the costs. Second, we must identify and remediate the means we have for paying for the interventions that we do identify as worthwhile. Taking on these issues is complex in the context of any population dealing with any serious condition. For the pediatric oncologist, without formal training in this area, thinking about these issues will not come naturally. Moreover, when faced with the urgency of the child's clinical needs, it is particularly challenging to weigh economic factors in clinical decision making. It will therefore be critical for society to confront these issues explicitly so that the physician and family are afforded the greatest support possible.

References

1. Population Division, U.S. Census Bureau. Projections of the population by selected age groups and sex for the United States: 2010 to 2050 (NP-2008-T2). http://www.census.gov/population/www/projections/summarytables.html. Accessed June 22, 2010.
2. Sisko A, Truffer C, Smith S, et al. Health spending projections through 2018: recession effects add uncertainty to the outlook. Health Aff 2009;28(2):w346–w357.
3. Smith BD, Smith GL, Hurria A, et al. Future of cancer incidence in the United States: burdens upon an aging, changing nation. J Clin Oncol 2009;27(17):2758–2765.
4. American Cancer Society. Cancer facts and figures 2009. Atlanta, GA: American Cancer Society, 2009.
5. Bach PB. Limits on medicare's ability to control rising spending on cancer drugs. N Engl J Med 2009;360(6):626.
6. Neumann PJ. Using cost-effectiveness analysis to improve health care: opportunities and barriers. Oxford, UK: Oxford University Press, 2005.
7. Neumann PJ. American exceptionalism and American health care: implications for the US debate on cost-effectiveness analysis. Office of Health Economics OHE Briefing 47, 2009.
8. NPR, Kaiser Family Foundation, and Harvard School of Public Health. The Public and the Health Care Delivery System. http://www.kff.org/kaiserpolls/7888.cfm. Accessed June 22, 2010.
9. Neumann PJ, Palmer JA, Nadler E, et al. Cancer therapy costs influence treatment: a national survey of oncologists. Health Aff 2010;29(1):196–202.
10. Hillner BE, Smith TJ. Efficacy does not necessarily translate to cost effectiveness: a case study in the challenges associated with 21st-Century cancer drug pricing. J Clin Oncol 2009;27(13):2111.
11. McFarlane J, Riggins J, Smith TJ. SPIKE$: a six-step protocol for delivering bad news about the cost of medical care. J Clin Oncol 2008;26(25):4200–4204.

12. Schnipper LE. Discussing the Cost of Care with Patients with Cancer: What Can We Tell Them? What is the Goal? In: Presentation at the Education Session, Geriatric Oncology track at 45th Annual Meeting of the American Society of Clinical Oncology; Orlando, Florida, 2009.
13. Drummond M, Stoddart G, Labelle R, et al. Health economics: An introduction for clinicians. Ann Intern Med 1987;107(1):88–92.
14. Drummond MF, Sculpher MJ, Torrance GW, et al. Methods for the economic evaluation of health care programmes: Third Edition. New York: Oxford University Press, 2005.
15. Drummond MF, O'Brien B, Stoddart GL, et al. Methods for the economic evaluation of health care programmes. Oxford, UK: Oxford University Press, 1997.
16. Green DM, Breslow NE, Beckwith B, et al. Effect of duration of treatment on treatment outcome and cost of treatment for Wilms' tumor: a report from the national Wilms' tumor study group. J Clin Oncol 1998;16(12):3744–3751.
17. Bennett CL, Stinson TJ, Lande D, et al. Cost analysis of filgrastim for the prevention of neutropenia in pediatric T-cell leukemia and advanced lymphoblastic lymphoma: a case for prospective economic analysis in cooperative group trials. Med Pediatr Oncol 2000;34(2):92–96.
18. Lipscomb J, Weinstein MC, Torrance GW. Time preference. In: Gold M, Siegel J, Russell L, et al., eds. Cost-effectiveness in health and medicine. New York: Oxford University Press, 1996:213.
19. Bennett CL, Armitage JL, LeSage S, et al. Economic analyses of clinical trials in cancer: are they helpful to policy makers? Stem Cells 1994;12(1):424–429.
20. Kievit W, de Bruin JH, Adang EM, et al. Cost effectiveness of a new strategy to identify HNPCC patients. Gut 2005;54(1):97–102.
21. Nelson AL, Cohen JT, Greenberg D, Kent DM. Much cheaper, almost as good: decrementally cost-effective medical innovation. Ann Intern Med 2009;151(9):662–667.
22. Grosse SD. Assessing cost-effectiveness in healthcare: history of the $50,000 per QALY threshold. Expert Rev Pharmacoecon Outcomes Res 2008;8(2):165–178.
23. Braithwaite RS, Meltzer DO, King JT Jr, Leslie D, Roberts MS. What does the value of modern medicine say about the $50,000 per quality-adjusted life-year decision rule? Med Care 2008;46(4):343–345.
24. Weinstein MC, Fineberg HV, Elstein AS, et al. Clinical decision analysis. Philadelphia, PA: Saunders, 1980.
25. Gilmore A, Milne R. Methylphenidate in children with hyperactivity: review and cost-utility analysis. Pharmacoepidemiol Drug Saf 2001;10(2):85–94.
26. Rowley PT, Loader S, Kaplan RM. Prenatal screening for cystic fibrosis carriers: an economic evaluation. Am J Hum Genet 1998;63(4):1160–1174.
27. Bell CM, Chapman RH, Stone PW, et al. An off-the-shelf help list: a comprehensive catalog of preference scores from published cost-utility analyses. Med Decis Making 2001; 21(4):288–294.
28. Ladapo JA, Neumann PJ, Keren R, et al. Valuing children's health: a comparison of cost-utility analyses for adult and paediatric health interventions in the US. Pharmacoeconomics 2007;25(10):817–828.
29. Feeny DH, Furlong W, Barr RD, et al. A comprehensive multiattribute system for classifying the health status of survivors of childhood cancer. J Clin Oncol 1992;10(6): 923–928.
30. Feeny D, Furlong W, Saigal S, et al. Comparing directly measured standard gamble scores to HUI2 and HUI3 utility scores: group- and individual-level comparisons. Soc Sci Med 2004;58(4):799–809.
31. Chapman RH, Berger M, Weinstein MC, et al. When does quality-adjusting life-years matter in cost-effectiveness analysis? Health Econ 2004;13(5):429–436.
32. Greenberg D, Earle C, Fang CH, et al. When is cancer care cost-effective? A systematic overview of cost-utility analyses in oncology. J Natl Cancer Inst 2010;102(2):82–88.
33. Zbrozek AS, Cantor SB, Cardenas MP, et al. Pharmacoeconomic analysis of ondansetron versus metoclopramide for cisplatin-induced nausea and vomiting. Am J Hosp Pharm 1994;51(12):1555–1563.
34. Lundkvist J, Ekman M, Ericsson S, et al. Cost-effectiveness of proton radiation in the treatment of childhood medulloblastoma. Cancer 2005;103(4):793–801.
35. Medina LS, Kuntz KM, Pomeroy S. Children with headache suspected of having a brain tumor: a cost-effectiveness analysis of diagnostic strategies. Pediatrics 2001;108(2): 255–263.
36. Goldie SJ, Kohli M, Grima D, et al. Projected clinical benefits and cost-effectiveness of a human papillomavirus 16/18 vaccine. J Natl Cancer Inst 2004;96(8):604–615.
37. Institute of Medicine of the National Academies. Beyond ratios: Ethical and nonquantifiable aspects of regulatory decisions. In: Miller W, Robinson L, Lawrence R, eds. Valuing health for regulatory cost-effectiveness analysis. Washington, D.C.: The National Academies Press, 2006.
38. Office of Information and Regulatory Affairs, US Office of Management and Budget. Advance notice of proposed rulemaking, extension of comment period and release of contegnet valuation methodology report. Fed Regist 1993;58(10):4602–4614.
39. Green M, Waitzman N. Cost analysis needs analyzing. New York: The New York Times, Feb 8, 1981.
40. American Cancer Society. Cancer facts and figures 2008. Atlanta, GA: American Cancer Society, 2008.
41. Martin S, Ulrich C, Munsell M, et al. Delays in cancer diagnosis in underinsured young adults and older adolescents. Oncologist 2007;12(7):816.
42. Halpern MT, Ward EM, Pavluck AL, et al. Association of insurance status and ethnicity with cancer stage at diagnosis for 12 cancer sites: a retrospective analysis. Lancet Oncol 2008;9(3):222–231.
43. Harlan LC, Greene AL, Clegg LX, et al. Insurance status and the use of guideline therapy in the treatment of selected cancers. J Clin Oncol 2005;23(36):9079.
44. Bach PB. Using practice guidelines to assess cancer care quality. J Clin Oncol 2005; 23(36):9041.
45. Virnig BA. Associating insurance status with cancer stage at diagnosis. Lancet Oncol 2008;9(3):189–191.
46. Liu J. Childhood survivors: cost of long term medical, rehabilitative, psychologic and social needs. Cancer 1993;71:3351–3353.
47. Nathan PC, Ford JS, Henderson TO, et al. Health behaviors, medical care, and interventions to promote healthy living in the Childhood Cancer Survivor Study cohort. J Clin Oncol 2009;27(14):2363–2373.
48. Schwartz K, Claxton G, Martin K, et al; Kaiser Family Foundation and American Cancer Society. Spending to survive: cancer patients confront holes in the health insurance system. 7851. Kaiser Family Foundation. http://www.kff.org/insurance/7851.cfm. Accessed June 22, 2010.
49. Park ER, Li FP, Liu Y, et al; and Childhood Cancer, Survivor Study. Health insurance coverage in survivors of childhood cancer: the Childhood Cancer Survivor Study. J Clin Oncol 2005;23(36):9187–9197.
50. Holahan J, Cook A. Changes in economic conditions and health insurance coverage, 2000–2004. Health Aff 2005;24(1):489–508.
51. DeNavas-Walt C, Proctor BD, Smith JC. Income, poverty, and health insurance coverage in the United States: 2007. Washington, DC: U.S. Government Printing Office, 2007.
52. The Henry J. Kaiser Family Foundation. Employer health benefits, 2008 summary of findings. http://ehbs.kff.org/images/abstract/7791.pdf. Accessed June 22, 2010.
53. Rasell E, Bernstein J, Tang K. The impact of health care financing on family budgets. Int J Health Serv 1994;24(4):691–714.
54. Konrad W. Health insurance with high deductibles isn't always a bargain. The New York Times May 30, 2009: B6.
55. Kaiser Commission on Medicaid and the Uninsured. Children's health insurance program reauthorization act of 2009 (CHIPRA) fact sheet. Washington DC: Kaiser Family Foundation, 2009.
56. Rowland, D. Health care and medicaid—weathering the recession. N Engl J Med 2009; 360(13):1273.
57. Vistnes JP, Schone BS. Pathways to coverage: the changing roles of public and private sources. Health Aff 2008;27(1):44–57.
58. Smith BM. Trends in health care coverage and financing and their implications for policy. N Engl J Med 1997;337(14):1000–1003.
59. Cunningham PJ. SCHIP making progress: increased take-up contributes to coverage gains. Health Aff (Millwood) 2003;22(4):163–172.
60. Cunningham PJ, Park MH. Recent trends in children's health insurance coverage: no gains for low-income children. Issue Brief Cent Stud Health Syst Change 2000;29(1): 1–6.
61. Strunk BC, Reschovsky JD. Trends in U.S. health insurance coverage, 2001–2003. Track Rep 2004;(9):1–5.
62. Cohen R, Hao C, Coriaty-Nelson Z. Health insurance coverage: estimates from the National Health Interview Survey, January–June 2004. Centers for disease control and prevention, http://www.cdc.gov/nchs/data/nhis/earlyrelease/insur200412.pdf. Accessed June 22, 2010.
63. Table HIA-6. Health insurance coverage status and type of coverage by state—persons under 65: 1999 to 2008. U.S. census bureau, current population survey, annual social and economic supplements. http://www.census.gov/hhes/www/hlthins/data/historical/files/hihistt6.xls. Accessed June 22, 2010.
64. Newacheck PW, Park MJ, Brindis CD, et al. Trends in private and public health insurance for adolescents. JAMA 2004;291(10):1231–1237.
65. Social Security Administration. SSI annual statistical report, 2007. http://www.socialsecurity.gov/policy/docs/statcomps/ssi_asr/#contact. Accessed June 22, 2010.
66. Kuhlthau K, Perrin JM, Ettner SL, et al. High-expenditure children with Supplemental Security Income. Pediatrics 1998;102(3 Pt 1):610–615.
67. U.S. Department of Health and Human Services. 2008 Indicators of Welfare Dependence. Appendix A: Program Data. http://aspe.hhs.gov/hsp/indicators08/apa.shtml#Supplemental. Accessed June 22, 2010.
68. Hoffman B. Cancer survivors' employment and insurance rights: a primer for oncologists. Oncology 1999;13(6):841–852.
69. Rothstein MA, Kennedy K, Ritchie KJ, et al. Are cancer patients subject to employment discrimination? Oncology 1995;9(12):1303–1306.
70. Cutler DM, Gelber AM. Changes in the incidence and duration of periods without insurance. N Engl J Med 2009;360(17):1740–1748.
71. Ziv A, Boulet JR, Slap GB. Emergency department utilization by adolescents in the United States. Pediatrics 1998;101(6):987–994.
72. Weissman J. Uncompensated hospital care: Will it be there if we need it? JAMA 1996; 276(10):823–828.
73. Pear R. Hospitals mobilizing to fight proposed charity care rules. The New York Times. June 1, 2009: A12.
74. Massachusetts Health Connector. http://www.mahealthconnector.org/portal/site/connector. Accessed June 22, 2010.
75. Hart MA. Massachusetts: expanding access to care: the health care access and affordability act. Am J Nurs 2006;106(10):38.
76. Long SK, Masi PB. Access and affordability: an update on health reform in Massachusetts, Fall 2008. Health Aff (Millwood) 2009;28:w578–w587.
77. Kim P. Cost of cancer care: the patient perspective. J Clin Oncol 2007;25(2):228.
78. Cunningham P, Miller C, Cassil A. Living on the edge. Center for Studying Health System Change, Research Brief # 10. http://www.hschange.com/CONTENT/1034/#ib1. Accessed June 22, 2010.
79. Banthin JS, Cunningham P, Bernard DM. Financial burden of health care, 2001–2004. Health Aff 2008;27(1):188–195.
80. Lansky SB, Cairns NU, Clark GM, et al. Childhood cancer: nonmedical costs of the illness. Cancer 1979;43(1):403–408.
81. Lansky SB, Black JL, Cairns NU. Childhood cancer: medical costs. Cancer 1983;52(4): 762–766.
82. Barr R, Furlong W, Henwood J, et al. Economic evaluation of allogeneic bone marrow transplantation: a rudimentary model to generate estimates for the timely formulation of clinical policy. J Clin Oncol 1996;14(5):1413–1420.
83. Eiser C, Upton P. Costs of caring for a child with cancer: a questionnaire survey. Child Care Health Dev 2007;33(4):455.
84. Houts PS, Lipton A, Harvey HA, et al. Nonmedical costs to patients and their families associated with outpatient chemotherapy. Cancer 1984;53(1):2388–2392.
85. Houts PS, Harvey HA, Simmonds MA, et al. Characteristics of patients at risk for financial burden because of cancer and its treatment. J Psychosoc Oncol 1985;3(2): 15–22.
86. Dicker, M, Sunshine JH. Determinants of financially burdensome family health expenses: United States, 1980. Natl Med Care Util Expend Surv C 1988;1–66.
87. Grumbach K, Bodenheimer T. Mechanisms for controlling costs. JAMA 1995;273(15): 1223–1230.
88. Bernard D, Banthin J. Family level expenditures on health care and insurance premiums among the nonelderly population, 2006. Research Findings No. 29. Rockville, MD: Agency for Healthcare Research and Quality, 2009.
89. Newacheck PW, Inkelas M, Kim SE. Health services use and health care expenditures for children with disabilities. Pediatrics 2004;114(1):79–85.
90. Connors AF, Dawson NV, Desbiens N, et al. A controlled trial to improve care for seriously ill hospitalized patients. The study to understand prognoses and preferences for outcomes and risks of treatments (SUPPORT). The SUPPORT Principal Investigators. JAMA 1995;274(20):1591–1598.
91. Covinsky KE, Goldman L, Cook EF, et al. The impact of serious illness on patients' families. SUPPORT Investigators. Study to Understand Prognoses and Preferences for Outcomes and Risks of Treatment. JAMA 1994;272(23):1839–1844.

92. Muurinen JM. The economics of informal care. Labor market effects in the National Hospice Study. Med Care 1986;24(11):1007–1017.

93. Birenbaum LK, Clarke-Steffen L. Terminal care costs in childhood cancer. Pediatr Nurs 1992;18(3):258.

94. Arno PS, Levine C, Memmott MM. The economic value of informal caregiving. Health Aff (Millwood) 1999;18(2):182–188.

95. Gibson MJ, Houser A. AARP Issue brief. Valuing the invaluable: a new look at the economic value of family caregiving. Washington, DC: American Association of Retired Persons, 2007.

96. National Family Caregivers Association and Fortis, Inc., Family caregiving demands recognition: caregiving across the lifecycle. Final report. Milwaukee, WI, 1998.

97. Jensen S, Given B. Fatigue affecting family caregivers of cancer patients. Support Care Cancer 1993;1(1):321–325.

98. Patterson JM, Leonard BJ, Titus JC. Home care for medically fragile children: impact on family health and well-being. J Dev Behav Pediatr 1992;13(4):248–255.

99. Schulz R, Beach SR. Caregiving as a risk factor for mortality: the caregiver health effects study. JAMA 1999;282(23):2215–2219.

100. Oliphant T. Saving home health care. The Boston Globe 2000. 3 Jul 2000: A13.

101. National Alliance for Caregiving. Evercare®/National Alliance for Caregiving survey of the economic downturn and its impact on family caregiving. Report of findings. April 28, 2009. Evercare and National Alliance for Caregiving, http://www.caregiving.org/data/EVC_Caregivers_Economy_Report%20FINAL_4-28-09.pdf. Accessed on June 22, 2010.

102. Stolberg S, Pear R. Democratic senators set to visit White House to discuss health care overhaul. The New York Times 2009. June 2, 2009: A14.

103. Meadows AT, McKee L, Kazak AE. Psychosocial status of young adult survivors of childhood cancer: a survey. Med Pediatr Oncol 1989;17(6):466–470.

104. Green DM, Zevon MA, Hall B. Achievement of life goals by adult survivors of modern treatment for childhood cancer. Cancer 1990;67(1):206–213.

105. de Boer AG, Taskila T, Ojajarvi A, et al. Cancer survivors and unemployment: a meta-analysis and meta-regression. JAMA 2009;301(7):753.

106. Monaco GP. Socioeconomic considerations in childhood cancer survival. Am J Pediatr Hematol Oncol 1987;9(1):92–98.

107. Hays DM, Landsverk J, Sallan SE, et al. Educational, occupational, and insurance status of childhood cancer survivors in their fourth and fifth decades of life. J Clin Oncol 1992;10(9):1397–1406.

108. Hays DM. Adult survivors of childhood cancer. Employment and insurance issues in different age groups. Cancer 1993;71(Suppl 10):3306–3309.

109. Hoffman B. Cancer survivors at work: a generation of progress. CA Cancer J Clin 2005;55(5):271–280.

110. Monaco GP, Smith G, Fiduccia D. The Rothstein et al article reviewed. Oncology 1995;9(1):1311–1312.

CHAPTER 51 ■ PEDIATRIC CANCER: ADVOCACY, INSURANCE, EDUCATION, AND EMPLOYMENT

SUSAN L. WEINER, GILBERT P. SMITH, GRACE P. MONACO, AND JOSEPH FAY

When you have the opportunity to join with other organizations and feel the collective power derived from uniting around a common goal, you become an advocate. When you observe a gap in services and recognize an opportunity for growth, you become an advocate.[1]

Each new family encountering a diagnosis of childhood cancer faces the challenge of how and what they are able do about these events. When the shock of diagnosis thrusts families into a new universe, advocacy begins with negotiating their individual child's treatment with a medical care team (MCT). These experiences of pediatric oncology care are the foundation from which program and policy ideas are generated to improve care and treatment.

This chapter on advocacy for oncology professionals is an analysis and update of some of the activities in which nonscientist advocates and health care professionals have partnered to improve the treatment, care, and well-being of children with cancer. It can serve to inform those interested in how, why, and where families act as resources to advance the pediatric oncology enterprise. Part I describes key priorities in childhood cancer policy and advocacy, including research funding, drug development, ethics, and health care reform. Part II offers resources and strategies for health care professionals to help individual families and survivors advocate for better access to health insurance, medical care, and support services for families, children in treatment, and long-term survivors.

I. CHILDHOOD CANCER ADVOCACY PRIORITIES

Each family has its cancer story—a set of experiences forming the basis of what for many becomes a continuing effort to improve not just their child's but often to go further to change similar experiences for other children and families. Cancer advocacy is defined here as an interaction: of the actions that families and survivors take to improve their own care and of the policies and practices that have an impact on childhood cancer experiences.

The continuum of personal, community, and national advocacy[2] depends for its validity on a feedback loop to the point of service delivery. Cancer advocacy had origins in the self-help movements of the 1970s that have grown into national action-oriented cancer advocacy organizations and coalitions.[2,3] The cancer community shares a core consensus: increased research funding, care that is based on the best scientific evidence, and health insurance that is accessible without discrimination based on condition, genetic background, age or cost.

Priorities for childhood cancer advocacy arise in part through working with adult oncology advocates. Collaboration among groups with common interests increases the impact of the smaller pediatric population and amplifies understanding about children's issues. Advocates necessarily must be both proactive and reactive to political and legislative events to have an impact on behalf of children. The political influence of well-placed individuals and the considerable fundraising capability of a few are also key factors. However, research and policy analysis can and should be the foundations for responsible advocacy. The priorities discussed later exemplify these influences on national childhood cancer policy priorities.

A. Advocacy for Research on Treatment

For families and friends of children with cancer, raising private money is a most satisfying advocacy activity. It gives people control in circumstances where there is little they can do to change events. It can give immediate feedback; it can bond a community; and it engenders hope that people have helped find treatments hopefully to cure children.

In the first decade of this century, the National Institutes of Health (NIH) budget, including that of the National Cancer Institute (NCI), flattened, effecting a research funding reduction, after a period of doubling in the 1990s. Cancer advocates reacted vigorously to this funding drought, pressuring Congress to act and articulating the implications of the decline in research funds, including on pediatric oncology clinical trials.

Coincident with the decline in funding, several large advocate-founded research fundraising organizations emerged, including St. Baldrick's Foundation,[4] Alex's Lemonade Stand Foundation,[5] and Hope Street Kids.[6] In 2008, for example, Alex's Lemonade Stand Foundation and St. Baldrick's Foundation gave away close to $17 million for pediatric oncology research.[7] Older private disease specific groups, such as the Leukemia and Lymphoma Society,[8] the Children's Brain Tumor Foundation,[9] the Pediatric Brain Tumor Foundation of the US,[10] and the Children's Tumor Foundation (for neurofibromatosis)[11] attempted to respond within their current grant programs to researchers' increased demand for research money.

Hope Street Kids, founded by former U.S. Representative Deborah Pryce, recently strengthened the fundraising efforts of CureSearch, the public face of the National Childhood Cancer Foundation and the Children's Oncology Group (COG).[12] CureSearch has expanded its fundraising efforts through social media (Twitter, Facebook, etc.) and online networking activities in addition to traditional fundraising events. CureSearch has also been successful in securing congressionally appropriated funds specifically for childhood cancer research. Working with Representative Pryce, CureSearch and its fundraising advocates lobbied successfully for the enactment of the Carolyn Pryce Walker Conquer Childhood Cancer Act of 2008.[13] The law authorizes $30 million annually over 5 years to NCI for childhood cancer cooperative group and translational research. It calls for a national childhood cancer registry and funds to increase awareness, educational and support services for patients and families. Congress is currently struggling with budget deficits and may appropriate only $10 million funds in 2010 for this measure.

Family advocates also recently created a nonprofit fundraising group for the NCI-supported pediatric brain tumor cooperative group, the Pediatric Brain Tumor Consortium (PBTC).[14] The PBTC Foundation raises funds and supports for PBTC research and collaborates with other private research funding groups, such as the St. Baldrick's Foundation.[15]

Internet interactivity, which has enabled far easier engagement of families with one another, has generated an even newer group of childhood cancer research organizations. Although most older groups' funding is for basic and translational pediatric oncology research, some of the very new groups are funding Phase 1 clinical trials outside of NCI's official clinical networks (e.g., Solve Kids Cancer and Magic Water).[16,17]

NIH received $8.6 billion from the American Recovery and Reinvestment Act of 2009 for extramural grants, $5 billion of which was recently awarded.[18] These funds, allocated outside of the normal annual federal budget, are an effort to retain and generate jobs and stimulate the economy. Grants are for 2 years and are expected to show scientific progress by the end of that period. As important as the new stimulus funding is, continued high levels of funding for biomedical research will be necessary to realize the potential of this extraordinary boost to advance research.

B. Advocates' Training and Participation in Federal Research Reviews and Planning Groups

Training in partnership with health care professionals is essential for nonscientist family members or survivors to move beyond being informed individual consumers and advocates to advocates who can effectively participate in scientific research and planning.

Patient/family advocacy committees in the both COG and the PBTC conduct workshops to assist members in understanding how cancer research is conducted and how their input can add value. These advocates participate in most the disease and discipline committees within their cooperative groups and provide input on issues such as the ethical challenges of trials, the practicality of trial designs, and the clarity of consent forms.

At NCI, advocates are part of research grant reviews, planning, and cancer communications activities. For example, childhood cancer advocates are advisors to the TARGET research project[19] and the NIH Institutional Review Board. Most advocates serving on NCI reviews are selected through the Consumer Advocates in Research and Related Activities (CARRA) program, administered by the Office of Advocacy Relations.[20,21] CARRA advocates represent various cancer types, age, and ethnic groups across the nation. In the past few years, NCI has expanded its educational resources for nonscientists through teleconference seminars, training curricula, and an enhanced web site. The Office of Liaison Activities now has a workshop to prepare nonscientists to participate in peer review and represent the views of survivors, patients, and family members in grant reviews.

Advocates also participate in the NCI Director's Consumer Liaison Group[22] and the NIH Director's Council of Public Representatives.[23] These forums are opportunities for advocates to guarantee that the implications of policy discussions, plans, and decisions take account of the needs of childhood patients with cancer, survivors, and families.

At the Food and Drug Administration (FDA), patient and family advocates provide input to the Center for Drug Evaluation and Research. Childhood cancer advocates are required members of the Pediatric Oncology Subcommittee of the Oncologic Drugs Advisory Committee (ODAC), the public advisory group which addresses the challenges in pediatric oncology drug development. Adult cancer advocates routinely participate in ODAC drug review meetings; pediatric advocates are infrequent participants due to the rarity with which pediatric cancer drugs come up for FDA approval.

FDA also has a mechanism for cancer advocates to participate in oncology drug development discussions prior to ODAC meetings. The Cancer Drug Development Patient Consultant Program offers training about FDA, the drug development process, and the patient consultant's role and responsibilities.[24]

Several nonprofit organizations have taken on the responsibility of training all types of cancer advocates so as to increase nonscientists' effectiveness as they participate in scientific activities. Although their materials are not designed for the specific concerns of pediatric oncology, the training materials can provide a reliable information base for childhood patient with cancer, survivor, and family advocates. For example, breast cancer advocates founded the Research Advocacy Network, which has an Advocate Institute[25] offering courses, training exercises, and publications on, for example, genomics in cancer, clinical trial design, and the importance of tissue sampling. Oncology professionals have created materials for advocate members of the Coalition of Cancer Cooperative Groups,[26] which encourages patients with cancer to enroll in clinical trials.

C. Advocacy for Childhood, Adolescent and Young Adult Survivors

Family and survivor advocates have been especially busy during the past 5 years designing new programs and support services for young survivors. The policy and research foundations for this work derived in part from the Institute of Medicine's (IOM) reports on childhood and adult survivorship[27,28] and in part from the Center for Disease Control's national action plan on survivorship.[29] Most important for direct care were the publication and dissemination of the COG guidelines for follow-up care[30] and the findings of dozens of studies from the Childhood Cancer Survivors' study.[31]

The Lance Armstrong Foundation, its LiveStrong public relations campaign and symbolic yellow bracelets, frequently brought the face of young survivors to the public eye.[32] The National Coalition for Cancer Survivorship (NCCS), pioneers in addressing survivorship, laid the groundwork in cancer advocacy. It redefined survivorship as starting at the time of diagnosis, and its mission was to include all types of cancer survivors in its community and national advocacy efforts.[33]

Regarding childhood cancer survivorship, program developments have been guided by policy recommendations from the IOM report and the results of studies from the Childhood Cancer Survivors Study. Programs typically responded to recommendations about survivors' need for education and social and emotional supports, as illustrated below:

■ The Children's Cause for Cancer Advocacy created Rise to Action, a national education and advocacy program to make survivors aware of potential late effects and to equip them to be better advocates for their care and quality of life as they grow.[34]

- The Children's Brain Tumor Foundation created a support program for young adult survivors to expand their career development and employment opportunities; bridge their social isolation through support groups and a peer mentoring; and strengthen their self-advocacy skills as they mature.[35]
- The Lance Armstrong Foundation published and disseminated worksheets to assist survivors retain and organize information about their medical treatment history, personal financial and legal circumstances, and their current health regimens.[36]
- Fertile Hope (now affiliated with the Lance Armstrong Foundation) brought strong support services and education services about fertility to a new generation of young adults whose disease or treatment may have compromised the ability to bear children.[37]
- The special needs of patients diagnosed as young adults has brought advocates together, galvanized by an NCI Adolescent and Young Adult Oncology Progress Review Group report, funded by the Lance Armstrong Foundation. This effort spawned the formation of the Young Adult Alliance, advocates and professionals together, who focus on clinical research, standards of care, and awareness of the needs of young adults diagnosed with cancer.[38]

The issues of posttreatment care, care summaries, and care planning are the focus of programmatic and legislative efforts. For example, the Passport for Care, an innovative Internet-based program that enables survivors and their caregivers' access to information about their treatment and an array of follow-up and educational material, was developed by Texas Children's Cancer Center with private funds.[39] A network of collaborating survivorship clinics at comprehensive cancer centers and their affiliates has emerged, initiated by seed money from the Lance Armstrong Foundation. Most large hospital based follow-up programs now provide treatment summaries and an array of privately funded service programs, for example, school transition, psychological services, recreational programs, and more, such as those through the Cure and Beyond at Tomorrows Children's Institute[40] and the After Completion of Therapy at St. Jude Children's Research Hospital.[41]

Although some families of long-term survivors realize that the stress of initial treatment decisions might prevent them from absorbing information about potential late treatment effects and the need to plan for them, other families are puzzled by why they did not receive such information around the time of treatment. NCCS, working with the Cancer Leadership Council (a coalition of 33 cancer patient organizations, professional societies, and research organizations), has been advocating for the Comprehensive Cancer Care Improvement Act of 2009.[42] This bill calls for Medicare to cover the costs of comprehensive cancer care planning services and the expansion of professional training, research, and services for symptom management and palliative care for patients with cancer. If Medicare can set the precedent for these services, childhood cancer advocates hope that private reimbursement for care planning, research, and training programs will extend equally to children.

Childhood cancer advocates have been working hard on other legislative efforts to improve survivors' lives. Bills pending in the 111th Congress are the direct result of advocates' efforts. The Pediatric, Adolescent, and Young Adult Cancer Survivorship Research and Quality of Life Act,[43] building on the recommendations of the pediatric IOM report, is the result of efforts by the Children's Cause for Cancer Advocacy

working with the Alliance for Childhood Cancer and its 20 national patient advocacy and professional group members.[44] This bill proposes that NIH fund pilot programs to develop, study, or evaluate model systems of follow-up care for childhood cancer survivors, expand training in survivorship, conduct research on minority or underserved survivors, and fund follow-up clinics to improve the well-being of survivors. They also pressed for childhood cancer survivorship funding in Senator Ted Kennedy's last cancer bill, the 21st Century Cancer ALERT (Access to Life-Saving Early detection, Research, and Treatment Act),[45] cosponsored by Senator Kay Bailey Hutchison.

D. Advocacy for New Treatments: Challenges, Ethics, and Proposals

Similar to adult cancer advocates, parent advocates have been keenly interested in the potential of personalized medicine and the idea that a child with cancer might not just be cured but have a normal life, free of late effects.

To help analyze this complex problem, the IOM's National Cancer Policy Board published *Making Better Drugs for Children with Cancer*, a careful review of federal resources available to develop drugs for children as well as a description of the considerable commercial and regulatory barriers in doing so.[46] Citing fragmented resources, lack of financial incentives, and federal regulatory hurdles, the IOM recommended a new and more comprehensive approach to discovering and developing oncology agents for children, in part in response to families' advocacy. The IOM recommended, "A new public–private partnership, involving government, industry, academic and other research institutions, advocacy groups, philanthropies, and others, should be formed to lead pediatric cancer drug discovery and development." Although its implementation is complex, the idea has attracted the interest of a number of major academic centers around the country. The lay press followed up the report with several articles, for example, in the *Wall Street Journal*[47] and *USA Today*,[48] which illustrated what the financial and ethical difficulties of developing new agents for low incidence pediatric malignances and very rare diseases and what that can mean for families.

During 2006 to 2007, childhood cancer advocates working with the American Academy of Pediatrics, lobbied congress to pass legislation that would reauthorize and refine incentives and requirements for pharmaceutical companies to conduct pediatric research studies of drugs.[49,50] However, this legislation offers an ineffective solutions to the economic challenges companies face in developing drugs for children and is only partially effective in improving clinical oncology care for children.[51]

The FDA law also reauthorized the Pediatric Subcommittee of ODAC for another 5 years, an important mechanism that keeps pediatric oncology challenges visible at the FDA and to the public.

Ethical review of pediatric oncology research, especially of early clinical trials, requires substantive input from families in weighing the risks and benefits of research in children. Patients, survivors, and families are active members of the committees of the NCI cooperative pediatric networks. They review and comment on protocols, including on trial designs, schedules of procedures, and language of consent forms. Advocates' input has resulted in a number of changes in how consent forms are presented. For example, the COG Patient Advocates Committee has shortened and the simplified consent process for families and clarified language distinguishing research procedures from standard care (M. Layfield, personal communication, June 24, 2009).

At the federal level, pediatric oncology advocates have served as members of the Department of Health and Human Services Secretary's Advisory Committee on Human Research Protections (SACHRP). The Pediatric Subcommittee of SACHRP conducted an in-depth analysis of the federal regulations related to research in children.[52]

Of particular interest to families and oncology researchers is the increasingly important issue of consents for tissue and specimen studies that are for research purposes only and offer no prospect of direct benefit to individual study participants.[53] Both COG and PBTC parent advocates have required that there are opt-out provisions for research-only procedures. This issue was debated in SACHRP, which recommended that protocol consents include such opt-out provisions. To date, the Secretary has not implemented SACHRP's pediatric recommendations, and IRBs vary from site to site as to whether they require families to agree to research-only studies when bundled into a single protocol consent.

Regarding children's assent, the COG Patient Advocates Committee developed guidelines for obtaining children's assent to participation in clinical trials. Advocates on the independent COG Pediatric Central Institutional Review Board have also created templates for assent that now must be included in the packet that local IRBs receive from the Pediatric Central Institutional Review Board (G. McMillan, personal communication, September 25, 2009). To help families decide about treatment options and understand what protocols entail, patient advocates in the COG and in the PBTC write abbreviated nontechnical summaries of trials that are posted on their respective web sites.

Off-Protocol, Single-Patient Use, and Expanded Access to Investigational Agents

Pressure from cancer and other advocates over the past few years has drawn the attention of the FDA to how it handles requests for patient access to investigational drugs outside of a clinical trial. For many families whose children are severely ill from cancer and who no longer have treatment options available within clinical trials, final hopes can rest on obtaining access to an early phase investigational drug whose safety and efficacy are still under investigation. Advocates, largely from the cancer community including the NCCS, the American Society of Clinical Oncology,[54] and the Abigail Alliance for Better Access to Developmental Drugs, have pressed FDA for clarity about such access.[55] FDA responded with revised regulations on expanded access, clarifying procedures and requirements that apply to "compassionate use" or "treatment IND." FDA also expanded the circumstances under which families may pay companies to access an unapproved agent. Perhaps the most important result is FDA's increased transparency about these issues and an enhanced web site.[56]

E. Health Care Reform: Coverage, Cost, and Quality

The Patient Protection and Affordable Care Act (PPACA)[57], which became law in March, 2010, represents major changes in health and insurance reform for the nation and brings important gains to children with cancer and surviving cancer. The new law was primarily intended to maximize the number of Americans required to have health insurance, increase its affordability, and improve the quality of healthcare.[58]

Childhood cancer advocates, through the Children's Cause for Cancer Advocacy and the Alliance for Childhood Cancer, actively worked with Congress to promote the interests of children with cancer, survivors and their families. As the legislation proceeded through congress, advocates emphasized the particular importance of timely access to affordable, quality care.

Coverage. Several provisions in the health care reform law offer new and important protections to survivors. Of particular interest is the prohibition of coverage denial for individuals with preexisting conditions. Previously, many survivors were excluded from private health insurance coverage because of the history of their disease and the late effects of treatment. Under pressure from President Obama[59] and many cancer advocates, survivors can no longer be denied health care coverage from any type of insurance plan because of a preexisting cancer diagnosis or its sequelae.

Health reform also provides new coverage for young adult childhood cancer survivors up to age 26. HHS drew special attention to this problem, documenting that 30 percent of young adults (under age 30) did not have health insurance as opposed to 17 percent of adults from 30–64 years.[60] Adult survivors of childhood cancer have had even lower rates of health insurance coverage and more problems obtaining coverage when compared to their siblings.[61] Young adults have had to go without coverage because they age out of their parents' plans, are unemployed or even if employed in a small business have not been able to obtain coverage. Now, coverage is available for all children and young adults up to age 26 as dependents under their parents' individual and group policies.

Childhood cancer advocates worked with Families USA and other groups to urge congress to pass the Children's Health Insurance Program Reauthorization Act of 2009 (CHIPRA)[62]. CHIPRA, now embedded in PPACP, covers children from families with incomes up to 300 percent of the poverty level, expanding the numbers of children covered. Expanding state coverage for more middle income families is especially important for those whose children have special health care needs, including children with cancer. HHS in 2009 also awarded states $40 million to increase the enrollment of eligible but uninsured minority children in CHIPRA.[63]

Costs of care. Because most children with cancer in the United States are treated in the context of clinical trials, coverage of the routine care costs in clinical trials has been an important advocacy issue.[64] Private insurers generally follow the reimbursement policies set by Medicare, the driving market force in US healthcare. For many years, childhood cancer advocates, following the lead of the adult cancer community, actively supported bills to cover the costs of clinical trial participation, hoping for a downstream impact on coverage for pediatric oncology care.[65] Advocacy efforts have recently been directed at prohibiting denials of coverage for routine care costs for federal employees and their families who are treated in the context of clinical trials[66]

Families of children with cancer frequently seek assistance from advocacy groups to help cover the substantial costs of co-pays and deductibles required for their children's care. Recent studies from the Kaiser Family Foundation dramatically illustrate how children and adults with special health care needs incur major out of pocket costs even when they have high quality health insurance plans.[67,68] Though none of the cases analyzed involved children with cancer, the gaps in services and continuing need for care are similar and highlight how families must cope with the complex coordination of care. While not providing immediate relief for co-pays and deductibles, health reform law does prohibit private insurers from charging higher premiums based on an individual's health status.

Health reform eliminates another important cost concern of parents and survivors by prohibiting individual and group health plans from placing lifetime limits on insurance coverage. Childhood cancer can be understood as a chronic disease, and late effects, including premature diseases of aging, are a reality for many survivors. For parents of very young children, whose cancer care can continue for a child's lifetime, this change is most welcome.

Quality of Care and Comparative Effectiveness Research. The standard of clinical care for children with cancer continues to be treatment in the context of Phase 3 clinical trials. Comparative effectiveness research (CER) is a descriptor for an obtaining an evidence-base for clinical practice. Because standard treatment of children with cancer evolves as a result of clinical research studies, by definition the pediatric oncology enterprise can be considered engaged in the practice of comparative effectiveness research.

Congress indicated its interest in improving quality care by requiring the IOM to propose a list of priorities for CER as part of the American Recovery and Reinvestment Act of 2009 (ARRA) legislation.[69] ASCO, in its background comments to IOM, made two points where the involvement of childhood cancer advocates is likely to be important in protecting the interests of children. ASCO emphasized the importance of engaging oncology experts and the cooperative group infrastructure as cancer effectiveness priorities are determined.[70]

Administrative and legislative approaches to CER that involve children need to take account of the critical differences between pediatric and adult oncology research, including the smaller size of the cooperative group structures, the small sizes of the patient populations and the large number of different types of pediatric cancers. Further, federal regulations on research in human subjects limit the types of research questions that can be asked when children are subjects. These factors and others make it more complex and more time consuming to conduct clinical research in children with cancer. Pediatric cancer treatments are a moving research target, and advocates must ensure that public and private reimbursement for care covers all phases of clinical research.

A second point made by ASCO concerns the importance of including correlative studies as part of CER. Data from correlative studies ensures that effects of drug regimens or targeted agents in patient subgroups (such as children) can be evaluated by biomarkers, imaging and other indicators. The ethical sensitivity of studies in children which are conducted for research purposes only (see above) will require continued attention and input from families and pediatric oncology bioethicists.

It is interesting to note that among the 100 priorities for CER cited by IOM, about 15 relate to maternal or child health, 7 relate directly to cancer treatment, and none relate to childhood cancer research.[71] This fact may suggest that comparative evaluations of treatment in childhood cancer may already in place. However, if comparative effectiveness of childhood cancer treatments become an active issue outside the academic pediatric oncology community, cancer advocates will need to work closely with researchers to make certain that cooperative group research continues to be the primary mechanism through which CER takes place.

II. CASE ADVOCACY FOR INDIVIDUAL PATIENTS AND SURVIVORS: INSURANCE, EDUCATION, AND EMPLOYMENT CHALLENGES

Childhood cancer groups founded and led by families provide a rich array of case advocacy services for patients, survivors, and families. For example, Candlelighters, the oldest childhood cancer organization, offers case advocacy support services for individuals and families across the country and has broad knowledge base about the burdens that families sustain in caring for their children. Many groups focus on a specific type of childhood cancer and have professionals on staff, such as the Children's Brain Tumor Foundation and the Leukemia and Lymphoma Society.

Health care professionals are key to helping patients and survivors overcome insurance, education, and employment barriers to care and appropriate services. There are abundant resources available to help the MCT help families and survivors with insurance, education, and employment issues.[72,73] For example, groups such as the Patient Advocate Foundation have case managers and *pro bono* attorneys to help resolve insurance, job discrimination, and debt crisis. The Cancer Legal Resource Center is also available for *pro bono* help.[74] Specific case advocacy assistance, particularly around insurance issues, is offered by the Childhood Cancer Ombudsman Program (CCOP) (part of the Childhood Brain Tumor Foundation) and specializes in *pro bono* case advocacy assistance and information to families and survivors.[75] CCOP is also an information resource about the rights of families and survivors for attorneys, physicians, and other health care professionals and school personnel. CCOP links patients and families nationwide with treatment, school, rehabilitation, health insurance, and employment problems with attorneys, regional, state, and local agencies, and committees that can assist them in exercising their rights and obtaining needed services. CCOP engages the services of volunteer specialists in psychology, social work, law, nursing, physical and occupational therapists, and physicians to help resolve families' and survivors' problems.

A. Private Insurance: Reimbursement Denials, Access to Health Care Coverage, Specialty, and Follow-Up Care

MCTs can assist patients and families manage financial problems with their health insurance through some of the suggestions in the following section.

Reimbursement Denials

Despite Medicare regulations and laws in many states, insurers may not cover the costs of routine care if patients are enrolled in clinical trials. Health plans are likely to cover clinical trial participation, however, if it is clear that the trials are cost effective, scientifically valuable, and expected to benefit a patient.

Patients whose health plans deny coverage of clinical trials, based on investigational or "experimental" exclusions or other coverage denials, may need to engage the MCT's assistance. When coverage of a medically necessary procedure or medication is denied, the following approaches may help.

Tips for Letters of Support

Some health care plans flag complex and expensive categories of treatment and automatically review pediatric cancer clinical trials. The MCT will need to send a detailed letter of support when care is denied and deemed experimental. Successful letters of support are concise and neutral in tone, focusing on the medical facts of the case and providing arguments to support the intervention. For crafting successful letters:

■ Conduct a careful review of a family's health care policy, especially related to exclusions; determine whether there is an 'individual managed care option,' permitting a patient to obtain treatment outside of coverage limitations if the plan finds it justifiable.

- Use a plan's own definition of experimental or investigational; state that the disputed procedure builds on the foundations of previous pediatric oncology treatments with known benefit, and that patients will receive baseline benefits established through previous clinical trials.
- State that the participation of childhood patients with cancer in clinical trials is the standard of care.
- Attach test relevant test results and peer-reviewed articles or other medical or scientific evidence, if a procedure is expensive or complicated or if a plan's treatment guidelines are misguided or obsolete.
- Inquire whether pediatric charges are typically included in the reasonable and customary charges for a procedure.

Tips for Conducting Investigations and Appeals

Obtaining a copy of the denial letter or documented phone call is the first step in an investigation. Below are some next steps for preparing a denial:

- Determine whether a health plan or state requires claims to be processed and resolved within a particular time period; some health plans or states respond more quickly if a patient is considered or presumed to be "terminal;" if a plan has not responded within the statutory limits or within their own stated time limits, they may be obligated to pay the costs associated with treatment.[76]
- Determine the rationale for why the contract language excludes the treatment in question.
- If a denial is based on lack of medical necessity, a letter from the MCT could:
  - Request whether the claim was reviewed by a pediatric oncology specialist and, if so, request a copy of the specialist's review, the literature relied on, and a description of the specialist qualifications.
  - Request any other contractual agreement or arrangement a plan has with the reviewer.

All denials should be appealed, first by taking full advantage of a plan's internal appeal process, and if necessary, taking advantage of any external review options, especially if mandated in the state.[77]

Tips for Conducting the Appeal itself

- Check the policy for details on the appeals process
- Inquire whether a lawyer or advocate can accompany the family or patient to the appeal hearing
- Request a description of the qualifications of the persons on the appeal panel
- Determine who makes the final reimbursement decision
- Request articles, statements, and any other materials used or referenced in the denial.

If possible, the family or patient should attend the appeal hearing or participate in a conference call along with a member of the MCT. In CCOP's experience, reasons for denial can be simple to remedy. For example, an "eligible" patient may be mistakenly declared ineligible for a protocol; or an intervention may be provided in error as standard treatment when the patient should have been in a protocol.

State-Mandated External Review

State-mandated external reviews offer an important strategy to remedy insurance reimbursement and coverage denials. Forty-four states and the District of Columbia offer the option of an independent external review. If a patient or survivor is not satisfied with a health plan's treatment, drug or service decision, and the plan's internal appeal process has been exhausted, an appeal can be made to a state's external review program.

External reviews are performed by Independent Review Organizations (IROs) that have no affiliation with the health plan. IROs are designed to monitor health insurers' coverage decisions and hold them accountable. IRO services are free to health plan enrollees and are overseen by states' Departments of Insurance.

States differ in their external review programs regarding the types of disputes that are eligible for appeal, the process used to resolve the appeal, and the time limits imposed at each step of the process. The Kaiser Family Foundation provides a state-by-state guide to these requirements and state contact information.[77]

Option for Out-of-Network Coverage

If a treatment requested cannot be adequately provided by a health plan's in-network or out-of-network specialists, patients may be eligible for coverage of care not normally provided out-of-network. An exceptional out-of-network coverage option is usually negotiated on a case-by-case basis. If successful, a plan will cover a procedure at the usual in-network or out-of-network treatment rate.

B. Access to Coverage

As described above, coverage for low income, Medicaid ineligible children, has expanded with the passage of CHIPRA. Insurance coverage for young adult survivors may be remedied as a result of health care reform (see earlier). There are additional federal protections that assist survivors and their families in obtaining health insurance coverage.

Health Insurance Portability Act and Accountability (HIPAA)[78] Act and Genetic Information Nondiscrimination Act (GINA)[79]

With the passage of health reform, patients with preexisting conditions cannot be denied coverage. HIPAA, in addition to helping people with preexisting conditions to secure comprehensive health insurance coverage, it also helps people maintain their coverage if they change jobs or insurance plans. At the time of this writing, it is not clear how the new health reform law interacts with HIPAA provisions. Under HIPAA, a health plan cannot

- Charge higher premiums among some workers
- Deny individual coverage to someone leaving a group health plan because of loss of employment or because the new employer does not offer insurance coverage
- Impose waiting periods or preexisting condition exclusions as long as the individual opted for and exhausted Consolidated Omnibus Budget Reconciliation Act (COBRA) continuation coverage; has had at least 18 months of prior health insurance coverage; and has had no gap in insurance coverage of more than 63 days, excluding employer waiting periods; however, the insurer can charge higher premiums under the individual coverage plan
- Refuse to provide credit for the time an individual was insured against the preexisting waiting period (e.g., if an individual had prior insurance but it was not in effect when he or she switched jobs)
- Refuse to renew group and individual plans

▥ Deny coverage for a disabled employee who switches group health insurance plan from one carrier to a succeeding carrier, if the individual was disabled when the original plan was terminated.

However, HIPAA allows a health plan to:

▥ Impose preexisting condition waiting periods on persons applying for individual plan coverage who have a break in their prior coverage for more than 63 days, excluding any employer-imposed waiting period (including Medicaid).

▥ Impose a preexisting condition waiting period of 12 months (up to 18 months for late enrollees) on persons applying for group insurance who have no prior insurance.

▥ Select, on a nondiscriminatory basis, the coverage and benefits they offer (e.g., they can exclude coverage for cancer treatment but would have to do so for all employees).

▥ Cap lifetime benefits.

Under HIPAA, insurers cannot deny enrollment based on health status, medical condition, claims history, medical history, or genetic information. GINA extends and clarifies the HIPAA law. Under GINA and its currently regulations[80], exclude consumers due to preexisting conditions or use an individual's genetic information. GINA also prohibits issuers from using genetic information to deny individual coverage, raise premiums, or impose preexisting condition exclusions.

GINA and its proposed rules will prohibit insurers from requesting, requiring, or buying genetic information, or asking individuals or family members to undergo a genetic test. The proposed rules hold the statutory definition of genetic testing, in which a test "provides an analysis of human DNA, RNA, chromosomes, proteins, or metabolites, if it detects genotypes, mutations, or chromosomal changes." Violation of GINA can also result in the imposition of fines on insurers.

Consolidated Omnibus Budget Reconciliation Act[81]

COBRA provides additional protection for survivors and families if they are insured through their employer and they lose their job. COBRA mandates that public and private employers, who employ 20 or more people on more than 50% of the working days in the previous calendar year, make insurance coverage available for a period of 18 months. Employees who have been fired or laid off have a right to continue their group health coverage at their own expense and at a rate no higher than 102% of the employer's group insurance premium. Since 1989, the same benefits have been available for people with disabilities for up to 29 months in order to bridge the gap to Medicare. The premium for people with disabilities from months 18 to 29 can increase up to 150% of the premium charged.

An employer must notify employees of their COBRA rights and the group health plan of an employee's change in employment status. Coverage may also extend to a spouse after the death of an eligible employee, after divorce or legal separation. It may extend to a dependent under the same conditions or to a child who is no longer dependent during the COBRA period. COBRA coverage may be terminated if an employer stops providing employee group health insurance, if the employee obtains coverage under another plan (including Medicare) or does not pay COBRA continuation premiums.

The American Recovery and Reinvestment Act of 2009 provides for premium reductions and additional election opportunities for health benefits under the COBRA. Eligible individuals pay only 35% of their COBRA premiums and the remaining 65% is reimbursed to the coverage provider through a tax credit. The premium reduction applies to periods of health care coverage beginning on or after February 17, 2009. The reduction lasts for up to 9 months for individuals eligible for COBRA during the period beginning September 1, 2008 and ending December 31, 2009 if an involuntary termination of employment occurred during that period. The TAA Health Coverage Improvement Act of 2009, enacted as part of ARRA, also made changes with regard to COBRA continuation coverage.[82]

C. Access to Specialty Care and Care for Late Effects

When survivors have late effects, access to specialty care and related services are critical to their continued health and well-being. Although some plans may have strict exceptions and exclusions for specialty care, plans typically have a procedure whereby members can access specialists for medically necessary care.

The MCT can help first by determining when a patient needs specialist intervention and then providing a letter of support to obtain that service. Federal laws are available to ensure that survivors can have access to specialty care, for example, the U.S. Department of Labor's actions with respect to Employee Retirement Income Security Act plans. The Department of Labor includes a "quality of services/provider" as a relevant factor in the choice of providers.[83] Medicaid provides children the right to reasonable, adequate, and prompt provision of specialty care services.[84] Lawsuits have also set precedents, fining health maintenance organizations (HMOs) for not referring pediatric patients with cancer to appropriate specialists in a timely manner.[85]

For nursing care, families eligible for Medicaid can apply for waivers to receive care in the home or community and not in an institution, if a state has applied for federal permission to amend their Medicaid programs.[48] In some states, the "Katie Beckett" waiver allows severely disabled children on Medicaid to receive care at home instead of in a hospital or nursing facility. States have experimented with other types of waivers that enable patients to receive care out of institutional settings.

For mental health services, HIPAA requires that such benefits be provided on an equal basis with physical health benefits. However, exceptions and limitations abound in the way the law is applied. To control costs, many county mental health agencies severely limit services to those who are suicidal or violent. When this is the case, it will take advocacy on the part of MCTs, Late Effects Program Staff, local parents of children with cancer, and parent groups concerned with mental health to encourage the development and allocation of sufficient resources to serve survivors' needs.

For personal assistant services, severely disabled adults may be covered for help with activities of daily living through Medicaid or Title XX of the Social Security Act. These services may also be available to nonbeneficiaries who pay a "share of cost" toward the service. Access to such services may allow disabled young survivors to live at home rather than in an institutional setting.

Supplemental Security Income (SSI) is another assistance program for low-income families with severely disabled children. However, having cancer alone does not qualify a child for SSI. SSI is not awarded for financial need alone, however. The Social Security Administration conducts a three-step evaluation to determine if a child has a disability.

The American Academy of Pediatrics has detailed recommendations about this evaluation process.[86]

TABLE 51.1

CHILDREN'S THREE STEP SEQUENTIAL EVALUATION PROCESS FOR SOCIAL SECURITY ELIGIBILITY[87]

Step 1	Is the child working (engaging in substantial gainful activity)? If yes, denied. If no, go to Step 2
Step 2	Does the child have a medically determinable impairment or combination of impairments that is severe? If no, the claim is denied. If yes, go to Step 3. For purposes of evaluation, "Severe" is defined as "more than a slight abnormality or a combination of slight abnormalities that cause more than minimal limitation in a child's ability to function independently, appropriately, and effectively in an age appropriate manner" (20 CFR §416.924[c]). This step is used to filter out children who either (a) do not have any medically determinable impairment, or (b) have medically determinable impairment, but those impairments do not impose more than minimum functional limitations
Step 3	Does the child's impairment(s) meet, is medically equal to, or functionally equal to any condition described in the Listing of Impairments. If no, the claim is denied. If yes, disability benefits are granted. The Listing of Impairments is at www.ssa.gov

Social security benefits are notoriously late at being approved and sent out. The Social Security Administration now has a program called "Compassionate Allowances," which fast-tracks benefits for those whose medical conditions are so severe that their cases would obviously be approved.[87] Compassionate Allowances permit people who have 1 of 50 highly serious conditions, including 25 types of cancer, to receive decisions on their applications for Social Security disability benefits in a matter of days, not months or years. However the beneficiaries must, by law, wait 5 months before they receive their first payment.

D. Education Rights for School-Age Children

Patients and young survivors of childhood cancer may need special education services or accommodations during treatment or over the long term. Children with defined special needs are entitled to a free appropriate public education and have rights to obtain needed services through a federal law, the Individuals with Disabilities Education Act (IDEA).[88] Under IDEA, students are eligible to receive a free and timely educational evaluation, resulting in an individual educational plan. Most states have free materials describing students' rights under IDEA that are available through a state's Department of Education.

Children with cancer may qualify as being "other health impaired," according to IDEA categories of disabling conditions. Survivors may have hearing impairments, learning disabilities, and other moderate or severe long-term effects of disease or treatment. Appropriate accommodations may include home instruction, resting during the school day, special resource room instruction, or health-related accommodations (see Chapter 48).

The MCT can substantiate in a letter the reasons for a pediatric patient with cancer need for special educational

accommodations. All students with disabilities have a right to attend school when they are medically able to do so, regardless of the nature or extent of the health-related services they may require during school hours, so long as a physician's services are not required.

Children who are off treatment and whose mental or physical condition does not strictly meet IDEA's categories may qualify for reasonable accommodations under Section 504 of the federal Rehabilitation Act of 1973.[89] The MCT can request that a school district's 504 coordinator be present at an individual educational plan meeting so that the school's child study team can develop a plan even if it is determined that the child does not qualify under IDEA.

For children who are physically and/or neurologically impaired as a result of cancer or treatment and are Medicaid eligible, they may receive assistance in school under Medicaid. The state Medicaid agency may not withdraw or change nursing support guidelines to eliminate this assistance. Beneficiaries have a right to notice and appeal before benefits are reduced. A family may file for a "fair hearing" with the state Medicaid office to maintain services until a judge issues a decision. If Medicaid coverage fails, school districts are required by law to provide nurses for "health" (not for "medical") services for students with disabilities. Resolving educational issues such as these can be protracted and complex, and families and the MCT should consider seeking outside expertise. There publications, professional organizations, and parents groups offer many resources to help patients with cancer, survivors, and their families negotiate educational challenges.[90]

Young adult survivors who are able to work part time can apply to their state rehabilitation agency to receive assessment, training, and counseling to find suitable employment settings. Rehabilitation agencies also may pay for state college tuition so that a survivor might get paid to go to school. The Work Incentives Improvement Act of 1999 can assist survivors on Social Security Administration benefits to maintain Medicaid or Medicare benefits as they return to work.

E. Employment Rights

Cancer survivors and their families have federal protections that may enable them to continue working during treatment and beyond.

Family and Medical Leave Act (FMLA)[91]

FMLA entitles eligible employees to take up to 12 weeks of unpaid, job-protected leave and continued benefits in a 12-month period for specified family and medical reasons, including a family medical emergency. Leave may be taken as needed and does not need to be consecutive ("intermittent leave").

FMLA applies to all state, local, and federal employers. It also applies to private-sector employers with 50 or more employees in 20 or more workweeks in the current or preceding calendar year. To be eligible for FMLA benefits, an employee must also (a) work for a covered employer, (b) have worked for the employer for a total of 12 months, (c) have worked at least 1250 hours over the previous 12 months, and (d) work for an employer whose worksite is within 75 miles.

A covered employer must grant a FMLA 12 workweek leave during any 12-month period to an individual to care for an immediate family member with a serious health condition or who is unable to work due to a serious health condition. A covered employer is required to maintain group health insurance coverage for an employee on FMLA leave on the same terms as before the leave was taken. Employees may have to pay their share of premiums while on leave. Additionally, on returning to work, an employee must be restored to his or her original job or its equivalent with equivalent pay and benefits.

In some instances, an employer can refuse to reinstate highly paid "key" employees after using FMLA leave when health insurance coverage was maintained. Eligible "key," employees must be among the highest paid 10% of employees. Some states also have laws to help working families who have a child with special needs. For example, California's Family Rights Act allows employees to take 4 months of leave every 2 years to care for a family member. Nonprofit organizations and federal resources are available to assist families and survivors with FMLA questions (M. Layfield, personal communication, June 24, 2009).

Americans with Disabilities Act (ADA)[91]

Young adult cancer survivors may receive protections under ADA, a federal civil rights law, mandating nondiscrimination against people with disabilities, including those with a history of childhood cancer. Some states provide greater legal protections than the minimum standards provided by the ADA. The ADA requires that persons with disabilities have equal access to benefits, such as health insurance, and be treated with equal opportunity in all stages of employment, from hiring through each promotion. It mandates that reasonable accommodations be granted to individuals with disabilities unless such accommodations will cause undue hardship on the employer. Reasonable accommodations include, but are not limited to, flextime, leave time, job restructuring, and the purchase of equipment so that the employee can perform the essential job functions. It also provides a cause of action for disability-based employer harassment.[92]

Employees with disabilities do not receive special job protection once they are hired. The ADA applies to any qualified individual who can perform the essential functions of the job, regardless of whether the job applicant needs a reasonable accommodation from the employer. A qualified individual with a disability means that the job applicant or employee has the requisite skills, education, and experience required for the position. The employer is not required to provide reasonable accommodations when doing so would cause an undue hardship for the employer, for example, causing administrative disruption or great expense.

The ADA covers companies with 15 or more employees, bringing most small businesses within the jurisdiction of the law. It also protects job applicants from disclosing medical information before being given a conditional job offer so that employers cannot use medical information as the basis for denying a job. It is important to note that confidential medical information in an employee's file is still protected even after the employee leaves a job or retires.

Medical examinations and inquiries are considered unlawful prior to a conditional offer of employment unless they apply to all applicants for that job. If an employer withdraws a job conditional offer after a medical examination, the employer must show that the company's medical standards are job related and consistent with business necessity. The ADA does permit an employer to require an examination to show that the applicant employee can perform the functions specified in the job description.[93]

The ADA also protects those who are associated with a person with disabilities. Insurance discrimination against dependents is prohibited, but the scope of coverage afforded dependents may be different from that afforded the employee. A covered employer may not refuse to hire an applicant or fire an employee if (a) that person has a dependent with a disability or (b) that person has a dependent who is either not covered by the employer's current health insurance plan or might cause increased health care costs. An employer is also prohibited from refusing to insure or providing different insurance conditions for a person solely because they have a dependent with a disability.

Accommodations may also apply to taking college entrance, postgraduate, and professional licensing examinations.[94] Survivors and patients with documented learning disabilities as a result of cancer or treatment can be eligible for reasonable accommodations, such as isolation or the use of a computer or other assistive device, when taking such examinations.

Perhaps most important for cancer survivors, ADA protects someone with a record of impairment. Every cancer survivor has a record of substantial impairment, so ADA protects survivors whether the cancer is cured, stable, or in remission, and this applies for the remainder of a survivor's life.

F. Employment in the Armed Forces, Police, and Fire Departments

Survivors of childhood cancer, who meet the physical requirements, may be eligible for a medical waiver to obtain admission to service academies and to serve in the Armed Forces, Reserves, and Reserve Officers' Training Corps. The general rule is that a survivor must be completely free of cancer and off therapy for at least 5 years.[95] For survivors of Wilms tumor and germ cell tumors of the testes, there is only a 2-year waiting period. These protections have been expanded to apply to the reenlistment of a disabled reservist.

Police and fire departments have their own physical admission standards. However, they usually focus on an applicant's current physical condition. Departments cannot ask questions about health or request medical histories until a conditional job offer has been made (see earlier).

CONCLUSION

Advances in care for children, survivors, and their families depend in large part on collaborations and shared definitions of quality care among pediatric oncology researchers, health care providers, and advocates. Not all interests overlap, however, and sometimes when these interests diverge, families and survivors can be especially valuable to physicians and researchers. As national advocates, families can offer perspectives in scientific discussions and policy debates about research, ethics, and care that are unconflicted by financial or career concerns can build on this partnership to improve both individuals' care and the systems of care. As new, Internet-savvy parents are told that their children have cancer, it is vital that they are able to use their new perspectives on life and death and their unprecedented access to medical information to assist MCTs to care for children with cancer. It is essential that parents of newly diagnosed children help advance pediatric oncology research to improve the long-term outlook for all children struggling with these diseases.

References

1. Larson J. Why i am an advocate. The Next Step. Children's Cause for Cancer Advocacy. Winter 2008;3;3.
2. Weiner SL, McCabe M, Smith G, et al. Pediatric cancer: advocacy, legal, insurance and employment issues. In: Pizzo P, Poplack D, eds. Principles and practice of pediatric oncology chapter. 5th ed. Philadelphia, PA: Lippincott Williams & Wilkins Publishers, 2005.
3. Hoffman B, Stovall E. Survivorship perspectives and advocacy. J Clin Oncol 2006; 24(32):5154–5159.
4. http://www.stbaldricks.org/. Accessed October 11, 2009.
5. http://www.alexslemonade.org/slideshow. Accessed October 11, 2009.
6. http://www.hopestreetkids.org/. Accessed October 11, 2009.
7. http://www.guidestar.org/. Accessed October 11, 2009.
8. http://lls.org/. Accessed June 24, 2010.
9. http://www.cbtf.org/. Accessed October 11, 2009.
10. http://www.pbtfus.org/. Accessed October 11, 2009.
11. http://www.ctf.org/. Accessed October 11, 2009.
12. http://www.curesearch.org/. Accessed October 11, 2009.
13. http://thomas.loc.gov/cgi-bin/bdquery/z?d110:HR01553:@@@L&summ2=m&. Accessed October 11, 2009
14. http://pbtc.org/
15. http://pbtcfoundation.org/. Accessed October 11, 2009.
16. http://solvingkidscancer.org/
17. http://www.magicwater.org/ Accessed October 11, 2009.
18. http://grants.nih.gov/recovery.
19. http://deainfo.nci.nih.gov/Advisory/bsa/sub-cmte/target/roster.pdf. Accessed October 11, 2009.
20. http://carra.cancer.gov/. Accessed October 11, 2010.
21. http://ola.cancer.gov/. Accessed October 11, 2009.
22. http://dclg.cancer.gov/. Accessed October 11, 2009.
23. http://copr.nih.gov/. Accessed October 11, 2009.
24. http://www.fda.gov/ForConsumers/ByAudience/ForPatientAdvocates/CancerLiaison Program/ucm127679.htm.
25. http://www.researchadvocacy.org/advocateInstitute/index.php.
26. http://www.cancertrialshelp.org/.
27. Hewitt M, Weiner SL, Simone J. Childhood cancer survivorship: improving care and quality of life. Report from the National Research Council and Institute of Medicine, National Academies of Science, 2003.
28. Hewitt M, Greenfield S, Stovall E, eds. From cancer patient to cancer survivor: lost in transition. Report from the National Research Council and Institute of Medicine, National Academies of Science, 2006.
29. http://www.cdc.gov/cancer/survivorship/pdf/plan.pdf.
30. http://www.survivorshipguidelines.org/pdf/LTFUGuidelines.pdf.
31. http://ccss.stjude.org/published-research/publications. Accessed June 24, 2010.
32. http://www.livestrong.org/. Accessed June 24, 2010.
33. http://www.canceradvocacy.org/.
34. http://www.childrenscause.org/programs/rta.
35. http://cbtf.org/cms/survivor.
36. http://www.livestrong.org/Get-Help/Learn-About-Cancer/LIVESTRONG-Guidebook. Accessed June 24, 2010.
37. http://www.fertilehope.org
38. http://www.livestrong.org/What-We-Do/Our-Actions/Programs-Partnerships/ LIVESTRONG-Young-Adult-Alliance. Accessed June 24, 2010.
39. http://www.txcccc.org/content.cfm?content_id=1643. Accessed June 24, 2010.
40. http://www.atcfkid.com/how_we_help.php.
41. http://www.stjude.org/stjude/v/index.jsp?vgnextoid=72850307f6e70110VgnVCM 1000001e0215acRCRD&vgnextchannel=4e27ef786d543110VgnVCM1000001e0215 acRCRD.
42. http://thomas.loc.gov/cgi-bin/bdquery/z?d111:H.R.1844:.
43. http://thomas.loc.gov/cgi-bin/bdquery/D?d111:1:./temp/~bd9in1::l/home/Legislative Data.php. Accessed June 24, 2010.
44. http://acc.stateaffiliates-asco.org/acc/Policy_Issues/.
45. http://thomas.loc.gov/cgi-bin/query/z?c111:S.717:.
46. Adamson PC, Weiner SL, Simone J, et al. Making better drugs for children with cancer. Report from the National Research Council and Institute of Medicine, National Academies of Science, 2005.
47. Marcus AD. Testing smart drugs on children with cancer. Wall Street Journal May 31, 2005:D1.
48. Szabo, L. Who's fighting cancer in kids? USA Today July 7, 2005; Health.
49. http://www.allianceforchildhoodcancer.org/acc/Policy_Issues/.
50. http://www.fda.gov/downloads/Drugs/DevelopmentApprovalProcess/Development Resources/UCM049870.pdf.

51. http://www.fda.gov/ohrms/dockets/ac/07/slides/2007-4303s1-02-FDA-Santana_ files/frame.htm.
52. http://www.hhs.gov/ohrp/sachrp/commsec.html.
53. Anderson BD, Adamson PC, Weiner SL, et al. Tissue collection for correlative studies in childhood cancer clinical trials: ethical considerations and special imperatives. J Clin Oncol 2004;22:4794–4798.
54. http://www.cancerleadership.org/policy/fda/061206.html.
55. http://abigail-alliance.org/WLF_FDA.pdf.
56. http://www.fda.gov/Drugs/DevelopmentApprovalProcess/HowDrugsareDevelopedand Approved/ApprovalApplications/InvestigationalNewDrugINDApplication/ucm172492.htm.
57. http://frwebgate.access.gpo.gov/cgi-bin/getdoc.cgi?dbname=111_cong_bills&docid= f:h3590enr.txt.pdf. Accessed June 25, 2010.
58. For a concise and updated summary, see http://www.kff.org/healthreform/upload/ 8061.pdf. Accessed June 25, 2010.
59. http://www.whitehouse.gov/issues/health_care/
60. http://healthreform.gov/reports/youngadults/youngamericans.pdf.pdf
61. Park ER, Li FP, Liu Y, Emmons KE, Ablin A, Robison L, & Mertens A. Health Insurance Coverage in Survivors of Childhood Cancer: The Childhood Cancer Survivor Study. J Clin Oncol; 23 (36) 9187–9197.
62. http://thomas.loc.gov/cgi-bin/query/z?c111:H.R.2:
63. http://www.hhs.gov/news/press/2009pres/09/20090930a.html
64. Weiner, S.L, McCabe, M., Smith, G., Monaco, G. (2005) Pediatric Cancer: Advocacy, Legal, Insurance and Employment Issues. In P. Pizzo and D. Poplack (Eds.). Principles and Practice of Pediatric Oncology Chapter, 5th Edition. Phila., PA, Lippincott Williams & Wilkins Publishers.
65. http://www.cancerleadership.org/policy/clinic_medicare/index.html.
66. http://www.cancerleadership.org/policy/clinic_privins/090428.html.
67. http://www.kff.org/healthreform/upload/7980.pdf.
68. http://www.kff.org/healthreform/7980.cfm.
69. http://frwebgate.access.gpo.gov/cgi-bin/getdoc.cgi?dbname=111_cong_bills&docid=f: h1enr.pdf.
70. http://www.asco.org/ASCO/Downloads/Cancer%20Policy%20and%20Clinical%20 Affairs/ASCO%20CER%20Testimony%20IOM%203%2009.pdf.
71. Initial Priorities for Comparative Effectiveness Research, Institute of Medicine; National Academies of Science: 2009.
72. http://www.patientadvocate.org/index.php?p=8.
73. http://www.canceradvocacy.org/resources/publications/.
74. http://www.cancerlegalresourcecenter.org/.
75. http://www.childhoodbraintumor.org/index.php/services.html.
76. Harrison v Aetna U.S. Healthcare, Inc., No. 2000CV194–69 (GA. Super. Ct., filed February 16, 2000).
77. http://www.statehealthfacts.org/comparecat.jsp?cat=7&rgn=6&rgn=1. Accessed June 24, 2010.
78. http://www.hipaa.org/.
79. http://www.genome.gov/24519851.
80. http://edocket.access.gpo.gov/2009/pdf/E9-22504.pdf. Accessed June 24, 2010.
81. http://www.dol.gov/dol/topic/health-plans/cobra.htm.
82. http://www.dol.gov/ebsa/cobra.html.
83. http://www.dol.gov/ebsa/compliance_assistance.html. Accessed june 24, 2010.
84. See Kirk T. v Housoun, HLD 27(12) 77–78 (December 1999), Docket No. CIV. A. 99–3253, 1999 WL 820201 (E.D. PA. Sept. 28, 1999); and Commissioner v TakeCare Health Plan, Inc. No. 933–0290, OAH No. N9412060, Decision of Administrative Law Judge Ruth S. Astle, accepted by Commissioner Keith Paul Bishop on October 29, 1996 (Department of Corporations, State of California, San Francisco).
85. See Nealy v U.S. Healthcare HMO, NY, 93 N.Y.2d 209, 711 N.E. 2d 621, 689 NYS 2d 406 (NY 1999), failure to expedite member's transfer to specialty center; Pappas v Asbel, 724 A.2d 889 (PA 1998), petition for cert. filed, 67 U.S.LW 3717 (May 13, 1999) (No. 98- 1836); and Mecca v PacifiCare of California, Inc., 87 Cal. Rtr. 2d. 784 (Cal. Ct. App 1999).
86. http://aappolicy.aappublications.org/cgi/content/full/pediatrics;107/4/790.
87. http://www.socialsecurity.gov/compassionateallowances/conditions.htm.
88. http://idea.ed.gov/.
89. http://www.ed.gov/about/offices/list/ocr/504faq.html.
90. http://www.nichcy.org/Pages/Home.aspx.
91. http://www.dol.gov/whd/fmla/index.htm
92. Flowers v Southern Reg"l Physician Servs., Inc., No. 99–31343, 2001 WL 314603 (5th Cir. Mar. 30, 2001).
93. Tice v Centre Area Transp. Auth., No. 00–1753 (3d Cir. Apr. 23, 2001).
94. Heath Resource Center. http://www.heath.gwu.edu/.
95. U.S. Department of Defense Directive No. 6130, March 31, 1986, physical standards for enlistment, appointment, and induction.

CHAPTER 52 ■ COMPLEMENTARY AND ALTERNATIVE MEDICAL THERAPIES IN PEDIATRIC ONCOLOGY

THOMAS W. MCLEAN AND KATHI J. KEMPER

INTRODUCTION

Clinicians confront a variety of questions about integrating complementary and alternative medical therapies with their ongoing oncology care:

- What kinds of complementary therapies might my patients be using, and how do I find out?
- How do I answer a parent's question about boosting the immune system with natural products?
- What are the potential risks and benefits of combining complementary and alternative medicine (CAM) and conventional treatments?
- How can I find a massage therapist or acupuncturist who can help my patients relax and have less anxiety and pain?
- What natural approaches can a family use to help reduce the child's side effects and optimize their overall health?
- Where do I turn for reliable, evidence-based information about complementary therapies?
- How can I help patients distinguish between legitimate and "quack" therapies?

Understandably, families want to do everything they can to help their child recover from cancer and to reduce their future health risks. Physicians need solid scientific evidence to provide comprehensive advice. We need to able to elicit a complete history of the different therapies families are considering (or are already using) for their child, understand basic information about CAM practices and CAM providers, and know where to turn for additional information. This chapter provides an overview of CAM in pediatric oncology. Other chapters in this text cover closely related topics such as nutrition (Chapter 41), symptom management (Chapter 42), psychosocial support (Chapter 45), and ethical considerations (Chapter 46).

DEFINITIONS

Complementary therapies are used *in conjunction with* mainstream medical therapies. Examples include dietary supplements, massage, guided imagery, biofeedback, and hypnosis. These therapies are not replacements for medical regimens for serious medical problems but are offered to support the patient and family. *Alternative* medicine refers to therapies used *in place of* mainstream medical therapies; for example, using prayer or spiritual healing to replace chemotherapy. *Folk medicine* refers to therapies that are provided as part of a family or cultural tradition. Examples include chicken soup for upper respiratory tract infections and "cold" foods for "hot" illnesses. The term *CAM* is used by the National Institutes of Health's (NIH's) National Center for Complementary and Alternative Medicine, but is being replaced in the popular media and some professional organizations (such as the Consortium of Academic Health Centers for Integrative Medicine) by the terms *holistic and integrative medicine*.

Holistic medicine refers to care of the whole patient—body, mind, emotions, spirit, and relationships—in the context of the patient's values, beliefs, family, culture, and community. *Integrative medicine* refers to health care that focuses on wellness and health promotion, combining complementary or folk remedies with mainstream therapies on the basis of scientific evidence in the context of patient- and family-centered comprehensive care. Families who use complementary therapies (prayer, massage, dietary changes, and guided imagery) along with chemotherapy are using an integrated approach.

EPIDEMIOLOGY

Approximately one in nine American children and adolescents use CAM; use is higher in clinical populations and among children with chronic, recurrent, or incurable condition.[1] Because cancer is life-threatening, clinicians caring for pediatric oncology patients are likely to encounter CAM use more frequently than do general pediatricians.[2] CAM use by pediatric oncology patients has been reported from many countries and cultures.[3–15] Geography and culture play important roles in CAM prevalence and types. For example, the most commonly reported CAM therapies in pediatric oncology include prayer/spiritual healing in the southeastern United States,[3] Traditional Chinese Medicines (TCMs) in Taiwan,[6] homeopathy in Germany,[8] herbs in Mexico,[10] stinging nettle in Turkey,[12] and water therapy in Malaysia.[11] Some studies, but not all, have associated CAM use with older patient age, poor prognosis, use of CAM by a parent or other family member, longer time since diagnosis, and higher parental education level. Religious families were more likely to use CAM in one study from the United States,[3] whereas nonreligious families were more likely to use CAM in another study from Israel.[9] The use of CAM use by children with cancer ranges from 21% to 84% depending on definitions of CAM and how the questions are asked (Table 52.1). CAM use is also common in adult survivors of pediatric cancer, often to alleviate long-term symptoms from the cancer or its treatment.[16]

Studies consistently report that many patients and families do not report CAM use spontaneously, so clinicians should inquire routinely about all the therapies patients are using. Many pediatric oncologists, however, do not ask about CAM use, primarily because of a lack of time and knowledge.[18] In addition, few institutions, state agencies, and professional organizations have policies regarding the use of CAM in children.[19,20] Many patients use more than one CAM therapy but

TABLE 52.1

PREVALENCE OF MOST FREQUENTLY USED CAM THERAPIES IN PEDIATRIC ONCOLOGY

CAM therapy	Prevalence (%)
Prayer	10–87
Relaxation/imagery	15–75
Dietary supplements	4–73
Herbal medicines/teas	9–69
Massage	7–66
Megavitamins/minerals	8–59
Special diet	3–49
Therapeutic touch	0–42
Lifestyle/exercise	16–37
Homeopathy	2–25
Chiropractic	1–20
Chinese medicines	0–20
Topical therapies	0–17
Spiritual healing	5–16
Energy healing	3–16
Hypnotherapy	0–15
Miscellaneous	7–10
Naturopathic medicine	5–8
Aromatherapy	0–6
Acupuncture	0–1
Biofeedback	0–1
Overall prevalence (all types)	*21–87*

CAM, complementary and alternative medicine.
Sources of statistics[3–7,9,10,12–15,17].
Note: No study assessed the prevalence of every treatment listed here, and definitions varied between studies.

may not consider their use of this therapy as "CAM." For example, many families pray, give back rubs, or drink herbal teas without thinking of these as CAM remedies. Prayer, mind-body therapies (MBTs) (such as relaxation and guided imagery), dietary supplements (including vitamins, minerals, and herbs), and massage are the most commonly used in North America.

Patients' and Families' Reasons for Using Complementary and Alternative Medicine

Families seek therapies that are consistent with their values and culture and seek care from therapists who respect them as individuals and who offer them time and attention. Patients prize the care they receive from compassionate, comprehensive, empathetic clinicians who provide individualized care. They seek additional information on healthy lifestyle choices, dietary supplements, music, aromatherapy, and other strategies over which they may exert some control and that may enhance the child's resilience and reduce side effects of treatment. Families who use CAM therapies rarely abandon mainstream care, and they value the opinion of knowledgeable physicians regarding the safety and efficacy of a variety of products and therapies.

Mainstream and complementary therapies tend to emphasize different primary outcomes or goals. Mainstream therapies are geared toward specific, problem-oriented outcomes such as curing the cancer, managing symptoms, and preventing specific problems (such as secondary infections). Many complementary therapies, on the other hand, promote the

patient's overall well-being and resilience, and thereby improving symptoms. While many mainstream physicians attend to patients' global goals for health promotion, and many complementary therapists treat specific symptoms, this simplified dichotomy may be helpful in understanding families' rationale for seeking different kinds of care.

Few children take supplements to prevent primary tumors. However, children who have one malignancy are at increased risk of later developing other malignancies, and as these children grow older, they may be interested in taking supplements to reduce their subsequent risks. Common and well-accepted cancer risk factors in adults include tobacco use, excessive alcohol use, excessive sun exposure, poor nutrition, obesity, physical inactivity, some infections (human papilloma virus, hepatitis B), and unsafe sex.[21,22] These well-established risk factors should definitely be avoided by patients hoping to avoid secondary malignancies.

Conventional therapies for children with cancer may be arduous and often have debilitating side effects. Treatment complications are accepted by most families because they are optimistic that standard treatments will cure the cancer. However, as treatments affect the child's quality of life, many parents look toward other therapies to help the child feel better. The most common reasons for CAM use include doing everything possible, to help with symptom management, to boost the immune system, and also to treat or cure the cancer itself.[23] If conventional therapies are unsuccessful, parents often begin searching for any therapy that might offer hope of a cure.[24]

Talking with Patients and Families

The primary reason that families do not communicate about their use of CAM therapies is that they are not asked. It is important for physicians to initiate discussions in a systematic fashion. The American Academy of Pediatrics (AAP) has published guidelines for counseling families who choose CAM therapies (Table 52.2).[1,25] Clinicians should assess the patients'/family's goals, types of therapies under consideration, source of recommendations and information, the family's opinion about and experience with it, and their interest in learning more or pursuing the therapy. For example, families may be most interested in efficacy, safety, cost, insurance reimbursement, or the names of reputable products or practitioners. Exploring the family's sense of expected end points of therapy and the timeline for achieving their goals can aid in developing realistic expectations and contingency plans.

Having a ready supply of patient information materials about the more commonly used therapies and therapists is valuable in addressing common concerns and helping patients distinguish between evidence-based and market-driven therapies. The AAP has published a brochure for families about complementary and integrative medicine; the pamphlet encourages families to talk with their clinician about all the therapies they are using.* Additional evidence-based resources are listed in Table 52.3. It is also helpful to collaborate with hospital and oncology center librarians, pharmacists, and nutritionists. There may be additional resources within the

---

*Posters to encourage families to talk with their clinician about CAM are available from the NIH NCCAM, http://nccam.nih.gov/timetotalk/; the Canadian Pediatric Society, http://www.pedcam.ca/index. php?resources; and the American Academy of Pediatrics Section for Complementary and Integrative Medicine, http://www.aap.org/sections/CHIM/ClinicianResources.html. The AAP also has a patient brochure on CAM: http://www.aap.org/healthtopics/complementarymedicine.cfm.

TABLE 52.2

COUNSELING FAMILIES WHO CHOOSE AN INTEGRATIVE APPROACH TO CANCER CARE[a]

1. Ask families systematically about different therapies the patient may be using. Use examples when possible. Rather than asking about "alternative" therapies, the clinician should ask about the use of "vitamins, herbs, supplements, teas, homemade remedies, back rubs, chiropractic, acupuncture, or other services" to enhance health. It is also useful to ask how the patient manages stress; examples may include exercise, prayer, music, or talking with friends or trusted adults.
2. Identify the health goals of the patient and family.
3. Be sensitive to and respectful of families' values, culture, and education level. Do not be dismissive about their interest in complementary therapies or folk remedies. Be empathetic and listen actively.
4. Recognize feelings of being threatened and guard against becoming defensive or confrontational.
5. Seek information from reliable sources about the therapies of interest.
6. Evaluate scientific merits of specific therapies for specific problems or specific outcomes. Do not "lump" all complementary therapies or all goals together. Herbs are not equivalent to massage. The goal of cure is not the same as a goal of knowing one has explored all reasonable options to help.
7. Identify risks or potential harmful effects including interactions with medications.
8. Provide information to families about a range of options including common use, evidence of benefits, and evidence of risk.
9. Regardless of the family's choices, offer to assist in monitoring and evaluating the response to treatment.
10. If feasible (and with the permission of the family) coordinate care of CAM providers in the overall care of the patient.

CAM, complementary and alternative medicine.
[a]Modified from Kemper KJ, Vohra S, Walls R; American Academy of Pediatrics. The use of complementary and alternative medicine in pediatrics. Pediatrics 2008;122(6):1374–1386; and Committee on Children with Disabilities. American Academy of Pediatrics: Counseling families who choose complementary and alternative medicine for their child with chronic illness or disability. Committee on Children With Disabilities. Pediatrics 2001;107(3):598–601.

TABLE 52.3

EVIDENCE-BASED INTERNET RESOURCES

American Academy of Pediatrics	Section on Complementary and Integrative Medicine http://www.aap.org/sections/CHIM/default.cfm
CAHCIM	Consortium of Academic Health Centers for Integrative Medicine http://www.imconsortium.org/home.html
Academic sites	M.D. Anderson Cancer Center site Complementary and Integrative Medicine Educational Resources: http://www.mdanderson.org/departments/cimer/ Memorial Sloan Kettering Information about Herbs, Botanicals and Other Products: http://www.mskcc.org/mskcc/html/11570.cfm Wake Forest University School of Medicine site, BestHealth: http://www.besthealth.com/cam/ Consortium of Academic Health Centers for Integrative Medicine http://www.imconsortium.org/
Government sites	National Cancer Institute's page on Complementary and Alternative Medicine: http://www3.cancer.gov/occam/ National Center for Complementary and Alternative Medicine: http://www.nccam.nih.gov/ National Library of Medicine page on dietary supplements and complementary medicine: http://www.nlm.nih.gov/services/dietsup.html NIH Office of Dietary Supplements http://ods.od.nih.gov/
Other nonprofit sites	The American Cancer Society – complementary and alternative therapies http://www.cancer.org/docroot/ETO/ETO_5.asp?sitearea=ETO Cancer Treatment Centers of America, Cancer Source Internet site, featuring Complementary and Integrative Medicine information pages http://www.cancercenter.com/cancer-treatments.cfm
Subscription information	ConsumerLab, independent testing of the quality of herbal and dietary supplement products: www.consumerlab.com Natural Medicine Comprehensive Database, produced by the publishers of Prescriber's Letter. Very comprehensive: http://www.naturaldatabase.com/

institution, such as nurses or physical therapists who practice massage or therapeutic touch (TT). Families have far more respect for a physician whose response to a question about an alternative therapy is "I don't know, but I'll do my best to find out to help your child," than to a physician who ignores, disparages, or dismisses their questions.

By better understanding the patient and family viewpoints, experiences, and expectations and by anticipating common questions and informational needs about specific treatments, the physician can offer better advice in a focused, efficient manner. Even after learning about a family's particular interest in complementary therapy, it is wise to step back and ask in a systematic fashion about all the other therapies the family may have considered before rushing in to offer advice. Frequently, the initial question raised by the family (e.g., Do you know a massage therapist who is skilled in working with children?) is a way of testing the waters of physician empathy and knowledge before raising questions about more challenging or sensitive issues.

Families facing a crisis may be more susceptible to testimonials, misleading claims, and quackery than do other families. The Internet can introduce families to deceptive claims, but it also is a rich source of evidence-based guidelines.[26–28] The resources included here (Table 52.3) should prove helpful to health care providers and families.

CAM THERAPIES

The types and number of potential therapies available to patients and promoted in the media can be overwhelming. It is helpful to use written forms to collect information systematically and to request families to bring all the medications and other remedies they are using to appointments so that they can be reviewed. It is essential to have a systematic approach when considering the potential risks and benefits of different therapies. Therapeutic options may be considered in four major categories: (a) biochemical, (b) lifestyle, (c) biomechanical, and (d) bioenergetic, which are distinguished by their purported mechanism of action or traditional use. Each of these major categories has several subcategories, some that may be considered mainstream and others that may be considered complementary, depending on cultural circumstances and definitions (Table 52.4). For example, within the general category of biochemical therapies are medications (both prescription and nonprescription), herbs, vitamins, and other dietary supplements. The quality and quantity of evidence about the different biochemical therapies varies, but the purported mechanism of action (biochemical effects) is similar. Preclinical evidence based on *in vitro* data does not always correlate to *in vivo* efficacy. Some therapies such as hydrazine sulfate, laetrile, and others have been disproven in good quality clinical trials.[29]

Lifestyle therapies include nutrition, exercise, sleep, stress management, and promoting healthy relationships and envi-

ronments. Biomechanical therapies include diverse treatments whose mechanism of action includes some mechanical effect; these include surgery, physical therapy, massage, and joint or soft tissue manipulation. Bioenergetic therapies are also diverse, but similar in terms of their belief in the relationship between a powerful invisible spirit (God) or life energy (chi) and health; these therapies include prayer, acupuncture, Reiki, TT, and homeopathy.

BIOCHEMICAL THERAPIES

Vitamins, minerals, herbs, hormones (such as melatonin), and other dietary supplements are commonly used natural products. One factor complicating care in this area is the dynamic and ever-changing nature of the therapies families are using as a result of information technology, economic forces, and popular culture. Oncology patients, desperate for a cure or "natural" therapy to complement conventional therapy, are particularly vulnerable to marketing claims of efficacy. Reliable sources of information are vital to address patient questions. Table 52.3 lists reliable, evidence-based sources of information.[28]

This section focuses on a few examples of the herbs and supplements used to (a) prevent cancer, (b) treat cancer itself, (c) treat/prevent symptoms and side effects of cancer therapy, and (d) those that may be contraindicated due to their toxicity and/or have been disproven. Several review articles explore the use of dietary supplements in the prevention and treatment of cancer. However, relatively little research has been done to rigorously assess their safety and efficacy for pediatric oncology patients. The vast majority of studies evaluating the efficacy and safety of these therapies may not apply to pediatric patients. Of note, even for randomized clinical trials published in the medical literature, caution must be exerted because most have not confirmed the quality of the supplement tested.[30]

Herbs and dietary supplements are among the most commonly used complementary therapy in pediatric oncology patients, with reported prevalence rates as high as 69%.[10] However, in many instances (up to 55%) parents administer CAM therapies to their children unbeknownst to the child's physician.[31]

This section focuses on a few examples of the herbs and supplements purported to prevent or treat cancer or to ameliorate the side effects of cancer therapy. Rather than a comprehensive review of each therapy, an overview of those therapies pertinent to pediatric oncology will be provided. Each of the natural compounds reviewed has several dietary sources, mechanisms of action, molecular targets, and potential interactions with other compounds.[32,33] Many are being actively investigated in clinical trials (www.clinicaltrials.gov).

Supplements Used to Prevent Cancer

Green tea, made from the dried leaves of *Camellia sinensis*, has long been used as a beverage in cultures worldwide, particularly in Asia. Tea polyphenols such as epigallocatechin-3-gallate induce apoptosis in some tumor cells and inhibit angiogenesis. Other *in vitro* actions that could potentially contribute to tea's cancer protective effects include antioxidation, inhibition of lipid peroxidation, and inhibition of transcription factors such as NK-kB.[33] Although several studies have suggested that the consumption of green tea may reduce the risk of some solid tumors in adults, when taken together the evidence for the role of green tea consumption in preventing cancer is insufficient and conflicting.[34] Green tea is generally safe when consumed as a beverage, although excessive intake may lead to caffeine-related toxicity or hepatotoxicity.[35]

TABLE 52.4

SYSTEMATIC APPROACH TO INQUIRING ABOUT PATIENTS' THERAPIES

1. Biochemical therapies
   Medications (prescription and nonprescription)
   Herbs (such as medicinal mushrooms, milk thistle, Essiac)
   Vitamins, minerals, and other dietary supplements (such as vitamin D, ginger, curcumin, Coenzyme Q_{10})
2. Lifestyle therapies
   Diet (such as macrobiotic)
   Exercise/rest (such as yoga, tai chi)
   Environmental therapies— music/quiet, light, aromas, colors, art, heat, cold
   Mind-body therapies (such as guided imagery, biofeedback, psychotherapy, meditation)
3. Biomechanical therapies
   Surgery
   Massage or other bodywork
   Spinal adjustments or joint adjustments through Chiropractic or Osteopathy
4. Bioenergetic therapies
   Acupuncture, acupressure
   Therapeutic or healing touch, Reiki, Qigong
   Prayer, religious, or spiritual healing or rituals
   Homeopathic remedies

Garlic and its constituents have properties that may help prevent certain adult cancers such as those arising in the prostate, colon, esophagus, and other sites.[36] Onions, leeks, shallots, and chives are other *Allium vegetables* that are widely consumed and may have similar chemopreventive properties although they have been studied less extensively than garlic. Garlic may cause bad breath and body odor, and excessive amounts may cause gastrointestinal symptoms. An antiplatelet effect could potentially increase bleeding risk of patients with thrombocytopenia or on anticoagulation.[37,38] Otherwise, the consumption of garlic (and other Allium vegetables) is not known to cause any adverse effects.

The polyphenol *resveratrol* is found in grape seeds, skins, juice, and red wine, and to a lesser extent in white wine, mulberries, and peanuts; the richest source is the root of *Polygonum cuspidatum*, which is used in traditional Chinese and Japanese medicine. Resveratrol has antioxidant, antitumor, antimutagenic, antiangiogenesis, and proapoptotic activity.[32,39,40] Resveratrol has some antiplatelet effects and could theoretically interact with anticoagulant or antiplatelet medications, but side effects are rare.

Dietary supplements with *multivitamins and minerals* are commonly used. The AAP recommends iron and vitamin D to prevent iron deficiency and rickets, but it is unknown if they have cancer preventing properties in children. In adults, vitamin D levels inversely correlate with the incidence of cancer of the colon, breast, prostate, and ovaries, suggesting that vitamin D supplementation may help prevent these cancers.[41] Because vitamin D can be synthesized by the skin in response to ultraviolet light, controversy has developed regarding the optimal amount and source of vitamin D (dietary vs. sun exposure).[42] As of 2008, the AAP recommends that infants have a minimum daily intake of at least 400 IU vitamin D daily beginning soon after birth and continuing through adolescence.[43] Similar to vitamin D, calcium may reduce the risk of incidence of colorectal cancer in adults.[44]

Most trials designed to assess cancer prevention by supplementation have not shown any benefit with the possible exception of selenium supplementation in men.[45,46] In one epidemiologic study in children, supplemental vitamin administration was associated with an increased risk of leukemia.[47] Supplemental synthetic vitamin E, vitamin A, and beta-carotene do not appear to prevent cancer and in fact may be dangerous for certain patients.[48–50] Vitamin C has long been used to treat numerous conditions, and it remains one of the most popular vitamin supplements. Controversy about the efficacy of vitamin C in preventing and treating cancer persists despite a lack of clear evidence to date.[51]

The consumption of soy products that contain the phytoestrogen genistein has been linked epidemiologically to decreased rates of some cancers.[32,52] Although soy products may be beneficial to cardiovascular and overall health, isolated soy protein supplements have not been shown to effectively prevent or treat cancer of the breast, endometrium, and prostate.[53] Other natural compounds with cancer-preventing properties *in vitro* include curcumin, luteolin, pomegranate, lycopene, ellagic acid, terpenes, n-3 polyunsaturated fatty acids, and ginkgolide B.[32,33]

Supplements Used to Augment the Effectiveness of Standard Chemotherapy or Radiation

Although it is most commonly used as a sleeping aid, *melatonin* has been studied in higher doses (10 to 50 mg) as an adjunctive therapy for adults with solid tumors. Melatonin appears to be helpful for some adult patients with metastatic disease in reducing chemotherapy-associated toxicities including cachexia, neuropathies, and anemia. It may prevent or treat cancer by several mechanisms including apoptosis, inhibiting angiogenesis, and augmenting NK cell activity.[54–56] Side effects are usually mild but may include sleepiness, headache, depression, mild tremor, confusion, nausea, vomiting, and hypotension. Theoretically, melatonin may enhance the effects of sedative and immunosuppressive medications.

Curcumin is a polyphenol from the root of *Curcuma longa*, commonly called turmeric and has long been used in Asian medicine to treat a number of ailments. Research has generated *in vitro* data about curcumin's anticancer properties. Its effects appear to stem from multiple mechanisms of action.[57] Turmeric also suppresses the proliferation of a wide variety of tumor cells, downregulates transcription factors, downregulates growth factor receptors, and functions as an antioxidant and anti-inflammatory agent.[58] Human studies of turmeric's cancer prevention and treatment efficacy are still in progress. Curcumin (turmeric) is widely used as a kitchen spice and has few side effects.

There are hundreds of *mushroom* species with purported immunomodulating and antitumor properties. Among the medicinal mushrooms are the Coriolus, Cordyceps, Maitake, Reishi, and Shiitake. Multiple mechanisms of action have been proposed on the basis of *in vitro* data.[59] Because mushrooms are often consumed as a food, side effects are generally mild but may include upset stomach, diarrhea, eosinophilia, allergies, and rash. Despite mushrooms' popularity and potential for the prevention and treatment of cancer and other conditions, limited data exist for children.

Antineoplastons are peptides and amino acid derivatives originally isolated from human blood and urine and are controversial cancer therapies. Several phase II trials involving pediatric patients with brain tumors have been published[60,61]; however, no phase III controlled trials utilizing antineoplastons in children have yet been published.

Essiac is a combination of several herbs (burdock, sheep's sorrel, medicinal rhubarb, and slippery elm bark), widely sold in the United States and Canada as an alternative cancer treatment. *In vitro* studies show cytotoxic effects against cancer cell lines.[62] Although high doses of its constituent herbs may be toxic, there are few reports of serious toxicity from Essiac itself. There are no randomized controlled trials suggesting that it is effective for any type of cancer.

Cat's claw (*Uncaria tomentosa*) extracts are popular in some countries. Studies of the *in vitro* effects of *U. tomentosa* are contradictory. Some data suggest that it has antiproliferative and apoptotic effects,[63] whereas other data suggest that it may stimulate leukemia cells to grow.[64] There are no published clinical trials demonstrating its effectiveness. Several herbs go by the name cat's claw, which increases the risk of misidentification/misuse, and toxicities have been reported.

Dietary Supplements to Help Manage Side Effects of Chemotherapy and Radiation

Ginger tea; candied ginger; and dried, powdered ginger are widely used to prevent and treat nausea and also used as a mild systemic anti-inflammatory agent. Randomized controlled trials in adults suggest it may be helpful in preventing nausea in early pregnancy, postoperative nausea, and chemotherapy-associated nausea, although some studies have found no benefit.[65] *In vitro*, ginger extracts inhibit thromboxane generation and platelet aggregation in a dose-dependent fashion. However, no clinically significant anticoagulant effects have been documented.

Coenzyme Q$_{10}$ (CoQ$_{10}$ or ubiquinone) is an antioxidant that purportedly protects the heart from anthracycline-induced cardiotoxicity. It is also used to ameliorate liver toxicity from cancer therapy, but its efficacy remains controversial and rigorous trials have not been conducted.[66] Few serious side effects have been reported.

Multivitamin/antioxidant use is common, although in theory antioxidants could counteract the cytotoxic effects of radiation therapy and some chemotherapy. Preliminary data suggest supplemental vitamins may reduce toxicities,[67,68] but more research is needed. Vitamin A deficiency in children with cancer may increase the risk of febrile neutropenia.[69] Supplementation with vitamin C, vitamin E, and selenium may decrease high-frequency hearing loss caused by cisplatin.[70]

Selenium is an essential mineral that has antioxidant properties; it is an important constituent of the enzyme glutathione peroxidase. Supplementation with selenium appears to help moderate the acute toxic effects of chemotherapy in adults and has also been shown to reduce the risk of prostate and gastrointestinal cancers.[48,71] Selenium deficiency is common among newly diagnosed pediatric cancer patients;[72] however, there are no studies evaluating its role as an adjunctive therapy. Food sources of selenium include fish, shellfish, red meat, grains, eggs, chicken, and garlic. Vegetables, such as broccoli, can also be a good source if grown in selenium-rich soils.

Milk thistle (*Silybinum marianum*) is an herbal remedy that has been shown in some adult studies to protect the liver and kidneys from chemotherapy toxicity.[73,74] Clinical trials are ongoing. Milk thistle is generally well tolerated; the most commonly adverse effects are a mild laxative effect and gastrointestinal upset.

In TCM, *ginseng* is included in many herbal tonic mixtures to restore vitality and reduce inflammation.[75] Ginseng has not undergone substantial research as an adjunctive therapy for oncology patients. There are several species of ginseng with slightly different effects. Panax ginseng is usually well tolerated, but insomnia, nausea, vomiting, and diarrhea have been reported; it may also increase the hypoglycemic effect of insulin and sulfonylureas, and possibly antagonize the effects of anticoagulants and interact with monoamine oxidase inhibitors.

Other Popular CAM Therapies

Noni juice is in part derived from various components of *Morinda citrifolia*, a tree found in Polynesia. Parts of the noni tree have long been used as herbal remedies for various conditions, and noni juice is a relatively popular complementary cancer therapy. *In vitro* and animal studies suggest that noni juice may have antitumor effects directly and also by stimulating the host's immune system.[76] No controlled trials have yet been conducted in humans, however. Similarly, *mangosteen juice* is currently marketed as an effective health-promoting product, but no data exist regarding its use in the oncology setting. Laetrile, a popular CAM therapy in the 1970s, has little to no evidence that it has beneficial effects for cancer patients.[77] Studies of shark cartilage have also shown no benefit.[78]

Toxicities and Other Risks

Side effects of various CAM therapies, including allergic reaction, are well known. Many products from developing countries, such as Ayurvedic medicines and traditional Chinese herbal combinations may be contaminated by other ingredients such as lead, mercury, arsenic, pesticides, and insecticides.[79-81] In addition, there are potential adverse interactions between natural health products and conventional medicines, including chemotherapy.[82,83] More worrisome is *in vitro* evidence that some herbs may actually promote proliferation of leukemia cells rather than kill them.[64] Practical strategies and algorithms have been devised that help practitioners, together with families, make informed decisions about combining CAM therapies with conventional treatments.[83-85]

LIFESTYLE THERAPIES

Diet

The vast majority of families ask their oncologist if any special food can benefit the patient during therapy. In one study of pediatric oncology patients, almost half of all respondents implemented dietary changes including increasing fruit and vegetable consumption, switching to organic foods, reducing fat intake, eliminating red meat, and adding specific foods to the diet.[17] Families frequently consult alternative health care providers, relatives, friends, neighbors, salespersons, books, and the Internet about specific diets.

It has been estimated that approximately 30% of adult cancers in developed counties are associated with dietary factors. In particular, obesity and excess alcohol consumption increase the risk of many adult cancers. In contrast, a diet rich in fruits and vegetables is almost certainly protective for some cancers.[86] There is evidence that breast feeding may reduce the risk of some childhood malignancies.[87-89] Thus, dietary factors are important in preventing certain cancers and may be helpful to a child's overall health, but there are no data that specific dietary changes can treat or cure pediatric cancer. Restrictive diets that limit intake of essential nutrients can be dangerous.[90]

Several dietary programs have been widely used to treat adults suffering from cancer. Generally, the diets are just one part of comprehensive lifestyle programs for adult cancer patients. Four such programs are the Block nutritional program, Gerson therapy, Livingston-Wheeler regimen, and macrobiotics. The Gerson and Livingston-Wheeler regimens also include coffee enemas and dietary supplements. Nearly all of these diets are low in fat; high in complex carbohydrates, fruits, and vegetables; and devoid of sugar, fats, and oils. Severe dietary restrictions run the risk of vitamin and mineral deficiencies, caloric deprivation, and reduced quality of life. For example, the restrictive forms of macrobiotic diets have been associated with cases of scurvy, anemia, and hypoproteinemia. Although there are numerous testimonials and case reports about the effectiveness of these diets in adult oncology patients, they have not been evaluated in pediatric patients.

Other diets used to promote cardiovascular health, lose weight, and avoid other adult health problems may also be adopted by families looking for healthy lifestyle approaches and for cancer treatment. These include low-fat (high carbohydrate), low-carbohydrate (high protein/fat), high-fiber, vegetarian, vegan, macrobiotic, and Mediterranean diets.[91] It is well recognized that pediatric oncology survivors are at risk for second malignant neoplasms (as a result of underlying genetic- and therapy-related factors). Although the consumption of particular foods has not been shown to reduce this risk, it is prudent to recommend a balanced diet with plenty of fruits and vegetables and little processed food or fast food. Fruits and vegetables provide vitamins, minerals, and fiber that may reduce subsequent cancer risk, and minimizing processed and fast foods helps combat obesity, a condition associated with an increased risk of certain cancers as well as other diseases.[86]

Diets rich in calcium and vitamin D may also help promote skeletal health, which is adversely affected by therapy in patients with acute lymphoblastic leukemia, Wilms' tumor, and some brain tumors.[92-95] To prevent weight loss during conventional therapy, drinking a protein and energy dense nutritional supplement containing eicosapentaenoic acid, an omega-3 fatty acid, appears effective.[96] Although controversial, no dietary restrictions have been proven to be protective for patients who have neutropenia.[97]

The approach to nutritional care in pediatric oncology varies widely.[98] Specific guidelines for children with cancer have been published by the AAP.[99] Pediatric oncology patients often need aggressive nutritional support, and in selected cases consultation with a pediatric dietitian may be helpful.

Exercise

Although exercise is an important part of a healthy child's life, physical activity in children with cancer may be limited by fatigue, pain, concerns about trauma/bleeding, altered neurological or limb function, feelings of self-consciousness, or diminished strength and endurance. Studies have documented an association between physical activity/exercise and improved psychological outcomes, including reduced depression and anxiety. Although intense exercise temporarily lowers NK cell activity, regular moderate physical exercise is associated with reduced rates of cancer and enhanced NK cytotoxicity. The interaction between exercise, immunity, and psychological effects are complex. For patients at risk of exercise-associated complications, exercise recommendations should be individualized. For cancer patients in general, however, the benefits of exercise far outweigh the risks.[100]

For patients receiving conventional cancer therapy, moderate exercise improves a number of symptoms, most notably physical function and fatigue.[101-103] Survivors of childhood cancer have reduced physical fitness compared with healthy control subjects, and these patients should be encouraged to exercise regularly.[104,105] A study in children with acute lymphoblastic leukemia showed benefits of a physical therapy and exercise intervention.[106] Similarly, studies in cancer survivors (mostly adults) suggest that exercise after completion of therapy improves functional capacity, fatigue ,and immune function, and lowers the percentage of body fat.[102,107,108] Exercise, along with adequate calcium and vitamin D, can help prevent and treat osteoporosis in children with cancer.[93,109]

There has also been a growing interest in Eastern meditative exercises such as yoga, tai chi, and chi kung (Qigong), and their potential therapeutic influences on chronic illnesses such as asthma and cancer. In adults, yoga and Qigong classes are popular and beneficial in terms of patients' self-evaluation of energy levels, stress reduction, more restful sleep, and sense of well-being. Because these exercises can be done slowly and noncompetitively and can be practiced in a group or individually at home, they may be useful for children in various stages of cancer therapy. Walking is perhaps the easiest and one of the safest exercises to perform. Its benefits are far reaching and it can be done with other family members or friends for additive benefits.[110]

Environment

Although oncologists pay close attention to the microbial aspects of the environment, particularly for patients undergoing transplants, patients experience a broad range of environmental influences as helpful or stressful. Boredom and depression commonly follow exposure to isolation and extremely restricted environments. A team meeting in consultation with the family, child life specialists, psychologists, social workers, clergy, and nursing staff may be helpful in anticipating and planning to meet the child's needs for appropriate and helpful stimulation and distraction during a prolonged hospitalization. Developing routines and a predictable schedule during hospitalization may help a child feel a greater sense of control in the face of an overwhelming disease. Medical and nursing routines may need to be modified to meet the child's needs for uninterrupted quiet and rest. One study highlighted the importance of minimizing noise to help hospitalized patients sleep. Interventions such as closing doors, moving the location of nursing reports, lowering monitor volumes, and using flashlights instead of overhead lights can all promote better sleep.[111]

Families may also be interested in a variety of other environmental strategies to help the child feel more comfortable during treatment. Most of these approaches rely on common sense and attention to individual preferences. Bright or dim lights; bright, pastel, or neutral colors; posters, photographs, and other visual art; sounds, music, and television; video games, books, and homework; aromatherapies and/or avoidance of noxious odors; crystals and magnets; hot and cold packs; and favorite pillows, blankets, and other objects can all contribute to comfort (when they fit with the child's perceived needs) or on the other hand to stress (when there is poor fit with the child's needs). Modifying patients' environments by the methods mentioned above generally entail few risks and modest costs. The benefits may be significant not only for the patients, but also for their families.

Music therapy has well-recognized benefits in the palliative care setting. For hospitalized adult oncology patients, music therapy reduces pain and mood disturbance, improves relaxation, and reduces anxiety, and for outpatient pediatric oncology patients music promotes relaxation.[112] Live music, ideally provided by music therapists, has been shown to be more effective than recorded music.[113,114] Although no randomized clinical trials have been performed in pediatric oncology patients, interactive music therapy has been shown to have a positive effect on the well-being of these patients, and music is well received by their parents.[115] Even in the absence of trained music therapists, recruiting skilled musicians or providing recorded music for patients may be beneficial.

Although evidence of biologic plausibility is limited, static and electromagnetic therapies have been evaluated for a number of conditions, most of which involve musculoskeletal pain. Results have been mixed to date,[116] and trials have not yet been done in pediatric oncology patients.

Mind-Body

In the past two decades, there has been increasing attention to the interaction between psychological states and somatic function. MBTs encompass a broad range of practices including relaxation techniques, meditation, guided imagery, hypnosis, and biofeedback; individual and group psychotherapy; and other support groups and psychosocial interventions. MBTs are designed to positively affect patients' emotional states, coping skills, and physical symptoms, that is, their morbidity rather than mortality. MBTs can positively affect patients' perceptions of symptoms including anxiety, depression, mood, quality of life, coping, nausea/vomiting, and pain.[117-119] Hypnosis and music therapy may be helpful in minimizing acute procedural pain in children, but more research is needed.[120,121]

The perception of social support also has a clear impact on the adjustment process, and studies have shown favorable effects of support groups for patients and families.[122,123] One study of adolescents showed a high need for information (especially on paper), face-to-face peer social support, and self-management therapy (preferably with the aid of a therapist), and that these needs are often not met.[124] Other studies have confirmed a relatively poor rate of referral or recommendation for cancer support services and other nonpharmacologic strategies. In addition to the patient, support groups for parents and siblings of children with cancer may enhance their own psychological well-being and indirectly aid the sick child.

Although most of this research has focused on adult cancer patients, elements of MBTs can be adapted for children of varying ages and levels of cognitive development. Because parents usually have a profound influence on the coping capabilities of their children, instruction in techniques that they can use to relax, distract, and comfort their children can greatly improve the child's tolerance and cooperation in diagnostic and therapeutic endeavors.

BIOMECHANICAL THERAPIES

Massage

Nearly every cultural group in the world has a historical tradition of massage therapy. There are many different types and variations of massage including Swedish, deep tissue, medical/orthopedic, sports, aromatherapy, shiatsu, reflexology, and Rolfing. Massage is often provided informally by parents and is one of the most commonly used complementary therapies. Massage can be provided alone or in conjunction with guided imagery, music therapy, aromatherapy, or Healing Touch.

Massage has proved useful for infants, children, and adolescents with diverse health conditions including cancer.[125,126] Massage provides tangible reassurance that the patient is cared for, enhancing self-esteem and a sense of psychological and emotional support. Randomized trials support its use in reducing symptoms such as nausea, anxiety, pain, depression, anger, stress, and fatigue.[127] Massage is cheap, noninvasive, and has very few contraindications. It can be helpful not only for the patient but also for parents.[125,128] Common sense precludes the use of vigorous massage over a solid tumor, a surgical wound, skin infections, abrasions, or burns. Individual adjustments are required for children who are restless or dislike being touched.

Chiropractic Therapy: Spinal and Cranial Adjustment

Chiropractors are licensed in all 50 states in the Unites States, and nearly all chiropractic schools now offer courses in pediatric care. Chiropractic therapy is mostly used for musculoskeletal symptoms.[129] Some feel that optimizing spinal alignment helps build resilience in the face of any health condition, resulting in fewer symptoms and a greater likelihood of healing. There are no randomized, controlled trials demonstrating chiropractic's effectiveness in preventing or treating pediatric malignancies. Acute significant adverse effects from chiropractic adjustments are very rare, and the rate of malpractice claims against chiropractors is much lower than that against medical doctors. Research is needed to better understand the use of chiropractic services by oncology patients, their satisfaction with care, and the cost-effectiveness of chiropractic in promoting patients' sense of well-being and quality of life.

BIOENERGETIC THERAPIES

Acupuncture

Acupuncture is one component of TCM that also includes herbal therapies, nutrition, exercise, and meditation practices. TCM is based on the theory of a vital energy, chi (qi) that circulates through the body in channels called *meridians*. When the flow of chi is blocked or disrupted, disease occurs; when the flow is balanced, harmonized, and restored, the patient experiences health. The flow of chi can be affected by stimulating specific points along the energy meridians.

Acupuncture is sometimes used as an adjunctive therapy to minimize nausea, anxiety, breathlessness, fatigue, and pain experienced by cancer patients. The NIH consensus conference on acupuncture concluded that acupuncture is effective in treating pain and nausea in adults,[130] although the evidence for cancer-related pain is less convincing.[131] Acupuncture research in pediatric oncology is limited. Although it appears safe, its efficacy for most symptoms is still largely unproven.[132,133] Pediatric patients who are referred for acupuncture generally find the process interesting, helpful, and much less painful or frightening than they had anticipated.[134]

Acupuncture is rarely covered by insurance. Side effects from acupuncture treatment, such as infections, broken or retained needles, pneumothorax, and cardiac tamponade, are rare.[135] Because acupuncturists may also recommend advice about diet, herbs, and lifestyle, physicians should discuss the appropriateness and risks of these therapies specifically with families who seek acupuncture care for their child.[136]

For needle-phobic children, acupressure can be used to minimize the risks and fears associated with needles. Acupressure is safe, noninvasive, and inexpensive. It has been shown to reduce nausea in adult cancer patients receiving radiation therapy,[137] and a pilot study has shown it to be safe and well accepted in pediatric cancer patients.[138]

Healing or Therapeutic Touch, Reiki and Qigong

Healing touch, TT, Reiki, and Qigong are different kinds of bioenergetic therapies in which the healer transmits a spiritual or invisible healing intention through his or her hands to help patients.[139] They are nonreligious forms of "laying on of hands" healing, and they are the most common types of secular healing techniques in the United States.

Although these kinds of energy healing techniques seem farfetched to many physicians, they can be profoundly meaningful to children and families. A family's request for information on herbs is often a way of testing the waters to determine how their questions or interest in biofield or spiritual healing will be received by the physician. These therapies are rarely used as a replacement for mainstream medicine, and they are safe. All of these therapies are provided with the patient fully clothed, and they may be provided in any clinical setting including outpatient clinics and intensive care units.

Studies in adult, adolescent, and pediatric populations support the use of TT to reduce pain and anxiety and to promote relaxation and a sense of well-being. Fewer studies have evaluated the effectiveness of TT in treating children, but they consistently report a sense of relaxation and comfort associated with the technique.[139]

Reiki is a similar practice that grew out of a Japanese tradition. Reiki practitioners are trained by a Reiki master through a workshop and an "empowerment" or "attunement." Reiki practitioners believe in a universal healing force that may be transmitted through the healer to patient through placing the hands on particular parts of the patient's body. In some cases, Reiki healers do long-distance healing in which the patient is visualized and energy is sent through intention rather than being transmitted by direct physical contact. There are no national certifying examinations, no state licensure, and no studies evaluating its effectiveness in treating children. There are no reported side effects.

Similarly, Qigong or external Qigong is part of TCM in which a Qigong master purportedly transmits Qi or vital energy to the patient, directing the Qi by the intention and the hands. Qigong can also refer to a set of exercises (internal Qigong) that are similar to Tai Chi, performed by the patients to enhance overall well-being. There are no reported side effects. Qigong is frequently used in China as a complementary therapy for cancer patients. In adult cancer patients, Qigong may improve quality of life, fatigue, positive mood status, and it may also reduce some side effects.[140] Systematic reviews suggest that additional high-quality clinical trials of Qigong and Tai Chi are needed.[141,142]

Prayer

As oncologists are well aware, every cancer diagnosis presents a potential spiritual crisis for a child and a family. Families are frequently eager to discuss the impact of the diagnosis on their spiritual or religious beliefs and often rely on these beliefs as an important coping strategy.[143–145] Many patients and physicians believe that spiritual well-being is an important component of overall health and strongly linked to functional status in cancer patients, yet many physicians feel poorly prepared to address families' questions and concerns in this area, particularly at the end of life.[146]

The classification of prayer or religion as a CAM therapy is controversial. Other terms used in the literature include faith healing and spiritual healing. In several surveys, prayer or spiritual healing are more commonly used than other CAM therapies in pediatric oncology patients (Table 52.1). In adults with advanced cancer, positive religious coping is associated with the use of intensive life-prolonging medical care in the last week of life.[147] Such a study has not been done in children. The goals of using religion and CAM may overlap in some areas and differ in others, but it is clear that many patients often use both.[148]

When used as an adjunctive therapy, intercessory prayer on behalf of patients is low in cost and free of side effects. Although some studies of prayer and other distant healing techniques suggest that they may offer tangible health benefits, most are equivocal or show no benefit.[149] Regardless of its impact on disease or symptom management, prayer often helps families feel that they are doing everything they can do to help the child; reinforces the family's sense of religion, culture, and meaning; and promotes a sense of peace and harmony.[143]

Occasionally, physicians are confronted with families who express concerns about medical care and their preference to rely on God or their faith for healing. It is helpful in working with such families to acknowledge their beliefs and to ask the family (and the family's spiritual community, if appropriate) to pray for the physicians, nurses, and other health professionals whose mission or calling is to help the child. Making analogies is also helpful—just as we would not expect God to warm our houses without electricity, coal, oil, or wood, we cannot expect God to work without the various tools and persons engaged in the prevention and treatment of disease. Oncologists who feel uncomfortable in these situations may

wish to hold a case conference including the family, the child's primary care physician and pastoral counselors to assist in addressing these issues before they reach the stage of requiring a court order to override family wishes. In some cases, the use of newer drugs or technologies (such as recombinant erythropoietin for Jehovah's Witness patients) may avoid potential conflicts.[150]

Homeopathy

Homeopathic remedies are commonly used in the United States and even more widely used in Canada, Europe, and India.[151] An estimated 12,000 homeopaths practice in the United States; of these, approximately 50% are lay practitioners; 35% are chiropractors; and approximately 15% are physicians, naturopaths, nurses, and other health professionals.

Homeopathy is based on two principles: (a) the law of similars or "like cures like" and (b) the law of dilutions. The law of similars means that a remedy that would cause a symptom in a healthy person is used to treat the same symptom in a sick person. For example, a homeopathic remedy made from Ipecac might be used to treat a child suffering from nausea. Although such remedies raise immediate concerns about safety, serious side effects from homeopathic treatment are rare due to the second principle of homeopathic treatment—the law of dilutions. This law says that the more the remedy is diluted, the more powerful it becomes. Homeopathic practitioners believe that these very dilute remedies contain an energy or information that is used by the patient to heal their symptoms; this energy is strengthened during the dilution process as the gross material is diluted out and the intention for healing is strengthened.

Although homeopathy is largely considered safe and a few randomized trials suggest efficacy for various conditions, the biologic plausibility and overall body of evidence for efficacy is weak.[152–154] Homeopathic remedies are available over the counter, through mail order catalogs, and through the Internet without a prescription at relatively low cost.

Ethical and Legal Considerations

The use of CAM therapies in children, especially unproven ones, obviously raises serious ethical and legal considerations.[20,155,156] This is particularly true when the patient or parent rejects mainstream medicine in favor of CAM. Several such cases have garnered considerable lay press, and others are certain to arise. Health care providers, policy makers, and legal professionals need to be aware of these considerations.[20] Regardless of the conflict, respectful communication between the family and health care team is crucial to a mutually satisfactory outcome.

A simple yet sound approach to medical therapies can be illustrated by a 2 × 2 table (Fig. 52.1). If a therapy is safe and effective, it can (and should) be recommended (e.g., antibiotics

		Effective	
		Yes	No
Safe	Yes	Use/recommend	Tolerate
	No	Monitor closely	Advise against

FIGURE 52.1 2 × 2 Table illustrating an approach to CAM therapies in children based on efficacy and safety.

for a bacterial infection). If a therapy is safe but has unknown or no effectiveness (e.g., aromatherapy to reduce stress), it should be reasonably tolerated by clinicians. If a therapy is unsafe or risky but effective (e.g., chemotherapy for acute lymphoblastic leukemia), it should be administered but the patient monitored closely. Finally, if a therapy is unsafe and ineffective, it should be avoided.

SUMMARY

The use of CAM in pediatric oncology patients is common, mostly to treat or ameliorate the symptoms associated with cancer and its therapies. There are little data to support the use of biological CAM therapies in children. Most studies on biological therapies have not been performed in humans, much less in children, and many biological agents may cause adverse effects or interactions with conventional medicines.

There is an ongoing need for well-designed clinical trials to evaluate the safety and efficacy of biological CAM therapies in children. Several lifestyle and biomechanical therapies are safe and helpful in providing supportive care. Bioenergetic therapies are safe but largely unproven. The best approach may be to reinforce those things that we unequivocally know are helpful: a well-balanced, nutritious diet with plenty of fruit and vegetables; adequate exercise; immunizations; and avoidance of overeating, tobacco, excess alcohol, unprotected sex, and excess sun exposure. Guidelines for advising pediatric patients about CAM therapies have been published. Clinicians should periodically ask all oncology patients if they are using CAM therapies, so they can offer evidence-based information to guide family choices. To provide truly comprehensive and compassionate care, pediatric oncologists need to be aware of the most common types of therapies, families' reasons and goals in using them, and reliable resources for more information.

References

1. Kemper KJ, Vohra S, Walls R; American Academy of Pediatrics. The use of complementary and alternative medicine in pediatrics. Pediatrics 2008;122(6):1374–1386.
2. Post-White J, Fitzgerald M, Hageness S, et al. Complementary and alternative medicine use in children with cancer and general and specialty pediatrics. J Pediatr Oncol Nurs 2009;26(1):7–15.
3. McCurdy EA, Spangler JG, Wofford MM, et al. Religiosity is associated with the use of complementary medical therapies by pediatric oncology patients. J Pediatr Hematol Oncol 2003;25(2):125–129.
4. Bold J, Leis A. Unconventional therapy use among children with cancer in Saskatchewan. J Pediatr Oncol Nurs 2001;18(1):16–25.
5. Neuhouser ML, Patterson RE, Schwartz SM, et al. Use of alternative medicine by children with cancer in Washington state. Prev Med 2001;33(5):347–354.
6. Yeh CH, Tsai JL, Li W, et al. Use of alternative therapy among pediatric oncology patients in Taiwan. Pediatr Hematol Oncol 2000;17(1):55–65.
7. Lim J, Wong M, Chan MY, et al. Use of complementary and alternative medicine in paediatric oncology patients in Singapore. Ann Acad Med Singapore 2006;35(11):753–758.
8. Laengler A, Spix C, Seifert G, et al. Complementary and alternative treatment methods in children with cancer: a population-based retrospective survey on the prevalence of use in Germany. Eur J Cancer 2008;44(15):2233–2240.
9. Weyl Ben Arush M, Geva H, Ofir R, et al. Prevalence and characteristics of complementary medicine used by pediatric cancer patients in a mixed western and middle-eastern population. J Pediatr Hematol Oncol 2006;28(3):141–146.
10. Gomez-Martinez R, Tlacuilo-Parra A, Garibaldi-Covarrubias R. Use of complementary and alternative medicine in children with cancer in Occidental, Mexico. Pediatr Blood Cancer 2007;49(6):820–823.
11. Hamidah A, Rustam ZA, Tamil AM, et al. Prevalence and parental perceptions of complementary and alternative medicine use by children with cancer in a multi-ethnic Southeast Asian population. Pediatr Blood Cancer 2009;52(1):70–74.
12. Karadeniz C, Pinarli FG, Oguz A, et al. Complementary/alternative medicine use in a pediatric oncology unit in Turkey. Pediatr Blood Cancer 2007;48(5):540–543.
13. Gozum S, Arikan D, Buyukavci M. Complementary and alternative medicine use in pediatric oncology patients in eastern Turkey. Cancer Nurs 2007;30(1):38–44.
14. Nathanson I, Sandler E, Ramirez-Garnica G, et al. Factors influencing complementary and alternative medicine use in a multisite pediatric oncology practice. J Pediatr Hematol Oncol 2007;29(10):705–708.
15. Martel D, Bussieres JF, Theoret Y, et al. Use of alternative and complementary therapies in children with cancer. Pediatr Blood Cancer 2005;44(7):660–668.
16. Mertens AC, Sencer S, Myers CD, et al. Complementary and alternative therapy use in adult survivors of childhood cancer: a report from the Childhood Cancer Survivor Study. Pediatr Blood Cancer 2008;50(1):90–97.
17. Kelly KM, Jacobson JS, Kennedy DD, et al. Use of unconventional therapies by children with cancer at an urban medical center. J Pediatr Hematol Oncol 2000;22(5):412–416.
18. Roth M, Lin J, Kim M, et al. Pediatric oncologists' views toward the use of complementary and alternative medicine in children with cancer. J Pediatr Hematol Oncol 2009;31(3):177–182.
19. Johnston DL, Nagel K, O'Halloran C, et al. Complementary and alternative medicine in pediatric oncology: availability and institutional policies in Canada–a report from the Children's Oncology Group. Pediatr Blood Cancer 2006;47(7):955–958.
20. Cohen MH, Kemper KJ, Stevens L, et al. Pediatric use of complementary therapies: ethical and policy choices. Pediatrics 2005;116(4):e568–e575.
21. Uauy R, Solomons N. Diet, nutrition, and the life-course approach to cancer prevention. J Nutr 2005;135(12 Suppl):2934S–2945S.
22. Danaei G, Vander Hoorn S, Lopez AD, et al. Causes of cancer in the world: comparative risk assessment of nine behavioural and environmental risk factors. Lancet 2005;366(9499):1784–1793.
23. Myers C, Stuber ML, Bonamer-Rheingans JI, et al. Complementary therapies and childhood cancer. Cancer Control 2005;12(3):172–180.
24. Bluebond-Langner M, Belasco JB, Goldman A, et al. Understanding parents' approaches to care and treatment of children with cancer when standard therapy has failed. J Clin Oncol 2007;25(17):2414–2419.
25. Committee on Children with Disabilities. American Academy of Pediatrics: Counseling families who choose complementary and alternative medicine for their child with chronic illness or disability. Committee on Children With Disabilities. Pediatrics 2001;107(3):598–601.
26. Aphinyanaphongs Y, Aliferis C. Text categorization models for identifying unproven cancer treatments on the web. Stud Health Technol Inform 2007;129(Pt 2):968–972.
27. Mazzini MJ, Glode LM. Internet oncology: increased benefit and risk for patients and oncologists. Hematol Oncol Clin North Am 2001;15(3):583–592.
28. Boddy K, Ernst E. Review of reliable information sources related to integrative oncology. Hematol Oncol Clin North Am 2008;22(4):619–630.
29. Vickers A, Cassileth B, Ernst E, et al. How should we research unconventional therapies? A panel report from the Conference on Complementary and Alternative Medicine Research Methodology, National Institutes of Health. Int J Technol Assess Health Care 1997;13(1):111–121.
30. Wolsko PM, Solondz DK, Phillips RS, et al. Lack of herbal supplement characterization in published randomized controlled trials. Am J Med 2005;118(10):1087–1093.
31. McLean TW, Kemper KJ. Complementary and alternative medicine therapies in pediatric oncology patients. J Soc Integr Oncol 2006;4(1):40–45.
32. Amin AR, Kucuk O, Khuri FR, et al. Perspectives for cancer prevention with natural compounds. J Clin Oncol 2009;27(16):2712–2725.
33. Melnick SJ. Developmental therapeutics: review of biologically based complementary and alternative medicine (CAM) therapies for potential application in children with cancer-part II. J Pediatr Hematol Oncol 2006;28(5):271–285.
34. Boehm K, Borrelli F, Ernst E, et al. Green tea (Camellia sinensis) for the prevention of cancer. Cochrane Database Syst Rev 2009(3):CD005004.
35. Schneider C, Segre T. Green tea: potential health benefits. Am Fam Physician 2009;79(7):591–594.
36. Kim JY, Kwon O. Garlic intake and cancer risk: an analysis using the Food and Drug Administration's evidence-based review system for the scientific evaluation of health claims. Am J Clin Nutr 2009;89(1):257–264.
37. Hassan HT. Ajoene (natural garlic compound): a new anti-leukaemia agent for AML therapy. Leuk Res 2004;28(7):667–671.
38. Tattelman E. Health effects of garlic. Am Fam Physician 2005;72(1):103–106.
39. Bhardwaj A, Sethi G, Vadhan-Raj S, et al. Resveratrol inhibits proliferation, induces apoptosis, and overcomes chemoresistance through down-regulation of STAT3 and nuclear factor-kappaB-regulated antiapoptotic and cell survival gene products in human multiple myeloma cells. Blood 2007;109(6):2293–2302.
40. Kundu JK, Surh YJ. Cancer chemopreventive and therapeutic potential of resveratrol: mechanistic perspectives. Cancer Lett 2008;269(2):243–261.
41. Giovannucci E. Vitamin D and cancer incidence in the Harvard cohorts. Ann Epidemiol 2009;19(2):84–88.
42. Holick MF. Sunlight, UV-radiation, vitamin D and skin cancer: how much sunlight do we need? Adv Exp Med Biol 2008;624:1–15.
43. Wagner CL, Greer FR. Prevention of rickets and vitamin D deficiency in infants, children, and adolescents. Pediatrics 2008;122(5):1142–1152.
44. Weingarten MA, Zalmanovici A, Yaphe J. Dietary calcium supplementation for preventing colorectal cancer and adenomatous polyps. Cochrane Database Syst Rev 2008(1):CD003548.
45. Bardia A, Tleyjeh IM, Cerhan JR, et al. Efficacy of antioxidant supplementation in reducing primary cancer incidence and mortality: systematic review and meta-analysis. Mayo Clin Proc 2008;83(1):23–34.
46. Huang HY, Caballero B, Chang S, et al. The efficacy and safety of multivitamin and mineral supplement use to prevent cancer and chronic disease in adults: a systematic review for a National Institutes of Health state-of-the-science conference. Ann Intern Med 2006;145(5):372–385.
47. MacArthur AC, McBride ML, Spinelli JJ, et al. Risk of childhood leukemia associated with vaccination, infection, and medication use in childhood: the Cross-Canada Childhood Leukemia Study. Am J Epidemiol 2008;167(5):598–606.
48. Bjelakovic G, Nikolova D, Simonetti RG, et al. Antioxidant supplements for preventing gastrointestinal cancers. Cochrane Database Syst Rev 2004(4):CD004183.
49. Lonn E, Bosch J, Yusuf S, et al. Effects of long-term vitamin E supplementation on cardiovascular events and cancer: a randomized controlled trial. JAMA 2005;293(11):1338–1347.
50. Pham DQ, Plakogiannis R. Vitamin E supplementation in cardiovascular disease and cancer prevention: Part 1. Ann Pharmacother 2005;39(11):1870–1878.

51. Verrax J, Calderon PB. The controversial place of vitamin C in cancer treatment. Biochem Pharmacol 2008;76(12):1644–1652.
52. Sarkar FH, Li Y. Soy isoflavones and cancer prevention. Cancer Invest 2003;21(5): 744–757.
53. Sacks FM, Lichtenstein A, Van Horn L, et al. Soy protein, isoflavones, and cardiovascular health. An American Heart Association Science Advisory for Professionals from the Nutrition Committee. Circulation 2006;113(7):1034–1044.
54. Srinivasan V, Spence DW, Pandi-Perumal SR, et al. Therapeutic actions of melatonin in cancer: possible mechanisms. Integr Cancer Ther 2008;7(3):189–203.
55. Mills E, Wu P, Seely D, et al. Melatonin in the treatment of cancer: a systematic review of randomized controlled trials and meta-analysis. J Pineal Res 2005;39(4):360–366.
56. Hoang BX, Shaw DG, Pham PT, et al. Neurobiological effects of melatonin as related to cancer. Eur J Cancer Prev 2007;16(6):511–516.
57. Kunnumakkara AB, Anand P, Aggarwal BB. Curcumin inhibits proliferation, invasion, angiogenesis and metastasis of different cancers through interaction with multiple cell signaling proteins. Cancer Lett 2008;269(2):199–225.
58. Kuttan G, Kumar KB, Guruvayoorappan C, et al. Antitumor, anti-invasion, and antimetastatic effects of curcumin. Adv Exp Med Biol 2007;595:173–184.
59. Mantovani MS, Bellini MF, Angeli JP, et al. Beta-glucans in promoting health: prevention against mutation and cancer. Mutat Res 2008;658(3):154–161.
60. Burzynski SR, Janicki TJ, Weaver RA, et al. Targeted therapy with antineoplastons A10 and AS2–1 of high-grade, recurrent, and progressive brainstem glioma. Integr Cancer Ther 2006;5(1):40–47.
61. Burzynski SR, Weaver RA, Janicki T, et al. Long-term survival of high-risk pediatric patients with primitive neuroectodermal tumors treated with antineoplastons A10 and AS2–1. Integr Cancer Ther 2005;4(2):168–177.
62. Seely D, Kennedy DA, Myers SP, et al. In vitro analysis of the herbal compound Essiac. Anticancer Res 2007;27(6B):3875–3882.
63. Bacher N, Tiefenthaler M, Sturm S, et al. Oxindole alkaloids from *Uncaria tomentosa* induce apoptosis in proliferating, G0/G1-arrested and bcl-2-expressing acute lymphoblastic leukaemia cells. Br J Haematol 2006;132(5):615–22.
64. Styczynski J, Wysocki M. Alternative medicine remedies might stimulate viability of leukemic cells. Pediatr Blood Cancer 2006;46(1):94–98.
65. Zick SM, Ruffin MT, Lee J, et al. Phase II trial of encapsulated ginger as a treatment for chemotherapy-induced nausea and vomiting. Support Care Cancer 2009;17(5): 563–572.
66. Roffe L, Schmidt K, Ernst E. Efficacy of coenzyme Q10 for improved tolerability of cancer treatments: a systematic review. J Clin Oncol 2004;22(21):4418–4424.
67. Kelly KM. Bringing evidence to complementary and alternative medicine in children with cancer: Focus on nutrition-related therapies. Pediatr Blood Cancer 2008;50(2 Suppl):490–493.
68. Dagdemir A, Yildirim H, Aliyazicioglu Y, et al. Does vitamin A prevent high-dose-methotrexate-induced D-xylose malabsorption in children with cancer? Support Care Cancer 2004;12(4):263–267.
69. Wessels G, Hesseling PB, Stefan DC, et al. The effect of vitamin A status in children treated for cancer. Pediatr Hematol Oncol 2008;25(4):283–290.
70. Weijl NI, Elsendoorn TJ, Lentjes EG, et al. Supplementation with antioxidant micronutrients and chemotherapy-induced toxicity in cancer patients treated with cisplatin-based chemotherapy: a randomised, double-blind, placebo-controlled study. Eur J Cancer 2004;40(11):1713–1723.
71. Ladas EJ, Jacobson JS, Kennedy DD, et al. Antioxidants and cancer therapy: a systematic review. J Clin Oncol 2004;22(3):517–528.
72. Postovsky S, Arush MW, Diamond E, et al. The prevalence of low selenium levels in newly diagnosed pediatric cancer patients. Pediatr Hematol Oncol 2003;20(4): 273–280.
73. Tamayo C, Diamond S. Review of clinical trials evaluating safety and efficacy of milk thistle (*Silybum marianum* [L.] Gaertn.). Integr Cancer Ther 2007;6(2):146–157.
74. Post-White J, Ladas EJ, Kelly KM. Advances in the use of milk thistle (*Silybum marianum*). Integr Cancer Ther 2007;6(2):104–109.
75. Hofseth LJ, Wargovich MJ. Inflammation, cancer, and targets of ginseng. J Nutr 2007;137(1 Suppl):183S–185S.
76. Li J, Stickel SL, Bouton-Verville H, et al. Fermented noni exudate (fNE): a mediator between immune system and anti-tumor activity. Oncol Rep 2008;20(6):1505–1509.
77. Milazzo S, Ernst E, Lejeune S, et al. Laetrile treatment for cancer. Cochrane Database Syst Rev 2006(2):CD005476.
78. Loprinzi CL, Levitt R, Barton DL, et al. Evaluation of shark cartilage in patients with advanced cancer: a North Central Cancer Treatment Group trial. Cancer 2005;104(1): 176–182.
79. Saper RB, Kales SN, Paquin J, et al. Heavy metal content of Ayurvedic herbal medicine products. JAMA 2004;292(23):2868–2873.
80. Ernst E. Serious adverse effects of unconventional therapies for children and adolescents: a systematic review of recent evidence. Eur J Pediatr 2003;162(2):72–80.
81. Ahmed MT, Loutfy N, Yousef Y. Contamination of medicinal herbs with organophosphorus insecticides. Bull Environ Contam Toxicol 2001;66(4):421–426.
82. Werneke U, Earl J, Seydel C, et al. Potential health risks of complementary alternative medicines in cancer patients. Br J Cancer 2004;90(2):408–413.
83. Seely D, Stempak D, Baruchel S. A strategy for controlling potential interactions between natural health products and chemotherapy: a review in pediatric oncology. J Pediatr Hematol Oncol 2007;29(1):32–47.
84. Renella R, Fanconi S. Decision-making in pediatrics: a practical algorithm to evaluate complementary and alternative medicine for children. Eur J Pediatr 2006;165(7): 437–441.
85. Jankovic M, Spinetta JJ, Martins AG, et al. Non-conventional therapies in childhood cancer: guidelines for distinguishing non-harmful from harmful therapies: a report of the SIOP Working Committee on Psychosocial Issues in Pediatric Oncology. Pediatr Blood Cancer 2004;42(1):106–108.
86. Key TJ, Allen NE, Spencer EA, et al. The effect of diet on risk of cancer. Lancet 2002;360(9336):861–868.
87. Guise JM, Austin D, Morris CD. Review of case-control studies related to breastfeeding and reduced risk of childhood leukemia. Pediatrics 2005;116(5):e724–e731.
88. Kwan ML, Buffler PA, Abrams B, et al. Breastfeeding and the risk of childhood leukemia: a meta-analysis. Public Health Rep 2004;119(6):521–535.
89. Mathur GP, Gupta N, Mathur S, et al. Breastfeeding and childhood cancer. Br J Cancer 2001;85(11):1685–1694.
90. Weitzman S. Complementary and alternative (CAM) dietary therapies for cancer. Pediatr Blood Cancer 2008;50(2 Suppl):494–497.
91. Sofi F, Cesari F, Abbate R, et al. Adherence to Mediterranean diet and health status: meta-analysis. BMJ 2008;337:a1344.
92. Bowden SA, Robinson RF, Carr R, et al. Prevalence of vitamin D deficiency and insufficiency in children with osteopenia or osteoporosis referred to a pediatric metabolic bone clinic. Pediatrics 2008;121(6):e1585–e1590.
93. Krishnamoorthy P, Freeman C, Bernstein ML, et al. Osteopenia in children who have undergone posterior fossa or craniospinal irradiation for brain tumors. Arch Pediatr Adolesc Med 2004;158(5):491–496.
94. van der Sluis IM, van den Heuvel-Eibrink MM, Hahlen K, et al. Altered bone mineral density and body composition, and increased fracture risk in childhood acute lymphoblastic leukemia. J Pediatr 2002;141(2):204–210.
95. Othman F, Guo CY, Webber C, et al. Osteopenia in survivors of Wilms' tumor. Int J Oncol 2002;20(4):827–833.
96. Bayram I, Erbey F, Celik N, et al. The use of a protein and energy dense eicosapentaenoic acid containing supplement for malignancy-related weight loss in children. Pediatr Blood Cancer 2009;52(5):571–574.
97. Moody K, Charlson ME, Finlay J. The neutropenic diet: what's the evidence? J Pediatr Hematol Oncol 2002;24(9):717–721.
98. Ladas EJ, Sacks N, Brophy P, et al. Standards of nutritional care in pediatric oncology: results from a nationwide survey on the standards of practice in pediatric oncology. A Children's Oncology Group study. Pediatr Blood Cancer 2006;46(3):339–344.
99. American Academy of Pediatrics. Nutritional management of children with cancer. In: Kleinman R, ed. Pediatric nutrition handbook. 6th ed. Elk Grove Village, IL: AAP, 2009:927–939.
100. Newton RU, Galvao DA. Exercise in prevention and management of cancer. Curr Treat Options Oncol 2008;9(2–3):135–146.
101. Mustian KM, Griggs JJ, Morrow GR, et al. Exercise and side effects among 749 patients during and after treatment for cancer: a University of Rochester Cancer Center Community Clinical Oncology Program Study. Support Care Cancer 2006;14(7): 732–741.
102. Galvao DA, Newton RU. Review of exercise intervention studies in cancer patients. J Clin Oncol 2005;23(4):899–909.
103. Lucia A, Earnest C, Perez M. Cancer-related fatigue: can exercise physiology assist oncologists? Lancet Oncol 2003;4(10):616–625.
104. van Brussel M, Takken T, Lucia A, et al. Is physical fitness decreased in survivors of childhood leukemia? A systematic review. Leukemia 2005;19(1):13–17.
105. Miller TL, Miller AM, Lopez-Mitnik G, et al. Exercise capacity in long-term survivors of pediatric cancer. J Clin Oncol 2009;27(15s):abstr 10026.
106. Marchese VG, Chiarello LA, Lange BJ. Effects of physical therapy intervention for children with acute lymphoblastic leukemia. Pediatr Blood Cancer 2004;42(2): 127–133.
107. Fairey AS, Courneya KS, Field CJ, et al. Physical exercise and immune system function in cancer survivors: a comprehensive review and future directions. Cancer 2002;94(2): 539–551.
108. Hayes S, Davies PS, Parker T, et al. Total energy expenditure and body composition changes following peripheral blood stem cell transplantation and participation in an exercise programme. Bone Marrow Transplant 2003;31(5):331–338.
109. van der Sluis IM, van den Heuvel-Eibrink MM. Osteoporosis in children with cancer. Pediatr Blood Cancer 2008;50(2 Suppl):474–478.
110. Blaauwbroek R, Bouma MJ, Tuinier W, et al. The effect of exercise counselling with feedback from a pedometer on fatigue in adult survivors of childhood cancer: a pilot study. Support Care Cancer 2009;17:1041–1048.
111. Cmiel CA, Karr DM, Gasser DM, et al. Noise control: a nursing team's approach to sleep promotion. Am J Nurs 2004;104(2):40–48.
112. Kemper KJ, Hamilton CA, McLean TW, et al. Impact of music on pediatric oncology outpatients. Pediatr Res 2008;64(1):105–109.
113. Holmes C, Knights A, Dean C, et al. Keep music live: music and the alleviation of apathy in dementia subjects. Int Psychogeriatr 2006;18(4):623–630.
114. Arnon S, Shapsa A, Forman L, et al. Live music is beneficial to preterm infants in the neonatal intensive care unit environment. Birth 2006;33(2):131–136.
115. Kemper KJ, McLean TW. Parents' attitudes and expectations about music's impact on pediatric oncology patients. J Soc Integr Oncol 2008;6(4):146–149.
116. Pittler MH, Brown EM, Ernst E. Static magnets for reducing pain: systematic review and meta-analysis of randomized trials. CMAJ 2007;177(7):736–742.
117. Post-White J, Hawks RG. Complementary and alternative medicine in pediatric oncology. Semin Oncol Nurs 2005;21(2):107–114.
118. Astin JA, Shapiro SL, Eisenberg DM, et al. Mind-body medicine: state of the science, implications for practice. J Am Board Fam Pract 2003;16(2):131–147.
119. Astin JA. Mind-body therapies for the management of pain. Clin J Pain 2004;20(1): 27–32.
120. Evans S, Tsao JC, Zeltzer LK. Complementary and alternative medicine for acute procedural pain in children. Altern Ther Health Med 2008;14(5):52–56.
121. Richardson J, Smith JE, McCall G, et al. Hypnosis for procedure-related pain and distress in pediatric cancer patients: a systematic review of effectiveness and methodology related to hypnosis interventions. J Pain Symptom Manage 2006;31(1): 70–84.
122. Weis J. Support groups for cancer patients. Support Care Cancer 2003;11(12): 763–768.
123. Rehse B, Pukrop R. Effects of psychosocial interventions on quality of life in adult cancer patients: meta analysis of 37 published controlled outcome studies. Patient Educ Couns 2003;50(2):179–186.
124. Ljungman G, McGrath PJ, Cooper E, et al. Psychosocial needs of families with a child with cancer. J Pediatr Hematol Oncol 2003;25(3):223–231.
125. Post-White J, Fitzgerald M, Savik K, et al. Massage therapy for children with cancer. J Pediatr Oncol Nurs 2009;26(1):16–28.
126. Hughes D, Ladas E, Rooney D, et al. Massage therapy as a supportive care intervention for children with cancer. Oncol Nurs Forum 2008;35(3):431–442.
127. Ernst E. Massage therapy for cancer palliation and supportive care: a systematic review of randomised clinical trials. Support Care Cancer 2009;17(4):333–337.
128. Iwasaki M. Interventional study on fatigue relief in mothers caring for hospitalized children–effect of massage incorporating techniques from oriental medicine. Kurume Med J 2005;52(1–2):19–27.
129. Bellas A, Lafferty WE, Lind B, et al. Frequency, predictors, and expenditures for pediatric insurance claims for complementary and alternative medical professionals in Washington State. Arch Pediatr Adolesc Med 2005;159(4):367–372.
130. NIH Consensus Conference. Acupuncture. JAMA 1998;280(17):1518–1524.

131. Lee H, Schmidt K, Ernst E. Acupuncture for the relief of cancer-related pain–a systematic review. Eur J Pain 2005;9(4):437–444.
132. Jindal V, Ge A, Mansky PJ. Safety and efficacy of acupuncture in children: a review of the evidence. J Pediatr Hematol Oncol 2008;30(6):431–442.
133. Ezzo JM, Richardson MA, Vickers A, et al. Acupuncture-point stimulation for chemotherapy-induced nausea or vomiting. Cochrane Database Syst Rev 2006(2):CD002285.
134. Kemper KJ, Sarah R, Silver-Highfield E, et al. On pins and needles? Pediatric pain patients' experience with acupuncture. Pediatrics 2000;105(4 Pt 2):941–947.
135. Ernst G, Strzyz H, Hagmeister H. Incidence of adverse effects during acupuncture therapy-a multicentre survey. Complement Ther Med 2003;11(2):93–97.
136. Sherman KJ, Cherkin DC, Eisenberg DM, et al. The practice of acupuncture: who are the providers and what do they do? Ann Fam Med 2005;3(2):151–158.
137. Roscoe JA, Bushunow P, Jean-Pierre P, et al. Acupressure bands are effective in reducing radiation therapy-related nausea. J Pain Symptom Manage 2009;27:27.
138. Jones E, Isom S, Kemper KJ, et al. Acupressure for chemotherapy-associated nausea and vomiting in children. J Soc Integr Oncol 2008;6(4):141–145.
139. Kemper KJ, Kelly EA. Treating children with therapeutic and healing touch. Pediatr Ann 2004;33(4):248–252.
140. Oh B, Butow P, Mullan B, et al. Randomized clinical trial of medical qigong on quality of life, fatigue, side effects, mood, status, and inflammation of cancer patients. J Clin Oncol 2009;27(15 s):abstr 9617.
141. Lee MS, Chen KW, Sancier KM, et al. Qigong for cancer treatment: a systematic review of controlled clinical trials. Acta Oncol 2007;46(6):717–722.
142. Lee MS, Pittler MH, Ernst E. Is Tai Chi an effective adjunct in cancer care? A systematic review of controlled clinical trials. Support Care Cancer 2007;15(6):597–601.
143. Elkin TD, Jensen SA, McNeil L, et al. Religiosity and coping in mothers of children diagnosed with cancer: an exploratory analysis. J Pediatr Oncol Nurs 2007;24(5):274–278.
144. Kristeller JL, Rhodes M, Cripe LD, et al. Oncologist Assisted Spiritual Intervention Study (OASIS): patient acceptability and initial evidence of effects. Int J Psychiatry Med 2005;35(4):329–347.
145. Ambs AH, Miller MF, Smith AW, et al. Religious and spiritual practices and identification among individuals living with cancer and other chronic disease. J Soc Integr Oncol 2007;5(2):53–60.
146. Lo B, Ruston D, Kates LW, et al. Discussing religious and spiritual issues at the end of life: a practical guide for physicians. JAMA 2002;287(6):749–754.
147. Phelps AC, Maciejewski PK, Nilsson M, et al. Religious coping and use of intensive life-prolonging care near death in patients with advanced cancer. JAMA 2009;301(11):1140–1147.
148. Tatsumura Y, Maskarinec G, Shumay DM, et al. Religious and spiritual resources, CAM, and conventional treatment in the lives of cancer patients. Altern Ther Health Med 2003;9(3):64–71.
149. Roberts L, Ahmed I, Hall S, et al. Intercessory prayer for the alleviation of ill health. Cochrane Database Syst Rev 2009(2):CD000368.
150. Mazza P, Palazzo G, Amurri B, et al. Acute leukemia in Jehovah's Witnesses: a challenge for hematologists. Haematologica 2000;85(11):1221–1222.
151. Lee AC, Kemper KJ. Homeopathy and naturopathy: practice characteristics and pediatric care. Arch Pediatr Adolesc Med 2000;154(1):75–80.
152. Altunc U, Pittler MH, Ernst E. Homeopathy for childhood and adolescence ailments: systematic review of randomized clinical trials. Mayo Clin Proc 2007;82(1):69–75.
153. Jonas WB, Kaptchuk TJ, Linde K. A critical overview of homeopathy. Ann Intern Med 2003;138(5):393–399.
154. Milazzo S, Russell N, Ernst E. Efficacy of homeopathic therapy in cancer treatment. Eur J Cancer 2006;42(3):282–289.
155. Cohen MH. Legal and ethical issues relating to use of complementary therapies in pediatric hematology/oncology. J Pediatr Hematol Oncol 2006;28(3):190–193.
156. Cohen MH, Kemper KJ. Complementary therapies in pediatrics: a legal perspective. Pediatrics 2005;115(3):774–780.

CHAPTER 53 ■ PEDIATRIC ONCOLOGY IN COUNTRIES WITH LIMITED RESOURCES

RONALD BARR, FEDERICO ANTILLON, BHARAT AGARWAL, PARTH MEHTA, AND RAUL RIBEIRO

Countries with limited resources are defined economically by the World Bank on the basis of gross national income (GNI) per capita.[1] Of those in the low-income category, 10 have a GNI per capita of less than U.S. $300 and 90% of those are in sub-Saharan Africa. The only other country at this end of the spectrum is Afghanistan. Unfortunately, the gap between rich and poor countries continues to grow, ranging from GNIs per capita of U.S. $110 in Burundi to U.S. $76,450 in Norway. All five countries with a GNI per capita of more than $50,000 are in Western Europe. In contrast, of the 25 countries in which the proportion of the population below the international poverty line (U.S. $1.25/d in 2005) was at least 50%, 21 are in sub-Saharan Africa. The others are Bangladesh, Haiti, Nepal, and Timor Leste.

In September 2000, the United Nations adopted the Millennium Declaration incorporating the Millennium Development Goals for 2015. Progress in meeting the component targets has been slow and uneven. The current global economic crisis threatens this trajectory further, and even limited gains risk reversal. What is the impact of such severe and prolonged financial limitations on public health? Some indicators of health resources are listed in Table 53.1, again illustrating disproportionate deficits in sub-Saharan Africa. Not surprisingly, these disadvantages are mirrored in indicators of poor health outcomes (Table 53.1), both now and in the future. It appears clear at least at the disadvantaged end of the spectrum (Fig. 53.1) that postulated 5-year survival rates for children with cancer are directly proportional to several health indicators, including GNI per capita, the number of physicians per 1,000 population, and, most significantly, the annual government expenditure on health care per capita.[2]

Where does cancer lie in the overall burden of disease that afflicts the world's population? Although it has been estimated by Dr. Charles Stiller (Stiller C. Personal communication, December 2006) of the Cancer Research Group in Oxford, United Kingdom that there are approximately 1 million new cases of malignant disease annually in the adolescent and young adult age group (15–39 years) alone, cancer is relegated to little more than a passing mention, with no separate consideration of cancer in children, in the most recent World Health Report,[3] that is dominated by infectious diseases, particularly human immunodeficiency virus (HIV) and acquired immunodeficiency syndrome (AIDS), malaria, and tuberculosis. Certainly, the global importance of these diseases dwarfs that of cancer. For example, in 2007, there were 15 million children (0–17 years) who have been orphaned by AIDS, more than 77% of them in sub-Saharan Africa.

Beset by such obstacles, how are we to respond to the pledge from the United Nations General Assembly in May 2002, at the close of its Special Session on Children, to build "a world fit for children"?[4] And how can we support pediatric oncology and the care of children with cancer given these limitations and constraints? Some of the issues that have to be addressed form the substance of this chapter, which seeks to inform the reader of the scope of the challenge in countries with limited resources.

We will examine cancer in children in countries with limited resources from several perspectives, as follows—Epidemiology; Barriers to Progress; Opportunities for Research; and Strategies for Change.

EPIDEMIOLOGY

Although there are few, truly population-based cancer registries in developing countries, it is clear (especially from the work of the International Agency for Research on Cancer—IARC)[5] that the reported annual cancer incidence rates in children are generally lower in low- and middle-income countries (as low as 45.6 per million in Namibia) than that in industrialized societies (all more than 100 per million), raising concerns about underdiagnosis and underreporting. A group of investigators at St. Jude Children's Research Hospital (SJCRH) has described the links in the chain of childhood cancer registration (Fig. 53.2) and noted that the greatest disparity in incidence rates is for acute leukemia (the commonest form of cancer worldwide and, arguably, among the most difficult to diagnose).[6] This challenge is compounded by the high prevalence of infectious diseases, the symptoms of which are similar to those of leukemia. In low-income countries in which the burden of infectious disease in childhood is high, the under 5 mortality rate (generally held to be the best indicator of child health in a population) correlates inversely with the reported frequency of leukemia but not of solid tumors.[6]

Despite these lower incidence rates, the absolute number of incident cases in developing countries is growing faster than the number in more privileged societies, reflecting the expanding population of the former and the projected contraction in and aging of the population of at least some of the latter, almost 80% of which are in Eastern Europe. Thus, the proportion of the childhood cancer burden borne in countries least able to deal with it continues to rise and now approximates 80%. However, it is also apparent that incidence rates vary among different ethnic groups in the same country and between the same ethnic groups in different countries. Regional differences in disease distribution are likely to reflect differences in biology, both in the host and environment. These have provided important opportunities for study and have led to enhanced understanding of disease processes. Among the best-known examples are the greater proportions and evidently higher incidence rates in low-income countries of non-Hodgkin lymphoma (especially Burkitt's lymphoma) and retinoblastoma such that, in some countries, these are the commonest forms of cancer in childhood.[7] Interactions between the host and the environment are well exemplified by the increasing incidence rates and the changing distribution of

TABLE 53.1

CURRENT INDICATORS OF PUBLIC HEALTH IN LOW- AND MIDDLE-INCOME COUNTRIES (2006)

Resource indicators	Sub Saharan African countries $n = 46$	Other countries
Annual expenditure on health per capita <$10	$n = 7$	Democratic Republic of Korea, Myanmar
<5% of central government expenditures allocated to health	$n = 9$	$n = 7$
<1 physician per 10,000 population[a]	$n = 25$	Bhutan, Timor Leste
Outcome indicators		
Maternal mortality		
>10 per 1,000 live births	$n = 13$	Afghanistan
Under 5 mortality rate		
>100 per 1,000 live births	$n = 35$	Afghanistan, Myanmar
Life expectancy at birth		
<50 years	$n = 26$	Afghanistan

World Development Indicators 2008, the World Bank.
[a]Data not available for numerous countries.

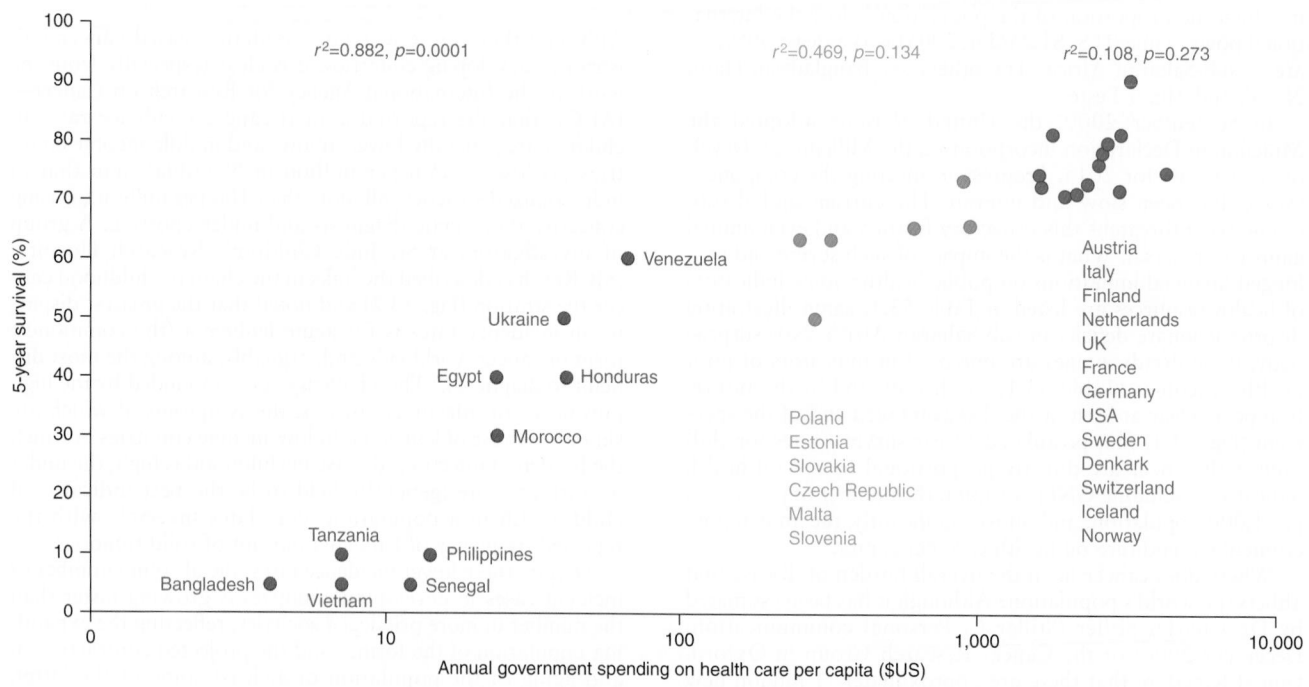

FIGURE 53.1 Childhood cancer survival and government annual health care spending per capita.

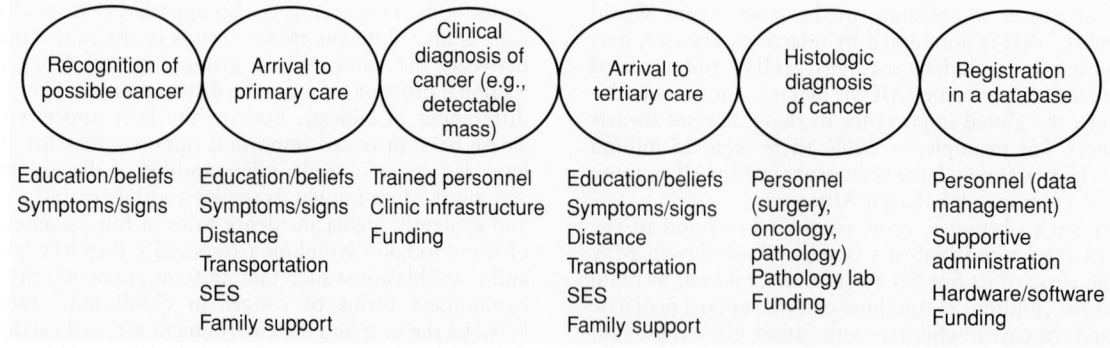

FIGURE 53.2 Links in the chain of childhood cancer diagnosis and registration in low-income countries.

diseases (notably Kaposi's sarcoma and Burkitt's lymphoma) and in their individual clinical presentations, in Malawi during the era of HIV infection.[8] By contrast, the occurrence of Ewing's sarcoma in certain populations (e.g., blacks and Chinese) is decidedly uncommon,[9] for reasons not yet obvious.

The epidemiology of brain tumors is more complex. Apparently, striking regional differences in the reported frequencies of primary tumors in the central nervous system seems likely to represent large negative ascertainment biases.[10] Underdiagnosis may reflect several phenomena, including misassessment and lack of neuroradiologic as well as neurosurgical resources.[11] In a curious inversion of this scenario, the supposed increase in the incidence of brain tumors in children in the United States has be attributed to a positive ascertainment bias due to the widespread availability and use of sophisticated neuroradiologic techniques.[12] A similar experience has been reported from Canada.[13] By contrast, there appears to be a real, striking deficit, unrelated to a disparity in neuroradiologic services, in children of Indian (but not Pakistani) origin living in the United Kingdom.[14]

Regional differences in the proportionality of subgroups of disease attest to geographic variation in biology. The most widely studied disease in this regard is acute lymphoblastic leukemia.[15] A higher proportion of cases of T-cell phenotypes are typical of the subgroup distribution in low-income countries.[15] Even regional variations in the categories within this phenotype have been described, for example, in Egypt[16] and Saudi Arabia.[17] Clues to causal relationships with subgroup distribution are perhaps strongest with acute lymphoblastic leukemia of "common" phenotype, for this appears to have become more frequent (and accompanied by an early age peak) in association with industrialization, on retrospective examination over a long period of time in the United Kingdom.[18] This recognition leads to two infection-based theories of leukemogenesis—the delayed infection hypothesis[19] and the population mixing hypothesis[20] that invoke abnormal immune responses to and defective immunosurveillance of common pathogens, respectively. A similar but much more abbreviated transition in phenotypes has been described in the Gaza Strip.[21]

Molecular genetic analyses may provide a partial explanation for the relative refractoriness of acute lymphoblastic leukemia in some developing countries to chemotherapy, as in the paucity of the RUNX1 translocation reported from India.[22]

BARRIERS TO PROGRESS

Although it is widely appreciated that enormous efforts, and correspondingly huge sums of money, are being expended to address the global control of HIV, tuberculosis, and malaria, it is much less well known that there are more deaths from cancer worldwide, in children and adults overall, than from these three infectious diseases combined.[23] As has been expressed, "cancer is set to become the newest epidemic in the developing world."[24] An effort to focus attention on this challenge in Africa led to the identification of numerous barriers to progress (Table 53.2); to the recognition that the conventional elements of cancer control require modification in this context (Table 53.3); and to the agreement that tackling the burden of cancer will require alignment of strategies to those in place for limiting the spread of HIV, tuberculosis, and malaria.[24] The barriers to progress that are particular to pediatric oncology are no less daunting and are reflected in the postulated 5% to 10% 5-year survival rates in Bangladesh, the Philippines, Senegal, Tanzania, and Vietnam.[2]

TABLE 53.2

BARRIERS TO EFFECTIVE CANCER PLANNING

- Insufficient political priority and funding among donor agencies and governments of developing countries, which have many competing priorities.
- Limited ability to counter life style changes following modernization and urbanization.
- Fragmented and underfinanced health care systems that have not been set up for chronic disease management.
- A lack of cancer awareness, knowledge, and capacity among health workers.
- Lack of diagnostic and treatment capacity.
- Too few effective cancer medicines that are easy to administer and do not require hospitalization.
- Weak referral systems.
- Limited data on cancer incidence and mortality in developing countries due to a lack of functioning cancer registries and limited death certification.

Population Dynamics

Some 25 years ago, the World Bank, in its World Development Report, noted that developing countries represented 78% of the global population in 1990, but that 86% of the world's children resided in these countries with limited resources, and that this figure was projected to increase to more than 90% by 2030.[25] The most recent World Development Report,[26] released officially on April 1, 2009, provided no modification of this projection but rather focuses on "Spatial Disparities and Development Policy."

In contrast to some industrialized nations, in which the birth rate is so low that there is projected to be negative population growth, many developing countries have much higher birth rates. Despite higher infant mortality rates and shorter life expectancies, these marked differences in birth and fertility rates account in large measure for disparate annual population growth rates and the inexorable increase in proportions of children and adults living in countries with limited resources.

However, the impact of these population dynamics is far from uniform within the developing world. For example, in much of the Middle East, health care services are highly developed, readily accessible, and "free" or heavily subsidized. This

---

TABLE 53.3

CONVENTIONAL AND MODIFIED ELEMENTS OF CANCER CONTROL FOR COUNTRIES WITH LIMITED RESOURCES

Conventional
- Prevention, screening, diagnosis, treatment, supportive care, palliation, and end-of-life care

Modified
- Cancer intelligence units/registries
- Tobacco control
- Early diagnosis and prevention
- Curing the curable
- Palliative care
- Training and education

is in stark contrast to most of sub-Saharan Africa. Consequently, it is no surprise that effective cancer control in childhood varies widely in countries with limited resources.

Political Realities

The late Dr. James Grant of UNICEF declared that "Family planning could bring more benefits to more people at less cost than any other technology now available to the human race."[27] This truism is exemplified by the impact of family planning on reducing the infant mortality rate by up to 50% if children are spaced by more than 2 years.[28] This is but one benefit of investing in the education of women. As deduced from the National Family Health Survey 1992 to 1993[29] in India, the population of which is soon to exceed that of China, there are strong associations between the education of women and fertility, infant and child mortality rates, and the nutritional status of children. Moreover, there is a "dose effect"—the more years women spend in school, the greater the impact on these outcome variables.[29]

Cultural Issues

Preferences for traditional forms of health care interventions are rooted deeply in developing countries and must be respected. For example, the government of India has elected to promote traditional health practices.[30] Indeed, there is much that "modern" practitioners can learn from these provider–consumer interactions, including the nature of the interpersonal bond (with its strong elements of trust and compliance) and the biologic effects of the interventions prescribed. Similar considerations underlie the widespread use of complementary and alternative medicines among the families of children with cancer in more privileged societies,[31] prompting calls for more rigorous evaluation of the putative efficacy of these (usually dietary) interventions.[32] It is salutary to observe the parallel and contemporaneous practices of traditional and modern health care in children's hospitals in China and to note that patients are referred easily and commonly from one form of practice to the other.

More troublesome is the custom of gender bias, favoring males, in referral for health care, including treatment of cancer in children,[33] even when gender ratios are adjusted for prevalent and male-dominated lymphomas (Table 53.4).[33] This is but one example of gender inequity, the most extreme forms of which include selective female feticide. Clearly, these practices must be targets for change, just as the male exclusivity with respect to educational opportunities and enfranchisement, which exists in some societies, is subject to legitimate criticism.

On a positive note, striking success has been achieved in another area that constrains the ability to effect cure in children with cancer in countries with limited resources; namely, the abandonment of therapy. This is a widespread problem[34] in some developing countries being the commonest cause of treatment failure. Yet, the phenomenon is amenable to change, as exemplified by the impact of a "twinning" program on the reduction of the abandonment rate in Recife, Brazil from 16% to 0.5%.[35] Similar improvements by an order of magnitude have been reported from several countries in Central America. Again, a national investment by the federal government of Mexico has limited the rate of abandonment by families of children with acute lymphoblastic leukemia to less than 1%.[36]

Comorbidities

The major killers of children in countries with limited resources remain infections (especially bacterial pneumonia, malaria, measles, and HIV/AIDS), malnutrition (including micronutrient deficiencies of iron, iodine, and vitamin A), and diarrheal dehydration. But these circumstances are undergoing considerable change. The impacts of immunization programs, treated mosquito netting, nutritional education, and the widespread availability of inexpensive oral rehydration solutions have been enormous when judged by the number of lives saved, as reflected by improvements in the under 5 mortality rates.

In considerable part as a consequence of these successes, there has been an increase in the relative importance of cancer in the spectrum of disease in childhood, in at least some developing countries. For example, cancer is now the most common cause of disease-related death in children of school age in China, and the same is true in parts of Latin America.

However, there are important interactions between infections, nutritional status, and cancer in early life. The contribution of Epstein-Barr virus to the pathogenesis of Burkitt's lymphoma, Hodgkin disease, and nasopharyngeal carcinoma are well known, as is the association between the hepatitis B virus (with or without co-exposure to aflatoxin) and hepatocellular carcinoma. More recently, it has become clear that the prevalence of carcinoma of the cervix in adolescent females in developing countries is a consequence of infection with human papilloma virus (HPV), especially HPV 16 and 18. The impact of the introduction of HPV vaccines at the population level is eagerly awaited.[37]

TABLE 53.4

GENDER RATIOS FOR CHILDHOOD CANCER REGISTRATIONS

Country	Childhood population gender ratio M:F	Cancer registration gender ratio M:F	Lymphoma registration gender ratio M:F	Other cancer registration gender ratio M:F
Bangladesh	1.07	1.97	2.88	1.88
Egypt	1.02	1.55	2.05	1.38
Hong Kong	1.08	1.46	2.26	1.39
India	1.06	1.65	2.87	1.49
Nigeria	0.99	1.68	2.30	1.38
Pakistan	n/a	2.05	3.83	1.79
Papua New Guinea	1.15	1.91	2.93	1.50
Uganda	0.09	1.41	1.53	1.37

Hepatitis B vaccination has had a measurable influence on the death rate from hepatocellular carcinoma,[38] although the vaccine is often not available in poor countries in which hepatitis B infection is prevalent.[39] Similarly, control of HIV infection must be a high priority, especially in African countries where there has been an increase in the numbers of cases of Kaposi's sarcoma in children,[8] with a shift in the lymphadenopathic form of the disease to that predominantly involving the skin.[40]

The World Health Organization (WHO)/AIDS Update in 2006 reported 650,000 new cases of HIV/AIDS in children worldwide, with even a country as small as Botswana having 32,000 children affected under the age of 15.[41] While the CDC Surveillance Report of 1996 indicated that 2% of 7,629 children with AIDS had cancer as the AIDS-defining illness,[42] this is likely an underestimate of the cancer burden as only the initial AIDS-defining illness was reported. Even this underestimate translates to about 13,000 cases of HIV-related malignancies in children per year worldwide.

Malnutrition is defined by the WHO as acute (wasting) or chronic (stunting) on the basis of weight for height (WFH) and height for age (HFA), respectively. However, these measures may not be appropriate for children with cancer, especially in countries with limited resources. In children with advanced disease (an all-too-common circumstance in the developing world), the size of the tumor may result in an overestimation of the WFH (and so of true nutritional status).[43] Some populations, such as the Mayans in Central America, may be constitutively shorter than children in Western Europe and North America, with a resultant overestimation of chronic malnutrition (Table 53.5). But there is little doubt on the importance of nutritional morbidity (Fig. 53.3) in children with malignant disease.[44] The second international workshop devoted to this topic was held in Puebla, Mexico in November 2006.[45]

Socioeconomic Status

Clearly, socioeconomic status is a multielement construct. As a result, definitions vary widely, according to the elements included. In Brazil, for example, one pragmatic approach used an amalgam of household income and quantified utilization of electricity.[46] This particular construct has demonstrable interrelationships with nutritional status and the prevalence of

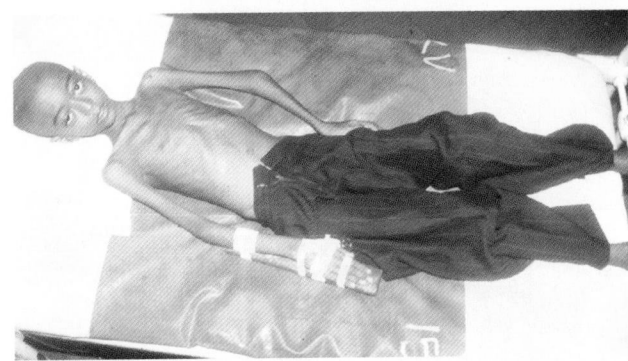

FIGURE 53.3 Child with metastatic neuroblastoma.

infectious diseases, which are matters of particular concern in the context of cancer in childhood. Indeed, as defined in the Brazilian scenario, there is a clear association between socioeconomic status and survival, as reported for acute lymphoblastic leukemia.[46] Interestingly, socioeconomic status has been linked to immunophenotype in this disease.[47]

By what mechanism does socioeconomic status impact morbidity and mortality in pediatric oncology? The particularly disadvantaged members of society are less likely to seek conventional health care (being more inclined to consult traditional healers) and have more difficulty accessing medical systems because of limited availability and maldistribution of services, as well as the need to undertake expensive travel, as exemplified in Mexico.[48] Yet, the convention on the Rights of the Child, adopted more than 15 years ago by the United Nations General Assembly, clearly states (Article 21): "State Parties recognize the right of the child to the enjoyment of the highest attainable standard of health and to facilities for the treatment of illness and rehabilitation of health. State Parties shall strive to ensure that no child is deprived of his or her right to access to such healthcare services"—clearly a particular challenge in the developing country context.

Even if access is achieved, affordability is often an issue; in Mumbai, India (Fig. 53.4) as many as one-third of families were forced to decline antineoplastic therapy for their children.[49] Similar experiences have been reported from Indonesia and Sudan, whereas the figure has reached 60% in Bangladesh.[50] In 1995, Chandy suggested[51] that there were

TABLE 53.5

MALNUTRITION IN CHILDREN IN CENTRAL AMERICA

Country	Wasting[a] (%)	Stunting[a] (%)	U5MR[b]	GNI per capita[c]	Indigenous population (%)	Mayan population (%)
Costa Rica	2	6	11	5,560	2	0
Dominican Republic	1	7	38	3,550	<1	0
El Salvador	1	19	24	2,850	8	<1
Guatemala	2	49	39	2,440	58	57.5
Honduras	1	25	24	1,600	8.5	<1
Nicaragua	1	17	35	980	7	0
Panama	1	18	23	5,510	10	0

[a]Moderate/severe aged 0–5 yrs, by WHO criteria.
[b]Under 5 mortality rate.
[c]U.S. $ per year.
U5MR is similar in Dominican Republic, Guatemala, and Nicaragua but the proportion of patients who are "stunted" is markedly higher in Guatemala. The countries with the lowest proportion of indigenous populations (Costa Rica and Dominican Republic) have the lowest rates of "stunting" despite markedly different U5MR.

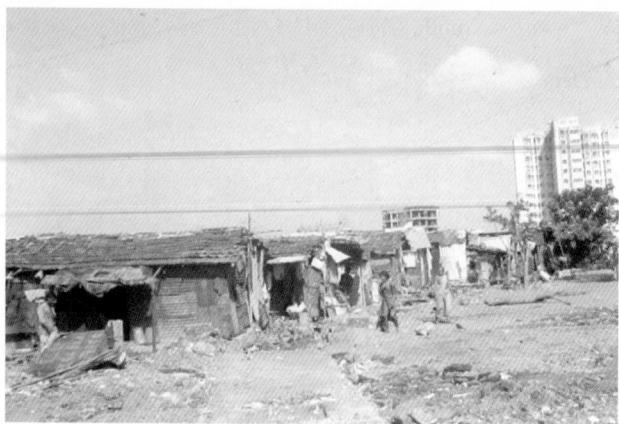

FIGURE 53.4 Urban slums (Mumbai).

three categories of families on the basis of income, educational status, and motivation to undergo treatment:

1. Illiterate parents, working as laborers with a monthly family income of less than $20, who have little motivation to treat a child with cancer. They constituted 70% of the population in the developing world at that time.
2. Literate parents with average incomes of U.S. $50 to 100 per month, who are well motivated but have considerable difficulty in finding the necessary resources. They constituted 25% of the population in the developing world.
3. Highly educated parents, with monthly incomes exceeding U.S. $1,000, who are strongly motivated and possess the resources necessary to support prolonged, intensive treatment. They constituted less than 5% of the population in the developing world.

However, overcoming the costs of treatment may not provide an adequate solution for subsequent abandonment of conventional care is all too common (described earlier). But this is only the most extreme form of reduced compliance with therapeutic protocols for, as was demonstrated in an Australian study,[52] there is a clear relationship between overall compliance and socioeconomic status. Moreover, such problems are not otherwise limited to countries listed as having limited resources. For example, there is persuasive evidence from Glasgow, Scotland (one of the poorest cities in Western Europe) that low socioeconomic status is linked to diminished nutritional status and predicts for compromised survival prospects in children with acute lymphoblastic leukemia.[53]

Resource Restriction and Malutilization

There are too few specialized physicians, and they are usually concentrated in big cities, although a large proportion of the population may live in the countryside and in smaller conurbations. Access to these well-trained and capable doctors is limited further by their need to spend the majority of their time in private practice to augment the grossly inadequate incomes provided by the public health care system. Efforts to increase the number of specialized physicians and to expand their availability are well exemplified by the programs of the Indian Academy of Pediatrics.[54] A regional approach has been adopted in Central America in which young physicians from several countries undertake fellowship training in pediatric oncology in Guatemala, returning thereafter to their homelands.

In many instances, nurses are undereducated and quite simply unable to meet the demands of providing complex care to children with cancer. This major deficit in a cornerstone of clinical practice is widely recognized, and it is now the target of numerous concentrated efforts to bridge the gap by implementing intensive training in local circumstances with the aid of expert nurses from larger centers in industrialized countries. The International Outreach Program of St. Jude Children's Research Hospital has engaged in such activities in Central America, as an example.[55]

Not surprisingly, many allied health professions are grievously under-represented in the clinical teams. Social workers, clinical pharmacists, dieticians, and child life specialists are seldom to be found. Psychologists, physiotherapists, and others are equally scarce. In the face of such shortages, it is especially troublesome to learn about different levels of care being provided according to the socioeconomic status, as has been described in Indonesia.[56]

A paucity of diagnostic capability, both quantitative and qualitative, regrettably characterizes the working conditions in many countries with limited resources. Within laboratories, there is very little in the way of immunohistochemistry, flow cytometry, ultrastructural analysis, karyotyping, and molecular genetics. Similarly, in radiology, the availability of computed tomography, magnetic resonance imaging, and the techniques of nuclear medicine is severely restricted, notably in much of Africa. These deficits impose major limitations on diagnostic accuracy, without which decisions on appropriate therapy are jeopardized. Solutions include the development of regional facilities and expertise, as exemplified by the flow cytometry center in Central America.[57]

Turning to therapeutic modalities, one has to give immediate attention to the resource-intensive and consumptive aspects of surgical and radiation oncology. The latter is virtually unavailable in much of sub-Saharan Africa (Fig. 53.5), while sophisticated neurosurgical techniques and limb salvage procedures are almost unknown in large areas of the developing world. A striking exception has been reported from Chile, with the successful delivery of multimodality care, including limb reconstruction, in patients with osteosarcoma;[58] and at an order of magnitude less cost than in Memphis, United States. Likewise, in the absence of radiotherapy in a much poorer country—Nicaragua—good results have been obtained in the treatment of Wilms' tumor[59] and Hodgkin disease.[60] This success has been extended to non-Hodgkin lymphoma.[61]

Perhaps the single most important constraint on progress in pediatric oncology in developing countries is the limited

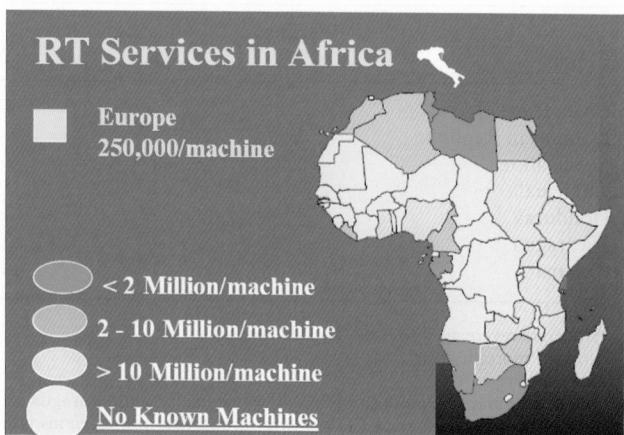

FIGURE 53.5 Radiotherapy services in Africa.

availability of effective chemotherapy. In large measure, this is often due to costs that are exorbitant by local standards. The problem is magnified by similar limitations in access to antibiotics (which are sometimes more expensive than antineoplastic drugs), antiemetics, and other agents used in supportive care. These difficulties may be compounded by cumbersome import regulations, expensive tariffs, and poor inventory control.[11] Attempts to overcome these obstacles by the local production of pharmaceuticals do not always meet acceptable standards of quality with respect to safety and efficacy.

Despite these impediments, progress can be made in the most challenging circumstances, as demonstrated in children with Burkitt's lymphoma in several African countries using a simplified protocol with a drug cost of less than $50 per patient.[62,63] Even patients with resistant disease or who relapse can be salvaged.[64] Such experience supports the WHO initiative to develop an evidence-based list of essential drugs for the treatment of malignant diseases in children (Hill S, personal communication, 2009), building on the "complementary list" associated with the list of essential medicines for children.[65] Inclusion on this list may increase the prospect of government-sponsored availability of individual drugs in countries with limited resources as the list is intended to be a guide and stimulus in this regard.

In the area of supportive care, there is a particularly difficult challenge regarding blood products. The seemingly simple matter of blood donation and collection may be complicated by a wide range of obstacles, from cultural taboos (a donation is viewed as losing part of oneself) to underfunding. Negative attitudes to donation also underlie the racial and ethnic imbalances in the pools of volunteer bone marrow donors in industrialized countries. Strategies to increase the supply of blood products have included the requirement for healthy relatives to provide undirected donations and contracts with commercial companies to provide packed red cells and platelet concentrates in exchange for fractionated plasma. Despite such initiatives, it has been estimated that, in India, with more than 1,000 blood banks, only 50% of the need for blood products is met.[66] Such challenges have been the subject of considerable debate centered on safety, efficacy, and cost.[67]

Concerns about safety abound and are well founded.[66] This is especially true with respect to the prevalence of hepatitis B and HIV infections in the apparently healthy population, which may be as high as 20% (in China) and 40% (in parts of Africa), respectively. Indeed, the HIV-1 seroprevalence in sex workers in Kenya, Uganda, and Zimbabwe exceeds 80%.[67] In India, a considerable fraction of the blood supply is obtained from paid "professional" donors who are mainly men of low socioeconomic status.[68] Testing for hepatitis B and HIV is limited and erratic, and it has been estimated that only about 50% of transfused blood is properly screened and safe.[69] In Botswana, directed donor transfusions are disallowed due to the high prevalence of HIV infection and the stigma of having a positive status become known within the family. Faced with these challenges, there is an evident need to be stringent in the use of blood products, for example, by setting conservative "transfusion triggers" for the correction of euvolemic anemia and the administration of prophylactic platelet concentrates. Strategies for addressing some of these difficulties have been proposed.[70]

The WHO convened World Blood Donor Day on June 14, 2007; noting that, in the half-million women who die every year during pregnancy (99% in developing countries), the commonest cause of death is hemorrhage. The minimum screening recommended is for HIV, hepatitis B and C, and syphilis. The majority of sub-Saharan African countries had not yet met the target in the WHO survey, but 10 countries with limited resources reported that they had achieved that goal—Benin, Burundi, Chile, Democratic Republic of Congo, Ecuador, Guinea-Bissau, Honduras, Mauritania, Uzbekistan, and Democratic Republic of Korea.[70]

Elements of Cancer Control

There are few opportunities to effect prevention of cancers that occur during childhood and adolescence, but the prospects are not entirely bleak. Educational programs aimed at reducing sun exposure, avoiding unprotected sex, and changing some regional habits (e.g., chewing of betel nuts and smokeless tobacco) could affect the prevalence of malignant melanoma, HIV-associated Kaposi's sarcoma, and oral cancer, respectively. Hepatitis B and HPV vaccination are additional strategies to pursue (described earlier). At least as importantly, global efforts to encourage young people not to smoke predictably will have a major impact on the incidences of tobacco-related cancers (and other illnesses) in adult life—surely an enormously worthwhile goal.

As to the issue of cancer screening, numerous challenges are presented. In the circumstance of familial retinoblastoma, the need for early and repeated examination of the eyes is obvious. Whether such a practice would have a role, in those parts of the world where the sporadic disease is most common, remains to be tested. It is unlikely that screening for neuroblastoma will be useful in countries with limited resources because the incidence of this disease in general is lower than in industrialized societies in which screening programs have not effected an appreciable reduction in morbidity or mortality.[71] By contrast, there is good evidence for the role of routine cervical smear examinations in reducing the burden of illness associated with carcinoma of the cervix, a disease that does occur among girls in developing countries.[72] It remains to be determined whether the training of primary health care workers in developing countries, in the Integrated Management of Childhood Illness, as advocated by the WHO,[73] will result in the earlier detection of more cases of cancer in children (Fig. 53.6). Experience in Brazil suggests that knowledge of symptoms and signs of cancer in children, among community health workers, is poor (not unexpectedly).[74]

Treatment is the most important component of cancer control in childhood. Although it is manifestly important to promote adherence to fundamental oncologic principles in surgical practice (as with needle biopsies, sampling of lymph nodes, and obtaining clear lines of resection), surgeons are ever more commonly facing the challenges of operating after neoadjuvant therapy. Because children with solid tumors often are

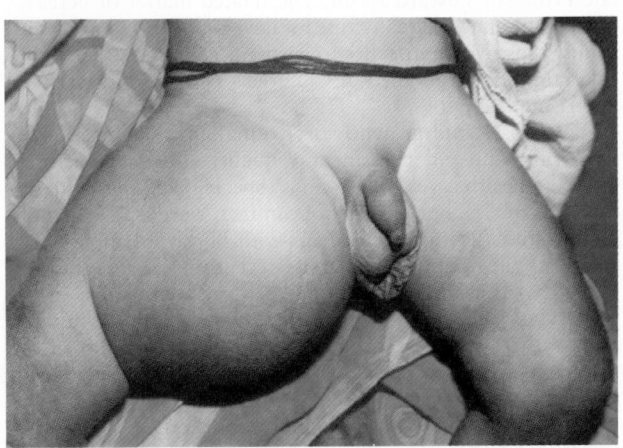

FIGURE 53.6 Infant with locally advanced fibrosarcoma.

referred initially to surgeons (who may be the only practitioners of oncology in some parts of the world), fostering modern surgical contributions to the care of children with cancer can be difficult, demanding a combination of patience, persistence, and continuing education. With radiotherapy, the challenges are materially different, relating more to issues of availability, equipment costs (including maintenance), quality control, and appropriate utilization. On the other hand, delivering cost-effective chemotherapy requires that close attention be paid to the therapeutic index—the often precarious balance between efficacy and toxicity. Walking this line can pose particular hazards in the context of comorbidities (described earlier), and simplification of chemotherapy may be important. Detailed knowledge of local circumstances can allow the elaboration of appropriate treatment strategies. In a thoughtful contribution,[75] Hunger and colleagues have outlined treatment protocols of graduated intensity for acute lymphoblastic leukemia in countries with limited resources.

Acceptable effectiveness may require considerable treatment intensity, especially if high-dose chemotherapy and multimodality approaches are employed, but treatment intensity comes at the price of toxicity. As a result, the importance of supportive care cannot be overstated and treatment-related mortality is a major challenge.[76] The essential components of infection control, pain management, antiemesis, blood product supply, and nutritional support must be in place. In countries with limited resources, provision of supportive care can be especially demanding, often generating imaginative and innovative solutions, which ought to be (and sometimes are) incorporated in the therapeutic armamentarium of less resource-restricted centers. Among these may be cited the safe and effective delivery of high-dose methotrexate with "rescue" on an ambulatory basis[77] (reported recently as having been adopted successfully at the Memorial Sloan Kettering Cancer Centre[78]), outpatient management of fever and neutropenia with oral antibiotics[79] (emulated cost effectively in the United States),[80] and the administration of supplemented candy bars as nutritional support.[81] Even allogeneic stem cell transplantation without myeloablative conditioning has been accomplished without hospital admission in the developing country setting.[82]

Palliative care for children outside of the hospital environment may seem like an insuperable problem in countries with limited resources, especially as it remains a major challenge even in the most privileged circumstances.[83] Yet, it is in these situations that the great majority of deaths from cancer in childhood will occur. When there is sufficient will to address the issue, surprising success may ensue, as in the case of the hospice established more than 20 years ago in Kenya by the late Professor Edward Kasili. The related matter of bereavement counseling is equally ripe for development, requiring culturally sensitive approaches to ensure acceptability. Such considerations are embodied in Children's Hospice International and related activities.[84]

For those children who survive malignant disease, long-term follow-up and assessment of quality of life become focal points in health care. Follow-up is especially difficult in developing countries, but persistence can be rewarded, as exemplified by studies of former patients with Burkitt's lymphoma in Uganda,[85] in Malawi[86] and more recently in Saudi Arabia.[87] Similarly, efforts to measure the health-related quality of life of survivors should not be viewed as a superfluous luxury. Such measurements can be made with ease and have been accomplished in countries with limited resources, with surprising positive results.[88,89] These achievements allow the calculation of disability-adjusted life years (DALYS), judged by the WHO to be important measures of the comprehensive health status of individuals and populations,[90] and provide a

basis for a more rigorous definition of cure in the form of quality-adjusted survival.[91]

OPPORTUNITIES FOR RESEARCH

Contrary to a prevalent supposition that countries with limited resources cannot afford to support and conduct research, the case for Essential National Health Research has been made persuasively.[92,93] This cogent argument is stimulated in part by the evident need to find locally appropriate, cost-effective solutions to local problems and opportunities. Among these is the challenge of caring for children with cancer, determined by the World Bank to be a cost-effective undertaking in developing countries.[94] Particularly expensive procedures, such as stem cell transplantation, are proper targets for economic evaluation.[95]

In this setting, there are particular prospects worthy of attention that should attract the investment of more privileged parties, notably in sophisticated technology. The epidemiologic evidence of widely disparate distributions of disease has prompted interest in genetic predisposition and molecular oncogenesis, especially with respect to viral etiology. Coupled with the markedly different circumstances of rural and urban populations, which provide fertile ground for investigations of potential environmental pathogenesis, such studies should shed new light on the biology of cancer in childhood around the world. Moreover, there is the added value of technology transfer in such "North–South" cooperative ventures and more recently in "South–South" partnerships in Asia.[96] A striking example is provided by the recent discovery of a novel, consistent, and germ-line mutation in children with adrenocortical tumors in Brazil.[97] Furthermore, good clinical epidemiology can contribute to advances in health care delivery.[6,98]

The survival advantage offered to children with cancer by participation in therapeutic trials, while receiving care in specialized centers in privileged societies, has its parallels in the developing country setting (as exemplified by the Indian experience with protocols for acute lymphoblastic leukemia[99,100]) and provides a sound rationale for fostering clinical research in pediatric oncology in countries with limited resources. At the same time, we must devote considerable attention also to the ethical responsibilities of investigators. Participation in such endeavors, which include the essentiality of good data management, enhances the discipline of health care delivery and establishes a higher standard of practice. These goals are promoted by the formation of cooperative groups. Successful examples of such enterprises exist in Latin America, within individual countries (such as the Wilms' tumor consortium in Brazil and PINDA in Chile) as well as multinationally (as with AHOPCA in Central America). These entities have built a solid track record, producing outcomes rivaling those reported from equivalent clinical trials in Europe and North America. Again, there is added value; in this instance, it is the building of knowledge and experience in networks of pediatric oncologists.

STRATEGIES FOR CHANGE

According to the Global Health Research Forum in 2002,[101] "Every year more than US$70 billion is spent on health research and development by the public and private sectors. But only about 10% of this is used for research into 90% of the world's health problems. This is what is called the 10/90 gap." A related gap exists between those with and those without access to effective health care services, which in some countries is widening. A forum to debate these issues has been established.[102]

As has been enunciated by others, setting and implementing the research agenda must occur at local or regional levels and not be imposed by paternalistic or colonial influences. The approach must be comprehensive yet appropriate to local country and community-level needs; it must capitalize on effective North–South, West–East partnerships (including public–private partnerships) yet engender local ownership, capacity strengthening, and institution building; it must encourage prioritization of limited resources yet enable sustainability; and it must be informed by the best available evidence and must be scientifically sound.[103]

Sharing experience and resources is the basis of the successful "twinning" programs between well-established pediatric oncology centers in developed countries and aspiring institutions in countries with limited resources,[103] as espoused in the Montevideo Document.[104] These programs must be real partnerships of equals, addressing objectives approved bilaterally, to be mutually rewarding. Such is the case between a consortium of centers in German-speaking countries and numerous institutions in Eastern Europe; between the International Network for Cancer Treatment and Research and a group of partners in India; between various centers in Italy and their one-to-one linkages in Latin America (one of the successful outcomes from the Monza International School for Pediatric Hematology-Oncology); and with the International Outreach Program of St. Jude Children's Research Hospital and its network, including institutions in the Middle East. Measurement of the effect of such programs has been made.[105] One of the most important platforms on which these programs have been built is the exchange of personnel with a focus on training. The long-term impact of these educational opportunities is enormous. In large measure, however, these have involved only physicians, laboratory scientists, and nurses so far. There is a major need to extend opportunities of this kind to data managers, clinical pharmacists, and other member groups of multidisciplinary pediatric oncology health care teams.

As stated by Magrath,[106] training oncology nurses will free doctors from many of the tasks they currently perform, such as the administration of chemotherapy, providing information to patients, and organizing follow-up visits. Training doctors in the conduct of clinical research, and developing a cadre of data managers, will make it possible to conduct clinical trials and provide incentive, in addition to the particular topic of research, to identify the reasons for late presentation and poor follow up, and to develop effective strategies to improve the situation. Ideally, such training should be conducted in the institutions in developing countries themselves.

Success in such ventures should lead to the establishment of pediatric oncology units, functioning as local centers of excellence. A prime example has been described from Recife, Brazil.[35] It is even possible to envision such centers engaging in shared care with nonspecialist health care professionals (such as general pediatricians) who work closer to the home of the child and family—a model proposed for the large and populous country of India.[107] A model for the progressive development of such capacity has been proposed.[108]

However, even these "twinning" programs have restricted scope. A broader, more inclusive alliance of stakeholders is needed. In particular, the value of involving parents has become obvious. Local and national organizations have formed the International Confederation of Childhood Cancer Parent Organizations (ICCCPO), established in 1994 and now with 43 member countries. This organization is affiliated with the International Society for Pediatric Oncology (SIOP), with which it holds contemporaneous annual meetings. The potential role for ICCCPO in advocating for increased resource allocation, to address the imminent needs of children with cancer and their families, is enormous. It is likely also that they could play important roles in the continuing debate about ethical standards in the conduct of clinical research in developing countries. However, in many countries with limited resources, parents alone do not have the skills to fulfill such roles; there, the establishment of community-based support groups can prove to be invaluable.

The remarkable progress in pediatric oncology, enjoyed in industrialized societies, has come at increasing cost. This escalating financial burden, on families as well as on health care systems,[109] highlights and serves to amplify the inadequacy of resources available in developing countries for the care of children with cancer. Such a widening gap strains the abilities of governments to meet the need and prompts consideration of alliances of associations of parents and volunteers with physicians and other health professionals to provide a realistic framework for progress in developing countries. Strategies to minimize drug costs have been reviewed,[110] and optimizing donated chemotherapeutic agents has been described.[111]

As governments are increasingly interested in economic evaluation of health care technologies, including clinical interventions, there are opportunities to perform cost analyses and match these with measurements of health status and health-related quality of life to better inform health care planning and policy development.[112] There are even emerging accounts of measures of the quality of care provided by hospitals in developing countries.[113] Others have contributed constructively to this debate,[114] and the My Child Matters program

---

TABLE 53.6

THE WORLD CANCER DECLARATION 2008 TARGETS: BY 2020

- Sustainable delivery systems will be in place to ensure that effective cancer control programs are available in all countries
- The measurement of the global cancer burden and the impact of cancer control interventions will have improved significantly
- Global tobacco consumption, obesity, and alcohol intake levels will have fallen significantly
- Populations in the areas affected by HPV and HBV will be covered by universal vaccination programs
- Public attitudes toward cancer will improve, and damaging myths and misconceptions about the disease will be dispelled
- Many more cancers will be diagnosed when still localized through the provision of screening and early detection programs and high levels of public and professional awareness about important cancer warning signs
- Access to accurate cancer diagnosis, appropriate cancer treatments, supportive care, rehabilitation services, and palliative care will have improved for all patients worldwide
- Effective pain control measures will be available universally to all cancer patients in pain
- The number of training opportunities available for health professionals in different aspects of cancer control will have improved significantly
- Emigration of health workers with specialist training in cancer control will have reduced dramatically
- There will be major improvements in cancer survival rates in all countries

orchestrated by the International Union Against Cancer (UICC) holds promise as an agent of change.[2,114]

Bringing all of these elements together will be facilitated by the tools of electronic communication (on-line journals, telemedicine, UNICEF Web sites, and the like). Providing these amenities and the training to use them is sure to foster the continuing development of pediatric oncology in countries with limited resources. "We will meet in the developing world a level of will, skill, and constancy that may put ours to shame. We may well find ourselves not the teachers we thought we were, but students of those who simply will not be stopped under circumstances that would have stopped us long ago."[113]

In its admittedly ambitious effort, the UICC developed The World Cancer Declaration 2008 that was adopted by the World Cancer Summit 2008 and endorsed by the World Cancer Congress 2008. Its lofty call to action from the global cancer community reads—"we the global cancer community call on governments, international governmental organizations, the international donor community, development agencies, professional organizations, the private sector and all civil society to take immediate steps to slow and ultimately reverse the growth in deaths from cancer, by committing to the targets set out below and providing resources and political backing for the priority actions needed to achieve them." The targets, to be attained by 2020, are listed in Table 53.6, an ambitious agenda indeed for the forthcoming decade. In making a start, the UICC has partnered with the Lance Armstrong Foundation to host a Global Cancer Summit in Dublin, Ireland.

References

1. The World Bank. Data and Statistics http://web.worldbank.org. Accessed March 24, 2009.
2. Ribeiro RC, Steliarova-Foucher E, Magrath I, et al. Baseline status of pediatric oncology care in ten low-income or mid-income countries receiving My Child Matters support: a descriptive study. Lancet Oncol 2008;9:721–729.
3. The World Health Report. World Health Organization http://www.who.int/whr/en/index.htm. Accessed March 24, 2009.
4. A world fit for children. Millennium development goals. Special session on children. Documents and the Convention on the Rights of the Child. New York, NY: UNICEF, 2002;14:16.
5. Parkin DM, Kramarova E, Draper GJ, et al. International incidence of childhood cancer Vol II. Lyon France: International Agency for Research on Cancer, 1998;1–391.
6. Howard SC, Metzger ML, Wilimas JA, et al. Childhood cancer epidemiology in low income countries. Cancer 2008;112:461–472.
7. Stiller CA, Parkin DM. Geographic and ethnic variations in the incidence of childhood cancer. Br Med Bull 1996;52:682–703.
8. Sinfield RL, Molyneux EM, Banda K. et al. Spectrum and presentation of pediatric malignancies in the HIV era: experience from Blantyre, Malawi 1998–2003. Pediatr Blood Cancer 2007;48:515–520.
9. Bernstein M, Kovar H, Paulussen M, et al. Ewing sarcoma family of tumors: Ewing sarcoma of bone and soft tissue and the peripheral primitive neuroectodermal tumors. In: Pizzo PA, Poplack DG, eds. Principles and practice of pediatric oncology. 5th ed. Philadelphia, PA: Lippincott Williams and Wilkins, 2006:1002–1032.
10. Barr RD. The challenge of childhood cancer in the developing world. East Afr Med J 1994;71:223–225.
11. Barr RD, Kasili EG. Caring for children with cancer in the developing world. In: Pochedly C, ed. Neoplastic diseases of childhood. Chur: Harwood Academic Publishers, 1994:1535–1558.
12. Smith MA, Friedlin B, Ries LA, et al. Trends in reported incidence of primary malignant brain tumors in children in the United States. J Natl Cancer Inst 1998;90:1269–1277.
13. Agha M, DiMonte B, Greenberg M, et al. Incidence trends and projections for childhood cancer in Ontario. Int J Cancer 2006;118:1939–1948.
14. Powell JE, Kelly AM, Parkes SE, et al. Cancer and congenital abnormalities in Asian children: a population-based study from the West Midlands. Br J Cancer 1995;72:1563–1569.
15. Greaves MF, Colman SM, Beard MEJ, et al. Geographical distribution of acute lymphoblastic leukemia subtypes: second report of the collaborative group study. Leukemia 1993;7:27–34.
16. Kamel AM, Ghaleb FM, Assem MM, et al. Phenotypic analysis of acute lymphoblastic leukemia in Egypt. Leukemia Res 1990;14:601–609.
17. Roberts GT, Aur RJ, Sheth KV. Immunophenotypic and age patterns of childhood acute lymphoblastic leukemia in Saudi Arabia. Leukemia Res 1990;14:667–672.
18. Court Brown WM, Doll R. Leukemia in childhood and young adult life. Trends in mortality in relation to aetiology. BMJ 1961;81:988–981.
19. Greaves M. Infection, immune responses and the aetiology of childhood leukaemia. Nature Rev Cancer 2006;6:193–203.
20. Kinlen L. Infections and immune factors in cancer: the role of epidemiology. Oncogene 2004;23:6341–6348.
21. Ramot B, Magrath I. Hypothesis: the environment is a major determinant of the immunological subtype of lymphoma and acute lymphoblastic leukemia in children. Br J Haematol 1982;52:183–189.
22. Sazawal S, Bhatia K, Gutierrez, MI, et al. Paucity of TEL-AML 1 translocation, by multiplex RT-PCR, in B-lineage acute lymphoblastic leukemia (ALL) in Indian patients. Am J Hematol 2004;76:80–82.
23. Stewart BW, Kleihues P, eds. World cancer report. Lyon: International Agency for Research on Cancer, 2005.
24. Lingwood RJ, Boyle P, Milburn A, et al. The challenge of cancer control in Africa. Nature Rev Cancer 2008;8:398–403.
25. World development report 1993. New York, NY: Oxford University Press, 1993.
26. http://www.worldbank.org/wdr 2009. Accessed April 7, 2009.
27. Grant J. The state of the world's children 1992. Oxford: Oxford University Press for UNICEF, 1993.
28. Fathalla M. Impact of family planning on health. In: Senanayake P, Kleinman R, eds. Family planning: meeting challenges, promoting choices. Carnforth: Parthenon, 1993:18–22.
29. International Institute for Population Studies. National family health survey 1992–1993: a summary report. Bombay: International Institute for Population Studies, 1995:36–39.
30. Kumar S. India's government promotes traditional health practices. Lancet 2000;355:1252.
31. Weitzman S. Complementary and alternative (CAM) dietary therapies for cancer. In: Barr RD, ed. Nutrition and cancer in children. The Second International Workshop. Pediatr Blood Cancer 2008;50:494–497.
32. Kelly K. Bringing evidence to complementary and alternative medicine in children with cancer: focus on nutrition-related therapies. In: Barr RD, ed. Nutrition and Cancer in Children. The Second International Workshop. Pediatr Blood Cancer 2008;50: 490–493.
33. Pearce MS, Parker L. Childhood cancer registrations in the developing world: Still more boys than girls. Int J Cancer 2001;91:402–406.
34. Arora RS, Eden T, Pizer B. The problem of treatment abandonment in children from developing countries with cancer. Pediatr Blood Cancer 2007;49:941–949.
35. Howard SC, Pedrosa M, Lins M, et al. Establishment of a pediatric oncology program and outcomes of childhood acute lymphoblastic leukemia in a resource-poor area. JAMA 2004;291:2471–2475.
36. Rivera-Luna R, Leal-Leal C, Rodriguez-Suarez R, et al. A national program for acute lymphoblastic leukemia from medically uninsured Mexican children: preliminary results [abstract PD 004]. Pediatr Blood Cancer 2006;47:428.
37. Kontsky L. The epidemiology behind the HPV vaccine discovery. Ann Epidemiol 2009;19:239–244.
38. Chang MH, Chen CJ, Lai MS, et al. Universal hepatitis B vaccination in Taiwan and incidence of hepatocellular carcinoma in children. N Engl J Med 1997;336:1855–1859.
39. Shann F, Steinhoff MC. Vaccines for children in rich and poor countries. Lancet 1999;354(Suppl 2):7–11.
40. Chintu C, Athale UH, Patil PS. Childhood cancers in Zambia before and after the HIV epidemic. Arch Dis Child 1995;73:100–104.
41. Epidemiology Facts Sheets on HIV/AIDS and Sexually Transmitted Diseases. 2006.
42. AIDS. Among children—United States 1996. MMWR 1996;45:1005–1010.
43. Smith DE, Stevenson MCG, Booth IW. Malnutrition at diagnosis of malignancy in childhood. Common but mostly missed. Eur J Pediatr 1991;150:318–322.
44. Sala A, Pencharz B, Barr RD. Children, cancer and nutrition—a dynamic triangle in review. Cancer 2004;100:677–687.
45. Barr RD, ed. Nutrition and cancer in children. The second international workshop. Pediatr Blood Cancer, 2008;50(Suppl):437–519.
46. Viana MB, Fernandes RA, De Carvalho RI, et al. How socio-economic status is a strong independent predictor of relapse in childhood acute lymphoblastic leukemia. Int J Cancer 1998;(Suppl 11):56–61.
47. Paes CA, Viana MB, Freire RV, et al. Direct association of socio-economic status with T cell acute lymphoblastic leukemia in children. Leukemia Res 2003;27:789.
48. Fajardo-Gutierrez A, Sandoval-Mex A, Mejia-Arangure JM, et al. Clinical and social factors that affect the time to diagnosis of Mexican children with cancer. Med Pediatr Oncol 2002;39:25–31.
49. Advani SH, Pai S, Venzon D, et al. ALL in India: an analysis of prognostic factors using a single treatment regimen. Ann Oncol 1999;10:167–176.
50. Mannan MA, Islam A, Gosh NK. Acute lymphoblastic leukemia—outcome of treatment with a "hybrid" protocol [abstract]. Ind J Pediar 2002;69:51.
51. Chandy M. Childhood acute lymphoblastic leukemia in India. An approach to management in a three–tier society. Med Pediatr Oncol 1995;25:197–203.
52. McWhirter WR, Smith IJ, McWhirter KM. Social class as a prognostic variable in acute lymphoblastic leukemia. Med J Aust 1983;ii:319–321.
53. Barr RD, Gibson BES. Nutritional status and cancer in childhood. J Pediatr Hematol Oncol 2000;22:491–494.
54. Agarwal BR, Marwaha RK, Kurkure PA, et al. Indian national training project practical paediatric oncology (INTPPPO): 2nd national teachers' meeting consensus report. Med Pediatr Oncol 2002;39:251.
55. Wilimas JA, Donahue N, Chammas G, et al. Training sub-specialty nurses in developing countries: methods, outcome and cost. Med Pediatr Oncol 2003;41:136–140.
56. Mostert S, Sitaresmi MN, Gundy CM, et al. Attitude of health care providers toward childhood leukemia patients with different socio-economic status. Pediatr Blood Cancer 2008;50:1001–1005.
57. Howard SC, Campana D, Coustan-Smith E, et al. Development of a regional flow cytometry centre for diagnosis of childhood leukemia in Central America. Leukemia 2005;19:323–325.
58. Rivera GK, Quintana J, Villarroel M, et al. Transfer of complex front-line anticancer therapy to a developing country: the St. Jude osetosarcoma experience in Chile. Pediatr Blood Cancer 2008;50:1143–1146.
59. Baez F, Fossati-Bellani F, Ocampo E, et al. Treatment of childhood Wilms' tumour without radiotherapy in Nicaragua. Ann Oncol 2002;13:944–948.

60. Baez F, Ocampo E, Conter V, et al. Treatment of childhood Hodgkin's disease with COPP or COPP-ABV (hybrid) without radiotherapy in Nicaragua. Ann Oncol 1997;8: 247–250.

61. Baez F, Pillon M, Manfredini L, et al. Treatment of pediatric non-Hodgkin lymphomas in a country with limited resources: results of the first national protocol in Nicaragua. Pediatr Blood Cancer 2008;50:148–152.

62. Harif M, Barsaoui S, Benchekroun S, et al. Treatment of B cell lymphoma with LMB modified protocols in Africa—report of the French-African pediatric oncology group (GFAOP). Pediatr Blood Cancer 2008;50:1138–1142.

63. Hesseling PB, Molyneux E, Tchintseme F, et al. Treating Burkitt's lymphoma in Malawi, Cameroon, and Ghana. Lancet Oncol 2008;9:512–513.

64. Hesseling PB, Molyneux E, Kamiza S, et al. Rescue chemotherapy for patients with resistant or relapsed endemic Burkitt lymphoma. Trans R Soc Trop Med Hyg 2008;102: 602–607.

65. World Health Organization. Essential Medicines http://www.who.int/medicines/services/essmedicines_def/en/print.html.

66. Dasgupta PR, Manoj K, Jain T, et al. Government response to HIV/AIDS in India. AIDS 1994;8(Suppl 2):S83–S90.

67. Bates I, Manyasi G, Medina LA. Reducing replacement donors in sub-Saharan Africa: challenges and affordability. Transfus Med 2007;17:434–442.

68. Jain MK, John TJ, Keusch GT. Epidemiology of HIV and AIDS in India. AIDS 1994; 8(Suppl 2):S61–S75.

69. World development indicators 1998. Washington DC: International Bank for Reconstruction and Development/The World Bank, 1998.

70. Improving blood safety worldwide. Editorial. Lancet 2007;370:361.

71. Woods WG, Tuchman M, Robison LL. A population-based study of the usefulness of screening for neuroblastoma. Lancet 1996;348:1682–1687.

72. Boring C, Squires TS, Tong T. Cancer statistics 1992. CA Cancer J Clin 1992;42:19–38.

73. Tulloch J. Integrated approach to child health in developing countries. Lancet 1999; 354(Suppl 2):16–20.

74. Workman GM, Ribeiro RC, Rai SN, et al. Pediatric cancer knowledge: assessment of knowledge of warning signs and symptoms for pediatric cancer among Brazilian community health workers. J Cancer Educ 2007;22:181–118.

75. Hunger SP, Sung L, Howard SC. Treatment strategies and regimens of graduated intensity for childhood acute lymphoblastic leukemia in low-income countries: a proposal. Pediatr Blood Cancer 2009;52:559–565.

76. Gupta S, Bonilla M, Fuentes SL, et al. Prevalence and predictors of treatment-related mortality in pediatric acute leukemia in El Salvador. Br J Cancer 2009;100:1026–1031.

77. Tanaka C, Goncalves-Diaz C, Ciolette A, et al. High dose methotrexate: multi-disciplinary support and ambulatorial care [abstract 252]. Med Pediatr Oncol 1996;27:274.

78. Zelcer S, Kellick M, Wexler LH, et al. The Memorial Sloan Kettering Cancer Centre experience with outpatient administration of high dose methotrexate with leucovorin rescue. Pediatr Blood Cancer 2008;50:1176–1180.

79. Petrilli AS, Dantas LS, Campos MC, et al. Oral ciprofloxacin vs. intravenous ceftriaxone administered in an outpatient setting for fever and neutropenia in low risk pediatric oncology patients: randomised prospective trial. Med Pediatr Oncol 2000;34:87–91.

80. Mullen CA, Petropoulos D, Roberts WM, et al. Economic and resource utilization analysis of outpatient management of fever and neutropenia in low risk pediatric patients with cancer. J Pediatr Hematol Oncol 1999;21:212–218.

81. Gomez-Almaguer D, Montemajor J, Gonzalez-Llano O, et al. Leukemia and nutrition IV. Improvement in the nutritional status of children with standard risk acute lymphoblastic leukemia is associated with better tolerance to continuation chemotherapy. Int J Pediatr Hematol Oncol 1995;2:53–56.

82. Gomez-Almaguer D, Ruiz-Arguelles GI, Ruiz-Arguelles A, et al. Hematopoietic stem cell allografts using a non-myeloablative conditioning regimen can be safely performed on an outpatient basis: report of four cases. Bone Marrow Transplant 2000;25:131–133.

83. Wolfe I, Grier HE, Klar N, et al. Symptoms and suffering at the end of life in children with cancer. N Engl J Med 2000;342:326–333.

84. Chambers L, McDowall J, Gelb B. A global children's hospice and palliative care website. Int J Palliat Nurs 2005;11:292–293.

85. Magrath IT. African Burkitt's lymphoma. History, biology, clinical features and treatment. Am J Pediatr Hematol Oncol 1991;13:222–246.

86. Kazembe P, Hesseling PB, Griffin BE, et al. Long-term survival of children with Burkitt lymphoma in Malawi after cyclophosphamide monotherapy. Med Pediatr Oncol 2003; 40:23–25.

87. Brown S, Belgaumi A, Kofide A, et al. Failure to attend appointments and loss to follow-up: a prospective study of patients with malignant lymphoma in Riyadh, Saudi Arabia. Eur J Cancer Care 2009;18:313–317.

88. Fluchel M, Horsman JR, Furlong W, et al. Self- and proxy-reported health status and health-related quality of life in survivors of childhood cancer in Uruguay. Pediatr Blood Cancer 2008;50:838–843.

89. Shimoda S, Horsman J, Furlong W, et al. Disability and health-related quality of life in long-term survivors of cancer in childhood in Brazil. J Pediat Hematol Oncol 2008;30: 563–570.

90. World Health Report 1999. Geneva: World Health Organization, 1999.

91. Barr RD, Sala A. Quality-adjusted survival: a rigorous assessment of cure after cancer during childhood and adolescence. Pediatr Blood Cancer 2005;44:201–204.

92. Evans J. Health research. Essential link to equity in research. New York, NY: Oxford University Press, 1990.

93. Lucas AO, Michaud C, Malina D. Essential national health research. A strategy for action in health and human development. Geneva: Task Force on Health Research for Development, 1991.

94. Barnum H, Greenberg R. Cancers: health sectors priorities review. Washington DC: World Bank, 1991.

95. Barr RD. Costs and consequences of stem cell transplantation in children. Pediatr Transplant 2003;7(Suppl 3):7–11.

96. Weatherall D. Ruminations of a geriatric emeritus regius professor of medicine. Clin Med 2009;9:104–107.

97. Ribeiro RC, Sandrini F, Figueiredo B, et al. An inherited p 53 mutation that contributes in a tissue-specific manner to pediatric adrenocortical carcinomas. Proc Natl Acad Sci USA 2001;98:9330–9335.

98. Valsecchi MG, Tognoni G, Bonilla M, et al. Clinical epidemiology of childhood cancer in Central America and Caribbean countries. Ann Oncol 2004;15:680–685.

99. Magrath I, Shanta V, Advani S, et al. Treatment of acute lymphoblastic leukemia in countries with limited resources; lessons from use of a single protocol in India over a twenty year period. Eur J Cancer 2005;41:1570–1583.

100. Bajel A, George B, Mathews V, et al. Treatment of children with acute lymphoblastic leukemia in India using a BFM protocol. Pediatr Blood Cancer 2008;51:621–625.

101. Global Forum for Health Research. The 10/90 report on health research 2001. Geneva: Global Forum for Health Research, 2002.

102. Flanagin A, Winker MA. Global health: targeting problems and achieving solutions. JAMA 2003;290:1382–1384.

103. Ribeiro RC, Pui CH. Saving the children—improving childhood cancer treatment in developing countries. N Engl J Med 2005;352:2158–2160.

104. International Society of Pediatric Oncology. Pediatric oncology in low income countries. The Montevideo Document, SIOP News, October 1995.

105. Sala A, Barr RD, Masera G. A survey of resources and activities in the MISPHO families of institutions in Latin America: a comparison of two eras. Pediatr Blood Cancer 2004;43:758–764.

106. Magrath I. Foreword. In: Tannenberger S, Cavalli F, Pannutti F, eds. Cancer in developing countries: the great challenge for oncology in the 21st century. Munich: W Zuchschwerdt Verlag, 2004:1–9.

107. Agarwal BR, Dalvi RB. Treatment of childhood leukemias in underprivileged countries. In: Pui CH, ed. Treatment of acute leukemias: New Directions for Clinical Research. Current clinical oncology series. New Jersey, The Humana Press Inc., 2003: 321–329.

108. Howard SC, Ribeiro RC, Pui C-H. Strategies to improve outcomes of children with cancer in low-income countries. Eur J Cancer 2005;41:1584–1587.

109. Barr RD, Furlong W, Horsman JR, et al. The monetary costs of childhood cancer to the families of patients. Int J Oncol 1996;8:933–940.

110. Steinbrook R. Closing the affordability gap for drugs in low income countries. N Engl J Med 2007;357:1996–1999.

111. Mostert S, Sitaresmi MN, Gundy CM, et al. Does aid reach the poor? Experiences of a childhood leukaemia outreach-programme. Eur J Cancer 2009;45:414–419.

112. Barr RD, Feeny D, Furlong W. Economic evaluation of childhood cancer care. Eur J Cancer 2004;40:1335–1345.

113. Berwick DM. Lessons from developing nations on improving health care. BMJ 2004; 328:1124–1129.

114. Kellie SJ, Howard SC. Global child health priorities: what role for paediatric oncologists? Eur J Cancer 2008;44:2388–2396.

CHAPTER 54 ■ PREVENTING CANCER IN ADULTHOOD: ADVICE FOR THE PEDIATRICIAN

BRAD H. POLLOCK AND GAIL E. TOMLINSON

Although the origins of cancer may begin at conception, the risk for cancer may be modified from preconception through adulthood. The premise of this chapter is that the risk of cancer during adulthood may be influenced by cancer prevention practices that are initiated during childhood. Pediatricians are in an optimal position to influence their patients' risk of preventable cancers during the lifespan. These practices include identifying constitutional risk factors as well as advancing behaviors designed to minimize the burden of cancer during adulthood. Prevention strategies should take full advantage of our knowledge about the origins of cancer as well as established evidence demonstrating the benefits of practices that reduce harmful exposures and increase protective exposures. General pediatricians, family practitioners, and other primary care providers have the ability to identify children at the greatest risk for adult cancers and initiate early detection surveillance. Preventive interventions using educational methods may be more effective in children as they may be more receptive to behavioral change than adults. This chapter describes principles and practice of cancer prevention for children with the goal of preventing cancers that occur in adulthood.

In the United States, pediatric malignancies are rare; in 2007, there were an estimated 10,400 new malignancies diagnosed in children aged 0 to 14 years, representing 0.72% of all diagnosed malignancies.[1] For both children and adults, cancer is the second leading cause of death in the United States. For adults, only deaths due to cardiovascular disease outnumber cancer deaths. However, the death rates from cardiovascular disease declined to 26.4% from 1995 to 2005,[2] and it is predicted that cancer will become the most common cause of death. Concern about the adult cancer burden is related not only to incidence and mortality but also to societal economic costs and the emotional toll that cancer has on its stricken patients and their family members.

Although pediatric malignancies are a small component of the U.S. cancer burden, they are scientifically significant. Our understanding that cancer is a genetic disease was derived from the observation of a small number of families with a defect in a single gene. These relatively rare single-gene mutations foreshadow a significantly increased risk of cancer occurrence in children, adults, or both age groups. The study of childhood cancer has contributed to our understanding of the basic biological mechanisms of cancer. More subtle but far more common genetic factors impact cancer susceptibility, albeit in a more complex manner than single-gene mutations. These other genetic factors modify the biological impact of environmental exposures. Such gene–environmental interactions are more commonly associated with adult cancers. In the United States, given cancer's incidence, mortality, and economic cost to the general population, prevention and control of adult malignancies will remain a top public health priority and will play a more prominent role as incidence and mortality from the most common cause of death, cardiovascular disease, continues to decline.

The etiology of cancer is associated with spontaneous somatic genetic events such as translocations and mutations. For childhood and adult cancer, germ line mutations also play a role, but to a lesser extent. In contrast, environmental exposures have a predominant role in the etiology of most of the common adult malignancies. The significant influence of environmental factors on cancer occurrence can be seen from the wide variation in adult cancer incidence rates across different geographic areas and from migration studies where individuals and their offspring acquire the cancer incidence patterns of their new environment, most often over several generations. These changes occur gradually because of the long latency between exposure and biological effect. Capitalizing on the relatively long latency period of most adult cancers, interventions aimed at reducing exposure to harmful exogenous substances can be initiated much earlier in life, including during childhood. Testing for constitutional genetic risk factors has the potential to identify subsets of children at particularly high risk of adult cancer. Thus, screening efforts can be initiated early when they are most likely to provide early detection benefit. Genetic risk factors for adult cancer can be identified at birth and theoretically even *in utero*, although it may not be appropriate in all instances to do so. Exposure to harmful exogenous agents that increase adult cancer risk can be identified in childhood. Health-promoting lifestyles that influence future cancer risk should begin in childhood. Preventive strategies targeted at children could have enormous impact on reducing the occurrence of adult cancers.

This chapter contains a description of many of the known determinants of adult malignancies and potentially applicable prevention strategies for children and adolescents, which may reduce the incidence, cancer-related morbidity, and mortality of adult cancer. Children are often more receptive to prevention messages than are adults. Children possess more "teachable moments" that can lead individuals to positive behavior change. Small lifestyle changes adopted during childhood can have dramatic effects on future cancer risk. Surveillance screening practices for high-risk children identified through genetic testing performed many years before the peak age incidence has the potential to reduce cancer burden and reduce economic cost of cancer treatment. The pediatrician and other primary care providers are in a unique position to encourage cancer prevention behaviors and practices that will yield public health benefits over many decades.

CHARACTERISTICS OF ADULT CANCER

Although in 2007 there were 10,400 estimated new cancer cases among individuals younger than 20, this is dwarfed by an estimated 1,444,902 new adult cancer cases. The spectrum of malignancies varies as a function of age. Most childhood cancers originate in the neuroectoderm and mesoderm-derived tissues and often arise in target cells no longer present in adults, as with retinoblastoma, neuroblastoma, medulloblastoma, nephroblastoma, hepatoblastoma, and infantile leukemia. Childhood cancers are primarily characterized by histological features. In contrast, adult malignancies are most often characterized by anatomic site of occurrence because most of these tumors are derived from epithelial tissue, all of which are actively renewing. This accounts for the steadily increasing incidences of epithelial-derived cancers with age. Table 54.1 shows the estimated new cancer cases and deaths in the United States for the year 2009.[3] For women, the most common adult malignancies are cancer of the breast, lung and bronchus, and uterine. For men, the most frequently occurring malignancies include cancer of the prostate (accounting for ~25% of cancers in males), followed by lung and bronchus, colon and rectum, and urinary bladder. For both sexes combined, the highest numbers of cancer deaths occur with lung and bronchus cancer followed by breast cancer and then colorectal cancer for women and prostate cancer followed by colorectal cancer for men.

METHODS OF CANCER PREVENTION

Overall cancer risk can be attributed to the complex interplay between genetic factors and environmental exposures, superimposed upon background mutations that result from defects in repair of spontaneous DNA damage that occurs during S phase of the cell cycle. The first evidence that cancer is a genetic disease was provided by the observation of an unusual clustering of cancer within families. Single-gene defects are the primary cause of unusual cancer occurrence within these families, only a small proportion of the overall general population incidence is attributable to these defects. Other more subtle forms of genetic susceptibility predispose to an increased risk of cancer but do so in an etiologically far more complex manner. Cumulative exposure to exogenous substances like tobacco smoke, occupational exposure to asbestos and chemicals, exposure to carcinogens in water and air pollutants, and harmful dietary exposures, together with constitutional or acquired genetic susceptibility, are usually required to cross a biological threshold for carcinogenesis. Although host genetic susceptibility factors, such as germ line mutations, can contribute to that process, they are usually insufficient to serve as solitary etiologic causes.

Effective cancer prevention strategies include reducing or eliminating exposure to known cancer-causing exogenous substances, thus slowing the rate of transition of accumulated cellular genetic changes. Alternatively, prevention strategies can include increasing exposure to protective exogenous agents. This latter approach has been validated with the successful prevention of breast[4,5] and prostate cancers.[6,7] Interventions designed to detect cancer at the earliest stages of development, although of no utility in preventing the onset of disease, can reduce consequent morbidity and mortality of cancer. Parents in some cancer-prone families might consider cancer susceptibility testing of their children as a prevention strategy. Genetic testing could be used to identify cancer predisposition factors during childhood but should always be done together with family genetic counseling. As described in more detail later in the chapter, for several cancer predisposition syndromes, such as the multiple endocrine neoplasias (MEN1 and MEN2), or Familial Adenomatous Polyposis, genetic testing of children can lead to enhanced surveillance and early detection of disease, whereas recognition of other syndromes may not have direct benefit to the child. Previous concerns of genetic testing have included the risks of stigmatization as well as uninsurability; however, the recent enaction in 2008 of the Genetic Information Nondiscrimination Act (GINA) prohibits the use of genetic information in determining insurability and also prohibits employment discrimination based on genetic information. When genetic testing is performed in childhood, the child should be involved in the consent or assent process in an age-appropriate manner. However, testing for genetic syndromes involving only adult cancers for which there is no early effective intervention in childhood is not recommended.

Although effective strategies to prevent common childhood malignancies do not exist at present, many adult cancers are amenable to prevention. Initiating cancer prevention practices during childhood and adolescence may reduce subsequent cancer risk in adulthood including interventions to reduce exposure to harmful agents and increase exposure to protective substances. Interventions may also include the implementation of screening and early detection practices in childhood or even during the prenatal period, with benefits accruing to individuals over many decades of life. Even earlier, genetic counseling prior to conception may provide a means to prevent future cancers.

Cancer control and prevention is defined as a research science aimed at reducing cancer incidence, morbidity, and mortality.[8] There is a significant body of research demonstrating the successful translation of prevention research into reductions of cancer incidence and mortality.[9] Prevention research builds upon laboratory and clinical investigation with emphasis on early detection and screening, clinical intervention, and health education, and evaluation in diverse groups including traditionally underserved and high-risk populations. Cancer control research priorities are partially influenced by the relative incidence and mortality rates in the population, availability of efficient methods to modify exposure to known risk factors, and availability of effective treatments. *Primary prevention* consists of blocking the initial onset of disease while *secondary prevention* includes methods to identify cancer in its earliest stage of development, typically long before the malignancy would come to medical attention. *Tertiary prevention* interventions enhance long-term outcomes, such as reducing the risk of treatment-related second malignant neoplasms and other treatment-related sequelae or improving health-related quality of life. The remainder of this chapter is focused on primary and secondary prevention to reduce adult cancer burden.

Primary Prevention

Reducing exposure to harmful substances or increasing exposure to beneficial agents can reduce cancer incidence. Usually, this is the most efficacious and cost-effective strategy to reduce cancer burden. From a public health perspective, interventions at this level are primary prevention. Primary prevention usually provides the most effective means of lowering cancer-related mortality and morbidity as well as reducing the consequent economic and psychosocial impact of disease. A causal association between one or more putative risk factors and disease must be demonstrated before primary preventive interventions can be applied. Effective and preferably cost-effective interventions to reduce exposure must be available. Because most childhood cancers are thought to result from spontaneous (background) rather than induced somatic mutations, primary prevention is not feasible with the current state of knowledge about their etiology. In contrast, for many of the common adult malignancies, such as lung cancer, head and neck cancer, and esophageal cancer, where tobacco use accounts for most of the incidence, effective primary prevention strategies are available.

TABLE 54.1

ESTIMATED NEW CANCER CASES AND DEATHS BY SEX, UNITED STATES, 2009[a]

	Estimated new cases			Estimated deaths		
	Both sexes	Male	Female	Both sexes	Male	Female
All sites	1,479,350	766,130	713,220	562,340	292,540	269,800
Oral cavity and pharynx	35,720	25,240	10,480	7,600	5,240	2,360
Tongue	10,530	7,470	3,060	1,910	1,240	670
Mouth	10,750	6,450	4,300	1,810	1,110	700
Pharynx	12,610	10,020	2,590	2,230	1,640	590
Other oral cavity	1,830	1,300	530	1,650	1,250	400
Digestive system	275,720	150,020	125,700	135,830	76,020	59,810
Esophagus	16,470	12,940	3,530	14,530	11,490	3,040
Stomach	21,130	12,820	8,310	10,620	6,320	4,300
Small intestine	6,230	3,240	2,990	1,110	580	530
Colon[b]	106,100	52,010	54,090	49,920	25,240	24,680
Rectum	40,870	23,580	17,290			
Anus, anal canal, and anorectum	5,290	2,100	3,190	710	260	450
Liver and intrahepatic bile duct	22,620	16,410	6,210	18,160	12,090	6,070
Gallbladder and other biliary	9,760	4,320	5,440	3,370	1,250	2,120
Pancreas	42,470	21,050	21,420	35,240	18,030	17,210
Other digestive organs	4,780	1,550	3,230	2,170	760	1,410
Respiratory system	236,990	129,710	107,280	163,790	92,240	71,550
Larynx	12,290	9,920	2,370	3,660	2,900	760
Lung and bronchus	219,440	116,090	103,350	159,390	88,900	70,490
Other respiratory organs	5,260	3,700	1,560	740	440	300
Bones and joints	2,570	1,430	1,140	1,470	800	670
Soft tissue (including heart)	10,660	5,780	4,880	3,820	1,960	1,860
Skin (excluding basal and squamous)	74,610	42,920	31,690	11,590	7,670	3,920
Melanoma-skin	68,720	39,080	29,640	8,650	5,550	3,100
Other nonepithelial skin	5,890	3,840	2,050	2,940	2,120	820
Breast	194,280	1,910	192,370	40,610	440	40,170
Genital system	282,690	201,970	80,720	56,160	28,040	28,120
Uterine cervix	11,270		11,270	4,070		4,070
Uterine corpus	42,160		42,160	7,780		7,780
Ovary	21,550		21,550	14,600		14,600
Vulva	3,580		3,580	900		900
Vagina and other genital, female	2,160		2,160	770		770
Prostate	192,280	192,280		27,360	27,360	
Testis	8,400	8,400		380	380	
Penis and other genital, male	1,290	1,290		300	300	
Urinary system	131,010	89,640	41,370	28,100	18,800	9,300
Urinary bladder	70,980	52,810	18,170	14,330	10,180	4,150
Kidney and renal pelvis	57,760	35,430	22,330	12,980	8,160	4,820
Ureter and other urinary organs	2,270	1,400	870	790	460	330
Eye and orbit	2,350	1,200	1,150	230	120	110
Brain and other nervous system	22,070	12,010	10,060	12,920	7,330	5,590
Endocrine system	39,330	11,070	28,260	2,470	1,100	1,370
Thyroid	37,200	10,000	27,200	1,630	690	940
Other endocrine	2,130	1,070	1,060	840	410	430
Lymphoma	74,490	40,630	33,860	20,790	10,630	10,160
Hodgkin lymphoma	8,510	4,640	3,870	1,290	800	490
Non-Hodgkin lymphoma	65,980	35,990	29,990	19,500	9,830	9,670
Myeloma	20,580	11,680	8,900	10,580	5,640	4,940
Leukemia	44,790	25,630	19,160	21,870	12,590	9,280
Acute lymphocytic leukemia	5,760	3,350	2,410	1,400	740	660
Chronic lymphocytic leukemia	15,490	9,200	6,290	4,390	2,630	1,760
Acute myeloid leukemia	12,810	6,920	5,890	9,000	5,170	3,830
Chronic myeloid leukemia	5,050	2,930	2,120	470	220	250
Other leukemia[c]	5,680	3,230	2,450	6,610	3,830	2,780
Other and unspecified primary sites[c]	31,490	15,290	16,200	44,510	23,920	20,590

[a]Rounded to the nearest 10; estimated new cases exclude basal and squamous cell skin cancers and *in situ* carcinomas except urinary bladder. About 62,280 female carcinoma *in situ* of the breast and 53,120 melanoma *in situ* will be newly diagnosed in 2009.
[b]Estimated deaths for colon and rectum cancers are combined.
[c]More deaths than cases may suggest lack of specificity in recording underlying cause of death on death certificates.
Source: Estimated new cases are based on 1995–2005 incidence rates from 41 states and the District of Columbia as reported by the North American Association of Central Cancer Registries (NAACCR), representing about 85% of the U.S. population. Estimated deaths are based on U.S. mortality data, 1969–2006, National Center for Health Statistics, Centers for Disease Control and Prevention, 2009.

Secondary Prevention

Secondary prevention is the detection of cancer in its earliest detectable stages of development. A prerequisite for secondary preventive interventions is that early diagnosis will result in reduced mortality and morbidity; that is, early detection requires less invasive therapy, treatment of early cancers is less costly, or the occurrence and severity of treatment-related sequelae is lower in less advanced malignancies. The benefits of screening and early detection interventions must be evaluated in relationship to the associated psychosocial and ethically negative impact that results from assignment of "high-risk" status. Alternatively, vigilance in awareness of cancer-relevant symptoms may be inappropriately relaxed as a result of a false-negative screening test. The effects of misclassification (false-negatives and false-positives) must be fully weighed in assessing the feasibility of administering an early detection screening program. Secondary prevention may offer the only practical means of positively influencing cancer outcome when primary prevention is not possible or practical. However, at present, this prevention strategy for children is impractical because of the relatively low yield of screening tests applied to pediatric and adolescent populations. Advancing technology has contributed to the development of more accurate methods to identify early stage adult cancer through the use of biomarkers and new imaging techniques. Both genomic as well as proteomic high-throughput technologies are beginning to be evaluated as more accurate screening assays. Expanded application of these methods is likely to delay or prevent the transition from early-to-late stage disease, thus improving outcomes.

Cancer Prevention Strategies

Cancer prevention and control research programs optimally make use of multidisciplinary investigators including oncologists, epidemiologists, molecular biologists, geneticists, toxicologists, psychologists, primary care providers, and health educators, as well as public policy specialists, health care economists, and lawmakers. These individuals must work in tandem to develop and evaluate strategies to identify determinants of cancer risk, reduce exposure to risk factors, encourage protective behaviors, and develop cost-effective early detection interventions. Evidence of efficacy as well as cost effectiveness for any prevention strategy must be obtained prior to widespread implementation. At present, the evidence base is lacking to specifically target children for adult cancer prevention purposes.

GENETIC BASIS FOR CANCER

Cancer results from a multistage process in which loss of control of cellular growth and differentiation occurs. There is a period of latency between the initial etiologic exposure and the occurrence of a malignancy; in the case of adult cancers, this is usually a long period of time. Table 54.2 depicts a theoretical model for the pathogenesis of colorectal cancer and has become a classic example of the process of accumulating events leading to malignancy.[10] The process begins with an inherited germ line mutation or acquired mutation or loss in the *APC* gene. This single-APC mutation leads to hyperproliferation of normal epithelium and subsequent formation of dysplastic aberrant cryptic foci and early adenomas in the colon, usually following mutation, inactivation, or loss of the second copy of the gene. Next, activation of the *KRAS* gene frequently occurs in one of the benign adenomas, allowing one of the cells to outgrow its sister cells to form a

TABLE 54.2

PATHOGENESIS OF COLORECTAL CANCER THROUGH ACCUMULATION OF SEQUENTIAL MUTATIONS

Tissue state	Genetic mutation
Normal epithelium	*APC*
↓	
Dysplastic aberrant cryptic foci	
↓	
Early adenoma	*KRAS*
↓	
Intermediate adenoma	*DCC, DPC4, MADR2/JV18–1*
↓	
Late adenoma	*TP53*
↓	
Carcinoma	
↓	
Metastasis	

larger intermediate, dysplastic adenoma with loss of *DCC*. Within this population of cells, further mutations or losses occur, including those in the TP53 tumor suppressor gene. Acquired *TP53* mutations lead to loss of apoptosis (programmed cell death) in turn transitioning into a carcinoma. Metastatic potential is attained when a cell acquires a sufficient number of mutations. The entire process may require four or more sequential mutations. Myriad factors can further affect cellular growth and proliferation of a malignant clone of cells including the microenvironment of an organ such as the colon. These may further serve to change the invasive potential (i.e., aggressiveness) of the tumor with subsequent metastasis. Malignancy formation is dependent on the sequential acquisition of mutations in oncogenes, inactivating mutations in recessive tumor suppressor genes, and epigenetic changes that modify the expression of these genes.[11]

On the basis of experimental observations on the effects of chemical and radiation exposure in inducing the development of malignancy, carcinogenesis involves several theoretical steps. *Initiation* is marked by the occurrence of the first cellular genetic abnormality, consisting of a mutation that can be transmitted to progeny cells. The period following initiation until the appearance of an observable neoplasm is *promotion* that is characterized by the development of benign tumors or focal proliferative lesions. *Progression* marks the conversion of these tumors or focal proliferative lesions into malignant tumors. Although initiation, promotion, and progression are well characterized in certain experimentally induced cancers, they are not usually directly observable. For adult malignancies, the often subtle nature of carcinogenesis makes it difficult to differentiate between discrete transition states, such as changes in normal cells through the stages of proliferation, dysplasia, and *in situ* carcinoma. At a cellular level, cancer can be envisioned as a genetic disease of somatic tissue. Eliminating or slowing the rate of transition through a multistage model of malignancy formation forms the basis for cancer control and prevention efforts.

Cancer Family Syndromes

Familial cancer syndromes, usually involving autosomal dominant inheritance of single-gene mutations, have provided important clues about the genetic basis for cancer. Retinoblastoma was the first identified genetic model explaining the distinction between the hereditary and nonhereditary forms of the same malignancy and the contribution of the same gene to both types. It had been noted early on that in some cases, chromosomal band 13q14 was completely or partially deleted in all cells of the body.[12] Friend et al.[13] cloned the *RB1* gene at this locus in 1986, confirming the mechanism of how tumor suppressor genes work. Mutations or deletions at tumor suppressor gene sites result in total reduction or production of dysfunctional proteins that normally regulate cellular growth and proliferation. In this case, the two alleles at the *RB1* locus produce the RB protein (pRb) that inhibits uncontrolled cellular proliferation. Children with a germ line mutation have only one of the two normal alleles that produce normal pRb. All retinoblast cells are deficient in pRb and are therefore more susceptible to development of cancer caused by a new second somatic mutation, knocking out the remaining normal allele and leading to the development of retinoblastoma. These cancers thus result from two hits. As children with the germ line *RB1* mutations become adults, they continue to carry an elevated risk of cancer; however, the tissue specificity will have broadened and no longer involves the retina. Survivors of retinoblastoma, who fall into the "heritable" and thus germ line mutation category, have a particularly high rate of sarcomas that appears to be exacerbated by the treatment of initial cancer with external beam therapy.[14–16] External beam treatment was largely abandoned by the late 1990s in favor of localized treatment combined with systemic chemotherapy. This is an excellent example of how the observation of late effects in adulthood substantially influenced the development of new therapies for the treatment of primary childhood cancers. However, even without the exposure to radiation, survivors of retinoblastoma are prone to develop both benign and malignant tumors at increased frequency, including lipomas and common tumors such as lung cancer.[16]

Another well-characterized tumor suppressor gene is *TP53*, which encodes for the protein p53. Mutation or loss of p53 leads to a decrease in apoptosis, resulting in a decreased death rate for cancer cells. Germ line *TP53* mutations are associated with the Li-Fraumeni cancer family syndrome.[17] Individuals from these families are predisposed to a wide spectrum of pediatric and adult malignancies, the most common of which are sarcomas of various types and very early onset breast cancer in women. Germ line *TP53* mutations predispose to the widest spectrum of cancer types of any cancer syndrome. In contrast, most familial cancer syndromes are associated with a relatively limited number of malignancies. Although testing minor children for germ line TP53 mutations remains controversial because of issues involving informed consent of minors and lack of interventions to reduce risk of many of the cancer types,[18] as children in Li-Fraumeni families become adults, an understanding of their risks can be beneficial particularly for young women who may be at risk of breast cancer in their twenties and for whom intervention with increased surveillance or even prophylactic surgery could be of benefit.[19]

Although Li-Fraumeni syndrome and hereditary retinoblastoma are associated largely with pediatric cancer, other familial cancer syndromes are associated primarily with adult onset tumors but have implications for pediatric patients as well. The alert pediatrician should recognize these syndromes by taking a careful family history. One such syndrome is Familial Adenomatous Polyposis (FAP) that is associated with the development of colonic polyps in adolescents and leads to the almost certain development of colonic neoplasia in early adulthood. Recognition of FAP syndrome in the family of a healthy child has two implications. First, screening for the development of colon polyps is recom-

mended in adolescence so that intervention is possible prior to the onset of symptoms or neoplasia.[20] Second, in FAP families, young children can be affected by other extracolonic tumors, including hepatoblastoma and medulloblastoma.[21] Older children and young adults in FAP families are also at risk of thyroid cancers.[22,23] Screening for thyroid cancer in such individuals has been suggested but needs further study.[24] Although under reexamination in light of reported toxicity, there is evidence of efficacy of both nonsteroidal anti-inflammatory agents and COX-2 inhibitors in reducing colonic polyp formation; hope exists that chemoprevention will play a major prevention role in this inherited cancer syndrome in the future.[25] Genetic counseling and testing should be undertaken with evaluation of all children in FAP families.[26]

Hereditary nonpolyposis colorectal cancer (HNPCC) can be associated with colorectal cancers in the absence of polyposis and is caused by defective DNA repair. The *MSH2*, *MLH1*, *MSH6*, *PMS1*, and *PMS2* genes code for proteins that are involved in correcting mismatch errors in DNA replication. A second hit in a repair gene produces a cell that has a thousand-fold increase in the mutation rate. HNPCC is associated with secondary sites such as endometrial cancer, gastric, and esophageal cancers.[18] Increased rates of somatic mutations increase the probability that critical events will accumulate and lead to cancer. Although pediatric tumors have been reported in HNPCC families, they are rare.[27,28] Screening guidelines for adults with HNPCC have been recommended, although often need to be adjusted on the basis of specific gene mutation or spectrum of cancers within a family.

Von-Hippel–Lindau syndrome is a disorder of angiogenesis, and although rarely associated with true malignancy in childhood, it is characterized by the development of renal cell carcinoma in adulthood. Manifestations in childhood most notably include ocular retinomas that can lead to loss of vision and cerebral hemangioblastomas. Recognition of the syndrome by family history will allow life-long surveillance for benign and malignant tumors, which can substantially reduce morbidity and mortality.[29]

The multiple endocrine neoplasias, including both MEN1 and MEN2, affect both children and adults. MEN2 is caused by mutation of the RET proto-oncogene and is characterized by both medullary thyroid cancer and pheochromocytoma.[26,30–32] Prophylactic thyroidectomy to achieve primary prevention of thyroid cancer is recommended for children with familial multiple endocrine neoplasia types IIA and IIB, and life-long yearly screening for pheochromocytoma with urinary catecholamines is recommended to achieve secondary prevention, that is, early detection of tumor growth.[33]

Other familial cancer syndromes, which when recognized in childhood aid in surveillance for tumors that typically manifest later in life, include Cowden syndrome, also known as Proteus syndrome or multiple hamartoma syndrome that can be associated with early-onset breast cancer and thyroid cancer.[34] These syndromes can be identified by a combination of family history of cancer as well as physical findings. A number of familiar cancer syndromes may affect the risk of developing adult malignancy. These syndromes are often recognizable in children or adolescents, and early recognition can lead to effective screening starting at the appropriate age and continuing throughout life (Table 54.3).

Cancers that almost exclusively appear in adulthood have also been associated with germ line mutations. Although they account for a relatively small proportion of breast cancers in the general population,[35] mutations in *BRCA1* and *BRCA2* are strongly associated with familial breast cancer[36] and may account for 40% of familial cases. Although fewer than 10% of ovarian cancers are familial, the majority of familial

TABLE 54.3

EXAMPLES OF MAJOR CANCER PREDISPOSITION SYNDROMES AFFECTING THE RISK OF CANCER IN ADULTHOOD THAT POTENTIALLY COULD BE SCREENED FOR AND ARE RECOGNIZABLE IN CHILDHOOD OR ADOLESCENCE

Gene	Syndrome	Benign physical stigmata	Childhood tumor types	Adult tumor types
TP53	Li-Fraumeni Cancer Family Syndrome/ Breast Sarcoma Family Cancer Syndrome	None	Sarcomas, brain, leukemia, adrenocortical, others	Breast, sarcoma, brain, others
RB1	Heritable retinoblastoma	Pinealoma, retinoma, facial abnormalities in rare cases of 13q deletion syndrome	Retinoblastoma, usually bilateral, pinealoblastoma, osteosarcoma	Sarcomas, lung, melanoma, lipomas, others
PTEN	Cowden/Bannayan–Riley–Ruvalcaba/ Proteus-like syndromes	Macrocephaly, skin tags, lipomas, hamartomas of various sites, acral or palmar keratoses, colonic polyps	Hamartoma, thyroid, benign masses	Breast, thyroid, endometrium, renal cell carcinoma
APC	Familial Adenomatous Polyposis/Gardner syndrome	Gastrointestinal polyps desmoid tumors, supernumery teeth epidermal cysts, osteomas	Hepatoblastoma, medulloblastoma (Turcot syndrome)	Colorectal cancer, upper gastrointestinal tract cancers, thyroid cancer
MENIN	Multiple endocrine neoplasia, type 1	Lipomas, endocrine abnormalities from benign tumors	Pituitary adenoma, pancreatic islet cell tumors, vasoactive intestinal peptide tumor (VIPoma)	Pituitary adenoma, parathyroid tumor, pancreatic islet cell, vasoactive intestinal peptide tumor (VIPoma)
RET	Multiple endocrine neoplasia, type 2B	MEN2B: Coarse facial features, mucosal neuromas, skeletal abnormalities of spine	Medullary thyroid cancer, pheochromocytoma	Medullary thyroid cancer, pheochromocytoma
NF1	Neurofibromatosis, type 1/von Recklinghausen's disease	Café au lait spots, axillary freckling Lisch nodules neurofibromas	Optic glioma, other CNS, peripheral nerve sheath tumors, JMML	Optic glioma, other CNS, peripheral nerve sheath tumor
NF2	Neurofibromatosis, type 2	Café au lait (but less prominent than in NF1), neurofibroma, cataracts	Acoustic neuroma, spinal cord schwannomas, meningiomas	Acoustic neuroma, spinal cord schwannomas, meningiomas
PTCH	Gorlin syndrome	Palmar pits, odontogenic cysts	Medulloblastoma	Basal cell carcinoma, medulloblastoma
STK11	Peutz–Jeghers	Mucocutaneous hyperpigmented lesions, hamartomatous polyps		Intestinal tumors, pancreatic, breast, ovarian cancers
TSC1	Tuberous sclerosis, type 1	Hypomelanic macules (ash-leaf spots), CNS tubers, subependymal nodules, angiolipoma, adenoma sebaceum, cardiac rhabdomyoma, hamartomas, renal cysts, pulmonary lymphangioleiomyomatosis, oncocytoma	Renal cell carcinoma, hamartoblastoma (rare)	Renal cell carcinoma
TSC2/ LAM	Tuberous sclerosis, type 2	Similar to TSC1, often more severe	Renal cell carcinoma hamartoblastoma (rare)	Renal cell carcinoma
VHL	Von Hippel–Lindau	Hemangioblastoma of retina, CNS, other hemangiomas, Renal and pancreatic cysts	Pheochromocytoma	Renal Carcinoma, pheochromocytoma
SMARCB1/ hSNF5/ INI1	Rhabdoid tumor syndrome; also schwannomatosis	Schwannomas	Rhabdoid tumors, choroid plexus tumors	Schwannomas, brain tumors, epithelioid sarcoma
MLH1, MSH2, MSH6, PMS1	Hereditary nonpolyposis colon cancer	Polyps (less numerous than in FAP)	CNS tumors, especially glial tumors	Colorectal, uterine, ovarian cancer
BRCA2	Breast–ovarian cancer family syndrome	± Features of Fanconi anemia in biallelic mutation carriers	Wilms, CNS, AML in biallelic mutations carriers	Breast, ovarian, prostate, pancreatic

Note: This is not intended to be a comprehensive listing.

cancers involve *BRCAI* or *BRCA2* mutations.[37] Childhood cancers have not been seen in *BRCA1*-mutation carriers but have been reported in *BRCA2*-affected families; however, these are rare and tend to occur in individuals with inherited biallelic mutations.[38,39] The prevalence of germ line *BRCA1* or *BRCA2* mutations is not equal in all populations. The Ashkenazi Jewish population has a particularly high incidence of *BRCA1*- and *BRCA2*-related breast and ovarian cancer such that a mutation in *BRCA1* or *BRCA2* is present in approximately 2% of individuals of Ashkenazi descent, a population that could benefit significantly from population screening.[40] This has implications for screening and risk reduction in adult women, although to date no effective interventions starting in childhood or adolescence are known. Nonetheless, risk counseling becomes relevant and important as adolescents enter adulthood. Given that hormones play a role in the development of breast cancer and may further increase the risk in mutation carriers, avoidance or minimization of hormonal use at any age in breast cancer-prone families may be prudent.

What can be done with knowledge that a child possesses or is at risk of carrying a germ line mutation associated with adult cancer? In certain syndromes, testing, screening, and interventions can be beneficial such as prophylactic surgery in FAP or MEN2 syndromes. Undoubtedly additional interventions will become available as knowledge of cancer predisposition and etiology continues to accumulate. Rather than attempt to become expert in the vast spectrum of familial cancers, the pediatrician should carefully note and update the family history and make appropriate referrals to cancer genetic counselors of families with histories of early onset adult cancers, multiple pediatric cancer, or multiple or recurring benign tumors.[41]

Not all inherited cancer syndromes are autosomal dominant. Ataxia telangiectasia (AT) is a rare autosomal recessive disorder and fatal neurological disease. The gene responsible for AT is ATM.[42,43] For heterozygote carriers, the AT gene is a genetic cancer predisposition factor. Carriers express significantly increased risk of breast cancer[44] due to increased sensitivity to ionizing radiation and defective DNA repair. The estimated prevalence of AT carriers is between 0.2% and 1.0%. The risk for breast cancer in female carriers is higher. Demonstrating a gene–environmental interaction, for female AT carriers, the cumulative lifetime breast cancer rates for smokers is four times higher than for carriers who never smoked.[45] Carriers could be identified through mass screening; given their increased sensitivity to radiation, these individuals may be counseled to strictly avoid all elective radiation exposures such as routine but nonessential medical or dental x-rays.

More subtle genetic effects are certain polymorphisms that can increase susceptibility to cancer without causing a defined familial cancer genetic syndrome. There are several classes of these polymorphisms, an important one being those that code for xenobiotic metabolizing enzymes such as cytochrome P-450, glutathione *S*-transferase, and *N*-acetyltransferase.[46,47] Polymorphisms of metabolizing enzymes are associated with detoxification of exogenous contaminants or metabolism of relatively inactive contaminants into active carcinogens. From a population perspective, cancer susceptibility from polymorphisms is likely to account for the observed interindividual variation in response to identical levels of carcinogen exposure. As more sensitive molecular toxicology and pharmacogenomic technology become more widely available, we are likely to develop more accurate predictive models of cancer risk. This would enhance our efforts to aim our more aggressive interventions, such as the avoidance of certain carcinogens, in high-risk individuals.

Characteristics of Adult Cancer Compared with Childhood Cancer

Adult malignancies are more likely to have a multifactorial etiology than are childhood malignancies. Geographically, the wider variation of incidence patterns as well as evidence from migrant studies support the notion that most adult malignancies have a multifactorial etiology involving environmental factors. Although cancer family syndromes are implicated as the primary etiologic source of cancer in a defined subset of the population, their overall impact on cancer incidence is very small. However, well-studied familial cancer cases reveal that the tumors often display the same changes found in the nonhereditary forms. This suggests that preventive measures that are efficacious for high-risk hereditary cases should be applicable to nonhereditary cases.

Far more is known about potentially modifiable risk factors for adult malignancies than for childhood malignancies. Adult malignancies typically require a greater number of sequence-dependent genetic "hits" (i.e., mutations) than those required for pediatric malignancies. Colorectal cancer probably requires four or more hits. Given the greater number of required hits, adult malignancies may be more amenable to interventions designed to block exposure to harmful, modifiable risk factors, or increase exposure to protective factors, thus providing more opportunities to block or delay the onset of adult cancers.

RISK FACTORS FOR ADULT CANCER

Although spontaneous mutations contribute to the development of cancer, exogenous factors are important determinants of cancer risk. Because the majority of harmful exogenous exposures are modifiable, much of the adult cancer burden is theoretically preventable. From a multifactorial etiologic perspective, the challenges are to identify these factors and their interactions to develop interventions that will reduce harmful exposure or decrease host susceptibility. The ultimate impact of preventive interventions is to reduce cancer incidence, mortality, and morbidity. Results from cancer prevention research should guide the formation of health policies and regulations to minimize public exposure to harmful substances or increase exposure to protective substances.

Genetic, hormonal, immunologic, and other endogenous factors play an important etiologic role. However, control over these factors, many of which are constitutional host characteristics, is impossible or impractical to manipulate. For example, it is currently impossible to repair germ line mutations in the *APC* locus for the purpose of reducing cancer risk. Gene therapy may someday offer a means to manipulate germ line mutations, but the only current means of lowering the risk for individuals with inherited cancer susceptibility is to control exogenous exposure or use secondary prevention methods for earlier detection, or, in some cases, to exercise prevention by surgical removal of the at-risk organ.

The response to environmental exposures and host factors is not limited to the first stage of cancer development—initiation. These factors can exert their effects on the later stages of promotion and progression. In addition, multiple etiologic pathways can exist for a single agent, and multiple agents can interact between themselves and with host characteristics. Carcinogenesis of breast, colon, and prostate are thought to involve alternate pathways for oncogenesis. The pathogenesis of cancers of the upper airway and digestive tract, such as oral, pharyngeal, esophageal, and lung cancer, may be simpler because tobacco use and alcohol consumption are known to be sufficient causes for the majority of these malignancies. Other host factors, such as constitutionally defective DNA repair mechanisms, unfavorable polymorphisms of metabolizing enzymes, tumor suppressor gene mutations, and immunodeficiency, may explain the wide variation in incidence among persons exposed to the same levels of tobacco and alcohol.

Other Host Characteristics

Host characteristics play a pivotal etiologic role in human cancer. Given the multifactorial nature of oncogenesis, constitutional factors mediate the harmful effects of some exogenous exposures significantly affecting cancer risk. Major categories of cancer-associated host characteristics are reviewed below.

Hormonal Factors

Endogenous hormones play a role in the etiology of breast cancer.[23] Estrogens are important risk factors for breast cancer. Hormones such as estradiol and progesterone, along with their age-dependent exposure pattern of use, influence breast cancer risk. Estrogen-related risk is thought to be mediated through the estrogen-receptor (ER), constitutional polymorphisms of which can affect estrogen biosynthesis. Other factors that influence breast cancer risk include early age at menarche, nulliparity, late age at menopause, and late age at first full-term pregnancy. Obesity has also been identified as a risk factor, especially in postmenopausal women. Excess fat stores in the body may effect endogenous aromatase modulation. Diet, physical activity, and smoking can mediate hormones related to breast cancer risk.

Immunologic Factors

Immunodeficiency, either inherited or acquired, is strongly associated with cancer risk. Cancer was a sentinel indicator for infection with human immunodeficiency virus (HIV).[48–50] Inherited immunodeficiency syndromes that are associated with cancer include AT, severe combined immunodeficiency syndrome, Wiskott–Aldrich syndrome, and Bloom syndrome. Autoimmune syndromes have also been implicated as risk factors. Aside from infection that induces immunodeficiency, other acquired immunodeficiencies can be related to thymectomy, chemotherapy, radiation exposure, or multimodal therapies such as bone marrow transplantation, all of which can predispose to cancer.

Other medical conditions, such as lupus or inflammatory bowel disease, which exert an effect through an autoimmune-mediated process, or infections with agents that impair T-cell-mediated immune surveillance, are associated with increased cancer risk. Although HIV is not directly involved in cellular transformation, it may impair normal immune function and may enhance the oncogenic potential of viral coinfections, such as Kaposi's sarcoma-associated herpesvirus (KSHV)[51] or Epstein–Barr virus (EBV).[52]

Exogenous Exposures

Although host characteristics alone account for a very small proportion of cancers, exposure to chemical, physical, and biologic factors plays an important role in the etiology of most common adult malignancies. The risk from exposure to an exogenous factor should be considered relative to the exposure dose, exposure duration, age of the individual, the biologic response, and interactions between these and other factors. Chemical exposures can act as initiators, promoters, or factors that aid progression alone or in combination. Genotoxic chemical carcinogens are highly reactive and can bind directly to DNA to form DNA adducts, in turn leading to base mispairing, small deletions, missense or nonsense mutations, chromosomal breaks, or large deletions. Nongenotoxic chemicals rarely interact directly with cellular DNA but can serve as effect modifiers for genotoxic agents or can act independently as endocrine or immune disruptors.

Chemical exposures can occur in both occupational and residential settings. Children can be exposed to high levels of pesticides if they live near agricultural areas, and they can be exposed to industrial contaminants if they live or play near polluted areas. They can also be exposed to contaminants through the public water supply. Personal exposure to tobacco smoke, which contains a complex mixture of many compounds that are known carcinogens, can increase cancer risk. Foods may contain artificial or naturally occurring substances that are harmful (e.g., aflatoxins). Because of the latency between exposure to these carcinogens in childhood and the effect on the development of cancer, increased incidence of cancers in adulthood is of primary concern.

Potentially harmful physical exposures include asbestos,[53,54] ionizing radiation (e.g., x-rays, nuclear fallout, and residential radon), ultraviolet radiation from sun exposure or artificial ultraviolet light sources,[55] and electromagnetic fields.[56] Given their widespread use, there has been concern about the cancer risks associated with radiofrequency radiation emitted by cellular telephones; however, an extended analysis of a large historic cohort study of 420,095 persons in Denmark failed to find significant associations between cell phone use and malignancy,[57] consistent with the findings of most but not all brain tumor case-control studies.[58–60]

The etiologic effects of high-dose ionizing radiation are well known from the atomic bombing of the cities Hiroshima and Nagasaki,[61] the formerly widespread use of fluoroscopy in fitting shoes and older high-dose medical radiographic imaging. Because of its latency of effect on the development of cancer, ionizing radiation exposure is thought to be an initiating event, leaving open the contributory carcinogenic effects of other exposures.

The single most important preventable known risk factor for adult cancer is tobacco use that includes using cigarettes, cigars, pipe tobacco, and smokeless tobacco products. A substantial proportion of all cancer deaths can be attributed to tobacco use. In particular, tobacco use is strongly associated with cancers of the upper airway and digestive system and moderately associated with cancer of the bladder, uterine cervix, pancreas, and kidney. In addition to its cancer effects, tobacco use is a major risk factor for the most common cause of death in the United States, cardiovascular disease as well as cerebrovascular disease, and respiratory illnesses such as chronic obstructive pulmonary disease and emphysema.

A number of viral agents have been associated with malignancy, including EBV, KSHV, and retroviruses such as the human T-cell lymphoproliferative viruses (HTLV-1 and HTLV-II) and HIV. The bacterium Helicobacter pylori is associated with gastric and esophageal cancers. The human papillomavirus (HPV) is strongly associated with cervical and anorectal cancers, while hepatitis B and hepatitis C are associated with hepatocellular carcinoma. Squamous cell carcinoma of the bladder is associated with Schistosomiasis,[55] but in the developed world, the overall incidence of bladder cancer is very low and tends to be of the transitional cell carcinoma subtype. Infectious agents account for a high proportion of malignancies in the developing world. Examples include Burkitt's lymphoma in equatorial Africa, nasopharyngeal carcinoma in China, and gastric cancer in Chile and Japan. Infectious agents can exert direct carcinogenic effects, or their effects can be indirect, such as stimulation of chronic cellular proliferation leading to an increase in the number of spontaneous accumulated mutations.

Host factors can modify the etiologic effect of infectious agents. For example, early age of infection with EBV and coinfection with malaria (Plasmodium falciparum) predispose to the endemic form of Burkitt's lymphoma. Acquired immunodeficiency syndrome-associated malignancies are the result of interaction between HIV-induced immunodeficiency and EBV-related lymphoproliferation.[52] Although nasopharyngeal carcinoma is associated with EBV infection, geographic-defined population genetic factors alter susceptibility such as with the higher rates in Southern China.

Obesity and Cancer Risks

Excess body weight has been identified as an independent risk factor for adult cancer. There is growing evidence that increased body mass is associated with the risk of all cancers combined[62,63] as well as site-specific malignancies, including endometrium, breast (in postmenopausal women), colon, and prostate.[62–66]

A recent study by the Million Women Study Collaboration in the United Kingdom demonstrated that increased body mass index was associated with a significant increase in 10 of 17 specific types of cancer.[67]

The specific mechanisms by which obesity influences the development of cancer have not been fully elucidated but may include alterations in endogenous hormonal patterns including sex hormones and insulin, the distribution of body fat, and changes in adiposity at different ages:[63,64,68] Diet high in fat and low in complex carbohydrates may lead to hyperinsulinemia, which in turn promotes the development of cancer.[69,70] Childhood obesity is associated with an earlier age of puberty, which in girls may increase the risk of breast cancer.[71]

In addition to increasing cancer risks, obesity is associated with a poorer outcome in several types of tumors in adults including breast, pancreatic, colon, and prostate.[72–76] The reasons for the poor outcomes in obese patients are just beginning to be understood and undoubtedly involve interplay with pharmacokinetic factors, other hormonal factors, and host genetic polymorphisms as well as other comorbidities observed in obese patients.

The prevalence of childhood obesity has doubled in the past 2 decades in the United States with 15.3% of children aged 6 to 11 and 15.5% of those aged 12 to 19, falling at or above the 95th percentile for body mass index.[77–79] The increase in prevalence has been particularly striking for both Hispanics and African Americans. Obesity prevention is currently a top public health priority.[80] Federal agencies have instituted programs focusing on public education, school- and community-based interventions in nutrition and physical activity, obesity-related disease surveillance, and clinical preventive services and therapeutics. Because childhood obesity is a strong determinant of obesity in adulthood, early childhood is an important period for interventions on weight reduction and obesity prevention.[80]

PREVENTION AND CONTROL STRATEGIES FOR ADULT CANCERS

Primary Prevention

Dietary Factors

From a wide range of observational studies, dietary factors appear to influence the risk of cancer.[81] A pooled analysis showed a significant reduction in the risk for renal cell carcinoma associated with higher consumption levels of fruits, vegetables, and carotenoids.[82] International ecologic correlations[83] and studies of Japanese migrants to Hawaii[84] have demonstrated increased breast cancer risk with adoption of a more Western lifestyle. There are several challenges to conducting studies that examine the health effects of diet on cancer, including difficulties in measuring nutrient intake and selection of intermediate biomarkers that are predictive of cancer incidence or mortality.[85]

There have been a number of randomized intervention trials assessing the effects of dietary supplements. The randomized Alpha-Tocopherol, Beta-Carotene Cancer Prevention (ATBC) Trial, which studied male cigarette smokers, was undertaken to determine the impact of these dietary supplements on cancer incidence and mortality with a focus on lung cancer.[86] The incidence of lung cancer after 5 to 8 years of dietary supplementation with alpha-tocopherol or beta carotene was not reduced. In the study groups receiving beta-carotene, the risk was increased for lung cancers but decreased for prostate cancers, while the overall all-cause mortality increased by 8%. In an updated analysis of the study cohort, Vitamin E supplementation was not associated with mortality however; the effects of Vitamin E interacted with age, smoking, and dietary vitamin C intake in a complex manner.[87] The Selenium and Vitamin E Cancer Prevention Trial (SELECT) found that selenium and vitamin E taken alone or together for an average of 5 and one-half years did not prevent prostate cancer.[88]

Dietary recommendations must be based on evidence of strong anticancer effects but must also consider costs as well as acceptability to individuals. Because of discordance, laboratory findings of protective effects in vitro or in vivo must be put to the appropriate test in human subjects. Aside from recommendations to regulate food intake to prevent obesity, associated with cancer risk, evidence of effectiveness of radical changes in diet or consumption of dietary supplements is lacking to shape recommendations and policies for cancer control.

Tobacco Use

Tobacco use represents the single most important modifiable risk factor for cancer. Overall, the prevalence of smoking for adults in the United States has gone from 41.9% in 1965 to 22.7% in 2001 and to 19.8% in 2007.[89] On the basis of the National Youth Risk Behavior Survey,[90] the rate of decline in tobacco use has slowed dramatically in more recent years. The overall smoking prevalence rate in 2007 among high-school students was 20%. Rates were of 23.2%, 16.7%, and 11.6% white non-Hispanics, Hispanics, and African American (non-Hispanic), respectively. In addition to cigarette use, smokeless tobacco use (defined as at least 1 day during the previous 30 days) was almost 8% among high-school students (13% male and 2% female). Smokeless tobacco products include chewing tobacco, snuff, or dip. There appears to be an increase in smokeless tobacco use among young people in the recent years.[91] For both adults and youth, tobacco use is associated with gender, race/ethnicity, and markers of socioeconomic status such as education. Over the past three decades, there has been an overall decrease in lung cancer incidence and mortality in the United States. The annual percentage change (APC) in lung and bronchus incidence rates went from 2.5% to −1.0% to −0.8% for the periods from 1975 to 1982, 1982 to 1991, and 1992 to 2006, respectively. There was a more dramatic decline in lung cancer incidence for males who went from an APC of 1.4% to −0.4% to −1.9% compared with females who went from 5.5% to 3.5% to 1.0% for the periods from 1975 to 1982, 1982 to 1991, and 1992 to 2006, respectively. Female lung cancer incidence continues to increase. Mortality patterns reflect the incidence patterns. Although the rate of increase has slowed, women continue to experience higher mortality rates from year to year. These differences may be related not only to sex-based differences in women's smoking behaviors[92] but also to differences in tobacco-related cancer biology.[93]

Antismoking research seeks to accurately characterize smoking patterns in the population, understand the etiology of smoking behaviors, develop effective strategies to prevent new individuals from beginning to smoke, and develop smoking cessation interventions. There are many factors that are associated with success in quitting smoking such as the magnitude of addiction or dependence (dose as well as duration of smoking), social influences including parents and peers smoking, academic performance and school commitment, youth depression, and personal coping styles.[94,95] There have been a number of programs aimed at reducing children and adolescent tobacco use, many of which have been administered through school-based interventions but most of which have targeted particular sociodemographic groups. Given their variable short-term effectiveness, new school-based programs need to continue to be developed.[96] Public policies regulating and restricting access to tobacco products for young persons have also impacted use.

Recent evidence has indicated that smoking habits may be influenced by genetic predisposition and that these are tightly associated with the development of lung cancer.[97-101] Genetic predisposition to smoking is associated with specific polymorphic loci in the region of chromosome 15q25 encoding subunits of the nicotinic acetylcholine receptor subunits. These subunits are expressed in alveolar epithelial cells and pulmonary neuroendocrine cells as well as lung cancer cell lines.[98] Persons with the at-risk genotype may have a high level of biological addiction to smoking, making smoking cessation difficult. Recognition of the heritable nature of smoking addiction and the inherent difficulties in smoking cessation may underscore the need for intervention by the means of education of children and parents *before* the child initiates smoking.

The Institute of Medicine convened the Committee on Reducing Tobacco Use: Strategies, Barriers, and Consequences with the ultimate goal of ending the tobacco problem; that is, reducing tobacco use so that it is no longer a significant public health problem.[102] Although this was stated as a goal that will take a very long time to achieve, the aim was to begin to set the nation irreversibly on a course that will ultimately achieve the goal. The strategy is to concentrate on implementing and strengthening traditional but effective tobacco control measures and making changes to the regulatory landscape including Federal regulation of tobacco products and their marketing and distribution. The Committee noted that while there have been dramatic reductions in smoking from the time that the 1964 Surgeon's General Report on the dangers of smoking, the current annual rate of cessation among smokers remains fairly low and the rate of decline in the initiation of smoking has started to level off. Therefore, strong new efforts are required to lower the overall smoking prevalence rate over the next several decades.

Pediatricians have an important responsibility to counsel their patients to avoid tobacco use. Preventing initiation of smoking is far more effective than achieving cessation of an established cigarette-smoking habit. There are a wide array of treatments to assist smoking cessation efforts.[103] In addition, identification of the most vulnerable children, that is, those in a household of family members who are smokers or those with certain nicotine receptor genotypes, can aid in targeting prevention efforts. These children through either genetic or social factors will be most inclined to take up smoking, and educational initiatives should be targeted at both smokers and nonsmokers in such households. Advertising campaigns that have emphasized social stigmatization, as well as outright bans on smoking in public places, will further these efforts.[104]

Vaccination and Cancers

For decades, providing vaccinations against life-threatening disease has been an area where pediatricians have traditionally played a paramount role. Researchers have long talked of vaccines for cancers. In 2006, a vaccine against HPV types 6, 11, 16, and 18 (Gardasil) became available and approved for use in girls and young women age 9 through 26.[105] Although technically not a vaccine against cancer per se, this vaccine prevents development of HPV, which is the major cause of both cervical cancer and genital warts. Vaccine use for males of similar age has been suggested in an effort to further achieve herd immunity[106] and potentially prevent genital warts. Two meta-analyses of six randomized controlled trials demonstrated a reduction in the frequency of high-grade cervical lesions.[107,108] In addition, not surprisingly, the vaccine demonstrated a decrease in other HPV-related illnesses including chronic infection and genital warts. The vaccine has a fairly good safety profile.[109] A second vaccine, Cervarix, is active against types 16 and 18 and is currently being used in Europe and other countries.[110]

Barriers in fully implementing HPV vaccinations have included not only cost and access but also patient and family acceptability. As HPV infection is sexually transmitted, concerns about giving the vaccine to adolescent girls has been viewed by some opponents as tacit acceptance of sexual activity in this young population. However, studies in limited populations have indicated that the vaccine is generally accepted by parents.[111-113] One such study involving nurses' attitudes toward vaccination of their own daughters suggested more enthusiasm for vaccination of older adolescents compared with girls of pubertal age.[112] On-going education and discussion with both parents and patients in the use as well as the limitations of the HPV vaccine will be the responsibility of the adolescent health provider. Professional organizations may also play a role in advocating the use of the vaccine.[114]

Early detection of cervical cancer by means of the Pap smear has reduced the mortality from this disease by 74% by over the past four decades. Still, however, in 2009 over 4,000 women are expected to die from this disease. Although the introduction of HPV vaccination is likely to further decrease mortality from cervical cancer, use of cervical cancer screening is still recommended in vaccinated women. As the risk of cervical cancer is life long, the true impact of vaccinating adolescents with the HPV vaccine in terms of maintenance of viral immunity and of further reducing the overall morbidity and mortality from cervical cancer will require additional long-term follow-up. Specific recommendations for continued use of Pap smear screening will undoubtedly evolve in the future.

Control of Cancer-Related Infectious Disease Exposure

Aside from the association between HPV and cervical cancer, the prevention or control of other infections may be an important means to prevent cancer. For example, screening for the presence of *H. pylori* and antibiotic treatment may reduce the risk of Barrett's esophagus and subsequent gastric cancer.[115] The now common universal vaccinations for hepatitis B for children will lower future hepatocellular carcinoma incidence rates. Malarial control along with improved hygiene may decrease the incidence of endemic Burkitt's lymphoma by shifting EBV infection to older ages. Aside from a vaccination, for sexually transmitted etiologic infectious agents, such as

HPV, implementing programs to promote safe sexual practices, such as the use of condoms and abstinence education, may reduce cancer incidence. These same safe sex practices will also lower the risk of transmission of HIV and KSHV.

Reducing Exposure to Sunlight

Exposure to sunlight and sunburn, especially during early childhood, are the principal causes of cutaneous malignant melanoma. Study of migrants from the United Kingdom to Australia suggests that exposure at young ages and duration of stay in Australia affected adult melanoma risk.[116] Known risk factors for melanoma other than sun exposure include light complexion, blond or red hair, and blue eyes.[117] Identified genetic factors include inherited mutations in the melanocortin-1 receptors[118] and other genetic susceptibility factors.[119] Techniques such as skin self-examination,[120] health education interventions aimed at increasing sun-protection behaviors,[121] and even chemoprevention[122] have the potential to improve skin cancer outcomes. The U.S. Preventive Services Task Force conducted a systematic review to assess the utility of skin cancer screening to improve health outcomes and concluded that limited evidence prevents accurate determination of the benefits of screening for skin cancer in the general population.[123]

Chemoprevention

A multibillion dollar industry has developed for chemopreventive agents that are intended to inhibit, delay, or reverse carcinogenesis. These agents include many classes of compounds such as antioxidants including both naturally occurring as well as synthetic compounds such as vitamin E, vitamin C, selenium, isoflavonoids, and retinoids; anti-inflammatory agents such as nonsteroidal anti-inflammatory drugs and Cyclooxygenase 2 (COX-2) inhibitors; and synthetic hormones or hormone modulators that are antiestrogenic such as tamoxifen and raloxifene. Finasteride, a drug developed to treat benign prostatic hyperplasia, has been shown to be effective at preventing or delaying the occurrence of prostate cancer[6] without impacting the risk of high-grade prostate cancer.[124] Potentially effective chemoprevention agents must be evaluated in the same manner as other therapeutic agents. Testing would include preclinical, phase I through III trials, as well as postmarketing evaluations. A major challenge for these efficacy trials is selecting an end point that is measurable within the time frame for a typical clinical trial. Given that the effect of chemotherapeutic agents on the incidence of cancer may not be seen for many decades, surrogate end points that can be measured over a relatively short duration are chosen. Often, however, these surrogate measures are not perfectly predictive of incidence and mortality end points; thus, the validity of some chemoprevention trials may be compromised. There is a continuous search for more valid intermediate biomarkers. Evolving methods such as high-throughput DNA microarray expression analysis, protein profiling, cell culture, and the development of transgenic and gene knockout mice are aiding the discovery of new targeted chemotherapeutic as well as chemopreventive agents. High-risk subjects are often used for early phase trials, that is, those with known *APC* mutations for a colorectal chemoprevention trial.

Secondary Prevention

The goal of secondary prevention is to identify cancer in earlier stages of its natural history. With existing techniques, early detection and screening can be advanced by means of simple personal educational efforts such as testicular self-examination, clinical examinations such as colonoscopy, radioimaging including routine mammography, image-guided biopsy, or detection of tumor biomarkers. Biomarkers are biochemical or cellular compounds that can be used to identify increased cancer susceptibility, the effects of tumorigenesis, or the presence of precancerous lesions or asymptomatic malignant tumors. Biomarkers for susceptibility can be used to identify high-risk subsets that can be targeted for increased screening surveillance. They can also be used to track the disappearance or regression of early lesions, including those that occur spontaneously and those induced from early therapeutic responses. Surrogate end points such as biomarkers that detect cellular changes within tumors (e.g., biomarkers for angiogenesis and apoptosis) can be used as proxy end point measures of effect to speed the conduct of prevention trials. Late steps of tumorigenesis are often marked by detectable *RAS* or *TP53* mutations. With the rapid advancement and deployment of bioinformatics methods used for genomic, proteomic as well as imaging analysis, the sensitivity and precision of early cancer detection should continue to improve over time.[125]

Secondary prevention requires the availability of an accurate method to detect cancer or a premalignant state and evidence that early therapeutic intervention will result in better outcomes. Early detection and screening methods must first be shown to be valid (i.e., high sensitivity and specificity) and cost-effective. Costs must be considered in terms of economic, physical (e.g., morbidity and mortality of invasive tests), and psychosocial impact. At present, there are no cost-effective mass screening tests to detect childhood cancer. In contrast, there is substantial evidence that screening is effective at lowering mortality for breast cancer and colon cancer. FAP screening provides an example of how early detection might be used in a pediatric setting. Screening for mutations in the *APC* locus would allow children to be identified who are at high risk for the development of colorectal cancer later in life. Although the onset of these malignancies can occur in the second decade of life, cancers typically do not develop until the third or fourth decades. Screening for prostate cancer using Prostate-Specific Antigen (PSA) testing has proven more controversial in that the test is somewhat nonspecific and that identification of disease is not strongly associated with mortality;[126,127] that is, many indolent prostate tumors are detected that would otherwise not impact an individual's mortality.

The baseline level of suspicion for genetic predisposition syndromes, such as *APC* mutations, is not high unless there is a remarkable family history of cancer. Detection of *APC* mutations in childhood could positively influence cancer prevention practices such as introduction of dietary modification, chemoprevention, and increased surveillance with annual colonoscopy and polypectomy starting in adolescence. For extremely high-risk cases, prophylactic colectomy may be a viable medical option.

HEALTH POLICY ISSUES RELATED TO PREVENTION DURING CHILDHOOD

Effective comprehensive cancer prevention strategies should include ready access to health care services including susceptibility screening to identify high-risk individuals, mass screening for early detection of new malignancies, educational efforts aimed at promoting healthy lifestyles (including tobacco use avoidance, obesity prevention with dietary and physical activity improvement), HPV and Hepatitis B vaccination, and the possible use of chemoprevention agents that can significantly decrease cancer incidence and mortality. Health policies must contain provisions to ensure that all applicable cancer prevention measures are available. Improvements in information technology not only have direct consequences for improving the health care delivery for individuals but will also facilitate the development of new prevention research.

Genetic testing for adult cancer susceptibility is only useful in rare families at present. The level of suspicion for cancer predisposition is higher for families that have experienced an unusual number of cancers affecting both children and adults, such as *TP53* germ line mutation (associated with childhood gliomas and soft tissue sarcomas and adult early onset breast cancers). However, the utility of genetic screening during childhood is less obvious for predisposition syndromes that affect only adults, such as *BRCA1*-related breast cancer. Theoretically, identifying adult cancer predisposition syndromes as well as more subtle genetic susceptibility factors at young ages should confer advantages over their identification in adulthood.

With the continuing improvements and deployment of high-throughput genomic screening, coupled with advanced bioinformatics methods for interpreting vast amounts of genetic data, more affordable and complete genotyping of individuals may soon be within the reach. Susceptibility assessment using genotype can become a major component of "personalized medicine" much like developing individualized therapies. Along with the opportunity to positively exploit genotype information for health gains come increased risks such as loss of confidentiality and potential commercial misuse of this information, including discrimination for employment and denial of health care insurance coverage. The U.S. Federal government recently signed into law the Genetic Information Nondiscrimination Act of 2008 (GINA).[128] Together with the nondiscrimination provisions of the Health Insurance Portability and Accountability Act, GINA will prohibit discrimination in health coverage and employment on the basis of genetic information. One of the intended effects of this legislation will be to remove barriers to more widespread genetic testing. The physician will have greater ability to genetically identify individuals most likely to benefit from primary prevention (e.g., chemoprevention and prophylactic surgery) or secondary prevention (e.g., screening only high-risk individuals that result in higher test yields).

From an economic perspective, identifying high-risk populations can greatly improve the efficacy of cancer surveillance and use limited health resources more efficiently. Expensive and invasive early screening tests can be reserved for those individuals predicted to be at highest risk for cancer. Prevention efforts could be directed to high-risk individuals who are most likely to benefit from avoidance of environmental, occupational, or lifestyle-determined exposures such as agrochemicals, low-dose radiation, tobacco, and sexually transmitted infectious organisms. Susceptibility assessment could also identify those who are most likely to benefit from a chemoprevention regimen.

Continuing efforts are needed to expand cancer prevention research infrastructure. Prevention activities will be enhanced through the identification of risk factors utilizing gene mapping information from the Human Genome Project and the Cancer Genome Atlas. The functional significance of genes as they relate to cancer risk can benefit from partnerships such as the International HapMap Project. Cancer Biomedical Grid (caBIG) will continue to more fully integrate vast stores of biological data with the assessment of new treatments and preventive interventions.

Expanded infrastructure is needed to support improvements in our capacity to conduct population-based research to identify determinants of cancer risk. Case-control studies have identified many important genetic and environmental risk factors for cancer. However, these studies are limited to identifying factors for a single disease and are more likely to suffer from differential recall bias between cases and control about previous exposures. In contrast, large prospective cohort studies directly quantitate the effect of etiologic factors on disease incidence and multiple diseases can be studied. It has been suggested that a large prospective cohort study using a representative sample of the U.S. population be conducted to study the effects of genes and environmental factors. This has been done in other countries such as the United Kingdom, Canada, Japan, and Iceland.[129] The National Children's Study (NCS) is currently being launched with a plan to study a representative population of 100,000 children from prebirth until the age of 21 in the United States. The NCS will collect information on pregnancy and childhood exposures as well as collect and bank biospecimens for future use. Although the overall goal of the NCS is to identify determinants of childhood health and development, childhood cancer is not a primary end point given the rarity of its occurrence. However, it is conceivable that this cohort could be used for future studies of adult cancer risk that focus on genetics and childhood exposures.

The Federal government is taking an active hand in guiding the development of an electronic health record (EHR) that will conform to common standards and will allow for some degree of interoperability and data exchange. A need exists to advance our medical informatics capacity and be able to track individuals as they move through different health care systems and providers, thus improving our ability to conduct prevention studies with long-term outcomes. The American Recovery and Reinvestment Act of 2009 provides funds to improve U.S. health care through health information technology.[130] The Federal government has recently agreed to reimburse states for 90% of the administrative costs of overseeing EHR incentive payments to doctors and hospitals for the administration of Medicaid state operations. Continued expansion of our informatics capabilities will allow for linkages of high-throughput genomic and proteomic information with clinical data from EHRs. When combined with advances in pharmacogenomics, bioinformatics, and clinical informatics, we will be able to increase the precision of cancer susceptibility screening and develop better targeted chemoprevention interventions.

The launch of the National Institutes of Health Clinical Translational Science Award (CTSA) network and the National Cancer Institute's caBIG are beginning to have a transformative effect on the development of translational research in which basic sciences are more fully integrated with the clinical- and population-based research framework. These translational research consortia are bringing multiple institutions together into common research networks that will accelerate research discoveries, reduce duplication of research resources, and have the potential of evaluating new hypotheses in larger, much more generalizable study populations. Enhanced translational research infrastructure will accelerate cancer prevention discoveries that will ultimately decrease cancer burden.

Although there is future hope for mass-screening techniques that can identify genetically derived cancer susceptibility, the societal implications need to be fully delineated before implementation. For example, for children with a history of FAP, there is evidence suggesting that genetic testing has minimal impact on causing psychological distress, although there is some increase in anxiety-related symptoms.

Lifestyle behavior interventions are challenging, especially in the adolescent and young adult population. The concept of adolescent "invulnerability" is a serious barrier to both adaption of healthful practices as well as adolescents' decisions to engage in potentially harmful behavior. There is evidence that innovative methods can overcome some adherence barriers in young persons.[131] Reduction in the prevalence of high-risk behaviors is more efficient if these can be prevented altogether rather than abated. Introduction of lifelong health-promoting behaviors including prevention of tobacco use, adherence to health lifestyle recommendations, reductions in infection with oncogenic viruses, and adherence to recommended screening and early detection guidelines should be started early in life. Parents have a responsibility to promote healthy behaviors in early childhood; school-aged children become more receptive to health-promotion messages. HPV vaccination provides one of the most important opportunities to prevent adult cancer. However, even with demonstrated efficacy of the vaccine, both economic as well as social barriers remain. Among the lay public, few individuals understand HPV and the consequences of infection; there are fears about vaccine safety and confusion about the respective roles of Pap smear screening and HPV vaccination, and parents have concerns about increased risk of sexual activity if their children are vaccinated.

RECOMMENDATIONS

Cancer prevention and control strategies introduced during childhood and adolescence have great potential to reduce subsequent cancer morbidity and mortality. The sequential and often lengthy process of carcinogenesis provides multiple targets and opportunities to block biological transitions required for the development of adult malignancies. Intervening much earlier in life should provide the most cost-effective means of preventing cancer. Exposures during childhood are known to be important determinants of certain adult cancers such as melanoma (i.e., repeated severe sunburns during childhood), cervical cancer (i.e., HPV exposure during adolescence), and breast cancer (i.e., hormone levels in late adolescence). Simple interventions, such as vaccination to prevent HPV infection, modifying the formulation of oral contraceptives (e.g., reduced steroid dose by use of a gonadotropin-releasing hormone agonist with very low-dose estrogens and intermittent

progestogens), using sunblock and adhering to safe-sunning practices, encouraging sexual abstinence or the use of condoms to reduce the sexual transmission of infectious oncogenic agents, and reducing exposure to tobacco, can significantly lower the likelihood of cancer later in life.

There are known disparities in cancer burden affecting certain subgroups that track with reduced access to routine health care, including access to preventive care. Individuals in groups defined by characteristics such as socioeconomic status, race, ethnicity, culture, or geography cannot or choose not to avail themselves of routine medical care including cancer prevention services. Although children are the exception, even pediatrician visits for recommended "well-care" greatly diminish throughout adolescence. Young adults are likely to receive no regular contact with health care providers except in cases of acute illnesses. For adolescents and young adults, the responsibility for providing routine medical care falls somewhere between the pediatrician and the internist or other primary care provider. Health care providers need to ensure that adolescents receive routine preventive care so that early detection for identified high-risk individuals as well as healthy lifestyle, including cancer-related, behaviors can be initiated and maintained at an early age.

The health care workforce has a duty to ensure that children receive the benefits from effective cancer prevention health practices and should insist on developing research needed to expand the evidence base for effective preventive interventions. Health education efforts have proven to be effective at lowering smoking prevalence as have regulatory restrictions in access to tobacco products. Targeted efforts should be made to reach out to traditionally underserved pediatric populations. A health care system that guarantees continuity of medical care from childhood through adolescence and into early adulthood could mandate the provision of cancer prevention services. Detection of increased cancer susceptibility during childhood can lead to more effective surveillance strategies. Pediatricians have a crucial role to play in educating their patients to choose healthy lifestyle behaviors that will ultimately have a dramatic impact on future cancer incidence and mortality.

References

1. American Cancer Society. Cancer Facts & Figures 2007. Atlanta, GA: American Cancer Society, 2007.
2. American Heart Association. Heart Disease and Stroke Statistics—2009 Update. Dallas, TX: American Heart Association, 2009.
3. Jemal A, Siegel R, Ward E, et al. Cancer statistics, 2009. CA Cancer J Clin 2009;59(4): 225–249.
4. Fisher B, Costantino JP, Wickerham DL, et al. Tamoxifen for prevention of breast cancer: report of the National Surgical Adjuvant Breast and Bowel Project P-1 Study. J Natl Cancer Inst 1998;90(18):1371–1388.
5. Vogel VG, Costantino JP, Wickerham DL, et al. Effects of tamoxifen vs raloxifene on the risk of developing invasive breast cancer and other disease outcomes: the NSABP study of tamoxifen and raloxifene (STAR) P-2 trial. JAMA 2006;295(23):2727–2741.
6. Thompson IM, Goodman PJ, Tangen CM, et al. The influence of finasteride on the development of prostate cancer. N Engl J Med 2003;349(3):215–224.
7. Lucia MS, Epstein JI, Goodman PJ, et al. Finasteride and high-grade prostate cancer in the Prostate Cancer Prevention Trial. J Natl Cancer Inst 2007;99(18):1375–1383.
8. Greenwald P. Introduction: history of cancer prevention and control. In: Greenwald P, Kramer BS, Weed DL, eds. Cancer prevention and control. New York, NY: Marcel Dekker, Inc., 1995:1–7.
9. Greenwald P, Dunn BK. Do we make optimal use of the potential of cancer prevention? Recent Results Cancer Res 2009;181:3–17.
10. Fearon ER, Vogelstein B. A genetic model for colorectal tumorigenesis. Cell 1990;61(5): 759–767.
11. Weinstein IB. Disorders in cell circuitry during multistage carcinogenesis: the role of homeostasis. Carcinogenesis. 2000;21(5):857–864.
12. Knudson AG, Meadows AT, Hill R, et al. Chromosomal deletion and retinoblastoma. N Engl J Med 1976;295(20):1120–1123.
13. Friend SH, Bernards R, Rogelj S, et al. A human DNA segment with properties of the gene that predisposes to retinoblastoma and osteosarcoma. Nature 1986;323:643–646.
14. Eng C, Li FP, Abramson DH, et al. Mortality from second tumors among long-term survivors of retinoblastoma. J Natl Cancer Inst 1993;85(14):1121–1128.
15. Wong FL, Boice JD Jr, Abramson DH, et al. Cancer incidence after retinoblastoma. Radiation dose and sarcoma risk. JAMA 1997;278(15):1262–1267.
16. Kleinerman RA, Tucker MA, Tarone RE, et al. Risk of new cancers after radiotherapy in long-term survivors of retinoblastoma: an extended follow-up. J Clin Oncol 2005; 23(10):2272–2279.
17. Quesnel S, Malkin D. Genetic predisposition to cancer and familial cancer syndromes. Pediatr Clin North Am 1997;44(4):791–808.
18. Geary J, Sasieni P, Houlston R, et al. Gene-related cancer spectrum in families with hereditary non-polyposis colorectal cancer (HNPCC). Fam Cancer 2008;7(2):163–172.
19. Frebourg T, Abel A, Bonaiti-Pellie C, et al. [Li-Fraumeni syndrome: update, new data and guidelines for clinical management]. Bull Cancer 2001;88(6):581–587.
20. Vasen HF, Moslein G, Alonso A, et al. Guidelines for the clinical management of familial adenomatous polyposis (FAP). Gut 2008;57(5):704–713.
21. Augustyn AM, Wallerstein R. The role of pediatricians in families with a history of familial adenomatous polyposis. Clin Pediatr 2009;48(6):623–626.
22. Cetta F, Toti P, Petracci M, et al. Thyroid carcinoma associated with familial adenomatous polyposis. Histopathology 1997;31(3):231–236.
23. Cetta F, Pelizzo MR, Curia MC, et al. Genetics and clinicopathological findings in thyroid carcinomas associated with familial adenomatous polyposis. Am J Pathol 1999; 155(1):7–9.
24. Herraiz M, Barbesino G, Faquin W, et al. Prevalence of thyroid cancer in familial adenomatous polyposis syndrome and the role of screening ultrasound examinations. Clin Gastroenterol Hepatol 2007;5(3):367–373.
25. Lynch PM. Chemoprevention with special reference to inherited colorectal cancer. Fam Cancer 2008;7(1):59–64.
26. Doxey BW, Kuwada SK, Burt RW. Inherited polyposis syndromes: molecular mechanisms, clinicopathology, and genetic testing. Clin Gastroenterol Hepatol 2005;3(7): 633–641.
27. Poley JW, Wagner A, Hoogmans MM, et al. Biallelic germline mutations of mismatch-repair genes: a possible cause for multiple pediatric malignancies. Cancer 2007;109(11): 2349–2356.
28. Tan TY, Orme LM, Lynch E, et al. Biallelic PMS2 mutations and a distinctive childhood cancer syndrome. J Pediatr Hematol Oncol 2008;30(3):254–257.
29. Joerger M, Koeberle D, Neumann HP, et al. Von Hippel-Lindau disease—a rare disease important to recognize. Onkologie 2005;28(3):159–163.

30. Szinnai G, Sarnacki S, Polak M. Hereditary medullary thyroid carcinoma: how molecular genetics made multiple endocrine neoplasia type 2 a paediatric disease. Endocr Dev 2007;10:173–187.
31. de Krijger RR. Endocrine tumor syndromes in infancy and childhood. Endocr Pathol 2004;15(3):223–226.
32. Johnston LB, Chew SL, Lowe D, et al. Investigating familial endocrine neoplasia syndromes in children. Horm Res 2001;55(Suppl 1):31–35.
33. Lakhani VT, You YN, Wells SA. The multiple endocrine neoplasia syndromes. Annu Rev Med 2007;58:253–265.
34. Gustafson S, Zbuk KM, Scacheri C, et al. Cowden syndrome. Semin Oncol 2007;34(5):428–434.
35. Newman B, Mu H, Butler LM, et al. Frequency of breast cancer attributable to BRCA1 in a population-based series of American women. JAMA 1998;279(12):915–921.
36. Malone KE, Daling JR, Neal C, et al. Frequency of BRCA1/BRCA2 mutations in a population-based sample of young breast carcinoma cases. Cancer 2000;88(6):1393–1402.
37. Holschneider CH, Berek JS. Ovarian cancer: epidemiology, biology, and prognostic factors. Semin Surg Oncol 2000;19(1):3–10.
38. Magnusson S, Borg A, Kristoffersson U, et al. Higher occurrence of childhood cancer in families with germline mutations in BRCA2, MMR and CDKN2 A genes. Fam Cancer 2008;7(4):331–337.
39. Reid S, Renwick A, Seal S, et al. Biallelic BRCA2 mutations are associated with multiple malignancies in childhood including familial Wilms tumour. J Med Genet 2005;42(2):147–151.
40. Rubinstein WS, Jiang H, Dellefave L, et al. Cost-effectiveness of population-based BRCA1/2 testing and ovarian cancer prevention for Ashkenazi Jews: A call for dialogue. Genet Med. 2009;11(9):629–639.
41. Eng C, Hampel H, de la Chapelle A. Genetic testing for cancer predisposition. Annu Rev Med 2001;52:371–400.
42. Savitsky K, Sfez S, Tagle DA, et al. The complete sequence of the coding region of the ATM gene reveals similarity to cell cycle regulators in different species. Hum Mol Genet 1995;4(11):2025–2032.
43. Savitsky K, Bar-Shira A, Gilad S, et al. A single ataxia telangiectasia gene with a product similar to PI-3 kinase. Science 1995;268(5218):1749–1753.
44. Olsen JH, Hahnemann JM, Borresen-Dale AL, et al. Cancer in patients with ataxia-telangiectasia and in their relatives in the nordic countries. J Natl Cancer Inst 2001;93(2):121–127.
45. Swift M, Lukin JL. Breast cancer incidence and the effect of cigarette smoking in heterozygous carriers of mutations in the ataxia-telangiectasia gene. Cancer Epidemiol Biomarkers Prev 2008;17(11):3188–3192.
46. Swinney R, Hsu S, Tomlinson G. Phase I and Phase II enzyme polymorphisms and childhood cancer. J Investig Med 2006;54(6):303–320.
47. Reszka E, Wasowicz W, Gromadzinska J. Genetic polymorphism of xenobiotic metabolising enzymes, diet and cancer susceptibility. Br J Nutr 2006;96(4):609–619.
48. Gottlieb MS, Schroff R, Schanker HM, et al. Pneumocystis carinii pneumonia and mucosal candidiasis in previously healthy homosexual men: evidence of a new acquired cellular immunodeficiency. N Engl J Med 1981;305(24):1425–1431.
49. Gail MH, Pluda JM, Rabkin CS, et al. Projections of the incidence of non-Hodgkin's lymphoma related to acquired immunodeficiency syndrome. J Natl Cancer Inst 1991;83(10):695–701.
50. McClain KL, Leach CT, Jenson HB, et al. Association of Epstein-Barr virus with leiomyosarcomas in children with AIDS. N Engl J Med 1995;332(1):12–18.
51. Moore PS, Boshoff C, Weiss RA, et al. Molecular mimicry of human cytokine and cytokine response pathway genes by KSHV. Science 1996;274(5293):1739–1744.
52. Pollock BH, Jenson HB, Leach CT, et al. Risk factors for pediatric human immunodeficiency virus-related malignancy. JAMA. 2003;289(18):2393–2399.
53. Azuma K, Uchiyama I, Chiba Y, et al. Mesothelioma risk and environmental exposure to asbestos: past and future trends in Japan. Int J Occup Environ Health 2009;15(2):166–172.
54. Richardson DB. Lung cancer in chrysotile asbestos workers: analyses based on the two-stage clonal expansion model. Cancer Causes Control 2009;20(6):917–923.
55. Wakeford R. The cancer epidemiology of radiation. Oncogene 2004;23(38):6404–6428.
56. Feychting M, Ahlbom A, Kheifets L. EMF and health. Annu Rev Public Health 2005;26:165–189.
57. Schuz J, Jacobsen R, Olsen JH, et al. Cellular telephone use and cancer risk: update of a nationwide Danish cohort. J Natl Cancer Inst 2006;98(23):1707–1713.
58. Lonn S, Ahlbom A, Hall P, et al. Long-term mobile phone use and brain tumor risk. Am J Epidemiol 2005;161(6):526–535.
59. Lahkola A, Auvinen A, Raitanen J, et al. Mobile phone use and risk of glioma in 5 North European countries. Int J Cancer 2007;120(8):1769–1775.
60. Inskip PD, Tarone RE, Hatch EE, et al. Cellular-telephone use and brain tumors. N Engl J Med 2001;344(2):79–86.
61. Land CE, Tokunaga M, Koyama K, et al. Incidence of female breast cancer among atomic bomb survivors, Hiroshima and Nagasaki, 1950–1990. Radiat Res 2003;160(6):707–717.
62. Bergstrom A, Pisani P, Tenet V, et al. Overweight as an avoidable cause of cancer in Europe. Int J Cancer 2001;91(3):421–430.
63. Calle EE, Rodriguez C, Walker-Thurmond K, et al. Overweight, obesity, and mortality from cancer in a prospectively studied cohort of U.S. adults. N Engl J Med 2003;348(17):1625–1638.
64. Carroll KK. Obesity as a risk factor for certain types of cancer. Lipids 1998;33(11):1055–1059.
65. Ford ES. Body mass index and colon cancer in a national sample of adult US men and women. Am J Epidemiol 1999;150(4):390–398.
66. Giovannucci E, Ascherio A, Rimm EB, et al. Physical activity, obesity, and risk for colon cancer and adenoma in men. Ann Intern Med 1995;122(5):327–334.
67. Reeves GK, Pirie K, Beral V, et al. Cancer incidence and mortality in relation to body mass index in the Million Women Study: cohort study. BMJ 2007;335(7630):1134.
68. Meyerhardt JA, Catalano PJ, Haller DG, et al. Impact of diabetes mellitus on outcomes in patients with colon cancer. J Clin Oncol 2003;21(3):433–440.
69. Bruce WR, Wolever TM, Giacca A. Mechanisms linking diet and colorectal cancer: the possible role of insulin resistance. Nutr Cancer 2000;37(1):19–26.
70. Giovannucci E. Insulin and colon cancer. Cancer Causes Control 1995;6(2):164–179.
71. Ahmed ML, Ong KK, Dunger DB. Childhood obesity and the timing of puberty. Trends Endocrinol Metab TEM 2009;20(5):237–242.
72. Jayachandran J, Banez LL, Aronson WJ, et al. Obesity as a predictor of adverse outcome across black and white race: results from the Shared Equal Access Regional Cancer Hospital (SEARCH) Database. Cancer 2009;115(22):5263–5271.
73. de Azambuja E, McCaskill-Stevens W, Francis P, et al. The effect of body mass index on overall and disease-free survival in node-positive breast cancer patients treated with docetaxel and doxorubicin-containing adjuvant chemotherapy: the experience of the BIG 02–98 trial. Breast Cancer Res Treat 2009;119(1):145–153.
74. Li D, Morris JS, Liu J, et al. Body mass index and risk, age of onset, and survival in patients with pancreatic cancer. JAMA 2009;301(24):2553–2562.
75. Ma J, Li H, Giovannucci E, et al. Prediagnostic body-mass index, plasma C-peptide concentration, and prostate cancer-specific mortality in men with prostate cancer: a long-term survival analysis. Lancet Oncol 2008;9(11):1039–1047.
76. Ogino S, Nosho K, Shima K, et al. p21 Expression in colon cancer and modifying effects of patient age and body mass index on prognosis. Canc Epidemiol Biomarkers Prev 2009;18(9):2513–2521.
77. Hedley AA, Ogden CL, Johnson CL, et al. Prevalence of overweight and obesity among US children, adolescents, and adults, 1999–2002. JAMA 2004;291(23):2847–2850.
78. Krebs NF, Jacobson MS. Prevention of pediatric overweight and obesity. Pediatrics 2003;112(2):424–430.
79. Deitel M. The Surgeon-General's call to action to prevent an increase in overweight and obesity. Released Dec. 13, 2001. Obes Surg 2002;12(1):3–4.
80. Gerberding JL, Marks JS. Making America fit and trim–steps big and small. Am J Public Health 2004;94(9):1478–1479.
81. McCullough ML, Giovannucci EL. Diet and cancer prevention. Oncogene 2004;23(38):6349–6364.
82. Lee JE, Mannisto S, Spiegelman D, et al. Intakes of fruit, vegetables, and carotenoids and renal cell cancer risk: a pooled analysis of 13 prospective studies. Cancer Epidemiol Biomarkers Prev 2009;18(6):1730–1739.
83. Armstrong B, Doll R. Environmental factors and cancer incidence and mortality in different countries, with special reference to dietary practices. Int J Cancer 1975;15(4):617–631.
84. Ziegler RG, Hoover RN, Pike MC, et al. Migration patterns and breast cancer risk in Asian-American women. J Natl Cancer Inst 1993;85(22):1819–1827.
85. Prentice RL, Willett WC, Greenwald P, et al. Nutrition and physical activity and chronic disease prevention: research strategies and recommendations. J Natl Cancer Inst 2004;96(17):1276–1287.
86. Alpha-Tocopherol BCCPSG. The effect of vitamin E and beta carotene on the incidence of lung cancer and other cancers in male smokers. N Engl J Med 1994;330(15):1029–1035.
87. Hemila H, Kaprio J. Modification of the effect of vitamin E supplementation on the mortality of male smokers by age and dietary vitamin C. Am J Epidemiol 2009;169(8):946–953.
88. Lippman SM, Klein EA, Goodman PJ, et al. Effect of selenium and vitamin E on risk of prostate cancer and other cancers: the Selenium and Vitamin E Cancer Prevention Trial (SELECT). JAMA 2009;301(1):39–51.
89. State-specific prevalence and trends in adult cigarette smoking–United States, 1998–2007. MMWR Morb Mortal Wkly Rep 2009;58(9):221–226.
90. Eaton DK, Kann L, Kinchen S, et al. Youth risk behavior surveillance–United States, 2007. MMWR Surveill Summ 2008;57(4):1–131.
91. Ramsey F, Ussery-Hall A, Garcia D, et al. Prevalence of selected risk behaviors and chronic diseases–Behavioral Risk Factor Surveillance System (BRFSS), 39 steps communities, United States, 2005. MMWR Surveill Summ 2008;57(11):1–20.
92. Zang EA, Wynder EL. Differences in lung cancer risk between men and women: examination of the evidence. J Natl Cancer Inst 1996;88(3,4):183–192.
93. Reid ME, Santella R, Ambrosone CB. Molecular epidemiology to better predict lung cancer risk. Clin Lung Cancer 2008;9(3):149–153.
94. Lichtenstein E. Behavioral research contributions and needs in cancer prevention and control: tobacco use prevention and cessation. Prev Med 1997;26(5):S57–S63.
95. Kim MJ, Fleming CB, Catalano RF. Individual and social influences on progression to daily smoking during adolescence. Pediatrics 2009;124:895–902.
96. Sherman EJ, Primack BA. What works to prevent adolescent smoking? A systematic review of the national cancer institute's research-tested intervention programs. J Sch Health 2009;79(9):391–399.
97. Caporaso N, Gu F, Chatterjee N, et al. Genome-wide and candidate gene association study of cigarette smoking behaviors. PloS one 2009;4(2):e4653.
98. Hung RJ, McKay JD, Gaborieau V, et al. A susceptibility locus for lung cancer maps to nicotinic acetylcholine receptor subunit genes on 15q25. Nature 2008;452(7187):633–637.
99. Liu P, Vikis HG, Wang D, et al. Familial aggregation of common sequence variants on 15q24–25.1 in lung cancer. J Natl Cancer Inst 2008;100(18):1326–1330.
100. Spitz MR, Amos CI, Dong Q, et al. The CHRNA5-A3 region on chromosome 15q24–25.1 is a risk factor both for nicotine dependence and for lung cancer. J Natl Cancer Inst 2008;100(21):1552–1556.
101. Wang Y, Broderick P, Webb E, et al. Common 5p15.33 and 6p21.33 variants influence lung cancer risk. Nat Genet 2008;40(12):1407–1409.
102. Bonnie RJ, Stratton K, Wallace RB, Committee on Reducing Tobacco Use: Strategies B, and Consequences, eds. Ending the Tobacco Problem: A Blueprint for the Nation: National Academies Press; 2007.
103. Hughes JR. New treatments for smoking cessation. CA Cancer J Clin. 2000;50(3):143–151; quiz 152–145.
104. Institute of Medicine. Ending the tobacco problem: A blueprint for the nation The National Academies Press; 2007.
105. Markowitz L, Dunne E, Saraiya M, et al. Quadrivalent human papillomavirus Vaccine: recommendations of the advisory committee on immunization practices (ACIP). MMWR Recomm Rep 2007;23(56):1–24.
106. Hull S, Caplan A. The case for vaccinating boys against human papillomavirus. Public Health Genomics 2009;12(5,6):362–367.
107. La Torre G, de Waure C, Chiaradia G, et al. HPV vaccine efficacy in preventing persistent cervical HPV infection: a systematic review and meta-analysis. Vaccine 2007;25(50):8352–8358.
108. Rambout L, Hopkins L, Hutton B, et al. Prophylactic vaccination against human papillomavirus infection and disease in women: a systematic review of randomized controlled trials. CMAJ 2007;177(5):469–479.
109. Slade BA, Leidel L, Vellozzi C, et al. Postlicensure safety surveillance for quadrivalent human papillomavirus recombinant vaccine. JAMA 2009;302(7):750–757.
110. Schwarz T. AS04-adjuvanted human papillomavirus-16/18 vaccination: recent advances in cervical cancer prevention. Expert Rev Vaccines 2008;7(10):1465–1473.

111. Dahlstrom L, Tran T, Lundholm C, et al. Attitudes to HPV vaccination among parents of children aged 12–15 years—a population-based survey in Sweden [published online ahead of print 2009]. Int J Cancer 2009;126(2):500–507.

112. Kahn J, Ding L, Huang B, et al. Mothers' intention for their daughters and themselves to receive the human papillomavirus vaccine: a national study of nurses. Pediatrics 2009;123(6):1439–1445.

113. Ogilvie G, Remple V, Marra F, et al. Parental intention to have daughters receive the human papillomavirus vaccine. CMAJ 2007;177:1506–1512.

114. Rothman S, Rothman D. Marketing HPV Vaccine: implications for adolescent health and medical professionalism. JAMA 2009;302(7):781–786.

115. Wisniewski RM, Peura DA. Helicobacter pylori: beyond peptic ulcer disease. Gastroenterologist 1997;5(4):295–305.

116. Khlat M, Vail A, Parkin M, et al. Mortality from melanoma in migrants to Australia: variation by age at arrival and duration of stay. Am J Epidemiol 1992;135(10):1103–1113.

117. Bliss JM, Ford D, Swerdlow AJ, et al. Risk of cutaneous melanoma associated with pigmentation characteristics and freckling: systematic overview of 10 case-control studies. The international melanoma analysis group (IMAGE). Int J Cancer 1995;62(4):367–376.

118. Rees JL. The genetics of sun sensitivity in humans. Am J Hum Genet 2004;75(5):739–751.

119. Landi MT, Goldstein AM, Tsang S, et al. Genetic susceptibility in familial melanoma from northeastern Italy. J Med Genet 2004;41(7):557–566.

120. Oliveria SA, Dusza SW, Phelan DL, et al. Patient adherence to skin self-examination: effect of nurse intervention with photographs. Am J Prev Med 2004;26(2):152–155.

121. Manganoni AM, Cainelli T, Zumiani G, et al. Study of sunbathing in children: the preliminary evaluation of a prevention program. Tumori 2005;91(2):116–120.

122. Einspahr JG, Stratton SP, Bowden GT, Alberts DS. Chemoprevention of human skin cancer. Crit Rev Oncol Hematol 2002;41(3):269–285.

123. Wolff T, Tai E, Miller T. Screening for skin cancer: an update of the evidence for the U.S. Preventive Services Task Force. Ann Intern Med 2009;150(3):194–198.

124. Redman MW, Tangen CM, Goodman PJ, et al. Finasteride does not increase the risk of high-grade prostate cancer: a bias-adjusted modeling approach. Cancer Prev Res 2008;1(3):174–181.

125. Kapetanovic IM, Umar A, Khan J. Proceedings: The Applications of Bioinformatics in Cancer Detection Workshop. Annals of the New York Academy of Sciences, 2004;1020 (The Applications of Bioinformatics in Cancer Detection):1–9.

126. Schroder FH, Hugosson J, Roobol MJ, et al. Screening and prostate-cancer mortality in a randomized European study. N Engl J Med 2009;360(13):1320–1328.

127. Andriole GL, Crawford ED, Grubb RL III, et al. Mortality results from a randomized prostate-cancer screening trial. N Engl J Med 2009;360(13):1310–1319.

128. Office for Human Research Protections. Guidance on the genetic information nondiscrimination act: implications for investigators and institutional review boards. 2009; http://www.hhs.gov/ohrp/humansubjects/guidance/gina.html. Accessed March 24, 2009.

129. Collins FS. The case for a US prospective cohort study of genes and environment. Nature 2004;429(6990):475–477.

130. Centers for Medicaid and Medicare Services. CMS information related to the economic recovery act of 2009: health information technology. http://www.cms.hhs.gov/Recovery/11_HealthIT.asp, 2009.

131. Kato PM, Cole SW, Bradlyn AS, et al. A video game improves behavioral outcomes in adolescents and young adults with cancer: a randomized trial. Pediatrics 2008;122(2):e305–e317.

CHAPTER 55 ■ RESOURCES FOR CHILDREN WITH CANCER, THEIR FAMILIES, AND PHYSICIANS

CHERYL C. RODGERS

Pediatric oncology is a specialty field that requires providers to have extensive knowledge and specialized skills. To adequately care for these children, a variety of resources should be available to assist with patient's needs, referrals, and networking opportunities from other cancer centers. This chapter provides information on many of the medical organizations around the world that provide support, diagnostic services, and treatment to children with cancer. Web addresses have been listed to facilitate communication and gain access to the most up-to-date information regarding these organizations. Organizations are listed alphabetically by country within the text.

ALGERIA

Mustapha Pacha Hospital
Algiers, ALGERIA
Tel: 213-2-67333

ARGENTINA

Hospital de Ninos
Buenos Aires, ARGENTINA
Web: http://www.guti.gov.ar/

Hospital de Ninos Sor Maria Ludovica
La Plata, ARGENTINA
Web: http://www.ludovica.org.ar/

Hospital de Ninos "Victor J. Vilela"
Rosario, ARGENTINA
Web: http://www.rosario.gov.ar/

**Hospital de Pediatria S.A.M.I.C.
"Prof. Dr. Juan P. Garrahan"**
Buenos Aires, ARGENTINA
Web: http://www.garrahan.gov.ar/docs/hospi.html

Hospital Pediátrico Dr. Humberto Notti Children's Hospital
Mendoza, ARGENTINA
Web: http://hospinotti.mendoza.gov.ar/

Hospital Privado Centro Medico De Cordoba
Cordoba, ARGENTINA
Web: http://www.hospitalprivadosa.com.ar/

Hospital Provincial del Centenario
Rosario, ARGENTINA
Tel: 54-341-4307320

AUSTRALIA

Peter MacCallum Cancer Centre
East Melbourne, AUSTRALIA
Web: http://www.petermac.org/

Princess Margaret Hospital—Child and Adolescent Health Service
Perth, AUSTRALIA
Web: http://www.pmh.health.wa.gov.au

Royal Children's Hospital and Health Services
Brisbane, AUSTRALIA
Web: http://www.health.qld.gov.au/rch/default.asp

Royal Children's Hospital—Melbourne
Parkville, AUSTRALIA
Web: http://www.rch.org.au

Sydney Children's Hospital
Randwick, AUSTRALIA
Web: http://www.sch.edu.au

The Children's Hospital at Westmead
Westmead, AUSTRALIA
Web: http://www.chw.edu.au

Women's and Children's Hospital Department of Clinical Haematology/Oncology
North Adelaide, AUSTRALIA
Web: http://www.wch.sa.gov.au/services/az/divisions/
paedm/clinhaem/index.html

AUSTRIA

St. Anna Kinderkrebsforschung Children's Cancer Research Institute
Vienna, AUSTRIA
Web: http://www.kinderkrebsforschung.at/science/

University Children's Hospital Division of Paediatric Haematology/Oncology
Graz, AUSTRIA
Web: http://www.medunigraz.at/kinderklinik/onko/
onkotitels.htm

Univiversität Kinderklinik
Innsbruck, AUSTRIA
Web: http://www.uibk.ac.at/c/c5/c517/

BANGLADESH

Bangabandhu Sheikh Mujib Medical University
Dhaka, BANGLADESH
Web: http://www.bsmmu.org/

Dhaka Shishu Hospital
Dhaka, BANGLADESH
Web: http://www.shishu-microbiology.org/dsh.html

Institute of Child and Mother Health
Dhaka, BANGLADESH
Web: http://www.icmh.org.bd/

BELARUS

Belarusian Research Centre for Paediatric Oncology and Haematology
Minsk, BELARUS
Tel: 375-17-2654861

BELGIUM

Centre Hospitalier Regional De La Citadelle
Liege, BELGIUM
Web: http://www.chrcitadelle.be/

Clinique de l'Espérance
Montegnée, BELGIUM
Web: http://www.chc.be/hopital/default.asp?id=27&hopital=3

Clinique Universitaires Saint Luc
Brussels, BELGIUM
Web: http://www.saintluc.be/

Hospital Universitaires Des Enfants
Brussels, BELGIUM
Web: http://www.huderf.be/

Oncologisch Centrum Antwerpen
Antwerpen, BELGIUM
Web: http://www.wijook.be/ocasite/

Queen Paola Children's Hospital Division of Haematology and Oncology
Antwerp, BELGIUM
Web: http://www.huderf.be/

University Hospital Klinik Voor Kinderziekten C. Hooft
Ghent, BELGIUM
Web: http://www.healthcarebelgium.com/index.php?id=158

University Hospitals Leuven
Leuven, BELGIUM
Web: http://www.uzleuven.be/en

Universitair Ziekenhuis Brussel
Brussels, BELGIUM
Web: http://www.uzbrussel.be/u/view

BOLIVIA

Instituto Oncológico del Oriente Boliviano—Servicio de Oncología Pediátrica
Santa Cruz, BOLIVIA
Web: http://www.afanic.com/Html/DondeActuamos/DA4.html

BRAZIL

A.C. Camargo Hospital
São Paulo, BRAZIL
Web: http://www.hcanc.org.br/

Centro de Estudos e Pesquisas Oncológicas de Minas Gerais
Belo Horizonte, BRAZIL
Web: http://www.ceomg.com.br/

Centro de Oncologia e Hematologia de Osasco
Osasco, BRAZIL
Web: http://www.cancerosasco.com.br/empresa.htm

Centro Infantil Boldrini
São Paulo, BRAZIL
Web: http://www.boldrini.org.br

Hospital De Clinicas De Porto Alegre
Porto Alegre, BRAZIL
Web: http://www.hcpa.ufrgs.br/

Hospital Infantil Darcy Vargas
São Paulo, BRAZIL
Web: http://www.cedarcyvargas.org.br/

Instituto De Oncologia Pediátrica
São Paulo, BRAZIL
Web: http://www.unifesp.br/dped/exten/iop.html

BULGARIA

Medical University—Plovdiv
Plovdiv, BULGARIA
Web: http://meduniversity-plovdiv.bg/index.php?lang_id=2&prm=about

Specialized Children's Oncohematology Hospital
Sofia, BULGARIA
Web: http://en.sbaldohz.com/

CAMEROON

University of Yaounde I
Yaoundé, CAMEROON
Web: http://www.utdallas.edu/~ett032000/yaounde.html

CANADA

Alberta Children's Hospital
Calgary, AB, CANADA
Web: http://www.calgaryhealthregion.ca/ACH/

British Columbia Children's Hospital Department of Oncology, Hematology, & BMT
Vancouver, BC, CANADA
Web: http://www.bcchildrens.ca/Services/OncHemBMT

Cancer Centre of Southwestern Ontario—Kingston General Hospital
Kingston, ON, CANADA
Web: http://www.krcc.on.ca/

Children's Hospital of Eastern Ontario
Ottawa, ON, CANADA
Web: http://www.cheo.on.ca/

Children's Hospital London Health Sciences Centre
London, ON, CANADA
Web: http://www.lhsc.on.ca/About_Us/Childrens_Hospital/

CHU Sainte-Justine Hospital
Montreal, QC, CANADA
Web: http://www.chu-sainte-justine.org/

Hamilton Health Sciences
Hamilton, ON, CANADA
Web: http://www.hamiltonhealthsciences.ca

Hospital for Sick Children
Toronto, ON, CANADA
Web: http://www.sickkids.ca/

IWK Health Care
Halifax, NS, CANADA
Web: http://www.iwk.nshealth.ca/

Janeway Child Health Center
St. John's, NF, CANADA
Web: http://www.easternhealth.ca/

Montreal Children's Hospital McGill University Health Centre
Montreal, QC, CANADA
Web: http://www.muhc.ca/pfv/mch/

Saskatchewan Cancer Agency—Allan Blair Cancer Centre
Regina, SK, CANADA
Web: http://www.saskcancer.ca/Default.aspx?DN=a9576f90-46da-410d-9772-8899b89f9ca7

Saskatoon Health Region
Saskatoon, SK, CANADA
Web: http://www.saskatoonhealthregion.ca/

CHILE

Clinica Las Condes
Santiago, CHILE
Web: http://www.clc.cl/home.cgi

Hospital de Ninos, Dr. Calvo Mackenna
Santiago, CHILE
Web: http://www.calvomackenna.cl/

Hospital Dr. Gustavo Fricke
Viña del Mar, CHILE
Web: http://www.hospitalfricke.cl/

Hospital Dr. Sotero Del Rio
Santiago, CHILE
Web: http://www.hospitalsoterodelrio.cl/

CHINA

Beijing Children's Hospital
Beijing, CHINA
Web: http://www.bch.com.cn/

Children's Hospital, Zhejiang University School of Medicine
Hangzhou, CHINA
Web: http://www.zjuch.cn/

GuangZhou Children's Hospital
Guangzhou, CHINA
Web: http://www.gzch.org/

JieShuiTan Hospital
Beijing, CHINA
Web: http://english.bjhb.gov.cn

Shanghai Children's Medical Center
Shanghai, CHINA
Web: http://www.scmc.com.cn/

Sun Yat-Sen Cancer Center
Guangzhou, CHINA
Web: http://www.sysucc.com/

TienTan Hospital
Beijing, CHINA
Web: http://www.bjtth.org

West China Hospital
Chengdu, CHINA
Web: http://www.cd120.com/

Xinhua Hospital
Shanghai, CHINA
Web: http://www.xinhua-scmc.com.cn/

COLOMBIA

Clinica Del Country
Bogotá, COLOMBIA
Web: http://www.clinicadelcountry.com/index.php

Hospital Unversitario del Valle
Cali, COLOMBIA
Web: http://www.huv.gov.co/

Hospital Universitario San Vincente de Paul
Medellin, COLOMBIA
Web: http://www.elhospital.org.co/

COSTA RICA

Hospital Nacional de Ninos
San José, COSTA RICA
Web: http://www.hnn.sa.cr/

CROATIA

Clinical Hospital Split
Split, CROATIA
Web: http://www.salus.hr/hrv/index.html

Children's Hospital Zagreb
Zagreb, CROATIA
Web: http://www.kdb.hr/

Klinicka Bolnica Dubrava
Zagreb, CROATIA
Web: http://www.kbd.hr/

Klinicka Bolnica Osijek
Osijek, CROATIA
Web: http://www.kbo.hr/

University Hospital "Sestre Milosrdnice"
Zagreb, CROATIA
Web: http://www.kbsm.hr/

University of Rijeka
Rijeka, CROATIA
Web: http://www.uniri.hr/

CUBA

Hospital Pediatrico—William Soler
Havanna, CUBA
Web: http://www.sld.cu/sitios/williamsoler/

Hospital Pediátrico Docente "Juan Manuel Márquez"
Havanna, CUBA
Web: http://www.jmm.sld.cu

CYPRUS

Makarios Hospital
Nicosia, CYPRUS
Tel: 357-22-405000

CZECH REPUBLIC

Faculty Hospital Brno—Children's Medical Center
Brno, CZECH REPUBLIC
Web: http://www.fnbrno.cz/

Hospital of Ceské Budejovice
Ceske Budejovice, CZECH REPUBLIC
Web: http://www.nemcb.cz/

Motol University Hospital
Prague, CZECH REPUBLIC
Web: http://fnmotol.cz/

University Hospital Ostrava
Vratimov, CZECH REPUBLIC
Web: http://www.fno.cz/

DENMARK

Odense University Hospital
Odense, DENMARK
Web: http://www.ouh.dk/wm122110

Rigshospitalet
Copenhagen, DENMARK
Web: http://www.rigshospitalet.dk

St Anna Hospital: Willkommen
Herne, DENMARK
Web: http://www.annahospital.de/

University Hospital of Aarhus
Aarhus, DENMARK
Web: https://www.sundhed.dk/Profil.aspx?id=
   29174.482.50671

ECUADOR

Hospital Metropolitano
Quito, ECUADOR
Web: http://www.hospitalmetropolitano.org/

EGYPT

Ain Shams University
Cairo, EGYPT
Web: http://net.shams.edu.eg/hospitals.asp

Children's Cancer Hospital
Cairo, EGYPT
Web: http://www.57357.com/

Mansoura University—Oncology Center
Manura, EGYPT
Web: http://www.mans.edu.eg/centers/ocmu/

Medical Research Institute—Alexandria University
Alexandria, EGYPT
Web: http://www.mri.edu.eg/

National Cancer Institute—Cairo University
Cairo, EGYPT
Web: http://www.nci.edu.eg/

South Egypt Cancer Institute
Assiut, EGYPT
Web: http://www.seci.info/

Zagazig University
Alexandria, EGYPT
Web: http://www.mohp.gov.eg/

El SALVADOR

"Benjamin Bloom" National Children's Hospital
San Salvador, EL SALVADOR
Web: http://quemaduras.org/clinics/
   national-childrens-hospital-benjamin-bloom.html

FINLAND

Helsinki University Central Hospital
Helsinki, FINLAND
Web: http://www.randburg.com/fi/huch.html

University of Oulu
Oulu, FINLAND
Web: http://www.ppshp.fi/page.asp?Section=6498

FRANCE

Centre Léon Berard
Lyon, FRANCE
Web: http://oncora1.lyon.fnclcc.fr/

Centre Oscar Lambret
Lille Cedex, FRANCE
Web: http://www.centreoscarlambret.fr/

C.H.R.U. Montpellier—Hôpital Arnaud de Villeneuve
Montpellier, FRANCE
Web: http://www.chu-montpellier.fr/
   fr/presentation_villeneuve.jsp

C.H.U. De Reims
Reims, FRANCE
Web: http://www.chu-reims.fr/

C.H.U. De Poitiers
Poitiers, FRANCE
Web: http://www.chu-poitiers.fr/

C.H.U. De Toulouse
Toulouse Cedex, FRANCE
Web: http://www.chu-toulouse.fr/

C.H.U. Saint-Etienne
Saint Etienne Cedex, FRANCE
Web: http://www.chu-st-etienne.fr/

Hôpital Brabois Enfants
Vandoeuvre les Nancy Cedex, FRANCE
Web: http://www.chu-nancy.fr/index.htm/page117langfr

Hôpital d'Enfants Armand Trousseau
Paris Cedex, FRANCE
Web: http://www.eurocran.org/content.asp?contentID=1042

Hôpital d'Enfants de la Timone
Marseille Cedex, FRANCE
Web: http://www.doctoralia.fr/centre-medical/hopital+d+
   enfants+de+la+timone-1116219

Hôpital d'Enfants Margency
Margercy, FRANCE
Web: http://ctp-margency.croix-rouge.fr/

Hôpital Dieu
Paris Cedex, FRANCE
Web: http://www.aphp.fr/index.php?module=
   hopital&action=hopitaux_detail&vue=
   hopital_detail&obj=20

Hôpital Jeanne de Flandre
Lillie Cedex, FRANCE
Web: http://www.doctoralia.fr/centre-medical/
   hopital+jeanne+de+flandre-1095700

Hôpital Necker Enfants Malades
Paris Cedex, FRANCE
Web: http://www.hopital-necker.aphp.fr/

Hôpital Saint Antoine
Paris Cedex, FRANCE
Web: http://www.clinique-saint-antoine.com/

Hôpital Saint Louis
Paris, FRANCE
Web: http://www.chu-stlouis.fr/

Hopitaux Universitaires de Strasbourg
Strasbourg Cedex, FRANCE
Web: http://www.chru-strasbourg.fr/Hus/

Institut Curie
Paris Cedex, FRANCE
Web: http://www.curie.fr/

Institut de cancérologie Gustave Roussy
Villejuif, FRANCE
Web: http://www.igr.fr/

University of Grenoble—Centre de Santé
Grenoble, FRANCE
Web: http://sante.grenoble-univ.fr/88221694/0/
   fiche_pagelibre/&RH=

GERMANY

Asklepios Klinik Sankt Augustin
St. Augustin, GERMANY
Web: http://www.asklepios-kinderklinik.de/

Charité—University Medicine Berlin
Berlin, GERMANY
Web: http://www.charite.de/

**Children's Hospital Medical Center of the University
of Bonn**
Bonn, GERMANY
Web: http://www.meb.uni-bonn.de/kinder/englpage.html

Deutsches Rotes Kreuz-Kinderklinik Siegen
Siegen, GERMANY
Web: http://www.drk-kinderklinik.de/index01.htm

Gemeinschaftskrankenhaus
Herdecke, GERMANY
Web: http://www.gemeinschaftskrankenhaus.de/

Klinik für Allgemeine Pädiatrie—Kiel
Kiel, GERMANY
Web: http://www.uk-sh.de/index.phtml?NavID=676.397.3&

Klinik für Kinder und Jugendklinik
Erlangen, GERMANY
Web: http://www.kinderklinik.med.uni-erlangen.de/

Kinderklinik der Universität München
München, GERMANY
Web: http://www.klinikum.uni-muenchen.de/de/

**Kinderklinik und Poliklinik des Universitätsklinikums
Würzburg**
Würzburg, GERMANY
Web: http://www.kinderklinik.uni-wuerzburg.de/

**Klinik und Poliklinik für Kinderheilkunde und
Jugendmedizin**
Berlin, GERMANY
Web: http://www.kind.med.tu-muenchen.de/cms/
front_content.php

Klinikum Augsburg
Ausburg, GERMANY
Web: http://www.klinikum-augsburg.de/

Kreiskrankenhause Gummersbach
Gummersbach, GERMANY
Web: http://www.kkh-gummersbach.de/

Martin Luther Universität Hospital
Halle, GERMANY
Web: http://www.medizin.uni-halle.de/index.php?id=35

**Medical School Hannover—Clinic for Haematology and
Oncology**
Hannover, GERMANY
Web: http://www.mh-hannover.de/250.html

Medical University of Lübeck
Lübeck, GERMANY
Web: http://www.mu-luebeck.de/

Olgahospital
Stuttgart, GERMANY
Web: http://www.olgahospital.de

Universitäts Klinikum
Freiburg, GERMANY
Web: http://www.uniklinik-freiburg.de/ip/live/index_
en.html

Universität of Tübingne
Tübingen, GERMANY
Web: http://www.medizin.uni-tuebingen.de/

Universitätsklinik des Saalandes
Homburg/Saar, GERMANY
Web: http://www.uniklinikum-saarland.de/de/
einrichtungen/kliniken_institute/kinderonkologie

Universitätsklinikum Essen
Essen, GERMANY
Web: http://www.uk-essen.de/
index.php?id=kinderheilkundeiii

Universitätsklinikum Hamburg-Eppendorf
Hamburg, GERMANY
Web: http://www.uke.de/

**Universitätsklinikum Jena Friedrich-Schiller-
Universität**
Jena, GERMANY
Web: http://www.uniklinikum-jena.de/Willkommen.html

Universitätsklinikum Leipzig
Leipzig, GERMANY
Web: http://kik.uniklinikum-leipzig.de/

Universitätsklinikum Münster
Münster, GERMANY
Web: http://www.klinikum.uni-muenster.de/

University of Düsseldorf Children's Hospital
Düsseldorf, GERMANY
Web: http://www.med.uni-duesseldorf.de/

GREECE

Agia Sophia Children's Hospital
Athens, GREECE
Web: http://www.paidon-agiasofia.gr/

**Ahepa General Hospital—Aristotle University of
Thessaloniki**
Thessaloniki, GREECE
Web: http://www.ahepahosp.gr/

Children's Hospital Aglaia Kyriakou
Athens, GREECE
Web: http://www.aglaiakyriakou.gr/

Ippokration Hospital
Thessaloniki, GREECE
Web: http://www.ippokratio.gr/

Metaxa Cancer Hospital
Piraeus, GREECE
Web: http://www.metaxa-hospital.gr/

University Hospital of Heraklion
Crete, GREECE
Web: http://www.pepagnh.gr/

GUATEMALA

Central Medico de la Ciudad de Guatemala
Cuidad de Guatemala, GUATEMALA
Web: http://www.centromedico.com.gt/

Hospital Herrera Llerandi
Cuidad de Guatemala, GUATEMALA
Web: http://www.herrerallerandi.com/

HONDURAS

Honduras Medical Center
Tegucigalpa, HONDURAS
Web: http://www.hmc.hn

HONG KONG

**Prince of Wales Hospital/The Chinese University of
Hong Kong**
Shatin Hong Kong, HONG KONG
Web: http://www13.ha.org.hk/pwh/index.htm

Queen Elizabeth Hospital
Kowloon, HONG KONG
Web: http://www.ha.org.hk/haho/ho/hesd/100149e.htm

Queen Mary Hospital
HONG KONG
Web: http://www3.ha.org.hk/qmh/index.htm

Tuen Mun Hospital
Tuen Mun New Territories, HONG KONG
Web: http://www.ha.org.hk/tmh/ewelcome.html

HUNGARY

Heim Pál Hospital for Sick Children
Budapest, HUNGARY
Web: http://hpgyk.hu/

Semmelweis University Medical School
Budapest, HUNGARY
Web: http://www.sote.hu/

**University of Debrecen Medical and
 Health Science Center**
Debrecen, HUNGARY
Web: http://www.ud-mhsc.org/

University of Szeged Faculty of Medicine
Szeged, HUNGARY
Web: http://www.szote.u-szeged.hu/angoltit/

University Medical School of Pecs
Pecs, HUNGARY
Web: http://www.pote.hu/

INDIA

All India Institute of Medical Sciences
New Delhi, INDIA
Web: http://www.aiims.edu/

Amala Cancer Hospital and Research Centre
Kerala, INDIA
Web: http://www.amala.com/

B.J. Wadia Hospital for Children
Bombay, INDIA
Web: http://www.wadiagroup.com/Grp_Cmp/
 bai_jerbai_wadia_hospital_profile.htm

Cancer Institute (WIA)
Chennai, INDIA
Web: http://www.cancerinstitutewia.org/

Christian Medical College and Hospital
Vellore, INDIA
Web: http://www.cmch-vellore.edu/

Dr. B. Borooah Cancer Institute
Assam, INDIA
Web: http://www.bbcionline.org/

Indraprastha Apollo Hospital
New Delhi, INDIA
Web: http://www.apollohospdelhi.com/

Kidwai Memorial Institute of Oncology
Bangalore, INDIA
Web: http://kidwai.kar.nic.in/

King George's Medical University
Lucknow, INDIA
Web: http://www.kgmcindia.edu/

**P.D. Hinduja National Hospital and Medical
 Research Centre**
Mumbai, INDIA
Web: http://www.hindujahospital.com/

**Post Graduate Institute of Medical
 Education and Research**
Chandigarh, INDIA
Web: http://pgimer.nic.in/

Rajiv Gandhi Cancer Institute and Research Centre
New Delhi, INDIA
Web: http://www.rgci.org/

Regional Cancer Centre, Thiruvananthapuram
Kerala, INDIA
Web: http://www.rcctvm.org/

Tata Memorial Hospital
Mumbai, INDIA
Web: http://www.tatamemorialcentre.com/

INDONESIA

Central Army Hospital (RSPAD)
Jakarta, INDONESIA
Tel: 62-21-3520643

Dharmais Cancer Hospital
Jakarta Barat, INDONESIA
Web: http://www.dharmais.co.id/

Hasan Sadikin Federal Hospital
Bandung, INDONESIA
Tel: 62-22-2034426

Kariadi Hospital—Diponegoro Hospital
Semarang, INDONESIA
Web: http://www.undip.ac.id/

**RSCM (Rumah Sakit Dr. Cipto Mangunkusmo)
 Hospital**
Jakarta, INDONESIA
Web: http://rscm.co.id/

Women and Children's Harapan Kita Hospital
Jakarta, INDONESIA
Web: http://rsab-harapankita.go.id/

IRAN

**Aliasghar Children's Hospital—Iran University of
 Medical Sciences**
Tehran, IRAN
Web: http://www.iums.ac.ir/

Cancer Institute of Iran
Teheran, IRAN
Web: http://cancer-institute.ac.ir/

**Children's Hospital (Markaz Tebbi Kodakan Hospital),
 Tehran University of Medical Services**
Tehran, IRAN
Web: http://www.tums.ac.ir/english/

Shaheed Beheshti Medical University
Tehran, IRAN
Web: http://www.sbmu.ac.ir/

IRELAND

Our Lady's Hospital for Sick Children
Dublin, IRELAND
Web: http://www.olhsc.ie/

ISRAEL

Hadassah Medical Organization
Jerusalem, ISRAEL
Web: http://www.hadassah.org.il/

Haemek Medical Center
Afula, ISRAEL
Web: http://www.clalit.org.il/haemek/

Rambam Health Care Campus
Haifa, ISRAEL
Web: http://www.rambam.org.il/

Schneider Children's Medical Center of Israel
Petah-Tiqva, ISRAEL
Web: http://www.schneider.org.il/

Soroka University Medical Center
Beer Sheva, ISRAEL
Web: http://www.clalit.org.il/soroka/

ITALY

Azienda Ospedaliera San Gerardo
Monza, ITALY
Web: http://www.hsgerardo.org/

Azienda Ospedaliera di Perugia
Perugia, ITALY
Web: http://www.ospedale.perugia.it

Azienda Ospedaliera "Santa Maria Degli Angeli"
Pordenone, ITALY
Web: http://www.aopn.sanita.fvg.it/

Azienda Ospedali Vittorio Emanuele Ferraotti S. Bambino
Catania, ITALY
Web: http://www.ao-ve.it/

Centro Servizi per il Volontariato—Napoli
Naples, ITALY
Web: http://www.csvnapoli.it/

Istituto Giannina Gaslini—Pediatric Hematology/ Oncology
Genova, ITALY
Web: http://www.gaslini.org/eng/schedauo.asp?liv= 1_4&dir=&id=107

Istituto Nazionale Dei Tumori
Milan, ITALY
Web: http://www.istitutotumori.mi.it/

Ospedale Pediatrico Bambino Gesu
Rome, ITALY
Web: http://www.ospedalebambinogesu.it/

Ospedale Infantile Burlo Garofolo
Trieste, ITALY
Web: http://www.burlo.trieste.it/

Palermo University—Faculty of Medicine
Palermo, ITALY
Web: http://www.medpa.it/

Policlinico di Bari—Ospedale Giovanni XXIII
Bari, ITALY
Web: http://www.policlinico.ba.it/sito/associazioni.php

Policlinico Gemelli—Universita Cattolica
Rome, ITALY
Web: http://www.policlinicogemelli.it/area/

Policlinico S. Orsola-Malpighi—Universita di Bologna
Bologna, ITALY
Web: http://www.aosp.bo.it/

Umberto I Policlinico di Roma
Rome, ITALY
Web: http://www.policlinicoumberto1.it/

IVORY COAST

Centre Hospitalier Universitaire de Treichville
Abidjan, IVORY COAST
Web: http://chu-treichville.org/

JAPAN

Chiba University Hospital
Chiba, JAPAN
Web: http://www.ho.chiba-u.ac.jp/

Gunma Children's Medical Center
Gunma, JAPAN
Web: http://www.gcmc.pref.gunma.jp/

Hamamatsu University School of Medicine—University Hospital
Hamamtsu City, JAPAN
Web: http://www.hama-med.ac.jp/

Ibaraki Children's Hospital
Ibaraki, JAPAN
Web: http://www.ibaraki-kodomo.com/

Keio University Hospital - School of Medicine
Tokyo, JAPAN
Web: http://www.med.keio.ac.jp/en-file/ e-school_of_medicine.html

University Hospital—Kyoto Prefectural University of Medicine
Kyoto, JAPAN
Web: http://www.h.kpu-m.ac.jp/

Kyorin University Hospital
Mitaka Shi, JAPAN
Web: http://www.kyorin-u.ac.jp/

Mie University, Graduate School of Medicine
Mie, JAPAN
Web: http://official.medic.mie-u.ac.jp/

National Cancer Center
Tokyo, JAPAN
Web: http://www.ncc.go.jp/

National Center for Child Health and Development
Tokyo, JAPAN
Web: http://www.ncchd.go.jp/

Osaka Medical Center for Maternal and Child Health
Osaka, JAPAN
Web: http://www.med.osaka-u.ac.jp/pub/inst-mch/ E_index.html

Saitama Medical Center, Jichi Medical University
Saitama, JAPAN
Web: http://www.jichi.ac.jp/index_e.html

Sapporo Medical Center
Sapporo, JAPAN
Web: http://hokuyu-aoth.org/

Tokyo Medical University Hospital
Tokyo, JAPAN
Web: http://hospinfo.tokyo-med.ac.jp/

Tsukuba University Hospital
Ibaraki, JAPAN
Web: http://www.s.hosp.tsukuba.ac.jp/

JORDAN

University of Jordan Hospital
Amman, JORDAN
Web: http://www.ju.edu.jo/medical/hospital/

KAZAKHSTAN

Kazakh National Medical University
Almaty, KAZAKHSTAN
Web: http://www.kaznmu.kz/en/kafdetbolen.htm

KENYA

Gertrude's Children's Hospital
Nairobi, KENYA
Web: http://www.gerties.org/

KOREA

Asan Medical Center
Seoul, KOREA
Web: http://eng.amc.seoul.kr/

Korea University Anam Hospital
Seoul, KOREA
Web: http://anam.kumc.or.kr/

Yongsei University Health System
Seoul, KOREA
Web: http://www.yuhs.or.kr/en/contents.asp?cat_no=14930

LEBANON

Hotel-Dieu de France Hospital
Beirut, LEBANON
Web: http://www.1stlebanon.net/lebanon/hoteldieu.html

LITHUANIA

Institute of Oncology Vilnius University
Vilnus, LITHUANIA
Web: http://www.loc.lt/

MACEDONIA

University St. Kiril I Metodij
Skopje, MACEDONIA
Web: http://www.ukim.edu.mk/

MALAYSIA

Kuala Lumpur General Hospital
Kuala Lumpur, MALAYSIA
Web: http://www.hkl.gov.my/

MALTA

Sir Paul Boffa Hospital Radiotherapy and Oncology Department
Floriana VLT, MALTA
Web: http://www.sahha.gov.mt/pages.aspx?page=286

MEXICO

Centenario Hospital Miguel Hidalgo
Aguascalientes, MEXICO
Web: http://www.aguascalientes.gob.mx/hospitalhidalgo/default.aspx

Centro Estatal de Cancerologia "Dr. Miguel Dorantes Mesa"
Veracruz, MEXICO
Tel: 228-840-0975

Centro Médico Nacional "20 de Noviembre"
Mexico City, MEXICO
Web: http://www.issste-cmn20n.gob.mx/

Centro Oncologico de Chihuahua
Chihuahua, MEXICO
Web: http://www.cochihuahua.com/

Centro Universitario Contra el Cancer, Hospital Universitario "Dr. Jose E. Gonzalez"
Monterrey, MEXICO
Web: http://hospitaluniversitario.org/

Clinica de Mérida
Merida, MEXICO
Web: http://www.clinicademerida.com.mx/

Hospital Angeles Ciudad Juarez
Chihuahua, MEXICO
Web: http://www.hospitalangelesciudadjuarez.com.mx/

Hospital Central "Dr. Ignacio Morones Prieto"
San Luis Potosi, MEXICO
Web: http://www.hospitalcentral.gob.mx/

Hospitales Civiles de Guadalajara
Guadalajara, MEXICO
Web: http://www.hcg.udg.mx/

Hospital de León
León, MEXICO
Web: http://www.hospitaldeleon.com/

Hospital del Nino DIF
Hidalgo, MEXICO
Web: http://dif.hidalgo.gob.mx/

Hospital del Nino Morelense
Morelos, MEXICO
Web: http://www.hnm.org.mx/

Hospital del Nino Poblano
Puebla, MEXICO
Web: http://www.hnp.pue.gob.mx/index.php

Hospital del Nino Rodolfo Nieto Padron
Tabasco, MEXICO
Tel: 993-351-1090

Hospital General de Mexico
Distrito Federal, MEXICO
Web: http://www.hgm.salud.gob.mx

Hospital General "Dr. Agustin O'Horan"
Yucatan, MEXICO
Tel: 999-924-4355

Hospital General "Dr. Aurelio Valdivieso"
Oaxaca, MEXICO
Tel: 951-515-1422

Hospital General Tijuana
Tijuana, MEXICO
Web: http://www.hospitalgeneraltijuana.org/

Hospital Infantil de Mexico Federico Gomez
Coahuila, MEXICO
Web: http://www.himfg.edu.mx

Hospital Infantil de Tamaulipas
Tamaulipas, MEXICO
Web: http://www.hospitalinfantiltamaulipas.gob.mx/default2.htm

Hospital Infantil del Estado
Chihuahua, MEXICO
Web: http://www.chihuahua.gob.mx/hospitalinfantil/

Hospital Infantil del Estado de Sonora
Sonora, MEXICO
Web: http://www.hies.gob.mx/

Hospital Subregional de Poza Rica
Veracruz, MEXICO
Tel: 782-823-3430

Instituto Nacional de Cancerología
Mexico City, MEXICO
Web: http://www.incan.edu.mx/

Instituto Nacional de Pediatria
Distrito Federal, MEXICO
Web: http://www.pediatria.gob.mx

UMAE Hospital de Pediatría Centro Médico Nacional
Siglo XXI
Mexico City, MEXICO
Web: http://edumed.imss.gob.mx/pediatria/index.htm

MOROCCO

Centre Hospitalier Ibn Sina, L'Hopital D'Enfants
Rabat, MOROCCO
Web: http://www.chisrabat.ma/

Hospital du 20 Aout 1953—Service of Pediatric
Hematology and Oncology
Casablanca, MOROCCO
Web: http://www.fmp-uh2c.ac.ma/hemato/shop.htm

NEPAL

Kanti Children's Hospital
Kathmandu, NEPAL
Web: http://www.kantihospital.org/np

NETHERLANDS

Beatrix Children's Hospital—University Medical Center
Groningen
Groningen, NETHERLANDS
Web: http://www.umcg.nl/azg/nl/kinderen/

Catharina Ziekenhuis
Eindhoven, NETHERLANDS
Web: http://www.cze.nl/

Emma Kinderziekenhuis
Amsterdam, NETHERLANDS
Web: http://www.amc.nl/?pid=815

Erasmus Medical Center—Sophia Children's Hospital
Rotterdam, NETHERLANDS
Web: http://www.erasmusmc.nl/sophia/?lang=en

Groot Ziekengasthuis (Great Sick Hospital)
Shertogenbosch, NETHERLANDS
Web: http://groetenuitdenbosch.nl/110.htm

Leiden University Medical Center
Leiden, NETHERLANDS
Web: http://www.lumc.nl/

Netherlands Cancer Institute
Breukelen, NETHERLANDS
Web: http://www.nki.nl/

Radboud University Nijmegen
Nijmegen, NETHERLANDS
Web: http://www.umcn.nl/

St. Elisabeth Ziekenhuis
Tilburg, NETHERLANDS
Web: http://www.elisabeth.nl/

Vrije Universiteit Medical Center
Amsterdam, NETHERLANDS
Web: http://www.vumc.nl/

Wilhelmina Kinderziekenhuis
Utrecht, NETHERLANDS
Web: http://www.hetwkz.nl/

NEW ZEALAND

Christchurch Hospital
Christchurch, NEW ZEALAND
Web: http://www.cdhb.govt.nz/chc/

Starship Children's Hospital
Auckland, NEW ZEALAND
Web: http://www.starship.org.nz/

NICARAGUA

Hospital Infantil Manuel Jesus Rivera
Managua, NICARAGUA
Web: http://www.minsa.gob.ni/

NIGERIA

Ahmadu Bello University Teaching Hospital
Zaria, NIGERIA
Web: http://www.abuth.org/

Lagos University Teaching Hospital
Lagos, NIGERIA
Web: http://www.lasuth.org/

Obafemi Awolowo University Teaching Hospital
Ile-Ife, NIGERIA
Web: http://oauthife.org/

University of Benin Teaching Hospital
Benin City, NIGERIA
Web: http://www.ubth.org/

University of Calabar Teaching Hospital
Calabar, NIGERIA
Tel: 234-8037183961

University of Ibadan Teaching Hospital
Ibadan, NIGERIA
Tel: 234-2-2410088

NORWAY

Helse Bergen—Haukeland Universitetssykehus—
Barneklinikken
Bergen, NORWAY
Web: http://www.helse-bergen.no/avd/barneklinikken/

Rikshospitalet University Hospital
Oslo, NORWAY
Web: http://www.rikshospitalet.no/ikbViewer/page/no/
pages/forsiden

St. Olav's Hospital Sykehuset
Trondheim, NORWAY
Web: http://www.stolav.no

Ullevål Universitetssykehus
Oslo, NORWAY
Web: http://www.ulleval.no/

Universitetssykehuset Nord-Norge HF—Tromsö
Tromso, NORWAY
Web: http://www.unn.no/unn-tromsoe/category20629.html

OMAN

Royal Hospital
Sultanate of Oman, OMAN
Web: http://www.royalhospital.med.om/

PAKISTAN

Aga Khan University Hospital
Karachi, PAKISTAN
Web: http://www.aku.edu/AKUH/

Shaukat Khanum Memorial Cancer Hospital and Research Centre
Lashore, PAKISTAN
Web: http://www.shaukatkhanum.org.pk/

Ziauddin Hospital
Karachi, PAKISTAN
Web: http://www.zu.edu.pk/

PANAMA

Hospital Del Nino
Panama City, PANAMA
Web: http://www.hden.sld.pa/

PARAGUAY

Sanatorio Santa Clara
Asunción, PARAGUAY
Web: http://www.santaclara.com.py/

PERU

Centro Medico Corpac
Lima, PERU
Web: http://www.doctorperu.com/
doctor-peru-3983-centro-medico-corpac.php

Hospital Nacional Edgardo Rebagliati Martins
Lima, PERU
Web: http://cuerpomedicorebagliati.org/

PHILIPPINES

Asian Hospital and Medical Center
Alabang, Multinlupa City, PHILIPPINES
Web: http://www.asianhospital.com/

East Avenue Medical Center
Quezon City, PHILIPPINES
Web: http://www.doh.gov.ph/eamc/

Makati Medical Center
Makati City, PHILIPPINES
Web: http://www.makatimed.net.ph/

Philippine Children's Medical Center
Quezon City, PHILIPPINES
Web: http://www.pcmc.gov.ph/

POLAND

Children's Memorial Health Institute
Warsaw, POLAND
Web: http://www.czd.waw.pl/

Children's University Hospital—Hematology/Oncology
Lublin, POLAND
Web: http://www.szpitalzdrowia.pl/

Dolnoslaskie Centrum Transplantacji Komorkowych
Wroclaw, POLAND
Web: http://www.dctk.wroc.pl/

National Research Institute of Mother and Child
Warsaw, POLAND
Web: http://www.imid.med.pl/

Pomeranian Academy of Medicine in Szczecin
Szczecin, POLAND
Web: http://www.pam.szczecin.pl/

University Children's Hospital of Krakow
Krakow, POLAND
Web: http://www.wssdzkrakow.hg.pl/

Universytecki Szpital Kliniczny
Poznan, POLAND
Web: http://spskam.bialystok.pl/

PORTUGAL

Hospital de São João
Porto, PORTUGAL
Web: http://www.hsjoao.min-saude.pt/

Hospital Dona Estefânia
Lisbon, PORTUGAL
Web: http://www.hdestefania.min-saude.pt/

Instituto Português de Oncologia de Lisboa
Lisbon, PORTUGAL
Web: http://www.ipolisboa.min-saude.pt/

ROMANIA

Institute of Oncology Bucharest
Bucharest, ROMANIA
Web: http://www.iob.ro/

Institutul Oncologic "Prof. Dr. I. Chiricuta"
Cluj-Napoca, ROMANIA
Web: http://www.iocn.ro/

University of Medicine and Pharmacie "Victor Babes"
Timisoara, ROMANIA
Web: http://www.umft.ro/

RUSSIA

Ekaterinburg Region Pediatric Cancer Research Center
Ekaterinburg, RUSSIA
Tel: 7-908-903-7736

Memorial R.M. Gorbacheva Institute of Children Hematology and Transplantation, St. Petersburg Pavlov State Medical University
St. Petersburg, RUSSIA
Tel: 7-812-233-8307

N.N. Blokhin Russian Cancer Research Center, Institute for Pediatric Oncology and Hematology
Moscow, RUSSIA
Web: http://www.ronc.ru/

N.N. Petrov Research Institute of Oncology
St. Petersburg, RUSSIA
Tel: 7-812-596-8936

Russian Children's Clinical Hospital
Moscow, RUSSIA
Web: http://www.rdkb.ru/

SAUDI ARABIA

King Abdulaziz Hospital
Jeddah, SAUDI ARABIA
Web: http://www.kau.edu.sa/

King Fahad National Centre for Children's Cancer and Research
Riyadh, SAUDI ARABIA
Web: http://www.bportal.kfshrc.edu.sa/wps/portal/bportal/KFNCCC

King Faisal Specialist Hospital and Research Institute
Riyadh, SAUDI ARABIA
Web: http://www.kfshrcj.org/KFSHRCJ/Clinics/Oncology/

Kingdom of Saudi Arabia National Guard Health Affairs
Jeddah, SAUDI ARABIA
Web: http://www.ngha.med.sa/

Riyadh Armed Forces Hospital
Riyadh, SAUDI ARABIA
Web: http://www.rkh.med.sa/

REPUBLIC OF SINGAPORE

K.K. Women's and Children's Hospital
Singapore, REPUBLIC OF SINGAPORE
Web: http://www.kkh.com.sg/

SLOVAK REPUBLIC

Children's Faculty Hospital
Bratislava, SLOVAK REPUBLIC
Tel: 421-02-59371111

Fakultná Nemocnica L. Pasteura Kosice
Kosice, SLOVAK REPUBLIC
Web: http://www.fnlp.sk/

University Children's Hospital
Banska Bystrica, SLOVAK REPUBLIC
Tel: 421-048-4726511

SLOVENIA

Institut of Oncology Ljubljana
Ljubljana, SLOVENIA
Web: http://www.onko-i.si/en/institute_of_oncology_
    ljubljana/

University Medical Centre Ljubljana
Ljubljana, SLOVENIA
Web: http://www3.kclj.si/ang/index.php?m=2&s=0

SOUTH AFRICA

Chris Hani Baragwanath Hospital
Johannesburg, SOUTH AFRICA
Web: http://www.chrishanibaragwanathhospital.co.za/

Johannesburg Academic Hospital
Johannesburg, SOUTH AFRICA
Web: http://www.johannesburghospital.org.za/

Kalafong Academic Hospital—University of Pretoria
Pretoria, SOUTH AFRICA
Web: http://www.up.ac.za/academic/medicine/campus/
    kalafong.htm

Red Cross Children's Hospital
Rondebosch, SOUTH AFRICA
Web: http://www.childrenshospitaltrust.org.za/

Tygerberg Hospital—University of Stellenbosch
Tygerberg, SOUTH AFRICA
Web: http://www.capegateway.gov.za/eng/your_gov/5987

SPAIN

**Complexo Hospitalario Universitario de Santiago de
    Compostela**
Santiago de Compostela, SPAIN
Web: http://www.chusantiago.sergas.es/

El Mundo Médico Pediatra—Puericultor
Madrid, SPAIN
Web: http://www.mundogaleno.com/especialidades/
    pediatria_puericultura.htm

Fundacion Jimenez Diaz
Madrid, SPAIN
Web: http://www.capiosanidad.es/fjd/

Hospital de Basurto
Bilbao, SPAIN
Web: http://www.hospitalbasurto.com/

Hospital de Cruces
Vizcaya, SPAIN
Web: http://www.hospitalcruces.com/

Hospital de La Santa Creu I Sant Pau
Barcelona, SPAIN
Web: http://www.santpau.es/

**Hospital General Universitario Gregoria Marañon—
    Hospital Materno Infantil**
Madrid, SPAIN
Web: http://www.hggm.es/webmaternoinfantil/
    Web_HMI/home.htm

Hospital Materno Infantil Vall d' Hebron
Barcelona, SPAIN
Web: http://www.vhebron.es/hmi/mainc.htm

Hospital Infantil La Paz
Madrid, SPAIN
Web: http://www.hospitalinfantillapaz.com/

Hospital Infantil Universitario Niño Jesús
Madrid, SPAIN
Web: http://www.madrid.org/cs/Satellite?pagename=
    HospitalNinoJesus/Page/HNIJ_home

Hospital San Rafael
Madrid, SPAIN
Web: http://www.hospitalsanrafael.es/

Hospital Universitari Infantil La Fe
Valencia, SPAIN
Web: http://www.dep7.san.gva.es/infoGeneral/
    infantil.asp

Hospital Universitario Miguel Servet
Zaragoza, SPAIN
Web: http://www.hmservet.es/

Hospital Universitario Virgen del Rocío
Sevilla, SPAIN
Web: http://www.huvr.es/

Hospital Virgin del Camino
Pamplona, SPAIN
Web: http://www.virgendelcamino.es/

**Unidad de Hematología y Oncología
    Pediátrica**
Madrid, SPAIN
Web: http://www.oncologiapediatricahm.es/

SWEDEN

**Akademiska Sjukhuset (Uppsala University
    Hospital)**
Uppsala, SWEDEN
Web: http://www.akademiska.se/

**Astrid Lindgrens Children's Hospital—Karolinska
    Universitetssjukhuset**
Stockholm, SWEDEN
Web: http://www.karolinska.se/

Lund University Hospital
Lund, SWEDEN
Web: http://www.skane.se/templates/
    Page.aspx?id=158344

Sahlgrenska University Hospital
Gothenburg, SWEDEN
Web: http://www.sahlgrenska.se/

University Hospital in Linköping
Linköping, SWEDEN
Web: http://www.lio.se/

SWITZERLAND

Centre Hospitalier Universitaire Vaudois (C.H.U.V.)
Lausanne, SWITZERLAND
Web: http://www.chuv.ch/

Hopital des enfants—Hopitaux Universitaires de Genéve
Geneva, SWITZERLAND
Web: http://www.hug-ge.ch/soins/hopital_enfants.html

Hospital de la Tour
Geneve, SWITZERLAND
Web: http://www.latour.ch/

Inselspital—Universitatsspital Bern
Bern, SWITZERLAND
Web: http://www.insel.ch/

Kinderspital Zürich
Zürich, SWITZERLAND
Web: http://www.kispi.unizh.ch/

Ospedale Regionale di Locarno La Carita
Locarno, SWITZERLAND
Web: http://www.eoc.ch/

Ostschweizer Kinderspital
St. Gallen, SWITZERLAND
Web: http://www.kispisg.ch/

Regionales Pflegeheim Gossau
Gossau, SWITZERLAND
Web: http://www.pflegeheim-gossau.ch/

Universitatsspital Basel
Basel, SWITZERLAND
Web: http://www.unispital-basel.ch/

TAIWAN

Chang-Gung Children's Hospital
Taoyuan Hsien, TAIWAN
Web: http://www.cgmh.org.tw/eng2002/intr_chd.htm

National Cheng Kung University Hospital
Tainan, TAIWAN
Web: http://www.ncku.edu.tw/

TANZANIA

Muhimbili University of Health and Allied Sciences
Dar Es Salaam, TANZANIA
Web: http://www.muchs.ac.tz/

THAILAND

Bumrungrad Hospital—Children's Center
Bangkok, THAILAND
Web: http://www.bumrungrad.com/thailand-expat/
    Medical-Services/clinics-and-centers/children-s-center.aspx

TUNESIA

Hospital d'Enfants de Tunis
Tunis, TUNESIA
Tel: 216-71-262987

TURKEY

Akdeniz Universitesi Hastanesi
Antalya, TURKEY
Web: http://www.hastane.akdeniz.edu.tr/

Dokuz Eylûl University Hospital
Izmir, TURKEY
Web: http://www.deu.edu.tr/

Ege University Hospital
Izmir, TURKEY
Web: http://www.medicine.ege.edu.tr/

Gülhane Military Medical Academy Hospital
Ankara, TURKEY
Web: http://www.gata.edu.tr/

Hacettepe University Institute of Oncology
Ankara, TURKEY
Web: http://www.onkoloji.hacettepe.edu.tr/

Istanbul University—Cerrahpasa Hospital
Istanbul, TURKEY
Web: http://www.ctf.edu.tr/erasmus/about.htm

Ssk Tepecik Hospital
Izmir, TURKEY
Web: http://www.tepecikhastanesi.gov.tr/

UKRAINE

Boris Clinic
Kiev, UKRAINE
Web: http://www.boris.kiev.ua/

Ministry of Health of Ukraine
Kiev, UKRAINE
Web: http://www.moz.gov.ua/

UNITED ARAB EMIRATES

Shaikh Khalifa Medical Center
Abu Dhabi, UNITED ARAB EMIRATES
Web: http://www.skmc.gov.ae/

Tawam Hospital
Abu Dhabi, UNITED ARAB EMIRATES
Web: http://www.tawamhospital.ae/

**United Arab Emirates University Faculty of Medicine
and Health Sciences**
Al Ain, UNITED ARAB EMIRATES
Web: http://www.fmhs.uaeu.ac.ae/Links.asp?n=2

UNITED KINGDOM

Alder Hey Children's Hospital
Liverpool, UNITED KINGDOM
Web: http://www.alderhey.com/

Barts and the Royal London NHS Trust
London, UNITED KINGDOM
Web: http://www.bartsandthelondon.org.uk/

Birmingham Children's Hospital
Birmingham, UNITED KINGDOM
Web: http://www.bch.org.uk/

Bristol Haematology and Oncology Centre
Bristol, UNITED KINGDOM
Web: http://www.uhbristol.nhs.uk/your-hospitals/
    bristol-haematology-and-oncology-centre.html

**Great Ormond Street Hospital for Children NHS
Trust—Institute of Child Health**
London, UNITED KINGDOM
Web: http://www.ich.ucl.ac.uk/

Manchester Children's Hospital NHS Trust
Manchester, UNITED KINGDOM
Web: http://www.cmft.nhs.uk/childrens-hospitals/home.aspx

**Queens Medical Centre—Nottingham University Hospital
NHS Trust**
Nottingham, UNITED KINGDOM
Web: http://www.qmc.nhs.uk/

Royal Hospital for Sick Children
Edinburgh, UNITED KINGDOM
Web: http://www.nhslothian.scot.nhs.uk/hospitals/
rhsc.asp

Royal Victoria Infirmary—The Newcastle upon Tyne Hospitals NHS Trust
Newcastle Upon Tyne, UNITED KINGDOM
Web: http://www.newcastle-hospitals.org.uk/hospitals/
royal-victoria-infirmary.aspx

Sheffield Children's Hospital NHS Trust
Sheffield, UNITED KINGDOM
Web: http://www.sheffieldchildrens.nhs.uk/

Southampton University Hospital NHS Trust
Southampton, UNITED KINGDOM
Web: http://www.suht.nhs.uk/

St. Bartholomew's (Barts) Hospital
West Smithfield, London, UNITED KINGDOM
Web: http://www.sbmc.org.uk/

St. James' University Hospital—The Leeds Teaching Hospital
Leeds, UNITED KINGDOM
Web: http://www.leedsth.nhs.uk/

The Beatson West of Scotland Cancer Centre
Glasgow, UNITED KINGDOM
Web: http://www.beatson.scot.nhs.uk/

The Christie Hospital NHS Trust
Manchester, UNITED KINGDOM
Web: http://www.christie.nhs.uk/

The Royal Marsden NHS Trust
Surrey, UNITED KINGDOM
Web: http://www.royalmarsden.org/

University Hospital Llandough
Llandough, UNITED KINGDOM
Web: http://www.cardiffandvale.wales.nhs.uk/

Western General Hospital
Edinburgh, UNITED KINGDOM
Web: http://www.nhslothian.scot.nhs.uk/hospitals/
wgh.asp

UNITED STATES OF AMERICA

Alabama

University of Alabama Comprehensive Cancer Center
Birmingham, AL
Web: http://www.ccc.uab.edu

Alaska

Children's Hospital at Providence
Anchorage, AK
Web: http://www.providence.org/alaska/services/
children/

Arizona

Phoenix Children's Hospital
Phoenix, AZ
Web: http://www.phoenixchildrens.com/

St. Joseph's Hospital and Medical Center
Phoenix, AZ
Web: http://www.stjosephs-phx.org/index.htm

University of Arizona Pediatric Hematology/Oncology
Tucson, AZ
Web: http://www.peds.arizona.edu

Arkansas

Arkansas Children's Hospital
Little Rock, AR
Web: http://www.archildrens.org/

California

Cedars-Sinai Medical Center
Los Angeles, CA
Web: http://www.cedars-sinai.edu/

Children's Hospital and Research Center Oakland
Oakland, CA
Web: http://www.childrenshospitaloakland.org/

Children's Hospital Center California
Madera, CA
Web: http://www.childrenscentralcal.org/

Childrens Hospital Los Angeles
Los Angeles, CA
Web: http://www.chla.org

Children's Hospital of Orange County
Orange, CA
Web: http://www.choc.org/

City of Hope
Duarte, CA
Web: http://www.cityofhope.org/

David Grant USAF Medical Center
Travis AFB, CA
Web: http://www.travis.af.mil/units/dgmc/
index.asp

Harbor/UCLA Medical Center
Torrance, CA
Web: http://www.humc.edu

Kaiser Permanente
Oakland and Santa Clara, CA
Web: https://www.kaiserpermanente.org/

Loma Linda University Children's Hospital
Loma Linda, CA
Web: http://lomalindahealth.org/childrens-hospital/

Lucille Packard Children's Hospital at Stanford
Palo Alto, CA
Web: http://www.lpch.org/

Mattel Children's Hospital University of California at Los Angeles
Los Angeles, CA
Web: http://www.uclahealth.org/homepage_mattel.
cfm?id=266

Memorial Miller Children's Hospital
Long Beach, CA
Web: http://www.memorialcare.org/miller/about.cfm

Naval Medical Center, San Diego
San Diego, CA
Web: http://www.nmcsd.med.navy.mil

Salk Institute Cancer Center
La Jolla, CA
Web: http://www.salk.edu/faculty/cancer_center.html

Stanford University School of Medicine
Stanford, CA
Web: http://med.stanford.edu/

The Burnham Institute
La Jolla, CA
Web: http://www.burnham.org

U.C. Davis Children's Hospital
Sacramento, CA
Web: http://www.ucdmc.ucdavis.edu/children/

University of California at Irvine Healthcare
Orange, CA
Web: http://www.healthcare.uci.edu/

University of California at San Francisco Children's Hospital
San Francisco, CA
Web: http://www.ucsfhealth.org/childrens/

U.S.C./Norris Comprehensive Cancer Center
Los Angeles, CA
Web: http://www.ccnt.hsc.usc.edu/

Colorado

Childhood Hematology/Oncology Associates
Colorado Springs, CO
Web: http://www.choa.net/

Presbyterian/St. Luke's Medical Center
Denver, CO
Web: http://www.pslmc.com/

The Children's Hospital of Denver
Denver, CO
Web: http://www.thechildrenshospital.org/

Connecticut

University of Connecticut Health Science Center
Hartford, CT
Web http://www.uchc.edu/

Yale University School of Medicine—Comprehensive Cancer Center
New Haven, CT
Web: http://www.medicine.yale.edu/

Delaware

Children's National Medical Center
Washington, DC
Web: http://www.childrensnational.org/

Georgetown University Medical Center
Washington, DC
Web: http://www.gumc.georgetown.edu/

Howard University Hospital
Washington, DC
Web: http://www.huhealthcare.com/

Nemours/Alfred I. duPont Hospital for Children
Wilmington, DE
Web: http://www.nemours.org

Walter Reed Army Medical Center
Washington, DC
Web: http://www.wramc.amedd.army.mil/

Florida

All Children's Hospital
St. Petersburg, FL
Web: http://www.allkids.org/

Arnold Palmer Hospital for Children
Orlando, FL
Web: http://orlandohealth.com/arnoldpalmerhospital/index.aspx

Florida Hospital Cancer Institute
Orlando, FL
Web: http://www.floridahospitalcancer.com/

Jackson Health System
Miami, FL
Web: http://www.jhsmiami.org/

Joe DiMaggio Children's Hospital at Memorial
Hollywood, FL
Web: http://www.jdch.com

Miami Children's Hospital
Miami, FL
Web: http://www.mch.com

Nemours Children's Clinic in Jacksonville
Jacksonville, FL
Web: http://www.nemours.org/clinic/fl/jax.html

Sacred Heart Children's Hospital
Pensacola, FL
Web: http://www.sacred-heart.org/childrenshospital/

Shands Children's Hospital/University of Florida
Gainesville, FL
Web: http://www.shands.org/hospitals/children/

St. Joseph's Children's Hospital of Tampa
Tampa, FL
Web: http://www.sjbhealth.org/home_childrens.cfm?id=585

Sylvester Comprehensive Cancer Center/University of Miami Health System
Miami, FL
Web: http://www.sylvester.org/

The Children's Hospital of Southwest Florida Lee Memorial
Fort Myers, FL
Web: http://www.leememorial.org/childrenhospital/

Georgia

Backus Children's Hospital at MHUMC
Savannah, GA
Web: http://www.memorialhealth.com/backus/

Children's Healthcare of Atlanta
Atlanta, GA
Web: http://www.choa.org/

Medical College of Georgia, Department of Pediatrics
Augusta, GA
Web: http://www.mcg.edu/pediatrics/

The Children's Hospital at the Medical Center of Central Georgia
Macon, GA
Web: http://www.mccg.org/services/childh.asp

Hawaii

Kapi'olani Medical Center for Women and Children
Honolulu, HI
Web: http://www.kapiolani.org/

Tripler Army Medical Center
Tripler AMC, HI
Web: http://www.tamc.amedd.army.mil/

Idaho

St. Luke's Regional Health System
Boise, ID
Web: http://www.stlukesonline.org/

Illinois

Advocate Lutheran General Hospital
Park Ridge, IL
Web: http://www.advocatehealth.com/luth/

Children's Memorial Hospital
Chicago, IL
Web: http://www.childrensmemorial.org/

John H. Stroger Jr. Hospital
Chicago, IL
Web: http://www.cchil.org/

Loyola University Medical Center
Maywood, IL
Web: http://loyolamedicine.org/

Rush University Medical Center
Chicago, IL
Web: http://www.rush.edu/

Southern Illinois University School of Medicine
Springfield, IL
Web: http://www.siumed.edu/

The University of Chicago Cancer Research Center
Chicago, IL
Web: http://uccrc.uchicago.edu/

The University of Chicago Comer Children's Hospital
Chicago, IL
Web: http://www.uchicagokidshospital.org/specialties/

University of Illinois Medical Center at Chicago
Chicago, IL
Web: http://uillinoismedcenter.org/

Indiana

Purdue University Cancer Center
West Lafayette, IN
Web: http://www.cancer.purdue.edu/

Riley Hospital for Children
Indianapolis, IN
Web: http://rileychildrenshospital.com/

St. Vincent Mercy Children's Hospital
Indianapolis, IN
Web: http://mercyweb.org/childrens/

Iowa

Blank Children's Hospital
Des Moines, IA
Web: http://www.blankchildrens.org

University of Iowa Hospitals and Clinics
Iowa City, Iowa
Web: http://www.uihealthcare.com/

Kansas

The University of Kansas Hospital
Kansas City, KS
Web: http://www.kumc.com/

Via Christi Health System
Wichita, KS
Web: http://www.via-christi.org/

Kentucky

Kosair Children's Hospital
Louisville, KY
Web: http://www.nortonhealthcare.com/locations/
hospitals/kosair/

University of Kentucky Children's Hospital
Lexington, KY
Web: http://ukhealthcare.uky.edu/KCH/

Louisiana

Children's Hospital of New Orleans
New Orleans, LA
Web: http://www.chnola.org/

Tulane Medical Center
New Orleans, LA
Web: http://www.tuhc.com/

Maine

Eastern Maine Medical Center
Bangor, ME
Web: http://www.emh.org/

Maine Medical Center
Portland, ME
Web: http://www.mmc.org/

Maryland

**Johns Hopkins/Sidney Kimmel Comprehensive
Cancer Center**
Baltimore, MD
Web: http://www.hopkinskimmelcancercenter.org/

National Cancer Institute
Bethesda, MD
Web: http://www.cancer.gov

National Naval Medical Center
Bethesda, MD
Web: http://www.bethesda.med.navy.mil/

**The Herman and Walter Samuelson Children's Hospital
at Sinai**
Baltimore, MD
Web: http://www.lifebridgehealth.org/chs.cfm?id=1620

University of Maryland Medical Center
Baltimore, MD
Web: http://www.umm.edu/pediatrics/ped-hemat.htm

Massachusetts

Baystate Children's Hospital
Springfield, MA
Web: http://www.baystatehealth.com/

Dana-Farber/Children's Hospital Cancer Care
Boston, MA
Web: http://www.danafarberchildrens.org/

Floating Hospital for Children at Tufts Medical Center
Boston, MA
Web: http://www.floatinghospital.org/

Massachusetts General Hospital Cancer Center
Boston, MA
Web: http://www.massgeneral.org/Cancer/

**The David H. Koch Institute for Integrative Cancer Research
at MIT**
Cambridge, MA
Web: http://web.mit.edu/ki/

**University of Massachusetts Memorial Children's Medical
Center**
Worcester, MA
Web: http://www.umassmed.edu/Pediatrics/

Michigan

**Barbara Ann Karmanos Cancer Institute/Wayne State
University**
Detroit, MI
Web: http://www.karmanos.org/

Children's Hospital of Michigan
Detroit, MI
Web: http://www.childrensdmc.org/

Grand Rapids Clinical Oncology Program
Grand Rapids, MI
Web: http://www.grcop.org/

Henry Ford Health System
Detroit, MI
Web: http://www.henryford.com/

Hurley Medical Center
Flint, MI
Web: http://www.hurleymc.com/

Michigan State University Health Team
East Lansing, MI
Web: http://healthteam.msu.edu/

St. John Health System
Warren, MI
Web: http://www.stjohn.org/

University of Michigan Comprehensive Cancer Center
Ann Arbor, MI
Web: http://www.cancer.med.umich.edu/

William Beaumont Hospital
Royal Oak, MI
Web: https://www.beaumonthospitals.com/

Minnesota

Cancer Center at Mayo Clinic
Rochester, MN
Web: http://cancercenter.mayo.edu/

St. Mary's Medical Center
Duluth, MN
Web: http://www.smdc.org/

University of Minnesota Hospital & Clinics
Minneapolis, MN
Web: http://www.childrensmn.org/

Mississippi

University of Mississippi Medical Center
Jackson, MS
Web: http://www.umc.edu

Missouri

Children's Mercy Hospital
Kansas City, MO
Web: http://www.childrens-mercy.org

SSM Cardinal Glennon Children's Medical Center
St. Louis, MO
Web: http://www.cardinalglennon.com

St. Louis Children's Hospital
St. Louis, MO
Web: http://www.stlouischildrens.org/

University of Missouri Health Care—Children's Hospital
Columbia, MO
Web: http://www.muhealth.org/children/

Nebraska

Children's Hospital and Medical Center
Omaha, NE
Web: http://www.chsomaha.org/

University of Nebraska Medical Center
Omaha, NE
Web: http://www.unmc.edu/

Nevada

Sunrise Hospital and Medical Center
Las Vegas, NV
Web: http://www.sunrisehospital.com

New Hampshire

Dartmouth-Hitchcock Medical Center
Lebanon, NH
Web: http://www.dhmc.org/

New Jersey

Bristol-Myers Squibb Children's Hospital
New Brunswick, NJ
Web: http://www.bmsch.org/

Children's Hospital of New Jersey at Newark Beth Israel Medical Center
Newark, NJ
Web: http://www.saintbarnabas.com/hospitals/
    childrens_hospital/index.html

Cooper University Hospital
Camden, NJ
Web: http://www.cooperhealth.org/

Hackensack Medical Center
Hackensack, NJ
Web: http://www.humed.com/

Overlook Hospital
Summit, NJ
Web: http://www.atlantichealth.org/Overlook/

St. Joseph's Healthcare System
Paterson, NJ
Web: http://www.stjosephshealth.org/

New Mexico

University of New Mexico Children's Hospital
Albuquerque, NM
Web: http://hospitals.unm.edu/UNMCH/

New York

Albany Medical Center
Albany, NY
Web: http://www.amc.edu/

Albert Einstein Cancer Center
Bronx, NY
Web: http://www.aecom.yu.edu/cancercenter/page.
    aspx

Babies and Children's Hospital of New York—Columbia University
New York, NY
Web: http://www.cumc.columbia.edu/dept/babies/

Brookdale University Hospital and Medical Center
Brooklyn, NY
Web: http://www.brookdale.edu/

Brooklyn Hospital Center
Brooklyn, NY
Web: http://www.tbh.org/

Golisano Children's Hospital—University of Rochester Medical Center
Rochester, NY
Web: http://www.urmc.rochester.edu/childrens-hospital/

Memorial Sloan Kettering Cancer Center
New York, NY
Web: http://www.mskcc.org/

Mount Sinai Jack Martin Division of Pediatric Hematology/Oncology
New York, NY
Web: http://www.mountsinai.org/Education/School%20of%20Medicine/Departments%20and%20Divisions/Pediatrics/Divisions/Hematology%20and%20Oncology

New York Presbyterian Hospital
New York, NY
Web: http://nyp.org/

Roswell Park Cancer Institute
Buffalo, NY
Web: http://www.roswellpark.org/

Schneider Children's Hospital
New Hyde Park, NY
Web: http://www.schneiderchildrenshospital.org/

Stephen D. Hassenfeld Children's Center for Cancer and Blood Disorders
New York, NY
Web: http://hassenfeld.med.nyu.edu/

SUNY Downstate Medical Center
Brooklyn, NY
Web: http://www.downstate.edu/

The Children's Hospital at Montefiore Hospital
Bronx, NY
Web: http://www.montekids.org/

University Hospital SUNY Health Science Center
Syracuse, NY
Web: http://www.upstate.edu/uh/

West Chester Medical Center
Valhalla, NY
Web: http://westchestermedcenter.com/

North Carolina

Carolinas Medical Center
Charlotte, NC
Web: http://www.carolinasmedicalcenter.org/

Duke University Health System
Durham, NC
Web: http://www.dukehealth.org/

Presbyterian Healthcare
Charlotte, NC
Web: http://www.presbyterian.org/

UNC Lineberger Comprehensive Cancer Center
Chapel Hill, NC
Web: http://cancer.unc.edu/

Wake Forest University Baptist Comprehensive Cancer Center
Winston-Salem, NC
Web: http://www1.wfubmc.edu/cancer/

North Dakota

St. Alexius Medical Center
Bismarck, ND
Web: http://www.st.alexius.org/

Roger Maris Cancer Center
Fargo, ND
Web: http://www.meritcare.com/medicalservices/specialties/cancer/rogermariscancercenter/

Ohio

Akron Children's Hospital
Akron, OH
Web: https://www.akronchildrens.org/

Cincinnati Children's Hospital Medical Center
Cincinnati, OH
Web: http://www.cincinnatichildrens.org/

Cleveland Clinic
Cleveland, OH
Web: http://my.clevelandclinic.org/

Nationwide Children's Hospital
Columbus, OH
Web: http://www.nationwidechildrens.org/

St. Vincent Mercy Children's Hospital
Toledo, OH
Web: http://mercyweb.org/childrens/

The Children's Medical Center of Dayton
Dayton, OH
Web: http://www.childrensdayton.org/

University Hospitals Rainbow Babies & Children's Hospital
Cleveland, OH
Web: http://www.uhhospitals.org/rainbowchildren/

Oklahoma

Saint Francis Health System – Natalie Warren Bryant Cancer Center
Tulsa, OK
Web: http://www.saintfrancis.com/locations/nwbcc/default.aspx

The Children's Hospital of OU Medical Center
Oklahoma City, OK
Web: http://www.ouphysicians.com/landing.cfm?id=454

Oregon

Legacy Health System
Portland, OR
Web: http://www.legacyhealth.org/

Oregon Health & Science University—Doernbecher Children's Hospital
Portland, OR
Web: http://www.ohsu.edu/health/clinics-and-services/doernbecher/

Pennsylvania

Abramson Cancer Center of the University of Pennsylvania
Philadelphia, PA
Web: http://www.penncancer.org/

Albert Einstein Healthcare Network
Philadelphia, PA
Web: http://www.einstein.edu/

Children's Hospital of Philadelphia
Philadelphia, PA
Web: http://www.chop.edu/

Children's Hospital of Pittsburgh
Pittsburgh, PA
Web: http://www.chp.edu/CHP/Home

Hospital of the University of
    Pennsylvania
Philadelphia, PA
Web: http://pennhealth.com/hup/

Fox Chase Cancer Center
Philadelphia, PA
Web: http://www.fccc.edu/

Janet Weis Children's Hospital
Danville, PA
Web: http://www.geisinger.org/services/jwch/
    index.html

Penn State Hershey Medical Center
Hershey, PA
Web: http://www.pennstatehershey.org/

St. Christopher's Hospital for Children
Philadelphia, PA
Web: http://www.stchristophershospital.com/

Temple University School of Medicine
Philadelphia, PA
Web: http://www.temple.edu/medicine/

University of Pittsburgh Medical Center Cancer
    Centers
Pittsburgh, PA
Web: http://www.upmccancercenters.com/

Puerto Rico

San Jorge Children's Hospital
Santurce, PR
Web: http://65.36.184.133/

Rhode Island

Hasbro Children's Hospital
Providence, RI
Web: http://www.lifespan.org/hch/

South Carolina

Greenville Hospital System
Greenville, SC
Web: http://www.ghs.org/

Medical University of South Carolina Children's
    Hospital
Charleston, SC
Web: http://www.musckids.com/

Palmetto-Richland Memorial Hospital
Columbia, SC
Web: http://www.palmettohealth.org/

South Dakota

Avera McKennan Hospital and Cancer
    Institute
Sioux Falls, SD
Web: http://www.mckennan.org/amck/cancer/
    index.aspx

Sanford Medical Center
Sioux Falls, SD
Web: http://www.sanfordhealth.org/

Tennessee

East Tennessee Children's Hospital
Knoxville, TN
Web: http://www.etch.com/

Monroe Carell Jr. Children's Hospital at Vanderbilt
Nashville, TN
Web: http://www.vanderbiltchildrens.com/

St. Jude Children's Research Hospital
Memphis, TN
Web: http://www.stjude.org/

T.C. Thompson Children's Hospital
Chattanooga, TN
Web: http://www.erlanger.org/body.cfm?id=32&fr=true

Texas

Children's Medical Center of Dallas
Dallas, TX
Web: http://www.childrens.com/

Cook Children's
Fort Worth, TX
Web: http://www.cookchildrens.org/

Dell Children's Medical Center of
    Central Texas
Austin, TX
Web: http://www.dellchildrens.net/

Driscoll Children's Hospital
Corpus Christi, TX
Web: http://www.driscollchildrens.org/

Cancer Therapy & Research Center
San Antonio, TX
Web: http://www.ctrc.net/

Northwest Texas Healthcare Systems
Amarillo, TX
Web: http://www.nwtexashealthcare.com/

San Antonio Military Medical Center
Fort Sam Houston, TX
Web: http://www.sammc.amedd.army.mil/

Scott & White Healthcare
Temple, TX
Web: http://www.sw.org/

Texas Children's Cancer Center and Hematology
    Service
Houston, TX
Web: http://www.txccc.org/

The University of Texas M. D. Anderson Children's
    Cancer Hospital
Houston, TX
Web: http://www.mdanderson.org/children/

University Medical Center Children's Hospital
Lubbock, TX
Web: https://www.umchealthsystem.com/Childrens
    Hospital/

University of Texas Health Sciences Center
    San Antonio
San Antonio, TX
Web: http://www.uthscsa.edu/

University of Texas Medical Branch at Galveston
Galveston, TX
Web: http://www.utmb.edu/

William Beaumont Army Medical Center
El Paso, TX
Web: http://www.wbamc.amedd.army.mil/

Utah

Huntsman Cancer Institute/University of Utah
Salt Lake City, UT
Web: http://www.huntsmancancer.org/

Primary Children's Medical Center
Salt Lake City, UT
Web: http://intermountainhealthcare.org/hospitals/
    primarychildrens/Pages/home.aspx

Vermont

Fletcher Allen Healthcare
Burlington, VT
Web: http://www.fahc.org/

Virginia

Carilion Clinic Children's Hospital
Roanoke, VA
Web: http://www.carilionclinic.org/Carilion/childrens

Children's Hospital of the King's Daughters
Norfolk, VA
Web: http://www.chkd.org/

Inova Health System—Pediatric Service
Falls Church, VA
Web: http://www.inova.com/healthcare-services/pediatrics/

**Naval Medical Center Portsmouth Pediatric
Hematology/Oncology**
Portsmouth, VA
Web: http://www-nmcp.mar.med.navy.mil/Pediatrics/
    hemeonc.asp

University of Virginia Children's Hospital
Charlottesville, VA
Web: http://www.healthsystem.virginia.edu/uvahealth/
    uvachildrenshospital/

**Virginia Commonwealth University Children's Medical
Center**
Richmond, VA
Web: http://www.vcuchildrens.org/

Washington

Deaconess Medical Center
Spokane, WA
Web: http://www.deaconess-spokane.org/

Fred Hutchinson Cancer Research Center
Seattle, WA
Web: http://www.fhcrc.org/

Madigan Army Medical Center
Tacoma, WA
Web: http://www.mamc.amedd.army.mil/

Mary Bridge Children's Hospital & Health Center
Tacoma, WA
Web: http://www.multicare.org/marybridge/

Sacred Heart Children's Hospital
Spokane, WA
Web: http://www.shmcchildren.org/

Seattle Children's Hospital & Research Foundation
Seattle, WA
Web: http://www.seattlechildrens.org/

West Virginia

Cabell Huntington Hospital
Huntington, WV
Web: http://cabellhuntington.org/

West Virginia University Children's Hospital
Charleston, WV
Web: http://www.wvukids.com/

Wisconsin

Children's Hospital of Wisconsin
Milwaukee, WI
Web: http://www.chw.org/

Dean Medical Center
Madison, WI
Web: http://www.deancare.com/

Gundersen Lutheran Pediatric Cancer & Blood Disorders
La Crosse, WI
Web: http://www.gundluth.com/?id=377&sid=1

Marshfield Clinic Children's Hematology-Oncology
Marshfield, WI
Web: http://www.marshfieldclinic.org/patients/
    default.aspx?page=childrens_hematology

St. Vincent Hospital
Green Bay, WI
Web: http://www.stvincenthospital.org/Scripts/

University of Wisconsin Comprehensive Cancer Center
Madison, WI
Web: http://www.cancer.wisc.edu/

URUGUAY

Hospital Pereira Rossell
Montevideo, URUGUAY
Web: http://www.pereirarossell.gub.uy/

VENEZUELA

Centro Medico de Caracas
Caracas, VENEZUELA
Web: http://centromedicodecaracas.com.ve/

Hospital de Niños J.M. de Los Rios
Caracas, VENEZUELA
Web: http://mipagina.cantv.net/hospitaljm/

Instituto Oncologica—Unidad de Oncología Pediátrica
Caracas, VENEZUELA
Web: http://www.oncoped.org.ve/

VIETNAM

Ho Chi Minh City Cho Ray Hospital
Ho Chi Minh City, VIETNAM
Web: http://www.choray.org.vn/

National Cancer Institute-Vietnam
Hanoi, VIETNAM
Web: http://nci.org.vn/

YUGOSLAVIA

Children's University Hospital
Belgrade, YUGOSLAVIA
Web: http://www.udk.bg.ac.yu/

Health Care Institute for Children and Youth
Novi Sad, YUGOSLAVIA
Web: http://www.izzzdiov.org/

Mother and Children Health Care Institute
of Serbia
Belgrade, YUGOSLAVIA
Web: http://www.imd.org.yu/

Institute of Oncology and Radiology of Serbia
Belgrade, YUGOSLAVIA
Web: http://www.ncrc.ac.yu

K.B.C Kragujevac
Kragujevac, YUGOSLAVIA
Web: http://www.kc-kg.co.yu/

ZAMBIA

University Teaching Hospital
Lusaka, ZAMBIA
Web: http://www.zambiandoctors.com/zambianhospitals/
uth.html

ZIMBABWE

Cancer Association of Zimbabwe
Harare, ZIMBABWE
E-mail: cancer.registry@healthnet.zw

INDEX

Note: Page numbers followed by "f" indicate figures, page numbers followed by "t" indicate tables.